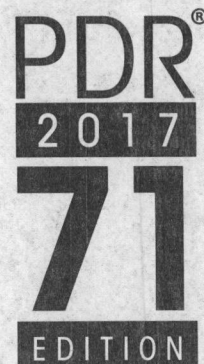

D1270966

PHYSICIANS' DESK REFERENCE®

Chief Executive Officer: Harry Totonis
President and Chief Commercial Officer: Rick Ratliff
Chief Technology Officer: David Cheng
Chief Operations Officer: Don Huonker
Senior Vice President, Digital Products: Eugene Lee
Senior Vice President, Product Marketing and Market Research:
  Barbara Senich, BSN, MBA, MPH
**Senior Vice President and Business Manager for Prescription
 Discount Programs:** Lisa Collins
Vice President, Clinical and Regulatory Solutions:
  Mukesh Mehta, DPh, MBA, RPh
**Director, Communications and Database Channel Lifecycle
 Management:** David Weatherbee

Director, Manufacturing and Distribution: Thomas Westburgh
Director, Operations: Noel Deloughery
Senior Content Operations Specialist: Allison O'Hare
Senior Production Coordinator: Yasmin Hernández
Production Coordinator: Eric Udina
Associate Director, Clinical Operations: Anila Patel, PharmD
Associate Manager, Clinical Operations: Pauline Lee, PharmD
Senior Director, Marketing: Kim Marich
Manager, Marketing Services: Livio Udina
Manager, Fulfillment and DMS Operations: Gary Lew
Customer Service Supervisor: Ricardo Plaisir
Managing Editor: Christa Mary Kronick, MA

Special thanks to the following contributors:
Jeffrey D. Schaefer; Demyana Farag, PharmD; Kristine Mecca, PharmD; Vanessa Azevedo, PharmD; Autri Sajedeen, PharmD; Caroline Gadalla, PharmD;
Jasmine Kim, PharmD

ISBN: 978-1-56363-838-1

FOREWORD TO THE 71st EDITION

About PDR, LLC (PDR®)

PDR has always been at the ready for prescribers from the first edition of the *Physicians' Desk Reference®* (*PDR®*) in 1947. Today, prescribers have a multitude of ways to access that same trusted information, all at their fingertips. Now in its 71st year, PDR remains committed to ensuring that prescribers have access to drug labeling, safety, and other clinically relevant information at the point-of-prescribing. PDR distributes this information through the PDR suite of digital and print services, which includes: (1) the *PDR*, the most highly trusted drug information reference available in the US; (2) PDR interactive drug information services for prescribers, embedded in their electronic medical record (EMR) systems; (3) PDR.net®, the online home of the *PDR*; (4) *mobile*PDR®, the official drug lookup and comparison app from PDR; (5) PDR Safety Communications; and (6) PDR Updates, print and electronic labeling updates sent directly to prescribers.

PDR's mission is to deliver actionable health information that matters. By improving the communication of important medication information and FDA-approved drug alerts, PDR's unique services enhance patient safety and may help to reduce prescribers' medical liability. For more information or to sign up for electronic PDR Safety Communications, visit PDR.net/registration.

About Product Information in the *PDR*

The *PDR* book and related products contain FDA-approved product labeling and are produced by PDR in cooperation with participating manufacturers. In accordance with current FDA policies, the *PDR* also includes prescribing information provided by manufacturers for products marketed without FDA approval, as well as information on some dietary supplements and other products. PDR makes this information available in multiple formats, including both the classic print edition and the *mobile*PDR.

For ease of use, the *PDR* includes color-coded indices (designated with white, pink, or blue pages at the front of the book). In addition, manufacturer-supplied information on dietary supplements is listed separately in Section 8.

Each full-length product information entry provides an exact, formatted copy of the product's FDA-approved or other manufacturer-supplied labeling. Under the Federal Food, Drug, and Cosmetic (FD&C) Act, a drug approved for marketing may be labeled, promoted, and advertised by the manufacturer for only those uses for which the drug's safety and effectiveness have been established. The Code of Federal Regulations [Title 21 Section 201.100(d)(1)] pertaining to labeling for prescription products requires that for *PDR* content, "indications, effects, dosages, routes, methods, and frequency and duration of administration, and any relevant warnings, hazards, contraindications, side effects, and precautions" must be the *same in language and emphasis* as the approved labeling for the products. The FDA regards the words *same in language and emphasis* as requiring VERBATIM use of the approved labeling when providing such information. Furthermore, information that is emphasized in the FDA-approved labeling by the use of type set in a box, or in capitals, boldface, or italics, must be given the same emphasis in the *PDR*.

The FDA has acknowledged that the FD&C Act does not limit the manner in which a prescriber may use an approved drug. Once a product has been approved for marketing, a prescriber may choose to order it for uses, treatment regimens, or patient populations that are not included in the approved labeling. The FDA also observed that accepted medical practice includes drug use that is not reflected in approved drug labeling. In addition, the dietary supplements listed in Section 8 are marketed under the Dietary Supplement Health and Education Act of 1994 (DSHEA). Products marketed under the DSHEA do not receive formal evaluation or approval from the FDA. The following disclaimer applies to all product information listed in Section 8, as mandated by the federal government: *These statements have not been evaluated by the Food and Drug Administration. This product is not intended to diagnose, treat, cure, or prevent any disease.*

The function of PDR is the compilation, organization, and distribution of this information. All product information appearing in the *PDR* is made possible through the courtesy of the manufacturers whose products appear in it. The information concerning each product has been provided by its manufacturer and in each instance is fully approved by such manufacturer prior to publication by PDR. In organizing and presenting the material in the *PDR*, PDR does not warrant or guarantee any of the products described, or perform any independent analysis in connection with any of the product information contained herein. PDR does not assume, and expressly disclaims, any obligation to obtain and include any information other than that provided to it by the manufacturers. It should be understood that by making this material available, PDR is not advocating the use of any product described herein, nor is PDR responsible for the use of a product, or the use and/or misuse of a product due to typographical error. Additional information on any product may be obtained from the manufacturer.

Updates to the *PDR*

The print edition of the *PDR* contains the latest information that was available when the edition closed for new material. As new drugs are released and new research data, clinical findings, and safety information emerge throughout the year, it is the responsibility of the manufacturer to provide that information to the medical community and revise that information accordingly in PDR's database. These revisions are distributed via monthly electronic drug updates, through our 60-day PDR Update (in print and electronic versions, sent six times a year), on PDR.net, within *mobile*PDR, and on-screen for those providers who use EMR systems that belong to PDR's network of EMR partners. To be certain that prescribers have the most current data, they should always consult these PDR sources before prescribing or administering any medications described in the following pages.

About Drug Summaries in the *PDR*

Two unique features of this edition are Section 9, Drug Summaries and Section 10, Specialty Drug Summaries, each of which includes a robust compendium of succinct monographs on a selection of prescribed drugs. Color-coded indices at the front of the book are included for each of these sections.

Electronic PDR Resources

PDR.net, a web portal designed specifically for prescribers, provides trusted, professional drug information, including full FDA-approved labeling, concise point-of-care drug information, as well as other relevant professional resources. **PDR.net** provides prescribers with online access to the authoritative drug information they need to support their treatment decisions.

*mobile*PDR is the official drug information and comparison app from PDR, allowing healthcare professionals free access to current drug prescribing information using an Apple® or Android™ device. Fast and easy to use, *mobile*PDR employs a simple, but powerful, search tool with access to thousands of drug summaries continually updated by PDR PharmDs. Also available is a drug comparison tool that allows users to compare characteristics of two or more drugs, a drug interaction tool that indicates the nature and severity of drug-drug interactions, and a pill identification tool. Registration is required. Please visit PDR.net/mobilePDR for more information.

PDR Services Within EMRs

PDR provides current prescribing information, patient education, and other services in eRx/EMR systems. These services for healthcare providers and their patients are convenient and readily accessible within clinical workflow at no cost to prescribers or their patients:

- **For Healthcare Providers:** In-EMR drug and condition messaging and prescribing information

- **For Patients:** In-EMR patient-friendly drug and condition information as well as patient savings opportunities

To request PDR's services in your EMR, email PDR at ehr@pdr.net telling us the name of your EMR vendor and we will contact them for you.

PDR Safety Communications

Critical communications are delivered electronically to physicians and other prescribers who register to receive them at PDR.net/registration, through participating medical societies, or by returning the verification form distributed with complimentary copies of the *PDR*.

Any portion of PDR's products that is reproduced, duplicated, copied, downloaded, sold, resold, or otherwise exploited for any commercial purpose without the express written consent of PDR is prohibited. Any use of trademarks, logos, or other proprietary information (including images, text, page layout, and form) of PDR's products and/or its affiliates without the express written consent of PDR is also prohibited. For more information about licensing PDR content, please call 800-232-7379.

Listed in this index are all manufacturers participating in the *Physicians' Desk Reference*®. It is through their courtesy that the *PDR*® is brought to the medical profession.

Each company's entry may include the address, phone, and fax number of its headquarters and regional offices, as well as email address, website, and contacts for inquiries, orders, and medical emergency information. Products with entries in the Product Information section are listed with their page numbers. Other products available from the

manufacturer are listed following the described products.

If an entry in the index lists multiple page numbers, the first one shown refers to images of the product; the last one refers to its prescribing information.

- **Bold page numbers** indicate full prescribing information.
- *Italic page numbers* signify partial information.
- The ◆ symbol marks drugs shown in the Product Identification Guide.

EDGEMONT   508, 952
PHARMACEUTICALS, LLC
1250 Capital of Texas Hwy, South
Building 3, Suite 400
Austin, TX 78746

Direct Inquiries to:
Toll Free: (888) 594-4332
Fax: (512) 329-2094
customerservice@edgemontpharma.com

Products Described:
◆Forfivo XL Extended-Release
  Tablets.......................508, 952

EGALET US INC.   508, 960
600 Lee Road, Suite 100
Wayne, PA 19087

Direct Inquiries to:
1-800-518-1084

Products Described:
◆Oxaydo Tablets 508, 960
◆Sprix Nasal Spray.............508, 964

ESSENTIA WATER, LLC   508, 1126
22833 Bothell Everett
  Highway, Suite 220
Bothell, WA 98021

Direct Inquiries to:
(425) 402-9555
or tolle free (877) 293-2239

Products Described:
◆Essentia Water...............508, 1126

GLENWOOD   508, 972
111 Cedar Lane
Englewood, NJ 07631

Direct Inquiries to:
Professional Services Department
(201) 569-0050
(800) 542-0772

For Medical Information Contact:
In Emergencies:
Professional Services Department
(201) 569-0050
(800) 542-0772

Products Described:
◆Potaba Capsules...............508, 972

GORDON LABORATORIES   509, 972
6801 Ludlow Street
Upper Darby, PA 19082

Direct Inquiries to:
Customer Service
(610) 734-2011
Fax: (610) 734-2049
Website: http://www.gordonlabs.net
E-mail: gordonlabs@att.net

For medical emergencies contact:
David Dercher
(610) 734-2011
Fax: (610) 734-2049

Products Described:
◆Formadon Solution............509, 972
◆Gordochom Solution 509, 972

Other Products Available:
Abscents Deodorizing Powder
Aloe Grande Creme
Aloe Grande Lotion
Anti-Rust Powder for Metal Instruments
Bromi-Lotion
Bromi-Talc Powder
Bromi-Talc Plus Powder
Calicylic Creme
Emollia Creme
Emollia Lotion
Forma-Ray Solution
GL-2 Skin Adherent
GL-7 Skin Adherent
Gordobalm Massage Lotion
Gordofilm Wart Remover
Gordomatic Crystals
Gordon's Boro-Packs
Gordon's No. Five Spray Foot Powder
Gordon's Vite A Creme
Gordon's Vite A Lotion
Gordon's Vite E Creme
Gordo-Pool Whirlpool Drops
Gormel Creme
Gormel Ten Lotion
Lugol's Strong Iodine Solution
Monsel's Ferric Subsulfate Solution
Mycomist Shoe & Boot Spray
Potassium Hydroxide Solution 5%
Silver Nitrate Solutions 10%, 25%, 50%
Sodium Hydroxide Solution 10%
Sorbidon Hydrate Creme

Stik It Skin Adherent Ampules
Tri-Chlor Solution
Vita-Ray Creme

IMMUNOTEC INC.   1126
300 Joseph Carrier
Vaudreuil-Dorion, QC
Canada J7V 5V5

For Direct Inquiries Contact:
(450) 424-9992 Ext 4453

Products Described:
Immunocal Powder Sachets 1126

INCYTE CORPORATION   973
1801 Augustine Cut-Off
Wilmington, DE 19803

Direct Inquiries to:
(855) 4-INCYTE (855-446-2983)
(302) 498-6700

Medical Information Contact:
(855)-4-MEDINFO (855-463-3463)
medinfo@incyte.com
Normal business hours: 8am to 8pm ET,
  Mon-Fri

Products Described:
Jakafi Tablets 973

JACOBUS PHARMACEUTICAL   982
CO., INC.
37 Cleveland Lane
P.O. Box 5290
Princeton, NJ 08540

Direct All Inquiries to:
(609) 921-7447
FAX: (609) 799-1176

Products Described:
Dapsone Tablets USP...............982
Paser Granules.....................983

KOWA   509, 985
PHARMACEUTICALS
AMERICA, INC.
530 Industrial Park Boulevard
Montgomery, AL 36117

Direct Inquiries:
(334) 288-1288
Fax: (334) 288-2788
info@kowapharma.com

Products Described:
◆Livalo Tablets..................509, 985

LIFEPHARM   509, 1127
32 Rancho Circle
Lake Forest, CA 92630

Direct Inquiries to:
(949) 216-9600
(800) 400-1287
Fax: (949) 216-9601
CustomerService@LifePharmGlobal.com

Products Described:
◆Laminine Capsules............509, 1127

NSE PRODUCTS, INC.   1130
(PHARMANEX)
75 West Center Street
Provo, UT 84601

For Information and Product Support:
1-(800) 487-1000
Website: www.nuskin.com

Products Described:
ageLOC R^2 Day Capsules..........1130
ageLOC R^2 Night Capsules 1130
ageLOC TR90 Control Capsules....1130
ageLOC TR90 Fit Capsules........1130
ageLOC TR90 JumpStart Powder ..1130
ageLOC TR90 TrimShake
  Powder 1130
ageLOC Youth Capsules 1131
g3 Juice 1131
LifePak Capsules 1131
ReishiMax GLp Capsules 1132
Tegreen 97 Capsules 1132

OREXIGEN   509, 990
THERAPEUTICS, INC.
3344 N. Torrey Pines Court,
  Suite 200
La Jolla, CA 92037

Direct Inquiries to:
(858) 875-8600
Fax: (858) 875-8650

Products Described:
◆Contrave Extended-Release
  Tablets....................509, 990

PERNIX THERAPEUTICS,   509, 1002
LLC
10 North Park Place
Suite 201
Morristown, NJ 07960

Products Described:
◆Silenor Tablets...............509, 1002
◆Treximet Tablets.............509, 1006

PERQUE INTEGRATIVE   1132
HEALTH
44621 Guilford Drive, Suite 150
Ashburn, VA 20147

Direct Inquiries to:
(800) 525-7372

Products Described:
Perque Life Guard Tabsules........1132
Perque Potent C Guard Powder.....1133
Perque Repair Guard Tabsules......1133
Perque Vessel Health Guard
  Lozenges.......................1133
Perque Whey Guard Repair
  Powder........................1133

PFIZER INC.   1016
235 East 42nd Street
New York, NY 10017-5755
For updates to the product information
  listed below, please check the Pfizer
  Web site http://www.pfizerpro.com
  or call (800) 438-1985.

For Medical Information, Contact:
(800) 438-1985
24 hours a day, 7 days a week

Distribution:
1855 Shelby Oaks Drive North
Memphis, TN 38134
(901) 387-5200

Customer Service:
(800) 533-4535

Pfizer Companies Include:
Agouron Pharmaceuticals
King Pharmaceuticals, Inc.
Parke-Davis
Pharmacia & Upjohn
G.D. Searle & Co.
Wyeth Pharmaceuticals

Products Described:
Viagra Tablets 1016
Xeljanz Tablets 1024
Xeljanz XR Extended-Release
  Tablets.........................1024

Other Products Available:
Accupril Tablets
Accuretic Tablets
Aldactazide Tablets
Alsuma Injection
Altace Capsules
Aromasin Tablets
Arthrotec Tablets
Atgam Sterile Solution
Avinza Capsules
Azulfidine Tablets, EN-Tabs
Bicillin L-A Injection
Bosulif Tablets
Caduet Tablets
Calan Tablets, SR Caplets
Camptosar for Injection
Cardura Tablets, XL Tablets
Caverject
Celebrex Capsules
Celontin Capsules
Chantix Tablets
Cleocin HCl Capsules
Cleocin Pediatric for Oral Solution, USP
Cleocin Phosphate Sterile Solution
Cleocin T Topical Gel, Lotion, Solution
Cleocin Vaginal Cream, Ovules
Colestid Tablets, Oral Suspension
Colestid/Flavored Colestid for Oral
  Suspension
Cortef Tablets
Daypro Caplets
Depo-Estradiol Injectable Solution
Depo-Medrol Injectable Suspension
Depo-Provera
depo-subQ provera Injectable Suspension
Depo-Testosterone Injection
Detrol Tablets
Detrol LA Capsules
Didrex Tablets
Diflucan

Dilantin
Elelyso Injection
Ellence Injection
Embeda Extended Release Capsules
Emcyt Capsules
Eraxis for Injection
Estring Vaginal Ring
Feldene Capsules
Flagyl
Flector Patch
Gelfilm Sterile Film
Gelfoam Sterile Powder, Sponge
Genotropin Lyophilized Powder
Geodon
Glucotrol Tablets, XL Tablets
Glynase PresTab Tablets
Glyset Tablets
Halcion Tablets
Hemabate Sterile Solution (Sales
  restricted to hospitals only)
Idamycin
Inlyta Tablets
Inspra Tablets
Levoxyl Tablets
Lincocin Sterile Solution
Lipitor Tablets
Lomotil Tablets
Lopid Tablets
Lyrica Capsules, Oral Solution
Medrol Tablets and Dosepak
Mycobutin Capsules
Nardil Tablets
Neurontin Capsules, Tablets, Oral
  Solution
Nitrostat Tablets
Norpace
Norvasc Tablets
Oxecta Tablets
Pfizerpen for Injection
Prepidil Gel
Procardia Capsules, XL Tablets
Prostin E2 Vaginal Suppository
Prostin VR Pediatric Sterile Solution
Provera Tablets
Relpax Tablets
Revatio Injection, Tablets
R-Gene 10 for Intravenous Use
Skelaxin Tablets
Solu-Cortef Injection
Solu-Medrol Injection
Somavert for Injection
Sutent Capsules
Tikosyn Capsules
Toviaz Extended-Release Tablets
Unasyn
VFEND
Vibramycin
Xalatan Sterile Ophthalmic Solution
Xalkori Capsules
Xanax Tablets, XR Tablets
Zithromax
Zmax for Oral Suspension
Zoloft
Zyvox

PURDUE PHARMA L.P.   509, 1032
One Stamford Forum
Stamford, CT 06901-3431

For Medical Inquiries:
(888) 726-7535

Adverse Drug Experiences:
(888) 726-7535

Customer Service:
(800) 877-5666
FAX: (203) 588-8850

Products Described:
◆Butrans Transdermal System .. 509, 1032
◆Hysingla ER Tablets..........509, 1042
◆OxyContin Tablets...........509, 1050

PURETRIM   509, 1134
1201 South Alma School Rd
Suite 8550
Mesa, AZ 85210

Direct Inquiries to:
800-69AWARE (9273)
http://www.puretrim.net

Products Described:
◆Boost Tea...................509, 1134
◆Experience Capsules........509, 1134
◆Liquid Daily Complete.......509, 1134
◆LiverMaster Capsules.......509, 1134
◆PureTrim Joint Tea.........509, 1134
◆PureTrim Mediterranean
  Wellness Shakes............509, 1134

RLC LABS, INC.   510, 1059
Cave Creek, AZ 85331

For Product Information:
(877) 797-7997
sales@rlclabs.com

◆ Shown in Product Identification Guide   *Italic Page Number* Indicates Brief Listing

CONTENTS

(Continued)

CONTENTS (Continued)

BRAND AND GENERIC NAME INDEX

◆ Shown in Product Identification Guide   Underline Denotes Generic Name   *Italic Page Number* **Indicates Brief Listing**

BRAND AND GENERIC NAME INDEX

SECTION 3

PRODUCT CATEGORY INDEX

This index lists products by prescribing category, allowing you to quickly and easily identify all agents with a given therapeutic use or mechanism of action. Categories are based on the latest medical terminology and are comprehensively cross-referenced. All fully described products in the Product Information section of the *PDR®* are included here.

If an entry in the index lists multiple page numbers, the first one shown refers to images of the product; the last one refers to its prescribing information.

A

ACE INHIBITORS
(see under:
CARDIOVASCULAR AGENTS
ANGIOTENSIN CONVERTING ENZYME
(ACE) INHIBITORS
ANGIOTENSIN CONVERTING ENZYME
(ACE) INHIBITORS WITH CALCIUM
CHANNEL BLOCKERS)

**ACQUIRED IMMUNE
DEFICIENCY SYNDROME
THERAPY**
(see under:
**ANTI-INFECTIVE AGENTS,
SYSTEMIC**
AIDS ADJUNCT ANTI-INFECTIVES
AIDS CHEMOTHERAPEUTIC AGENTS)

AIDS THERAPY
(see under:
**ANTI-INFECTIVE AGENTS,
SYSTEMIC**
AIDS ADJUNCT ANTI-INFECTIVES
AIDS CHEMOTHERAPEUTIC AGENTS)

AIDS/HIV ADJUNCT AGENTS
(see under:
**ANTI-INFECTIVE AGENTS,
SYSTEMIC**
AIDS ADJUNCT ANTI-INFECTIVES)

ALTERNATIVE MEDICINE
(see under:
HOMEOPATHIC REMEDIES)

AMINO ACIDS
(see under:
DIETARY SUPPLEMENTS
AMINO ACIDS & COMBINATIONS)

ANALGESICS
(see also under:
**GOUT PREPARATIONS
MIGRAINE PREPARATIONS
NASAL PREPARATIONS**
ANALGESICS)
**ACETAMINOPHEN &
COMBINATIONS**
Vicodin/Vicodin ES/
Vicodin HP Tablets
(AbbVie) **506, 507, 833**
NARCOTICS
**NARCOTIC
AGONIST-ANTAGONIST &
COMBINATIONS**
Butrans Transdermal System
(Purdue) **509, 1032**
NARCOTICS & COMBINATIONS
Hysingla ER Tablets *(Purdue)* **509, 1042**
Oxaydo Tablets *(Egalet)* **508, 960**
OxyContin Tablets *(Purdue)* **509, 1050**
Vicodin/Vicodin ES/
Vicodin HP Tablets
(AbbVie) **506, 507, 833**
Vicoprofen Tablets *(AbbVie)* **507, 835**
**NONSTEROIDAL
ANTI-INFLAMMATORY DRUGS
(NSAIDS) & COMBINATIONS**
Sprix Nasal Spray *(Egalet)* **508, 964**
Treximet Tablets *(Pernix)* **509, 1006**
Vicoprofen Tablets *(AbbVie)* **507, 835**

ANESTHETICS
GENERAL ANESTHETICS
Ultane Volatile Liquid for Inhalation
(AbbVie) **506, 822**

**ANGIOTENSIN CONVERTING
ENZYME INHIBITORS**
(see under:
CARDIOVASCULAR AGENTS
ANGIOTENSIN CONVERTING ENZYME
(ACE) INHIBITORS
ANGIOTENSIN CONVERTING ENZYME
(ACE) INHIBITORS WITH CALCIUM
CHANNEL BLOCKERS)

ANORECTICS
(see under:
OBESITY MANAGEMENT)

ANOREXIANTS
(see under:
OBESITY MANAGEMENT)

ANTACIDS
(see under:
GASTROINTESTINAL AGENTS
ANTACIDS)

ANTIARTHRITICS
(see under:
ANALGESICS
NONSTEROIDAL ANTI-INFLAMMATORY
DRUGS (NSAIDS) & COMBINATIONS
**ANTIRHEUMATIC AGENTS
GOUT PREPARATIONS
HORMONES**
GLUCOCORTICOIDS)

ANTIBIOTICS
(see under:
**ANTI-INFECTIVE AGENTS,
SYSTEMIC**
ANTIBIOTICS
**SKIN & MUCOUS MEMBRANE
AGENTS**
ANTI-INFECTIVES
ANTIBIOTICS & COMBINATIONS)

ANTICONVULSANTS
**MISCELLANEOUS
ANTICONVULSANTS**
Depakote ER Tablet, Extended
Release for Oral Use *(AbbVie)* ... **505, 632**
Oxtellar XR Extended-Release
Tablets *(Supernus)* **510, 1063**
Trokendi XR Extended-Release
Capsules *(Supernus)* **510, 1071**
Zonegran Capsules *(Concordia)*. **508, 919**

ANTIDEPRESSANTS
(see under:
PSYCHOTHERAPEUTIC AGENTS
ANTIDEPRESSANTS)

ANTIDOTES
MISCELLANEOUS ANTIDOTES
Kcentra Lyophilized Powder
(CSL Behring) **508, 944**

ANTIFIBRINOLYTIC AGENTS
(see under:
BLOOD MODIFIERS
HEMOSTATICS)

**ANTIFIBROSIS THERAPY,
SYSTEMIC**
Potaba Capsules *(Glenwood)* **508, 972**

ANTIFUNGALS
(see under:
**SKIN & MUCOUS MEMBRANE
AGENTS**
ANTI-INFECTIVES
ANTIFUNGALS & COMBINATIONS)

**ANTIHYPERTENSIVE
MEDICATIONS**
(see under:
CARDIOVASCULAR AGENTS
ANGIOTENSIN CONVERTING ENZYME
(ACE) INHIBITORS
ANGIOTENSIN CONVERTING ENZYME
(ACE) INHIBITORS WITH CALCIUM
CHANNEL BLOCKERS
BETA ADRENERGIC BLOCKING AGENTS
WITH DIURETICS
DIURETICS)

ANTI-INFECTIVE AGENTS
(see under:
**ANTI-INFECTIVE AGENTS,
SYSTEMIC**
**SKIN & MUCOUS MEMBRANE
AGENTS**
ANTI-INFECTIVES)

**ANTI-INFECTIVE AGENTS,
SYSTEMIC**
AIDS ADJUNCT ANTI-INFECTIVES
Biaxin Filmtab Tablets *(AbbVie)* **505, 615**
Biaxin Granules *(AbbVie)* **505, 615**
**AIDS CHEMOTHERAPEUTIC
AGENTS**
**PROTEASE INHIBITORS &
COMBINATIONS**
Kaletra Oral Solution *(AbbVie)*. **505, 687**
Kaletra Tablets *(AbbVie)* **505, 687**
Norvir Oral Solution *(AbbVie)* **506, 769**
Norvir Tablets *(AbbVie)* **506, 769**
ANTIBIOTICS
MACROLIDES & COMBINATIONS
Biaxin Filmtab Tablets *(AbbVie)*. ... **505, 615**
Biaxin Granules *(AbbVie)*. **505, 615**
Biaxin XL Filmtab Tablets *(AbbVie)* **615**
ANTIMALARIAL AGENTS
Plaquenil Tablets *(Concordia)* **508, 913**
ANTITUBERCULOSIS AGENTS
Paser Granules *(Jacobus)* **983**
ANTIVIRALS
Kaletra Oral Solution *(AbbVie)*. **505, 687**
Kaletra Tablets *(AbbVie)* **505, 687**
Moderiba Tablets *(AbbVie)* **506, 749**
Norvir Oral Solution *(AbbVie)* **506, 769**
Norvir Tablets *(AbbVie)* **506, 769**
Technivie Tablets *(AbbVie)* **800**
Viekira Pak *(AbbVie)*. **507, 839**
Viekira XR Extended-Release
Tablets *(AbbVie)* **507, 856**
LEPROSTATICS
Dapsone Tablets USP *(Jacobus)*. **982**

ANTI-INFLAMMATORY AGENTS
(see under:
ANALGESICS
NONSTEROIDAL ANTI-INFLAMMATORY
DRUGS (NSAIDS) & COMBINATIONS
**ANTIRHEUMATIC AGENTS
GASTROINTESTINAL AGENTS**
ANTI-INFLAMMATORY AGENTS
**GOUT PREPARATIONS
HORMONES**
GLUCOCORTICOIDS
NASAL PREPARATIONS
ANTI-INFLAMMATORY AGENTS
**SKIN & MUCOUS MEMBRANE
AGENTS**
STEROIDS & COMBINATIONS)

**ANTI-INFLAMMATORY AGENTS,
SKIN AND MUCOUS
MEMBRANE**
Orapred ODT Orally Disintegrating
Tablets *(Concordia)* **508, 906**

ANTILIPEMIC AGENTS
(see under:
CARDIOVASCULAR AGENTS
ANTILIPIDEMIC AGENTS)

ANTIMYCOTICS
(see under:
**SKIN & MUCOUS MEMBRANE
AGENTS**
ANTI-INFECTIVES
ANTIFUNGALS & COMBINATIONS)

ANTINEOPLASTICS
ADJUNCT THERAPY
Nature-Throid Tablets *(RLC)* **510, 1059**
Synthroid Tablets *(AbbVie)*. **506, 789**
WP Thyroid Tablets *(RLC)*. **510, 1061**
**HORMONAL AGONISTS/
ANTAGONISTS**
ANTIANDROGENS
Nilandron Tablets *(Concordia)*. **508, 904**
**GONADOTROPIN RELEASING
HORMONE (GNRH) ANALOGUES**
Lupron Depot 7.5 mg for 1-Month
Administration *(AbbVie)*. **506, 728**
Lupron Depot— 22.5 mg for
3-Month Administration
(AbbVie) **506, 728**
Lupron Depot— 30 mg for
4-Month Administration
(AbbVie) **506, 728**
Lupron Depot— 45 mg for
6-Month Administration
(AbbVie) **728**
KINASE INHIBITORS
Jakafi Tablets *(Incyte)*. **973**
**MISCELLANEOUS
ANTINEOPLASTICS**
Imlygic Suspension for Intralesional
Injection *(Amgen)* **507, 880**
Venclexta Tablets *(AbbVie)*. **506, 827**
**SKIN & MUCOUS MEMBRANE
AGENTS**
(see under:
**SKIN & MUCOUS MEMBRANE
AGENTS**
ANTINEOPLASTICS)
STEROIDS & COMBINATIONS
Orapred ODT Orally Disintegrating
Tablets *(Concordia)* **508, 906**

ANTIPARKINSONIAN AGENTS
**DOPAMINERGIC AGENTS &
COMBINATIONS**
Duopa Enteral Suspension *(AbbVie)*. .. **505, 644**

ANTIPERSPIRANTS
(see under:
**SKIN & MUCOUS MEMBRANE
AGENTS**
ANTIPERSPIRANTS)

ANTIPSYCHOTIC MEDICATIONS
(see under:
PSYCHOTHERAPEUTIC AGENTS
ANTIPSYCHOTIC AGENTS)

ANTIPYRETICS
(see under:
ANALGESICS
ACETAMINOPHEN & COMBINATIONS
NONSTEROIDAL ANTI-INFLAMMATORY
DRUGS (NSAIDS) & COMBINATIONS)

SECTION 4

BRAND AND GENERIC NAME INDEX FOR DRUG SUMMARIES

This index includes the brand and generic names of each drug in the Drug Summaries section. The main monograph names are fully capitalized (eg, ABILIFY) and generic names begin with initial caps (eg, Abacavir sulfate). Any brand name associated with an entry is listed under the product.

SECTION 4A

BRAND AND GENERIC NAME INDEX FOR SPECIALTY DRUG SUMMARIES

This index includes the brand and generic names of each drug in the Specialty Drug Summaries section. The main monograph names are fully capitalized (eg, | ABRAXANE) and generic names begin with initial caps (eg, Paclitaxel protein-bound). Any brand name associated with an entry is listed under the product.

SECTION 5

PRODUCT CATEGORY INDEX FOR DRUG SUMMARIES

Organized alphabetically, this index includes the product category (therapeutic class) of each drug in the Drug Summaries section. Product category headings are based on information provided in the drug monographs. The drug entries listed under each bold product category are organized alphabetically by brand name or monograph title (shown in capitalized letters), followed by the generic name in parentheses.

PRODUCT CATEGORY INDEX FOR DRUG SUMMARIES

PRODUCT CATEGORY INDEX FOR DRUG SUMMARIES

PRODUCT CATEGORY INDEX FOR DRUG SUMMARIES

SECTION 5A

PRODUCT CATEGORY INDEX FOR SPECIALTY DRUG SUMMARIES

Organized alphabetically, this index includes the product category (therapeutic class) of each drug in the Specialty Drug Summaries section. Product category headings are based on information provided in the drug monographs. The drug entries listed under each bold product category are organized alphabetically by brand name or monograph title (shown in capitalized letters), followed by the generic name in parentheses.

4-HYDROXYPHENYLPYRUVATE DIOXYGENASE (HPPD) INHIBITOR
ORFADIN
(nitisinone)...................................S-1297

5-HT$_{1B/1D}$ AGONIST (TRIPTANS)
ZECUITY
(sumatriptan)................................S-1432

A

ACETYLCHOLINE RELEASE INHIBITOR
BOTOX
(onabotulinumtoxinA).................S-1093
DYSPORT
(abobotulinumtoxinA)..................S-1137
MYOBLOC
(rimabotulinumtoxinB)................S-1266
XEOMIN
(incobotulinumtoxinA)................S-1422

ACTINOMYCIN ANTIBIOTIC
COSMEGEN
(dactinomycin).............................S-1117

ADENOSINE DEAMINASE (ADA) INHIBITOR
NIPENT
(pentostatin)................................S-1277

ALKYLATING AGENT
BENDEKA
(bendamustine hydrochloride)....S-1085
BUSULFEX
(busulfan)....................................S-1096
DACARBAZINE
(dacarbazine)...............................S-1126
EVOMELA
(melphalan)..................................S-1156
TEMODAR
(temozolomide)...........................S-1377
TREANDA
(bendamustine hydrochloride)....S-1384
YONDELIS
(trabectedin)................................S-1428

ALLERGEN EXTRACT
ORALAIR
(sweet vernal/orchard/perennial rye/
timothy/kentucky bluegrass mixed
pollens allergen extract)..............S-1295

ALPHA$_1$-PROTEINASE INHIBITOR (A$_1$PI)
ARALAST NP
(alpha1-proteinase inhibitor
(human))......................................S-1072
GLASSIA
(alpha1-proteinase inhibitor
(human))......................................S-1189
PROLASTIN-C
(alpha1-proteinase inhibitor
(human))......................................S-1319
ZEMAIRA
(alpha1-proteinase inhibitor
(human))......................................S-1434

ALPHA/BETA ADRENERGIC AGONIST
NORTHERA
(droxidopa)..................................S-1278

ALPHA-L-IDURONIDASE
ALDURAZYME
(laronidase).................................S-1064

AMINOGLYCOSIDE
BETHKIS
(tobramycin)................................S-1089
KITABIS PAK
(tobramycin)................................S-1237
TOBI
(tobramycin)................................S-1382

ANDROGEN
AVEED
(testosterone undecanoate).........S-1082

ANTHRACYCLINE
DAUNORUBICIN
(daunorubicin hydrochloride)........S-1129
DOXIL
(doxorubicin hydrochloride
liposome)....................................S-1134
DOXORUBICIN
(doxorubicin hydrochloride).........S-1135
ELLENCE
(epirubicin hydrochloride)............S-1142
IDAMYCIN PFS
(idarubicin hydrochloride)............S-1211
VALSTAR
(valrubicin)..................................S-1397

ANTIANDROGEN
XTANDI
(enzalutamide)............................S-1426
ZYTIGA
(abiraterone acetate)...................S-1444

ANTICOAGULANT PROTEIN
CEPROTIN
(protein C concentrate
(human))......................................S-1104

ANTIFOLATE
ALIMTA
(pemetrexed disodium)................S-1066

ANTIHEMOPHILIC AGENT
ALPHANATE
(antihemophilic factor/von Willebrand
factor complex (human)).............S-1068
ALPHANINE SD
(coagulation factor IX (human))....S-1068
BEBULIN
(factor IX complex).....................S-1084
FEIBA NF
(anti-inhibitor coagulant
complex)......................................S-1164
HEMOFIL M
(antihemophilic factor (human))....S-1197
HUMATE-P
(antihemophilic factor/von Willebrand
factor complex (human))..............S-1201
KOATE-DVI
(antihemophilic factor (human))....S-1237
MONOCLATE-P
(antihemophilic factor (human))....S-1262
MONONINE
(coagulation factor IX (human))....S-1262
NOVOSEVEN RT
(coagulation factor VIIa
(recombinant))............................S-1281
PROFILNINE
(factor IX complex).....................S-1317

ANTIHEMOPHILIC FACTOR (RECOMBINANT)
ADVATE
(antihemophilic factor
(recombinant))............................S-1061
ADYNOVATE
(antihemophilic factor (recombinant),
pegylated)...................................S-1061
ALPROLIX
(coagulation factor IX (recombinant),
Fc fusion protein).......................S-1069
BENEFIX
(coagulation factor IX
(recombinant))............................S-1086
ELOCTATE
(antihemophilic factor (recombinant),
fc fusion protein)........................S-1143

HELIXATE FS
(antihemophilic factor
(recombinant))............................S-1196
IXINITY
(coagulation factor IX
(recombinant))............................S-1224
KOGENATE FS
(antihemophilic factor
(recombinant))............................S-1238
KOVALTRY
(antihemophilic factor
(recombinant))............................S-1239
NOVOEIGHT
(antihemophilic factor
(recombinant))............................S-1280
NUWIQ
(antihemophilic factor
(recombinant))............................S-1285
OBIZUR
(antihemophilic factor (recombinant),
porcine sequence).......................S-1286
RECOMBINATE
(antihemophilic factor
(recombinant))............................S-1330
RIXUBIS
(coagulation factor IX
(recombinant))............................S-1343
XYNTHA
(antihemophilic factor
(recombinant))............................S-1426

ANTIMETABOLITE
ADRUCIL
(fluorouracil)...............................S-1060
CLOLAR
(clofarabine)................................S-1110
CYTARABINE
(cytarabine).................................S-1124
DEPOCYT
(cytarabine liposome).................S-1130
FLOXURIDINE
(floxuridine)................................S-1169
FLUDARABINE
(fludarabine phosphate)...............S-1169
FLUOROPLEX
(fluorouracil)...............................S-1170

ANTIMICROTUBULE AGENT
ABRAXANE
(paclitaxel protein-bound)...........S-1054
DOCEFREZ
(docetaxel)..................................S-1131
DOCETAXEL
(docetaxel)..................................S-1133
HALAVEN
(eribulin mesylate).......................S-1195
IXEMPRA
(ixabepilone)...............................S-1223
JEVTANA
(cabazitaxel)...............................S-1228
PACLITAXEL
(paclitaxel)..................................S-1302

ANTISENSE OLIGONUCLEOTIDE
EXONDYS 51
(eteplirsen).................................S-1159

ARGININE VASOPRESSIN ANTAGONIST
SAMSCA
(tolvaptan)..................................S-1346

ATTENUATED LIVE BCG CULTURE
BCG VACCINE
(BCG live)...................................S-1083
THERACYS
(BCG live)...................................S-1379

ATYPICAL ANTIPSYCHOTIC
NUPLAZID
(pimavanserin)............................S-1284

B

BCL-2 INHIBITOR
VENCLEXTA
(venetoclax).................................S-1402

BENZOTHIAZOLE
RILUTEK
(riluzole).....................................S-1342

BILE ACID
CHOLBAM
(cholic acid)................................S-1106

BIOLOGICAL RESPONSE MODIFIER
ACTIMMUNE
(interferon gamma-1b).................S-1057
ALFERON N
(interferon alfa-n3 (human leukocyte
derived))......................................S-1065
AVONEX
(interferon beta-1a).....................S-1082
BETASERON
(interferon beta-1b).....................S-1088
EXTAVIA
(interferon beta-1b).....................S-1160
INFERGEN
(interferon alfacon-1)..................S-1216
INTRON A
(interferon alfa-2b,
recombinant)...............................S-1219
PEGASYS
(peginterferon alfa-2a)................S-1305
PEGINTRON
(peginterferon alfa-2b)................S-1306
PLEGRIDY
(peginterferon beta-1a)...............S-1308
PROLEUKIN
(aldesleukin)...............................S-1319
REBIF
(interferon beta-1a).....................S-1328
SYLATRON
(peginterferon alfa-2b)................S-1366

BISPHOSPHONATE
PAMIDRONATE
(pamidronate disodium)...............S-1303
RECLAST
(zoledronic acid).........................S-1329
ZOMETA
(zoledronic acid).........................S-1440

BRADYKININ B$_2$-RECEPTOR ANTAGONIST
FIRAZYR
(icatibant)...................................S-1165

C

C1 ESTERASE INHIBITOR
BERINERT
(C1 esterase inhibitor (human)).....S-1088
CINRYZE
(C1 esterase inhibitor (human)).....S-1108
RUCONEST
(C1 esterase inhibitor
(recombinant))............................S-1344

CALCIMIMETIC AGENT
SENSIPAR
(cinacalcet)................................S-1350

CALCINEURIN-INHIBITOR IMMUNOSUPPRESSANT
ASTAGRAF XL
(tacrolimus)................................S-1077

PRODUCT CATEGORY INDEX FOR SPECIALTY DRUG SUMMARIES

Key to Controlled Substances Schedule

Products listed with the symbols shown below are subject to the Controlled Substances Act of 1970. These drugs are categorized according to their potential for abuse. The greater the potential, the more severe the limitations on their prescription.

SCHEDULE   INTERPRETATION

Ⓒ II   **HIGH POTENTIAL FOR ABUSE.** Use may lead to severe physical or psychological dependence.

Ⓒ III   **POTENTIAL FOR ABUSE LESS THAN THE DRUGS OR OTHER SUBSTANCES IN C-II.** Use may lead to low-to-moderate physical dependence or high psychological dependence.

Ⓒ IV   **LOW POTENTIAL FOR ABUSE RELATIVE TO DRUGS OR OTHER SUBSTANCES IN C-III.** Use may lead to limited physical or psychological dependence relative to the drugs or other substances in C-III.

Ⓒ V   **LOW POTENTIAL FOR ABUSE RELATIVE TO DRUGS OR OTHER SUBSTANCES IN C-IV.** Use may lead to limited physical or psychological dependence relative to the drugs or other substances in C-IV.

FDA Requirements for Pregnancy and Lactation Labeling

The FDA has amended its regulations governing the content and format of the "Pregnancy," "Labor and delivery," and "Nursing mothers" subsections of the "Use in Specific Populations" section of the labeling for human prescription drug and biological products. The Pregnancy and Lactation Labeling Rule (PLLR) requires changes to the content and format for information presented in prescription drug labeling in the Physician Labeling Rule format to assist healthcare providers in assessing benefit versus risk and in subsequent counseling of pregnant women and nursing mothers who need to take medication, thus allowing them to make informed and educated decisions for themselves and their children. The PLLR removes pregnancy letter categories – A, B, C, D, and X. The PLLR also requires the label to be updated when information becomes outdated. This rule became effective June 30, 2015. The changes are as follows:

Pregnancy (8.1) – The **Pregnancy** subsection now includes information on labor and delivery and other content including:

- information for a **pregnancy exposure registry** (when one is available) that collects and maintains data on the effects of approved drugs that are prescribed to and used by pregnant women;

- a **Risk Summary** subheading that provides information on all the available data regarding risk of adverse developmental outcomes;

- a **Clinical Considerations** subheading that provides information to further inform prescribing and risk-benefit counseling; and

- a **Data** subheading that includes the human or animal data available that is discussed in the Risk Summary and Clinical Considerations sections.

Lactation (8.2) – The "Nursing mothers" subsection was renamed the **Lactation** subsection and provides information about using the drug while breastfeeding, such as the amount of drug in breast milk and potential effects on the breastfed child. Information is presented under the following subheadings:

- **Risk Summary** subheading that provides information on the effects of the drug and/or its active metabolite on a breastfed child and on milk production

- **Clinical Considerations** subheading that discusses ways to minimize exposure to the breastfed child and monitor for adverse reactions

- **Data** subheading that describes the data on which the Risk Summary and Clinical Considerations are based

Females and Males of Reproductive Potential (8.3) – This is a new subsection that is required to include information on recommendations or requirements for pregnancy testing and/or contraception before, during, or after drug therapy and/or if there are human and/or animal data suggesting drug-associated effects on fertility and/or preimplantation loss effects.

Prior Use-in-Pregnancy Ratings

The FDA use-in-pregnancy rating system was previously used to weigh the degree to which available information has ruled out risk to the fetus against the drug's potential benefit to the patient. The ratings, and their interpretations, are as follows:

SCHEDULE	INTERPRETATION
A	**CONTROLLED STUDIES SHOW NO RISK.** Adequate, well-controlled studies in pregnant women have failed to demonstrate a risk to the fetus in the first trimester of pregnancy (and there is no evidence of a risk in later trimesters).
B	**NO EVIDENCE OF RISK IN HUMANS.** Adequate, well-controlled studies in pregnant women are lacking, and animal studies have not shown increased risk of fetal abnormalities. The chance of fetal harm is remote, but remains a possibility.
C	**RISK CANNOT BE RULED OUT.** Adequate, well-controlled human studies in pregnant women are lacking, and animal studies have shown a risk to the fetus. There is a chance of fetal harm if the drug is administered during pregnancy, but the potential benefits may outweigh the potential risk.
D	**POSITIVE EVIDENCE OF RISK.** Studies in humans, or investigational or postmarketing data, have demonstrated fetal risk. Nevertheless, potential benefits from the use of the drug may outweigh the potential risk. For example, the drug may be acceptable if needed in a life-threatening situation or serious disease for which safer drugs cannot be used or are ineffective.
X	**CONTRAINDICATED IN PREGNANCY.** Studies in animals or humans have demonstrated fetal abnormalities or if there is positive evidence of fetal risk based on adverse reaction reports from investigational or marketing experience, or both, and risk of use clearly outweighs any possible benefit.

SECTION 6

PRODUCT IDENTIFICATION GUIDE

To aid in quick identification, this section provides full-color, actual-sized images of tablets and capsules. A variety of other dosage forms and packages are shown at less than actual size.

Products in this section are arranged alphabetically by manufacturer. Some exceptions, however, have been made based on space available in this section. In some instances, not all dosage forms and sizes are pictured. If others are available, a † symbol precedes the product's name. Letters or numbers representing the manufacturer's identification code are followed by a * symbol.

For more information on any of the products in this section, please turn to the Product Information section, or check directly with the manufacturer. The page number of each product's text entry appears with its images.

While every effort has been made to guarantee faithful reproduction of the images in this section, changes in size, color, and design are always a possibility. Be sure to confirm a product's identity with the manufacturer or a pharmacist.

INDEX BY MANUFACTURER

This section is made possible through the courtesy of the manufacturers whose products appear on the following pages.

4LIFE

DS   4LIFE   P. 1118

**4Life Transfer Factor®
Tri-Factor® Formula**

A&Z PHARMACEUTICAL

OTC   A&Z PHARMACEUTICAL   P. 602

D-Cal®
(calcium carbonate/vitamin D₃)

Calcium 300 mg/vitamin D_3 100 IU

60 Chewable Tablets

OTC   A&Z PHARMACEUTICAL   P. 602

D-Cal®
(calcium carbonate/vitamin D₃)

Calcium 300 mg/vitamin D_3 100 IU

30 Chewable Tablets

D-Cal® Kids
(calcium carbonate/vitamin D₃)

While every effort has been
made to reproduce products
faithfully, this section is to be
considered a quick reference
identification aid. In cases of
suspected overdosing, etc.,
chemical analysis should
be done.

OTC   A&Z PHARMACEUTICAL   P. 602

Calcium 300 mg/vitamin D_3 100 IU
10 pouches

Granules

D-Cal® Kids Granules
(calcium carbonate/vitamin D₃)

ABBVIE INC.

**For description of
Abbo-Code Identifications,
see Abbo-Code index at the
beginning of the AbbVie
Information Section.**

C-III   AbbVie Inc.   P. 603

AndroGel® 1%
(testosterone gel)

C-III   AbbVie Inc.   P. 609

AndroGel® 1.62%
(testosterone gel)

RX   AbbVie Inc.   P. 615

KT* 250 mg

KL* 500 mg

Biaxin® Filmtab®
(clarithromycin tablets, USP)

RX   AbbVie Inc.   P. 615

250 mg/5 mL

†Biaxin® Granules
(clarithromycin for oral suspension, USP)

RX   AbbVie Inc.   P. 628

Creon®
(pancrelipase)
Delayed-Release Capsules

RX   AbbVie Inc.   P. 632

250 mg

†Depakene®
(valproic acid)
Capsules and Oral Solution

RX   AbbVie Inc.   P. 632

NT* 125 mg

NR* 250 mg

NS* 500 mg

Depakote®
(divalproex sodium)
Tablets for Oral Use

RX   AbbVie Inc.   P. 632

HF* 250 mg

HC* 500 mg

Depakote® ER
(divalproex sodium)
Tablets, Extended-Release for Oral Use

RX   AbbVie Inc.   P. 632

125 mg

**Depakote® Sprinkle
Capsules**
(divalproex sodium
delayed release capsules)

RX   AbbVie Inc.   P. 644

4.63 mg and 20 mg/mL

Duopa™
(carbidopa and levodopa)

Products in this section are
arranged alphabetically by
manufacturer. In some instances,
not all dosage forms and/or
sizes are pictured. If others are
available, a † symbol precedes
the product's name. Letters or
numbers representing the
manufacturer's identification code
are followed by a * symbol.

RX   AbbVie Inc.   P. 655

OR* 25 mg

OS* 50 mg

OT* 100 mg

Gengraf® Capsules
(cyclosporine capsules, USP [MODIFIED])

RX   AbbVie Inc.   P. 665

prefilled syringe

40 mg/0.4 mL
pen

prefilled syringe

40 mg/0.8 mL
pen

†HUMIRA®
(adalimumab)

RX   AbbVie Inc.   P. 687

80 mg-20 mg/mL
160 mL bottle

Kaletra®
(lopinavir/ritonavir)
Solution for Oral Use

RX   AbbVie Inc.   P. 687

100 mg/25 mg

Kaletra®
(lopinavir/ritonavir)
Tablet Film-Coated for Oral Use

RX   AbbVie Inc.   P. 687

200 mg/50 mg

Kaletra®
(lopinavir/ritonavir)
Tablet Film-Coated for Oral Use

RX   AbbVie Inc.   P. 704, 711

1-Month 3.75 mg/5 mg

3-Month 11.25 mg/5 mg

Lupaneta Pack®
(leuprolide acetate for depot suspension
and norethindrone acetate tablets)

RX   AbbVie Inc.   P. 718, 723

1-Month 3.75 mg

3-Month 11.25 mg

Lupron Depot® GYN
(leuprolide acetate for depot suspension)

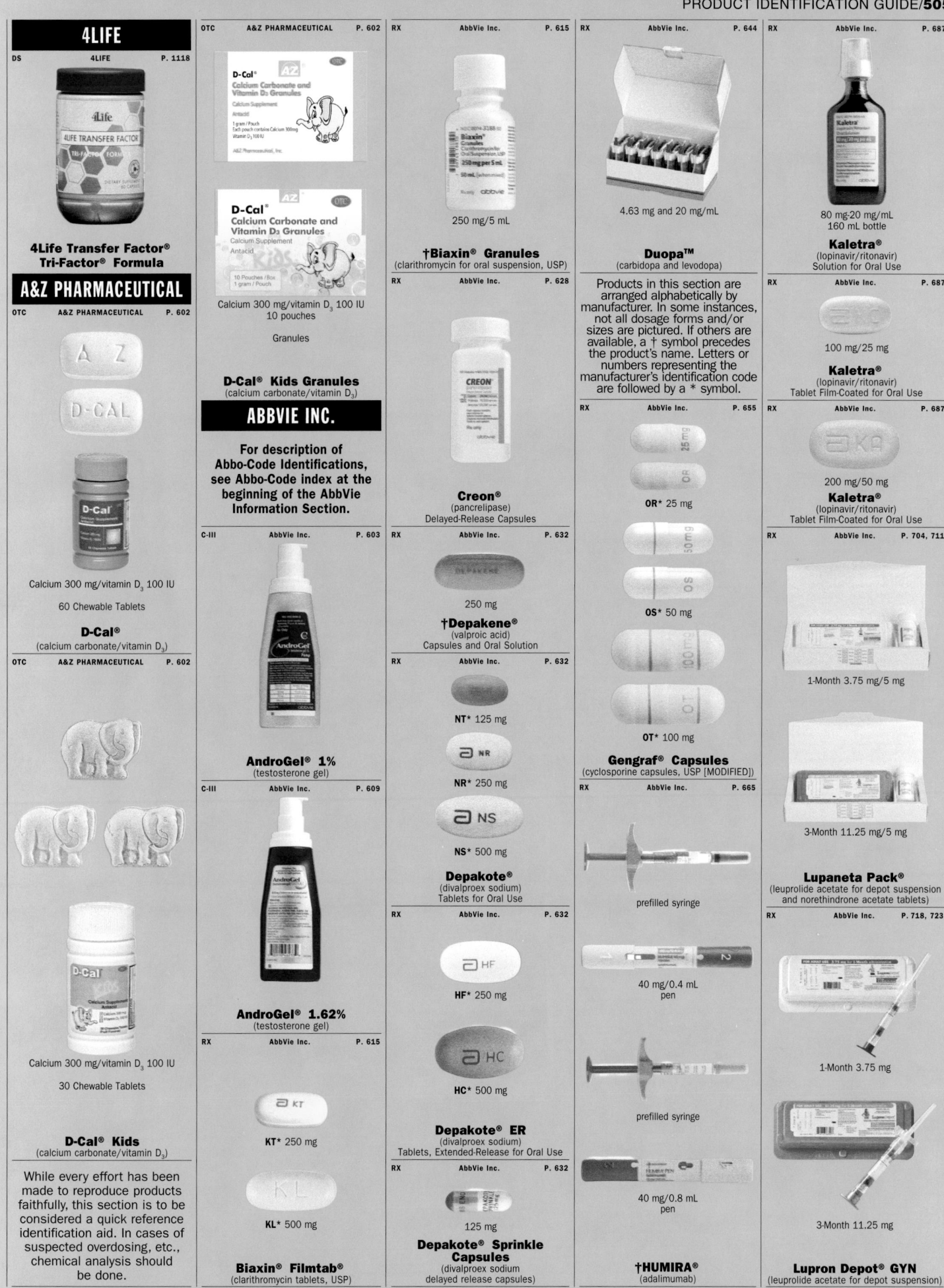

*AbbVie Abbo-Code identification letters. Filmtab® Film-sealed tablets, AbbVie.

†Additional dosage forms and sizes available.

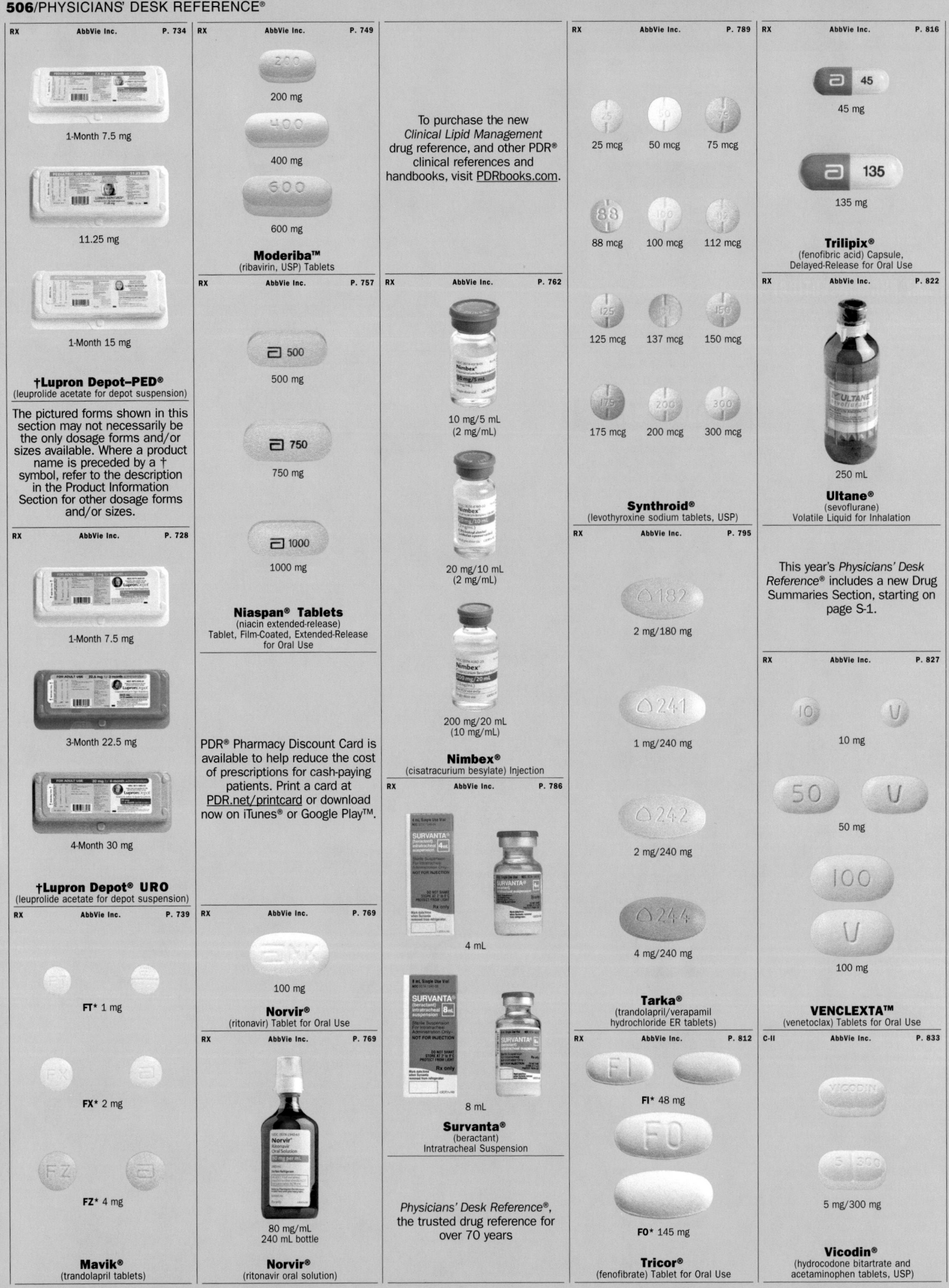

RX   AbbVie Inc.   P. 734

1-Month 7.5 mg

11.25 mg

1-Month 15 mg

†Lupron Depot–PED®
(leuprolide acetate for depot suspension)

The pictured forms shown in this section may not necessarily be the only dosage forms and/or sizes available. Where a product name is preceded by a † symbol, refer to the description in the Product Information Section for other dosage forms and/or sizes.

RX   AbbVie Inc.   P. 728

1-Month 7.5 mg

3-Month 22.5 mg

4-Month 30 mg

†Lupron Depot® URO
(leuprolide acetate for depot suspension)

RX   AbbVie Inc.   P. 739

FT* 1 mg

FX* 2 mg

FZ* 4 mg

Mavik®
(trandolapril tablets)

RX   AbbVie Inc.   P. 749

200 mg

400 mg

600 mg

Moderiba™
(ribavirin, USP) Tablets

RX   AbbVie Inc.   P. 757

500 mg

750 mg

1000 mg

Niaspan® Tablets
(niacin extended-release)
Tablet, Film-Coated, Extended-Release for Oral Use

PDR® Pharmacy Discount Card is available to help reduce the cost of prescriptions for cash-paying patients. Print a card at PDR.net/printcard or download now on iTunes® or Google Play™.

RX   AbbVie Inc.   P. 769

100 mg

Norvir®
(ritonavir) Tablet for Oral Use

RX   AbbVie Inc.   P. 769

80 mg/mL
240 mL bottle

Norvir®
(ritonavir oral solution)

To purchase the new *Clinical Lipid Management* drug reference, and other PDR® clinical references and handbooks, visit PDRbooks.com.

RX   AbbVie Inc.   P. 762

10 mg/5 mL
(2 mg/mL)

20 mg/10 mL
(2 mg/mL)

200 mg/20 mL
(10 mg/mL)

Nimbex®
(cisatracurium besylate) Injection

RX   AbbVie Inc.   P. 786

4 mL

8 mL

Survanta®
(beractant)
Intratracheal Suspension

Physicians' Desk Reference®, the trusted drug reference for over 70 years

---

RX   AbbVie Inc.   P. 789

25 mcg   50 mcg   75 mcg

88 mcg   100 mcg   112 mcg

125 mcg   137 mcg   150 mcg

175 mcg   200 mcg   300 mcg

Synthroid®
(levothyroxine sodium tablets, USP)

RX   AbbVie Inc.   P. 795

2 mg/180 mg

1 mg/240 mg

2 mg/240 mg

4 mg/240 mg

Tarka®
(trandolapril/verapamil hydrochloride ER tablets)

RX   AbbVie Inc.   P. 812

FI* 48 mg

FO* 145 mg

Tricor®
(fenofibrate) Tablet for Oral Use

RX   AbbVie Inc.   P. 816

45 mg

135 mg

Trilipix®
(fenofibric acid) Capsule,
Delayed-Release for Oral Use

RX   AbbVie Inc.   P. 822

250 mL

Ultane®
(sevoflurane)
Volatile Liquid for Inhalation

This year's *Physicians' Desk Reference®* includes a new Drug Summaries Section, starting on page S-1.

RX   AbbVie Inc.   P. 827

10 mg

50 mg

100 mg

VENCLEXTA™
(venetoclax) Tablets for Oral Use

C-II   AbbVie Inc.   P. 833

5 mg/300 mg

Vicodin®
(hydrocodone bitartrate and acetaminophen tablets, USP)

---

*AbbVie Abbo-Code identification letters. Filmtab® Film-sealed tablets, AbbVie.   †Additional dosage forms and sizes available.

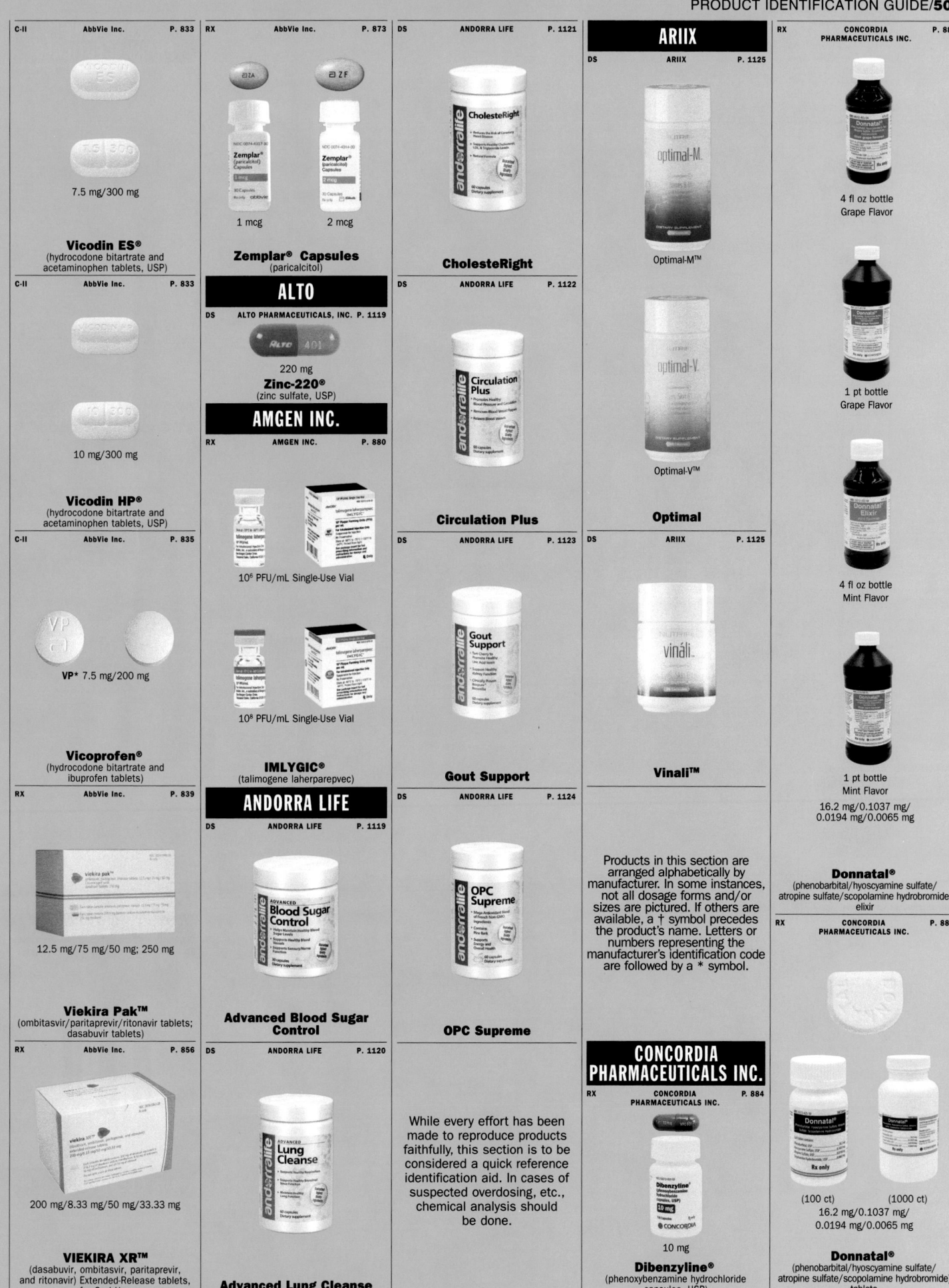

C-II AbbVie Inc. P. 833	RX AbbVie Inc. P. 873	DS ANDORRA LIFE P. 1121	**ARIIX** DS ARIIX P. 1125	RX CONCORDIA PHARMACEUTICALS INC. P. 885

7.5 mg/300 mg

Vicodin ES®
(hydrocodone bitartrate and acetaminophen tablets, USP)

1 mcg 2 mcg

Zemplar® Capsules
(paricalcitol)

ALTO

DS ALTO PHARMACEUTICALS, INC. P. 1119

220 mg

Zinc-220®
(zinc sulfate, USP)

AMGEN INC.

RX AMGEN INC. P. 880

10⁶ PFU/mL Single-Use Vial

10⁸ PFU/mL Single-Use Vial

IMLYGIC®
(talimogene laherparepvec)

ANDORRA LIFE

DS ANDORRA LIFE P. 1119

Advanced Blood Sugar Control

DS ANDORRA LIFE P. 1120

Advanced Lung Cleanse

CholesteRight

DS ANDORRA LIFE P. 1122

Circulation Plus

DS ANDORRA LIFE P. 1123

Gout Support

DS ANDORRA LIFE P. 1124

OPC Supreme

Products in this section are arranged alphabetically by manufacturer. In some instances, not all dosage forms and/or sizes are pictured. If others are available, a † symbol precedes the product's name. Letters or numbers representing the manufacturer's identification code are followed by a * symbol.

While every effort has been made to reproduce products faithfully, this section is to be considered a quick reference identification aid. In cases of suspected overdosing, etc., chemical analysis should be done.

Optimal-M™

Optimal-V™

Optimal

Vinali™

CONCORDIA PHARMACEUTICALS INC.

RX CONCORDIA PHARMACEUTICALS INC. P. 884

10 mg

Dibenzyline®
(phenoxybenzamine hydrochloride capsules, USP)

4 fl oz bottle Grape Flavor

1 pt bottle Grape Flavor

4 fl oz bottle Mint Flavor

1 pt bottle Mint Flavor
16.2 mg/0.1037 mg/ 0.0194 mg/0.0065 mg

Donnatal®
(phenobarbital/hyoscyamine sulfate/ atropine sulfate/scopolamine hydrobromide) elixir

RX CONCORDIA PHARMACEUTICALS INC. P. 886

(100 ct) (1000 ct)
16.2 mg/0.1037 mg/ 0.0194 mg/0.0065 mg

Donnatal®
(phenobarbital/hyoscyamine sulfate/ atropine sulfate/scopolamine hydrobromide) tablets

VP* 7.5 mg/200 mg

Vicoprofen®
(hydrocodone bitartrate and ibuprofen tablets)

RX AbbVie Inc. P. 839

12.5 mg/75 mg/50 mg; 250 mg

Viekira Pak™
(ombitasvir/paritaprevir/ritonavir tablets; dasabuvir tablets)

RX AbbVie Inc. P. 856

200 mg/8.33 mg/50 mg/33.33 mg

VIEKIRA XR™
(dasabuvir, ombitasvir, paritaprevir, and ritonavir) Extended-Release tablets, for Oral Use

10 mg/300 mg

Vicodin HP®
(hydrocodone bitartrate and acetaminophen tablets, USP)

*AbbVie Abbo-Code identification letters. Filmtab® Film-sealed tablets, AbbVie.

The pictured forms shown in this section may not necessarily be the only dosage forms and/or sizes available. Where a product name is preceded by a † symbol, refer to the description in the Product Information Section for other dosage forms and/or sizes.

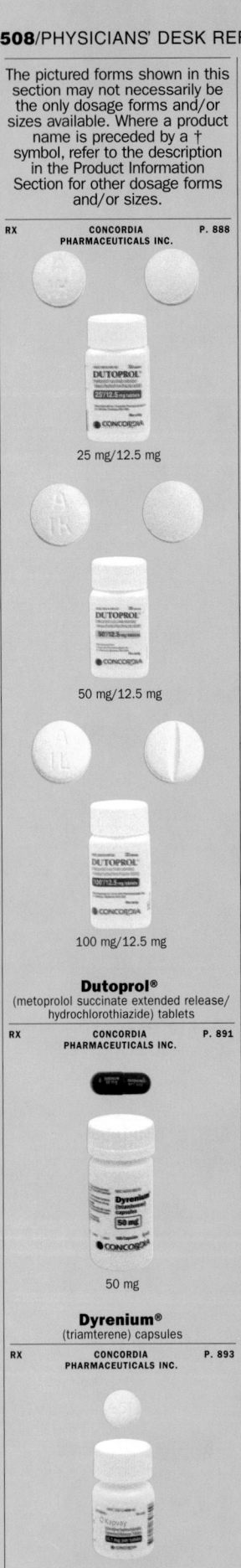

RX   CONCORDIA PHARMACEUTICALS INC.   P. 888

25 mg/12.5 mg

50 mg/12.5 mg

100 mg/12.5 mg

Dutoprol®
(metoprolol succinate extended release/
hydrochlorothiazide) tablets

RX   CONCORDIA PHARMACEUTICALS INC.   P. 891

50 mg

Dyrenium®
(triamterene) capsules

RX   CONCORDIA PHARMACEUTICALS INC.   P. 893

0.1 mg
Also available as 0.2 mg tablets

Kapvay®
(clonidine hydrochloride)
extended-release tablets

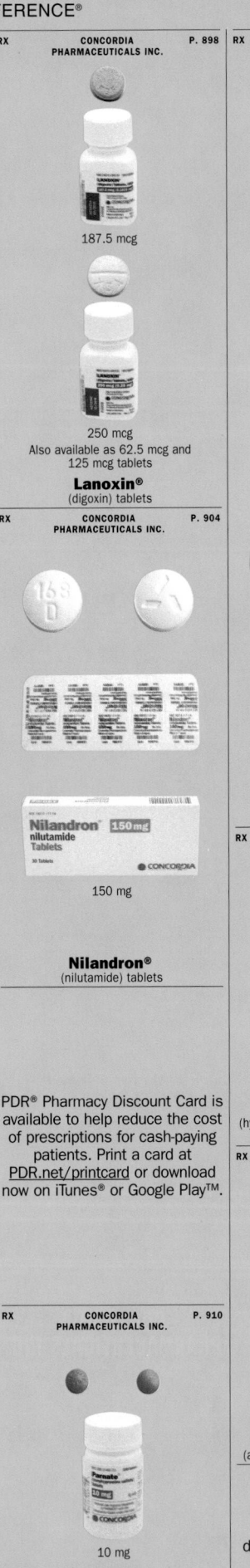

RX   CONCORDIA PHARMACEUTICALS INC.   P. 898

187.5 mcg

250 mcg
Also available as 62.5 mcg and
125 mcg tablets

Lanoxin®
(digoxin) tablets

RX   CONCORDIA PHARMACEUTICALS INC.   P. 904

Nilandron nilutamide Tablets

150 mg

Nilandron®
(nilutamide) tablets

PDR® Pharmacy Discount Card is available to help reduce the cost of prescriptions for cash-paying patients. Print a card at PDR.net/printcard or download now on iTunes® or Google Play™.

RX   CONCORDIA PHARMACEUTICALS INC.   P. 910

10 mg

Parnate®
(tranylcypromine sulfate) tablets

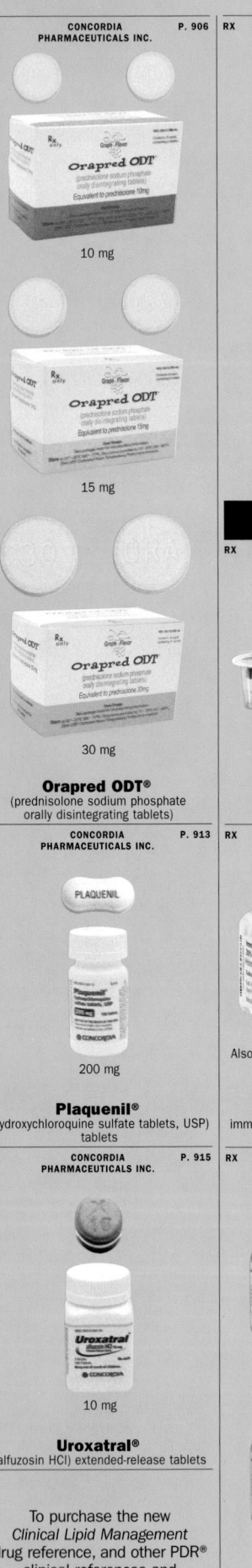

RX   CONCORDIA PHARMACEUTICALS INC.   P. 906

Orapred ODT
10 mg

Orapred ODT
15 mg

Orapred ODT
30 mg

Orapred ODT®
(prednisolone sodium phosphate
orally disintegrating tablets)

RX   CONCORDIA PHARMACEUTICALS INC.   P. 913

PLAQUENIL

200 mg

Plaquenil®
(hydroxychloroquine sulfate tablets, USP)
tablets

RX   CONCORDIA PHARMACEUTICALS INC.   P. 915

Uroxatral
10 mg

Uroxatral®
(alfuzosin HCl) extended-release tablets

To purchase the new
Clinical Lipid Management
drug reference, and other PDR®
clinical references and
handbooks, visit PDRbooks.com.

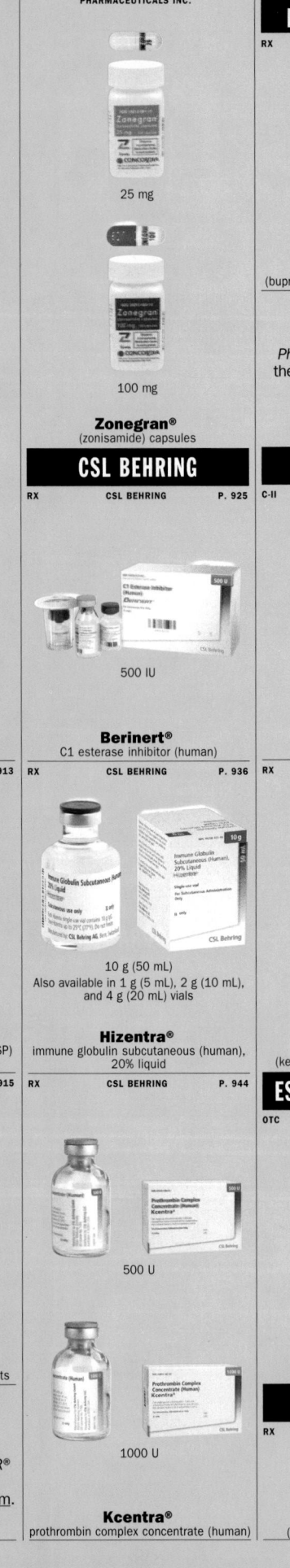

RX   CONCORDIA PHARMACEUTICALS INC.   P. 919

Zonegran
25 mg

Zonegran
100 mg

Zonegran®
(zonisamide) capsules

CSL BEHRING

RX   CSL BEHRING   P. 925

500 IU

Berinert®
C1 esterase inhibitor (human)

RX   CSL BEHRING   P. 936

10 g (50 mL)
Also available in 1 g (5 mL), 2 g (10 mL),
and 4 g (20 mL) vials

Hizentra®
immune globulin subcutaneous (human),
20% liquid

RX   CSL BEHRING   P. 944

500 U

1000 U

Kcentra®
prothrombin complex concentrate (human)

EDGEMONT PHARMACEUTICALS

RX   EDGEMONT PHARMACEUTICALS   P. 952

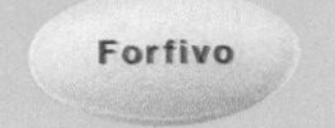

Forfivo
450 mg

Forfivo XL®
(bupropion HCl extended-release tablets)

Physicians' Desk Reference®,
the trusted drug reference for
over 70 years

EGALET US INC.

C-II   EGALET US INC.   P. 960

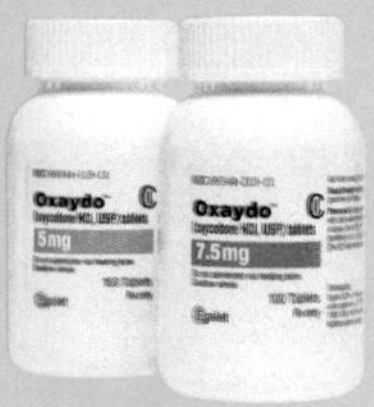

5 mg   7.5 mg

Oxaydo™
(oxycodone HCl, USP) tablets

RX   EGALET US INC.   P. 964

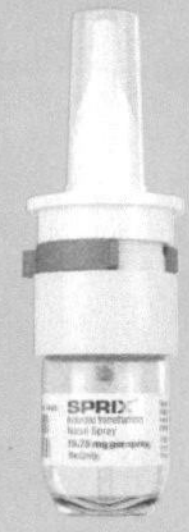

15.75 mg/spray

Sprix®
(ketorolac tromethamine) nasal spray

ESSENTIA WATER, LLC

OTC   ESSENTIA WATER, LLC   P. 1126

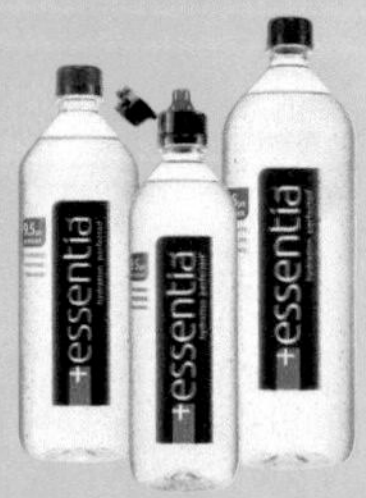

Essentia® Water

GLENWOOD

RX   GLENWOOD   P. 972

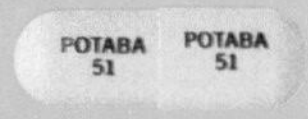

POTABA 51   POTABA 51

500 mg

Potaba®
(aminobenzoate potassium, USP)

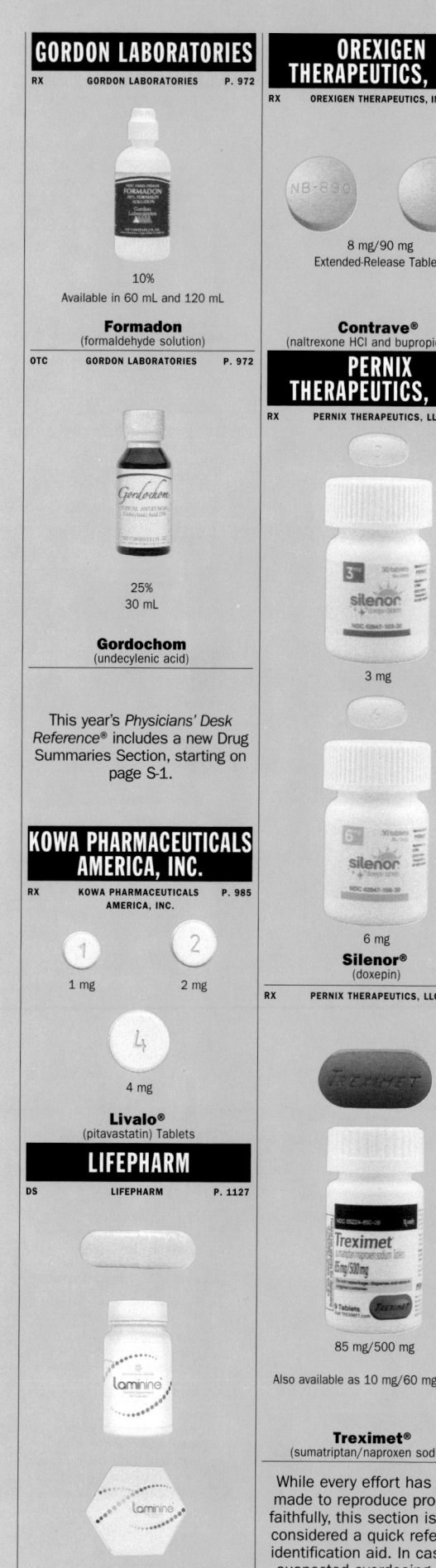

GORDON LABORATORIES

RX   GORDON LABORATORIES   P. 972

10%
Available in 60 mL and 120 mL

Formadon
(formaldehyde solution)

OTC   GORDON LABORATORIES   P. 972

25%
30 mL

Gordochom
(undecylenic acid)

This year's *Physicians' Desk Reference*® includes a new Drug Summaries Section, starting on page S-1.

KOWA PHARMACEUTICALS AMERICA, INC.

RX   KOWA PHARMACEUTICALS   P. 985
AMERICA, INC.

1 mg   2 mg

4 mg

Livalo®
(pitavastatin) Tablets

LIFEPHARM

DS   LIFEPHARM   P. 1127

Laminine®

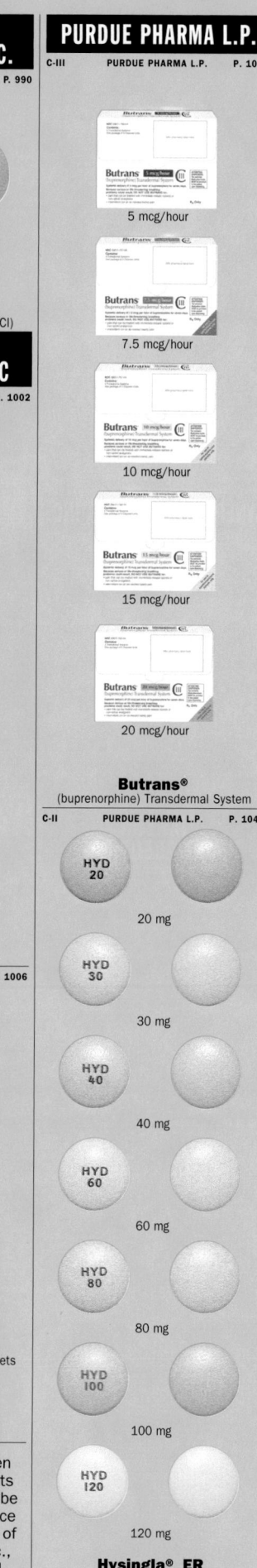

OREXIGEN THERAPEUTICS, INC.

RX   OREXIGEN THERAPEUTICS, INC.   P. 990

8 mg/90 mg
Extended-Release Tablets

Contrave®
(naltrexone HCl and bupropion HCl)

PERNIX THERAPEUTICS, LLC

RX   PERNIX THERAPEUTICS, LLC   P. 1002

3 mg

6 mg

Silenor®
(doxepin)

RX   PERNIX THERAPEUTICS, LLC   P. 1006

85 mg/500 mg

Also available as 10 mg/60 mg tablets

Treximet®
(sumatriptan/naproxen sodium)

While every effort has been made to reproduce products faithfully, this section is to be considered a quick reference identification aid. In cases of suspected overdosing, etc., chemical analysis should be done.

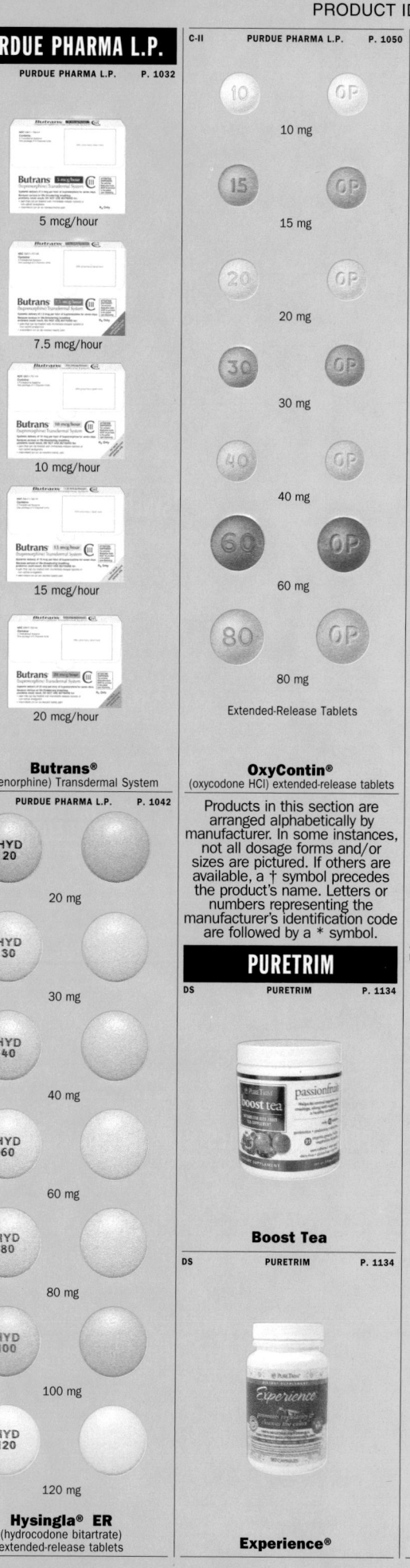

PURDUE PHARMA L.P.

C-III   PURDUE PHARMA L.P.   P. 1032

5 mcg/hour

7.5 mcg/hour

10 mcg/hour

15 mcg/hour

20 mcg/hour

Butrans®
(buprenorphine) Transdermal System

C-II   PURDUE PHARMA L.P.   P. 1042

HYD 20   20 mg

HYD 30   30 mg

HYD 40   40 mg

HYD 60   60 mg

HYD 80   80 mg

HYD 100   100 mg

HYD 120   120 mg

Hysingla® **ER**
(hydrocodone bitartrate)
extended-release tablets

C-II   PURDUE PHARMA L.P.   P. 1050

10   OP   10 mg

15   OP   15 mg

20   OP   20 mg

30   OP   30 mg

40   OP   40 mg

60   OP   60 mg

80   OP   80 mg

Extended-Release Tablets

OxyContin®
(oxycodone HCl) extended-release tablets

Products in this section are arranged alphabetically by manufacturer. In some instances, not all dosage forms and/or sizes are pictured. If others are available, a † symbol precedes the product's name. Letters or numbers representing the manufacturer's identification code are followed by a * symbol.

PURETRIM

DS   PURETRIM   P. 1134

Boost Tea

DS   PURETRIM   P. 1134

Experience®

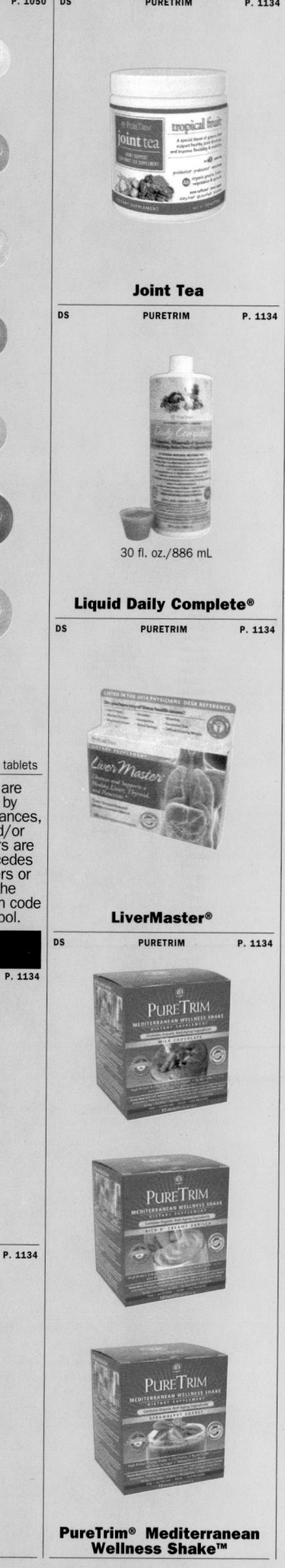

DS   PURETRIM   P. 1134

Joint Tea

DS   PURETRIM   P. 1134

30 fl. oz./886 mL

Liquid Daily Complete®

DS   PURETRIM   P. 1134

LiverMaster®

DS   PURETRIM   P. 1134

PureTrim® **Mediterranean Wellness Shake**™

RLC LABS, INC.

RX   RLC LABS, INC.   P. 1059

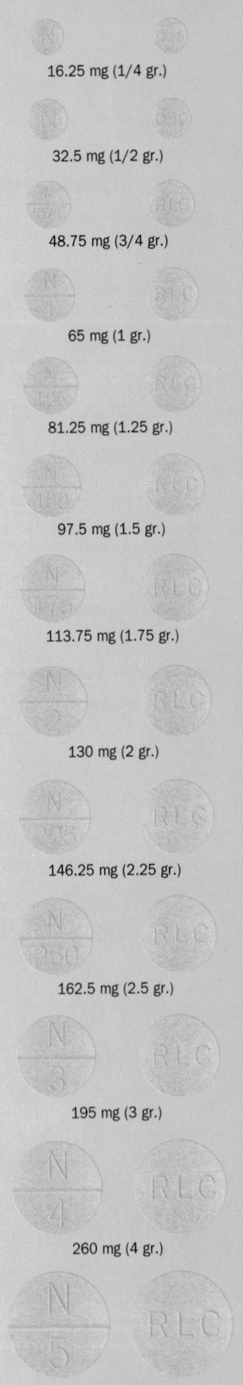

16.25 mg (1/4 gr.)

32.5 mg (1/2 gr.)

48.75 mg (3/4 gr.)

65 mg (1 gr.)

81.25 mg (1.25 gr.)

97.5 mg (1.5 gr.)

113.75 mg (1.75 gr.)

130 mg (2 gr.)

146.25 mg (2.25 gr.)

162.5 mg (2.5 gr.)

195 mg (3 gr.)

260 mg (4 gr.)

325 mg (5 gr.)

Nature-Throid®
(Thyroid USP) tablets

The pictured forms shown in this section may not necessarily be the only dosage forms and/or sizes available. Where a product name is preceded by a † symbol, refer to the description in the Product Information Section for other dosage forms and/or sizes.

RX   RLC LABS, INC.   P. 1061

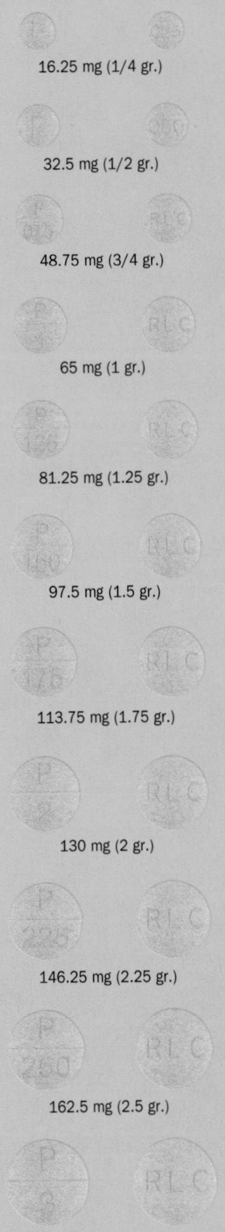

16.25 mg (1/4 gr.)

32.5 mg (1/2 gr.)

48.75 mg (3/4 gr.)

65 mg (1 gr.)

81.25 mg (1.25 gr.)

97.5 mg (1.5 gr.)

113.75 mg (1.75 gr.)

130 mg (2 gr.)

146.25 mg (2.25 gr.)

162.5 mg (2.5 gr.)

195 mg (3 gr.)

WP Thyroid®
(Thyroid USP) tablets

SUPERNUS PHARMACEUTICALS

RX   SUPERNUS PHARMACEUTICALS P. 1063

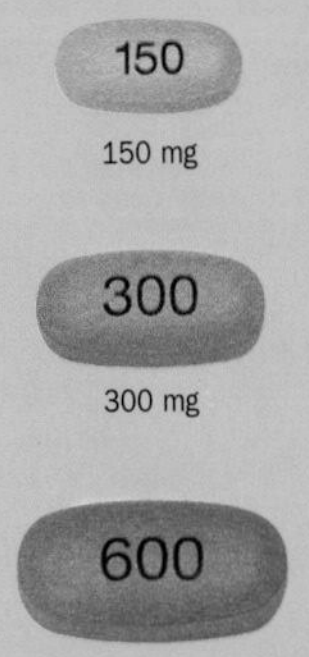

150
150 mg

300
300 mg

600
600 mg
Extended-Release Tablets

Oxtellar XR®
(oxcarbazepine)
extended-release tablets

RX   SUPERNUS PHARMACEUTICALS P. 1071

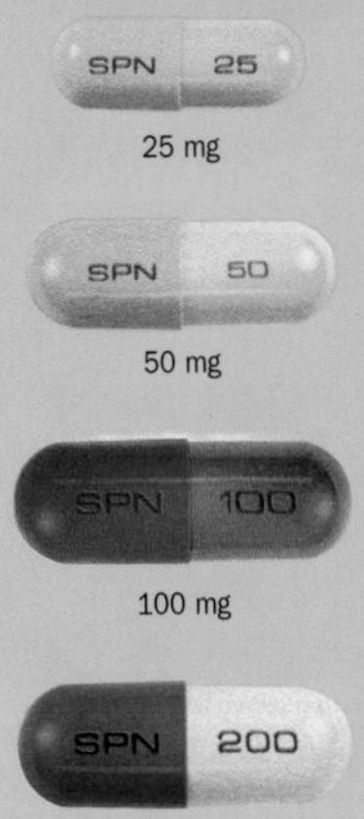

SPN 25
25 mg

SPN 50
50 mg

SPN 100
100 mg

SPN 200
200 mg
Extended-Release Capsules

Trokendi XR®
(topiramate)
extended-release capsules

SYNERGY WORLDWIDE, INC.

DS   SYNERGY WORLDWIDE, INC.   P. 1135

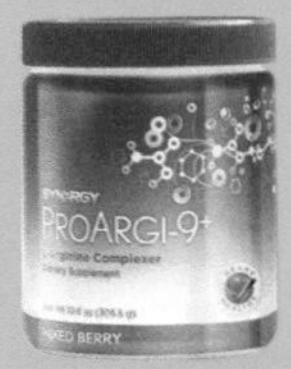

ProArgi-9⁺
(l-arginine complexer)

TAKEDA PHARMACEUTICALS

RX   TAKEDA PHARMACEUTICALS   P. 1087

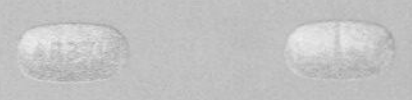

0.6 mg

Colcrys®
(colchicine, USP) tablets

RX   TAKEDA PHARMACEUTICALS   P. 1094

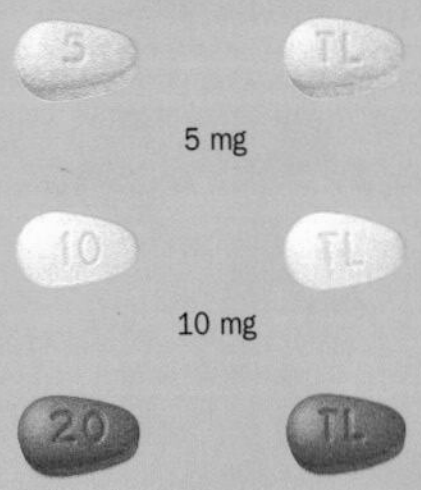

5 TL
5 mg

10 TL
10 mg

20 TL
20 mg
Also available as 15 mg tablet

Trintellix®
(vortioxetine)

RX   TAKEDA PHARMACEUTICALS   P. 1102

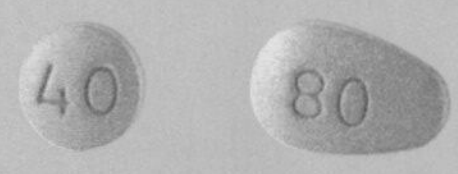

40
40 mg

80
80 mg

Uloric®
(febuxostat)

PDR® Pharmacy Discount Card is available to help reduce the cost of prescriptions for cash-paying patients. Print a card at PDR.net/printcard or download now on iTunes® or Google Play™.

UNICITY INTERNATIONAL, INC.

DS   UNICITY INTERNATIONAL, INC.   P. 1135

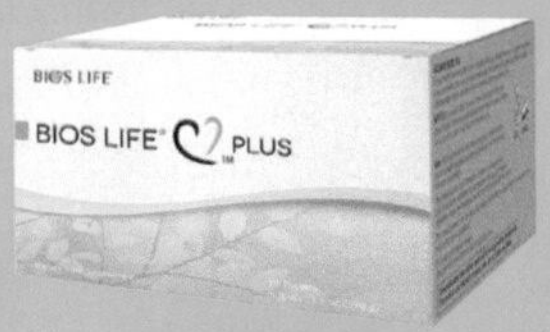

Dietary Supplement

Bios Life® C Plus

DS   UNICITY INTERNATIONAL, INC.   P. 1137

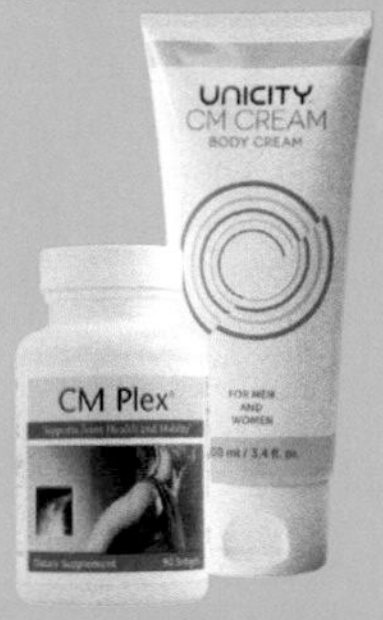

Dietary Supplement

CM Plex®

DS   UNICITY INTERNATIONAL, INC.   P. 1138

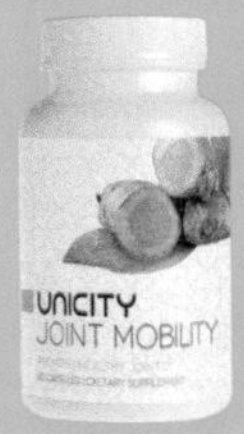

Dietary Supplement

Joint Mobility™

DS   UNICITY INTERNATIONAL, INC.   P. 1139

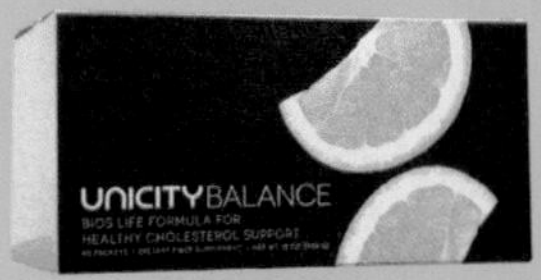

Dietary Supplement

Unicity Balance™

UNILEVER THAI TRADING LIMITED

DS   UNILEVER THAI TRADING LIMITED P. 1139

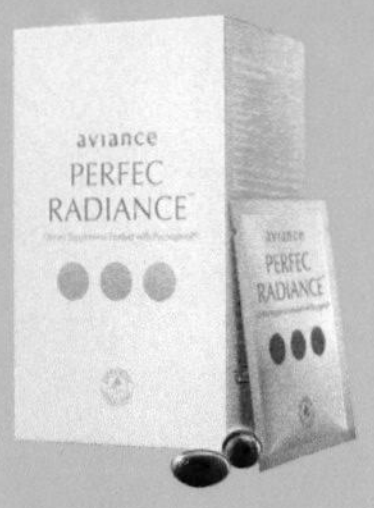

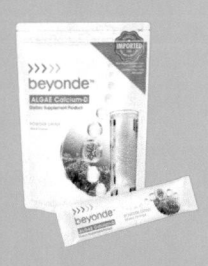

aviance Perfec Radiance™

DS   UNILEVER THAI TRADING LIMITED P. 1140

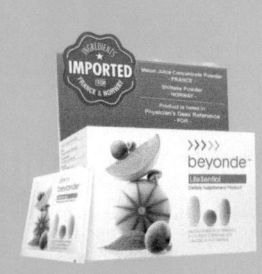

beyonde™ Algae Calcium-D

DS   UNILEVER THAI TRADING LIMITED P. 1141

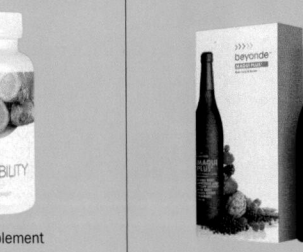

beyonde™ Life Sential

DS   UNILEVER THAI TRADING LIMITED P. 1141

beyonde™ Maqui Plus⁺
Multi Fruits & Berries

To purchase the new *Clinical Lipid Management* drug reference, and other PDR® clinical references and handbooks, visit PDRbooks.com.

VANDA PHARMACEUTICALS

RX   **VANDA PHARMACEUTICALS**   P. 1107

1 mg

2 mg

4 mg

6 mg

8 mg

10 mg

12 mg

DOSAGE INSTRUCTIONS:

Titration Pack

Fanapt®
(iloperidone) Tablets

RX   **VANDA PHARMACEUTICALS**   P. 1113

Hetlioz™
(tasimelteon) capsule
20 mg

20 mg

Hetlioz®
(tasimelteon) Capsules

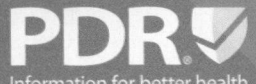
PDR⦿
Information for better health

You are seconds away from saving on prescription medication

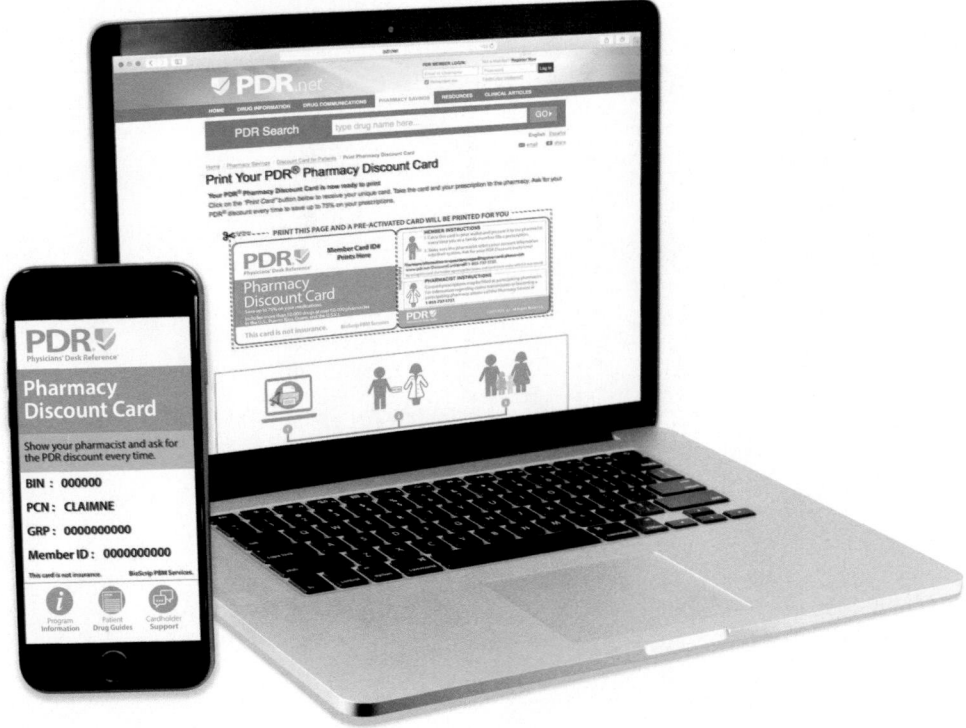

The PDR Pharmacy Discount Card is available to help reduce the cost of prescriptions for individuals paying the cash price for prescriptions.

- Free program
- Pre-activated and ready to use
- No registration
- No pre-approvals
- No personal information needed

At the pharmacy, the cardholder needs only show their printed card or mobile card account numbers to the pharmacist and ask for their PDR discount.

To learn more, print cards, or get the app
visit PDR.net/DiscountCard

SECTION 7

PRODUCT INFORMATION

This section of the PDR contains the latest full label product information available when the book went to press. As new drugs are released, and new reseach data, clinical findings, and safety information emerge throughout the year, it is the responsibility of the manufacturer to provide that information to the medical community and to revise that information in the PDR database.

Revisions are released throughout the year in the *PDR Update,* on PDR.net, and on *mobile*PDR, as well as emailed via the *PDR eDrug Update* and *PDR Safety Communications.* These updates can also be found on-screen for those healthcare providers who use electronic health record (EHR) systems that belong to PDR's network of EHR partners. To be certain that you have the most current information, always consult these products before prescribing or administering any medications described in the following pages.

A&Z Pharmaceutical Inc.
180 OSER AVENUE, SUITE 300
HAUPPAUGE, NY 11788

Direct Inquiries to:
Telephone: (631) 952-3800
Fax: (631) 952-3900
E-Mail: info@azpharmaceutical.com
Website: www.azpharmaceutical.com

D-Cal®   OTC
Calcium Supplement Antacid
Calcium 300 mg
Vitamin D₃ 100 IU

60 Chewable Tablets

Supplement Facts

	Adults	Children
■ Serving Size	2	1
■ Serving per Container	30	60
■ Amount per Serving		
Calories	4	2
Calcium (as calcium	600 mg	300 mg
carbonate)	(60% DV)	(30% DV)
Vitamin D₃	200 IU	100 IU
	(50% DV)	(25% DV)

Drug Facts

Active Ingredient (in each tablet)	Purpose
Calcium Carbonate 750 mg	Antacid

Uses
relieves ■ heartburn ■ acid indigestion ■ sour stomach ■ upset stomach due to these symptoms

Warnings
Ask a doctor or pharmacist before use if you are taking a prescription drug. Antacids may interact with certain prescription drugs.
When using this product ■ do not take more than 10 tablets for adults and 5 tablets for children in a 24 hour period.
Keep out of reach of children.

Directions
■ **Adults:** chew 2 tablets daily. ■ **Children:** chew 1 tablet daily.
If symptoms persist, ask a doctor.

Other Information
■ store in a dry place
■ do not use if imprinted seal under cap is torn or open
Inactive Ingredients cholecalciferol, D&C red #27, flavors, magnesium stearate, sorbitol
Manufactured by:
A&Z Pharmaceutical, Inc.
Hauppauge, NY 11788
Shown in Product Identification Guide, page 505

D-Cal® Kids   OTC
Calcium Supplement Antacid
Calcium 300 mg
Vitamin D₃ 100 IU

30 Chewable Tablets

Supplement Facts

■ Serving Size	1
■ Serving per Container	30
■ Amount per Serving	
Calories	2
Calcium (as calcium carbonate)	300 mg (30% DV)
Vitamin D₃	100 IU (25% DV)

Drug Facts

Active Ingredient (in each tablet)	Purpose
Calcium Carbonate 750 mg	Antacid

Uses
relieves ■ heartburn ■ acid indigestion ■ sour stomach ■ upset stomach due to these symptoms

Warnings
Ask a doctor or pharmacist before use if you are taking a prescription drug. Antacids may interact with certain prescription drugs.
When using this product ■ do not take more than 5 tablets in a 24 hour period.
Keep out of reach of children.

Directions
■ chew one tablet daily. If symptoms persist, ask a doctor.

Other Information
■ store in a dry place ■ do not use if imprinted seal under cap is torn or open
Inactive Ingredients cholecalciferol, aspartame, citric acid, D&C Yellow #6, FD&C Blue #1, FD&C Red #40, FD&C Yellow #5, D&C Yellow #10, flavors, magnesium stearate, sorbitol
Manufactured by:
A&Z Pharmaceutical, Inc.
Hauppauge, NY 11788
Shown in Product Identification Guide, page 505

D-Cal®   OTC
Calcium Carbonate and Vitamin D₃ Granules
Calcium Supplement Antacid
Calcium 300 mg
Vitamin D₃ 100 IU

10 Pouches / Box
1 gram / Pouch

Supplement Facts

■ Serving Size	1g
■ Serving per Container	10
■ Amount per Serving	
Calories	1
Calcium (as calcium carbonate)	300 mg (37.5% DV)
Vitamin D₃	100 IU (25% DV)

Drug Facts

Active Ingredient (in each pouch)	Purpose
Calcium Carbonate 750 mg	Antacid

Uses
relieves ■ heartburn ■ acid indigestion ■ sour stomach ■ upset stomach due to these symptoms

Warnings
Ask a doctor or pharmacist before use if you are taking a prescription drug. Antacids may interact with certain prescription drugs.
When using this product ■ do not take more than 1 pouch in a 24 hour period.
Keep out of reach of children.

Directions
■ find the right dose on chart below based on weight, otherwise use age.
■ pour powder into cup and add 15 mL (0.51 oz.) of water, stir and drink.

Dosing Chart

Weight (lbs)	Age	Dose
Under 24	Under 2 yrs	Ask a doctor
24-47	2-5 yrs	1/2 pouch
48-95	6-11 yrs	1 pouch

Other Information
■ store in a dry place ■ do not use if pouch is open or torn
Inactive Ingredients cholecalciferol, dextrose, maltodextrin, sodium citrate
Manufactured by:
A&Z Pharmaceutical, Inc.
Hauppauge, NY 11788
Shown in Product Identification Guide, page 505

PDR® Pharmacy Discount Card is available to help reduce the cost of prescriptions for cash-paying patients. Print a card at PDR.net/printcard or download now on iTunes® or Google Play™.

AbbVie Inc.
1 NORTH WAUKEGAN ROAD
NORTH CHICAGO, IL 60064

Direct Inquiries to:
Customer Service:
(800) 255-5162
Patient Assistance Program:
(800) 441-4987
For Medical Services Department:
(800) 633-9110 or www.abbviemedinfo.com
Adverse experiences or side effects
(for all AbbVie drug products):
(800) 633-9110 or www.abbviemedinfo.com
Sales and Ordering:
(800) 255-5162

ABBO–CODE™ INDEX

The Abbo-Code identification system provides positive identification of a drug and dosage strength. The following AbbVie products are imprinted or debossed with an Abbo-Code designation:

PRODUCT	ABBO-CODE
Biaxin® Filmtab® Tablets (clarithromycin tablets, USP)	
250 mg	KT
500 mg	KL
Biaxin® XL Filmtab® Tablets (clarithromycin extended-release tablets)	
500 mg	KJ
Creon (pancrelipase) delayed-release capsules for oral use	
CREON 3000	Creon 1203
CREON 6000	Creon 1206
CREON 12000	Creon 1212
CREON 24000	Creon 1224
CREON 36000	Creon 1236
Depakene® Capsules (valproic acid capsules, USP)	
250 mg	DEPAKENE
Depakote® ER Tablets (divalproex sodium EXTENDED-RELEASE tablets)	
500 mg	HC
250 mg	HF
Depakote® Sprinkle Capsules (divalproex sodium coated particles in capsules)	
125 mg	↑THIS END UP DEPAKOTE SPRINKLE 125 mg
Depakote® Tablets (divalproex sodium delayed-release tablets)	
125 mg	NT
250 mg	NR
500 mg	NS
Gengraf® Capsules (cyclosporine capsules, USP [MODIFIED])	
25 mg	OR 25 mg
100 mg	OT 100 mg
Kaletra® (lopinavir/ritonavir)	
133.3 mg lopinavir/33.3 mg ritonavir	PK
Kaletra® Tablet (lopinavir/ritonavir)	
100 mg lopinavir/25 mg ritonavir	KC
200 mg lopinavir/50 mg ritonavir	KA
K-Tab® Filmtab® Tablets (potassium chloride extended-release tablets, USP)	
10 mEq (750 mg)	K-TAB
Marinol® (dronabinal capsules)	
2.5 mg	UM
5 mg	UM
10 mg	UM
Mavik® Tablets (trandolapril)	
1 mg	FT
2 mg	FX
4 mg	FZ
Niaspan® (niacin extended-release tablets) [film-coated]	
500 mg	Niaspan 500

ANDROGEL® 1%

Ⓒ ℞

[an drow jel]
(testosterone gel) for topical use

HIGHLIGHTS OF PRESCRIBING INFORMATION

These highlights do not include all the information needed to use AndroGel 1% safely and effectively. See full prescribing information for AndroGel 1%.
AndroGel® (testosterone gel) 1% for topical use CIII
Initial U.S. Approval: 1953

WARNING: SECONDARY EXPOSURE TO TESTOSTERONE

See full prescribing information for complete boxed warning.

- Virilization has been reported in children who were secondarily exposed to testosterone gel. (5.2, 6.2)
- **Children should avoid contact with unwashed or unclothed application sites in men using testosterone gel. (2.2, 5.2)**
- **Healthcare providers should advise patients to strictly adhere to recommended instructions for use. (2.2, 5.2, 17)**

RECENT MAJOR CHANGES

Indications and Usage (1)	5/2015
Dosage and Administration (2)	5/2015
Dosage and Administration (2.2)	11/2014
Warnings and Precautions (5.4)	6/2014
Warnings and Precautions (5.5)	5/2015

INDICATIONS AND USAGE

AndroGel 1% is indicated for replacement therapy in males for conditions associated with a deficiency or absence of endogenous testosterone:
- Primary hypogonadism (congenital or acquired). (1)
- Hypogonadotropic hypogonadism (congenital or acquired). (1)

Limitations of use:
- Safety and efficacy of AndroGel 1% in men with "age-related hypogonadism" have not been established. (1)
- Safety and efficacy of AndroGel 1% in males less than 18 years old have not been established. (8.4)
- Topical testosterone products may have different doses, strengths or application instructions that may result in different systemic exposure. (1, 12.3)

DOSAGE AND ADMINISTRATION

- **Dosage and Administration for AndroGel 1% differs from AndroGel 1.62 %. For dosage and administration of AndroGel 1.62% refer to its full prescribing information. (2)**
- Prior to initiating AndroGel 1%., confirm the diagnosis of hypogonadism by ensuring that serum testosterone has been measured in the morning on at least two separate days and that these concentrations are below the normal range (2).
- Starting dose of AndroGel 1% is 50 mg of testosterone (4 pump actuations, two 25 mg packets, or one 50 mg packet), applied once daily in the morning. (2.1)
- Apply to clean, dry, intact skin of shoulders and upper arms and/or abdomen. Do NOT apply AndroGel 1% to any other parts of the body including the genitals, chest, armpits (axillae), knees, or back. (2.2)
- Dose adjustment: AndroGel 1% can be dose adjusted using 50 mg, 75 mg, or 100 mg of testosterone on the basis of total serum testosterone concentration. The dose should be titrated based on the serum testosterone concentration. Additionally, serum testosterone concentration should be assessed periodically. (2.1)
- Patients should wash hands immediately with soap and water after applying AndroGel 1% and cover the application site(s) with clothing after the gel has dried. Wash the application site thoroughly with soap and water prior to any situation where skin-to-skin contact of the application site with another person is anticipated. (2.2)

DOSAGE FORMS AND STRENGTHS

AndroGel (testosterone gel) 1% for topical use is available as follows:
- Metered-dose pump that delivers 12.5 mg of testosterone per actuation. (3)
- Packets containing 25 mg of testosterone. (3)
- Packets containing 50 mg of testosterone. (3)

CONTRAINDICATIONS

- Men with carcinoma of the breast or known or suspected prostate cancer. (4, 5.1)
- Pregnant or breastfeeding women. Testosterone may cause fetal harm. (4, 8.1, 8.3)

WARNINGS AND PRECAUTIONS

- Monitor patients with benign prostatic hyperplasia (BPH) for worsening of signs and symptoms of BPH. (5.1)
- Avoid unintentional exposure of women or children to AndroGel 1%. Secondary exposure to testosterone can produce signs of virilization. AndroGel 1% should be discontinued until the cause of virilization is identified. (5.2)
- Venous thromboembolism (VTE), including deep vein thrombosis (DVT) and pulmonary embolism (PE) have been reported in patients using testosterone products. Evaluate patients with signs or symptoms consistent with DVT or PE. (5.4)
- Some postmarketing studies have shown an increased risk of myocardial infarction and stroke associated with use of testosterone replacement therapy. (5.5)
- Exogenous administration of androgens may lead to azoospermia. (5.7)
- Edema, with or without congestive heart failure (CHF), may be a complication in patients with preexisting cardiac, renal, or hepatic disease. (5.9, 6.2)
- Sleep apnea may occur in those with risk factors. (5.11)
- Monitor serum testosterone, prostate specific antigen (PSA), hemoglobin, hematocrit, liver function tests, and lipid concentrations periodically. (5.1, 5.3, 5.8, 5.12)
- AndroGel 1% is flammable until dry. (5.15)

ADVERSE REACTIONS

Most common adverse reactions (incidence ≥ 5%) are acne, application site reaction, abnormal lab tests, and prostatic disorders. (6.1)

To report SUSPECTED ADVERSE REACTIONS, contact AbbVie Inc. at 1-800-633-9110 or FDA at 1-800-FDA-1088 or *www.fda.gov/medwatch.*

DRUG INTERACTIONS

- Androgens may decrease blood glucose and therefore may decrease insulin requirements in diabetic patients. (7.1)
- Changes in anticoagulant activity may be seen with androgens. More frequent monitoring of INR and prothrombin time is recommended. (7.2)
- Use of testosterone with adrenocorticotrophic hormone (ACTH) or corticosteroids may result in increased fluid retention. Use with caution, particularly in patients with cardiac, renal, or hepatic disease. (7.3)

USE IN SPECIFIC POPULATIONS

There are insufficient long-term safety data in geriatric patients using AndroGel 1% to assess the potential risks of cardiovascular disease and prostate cancer. (8.5)
See 17 for PATIENT COUNSELING INFORMATION and Medication Guide.

Revised: 5/2015

FULL PRESCRIBING INFORMATION: CONTENTS*
WARNING: SECONDARY EXPOSURE TO TESTOSTERONE

Continued on next page

Information on the AbbVie, Inc. products listed on these pages is from the prescribing information in use as of July 31, 2016. For more information, please visit rxabbvie.com or call 1-800-633-9110.

* Sections or subsections omitted from the full prescribing information are not listed.

FULL PRESCRIBING INFORMATION

> **WARNING: SECONDARY EXPOSURE TO TESTOSTERONE**
> - Virilization has been reported in children who were secondarily exposed to testosterone gel *[see Warnings and Precautions (5.2) and Adverse Reactions (6.2)]*.
> - Children should avoid contact with unwashed or unclothed application sites in men using testosterone gel *[see Dosage and Administration (2.2) and Warnings and Precautions (5.2)]*.
> - Healthcare providers should advise patients to strictly adhere to recommended instructions for use *[see Dosage and Administration (2.2), Warnings and Precautions (5.2) and Patient Counseling Information (17)]*.

1   INDICATIONS AND USAGE

AndroGel 1% is indicated for replacement therapy in adult males for conditions associated with a deficiency or absence of endogenous testosterone:

- Primary hypogonadism (congenital or acquired): testicular failure due to conditions such as cryptorchidism, bilateral torsion, orchitis, vanishing testis syndrome, orchiectomy, Klinefelter's syndrome, chemotherapy, or toxic damage from alcohol or heavy metals. These men usually have low serum testosterone concentrations and gonadotropins (follicle-stimulating hormone [FSH], luteinizing hormone [LH]) above the normal range.
- Hypogonadotropic hypogonadism (congenital or acquired): gonadotropin or luteinizing hormone-releasing hormone (LHRH) deficiency or pituitary-hypothalamic injury from tumors, trauma, or radiation. These men have low testosterone serum concentrations, but have gonadotropins in the normal or low range.

Limitations of use:
- Safety and efficacy of AndroGel 1% in men with "age-related hypogonadism" (also referred to as "late-onset hypogonadism") have not been established.
- Safety and efficacy of AndroGel 1% in males less than 18 years old have not been established *[see Use in Specific Populations (8.4)]*.
- Topical testosterone products may have different doses, strengths or application instructions that may result in different systemic exposure (1, 12.3).

2   DOSAGE AND ADMINISTRATION

Dosage and Administration for AndroGel 1% differs from AndroGel 1.62%. For dosage and administration of AndroGel 1.62% refer to its full prescribing information. (2)
Prior to initiating AndroGel 1%, confirm the diagnosis of hypogonadism by ensuring that serum testosterone concentrations have been measured in the morning on at least two separate days and that these serum testosterone concentrations are below the normal range.

2.1   Dosing and Dose Adjustment

The recommended starting dose of AndroGel 1% is 50 mg of testosterone (4 pump actuations, two 25 mg packets, or one 50 mg packet), applied topically once daily in the morning to the shoulders and upper arms and/or abdomen area (preferably at the same time every day).

Dose Adjustment
To ensure proper dosing, serum testosterone concentrations should be measured at intervals. If the serum testosterone concentration is below the normal range, the daily AndroGel 1% dose may be increased from 50 mg to 75 mg and from 75 mg to 100 mg for adult males as instructed by the physician (see Table 1, Dosing Information for AndroGel 1%). If the serum testosterone concentration exceeds the normal range, the daily AndroGel 1% dose may be decreased. If the serum testosterone concentration consistently exceeds the normal range at a daily dose of 50 mg, AndroGel 1% therapy should be discontinued. In addition, serum testosterone concentrations should be assessed periodically.

The application site and dose of AndroGel 1% are not interchangeable with other topical testosterone products.

2.2   Administration Instructions

AndroGel 1% should be applied to clean, dry, healthy, intact skin of the right and left upper arms/shoulders and/or right and left abdomen. Area of application should be limited to the area that will be covered by the patient's short sleeve T-shirt. Do not apply AndroGel 1% to any other part of the body including the genitals, chest, armpits (axillae), knees, or back. AndroGel 1% should be evenly distributed between the right and left upper arms/shoulders or both sides of the abdomen.

The prescribed daily dose of AndroGel 1% should be applied to the right and left upper arms/shoulders and/or right/left abdomen as shown in the shaded areas in the figure below.

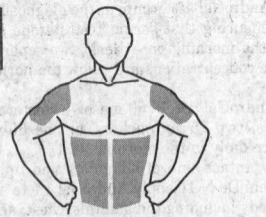

After applying the gel, the application site should be allowed to dry prior to dressing. Hands should be washed thoroughly with soap and water after application. Avoid fire, flames or smoking until the gel has dried since alcohol based products, including AndroGel 1%, are flammable.
The patient should be advised to avoid swimming or showering for at least 5 hours after the application of AndroGel 1%.

Multi-Dose Pump
To obtain a full first dose, it is necessary to prime the canister pump. To do so, with the canister in the upright position, slowly and fully depress the actuator three times. Safely discard the gel from the first three actuations. It is only necessary to prime the pump before the first dose. After the priming procedure, patients should completely depress the pump one time actuation for every 12.5 mg of testosterone required to achieve the daily prescribed dosage. The product should be delivered directly into the palm of the hand and then applied to the desired application sites. Alternatively, AndroGel 1% can be applied directly to the application sites. Table 1 provides dosing information for adult males.

Table 1: Dosing Information for AndroGel 1%

Amount of Testosterone	Number of Pump Actuations
50 mg	4 (once daily)
75 mg	6 (once daily)
100 mg	8 (once daily)

Packets
The entire contents should be squeezed into the palm of the hand and immediately applied to the application sites. Alternately, patients may squeeze a portion of the gel from the packet into the palm of the hand and apply to application sites. Repeat until entire contents have been applied.
Strict adherence to the following precautions is advised in order to minimize the potential for secondary exposure to testosterone from AndroGel 1%-treated skin:

- Children and women should avoid contact with unwashed or unclothed application site(s) of men using AndroGel 1%.
- Patients should wash hands with soap and water immediately after application of AndroGel 1%.
- Patients should cover the application site(s) with clothing (e.g., a T-shirt) after the gel has dried.
- Prior to situation in which direct skin-to-skin contact is anticipated, patients should wash the application site thoroughly with soap and water to remove any testosterone residue.
- In the event that unwashed or unclothed skin to which AndroGel 1% has been applied comes in direct contact with the skin of another person, the general area of contact on the other person should be washed with soap and water as soon as possible.

3   DOSAGE FORMS AND STRENGTHS

AndroGel (testosterone gel) 1% for topical use is available as follows:
- A metered-dose pump. Each pump actuation delivers 12.5 mg of testosterone in 1.25 g of gel.
- A unit dose packet containing 25 mg of testosterone provided in 2.5 g of gel.
- A unit dose packet containing 50 mg of testosterone provided in 5 g of gel.

4   CONTRAINDICATIONS

- AndroGel 1% is contraindicated in men with carcinoma of the breast or known or suspected carcinoma of the prostate *[see Warnings and Precautions (5.1), Adverse Reactions (6.1), and Nonclinical Toxicology (13.1)]*.
- AndroGel 1% is contraindicated in women who are or may become pregnant, or who are breastfeeding. AndroGel 1% may cause fetal harm when administered to a pregnant woman. AndroGel 1% may cause serious adverse reactions in nursing infants. Exposure of a female fetus or nursing infant to androgens may result in varying degrees of virilization. Pregnant women or those who may become pregnant need to be aware of the potential for transfer of testosterone from men treated with AndroGel 1%. If a pregnant woman is exposed to AndroGel 1%, she should be apprised of the potential hazard to the fetus *[see Warnings and Precautions (5.2) and Use in Specific Populations (8.1, 8.3)]*.

5   WARNINGS AND PRECAUTIONS

5.1   Worsening of Benign Prostatic Hyperplasia (BPH) and Potential Risk of Prostate Cancer

- Patients with BPH treated with androgens are at an increased risk for worsening of signs and symptoms of BPH. Monitor patients with BPH for worsening signs and symptoms.
- Patients treated with androgens may be at increased risk for prostate cancer. Evaluate patients for prostate cancer prior to initiating and during treatment with androgens *[see Contraindications (4), Adverse Reactions (6.1) and Nonclinical Toxicology (13.1)]*.

5.2   Potential for Secondary Exposure to Testosterone

Cases of secondary exposure resulting in virilization of children have been reported in postmarketing surveillance. Signs and symptoms have included enlargement of the penis or clitoris, development of pubic hair, increased erections and libido, aggressive behavior, and advanced bone age. In most cases, these signs and symptoms regressed with removal of the exposure to testosterone gel. In a few cases, however, enlarged genitalia did not fully return to age-appropriate normal size, and bone age remained modestly greater than chronological age. The risk of transfer was increased in some of these cases by not adhering to precautions for the appropriate use of the topical testosterone product. Children and women should avoid contact with unwashed or unclothed application sites in men using AndroGel 1% *[see Dosage and Administration (2.2), Use in Specific Populations (8.1) and Clinical Pharmacology (12.3)]*.

Inappropriate changes in genital size or development of pubic hair or libido in children, or changes in body hair distribution, significant increase in acne, or other signs of virilization in adult women should be brought to the attention of a physician and the possibility of secondary exposure to testosterone gel should also be brought to the attention of a physician. Testosterone gel should be promptly discontinued until the cause of virilization has been identified.

5.3   Polycythemia

Increases in hematocrit, reflective of increases in red blood cell mass, may require lowering or discontinuation of testosterone. Check hematocrit prior to initiating treatment. It would also be appropriate to re-evaluate the hematocrit 3 to 6 months after starting treatment, and then annually. If hematocrit becomes elevated, stop therapy until hematocrit decreases to an acceptable concentration. An increase in red blood cell mass may increase the risk of thromboembolic events.

5.4 Venous Thromboembolism

There have been postmarketing reports of venous thromboembolic events, including deep vein thrombosis (DVT) and pulmonary embolism (PE), in patients using testosterone products such as AndroGel 1%. Evaluate patients who report symptoms of pain, edema, warmth and erythema in the lower extremity for DVT and those who present with acute shortness of breath for PE. If a venous thromboembolic event is suspected, discontinue treatment with AndroGel 1% and initiate appropriate workup and management [see Adverse Reactions (6.2)].

5.5 Cardiovascular Risk

Long term clinical safety trials have not been conducted to assess the cardiovascular outcomes of testosterone replacement therapy in men. To date, epidemiologic studies and randomized controlled trials have been inconclusive for determining the risk of major adverse cardiovascular events (MACE), such as non-fatal myocardial infarction, non-fatal stroke, and cardiovascular death, with the use of testosterone compared to non-use. Some studies, but not all, have reported an increased risk of MACE in association with use of testosterone replacement therapy in men.

Patients should be informed of this possible risk when deciding whether to use or to continue to use AndroGel 1%.

5.6 Use in Women

Due to lack of controlled evaluations in women and potential virilizing effects, AndroGel 1% is not indicated for use in women [see Contraindications (4) and Use in Specific Populations (8.1, 8.3)].

5.7 Potential for Adverse Effects on Spermatogenesis

With large doses of exogenous androgens, including AndroGel 1%, spermatogenesis may be suppressed through feedback inhibition of pituitary follicle-stimulating hormone (FSH) which could possibly lead to adverse effects on semen parameters including sperm count.

5.8 Hepatic Adverse Effects

Prolonged use of high doses of orally active 17-alpha-alkyl androgens (e.g., methyltestosterone) has been associated with serious hepatic adverse effects (peliosis hepatis, hepatic neoplasms, cholestatic hepatitis, and jaundice). Peliosis hepatis can be a life-threatening or fatal complication. Long-term therapy with intramuscular testosterone enanthate has produced multiple hepatic adenomas. AndroGel 1% is not known to cause these adverse effects.

5.9 Edema

Androgens, including AndroGel 1%, may promote retention of sodium and water. Edema, with or without congestive heart failure, may be a serious complication in patients with preexisting cardiac, renal, or hepatic disease [see Adverse Reactions (6.2)].

5.10 Gynecomastia

Gynecomastia may develop and persist in patients being treated with androgens, including AndroGel 1%, for hypogonadism.

5.11 Sleep Apnea

The treatment of hypogonadal men with testosterone may potentiate sleep apnea in some patients, especially those with risk factors such as obesity or chronic lung diseases [see Adverse Reactions (6.2)].

5.12 Lipids

Changes in serum lipid profile may require dose adjustment or discontinuation of testosterone therapy.

5.13 Hypercalcemia

Androgens, including AndroGel 1%, should be used with caution in cancer patients at risk of hypercalcemia (and associated hypercalciuria). Regular monitoring of serum calcium concentrations is recommended in these patients.

5.14 Decreased Thyroxine-binding Globulin

Androgens, including AndroGel 1%, may decrease concentrations of thyroxin-binding globulins, resulting in decreased total T4 serum concentrations and increased resin uptake of T3 and T4. Free thyroid hormone concentrations remain unchanged, however, and there is no clinical evidence of thyroid dysfunction.

5.15 Flammability

Alcohol based products, including AndroGel 1%, are flammable; therefore, patients should be advised to avoid fire, flame or smoking until the AndroGel 1% has dried.

6 ADVERSE REACTIONS

6.1 Clinical Trial Experience

Because clinical trials are conducted under widely varying conditions, adverse reaction rates observed in the clinical trials of a drug cannot be directly compared to rates in the clinical trials of another drug and may not reflect the rates observed in practice.

Clinical Trials in Hypogonadal Men

Table 2 shows the incidence of all adverse events judged by the investigator to be at least possibly related to treatment with AndroGel 1% and reported by >1% of patients in a 180 Day, Phase 3 study.

Table 2: Adverse Events Possibly, Probably or Definitely Related to Use of AndroGel 1% in the 180-Day Controlled Clinical Trial

Adverse Event	Dose of AndroGel 1%		
	50 mg	75 mg	100 mg
	N = 77	N = 40	N = 78
Acne	1%	3%	8%
Alopecia	1%	0%	1%
Application Site Reaction	5%	3%	4%
Asthenia	0%	3%	1%
Depression	1%	0%	1%
Emotional Lability	0%	3%	3%
Gynecomastia	1%	0%	3%
Headache	4%	3%	0%
Hypertension	3%	0%	3%
Lab Test Abnormal*	6%	5%	3%
Libido Decreased	0%	3%	1%
Nervousness	0%	3%	1%
Pain Breast	1%	3%	1%
Prostate Disorder**	3%	3%	5%
Testis Disorder***	3%	0%	0%

*Lab test abnormal occurred in nine patients with one or more of the following events reported: elevated hemoglobin or hematocrit, hyperlipidemia, elevated triglycerides, hypokalemia, decreased HDL, elevated glucose, elevated creatinine, elevated total bilirubin.

**Prostate disorders included five patients with enlarged prostate, one with BPH, and one with elevated PSA results.

***Testis disorders were reported in two patients: one with left varicocele and one with slight sensitivity of left testis.

Other less common adverse reactions, reported in fewer than 1% of patients included: amnesia, anxiety, discolored hair, dizziness, dry skin, hirsutism, hostility, impaired urination, paresthesia, penis disorder, peripheral edema, sweating, and vasodilation.

In this 180 day clinical trial, skin reactions at the site of application were reported with AndroGel 1%, but none was severe enough to require treatment or discontinuation of drug.

Six patients (4%) in this trial had adverse events that led to discontinuation of AndroGel 1%. These events included: cerebral hemorrhage, convulsion (neither of which were considered related to AndroGel 1% administration), depression, sadness, memory loss, elevated prostate specific antigen, and hypertension. No AndroGel 1% patient discontinued due to skin reactions.

In a separate uncontrolled pharmacokinetic study of 10 patients, two had adverse events associated with AndroGel 1%; these were asthenia and depression in one patient and increased libido and hyperkinesia in the other.

In a 3 year, flexible dose, extension study, the incidence of all adverse events judged by the investigator to be at least possibly related to treatment with AndroGel 1% and reported by > 1% of patients is shown in Table 3.

Table 3: Adverse Events Possibly, Probably or Definitely Related to Use of AndroGel 1% in the 3 Year, Flexible Dose, Extension Study

Adverse Event	Percent of Subjects
	(N = 162)
Lab Test Abnormal+	9.3
Skin dry	1.9
Application Site Reaction	5.6
Acne	3.1
Pruritus	1.9
Enlarged Prostate	11.7
Carcinoma of Prostate	1.2
Urinary Symptoms*	3.7
Testis Disorder**	1.9
Gynecomastia	2.5
Anemia	2.5

+Lab test abnormal occurred in 15 patients with one or more of the following events reported: elevated AST, elevated ALT, elevated testosterone, elevated hemoglobin or hematocrit, elevated cholesterol, elevated cholesterol/LDL ratio, elevated triglycerides, elevated HDL, elevated serum creatinine.

*Urinary symptoms included nocturia, urinary hesitancy, urinary incontinence, urinary retention, urinary urgency and weak urinary stream.

**Testis disorders included three patients. There were two with a non-palpable testis and one with slight right testicular tenderness.

Two patients reported serious adverse events considered possibly related to treatment: deep vein thrombosis (DVT) and prostate disorder requiring a transurethral resection of the prostate (TURP).

Discontinuation for adverse events in this study included: two patients with application site reactions, one with kidney failure, and five with prostate disorders (including increase in serum PSA in 4 patients, and increase in PSA with prostate enlargement in a fifth patient).

Increases in Serum PSA Observed in Clinical Trials of Hypogonadal Men

During the initial 6-month study, the mean change in PSA values had a statistically significant increase of 0.26 ng/mL. Serum PSA was measured every 6 months thereafter in the 162 hypogonadal men on AndroGel 1% in the 3-year extension study. There was no additional statistically significant increase observed in mean PSA from 6 months through 36 months. However, there were increases in serum PSA observed in approximately 18% of individual patients. The overall mean change from baseline in serum PSA values for the entire group from month 6 to 36 was 0.11 ng/mL.

Twenty-nine patients (18%) met the per-protocol criterion for increase in serum PSA, defined as >2X the baseline or any single serum PSA >6 ng/mL. Most of these (25/29) met this criterion by at least doubling of their PSA from baseline. In most cases where PSA at least doubled (22/25), the maximum serum PSA value was still <2 ng/mL. The first occurrence of a pre-specified, post-baseline increase in serum PSA was seen at or prior to Month 12 in most of the patients who met this criterion (23 of 29; 79%).

Four patients met this criterion by having a serum PSA >6 ng/mL and in these, maximum serum PSA values were 6.2 ng/mL, 6.6 ng/mL, 6.7 ng/mL, and 10.7 ng/mL. In two of these patients, prostate cancer was detected on biopsy. The first patient's PSA levels were 4.7 ng/mL and 6.2 ng/mL at baseline and at Month 6/Final, respectively. The second patient's PSA levels were 4.2 ng/mL, 5.2 ng/mL, 5.8 ng/mL, and 6.6 ng/mL at baseline, Month 6, Month 12, and Final, respectively.

6.2 Postmarketing Experience

The following adverse reactions have been identified during post approval use of AndroGel 1%. Because the reactions are reported voluntarily from a population of uncertain size, it is not always possible to reliably estimate their frequency or establish a causal relationship to drug exposure (Table 4).

Table 4: Adverse Drug Reactions from Postmarketing Experience of AndroGel 1% by MedDRA System Organ Class

Blood and the lymphatic system disorders:	Elevated Hgb, Hct (polycythemia)
Cardiovascular disorders:	Myocardial infarction, stroke
Endocrine disorders:	Hirsutism
Gastrointestinal disorders:	Nausea
General disorders and administration site reactions:	Asthenia, edema, malaise
Genitourinary disorders:	Impaired urination

Continued on next page

Information on the AbbVie, Inc. products listed on these pages is from the prescribing information in use as of July 31, 2016. For more information, please visit rxabbvie.com or call 1-800-633-9110.

Hepatobiliary disorders:	Abnormal liver function tests (e.g. transaminases, elevated GGTP, bilirubin)
Investigations:	Elevated PSA, electrolyte changes (nitrogen, calcium, potassium, phosphorus, sodium), changes in serum lipids (hyperlipidemia, elevated triglycerides, decreased HDL), impaired glucose tolerance, fluctuating testosterone concentrations, weight increase
Neoplasms benign, malignant and unspecified (cysts and polyps):	Prostate cancer
Nervous system:	Headache, dizziness, sleep apnea, insomnia
Psychiatric disorders:	Depression, emotional lability, decreased libido, nervousness, hostility, amnesia, anxiety
Reproductive system and breast disorders:	Gynecomastia, mastodynia, prostatic enlargement, testicular atrophy, oligospermia, priapism (frequent or prolonged erections)
Respiratory disorders:	Dyspnea
Skin and subcutaneous tissue disorders:	Acne, alopecia, application site reaction (pruritus, dry skin, erythema, rash, discolored hair, paresthesia), sweating
Vascular disorders:	Hypertension, vasodilation (hot flushes), venous thromboembolism

Secondary Exposure to Testosterone in Children
Cases of secondary exposure to testosterone resulting in virilization of children have been reported in postmarket surveillance. Signs and symptoms of these reported cases have included enlargement of the clitoris (with surgical intervention) or the penis, development of pubic hair, increased erections and libido, aggressive behavior, and advanced bone age. In most cases with a reported outcome, these signs and symptoms were reported to have regressed with removal of the testosterone gel exposure. In a few cases, however, enlarged genitalia did not fully return to age appropriate normal size, and bone age remained modestly greater than chronological age. In some of the cases, direct contact with the sites of application on the skin of men using testosterone gel was reported. In at least one reported case, the reporter considered the possibility of secondary exposure from items such as the testosterone gel user's shirts and/or other fabric, such as towels and sheets [*see Warnings and Precautions (5.2)*].

7   DRUG INTERACTIONS
7.1   Insulin
Changes in insulin sensitivity or glycemic control may occur in patients treated with androgens. In diabetic patients, the metabolic effects of androgens may decrease blood glucose and, therefore, may decrease insulin requirements.
7.2   Oral Anticoagulants
Changes in anticoagulant activity may be seen with androgens, therefore more frequent monitoring of international normalized ratio (INR) and prothrombin time are recommended in patients taking anticoagulants, especially at the initiation and termination of androgen therapy.
7.3   Corticosteroids
The concurrent use of testosterone with adrenocorticotropic hormone (ACTH) or corticosteroids may result in increased fluid retention and requires careful monitoring particularly in patients with cardiac, renal or hepatic disease.

8   USE IN SPECIFIC POPULATIONS
8.1   Pregnancy
Pregnancy Category X [*see Contraindications (4)*]:
AndroGel 1% is contraindicated during pregnancy or in women who may become pregnant. Testosterone is teratogenic and may cause fetal harm. Exposure to androgens may result in varying degrees of virilization. If this drug is used during pregnancy, or if the patient becomes pregnant while taking this drug, the patient should be apprised of the potential hazard to a fetus.
8.3   Nursing Mothers
Although it is not known how much testosterone transfers into human milk, AndroGel 1% is contraindicated in nursing women because of the potential for serious adverse reactions in nursing infants. Testosterone and other androgens may adversely affect lactation [*see Contraindications (4)*].
8.4   Pediatric Use
The safety and efficacy of AndroGel 1% in pediatric patients less than 18 years old has not been established. Improper use may result in acceleration of bone age and premature closure of epiphyses.
8.5   Geriatric Use
There have not been sufficient numbers of geriatric patients involved in controlled clinical studies utilizing AndroGel 1% to determine whether efficacy in those over 65 years of age differs from younger subjects. Additionally, there is insufficient long-term safety data in geriatric patients to assess the potential risks of cardiovascular disease and prostate cancer.
Geriatric patients treated with androgens may also be at risk for worsening of signs and symptoms of BPH.
8.6   Renal Impairment
No studies were conducted in patients with renal impairment.
8.7   Hepatic Impairment
No studies were conducted in patients with hepatic impairment.

9   DRUG ABUSE AND DEPENDENCE
9.1   Controlled Substance
AndroGel 1% contains testosterone, a Schedule III controlled substance in the Controlled Substances Act.
9.2   Abuse
Anabolic steroids, such as testosterone, are abused. Abuse is often associated with adverse physical and psychological effects.
9.3   Dependence
Although drug dependence is not documented in individuals using therapeutic doses of anabolic steroids for approved indications, dependence is observed in some individuals abusing high doses of anabolic steroids. In general, anabolic steroid dependence is characterized by any three of the following:
- Taking more drug than intended
- Continued drug use despite medical and social problems
- Significant time spent in obtaining adequate amounts of drug
- Desire for anabolic steroids when supplies of the drugs are interrupted
- Difficulty in discontinuing use of the drug despite desires and attempts to do so
- Experience of a withdrawal syndrome upon discontinuation of anabolic steroid use

10   OVERDOSAGE
There is one report of acute overdosage with use of an approved injectable testosterone product: this subject had serum testosterone concentrations of up to 11,400 ng/dL with a cerebrovascular accident.
Treatment of overdosage would consist of discontinuation of AndroGel 1%, washing the application site with soap and water, and appropriate symptomatic and supportive care.

11   DESCRIPTION
AndroGel (testosterone gel) 1% is a clear, colorless hydroalcoholic gel containing testosterone.
The active pharmacologic ingredient in AndroGel 1% is testosterone, an androgen. Testosterone USP is a white to practically white crystalline powder chemically described as 17-beta hydroxyandrost-4-en-3-one. The structural formula is:

Testosterone

$C_{19}H_{28}O_2$ MW 288.42

Pharmacologically inactive ingredients in AndroGel 1% are carbomer 980, ethanol 67.0%, isopropyl myristate, purified water, and sodium hydroxide. These ingredients are not pharmacologically active.

12   CLINICAL PHARMACOLOGY
12.1   Mechanism of Action
Endogenous androgens, including testosterone and dihydrotestosterone (DHT), are responsible for the normal growth and development of the male sex organs and for maintenance of secondary sex characteristics. These effects include the growth and maturation of prostate, seminal vesicles, penis and scrotum; the development of male hair distribution, such as facial, pubic, chest and axillary hair; laryngeal enlargement, vocal chord thickening, alterations in body musculature and fat distribution. Testosterone and DHT are necessary for the normal development of secondary sex characteristics.
Male hypogonadism, a clinical syndrome resulting from insufficient secretion of testosterone, has two main etiologies. Primary hypogonadism is caused by defects of the gonads, such as Klinefelter's syndrome or Leydig cell aplasia, whereas secondary hypogonadism is the failure of the hypothalamus (or pituitary) to produce sufficient gonadotropins (FSH, LH).
12.2   Pharmacodynamics
No specific pharmacodynamic studies were conducted using AndroGel 1%.
12.3   Pharmacokinetics
Absorption
AndroGel 1% delivers physiologic amounts of testosterone, producing circulating testosterone concentrations that approximate normal concentrations (298 - 1043 ng/dL) seen in healthy men. AndroGel 1% provides continuous transdermal delivery of testosterone for 24 hours following a single application to intact, clean, dry skin of the shoulders, upper arms and/or abdomen.
AndroGel 1% is a hydroalcoholic formulation that dries quickly when applied to the skin surface. The skin serves as a reservoir for the sustained release of testosterone into the systemic circulation. Approximately 10% of the testosterone dose applied on the skin surface from AndroGel is absorbed into systemic circulation. In a study with AndroGel 1% 100 mg , all patients showed an increase in serum testosterone within 30 minutes, and eight of nine patients had a serum testosterone concentration within normal range by 4 hours after the initial application. Absorption of testosterone into the blood continues for the entire 24-hour dosing interval. Serum concentrations approximate the steady-state concentration by the end of the first 24 hours and are at steady state by the second or third day of dosing. With single daily applications of AndroGel 1%, follow-up measurements 30, 90 and 180 days after starting treatment have confirmed that serum testosterone concentrations are generally maintained within the eugonadal range. Figure 1 summarizes the 24-hour pharmacokinetic profiles of testosterone for hypogonadal men (less than 300 ng/dL) maintained on AndroGel 1% 50 mg or 100 mg for 30 days. The average (± SD) daily testosterone concentration produced by AndroGel 1% 100 mg on Day 30 was 792 (± 294) ng/dL and by AndroGel 1% 50 mg 566 (± 262) ng/dL.

Figure 1: Mean (± SD) Steady-State Serum Testosterone Concentrations on Day 30 in Patients Applying AndroGel 1% Once Daily

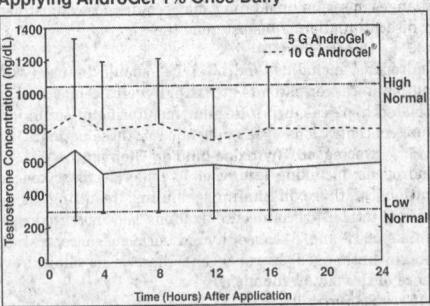

Distribution
Circulating testosterone is primarily bound in the serum to sex hormone-binding globulin (SHBG) and albumin. Approximately 40% of testosterone in plasma is bound to SHBG, 2% remains unbound (free) and the rest is bound to albumin and other proteins.

Metabolism

Testosterone is metabolized to various 17-keto steroids through two different pathways. The major active metabolites of testosterone are estradiol and dihydrotestosterone (DHT).

DHT concentrations increased in parallel with testosterone concentrations during AndroGel 1% treatment. The mean steady-state DHT/T ratio during 180 days of AndroGel 1%/day) and from 0.27 to 0.33 (100 mg of AndroGel 1%/day).

Excretion

There is considerable variation in the half-life of testosterone concentration as reported in the literature, ranging from 10 to 100 minutes. About 90% of a dose of testosterone given intramuscularly is excreted in the urine as glucuronic and sulfuric acid conjugates of testosterone and its metabolites. About 6% of a dose is excreted in the feces, mostly in the unconjugated form. Inactivation of testosterone occurs primarily in the liver.

When AndroGel 1% treatment is discontinued after achieving steady state, serum testosterone concentrations remain in the normal range for 24 to 48 hours but return to their pretreatment concentrations by the fifth day after the last application.

Testosterone Transfer from Male Patients to Female Partners

The potential for dermal testosterone transfer following AndroGel 1% use was evaluated in a clinical study between males dosed with AndroGel 1% and their untreated female partners. Two (2) to 12 hours after application of 100 mg of testosterone administered as AndroGel 1% by the male subjects, the couples (N = 38 couples) engaged in daily, 15-minute sessions of vigorous skin-to-skin contact so that the female partners gained maximum exposure to the AndroGel 1% application sites. Under these study conditions, all unprotected female partners had a serum testosterone concentration >2 times the baseline value at some time during the study. When a shirt covered the application site(s), the transfer of testosterone from the males to the female partners was completely prevented.

13 NONCLINICAL TOXICOLOGY

13.1 Carcinogenesis, Mutagenesis, Impairment of Fertility

Testosterone has been tested by subcutaneous injection and implantation in mice and rats. In mice, the implant induced cervical-uterine tumors which metastasized in some cases. There is suggestive evidence that injection of testosterone into some strains of female mice increases their susceptibility to hepatoma. Testosterone is also known to increase the number of tumors and decrease the degree of differentiation of chemically induced carcinomas of the liver in rats. Testosterone was negative in the *in vitro* Ames and in the *in vivo* mouse micronucleus assays. The administration of exogenous testosterone has been reported to suppress spermatogenesis in the rat, dog and non-human primates, which was reversible on cessation of the treatment.

14 CLINICAL STUDIES

14.1 Clinical Trials in Adult Hypogonadal Males

AndroGel 1% was evaluated in a multi-center, randomized, parallel-group, active-controlled, 180-day trial in 227 hypogonadal men. The study was conducted in 2 phases. During the Initial Treatment Period (Days 1-90), 73 patients were randomized to AndroGel 1% 50 mg daily, 78 patients to AndroGel 1% 100 mg daily, and 76 patients to a non-scrotal testosterone transdermal system. The study was double-blind for dose of AndroGel 1% but open-label for active control. Patients who were originally randomized to AndroGel 1% and who had single-sample serum testosterone concentrations above or below the normal range on Day 60 were titrated to 75 mg daily on Day 91. During the Extended Treatment Period (Days 91-180), 51 patients continued on AndroGel 1% 50 mg daily, 52 patients continued on AndroGel 1% 100 mg daily, 41 patients continued on a non-scrotal testosterone transdermal system (5 mg daily), and 40 patients received AndroGel 1% 75 mg daily. Upon completion of the initial study, 163 enrolled and 162 patients received treatment in an open-label extension study of AndroGel 1% for an additional period of up to 3 years.

Mean peak, trough and average serum testosterone concentrations within the normal range (298-1043 ng/dL) were achieved on the first day of treatment with doses of 50 mg and 100 mg of AndroGel 1%. In patients continuing on AndroGel 1% 50 mg and 100 mg, these mean testosterone concentrations were maintained within the normal range for the 180-day duration of the original study. Figure 2 summarizes the 24-hour pharmacokinetic profiles of testosterone administered as AndroGel 1% for 30, 90 and 180 days. Testosterone concentrations were maintained as long as the patient continued to properly apply the prescribed AndroGel 1% treatment.

Figure 2: Mean Steady-State Testosterone Concentrations in Patients with Once-Daily AndroGel 1% Therapy

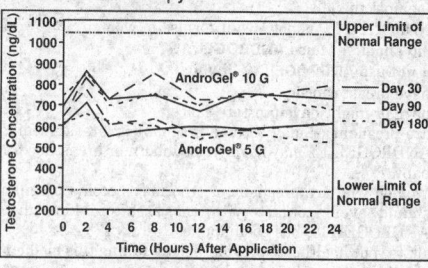

Table 5 summarizes the mean testosterone concentrations on Treatment Day 180 for patients receiving 50 mg, 75 mg, or 100 mg of AndroGel 1%. The 75 mg dose produced mean concentrations intermediate to those produced by 50 mg and 100 mg of AndroGel 1%.

Table 5: Mean (± SD) Steady-State Serum Testosterone Concentrations During Therapy (Day 180)

	50 mg N = 44	75 mg N = 37	100 mg N = 48
C_{avg}	555 ± 225	601 ± 309	713 ± 209
C_{max}	830 ± 347	901 ± 471	1083 ± 434
C_{min}	371 ± 165	406 ± 220	485 ± 156

Of 129 hypogonadal men who were appropriately titrated with AndroGel 1% and who had sufficient data for analysis, 87% achieved an average serum testosterone concentration within the normal range on Treatment Day 180.

In patients treated with AndroGel 1%, there were no observed differences in the average daily serum testosterone concentrations at steady-state based on age, cause of hypogonadism, or body mass index.

DHT concentrations increased in parallel with testosterone concentrations at AndroGel 1% doses of 50 mg/day and 100 mg/day, but the DHT/T ratio stayed within the normal range, indicating enhanced availability of the major physiologically active androgen. Serum estradiol (E2) concentrations increased significantly within 30 days of starting treatment with AndroGel 1% 50 or 100 mg/day and remained elevated throughout the treatment period but remained within the normal range for eugonadal men. Serum levels of SHBG decreased very slightly (1 to 11%) during AndroGel 1% treatment. In men with hypergonadotropic hypogonadism, serum levels of LH and FSH fell in a dose- and time-dependent manner during treatment with AndroGel 1%.

14.2 Phototoxicity in Humans

The phototoxic potential of AndroGel 1% was evaluated in a double-blind, single-dose study in 27 subjects with photosensitive skin types. The Minimal Erythema Dose (MED) of ultraviolet radiation was determined for each subject. A single 24 (+1) hour application of duplicate patches containing test articles (placebo gel, testosterone gel, or saline) was made to naive skin sites on Day 1. On Day 2, each subject received five exposure times of ultraviolet radiation, each exposure being 25% greater than the previous one. Skin evaluations were made on Days 2 to 5. Exposure of test and control article application sites to ultraviolet light did not produce increased inflammation relative to non-irradiated sites, indicating no phototoxic effect.

16 HOW SUPPLIED/STORAGE AND HANDLING

AndroGel 1% is supplied in non-aerosol, metered-dose pumps that deliver 12.5 mg of testosterone per complete pump actuation. The pumps are composed of plastic and stainless steel and an LDPE/aluminum foil inner liner encased in rigid plastic with a polypropylene cap. Each 88 g metered-dose pump is capable of dispensing 75 g of gel or 60-metered pump actuations; each pump actuation dispenses 1.25 g of gel.

AndroGel 1% is also supplied in unit-dose aluminum foil packets in cartons of 30. Each packet of 2.5 g or 5 g gel contains 25 mg or 50 mg testosterone, respectively.

NDC Number	Package Size
0051-8488-88	2 × 75 g pump (each pump dispenses 60 metered pump actuations with each pump actuation containing 12.5 mg of testosterone in 1.25 g of gel)
0051-8425-30	30 packets (a unit dose packet containing 25 mg of testosterone provided in 2.5 g of gel)
0051-8450-30	30 packets (a unit dose packet containing 50 mg of testosterone provided in 5 g of gel)

Storage

Store at 25°C (77°F); excursions permitted to 15° to 30°C (59° to 86°F) [see USP Controlled Room Temperature].

Disposal

Used AndroGel 1% pumps or used AndroGel 1% packets should be discarded in household trash in a manner that prevents accidental application or ingestion by children or pets.

17 PATIENT COUNSELING INFORMATION

See FDA-Approved Patient Labeling (Medication Guide)
Patients should be informed of the following:

17.1 Use in Men with Known or Suspected Prostate or Breast Cancer

Men with known or suspected prostate or breast cancer should not use AndroGel 1% *[see Contraindications (4) and Warnings and Precautions (5.1)]*.

17.2 Potential for Secondary Exposure to Testosterone and Steps to Prevent Secondary Exposure

Secondary exposure to testosterone in children and women can occur with the use of testosterone gel in men. Cases of secondary exposure to testosterone have been reported in children.

Physicians should advise patients of the reported signs and symptoms of secondary exposure which may include the following:

- In children; unexpected sexual development including inappropriate enlargement of the penis or clitoris, premature development of pubic hair, increased erections, and aggressive behavior
- In women; changes in hair distribution, increase in acne, or other signs of testosterone effects
- The possibility of secondary exposure to testosterone gel should be brought to the attention of a healthcare provider
- AndroGel 1% should be promptly discontinued until the cause of virilization is identified

Strict adherence to the following precautions is advised to minimize the potential for secondary exposure to testosterone from testosterone gel in men *[see Medication Guide]*:

- Children and women should avoid contact with unwashed or unclothed application site(s) of men using testosterone gel
- Patients using AndroGel 1% should apply the product as directed and strictly adhere to the following:
  - **Wash hands** with soap and water after application
  - **Cover the application site(s)** with clothing after the gel has dried
  - **Wash the application site(s) thoroughly** with soap and water prior to any situation where skin-to-skin contact of the application site with another person is anticipated
  - In the event that unwashed or unclothed skin to which AndroGel 1% has been applied comes in contact with the skin of another person, the general area of contact on the other person should be washed with soap and water as soon as possible *[see Dosage and Administration (2.2), Warnings and Precautions (5.2) and Clinical Pharmacology (12.3)]*.

17.3 Potential Adverse Reactions with Androgens

Patients should be informed that treatment with androgens may lead to adverse reactions which include:

- Changes in urinary habits such as increased urination at night, trouble starting your urine stream, passing urine

Continued on next page

many times during the day, having an urge that you have to go to the bathroom right away, having a urine accident, being unable to pass urine and weak urine flow.
- Breathing disturbances, including those associated with sleep, or excessive daytime sleepiness.
- Too frequent or persistent erections of the penis.
- Nausea, vomiting, changes in skin color, or ankle swelling.

17.4   Patients Should Be Advised of the Following Instructions for Use:
- **Read the Medication Guide before starting AndroGel 1% therapy and to reread it each time the prescription is renewed**
- **AndroGel 1% should be applied and used appropriately to maximize the benefits and to minimize the risk of secondary exposure in children and women**
- **Keep AndroGel 1% out of the reach of children**
- **AndroGel 1% is an alcohol based product and is flammable; therefore avoid fire, flame or smoking until the gel has dried**
- **It is important to adhere to all recommended monitoring**
- **Report any changes in their state of health, such as changes in urinary habits, breathing, sleep, and mood**
- AndroGel 1% is prescribed to meet the patient's specific needs; therefore, the patient should never share AndroGel 1% with anyone.
- Wait 5 hours before swimming or washing following application of AndroGel 1%. This will ensure that the greatest amount of AndroGel 1% is absorbed into their system.

Medication Guide
ANDROGEL® (AN DROW JEL) ⑩
(testosterone gel) 1%
Read this Medication Guide that comes with ANDROGEL 1% before you start taking it and each time you get a refill. There may be new information. This Medication Guide does not take the place of talking to your healthcare provider about your medical condition or your treatment.

What is the most important information I should know about ANDROGEL 1%?
1. **Early signs and symptoms of puberty have happened in young children who were accidentally exposed to testosterone through contact with men using ANDROGEL 1%.**
   Signs and symptoms of early puberty in a child may include:
   - enlarged penis or clitoris
   - early development of pubic hair
   - increased erections or sex drive
   - aggressive behavior
   ANDROGEL 1% can transfer from your body to others.
2. **Women and children should avoid contact with the unwashed or unclothed area where ANDROGEL 1% has been applied to your skin.**
   Stop using ANDROGEL 1% and call your healthcare provider right away if you see any signs and symptoms in a child or a woman that may have occurred through accidental exposure to ANDROGEL 1%.
   Signs and symptoms of exposure to ANDROGEL 1% in children may include:
   - enlarged penis or clitoris
   - early development of pubic hair
   - increased erections or sex drive
   - aggressive behavior
   Signs and symptoms of exposure to ANDROGEL 1% in women may include:
   - changes in body hair
   - a large increase in acne
- **To lower the risk of transfer of ANDROGEL 1% from your body to others, you should follow these important instructions:**
   ○ Apply ANDROGEL 1% **only** to areas that will be covered by a short sleeve T-shirt. These areas are your shoulders and upper arms, or stomach area (abdomen), or shoulders, upper arms and stomach area.
   ○ Wash your hands **right away** with soap and water after applying ANDROGEL 1%.
   ○ After the gel has dried, **cover the application area with clothing.** Keep the area covered until you have washed the application area well or have showered.
   ○ **If you expect to have skin-to-skin contact with another person, first wash the application area well with soap and water.**
   ○ **If a woman or child makes contact with the ANDROGEL 1% application area,** that area on the woman or child should be washed well with soap and water right away.

What is ANDROGEL 1%?
ANDROGEL 1% is a prescription medicine that contains testosterone. ANDROGEL 1% is used to treat adult males who have low or no testosterone due to certain medical conditions.
Your healthcare provider will test your blood before you start and while you are taking ANDROGEL 1%.

It is not known if ANDROGEL 1% is safe or effective to treat men who have low testosterone due to aging.
It is not known if ANDROGEL 1% is safe or effective in children younger than 18 years old. Improper use of ANDROGEL 1% may affect bone growth in children.
ANDROGEL 1% is a controlled substance (CIII) because it contains testosterone that can be a target for people who abuse prescription medicines. Keep your ANDROGEL 1% in a safe place to protect it. Never give your ANDROGEL 1% to anyone else, even if they have the same symptoms you have. Selling or giving away this medicine may harm others and is against the law.
ANDROGEL 1% is not meant for use in women.

Who should not use ANDROGEL 1%?
Do not use ANDROGEL 1% if you:
- have breast cancer
- have or might have prostate cancer
- are pregnant or may become pregnant or breast-feeding. ANDROGEL 1% may harm your unborn or breast-feeding baby.
  Women who are pregnant or who may become pregnant should avoid contact with the area of skin where ANDROGEL 1% has been applied.
Talk to your healthcare provider before taking this medicine if you have any of the above conditions.

What should I tell my healthcare provider before using ANDROGEL 1%?
Before you use ANDROGEL 1%, tell your healthcare provider if you:
- have breast cancer
- have or might have prostate cancer
- have urinary problems due to an enlarged prostate
- have heart problems
- have liver or kidney problems
- have problems breathing while you sleep (sleep apnea)
- have any other medical conditions
Tell your healthcare provider about all the medicines you take, including prescription and non-prescription medicines, vitamins, and herbal supplements.
Using ANDROGEL 1% with certain other medicines can affect each other.
Especially, tell your healthcare provider if you take:
- insulin
- corticosteroids
- medicines that decrease blood clotting
Know the medicines you take. Ask your healthcare provider or pharmacist for a list of these medicines, if you are not sure. Keep a list of them and show it to your healthcare provider and pharmacist when you get a new medicine.

How should I use ANDROGEL 1%?
- It is important that you apply ANDROGEL 1% exactly as your healthcare provider tells you to.
- Your healthcare provider will tell you how much ANDROGEL 1% to apply and when to apply it.
- Your healthcare provider may change your ANDROGEL 1% dose. **Do not** change your ANDROGEL 1% dose without talking to your healthcare provider.
- **ANDROGEL 1% is to be applied to the area of your shoulders, upper arms, or abdomen that will be covered by a short sleeve t-shirt.** Do not apply ANDROGEL 1% to any other parts of your body such as your penis, scrotum, chest, armpits (axillae), knees, or back.
- Apply AndroGel 1% at the same time each morning. ANDROGEL 1% should be applied after showering or bathing.
- **Wash your hands right away** with soap and water after applying ANDROGEL 1%.
- Avoid showering, swimming, or bathing for at least 5 hours after you apply ANDROGEL 1%.
- ANDROGEL 1% is flammable until dry. Let ANDROGEL 1% dry before smoking or going near an open flame.
- Let the application areas dry completely before putting on a t-shirt.

Applying ANDROGEL 1%:
ANDROGEL 1% comes in a pump or in packets.
- **Before applying ANDROGEL 1%, make sure that your shoulders, upper arms, and abdomen are clean, dry, and there is no broken skin.**
- The application sites for ANDROGEL 1% are the shoulders, upper arms, or abdomen that will be covered by a short sleeve t-shirt (See Figure A).

If you are using the ANDROGEL 1% pump:
- Before using a new bottle of ANDROGEL 1% for the first time, you will need to prime the pump. To prime the ANDROGEL 1% pump, slowly push the pump all the way down 3 times. **Do not** use any ANDROGEL 1% that came out while priming. Wash it down the sink to avoid accidental exposure to others. Your ANDROGEL 1% pump is ready to use.

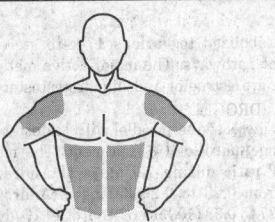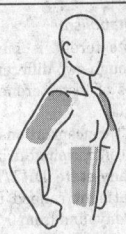

(Figure A)

- Remove the cap from the pump. Then, position the nozzle over the palm of your hand and slowly push the pump all the way down. Apply ANDROGEL 1% to the application site. You may also apply ANDROGEL 1% directly to the application site.
- **Wash your hands with soap and water right away.**
- Your healthcare provider will tell you the number of times to press the pump for each dose.

If you are using ANDROGEL 1% packets:
- Tear open the packet completely at the dotted line. Squeeze from the bottom of the packet to the top.
- Squeeze all of the ANDROGEL 1% out of the packet into the palm of your hand. Apply ANDROGEL 1% to the application site. You may also apply ANDROGEL 1% from the packet directly to the application site.
- ANDROGEL 1% should be applied right away.
- **Wash your hands with soap and water right away.**

What are the possible side effects of ANDROGEL 1%?
See "**What is the most important information I should know about ANDROGEL 1%?**"
ANDROGEL 1% can cause serious side effects including:
- **If you already have enlargement of your prostate gland your signs and symptoms can get worse while using ANDROGEL 1%.** This can include:
   ○ increased urination at night
   ○ trouble starting your urine stream
   ○ having to pass urine many times during the day
   ○ having an urge that you have to go to the bathroom right away
   ○ having a urine accident
   ○ being unable to pass urine or weak urine flow
- **Possible increased risk of prostate cancer.** Your healthcare provider should check you for prostate cancer or any other prostate problems before you start and while you use ANDROGEL 1%.
- **Blood clots in the legs or lungs.** Signs and symptoms of a blood clot in your leg can include leg pain, swelling or redness. Signs and symptoms of a blood clot in your lungs can include difficulty breathing or chest pain.
- **Possible increased risk of heart attack or stroke**
- **In large doses ANDROGEL 1% may lower your sperm count.**
- **Swelling of your ankles, feet, or body, with or without heart failure.**
- **Enlarged or painful breasts.**
- **Have problems breathing while you sleep (sleep apnea).**
Call your healthcare provider right away if you have any of the serious side effects listed above.
The most common side effects of ANDROGEL 1% include:
- acne
- skin irritation where ANDROGEL 1% is applied
- lab test changes
- increased prostate specific antigen (a test used to screen for prostate cancer)
Other side effects include more erections than are normal for you or erections that last a long time.
Tell your healthcare provider if you have any side effect that bothers you or that does not go away.
These are not all the possible side effects of ANDROGEL 1%. For more information, ask your healthcare provider or pharmacist.
Call your doctor for medical advice about side effects. You may report side effects to FDA at 1-800-FDA-1088.

How should I store ANDROGEL 1%?
- Store ANDROGEL 1% between 59°F to 86°F (15°C to 30°C).
- Safely throw away used ANDROGEL 1% in household trash. Be careful to prevent accidental exposure of children or pets.
- Keep ANDROGEL 1% away from fire.
Keep ANDROGEL 1% and all medicines out of the reach of children.

General information about the safe and effective use of ANDROGEL 1%
Medicines are sometimes prescribed for purposes other than those listed in a Medication Guide. Do not use ANDROGEL

1% for a condition for which it was not prescribed. Do not give ANDROGEL 1% to other people, even if they have the same symptoms you have. It may harm them.

This Medication Guide summarizes the most important information about ANDROGEL 1%. If you would like more information, talk to your healthcare provider. You can ask your pharmacist or healthcare provider for information about ANDROGEL 1% that is written for health professionals.

For more information, go to www.ANDROGEL.com or call 1-800-633-9110.

What are the ingredients in ANDROGEL 1%?
Active ingredient: testosterone
Inactive ingredients: carbomer 980, ethyl alcohol 67.0%, isopropyl myristate, purified water and sodium hydroxide. This Medication Guide has been approved by the U.S. Food and Drug Administration.
Marketed by:
AbbVie Inc.
North Chicago, IL 60064, USA
© 2015 AbbVie Inc.
Ref. A090630059176-Revised May, 2015
Shown in Product Identification Guide, page 505

ANDROGEL® 1.62%
[AN DROW JEL]
(testosterone gel)
for topical use

Rx ℞

HIGHLIGHTS OF PRESCRIBING INFORMATION
These highlights do not include all the information needed to use ANDROGEL 1.62% safely and effectively. See full prescribing information for ANDROGEL 1.62%.
AndroGel® (testosterone gel) 1.62% for topical use CIII
Initial U.S. Approval: 1953

WARNING: SECONDARY EXPOSURE TO TESTOSTERONE

See full prescribing information for complete boxed warning.

- **Virilization has been reported in children who were secondarily exposed to testosterone gel (5.2, 6.2).**
- **Children should avoid contact with unwashed or unclothed application sites in men using testosterone gel (2.2, 5.2).**
- **Healthcare providers should advise patients to strictly adhere to recommended instructions for use (2.2, 5.2, 17).**

RECENT MAJOR CHANGES
Indications and Usage (1)	5/2015
Dosage and Administration (2)	5/2015
Dosage and Administration (2.2)	11/2014
Warnings and Precautions (5.4)	6/2014
Warnings and Precautions (5.5)	5/2015

INDICATIONS AND USAGE
AndroGel 1.62% is indicated for replacement therapy in males for conditions associated with a deficiency or absence of endogenous testosterone:
- Primary hypogonadism (congenital or acquired) (1)
- Hypogonadotropic hypogonadism (congenital or acquired) (1)

Limitations of use:
- Safety and efficacy of AndroGel 1.62% in men with "age-related hypogonadism" have not been established. (1)
- Safety and efficacy of AndroGel 1.62% in males less than 18 years old have not been established. (1, 8.4)
- Topical testosterone products may have different doses, strengths, or application instructions that may result in different systemic exposure. (1, 12.3)

DOSAGE AND ADMINISTRATION
- **Dosage and Administration for AndroGel 1.62% differs from AndroGel 1%. For dosage and administration of AndroGel 1% refer to its full prescribing information. (2)**
- Prior to initiating AndroGel 1.62%, confirm the diagnosis of hypogonadism by ensuring that serum testosterone has been measured in the morning on at least two separate days and that these concentrations are below the normal range (2).
- Starting dose of AndroGel 1.62% is 40.5 mg of testosterone (2 pump actuations or a single 40.5 mg packet), applied topically once daily in the morning. (2.1)

- Apply to clean, dry, intact skin of the shoulders and upper arms. Do not apply AndroGel 1.62% to any other parts of the body including the abdomen, genitals, chest, armpits (axillae), or knees. (2.2, 12.3)
- Dose adjustment: AndroGel 1.62% can be dose adjusted between a minimum of 20.25 mg of testosterone (1 pump actuation or a single 20.25 mg packet) and a maximum of 81 mg of testosterone (4 pump actuations or two 40.5 mg packets). The dose should be titrated based on the pre-dose morning serum testosterone concentration at approximately 14 days and 28 days after starting treatment or following dose adjustment. Additionally, serum testosterone concentration should be assessed periodically thereafter. (2.1)
- Patients should wash hands immediately with soap and water after applying AndroGel 1.62% and cover the application site(s) with clothing after the gel has dried. Wash the application site thoroughly with soap and water prior to any situation where skin-to-skin contact of the application site with another person is anticipated. (2.2)

DOSAGE FORMS AND STRENGTHS
AndroGel (testosterone gel) 1.62% for topical use is available as follows:
- a metered-dose pump that delivers 20.25 mg testosterone per actuation. (3)
- packets containing 20.25 mg testosterone. (3)
- packets containing 40.5 mg testosterone. (3)

CONTRAINDICATIONS
- Men with carcinoma of the breast or known or suspected prostate cancer (4, 5.1)
- Pregnant or breast-feeding women. Testosterone may cause fetal harm (4, 8.1, 8.3)

WARNINGS AND PRECAUTIONS
- Monitor patients with benign prostatic hyperplasia (BPH) for worsening of signs and symptoms of BPH (5.1)
- Avoid unintentional exposure of women or children to AndroGel 1.62%. Secondary exposure to testosterone can produce signs of virilization. AndroGel 1.62% should be discontinued until the cause of virilization is identified (5.2)
- Venous thromboembolism (VTE), including deep vein thrombosis (DVT) and pulmonary embolism (PE) have been reported in patients using testosterone products. Evaluate patients with signs or symptoms consistent with DVT or PE. (5.4)
- Some postmarketing studies have shown an increased risk of myocardial infarction and stroke associated with use of testosterone replacement therapy. (5.5)
- Exogenous administration of androgens may lead to azoospermia (5.7)
- Edema with or without congestive heart failure (CHF) may be a complication in patients with preexisting cardiac, renal, or hepatic disease (5.9)
- Sleep apnea may occur in those with risk factors (5.11)
- Monitor serum testosterone, prostate specific antigen (PSA), hemoglobin, hematocrit, liver function tests and lipid concentrations periodically (5.1, 5.3, 5.8, 5.12)
- AndroGel 1.62% is flammable until dry (5.15)

ADVERSE REACTIONS
The most common adverse reaction (incidence ≥ 5%) is an increase in prostate specific antigen (PSA). (6.1)
To report SUSPECTED ADVERSE REACTIONS, contact AbbVie Inc. at 1-800-633-9110 or FDA at 1-800-FDA-1088 or www.fda.gov/medwatch.

DRUG INTERACTIONS
- Androgens may decrease blood glucose and therefore may decrease insulin requirements in diabetic patients (7.1)
- Changes in anticoagulant activity may be seen with androgens. More frequent monitoring of International Normalized Ratio (INR) and prothrombin time is recommended (7.2)
- Use of testosterone with adrenocorticotrophic hormone (ACTH) or corticosteroids may result in increased fluid retention. Use with caution, particularly in patients with cardiac, renal, or hepatic disease (7.3)

USE IN SPECIFIC POPULATIONS
There are insufficient long-term safety data in geriatric patients using AndroGel 1.62% to assess the potential risks of cardiovascular disease and prostate cancer. (8.5)

See 17 for PATIENT COUNSELING INFORMATION and Medication Guide.

Revised: 5/2015

FULL PRESCRIBING INFORMATION

WARNING: SECONDARY EXPOSURE TO TESTOSTERONE
- Virilization has been reported in children who were secondarily exposed to testosterone gel [see Warnings and Precautions (5.2) and Adverse Reactions (6.2)].
- Children should avoid contact with unwashed or unclothed application sites in men using testosterone gel [see Dosage and Administration (2.2) and Warnings and Precautions (5.2)].

Continued on next page

- Healthcare providers should advise patients to strictly adhere to recommended instructions for use [see Dosage and Administration (2.2), Warnings and Precautions (5.2) and Patient Counseling Information (17)].

1 INDICATIONS AND USAGE

AndroGel 1.62% is indicated for replacement therapy in adult males for conditions associated with a deficiency or absence of endogenous testosterone:

- Primary hypogonadism (congenital or acquired): testicular failure due to conditions such as cryptorchidism, bilateral torsion, orchitis, vanishing testis syndrome, orchiectomy, Klinefelter's syndrome, chemotherapy, or toxic damage from alcohol or heavy metals. These men usually have low serum testosterone concentrations and gonadotropins (follicle-stimulating hormone [FSH], luteinizing hormone [LH]) above the normal range.
- Hypogonadotropic hypogonadism (congenital or acquired): gonadotropin or luteinizing hormone-releasing hormone (LHRH) deficiency or pituitary-hypothalamic injury from tumors, trauma, or radiation. These men have low testosterone serum concentrations, but have gonadotropins in the normal or low range.

Limitations of use:

- Safety and efficacy of AndroGel 1.62% in men with "age-related hypogonadism" (also referred to as "late-onset hypogonadism") have not been established.
- Safety and efficacy of AndroGel 1.62% in males less than 18 years old have not been established [see Use in Specific Populations (8.4)].
- Topical testosterone products may have different doses, strengths, or application instructions that may result in different systemic exposure [see Indications and Usage (1), and Clinical Pharmacology (12.3)].

2 DOSAGE AND ADMINISTRATION

Dosage and Administration for AndroGel 1.62% differs from AndroGel 1%. For dosage and administration of AndroGel 1% refer to its full prescribing information. (2)

Prior to initiating AndroGel 1.62%, confirm the diagnosis of hypogonadism by ensuring that serum testosterone concentrations have been measured in the morning on at least two separate days and that these serum testosterone concentrations are below the normal range.

2.1 Dosing and Dose Adjustment

The recommended starting dose of AndroGel 1.62% is 40.5 mg of testosterone (2 pump actuations or a single 40.5 mg packet) applied topically once daily in the morning to the shoulders and upper arms.

The dose can be adjusted between a minimum of 20.25 mg of testosterone (1 pump actuation or a single 20.25 mg packet) and a maximum of 81 mg of testosterone (4 pump actuations or two 40.5 mg packets). To ensure proper dosing, the dose should be titrated based on the pre-dose morning serum testosterone concentration from a single blood draw at approximately 14 days and 28 days after starting treatment or following dose adjustment. In addition, serum testosterone concentration should be assessed periodically thereafter. Table 1 describes the dose adjustments required at each titration step.

Table 1: Dose Adjustment Criteria

Pre-Dose Morning Total Serum Testosterone Concentration	Dose Titration
Greater than 750 ng/dL	Decrease daily dose by 20.25 mg (1 pump actuation or the equivalent of one 20.25 mg packet)
Equal to or greater than 350 and equal to or less than 750 ng/dL	No change: continue on current dose
Less than 350 ng/dL	Increase daily dose by 20.25 mg (1 pump actuation or the equivalent of one 20.25 mg packet)

The application site and dose of AndroGel 1.62% are not interchangeable with other topical testosterone products.

2.2 Administration Instructions

AndroGel 1.62% should be applied to clean, dry, intact skin of the upper arms and shoulders. Do not apply AndroGel 1.62% to any other parts of the body, including the abdomen, genitals, chest, armpits (axillae), or knees [see Clinical Pharmacology (12.3)]. Area of application should be limited to the area that will be covered by the patient's short sleeve t-shirt. Patients should be instructed to use the palm of the hand to apply AndroGel 1.62% and spread across the maximum surface area as directed in Table 2 (for pump) and Table 3 (for packets) and in Figure 1.

Table 2: Application Sites for AndroGel 1.62%, Pump

Total Dose of Testosterone	Total Pump Actuations	Pump Actuations Per Upper Arm and Shoulder	
		Upper Arm and Shoulder #1	Upper Arm and Shoulder #2
20.25 mg	1	1	0
40.5 mg	2	1	1
60.75 mg	3	2	1
81 mg	4	2	2

[See table 3 below]

The prescribed daily dose of AndroGel 1.62% should be applied to the right and left upper arms and shoulders as shown in the shaded areas in Figure 1.

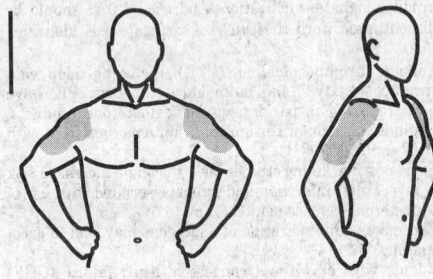

Figure 1. Application Sites for AndroGel 1.62%

Once the application site is dry, the site should be covered with clothing [see Clinical Pharmacology (12.3)]. Wash hands thoroughly with soap and water. Avoid fire, flames or smoking until the gel has dried since alcohol based products, including AndroGel 1.62%, are flammable.

The patient should avoid swimming or showering or washing the administration site for a minimum of 2 hours after application [see Clinical Pharmacology (12.3)].

To obtain a full first dose, it is necessary to prime the canister pump. To do so, with the canister in the upright position, slowly and fully depress the actuator three times. Safely discard the gel from the first three actuations. It is only necessary to prime the pump before the first dose. After the priming procedure, fully depress the actuator once for every 20.25 mg of AndroGel 1.62%. AndroGel 1.62% should be delivered directly into the palm of the hand and then applied to the application sites.

When using packets, the entire contents should be squeezed into the palm of the hand and immediately applied to the application sites. When 40.5 mg packets need to be split between the left and right shoulder, patients may squeeze a portion of the gel from the packet into the palm of the hand and apply to application sites. Repeat until entire contents have been applied. Alternatively, AndroGel 1.62% can be applied directly to the application sites from the pump or packets.

Strict adherence to the following precautions is advised in order to minimize the potential for secondary exposure to testosterone from AndroGel 1.62%-treated skin:

- Children and women should avoid contact with unwashed or unclothed application site(s) of men using AndroGel 1.62%.
- AndroGel 1.62% should only be applied to the upper arms and shoulders. The area of application should be limited to the area that will be covered by a short sleeve t-shirt.
- Patients should wash their hands with soap and water immediately after applying AndroGel 1.62%.
- Patients should cover the application site(s) with clothing (e.g., a t-shirt) after the gel has dried.
- Prior to situations in which direct skin-to-skin contact is anticipated, patients should wash the application site(s) thoroughly with soap and water to remove any testosterone residue.
- In the event that unwashed or unclothed skin to which AndroGel 1.62% has been applied comes in direct contact with the skin of another person, the general area of contact on the other person should be washed with soap and water as soon as possible.

3 DOSAGE FORMS AND STRENGTHS

AndroGel (testosterone gel) 1.62% for topical use only, is available as follows:

- A metered-dose pump. Each pump actuation delivers 20.25 mg of testosterone in 1.25 g of gel.
- A unit dose packet containing 20.25 mg of testosterone in 1.25 g of gel.
- A unit dose packet containing 40.5 mg of testosterone in 2.5 g of gel.

4 CONTRAINDICATIONS

- AndroGel 1.62% is contraindicated in men with carcinoma of the breast or known or suspected carcinoma of the prostate [see Warnings and Precautions (5.1) and Adverse Reactions (6.1)].
- AndroGel 1.62% is contraindicated in women who are or may become pregnant, or who are breastfeeding. AndroGel 1.62% may cause fetal harm when administered to a pregnant woman. AndroGel 1.62% may cause serious adverse reactions in nursing infants. Exposure of a fetus or nursing infant to androgens may result in varying degrees of virilization. Pregnant women or those who may become pregnant need to be aware of the potential for transfer of testosterone from men treated with AndroGel 1.62%. If a pregnant woman is exposed to AndroGel 1.62%, she should be apprised of the potential hazard to the fetus [see Warnings and Precautions (5.2) and Use in Specific Populations (8.1, 8.3)].

5 WARNINGS AND PRECAUTIONS

5.1 Worsening of Benign Prostatic Hyperplasia (BPH) and Potential Risk of Prostate Cancer

- Patients with BPH treated with androgens are at an increased risk for worsening of signs and symptoms of BPH. Monitor patients with BPH for worsening signs and symptoms.
- Patients treated with androgens may be at increased risk for prostate cancer. Evaluation of patients for prostate cancer prior to initiating and during treatment with androgens is appropriate [see Contraindications (4)].

5.2 Potential for Secondary Exposure to Testosterone

Cases of secondary exposure resulting in virilization of children have been reported in postmarketing surveillance of testosterone gel products. Signs and symptoms have included enlargement of the penis or clitoris, development of pubic hair, increased erections and libido, aggressive behavior, and advanced bone age. In most cases, these signs and symptoms regressed with removal of the exposure to testosterone gel. In a few cases, however, enlarged genitalia did not fully return to age-appropriate normal size, and bone age remained modestly greater than chronological age. The risk of transfer was increased in some of these cases by not adhering to precautions for the appropriate use of the topical testosterone product. Children and women should avoid contact with unwashed or unclothed application sites in men using AndroGel 1.62% [see Dosage and Administration (2.2), Use in Specific Populations (8.1) and Clinical Pharmacology (12.3)].

Inappropriate changes in genital size or development of pubic hair or libido in children, or changes in body hair distri-

Table 3: Application Sites for AndroGel 1.62%, Packets

Total Dose of Testosterone	Total packets	Gel Applications Per Upper Arm and Shoulder	
		Upper Arm and Shoulder #1	Upper Arm and Shoulder #2
20.25 mg	One 20.25 mg packet	One 20.25 mg packet	0
40.5 mg	One 40.5 mg packet	Half of contents of One 40.5 mg packet	Half of contents of One 40.5 mg packet
60.75 mg	One 20.25 mg packet AND One 40.5 mg packet	One 40.5 mg packet	One 20.25 mg packet
81 mg	Two 40.5 mg packets	One 40.5 mg packet	One 40.5 mg packet

bution, significant increase in acne, or other signs of virilization in adult women should be brought to the attention of a physician and the possibility of secondary exposure to testosterone gel should also be brought to the attention of a physician. Testosterone gel should be promptly discontinued until the cause of virilization has been identified.

5.3 Polycythemia
Increases in hematocrit, reflective of increases in red blood cell mass, may require lowering or discontinuation of testosterone. Check hematocrit prior to initiating treatment. It would also be appropriate to re-evaluate the hematocrit 3 to 6 months after starting treatment, and then annually. If hematocrit becomes elevated, stop therapy until hematocrit decreases to an acceptable concentration. An increase in red blood cell mass may increase the risk of thromboembolic events.

5.4 Venous Thromboembolism
There have been postmarketing reports of venous thromboembolic events, including deep vein thrombosis (DVT) and pulmonary embolism (PE), in patients using testosterone products such as AndroGel 1.62%. Evaluate patients who report symptoms of pain, edema, warmth and erythema in the lower extremity for DVT and those who present with acute shortness of breath for PE. If a venous thromboembolic event is suspected, discontinue treatment with AndroGel 1.62% and initiate appropriate workup and management *[see Adverse Reactions (6.2)]*.

5.5 Cardiovascular Risk
Long term clinical safety trials have not been conducted to assess the cardiovascular outcomes of testosterone replacement therapy in men. To date, epidemiologic studies and randomized controlled trials have been inconclusive for determining the risk of major adverse cardiovascular events (MACE), such as non-fatal myocardial infarction, non-fatal stroke, and cardiovascular death, with the use of testosterone compared to non-use. Some studies, but not all, have reported an increased risk of MACE in association with use of testosterone replacement therapy in men.
Patients should be informed of this possible risk when deciding whether to use or to continue to use AndroGel 1.62%.

5.6 Use in Women
Due to the lack of controlled evaluations in women and potential virilizing effects, AndroGel 1.62% is not indicated for use in women *[see Contraindications (4) and Use in Specific Populations (8.1, 8.3)]*.

5.7 Potential for Adverse Effects on Spermatogenesis
With large doses of exogenous androgens, including AndroGel 1.62%, spermatogenesis may be suppressed through feedback inhibition of pituitary FSH possibly leading to adverse effects on semen parameters including sperm count.

5.8 Hepatic Adverse Effects
Prolonged use of high doses of orally active 17-alpha-alkyl androgens (e.g., methyltestosterone) has been associated with serious hepatic adverse effects (peliosis hepatis, hepatic neoplasms, cholestatic hepatitis, and jaundice). Peliosis hepatis can be a life-threatening or fatal complication. Long-term therapy with intramuscular testosterone enanthate has produced multiple hepatic adenomas. AndroGel 1.62% is not known to cause these adverse effects.

5.9 Edema
Androgens, including AndroGel 1.62%, may promote retention of sodium and water. Edema, with or without congestive heart failure, may be a serious complication in patients with preexisting cardiac, renal, or hepatic disease *[see Adverse Reactions (6.2)]*.

5.10 Gynecomastia
Gynecomastia may develop and persist in patients being treated with androgens, including AndroGel 1.62%, for hypogonadism.

5.11 Sleep Apnea
The treatment of hypogonadal men with testosterone may potentiate sleep apnea in some patients, especially those with risk factors such as obesity or chronic lung diseases.

5.12 Lipids
Changes in serum lipid profile may require dose adjustment or discontinuation of testosterone therapy.

5.13 Hypercalcemia
Androgens, including AndroGel 1.62 %, should be used with caution in cancer patients at risk of hypercalcemia (and associated hypercalciuria). Regular monitoring of serum calcium concentrations is recommended in these patients.

5.14 Decreased Thyroxine-binding Globulin
Androgens, including AndroGel 1.62%, may decrease concentrations of thyroxin-binding globulins, resulting in decreased total T4 serum concentrations and increased resin uptake of T3 and T4. Free thyroid hormone concentrations remain unchanged, however, and there is no clinical evidence of thyroid dysfunction.

5.15 Flammability
Alcohol based products, including AndroGel 1.62%, are flammable; therefore, patients should be advised to avoid fire, flame or smoking until the AndroGel 1.62% has dried.

6 ADVERSE REACTIONS
6.1 Clinical Trial Experience
Because clinical trials are conducted under widely varying conditions, adverse reaction rates observed in the clinical trials of a drug cannot be directly compared to rates in the clinical trials of another drug and may not reflect the rates observed in practice.
AndroGel 1.62% was evaluated in a two-phase, 364-day, controlled clinical study. The first phase was a multi-center, randomized, double-blind, parallel-group, placebo-controlled period of 182 days, in which 234 hypogonadal men were treated with AndroGel 1.62% and 40 received placebo. Patients could continue in an open-label, non-comparative, maintenance period for an additional 182 days *[see Clinical Studies (14.1)]*.
The most common adverse reaction reported in the double-blind period was increased prostate specific antigen (PSA) reported in 26 AndroGel 1.62%-treated patients (11.1%). In 17 patients, increased PSA was considered an adverse event by meeting one of the two pre-specified criteria for abnormal PSA values, defined as (1) average serum PSA >4 ng/mL based on two separate determinations, or (2) an average change from baseline in serum PSA of greater than 0.75 ng/mL on two determinations.
During the 182-day, double-blind period of the clinical trial, the mean change in serum PSA value was 0.14 ng/mL for patients receiving AndroGel 1.62% and -0.12 ng/mL for the patients in the placebo group. During the double-blind period, seven patients had a PSA value >4.0 ng/mL, four of these seven patients had PSA less than or equal to 4.0 ng/mL upon repeat testing. The other three patients did not undergo repeat PSA testing.
During the 182-day, open-label period of the study, the mean change in serum PSA values was 0.10 ng/mL for both patients continuing on active therapy and patients transitioning onto active from placebo. During the open-label period, three patients had a serum PSA value > 4.0 ng/mL, two of whom had a serum PSA less than or equal to 4.0 ng/mL upon repeated testing. The other patient did not undergo repeat PSA testing. Among previous placebo patients, 3 of 28 (10.7%), had increased PSA as an adverse event in the open-label period.
Table 4 shows adverse reactions reported by >2% of patients in the 182-day, double-blind period of the AndroGel 1.62% clinical trial and more frequent in the AndroGel 1.62% treated group versus placebo.

Table 4: Adverse Reactions Reported in >2% of Patients in the 182-Day, Double-Blind Period of AndroGel 1.62% Clinical Trial

Adverse Reaction	Number (%) of Patients	
	AndroGel 1.62% N=234	Placebo N=40
PSA increased*	26 (11.1%)	0%
Emotional lability**	6 (2.6%)	0%
Hypertension	5 (2.1%)	0%
Hematocrit or hemoglobin increased	5 (2.1%)	0%
Contact dermatitis***	5 (2.1%)	0%

***PSA increased** includes: PSA values that met pre-specified criteria for abnormal PSA values (an average change from baseline > 0.75 ng/mL and/or an average PSA value >4.0 ng/mL based on two measurements) as well as those reported as adverse events.
****Emotional lability** includes: mood swings, affective disorder, impatience, anger, and aggression.
*****Contact dermatitis** includes: 4 patients with dermatitis at non-application sites.

Other adverse reactions occurring in less than or equal to 2% of AndroGel 1.62%-treated patients and more frequently than placebo included: frequent urination, and hyperlipidemia.

In the open-label period of the study (N=191), the most commonly reported adverse reaction (experienced by greater than 2% of patients) was increased PSA (n=13; 6.2%) and sinusitis. Other adverse reactions reported by less than or equal to 2% of patients included increased hemoglobin or hematocrit, hypertension, acne, libido decreased, insomnia, and benign prostatic hypertrophy.
During the 182-day, double-blind period of the clinical trial, 25 AndroGel 1.62%-treated patients (10.7%) discontinued treatment because of adverse reactions. These adverse reactions included 17 patients with PSA increased and 1 report each of: hematocrit increased, blood pressure increased, frequent urination, diarrhea, fatigue, pituitary tumor, dizziness, skin erythema and skin nodule (same patient – neither at application site), vasovagal syncope, and diabetes mellitus. During the 182-day, open-label period, 9 patients discontinued treatment because of adverse reactions. These adverse reactions included 6 reports of PSA increased, 2 of hematocrit increased, and 1 each of triglycerides increased and prostate cancer.

Application Site Reactions
In the 182-day double-blind period of the study, application site reactions were reported in two (2/234; 0.9%) patients receiving AndroGel 1.62%, both of which resolved. Neither of these patients discontinued the study due to application site adverse reactions. In the open-label period of the study, application site reactions were reported in three (3/219; 1.4%) additional patients that were treated with AndroGel 1.62%. None of these subjects were discontinued from the study due to application site reactions.

6.2 Postmarketing Experience
The following adverse reactions have been identified during post approval use of AndroGel 1%. Because the reactions are reported voluntarily from a population of uncertain size, it is not always possible to reliably estimate their frequency or establish a causal relationship to drug exposure (Table 5).

Table 5: Adverse Reactions from Post Approval Experience of AndroGel 1% by System Organ Class

System Organ Class	Adverse Reaction
Blood and lymphatic system disorders:	Elevated hemoglobin or hematocrit, polycythemia, anemia
Cardiovascular disorders:	Myocardial infarction, stroke
Endocrine disorders:	Hirsutism
Gastrointestinal disorders:	Nausea
General disorders:	Asthenia, edema, malaise
Genitourinary disorders:	Impaired urination*
Hepatobiliary disorders:	Abnormal liver function tests
Investigations:	Lab test abnormal**, elevated PSA, electrolyte changes (nitrogen, calcium, potassium [includes hypokalemia], phosphorus, sodium), impaired glucose tolerance, hyperlipidemia, HDL, fluctuating testosterone levels, weight increase
Neoplasms:	Prostate cancer
Nervous system disorders:	Dizziness, headache, insomnia, sleep apnea
Psychiatric disorders:	Amnesia, anxiety, depression, hostility, emotional lability, decreased libido, nervousness

Continued on next page

Information on the AbbVie, Inc. products listed on these pages is from the prescribing information in use as of July 31, 2016. For more information, please visit rxabbvie.com or call 1-800-633-9110.

Reproductive system and breast disorders:	Gynecomastia, mastodynia, oligospermia, priapism (frequent or prolonged erections), prostate enlargement, BPH, testis disorder***
Respiratory disorders:	Dyspnea
Skin and subcutaneous tissue disorders:	Acne, alopecia, application site reaction (discolored hair, dry skin, erythema, paresthesia, pruritus, rash), skin dry, pruritus, sweating
Vascular disorders:	Hypertension, vasodilation (hot flushes), venous thromboembolism

* *Impaired urination* includes nocturia, urinary hesitancy, urinary incontinence, urinary retention, urinary urgency and weak urinary stream

***Lab test abnormal* includes elevated AST, elevated ALT, elevated testosterone, elevated hemoglobin or hematocrit, elevated cholesterol, elevated cholesterol/LDL ratio, elevated triglycerides, or elevated serum creatinine

***Testis disorder includes atrophy or non-palpable testis, varicocele, testis sensitivity or tenderness

Secondary Exposure to Testosterone in Children
Cases of secondary exposure to testosterone resulting in virilization of children have been reported in postmarketing surveillance of testosterone gel products. Signs and symptoms of these reported cases have included enlargement of the clitoris (with surgical intervention) or the penis, development of pubic hair, increased erections and libido, aggressive behavior, and advanced bone age. In most cases with a reported outcome, these signs and symptoms were reported to have regressed with removal of the testosterone gel exposure. In a few cases, however, enlarged genitalia did not fully return to age appropriate normal size, and bone age remained modestly greater than chronological age. In some of the cases, direct contact with the sites of application on the skin of men using testosterone gel was reported. In at least one reported case, the reporter considered the possibility of secondary exposure from items such as the testosterone gel user's shirts and/or other fabric, such as towels and sheets *[see Warnings and Precautions (5.2)]*.

7   DRUG INTERACTIONS
7.1   Insulin
Changes in insulin sensitivity or glycemic control may occur in patients treated with androgens. In diabetic patients, the metabolic effects of androgens may decrease blood glucose and, therefore, may decrease insulin requirements.

7.2   Oral Anticoagulants
Changes in anticoagulant activity may be seen with androgens, therefore more frequent monitoring of international normalized ratio (INR) and prothrombin time are recommended in patients taking anticoagulants, especially at the initiation and termination of androgen therapy.

7.3   Corticosteroids
The concurrent use of testosterone with adrenocorticotropic hormone (ACTH) or corticosteroids may result in increased fluid retention and requires careful monitoring particularly in patients with cardiac, renal or hepatic disease.

8   USE IN SPECIFIC POPULATIONS
8.1   Pregnancy
Pregnancy Category X *[see Contraindications (4)]*: AndroGel 1.62% is contraindicated during pregnancy or in women who may become pregnant. Testosterone is teratogenic and may cause fetal harm. Exposure of a fetus to androgens may result in varying degrees of virilization. If this drug is used during pregnancy, or if the patient becomes pregnant while taking this drug, the patient should be made aware of the potential hazard to the fetus.

8.3   Nursing Mothers
Although it is not known how much testosterone transfers into human milk, AndroGel 1.62% is contraindicated in nursing women because of the potential for serious adverse reactions in nursing infants. Testosterone and other androgens may adversely affect lactation *[see Contraindications (4)]*.

8.4   Pediatric Use
The safety and effectiveness of AndroGel 1.62% in pediatric patients less than 18 years old has not been established. Improper use may result in acceleration of bone age and premature closure of epiphyses.

8.5   Geriatric Use
There have not been sufficient numbers of geriatric patients involved in controlled clinical studies utilizing AndroGel 1.62% to determine whether efficacy in those over 65 years of age differs from younger subjects. Of the 234 patients enrolled in the clinical trial utilizing AndroGel 1.62%, 21 were over 65 years of age. Additionally, there is insufficient long-term safety data in geriatric patients to assess the potentially increased risks of cardiovascular disease and prostate cancer.
Geriatric patients treated with androgens may also be at risk for worsening of signs and symptoms of BPH.

8.6   Renal Impairment
No studies were conducted involving patients with renal impairment.

8.7   Hepatic Impairment
No studies were conducted in patients with hepatic impairment.

9   DRUG ABUSE AND DEPENDENCE
9.1   Controlled Substance
AndroGel 1.62% contains testosterone, a Schedule III controlled substance in the Controlled Substances Act.

9.2   Abuse
Anabolic steroids, such as testosterone, are abused. Abuse is often associated with adverse physical and psychological effects.

9.3   Dependence
Although drug dependence is not documented in individuals using therapeutic doses of anabolic steroids for approved indications, dependence is observed in some individuals abusing high doses of anabolic steroids. In general, anabolic steroid dependence is characterized by any three of the following:
• Taking more drug than intended
• Continued drug use despite medical and social problems
• Significant time spent in obtaining adequate amounts of drug
• Desire for anabolic steroids when supplies of the drugs are interrupted
• Difficulty in discontinuing use of the drug despite desires and attempts to do so
• Experience of a withdrawal syndrome upon discontinuation of anabolic steroid use

10   OVERDOSAGE
There is a single report of acute overdosage after parenteral administration of an approved testosterone product in the literature. This subject had serum testosterone concentrations of up to 11,400 ng/dL, which were implicated in a cerebrovascular accident. There were no reports of overdosage in the AndroGel 1.62% clinical trial.
Treatment of overdosage would consist of discontinuation of AndroGel 1.62%, washing the application site with soap and water, and appropriate symptomatic and supportive care.

11   DESCRIPTION
AndroGel 1.62% for topical use is a clear, colorless gel containing testosterone. Testosterone is an androgen. AndroGel 1.62% is available in a metered-dose pump or unit dose packets.
The active pharmacologic ingredient in AndroGel 1.62% is testosterone. Testosterone USP is a white to almost white powder chemically described as 17-beta hydroxyandrost-4-en-3-one. The structural formula is:

Testosterone

$C_{19}H_{28}O_2$ MW 288.42

The inactive ingredients in AndroGel 1.62% are: carbopol 980, ethyl alcohol, isopropyl myristate, purified water, and sodium hydroxide.

12   CLINICAL PHARMACOLOGY
12.1   Mechanism of Action
Endogenous androgens, including testosterone and dihydrotestosterone (DHT), are responsible for the normal growth and development of the male sex organs and for maintenance of secondary sex characteristics. These effects include the growth and maturation of prostate, seminal vesicles, penis and scrotum; the development of male hair distribution, such as facial, pubic, chest and axillary hair; laryngeal enlargement; vocal chord thickening; and alterations in body musculature and fat distribution. Testosterone and DHT are necessary for the normal development of secondary sex characteristics.
Male hypogonadism, a clinical syndrome resulting from insufficient secretion of testosterone, has two main etiologies. Primary hypogonadism is caused by defects of the gonads, such as Klinefelter's syndrome or Leydig cell aplasia, whereas secondary hypogonadism is the failure of the hypothalamus (or pituitary) to produce sufficient gonadotropins (FSH, LH).

12.2   Pharmacodynamics
No specific pharmacodynamic studies were conducted using AndroGel 1.62%.

12.3   Pharmacokinetics
Absorption
AndroGel 1.62% delivers physiologic amounts of testosterone, producing circulating testosterone concentrations that approximate normal levels (300 – 1000 ng/dL) seen in healthy men. AndroGel 1.62% provides continuous transdermal delivery of testosterone for 24 hours following once daily application to clean, dry, intact skin of the shoulders and upper arms. Average serum testosterone concentrations over 24 hours (C_{avg}) observed when AndroGel 1.62% was applied to the upper arms/shoulders were comparable to average serum testosterone concentrations (C_{avg}) when AndroGel 1.62% was applied using a rotation method utilizing the abdomen and upper arms/shoulders. The rotation of abdomen and upper arms/shoulders was a method used in the pivotal clinical trial *[see Clinical Studies (14.1)]*.

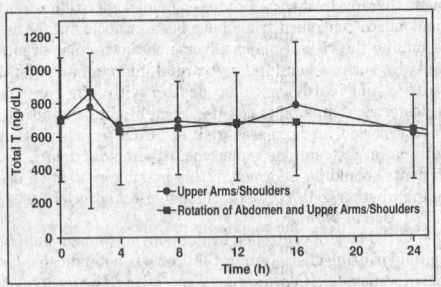

Figure 2: Mean (±SD) Serum Total Testosterone Concentrations on Day 7 in Patients Following AndroGel 1.62% Once-Daily Application of 81 mg of Testosterone (N=33) for 7 Days

Distribution
Circulating testosterone is primarily bound in the serum to sex hormone-binding globulin (SHBG) and albumin. Approximately 40% of testosterone in plasma is bound to SHBG, 2% remains unbound (free) and the rest is loosely bound to albumin and other proteins.

Metabolism
Testosterone is metabolized to various 17-keto steroids through two different pathways. The major active metabolites of testosterone are estradiol and DHT.

Excretion
There is considerable variation in the half-life of testosterone concentration as reported in the literature, ranging from 10 to 100 minutes. About 90% of a dose of testosterone given intramuscularly is excreted in the urine as glucuronic acid and sulfuric acid conjugates of testosterone and its metabolites. About 6% of a dose is excreted in the feces, mostly in the unconjugated form. Inactivation of testosterone occurs primarily in the liver.
When AndroGel 1.62% treatment is discontinued, serum testosterone concentrations return to approximately baseline concentrations within 48-72 hours after administration of the last dose.

Potential for testosterone transfer
The potential for testosterone transfer following administration of AndroGel 1.62% when it was applied only to upper arms/shoulders was evaluated in two clinical studies of males dosed with AndroGel 1.62% and their untreated female partners. In one study, 8 male subjects applied a single dose of AndroGel 1.62% 81 mg to their shoulders and upper arms. Two (2) hours after application, female subjects rubbed their hands, wrists, arms, and shoulders to the application site of the male subjects for 15 minutes. Serum concentrations of testosterone were monitored in female subjects for 24 hours after contact occurred. After direct skin-to-skin contact with the site of application, mean

testosterone C_{avg} and C_{max} in female subjects increased by 280% and 267%, respectively, compared to mean baseline testosterone concentrations. In a second study evaluating transfer of testosterone, 12 male subjects applied a single dose of AndroGel 1.62% 81 mg to their shoulders and upper arms. Two (2) hours after application, female subjects rubbed their hands, wrists, arms, and shoulders to the application site of the male subjects for 15 minutes while the site of application was covered by a t-shirt. When a t-shirt was used to cover the site of application, mean testosterone C_{avg} and C_{max} in female subjects increased by 6% and 11%, respectively, compared to mean baseline testosterone concentrations.

A separate study was conducted to evaluate the potential for testosterone transfer from 16 males dosed with AndroGel 1.62% 81 mg when it was applied to abdomen only for 7 days, a site of application not approved for AndroGel 1.62%. Two (2) hours after application to the males on each day, the female subjects rubbed their abdomens for 15 minutes to the abdomen of the males. The males had covered the application area with a T-shirt. The mean testosterone C_{avg} and C_{max} in female subjects on day 1 increased by 43% and 47%, respectively, compared to mean baseline testosterone concentrations. The mean testosterone C_{avg} and C_{max} in female subjects on day 7 increased by 60% and 58%, respectively, compared to mean baseline testosterone concentrations.

Effect of showering
In a randomized, 3-way (3 treatment periods without washout period) crossover study in 24 hypogonadal men, the effect of showering on testosterone exposure was assessed after once daily application of AndroGel 1.62% 81 mg to upper arms/shoulders for 7 days in each treatment period. On the 7th day of each treatment period, hypogonadal men took a shower with soap and water at either 2, 6, or 10 hours after drug application. The effect of showering at 2 or 6 hours post-dose on Day 7 resulted in 13% and 12% decreases in mean C_{avg}, respectively, compared to Day 6 when no shower was taken after drug application. Showering at 10 hours after drug application had no effect on bioavailability. The amount of testosterone remaining in the outer layers of the skin at the application site on the 7th day was assessed using a tape stripping procedure and was reduced by at least 80% after showering 2-10 hours post-dose compared to on the 6th day when no shower was taken after drug application.

Effect of hand washing
In a randomized, open-label, single-dose, 2-way crossover study in 16 healthy male subjects, the effect of hand washing on the amount of residual testosterone on the hands was evaluated. Subjects used their hands to apply the maximum dose (81 mg testosterone) of AndroGel 1.62% to their upper arms and shoulders. Within 1 minute of applying the gel, subjects either washed or did not wash their hands prior to study personnel wiping the subjects' hands with ethanol dampened gauze pads. The gauze pads were then analyzed for residual testosterone content. A mean (SD) of 0.1 (0.04) mg of residual testosterone (0.12% of the actual applied dose of testosterone, and a 96% reduction compared to when hands were not washed) was recovered after washing hands with water and soap.

Effect of sunscreen or moisturizing lotion on absorption of testosterone
In a randomized, 3-way (3 treatment periods without washout period) crossover study in 18 hypogonadal males, the effect of applying a moisturizing lotion or a sunscreen on the absorption of testosterone was evaluated with the upper arms/shoulders as application sites. For 7 days, moisturizing lotion or sunscreen (SPF 50) was applied daily to the AndroGel 1.62% application site 1 hour after the application of AndroGel 1.62% 40.5 mg. Application of moisturizing lotion increased mean testosterone C_{avg} and C_{max} by 14% and 17%, respectively, compared to AndroGel 1.62% administered alone. Application of sunscreen increased mean testosterone C_{avg} and C_{max} by 8% and 13%, respectively, compared to AndroGel 1.62% applied alone.

13 NONCLINICAL TOXICOLOGY
13.1 Carcinogenesis, Mutagenesis, Impairment of Fertility
Testosterone has been tested by subcutaneous injection and implantation in mice and rats. In mice, the implant induced cervical-uterine tumors which metastasized in some cases. There is suggestive evidence that injection of testosterone into some strains of female mice increases their susceptibility to hepatoma. Testosterone is also known to increase the number of tumors and decrease the degree of differentiation of chemically induced carcinomas of the liver in rats. Testosterone was negative in the *in vitro* Ames and in the *in vivo* mouse micronucleus assays. The administration of exogenous testosterone has been reported to suppress spermatogenesis in the rat, dog and non-human primates, which was reversible on cessation of the treatment.

14 CLINICAL STUDIES
14.1 Clinical Trials in Hypogonadal Males
AndroGel 1.62% was evaluated in a multi-center, randomized, double-blind, parallel-group, placebo-controlled study (182-day double-blind period) in 274 hypogonadal men with body mass index (BMI) 18-40 kg/m^2 and 18-80 years of age (mean age 53.8 years). The patients had an average serum testosterone concentration of <300 ng/dL, as determined by two morning samples collected on the same visit. Patients were Caucasian 83%, Black 13%, Asian or Native American 4%. 7.5% of patients were Hispanic.

Patients were randomized to receive active treatment or placebo using a rotation method utilizing the abdomen and upper arms/shoulders for 182 days. All patients were started at a daily dose of 40.5 mg (two pump actuations) AndroGel 1.62% or matching placebo on Day 1 of the study. Patients returned to the clinic on Day 14, Day 28, and Day 42 for predose serum total testosterone assessments. The patient's daily dose was titrated up or down in 20.25 mg increments if the predose serum testosterone value was outside the range of 350-750 ng/dL. The study included four active AndroGel 1.62% doses: 20.25 mg, 40.5 mg, 60.75 mg, and 81 mg daily.

The primary endpoint was the percentage of patients with C_{avg} within the normal range of 300-1000 ng/dL on Day 112. In patients treated with AndroGel 1.62%, 81.6% (146/179) had C_{avg} within the normal range at Day 112. The secondary endpoint was the percentage of patients, with C_{max} above three pre-determined limits. The percentages of patients with C_{max} greater than 1500 ng/dL, and between 1800 and 2499 ng/dL on Day 112 were 11.2% and 5.5%, respectively. Two patients had a C_{max} >2500 ng/dL on Day 112 (2510 ng/dL and 2550 ng/dL, respectively); neither of these 2 patients demonstrated an abnormal C_{max} on prior or subsequent assessments at the same dose.

Patients could agree to continue in an open-label, active treatment maintenance period of the study for an additional 182 days.

Dose titrations on Days 14, 28, and 42 resulted in final doses of 20.25 mg – 81 mg on Day 112 as shown in Table 6.
[See table 6 above]

Figure 3 summarizes the pharmacokinetic profile of total testosterone in patients completing 112 days of AndroGel 1.62% treatment administered as a starting dose of 40.5 mg of testosterone (2 pump actuations) for the initial 14 days followed by possible titration according to the follow-up testosterone measurements.

Efficacy was maintained in the group of men that received AndroGel 1.62% for one full year. In that group, 78% (106/136) had average serum testosterone concentrations in the normal range at Day 364. Figure 4 summarizes the mean total testosterone profile for these patients on Day 364.

The mean estradiol and DHT concentration profiles paralleled the changes observed in testosterone. The levels of LH and FSH decreased with testosterone treatment. The decreases in levels of LH and FSH are consistent with reports published in the literature of long-term treatment with testosterone.

16 HOW SUPPLIED/STORAGE AND HANDLING
AndroGel 1.62% is supplied in non-aerosol, metered-dose pumps that deliver 20.25 mg of testosterone per complete pump actuation. The pumps are composed of plastic and stainless steel and an LDPE/aluminum foil inner liner encased in rigid plastic with a polypropylene cap. Each 88 g metered-dose pump is capable of dispensing 75 g of gel or 60-metered pump actuations; each pump actuation dispenses 1.25 g of gel.
AndroGel 1.62% is also supplied in unit-dose aluminum foil packets in cartons of 30. Each packet of 1.25 g or 2.5 g gel contains 20.25 mg or 40.5 mg testosterone, respectively.

Continued on next page

Table 6: Mean (SD) Testosterone Concentrations (C_{avg} and C_{max}) by final dose on Days 112 and 364

Parameter	Final Dose on Day 112					
	Placebo (n=27)	20.25 mg (n=12)	40.5 mg (n=34)	60.75 mg (n=54)	81 mg (n=79)	All Active (n=179)
C_{avg} (ng/dL)	303 (135)	457 (275)	524 (228)	643 (285)	537 (240)	561 (259)
C_{max} (ng/dL)	450 (349)	663 (473)	798 (439)	958 (497)	813 (479)	845 (480)
	Final Dose on Day 364					
		20.25 mg (n=7)	40.5 mg (n=26)	60.75 mg (n=29)	81 mg (n=74)	Continuing Active (n=136)
C_{avg} (ng/dL)		386 (130)	474 (176)	513 (222)	432 (186)	455 (192)
C_{max} (ng/dL)		562 (187)	715 (306)	839 (568)	649 (329)	697 (389)

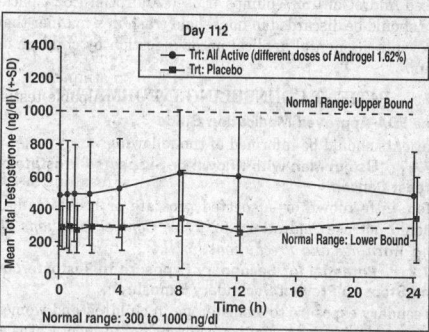

Figure 3: Mean (±SD) Steady-State Serum Total Testosterone Concentrations on Day 112

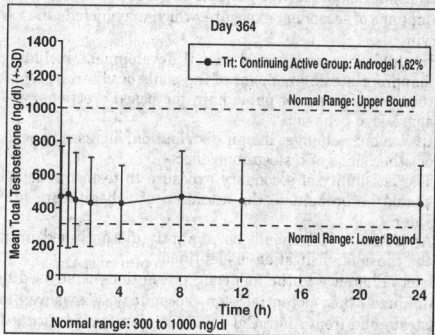

Figure 4: Mean (±SD) Steady-State Serum Total Testosterone Concentrations on Day 364

Information on the AbbVie, Inc. products listed on these pages is from the prescribing information in use as of July 31, 2016. For more information, please visit rxabbvie.com or call 1-800-633-9110.

NDC Number	Package Size
0051-8462-33	88 g pump (each pump dispenses 60 metered pump actuations with each pump actuation containing 20.25 mg of testosterone in 1.25 g of gel)
0051-8462-12	Each unit dose packet contains 20.25 mg of testosterone provided in 1.25 g of gel
0051-8462-31	30 packets (each unit dose packet contains 20.25 mg of testosterone provided in 1.25 g of gel)
0051-8462-01	Each unit dose packet contains 40.5 mg of testosterone provided in 2.5 g of gel
0051-8462-30	30 packets (each unit dose packet contains 40.5 mg of testosterone provided in 2.5 g of gel)

Store at controlled room temperature 20°-25°C (68°-77°F); excursions permitted to 15°-30°C (59°-86°F) [see USP Controlled Room Temperature].

Used AndroGel 1.62% pumps or used AndroGel 1.62% packets should be discarded in household trash in a manner that prevents accidental application or ingestion by children or pets.

17   PATIENT COUNSELING INFORMATION

See FDA-Approved Medication Guide

Patients should be informed of the following:

17.1   Use in Men with Known or Suspected Prostate or Breast Cancer

Men with known or suspected prostate or breast cancer should not use AndroGel 1.62% [see Contraindications (4) and Warnings and Precautions (5.1)].

17.2   Potential for Secondary Exposure to Testosterone and Steps to Prevent Secondary Exposure

Secondary exposure to testosterone in children and women can occur with the use of testosterone gel in men. Cases of secondary exposure to testosterone have been reported in children.

Physicians should advise patients of the reported signs and symptoms of secondary exposure, which may include the following:

- In children: unexpected sexual development including inappropriate enlargement of the penis or clitoris, premature development of pubic hair, increased erections, and aggressive behavior.
- In women: changes in hair distribution, increase in acne, or other signs of testosterone effects.
- The possibility of secondary exposure to testosterone gel should be brought to the attention of a healthcare provider.
- AndroGel 1.62% should be promptly discontinued until the cause of virilization is identified.

Strict adherence to the following precautions is advised to minimize the potential for secondary exposure to testosterone from AndroGel 1.62% in men [see Medication Guide]:

- **Children and women should avoid contact with unwashed or unclothed application site(s)** of men using AndroGel 1.62%.
- Patients using AndroGel 1.62% should apply the product as directed and strictly adhere to the following:
  - **Wash hands** with soap and water immediately after application.
  - **Cover the application site(s)** with clothing after the gel has dried.
  - **Wash the application site(s) thoroughly** with soap and water prior to any situation where skin-to-skin contact of the application site with another person is anticipated.
- In the event that unwashed or unclothed skin to which AndroGel 1.62% has been applied comes in contact with the skin of another person, the general area of contact on the other person should be washed with soap and water as soon as possible [see Dosage and Administration (2.2), Warnings and Precautions (5.2) and Clinical Pharmacology (12.3)].

17.3   Potential Adverse Reactions with Androgens

Patients should be informed that treatment with androgens may lead to adverse reactions which include:

- Changes in urinary habits such as increased urination at night, trouble starting the urine stream, passing urine many times during the day, having an urge to go to the bathroom right away, having a urine accident, being unable to pass urine and weak urine flow.
- Breathing disturbances, including those associated with sleep, or excessive daytime sleepiness.
- Too frequent or persistent erections of the penis.
- Nausea, vomiting, changes in skin color, or ankle swelling.

17.4   Patients Should Be Advised of the Following Instructions for Use

- Read the Medication Guide before starting AndroGel 1.62% therapy and to reread it each time the prescription is renewed.
- AndroGel 1.62% should be applied and used appropriately to maximize the benefits and to minimize the risk of secondary exposure in children and women.
- Keep AndroGel 1.62% out of the reach of children.
- AndroGel 1.62% is an alcohol based product and is flammable; therefore avoid fire, flame or smoking until the gel has dried.
- It is important to adhere to all recommended monitoring.
- Report any changes in their state of health, such as changes in urinary habits, breathing, sleep, and mood.
- AndroGel 1.62% is prescribed to meet the patient's specific needs; therefore, the patient should never share AndroGel 1.62% with anyone.
- Wait 2 hours before swimming or washing following application of AndroGel 1.62%. This will ensure that the greatest amount of AndroGel 1.62% is absorbed into their system.

Medication Guide
ANDROGEL® (AN DROW JEL) ⟨III⟩
(testosterone gel) 1.62%

Read this Medication Guide before you start using ANDROGEL 1.62% and each time you get a refill. There may be new information. This information does not take the place of talking with your healthcare provider about your medical condition or treatment.

What is the most important information I should know about ANDROGEL 1.62%?

1. **Early signs and symptoms of puberty have happened in young children who were accidentally exposed to testosterone through contact with men using ANDROGEL 1.62%.**
   Signs and symptoms of early puberty in a child may include:
   - enlarged penis or clitoris
   - early development of pubic hair
   - increased erections or sex drive
   - aggressive behavior
   ANDROGEL 1.62% can transfer from your body to others.
2. **Women and children should avoid contact with the unwashed or unclothed area where ANDROGEL 1.62% has been applied to your skin.**
   Stop using ANDROGEL 1.62% and call your healthcare provider right away if you see any signs and symptoms in a child or a woman that may have occurred through accidental exposure to ANDROGEL 1.62%.
   Signs and symptoms of exposure to ANDROGEL 1.62% in children may include:
   - enlarged penis or clitoris
   - early development of pubic hair
   - increased erections or sex drive
   - aggressive behavior
   Signs and symptoms of exposure to ANDROGEL 1.62% in women may include:
   - changes in body hair
   - a large increase in acne
- **To lower the risk of transfer of ANDROGEL 1.62% from your body to others, you should follow these important instructions:**
   - Apply ANDROGEL 1.62% **only** to your shoulders and upper arms that will be covered by a short sleeve t-shirt.
   - Wash your hands **right away** with soap and water after applying ANDROGEL 1.62%.
   - After the gel has dried, **cover the application area with clothing.** Keep the area covered until you have washed the application area well or have showered.
   - If you expect to have skin-to-skin contact with another person, first wash the application area well with soap and water.
   - If a woman or child makes contact with the ANDROGEL 1.62% application area, that area on the woman or child should be washed well with soap and water right away.

What is ANDROGEL 1.62%?

ANDROGEL 1.62% is a prescription medicine that contains testosterone. ANDROGEL 1.62% is used to treat adult males who have low or no testosterone due to certain medical conditions.

Your healthcare provider will test your blood before you start and while you are taking ANDROGEL 1.62%.

It is not known if AndroGel 1.62% is safe or effective to treat men who have low testosterone due to aging.

It is not known if ANDROGEL 1.62% is safe or effective in children younger than 18 years old. Improper use of ANDROGEL 1.62% may affect bone growth in children.

ANDROGEL 1.62% is a controlled substance (CIII) because it contains testosterone that can be a target for people who abuse prescription medicines. Keep your ANDROGEL 1.62% in a safe place to protect it. Never give your ANDROGEL 1.62% to anyone else, even if they have the same symptoms you have. Selling or giving away this medicine may harm others and is against the law.

ANDROGEL 1.62% is not meant for use in women.

Who should not use ANDROGEL 1.62%?

Do not use ANDROGEL 1.62% if you:

- have breast cancer
- have or might have prostate cancer
- are pregnant or may become pregnant or are breast-feeding. ANDROGEL 1.62% may harm your unborn or breast-feeding baby.
  Women who are pregnant or who may become pregnant should avoid contact with the area of skin where ANDROGEL 1.62% has been applied.

Talk to your healthcare provider before taking this medicine if you have any of the above conditions.

What should I tell my healthcare provider before using ANDROGEL 1.62%?

Before you use ANDROGEL 1.62%, tell your healthcare provider if you:

- have breast cancer
- have or might have prostate cancer
- have urinary problems due to an enlarged prostate
- have heart problems
- have kidney or liver problems
- have problems breathing while you sleep (sleep apnea)
- have any other medical conditions

Tell your healthcare provider about all the medicines you take, including prescription and non-prescription medicines, vitamins, and herbal supplements.

Using ANDROGEL 1.62% with certain other medicines can affect each other.

Especially, tell your healthcare provider if you take:

- insulin
- medicines that decrease blood clotting
- corticosteroids

Know the medicines you take. Ask your healthcare provider or pharmacist for a list of all of your medicines, if you are not sure. Keep a list of them and show it to your healthcare provider and pharmacist when you get a new medicine.

How should I use ANDROGEL 1.62%?

- It is important that you apply ANDROGEL 1.62% exactly as your healthcare provider tells you to.
- Your healthcare provider will tell you how much ANDROGEL 1.62% to apply and when to apply it.
- Your healthcare provider may change your ANDROGEL 1.62% dose. **Do not** change your ANDROGEL 1.62% dose without talking to your healthcare provider.
- **ANDROGEL 1.62% is to be applied to the area of your shoulders and upper arms that will be covered by a short sleeve t-shirt. Do not** apply ANDROGEL 1.62% to any other parts of your body such as your stomach area (abdomen), penis, scrotum, chest, armpits (axillae), or knees.
- Apply ANDROGEL 1.62% at the same time each morning. ANDROGEL 1.62% should be applied after showering or bathing.
- **Wash your hands right away** with soap and water after applying ANDROGEL 1.62%.
- Avoid showering, swimming or bathing for at least 2 hours after you apply ANDROGEL 1.62%.
- ANDROGEL 1.62% is flammable until dry. Let ANDROGEL 1.62% dry before smoking or going near an open flame.
- Let the application site dry completely before putting on a t-shirt.

Applying ANDROGEL 1.62%:

ANDROGEL 1.62% comes in a pump or in packets.

- Before applying ANDROGEL 1.62% make sure that your shoulders and upper arms are clean, dry, and that there is no broken skin.
- The application sites for ANDROGEL 1.62% are the upper arms and shoulders that will be covered by a short sleeve t-shirt (See Figure A).

If you are using ANDROGEL 1.62% pump:

- Before using a new bottle of ANDROGEL 1.62 % for the first time, you will need to prime the pump. To prime the ANDROGEL 1.62% pump, slowly push the pump all the way down 3 times. **Do not** use any ANDROGEL 1.62% that came out while priming. Wash it down the sink to avoid accidental exposure to others. Your ANDROGEL 1.62% pump is now ready to use.
- Remove the cap from the pump. Then, position the nozzle over the palm of your hand and slowly push the pump all the way down. Apply ANDROGEL 1.62% to the application site. You may also apply ANDROGEL 1.62% directly to the application site.

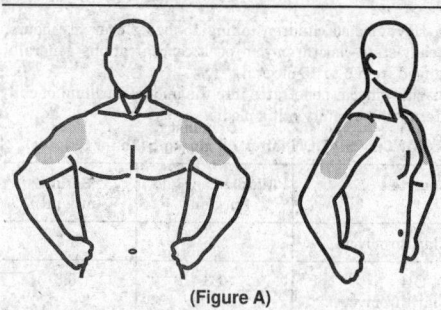

(Figure A)

- **Wash your hands with soap and water right away.**
[See first table above]

If you are using ANDROGEL 1.62% packets:
- Tear open the packet completely at the dotted line. Squeeze from the bottom of the packet to the top.
- Squeeze all of the ANDROGEL 1.62% out of the packet into the palm of your hand. Apply ANDROGEL 1.62% to the application site. You may also apply ANDROGEL 1.62% directly to the application site.
- ANDROGEL 1.62% should be applied right away.
- **Wash your hands with soap and water right away.**
[See second table above]

What are the possible side effects of ANDROGEL 1.62%?
See "What is the most important information I should know about ANDROGEL 1.62%?"
ANDROGEL 1.62% can cause serious side effects including:
- **If you already have enlargement of your prostate gland your signs and symptoms can get worse while using ANDROGEL 1.62%.** This can include:
  ○ increased urination at night
  ○ trouble starting your urine stream
  ○ having to pass urine many times during the day
  ○ having an urge that you have to go to the bathroom right away
  ○ having a urine accident
  ○ being unable to pass urine or weak urine flow
- **Possible increased risk of prostate cancer.** Your healthcare provider should check you for prostate cancer or any other prostate problems before you start and while you use ANDROGEL 1.62%.
- **Blood clots in the legs or lungs.** Signs and symptoms of a blood clot in your leg can include leg pain, swelling, or redness. Signs and symptoms of a blood clot in your lungs can include difficulty breathing or chest pain.
- **Possible increased risk of heart attack or stroke.**
- **In large doses ANDROGEL 1.62% may lower your sperm count.**
- **Swelling of your ankles, feet, or body, with or without heart failure.**
- **Enlarged or painful breasts.**
- **Have problems breathing while you sleep (sleep apnea).**
Call your healthcare provider right away if you have any of the serious side effects listed above.
The most common side effects of ANDROGEL 1.62% include:
- increased prostate specific antigen (a test used to screen for prostate cancer)
- mood swings
- hypertension
- increased red blood cell count
- skin irritation where ANDROGEL 1.62% is applied
Other side effects include more erections than are normal for you or erections that last a long time.
Tell your healthcare provider if you have any side effect that bothers you or that does not go away.
These are not all the possible side effects of ANDROGEL 1.62%. For more information, ask your healthcare provider or pharmacist.
Call your doctor for medical advice about side effects. You may report side effects to FDA at 1-800-FDA-1088.
How should I store ANDROGEL 1.62%?
- Store ANDROGEL 1.62% at 59°F to 86°F (15°C to 30°C).
- When it is time to throw away the pump or packets, safely throw away used ANDROGEL 1.62% in household trash. Be careful to prevent accidental exposure of children or pets.
- Keep ANDROGEL 1.62% away from fire.
Keep ANDROGEL 1.62% and all medicines out of the reach of children.
General information about the safe and effective use of ANDROGEL 1.62%
Medicines are sometimes prescribed for purposes other than those listed in a Medication Guide. Do not use ANDROGEL

Find Your Dose as Prescribed by Your Healthcare Provider		Application Method
1 PUMP DEPRESSION	20.25 mg	Apply 1 pump depression of ANDROGEL 1.62% to 1 upper arm and shoulder.
2 PUMP DEPRESSIONS	40.5 mg	Apply 1 pump depression of ANDROGEL 1.62% to 1 upper arm and shoulder and then apply 1 pump depression of ANDROGEL 1.62% to the opposite upper arm and shoulder.
3 PUMP DEPRESSIONS	60.75 mg	Apply 2 pump depressions of ANDROGEL 1.62% to 1 upper arm and shoulder and then apply 1 pump depression of ANDROGEL 1.62% to the opposite upper arm and shoulder.
4 PUMP DEPRESSIONS	81 mg	Apply 2 pump depressions of ANDROGEL 1.62% to 1 upper arm and shoulder and then apply 2 pump depressions of ANDROGEL 1.62% to the opposite upper arm and shoulder.

Find Your Dose as Prescribed by Your Healthcare Provider		Application Method
One 20.25 mg packet	20.25 mg	Apply 1 packet of ANDROGEL 1.62% to 1 upper arm and shoulder.
One 40.5 mg packet	40.5 mg	Apply half of the 40.5 mg packet of ANDROGEL 1.62% to 1 upper arm and shoulder and then apply the remaining packet contents to the opposite upper arm and shoulder.
One 40.5 mg packet and one 20.25 mg packet	60.75 mg	Apply one 40.5 mg packet of ANDROGEL 1.62% to 1 upper arm and shoulder and then apply one 20.25 mg packet of ANDROGEL 1.62% to the opposite upper arm and shoulder.
Two 40.5 mg packets	81 mg	Apply one 40.5 mg packet of ANDROGEL 1.62% to 1 upper arm and shoulder and then apply one 40.5 mg packet of ANDROGEL 1.62% to the opposite upper arm and shoulder.

1.62% for a condition for which it was not prescribed. Do not give ANDROGEL 1.62% to other people, even if they have the same symptoms you have. It may harm them.
This Medication Guide summarizes the most important information about ANDROGEL 1.62%. If you would like more information, talk to your healthcare provider. You can ask your pharmacist or healthcare provider for information about ANDROGEL 1.62% that is written for health professionals.
For more information, go to www.androgel.com or call 1-800-633-9110.
What are the ingredients in ANDROGEL 1.62%?
Active ingredient: testosterone
Inactive ingredients: carbopol 980, ethyl alcohol, isopropyl myristate, purified water and sodium hydroxide.
This Medication Guide has been approved by the U.S. Food and Drug Administration.
Marketed by:
AbbVie Inc.
North Chicago, IL 60064, USA
© 2015 AbbVie Inc.
Ref. A090630059177-Revised May, 2015
Shown in Product Identification Guide, page 505

BIAXIN® Filmtab®   ℞
[bī ax ən]
(clarithromycin tablets, USP)
BIAXIN® XL Filmtab®
(clarithromycin extended-release tablets)
BIAXIN® Granules
(clarithromycin for oral suspension, USP)

To reduce the development of drug-resistant bacteria and maintain the effectiveness of BIAXIN and other antibacterial drugs, BIAXIN should be used only to treat or prevent infections that are proven or strongly suspected to be caused by bacteria.

DESCRIPTION
Clarithromycin is a semi-synthetic macrolide antibiotic. Chemically, it is 6-0-methylerythromycin. The molecular formula is $C_{38}H_{69}NO_{13}$, and the molecular weight is 747.96. The structural formula is:
[See structural formula in next column]
Clarithromycin is a white to off-white crystalline powder. It is soluble in acetone, slightly soluble in methanol, ethanol, and acetonitrile, and practically insoluble in water.
BIAXIN is available as immediate-release tablets, extended-release tablets, and granules for oral suspension. Each yellow oval film-coated immediate-release BIAXIN tablet (clarithromycin tablets, USP) contains 250 mg or 500 mg of clarithromycin and the following inactive ingredients:

250 mg tablets: hypromellose, hydroxypropyl cellulose, croscarmellose sodium, D&C Yellow No. 10, FD&C Blue No. 1, magnesium stearate, microcrystalline cellulose, povidone, pregelatinized starch, propylene glycol, silicon dioxide, sorbic acid, sorbitan monooleate, stearic acid, talc, titanium dioxide, and vanillin.
500 mg tablets: hypromellose, hydroxypropyl cellulose, colloidal silicon dioxide, croscarmellose sodium, D&C Yellow No. 10, magnesium stearate, microcrystalline cellulose, povidone, propylene glycol, sorbic acid, sorbitan monooleate, titanium dioxide, and vanillin.
Each yellow oval film-coated BIAXIN XL tablet (clarithromycin extended-release tablets) contains 500 mg of clarithromycin and the following inactive ingredients: cellulosic polymers, D&C Yellow No. 10, lactose monohydrate, magnesium stearate, propylene glycol, sorbic acid, sorbitan monooleate, talc, titanium dioxide, and vanillin.
After constitution, each 5 mL of BIAXIN suspension (clarithromycin for oral suspension, USP) contains 125 mg or 250 mg of clarithromycin. Each bottle of BIAXIN granules contains 1250 mg (50 mL size), 2500 mg (50 and 100 mL sizes) or 5000 mg (100 mL size) of clarithromycin and the following inactive ingredients: carbomer, castor oil, citric acid, hypromellose phthalate, maltodextrin, potassium sorbate, povidone, silicon dioxide, sucrose, xanthan gum, titanium dioxide and fruit punch flavor.

CLINICAL PHARMACOLOGY
Pharmacokinetics
Clarithromycin is rapidly absorbed from the gastrointestinal tract after oral administration. The absolute bioavailability of 250 mg clarithromycin tablets was approximately 50%. For a single 500 mg dose of clarithromycin, food

Continued on next page

Information on the AbbVie, Inc. products listed on these pages is from the prescribing information in use as of July 31, 2016. For more information, please visit rxabbvie.com or call 1-800-633-9110.

slightly delays the onset of clarithromycin absorption, increasing the peak time from approximately 2 to 2.5 hours. Food also increases the clarithromycin peak plasma concentration by about 24%, but does not affect the extent of clarithromycin bioavailability. Food does not affect the onset of formation of the antimicrobially active metabolite, 14-OH clarithromycin or its peak plasma concentration but does slightly decrease the extent of metabolite formation, indicated by an 11% decrease in area under the plasma concentration-time curve (AUC). Therefore, BIAXIN tablets may be given without regard to food.

In nonfasting healthy human subjects (males and females), peak plasma concentrations were attained within 2 to 3 hours after oral dosing. Steady-state peak plasma clarithromycin concentrations were attained within 3 days and were approximately 1 to 2 mcg/mL with a 250 mg dose administered every 12 hours and 3 to 4 mcg/mL with a 500 mg dose administered every 8 to 12 hours. The elimination half-life of clarithromycin was about 3 to 4 hours with 250 mg administered every 12 hours but increased to 5 to 7 hours with 500 mg administered every 8 to 12 hours. The nonlinearity of clarithromycin pharmacokinetics is slight at the recommended doses of 250 mg and 500 mg administered every 8 to 12 hours. With a 250 mg every 12 hours dosing, the principal metabolite, 14-OH clarithromycin, attains a peak steady-state concentration of about 0.6 mcg/mL and has an elimination half-life of 5 to 6 hours. With a 500 mg every 8 to 12 hours dosing, the peak steady-state concentration of 14-OH clarithromycin is slightly higher (up to 1 mcg/mL), and its elimination half-life is about 7 to 9 hours. With any of these dosing regimens, the steady-state concentration of this metabolite is generally attained within 3 to 4 days.

After a 250 mg tablet every 12 hours, approximately 20% of the dose is excreted in the urine as clarithromycin, while after a 500 mg tablet every 12 hours, the urinary excretion of clarithromycin is somewhat greater, approximately 30%. In comparison, after an oral dose of 250 mg (125 mg/5 mL) suspension every 12 hours, approximately 40% is excreted in urine as clarithromycin. The renal clearance of clarithromycin is, however, relatively independent of the dose size and approximates the normal glomerular filtration rate. The major metabolite found in urine is 14-OH clarithromycin, which accounts for an additional 10% to 15% of the dose with either a 250 mg or a 500 mg tablet administered every 12 hours.

Steady-state concentrations of clarithromycin and 14-OH clarithromycin observed following administration of 500 mg doses of clarithromycin every 12 hours to adult patients with HIV infection were similar to those observed in healthy volunteers. In adult HIV-infected patients taking 500- or 1000-mg doses of clarithromycin every 12 hours, steady-state clarithromycin C_{max} values ranged from 2 to 4 mcg/mL and 5 to 10 mcg/mL, respectively.

The steady-state concentrations of clarithromycin in subjects with impaired hepatic function did not differ from those in normal subjects; however, the 14-OH clarithromycin concentrations were lower in the hepatically impaired subjects. The decreased formation of 14-OH clarithromycin was at least partially offset by an increase in renal clearance of clarithromycin in the subjects with impaired hepatic function when compared to healthy subjects. The pharmacokinetics of clarithromycin was also altered in subjects with impaired renal function (see **PRECAUTIONS** and **DOSAGE AND ADMINISTRATION**).

Clarithromycin and the 14-OH clarithromycin metabolite distribute readily into body tissues and fluids. There are no data available on cerebrospinal fluid penetration. Because of high intracellular concentrations, tissue concentrations are higher than serum concentrations. Examples of tissue and serum concentrations are presented below.

CONCENTRATION (after 250 mg q12h)

Tissue Type	Tissue (mcg/g)	Serum (mcg/mL)
Tonsil	1.6	0.8
Lung	8.8	1.7

Clarithromycin extended-release tablets provide extended absorption of clarithromycin from the gastrointestinal tract after oral administration. Relative to an equal total daily dose of immediate-release clarithromycin tablets, clarithromycin extended-release tablets provide lower and later steady-state peak plasma concentrations but equivalent 24-hour AUC's for both clarithromycin and its microbiologically-active metabolite, 14-OH clarithromycin. While the extent of formation of 14-OH clarithromycin following administration of BIAXIN XL tablets (2 × 500 mg once daily) is not affected by food, administration under fasting conditions is associated with approximately 30% lower clarithromycin AUC relative to administration with food. Therefore, BIAXIN XL tablets should be taken with food.

Steady-State Clarithromycin Plasma Concentration-Time Profiles

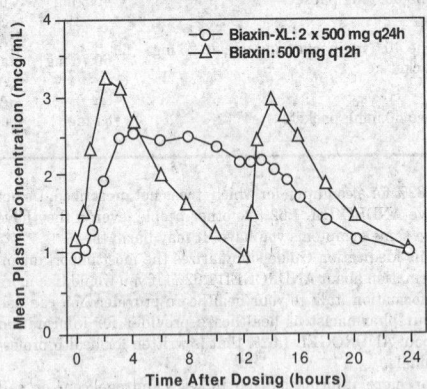

In healthy human subjects, steady-state peak plasma clarithromycin concentrations of approximately 2 to 3 mcg/mL were achieved about 5 to 8 hours after oral administration of 2 × 500 mg BIAXIN XL tablets once daily; for 14-OH clarithromycin, steady-state peak plasma concentrations of approximately 0.8 mcg/mL were attained about 6 to 9 hours after dosing. Steady-state peak plasma clarithromycin concentrations of approximately 1 to 2 mcg/mL were achieved about 5 to 6 hours after oral administration of a single 500 mg BIAXIN XL tablet once daily; for 14-OH clarithromycin, steady-state peak plasma concentrations of approximately 0.6 mcg/mL were attained about 6 hours after dosing.

When 250 mg doses of clarithromycin as BIAXIN suspension were administered to fasting healthy adult subjects, peak plasma concentrations were attained around 3 hours after dosing. Steady-state peak plasma concentrations were attained in 2 to 3 days and were approximately 2 mcg/mL for clarithromycin and 0.7 mcg/mL for 14-OH clarithromycin when 250-mg doses of the clarithromycin suspension were administered every 12 hours. Elimination half-life of clarithromycin (3 to 4 hours) and that of 14-OH clarithromycin (5 to 7 hours) were similar to those observed at steady state following administration of equivalent doses of BIAXIN tablets.

For adult patients, the bioavailability of 10 mL of the 125 mg/5 mL suspension or 10 mL of the 250 mg/5 mL suspension is similar to a 250 mg or 500 mg tablet, respectively.

In children requiring antibiotic therapy, administration of 7.5 mg/kg q12h doses of clarithromycin as the suspension generally resulted in steady-state peak plasma concentrations of 3 to 7 mcg/mL for clarithromycin and 1 to 2 mcg/mL for 14-OH clarithromycin.

In HIV-infected children taking 15 mg/kg every 12 hours, steady-state clarithromycin peak concentrations generally ranged from 6 to 15 mcg/mL.

Clarithromycin penetrates into the middle ear fluid of children with secretory otitis media.

CONCENTRATION (after 7.5 mg/kg q12h for 5 doses)

Analyte	Middle Ear Fluid (mcg/mL)	Serum (mcg/mL)
Clarithromycin	2.5	1.7
14-OH Clarithromycin	1.3	0.8

In adults given 250 mg clarithromycin as suspension (n = 22), food appeared to decrease mean peak plasma clarithromycin concentrations from 1.2 (± 0.4) mcg/mL to 1.0 (± 0.4) mcg/mL and the extent of absorption from 7.2 (± 2.5) hr•mcg/mL to 6.5 (± 3.7) hr•mcg/mL.

When children (n = 10) were administered a single oral dose of 7.5 mg/kg suspension, food increased mean peak plasma clarithromycin concentrations from 3.6 (± 1.5) mcg/mL to 4.6 (± 2.8) mcg/mL and the extent of absorption from 10.0 (± 5.5) hr•mcg/mL to 14.2 (± 9.4) hr•mcg/mL.

Clarithromycin 500 mg every 8 hours was given in combination with omeprazole 40 mg daily to healthy adult males. The plasma levels of clarithromycin and 14-hydroxy-clarithromycin were increased by the concomitant administration of omeprazole. For clarithromycin, the mean C_{max} was 10% greater, the mean C_{min} was 27% greater, and the mean AUC_{0-8} was 15% greater when clarithromycin was administered with omeprazole than when clarithromycin was administered alone. Similar results were seen for 14-hydroxy-clarithromycin, the mean C_{max} was 45% greater, the mean C_{min} was 57% greater, and the mean AUC_{0-8} was 45% greater. Clarithromycin concentrations in the gastric tissue and mucus were also increased by concomitant administration of omeprazole.

[See table below]

For information about other drugs indicated in combination with BIAXIN, refer to the **CLINICAL PHARMACOLOGY** section of their package inserts.

Microbiology

Clarithromycin exerts its antibacterial action by binding to the 50S ribosomal subunit of susceptible bacteria resulting in inhibition of protein synthesis.

Clarithromycin is active *in vitro* against a variety of aerobic and anaerobic Gram-positive and Gram-negative bacteria as well as most *Mycobacterium avium* complex (MAC) bacteria.

Additionally, the 14-OH clarithromycin metabolite also has clinically significant antimicrobial activity. The 14-OH clarithromycin is twice as active against *Haemophilus influenzae* microorganisms as the parent compound. However, for *Mycobacterium avium* complex (MAC) isolates the 14-OH metabolite is 4 to 7 times less active than clarithromycin. The clinical significance of this activity against *Mycobacterium avium* complex is unknown.

Clarithromycin has been shown to be active against most strains of the following microorganisms both *in vitro* and in clinical infections as described in the **INDICATIONS AND USAGE** section:

Gram-Positive Microorganisms
Staphylococcus aureus
Streptococcus pneumoniae
Streptococcus pyogenes
Gram-Negative Microorganisms
Haemophilus influenzae
Haemophilus parainfluenzae
Moraxella catarrhalis
Other Microorganisms
Mycoplasma pneumoniae
Chlamydophila pneumoniae (TWAR) [previously *Chlamydia pneumoniae*]
Mycobacteria
Mycobacterium avium complex (MAC) consisting of:
Mycobacterium avium
Mycobacterium intracellulare
Beta-lactamase production should have no effect on clarithromycin activity.
NOTE: Most isolates of methicillin-resistant and oxacillin-resistant staphylococci are resistant to clarithromycin.
Omeprazole/clarithromycin dual therapy; ranitidine bismuth citrate/clarithromycin dual therapy; omeprazole/

Clarithromycin Tissue Concentrations 2 hours after Dose (mcg/mL)/(mcg/g)					
Treatment	N	antrum	fundus	N	mucus
Clarithromycin	5	10.48 ± 2.01	20.81 ± 7.64	4	4.15 ± 7.74
Clarithromycin + Omeprazole	5	19.96 ± 4.71	24.25 ± 6.37	4	39.29 ± 32.79

clarithromycin/amoxicillin triple therapy; and lansoprazole/clarithromycin/amoxicillin triple therapy have been shown to be active against most strains of *Helicobacter pylori in vitro* and in clinical infections as described in the **INDICATIONS AND USAGE** section.

Helicobacter

Helicobacter pylori

Pretreatment Resistance

Clarithromycin pretreatment resistance rates were 3.5% (4/113) in the omeprazole/clarithromycin dual therapy studies (M93-067, M93-100) and 9.3% (41/439) in the omeprazole/clarithromycin/amoxicillin triple therapy studies (126, 127, M96-446). Clarithromycin pretreatment resistance was 12.6% (44/348) in the ranitidine bismuth citrate/clarithromycin b.i.d. versus t.i.d. clinical study (H2BA3001). Clarithromycin pretreatment resistance rates were 9.5% (91/960) by E-test and 11.3% (12/106) by agar dilution in the lansoprazole/clarithromycin/amoxicillin triple therapy clinical trials (M93-125, M93-130, M93-131, M95-392, and M95-399).

Amoxicillin pretreatment susceptible isolates (< 0.25 mcg/mL) were found in 99.3% (436/439) of the patients in the omeprazole/clarithromycin/amoxicillin clinical studies (126, 127, M96-446). Amoxicillin pretreatment minimum inhibitory concentrations (MICs) > 0.25 mcg/mL occurred in 0.7% (3/439) of the patients, all of whom were in the clarithromycin/amoxicillin study arm. Amoxicillin pretreatment susceptible isolates (< 0.25 mcg/mL) occurred in 97.8% (936/957) and 98.0% (98/100) of the patients in the lansoprazole/clarithromycin/amoxicillin triple-therapy clinical trials by E-test and agar dilution, respectively. Twenty-one of the 957 patients (2.2%) by E-test and 2 of 100 patients (2.0%) by agar dilution had amoxicillin pretreatment MICs of > 0.25 mcg/mL. Two patients had an unconfirmed pretreatment amoxicillin minimum inhibitory concentration (MIC) of > 256 mcg/mL by E-test.

[See table below]

Patients not eradicated of *H. pylori* following omeprazole/clarithromycin, ranitidine bismuth citrate/clarithromycin, omeprazole/clarithromycin/amoxicillin, or lansoprazole/clarithromycin/ amoxicillin therapy would likely have clarithromycin resistant *H. pylori* isolates. Therefore, for patients who fail therapy, clarithromycin susceptibility testing should be done, if possible. Patients with clarithromycin resistant *H. pylori* should not be treated with any of the following: omeprazole/clarithromycin dual therapy; ranitidine bismuth citrate/clarithromycin dual therapy; omeprazole/clarithromycin/amoxicillin triple therapy; lansoprazole/clarithromycin/amoxicillin triple therapy; or other regimens which include clarithromycin as the sole antimicrobial agent.

Amoxicillin Susceptibility Test Results and Clinical/Bacteriological Outcomes

In the omeprazole/clarithromycin/amoxicillin triple-therapy clinical trials, 84.9% (157/185) of the patients who had pretreatment amoxicillin susceptible MICs (< 0.25 mcg/mL) were eradicated of *H. pylori* and 15.1% (28/185) failed therapy. Of the 28 patients who failed triple therapy, 11 had no post-treatment susceptibility test results, and 17 had post-treatment *H. pylori* isolates with amoxicillin susceptible MICs. Eleven of the patients who failed triple therapy also had post-treatment *H. pylori* isolates with clarithromycin resistant MICs.

In the lansoprazole/clarithromycin/amoxicillin triple-therapy clinical trials, 82.6% (195/236) of the patients that had pretreatment amoxicillin susceptible MICs (< 0.25 mcg/mL) were eradicated of *H. pylori*. Of those with pretreatment amoxicillin MICs of > 0.25 mcg/mL, three of six had the *H. pylori* eradicated. A total of 12.8% (22/172) of the patients failed the 10- and 14-day triple-therapy regimens. Post-treatment susceptibility results were not obtained on 11 of the patients who failed therapy. Nine of the 11 patients with amoxicillin post-treatment MICs that failed the triple-therapy regimen also had clarithromycin resistant *H. pylori* isolates.

The following *in vitro* data are available, **but their clinical significance is unknown**. Clarithromycin exhibits *in vitro* activity against most isolates of the following bacteria; however, the safety and effectiveness of clarithromycin in treating clinical infections due to these bacteria have not been established in adequate and well-controlled clinical trials.

Gram-Positive Bacteria
Streptococcus agalactiae
Streptococci (Groups C, F, G)
Viridans group streptococci

Clarithromycin Susceptibility Test Results and Clinical/Bacteriological Outcomes[a]

Clarithromycin Pretreatment Results	Clarithromycin Post-treatment Results				
	H. pylori negative - eradicated	*H. pylori* positive - not eradicated Post-treatment susceptibility results			
		S[b]	I[b]	R[b]	No MIC
Omeprazole 40 mg q.d./clarithromycin 500 mg t.i.d. for 14 days followed by omeprazole 20 mg q.d. for another 14 days (M93-067, M93-100)					
Susceptible[b]	108	72	1		26	9
Intermediate[b]	1				1	
Resistant[b]	4				4	
Ranitidine bismuth citrate 400 mg b.i.d./clarithromycin 500 mg t.i.d. for 14 days followed by ranitidine bismuth citrate 400 mg b.i.d. for another 14 days (H2BA3001)					
Susceptible[b]	124	98	4		14	8
Intermediate[b]	3	2				1
Resistant[b]	17	1			15	1
Ranitidine bismuth citrate 400 mg b.i.d./clarithromycin 500 mg b.i.d. for 14 days followed by ranitidine bismuth citrate 400 mg b.i.d. for another 14 days (H2BA3001)					
Susceptible[b]	125	106	1	1	12	5
Intermediate[b]	2	2				
Resistant[b]	20	1			19	
Omeprazole 20 mg b.i.d./clarithromycin 500 mg b.i.d./amoxicillin 1 g b.i.d. for 10 days (126, 127, M96-446)					
Susceptible[b]	171	153	7		3	8
Intermediate[b]						
Resistant[b]	14	4	1		6	3
Lansoprazole 30 mg b.i.d./clarithromycin 500 mg b.i.d./amoxicillin 1 g b.i.d. for 14 days (M95-399, M93-131, M95-392)					
Susceptible[b]	112	105				7
Intermediate[b]	3	3				
Resistant[b]	17	6			7	4
Lansoprazole 30 mg b.i.d./clarithromycin 500 mg b.i.d./amoxicillin 1 g b.i.d. for 10 days (M95-399)					
Susceptible[b]	42	40	1		1	
Intermediate[b]						
Resistant[b]	4	1			3	

a Includes only patients with pretreatment clarithromycin susceptibility tests
b Breakpoints for antimicrobial susceptibility testing at the time of studies were: Susceptible (S) MIC < 0.25 mcg/mL, Intermediate (I) MIC 0.5-1.0 mcg/mL, Resistant (R) MIC > 2 mcg/mL. For current antimicrobial susceptibility testing guidelines see reference 4. For current susceptibility test interpretive criteria, see Susceptibility Test for *Helicobacter pylori* below.

Gram-Negative Bacteria
Bordetella pertussis
Legionella pneumophila
Pasteurella multocida
Gram-Positive Bacteria
Clostridium perfringens
Peptococcus niger
Propionibacterium acnes
Gram-Negative Anaerobic Bacteria
Prevotella melaninogenica (formerly *Bacteriodes melaninogenicus*)

Susceptibility Testing Methods (Excluding Mycobacteria and Helicobacter)

Dilution Techniques

Quantitative methods are used to determine antimicrobial minimum inhibitory concentrations (MICs). These MICs provide estimates of the susceptibility of bacteria to antimicrobial compounds. The MICs should be determined using a standardized procedure. Standardized procedures are based on a dilution method[1] (broth or agar) or equivalent with standardized inoculum concentrations and standardized concentrations of clarithromycin powder. The MIC values should be interpreted according to the following criteria[2]:

Susceptibility Test Interpretive Criteria for *Staphylococcus aureus*

MIC (mcg/mL)	Interpretation
≤ 2.0	Susceptible (S)
4.0	Intermediate (I)
≥ 8.0	Resistant (R)

Susceptibility Test Interpretive Criteria for *Streptococcus pyogenes* and *Streptococcus pneumoniae*[a]

MIC (mcg/mL)	Interpretation

Continued on next page

Information on the AbbVie, Inc. products listed on these pages is from the prescribing information in use as of July 31, 2016. For more information, please visit rxabbvie.com or call 1-800-633-9110.

≤ 0.25	Susceptible (S)
0.5	Intermediate (I)
≥ 1.0	Resistant (R)

a These interpretive standards are applicable only to broth microdilution susceptibility tests using cation-adjusted Mueller-Hinton broth with 2-5% lysed horse blood.

For testing *Haemophilus spp.*[b]

MIC (mcg/mL)	Interpretation
≤ 8.0	Susceptible (S)
16.0	Intermediate (I)
≥ 32.0	Resistant (R)

b These interpretive standards are applicable only to broth microdilution susceptibility tests with *Haemophilus spp.* using Haemophilus Testing Medium (HTM).[1]

Note: When testing *Streptococcus pyogenes* and *Streptococcus pneumoniae*, susceptibility and resistance to clarithromycin can be predicted using erythromycin.

A report of "Susceptible" indicates that the pathogen is likely to be inhibited if the antimicrobial compound in the blood reaches the concentrations usually achievable. A report of "Intermediate" indicates that the result should be considered equivocal, and, if the microorganism is not fully susceptible to alternative, clinically feasible drugs, the test should be repeated. This category implies possible clinical applicability in body sites where the drug is physiologically concentrated or in situations where high dosage of drug can be used. This category also provides a buffer zone which prevents small uncontrolled technical factors from causing major discrepancies in interpretation. A report of "Resistant" indicates that the pathogen is not likely to be inhibited if the antimicrobial compound in the blood reaches the concentrations usually achievable; other therapy should be selected.

Quality Control
Standardized susceptibility test procedures require the use of laboratory control bacteria to monitor and ensure the accuracy and precision of supplies and reagents in the assay, and the techniques of the individual performing the test.[1,2] Standard clarithromycin powder should provide the following MIC ranges.

QC Strain		MIC (mcg/mL)
S. aureus	ATCC® 29213[c]	0.12 to 0.5
S. pneumoniae[d]	ATCC 49619	0.03 to 0.12
Haemophilus influenzae[e]	ATCC 49247	4 to 16

c ATCC is a registered trademark of the American Type Culture Collection.
d This quality control range is applicable only to *S. pneumoniae* ATCC 49619 tested by a microdilution procedure using cation-adjusted Mueller-Hinton broth with 2-5% lysed horse blood.
e This quality control range is applicable only to *H. influenzae* ATCC 49247 tested by a microdilution procedure using HTM[1].

Diffusion Techniques
Quantitative methods that require measurement of zone diameters also provide reproducible estimates of the susceptibility of bacteria to antimicrobial compounds. The zone size provides an estimate of the susceptibility of bacteria to antimicrobial compounds. The zone size should be determined using a standardized method.[2,3] The procedure uses paper disks impregnated with 15 mcg of clarithromycin to test the susceptibility of bacteria. The disk diffusion interpretive criteria are provided below.

Susceptibility Test Interpretive Criteria for *Staphylococcus aureus*

Zone diameter (mm)	Interpretation
≥ 18	Susceptible (S)
14 to 17	Intermediate (I)
≤ 13	Resistant (R)

Susceptibility Test Interpretive Criteria for *Streptococcus pyogenes* and *Streptococcus pneumoniae*[f]

Zone diameter (mm)	Interpretation
≥ 21	Susceptible (S)
17 to 20	Intermediate (I)
≤ 16	Resistant (R)

f These zone diameter standards only apply to tests performed using Mueller-Hinton agar supplemented with 5% sheep blood incubated in 5% CO_2.

For testing *Haemophilus spp.*[g]

Zone diameter (mm)	Interpretation
≥ 13	Susceptible (S)
11 to 12	Intermediate (I)
≤ 10	Resistant (R)

g These zone diameter standards are applicable only to tests with *Haemophilus spp.* using HTM[2].

Note: When testing *Streptococcus pyogenes* and *Streptococcus pneumoniae*, susceptibility and resistance to clarithromycin can be predicted using erythromycin.

Quality Control
Standardized susceptibility test procedures require the use of laboratory control bacteria to monitor and ensure the accuracy and precision of supplies and reagents in the assay, and the techniques of the individual performing the test.[2,3] For the diffusion technique using the 15 mcg disk, the criteria in the following table should be achieved.

Acceptable Quality Control Ranges for Clarithromycin

QC Strain		Zone diameter (mm)
S. aureus	ATCC 25923	26 to 32
S. pneumoniae[h]	ATCC 49619	25 to 31
Haemophilus influenzae[i]	ATCC 49247	11 to 17

h This quality control range is applicable only to tests performed by disk diffusion using Mueller-Hinton agar supplemented with 5% defibrinated sheep blood.
i This quality control limit applies to tests conducted with *Haemophilus influenzae* ATCC 49247 using HTM[2].

In vitro Activity of Clarithromycin against Mycobacteria
Clarithromycin has demonstrated *in vitro* activity against *Mycobacterium avium* complex (MAC) microorganisms isolated from both AIDS and non-AIDS patients. While gene probe techniques may be used to distinguish *M. avium* species from *M. intracellulare*, many studies only reported results on *M. avium* complex (MAC) isolates.
Various *in vitro* methodologies employing broth or solid media at different pH's, with and without oleic acid-albumin-dextrose-catalase (OADC), have been used to determine clarithromycin MIC values for mycobacterial species. In general, MIC values decrease more than 16-fold as the pH of Middlebrook 7H12 broth media increases from 5.0 to 7.4. At pH 7.4, MIC values determined with Mueller-Hinton agar were 4- to 8-fold higher than those observed with Middlebrook 7H12 media. Utilization of oleic acid-albumin-dextrose-catalase (OADC) in these assays has been shown to further alter MIC values.

Clarithromycin activity against 80 MAC isolates from AIDS patients and 211 MAC isolates from non-AIDS patients was evaluated using a microdilution method with Middlebrook 7H9 broth. Results showed an MIC value of ≤ 4.0 mcg/mL in 81% and 89% of the AIDS and non-AIDS MAC isolates, respectively. Twelve percent of the non-AIDS isolates had an MIC value ≤ 0.5 mcg/mL. Clarithromycin was also shown to be active against phagocytized *M. avium* complex (MAC) in mouse and human macrophage cell cultures as well as in the beige mouse infection model.
Clarithromycin activity was evaluated against *Mycobacterium tuberculosis* microorganisms. In one study utilizing the agar dilution method with Middlebrook 7H10 media, 3 of 30 clinical isolates had an MIC of 2.5 mcg/mL. Clarithromycin inhibited all isolates at > 10.0 mcg/mL.
Susceptibility Testing for *Mycobacterium avium* Complex (MAC)
The disk diffusion and dilution techniques for susceptibility testing against gram-positive and gram-negative bacteria should not be used for determining clarithromycin MIC values against mycobacteria. *In vitro* susceptibility testing methods and diagnostic products currently available for determining minimum inhibitory concentration (MIC) values against *Mycobacterium avium* complex (MAC) organisms have not been standardized or validated. Clarithromycin MIC values will vary depending on the susceptibility testing method employed, composition and pH of the media, and the utilization of nutritional supplements. Breakpoints to determine whether clinical isolates of *M. avium* or *M. intracellulare* are susceptible or resistant to clarithromycin have not been established.
Susceptibility Test for *Helicobacter pylori*
The reference methodology for susceptibility testing of *H. pylori* is agar dilution MICs.[4] One to three microliters of an inoculum equivalent to a No. 2 McFarland standard (1×10^7-1×10^8 CFU/mL for *H. pylori*) are inoculated directly onto freshly prepared antimicrobial containing Mueller-Hinton agar plates with 5% aged defibrinated sheep blood (> 2-weeks old). The agar dilution plates are incubated at 35°C in a microaerobic environment produced by a gas generating system suitable for *Campylobacter* species. After 3 days of incubation, the MICs are recorded as the lowest concentration of antimicrobial agent required to inhibit growth of the organism. The clarithromycin and amoxicillin MIC values should be interpreted according to the following criteria:

Susceptibility Test Interpretive Criteria for *H. pylori*

Clarithromycin MIC (mcg/mL) [i]	Interpretation
≤ 0.25	Susceptible (S)
0.5	Intermediate (I)
≥ 1.0	Resistant (R)

Susceptibility Test Interpretive Criteria for *H. pylori*

Amoxicillin MIC (mcg/mL) [j,k]	Interpretation
< 0.25	Susceptible (S)

j These are tentative breakpoints for the agar dilution methodology, and should not be used to interpret results obtained using alternative methods.
k There were not enough organisms with MICs > 0.25 mcg/mL to determine a resistance breakpoint.

Standardized susceptibility test procedures require the use of laboratory control bacteria to monitor and ensure the accuracy and precision of supplies and reagents in the assay, and the techniques of the individual performing the test. Standard clarithromycin or amoxicillin powder should provide the following MIC ranges.
[See table at top of next page]

INDICATIONS AND USAGE

BIAXIN Filmtab (clarithromycin tablets, USP) and BIAXIN Granules (clarithromycin for oral suspension, USP) are indicated for the treatment of mild to moderate infections caused by susceptible isolates of the designated bacteria in the conditions as listed below:
Adults (BIAXIN Filmtab Tablets and Granules for Oral Suspension)
Pharyngitis/Tonsillitis due to *Streptococcus pyogenes* (The usual drug of choice in the treatment and prevention of

Acceptable Quality Control Ranges		Antimicrobial Agent	MIC (mcg/mL)[1]
H. pylori	ATCC 43504	Clarithromycin	0.015-0.12 mcg/mL
H. pylori	ATCC 43504	Amoxicillin	0.015-0.12 mcg/mL

1 These are quality control ranges for the agar dilution methodology and should not be used to control test results obtained using alternative methods.

streptococcal infections and the prophylaxis of rheumatic fever is penicillin administered by either the intramuscular or the oral route. Clarithromycin is generally effective in the eradication of *S. pyogenes* from the nasopharynx; however, data establishing the efficacy of clarithromycin in the subsequent prevention of rheumatic fever are not available at present).

Acute maxillary sinusitis due to *Haemophilus influenzae*, *Moraxella catarrhalis*, or *Streptococcus pneumoniae*.

Acute bacterial exacerbation of chronic bronchitis due to *Haemophilus influenzae*, *Haemophilus parainfluenzae*, *Moraxella catarrhalis*, or *Streptococcus pneumoniae*.

Community-Acquired Pneumonia due to *Haemophilus influenzae*, *Mycoplasma pneumoniae*, *Streptococcus pneumoniae*, or *Chlamydophila pneumoniae* (TWAR).

Uncomplicated skin and skin structure infections due to *Staphylococcus aureus*, or *Streptococcus pyogenes* (Abscesses usually require surgical drainage).

Disseminated mycobacterial infections due to *Mycobacterium avium*, or *Mycobacterium intracellulare*

BIAXIN (clarithromycin) Filmtab tablets in combination with amoxicillin and PREVACID (lansoprazole) or PRILOSEC (omeprazole) Delayed-Release Capsules, as triple therapy, are indicated for the treatment of patients with *Helicobacter pylori* infection and duodenal ulcer disease (active or five-year history of duodenal ulcer) to eradicate *H. pylori*.

BIAXIN Filmtab tablets in combination with PRILOSEC (omeprazole) capsules or TRITEC (ranitidine bismuth citrate) tablets are also indicated for the treatment of patients with an active duodenal ulcer associated with *H. pylori* infection. However, regimens which contain clarithromycin as the single antimicrobial agent are more likely to be associated with the development of clarithromycin resistance among patients who fail therapy. Clarithromycin-containing regimens should not be used in patients with known or suspected clarithromycin resistant isolates because the efficacy of treatment is reduced in this setting.

In patients who fail therapy, susceptibility testing should be done if possible. If resistance to clarithromycin is demonstrated, a non-clarithromycin-containing therapy is recommended. (For information on development of resistance see **Microbiology** section.) The eradication of *H. pylori* has been demonstrated to reduce the risk of duodenal ulcer recurrence.

Children (BIAXIN Filmtab Tablets and Granules for Oral Suspension)
Pharyngitis/Tonsillitis due to *Streptococcus pyogenes*.

Community-Acquired Pneumonia due to *Mycoplasma pneumoniae*, *Streptococcus pneumoniae*, or *Chlamydophila pneumoniae* (TWAR)

Acute maxillary sinusitis due to *Haemophilus influenzae*, *Moraxella catarrhalis*, or *Streptococcus pneumoniae*

Acute otitis media due to *Haemophilus influenzae*, *Moraxella catarrhalis*, or *Streptococcus pneumoniae*

NOTE: For information on otitis media, see **CLINICAL STUDIES - Otitis Media.**

Uncomplicated skin and skin structure infections due to *Staphylococcus aureus*, or *Streptococcus pyogenes* (Abscesses usually require surgical drainage).

Disseminated mycobacterial infections due to *Mycobacterium avium*, or *Mycobacterium intracellulare*

Adults (BIAXIN XL Filmtab Tablets)
BIAXIN XL Filmtab (clarithromycin extended-release tablets) are indicated for the treatment of adults with mild to moderate infection caused by susceptible strains of the designated microorganisms in the conditions listed below:

Acute maxillary sinusitis due to *Haemophilus influenzae*, *Moraxella catarrhalis*, or *Streptococcus pneumoniae*

Acute bacterial exacerbation of chronic bronchitis due to *Haemophilus influenzae*, *Haemophilus parainfluenzae*, *Moraxella catarrhalis*, or *Streptococcus pneumoniae*

Community-Acquired Pneumonia due to *Haemophilus influenzae*, *Haemophilus parainfluenzae*, *Moraxella catarrhalis*, *Streptococcus pneumoniae*, *Chlamydophila pneumoniae* (TWAR), or *Mycoplasma pneumoniae*

THE EFFICACY AND SAFETY OF BIAXIN XL IN TREATING OTHER INFECTIONS FOR WHICH OTHER FORMULATIONS OF BIAXIN ARE APPROVED HAVE NOT BEEN ESTABLISHED.
Prophylaxis
BIAXIN Filmtab tablets and BIAXIN Granules for oral suspension are indicated for the prevention of disseminated *Mycobacterium avium* complex (MAC) disease in patients with advanced HIV infection.

To reduce the development of drug-resistant bacteria and maintain the effectiveness of BIAXIN and other antibacterial drugs, BIAXIN should be used only to treat or prevent infections that are proven or strongly suspected to be caused by susceptible bacteria. When culture and susceptibility information are available, they should be considered in selecting or modifying antibacterial therapy. In the absence of such data, local epidemiology and susceptibility patterns may contribute to the empiric selection of therapy.

CONTRAINDICATIONS
Clarithromycin is contraindicated in patients with a known hypersensitivity to clarithromycin or any of its excipients, erythromycin, or any of the macrolide antibiotics.

Clarithromycin is contraindicated in patients with a history of cholestatic jaundice/hepatic dysfunction associated with prior use of clarithromycin.

Concomitant administration of clarithromycin and any of the following drugs is contraindicated: cisapride, pimozide, astemizole, terfenadine, and ergotamine or dihydroergotamine (see **Drug Interactions**). There have been postmarketing reports of drug interactions when clarithromycin and/or erythromycin are coadministered with cisapride, pimozide, astemizole, or terfenadine resulting in cardiac arrhythmias (QT prolongation, ventricular tachycardia, ventricular fibrillation, and torsades de pointes) most likely due to inhibition of metabolism of these drugs by erythromycin and clarithromycin. Fatalities have been reported.

Concomitant administration of clarithromycin and colchicine is contraindicated in patients with renal or hepatic impairment.

Clarithromycin should not be given to patients with history of QT prolongation or ventricular cardiac arrhythmia, including *torsades de pointes*.

Clarithromycin should not be used concomitantly with HMG-CoA reductase inhibitors (statins) that are extensively metabolized by CYP3A4 (lovastatin or simvastatin), due to the increased risk of myopathy, including rhabdomyolysis (see **WARNINGS**).

For information about contraindications of other drugs indicated in combination with BIAXIN, refer to the **CONTRAINDICATIONS** section of their package inserts.

WARNINGS
Use In Pregnancy
CLARITHROMYCIN SHOULD NOT BE USED IN PREGNANT WOMEN EXCEPT IN CLINICAL CIRCUMSTANCES WHERE NO ALTERNATIVE THERAPY IS APPROPRIATE. IF PREGNANCY OCCURS WHILE TAKING THIS DRUG, THE PATIENT SHOULD BE APPRISED OF THE POTENTIAL HAZARD TO THE FETUS. CLARITHROMYCIN HAS DEMONSTRATED ADVERSE EFFECTS OF PREGNANCY OUTCOME AND/OR EMBRYO-FETAL DEVELOPMENT IN MONKEYS, RATS, MICE, AND RABBITS AT DOSES THAT PRODUCED PLASMA LEVELS 2 TO 17 TIMES THE SERUM LEVELS ACHIEVED IN HUMANS TREATED AT THE MAXIMUM RECOMMENDED HUMAN DOSES (see PRECAUTIONS - Pregnancy).
Hepatotoxicity
Hepatic dysfunction, including increased liver enzymes, and hepatocellular and/or cholestatic hepatitis, with or without jaundice, has been reported with clarithromycin. This hepatic dysfunction may be severe and is usually reversible. In some instances, hepatic failure with fatal outcome has been reported and generally has been associated with serious underlying diseases and/or concomitant medications. Symptoms of hepatitis can include anorexia, jaundice, dark urine, pruritus, or tender abdomen. Discontinue clarithromycin immediately if signs and symptoms of hepatitis occur.

QT Prolongation
Clarithromycin has been associated with prolongation of the QT interval and infrequent cases of arrhythmia. Cases of *torsades de pointes* have been spontaneously reported during postmarketing surveillance in patients receiving clarithromycin. Fatalities have been reported. Clarithromycin should be avoided in patients with ongoing proarrhythmic conditions such as uncorrected hypokalemia or hypomagnesemia, clinically significant bradycardia (see **CONTRAINDICATIONS**) and in patients receiving Class IA (quinidine, procainamide) or Class III (dofetilide, amiodarone, sotalol) antiarrhythmic agents. Elderly patients may be more susceptible to drug-associated effects on the QT interval.
Drug Interactions
Serious adverse reactions have been reported in patients taking clarithromycin concomitantly with CYP3A4 substrates. These include colchicine toxicity with colchicine; rhabdomyolysis with simvastatin, lovastatin, and atorvastatin; hypoglycemia with disopyramide; and hypotension and acute kidney injury with calcium channel blockers metabolized by CYP3A4 (e.g., verapamil, amlodipine, diltiazem, nifedipine). Most reports of acute kidney injury with calcium channel blockers metabolized by CYP3A4 involved elderly patients 65 years of age or older (see **CONTRAINDICATIONS** and **PRECAUTIONS – Drug Interactions**). Clarithromycin should be used with caution when administered concurrently with medications that induce the cytochrome CYP3A4 enzyme (see **PRECAUTIONS - Drug Interactions**).
Colchicine
Life-threatening and fatal drug interactions have been reported in patients treated with clarithromycin and colchicine. Clarithromycin is a strong CYP3A4 inhibitor and this interaction may occur while using both drugs at their recommended doses. If co-administration of clarithromycin and colchicine is necessary in patients with normal renal and hepatic function, the dose of colchicine should be reduced. Patients should be monitored for clinical symptoms of colchicine toxicity. Concomitant administration of clarithromycin and colchicine is contraindicated in patients with renal or hepatic impairment (see **CONTRAINDICATIONS** and **PRECAUTIONS – Drug Interactions**).
Benzodiazepines
Increased sedation and prolongation of sedation have been reported with concomitant administration of clarithromycin and triazolobenzodiazepines, such as triazolam, and midazolam.
Quetiapine
Use quetiapine and clarithromycin concomitantly with caution. Co-administration could result in increased quetiapine exposure and quetiapine related toxicities such as somnolence, orthostatic hypotension, altered state of consciousness, neuroleptic malignant syndrome, and QT prolongation. Refer to quetiapine prescribing information for recommendations on dose reduction if co-administered with CYP3A4 inhibitors such as clarithromycin.
Oral Hypoglycemic Agents/Insulin
The concomitant use of clarithromycin and oral hypoglycemic agents and/or insulin can result in significant hypoglycemia. With certain hypoglycemic drugs such as nateglinide, pioglitazone, repaglinide and rosiglitazone, inhibition of CYP3A enzyme by clarithromycin may be involved and could cause hypoglycemia when used concomitantly. Careful monitoring of glucose is recommended.
Oral Anticoagulants
There is a risk of serious hemorrhage and significant elevations in INR and prothrombin time when clarithromycin is co-administered with warfarin. INR and prothrombin times should be frequently monitored while patients are receiving clarithromycin and oral anticoagulants concurrently.
HMG-CoA Reductase Inhibitors (statins)
Concomitant use of clarithromycin with lovastatin or simvastatin is contraindicated (see **CONTRAINDICATIONS**) as these statins are extensively metabolized by CYP3A4, and concomitant treatment with clarithromycin increases their plasma concentration, which increases the risk of my-

Continued on next page

Information on the AbbVie, Inc. products listed on these pages is from the prescribing information in use as of July 31, 2016. For more information, please visit rxabbvie.com or call 1-800-633-9110.

opathy, including rhabdomyolysis. Cases of rhabdomyolysis have been reported in patients taking clarithromycin concomitantly with these statins. If treatment with clarithromycin cannot be avoided, therapy with lovastatin or simvastatin must be suspended during the course of treatment.

Caution should be exercised when prescribing clarithromycin with statins. In situations where the concomitant use of clarithromycin with atorvastatin or pravastatin cannot be avoided, atorvastatin dose should not exceed 20 mg daily and pravastatin dose should not exceed 40 mg daily. Use of a statin that is not dependent on CYP3A metabolism (e.g.fluvastatin) can be considered. It is recommended to prescribe the lowest registered dose if concomitant use cannot be avoided.

Clostridium difficile Associated Diarrhea

Clostridium difficile associated diarrhea (CDAD) has been reported with use of nearly all antibacterial agents, including BIAXIN, and may range in severity from mild diarrhea to fatal colitis. Treatment with antibacterial agents alters the normal flora of the colon leading to overgrowth of *C. difficile.*

C. difficile produces toxins A and B which contribute to the development of CDAD. Hypertoxin producing strains of *C. difficile* cause increased morbidity and mortality, as these infections can be refractory to antimicrobial therapy and may require colectomy. CDAD must be considered in all patients who present with diarrhea following antibiotic use. Careful medical history is necessary since CDAD has been reported to occur over two months after the administration of antibacterial agents.

If CDAD is suspected or confirmed, ongoing antibiotic use not directed against *C. difficile* may need to be discontinued. Appropriate fluid and electrolyte management, protein supplementation, antibiotic treatment of *C. difficile*, and surgical evaluation should be instituted as clinically indicated.

Acute Hypersensitivity Reactions

In the event of severe acute hypersensitivity reactions, such as anaphylaxis, Stevens-Johnson Syndrome, toxic epidermal necrolysis, drug rash with eosinophilia and systemic symptoms (DRESS), and Henoch-Schonlein purpura clarithromycin therapy should be discontinued immediately and appropriate treatment should be urgently initiated.

Combination Therapy with Other Drugs

For information about warnings of other drugs indicated in combination with BIAXIN, refer to the **WARNINGS** section of their package inserts.

PRECAUTIONS
General

Prescribing BIAXIN in the absence of a proven or strongly suspected bacterial infection or a prophylactic indication is unlikely to provide benefit to the patient and increases the risk of the development of drug-resistant bacteria.

Clarithromycin is principally excreted via the liver and kidney. Clarithromycin may be administered without dosage adjustment to patients with hepatic impairment and normal renal function. However, in the presence of severe renal impairment with or without coexisting hepatic impairment, decreased dosage or prolonged dosing intervals may be appropriate.

Clarithromycin in combination with ranitidine bismuth citrate therapy is not recommended in patients with creatinine clearance less than 25 mL/min (see **DOSAGE AND ADMINISTRATION**).

Clarithromycin in combination with ranitidine bismuth citrate should not be used in patients with a history of acute porphyria.

Exacerbation of symptoms of myasthenia gravis and new onset of symptoms of myasthenic syndrome has been reported in patients receiving clarithromycin therapy.

For information about precautions of other drugs indicated in combination with BIAXIN, refer to the **PRECAUTIONS** section of their package inserts.

Information to Patients

Patients should be counseled that antibacterial drugs including BIAXIN should only be used to treat bacterial infections. They do not treat viral infections (e.g., the common cold). When BIAXIN is prescribed to treat a bacterial infection, patients should be told that although it is common to feel better early in the course of therapy, the medication should be taken exactly as directed. Skipping doses or not completing the full course of therapy may (1) decrease the effectiveness of the immediate treatment and (2) increase the likelihood that bacteria will develop resistance and will not be treatable by BIAXIN or other antibacterial drugs in the future.

Diarrhea is a common problem caused by antibiotics which usually ends when the antibiotic is discontinued. Sometimes after starting treatment with antibiotics, patients can develop watery and bloody stools (with or without stomach cramps and fever) even as late as two or more months after having taken the last dose of the antibiotic. If this occurs, patients should contact their physician as soon as possible. BIAXIN may interact with some drugs; therefore patients should be advised to report to their doctor the use of any other medications.

BIAXIN tablets and oral suspension can be taken with or without food and can be taken with milk; however, BIAXIN XL tablets should be taken with food. Do **NOT** refrigerate the suspension.

Drug Interactions

Clarithromycin use in patients who are receiving theophylline may be associated with an increase of serum theophylline concentrations. Monitoring of serum theophylline concentrations should be considered for patients receiving high doses of theophylline or with baseline concentrations in the upper therapeutic range. In two studies in which theophylline was administered with clarithromycin (a theophylline sustained-release formulation was dosed at either 6.5 mg/kg or 12 mg/kg together with 250 or 500 mg q12h clarithromycin), the steady-state levels of C_{max}, C_{min}, and the area under the serum concentration time curve (AUC) of theophylline increased about 20%.

Hypotension, bradyarrhythmias, and lactic acidosis have been observed in patients receiving concurrent verapamil, belonging to the calcium channel blockers drug class.

Concomitant administration of single doses of clarithromycin and carbamazepine has been shown to result in increased plasma concentrations of carbamazepine. Blood level monitoring of carbamazepine may be considered.

When clarithromycin and terfenadine were coadministered, plasma concentrations of the active acid metabolite of terfenadine were threefold higher, on average, than the values observed when terfenadine was administered alone. The pharmacokinetics of clarithromycin and the 14-OH-clarithromycin were not significantly affected by coadministration of terfenadine once clarithromycin reached steady-state conditions. Concomitant administration of clarithromycin with terfenadine is contraindicated (see **CONTRAINDICATIONS**).

Clarithromycin 500 mg every 8 hours was given in combination with omeprazole 40 mg daily to healthy adult subjects. The steady-state plasma concentrations of omeprazole were increased (C_{max}, AUC_{0-24}, and $t_{1/2}$ increases of 30%, 89%, and 34%, respectively), by the concomitant administration of clarithromycin. The mean 24-hour gastric pH value was 5.2 when omeprazole was administered alone and 5.7 when coadministered with clarithromycin.

Coadministration of clarithromycin with ranitidine bismuth citrate resulted in increased plasma ranitidine concentrations (57%), increased plasma bismuth trough concentrations (48%), and increased 14-hydroxy-clarithromycin plasma concentrations (31%). These effects are clinically insignificant.

Simultaneous oral administration of BIAXIN tablets and zidovudine to HIV-infected adult patients may result in decreased steady-state zidovudine concentrations. Following administration of clarithromycin 500 mg tablets twice daily with zidovudine 100 mg every 4 hours, the steady-state zidovudine AUC decreased 12% compared to administration of zidovudine alone (n=4). Individual values ranged from a decrease of 34% to an increase of 14%. When clarithromycin tablets were administered two to four hours prior to zidovudine, the steady-state zidovudine C_{max} increased 100% whereas the AUC was unaffected (n=24). Administration of clarithromycin and zidovudine should be separated by at least two hours. The impact of co-administration of clarithromycin extended-release tablets and zidovudine has not been evaluated.

Simultaneous administration of BIAXIN tablets and didanosine to 12 HIV-infected adult patients resulted in no statistically significant change in didanosine pharmacokinetics.

Following administration of fluconazole 200 mg daily and clarithromycin 500 mg twice daily to 21 healthy volunteers, the steady-state clarithromycin C_{min} and AUC increased 33% and 18%, respectively. Steady-state concentrations of 14-OH clarithromycin were not significantly affected by concomitant administration of fluconazole. No dosage adjustment of clarithromycin is necessary when co-administered with fluconazole.

Ritonavir

Concomitant administration of clarithromycin and ritonavir (n = 22) resulted in a 77% increase in clarithromycin AUC and a 100% decrease in the AUC of 14-OH clarithromycin. Clarithromycin may be administered without dosage adjustment to patients with normal renal function taking ritonavir. Since concentrations of 14-OH clarithromycin are significantly reduced when clarithromycin is co-administered with ritonavir, alternative antibacterial therapy should be considered for indications other than infections due to *Mycobacterium avium* complex (see **PRECAUTIONS – Drug Interactions**). Doses of clarithromycin greater than 1000 mg per day should not be co-administered with protease inhibitors.

Spontaneous reports in the post-marketing period suggest that concomitant administration of clarithromycin and oral anticoagulants may potentiate the effects of the oral anticoagulants. Prothrombin times should be carefully monitored while patients are receiving clarithromycin and oral anticoagulants simultaneously.

Digoxin is a substrate for P-glycoprotein (Pgp) and clarithromycin is known to inhibit Pgp. When clarithromycin and digoxin are co-administered, inhibition of Pgp by clarithromycin may lead to increased exposure of digoxin. Elevated digoxin serum concentrations in patients receiving clarithromycin and digoxin concomitantly have been reported in post-marketing surveillance. Some patients have shown clinical signs consistent with digoxin toxicity, including potentially fatal arrhythmias. Monitoring of serum digoxin concentrations should be considered, especially for patients with digoxin concentrations in the upper therapeutic range.

Co-administration of clarithromycin, known to inhibit CYP3A, and a drug primarily metabolized by CYP3A may be associated with elevations in drug concentrations that could increase or prolong both therapeutic and adverse effects of the concomitant drug.

Clarithromycin should be used with caution in patients receiving treatment with other drugs known to be CYP3A enzyme substrates, especially if the CYP3A substrate has a narrow safety margin (e.g., carbamazepine) and/or the substrate is extensively metabolized by this enzyme. Dosage adjustments may be considered, and when possible, serum concentrations of drugs primarily metabolized by CYP3A should be monitored closely in patients concurrently receiving clarithromycin.

The following are examples of some clinically significant CYP3A based drug interactions. Interactions with other drugs metabolized by the CYP3A isoform are also possible.

Carbamazepine and Terfenadine

Increased serum concentrations of carbamazepine and the active acid metabolite of terfenadine were observed in clinical trials with clarithromycin.

Colchicine

Colchicine is a substrate for both CYP3A and the efflux transporter, P-glycoprotein (Pgp). Clarithromycin and other macrolides are known to inhibit CYP3A and Pgp. When a single dose of colchicine 0.6 mg was administered with clarithromycin 250 mg BID for 7 days, the colchicine C_{max} increased 197% and the $AUC_{0-\infty}$ increased 239% compared to administration of colchicine alone. The dose of colchicine should be reduced when co-administered with clarithromycin in patients with normal renal and hepatic function. Concomitant use of clarithromycin and colchicine is contraindicated in patients with renal or hepatic impairment (see **WARNINGS**).

Efavirenz, Nevirapine, Rifampicin, Rifabutin, and Rifapentine

Inducers of CYP3A enzymes, such as efavirenz, nevirapine, rifampicin, rifabutin, and rifapentine will increase the metabolism of clarithromycin, thus decreasing plasma concentrations of clarithromycin, while increasing those of 14-OH-clarithromycin. Since the microbiological activities of clarithromycin and 14-OH-clarithromycin are different for different bacteria, the intended therapeutic effect could be impaired during concomitant administration of clarithromycin and enzyme inducers. Alternative antibacterial treatment should be considered when treating patients receiving inducers of CYP3A. Concomitant administration of rifabutin and clarithromycin resulted in an increase in rifabutin, and decrease in clarithromycin serum levels together with an increased risk of uveitis.

Etravirine

Clarithromycin exposure was decreased by etravirine; however, concentrations of the active metabolite, 14-OH-clarithromycin, were increased. Because 14-OH-clarithromycin has reduced activity against *Mycobacterium avium* complex (MAC), overall activity against this pathogen may be altered; therefore alternatives to clarithromycin should be considered for the treatment of MAC.

Sildenafil, Tadalafil, and Vardenafil

Each of these phosphodiesterase inhibitors is primarily metabolized by CYP3A, and CYP3A will be inhibited by concomitant administration of clarithromycin. Co-administration of clarithromycin with sildenafil, tadalafil, or vardenafil will result in increased exposure of these phosphodiesterase inhibitors. Co-administration of these phosphodiesterase inhibitors with clarithromycin is not recommended.

Tolterodine

The primary route of metabolism for tolterodine is via CYP2D6. However, in a subset of the population devoid of CYP2D6, the identified pathway of metabolism is via CYP3A. In this population subset, inhibition of CYP3A results in significantly higher serum concentrations of tolterodine. Tolterodine 1 mg twice daily is recommended in patients deficient in CYP2D6 activity (poor metabolizers) when co-administered with clarithromycin.

Triazolobenzodiazepines (e.g., alprazolam, midazolam, triazolam)

When a single dose of midazolam was co-administered with clarithromycin tablets (500 mg twice daily for 7 days), midazolam AUC increased 174% after intravenous administration of midazolam and 600% after oral administration. When oral midazolam is co-administered with clarithromycin, dose adjustments may be necessary and possible prolongation and intensity of effect should be anticipated. Caution and appropriate dose adjustments should be considered when triazolam or alprazolam is co-administered with clarithromycin. For benzodiazepines which are not metabolized by CYP3A (e.g., temazepam, nitrazepam, lorazepam), a clinically important interaction with clarithromycin is unlikely.

There have been post-marketing reports of drug interactions and central nervous system (CNS) effects (e.g., somnolence and confusion) with the concomitant use of clarithromycin and triazolam. Monitoring the patient for increased CNS pharmacological effects is suggested.

Atazanavir

Both clarithromycin and atazanavir are substrates and inhibitors of CYP3A, and there is evidence of a bi-directional drug interaction. Following administration of clarithromycin (500 mg twice daily) with atazanavir (400 mg once daily), the clarithromycin AUC increased 94%, the 14-OH clarithromycin AUC decreased 70% and the atazanavir AUC increased 28%. When clarithromycin is co-administered with atazanavir, the dose of clarithromycin should be decreased by 50%. Since concentrations of 14-OH clarithromycin are significantly reduced when clarithromycin is co-administered with atazanavir, alternative antibacterial therapy should be considered for indications other than infections due to *Mycobacterium avium* complex (see **PRECAUTIONS – Drug Interactions**). Doses of clarithromycin greater than 1000 mg per day should not be co-administered with protease inhibitors.

Itraconazole

Both clarithromycin and itraconazole are substrates and inhibitors of CYP3A, potentially leading to a bi-directional drug interaction when administered concomitantly. Clarithromycin may increase the plasma concentrations of itraconazole, while itraconazole may increase the plasma concentrations of clarithromycin. Patients taking itraconazole and clarithromycin concomitantly should be monitored closely for signs or symptoms of increased or prolonged adverse reactions.

Saquinavir

Both clarithromycin and saquinavir are substrates and inhibitors of CYP3A and there is evidence of a bi-directional drug interaction. Following administration of clarithromycin (500 mg bid) and saquinavir (soft gelatin capsules, 1200 mg tid) to 12 healthy volunteers, the steady-state saquinavir AUC and C_{max} increased 177% and 187% respectively compared to administration of saquinavir alone. Clarithromycin AUC and C_{max} increased 45% and 39% respectively, whereas the 14–OH clarithromycin AUC and C_{max} decreased 24% and 34% respectively, compared to administration with clarithromycin alone. No dose adjustment of clarithromycin is necessary when clarithromycin is co-administered with saquinavir in patients with normal renal function. When saquinavir is co-administered with rito-

navir, consideration should be given to the potential effects of ritonavir on clarithromycin (refer to interaction between clarithromycin and ritonavir) (see **PRECAUTIONS – Drug Interactions**).

The following CYP3A based drug interactions have been observed with erythromycin products and/or with clarithromycin in post-marketing experience:

Antiarrhythmics

There have been post-marketing reports of torsades de pointes occurring with concurrent use of clarithromycin and quinidine or disopyramide. Electrocardiograms should be monitored for QTc prolongation during coadministration of clarithromycin with these drugs. Serum concentrations of these medications should also be monitored.

There have been post marketing reports of hypoglycemia with the concomitant administration of clarithromycin and disopyramide. Therefore, blood glucose levels should be monitored during concomitant administration of clarithromycin and disopyramide.

Ergotamine/Dihydroergotamine

Post-marketing reports indicate that coadministration of clarithromycin with ergotamine or dihydroergotamine has been associated with acute ergot toxicity characterized by vasospasm and ischemia of the extremities and other tissues including the central nervous system. Concomitant administration of clarithromycin with ergotamine or dihydroergotamine is contraindicated (see **CONTRAINDICATIONS**).

Triazolobenzodiazepines (Such as Triazolam and Alprazolam) and Related Benzodiazepines (Such as Midazolam)

Erythromycin has been reported to decrease the clearance of triazolam and midazolam, and thus, may increase the pharmacologic effect of these benzodiazepines. There have been post-marketing reports of drug interactions and CNS effects (e.g., somnolence and confusion) with the concomitant use of clarithromycin and triazolam.

Quetiapine

Quetiapine is a substrate for CYP3A4, which is inhibited by clarithromycin. Co-administration with clarithromycin could result in increased quetiapine exposure and possible quetiapine related toxicities. There have been post-marketing reports of somnolence, orthostatic hypotension, altered state of consciousness, neuroleptic malignant syndrome, and QT prolongation during concomitant administration. Refer to quetiapine prescribing information for recommendations on dose reduction if co-administered with CYP3A4 inhibitors such as clarithromycin.

Sildenafil (Viagra)

Erythromycin has been reported to increase the systemic exposure (AUC) of sildenafil. A similar interaction may occur with clarithromycin; reduction of sildenafil dosage should be considered. (See Viagra package insert.)

There have been spontaneous or published reports of CYP3A based interactions of erythromycin and/or clarithromycin with cyclosporine, carbamazepine, tacrolimus, alfentanil, disopyramide, rifabutin, quinidine, methylprednisolone, cilostazol, bromocriptine, vinblastine, phenobarbital and St. John's Wort.

Concomitant administration of clarithromycin with cisapride, pimozide, astemizole, or terfenadine is contraindicated (see **CONTRAINDICATIONS**).

In addition, there have been reports of interactions of erythromycin or clarithromycin with drugs not thought to be metabolized by CYP3A, including hexobarbital, phenytoin, and valproate.

Carcinogenesis, Mutagenesis, Impairment of Fertility

The following *in vitro* mutagenicity tests have been conducted with clarithromycin:

Salmonella/Mammalian Microsomes Test

Bacterial Induced Mutation Frequency Test

In Vitro Chromosome Aberration Test

Rat Hepatocyte DNA Synthesis Assay

Mouse Lymphoma Assay

Mouse Dominant Lethal Study

Mouse Micronucleus Test

All tests had negative results except the *In Vitro* Chromosome Aberration Test which was weakly positive in one test and negative in another.

In addition, a Bacterial Reverse-Mutation Test (Ames Test) has been performed on clarithromycin metabolites with negative results.

Fertility and reproduction studies have shown that daily doses of up to 160 mg/kg/day (1.3 times the recommended maximum human dose based on mg/m²) to male and female

rats caused no adverse effects on the estrous cycle, fertility, parturition, or number and viability of offspring. Plasma levels in rats after 150 mg/kg/day were 2 times the human serum levels.

In the 150 mg/kg/day monkey studies, plasma levels were 3 times the human serum levels. When given orally at 150 mg/kg/day (2.4 times the recommended maximum human dose based on mg/m²), clarithromycin was shown to produce embryonic loss in monkeys. This effect has been attributed to marked maternal toxicity of the drug at this high dose.

In rabbits, *in utero* fetal loss occurred at an intravenous dose of 33 mg/m², which is 17 times less than the maximum proposed human oral daily dose of 618 mg/m².

Long-term studies in animals have not been performed to evaluate the carcinogenic potential of clarithromycin.

Pregnancy

Teratogenic Effects

Pregnancy Category C

Four teratogenicity studies in rats (three with oral doses and one with intravenous doses up to 160 mg/kg/day administered during the period of major organogenesis) and two in rabbits at oral doses up to 125 mg/kg/day (approximately 2 times the recommended maximum human dose based on mg/m²) or intravenous doses of 30 mg/kg/day administered during gestation days 6 to 18 failed to demonstrate any teratogenicity from clarithromycin. Two additional oral studies in a different rat strain at similar doses and similar conditions demonstrated a low incidence of cardiovascular anomalies at doses of 150 mg/kg/day administered during gestation days 6 to 15. Plasma levels after 150 mg/kg/day were 2 times the human serum levels. Four studies in mice revealed a variable incidence of cleft palate following oral doses of 1000 mg/kg/day (2 and 4 times the recommended maximum human dose based on mg/m², respectively) during gestation days 6 to 15. Cleft palate was also seen at 500 mg/kg/day. The 1000 mg/kg/day exposure resulted in plasma levels 17 times the human serum levels. In monkeys, an oral dose of 70 mg/kg/day (an approximate equidose of the recommended maximum human dose based on mg/m²) produced fetal growth retardation at plasma levels that were 2 times the human serum levels.

There are no adequate and well-controlled studies in pregnant women. Clarithromycin should be used during pregnancy only if the potential benefit justifies the potential risk to the fetus (see **WARNINGS**).

Nursing Mothers

Clarithromycin and its active metabolite 14-hydroxy clarithromycin are excreted in human milk. Serum and milk samples were obtained after 3 days of treatment, at steady state, from one published study of 12 lactating women who were taking clarithromycin 250 mg orally twice daily. Based on the limited data from this study, and assuming milk consumption of 150 mL/kg/day, an exclusively human milk fed infant would receive an estimated average of 136 mcg/kg/day of clarithromycin and its active metabolite, with this maternal dosage regimen. This is less than 2% of the maternal weight-adjusted dose (7.8 mg/kg/day, based on the average maternal weight of 64 kg), and less than 1% of the pediatric dose (15 mg/kg/day) for children greater than 6 months of age.

A prospective observational study of 55 breastfed infants of mothers taking a macrolide antibiotic (6 were exposed to clarithromycin) were compared to 36 breastfed infants of mothers taking amoxicillin. Adverse reactions were comparable in both groups. Adverse reactions occurred in 12.7% of infants exposed to macrolides and included rash, diarrhea, loss of appetite, and somnolence.

Caution should be exercised when clarithromycin is administered to nursing women. The development and health benefits of human milk feeding should be considered along with the mother's clinical need for Biaxin and any potential adverse effects on the human milk fed child from the drug or from the underlying maternal condition.

Pediatric Use

Safety and effectiveness of clarithromycin in pediatric patients under 6 months of age have not been established. The

Continued on next page

Information on the AbbVie, Inc. products listed on these pages is from the prescribing information in use as of July 31, 2016. For more information, please visit rxabbvie.com or call 1-800-633-9110.

safety of clarithromycin has not been studied in MAC patients under the age of 20 months. Neonatal and juvenile animals tolerated clarithromycin in a manner similar to adult animals. Young animals were slightly more intolerant to acute overdosage and to subtle reductions in erythrocytes, platelets and leukocytes but were less sensitive to toxicity in the liver, kidney, thymus, and genitalia.

Geriatric Use

In a steady-state study in which healthy elderly subjects (age 65 to 81 years old) were given 500 mg every 12 hours, the maximum serum concentrations and area under the curves of clarithromycin and 14-OH clarithromycin were increased compared to those achieved in healthy young adults. These changes in pharmacokinetics parallel known age-related decreases in renal function. In clinical trials, elderly patients did not have an increased incidence of adverse events when compared to younger patients. Dosage adjustment should be considered in elderly patients with severe renal impairment. Elderly patients may be more susceptible to development of *torsades de pointes* arrhythmias than younger patients (see **WARNINGS** and **PRECAUTIONS**).

Most reports of acute kidney injury with calcium channel blockers metabolized by CYP3A4 (e.g., verapamil, amlodipine, diltiazem, nifedipine) involved elderly patients 65 years of age or older (see **WARNINGS**).

ADVERSE REACTIONS

The most frequent and common adverse reactions related to clarithromycin therapy for both adult and pediatric populations are abdominal pain, diarrhea, nausea, vomiting and dysgeusia. These adverse reactions are consistent with the known safety profile of macrolide antibiotics.

There is no significant difference in the incidence of these gastrointestinal adverse reactions during clinical trials between the patient population with or without preexisting mycobacterial infections.

Adverse Reactions Observed During Clinical Trials of Clarithromycin

The following adverse reactions were observed in clinical trials with clarithromycin at a rate greater than or equal to 1%:

Gastrointestinal Disorders

Diarrhea, vomiting, dyspepsia, nausea, abdominal pain

Hepatobiliary Disorders

Liver function test abnormal

Immune System Disorders

Anaphylactoid reaction

Infection and Infestations

Candidiasis

Nervous System Disorders

Dysgeusia, headache

Psychiatric Disorders

Insomnia

Skin and Subcutaneous Tissue Disorders

Rash

Other Adverse Reactions Observed During Clinical Trials of Clarithromycin

The following adverse reactions were observed in clinical trials with clarithromycin at a rate less than 1%:

Blood and Lymphatic System Disorders

Leukopenia, neutropenia, thrombocythemia, eosinophilia

Cardiac Disorders

Electrocardiogram QT prolonged, cardiac arrest, atrial fibrillation, extrasystoles, palpitations

Ear and Labyrinth Disorders

Vertigo, tinnitus, hearing impaired

Gastrointestinal Disorders

Stomatitis, glossitis, esophagitis, gastrooesophageal reflux disease, gastritis, proctalgia, abdominal distension, constipation, dry mouth, eructation, flatulence

General Disorders and Administration Site Conditions

Malaise, pyrexia, asthenia, chest pain, chills, fatigue

Hepatobiliary Disorders

Cholestasis, hepatitis

Immune System Disorders

Hypersensitivity

Infections and Infestations

Cellulitis, gastroenteritis, infection, vaginal infection

Investigations

Blood bilirubin increased, blood alkaline phosphatase increased, blood lactate dehydrogenase increased, albumin globulin ratio abnormal

Metabolism and Nutrition Disorders

Anorexia, decreased appetite

Musculoskeletal and Connective Tissue Disorders

Myalgia, muscle spasms, nuchal rigidity

Nervous System Disorders

Dizziness, tremor, loss of consciousness, dyskinesia, somnolence

Psychiatric Disorders

Anxiety, nervousness

Renal and Urinary Disorders

Blood creatinine increased, blood urea increased

Respiratory, Thoracic and Mediastinal Disorders

Asthma, epistaxis, pulmonary embolism

Skin and Subcutaneous Tissue Disorders

Urticaria, dermatitis bullous, pruritus, hyperhidrosis, rash maculo-papular

In the acute exacerbation of chronic bronchitis and acute maxillary sinusitis studies overall gastrointestinal adverse events were reported by a similar proportion of patients taking either BIAXIN tablets or BIAXIN XL tablets; however, patients taking BIAXIN XL tablets reported significantly less severe gastrointestinal symptoms compared to patients taking BIAXIN tablets. In addition, patients taking BIAXIN XL tablets had significantly fewer premature discontinuations for drug-related gastrointestinal or abnormal taste adverse events compared to BIAXIN tablets.

In community-acquired pneumonia studies conducted in adults comparing clarithromycin to erythromycin base or erythromycin stearate, there were fewer adverse events involving the digestive system in clarithromycin-treated patients compared to erythromycin-treated patients (13% vs 32%; p < 0.01). Twenty percent of erythromycin-treated patients discontinued therapy due to adverse events compared to 4% of clarithromycin-treated patients.

In two U.S. studies of acute otitis media comparing clarithromycin to amoxicillin/potassium clavulanate in pediatric patients, there were fewer adverse events involving the digestive system in clarithromycin-treated patients compared to amoxicillin/potassium clavulanate-treated patients (21% vs. 40%, p < 0.001). One-third as many clarithromycin-treated patients reported diarrhea as did amoxicillin/potassium clavulanate-treated patients.

Post-Marketing Experience

The following adverse reactions have been identified during post approval use of clarithromycin. Because these reactions are reported voluntarily from a population of uncertain size, it is not always possible to reliably estimate their frequency or establish a causal relationship to drug exposure.

Blood and Lymphatic System Disorders

Thrombocytopenia, agranulocytosis

Cardiac Disorders

Torsades de pointes, ventricular tachycardia, ventricular arrhythmia

Ear and Labyrinth Disorders

Deafness was reported chiefly in elderly women and was usually reversible.

Gastrointestinal Disorders

Pancreatitis acute, tongue discoloration, tooth discoloration was reported and was usually reversible with professional cleaning upon discontinuation of the drug. There have been reports of BIAXIN XL tablets in the stool, many of which have occurred in patients with anatomic (including ileostomy or colostomy) or functional gastrointestinal disorders with shortened GI transit times. In several reports, tablet residues have occurred in the context of diarrhea. It is recommended that patients who experience tablet residue in the stool and no improvement in their condition should be switched to a different clarithromycin formulation (e.g. suspension) or another antibacterial drug.

Hepatobiliary Disorders

Hepatic failure, jaundice hepatocellular. Adverse reactions related to hepatic dysfunction have been reported with clarithromycin (see **WARNINGS - Hepatotoxicity**).

Immune System Disorders

Anaphylactic reaction, angioedema

Infections and Infestations

Pseudomembranous colitis

Investigations

Prothrombin time prolonged, white blood cell count decreased, international normalized ratio increased. Abnormal urine color has been reported, associated with hepatic failure.

Metabolism and Nutrition Disorders

Hypoglycemia has been reported in patients taking oral hypoglycemic agents or insulin.

Musculoskeletal and Connective Tissue Disorders

Myopathy, rhabdomyolysis was reported and in some of the reports, clarithromycin was administered concomitantly with statins, fibrates, colchicine or allopurinol (see **CONTRAINDICATIONS** and **WARNINGS**).

Nervous System Disorders

Convulsion, ageusia, parosmia, anosmia, paraesthesia

Psychiatric Disorders

Psychotic disorder, confusional state, depersonalization, depression, disorientation, manic behavior, hallucination, abnormal behavior, abnormal dreams. These disorders usually resolve upon discontinuation of the drug.

There are no data on the effect of clarithromycin on the ability to drive or use machines. The potential for dizziness, vertigo, confusion and disorientation, which may occur with the medication, should be taken into account before patients drive or use machines.

Renal and Urinary Disorders

Nephritis interstitial, renal failure

Skin and Subcutaneous Tissue Disorders

Stevens-Johnson syndrome, toxic epidermal necrolysis, drug rash with eosinophilia and systemic symptoms (DRESS), Henoch-Schonlein purpura, acne

Vascular Disorders

Hemorrhage

There have been reports of colchicine toxicity with concomitant use of clarithromycin and colchicine, especially in the elderly, some of which occurred in patients with renal insufficiency. Deaths have been reported in some such patients (see **WARNINGS** and **PRECAUTIONS**).

OVERDOSAGE

Overdosage of clarithromycin can cause gastrointestinal symptoms such as abdominal pain, vomiting, nausea, and diarrhea.

Adverse reactions accompanying overdosage should be treated by the prompt elimination of unabsorbed drug and supportive measures. As with other macrolides, clarithromycin serum concentrations are not expected to be appreciably affected by hemodialysis or peritoneal dialysis.

DOSAGE AND ADMINISTRATION

BIAXIN® Filmtab® (clarithromycin tablets, USP) and BIAXIN® Granules (clarithromycin for oral suspension, USP) may be given with or without food. BIAXIN® XL Filmtab® (clarithromycin extended-release tablets) should be taken with food. BIAXIN XL tablets should be swallowed whole and not chewed, broken or crushed.

Clarithromycin may be administered without dosage adjustment in the presence of hepatic impairment if there is normal renal function. In patients with severe renal impairment ($CL_{CR} < 30$ mL/min), the dose of clarithromycin should be reduced by 50%. However, when patients with moderate or severe renal impairment are taking clarithromycin concomitantly with atazanavir or ritonavir, the dose of clarithromycin should be reduced by 50% or 75% for patients with CL_{CR} of 30 to 60 mL/min or < 30 mL/min, respectively.

[See table at top of next page]

H. pylori **Eradication to Reduce the Risk of Duodenal Ulcer Recurrence**

Triple therapy: BIAXIN/lansoprazole/amoxicillin

The recommended adult dose is 500 mg BIAXIN, 30 mg lansoprazole, and 1 gram amoxicillin, all given twice daily (q12h) for 10 or 14 days (see **INDICATIONS AND USAGE** and **CLINICAL STUDIES** sections).

Triple therapy: BIAXIN/omeprazole/amoxicillin

The recommended adult dose is 500 mg BIAXIN, 20 mg omeprazole, and 1 gram amoxicillin, all given twice daily (q12h) for 10 days (see **INDICATIONS AND USAGE** and **CLINICAL STUDIES** sections). In patients with an ulcer present at the time of initiation of therapy, an additional 18 days of omeprazole 20 mg once daily is recommended for ulcer healing and symptom relief.

Dual therapy: BIAXIN/omeprazole

The recommended adult dose is 500 mg BIAXIN given three times daily (q8h) and 40 mg omeprazole given once daily (qAM) for 14 days (see **INDICATIONS AND USAGE** and **CLINICAL STUDIES** sections). An additional 14 days of omeprazole 20 mg once daily is recommended for ulcer healing and symptom relief.

Dual therapy: BIAXIN/ranitidine bismuth citrate

The recommended adult dose is 500 mg BIAXIN given twice daily (q12h) or three times daily (q8h) and 400 mg ranitidine bismuth citrate given twice daily (q12h) for 14 days. An additional 14 days of 400 mg twice daily is recommended for

ADULT DOSAGE GUIDELINES

Infection	BIAXIN Tablets		BIAXIN XL Tablets	
	Dosage (q12h)	Duration (days)	Dosage (q24h)	Duration (days)
Pharyngitis/Tonsillitis due to				
S. pyogenes	250 mg	10	-	-
Acute maxillary sinusitis due to	500 mg	14	2 × 500 mg	14
H. influenzae				
M. catarrhalis				
S. pneumoniae				
Acute exacerbation of chronic bronchitis due to				
H. influenzae	500 m'g	7-14	2 × 500 mg	7
H. parainfluenzae	500 mg	7	2 × 500 mg	7
M. catarrhalis	250 mg	7-14	2 × 500 mg	7
S. pneumoniae	250 mg	7-14	2 × 500 mg	7
Community-Acquired Pneumonia due to				
H. influenzae	250 mg	7	2 × 500 mg	7
H. parainfluenzae	-	-	2 × 500 mg	7
M. catarrhalis	-	-	2 × 500 mg	7
S. pneumoniae	250 mg	7-14	2 × 500 mg	7
C. pneumoniae	250 mg	7-14	2 × 500 mg	7
M. pneumoniae	250 mg	7-14	2 × 500 mg	7
Uncomplicated skin and skin structure	250 mg	7-14	-	-
S. aureus				
S. pyogenes				

ulcer healing and symptom relief. BIAXIN and ranitidine bismuth citrate combination therapy is not recommended in patients with creatinine clearance less than 25 mL/min (see **INDICATIONS AND USAGE** and **CLINICAL STUDIES** sections).

Children
The usual recommended daily dosage is 15 mg/kg/day divided q12h for 10 days.

PEDIATRIC DOSAGE GUIDELINES

Based on Body Weight

Dosing Calculated on 7.5 mg/kg q12h

Weight		Dose		
Kg	lbs	(q12h)	125 mg/5 mL	250 mg/5 mL
9	20	62.5 mg	2.5 mL q12h	1.25 mL q12h
17	37	125 mg	5 mL q12h	2.5 mL q12h
25	55	187.5 mg	7.5 mL q12h	3.75 mL q12h
33	73	250 mg	10 mL q12h	5 mL q12h

Mycobacterial Infections
Prophylaxis
The recommended dose of BIAXIN for the prevention of disseminated *Mycobacterium avium* disease is 500 mg b.i.d. In children, the recommended dose is 7.5 mg/kg b.i.d. up to 500 mg b.i.d. No studies of clarithromycin for MAC prophylaxis have been performed in pediatric populations and the doses recommended for prophylaxis are derived from MAC treatment studies in children. Dosing recommendations for children are in the table above.
Treatment
Clarithromycin is recommended as the primary agent for the treatment of disseminated infection due to *Mycobacterium avium* complex. Clarithromycin should be used in combination with other antimycobacterial drugs that have shown *in vitro* activity against MAC or clinical benefit in MAC treatment (see **CLINICAL STUDIES**). The recom-

mended dose for mycobacterial infections in adults is 500 mg b.i.d. In children, the recommended dose is 7.5 mg/kg b.i.d. up to 500 mg b.i.d. Dosing recommendations for children are in the table above.
Clarithromycin therapy should continue if clinical response is observed. Clarithromycin can be discontinued when the patient is considered at low risk of disseminated infection.
Constituting Instructions
The table below indicates the volume of water to be added when constituting:

Total Volume After Constitution	Clarithromycin Concentration After Constitution	Amount of Water to be Added*
50 mL	125 mg/5 mL	27 mL
100 mL	125 mg/5 mL	55 mL
50 mL	250 mg/5 mL	27 mL
100 mL	250 mg/5 mL	55 mL

* see instructions below.

Add half the volume of water to the bottle and shake vigorously. Add the remainder of water to the bottle and shake. Shake well before each use. Oversize bottle provides shake space. Keep tightly closed. Do not refrigerate. After mixing, store below 25°C (77°F) and use within 14 days.

HOW SUPPLIED
BIAXIN® Filmtab® (clarithromycin tablets, USP) are supplied as yellow oval film-coated tablets in the following packaging sizes:
250 mg tablets: (imprinted in blue with the "a" logo and code KT)
Bottles of 60 (**NDC** 0074-3368-60) and unit dose strip packages of 100 (**NDC** 0074-3368-11).

Store BIAXIN 250 mg tablets at controlled room temperature 15° to 30°C (59° to 86°F) in a well-closed container. Protect from light.
500 mg tablets: (debossed with the "a" logo on one side and code KL on the opposite side)
Bottles of 60 (**NDC** 0074-2586-60) and unit dose strip packages of 100 (**NDC** 0074-2586-11).
Store BIAXIN 500 mg tablets at controlled room temperature 20° to 25°C (68° to 77°F) in a well-closed container.
BIAXIN® XL Filmtab® (clarithromycin extended-release tablets) are supplied as yellow oval film-coated 500 mg tablets debossed (on one side) with the "a" logo and a two-letter code designation, KJ in the following packaging sizes:
500 mg tablets:
Bottles of 60 (**NDC** 0074-3165-60), unit dose strip packages of 100 (**NDC** 0074-3165-11), and BIAXIN® XL PAC carton of 4 blister packages 14 tablets each (**NDC** 0074-3165-41).
Store BIAXIN XL tablets at 20° to 25°C (68° to 77°F). Excursions permitted to 15° to 30°C (59° to 86°F). [See USP Controlled Room Temperature.]
BIAXIN® Granules (clarithromycin for oral suspension, USP) is supplied in the following strengths and sizes:
[See table at top of next page]
Store BIAXIN granules for oral suspension below 25°C (77°F) in a well-closed container. Do not refrigerate BIAXIN suspension.

CLINICAL STUDIES
Mycobacterial Infections
Prophylaxis
A randomized, double-blind study (561) compared clarithromycin 500 mg b.i.d. to placebo in patients with CDC-defined AIDS and CD_4 counts < 100 cells/μL. This study accrued 682 patients from November 1992 to January 1994, with a median CD_4 cell count at study entry of 30 cells/μL. Median duration of clarithromycin was 10.6 months vs. 8.2 months for placebo. More patients in the placebo arm than the clarithromycin arm discontinued prematurely from the study (75.6% and 67.4%, respectively). However, if premature discontinuations due to MAC or death are excluded, approximately equal percentages of patients on each arm (54.8% on clarithromycin and 52.5% on placebo) discontinued study drug early for other reasons. The study was designed to evaluate the following endpoints:
1. MAC bacteremia, defined as at least one positive culture for *M. avium* complex bacteria from blood or another normally sterile site.
2. Survival.
3. Clinically significant disseminated MAC disease, defined as MAC bacteremia accompanied by signs or symptoms of serious MAC infection, including fever, night sweats, weight loss, anemia, or elevations in liver function tests.
MAC Bacteremia
In patients randomized to clarithromycin, the risk of MAC bacteremia was reduced by 69% compared to placebo. The difference between groups was statistically significant (p < 0.001). On an intent-to-treat basis, the one-year cumulative incidence of MAC bacteremia was 5.0% for patients randomized to clarithromycin and 19.4% for patients randomized to placebo. While only 19 of the 341 patients randomized to clarithromycin developed MAC, 11 of these cases were resistant to clarithromycin. The patients with resistant MAC bacteremia had a median baseline CD_4 count of 10 cells/mm³ (range 2 to 25 cells/mm³). Information regarding the clinical course and response to treatment of the patients with resistant MAC bacteremia is limited. The 8 patients who received clarithromycin and developed susceptible MAC bacteremia had a median baseline CD_4 count of 25 cells/mm³ (range 10 to 80 cells/mm³). Comparatively, 53 of the 341 placebo patients developed MAC; none of these isolates were resistant to clarithromycin. The median baseline CD_4 count was 15 cells/mm³ (range 2 to 130 cells/mm³) for placebo patients that developed MAC.
Survival
A statistically significant survival benefit was observed.

	Mortality		Reduction in
	Placebo	Clarithromycin	Mortality on Clarithromycin

Continued on next page

Information on the AbbVie, Inc. products listed on these pages is from the prescribing information in use as of July 31, 2016. For more information, please visit rxabbvie.com or call 1-800-633-9110.

Survival All Randomized Patients

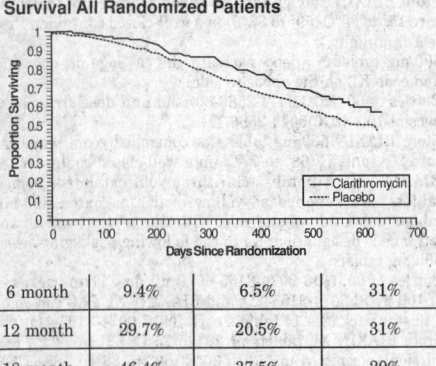

6 month	9.4%	6.5%	31%
12 month	29.7%	20.5%	31%
18 month	46.4%	37.5%	20%

Since the analysis at 18 months includes patients no longer receiving prophylaxis the survival benefit of clarithromycin may be underestimated.

Clinically Significant Disseminated MAC Disease
In association with the decreased incidence of bacteremia, patients in the group randomized to clarithromycin showed reductions in the signs and symptoms of disseminated MAC disease, including fever, night sweats, weight loss, and anemia.

Safety
In AIDS patients treated with clarithromycin over long periods of time for prophylaxis against *M. avium*, it was often difficult to distinguish adverse events possibly associated with clarithromycin administration from underlying HIV disease or intercurrent illness. Median duration of treatment was 10.6 months for the clarithromycin group and 8.2 months for the placebo group.

Treatment-related* Adverse Event Incidence Rates (%) in Immunocompromised Adult Patients Receiving Prophylaxis Against *M. avium* Complex

Body System[‡] Adverse Event	Clarithromycin (n = 339) %	Placebo (n = 339) %
Body as a Whole		
Abdominal pain	5.0%	3.5%
Headache	2.7%	0.9%
Digestive		
Diarrhea	7.7%	4.1%
Dyspepsia	3.8%	2.7%
Flatulence	2.4%	0.9%
Nausea	11.2%	7.1%
Vomiting	5.9%	3.2%
Skin & Appendages		
Rash	3.2%	3.5%
Special Senses		
Taste Perversion	8.0%	0.3%

* Includes those events possibly or probably related to study drug and excludes concurrent conditions.
‡ > 2% Adverse Event Incidence Rates for either treatment group.

Among these events, taste perversion was the only event that had significantly higher incidence in the clarithromycin-treated group compared to the placebo-treated group.
Discontinuation due to adverse events was required in 18% of patients receiving clarithromycin compared to 17% of patients receiving placebo in this trial. Primary reasons for discontinuation in clarithromycin treated patients include headache, nausea, vomiting, depression and taste perversion.
Changes in Laboratory Values of Potential Clinical Importance

Total Volume After Constitution	Clarithromycin Concentration After Constitution	Clarithromycin Contents Per Bottle	NDC
50 mL	125 mg/5 mL	1250 mg	0074-3163-50
100 mL	125 mg/5 mL	2500 mg	0074-3163-13
50 mL	250 mg/5 mL	2500 mg	0074-3188-50
100 mL	250 mg/5 mL	5000 mg	0074-3188-13

In immunocompromised patients receiving prophylaxis against *M. avium*, evaluations of laboratory values were made by analyzing those values outside the seriously abnormal value (i.e., the extreme high or low limit) for the specified test.

Percentage of Patients[a] Exceeding Extreme Laboratory Value in Patients Receiving Prophylaxis Against *M. avium* Complex

		Clarithromycin 500 mg b.i.d.	Placebo
Hemoglobin	< 8 g/dL	4/118 3%	5/103 5%
Platelet Count	< 50 × 10⁹/L	11/249 4%	12/250 5%
WBC Count	< 1 × 10⁹/L	2/103 4%	0/95 0%
SGOT	> 5 × ULN[b]	7/196 4%	5/208 2%
SGPT	> 5 × ULN[b]	6/217 3%	4/232 2%
Alk. Phos.	> 5 × ULN[b]	5/220 2%	5/218 2%

(a) Includes only patients with baseline values within the normal range or borderline high (hematology variables) and within the normal range or borderline low (chemistry variables).
(b) ULN = Upper Limit of Normal

Treatment
Three randomized studies (500, 577, and 521) compared different dosages of clarithromycin in patients with CDC-defined AIDS and CD$_4$ counts < 100 cells/µL. These studies accrued patients from May 1991 to March 1992. Study 500 was randomized, double-blind; Study 577 was open-label compassionate use. Both studies used 500 and 1000 mg b.i.d. doses; Study 500 also had a 2000 mg b.i.d. dose. Study 521 was a pediatric study at 3.75, 7.5, and 15 mg/kg b.i.d. Study 500 enrolled 154 adult patients, Study 577 enrolled 469 adult patients, and Study 521 enrolled 25 patients between the ages of 1 to 20. The majority of patients had CD$_4$ cell counts <50/µL at study entry. The studies were designed to evaluate the following end points:
1. Change in MAC bacteremia or blood cultures negative for *M. avium*.
2. Change in clinical signs and symptoms of MAC infection including one or more of the following: fever, night sweats, weight loss, diarrhea, splenomegaly, and hepatomegaly.
The results for the 500 study are described below. The 577 study results were similar to the results of the 500 study. Results with the 7.5 mg/kg b.i.d. dose in the pediatric study were comparable to those for the 500 mg b.i.d. regimen in the adult studies.
Study 069 compared the safety and efficacy of clarithromycin in combination with ethambutol versus clarithromycin in combination with ethambutol and clofazimine for the treatment of disseminated MAC (dMAC) infection.[4,5] This 24-week study enrolled 106 patients with AIDS and dMAC, with 55 patients randomized to receive clarithromycin and ethambutol, and 51 patients randomized to receive clarithromycin, ethambutol, and clofazimine. Baseline characteristics between study arms were similar with the exception of median CFU counts being at least 1 log higher in the clarithromycin, ethambutol, and clofazimine arm.
Compared to prior experience with clarithromycin monotherapy, the two-drug regimen of clarithromycin and ethambutol was well tolerated and extended the time to microbiologic relapse, largely through suppressing the emergence of clarithromycin resistant strains. However, the addition of clofazimine to the regimen added no additional microbio-

logic or clinical benefit. Tolerability of both multidrug regimens was comparable with the most common adverse events being gastrointestinal in nature. Patients receiving the clofazimine-containing regimen had reduced survival rates; however, their baseline mycobacterial colony counts were higher. The results of this trial support the addition of ethambutol to clarithromycin for the treatment of initial dMAC infections but do not support adding clofazimine as a third agent.
MAC Bacteremia
Decreases in MAC bacteremia or negative blood cultures were seen in the majority of patients in all dose groups. Mean reductions in colony forming units (CFU) are shown below. Included in the table are results from a separate study with a four drug regimen[6] (ciprofloxacin, ethambutol, rifampicin, and clofazimine). Since patient populations and study procedures may vary between these two studies, comparisons between the clarithromycin results and the combination therapy results should be interpreted cautiously.

Mean Reductions in Log CFU from Baseline (After 4 Weeks of Therapy)

500 mg b.i.d. (N = 35)	1000 mg b.i.d. (N = 32)	2000 mg b.i.d. (N = 26)	Four Drug Regimen (N = 24)
1.5	2.3	2.3	1.4

Although the 1000 mg and 2000 mg b.i.d. doses showed significantly better control of bacteremia during the first four weeks of therapy, no significant differences were seen beyond that point. The percent of patients whose blood was sterilized as shown by one or more negative cultures at any time during acute therapy was 61% (30/49) for the 500 mg b.i.d. group and 59% (29/49) and 52% (25/48) for the 1000 and 2000 mg b.i.d. groups, respectively. The percent of patients who had 2 or more negative cultures during acute therapy that were sustained through study Day 84 was 25% (12/49) in both the 500 and 1000 mg b.i.d. groups and 8% (4/48) for the 2000 mg b.i.d. group. By Day 84, 23% (11/49), 37% (18/49), and 56% (27/48) of patients had died or discontinued from the study, and 14% (7/49), 12% (6/49), and 13% (6/48) of patients had relapsed in the 500, 1000, and 2000 mg b.i.d. dose groups, respectively. All of the isolates had an MIC < 8 mcg/mL at pre-treatment. Relapse was almost always accompanied by an increase in MIC. The median time to first negative culture was 54, 41, and 29 days for the 500, 1000, and 2000 mg b.i.d. groups, respectively. The time to first decrease of at least 1 log in CFU count was significantly shorter with the 1000 and 2000 mg b.i.d. doses (median equal to 16 and 15 days, respectively) in comparison to the 500 mg b.i.d. group (median equal to 29 days). The median time to first positive culture or study discontinuation following the first negative culture was 43, 59 and 43 days for the 500, 1000, and 2000 mg b.i.d. groups, respectively.
Clinically Significant Disseminated MAC Disease
Among patients experiencing night sweats prior to therapy, 84% showed resolution or improvement at some point during the 12 weeks of clarithromycin at 500 to 2000 mg b.i.d. doses. Similarly, 77% of patients reported resolution or improvement in fevers at some point. Response rates for clinical signs of MAC are given below:
[See table at top of next page]
[See first table at top of page 626]
The median duration of response, defined as improvement or resolution of clinical signs and symptoms, was 2 to 6 weeks.
Since the study was not designed to determine the benefit of monotherapy beyond 12 weeks, the duration of response may be underestimated for the 25 to 33% of patients who continued to show clinical response after 12 weeks.

Resolution of Fever			Resolution of Night Sweats		
b.i.d. dose (mg)	% ever afebrile	% afebrile ≥ 6 weeks	b.i.d. dose (mg)	% ever resolving	% resolving ≥ 6 weeks
500	67%	23%	500	85%	42%
1000	67%	12%	1000	70%	33%
2000	62%	22%	2000	72%	36%

Survival

Median survival time from study entry (Study 500) was 249 days at the 500 mg b.i.d. dose compared to 215 days with the 1000 mg b.i.d. dose. However, during the first 12 weeks of therapy, there were 2 deaths in 53 patients in the 500 mg b.i.d. group versus 13 deaths in 51 patients in the 1000 mg b.i.d. group. The reason for this apparent mortality difference is not known. Survival in the two groups was similar beyond 12 weeks. The median survival times for these dosages were similar to recent historical controls with MAC when treated with combination therapies.[6]

Median survival time from study entry in Study 577 was 199 days for the 500 mg b.i.d. dose and 179 days for the 1000 mg b.i.d. dose. During the first four weeks of therapy, while patients were maintained on their originally assigned dose, there were 11 deaths in 255 patients taking 500 mg b.i.d. and 18 deaths in 214 patients taking 1000 mg b.i.d.

Safety

The adverse event profiles showed that both the 500 and 1000 mg b.i.d. doses were well tolerated. The 2000 mg b.i.d. dose was poorly tolerated and resulted in a higher proportion of premature discontinuations.

In AIDS patients and other immunocompromised patients treated with the higher doses of clarithromycin over long periods of time for mycobacterial infections, it was often difficult to distinguish adverse events possibly associated with clarithromycin administration from underlying signs of HIV disease or intercurrent illness.

The following analyses summarize experience during the first 12 weeks of therapy with clarithromycin. Data are reported separately for Study 500 (randomized, double-blind) and Study 577 (open-label, compassionate use) and also combined. Adverse events were reported less frequently in Study 577, which may be due in part to differences in monitoring between the two studies. In adult patients receiving clarithromycin 500 mg b.i.d., the most frequently reported adverse events, considered possibly or probably related to study drug, with an incidence of 5% or greater, are listed below. Most of these events were mild to moderate in severity, although 5% (Study 500: 8%; Study 577: 4%) of patients receiving 500 mg b.i.d. and 5% (Study 500: 4%; Study 577: 6%) of patients receiving 1000 mg b.i.d. reported severe adverse events. Excluding those patients who discontinued therapy or died due to complications of their underlying non-mycobacterial disease, approximately 8% (Study 500: 15%; Study 577: 7%) of the patients who received 500 mg b.i.d. and 12% (Study 500: 14%; Study 577: 12%) of the patients who received 1000 mg b.i.d. discontinued therapy due to drug-related events during the first 12 weeks of therapy. Overall, the 500 and 1000 mg b.i.d. doses had similar adverse event profiles.

Treatment-related* Adverse Event Incidence Rates (%) in Immunocompromised Adult Patients During the First 12 Weeks of Therapy with 500 mg b.i.d. Clarithromycin Dose

Adverse Event	Study 500 (n = 53)	Study 577 (n = 255)	Combined (n = 308)
Abdominal Pain	7.5	2.4	3.2
Diarrhea	9.4	1.6	2.9
Flatulence	7.5	0.0	1.3
Headache	7.5	0.4	1.6
Nausea	28.3	9.0	12.3
Rash	9.4	2.0	3.2
Taste Perversion	18.9	0.4	3.6
Vomiting	24.5	3.9	7.5

* Includes those events possibly or probably related to study drug and excludes concurrent conditions.

A limited number of pediatric AIDS patients have been treated with clarithromycin suspension for mycobacterial infections. The most frequently reported adverse events, excluding those due to the patient's concurrent condition, were consistent with those observed in adult patients.

Changes in Laboratory Values

In immunocompromised patients treated with clarithromycin for mycobacterial infections, evaluations of laboratory values were made by analyzing those values outside the seriously abnormal level (i.e., the extreme high or low limit) for the specified test.

Percentage of Patients[a] Exceeding Extreme Laboratory Value Limits During First 12 Weeks of Treatment 500 mg b.i.d. Dose[b]

		Study 500	Study 577	Combined
BUN	> 50 mg/dL	0%	< 1%	< 1%
Platelet Count	< 50 × 10⁹/L	0%	< 1%	< 1%
SGOT	> 5 × ULN[c]	0%	3%	2%
SGPT	> 5 × ULN[c]	0%	2%	1%
WBC	< 1 × 10⁹/L	0%	1%	1%

(a) Includes only patients with baseline values within the normal range or borderline high (hematology variables) and within the normal range or borderline low (chemistry variables).
(b) Includes all values within the first 12 weeks for patients who start on 500 mg b.i.d.
(c) ULN = Upper Limit of Normal

Otitis Media

In a controlled clinical study of acute otitis media performed in the United States, where significant rates of beta-lactamase producing organisms were found, clarithromycin was compared to an oral cephalosporin. In this study, very strict evaluability criteria were used to determine clinical response. For the 223 patients who were evaluated for clinical efficacy, the clinical success rate (i.e., cure plus improvement) at the post-therapy visit was 88% for clarithromycin and 91% for the cephalosporin.

In a smaller number of patients, microbiologic determinations were made at the pre-treatment visit. The following presumptive bacterial eradication/clinical cure outcomes (i.e., clinical success) were obtained:

U.S. Acute Otitis Media Study Clarithromycin vs. Oral Cephalosporin EFFICACY RESULTS

PATHOGEN	OUTCOME
S. pneumoniae	clarithromycin success rate, 13/15 (87%), control 4/5
H. influenzae*	clarithromycin success rate, 10/14 (71%), control 3/4
M. catarrhalis	clarithromycin success rate, 4/5, control 1/1
S. pyogenes	clarithromycin success rate, 3/3, control 0/1
Overall	clarithromycin success rate, 30/37 (81%), control 8/11 (73%)

* None of the *H. influenzae* isolated pre-treatment was resistant to clarithromycin; 6% were resistant to the control agent.

Safety

The incidence of adverse events in all patients treated, primarily diarrhea and vomiting, did not differ clinically or statistically for the two agents.

In two other controlled clinical trials of acute otitis media performed in the United States, where significant rates of beta-lactamase producing organisms were found, clarithromycin was compared to an oral antimicrobial agent that contained a specific beta-lactamase inhibitor. In these studies, very strict evaluability criteria were used to determine the clinical responses. In the 233 patients who were evaluated for clinical efficacy, the combined clinical success rate (i.e., cure and improvement) at the post-therapy visit was 91% for both clarithromycin and the control.

For the patients who had microbiologic determinations at the pre-treatment visit, the following presumptive bacterial eradication/clinical cure outcomes (i.e., clinical success) were obtained:

Two U.S. Acute Otitis Media Studies Clarithromycin vs. Antimicrobial/Beta-lactamase Inhibitor EFFICACY RESULTS

PATHOGEN	OUTCOME
S. pneumoniae	clarithromycin success rate, 43/51 (84%), control 55/56 (98%)
H. influenzae*	clarithromycin success rate, 36/45 (80%), control 31/33 (94%)
M. catarrhalis	clarithromycin success rate, 9/10 (90%), control 6/6
S. pyogenes	clarithromycin success rate, 3/3, control 5/5
Overall	clarithromycin success rate, 91/109 (83%), control 97/100 (97%)

* Of the *H. influenzae* isolated pre-treatment, 3% were resistant to clarithromycin and 10% were resistant to the control agent.

Safety

The incidence of adverse events in all patients treated, primarily diarrhea (15% vs. 38%) and diaper rash (3% vs. 11%) in young children, was clinically and statistically lower in the clarithromycin arm versus the control arm.

Duodenal Ulcer Associated with *H. pylori* Infection

Clarithromycin + Lansoprazole and Amoxicillin

H. pylori Eradication for Reducing the Risk of Duodenal Ulcer Recurrence

Two U.S. randomized, double-blind clinical studies in patients with *H. pylori* and duodenal ulcer disease (defined as an active ulcer or history of an active ulcer within one year) evaluated the efficacy of clarithromycin in combination with lansoprazole and amoxicillin capsules as triple 14-day therapy for eradication of *H. pylori*. Based on the results of these studies, the safety and efficacy of the following eradication regimen were established:

Triple therapy: BIAXIN (clarithromycin) 500 mg b.i.d. + lansoprazole 30 mg b.i.d. + amoxicillin 1 gm b.i.d.

Treatment was for 14 days. *H. pylori* eradication was defined as two negative tests (culture and histology) at 4 to 6 weeks following the end of treatment.

The combination of BIAXIN plus lansoprazole and amoxicillin as triple therapy was effective in eradicating *H. pylori*. Eradication of *H. pylori* has been shown to reduce the risk of duodenal ulcer recurrence.

A randomized, double-blind clinical study performed in the U.S. in patients with *H. pylori* and duodenal ulcer disease (defined as an active ulcer or history of an ulcer within one year) compared the efficacy of clarithromycin in combination with lansoprazole and amoxicillin as triple therapy for

Continued on next page

Information on the AbbVie, Inc. products listed on these pages is from the prescribing information in use as of July 31, 2016. For more information, please visit rxabbvie.com or call 1-800-633-9110.

10 and 14 days. This study established that the 10-day triple therapy was equivalent to the 14-day triple therapy in eradicating *H. pylori*.
[See second table at right]

Clarithromycin + Omeprazole and Amoxicillin Therapy

H. pylori Eradication for Reducing the Risk of Duodenal Ulcer Recurrence

Three U.S., randomized, double-blind clinical studies in patients with *H. pylori* infection and duodenal ulcer disease (n = 558) compared clarithromycin plus omeprazole and amoxicillin to clarithromycin plus amoxicillin. Two studies (Studies 126 and 127) were conducted in patients with an active duodenal ulcer, and the third study (Study 446) was conducted in patients with a duodenal ulcer in the past 5 years, but without an ulcer present at the time of enrollment. The dosage regimen in the studies was clarithromycin 500 mg b.i.d. plus omeprazole 20 mg b.i.d. plus amoxicillin 1 gram b.i.d. for 10 days. In Studies 126 and 127, patients who took the omeprazole regimen also received an additional 18 days of omeprazole 20 mg q.d. Endpoints studied were eradication of *H. pylori* and duodenal ulcer healing (studies 126 and 127 only). *H. pylori* status was determined by CLOtest®, histology, and culture in all three studies. For a given patient, *H. pylori* was considered eradicated if at least two of these tests were negative, and none was positive. The combination of clarithromycin plus omeprazole and amoxicillin was effective in eradicating *H. pylori*.
[See table below]

Safety

In clinical trials using combination therapy with clarithromycin plus omeprazole and amoxicillin, no adverse reactions peculiar to the combination of these drugs have been observed. Adverse reactions that have occurred have been limited to those that have been previously reported with clarithromycin, omeprazole, or amoxicillin.

The most frequent adverse experiences observed in clinical trials using combination therapy with clarithromycin plus omeprazole and amoxicillin (n = 274) were diarrhea (14%), taste perversion (10%), and headache (7%).

For information about adverse reactions with omeprazole or amoxicillin, refer to the **ADVERSE REACTIONS** section of their package inserts.

Clarithromycin + Omeprazole Therapy

Four randomized, double-blind, multi-center studies (067, 100, 812b, and 058) evaluated clarithromycin 500 mg t.i.d. plus omeprazole 40 mg q.d. for 14 days, followed by omeprazole 20 mg q.d. (067, 100, and 058) or by omeprazole 40 mg q.d. (812b) for an additional 14 days in patients with active duodenal ulcer associated with *H. pylori*. Studies 067 and 100 were conducted in the U.S. and Canada and enrolled 242 and 256 patients, respectively. *H. pylori* infection and duodenal ulcer were confirmed in 219 patients in Study 067 and 228 patients in Study 100. These studies compared the combination regimen to omeprazole and clarithromycin monotherapies. Studies 812b and 058 were conducted in Europe and enrolled 154 and 215 patients, respectively. *H. pylori* infection and duodenal ulcer were confirmed in 148 patients in Study 812b and 208 patients in Study 058.

Weight Gain > 3%			Hemoglobin Increase > 1 gm		
b.i.d. dose (mg)	% ever gaining	% gaining ≥ 6 weeks	b.i.d. dose (mg)	% ever increasing	% increasing ≥ 6 weeks
500	33%	14%	500	58%	26%
1000	26%	17%	1000	37%	6%
2000	26%	12%	2000	62%	18%

H. pylori Eradication Rates-Triple Therapy (BIAXIN/lansoprazole/amoxicillin) Percent of Patients Cured [95% Confidence Interval] (number of patients)

Study	Duration	Triple Therapy Evaluable Analysis*	Triple Therapy Intent-to-Treat Analysis#
M93-131	14 days	92[†] [80.0-97.7] (n = 48)	86[†] [73.3-93.5] (n = 55)
M95-392	14 days	86[‡] [75.7-93.6] (n = 66)	83[‡] [72.0-90.8] (n = 70)
M95-399[¶]	14 days	85 [77.0-91.0] (N = 113)	82 [73.9-88.1] (N = 126)
	10 days	84 [76.0-89.8] (N = 123)	81 [73.9-87.6] (N = 135)

* Based on evaluable patients with confirmed duodenal ulcer (active or within one year) and *H. pylori* infection at baseline defined as at least two of three positive endoscopic tests from CLOtest (Delta West LTD., Bentley, Australia), histology, and/or culture. Patients were included in the analysis if they completed the study. Additionally, if patients were dropped out of the study due to an adverse event related to the study drug, they were included in the analysis as evaluable failures of therapy.

\# Patients were included in the analysis if they had documented *H. pylori* infection at baseline as defined above and had a confirmed duodenal ulcer (active or within one year). All dropouts were included as failures of therapy.

† (p < 0.05) versus BIAXIN/lansoprazole and lansoprazole/amoxicillin dual therapy.

‡ (p < 0.05) versus BIAXIN/amoxicillin dual therapy.

¶ The 95% confidence interval for the difference in eradication rates, 10-day minus 14-day, is (-10.5, 8.1) in the evaluable analysis and (-9.7, 9.1) in the intent-to-treat analysis.

These studies compared the combination regimen to omeprazole monotherapy. The results for the efficacy analyses for these studies are described below.

Duodenal Ulcer Healing

The combination of clarithromycin and omeprazole was as effective as omeprazole alone for healing duodenal ulcer.
[See first table at the top of next page]

Eradication of H. pylori Associated with Duodenal Ulcer

The combination of clarithromycin and omeprazole was effective in eradicating *H. pylori*.
[See second table at the top of next page]

H. pylori eradication was defined as no positive test (culture or histology) at 4 weeks following the end of treatment, and two negative tests were required to be considered eradicated. In the per-protocol analysis, the following patients were excluded: dropouts, patients with major protocol violations, patients with missing *H. pylori* tests post-treatment, and patients that were not assessed for *H. pylori* eradica-

tion at 4 weeks after the end of treatment because they were found to have an unhealed ulcer at the end of treatment. Ulcer recurrence at 6-months following the end of treatment was assessed for patients in whom ulcers were healed post-treatment.

Ulcer Recurrence at 6 months by H. pylori Status at 4-6 Weeks

	H. pylori Negative	H. pylori Positive
U.S. Studies		
Study 100		
Clarithromycin + Omeprazole	6% (2/34)	56% (9/16)
Omeprazole	- (0/0)	71% (35/49)
Clarithromycin	12% (2/17)	32% (7/22)
Study 067		
Clarithromycin + Omeprazole	38% (11/29)	50% (6/12)
Omeprazole	- (0/0)	67% (31/46)
Clarithromycin	18% (2/11)	52% (14/27)
Non-U.S. Studies		
Study 058		
Clarithromycin + Omeprazole	6% (3/53)	24% (4/17)
Omeprazole	0% (0/3)	55% (39/71)
Study 812b*		
Clarithromycin + Omeprazole	5% (2/42)	0% (0/7)
Omeprazole	0% (0/1)	54% (32/59)

Per-Protocol and Intent-to-Treat H. pylori Eradication Rates % of Patients Cured [95% Confidence Interval]

	Clarithromycin + omeprazole + amoxicillin		Clarithromycin + amoxicillin	
	Per-Protocol [†]	Intent-to-Treat [‡]	Per-Protocol [†]	Intent-to-Treat [‡]
Study 126	*77 [64, 86] (n = 64)	69 [57, 79] (n = 80)	43 [31, 56] (n = 67)	37 [27, 48] (n = 84)
Study 127	*78 [67, 88] (n = 65)	73 [61, 82] (n = 77)	41 [29, 54] (n = 68)	36 [26, 47] (n = 84)
Study M96-446	*90 [80, 96] (n = 69)	83 [74, 91] (n = 84)	33 [24, 44] (n = 93)	32 [23, 42] (n = 99)

† Patients were included in the analysis if they had confirmed duodenal ulcer disease (active ulcer studies 126 and 127; history of ulcer within 5 years, study M96-446) and *H. pylori* infection at baseline defined as at least two of three positive endoscopic tests from CLOtest®, histology, and/or culture. Patients were included in the analysis if they completed the study. Additionally, if patients dropped out of the study due to an adverse event related to the study drug, they were included in the analysis as failures of therapy. The impact of eradication on ulcer recurrence has not been assessed in patients with a past history of ulcer.

‡ Patients were included in the analysis if they had documented *H. pylori* infection at baseline and had confirmed duodenal ulcer disease. All dropouts were included as failures of therapy.

* p < 0.05 versus clarithromycin plus amoxicillin.

*12-month recurrence rates:		
Clarithromycin + Omeprazole	3% (1/40)	0% (0/6)
Omeprazole	0% (0/1)	67% (29/43)

Thus, in patients with duodenal ulcer associated with *H. pylori* infection, eradication of *H. pylori* reduced ulcer recurrence.

Safety

The adverse event profiles for the four studies showed that the combination of clarithromycin 500 mg t.i.d. and omeprazole 40 mg q.d. for 14 days, followed by omeprazole 20 mg q.d. (067, 100, and 058) or 40 mg q.d. (812b) for an additional 14 days was well tolerated. Of the 346 patients who received the combination, 12 (3.5%) patients discontinued study drug due to adverse events.

[See third table at right]

Most of these events were mild to moderate in severity.

Changes in Laboratory Values

Changes in laboratory values with possible clinical significance in patients taking clarithromycin and omeprazole were as follows:

Hepatic - elevated direct bilirubin < 1%; GGT < 1%; SGOT (AST) < 1%; SGPT (ALT) < 1%.

Renal - elevated serum creatinine < 1%.

For information on omeprazole, refer to the **ADVERSE RE-ACTIONS** section of the PRILOSEC package insert.

Clarithromycin + Ranitidine Bismuth Citrate Therapy

In a U.S. double-blind, randomized, multicenter, dose-comparison trial, ranitidine bismuth citrate 400 mg b.i.d. for 4 weeks plus clarithromycin 500 mg b.i.d. for the first 2 weeks was found to have an equivalent *H. pylori* eradication rate (based on culture and histology) when compared to ranitidine bismuth citrate 400 mg b.i.d. for 4 weeks plus clarithromycin 500 mg t.i.d. for the first 2 weeks. The intent-to-treat *H. pylori* eradication rates are shown below:

[See fourth table at right]

H. pylori eradication was defined as no positive test at 4 weeks following the end of treatment. Patients must have had two tests performed, and these must have been negative to be considered eradicated of *H. pylori*. The following patients were excluded from the per-protocol analysis: patients not infected with *H. pylori* prestudy, dropouts, patients with major protocol violations, patients with missing *H. pylori* tests. Patients excluded from the intent-to-treat analysis included those not infected with *H. pylori* prestudy and those with missing *H. pylori* tests prestudy. Patients were assessed for *H. pylori* eradication (4 weeks following treatment) regardless of their healing status (at the end of treatment).

The relationship between *H. pylori* eradication and duodenal ulcer recurrence was assessed in a combined analysis of six U.S. randomized, double-blind, multicenter, placebo-controlled trials using ranitidine bismuth citrate with or without antibiotics. The results from approximately 650 U.S. patients showed that the risk of ulcer recurrence within 6 months of completing treatment was two times less likely in patients whose *H. pylori* infection was eradicated compared to patients in whom *H. pylori* infection was not eradicated.

Safety

In clinical trials using combination therapy with clarithromycin plus ranitidine bismuth citrate, no adverse reactions peculiar to the combination of these drugs (using clarithromycin twice daily or three times a day) were observed. Adverse reactions that have occurred have been limited to those reported with clarithromycin or ranitidine bismuth citrate. (See **ADVERSE REACTIONS** section of the Tritec package insert.) The most frequent adverse experiences observed in clinical trials using combination therapy with clarithromycin (500 mg three times a day) with ranitidine bismuth citrate (n = 329) were taste disturbance (11%), diarrhea (5%), nausea and vomiting (3%). The most frequent adverse experiences observed in clinical trials using combination therapy with clarithromycin (500 mg twice daily) with ranitidine bismuth citrate (n = 196) were taste disturbance (8%), nausea and vomiting (5%), and diarrhea (4%).

ANIMAL PHARMACOLOGY AND TOXICOLOGY

Clarithromycin is rapidly and well-absorbed with dose-linear kinetics, low protein binding, and a high volume of distribution. Plasma half-life ranged from 1 to 6 hours and

End-of-Treatment Ulcer Healing Rates Percent of Patients Healed (n/N)			
Study	Clarithromycin + Omeprazole	Omeprazole	Clarithromycin
U.S. Studies			
Study 100	94% (58/62)[†]	88% (60/68)	71% (49/69)
Study 067	88% (56/64)[†]	85% (55/65)	64% (44/69)
Non-U.S. Studies			
Study 058	99% (84/85)	95% (82/86)	N/A
Study 812b[1]	100% (64/64)	99% (71/72)	N/A

† p < 0.05 for clarithromycin + omeprazole versus clarithromycin monotherapy.
1 In Study 812b patients received omeprazole 40 mg daily for days 15 to 28.

H. pylori Eradication Rates (Per-Protocol Analysis) at 4 to 6 weeks Percent of Patients Cured (n/N)			
Study	Clarithromycin + Omeprazole	Omeprazole	Clarithromycin
U.S. Studies			
Study 100	64% (39/61)[†‡]	0% (0/59)	39% (17/44)
Study 067	74% (39/53)[†‡]	0% (0/54)	31% (13/42)
Non-U.S. Studies			
Study 058	74% (64/86)[‡]	1% (1/90)	N/A
Study 812b	83% (50/60)[‡]	1% (1/74)	N/A

† Statistically significantly higher than clarithromycin monotherapy (p < 0.05).
‡ Statistically significantly higher than omeprazole monotherapy (p < 0.05).

Adverse Events with an Incidence of 3% or Greater			
Adverse Event	Clarithromycin + Omeprazole (N = 346) % of Patients	Omeprazole (N = 355) % of Patients	Clarithromycin (N = 166) % of Patients*
Taste Perversion	15%	1%	16%
Nausea	5%	1%	3%
Headache	5%	6%	9%
Diarrhea	4%	3%	7%
Vomiting	4%	< 1%	1%
Abdominal Pain	3%	2%	1%
Infection	3%	4%	2%

* Studies 067 and 100, only.

H. pylori Eradication Rates in Study H2BA-3001			
Analysis	RBC 400 mg + Clarithromycin 500 mg b.i.d.	RBC 400 mg + Clarithromycin 500 mg t.i.d.	95% CI Rate Difference
ITT	65% (122/188) [58%, 72%]	63% (122/195) [55%, 69%]	(-8%, 12%)
Per-Protocol	72% (117/162) [65%, 79%]	71% (120/170) [63%, 77%]	(-9%, 12%)

was species dependent. High tissue concentrations were achieved, but negligible accumulation was observed. Fecal clearance predominated. Hepatotoxicity occurred in all species tested (i.e., in rats and monkeys at doses 2 times greater than and in dogs at doses comparable to the maximum human daily dose, based on mg/m^2). Renal tubular degeneration (calculated on a mg/m^2 basis) occurred in rats at doses 2 times, in monkeys at doses 8 times, and in dogs at doses 12 times greater than the maximum human daily dose. Testicular atrophy (on a mg/m^2 basis) occurred in rats at doses 7 times, in dogs at doses 3 times, and in monkeys at doses 8 times greater than the maximum human daily dose. Corneal opacity (on a mg/m^2 basis) occurred in dogs at doses 12 times and in monkeys at doses 8 times greater than the

maximum human daily dose. Lymphoid depletion (on a mg/m^2 basis) occurred in dogs at doses 3 times greater than and in monkeys at doses 2 times greater than the maximum human daily dose. These adverse events were absent during clinical trials.

Continued on next page

REFERENCES

1. Clinical and Laboratory Standards Institute (CLSI). Methods for Dilution Antimicrobial Susceptibility Tests for Bacteria that Grow Aerobically – 9th edition. Approved Standard. CLSI Document M07-A9, CLSI. 950 West Valley Rd, Suite 2500, Wayne, PA 19087, 2012.
2. CLSI. Performance Standards for Antimicrobial Susceptibility Testing, 23rd Informational Supplement, CLSI Document M100-S23, 2013.
3. CLSI. Performance Standards for Antimicrobial Disk Susceptibility Tests, 11th edition. Approved Standard CLSI Document M02-A11, 2012.
4. CLSI. Methods for Antimicrobial Dilution and Disk Diffusion Susceptibility Testing of Infrequently Isolated or Fastidious Bacteria – 2nd edition. CLSI document M45-A2, 2010.
5. Chaisson RE, et al. Clarithromycin and Ethambutol with or without Clofazimine for the Treatment of Bacteremic *Mycobacterium avium* Complex Disease in Patients with HIV Infection. AIDS. 1997;11:311-317.
6. Kemper CA, et al. Treatment of *Mycobacterium avium* Complex Bacteremia in AIDS with a Four-Drug Oral Regimen. *Ann Intern Med.* 1992;116:466-472.

Filmtab® – Film-sealed tablets, AbbVie Inc.

Biaxin Filmtab 250 mg and 500 mg and Biaxin XL 500 mg Mfd. by AbbVie LTD, Barceloneta, PR 00617

Biaxin Granules for Oral Suspension, 125 mg/5 mL and 250 mg/5 mL

Mfd. by AbbVie Inc., North Chicago, IL 60064

For AbbVie Inc., North Chicago, IL 60064, U.S.A.

03-B176 October, 2015

Shown in Product Identification Guide, page 505

CREON®   ℞

[krē'ŏn]

(pancrelipase)

delayed-release capsules for oral use

HIGHLIGHTS OF PRESCRIBING INFORMATION

These highlights do not include all the information needed to use CREON safely and effectively. See full prescribing information for CREON.

CREON (pancrelipase) delayed-release capsules for oral use
Initial U.S. Approval: 2009

——————INDICATIONS AND USAGE——————

CREON is a combination of porcine-derived lipases, proteases, and amylases indicated for the treatment of exocrine pancreatic insufficiency due to cystic fibrosis, chronic pancreatitis, pancreatectomy, or other conditions. (1)

——————DOSAGE AND ADMINISTRATION——————

CREON is not interchangeable with any other pancrelipase product. (2.1)

Do not crush or chew capsules and capsule contents. For infants or patients unable to swallow intact capsules, the contents may be sprinkled on soft acidic food, e.g., applesauce. (2.1) Dosing should not exceed the recommended maximum dosage set forth by the Cystic Fibrosis Foundation Consensus Conferences Guidelines. (2.2)

Infants (up to 12 months)
• Prior to each feeding, infants may be given 3,000 lipase units (one capsule) per 120 mL of formula or per breast-feeding. (2.1)
• Do not mix CREON capsule contents directly into formula or breast milk prior to administration. (2.1)

Children Older than 12 Months and Younger than 4 Years
• Begin with 1,000 lipase units/kg of body weight per meal for children less than age 4 years to a maximum of 2,500 lipase units/kg of body weight per meal (or less than or equal to 10,000 lipase units/kg of body weight per day), or less than 4,000 lipase units/g fat ingested per day. (2.2)

Children 4 Years and Older and Adults
• Begin with 500 lipase units/kg of body weight per meal for those older than age 4 years to a maximum of 2,500 lipase units/kg of body weight per meal (or less than or equal to 10,000 lipase units/kg of body weight per day), or less than 4,000 lipase units/g fat ingested per day. (2.2)

Adults with Exocrine Pancreatic Insufficiency Due to Chronic Pancreatitis or Pancreatectomy
• Individualize dosage based on clinical symptoms, the degree of steatorrhea present and the fat content of the diet. (2.2)

——————DOSAGE FORMS AND STRENGTHS——————

• Delayed-Release Capsules: 3,000 USP units of lipase; 9,500 USP units of protease; 15,000 USP units of amylase (3)
• Delayed-Release Capsules: 6,000 USP units of lipase; 19,000 USP units of protease; 30,000 USP units of amylase (3)
• Delayed-Release Capsules: 12,000 USP units of lipase; 38,000 USP units of protease; 60,000 USP units of amylase (3)
• Delayed-Release Capsules: 24,000 USP units of lipase; 76,000 USP units of protease; 120,000 USP units of amylase (3)
• Delayed-Release Capsules: 36,000 USP units of lipase; 114,000 USP units of protease; 180,000 USP units of amylase (3)

——————CONTRAINDICATIONS——————

None (4)

——————WARNINGS AND PRECAUTIONS——————

• Fibrosing colonopathy is associated with high-dose use of pancreatic enzyme replacement in the treatment of cystic fibrosis patients. Exercise caution when doses of CREON exceed 2,500 lipase units/kg of body weight per meal (or greater than 10,000 lipase units/kg of body weight per day). (5.1)
• To avoid irritation of oral mucosa, do not chew CREON or retain in the mouth. (5.2)
• Exercise caution when prescribing CREON to patients with gout, renal impairment, or hyperuricemia. (5.3)
• There is theoretical risk of viral transmission with all pancreatic enzyme products including CREON. (5.4)
• Exercise caution when administering pancrelipase to a patient with a known allergy to proteins of porcine origin. (5.5)

——————ADVERSE REACTIONS——————

• Adverse reactions occurring in at least 2 cystic fibrosis patients (greater than or equal to 4%) receiving CREON are vomiting, dizziness, and cough. (6.1)
• Adverse reactions that occurred in at least 1 chronic pancreatitis or pancreatectomy patient (greater than or equal to 4%) receiving CREON are hyperglycemia, hypoglycemia, abdominal pain, abnormal feces, flatulence, frequent bowel movements, and nasopharyngitis. (6.1)

To report SUSPECTED ADVERSE REACTIONS, contact AbbVie Inc. at 1-800-633-9110 or FDA at 1-800-FDA-1088 or www.fda.gov/medwatch.

See 17 for PATIENT COUNSELING INFORMATION and Medication Guide.

Revised: 3/2015

FULL PRESCRIBING INFORMATION: CONTENTS*

FULL PRESCRIBING INFORMATION

1   INDICATIONS AND USAGE

CREON® (pancrelipase) is indicated for the treatment of exocrine pancreatic insufficiency due to cystic fibrosis, chronic pancreatitis, pancreatectomy, or other conditions.

2   DOSAGE AND ADMINISTRATION

CREON is not interchangeable with other pancrelipase products.

CREON is orally administered. Therapy should be initiated at the lowest recommended dose and gradually increased. The dosage of CREON should be individualized based on clinical symptoms, the degree of steatorrhea present, and the fat content of the diet as described in the Limitations on Dosing below [see Dosage and Administration (2.2) and Warnings and Precautions (5.1)].

2.1   Administration

Infants (up to 12 months)

CREON should be administered to infants immediately prior to each feeding, using a dosage of 3,000 lipase units per 120 mL of formula or prior to breast-feeding. Contents of the capsule may be administered directly to the mouth or with a small amount of applesauce. Administration should be followed by breast milk or formula. Contents of the capsule should not be mixed directly into formula or breast milk as this may diminish efficacy. Care should be taken to ensure that CREON is not crushed or chewed or retained in the mouth, to avoid irritation of the oral mucosa.

Children and Adults

CREON should be taken during meals or snacks, with sufficient fluid. CREON capsules and capsule contents should not be crushed or chewed. Capsules should be swallowed whole.

For patients who are unable to swallow intact capsules, the capsules may be carefully opened and the contents added to a small amount of acidic soft food with a pH of 4.5 or less, such as applesauce, at room temperature. The CREON-soft food mixture should be swallowed immediately without crushing or chewing, and followed with water or juice to ensure complete ingestion. Care should be taken to ensure that no drug is retained in the mouth.

2.2   Dosage

Dosage recommendations for pancreatic enzyme replacement therapy were published following the Cystic Fibrosis Foundation Consensus Conferences.[1, 2, 3] CREON should be administered in a manner consistent with the recommendations of the Cystic Fibrosis Foundation Consensus Conferences (also known as Conferences) provided in the following paragraphs, except for infants. Although the Conferences recommend doses of 2,000 to 4,000 lipase units in infants up to 12 months, CREON is available in a 3,000 lipase unit capsule. Therefore, the recommended dose of CREON in infants up to 12 months is 3,000 lipase units per 120 mL of formula or per breast-feeding. Patients may be dosed on a fat ingestion-based or actual body weight-based dosing scheme.

Additional recommendations for pancreatic enzyme therapy in patients with exocrine pancreatic insufficiency due to chronic pancreatitis or pancreatectomy are based on a clinical trial conducted in these populations.

Infants (up to 12 months)

CREON is available in the strength of 3,000 USP units of lipase thus infants may be given 3,000 lipase units (one capsule) per 120 mL of formula or per breast-feeding. Do not mix CREON capsule contents directly into formula or breast milk prior to administration [see Administration (2.1)].

Children Older than 12 Months and Younger than 4 Years

Enzyme dosing should begin with 1,000 lipase units/kg of body weight per meal for children less than age 4 years to a maximum of 2,500 lipase units/kg of body weight per meal (or less than or equal to 10,000 lipase units/kg of body weight per day), or less than 4,000 lipase units/g fat ingested per day.

Children 4 Years and Older and Adults

Enzyme dosing should begin with 500 lipase units/kg of body weight per meal for those older than age 4 years to a maximum of 2,500 lipase units/kg of body weight per meal (or less than or equal to 10,000 lipase units/kg of body weight per day), or less than 4,000 lipase units/g fat ingested per day.

Usually, half of the prescribed CREON dose for an individualized full meal should be given with each snack. The total daily dose should reflect approximately three meals plus two or three snacks per day.

Enzyme doses expressed as lipase units/kg of body weight per meal should be decreased in older patients because they weigh more but tend to ingest less fat per kilogram of body weight.

Adults with Exocrine Pancreatic Insufficiency Due to Chronic Pancreatitis or Pancreatectomy

The initial starting dose and increases in the dose per meal should be individualized based on clinical symptoms, the degree of steatorrhea present, and the fat content of the diet.

In one clinical trial, patients received CREON at a dose of 72,000 lipase units per meal while consuming at least 100 g of fat per day *[see Clinical Studies (14.2)]*. Lower starting doses recommended in the literature are consistent with the 500 lipase units/kg of body weight per meal lowest starting dose recommended for adults in the Cystic Fibrosis Foundation Consensus Conferences Guidelines.[1, 2, 3, 4] Usually, half of the prescribed CREON dose for an individualized full meal should be given with each snack.

Limitations on Dosing

Dosing should not exceed the recommended maximum dosage set forth by the Cystic Fibrosis Foundation Consensus Conferences Guidelines.[1, 2, 3] If symptoms and signs of steatorrhea persist, the dosage may be increased by the healthcare professional. Patients should be instructed not to increase the dosage on their own. There is great interindividual variation in response to enzymes; thus, a range of doses is recommended. Changes in dosage may require an adjustment period of several days. If doses are to exceed 2,500 lipase units/kg of body weight per meal, further investigation is warranted. Doses greater than 2,500 lipase units/kg of body weight per meal (or greater than 10,000 lipase units/kg of body weight per day) should be used with caution and only if they are documented to be effective by 3-day fecal fat measures that indicate a significantly improved coefficient of fat absorption. Doses greater than 6,000 lipase units/kg of body weight per meal have been associated with colonic stricture, indicative of fibrosing colonopathy, in children less than 12 years of age *[see Warnings and Precautions (5.1)]*. Patients currently receiving higher doses than 6,000 lipase units/kg of body weight per meal should be examined and the dosage either immediately decreased or titrated downward to a lower range.

3 DOSAGE FORMS AND STRENGTHS

The active ingredient in CREON evaluated in clinical trials is lipase. CREON is dosed by lipase units.

Other active ingredients include protease and amylase. Each CREON delayed-release capsule strength contains the specified amounts of lipase, protease, and amylase as follows:

- 3,000 USP units of lipase; 9,500 USP units of protease; 15,000 USP units of amylase delayed-release capsules have a white opaque cap with imprint "CREON 1203" and a white opaque body.
- 6,000 USP units of lipase; 19,000 USP units of protease; 30,000 USP units of amylase delayed-release capsules have an orange opaque cap with imprint "CREON 1206" and a blue opaque body.
- 12,000 USP units of lipase; 38,000 USP units of protease; 60,000 USP units of amylase delayed-release capsules have a brown opaque cap with imprint "CREON 1212" and a colorless transparent body.
- 24,000 USP units of lipase; 76,000 USP units of protease; 120,000 USP units of amylase delayed-release capsules have an orange opaque cap with imprint "CREON 1224" and a colorless transparent body.
- 36,000 USP units of lipase; 114,000 USP units of protease; 180,000 USP units of amylase delayed-release capsules have a blue opaque cap with imprint "CREON 1236" and a colorless transparent body.

4 CONTRAINDICATIONS

None.

5 WARNINGS AND PRECAUTIONS

5.1 Fibrosing Colonopathy

Fibrosing colonopathy has been reported following treatment with different pancreatic enzyme products.[5, 6] Fibrosing colonopathy is a rare, serious adverse reaction initially described in association with high-dose pancreatic enzyme use, usually over a prolonged period of time and most commonly reported in pediatric patients with cystic fibrosis. The underlying mechanism of fibrosing colonopathy re-

mains unknown. Doses of pancreatic enzyme products exceeding 6,000 lipase units/kg of body weight per meal have been associated with colonic stricture in children less than 12 years of age.[1] Patients with fibrosing colonopathy should be closely monitored because some patients may be at risk of progressing to stricture formation. It is uncertain whether regression of fibrosing colonopathy occurs.[1] It is generally recommended, unless clinically indicated, that enzyme doses should be less than 2,500 lipase units/kg of body weight per meal (or less than 10,000 lipase units/kg of body weight per day) or less than 4,000 lipase units/g fat ingested per day *[see Dosage and Administration (2.1)]*.

Doses greater than 2,500 lipase units/kg of body weight per meal (or greater than 10,000 lipase units/kg of body weight per day) should be used with caution and only if they are documented to be effective by 3-day fecal fat measures that indicate a significantly improved coefficient of fat absorption. Patients receiving higher doses than 6,000 lipase units/kg of body weight per meal should be examined and the dosage either immediately decreased or titrated downward to a lower range.

5.2 Potential for Irritation to Oral Mucosa

Care should be taken to ensure that no drug is retained in the mouth. CREON should not be crushed or chewed or mixed in foods having a pH greater than 4.5. These actions can disrupt the protective enteric coating resulting in early release of enzymes, irritation of oral mucosa, and/or loss of enzyme activity *[see Dosage and Administration (2.2) and Patient Counseling Information (17.1)]*. For patients who are unable to swallow intact capsules, the capsules may be carefully opened and the contents added to a small amount of acidic soft food with a pH of 4.5 or less, such as applesauce, at room temperature. The CREON-soft food mixture should be swallowed immediately and followed with water or juice to ensure complete ingestion.

5.3 Potential for Risk of Hyperuricemia

Caution should be exercised when prescribing CREON to patients with gout, renal impairment, or hyperuricemia. Porcine-derived pancreatic enzyme products contain purines that may increase blood uric acid levels.

5.4 Potential Viral Exposure from the Product Source

CREON is sourced from pancreatic tissue from swine used for food consumption. Although the risk that CREON will transmit an infectious agent to humans has been reduced by testing for certain viruses during manufacturing and by inactivating certain viruses during manufacturing, there is a theoretical risk for transmission of viral disease, including diseases caused by novel or unidentified viruses. Thus, the presence of porcine viruses that might infect humans cannot be definitely excluded. However, no cases of transmission of an infectious illness associated with the use of porcine pancreatic extracts have been reported.

5.5 Allergic Reactions

Caution should be exercised when administering pancrelipase to a patient with a known allergy to proteins of porcine origin. Rarely, severe allergic reactions including anaphylaxis, asthma, hives, and pruritus, have been reported with other pancreatic enzyme products with different formulations of the same active ingredient (pancrelipase). The risks and benefits of continued CREON treatment in patients with severe allergy should be taken into consideration with the overall clinical needs of the patient.

6 ADVERSE REACTIONS

The most serious adverse reactions reported with different pancreatic enzyme products of the same active ingredient (pancrelipase) that are described elsewhere in the label include fibrosing colonopathy, hyperuricemia and allergic reactions *[see Warnings and Precautions (5)]*.

6.1 Clinical Trials Experience

Because clinical trials are conducted under widely varying conditions, adverse reaction rates observed in the clinical trials of a drug cannot be directly compared to the rates in the clinical trials of another drug and may not reflect the rates observed in practice.

The short-term safety of CREON was assessed in clinical trials conducted in 121 patients with exocrine pancreatic insufficiency (EPI): 67 patients with EPI due to cystic fibrosis (CF) and 25 patients with EPI due to chronic pancreatitis or pancreatectomy were treated with CREON.

Cystic Fibrosis

Studies 1 and 2 were randomized, double-blind, placebo-controlled, crossover studies of 49 patients, ages 7 to 43 years, with EPI due to CF. Study 1 included 32 patients ages 12 to 43 years and Study 2 included 17 patients ages 7 to 11 years. In these studies, patients were randomized to

receive CREON at a dose of 4,000 lipase units/g fat ingested per day or matching placebo for 5 to 6 days of treatment, followed by crossover to the alternate treatment for an additional 5 to 6 days. The mean exposure to CREON during these studies was 5 days.

In Study 1, one patient experienced duodenitis and gastritis of moderate severity 16 days after completing treatment with CREON. Transient neutropenia without clinical sequelae was observed as an abnormal laboratory finding in one patient receiving CREON and a macrolide antibiotic.

In Study 2, adverse reactions that occurred in at least 2 patients (greater than or equal to 12%) treated with CREON were vomiting and headache. Vomiting occurred in 2 patients treated with CREON and did not occur in patients treated with placebo; headache occurred in 2 patients treated with CREON and did not occur in patients treated with placebo.

The most common adverse reactions (greater than or equal to 4%) in Studies 1 and 2 were vomiting, dizziness, and cough. Table 1 enumerates adverse reactions that occurred in at least 2 patients (greater than or equal to 4%) treated with CREON at a higher rate than with placebo in Studies 1 and 2.

Table 1: Adverse Reactions Occurring in at Least 2 Patients (greater than or equal to 4%) in Cystic Fibrosis (Studies 1 and 2)

Adverse Reaction	CREON Capsules n = 49 (%)	Placebo n = 47 (%)
Vomiting	3 (6)	1 (2)
Dizziness	2 (4)	1 (2)
Cough	2 (4)	0

An additional open-label, single-arm study assessed the short-term safety and tolerability of CREON in 18 infants and children, ages 4 months to 6 years, with EPI due to cystic fibrosis. Patients received their usual pancreatic enzyme replacement therapy (mean dose of 7,000 lipase units/kg/day for a mean duration of 18.2 days) followed by CREON (mean dose of 7,500 lipase units/kg/day for a mean duration of 12.6 days). There were no serious adverse reactions. Adverse reactions that occurred in patients during treatment with CREON were vomiting, irritability, and decreased appetite, each occurring in 6% of patients.

Chronic Pancreatitis or Pancreatectomy

A randomized, double-blind, placebo-controlled, parallel group study was conducted in 54 adult patients, ages 32 to 75 years, with EPI due to chronic pancreatitis or pancreatectomy. Patients received single-blind placebo treatment during a 5-day run-in period followed by an intervening period of up to 16 days of investigator-directed treatment with no restrictions on pancreatic enzyme replacement therapy. Patients were then randomized to receive CREON or matching placebo for 7 days. The CREON dose was 72,000 lipase units per main meal (3 main meals) and 36,000 lipase units per snack (2 snacks). The mean exposure to CREON during this study was 6.8 days in the 25 patients that received CREON.

The most common adverse reactions reported during the study were related to glycemic control and were reported more commonly during CREON treatment than during placebo treatment.

Table 2 enumerates adverse reactions that occurred in at least 1 patient (greater than or equal to 4%) treated with CREON at a higher rate than with placebo.

Table 2: Adverse Reactions in at Least 1 Patient (greater than or equal to 4%) in the Chronic Pancreatitis or Pancreatectomy Trial

Adverse Reaction	CREON Capsules n = 25 (%)	Placebo n = 29 (%)
Hyperglycemia	2 (8)	2 (7)

Continued on next page

Information on the AbbVie, Inc. products listed on these pages is from the prescribing information in use as of July 31, 2016. For more information, please visit rxabbvie.com or call 1-800-633-9110.

Hypoglycemia	1 (4)	1 (3)
Abdominal Pain	1 (4)	1 (3)
Abnormal Feces	1 (4)	0
Flatulence	1 (4)	0
Frequent Bowel Movements	1 (4)	0
Nasopharyngitis	1 (4)	0

6.2 Postmarketing Experience

Postmarketing data from this formulation of CREON have been available since 2009. The following adverse reactions have been identified during post approval use of this formulation of CREON. Because these reactions are reported voluntarily from a population of uncertain size, it is not always possible to reliably estimate their frequency or establish a causal relationship to drug exposure.

Gastrointestinal disorders (including abdominal pain, diarrhea, flatulence, constipation and nausea), skin disorders (including pruritus, urticaria and rash), blurred vision, myalgia, muscle spasm, and asymptomatic elevations of liver enzymes have been reported with this formulation of CREON.

Delayed- and immediate-release pancreatic enzyme products with different formulations of the same active ingredient (pancrelipase) have been used for the treatment of patients with exocrine pancreatic insufficiency due to cystic fibrosis and other conditions, such as chronic pancreatitis. The long-term safety profile of these products has been described in the medical literature. The most serious adverse reactions included fibrosing colonopathy, distal intestinal obstruction syndrome (DIOS), recurrence of pre-existing carcinoma, and severe allergic reactions including anaphylaxis, asthma, hives, and pruritus.

7 DRUG INTERACTIONS

No drug interactions have been identified. No formal interaction studies have been conducted.

8 USE IN SPECIFIC POPULATIONS

8.1 Pregnancy

Teratogenic effects

Pregnancy Category C: Animal reproduction studies have not been conducted with pancrelipase. It is also not known whether pancrelipase can cause fetal harm when administered to a pregnant woman or can affect reproduction capacity. CREON should be given to a pregnant woman only if clearly needed. The risk and benefit of pancrelipase should be considered in the context of the need to provide adequate nutritional support to a pregnant woman with exocrine pancreatic insufficiency. Adequate caloric intake during pregnancy is important for normal maternal weight gain and fetal growth. Reduced maternal weight gain and malnutrition can be associated with adverse pregnancy outcomes.

8.3 Nursing Mothers

It is not known whether this drug is excreted in human milk. Because many drugs are excreted in human milk, caution should be exercised when CREON is administered to a nursing woman. The risk and benefit of pancrelipase should be considered in the context of the need to provide adequate nutritional support to a nursing mother with exocrine pancreatic insufficiency.

8.4 Pediatric Use

The short-term safety and effectiveness of CREON were assessed in two randomized, double-blind, placebo-controlled, crossover studies of 49 patients with EPI due to cystic fibrosis, 25 of whom were pediatric patients. Study 1 included 8 adolescents between 12 and 17 years of age. Study 2 included 17 children between 7 and 11 years of age. The safety and efficacy in pediatric patients in these studies were similar to adult patients [see Adverse Reactions (6.1) and Clinical Studies (14)].

An open-label, single-arm, short-term study of CREON was conducted in 18 infants and children, ages 4 months to six years of age, with EPI due to cystic fibrosis. Patients received their usual pancreatic enzyme replacement therapy (mean dose of 7,000 lipase units/kg/day for a mean duration of 18.2 days) followed by CREON (mean dose of 7,500 lipase units/kg/day for a mean duration of 12.6 days). The mean daily fat intake was 48 grams during treatment with usual pancreatic enzyme replacement therapy and 47 grams during treatment with CREON. When patients were switched from their usual pancreatic enzyme replacement therapy to CREON, they demonstrated similar spot fecal fat testing re-

sults; the clinical relevance of spot fecal fat testing has not been demonstrated. Adverse reactions that occurred in patients during treatment with CREON were vomiting, irritability, and decreased appetite [see Adverse Reactions (6.1)]. The safety and efficacy of pancreatic enzyme products with different formulations of pancrelipase consisting of the same active ingredient (lipases, proteases, and amylases) for treatment of children with exocrine pancreatic insufficiency due to cystic fibrosis have been described in the medical literature and through clinical experience.

Dosing of pediatric patients should be in accordance with recommended guidance from the Cystic Fibrosis Foundation Consensus Conferences [see Dosage and Administration (2.1)]. Doses of other pancreatic enzyme products exceeding 6,000 lipase units/kg of body weight per meal have been associated with fibrosing colonopathy and colonic strictures in children less than 12 years of age [see Warnings and Precautions (5.1)].

8.5 Geriatric Use

Clinical studies of CREON did not include sufficient numbers of subjects aged 65 and over to determine whether they respond differently from younger subjects. Other reported clinical experience has not identified differences in responses between the elderly and younger patients.

10 OVERDOSAGE

There have been no reports of overdose in clinical trials or postmarketing surveillance with this formulation of CREON. Chronic high doses of pancreatic enzyme products have been associated with fibrosing colonopathy and colonic strictures [see Dosage and Administration (2.2) and Warnings and Precautions (5.1)]. High doses of pancreatic enzyme products have been associated with hyperuricosuria and hyperuricemia, and should be used with caution in patients with a history of hyperuricemia, gout, or renal impairment [see Warnings and Precautions (5.3)].

11 DESCRIPTION

CREON is a pancreatic enzyme preparation consisting of pancrelipase, an extract derived from porcine pancreatic glands. Pancrelipase contains multiple enzyme classes, including porcine-derived lipases, proteases, and amylases. Pancrelipase is a beige-white amorphous powder. It is miscible in water and practically insoluble or insoluble in alcohol and ether.

Each delayed-release capsule for oral administration contains enteric-coated spheres (0.71–1.60 mm in diameter). The active ingredient evaluated in clinical trials is lipase. CREON is dosed by lipase units.

Other active ingredients include protease and amylase.

CREON contains the following inactive ingredients: cetyl alcohol, dimethicone, hypromellose phthalate, polyethylene glycol, and triethyl citrate.

3,000 USP units of lipase; 9,500 USP units of protease; 15,000 USP units of amylase delayed-release capsules have a white opaque cap with imprint "CREON 1203" and a white opaque body. The shells contain titanium dioxide and hypromellose.

6,000 USP units of lipase; 19,000 USP units of protease; 30,000 USP units of amylase delayed-release capsules have a Swedish-orange opaque cap with imprint "CREON 1206" and a blue opaque body. The shells contain FD&C Blue No. 2, gelatin, red iron oxide, sodium lauryl sulfate, titanium dioxide, and yellow iron oxide.

12,000 USP units of lipase; 38,000 USP units of protease; 60,000 USP units of amylase delayed-release capsules have a brown opaque cap with imprint "CREON 1212" and a colorless transparent body. The shells contain black iron oxide, gelatin, red iron oxide, sodium lauryl sulfate, titanium dioxide, and yellow iron oxide.

24,000 USP units of lipase; 76,000 USP units of protease; 120,000 USP units of amylase delayed-release capsules have a Swedish-orange opaque cap with imprint "CREON 1224" and a colorless transparent body. The shells contain gelatin, red iron oxide, sodium lauryl sulfate, titanium dioxide, and yellow iron oxide.

36,000 USP units of lipase; 114,000 USP units of protease; 180,000 USP units of amylase delayed-release capsules have a blue opaque cap with imprint "CREON 1236" and a colorless transparent body. The shells contain gelatin, titanium dioxide, FD&C Blue No. 2 and sodium lauryl sulfate.

12 CLINICAL PHARMACOLOGY

12.1 Mechanism of Action

The pancreatic enzymes in CREON catalyze the hydrolysis of fats to monoglyceride, glycerol and free fatty acids, proteins into peptides and amino acids, and starches into dex-

trins and short chain sugars such as maltose and maltriose in the duodenum and proximal small intestine, thereby acting like digestive enzymes physiologically secreted by the pancreas.

12.3 Pharmacokinetics

The pancreatic enzymes in CREON are enteric-coated to minimize destruction or inactivation in gastric acid. CREON is designed to release most of the enzymes *in vivo* at an approximate pH of 5.5 or greater. Pancreatic enzymes are not absorbed from the gastrointestinal tract in appreciable amounts.

13 NONCLINICAL TOXICOLOGY

13.1 Carcinogenesis, Mutagenesis, Impairment of Fertility

Carcinogenicity, genetic toxicology, and animal fertility studies have not been performed with pancrelipase.

14 CLINICAL STUDIES

The short-term efficacy of CREON was evaluated in three studies conducted in 103 patients with exocrine pancreatic insufficiency (EPI). Two studies were conducted in 49 patients with EPI due to cystic fibrosis (CF); one study was conducted in 54 patients with EPI due to chronic pancreatitis or pancreatectomy.

14.1 Cystic Fibrosis

Studies 1 and 2 were randomized, double-blind, placebo-controlled, crossover studies in 49 patients, ages 7 to 43 years, with exocrine pancreatic insufficiency due to cystic fibrosis. Study 1 included patients aged 12 to 43 years (n = 32). The final analysis population was limited to 29 patients; 3 patients were excluded due to protocol deviations. Study 2 included patients aged 7 to 11 years (n = 17). The final analysis population was limited to 16 patients; 1 patient withdrew consent prior to stool collection during treatment with CREON. In each study, patients were randomized to receive CREON at a dose of 4,000 lipase units/g fat ingested per day or matching placebo for 5 to 6 days of treatment, followed by crossover to the alternate treatment for an additional 5 to 6 days. All patients consumed a high-fat diet (greater than or equal to 90 grams of fat per day, 40% of daily calories derived from fat) during the treatment periods.

The coefficient of fat absorption (CFA) was determined by a 72-hour stool collection during both treatments, when both fat excretion and fat ingestion were measured. Each patient's CFA during placebo treatment was used as their no-treatment CFA value.

In Study 1, mean CFA was 89% with CREON treatment compared to 49% with placebo treatment. The mean difference in CFA was 41 percentage points in favor of CREON treatment with 95% CI: (34, 47) and p<0.001.

In Study 2, mean CFA was 83% with CREON treatment compared to 47% with placebo treatment. The mean difference in CFA was 35 percentage points in favor of CREON treatment with 95% CI: (27, 44) and p<0.001.

Subgroup analyses of the CFA results in Studies 1 and 2 showed that mean change in CFA with CREON treatment was greater in patients with lower no-treatment (placebo) CFA values than in patients with higher no-treatment (placebo) CFA values. There were no differences in response to CREON by age or gender, with similar responses to CREON observed in male and female patients, and in younger (under 18 years of age) and older patients.

The coefficient of nitrogen absorption (CNA) was determined by a 72-hour stool collection during both treatments, when nitrogen excretion was measured and nitrogen ingestion from a controlled diet was estimated (based on the assumption that proteins contain 16% nitrogen). Each patient's CNA during placebo treatment was used as their no-treatment CNA value.

In Study 1, mean CNA was 86% with CREON treatment compared to 49% with placebo treatment. The mean difference in CNA was 37 percentage points in favor of CREON treatment with 95% CI: (31, 42) and p<0.001.

In Study 2, mean CNA was 80% with CREON treatment compared to 45% with placebo treatment. The mean difference in CNA was 35 percentage points in favor of CREON treatment with 95% CI: (26, 45) and p<0.001.

14.2 Chronic Pancreatitis or Pancreatectomy

A randomized, double-blind, placebo-controlled, parallel group study was conducted in 54 adult patients, ages 32 to 75 years, with EPI due to chronic pancreatitis or pancreatectomy. The final analysis population was limited to 52 patients; 2 patients were excluded due to protocol violations. Ten patients had a history of pancreatectomy (7 were treated with CREON). In this study, patients received placebo for 5 days (run-in period), followed by pancreatic enzyme replacement therapy as directed by the investigator for 16 days; this was followed by randomization to CREON or matching placebo for 7 days of treatment (double-blind period). Only patients with CFA less than 80% in the run-in period were randomized to the double-blind period. The dose of CREON during the double-blind period was 72,000 lipase units per main meal (3 main meals) and 36,000 lipase units per snack (2 snacks). All patients consumed a high-fat diet (greater than or equal to 100 grams of fat per day) during the treatment period.

The CFA was determined by a 72-hour stool collection during the run-in and double-blind treatment periods, when both fat excretion and fat ingestion were measured. The mean change in CFA from the run-in period to the end of the double-blind period in the CREON and Placebo groups is shown in Table 3.

Table 3: Change in CFA in the Chronic Pancreatitis and Pancreatectomy Trial (Run-in Period to End of Double-Blind Period)

	CREON n = 24	Placebo n = 28
CFA [%]		
Run-in Period (Mean, SD)	54 (19)	57 (21)
End of Double-Blind Period (Mean, SD)	86 (6)	66 (20)
Change in CFA * [%]		
Run-in Period to End of Double-Blind Period (Mean, SD)	32 (18)	9 (13)
Treatment Difference (95% CI)	21 (14, 28)	

*$p < 0.0001$

Subgroup analyses of the CFA results showed that mean change in CFA was greater in patients with lower run-in period CFA values than in patients with higher run-in period CFA values. Only 1 of the patients with a history of total pancreatectomy was treated with CREON in the study. That patient had a CFA of 26% during the run-in period and a CFA of 73% at the end of the double-blind period. The remaining 6 patients with a history of partial pancreatectomy treated with CREON on the study had a mean CFA of 42% during the run-in period and a mean CFA of 84% at the end of the double-blind period.

15 REFERENCES

[1] Borowitz DS, Grand RJ, Durie PR, et al. Use of pancreatic enzyme supplements for patients with cystic fibrosis in the context of fibrosing colonopathy. *Journal of Pediatrics.* 1995; 127: 681-684.

[2] Borowitz DS, Baker RD, Stallings V. Consensus report on nutrition for pediatric patients with cystic fibrosis. *Journal of Pediatric Gastroenterology Nutrition.* 2002 Sep; 35: 246-259.

[3] Stallings VA, Stark LJ, Robinson KA, et al. Evidence-based practice recommendations for nutrition-related management of children and adults with cystic fibrosis and pancreatic insufficiency: results of a systematic review. *Journal of the American Dietetic Association.* 2008; 108: 832-839.

[4] Dominguez-Munoz JE. Pancreatic enzyme therapy for pancreatic exocrine insufficiency. *Current Gastroenterology Reports.* 2007; 9: 116-122.

[5] Smyth RL, Ashby D, O'Hea U, et al. Fibrosing colonopathy in cystic fibrosis: results of a case-control study. *Lancet.* 1995; 346: 1247-1251.

[6] FitzSimmons SC, Burkhart GA, Borowitz DS, et al. High-dose pancreatic-enzyme supplements and fibrosing colonopathy in children with cystic fibrosis. *New England Journal of Medicine.* 1997; 336: 1283-1289.

16 HOW SUPPLIED/STORAGE AND HANDLING

CREON (pancrelipase) Delayed-Release Capsules
3,000 USP units of lipase; 9,500 USP units of protease; 15,000 USP units of amylase

Each CREON capsule is available as a two piece hypromellose capsule with a white opaque cap with imprint "CREON 1203" and a white opaque body that contains tan colored, delayed-release pancrelipase supplied in bottles of:
• 70 capsules (NDC 0032-1203-70)
CREON (pancrelipase) Delayed-Release Capsules
6,000 USP units of lipase; 19,000 USP units of protease; 30,000 USP units of amylase

Each CREON capsule is available as a two-piece gelatin capsule with orange opaque cap with imprint "CREON 1206" and a blue opaque body that contains tan-colored, delayed-release pancrelipase supplied in bottles of:
• 100 capsules (NDC 0032-1206-01)
• 250 capsules (NDC 0032-1206-07)
CREON (pancrelipase) Delayed-Release Capsules
12,000 USP units of lipase; 38,000 USP units of protease; 60,000 USP units of amylase

Each CREON capsule is available as a two-piece gelatin capsule with a brown opaque cap with imprint "CREON 1212" and a colorless transparent body that contains tan-colored, delayed-release pancrelipase supplied in bottles of:
• 100 capsules (NDC 0032-1212-01)
• 250 capsules (NDC 0032-1212-07)
CREON (pancrelipase) Delayed-Release Capsules
24,000 USP units of lipase; 76,000 USP units of protease; 120,000 USP units of amylase

Each CREON capsule is available as a two-piece gelatin capsule with orange opaque cap with imprint "CREON 1224" and a colorless transparent body that contains tan-colored, delayed-release pancrelipase supplied in bottles of:
• 100 capsules (NDC 0032-1224-01)
• 250 capsules (NDC 0032-1224-07)
CREON (pancrelipase) Delayed-Release Capsules
36,000 USP units of lipase; 114,000 USP units of protease; 180,000 USP units of amylase

Each CREON capsule is available as a two-piece gelatin capsule with blue opaque cap with imprint "CREON 1236" and a colorless transparent body that contains tan-colored, delayed-release pancrelipase supplied in bottles of:
• 100 capsules (NDC 0032-3016-13)
• 250 capsules (NDC 0032-3016-28)
Storage and Handling
CREON must be stored at room temperature up to 25°C (77°F) and protected from moisture. Temperature excursions are permitted between 25°C to 40°C (77°F and 104°F) for up to 30 days. Product should be discarded if exposed to higher temperature and moisture conditions higher than 70%. After opening, keep bottle tightly closed between uses to protect from moisture.

Bottles of CREON 3,000 USP units of lipase must be stored and dispensed in the original container.

Do not crush CREON delayed-release capsules or the capsule contents.

17 PATIENT COUNSELING INFORMATION

See FDA-approved patient labeling (Medication Guide)
17.1 Dosing and Administration
• Instruct patients and caregivers that CREON should only be taken as directed by their healthcare professional. Patients should be advised that the total daily dose should not exceed 10,000 lipase units/kg body weight/day unless clinically indicated. This needs to be especially emphasized for patients eating multiple snacks and meals per day. Patients should be informed that if a dose is missed, the next dose should be taken with the next meal or snack as directed. Doses should not be doubled *[see Dosage and Administration (2)].*
• Instruct patients and caregivers that CREON should always be taken with food. Patients should be advised that CREON delayed-release capsules and the capsule contents must not be crushed or chewed as doing so could cause early release of enzymes and/or loss of enzymatic activity. Patients should swallow the intact capsules with adequate amounts of liquid at mealtimes. If necessary, the capsule contents can also be sprinkled on soft acidic foods *[see Dosage and Administration (2)].*
17.2 Fibrosing Colonopathy
Advise patients and caregivers to follow dosing instructions carefully, as doses of pancreatic enzyme products exceeding 6,000 lipase units/kg of body weight per meal have been associated with colonic strictures in children below the age of 12 years *[see Dosage and Administration (2)].*
17.3 Allergic Reactions
Advise patients and caregivers to contact their healthcare professional immediately if allergic reactions to CREON develop *[see Warnings and Precautions (5.5)].*
17.4 Pregnancy and Breast Feeding
• Instruct patients to notify their healthcare professional if they are pregnant or are thinking of becoming pregnant during treatment with CREON *[see Use in Specific Populations (8.1)].*
• Instruct patients to notify their healthcare professional if they are breast feeding or are thinking of breast feeding during treatment with CREON *[see Use in Specific Populations (8.3)].*

Manufactured by:
Abbott Laboratories GmbH
Hannover, Germany
Marketed by:
AbbVie Inc.
North Chicago, IL 60064, U.S.A.
© 2015 AbbVie Inc.
03-B115 March, 2015

MEDICATION GUIDE
CREON® (krē'ŏn)
(pancrelipase)
Delayed-Release Capsules

Read this Medication Guide before you start taking CREON and each time you get a refill. There may be new information. This information does not take the place of talking to your doctor about your medical condition or treatment.
What is the most important information I should know about CREON?
CREON® (pancrelipase) may increase your chance of having a rare bowel disorder called fibrosing colonopathy. This condition is serious and may require surgery. The risk of having this condition may be reduced by following the dosing instructions that your doctor gave you. **Call your doctor right away if you have any unusual or severe:**
• stomach area (abdominal) pain
• bloating
• trouble passing stool (having bowel movements)
• nausea, vomiting, or diarrhea
Take CREON exactly as prescribed. Do not take more or less CREON than directed by your doctor.
What is CREON?
CREON is a prescription medicine used to treat people who cannot digest food normally because their pancreas does not make enough enzymes due to cystic fibrosis, swelling of the pancreas that lasts a long time (chronic pancreatitis), removal of some or all of the pancreas (pancreatectomy), or other conditions. CREON may help your body use fats, proteins, and sugars from food.
CREON contains a mixture of digestive enzymes including lipases, proteases, and amylases from pig pancreas.
What should I tell my doctor before taking CREON?
Before taking CREON, tell your doctor about all your medical conditions, including if you:
• are allergic to pork (pig) products
• have a history of intestinal blockage of your intestines, or scarring or thickening of your bowel wall (fibrosing colonopathy)
• have gout, kidney disease, or high blood uric acid (hyperuricemia)
• have trouble swallowing capsules
• have any other medical condition
• are pregnant or plan to become pregnant. It is not known if CREON will harm your unborn baby.
• are breast-feeding or plan to breast-feed. It is not known if CREON passes into your breast milk.
Tell your doctor about all the medicines you take, including prescription and nonprescription medicines, vitamins, and herbal supplements.
Know the medicines you take. Keep a list of them and show it to your doctor and pharmacist when you get a new medicine.
How should I take CREON?
• **Take CREON exactly as your doctor tells you.**
• You should not switch CREON with any other pancreatic enzyme product without first talking to your doctor.
• Do not take more capsules in a day than the number your doctor tells you to take (total daily dose).
• Always take CREON with a meal or snack and enough liquid to swallow CREON completely. If you eat a lot of meals or snacks in a day, be careful not to go over your total daily dose.
• Your doctor may change your dose based on the amount of fatty foods you eat or based on your weight.
• **Do not crush or chew CREON capsules or its contents, and do not hold the capsule or capsule contents in your mouth.** Crushing, chewing or holding the CREON capsules in your mouth may cause irritation in your mouth or change the way CREON works in your body.
Giving CREON to infants (children up to 12 months)

Continued on next page

Information on the AbbVie, Inc. products listed on these pages is from the prescribing information in use as of July 31, 2016. For more information, please visit rxabbvie.com or call 1-800-633-9110.

1. Give CREON right before each feeding of formula or breast milk.
2. Do not mix CREON capsule contents directly into formula or breast milk.
3. Open the capsules and sprinkle the contents directly into your infant's mouth or mix the contents in a small amount of room temperature acidic soft food such as applesauce. These foods should be the kind found in baby food jars that you buy at the store, or other food recommended by your doctor.
4. If you sprinkle the CREON on food, give the CREON and food mixture to your child right away. Do not store CREON that is mixed with food.
5. Give your child enough liquid to completely swallow the CREON contents or the CREON and food mixture.
6. Look in your child's mouth to make sure that all of the medicine has been swallowed.

Giving CREON to children and adults

1. Swallow CREON capsules whole and take them with enough liquid to swallow them right away.
2. If you have trouble swallowing capsules, open the capsules and sprinkle the contents on a small amount of room temperature acidic food such as applesauce. Ask your doctor about other foods you can mix with CREON.
3. If you sprinkle CREON on food, swallow it right after you mix it and drink enough water or juice to make sure the medicine is swallowed completely. Do not store CREON that is mixed with food.
4. If you forget to take CREON, call your doctor or wait until your next meal and take your usual number of capsules. Take your next dose at your usual time. **Do not make up for missed doses.**

What are the possible side effects of CREON?

CREON may cause serious side effects, including:

- See "What is the most important information I should know about CREON?"
- **Irritation of the inside of your mouth.** This can happen if CREON is not swallowed completely.
- **Increase in blood uric acid levels.** This may cause worsening of swollen, painful joints (gout) caused by an increase in your blood uric acid levels.
- **Allergic reactions, including trouble with breathing, skin rashes, or swollen lips.**

Call your doctor right away if you have any of these symptoms.

The most common side effects of CREON include:

- Blood sugar increase (hyperglycemia) or decrease (hypoglycemia)
- Pain in your stomach (abdominal area)
- Frequent or abnormal bowel movements
- Gas
- Vomiting
- Dizziness
- Sore throat and cough

Other Possible Side Effects:

CREON and other pancreatic enzyme products are made from the pancreas of pigs, the same pigs people eat as pork. These pigs may carry viruses. Although it has never been reported, it may be possible for a person to get a viral infection from taking pancreatic enzyme products that come from pigs.

Tell your doctor if you have any side effect that bothers you or that does not go away.

These are not all the side effects of CREON. For more information, ask your doctor or pharmacist.

Call your doctor for medical advice about side effects. You may report side effects to the FDA at 1-800-FDA-1088.

You may also report side effects to AbbVie Inc. at 1-800-633-9110.

How should I store CREON?

- Store CREON at room temperature below 77°F (25°C). Avoid heat.
- You may store CREON at a temperature between 77°F to 104°F (25°C to 40°C) for up to 30 days. Throw away any CREON stored at these temperatures for more than 30 days.
- Keep CREON in a dry place and in the original container.
- After opening the bottle, keep it closed tightly between uses to protect from moisture.

Keep CREON and all medicines out of the reach of children.

General information about CREON

Medicines are sometimes prescribed for purposes other than those listed in a Medication Guide. Do not use CREON for a condition for which it was not prescribed. Do not give CREON to other people to take, even if they have the same symptoms you have. It may harm them.

This Medication Guide summarizes the most important information about CREON. If you would like more informa-

tion, talk to your doctor. You can ask your doctor or pharmacist for information about CREON that is written for healthcare professionals. For more information, go to www.creon-us.com or call toll-free [1-800-633-9110].

What are the ingredients in CREON?

Active Ingredient: lipase, protease, amylase

Inactive Ingredients: cetyl alcohol, dimethicone, hypromellose phthalate, polyethylene glycol, and triethyl citrate.

The shells of the CREON 6,000 USP units of lipase, 12,000 USP units of lipase, and 24,000 USP units of lipase strengths contain: gelatin, red iron oxide, sodium lauryl sulfate, titanium dioxide, and yellow iron oxide.

In addition:

The shells for the CREON 3,000 USP units of lipase strength capsules contain titanium dioxide and hypromellose.

The shells of the CREON 6,000 USP units of lipase strength capsules contain FD&C Blue No. 2.

The shells of the CREON 12,000 USP units of lipase strength capsules contain black iron oxide.

The shells of the CREON 36,000 USP units of lipase strength capsules contain gelatin, titanium dioxide, sodium lauryl sulfate and FD&C Blue No. 2.

This Medication Guide has been approved by the U.S. Food and Drug Administration.

Manufactured for:

AbbVie Inc.

North Chicago, IL 60064, U.S.A.

© 2015 AbbVie Inc.

03-B115 March, 2015

Shown in Product Identification Guide, page 505

DEPAKOTE® ER   ℞

[*dĕp'ă-kōte*]

(divalproex sodium)

extended-release tablets

HIGHLIGHTS OF PRESCRIBING INFORMATION

These highlights do not include all the information needed to use Depakote ER safely and effectively. See full prescribing information for Depakote ER.

Depakote ER (divalproex sodium) extended-release tablets, for oral use

Initial U.S. Approval: 2000

WARNING: LIFE THREATENING ADVERSE REACTIONS

See full prescribing information for complete boxed warning.

- **Hepatotoxicity, including fatalities, usually during first 6 months of treatment. Children under the age of two years and patients with mitochondrial disorders are at higher risk. Monitor patients closely, and perform serum liver testing prior to therapy and at frequent intervals thereafter (5.1)**
- **Fetal Risk, particularly neural tube defects, other major malformations, and decreased IQ (5.2, 5.3, 5.4)**
- **Pancreatitis, including fatal hemorrhagic cases (5.5)**

RECENT MAJOR CHANGES

Dosage and Administration, Dosing in Patients Taking Rufinamide (2.6)	2/2016

INDICATIONS AND USAGE

Depakote ER is an anti-epileptic drug indicated for:

- Acute treatment of manic or mixed episodes associated with bipolar disorder, with or without psychotic features (1.1)
- Monotherapy and adjunctive therapy of complex partial seizures and simple and complex absence seizures; adjunctive therapy in patients with multiple seizure types that include absence seizures (1.2)
- Prophylaxis of migraine headaches (1.3)

DOSAGE AND ADMINISTRATION

- Depakote ER is intended for once-a-day oral administration. Depakote ER should be swallowed whole and should not be crushed or chewed (2.1, 2.2).
- Mania: Initial dose is 25 mg/kg/day, increasing as rapidly as possible to achieve therapeutic response or desired plasma level (2.1). The maximum recommended dosage is 60 mg/kg/day (2.1, 2.2).
- Complex Partial Seizures: Start at 10 to 15 mg/kg/day, increasing at 1 week intervals by 5 to 10 mg/kg/day to

achieve optimal clinical response; if response is not satisfactory, check valproate plasma level; see full prescribing information for conversion to monotherapy (2.2). The maximum recommended dosage is 60 mg/kg/day (2.1, 2.2).
- Absence Seizures: Start at 15 mg/kg/day, increasing at 1 week intervals by 5 to 10 mg/kg/day until seizure control or limiting side effects (2.2). The maximum recommended dosage is 60 mg/kg/day (2.1, 2.2).
- Migraine: The recommended starting dose is 500 mg/day for 1 week, thereafter increasing to 1000 mg/day (2.3).

DOSAGE FORMS AND STRENGTHS

Tablets: 250 mg and 500 mg (3)

CONTRAINDICATIONS

- Hepatic disease or significant hepatic dysfunction (4, 5.1)
- Known mitochondrial disorders caused by mutations in mitochondrial DNA polymerase γ (POLG) (4, 5.1)
- Suspected POLG-related disorder in children under two years of age (4, 5.1)
- Known hypersensitivity to the drug (4, 5.12)
- Urea cycle disorders (4, 5.6)
- Pregnant patients treated for prophylaxis of migraine headaches (4, 8.1)

WARNINGS AND PRECAUTIONS

- Hepatotoxicity; evaluate high risk populations and monitor serum liver tests (5.1)
- Birth defects and decreased IQ following *in utero* exposure; only use to treat pregnant women with epilepsy or bipolar disorder if other medications are unacceptable; should not be administered to a woman of childbearing potential unless essential (5.2, 5.3, 5.4)
- Pancreatitis; Depakote ER should ordinarily be discontinued (5.5)
- Suicidal behavior or ideation; Antiepileptic drugs, including Depakote ER, increase the risk of suicidal thoughts or behavior (5.7)
- Bleeding and other hematopoietic disorders; monitor platelet counts and coagulation tests (5.8)
- Hyperammonemia and hyperammonemic encephalopathy; measure ammonia level if unexplained lethargy and vomiting or changes in mental status, and also with concomitant topiramate use; consider discontinuation of valproate therapy (5.6, 5.9, 5.10)
- Hypothermia; Hypothermia has been reported during valproate therapy with or without associated hyperammonemia. This adverse reaction can also occur in patients using concomitant topiramate (5.11)
- Drug Reaction with Eosinophilia and Systemic Symptoms (DRESS)/Multiorgan hypersensitivity reaction; discontinue Depakote ER (5.12)
- Somnolence in the elderly can occur. Depakote ER dosage should be increased slowly and with regular monitoring for fluid and nutritional intake (5.14)

ADVERSE REACTIONS

- Most common adverse reactions (reported >5%) reported in adult studies are nausea, somnolence, dizziness, vomiting, asthenia, abdominal pain, dyspepsia, rash, diarrhea, increased appetite, tremor, weight gain, back pain, alopecia, headache, fever, anorexia, constipation, diplopia, amblyopia/blurred, ataxia, nystagmus, emotional lability, thinking abnormal, amnesia, flu syndrome, infection, bronchitis, rhinitis, ecchymosis, peripheral edema, insomnia, nervousness, depression, pharyngitis, dyspnea, tinnitus (6.1, 6.2, 6.3, 6.4).
- The safety and tolerability of valproate in pediatric patients were shown to be comparable to those in adults (8.4).

To report SUSPECTED ADVERSE REACTIONS, contact AbbVie Inc. at 1-800-633-9110 or FDA at 1-800-FDA-1088 or www.fda.gov/medwatch

DRUG INTERACTIONS

- Hepatic enzyme-inducing drugs (e.g., phenytoin, carbamazepine, primidone, phenobarbital, rifampin) can increase valproate clearance, while enzyme inhibitors (e.g., felbamate) can decrease valproate clearance. Therefore increased monitoring of valproate and concomitant drug concentrations and dose adjustment is indicated whenever enzyme-inducing or inhibiting drugs are introduced or withdrawn (7.1)
- Aspirin, carbapenem antibiotics: Monitoring of valproate concentrations are recommended (7.1)
- Co-administration of valproate can affect the pharmacokinetics of other drugs (e.g. diazepam, ethosuximide, lamotrigine, phenytoin) by inhibiting their metabolism or protein binding displacement (7.2)
- Patients stabilized on rufinamide should begin valproate therapy at a low dose, and titrate to clinically effective dose (7.2)

- Dosage adjustment of amitriptyline/nortriptyline, warfarin, and zidovudine may be necessary if used concomitantly with Depakote ER (7.2)
- Topiramate: Hyperammonemia and encephalopathy (5.10, 7.3)

---USE IN SPECIFIC POPULATIONS---

- Pregnancy: Depakote ER can cause congenital malformations including neural tube defects and decreased IQ. (5.2, 5.3, 8.1)
- Pediatric: Children under the age of two years are at considerably higher risk of fatal hepatotoxicity (5.1, 8.4)
- Geriatric: Reduce starting dose; increase dosage more slowly; monitor fluid and nutritional intake, and somnolence (5.14, 8.5)

See 17 for PATIENT COUNSELING INFORMATION and Medication Guide.

Revised: 2/2016

FULL PRESCRIBING INFORMATION: CONTENTS*
WARNING: LIFE THREATENING ADVERSE REACTIONS

* Sections or subsections omitted from the full prescribing information are not listed.

FULL PRESCRIBING INFORMATION

WARNING: LIFE THREATENING ADVERSE REACTIONS

Hepatotoxicity

General Population: Hepatic failure resulting in fatalities has occurred in patients receiving valproate and its derivatives. These incidents usually have occurred during the first six months of treatment. Serious or fatal hepatotoxicity may be preceded by nonspecific symptoms such as malaise, weakness, lethargy, facial edema, anorexia, and vomiting. In patients with epilepsy, a loss of seizure control may also occur. Patients should be monitored closely for appearance of these symptoms. Serum liver tests should be performed prior to therapy and at frequent intervals thereafter, especially during the first six months [see Warnings and Precautions (5.1)].

Children under the age of two years are at a considerably increased risk of developing fatal hepatotoxicity, especially those on multiple anticonvulsants, those with congenital metabolic disorders, those with severe seizure disorders accompanied by mental retardation, and those with organic brain disease. When Depakote ER is used in this patient group, it should be used with extreme caution and as a sole agent. The benefits of therapy should be weighed against the risks. The incidence of fatal hepatotoxicity decreases considerably in progressively older patient groups.

Patients with Mitochondrial Disease: There is an increased risk of valproate-induced acute liver failure and resultant deaths in patients with hereditary neurometabolic syndromes caused by DNA mutations of the mitochondrial DNA Polymerase γ (POLG) gene (e.g. Alpers Huttenlocher Syndrome). Depakote ER is contraindicated in patients known to have mitochondrial disorders caused by POLG mutations and children under two years of age who are clinically suspected of having a mitochondrial disorder [see Contraindications (4)]. In patients over two years of age who are clinically suspected of having a hereditary mitochondrial disease, Depakote ER should only be used after other anticonvulsants have failed. This older group of patients should be closely monitored during treatment with Depakote ER for the development of acute liver injury with regular clinical assessments and serum liver testing. POLG mutation screening should be performed in accordance with current clinical practice [see Warnings and Precautions (5.1)].

Fetal Risk

Valproate can cause major congenital malformations, particularly neural tube defects (e.g., spina bifida). In addition, valproate can cause decreased IQ scores following in utero exposure.

Valproate is therefore contraindicated in pregnant women treated for prophylaxis of migraine [see Contraindications (4)]. Valproate should only be used to treat pregnant women with epilepsy or bipolar disorder if other medications have failed to control their symptoms or are otherwise unacceptable.

Valproate should not be administered to a woman of childbearing potential unless the drug is essential to the management of her medical condition. This is especially important when valproate use is considered for a condition not usually associated with permanent injury or death (e.g., migraine). Women should use effective contraception while using valproate [see Warnings and Precautions (5.2, 5.3, 5.4)].

A Medication Guide describing the risks of valproate is available for patients [see Patient Counseling Information (17)].

Pancreatitis

Cases of life-threatening pancreatitis have been reported in both children and adults receiving valproate. Some of the cases have been described as hemorrhagic with a rapid progression from initial symptoms to death. Cases have been reported shortly after initial use as well as after several years of use. Patients and guardians should be warned that abdominal pain, nausea, vomiting and/or anorexia can be symptoms of pancreatitis that require prompt medical evaluation. If pancreatitis is diagnosed, val-

proate should ordinarily be discontinued. Alternative treatment for the underlying medical condition should be initiated as clinically indicated [see Warnings and Precautions (5.5)].

1 INDICATIONS AND USAGE
1.1 Mania

Depakote ER is a valproate and is indicated for the treatment of acute manic or mixed episodes associated with bipolar disorder, with or without psychotic features. A manic episode is a distinct period of abnormally and persistently elevated, expansive, or irritable mood. Typical symptoms of mania include pressure of speech, motor hyperactivity, reduced need for sleep, flight of ideas, grandiosity, poor judgment, aggressiveness, and possible hostility. A mixed episode is characterized by the criteria for a manic episode in conjunction with those for a major depressive episode (depressed mood, loss of interest or pleasure in nearly all activities).

The efficacy of Depakote ER is based in part on studies of Depakote (divalproex sodium delayed release tablets) in this indication, and was confirmed in a 3-week trial with patients meeting DSM-IV TR criteria for bipolar I disorder, manic or mixed type, who were hospitalized for acute mania [see Clinical Studies (14.1)].

The effectiveness of valproate for long-term use in mania, i.e., more than 3 weeks, has not been demonstrated in controlled clinical trials. Therefore, healthcare providers who elect to use Depakote ER for extended periods should continually reevaluate the long-term risk-benefits of the drug for the individual patient.

1.2 Epilepsy

Depakote ER is indicated as monotherapy and adjunctive therapy in the treatment of adult patients and pediatric patients down to the age of 10 years with complex partial seizures that occur either in isolation or in association with other types of seizures. Depakote ER is also indicated for use as sole and adjunctive therapy in the treatment of simple and complex absence seizures in adults and children 10 years of age or older, and adjunctively in adults and children 10 years of age or older with multiple seizure types that include absence seizures.

Simple absence is defined as very brief clouding of the sensorium or loss of consciousness accompanied by certain generalized epileptic discharges without other detectable clinical signs. Complex absence is the term used when other signs are also present.

1.3 Migraine

Depakote ER is indicated for prophylaxis of migraine headaches. There is no evidence that Depakote ER is useful in the acute treatment of migraine headaches.

1.4 Important Limitations

Because of the risk to the fetus of decreased IQ, neural tube defects, and other major congenital malformations, which may occur very early in pregnancy, valproate should not be administered to a woman of childbearing potential unless the drug is essential to the management of her medical condition [see Warnings and Precautions (5.2, 5.3, 5.4), Use in Specific Populations (8.1), and Patient Counseling Information (17)].

Depakote ER is contraindicated for prophylaxis of migraine headaches in women who are pregnant.

2 DOSAGE AND ADMINISTRATION

Depakote ER is an extended-release product intended for once-a-day oral administration. Depakote ER tablets should be swallowed whole and should not be crushed or chewed.

2.1 Mania

Depakote ER tablets are administered orally. The recommended initial dose is 25 mg/kg/day given once daily. The dose should be increased as rapidly as possible to achieve the lowest therapeutic dose which produces the desired clinical effect or the desired range of plasma concentrations. In a placebo-controlled clinical trial of acute mania or mixed type, patients were dosed to a clinical response with a trough plasma concentration between 85 and 125 mcg/mL. The maximum recommended dosage is 60 mg/kg/day.

Continued on next page

Information on the AbbVie, Inc. products listed on these pages is from the prescribing information in use as of July 31, 2016. For more information, please visit rxabbvie.com or call 1-800-633-9110.

There is no body of evidence available from controlled trials to guide a clinician in the longer term management of a patient who improves during Depakote ER treatment of an acute manic episode. While it is generally agreed that pharmacological treatment beyond an acute response in mania is desirable, both for maintenance of the initial response and for prevention of new manic episodes, there are no data to support the benefits of Depakote ER in such longer-term treatment (i.e., beyond 3 weeks).

2.2 Epilepsy

Depakote ER (divalproex sodium) extended release tablets are administered orally, and must be swallowed whole. As Depakote ER dosage is titrated upward, concentrations of clonazepam, diazepam, ethosuximide, lamotrigine, tolbutamide, phenobarbital, carbamazepine, and/or phenytoin may be affected *[see Drug Interactions (7.2)]*.

Complex Partial Seizures

For adults and children 10 years of age or older.

Monotherapy (Initial Therapy)

Depakote ER has not been systematically studied as initial therapy. Patients should initiate therapy at 10 to 15 mg/kg/day. The dosage should be increased by 5 to 10 mg/kg/week to achieve optimal clinical response. Ordinarily, optimal clinical response is achieved at daily doses below 60 mg/kg/day. If satisfactory clinical response has not been achieved, plasma levels should be measured to determine whether or not they are in the usually accepted therapeutic range (50 to 100 mcg/mL). No recommendation regarding the safety of valproate for use at doses above 60 mg/kg/day can be made.

The probability of thrombocytopenia increases significantly at total trough valproate plasma concentrations above 110 mcg/mL in females and 135 mcg/mL in males. The benefit of improved seizure control with higher doses should be weighed against the possibility of a greater incidence of adverse reactions.

Conversion to Monotherapy

Patients should initiate therapy at 10 to 15 mg/kg/day. The dosage should be increased by 5 to 10 mg/kg/week to achieve optimal clinical response. Ordinarily, optimal clinical response is achieved at daily doses below 60 mg/kg/day. If satisfactory clinical response has not been achieved, plasma levels should be measured to determine whether or not they are in the usually accepted therapeutic range (50 - 100 mcg/mL). No recommendation regarding the safety of valproate for use at doses above 60 mg/kg/day can be made. Concomitant antiepilepsy drug (AED) dosage can ordinarily be reduced by approximately 25% every 2 weeks. This reduction may be started at initiation of Depakote ER therapy, or delayed by 1 to 2 weeks if there is a concern that seizures are likely to occur with a reduction. The speed and duration of withdrawal of the concomitant AED can be highly variable, and patients should be monitored closely during this period for increased seizure frequency.

Adjunctive Therapy

Depakote ER may be added to the patient's regimen at a dosage of 10 to 15 mg/kg/day. The dosage may be increased by 5 to 10 mg/kg/week to achieve optimal clinical response. Ordinarily, optimal clinical response is achieved at daily doses below 60 mg/kg/day. If satisfactory clinical response has not been achieved, plasma levels should be measured to determine whether or not they are in the usually accepted therapeutic range (50 to 100 mcg/mL). No recommendation regarding the safety of valproate for use at doses above 60 mg/kg/day can be made.

In a study of adjunctive therapy for complex partial seizures in which patients were receiving either carbamazepine or phenytoin in addition to valproate, no adjustment of carbamazepine or phenytoin dosage was needed *[see Clinical Studies (14.2)]*. However, since valproate may interact with these or other concurrently administered AEDs as well as other drugs, periodic plasma concentration determinations of concomitant AEDs are recommended during the early course of therapy *[see Drug Interactions (7)]*.

Simple and Complex Absence Seizures

The recommended initial dose is 15 mg/kg/day, increasing at one week intervals by 5 to 10 mg/kg/day until seizures are controlled or side effects preclude further increases. The maximum recommended dosage is 60 mg/kg/day.

A good correlation has not been established between daily dose, serum concentrations, and therapeutic effect. However, therapeutic valproate serum concentration for most patients with absence seizures is considered to range from 50 to 100 mcg/mL. Some patients may be controlled with lower or higher serum concentrations *[see Clinical Pharmacology (12.3)]*.

As Depakote ER dosage is titrated upward, blood concentrations of phenobarbital and/or phenytoin may be affected *[see Drug Interactions (7.2)]*.

Antiepilepsy drugs should not be abruptly discontinued in patients in whom the drug is administered to prevent major seizures because of the strong possibility of precipitating status epilepticus with attendant hypoxia and threat to life.

2.3 Migraine

Depakote ER is indicated for prophylaxis of migraine headaches in adults.

The recommended starting dose is 500 mg once daily for 1 week, thereafter increasing to 1000 mg once daily. Although doses other than 1000 mg once daily of Depakote ER have not been evaluated in patients with migraine, the effective dose range of Depakote (divalproex sodium delayed-release tablets) in these patients is 500-1000 mg/day. As with other valproate products, doses of Depakote ER should be individualized and dose adjustment may be necessary. If a patient requires smaller dose adjustments than that available with Depakote ER, Depakote should be used instead.

2.4 Conversion from Depakote to Depakote ER

In adult patients and pediatric patients 10 years of age or older with epilepsy previously receiving Depakote, Depakote ER should be administered once-daily using a dose 8 to 20% higher than the total daily dose of Depakote (Table 1). For patients whose Depakote total daily dose cannot be directly converted to Depakote ER, consideration may be given at the clinician's discretion to increase the patient's Depakote total daily dose to the next higher dosage before converting to the appropriate total daily dose of Depakote ER.

Table 1. Dose Conversion

Depakote Total Daily Dose (mg)	Depakote ER (mg)
500* - 625	750
750* - 875	1000
1000*-1125	1250
1250-1375	1500
1500-1625	1750
1750	2000
1875-2000	2250
2125-2250	2500
2375	2750
2500-2750	3000
2875	3250
3000-3125	3500

* These total daily doses of Depakote cannot be directly converted to an 8 to 20% higher total daily dose of Depakote ER because the required dosing strengths of Depakote ER are not available. Consideration may be given at the clinician's discretion to increase the patient's Depakote total daily dose to the next higher dosage before converting to the appropriate total daily dose of Depakote ER.

There is insufficient data to allow a conversion factor recommendation for patients with DEPAKOTE doses above 3125 mg/day. Plasma valproate C_{min} concentrations for DEPAKOTE ER on average are equivalent to DEPAKOTE, but may vary across patients after conversion. If satisfactory clinical response has not been achieved, plasma levels should be measured to determine whether or not they are in the usually accepted therapeutic range (50 to 100 mcg/mL) *[see Clinical Pharmacology (12.2)]*.

2.5 General Dosing Advice

Dosing in Elderly Patients

Due to a decrease in unbound clearance of valproate and possibly a greater sensitivity to somnolence in the elderly, the starting dose should be reduced in these patients. Starting doses in the elderly lower than 250 mg can only be achieved by the use of Depakote. Dosage should be increased more slowly and with regular monitoring for fluid and nutritional intake, dehydration, somnolence, and other adverse reactions. Dose reductions or discontinuation of valproate should be considered in patients with decreased food or fluid intake and in patients with excessive somnolence. The ultimate therapeutic dose should be achieved on the basis of both tolerability and clinical response *[see Warnings and Precautions (5.14), Use in Specific Populations (8.5) and Clinical Pharmacology (12.3)]*.

Dose-Related Adverse Reactions

The frequency of adverse effects (particularly elevated liver enzymes and thrombocytopenia) may be dose-related. The probability of thrombocytopenia appears to increase significantly at total valproate concentrations of ≥ 110 mcg/mL (females) or ≥ 135 mcg/mL (males) *[see Warnings and Precautions (5.8)]*. The benefit of improved therapeutic effect with higher doses should be weighed against the possibility of a greater incidence of adverse reactions.

G.I. Irritation

Patients who experience G.I. irritation may benefit from administration of the drug with food or by slowly building up the dose from an initial low level.

Compliance

Patients should be informed to take Depakote ER every day as prescribed. If a dose is missed it should be taken as soon as possible, unless it is almost time for the next dose. If a dose is skipped, the patient should not double the next dose.

2.6 Dosing in Patients Taking Rufinamide

Patients stabilized on rufinamide before being prescribed valproate should begin valproate therapy at a low dose, and titrate to a clinically effective dose *[see Drug Interactions (7.2)]*.

3 DOSAGE FORMS AND STRENGTHS

Depakote ER 250 mg is available as white ovaloid tablets with the "a" logo and the code (HF). Each Depakote ER tablet contains divalproex sodium equivalent to 250 mg of valproic acid.

Depakote ER 500 mg is available as gray ovaloid tablets with the "a" logo and the code HC. Each Depakote ER tablet contains divalproex sodium equivalent to 500 mg of valproic acid.

4 CONTRAINDICATIONS

- Depakote ER should not be administered to patients with hepatic disease or significant hepatic dysfunction *[see Warnings and Precautions (5.1)]*.
- Depakote ER is contraindicated in patients known to have mitochondrial disorders caused by mutations in mitochondrial DNA polymerase γ (POLG; e.g., Alpers-Huttenlocher Syndrome) and children under two years of age who are suspected of having a POLG-related disorder *[see Warnings and Precautions (5.1)]*.
- Depakote ER is contraindicated in patients with known hypersensitivity to the drug *[see Warnings and Precautions (5.12)]*.
- Depakote ER is contraindicated in patients with known urea cycle disorders *[see Warnings and Precautions (5.6)]*.
- Depakote ER is contraindicated for use in prophylaxis of migraine headaches in pregnant women *[see Warnings and Precautions (5.3) and Use in Specific Populations (8.1)]*.

5 WARNINGS AND PRECAUTIONS

5.1 Hepatotoxicity

General Information on Hepatotoxicity

Hepatic failure resulting in fatalities has occurred in patients receiving valproate. These incidents usually have occurred during the first six months of treatment. Serious or fatal hepatotoxicity may be preceded by non-specific symptoms such as malaise, weakness, lethargy, facial edema, anorexia, and vomiting. In patients with epilepsy, a loss of seizure control may also occur. Patients should be monitored closely for appearance of these symptoms. Serum liver tests should be performed prior to therapy and at frequent intervals thereafter, especially during the first six months. However, healthcare providers should not rely totally on serum biochemistry since these tests may not be abnormal in all instances, but should also consider the results of careful interim medical history and physical examination.

Caution should be observed when administering valproate products to patients with a prior history of hepatic disease. Patients on multiple anticonvulsants, children, those with congenital metabolic disorders, those with severe seizure disorders accompanied by mental retardation, and those with organic brain disease may be at particular risk. See below, "Patients with Known or Suspected Mitochondrial Disease."

Experience has indicated that children under the age of two years are at a considerably increased risk of developing fatal hepatotoxicity, especially those with the aforementioned conditions. When Depakote ER is used in this patient group, it should be used with extreme caution and as a sole agent. The benefits of therapy should be weighed against the risks. In progressively older patient groups experience in epilepsy has indicated that the incidence of fatal hepatotoxicity decreases considerably.

Patients with Known or Suspected Mitochondrial Disease

Depakote ER is contraindicated in patients known to have mitochondrial disorders caused by POLG mutations and children under two years of age who are clinically suspected of having a mitochondrial disorder *[see Contraindications (4)]*. Valproate-induced acute liver failure and liver-related deaths have been reported in patients with hereditary neurometabolic syndromes caused by mutations in the gene for mitochondrial DNA polymerase γ (POLG) (e.g., Alpers-Huttenlocher Syndrome) at a higher rate than those without these syndromes. Most of the reported cases of liver failure in patients with these syndromes have been identified in children and adolescents.

POLG-related disorders should be suspected in patients with a family history or suggestive symptoms of a POLG-related disorder, including but not limited to unexplained encephalopathy, refractory epilepsy (focal, myoclonic), status epilepticus at presentation, developmental delays, psychomotor regression, axonal sensorimotor neuropathy, myopathy cerebellar ataxia, opthalmoplegia, or complicated migraine with occipital aura. POLG mutation testing should be performed in accordance with current clinical practice for the diagnostic evaluation of such disorders. The A467T and W748S mutations are present in approximately 2/3 of patients with autosomal recessive POLG-related disorders.

In patients over two years of age who are clinically suspected of having a hereditary mitochondrial disease, Depakote ER should only be used after other anticonvulsants have failed. This older group of patients should be closely monitored during treatment with Depakote ER for the development of acute liver injury with regular clinical assessments and serum liver test monitoring.

The drug should be discontinued immediately in the presence of significant hepatic dysfunction, suspected or apparent. In some cases, hepatic dysfunction has progressed in spite of discontinuation of drug *[see Boxed Warning and Contraindications (4)]*.

5.2 Birth Defects

Valproate can cause fetal harm when administered to a pregnant woman. Pregnancy registry data show that maternal valproate use can cause neural tube defects and other structural abnormalities (e.g., craniofacial defects, cardiovascular malformations, hypospadias, limb malformations). The rate of congenital malformations among babies born to mothers using valproate is about four times higher than the rate among babies born to epileptic mothers using other anti-seizure monotherapies. Evidence suggests that folic acid supplementation prior to conception and during the first trimester of pregnancy decreases the risk for congenital neural tube defects in the general population.

5.3 Decreased IQ Following *in utero* Exposure

Valproate can cause decreased IQ scores following *in utero* exposure. Published epidemiological studies have indicated that children exposed to valproate *in utero* have lower cognitive test scores than children exposed *in utero* to either another antiepileptic drug or to no antiepileptic drugs. The largest of these studies[1] is a prospective cohort study conducted in the United States and United Kingdom that found that children with prenatal exposure to valproate (n=62) had lower IQ scores at age 6 (97 [95% C.I. 94-101]) than children with prenatal exposure to the other antiepileptic drug monotherapy treatments evaluated: lamotrigine (108 [95% C.I. 105–110]), carbamazepine (105 [95% C.I. 102–108]), and phenytoin (108 [95% C.I. 104–112]). It is not known when during pregnancy cognitive effects in valproate-exposed children occur. Because the women in this study were exposed to antiepileptic drugs throughout pregnancy, whether the risk for decreased IQ was related to a particular time period during pregnancy could not be assessed.

Although all of the available studies have methodological limitations, the weight of the evidence supports the conclusion that valproate exposure *in utero* can cause decreased IQ in children.

In animal studies, offspring with prenatal exposure to valproate had malformations similar to those seen in humans and demonstrated neurobehavioral deficits *[see Use in Specific Populations (8.1)]*.

Valproate use is contraindicated during pregnancy in women being treated for prophylaxis of migraine headaches. Women with epilepsy or bipolar disorder who are pregnant or who plan to become pregnant should not be treated with valproate unless other treatments have failed to provide adequate symptom control or are otherwise unacceptable. In such women, the benefits of treatment with valproate during pregnancy may still outweigh the risks.

5.4 Use in Women of Childbearing Potential

Because of the risk to the fetus of decreased IQ and major congenital malformations (including neural tube defects), which may occur very early in pregnancy, valproate should not be administered to a woman of childbearing potential unless the drug is essential to the management of her medical condition. This is especially important when valproate use is considered for a condition not usually associated with permanent injury or death (e.g., migraine). Women should use effective contraception while using valproate. Women who are planning a pregnancy should be counseled regarding the relative risks and benefits of valproate use during pregnancy, and alternative therapeutic options should be considered for these patients *[see Boxed Warning and Use in Specific Populations (8.1)]*.

To prevent major seizures, valproate should not be discontinued abruptly, as this can precipitate status epilepticus with resulting maternal and fetal hypoxia and threat to life.

Evidence suggests that folic acid supplementation prior to conception and during the first trimester of pregnancy decreases the risk for congenital neural tube defects in the general population. It is not known whether the risk of neural tube defects or decreased IQ in the offspring of women receiving valproate is reduced by folic acid supplementation. Dietary folic acid supplementation both prior to conception and during pregnancy should be routinely recommended for patients using valproate.

5.5 Pancreatitis

Cases of life-threatening pancreatitis have been reported in both children and adults receiving valproate. Some of the cases have been described as hemorrhagic with rapid progression from initial symptoms to death. Some cases have occurred shortly after initial use as well as after several years of use. The rate based upon the reported cases exceeds that expected in the general population and there have been cases in which pancreatitis recurred after rechallenge with valproate. In clinical trials, there were 2 cases of pancreatitis without alternative etiology in 2416 patients, representing 1044 patient-years experience. Patients and guardians should be warned that abdominal pain, nausea, vomiting, and/or anorexia can be symptoms of pancreatitis that require prompt medical evaluation. If pancreatitis is diagnosed, Depakote ER should ordinarily be discontinued. Alternative treatment for the underlying medical condition should be initiated as clinically indicated *[see Boxed Warning]*.

5.6 Urea Cycle Disorders

Depakote ER is contraindicated in patients with known urea cycle disorders (UCD). Hyperammonemic encephalopathy, sometimes fatal, has been reported following initiation of valproate therapy in patients with urea cycle disorders, a group of uncommon genetic abnormalities, particularly ornithine transcarbamylase deficiency. Prior to the initiation of Depakote ER therapy, evaluation for UCD should be considered in the following patients: 1) those with a history of unexplained encephalopathy or coma, encephalopathy associated with a protein load, pregnancy-related or postpartum encephalopathy, unexplained mental retardation, or history of elevated plasma ammonia or glutamine; 2) those with cyclical vomiting and lethargy, episodic extreme irritability, ataxia, low BUN, or protein avoidance; 3) those with a family history of UCD or a family history of unexplained infant deaths (particularly males); 4) those with other signs or symptoms of UCD. Patients who develop symptoms of unexplained hyperammonemic encephalopathy while receiving valproate therapy should receive prompt treatment (including discontinuation of valproate therapy) and be evaluated for underlying urea cycle disorders *[see Contraindications (4) and Warnings and Precautions (5.10)]*.

5.7 Suicidal Behavior and Ideation

Antiepileptic drugs (AEDs), including Depakote ER, increase the risk of suicidal thoughts or behavior in patients taking these drugs for any indication. Patients treated with any AED for any indication should be monitored for the emergence or worsening of depression, suicidal thoughts or behavior, and/or any unusual changes in mood or behavior.

Pooled analyses of 199 placebo-controlled clinical trials (mono- and adjunctive therapy) of 11 different AEDs showed that patients randomized to one of the AEDs had approximately twice the risk (adjusted Relative Risk 1.8, 95% CI:1.2, 2.7) of suicidal thinking or behavior compared to patients randomized to placebo. In these trials, which had a median treatment duration of 12 weeks, the estimated incidence rate of suicidal behavior or ideation among 27,863 AED-treated patients was 0.43%, compared to 0.24% among 16,029 placebo-treated patients, representing an increase of approximately one case of suicidal thinking or behavior for every 530 patients treated. There were four suicides in drug-treated patients in the trials and none in placebo-treated patients, but the number is too small to allow any conclusion about drug effect on suicide.

The increased risk of suicidal thoughts or behavior with AEDs was observed as early as one week after starting drug treatment with AEDs and persisted for the duration of treatment assessed. Because most trials included in the analysis did not extend beyond 24 weeks, the risk of suicidal thoughts or behavior beyond 24 weeks could not be assessed.

The risk of suicidal thoughts or behavior was generally consistent among drugs in the data analyzed. The finding of increased risk with AEDs of varying mechanisms of action and across a range of indications suggests that the risk applies to all AEDs used for any indication. The risk did not vary substantially by age (5-100 years) in the clinical trials analyzed.

Table 2 shows absolute and relative risk by indication for all evaluated AEDs.

[See table 2 below]

The relative risk for suicidal thoughts or behavior was higher in clinical trials for epilepsy than in clinical trials for psychiatric or other conditions, but the absolute risk differences were similar for the epilepsy and psychiatric indications.

Anyone considering prescribing Depakote ER or any other AED must balance the risk of suicidal thoughts or behavior with the risk of untreated illness. Epilepsy and many other illnesses for which AEDs are prescribed are themselves associated with morbidity and mortality and an increased risk of suicidal thoughts and behavior. Should suicidal thoughts and behavior emerge during treatment, the prescriber needs to consider whether the emergence of these symptoms in any given patient may be related to the illness being treated.

Continued on next page

Table 2. Risk by indication for antiepileptic drugs in the pooled analysis

Indication	Placebo Patients with Events Per 1000 Patients	Drug Patients with Events Per 1000 Patients	Relative Risk: Incidence of Events in Drug Patients/ Incidence in Placebo Patients	Risk Difference: Additional Drug Patients with Events Per 1000 Patients
Epilepsy	1.0	3.4	3.5	2.4
Psychiatric	5.7	8.5	1.5	2.9
Other	1.0	1.8	1.9	0.9
Total	2.4	4.3	1.8	1.9

Information on the AbbVie, Inc. products listed on these pages is from the prescribing information in use as of July 31, 2016. For more information, please visit rxabbvie.com or call 1-800-633-9110.

Patients, their caregivers, and families should be informed that AEDs increase the risk of suicidal thoughts and behavior and should be advised of the need to be alert for the emergence or worsening of the signs and symptoms of depression, any unusual changes in mood or behavior, or the emergence of suicidal thoughts, behavior, or thoughts about self-harm. Behaviors of concern should be reported immediately to healthcare providers.

5.8 Bleeding and Other Hematopoietic Disorders

Valproate is associated with dose-related thrombocytopenia. In a clinical trial of valproate as monotherapy in patients with epilepsy, 34/126 patients (27%) receiving approximately 50 mg/kg/day on average, had at least one value of platelets $\leq 75 \times 10^9$/L. Approximately half of these patients had treatment discontinued, with return of platelet counts to normal. In the remaining patients, platelet counts normalized with continued treatment. In this study, the probability of thrombocytopenia appeared to increase significantly at total valproate concentrations of ≥ 110 mcg/mL (females) or ≥ 135 mcg/mL (males). The therapeutic benefit which may accompany the higher doses should therefore be weighed against the possibility of a greater incidence of adverse effects. Valproate use has also been associated with decreases in other cell lines and myelodysplasia.

Because of reports of cytopenias, inhibition of the secondary phase of platelet aggregation, and abnormal coagulation parameters, (e.g., low fibrinogen, coagulation factor deficiencies, acquired von Willebrand's disease), measurements of complete blood counts and coagulation tests are recommended before initiating therapy and at periodic intervals. It is recommended that patients receiving Depakote ER be monitored for blood counts and coagulation parameters prior to planned surgery and during pregnancy *[see Use in Specific Populations (8.1)]*. Evidence of hemorrhage, bruising, or a disorder of hemostasis/coagulation is an indication for reduction of the dosage or withdrawal of therapy.

5.9 Hyperammonemia

Hyperammonemia has been reported in association with valproate therapy and may be present despite normal liver function tests. In patients who develop unexplained lethargy and vomiting or changes in mental status, hyperammonemic encephalopathy should be considered and an ammonia level should be measured. Hyperammonemia should also be considered in patients who present with hypothermia *[see Warnings and Precautions (5.11)]*. If ammonia is increased, valproate therapy should be discontinued. Appropriate interventions for treatment of hyperammonemia should be initiated, and such patients should undergo investigation for underlying urea cycle disorders *[see Contraindications (4) and Warnings and Precautions (5.6, 5.10)]*.

During the placebo controlled pediatric mania trial, one (1) in twenty (20) adolescents (5%) treated with valproate developed increased plasma ammonia levels compared to no (0) patients treated with placebo.

Asymptomatic elevations of ammonia are more common and when present, require close monitoring of plasma ammonia levels. If the elevation persists, discontinuation of valproate therapy should be considered.

5.10 Hyperammonemia and Encephalopathy associated with Concomitant Topiramate Use

Concomitant administration of topiramate and valproate has been associated with hyperammonemia with or without encephalopathy in patients who have tolerated either drug alone. Clinical symptoms of hyperammonemic encephalopathy often include acute alterations in level of consciousness and/or cognitive function with lethargy or vomiting. Hypothermia can also be a manifestation of hyperammonemia *[see Warnings and Precautions (5.11)]*. In most cases, symptoms and signs abated with discontinuation of either drug. This adverse event is not due to a pharmacokinetic interaction. Patients with inborn errors of metabolism or reduced hepatic mitochondrial activity may be at an increased risk for hyperammonemia with or without encephalopathy. Although not studied, an interaction of topiramate and valproate may exacerbate existing defects or unmask deficiencies in susceptible persons. In patients who develop unexplained lethargy, vomiting, or changes in mental status, hyperammonemic encephalopathy should be considered and an ammonia level should be measured *[see Contraindications (4) and Warnings and Precautions (5.6, 5.9)]*.

5.11 Hypothermia

Hypothermia, defined as an unintentional drop in body core temperature to < 35°C (95°F), has been reported in association with valproate therapy both in conjunction with and in the absence of hyperammonemia. This adverse reaction can also occur in patients using concomitant topiramate with valproate after starting topiramate treatment or after increasing the daily dose of topiramate *[see Drug Interactions (7.3)]*. Consideration should be given to stopping valproate in patients who develop hypothermia, which may be manifested by a variety of clinical abnormalities including lethargy, confusion, coma, and significant alterations in other major organ systems such as the cardiovascular and respiratory systems. Clinical management and assessment should include examination of blood ammonia levels.

5.12 Drug Reaction with Eosinophilia and Systemic Symptoms (DRESS)/Multiorgan Hypersensitivity Reactions

Drug Reaction with Eosinophilia and Systemic Symptoms (DRESS), also known as Multiorgan Hypersensitivity, has been reported in patients taking valproate. DRESS may be fatal or life-threatening. DRESS typically, although not exclusively, presents with fever, rash, and/or lymphadenopathy, in association with other organ system involvement, such as hepatitis, nephritis, hematological abnormalities, myocarditis, or myositis sometimes resembling an acute viral infection. Eosinophilia is often present. Because this disorder is variable in its expression, other organ systems not noted here may be involved. It is important to note that early manifestations of hypersensitivity, such as fever or lymphadenopathy, may be present even though rash is not evident. If such signs or symptoms are present, the patient should be evaluated immediately. Valproate should be discontinued and not be resumed if an alternative etiology for the signs or symptoms cannot be established.

5.13 Interaction with Carbapenem Antibiotics

Carbapenem antibiotics (for example, ertapenem, imipenem, meropenem; this is not a complete list) may reduce serum valproate concentrations to subtherapeutic levels, resulting in loss of seizure control. Serum valproate concentrations should be monitored frequently after initiating carbapenem therapy. Alternative antibacterial or anticonvulsant therapy should be considered if serum valproate concentrations drop significantly or seizure control deteriorates *[see Drug Interactions (7.1)]*.

5.14 Somnolence in the Elderly

In a double-blind, multicenter trial of valproate in elderly patients with dementia (mean age = 83 years), doses were increased by 125 mg/day to a target dose of 20 mg/kg/day. A significantly higher proportion of valproate patients had somnolence compared to placebo, and although not statistically significant, there was a higher proportion of patients with dehydration. Discontinuations for somnolence were also significantly higher than with placebo. In some patients with somnolence (approximately one-half), there was associated reduced nutritional intake and weight loss. There was a trend for the patients who experienced these events to have a lower baseline albumin concentration, lower valproate clearance, and a higher BUN. In elderly patients, dosage should be increased more slowly and with regular monitoring for fluid and nutritional intake, dehydration, somnolence, and other adverse reactions. Dose reductions or discontinuation of valproate should be considered in patients with decreased food or fluid intake and in patients with excessive somnolence *[see Dosage and Administration (2.4)]*.

5.15 Monitoring: Drug Plasma Concentration

Since valproate may interact with concurrently administered drugs which are capable of enzyme induction, periodic plasma concentration determinations of valproate and concomitant drugs are recommended during the early course of therapy *[see Drug Interactions (7)]*.

5.16 Effect on Ketone and Thyroid Function Tests

Valproate is partially eliminated in the urine as a keto-metabolite which may lead to a false interpretation of the urine ketone test.

There have been reports of altered thyroid function tests associated with valproate. The clinical significance of these is unknown.

5.17 Effect on HIV and CMV Viruses Replication

There are *in vitro* studies that suggest valproate stimulates the replication of the HIV and CMV viruses under certain experimental conditions. The clinical consequence, if any, is not known. Additionally, the relevance of these *in vitro* findings is uncertain for patients receiving maximally suppressive antiretroviral therapy. Nevertheless, these data should be borne in mind when interpreting the results from regular monitoring of the viral load in HIV infected patients receiving valproate or when following CMV infected patients clinically.

5.18 Medication Residue in the Stool

There have been rare reports of medication residue in the stool. Some patients have had anatomic (including ileostomy or colostomy) or functional gastrointestinal disorders with shortened GI transit times. In some reports, medication residues have occurred in the context of diarrhea. It is recommended that plasma valproate levels be checked in patients who experience medication residue in the stool, and patients' clinical condition should be monitored. If clinically indicated, alternative treatment may be considered.

6 ADVERSE REACTIONS

The following serious adverse reactions are described below and elsewhere in the labeling:

- Hepatic failure *[see Warnings and Precautions (5.1)]*
- Birth defects *[see Warnings and Precautions (5.2)]*
- Decreased IQ following *in utero* exposure *[see Warnings and Precautions (5.3)]*
- Pancreatitis *[see Warnings and Precautions (5.5)]*
- Hyperammonemic encephalopathy *[see Warnings and Precautions (5.6, 5.9, 5.10)]*
- Suicidal behavior and ideation *[see Warnings and Precautions (5.7)]*
- Bleeding and other hematopoietic disorders *[see Warnings and Precautions (5.8)]*
- Hypothermia *[see Warnings and Precautions (5.11)]*
- Drug Reaction with Eosinophilia and Systemic Symptoms (DRESS)/Multiorgan hypersensitivity reactions *[see Warnings and Precautions (5.12)]*
- Somnolence in the elderly *[see Warnings and Precautions (5.14)]*

Because clinical studies are conducted under widely varying conditions, adverse reaction rates observed in the clinical studies of a drug cannot be directly compared to rates in the clinical studies of another drug and may not reflect the rates observed in practice.

Information on pediatric adverse reactions is presented in section 8.

6.1 Mania

The incidence of treatment-emergent events has been ascertained based on combined data from two three week placebo-controlled clinical trials of Depakote ER in the treatment of manic episodes associated with bipolar disorder.

Table 3 summarizes those adverse reactions reported for patients in these trials where the incidence rate in the Depakote ER-treated group was greater than 5% and greater than the placebo incidence.

Table 3. Adverse Reactions Reported by > 5% of Depakote-Treated Patients During Placebo-Controlled Trials of Acute Mania[1]

Adverse Event	Depakote ER (n=338)	Placebo (n=263)
Somnolence	26%	14%
Dyspepsia	23%	11%
Nausea	19%	13%
Vomiting	13%	5%
Diarrhea	12%	8%
Dizziness	12%	7%
Pain	11%	10%
Abdominal pain	10%	5%
Accidental injury	6%	5%
Asthenia	6%	5%
Pharyngitis	6%	5%

1. The following adverse reactions/event occurred at an equal or greater incidence for placebo than for Depakote ER: headache

The following additional adverse reactions were reported by greater than 1% of the Depakote ER-treated patients in controlled clinical trials:

Body as a Whole: Back Pain, Chills, Chills and Fever, Drug Level Increased, Flu Syndrome, Infection, Infection Fungal, Neck Rigidity.

Cardiovascular System: Arrhythmia, Hypertension, Hypotension, Postural Hypotension.

Digestive System: Constipation, Dry Mouth, Dysphagia, Fecal Incontinence, Flatulence, Gastroenteritis, Glossitis, Gum Hemorrhage, Mouth Ulceration.

Hemic and Lymphatic System: Anemia, Bleeding Time Increased, Ecchymosis, Leucopenia.

Metabolic and Nutritional Disorders: Hypoproteinemia, Peripheral Edema.

Musculoskeletal System: Arthrosis, Myalgia.

Nervous System: Abnormal Gait, Agitation, Catatonic Reaction, Dysarthria, Hallucinations, Hypertonia, Hypokinesia, Psychosis, Reflexes Increased, Sleep Disorder, Tardive Dyskinesia, Tremor.

Respiratory System: Hiccup, Rhinitis.

Skin and Appendages: Discoid Lupus Erythematosus, Erythema Nodosum, Furunculosis, Maculopapular Rash, Pruritus, Rash, Seborrhea, Sweating, Vesiculobullous Rash.

Special Senses: Conjunctivitis, Dry Eyes, Eye Disorder, Eye Pain, Photophobia, Taste Perversion.

Urogenital System: Cystitis, Urinary Tract Infection, Menstrual Disorder, Vaginitis.

6.2 Epilepsy

Based on a placebo-controlled trial of adjunctive therapy for treatment of complex partial seizures, Depakote was generally well tolerated with most adverse reactions rated as mild to moderate in severity. Intolerance was the primary reason for discontinuation in the Depakote-treated patients (6%), compared to 1% of placebo-treated patients.

Table 4 lists treatment-emergent adverse reactions which were reported by ≥ 5% of Depakote-treated patients and for which the incidence was greater than in the placebo group, in the placebo-controlled trial of adjunctive therapy for treatment of complex partial seizures. Since patients were also treated with other antiepilepsy drugs, it is not possible, in most cases, to determine whether the following adverse reactions can be ascribed to Depakote alone, or the combination of Depakote and other antiepilepsy drugs.

Table 4. Adverse Reactions Reported by ≥ 5% of Patients Treated with Valproate During Placebo-Controlled Trial of Adjunctive Therapy for Complex Partial Seizures

Body System/Event	Depakote (%) (N=77)	Placebo (%) (N=70)
Body as a Whole		
Headache	31	21
Asthenia	27	7
Fever	6	4
Gastrointestinal System		
Nausea	48	14
Vomiting	27	7
Abdominal pain	23	6
Diarrhea	13	6
Anorexia	12	0
Dyspepsia	8	4
Constipation	5	1
Nervous System		
Somnolence	27	11
Tremor	25	6
Dizziness	25	13
Diplopia	16	9
Amblyopia/Blurred Vision	12	9
Ataxia	8	1
Nystagmus	8	1
Emotional Lability	6	4
Thinking Abnormal	6	0
Amnesia	5	1

Respiratory System

Flu Syndrome	12	9
Infection	12	6
Bronchitis	5	1
Rhinitis	5	4
Other		
Alopecia	6	1
Weight Loss	6	0

Table 5 lists treatment-emergent adverse reactions which were reported by ≥ 5% of patients in the high dose valproate group, and for which the incidence was greater than in the low dose group, in a controlled trial of Depakote monotherapy treatment of complex partial seizures. Since patients were being titrated off another antiepilepsy drug during the first portion of the trial, it is not possible, in many cases, to determine whether the following adverse reactions can be ascribed to Depakote alone, or the combination of valproate and other antiepilepsy drugs.

Table 5. Adverse Reactions Reported by ≥ 5% of Patients in the High Dose Group in the Controlled Trial of Valproate Monotherapy for Complex Partial Seizures[1]

Body System/Event	High Dose (%) (n=131)	Low Dose (%) (n=134)
Body as a Whole		
Asthenia	21	10
Digestive System		
Nausea	34	26
Diarrhea	23	19
Vomiting	23	15
Abdominal pain	12	9
Anorexia	11	4
Dyspepsia	11	10
Hemic/Lymphatic System		
Thrombocytopenia	24	1
Ecchymosis	5	4
Metabolic/Nutritional		
Weight Gain	9	4
Peripheral Edema	8	3
Nervous System		
Tremor	57	19
Somnolence	30	18
Dizziness	18	13
Insomnia	15	9
Nervousness	11	7
Amnesia	7	4
Nystagmus	7	1
Depression	5	4
Respiratory System		
Infection	20	13
Pharyngitis	8	2
Dyspnea	5	1

Skin and Appendages

Alopecia	24	13
Special Senses		
Amblyopia/Blurred Vision	8	4
Tinnitus	7	1

1. Headache was the only adverse event that occurred in ≥5% of patients in the high dose group and at an equal or greater incidence in the low dose group.

The following additional adverse reactions were reported by greater than 1% but less than 5% of the 358 patients treated with valproate in the controlled trials of complex partial seizures:

Body as a Whole: Back pain, chest pain, malaise.

Cardiovascular System: Tachycardia, hypertension, palpitation.

Digestive System: Increased appetite, flatulence, hematemesis, eructation, pancreatitis, periodontal abscess.

Hemic and Lymphatic System: Petechia.

Metabolic and Nutritional Disorders: SGOT increased, SGPT increased.

Musculoskeletal System: Myalgia, twitching, arthralgia, leg cramps, myasthenia.

Nervous System: Anxiety, confusion, abnormal gait, paresthesia, hypertonia, incoordination, abnormal dreams, personality disorder.

Respiratory System: Sinusitis, cough increased, pneumonia, epistaxis.

Skin and Appendages: Rash, pruritus, dry skin.

Special Senses: Taste perversion, abnormal vision, deafness, otitis media.

Urogenital System: Urinary incontinence, vaginitis, dysmenorrhea, amenorrhea, urinary frequency.

6.3 Migraine

Based on two placebo-controlled clinical trials and their long term extension, valproate was generally well tolerated with most adverse reactions rated as mild to moderate in severity. Of the 202 patients exposed to valproate in the placebo-controlled trials, 17% discontinued for intolerance. This is compared to a rate of 5% for the 81 placebo patients. Including the long term extension study, the adverse reactions reported as the primary reason for discontinuation by ≥ 1% of 248 valproate-treated patients were alopecia (6%), nausea and/or vomiting (5%), weight gain (2%), tremor (2%), somnolence (1%), elevated SGOT and/or SGPT (1%), and depression (1%).

Table 6 includes those adverse reactions reported for patients in the placebo-controlled trial where the incidence rate in the Depakote ER-treated group was greater than 5% and was greater than that for placebo patients.

Table 6. Adverse Reactions Reported by >5% of Depakote ER-Treated Patients During the Migraine Placebo-Controlled Trial with a Greater Incidence than Patients Taking Placebo[1]

Body System Event	Depakote ER (n=122)	Placebo (n=115)
Gastrointestinal System		
Nausea	15%	9%
Dyspepsia	7%	4%
Diarrhea	7%	3%
Vomiting	7%	2%
Abdominal Pain	7%	5%

Continued on next page

Information on the AbbVie, Inc. products listed on these pages is from the prescribing information in use as of July 31, 2016. For more information, please visit rxabbvie.com or call 1-800-633-9110.

Nervous System

Somnolence	7%	2%

Other

Infection	15%	14%

1. The following adverse reactions occurred in greater than 5% of Depakote ER-treated patients and at a greater incidence for placebo than for Depakote ER: asthenia and flu syndrome.

The following additional adverse reactions were reported by greater than 1% but not more than 5% of Depakote ER-treated patients and with a greater incidence than placebo in the placebo-controlled clinical trial for migraine prophylaxis:

Body as a Whole: Accidental injury, viral infection.
Digestive System: Increased appetite, tooth disorder.
Metabolic and Nutritional Disorders: Edema, weight gain.
Nervous System: Abnormal gait, dizziness, hypertonia, insomnia, nervousness, tremor, vertigo.
Respiratory System: Pharyngitis, rhinitis.
Skin and Appendages: Rash.
Special Senses: Tinnitus.

Table 7 includes those adverse reactions reported for patients in the placebo-controlled trials where the incidence rate in the valproate-treated group was greater than 5% and was greater than that for placebo patients.

Table 7. Adverse Reactions Reported by > 5% of Valproate-Treated Patients During Migraine Placebo-Controlled Trials with a Greater Incidence than Patients Taking Placebo[1]

Body System Reaction	Depakote (n=202)	Placebo (n=81)
Gastrointestinal System		
Nausea	31%	10%
Dyspepsia	13%	9%
Diarrhea	12%	7%
Vomiting	11%	1%
Abdominal pain	9%	4%
Increased appetite	6%	4%
Nervous System		
Asthenia	20%	9%
Somnolence	17%	5%
Dizziness	12%	6%
Tremor	9%	0%
Other		
Weight gain	8%	2%
Back pain	8%	6%
Alopecia	7%	1%

1. The following adverse reactions occurred in greater than 5% of Depakote-treated patients and at a greater incidence for placebo than for Depakote: flu syndrome and pharyngitis.

The following additional adverse reactions were reported by greater than 1% but not more than 5% of the 202 valproate-treated patients in the controlled clinical trials:

Body as a Whole: Chest pain.
Cardiovascular System: Vasodilatation.
Digestive System: Constipation, dry mouth, flatulence, and stomatitis.
Hemic and Lymphatic System: Ecchymosis.
Metabolic and Nutritional Disorders: Peripheral edema.
Musculoskeletal System: Leg cramps.
Nervous System: Abnormal dreams, confusion, paresthesia, speech disorder, and thinking abnormalities.
Respiratory System: Dyspnea, and sinusitis.

Skin and Appendages: Pruritus.
Urogenital System: Metrorrhagia.

6.4   Post-Marketing Experience

The following adverse reactions have been identified during post approval use of Depakote. Because these reactions are reported voluntarily from a population of uncertain size, it is not always possible to reliably estimate their frequency or establish a causal relationship to drug exposure.

Dermatologic: Hair texture changes, hair color changes, photosensitivity, erythema multiforme, toxic epidermal necrolysis, nail and nail bed disorders, and Stevens-Johnson syndrome.
Psychiatric: Emotional upset, psychosis, aggression, psychomotor hyperactivity, hostility, disturbance in attention, learning disorder, and behavioral deterioration.
Neurologic: There have been several reports of acute or subacute cognitive decline and behavioral changes (apathy or irritability) with cerebral pseudoatrophy on imaging associated with valproate therapy; both the cognitive/behavioral changes and cerebral pseudoatrophy reversed partially or fully after valproate discontinuation.
Musculoskeletal: Fractures, decreased bone mineral density, osteopenia, osteoporosis, and weakness.
Hematologic: Relative lymphocytosis, macrocytosis, leukopenia, anemia including macrocytic with or without folate deficiency, bone marrow suppression, pancytopenia, aplastic anemia, agranulocytosis, and acute intermittent porphyria.
Endocrine: Irregular menses, secondary amenorrhea, hyperandrogenism, hirsutism, elevated testosterone level, breast enlargement, galactorrhea, parotid gland swelling, polycystic ovary disease, decrease carnitine concentrations, hyponatremia, hyperglycinemia, and inappropriate ADH secretion.
There have been rare reports of Fanconi's syndrome occurring chiefly in children.
Metabolism and nutrition: Weight gain.
Reproductive: Aspermia, azoospermia, decreased sperm count, decreased spermatozoa motility, male infertility, and abnormal spermatozoa morphology.
Genitourinary: Enuresis and urinary tract infection.
Special Senses: Hearing loss.
Other: Allergic reaction, anaphylaxis, developmental delay, bone pain, bradycardia, and cutaneous vasculitis.

7   DRUG INTERACTIONS

7.1   Effects of Co-Administered Drugs on Valproate Clearance

Drugs that affect the level of expression of hepatic enzymes, particularly those that elevate levels of glucuronosyltransferases (such as ritonavir), may increase the clearance of valproate. For example, phenytoin, carbamazepine, and phenobarbital (or primidone) can double the clearance of valproate. Thus, patients on monotherapy will generally have longer half-lives and higher concentrations than patients receiving polytherapy with antiepilepsy drugs.

In contrast, drugs that are inhibitors of cytochrome P450 isozymes, e.g., antidepressants, may be expected to have little effect on valproate clearance because cytochrome P450 microsomal mediated oxidation is a relatively minor secondary metabolic pathway compared to glucuronidation and beta-oxidation.

Because of these changes in valproate clearance, monitoring of valproate and concomitant drug concentrations should be increased whenever enzyme inducing drugs are introduced or withdrawn.

The following list provides information about the potential for an influence of several commonly prescribed medications on valproate pharmacokinetics. The list is not exhaustive nor could it be, since new interactions are continuously being reported.

Drugs for which a potentially important interaction has been observed

Aspirin

A study involving the co-administration of aspirin at antipyretic doses (11 to 16 mg/kg) with valproate to pediatric patients (n=6) revealed a decrease in protein binding and an inhibition of metabolism of valproate. Valproate free fraction was increased 4-fold in the presence of aspirin compared to valproate alone. The β-oxidation pathway consisting of 2-E-valproic acid, 3-OH-valproic acid, and 3-keto valproic acid was decreased from 25% of total metabolites excreted on valproate alone to 8.3% in the presence of aspirin. Whether or not the interaction observed in this study applies to adults is unknown, but caution should be observed if valproate and aspirin are to be co-administered.

Carbapenem Antibiotics

A clinically significant reduction in serum valproic acid concentration has been reported in patients receiving carbapenem antibiotics (for example, ertapenem, imipenem, meropenem; this is not a complete list) and may result in loss of seizure control. The mechanism of this interaction in not well understood. Serum valproic acid concentrations should be monitored frequently after initiating carbapenem therapy. Alternative antibacterial or anticonvulsant therapy should be considered if serum valproic acid concentrations drop significantly or seizure control deteriorates *[see Warnings and Precautions (5.13)]*.

Felbamate

A study involving the co-administration of 1200 mg/day of felbamate with valproate to patients with epilepsy (n=10) revealed an increase in mean valproate peak concentration by 35% (from 86 to 115 mcg/mL) compared to valproate alone. Increasing the felbamate dose to 2400 mg/day increased the mean valproate peak concentration to 133 mcg/mL (another 16% increase). A decrease in valproate dosage may be necessary when felbamate therapy is initiated.

Rifampin

A study involving the administration of a single dose of valproate (7 mg/kg) 36 hours after 5 nights of daily dosing with rifampin (600 mg) revealed a 40% increase in the oral clearance of valproate. Valproate dosage adjustment may be necessary when it is co-administered with rifampin.

Drugs for which either no interaction or a likely clinically unimportant interaction has been observed

Antacids

A study involving the co-administration of valproate 500 mg with commonly administered antacids (Maalox, Trisogel, and Titralac - 160 mEq doses) did not reveal any effect on the extent of absorption of valproate.

Chlorpromazine

A study involving the administration of 100 to 300 mg/day of chlorpromazine to schizophrenic patients already receiving valproate (200 mg BID) revealed a 15% increase in trough plasma levels of valproate.

Haloperidol

A study involving the administration of 6 to 10 mg/day of haloperidol to schizophrenic patients already receiving valproate (200 mg BID) revealed no significant changes in valproate trough plasma levels.

Cimetidine and Ranitidine

Cimetidine and ranitidine do not affect the clearance of valproate.

7.2   Effects of Valproate on Other Drugs

Valproate has been found to be a weak inhibitor of some P450 isozymes, epoxide hydrase, and glucuronosyltransferases.

The following list provides information about the potential for an influence of valproate co-administration on the pharmacokinetics or pharmacodynamics of several commonly prescribed medications. The list is not exhaustive, since new interactions are continuously being reported.

Drugs for which a potentially important valproate interaction has been observed

Amitriptyline/Nortriptyline

Administration of a single oral 50 mg dose of amitriptyline to 15 normal volunteers (10 males and 5 females) who received valproate (500 mg BID) resulted in a 21% decrease in plasma clearance of amitriptyline and a 34% decrease in the net clearance of nortriptyline. Rare postmarketing reports of concurrent use of valproate and amitriptyline resulting in an increased amitriptyline level have been received. Concurrent use of valproate and amitriptyline has rarely been associated with toxicity. Monitoring of amitriptyline levels should be considered for patients taking valproate concomitantly with amitriptyline. Consideration should be given to lowering the dose of amitriptyline/nortriptyline in the presence of valproate.

Carbamazepine/carbamazepine-10,11-Epoxide

Serum levels of carbamazepine (CBZ) decreased 17% while that of carbamazepine-10,11-epoxide (CBZ-E) increased by 45% upon co-administration of valproate and CBZ to epileptic patients.

Clonazepam

The concomitant use of valproate and clonazepam may induce absence status in patients with a history of absence type seizures.

Diazepam

Valproate displaces diazepam from its plasma albumin binding sites and inhibits its metabolism. Co-administration of valproate (1500 mg daily) increased the free fraction of diazepam (10 mg) by 90% in healthy volunteers (n=6). Plasma clearance and volume of distribution for free diazepam were reduced by 25% and 20%, respectively, in the presence of valproate. The elimination half-life of diazepam remained unchanged upon addition of valproate.

Ethosuximide

Valproate inhibits the metabolism of ethosuximide. Administration of a single ethosuximide dose of 500 mg with valproate (800 to 1600 mg/day) to healthy volunteers (n=6) was accompanied by a 25% increase in elimination half-life of ethosuximide and a 15% decrease in its total clearance as compared to ethosuximide alone. Patients receiving valproate and ethosuximide, especially along with other anticonvulsants, should be monitored for alterations in serum concentrations of both drugs.

Lamotrigine

In a steady-state study involving 10 healthy volunteers, the elimination half-life of lamotrigine increased from 26 to 70 hours with valproate co-administration (a 165% increase). The dose of lamotrigine should be reduced when co-administered with valproate. Serious skin reactions (such as Stevens-Johnson syndrome and toxic epidermal necrolysis) have been reported with concomitant lamotrigine and valproate administration. See lamotrigine package insert for details on lamotrigine dosing with concomitant valproate administration.

Phenobarbital

Valproate was found to inhibit the metabolism of phenobarbital. Co-administration of valproate (250 mg BID for 14 days) with phenobarbital to normal subjects (n=6) resulted in a 50% increase in half-life and a 30% decrease in plasma clearance of phenobarbital (60 mg single-dose). The fraction of phenobarbital dose excreted unchanged increased by 50% in presence of valproate.

There is evidence for severe CNS depression, with or without significant elevations of barbiturate or valproate serum concentrations. All patients receiving concomitant barbiturate therapy should be closely monitored for neurological toxicity. Serum barbiturate concentrations should be obtained, if possible, and the barbiturate dosage decreased, if appropriate.

Primidone, which is metabolized to a barbiturate, may be involved in a similar interaction with valproate.

Phenytoin

Valproate displaces phenytoin from its plasma albumin binding sites and inhibits its hepatic metabolism. Co-administration of valproate (400 mg TID) with phenytoin (250 mg) in normal volunteers (n=7) was associated with a 60% increase in the free fraction of phenytoin. Total plasma clearance and apparent volume of distribution of phenytoin increased 30% in the presence of valproate. Both the clearance and apparent volume of distribution of free phenytoin were reduced by 25%.

In patients with epilepsy, there have been reports of breakthrough seizures occurring with the combination of valproate and phenytoin. The dosage of phenytoin should be adjusted as required by the clinical situation.

Rufinamide

Based on a population pharmacokinetic analysis, rufinamide clearance was decreased by valproate. Rufinamide concentrations were increased by <16% to 70%, dependent on concentration of valproate (with the larger increases being seen in pediatric patients at high doses or concentrations of valproate). Patients stabilized on rufinamide before being prescribed valproate should begin valproate therapy at a low dose, and titrate to a clinically effective dose *[see Dosage and Administration (2.6)]*. Similarly, patients on valproate should begin at a rufinamide dose lower than 10 mg/kg per day (pediatric patients) or 400 mg per day (adults).

Tolbutamide

From *in vitro* experiments, the unbound fraction of tolbutamide was increased from 20% to 50% when added to plasma samples taken from patients treated with valproate. The clinical relevance of this displacement is unknown.

Warfarin

In an *in vitro* study, valproate increased the unbound fraction of warfarin by up to 32.6%. The therapeutic relevance of this is unknown; however, coagulation tests should be monitored if valproate therapy is instituted in patients taking anticoagulants.

Zidovudine

In six patients who were seropositive for HIV, the clearance of zidovudine (100 mg q8h) was decreased by 38% after administration of valproate (250 or 500 mg q8h); the half-life of zidovudine was unaffected.

Drugs for which either no interaction or a likely clinically unimportant interaction has been observed

Acetaminophen

Valproate had no effect on any of the pharmacokinetic parameters of acetaminophen when it was concurrently administered to three epileptic patients.

Clozapine

In psychotic patients (n=11), no interaction was observed when valproate was co-administered with clozapine.

Lithium

Co-administration of valproate (500 mg BID) and lithium carbonate (300 mg TID) to normal male volunteers (n=16) had no effect on the steady-state kinetics of lithium.

Lorazepam

Concomitant administration of valproate (500 mg BID) and lorazepam (1 mg BID) in normal male volunteers (n=9) was accompanied by a 17% decrease in the plasma clearance of lorazepam.

Olanzapine

No dose adjustment for olanzapine is necessary when olanzapine is administered concomitantly with valproate. Co-administration of valproate (500 mg BID) and olanzapine (5 mg) to healthy adults (n=10) caused 15% reduction in C_{max} and 35% reduction in AUC of olanzapine.

Oral Contraceptive Steroids

Administration of a single-dose of ethinyloestradiol (50 mcg)/levonorgestrel (250 mcg) to 6 women on valproate (200 mg BID) therapy for 2 months did not reveal any pharmacokinetic interaction.

7.3 Topiramate

Concomitant administration of valproate and topiramate has been associated with hyperammonemia with and without encephalopathy *[see Contraindications (4) and Warnings and Precautions (5.6, 5.9, 5.10)]*. Concomitant administration of topiramate with valproate has also been associated with hypothermia in patients who have tolerated either drug alone. It may be prudent to examine blood ammonia levels in patients in whom the onset of hypothermia has been reported *[see Warnings and Precautions (5.9, 5.11)]*.

8 USE IN SPECIFIC POPULATIONS

8.1 Pregnancy

Pregnancy Category D for epilepsy and for manic episodes associated with bipolar disorder *[see Warnings and Precautions (5.2, 5.3)]*.

Pregnancy Category X for prophylaxis of migraine headaches *[see Contraindications (4)]*.

Pregnancy Registry

To collect information on the effects of *in utero* exposure to Depakote, physicians should encourage pregnant patients taking Depakote to enroll in the North American Antiepileptic Drug (NAAED) Pregnancy Registry. This can be done by calling toll free 1-888-233-2334, and must be done by the patients themselves. Information on the registry can be found at the website, http://www.aedpregnancyregistry.org/.

Fetal Risk Summary

All pregnancies have a background risk of birth defects (about 3%), pregnancy loss (about 15%), or other adverse outcomes regardless of drug exposure. Maternal valproate use during pregnancy for any indication increases the risk of congenital malformations, particularly neural tube defects, but also malformations involving other body systems (e.g., craniofacial defects, cardiovascular malformations, hypospadias, limb malformations). The risk of major structural abnormalities is greatest during the first trimester; however, other serious developmental effects can occur with valproate use throughout pregnancy. The rate of congenital malformations among babies born to epileptic mothers who used valproate during pregnancy has been shown to be about four times higher than the rate among babies born to epileptic mothers who used other anti-seizure monotherapies *[see Warnings and Precautions (5.3)]*.

Several published epidemiological studies have indicated that children exposed to valproate *in utero* have lower IQ scores than children exposed to either another antiepileptic drug *in utero* or to no antiepileptic drugs *in utero [see Warnings and Precautions (5.3)]*.

An observational study has suggested that exposure to valproate products during pregnancy may increase the risk of autism spectrum disorders. In this study, children born to mothers who had used valproate products during pregnancy had 2.9 times the risk (95% confidence interval [CI]: 1.7-4.9) of developing autism spectrum disorders compared to children born to mothers not exposed to valproate products during pregnancy. The absolute risks for autism spectrum dis-

orders were 4.4% (95% CI: 2.6%-7.5%) in valproate-exposed children and 1.5% (95% CI: 1.5%-1.6%) in children not exposed to valproate products. Because the study was observational in nature, conclusions regarding a causal association between *in utero* valproate exposure and an increased risk of autism spectrum disorder cannot be considered definitive.

In animal studies, offspring with prenatal exposure to valproate had structural malformations similar to those seen in humans and demonstrated neurobehavioral deficits.

Clinical Considerations

- Neural tube defects are the congenital malformation most strongly associated with maternal valproate use. The risk of spina bifida following *in utero* valproate exposure is generally estimated as 1-2%, compared to an estimated general population risk for spina bifida of about 0.06 to 0.07% (6 to 7 in 10,000 births).
- Valproate can cause decreased IQ scores in children whose mothers were treated with valproate during pregnancy.
- Because of the risks of decreased IQ, neural tube defects, and other fetal adverse events, which may occur very early in pregnancy:
- Valproate should not be administered to a woman of childbearing potential unless the drug is essential to the management of her medical condition. This is especially important when valproate use is considered for a condition not usually associated with permanent injury or death (e.g., migraine).
- Valproate is contraindicated during pregnancy in women being treated for prophylaxis of migraine headaches.
- Valproate should not be used to treat women with epilepsy or bipolar disorder who are pregnant or who plan to become pregnant unless other treatments have failed to provide adequate symptom control or are otherwise unacceptable. In such women, the benefits of treatment with valproate during pregnancy may still outweigh the risks. When treating a pregnant woman or a woman of childbearing potential, carefully consider both the potential risks and benefits of treatment and provide appropriate counseling.
- To prevent major seizures, women with epilepsy should not discontinue valproate abruptly, as this can precipitate status epilepticus with resulting maternal and fetal hypoxia and threat to life. Even minor seizures may pose some hazard to the developing embryo or fetus. However, discontinuation of the drug may be considered prior to and during pregnancy in individual cases if the seizure disorder severity and frequency do not pose a serious threat to the patient.
- Available prenatal diagnostic testing to detect neural tube and other defects should be offered to pregnant women using valproate.
- Evidence suggests that folic acid supplementation prior to conception and during the first trimester of pregnancy decreases the risk for congenital neural tube defects in the general population. It is not known whether the risk of neural tube defects or decreased IQ in the offspring of women receiving valproate is reduced by folic acid supplementation. Dietary folic acid supplementation both prior to conception and during pregnancy should be routinely recommended for patients using valproate.
- Pregnant women taking valproate may develop clotting abnormalities including thrombocytopenia, hypofibrinogenemia, and/or decrease in other coagulation factors, which may result in hemorrhagic complications in the neonate including death *[see Warnings and Precautions (5.8)]*. If valproate is used in pregnancy, the clotting parameters should be monitored carefully in the mother. If abnormal in the mother, then these parameters should also be monitored in the neonate.
- Patients taking valproate may develop hepatic failure *[see Boxed Warning and Warnings and Precautions (5.1)]*. Fatal cases of hepatic failure in infants exposed to valproate *in utero* have also been reported following maternal use of valproate during pregnancy.
- Hypoglycemia has been reported in neonates whose mothers have taken valproate during pregnancy.

Data

Human

There is an extensive body of evidence demonstrating that exposure to valproate *in utero* increases the risk of neural tube defects and other structural abnormalities. Based on

Continued on next page

Information on the AbbVie, Inc. products listed on these pages is from the prescribing information in use as of July 31, 2016. For more information, please visit rxabbvie.com or call 1-800-633-9110.

published data from the CDC's National Birth Defects Prevention Network, the risk of spina bifida in the general population is about 0.06 to 0.07%. The risk of spina bifida following *in utero* valproate exposure has been estimated to be approximately 1 to 2%.

The NAAED Pregnancy Registry has reported a major malformation rate of 9-11% in the offspring of women exposed to an average of 1,000 mg/day of valproate monotherapy during pregnancy. These data show up to a five-fold increased risk for any major malformation following valproate exposure *in utero* compared to the risk following exposure *in utero* to other antiepileptic drugs taken in monotherapy. The major congenital malformations included cases of neural tube defects, cardiovascular malformations, craniofacial defects (e.g., oral clefts, craniosynostosis), hypospadias, limb malformations (e.g., clubfoot, polydactyly), and malformations of varying severity involving other body systems.

Published epidemiological studies have indicated that children exposed to valproate *in utero* have lower IQ scores than children exposed to either another antiepileptic drug *in utero* or to no antiepileptic drugs *in utero*. The largest of these studies is a prospective cohort study conducted in the United States and United Kingdom that found that children with prenatal exposure to valproate (n=62) had lower IQ scores at age 6 (97 [95% C.I. 94-101]) than children with prenatal exposure to the other anti-epileptic drug monotherapy treatments evaluated: lamotrigine (108 [95% C.I. 105–110]), carbamazepine (105 [95% C.I. 102–108]) and phenytoin (108 [95% C.I. 104–112]). It is not known when during pregnancy cognitive effects in valproate-exposed children occur. Because the women in this study were exposed to antiepileptic drugs throughout pregnancy, whether the risk for decreased IQ was related to a particular time period during pregnancy could not be assessed.

Although all of the available studies have methodological limitations, the weight of the evidence supports a causal association between valproate exposure *in utero* and subsequent adverse effects on cognitive development.

There are published case reports of fatal hepatic failure in offspring of women who used valproate during pregnancy.

Animal

In developmental toxicity studies conducted in mice, rats, rabbits, and monkeys, increased rates of fetal structural abnormalities, intrauterine growth retardation, and embryo-fetal death occurred following treatment of pregnant animals with valproate during organogenesis at clinically relevant doses (calculated on a body surface area basis). Valproate induced malformations of multiple organ systems, including skeletal, cardiac, and urogenital defects. In mice, in addition to other malformations, fetal neural tube defects have been reported following valproate administration during critical periods of organogenesis, and the teratogenic response correlated with peak maternal drug levels. Behavioral abnormalities (including cognitive, locomotor, and social interaction deficits) and brain histopathological changes have also been reported in mice and rat offspring exposed prenatally to clinically relevant doses of valproate.

8.3 Nursing Mothers

Valproate is excreted in human milk. Caution should be exercised when valproate is administered to a nursing woman.

8.4 Pediatric Use

Experience has indicated that pediatric patients under the age of two years are at a considerably increased risk of developing fatal hepatotoxicity, especially those with the aforementioned conditions *[see Boxed Warning and Warnings and Precautions (5.1)]*. When valproate is used in this patient group, it should be used with extreme caution and as a sole agent. The benefits of therapy should be weighed against the risks. Above the age of 2 years, experience in epilepsy has indicated that the incidence of fatal hepatotoxicity decreases considerably in progressively older patient groups.

Younger children, especially those receiving enzyme inducing drugs, will require larger maintenance doses to attain targeted total and unbound valproate concentrations. Pediatric patients (i.e., between 3 months and 10 years) have 50% higher clearances expressed on weight (i.e., mL/min/kg) than do adults. Over the age of 10 years, children have pharmacokinetic parameters that approximate those of adults.

The variability in free fraction limits the clinical usefulness of monitoring total serum valproic acid concentration. Interpretation of valproic acid concentrations in children should include consideration of factors that affect hepatic metabolism and protein binding.

Pediatric Clinical Trials

Depakote was studied in seven pediatric clinical trials.

Two of the pediatric studies were double-blinded placebo-controlled trials to evaluate the efficacy of Depakote ER for the indications of mania (150 patients aged 10 to 17 years, 76 of whom were on Depakote ER) and migraine (304 patients aged 12 to 17 years, 231 of whom were on Depakote ER). Efficacy was not established for either the treatment of migraine or the treatment of mania. The most common drug-related adverse reactions (reported >5% and twice the rate of placebo) reported in the controlled pediatric mania study were nausea, upper abdominal pain, somnolence, increased ammonia, gastritis and rash.

The remaining five trials were long term safety studies. Two six-month pediatric studies were conducted to evaluate the long-term safety of Depakote ER for the indication of mania (292 patients aged 10 to 17 years). Two twelve-month pediatric studies were conducted to evaluate the long-term safety of Depakote ER for the indication of migraine (353 patients aged 12 to 17 years). One twelve-month study was conducted to evaluate the safety of Depakote Sprinkle Capsules in the indication of partial seizures (169 patients aged 3 to 10 years).

In these seven clinical trials, the safety and tolerability of Depakote in pediatric patients were shown to be comparable to those in adults *[see Adverse Reactions (6)]*.

Juvenile Animal Toxicology

In studies of valproate in immature animals, toxic effects not observed in adult animals included retinal dysplasia in rats treated during the neonatal period (from postnatal day 4) and nephrotoxicity in rats treated during the neonatal and juvenile (from postnatal day 14) periods. The no-effect dose for these findings was less than the maximum recommended human dose on a mg/m^2 basis.

8.5 Geriatric Use

No patients above the age of 65 years were enrolled in double-blind prospective clinical trials of mania associated with bipolar illness. In a case review study of 583 patients, 72 patients (12%) were greater than 65 years of age. A higher percentage of patients above 65 years of age reported accidental injury, infection, pain, somnolence, and tremor. Discontinuation of valproate was occasionally associated with the latter two events. It is not clear whether these events indicate additional risk or whether they result from preexisting medical illness and concomitant medication use among these patients.

A study of elderly patients with dementia revealed drug related somnolence and discontinuation for somnolence *[see Warnings and Precautions (5.14)]*. The starting dose should be reduced in these patients, and dosage reductions or discontinuation should be considered in patients with excessive somnolence *[see Dosage and Administration (2.5)]*.

There is insufficient information available to discern the safety and effectiveness of valproate for the prophylaxis of migraines in patients over 65.

The capacity of elderly patients (age range: 68 to 89 years) to eliminate valproate has been shown to be reduced compared to younger adults (age range: 22 to 26 years) *[see Clinical Pharmacology (12.3)]*.

8.6 Effect of Disease

Liver Disease

[(See Boxed Warning, Contraindications (4), Warnings and Precautions (5), and Clinical Pharmacology (12.3)]. Liver disease impairs the capacity to eliminate valproate.

10 OVERDOSAGE

Overdosage with valproate may result in somnolence, heart block, deep coma, and hypernatremia. Fatalities have been reported; however patients have recovered from valproate levels as high as 2120 mcg/mL.

In overdose situations, the fraction of drug not bound to protein is high and hemodialysis or tandem hemodialysis plus hemoperfusion may result in significant removal of drug. The benefit of gastric lavage or emesis will vary with the time since ingestion. General supportive measures should be applied with particular attention to the maintenance of adequate urinary output.

Naloxone has been reported to reverse the CNS depressant effects of valproate overdosage. Because naloxone could theoretically also reverse the antiepileptic effects of valproate, it should be used with caution in patients with epilepsy.

11 DESCRIPTION

Divalproex sodium is a stable co-ordination compound comprised of sodium valproate and valproic acid in a 1:1 molar relationship and formed during the partial neutralization of valproic acid with 0.5 equivalent of sodium hydroxide. Chemically it is designated as sodium hydrogen bis (2-propylpentanoate). Divalproex sodium has the following structure:

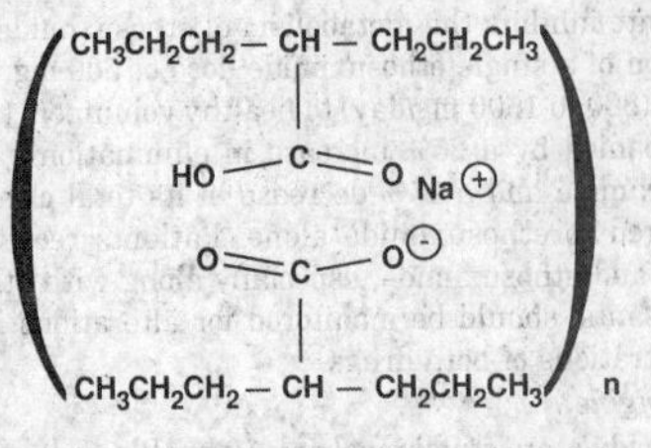

Divalproex sodium occurs as a white powder with a characteristic odor.

Depakote ER 250 and 500 mg tablets are for oral administration. Depakote ER tablets contain divalproex sodium in a once-a-day extended-release formulation equivalent to 250 and 500 mg of valproic acid.

Inactive Ingredients

Depakote ER 250 and 500 mg tablets: FD&C Blue No. 1, hypromellose, lactose, microcrystalline cellulose, polyethylene glycol, potassium sorbate, propylene glycol, silicon dioxide, titanium dioxide, and triacetin.

In addition, 500 mg tablets contain iron oxide and polydextrose.

Meets USP Dissolution Test 2.

12 CLINICAL PHARMACOLOGY

12.1 Mechanism of Action

Divalproex sodium dissociates to the valproate ion in the gastrointestinal tract. The mechanisms by which valproate exerts its therapeutic effects have not been established. It has been suggested that its activity in epilepsy is related to increased brain concentrations of gamma-aminobutyric acid (GABA).

12.2 Pharmacodynamics

The relationship between plasma concentration and clinical response is not well documented. One contributing factor is the nonlinear, concentration dependent protein binding of valproate which affects the clearance of the drug. Thus, monitoring of total serum valproate may not provide a reliable index of the bioactive valproate species.

For example, because the plasma protein binding of valproate is concentration dependent, the free fraction increases from approximately 10% at 40 mcg/mL to 18.5% at 130 mcg/mL. Higher than expected free fractions occur in the elderly, in hyperlipidemic patients, and in patients with hepatic and renal diseases.

Epilepsy

The therapeutic range in epilepsy is commonly considered to be 50 to 100 mcg/mL of total valproate, although some patients may be controlled with lower or higher plasma concentrations.

Mania

In placebo-controlled clinical trials of acute mania, patients were dosed to clinical response with trough plasma concentrations between 85 and 125 mcg/mL *[see Dosage and Administration (2.1)]*.

12.3 Pharmacokinetics

Absorption/Bioavailability

The absolute bioavailability of Depakote ER tablets administered as a single dose after a meal was approximately 90% relative to intravenous infusion.

When given in equal total daily doses, the bioavailability of Depakote ER is less than that of Depakote (divalproex sodium delayed-release tablets). In five multiple-dose studies in healthy subjects (N=82) and in subjects with epilepsy (N=86), when administered under fasting and nonfasting conditions, Depakote ER given once daily produced an average bioavailability of 89% relative to an equal total daily dose of Depakote given BID, TID, or QID. The median time to maximum plasma valproate concentrations (C_{max}) after Depakote ER administration ranged from 4 to 17 hours. After multiple once-daily dosing of Depakote ER, the peak-to-trough fluctuation in plasma valproate concentrations was 10-20% lower than that of regular Depakote given BID, TID, or QID.

Conversion from Depakote to Depakote ER

When Depakote ER is given in doses 8 to 20% higher than the total daily dose of Depakote, the two formulations are bioequivalent. In two randomized, crossover studies, multiple daily doses of Depakote were compared to 8 to 20% higher once-daily doses of Depakote ER. In these two studies, Depakote ER and Depakote regimens were equivalent with respect to area under the curve (AUC; a measure of the extent of bioavailability). Additionally, valproate C_{max} was lower, and C_{min} was either higher or not different, for Depakote ER relative to Depakote regimens (see Table 8). [See table 8]

Concomitant antiepilepsy drugs (topiramate, phenobarbital, carbamazepine, phenytoin, and lamotrigine were evaluated) that induce the cytochrome P450 isozyme system did not significantly alter valproate bioavailability when converting between Depakote and Depakote ER.

Distribution
Protein Binding

The plasma protein binding of valproate is concentration dependent and the free fraction increases from approximately 10% at 40 mcg/mL to 18.5% at 130 mcg/mL. Protein binding of valproate is reduced in the elderly, in patients with chronic hepatic diseases, in patients with renal impairment, and in the presence of other drugs (e.g., aspirin). Conversely, valproate may displace certain protein-bound drugs (e.g., phenytoin, carbamazepine, warfarin, and tolbutamide) *[see Drug Interactions (7.2) for more detailed information on the pharmacokinetic interactions of valproate with other drugs]*.

CNS Distribution

Valproate concentrations in cerebrospinal fluid (CSF) approximate unbound concentrations in plasma (about 10% of total concentration).

Metabolism

Valproate is metabolized almost entirely by the liver. In adult patients on monotherapy, 30-50% of an administered dose appears in urine as a glucuronide conjugate. Mitochondrial β-oxidation is the other major metabolic pathway, typically accounting for over 40% of the dose. Usually, less than 15-20% of the dose is eliminated by other oxidative mechanisms. Less than 3% of an administered dose is excreted unchanged in urine.

The relationship between dose and total valproate concentration is nonlinear; concentration does not increase proportionally with the dose, but rather, increases to a lesser extent due to saturable plasma protein binding. The kinetics of unbound drug are linear.

Elimination

Mean plasma clearance and volume of distribution for total valproate are 0.56 L/hr/1.73 m^2 and 11 L/1.73 m^2, respectively. Mean plasma clearance and volume of distribution for free valproate are 4.6 L/hr/1.73 m^2 and 92 L/1.73 m^2. Mean terminal half-life for valproate monotherapy ranged from 9 to 16 hours following oral dosing regimens of 250 to 1000 mg.

The estimates cited apply primarily to patients who are not taking drugs that affect hepatic metabolizing enzyme systems. For example, patients taking enzyme-inducing antiepileptic drugs (carbamazepine, phenytoin, and phenobarbital) will clear valproate more rapidly. Because of these changes in valproate clearance, monitoring of antiepileptic concentrations should be intensified whenever concomitant antiepileptics are introduced or withdrawn.

Special Populations
Effect of Age
Pediatric

The valproate pharmacokinetic profile following administration of Depakote ER was characterized in a multiple-dose, non-fasting, open label, multi-center study in children and adolescents. Depakote ER once daily doses ranged from 250-1750 mg. Once daily administration of Depakote ER in pediatric patients (10-17 years) produced plasma VPA concentration-time profiles similar to those that have been observed in adults.

Elderly

The capacity of elderly patients (age range: 68 to 89 years) to eliminate valproate has been shown to be reduced compared to younger adults (age range: 22 to 26). Intrinsic clearance is reduced by 39%; the free fraction is increased by 44%. Accordingly, the initial dosage should be reduced in the elderly *[see Dosage and Administration (2.4)]*.

Effect of Sex

There are no differences in the body surface area adjusted unbound clearance between males and females (4.8±0.17 and 4.7±0.07 L/hr per 1.73 m^2, respectively).

Effect of Race

The effects of race on the kinetics of valproate have not been studied.

Effect of Disease
Liver Disease

Table 8. Bioavailability of Depakote ER Tablets Relative to Depakote When Depakote ER Dose is 8 to 20% Higher

Study Population	Regimens	Relative Bioavailability		
	Depakote ER vs. Depakote	AUC_{24}	C_{max}	C_{min}
Healthy Volunteers (N=35)	1000 & 1500 mg Depakote ER vs. 875 & 1250 mg Depakote	1.059	0.882	1.173
Patients with epilepsy on concomitant enzyme-inducing antiepilepsy drugs (N = 64)	1000 to 5000 mg Depakote ER vs. 875 to 4250 mg Depakote	1.008	0.899	1.022

Liver disease impairs the capacity to eliminate valproate. In one study, the clearance of free valproate was decreased by 50% in 7 patients with cirrhosis and by 16% in 4 patients with acute hepatitis, compared with 6 healthy subjects. In that study, the half-life of valproate was increased from 12 to 18 hours. Liver disease is also associated with decreased albumin concentrations and larger unbound fractions (2 to 2.6 fold increase) of valproate. Accordingly, monitoring of total concentrations may be misleading since free concentrations may be substantially elevated in patients with hepatic disease whereas total concentrations may appear to be normal *[see Boxed Warning, Contraindications (4), and Warnings and Precautions (5.1)]*.

Renal Disease

A slight reduction (27%) in the unbound clearance of valproate has been reported in patients with renal failure (creatinine clearance < 10 mL/minute); however, hemodialysis typically reduces valproate concentrations by about 20%. Therefore, no dosage adjustment appears to be necessary in patients with renal failure. Protein binding in these patients is substantially reduced; thus, monitoring total concentrations may be misleading.

13 NONCLINICAL TOXICOLOGY
13.1 Carcinogenesis, Mutagenesis, and Impairment of Fertility
Carcinogenesis

Valproate was administered orally to rats and mice at doses of 80 and 170 mg/kg/day (less than the maximum recommended human dose on a mg/m^2 basis) for two years. The primary findings were an increase in the incidence of subcutaneous fibrosarcomas in high-dose male rats receiving valproate and a dose-related trend for benign pulmonary adenomas in male mice receiving valproate. The significance of these findings for humans is unknown.

Mutagenesis

Valproate was not mutagenic in an *in vitro* bacterial assay (Ames test), did not produce dominant lethal effects in mice, and did not increase chromosome aberration frequency in an *in vivo* cytogenetic study in rats. Increased frequencies of sister chromatid exchange (SCE) have been reported in a study of epileptic children taking valproate, but this association was not observed in another study conducted in adults. There is some evidence that increased SCE frequencies may be associated with epilepsy. The biological significance of an increase in SCE frequency is not known.

Impairment of Fertility

Chronic toxicity studies of valproate in juvenile and adult rats and dogs demonstrated reduced spermatogenesis and testicular atrophy at oral doses of 400 mg/kg/day or greater in rats (approximately equivalent to or greater than the maximum recommended human dose (MRHD) on a mg/m^2 basis) and 150 mg/kg/day or greater in dogs (approximately 1.4 times the MRHD or greater on a mg/m^2 basis). Fertility studies in rats have shown no effect on fertility at oral doses of valproate up to 350 mg/kg/day (approximately equal to the MRHD on a mg/m^2 basis) for 60 days. The effect of valproate on testicular development and on sperm parameters and fertility in humans is unknown.

14 CLINICAL STUDIES
14.1 Mania

The effectiveness of Depakote ER for the treatment of acute mania is based in part on studies establishing the effectiveness of Depakote (divalproex sodium delayed release tablets) for this indication. Depakote ER's effectiveness was confirmed in one randomized, double-blind, placebo-controlled, parallel group, 3-week, multicenter study. The study was designed to evaluate the safety and efficacy of Depakote ER in the treatment of bipolar I disorder, manic or mixed type, in adults. Adult male and female patients who had a current DSM-IV TR primary diagnosis of bipolar

I disorder, manic or mixed type, and who were hospitalized for acute mania, were enrolled into this study. Depakote ER was initiated at a dose of 25 mg/kg/day given once daily, increased by 500 mg/day on Day 3, then adjusted to achieve plasma valproate concentrations in the range of 85-125 mcg/mL. Mean daily Depakote ER doses for observed cases were 2362 mg (range: 500-4000), 2874 mg (range: 1500-4500), 2993 mg (range: 1500-4500), 3181 mg (range: 1500-5000), and 3353 mg (range: 1500-5500) at Days 1, 5, 10, 15, and 21, respectively. Mean valproate concentrations were 96.5 mcg/mL, 102.1 mcg/mL, 98.5 mcg/mL, 89.5 mcg/mL at Days 5, 10, 15 and 21, respectively. Patients were assessed on the Mania Rating Scale (MRS; score ranges from 0-52).

Depakote ER was significantly more effective than placebo in reduction of the MRS total score.

14.2 Epilepsy

The efficacy of valproate in reducing the incidence of complex partial seizures (CPS) that occur in isolation or in association with other seizure types was established in two controlled trials.

In one, multi-clinic, placebo controlled study employing an add-on design, (adjunctive therapy) 144 patients who continued to suffer eight or more CPS per 8 weeks during an 8 week period of monotherapy with doses of either carbamazepine or phenytoin sufficient to assure plasma concentrations within the "therapeutic range" were randomized to receive, in addition to their original antiepilepsy drug (AED), either Depakote or placebo. Randomized patients were to be followed for a total of 16 weeks. The following Table presents the findings.

Table 9. Adjunctive Therapy Study Median Incidence of CPS per 8 Weeks

Add-on Treatment	Number of Patients	Baseline Incidence	Experimental Incidence
Depakote	75	16.0	8.9*
Placebo	69	14.5	11.5

* Reduction from baseline statistically significantly greater for valproate than placebo at p ≤ 0.05 level.

Figure 1 presents the proportion of patients (X axis) whose percentage reduction from baseline in complex partial seizure rates was at least as great as that indicated on the Y axis in the adjunctive therapy study. A positive percent reduction indicates an improvement (i.e., a decrease in seizure frequency), while a negative percent reduction indicates worsening. Thus, in a display of this type, the curve for an effective treatment is shifted to the left of the curve for placebo. This Figure shows that the proportion of patients achieving any particular level of improvement was consistently higher for valproate than for placebo. For example, 45% of patients treated with valproate had a ≥ 50% reduction in complex partial seizure rate compared to 23% of patients treated with placebo.

The second study assessed the capacity of valproate to reduce the incidence of CPS when administered as the sole AED. The study compared the incidence of CPS among patients randomized to either a high or low dose treatment arm. Patients qualified for entry into the randomized comparison phase of this study only if 1) they continued to ex-

Continued on next page

Information on the AbbVie, Inc. products listed on these pages is from the prescribing information in use as of July 31, 2016. For more information, please visit rxabbvie.com or call 1-800-633-9110.

Figure 1

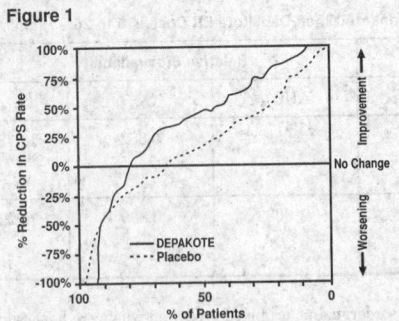

perience 2 or more CPS per 4 weeks during an 8 to 12 week long period of monotherapy with adequate doses of an AED (i.e., phenytoin, carbamazepine, phenobarbital, or primidone) and 2) they made a successful transition over a two week interval to valproate. Patients entering the randomized phase were then brought to their assigned target dose, gradually tapered off their concomitant AED and followed for an interval as long as 22 weeks. Less than 50% of the patients randomized, however, completed the study. In patients converted to Depakote monotherapy, the mean total valproate concentrations during monotherapy were 71 and 123 mcg/mL in the low dose and high dose groups, respectively.

The following Table presents the findings for all patients randomized who had at least one post-randomization assessment.

Table 10. Monotherapy Study Median Incidence of CPS per 8 Weeks

Treatment	Number of Patients	Baseline Incidence	Randomized Phase Incidence
High dose Valproate	131	13.2	10.7*
Low dose Valproate	134	14.2	13.8

* Reduction from baseline statistically significantly greater for high dose than low dose at p ≤ 0.05 level.

Figure 2 presents the proportion of patients (X axis) whose percentage reduction from baseline in complex partial seizure rates was at least as great as that indicated on the Y axis in the monotherapy study. A positive percent reduction indicates an improvement (i.e., a decrease in seizure frequency), while a negative percent reduction indicates worsening. Thus, in a display of this type, the curve for a more effective treatment is shifted to the left of the curve for a less effective treatment. This Figure shows that the proportion of patients achieving any particular level of reduction was consistently higher for high dose valproate than for low dose valproate. For example, when switching from carbamazepine, phenytoin, phenobarbital or primidone monotherapy to high dose valproate monotherapy, 63% of patients experienced no change or a reduction in complex partial seizure rates compared to 54% of patients receiving low dose valproate.

Figure 2

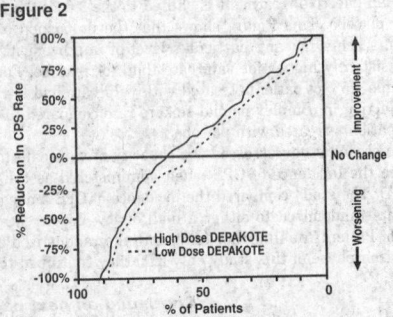

Information on pediatric studies are presented in section 8.

14.3   Migraine

The results of a multicenter, randomized, double-blind, placebo-controlled, parallel-group clinical trial demonstrated the effectiveness of Depakote ER in the prophylactic treatment of migraine headache. This trial recruited patients with a history of migraine headaches with or without aura occurring on average twice or more a month for the preceding three months. Patients with cluster or chronic daily headaches were excluded. Women of childbearing potential were allowed in the trial if they were deemed to be practicing an effective method of contraception.

Patients who experienced ≥ 2 migraine headaches in the 4-week baseline period were randomized in a 1:1 ratio to Depakote ER or placebo and treated for 12 weeks. Patients initiated treatment on 500 mg once daily for one week, and were then increased to 1000 mg once daily with an option to permanently decrease the dose back to 500 mg once daily during the second week of treatment if intolerance occurred. Ninety-eight of 114 Depakote ER-treated patients (86%) and 100 of 110 placebo-treated patients (91%) treated at least two weeks maintained the 1000 mg once daily dose for the duration of their treatment periods. Treatment outcome was assessed on the basis of reduction in 4-week migraine headache rate in the treatment period compared to the baseline period.

Patients (50 male, 187 female) ranging in age from 16 to 69 were treated with Depakote ER (N=122) or placebo (N=115). Four patients were below the age of 18 and 3 were above the age of 65. Two hundred and two patients (101 in each treatment group) completed the treatment period. The mean reduction in 4-week migraine headache rate was 1.2 from a baseline mean of 4.4 in the Depakote ER group, versus 0.6 from a baseline mean of 4.2 in the placebo group. The treatment difference was statistically significant (see Figure 3).

Figure 3 Mean Reduction In 4-Week Migraine Headache Rates

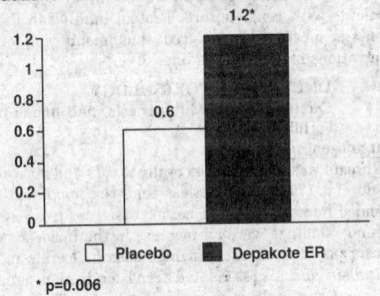

* p=0.006

15   REFERENCES

1. Meador KJ, Baker GA, Browning N, et al. Fetal antiepileptic drug exposure and cognitive outcomes at age 6 years (NEAD study): a prospective observational study. Lancet Neurology 2013; 12 (3):244-252.

16   HOW SUPPLIED/STORAGE AND HANDLING

Depakote ER 250 mg is available as white ovaloid tablets with the "a" logo and the code (HF). Each Depakote ER tablet contains divalproex sodium equivalent to 250 mg of valproic acid in the following package sizes:

Bottles of 100 ....(NDC 0074-3826-13).
Unit Dose Packages of 100...................(NDC 0074-3826-11).
Depakote ER 500 mg is available as gray ovaloid tablets with the "a" logo and the code HC. Each Depakote ER tablet contains divalproex sodium equivalent to 500 mg of valproic acid in the following packaging sizes:

Bottles of 100 ....(NDC 0074-7126-13).
Bottles of 500 ....(NDC 0074-7126-53).
Unit Dose Packages of 100...................(NDC 0074-7126-11).
Recommended Storage
Store tablets at 25°C (77°F); excursions permitted to 15-30°C (59-86°F) [see USP Controlled Room Temperature].

17   PATIENT COUNSELING INFORMATION

Advise the patient to read the FDA-approved patient labeling (Medication Guide).

Hepatotoxicity
Warn patients and guardians that nausea, vomiting, abdominal pain, anorexia, diarrhea, asthenia, and/or jaundice can be symptoms of hepatotoxicity and, therefore, require further medical evaluation promptly [see Warnings and Precautions (5.1)].

Pancreatitis
Warn patients and guardians that abdominal pain, nausea, vomiting, and/or anorexia can be symptoms of pancreatitis and, therefore, require further medical evaluation promptly [see Warnings and Precautions (5.5)].

Birth Defects and Decreased IQ
Inform pregnant women and women of childbearing potential that use of valproate during pregnancy increases the risk of birth defects and decreased IQ in children who were exposed. Advise women to use effective contraception while using valproate. When appropriate, counsel these patients about alternative therapeutic options. This is particularly important when valproate use is considered for a condition not usually associated with permanent injury or death. Advise patients to read the Medication Guide, which appears as the last section of the labeling [see Warnings and Precautions (5.2, 5.3, 5.4) and Use in Specific Populations (8.1)]. Advise women of childbearing potential to discuss pregnancy planning with their doctor and to contact their doctor immediately if they think they are pregnant.

Encourage patients to enroll in the NAAED Pregnancy Registry if they become pregnant. This registry is collecting information about the safety of antiepileptic drugs during pregnancy. To enroll, patients can call the toll free number 1-888-233-2334 [see Use in Specific Populations (8.1)].

Suicidal Thinking and Behavior
Counsel patients, their caregivers, and families that AEDs, including Depakote ER, may increase the risk of suicidal thoughts and behavior and should be advised of the need to be alert for the emergence or worsening of symptoms of depression, any unusual changes in mood or behavior, or the emergence of suicidal thoughts, behavior, or thoughts about self-harm. Instruct patients, caregivers, and families to report behaviors of concern immediately to the healthcare providers [see Warnings and Precautions (5.7)].

Hyperammonemia
Inform patients of the signs and symptoms associated with hyperammonemic encephalopathy and be told to inform the prescriber if any of these symptoms occur [see Warnings and Precautions (5.9, 5.10)].

CNS Depression
Since valproate products may produce CNS depression, especially when combined with another CNS depressant (e.g., alcohol), advise patients not to engage in hazardous activities, such as driving an automobile or operating dangerous machinery, until it is known that they do not become drowsy from the drug.

Multiorgan Hypersensitivity Reaction
Instruct patients that a fever associated with other organ system involvement (rash, lymphadenopathy, etc.) may be drug-related and should be reported to the physician immediately [see Warnings and Precautions (5.12)].

Medication Residue in the Stool
Instruct patients to notify their healthcare provider if they notice a medication residue in the stool [see Warnings and Precautions (5.18)].

250 mg is Mfd. by AbbVie LTD, Barceloneta, PR 00617
500 mg is Mfd. by AbbVie Inc., North Chicago, IL 60064 U.S.A. or
AbbVie LTD, Barceloneta, PR 00617
For AbbVie Inc., North Chicago, IL 60064 U.S.A.
©2016 AbbVie Inc.
Revised: February 2016
03-B304

MEDICATION GUIDE
DEPAKOTE ER (dep-a-kOte)
(divalproex sodium)
Extended Release Tablets
DEPAKOTE (dep-a-kOte)
(divalproex sodium)
Tablets
DEPAKOTE (dep-a-kOte)
(divalproex sodium delayed release capsules)
Sprinkle Capsules
DEPAKENE (dep-a-keen)
(valproic acid)
Capsules and Oral Solution

Read this Medication Guide before you start taking Depakote or Depakene and each time you get a refill. There may be new information. This information does not take the place of talking to your healthcare provider about your medical condition or treatment.
What is the most important information I should know about Depakote and Depakene?
Do not stop taking Depakote or Depakene without first talking to your healthcare provider.
Stopping Depakote or Depakene suddenly can cause serious problems.
Depakote and Depakene can cause serious side effects, including:

1. **Serious liver damage that can cause death, especially in children younger than 2 years old.** The risk of getting this serious liver damage is more likely to happen within the first 6 months of treatment.
   Call your healthcare provider right away if you get any of the following symptoms:
   - nausea or vomiting that does not go away
   - loss of appetite
   - pain on the right side of your stomach (abdomen)
   - dark urine
   - swelling of your face
   - yellowing of your skin or the whites of your eyes

   In some cases, liver damage may continue despite stopping the drug.

2. **Depakote or Depakene may harm your unborn baby.**
   - If you take Depakote or Depakene during pregnancy for any medical condition, your baby is at risk for serious birth defects that affect the brain and spinal cord and are called spina bifida or neural tube defects. These defects occur in 1 to 2 out of every 100 babies born to mothers who use this medicine during pregnancy. These defects can begin in the first month, even before you know you are pregnant. Other birth defects that affect the structures of the heart, head, arms, legs, and the opening where the urine comes out (urethra) on the bottom of the penis can also happen.
   - Birth defects may occur even in children born to women who are not taking any medicines and do not have other risk factors.
   - Taking folic acid supplements before getting pregnant and during early pregnancy can lower the chance of having a baby with a neural tube defect.
   - If you take Depakote or Depakene during pregnancy for any medical condition, your child is at risk for having a lower IQ.
   - There may be other medicines to treat your condition that have a lower chance of causing birth defects and decreased IQ in your child.
   - Women who are pregnant must not take Depakote or Depakene to prevent migraine headaches.
   - **All women of child-bearing age should talk to their healthcare provider about using other possible treatments instead of Depakote or Depakene. If the decision is made to use Depakote or Depakene, you should use effective birth control (contraception).**
   - Tell your healthcare provider right away if you become pregnant while taking Depakote or Depakene. You and your healthcare provider should decide if you will continue to take Depakote or Depakene while you are pregnant.

   Pregnancy Registry: If you become pregnant while taking Depakote or Depakene, talk to your healthcare provider about registering with the North American Antiepileptic Drug Pregnancy Registry. You can enroll in this registry by calling 1-888-233-2334. The purpose of this registry is to collect information about the safety of antiepileptic drugs during pregnancy.

3. **Inflammation of your pancreas that can cause death.**
   Call your healthcare provider right away if you have any of these symptoms:
   - severe stomach pain that you may also feel in your back
   - nausea or vomiting that does not go away

4. **Like other antiepileptic drugs, Depakote or Depakene may cause suicidal thoughts or actions in a very small number of people, about 1 in 500.**
   Call a healthcare provider right away if you have any of these symptoms, especially if they are new, worse, or worry you:
   - thoughts about suicide or dying
   - attempts to commit suicide
   - new or worse depression
   - new or worse anxiety
   - feeling agitated or restless
   - panic attacks
   - trouble sleeping (insomnia)
   - new or worse irritability
   - acting aggressive, being angry, or violent
   - acting on dangerous impulses
   - an extreme increase in activity and talking (mania)
   - other unusual changes in behavior or mood

   How can I watch for early symptoms of suicidal thoughts and actions?
   - Pay attention to any changes, especially sudden changes in mood, behaviors, thoughts, or feelings.
   - Keep all follow-up visits with your healthcare provider as scheduled.

   Call your healthcare provider between visits as needed, especially if you are worried about symptoms.
   Do not stop Depakote or Depakene without first talking to a healthcare provider. Stopping Depakote or Depakene suddenly can cause serious problems. Stopping a seizure medicine suddenly in a patient who has epilepsy can cause seizures that do not stop (status epilepticus).

   Suicidal thoughts or actions can be caused by things other than medicines. If you have suicidal thoughts or actions, your healthcare provider may check for other causes.

What are Depakote and Depakene?

Depakote and Depakene come in different dosage forms with different usages.

Depakote Tablets and Depakote Extended Release Tablets are prescription medicines used:
- to treat manic episodes associated with bipolar disorder.
- alone or with other medicines to treat:
  - complex partial seizures in adults and children 10 years of age and older
  - simple and complex absence seizures, with or without other seizure types
- to prevent migraine headaches

Depakene (solution and liquid capsules) and Depakote Sprinkles are prescription medicines used alone or with other medicines, to treat:
- complex partial seizures in adults and children 10 years of age and older
- simple and complex absence seizures, with or without other seizure types

Who should not take Depakote or Depakene?

Do not take Depakote or Depakene if you:
- have liver problems
- have or think you have a genetic liver problem caused by a mitochondrial disorder (e.g. Alpers-Huttenlocher syndrome)
- are allergic to divalproex sodium, valproic acid, sodium valproate, or any of the ingredients in Depakote or Depakene. See the end of this leaflet for a complete list of ingredients in Depakote and Depakene.
- have a genetic problem called urea cycle disorder
- are pregnant for the prevention of migraine headaches

What should I tell my healthcare provider before taking Depakote or Depakene?

Before you take Depakote or Depakene, tell your healthcare provider if you:
- have a genetic liver problem caused by a mitochondrial disorder (e.g. Alpers-Huttenlocher syndrome)
- drink alcohol
- are pregnant or breastfeeding. Depakote or Depakene can pass into breast milk. Talk to your healthcare provider about the best way to feed your baby if you take Depakote or Depakene.
- have or have had depression, mood problems, or suicidal thoughts or behavior
- have any other medical conditions

Tell your healthcare provider about all the medicines you take, including prescription and non-prescription medicines, vitamins, herbal supplements and medicines that you take for a short period of time.

Taking Depakote or Depakene with certain other medicines can cause side effects or affect how well they work. Do not start or stop other medicines without talking to your healthcare provider.

Know the medicines you take. Keep a list of them and show it to your healthcare provider and pharmacist each time you get a new medicine.

How should I take Depakote or Depakene?
- Take Depakote or Depakene exactly as your healthcare provider tells you. Your healthcare provider will tell you how much Depakote or Depakene to take and when to take it.
- Your healthcare provider may change your dose.
- Do not change your dose of Depakote or Depakene without talking to your healthcare provider.
- **Do not stop taking Depakote or Depakene without first talking to your healthcare provider.** Stopping Depakote or Depakene suddenly can cause serious problems.
- Swallow Depakote tablets, Depakote ER tablets or Depakene capsules whole. Do not crush or chew Depakote tablets, Depakote ER tablets, or Depakene capsules. Tell your healthcare provider if you cannot swallow Depakote or Depakene whole. You may need a different medicine.
- Depakote Sprinkle Capsules may be swallowed whole, or they may be opened and the contents may be sprinkled on a small amount of soft food, such as applesauce or pudding. See the Patient Instructions for Use at the end of this Medication Guide for detailed instructions on how to use Depakote Sprinkle Capsules.
- If you take too much Depakote or Depakene, call your healthcare provider or local Poison Control Center right away.

What should I avoid while taking Depakote or Depakene?
- Depakote and Depakene can cause drowsiness and dizziness. Do not drink alcohol or take other medicines that make you sleepy or dizzy while taking Depakote or Depakene, until you talk with your doctor. Taking Depakote or Depakene with alcohol or drugs that cause sleepiness or dizziness may make your sleepiness or dizziness worse.
- Do not drive a car or operate dangerous machinery until you know how Depakote or Depakene affect you. Depakote and Depakene can slow your thinking and motor skills.

What are the possible side effects of Depakote or Depakene?
- See "What is the most important information I should know about Depakote or Depakene?"

Depakote or Depakene may cause other serious side effects including:
- **Bleeding problems:** red or purple spots on your skin, bruising, pain and swelling into your joints due to bleeding or bleeding from your mouth or nose.
- **High ammonia levels in your blood:** feeling tired, vomiting, changes in mental status.
- **Low body temperature (hypothermia):** drop in your body temperature to less than 95°F, feeling tired, confusion, coma.
- **Allergic (hypersensitivity) reactions:** fever, skin rash, hives, sores in your mouth, blistering and peeling of your skin, swelling of your lymph nodes, swelling of your face, eyes, lips, tongue, or throat, trouble swallowing or breathing.
- **Drowsiness or sleepiness in the elderly.** This extreme drowsiness may cause you to eat or drink less than you normally would. Tell your doctor if you are not able to eat or drink as you normally do. Your doctor may start you at a lower dose of Depakote or Depakene.

Call your healthcare provider right away, if you have any of the symptoms listed above.

The common side effects of Depakote and Depakene include:
- nausea
- headache
- sleepiness
- vomiting
- weakness
- tremor
- dizziness
- stomach pain
- blurry vision
- double vision
- diarrhea
- increased appetite
- weight gain
- hair loss
- loss of appetite
- problems with walking or coordination

These are not all of the possible side effects of **Depakote or Depakene.** For more information, ask your healthcare provider or pharmacist.

Tell your healthcare provider if you have any side effect that bothers you or that does not go away.

Call your doctor for medical advice about side effects. You may report side effects to FDA at 1-800-FDA-1088.

How should I store Depakote or Depakene?
- Store Depakote Extended Release Tablets between 59°F to 86°F (15°C to 30°C).
- Store Depakote Delayed Release Tablets below 86°F (30°C).
- Store Depakote Sprinkle Capsules below 77°F (25°C).
- Store Depakene Capsules at 59°F to 77°F (15°C to 25°C).
- Store Depakene Oral Solution below 86°F (30°C).

Keep Depakote or Depakene and all medicines out of the reach of children.

General information about the safe and effective use of Depakote or Depakene

Medicines are sometimes prescribed for purposes other than those listed in a Medication Guide. Do not use Depakote or Depakene for a condition for which it was not prescribed. Do not give Depakote or Depakene to other people, even if they have the same symptoms that you have. It may harm them.

This Medication Guide summarizes the most important information about Depakote or Depakene. If you would like

Continued on next page

Information on the AbbVie, Inc. products listed on these pages is from the prescribing information in use as of July 31, 2016. For more information, please visit rxabbvie.com or call 1-800-633-9110.

more information, talk with your healthcare provider. You can ask your pharmacist or healthcare provider for information about Depakote or Depakene that is written for health professionals.

For more information, go to www.rxabbvie.com or call 1-800-633-9110.

What are the ingredients in Depakote or Depakene?

Depakote:

Active ingredient: divalproex sodium

Inactive ingredients:

• **Depakote Extended Release Tablets:** FD&C Blue No. 1, hypromellose, lactose, microcrystalline cellulose, polyethylene glycol, potassium sorbate, propylene glycol, silicon dioxide, titanium dioxide, and triacetin. The 500 mg tablets also contain iron oxide and polydextrose.

• **Depakote Tablets:** cellulosic polymers, diacetylated monoglycerides, povidone, pregelatinized starch (contains corn starch), silica gel, talc, titanium dioxide, and vanillin. Individual tablets also contain:

  125 mg tablets: FD&C Blue No. 1 and FD&C Red No. 40,

  250 mg tablets: FD&C Yellow No. 6 and iron oxide,

  500 mg tablets: D&C Red No. 30, FD&C Blue No. 2, and iron oxide.

• **Depakote Sprinkle Capsules:** cellulosic polymers, D&C Red No. 28, FD&C Blue No. 1 gelatin, iron oxide, magnesium stearate, silica gel, titanium dioxide, and triethyl citrate.

Depakene:

Active ingredient: valproic acid

Inactive ingredients:

• **Depakene Capsules:** corn oil, FD&C Yellow No. 6, gelatin, glycerin, iron oxide, methylparaben, propylparaben, and titanium dioxide.

• **Depakene Oral Solution:** FD&C Red No. 40, glycerin, methylparaben, propylparaben, sorbitol, sucrose, water, and natural and artificial flavors.

Depakote ER:

250 mg is Mfd. by AbbVie LTD, Barceloneta, PR 00617

500 mg is Mfd. by AbbVie Inc., North Chicago, IL 60064 U.S.A. or

AbbVie LTD, Barceloneta, PR 00617

For AbbVie Inc., North Chicago, IL 60064 U.S.A.

Depakote Tablets:

Mfd. by AbbVie LTD, Barceloneta, PR 00617

For AbbVie Inc., North Chicago, IL 60064, U.S.A.

Depakote Sprinkle Capsules:

AbbVie Inc., North Chicago, IL 60064, U.S.A.

Depakene Capsules:

Mfd. by Banner Pharmacaps, Inc., High Point, NC 27265 U.S.A.

For AbbVie Inc., North Chicago, IL 60064, U.S.A.

Depakene Oral solution:

Mfd. by AbbVie Inc., North Chicago, IL 60064, U.S.A.

OR by DPT Laboratories, Ltd., San Antonio, TX 78215, U.S.A.

For AbbVie Inc., North Chicago, IL 60064, U.S.A.

This Medication Guide has been approved by the U.S. Food and Drug Administration.

©2016 AbbVie Inc.

Revised: February 2016

03-B304

Shown in Product Identification Guide, page 505

DUOPA   ℞

[Do-oh-pa]

(carbidopa and levodopa)

enteral suspension

HIGHLIGHTS OF PRESCRIBING INFORMATION

These highlights do not include all the information needed to use DUOPA safely and effectively. See full prescribing information for DUOPA.

DUOPA (carbidopa and levodopa) enteral suspension

Initial U.S. Approval: 1975

──────INDICATIONS AND USAGE──────

DUOPA is a combination of carbidopa (an aromatic amino acid decarboxylation inhibitor) and levodopa (an aromatic amino acid) indicated for the treatment of motor fluctuations in patients with advanced Parkinson's disease (1)

──────DOSAGE AND ADMINISTRATION──────

• The maximum recommended daily dose of DUOPA is 2000 mg of levodopa (i.e., one cassette per day) administered over 16 hours (2.1)

• Prior to initiating DUOPA, convert patients from all forms of levodopa to oral immediate-release carbidopa-levodopa tablets (1:4 ratio) (2.2)

• Titrate total daily dose based on clinical response for the patient (2.2)

• Administer DUOPA into the jejunum through a percutaneous endoscopic gastrostomy with jejunal tube (PEG-J) with the CADD®-Legacy 1400 portable infusion pump (2.3)

──────DOSAGE FORMS AND STRENGTHS──────

Enteral Suspension: 4.63 mg carbidopa and 20 mg levodopa per mL (3)

──────CONTRAINDICATIONS──────

DUOPA is contraindicated in patients taking nonselective monoamine oxidase (MAO) inhibitors (4)

──────WARNINGS AND PRECAUTIONS──────

• Gastrointestinal procedure-related complications may result in serious outcomes, such as need for surgery or death (5.1)

• May cause falling asleep during activities of daily living (5.2)

• Monitor patients for orthostatic hypotension, especially after starting DUOPA or increasing the dose (5.3)

• Hallucinations/Psychosis/Confusion: May respond to dose reduction in levodopa (5.4)

• Impulse Control Disorders: Consider dose reductions or stopping DUOPA (5.5)

• Monitor patients for depression and suicidality (5.6)

• Avoid sudden discontinuation or rapid dose reduction to reduce the risk of withdrawal-emergent hyperpyrexia and confusion (5.7)

• May cause or exacerbate dyskinesia: Consider dose reduction (5.8)

• Monitor patients for signs and symptoms of peripheral neuropathy (5.9)

──────ADVERSE REACTIONS──────

Most common adverse reactions for DUOPA (DUOPA incidence at least 7% greater than oral carbidopa-levodopa incidence) were: complication of device insertion, nausea, depression, peripheral edema, hypertension, upper respiratory tract infection, oropharyngeal pain, atelectasis, and incision site erythema. (6.1)

To report SUSPECTED ADVERSE REACTIONS, contact AbbVie Inc. at 1-800-633-9110 or FDA at 1-800-FDA-1088 or www.fda.gov/medwatch.

──────DRUG INTERACTIONS──────

• Selective MAO-B inhibitors: May cause orthostatic hypotension (7.1)

• Antihypertensive drugs: May cause symptomatic postural hypotension. Dosage adjustment of the antihypertensive drug may be needed (7.2)

• Dopamine D2 receptor antagonists, isoniazid, iron salts, and high-protein diet may reduce the effectiveness of DUOPA (7.3, 7.4, 7.5)

──────USE IN SPECIFIC POPULATIONS──────

Pregnancy: Based on animal data, may cause fetal harm (8.1)

See 17 for PATIENT COUNSELING INFORMATION and Medication Guide.

Revised: 2/2016

FULL PRESCRIBING INFORMATION

1   INDICATIONS AND USAGE

DUOPA is indicated for the treatment of motor fluctuations in patients with advanced Parkinson's disease.

2   DOSAGE AND ADMINISTRATION

2.1   DUOPA Daily Dose

DUOPA is administered over a 16-hour infusion period. The daily dose is determined by individualized patient titration and composed of:

• A Morning Dose

• A Continuous Dose

• Extra Doses

The maximum recommended daily dose of DUOPA is 2000 mg of the levodopa component (i.e., one cassette per day) administered over 16 hours. At the end of the daily 16-hour infusion, patients will disconnect the pump from the PEG-J and take their night-time dose of oral immediate-release carbidopa-levodopa tablets.

Treatment with DUOPA is initiated in 3 steps *[see Dosage and Administration (2.2)]*:

1. Conversion of patients to oral immediate-release carbidopa-levodopa tablets in preparation for DUOPA treatment.

2. Calculation and administration of the DUOPA starting dose (Morning Dose and Continuous Dose) for Day 1.

3. Titration of the dose as needed based on individual clinical response and tolerability.

Extra Doses

DUOPA has an extra dose function that can be used to manage acute "Off" symptoms that are not controlled by the Morning Dose and the Continuous Dose administered over 16 hours. The extra dose function should be set at 1 mL (20 mg of levodopa) when starting DUOPA. If the amount of the extra dose needs to be adjusted, it is typically done in 0.2 mL increments. The extra dose frequency should be limited to one extra dose every 2 hours. Administration of frequent extra doses may cause or worsen dyskinesias.

Once no further adjustments are required to the DUOPA Morning Dose, Continuous Dose, or Extra Dose, this dosing regimen should be administered daily. Over time, additional changes may be necessary based on the patient's clinical response and tolerability.

2.2   Initiation and Titration Instructions

Prepare for DUOPA Treatment

Prior to initiating DUOPA, convert patients from all other forms of levodopa to oral immediate-release carbidopa-levodopa tablets (1:4 ratio). Patients should remain on a stable dose of their concomitant medications taken for the treatment of Parkinson's disease before initiation of DUOPA infusion.

Healthcare providers should ensure patients take their oral Parkinson's disease medications the morning of the PEG-J procedure.

Determine the DUOPA Starting Dose for Day 1

The steps for determining the initial DUOPA daily dosing (Morning Dose and Continuous Dose) for Day 1 are outlined below.

Step 1: Calculate and administer the DUOPA Morning Dose for Day 1

a.	Determine the total amount of levodopa (in milligrams) in the first dose of oral immediate-release carbidopa-levodopa that was taken by the patient on the previous day.
b.	Convert the oral levodopa dose from milligrams to milliliters by multiplying the oral dose by 0.8 and dividing by 20 mg/mL. This calculation will provide the Morning Dose of DUOPA in milliliters.
c.	Add 3 milliliters to the Morning Dose to fill (prime) the intestinal tube to obtain the Total Morning Dose.
d.	The Total Morning Dose is usually administered over 10 to 30 minutes.
e.	Program the pump to deliver the Total Morning Dose.

Step 2: Calculate and administer the DUOPA Continuous Dose for Day 1

a.	Determine the amount of oral immediate-release levodopa that the patient received from oral immediate-release carbidopa-levodopa doses throughout the previous day (16 waking hours), in milligrams. Do not include the doses of oral immediate-release carbidopa-levodopa taken at night when calculating the levodopa amount.
b.	Subtract the first oral levodopa dose in milligrams taken by the patient on the previous day (determined in Step 1 (a)) from the total oral levodopa dose in milligrams taken over 16 waking hours (determined in Step 2 (a)). Divide the result by 20 mg/mL. This is the dose of DUOPA administered as a Continuous Dose (in mL) over 16 hours.
c.	The hourly infusion rate (mL per hour) is obtained by dividing the Continuous Dose by 16 (hours). This value will be programmed into the pump as the continuous rate.
d.	If persistent or numerous "Off" periods occur during the 16-hour infusion, consider increasing the Continuous Dose or using the Extra Dose function. If dyskinesia or DUOPA-related adverse reactions occur, consider decreasing the Continuous Dose or stopping the infusion until the adverse reactions subside.

DUOPA Titration

The daily dose of DUOPA can be titrated as needed, based on the patient's individual clinical response and tolerability after Day 1 of DUOPA treatment and until a stable daily dose is maintained. Adjustments to concomitant Parkinson's disease medications may be needed. In the controlled trial, the average number of titration days required to establish a stable Morning and Continuous Dose was 5 days. Additional dose adjustments may be necessary over time based on the patient level of activity and disease progression.

The recommendations for adjusting the DUOPA Morning and Continuous Doses are provided below.

Morning Dose Adjustment

If there was an inadequate clinical response within 1 hour of the Morning Dose on the preceding day, adjust the Morning Dose (excluding the 3 mL to fill the tube) as follows:

• If the Morning Dose on the preceding day was less than or equal to 6 mL, increase the Morning Dose by 1 mL.
• If the Morning Dose on the preceding day was greater than 6 mL, increase the Morning Dose by 2 mL.

If the patient experienced dyskinesias or DUOPA-related adverse reactions within 1 hour of the Morning Dose on the preceding day, decrease the Morning Dose by 1 mL.

Continuous Dose Adjustment

Consider increasing the Continuous Dose based on the number and volume of Extra Doses of DUOPA (i.e., total amount of levodopa component) that were needed for the previous day and the patient's clinical response.

Consider decreasing the Continuous Dose if the patient experienced troublesome dyskinesia, or other troublesome DUOPA-related adverse reactions on the preceding day:

• For troublesome adverse reactions lasting for a period of one hour or more, decrease the Continuous Dose by 0.3 mL per hour.
• For troublesome adverse reactions lasting for two or more periods of one hour or more, decrease the Continuous Dose by 0.6 mL per hour.

2.3   Administration Information

• DUOPA should be used at room temperature. Take one DUOPA cassette out of the refrigerator and out of the carton 20 minutes prior to use; failure to use the product at room temperature may result in the patient not receiving the right amount of medication.
• DUOPA is delivered as a 16-hour infusion through either a naso-jejunal tube for short-term administration or through a PEG-J for long-term administration.
• The cassettes are for single-use only and should not be used for longer than 16 hours, even if some drug product remains.
• An opened cassette should not be re-used.
• The PEG-J should be disconnected from the pump at the end of the daily 16-hour administration period and flushed with room temperature potable water with a syringe.

Long-term administration of DUOPA requires placement of a PEG-J outer transabdominal tube and inner jejunal tube by percutaneous endoscopic gastrostomy. DUOPA is dispensed from medication cassette reservoirs that are specifically designed to be connected to the CADD®-Legacy 1400 pump.

Establishment of the transabdominal port should be performed by a gastroenterologist or other healthcare provider experienced in this procedure. See Table 1 for the recommended tubing sets for PEG-J administration.

For short-term, temporary administration of DUOPA prior to PEG-J tube placement, treatment may be initiated by a naso-jejunal tube with observation of the patient's clinical response. See Table 2 for the recommended tubing sets for naso-jejunal administration.

Table 1. Recommended Tubing Sets for Long-Term PEG-J DUOPA Administration

Product Name	Manufacturer
AbbVie PEG 15 and 20 Fr	AbbVie Inc.
AbbVie J	AbbVie Inc.

Table 2. Recommended Tubing Sets for Short-Term Naso-Jejunal DUOPA Administration

Product Name	Manufacturer
AbbVie NJ	AbbVie Inc.
NJFT-10	Wilson-Cook Medical, Inc.
Kangaroo™ Naso-Jejunal Feeding Tube	Covidien
Kangaroo™	Covidien

2.4   Discontinuation of DUOPA

Avoid sudden discontinuation or rapid dose reduction in patients taking DUOPA.

If patients need to discontinue DUOPA, the dose should be tapered or patients should be switched to oral immediate-release carbidopa-levodopa tablets *[see Warnings and Precautions (5.7)]*.

When using a PEG-J tube, DUOPA can be discontinued by withdrawing the tube and letting the stoma heal. The removal of the tube should only be performed by a qualified healthcare provider.

3   DOSAGE FORMS AND STRENGTHS

Enteral suspension: 4.63 mg carbidopa and 20 mg levodopa per mL in a single-use cassette. Each cassette contains approximately 100 mL of suspension.

4   CONTRAINDICATIONS

DUOPA is contraindicated in patients who are currently taking a nonselective monoamine oxidase (MAO) inhibitor (e.g., phenelzine and tranylcypromine) or have recently (within 2 weeks) taken a nonselective MAO inhibitor. Hypertension can occur if these drugs are used concurrently *[see Drug Interactions (7.1 and 7.2)]*.

5   WARNINGS AND PRECAUTIONS

5.1   Gastrointestinal and Gastrointestinal Procedure-Related Risks

Because DUOPA is administered using a PEG-J or naso-jejunal tube, gastrointestinal complications can occur.

These complications include bezoar, ileus, implant site erosion/ulcer, intestinal hemorrhage, intestinal ischemia, intestinal obstruction, intestinal perforation, pancreatitis, peritonitis, pneumoperitoneum, and post-operative wound infection. These complications may result in serious outcomes, such as the need for surgery or death.

Instruct patients to notify their healthcare provider immediately if they experience abdominal pain, prolonged constipation, nausea, vomiting, fever, or melanotic stool *[see Patient Counseling Information (17)]*.

5.2   Falling Asleep During Activities of Daily Living and Somnolence

Patients treated with levodopa, a component of DUOPA, have reported falling asleep while engaged in activities of daily living, including the operation of motor vehicles, which sometimes resulted in accidents. Although many of these patients reported somnolence while on levodopa, some perceived that they had no warning signs (sleep attack), such as excessive drowsiness, and believed that they were alert immediately prior to the event. Some of these events have been reported more than one year after initiation of treatment.

Falling asleep while engaged in activities of daily living usually occurs in patients experiencing preexisting somnolence, although patients may not give such a history. For this reason, prescribers should reassess patients for drowsiness or sleepiness in DUOPA-treated patients, especially since some of the events occur well after the start of treatment. Prescribers should be aware that patients may not acknowledge drowsiness or sleepiness until directly questioned about drowsiness or sleepiness during specific activities. Patients who have already experienced somnolence or an episode of sudden sleep onset should not participate in these activities while taking DUOPA.

Before initiating treatment with DUOPA, advise patients about the potential to develop drowsiness and specifically ask about factors that may increase the risk for somnolence with DUOPA such as the use of concomitant sedating medications or the presence of sleep disorders. Consider discontinuing DUOPA in patients who report significant daytime sleepiness or episodes of falling asleep during activities that require active participation (e.g., conversations, eating). If DUOPA is continued, they should be advised to avoid driving and other potentially dangerous activities that might result in harm if the patient becomes somnolent.

5.3   Orthostatic Hypotension

DUOPA-treated patients were more likely to experience a decline in orthostatic blood pressure than patients treated with oral immediate-release carbidopa-levodopa in the controlled clinical study. Orthostatic systolic hypotension (≥30 mm Hg decrease) occurred in 73% of DUOPA-treated patients compared to 68% of patients treated with oral immediate-release carbidopa-levodopa in the controlled clinical study. Orthostatic diastolic hypotension (≥20 mm Hg decrease) occurred in 70% of DUOPA-treated patients compared to 62% of patients treated with oral immediate-release carbidopa-levodopa. Inform patients about the risk for hypotension and syncope. Monitor patients for orthostatic hypotension, especially after starting DUOPA or increasing the dose.

5.4   Hallucinations/Psychosis/Confusion

There is an increased risk for hallucinations and psychosis in patients taking DUOPA. In the controlled clinical trial, hallucinations occurred in 5% of DUOPA-treated patients compared to 3% of patients treated with oral immediate-release carbidopa-levodopa. Confusion occurred in 8% of DUOPA-treated patients compared to 3% of patients treated with oral immediate-release carbidopa-levodopa, and psychotic disorder occurred in 5% of DUOPA-treated patients compared to 3% of patients treated with oral immediate-release carbidopa-levodopa.

Hallucinations associated with levodopa may present shortly after the initiation of therapy and may be responsive to dose reduction in levodopa. Confusion, insomnia, and excessive dreaming may accompany hallucinations. Abnormal thinking and behavior may present with one or more symptoms, including paranoid ideation, delusions, hallucinations, confusion, psychosis, disorientation, aggressive behavior, agitation, and delirium.

Continued on next page

Information on the AbbVie, Inc. products listed on these pages is from the prescribing information in use as of July 31, 2016. For more information, please visit rxabbvie.com or call 1-800-633-9110.

Because of the risk of exacerbating psychosis, patients with a major psychotic disorder should not be treated with DUOPA. In addition, medications that antagonize the effects of dopamine used to treat psychosis may exacerbate the symptoms of Parkinson's disease and may decrease the effectiveness of DUOPA [see Drug Interactions (7.3)].

5.5 Impulse Control/Compulsive Behaviors

Patients may experience intense urges to gamble, increased sexual urges, intense urges to spend money, binge or compulsive eating, and/or other intense urges, and the inability to control these urges while taking one or more of the medications, including DUOPA, that increase central dopaminergic tone and that are generally used for the treatment of Parkinson's disease. In some cases, although not all, these urges were reported to have stopped when the dose was reduced or the medication was discontinued.

Because patients may not recognize these behaviors as abnormal, it is important for prescribers to ask patients or their caregivers specifically about the development of new or increased gambling urges, sexual urges, uncontrolled spending, binge or compulsive eating, or other urges while being treated with DUOPA. Consider reducing the dose or discontinuing DUOPA if a patient develops such urges.

5.6 Depression and Suicidality

In the controlled clinical trial, 11% of DUOPA-treated patients developed depression compared to 3% of oral immediate-release carbidopa-levodopa-treated patients. Monitor patients for the development of depression and concomitant suicidal tendencies.

5.7 Withdrawal-Emergent Hyperpyrexia and Confusion

A symptom complex that resembles neuroleptic malignant syndrome (characterized by elevated temperature, muscular rigidity, altered consciousness, and autonomic instability), with no other obvious etiology, has been reported in association with rapid dose reduction, withdrawal of, or changes in dopaminergic therapy. Avoid sudden discontinuation or rapid dose reduction in patients taking DUOPA. If DUOPA is discontinued, the dose should be tapered to reduce the risk of hyperpyrexia and confusion [see Dosage and Administration (2.4)].

5.8 Dyskinesia

DUOPA may cause or exacerbate dyskinesias. In the controlled clinical trial, dyskinesia occurred in 14% of DUOPA-treated patients compared to 12% of patients treated with oral immediate-release carbidopa-levodopa. The occurrence of dyskinesias may require a dosage reduction of DUOPA or other medications used to treat Parkinson's disease.

5.9 Neuropathy

In clinical studies, 19 of 412 (5%) patients treated with DUOPA developed a generalized polyneuropathy. The onset of neuropathy could be determined in 13 of 19 patients. Most cases (12/19) were classified as subacute or chronic in onset. The neuropathy was most often characterized as sensory or sensorimotor. Electrodiagnostic testing performed in 16 patients was most often (15/16) consistent with an axonal polyneuropathy, and one patient was classified as having a demyelinating neuropathy. There was insufficient information to determine the potential role of vitamin deficiencies in the etiology of neuropathy associated with DUOPA.

Patients should have clinical assessments for the signs and symptoms of peripheral neuropathy before starting DUOPA. Monitor patients periodically for signs of neuropathy after starting DUOPA, especially in patients with pre-existing neuropathy and in patients taking medications or those who have medical conditions that are also associated with neuropathy.

5.10 Cardiovascular Ischemic Events

In clinical studies, myocardial infarction and arrhythmia were reported in patients taking carbidopa-levodopa. Ask patients about symptoms of ischemic heart disease and arrhythmia, especially those with a history of myocardial infarction or cardiac arrhythmias.

5.11 Melanoma

Epidemiological studies have shown that patients with Parkinson's disease have a higher risk (2 to approximately 6-fold higher) of developing melanoma than the general population. Whether the increased risk observed was due to Parkinson's disease or other factors, such as drugs used to treat Parkinson's disease, is unclear. In the clinical studies, 2 of 416 (0.5%) DUOPA-treated patients developed melanoma.

Appropriately qualified health care providers (e.g., dermatologists) should perform periodic skin examinations to monitor for melanoma in patients receiving DUOPA.

5.12 Laboratory Test Abnormalities

DUOPA may increase the risk for elevated (above the upper limit of normal for the reference range) blood urea nitrogen (BUN) and creatine phosphokinase (CPK). In the controlled clinical trial, the shift from a low or normal value at baseline to an increased BUN value was greater for DUOPA-treated patients (13%) than for patients treated with oral immediate-release carbidopa-levodopa (4%). The shift from a low or normal value at baseline to an increased CPK value was greater for DUOPA-treated patients (17%) than for patients treated with oral immediate-release carbidopa-levodopa (7%). The incidence of patients with a markedly increased BUN (≥10 mmol/L; ≥28 mg/dL) was greater for patients treated with DUOPA (11%) than that for patients treated with oral immediate-release carbidopa-levodopa (0%). The incidence of patients with an increased CPK (>3 times the upper limit of normal) was greater for patients treated with DUOPA (9%) than that for patients treated with oral immediate-release carbidopa-levodopa (0%). Patients taking levodopa or carbidopa-levodopa may have increased levels of catecholamines and their metabolites in plasma and urine giving false positive results suggesting the diagnosis of pheochromocytoma in patients on levodopa and carbidopa-levodopa.

5.13 Glaucoma

Carbidopa-levodopa may cause increased intraocular pressure in patients with glaucoma. Monitor intraocular pressure in patients with glaucoma after starting DUOPA.

6 ADVERSE REACTIONS

The following serious adverse reactions are discussed below and elsewhere in labeling:

- Gastrointestinal and Gastrointestinal Procedure-Related Risks [see Warnings and Precautions (5.1)]
- Falling Asleep During Activities of Daily Living and Somnolence [see Warnings and Precautions (5.2)]
- Orthostatic Hypotension [see Warnings and Precautions (5.3)]
- Hallucinations/Psychosis/Confusion [see Warnings and Precautions (5.4)]
- Impulse Control/Compulsive Behaviors [see Warnings and Precautions (5.5)]
- Depression and Suicidality [see Warnings and Precautions (5.6)]
- Withdrawal-Emergent Hyperpyrexia and Confusion [see Warnings and Precautions (5.7)]
- Dyskinesia [see Warnings and Precautions (5.8)]
- Neuropathy [see Warnings and Precautions (5.9)]
- Cardiovascular Ischemic Events [see Warnings and Precautions (5.10)]
- Melanoma [see Warnings and Precautions (5.11)]
- Laboratory Test Abnormalities [see Warnings and Precautions (5.12)]
- Glaucoma [see Warnings and Precautions (5.13)]

6.1 Clinical Trials Experience

Because clinical studies are run under widely varying conditions, the incidence of adverse reactions observed in the clinical trials of a drug cannot be directly compared to rates in the clinical trials of another drug and may not reflect the rates observed in practice.

In clinical studies, 416 patients with advanced Parkinson's disease received DUOPA. 338 patients were treated with DUOPA for more than 1 year, 233 patients were treated with DUOPA for more than 2 years, and 162 patients were treated with DUOPA for more than 3 years.

In a 12-week, active-controlled clinical trial (Study 1), a total of 71 patients with advanced Parkinson's disease were enrolled and had a PEG-J procedure. Of these, 37 patients received DUOPA and 34 received oral immediate-release carbidopa-levodopa.

The most common adverse reactions for DUOPA (incidence at least 7% greater than oral immediate-release carbidopa-levodopa) were: complication of device insertion, nausea, depression, peripheral edema, hypertension, upper respiratory tract infection, oropharyngeal pain, atelectasis, and incision site erythema.

Table 3 lists the incidence of adverse reactions occurring in the DUOPA-treated group (requiring at least 2 patients in this group) in Study 1 when the incidence was numerically greater than that for oral immediate-release carbidopa-levodopa.

Table 3. Adverse Reactions in Study 1 for DUOPA in Patients with Advanced Parkinson's disease

Preferred Term	DUOPA (n = 37) %	Oral immediate-release carbidopa-levodopa[a] (n = 34) %
Complication of device insertion	57	44
Nausea	30	21
Constipation	22	21
Incision site erythema	19	12
Dyskinesia	14	12
Depression	11	3
Post procedural discharge	11	9
Peripheral edema	8	0
Hypertension	8	0
Upper respiratory tract infection	8	0
Oropharyngeal pain	8	0
Atelectasis	8	0
Confusional state	8	3
Anxiety	8	3
Dizziness	8	6
Hiatal hernia	8	6
Postoperative ileus	5	0
Sleep disorder	5	0
Pyrexia	5	0
Excessive granulation tissue	5	0
Rash	5	0
Bacteriuria	5	0
White blood cells urine positive	5	0
Hallucination	5	3
Psychotic disorder	5	3
Diarrhea	5	3
Dyspepsia	5	3

[a] All patients in the clinical trial regardless of treatment arm received a PEG-J.

Procedure and Device-Related Adverse Reactions

The most common adverse reactions associated with complications due to naso-jejunal (NJ) insertion were: oropharyngeal pain, abdominal distention, abdominal pain, abdominal discomfort, pain, throat irritation, gastrointestinal injury, esophageal hemorrhage, anxiety, dysphagia, and vomiting. The most common adverse reactions associated with complications due to PEG-J insertion were: abdominal pain, abdominal discomfort, abdominal distension, flatulence, or pneumoperitoneum.

Additional adverse reactions that were co-reported with complication of naso-jejunal and PEG-J insertion included upper abdominal pain, duodenal ulcer, duodenal ulcer hemorrhage, erosive duodenitis, erosive gastritis, gastrointestinal hemorrhage, peritonitis, post-operative abscess, and small intestine ulcer.

7 DRUG INTERACTIONS

7.1 Monoamine Oxidase (MAO) Inhibitors

The use of nonselective MAO inhibitors with DUOPA is contraindicated [see Contraindications (4)]. Discontinue use of any nonselective MAO inhibitors at least two weeks prior to initiating DUOPA.

The use of selective MAO-B inhibitors (e.g., rasagiline and selegiline) with DUOPA may be associated with orthostatic hypotension. Monitor patients who are taking these drugs.

7.2 Antihypertensive Drugs

The concurrent use of DUOPA with antihypertensive medications can cause symptomatic postural hypotension. A dose reduction of the antihypertensive medication may be needed after starting or increasing the dose of DUOPA.

7.3 Dopamine D2 Receptor Antagonists and Isoniazid

Dopamine D2 receptor antagonists (e.g., phenothiazines, butyrophenones, risperidone, metoclopramide, papaverine) and isoniazid may reduce the effectiveness of levodopa. Monitor patients for worsening Parkinson's symptoms.

7.4 Iron Salts

Iron salts or multi-vitamins containing iron salts can form chelates with levodopa, carbidopa, and can cause a reduction in the bioavailability of DUOPA. If iron salts or multi-vitamins containing iron salts are co-administered with DUOPA, monitor patients for worsening Parkinson's symptoms.

7.5 High-Protein Diet

Because levodopa competes with certain amino acids for transport across the gut wall, the absorption of levodopa may be decreased in patients on a high-protein diet. Advise patients that a high-protein diet may reduce the effectiveness of DUOPA.

8 USE IN SPECIFIC POPULATIONS

8.1 Pregnancy

Pregnancy Category C.

There are no adequate or well-controlled studies in pregnant women. It has been reported from individual cases that levodopa crosses the human placental barrier, enters the fetus, and is metabolized. In animal studies, carbidopa-levodopa has been shown to be developmentally toxic (including teratogenic effects) at clinically relevant doses. DUOPA should be used during pregnancy only if the potential benefit justifies the potential risk to the fetus.

When administered to pregnant rabbits throughout organogenesis, carbidopa-levodopa caused both visceral and skeletal malformations in fetuses at all doses and ratios of carbidopa-levodopa tested. No teratogenic effects were observed when carbidopa-levodopa was administered to pregnant mice throughout organogenesis.

There was a decrease in the number of live pups delivered by rats receiving carbidopa-levodopa during organogenesis.

8.3 Nursing Mothers

Carbidopa is excreted in rat milk. In a study of one nursing mother with Parkinson's disease, excretion of levodopa in human milk was reported. Caution should be exercised when DUOPA is administered to a nursing woman.

8.4 Pediatric Use

Safety and effectiveness in pediatric patients have not been established.

8.5 Geriatric Use

In the controlled clinical trial, 49% of patients were 65 years and older, and 8% were 75 years and older. In patients 65 years and older, there was an increased risk for elevation of BUN and CPK (above the upper limit of the normal reference range for these laboratory analytes) during treatment with DUOPA compared to the risk for patients less than 65 years.

10 OVERDOSAGE

Management of acute overdosage with DUOPA is the same as management of acute overdosage with levodopa. Pyridoxine is not effective in reversing the actions of oral immediate-release carbidopa-levodopa.

In the event of an overdosage with DUOPA, the infusion should be stopped and the pump disconnected immediately. Administer intravenous fluids and maintain an adequate airway. Patients should receive electrocardiographic monitoring for arrhythmias and hypotension.

11 DESCRIPTION

DUOPA is a combination of carbidopa, an inhibitor of aromatic amino acid decarboxylation, and levodopa, an aromatic amino acid.

Carbidopa is a white, crystalline compound, slightly soluble in water, with a molecular weight of 244.2. It is designated chemically as (2S)-3-(3,4-dihydroxyphenyl)-2-hydrazino-2-methylpropanoic acid monohydrate. Its empirical formula is $C_{10}H_{14}N_2O_4 \cdot H_2O$, and its structural formula is:

The content of carbidopa in DUOPA is expressed in terms of anhydrous carbidopa which has a molecular weight of 226.3. The 4.63 mg/mL of anhydrous carbidopa is equivalent to 5.0 mg/mL of carbidopa.

Levodopa is a white, crystalline compound, slightly soluble in water, with a molecular weight of 197.2. It is designated chemically as (2S)-2-Amino-3-(3,4-dihydroxyphenyl) propanoic acid. Its empirical formula is $C_9H_{11}NO_4$, and its structural formula is:

The inactive ingredients in DUOPA are carmellose sodium and purified water.

12 CLINICAL PHARMACOLOGY

12.1 Mechanism of Action

Carbidopa

When levodopa is administered orally, it is rapidly decarboxylated to dopamine in extracerebral tissues so that only a small portion of a given dose is transported unchanged to the central nervous system. Carbidopa inhibits the decarboxylation of peripheral levodopa, making more levodopa available for delivery to the brain.

Levodopa

Levodopa is the metabolic precursor of dopamine, does cross the blood-brain barrier, and presumably is converted to dopamine in the brain. This is thought to be the mechanism whereby levodopa treats the symptoms of Parkinson's disease.

12.2 Pharmacodynamics

Because its decarboxylase inhibiting activity is limited to extracerebral tissues, administration of carbidopa with levodopa makes more levodopa available to the brain. The addition of carbidopa to levodopa reduces the peripheral effects (e.g., nausea and vomiting) due to decarboxylation of levodopa; however, carbidopa does not decrease the adverse reactions due to the central effects of levodopa.

12.3 Pharmacokinetics

The pharmacokinetics of carbidopa and levodopa with 16-hour intrajejunal infusion of DUOPA was evaluated in 18 patients with advanced Parkinson's disease who had been on DUOPA therapy for 30 days or longer. Patients remained on their individualized DUOPA doses.

The plasma concentrations versus time profile for levodopa with DUOPA 16-hour intrajejunal infusion is presented in Figure 1.

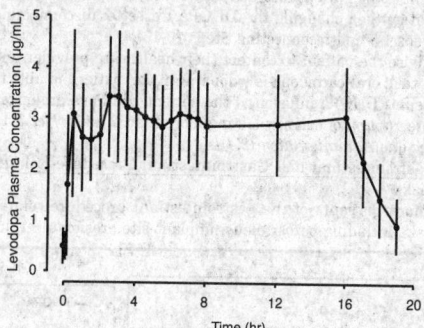

Figure 1. Plasma Concentrations (mean ± standard deviation) versus Time Profile of Levodopa with DUOPA (levodopa, 1580 ± 403 mg; carbidopa, 366 ± 92 mg) 16-Hour Infusion

Absorption and Bioavailability

Following initiation of the 16-hour intrajejunal infusion of DUOPA, peak plasma levels of levodopa is reached at 2.5 hours. The absorption of levodopa may be decreased in patients on a high-protein diet because levodopa competes with certain amino acids for transport across the gut wall. The gastric emptying rate does not influence the absorption of DUOPA since it is administered by continuous intestinal infusion. In a cross-study population pharmacokinetic analysis, DUOPA had comparable bioavailability to the oral immediate-release carbidopa-levodopa (25/100 mg) tablets (over-encapsulated tablets). The estimated bioavailability for levodopa from DUOPA relative to oral immediate-release carbidopa-levodopa tablets was 97% (95% confidence interval; 95% to 98%).

In the controlled clinical trial, the intra-subject variability in carbidopa and levodopa plasma concentrations were lower for patients treated with DUOPA (N=33, 25% and 21%, respectively) than in patients treated with oral immediate-release carbidopa-levodopa (25/100 mg) tablets (N=28, 39% and 67%, respectively).

Distribution

Carbidopa is approximately 36% bound to plasma proteins. Levodopa is approximately 10-30% bound to plasma proteins.

Metabolism and Elimination

Carbidopa

Carbidopa is metabolized to two main metabolites (α-methyl-3-methoxy-4-hydroxyphenylpropionic acid and α-methyl-3,4-dihydroxyphenylpropionic acid). These 2 metabolites are primarily eliminated in the urine unchanged or as glucuronide conjugates. Unchanged carbidopa accounts for 30% of the total urinary excretion. The elimination half-life of carbidopa is approximately 2 hours.

Levodopa

Levodopa is mainly eliminated via metabolism by the aromatic amino acid decarboxylase (AAAD) and the catechol-O-methyl-transferase (COMT) enzymes. Other routes of metabolism are transamination and oxidation. The decarboxylation of levodopa to dopamine by AAAD is the major enzymatic pathway when no enzyme inhibitor is co-administered. O-methylation of levodopa by COMT forms 3-O-methyldopa. When administered with carbidopa, the elimination half-life of levodopa is approximately 1.5 hours (see Figure 1).

Drug Interaction Studies

COMT Inhibitors

Systemic exposure of levodopa is expected to increase in the presence of entacapone.

13 NONCLINICAL TOXICOLOGY

13.1 Carcinogenesis, Mutagenesis, Impairment of Fertility

Carcinogenesis

In rat, oral administration of carbidopa-levodopa for two years resulted in no evidence of carcinogenicity. DUOPA contains hydrazine, a degradation product of carbidopa. In published studies, hydrazine has been demonstrated to be carcinogenic in multiple animal species. Increases in liver (adenoma, carcinoma) and lung (adenoma, adenocarcinoma) tumors have been reported with oral administration of hydrazine in mouse, rat, and hamster.

Mutagenesis

Carbidopa was positive in the *in vitro* Ames test, in the presence and absence of metabolic activation, and the *in vitro* mouse lymphoma *tk* assay in the absence of metabolic activation but was negative in the *in vivo* mouse micronucleus assay.

In published studies, hydrazine was reported to be positive in *in vitro* genotoxicity (Ames, chromosomal aberration in mammalian cells, and mouse lymphoma *tk*) assays and in the *in vivo* mouse micronucleus assay.

Impairment of Fertility

In reproduction studies, no effects on fertility were observed in rats receiving carbidopa -levodopa.

14 CLINICAL STUDIES

The efficacy of DUOPA was established in a randomized, double-blind, double-dummy, active-controlled, parallel group, 12-week study (Study 1) in patients with advanced Parkinson's disease who were levodopa-responsive and had persistent motor fluctuations while on treatment with oral immediate-release carbidopa-levodopa and other Parkinson's disease medications.

Patients were eligible for participation in the studies if they were experiencing 3 hours or more of "Off" time on their current Parkinson's disease drug treatment and they demonstrated a clear responsiveness to treatment with levodopa. Seventy-one (71) patients enrolled in the study and 66 patients completed the treatment (3 patients discontinued treatment because of adverse reactions, 1 patient for lack of effect, and 1 patient for non-compliance).

Continued on next page

Information on the AbbVie, Inc. products listed on these pages is from the prescribing information in use as of July 31, 2016. For more information, please visit rxabbvie.com or call 1-800-633-9110.

Patients enrolled in this study had a mean age of 64 years and disease duration of 11 years. Most patients (89%) were taking at least one concomitant medication for Parkinson's disease (e.g., dopaminergic agonist, COMT-inhibitor, MAO-B inhibitor) in addition to oral immediate-release carbidopa-levodopa. Thirty nine percent of patients were taking two or more of such concomitant medications.

Patients were randomized to either DUOPA and placebo capsules or placebo suspension and oral immediate-release carbidopa-levodopa 25/100 mg capsules. Patients in both treatment arms had a PEG-J device placement. DUOPA or placebo-suspension was infused over 16 hours daily through a PEG-J tube via the CADD®-Legacy 1400 model ambulatory infusion pump. The mean daily levodopa dose was 1117 mg/day in the DUOPA group and 1351 mg/day in the oral immediate-release carbidopa-levodopa group.

The clinical outcome measure in Study 1 was the mean change from baseline to Week 12 in the total daily mean "Off" time, based on a Parkinson's disease diary. The "Off" time was normalized to a 16-hour awake period, based on a typical person's waking day and the daily infusion duration of 16 hours. The mean score decrease (i.e., improvement) in "Off" time from baseline to Week 12 for DUOPA was significantly greater (p=0.0015) than for oral immediate-release carbidopa-levodopa. Additionally, the mean score increase (i.e., improvement) in "On" time without troublesome dyskinesia from baseline to Week 12 was significantly greater (p=0.0059) for DUOPA than for oral immediate-release carbidopa-levodopa. The treatment difference (DUOPA – oral immediate release carbidopa-levodopa) for decrease in "Off" time was approximately 1.9 hours and the treatment difference for the increase in "On" time without troublesome dyskinesia was approximately 1.9 hours. Results of Study 1 are shown in Table 4.

Table 4. Change from Baseline to Week 12 in "Off" Time and in "On" Time Without Troublesome Dyskinesia in Patients with Advanced Parkinson's Disease

Treatment Group	Baseline (hours)	LS Mean Change from Baseline at Week 12 (hours)
"Off" time		
Oral immediate-release carbidopa-levodopa	6.9	-2.1
DUOPA	6.3	-4.0*
"On" time without troublesome dyskinesia		
Oral immediate-release carbidopa-levodopa	8.0	2.2
DUOPA	8.7	4.1*

LS Mean Change from Baseline based on Analysis of Covariance (ANCOVA).
*=Statistically Significant.

Figure 2 shows results over time according to treatment for the efficacy variable (change from baseline in "Off" time) that served as the clinical outcome measure at the end of the trial at 12 weeks.
[See Figure 2 below]

16 HOW SUPPLIED/STORAGE AND HANDLING

16.1 How Supplied

Single-use cassettes containing 4.63 mg carbidopa (as 5 mg of the monohydrate) and 20 mg levodopa per mL of enteral suspension. Each cassette contains approximately 100 mL of suspension.

Carton of 7 DUOPA cassettes: NDC 0074-3012-07

16.2 Storage and Handling

Store in freezer at -20°C (-4°F). Thaw in refrigerator at 2°C to 8°C (36°F to 46°F) prior to dispensing. Cassettes should be protected from light and kept in the carton prior to use.

Thawing instructions for pharmacies
• Assign a 12 week "Use By" date based on the time the cartons are put into the refrigerator to thaw.
• Fully thaw DUOPA in the refrigerator prior to dispensing.
• In order to ensure controlled thawing of DUOPA, take the cartons containing the seven individual cassettes out of the transport box and separate the cartons from each other.
• Thawing may take up to 96 hours when the cartons are taken out of the transport box.
• Once the product has thawed, the individual cartons may be packed in a closer configuration within the refrigerator.

17 PATIENT COUNSELING INFORMATION

Advise the patient to read the FDA-approved patient labeling (Medication Guide and Instructions for Use).

Administration Information
Ask patients if they have had any previous surgery in the upper part of their abdomen that may lead to difficulty in performing the gastrostomy or jejunostomy [see Dosage and Administration (2.3)].
Advise patients that foods that are high in protein may reduce the effectiveness of DUOPA [see Drug Interactions (7.5) and Clinical Pharmacology (12.3)].

Interruption of DUOPA Infusion
If the patient anticipates disconnecting the pump for a short period of time (less than 2 hours such as to swim, shower, or short medical procedure), no supplemental oral medication is needed, but the patient may be advised to take an extra-dose of DUOPA before disconnecting. Instruct the patient to stop the continuous rate, turn off the pump, clamp the cassette tube, disconnect the tubing, and replace the red cap on the cassette tube. The DUOPA cassette can remain attached to the pump until the tubing is reconnected. Refer the patient to the Patient Instructions for Use for additional information (i.e., changing the DUOPA Cassette: disconnecting Steps 1-5 and reconnecting Steps 10-16).
Advise the patient to contact their healthcare provider and to take oral carbidopa-levodopa until the patient is able to resume DUOPA infusion, if the patient will have prolonged interruption of therapy lasting more than 2 hours [see Dosage and Administration (2.4)].

Gastrointestinal and Gastrointestinal Procedure-Related Risks
Inform patients of the gastrointestinal procedure-related risks including bezoar, ileus, implant site erosion/ulcer, intestinal hemorrhage, intestinal ischemia, intestinal obstruction, intestinal perforation, pancreatitis, peritonitis, pneumoperitoneum, post-operative wound infection and sepsis. Advise patients of the symptoms of the above listed complications and instruct them to contact their healthcare provider if they experience any of these symptoms [see Warnings and Precautions (5.1)].

Falling Asleep during Activities of Daily Living and Somnolence
Alert patients to the potential sedating effects caused by DUOPA, including somnolence and the possibility of falling asleep while engaged in activities of daily living. Because somnolence is a common adverse reaction with potentially serious consequences, patients should not drive a car, operate machinery, or engage in other potentially dangerous activities until they have gained sufficient experience with DUOPA to gauge whether or not it affects their mental and/or motor performance adversely. Advise patients that if increased somnolence or episodes of falling asleep during activities of daily living (e.g., conversations, eating, driving a motor vehicle, etc.) are experienced at any time during treatment, they should not drive or participate in potentially dangerous activities until they have contacted their physician.
Advise patients of possible additive effects when patients are taking other sedating medications, alcohol, or other central nervous system depressants (e.g., benzodiazepines, antipsychotics, antidepressants, etc.) in combination with DUOPA or when taking a concomitant medication that increases plasma levels of levodopa [see Warnings and Precautions (5.2)].

Orthostatic Hypotension
Advise patients that they may experience syncope and may develop hypotension with or without symptoms such as dizziness, nausea, syncope, and sometimes sweating while taking DUOPA. Accordingly, caution patients against standing rapidly after sitting or lying down, especially if they have been doing so for prolonged periods and especially at the initiation of treatment with DUOPA [see Warnings and Precautions (5.3)].

Hallucinations/Psychosis/Confusion
Inform patients that they may experience hallucinations (unreal visions, sounds, or sensations) and other symptoms of psychosis can occur while taking DUOPA. Tell patients to report hallucinations, abnormal thinking, psychotic behavior or confusion to their healthcare provider promptly should they develop [see Warnings and Precautions (5.4)].

Impulse Control/Compulsive Behaviors
Advise patients that they may experience impulse control and/or compulsive behaviors while taking DUOPA. Advise patients to inform their physician or healthcare provider if they develop new or increased gambling urges, sexual urges, uncontrolled spending, binge or compulsive eating, or other urges while being treated with DUOPA [see Warnings and Precautions (5.5)].

Depression and Suicidality
Inform patients that they may develop depression or experience worsening of depression while taking DUOPA. Instruct patients to contact their healthcare provider if they experience depression, worsening of depression, or suicidal thoughts [see Warnings and Precautions (5.6)].

Withdrawal-Emergent Hyperpyrexia and Confusion
Advise patients to contact their healthcare provider before stopping DUOPA. Tell patients to inform their healthcare provider if they develop withdrawal symptoms such as fever, confusion, or severe muscle stiffness [see Warnings and Precautions (5.7)].

Dyskinesia
Inform patients that DUOPA may cause or exacerbate pre-existing dyskinesias [see Warnings and Precautions (5.8)].

Neuropathy
Inform patients that neuropathy may develop or they may experience worsening neuropathy on DUOPA, and to contact their healthcare provider if they develop any symptoms or features suggesting neuropathy [see Warnings and Precautions (5.9)].

Melanoma
Advise patients with Parkinson's disease that they have a higher risk of developing melanoma. Advise patients to have their skin examined on a regular basis by a qualified healthcare provider (e.g., dermatologist) when using DUOPA [see Warnings and Precautions (5.11)].

Nursing Mothers
Because of the possibility that carbidopa or levodopa may be excreted in human milk, a decision should be made whether

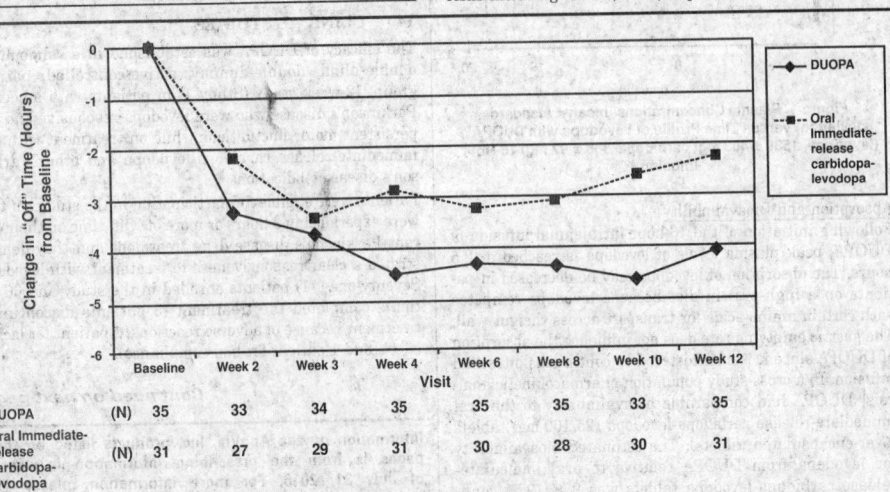

		Baseline	Week 2	Week 3	Week 4	Week 6	Week 8	Week 10	Week 12
DUOPA	(N)	35	33	34	35	35	35	33	35
Oral Immediate-release carbidopa-levodopa	(N)	31	27	29	31	30	28	30	31

Figure 2. Change in "Off" Time Over 12 Weeks.

to discontinue nursing or to discontinue the drug, taking into account the importance of the drug to the mother [see Use in Specific Populations (8.3)].
Manufactured by AbbVie Inc., North Chicago, IL 60064, USA
or by Fresenius Kabi Norge AS, 1788 Halden, Norway
For AbbVie Inc.
North Chicago, IL 60064, USA
03-B152 February 2016

MEDICATION GUIDE
DUOPA (Do-oh-pa)
(carbidopa and levodopa) enteral suspension
Read this Medication Guide before you start using DUOPA and each time you get a refill. There may be new information. This information does not take the place of talking to your healthcare provider about your medical condition or treatment.

What is the most important information I should know about DUOPA?
DUOPA can cause serious side effects, including:
- **Stomach and intestine (gastrointestinal) problems and problems from the procedure you will need to have to receive DUOPA (gastrointestinal procedure-related problems).**
  Some of these problems may require surgery and may lead to death.
  ○ a blockage of your stomach or intestines (bezoar)
  ○ stopping movement through intestines (ileus)
  ○ drainage, redness, swelling, pain, feeling of warmth around the small hole in your stomach wall (stoma)
  ○ bleeding from stomach ulcers or your intestines
  ○ inflammation of your pancreas (pancreatitis)
  ○ air or gas in your abdominal cavity
  ○ skin infection around the intestinal tube, infection in your blood or abdominal cavity may occur, after surgery
  ○ stomach pain, nausea or vomiting
- **Tell your healthcare provider right away if you have any of the following symptoms of stomach and intestine problems and gastrointestinal procedure-related problems:**
  ○ stomach (abdominal) pain
  ○ constipation that does not go away
  ○ nausea or vomiting
  ○ fever
  ○ blood in your stool or a dark tarry stool (melanotic stool)
You will need to have a procedure to make a small hole (called a "stoma") in your stomach wall to place a gastrojejunostomy tube (called a PEG-J tube) in an area of your small intestine called the jejunum. DUOPA is delivered directly to your small intestine through this tube. Your healthcare provider will talk to you about the stoma procedure. Before the stoma procedure, tell your healthcare provider if you have ever had a surgery or problems with your stomach.
Talk to your healthcare provider about what you need to do to care for your stoma. After the procedure, you and your healthcare provider will need to regularly check the stoma for any signs of infection.
If your PEG-J tube becomes kinked, knotted, or blocked this may cause you to have worsening of your Parkinson's symptoms or recurring movement problems (motor fluctuations). Call your healthcare provider if your Parkinson's symptoms get worse or you have slow movement while you are treated with DUOPA.

What is DUOPA?
DUOPA is a prescription medicine used for treatment of advanced Parkinson's disease. DUOPA contains 2 medicines, carbidopa and levodopa.
DUOPA should not be given to children (younger than 18 years).

Who should not use DUOPA?
Do not use DUOPA if you:
- take a medicine called a nonselective Monoamine Oxidase (MAO) Inhibitor (such as phenelzine or tranylcypromine) or have taken a nonselective MAO Inhibitor within the last 14 days.
Ask your healthcare provider or pharmacist if you are not sure if you take an MAO Inhibitor.

What should I tell my healthcare provider before using DUOPA?
Before you use DUOPA, tell your healthcare provider if you:
- have or have had stomach ulcers or stomach surgery
- have low blood pressure (hypotension) or if you feel dizzy or faint, especially when getting up from sitting or lying down
- have had problems with fainting (syncope)
- feel sleepy or have fallen asleep suddenly during the day

- have or have had depression (feelings of hopelessness or sadness) or any mental problems
- drink alcohol. Alcohol can increase the chance that DUOPA will make you feel sleepy or fall asleep when you should be awake
- have trouble controlling your muscles (dyskinesia)
- have nerve problems (peripheral neuropathy)
- have or have had heart problems, an abnormal heart rate or have had a heart attack in the past
- have or have had a type of skin cancer called melanoma
- have or have had high blood pressure (hypertension)
- have eye problems that cause increased pressure in your eye (glaucoma)
- have a history of attacks of suddenly falling asleep without warning
- have any other medical conditions
- are pregnant or planning to become pregnant. It is not known if DUOPA will harm your unborn baby
- are breastfeeding or plan to breastfeed. DUOPA can pass into your milk and may harm your baby. Talk to your healthcare provider about the best way to feed your baby if you take DUOPA

Tell your healthcare provider about all the medicines you take, including prescription and over-the-counter medicines, vitamins, herbal supplements.
Using DUOPA with certain other medicines may affect each other and cause serious side effects.
Especially tell your healthcare provider if you take:
- medicines used to treat high blood pressure (hypertension)
- medicines used to treat depression called nonselective Monoamine Oxidase (MAO) Inhibitor (such as phenelzine or tranylcypromine) or have taken one within the last 14 days
- dopamine D2 receptor antagonists (antipsychotics or metoclopramide), and isoniazid
- iron or multivitamins with iron
Eating high protein foods may affect how DUOPA works. Tell your healthcare provider if you change your diet.
Ask your healthcare provider or pharmacist for a list of these medicines or foods if you are not sure.
Know the medicines you take. Keep a list of them to show your healthcare provider and pharmacist when you get a new medicine.

How should I use DUOPA?
- Use DUOPA exactly as your healthcare provider tells you to use it.
- Your healthcare provider should show you how to use DUOPA before you use it for the first time. Ask your healthcare provider or pharmacist if you have any questions.
- Your prescribed dose of DUOPA will be programmed into your pump by a healthcare provider and should only be changed by your healthcare provider or while you are with your healthcare provider.
- **Do not** stop using DUOPA or change your dose unless you are told to do so by your healthcare provider. Tell your healthcare provider if you develop withdrawal symptoms such as fever, confusion, or severe muscle stiffness.
- Keep a supply of oral carbidopa-levodopa immediate release (IR) tablets with you in case you are unable to give your DUOPA infusion.
- DUOPA is given continuously over 16 hours through a tube that is put into your stomach called a PEG-J. A small pump (CADD-Legacy 1400) is used to move DUOPA from the medication cassette through your PEG-J tube.
- Your DUOPA dose has three parts:
  ○ a morning dose
  ○ a continuous dose
  ○ extra doses
- DUOPA can also be given for a short time (short-term) through a tube put into your nose called a naso-jejunal (NJ) tube.
- The CADD-Legacy 1400 portable infusion pump should be used to give DUOPA through your PEG-J tube. See the Instructions for Use that comes with your CADD-Legacy 1400 portable infusion pump for complete instructions on how to use the pump.
- DUOPA comes in a small plastic container (cassette) that you connect to the pump to get your medicine.
  ○ Each cassette can only be used **1** time. An opened cassette should not be reused.
  ○ The cassette should not be used for longer than **16** hours.
  ○ The cassette should be thrown away at the end of the infusion, even if there is some medicine still in the cassette.
- Disconnect the pump from your PEG-J tube after the **16** hour dosing time is finished. Use a syringe filled with room temperature water to flush your PEG-J tube. See the "Instructions for Use" for more information about how to flush your PEG-J tube with a syringe.

- After your daily DUOPA infusion, you should take your usual night-time dose of oral carbidopa-levodopa tablets as prescribed.
- If you stop your DUOPA infusion for more than 2 hours during your **16** hour dosing time for any reason, call your healthcare provider and take oral carbidopa-levodopa as prescribed until you are able to restart your DUOPA infusion.
- If you stop your DUOPA infusion for less than 2 hours, you do not need to take oral carbidopa-levodopa, but your healthcare provider may tell you to take an extra dose of DUOPA.

What should I avoid while using DUOPA?
- **Do not** drive, operate machinery, or do other activities until you know how DUOPA affects you. Sleepiness and falling asleep suddenly caused by DUOPA can happen as late as 1 year after you start your treatment.

What are the possible side effects of DUOPA?
DUOPA may cause serious side effects, including:
- See "What is the most important information I should know about DUOPA?"
- **Falling asleep during normal daily activities.** DUOPA may cause you to fall asleep while you are doing daily activities such as driving, talking with other people, or eating.
  ○ You could fall asleep without any warning.
  ○ Some people using DUOPA have had car accidents because they fell asleep while driving.
  Do not drive or operate machinery until you are sure how DUOPA affects you.
  Tell your healthcare provider if you take other medicines that can make you sleepy such as sleep medicines, antidepressants, or antipsychotics.
- **Low blood pressure when you sit or stand up quickly.** After you have been sitting or lying down, stand up slowly until you know how DUOPA affects you. This may help reduce the following symptoms while you are using DUOPA:
  ○ dizziness
  ○ nausea
  ○ sweating
  ○ fainting
- **Seeing things that are not there, hearing sounds or feeling sensations that are not real (hallucinations).** Hallucinations can happen in people who use DUOPA. Tell your healthcare provider if you have hallucinations.
- **Unusual urges.** Some people taking certain medicines to treat Parkinson's disease, including DUOPA, have reported problems, such as gambling, compulsive eating, compulsive shopping, and increased sex drive.
  If you or your family members notice that you are having unusual urges or behaviors, talk to your healthcare provider.
- **Depression and suicide.** DUOPA can cause depression or make your depression worse. Pay close attention to sudden changes in your mood, behavior, thoughts, or feelings. Call your healthcare provider right away if you feel depressed or have thoughts of suicide.
- **Uncontrolled sudden movements (dyskinesia).** If you have new dyskinesia, or your dyskinesia gets worse, tell your healthcare provider. This may be a sign that your dose of DUOPA or other medicines to control your Parkinson's disease may need to be adjusted.
- **Progressive weakness or numbness or loss of sensation in the fingers or feet (neuropathy).**
- **Heart attack or other heart problems. Tell your healthcare provider if you have experienced increased blood pressure, a fast or irregular heartbeat or chest pain.**
- **Skin cancer (melanoma).** Parkinson's disease may be associated with a higher chance of having melanoma than people who do not have Parkinson's disease. It is not known if the chance of having melanoma is higher because of the medicines used to treat Parkinson's disease, like DUOPA, or from the Parkinson's disease. People who use DUOPA should have their skin checked regularly for melanoma by a qualified healthcare professional.
- **Abnormal blood tests.** DUOPA may cause changes in certain blood tests, especially certain hormone and kidney function blood tests.

Continued on next page

Information on the AbbVie, Inc. products listed on these pages is from the prescribing information in use as of July 31, 2016. For more information, please visit rxabbvie.com or call 1-800-633-9110.

- **Worsening of the increased pressure in your eyes (glaucoma).** The pressure in your eyes should be checked after starting DUOPA.
- **The most common side effects of DUOPA include:**
  - swelling of legs and feet
  - nausea
  - high blood pressure (hypertension)
  - depression
  - mouth and throat pain

Call your healthcare provider or get medical care right away if you have any of the above symptoms. Your healthcare provider will tell you if you should stop treatment with DUOPA and if needed, tell you how to discontinue DUOPA.

Tell your healthcare provider if you have any side effect that bothers you or does not go away.

These are not all of the possible side effects of DUOPA. For more information, ask your healthcare provider or pharmacist.

Call your doctor for medical advice about side effects. You may report side effects to FDA at 1-800-FDA-1088.

How should I store DUOPA?
- Store DUOPA in the refrigerator between 36°F to 46°F (2°C to 8°C). Do not freeze.
- Use at room temperature. Take one DUOPA cassette out of the carton and out of the refrigerator 20 minutes prior to use. Use the product at room temperature or you may not get the right amount of medication.
- Protect the cassette from light and keep it in the carton before using.
- Use DUOPA before the expiration date printed on the cassette.

Keep DUOPA and all medicines out of the reach of children.

General information about the safe and effective use of DUOPA.

Medicines are sometimes prescribed for purposes other than those listed in a Medication Guide. Do not use DUOPA for a condition for which it was not prescribed. Do not give DUOPA to other people, even if they have the same symptoms that you have. It may harm them.

This Medication Guide summarizes the most important information about DUOPA. If you would like more information, talk with your healthcare provider. You can ask your healthcare provider or pharmacist for information about DUOPA that was written for healthcare professionals.

For more information go to www.DUOPA.com or call 1-844-386-4968.

What are the ingredients in DUOPA?

Active ingredients: carbidopa and levodopa

Inactive ingredients: carmellose sodium and purified water

This Medication Guide has been approved by the U.S. Food and Drug Administration.

Manufactured by AbbVie Inc., North Chicago, IL 60064, USA or by Fresenius Kabi Norge AS, 1788 Halden, Norway

For AbbVie Inc.
North Chicago, IL 60064, USA
03-B152 Revised: February 2016

INSTRUCTIONS FOR USE

[See Figure A at top of next page]
[See Figure at top of page 652]

WARNINGS and CAUTIONS

Failure to follow the Warnings and Cautions below could cause return of your symptoms, damage to the pump, serious injury, or may lead to death in rare cases.

WARNINGS
- Only use the pump in a manner described in this Instructions for Use, after you have received training by your healthcare provider.
- To avoid explosion hazard, **do not** use the pump near flammable explosive gases.
- Only use extension sets that are approved for use with DUOPA (See the Full Prescribing Information for DUOPA), pay attention to all warnings and cautions associated with their use.
- Always have new batteries available for replacement. If power is lost, DUOPA will not be delivered.

- If the pump is dropped or hit, the battery door or tabs may break. **Do not** use the pump if the battery door or tabs are damaged because the batteries will not be correctly secured. This may cause loss of power and DUOPA will not be delivered.
- If the pump is dropped or hit, look at the pump for damage. **Do not** use a pump that is damaged or is not functioning correctly.
- If a gap is present between the battery door and the pump housing, this means the door is not correctly latched. If the battery door becomes detached or loose, the batteries will not be correctly secured. This could cause loss of power and DUOPA will not be delivered.
- Use only DUOPA cassettes for pump accuracy and to make sure the pump works correctly. Attach the DUOPA cassette correctly. A detached or incorrectly attached DUOPA cassette could cause a problem with getting your DUOPA.

CAUTIONS
- Use only Smiths Medical accessories and replacement parts for the pump as using other brands may adversely affect the operation of the pump.
- **Do not** operate the pump at temperatures below 36°F (2°C) or above 104°F (40°C).
- **Do not** store the pump at temperatures below -4°F (-20°C) or above 140°F (60°C). **Do not** store the pump with a DUOPA cassette attached. Use the protective cassette provided when storing the pump.
- **Do not** keep the pump in humidity levels below 20% or above 90% relative humidity.
- **Do not** place the pump in cleaning fluid or water, or allow solution to soak into the pump, keypad, or battery compartment.
- **Do not** clean the pump with acetone, other plastic solvents, or abrasive cleaners.
- **Do not** use rechargeable NiCd or nickel metal hydride (NiMH) batteries. **Do not** use carbon zinc (heavy duty) batteries. They do not provide enough power for the pump to operate correctly.
- **Do not** store the pump for long periods of time with the batteries installed. Battery leakage could damage the pump.

Morning Procedure

- **Take the DUOPA carton containing the DUOPA cassettes out of the refrigerator. Check the expiration date on the carton. Do not use any of the cassettes if the expiration date has passed.**
- **Take a DUOPA cassette out of the carton.** Return the carton with the remaining cassettes to the refrigerator. **Do not** use the cassette if the expiration date has passed or the cassette is damaged or empty. **Leave the DUOPA cassette at room temperature for 20 minutes before using.**
- Each DUOPA cassette may be used for up to **16** hours after removal from the refrigerator.

WARNING: Use only DUOPA cassettes to make sure the pump works correctly.

1) Remove the cassette clip (see Figure B):

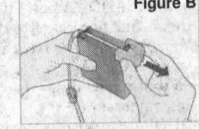

Figure B

- Remove the cassette tube from its slot in the clip.
- Pull the clip from cassette to slide it off of the cassette top.

2) Attach the DUOPA cassette to the pump (see Figure C):

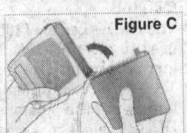

Figure C

- Hold the pump so the latch faces up.
- Hold the DUOPA cassette so the tube points down.
- Insert the DUOPA cassette hooks into the hinge pins at the base of the pump.

3) Latch the DUOPA cassette into the pump:

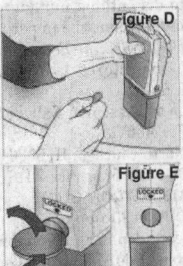

Figure D

- Hold the pump and DUOPA cassette upright against a flat surface.
- Press down on the pump, until the DUOPA cassette fits tightly against the pump (see Figure D).

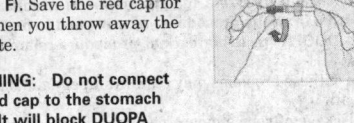

Figure E

- Use a coin to twist the latch counterclockwise until the latch lines up straight with the arrow (see Figure E).

WARNING: Attach the DUOPA cassette correctly. A detached or incorrectly attached cassette could cause a problem with getting your DUOPA.

4) Remove the red cap on the end of the cassette tube (see Figure F). Save the red cap for use when you throw away the cassette.

Figure F

WARNING: Do not connect the red cap to the stomach tube. It will block DUOPA flow.

5) Connect the stomach tube to the cassette tube:

Figure G

- While holding the stomach tube steady, twist off the white cap on the end of the longer colored connector (see Figure G). **WARNING: Do not twist the stomach tube.**

Figure H

- Connect the cassette tube to the end of the longer colored connector (see Figure H). Do not connect to the shorter white connector.

6) Turn the pump on:
- Press and hold

ON/OFF

until the display turns on.
- Wait approximately **30** seconds for the pump to review settings.
- Check for

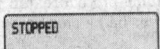

STOPPED

on the screen.

PUMP STATUS: The pump is now on but not yet delivering DUOPA.

7) Inspect the tubing for kinks or closed clamps. If needed straighten kinks or open clamps (see Figure I).

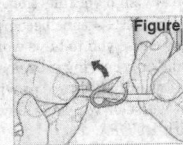

Figure I

8) Start the pump:
- Press and hold

STOP/START

until **3** dashes appear and then disappear from the screen.
- Wait approximately **15** seconds for the pump to start running.
- Check for

RUN

on the display.

PUMP STATUS: The pump is now running. DUOPA delivery will begin as programmed by your healthcare provider. If the pump will not start, a message should appear on the display. Refer to the **Alarms and Messages** section.

It will take between 10 minutes and 30 minutes to deliver your morning dose. To start delivery of your Morning Dose you will need to press the Morning Dose key 2 times.

NOTE: If you are unable to deliver your Morning Dose, it may be too soon since the last Morning Dose to deliver another dose. You may need to wait longer. The time between Morning Doses is decided by your healthcare provider.

9) The first key press shows the Morning Dose on the display.
• Press

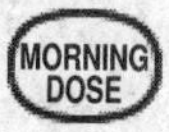

• Check for

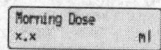

on the display. The number on your display is the Morning Dose of DUOPA your healthcare provider prescribed for you.

10) The second key press starts Morning Dose delivery.
• Press

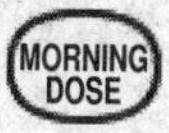

a second time to deliver the Morning Dose.

• The display

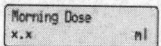

shows a countdown of your Morning Dose.

PUMP STATUS: After the Morning Dose finishes, the pump will automatically begin delivering the Continuous Rate. **RUN** will appear on the display. This completes DUOPA delivery for your Morning Procedure.

11) Insert pump into the carrying bag (see Figure J).
• Other carrying cases are also available. Refer to the specific Instructions for Use, which accompanies your carrying case.

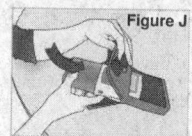
Figure J

12) Wear the bag over your shoulder or neck:

• Place the bag strap over your shoulder or neck (see **Figure K**).
• Make sure the pump is in correct position (see **Figure L**).

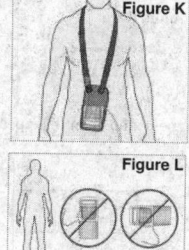
Figure K

Figure L

DUOPA
(carbidopa and levodopa) enteral suspension
These instructions are for use along with any other instructions your healthcare provider gives you.
Please read the Medication Guide before you start using DUOPA and each time you get a refill.
For questions or problems, call DUOPA support toll free at **1-844-386-4968**.

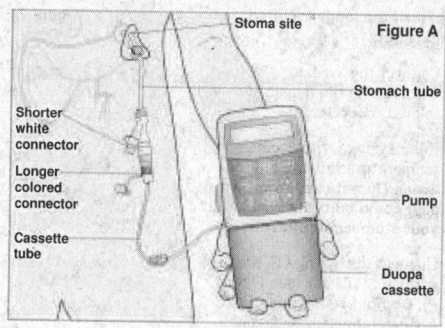
Figure A — Stoma site, Stomach tube, Shorter white connector, Longer colored connector, Cassette tube, Pump, Duopa cassette

The CADD-Legacy® 1400 pump is used for delivery of DUOPA through a tube into your stomach attached to the longer colored connector. Enteral nutrition should only be given by the shorter white connector (see **Figure A**).
This Instructions for Use provides information for the CADD-Legacy® model 1400 pump only. There are other CADD-Legacy® pump models available. Read the label on the back of the pump to make sure it is a model 1400 pump. Your healthcare provider prescribed DUOPA for you. Your healthcare provider programs your prescription into the CADD-Legacy® 1400 pump. The CADD-Legacy® 1400 pump is approved for use with DUOPA. DUOPA is provided as medication inside cassettes that connect to the CADD-Legacy®1400 pump.
The pump delivers DUOPA in **3** ways:
• Continuous Rate: Steady delivery of DUOPA delivered throughout the day while pump is on
• Morning Dose: A large dose of DUOPA given each morning
• Extra Dose: A small dose of DUOPA given as needed during the day
You will need the following items to complete these steps:
• Pump
• DUOPA cassette
• Coin, like a quarter
• Carrying bag
• Syringe
• Syringe connector
• Room temperature water

Extra Dose

1) Give an Extra Dose of DUOPA:
NOTE: If you are unable to deliver the Extra Dose, it may be too soon since the last Extra Dose to deliver another and you may need to wait longer. The time between Extra Doses and the amount of DUOPA in the Extra Dose is decided by your healthcare provider.
• Check for

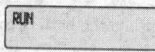

on the display.
• Press

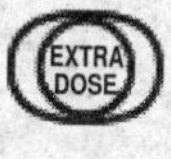

• Listen for **2** beeps.
• The display will show

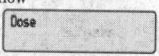

PUMP STATUS: The pump is now delivering the Extra Dose. When it finishes, **RUN** will appear on the display and the Continuous Rate will continue to run.

For instructions on changing a DUOPA cassette, see **Changing the Cassette.**

Evening Procedure

You will need:
• 1 Syringe
• 1 Syringe connector
• Room temperature water
• 1 Coin, like a quarter

1) Remove the pump from the carrying bag (see Figure M).

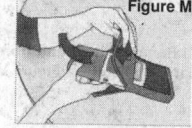
Figure M

2) Stop the Continuous Rate:
• Press and **hold**

until **3** dashes appear and then disappear from the display.
• Check for

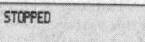

on the display.

3) Turn the pump off:
• Press and **hold**

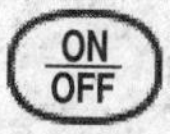

until **3** sets of dots appear and then disappear from the display and the display turns off.
• Check that the display is off.

4) Clamp the cassette tube (see Figure N).

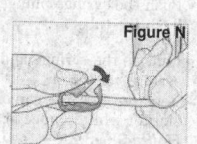
Figure N

5) Disconnect the tubing:
• Twist the cassette tube to disconnect it from the longer colored connector (see **Figure O**). **WARNING:** Do not twist the stomach tube.
• Replace the red cap on the cassette tube.

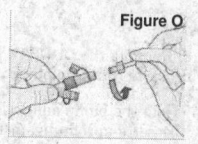
Figure O

Continued on next page

Information on the AbbVie, Inc. products listed on these pages is from the prescribing information in use as of July 31, 2016. For more information, please visit rxabbvie.com or call 1-800-633-9110.

6) Flush the longer colored connector:

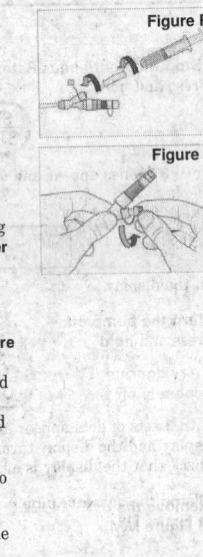

- Connect the syringe connector to the longer colored connector.

- Fill a syringe with room temperature tap or drinking water. **Do not use hot water as it could burn the wall of your stomach or intestine.**

- Connect the syringe to the syringe connector **(see Figure P)**. **Do not** over-tighten the syringe connector or it could break. **Do not** use the syringe connector if it is cracked or broken.

- Push the syringe plunger to flush the tube. **Do not** force the syringe if flushing the tube is difficult. Call your healthcare provider if you are unable or have difficulty flushing your tube.

- Remove the syringe and the syringe connector.

- Replace the white cap on the longer colored connector **(see Figure Q)**.

7) Flush the shorter white connector:

- Twist the white cap off the shorter white connector.

- Connect the syringe connector to the shorter white connector.

- Fill a syringe with room temperature tap or drinking water. **Do not use hot water as it could burn the wall of your stomach or intestine.**

- Connect the syringe to the syringe connector **(see Figure R)**. **Do not** over-tighten the syringe connector or it could break. **Do not** use the syringe connector if cracked or broken.

- Push the syringe plunger to flush the tube.

- Remove the syringe and the syringe connector. Replace the white cap on the shorter white connector **(see Figure S)**.

8) Remove the DUOPA cassette from the pump:

- Hold the pump and DUOPA cassette upright against a flat surface **(see Figure T)**.

- Use a coin to twist the latch clockwise until the latch pops out **(see Figure U)**.

- Remove the DUOPA cassette from the pump.

CADD-Legacy®-1400 Pump

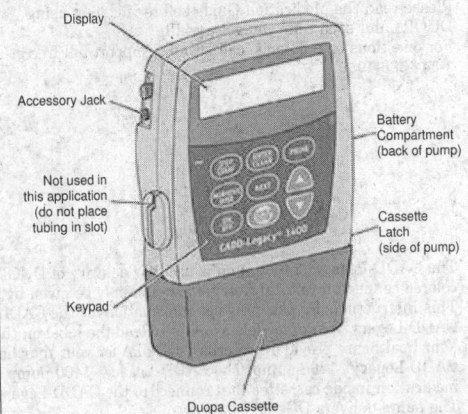

CADD-Legacy • 1400 Pump

- Display
- Accessory Jack
- Not used in this application (do not place tubing in slot)
- Keypad
- Battery Compartment (back of pump)
- Cassette Latch (side of pump)
- Duopa Cassette

Display
The display shows programming information and messages. The main screen, which the pump displays most of the time, shows the following:

When running:
Status of pump — RUN

Battery Status (for example, LowBat appears when battery power becomes low)

When stopped:
Status of pump — STOPPED

DUOPA Cassette
The single-use DUOPA cassette is for use with the CADD-Legacy® 1400 pump.
Battery Compartment
Two **AA** batteries fit into the battery compartment.
Cassette Latch
The cassette latch secures the DUOPA cassette to the pump.

Changing the DUOPA Cassette

- **Take the DUOPA carton containing the DUOPA cassette out of the refrigerator. Check the expiration date on the carton. Do not use any of the cassettes if the expiration date has passed.**

- **Take a DUOPA cassette out of the carton.** Return the carton with the remaining cassettes to the refrigerator. **Do not** use the cassette if the expiration date has passed or the cassette is damaged or empty. **Leave the DUOPA cassette at room temperature for 20 minutes before using.**

- Each DUOPA cassette may be used for up to **16** hours after removal from the refrigerator.
WARNING: Use only DUOPA cassettes to make sure the pump works correctly.

1) Remove the pump from the carrying bag (see Figure V).

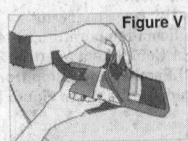

Description of the Keys

- (STOP START) Used to start and stop the pump. Also used to silence alarms.

- (ENTER CLEAR) Used to save new values when programming.

- (PRIME) Used to fill the tubing with Duopa.

   NOTE: *The PRIME key is intended for use **only** by healthcare providers.*

- (MORNING DOSE) Used to deliver the **Morning Dose.**

- (NEXT) Used to advance from one screen to the next. Also used to silence alarms.

- (▲) Used to increase a value.

- (▼) Used to decrease a value.

- (ON OFF) Used to put the pump into a low power state when not in use or back into full power.

- (EXTRA DOSE) Used to deliver extra doses of Duopa, if allowed.

2) Stop the Continuous Rate:
- Press and hold

until **3** dashes appear and then disappear from the display.

- Check for

STOPPED

on the display.

3) Turn the pump off:
- Press and hold

until **3** sets of dots appear and then disappear from the display and the display turns off.

- Check that the display is off.

4) Clamp the cassette tube (see Figure W).

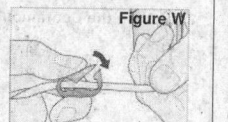

Figure W

5) Disconnect the tubing:

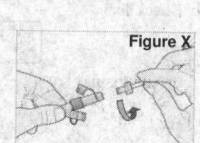

Figure X

• Twist the cassette tube to disconnect it from the longer colored connector **(see Figure X). WARNING: Do not twist the stomach tube.**

• Replace the red cap on the cassette tube.

6) Remove the DUOPA cassette from the pump:

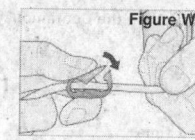

Figure Y

• Hold the pump and DUOPA cassette upright against a flat surface **(see Figure Y).**

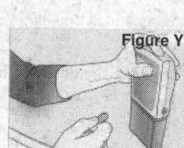

Figure Z

• Use a coin to twist the latch clockwise until the latch pops out **(see Figure Z).**

• Remove the DUOPA cassette from the pump.

7) Remove the cassette clip on the new DUOPA cassette (see Figure AA):

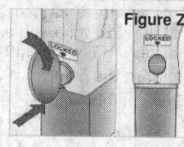

Figure AA

• Remove the cassette tube from its secured slot in the clip.

• Pull the clip from the cassette to slide it off of the cassette top.

8) Attach the new DUOPA cassette to the pump (see Figure BB):

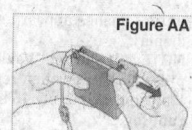

Figure BB

• Hold the pump so that the latch faces up.
• Hold the DUOPA cassette so that the tube points down.
• Insert the DUOPA cassette hooks into the hinge pins at the base of the pump.

9) Latch the new DUOPA cassette into the pump:

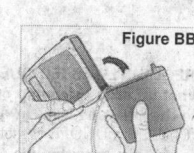

Figure CC

• Hold the pump and DUOPA cassette upright against a flat surface.
• Press down on the pump until the DUOPA cassette fits tightly against the pump **(see Figure CC).**

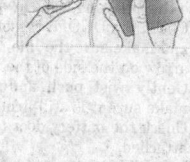

Figure DD

• Use a coin to twist the latch counterclockwise until the latch lines up straight with the arrow **(see Figure DD).**

WARNING: Attach the DUOPA cassette correctly. A detached or incorrectly attached cassette could cause a problem with getting your DUOPA.

10) Remove the red cap on the end of the cassette tube (see Figure EE).

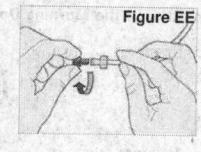

Figure EE

Save the red cap to use when discarding the cassette.
WARNING: Do not connect the red cap to the stomach tube as it will block DUOPA flow.

11) Connect the stomach tube to the cassette tube:

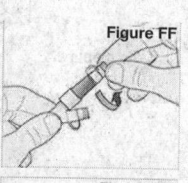

Figure FF

• While holding the stomach tube steady, twist off the white cap on the end of the longer colored connector **(see Figure FF). WARNING: Do not twist the stomach tube.**

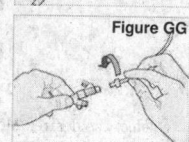

Figure GG

• Connect the cassette tube to the end of the longer colored connector **(see Figure GG). Do not connect to the shorter white connector.**

12) Turn the pump on:

• Press and **hold**

ON OFF

until the display turns on.
• Wait approximately **30** seconds for the pump to review settings.
• Check for

STOPPED

on the display.

PUMP STATUS: The pump is now on but not delivering DUOPA.

13) Inspect the tubing for kinks or closed clamps. If needed straighten kinks or open clamps (see Figure HH).

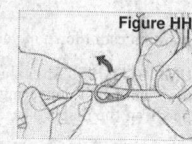

Figure HH

14) Start the pump:
• Press and **hold**

STOP START

until **3** dashes appear and then disappear from the display.

• Wait approximately **15** seconds for pump to start running.

• Check for

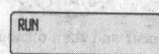
RUN

on the display.

PUMP STATUS: The pump is now running.

15) Insert the pump into the carrying bag (See Figure II).

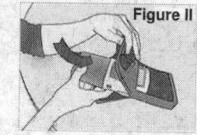

Figure II

16) Wear the bag on your shoulder or neck:

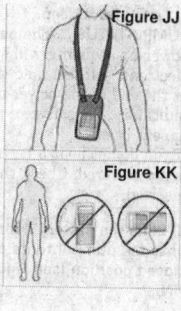

Figure JJ

Figure KK

• Place the bag strap over your shoulder or neck **(see Figure JJ).**

• Make sure the pump is in correct position **(see Figure KK).**

Changing the Batteries:

If you see **LowBat** or **Battery Depleted** on the display, change the batteries. Use **2** new **AA** alkaline batteries such as DURACELL® or EVEREADY® ENERGIZER®. The pump keeps all the important information when the batteries are removed.

WARNING:

• **Always have new batteries available for replacement. If** power is lost, DUOPA will not be delivered.

• **If the pump is dropped or hit, the battery door or tabs may break. Do not** use the pump if the battery door or tabs are damaged because the batteries will not be correctly secured. This may lead to loss of power and DUOPA will not be delivered.

• **If a gap is present anywhere between the battery door and the pump housing, the door is not correctly latched. If the battery door becomes detached or loose,** the batteries will not be correctly secured. This could cause loss of power and DUOPA will not be delivered.

CAUTION:

• **Do not use rechargeable NiCd or nickel metal hydride (NiMH) batteries. Do not use carbon zinc ("heavy duty")** batteries. They do not provide enough power for the pump to operate correctly.

• **Do not store the pump for prolonged periods of time with the batteries installed.** Battery leakage could damage the pump.

1) Ensure the pump is stopped.

2) Push and hold the arrow button while sliding the battery door until it comes completely off the pump (see Figure LL).

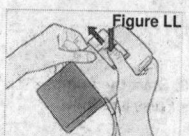

Figure LL

3) Remove the used batteries (see Figure MM).

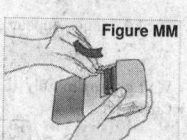

Figure MM

4) Install new batteries into the battery compartment. NOTE: Insert the batteries correctly based on the picture in the battery compartment. If you insert the batteries backwards, the display will remain blank. Reinsert the batteries, making sure to match the + and – markings with the battery compartment picture.

Continued on next page

5) Listen for a beep.
PUMP STATUS: The pump is now powered. The power-up sequence will start, the pump will go through an electronic self-test, and then the pump will beep **6** times at the end of the power-up sequence. All of the display indicators, the software revision, and each setting will appear briefly.
If you do not hear a beep, and the display is off, the pump is not powered. Check that the batteries are correctly inserted.

6) Slide the battery door back onto the pump into its original closed position (see Figure NN).

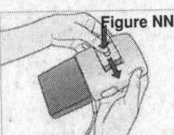

Figure NN

Your healthcare provider may have set your pump to allow for dose changes to your Morning Dose and Continuous Rate (Lock Level 1). **Do not** change your medicine dose without approval and training from your healthcare provider.
Talk with your healthcare provider to decide when to change your Morning Dose and Continuous Rate. **Do not** change your Extra Dose unless your healthcare provider tells you to. If your Extra Dose requires changes, your healthcare provider will provide instructions.

Change the Morning Dose
WARNING: Do not use the Prime button. Priming is for use by your healthcare provider only.

1) Turn the pump on:
• Press and **hold**

until the display turns on.
• Wait approximately **30** seconds for pump to review settings.
• Check for

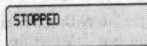

on the display.
PUMP STATUS: The pump is now on but not yet delivering DUOPA.

2) Inspect the tubing for kinks or closed clamps. If needed, straighten kinks or open clamps (see Figure OO).

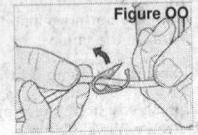

Figure OO

3) Start the pump:
• Press and **hold**

until **3** dashes appear and then disappear from the display.

• Wait approximately **15** seconds for pump to start running.
• Check for

on the display.
PUMP STATUS: The pump is now running.

---

4) Change the Morning Dose:
a. Press

1 time.
b. Check for

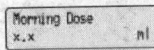

on the display.
c. Press

or

to select the desired Morning Dose.
d. Press

to store the Morning Dose.
e. Make sure you see the correct Morning Dose on the display. If not, repeat **Steps 4c to 4e.**

5) Deliver the Morning Dose:
• Press

1 time.
NOTE: If you see "**Value not saved**" on the display, press **NEXT** and then repeat **Steps 4c to 4e.**
• The display

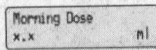

shows a countdown of your Morning Dose.

PUMP STATUS: After the Morning Dose finishes, the pump will begin delivering the Continuous Rate. **RUN** will appear on the display.

NOTE: If you are unable to deliver a Morning Dose, it may be too soon since the last Morning Dose to deliver another and you may need to wait longer. The time between Morning Doses is decided by your healthcare provider.

Change the Continuous Rate

1) Stop the Continuous Rate:
• Press and **hold**

until **3** dashes appear and then disappear from the display.
• Check for

on the display.

---

2) Change the Continuous Rate:
a. Press

2 times.
b. Check for

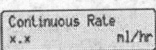

on the display.
c. Press

or

to select the desired Continuous Rate.
d. Press

to store the Continuous Rate.
e. Make sure you see the desired Continuous Rate on the display. If not, repeat **Steps 2c to 2e.**

3) Start the pump:
• Press and **hold**

until **3** dashes appear and then disappear from the display.
NOTE: If you see "**Value not saved**" on the display, press **NEXT** and then repeat **Steps 2c to 2e.**
• Wait approximately **15** seconds for the pump to start running.
• The display will show

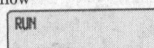

PUMP STATUS: The pump is now running.

[See table at top of next page]

FREQUENTLY ASKED QUESTIONS
What if I drop the pump or hit it against a hard surface?
Do the following right away:
• Check the DUOPA cassette latch on the side of the pump and make sure the line on the latch lines up with the arrow on the side of the pump.
• Gently twist, push, and pull on the DUOPA cassette to make sure it is still firmly attached.
• Check the battery door to make sure it is still firmly attached.
If the DUOPA cassette or the battery door is loose or damaged, do not use the pump.
Stop the pump right away, close the tubing clamp, and contact your healthcare provider.
What should I do if I drop the pump in water?
If you accidentally drop the pump in water, pick it up quickly, dry it off with a towel, and call your healthcare provider.
WARNING: If the pump is dropped or hit, look at the pump for damage. Do not use a pump that is damaged or is not working correctly.

Alarms and Messages
The table below shows some of the common alarms that you may hear from the pump. With all alarms, read the display before pressing

NEXT

to silence the alarm.

What you see:	What you hear:	Meaning	Response
Error	Two-Tone Alarm	An error with the pump has occurred.	Contact your healthcare provider.
High Pressure	Two-Tone Alarm	There is pressure backed up in the tubing.	Check tubing for clamps, kinks, or blockages. Make sure the red cap has been removed from the DUOPA cassette tube. Flush connectors if necessary. If it is not possible to flush the tubes, contact your healthcare provider as your tube may be blocked.
LowBat	3 Two-Tone Beeps Every 5 minutes	The pump batteries are low.	Change the batteries right away.
Upstream Occlusion	Two-Tone Alarm	If your healthcare provider has the Upstream Occlusion Sensor set to ON and a blockage in the DUOPA cassette is detected, this alarm will sound.	Detach the DUOPA cassette. Check if the DUOPA cassette is empty. If not empty, reattach the DUOPA cassette. Restart the pump to continue delivery. Contact your healthcare provider if the alarm continues.
No message on display	Two-Tone Alarm	Batteries were removed within approximately 15 seconds after stopping the pump.	Install new batteries to silence the alarm. Otherwise, the alarm will stop within a short period of time.
Display shows current pump status	2 Beeps (Long-Short)	The DUOPA cassette is not lined up with the pump or DUOPA is not flowing from the DUOPA cassette to the pumping mechanism. Very cold or extremely thick DUOPA may cause this alarm as well.	Press NEXT to silence the alarm. The pump continues to run. Make sure the DUOPA cassette is correctly lined up with the pump and DUOPA is flowing. Take the DUOPA cassette out of the refrigerator for 20 minutes before attaching to the pump.
Battery Depleted	Two-Tone Alarm	Batteries are dead.	Install new batteries. To continue delivery, restart the pump when completed.
Key pressed, Please release	Two-Tone Alarm	Key is being held down.	Stop pressing key. If the alarm persists, close the cassette tube clamp and remove the pump from use. Contact your healthcare provider.
No Disposable, Clamp Tubing	Two-Tone Alarm	**Disposable** refers to the DUOPA Cassette. **No Disposable** means the DUOPA cassette was removed. The pump is not sensing proper cassette attachment.	Clamp the cassette tube and disconnect it from your stomach tube. A DUOPA cassette must be correctly attached in order for the pump to run. Press NEXT to silence the alarm.
No Disposable, Pump won't run	Two-Tone Alarm	**Disposable** refers to the DUOPA Cassette. You have tried to start the pump without a disposable DUOPA cassette attached.	Press NEXT to silence the alarm. A DUOPA cassette must be correctly attached for the pump to run.
Service Due See manual	Two-Tone Alarm	The pump is scheduled for service.	Press NEXT to silence the alarm. The pump is still working, but contact your healthcare provider for further instructions.

What should I do if I need to bathe while wearing the pump?
You'll need to detach the pump before you shower, bathe, or swim. Reattach the pump to the stomach tubing afterwards and restart it.

What should I do if I need to have a medical test while wearing the pump?
The pump may need to be removed prior to certain medical tests. Be sure to talk to your doctor about your DUOPA pump before you take these tests.

STORAGE and DISPOSAL
Storage
• Store DUOPA in the refrigerator with the temperature between 36°F to 46°F (2°C to 8°C).
• When the DUOPA cassette has been removed from the refrigerator, DUOPA should be used within **16** hours.
• The DUOPA cassettes are for single use only and should not be used for longer than **16** hours, even if some of the medicine remains. An opened cassette should not be re-used.
• Protect the cassette from light and keep it in the carton before using.
Throwing away your DUOPA cassette or batteries
• Throw away the DUOPA cassette as your healthcare provider tells you to.
• Throw away used batteries in a manner safe for the environment, and according to any regulations that apply.

This Instructions for Use has been approved by the U.S. Food and Drug Administration.

AbbVie Inc.   abbvie
North Chicago, IL 60064, U.S.A.
For DUOPA Support: 1-844-386-4968

Pump manufactured by:
Smiths Medical ASD, Inc.
1265 Grey Fox Road
St. Paul, MN 55112 USA
Tel: 1-800-258-5361
www.smiths-medical.com
03-B169 Revised: May 2015
Shown in Product Identification Guide, page 505

GENGRAF® CAPSULES   ℞
[jen-graf]
(cyclosporine capsules, USP [MODIFIED])

> **WARNING**
> Only physicians experienced in management of systemic immunosuppressive therapy for the indicated disease should prescribe Gengraf® Capsules (cyclosporine capsules, USP [MODIFIED]). At doses used in solid organ transplantation, only physicians experienced in immunosuppressive therapy and management of organ transplant recipients should prescribe Gengraf®. Patients receiving the drug should be managed in facilities equipped and staffed with adequate laboratory and supportive medical resources. The physician responsible for maintenance therapy should have complete information requisite for the follow-up of the patient.
> Gengraf®, a systemic immunosuppressant, may increase the susceptibility to infection and the development of neoplasia. In kidney, liver, and heart transplant patients Gengraf® may be administered with other immunosuppressive agents. Increased susceptibility to infection and the possible development of lymphoma and other neoplasms may result from the increase in the degree of immunosuppression in transplant patients.
> Gengraf® Capsules (cyclosporine capsules, USP [MODIFIED]) has increased bioavailability in compari-

Continued on next page

Information on the AbbVie, Inc. products listed on these pages is from the prescribing information in use as of July 31, 2016. For more information, please visit rxabbvie.com or call 1-800-633-9110.

son to Sandimmune® Soft Gelatin Capsules (cyclosporine capsules, USP). Gengraf® and Sandimmune® are not bioequivalent and cannot be used interchangeably without physician supervision. For a given trough concentration, cyclosporine exposure will be greater with Gengraf® than with Sandimmune®. If a patient who is receiving exceptionally high doses of Sandimmune® is converted to Gengraf®, particular caution should be exercised. Cyclosporine blood concentrations should be monitored in transplant and rheumatoid arthritis patients taking Gengraf® to avoid toxicity due to high concentrations. Dose adjustments should be made in transplant patients to minimize possible organ rejection due to low concentrations. Comparison of blood concentrations in the published literature with blood concentrations obtained using current assays must be done with detailed knowledge of the assay methods employed.

For Psoriasis Patients (See also BOXED WARNING above)

Psoriasis patients previously treated with PUVA and to a lesser extent, methotrexate or other immunosuppressive agents, UVB, coal tar, or radiation therapy, are at an increased risk of developing skin malignancies when taking Gengraf® Capsules (cyclosporine capsules, USP [**MODIFIED**]).

Cyclosporine, the active ingredient in Gengraf®, in recommended dosages, can cause systemic hypertension and nephrotoxicity. The risk increases with increasing dose and duration of cyclosporine therapy. Renal dysfunction, including structural kidney damage, is a potential consequence of cyclosporine, and therefore, renal function must be monitored during therapy.

DESCRIPTION

Gengraf® Capsules (cyclosporine capsules, USP [**MODIFIED**]) is a modified oral formulation of cyclosporine that forms an aqueous dispersion in an aqueous environment.

Cyclosporine, the active principle in Gengraf®, is a cyclic polypeptide immunosuppressant agent consisting of 11 amino acids. It is produced as a metabolite by the fungus species *Aphanocladium album*.

Chemically, cyclosporine is designated as [R-[R*,R*-(E)]]-cyclic-(L-alanyl-D-alanyl-*N*-methyl-L-leucyl-*N*-methyl-L-leucyl-*N*-methyl-L-valyl-3-hydroxy-*N*,4-dimethyl-L-2-amino-6-octenoyl-L-α-amino-butyryl-*N*-methylglycyl-*N*-methyl-L-leucyl-L-valyl-*N*-methyl-L-leucyl).

Gengraf® Capsules (cyclosporine capsules, USP [**MODIFIED**]) are available in 25 mg, 50 mg, and 100 mg strengths.

Each 25 mg capsule contains

cyclosporine, 25 mg, alcohol, USP, absolute, 12.8% v/v (10.1% wt/vol.).

Each 50 mg capsule contains

cyclosporine, 50 mg, alcohol, USP, absolute, 12.8% v/v (10.1% wt/vol.).

Each 100 mg capsule contains

cyclosporine, 100 mg, alcohol, USP, absolute, 12.8% v/v (10.1% wt/vol.).

Inactive Ingredients

FD&C Blue No. 2, gelatin NF, polyethylene glycol NF, polyoxyl 35 castor oil NF, polysorbate 80 NF, propylene glycol USP, sorbitan monooleate NF, titanium dioxide.

The chemical structure for cyclosporine USP is:

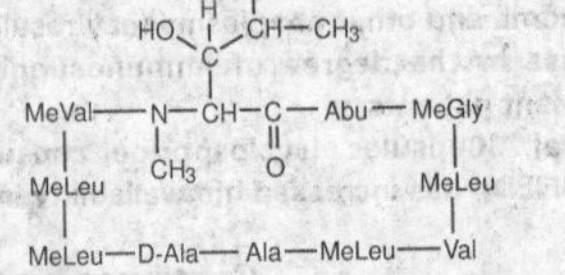

$C_{62}H_{111}N_{11}O_{12}$ Mol. Wt. 1202.61

CLINICAL PHARMACOLOGY

Cyclosporine is a potent immunosuppressive agent that in animals prolongs survival of allogeneic transplants involving skin, kidney, liver, heart, pancreas, bone marrow, small intestine, and lung. Cyclosporine has been demonstrated to suppress some humoral immunity and to a greater extent, cell-mediated immune reactions such as allograft rejection, delayed hypersensitivity, experimental allergic encephalomyelitis, Freund's adjuvant arthritis, and graft versus host disease in many animal species for a variety of organs.

The effectiveness of cyclosporine results from specific and reversible inhibition of immunocompetent lymphocytes in the G_0- and G_1-phase of the cell cycle. T-lymphocytes are preferentially inhibited. The T-helper cell is the main target, although the T-suppressor cell may also be suppressed. Cyclosporine also inhibits lymphokine production and release including interleukin-2.

No effects on phagocytic function (changes in enzyme secretions, chemotactic migration of granulocytes, macrophage migration, carbon clearance *in vivo*) have been detected in animals. Cyclosporine does not cause bone marrow suppression in animal models or man.

Pharmacokinetics

The immunosuppressive activity of cyclosporine is primarily due to parent drug. Following oral administration, absorption of cyclosporine is incomplete. The extent of absorption of cyclosporine is dependent on the individual patient, the patient population, and the formulation. Elimination of cyclosporine is primarily biliary with only 6% of the dose (parent drug and metabolites) excreted in urine. The disposition of cyclosporine from blood is generally biphasic, with a terminal half-life of approximately 8.4 hours (range 5 to 18 hours). Following intravenous administration, the blood clearance of cyclosporine (assay: HPLC) is approximately 5 to 7 mL/min/kg in adult recipients of renal or liver allografts. Blood cyclosporine clearance appears to be slightly slower in cardiac transplant patients.

The Gengraf® Capsules (cyclosporine capsules, USP [**MODIFIED**]) and Gengraf® Oral Solution (cyclosporine oral solution, USP [**MODIFIED**]) are bioequivalent.

The relationship between administered dose and exposure (area under the concentration versus time curve, AUC) is linear within the therapeutic dose range. The intersubject variability (total, %CV) of cyclosporine exposure (AUC) when cyclosporine (**MODIFIED**) or Sandimmune® is administered ranges from approximately 20% to 50% in renal transplant patients. This intersubject variability contributes to the need for individualization of the dosing regimen for optimal therapy (See **DOSAGE AND ADMINISTRATION**). Intrasubject variability of AUC in renal transplant recipients (%CV) was 9% to 21% for cyclosporine (**MODIFIED**) and 19% to 26% for Sandimmune®. In the same studies, intrasubject variability of trough concentrations (%CV) was 17% to 30% for cyclosporine (**MODIFIED**) and 16% to 38% for Sandimmune®.

Absorption

Cyclosporine (**MODIFIED**) has increased bioavailability compared to Sandimmune®. The absolute bioavailability of cyclosporine administered as Sandimmune® is dependent on the patient population, estimated to be less than 10% in liver transplant patients and as great as 89% in some renal transplant patients. The absolute bioavailability of cyclosporine administered as cyclosporine (**MODIFIED**) has not been determined in adults. In studies of renal transplant, rheumatoid arthritis and psoriasis patients, the mean cyclosporine AUC was approximately 20% to 50% greater and the peak blood cyclosporine concentration (C_{max}) was approximately 40% to 106% greater following administration of cyclosporine (**MODIFIED**) compared to following administration of Sandimmune®. The dose normalized AUC in *de novo* liver transplant patients administered cyclosporine (**MODIFIED**) 28 days after transplantation was 50% greater and C_{max} was 90% greater than in those patients administered Sandimmune®. AUC and C_{max} are also increased (cyclosporine [**MODIFIED**] relative to Sandimmune®) in heart transplant patients, but data are very limited. Although the AUC and C_{max} values are higher on cyclosporine (**MODIFIED**) relative to Sandimmune®, the predose trough concentrations (dose-normalized) are similar for the two formulations.

Following oral administration of cyclosporine (**MODIFIED**), the time to peak blood cyclosporine concentrations (T_{max}) ranged from 1.5 to 2.0 hours. The administration of food with cyclosporine (**MODIFIED**) decreases the cyclosporine AUC and C_{max}. A high fat meal (669 kcal, 45 grams fat) consumed within one-half hour before cyclosporine (**MODIFIED**) administration decreased the AUC by 13% and C_{max} by 33%. The effects of a low fat meal (667 kcal, 15 grams fat) were similar.

The effect of T-tube diversion of bile on the absorption of cyclosporine from cyclosporine (**MODIFIED**) was investigated in eleven *de novo* liver transplant patients. When the patients were administered cyclosporine (**MODIFIED**) with and without T-tube diversion of bile, very little difference in absorption was observed, as measured by the change in maximal cyclosporine blood concentrations from pre-dose values with the T-tube closed relative to when it was open: 6.9±41% (range -55% to 68%).

[See table at top of next page]

Distribution

Cyclosporine is distributed largely outside the blood volume. The steady state volume of distribution during intravenous dosing has been reported as 3 to 5 L/kg in solid organ transplant recipients. In blood, the distribution is concentration dependent. Approximately 33% to 47% is in plasma, 4% to 9% in lymphocytes, 5% to 12% in granulocytes, and 41% to 58% in erythrocytes. At high concentrations, the binding capacity of leukocytes and erythrocytes becomes saturated. In plasma, approximately 90% is bound to proteins, primarily lipoproteins. Cyclosporine is excreted in human milk. (See **PRECAUTIONS, Nursing Mothers**)

Metabolism

Cyclosporine is extensively metabolized by the cytochrome P-450 3A enzyme system in the liver, and to a lesser degree in the gastrointestinal tract, and the kidney. The metabolism of cyclosporine can be altered by the coadministration of a variety of agents. (See **PRECAUTIONS, Drug Interactions**) At least 25 metabolites have been identified from human bile, feces, blood, and urine. The biological activity of the metabolites and their contributions to toxicity are considerably less than those of the parent compound. The major metabolites (M1, M9, and M4N) result from oxidation at the 1-beta, 9-gamma, and 4-N-demethylated positions, respectively. At steady state following the oral administration of Sandimmune®, the mean AUCs for blood concentrations of M1, M9, and M4N are about 70%, 21%, and 7.5% of the AUC for blood cyclosporine concentrations, respectively. Based on blood concentration data from stable renal transplant patients (13 patients administered cyclosporine [**MODIFIED**] and Sandimmune® in a crossover study), and bile concentration data from *de novo* liver transplant patients (4 administered cyclosporine [**MODIFIED**], 3 administered Sandimmune®), the percentage of dose present as M1, M9, and M4N metabolites is similar when either cyclosporine (**MODIFIED**) or Sandimmune® is administered.

Excretion

Only 0.1% of a cyclosporine dose is excreted unchanged in the urine. Elimination is primarily biliary with only 6% of the dose (parent drug and metabolites) excreted in the urine. Neither dialysis nor renal failure alters cyclosporine clearance significantly.

Drug Interactions

(See **PRECAUTIONS, Drug Interactions**) When diclofenac or methotrexate was coadministered with cyclosporine in rheumatoid arthritis patients, the AUC of diclofenac and methotrexate, each was significantly increased. (See **PRECAUTIONS, Drug Interactions**) No clinically significant pharmacokinetic interactions occurred between cyclosporine and aspirin, ketoprofen, piroxicam, or indomethacin.

Specific Populations

Renal Impairment

In a study performed in 4 subjects with end-stage renal disease (creatinine clearance <5 mL/min), an intravenous infusion of 3.5 mg/kg of cyclosporine over 4 hours administered at the end of a hemodialysis session resulted in a mean volume of distribution (Vdss) of 3.49 L/kg and systemic clearance (CL) of 0.369 L/hr/kg. This systemic CL (0.369 L/hr/kg) was approximately two thirds of the mean systemic CL (0.56 L/hr/kg) of cyclosporine in historical control subjects with normal renal function. In 5 liver transplant patients, the mean clearance of cyclosporine on and off hemodialysis was 463 mL/min and 398 mL/min, respectively. Less than 1% of the dose of cyclosporine was recovered in the dialysate.

Hepatic Impairment

Cyclosporine is extensively metabolized by the liver. Since severe hepatic impairment may result in significantly increased cyclosporine exposures, the dosage of cyclosporine may need to be reduced in these patients.

Pediatric Population

Pharmacokinetic data from pediatric patients administered cyclosporine (**MODIFIED**) or Sandimmune® are very limited. In 15 renal transplant patients aged 3-16 years,

Patient Population	Dose/day[1] (mg/d)	Dose/weight (mg/kg/d)	AUC[2] (ng·hr/mL)	C_max (ng/mL)	Trough[3] (ng/mL)	CL/F (mL/min)	CL/F (mL/min/kg)
De novo renal transplant[4] Week 4 (N=37)	597±174	7.95±2.81	8772±2089	1802±428	361±129	593±204	7.8±2.9
Stable renal transplant[4] (N=55)	344±122	4.10±1.58	6035±2194	1333±469	251±116	492±140	5.9±2.1
De novo liver transplant[5] Week 4 (N=18)	458±190	6.89±3.68	7187±2816	1555±740	268±101	577±309	8.6±5.7
De novo rheumatoid arthritis[6] (N=23)	182±55.6	2.37±0.36	2641±877	728±263	96.4±37.7	613±196	8.3±2.8
De novo psoriasis[6] Week 4 (N=18)	189±69.8	2.48±0.65	2324±1048	655±186	74.9±46.7	723±186	10.2±3.9

[1]Total daily dose was divided into two doses administered every 12 hours
[2]AUC was measured over one dosing interval
[3]Trough concentration was measured just prior to the morning cyclosporine (**MODIFIED**) dose, approximately 12 hours after the previous dose
[4]Assay: TDx specific monoclonal fluorescence polarization immunoassay
[5]Assay: Cyclo-trac specific monoclonal radioimmunoassay
[6]Assay: INCSTAR specific monoclonal radioimmunoassay

cyclosporine whole blood clearance after IV administration of Sandimmune® was 10.6±3.7 mL/min/kg (assay: Cyclo-trac specific RIA). In a study of 7 renal transplant patients aged 2-16, the cyclosporine clearance ranged from 9.8-15.5 mL/min/kg. In 9 liver transplant patients aged 0.6-5.6 years, clearance was 9.3±5.4 mL/min/kg (assay: HPLC).
In the pediatric population, cyclosporine (**MODIFIED**) also demonstrates an increased bioavailability as compared to Sandimmune®. In 7 liver _de novo_ transplant patients aged 1.4-10 years, the absolute bioavailability of cyclosporine (**MODIFIED**) was 43% (range 30%-68%) and for Sandimmune® in the same individuals absolute bioavailability was 28% (range 17%-42%).
[See table at top of page 659]
Geriatric Population
Comparison of single dose data from both normal elderly volunteers (N=18, mean age 69 years) and elderly rheumatoid arthritis patients (N=16, mean age 68 years) to single dose data in young adult volunteers (N=16, mean age 26 years) showed no significant difference in the pharmacokinetic parameters.

CLINICAL TRIALS
Rheumatoid Arthritis
The effectiveness of Sandimmune® and cyclosporine (**MODIFIED**) in the treatment of severe rheumatoid arthritis was evaluated in 5 clinical studies involving a total of 728 cyclosporine treated patients and 273 placebo treated patients.
A summary of the results is presented for the "responder" rates per treatment group, with a responder being defined as a patient having _completed_ the trial with a 20% improvement in the tender and the swollen joint count and a 20% improvement in 2 of 4 of investigator global, patient global, disability, and erythrocyte sedimentation rates (ESR) for the Studies 651 and 652 and 3 of 5 of investigator global, patient global, disability, visual analog pain, and ESR for Studies 2008, 654 and 302.
Study 651 enrolled 264 patients with active rheumatoid arthritis with at least 20 involved joints, who had failed at least one major RA drug, using a 3:3:2 randomization to one of the following three groups: (1) cyclosporine dosed at 2.5 to 5 mg/kg/day, (2) methotrexate at 7.5 to 15 mg/week, or (3) placebo. Treatment duration was 24 weeks. The mean cyclosporine dose at the last visit was 3.1 mg/kg/day. See Graph below.
Study 652 enrolled 250 patients with active RA with >6 active painful or tender joints who had failed at least one major RA drug. Patients were randomized using a 3:3:2 randomization to 1 of 3 treatment arms: (1) 1.5 to 5 mg/kg/day of cyclosporine, (2) 2.5 to 5 mg/kg/day of cyclosporine, and (3) placebo. Treatment duration was 16 weeks. The mean cyclosporine dose for group 2 at the last visit was 2.92 mg/kg/day. See Graph below.

Study 2008 enrolled 144 patients with active RA and >6 active joints who had unsuccessful treatment courses of aspirin and gold or Penicillamine. Patients were randomized to 1 of 2 treatment groups (1) cyclosporine 2.5 to 5 mg/kg/day with adjustments after the first month to achieve a target trough level and (2) placebo. Treatment duration was 24 weeks. The mean cyclosporine dose at the last visit was 3.63 mg/kg/day. See Graph below.
Study 654 enrolled 148 patients who remained with active joint counts of 6 or more despite treatment with maximally tolerated methotrexate doses for at least three months. Patients continued to take their current dose of methotrexate and were randomized to receive, in addition, one of the following medications: (1) cyclosporine 2.5 mg/kg/day with dose increases of 0.5 mg/kg/day at weeks 2 and 4 if there was no evidence of toxicity and further increases of 0.5 mg/kg/day at weeks 8 and 16 if a <30% decrease in active joint count occurred without any significant toxicity; dose decreases could be made at any time for toxicity or (2) placebo. Treatment duration was 24 weeks. The mean cyclosporine dose at the last visit was 2.8 mg/kg/day (range: 1.3-4.1). See Graph below.
Study 302 enrolled 299 patients with severe active RA, 99% of whom were unresponsive or intolerant to at least one prior major RA drug. Patients were randomized to 1 of 2 treatment groups (1) cyclosporine (**MODIFIED**) and (2) Sandimmune®, both of which were started at 2.5 mg/kg/day and increased after 4 weeks for inefficacy in increments of 0.5 mg/kg/day to a maximum of 5 mg/kg/day and decreased at any time for toxicity. Treatment duration was 24 weeks. The mean cyclosporine dose at the last visit was 2.91 mg/kg/day (range: 0.72 to 5.17) for cyclosporine (**MODIFIED**) and 3.27 mg/kg/day (range: 0.73 to 5.68) for Sandimmune®. See Graph below.

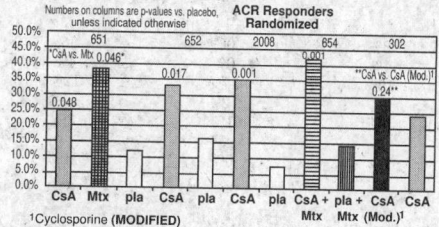

Numbers on columns are p-values vs. placebo, unless indicated otherwise
ACR Responders Randomized

[1]Cyclosporine (**MODIFIED**)

INDICATIONS AND USAGE
Kidney, Liver, and Heart Transplantation
Gengraf® Capsules (cyclosporine capsules, USP [**MODIFIED**]) is indicated for the prophylaxis of organ rejection in kidney, liver, and heart allogeneic transplants. Cyclosporine (**MODIFIED**) has been used in combination with azathioprine and corticosteroids.

Rheumatoid Arthritis
Gengraf® Capsules (cyclosporine capsules, USP [**MODIFIED**]) is indicated for the treatment of patients with severe active, rheumatoid arthritis where the disease has not adequately responded to methotrexate. Gengraf® can be used in combination with methotrexate in rheumatoid arthritis patients who do not respond adequately to methotrexate alone.
Psoriasis
Gengraf® Capsules (cyclosporine capsules, USP [**MODIFIED**]) is indicated for the treatment of _adult, nonimmunocompromised_ patients with severe (i.e., extensive and/or disabling), recalcitrant, plaque psoriasis who have failed to respond to at least one systemic therapy (e.g., PUVA, retinoids, or methotrexate) or in patients for whom other systemic therapies are contraindicated, or cannot be tolerated. While rebound rarely occurs, most patients will experience relapse with Gengraf® as with other therapies upon cessation of treatment.

CONTRAINDICATIONS
General
Gengraf® Capsules (cyclosporine capsules, USP [**MODIFIED**]) is contraindicated in patients with a hypersensitivity to cyclosporine or to any of the ingredients of the formulation.
Rheumatoid Arthritis
Rheumatoid arthritis patients with abnormal renal function, uncontrolled hypertension, or malignancies should not receive Gengraf® Capsules (cyclosporine capsules, USP [**MODIFIED**]).
Psoriasis
Psoriasis patients who are treated with Gengraf® Capsules (cyclosporine capsules, USP [**MODIFIED**]) should not receive concomitant PUVA or UVB therapy, methotrexate or other immunosuppressive agents, coal tar or radiation therapy. Psoriasis patients with abnormal renal function, uncontrolled hypertension, or malignancies should not receive Gengraf®.

WARNINGS
(See also **BOXED WARNING**)
All Patients
Cyclosporine, the active ingredient of Gengraf® Capsules (cyclosporine capsules, USP [**MODIFIED**]), can cause nephrotoxicity and hepatotoxicity. The risk increases with increasing doses of cyclosporine. Renal dysfunction including structural kidney damage is a potential consequence of Gengraf® and therefore renal function must be monitored during therapy. **Care should be taken in using cyclosporine with nephrotoxic drugs. (See PRECAUTIONS)**
Patients receiving Gengraf® require frequent monitoring of serum creatinine. (See Special Monitoring under **DOSAGE AND ADMINISTRATION**) Elderly patients should be monitored with particular care, since decreases in renal function also occur with age. If patients are not properly monitored and doses are not properly adjusted, cyclosporine therapy can be associated with the occurrence of structural kidney damage and persistent renal dysfunction.
An increase in serum creatinine and BUN may occur during Gengraf® therapy and reflect a reduction in the glomerular filtration rate. Impaired renal function at any time requires close monitoring, and frequent dosage adjustment may be indicated. The frequency and severity of serum creatinine elevations increase with dose and duration of cyclosporine therapy. These elevations are likely to become more pronounced without dose reduction or discontinuation.
Because Gengraf® Capsules (cyclosporine capsules, USP [MODIFIED]) is not bioequivalent to Sandimmune® Soft Gelatin Capsules (cyclosporine capsules, USP), conversion from Gengraf® to Sandimmune® using a 1:1 ratio (mg/kg/day) may result in lower cyclosporine blood concentrations. Conversion from Gengraf® to Sandimmune® should be made with increased monitoring to avoid the potential of underdosing.
Kidney, Liver, and Heart Transplant
Nephrotoxicity
Cyclosporine, the active ingredient of Gengraf® Capsules (cyclosporine capsules, USP [**MODIFIED**]), can cause neph-

Continued on next page

Cyclosporine (MODIFIED)/Sandimmune® Rheumatoid Arthritis Percentage of Patients with Adverse Events ≥3% in any Cyclosporine Treated Group

Body System	Preferred Term	Studies 651+652 +2008 Sandimmune®† (N=269)	Study 302 Sand-immune® (N=155)	Study 654 Metho-trexate & Sandimmune® (N=74)	Study 654 Metho-trexate & Placebo (N=73)	Study 302 Cyclosporine (MODIFIED) (N=143)	Studies 651+652 +2008 Placebo (N=201)
Autonomic Nervous System Disorders							
	Flushing	2%	2%	3%	0%	5%	2%
Body As A Whole–General Disorders							
	Accidental Trauma	0%	1%	10%	4%	4%	0%
	Edema NOS*	5%	14%	12%	4%	10%	<1%
	Fatigue	6%	3%	8%	12%	3%	7%
	Fever	2%	3%	0%	0%	2%	4%
	Influenza-like symptoms	<1%	6%	1%	0%	3%	2%
	Pain	6%	9%	10%	15%	13%	4%
	Rigors	1%	1%	4%	0%	3%	1%
Cardiovascular Disorders							
	Arrhythmia	2%	5%	5%	6%	2%	1%
	Chest Pain	4%	5%	1%	1%	6%	1%
	Hypertension	8%	26%	16%	12%	25%	2%
Central and Peripheral Nervous System Disorders							
	Dizziness	8%	6%	7%	3%	8%	3%
	Headache	17%	23%	22%	11%	25%	9%
	Migraine	2%	3%	0%	0%	3%	1%
	Paresthesia	8%	7%	8%	4%	11%	1%
	Tremor	8%	7%	7%	3%	13%	4%
Gastrointestinal System Disorders							
	Abdominal Pain	15%	15%	15%	7%	15%	10%
	Anorexia	3%	3%	1%	0%	3%	3%
	Diarrhea	12%	12%	18%	15%	13%	8%
	Dyspepsia	12%	12%	10%	8%	8%	4%
	Flatulence	5%	5%	5%	4%	4%	1%
	Gastrointestinal Disorder NOS*	0%	2%	1%	4%	4%	0%
	Gingivitis	4%	3%	0%	0%	0%	1%
	Gum Hyperplasia	2%	4%	1%	3%	4%	1%
	Nausea	23%	14%	24%	15%	18%	14%
	Rectal Hemorrhage	0%	3%	0%	0%	1%	1%
	Stomatitis	7%	5%	16%	12%	6%	8%
	Vomiting	9%	8%	14%	7%	6%	5%
Hearing and Vestibular Disorders							
	Ear Disorder NOS*	0%	5%	0%	0%	1%	0%
Metabolic and Nutritional Disorders							
	Hypomagnesemia	0%	4%	0%	0%	6%	0%
Musculoskeletal System Disorders							
	Arthropathy	0%	5%	0%	1%	4%	0%
	Leg Cramps / Involuntary Muscle Contractions	2%	11%	11%	3%	12%	1%
Psychiatric Disorders							
	Depression	3%	6%	3%	1%	1%	2%
	Insomnia	4%	1%	1%	0%	3%	2%
Renal							
	Creatinine elevations ≥30%	43%	39%	55%	19%	48%	13%
	Creatinine elevations ≥50%	24%	18%	26%	8%	18%	3%
Reproductive Disorders, Female							
	Leukorrhea	1%	0%	4%	0%	1%	0%
	Menstrual Disorder	3%	2%	1%	0%	1%	1%
Respiratory System Disorders							
	Bronchitis	1%	3%	1%	0%	1%	3%
	Coughing	5%	3%	5%	7%	4%	4%
	Dyspnea	5%	1%	3%	3%	1%	2%
	Infection NOS*	9%	5%	0%	7%	3%	10%
	Pharyngitis	3%	5%	5%	6%	4%	4%
	Pneumonia	1%	0%	4%	0%	1%	1%
	Rhinitis	0%	3%	11%	10%	1%	0%
	Sinusitis	4%	4%	8%	4%	3%	3%
	Upper Respiratory Tract	0%	14%	23%	15%	13%	0%
Skin and Appendages Disorders							
	Alopecia	3%	0%	1%	1%	4%	4%
	Bullous Eruption	1%	0%	4%	1%	1%	1%
	Hypertrichosis	19%	17%	12%	0%	15%	3%
	Rash	7%	12%	10%	7%	8%	10%
	Skin Ulceration	1%	1%	3%	4%	0%	2%
Urinary System Disorders							
	Dysuria	0%	0%	11%	3%	1%	2%
	Micturition Frequency	2%	4%	3%	1%	2%	2%
	NPN, Increased	0%	19%	12%	0%	18%	0%
	Urinary Tract Infection	0%	3%	5%	4%	3%	0%
Vascular (Extracardiac) Disorders							
	Purpura	3%	4%	1%	1%	2%	0%

† Includes patients in 2.5 mg/kg/day dose group only.
*NOS=Not Otherwise Specified.

Patient Population	Pediatric Pharmacokinetic Parameters (mean±SD) Dose/day (mg/d)	Dose/weight (mg/kg/d)	AUC[1] (ng•hr/mL)	C_{max} (ng/mL)	CL/F (mL/min)	CL/F (mL/min/kg)
Stable liver transplant[2]						
Age 2-8, Dosed TID (N=9)	101±25	5.95±1.32	2163±801	629±219	285±94	16.6±4.3
Age 8-15, Dosed BID (N=8)	188±55	4.96±2.09	4272±1462	975±281	378±80	10.2±4.0
Stable liver transplant[3]						
Age 3, Dosed BID (N=1)	120	8.33	5832	1050	171	11.9
Age 8-15, Dosed BID (N=5)	158±55	5.51±1.91	4452±2475	1013±635	328±121	11.0±1.9
Stable renal transplant[3]						
Age 7-15, Dosed BID (N=5)	328±83	7.37±4.11	6922±1988	1827±487	418±143	8.7±2.9

[1]AUC was measured over one dosing interval
[2]Assay: Cyclo-trac specific monoclonal radioimmunoassay
[3]Assay: TDx specific monoclonal fluorescence polarization immunoassay

rotoxicity and hepatotoxicity when used in high doses. It is not unusual for serum creatinine and BUN levels to be elevated during cyclosporine therapy. These elevations in renal transplant patients do not necessarily indicate rejection, and each patient must be fully evaluated before dosage adjustment is initiated.

Based on the historical Sandimmune® experience with oral solution, nephrotoxicity associated with cyclosporine had been noted in 25% of cases of renal transplantation, 38% of cases of cardiac transplantation, and 37% of cases of liver transplantation. Mild nephrotoxicity was generally noted 2 to 3 months after renal transplant and consisted of an arrest in the fall of the pre-operative elevations of BUN and creatinine at a range of 35 to 45 mg/dL and 2.0 to 2.5 mg/dL respectively. These elevations were often responsive to cyclosporine dosage reduction.

More overt nephrotoxicity was seen early after transplantation and was characterized by a rapidly rising BUN and creatinine. Since these events are similar to renal rejection episodes, care must be taken to differentiate between them. This form of nephrotoxicity is usually responsive to cyclosporine dosage reduction.

Although specific diagnostic criteria which reliably differentiate renal graft rejection from drug toxicity have not been found, a number of parameters have been significantly associated with one or the other. It should be noted however, that up to 20% of patients may have simultaneous nephrotoxicity and rejection.

[See table at top of next page]

A form of a cyclosporine-associated nephropathy is characterized by serial deterioration in renal function and morphologic changes in the kidneys. From 5% to 15% of transplant recipients who have received cyclosporine will fail to show a reduction in rising serum creatinine despite a decrease or discontinuation of cyclosporine therapy. Renal biopsies from these patients will demonstrate one or several of the following alterations: tubular vacuolization, tubular microcalcifications, peritubular capillary congestion, arteriolopathy, and a striped form of interstitial fibrosis with tubular atrophy. Though none of these morphologic changes is entirely specific, a diagnosis of cyclosporine-associated structural nephrotoxicity requires evidence of these findings.

When considering the development of cyclosporine-associated nephropathy, it is noteworthy that several authors have reported an association between the appearance of interstitial fibrosis and higher cumulative doses or persistently high circulating trough concentrations of cyclosporine. This is particularly true during the first 6 post-transplant months when the dosage tends to be highest and when, in kidney recipients, the organ appears to be most vulnerable to the toxic effects of cyclosporine. Among other contributing factors to the development of interstitial fibrosis in these patients are prolonged perfusion time, warm ischemia time, as well as episodes of acute toxicity, and acute and chronic rejection. The reversibility of interstitial fibrosis and its correlation to renal function have not yet been determined. Reversibility of arteriolopathy has been reported after stopping cyclosporine or lowering the dosage.

Impaired renal function at any time requires close monitoring, and frequent dosage adjustment may be indicated.

In the event of severe and unremitting rejection, when rescue therapy with pulse steroids and monoclonal antibodies fail to reverse the rejection episode, it may be preferable to switch to alternative immunosuppressive therapy rather than increase the Gengraf® dose to excessive blood concentrations.

Due to the potential for additive or synergistic impairment of renal function, caution should be exercised when coadministering Gengraf® with other drugs that may impair renal function. (See **PRECAUTIONS, Drug Interactions**)

Thrombotic Microangiopathy

Occasionally patients have developed a syndrome of thrombocytopenia and microangiopathic hemolytic anemia which may result in graft failure. The vasculopathy can occur in the absence of rejection and is accompanied by avid platelet consumption within the graft as demonstrated by Indium 111 labeled platelet studies. Neither the pathogenesis nor the management of this syndrome is clear. Though resolution has occurred after reduction or discontinuation of cyclosporine and 1) administration of streptokinase and heparin or 2) plasmapheresis, this appears to depend upon early detection with Indium 111 labeled platelet scans. (See **ADVERSE REACTIONS**)

Hyperkalemia

Significant hyperkalemia (sometimes associated with hyperchloremic metabolic acidosis) and hyperuricemia have been seen occasionally in individual patients.

Hepatotoxicity

Cases of hepatotoxicity and liver injury including cholestasis, jaundice, hepatitis, and liver failure have been reported in patients treated with cyclosporine. Most reports included patients with significant co-morbidities, underlying conditions and other confounding factors including infectious complications and comedications with hepatotoxic potential. In some cases, mainly in transplant patients, fatal outcomes have been reported. (See **ADVERSE REACTIONS, Postmarketing Experience, Kidney, Liver and Heart Transplantation**)

Hepatotoxicity, usually manifested by elevations in hepatic enzymes and bilirubin, was reported in patients treated with cyclosporine in clinical trials: 4% in renal transplantation, 7% in cardiac transplantation, and 4% in liver transplantation. This was usually noted during the first month of therapy when high doses of cyclosporine were used. The chemistry elevations usually decreased with a reduction in dosage.

Malignancies

As in patients receiving other immunosuppressants, those patients receiving cyclosporine are at increased risk for development of lymphomas and other malignancies, particularly those of the skin. Patients taking cyclosporine should be warned to avoid excess ultraviolet light exposure. The increased risk appears related to the intensity and duration of immunosuppression rather than to the use of specific agents. Because of the danger of oversuppression of the immune system resulting in increased risk of infection or malignancy, a treatment regimen containing multiple immunosuppressants should be used with caution. Some malignancies may be fatal. Transplant patients receiving cyclosporine are at increased risk for serious infection with fatal outcome.

Serious Infections

Patients receiving immunosuppressants, including Gengraf®, are at increased risk of developing bacterial, viral, fungal, and protozoal infections, including opportunistic infections. These infections may lead to serious, including fatal, outcomes. (See **BOXED WARNING** and **ADVERSE REACTIONS**)

Polyoma Virus Infections

Patients receiving immunosuppressants, including Gengraf®, are at increased risk for opportunistic infections, including polyoma virus infections. Polyoma virus infections in transplant patients may have serious, and sometimes, fatal outcomes. These include cases of JC virus-associated progressive multifocal leukoencephalopathy (PML), and polyoma virus-associated nephropathy (PVAN), especially due to BK virus infection, which have been observed in patients receiving cyclosporine. PVAN is associated with serious outcomes, including deteriorating renal function and renal graft loss, (See **ADVERSE REACTIONS, Postmarketing Experience, Kidney, Liver and Heart Transplantation**). Patient monitoring may help detect patients at risk for PVAN.

Cases of PML have been reported in patients treated with Gengraf®. PML, which is sometimes fatal, commonly presents with hemiparesis, apathy, confusion, cognitive deficiencies and ataxia. Risk factors for PML include treatment with immunosuppressant therapies and impairment of immune function. In immunosuppressed patients, physicians should consider PML in the differential diagnosis in patients reporting neurological symptoms and consultation with a neurologist should be considered as clinically indicated.

Consideration should be given to reducing the total immunosuppression in transplant patients who develop PML or PVAN. However, reduced immunosuppression may place the graft at risk.

Neurotoxicity

There have been reports of convulsions in adult and pediatric patients receiving cyclosporine, particularly in combination with high dose methylprednisolone.

Encephalopathy, including Posterior Reversible Encephalopathy Syndrome (PRES), has been described both in postmarketing reports and in the literature. Manifestations include impaired consciousness, convulsions, visual disturbances (including blindness), loss of motor function, movement disorders and psychiatric disturbances. In many cases, changes in the white matter have been detected using imaging techniques and pathologic specimens. Predisposing factors such as hypertension, hypomagnesemia, hypocholesterolemia, high-dose corticosteroids, high cyclosporine blood concentrations, and graft-versus-host disease have been noted in many but not all of the reported cases. The changes in most cases have been reversible upon discontinuation of cyclosporine, and in some cases improvement was noted after reduction of dose. It appears that patients receiving liver transplant are more susceptible to encephalopathy than those receiving kidney transplant. Another rare manifestation of cyclosporine-induced neurotoxicity, occurring in transplant patients more frequently than in other indications, is optic disc edema including papilloedema, with possible visual impairment, secondary to benign intracranial hypertension.

Care should be taken in using cyclosporine with nephrotoxic drugs. (See **PRECAUTIONS**)

Rheumatoid Arthritis

Cyclosporine nephropathy was detected in renal biopsies of 6 out of 60 (10%) rheumatoid arthritis patients after the average treatment duration of 19 months. Only one patient, out of these 6 patients, was treated with a dose ≤4 mg/kg/day. Serum creatinine improved in all but one patient after discontinuation of cyclosporine. The "maximal creatinine increase" appears to be a factor in predicting cyclosporine nephropathy.

There is a potential, as with other immunosuppressive agents, for an increase in the occurrence of malignant lymphomas with cyclosporine. It is not clear whether the risk with cyclosporine is greater than that in rheumatoid arthritis patients or in rheumatoid arthritis patients on cytotoxic treatment for this indication. Five cases of lymphoma were detected: four in a survey of approximately 2,300 patients treated with cyclosporine for rheumatoid arthritis, and another case of lymphoma was reported in a clinical trial. Although other tumors (12 skin cancers, 24 solid tumors of diverse types, and 1 multiple myeloma) were also reported in this survey, epidemiologic analyses did not support a relationship to cyclosporine other than for malignant lymphomas.

Patients should be thoroughly evaluated before and during Gengraf® Capsules (cyclosporine capsules, USP [**MODIFIED**]) treatment for the development of malignancies.

Continued on next page

Information on the AbbVie, Inc. products listed on these pages is from the prescribing information in use as of July 31, 2016. For more information, please visit rxabbvie.com or call 1-800-633-9110.

Moreover, use of Gengraf® therapy with other immunosuppressive agents may induce an excessive immunosuppression which is known to increase the risk of malignancy.

Psoriasis
(See also **BOXED WARNING** for Psoriasis)

Since cyclosporine is a potent immunosuppressive agent with a number of potentially serious side effects, the risks and benefits of using Gengraf® Capsules (cyclosporine capsules, USP [**MODIFIED**]) should be considered before treatment of patients with psoriasis. Cyclosporine, the active ingredient in Gengraf®, can cause nephrotoxicity and hypertension (See **PRECAUTIONS**) and the risk increases with increasing dose and duration of therapy. Patients who may be at increased risk such as those with abnormal renal function, uncontrolled hypertension or malignancies, should not receive Gengraf®.

Renal dysfunction is a potential consequence of Gengraf®, therefore renal function must be monitored during therapy. Patients receiving Gengraf® require frequent monitoring of serum creatinine. (See Special Monitoring under **DOSAGE AND ADMINISTRATION**) Elderly patients should be monitored with particular care, since decreases in renal function also occur with age. If patients are not properly monitored and doses are not properly adjusted, cyclosporine therapy can cause structural kidney damage and persistent renal dysfunction.

An increase in serum creatinine and BUN may occur during Gengraf® therapy and reflects a reduction in the glomerular filtration rate.

Kidney biopsies from 86 psoriasis patients treated for a mean duration of 23 months with 1.2 to 7.6 mg/kg/day of cyclosporine showed evidence of cyclosporine nephropathy in 18/86 (21%) of the patients. The pathology consisted of renal tubular atrophy and interstitial fibrosis. On repeat biopsy of 13 of these patients maintained on various dosages of cyclosporine for a mean of 2 additional years, the number with cyclosporine induced nephropathy rose to 26/86 (30%). The majority of patients (19/26) were on a dose of ≥5.0 mg/kg/day (the highest recommended dose is 4 mg/kg/day). The patients were also on cyclosporine for greater than 15 months (18/26) and/or had a clinically significant increase in serum creatinine for greater than 1 month (21/26). Creatinine levels returned to normal range in 7 of 11 patients in whom cyclosporine therapy was discontinued.

There is an increased risk for the development of skin and lymphoproliferative malignancies in cyclosporine-treated psoriasis patients. The relative risk of malignancies is comparable to that observed in psoriasis patients treated with other immunosuppressive agents.

Tumors were reported in 32 (2.2%) of 1439 psoriasis patients treated with cyclosporine worldwide from clinical trials. Additional tumors have been reported in 7 patients in cyclosporine postmarketing experience. Skin malignancies were reported in 16 (1.1%) of these patients; all but 2 of them had previously received PUVA therapy. Methotrexate was received by 7 patients. UVB and coal tar had been used by 2 and 3 patients, respectively. Seven patients had either a history of previous skin cancer or a potentially predisposing lesion was present prior to cyclosporine exposure. Of the 16 patients with skin cancer, 11 patients had 18 squamous cell carcinomas and 7 patients had 10 basal cell carcinomas. There were two lymphoproliferative malignancies; one case of non-Hodgkin's lymphoma which required chemotherapy, and one case of mycosis fungoides which regressed spontaneously upon discontinuation of cyclosporine. There were four cases of benign lymphocytic infiltration: 3 regressed spontaneously upon discontinuation of cyclosporine, while the fourth regressed despite continuation of the drug. The remainder of the malignancies, 13 cases (0.9%), involved various organs.

Patients should not be treated concurrently with cyclosporine and PUVA or UVB, other radiation therapy, or

Nephrotoxicity vs. Rejection

Parameter	Nephrotoxicity	Rejection
History	Donor >50 years old or hypotensive Prolonged kidney preservation Prolonged anastomosis time Concomitant nephrotoxic drugs	Anti-donor immune response Retransplant patient
Clinical	Often >6 weeks postop[b] Prolonged initial nonfunction (acute tubular necrosis)	Often <4 weeks postop[b] Fever >37.5°C Weight gain >0.5 kg Graft swelling and tenderness Decrease in daily urine volume >500 mL (or 50%)
Laboratory	CyA serum trough level >200 ng/mL Gradual rise in Cr (<0.15 mg/dL/day)[a] Cr plateau <25% above baseline BUN/Cr ≥20	CyA serum trough level <150 ng/mL Rapid rise in Cr (>0.3 mg/dL/day)[a] Cr >25% above baseline BUN/Cr <20
Biopsy	Arteriolopathy (medial hypertrophy[a], hyalinosis, nodular deposits, intimal thickening, endothelial vacuolization, progressive scarring) Tubular atrophy, isometric vacuolization, isolated calcifications Minimal edema Mild focal infiltrates[c] Diffuse interstitial fibrosis, often striped form	Endovasculitis[c] (proliferation[a], intimal arteritis[b], necrosis, sclerosis) Tubulitis with RBC[b] and WBC[b] casts, some irregular vacuolization Interstitial edema[c] and hemorrhage[b] Diffuse moderate to severe mononuclear infiltrates[d] Glomerulitis (mononuclear cells)[c]
Aspiration Cytology	CyA deposits in tubular and endothelial cells Fine isometric vacuolization of tubular cells	Inflammatory infiltrate with mononuclear phagocytes, macrophages, lymphoblastoid cells, and activated T-cells These strongly express HLA-DR antigens
Urine Cytology	Tubular cells with vacuolization and granularization	Degenerative tubular cells, plasma cells, and lymphocyturia >20% of sediment
Manometry Ultrasonography	Intracapsular pressure <40 mm Hg[b] Unchanged graft cross sectional area	Intracapsular pressure >40 mm Hg[b] Increase in graft cross sectional area AP diameter ≥ Transverse diameter
Magnetic Resonance Imagery	Normal appearance	Loss of distinct corticomedullary junction, swelling image intensity of parachyma approaching that of psoas, loss of hilar fat
Radionuclide Scan	Normal or generally decreased perfusion Decrease in tubular function (^{131}I-hippuran) > decrease in perfusion (^{99m}Tc DTPA)	Patchy arterial flow Decrease in perfusion > decrease in tubular function Increased uptake of Indium 111 labeled platelets or Tc-99m in colloid
Therapy	Responds to decreased cyclosporine	Responds to increased steroids or antilymphocyte globulin

[a]p <0.05, [b]p <0.01, [c]p <0.001, [d]p <0.0001

---

other immunosuppressive agents, because of the possibility of excessive immunosuppression and the subsequent risk of malignancies. (See **CONTRAINDICATIONS**) Patients should also be warned to protect themselves appropriately when in the sun, and to avoid excessive sun exposure. Patients should be thoroughly evaluated before and during treatment for the presence of malignancies remembering that malignant lesions may be hidden by psoriatic plaques. Skin lesions not typical of psoriasis should be biopsied before starting treatment. Patients should be treated with Gengraf® Capsules (cyclosporine capsules, USP [**MODIFIED**]) only after complete resolution of suspicious lesions, and only if there are no other treatment options. (See **Special Monitoring for Psoriasis Patients**)

Special Excipients
Alcohol (ethanol)
The alcohol content (See **DESCRIPTION**) of Gengraf® should be taken into account when given to patients in whom alcohol intake should be avoided or minimized, e.g., pregnant or breastfeeding women, in patients presenting with liver disease or epilepsy, in alcoholic patients, or pediatric patients. For an adult weighing 70 kg, the maximum daily oral dose would deliver about 1 gram of alcohol which is approximately 6% of the amount of alcohol contained in a standard drink.

Antibiotics	Antineoplastics	Anti-inflammatory Drugs	Gastrointestinal Agents
ciprofloxacin	melphalan	azapropazon	cimetidine
gentamicin		colchicine	ranitidine
tobramycin	**Antifungals**	diclofenac	
vancomycin	amphotericin B	naproxen	**Immunosuppressives**
trimethoprim with	ketoconazole	sulindac	tacrolimus
sulfamethoxazole			

Other Drugs
fibric acid derivatives
(e.g.,bezafibrate, fenofibrate)
methotrexate

PRECAUTIONS
General
Hypertension
Cyclosporine is the active ingredient of Gengraf® Capsules (cyclosporine capsules, USP [**MODIFIED**]). Hypertension is a common side effect of cyclosporine therapy which may persist. (See **ADVERSE REACTIONS** and **DOSAGE AND ADMINISTRATION** for monitoring recommendations) Mild or moderate hypertension is encountered more frequently than severe hypertension and the incidence decreases over time. In recipients of kidney, liver, and heart allografts treated with cyclosporine, antihypertensive therapy may be required. (See **Special Monitoring of Rheumatoid Arthritis and Psoriasis Patients**) However, since cyclosporine may cause hyperkalemia, potassium-sparing diuretics should not be used. While calcium antagonists can be effective agents in treating cyclosporine-associated hypertension, they can interfere with cyclosporine metabolism. (See **Drug Interactions**)

Vaccination
During treatment with cyclosporine, vaccination may be less effective; and the use of live attenuated vaccines should be avoided.

Special Monitoring of Rheumatoid Arthritis Patients
Before initiating treatment, a careful physical examination, including blood pressure measurements (on at least two occasions) and two creatinine levels to estimate baseline should be performed. Blood pressure and serum creatinine should be evaluated every 2 weeks during the initial 3 months and then monthly if the patient is stable. It is advisable to monitor serum creatinine and blood pressure always after an increase of the dose of nonsteroidal anti-inflammatory drugs (NSAIDs) and after initiation of new NSAID therapy during Gengraf® Capsules (cyclosporine capsules, USP [**MODIFIED**]) treatment. If coadministered with methotrexate, CBC and liver function tests are recommended to be monitored monthly. (See also **PRECAUTIONS, General, Hypertension**)

In patients who are receiving cyclosporine, the dose of Gengraf® should be decreased by 25% to 50% if hypertension occurs. If hypertension persists, the dose of Gengraf® should be further reduced or blood pressure should be controlled with antihypertensive agents. In most cases, blood pressure has returned to baseline when cyclosporine was discontinued.

In placebo-controlled trials of rheumatoid arthritis patients, systolic hypertension (defined as an occurrence of two systolic blood pressure readings >140 mmHg) and diastolic hypertension (defined as two diastolic blood pressure readings >90 mmHg) occurred in 33% and 19% of patients treated with cyclosporine, respectively. The corresponding placebo rates were 22% and 8%.

Special Monitoring for Psoriasis Patients

Before initiating treatment, a careful dermatological and physical examination, including blood pressure measurements (on at least two occasions) should be performed. Since Gengraf® (cyclosporine capsules, USP [MODIFIED]) is an immunosuppressive agent, patients should be evaluated for the presence of occult infection on their first physical examination and for the presence of tumors initially, and throughout treatment with Gengraf®. Skin lesions not typical for psoriasis should be biopsied before starting Gengraf®. Patients with malignant or premalignant changes of the skin should be treated with Gengraf® only after appropriate treatment of such lesions and if no other treatment option exists.

Baseline laboratories should include serum creatinine (on two occasions), BUN, CBC, serum magnesium, potassium, uric acid, and lipids.

The risk of cyclosporine nephropathy is reduced when the starting dose is low (2.5 mg/kg/day), the maximum dose does not exceed 4.0 mg/kg/day, serum creatinine is monitored regularly while cyclosporine is administered, and the dose of Gengraf® is decreased when the rise in creatinine is greater than or equal to 25% above the patient's pretreatment level. The increase in creatinine is generally reversible upon timely decrease of the dose of Gengraf® or its discontinuation.

Serum creatinine and BUN should be evaluated every 2 weeks during the initial 3 months of therapy and then monthly if the patient is stable. If the serum creatinine is greater than or equal to 25% above the patient's pretreatment level, serum creatinine should be repeated within two weeks. If the change in serum creatinine remains greater than or equal to 25% above baseline, Gengraf® should be reduced by 25% to 50%. If at **any time** the serum creatinine increases by greater than or equal to 50% above pretreatment level, Gengraf® should be reduced by 25% to 50%. Gengraf® should be discontinued if reversibility (within 25% of baseline) of serum creatinine is not achievable after two dosage modifications. It is advisable to monitor serum creatinine after an increase of the dose of nonsteroidal anti-inflammatory drug and after initiation of new nonsteroidal anti-inflammatory therapy during Gengraf® treatment.

Blood pressure should be evaluated every 2 weeks during the initial 3 months of therapy and then monthly if the patient is stable, or more frequently when dosage adjustments are made. Patients without a history of previous hypertension before initiation of treatment with Gengraf®, should have the drug reduced by 25%-50% if found to have sustained hypertension. If the patient continues to be hypertensive despite multiple reductions of Gengraf®, then Gengraf® should be discontinued. For patients with treated hypertension, before the initiation of Gengraf® therapy, their medication should be adjusted to control hypertension while on Gengraf®. Gengraf® should be discontinued if a change in hypertension management is not effective or tolerable.

CBC, uric acid, potassium, lipids, and magnesium should also be monitored every 2 weeks for the first 3 months of therapy, and then monthly if the patient is stable or more frequently when dosage adjustments are made. Gengraf® dosage should be reduced by 25%-50% for any abnormality of clinical concern.

In controlled trials of cyclosporine in psoriasis patients, cyclosporine blood concentrations did not correlate well with either improvement or with side effects such as renal dysfunction.

Information for Patients: Patients should be advised that any change of cyclosporine formulation should be made cautiously and only under physician supervision because it may result in the need for a change in dosage.

Patients should be informed of the necessity of repeated laboratory tests while they are receiving cyclosporine. Patients should be advised of the potential risks during pregnancy and informed of the increased risk of neoplasia. Patients should also be informed of the risk of hypertension and renal dysfunction.

Patients should be advised that during treatment with cyclosporine, vaccination may be less effective and the use of live attenuated vaccines should be avoided.

Patients should be advised to take Gengraf® on a consistent schedule with regard to time of day and relation to meals. Grapefruit and grapefruit juice affect metabolism, increasing blood concentration of cyclosporine, thus should be avoided.

Laboratory Tests

In all patients treated with cyclosporine, renal and liver functions should be assessed repeatedly by measurement of serum creatinine, BUN, serum bilirubin, and liver enzymes. Serum lipids, magnesium, and potassium should also be monitored. Cyclosporine blood concentrations should be routinely monitored in transplant patients (See **DOSAGE AND ADMINISTRATION, Blood Concentration Monitoring in Transplant Patients**), and periodically monitored in rheumatoid arthritis patients.

Drug Interactions

A. Effect of Drugs and Other Agents on Cyclosporine Pharmacokinetics and/or Safety

All of the individual drugs cited below are well substantiated to interact with cyclosporine. In addition, concomitant use of NSAIDs with cyclosporine, particularly in the setting of dehydration, may potentiate renal dysfunction. Caution should be exercised when using other drugs which are known to impair renal function. (See **WARNINGS, Nephrotoxicity**)

Drugs That May Potentiate Renal Dysfunction
[See table at bottom of previous page]
During the concomitant use of a drug that may exhibit additive or synergistic renal impairment with cyclosporine, close monitoring of renal function (in particular serum creatinine) should be performed. If a significant impairment of renal function occurs, the dosage of the coadministered drug should be reduced or an alternative treatment considered. Cyclosporine is extensively metabolized by CYP 3A isoenzymes, in particular CYP3A4, and is a substrate of the multidrug efflux transporter P-glycoprotein. Various agents are known to either increase or decrease plasma or whole blood concentrations of cyclosporine usually by inhibition or induction of CYP3A4 or P-glycoprotein transporter or both. Compounds that decrease cyclosporine absorption such as orlistat should be avoided. Appropriate Gengraf® dosage adjustment to achieve the desired cyclosporine concentrations is essential when drugs that significantly alter cyclosporine concentrations are used concomitantly. (See **Blood Concentration Monitoring**)

1. Drugs That Increase Cyclosporine Concentrations
[See table above]
HIV Protease inhibitors
The HIV protease inhibitors (e.g., indinavir, nelfinavir, ritonavir, and saquinavir) are known to inhibit cytochrome P-450 3A and thus could potentially increase the concentrations of cyclosporine, however no formal studies of the interaction are available. Care should be exercised when these drugs are administered concomitantly.
Grapefruit juice
Grapefruit and grapefruit juice affect metabolism, increasing blood concentrations of cyclosporine, thus should be avoided.

2. Drugs/Dietary Supplements That Decrease Cyclosporine Concentrations

Antibiotics	Anticonvulsants	Other Drugs/Dietary Supplements
nafcillin	carbamazepine	bosentan

Calcium Channel Blockers	Antifungals	Antibiotics	Glucocorticoids	Other Drugs
diltiazem	fluconazole	azithromycin	methylprednisolone	Allopurinol
nicardipine	itraconazole	clarithromycin		Amiodarone
verapamil	ketoconazole	erythromycin		Bromocriptine
	voriconazole	quinupristin/ dalfopristin		colchicine
				danazol
				imatinib
				metoclopramide
				nefazodone
				oral contraceptives

rifampin	oxcarbazepine	octreotide
	phenobarbital	orlistat
	phenytoin	sulfinpyrazone
		St. John's Wort
		terbinafine
		ticlopidine

Bosentan
Coadministration of bosentan (250 to 1000 mg every 12 hours based on tolerability) and cyclosporine (300 mg every 12 hours for 2 days then dosing to achieve a C_{min} of 200 to 250 ng/mL) for 7 days in healthy subjects resulted in decreases in the cyclosporine mean dose-normalized AUC, C_{max}, and trough concentration of approximately 50%, 30%, and 60%, respectively, compared to when cyclosporine was given alone (See also *Effect of Cyclosporine on the Pharmacokinetics and/or Safety of Other Drugs or Agents*). Coadministration of cyclosporine with bosentan should be avoided.
Boceprevir
Coadministration of boceprevir (800 mg three times daily for 7 days) and cyclosporine (100 mg single dose) in healthy subjects resulted in increases in the mean AUC and C_{max} of cyclosporine approximately 2.7-fold and 2-fold, respectively, compared to when cyclosporine was given alone.
Telaprevir
Coadministration of telaprevir (750 mg every 8 hours for 11 days) with cyclosporine (10 mg on day 8) in healthy subjects resulted in increases in the mean dose-normalized AUC and C_{max} of cyclosporine approximately 4.5-fold and 1.3-fold, respectively, compared to when cyclosporine (100 mg single dose) was given alone.

St. John's Wort
There have been reports of a serious drug interaction between cyclosporine and the herbal dietary supplement St. John's Wort. This interaction has been reported to produce a marked reduction in the blood concentrations of cyclosporine, resulting in subtherapeutic levels, rejection of transplanted organs, and graft loss.
Rifabutin
Rifabutin is known to increase the metabolism of other drugs metabolized by the cytochrome P-450 system. The interaction between rifabutin and cyclosporine has not been studied. Care should be exercised when these two drugs are administered concomitantly.
B. Effect of Cyclosporine on the Pharmacokinetics and/or Safety of Other Drugs or Agents
Cyclosporine is an inhibitor of CYP3A4 and of multiple drug efflux transporters (e.g., P-glycoprotein) and may increase plasma concentrations of comedications that are substrates of CYP3A4, P-glycoprotein or organic anion transporter proteins.
Cyclosporine may reduce the clearance of digoxin, colchicine, prednisolone, HMG-CoA reductase inhibitors (statins), and, aliskiren, bosentan, dabigatran, repaglinide, NSAIDs, sirolimus, etoposide, and other drugs.
See the full prescribing information of the other drug for further information and specific recommendations. The decision on coadministration of cyclosporine with other drugs or agents should be made by the healthcare provider following the careful assessment of benefits and risks.
Digoxin
Severe digitalis toxicity has been seen within days of starting cyclosporine in several patients taking digoxin. If digoxin is used concurrently with cyclosporine, serum digoxin concentrations should be monitored.

Continued on next page

Information on the AbbVie, Inc. products listed on these pages is from the prescribing information in use as of July 31, 2016. For more information, please visit rxabbvie.com or call 1-800-633-9110.

Colchicine
There are reports on the potential of cyclosporine to enhance the toxic effects of colchicine such as myopathy and neuropathy, especially in patients with renal dysfunction. Concomitant administration of cyclosporine and colchicine results in significant increases in colchicine plasma concentrations. If colchicine is used concurrently with cyclosporine, a reduction in the dosage of colchicine is recommended.
HMG-CoA reductase inhibitors (statins)
Literature and postmarketing cases of myotoxicity, including muscle pain and weakness, myositis, and rhabdomyolysis, have been reported with concomitant administration of cyclosporine with lovastatin, simvastatin, atorvastatin, pravastatin, and, rarely fluvastatin. When concurrently administered with cyclosporine, the dosage of these statins should be reduced according to label recommendations. Statin therapy needs to be temporarily withheld or discontinued in patients with signs and symptoms of myopathy or those with risk factors predisposing to severe renal injury, including renal failure, secondary to rhabdomyolysis.
Repaglinide
Cyclosporine may increase the plasma concentrations of repaglinide and thereby increase the risk of hypoglycemia. In 12 healthy male subjects who received two doses of 100 mg cyclosporine capsule orally 12 hours apart with a single dose of 0.25 mg repaglinide tablet (one-half of a 0.5mg tablet) orally 13 hours after the cyclosporine initial dose, the repaglinide mean C_{max} and AUC were increased 1.8 fold (range: 0.6 to 3.7 fold) and 2.4 fold (range 1.2 to 5.3 fold), respectively. Close monitoring of blood glucose level is advisable for a patient taking cyclosporine and repaglinide concomitantly.
Ambrisentan
Coadministration of ambrisentan (5 mg daily) and cyclosporine (100 to 150 mg twice daily initially, then dosing to achieve C_{min} 150 to 200 ng/mL) for 8 days in healthy subjects resulted in mean increases in ambrisentan AUC and C_{max} of approximately 2-fold and 1.5-fold, respectively, compared to ambrisentan alone. When coadministering ambrisentan with cyclosporine, the ambrisentan dose should not be titrated to the recommended maximum daily dose.
Anthracycline antibiotics
High doses of cyclosporine (e.g., at starting intravenous dose of 16 mg/kg/day) may increase the exposure to anthracycline antibiotics (e.g., doxorubicin, mitoxantrone, daunorubicin) in cancer patients.
Aliskiren
Cyclosporine alters the pharmacokinetics of aliskiren, a substrate of P-glycoprotein and CYP3A4. In 14 healthy subjects who received concomitantly single doses of cyclosporine (200 mg) and reduced dose aliskiren (75 mg), the mean C_{max} of aliskiren was increased by approximately 2.5-fold (90% CI: 1.96 to 3.17) and the mean AUC by approximately 4.3 fold (90% CI: 3.52 to 5.21), compared to when these subjects received aliskiren alone. The concomitant administration of aliskiren with cyclosporine prolonged the median aliskiren elimination half-life (26 hours versus 43 to 45 hours) and the T_{max} (0.5 hours versus 1.5 to 2.0 hours). The mean AUC and C_{max} of cyclosporine were comparable to reported literature values. Coadministration of cyclosporine and aliskiren in these subjects also resulted in an increase in the number and/or intensity of adverse events, mainly headache, hot flush, nausea, vomiting, and somnolence. The coadministration of cyclosporine with aliskiren is not recommended.
Bosentan
In healthy subjects, coadministration of bosentan and cyclosporine resulted in time-dependent mean increases in dose-normalized bosentan trough concentrations (i.e., approximately 21-fold on day 1 and 2-fold on day 8 (steady state)) compared to when bosentan was given alone as a single dose on day 1. (See also *Effect of Drugs and Other Agents on Cyclosporine Pharmacokinetics and/or Safety*) Coadministration of cyclosporine with bosentan should be avoided.
Dabigatran
The effect of cyclosporine on dabigatran concentrations had not been formally studied. Concomitant administration of dabigatran and cyclosporine may result in increased plasma dabigatran concentrations due to the P-gp inhibitory activity of cyclosporine. Coadministration of cyclosporine with dabigatran should be avoided.
Potassium-Sparing Diuretics
Cyclosporine should not be used with potassium-sparing diuretics because hyperkalemia can occur. Caution is also required when cyclosporine is coadministered with potassium sparing drugs (e.g., angiotensin converting enzyme inhibitors, angiotensin II receptor antagonists), potassium-containing drugs as well as in patients on a potassium rich diet. Control of potassium levels in these situations is advisable.
Nonsteroidal Anti-inflammatory Drug (NSAID) Interactions
Clinical status and serum creatinine should be closely monitored when cyclosporine is used with NSAIDs in rheumatoid arthritis patients. (See **WARNINGS**)
Pharmacodynamic interactions have been reported to occur between cyclosporine and both naproxen and sulindac, in that concomitant use is associated with additive decreases in renal function, as determined by ^{99m}Tc-diethylenetriaminepentaacetic acid (DTPA) and (*p*-aminohippuric acid) PAH clearances. Although concomitant administration of diclofenac does not affect blood concentrations of cyclosporine, it has been associated with approximate doubling of diclofenac blood concentrations and occasional reports of reversible decreases in renal function. Consequently, the dose of diclofenac should be in the lower end of the therapeutic range.
Methotrexate Interaction
Preliminary data indicate that when methotrexate and cyclosporine were coadministered to rheumatoid arthritis patients (N=20), methotrexate concentrations (AUCs) were increased approximately 30% and the concentrations (AUCs) of its metabolite, 7-hydroxy methotrexate, were decreased by approximately 80%. The clinical significance of this interaction is not known. Cyclosporine concentrations do not appear to have been altered (N=6).
Sirolimus
Elevations in serum creatinine were observed in studies using sirolimus in combination with full-dose cyclosporine. This effect is often reversible with cyclosporine dose reduction. Simultaneous coadministration of cyclosporine significantly increases blood levels of sirolimus. To minimize increases in sirolimus concentrations, it is recommended that sirolimus be given 4 hours after cyclosporine administration.
Nifedipine
Frequent gingival hyperplasia when nifedipine is given concurrently with cyclosporine has been reported. The concomitant use of nifedipine should be avoided in patients in whom gingival hyperplasia develops as a side effect of cyclosporine.
Methylprednisolone
Convulsions when high dose methylprednisolone is given concurrently with cyclosporine have been reported.
Other Immunosuppressive Drugs and Agents
Psoriasis patients receiving other immunosuppressive agents or radiation therapy (including PUVA and UVB) should not receive concurrent cyclosporine because of the possibility of excessive immunosuppression.
C. Effect of Cyclosporine on the Efficacy of Live Vaccines
During treatment with cyclosporine, vaccination may be less effective. The use of live vaccines should be avoided.
For additional information on Cyclosporine Drug Interactions please contact AbbVie Inc. Medical Information Department at 1-800-633-9110.

Carcinogenesis, Mutagenesis, and Impairment of Fertility
Carcinogenicity studies were carried out in male and female rats and mice. In the 78-week mouse study, evidence of a statistically significant trend was found for lymphocytic lymphomas in females, and the incidence of hepatocellular carcinomas in mid-dose males significantly exceeded the control value. In the 24-month rat study, pancreatic islet cell adenomas significantly exceeded the control rate in the low dose level. Doses used in the mouse and rat studies were 0.01 to 0.16 times the clinical maintenance dose (6 mg/kg). The hepatocellular carcinomas and pancreatic islet cell adenomas were not dose related. Published reports indicate that co-treatment of hairless mice with UV irradiation and cyclosporine or other immunosuppressive agents shorten the time to skin tumor formation compared to UV irradiation alone.
Cyclosporine was not mutagenic in appropriate test systems. Cyclosporine has not been found to be mutagenic/genotoxic in the Ames Test, the V79-HGPRT Test, the micronucleus test in mice and Chinese hamsters, the chromosome-aberration tests in Chinese hamster bone-marrow, the mouse dominant lethal assay, and the DNA-repair test in sperm from treated mice. A recent study analyzing sister chromatid exchange (SCE) induction by cyclosporine using human lymphocytes *in vitro* gave indication of a positive effect (i.e., induction of SCE), at high concentrations in this system. In two published research studies, rabbits exposed to cyclosporine *in utero* (10 mg/kg/day subcutaneously) demonstrated reduced numbers of nephrons, renal hypertrophy, systemic hypertension and progressive renal insufficiency up to 35 weeks of age. Pregnant rats which received 12 mg/kg/day of cyclosporine intravenously (twice the recommended human intravenous dose) had fetuses with an increased incidence of ventricular septal defect. These findings have not been demonstrated in other species and their relevance for humans is unknown. No impairment in fertility was demonstrated in studies in male and female rats.
Widely distributed papillomatosis of the skin was observed after chronic treatment of dogs with cyclosporine at 9 times the human initial psoriasis treatment dose of 2.5 mg/kg, where doses are expressed on a body surface area basis. This papillomatosis showed a spontaneous regression upon discontinuation of cyclosporine.
An increased incidence of malignancy is a recognized complication of immunosuppression in recipients of organ transplants and patients with rheumatoid arthritis and psoriasis. The most common forms of neoplasms are non-Hodgkin's lymphoma and carcinomas of the skin. The risk of malignancies in cyclosporine recipients is higher than in the normal, healthy population but similar to that in patients receiving other immunosuppressive therapies. Reduction or discontinuance of immunosuppression may cause the lesions to regress.
In psoriasis patients on cyclosporine, development of malignancies, especially those of the skin has been reported. (See **WARNINGS**) Skin lesions not typical for psoriasis should be biopsied before starting cyclosporine treatment. Patients with malignant or premalignant changes of the skin should be treated with cyclosporine only after appropriate treatment of such lesions and if no other treatment option exists.

Pregnancy
Pregnancy Category C
Animal studies have shown reproductive toxicity in rats and rabbits. Cyclosporine gave no evidence of mutagenic or teratogenic effects in the standard test systems with oral application (rats up to 17 mg/kg and rabbits up to 30 mg/kg per day orally). Only at dose levels toxic to dams, were adverse effects seen in reproduction studies in rats. Cyclosporine has been shown to be embryo- and fetotoxic in rats and rabbits following oral administration at maternally toxic doses. Fetal toxicity was noted in rats at 0.8 and rabbits at 5.4 times the transplant doses in humans of 6.0 mg/kg, where dose corrections are based on body surface area. Cyclosporine was embryo- and fetotoxic as indicated by increased pre- and postnatal mortality and reduced fetal weight together with related skeletal retardation.
There are no adequate and well-controlled studies in pregnant women and, therefore, Gengraf® Capsules (cyclosporine capsules, USP [**MODIFIED**]) should not be used during pregnancy unless the potential benefit to the mother justifies the potential risk to the fetus.
In pregnant transplant recipients who are being treated with immunosuppressants the risk of premature birth is increased. The following data represent the reported outcomes of 116 pregnancies in women receiving cyclosporine during pregnancy, 90% of whom were transplant patients, and most of whom received cyclosporine throughout the entire gestational period. The only consistent patterns of abnormality were premature birth (gestational period of 28 to 36 weeks) and low birth weight for gestational age. Sixteen fetal losses occurred. Most of the pregnancies (85 of 100) were complicated by disorders; including, preeclampsia, eclampsia, premature labor, abruptio placentae, oligohydramnios, Rh incompatibility, and fetoplacental dysfunction. Pre-term delivery occurred in 47%. Seven malformations were reported in 5 viable infants and in 2 cases of fetal loss. Twenty-eight percent of the infants were small for gestational age. Neonatal complications occurred in 27%. Therefore, the risks and benefits of using Gengraf® during pregnancy should be carefully weighed.
A limited number of observations in children exposed to cyclosporine *in utero* are available, up to an age of approximately 7 years. Renal function and blood pressure in these children were normal.
Because of the possible disruption of maternal-fetal interaction, the risk/benefit ratio of using Gengraf® in psoriasis patients during pregnancy should carefully be weighed with serious consideration for discontinuation of Gengraf®.

The alcohol content of the Gengraf® formulations should also be taken into account in pregnant women. (See **WARNINGS, Special Excipients**)

Nursing Mothers
Cyclosporine is present in breast milk. Because of the potential for serious adverse drug reactions in nursing infants from Gengraf®, a decision should be made whether to discontinue nursing or to discontinue the drug, taking into account the importance of the drug to the mother. Gengraf® contains ethanol. Ethanol will be present in human milk at levels similar to that found in maternal serum and if present in breast milk will be orally absorbed by a nursing infant (See **WARNINGS**).

Pediatric Use
Although no adequate and well-controlled studies have been completed in children, transplant recipients as young as one year of age have received cyclosporine (**MODIFIED**) with no unusual adverse effects. The safety and efficacy of cyclosporine (**MODIFIED**) treatment in children with juvenile rheumatoid arthritis or psoriasis below the age of 18 have not been established.

Geriatric Use
In rheumatoid arthritis clinical trials with cyclosporine, 17.5% of patients were age 65 or older. These patients were more likely to develop systolic hypertension on therapy, and more likely to show serum creatinine rises ≥50% above the baseline after 3 to 4 months of therapy.
Clinical studies of cyclosporine oral solution (modified) in transplant and psoriasis patients did not include a sufficient number of subjects aged 65 and over to determine whether they respond differently from younger subjects. Other reported clinical experiences have not identified differences in response between the elderly and younger patients. In general, dose selection for an elderly patient should be cautious, usually starting at the low end of the dosing range, reflecting the greater frequency of decreased hepatic, renal, or cardiac function, and of concomitant disease or other drug therapy.

ADVERSE REACTIONS
Kidney, Liver, and Heart Transplantation
The principal adverse reactions of cyclosporine therapy are renal dysfunction, tremor, hirsutism, hypertension, and gum hyperplasia.

Hypertension
Hypertension, which is usually mild to moderate, may occur in approximately 50% of patients following renal transplantation and in most cardiac transplant patients.

Glomerular Capillary Thrombosis
Glomerular capillary thrombosis has been found in patients treated with cyclosporine and may progress to graft failure. The pathologic changes resembled those seen in the hemolytic-uremic syndrome and included thrombosis of the renal microvasculature, with platelet-fibrin thrombi occluding glomerular capillaries and afferent arterioles, microangiopathic hemolytic anemia, thrombocytopenia, and decreased renal function. Similar findings have been observed when other immunosuppressives have been employed post-transplantation.

Hypomagnesemia
Hypomagnesemia has been reported in some, but not all, patients exhibiting convulsions while on cyclosporine therapy. Although magnesium-depletion studies in normal subjects suggest that hypomagnesemia is associated with neurologic disorders, multiple factors, including hypertension, high dose methylprednisolone, hypocholesterolemia, and nephrotoxicity associated with high plasma concentrations of cyclosporine appear to be related to the neurological manifestations of cyclosporine toxicity.

Clinical Studies
In controlled studies, the nature, severity, and incidence of the adverse events that were observed in 493 transplanted patients treated with cyclosporine (**MODIFIED**) were comparable with those observed in 208 transplanted patients who received Sandimmune® in these same studies when the dosage of the two drugs was adjusted to achieve the same cyclosporine blood trough concentrations.
Based on the historical experience with Sandimmune®, the following reactions occurred in 3% or greater of 892 patients involved in clinical trials of kidney, heart, and liver transplants.

[See table above]

Among 705 kidney transplant patients treated with cyclosporine oral solution (Sandimmune®) in clinical trials, the reason for treatment discontinuation was renal toxicity in 5.4%, infection in 0.9%, lack of efficacy in 1.4%, acute tu-

Body System	Adverse Reactions	Randomized Kidney Patients		Cyclosporine Patients (Sandimmune®)		
		Sandimmune® (N = 227) %	Azathioprine (N = 228) %	Kidney (N = 705) %	Heart (N = 112) %	Liver (N = 75) %
Genitourinary						
	Renal Dysfunction	32	6	25	38	37
Cardiovascular						
	Hypertension	26	18	13	53	27
	Cramps	4	<1	2	<1	0
Skin						
	Hirsutism	21	<1	21	28	45
	Acne	6	8	2	2	1
Central Nervous System						
	Tremor	12	0	21	31	55
	Convulsions	3	1	1	4	5
	Headache	2	<1	2	15	4
Gastrointestinal						
	Gum Hyperplasia	4	0	9	5	16
	Diarrhea	3	<1	3	4	8
	Nausea/Vomiting	2	<1	4	10	4
	Hepatotoxicity	<1	<1	4	7	4
	Abdominal Discomfort	<1	0	<1	7	0
Autonomic Nervous System						
	Paresthesia	3	0	1	2	1
	Flushing	<1	0	4	0	4
Hematopoietic						
	Leukopenia	2	19	<1	6	0
	Lymphoma	<1	0	1	6	1
Respiratory						
	Sinusitis	<1	0	4	3	7
Miscellaneous						
	Gynecomastia	<1	0	<1	4	4

bular necrosis in 1.0%, lymphoproliferative disorders in 0.3%, hypertension in 0.3%, and other reasons in 0.7% of the patients.
The following reactions occurred in 2% or less of cyclosporine-treated patients: allergic reactions, anemia, anorexia, confusion, conjunctivitis, edema, fever, brittle fingernails, gastritis, hearing loss, hiccups, hyperglycemia, migraine (Gengraf®), muscle pain, peptic ulcer, thrombocytopenia, tinnitus.
The following reactions occurred rarely: anxiety, chest pain, constipation, depression, hair breaking, hematuria, joint pain, lethargy, mouth sores, myocardial infarction, night sweats, pancreatitis, pruritus, swallowing difficulty, tingling, upper GI bleeding, visual disturbance, weakness, weight loss.
Patients receiving immunosuppressive therapies, including cyclosporine and cyclosporine - containing regimens, are at increased risk of infections (viral, bacterial, fungal, parasitic). Both generalized and localized infections can occur. Pre-existing infections may also be aggravated. Fatal outcomes have been reported. (See **WARNINGS**)

Infectious Complications in Historical Randomized Studies in Renal Transplant Patients Using Sandimmune®

Complication	Cyclosporine Treatment (N=227) % of Complications	Azathioprine with Steroids* (N=228) % of Complications
Septicemia	5.3	4.8
Abscesses	4.4	5.3
Systemic Fungal Infection	2.2	3.9
Local Fungal Infection	7.5	9.6
Cytomegalovirus	4.8	12.3
Other Viral Infections	15.9	18.4
Urinary Tract Infections	21.1	20.2
Wound and Skin Infections	7.0	10.1
Pneumonia	6.2	9.2

*Some patients also received ALG.

Postmarketing Experience, Kidney, Liver and Heart Transplantation
Hepatotoxicity
Cases of hepatotoxicity and liver injury including cholestasis, jaundice, hepatitis and liver failure; serious and/or fatal outcomes have been reported. (See **WARNINGS, Hepatotoxicity**)

Increased Risk of Infections
Cases of JC virus-associated progressive multifocal leukoencephalopathy (PML), sometimes fatal; and polyoma virus-associated nephropathy (PVAN), especially BK virus resulting in graft loss have been reported. (See **WARNINGS, Polyoma Virus Infection**)
Headache, including Migraine
Cases of migraine have been reported. In some cases, patients have been unable to continue cyclosporine. Pain of treatment discontinuation should be made by the treating physician following the careful assessment of benefits versus risks.
Pain of lower extremities
Isolated cases of pain of lower extremities have been reported in association with cyclosporine. Pain of lower extremities has also been noted as part of Calcineurin-Inhibitor Induced Pain Syndrome (CIPS) as described in the literature.

Rheumatoid Arthritis
The principal adverse reactions associated with the use of cyclosporine in rheumatoid arthritis are renal dysfunction (See **WARNINGS**), hypertension (See **PRECAUTIONS**), headache, gastrointestinal disturbances, and hirsutism/hypertrichosis.
In rheumatoid arthritis patients treated in clinical trials within the recommended dose range, cyclosporine therapy was discontinued in 5.3% of the patients because of hypertension and in 7% of the patients because of increased creatinine. These changes are usually reversible with timely dose decrease or drug discontinuation. The frequency and severity of serum creatinine elevations increase with dose and duration of cyclosporine therapy. These elevations are likely to become more pronounced without dose reduction or discontinuation.
The following adverse events occurred in controlled clinical trials:
[See table on page 658]
In addition, the following adverse events have been reported in 1% to <3% of the rheumatoid arthritis patients in the cyclosporine treatment group in controlled clinical trials.
Autonomic Nervous System: dry mouth, increased sweating
Body as a Whole: allergy, asthenia, hot flushes, malaise, overdose, procedure NOS*, tumor NOS*, weight decrease, weight increase

Continued on next page

Information on the AbbVie, Inc. products listed on these pages is from the prescribing information in use as of July 31, 2016. For more information, please visit rxabbvie.com or call 1-800-633-9110.

Cardiovascular: abnormal heart sounds, cardiac failure, myocardial infarction, peripheral ischemia

Central and Peripheral Nervous System: hypoesthesia, neuropathy, vertigo

Endocrine: goiter

Gastrointestinal: constipation, dysphagia, enanthema, eructation, esophagitis, gastric ulcer, gastritis, gastroenteritis, gingival bleeding, glossitis, peptic ulcer, salivary gland enlargement, tongue disorder, tooth disorder

Infection: abscess, bacterial infection, cellulitis, folliculitis, fungal infection, herpes simplex, herpes zoster, renal abscess, moniliasis, tonsillitis, viral infection

Hematologic: anemia, epistaxis, leukopenia, lymphadenopathy

Liver and Biliary System: bilirubinemia

Metabolic and Nutritional: diabetes mellitus, hyperkalemia, hyperuricemia, hypoglycemia

Musculoskeletal System: arthralgia, bone fracture, bursitis, joint dislocation, myalgia, stiffness, synovial cyst, tendon disorder

Neoplasms: breast fibroadenosis, carcinoma

Psychiatric: anxiety, confusion, decreased libido, emotional lability, impaired concentration, increased libido, nervousness, paroniria, somnolence

Reproductive (Female): breast pain, uterine hemorrhage

Respiratory System: abnormal chest sounds, bronchospasm

Skin and Appendages: abnormal pigmentation, angioedema, dermatitis, dry skin, eczema, nail disorder, pruritus, skin disorder, urticaria

Special Senses: abnormal vision, cataract, conjunctivitis, deafness, eye pain, taste perversion, tinnitus, vestibular disorder

Urinary System: abnormal urine, hematuria, increased BUN, micturition urgency, nocturia, polyuria, pyelonephritis, urinary incontinence

*NOS=Not Otherwise Specified

Psoriasis

The principal adverse reactions associated with the use of cyclosporine in patients with psoriasis are renal dysfunction, headache, hypertension, hypertriglyceridemia, hirsutism/hypertrichosis, paresthesia or hyperesthesia, influenza-like symptoms, nausea/vomiting, diarrhea, abdominal discomfort, lethargy, and musculoskeletal or joint pain.

In psoriasis patients treated in US controlled clinical studies within the recommended dose range, cyclosporine therapy was discontinued in 1.0% of the patients because of hypertension and in 5.4% of the patients because of increased creatinine. In the majority of cases, these changes were reversible after dose reduction or discontinuation of cyclosporine.

There has been one reported death associated with the use of cyclosporine in psoriasis. A 27-year-old male developed renal deterioration and was continued on cyclosporine. He had progressive renal failure leading to death.

Frequency and severity of serum creatinine increases with dose and duration of cyclosporine therapy. These elevations are likely to become more pronounced and may result in irreversible renal damage without dose reduction or discontinuation.

[See table below]

The following events occurred in 1% to less than 3% of psoriasis patients treated with cyclosporine:

Body as a Whole: fever, flushes, hot flushes

Cardiovascular: chest pain

Central and Peripheral Nervous System: appetite increased, insomnia, dizziness, nervousness, vertigo

Gastrointestinal: abdominal distention, constipation, gingival bleeding

Liver and Biliary System: hyperbilirubinemia

Neoplasms: skin malignancies [squamous cell (0.9%) and basal cell (0.4%) carcinomas]

Reticuloendothelial: platelet, bleeding, and clotting disorders, red blood cell disorder

Respiratory: infection, viral and other infection

Skin and Appendages: acne, folliculitis, keratosis, pruritus, rash, dry skin

Urinary System: micturition frequency

Vision: abnormal vision

Mild hypomagnesemia and hyperkalemia may occur but are asymptomatic. Increases in uric acid may occur and attacks of gout have been rarely reported. A minor and dose related hyperbilirubinemia has been observed in the absence of hepatocellular damage. Cyclosporine therapy may be associated with a modest increase of serum triglycerides or cholesterol. Elevations of triglycerides (>750 mg/dL) occur in about 15% of psoriasis patients; elevations of cholesterol (>300 mg/dL) are observed in less than 3% of psoriasis patients. Generally these laboratory abnormalities are reversible upon dose reduction or discontinuation of cyclosporine.

Postmarketing Experience, Psoriasis

Cases of transformation to erythrodermic psoriasis or generalized pustular psoriasis upon either withdrawal or reduction of cyclosporine in patients with chronic plaque psoriasis have been reported.

OVERDOSAGE

There is a minimal experience with cyclosporine overdosage. Forced emesis and gastric lavage can be of value up to 2 hours after administration of Gengraf® Capsules (cyclosporine capsules, USP [MODIFIED]). Transient hepatotoxicity and nephrotoxicity may occur which should resolve following drug withdrawal. Oral doses of cyclosporine up to 10 g (about 150 mg/kg) have been tolerated with relatively minor clinical consequences, such as vomiting, drowsiness, headache, tachycardia and, in a few patients, moderately severe, reversible impairment of renal function. However, serious symptoms of intoxication have been reported following accidental parenteral overdosage with cyclosporine in premature neonates. General supportive measures and symptomatic treatment should be followed in all cases of overdosage. Cyclosporine is not dialyzable to any great extent, nor is it cleared well by charcoal hemoperfusion. The oral dosage at which half of experimental animals are estimated to die is 31 times, 39 times, and >54 times the human maintenance dose for transplant patients (6mg/kg; corrections based on body surface area) in mice, rats, and rabbits.

DOSAGE AND ADMINISTRATION

Gengraf® Capsules (cyclosporine capsules, USP [MODIFIED]) has increased bioavailability in comparison to Sandimmune® Soft Gelatin Capsules (cyclosporine capsules, USP). Gengraf® and Sandimmune® are not bioequivalent and cannot be used interchangeably without physician supervision.

The daily dose of Gengraf® Capsules (cyclosporine capsules, USP [MODIFIED]) should always be given in two divided doses (BID). It is recommended that Gengraf® be administered on a consistent schedule with regard to time of day and relation to meals. Grapefruit and grapefruit juice affect metabolism, increasing blood concentration of cyclosporine, thus should be avoided.

Specific Populations

Renal Impairment in Kidney, Liver, and Heart Transplantation

Cyclosporine undergoes minimal renal elimination and its pharmacokinetics do not appear to be significantly altered in patients with end-stage renal disease who receive routine hemodialysis treatments (See **CLINICAL PHARMACOLOGY**). However, due to its nephrotoxic potential (See **WARNINGS**), careful monitoring of renal function is recommended; cyclosporine dosage should be reduced if indicated. (See **WARNINGS** and **PRECAUTIONS**)

Renal Impairment in Rheumatoid Arthritis and Psoriasis

Patients with impaired renal function should not receive cyclosporine. (See **CONTRAINDICATIONS, WARNINGS** and **PRECAUTIONS**)

Hepatic Impairment

The clearance of cyclosporine may be significantly reduced in severe liver disease patients (See **CLINICAL PHARMACOLOGY**). Dose reduction may be necessary in patients with severe liver impairment to maintain blood concentrations within the recommended target range (See **WARNINGS** and **PRECAUTIONS**)

Newly Transplanted Patients

The initial oral dose of Gengraf® Capsules (cyclosporine capsules, USP [MODIFIED]) can be given 4 to 12 hours prior to transplantation or be given postoperatively. The initial dose of Gengraf® varies depending on the transplanted organ and the other immunosuppressive agents included in the immunosuppressive protocol. In newly transplanted patients, the initial oral dose of Gengraf® is the same as the initial oral dose of Sandimmune®. Suggested initial doses are available from the results of a 1994 survey of the use of Sandimmune® in US transplant centers. The mean ± SD initial doses were 9±3 mg/kg/day for renal transplant patients (75 centers), 8±4 mg/kg/day for liver transplant patients (30 centers), and 7±3 mg/kg/day for heart transplant patients (24 centers). Total daily doses were divided into two equal daily doses. The Gengraf® dose is subsequently adjusted to achieve a pre-defined cyclosporine blood concentration. (See **Blood Concentration Monitoring in Transplant Patients**, below) If cyclosporine trough blood concentrations are used,

Adverse Events Occurring in 3% or More of Psoriasis Patients in Controlled Clinical Trials			
Body System*	Preferred Term	Cyclosporine (MODIFIED) (N=182)	Sandimmune® (N=185)
Infection or Potential Infection		24.7%	24.3%
	Influenza-Like Symptoms	9.9%	8.1%
	Upper Respiratory Tract Infections	7.7%	11.3%
Cardiovascular System		28.0%	25.4%
	Hypertension**	27.5%	25.4%
Urinary System		24.2%	16.2%
	Increased Creatinine	19.8%	15.7%
Central and Peripheral Nervous System		26.4%	20.5%
	Headache	15.9%	14.0%
	Paresthesia	7.1%	4.8%
Musculoskeletal System		13.2%	8.7%
	Arthralgia	6.0%	1.1%
Body As a Whole–General		29.1%	22.2%
	Pain	4.4%	3.2%
Metabolic and Nutritional		9.3%	9.7%
Reproductive, Female		8.5% (4 of 47 females)	11.5% (6 of 52 females)
Resistance Mechanism		18.7%	21.1%
Skin and Appendages		17.6%	15.1%
	Hypertrichosis	6.6%	5.4%
Respiratory System		5.0%	6.5%
	Bronchospasm, Coughing, Dyspnea, Rhinitis	5.0%	4.9%
Psychiatric		5.0%	3.8%
Gastrointestinal System		19.8%	28.7%
	Abdominal Pain	2.7%	6.0%
	Diarrhea	5.0%	5.9%
	Dyspepsia	2.2%	3.2%
	Gum Hyperplasia	3.8%	6.0%
	Nausea	5.5%	5.9%
White cell and RES		4.4%	2.7%

*Total percentage of events within the system
**Newly occurring hypertension=SBP ≥160 mm Hg and/or DBP ≥90 mm Hg

the target range is the same for Gengraf® as for Sandimmune®. Using the same trough concentration target range for Gengraf® as for Sandimmune® results in greater cyclosporine exposure when Gengraf® is administered. (See **Pharmacokinetics, Absorption**) Dosing should be titrated based on clinical assessments of rejection and tolerability. Lower Gengraf® doses may be sufficient as maintenance therapy.

Adjunct therapy with adrenal corticosteroids is recommended initially. Different tapering dosage schedules of prednisone appear to achieve similar results. A representative dosage schedule based on the patient's weight started with 2.0 mg/kg/day for the first 4 days tapered to 1.0 mg/kg/day by 1 week, 0.6 mg/kg/day by 2 weeks, 0.3 mg/kg/day by 1 month, and 0.15 mg/kg/day by 2 months and thereafter as a maintenance dose. Steroid doses may be further tapered on an individualized basis depending on status of patient and function of graft. Adjustments in dosage of prednisone must be made according to the clinical situation.

Conversion from Sandimmune® (Cyclosporine) to Gengraf® Capsules (Cyclosporine Capsules, USP [MODIFIED]) in Transplant Patients

In transplanted patients who are considered for conversion to Gengraf® from Sandimmune® (cyclosporine), Gengraf® should be started with the same daily dose as was previously used with Sandimmune® (cyclosporine) (1:1 dose conversion). The Gengraf® dose should subsequently be adjusted to attain the pre-conversion cyclosporine blood trough concentration. Using the same trough concentration target range for Gengraf® as for Sandimmune® (cyclosporine) results in greater cyclosporine exposure when Gengraf® is administered. (See **Pharmacokinetics, Absorption**) Patients with suspected poor absorption of Sandimmune® (cyclosporine) require different dosing strategies. (See **Transplant Patients with Poor Absorption of Sandimmune® (cyclosporine)**, below) In some patients, the increase in blood trough concentration is more pronounced and may be of clinical significance.

Until the blood trough concentration attains the pre-conversion value, it is strongly recommended that the cyclosporine blood trough concentration be monitored every 4 to 7 days after conversion to Gengraf®. In addition, clinical safety parameters such as serum creatinine and blood pressure should be monitored every two weeks during the first two months after conversion. If the blood trough concentrations are outside the desired range and/or if the clinical safety parameters worsen, the dosage of Gengraf® must be adjusted accordingly.

Transplant Patients with Poor Absorption of Sandimmune® (Cyclosporine)

Patients with lower than expected cyclosporine blood trough concentrations in relation to the oral dose of Sandimmune® (cyclosporine) may have poor or inconsistent absorption of cyclosporine from Sandimmune® (cyclosporine). After conversion to Gengraf® Capsules (cyclosporine capsules, USP [**MODIFIED**]), patients tend to have higher cyclosporine concentrations. **Due to the increase in bioavailability of cyclosporine following conversion to Gengraf®, the cyclosporine blood trough concentration may exceed the target range. Particular caution should be exercised when converting patients to Gengraf® at doses greater than 10 mg/kg/day.** The dose of Gengraf® should be titrated individually based on cyclosporine trough concentrations, tolerability, and clinical response. In this population the cyclosporine blood trough concentration should be measured more frequently, at least twice a week (daily, if initial dose exceeds 10 mg/kg/day) until the concentration stabilizes within the desired range.

Rheumatoid Arthritis

The initial dose of Gengraf® Capsules (cyclosporine capsules, USP [**MODIFIED**]) is 2.5 mg/kg/day, taken twice daily as a divided (BID) oral dose. Salicylates, NSAIDs, and oral corticosteroids may be continued. (See **WARNINGS** and **PRECAUTIONS, Drug Interactions**) Onset of action generally occurs between 4 and 8 weeks. If insufficient clinical benefit is seen and tolerability is good (including serum creatinine less than 30% above baseline), the dose may be increased by 0.5-0.75 mg/kg/day after 8 weeks and again after 12 weeks to a maximum of 4 mg/kg/day. If no benefit is seen by 16 weeks of therapy, Gengraf® therapy should be discontinued.

Dose decreases by 25%-50% should be made at any time to control adverse events, e.g., hypertension elevations in serum creatinine (30% above patient's pretreatment level) or clinically significant laboratory abnormalities. (See **WARNINGS** and **PRECAUTIONS**)

If dose reduction is not effective in controlling abnormalities or if the adverse event or abnormality is severe, Gengraf® should be discontinued. The same initial dose and dosage range should be used if Gengraf® is combined with the recommended dose of methotrexate. Most patients can be treated with Gengraf® doses of 3 mg/kg/day or below when combined with methotrexate doses of up to 15 mg/week. (See **CLINICAL PHARMACOLOGY, Clinical Trials**)

There is limited long-term treatment data. Recurrence of rheumatoid arthritis disease activity is generally apparent within 4 weeks after stopping cyclosporine.

Psoriasis

The initial dose of Gengraf® Capsules (cyclosporine capsules, USP [**MODIFIED**]) should be 2.5 mg/kg/day. Gengraf® should be taken twice daily, as a divided (1.25 mg/kg BID) oral dose. Patients should be kept at that dose for at least 4 weeks, barring adverse events. If significant clinical improvement has not occurred in patients by that time, the patient's dosage should be increased at 2-week intervals. Based on patient response, dose increases of approximately 0.5 mg/kg/day should be made to a maximum of 4.0 mg/kg/day.

Dose decreases by 25% to 50% should be made at any time to control adverse events, e.g., hypertension, elevations in serum creatinine (≥25% above the patient's pretreatment level), or clinically significant laboratory abnormalities.

If dose reduction is not effective in controlling abnormalities, or if the adverse event or abnormality is severe, Gengraf® should be discontinued. (See **Special Monitoring of Psoriasis Patients**)

Patients generally show some improvement in the clinical manifestations of psoriasis in 2 weeks. Satisfactory control and stabilization of the disease may take 12 to 16 weeks to achieve. Results of a dose-titration clinical trial with Gengraf® indicate that an improvement of psoriasis by 75% or more (based on PASI) was achieved in 51% of the patients after 8 weeks and in 79% of the patients after 16 weeks. Treatment should be discontinued if satisfactory response cannot be achieved after 6 weeks at 4 mg/kg/day or the patient's maximum tolerated dose. Once a patient is adequately controlled and appears stable the dose of Gengraf® should be lowered, and the patient treated with the lowest dose that maintains an adequate response (this should not necessarily be total clearing of the patient). In clinical trials, cyclosporine doses at the lower end of the recommended dosage range were effective in maintaining a satisfactory response in 60% of the patients. Doses below 2.5 mg/kg/day may also be equally effective.

Upon stopping treatment with cyclosporine, relapse will occur in approximately 6 weeks (50% of the patients) to 16 weeks (75% of the patients). In the majority of patients rebound does not occur after cessation of treatment with cyclosporine. Thirteen cases of transformation of chronic plaque psoriasis to more severe forms of psoriasis have been reported. There were 9 cases of pustular and 4 cases of erythrodermic psoriasis. Long term experience with Gengraf® in psoriasis patients is limited and continuous treatment for extended periods greater than one year is not recommended. Alternation with other forms of treatment should be considered in the long term management of patients with this life long disease.

Blood Concentration Monitoring in Transplant Patients

Transplant centers have found blood concentration monitoring of cyclosporine to be an essential component of patient management. Of importance to blood concentration analysis are the type of assay used, the transplanted organ, and other immunosuppressant agents being administered. While no fixed relationship has been established, blood concentration monitoring may assist in the clinical evaluation of rejection and toxicity, dose adjustments, and the assessment of compliance.

Various assays have been used to measure blood concentrations of cyclosporine. Older studies using a nonspecific assay often cited concentrations that were roughly twice those of the specific assays. Therefore, comparison between concentrations in the published literature and an individual patient concentration using current assays must be made with detailed knowledge of the assay methods employed. Current assay results are also not interchangeable and their use should be guided by their approved labeling. A discussion of the different assay methods is contained in Annals of Clinical Biochemistry 1994;31:420-446. While several assays and assay matrices are available, there is a consensus that parent-compound-specific assays correlate best with clinical events. Of these, HPLC is the standard reference, but the monoclonal antibody RIAs and the monoclonal antibody FPIA offer sensitivity, reproducibility, and convenience. Most clinicians base their monitoring on trough cyclosporine concentrations. Applied Pharmacokinetics, Principles of Therapeutic Drug Monitoring (1992) contains a broad discussion of cyclosporine pharmacokinetics and drug monitoring techniques. Blood concentration monitoring is not a replacement for renal function monitoring or tissue biopsies.

HOW SUPPLIED

Gengraf® Capsules (cyclosporine capsules, USP [MODIFIED])

25 mg

Oval, white imprinted in blue, 25 mg, and the code OR. Packages of 30 unit-dose blisters. (**NDC** 0074-3108-32).

Oval, white imprinted in blue, the **"a"** logo, 25 mg, and the code OR. Packages of 30 unit-dose blisters. (**NDC** 0074-6463-32).

50 mg

Oval, white, with one blue stripe, imprinted in blue, 50 mg, and the code OS. Packages of 30 unit-dose blisters. (**NDC** 0074-0541-30).

100 mg

Oval, white, with two blue stripes, imprinted in blue, 100 mg, and the code OT. Packages of 30 unit-dose blisters. (**NDC** 0074-3109-32).

Oval, white, with two blue stripes, imprinted in blue, the **"a"** logo, 100 mg, and the code OT. Packages of 30 unit-dose blisters. (**NDC** 0074-6479-32).

Store and Dispense

In the original unit-dose container at controlled room temperature

68°-77°F (20°-25°C). (See USP Controlled Room Temperature).

Sandimmune® is a registered trademark of Novartis Pharmaceuticals Corporation.

AbbVie Inc., North Chicago, IL 60064, U.S.A.

03-B247 December, 2015

Shown in Product Identification Guide, page 505

HUMIRA® ℞

[hu-mare-ah]

(adalimumab)

injection, for subcutaneous use

HIGHLIGHTS OF PRESCRIBING INFORMATION

These highlights do not include all the information needed to use HUMIRA® (adalimumab) safely and effectively. See full prescribing information for HUMIRA.

HUMIRA (adalimumab) injection, for subcutaneous use

Initial U.S. Approval: 2002

WARNING: SERIOUS INFECTIONS AND MALIGNANCY

See full prescribing information for complete boxed warning.

SERIOUS INFECTIONS (5.1, 6.1):

- **Increased risk of serious infections leading to hospitalization or death, including tuberculosis (TB), bacterial sepsis, invasive fungal infections (such as histoplasmosis), and infections due to other opportunistic pathogens.**
- **Discontinue HUMIRA if a patient develops a serious infection or sepsis during treatment.**
- **Perform test for latent TB; if positive, start treatment for TB prior to starting HUMIRA.**
- **Monitor all patients for active TB during treatment, even if initial latent TB test is negative.**

MALIGNANCY (5.2):

- **Lymphoma and other malignancies, some fatal, have been reported in children and adolescent patients treated with TNF blockers including HUMIRA.**

Continued on next page

Information on the AbbVie, Inc. products listed on these pages is from the prescribing information in use as of July 31, 2016. For more information, please visit rxabbvie.com or call 1-800-633-9110.

- Post-marketing cases of hepatosplenic T-cell lymphoma (HSTCL), a rare type of T-cell lymphoma, have occurred in adolescent and young adults with inflammatory bowel disease treated with TNF blockers including HUMIRA.

RECENT MAJOR CHANGES

Indications and Usage, Hidradenitis Suppurativa (1.9)	9/2015
Indications and Usage, Uveitis (1.10)	6/2016
Dosage and Administration, Plaque Psoriasis and Uveitis (2.6)	6/2016
Dosage and Administration, Hidradenitis Suppurativa (2.7)	9/2015
Dosage and Administration, General Considerations for Administration (2.9)	11/2015
Warnings and Precautions, Malignancies (5.2)	6/2016
Warnings and Precautions, Neurologic Reactions (5.5)	6/2016
Warnings and Precautions, Immunizations (5.10)	6/2016

INDICATIONS AND USAGE

HUMIRA is a tumor necrosis factor (TNF) blocker indicated for treatment of:

- **Rheumatoid Arthritis (RA) (1.1):** Reducing signs and symptoms, inducing major clinical response, inhibiting the progression of structural damage, and improving physical function in adult patients with moderately to severely active RA.
- **Juvenile Idiopathic Arthritis (JIA) (1.2):** Reducing signs and symptoms of moderately to severely active polyarticular JIA in patients 2 years of age and older.
- **Psoriatic Arthritis (PsA) (1.3):** Reducing signs and symptoms, inhibiting the progression of structural damage, and improving physical function in adult patients with active PsA.
- **Ankylosing Spondylitis (AS) (1.4):** Reducing signs and symptoms in adult patients with active AS.
- **Adult Crohn's Disease (CD) (1.5):** Reducing signs and symptoms and inducing and maintaining clinical remission in adult patients with moderately to severely active Crohn's disease who have had an inadequate response to conventional therapy. Reducing signs and symptoms and inducing clinical remission in these patients if they have also lost response to or are intolerant to infliximab.
- **Pediatric Crohn's Disease (1.6):** Reducing signs and symptoms and inducing and maintaining clinical remission in patients 6 years of age and older with moderately to severely active Crohn's disease who have had an inadequate response to corticosteroids or immunomodulators such as azathioprine, 6-mercaptopurine, or methotrexate.
- **Ulcerative Colitis (UC) (1.7):** Inducing and sustaining clinical remission in adult patients with moderately to severely active ulcerative colitis who have had an inadequate response to immunosuppressants such as corticosteroids, azathioprine or 6-mercaptopurine (6-MP). The effectiveness of HUMIRA has not been established in patients who have lost response to or were intolerant to TNF blockers.
- **Plaque Psoriasis (Ps) (1.8):** The treatment of adult patients with moderate to severe chronic plaque psoriasis who are candidates for systemic therapy or phototherapy, and when other systemic therapies are medically less appropriate.
- **Hidradenitis Suppurativa (HS) (1.9):** The treatment of moderate to severe hidradenitis suppurativa.
- **Uveitis (UV) (1.10):** The treatment of non-infectious intermediate, posterior and panuveitis in adult patients.

DOSAGE AND ADMINISTRATION

- Administered by subcutaneous injection (2)

Rheumatoid Arthritis, Psoriatic Arthritis, Ankylosing Spondylitis (2.1):
- 40 mg every other week.
  - Some patients with RA not receiving methotrexate may benefit from increasing the frequency to 40 mg every week.

Juvenile Idiopathic Arthritis (2.2):
- *10 kg (22 lbs) to <15 kg (33 lbs):* 10 mg every other week
- *15 kg (33 lbs) to < 30 kg (66 lbs):* 20 mg every other week
- *≥30 kg (66 lbs):* 40 mg every other week

Adult Crohn's Disease and Ulcerative Colitis (2.3, 2.5):
- Initial dose (Day 1): 160 mg (four 40 mg injections in one day or two 40 mg injections per day for two consecutive days)
- Second dose two weeks later (Day 15): 80 mg
  - Two weeks later (Day 29): Begin a maintenance dose of 40 mg every other week.

- For patients with Ulcerative Colitis only: Only continue HUMIRA in patients who have shown evidence of clinical remission by eight weeks (Day 57) of therapy.

Pediatric Crohn's Disease (2.4):
- *17 kg (37 lbs) to < 40 kg (88 lbs):*
- Initial dose (Day 1): 80 mg (two 40 mg injections in one day)
- Second dose two weeks later (Day 15): 40 mg
  - Two weeks later (Day 29): Begin a maintenance dose of 20 mg every other week.
- *≥ 40 kg (88 lbs):*
- Initial dose (Day 1): 160 mg (four 40 mg injections in one day or two 40 mg injections per day for two consecutive days)
- Second dose two weeks later (Day 15): 80 mg (two 40 mg injections in one day)
  - Two weeks later (Day 29): Begin a maintenance dose of 40 mg every other week.

Plaque Psoriasis or Uveitis (2.6):
- 80 mg initial dose, followed by 40 mg every other week starting one week after initial dose.

Hidradenitis Suppurativa (2.7):
- Initial dose (Day 1): 160 mg (given as four 40 mg injections on Day 1 or as two 40 mg injections per day on Days 1 and 2)
- Second dose two weeks later (Day 15): 80 mg (two 40 mg injections in one day)
- Third (Day 29) and subsequent doses: 40 mg every week.

DOSAGE FORMS AND STRENGTHS

- Injection: 40 mg/0.8 mL in a single-use prefilled pen (HUMIRA Pen) (3)
- Injection: 40 mg/0.4 mL in a single-use prefilled pen (HUMIRA Pen) (3)
- Injection: 40 mg/0.8 mL in a single-use prefilled glass syringe (3)
- Injection: 40 mg/0.4 mL in a single-use prefilled glass syringe (3)
- Injection: 20 mg/0.4 mL in a single-use prefilled glass syringe (3)
- Injection: 10 mg/0.2 mL in a single-use prefilled glass syringe (3)
- Injection: 40 mg/0.8 mL in a single-use glass vial for institutional use only (3)

CONTRAINDICATIONS

None (4)

WARNINGS AND PRECAUTIONS

- *Serious infections:* Do not start HUMIRA during an active infection. If an infection develops, monitor carefully, and stop HUMIRA if infection becomes serious (5.1)
- *Invasive fungal infections:* For patients who develop a systemic illness on HUMIRA, consider empiric antifungal therapy for those who reside or travel to regions where mycoses are endemic (5.1)
- *Malignancies:* Incidence of malignancies was greater in HUMIRA-treated patients than in controls (5.2)
- *Anaphylaxis or serious allergic reactions* may occur (5.3)
- *Hepatitis B virus reactivation:* Monitor HBV carriers during and several months after therapy. If reactivation occurs, stop HUMIRA and begin anti-viral therapy (5.4)
- *Demyelinating disease:* Exacerbation or new onset, may occur (5.5)
- *Cytopenias, pancytopenia:* Advise patients to seek immediate medical attention if symptoms develop, and consider stopping HUMIRA (5.6)
- *Heart failure:* Worsening or new onset, may occur (5.8)
- *Lupus-like syndrome:* Stop HUMIRA if syndrome develops (5.9)

ADVERSE REACTIONS

Most common adverse reactions (incidence >10%): infections (e.g. upper respiratory, sinusitis), injection site reactions, headache and rash (6.1)

To report SUSPECTED ADVERSE REACTIONS, contact AbbVie Inc. at 1-800-633-9110 or FDA at 1-800-FDA-1088 or www.fda.gov/medwatch

DRUG INTERACTIONS

- *Abatacept:* Increased risk of serious infection (5.1, 5.11, 7.2)
- *Anakinra:* Increased risk of serious infection (5.1, 5.7, 7.2)
- *Live vaccines:* Avoid use with HUMIRA (5.10, 7.3)

See 17 for PATIENT COUNSELING INFORMATION and Medication Guide.

Revised: 7/2016

FULL PRESCRIBING INFORMATION: CONTENTS*
WARNING: SERIOUS INFECTIONS AND MALIGNANCY

* Sections or subsections omitted from the full prescribing information are not listed.

FULL PRESCRIBING INFORMATION

WARNING: SERIOUS INFECTIONS AND MALIGNANCY

SERIOUS INFECTIONS

Patients treated with HUMIRA are at increased risk for developing serious infections that may lead to hospitalization or death *[see Warnings and Precautions (5.1)]*. Most patients who developed these infections were taking concomitant immunosuppressants such as methotrexate or corticosteroids.

Discontinue HUMIRA if a patient develops a serious infection or sepsis.

Reported infections include:
- Active tuberculosis (TB), including reactivation of latent TB. Patients with TB have frequently presented

with disseminated or extrapulmonary disease. Test patients for latent TB before HUMIRA use and during therapy. Initiate treatment for latent TB prior to HUMIRA use.
- Invasive fungal infections, including histoplasmosis, coccidioidomycosis, candidiasis, aspergillosis, blastomycosis, and pneumocystosis. Patients with histoplasmosis or other invasive fungal infections may present with disseminated, rather than localized, disease. Antigen and antibody testing for histoplasmosis may be negative in some patients with active infection. Consider empiric anti-fungal therapy in patients at risk for invasive fungal infections who develop severe systemic illness.
- Bacterial, viral and other infections due to opportunistic pathogens, including Legionella and Listeria.

Carefully consider the risks and benefits of treatment with HUMIRA prior to initiating therapy in patients with chronic or recurrent infection.

Monitor patients closely for the development of signs and symptoms of infection during and after treatment with HUMIRA, including the possible development of TB in patients who tested negative for latent TB infection prior to initiating therapy *[see Warnings and Precautions (5.1) and Adverse Reactions (6.1)]*.

MALIGNANCY

Lymphoma and other malignancies, some fatal, have been reported in children and adolescent patients treated with TNF blockers including HUMIRA *[see Warnings and Precautions (5.2)]*. Post-marketing cases of hepatosplenic T-cell lymphoma (HSTCL), a rare type of T-cell lymphoma, have been reported in patients treated with TNF blockers including HUMIRA. These cases have had a very aggressive disease course and have been fatal. The majority of reported TNF blocker cases have occurred in patients with Crohn's disease or ulcerative colitis and the majority were in adolescent and young adult males. Almost all these patients had received treatment with azathioprine or 6-mercaptopurine (6–MP) concomitantly with a TNF blocker at or prior to diagnosis. It is uncertain whether the occurrence of HSTCL is related to use of a TNF blocker or a TNF blocker in combination with these other immunosuppressants *[see Warnings and Precautions (5.2)]*.

1 INDICATIONS AND USAGE

1.1 Rheumatoid Arthritis
HUMIRA is indicated for reducing signs and symptoms, inducing major clinical response, inhibiting the progression of structural damage, and improving physical function in adult patients with moderately to severely active rheumatoid arthritis. HUMIRA can be used alone or in combination with methotrexate or other non-biologic disease-modifying anti-rheumatic drugs (DMARDs).

1.2 Juvenile Idiopathic Arthritis
HUMIRA is indicated for reducing signs and symptoms of moderately to severely active polyarticular juvenile idiopathic arthritis in patients 2 years of age and older. HUMIRA can be used alone or in combination with methotrexate.

1.3 Psoriatic Arthritis
HUMIRA is indicated for reducing signs and symptoms, inhibiting the progression of structural damage, and improving physical function in adult patients with active psoriatic arthritis. HUMIRA can be used alone or in combination with non-biologic DMARDs.

1.4 Ankylosing Spondylitis
HUMIRA is indicated for reducing signs and symptoms in adult patients with active ankylosing spondylitis.

1.5 Adult Crohn's Disease
HUMIRA is indicated for reducing signs and symptoms and inducing and maintaining clinical remission in adult patients with moderately to severely active Crohn's disease who have had an inadequate response to conventional therapy. HUMIRA is indicated for reducing signs and symptoms and inducing clinical remission in these patients if they have also lost response to or are intolerant to infliximab.

1.6 Pediatric Crohn's Disease
HUMIRA is indicated for reducing signs and symptoms and inducing and maintaining clinical remission in pediatric patients 6 years of age and older with moderately to severely active Crohn's disease who have had an inadequate response to corticosteroids or immunomodulators such as azathioprine, 6-mercaptopurine, or methotrexate.

Pediatric Patients	Induction Dose	Maintenance Dose Starting at Week 4 (Day 29)
17 kg (37 lbs) to < 40 kg (88 lbs)	• 80 mg on Day 1 (administered as two 40 mg injections in one day); and • 40 mg two weeks later (on Day 15)	• 20 mg every other week
≥ 40 kg (88 lbs)	• 160 mg on Day 1 (administered as four injections in one day or as two 40 mg injections per day for two consecutive days); and • 80 mg two weeks later (on Day 15) (administered as two 40 mg injections in one day)	• 40 mg every other week

1.7 Ulcerative Colitis
HUMIRA is indicated for inducing and sustaining clinical remission in adult patients with moderately to severely active ulcerative colitis who have had an inadequate response to immunosuppressants such as corticosteroids, azathioprine or 6-mercaptopurine (6-MP). The effectiveness of HUMIRA has not been established in patients who have lost response to or were intolerant to TNF blockers *[see Clinical Studies (14.7)]*.

1.8 Plaque Psoriasis
HUMIRA is indicated for the treatment of adult patients with moderate to severe chronic plaque psoriasis who are candidates for systemic therapy or phototherapy, and when other systemic therapies are medically less appropriate. HUMIRA should only be administered to patients who will be closely monitored and have regular follow-up visits with a physician *[see Boxed Warning and Warnings and Precautions (5)]*.

1.9 Hidradenitis Suppurativa
HUMIRA is indicated for the treatment of moderate to severe hidradenitis suppurativa.

1.10 Uveitis
HUMIRA is indicated for the treatment of non-infectious intermediate, posterior and panuveitis in adult patients.

2 DOSAGE AND ADMINISTRATION
HUMIRA is administered by subcutaneous injection.

2.1 Rheumatoid Arthritis, Psoriatic Arthritis, and Ankylosing Spondylitis
The recommended dose of HUMIRA for adult patients with rheumatoid arthritis (RA), psoriatic arthritis (PsA), or ankylosing spondylitis (AS) is 40 mg administered every other week. Methotrexate (MTX), other non-biologic DMARDS, glucocorticoids, nonsteroidal anti-inflammatory drugs (NSAIDs), and/or analgesics may be continued during treatment with HUMIRA. In the treatment of RA, some patients not taking concomitant MTX may derive additional benefit from increasing the dosing frequency of HUMIRA to 40 mg every week.

2.2 Juvenile Idiopathic Arthritis
The recommended dose of HUMIRA for patients 2 years of age and older with polyarticular juvenile idiopathic arthritis (JIA) is based on weight as shown below. MTX, glucocorticoids, NSAIDs, and/or analgesics may be continued during treatment with HUMIRA.

Patients (2 years of age and older)	Dose
10 kg (22 lbs) to <15 kg (33 lbs)	10 mg every other week (10 mg Prefilled Syringe)
15 kg (33 lbs) to <30 kg (66 lbs)	20 mg every other week (20 mg Prefilled Syringe)
≥30 kg (66 lbs)	40 mg every other week (HUMIRA Pen or 40 mg Prefilled Syringe)

HUMIRA has not been studied in patients with polyarticular JIA less than 2 years of age or in patients with a weight below 10 kg.

2.3 Adult Crohn's Disease
The recommended HUMIRA dose regimen for adult patients with Crohn's disease (CD) is 160 mg initially on Day 1 (given as four 40 mg injections in one day or as two 40 mg injections per day for two consecutive days), followed by 80 mg two weeks later (Day 15). Two weeks later (Day 29) begin a maintenance dose of 40 mg every other week. Aminosalicylates and/or corticosteroids may be continued during treatment with HUMIRA. Azathioprine, 6-mercaptopurine (6-MP) *[see Warnings and Precautions (5.2)]* or MTX may be continued during treatment with HUMIRA if necessary. The use of HUMIRA in CD beyond one year has not been evaluated in controlled clinical studies.

2.4 Pediatric Crohn's Disease
The recommended HUMIRA dose regimen for pediatric patients 6 years of age and older with Crohn's disease (CD) is based on body weight as shown below:
[See table above]

2.5 Ulcerative Colitis
The recommended HUMIRA® (adalimumab) dose regimen for adult patients with ulcerative colitis (UC) is 160 mg initially on Day 1 (given as four 40 mg injections in one day or as two 40 mg injections per day for two consecutive days), followed by 80 mg two weeks later (Day 15). Two weeks later (Day 29) continue with a dose of 40 mg every other week.

Only continue HUMIRA in patients who have shown evidence of clinical remission by eight weeks (Day 57) of therapy. Aminosalicylates and/or corticosteroids may be continued during treatment with HUMIRA. Azathioprine and 6-mercaptopurine (6-MP) *[see Warnings and Precautions (5.2)]* may be continued during treatment with HUMIRA if necessary.

2.6 Plaque Psoriasis or Uveitis
The recommended dose of HUMIRA for adult patients with plaque psoriasis (Ps) or Uveitis (UV) is an initial dose of 80 mg, followed by 40 mg given every other week starting one week after the initial dose. The use of HUMIRA in moderate to severe chronic Ps beyond one year has not been evaluated in controlled clinical studies.

2.7 Hidradenitis Suppurativa
The recommended dose of HUMIRA for adult patients with hidradenitis suppurativa (HS) is 160 mg (given as four 40 mg injections on Day 1 or as two 40 mg injections per day on Days 1 and 2), followed by 80 mg two weeks later (Day 15). Begin 40 mg weekly dosing two weeks later (Day 29).

2.8 Monitoring to Assess Safety
Prior to initiating HUMIRA and periodically during therapy, evaluate patients for active tuberculosis and test for latent infection *[see Warnings and Precautions (5.1)]*.

2.9 General Considerations for Administration
HUMIRA is intended for use under the guidance and supervision of a physician. A patient may self-inject HUMIRA or a caregiver may inject HUMIRA using either the HUMIRA Pen or prefilled syringe if a physician determines that it is appropriate, and with medical follow-up, as necessary, after proper training in subcutaneous injection technique.

You may leave HUMIRA at room temperature for about 15 to 30 minutes before injecting. Do not remove the cap or cover while allowing it to reach room temperature. Carefully inspect the solution in the HUMIRA Pen, prefilled syringe, or single-use institutional use vial for particulate matter and discoloration prior to subcutaneous administration. If particulates and discolorations are noted, do not use the product. HUMIRA does not contain preservatives; therefore, discard unused portions of drug remaining from the syringe. NOTE: Instruct patients sensitive to latex not to handle the gray needle cover of the 27 gauge HUMIRA Pen and prefilled syringe because it contains natural rubber latex *[see How Supplied/Storage and Handling (16) for specific information]*.

Continued on next page

Information on the AbbVie, Inc. products listed on these pages is from the prescribing information in use as of July 31, 2016. For more information, please visit rxabbvie.com or call 1-800-633-9110.

Instruct patients using the HUMIRA Pen or prefilled syringe to inject the full amount in the syringe, according to the directions provided in the Instructions for Use *[see Instructions for Use]*.

Injections should occur at separate sites in the thigh or abdomen. Rotate injection sites and do not give injections into areas where the skin is tender, bruised, red or hard.

The HUMIRA single-use institutional use vial is for administration within an institutional setting only, such as a hospital, physician's office or clinic. Withdraw the dose using a sterile needle and syringe and administer promptly by a healthcare provider within an institutional setting. Only administer one dose per vial. The vial does not contain preservatives; therefore, discard unused portions.

3   DOSAGE FORMS AND STRENGTHS

• Pen

Injection: 40 mg/0.8 mL of HUMIRA is provided by a single-use pen (HUMIRA Pen), containing a 1 mL prefilled glass syringe with a fixed 27 gauge, ½ inch needle and a gray needle cover.

Injection: 40 mg/0.4 mL of HUMIRA is provided by a single-use pen (HUMIRA Pen), containing a 1 mL prefilled glass syringe with a fixed 29 gauge thin wall, ½ inch needle and a black needle cover.

• Prefilled Syringe

Injection: 40 mg/0.8 mL of HUMIRA is provided by a single-use, 1 mL prefilled glass syringe with a fixed 27 gauge, ½ inch needle and a gray needle cover.

Injection: 40 mg/0.4 mL of HUMIRA is provided by a single-use, 1 mL prefilled glass syringe with a fixed 29 gauge thin wall, ½ inch needle and a black needle cover.

Injection: 20 mg/0.4 mL of HUMIRA is provided by a single-use, 1 mL prefilled glass syringe with a fixed 27 gauge, ½ inch needle and a gray needle cover.

Injection: 10 mg/0.2 mL of HUMIRA is provided by a single-use, 1 mL prefilled glass syringe with a fixed 27 gauge, ½ inch needle and a gray needle cover.

• Single-Use Institutional Use Vial

Injection: 40 mg/0.8 mL of HUMIRA is provided by a single-use, glass vial for institutional use only.

4   CONTRAINDICATIONS

None.

5   WARNINGS AND PRECAUTIONS

5.1   Serious Infections

Patients treated with HUMIRA are at increased risk for developing serious infections involving various organ systems and sites that may lead to hospitalization or death *[see Boxed Warning]*. Opportunistic infections due to bacterial, mycobacterial, invasive fungal, viral, parasitic, or other opportunistic pathogens including aspergillosis, blastomycosis, candidiasis, coccidioidomycosis, histoplasmosis, legionellosis, listeriosis, pneumocystosis and tuberculosis have been reported with TNF blockers. Patients have frequently presented with disseminated rather than localized disease.

The concomitant use of a TNF blocker and abatacept or anakinra was associated with a higher risk of serious infections in patients with rheumatoid arthritis (RA); therefore, the concomitant use of HUMIRA and these biologic products is not recommended in the treatment of patients with RA *[see Warnings and Precautions (5.7, 5.11) and Drug Interactions (7.2)]*.

Treatment with HUMIRA should not be initiated in patients with an active infection, including localized infections. Patients greater than 65 years of age, patients with co-morbid conditions and/or patients taking concomitant immunosuppressants (such as corticosteroids or methotrexate), may be at greater risk of infection. Consider the risks and benefits of treatment prior to initiating therapy in patients:

• with chronic or recurrent infection;
• who have been exposed to tuberculosis;
• with a history of an opportunistic infection;
• who have resided or traveled in areas of endemic tuberculosis or endemic mycoses, such as histoplasmosis, coccidioidomycosis, or blastomycosis; or
• with underlying conditions that may predispose them to infection.

Tuberculosis

Cases of reactivation of tuberculosis and new onset tuberculosis infections have been reported in patients receiving HUMIRA, including patients who have previously received treatment for latent or active tuberculosis. Reports included cases of pulmonary and extrapulmonary (i.e., disseminated) tuberculosis. Evaluate patients for tuberculosis risk factors and test for latent infection prior to initiating HUMIRA and periodically during therapy.

Treatment of latent tuberculosis infection prior to therapy with TNF blocking agents has been shown to reduce the risk of tuberculosis reactivation during therapy. Prior to initiating HUMIRA, assess if treatment for latent tuberculosis is needed; and consider an induration of ≥ 5 mm a positive tuberculin skin test result, even for patients previously vaccinated with Bacille Calmette-Guerin (BCG).

Consider anti-tuberculosis therapy prior to initiation of HUMIRA in patients with a past history of latent or active tuberculosis in whom an adequate course of treatment cannot be confirmed, and for patients with a negative test for latent tuberculosis but having risk factors for tuberculosis infection. Despite prophylactic treatment for tuberculosis, cases of reactivated tuberculosis have occurred in patients treated with HUMIRA. Consultation with a physician with expertise in the treatment of tuberculosis is recommended to aid in the decision whether initiating anti-tuberculosis therapy is appropriate for an individual patient.

Strongly consider tuberculosis in the differential diagnosis in patients who develop a new infection during HUMIRA treatment, especially in patients who have previously or recently traveled to countries with a high prevalence of tuberculosis, or who have had close contact with a person with active tuberculosis.

Monitoring

Closely monitor patients for the development of signs and symptoms of infection during and after treatment with HUMIRA, including the development of tuberculosis in patients who tested negative for latent tuberculosis infection prior to initiating therapy. Tests for latent tuberculosis infection may also be falsely negative while on therapy with HUMIRA.

Discontinue HUMIRA if a patient develops a serious infection or sepsis. For a patient who develops a new infection during treatment with HUMIRA, closely monitor them, perform a prompt and complete diagnostic workup appropriate for an immunocompromised patient, and initiate appropriate antimicrobial therapy.

Invasive Fungal Infections

If patients develop a serious systemic illness and they reside or travel in regions where mycoses are endemic, consider invasive fungal infection in the differential diagnosis. Antigen and antibody testing for histoplasmosis may be negative in some patients with active infection. Consider appropriate empiric antifungal therapy, taking into account both the risk for severe fungal infection and the risks of antifungal therapy, while a diagnostic workup is being performed. To aid in the management of such patients, consider consultation with a physician with expertise in the diagnosis and treatment of invasive fungal infections.

5.2   Malignancies

Consider the risks and benefits of TNF-blocker treatment including HUMIRA prior to initiating therapy in patients with a known malignancy other than a successfully treated non-melanoma skin cancer (NMSC) or when considering continuing a TNF blocker in patients who develop a malignancy.

Malignancies in Adults

In the controlled portions of clinical trials of some TNF-blockers, including HUMIRA, more cases of malignancies have been observed among TNF-blocker-treated adult patients compared to control-treated adult patients. During the controlled portions of 39 global HUMIRA clinical trials in adult patients with rheumatoid arthritis (RA), psoriatic arthritis (PsA), ankylosing spondylitis (AS), Crohn's disease (CD), ulcerative colitis (UC), plaque psoriasis (Ps), hidradenitis suppurativa (HS) and uveitis (UV), malignancies, other than non-melanoma (basal cell and squamous cell) skin cancer, were observed at a rate (95% confidence interval) of 0.7 (0.48, 1.03) per 100 patient-years among 7973 HUMIRA-treated patients versus a rate of 0.7 (0.41, 1.17) per 100 patient-years among 4848 control-treated patients (median duration of treatment of 4 months for HUMIRA-treated patients and 4 months for control-treated patients). In 52 global controlled and uncontrolled clinical trials of HUMIRA in adult patients with RA, PsA, AS, CD, UC, Ps, HS and UV the most frequently observed malignancies, other than lymphoma and NMSC, were breast, colon, prostate, lung, and melanoma. The malignancies in HUMIRA-treated patients in the controlled and uncontrolled portions of the studies were similar in type and number to what would be expected in the general U.S. population according to the SEER database (adjusted for age, gender, and race).[1]

In controlled trials of other TNF blockers in adult patients at higher risk for malignancies (i.e., patients with COPD

with a significant smoking history and cyclophosphamide-treated patients with Wegener's granulomatosis), a greater portion of malignancies occurred in the TNF blocker group compared to the control group.

Non-Melanoma Skin Cancer

During the controlled portions of 39 global HUMIRA clinical trials in adult patients with RA, PsA, AS, CD, UC, Ps, HS and UV, the rate (95% confidence interval) of NMSC was 0.8 (0.52, 1.09) per 100 patient-years among HUMIRA-treated patients and 0.2 (0.10, 0.59) per 100 patient-years among control-treated patients. Examine all patients, and in particular patients with a medical history of prior prolonged immunosuppressant therapy or psoriasis patients with a history of PUVA treatment for the presence of NMSC prior to and during treatment with HUMIRA.

Lymphoma and Leukemia

In the controlled portions of clinical trials of all the TNF-blockers in adults, more cases of lymphoma have been observed among TNF-blocker-treated patients compared to control-treated patients. In the controlled portions of 39 global HUMIRA clinical trials in adult patients with RA, PsA, AS, CD, UC, Ps, HS and UV, 2 lymphomas occurred among 7973 HUMIRA-treated patients versus 1 among 4848 control-treated patients. In 52 global controlled and uncontrolled clinical trials of HUMIRA in adult patients with RA, PsA, AS, CD, UC, Ps, HS and UV with a median duration of approximately 0.7 years, including 24,605 patients and over 40,215 patient-years of HUMIRA, the observed rate of lymphomas was approximately 0.11 per 100 patient-years. This is approximately 3-fold higher than expected in the general U.S. population according to the SEER database (adjusted for age, gender, and race).[1] Rates of lymphoma in clinical trials of HUMIRA cannot be compared to rates of lymphoma in clinical trials of other TNF blockers and may not predict the rates observed in a broader patient population. Patients with RA and other chronic inflammatory diseases, particularly those with highly active disease and/or chronic exposure to immunosuppressant therapies, may be at a higher risk (up to several fold) than the general population for the development of lymphoma, even in the absence of TNF blockers. Post-marketing cases of acute and chronic leukemia have been reported in association with TNF-blocker use in RA and other indications. Even in the absence of TNF-blocker therapy, patients with RA may be at a higher risk (approximately 2-fold) than the general population for the development of leukemia.

Malignancies in Pediatric Patients and Young Adults

Malignancies, some fatal, have been reported among children, adolescents, and young adults who received treatment with TNF-blockers (initiation of therapy ≤ 18 years of age), of which HUMIRA is a member *[see Boxed Warning]*. Approximately half the cases were lymphomas, including Hodgkin's and non-Hodgkin's lymphoma. The other cases represented a variety of different malignancies and included rare malignancies usually associated with immunosuppression and malignancies that are not usually observed in children and adolescents. The malignancies occurred after a median of 30 months of therapy (range 1 to 84 months). Most of the patients were receiving concomitant immunosuppressants. These cases were reported post-marketing and are derived from a variety of sources including registries and spontaneous postmarketing reports.

Postmarketing cases of hepatosplenic T-cell lymphoma (HSTCL), a rare type of T-cell lymphoma, have been reported in patients treated with TNF blockers including HUMIRA *[see Boxed Warning]*. These cases have had a very aggressive disease course and have been fatal. The majority of reported TNF blocker cases have occurred in patients with Crohn's disease or ulcerative colitis and the majority were in adolescent and young adult males. Almost all of these patients had received treatment with the immunosuppressants azathioprine or 6-mercaptopurine (6–MP) concomitantly with a TNF blocker at or prior to diagnosis. It is uncertain whether the occurrence of HSTCL is related to use of a TNF blocker or a TNF blocker in combination with these other immunosuppressants. The potential risk with the combination of azathioprine or 6-mercaptopurine and HUMIRA should be carefully considered.

5.3   Hypersensitivity Reactions

Anaphylaxis and angioneurotic edema have been reported following HUMIRA administration. If an anaphylactic or other serious allergic reaction occurs, immediately discontinue administration of HUMIRA and institute appropriate therapy. In clinical trials of HUMIRA in adults, allergic reactions (e.g., allergic rash, anaphylactoid reaction, fixed drug reaction, non-specified drug reaction, urticaria) have been observed.

5.4 Hepatitis B Virus Reactivation

Use of TNF blockers, including HUMIRA, may increase the risk of reactivation of hepatitis B virus (HBV) in patients who are chronic carriers of this virus. In some instances, HBV reactivation occurring in conjunction with TNF blocker therapy has been fatal. The majority of these reports have occurred in patients concomitantly receiving other medications that suppress the immune system, which may also contribute to HBV reactivation. Evaluate patients at risk for HBV infection for prior evidence of HBV infection before initiating TNF blocker therapy. Exercise caution in prescribing TNF blockers for patients identified as carriers of HBV. Adequate data are not available on the safety or efficacy of treating patients who are carriers of HBV with anti-viral therapy in conjunction with TNF blocker therapy to prevent HBV reactivation. For patients who are carriers of HBV and require treatment with TNF blockers, closely monitor such patients for clinical and laboratory signs of active HBV infection throughout therapy and for several months following termination of therapy. In patients who develop HBV reactivation, stop HUMIRA and initiate effective anti-viral therapy with appropriate supportive treatment. The safety of resuming TNF blocker therapy after HBV reactivation is controlled is not known. Therefore, exercise caution when considering resumption of HUMIRA therapy in this situation and monitor patients closely.

5.5 Neurologic Reactions

Use of TNF blocking agents, including HUMIRA, has been associated with rare cases of new onset or exacerbation of clinical symptoms and/or radiographic evidence of central nervous system demyelinating disease, including multiple sclerosis (MS) and optic neuritis, and peripheral demyelinating disease, including Guillain-Barré syndrome. Exercise caution in considering the use of HUMIRA in patients with preexisting or recent-onset central or peripheral nervous system demyelinating disorders; discontinuation of HUMIRA should be considered if any of these disorders develop. There is a known association between intermediate uveitis and central demyelinating disorders.

5.6 Hematological Reactions

Rare reports of pancytopenia including aplastic anemia have been reported with TNF blocking agents. Adverse reactions of the hematologic system, including medically significant cytopenia (e.g., thrombocytopenia, leukopenia) have been infrequently reported with HUMIRA. The causal relationship of these reports to HUMIRA remains unclear. Advise all patients to seek immediate medical attention if they develop signs and symptoms suggestive of blood dyscrasias or infection (e.g., persistent fever, bruising, bleeding, pallor) while on HUMIRA. Consider discontinuation of HUMIRA therapy in patients with confirmed significant hematologic abnormalities.

5.7 Use with Anakinra

Concurrent use of anakinra (an interleukin-1 antagonist) and another TNF-blocker, was associated with a greater proportion of serious infections and neutropenia and no added benefit compared with the TNF-blocker alone in patients with RA. Therefore, the combination of HUMIRA and anakinra is not recommended [see Drug Interactions (7.2)].

5.8 Heart Failure

Cases of worsening congestive heart failure (CHF) and new onset CHF have been reported with TNF blockers. Cases of worsening CHF have also been observed with HUMIRA. HUMIRA has not been formally studied in patients with CHF; however, in clinical trials of another TNF blocker, a higher rate of serious CHF-related adverse reactions was observed. Exercise caution when using HUMIRA in patients who have heart failure and monitor them carefully.

5.9 Autoimmunity

Treatment with HUMIRA may result in the formation of autoantibodies and, rarely, in the development of a lupus-like syndrome. If a patient develops symptoms suggestive of a lupus-like syndrome following treatment with HUMIRA, discontinue treatment [see Adverse Reactions (6.1)].

5.10 Immunizations

In a placebo-controlled clinical trial of patients with RA, no difference was detected in anti-pneumococcal antibody response between HUMIRA and placebo treatment groups when the pneumococcal polysaccharide vaccine and influenza vaccine were administered concurrently with HUMIRA. Similar proportions of patients developed protective levels of anti-influenza antibodies between HUMIRA

and placebo treatment groups; however, titers in aggregate to influenza antigens were moderately lower in patients receiving HUMIRA. The clinical significance of this is unknown. Patients on HUMIRA may receive concurrent vaccinations, except for live vaccines. No data are available on the secondary transmission of infection by live vaccines in patients receiving HUMIRA.

It is recommended that pediatric patients, if possible, be brought up to date with all immunizations in agreement with current immunization guidelines prior to initiating HUMIRA therapy. Patients on HUMIRA may receive concurrent vaccinations, except for live vaccines.

The safety of administering live or live-attenuated vaccines in infants exposed to HUMIRA *in utero* is unknown. Risks and benefits should be considered prior to vaccinating (live or live-attenuated) exposed infants [see Use in Specific Populations (8.1, 8.4)].

5.11 Use with Abatacept

In controlled trials, the concurrent administration of TNF-blockers and abatacept was associated with a greater proportion of serious infections than the use of a TNF-blocker alone; the combination therapy, compared to the use of a TNF-blocker alone, has not demonstrated improved clinical benefit in the treatment of RA. Therefore, the combination of abatacept with TNF-blockers including HUMIRA is not recommended [see Drug Interactions (7.2)].

6 ADVERSE REACTIONS

The most serious adverse reactions described elsewhere in the labeling include the following:
• Serious Infections [see Warnings and Precautions (5.1)]
• Malignancies [see Warnings and Precautions (5.2)]

6.1 Clinical Trials Experience

Because clinical trials are conducted under widely varying conditions, adverse reaction rates observed in the clinical trials of a drug cannot be directly compared to rates in the clinical trials of another drug and may not reflect the rates observed in practice.

The most common adverse reaction with HUMIRA® (adalimumab) was injection site reactions. In placebo-controlled trials, 20% of patients treated with HUMIRA developed injection site reactions (erythema and/or itching, hemorrhage, pain or swelling), compared to 14% of patients receiving placebo. Most injection site reactions were described as mild and generally did not necessitate drug discontinuation.

The proportion of patients who discontinued treatment due to adverse reactions during the double-blind, placebo-controlled portion of studies in patients with RA (i.e., Studies RA-I, RA-II, RA-III and RA-IV) was 7% for patients taking HUMIRA and 4% for placebo-treated patients. The most common adverse reactions leading to discontinuation of HUMIRA in these RA studies were clinical flare reaction (0.7%), rash (0.3%) and pneumonia (0.3%).

Infections

In the controlled portions of the 39 global HUMIRA clinical trials in adult patients with RA, PsA, AS, CD, UC, Ps, HS and UV, the rate of serious infections was 4.3 per 100 patient-years in 7973 HUMIRA-treated patients versus a rate of 2.9 per 100 patient-years in 4848 control-treated patients. Serious infections observed included pneumonia, septic arthritis, prosthetic and post-surgical infections, erysipelas, cellulitis, diverticulitis, and pyelonephritis [see Warnings and Precautions (5.1)].

Tuberculosis and Opportunistic Infections

In 52 global controlled and uncontrolled clinical trials in RA, PsA, AS, CD, UC, Ps, HS and UV that included 24,605 HUMIRA-treated patients, the rate of reported active tuberculosis was 0.20 per 100 patient-years and the rate of positive PPD conversion was 0.09 per 100 patient-years. In a subgroup of 10,113 U.S. and Canadian HUMIRA-treated patients, the rate of reported active TB was 0.05 per 100 patient-years and the rate of positive PPD conversion was 0.07 per 100 patient-years. These trials included reports of miliary, lymphatic, peritoneal, and pulmonary TB. Most of the TB cases occurred within the first eight months after initiation of therapy and may reflect recrudescence of latent disease. In these global clinical trials, cases of serious opportunistic infections have been reported at an overall rate of 0.05 per 100 patient-years. Some cases of serious opportunistic infections and TB have been fatal [see Warnings and Precautions (5.1)].

Autoantibodies

In the rheumatoid arthritis controlled trials, 12% of patients treated with HUMIRA and 7% of placebo-treated patients that had negative baseline ANA titers developed pos-

itive titers at week 24. Two patients out of 3046 treated with HUMIRA developed clinical signs suggestive of new-onset lupus-like syndrome. The patients improved following discontinuation of therapy. No patients developed lupus nephritis or central nervous system symptoms. The impact of long-term treatment with HUMIRA on the development of autoimmune diseases is unknown.

Liver Enzyme Elevations

There have been reports of severe hepatic reactions including acute liver failure in patients receiving TNF-blockers. In controlled Phase 3 trials of HUMIRA (40 mg SC every other week) in patients with RA, PsA, and AS with control period duration ranging from 4 to 104 weeks, ALT elevations ≥ 3 × ULN occurred in 3.5% of HUMIRA-treated patients and 1.5% of control-treated patients. Since many of these patients in these trials were also taking medications that cause liver enzyme elevations (e.g., NSAIDS, MTX), the relationship between HUMIRA and the liver enzyme elevations is not clear. In a controlled Phase 3 trial of HUMIRA in patients with polyarticular JIA who were 4 to 17 years, ALT elevations ≥ 3 × ULN occurred in 4.4% of HUMIRA-treated patients and 1.5% of control-treated patients (ALT more common than AST); liver enzyme test elevations were more frequent among those treated with the combination of HUMIRA and MTX than those treated with HUMIRA alone. In general, these elevations did not lead to discontinuation of HUMIRA treatment. No ALT elevations ≥ 3 × ULN occurred in the open-label study of HUMIRA in patients with polyarticular JIA who were 2 to <4 years.

In controlled Phase 3 trials of HUMIRA (initial doses of 160 mg and 80 mg, or 80 mg and 40 mg on Days 1 and 15, respectively, followed by 40 mg every other week) in adult patients with CD with a control period duration ranging from 4 to 52 weeks, ALT elevations ≥ 3 × ULN occurred in 0.9% of HUMIRA-treated patients and 0.9% of control-treated patients. In the Phase 3 trial of HUMIRA in pediatric patients with Crohn's disease which evaluated efficacy and safety of two body weight based maintenance dose regimens following body weight based induction therapy up to 52 weeks of treatment, ALT elevations ≥ 3 × ULN occurred in 2.6% (5/192) of patients, of whom 4 were receiving concomitant immunosuppressants at baseline; none of these patients discontinued due to abnormalities in ALT tests. In controlled Phase 3 trials of HUMIRA (initial doses of 160 mg and 80 mg on Days 1 and 15 respectively, followed by 40 mg every other week) in patients with UC with control period duration ranging from 1 to 52 weeks, ALT elevations ≥3 × ULN occurred in 1.5% of HUMIRA-treated patients and 1.0% of control-treated patients. In controlled Phase 3 trials of HUMIRA (initial dose of 80 mg then 40 mg every other week) in patients with Ps with control period duration ranging from 12 to 24 weeks, ALT elevations ≥ 3 × ULN occurred in 1.8% of HUMIRA-treated patients and 1.8% of control-treated patients. In controlled trials of HUMIRA (initial doses of 160 mg at Week 0 and 80 mg at Week 2, followed by 40 mg every week starting at Week 4), in subjects with HS with a control period duration ranging from 12 to 16 weeks, ALT elevations ≥ 3 × ULN occurred in 0.3% of HUMIRA-treated subjects and 0.6% of control-treated subjects. In controlled trials of HUMIRA (initial doses of 80 mg at Week 0 followed by 40 mg every other week starting at Week 1) in patients with uveitis with an exposure of 165.4 PYs and 119.8 PYs in HUMIRA-treated and control-treated patients, respectively, ALT elevations ≥ 3 × ULN occurred in 2.4% of HUMIRA-treated patients and 2.4% of control-treated patients.

Immunogenicity

Patients in Studies RA-I, RA-II, and RA-III were tested at multiple time points for antibodies to adalimumab during the 6- to 12-month period. Approximately 5% (58 of 1062) of adult RA patients receiving HUMIRA developed low-titer antibodies to adalimumab at least once during treatment, which were neutralizing *in vitro*. Patients treated with concomitant methotrexate (MTX) had a lower rate of antibody development than patients on HUMIRA monotherapy (1% versus 12%). No apparent correlation of antibody development to adverse reactions was observed. With monotherapy,

Continued on next page

Information on the AbbVie, Inc. products listed on these pages is from the prescribing information in use as of July 31, 2016. For more information, please visit rxabbvie.com or call 1-800-633-9110.

patients receiving every other week dosing may develop antibodies more frequently than those receiving weekly dosing. In patients receiving the recommended dosage of 40 mg every other week as monotherapy, the ACR 20 response was lower among antibody-positive patients than among antibody-negative patients. The long-term immunogenicity of HUMIRA is unknown.

In patients with polyarticular JIA who were 4 to 17 years of age, adalimumab antibodies were identified in 16% of HUMIRA-treated patients. In patients receiving concomitant MTX, the incidence was 6% compared to 26% with HUMIRA monotherapy. In patients with polyarticular JIA who were 2 to <4 years of age or 4 years of age and older weighing <15 kg, adalimumab antibodies were identified in 7% (1 of 15) of HUMIRA-treated patients, and the one patient was receiving concomitant MTX.

In patients with AS, the rate of development of antibodies to adalimumab in HUMIRA-treated patients was comparable to patients with RA.

In patients with PsA, the rate of antibody development in patients receiving HUMIRA monotherapy was comparable to patients with RA; however, in patients receiving concomitant MTX the rate was 7% compared to 1% in RA.

In adult patients with CD, the rate of antibody development was 3%.

In pediatric patients with Crohn's disease, the rate of antibody development in patients receiving HUMIRA was 3%. However, due to the limitation of the assay conditions, antibodies to adalimumab could be detected only when serum adalimumab levels were < 2 mcg/mL. Among the patients whose serum adalimumab levels were < 2 mcg/mL (approximately 32% of total patients studied), the immunogenicity rate was 10%.

In patients with moderately to severely active UC, the rate of antibody development in patients receiving HUMIRA was 5%. However, due to the limitation of the assay conditions, antibodies to adalimumab could be detected only when serum adalimumab levels were < 2 mcg/mL. Among the patients whose serum adalimumab levels were < 2 mcg/mL (approximately 25% of total patients studied), the immunogenicity rate was 20.7%.

In patients with Ps, the rate of antibody development with HUMIRA monotherapy was 8%. However, due to the limitation of the assay conditions, antibodies to adalimumab could be detected only when serum adalimumab levels were < 2 mcg/mL. Among the patients whose serum adalimumab levels were < 2 mcg/mL (approximately 40% of total patients studied), the immunogenicity rate was 20.7%. In Ps patients who were on HUMIRA monotherapy and subsequently withdrawn from the treatment, the rate of antibodies to adalimumab after retreatment was similar to the rate observed prior to withdrawal.

In subjects with moderate to severe HS, the rate of anti-adalimumab antibody development in subjects treated with HUMIRA was 6.5%. However, because of the limitation of the assay conditions, antibodies to adalimumab could be detected only when serum adalimumab levels were < 2 mcg/mL. Among subjects who stopped HUMIRA treatment for up to 24 weeks and in whom adalimumab serum levels subsequently declined to < 2 mcg/mL (approximately 22% of total subjects studied), the immunogenicity rate was 28%.

In patients with non-infectious uveitis, anti-adalimumab antibodies were identified in 4.8% (12/249) of patients treated with adalimumab. However, due to the limitation of the assay conditions, antibodies to adalimumab could be detected only when serum adalimumab levels were < 2 mcg/mL. Among the patients whose serum adalimumab levels were < 2 mcg/mL (approximately 23% of total patients studied), the immunogenicity rate was 21.1%. Using an assay which could measure an anti-adalimumab antibody titer in all patients, titers were measured in 39.8% (99/249) of non-infectious uveitis patients treated with adalimumab. No correlation of antibody development to safety or efficacy outcomes was observed.

The data reflect the percentage of patients whose test results were considered positive for antibodies to adalimumab or titers, and are highly dependent on the assay. The observed incidence of antibody (including neutralizing antibody) positivity in an assay is highly dependent on several factors including assay sensitivity and specificity, assay methodology, sample handling, timing of sample collection, concomitant medications, and underlying disease. For these reasons, comparison of the incidence of antibodies to adalimumab with the incidence of antibodies to other products may be misleading.

Other Adverse Reactions
Rheumatoid Arthritis Clinical Studies
The data described below reflect exposure to HUMIRA in 2468 patients, including 2073 exposed for 6 months, 1497 exposed for greater than one year and 1380 in adequate and well-controlled studies (Studies RA-I, RA-II, RA-III, and RA-IV). HUMIRA was studied primarily in placebo-controlled trials and in long-term follow up studies for up to 36 months duration. The population had a mean age of 54 years, 77% were female, 91% were Caucasian and had moderately to severely active rheumatoid arthritis. Most patients received 40 mg HUMIRA every other week.

Table 1 summarizes reactions reported at a rate of at least 5% in patients treated with HUMIRA 40 mg every other week compared to placebo and with an incidence higher than placebo. In Study RA-III, the types and frequencies of adverse reactions in the second year open-label extension were similar to those observed in the one-year double-blind portion.

Table 1. Adverse Reactions Reported by ≥5% of Patients Treated with HUMIRA During Placebo-Controlled Period of Pooled RA Studies (Studies RA-I, RA-II, RA-III, and RA-IV)

Adverse Reaction (Preferred Term)	HUMIRA 40 mg subcutaneous Every Other Week (N=705)	Placebo (N=690)
Respiratory		
Upper respiratory infection	17%	13%
Sinusitis	11%	9%
Flu syndrome	7%	6%
Gastrointestinal		
Nausea	9%	8%
Abdominal pain	7%	4%
Laboratory Tests*		
Laboratory test abnormal	8%	7%
Hypercholesterolemia	6%	4%
Hyperlipidemia	7%	5%
Hematuria	5%	4%
Alkaline phosphatase increased	5%	3%
Other		
Headache	12%	8%
Rash	12%	6%
Accidental injury	10%	8%
Injection site reaction **	8%	1%
Back pain	6%	4%
Urinary tract infection	8%	5%
Hypertension	5%	3%

* Laboratory test abnormalities were reported as adverse reactions in European trials
** Does not include injection site erythema, itching, hemorrhage, pain or swelling

Less Common Adverse Reactions in Rheumatoid Arthritis Clinical Studies
Other infrequent serious adverse reactions that do not appear in the Warnings and Precautions or Adverse Reaction sections that occurred at an incidence of less than 5% in HUMIRA-treated patients in RA studies were:

Body As A Whole: Pain in extremity, pelvic pain, surgery, thorax pain
Cardiovascular System: Arrhythmia, atrial fibrillation, chest pain, coronary artery disorder, heart arrest, hypertensive encephalopathy, myocardial infarct, palpitation, pericardial effusion, pericarditis, syncope, tachycardia
Digestive System: Cholecystitis, cholelithiasis, esophagitis, gastroenteritis, gastrointestinal hemorrhage, hepatic necrosis, vomiting
Endocrine System: Parathyroid disorder
Hemic And Lymphatic System: Agranulocytosis, polycythemia
Metabolic And Nutritional Disorders: Dehydration, healing abnormal, ketosis, paraproteinemia, peripheral edema
Musculo-Skeletal System: Arthritis, bone disorder, bone fracture (not spontaneous), bone necrosis, joint disorder, muscle cramps, myasthenia, pyogenic arthritis, synovitis, tendon disorder
Neoplasia: Adenoma

Nervous System: Confusion, paresthesia, subdural hematoma, tremor
Respiratory System: Asthma, bronchospasm, dyspnea, lung function decreased, pleural effusion
Special Senses: Cataract
Thrombosis: Thrombosis leg
Urogenital System: Cystitis, kidney calculus, menstrual disorder

Juvenile Idiopathic Arthritis Clinical Studies
In general, the adverse reactions in the HUMIRA-treated patients in the polyarticular juvenile idiopathic arthritis (JIA) trials (Studies JIA-I and JIA-II) were similar in frequency and type to those seen in adult patients *[see Warnings and Precautions (5), Adverse Reactions (6)]*. Important findings and differences from adults are discussed in the following paragraphs.

In Study JIA-I, HUMIRA was studied in 171 patients who were 4 to 17 years of age, with polyarticular JIA. Severe adverse reactions reported in the study included neutropenia, streptococcal pharyngitis, increased aminotransferases, herpes zoster, myositis, metrorrhagia, and appendicitis. Serious infections were observed in 4% of patients within approximately 2 years of initiation of treatment with HUMIRA and included cases of herpes simplex, pneumonia, urinary tract infection, pharyngitis, and herpes zoster.

In Study JIA-I, 45% of patients experienced an infection while receiving HUMIRA with or without concomitant MTX in the first 16 weeks of treatment. The types of infections reported in HUMIRA-treated patients were generally similar to those commonly seen in polyarticular JIA patients who are not treated with TNF blockers. Upon initiation of treatment, the most common adverse reactions occurring in this patient population treated with HUMIRA were injection site pain and injection site reaction (19% and 16%, respectively). A less commonly reported adverse event in patients receiving HUMIRA was granuloma annulare which did not lead to discontinuation of HUMIRA treatment.

In the first 48 weeks of treatment in Study JIA-I, non-serious hypersensitivity reactions were seen in approximately 6% of patients and included primarily localized allergic hypersensitivity reactions and allergic rash.

In Study JIA-I, 10% of patients treated with HUMIRA who had negative baseline anti-dsDNA antibodies developed positive titers after 48 weeks of treatment. No patient developed clinical signs of autoimmunity during the clinical trial.

Approximately 15% of patients treated with HUMIRA developed mild-to-moderate elevations of creatine phosphokinase (CPK) in Study JIA-I. Elevations exceeding 5 times the upper limit of normal were observed in several patients. CPK levels decreased or returned to normal in all patients. Most patients were able to continue HUMIRA without interruption.

In Study JIA-II, HUMIRA was studied in 32 patients who were 2 to <4 years of age or 4 years of age and older weighing <15 kg with polyarticular JIA. The safety profile for this patient population was similar to the safety profile seen in patients 4 to 17 years of age with polyarticular JIA.

In Study JIA-II, 78% of patients experienced an infection while receiving HUMIRA. These included nasopharyngitis, bronchitis, upper respiratory tract infection, otitis media, and were mostly mild to moderate in severity. Serious infections were observed in 9% of patients receiving HUMIRA in the study and included dental caries, rotavirus gastroenteritis, and varicella.

In Study JIA-II, non-serious allergic reactions were observed in 6% of patients and included intermittent urticaria and rash, which were all mild in severity.

Psoriatic Arthritis and Ankylosing Spondylitis Clinical Studies
HUMIRA has been studied in 395 patients with psoriatic arthritis (PsA) in two placebo-controlled trials and in an open label study and in 393 patients with ankylosing spondylitis (AS) in two placebo-controlled studies. The safety profile for patients with PsA and AS treated with HUMIRA 40 mg every other week was similar to the safety profile seen in patients with RA, HUMIRA Studies RA-I through IV.

Adult Crohn's Disease Clinical Studies
HUMIRA has been studied in 1478 adult patients with Crohn's disease (CD) in four placebo-controlled and two open-label extension studies. The safety profile for adult patients with CD treated with HUMIRA was similar to the safety profile seen in patients with RA.

Pediatric Crohn's Disease Clinical Studies

HUMIRA has been studied in 192 pediatric patients with Crohn's disease in one double-blind study (Study PCD-I) and one open-label extension study. The safety profile for pediatric patients with Crohn's disease treated with HUMIRA was similar to the safety profile seen in adult patients with Crohn's disease.

During the 4 week open label induction phase of Study PCD-I, the most common adverse reactions occurring in the pediatric population treated with HUMIRA were injection site pain and injection site reaction (6% and 5%, respectively).

A total of 67% of children experienced an infection while receiving HUMIRA in Study PCD-I. These included upper respiratory tract infection and nasopharyngitis.

A total of 5% of children experienced a serious infection while receiving HUMIRA in Study PCD-I. These included viral infection, device related sepsis (catheter), gastroenteritis, H1N1 influenza, and disseminated histoplasmosis.

In Study PCD-I, allergic reactions were observed in 5% of children which were all non-serious and were primarily localized reactions.

Ulcerative Colitis Clinical Studies

HUMIRA has been studied in 1010 patients with ulcerative colitis (UC) in two placebo-controlled studies and one open-label extension study. The safety profile for patients with UC treated with HUMIRA was similar to the safety profile seen in patients with RA.

Plaque Psoriasis Clinical Studies

HUMIRA has been studied in 1696 subjects with plaque psoriasis (Ps) in placebo-controlled and open-label extension studies. The safety profile for subjects with Ps treated with HUMIRA was similar to the safety profile seen in subjects with RA with the following exceptions. In the placebo-controlled portions of the clinical trials in Ps subjects, HUMIRA-treated subjects had a higher incidence of arthralgia when compared to controls (3% *vs.* 1%).

Hidradenitis Suppurativa Clinical Studies

HUMIRA has been studied in 727 subjects with hidradenitis suppurativa (HS) in three placebo-controlled studies and one open-label extension study. The safety profile for subjects with HS treated with HUMIRA weekly was consistent with the known safety profile of HUMIRA.

Flare of HS, defined as ≥25% increase from baseline in abscesses and inflammatory nodule counts and with a minimum of 2 additional lesions, was documented in 22 (22%) of the 100 subjects who were withdrawn from HUMIRA treatment following the primary efficacy timepoint in two studies.

Uveitis Clinical Studies

HUMIRA has been studied in 464 patients with uveitis (UV) in placebo-controlled and open-label extension studies. The safety profile for patients with UV treated with HUMIRA was similar to the safety profile seen in patients with RA.

6.2 Postmarketing Experience

The following adverse reactions have been identified during post-approval use of HUMIRA. Because these reactions are reported voluntarily from a population of uncertain size, it is not always possible to reliably estimate their frequency or establish a causal relationship to HUMIRA exposure.

Gastrointestinal disorders: Diverticulitis, large bowel perforations including perforations associated with diverticulitis and appendiceal perforations associated with appendicitis, pancreatitis

General disorders and administration site conditions: Pyrexia

Hepato-biliary disorders: Liver failure, hepatitis

Immune system disorders: Sarcoidosis

Neoplasms benign, malignant and unspecified (including cysts and polyps): Merkel Cell Carcinoma (neuroendocrine carcinoma of the skin)

Nervous system disorders: Demyelinating disorders (e.g., optic neuritis, Guillain-Barré syndrome), cerebrovascular accident

Respiratory disorders: Interstitial lung disease, including pulmonary fibrosis, pulmonary embolism

Skin reactions: Stevens Johnson Syndrome, cutaneous vasculitis, erythema multiforme, new or worsening psoriasis (all sub-types including pustular and palmoplantar), alopecia

Vascular disorders: Systemic vasculitis, deep vein thrombosis

7   DRUG INTERACTIONS

7.1   Methotrexate

HUMIRA has been studied in rheumatoid arthritis (RA) patients taking concomitant methotrexate (MTX). Although MTX reduced the apparent adalimumab clearance, the data do not suggest the need for dose adjustment of either HUMIRA or MTX *[see Clinical Pharmacology (12.3)]*.

7.2   Biological Products

In clinical studies in patients with RA, an increased risk of serious infections has been seen with the combination of TNF blockers with anakinra or abatacept, with no added benefit; therefore, use of HUMIRA with abatacept or anakinra is not recommended in patients with RA *[see Warnings and Precautions (5.7 and 5.11)]*. A higher rate of serious infections has also been observed in patients with RA treated with rituximab who received subsequent treatment with a TNF blocker. There is insufficient information regarding the concomitant use of HUMIRA and other biologic products for the treatment of RA, PsA, AS, CD, UC, Ps, HS and UV. Concomitant administration of HUMIRA with other biologic DMARDS (e.g., anakinra and abatacept) or other TNF blockers is not recommended based upon the possible increased risk for infections and other potential pharmacological interactions.

7.3   Live Vaccines

Avoid the use of live vaccines with HUMIRA *[see Warnings and Precautions (5.10)]*.

7.4   Cytochrome P450 Substrates

The formation of CYP450 enzymes may be suppressed by increased levels of cytokines (e.g., TNFα, IL-6) during chronic inflammation. It is possible for a molecule that antagonizes cytokine activity, such as adalimumab, to influence the formation of CYP450 enzymes. Upon initiation or discontinuation of HUMIRA in patients being treated with CYP450 substrates with a narrow therapeutic index, monitoring of the effect (e.g., warfarin) or drug concentration (e.g., cyclosporine or theophylline) is recommended and the individual dose of the drug product may be adjusted as needed.

8   USE IN SPECIFIC POPULATIONS

8.1   Pregnancy

Risk Summary

Limited clinical data are available from the Humira Pregnancy Registry. Excluding lost-to-follow-up, data from the registry reports a rate of 5.6% for major birth defects with first trimester use of adalimumab in pregnant women with rheumatoid arthritis (RA), and a rate of 7.8% and 5.5% for major birth defects in the disease-matched and non-diseased comparison groups *[see Data]*. Adalimumab is actively transferred across the placenta during the third trimester of pregnancy and may affect immune response in the *in-utero* exposed infant *[see Clinical Considerations]*. In an embryo-fetal perinatal development study conducted in cynomolgus monkeys, no fetal harm or malformations were observed with intravenous administration of adalimumab during organogenesis and later in gestation, at doses that produced exposures up to approximately 373 times the maximum recommended human dose (MRHD) of 40 mg subcutaneous without methotrexate *[see Data]*.

The estimated background risk of major birth defects and miscarriage for the indicated populations is unknown. In the U.S. general population, the estimated background risk of major birth defects and miscarriage in clinically recognized pregnancies is 2-4% and miscarriage is 15-20%, respectively.

Clinical Considerations

Fetal/Neonatal adverse reactions

Monoclonal antibodies are increasingly transported across the placenta as pregnancy progresses, with the largest amount transferred during the third trimester *[see Data]*. Risks and benefits should be considered prior to administering live or live-attenuated vaccines to infants exposed to HUMIRA *in utero [see Use in Specific Populations (8.4)]*.

Data

Human Data

In a prospective cohort pregnancy exposure registry conducted in the U.S. and Canada between 2004 and 2013, 74 women with RA treated with adalimumab at least during the first trimester, 80 women with RA not treated with adalimumab and 218 women without RA (non-diseased) were enrolled. Excluding lost-to-follow-up, the rate of major defects in the adalimumab-exposed pregnancies (N=72), disease-matched (N=77), and non-diseased comparison groups (N=201) was 5.6%, 7.8% and 5.5%, respectively. However, this study cannot definitely establish the absence of any risk because of methodological limitations, including small sample size and non-randomized study design. Data from the Crohn's disease portion of the study is in the follow-up phase and the analysis is ongoing.

In an independent clinical study conducted in ten pregnant women with inflammatory bowel disease treated with HUMIRA, adalimumab concentrations were measured in maternal serum as well as in cord blood (n=10) and infant serum (n=8) on the day of birth. The last dose of HUMIRA was given between 1 and 56 days prior to delivery. Adalimumab concentrations were 0.16-19.7 µg/mL in cord blood, 4.28-17.7 µg/mL in infant serum, and 0-16.1 µg/mL in maternal serum. In all but one case, the cord blood level of adalimumab was higher than the maternal serum level, suggesting adalimumab actively crosses the placenta. In addition, one infant had serum levels at each of the following: 6 weeks (1.94 µg/mL), 7 weeks (1.31 µg/mL), 8 weeks (0.93 µg/mL), and 11 weeks (0.53 µg/mL), suggesting adalimumab can be detected in the serum of infants exposed *in utero* for at least 3 months from birth.

Animal Data

In an embryo-fetal perinatal development study, pregnant cynomolgus monkeys received adalimumab from gestation days 20 to 97 at doses that produced exposures up to 373 times that achieved with the MRHD without methotrexate (on an AUC basis with maternal IV doses up to 100 mg/kg/week). Adalimumab did not elicit harm to the fetuses or malformations.

8.2   Lactation

Risk Summary

Limited data from case reports in the published literature describe the presence of adalimumab in human milk at infant doses of 0.1% to 1% of the maternal serum level. There are no reports of adverse effects of adalimumab on the breastfed infant and no effects on milk production. The developmental and health benefits of breastfeeding should be considered along with the mother's clinical need for HUMIRA and any potential adverse effects on the breastfed child from HUMIRA or from the underlying maternal condition.

8.4   Pediatric Use

Safety and efficacy of HUMIRA in pediatric patients for uses other than polyarticular juvenile idiopathic arthritis (JIA) and pediatric Crohn's disease have not been established. Due to its inhibition of TNFα, HUMIRA administered during pregnancy could affect immune response in the *in utero*-exposed newborn and infant. Data from eight infants exposed to HUMIRA *in utero* suggest adalimumab crosses the placenta *[see Use in Specific Populations (8.1)]*. The clinical significance of elevated adalimumab levels in infants is unknown. The safety of administering live or live-attenuated vaccines in exposed infants is unknown. Risks and benefits should be considered prior to vaccinating (live or live-attenuated) exposed infants.

Post-marketing cases of lymphoma, including hepatosplenic T-cell lymphoma and other malignancies, some fatal, have been reported among children, adolescents, and young adults who received treatment with TNF-blockers including HUMIRA *[see Boxed Warning and Warnings and Precautions (5.2)]*.

Juvenile Idiopathic Arthritis

In Study JIA-I, HUMIRA was shown to reduce signs and symptoms of active polyarticular JIA in patients 4 to 17 years of age *[see Clinical Studies (14.2)]*. In Study JIA-II, the safety profile for patients 2 to <4 years of age was similar to the safety profile for patients 4 to 17 years of age with polyarticular JIA *[see Adverse Reactions (6.1)]*. HUMIRA has not been studied in patients with polyarticular JIA less than 2 years of age or in patients with a weight below 10 kg. The safety of HUMIRA in patients in the polyarticular JIA trials was generally similar to that observed in adults with certain exceptions *[see Adverse Reactions (6.1)]*.

Pediatric Crohn's Disease

The safety and effectiveness of HUMIRA for reducing signs and symptoms and inducing and maintaining clinical remission have been established in pediatric patients 6 years of age and older with moderately to severely active Crohn's disease who have had an inadequate response to corticosteroids or immunomodulators such as azathioprine, 6-mercaptopurine, or methotrexate. Use of HUMIRA in this age group is supported by evidence from adequate and well-

Continued on next page

Information on the AbbVie, Inc. products listed on these pages is from the prescribing information in use as of July 31, 2016. For more information, please visit rxabbvie.com or call 1-800-633-9110.

controlled studies of HUMIRA in adults with additional data from a randomized, double-blind, 52-week clinical study of two dose levels of HUMIRA in 192 pediatric patients (6 to 17 years of age) with moderately to severely active Crohn's disease *[see Clinical Studies (14.6)]*. The safety and effectiveness of HUMIRA has not been established in pediatric patients with Crohn's disease less than 6 years of age.

8.5   Geriatric Use

A total of 519 RA patients 65 years of age and older, including 107 patients 75 years of age and older, received HUMIRA in clinical studies RA-I through IV. No overall difference in effectiveness was observed between these patients and younger patients. The frequency of serious infection and malignancy among HUMIRA treated patients over 65 years of age was higher than for those under 65 years of age. Because there is a higher incidence of infections and malignancies in the elderly population, use caution when treating the elderly.

10   OVERDOSAGE

Doses up to 10 mg/kg have been administered to patients in clinical trials without evidence of dose-limiting toxicities. In case of overdosage, it is recommended that the patient be monitored for any signs or symptoms of adverse reactions or effects and appropriate symptomatic treatment instituted immediately.

11   DESCRIPTION

HUMIRA® (adalimumab) is a recombinant human IgG1 monoclonal antibody specific for human tumor necrosis factor (TNF). HUMIRA was created using phage display technology resulting in an antibody with human derived heavy and light chain variable regions and human IgG1:k constant regions. Adalimumab is produced by recombinant DNA technology in a mammalian cell expression system and is purified by a process that includes specific viral inactivation and removal steps. It consists of 1330 amino acids and has a molecular weight of approximately 148 kilodaltons.

HUMIRA is supplied as a sterile, preservative-free solution of adalimumab for subcutaneous administration. The drug product is supplied as either a single-use, prefilled pen (HUMIRA Pen), as a single-use, 1 mL prefilled glass syringe, or as a single-use institutional use vial. Enclosed within the pen is a single-use, 1 mL prefilled glass syringe. The solution of HUMIRA is clear and colorless, with a pH of about 5.2.

Each 40 mg/0.4 mL prefilled syringe or prefilled pen delivers 0.4 mL (40 mg) of drug product. Each 0.4 mL of HUMIRA contains adalimumab 40 mg, mannitol 16.8 mg, polysorbate 80 0.4 mg, and Water for Injection, USP.

Each 40 mg/0.8 mL prefilled syringe, prefilled pen, or single-use institutional use vial delivers 0.8 mL (40 mg) of drug product. Each 0.8 mL of HUMIRA contains adalimumab 40 mg, citric acid monohydrate 1.04 mg, dibasic sodium phosphate dihydrate 1.22 mg, mannitol 9.6 mg, monobasic sodium phosphate dihydrate 0.69 mg, polysorbate 80 0.8 mg, sodium chloride 4.93 mg, sodium citrate 0.24 mg and Water for Injection, USP. Sodium hydroxide is added as necessary to adjust pH.

Each 20 mg/0.4 mL prefilled syringe delivers 0.4 mL (20 mg) of drug product. Each 0.4 mL of HUMIRA contains adalimumab 20 mg, citric acid monohydrate 0.52 mg, dibasic sodium phosphate dihydrate 0.61 mg, mannitol 4.8 mg, monobasic sodium phosphate dihydrate 0.34 mg, polysorbate 80 0.4 mg, sodium chloride 2.47 mg, sodium citrate 0.12 mg and Water for Injection, USP. Sodium hydroxide is added as necessary to adjust pH.

Each 10 mg/0.2 mL prefilled syringe delivers 0.2 mL (10 mg) of drug product. Each 0.2 mL of HUMIRA contains adalimumab 10 mg, citric acid monohydrate 0.26 mg, dibasic sodium phosphate dihydrate 0.31 mg, mannitol 2.4 mg, monobasic sodium phosphate dihydrate 0.17 mg, polysorbate 80 0.2 mg, sodium chloride 1.23 mg, sodium citrate 0.06 mg and Water for Injection, USP. Sodium hydroxide is added as necessary to adjust pH.

12   CLINICAL PHARMACOLOGY

12.1   Mechanism of Action

Adalimumab binds specifically to TNF-alpha and blocks its interaction with the p55 and p75 cell surface TNF receptors. Adalimumab also lyses surface TNF expressing cells *in vitro* in the presence of complement. Adalimumab does not bind or inactivate lymphotoxin (TNF-beta). TNF is a naturally occurring cytokine that is involved in normal inflammatory and immune responses. Elevated levels of TNF are found in

the synovial fluid of patients with RA, JIA, PsA, and AS and play an important role in both the pathologic inflammation and the joint destruction that are hallmarks of these diseases. Increased levels of TNF are also found in psoriasis plaques. In Ps, treatment with HUMIRA may reduce the epidermal thickness and infiltration of inflammatory cells. The relationship between these pharmacodynamic activities and the mechanism(s) by which HUMIRA exerts its clinical effects is unknown.

Adalimumab also modulates biological responses that are induced or regulated by TNF, including changes in the levels of adhesion molecules responsible for leukocyte migration (ELAM-1, VCAM-1, and ICAM-1 with an IC_{50} of 1-2 X 10^{-10}M).

12.2   Pharmacodynamics

After treatment with HUMIRA, a decrease in levels of acute phase reactants of inflammation (C-reactive protein [CRP] and erythrocyte sedimentation rate [ESR]) and serum cytokines (IL-6) was observed compared to baseline in patients with rheumatoid arthritis. A decrease in CRP levels was also observed in patients with Crohn's disease, ulcerative colitis and hidradenitis suppurativa. Serum levels of matrix metalloproteinases (MMP-1 and MMP-3) that produce tissue remodeling responsible for cartilage destruction were also decreased after HUMIRA administration.

12.3   Pharmacokinetics

The maximum serum concentration (C_{max}) and the time to reach the maximum concentration (T_{max}) were 4.7 ± 1.6 µg/mL and 131 ± 56 hours respectively, following a single 40 mg subcutaneous administration of HUMIRA to healthy adult subjects. The average absolute bioavailability of adalimumab estimated from three studies following a single 40 mg subcutaneous dose was 64%. The pharmacokinetics of adalimumab were linear over the dose range of 0.5 to 10.0 mg/kg following a single intravenous dose.

The single dose pharmacokinetics of adalimumab in RA patients were determined in several studies with intravenous doses ranging from 0.25 to 10 mg/kg. The distribution volume (V_{ss}) ranged from 4.7 to 6.0 L. The systemic clearance of adalimumab is approximately 12 mL/hr. The mean terminal half-life was approximately 2 weeks, ranging from 10 to 20 days across studies. Adalimumab concentrations in the synovial fluid from five rheumatoid arthritis patients ranged from 31 to 96% of those in serum.

In RA patients receiving 40 mg HUMIRA every other week, adalimumab mean steady-state trough concentrations of approximately 5 µg/mL and 8 to 9 µg/mL, were observed without and with methotrexate (MTX), respectively. MTX reduced adalimumab apparent clearance after single and multiple dosing by 29% and 44% respectively, in patients with RA. Mean serum adalimumab trough levels at steady state increased approximately proportionally with dose following 20, 40, and 80 mg every other week and every week subcutaneous dosing. In long-term studies with dosing more than two years, there was no evidence of changes in clearance over time.

Adalimumab mean steady-state trough concentrations were slightly higher in psoriatic arthritis patients treated with 40 mg HUMIRA every other week (6 to 10 µg/mL and 8.5 to 12 µg/mL, without and with MTX, respectively) compared to the concentrations in RA patients treated with the same dose.

The pharmacokinetics of adalimumab in patients with AS were similar to those in patients with RA.

In patients with CD, the loading dose of 160 mg HUMIRA on Week 0 followed by 80 mg HUMIRA on Week 2 achieves mean serum adalimumab trough levels of approximately 12 µg/mL at Week 2 and Week 4. Mean steady-state trough levels of approximately 7 µg/mL were observed at Week 24 and Week 56 in CD patients after receiving a maintenance dose of 40 mg HUMIRA every other week.

In patients with UC, the loading dose of 160 mg HUMIRA on Week 0 followed by 80 mg HUMIRA on Week 2 achieves mean serum adalimumab trough levels of approximately 12 µg/mL at Week 2 and Week 4. Mean steady-state trough level of approximately 8 µg/mL was observed at Week 52 in UC patients after receiving a dose of 40 mg HUMIRA every other week, and approximately 15 µg/mL at Week 52 in UC patients who increased to a dose of 40 mg HUMIRA every week.

In patients with Ps, the mean steady-state trough concentration was approximately 5 to 6 µg/mL during HUMIRA 40 mg every other week monotherapy treatment.

In subjects with HS, a dose of 160 mg HUMIRA on Week 0 followed by 80 mg on Week 2 achieved serum adalimumab

trough concentrations of approximately 7 to 8 µg/mL at Week 2 and Week 4. The mean steady-state trough concentrations at Week 12 through Week 36 were approximately 7 to 11 µg/mL during HUMIRA 40 mg every week treatment. In patients with UV, the mean steady concentration was approximately 8 to 10 µg/mL during HUMIRA 40 mg every other week treatment.

Population pharmacokinetic analyses in patients with RA revealed that there was a trend toward higher apparent clearance of adalimumab in the presence of anti-adalimumab antibodies, and lower clearance with increasing age in patients aged 40 to >75 years.

Minor increases in apparent clearance were also predicted in RA patients receiving doses lower than the recommended dose and in RA patients with high rheumatoid factor or CRP concentrations. These increases are not likely to be clinically important.

No gender-related pharmacokinetic differences were observed after correction for a patient's body weight. Healthy volunteers and patients with rheumatoid arthritis displayed similar adalimumab pharmacokinetics.

No pharmacokinetic data are available in patients with hepatic or renal impairment.

In Study JIA-I for patients with polyarticular JIA who were 4 to 17 years of age, the mean steady-state trough serum adalimumab concentrations for patients weighing <30 kg receiving 20 mg HUMIRA subcutaneously every other week as monotherapy or with concomitant MTX were 6.8 µg/mL and 10.9 µg/mL, respectively. The mean steady-state trough serum adalimumab concentrations for patients weighing ≥30 kg receiving 40 mg HUMIRA subcutaneously every other week as monotherapy or with concomitant MTX were 6.6 µg/mL and 8.1 µg/mL, respectively. In Study JIA-II for patients with polyarticular JIA who were 2 to <4 years of age or 4 years of age and older weighing <15 kg, the mean steady-state trough serum adalimumab concentrations for patients receiving HUMIRA subcutaneously every other week as monotherapy or with concomitant MTX were 6.0 µg/mL and 7.9 µg/mL, respectively.

In pediatric subjects with CD weighing ≥ 40 kg, the mean ±SD serum adalimumab concentrations were 15.7±6.5 mcg/mL at Week 4 following subcutaneous doses of 160 mg at Week 0 and 80 mg at Week 2 and the mean ±SD steady-state trough serum adalimumab concentrations were 10.5±6.0 mcg/mL at Week 52 following subcutaneous doses of 40 mg every other week. In pediatric subjects with CD weighing < 40 kg, the mean ±SD serum adalimumab concentrations were 10.6±6.1 mcg/mL at Week 4 following subcutaneous doses of 80 mg at Week 0 and 40 mg at Week 2 and the mean ±SD steady-state trough serum adalimumab concentrations were 6.9±3.6 mcg/mL at Week 52 following subcutaneous doses of 20 mg every other week.

13   NONCLINICAL TOXICOLOGY

13.1   Carcinogenesis, Mutagenesis, Impairment of Fertility

Long-term animal studies of HUMIRA have not been conducted to evaluate the carcinogenic potential or its effect on fertility.

14   CLINICAL STUDIES

14.1   Rheumatoid Arthritis

The efficacy and safety of HUMIRA were assessed in five randomized, double-blind studies in patients ≥18 years of age with active rheumatoid arthritis (RA) diagnosed according to American College of Rheumatology (ACR) criteria. Patients had at least 6 swollen and 9 tender joints. HUMIRA was administered subcutaneously in combination with methotrexate (MTX) (12.5 to 25 mg, Studies RA-I, RA-III and RA-V) or as monotherapy (Studies RA-II and RA-V) or with other disease-modifying anti-rheumatic drugs (DMARDs) (Study RA-IV).

Study RA-I evaluated 271 patients who had failed therapy with at least one but no more than four DMARDs and had inadequate response to MTX. Doses of 20, 40 or 80 mg of HUMIRA or placebo were given every other week for 24 weeks.

Study RA-II evaluated 544 patients who had failed therapy with at least one DMARD. Doses of placebo, 20 or 40 mg of HUMIRA were given as monotherapy every other week or weekly for 26 weeks.

Study RA-III evaluated 619 patients who had an inadequate response to MTX. Patients received placebo, 40 mg of HUMIRA every other week with placebo injections on alternate weeks, or 20 mg of HUMIRA weekly for up to 52 weeks. Study RA-III had an additional primary endpoint at 52 weeks of inhibition of disease progression (as detected by X-ray results). Upon completion of the first 52 weeks, 457 patients enrolled in an open-label extension phase in which 40 mg of HUMIRA was administered every other week for up to 5 years.

Study RA-IV assessed safety in 636 patients who were either DMARD-naive or were permitted to remain on their pre-existing rheumatologic therapy provided that therapy was stable for a minimum of 28 days. Patients were randomized to 40 mg of HUMIRA or placebo every other week for 24 weeks.

Study RA-V evaluated 799 patients with moderately to severely active RA of less than 3 years duration who were ≥18 years old and MTX naïve. Patients were randomized to receive either MTX (optimized to 20 mg/week by week 8), HUMIRA 40 mg every other week or HUMIRA/MTX combination therapy for 104 weeks. Patients were evaluated for signs and symptoms, and for radiographic progression of joint damage. The median disease duration among patients enrolled in the study was 5 months. The median MTX dose achieved was 20 mg.

Clinical Response

The percent of HUMIRA treated patients achieving ACR 20, 50 and 70 responses in Studies RA-II and III are shown in Table 2.

[See table 2 above]

The results of Study RA-I were similar to Study RA-III; patients receiving HUMIRA 40 mg every other week in Study RA-I also achieved ACR 20, 50 and 70 response rates of 65%, 52% and 24%, respectively, compared to placebo responses of 13%, 7% and 3% respectively, at 6 months (p<0.01).

The results of the components of the ACR response criteria for Studies RA-II and RA-III are shown in Table 3. ACR response rates and improvement in all components of ACR response were maintained to week 104. Over the 2 years in Study RA-III, 20% of HUMIRA patients receiving 40 mg every other week (EOW) achieved a major clinical response, defined as maintenance of an ACR 70 response over a 6-month period. ACR responses were maintained in similar proportions of patients for up to 5 years with continuous HUMIRA treatment in the open-label portion of Study RA-III.

[See table 3 at top of next page]

The time course of ACR 20 response for Study RA-III is shown in Figure 1.

In Study RA-III, 85% of patients with ACR 20 responses at week 24 maintained the response at 52 weeks. The time course of ACR 20 response for Study RA-I and Study RA-II were similar.

Figure 1. Study RA-III ACR 20 Responses over 52 Weeks

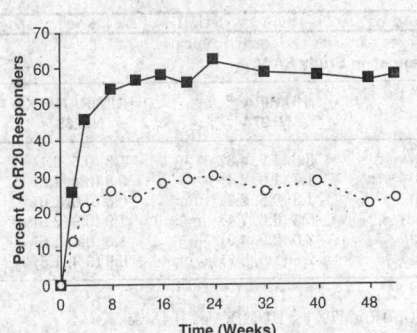

In Study RA-IV, 53% of patients treated with HUMIRA 40 mg every other week plus standard of care had an ACR 20 response at week 24 compared to 35% on placebo plus standard of care (p<0.001). No unique adverse reactions related to the combination of HUMIRA (adalimumab) and other DMARDs were observed.

In Study RA-V with MTX naïve patients with recent onset RA, the combination treatment with HUMIRA plus MTX led to greater percentages of patients achieving ACR responses than either MTX monotherapy or HUMIRA monotherapy at Week 52 and responses were sustained at Week 104 (see Table 4).

[See table 4 on next page]

At Week 52, all individual components of the ACR response criteria for Study RA-V improved in the HUMIRA/MTX group and improvements were maintained to Week 104.

Radiographic Response

In Study RA-III, structural joint damage was assessed radiographically and expressed as change in Total Sharp Score (TSS) and its components, the erosion score and Joint Space Narrowing (JSN) score, at month 12 compared to baseline. At baseline, the median TSS was approximately 55 in the placebo and 40 mg every other week groups. The results are shown in Table 5. HUMIRA/MTX treated patients demonstrated less radiographic progression than patients receiving MTX alone at 52 weeks.

[See table 5 on next page]

In the open-label extension of Study RA-III, 77% of the original patients treated with any dose of HUMIRA were evaluated radiographically at 2 years. Patients maintained inhibition of structural damage, as measured by the TSS. Fifty-four percent had no progression of structural damage as defined by a change in the TSS of zero or less. Fifty-five percent (55%) of patients originally treated with 40 mg HUMIRA every other week have been evaluated radiographically at 5 years. Patients had continued inhibition of structural damage with 50% showing no progression of structural damage defined by a change in the TSS of zero or less.

In Study RA-V, structural joint damage was assessed as in Study RA-III. Greater inhibition of radiographic progression, as assessed by changes in TSS, erosion score and JSN was observed in the HUMIRA/MTX combination group as compared to either the MTX or HUMIRA monotherapy group at Week 52 as well as at Week 104 (see Table 6).

[See table 6 on next page]

Physical Function Response

In studies RA-I through IV, HUMIRA® (adalimumab) showed significantly greater improvement than placebo in the disability index of Health Assessment Questionnaire (HAQ-DI) from baseline to the end of study, and significantly greater improvement than placebo in the health-outcomes as assessed by The Short Form Health Survey (SF 36). Improvement was seen in both the Physical Component Summary (PCS) and the Mental Component Summary (MCS).

In Study RA-III, the mean (95% CI) improvement in HAQ-DI from baseline at week 52 was 0.60 (0.55, 0.65) for the HUMIRA patients and 0.25 (0.17, 0.33) for placebo/MTX (p<0.001) patients. Sixty-three percent of HUMIRA-treated patients achieved a 0.5 or greater improvement in HAQ-DI at week 52 in the double-blind portion of the study. Eighty-two percent of these patients maintained that improvement through week 104 and a similar proportion of patients maintained this response through week 260 (5 years) of open-label treatment. Mean improvement in the SF-36 was maintained through the end of measurement at week 156 (3 years).

In Study RA-V, the HAQ-DI and the physical component of the SF-36 showed greater improvement (p<0.001) for the HUMIRA/MTX combination therapy group versus either the MTX monotherapy or the HUMIRA monotherapy group at Week 52, which was maintained through Week 104.

14.2   Juvenile Idiopathic Arthritis

The safety and efficacy of HUMIRA was assessed in two studies (Studies JIA-I and JIA-II) in patients with active polyarticular juvenile idiopathic arthritis (JIA).

Study JIA-I

The safety and efficacy of HUMIRA were assessed in a multicenter, randomized, withdrawal, double-blind, parallel-group study in 171 patients who were 4 to 17 years of age with polyarticular JIA. In the study, the patients were stratified into two groups: MTX-treated or non-MTX-treated. All patients had to show signs of active moderate or severe disease despite previous treatment with NSAIDs, analgesics, corticosteroids, or DMARDS. Patients who received prior treatment with any biologic DMARDS were excluded from the study.

The study included four phases: an open-label lead in phase (OL-LI; 16 weeks), a double-blind randomized withdrawal phase (DB; 32 weeks), an open-label extension phase (OLE-BSA; up to 136 weeks), and an open-label fixed dose phase (OLE-FD; 16 weeks). In the first three phases of the study, HUMIRA was administered based on body surface area at a dose of 24 mg/m² up to a maximum total body dose of 40 mg subcutaneously (SC) every other week. In the OLE-FD phase, the patients were treated with 20 mg of HUMIRA SC every other week if their weight was less than 30 kg and with 40 mg of HUMIRA SC every other week if their weight was 30 kg or greater. Patients remained on stable doses of NSAIDs and or prednisone (≤0.2 mg/kg/day or 10 mg/day maximum).

Patients demonstrating a Pediatric ACR 30 response at the end of OL-LI phase were randomized into the double blind (DB) phase of the study and received either HUMIRA or placebo every other week for 32 weeks or until disease flare. Disease flare was defined as a worsening of ≥30% from baseline in ≥3 of 6 Pediatric ACR core criteria, ≥2 active joints, and improvement of >30% in no more than 1 of the 6 criteria. After 32 weeks or at the time of disease flare during the DB phase, patients were treated in the open-label extension phase based on the BSA regimen (OLE-BSA), before converting to a fixed dose regimen based on body weight (OLE-FD phase).

Study JIA-I Clinical Response

At the end of the 16-week OL-LI phase, 94% of the patients in the MTX stratum and 74% of the patients in the non-MTX stratum were Pediatric ACR 30 responders. In the DB phase significantly fewer patients who received HUMIRA experienced disease flare compared to placebo, both without MTX (43% vs. 71%) and with MTX (37% vs. 65%). More patients treated with HUMIRA continued to show pediatric ACR 30/50/70 responses at Week 48 compared to patients treated with placebo. Pediatric ACR responses were maintained for up to two years in the OLE phase in patients who received HUMIRA throughout the study.

Continued on next page

Information on the AbbVie, Inc. products listed on these pages is from the prescribing information in use as of July 31, 2016. For more information, please visit rxabbvie.com or call 1-800-633-9110.

Table 2. ACR Responses in Studies RA-II and RA-III (Percent of Patients)

Response	Study RA-II Monotherapy (26 weeks)		Study RA-III Methotrexate Combination (24 and 52 weeks)	
	Placebo	HUMIRA 40 mg every other week	HUMIRA 40 mg weekly	Placebo/MTX	HUMIRA/MTX 40 mg every other week
	N=110	N=113	N=103	N=200	N=207
ACR20					
Month 6	19%	46%*	53%*	30%	63%*
Month 12	NA	NA	NA	24%	59%*
ACR50					
Month 6	8%	22%*	35%*	10%	39%*
Month 12	NA	NA	NA	10%	42%*
ACR70					
Month 6	2%	12%*	18%*	3%	21%*
Month 12	NA	NA	NA	5%	23%*

* p<0.01, HUMIRA *vs.* placebo

Study JIA-II
HUMIRA was assessed in an open-label, multicenter study in 32 patients who were 2 to <4 years of age or 4 years of age and older weighing <15 kg with moderately to severely active polyarticular JIA. Most patients (97%) received at least 24 weeks of HUMIRA treatment dosed 24 mg/m² up to a maximum of 20 mg every other week as a single SC injection up to a maximum of 120 weeks duration. During the study, most patients used concomitant MTX, with fewer reporting use of corticosteroids or NSAIDs. The primary objective of the study was evaluation of safety *[see Adverse Reactions (6.1)]*.

14.3   Psoriatic Arthritis
The safety and efficacy of HUMIRA was assessed in two randomized, double-blind, placebo controlled studies in 413 patients with psoriatic arthritis (PsA). Upon completion of both studies, 383 patients enrolled in an open-label extension study, in which 40 mg HUMIRA was administered every other week.

Study PsA-I enrolled 313 adult patients with moderately to severely active PsA (>3 swollen and >3 tender joints) who had an inadequate response to NSAID therapy in one of the following forms: (1) distal interphalangeal (DIP) involvement (N=23); (2) polyarticular arthritis (absence of rheumatoid nodules and presence of plaque psoriasis) (N=210); (3) arthritis mutilans (N=1); (4) asymmetric PsA (N=77); or (5) AS-like (N=2). Patients on MTX therapy (158 of 313 patients) at enrollment (stable dose of ≤30 mg/week for >1 month) could continue MTX at the same dose. Doses of HUMIRA 40 mg or placebo every other week were administered during the 24-week double-blind period of the study. Compared to placebo, treatment with HUMIRA resulted in improvements in the measures of disease activity (see Tables 7 and 8). Among patients with PsA who received HUMIRA, the clinical responses were apparent in some patients at the time of the first visit (two weeks) and were maintained up to 88 weeks in the ongoing open-label study. Similar responses were seen in patients with each of the subtypes of psoriatic arthritis, although few patients were enrolled with the arthritis mutilans and ankylosing spondylitis-like subtypes. Responses were similar in patients who were or were not receiving concomitant MTX therapy at baseline.

Patients with psoriatic involvement of at least three percent body surface area (BSA) were evaluated for Psoriatic Area and Severity Index (PASI) responses. At 24 weeks, the proportions of patients achieving a 75% or 90% improvement in the PASI were 59% and 42% respectively, in the HUMIRA group (N=69), compared to 1% and 0% respectively, in the placebo group (N=69) (p<0.001). PASI responses were apparent in some patients at the time of the first visit (two weeks). Responses were similar in patients who were or were not receiving concomitant MTX therapy at baseline.

Table 7. ACR Response in Study PsA-I (Percent of Patients)

	Placebo N=162	HUMIRA* N=151
ACR20	14%	58%
Week 12	15%	57%
Week 24		
ACR50	4%	36%
Week 12	6%	39%
Week 24		
ACR70	1%	20%
Week 12	1%	23%
Week 24		

* p<0.001 for all comparisons between HUMIRA and placebo

[See table 8 at top of next page]
Similar results were seen in an additional, 12-week study in 100 patients with moderate to severe psoriatic arthritis who had suboptimal response to DMARD therapy as manifested by ≥3 tender joints and ≥3 swollen joints at enrollment.
Radiographic Response
Radiographic changes were assessed in the PsA studies. Radiographs of hands, wrists, and feet were obtained at baseline and Week 24 during the double-blind period when patients were on HUMIRA or placebo and at Week 48 when all patients were on open-label HUMIRA. A modified Total Sharp Score (mTSS), which included distal interphalangeal joints (i.e., not identical to the TSS used for rheumatoid arthritis), was used by readers blinded to treatment group to assess the radiographs.

Table 3. Components of ACR Response in Studies RA-II and RA-III

Parameter (median)	Study RA-II				Study RA-III			
	Placebo N=110		HUMIRA[a] N=113		Placebo/MTX N=200		HUMIRA[a]/MTX N=207	
	Baseline	Wk 26	Baseline	Wk 26	Baseline	Wk 24	Baseline	Wk 24
Number of tender joints (0-68)	35	26	31	16*	26	15	24	8*
Number of swollen joints (0-66)	19	16	18	10*	17	11	18	5*
Physician global assessment[b]	7.0	6.1	6.6	3.7*	6.3	3.5	6.5	2.0*
Patient global assessment[b]	7.5	6.3	7.5	4.5*	5.4	3.9	5.2	2.0*
Pain[b]	7.3	6.1	7.3	4.1*	6.0	3.8	5.8	2.1*
Disability index (HAQ)[c]	2.0	1.9	1.9	1.5*	1.5	1.3	1.5	0.8*
CRP (mg/dL)	3.9	4.3	4.6	1.8*	1.0	0.9	1.0	0.4*

[a] 40 mg HUMIRA administered every other week
[b] Visual analogue scale; 0 = best, 10 = worst
[c] Disability Index of the Health Assessment Questionnaire; 0 = best, 3 = worst, measures the patient's ability to perform the following: dress/groom, arise, eat, walk, reach, grip, maintain hygiene, and maintain daily activity
* p<0.001, HUMIRA *vs.* placebo, based on mean change from baseline

Table 4. ACR Response in Study RA-V (Percent of Patients)

Response	MTX[b] N=257	HUMIRA[c] N=274	HUMIRA/MTX N=268
ACR20	63%	54%	73%
Week 52	56%	49%	69%
Week 104			
ACR50	46%	41%	62%
Week 52	43%	37%	59%
Week 104			
ACR70	27%	26%	46%
Week 52	28%	28%	47%
Week 104			
Major Clinical Response[a]	28%	25%	49%

[a] Major clinical response is defined as achieving an ACR70 response for a continuous six month period
[b] p<0.05, HUMIRA/MTX *vs.* MTX for ACR 20
  p<0.001, HUMIRA/MTX *vs.* MTX for ACR 50 and 70, and Major Clinical Response
[c] p<0.001, HUMIRA/MTX *vs.* HUMIRA

Table 5. Radiographic Mean Changes Over 12 Months in Study RA-III

	Placebo/MTX	HUMIRA/MTX 40 mg every other week	Placebo/MTX-HUMIRA/MTX (95% Confidence Interval*)	P-value**
Total Sharp score	2.7	0.1	2.6 (1.4, 3.8)	<0.001
Erosion score	1.6	0.0	1.6 (0.9, 2.2)	<0.001
JSN score	1.0	0.1	0.9 (0.3, 1.4)	0.002

*95% confidence intervals for the differences in change scores between MTX and HUMIRA.
**Based on rank analysis

Table 6. Radiographic Mean Change* in Study RA-V

		MTX[a] N=257	HUMIRA[a,b] N=274	HUMIRA/MTX N=268
52 Weeks	Total Sharp score	5.7 (4.2, 7.3)	3.0 (1.7, 4.3)	1.3 (0.5, 2.1)
	Erosion score	3.7 (2.7, 4.8)	1.7 (1.0, 2.4)	0.8 (0.4, 1.2)
	JSN score	2.0 (1.2, 2.8)	1.3 (0.5, 2.1)	0.5 (0.0, 1.0)
104 Weeks	Total Sharp score	10.4 (7.7, 13.2)	5.5 (3.6, 7.4)	1.9 (0.9, 2.9)
	Erosion score	6.4 (4.6, 8.2)	3.0 (2.0, 4.0)	1.0 (0.4, 1.6)
	JSN score	4.1 (2.7, 5.4)	2.6 (1.5, 3.7)	0.9 (0.3, 1.5)

* mean (95% confidence interval)
[a] p<0.001, HUMIRA/MTX *vs.* MTX at 52 and 104 weeks and for HUMIRA/MTX *vs.* HUMIRA at 104 weeks
[b] p<0.01, for HUMIRA/MTX *vs.* HUMIRA at 52 weeks

HUMIRA-treated patients demonstrated greater inhibition of radiographic progression compared to placebo-treated patients and this effect was maintained at 48 weeks (see Table 9).

Table 9. Change in Modified Total Sharp Score in Psoriatic Arthritis

	Placebo N=141	HUMIRA N=133	
	Week 24	Week 24	Week 48
Baseline mean	22.1	23.4	23.4
Mean Change ± SD	0.9 ± 3.1	-0.1 ± 1.7	-0.2 ± 4.9*

* <0.001 for the difference between HUMIRA, Week 48 and Placebo, Week 24 (primary analysis)

Physical Function Response
In Study PsA-I, physical function and disability were assessed using the HAQ Disability Index (HAQ-DI) and the SF-36 Health Survey. Patients treated with 40 mg of HUMIRA every other week showed greater improvement from baseline in the HAQ-DI score (mean decreases of 47% and 49% at Weeks 12 and 24 respectively) in comparison to placebo (mean decreases of 1% and 3% at Weeks 12 and 24 respectively). At Weeks 12 and 24, patients treated with

Table 8. Components of Disease Activity in Study PsA-I

Parameter: median	Placebo N=162 Baseline	24 weeks	HUMIRA* N=151 Baseline	24 weeks
Number of tender joints[a]	23.0	17.0	20.0	5.0
Number of swollen joints[b]	11.0	9.0	11.0	3.0
Physician global assessment[c]	53.0	49.0	55.0	16.0
Patient global assessment[c]	49.5	49.0	48.0	20.0
Pain[c]	49.0	49.0	54.0	20.0
Disability index (HAQ)[d]	1.0	0.9	1.0	0.4
CRP (mg/dL)[e]	0.8	0.7	0.8	0.2

* p<0.001 for HUMIRA *vs.* placebo comparisons based on median changes
[a] Scale 0-78
[b] Scale 0-76
[c] Visual analog scale; 0=best, 100=worst
[d] Disability Index of the Health Assessment Questionnaire; 0=best, 3=worst; measures the patient's ability to perform the following: dress/groom, arise, eat, walk, reach, grip, maintain hygiene, and maintain daily activity.
[e] Normal range: 0-0.287 mg/dL

HUMIRA showed greater improvement from baseline in the SF-36 Physical Component Summary score compared to patients treated with placebo, and no worsening in the SF-36 Mental Component Summary score. Improvement in physical function based on the HAQ-DI was maintained for up to 84 weeks through the open-label portion of the study.

14.4 Ankylosing Spondylitis

The safety and efficacy of HUMIRA 40 mg every other week was assessed in 315 adult patients in a randomized, 24 week double-blind, placebo-controlled study in patients with active ankylosing spondylitis (AS) who had an inadequate response to glucocorticoids, NSAIDs, analgesics, methotrexate or sulfasalazine. Active AS was defined as patients who fulfilled at least two of the following three criteria: (1) a Bath AS disease activity index (BASDAI) score ≥4 cm, (2) a visual analog score (VAS) for total back pain ≥ 40 mm, and (3) morning stiffness ≥ 1 hour. The blinded period was followed by an open-label period during which patients received HUMIRA 40 mg every other week subcutaneously for up to an additional 28 weeks.

Improvement in measures of disease activity was first observed at Week 2 and maintained through 24 weeks as shown in Figure 2 and Table 10.

Responses of patients with total spinal ankylosis (n=11) were similar to those without total ankylosis.

Figure 2. ASAS 20 Response By Visit, Study AS-I

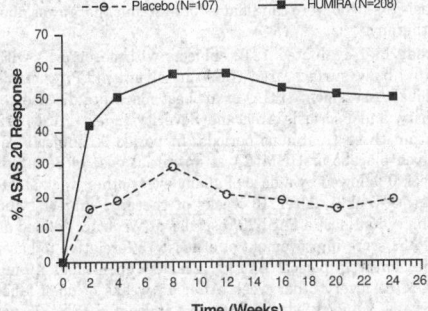

At 12 weeks, the ASAS 20/50/70 responses were achieved by 58%, 38%, and 23%, respectively, of patients receiving HUMIRA, compared to 21%, 10%, and 5% respectively, of patients receiving placebo (p <0.001). Similar responses were seen at Week 24 and were sustained in patients receiving open-label HUMIRA for up to 52 weeks.

A greater proportion of patients treated with HUMIRA (22%) achieved a low level of disease activity at 24 weeks (defined as a value <20 [on a scale of 0 to 100 mm] in each of the four ASAS response parameters) compared to patients treated with placebo (6%).

[See table 10 at top of next page]

A second randomized, multicenter, double-blind, placebo-controlled study of 82 patients with ankylosing spondylitis showed similar results.

Patients treated with HUMIRA achieved improvement from baseline in the Ankylosing Spondylitis Quality of Life Questionnaire (ASQoL) score (-3.6 *vs.* -1.1) and in the Short Form Health Survey (SF-36) Physical Component Summary (PCS) score (7.4 *vs.* 1.9) compared to placebo-treated patients at Week 24.

14.5 Adult Crohn's Disease

The safety and efficacy of multiple doses of HUMIRA were assessed in adult patients with moderately to severely active Crohn's disease, CD, (Crohn's Disease Activity Index (CDAI) ≥ 220 and ≤ 450) in randomized, double-blind, placebo-controlled studies. Concomitant stable doses of aminosalicylates, corticosteroids, and/or immunomodulatory agents were permitted, and 79% of patients continued to receive at least one of these medications.

Induction of clinical remission (defined as CDAI < 150) was evaluated in two studies. In Study CD-I, 299 TNF-blocker naïve patients were randomized to one of four treatment groups: the placebo group received placebo at Weeks 0 and 2, the 160/80 group received 160 mg HUMIRA at Week 0 and 80 mg at Week 2, the 80/40 group received 80 mg at Week 0 and 40 mg at Week 2, and the 40/20 group received 40 mg at Week 0 and 20 mg at Week 2. Clinical results were assessed at Week 4.

In the second induction study, Study CD-II, 325 patients who had lost response to, or were intolerant to, previous infliximab therapy were randomized to receive either 160 mg HUMIRA at Week 0 and 80 mg at Week 2, or placebo at Weeks 0 and 2. Clinical results were assessed at Week 4.

Maintenance of clinical remission was evaluated in Study CD-III. In this study, 854 patients with active disease received open-label HUMIRA, 80 mg at week 0 and 40 mg at Week 2. Patients were then randomized at Week 4 to 40 mg HUMIRA every other week, 40 mg HUMIRA every week, or placebo. The total study duration was 56 weeks. Patients in clinical response (decrease in CDAI ≥70) at Week 4 were stratified and analyzed separately from those not in clinical response at Week 4.

Induction of Clinical Remission

A greater percentage of the patients treated with 160/80 mg HUMIRA achieved induction of clinical remission versus placebo at Week 4 regardless of whether the patients were TNF blocker naïve (CD-I), or had lost response to or were intolerant to infliximab (CD-II) (see Table 11).

[See table 11 at top of next page]

Maintenance of Clinical Remission

In Study CD-III at Week 4, 58% (499/854) of patients were in clinical response and were assessed in the primary analysis. At Weeks 26 and 56, greater proportions of patients who were in clinical response at Week 4 achieved clinical remission in the HUMIRA 40 mg every other week maintenance group compared to patients in the placebo maintenance group (see Table 12). The group that received HUMIRA therapy every week did not demonstrate significantly higher remission rates compared to the group that received HUMIRA every other week.

Table 12. Maintenance of Clinical Remission in CD-III (Percent of Patients)

	Placebo N=170	40 mg HUMIRA every other week N=172
Week 26		
Clinical remission	17%	40%*
Clinical response	28%	54%*
Week 56		
Clinical remission	12%	36%*
Clinical response	18%	43%*

Clinical remission is CDAI score < 150; clinical response is decrease in CDAI of at least 70 points.
*p<0.001 for HUMIRA vs. placebo pairwise comparisons of proportions

Of those in response at Week 4 who attained remission during the study, patients in the HUMIRA every other week group maintained remission for a longer time than patients in the placebo maintenance group. Among patients who were not in response by Week 12, therapy continued beyond 12 weeks did not result in significantly more responses.

14.6 Pediatric Crohn's Disease

A randomized, double-blind, 52-week clinical study of 2 dose levels of HUMIRA (Study PCD-I) was conducted in 192 pediatric patients (6 to 17 years of age) with moderately to severely active Crohn's disease (defined as Pediatric Crohn's Disease Activity Index (PCDAI) score > 30).[2] Enrolled patients had over the previous two year period an inadequate response to corticosteroids or an immunomodulator (i.e., azathioprine, 6-mercaptopurine, or methotrexate). Patients who had previously received a TNF blocker were allowed to enroll if they had previously had loss of response or intolerance to that TNF blocker.

Patients received open-label induction therapy at a dose based on their body weight (≥40 kg and <40 kg). Patients weighing ≥40 kg received 160 mg (at Week 0) and 80 mg (at Week 2). Patients weighing <40 kg received 80 mg (at Week 0) and 40 mg (at Week 2). At Week 4, patients within each body weight category (≥40 kg and <40 kg) were randomized 1:1 to one of two maintenance dose regimens (high dose and low dose). The high dose was 40 mg every other week for patients weighing ≥40 kg and 20 mg every other week for patients weighing <40 kg. The low dose was 20 mg every other week for patients weighing ≥40 kg and 10 mg every other week for patients weighing <40 kg.

Concomitant stable dosages of corticosteroids (prednisone dosage ≤40 mg/day or equivalent) and immunomodulators (azathioprine, 6-mercaptopurine, or methotrexate) were permitted throughout the study.

At Week 12, patients who experienced a disease flare (increase in PCDAI of ≥ 15 from Week 4 and absolute PCDAI > 30) or who were non-responders (did not achieve a decrease in the PCDAI of ≥ 15 from baseline for 2 consecutive visits at least 2 weeks apart) were allowed to dose-escalate (i.e., switch from blinded every other week dosing to blinded every week dosing); patients who dose-escalated were considered treatment failures.

At baseline, 38% of patients were receiving corticosteroids, and 62% of patients were receiving an immunomodulator. Forty-four percent (44%) of patients had previously lost response or were intolerant to a TNF blocker. The median baseline PCDAI score was 40.

Of the 192 patients total, 188 patients completed the 4 week induction period, 152 patients completed 26 weeks of treatment, and 124 patients completed 52 weeks of treatment. Fifty-one percent (51%) (48/95) of patients in the low maintenance dose group dose-escalated, and 38% (35/93) of patients in the high maintenance dose group dose-escalated.

At Week 4, 28% (52/188) of patients were in clinical remission (defined as PCDAI ≤ 10).

The proportions of patients in clinical remission (defined as PCDAI ≤ 10) and clinical response (defined as reduction in PCDAI of at least 15 points from baseline) were assessed at Weeks 26 and 52.

At both Weeks 26 and 52, the proportion of patients in clinical remission and clinical response was numerically higher in the high dose group compared to the low dose group (Table 13). The recommended maintenance regimen is 20 mg every other week for patients weighing < 40 kg and 40 mg every other week for patients weighing ≥ 40 kg. Every week dosing is not the recommended maintenance dosing regimen *[see Dosage and Administration (2.4)]*.

Table 13. Clinical Remission and Clinical Response in Study PCD-I

	Low Maintenance Dose[†] (20 or 10 mg every other week) N = 95	High Maintenance Dose[#] (40 or 20 mg every other week) N = 93

Continued on next page

Week 26

Clinical Remission[‡]	28%	39%
Clinical Response[§]	48%	59%

Week 52

Clinical Remission[‡]	23%	33%
Clinical Response[§]	28%	42%

[†]The low maintenance dose was 20 mg every other week for patients weighing ≥ 40 kg and 10 mg every other week for patients weighing < 40 kg.

[#]The high maintenance dose was 40 mg every other week for patients weighing ≥ 40 kg and 20 mg every other week for patients weighing < 40 kg.

[‡]Clinical remission defined as PCDAI ≤ 10.

[§]Clinical response defined as reduction in PCDAI of at least 15 points from baseline.

14.7 Ulcerative Colitis

The safety and efficacy of HUMIRA® (adalimumab) were assessed in adult patients with moderately to severely active ulcerative colitis (Mayo score 6 to 12 on a 12 point scale, with an endoscopy subscore of 2 to 3 on a scale of 0 to 3) despite concurrent or prior treatment with immunosuppressants such as corticosteroids, azathioprine, or 6-MP in two randomized, double-blind, placebo-controlled clinical studies (Studies UC-I and UC-II). Both studies enrolled TNF-blocker naïve patients, but Study UC-II also allowed entry of patients who lost response to or were intolerant to TNF-blockers. Forty percent (40%) of patients enrolled in Study UC-II had previously used another TNF-blocker.

Concomitant stable doses of aminosalicylates and immunosuppressants were permitted. In Studies UC-I and II, patients were receiving aminosalicylates (69%), corticosteroids (59%) and/or azathioprine or 6-MP (37%) at baseline. In both studies, 92% of patients received at least one of these medications.

Induction of clinical remission (defined as Mayo score ≤ 2 with no individual subscores > 1) at Week 8 was evaluated in both studies. Clinical remission at Week 52 and sustained clinical remission (defined as clinical remission at both Weeks 8 and 52) were evaluated in Study UC-II.

In Study UC-I, 390 TNF-blocker naïve patients were randomized to one of three treatment groups for the primary efficacy analysis. The placebo group received placebo at Weeks 0, 2, 4 and 6. The 160/80 group received 160 mg HUMIRA at Week 0 and 80 mg at Week 2, and the 80/40 group received 80 mg HUMIRA at Week 0 and 40 mg at Week 2. After Week 2, patients in both HUMIRA treatment groups received 40 mg every other week (eow).

In Study UC-II, 518 patients were randomized to receive either HUMIRA 160 mg at Week 0, 80 mg at Week 2, and 40 mg eow starting at Week 4 through Week 50, or placebo starting at Week 0 and eow through Week 50. Corticosteroid taper was permitted starting at Week 8.

In both Studies UC-I and UC-II, a greater percentage of the patients treated with 160/80 mg of HUMIRA compared to patients treated with placebo achieved induction of clinical remission. In Study UC-II, a greater percentage of the patients treated with 160/80 mg of HUMIRA compared to patients treated with placebo achieved sustained clinical remission (clinical remission at both Weeks 8 and 52) (Table 14).

[See table 14 below]

In Study UC-I, there was no statistically significant difference in clinical remission observed between the HUMIRA 80/40 mg group and the placebo group at Week 8.

In Study UC-II, 17.3% (43/248) in the HUMIRA group were in clinical remission at Week 52 compared to 8.5% (21/246) in the placebo group (treatment difference: 8.8%; 95% confidence interval (CI): [2.8%, 14.5%]; p<0.05).

In the subgroup of patients in Study UC-II with prior TNF-blocker use, the treatment difference for induction of clinical remission appeared to be lower than that seen in the whole study population, and the treatment differences for sustained clinical remission and clinical remission at Week 52 appeared to be similar to those seen in the whole study population. The subgroup of patients with prior TNF-blocker use achieved induction of clinical remission at 9% (9/98) in the HUMIRA group versus 7% (7/101) in the placebo group, and sustained clinical remission at 5% (5/98) in the HUMIRA group versus 1% (1/101) in the placebo group. In the subgroup of patients with prior TNF-blocker use, 10% (10/98) were in clinical remission at Week 52 in the HUMIRA group versus 3% (3/101) in the placebo group.

14.8 Plaque Psoriasis

The safety and efficacy of HUMIRA were assessed in randomized, double-blind, placebo-controlled studies in 1696 adult subjects with moderate to severe chronic plaque psoriasis (Ps) who were candidates for systemic therapy or phototherapy.

Study Ps-I evaluated 1212 subjects with chronic Ps with ≥10% body surface area (BSA) involvement, Physician's Global Assessment (PGA) of at least moderate disease severity, and Psoriasis Area and Severity Index (PASI) ≥12 within three treatment periods. In period A, subjects received placebo or HUMIRA at an initial dose of 80 mg at Week 0 followed by doses of 40 mg every other week starting at Week 1. After 16 weeks of therapy, subjects who achieved at least a PASI 75 response at Week 16, defined as a PASI score improvement of at least 75% relative to baseline, entered period B and received open-label 40 mg HUMIRA every other week. After 17 weeks of open label therapy, subjects who maintained at least a PASI 75 response at Week 33 and were originally randomized to active therapy in period A were re-randomized in period C to receive 40 mg HUMIRA every other week or placebo for an additional 19 weeks. Across all treatment groups the mean baseline PASI score was 19 and the baseline Physician's Global Assessment score ranged from "moderate" (53%) to "severe" (41%) to "very severe" (6%).

Study Ps-II evaluated 99 subjects randomized to HUMIRA and 48 subjects randomized to placebo with chronic plaque psoriasis with ≥10% BSA involvement and PASI ≥12. Subjects received placebo, or an initial dose of 80 mg HUMIRA at Week 0 followed by 40 mg every other week starting at Week 1 for 16 weeks. Across all treatment groups the mean baseline PASI score was 21 and the baseline PGA score ranged from "moderate" (41%) to "severe" (51%) to "very severe" (8%).

Studies Ps-I and II evaluated the proportion of subjects who achieved "clear" or "minimal" disease on the 6-point PGA scale and the proportion of subjects who achieved a reduction in PASI score of at least 75% (PASI 75) from baseline at Week 16 (see Table 15 and 16).

Table 10. Components of Ankylosing Spondylitis Disease Activity

	Placebo N=107		HUMIRA N=208	
	Baseline mean	Week 24 mean	Baseline mean	Week 24 mean
ASAS 20 Response Criteria*				
Patient's Global Assessment of Disease Activity[a]*	65	60	63	38
Total back pain*	67	58	65	37
Inflammation[b]*	6.7	5.6	6.7	3.6
BASFI[c]*	56	51	52	34
BASDAI[d] score*	6.3	5.5	6.3	3.7
BASMI[e] score*	4.2	4.1	3.8	3.3
Tragus to wall (cm)	15.9	15.8	15.8	15.4
Lumbar flexion (cm)	4.1	4.0	4.2	4.4
Cervical rotation (degrees)	42.2	42.1	48.4	51.6
Lumbar side flexion (cm)	8.9	9.0	9.7	11.7
Intermalleolar distance (cm)	92.9	94.0	93.5	100.8
CRP[f]*	2.2	2.0	1.8	0.6

[a] Percent of subjects with at least a 20% and 10-unit improvement measured on a Visual Analog Scale (VAS) with 0 = "none" and 100 = "severe"

[b] mean of questions 5 and 6 of BASDAI (defined in 'd')

[c] Bath Ankylosing Spondylitis Functional Index

[d] Bath Ankylosing Spondylitis Disease Activity Index

[e] Bath Ankylosing Spondylitis Metrology Index

[f] C-Reactive Protein (mg/dL)

* statistically significant for comparisons between HUMIRA and placebo at Week 24

Table 11. Induction of Clinical Remission in Studies CD-I and CD-II (Percent of Patients)

	CD-I		CD-II	
	Placebo N=74	HUMIRA 160/80 mg N=76	Placebo N=166	HUMIRA 160/80 mg N=159
Week 4				
Clinical remission	12%	36%[*]	7%	21%[*]
Clinical response	34%	58%[**]	34%	52%[**]

Clinical remission is CDAI score < 150; clinical response is decrease in CDAI of at least 70 points.

[*] p<0.001 for HUMIRA *vs.* placebo pairwise comparison of proportions

[**] p<0.01 for HUMIRA *vs.* placebo pairwise comparison of proportions

Table 14. Induction of Clinical Remission in Studies UC-I and UC-II and Sustained Clinical Remission in Study UC-II (Percent of Patients)

	Study UC-I			Study UC-II		
	Placebo N=130	HUMIRA 160/80 mg N=130	Treatment Difference (95% CI)	Placebo N=246	HUMIRA 160/80 mg N=248	Treatment Difference (95% CI)
Induction of Clinical Remission (Clinical Remission at Week 8)	9.2%	18.5%	9.3%* (0.9%, 17.6%)	9.3%	16.5%	7.2%* (1.2%, 12.9%)
Sustained Clinical Remission (Clinical Remission at both Weeks 8 and 52)	N/A	N/A	N/A	4.1%	8.5%	4.4%* (0.1%, 8.6%)

Clinical remission is defined as Mayo score ≤ 2 with no individual subscores > 1.

CI=Confidence interval

* p<0.05 for HUMIRA *vs.* placebo pairwise comparison of proportions

Additionally, Study Ps-I evaluated the proportion of subjects who maintained a PGA of "clear" or "minimal" disease or a PASI 75 response after Week 33 and on or before Week 52.

Table 15. Efficacy Results at 16 Weeks in Study Ps-I Number of Subjects (%)

	HUMIRA 40 mg every other week N = 814	Placebo N = 398
PGA: Clear or minimal*	506 (62%)	17 (4%)
PASI 75	578 (71%)	26 (7%)

* Clear = no plaque elevation, no scale, plus or minus hyperpigmentation or diffuse pink or red coloration
Minimal = possible but difficult to ascertain whether there is slight elevation of plaque above normal skin, plus or minus surface dryness with some white coloration, plus or minus up to red coloration

Table 16. Efficacy Results at 16 Weeks in Study Ps-II Number of Subjects (%)

	HUMIRA 40 mg every other week N = 99	Placebo N = 48
PGA: Clear or minimal*	70 (71%)	5 (10%)
PASI 75	77 (78%)	9 (19%)

* Clear = no plaque elevation, no scale, plus or minus hyperpigmentation or diffuse pink or red coloration
Minimal = possible but difficult to ascertain whether there is slight elevation of plaque above normal skin, plus or minus surface dryness with some white coloration, plus or minus up to red coloration

Additionally, in Study Ps-I, subjects on HUMIRA who maintained a PASI 75 were re-randomized to HUMIRA (N = 250) or placebo (N = 240) at Week 33. After 52 weeks of treatment with HUMIRA, more subjects on HUMIRA maintained efficacy when compared to subjects who were re-randomized to placebo based on maintenance of PGA of "clear" or "minimal" disease (68% *vs.* 28%) or a PASI 75 (79% *vs.* 43%).

A total of 347 stable responders participated in a withdrawal and retreatment evaluation in an open-label extension study. Median time to relapse (decline to PGA "moderate" or worse) was approximately 5 months. During the withdrawal period, no subject experienced transformation to either pustular or erythrodermic psoriasis. A total of 178 subjects who relapsed re-initiated treatment with 80 mg of HUMIRA, then 40 mg eow beginning at week 1. At week 16, 69% (123/178) of subjects had a response of PGA "clear" or "minimal".

14.9   Hidradenitis Suppurativa
Two randomized, double-blind, placebo-controlled studies (Studies HS-I and II) evaluated the safety and efficacy of HUMIRA in a total of 633 adult subjects with moderate to severe hidradenitis suppurativa (HS) with Hurley Stage II or III disease and with at least 3 abscesses or inflammatory nodules. In both studies, subjects received placebo or HUMIRA at an initial dose of 160 mg at Week 0, 80 mg at Week 2, and 40 mg every week starting at Week 4 and continued through Week 11. Subjects used topical antiseptic wash daily. Concomitant oral antibiotic use was allowed in Study HS-II.
Both studies evaluated Hidradenitis Suppurativa Clinical Response (HiSCR) at Week 12. HiSCR was defined as at least a 50% reduction in total abscess and inflammatory nodule count with no increase in abscess count and no increase in draining fistula count relative to baseline (see Table 17). Reduction in HS-related skin pain was assessed using a Numeric Rating Scale in patients who entered the study with an initial baseline score of 3 or greater on a 11 point scale.
In both studies, a higher proportion of HUMIRA- than placebo-treated subjects achieved HiSCR (see Table 17).
[See table 17 above]
In both studies, from Week 12 to Week 35 (Period B), subjects who had received HUMIRA were re-randomized to 1 of 3 treatment groups (HUMIRA 40 mg every week, HUMIRA 40 mg every other week, or placebo). Subjects who had been randomized to placebo were assigned to receive HUMIRA 40 mg every week (Study HS-I) or placebo (Study HS-II).

Table 17. Efficacy Results at 12 Weeks in Subjects with Moderate to Severe Hidradenitis Suppurativa

	HS Study I		HS Study II*	
	Placebo	Humira 40 mg Weekly	Placebo	Humira 40 mg Weekly
Hidradenitis Suppurativa Clinical Response (HiSCR)	N = 154 40 (26%)	N = 153 64 (42%)	N=163 45 (28%)	N=163 96 (59%)

*19.3% of subjects in Study HS-II continued baseline oral antibiotic therapy during the study.

During Period B, flare of HS, defined as ≥25% increase from baseline in abscesses and inflammatory nodule counts and with a minimum of 2 additional lesions, was documented in 22 (22%) of the 100 subjects who were withdrawn from HUMIRA treatment following the primary efficacy timepoint in two studies.

14.10   Uveitis
The safety and efficacy of HUMIRA were assessed in adult patients with non-infectious intermediate, posterior and panuveitis excluding patients with isolated anterior uveitis, in two randomized, double-masked, placebo-controlled studies (UV I and II). Patients received placebo or HUMIRA at an initial dose of 80 mg followed by 40 mg every other week starting one week after the initial dose. The primary efficacy endpoint in both studies was 'time to treatment failure'.
Treatment failure was a multi-component outcome defined as the development of new inflammatory chorioretinal and/or inflammatory retinal vascular lesions, an increase in anterior chamber (AC) cell grade or vitreous haze (VH) grade or a decrease in best corrected visual acuity (BCVA). Study UV I evaluated 217 patients with active uveitis while being treated with corticosteroids (oral prednisone at a dose of 10 to 60 mg/day). All patients received a standardized dose of prednisone 60 mg/day at study entry followed by a mandatory taper schedule, with complete corticosteroid discontinuation by Week 15.
Study UV II evaluated 226 patients with inactive uveitis while being treated with corticosteroids (oral prednisone 10 to 35 mg/day) at baseline to control their disease. Patients subsequently underwent a mandatory taper schedule, with complete corticosteroid discontinuation by Week 19.
Clinical Response
Results from both studies demonstrated statistically significant reduction of the risk of treatment failure in patients treated with HUMIRA versus patients receiving placebo. In both studies, all components of the primary endpoint contributed cumulatively to the overall difference between HUMIRA and placebo groups (Table 18).
[See table 18 at top of next page]
[See Figure 3 on next page]

15   REFERENCES
1. National Cancer Institute. Surveillance, Epidemiology, and End Results Database (SEER) Program. SEER Incidence Crude Rates, 17 Registries, 2000-2007.
2. Hyams JS, Ferry GD, Mandel FS, et al. Development and validation of a pediatric Crohn's disease activity index. J Pediatr Gastroenterol Nutr. 1991;12:439-447.

16   HOW SUPPLIED/STORAGE AND HANDLING
HUMIRA® (adalimumab) is supplied as a preservative-free, sterile solution for subcutaneous administration. The following packaging configurations are available.

• **HUMIRA Pen Carton - 40 mg/0.8 mL**
HUMIRA is dispensed in a carton containing two alcohol preps and two dose trays. Each dose tray consists of a single-use pen, containing a 1 mL prefilled glass syringe with a fixed 27 gauge, ½ inch needle, providing 40 mg/0.8 mL of HUMIRA. The gray needle cover contains natural rubber latex. The NDC number is 0074-4339-02.

• **HUMIRA Pen Carton - 40 mg/0.4 mL**
HUMIRA is dispensed in a carton containing two alcohol preps and two dose trays. Each dose tray consists of a single-use pen, containing a 1 mL prefilled glass syringe with a fixed 29 gauge thin wall, ½ inch needle, providing 40 mg/0.4 mL of HUMIRA. The black needle cover is not made with natural rubber latex. The NDC number is 0074-0554-02.

• **HUMIRA Pen 40 mg/0.8 mL - Starter Package for Crohn's Disease, Ulcerative Colitis or Hidradenitis Suppurativa**
HUMIRA is dispensed in a carton containing 6 alcohol preps and 6 dose trays (Starter Package for Crohn's Disease, Ulcerative Colitis or Hidradenitis Suppurativa). Each dose tray consists of a single-use pen, containing a 1 mL prefilled glass syringe with a fixed 27 gauge, ½ inch

needle, providing 40 mg/0.8 mL of HUMIRA. The gray needle cover contains natural rubber latex. The NDC number is 0074-4339-06.

• **HUMIRA Pen 40 mg/0.4 mL - Starter Package for Crohn's Disease, Ulcerative Colitis or Hidradenitis Suppurativa**
HUMIRA is dispensed in a carton containing 6 alcohol preps and 6 dose trays (Starter Package for Crohn's Disease, Ulcerative Colitis or Hidradenitis Suppurativa). Each dose tray consists of a single-use pen, containing a 1 mL prefilled glass syringe with a fixed 29 gauge thin wall, ½ inch needle, providing 40 mg/0.4 mL of HUMIRA. The black needle cover is not made with natural rubber latex. The NDC number is 0074-0554-06.

• **HUMIRA Pen 40 mg/0.8 mL - Psoriasis/Uveitis Starter Package**
HUMIRA is dispensed in a carton containing 4 alcohol preps and 4 dose trays (Psoriasis/Uveitis Starter Package). Each dose tray consists of a single-use pen, containing a 1 mL prefilled glass syringe with a fixed 27 gauge, ½ inch needle, providing 40 mg/0.8 mL of HUMIRA. The gray needle cover contains natural rubber latex. The NDC number is 0074-4339-07.

• **HUMIRA Pen 40 mg/0.4 mL - Psoriasis/Uveitis Starter Package**
HUMIRA is dispensed in a carton containing 4 alcohol preps and 4 dose trays (Psoriasis/Uveitis Starter Package). Each dose tray consists of a single-use pen, containing a 1 mL prefilled glass syringe with a fixed 29 gauge thin wall, ½ inch needle, providing 40 mg/0.4 mL of HUMIRA. The black needle cover is not made with natural rubber latex. The NDC number is 0074-0554-04.

• **Prefilled Syringe Carton - 40 mg/0.8 mL**
HUMIRA is dispensed in a carton containing two alcohol preps and two dose trays. Each dose tray consists of a single-use, 1 mL prefilled glass syringe with a fixed 27 gauge, ½ inch needle, providing 40 mg/0.8 mL of HUMIRA. The gray needle cover contains natural rubber latex. The NDC number is 0074-3799-02.

• **Prefilled Syringe Carton - 40 mg/0.4 mL**
HUMIRA is dispensed in a carton containing two alcohol preps and two dose trays. Each dose tray consists of a single-use, 1 mL prefilled glass syringe with a fixed 29 gauge thin wall, ½ inch needle, providing 40 mg/0.4 mL of HUMIRA. The black needle cover is not made with natural rubber latex. The NDC number is 0074-0243-02.

• **Prefilled Syringe Carton - 20 mg/0.4 mL**
HUMIRA is supplied in a carton containing two alcohol preps and two dose trays. Each dose tray consists of a single-use, 1 mL pre-filled glass syringe with a fixed 27 gauge, ½ inch needle, providing 20 mg/0.4 mL of HUMIRA. The gray needle cover contains natural rubber latex. The NDC number is 0074-9374-02.

• **Prefilled Syringe Carton - 10 mg/0.2 mL**
HUMIRA is supplied in a carton containing two alcohol preps and two dose trays. Each dose tray consists of a single-use, 1 mL pre-filled glass syringe with a fixed 27 gauge, ½ inch needle, providing 10 mg/0.2 mL of HUMIRA. The gray needle cover contains natural rubber latex. The NDC number is 0074-6347-02.

• **HUMIRA Prefilled Syringe 40 mg/0.8 mL - Pediatric Crohn's Disease Starter Package (6 count)**
HUMIRA is dispensed in a carton containing 6 alcohol preps and 6 dose trays (Pediatric Starter Package). Each dose tray consists of a single-use, 1 mL prefilled glass syringe with a fixed 27 gauge, ½ inch needle, providing 40 mg/0.8 mL of HUMIRA. The gray needle cover contains natural rubber latex. The NDC number is 0074-3799-06.

• **HUMIRA Prefilled Syringe 40 mg/0.8 mL - Pediatric Crohn's Disease Starter Package (3 count)**

Continued on next page

Information on the AbbVie, Inc. products listed on these pages is from the prescribing information in use as of July 31, 2016. For more information, please visit rxabbvie.com or call 1-800-633-9110.

HUMIRA is dispensed in a carton containing 4 alcohol preps and 3 dose trays (Pediatric Starter Package). Each dose tray consists of a single-use, 1 mL prefilled glass syringe with a fixed 27 gauge, ½ inch needle, providing 40 mg/0.8 mL of HUMIRA. The gray needle cover contains natural rubber latex. The NDC number is 0074-3799-03.

- **Single-Use Institutional Use Vial Carton - 40 mg/0.8 mL**
HUMIRA is supplied for institutional use only in a carton containing a single-use, glass vial, providing 40 mg/0.8 mL of HUMIRA. The vial stopper is not made with natural rubber latex. The NDC number is 0074-3797-01.

Storage and Stability

Do not use beyond the expiration date on the container. HUMIRA must be refrigerated at 36°F to 46°F (2°C to 8°C). DO NOT FREEZE. Do not use if frozen even if it has been thawed.

Store in original carton until time of administration to protect from light.

If needed, for example when traveling, HUMIRA may be stored at room temperature up to a maximum of 77°F (25°C) for a period of up to 14 days, with protection from light. HUMIRA should be discarded if not used within the 14-day period. Record the date when HUMIRA is first removed from the refrigerator in the spaces provided on the carton and dose tray.

Do not store HUMIRA in extreme heat or cold.

17   PATIENT COUNSELING INFORMATION

See FDA-approved patient labeling (Medication Guide and Instructions for Use).

Patient Counseling

Provide the HUMIRA "Medication Guide" to patients or their caregivers, and provide them an opportunity to read it and ask questions prior to initiation of therapy and prior to each time the prescription is renewed. If patients develop signs and symptoms of infection, instruct them to seek medical evaluation immediately.

Advise patients of the potential benefits and risks of HUMIRA.

- **Infections**
Inform patients that HUMIRA may lower the ability of their immune system to fight infections. Instruct patients of the importance of contacting their doctor if they develop any symptoms of infection, including tuberculosis, invasive fungal infections, and reactivation of hepatitis B virus infections.

- **Malignancies**
Counsel patients about the risk of malignancies while receiving HUMIRA.

- **Allergic Reactions**
Advise patients to seek immediate medical attention if they experience any symptoms of severe allergic reactions. Advise latex-sensitive patients that the gray needle cap of the 27 gauge HUMIRA Pen and prefilled syringe contains natural rubber latex *[see How Supplied/Storage and Handling (16) for specific information]*.

- **Other Medical Conditions**
Advise patients to report any signs of new or worsening medical conditions such as congestive heart failure, neurological disease, autoimmune disorders, or cytopenias. Advise patients to report any symptoms suggestive of a cytopenia such as bruising, bleeding, or persistent fever.

Instructions on Injection Technique

Inform patients that the first injection is to be performed under the supervision of a qualified health care professional. If a patient or caregiver is to administer HUMIRA, instruct them in injection techniques and assess their ability to inject subcutaneously to ensure the proper administration of HUMIRA *[see Instructions for Use]*.

For patients who will use the HUMIRA Pen, tell them that they:

- Will hear a **loud 'click'** when the plum-colored activator button is pressed. The loud click means the **start** of the injection.
- Must keep holding the HUMIRA Pen against their squeezed, raised skin until all of the medicine is injected. This can take up to 10 seconds.
- Will know that the injection has finished when the yellow marker fully appears in the window view and stops moving.

Instruct patients to dispose of their used needles and syringes or used Pen in a FDA-cleared sharps disposal container immediately after use. **Instruct patients not to dispose of loose needles and syringes or Pen in their household trash.**

Instruct patients that if they do not have a FDA-cleared sharps disposal container, they may use a household container that is made of a heavy-duty plastic, can be closed with a tight-fitting and puncture-resistant lid without sharps being able to come out, upright and stable during use, leak-resistant, and properly labeled to warn of hazardous waste inside the container.

Instruct patients that when their sharps disposal container is almost full, they will need to follow their community guidelines for the correct way to dispose of their sharps disposal container. Instruct patients that there may be state or local laws regarding disposal of used needles and syringes. Refer patients to the FDA's website at http://www.fda.gov/safesharpsdisposal for more information about safe sharps disposal, and for specific information about sharps disposal in the state that they live in.

Instruct patients not to dispose of their used sharps disposal container in their household trash unless their community guidelines permit this. Instruct patients not to recycle their used sharps disposal container.

AbbVie Inc.
North Chicago, IL 60064, U.S.A.
US License Number 1889
03-B374 07/2016

MEDICATION GUIDE
HUMIRA® (Hu-MARE-ah)
(adalimumab)
injection

Read the Medication Guide that comes with HUMIRA before you start taking it and each time you get a refill. There may be new information. This Medication Guide does not take the place of talking with your doctor about your medical condition or treatment.

What is the most important information I should know about HUMIRA?

HUMIRA is a medicine that affects your immune system. HUMIRA can lower the ability of your immune system to fight infections. **Serious infections have happened in people taking HUMIRA. These serious infections include tuberculosis (TB) and infections caused by viruses, fungi or bacteria that have spread throughout the body. Some people have died from these infections.**

- Your doctor should test you for TB before starting HUMIRA.
- Your doctor should check you closely for signs and symptoms of TB during treatment with HUMIRA.

You should not start taking HUMIRA® (adalimumab) if you have any kind of infection unless your doctor says it is okay.

Before starting HUMIRA, tell your doctor if you:

- think you have an infection or have symptoms of infection such as:

Table 18. Time to Treatment Failure in Studies UV I and UV II

| | UV I | | | | UV II | |
	Placebo (N = 107)	HUMIRA (N = 110)	HR [95% CI][a]	Placebo (N = 111)	HUMIRA (N = 115)	HR [95% CI][a]
Failure[b] n (%)	84 (78.5)	60 (54.5)	0.50 [0.36, 0.70]	61 (55.0)	45 (39.1)	0.57 [0.39, 0.84]
Median Time to Failure (Months) [95% CI]	3.0 [2.7, 3.7]	5.6 [3.9, 9.2]	N/A	8.3 [4.8, 12.0]	NE[c]	N/A

[a] HR of HUMIRA versus placebo from proportional hazards regression with treatment as factor.
[b] Treatment failure at or after Week 6 in Study UV I, or at or after Week 2 in Study UV II, was counted as event. Subjects who discontinued the study were censored at the time of dropping out.
[c] NE = not estimable. Fewer than half of at-risk subjects had an event.

Figure 3: Kaplan-Meier Curves Summarizing Time to Treatment Failure on or after Week 6 (Study UV I) or Week 2 (Study UV II)

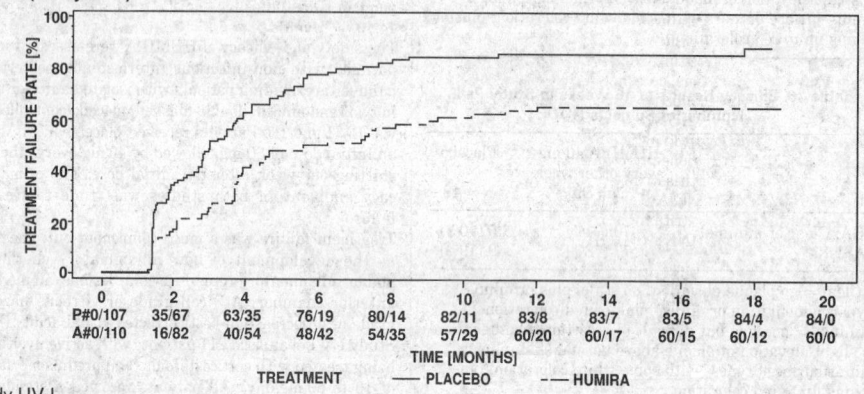

Study UV I

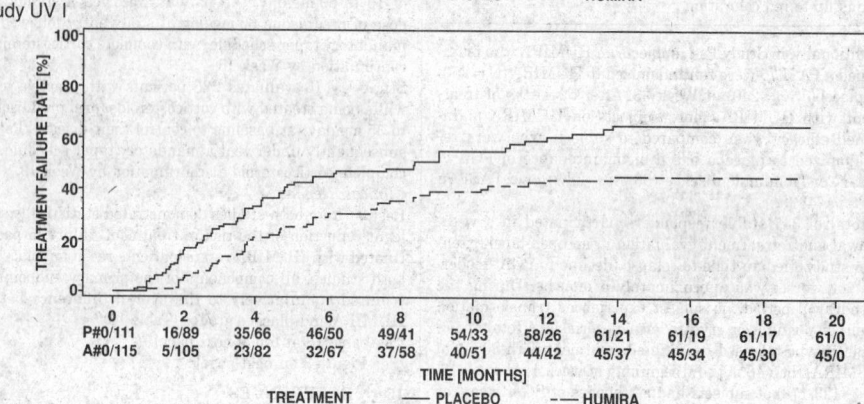

Study UV II

Note: P# = Placebo (Number of Events/Number at Risk); A# = HUMIRA (Number of Events/Number at Risk).

- ○ fever, sweats, or chills
- ○ muscle aches
- ○ cough
- ○ shortness of breath
- ○ blood in phlegm

- ○ warm, red, or painful skin or sores on your body
- ○ diarrhea or stomach pain
- ○ burning when you urinate or urinate more often than normal
- ○ feel very tired
- ○ weight loss

- are being treated for an infection
- get a lot of infections or have infections that keep coming back
- have diabetes
- have TB, or have been in close contact with someone with TB
- were born in, lived in, or traveled to countries where there is more risk for getting TB. Ask your doctor if you are not sure.
- live or have lived in certain parts of the country (such as the Ohio and Mississippi River valleys) where there is an increased risk for getting certain kinds of fungal infections (histoplasmosis, coccidioidomycosis, or blastomycosis). These infections may happen or become more severe if you use HUMIRA® (adalimumab). Ask your doctor if you do not know if you have lived in an area where these infections are common.
- have or have had hepatitis B
- use the medicine ORENCIA® (abatacept), KINERET® (anakinra), RITUXAN® (rituximab), IMURAN® (azathioprine), or PURINETHOL® (6–mercaptopurine, 6-MP).
- are scheduled to have major surgery

After starting HUMIRA, call your doctor right away if you have an infection, or any sign of an infection. HUMIRA can make you more likely to get infections or make any infection that you may have worse.

Cancer
- For children and adults taking TNF-blockers, including HUMIRA, the chances of getting cancer may increase.
- There have been cases of unusual cancers in children, teenagers, and young adults using TNF-blockers.
- People with RA, especially more serious RA, may have a higher chance for getting a kind of cancer called lymphoma.
- If you use TNF blockers including HUMIRA® (adalimumab) your chance of getting two types of skin cancer may increase (basal cell cancer and squamous cell cancer of the skin). These types of cancer are generally not life-threatening if treated. Tell your doctor if you have a bump or open sore that doesn't heal.
- Some people receiving TNF blockers including HUMIRA developed a rare type of cancer called hepatosplenic T-cell lymphoma. This type of cancer often results in death. Most of these people were male teenagers or young men. Also, most people were being treated for Crohn's disease or ulcerative colitis with another medicine called IMURAN® (azathioprine) or PURINETHOL® (6-mercaptopurine, 6–MP).

What is HUMIRA?
HUMIRA is a medicine called a Tumor Necrosis Factor (TNF) blocker. HUMIRA® (adalimumab) is used:
- To reduce the signs and symptoms of:
  - ○ **moderate to severe rheumatoid arthritis (RA) in adults.** HUMIRA can be used alone, with methotrexate, or with certain other medicines.
  - ○ **moderate to severe polyarticular juvenile idiopathic arthritis (JIA) in children** 2 years and older. HUMIRA can be used alone, with methotrexate, or with certain other medicines.
  - ○ **psoriatic arthritis (PsA) in adults.** HUMIRA can be used alone or with certain other medicines.
  - ○ **ankylosing spondylitis (AS) in adults.**
  - ○ **moderate to severe Crohn's disease (CD) in adults** when other treatments have not worked well enough.
  - ○ **moderate to severe Crohn's disease (CD) in children** 6 years and older when other treatments have not worked well enough.
  - ○ **moderate to severe hidradenitis suppurativa (HS) in adults.**
- In adults, to help get **moderate to severe ulcerative colitis (UC)** under control (induce remission) and keep it under control (sustain remission) when certain other medicines have not worked well enough. It is not known if HUMIRA® (adalimumab) is effective in people who stopped responding to or could not tolerate TNF-blocker medicines.
- To treat **moderate to severe chronic (lasting a long time) plaque psoriasis (Ps) in adults** who have the condition in many areas of their body and who may benefit from taking injections or pills (systemic therapy) or phototherapy (treatment using ultraviolet light alone or with pills).

- To treat **non-infectious intermediate, posterior and panu-veitis (UV) in adults.**

What should I tell my doctor before taking HUMIRA?
HUMIRA may not be right for you. Before starting HUMIRA, tell your doctor about all of your health conditions, including if you:
- have an infection. See **"What is the most important information I should know about HUMIRA?"**
- have or have had cancer.
- have any numbness or tingling or have a disease that affects your nervous system such as multiple sclerosis or Guillain-Barré syndrome.
- have or had heart failure.
- have recently received or are scheduled to receive a vaccine. You may receive vaccines, except for live vaccines while using HUMIRA® (adalimumab). Children should be brought up to date with all vaccines before starting HUMIRA.
- are allergic to rubber or latex. Tell your doctor if you have any allergies to rubber or latex.
  - ○ The gray needle cover for the HUMIRA Pen 40 mg/0.8 mL, HUMIRA 40 mg/0.8 mL prefilled syringe, HUMIRA 20 mg/0.4 mL prefilled syringe, and HUMIRA 10 mg/0.2 mL prefilled syringe contains natural rubber or latex.
  - ○ The black needle cover for the HUMIRA Pen 40 mg/0.4 mL, HUMIRA 40 mg/0.4 mL prefilled syringe and the vial stopper on the HUMIRA institutional use vial are not made with natural rubber or latex.
- are allergic to HUMIRA or to any of its ingredients. See the end of this Medication Guide for a list of ingredients in HUMIRA.
- are pregnant or plan to become pregnant. It is not known if HUMIRA will harm your unborn baby. HUMIRA should only be used during a pregnancy if needed.
- have a baby and you were using HUMIRA during your pregnancy. Tell your baby's doctor before your baby receives any vaccines.
- breastfeeding or plan to breastfeed. You and your doctor should decide if you will breastfeed or use HUMIRA® (adalimumab). You should not do both.

Tell your doctor about all the medicines you take, including prescription and over-the-counter medicines, vitamins, and herbal supplements.

Especially tell your doctor if you use:
- ORENCIA® (abatacept), KINERET® (anakinra), REMICADE® (infliximab), ENBREL® (etanercept), CIMZIA® (certolizumab pegol) or SIMPONI® (golimumab), because you should not use HUMIRA while you are also using one of these medicines.
- RITUXAN® (rituximab). Your doctor may not want to give you HUMIRA if you have received RITUXAN® (rituximab) recently.
- IMURAN® (azathioprine) or PURINETHOL® (6–mercaptopurine, 6-MP).

Keep a list of your medicines with you to show your doctor and pharmacist each time you get a new medicine.

How should I take HUMIRA?
- HUMIRA® (adalimumab) is given by an injection under the skin. Your doctor will tell you how often to take an injection of HUMIRA. This is based on your condition to be treated. **Do not inject HUMIRA more often than you were prescribed.**
- See the Instructions for Use inside the carton for complete instructions for the right way to prepare and inject HUMIRA® (adalimumab).
- Make sure you have been shown how to inject HUMIRA before you do it yourself. You can call your doctor or 1-800-4HUMIRA (1-800-448-6472) if you have any questions about giving yourself an injection. Someone you know can also help you with your injection after they have been shown how to prepare and inject HUMIRA.
- **Do not** try to inject HUMIRA yourself until you have been shown the right way to give the injections. If your doctor decides that you or a caregiver may be able to give your injections of HUMIRA at home, you should receive training on the right way to prepare and inject HUMIRA.
- Do not miss any doses of HUMIRA unless your doctor says it is okay. If you forget to take HUMIRA, inject a dose as soon as you remember. Then, take your next dose at your regular scheduled time. This will put you back on schedule. In case you are not sure when to inject HUMIRA, call your doctor or pharmacist.
- If you take more HUMIRA than you were told to take, call your doctor.

What are the possible side effects of HUMIRA?
HUMIRA can cause serious side effects, including:
See "What is the most important information I should know about HUMIRA?"
- **Serious Infections.**
  Your doctor will examine you for TB and perform a test to see if you have TB. If your doctor feels that you are at risk for TB, you may be treated with medicine for TB before you begin treatment with HUMIRA® (adalimumab) and during treatment with HUMIRA. Even if your TB test is negative your doctor should carefully monitor you for TB infections while you are taking HUMIRA. People who had a negative TB skin test before receiving HUMIRA have developed active TB. Tell your doctor if you have any of the following symptoms while taking or after taking HUMIRA:
  - ○ cough that does not go away
  - ○ low grade fever
  - ○ weight loss
  - ○ loss of body fat and muscle (wasting)
- **Hepatitis B infection in people who carry the virus in their blood.**
  If you are a carrier of the hepatitis B virus (a virus that affects the liver), the virus can become active while you use HUMIRA® (adalimumab). Your doctor should do blood tests before you start treatment, while you are using HUMIRA, and for several months after you stop treatment with HUMIRA. Tell your doctor if you have any of the following symptoms of a possible hepatitis B infection:
  - ○ muscle aches
  - ○ feel very tired
  - ○ dark urine
  - ○ skin or eyes look yellow
  - ○ little or no appetite
  - ○ vomiting
  - ○ clay-colored bowel movements
  - ○ fever
  - ○ chills
  - ○ stomach discomfort
  - ○ skin rash
- **Allergic reactions.** Allergic reactions can happen in people who use HUMIRA. Call your doctor or get medical help right away if you have any of these symptoms of a serious allergic reaction:
  - ○ hives
  - ○ trouble breathing
  - ○ swelling of your face, eyes, lips or mouth
- **Nervous system problems.** Signs and symptoms of a nervous system problem include: numbness or tingling, problems with your vision, weakness in your arms or legs, and dizziness.
- **Blood problems.** Your body may not make enough of the blood cells that help fight infections or help to stop bleeding. Symptoms include a fever that does not go away, bruising or bleeding very easily, or looking very pale.
- **New heart failure or worsening of heart failure you already have.** Call your doctor right away if you get new worsening symptoms of heart failure while taking HUMIRA® (adalimumab), including:
  - ○ shortness of breath
  - ○ sudden weight gain
  - ○ swelling of your ankles or feet
- **Immune reactions including a lupus-like syndrome.** Symptoms include chest discomfort or pain that does not go away, shortness of breath, joint pain, or a rash on your cheeks or arms that gets worse in the sun. Symptoms may improve when you stop HUMIRA® (adalimumab).
- **Liver Problems.** Liver problems can happen in people who use TNF-blocker medicines. These problems can lead to liver failure and death. Call your doctor right away if you have any of these symptoms:
  - ○ feel very tired
  - ○ poor appetite or vomiting
  - ○ skin or eyes look yellow
  - ○ pain on the right side of your stomach (abdomen)

Continued on next page

Information on the AbbVie, Inc. products listed on these pages is from the prescribing information in use as of July 31, 2016. For more information, please visit rxabbvie.com or call 1-800-633-9110.

- **Psoriasis.** Some people using HUMIRA had new psoriasis or worsening of psoriasis they already had. Tell your doctor if you develop red scaly patches or raised bumps that are filled with pus. Your doctor may decide to stop your treatment with HUMIRA.

Call your doctor or get medical care right away if you develop any of the above symptoms. Your treatment with HUMIRA may be stopped.

Common side effects with HUMIRA include:

- injection site reactions: redness, rash, swelling, itching, or bruising. These symptoms usually will go away within a few days. Call your doctor right away if you have pain, redness or swelling around the injection site that does not go away within a few days or gets worse.
- upper respiratory infections (including sinus infections)
- headaches
- rash

These are not all the possible side effects with HUMIRA® (adalimumab). Tell your doctor if you have any side effect that bothers you or that does not go away. Ask your doctor or pharmacist for more information.

Call your doctor for medical advice about side effects. You may report side effects to FDA at 1-800-FDA-1088

How should I store HUMIRA?

- Store HUMIRA in the refrigerator at 36°F to 46°F (2°C to 8°C). Store HUMIRA in the original carton until use to protect it from light.
- **Do not freeze HUMIRA.** Do not use HUMIRA if frozen, even if it has been thawed.
- Refrigerated HUMIRA may be used until the expiration date printed on the HUMIRA carton, dose tray, Pen or prefilled syringe. Do not use HUMIRA after the expiration date.
- If needed, for example when you are traveling, you may also store HUMIRA at room temperature up to 77°F (25°C) for up to 14 days. Store HUMIRA in the original carton until use to protect it from light.
- Throw away HUMIRA® (adalimumab) if it has been kept at room temperature and not been used within 14 days.
- Record the date you first remove HUMIRA from the refrigerator in the spaces provided on the carton and dose tray.
- Do not store HUMIRA in extreme heat or cold.
- Do not use a Pen or prefilled syringe if the liquid is cloudy, discolored, or has flakes or particles in it.
- Do not drop or crush HUMIRA. The prefilled syringe is glass.

Keep HUMIRA, injection supplies, and all other medicines out of the reach of children.

General information about the safe and effective use of HUMIRA

Medicines are sometimes prescribed for purposes other than those listed in a Medication Guide. Do not use HUMIRA for a condition for which it was not prescribed. Do not give HUMIRA to other people, even if they have the same condition. It may harm them.

This Medication Guide summarizes the most important information about HUMIRA. If you would like more information, talk with your doctor. You can ask your doctor or pharmacist for information about HUMIRA® (adalimumab) that is written for health professionals. For more information go to www.HUMIRA.com or you can enroll in a patient support program by calling 1-800-4HUMIRA (1-800-448-6472).

What are the ingredients in HUMIRA?

Active ingredient: adalimumab

HUMIRA Pen 40 mg/0.8 mL, HUMIRA 40 mg/0.8 mL prefilled syringe, HUMIRA 20 mg/0.4 mL prefilled syringe, HUMIRA 10 mg/0.2 mL prefilled syringe, and HUMIRA 40 mg/0.8 mL institutional use vial:

Inactive ingredients: citric acid monohydrate, dibasic sodium phosphate dihydrate, mannitol, monobasic sodium phosphate dihydrate, polysorbate 80, sodium chloride, sodium citrate and Water for Injection. Sodium hydroxide is added as necessary to adjust pH.

HUMIRA Pen 40 mg/0.4 mL and HUMIRA® (adalimumab) 40 mg/0.4 mL prefilled syringe:

Inactive ingredients: mannitol, polysorbate 80, and Water for Injection.

Manufactured by:

AbbVie Inc.
North Chicago, IL 60064, U.S.A.
US License Number 1889

This Medication Guide has been approved by the U.S. Food and Drug Administration.   Revised: 06/2016
03-B352

INSTRUCTIONS FOR USE
HUMIRA® (Hu-MARE-ah)
(adalimumab)
40 MG/0.8 ML
SINGLE-USE PEN

Do not try to inject HUMIRA yourself until you have been shown the right way to give the injections and have read and understand this Instructions for Use. If your doctor decides that you or a caregiver may be able to give your injections of HUMIRA at home, you should receive training on the right way to prepare and inject HUMIRA. It is important that you read, understand, and follow these instructions so that you inject HUMIRA the right way. It is also important to talk to your doctor to be sure you understand your HUMIRA dosing instructions. To help you remember when to inject HUMIRA, you can mark your calendar ahead of time. Call your healthcare provider if you or your caregiver have any questions about the right way to inject HUMIRA.

IMPORTANT:

- Do not use HUMIRA if frozen, even if it has been thawed.
- The HUMIRA Pen contains glass. Do not drop or crush the Pen because the glass inside may break.
- Do not remove the gray cap or the plum-colored cap until right before your injection.
- When the plum-colored button on the HUMIRA Pen is pressed to give your dose of HUMIRA® (adalimumab), you will hear a loud "click" sound.
  - You must practice injecting HUMIRA with your doctor or nurse so that you are not startled by this click when you start giving yourself the injections at home.
  - The loud click sound means the start of the injection.
  - You will know that the injection has finished when the yellow marker appears fully in the window view and stops moving.

See the section below called **"Prepare the HUMIRA Pen"**.

Gather the Supplies for Your Injection

- You will need the following supplies for each injection of HUMIRA.

Find a clean, flat surface to place the supplies on.

- 1 alcohol swab
- 1 cotton ball or gauze pad (not included in your HUMIRA carton)
- 1 HUMIRA Pen (See Figure A)
- FDA-cleared sharps disposal container for HUMIRA Pen disposal (not included in your HUMIRA carton)

If more comfortable, take your HUMIRA Pen out of the refrigerator **15 to 30 minutes** before injecting to allow the liquid to reach room temperature. **Do not** remove the gray or plum-colored caps while allowing it to reach room temperature. **Do not** warm HUMIRA® (adalimumab) in any other way (for example, **do not** warm it in a microwave or in hot water).

If you do not have all of the supplies you need to give yourself an injection, go to a pharmacy or call your pharmacist. The diagram below shows what the HUMIRA Pen looks like. See Figure A.

[See Figure A at top of next column]

Check the carton, dose tray, and HUMIRA Pen.

1. Make sure the name HUMIRA® (adalimumab) appears on the carton, dose tray, and HUMIRA Pen label.

2. **Do not use** and **do call** your doctor or pharmacist if:

- you drop or crush your HUMIRA Pen.
- the seals on the top or bottom of the carton are broken or missing.
- the expiration date on the carton, dose tray, and Pen has passed.
- the HUMIRA Pen has been frozen or left in direct sunlight.
- HUMIRA has been kept at room temperature for longer than **14** days or HUMIRA has been stored above 77°F (25°C).

See the **"How should I store HUMIRA?"** section at the end of this Instructions for Use.

3. Hold the Pen with the gray cap (Cap # 1) pointed down.

4. Make sure the amount of liquid in the Pen is at the fill line or close to the fill line seen through the window. This is the full dose of HUMIRA that you will inject. See Figure B.

[See Figure A at top of next column]

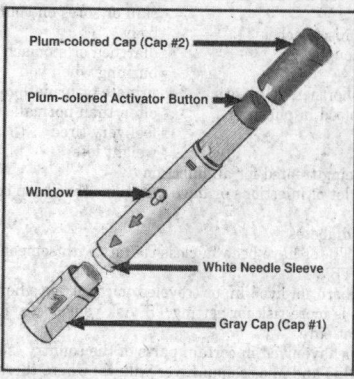

Figure A

Plum-colored Cap (Cap #2)
Plum-colored Activator Button
Window
White Needle Sleeve
Gray Cap (Cap #1)

5. If the Pen does not have the full amount of liquid, **do not use that Pen**. Call your pharmacist.

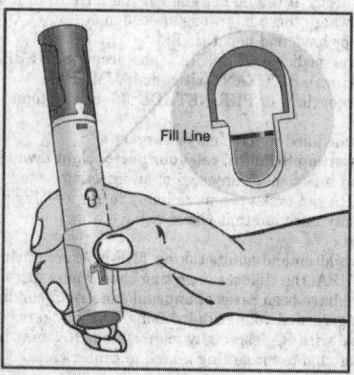

Figure B

Fill Line

6. Turn the Pen over and hold the Pen with the gray cap (Cap # 1) pointed up. See Figure C.

7. Check the solution through the windows on the side of the Pen to make sure the liquid is clear and colorless. **Do not use** your HUMIRA® (adalimumab) Pen if the liquid is cloudy, discolored, or if it has flakes or particles in it. Call your pharmacist. It is normal to see one or more bubbles in the window.

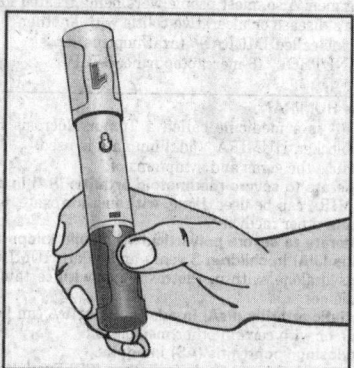

Figure C

Choose the Injection Site

8. Wash and dry your hands well.

9. Choose an injection site on:

- the front of your thighs or
- your lower abdomen (belly). If you choose your abdomen, do not use the area 2 inches around your belly button (navel). See Figure D.

[See Figure D at top of next column]

- Choose a different site each time you give yourself an injection. Each new injection should be given at least one inch from a site you used before.
- **Do not** inject HUMIRA® (adalimumab) into skin that is:

Figure D

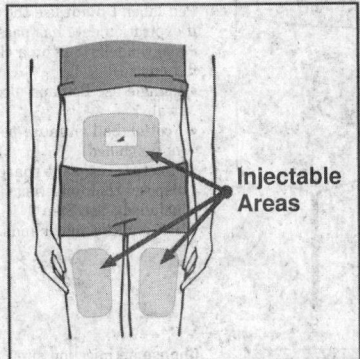

Injectable Areas

- sore (tender)
- bruised
- red
- hard
- scarred or where you have stretch marks
- If you have psoriasis, **do not** inject directly into any raised, thick, red or scaly skin patches or lesions on your skin.
- Do not inject through your clothes.

Prepare the Injection Site

10. Wipe the injection site with an alcohol prep (swab) using a circular motion.
- **Do not** touch this area again before giving the injection. Allow the skin to dry before injecting. **Do not** fan or blow on the clean area.

Preparing the HUMIRA Pen

11. **Do not remove the gray cap (Cap # 1) or the plum-colored cap (Cap # 2) until right before your injection.**

12. Hold the middle of the Pen (gray body) with one hand so that you are not touching the gray cap (Cap # 1) or the plum-colored cap (Cap # 2). Turn the Pen so that the gray cap (Cap # 1) is pointing up. See Figure E.

Figure E

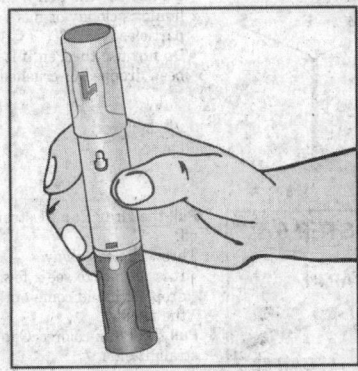

13. With your other hand, pull the gray cap (Cap # 1) straight off (do not twist the cap). Make sure the small gray needle cover of the syringe has come off with the gray cap (Cap # 1). See Figure F.
[See Figure F at top of next column]

14. Throw away the gray cap (Cap # 1).
- **Do not** put the gray cap (Cap # 1) back on the Pen. Putting the gray cap (Cap # 1) back on may damage the needle.
- The white needle sleeve, which covers the needle, can now be seen.
- **Do not** touch the needle with your fingers or let the needle touch anything.
- You may see a few drops of liquid come out of the needle. This is normal.

15. Remove the plum-colored cap (Cap # 2) from the bottom of the Pen by pulling it straight off (do not twist the cap). The Pen is now activated. Throw away the plum-colored cap.
- Do not put the plum-colored cap (Cap # 2) back on the Pen because it could cause medicine to come out of the syringe.

The plum-colored activator button:
- Turn the Pen so the plum-colored activator button is pointed up. See Figure G.
[See Figure G in next column]
- **Do not** press the plum-colored activator button until you are ready to inject HUMIRA® (adalimumab). Pressing the plum-colored activator button will release the medicine from the Pen.

Figure F

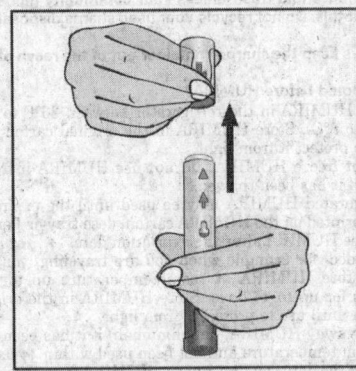

Figure G

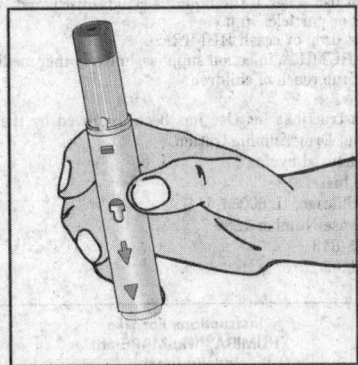

- Hold the Pen so that you can see the window. See Figure H. It is normal to see one or more bubbles in the window.

Figure H

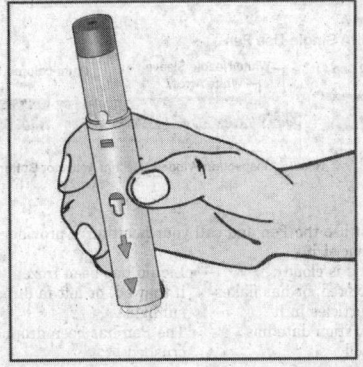

Position the Pen and Inject HUMIRA® (adalimumab)

16. Position the Pen:
- Gently squeeze the area of the cleaned skin and hold it firmly. See Figure I. You will inject into this raised area of skin.
[See Figure I at top of next column]

17. Place the white end of the Pen straight (at a 90° angle) and flat against the raised area of your skin that you are squeezing. Place the Pen so that it will not inject the needle into your fingers that are holding the raised skin. See Figure J.
[See Figure J in next column]

18. Inject HUMIRA® (adalimumab)
- With your index finger or your thumb, press the plum-colored activator button to begin the injection. Try not to cover the window. See Figure K.
[See Figure K in next column]
- You will hear a loud 'click' when you press the plum-colored activator button. The loud click means the start of the injection.
- Keep pressing the plum-colored activator button and continue to hold the Pen against your squeezed, raised skin until all of the medicine is injected. This can take up to 10 seconds, so count slowly to ten. Keep holding the Pen against the squeezed, raised skin of your injection site for the whole time so you get the full dose of medicine.

Figure I

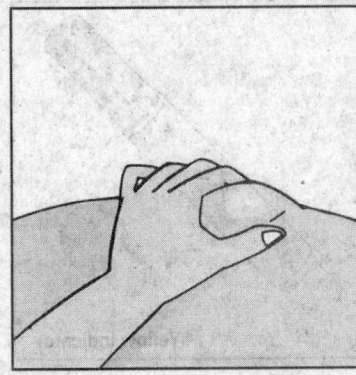

Figure J

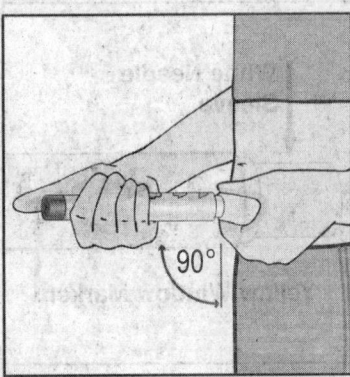

90°

Figure K

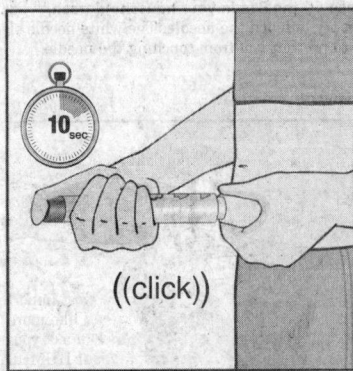

10 sec

((click))

- You will know that the injection has finished when the yellow marker fully appears in the window view and stops moving. See Figure L.
[See Figure L at top of next column]

19. When the injection is finished, slowly pull the Pen from your skin. The white needle sleeve will move to cover the needle tip. See Figure M.
- Do not touch the needle. The white needle sleeve is there to prevent you from touching the needle.
[See Figure M on next column]
- Press a cotton ball or gauze pad over the injection site and hold it for 10 seconds. Do **not** rub the injection site. You may have slight bleeding. This is normal.

20. Dispose of your used HUMIRA® (adalimumab) Pen. See the section **"How should I dispose of the used HUMIRA Pen?"**

21. Keep a record of the dates and location of your injection sites. To help you remember when to take HUMIRA, you can mark your calendar ahead of time.

How should I dispose of the used HUMIRA Pen?

Continued on next page

Information on the AbbVie, Inc. products listed on these pages is from the prescribing information in use as of July 31, 2016. For more information, please visit rxabbvie.com or call 1-800-633-9110.

Figure L

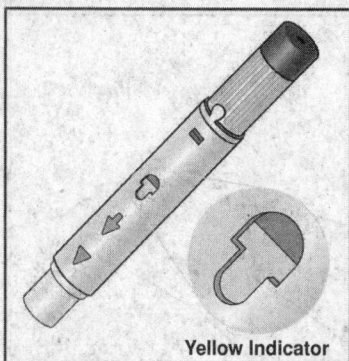

Yellow Indicator

Figure M

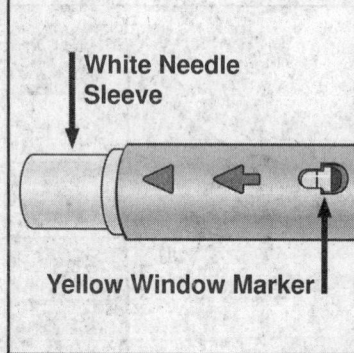

White Needle Sleeve

Yellow Window Marker

- Put your Pen in a FDA-cleared sharps disposal container right away after use. See Figure N. **Do not throw away (dispose of) the Pen in your household trash.**
- Do not try to touch the needle. The white needle sleeve is there to prevent you from touching the needle.

Figure N

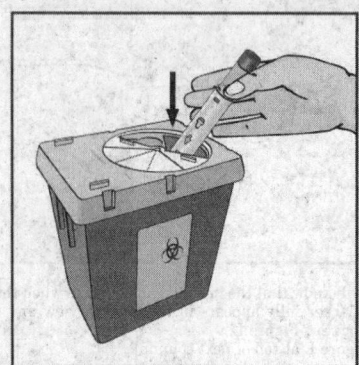

- If you do not have a FDA-cleared sharps disposal container, you may use a household container that is:
  ○ made of a heavy-duty plastic,
  ○ can be closed with a tight-fitting, puncture-resistant lid, without sharps being able to come out,
  ○ upright and stable during use,
  ○ leak-resistant, and
  ○ properly labeled to warn of hazardous waste inside the container.
- When your sharps disposal container is almost full, you will need to follow your community guidelines for the right way to dispose of your sharps disposal container. There may be state or local laws about how you should throw away used needles and syringes. For more information about safe sharps disposal, and for specific information about sharps disposal in the state that you live in, go to the FDA's website at: http://www.fda.gov/safesharpsdisposal.
- For the safety and health of you and others, never re-use your HUMIRA® (adalimumab) Pens.
- The used alcohol pads, cotton balls, dose trays and packaging may be placed in your household trash.

- Do not dispose of your used sharps disposal container in your household trash unless your community guidelines permit this. Do not recycle your used sharps disposal container.
- Always keep the sharps container out of the reach of children.

How should I store HUMIRA?
- Store HUMIRA in the refrigerator between 36°F to 46°F (2°C to 8°C). Store HUMIRA in the original carton until use to protect it from light.
- **Do not** freeze HUMIRA. **Do not** use HUMIRA if frozen, even if it has been thawed.
- Refrigerated HUMIRA may be used until the expiration date printed on the HUMIRA carton, dose tray or Pen. **Do not** use HUMIRA after the expiration date.
- If needed, for example when you are traveling, you may also store HUMIRA at room temperature up to 77°F (25°C) for up to **14** days. Store HUMIRA in the original carton until use to protect it from light.
- Throw away HUMIRA® (adalimumab) if it has been kept at room temperature and not been used within **14** days.
- Record the date you first remove HUMIRA from the refrigerator in the spaces provided on the carton and dose tray.
- Do not store HUMIRA in extreme heat or cold.
- Do not use a Pen if the sharps disposal container has flakes or particles in it.
- Do not drop or crush HUMIRA.
- Keep HUMIRA, injection supplies, and all other medicines out of the reach of children.

This Instructions for Use has been approved by the U.S. Food and Drug Administration.
Manufactured by:
AbbVie Inc.
North Chicago, IL 60064, U.S.A.
US License Number 1889
03-B355-R13
Revised: 06/2016

Instructions For Use
HUMIRA® (Hu-MARE-ah)
(adalimumab)
40 mg/0.4 mL
Single-Use Pen

Before Injecting: Your healthcare provider should show you how to use HUMIRA before you use it for the first time. Call your healthcare provider or **1-800-4HUMIRA** (1-800-448-6472) if you need help.

Figure A
HUMIRA Single-Use Pen

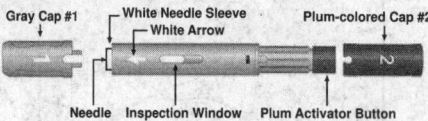

Gray Cap #1 · White Needle Sleeve · White Arrow · Plum-colored Cap #2
Needle · Inspection Window · Plum Activator Button

Do not use the Pen and call your healthcare provider or pharmacist if:
- Liquid is cloudy, discolored, or has flakes or particles in it
- Expiration date has passed
- Liquid has been frozen (even if thawed) or left in direct sunlight
- The Pen has been dropped or crushed

Keep the caps on until right before injection. Keep HUMIRA out of reach of children.
Read Instructions on All Pages Before Using the HUMIRA Pen

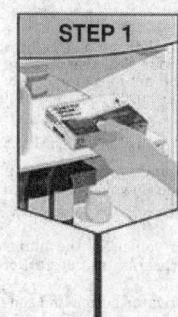
STEP 1

Take HUMIRA out of the refrigerator.
Leave HUMIRA at room temperature for **15 to 30 minutes** before injecting.
- **Do not** remove the Gray or Plum-colored Caps while allowing HUMIRA to reach room temperature
- **Do not** warm HUMIRA in any other way. For example, **do not** warm it in a microwave or in hot water.
- **Do not** use the Pen if liquid has been frozen (even if thawed)

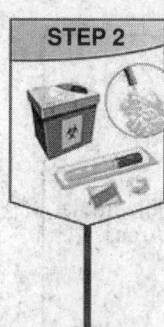
STEP 2

Check expiration date on the Pen label. **Do not** use the Pen if expiration date has passed.
Place the following on a clean, flat surface:
- 1 single-use Pen and alcohol swab
- 1 cotton ball or gauze pad (not included)
- Puncture-resistant sharps disposal container (not included). See Step 9
Wash and dry your hands.

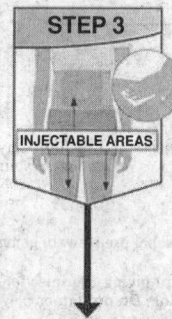
STEP 3
INJECTABLE AREAS

Choose an injection site:
- On the front of your thighs or
- Your abdomen (belly) at least 2 inches from your navel (belly button)
- Different from your last injection site
Wipe the injection site in a circular motion with the alcohol swab.
- **Do not** inject through clothes
- **Do not** inject into skin that is sore, bruised, red, hard, scarred, has stretch marks, or areas with psoriasis plaques

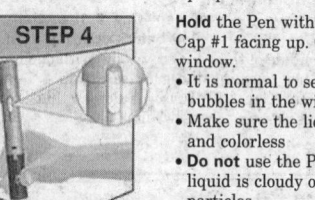
STEP 4

Hold the Pen with the Gray Cap #1 facing up. **Check** the window.
- It is normal to see 1 or more bubbles in the window
- Make sure the liquid is clear and colorless
- **Do not** use the Pen if the liquid is cloudy or has particles
- **Do not** use the Pen if it has been dropped or crushed

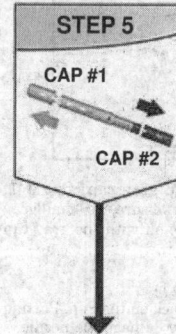
STEP 5
CAP #1
CAP #2

Pull the Gray Cap #1 straight off.
Throw the cap away.
- It is normal to see a few drops of liquid come out of the needle
Pull the Plum-colored Cap #2 straight off.
Throw the cap away.
Turn the Pen so that the white arrow points toward the injection site.

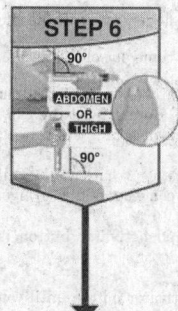
STEP 6
90°
ABDOMEN OR THIGH
90°

Squeeze the skin at your injection site to make a raised area and hold it firmly.
Point the white arrow toward the injection site.
Place the white needle sleeve straight (**90° angle**) against the injection site.
Hold the Pen so that you can see the inspection window.

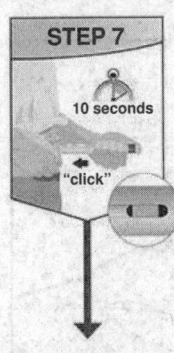

STEP 7

10 seconds

"click"

Push and keep pushing the Pen **down** against the injection site.
Press the plum activator button and count slowly for **10** seconds.
- A loud "click" will signal the **start** of the injection
- **Keep pushing** the Pen **down** against the injection site
- Injection is complete when the yellow indicator has stopped moving

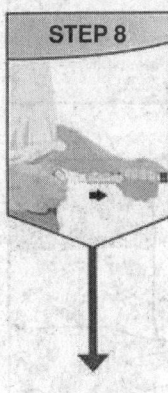

STEP 8

When the injection is completed, slowly pull the Pen from the skin. The white needle sleeve will cover the needle tip.
If there are more than a few drops of liquid on the injection site, call **1-800-4HUMIRA** (1-800-448-6472) for help.
After completing the injection, place a cotton ball or gauze pad on the skin of the injection site.
- **Do not** rub
- Slight bleeding at the injection site is normal

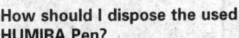

How should I dispose the used HUMIRA Pen?
- Put your used needles, Pens, and sharps in a FDA cleared sharps disposal container right away after use. **Do not throw away (dispose of) loose needles, syringes, and the Pen in the household trash.**
- If you do not have a FDA-cleared sharps disposal container, you may use a household container that is:
  - made of a heavy-duty plastic,
  - can be closed with a tight-fitting, puncture-resistant lid, without sharps being able to come out,
  - upright and stable during use,
  - leak-resistant, and
  - properly labeled to warn of hazardous waste inside the container.
- When your sharps disposal container is almost full, you will need to follow your community guidelines for the right way to dispose of your sharps disposal container. There may be state or local laws about how you should throw away used needles and syringes. For more information about safe sharps disposal, and for specific information about sharps disposal in the state that you live in, go to the FDA's website at: http://www.fda.gov/safesharpsdisposal.
- Do not dispose of your used sharps disposal container in your household trash unless your community guidelines permit this. Do not recycle your used sharps disposal container.

STEP 9

The Pen caps, alcohol swab, cotton ball or gauze pad, dose tray, and packaging may be placed in your household trash.

Questions About Using the HUMIRA Pen
What if I have not received in-person training from a healthcare provider?
- Call your healthcare provider or **1-800-4HUMIRA (1-800-448-6472)** or visit www.HUMIRA.com if you need help How do I know when the injection is complete?
- The yellow indicator has stopped moving. This takes up to 10 seconds **What should I do if there are more than a few drops of liquid on the injection site?**
- Call **1-800-4HUMIRA (1-800-448-6472)** for help
What if I do not have an FDA-cleared sharps disposal container or proper household container?
What if I do not have an FDA-cleared sharps disposal container or proper household container?
- Call **1-800-4HUMIRA (1-800-448-6472)** for a free FDA-cleared sharps disposal container

MONTH

Always keep the Pen and the sharps disposal container out of reach of children.
Keep a record of the dates and locations of your injections. To help remember when to take HUMIRA, mark your calendar ahead of time.

This Instructions For Use has been approved by the U.S. Food and Drug Administration.
Manufactured by AbbVie Inc. North Chicago, IL 60064 U.S.A.
US License Number 1889
03-B356
Revised 06/2016

INSTRUCTIONS FOR USE
HUMIRA® (Hu-MARE-ah)
(adalimumab)
40 MG/0.8 ML, 20 MG/0.4 ML AND 10 MG/0.2 ML
SINGLE-USE PREFILLED SYRINGE

Do not try to inject HUMIRA yourself until you have been shown the right way to give the injections and have read and understand this Instructions for Use. If your doctor decides that you or a caregiver may be able to give your injections of HUMIRA at home, you should receive training on the right way to prepare and inject HUMIRA. It is important that you read, understand, and follow these instructions so that you inject HUMIRA the right way. It is also important to talk to your doctor to be sure you understand your HUMIRA dosing instructions. To help you remember when to inject HUMIRA, you can mark your calendar ahead of time. Call your healthcare provider if you or your caregiver have any questions about the right way to inject HUMIRA.

Gather the Supplies for Your Injection
- You will need the following supplies for each injection of HUMIRA.
  Find a clean, flat surface to place the supplies on.
- 1 alcohol swab
- 1 cotton ball or gauze pad (not included in your HUMIRA carton)
- 1 HUMIRA prefilled syringe (See Figure A)
- FDA-cleared sharps disposal container for HUMIRA prefilled syringe disposal (not included in your HUMIRA carton)

If more comfortable, take your HUMIRA® (adalimumab) prefilled syringe out of the refrigerator **15 to 30 minutes** before injecting to allow the liquid to reach room temperature. **Do not** remove the needle cover while allowing it to reach room temperature. **Do not** warm HUMIRA in any other way (for example, **do not** warm it in a microwave or in hot water).

If you do not have all of the supplies you need to give yourself an injection, go to a pharmacy or call your pharmacist. The diagram below shows what a prefilled syringe looks like. See Figure A.

Check the carton, dose tray, and prefilled syringe
1. Make sure the name HUMIRA® (adalimumab) appears on the dose tray and prefilled syringe label.
2. **Do not use** and **do call** your doctor or pharmacist if:
- the seals on top or bottom of the carton are broken or missing.

Figure A

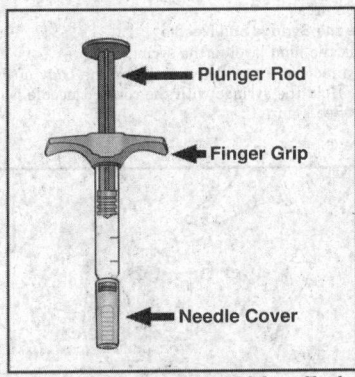

Plunger Rod

Finger Grip

Needle Cover

- the HUMIRA labeling has an expired date. Check the expiration date on your HUMIRA carton and **do not** use if the date has passed.
- the prefilled syringe that has been frozen or left in direct sunlight.
- HUMIRA has been kept at room temperature for longer than **14** days or HUMIRA has been stored above 77°F (25°C).
- the liquid in the prefilled syringe is cloudy, discolored or has flakes or particles in it. Make sure the liquid is clear and colorless.
See the **"How should I store HUMIRA® (adalimumab)?"** section at the end of this Instructions for Use.

Choose the Injection Site
3. Wash and dry your hands well.
4. Choose an injection site on:
- the front of your thighs or
- your lower abdomen (belly). If you choose your abdomen, do not use the area 2 inches around your belly button (navel). See Figure B.

Figure B

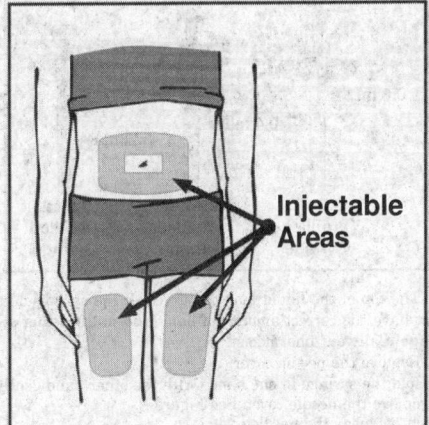

Injectable Areas

- Choose a different site each time you give yourself an injection. Each new injection should be given at least one inch from a site you used before.
- **Do not** inject into skin that is:
- sore (tender)
- bruised
- red
- hard
- scarred or where you have stretch marks
- If you have psoriasis, do not inject directly into any raised, thick, red or scaly skin patches or lesions on your skin.
- Do not inject through your clothes.

Prepare the Injection Site
5. Wipe the injection site with an alcohol prep (swab) using a circular motion.

Continued on next page

Information on the AbbVie, Inc. products listed on these pages is from the prescribing information in use as of July 31, 2016. For more information, please visit rxabbvie.com or call 1-800-633-9110.

6. Do **not** touch this area again before giving the injection. Allow the skin to dry before injecting. Do not fan or blow on the clean area.

Prepare the Syringe and Needle

7. Check the fluid level in the syringe:

• Always hold the prefilled syringe by the body of the syringe. Hold the syringe with the covered needle pointing down. See Figure C.

Figure C

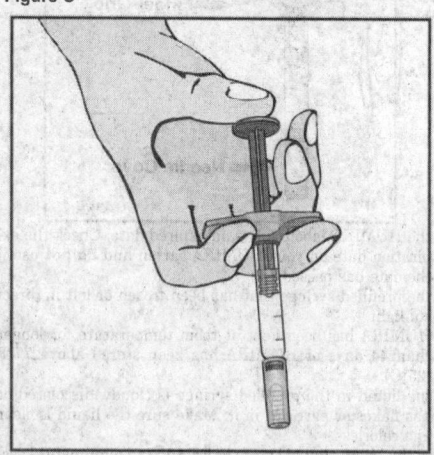

• Hold the syringe at eye level. Look closely to make sure that the amount of liquid in the syringe is the same or close to the:
  • 0.8 mL line for the 40 mg prefilled syringe. See Figure D.
  • 0.4 mL line for the 20 mg prefilled syringe. See Figure D.
  • 0.2 mL line for the 10 mg prefilled syringe. See Figure D.

Figure D

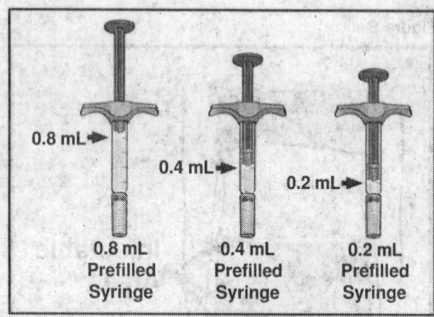

0.8 mL

0.4 mL

0.2 mL

0.8 mL
Prefilled
Syringe

0.4 mL
Prefilled
Syringe

0.2 mL
Prefilled
Syringe

8. The top of the liquid may be curved. If the syringe does not have the correct amount of liquid, **do not use that syringe**. Call your pharmacist.

9. Remove the needle cover:

• Hold the syringe in one hand. With the other hand gently remove the needle cover. See Figure E.
• Throw away the needle cover.

Figure E

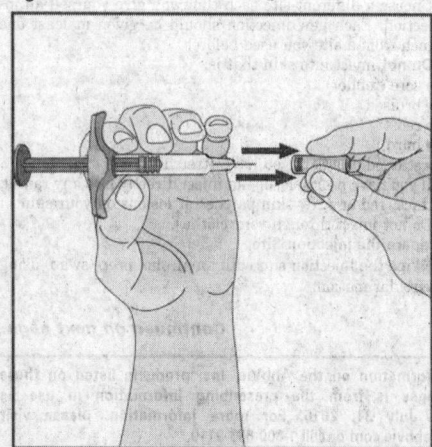

• Do not touch the needle with your fingers or let the needle touch anything.

10. Turn the syringe so the needle is facing up and hold the syringe at eye level with one hand so you can see the air in the syringe. Using your other hand, slowly push the plunger in to push the air out through the needle. See Figure F.

Figure F

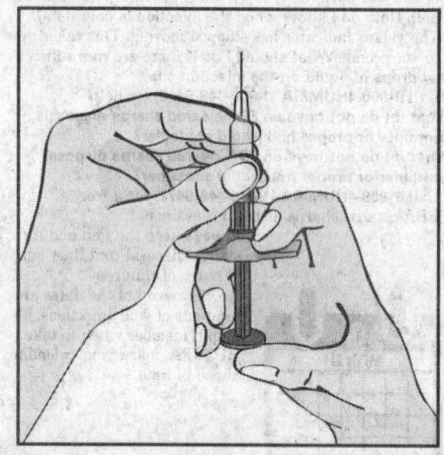

• You may see a drop of liquid at the end of the needle. This is normal.

Position the Prefilled Syringe and Inject HUMIRA® (adalimumab)

Position the Syringe

11. Hold the body of the prefilled syringe in one hand between the thumb and index finger. Hold the syringe in your hand like a pencil. See Figure G.

Figure G

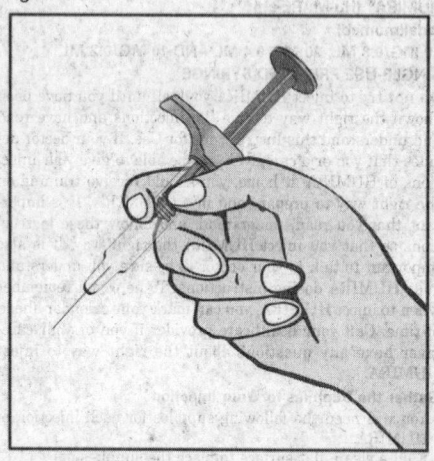

• **Do not** pull back on the plunger at any time.
• With your other hand, gently squeeze the area of the cleaned skin and hold it firmly. See Figure H.

[See Figure H at top of next column]

Inject HUMIRA® (adalimumab)

12. Using a quick, dart-like motion, insert the needle into the squeezed skin at about a **45-degree angle**. See Figure I.

[See Figure I at top of next column]

• After the needle is in, let go of the skin. Pull back gently on the plunger.

If blood appears in the syringe:

• It means that you have entered a blood vessel.
• **Do not inject HUMIRA.**
• Pull the needle out of the skin while keeping the syringe at the same angle.
• Press a cotton ball or gauze pad over the injection site and hold it for 10 seconds. See Figure J.

[See Figure J at top of next page]

• **Do not** use the same syringe and needle again. Throw away the needle and syringe in your special sharps container.
• **Do not** rub the injection site. You may have slight bleeding. This is normal.
• Repeat Steps 1 through 12 with a new prefilled syringe.

If no blood appears in the syringe:

Figure H

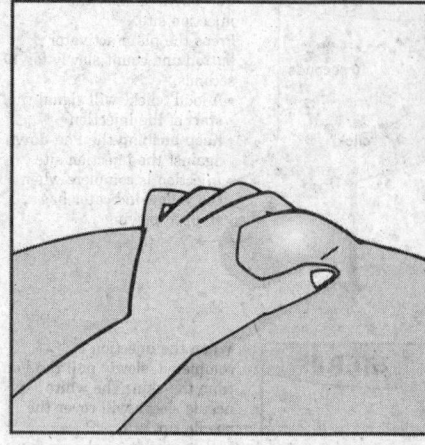

Figure I

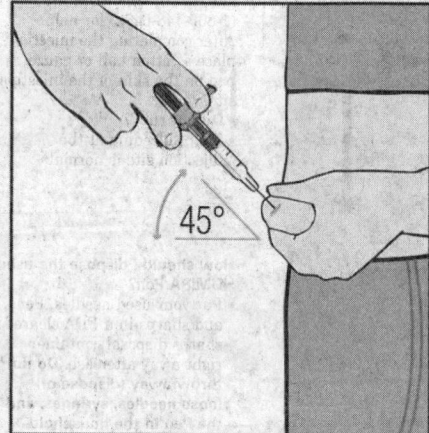

45°

• Slowly push the plunger all the way in until all of the liquid is injected and the syringe is empty.
• Pull the needle out of the skin while keeping the syringe at the same angle.
• Press a cotton ball or gauze pad over the injection site and hold it for 10 seconds. Do **not** rub the injection site. You may have slight bleeding. This is normal.

13. Throw away the used prefilled syringe and needle. See **"How should I dispose of used prefilled syringes and needles?"**

14. Keep a record of the dates and location of your injection sites. To help you remember when to take HUMIRA® (adalimumab), you can mark your calendar ahead of time.

How should I dispose of used prefilled syringes and needles?

• **Put your used needles and syringes in a FDA-cleared sharps disposal container right away after use.** See Figure K. **Do not throw away (dispose of) loose needles and syringes in your household trash.**
• Do not try to touch the needle.

[See Figure K at top of next page]

• If you do not have a FDA-cleared sharps disposal container, you may use a household container that is:
  ○ made of a heavy-duty plastic,
  ○ can be closed with a tight-fitting, puncture-resistant lid, without sharps being able to come out,
  ○ upright and stable during use,
  ○ leak-resistant, and
  ○ properly labeled to warn of hazardous waste inside the container.
• When your sharps disposal container is almost full, you will need to follow your community guidelines for the right way to dispose of your sharps disposal container. There may be state or local laws about how you should throw away used needles and syringes. For more information about safe sharps disposal, and for specific information about sharps disposal in the state that you live in, go to the FDA's website at: http://www.fda.gov/safesharpsdisposal.
• For the safety and health of you and others, needles and used syringes **must never** be re-used.

Figure J

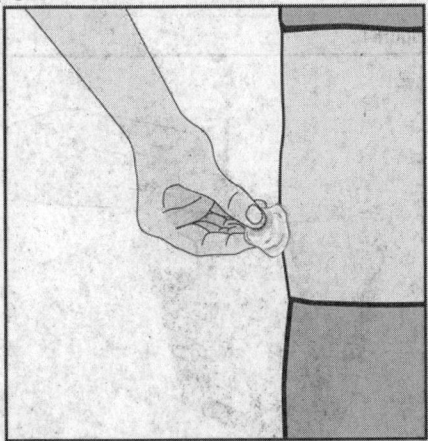

Figure K

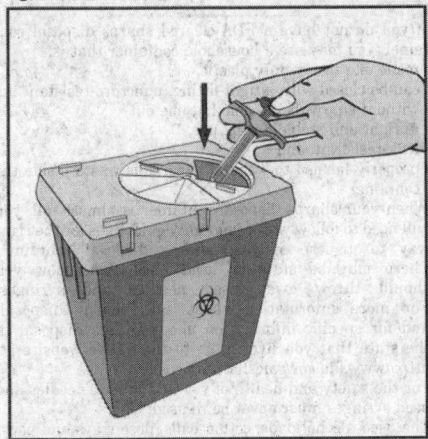

- The used alcohol pads, cotton balls, dose trays and packaging may be placed in your household trash.
- **Do not dispose of your used sharps disposal container in your household trash unless your community guidelines permit this. Do not recycle your used sharps disposal container.**
- **Always keep the sharps container out of the reach of children.**

How should I store HUMIRA?
- Store HUMIRA® (adalimumab) in the refrigerator between 36°F to 46°F (2°C to 8°C). Store HUMIRA in the original carton until use to protect it from light.
- **Do not** freeze HUMIRA. **Do not** use HUMIRA if frozen, even if it has been thawed.
- Refrigerated HUMIRA may be used until the expiration date printed on the HUMIRA carton, dose tray or prefilled syringe. **Do not** use HUMIRA after the expiration date.
- If needed, for example when you are traveling, you may also store HUMIRA at room temperature up to 77°F (25°C) for up to **14** days. Store HUMIRA in the original carton until use to protect it from light.
- Throw away HUMIRA® (adalimumab) if it has been kept at room temperature and not been used within **14** days.
- Record the date you first remove HUMIRA from the refrigerator in the spaces provided on the carton and dose tray.
- Do not store HUMIRA in extreme heat or cold.
- Do not use a prefilled syringe if the liquid is cloudy, discolored, or has flakes or particles in it.
- Do not drop or crush HUMIRA. The prefilled syringe is glass.
- Keep HUMIRA, injection supplies, and all other medicines out of the reach of children.

This Instructions for Use has been approved by the U.S. Food and Drug Administration.
Manufactured by:
AbbVie Inc.
North Chicago, IL 60064, U.S.A.
US License Number 1889
03-B353-R12
Revised: 06/2016

INSTRUCTIONS FOR USE
HUMIRA® (Hu-MARE-ah)
(adalimumab)
40 MG/0.4 ML
SINGLE-USE PREFILLED SYRINGE

Do not try to inject HUMIRA yourself until you have been shown the right way to give the injections and have read and understand this Instructions for Use. If your doctor decides that you or a caregiver may be able to give your injections of HUMIRA at home, you should receive training on the right way to prepare and inject HUMIRA. It is important that you read, understand, and follow these instructions so that you inject HUMIRA the right way. It is also important to talk to your doctor to be sure you understand your HUMIRA dosing instructions. To help you remember when to inject HUMIRA, you can mark your calendar ahead of time. Call your healthcare provider if you or your caregiver have any questions about the right way to inject HUMIRA.

Gather the Supplies for Your Injection
- You will need the following supplies for each injection of HUMIRA.
- Find a clean, flat surface to place the supplies on.
  - 1 alcohol swab
  - 1 cotton ball or gauze pad (not included in your HUMIRA carton)
  - 1 HUMIRA prefilled syringe (See Figure A)
  - FDA-cleared sharps disposal container for HUMIRA prefilled syringe disposal (not included in your HUMIRA carton)

If more comfortable, take your HUMIRA® (adalimumab) prefilled syringe out of the refrigerator **15 to 30 minutes** before injecting to allow the liquid to reach room temperature. **Do not** remove the needle cover while allowing it to reach room temperature. **Do not** warm HUMIRA in any other way (for example, **do not** warm it in a microwave or in hot water).

If you do not have all of the supplies you need to give yourself an injection, go to a pharmacy or call your pharmacist. The diagram below shows what a prefilled syringe looks like. See Figure A.

Figure A

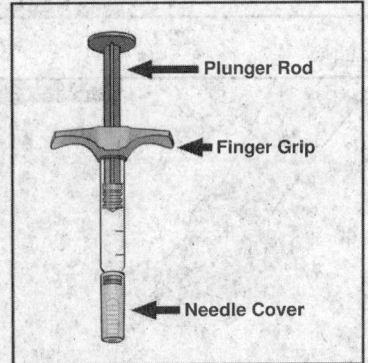

- Plunger Rod
- Finger Grip
- Needle Cover

Check the carton, dose tray, and prefilled syringe
1. Make sure the name HUMIRA® (adalimumab) appears on the dose tray and prefilled syringe label.
2. **Do not use** and **do call** your doctor or pharmacist if:
- the seals on top or bottom of the carton are broken or missing.
- the HUMIRA labeling has an expired date. Check the expiration date on your HUMIRA carton and **do not use** if the date has passed.
- the prefilled syringe that has been frozen or left in direct sunlight.
- HUMIRA has been kept at room temperature for longer than **14** days or HUMIRA has been stored above 77°F (25°C).
- the liquid in the prefilled syringe is cloudy, discolored or has flakes or particles in it. Make sure the liquid is clear and colorless.
See the **"How should I store HUMIRA® (adalimumab)?"** section at the end of this Instructions for Use.

Choose the Injection Site
3. Wash and dry your hands well.
4. Choose an injection site on:
- the front of your thighs or

- your lower abdomen (belly). If you choose your abdomen, do not use the area 2 inches around your belly button (navel). See Figure B.

Figure B

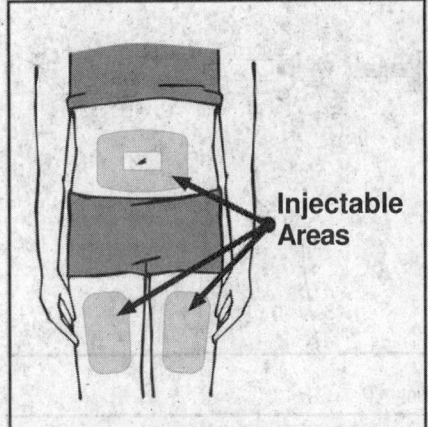

Injectable Areas

- Choose a different site each time you give yourself an injection. Each new injection should be given at least one inch from a site you used before.
- **Do not** inject into skin that is:
  - sore (tender)
  - bruised
  - red
  - hard
  - scarred or where you have stretch marks
- If you have psoriasis, do not inject directly into any raised, thick, red or scaly skin patches or lesions on your skin.
- Do not inject through your clothes.

Prepare the Injection Site
5. Wipe the injection site with an alcohol prep (swab) using a circular motion.
6. Do **not** touch this area again before giving the injection. Allow the skin to dry before injecting. Do not fan or blow on the clean area.

Prepare the Syringe and Needle
7. Remove the needle cover:
- Always hold the prefilled syringe by the body of the syringe.
- Hold the syringe in one hand. With the other hand gently remove the needle cover. See Figure C.
- Throw away the needle cover.
[See Figure C at top of next column]
- Do not touch the needle with your fingers or let the needle touch anything.
8. Turn the syringe so the needle is facing up and hold the syringe at eye level with one hand so you can see the air in the syringe. Using your other hand, slowly push the plunger in to push the air out through the needle. See Figure D.
[See Figure D in next column]
- You may see a drop of liquid at the end of the needle. This is normal.

Position the Prefilled Syringe and Inject HUMIRA® (adalimumab)
Position the Syringe
9. Hold the body of the prefilled syringe in one hand between the thumb and index finger. Hold the syringe in your hand like a pencil. See Figure E.
[See Figure E at next column]
- **Do not** pull back on the plunger at any time.
- With your other hand, gently squeeze the area of the cleaned skin and hold it firmly. See Figure F.
[See Figure F on next page]
Inject HUMIRA® (adalimumab)
10. Using a quick, dart-like motion, insert the needle into the squeezed skin at about a **45-degree angle**. See Figure G.
[See Figure G on next page]
- After the needle is in, let go of the skin. Pull back gently on the plunger.
If blood appears in the syringe:
- It means that you have entered a blood vessel.

Continued on next page

Information on the AbbVie, Inc. products listed on these pages is from the prescribing information in use as of July 31, 2016. For more information, please visit rxabbvie.com or call 1-800-633-9110.

Figure C

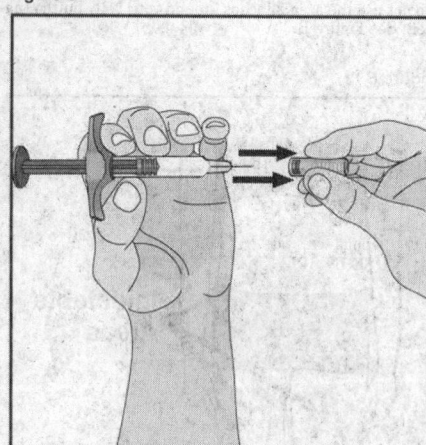

Figure D

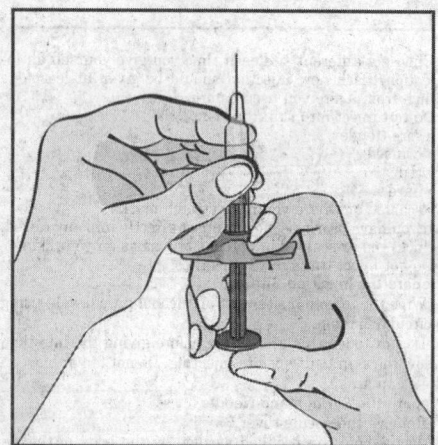

Figure E

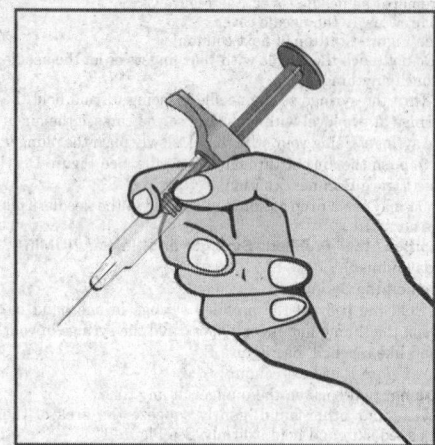

- **Do not** inject HUMIRA.
- Pull the needle out of the skin while keeping the syringe at the same angle.
- Press a cotton ball or gauze pad over the injection site and hold it for 10 seconds. See Figure H.

[See Figure H in next column]

- **Do not** use the same syringe and needle again. Throw away the needle and syringe in your special sharps container.
- **Do not** rub the injection site. You may have slight bleeding. This is normal.
- Repeat Steps 1 through 10 with a new prefilled syringe.

If no blood appears in the syringe:

- Slowly push the plunger all the way in until all of the liquid is injected and the syringe is empty.

Figure F

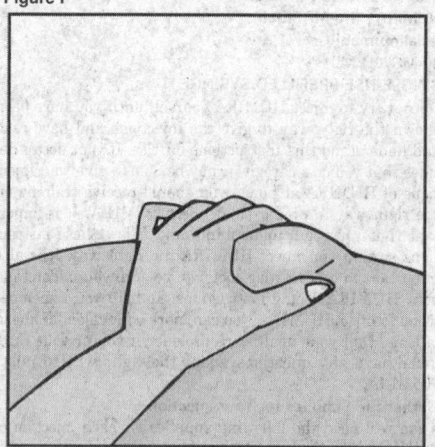

Figure G

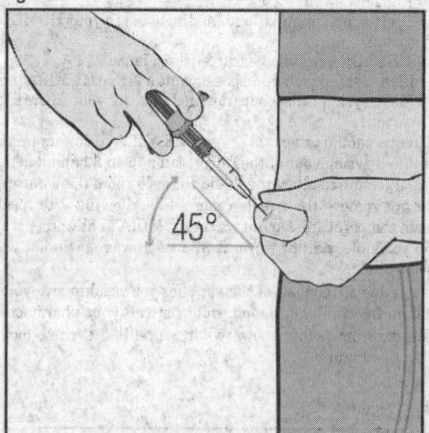

Figure H

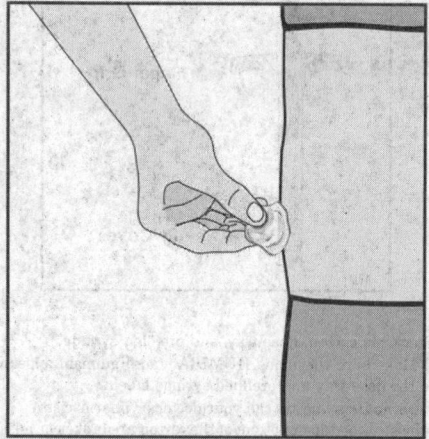

- Pull the needle out of the skin while keeping the syringe at the same angle.
- Press a cotton ball or gauze pad over the injection site and hold it for 10 seconds. Do **not** rub the injection site. You may have slight bleeding. This is normal.

11. Throw away the used prefilled syringe and needle. See "How should I dispose of used prefilled syringes and needles?"

12. Keep a record of the dates and location of your injection sites. To help you remember when to take HUMIRA® (adalimumab), you can mark your calendar ahead of time.

How should I dispose of used prefilled syringes and needles?

- **Put your used needles and syringes in a FDA-cleared sharps disposal container right away after use.** See Figure I. **Do not throw away (dispose of) loose needles and syringes in your household trash.**

- Do not try to touch the needle.

Figure I

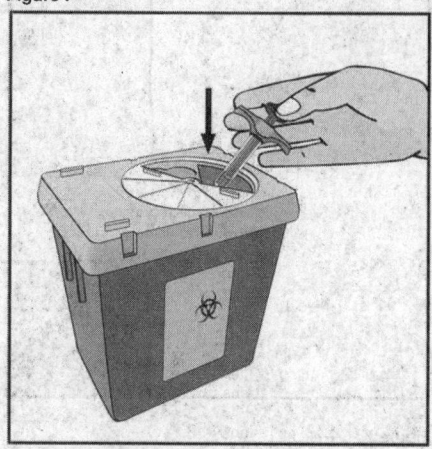

- If you do not have a FDA-cleared sharps disposal container, you may use a household container that is:
  - made of a heavy-duty plastic,
  - can be closed with a tight-fitting, puncture-resistant lid, without sharps being able to come out,
  - upright and stable during use,
  - leak-resistant, and
  - properly labeled to warn of hazardous waste inside the container.
- When your sharps disposal container is almost full, you will need to follow your community guidelines for the right way to dispose of your sharps disposal container. There may be state or local laws about how you should throw away used needles and syringes. For more information about safe sharps disposal, and for specific information about sharps disposal in the state that you live in, go to the FDA's website at: http://www.fda.gov/safesharpsdisposal.
- For the safety and health of you and others, needles and used syringes **must never** be re-used.
- The used alcohol pads, cotton balls, dose trays and packaging may be placed in your household trash.
- **Do not dispose of your used sharps disposal container in your household trash unless your community guidelines permit this. Do not recycle your used sharps disposal container.**
- **Always keep the sharps container out of the reach of children.**

How should I store HUMIRA?

- Store HUMIRA in the refrigerator between 36°F to 46°F (2°C to 8°C). Store HUMIRA in the original carton until use to protect it from light.
- **Do not** freeze HUMIRA. **Do not** use HUMIRA if frozen, even if it has been thawed.
- Refrigerated HUMIRA® (adalimumab) may be used until the expiration date printed on the HUMIRA carton, dose tray or prefilled syringe. **Do not** use HUMIRA after the expiration date.
- If needed, for example when you are traveling, you may also store HUMIRA at room temperature up to 77°F (25°C) for up to **14** days. Store HUMIRA in the original carton until use to protect it from light.
- Throw away HUMIRA® (adalimumab) if it has been kept at room temperature and not been used within **14** days.
- Record the date you first remove HUMIRA from the refrigerator in the spaces provided on the carton and dose tray.
- Do not store HUMIRA in extreme heat or cold.
- Do not use a prefilled syringe if the liquid is cloudy, discolored, or has flakes or particles in it.
- Do not drop or crush HUMIRA. The prefilled syringe is glass.
- Keep HUMIRA, injection supplies, and all other medicines out of the reach of children.

This Instructions for Use has been approved by the U.S. Food and Drug Administration.

Manufactured by:
AbbVie Inc.
North Chicago, IL 60064, U.S.A.
US License Number 1889
03-B354-R3
Revised: 06/2016

Shown in Product Identification Guide, page 505

KALETRA® ℞

[*kuh-LEE-tra*]
(lopinavir and ritonavir)
tablet, for oral use

KALETRA
(lopinavir and ritonavir)
oral solution

HIGHLIGHTS OF PRESCRIBING INFORMATION
These highlights do not include all the information needed to use KALETRA safely and effectively. See full prescribing information for KALETRA.
KALETRA (lopinavir and ritonavir) tablet, for oral use
KALETRA (lopinavir and ritonavir) oral solution
Initial U.S. Approval: 2000

———RECENT MAJOR CHANGES———

Dosage and Administration	
General Administration Recommendations (2.1)	01/2015
Dosage Recommendations in Adults (2.2)	01/2015
Dosage Recommendations in Pediatric Patients (2.3)	01/2015
Dosage Recommendations in Pregnancy (2.4)	01/2015
Warnings and Precautions	
Risk of Serious Adverse Reactions Due to Drug Interactions (5.1)	03/2015

———INDICATIONS AND USAGE———
KALETRA is an HIV-1 protease inhibitor indicated in combination with other antiretroviral agents for the treatment of HIV-1 infection in adults and pediatric patients (14 days and older). (1)

———DOSAGE AND ADMINISTRATION———
Tablets: May be taken with or without food, swallowed whole and not chewed, broken, or crushed. (2.1)
Oral solution: must be taken with food. (2.1)
Adults (2.2):
• Total recommended daily dosage is 800/200 mg given once or twice daily.
• KALETRA can be given as once daily or twice daily regimen. See Full Prescribing Information for details.
• KALETRA once daily dosing regimen is not recommended in:
  • Adult patients with three or more of the following lopinavir resistance-associated substitutions: L10F/I/R/V, K20M/N/R, L24I, L33F, M36I, I47V, G48V, I54L/T/V, V82A/C/F/S/T, and I84V. (12.4)
  • In combination with carbamazepine, phenobarbital, or phenytoin. (7.3)
  • In combination with efavirenz, nevirapine, or nelfinavir. (12.3)
  • In pregnant women. (2.4, 8.1, 12.3)
Pediatric Patients (14 days and older) (2.3):
• KALETRA once daily dosing regimen is not recommended in pediatric patients.
• Twice daily dose is based on body weight or body surface area.
Concomitant Therapy in Adults and Pediatric Patients:
• Dose adjustments of KALETRA may be needed when co-administering with efavirenz, nevirapine, or nelfinavir. (2.2, 2.3, 7.3)
• KALETRA oral solution should not be administered to neonates before a postmenstrual age (first day of the mother's last menstrual period to birth plus the time elapsed after birth) of 42 weeks and a postnatal age of at least 14 days has been attained (2.3, 5.2)
Pregnancy (2.4):
• 400/100 mg twice daily in pregnant patients with no documented lopinavir-associated resistance substitutions.
• There are insufficient data to recommend a KALETRA dose for pregnant patients with any documented KALETRA-associated resistance substitutions.
• No dose adjustment of KALETRA is required for patients during the postpartum period.

———DOSAGE FORMS AND STRENGTHS———
• Tablets: 200 mg lopinavir and 50 mg ritonavir (3)
• Tablets: 100 mg lopinavir and 25 mg ritonavir (3)
• Oral solution: 80 mg lopinavir and 20 mg ritonavir per milliliter (3)

———CONTRAINDICATIONS———
• Hypersensitivity to KALETRA (e.g., toxic epidermal necrolysis, Stevens-Johnson syndrome, erythema multiforme, urticaria, angioedema) or any of its ingredients, including ritonavir. (4)
• Co-administration with drugs highly dependent on CYP3A for clearance and for which elevated plasma levels may result in serious and/or life-threatening events. (4)
• Co-administration with potent CYP3A inducers where significantly reduced lopinavir plasma concentrations may be associated with the potential for loss of virologic response and possible resistance and cross resistance. (4)

———WARNINGS AND PRECAUTIONS———
The following have been observed in patients receiving KALETRA:
• The concomitant use of KALETRA and certain other drugs may result in known or potentially significant drug interactions. Consult the full prescribing information prior to and during treatment for potential drug interactions. (5.1, 7.3)
• Toxicity in preterm neonates: KALETRA oral solution should not be used in preterm neonates in the immediate postnatal period because of possible toxicities. A safe and effective dose of KALETRA oral solution in this patient population has not been established. (2.3, 5.2)
• Pancreatitis: Fatalities have occurred; suspend therapy as clinically appropriate. (5.3)
• Hepatotoxicity: Fatalities have occurred. Monitor liver function before and during therapy, especially in patients with underlying hepatic disease, including hepatitis B and hepatitis C, or marked transaminase elevations. (5.4, 8.6)
• QT interval prolongation and isolated cases of torsade de pointes have been reported although causality could not be established. Avoid use in patients with congenital long QT syndrome, those with hypokalemia, and with other drugs that prolong the QT interval. (5.1, 5.5, 12.3)
• PR interval prolongation may occur in some patients. Cases of second and third degree heart block have been reported. Use with caution in patients with pre-existing conduction system disease, ischemic heart disease, cardiomyopathy, underlying structural heart disease or when administering with other drugs that may prolong the PR interval. (5.1, 5.6, 12.3)
• Patients may develop new onset or exacerbations of diabetes mellitus, hyperglycemia (5.7), immune reconstitution syndrome. (5.8), redistribution/accumulation of body fat. (5.10)
• Total cholesterol and triglycerides elevations. Monitor prior to therapy and periodically thereafter. (5.9)
• Hemophilia: Spontaneous bleeding may occur, and additional factor VIII may be required. (5.11)

———ADVERSE REACTIONS———
Commonly reported adverse reactions to KALETRA included diarrhea, nausea, vomiting, hypertriglyceridemia and hypercholesterolemia. (6.1)
To report SUSPECTED ADVERSE REACTIONS, contact AbbVie Inc. at 1-800-633-9110 or FDA at 1-800-FDA-1088 or www.fda.gov/medwatch

———DRUG INTERACTIONS———
Co-administration of KALETRA can alter the plasma concentrations of other drugs and other drugs may alter the plasma concentrations of lopinavir. The potential for drug-drug interactions must be considered prior to and during therapy. (4, 5.1, 7, 12.3)

———USE IN SPECIFIC POPULATIONS———
Lactation: Breastfeeding not recommended. (8.2)
See 17 for PATIENT COUNSELING INFORMATION and Medication Guide.

Revised: 11/2015

FULL PRESCRIBING INFORMATION: CONTENTS*

FULL PRESCRIBING INFORMATION

1   INDICATIONS AND USAGE
KALETRA is indicated in combination with other antiretroviral agents for the treatment of HIV-1 infection in adults and pediatric patients (14 days and older).
The following points should be considered when initiating therapy with KALETRA:
• The use of other active agents with KALETRA is associated with a greater likelihood of treatment response [*see Microbiology (12.4)* and *Clinical Studies (14)*].
• Genotypic or phenotypic testing and/or treatment history should guide the use of KALETRA [*see Microbiology (12.4)*]. The number of baseline lopinavir resistance-associated substitutions affects the virologic response to KALETRA [*see Microbiology (12.4)*].

2   DOSAGE AND ADMINISTRATION
2.1   General Administration Recommendations
KALETRA tablets may be taken with or without food. The tablets should be swallowed whole and not chewed, broken, or crushed. KALETRA oral solution must be taken with food.
2.2   Dosage Recommendations in Adults
Considerations in Determining KALETRA Once Daily vs. Twice Daily Dosing Regimen:
• KALETRA can be given as once daily or twice daily dosing regimen in patients with less than three lopinavir resistance-associated substitutions.
• KALETRA must be given as twice daily dosing regimen in patients with three or more resistance-associated substitutions.
• Table 1 includes the recommended once daily dosing regimen and Tables 2 and 3 include the recommended twice daily dosing regimen.

Continued on next page

Information on the AbbVie, Inc. products listed on these pages is from the prescribing information in use as of July 31, 2016. For more information, please visit rxabbvie.com or call 1-800-633-9110.

KALETRA once daily dosing regimen is not recommended in:
- Adult patients with three or more of the following lopinavir resistance-associated substitutions: L10F/I/R/V, K20M/N/R, L24I, L33F, M36I, I47V, G48V, I54L/T/V, V82A/C/F/S/T, and I84V *[see Microbiology (12.4)]*.
- In combination with carbamazepine, phenobarbital, or phenytoin *[see Drug Interactions (7.3)]*.
- In combination with efavirenz, nevirapine, or nelfinavir *[see Drug Interactions (7.3) and Clinical Pharmacology (12.3)]*.
- In pregnant women *[see Dosage and Administration (2.4), Use in Specific Populations (8.1) and Clinical Pharmacology (12.3)]*.

The dose of KALETRA must be increased when administered in combination with efavirenz, nevirapine or nelfinavir.

Table 3 outlines the dosage recommendations for twice daily dosing when KALETRA is taken in combination with efavirenz, nevirapine or nelfinavir.

Table 1. Recommended Dosage in Adults- KALETRA Once Daily Regimen

KALETRA Dosage Form	Recommended Dosage
200 mg/50 mg Tablets	800 mg/200 mg (4 tablets) once daily
80 mg/20 mg per mL Oral Solution	800 mg/200 mg (10 mL) once daily

Table 2. Recommended Dosage in Adults - KALETRA Twice Daily Regimen

KALETRA Dosage Form	Recommended Dosage
200 mg/50 mg Tablets	400 mg/100 mg (2 tablets) twice daily
80 mg/20 mg per mL Oral Solution	400 mg/100 mg (5 mL) twice daily

Table 3. Recommended Dosage in Adults - KALETRA Twice Daily Regimen in Combination with Efavirenz, Nevirapine, or Nelfinavir

KALETRA Dosage Form	Recommended Dosage
200 mg/50 mg Tablets and 100 mg/25 mg Tablets	500 mg/125 mg (2 tablets of 200 mg/50 mg + 1 tablet of 100 mg/25 mg) twice daily
80 mg/20 mg per mL Oral Solution	520 mg/130 mg (6.5 mL) twice daily

2.3   Dosage Recommendations in Pediatric Patients
KALETRA® (lopinavir and ritonavir) tablets and oral solution should not be administered once daily in pediatric patients < 18 years of age. The dose of the oral solution should be administered using a calibrated dosing syringe.

Before prescribing KALETRA 100/25 mg tablets, children should be assessed for the ability to swallow intact tablets. If a child is unable to reliably swallow a KALETRA tablet, the KALETRA oral solution formulation should be prescribed.

KALETRA oral solution should not be administered to neonates before a postmenstrual age (first day of the mother's last menstrual period to birth plus the time elapsed after birth) of 42 weeks and a postnatal age of at least 14 days has been attained *[see Warnings and Precautions (5.2)]*.

KALETRA oral solution contains 42.4% (v/v) alcohol and 15.3% (w/v) propylene glycol. Special attention should be given to accurate calculation of the dosage of KALETRA, transcription of the medication order, dispensing information and dosing instructions to minimize the risk for medication errors, and overdose. This is especially important for infants and young children. Total amounts of alcohol and propylene glycol from all medicines that are to be given to pediatric patients 14 days to 6 months of age should be taken into account in order to avoid toxicity from these excipients *[see Warnings and Precautions (5.2) and Overdosage (10)]*.

Pediatric Dosage Calculations
Calculate the appropriate dose of KALETRA for each individual pediatric patient based on body weight (kg) or body surface area (BSA) to avoid underdosing or exceeding the recommended adult dose.

Body surface area (BSA) can be calculated as follows:

$$\text{* BSA (m}^2\text{)} = \sqrt{\frac{\text{Ht (Cm) x Wt (kg)}}{3600}}$$

The KALETRA dose can be calculated based on weight or BSA:

Based on Weight:
Patient Weight (kg) × Prescribed lopinavir dose (mg/kg) = Administered lopinavir dose (mg)

Based on BSA:
Patient BSA (m²) × Prescribed lopinavir dose (mg/m²) = Administered lopinavir dose (mg)

If KALETRA oral solution is used, the volume (mL) of KALETRA solution can be determined as follows:
Volume of KALETRA solution (mL) = Administered lopinavir dose (mg) ÷ 80 (mg/mL)

Dosage Recommendation in Pediatric Patients 14 Days to 6 Months:
In pediatric patients 14 days to 6 months of age, the recommended dosage of lopinavir/ritonavir using KALETRA oral solution is 16/4 mg/kg or 300/75 mg/m² twice daily. Prescribers should calculate the appropriate dose based on body weight or body surface area. Table 4 summarizes the recommended daily dosing regimen for pediatric patients 14 days to 6 months.

It is recommended that KALETRA not be administered in combination with efavirenz, nevirapine, or nelfinavir in patients < 6 months of age.

Table 4. Recommended KALETRA Oral Daily Dosage in Pediatric Patients 14 days to 6 months

Patient Age	Based on Weight (mg/kg)	Based on BSA (mg/m²)	Frequency
14 days to 6 months	16/4	300/75	Given twice daily

Dosage Recommendation in Pediatric Patients 6 Months to 18 Years:
Without Concomitant Efavirenz, Nevirapine, or Nelfinavir
Dosing recommendations using oral solution
In children 6 months to 18 years of age, the recommended dosage of lopinavir/ritonavir using KALETRA oral solution without concomitant efavirenz, nevirapine, or nelfinavir is 230/57.5 mg/m² given twice daily, not to exceed the recommended adult dose (400/100 mg [5 mL] twice daily). If weight-based dosing is preferred, the recommended dosage of lopinavir/ritonavir for patients < 15 kg is 12/3 mg/kg given twice daily and the dosage for patients ≥ 15 kg to 40 kg is 10/2.5 mg/kg given twice daily. Table 5 summarizes the recommended daily dosing regimen for pediatric patients 6 months to 18 years.

Table 5. Recommended KALETRA Oral Daily Dosage in Pediatric Patients 6 months to 18 years

Patient Age	Based on Weight (mg/kg)		Based on BSA (mg/m²)	Frequency
6 months to 18 years	<15 kg	12/3	230/57.5	Given twice daily
	≥15 kg to 40 kg	10/2.5		

Dosing recommendations using tablets
Table 6 provides the dosing recommendations for pediatric patients 6 months to 18 years of age based on body weight or body surface area for KALETRA tablets.

Table 6. Pediatric Dosing Recommendations for Patients 6 Months to 18 Years of Age Based on Body Weight or Body Surface Area for KALETRA Tablets Without Concomitant Efavirenz, Nevirapine, or Nelfinavir

Body Weight (kg)	Body Surface Area (m²)*	Recommended number of 100/25 mg Tablets Twice Daily
15 to 25	≥0.6 to < 0.9	2
>25 to 35	≥0.9 to < 1.4	3
>35	≥1.4	4 (or two 200/50 mg tablets)

* KALETRA oral solution is available for children with a BSA less than 0.6 m² or those who are unable to reliably swallow a tablet.

Concomitant Therapy: Efavirenz, Nevirapine, or Nelfinavir
Dosing recommendations using oral solution
A dose increase of KALETRA to 300/75 mg/m² using KALETRA oral solution is needed when co-administered with efavirenz, nevirapine, or nelfinavir in children (both treatment-naïve and treatment-experienced) 6 months to 18 years of age, not to exceed the recommended adult dose (533/133 mg [6.5 mL] twice daily). If weight-based dosing is preferred, the recommended dosage for patients <15 kg is 13/3.25 mg/kg given twice daily and the dosage for patients >15 kg to 45 kg is 11/2.75 mg/kg given twice daily.
Dosing recommendations using tablets
Table 7 provides the dosing recommendations for pediatric patients 6 months to 18 years of age based on body weight or body surface area for KALETRA tablets when given in combination with efavirenz, nevirapine, or nelfinavir.

Table 7. Pediatric Dosing Recommendations for Patients 6 Months to 18 Years of Age Based on Body Weight or Body Surface Area for KALETRA Tablets With Concomitant Efavirenz[†], Nevirapine, or Nelfinavir[†]

Body Weight (kg)	Body Surface Area (m²)*	Recommended number of 100/25 mg Tablets Twice Daily
15 to 20	≥0.6 to < 0.8	2
>20 to 30	≥0.8 to < 1.2	3
>30 to 45	≥1.2 to < 1.7	4 (or two 200/50 mg tablets)
>45	≥1.7	5 *[see Dosage and Administration (2.2)]*

* KALETRA oral solution is available for children with a BSA less than 0.6 m² or those who are unable to reliably swallow a tablet.
† Please refer to the individual product labels for appropriate dosing in children.

2.4   Dosage Recommendations in Pregnancy
Administer 400/100 mg of KALETRA twice daily in pregnant patients with no documented lopinavir-associated resistance substitutions. Once daily KALETRA dosing is not recommended in pregnancy *[see Use in Specific Populations (8.1) and Clinical Pharmacology (12.3)]*.
- There are insufficient data to recommend dosing in pregnant women with any documented lopinavir-associated resistance substitutions.
- No dosage adjustment of KALETRA is required for patients during the postpartum period.
- Avoid use of KALETRA oral solution in pregnant women *[see Use in Specific Populations (8.1)]*.

3   DOSAGE FORMS AND STRENGTHS
- *Tablets, 200 mg lopinavir, 50 mg ritonavir:* Yellow, film-coated, ovaloid, debossed with the "a" logo and the code KA providing 200 mg lopinavir and 50 mg ritonavir.
- *Tablets, 100 mg lopinavir, 25 mg ritonavir:* Pale yellow, film-coated, ovaloid, debossed with the "a" logo and the code KC providing 100 mg lopinavir and 25 mg ritonavir.
- *Oral Solution:* Light yellow to orange colored liquid containing 400 mg lopinavir and 100 mg ritonavir per 5 mL (80 mg lopinavir and 20 mg ritonavir per mL).

4   CONTRAINDICATIONS
- KALETRA is contraindicated in patients with previously demonstrated clinically significant hypersensitivity (e.g., toxic epidermal necrolysis, Stevens-Johnson syndrome, erythema multiforme, urticaria, angioedema) to any of its ingredients, including ritonavir.
- Co-administration of KALETRA is contraindicated with drugs that are highly dependent on CYP3A for clearance and for which elevated plasma concentrations are associated with serious and/or life-threatening reactions.
- Co-administration of KALETRA is contraindicated with potent CYP3A inducers where significantly reduced lopinavir plasma concentrations may be associated with

the potential for loss of virologic response and possible resistance and cross-resistance. These drugs are listed in Table 8.

[See table above]

5 WARNINGS AND PRECAUTIONS

5.1 Risk of Serious Adverse Reactions Due to Drug Interactions

Initiation of KALETRA, a CYP3A inhibitor, in patients receiving medications metabolized by CYP3A or initiation of medications metabolized by CYP3A in patients already receiving KALETRA, may increase plasma concentrations of medications metabolized by CYP3A. Initiation of medications that inhibit or induce CYP3A may increase or decrease concentrations of KALETRA, respectively. These interactions may lead to:

- Clinically significant adverse reactions, potentially leading to severe, life-threatening, or fatal events from greater exposures of concomitant medications.
- Clinically significant adverse reactions from greater exposures of KALETRA.
- Loss of therapeutic effect of KALETRA and possible development of resistance.

See Table 13 for steps to prevent or manage these possible and known significant drug interactions, including dosing recommendations *[see Drug Interactions (7)]*. Consider the potential for drug interactions prior to and during KALETRA therapy; review concomitant medications during KALETRA therapy, and monitor for the adverse reactions associated with the concomitant medications *[see Contraindications (4) and Drug Interactions (7)]*.

5.2 Toxicity in Preterm Neonates

KALETRA oral solution contains the excipients alcohol (42.4% v/v) and propylene glycol (15.3% w/v). When administered concomitantly with propylene glycol, ethanol competitively inhibits the metabolism of propylene glycol, which may lead to elevated concentrations. Preterm neonates may be at increased risk of propylene glycol-associated adverse events due to diminished ability to metabolize propylene glycol, thereby leading to accumulation and potential adverse events. Postmarketing life-threatening cases of cardiac toxicity (including complete AV block, bradycardia, and cardiomyopathy), lactic acidosis, acute renal failure, CNS depression and respiratory complications leading to death have been reported, predominantly in preterm neonates receiving KALETRA oral solution.

KALETRA oral solution should not be used in preterm neonates in the immediate postnatal period because of possible toxicities. A safe and effective dose of KALETRA oral solution in this patient population has not been established. However, if the benefit of using KALETRA oral solution to treat HIV infection in infants immediately after birth outweighs the potential risks, infants should be monitored closely for increases in serum osmolality and serum creatinine, and for toxicity related to KALETRA oral solution including: hyperosmolality, with or without lactic acidosis, renal toxicity, CNS depression (including stupor, coma, and apnea), seizures, hypotonia, cardiac arrhythmias and ECG changes, and hemolysis. Total amounts of alcohol and propylene glycol from all medicines that are to be given to infants should be taken into account in order to avoid toxicity from these excipients *[see Dosage and Administration (2.3) and Overdosage (10)]*.

5.3 Pancreatitis

Pancreatitis has been observed in patients receiving KALETRA therapy, including those who developed marked triglyceride elevations. In some cases, fatalities have been observed. Although a causal relationship to KALETRA has not been established, marked triglyceride elevations are a risk factor for development of pancreatitis *[see Warnings and Precautions (5.9)]*. Patients with advanced HIV-1 disease may be at increased risk of elevated triglycerides and pancreatitis, and patients with a history of pancreatitis may be at increased risk for recurrence during KALETRA therapy.

Pancreatitis should be considered if clinical symptoms (nausea, vomiting, abdominal pain) or abnormalities in laboratory values (such as increased serum lipase or amylase values) suggestive of pancreatitis occur. Patients who exhibit these signs or symptoms should be evaluated and KALETRA and/or other antiretroviral therapy should be suspended as clinically appropriate.

5.4 Hepatotoxicity

Patients with underlying hepatitis B or C or marked elevations in transaminase prior to treatment may be at increased risk for developing or worsening of transaminase elevations or hepatic decompensation with use of KALETRA.

Table 8. Drugs That are Contraindicated with KALETRA

Drug Class	Drugs Within Class That are Contraindicated with KALETRA	Clinical Comments
Alpha 1- Adrenoreceptor Antagonist	Alfuzosin	Potentially increased alfuzosin concentrations can result in hypotension.
Antimycobacterial	Rifampin	May lead to loss of virologic response and possible resistance to KALETRA or to the class of protease inhibitors or other co-administered antiretroviral agents *[see Drug Interactions (7)]*.
Ergot Derivatives	Dihydroergotamine, ergotamine, methylergonovine	Potential for acute ergot toxicity characterized by peripheral vasospasm and ischemia of the extremities and other tissues.
GI Motility Agent	Cisapride	Potential for cardiac arrhythmias.
Herbal Products	St. John's Wort (hypericum perforatum)	May lead to loss of virologic response and possible resistance to KALETRA or to the class of protease inhibitors.
HMG-CoA Reductase Inhibitors	Lovastatin, simvastatin	Potential for myopathy including rhabdomyolysis.
PDE5 Enzyme Inhibitor	Sildenafil[a] (Revatio®) when used for the treatment of pulmonary arterial hypertension	A safe and effective dose has not been established when used with KALETRA. There is an increased potential for sildenafil-associated adverse events, including visual abnormalities, hypotension, prolonged erection, and syncope *[see Drug Interactions (7)]*.
Neuroleptic	Pimozide	Potential for cardiac arrhythmias.
Sedative/Hypnotics	Triazolam; orally administered midazolam[b]	Prolonged or increased sedation or respiratory depression.

[a] see Drug Interactions (7), *Table 13* for co-administration of sildenafil in patients with erectile dysfunction.
[b] see Drug Interactions (7), *Table 13* for parenterally administered midazolam.

There have been postmarketing reports of hepatic dysfunction, including some fatalities. These have generally occurred in patients with advanced HIV-1 disease taking multiple concomitant medications in the setting of underlying chronic hepatitis or cirrhosis. A causal relationship with KALETRA therapy has not been established.

Elevated transaminases with or without elevated bilirubin levels have been reported in HIV-1 mono-infected and uninfected patients as early as 7 days after the initiation of KALETRA in conjunction with other antiretroviral agents. In some cases, the hepatic dysfunction was serious; however, a definitive causal relationship with KALETRA therapy has not been established.

Appropriate laboratory testing should be conducted prior to initiating therapy with KALETRA and patients should be monitored closely during treatment. Increased AST/ALT monitoring should be considered in the patients with underlying chronic hepatitis or cirrhosis, especially during the first several months of KALETRA treatment *[see Use in Specific Populations (8.6)]*.

5.5 QT Interval Prolongation

Postmarketing cases of QT interval prolongation and torsade de pointes have been reported although causality of KALETRA could not be established. Avoid use in patients with congenital long QT syndrome, those with hypokalemia, and with other drugs that prolong the QT interval *[see Clinical Pharmacology (12.3)]*.

5.6 PR Interval Prolongation

Lopinavir/ritonavir prolongs the PR interval in some patients. Cases of second or third degree atrioventricular block have been reported. KALETRA should be used with caution in patients with underlying structural heart disease, preexisting conduction system abnormalities, ischemic heart disease or cardiomyopathies, as these patients may be at increased risk for developing cardiac conduction abnormalities.

The impact on the PR interval of co-administration of KALETRA with other drugs that prolong the PR interval (including calcium channel blockers, beta-adrenergic blockers, digoxin and atazanavir) has not been evaluated. As a result, co-administration of KALETRA with these drugs should be undertaken with caution, particularly with those drugs metabolized by CYP3A. Clinical monitoring is recommended *[see Clinical Pharmacology (12.3)]*.

5.7 Diabetes Mellitus/Hyperglycemia

New onset diabetes mellitus, exacerbation of pre-existing diabetes mellitus, and hyperglycemia have been reported during post-marketing surveillance in HIV-1 infected patients receiving protease inhibitor therapy. Some patients required either initiation or dose adjustments of insulin or oral hypoglycemic agents for treatment of these events. In some cases, diabetic ketoacidosis has occurred. In those patients who discontinued protease inhibitor therapy, hyperglycemia persisted in some cases. Because these events have been reported voluntarily during clinical practice, estimates of frequency cannot be made and a causal relationship between protease inhibitor therapy and these events has not been established.

5.8 Immune Reconstitution Syndrome

Immune reconstitution syndrome has been reported in patients treated with combination antiretroviral therapy, including KALETRA. During the initial phase of combination antiretroviral treatment, patients whose immune system responds may develop an inflammatory response to indolent or residual opportunistic infections (such as *Mycobacterium avium* infection, cytomegalovirus, *Pneumocystis jirovecii* pneumonia [PCP], or tuberculosis) which may necessitate further evaluation and treatment.

Autoimmune disorders (such as Graves' disease, polymyositis, and Guillain-Barré syndrome) have also been reported to occur in the setting of immune reconstitution, however, the time to onset is more variable, and can occur many months after initiation of treatment.

5.9 Lipid Elevations

Treatment with KALETRA® (lopinavir and ritonavir) has resulted in large increases in the concentration of total cholesterol and triglycerides *[see Adverse Reactions (6.1)]*. Triglyceride and cholesterol testing should be performed prior to initiating KALETRA therapy and at periodic intervals during therapy. Lipid disorders should be managed as clinically appropriate, taking into account any potential drug-drug interactions with KALETRA and HMG-CoA reductase inhibitors *[see Contraindications (4) and Drug Interactions (7.3)]*.

5.10 Fat Redistribution

Redistribution/accumulation of body fat including central obesity, dorsocervical fat enlargement (buffalo hump), pe-

Continued on next page

Information on the AbbVie, Inc. products listed on these pages is from the prescribing information in use as of July 31, 2016. For more information, please visit rxabbvie.com or call 1-800-633-9110.

ripheral wasting, facial wasting, breast enlargement, and "cushingoid appearance" have been observed in patients receiving antiretroviral therapy. The mechanism and long-term consequences of these events are currently unknown. A causal relationship has not been established.

5.11   Patients with Hemophilia
Increased bleeding, including spontaneous skin hematomas and hemarthrosis have been reported in patients with hemophilia type A and B treated with protease inhibitors. In some patients additional factor VIII was given. In more than half of the reported cases, treatment with protease inhibitors was continued or reintroduced. A causal relationship between protease inhibitor therapy and these events has not been established.

5.12   Resistance/Cross-resistance
Because the potential for HIV cross-resistance among protease inhibitors has not been fully explored in KALETRA-treated patients, it is unknown what effect therapy with KALETRA will have on the activity of subsequently administered protease inhibitors [see Microbiology (12.4)].

6   ADVERSE REACTIONS
The following adverse reactions are discussed in greater detail in other sections of the labeling.
• QT Interval Prolongation, PR Interval Prolongation [see Warnings and Precautions (5.5, 5.6)]
• Drug Interactions [see Warnings and Precautions (5.1)]
• Pancreatitis [see Warnings and Precautions (5.3)]
• Hepatotoxicity [see Warnings and Precautions (5.4)]

6.1   Clinical Trials Experience
Because clinical trials are conducted under widely varying conditions, adverse reactions rates observed in the clinical trials of a drug cannot be directly compared to rates in the clinical trials of another drug and may not reflect the rates observed in clinical practice.

Adverse Reactions in Adults
The safety of KALETRA has been investigated in about 2,600 patients in Phase II-IV clinical trials, of which about 700 have received a dose of 800/200 mg (6 capsules or 4 tablets) once daily. Along with nucleoside reverse transcriptase inhibitors (NRTIs), in some studies, KALETRA was used in combination with efavirenz or nevirapine.

In clinical studies the incidence of diarrhea in patients treated with either KALETRA capsules or tablets was greater in those patients treated once daily than in those patients treated twice daily. Any grade of diarrhea was reported by at least half of patients taking once daily Kaletra capsules or tablets. At the time of treatment discontinuation, 4.2-6.3% of patients taking once daily Kaletra and 1.8-3.7% of those taking twice daily Kaletra reported ongoing diarrhea.

Commonly reported adverse reactions to KALETRA included diarrhea, nausea, vomiting, hypertriglyceridemia and hypercholesterolemia. Diarrhea, nausea and vomiting may occur at the beginning of the treatment while hypertriglyceridemia and hypercholesterolemia may occur later. The following have been identified as adverse reactions of moderate or severe intensity (Table 9):

Table 9. Adverse Reactions of Moderate or Severe Intensity Occurring in at Least 0.1% of Adult Patients Receiving KALETRA in Combined Phase II/IV Studies (N=2,612)

System Organ Class (SOC) and Adverse Reaction	n	%
BLOOD AND LYMPHATIC SYSTEM DISORDERS		
anemia*	54	2.1
leukopenia and neutropenia*	44	1.7
lymphadenopathy*	35	1.3
CARDIAC DISORDERS		
atherosclerosis such as myocardial infarction*	10	0.4
atrioventricular block*	3	0.1
tricuspid valve incompetence*	3	0.1
EAR AND LABYRINTH DISORDERS		
vertigo*	7	0.3
tinnitus	6	0.2
ENDOCRINE DISORDERS		
hypogonadism*	16	0.8[1]
EYE DISORDERS		
visual impairment*	8	0.3
GASTROINTESTINAL DISORDERS		
diarrhea*	510	19.5
nausea	269	10.3
vomiting*	177	6.8
abdominal pain (upper and lower)*	160	6.1
gastroenteritis and colitis*	66	2.5
dyspepsia	53	2.0
pancreatitis*	45	1.7
Gastroesophageal Reflux Disease (GERD)*	40	1.5
hemorrhoids	39	1.5
flatulence	36	1.4
abdominal distension	34	1.3
constipation*	26	1.0
stomatitis and oral ulcers*	24	0.9
duodenitis and gastritis*	20	0.8
gastrointestinal hemorrhage including rectal hemorrhage*	13	0.5
dry mouth	9	0.3
gastrointestinal ulcer*	6	0.2
fecal incontinence	5	0.2
GENERAL DISORDERS AND ADMINISTRATION SITE CONDITIONS		
fatigue including asthenia*	198	7.6
HEPATOBILIARY DISORDERS		
hepatitis including AST, ALT, and GGT increases*	91	3.5
hepatomegaly	5	0.2
cholangitis	3	0.1
hepatic steatosis	3	0.1
IMMUNE SYSTEM DISORDERS		
hypersensitivity including urticaria and angioedema*	70	2.7
immune reconstitution syndrome	3	0.1
INFECTIONS AND INFESTATIONS		
upper respiratory tract infection*	363	13.9
lower respiratory tract infection*	202	7.7
skin infections including cellulitis, folliculitis, and furuncle*	86	3.3
METABOLISM AND NUTRITION DISORDERS		
hypercholesterolemia*	192	7.4
hypertriglyceridemia*	161	6.2
weight decreased*	61	2.3
decreased appetite	52	2.0
blood glucose disorders including diabetes mellitus*	30	1.1
weight increased*	20	0.8
lactic acidosis*	11	0.4
increased appetite	5	0.2
MUSCULOSKELETAL AND CONNECTIVE TISSUE DISORDERS		
musculoskeletal pain including arthralgia and back pain*	166	6.4
myalgia*	46	1.8
muscle disorders such as weakness and spasms*	34	1.3
rhabdomyolysis*	18	0.7
osteonecrosis	3	0.1
NERVOUS SYSTEM DISORDERS		
headache including migraine*	165	6.3
insomnia*	99	3.8
neuropathy and peripheral neuropathy*	51	2.0
dizziness*	45	1.7
ageusia*	19	0.7
convulsion*	9	0.3
tremor*	9	0.3
cerebral vascular event*	6	0.2
PSYCHIATRIC DISORDERS		
anxiety*	101	3.9
abnormal dreams*	19	0.7
libido decreased	19	0.7
RENAL AND URINARY DISORDERS		
renal failure*	31	1.2
hematuria*	20	0.8
nephritis*	3	0.1
REPRODUCTIVE SYSTEM AND BREAST DISORDERS		
erectile dysfunction*	34	1.7[1]
menstrual disorders - amenorrhea, menorrhagia*	10	1.7[2]
SKIN AND SUBCUTANEOUS TISSUE DISORDERS		
rash including maculopapular rash*	99	3.8
lipodystrophy acquired including facial wasting*	58	2.2
dermatitis/rash including eczema and seborrheic dermatitis*	50	1.9
night sweats*	42	1.6
pruritus*	29	1.1
alopecia	10	0.4
capillaritis and vasculitis*	3	0.1
VASCULAR DISORDERS		
hypertension*	47	1.8
deep vein thrombosis*	17	0.7

*Represents a medical concept including several similar MedDRA PTs
[1] Percentage of male population (N=2,038)
[2] Percentage of female population (N=574)

Laboratory Abnormalities in Adults
The percentages of adult patients treated with combination therapy with Grade 3-4 laboratory abnormalities are presented in Table 10 (treatment-naïve patients) and Table 11 (treatment-experienced patients).
[See table 10 above]
[See table 11 at top of next page]

Adverse Reactions in Pediatric Patients
KALETRA oral solution dosed up to 300/75 mg/m² has been studied in 100 pediatric patients 6 months to 12 years of age. The adverse reaction profile seen during Study 940 was similar to that for adult patients.

Dysgeusia (22%), vomiting (21%), and diarrhea (12%) were the most common adverse reactions of any severity reported in pediatric patients treated with combination therapy for up to 48 weeks in Study 940. A total of 8 patients experienced adverse reactions of moderate to severe intensity. The adverse reactions meeting these criteria and reported for the 8 subjects include: hypersensitivity (characterized by fever, rash and jaundice), pyrexia, viral infection, constipation, hepatomegaly, pancreatitis, vomiting, alanine aminotransferase increased, dry skin, rash, and dysgeusia. Rash was the only event of those listed that occurred in 2 or more subjects (N = 3).

KALETRA oral solution dosed at 300/75 mg/m² has been studied in 31 pediatric patients 14 days to 6 months of age. The adverse reaction profile in Study 1030 was similar to that observed in older children and adults. No adverse reaction was reported in greater than 10% of subjects. Adverse drug reactions of moderate to severe intensity occurring in 2 or more subjects included decreased neutrophil count (N=3), anemia (N=2), high potassium (N=2), and low sodium (N=2).

KALETRA oral solution and soft gelatin capsules dosed at higher than recommended doses including 400/100 mg/m² (without concomitant NNRTI) and 480/120 mg/m² (with concomitant NNRTI) have been studied in 26 pediatric patients 7 to 18 years of age in Study 1038. Patients also had saquinavir mesylate added to their regimen at Week 4. Rash (12%), blood cholesterol abnormal (12%) and blood triglycerides abnormal (12%) were the only adverse reactions reported in greater than 10% of subjects. Adverse drug reactions of moderate to severe intensity occurring in 2 or more subjects included rash (N=3), blood triglycerides abnormal (N=3), and electrocardiogram QT prolonged (N=2). Both subjects with QT prolongation had additional predisposing conditions such as electrolyte abnormalities, concomitant medications, or pre-existing cardiac abnormalities.

Laboratory Abnormalities in Pediatric Patients
The percentages of pediatric patients treated with combination therapy including KALETRA with Grade 3-4 laboratory abnormalities are presented in Table 12.

Table 12. Grade 3-4 Laboratory Abnormalities Reported in ≥ 2% Pediatric Patients in Study 940

Variable	Limit[1]	KALETRA Twice Daily + RTIs (N = 100)
Chemistry	**High**	
Sodium	> 149 mEq/L	3%
Total Bilirubin	≥ 3.0 × ULN	3%
SGOT/AST	> 180 U/L	8%
SGPT/ALT	> 215 U/L	7%
Total Cholesterol	> 300 mg/dL	3%
Amylase	> 2.5 × ULN	7%[2]
Chemistry	**Low**	
Sodium	< 130 mEq/L	3%
Hematology	**Low**	
Platelet Count	< 50 × 10⁹/L	4%

Table 10. Grade 3-4 Laboratory Abnormalities Reported in ≥ 2% of Adult Antiretroviral-Naïve Patients

| Variable | Limit[1] | Study 863 (48 Weeks) | | Study 720 (360 Weeks) | Study 730 (48 Weeks) | |
		KALETRA 400/100 mg Twice Daily + d4T +3TC (N = 326)	Nelfinavir 750 mg Three Times Daily + d4T + 3TC (N = 327)	KALETRA Twice Daily + d4T + 3TC (N = 100)	KALETRA Once Daily + TDF +FTC (N = 333)	KALETRA Twice Daily + TDF +FTC (N = 331)
Chemistry	**High**					
Glucose	> 250 mg/dL	2%	2%	4%	0%	<1%
Uric Acid	> 12 mg/dL	2%	2%	5%	<1%	1%
SGOT/AST[2]	> 180 U/L	2%	4%	10%	1%	2%
SGPT/ALT[2]	>215 U/L	4%	4%	11%	1%	1%
GGT	>300 U/L	N/A	N/A	10%	N/A	N/A
Total Cholesterol	>300 mg/dL	9%	5%	27%	4%	3%
Triglycerides	>750 mg/dL	9%	1%	29%	3%	6%
Amylase	>2 × ULN	3%	2%	4%	N/A	N/A
Lipase	>2 × ULN	N/A	N/A	N/A	3%	5%
Chemistry	**Low**					
Calculated Creatinine Clearance	<50 mL/min	N/A	N/A	N/A	2%	2%
Hematology	**Low**					
Neutrophils	<0.75 × 10⁹/L	1%	3%	5%	2%	1%

1 ULN = upper limit of the normal range; N/A = Not Applicable.
2 Criterion for Study 730 was >5× ULN (AST/ALT).

Neutrophils	< 0.40 × 10⁹/L	2%

1 ULN = upper limit of the normal range.
2 Subjects with Grade 3-4 amylase confirmed by elevations in pancreatic amylase.

6.2   Postmarketing Experience
The following adverse reactions have been reported during postmarketing use of KALETRA® (lopinavir and ritonavir). Because these reactions are reported voluntarily from a population of unknown size, it is not possible to reliably estimate their frequency or establish a causal relationship to KALETRA exposure.
Body as a Whole
Redistribution/accumulation of body fat has been reported [see Warnings and Precautions (5.10)].
Cardiovascular
Bradyarrhythmias. First-degree AV block, second-degree AV block, third-degree AV block, QTc interval prolongation, torsades (torsade) de pointes [see Warnings and Precautions (5.5, 5.6)].
Skin and Appendages
Toxic epidermal necrolysis (TEN), Stevens-Johnson syndrome and erythema multiforme.

7   DRUG INTERACTIONS
See also Contraindications (4), Warnings and Precautions (5.1), Clinical Pharmacology (12.3)
7.1   Potential for KALETRA to Affect Other Drugs
Lopinavir/ritonavir is an inhibitor of CYP3A and may increase plasma concentrations of agents that are primarily metabolized by CYP3A. Agents that are extensively metabolized by CYP3A and have high first pass metabolism appear to be the most susceptible to large increases in AUC (> 3-fold) when co-administered with KALETRA. Thus, co-administration of KALETRA with drugs highly dependent on CYP3A for clearance and for which elevated plasma concentrations are associated with serious and/or life-threatening events is contraindicated. Co-administration with other CYP3A substrates may require a dose adjustment or additional monitoring as shown in Table 13.

Additionally, KALETRA induces glucuronidation.
7.2   Potential for Other Drugs to Affect Lopinavir
Lopinavir/ritonavir is a CYP3A substrate; therefore, drugs that induce CYP3A may decrease lopinavir plasma concentrations and reduce KALETRA's therapeutic effect. Although not observed in the KALETRA/ketoconazole drug interaction study, co-administration of KALETRA and other drugs that inhibit CYP3A may increase lopinavir plasma concentrations.
7.3   Established and Other Potentially Significant Drug Interactions
Table 13 provides a listing of established or potentially clinically significant drug interactions. Alteration in dose or regimen may be recommended based on drug interaction studies or predicted interaction [see Clinical Pharmacology (12.3) for magnitude of interaction].
[See table at top of page 693]
7.4   Drugs with No Observed or Predicted Interactions with KALETRA
Drug interaction or clinical studies reveal no clinically significant interaction between KALETRA and desipramine (CYP2D6 probe), pitavastatin, pravastatin, stavudine, lamivudine, omeprazole, raltegravir, or ranitidine.
Based on known metabolic profiles, clinically significant drug interactions are not expected between KALETRA and dapsone, trimethoprim/sulfamethoxazole, azithromycin, erythromycin, or fluconazole.

8   USE IN SPECIFIC POPULATIONS
8.1   Pregnancy
Pregnancy Exposure Registry
There is a pregnancy exposure registry that monitors pregnancy outcomes in women exposed to KALETRA® (lopinavir and ritonavir) during pregnancy. Physicians are encouraged to register patients by calling the Antiretroviral Pregnancy Registry at 1-800-258-4263.

Continued on next page

Information on the AbbVie, Inc. products listed on these pages is from the prescribing information in use as of July 31, 2016. For more information, please visit rxabbvie.com or call 1-800-633-9110.

Risk Summary

Available data from the Antiretroviral Pregnancy Registry show no difference in the risk of overall major birth defects compared to the background rate for major birth defects of 2.7% in the U.S. reference population of the Metropolitan Atlanta Congenital Defects Program (MACDP). No treatment-related malformations were observed when lopinavir in combination with ritonavir was administered to pregnant rats or rabbits; however embryonic and fetal developmental toxicities occurred in rats administered maternally toxic doses.

Clinical Considerations

Dose Adjustments During Pregnancy and the Postpartum Period

Administer 400/100 mg of KALETRA twice daily in pregnant patients with no documented lopinavir-associated resistance substitutions *[see Dosage and Administration (2.4) and Clinical Pharmacology (12.3)].* There are insufficient data to recommend KALETRA dosing for pregnant patients with any documented lopinavir-associated resistance substitutions. No dose adjustment of KALETRA is required for patients during the postpartum period.

Once daily KALETRA dosing is not recommended in pregnancy.

Avoid use of KALETRA oral solution during pregnancy due to the alcohol content. KALETRA oral solution contains the excipients alcohol (42.4% v/v) and propylene glycol (15.3% w/v).

Data

Human Data

KALETRA was evaluated in 12 HIV-infected pregnant women in an open-label pharmacokinetic trial *[see Clinical Pharmacology (12.3)].* No new trends in the safety profile were identified in pregnant women dosed with KALETRA compared to the safety described in non-pregnant adults, based on the review of these limited data.

Antiretroviral Pregnancy Registry Data: Based on prospective reports from the Antiretroviral Pregnancy Registry (APR) of over 3,000 exposures to lopinavir containing regimens (including over 1,000 exposed in the first trimester), there was no difference between lopinavir and overall birth defects compared with the background birth defect rate of 2.7% in the U.S. reference population of the Metropolitan Atlanta Congenital Defects Program. Based on prospective reports from the APR of over 5,000 exposures to ritonavir containing regimens (including over 2,000 exposures in the first trimester) there was no difference between ritonavir and overall birth defects compared with the U.S. background rate (MACDP). For both lopinavir and ritonavir, sufficient numbers of first trimester exposures have been monitored to detect at least a 1.5 fold increase in risk of overall birth defects and a 2 fold increase in risk of birth defects in the cardiovascular and genitourinary systems.

Animal Data

Embryonic and fetal developmental toxicities (early resorption, decreased fetal viability, decreased fetal body weight, increased incidence of skeletal variations and skeletal ossification delays) occurred in rats at a maternally toxic dosage. Based on AUC measurements, the drug exposures in rats at the toxic doses were approximately 0.7-fold for lopinavir and 1.8-fold for ritonavir for males and females that of the exposures in humans at the recommended therapeutic dose (400/100 mg twice daily). In a peri- and postnatal study in rats, a developmental toxicity (a decrease in survival in pups between birth and postnatal Day 21) occurred.

No embryonic and fetal developmental toxicities were observed in rabbits at a maternally toxic dosage. Based on AUC measurements, the drug exposures in rabbits at the toxic doses were approximately 0.6-fold for lopinavir and 1.0-fold for ritonavir that of the exposures in humans at the recommended therapeutic dose (400/100 mg twice daily).

8.2 Lactation

Risk Summary

The Centers for Disease Control and Prevention recommend that HIV-1 infected mothers not breastfeed their infants to avoid risking postnatal transmission of HIV-1. Because of the potential for HIV-1 transmission in breastfed infants, advise women not to breastfeed.

8.4 Pediatric Use

The safety, efficacy, and pharmacokinetic profiles of KALETRA in pediatric patients below the age of 14 days have not been established. KALETRA should not be administered once daily in pediatric patients.

Table 11. Grade 3-4 Laboratory Abnormalities Reported in ≥ 2% of Adult Protease Inhibitor-Experienced Patients

Variable	Limit[1]	Study 888 (48 Weeks)		Study 957[2] and Study 765[3] (84-144 Weeks)	Study 802 (48 Weeks)	
		KALETRA 400/100 mg Twice Daily + NVP + NRTIs (N = 148)	Investigator-Selected Protease Inhibitor(s) + NVP + NRTIs (N = 140)	KALETRA Twice Daily + NNRTI + NRTIs (N = 127)	KALETRA 800/200 mg Once Daily + NRTIs (N = 300)	KALETRA 400/100 mg Twice Daily + NRTIs (N = 299)
Chemistry	**High**					
Glucose	>250 mg/dL	1%	2%	5%	2%	2%
Total Bilirubin	>3.48 mg/dL	1%	3%	1%	1%	1%
SGOT/AST[4]	>180 U/L	5%	11%	8%	3%	2%
SGPT/ALT[4]	>215 U/L	6%	13%	10%	2%	2%
GGT	>300 U/L	N/A	N/A	29%	N/A	N/A
Total Cholesterol	>300 mg/dL	20%	21%	39%	6%	7%
Triglycerides	>750 mg/dL	25%	21%	36%	5%	6%
Amylase	>2 × ULN	4%	8%	8%	4%	4%
Lipase	>2 × ULN	N/A	N/A	N/A	4%	1%
Creatine Phosphokinase	>4 × ULN	N/A	N/A	N/A	4%	5%
Chemistry	**Low**					
Calculated Creatinine Clearance	<50 mL/min	N/A	N/A	N/A	3%	3%
Inorganic Phosphorus	<1.5 mg/dL	1%	0%	2%	1%	<1%
Hematology	**Low**					
Neutrophils	<0.75 × 10⁹/L	1%	2%	4%	3%	4%
Hemoglobin	<80 g/L	1%	1%	1%	1%	2%

1 ULN = upper limit of the normal range; N/A = Not Applicable.
2 Includes clinical laboratory data from patients receiving 400/100 mg twice daily (n = 29) or 533/133 mg twice daily (n = 28) for 84 weeks. Patients received KALETRA in combination with NRTIs and efavirenz.
3 Includes clinical laboratory data from patients receiving 400/100 mg twice daily (n = 36) or 400/200 mg twice daily (n = 34) for 144 weeks. Patients received KALETRA in combination with NRTIs and nevirapine.
4 Criterion for Study 802 was >5× ULN (AST/ALT).

An open-label, multi-center, dose-finding trial was performed to evaluate the pharmacokinetic profile, tolerability, safety and efficacy of KALETRA oral solution containing lopinavir 80 mg/mL and ritonavir 20 mg/mL at a dose of 300/75 mg/m² twice daily plus two NRTIs in HIV-infected infants ≥14 days and < 6 months of age. Results revealed that infants younger than 6 months of age generally had lower lopinavir AUC$_{12}$ than older children (6 months to 12 years of age), however, despite the lower lopinavir drug exposure observed, antiviral activity was demonstrated as reflected in the proportion of subjects who achieved HIV-1 RNA <400 copies/mL at Week 24 *[see Adverse Reactions (6.2), Clinical Pharmacology (12.3), Clinical Studies (14.4)].* Safety and efficacy in pediatric patients > 6 months of age was demonstrated in a clinical trial in 100 patients. The clinical trial was an open-label, multicenter trial evaluating the pharmacokinetic profile, tolerability, safety, and efficacy of KALETRA oral solution containing lopinavir 80 mg/mL and ritonavir 20 mg/mL in 100 antiretroviral naïve and experienced pediatric patients ages 6 months to 12 years. Dose selection for patients 6 months to 12 years of age was based on the following results. The 230/57.5 mg/m² oral solution twice daily regimen without nevirapine and the 300/75 mg/m² oral solution twice daily regimen with nevirapine provided lopinavir plasma concentrations similar to those obtained in adult patients receiving the 400/100 mg twice daily regimen (without nevirapine) *[see Adverse Reactions (6.2), Clinical Pharmacology (12.3), Clinical Studies (14.4)].*

A prospective multicenter, open-label trial evaluated the pharmacokinetic profile, tolerability, safety and efficacy of high-dose KALETRA with or without concurrent NNRTI therapy (Group 1: 400/100 mg/m² twice daily + ≥ 2 NRTIs; Group 2: 480/120 mg/m² twice daily + ≥ 1 NRTI + 1 NNRTI) in 26 children and adolescents ≥ 2 years to < 18 years of age who had failed prior therapy. Patients also had saquinavir mesylate added to their regimen. This strategy was intended to assess whether higher than approved doses of KALETRA could overcome protease inhibitor cross-resistance. High doses of KALETRA exhibited a safety profile similar to those observed in previous trials; changes in HIV-1 RNA were less than anticipated; three patients had HIV-1 RNA <400 copies/mL at Week 48. CD4+ cell count increases were noted in the eight patients who remained on treatment for 48 weeks *[see Adverse Reactions (6.2), Clinical Pharmacology (12.3)].*

A prospective multicenter, randomized, open-label study evaluated the efficacy and safety of twice-daily versus once-daily dosing of KALETRA tablets dosed by weight as part of combination antiretroviral therapy (cART) in virologically suppressed HIV-1 infected children (n=173). Children were eligible when they were aged < 18 years, ≥ 15 kg in weight, receiving cART that included KALETRA, HIV-1 ribonucleic

Table 13. Established and Other Potentially Significant Drug Interactions

Concomitant Drug Class: Drug Name	Effect on Concentration of Lopinavir or Concomitant Drug	Clinical Comments
HIV-1 Antiviral Agents		
HIV-1 Protease Inhibitor: fosamprenavir/ritonavir	↓ amprenavir ↓ lopinavir	An increased rate of adverse reactions has been observed with co-administration of these medications. Appropriate doses of the combinations with respect to safety and efficacy have not been established.
HIV-1 Protease Inhibitor: indinavir*	↑ indinavir	Decrease indinavir dose to 600 mg twice daily, when co-administered with KALETRA 400/100 mg twice daily *[see Clinical Pharmacology (12.3)]*. KALETRA once daily has not been studied in combination with indinavir.
HIV-1 Protease Inhibitor: nelfinavir*	↑ nelfinavir ↑ M8 metabolite of nelfinavir ↓ lopinavir	KALETRA should not be administered once daily in combination with nelfinavir *[see Dosage and Administration (2) and Clinical Pharmacology (12.3)]*.
HIV-1 Protease Inhibitor: ritonavir*	↑ lopinavir	Appropriate doses of additional ritonavir in combination with KALETRA with respect to safety and efficacy have not been established.
HIV-1 Protease Inhibitor: saquinavir*	↑ saquinavir	The saquinavir dose is 1000 mg twice daily, when co-administered with KALETRA 400/100 mg twice daily. KALETRA once daily has not been studied in combination with saquinavir.
HIV-1 Protease Inhibitor: tipranavir	↓ lopinavir AUC and C_{min}	KALETRA should not be administered with tipranavir (500 mg twice daily) co-administered with ritonavir (200 mg twice daily).
HIV CCR5 - Antagonist: maraviroc	↑ maraviroc	Concurrent administration of maraviroc with KALETRA will increase plasma levels of maraviroc. When co-administered, patients should receive 150 mg twice daily of maraviroc. For further details see complete prescribing information for Selzentry® (maraviroc).
Non-nucleoside Reverse Transcriptase Inhibitor: etravirine	↓ etravirine	Because the reduction in the mean systemic exposures of etravirine in the presence of lopinavir/ritonavir is similar to the reduction in mean systemic exposures of etravirine in the presence of darunavir/ritonavir, no dose adjustment is required.
Non-nucleoside Reverse Transcriptase Inhibitors: efavirenz*, nevirapine*	↓ lopinavir	KALETRA dose increase is recommended in all patients *[see Dosage and Administration (2) and Clinical Pharmacology (12.3)]*. Increasing the dose of KALETRA tablets to 500/125 mg (given as two 200/50 mg tablets and one 100/25 mg tablet) twice daily co-administered with efavirenz resulted in similar lopinavir concentrations compared to KALETRA tablets 400/100 mg (given as two 200/50 mg tablets) twice daily without efavirenz. Increasing the dose of KALETRA tablets to 600/150 mg (given as three 200/50 mg tablets) twice daily co-administered with efavirenz resulted in significantly higher lopinavir plasma concentrations compared to KALETRA tablets 400/100 mg twice daily without efavirenz. KALETRA should not be administered once daily in combination with efavirenz or nevirapine *[see Dosage and Administration (2) and Clinical Pharmacology (12.3)]*.
Non-nucleoside Reverse Transcriptase Inhibitor: delavirdine	↑ lopinavir	Appropriate doses of the combination with respect to safety and efficacy have not been established.
Non-nucleoside Reverse Transcriptase Inhibitor: rilpivirine	↑ rilpivirine	No dose adjustment is required.
Nucleoside Reverse Transcriptase Inhibitor: didanosine		KALETRA tablets can be administered simultaneously with didanosine without food. For KALETRA oral solution, it is recommended that didanosine be administered on an empty stomach; therefore, didanosine should be given one hour before or two hours after KALETRA oral solution (given with food).
Nucleoside Reverse Transcriptase Inhibitor: tenofovir	↑ tenofovir	KALETRA increases tenofovir concentrations. The mechanism of this interaction is unknown. Patients receiving KALETRA and tenofovir should be monitored for adverse reactions associated with tenofovir.

This table is continued on next page

acid (RNA) < 50 copies/mL for at least 24 weeks and able to swallow tablets. At week 24, efficacy (defined as the proportion of subjects with plasma HIV-1 RNA less than 50 copies per mL) was significantly higher in subjects receiving twice daily dosing compared to subjects receiving once daily dosing. The safety profile was similar between the two treatment arms although there was a greater incidence of diarrhea in the once daily treated subjects.

8.5   Geriatric Use
Clinical studies of KALETRA did not include sufficient numbers of subjects aged 65 and over to determine whether they respond differently from younger subjects. In general, appropriate caution should be exercised in the administration and monitoring of KALETRA in elderly patients reflecting the greater frequency of decreased hepatic, renal, or cardiac function, and of concomitant disease or other drug therapy.

8.6   Hepatic Impairment
KALETRA is principally metabolized by the liver; therefore, caution should be exercised when administering this drug to patients with hepatic impairment, because lopinavir concentrations may be increased *[see Warnings and Precautions (5.4) and Clinical Pharmacology (12.3)]*.

10   OVERDOSAGE
Overdoses with KALETRA oral solution have been reported, One of these reports described fatal cardiogenic shock in a 2.1 kg infant who received a single dose of 6.5 mL of KALETRA oral solution (520 mg lopinavir, approximately 10-fold above the recommended lopinavir dose) nine days prior. The following events have been reported in association with unintended overdoses in preterm neonates: complete AV block, cardiomyopathy, lactic acidosis, and acute renal failure *[see Warnings and Precautions (5.2)]*. Healthcare professionals should be aware that KALETRA oral solution is highly concentrated and therefore, should pay special attention to accurate calculation of the dose of KALETRA, transcription of the medication order, dispensing information and dosing instructions to minimize the risk for medication errors and overdose. This is especially important for infants and young children.
KALETRA oral solution contains 42.4% alcohol (v/v) and 15.3% propylene glycol (w/v). Ingestion of the product over the recommended dose by an infant or a young child could result in significant toxicity and could potentially be lethal. Human experience of acute overdosage with KALETRA is limited. Treatment of overdose with KALETRA should consist of general supportive measures including monitoring of vital signs and observation of the clinical status of the patient. There is no specific antidote for overdose with KALETRA. If indicated, elimination of unabsorbed drug should be achieved by gastric lavage. Administration of activated charcoal may also be used to aid in removal of unabsorbed drug. Since lopinavir is highly protein bound, dialysis is unlikely to be beneficial in significant removal of the drug. However, dialysis can remove both alcohol and propylene glycol in the case of overdose with KALETRA oral solution.

11   DESCRIPTION
KALETRA is a co-formulation of lopinavir and ritonavir. Lopinavir is an inhibitor of the HIV-1 protease. As co-formulated in KALETRA, ritonavir inhibits the CYP3A-mediated metabolism of lopinavir, thereby providing increased plasma levels of lopinavir.
Lopinavir is chemically designated as [1S-[1R*,(R*), 3R*, 4R*]]-N-[4-[[(2,6-dimethylphenoxy)acetyl]amino]-3-hydroxy-5-phenyl-1-(phenylmethyl)pentyl]tetrahydro-alpha-(1-methylethyl)-2-oxo-1(2H)-pyrimidineacetamide. Its molecular formula is $C_{37}H_{48}N_4O_5$, and its molecular weight is 628.80. Lopinavir is a white to light tan powder. It is freely soluble in methanol and ethanol, soluble in isopropanol and practically insoluble in water. Lopinavir has the following structural formula:
[See first chemical structure on page 698]
Ritonavir is chemically designated as 10-hydroxy-2-methyl-5-(1-methylethyl)-1- [2-(1-methylethyl)-4-thiazolyl]-3,6-dioxo-8,11-bis(phenylmethyl)-2,4,7,12-tetraazatridecan-13-oic acid, 5-thiazolylmethyl ester, [5S-(5R*,8R*,10R*,11R*)]. Its

Continued on next page

Information on the AbbVie, Inc. products listed on these pages is from the prescribing information in use as of July 31, 2016. For more information, please visit rxabbvie.com or call 1-800-633-9110.

molecular formula is $C_{37}H_{48}N_6O_5S_2$, and its molecular weight is 720.95. Ritonavir is a white to light tan powder. It is freely soluble in methanol and ethanol, soluble in isopropanol and practically insoluble in water. Ritonavir has the following structural formula:
[See second chemical structure on page 698]
KALETRA tablets are available for oral administration in two strengths:
• Yellow tablets containing 200 mg of lopinavir and 50 mg of ritonavir
• Pale yellow tablets containing 100 mg of lopinavir and 25 mg of ritonavir.
The yellow, 200 mg lopinavir and 50 mg ritonavir, tablets contain the following inactive ingredients: copovidone, sorbitan monolaurate, colloidal silicon dioxide, and sodium stearyl fumarate. The following are the ingredients in the film coating: hypromellose, titanium dioxide, polyethylene glycol 400, hydroxypropyl cellulose, talc, colloidal silicon dioxide, polyethylene glycol 3350, yellow ferric oxide E172, and polysorbate 80.
The pale yellow, 100 mg lopinavir and 25 mg ritonavir, tablets contain the following inactive ingredients: copovidone, sorbitan monolaurate, colloidal silicon dioxide, and sodium stearyl fumarate. The following are the ingredients in the film coating: polyvinyl alcohol, titanium dioxide, talc, polyethylene glycol 3350, and yellow ferric oxide E172.
KALETRA oral solution is available for oral administration as 80 mg lopinavir and 20 mg ritonavir per milliliter with the following inactive ingredients: acesulfame potassium, alcohol, artificial cotton candy flavor, citric acid, glycerin, high fructose corn syrup, Magnasweet-110 flavor, menthol, natural & artificial vanilla flavor, peppermint oil, polyoxyl 40 hydrogenated castor oil, povidone, propylene glycol, saccharin sodium, sodium chloride, sodium citrate, and water. KALETRA oral solution contains 42.4% alcohol (v/v).

12   CLINICAL PHARMACOLOGY
12.1   Mechanism of Action
Lopinavir is an antiviral drug *[see Microbiology (12.4)]*. As co-formulated in KALETRA, ritonavir inhibits the CYP3A-mediated metabolism of lopinavir, thereby providing increased plasma levels of lopinavir.
12.3   Pharmacokinetics
The pharmacokinetic properties of lopinavir co-administered with ritonavir have been evaluated in healthy adult volunteers and in HIV-1 infected patients; no substantial differences were observed between the two groups. Lopinavir is essentially completely metabolized by CYP3A. Ritonavir inhibits the metabolism of lopinavir, thereby increasing the plasma levels of lopinavir. Across studies, administration of KALETRA 400/100 mg twice daily yields mean steady-state lopinavir plasma concentrations 15- to 20-fold higher than those of ritonavir in HIV-1 infected patients. The plasma levels of ritonavir are less than 7% of those obtained after the ritonavir dose of 600 mg twice daily. The *in vitro* antiviral EC_{50} of lopinavir is approximately 10-fold lower than that of ritonavir. Therefore, the antiviral activity of KALETRA is due to lopinavir.
Figure 1 displays the mean steady-state plasma concentrations of lopinavir and ritonavir after KALETRA 400/100 mg twice daily with food for 3 weeks from a pharmacokinetic study in HIV-1 infected adult subjects (n = 19).
[See figure 1 on page 698]
Absorption
In a pharmacokinetic study in HIV-1 positive subjects (n = 19), multiple dosing with 400/100 mg KALETRA twice daily with food for 3 weeks produced a mean ± SD lopinavir peak plasma concentration (C_{max}) of 9.8 ± 3.7 µg/mL, occurring approximately 4 hours after administration. The mean steady-state trough concentration prior to the morning dose was 7.1 ± 2.9 µg/mL and minimum concentration within a dosing interval was 5.5 ± 2.7 µg/mL. Lopinavir AUC over a 12 hour dosing interval averaged 92.6 ± 36.7 µg•h/mL. The absolute bioavailability of lopinavir co-formulated with ritonavir in humans has not been established. Under non-fasting conditions (500 kcal, 25% from fat), lopinavir concentrations were similar following administration of KALETRA co-formulated capsules and oral solution. When administered under fasting conditions, both the mean AUC and C_{max} of lopinavir were 22% lower for the KALETRA oral solution relative to the capsule formulation.
Plasma concentrations of lopinavir and ritonavir after administration of two 200/50 mg KALETRA tablets are similar to three 133.3/33.3 mg KALETRA capsules under fed conditions with less pharmacokinetic variability.
Effects of Food on Oral Absorption
KALETRA Tablets

Table 13 *(cont.)* Established and Other Potentially Significant Drug Interactions

Concomitant Drug Class: Drug Name	Effect on Concentration of Lopinavir or Concomitant Drug	Clinical Comments
Nucleoside Reverse Transcriptase Inhibitors: abacavir zidovudine	↓ abacavir ↓ zidovudine	KALETRA induces glucuronidation; therefore, KALETRA has the potential to reduce zidovudine and abacavir plasma concentrations. The clinical significance of this potential interaction is unknown.
Other Agents		
Antiarrhythmics e.g.: amiodarone, bepridil, lidocaine (systemic), quinidine	↑ antiarrhythmics	Caution is warranted and therapeutic concentration monitoring (if available) is recommended for antiarrhythmics when co-administered with KALETRA.
Anticancer Agents: vincristine, vinblastine, dasatinib, nilotinib	↑ anticancer agents	Concentrations of these drugs may be increased when co-administered with KALETRA resulting in the potential for increased adverse events usually associated with these anticancer agents. For vincristine and vinblastine, consideration should be given to temporarily withholding the ritonavir-containing antiretroviral regimen in patients who develop significant hematologic or gastrointestinal side effects when KALETRA is administered concurrently with vincristine or vinblastine. If the antiretroviral regimen must be withheld for a prolonged period, consideration should be given to initiating a revised regimen that does not include a CYP3A or P-gp inhibitor. A decrease in the dosage or an adjustment of the dosing interval of nilotinib and dasatinib may be necessary for patients requiring co-administration with strong CYP3A inhibitors such as KALETRA. Please refer to the nilotinib and dasatinib prescribing information for dosing instructions.
Anticoagulants: warfarin, rivaroxaban	↑ rivaroxaban	Concentrations of warfarin may be affected. It is recommended that INR (international normalized ratio) be monitored. Avoid concomitant use of rivaroxaban and KALETRA. Co-administration of KALETRA and rivaroxaban is expected to result in increased exposure of rivaroxaban which may lead to risk of increased bleeding.
Anticonvulsants: carbamazepine, phenobarbital, phenytoin	↓ lopinavir ↓ phenytoin	KALETRA may be less effective due to decreased lopinavir plasma concentrations in patients taking these agents concomitantly and should be used with caution. KALETRA should not be administered once daily in combination with carbamazepine, phenobarbital, or phenytoin. In addition, co-administration of phenytoin and KALETRA may cause decreases in steady-state phenytoin concentrations. Phenytoin levels should be monitored when co-administering with KALETRA.
Anticonvulsants: lamotrigine, valproate	↓ lamotrigine ↓ or ↔ valproate	Co-administration of KALETRA and lamotrigine or valproate may decrease the exposure of lamotrigine or valproate. A dose increase of lamotrigine or valproate may be needed when co-administered with KALETRA and therapeutic concentration monitoring for lamotrigine may be indicated; particularly during dosage adjustments.
Antidepressant: bupropion	↓ bupropion ↓ active metabolite, hydroxybupropion	Concurrent administration of bupropion with KALETRA may decrease plasma levels of both bupropion and its active metabolite (hydroxybupropion). Patients receiving KALETRA and bupropion concurrently should be monitored for an adequate clinical response to bupropion.
Antidepressant: trazodone	↑ trazodone	Concomitant use of trazodone and KALETRA may increase concentrations of trazodone. Adverse reactions of nausea, dizziness, hypotension and syncope have been observed following co-administration of trazodone and ritonavir. If trazodone is used with a CYP3A4 inhibitor such as ritonavir, the combination should be used with caution and a lower dose of trazodone should be considered.

This table is continued on next page

No clinically significant changes in C_{max} and AUC were observed following administration of KALETRA tablets under fed conditions compared to fasted conditions. Relative to fasting, administration of KALETRA tablets with a moderate fat meal (500 - 682 Kcal, 23 to 25% calories from fat) increased lopinavir AUC and C_{max} by 26.9% and 17.6%, respectively. Relative to fasting, administration of KALETRA

tablets with a high fat meal (872 Kcal, 56% from fat) increased lopinavir AUC by 18.9% but not C_{max}. Therefore, KALETRA tablets may be taken with or without food.
KALETRA Oral Solution
Relative to fasting, administration of KALETRA oral solution with a moderate fat meal (500 - 682 Kcal, 23 to 25%

Table 13 (cont.) Established and Other Potentially Significant Drug Interactions

Concomitant Drug Class: Drug Name	Effect on Concentration of Lopinavir or Concomitant Drug	Clinical Comments
Anti-infective: clarithromycin	↑ clarithromycin	For patients with renal impairment, the following dosage adjustments should be considered: • For patients with CL_{CR} 30 to 60 mL/min the dose of clarithromycin should be reduced by 50%. • For patients with CL_{CR} < 30 mL/min the dose of clarithromycin should be decreased by 75%. No dose adjustment for patients with normal renal function is necessary.
Antifungals: ketoconazole*, itraconazole, voriconazole	↑ ketoconazole ↑ itraconazole ↓ voriconazole	High doses of ketoconazole (>200 mg/day) or itraconazole (> 200 mg/day) are not recommended. Co-administration of voriconazole with KALETRA has not been studied. However, a study has been shown that administration of voriconazole with ritonavir 100 mg every 12 hours decreased voriconazole steady-state AUC by an average of 39%; therefore, co-administration of KALETRA and voriconazole may result in decreased voriconazole concentrations and the potential for decreased voriconazole effectiveness and should be avoided, unless an assessment of the benefit/risk to the patient justifies the use of voriconazole. Otherwise, alternative antifungal therapies should be considered in these patients.
Anti-gout: colchicine	↑ colchicine	Patients with renal or hepatic impairment should not be given colchicine with KALETRA. Treatment of gout flares-co-administration of colchicine in patients on KALETRA: 0.6 mg (1 tablet) × 1 dose, followed by 0.3 mg (half tablet) 1 hour later. Dose to be repeated no earlier than 3 days. Prophylaxis of gout flares-co-administration of colchicine in patients on KALETRA: If the original colchicine regimen was 0.6 mg twice a day, the regimen should be adjusted to 0.3 mg once a day. If the original colchicine regimen was 0.6 mg once a day, the regimen should be adjusted to 0.3 mg once every other day. Treatment of familial Mediterranean fever (FMF)-co-administration of colchicine in patients on KALETRA: Maximum daily dose of 0.6 mg (may be given as 0.3 mg twice a day).
Antimycobacterial: bedaquiline	↑ bedaquiline	Bedaquiline should only be used with KALETRA if the benefit of co-administration outweighs the risk [see Pharmacokinetics (12.3)].
Antimycobacterial: rifabutin*	↑ rifabutin and rifabutin metabolite	Dosage reduction of rifabutin by at least 75% of the usual dose of 300 mg/day is recommended (i.e., a maximum dose of 150 mg every other day or three times per week). Increased monitoring for adverse reactions is warranted in patients receiving the combination. Further dosage reduction of rifabutin may be necessary.
Antimycobacterial: rifampin	↓ lopinavir	May lead to loss of virologic response and possible resistance to KALETRA or to the class of protease inhibitors or other co-administered antiretroviral agents. A study evaluated combination of rifampin 600 mg once daily, with KALETRA 800/200 mg twice daily or KALETRA 400/100 mg + ritonavir 300 mg twice daily. Pharmacokinetic and safety results from this study do not allow for a dose recommendation. Nine subjects (28%) experienced a ≥ grade 2 increase in ALT/AST, of which seven (21%) prematurely discontinued study per protocol. Based on the study design, it is not possible to determine whether the frequency or magnitude of the ALT/AST elevations observed is higher than what would be seen with rifampin alone [see Clinical Pharmacology (12.3) for magnitude of interaction]. *This table is continued on next page.*

calories from fat) increased lopinavir AUC and C_{max} by 80 and 54%, respectively. Relative to fasting, administration of KALETRA oral solution with a high fat meal (872 Kcal, 56% from fat) increased lopinavir AUC and C_{max} by 130% and 56%, respectively. To enhance bioavailability and minimize pharmacokinetic variability KALETRA oral solution should be taken with food.

Distribution

At steady state, lopinavir is approximately 98-99% bound to plasma proteins. Lopinavir binds to both alpha-1-acid glycoprotein (AAG) and albumin; however, it has a higher affinity for AAG. At steady state, lopinavir protein binding remains constant over the range of observed concentrations after 400/100 mg KALETRA twice daily, and is similar between healthy volunteers and HIV-1 positive patients.

Metabolism

In vitro experiments with human hepatic microsomes indicate that lopinavir primarily undergoes oxidative metabolism. Lopinavir is extensively metabolized by the hepatic cytochrome P450 system, almost exclusively by the CYP3A isozyme. Ritonavir is a potent CYP3A inhibitor which inhibits the metabolism of lopinavir, and therefore increases plasma levels of lopinavir. A ^{14}C-lopinavir study in humans showed that 89% of the plasma radioactivity after a single 400/100 mg KALETRA dose was due to parent drug. At least 13 lopinavir oxidative metabolites have been identified in man. Ritonavir has been shown to induce metabolic enzymes, resulting in the induction of its own metabolism. Pre-dose lopinavir concentrations decline with time during multiple dosing, stabilizing after approximately 10 to 16 days.

Elimination

Following a 400/100 mg ^{14}C-lopinavir/ritonavir dose, approximately 10.4 ± 2.3% and 82.6 ± 2.5% of an administered dose of ^{14}C-lopinavir can be accounted for in urine and feces, respectively, after 8 days. Unchanged lopinavir accounted for approximately 2.2 and 19.8% of the administered dose in urine and feces, respectively. After multiple dosing, less than 3% of the lopinavir dose is excreted unchanged in the urine. The apparent oral clearance (CL/F) of lopinavir is 5.98 ± 5.75 L/hr (mean ± SD, n = 19).

Once Daily Dosing

The pharmacokinetics of once daily KALETRA have been evaluated in HIV-1 infected subjects naïve to antiretroviral treatment. KALETRA 800/200 mg was administered in combination with emtricitabine 200 mg and tenofovir DF 300 mg as part of a once daily regimen. Multiple dosing of 800/200 mg KALETRA once daily for 4 weeks with food (n = 24) produced a mean ± SD lopinavir peak plasma concentration (C_{max}) of 11.8 ± 3.7 µg/mL, occurring approximately 6 hours after administration. The mean steady-state lopinavir trough concentration prior to the morning dose was 3.2 ± 2.1 µg/mL and minimum concentration within a dosing interval was 1.7 ± 1.6 µg/mL. Lopinavir AUC over a 24 hour dosing interval averaged 154.1 ± 61.4 µg• h/mL.

The pharmacokinetics of once daily KALETRA has also been evaluated in treatment experienced HIV-1 infected subjects. Lopinavir exposure (C_{max}, $AUC_{[0-24h]}$, C_{trough}) with once daily KALETRA administration in treatment experienced subjects is comparable to the once daily lopinavir exposure in treatment naïve subjects.

Effects on Electrocardiogram

QTcF interval was evaluated in a randomized, placebo and active (moxifloxacin 400 mg once daily) controlled crossover study in 39 healthy adults, with 10 measurements over 12 hours on Day 3. The maximum mean time-matched (95% upper confidence bound) differences in QTcF interval from placebo after baseline-correction were 5.3 (8.1) and 15.2 (18.0) mseconds (msec) for 400/100 mg twice daily and supratherapeutic 800/200 mg twice daily KALETRA, respectively. KALETRA 800/200 mg twice daily resulted in a Day 3 mean C_{max} approximately 2-fold higher than the mean C_{max} observed with the approved once daily and twice daily KALETRA doses at steady state.

PR interval prolongation was also noted in subjects receiving KALETRA in the same study on Day 3. The maximum mean (95% upper confidence bound) difference from placebo in the PR interval after baseline-correction were 24.9 (21.5, 28.3) and 31.9 (28.5, 35.3) msec for 400/100 mg twice daily and supratherapeutic 800/200 mg twice daily KALETRA, respectively [see Warnings and Precautions (5.5, 5.6)].

Special Populations

Gender, Race and Age

No gender related pharmacokinetic differences have been observed in adult patients. No clinically important pharmacokinetic differences due to race have been identified. Lopinavir pharmacokinetics have not been studied in elderly patients.

Pediatric Patients

The pharmacokinetics of KALETRA oral solution 300/75 mg/m^2 twice daily and 230/57.5 mg/m^2 twice daily have been studied in a total of 53 pediatric patients in Study 940, ranging in age from 6 months to 12 years [see Clinical Studies (14.4)]. The 230/57.5 mg/m^2 twice daily regimen without nevirapine and the 300/75 mg/m^2 twice daily regimen with nevirapine provided lopinavir plasma concentrations similar to those obtained in adult patients receiving the 400/100 mg twice daily regimen (without nevirapine). The mean steady-state lopinavir AUC, C_{max}, and C_{min} were 72.6 ± 31.1 µg•h/mL, 8.2 ± 2.9 and 3.4 ± 2.1 µg/mL, respectively after KALETRA oral solution 230/57.5 mg/m^2 twice daily without nevirapine (n = 12), and were 85.8 ± 36.9 µg• h/mL, 10.0 ± 3.3 and 3.6 ± 3.5 µg/mL, respectively, after 300/75 mg/m^2 twice daily with nevirapine (n = 12). The nevirapine regimen was 7 mg/kg twice daily (6 months to 8 years) or 4 mg/kg twice daily (> 8 years).

Continued on next page

Information on the AbbVie, Inc. products listed on these pages is from the prescribing information in use as of July 31, 2016. For more information, please visit rxabbvie.com or call 1-800-633-9110.

The pharmacokinetics of KALETRA oral solution at approximately 300/75 mg/m² twice daily have also been evaluated in infants at approximately 6 weeks of age (n = 9) and between 6 weeks and 6 months of age (n = 18) in Study 1030. The mean steady-state lopinavir AUC_{12}, C_{max}, and C_{12} were 43.4 ± 14.8 µg• h/mL, 5.2 ± 1.8 µg/mL and 1.9 ± 1.1 µg/mL, respectively, in infants at approximately 6 weeks of age, and 74.5 ± 37.9 µg• h/mL, 9.4 ± 4.9 and 3.1 ± 1.8 µg/mL, respectively, in infants between 6 weeks and 6 months of age after KALETRA oral solution was administered at approximately 300/75 mg/m² twice daily without concomitant NNRTI therapy.

The pharmacokinetics of KALETRA soft gelatin capsule and oral solution (Group 1: 400/100 mg/m² twice daily + 2 NRTIs; Group 2: 480/120 mg/m² twice daily + ≥ 1 NRTI + 1 NNRTI) have been evaluated in children and adolescents age ≥ 2 years to < 18 years of age who had failed prior therapy (n=26) in Study 1038. KALETRA doses of 400/100 and 480/120 mg/m² resulted in high lopinavir exposure, as almost all subjects had lopinavir AUC_{12} above 100 µg•h/mL. Both groups of subjects also achieved relatively high average minimum lopinavir concentrations.

Pregnancy
In an open-label pharmacokinetic study, 12 HIV-infected pregnant women received KALETRA 400 mg/100 mg (two 200/50 mg tablets) twice daily as part of an antiretroviral regimen. Plasma concentrations of lopinavir were measured over 12-hour periods during the second trimester (20-24 weeks gestation), the third trimester (30 weeks gestation) and at 8 weeks post-partum. The C_{12h} values of lopinavir were lower during the second and third trimester by approximately 40% as compared to post-partum, but this decrease is not considered clinically relevant in patients with no documented KALETRA-associated resistance substitutions receiving 400 mg/100 mg twice daily.

Renal Impairment
Lopinavir pharmacokinetics have not been studied in patients with renal impairment; however, since the renal clearance of lopinavir is negligible, a decrease in total body clearance is not expected in patients with renal impairment.

Hepatic Impairment
Lopinavir is principally metabolized and eliminated by the liver. Multiple dosing of KALETRA 400/100 mg twice daily to HIV-1 and HCV co-infected patients with mild to moderate hepatic impairment (n = 12) resulted in a 30% increase in lopinavir AUC and 20% increase in C_{max} compared to HIV-1 infected subjects with normal hepatic function (n = 12). Additionally, the plasma protein binding of lopinavir was statistically significantly lower in both mild and moderate hepatic impairment compared to controls (99.09 vs. 99.31%, respectively). Caution should be exercised when administering KALETRA to subjects with hepatic impairment. KALETRA has not been studied in patients with severe hepatic impairment *[see Warnings and Precautions (5.4) and Use in Specific Populations (8.6)]*.

Drug Interactions
KALETRA® (lopinavir and ritonavir) is an inhibitor of the P450 isoform CYP3A *in vitro*. Co-administration of KALETRA and drugs primarily metabolized by CYP3A may result in increased plasma concentrations of the other drug, which could increase or prolong its therapeutic and adverse effects *[see Contraindications (4) and Drug Interactions (7)]*. KALETRA does not inhibit CYP2D6, CYP2C9, CYP2C19, CYP2E1, CYP2B6 or CYP1A2 at clinically relevant concentrations.

KALETRA has been shown *in vivo* to induce its own metabolism and to increase the biotransformation of some drugs metabolized by cytochrome P450 enzymes and by glucuronidation.

KALETRA is metabolized by CYP3A. Drugs that induce CYP3A activity would be expected to increase the clearance of lopinavir, resulting in lowered plasma concentrations of lopinavir. Although not noted with concurrent ketoconazole, co-administration of KALETRA and other drugs that inhibit CYP3A may increase lopinavir plasma concentrations.

Drug interaction studies were performed with KALETRA and other drugs likely to be co-administered and some drugs commonly used as probes for pharmacokinetic interactions. The effects of co-administration of KALETRA on the AUC, C_{max} and C_{min} are summarized in Table 14 (effect of other drugs on lopinavir) and Table 15 (effect of KALETRA on other drugs). The effects of other drugs on ritonavir are not shown since they generally correlate with those observed with lopinavir (if lopinavir concentrations are decreased, ritonavir concentrations are decreased) unless otherwise indicated in the table footnotes. For information regarding clinical recommendations, see Table 13 in *Drug Interactions (7)*.

Table 13 *(cont)*. Established and Other Potentially Significant Drug Interactions

Concomitant Drug Class: Drug Name	Effect on Concentration of Lopinavir or Concomitant Drug	Clinical Comments
Antiparasitic: atovaquone	↓ atovaquone	Clinical significance is unknown; however, increase in atovaquone doses may be needed.
Antipsychotics: quetiapine	↑ quetiapine	Initiation of KALETRA in patients taking quetiapine: Consider alternative antiretroviral therapy to avoid increases in quetiapine exposures. If coadministration is necessary, reduce the quetiapine dose to 1/6 of the current dose and monitor for quetiapine-associated adverse reactions. Refer to the quetiapine prescribing information for recommendations on adverse reaction monitoring. Initiation of quetiapine in patients taking KALETRA: Refer to the quetiapine prescribing information for initial dosing and titration of quetiapine.
Benzodiazepines: parenterally administered midazolam	↑ midazolam	Midazolam is extensively metabolized by CYP3A4. Increases in the concentration of midazolam are expected to be significantly higher with oral than with parenteral administration. Therefore, KALETRA should not be given with orally administered midazolam *[see Contraindications (4)]*. If KALETRA is co-administered with parenteral midazolam, close clinical monitoring for respiratory depression and/or prolonged sedation should be exercised and dosage adjustment should be considered.
Contraceptive: ethinyl estradiol*	↓ ethinyl estradiol	Because contraceptive steroid concentrations may be altered when KALETRA is co-administered with oral contraceptives or with the contraceptive patch, alternative methods of nonhormonal contraception are recommended.
Corticosteroids (systemic): e.g. budesonide, dexamethasone, prednisone	↓ lopinavir ↑ glucocorticoids	Use with caution. KALETRA may be less effective due to decreased lopinavir plasma concentrations in patients taking these agents concomitantly. Concomitant use may result in increased steroid concentrations and reduced serum cortisol concentrations. Concomitant use of glucocorticoids that are metabolized by CYP3A, particularly for long-term use, should consider the potential benefit of treatment versus the risk of systemic corticosteroid effects. Concomitant use may increase the risk for development of systemic corticosteroid effects including Cushing's syndrome and adrenal suppression.
Dihydropyridine Calcium Channel Blockers: e.g. felodipine, nifedipine, nicardipine	↑ dihydropyridine calcium channel blockers	Caution is warranted and clinical monitoring of patients is recommended.
Disulfiram/metronidazole		KALETRA oral solution contains alcohol, which can produce disulfiram-like reactions when co-administered with disulfiram or other drugs that produce this reaction (e.g., metronidazole).
Endothelin Receptor Antagonists: bosentan	↑ bosentan	Co-administration of bosentan in patients on KALETRA: In patients who have been receiving KALETRA for at least 10 days, start bosentan at 62.5 mg once daily or every other day based upon individual tolerability. Co-administration of KALETRA in patients on bosentan: Discontinue use of bosentan at least 36 hours prior to initiation of KALETRA. After at least 10 days following the initiation of KALETRA, resume bosentan at 62.5 mg once daily or every other day based upon individual tolerability. *This table is continued on next page*

[See table 14 on pages 698 + 699]
[See table 15 on pages 701 + 702]

12.4   Microbiology
Mechanism of Action
Lopinavir, an inhibitor of the HIV-1 protease, prevents cleavage of the Gag-Pol polyprotein, resulting in the production of immature, non-infectious viral particles.

Antiviral Activity
The antiviral activity of lopinavir against laboratory HIV strains and clinical HIV-1 isolates was evaluated in acutely infected lymphoblastic cell lines and peripheral blood lymphocytes, respectively. In the absence of human serum, the mean 50% effective concentration (EC_{50}) values of lopinavir against five different HIV-1 subtype B laboratory strains ranged from 10-27 nM (0.006-0.017 µg/mL, 1 µg/mL = 1.6 µM) and ranged from 4-11 nM (0.003-0.007 µg/mL) against several HIV-1 subtype B clinical isolates (n = 6). In the presence of 50% human serum, the mean EC_{50} values of lopinavir against these five HIV-1 laboratory strains ranged from 65-289 nM (0.04-0.18 µg/mL), representing a 7 to 11-fold attenuation. Combination antiviral drug activity studies with lopinavir in cell cultures demonstrated additive to antagonistic activity with nelfinavir and additive to synergistic activity with amprenavir, atazanavir, indinavir, saquinavir and tipranavir. The EC_{50} values of lopinavir against three different HIV-2 strains ranged from 12-180 nM (0.008-113 µg/mL).

Resistance
HIV-1 isolates with reduced susceptibility to lopinavir have been selected in cell culture. The presence of ritonavir does not appear to influence the selection of lopinavir-resistant viruses in cell culture.

The selection of resistance to KALETRA in antiretroviral treatment naïve patients has not yet been characterized. In a study of 653 antiretroviral treatment naïve patients (Study 863), plasma viral isolates from each patient on

Table 13 *(cont).* **Established and Other Potentially Significant Drug Interactions**

Concomitant Drug Class: Drug Name	Effect on Concentration of Lopinavir or Concomitant Drug	Clinical Comments
HCV-Protease Inhibitor: boceprevir	↓ lopinavir ↓ boceprevir ↓ ritonavir	It is not recommended to co-administer KALETRA and boceprevir. Concomitant administration of KALETRA and boceprevir reduced boceprevir, lopinavir and ritonavir steady-state exposures *[see Clinical Pharmacology (12.3)].*
HCV-Protease Inhibitor: simeprevir	↑ simeprevir	It is not recommended to co-administer KALETRA and simeprevir.
HMG-CoA Reductase Inhibitors: atorvastatin rosuvastatin	↑ atorvastatin ↑ rosuvastatin	Use atorvastatin with caution and at the lowest necessary dose. Titrate rosuvastatin dose carefully and use the lowest necessary dose; do not exceed rosuvastatin 10 mg/day. See Drugs with No Observed or Predicted Interactions with KALETRA *(7.4)* and Clinical Pharmacology *(12.3)* for drug interaction data with other HMG-CoA reductase inhibitors.
Immunosuppressants: e.g. cyclosporine, tacrolimus, sirolimus	↑ immunosuppressants	Therapeutic concentration monitoring is recommended for immunosuppressant agents when co-administered with KALETRA.
Inhaled or Intranasal Steroids e.g.: fluticasone, budesonide	↑ glucocorticoids	Concomitant use of KALETRA and fluticasone or other glucocorticoids that are metabolized by CYP3A is not recommended unless the potential benefit of treatment outweighs the risk of systemic corticosteroid effects. Concomitant use may result in increased steroid concentrations and reduce serum cortisol concentrations. Systemic corticosteroid effects including Cushing's syndrome and adrenal suppression have been reported during postmarketing use in patients when certain ritonavir-containing products have been co-administered with fluticasone propionate or budesonide.
Long-acting beta-adrenoceptor Agonist: salmeterol	↑ salmeterol	Concurrent administration of salmeterol and KALETRA is not recommended. The combination may result in increased risk of cardiovascular adverse events associated with salmeterol, including QT prolongation, palpitations and sinus tachycardia.
Narcotic Analgesics: methadone,* fentanyl	↓ methadone ↑ fentanyl	Dosage of methadone may need to be increased when co-administered with KALETRA. Concentrations of fentanyl are expected to increase. Careful monitoring of therapeutic and adverse effects (including potentially fatal respiratory depression) is recommended when fentanyl is concomitantly administered with KALETRA. *This table is continued on next page*

treatment with plasma HIV-1 RNA > 400 copies/mL at Week 24, 32, 40 and/or 48 were analyzed. No evidence of resistance to KALETRA was observed in 37 evaluable KALETRA-treated patients (0%). Evidence of genotypic resistance to nelfinavir, defined as the presence of the D30N and/or L90M substitution in HIV-1 protease, was observed in 25/76 (33%) of evaluable nelfinavir-treated patients. The selection of resistance to KALETRA in antiretroviral treatment naïve pediatric patients (Study 940) appears to be consistent with that seen in adult patients (Study 863).

Resistance to KALETRA has been noted to emerge in patients treated with other protease inhibitors prior to KALETRA therapy. In studies of 227 antiretroviral treatment naïve and protease inhibitor experienced patients, isolates from 4 of 23 patients with quantifiable (> 400 copies/mL) viral RNA following treatment with KALETRA for 12 to 100 weeks displayed significantly reduced susceptibility to lopinavir compared to the corresponding baseline viral isolates. Three of these patients had previously received treatment with a single protease inhibitor (indinavir, nelfinavir, or saquinavir) and one patient had received treatment with multiple protease inhibitors (indinavir, ritonavir, and saquinavir). All four of these patients had at least 4 substitutions associated with protease inhibitor resistance immediately prior to KALETRA therapy. Following viral rebound, isolates from these patients all contained additional substitutions, some of which are recognized to be associated with protease inhibitor resistance. However, there are insufficient data at this time to identify patterns of lopinavir resistance-associated substitutions in isolates from patients on KALETRA therapy. The assessment of these patterns is under study.

Cross-resistance - Preclinical Studies
Varying degrees of cross-resistance have been observed among HIV-1 protease inhibitors. Little information is available on the cross-resistance of viruses that developed decreased susceptibility to lopinavir during KALETRA therapy.

The antiviral activity in cell culture of lopinavir against clinical isolates from patients previously treated with a single protease inhibitor was determined. Isolates that displayed > 4-fold reduced susceptibility to nelfinavir (n = 13) and saquinavir (n = 4), displayed < 4-fold reduced susceptibility to lopinavir. Isolates with > 4-fold reduced susceptibility to indinavir (n = 16) and ritonavir (n = 3) displayed a mean of 5.7- and 8.3-fold reduced susceptibility to lopinavir, respectively. Isolates from patients previously treated with two or more protease inhibitors showed greater reductions in susceptibility to lopinavir, as described in the following paragraph.

Clinical Studies - Antiviral Activity of KALETRA in Patients with Previous Protease Inhibitor Therapies
The clinical relevance of reduced susceptibility in cell culture to lopinavir has been examined by assessing the virologic response to KALETRA therapy in treatment-experienced patients, with respect to baseline viral genotype in three studies and baseline viral phenotype in one study.

Virologic response to KALETRA has been shown to be affected by the presence of three or more of the following amino acid substitutions in protease at baseline: L10F/I/R/V, K20M/N/R, L24I, L33F, M36I, I47V, G48V, I54L/T/V, V82A/C/F/S/T, and I84V. Table 16 shows the 48-week virologic response (HIV-1 RNA <400 copies/mL) according to the

number of the above protease inhibitor resistance-associated substitutions at baseline in studies 888 and 765 *[see Clinical Studies (14.2)* and *(14.3)]* and study 957 (see below). Once daily administration of KALETRA for adult patients with three or more of the above substitutions is not recommended.

[See table 16 on page 702]

Virologic response to KALETRA therapy with respect to phenotypic susceptibility to lopinavir at baseline was examined in Study 957. In this study 56 NNRTI-naïve patients with HIV-1 RNA >1,000 copies/mL despite previous therapy with at least two protease inhibitors selected from indinavir, nelfinavir, ritonavir, and saquinavir were randomized to receive one of two doses of KALETRA in combination with efavirenz and nucleoside reverse transcriptase inhibitors (NRTIs). The EC_{50} values of lopinavir against the 56 baseline viral isolates ranged from 0.5- to 96-fold the wild-type EC_{50} value. Fifty-five percent (31/56) of these baseline isolates displayed >4-fold reduced susceptibility to lopinavir. These 31 isolates had a median reduction in lopinavir susceptibility of 18-fold. Response to therapy by baseline lopinavir susceptibility is shown in Table 17.

Table 17. HIV-1 RNA Response at Week 48 by Baseline Lopinavir Susceptibility[1]

Lopinavir susceptibility[2] at baseline	HIV-1 RNA <400 copies/mL (%)	HIV-1 RNA <50 copies/mL (%)
< 10 fold	25/27 (93%)	22/27 (81%)
> 10 and < 40 fold	11/15 (73%)	9/15 (60%)
≥ 40 fold	2/8 (25%)	2/8 (25%)

1 Lopinavir susceptibility was determined by recombinant phenotypic technology performed by Virologic.
2 Fold change in susceptibility from wild type.

13   NONCLINICAL TOXICOLOGY
13.1   Carcinogenesis, Mutagenesis, Impairment of Fertility
Carcinogenesis
Lopinavir/ritonavir combination was evaluated for carcinogenic potential by oral gavage administration to mice and rats for up to 104 weeks. Results showed an increase in the incidence of benign hepatocellular adenomas and an increase in the combined incidence of hepatocellular adenomas plus carcinoma in both males and females in mice and males in rats at doses that produced approximately 1.6-2.2 times (mice) and 0.5 times (rats) the human exposure (based on AUC_{0-24hr} measurement) at the recommended dose of 400/100 mg KALETRA twice daily. Administration of lopinavir/ritonavir did not cause a statistically significant increase in the incidence of any other benign or malignant neoplasm in mice or rats.

Carcinogenicity studies in mice and rats have been carried out on ritonavir. In male mice, there was a dose dependent increase in the incidence of both adenomas and combined adenomas and carcinomas in the liver. Based on AUC measurements, the exposure at the high dose was approximately 4-fold for males that of the exposure in humans with the recommended therapeutic dose (400/100 mg KALETRA twice daily). There were no carcinogenic effects seen in females at the dosages tested. The exposure at the high dose was approximately 9-fold for the females that of the exposure in humans. There were no carcinogenic effects in rats. In this study, the exposure at the high dose was approximately 0.7-fold that of the exposure in humans with the 400/100 mg KALETRA twice daily regimen. Based on the exposures achieved in the animal studies, the significance of the observed effects is not known.

Mutagenesis
Neither lopinavir nor ritonavir was found to be mutagenic or clastogenic in a battery of *in vitro* and *in vivo* assays including the Ames bacterial reverse mutation assay using *S. typhimurium* and *E. coli*, the mouse lymphoma assay, the mouse micronucleus test and chromosomal aberration assays in human lymphocytes.

Continued on next page

Information on the AbbVie, Inc. products listed on these pages is from the prescribing information in use as of July 31, 2016. For more information, please visit rxabbvie.com or call 1-800-633-9110.

Impairment of Fertility

Lopinavir in combination with ritonavir at a 2:1 ratio produced no effects on fertility in male and female rats at levels of 10/5, 30/15 or 100/50 mg/kg/day. Based on AUC measurements, the exposures in rats at the high doses were approximately 0.7-fold for lopinavir and 1.8-fold for ritonavir of the exposures in humans at the recommended therapeutic dose (400/100 mg twice daily).

14 CLINICAL STUDIES

14.1 Adult Patients without Prior Antiretroviral Therapy

Study 863: KALETRA Capsules twice daily + stavudine + lamivudine compared to nelfinavir three times daily + stavudine + lamivudine

Study 863 was a randomized, double-blind, multicenter trial comparing treatment with KALETRA capsules (400/100 mg twice daily) plus stavudine and lamivudine versus nelfinavir (750 mg three times daily) plus stavudine and lamivudine in 653 antiretroviral treatment naïve patients. Patients had a mean age of 38 years (range: 19 to 84), 57% were Caucasian, and 80% were male. Mean baseline CD4+ cell count was 259 cells/mm^3 (range: 2 to 949 cells/mm^3) and mean baseline plasma HIV-1 RNA was 4.9 log$_{10}$ copies/mL (range: 2.6 to 6.8 log$_{10}$ copies/mL).

Treatment response and outcomes of randomized treatment are presented in Table 18.

[See table 18 on page 703]

Through 48 weeks of therapy, there was a statistically significantly higher proportion of patients in the KALETRA arm compared to the nelfinavir arm with HIV-1 RNA < 400 copies/mL (75% vs. 62%, respectively) and HIV-1 RNA < 50 copies/mL (67% vs. 52%, respectively). Treatment response by baseline HIV-1 RNA level subgroups is presented in Table 19.

[See table 19 on page 704]

Through 48 weeks of therapy, the mean increase from baseline in CD4+ cell count was 207 cells/mm^3 for the KALETRA arm and 195 cells/mm^3 for the nelfinavir arm.

Study 730: KALETRA Tablets once daily + tenofovir DF + emtricitabine compared to KALETRA Tablets twice daily + tenofovir DF + emtricitabine

Study 730 was a randomized, open-label, multicenter trial comparing treatment with KALETRA 800/200 mg once daily plus tenofovir DF and emtricitabine versus KALETRA 400/100 mg twice daily plus tenofovir DF and emtricitabine in 664 antiretroviral treatment-naïve patients. Patients were randomized in a 1:1 ratio to receive either KALETRA 800/200 mg once daily (n = 333) or KALETRA 400/100 mg twice daily (n = 331). Further stratification within each group was 1:1 (tablet vs. capsule). Patients administered the capsule were switched to the tablet formulation at Week 8 and maintained on their randomized dosing schedule. Patients were administered emtricitabine 200 mg once daily and tenofovir DF 300 mg once daily. Mean age of patients enrolled was 39 years (range: 19 to 71); 75% were Caucasian, and 78% were male. Mean baseline CD4+ cell count was 216 cells/mm^3 (range: 20 to 775 cells/mm^3) and mean baseline plasma HIV-1 RNA was 5.0 log$_{10}$ copies/mL (range: 1.7 to 7.0 log$_{10}$ copies/mL).

Treatment response and outcomes of randomized treatment through Week 48 are presented in Table 20.

Table 13 (cont). Established and Other Potentially Significant Drug Interactions

Concomitant Drug Class: Drug Name	Effect on Concentration of Lopinavir or Concomitant Drug	Clinical Comments
PDE5 inhibitors: avanafil, sildenafil, tadalafil, vardenafil	↑ avanafil ↑ sildenafil ↑ tadalafil ↑ vardenafil	Do not use KALETRA with avanafil because a safe and effective avanafil dosage regimen has not been established. Particular caution should be used when prescribing sildenafil, tadalafil, or vardenafil in patients receiving KALETRA. Co-administration of KALETRA with these drugs is expected to substantially increase their concentrations and may result in an increase in PDE5 inhibitor associated adverse reactions including hypotension, syncope, visual changes and prolonged erection. Use of PDE5 inhibitors for pulmonary arterial hypertension (PAH): Sildenafil (Revatio®) is contraindicated when used for the treatment of pulmonary arterial hypertension (PAH) because a safe and effective dose has not been established when used with KALETRA [see Contraindications (4)]. The following dose adjustments are recommended for use of tadalafil (Adcirca®) with KALETRA: Co-administration of ADCIRCA in patients on KALETRA: In patients receiving KALETRA for at least one week, start ADCIRCA at 20 mg once daily. Increase to 40 mg once daily based upon individual tolerability. Co-administration of KALETRA in patients on ADCIRCA: Avoid use of ADCIRCA during the initiation of KALETRA. Stop ADCIRCA at least 24 hours prior to starting KALETRA. After at least one week following the initiation of KALETRA, resume ADCIRCA at 20 mg once daily. Increase to 40 mg once daily based upon individual tolerability. Use of PDE5 inhibitors for erectile dysfunction: It is recommended not to exceed the following doses: • Sildenafil: 25 mg every 48 hours • Tadalafil: 10 mg every 72 hours • Vardenafil: 2.5 mg every 72 hours Use with increased monitoring for adverse events.

* see *Clinical Pharmacology (12.3)* for magnitude of interaction.

Table 20. Outcomes of Randomized Treatment Through Week 48 (Study 730)

Outcome	KALETRA Once Daily + TDF + FTC (n = 333)	KALETRA Twice Daily + TDF + FTC (n = 331)
Responder[1]	78%	77%

Virologic failure[2]
  Rebound
  Never suppressed through Week 48
	10%
	5%
	5%
		8%
		5%
		3%

Death	1%	<1%
Discontinued due to adverse events	4%	3%
Discontinued for other reasons[3]	8%	11%

1 Patients achieved and maintained confirmed HIV-1 RNA < 50 copies/mL through Week 48.
2 Includes confirmed viral rebound and failure to achieve confirmed < 50 copies/mL through Week 48.
3 Includes lost to follow-up, patient's withdrawal, non-compliance, protocol violation and other reasons.

Through 48 weeks of therapy, 78% in the KALETRA once daily arm and 77% in the KALETRA twice daily arm achieved and maintained HIV-1 RNA < 50 copies/mL (95% confidence interval for the difference, -5.9% to 6.8%). Mean CD4+ cell count increases at Week 48 were 186 cells/mm^3 for the KALETRA once daily arm and 198 cells/mm^3 for the KALETRA twice daily arm.

14.2 Adult Patients with Prior Antiretroviral Therapy

Study 888: KALETRA Capsules twice daily + nevirapine + NRTIs compared to investigator-selected protease inhibitor(s) + nevirapine + NRTIs

Study 888 was a randomized, open-label, multicenter trial comparing treatment with KALETRA capsules (400/100 mg

Figure 1. Mean Steady-State Plasma Concentrations with 95% Confidence Intervals (CI) for HIV-1 Infected Adult Subjects (N = 19)

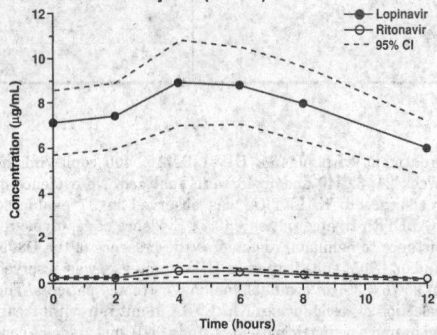

twice daily) plus nevirapine and nucleoside reverse transcriptase inhibitors versus investigator-selected protease inhibitor(s) plus nevirapine and nucleoside reverse transcriptase inhibitors in 288 single protease inhibitor-experienced, non-nucleoside reverse transcriptase inhibitor (NNRTI)-naïve patients. Patients had a mean age of 40 years (range: 18 to 74), 68% were Caucasian, and 86% were male. Mean baseline CD4+ cell count was 322 cells/mm^3 (range: 10 to 1059 cells/mm^3) and mean baseline plasma HIV-1 RNA was 4.1 log$_{10}$ copies/mL (range: 2.6 to 6.0 log$_{10}$ copies/mL).

Treatment response and outcomes of randomized treatment through Week 48 are presented in Table 21.

Table 21. Outcomes of Randomized Treatment Through Week 48 (Study 888)

Outcome	KALETRA + nevirapine + NRTIs (n = 148)	Investigator-Selected Protease Inhibitor(s) + nevirapine + NRTIs (n = 140)

Table 14. Drug Interactions: Pharmacokinetic Parameters for Lopinavir in the Presence of the Co-administered Drug for Recommended Alterations in Dose or Regimen

Co-administered Drug	Dose of Co-administered Drug (mg)	Dose of KALETRA (mg)	n	Ratio (in combination with Co-administered drug/alone) of Lopinavir Pharmacokinetic Parameters (90% CI); No Effect = 1.00		
				C_{max}	AUC	C_{min}
Boceprevir	800 q8h, 6 d	400/100 tablet twice daily, 22 d	13	0.70 (0.65, 0.77)	0.66[12] (0.60, 0.72)	0.57 (0.49, 0.65)
Efavirenz[1,2]	600 at bedtime, 9 d	400/100 capsule twice daily, 9 d	11, 7*	0.97 (0.78, 1.22)	0.81 (0.64, 1.03)	0.61 (0.38, 0.97)
	600 at bedtime, 9 d	500/125 tablet twice daily, 10 d	19	1.12 (1.02, 1.23)	1.06 (0.96, 1.17)	0.90 (0.78, 1.04)
	600 at bedtime, 9 d	600/150 tablet twice daily, 10 d	23	1.36 (1.28, 1.44)	1.36 (1.28, 1.44)	1.32 (1.21, 1.44)
Etravirine	200 twice daily	400/100 mg twice day (tablets)	16	0.89 (0.82-0.96)	0.87 (0.83-0.92)	0.80 (0.73-0.88)
Fosamprenavir[3]	700 twice daily plus ritonavir 100 twice daily, 14 d	400/100 capsule twice daily, 14 d	18	1.30 (0.85, 1.47)	1.37 (0.80, 1.55)	1.52 (0.72, 1.82)
Ketoconazole	200 single dose	400/100 capsule twice daily, 16 d	12	0.89 (0.80, 0.99)	0.87 (0.75, 1.00)	0.75 (0.55, 1.00)
Nelfinavir	1000 twice daily, 10 d	400/100 capsule twice daily, 21 d	13	0.79 (0.70, 0.89)	0.73 (0.63, 0.85)	0.62 (0.49, 0.78)
Nevirapine	200 twice daily, steady-state (> 1 yr)[4#]	400/100 capsule twice daily, steady-state	22, 19*	0.81 (0.62, 1.05)	0.73 (0.53, 0.98)	0.49 (0.28, 0.74)
	7 mg/kg or 4 mg/kg once daily, 2 wk; twice daily 1 wk[5]	(> 1 yr) 300/75 mg/m² oral solution twice daily, 3 wk	12, 15*	0.86 (0.64, 1.16)	0.78 (0.56, 1.09)	0.45 (0.25, 0.81)
Omeprazole	40 once daily, 5 d	400/100 tablet twice daily, 10 d	12	1.08 (0.99, 1.17)	1.07 (0.99, 1.15)	1.03 (0.90, 1.18)
	40 once daily, 5 d	800/200 tablet once daily, 10 d	12	0.94 (0.88, 1.00)	0.92 (0.86, 0.99)	0.71 (0.57, 0.89)

This table is continued on the next page.

Responder[1]	57%	33%
Virologic failure[2]	24%	41%
Rebound	11%	19%
Never suppressed through Week 48	13%	23%
Death	1%	2%
Discontinued due to adverse events	5%	11%
Discontinued for other reasons[3]	14%	13%

1 Patients achieved and maintained confirmed HIV-1 RNA < 400 copies/mL through Week 48.
2 Includes confirmed viral rebound and failure to achieve confirmed < 400 copies/mL through Week 48.
3 Includes lost to follow-up, patient's withdrawal, non-compliance, protocol violation and other reasons.

Through 48 weeks of therapy, there was a statistically significantly higher proportion of patients in the KALETRA arm compared to the investigator-selected protease inhibitor(s) arm with HIV-1 RNA < 400 copies/mL (57% vs. 33%, respectively).

Through 48 weeks of therapy, the mean increase from baseline in CD4 + cell count was 111 cells/mm³ for the KALETRA arm and 112 cells/mm³ for the investigator-selected protease inhibitor(s) arm.
Study 802: *KALETRA Tablets 800/200 mg Once Daily Versus 400/100 mg Twice Daily when Co-administered with Nucleoside/Nucleotide Reverse Transcriptase Inhibitors in Antiretroviral-Experienced, HIV-1 Infected Subjects*
M06-802 was a randomized open-label study comparing the safety, tolerability, and antiviral activity of once daily and twice daily dosing of KALETRA tablets in 599 subjects with detectable viral loads while receiving their current antiviral therapy. Of the enrolled subjects, 55% on both treatment arms had not been previously treated with a protease inhibitor and 81 – 88% had received prior NNRTIs as part of their anti-HIV treatment regimen. Patients were randomized in a 1:1 ratio to receive either KALETRA 800/200 mg once daily (n = 300) or KALETRA 400/100 mg twice daily (n = 299). Patients were administered at least two nucleoside/nucleotide reverse transcriptase inhibitors selected by the investigator. Mean age of patients enrolled was 41 years (range: 21 to 73); 51% were Caucasian, and 66% were male. Mean baseline CD4+ cell count was 254 cells/mm³ (range: 4 to 952 cells/mm³) and mean baseline plasma HIV-1 RNA was 4.3 log₁₀ copies/mL (range: 1.7 to 6.6 log₁₀ copies/mL). Treatment response and outcomes of randomized treatment through Week 48 are presented in Table 22.

Table 22. Outcomes of Randomized Treatment Through Week 48 (Study 802)

Outcome	KALETRA Once Daily + NRTIs (n = 300)	KALETRA Twice Daily + NRTIs (n = 299)
Virologic Success (HIV-1 RNA <50 copies/mL)	57%	54%
Virologic failure[1]	22%	24%
No virologic data in Week 48 window		
Discontinued study due to adverse event or death[2]	5%	7%
Discontinued study for other reasons[3]	13%	12%
Missing data during window but on study	3%	3%

1 Includes patients who discontinued prior to Week 48 for lack or loss of efficacy and patients with HIV-1 RNA ≥ 50 copies/mL at Week 48.
2 Includes patients who discontinued due to adverse events or death at any time from Day 1 through Week 48 if this resulted in no virologic data on treatment at Week 48.
3 Includes withdrawal of consent, loss to follow-up, non-compliance, protocol violation and other reasons.

Through 48 weeks of treatment, the mean change from baseline for CD4 + cell count was 135 cells/mm³ for the once daily group and 122 cells/mm³ for the twice daily group.

14.3 Other Studies Supporting Approval in Adult Patients

Study 720: KALETRA twice daily + stavudine + lamivudine
Study 765: KALETRA twice daily + nevirapine + NRTIs
Study 720 (patients without prior antiretroviral therapy) and study 765 (patients with prior protease inhibitor therapy) were randomized, blinded, multi-center trials evaluating treatment with KALETRA at up to three dose levels (200/100 mg twice daily [720 only], 400/100 mg twice daily, and 400/200 mg twice daily). In Study 720, all patients switched to 400/100 mg twice daily between Weeks 48-72. Patients in study 720 had a mean age of 35 years, 70% were Caucasian, and 96% were male, while patients in study 765 had a mean age of 40 years, 73% were Caucasian, and 90% were male. Mean (range) baseline CD4+ cell counts for patients in study 720 and study 765 were 338 (3-918) and 372 (72-807) cells/mm³, respectively. Mean (range) baseline plasma HIV-1 RNA levels for patients in study 720 and study 765 were 4.9 (3.3 to 6.3) and 4.0 (2.9 to 5.8) log₁₀ copies/mL, respectively.

Through 360 weeks of treatment in study 720, the proportion of patients with HIV-1 RNA < 400 (< 50) copies/mL was 61% (59%) [n = 100]. Among patients completing 360 weeks of treatment with CD4+ cell count measurements [n=60], the mean (median) increase in CD4+ cell count was 501 (457) cells/mm³. Thirty-nine patients (39%) discontinued the study, including 13 (13%) discontinuations due to adverse reactions and 1 (1%) death.

Through 144 weeks of treatment in study 765, the proportion of patients with HIV-1 RNA < 400 (< 50) copies/mL was 54% (50%) [n = 70], and the corresponding mean increase in CD4+ cell count was 212 cells/mm³. Twenty-seven patients (39%) discontinued the study, including 5 (7%) discontinuations secondary to adverse reactions and 2 (3%) deaths.

14.4 Pediatric Studies

Study 1030 was an open-label, multicenter, dose-finding trial evaluating the pharmacokinetic profile, tolerability, safety and efficacy of KALETRA oral solution containing

Continued on next page

lopinavir 80 mg/mL and ritonavir 20 mg/mL at a dose of 300/75 mg/m² twice daily plus 2 NRTIs in HIV-1 infected infants ≥14 days and <6 months of age.

Ten infants, ≥14 days and <6 wks of age, were enrolled at a median (range) age of 5.7 (3.6-6.0) weeks and all completed 24 weeks. At entry, median (range) HIV-1 RNA was 6.0 (4.7-7.2) $\log_{10}$ copies/mL. Seven of 10 infants had HIV-1 RNA <400 copies/mL at Week 24. At entry, median (range) CD4+ percentage was 41 (16-59) with a median decrease of 1% (95% CI: -10, 18) from baseline to week 24 in 6 infants with available data.

Twenty-one infants, between 6 weeks and 6 months of age, were enrolled at a median (range) age of 14.7 (6.9-25.7) weeks and 19 of 21 infants completed 24 weeks. At entry, median (range) HIV RNA level was 5.8 (3.7-6.9) $\log_{10}$ copies/mL. Ten of 21 infants had HIV RNA <400 copies/mL at Week 24. At entry, the median (range) CD4+ percentage was 32 (11-54) with a median increase of 4% (95% CI: -1, 9) from baseline to week 24 in 19 infants with available data.

See Clinical Pharmacology (12.3) for pharmacokinetic results.

Study 940 was an open-label, multicenter trial evaluating the pharmacokinetic profile, tolerability, safety and efficacy of KALETRA oral solution containing lopinavir 80 mg/mL and ritonavir 20 mg/mL in 100 antiretroviral naïve (44%) and experienced (56%) pediatric patients. All patients were non-nucleoside reverse transcriptase inhibitor naïve. Patients were randomized to either 230 mg lopinavir/57.5 mg ritonavir per m² or 300 mg lopinavir/75 mg ritonavir per m². Naïve patients also received lamivudine and stavudine. Experienced patients received nevirapine plus up to two nucleoside reverse transcriptase inhibitors.

Safety, efficacy and pharmacokinetic profiles of the two dose regimens were assessed after three weeks of therapy in each patient. After analysis of these data, all patients were continued on the 300 mg lopinavir/75 mg ritonavir per m² dose. Patients had a mean age of 5 years (range 6 months to 12 years) with 14% less than 2 years. Mean baseline CD4+ cell count was 838 cells/mm³ and mean baseline plasma HIV-1 RNA was 4.7 $\log_{10}$ copies/mL.

Through 48 weeks of therapy, the proportion of patients who achieved and sustained an HIV-1 RNA < 400 copies/mL was 80% for antiretroviral naïve patients and 71% for antiretroviral experienced patients. The mean increase from baseline in CD4+ cell count was 404 cells/mm³ for antiretroviral naïve and 284 cells/mm³ for antiretroviral experienced patients treated through 48 weeks. At 48 weeks, two patients (2%) had prematurely discontinued the study. One antiretroviral naïve patient prematurely discontinued secondary to an adverse reaction, while one antiretroviral experienced patient prematurely discontinued secondary to an HIV-1 related event.

Dose selection in pediatric patients was based on the following:

• Among patients 14 days to 6 months of age receiving 300/75 mg/m² twice daily without nevirapine, plasma concentrations were lower than those observed in adults or in older children. This dose resulted in HIV-1 RNA < 400 copies/mL in 55% of patients (70% in those initiating treatment at <6 weeks of age).

• Among patients 6 months to 12 years of age, the 230/57.5 mg/m² oral solution twice daily regimen without nevirapine and the 300/75 mg/m² oral solution twice daily regimen with nevirapine provided lopinavir plasma concentrations similar to those obtained in adult patients receiving the 400/100 mg twice daily regimen (without nevirapine). These doses resulted in treatment benefit (proportion of patients with HIV-1 RNA < 400 copies/mL) similar to that seen in the adult clinical trials.

• Among patients 12 to 18 years of age receiving 400/100 mg/m² or 480/120 mg/m² (with efavirenz) twice daily, plasma concentrations were 60-100% higher than among 6 to 12 year old patients receiving 230/57.5 mg/m². Mean apparent clearance was similar to that observed in adult patients receiving standard dose and in patients 6 to 12 years of age. Although changes in HIV-1 RNA in patients with prior treatment failure were less than anticipated, the pharmacokinetic data supports use of similar dosing as in patients 6 to 12 years of age, not to exceed the recommended adult dose.

• For all age groups, the body surface area dosing was converted to body weight dosing using the patient's prescribed lopinavir dose.

16   HOW SUPPLIED/STORAGE AND HANDLING

KALETRA® (lopinavir and ritonavir) tablets and oral solution are available in the following strengths and package sizes:

Table 14 (cont.) Drug Interactions: Pharmacokinetic Parameters for Lopinavir in the Presence of the Co-administered Drug for Recommended Alterations in Dose or Regimen

Co-administered Drug	Dose of Co-administered Drug (mg)	Dose of KALETRA (mg)	n	Ratio (in combination with Co-administered drug/alone) of Lopinavir Pharmacokinetic Parameters (90% CI); No Effect = 1.00		
				C_{max}	AUC	C_{min}
Pitavastatin[6]	4 once daily, 5 d	400/100 tablet twice daily, 16 d	23	0.93 (0.88-0.98)	0.91 (0.86-0.97)	N/A
Pravastatin	20 once daily, 4 d	400/100 capsule twice daily, 14 d	12	0.98 (0.89, 1.08)	0.95 (0.85, 1.05)	0.88 (0.77, 1.02)
Rifabutin	150 once daily, 10 d	400/100 capsule twice daily, 20 d	14	1.08 (0.97, 1.19)	1.17 (1.04, 1.31)	1.20 (0.96, 1.65)
Ranitidine	150 single dose	400/100 tablet twice daily, 10 d	12	0.99 (0.95, 1.03)	0.97 (0.93, 1.01)	0.90 (0.85, 0.95)
	150 single dose	800/200 tablet once daily, 10 d	10	0.97 (0.95, 1.00)	0.95 (0.91, 0.99)	0.82 (0.74, 0.91)
Rifampin	600 once daily, 10 d	400/100 capsule twice daily, 20 d	22	0.45 (0.40, 0.51)	0.25 (0.21, 0.29)	0.01 (0.01, 0.02)
	600 once daily, 14 d	800/200 capsule twice daily, 9 d[7]	10	1.02 (0.85, 1.23)	0.84 (0.64, 1.10)	0.43 (0.19, 0.96)
	600 once daily, 14 d	400/400 capsule twice daily, 9 d[8]	9	0.93 (0.81, 1.07)	0.98 (0.81, 1.17)	1.03 (0.68, 1.56)
Rilpivirine	150 once daily[13]	400/100 twice daily (capsules)	15	0.96 (0.88-1.05)	0.99 (0.89-1.10)	0.89 (0.73-1.08)
Ritonavir[4]	100 twice daily, 3-4 wk[#]	400/100 capsule twice daily, 3-4 wk	8, 21*	1.28 (0.94, 1.76)	1.46 (1.04, 2.06)	2.16 (1.29, 3.62)
Tenofovir[9]	300 once daily, 14 d	400/100 capsule twice daily, 14 d	24	NC†	NC†	NC†
Tipranavir/ ritonavir[4]	500/200 twice daily (28 doses)[#]	400/100 capsule twice daily (27 doses)	21 69	0.53 (0.40, 0.69)[10]	0.45 (0.32, 0.63)[10]	0.30 (0.17, 0.51)[10] 0.48 (0.40, 0.58)[11]

All interaction studies conducted in healthy, HIV-1 negative subjects unless otherwise indicated.
1 The pharmacokinetics of ritonavir are unaffected by concurrent efavirenz.
2 Reference for comparison is lopinavir/ritonavir 400/100 mg twice daily without efavirenz.
3 Data extracted from the fosamprenavir package insert.
4 Study conducted in HIV-1 positive adult subjects.
5 Study conducted in HIV-1 positive pediatric subjects ranging in age from 6 months to 12 years.
6 Data extracted from the pitavastatin package insert and results presented at the 2011 International AIDS Society Conference on HIV Pathogenesis, Treatment and Prevention (Morgan, *et al, poster #MOPE170*).
7 Titrated to 800/200 twice daily as 533/133 twice daily × 1 d, 667/167 twice daily × 1 d, then 800/200 twice daily × 7 d, compared to 400/100 twice daily × 10 days alone.
8 Titrated to 400/400 twice daily as 400/200 twice daily × 1 d, 400/300 twice daily × 1 d, then 400/400 twice daily × 7 d, compared to 400/100 twice daily × 10 days alone.
9 Data extracted from the tenofovir package insert.
10 Intensive PK analysis.
11 Drug levels obtained at 8-16 hrs post-dose.
12 AUC parameter is $AUC_{(0-last)}$
13 This interaction study has been performed with a dose higher than the recommended dose for rilpivirine (25 mg once daily) assessing the maximal effect on the co-administered drug.
* Parallel group design; n for KALETRA + co-administered drug, n for KALETRA alone.
N/A = Not available.
† NC = No change.
# For the nevirapine 200 mg twice daily study, ritonavir, and tipranavir/ritonavir studies, KALETRA was administered with or without food. For all other studies, KALETRA was administered with food.

16.1   KALETRA Tablets, 200 mg lopinavir and 50 mg ritonavir

Yellow film-coated ovaloid tablets debossed with the "a" logo and the code KA:

Bottles of 120 tablets.............................(NDC 0074-6799-22)
Recommended Storage

Store KALETRA tablets at 20°-25°C (68°-77°F); excursions permitted to 15°-30°C (59° to 86°F) [see USP controlled room temperature]. Dispense in original container or USP equivalent tight container (250 mL or less). For patient use:

Continued on next page

Table 15. Drug Interactions: Pharmacokinetic Parameters for Co-administered Drug in the Presence of KALETRA for Recommended Alterations in Dose or Regimen

Co-administered Drug	Dose of Co-administered Drug (mg)	Dose of KALETRA (mg)	n	Ratio (in combination with KALETRA/alone) of Co-administered Drug Pharmacokinetic Parameters (90% CI); No Effect = 1.00		
				C_{max}	AUC	C_{min}
Bedaquiline[1]	400 single dose	400/100 tablet twice daily, 24 d	N/A	N/A	1.22 (1.11, 1.34)	N/A
Boceprevir	800 q8h, 6 d	400/100 tablet twice daily, 22 d	13[9]	0.50 (0.45, 0.55)	0.55 (0.49, 0.61)	0.43 (0.36, 0.53)
Desipramine[3]	100 single dose	400/100 capsule twice daily, 10 d	15	0.91 (0.84, 0.97)	1.05 (0.96, 1.16)	N/A
Efavirenz	600 at bedtime, 9 d	400/100 capsule twice daily, 9 d	11, 12*	0.91 (0.72, 1.15)	0.84 (0.62, 1.15)	0.84 (0.58, 1.20)
Ethinyl Estradiol	35 µg once daily, 21 d (Ortho Novum®)	400/100 capsule twice daily, 14 d	12	0.59 (0.52, 0.66)	0.58 (0.54, 0.62)	0.42 (0.36, 0.49)
Etravirine	200 twice daily	400/100 mg twice day (tablets)	16	0.70 (0.64-0.78)	0.65 (0.59-0.71)	0.55 (0.49-0.62)
Fosamprenavir[4]	700 twice daily plus ritonavir 100 twice daily, 14 d	400/100 capsule twice daily, 14 d	18	0.42 (0.30, 0.58)	0.37 (0.28, 0.49)	0.35 (0.27, 0.46)
Indinavir[2]	600 twice daily, 10 d combo nonfasting vs. 800 three times daily, 5 d alone fasting	400/100 capsule twice daily, 15 d	13	0.71 (0.63, 0.81)	0.91 (0.75, 1.10)	3.47 (2.60, 4.64)
Ketoconazole	200 single dose	400/100 capsule twice daily, 16 d	12	1.13 (0.91, 1.40)	3.04 (2.44, 3.79)	N/A
Methadone	5 single dose	400/100 capsule twice daily, 10 d	11	0.55 (0.48, 0.64)	0.47 (0.42, 0.53)	N/A
Nelfinavir[2]	1000 twice daily, 10 d combo vs. 1250 twice daily 14 d alone	400/100 capsule twice daily, 21 d	13	0.93 (0.82, 1.05)	1.07 (0.95, 1.19)	1.86 (1.57, 2.22)
M8 metabolite				2.36 (1.91, 2.91)	3.46 (2.78, 4.31)	7.49 (5.85, 9.58)

This table is continued on the next page.

exposure of this product to high humidity outside the original container or USP equivalent tight container (250 mL or less) for longer than 2 weeks is not recommended.

16.2   KALETRA Tablets, 100 mg lopinavir and 25 mg ritonavir
Pale yellow film-coated ovaloid tablets debossed with the "a" logo and the code KC:
Bottles of 60 tablets...............................(NDC 0074-0522-60)
Recommended Storage
Store KALETRA tablets at 20°-25°C (68°-77°F); excursions permitted to 15°-30°C (59° to 86°F) [see USP controlled room temperature]. Dispense in original container or USP equivalent tight container (100 mL or less). For patient use: exposure of this product to high humidity outside the original container or USP equivalent tight container (100 mL or less) for longer than 2 weeks is not recommended.

16.3   KALETRA Oral Solution
KALETRA (lopinavir and ritonavir) oral solution is a light yellow to orange colored liquid supplied in amber-colored multiple-dose bottles containing 400 mg lopinavir and 100 mg ritonavir per 5 mL (80 mg lopinavir and 20 mg ritonavir per mL) packaged with a marked dosing cup in the following size:
160 mL bottle ....(NDC 0074-3956-46)
Recommended Storage
Store KALETRA oral solution at 2°-8°C (36°-46°F) until dispensed. Avoid exposure to excessive heat. For patient use, refrigerated KALETRA oral solution remains stable until the expiration date printed on the label. If stored at room temperature up to 25°C (77°F), oral solution should be used within 2 months.

17   PATIENT COUNSELING INFORMATION
Advise the patient to read the FDA-approved patient labeling (Medication Guide)
Patients or parents of patients should be informed that:
General Information
❏ They should pay special attention to accurate administration of their dose to minimize the risk of accidental overdose or underdose of KALETRA.
❏ They should inform their healthcare provider if their children's weight changes in order to make sure that the child's KALETRA dose is the correct one.
❏ They should take the prescribed dose of KALETRA as directed and to set up a daily routine in order to do so.
❏ KALETRA tablets may be taken with or without food. KALETRA oral solution should be taken with food to enhance absorption.
❏ Sustained decreases in plasma HIV-1 RNA have been associated with a reduced risk of progression to AIDS and death. Patients should remain under the care of a physician while using KALETRA. Patients should be advised to take KALETRA and other concomitant antiretroviral therapy every day as prescribed. KALETRA must always be used in combination with other antiretroviral drugs. Patients should not alter the dose or discontinue therapy without consulting with their doctor. If a dose of

KALETRA is missed patients should take the dose as soon as possible and then return to their normal schedule. However, if a dose is skipped the patient should not double the next dose. The amount of HIV-1 virus in their blood may increase if the medicine is stopped for even a short time. The virus may become resistant to KALETRA and become harder to treat.
❏ KALETRA is not a cure for HIV-1 infection and patients may continue to experience illnesses associated with HIV-1 infection, including opportunistic infections. Patients should remain under the care of a physician when using KALETRA.
Patients should be advised to avoid doing things that can spread HIV-1 infection to others.
• **Do not share needles or other injection equipment.**
• **Do not share personal items that can have blood or body fluids on them, like toothbrushes and razor blades.**
• **Do not have any kind of sex without protection.** Always practice safe sex by using a latex or polyurethane condom to lower the chance of sexual contact with semen, vaginal secretions, or blood.
• **Do not breastfeed.** Mothers with HIV-1 should not breastfeed because HIV-1 can be passed to the baby in the breast milk.
Drug Interactions
❏ KALETRA may interact with some drugs; therefore, patients should be advised to report to their doctor the use of any other prescription, non-prescription medication or herbal products, particularly St. John's Wort.
❏ KALETRA tablets can be taken at the same time as didanosine without food. Patients taking didanosine should take didanosine one hour before or two hours after KALETRA oral solution.
❏ If they are receiving avanafil, sildenafil, tadalafil, or vardenafil for the treatment of erectile dysfunction, there may be an increased risk of associated adverse reactions including hypotension, visual changes, and sustained erection, and should promptly report any symptoms to their doctor. If they are currently using or planning to use avanafil or tadalafil (for the treatment of pulmonary arterial hypertension) they should ask their doctor about potential adverse reactions these medications may cause when taken with KALETRA. The doctor may choose not to keep them on avanafil, or may adjust the dose of tadalafil while initiating treatment with KALETRA.
❏ If they are receiving estrogen-based hormonal contraceptives, additional or alternate contraceptive measures should be used during therapy with KALETRA.
❏ If they are taking or before they begin using Serevent® (salmeterol) and KALETRA, they should talk to their doctor about problems these two medications may cause when taken together. The doctor may choose not to keep someone on Serevent® (salmeterol).
❏ If they are taking or before they begin taking Advair® (salmeterol in combination with fluticasone propionate) and KALETRA, they should talk to their doctor about problems these two medications may cause when taken together. The doctor may choose not to keep someone on Advair® (salmeterol in combination with fluticasone propionate).
Potential Adverse Effects
❏ Skin rashes ranging in severity from mild to toxic epidermal necrolysis (TEN), Stevens-Johnson syndrome, erythema multiforme, urticaria, and angioedema have been reported in patients receiving KALETRA or its components lopinavir and/or ritonavir. Patients should be advised to contact their healthcare provider if they develop a rash while taking KALETRA. The healthcare provider will determine if treatment should be continued or an alternative antiretroviral regimen used.
❏ Patients should be advised that appropriate liver function testing will be conducted prior to initiating and during therapy with KALETRA. Pre-existing liver disease including Hepatitis B or C can worsen with use of KALETRA. This can be seen as worsening of transaminase elevations or hepatic decompensation. Patients should be advised that their liver function tests will need to be monitored closely especially during the first several months of KALETRA treatment and that they should notify their healthcare provider if they develop the signs and symptoms of worsening liver disease including loss of appetite, abdominal pain, jaundice, and itchy skin.
❏ New onset of diabetes or exacerbation of pre-existing diabetes mellitus, and hyperglycemia have been reported

during KALETRA use. Patients should be advised to notify their healthcare provider if they develop the signs and symptoms of diabetes mellitus including frequent urination, excessive thirst, extreme hunger or unusual weight loss and/or an increased blood sugar while on KALETRA as they may require a change in their diabetes treatment or new treatment.

❑ KALETRA might produce changes in the electrocardiogram (e.g., PR and/or QT prolongation). Patients should consult their physician if they experience symptoms such as dizziness, lightheadedness, abnormal heart rhythm or loss of consciousness.

❑ They should seek medical assistance immediately if they develop a sustained penile erection lasting more than 4 hours while taking KALETRA® (lopinavir and ritonavir) and a PDE 5 Inhibitor such as Viagra, Cialis or Levitra.

❑ Redistribution or accumulation of body fat may occur in patients receiving antiretroviral therapy and that the cause and long term health effects of these conditions are not known at this time.

❑ Patients should be informed that there may be a greater chance of developing diarrhea with the once daily regimen as compared with the twice daily regimen.

KALETRA Tablets, 200 mg lopinavir and 50 mg ritonavir Manufactured by AbbVie LTD, Barceloneta, PR 00617 for AbbVie Inc., North Chicago, IL 60064 USA
KALETRA Tablets, 100 mg lopinavir and 25 mg ritonavir and KALETRA Oral Solution
AbbVie Inc., North Chicago, IL 60064 USA
The brands listed are trademarks of their respective owners and are not trademarks of AbbVie Inc. The makers of these brands are not affiliated with and do not endorse AbbVie Inc. or its products.
© 2015 AbbVie Inc. All rights reserved.
03-B238

MEDICATION GUIDE
KALETRA® (kuh-LEE-tra)
(lopinavir and ritonavir)
tablets
KALETRA® (kuh-LEE-tra)
(lopinavir and ritonavir)
oral solution

Read this Medication Guide before you start taking KALETRA and each time you get a refill. There may be new information. This information does not take the place of talking with your doctor about your medical condition or treatment. You and your doctor should talk about your treatment with KALETRA before you start taking it and at regular check-ups. You should stay under your doctor's care when taking KALETRA.

What is the most important information I should know about KALETRA?

KALETRA may cause serious side effects, including:

• **Interactions with other medicines. It is important to know the medicines that should not be taken with KALETRA.** For more information, see "Who should not take KALETRA?"

• **Changes in your heart rhythm and the electrical activity of your heart.** These changes may be seen on an EKG (electrocardiogram) and can lead to serious heart problems. Your risk for these problems may be higher if you:
  ◦ already have a history of abnormal heart rhythm or other types of heart disease.
  ◦ take other medicines that can affect your heart rhythm while you take KALETRA.

Tell your doctor right away if you have any of these symptoms while taking KALETRA:
• dizziness
• lightheadedness
• fainting
• sensation of abnormal heartbeats

See "What are the possible side effects of KALETRA?" for more information about serious side effects.

What is KALETRA?

KALETRA® (lopinavir and ritonavir) is a prescription HIV-1 medicine that used with other HIV medicines to treat HIV-1 (Human Immunodeficiency Virus) infection in adults and children 14 days of age and older. HIV is the virus that causes AIDS (Acquired Immune Deficiency Syndrome). KALETRA is a type of HIV medicine called a protease inhibitor. KALETRA contains two medicines: lopinavir and ritonavir.

When used with other HIV medicines, KALETRA may help to reduce the amount of HIV in your blood (called "viral load"). KALETRA may also help to increase the number of white blood cells called CD4 (T) cell which help fight off other infections. Reducing the amount of HIV and increas-

ing the CD4 (T) cell count may improve your immune system. This may reduce your risk of death or infections that can happen when your immune system is weak (opportunistic infections).

It is not known if KALETRA is safe and effective in children under 14 days old.

Table 15 *(Cont.)* **Drug Interactions: Pharmacokinetic Parameters for Co-administered Drug in the Presence of KALETRA for Recommended Alterations in Dose or Regimen**

Co-administered Drug	Dose of Co-administered Drug (mg)	Dose of KALETRA (mg)	n	Ratio (in combination with KALETRA/alone) of Co-administered Drug Pharmacokinetic Parameters (90% CI); No Effect = 1.00		
				C_{max}	AUC	C_{min}
Nevirapine	200 once daily, 14 d; twice daily, 6 d	400/100 capsule twice daily, 20 d	5, 6*	1.05 (0.72, 1.52)	1.08 (0.72, 1.64)	1.15 (0.71, 1.86)
Norethindrone	1 once daily, 21 d (Ortho Novum®)	400/100 capsule twice daily, 14 d	12	0.84 (0.75, 0.94)	0.83 (0.73, 0.94)	0.68 (0.54, 0.85)
Pitavastatin[5]	4 once daily, 5 d	400/100 tablet twice daily, 16 d	23	0.96 (0.84-1.10)	0.80 (0.73-0.87)	N/A
Pravastatin	20 once daily, 4 d	400/100 capsule twice daily, 14 d	12	1.26 (0.87, 1.83)	1.33 (0.91, 1.94)	N/A
Rifabutin	150 once daily, 10 d; combo vs. 300 once daily, 10 d; alone	400/100 capsule twice daily, 10 d	12	2.12 (1.89, 2.38)	3.03 (2.79, 3.30)	4.90 (3.18, 5.76)
25-*O*-desacetyl rifabutin				23.6 (13.7, 25.3)	47.5 (29.3, 51.8)	94.9 (74.0, 122)
Rifabutin + 25-*O*-desacetyl rifabutin[6]				3.46 (3.07, 3.91)	5.73 (5.08, 6.46)	9.53 (7.56, 12.01)
Rilpivirine	150 once daily[10]	400/100 twice daily (capsules)	15	1.29 (1.18-1.40)	1.52 (1.36-1.70)	1.74 (1.46-2.08)
Rosuvastatin[7]	20 once daily, 7 d	400/100 tablet twice daily, 7 d	15	4.66 (3.4, 6.4)	2.08 (1.66, 2.6)	1.04 (0.9, 1.2)
Tenofovir[8]	300 once daily, 14 d	400/100 capsule twice daily, 14 d	24	NC†	1.32 (1.26, 1.38)	1.51 (1.32, 1.66)

All interaction studies conducted in healthy, HIV-1 negative subjects unless otherwise indicated.
1 Data extracted from the bedaquiline package insert.
2 Ratio of parameters for indinavir, and nelfinavir, are not normalized for dose.
3 Desipramine is a probe substrate for assessing effects on CYP2D6-mediated metabolism.
4 Data extracted from the fosamprenavir package insert.
5 Data extracted from the pitavastatin package insert and results presented at the 2011 International AIDS Society Conference on HIV Pathogenesis, Treatment and Prevention (Morgan, *et al*, poster *#MOPE170*).
6 Effect on the dose-normalized sum of rifabutin parent and 25-*O*-desacetyl rifabutin active metabolite.
7 Kiser, et al. J Acquir Immune Defic Syndr. 2008 Apr 15;47(5):570-8.
8 Data extracted from the tenofovir package insert.
9 N=12 for C_{min} (test arm)
10 This interaction study has been performed with a dose higher than the recommended dose for rilpivirine (25 mg once daily) assessing the maximal effect on the co-administered drug.
* Parallel group design; n for KALETRA + co-administered drug, n for co-administered drug alone.
N/A = Not available.
† NC = No change.

Table 16. Virologic Response (HIV-1 RNA <400 copies/mL) at Week 48 by Baseline KALETRA Susceptibility and by Number of Protease Substitutions Associated with Reduced Response to KALETRA[1]

Number of protease inhibitor substitutions at baseline[1]	Study 888 (Single protease inhibitor-experienced[2], NNRTI-naïve) n=130	Study 765 (Single protease inhibitor-experienced[3], NNRTI-naïve) n=56	Study 957 (Multiple protease inhibitor-experienced[4], NNRTI-naïve) n=50
0-2	76/103 (74%)	34/45 (76%)	19/20 (95%)
3-5	13/26 (50%)	8/11 (73%)	18/26 (69%)
6 or more	0/1 (0%)	N/A	1/4 (25%)

1 Substitutions considered in the analysis included L10F/I/R/V, K20M/N/R, L24I, L33F, M36I, I47V, G48V, I54L/T/V, V82A/C/F/S/T, and I84V.
2 43% indinavir, 42% nelfinavir, 10% ritonavir, 15% saquinavir.
3 41% indinavir, 38% nelfinavir, 4% ritonavir, 16% saquinavir.
4 86% indinavir, 54% nelfinavir, 80% ritonavir, 70% saquinavir.

KALETRA does not cure HIV infection or AIDS. People taking KALETRA may develop infections or other conditions associated with HIV infection, including opportunistic infections (for example, pneumonia and herpes virus infections).

Continued on next page

Table 18. Outcomes of Randomized Treatment Through Week 48 (Study 863)

Outcome	KALETRA+d4T+3TC (N = 326)	Nelfinavir+d4T+3TC (N = 327)
Responder[1]	75%	62%
Virologic failure[2]	9%	25%
Rebound	7%	15%
Never suppressed through Week 48	2%	9%
Death	2%	1%
Discontinued due to adverse events	4%	4%
Discontinued for other reasons[3]	10%	8%

1 Patients achieved and maintained confirmed HIV-1 RNA < 400 copies/mL through Week 48.
2 Includes confirmed viral rebound and failure to achieve confirmed < 400 copies/mL through Week 48.
3 Includes lost to follow-up, patient's withdrawal, non-compliance, protocol violation and other reasons. Overall discontinuation through Week 48, including patients who discontinued subsequent to virologic failure, was 17% in the KALETRA arm and 24% in the nelfinavir arm.

Avoid doing things that can spread HIV-1 infection to others:
• **Do not share needles or other injection equipment.**
• **Do not share personal items that can have blood or body fluids on them, like toothbrushes and razor blades.**
• **Do not have any kind of sex without protection.** Always practice safer sex by using a latex or polyurethane condom to lower the chance of sexual contact with semen, vaginal secretions, or blood.
Ask your doctor if you have any questions on how to prevent passing HIV to other people.

Who should not take KALETRA?
Do not take KALETRA if you take any of the following medicines:
• alfuzosin (Uroxatral®)
• cisapride (Propulsid®, Quicksolv®)
• ergot containing medicines including
  ○ ergotamine tartrate (Cafergot®, Migergot®, Ergomar®, Ergostat®, Medihaler®, Ergotamine, Wigraine®, Wigrettes®)
  ○ dihydroergotamine mesylate (D.H.E. 45®, Migranal®)
  ○ methylergonovine (Methergine®)
• lovastatin (Advicor®, Altoprev®, Mevacor®)
• midazolam oral syrup
• pimozide (Orap®)
• rifampin (Rifadin®, Rifamate®, Rifater®, Rimactane®)
• sildenafil (Revatio®), when used for the treatment of pulmonary arterial hypertension
• simvastatin (Zocor®, Vytorin®, Simcor®)
• St. John's Wort (Hypericum perforatum)
• triazolam (Halcion®)
Serious problems can happen if you or your child take any of the medicines listed above with KALETRA.
• **Do not take KALETRA if you are allergic** to lopinavir, ritonavir or any of the ingredients in KALETRA. See the end of this Medication Guide for a complete list of ingredients in KALETRA.
What should I tell my doctor before taking KALETRA?
KALETRA may not be right for you. Tell your doctor about all your medical conditions, including if you:
• have any heart problems, including if you have a condition called Congenital Long QT Syndrome.
• have or had pancreas problems.
• have liver problems, including Hepatitis B or Hepatitis C.
• have diabetes.
• have hemophilia. People who take KALETRA may have increased bleeding.
• have low potassium in your blood.
• are pregnant or plan to become pregnant. Taking KALETRA during pregnancy has not been associated with an increased risk of birth defects. You and your doctor should decide if KALETRA is right for you.
Pregnancy Registry. There is a pregnancy registry for women who take antiretroviral medicines during pregnancy. The purpose of the pregnancy registry is to collect information about the health of you and your baby. Talk to your doctor about how you can take part in this registry.
• are breastfeeding or plan to breastfeed. **Do not breastfeed if you take KALETRA.**
  • You should not breastfeed if you have HIV-1 because of the risk of passing HIV-1 to your baby.
  • Talk to your doctor about the best way to feed your baby.
Tell your doctor about all the medicines you take, including prescription and over-the-counter medicines, vitamins, and herbal supplements. Many medicines interact with KALETRA. Do not start taking a new medicine without tell-

ing your doctor or pharmacist. Your doctor can tell you if it is safe to take KALETRA with other medicines. Your doctor may need to change the dose of other medicines while you take KALETRA.
Especially tell your doctor if you take:
• medicine to treat HIV
• estrogen-based contraceptives (birth control pills and patches). KALETRA may reduce the effectiveness of estrogen-based contraceptives. During treatment with KALETRA, you should use a different type or an extra form of birth control. Talk to your doctor about what types of birth control you can use to prevent pregnancy while taking KALETRA.
• medicines to prevent organ transplant rejection
• medicines to treat cancer
• amiodarone (Cordarone®, Pacerone®)
• atorvastatin (Lipitor®)
• atovaquone (Marlarone®, Mepron®)
• avanafil (Stendra®), sildenafil (Viagra®), tadalafil (Cialis®), or vardenafil (Levitra®) for the treatment of erectile dysfunction (ED). If you get dizzy or faint (low blood pressure), have vision changes or have an erection that last longer than 4 hours, call your doctor or get medical help right away.
• bedaquiline (Sirturo®)
• bepridil (Bepadin®, Vascor®)
• boceprevir (Victrelis®)
• bosentan (Tracleer®)
• budesonide (Rhinocort®, Symbicort®, Pulmicort®, Entocort EC®)
• bupropion (Aplenzin®, Forfivo XL®, Wellbutrin®, Zyban®)
• carbamazepine (Carbatrol®, Epitol®, Equetro®, Tegretol®)
• clarithromycin (Biaxin®, Prevpac®)
• colchicine (Colcrys®)
• dexamethasone (Maxidex®, Ozurdex®)
• disulfiram
• felodipine
• fentanyl (Abstral®, Actiq®, Duragesic®, Fentora®, Lazanda®, Onsolis®, Subsys®)
• fluticasone (Cutivate®, Flonase®, Flovent®, Flovent Diskus®, Flovent HFA®, Veramyst®)
• itraconazole (Onmel®, Sporanox®)
• ketoconazole (Extina®, Ketozole®, Nizoral®, Xolegel®)
• lamotrigine (Lamictal®)
• lidocaine
• methadone hydrochloride (Dolphine hydrochloride, Methadose®)
• metronidazole
• nicardipine (Cardene®)
• nifedipine (Adalat CC®, Afeditab CR®, Procardia®)
• phenobarbital
• phenytoin (Dilantin®, Phenytek®)
• prednisone
• quinidine (Quinidex®)
• quetiapine (Seroquel®)
• rifabutin (Mycobutin®)
• rivaroxaban (Xarelto®)
• rosuvastatin (Crestor®)
• salmeterol (Serevent®) or salmeterol when taken in combination with fluticasone (Advair Diskus®, Advair HFA®)
• simeprevir (Olysio®)
• tadalafil (Adcirca®) for the treatment of pulmonary arterial hypertension
• trazodone (Oleptro®)
• valproate (Depakote®, Depakene®, Depacon®)
• voriconazole (Vfend®)
• warfarin (Coumadin®, Jantoven®)

KALETRA should not be administered once daily in combination with carbamazepine (Carbatrol®, Epitol®, Equetro®, Tegretol®), phenobarbital, or phenytoin (Dilantin®, Phenytek®)
Ask your doctor or pharmacist if you are not sure if your medicine is one that is listed above.
Know all the medicines that you take. Keep a list of them with you to show doctors and pharmacists when you get a new medicine.
If you are not sure if you are taking a medicine above, ask your doctor.
How should I take KALETRA?
• Take KALETRA every day exactly as prescribed by your doctor.
• It is very important to set up a dosing schedule and follow it every day.
• Do not change your treatment or stop treatment without first talking with your doctor.
• KALETRA tablets **should not** be taken 1 time each day if you are pregnant. You **should not** take KALETRA oral solution if you are pregnant.
• Swallow KALETRA tablets whole. Do not chew, break, or crush KALETRA tablets.
• KALETRA tablets can be taken with or without food.
• If you are taking both didanosine (Videx®) and KALETRA:
  ○ didanosine can be taken at the same time as KALETRA tablets, without food.
  ○ take didanosine either one hour before or two hours after taking KALETRA oral solution.
• Do not miss a dose of KALETRA. This could make the virus harder to treat. If you forget to take KALETRA, take the missed dose right away. If it is almost time for your next dose, do not take the missed dose. Instead, follow your regular dosing schedule by taking your next dose at its regular time. Do not take more than one dose of KALETRA at one time.
• If you take more than the prescribed dose of KALETRA, call your doctor or go to the nearest emergency room right away.
• Take KALETRA oral solution with food to help it work better.
• If your child is prescribed KALETRA, tell your doctor if your child's weight changes.
• KALETRA **should not** be given one time each day in children. When giving KALETRA to your child, give KALETRA exactly as prescribed.
• KALETRA oral solution contains propylene glycol and a large amount of alcohol. KALETRA oral solution **should not** be given to babies younger than 14 days of age unless your doctor thinks it is right for your baby.
  ○ If a young child drinks more than the recommended dose, it could make them sick. Contact your local poison control center or emergency room right away.
  ○ Talk with your doctor if you take or plan to take metronidazole or disulfiram. You can have severe nausea and vomiting if you take these medicines with KALETRA.
• When your KALETRA supply starts to run low, get more from your doctor or pharmacy. It is important not to run out of KALETRA. The amount of HIV-1 virus in your blood may increase if the medicine is stopped for even a short time. The virus may become resistant to KALETRA and become harder to treat.

What are the possible side effects of KALETRA?
KALETRA can cause serious side effects, including:
• See "What is the most important information I should know about KALETRA?"
• **Inflammation of the pancreas (pancreatitis).** Some people who take KALETRA get inflammation of the pancreas which may be serious and cause death. You have a higher chance of getting pancreatitis if you have had it before. Tell your doctor if you have nausea, vomiting, or abdominal pain while taking KALETRA. These may be signs of pancreatitis.
• **Liver problems.** Liver problems, including death, can happen in people who take KALETRA. Your doctor should do blood tests before and during your treatment with KALETRA to check your liver function. Some people with liver disease such as Hepatitis B and Hepatitis C who take KALETRA may have worsening liver disease. Tell your doctor right away if you have any of these signs and symptoms of liver problems:
  ○ loss of appetite
  ○ yellow skin and whites of eyes (jaundice)

Information on the AbbVie, Inc. products listed on these pages is from the prescribing information in use as of July 31, 2016. For more information, please visit rxabbvie.com or call 1-800-633-9110.

○ dark-colored urine
○ pale colored stools
○ itchy skin
○ stomach area (abdominal) pain.
- **Diabetes and high blood sugar (hyperglycemia).** Some people who take protease inhibitors including KALETRA get new or more serious diabetes, or high blood sugar. Tell your doctor if you notice an increase in thirst or urinate often while taking KALETRA.
- **Changes in your immune system (Immune Reconstitution Syndrome)** can happen when you start taking HIV medicines. Your immune system may get stronger and begin to fight infections that have been hidden in your body for a long time. Call your doctor right away if you start having new symptoms after starting your HIV medicine.
- **Increases in certain fat (triglycerides and cholesterol) levels in your blood.** Large increases of triglycerides and cholesterol can be seen in blood test results of some people who take KALETRA. Your doctor should do blood tests to check your cholesterol and triglyceride levels before you start taking KALETRA and during your treatment.
- **Changes in body fat.** Changes in body fat in some people who take antiretroviral therapy. These changes may include increased amount of fat in the upper back and neck ("buffalo hump"), breast, and around the trunk. Loss of fat from the legs, arms and face may also happen. The cause and long-term health effects of these conditions are not known at this time.
- **Increased bleeding for hemophiliacs.** Some people with hemophilia have increased bleeding with protease inhibitors including KALETRA.
- **Allergic reactions.** Skin rashes, some of them severe, can occur in people who take KALETRA. Tell your doctor if you had a rash when you took another medicine for your HIV-1 infection or if you notice any skin rash when you take KALETRA.
- **Babies taking KALETRA oral solution may have side effects.** KALETRA oral solution contains alcohol and propylene glycol. Call your doctor right away if your baby appears too sleepy or their breathing has changed.

Common side effects of KALETRA include:
- diarrhea
- nausea
- increased fats in blood (triglycerides or cholesterol)
- vomiting

Tell your doctor about any side effect that bothers you or that does not go away.

These are not all of the possible side effects of KALETRA. For more information, ask your doctor or pharmacist.

Call your doctor for medical advice about side effects. You may report side effects to FDA at 1-800-FDA-1088.

How should I store KALETRA?
KALETRA tablets:
- Store KALETRA tablets at room temperature, between 59°F to 86°F (15°C to 30°C).
- Do not keep KALETRA tablets out of the container it comes in for longer than 2 weeks, especially in areas where there is a lot of humidity. Keep the container closed tightly.

KALETRA oral solution:
- Store KALETRA oral solution in a refrigerator, between 36°F to 46°F (2°C to 8°C). KALETRA oral solution that is kept refrigerated may be used until the expiration date printed on the label.
- KALETRA oral solution that is stored at room temperature (less than 77°F or 25°C) should be used within 2 months.
- Keep KALETRA away from high heat.

Throw away any medicine that is out of date or that you no longer need.

Keep KALETRA and all medicines out of the reach of children.

General information about KALETRA

Medicines are sometimes prescribed for purposes other than those listed in a Medication Guide. Do not use KALETRA® (lopinavir and ritonavir) for a condition for which it was not prescribed. Do not give KALETRA to other people, even if they have the same condition you have. It may harm them.

This Medication Guide summarizes the most important information about KALETRA. If you would like more information, talk with your doctor. You can ask your pharmacist or doctor for information about KALETRA that is written for health professionals.

For more information about KALETRA call 1-800-633-9110 or go to www.KALETRA.com.

What are the ingredients in KALETRA?

Active ingredients: lopinavir and ritonavir
Inactive ingredients:

Table 19. Proportion of Responders Through Week 48 by Baseline Viral Load (Study 863)

Baseline Viral Load (HIV-1 RNA copies/mL)	KALETRA +d4T+3TC			Nelfinavir +d4T+3TC		
	<400 copies/mL [1]	<50 copies/mL [2]	n	<400 copies/mL [1]	<50 copies/mL [2]	n
< 30,000	74%	71%	82	79%	72%	87
≥ 30,000 to < 100,000	81%	73%	79	67%	54%	79
≥ 100,000 to < 250,000	75%	64%	83	60%	47%	72
≥ 250,000	72%	60%	82	44%	33%	89

1 Patients achieved and maintained confirmed HIV-1 RNA < 400 copies/mL through Week 48.
2 Patients achieved HIV-1 RNA < 50 copies/mL at Week 48.

KALETRA 200 mg lopinavir and 50 mg ritonavir tablets: copovidone, sorbitan monolaurate, colloidal silicon dioxide, and sodium stearyl fumarate. The film coating contains: hypromellose, titanium dioxide, polyethylene glycol 400, hydroxypropyl cellulose, talc, colloidal silicon dioxide, polyethylene glycol 3350, yellow ferric oxide 172, and polysorbate 80.

KALETRA 100 mg lopinavir and 25 mg ritonavir tablets: copovidone, sorbitan monolaurate, colloidal silicon dioxide, and sodium stearyl fumarate. The film coating contains: polyvinyl alcohol, titanium dioxide, talc, polytheylene glycol 3350, and yellow ferric oxide E172.

KALETRA oral solution: acesulfame potassium, alcohol, artificial cotton candy flavor, citric acid, glycerin, high fructose corn syrup, Magnasweet-110 flavor, menthol, natural and artificial vanilla flavor, peppermint oil, polyoxyl 40 hydrogenated castor oil, povidone, propylene glycol, saccharin sodium, sodium chloride, sodium citrate, and water.

KALETRA oral solution contains 42.4% alcohol (v/v). "See How should I take KALETRA?".

This Medication Guide has been approved by the U.S. Food and Drug Administration.

KALETRA Tablets, 200 mg lopinavir and 50 mg ritonavir
Manufactured by AbbVie LTD, Barceloneta, PR 00617
for AbbVie Inc., North Chicago, IL 60064 USA
KALETRA Tablets, 100 mg lopinavir and 25 mg ritonavir
and KALETRA Oral Solution
AbbVie Inc., North Chicago, IL 60064 USA
Revised: November 2015

The brands listed are trademarks of their respective owners and are not trademarks of AbbVie Inc. The makers of these brands are not affiliated with and do not endorse AbbVie Inc. or its products.

© 2015 AbbVie Inc. All rights reserved.
03-B238

Shown in Product Identification Guide, page 505

LUPANETA PACK® ℞
[loo-pan-e-tə pæk]
(leuprolide acetate for depot suspension, 3.75 mg for intramuscular injection only and norethindrone acetate tablets, 5 mg for oral administration)

HIGHLIGHTS OF PRESCRIBING INFORMATION
These highlights do not include all the information needed to use LUPANETA PACK safely and effectively. See full prescribing information for LUPANETA PACK.

LUPANETA PACK (leuprolide acetate for depot suspension; norethindrone acetate tablets), co-packaged for intramuscular use and for oral use, respectively
Initial U.S. Approval: 2012

INDICATIONS AND USAGE

LUPANETA PACK contains leuprolide acetate, a gonadotropin-releasing hormone (GnRH) agonist and norethindrone acetate, a progestin, indicated for
- Initial management of the painful symptoms of endometriosis (1)
- Management of recurrence of symptoms (1)

Limitations of Use: Initial treatment course is limited to 6 months and use is not recommended longer than a total of 12 months due to concerns about adverse impact on bone mineral density. (1, 2.1, 5.1)

DOSAGE AND ADMINISTRATION
- Leuprolide acetate for depot suspension 3.75 mg given by a healthcare provider as a single intramuscular injection every month for up to six injections (6 months of therapy) (2.1)

- Norethindrone acetate 5 mg tablets taken orally by the patient once per day for up to 6 months (2.1)
- If endometriosis symptoms recur after initial course of therapy, consider retreatment for up to another six months (2.1)
- Assess bone density before retreatment begins (2.1, 5.1)
- Reconstitute leuprolide acetate prior to use, see important administration instructions (2.3)

DOSAGE FORMS AND STRENGTHS
- Leuprolide acetate for depot suspension 3.75 mg syringe (3)
- Norethindrone acetate 5 mg tablets; 30 count bottle (3)

CONTRAINDICATIONS
- Hypersensitivity to GnRH, GnRH agonist or any of the excipients in leuprolide acetate for depot suspension or norethindrone acetate (4)
- Undiagnosed abnormal uterine bleeding (4)
- Pregnancy or suspected pregnancy (4, 8.1)
- Women who are breast-feeding (4)
- Known, suspected or history of breast or other hormone-sensitive cancer (4)
- Thrombotic or thromboembolic disorders (4)
- Liver tumors or liver disease (4)

WARNINGS AND PRECAUTIONS
- Loss of bone mineral density: do not use for more than two six-month treatment courses. (1, 2.1, 5.1)
- Exclude pregnancy before starting treatment and discontinue use if pregnancy occurs; use non-hormonal methods of contraception only. (5.2)
- Discontinue in case of sudden loss of vision or onset of proptosis, diplopia or migraine. (5.3)
- Carefully observe patients with history of depression and discontinue the drug if the depression recurs to a serious degree. (5.4)
- Assess and manage risk factors for cardiovascular disease before starting LUPANETA PACK. (5.6)

ADVERSE REACTIONS
Leuprolide acetate for depot suspension: Most common related adverse reactions (>10%) were hot flashes/sweats, headache/migraine, depression/emotional lability, nausea/vomiting, nervousness/anxiety, insomnia, pain, acne, asthenia, vaginitis, weight gain, constipation/diarrhea (6.1)
Progestins: breakthrough bleeding, spotting (6.1)
To report SUSPECTED ADVERSE REACTIONS, contact AbbVie Inc. at 1-800-633-9110 or FDA at 1-800-FDA-1088 or www.fda.gov/medwatch

USE IN SPECIFIC POPULATIONS
Pediatric: Safety and effectiveness of LUPANETA PACK has not been established in pediatric patients. (8.4)
Geriatric: LUPANETA PACK has not been studied in women over 65 years of age and is not indicated in this population. (8.5)
See 17 for PATIENT COUNSELING INFORMATION and FDA-approved patient labeling.

Revised: 6/2015

FULL PRESCRIBING INFORMATION: CONTENTS*
1   **INDICATIONS AND USAGE**
2   **DOSAGE AND ADMINISTRATION**
   2.1   Dosing Information
   2.2   Different Formulations of Leuprolide Acetate
   2.3   Reconstitution and Administration for Injection of Leuprolide Acetate

Continued on next page

FULL PRESCRIBING INFORMATION

1   INDICATIONS AND USAGE

LUPANETA PACK (leuprolide acetate for depot suspension and norethindrone acetate tablets) is indicated for initial management of the painful symptoms of endometriosis and for management of recurrence of symptoms.

Limitation of Use: Duration of use is limited due to concerns about adverse impact on bone mineral density *[see Warnings and Precautions (5.1)]*. The initial treatment course of LUPANETA PACK is limited to six months. A single retreatment course of not more than six months may be administered after the initial course of treatment if symptoms recur. Use of LUPANETA PACK for longer than a total of 12 months is not recommended.

2   DOSAGE AND ADMINISTRATION

2.1   Dosing Information

LUPANETA PACK is a co-packaging of leuprolide acetate for depot suspension for intramuscular use and norethindrone acetate tablets for oral use. Administer as follows:

• 3.75 mg of leuprolide acetate by intramuscular injection once a month for up to six injections (6 months of therapy); to be administered by a healthcare provider
• 5 mg of norethindrone acetate orally once daily for up to 6 months of therapy

The initial course of treatment with leuprolide acetate for depot suspension 3.75 mg in combination with norethindrone acetate 5 mg daily is not to exceed six months.

If the symptoms of endometriosis recur after the initial course of therapy, consider retreatment with LUPANETA PACK for up to another six months. It is recommended that bone density be assessed before retreatment begins *[see Warnings and Precautions (5.1)]*.

Treatment beyond two six-month courses has not been studied and is not recommended due to concerns about adverse impact on bone mineral density.

2.2   Different Formulations of Leuprolide Acetate

Due to the specific release characteristics of the 1-month depot formulation, HCPs should not administer 3 doses of the 3.75 mg 1-month formulation simultaneously to mimic the pharmacological profile of the 11.25 mg 3-month formulation.

2.3   Reconstitution and Administration for Injection of Leuprolide Acetate

• Reconstitute and administer the lyophilized microspheres as a single intramuscular injection.
• Inject the suspension immediately or discard if not used within two hours, because leuprolide acetate for depot suspension does not contain a preservative.

1. Visually inspect the leuprolide acetate for depot suspension powder. DO NOT USE the syringe if clumping or caking is evident. A thin layer of powder on the wall of the syringe is considered normal prior to mixing with the diluent. The diluent should appear clear.
2. To prepare for injection, screw the white plunger into the end stopper until the stopper begins to turn (see Figure 1 and Figure 2).
[See Figure 1 at the bottom of page 706]

Figure 2:

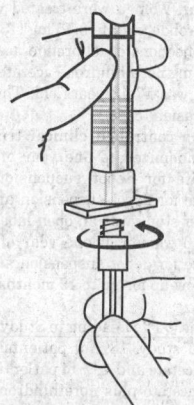

3. Hold the syringe UPRIGHT. Release the diluent by SLOWLY PUSHING (6 to 8 seconds) the plunger until the first middle stopper is at the blue line in the middle of the barrel (see Figure 3).

Figure 3:

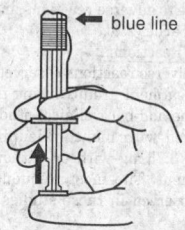

← blue line

4. Keep the syringe UPRIGHT. Mix the microspheres (powder) thoroughly by gently shaking the syringe until the powder forms a uniform suspension. The suspension will appear milky. If the powder adheres to the stopper or caking/clumping is present, tap the syringe with your finger to disperse. DO NOT USE if any of the powder has not gone into suspension (see Figure 4).

Figure 4:

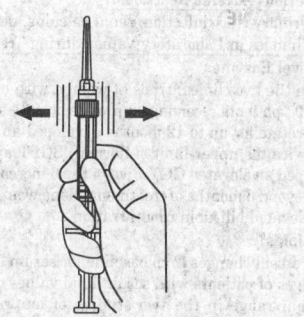

5. Keep the syringe UPRIGHT. With the opposite hand pull the needle cap upward without twisting.
6. Keep the syringe UPRIGHT. Advance the plunger to expel the air from the syringe. Now the syringe is ready for injection.
7. After cleaning the injection site with an alcohol swab, administer the intramuscular injection by inserting the needle at a 90 degree angle into the gluteal area, anterior thigh, or deltoid (see Figure 5). Alternate injection sites.
[See Figure 5 at top of next column]
NOTE: If a blood vessel is accidentally penetrated, aspirated blood will be visible just below the luer lock (see Figure 6) and can be seen through the transparent LuproLoc safety device. If blood is present, remove the needle immediately. Do not inject the medication.

Figure 5:

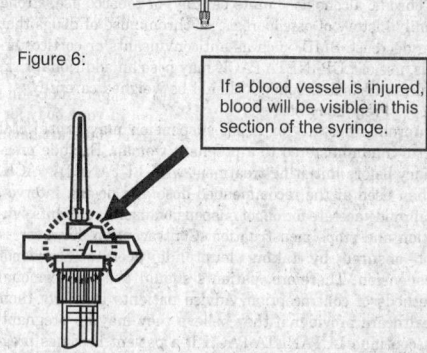

Figure 6:

If a blood vessel is injured, blood will be visible in this section of the syringe.

8. Inject the entire contents of the syringe intramuscularly.
9. Withdraw the needle. Once the syringe has been withdrawn, immediately activate the LuproLoc® safety device by pushing the arrow on the lock upward towards the needle tip with the thumb or finger, as illustrated, until the needle cover of the safety device over the needle is fully extended and a CLICK is heard or felt (see Figure 7).

Figure 7:

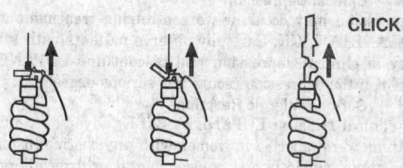

CLICK

10. Dispose of the syringe according to local regulations/procedures *[see References (15)]*.

3   DOSAGE FORMS AND STRENGTHS

LUPANETA PACK 1-month copackaged kit contains two separate components:

• Leuprolide acetate for depot suspension 3.75 mg for 1-month administration: Leuprolide acetate lyophilized powder for reconstitution with supplied diluent in a prefilled dual chamber syringe
• Norethindrone acetate 5 mg tablets: White to off-white oval, flat-faced beveled edged, uncoated debossed with 'G with breakline' on one side and 304 on other side

4   CONTRAINDICATIONS

LUPANETA PACK is contraindicated in women with the following:

• Hypersensitivity to gonadotropin-releasing hormone (GnRH), GnRH agonist analogs, any of the excipients in leuprolide acetate for depot suspension, or norethindrone acetate
• Undiagnosed abnormal uterine bleeding
• Known, suspected or planned pregnancy during the course of therapy *[see Use in Specific Populations (8.1)]*
• Lactating women *[see Use in Specific Populations (8.3)]*
• Known, suspected or history of breast cancer or other hormone-sensitive cancer
• Current or history of thrombotic or thromboembolic disorder
• Liver tumors or liver disease

5   WARNINGS AND PRECAUTIONS
5.1   Loss of Bone Mineral Density

Leuprolide acetate for depot suspension induces a hypoestrogenic state that results in loss of bone mineral density (BMD), some of which may not be reversible. Concurrent use of norethindrone acetate is effective in reducing the loss of BMD that occurs with leuprolide acetate *[see Clinical Studies (14)]*. Nonetheless, duration of use of LUPANETA

Continued on next page

Information on the AbbVie, Inc. products listed on these pages is from the prescribing information in use as of July 31, 2016. For more information, please visit rxabbvie.com or call 1-800-633-9110.

PACK is limited to two six-month courses of treatment due to concerns about the adverse impact on BMD. It is recommended that BMD be assessed before retreatment. Retreatment with leuprolide acetate for depot suspension alone is not recommended.

In women with major risk factors for decreased BMD such as chronic alcohol (> 3 units per day) or tobacco use, strong family history of osteoporosis, or chronic use of drugs that can decrease BMD, such as anticonvulsants or corticosteroids, use of LUPANETA PACK may pose an additional risk, and the risks and benefits should be weighed carefully.

5.2   Pregnancy Risk

Leuprolide acetate for depot suspension may cause fetal harm if administered to a pregnant woman. Exclude pregnancy before initiating treatment with LUPANETA PACK. When used at the recommended dose and dosing interval, leuprolide acetate for depot suspension usually inhibits ovulation and stops menstruation. Contraception, however, is not ensured by taking leuprolide acetate for depot suspension. Therefore, patients should use nonhormonal methods of contraception. Advise patients to notify their healthcare provider if they believe they may be pregnant. Discontinue LUPANETA PACK if a patient becomes pregnant during treatment and inform the patient of potential risk to the fetus *[see Contraindications (4) and Use in Specific Populations (8.1)]*.

5.3   Visual Abnormalities

Discontinue norethindrone acetate tablets in the LUPANETA PACK pending examination if there is a sudden partial or complete loss of vision or if there is sudden onset of proptosis, diplopia, or migraine. Discontinue LUPANETA PACK if examination reveals papilledema or retinal vascular lesions.

5.4   Clinical Depression

Depression may occur or worsen during treatment with LUPANETA PACK. Carefully observe patients with a history of clinical depression and discontinue LUPANETA PACK if the depression recurs to a serious degree.

5.5   Serious Allergic Reactions

In clinical trials of LUPANETA PACK, adverse events of asthma were reported in women with pre-existing histories of asthma, sinusitis and environmental or drug allergies. Symptoms consistent with an anaphylactoid or asthmatic process have been reported postmarketing.

5.6   Cardiovascular and Metabolic Disorders

Assess and manage risk factors for cardiovascular disease before starting LUPANETA PACK. Closely monitor women on norethindrone acetate who have risk factors for arterial vascular disease (e.g., hypertension, diabetes mellitus, tobacco use, hypercholesterolemia, and obesity) and/or venous thromboembolism (e.g., family history of VTE, obesity, and smoking) when using LUPANETA PACK. *[see Contraindications (4)]*.

5.7   Initial Flare of Symptoms

Following the first dose of leuprolide acetate, sex steroids temporarily rise above baseline because of the physiologic effect of the drug. Therefore, an increase in symptoms associated with endometriosis may be observed during the initial days of therapy, but these should dissipate with continued therapy.

5.8   Fluid Retention

Because norethindrone acetate may cause some degree of fluid retention, carefully observe women with conditions that might be influenced by this effect, such as epilepsy, migraine, cardiac or renal dysfunctions.

5.9   Convulsions

There have been postmarketing reports of convulsions in patients on leuprolide acetate therapy. These included patients with and without concurrent medications and comorbid conditions.

6   ADVERSE REACTIONS
6.1   Clinical Trials Experience

Because clinical trials are conducted under widely varying conditions, adverse reaction rates observed in the clinical trials of a drug cannot be directly compared to rates in the clinical trials of another drug and may not reflect the rates observed in clinical practice.

The safety of co-administering leuprolide acetate for depot suspension and norethindrone acetate was evaluated in two clinical studies in which a total of 242 women were treated for up to one year. Women were treated with monthly IM injections of leuprolide acetate 3.75 mg (13 injections) alone or monthly IM injections of leuprolide acetate 3.75 mg (13 injections) and 5 mg norethindrone acetate daily. The population age range was 17-43 years old. The majority of patients were Caucasian (87%).

One study was a controlled clinical trial in which 106 women were randomized to one year of treatment with leuprolide acetate for depot suspension alone or with leuprolide acetate for depot suspension and norethindrone acetate. The other study was an open-label single arm clinical study in 136 women of one year of treatment with leuprolide acetate for depot suspension and norethindrone acetate, with follow-up for up to 12 months after completing treatment.

Adverse Reactions (>1%) Leading to Study Discontinuation: In the controlled study, 18% of patients treated monthly with leuprolide acetate and 18% of patients treated monthly with leuprolide acetate plus norethindrone acetate discontinued therapy due to adverse reactions, most commonly hot flashes (6%) and insomnia (4%) in the leuprolide acetate alone group and hot flashes and emotional lability (4% each) in the leuprolide acetate and norethindrone group.

In the open label study, 13% of patients treated monthly with leuprolide acetate plus norethindrone acetate discontinued therapy due to adverse reactions, most commonly depression (4%) and acne (2%).

Common Adverse Reactions:

Table 1 lists the adverse reactions observed in at least 5% of patients in any treatment group, during the first 6 months of treatment in the add-back clinical studies, in which patients were treated with monthly leuprolide acetate for depot suspension 3.75 mg with or without norethindrone acetate co-treatment. The most frequently-occurring adverse reactions observed in these studies were hot flashes and headaches.

[See table 1 on next page]

In the controlled clinical trial, 50 of 51 (98%) patients in the leuprolide acetate alone group and 48 of 55 (87%) patients in the leuprolide acetate and norethindrone group reported experiencing hot flashes on one or more occasions during treatment. Table 2 presents hot flash data in the sixth month of treatment.

[See table 2 on page 708]

Serious Adverse Reactions:

Urinary tract infection, renal calculus, depression

Changes in Laboratory Values during Treatment:

Liver Enzymes

In the two clinical trials of women with endometriosis, 4 of 191 patients receiving leuprolide acetate and norethindrone acetate for up to 12 months developed an elevated (at least twice the upper limit of normal) SGPT and 2 of 136 developed an elevated GGT. Five of the 6 increases were observed beyond 6 months of treatment. None was associated with an elevated bilirubin concentration.

Lipids

Percent changes from baseline for serum lipids and percentages of patients with serum lipid values outside of the normal range in the two studies of leuprolide acetate and norethindrone acetate are summarized in the tables below. The major impact of adding norethindrone acetate to treatment with leuprolide acetate for depot suspension was a decrease in serum HDL cholesterol and an increase in the LDL/HDL ratio.

[See table 3 on page 708]

Changes from baseline tended to be greater at Week 52. After treatment, mean serum lipid levels from patients with follow up data (105 of 158 patients) returned to pretreatment values.

[See table 4 on page 708]

6.2   Postmarketing Experience

The following adverse reactions have been identified during postapproval use of leuprolide acetate for depot suspension or norethindrone acetate. Because these reactions are reported voluntarily from a population of uncertain size, it is not always possible to reliably estimate their frequency or establish a causal relationship to drug exposure.

Leuprolide Acetate for Depot Suspension

During postmarketing surveillance with other dosage forms and in the same or different populations, the following adverse reactions were reported:

- Allergic reactions (anaphylactic, rash, urticaria, and photosensitivity reactions)
- Mood swings, including depression
- Suicidal ideation and attempt
- Symptoms consistent with an anaphylactoid or asthmatic process
- Localized reactions including induration and abscess at the site of injection
- Symptoms consistent with fibromyalgia (e.g., joint and muscle pain, headaches, sleep disorders, gastrointestinal distress, and shortness of breath), individually and collectively

Other adverse reactions reported are:

Hepato-biliary disorder - Serious liver injury

Injury, poisoning and procedural complications - Spinal fracture

Investigations - Decreased white blood count

Musculoskeletal and connective tissue disorder - Tenosynovitis-like symptoms

Nervous System disorder - Convulsion, peripheral neuropathy, paralysis

Vascular disorder - Hypotension, Hypertension

Serious venous and arterial thrombotic and thromboembolic events, including deep vein thrombosis, pulmonary embolism, myocardial infarction, stroke, and transient ischemic attack

Pituitary apoplexy

During post-marketing surveillance, cases of pituitary apoplexy (a clinical syndrome secondary to infarction of the pituitary gland) have been reported after the administration of leuprolide acetate and other GnRH agonists. In a majority of these cases, a pituitary adenoma was diagnosed, with a majority of pituitary apoplexy cases occurring within 2 weeks of the first dose, and some within the first hour. In these cases, pituitary apoplexy has presented as sudden headache, vomiting, visual changes, ophthalmoplegia, altered mental status, and sometimes cardiovascular collapse. Immediate medical attention has been required.

7   DRUG INTERACTIONS
7.1   Drug-Drug Interactions

Leuprolide Acetate for Depot Suspension

No pharmacokinetic-based drug-drug interaction studies have been conducted with leuprolide acetate for depot suspension. However, drug interactions associated with cytochrome P-450 enzymes or protein binding would not be expected to occur *[see Clinical Pharmacology (12.3)]*.

Norethindrone Acetate

No pharmacokinetic drug interaction studies investigating any drug-drug interactions with norethindrone acetate have been conducted. Drugs or herbal products that induce or inhibit certain enzymes, including CYP3A4, may decrease or increase the serum concentrations of norethindrone.

7.2   Drug/Laboratory Test Interactions

Leuprolide Acetate for Depot Suspension

Administration of leuprolide acetate for depot suspension in therapeutic doses results in suppression of the pituitary-gonadal system. Normal function is usually restored within three months after treatment is discontinued. Therefore, diagnostic tests of pituitary gonadotropic and gonadal functions conducted during treatment and for up to three months after discontinuation of leuprolide acetate for depot suspension may be affected.

Figure 1:

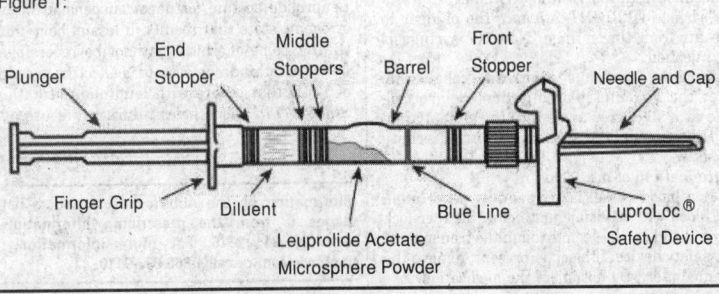

Plunger — End Stopper — Middle Stoppers — Barrel — Front Stopper — Needle and Cap — Finger Grip — Diluent — Leuprolide Acetate Microsphere Powder — Blue Line — LuproLoc® Safety Device

Table 1. Adverse Reactions Occurring in the First Six Months of Treatment in ≥ 5% of Patients with Endometriosis

	Controlled Study				Open Label Study	
	LA-Only*		LA/N†		LA/N†	
	N=51		N=55		N=136	
Adverse Reactions	N	%	N	%	N	%
Any Adverse Reaction	50	98	53	96	126	93
Body as a Whole						
Asthenia		18		18		11
Headache/Migraine		65		51		46
Injection Site Reaction		2		9		3
Pain		24		29		21
Cardiovascular System						
Hot flashes/Sweats		98		87		57
Digestive System						
Altered Bowel Function (constipation, diarrhea)		14		15		10
Changes in Appetite		4		0		6
GI Disturbance (dyspepsia, flatulence)		4		7		4
Nausea/Vomiting		25		29		13
Metabolic and Nutritional Disorders						
Edema		0		9		7
Weight Gain		12		13		4
Nervous System						
Depression/Emotional Lability		31		27		34
Dizziness/Vertigo		16		11		7
Insomnia/Sleep Disorder		31		13		15
Decreased Libido		10		4		7
Memory Disorder		6		2		4
Nervousness/Anxiety		8		4		11
Neuromuscular Disorder (leg cramps, paresthesia)		2		9		3
Skin and Appendages						
Androgen-Like Effects (acne, alopecia)		4		5		18
Skin/Mucous Membrane Reaction		4		9		11
Urogenital System						
Breast Changes/Pain/Tenderness		6		13		8
Menstrual Disorders		2		0		5
Vaginitis		20		15		8

* LA-Only = leuprolide acetate 3.75 mg
† LA/N = leuprolide acetate 3.75 mg plus norethindrone acetate 5 mg

8   USE IN SPECIFIC POPULATIONS
8.1   Pregnancy
Pregnancy Category X – *[See Contraindications (4)]*
Teratogenic Effects
LUPANETA PACK is contraindicated in women who are or may become pregnant while receiving the drug *[see Contraindications (4)]*. Before starting and during treatment with leuprolide acetate for depot suspension, establish whether the patient is pregnant. Leuprolide acetate for depot suspension is not a contraceptive. In reproductively capable women, a non-hormonal method of contraception should be used *[see Warnings and Precautions (5.4)]*.
Leuprolide acetate for depot suspension may cause fetal harm when administered to a pregnant woman.

When administered on day 6 of pregnancy at test dosages of 0.00024, 0.0024, and 0.024 mg/kg (1/300 to 1/3 of the human dose) to rabbits, leuprolide acetate for depot suspension produced a dose-related increase in major fetal abnormalities. Similar studies in rats failed to demonstrate an increase in fetal malformations. There was increased fetal mortality and decreased fetal weights with the two higher doses of leuprolide acetate for depot suspension in rabbits and with the highest dose (0.024 mg/kg) in rats.
8.3   Nursing Mothers
Do not use LUPANETA PACK in nursing mothers because the effects of leuprolide acetate for depot suspension on lactation and/or the breast-fed child have not been determined.

It is not known whether leuprolide acetate for depot suspension is excreted in human milk.
Detectable amounts of progestins have been identified in the milk of mothers receiving them *[see Contraindications (4)]*.
8.4   Pediatric Use
LUPANETA PACK is not indicated in premenarcheal adolescents. Safety and effectiveness of LUPANETA PACK have not been established in pediatric patients. Experience with LUPANETA PACK for treatment of endometriosis has been limited to women 18 years of age and older.
8.5   Geriatric Use
LUPANETA PACK is not indicated in postmenopausal women and has not been studied in women over 65 years of age.

11   DESCRIPTION
LUPANETA PACK (leuprolide acetate for depot suspension; norethindrone acetate tablets) 1-month contains one dual chamber syringe with leuprolide acetate for depot suspension 3.75 mg and norethindrone acetate tablets USP: 5 mg (bottle of 30 tablets).
Leuprolide Acetate for Depot Suspension
Leuprolide acetate for depot suspension is a synthetic non-apeptide analog of gonadotropin-releasing hormone (GnRH or LH-RH), a GnRH agonist. The chemical name is 5- oxo-L-prolyl-L-histidyl-L-tryptophyl-L-seryl-L-tyrosyl-D-leucyl-L-leucyl-L-arginyl-N-ethyl-L-prolinamide acetate (salt) with the following structural formula:
[See structural formula on next page]
Leuprolide acetate for depot suspension 3.75 mg is available in a prefilled dual-chamber syringe containing sterile lyophilized microspheres which, when mixed with diluent, become a suspension intended as an intramuscular injection. The front chamber of leuprolide acetate for depot suspension 3.75 mg prefilled dual-chamber syringe contains leuprolide acetate for depot suspension (3.75 mg), gelatin (0.65 mg), DL-lactic and glycolic acids copolymer (33.1 mg), and D-mannitol (6.6 mg). The second chamber of diluent contains carboxymethylcellulose sodium (5 mg), D-mannitol (50 mg), polysorbate 80 (1 mg), water for injection, USP, and glacial acetic acid, USP to control pH.
During the manufacture of leuprolide acetate for depot suspension, acetic acid is lost, leaving the peptide.
Norethindrone Acetate
Norethindrone acetate tablets USP - 5 mg oral tablets.
Norethindrone acetate USP, (17-hydroxy-19-nor-17α-pregn-4-en-20-yn-3-one acetate), a synthetic, orally active progestin, is the acetic acid ester of norethindrone. It is a white, or creamy white, crystalline powder.

Norethindrone acetate tablets USP, 5 mg contain the following inactive ingredients: colloidal silicon dioxide, lactose monohydrate, magnesium stearate, microcrystalline cellulose and talc.

12   CLINICAL PHARMACOLOGY
12.1   Mechanism of Action
Leuprolide Acetate for Depot Suspension
Leuprolide acetate for depot suspension is a long-acting GnRH analog. A single injection of leuprolide acetate for depot suspension results in an initial elevation followed by a prolonged suppression of pituitary gonadotropins. Repeated dosing at quarterly intervals results in decreased secretion of gonadal steroids; consequently, tissues and functions that depend on gonadal steroids for their maintenance become quiescent. This effect is reversible on discontinuation of drug therapy.
Leuprolide acetate is not active when given orally.
Norethindrone Acetate
Norethindrone acetate induces secretory changes in an estrogen-primed endometrium.

Continued on next page

12.2 Pharmacodynamics

In a pharmacokinetic/pharmacodynamic study of leuprolide acetate 11.25 mg for 3-month administration in healthy female subjects (N=20), the onset of estradiol suppression was observed for individual subjects between day 4 and week 4 after dosing. By the third week following the injection, the mean estradiol concentration (8 pg/mL) was in the menopausal range. Throughout the remainder of the dosing period, mean serum estradiol levels ranged from the menopausal to the early follicular range.

Serum estradiol was suppressed to ≤20 pg/mL in all subjects within four weeks and remained suppressed (≤40 pg/mL) in 80% of subjects until the end of the 12-week dosing interval, at which time two of these subjects had a value between 40 and 50 pg/mL. Four additional subjects had at least two consecutive elevations of estradiol (range 43-240 pg/mL) levels during the 12-week dosing interval, but there was no indication of luteal function for any of the subjects during this period.

12.3 Pharmacokinetics

Absorption

Leuprolide Acetate for Depot Suspension

Following a single injection of the three month formulation of leuprolide acetate for depot suspension (11.25 mg) in female subjects, a mean plasma leuprolide concentration of 36.3 ng/mL was observed at 4 hours. Leuprolide appeared to be released at a constant rate following the onset of steady-state levels during the third week after dosing and mean levels then declined gradually to near the lower limit of detection by 12 weeks. The mean (± standard deviation) leuprolide concentration from 3 to 12 weeks was 0.23 ± 0.09 ng/mL. However, intact leuprolide and an inactive major metabolite could not be distinguished by the assay which was employed in the study. The initial burst, followed by the rapid decline to a steady-state level, was similar to the release pattern seen with the monthly formulation.

Norethindrone Acetate

Norethindrone acetate is deacetylated to norethindrone after oral administration, and the disposition of norethindrone acetate is indistinguishable from that of orally administered norethindrone. Norethindrone acetate is absorbed from norethindrone acetate tablets, with maximum plasma concentration of norethindrone generally occurring at about 2 hours post-dose (see Figure 8). The pharmacokinetic parameters of norethindrone following single oral administration of 5 mg norethindrone acetate under fasting conditions in 29 healthy female volunteers are summarized in Table 5.

Table 5. Pharmacokinetic Parameters after a Single Dose of Norethindrone Acetate in Healthy Women

Norethindrone Acetate (n=29) Arithmetic Mean ± SD	
Norethindrone	
AUC (0-inf) (ng/ml*h)	166.90 ± 56.28
C_{max} (ng/ml)	26.19 ± 6.19
t_{max} (h)	1.83 ± 0.58
$t_{1/2}$ (h)	8.51 ± 2.19

AUC = area under the curve,
C_{max} = maximum plasma concentration,
t_{max} = time at maximum plasma concentration,
$t_{1/2}$ = half-life,
SD = standard deviation

[See Figure 8 on page 709]

Effect of Food:
The effect of food administration on the pharmacokinetics of norethindrone acetate has not been studied.

Distribution

Leuprolide Acetate for Depot Suspension

The mean steady-state volume of distribution of leuprolide following intravenous bolus administration to healthy male volunteers was 27 L. *In vitro* binding to human plasma proteins ranged from 43% to 49%.

Norethindrone Acetate

Norethindrone is 36% bound to sex hormone-binding globulin (SHBG) and 61% bound to albumin. Volume of distribution of norethindrone is about 4 L/kg.

Metabolism

Leuprolide Acetate for Depot Suspension

In healthy male volunteers, a 1 mg bolus of leuprolide administered intravenously revealed that the mean systemic clearance was 7.6 L/h, with a terminal elimination half-life of approximately 3 hours based on a two compartment model.

In rats and dogs, administration of ^{14}C-labeled leuprolide was shown to be metabolized to smaller inactive peptides, a pentapeptide (Metabolite I), tripeptides (Metabolites II and III) and a dipeptide (Metabolite IV). These fragments may be further catabolized.

Table 2. Hot Flashes in the Month Prior to the Assessment Visit (Controlled Study)

Assessment Visit	Treatment Group	Number of Patients Reporting Hot Flashes		Number of Days with Hot Flashes		Maximum Number of Hot Flashes in 24 Hours	
		N	(%)	N^2	Mean	N^2	Mean
Week 24	LA-Only*	32/37	86	37	19	36	5.8
	LA/N†	22/38	58[1]	38	7[1]	38	1.9[1]

* LA-Only = leuprolide acetate 3.75 mg
† LA/N = leuprolide acetate 3.75 mg plus norethindrone acetate 5 mg
[1]Statistically significantly less than the LA-Only group (p<0.01)
[2]Number of patients assessed.

Table 3. Serum Lipids: Mean Percent Changes from Baseline Values at Treatment Week 24

	leuprolide acetate 3.75 mg		leuprolide acetate for depot suspension 3.75 mg plus norethindrone acetate 5 mg daily			
	Controlled Study (n=39)		Controlled Study (n=41)		Open Label Study (n=117)	
	Baseline Value*	Wk 24% Change	Baseline Value*	Wk 24% Change	Baseline Value*	Wk 24% Change
Total Cholesterol	170.5	9.2%	179.3	0.2%	181.2	2.8%
HDL Cholesterol	52.4	7.4%	51.8	-18.8%	51.0	-14.6%
LDL Cholesterol	96.6	10.9%	101.5	14.1%	109.1	13.1%
LDL/HDL Ratio	2.0†	5.0%	2.1†	43.4%	2.3†	39.4%
Triglycerides	107.8	17.5%	130.2	9.5%	105.4	13.8%

* mg/dL
† ratio

Table 4. Percent of Patients with Serum Lipid Values Outside of the Normal Range

	leuprolide acetate for depot suspension 3.75 mg plus norethindrone acetate 5 mg daily			
	Controlled Study (n=41)		Open Label Study (n=117)	
	Baseline	Wk 24*	Baseline	Wk 24*
Total Cholesterol (>240 mg/dL)	15%	20%	6%	7%
HDL Cholesterol (<40 mg/dL)	15%	44%	15%	41%
LDL Cholesterol (>160 mg/dL)	5%	7%	9%	11%
LDL/HDL Ratio (>4.0)	2%	15%	7%	21%
Triglycerides (>200 mg/dL)	12%	10%	5%	9%

* Includes all patients regardless of baseline value.

In a pharmacokinetic/pharmacodynamic study of endometriosis patients, intramuscular 11.25 mg leuprolide acetate for depot suspension (n=19) every 12 weeks or intramuscular 3.75 mg leuprolide acetate for depot suspension (n=15) every 4 weeks was administered for 24 weeks. There was no statistically significant difference in changes of serum estradiol concentration from baseline between the 2 treatment groups.

Figure 8. Mean Norethindrone Plasma Concentration Profile after a Single Dose of 5 mg Norethindrone Acetate Administered to 29 Healthy Female Volunteers under Fasting Conditions

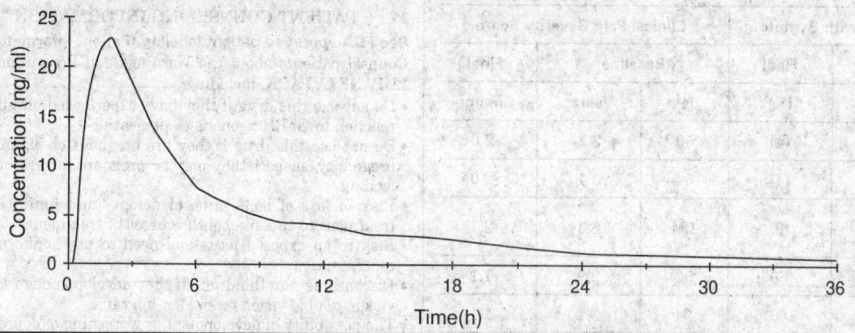

M-I plasma concentrations measured in 5 prostate cancer patients reached maximum concentration 2 to 6 hours after dosing and were approximately 6% of the peak parent drug concentration. One week after dosing, mean plasma M-I concentrations were approximately 20% of mean leuprolide concentrations.

Norethindrone Acetate
Norethindrone undergoes extensive biotransformation, primarily via reduction, followed by sulfate and glucuronide conjugation. The majority of metabolites in the circulation are sulfates, with glucuronides accounting for most of the urinary metabolites.

Excretion
Leuprolide Acetate for Depot Suspension
Following administration of leuprolide acetate for depot suspension 3.75 mg for 1-month administration to 3 patients, less than 5% of the dose was recovered as parent and M-I metabolite in the urine.

Norethindrone Acetate
Plasma clearance value for norethindrone is approximately 0.4 L/hr/kg. Norethindrone is excreted in both urine and feces, primarily as metabolites. The mean terminal elimination half-life of norethindrone following a single dose administration of norethindrone acetate is approximately 9 hours.

Specific Populations
Hepatic Impairment
The effect of hepatic disease on the disposition of norethindrone after norethindrone acetate administration has not been evaluated. However, norethindrone acetate is contraindicated in markedly impaired liver function or liver disease *[see Contraindications (4)]*.
The pharmacokinetics of the leuprolide acetate for depot suspension in hepatically impaired patients has not been determined.

Renal Impairment
The effect of renal disease on the disposition of norethindrone after norethindrone acetate administration has not been evaluated. In pre-menopausal women with chronic renal failure undergoing peritoneal dialysis who received multiple doses of an oral contraceptive containing ethinyl estradiol and norethindrone, plasma norethindrone concentration was unchanged compared to concentrations in pre-menopausal women with normal renal function.
The pharmacokinetics of the leuprolide acetate for depot suspension in renally impaired patients has not been determined.

Race
The effect of race on the disposition of norethindrone after norethindrone acetate administration has not been evaluated.

Drug Interactions
Leuprolide Acetate for Depot Suspension
Leuprolide acetate for depot suspension is a peptide that is primarily degraded by peptidase and not by cytochrome P-450 enzymes as noted in specific studies, and the drug is only about 46% bound to plasma proteins, drug interactions would not be expected to occur.

13 NONCLINICAL TOXICOLOGY
13.1 Carcinogenesis, Mutagenesis, Impairment of Fertility
Leuprolide Acetate for Depot Suspension
A two-year carcinogenicity study was conducted in rats and mice. In rats, a dose-related increase of benign pituitary hyperplasia and benign pituitary adenomas was noted at 24 months when the drug was administered subcutaneously

at high daily doses (0.6 to 4 mg/kg). There was a significant but not dose-related increase of pancreatic islet-cell adenomas in females and of testicular interstitial cell adenomas in males (highest incidence in the low dose group). In mice, no leuprolide acetate-induced tumors or pituitary abnormalities were observed at a dose as high as 60 mg/kg for two years. Patients have been treated with leuprolide acetate for up to three years with doses as high as 10 mg/day and for two years with doses as high as 20 mg/day without demonstrable pituitary abnormalities.
Mutagenicity studies have been performed with leuprolide acetate using bacterial and mammalian systems. These studies provided no evidence of a mutagenic potential.
Clinical and pharmacologic studies in adults (>18 years) with leuprolide acetate and similar analogs have shown reversibility of fertility suppression when the drug is discontinued after continuous administration for periods of up to 24 weeks. Although no clinical studies have been completed in children to assess the full reversibility of fertility suppression, animal studies (prepubertal and adult rats and monkeys) with leuprolide acetate and other GnRH analogs have shown functional recovery.

14 CLINICAL STUDIES
Leuprolide Acetate for Depot Suspension
Initial endometriosis efficacy data for leuprolide acetate for depot suspension were based on the 3.75 mg dose administered once monthly.
A pharmacokinetic/pharmacodynamic study in 41 women that included both the 3.75 mg dose administered once monthly and the 11.25 mg dose administered once every three months did not reveal clinically significant differences in terms of efficacy in reducing painful symptoms of endometriosis or magnitude of the decrease in bone mineral density (BMD) associated with use of leuprolide acetate.

Leuprolide Acetate for Depot Suspension Plus Norethindrone Acetate
Two clinical studies with treatment duration of 12 months were conducted to evaluate the effect of coadministration of leuprolide acetate for depot suspension and norethindrone acetate on the loss of bone mineral density (BMD) associated with leuprolide acetate for depot suspension and on the efficacy of leuprolide acetate for depot suspension in relieving symptoms of endometriosis. (All patients in these studies received calcium supplementation with 1000 mg elemental calcium). A total of 242 women were treated with monthly administration of leuprolide acetate 3.75 mg (13 injections) and with 5 mg norethindrone acetate taken daily. The population age range was 17-43 years old. The majority of patients were Caucasian (87%).
One coadministration study was a controlled, randomized and double-blind study included 51 women treated monthly with leuprolide acetate for depot suspension alone and 55 women treated monthly with leuprolide acetate for depot suspension plus norethindrone acetate daily. Women in this trial were followed for up to 24 months after completing one year of treatment. The other study was an open-label single arm clinical study in 136 women of one year of treatment with leuprolide acetate for depot suspension and norethindrone acetate, with follow-up for up to 12 months after completing treatment.
The second study was an open label, single arm study in which 136 women were treated monthly with leuprolide acetate for depot suspension plus norethindrone acetate daily, with follow-up for up to 12 months after completing treatment.

The assessment of efficacy was based on the investigator's or the patient's monthly assessment of five signs or symptoms of endometriosis (dysmenorrhea, pelvic pain, deep dyspareunia, pelvic tenderness and pelvic induration).
Table 6 below provides detailed efficacy data regarding relief of symptoms of endometriosis based on the two studies of coadministration of leuprolide acetate and norethindrone acetate.
[See table 6 on next page]
Suppression of menses (menses was defined as three or more consecutive days of menstrual bleeding) was maintained throughout treatment in 84% and 73% of patients receiving leuprolide acetate and norethindrone acetate, in the controlled study and open label study, respectively. The median time for menses resumption after treatment with leuprolide acetate and norethindrone acetate was 8 weeks.
Changes in Bone Density
The effect of leuprolide acetate for depot suspension and norethindrone acetate on bone mineral density was evaluated by dual energy x-ray absorptiometry (DXA) scan in the two clinical trials. For the open-label study, success in mitigating BMD loss was defined as the lower bound of the 95% confidence interval around the change from baseline at one year of treatment not to exceed –2.2%. The bone mineral density data of the lumbar spine from these two studies are presented in Table 7.
[See table 7 on page 710]
The change in BMD following discontinuation of treatment is shown in Table 8.
[See table 8 on page 710]
These clinical studies demonstrated that coadministration of leuprolide acetate and norethindrone acetate 5 mg daily is effective in significantly reducing the loss of bone mineral density that occurs with leuprolide acetate for depot suspension treatment, and in relieving symptoms of endometriosis.

15 REFERENCES
Leuprolide Acetate for Depot Suspension
1. NIOSH Alert: Preventing occupational exposures to antineoplastic and other hazardous drugs in healthcare settings. 2004. U.S. Department of Health and Human Services, Public Health Service, Centers for Disease Control and Prevention, National Institute for Occupational Safety and Health, DHHS (NIOSH) Publication No. 2004-165.
2. OSHA Technical Manual, TED 1-0.15A, Section VI: Chapter 2. Controlling Occupational Exposure to Hazardous Drugs. OSHA, 1999. http://www.osha.gov/dts/osta/otm/otm_vi/otm_vi_2.html
3. American Society of Health-System Pharmacists. ASHP guidelines on handling hazardous drugs. *Am J Health-Syst Pharm.* 2006; 63; 1172-1193.
4. Polovich, M., White, J.M., & Kelleher, L.O. (eds.) 2005. Chemotherapy and biotherapy guidelines and recommendations for practice (2nd. Ed.) Pittsburgh, PA: Oncology Nursing Society.

16 HOW SUPPLIED/STORAGE AND HANDLING
LUPANETA PACK for 1-month copackaged kit (NDC 0074-1052-05) is available in
cartons containing: leuprolide acetate for depot suspension 3.75 mg for 1-month administration Kit (NDC 0074-3641-04)
norethindrone acetate 5 mg tablets; 30 count bottle (NDC 0074-1049-02)
1. Leuprolide acetate for depot suspension 3.75 mg for 1-month administration kit contains:
   • one prefilled dual-chamber syringe
   • one plunger
   • two alcohol swab
   Each syringe contains sterile lyophilized microspheres of leuprolide acetate incorporated in a biodegradable copolymer of lactic and glycolic acids. When mixed with diluent, leuprolide acetate for depot suspension 3.75 mg for 1-month administration is administered as a single intramuscular injection.
2. Norethindrone acetate 5 mg 30 count bottle
   White to off-white oval, flat faced beveled edged, uncoated tablets debossed with 'G with breakline' on one side and 304 on other side.

Continued on next page

Table 6. Percentages of Patients with Symptoms of Endometriosis and Mean Clinical Severity Scores

| Variable | Study | Group | Percent of Patients with Symptom | | | | Clinical Pain Severity Score | | |
| | | | Baseline | | Final | | Baseline | | Final |
			N[1]	(%)[2]	(%)		N[1]	Value[3]	Change
Dysmenorrhea	Controlled Study	LA*	51	(100)	(4)		50	3.2	-2.0
		LA/N†	55	(100)	(4)		54	3.1	-2.0
	Open Label Study	LA/N	136	(99)	(9)		134	3.3	-2.1
Pelvic Pain	Controlled Study	LA	51	(100)	(66)		50	2.9	-1.1
		LA/N	55	(96)	(56)		54	3.1	-1.1
	Open Label Study	LA/N	136	(99)	(63)		134	3.2	-1.2
Deep Dyspareunia	Controlled Study	LA	42	(83)	(37)		25	2.4	-1.0
		LA/N	43	(84)	(45)		30	2.7	-0.8
	Open Label Study	LA/N	102	(91)	(53)		94	2.7	-1.0
Pelvic Tenderness	Controlled Study	LA	51	(94)	(34)		50	2.5	-1.0
		LA/N	54	(91)	(34)		52	2.6	-0.9
	Open Label Study	LA/N	136	(99)	(39)		134	2.9	-1.4
Pelvic Induration	Controlled Study	LA	51	(51)	(12)		50	1.9	-0.4
		LA/N	54	(46)	(17)		52	1.6	-0.4
	Open Label Study	LA/N	136	(75)	(21)		134	2.2	-0.9

* LA = leuprolide acetate 3.75 mg
† LA/N = leuprolide acetate 3.75 mg plus norethindrone acetate 5 mg
[1] Number of patients that were included in the assessment
[2] Percentage of patients with the symptom/sign
[3] Value description: 1=none; 2= mild; 3= moderate; 4= severe

Table 7. Mean Percent Change from Baseline in BMD of Lumbar Spine

| | leuprolide acetate for depot suspension 3.75 mg | | leuprolide acetate for depot suspension 3.75 mg plus norethindrone acetate 5 mg daily | | | |
| | Controlled Study | | Controlled Study | | Open Label Study | |
	N	Change (Mean, 95% CI)#	N	Change (Mean, 95% CI)#	N	Change (Mean, 95% CI)#
Week 24*	41	-3.2% (-3.8, -2.6)	42	-0.3% (-0.8, 0.3)	115	-0.2% (-0.6, 0.2)
Week 52†	29	-6.3% (-7.1, -5.4)	32	-1.0% (-1.9, -0.1)	84	-1.1% (-1.6, -0.5)

* Includes on-treatment measurements that fell within 2-252 days after the first day of treatment.
† Includes on-treatment measurements >252 days after the first day of treatment.
# 95% CI: 95% Confidence Interval

Table 8. Mean Percent Change from Baseline in BMD of Lumbar Spine in Post-Treatment Follow-up Period

| Post Treatment Measurement | Controlled Study | | | | | | Open Label Study | | |
| | LA-Only | | | LA/N | | | LA/N | | |
	N	Mean % Change	95% CI (%)	N	Mean % Change	95% CI (%)	N	Mean % Change	95% CI (%)[2]
Month 8	19	-3.3	(-4.9, -1.8)	23	-0.9	(-2.1, 0.4)	89	-0.6	(-1.2, 0.0)
Month 12	16	-2.2	(-3.3, -1.1)	12	-0.7	(-2.1, 0.6)	65	0.1	(-0.6, 0.7)

[1] Patients with post treatment measurements
[2] 95% CI (2-sided) of percent change in BMD values from baseline

Store at 25°C (77°F); excursions permitted to 15 to 30°C (59 to 86°F) [See USP Controlled Room Temperature]

17   PATIENT COUNSELING INFORMATION

See FDA-approved patient labeling (Patient Information)
Counsel patients about the Warnings and Precautions for LUPANETA PACK, including:
- Do not use this drug if they have experienced an allergic reaction to GnRH agonists or progestins
- Do not use this drug if they are pregnant or planning a pregnancy, suspect they may be pregnant, or are breast-feeding
- Risk of loss of bone mineral density and limitation of treatment to two six-month courses of treatment
- Risk to an exposed fetus and need to use nonhormonal contraception
- Discontinue norethindrone if they develop sudden loss of vision, double vision or sudden migraine
- The possibility of development or worsening of depression during treatment with leuprolide acetate for depot suspension
- Need for close monitoring if they have cardiovascular risk factors, or conditions like epilepsy, migraine or renal dysfunction
- Notify their healthcare provider if they develop new or worsened symptoms after beginning treatment

PATIENT INFORMATION
LUPANETA PACK®
(loo-pan-e-tə pæk)
(leuprolide acetate for depot suspension and norethindrone acetate tablets)
Read this Patient Information before you start taking LUPANETA PACK and each time you get a refill. There may be new information. This information does not take the place of talking with your doctor about your medical condition or your treatment.
What is LUPANETA PACK?
LUPANETA PACK contains 2 different prescription medicines:
- **leuprolide acetate for depot suspension** is a medicine injected into your muscle and used to treat pain due to endometriosis.
- **norethindrone acetate tablets** is a medicine taken by mouth and used to help lower the side effect of bone thinning that is caused by leuprolide acetate for depot suspension.
LUPANETA PACK should not be used longer than 6 months at a time after you first start treatment for your endometriosis symptoms. LUPANETA PACK should not be used for more than a total of 12 months during your treatment.
It is not known if LUPANETA PACK is safe and effective in children under 18 years of age.
Who should not take LUPANETA PACK?
Do not take LUPANETA PACK if you:
- have had an allergic reaction to medicines like leuprolide acetate for depot suspension or norethindrone acetate tablets. See the end of this leaflet for a complete list of ingredients in LUPANETA PACK.
- have uterine bleeding for which a cause has not been found.
- are pregnant or may be pregnant. LUPANETA PACK may harm your unborn baby.
- are breast-feeding or plan to breast-feed. It is not known if LUPANETA PACK passes into your breast milk.
- had or have breast cancer or other cancers that are sensitive to hormones.
- have problems with blood clots, a stroke or a heart attack.
- have liver problems.
What should I tell my doctor before taking LUPANETA PACK?
Before you take LUPANETA PACK, tell your doctor if you:
- drink alcohol
- have a family history of bone loss (osteoporosis)
- have high cholesterol
- have migraine headaches
- have epilepsy
- smoke
- have depression
- have had blood clots, a stroke or a heart attack
- have diabetes
- have kidney problems
Tell your doctor about all the medicines you take, including prescription and non-prescription medicines, vitamins, and herbal supplements.
Especially tell your doctor if you take anticonvulsant (seizure) or corticosteroid medicines.
Ask your doctor for a list of these medicines if you are not sure.
Know the medicines you take. Keep a list of them to show your doctor and pharmacist when you get a new medicine.

How should I take LUPANETA PACK?

- **Leuprolide acetate for depot suspension** for 1 month administration is injected into your muscle 1 time every month by a healthcare professional in your doctor's office.
- **Take norethindrone acetate tablets** exactly as your doctor tells you to take them. Take 1 norethindrone acetate tablet by mouth every day for 1 month after you receive your injection.
- Talk to your doctor about the birth control method that is right for you before you start taking LUPANETA PACK. You will need to use a form of birth control that does not contain hormones, such as:
  ○ a diaphragm with spermicide
  ○ condoms with spermicide
  ○ a copper IUD
- If you become pregnant while taking LUPANETA PACK, stop taking the norethindrone acetate tablets and call your doctor right away.

How well does LUPANETA PACK work?

LUPANETA PACK is used to treat pain due to endometriosis. The pain from endometriosis can happen when you have your period, during other times of the month, or during intercourse (sex). Most women feel some relief from their endometriosis pain after taking both drugs in LUPANETA PACK.

The tablets in LUPANETA PACK help lower the side effect of bone thinning that is caused by leuprolide acetate for depot suspension. Women taking both drugs in LUPANETA PACK lost an average of 1% of their bone density after about 1 year of treatment. Women regained some of their bone density about 1 year after they stopped treatment with LUPANETA PACK.

What are the possible side effects of LUPANETA PACK?

LUPANETA PACK may cause serious side effects, including:

- **bone thinning (decreased bone mineral density)**
- **harm to your unborn baby**
- **vision problems.** Call your doctor right away if you have sudden loss of vision, double vision, bulging eyes, or migraine headaches.
- **depression or worsening depression**
- **allergic reactions.** Get medical help right away if you have any of these symptoms of a serious allergic reaction:
  ○ swelling of your face, lips, mouth, or tongue
  ○ trouble breathing
  ○ wheezing
  ○ severe itching
  ○ skin rash, redness, or swelling
  ○ dizziness or fainting
  ○ fast heartbeat or pounding in your chest (tachycardia)
  ○ sweating
- **worsening endometriosis symptoms when you start taking LUPANETA PACK**
- **swelling (fluid retention)**

The most common side effects of LUPANETA PACK include:

- hot flashes and sweats
- headaches or migraine headaches
- depression and mood swings
- nausea and vomiting
- problems sleeping
- nervousness or feeling anxious
- pain
- acne
- weakness
- vaginal infection or inflammation
- weight gain
- constipation or diarrhea

Tell your doctor if you have any side effect that bothers you or that does not go away.

These are not all the possible side effects of LUPANETA PACK. For more information, ask your doctor or pharmacist.

Call your doctor for medical advice about side effects. You may report side effects to FDA at 1-800-FDA-1088.

How should I store norethindrone acetate tablets in the LUPANETA PACK?

- Store norethindrone acetate tablets at room temperature between 68°F to 77°F (20°C to 25°C).

Keep LUPANETA PACK and all medicines out of the reach of children.

General information about the safe and effective use of LUPANETA PACK.

Medicines are sometimes prescribed for purposes other than those listed in a Patient Information leaflet. Do not use LUPANETA PACK for a condition for which it was not prescribed. Do not give LUPANETA PACK to other people, even if they have the same symptoms that you have. It may harm them.

This Patient Information leaflet summarizes the most important information about LUPANETA PACK. If you would like more information, talk with your doctor. You can ask your pharmacist or doctor for information about LUPANETA PACK that is written for health professionals. For more information, go to www.lupanetapack.com or call 1-800-633-9110.

What are the ingredients in LUPANETA PACK?

leuprolide acetate for depot suspension:

Active Ingredients: leuprolide acetate for depot suspension

Inactive Ingredients: gelatin, DL-lactic and glycolic acids copolymer, D-mannitol, carboxymethylcellulose sodium, polysorbate 80, water for injection, USP,

and glacial acetic acid, USP to control pH.

norethindrone acetate tablets:

Active Ingredients: norethindrone acetate USP

Inactive Ingredients: colloidal silicon dioxide, lactose monohydrate, magnesium stearate, microcrystalline cellulose and talc.

This Patient Information has been approved by the U.S. Food and Drug Administration.

Leuprolide Acetate for Depot Suspension 3.75 mg:

Manufactured for

AbbVie Inc.

North Chicago, IL 60064

By Takeda Pharmaceutical Company Limited

Osaka, Japan 540–8645

Norethindrone Acetate:

Manufactured for

AbbVie Inc.

North Chicago, IL 60064

Manufactured by

Glenmark Pharmaceuticals Ltd.

Colvale-Bardez, Goa

403 513, India

LUPANETA PACK

Packaged by:

AbbVie Inc.

North Chicago, IL 60064

™-Trademark

® – Registered Trademark

©AbbVie Inc. 2015

03-B096-R3 June, 2015

Shown in Product Identification Guide, page 505

LUPANETA PACK®   ℞

[loo-pan-e-tə pæk]

(Leuprolide Acetate for Depot Suspension, 11.25 mg for intramuscular injection only and Norethindrone Acetate tablets, 5 mg for oral administration)

HIGHLIGHTS OF PRESCRIBING INFORMATION

These highlights do not include all the information needed to use LUPANETA PACK safely and effectively. See full prescribing information for LUPANETA PACK.

LUPANETA PACK (leuprolide acetate for depot suspension; norethindrone acetate tablets), co-packaged for intramuscular use and for oral use, respectively

Initial U.S. Approval: 2012

──────INDICATIONS AND USAGE──────

LUPANETA PACK contains leuprolide acetate, a gonadotropin-releasing hormone (GnRH) agonist and norethindrone acetate, a progestin, indicated for

- Initial management of the painful symptoms of endometriosis (1)
- Management of recurrence of symptoms (1)

Limitations of Use: Initial treatment course is limited to 6 months and use is not recommended longer than a total of 12 months due to concerns about adverse impact on bone mineral density. (1, 2.1, 5.1)

────DOSAGE AND ADMINISTRATION────

- Leuprolide acetate for depot suspension 11.25 mg given by a healthcare provider as a single intramuscular injection every 3 months for up to two injections (6 months of therapy) (2.1)
- Norethindrone acetate 5 mg tablets taken orally by the patient once per day for up to 6 months (2.1)
- If endometriosis symptoms recur after initial course of therapy, consider retreatment for up to another six months (2.1)
- Assess bone density before retreatment begins (2.1, 5.1)

- Reconstitute leuprolide acetate prior to use, see important administration instructions (2.3)

────DOSAGE FORMS AND STRENGTHS────

- Leuprolide acetate for depot suspension 11.25 mg syringe (3)
- Norethindrone acetate 5 mg tablets; 90 count bottle (3)

──────CONTRAINDICATIONS──────

- Hypersensitivity to GnRH, GnRH agonist or any of the excipients in leuprolide acetate for depot suspension or norethindrone acetate (4)
- Undiagnosed abnormal uterine bleeding (4)
- Pregnancy or suspected pregnancy (4, 8.1)
- Women who are breast-feeding (4)
- Known, suspected or history of breast or other hormone-sensitive cancer (4)
- Thrombotic or thromboembolic disorders (4)
- Liver tumors or liver disease (4)

────WARNINGS AND PRECAUTIONS────

- Loss of bone mineral density: do not use for more than two six-month treatment courses. (1, 2.1, 5.1)
- Exclude pregnancy before starting treatment and discontinue use if pregnancy occurs; use non-hormonal methods of contraception only. (5.2)
- Discontinue in case of sudden loss of vision or onset of proptosis, diplopia or migraine. (5.3)
- Carefully observe patients with history of depression and discontinue the drug if the depression recurs to a serious degree. (5.4)
- Assess and manage risk factors for cardiovascular disease before starting LUPANETA PACK. (5.6)

──────ADVERSE REACTIONS──────

Leuprolide acetate for depot suspension: Most common related adverse reactions (>10%) were hot flashes/sweats, headache/migraine, depression/emotional lability, nausea/vomiting, nervousness/anxiety, insomnia, pain, acne, asthenia, vaginitis, weight gain, constipation/diarrhea (6.1)

Progestins: breakthrough bleeding, spotting (6.1)

To report SUSPECTED ADVERSE REACTIONS, contact AbbVie Inc. at 1-800-633-9110 or FDA at 1-800-FDA-1088 or www.fda.gov/medwatch

────USE IN SPECIFIC POPULATIONS────

Pediatric: Safety and effectiveness of LUPANETA PACK has not been established in pediatric patients. (8.4)

Geriatric: LUPANETA PACK has not been studied in women over 65 years of age and is not indicated in this population. (8.5)

See 17 for PATIENT COUNSELING INFORMATION and FDA-approved patient labeling.

Revised: 6/2015

Continued on next page

Information on the AbbVie, Inc. products listed on these pages is from the prescribing information in use as of July 31, 2016. For more information, please visit rxabbvie.com or call 1-800-633-9110.

FULL PRESCRIBING INFORMATION

1   INDICATIONS AND USAGE

LUPANETA PACK (leuprolide acetate for depot suspension and norethindrone acetate tablets) is indicated for initial management of the painful symptoms of endometriosis and for management of recurrence of symptoms.

Limitation of Use: Duration of use is limited due to concerns about adverse impact on bone mineral density *[see Warnings and Precautions (5.1)]*. The initial treatment course of LUPANETA PACK is limited to six months. A single retreatment course of not more than six months may be administered after the initial course of treatment if symptoms recur. Use of LUPANETA PACK for longer than a total of 12 months is not recommended.

2   DOSAGE AND ADMINISTRATION

2.1   Dosing Information

LUPANETA PACK is a co-packaging of leuprolide acetate for depot suspension for intramuscular use and norethindrone acetate tablets for oral use. Administer as follows:

- 11.25 mg of leuprolide acetate by intramuscular injection once every three months for up to two injections (6 months of therapy); to be administered by a healthcare provider
- 5 mg of norethindrone acetate orally once daily for up to 6 months of therapy

The initial course of treatment with leuprolide acetate for depot suspension 11.25 mg in combination with norethindrone acetate 5 mg daily is not to exceed six months.

If the symptoms of endometriosis recur after the initial course of therapy, consider retreatment with LUPANETA PACK for up to another six months. It is recommended that bone density be assessed before retreatment begins *[see Warnings and Precautions (5.1)]*.

Treatment beyond two six-month courses has not been studied and is not recommended due to concerns about adverse impact on bone mineral density.

2.2   Different Formulations of Leuprolide Acetate

Due to different release characteristics, a fractional dose of the leuprolide acetate for depot suspension 3-month depot formulation is not equivalent to the same dose of the monthly formulation and should not be given.

2.3   Reconstitution and Administration for Injection of Leuprolide Acetate

- Reconstitute and administer the lyophilized microspheres as a single intramuscular injection.
- Inject the suspension immediately or discard if not used within two hours, because leuprolide acetate for depot suspension does not contain a preservative.

1. Visually inspect the leuprolide acetate for depot suspension powder. DO NOT USE the syringe if clumping or caking is evident. A thin layer of powder on the wall of the syringe is considered normal prior to mixing with the diluent. The diluent should appear clear.

2. To prepare for injection, screw the white plunger into the end stopper until the stopper begins to turn (see Figure 1 and Figure 2).
[See Figure 1 below]

Figure 2:

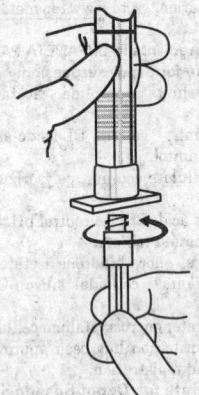

3. Hold the syringe UPRIGHT. Release the diluent by SLOWLY PUSHING (6 to 8 seconds) the plunger until the first middle stopper is at the blue line in the middle of the barrel (see Figure 3).

Figure 3:

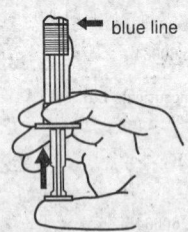

      ← blue line

4. Keep the syringe UPRIGHT. Mix the microspheres (powder) thoroughly by gently shaking the syringe until the powder forms a uniform suspension. The suspension will appear milky. If the powder adheres to the stopper or caking/clumping is present, tap the syringe with your finger to disperse. DO NOT USE if any of the powder has not gone into suspension (see Figure 4).

Figure 4:

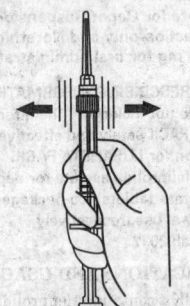

5. Keep the syringe UPRIGHT. With the opposite hand pull the needle cap upward without twisting.
6. Keep the syringe UPRIGHT. Advance the plunger to expel the air from the syringe. Now the syringe is ready for injection.

7. After cleaning the injection site with an alcohol swab, administer the intramuscular injection by inserting the needle at a 90 degree angle into the gluteal area, anterior thigh, or deltoid (see Figure 5).

Figure 5:

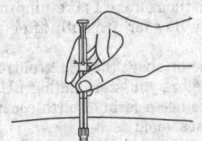

NOTE: If a blood vessel is accidentally penetrated, aspirated blood will be visible just below the luer lock (see Figure 6) and can be seen through the transparent LuproLoc safety device. If blood is present, remove the needle immediately. Do not inject the medication.

Figure 6:

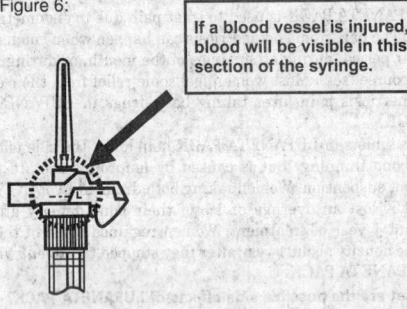

If a blood vessel is injured, blood will be visible in this section of the syringe.

8. Inject the entire contents of the syringe intramuscularly.
9. Withdraw the needle. Once the syringe has been withdrawn, immediately activate the LuproLoc® safety device by pushing the arrow on the lock upward towards the needle tip with the thumb or finger, as illustrated, until the needle cover of the safety device over the needle is fully extended and a CLICK is heard or felt (see Figure 7).
[See Figure 7 below]

Figure 7:

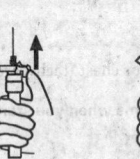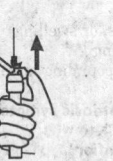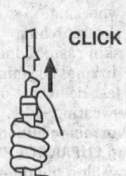   **CLICK**

10. Dispose of the syringe according to local regulations/procedures *[see References (15)]*.

3   DOSAGE FORMS AND STRENGTHS

LUPANETA PACK 3-month copackaged kit contains two separate components:

- Leuprolide acetate for depot suspension 11.25 mg for 3-month administration: Leuprolide acetate lyophilized powder for reconstitution with supplied diluent in a prefilled dual chamber syringe
- Norethindrone acetate 5 mg tablets: White to off-white oval, flat-faced beveled edged, uncoated debossed with 'G with breakline' on one side and 304 on other side

4   CONTRAINDICATIONS

LUPANETA PACK is contraindicated in women with the following:

- Hypersensitivity to gonadotropin-releasing hormone (GnRH), GnRH agonist analogs, any of the excipients in leuprolide acetate for depot suspension, or norethindrone acetate
- Undiagnosed abnormal uterine bleeding
- Known, suspected or planned pregnancy during the course of therapy *[see Use in Specific Populations (8.1)]*
- Lactating women *[see Use in Specific Populations (8.3)]*
- Known, suspected or history of breast cancer or other hormone-sensitive cancer
- Current or history of thrombotic or thromboembolic disorder
- Liver tumors or liver disease

5   WARNINGS AND PRECAUTIONS

5.1   Loss of Bone Mineral Density

Leuprolide acetate for depot suspension induces a hypoestrogenic state that results in loss of bone mineral density (BMD), some of which may not be reversible. Concurrent

Figure 1:

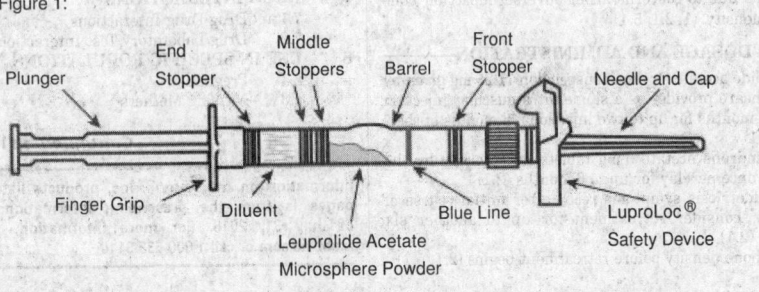

Plunger   End Stopper   Middle Stoppers   Barrel   Front Stopper   Needle and Cap

Finger Grip   Diluent   Leuprolide Acetate Microsphere Powder   Blue Line   LuproLoc® Safety Device

use of norethindrone acetate is effective in reducing the loss of BMD that occurs with leuprolide acetate *[see Clinical Studies (14)]*. Nonetheless, duration of use of LUPANETA PACK is limited to two six-month courses of treatment due to concerns about the adverse impact on BMD. It is recommended that BMD be assessed before retreatment. Retreatment with leuprolide acetate for depot suspension alone is not recommended.

In women with major risk factors for decreased BMD such as chronic alcohol (> 3 units per day) or tobacco use, strong family history of osteoporosis, or chronic use of drugs that can decrease BMD, such as anticonvulsants or corticosteroids, use of LUPANETA PACK may pose an additional risk, and the risks and benefits should be weighed carefully.

5.2   Pregnancy Risk

Leuprolide acetate for depot suspension may cause fetal harm if administered to a pregnant woman. Exclude pregnancy before initiating treatment with LUPANETA PACK. When used at the recommended dose and dosing interval, leuprolide acetate for depot suspension usually inhibits ovulation and stops menstruation. Contraception, however, is not ensured by taking leuprolide acetate for depot suspension. Therefore, patients should use nonhormonal methods of contraception. Advise patients to notify their healthcare provider if they believe they may be pregnant. Discontinue LUPANETA PACK if a patient becomes pregnant during treatment and inform the patient of potential risk to the fetus *[see Contraindications (4) and Use in Specific Populations (8.1)]*.

5.3   Visual Abnormalities

Discontinue norethindrone acetate tablets in the LUPANETA PACK pending examination if there is a sudden partial or complete loss of vision or if there is sudden onset of proptosis, diplopia, or migraine. Discontinue LUPANETA PACK if examination reveals papilledema or retinal vascular lesions.

5.4   Clinical Depression

Depression may occur or worsen during treatment with LUPANETA PACK. Carefully observe patients with a history of clinical depression and discontinue LUPANETA PACK if the depression recurs to a serious degree.

5.5   Serious Allergic Reactions

In clinical trials of LUPANETA PACK, adverse events of asthma were reported in women with pre-existing histories of asthma, sinusitis and environmental or drug allergies. Symptoms consistent with an anaphylactoid or asthmatic process have been reported postmarketing.

5.6   Cardiovascular and Metabolic Disorders

Assess and manage risk factors for cardiovascular disease before starting LUPANETA PACK. Closely monitor women on norethindrone acetate who have risk factors for arterial vascular disease (e.g., hypertension, diabetes mellitus, tobacco use, hypercholesterolemia, and obesity) and/or venous thromboembolism (e.g., family history of VTE, obesity, and smoking) when using LUPANETA PACK *[see Contraindications (4)]*.

5.7   Initial Flare of Symptoms

Following the first dose of leuprolide acetate, sex steroids temporarily rise above baseline because of the physiologic effect of the drug. Therefore, an increase in symptoms associated with endometriosis may be observed during the initial days of therapy, but these should dissipate with continued therapy.

5.8   Fluid Retention

Because norethindrone acetate may cause some degree of fluid retention, carefully observe women with conditions that might be influenced by this effect, such as epilepsy, migraine, cardiac or renal dysfunctions.

5.9   Convulsions

There have been postmarketing reports of convulsions in patients on leuprolide acetate therapy. These included patients with and without concurrent medications and comorbid conditions.

6   ADVERSE REACTIONS

6.1   Clinical Trials Experience

Because clinical trials are conducted under widely varying conditions, adverse reaction rates observed in the clinical trials of a drug cannot be directly compared to rates in the clinical trials of another drug and may not reflect the rates observed in clinical practice.

The safety of co-administering leuprolide acetate for depot suspension and norethindrone acetate was evaluated in two clinical studies in which a total of 242 women were treated for up to one year. Women were treated with monthly IM injections of leuprolide acetate 3.75 mg (13 injections) alone

Table 1. Adverse Reactions Occurring in the First Six Months of Treatment in ≥ 5% of Patients with Endometriosis

Adverse Reactions	Controlled Study				Open Label Study	
	LA-Only*		LA/N†		LA/N†	
	N=51		N=55		N=136	
	N	%	N	%	N	%
Any Adverse Reaction	50	98	53	96	126	93
Body as a Whole						
Asthenia		18		18		11
Headache/Migraine		65		51		46
Injection Site Reaction		2		9		3
Pain		24		29		21
Cardiovascular System						
Hot flashes/Sweats		98		87		57
Digestive System						
Altered Bowel Function (constipation, diarrhea)		14		15		10
Changes in Appetite		4		0		6
GI Disturbance (dyspepsia, flatulence)		4		7		4
Nausea/Vomiting		25		29		13
Metabolic and Nutritional Disorders						
Edema		0		9		7
Weight Gain		12		13		4
Nervous System						
Depression/Emotional Lability		31		27		34
Dizziness/Vertigo		16		11		7
Insomnia/Sleep Disorder		31		13		15
Decreased Libido		10		4		7
Memory Disorder		6		2		4
Nervousness/Anxiety		8		4		11
Neuromuscular Disorder (leg cramps, paresthesia)		2		9		3
Skin and Appendages						
Androgen-Like Effects (acne, alopecia)		4		5		18
Skin/Mucous Membrane Reaction		4		9		11
Urogenital System						
Breast Changes/Pain/Tenderness		6		13		8
Menstrual Disorders		2		0		5
Vaginitis		20		15		8

* LA-Only = leuprolide acetate 3.75 mg
† LA/N = leuprolide acetate 3.75 mg plus norethindrone acetate 5 mg

or monthly IM injections of leuprolide acetate 3.75 mg (13 injections) and 5 mg norethindrone acetate daily. The population age range was 17-43 years old. The majority of patients were Caucasian (87%).

One study was a controlled clinical trial in which 106 women were randomized to one year of treatment with leuprolide acetate for depot suspension alone or with leuprolide acetate for depot suspension and norethindrone acetate. The other study was an open-label single arm clinical study in 136 women of one year of treatment with leuprolide acetate for depot suspension and norethindrone acetate, with follow-up for up to 12 months after completing treatment.

Adverse Reactions (>1%) Leading to Study Discontinuation: In the controlled study, 18% of patients treated monthly with leuprolide acetate and 18% of patients treated monthly

with leuprolide acetate plus norethindrone acetate discontinued therapy due to adverse reactions, most commonly hot flashes (6%) and insomnia (4%) in the leuprolide acetate alone group and hot flashes and emotional lability (4% each) in the leuprolide acetate and norethindrone group.

Continued on next page

In the open label study, 13% of patients treated monthly with leuprolide acetate plus norethindrone acetate discontinued therapy due to adverse reactions, most commonly depression (4%) and acne (2%).

Common Adverse Reactions:

Table 1 lists the adverse reactions observed in at least 5% of patients in any treatment group, during the first 6 months of treatment in the add-back clinical studies, in which patients were treated with monthly leuprolide acetate for depot suspension 3.75 mg with or without norethindrone acetate co-treatment. The most frequently-occurring adverse reactions observed in these studies were hot flashes and headaches.

[See table on page 713]

In the controlled clinical trial, 50 of 51 (98%) patients in the leuprolide acetate alone group and 48 of 55 (87%) patients in the leuprolide acetate and norethindrone group reported experiencing hot flashes on one or more occasions during treatment. Table 2 presents hot flash data in the sixth month of treatment.

[See table 2 below]

Serious Adverse Reactions:

Urinary tract infection, renal calculus, depression

Changes in Laboratory Values during Treatment:

Liver Enzymes

In the two clinical trials of women with endometriosis, 4 of 191 patients receiving leuprolide acetate and norethindrone acetate for up to 12 months developed an elevated (at least twice the upper limit of normal) SGPT and 2 of 136 developed an elevated GGT. Five of the 6 increases were observed beyond 6 months of treatment. None was associated with an elevated bilirubin concentration.

Lipids

Percent changes from baseline for serum lipids and percentages of patients with serum lipid values outside of the normal range in the two studies of leuprolide acetate and norethindrone acetate are summarized in the tables below. The major impact of adding norethindrone acetate to treatment with leuprolide acetate for depot suspension was a decrease in serum HDL cholesterol and an increase in the LDL/HDL ratio.

[See table 3 on next page]

Changes from baseline tended to be greater at Week 52. After treatment, mean serum lipid levels from patients with follow up data (105 of 158 patients) returned to pretreatment values.

Table 4. Percent of Patients with Serum Lipid Values Outside of the Normal Range

	leuprolide acetate for depot suspension 3.75 mg plus norethindrone acetate 5 mg daily			
	Controlled Study (n=41)		Open Label Study (n=117)	
	Baseline	Wk 24*	Baseline	Wk 24*
Total Cholesterol (>240 mg/dL)	15%	20%	6%	7%
HDL Cholesterol (<40 mg/dL)	15%	44%	15%	41%
LDL Cholesterol (>160 mg/dL)	5%	7%	9%	11%
LDL/HDL Ratio (>4.0)	2%	15%	7%	21%

Triglycerides (>200 mg/dL)	12%	10%	5%	9%

* Includes all patients regardless of baseline value.

6.2   Postmarketing Experience

The following adverse reactions have been identified during postapproval use of leuprolide acetate for depot suspension or norethindrone acetate. Because these reactions are reported voluntarily from a population of uncertain size, it is not always possible to reliably estimate their frequency or establish a causal relationship to drug exposure.

Leuprolide Acetate for Depot Suspension

During postmarketing surveillance with other dosage forms and in the same or different populations, the following adverse reactions were reported:

• Allergic reactions (anaphylactic, rash, urticaria, and photosensitivity reactions)
• Mood swings, including depression
• Suicidal ideation and attempt
• Symptoms consistent with an anaphylactoid or asthmatic process
• Localized reactions including induration and abscess at the site of injection
• Symptoms consistent with fibromyalgia (e.g., joint and muscle pain, headaches, sleep disorders, gastrointestinal distress, and shortness of breath), individually and collectively

Other adverse reactions reported are:

Hepato-biliary disorder - Serious liver injury

Injury, poisoning and procedural complications - Spinal fracture

Investigations - Decreased white blood count

Musculoskeletal and connective tissue disorder - Tenosynovitis-like symptoms

Nervous System disorder - Convulsion, peripheral neuropathy, paralysis

Vascular disorder - Hypotension, Hypertension

Serious venous and arterial thrombotic and thromboembolic events, including deep vein thrombosis, pulmonary embolism, myocardial infarction, stroke, and transient ischemic attack

Pituitary apoplexy

During post-marketing surveillance, cases of pituitary apoplexy (a clinical syndrome secondary to infarction of the pituitary gland) have been reported after the administration of leuprolide acetate and other GnRH agonists. In a majority of these cases, a pituitary adenoma was diagnosed, with a majority of pituitary apoplexy cases occurring within 2 weeks of the first dose, and some within the first hour. In these cases, pituitary apoplexy has presented as sudden headache, vomiting, visual changes, ophthalmoplegia, altered mental status, and sometimes cardiovascular collapse. Immediate medical attention has been required.

7   DRUG INTERACTIONS

7.1   Drug-Drug Interactions

Leuprolide Acetate for Depot Suspension

No pharmacokinetic-based drug-drug interaction studies have been conducted with leuprolide acetate for depot suspension. However, drug interactions associated with cytochrome P-450 enzymes or protein binding would not be expected to occur *[see Clinical Pharmacology (12.3)]*.

Norethindrone Acetate

No pharmacokinetic drug interaction studies investigating any drug-drug interactions with norethindrone acetate have been conducted. Drugs or herbal products that induce or inhibit certain enzymes, including CYP3A4, may decrease or increase the serum concentrations of norethindrone.

7.2   Drug/Laboratory Test Interactions

Leuprolide Acetate for Depot Suspension

Administration of leuprolide acetate for depot suspension in therapeutic doses results in suppression of the pituitary-gonadal system. Normal function is usually restored within three months after treatment is discontinued. Therefore, diagnostic tests of pituitary gonadotropic and gonadal functions conducted during treatment and for up to three months after discontinuation of leuprolide acetate for depot suspension may be affected.

8   USE IN SPECIFIC POPULATIONS

8.1   Pregnancy

Pregnancy Category X – *[See Contraindications (4)]*

Teratogenic Effects

LUPANETA PACK is contraindicated in women who are or may become pregnant while receiving the drug *[see Contraindications (4)]*. Before starting and during treatment with leuprolide acetate for depot suspension, establish whether the patient is pregnant. Leuprolide acetate for depot suspension is not a contraceptive. In reproductively capable women, a non-hormonal method of contraception should be used *[see Warnings and Precautions (5.4)]*.

Leuprolide acetate for depot suspension may cause fetal harm when administered to a pregnant woman.

When administered on day 6 of pregnancy at test dosages of 0.00024, 0.0024, and 0.024 mg/kg (1/300 to 1/3 of the human dose) to rabbits, leuprolide acetate for depot suspension produced a dose-related increase in major fetal abnormalities. Similar studies in rats failed to demonstrate an increase in fetal malformations. There was increased fetal mortality and decreased fetal weights with the two higher doses of leuprolide acetate for depot suspension in rabbits and with the highest dose (0.024 mg/kg) in rats.

8.3   Nursing Mothers

Do not use LUPANETA PACK in nursing mothers because the effects of leuprolide acetate for depot suspension on lactation and/or the breast-fed child have not been determined. It is not known whether leuprolide acetate for depot suspension is excreted in human milk.

Detectable amounts of progestins have been identified in the milk of mothers receiving them *[see Contraindications (4)]*.

8.4   Pediatric Use

LUPANETA PACK is not indicated in premenarcheal adolescents. Safety and effectiveness of LUPANETA PACK have not been established in pediatric patients. Experience with LUPANETA PACK for treatment of endometriosis has been limited to women 18 years of age and older.

8.5   Geriatric Use

LUPANETA PACK is not indicated in postmenopausal women and has not been studied in women over 65 years of age.

11   DESCRIPTION

LUPANETA PACK (leuprolide acetate for depot suspension; norethindrone acetate tablets) 3-month contains one dual chamber syringe with leuprolide acetate for depot suspension 11.25 mg and norethindrone acetate tablets USP: 5 mg (bottle of 90 tablets).

Leuprolide Acetate for Depot Suspension

Leuprolide acetate for depot suspension is a synthetic nonapeptide analog of gonadotropin-releasing hormone (GnRH or LH-RH), a GnRH agonist. The chemical name is 5- oxo-L-prolyl-L-histidyl-L-tryptophyl-L-seryl-L-tyrosyl-D-leucyl-L-leucyl-L-arginyl-N-ethyl-L-prolinamide acetate (salt) with the following structural formula:

[See structural formula on the next page]

Leuprolide acetate for depot suspension 11.25 mg is available in a prefilled dual-chamber syringe containing sterile lyophilized microspheres which, when mixed with diluent, become a suspension intended as an intramuscular injection.

The front chamber of leuprolide acetate for depot suspension 11.25 mg for 3-month administration prefilled dual-chamber syringe contains leuprolide acetate for depot suspension (11.25 mg), polylactic acid (99.3 mg) and D-mannitol (19.45 mg). The second chamber of diluent contains carboxymethylcellulose sodium (7.5 mg), D-mannitol (75 mg), polysorbate 80 (1.5 mg), water for injection, USP, and glacial acetic acid, USP to control pH.

During the manufacture of leuprolide acetate for depot suspension, acetic acid is lost, leaving the peptide.

Table 2. Hot Flashes in the Month Prior to the Assessment Visit (Controlled Study)

Assessment Visit	Treatment Group	Number of Patients Reporting Hot Flashes		Number of Days with Hot Flashes		Maximum Number of Hot Flashes in 24 Hours	
		N	(%)	N[2]	Mean	N[2]	Mean
Week 24	LA-Only*	32/37	86	37	19	36	5.8
	LA/N†	22/38	58[1]	38	7[1]	38	1.9[1]

* LA-Only = leuprolide acetate 3.75 mg
† LA/N = leuprolide acetate 3.75 mg plus norethindrone acetate 5 mg
[1] Statistically significantly less than the LA-Only group (p<0.01)
[2] Number of patients assessed.

Table 3. Serum Lipids: Mean Percent Changes from Baseline Values at Treatment Week 24

| | leuprolide acetate 3.75 mg | | leuprolide acetate for depot suspension 3.75 mg plus norethindrone acetate 5 mg daily | | | |
| | Controlled Study (n=39) | | Controlled Study (n=41) | | Open Label Study (n=117) | |
	Baseline Value*	Wk 24 % Change	Baseline Value*	Wk 24 % Change	Baseline Value*	Wk 24 % Change
Total Cholesterol	170.5	9.2%	179.3	0.2%	181.2	2.8%
HDL Cholesterol	52.4	7.4%	51.8	-18.8%	51.0	-14.6%
LDL Cholesterol	96.6	10.9%	101.5	14.1%	109.1	13.1%
LDL/HDL Ratio	2.0†	5.0%	2.1†	43.4%	2.3†	39.4%
Triglycerides	107.8	17.5%	130.2	9.5%	105.4	13.8%

* mg/dL
† ratio

Norethindrone Acetate

Norethindrone acetate tablets USP - 5 mg oral tablets. Norethindrone acetate USP, (17-hydroxy-19-nor-17α-pregn-4-en-20-yn-3-one acetate), a synthetic, orally active progestin, is the acetic acid ester of norethindrone. It is a white, or creamy white, crystalline powder.

Norethindrone acetate tablets USP, 5 mg contain the following inactive ingredients: colloidal silicon dioxide, lactose monohydrate, magnesium stearate, microcrystalline cellulose and talc.

12   CLINICAL PHARMACOLOGY

12.1   Mechanism of Action

Leuprolide Acetate for Depot Suspension

Leuprolide acetate for depot suspension is a long-acting GnRH analog. A single injection of leuprolide acetate for depot suspension results in an initial elevation followed by a prolonged suppression of pituitary gonadotropins. Repeated dosing at quarterly intervals results in decreased secretion of gonadal steroids; consequently, tissues and functions that depend on gonadal steroids for their maintenance become quiescent. This effect is reversible on discontinuation of drug therapy.

Leuprolide acetate is not active when given orally.

Norethindrone Acetate

Norethindrone acetate induces secretory changes in an estrogen-primed endometrium.

12.2   Pharmacodynamics

In a pharmacokinetic/pharmacodynamic study of leuprolide acetate 11.25 mg for 3-month administration in healthy female subjects (N=20), the onset of estradiol suppression was observed for individual subjects between day 4 and week 4 after dosing. By the third week following the injection, the mean estradiol concentration (8 pg/mL) was in the menopausal range. Throughout the remainder of the dosing period, mean serum estradiol levels ranged from the menopausal to the early follicular range.

Serum estradiol was suppressed to ≤20 pg/mL in all subjects within four weeks and remained suppressed (≤40 pg/mL) in 80% of subjects until the end of the 12-week dosing interval, at which time two of these subjects had a value between 40 and 50 pg/mL. Four additional subjects had at least two consecutive elevations of estradiol (range 43-240 pg/mL) levels during the 12-week dosing interval, but there was no indication of luteal function for any of the subjects during this period.

12.3   Pharmacokinetics

Absorption

Leuprolide Acetate for Depot Suspension

Following a single injection of the three month formulation of leuprolide acetate for depot suspension (11.25 mg) in female subjects, a mean plasma leuprolide concentration of 36.3 ng/mL was observed at 4 hours. Leuprolide appeared to be released at a constant rate following the onset of steady-state levels during the third week after dosing and mean levels then declined gradually to near the lower limit of detection by 12 weeks. The mean (± standard deviation) leuprolide concentration from 3 to 12 weeks was 0.23 ± 0.09 ng/mL. However, intact leuprolide and an inactive major metabolite could not be distinguished by the assay which was employed in the study. The initial burst, followed by the rapid decline to a steady-state level, was similar to the release pattern seen with the monthly formulation.

Norethindrone Acetate

Norethindrone acetate is deacetylated to norethindrone after oral administration, and the disposition of norethindrone acetate is indistinguishable from that of orally administered norethindrone. Norethindrone acetate is absorbed from norethindrone acetate tablets, with maximum plasma concentration of norethindrone generally occurring at about 2 hours post-dose (see Figure 8). The pharmacokinetic parameters of norethindrone following single oral administration of 5 mg norethindrone acetate under fasting conditions in 29 healthy female volunteers are summarized in Table 5.

Table 5. Pharmacokinetic Parameters after a Single Dose of Norethindrone Acetate in Healthy Women

Norethindrone Acetate (n=29)	Arithmetic Mean ± SD
Norethindrone	
AUC (0-inf) (ng/ml*h)	166.90 ± 56.28
C_{max} (ng/ml)	26.19 ± 6.19
t_{max} (h)	1.83 ± 0.58
$t_{1/2}$ (h)	8.51 ± 2.19

AUC = area under the curve,
C_{max} = maximum plasma concentration,
t_{max} = time at maximum plasma concentration,
$t_{1/2}$ = half-life,
SD = standard deviation

[See Figure 8 on next page]

Effect of Food:

The effect of food administration on the pharmacokinetics of norethindrone acetate has not been studied.

Distribution

Leuprolide Acetate for Depot Suspension

The mean steady-state volume of distribution of leuprolide following intravenous bolus administration to healthy male volunteers was 27 L. *In vitro* binding to human plasma proteins ranged from 43% to 49%.

Norethindrone Acetate

Norethindrone is 36% bound to sex hormone-binding globulin (SHBG) and 61% bound to albumin. Volume of distribution of norethindrone is about 4 L/kg.

Metabolism

Leuprolide Acetate for Depot Suspension

In healthy male volunteers, a 1 mg bolus of leuprolide administered intravenously revealed that the mean systemic clearance was 7.6 L/h, with a terminal elimination half-life of approximately 3 hours based on a two compartment model.

In rats and dogs, administration of ^{14}C-labeled leuprolide was shown to be metabolized to smaller inactive peptides, a pentapeptide (Metabolite I), tripeptides (Metabolites II and III) and a dipeptide (Metabolite IV). These fragments may be further catabolized.

In a pharmacokinetic/pharmacodynamic study of endometriosis patients, intramuscular 11.25 mg leuprolide acetate for depot suspension (n=19) every 12 weeks or intramuscular 3.75 mg leuprolide acetate for depot suspension (n=15) every 4 weeks was administered for 24 weeks. There was no statistically significant difference in changes of serum estradiol concentration from baseline between the 2 treatment groups.

M-I plasma concentrations measured in 5 prostate cancer patients reached maximum concentration 2 to 6 hours after dosing and were approximately 6% of the peak parent drug concentration. One week after dosing, mean plasma M-I concentrations were approximately 20% of mean leuprolide concentrations.

Norethindrone Acetate

Norethindrone undergoes extensive biotransformation, primarily via reduction, followed by sulfate and glucuronide conjugation. The majority of metabolites in the circulation are sulfates, with glucuronides accounting for most of the urinary metabolites.

Excretion

Leuprolide Acetate for Depot Suspension

Following administration of leuprolide acetate for depot suspension 3.75 mg for 1-month administration to 3 patients, less than 5% of the dose was recovered as parent and M-I metabolite in the urine.

Norethindrone Acetate

Plasma clearance value for norethindrone is approximately 0.4 L/hr/kg. Norethindrone is excreted in both urine and feces, primarily as metabolites. The mean terminal elimination half-life of norethindrone following a single dose administration of norethindrone acetate is approximately 9 hours.

Specific Populations

Hepatic Impairment

The effect of hepatic disease on the disposition of norethindrone after norethindrone acetate administration has not been evaluated. However, norethindrone acetate is contraindicated in markedly impaired liver function or liver disease *[see Contraindications (4)]*.

The pharmacokinetics of the leuprolide acetate for depot suspension in hepatically impaired patients has not been determined.

Renal Impairment

The effect of renal disease on the disposition of norethindrone after norethindrone acetate administration has not been evaluated. In pre-menopausal women with chronic renal failure undergoing peritoneal dialysis who received multiple doses of an oral contraceptive containing ethinyl estradiol and norethindrone, plasma norethindrone concentration was unchanged compared to concentrations in pre-menopausal women with normal renal function.

The pharmacokinetics of the leuprolide acetate for depot suspension in renally impaired patients has not been determined.

Race

The effect of race on the disposition of norethindrone after norethindrone acetate administration has not been evaluated.

Drug Interactions

Leuprolide Acetate for Depot Suspension

Leuprolide acetate for depot suspension is a peptide that is primarily degraded by peptidase and not by cytochrome P-450 enzymes as noted in specific studies, and the drug is only about 46% bound to plasma proteins, drug interactions would not be expected to occur.

Continued on next page

13 NONCLINICAL TOXICOLOGY

13.1 Carcinogenesis, Mutagenesis, Impairment of Fertility

Leuprolide Acetate for Depot Suspension

A two-year carcinogenicity study was conducted in rats and mice. In rats, a dose-related increase of benign pituitary hyperplasia and benign pituitary adenomas was noted at 24 months when the drug was administered subcutaneously at high daily doses (0.6 to 4 mg/kg). There was a significant but not dose-related increase of pancreatic islet-cell adenomas in females and of testicular interstitial cell adenomas in males (highest incidence in the low dose group). In mice, no leuprolide acetate-induced tumors or pituitary abnormalities were observed at a dose as high as 60 mg/kg for two years. Patients have been treated with leuprolide acetate for up to three years with doses as high as 10 mg/day and for two years with doses as high as 20 mg/day without demonstrable pituitary abnormalities.

Mutagenicity studies have been performed with leuprolide acetate using bacterial and mammalian systems. These studies provided no evidence of a mutagenic potential. Clinical and pharmacologic studies in adults (> 18 years) with leuprolide acetate and similar analogs have shown reversibility of fertility suppression when the drug is discontinued after continuous administration for periods of up to 24 weeks. Although no clinical studies have been completed in children to assess the full reversibility of fertility suppression, animal studies (prepubertal and adult rats and monkeys) with leuprolide acetate and other GnRH analogs have shown functional recovery.

14 CLINICAL STUDIES

Leuprolide Acetate for Depot Suspension

Initial endometriosis efficacy data for leuprolide acetate for depot suspension were based on the 3.75 mg dose administered once monthly.

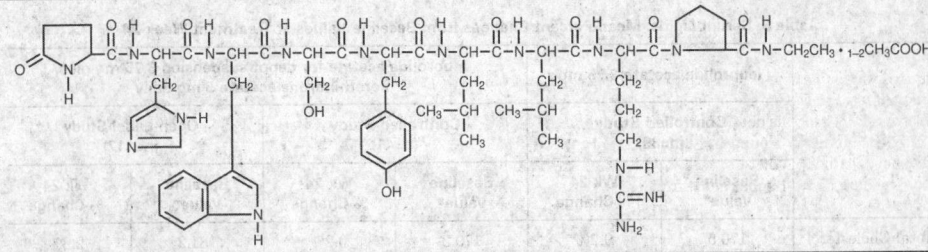

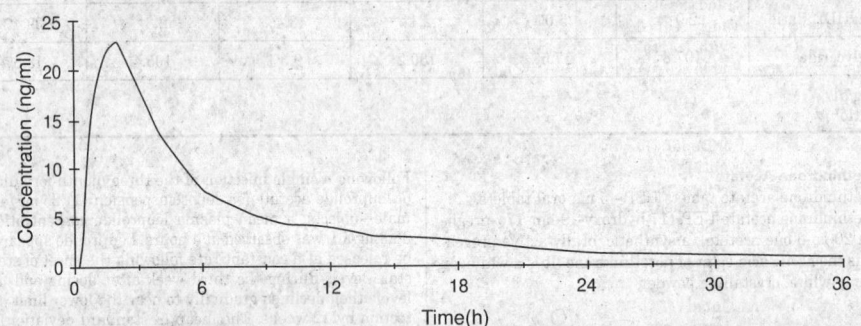

Figure 8. Mean Norethindrone Plasma Concentration Profile after a Single Dose of 5 mg Norethindrone Acetate Administered to 29 Healthy Female Volunteers under Fasting Conditions

A pharmacokinetic/pharmacodynamic study in 41 women that included both the 3.75 mg dose administered once monthly and the 11.25 mg dose administered once every three months did not reveal clinically significant differences in terms of efficacy in reducing painful symptoms of endometriosis or magnitude of the decrease in bone mineral density (BMD) associated with use of leuprolide acetate.

Leuprolide Acetate for Depot Suspension Plus Norethindrone Acetate

Two clinical studies with treatment duration of 12 months were conducted to evaluate the effect of coadministration of leuprolide acetate for depot suspension and norethindrone acetate on the loss of bone mineral density (BMD) associated with leuprolide acetate for depot suspension and on the efficacy of leuprolide acetate for depot suspension in relieving symptoms of endometriosis. (All patients in these studies received calcium supplementation with 1000 mg elemental calcium). A total of 242 women were treated with monthly administration of leuprolide acetate 3.75 mg (13 injections) and with 5 mg norethindrone acetate taken daily. The population age range was 17-43 years old. The majority of patients were Caucasian (87%).

One coadministration study was a controlled, randomized and double-blind study included 51 women treated monthly with leuprolide acetate for depot suspension alone and 55 women treated monthly with leuprolide acetate for depot suspension plus norethindrone acetate daily. Women in this trial were followed for up to 24 months after completing one year of treatment. The other study was an open-label single arm clinical study in 136 women of one year of treatment with leuprolide acetate for depot suspension and norethindrone acetate, with follow-up for up to 12 months after completing treatment.

The second study was an open label, single arm study in which 136 women were treated monthly with leuprolide acetate for depot suspension plus norethindrone acetate daily, with follow-up for up to 12 months after completing treatment.

The assessment of efficacy was based on the investigator's or the patient's monthly assessment of five signs or symptoms of endometriosis (dysmenorrhea, pelvic pain, deep dyspareunia, pelvic tenderness and pelvic induration).

Table 6 below provides detailed efficacy data regarding relief of symptoms of endometriosis based on the two studies of coadministration of leuprolide acetate and norethindrone acetate.

[See table 6 in the previous column]

Suppression of menses (menses was defined as three or more consecutive days of menstrual bleeding) was maintained throughout treatment in 84% and 73% of patients receiving leuprolide acetate and norethindrone acetate, in the controlled study and open label study, respectively. The median time for menses resumption after treatment with leuprolide acetate and norethindrone acetate was 8 weeks.

Table 6. Percentages of Patients with Symptoms of Endometriosis and Mean Clinical Severity Scores

Variable	Study	Group	Percent of Patients with Symptom — Baseline N[1]	Percent of Patients with Symptom — Baseline (%)[2]	Percent of Patients with Symptom — Final (%)	Clinical Pain Severity Score — Baseline N[1]	Clinical Pain Severity Score — Baseline Value[3]	Clinical Pain Severity Score — Final Change
Dysmenorrhea	Controlled Study	LA*	51	(100)	(4)	50	3.2	-2.0
		LA/N†	55	(100)	(4)	54	3.1	-2.0
	Open Label Study	LA/N	136	(99)	(9)	134	3.3	-2.1
Pelvic Pain	Controlled Study	LA	51	(100)	(66)	50	2.9	-1.1
		LA/N	55	(96)	(56)	54	3.1	-1.1
	Open Label Study	LA/N	136	(99)	(63)	134	3.2	-1.2
Deep Dyspareunia	Controlled Study	LA	42	(83)	(37)	25	2.4	-1.0
		LA/N	43	(84)	(45)	30	2.7	-0.8
	Open Label Study	LA/N	102	(91)	(53)	94	2.7	-1.0
Pelvic Tenderness	Controlled Study	LA	51	(94)	(34)	50	2.5	-1.0
		LA/N	54	(91)	(34)	52	2.6	-0.9
	Open Label Study	LA/N	136	(99)	(39)	134	2.9	-1.4
Pelvic Induration	Controlled Study	LA	51	(51)	(12)	50	1.9	-0.4
		LA/N	54	(46)	(17)	52	1.6	-0.4
	Open Label Study	LA/N	136	(75)	(21)	134	2.2	-0.9

* LA = leuprolide acetate 3.75 mg assessment
† LA/N = leuprolide acetate 3.75 mg plus norethindrone acetate 5 mg
[1] Number of patients that were included in the assessment
[2] Percentage of patients with the symptom/sign
[3] Value description: 1=none; 2= mild; 3= moderate; 4= severe

Changes in Bone Density

The effect of leuprolide acetate for depot suspension and norethindrone acetate on bone mineral density was evaluated by dual energy x-ray absorptiometry (DXA) scan in the two clinical trials. For the open-label study, success in mitigating BMD loss was defined as the lower bound of the 95% confidence interval around the change from baseline at one year of treatment not to exceed -2.2%. The bone mineral density data of the lumbar spine from these two studies are presented in Table 7.

[See table 7 above]

The change in BMD following discontinuation of treatment is shown in Table 8.

[See table 8 at top of next page]

These clinical studies demonstrated that coadministration of leuprolide acetate and norethindrone acetate 5 mg daily is effective in significantly reducing the loss of bone mineral density that occurs with leuprolide acetate for depot suspension treatment, and in relieving symptoms of endometriosis.

15   REFERENCES

Leuprolide Acetate for Depot Suspension

1. NIOSH Alert: Preventing occupational exposures to antineoplastic and other hazardous drugs in healthcare settings. 2004. U.S. Department of Health and Human Services, Public Health Service, Centers for Disease Control and Prevention, National Institute for Occupational Safety and Health, DHHS (NIOSH) Publication No. 2004-165.
2. OSHA Technical Manual, TED 1-0.15A, Section VI: Chapter 2. Controlling Occupational Exposure to Hazardous Drugs. OSHA, 1999. http://www.osha.gov/dts/osta/otm/otm_vi/otm_vi_2.html
3. American Society of Health-System Pharmacists. ASHP guidelines on handling hazardous drugs. *Am J Health-Syst Pharm.* 2006; 63; 1172-1193.
4. Polovich, M., White, J.M., & Kelleher, L.O. (eds.) 2005. Chemotherapy and biotherapy guidelines and recommendations for practice (2nd. Ed.) Pittsburgh, PA: Oncology Nursing Society.

16   HOW SUPPLIED/STORAGE AND HANDLING

LUPANETA PACK for 3-month copackaged kit (NDC 0074-1053-05) is available in cartons containing:

leuprolide acetate for depot suspension 11.25 mg for 3-month administration Kit (NDC 0074-3663-04)

norethindrone acetate 5 mg tablets; 90 count bottle (NDC 0074-1049-04)

1. Leuprolide acetate for depot suspension 11.25 mg for 3-month administration kit contains:
   • one prefilled dual-chamber syringe
   • one plunger
   • two alcohol swabs

Each syringe contains sterile lyophilized microspheres of leuprolide acetate incorporated in a biodegradable polymer of polylactic acid. When mixed with 1.5 mL of the diluent, leuprolide acetate for depot suspension 11.25 mg for 3-month administration is administered as a single intramuscular injection.

2. Norethindrone acetate 5 mg 90 count bottle
   White to off-white oval, flat faced beveled edged, uncoated tablets debossed with 'G with breakline' on one side and 304 on other side.

Store at 25°C (77°F); excursions permitted to 15 to 30°C (59 to 86°F) [See USP Controlled Room Temperature]

17   PATIENT COUNSELING INFORMATION

See FDA-approved patient labeling (Patient Information)

Counsel patients about the Warnings and Precautions for LUPANETA PACK, including:

• Do not use this drug if they have experienced an allergic reaction to GnRH agonists or progestins
• Do not use this drug if they are pregnant or planning a pregnancy, suspect they may be pregnant, or are breastfeeding
• Risk of loss of bone mineral density and limitation of treatment to two six-month courses of treatment
• Risk to an exposed fetus and need to use nonhormonal contraception
• Discontinue norethindrone if they develop sudden loss of vision, double vision or sudden migraine
• The possibility of development or worsening of depression during treatment with leuprolide acetate for depot suspension
• Need for close monitoring if they have cardiovascular risk factors, or conditions like epilepsy, migraine or renal dysfunction

Table 7. Mean Percent Change from Baseline In BMD of Lumbar Spine

| | leuprolide acetate for depot suspension 3.75 mg | | leuprolide acetate for depot suspension 3.75 mg plus norethindrone acetate 5 mg daily | | | |
| | Controlled Study | | Controlled Study | | Open Label Study | |
	N	Change (Mean, 95% CI)#	N	Change (Mean, 95% CI)#	N	Change (Mean, 95% CI)#
Week 24*	41	-3.2% (-3.8, -2.6)	42	-0.3% (-0.8, 0.3)	115	-0.2% (-0.6, 0.2)
Week 52†	29	-6.3% (-7.1, -5.4)	32	-1.0% (-1.9, -0.1)	84	-1.1% (-1.6, -0.5)

* Includes on-treatment measurements that fell within 2-252 days after the first day of treatment.
† Includes on-treatment measurements >252 days after the first day of treatment.
# 95% CI: 95% Confidence Interval

• Notify their healthcare provider if they develop new or worsened symptoms after beginning treatment

PATIENT INFORMATION
LUPANETA PACK®
(loo-pan-e-tə pæk)
(leuprolide acetate for depot suspension and norethindrone acetate tablets)

Read this Patient Information before you start taking LUPANETA PACK and each time you get a refill. There may be new information. This information does not take the place of talking with your doctor about your medical condition or your treatment.

What is LUPANETA PACK?

LUPANETA PACK contains 2 different prescription medicines:

• **leuprolide acetate for depot suspension** is a medicine injected into your muscle and used to treat pain due to endometriosis.
• **norethindrone acetate tablets** is a medicine taken by mouth and used to help lower the side effect of bone thinning that is caused by leuprolide acetate for depot suspension.

LUPANETA PACK should not be used longer than 6 months at a time after you first start treatment for your endometriosis symptoms. LUPANETA PACK should not be used for more than a total of 12 months during your treatment.

It is not known if LUPANETA PACK is safe and effective in children under 18 years of age.

Who should not take LUPANETA PACK?

Do not take LUPANETA PACK if you:

• have had an allergic reaction to medicines like leuprolide acetate for depot suspension or norethindrone acetate tablets. See the end of this leaflet for a complete list of ingredients in LUPANETA PACK.
• have uterine bleeding for which a cause has not been found
• are pregnant or may be pregnant. LUPANETA PACK may harm your unborn baby.
• are breastfeeding or plan to breastfeed. It is not known if LUPANETA PACK passes into your breast milk.
• had or have breast cancer or other cancers that are sensitive to hormones
• have problems with blood clots, a stroke or a heart attack
• have liver problems

What should I tell my doctor before taking LUPANETA PACK?

Before you take LUPANETA PACK, tell your doctor if you:

• drink alcohol
• have a family history of bone loss (osteoporosis)
• have high cholesterol
• have migraine headaches
• have epilepsy
• smoke
• have depression
• have had blood clots, a stroke or a heart attack
• have diabetes
• have kidney problems

Tell your doctor about all the medicines you take, including prescription and non-prescription medicines, vitamins, and herbal supplements.

Especially tell your doctor if you take anticonvulsant (seizure) or corticosteroid medicines.

Ask your doctor for a list of these medicines if you are not sure.

Know the medicines you take. Keep a list of them to show your doctor and pharmacist when you get a new medicine.

How should I take LUPANETA PACK?

• **Leuprolide acetate for depot suspension** for 3-month administration is injected into your muscle 1 time every 3 months by a healthcare professional in your doctor's office.

• **Take norethindrone acetate tablets** exactly as your doctor tells you to take them. Take 1 norethindrone acetate tablet by mouth every day for 3 months after you receive your injection.
• Talk to your doctor about the birth control method that is right for you before you start taking LUPANETA PACK. You will need to use a form of birth control that does not contain hormones, such as:
   ○ a diaphragm with spermicide
   ○ condoms with spermicide
   ○ a copper IUD
• If you become pregnant while taking LUPANETA PACK, stop taking the norethindrone acetate tablets and call your doctor right away.

How well does LUPANETA PACK work?

LUPANETA PACK is used to treat pain due to endometriosis. The pain from endometriosis can happen when you have your period, during other times of the month, or during intercourse (sex). Most women feel some relief from their endometriosis pain after taking both drugs in LUPANETA PACK.

The tablets in LUPANETA PACK help lower the side effect of bone thinning that is caused by leuprolide acetate for depot suspension. Women taking both drugs in LUPANETA PACK lost an average of 1% of their bone density after about 1 year of treatment. Women regained some of their bone density about 1 year after they stopped treatment with LUPANETA PACK.

What are the possible side effects of LUPANETA PACK?

LUPANETA PACK may cause serious side effects, including:

• **bone thinning (decreased bone mineral density)**
• **harm to your unborn baby**
• **vision problems.** Call your doctor right away if you have sudden loss of vision, double vision, bulging eyes, or migraine headaches.
• **depression or worsening depression**
• **allergic reactions.** Get medical help right away if you have any of these symptoms of a serious allergic reaction:
   ○ swelling of your face, lips, mouth, or tongue
   ○ trouble breathing
   ○ wheezing
   ○ severe itching
   ○ skin rash, redness, or swelling
   ○ dizziness or fainting
   ○ fast heartbeat or pounding in your chest (tachycardia)
   ○ sweating
• **worsening endometriosis symptoms when you start taking LUPANETA PACK**
• **swelling (fluid retention)**

The most common side effects of LUPANETA PACK include:

• hot flashes and sweats
• headaches or migraine headaches
• depression and mood swings
• nausea and vomiting
• problems sleeping
• nervousness or feeling anxious
• pain
• acne
• weakness
• vaginal infection or inflammation
• weight gain

Continued on next page

Table 8. Mean Percent Change from Baseline in BMD of Lumbar Spine in Post-Treatment Follow-up Period

Post Treatment Measurement	Controlled Study						Open Label Study		
	LA-Only			LA/N			LA/N		
	N	Mean % Change	95% CI (%)	N	Mean % Change	95% CI (%)	N	Mean % Change	95% CI (%)[2]
Month 8	19	-3.3	(-4.9, -1.8)	23	-0.9	(-2.1, 0.4)	89	-0.6	(-1.2, 0.0)
Month 12	16	-2.2	(-3.3, -1.1)	12	-0.7	(-2.1, 0.6)	65	0.1	(-0.6, 0.7)

[1] Patients with post treatment measurements
[2] 95% CI (2-sided) of percent change in BMD values from baseline

• constipation or diarrhea

Tell your doctor if you have any side effect that bothers you or that does not go away.

These are not all the possible side effects of LUPANETA PACK. For more information, ask your doctor or pharmacist.

Call your doctor for medical advice about side effects. You may report side effects to FDA at 1-800-FDA-1088.

How should I store norethindrone acetate tablets in the LUPANETA PACK?

• Store norethindrone acetate tablets at room temperature between 68°F to 77°F (20°C to 25°C).

Keep LUPANETA PACK and all medicines out of the reach of children.

General information about the safe and effective use of LUPANETA PACK.

Medicines are sometimes prescribed for purposes other than those listed in a Patient Information leaflet. Do not use LUPANETA PACK for a condition for which it was not prescribed. Do not give LUPANETA PACK to other people, even if they have the same symptoms that you have. It may harm them.

This Patient Information leaflet summarizes the most important information about LUPANETA PACK. If you would like more information, talk with your doctor. You can ask your pharmacist or doctor for information about LUPANETA PACK that is written for health professionals. For more information, go to www.lupanetapack.com or call 1-800-633-9110.

What are the ingredients in LUPANETA PACK?

leuprolide acetate for depot suspension:

Active Ingredients: leuprolide acetate for depot suspension

Inactive Ingredients: polylactic acid, D-mannitol, carboxymethylcellulose sodium, polysorbate 80, water for injection, USP, and glacial acetic acid, USP

norethindrone acetate tablets:

Active Ingredients: norethindrone acetate USP

Inactive Ingredients: colloidal silicon dioxide, lactose monohydrate, magnesium stearate, microcrystalline cellulose and talc.

This Patient Information has been approved by the U.S. Food and Drug Administration.

Leuprolide Acetate for Depot Suspension 11.25 mg:

Manufactured for
AbbVie Inc.
North Chicago, IL 60064
By Takeda Pharmaceutical Company Limited
Osaka, Japan 540-8645

Norethindrone Acetate:

Manufactured for
AbbVie Inc.
North Chicago, IL 60064
Manufactured by
Glenmark Pharmaceuticals Ltd.
Colvale-Bardez, Goa
403 513, India

LUPANETA PACK
Packaged by:
AbbVie Inc.
North Chicago, IL 60064
™-Trademark
® – Registered Trademark
©2015 AbbVie Inc.
03-B184-R3 June, 2015
Shown in Product Identification Guide, page 505

LUPRON DEPOT® 3.75 mg ℞

[lew-prŏn]

(leuprolide acetate for depot suspension)

Rx only

This is combined labeling. Examples of different fonts and colors appear below.

• General information
• Information on endometriosis
• Information on uterine fibroids

DESCRIPTION

Leuprolide acetate is a synthetic nonapeptide analog of naturally occurring gonadotropin-releasing hormone (GnRH or LH-RH). The analog possesses greater potency than the natural hormone. The chemical name is 5-oxo-L-prolyl-L-histidyl-L-tryptophyl-L-seryl-L-tyrosyl-D-leucyl-L-leucyl-L-arginyl-N-ethyl-L-prolinamide acetate (salt) with the following structural formula:

[See structured formula below]

LUPRON DEPOT is available in a prefilled dual-chamber syringe containing sterile lyophilized microspheres which, when mixed with diluent, become a suspension intended as a monthly intramuscular injection.

The front chamber of LUPRON DEPOT 3.75 mg prefilled dual-chamber syringe contains leuprolide acetate (3.75 mg), purified gelatin (0.65 mg), DL-lactic and glycolic acids copolymer (33.1 mg), and D-mannitol (6.6 mg). The second chamber of diluent contains carboxymethylcellulose sodium (5 mg), D-mannitol (50 mg), polysorbate 80 (1 mg), water for injection, USP, and glacial acetic acid, USP to control pH. During the manufacture of LUPRON DEPOT 3.75 mg, acetic acid is lost, leaving the peptide.

CLINICAL PHARMACOLOGY

Leuprolide acetate is a long-acting GnRH analog. A single monthly injection of LUPRON DEPOT 3.75 mg results in an initial stimulation followed by a prolonged suppression of pituitary gonadotropins.

Repeated dosing at monthly intervals results in decreased secretion of gonadal steroids; consequently, tissues and functions that depend on gonadal steroids for their maintenance become quiescent. This effect is reversible on discontinuation of drug therapy.

Leuprolide acetate is not active when given orally. Intramuscular injection of the depot formulation provides plasma concentrations of leuprolide over a period of one month.

Pharmacokinetics

Absorption

A single dose of LUPRON DEPOT 3.75 mg was administered by intramuscular injection to healthy female volunteers. The absorption of leuprolide was characterized by an initial increase in plasma concentration, with peak concentration ranging from 4.6 to 10.2 ng/mL at four hours postdosing. However, intact leuprolide and an inactive metabolite could not be distinguished by the assay used in the study. Following the initial rise, leuprolide concentrations started to plateau within two days after dosing and remained relatively stable for about four to five weeks with plasma concentrations of about 0.30 ng/mL.

Distribution

The mean steady-state volume of distribution of leuprolide following intravenous bolus administration to healthy male volunteers was 27 L. *In vitro* binding to human plasma proteins ranged from 43% to 49%.

Metabolism

In healthy male volunteers, a 1 mg bolus of leuprolide administered intravenously revealed that the mean systemic clearance was 7.6 L/h, with a terminal elimination half-life of approximately 3 hours based on a two compartment model.

In rats and dogs, administration of ^{14}C-labeled leuprolide was shown to be metabolized to smaller inactive peptides, a pentapeptide (Metabolite I), tripeptides (Metabolites II and III) and a dipeptide (Metabolite IV). These fragments may be further catabolized.

The major metabolite (M-I) plasma concentrations measured in 5 prostate cancer patients reached maximum concentration 2 to 6 hours after dosing and were approximately 6% of the peak parent drug concentration. One week after dosing, mean plasma M-I concentrations were approximately 20% of mean leuprolide concentrations.

Excretion

Following administration of LUPRON DEPOT 3.75 mg to 3 patients, less than 5% of the dose was recovered as parent and M-I metabolite in the urine.

Special Populations

The pharmacokinetics of the drug in hepatically and renally impaired patients have not been determined.

Drug Interactions

No pharmacokinetic-based drug-drug interaction studies have been conducted with LUPRON DEPOT. However, because leuprolide acetate is a peptide that is primarily degraded by peptidase and not by cytochrome P-450 enzymes as noted in specific studies, and the drug is only about 46% bound to plasma proteins, drug interactions would not be expected to occur.

CLINICAL STUDIES

Endometriosis

In controlled clinical studies, LUPRON DEPOT 3.75 mg monthly for six months was shown to be comparable to danazol 800 mg/day in relieving the clinical sign/symptoms of endometriosis (pelvic pain, dysmenorrhea, dyspareunia, pelvic tenderness, and induration) and in reducing the size of endometrial implants as evidenced by laparoscopy. The clinical significance of a decrease in endometriotic lesions is not known at this time, and in addition laparoscopic staging of endometriosis does not necessarily correlate with the severity of symptoms.

LUPRON DEPOT 3.75 mg monthly induced amenorrhea in 74% and 98% of the patients after the first and second treatment months respectively. Most of the remaining patients reported episodes of only light bleeding or spotting. In the first, second and third posttreatment months, normal menstrual cycles resumed in 7%, 71% and 95% of patients, respectively, excluding those who became pregnant.

Figure 1 illustrates the percent of patients with symptoms at baseline, final treatment visit and sustained relief at 6 and 12 months following discontinuation of treatment for the various symptoms evaluated during two controlled clinical studies. This included all patients at end of treatment and those who elected to participate in the follow-up period. This might provide a slight bias in the results at follow-up as 75% of the original patients entered the follow-up study, and 36% were evaluated at 6 months and 26% at 12 months.

[See Figure 1 on top of next page]

Hormonal replacement therapy

Two clinical studies with a treatment duration of 12 months indicate that concurrent hormonal therapy (norethindrone acetate 5 mg daily) is effective in significantly reducing the loss of bone mineral density associated with LUPRON, without compromising the efficacy of LUPRON in relieving symptoms of endometriosis. (All patients in these studies received calcium supplementation with

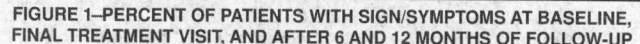

FIGURE 1–PERCENT OF PATIENTS WITH SIGN/SYMPTOMS AT BASELINE, FINAL TREATMENT VISIT, AND AFTER 6 AND 12 MONTHS OF FOLLOW-UP

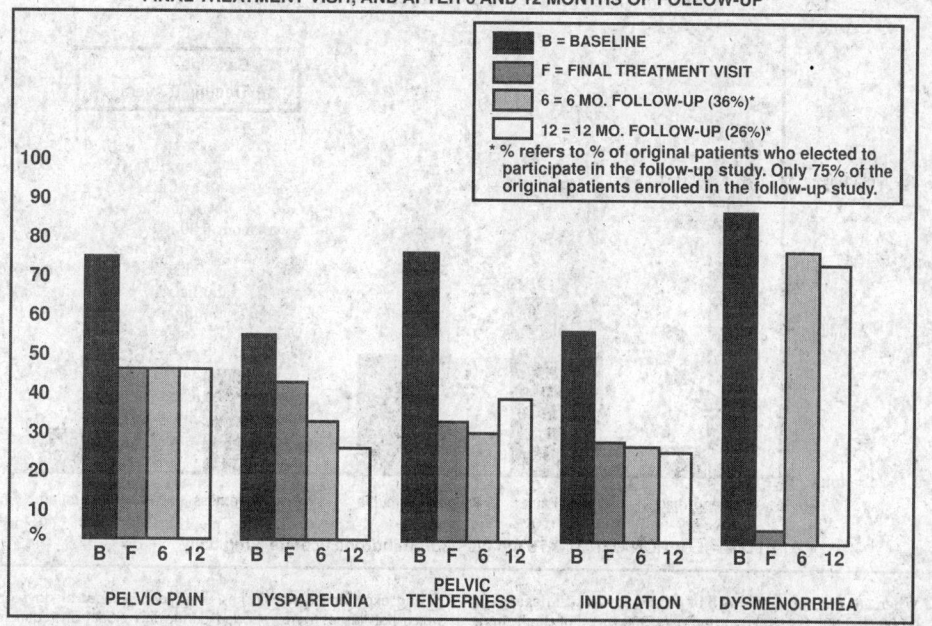

B = BASELINE
F = FINAL TREATMENT VISIT
6 = 6 MO. FOLLOW-UP (36%)*
12 = 12 MO. FOLLOW-UP (26%)*

* % refers to % of original patients who elected to participate in the follow-up study. Only 75% of the original patients enrolled in the follow-up study.

PELVIC PAIN DYSPAREUNIA PELVIC TENDERNESS INDURATION DYSMENORRHEA

1000 mg elemental calcium). One controlled, randomized and double-blind study included 51 women treated with LUPRON DEPOT alone and 55 women treated with LUPRON plus norethindrone acetate 5 mg daily. The second study was an open label study in which 136 women were treated with LUPRON plus norethindrone acetate 5 mg daily. This study confirmed the reduction in loss of bone mineral density that was observed in the controlled study. Suppression of menses was maintained throughout treatment in 84% and 73% of patients receiving LD/N in the controlled study and open label study, respectively. The median time for menses resumption after treatment with LD/N was 8 weeks.

Figure 2 illustrates the mean pain scores for the LD/N group from the controlled study.

[See Figure 2 on top of page 720]

Uterine Leiomyomata (Fibroids)

In controlled clinical trials, administration of LUPRON DEPOT 3.75 mg for a period of three or six months was shown to decrease uterine and fibroid volume, thus allowing for relief of clinical symptoms (abdominal bloating, pelvic pain, and pressure). Excessive vaginal bleeding (menorrhagia and menometrorrhagia) decreased, resulting in improvement in hematologic parameters.

In three clinical trials, enrollment was not based on hematologic status. Mean uterine volume decreased by 41% and myoma volume decreased by 37% at final visit as evidenced by ultrasound or MRI. These patients also experienced a decrease in symptoms including excessive vaginal bleeding and pelvic discomfort. Benefit occurred by three months of therapy, but additional gain was observed with an additional three months of LUPRON DEPOT 3.75 mg. Ninety-five percent of these patients became amenorrheic with 61%, 25%, and 4% experiencing amenorrhea during the first, second, and third treatment months respectively.

Post-treatment follow-up was carried out for a small percentage of LUPRON DEPOT 3.75 mg patients among the 77% who demonstrated a ≥ 25% decrease in uterine volume while on therapy. Menses usually returned within two months of cessation of therapy. Mean time to return to pretreatment uterine size was 8.3 months. Regrowth did not appear to be related to pretreatment uterine volume.

In another controlled clinical study, enrollment was based on hematocrit ≤ 30% and/or hemoglobin ≤ 10.2 g/dL. Administration of LUPRON DEPOT 3.75 mg, concomitantly with iron, produced an increase of ≥ 6% hematocrit and ≥ 2 g/dL hemoglobin in 77% of patients at three months of therapy. The mean change in hematocrit was 10.1% and the mean change in hemoglobin was 4.2 g/dL. Clinical response was judged to be a hematocrit of ≥ 36% and hemoglobin of ≥ 12 g/dL, thus allowing for autologous blood donation prior to surgery. At three months, 75% of patients met this criterion.

At three months, 80% of patients experienced relief from either menorrhagia or menometrorrhagia. As with the previous studies, episodes of spotting and menstrual-like bleeding were noted in some patients.

In this same study, a decrease of ≥ 25% was seen in uterine and myoma volumes in 60% and 54% of patients respectively. LUPRON DEPOT 3.75 mg was found to relieve symptoms of bloating, pelvic pain, and pressure.

There is no evidence that pregnancy rates are enhanced or adversely affected by the use of LUPRON DEPOT 3.75 mg.

INDICATIONS AND USAGE

Endometriosis

LUPRON DEPOT 3.75 mg is indicated for management of endometriosis, including pain relief and reduction of endometriotic lesions. LUPRON DEPOT monthly with norethindrone acetate 5 mg daily is also indicated for initial management of endometriosis and for management of recurrence of symptoms. (Refer also to norethindrone acetate prescribing information for WARNINGS, PRECAUTIONS, CONTRAINDICATIONS and ADVERSE REACTIONS associated with norethindrone acetate). Duration of initial treatment or retreatment should be limited to 6 months.

Uterine Leiomyomata (Fibroids)

LUPRON DEPOT 3.75 mg concomitantly with iron therapy is indicated for the preoperative hematologic improvement of patients with anemia caused by uterine leiomyomata. The clinician may wish to consider a one-month trial period on iron alone inasmuch as some of the patients will respond to iron alone. (See **Table 1**.) LUPRON may be added if the response to iron alone is considered inadequate. Recommended duration of therapy with LUPRON DEPOT 3.75 mg is **up to** three months.

Experience with LUPRON DEPOT in females has been limited to women 18 years of age and older.

Table 1 PERCENT OF PATIENTS ACHIEVING HEMOGLOBIN ≥ 12 GM/DL

Treatment Group	Week 4	Week 8	Week 12
LUPRON DEPOT 3.75 mg with Iron	41*	71†	79*
Iron Alone	17	40	56

* P-Value < 0.01
† P-Value < 0.001

CONTRAINDICATIONS

1. Hypersensitivity to GnRH, GnRH agonist analogs or any of the excipients in LUPRON DEPOT.
2. Undiagnosed abnormal vaginal bleeding.
3. LUPRON DEPOT is contraindicated in women who are or may become pregnant while receiving the drug. LUPRON DEPOT may cause fetal harm when administered to a pregnant woman. Major fetal abnormalities were observed in rabbits but not in rats after administration of LUPRON DEPOT throughout gestation. There was increased fetal mortality and decreased fetal weights

in rats and rabbits. (See **Pregnancy** section.) The effects on fetal mortality are expected consequences of the alterations in hormonal levels brought about by the drug. If this drug is used during pregnancy, or if the patient becomes pregnant while taking this drug, the patient should be apprised of the potential hazard to the fetus.
4. Use in women who are breast-feeding. (See **Nursing Mothers** section.)
5. Norethindrone acetate is contraindicated in women with the following conditions:
   ○ Thrombophlebitis, thromboembolic disorders, cerebral apoplexy, or a past history of these conditions
   ○ Markedly impaired liver function or liver disease
   ○ Known or suspected carcinoma of the breast

WARNINGS

Safe use of leuprolide acetate or norethindrone acetate in pregnancy has not been established clinically. Before starting treatment with LUPRON DEPOT, pregnancy must be excluded.

When used monthly at the recommended dose, LUPRON DEPOT usually inhibits ovulation and stops menstruation. Contraception is not insured, however, by taking LUPRON DEPOT. Therefore, patients should use non-hormonal methods of contraception.

Patients should be advised to see their physician if they believe they may be pregnant. If a patient becomes pregnant during treatment, the drug must be discontinued and the patient must be apprised of the potential risk to the fetus. During the early phase of therapy, sex steroids temporarily rise above baseline because of the physiologic effect of the drug. Therefore, an increase in clinical signs and symptoms may be observed during the initial days of therapy, but these will dissipate with continued therapy.

Symptoms consistent with an anaphylactoid or asthmatic process have been rarely reported post-marketing.

The following applies to co-treatment with LUPRON and norethindrone acetate:

Norethindrone acetate treatment should be discontinued if there is a sudden partial or complete loss of vision or if there is sudden onset of proptosis, diplopia, or migraine. If examination reveals papilledema or retinal vascular lesions, medication should be withdrawn.

Because of the occasional occurrence of thrombophlebitis and pulmonary embolism in patients taking progestogens, the physician should be alert to the earliest manifestations of the disease in women taking norethindrone acetate.

Assessment and management of risk factors for cardiovascular disease is recommended prior to initiation of add-back therapy with norethindrone acetate. Norethindrone acetate should be used with caution in women with risk factors, including lipid abnormalities or cigarette smoking.

PRECAUTIONS

Information for Patients

Patients should be aware of the following information:

1. Since menstruation usually stops with effective doses of LUPRON DEPOT, the patient should notify her physician if regular menstruation persists. Patients missing successive doses of LUPRON DEPOT may experience breakthrough bleeding.
2. Patients should not use LUPRON DEPOT if they are pregnant, breast feeding, have undiagnosed abnormal vaginal bleeding, or are allergic to any of the ingredients in LUPRON DEPOT.
3. Safe use of the drug in pregnancy has not been established clinically. Therefore, a non-hormonal method of contraception should be used during treatment. Patients should be advised that if they miss successive doses of LUPRON DEPOT, breakthrough bleeding or ovulation may occur with the potential for conception. If a patient becomes pregnant during treatment, she should discontinue treatment and consult her physician.
4. Adverse events occurring in clinical studies with LUPRON DEPOT that are associated with hypoestrogenism include: hot flashes, headaches, emotional lability, decreased libido, acne, myalgia, reduction in breast size, and vaginal dryness. Estrogen levels returned to normal after treatment was discontinued.
5. Patients should be counseled on the possibility of the development or worsening of depression and the occurrence of memory disorders.

Continued on next page

6. The induced hypoestrogenic state **also** results in a loss in bone density over the course of treatment, some of which may not be reversible. Clinical studies show that concurrent hormonal therapy with norethindrone acetate 5 mg daily is effective in reducing loss of bone mineral density that occurs with LUPRON. (All patients received calcium supplementation with 1000 mg elemental calcium.) (See *Changes in Bone Density* section).

7. If the symptoms of endometriosis recur after a course of therapy, retreatment with a six-month course of LUPRON DEPOT and norethindrone acetate 5 mg daily may be considered. Retreatment beyond this one six month course cannot be recommended. It is recommended that bone density be assessed before retreatment begins to ensure that values are within normal limits. Retreatment with LUPRON DEPOT alone is not recommended.

8. In patients with major risk factors for decreased bone mineral content such as chronic alcohol and/or tobacco use, strong family history of osteoporosis, or chronic use of drugs that can reduce bone mass such as anticonvulsants or corticosteroids, LUPRON DEPOT therapy may pose an additional risk. In these patients, the risks and benefits must be weighed carefully before therapy with LUPRON DEPOT alone is instituted, and concomitant treatment with norethindrone acetate 5 mg daily should be considered. Retreatment with gonadotropin-releasing hormone analogs, including LUPRON is not advisable in patients with major risk factors for loss of bone mineral content.

9. Because norethindrone acetate may cause some degree of fluid retention, conditions which might be influenced by this factor, such as epilepsy, migraine, asthma, cardiac or renal dysfunctions require careful observation during norethindrone acetate add-back therapy.

10. Patients who have a history of depression should be carefully observed during treatment with norethindrone acetate and norethindrone acetate should be discontinued if severe depression occurs.

Convulsions
There have been postmarketing reports of convulsions in patients on leuprolide acetate therapy. These included patients with and without concurrent medications and comorbid conditions.
Laboratory Tests
See **ADVERSE REACTIONS** section.
Drug Interactions
See **CLINICAL PHARMACOLOGY, Pharmacokinetics**.
Drug/Laboratory Test Interactions
Administration of LUPRON DEPOT in therapeutic doses results in suppression of the pituitary-gonadal system. Normal function is usually restored within three months after treatment is discontinued. Therefore, diagnostic tests of pituitary gonadotropic and gonadal functions conducted during treatment and for up to three months after discontinuation of LUPRON DEPOT may be misleading.
Carcinogenesis, Mutagenesis, Impairment of Fertility
A two-year carcinogenicity study was conducted in rats and mice. In rats, a dose-related increase of benign pituitary hyperplasia and benign pituitary adenomas was noted at 24 months when the drug was administered subcutaneously at high daily doses (0.6 to 4 mg/kg). There was a significant but not dose-related increase of pancreatic islet-cell adenomas in females and of testicular interstitial cell adenomas in males (highest incidence in the low dose group). In mice, no leuprolide acetate-induced tumors or pituitary abnormalities were observed at a dose as high as 60 mg/kg for two years. Patients have been treated with leuprolide acetate for up to three years with doses as high as 10 mg/day and for two years with doses as high as 20 mg/day without demonstrable pituitary abnormalities.
Mutagenicity studies have been performed with leuprolide acetate using bacterial and mammalian systems. These studies provided no evidence of a mutagenic potential.
Clinical and pharmacologic studies in adults (>18 years) with leuprolide acetate and similar analogs have shown reversibility of fertility suppression when the drug is discontinued after continuous administration for periods of up to 24 weeks. Although no clinical studies have been completed in children to assess the full reversibility of fertility suppression, animal studies (prepubertal and adult rats and monkeys) with leuprolide acetate and other GnRH analogs have shown functional recovery.
Pregnancy
Teratogenic Effects
Pregnancy Category X (see **CONTRAINDICATIONS** section).

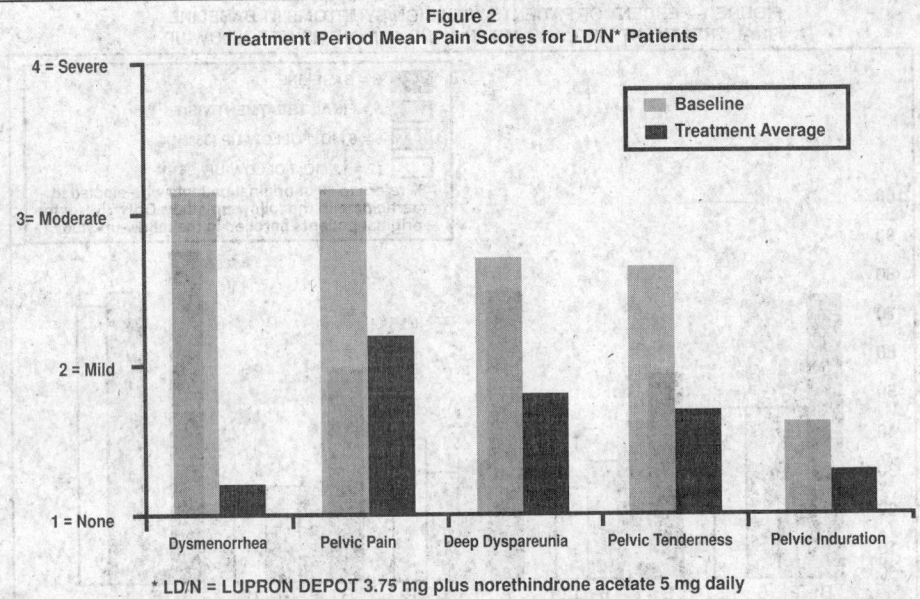

Figure 2
Treatment Period Mean Pain Scores for LD/N* Patients

* LD/N = LUPRON DEPOT 3.75 mg plus norethindrone acetate 5 mg daily

When administered on day 6 of pregnancy at test dosages of 0.00024, 0.0024, and 0.024 mg/kg (1/300 to 1/3 of the human dose) to rabbits, LUPRON DEPOT produced a dose-related increase in major fetal abnormalities. Similar studies in rats failed to demonstrate an increase in fetal malformations. There was increased fetal mortality and decreased fetal weights with the two higher doses of LUPRON DEPOT in rabbits and with the highest dose (0.024 mg/kg) in rats.
Nursing Mothers
It is not known whether LUPRON DEPOT is excreted in human milk. Because many drugs are excreted in human milk, and because the effects of LUPRON DEPOT on lactation and/or the breast-fed child have not been determined, LUPRON DEPOT should not be used by nursing mothers.
Pediatric Use
Experience with LUPRON DEPOT 3.75 mg for treatment of endometriosis has been limited to women 18 years of age and older. See LUPRON DEPOT-PED® (leuprolide acetate for depot suspension) labeling for the safety and effectiveness in children with central precocious puberty.
Geriatric Use
This product has not been studied in women over 65 years of age and is not indicated in this population.

ADVERSE REACTIONS
Clinical Trials
Estradiol levels may increase during the first weeks following the initial injection of LUPRON, but then decline to menopausal levels. This transient increase in estradiol can be associated with a temporary worsening of signs and symptoms (see **WARNINGS** section).
As would be expected with a drug that lowers serum estradiol levels, the most frequently reported adverse reactions were those related to hypoestrogenism.
The **monthly formulation of LUPRON DEPOT 3.75 mg** was utilized in controlled clinical trials that studied the drug in 166 endometriosis and 166 uterine fibroids patients. Adverse events reported in ≥5% of patients in either of these populations and thought to be potentially related to drug are noted in the following table.
[See table 2 at top of next page]
In one controlled clinical trial utilizing the monthly formulation of LUPRON DEPOT, patients diagnosed with uterine fibroids received a higher dose (7.5 mg) of LUPRON DEPOT. Events seen with this dose that were thought to be potentially related to drug and were not seen at the lower dose included glossitis, hypesthesia, lactation, pyelonephritis, and urinary disorders. Generally, a higher incidence of hypoestrogenic effects was observed at the higher dose.
Table 3 lists the potentially drug-related adverse events observed in at least 5% of patients in any treatment group during the first 6 months of treatment in the add-back clinical studies.
In the controlled clinical trial, 50 of 51 (98%) patients in the LD group and 48 of 55 (87%) patients in the LD/N group reported experiencing hot flashes on one or more occasions during treatment. During Month 6 of treatment, 32 of 37 (86%) patients in the LD group and 22 of 38 (58%) patients in the LD/N group reported

having experienced hot flashes. The mean number of days on which hot flashes were reported during this month of treatment was 19 and 7 in the LD and LD/N treatment groups, respectively. The mean maximum number of hot flashes in a day during this month of treatment was 5.8 and 1.9 in the LD and LD/N treatment groups, respectively.
[See table 3 on page 722]
Changes in Bone Density
In controlled clinical studies, patients with endometriosis (six months of therapy) or uterine fibroids (three months of therapy) were treated with LUPRON DEPOT 3.75 mg. In endometriosis patients, vertebral bone density as measured by dual energy x-ray absorptiometry (DEXA) decreased by an average of 3.2% at six months compared with the pre-treatment value. Clinical studies demonstrate that concurrent hormonal therapy (norethindrone acetate 5 mg daily) and calcium supplementation is effective in significantly reducing the loss of bone mineral density that occurs with LUPRON treatment, without compromising the efficacy of LUPRON in relieving symptoms of endometriosis.
LUPRON DEPOT 3.75 mg plus norethindrone acetate 5 mg daily was evaluated in two clinical trials. The results from this regimen were similar in both studies. LUPRON DEPOT 3.75 mg was used as a control group in one study. The bone mineral density data of the lumbar spine from these two studies are presented in Table 4.
[See table 4 on page 722]
When LUPRON DEPOT 3.75 mg was administered for three months in uterine fibroid patients, vertebral trabecular bone mineral density as assessed by quantitative digital radiography (QDR) revealed a mean decrease of 2.7% compared with baseline. Six months after discontinuation of therapy, a trend toward recovery was observed. Use of LUPRON DEPOT for longer than three months (uterine fibroids) or six months (endometriosis) or in the presence of other known risk factors for decreased bone mineral content may cause additional bone loss **and is not recommended**.
Changes in Laboratory Values During Treatment
Plasma Enzymes
Endometriosis
During early clinical trials with LUPRON DEPOT 3.75 mg, regular laboratory monitoring revealed that AST levels were more than twice the upper limit of normal in only one patient. There was no clinical or other laboratory evidence of abnormal liver function.
In two other clinical trials, 6 of 191 patients receiving LUPRON DEPOT 3.75 mg plus norethindrone acetate 5 mg daily for up to 12 months developed an elevated (at least twice the upper limit of normal) SGPT or GGT. Five of the 6 increases were observed beyond 6 months of treatment. None were associated with elevated bilirubin concentration.
Uterine Leiomyomata (Fibroids)
In clinical trials with LUPRON DEPOT 3.75 mg, five (3%) patients had a post-treatment transaminase value that was at least twice the baseline value and above the upper limit of the normal range. None of the laboratory increases were associated with clinical symptoms.

Table 2 ADVERSE EVENTS REPORTED TO BE CAUSALLY RELATED TO DRUG IN ≥ 5% OF PATIENTS

| | Endometriosis (2 Studies) | | | | | | Uterine Fibroids (4 Studies) | | | |
| | LUPRON DEPOT 3.75 mg N=166 | | Danazol N=136 | | Placebo N=31 | | LUPRON DEPOT 3.75 mg N=166 | | Placebo N=163 | |
	N	(%)	N	(%)	N	(%)	N	(%)	N	(%)
Body as a Whole										
Asthenia	5	(3)	9	(7)	0	(0)	14	(8.4)	8	(4.9)
General pain	31	(19)	22	(16)	1	(3)	14	(8.4)	10	(6.1)
Headache*	53	(32)	30	(22)	2	(6)	43	(25.9)	29	(17.8)
Cardiovascular System										
Hot flashes/sweats*	139	(84)	77	(57)	9	(29)	121	(72.9)	29	(17.8)
Gastrointestinal System										
Nausea/vomiting	21	(13)	17	(13)	1	(3)	8	(4.8)	6	(3.7)
GI disturbances*	11	(7)	8	(6)	1	(3)	5	(3.0)	2	(1.2)
Metabolic and Nutritional Disorders										
Edema	12	(7)	17	(13)	1	(3)	9	(5.4)	2	(1.2)
Weight gain/loss	22	(13)	36	(26)	0	(0)	5	(3.0)	2	(1.2)
Endocrine System										
Acne	17	(10)	27	(20)	0	(0)	0	(0)	0	(0)
Hirsutism	2	(1)	9	(7)	1	(3)	1	(0.6)	0	(0)
Musculoskeletal System										
Joint disorder*	14	(8)	11	(8)	0	(0)	13	(7.8)	5	(3.1)
Myalgia*	1	(1)	7	(5)	0	(0)	1	(0.6)	0	(0)
Nervous System										
Decreased libido*	19	(11)	6	(4)	0	(0)	3	(1.8)	0	(0)
Depression/emotional lability*	36	(22)	27	(20)	1	(3)	18	(10.8)	7	(4.3)
Dizziness	19	(11)	4	(3)	0	(0)	3	(1.8)	6	(3.7)
Nervousness*	8	(5)	11	(8)	0	(0)	8	(4.8)	1	(0.6)
Neuromuscular disorders*	11	(7)	17	(13)	0	(0)	3	(1.8)	0	(0)
Paresthesias	12	(7)	11	(8)	0	(0)	2	(1.2)	1	(0.6)
Skin and Appendages										
Skin reactions	17	(10)	20	(15)	1	(3)	5	(3.0)	2	(1.2)
Urogenital System										
Breast changes/tenderness/pain*	10	(6)	12	(9)	0	(0)	3	(1.8)	7	(4.3)
Vaginitis*	46	(28)	23	(17)	0	(0)	19	(11.4)	3	(1.8)

In these same studies, symptoms reported in <5% of patients included: *Body as a Whole* - Body odor, Flu syndrome, Injection site reactions; *Cardiovascular System* - Palpitations, Syncope, Tachycardia; *Digestive System* - Appetite changes, Dry mouth, Thirst; *Endocrine System* - Androgen-like effects; *Hemic and Lymphatic System* - Ecchymosis, Lymphadenopathy; *Nervous System* – Anxiety*, Insomnia/Sleep disorders*, Delusions, Memory disorder, Personality disorder; *Respiratory System* - Rhinitis; *Skin and Appendages* - Alopecia, Hair disorder, Nail disorder; *Special Senses* - Conjunctivitis, Ophthalmologic disorders*, Taste perversion; *Urogenital System* - Dysuria*, Lactation, Menstrual disorders.
* = Possible effect of decreased estrogen.

Lipids
Endometriosis
In earlier clinical studies, 4% of the LUPRON DEPOT 3.75 mg patients and 1% of the danazol patients had total cholesterol values above the normal range at enrollment. These patients also had cholesterol values above the normal range at the end of treatment. Of those patients whose pretreatment cholesterol values were in the normal range, 7% of the LUPRON DEPOT 3.75 mg patients and 9% of the danazol patients had post-treatment values above the normal range.
The mean (±SEM) pretreatment values for total cholesterol from all patients were 178.8 (2.9) mg/dL in the LUPRON DEPOT 3.75 mg groups and 175.3 (3.0) mg/dL in the danazol group. At the end of treatment, the mean values for total cholesterol from all patients were 193.3 mg/dL in the LUPRON DEPOT 3.75 mg group and 194.4 mg/dL in the danazol group. These increases from the pretreatment values were statistically significant (p<0.03) in both groups.
Triglycerides were increased above the upper limit of normal in 12% of the patients who received LUPRON DEPOT 3.75 mg and in 6% of the patients who received danazol.
At the end of treatment, HDL cholesterol fractions decreased below the lower limit of the normal range in 2% of the LUPRON DEPOT 3.75 mg patients compared with 54% of those receiving danazol. LDL cholesterol fractions increased above the upper limit of the normal range in 6% of the patients receiving LUPRON DEPOT 3.75 mg compared with 23% of those receiving danazol. There was no increase in the LDL/HDL ratio in patients receiving LUPRON DEPOT 3.75 mg but there was approximately a two-fold increase in the LDL/HDL ratio in patients receiving danazol.
In two other clinical trials, LUPRON DEPOT 3.75 mg plus norethindrone acetate 5 mg daily was evaluated for 12 months of treatment. LUPRON DEPOT 3.75 mg was used as a control group in one study. Percent changes from baseline for serum lipids and percentages of patients with serum lipid values outside of the normal range in the two studies are summarized in the tables below.
[See table 5 on next page]

Changes from baseline tended to be greater at Week 52. After treatment, mean serum lipid levels from patients with follow up data returned to pretreatment values.
[See table 6 at top of page 723]
Low HDL-cholesterol (<40 mg/dL) and elevated LDL-cholesterol (>160 mg/dL) are recognized risk factors for cardiovascular disease. The long-term significance of the observed treatment-related changes in serum lipids in women with endometriosis is unknown. Therefore assessment of cardiovascular risk factors should be considered prior to initiation of concurrent treatment with LUPRON and norethindrone acetate.
Uterine Leiomyomata (Fibroids)
In patients receiving LUPRON DEPOT 3.75 mg, mean changes in cholesterol (+11 mg/dL to +29 mg/dL), LDL cholesterol (+8 mg/dL to +22 mg/dL), HDL cholesterol (0 to +6 mg/dL), and the LDL/HDL ratio (-0.1 to +0.5) were observed across studies. In the one study in which triglycerides were determined, the mean increase from baseline was 32 mg/dL.
Other Changes
Endometriosis
The following changes were seen in approximately 5% to 8% of patients. In the earlier comparative studies, LUPRON DEPOT 3.75 mg was associated with elevations of LDH and phosphorus, and decreases in WBC counts. Danazol therapy was associated with increases in hematocrit, platelet count, and LDH. In the hormonal add-back studies LUPRON DEPOT in combination with norethindrone acetate was associated with elevations of GGT and SGPT.
Uterine Leiomyomata (Fibroids)
Hematology: (see **CLINICAL STUDIES** section) In LUPRON DEPOT 3.75 mg treated patients, although there were statistically significant mean decreases in platelet counts from baseline to final visit, the last mean platelet counts were within the normal range. Decreases in total WBC count and neutrophils were observed, but were not clinically significant.

Chemistry: Slight to moderate mean increases were noted for glucose, uric acid, BUN, creatinine, total protein, albumin, bilirubin, alkaline phosphatase, LDH, calcium, and phosphorus. None of these increases were clinically significant.
Postmarketing
The following adverse reactions have been identified during postapproval use of LUPRON DEPOT. Because these reactions are reported voluntarily from a population of uncertain size, it is not always possible to reliably estimate their frequency or establish a causal relationship to drug exposure.
During postmarketing surveillance, the following adverse events were reported. Like other drugs in this class, mood swings, including depression, have been reported. There have been rare reports of suicidal ideation and attempt. Many, but not all, of these patients had a history of depression or other psychiatric illness. Patients should be counseled on the possibility of development or worsening of depression during treatment with LUPRON.
Symptoms consistent with an anaphylactoid or asthmatic process have been rarely reported. Rash, urticaria, and photosensitivity reactions have also been reported.
Localized reactions including induration and abscess have been reported at the site of injection. Symptoms consistent with fibromyalgia (eg: joint and muscle pain, headaches, sleep disorder, gastrointestinal distress, and shortness of breath) have been reported individually and collectively.
Other events reported are:
Hepato-biliary disorder: Rarely reported serious liver injury
Injury, poisoning and procedural complications: Spinal fracture
Investigations: Decreased WBC
Musculoskeletal and Connective tissue disorder: Tenosynovitis-like symptoms
Nervous System Disorder: Convulsion, peripheral neuropathy, paralysis
Vascular Disorder: Hypotension
Cases of serious venous and arterial thromboembolism have been reported, including deep vein thrombosis, pulmonary embolism, myocardial infarction, stroke, and transient ischemic attack. Although a temporal relationship was reported in some cases, most cases were confounded by risk factors or concomitant medication use. It is unknown if there is a causal association between the use of GnRH analogs and these events.
Pituitary apoplexy
During post-marketing surveillance, rare cases of pituitary apoplexy (a clinical syndrome secondary to infarction of the pituitary gland) have been reported after the administration of gonadotropin-releasing hormone agonists. In a majority of these cases, a pituitary adenoma was diagnosed, with a majority of pituitary apoplexy cases occurring within 2 weeks of the first dose, and some within the first hour. In these cases, pituitary apoplexy has presented as sudden headache, vomiting, visual changes, ophthalmoplegia, altered mental status, and sometimes cardiovascular collapse. Immediate medical attention has been required.
See other LUPRON DEPOT and LUPRON Injection package inserts for other events reported in different patient populations.

OVERDOSAGE

In rats subcutaneous administration of 250 to 500 times the recommended human dose, expressed on a per body weight basis, resulted in dyspnea, decreased activity, and local irritation at the injection site. There is no evidence that there is a clinical counterpart of this phenomenon. In early clinical trials using daily subcutaneous leuprolide acetate in patients with prostate cancer, doses as high as 20 mg/day for up to two years caused no adverse effects differing from those observed with the 1 mg/day dose.

DOSAGE AND ADMINISTRATION

LUPRON DEPOT Must Be Administered Under The Supervision Of A Physician.
Endometriosis
The recommended duration of treatment with LUPRON DEPOT 3.75 mg alone or in combination with norethindrone acetate is six

Continued on next page

Information on the AbbVie, Inc. products listed on these pages is from the prescribing information in use as of July 31, 2016. For more information, please visit rxabbvie.com or call 1-800-633-9110.

months. The choice of LUPRON DEPOT alone or LUPRON DEPOT plus norethindrone acetate therapy for initial management of the symptoms and signs of endometriosis should be made by the health care professional in consultation with the patient and should take into consideration the risks and benefits of the addition of norethindrone to LUPRON DEPOT alone.

If the symptoms of endometriosis recur after a course of therapy, retreatment with a six-month course of LUPRON DEPOT administered monthly and norethindrone acetate 5 mg daily may be considered. Retreatment beyond this one six-month course cannot be recommended. It is recommended that bone density be assessed before retreatment begins to ensure that values are within normal limits. LUPRON DEPOT alone is not recommended for retreatment. If norethindrone acetate is contraindicated for the individual patient, then retreatment is not recommended.

An assessment of cardiovascular risk and management of risk factors such as cigarette smoking is recommended before beginning treatment with LUPRON DEPOT and norethindrone acetate.

Uterine Leiomyomata (Fibroids)
*Recommended duration of therapy with LUPRON DEPOT 3.75 mg is **up to** 3 months. The symptoms associated with uterine leiomyomata will recur following discontinuation of therapy. If additional treatment with LUPRON DEPOT 3.75 mg is contemplated, bone density should be assessed prior to initiation of therapy to ensure that values are within normal limits.*
The recommended dose of LUPRON DEPOT is 3.75 mg, incorporated in a depot formulation.

For optimal performance of the prefilled dual chamber syringe (PDS), read and follow the following instructions:
Reconstitution and Administration Instructions
• The lyophilized microspheres are to be reconstituted and administered as a single intramuscular injection.
• Since LUPRON DEPOT does not contain a preservative, the suspension should be injected immediately or discarded if not used within two hours.
• As with other drugs administered by injection, the injection site should be varied periodically.
1. The LUPRON DEPOT powder should be visually inspected and the syringe should NOT BE USED if clumping or caking is evident. A thin layer of powder on the wall of the syringe is considered normal prior to mixing with the diluent. The diluent should appear clear.
2. To prepare for injection, screw the white plunger into the end stopper until the stopper begins to turn.

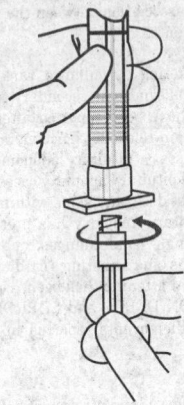

3. Hold the syringe UPRIGHT. Release the diluent by SLOWLY PUSHING (6 to 8 seconds) the plunger until the first stopper is at the blue line in the middle of the barrel.

← blue line

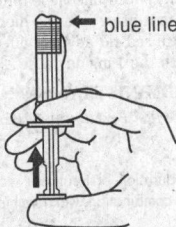

4. Keep the syringe UPRIGHT. Mix the microspheres (powder) thoroughly by gently shaking the syringe until the powder forms a uniform suspension. The suspension will appear milky. If the powder adheres to the stopper or cak-

ing/clumping is present, tap the syringe with your finger to disperse. DO NOT USE if any of the powder has not gone into suspension.
[See first figure at top of next page]
5. Hold the syringe UPRIGHT. With the opposite hand pull the needle cap upward without twisting.
6. Keep the syringe UPRIGHT. Advance the plunger to expel the air from the syringe. Now the syringe is ready for injection.

7. After cleaning the injection site with an alcohol swab, the intramuscular injection should be performed by inserting the needle at a 90 degree angle into the gluteal area, anterior thigh, or deltoid; injection sites should be alternated.
[See Figure at top of next column]
[See second figure at top of next page]
NOTE: Aspirated blood would be visible just below the luer lock connection if a blood vessel is accidentally penetrated. If present, blood can be seen through the trans-

Table 3 TREATMENT-RELATED ADVERSE EVENTS OCCURRING IN ≥5% OF PATIENTS

| | Controlled Study | | | | Open Label Study | |
| | LD - Only* N=51 | | LD/N† N=55 | | LD/N† N=136 | |
Adverse Events	N	(%)	N	(%)	N	(%)
Any Adverse Event	50	(98)	53	(96)	126	(93)
Body as a Whole						
Asthenia	9	(18)	10	(18)	15	(11)
Headache/Migraine	33	(65)	28	(51)	63	(46)
Injection Site Reaction	1	(2)	5	(9)	4	(3)
Pain	12	(24)	16	(29)	29	(21)
Cardiovascular System						
Hot flashes/sweats	50	(98)	48	(87)	78	(57)
Digestive System						
Altered Bowel Function	7	(14)	8	(15)	14	(10)
Changes in Appetite	2	(4)	0	(0)	8	(6)
GI Disturbance	2	(4)	4	(7)	6	(4)
Nausea/Vomiting	13	(25)	16	(29)	17	(13)
Metabolic and Nutritional Disorders						
Edema	0	(0)	5	(9)	9	(7)
Weight Changes	6	(12)	7	(13)	6	(4)
Nervous System						
Anxiety	3	(6)	0	(0)	11	(8)
Depression/Emotional Lability	16	(31)	15	(27)	46	(34)
Dizziness/Vertigo	8	(16)	6	(11)	10	(7)
Insomnia/Sleep Disorder	16	(31)	7	(13)	20	(15)
Libido Changes	5	(10)	2	(4)	10	(7)
Memory Disorder	3	(6)	1	(2)	6	(4)
Nervousness	4	(8)	2	(4)	15	(11)
Neuromuscular Disorder	1	(2)	5	(9)	4	(3)
Skin and Appendages						
Alopecia	0	(0)	5	(9)	4	(3)
Androgen-Like Effects	2	(4)	3	(5)	24	(18)
Skin/Mucous Membrane Reaction	2	(4)	5	(9)	15	(11)
Urogenital System						
Breast Changes/Pain/Tenderness	3	(6)	7	(13)	11	(8)
Menstrual Disorders	1	(2)	0	(0)	7	(5)
Vaginitis	10	(20)	8	(15)	11	(8)

* LD-Only = LUPRON DEPOT 3.75 mg
† LD/N = LUPRON DEPOT 3.75 mg plus norethindrone acetate 5 mg

Table 4 MEAN PERCENT CHANGE FROM BASELINE IN BONE MINERAL DENSITY OF LUMBAR SPINE

| | LUPRON DEPOT 3.75 mg Controlled Study | | LUPRON DEPOT 3.75 mg plus norethindrone acetate 5 mg daily Controlled Study | | Open Label Study | |
	N	Change (Mean, 95% CI)#	N	Change (Mean, 95% CI)#	N	Change (Mean, 95% CI)#
Week 24*	41	-3.2% (-3.8, -2.6)	42	-0.3% (-0.8, 0.3)	115	-0.2% (-0.6, 0.2)
Week 52†	29	-6.3% (-7.1, -5.4)	32	-1.0% (-1.9, -0.1)	84	-1.1% (-1.6, -0.5)

* Includes on-treatment measurements that fell within 2–252 days after the first day of treatment.
† Includes on-treatment measurements >252 days after the first day of treatment.
\# 95% CI: 95% Confidence Interval

Table 5 SERUM LIPIDS: MEAN PERCENT CHANGES FROM BASELINE VALUES AT TREATMENT WEEK 24

| | LUPRON Controlled Study (n=39) | | LUPRON plus norethindrone acetate 5 mg daily Controlled Study (n=41) | | Open Label Study (n=117) | |
	Baseline Value*	Wk 24 % Change	Baseline Value*	Wk 24 % Change	Baseline Value*	Wk 24 % Change
Total Cholesterol	170.5	9.2%	179.3	0.2%	181.2	2.8%
HDL Cholesterol	52.4	7.4%	51.8	-18.8%	51.0	-14.6%
LDL Cholesterol	96.6	10.9%	101.5	14.1%	109.1	13.1%
LDL/HDL Ratio	2.0†	5.0%	2.1†	43.4%	2.3†	39.4%
Triglycerides	107.8	17.5%	130.2	9.5%	105.4	13.8%

* mg/dL
† ratio

Table 6 PERCENTAGE OF PATIENTS WITH SERUM LIPID VALUES OUTSIDE OF THE NORMAL RANGE

| | LUPRON Controlled Study (n=39) | | LUPRON plus norethindrone acetate 5 mg daily | | | |
| | | | Controlled Study (n=41) | | Open Label Study (n=117) | |
	Wk 0	Wk 24*	Wk 0	Wk 24*	Wk 0	Wk 24*
Total Cholesterol (>240 mg/dL)	15%	23%	15%	20%	6%	7%
HDL Cholesterol (<40 mg/dL)	15%	10%	15%	44%	15%	41%
LDL Cholesterol (>160 mg/dL)	0%	8%	5%	7%	9%	11%
LDL/HDL Ratio (>4.0)	0%	3%	2%	15%	7%	21%
Triglycerides (>200 mg/dL)	13%	13%	12%	10%	5%	9%

* Includes all patients regardless of baseline value.

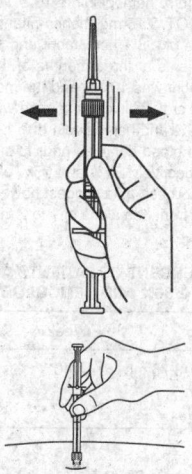

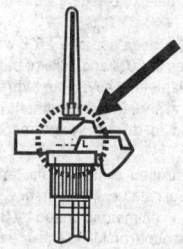

parent LuproLoc® safety device. If blood is present remove the needle immediately. Do not inject the medication.

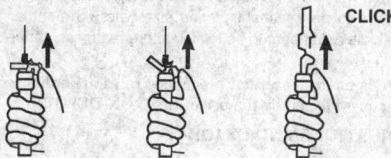

8. Inject the entire contents of the syringe intramuscularly at the time of reconstitution. The suspension settles very quickly following reconstitution; therefore, LUPRON DEPOT should be mixed and used immediately.

AFTER INJECTION

9. Withdraw the needle. Once the syringe has been withdrawn, activate immediately the LuproLoc® safety device by pushing the arrow on the lock upward towards the needle tip with the thumb or finger, as illustrated, until the needle cover of the safety device over the needle is fully extended and a CLICK is heard or felt.

CLICK

ADDITIONAL INFORMATION
• Dispose of the syringe according to local regulations/procedures.

HOW SUPPLIED
Each LUPRON DEPOT 3.75 mg kit (NDC 0074-3641-03) contains:
• one prefilled dual-chamber syringe
• one plunger
• two alcohol swabs
• a complete prescribing information enclosure
Each syringe contains sterile lyophilized microspheres, which is leuprolide incorporated in a biodegradable copoly-mer of lactic and glycolic acids. When mixed with diluent, LUPRON DEPOT 3.75 mg is administered as a single monthly IM injection.
Store at 25°C (77°F); excursions permitted to 15-30°C (59-86°F) [See USP Controlled Room Temperature]

REFERENCES
1. NIOSH Alert: Preventing occupational exposures to antineoplastic and other hazardous drugs in healthcare settings. 2004. U.S. Department of Health and Human Services, Public Health Service, Centers for Disease Control and Prevention, National Institute for Occupational Safety and Health, DHHS (NIOSH) Publication No. 2004-165.
2. OSHA Technical Manual, TED 1-0.15A, Section VI: Chapter 2. Controlling Occupational Exposure to Hazardous Drugs. OSHA, 1999. http://www.osha.gov/dts/osta/otm/otm_vi/otm_vi_2.html
3. American Society of Health-System Pharmacists. ASHP guidelines on handling hazardous drugs. *Am J Health-Syst Pharm.* 2006; 63; 1172-1193.
4. Polovich, M., White, J.M., & Kelleher, L.O. (eds.) 2005. Chemotherapy and biotherapy guidelines and recommendations for practice (2nd. Ed.) Pittsburgh, PA: Oncology Nursing Society.
Manufactured for
AbbVie Inc.
North Chicago, IL 60064
by Takeda Pharmaceutical Company Limited
Osaka, Japan 540-8645
™ - Trademark
® - Registered Trademark
(No. 3641)
Ref: 03-A891-Revised October, 2013
© 2013 AbbVie Inc.
Shown in Product Identification Guide, page 505

LUPRON DEPOT® -3 MONTH 11.25 MG   ℞
[lew-prŏn]
(leuprolide acetate for depot suspension)
3-MONTH FORMULATION

Rx only
This is combined labeling. Examples of different fonts and colors appear below.
• General information
• Information on endometriosis
• Information on uterine fibroids

DESCRIPTION
Leuprolide acetate is a synthetic nonapeptide analog of naturally occurring gonadotropin-releasing hormone (GnRH or LH-RH). The analog possesses greater potency than the natural hormone. The chemical name is 5-oxo-L-prolyl-L-histidyl-L-tryptophyl-L-seryl-L-tyrosyl-D-leucyl-L-leucyl-L-arginyl-N-ethyl-L-prolinamide acetate (salt) with the following structural formula:
[See structural formula at top of next page]
LUPRON DEPOT–3 Month 11.25 mg is available in a prefilled dual-chamber syringe containing sterile lyophilized microspheres which, when mixed with diluent, become a suspension intended as an intramuscular injection to be given **ONCE EVERY THREE MONTHS**.
The front chamber of LUPRON DEPOT–3 Month 11.25 mg prefilled dual-chamber syringe contains leuprolide acetate (11.25 mg), polylactic acid (99.3 mg) and D-mannitol (19.45 mg). The second chamber of diluent contains carboxymethylcellulose sodium (7.5 mg), D-mannitol (75.0 mg), polysorbate 80 (1.5 mg), water for injection, USP, and glacial acetic acid, USP to control pH.
During the manufacture of LUPRON DEPOT–3 Month 11.25 mg, acetic acid is lost, leaving the peptide.

CLINICAL PHARMACOLOGY
Leuprolide acetate is a long-acting GnRH analog. A single injection of LUPRON DEPOT–3 Month 11.25 mg will result in an initial stimulation followed by a prolonged suppression of pituitary gonadotropins. Repeated dosing at quarterly (LUPRON DEPOT–3 Month 11.25 mg) intervals results in decreased secretion of gonadal steroids; consequently, tissues and functions that depend on gonadal steroids for their maintenance become quiescent. This effect is reversible on discontinuation of drug therapy.
Leuprolide acetate is not active when given orally.

Pharmacokinetics
Absorption
Following a single injection of the three month formulation of LUPRON DEPOT–3 Month 11.25 mg in female subjects, a mean plasma leuprolide concentration of 36.3 ng/mL was observed at 4 hours. Leuprolide appeared to be released at a constant rate following the onset of steady-state levels during the third week after dosing and mean levels then declined gradually to near the lower limit of detection by 12 weeks. The mean (± standard deviation) leuprolide concentration from 3 to 12 weeks was 0.23 ± 0.09 ng/mL. However, intact leuprolide and an inactive major metabolite could not be distinguished by the assay which was employed in the study. The initial burst, followed by the rapid decline to a steady-state level, was similar to the release pattern seen with the monthly formulation.
Distribution
The mean steady-state volume of distribution of leuprolide following intravenous bolus administration to healthy male volunteers was 27 L. *In vitro* binding to human plasma proteins ranged from 43% to 49%.
Metabolism
In healthy male volunteers, a 1 mg bolus of leuprolide administered intravenously revealed that the mean systemic clearance was 7.6 L/h, with a terminal elimination half-life of approximately 3 hours based on a two compartment model.
In rats and dogs, administration of ^{14}C-labeled leuprolide was shown to be metabolized to smaller inactive peptides, a pentapeptide (Metabolite I), tripeptides (Metabolites II and III) and a dipeptide (Metabolite IV). These fragments may be further catabolized.
In a pharmacokinetic/pharmacodynamic study of endometriosis patients, intramuscular 11.25 mg LUPRON DEPOT (n=19) every 12 weeks or intramuscular 3.75 mg LUPRON DEPOT (n=15) every 4 weeks was administered for 24 weeks. There was no statistically significant difference in changes of serum estradiol concentration from baseline between the 2 treatment groups.
M-I plasma concentrations measured in 5 prostate cancer patients reached maximum concentration 2 to 6 hours after dosing and were approximately 6% of the peak parent drug concentration. One week after dosing, mean plasma M-I concentrations were approximately 20% of mean leuprolide concentrations.
Excretion
Following administration of LUPRON DEPOT 3.75 mg to 3 patients, less than 5% of the dose was recovered as parent and M-I metabolite in the urine.
Special Populations
The pharmacokinetics of the drug in hepatically and renally impaired patients have not been determined.
Drug Interactions
No pharmacokinetic-based drug-drug interaction studies have been conducted with LUPRON DEPOT. However, because leuprolide acetate is a peptide that is primarily degraded by peptidase and not by cytochrome P-450 enzymes as noted in specific studies, and the drug is only about 46% bound to plasma proteins, drug interactions would not be expected to occur.

CLINICAL STUDIES
In a pharmacokinetic/pharmacodynamic study of healthy female subjects (N=20), the onset of estradiol suppression was observed for individual subjects between day 4 and week 4 after dosing. By the third week following the injection, the mean estradiol concentration (8 pg/mL) was in the

Continued on next page

menopausal range. Throughout the remainder of the dosing period, mean serum estradiol levels ranged from the menopausal to the early follicular range.

Serum estradiol was suppressed to ≤20 pg/mL in all subjects within four weeks and remained suppressed (≤40 pg/mL) in 80% of subjects until the end of the 12-week dosing interval, at which time two of these subjects had a value between 40 and 50 pg/mL. Four additional subjects had at least two consecutive elevations of estradiol (range 43-240 pg/mL) levels during the 12-week dosing interval, but there was no indication of luteal function for any of the subjects during this period.

LUPRON DEPOT–3 Month 11.25 mg induced amenorrhea in 85% (N=17) of subjects during the initial month and 100% during the second month following the injection. All subjects remained amenorrheic through the remainder of the 12-week dosing interval. Episodes of light bleeding and spotting were reported by a majority of subjects during the first month after the injection and in a few subjects at later time-points. Menses resumed on average 12 weeks (range 2.9 to 20.4 weeks) following the end of the 12-week dosing interval.

LUPRON DEPOT–3 Month 11.25 mg produced similar pharmacodynamic effects in terms of hormonal and menstrual suppression to those achieved with monthly injections of LUPRON DEPOT 3.75 mg during the controlled clinical trials for the management of endometriosis and the anemia caused by uterine fibroids.

Endometriosis

In a Phase IV pharmacokinetic/pharmacodynamic study of patients, LUPRON DEPOT–3 Month 11.25 mg (N=21) was shown to be comparable to monthly LUPRON DEPOT 3.75 mg (N=20) in relieving the clinical signs/symptoms of endometriosis (dysmenorrhea, non-menstrual pelvic pain, pelvic tenderness and pelvic induration). In both treatment groups, suppression of menses was achieved in 100% of the patients who remained in the study for at least 60 days. Suppression is defined as no new menses for at least 60 consecutive days.

In controlled clinical studies, LUPRON DEPOT 3.75 mg monthly for six months was shown to be comparable to danazol 800 mg/day in relieving the clinical sign/symptoms of endometriosis (pelvic pain, dysmenorrhea, dyspareunia, pelvic tenderness, and induration) and in reducing the size of endometrial implants as evidenced by laparoscopy.

The clinical significance of a decrease in endometriotic lesions is not known at this time, and in addition laparoscopic staging of endometriosis does not necessarily correlate with the severity of symptoms.

LUPRON DEPOT 3.75 mg monthly induced amenorrhea in 74% and 98% of the patients after the first and second treatment months respectively. Most of the remaining patients reported episodes of only light bleeding or spotting. In the first, second and third post-

treatment months, normal menstrual cycles resumed in 7%, 71% and 95% of patients, respectively, excluding those who became pregnant.

Figure 1 illustrates the percent of patients with symptoms at baseline, final treatment visit and sustained relief at 6 and 12 months following discontinuation of treatment for the various symptoms evaluated during the two controlled clinical studies. A total of 166 patients received LUPRON DEPOT 3.75 mg. Seventy-five percent (N=125) of these elected to participate in the follow-up period. Of these patients, 36% and 24% are included in the 6 month and 12 month follow-up analysis, respectively. All the patients who had a pain evaluation at baseline and at a minimum of one treatment visit, are included in the Baseline (B) and final treatment visit (F) analysis.

[See Figure 1 below]

Hormonal add-back therapy

Two clinical studies with a treatment duration of 12 months indicate that concurrent hormonal therapy (norethindrone acetate 5 mg daily) is effective in significantly reducing the loss of bone mineral density associated with LUPRON, without compromising the efficacy of LUPRON in relieving symptoms of endometriosis. (All patients in these studies received calcium supplementation with 1000 mg elemental calcium). One controlled, randomized and double-blind study included 51 women treated with LUPRON DEPOT 3.75 mg alone and 55 women treated with LUPRON DEPOT 3.75 mg plus norethindrone acetate 5 mg (LD/N) daily. The second study was an open label study in which 136 women were treated with monthly LUPRON DEPOT 3.75 mg plus norethindrone acetate 5 mg daily. This study confirmed the reduction in loss of bone mineral density that was observed in the controlled study. Suppression of menses was maintained throughout treatment in 84% and 73% of patients receiving LD/N, in the controlled study and open label study, respectively. The median time for menses resumption after treatment with LD/N was 8 weeks.

Figure 2 Illustrates the mean pain scores for the LD/N group from the controlled study.

[See Figure 2 at top of next page]

Uterine Leiomyomata (Fibroids)

LUPRON DEPOT 3.75 mg for a period of three to six months was studied in four controlled clinical trials.

In one of these clinical studies, enrollment was based on hematocrit ≤ 30% and/or hemoglobin ≤ 10.2 g/dL. Administration of LUPRON DEPOT 3.75 mg, concomitantly with iron, produced an increase of ≥ 6% hematocrit and ≥ 2 g/dL hemoglobin in 77% of patients at three months of therapy. The mean change in hematocrit was 10.1% and the mean change in hemoglobin was 4.2 g/dL. Clinical response was judged to be a hematocrit of ≥ 36% and hemoglobin of ≥ 12 g/dL, thus allowing for autologous blood donation prior to surgery. At two and three months respectively, 71% and 75% of patients met this criterion (Table 1). These data suggest however, that some patients may benefit from iron alone or 1 to 2 months of LUPRON DEPOT 3.75 mg.

Table 1 PERCENT OF PATIENTS ACHIEVING HEMATOCRIT ≥ 36% AND HEMOGLOBIN ≥ 12 GM/DL

Treatment Group	Week 4	Week 8	Week 12
LUPRON DEPOT 3.75 mg with Iron (N=104)	40*	71†	75*
Iron Alone (N=98)	17	39	49

* P-Value < 0.01
† P-Value < 0.001

Excessive vaginal bleeding (menorrhagia or menometrorrhagia) decreased in 80% of patients at three months. Episodes of spotting and menstrual-like bleeding were noted in 16% of patients at final visit.

In this same study, a decrease of ≥ 25% was seen in uterine and myoma volumes in 60% and 54% of patients respectively. The mean fibroid diameter was 6.3 cm at pretreatment and decreased to 5.6 cm at the end of treatment. LUPRON DEPOT 3.75 mg was found to relieve symptoms of bloating, pelvic pain, and pressure.

In three other controlled clinical trials, enrollment was not based on hematologic status. Mean uterine volume decreased by 41% and myoma volume decreased by 37% at final visit as evidenced by ultrasound or MRI. The mean fibroid diameter was 5.6 cm at pretreatment and decreased to 4.7 cm at the end of treatment. These patients also experienced a decrease in symptoms including excessive vaginal bleeding and pelvic discomfort. Ninety-five percent of these patients became amenorrheic with 61%, 25%, and 4% experiencing amenorrhea during the first, second, and third treatment months respectively.

In addition, posttreatment follow-up was carried out in one clinical trial for a small percentage of LUPRON DEPOT 3.75 mg patients (N=46) among the 77% who demonstrated a ≥ 25% decrease in uterine volume while on therapy. Menses usually returned within two months of cessation of therapy. Mean time to return to pretreatment uterine size was 8.3 months. Regrowth did not appear to be related to pretreatment uterine volume.

There is no evidence that pregnancy rates are enhanced or adversely affected by the use of LUPRON DEPOT.

INDICATIONS AND USAGE

Endometriosis

LUPRON DEPOT–3 Month 11.25 mg is indicated for management of endometriosis, including pain relief and reduction of endometriotic lesions. LUPRON DEPOT with norethindrone acetate 5 mg daily is also indicated for initial management of endometriosis and for management of recurrence of symptoms. (Refer also to norethindrone acetate prescribing information for **WARNINGS, PRECAUTIONS, CONTRAINDICATIONS** and **ADVERSE REACTIONS** associated with norethindrone acetate). Duration of initial treatment or retreatment should be limited to 6 months.

Uterine Leiomyomata (Fibroids)

LUPRON DEPOT–3 Month 11.25 mg concomitantly with iron therapy is indicated for the preoperative hematologic improve-

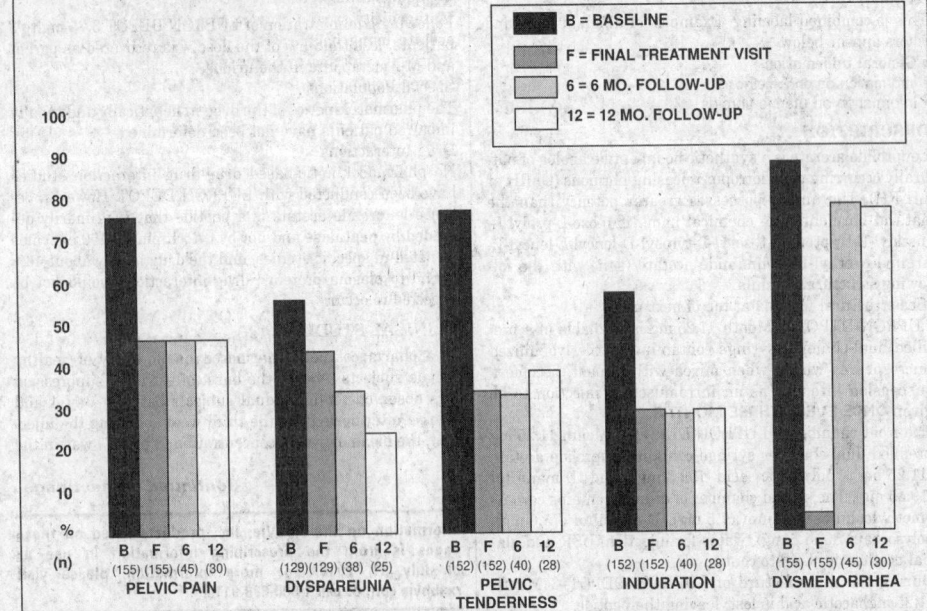

FIGURE 1 – PERCENT OF PATIENTS WITH SIGN/SYMPTOMS OF ENDOMETRIOSIS AT BASELINE, FINAL TREATMENT VISIT, AND AFTER 6 AND 12 MONTHS OF FOLLOW-UP

B = BASELINE
F = FINAL TREATMENT VISIT
6 = 6 MO. FOLLOW-UP
12 = 12 MO. FOLLOW-UP

PELVIC PAIN (155)(155)(45)(30)
DYSPAREUNIA (129)(129)(38)(25)
PELVIC TENDERNESS (152)(152)(40)(28)
INDURATION (152)(152)(40)(28)
DYSMENORRHEA (155)(155)(45)(30)

Figure 2
Treatment Period Mean Pain Scores For LD/N* Patients

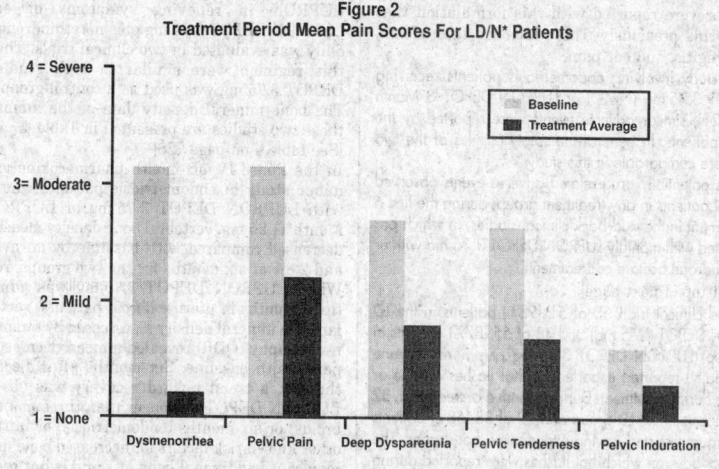

* LD/N = LUPRON DEPOT 3.75 mg plus norethindrone acetate 5 mg daily

ment of patients with anemia caused by uterine leiomyomata. The clinician may wish to consider a one-month trial period on iron alone inasmuch as some of the patients will respond to iron alone. (See **Table 1, CLINICAL STUDIES** section.) LUPRON may be added if the response to iron alone is considered inadequate. Recommended therapy is a single injection of LUPRON DEPOT–3 Month 11.25 mg. This dosage form is indicated only for women for whom three months of hormonal suppression is deemed necessary.

Experience with LUPRON DEPOT–3 Month 11.25 mg in females has been limited to women 18 years of age and older treated for no more than 6 months.

CONTRAINDICATIONS

1. Hypersensitivity to GnRH, GnRH agonist analogs or any of the excipients in LUPRON DEPOT.
2. Undiagnosed abnormal vaginal bleeding.
3. LUPRON DEPOT is contraindicated in women who are or may become pregnant while receiving the drug. LUPRON DEPOT may cause fetal harm when administered to a pregnant woman. Major fetal abnormalities were observed in rabbits but not in rats after administration of LUPRON DEPOT throughout gestation. There was increased fetal mortality and decreased fetal weights in rats and rabbits. (See **Pregnancy** section.) The effects on fetal mortality are expected consequences of the alterations in hormonal levels brought about by the drug. If this drug is used during pregnancy or if the patient becomes pregnant while taking this drug, the patient should be apprised of the potential hazard to the fetus.
4. Use in women who are breast-feeding. (See **Nursing Mothers** section.)
5. Norethindrone acetate is contraindicated in women with the following conditions:
   ○ Thrombophlebitis, thromboembolic disorders, cerebral apoplexy, or a past history of these conditions
   ○ Markedly impaired liver function or liver disease
   ○ Known or suspected carcinoma of the breast

WARNINGS

1. As the effects of LUPRON DEPOT–3 Month 11.25 mg are present throughout the course of therapy, the drug should only be used in patients who require hormonal suppression for at least three months.
2. Experience with LUPRON DEPOT–3 Month 11.25 mg in females has been limited to six months; therefore, exposure should be limited to six months of therapy.
3. Safe use of leuprolide acetate or norethindrone acetate in pregnancy has not been established clinically. Before starting treatment with LUPRON DEPOT pregnancy must be excluded.
4. When used at the recommended dose and dosing interval, LUPRON DEPOT usually inhibits ovulation and stops menstruation. Contraception is not insured, however, by taking LUPRON DEPOT. Therefore, patients should use non-hormonal methods of contraception. Patients should be advised to see their physician if they believe they may be pregnant. If a patient becomes pregnant during treatment, the drug must be discontinued and the patient must be apprised of the potential risk to the fetus. (See **CONTRAINDICATIONS** section.)
5. During the early phase of therapy, sex steroids temporarily rise above baseline because of the physiologic effect of the drug. Therefore, an increase in clinical signs and

symptoms may be observed during the initial days of therapy, but these will dissipate with continued therapy.
6. Symptoms consistent with an anaphylactoid or asthmatic process have been rarely reported post-marketing.
7. The following applies to co-treatment with LUPRON and norethindrone acetate:

Norethindrone acetate treatment should be discontinued if there is a sudden partial or complete loss of vision or if there is sudden onset of proptosis, diplopia, or migraine. If examination reveals papilledema or retinal vascular lesions, medication should be withdrawn.

Because of the occasional occurrence of thrombophlebitis and pulmonary embolism in patients taking progestogens, the physician should be alert to the earliest manifestations of the disease in women taking norethindrone acetate.

Assessment and management of risk factors for cardiovascular disease is recommended prior to initiation of add-back therapy with norethindrone acetate. Norethindrone acetate should be used with caution in women with risk factors, including lipid abnormalities or cigarette smoking.

PRECAUTIONS
Information for Patients
Patients should be aware of the following information:

1. Since menstruation usually stops with effective doses of LUPRON DEPOT, the patient should notify her physician if regular menstruation persists. Patients missing successive doses of LUPRON DEPOT may experience breakthrough bleeding.
2. Patients should not use LUPRON DEPOT if they are pregnant, breast feeding, have undiagnosed abnormal vaginal bleeding, or are allergic to any of the ingredients in LUPRON DEPOT.
3. LUPRON DEPOT is contraindicated for use during pregnancy. Therefore, a non-hormonal method of contraception should be used during treatment. Patients should be advised that if they miss successive doses of LUPRON DEPOT, breakthrough bleeding or ovulation may occur with the potential for conception. If a patient becomes pregnant during treatment, she should discontinue treatment and consult her physician.
4. Adverse events occurring in clinical studies with LUPRON DEPOT that are associated with hypoestrogenism include: hot flashes, headaches, emotional lability, decreased libido, acne, myalgia, reduction in breast size, and vaginal dryness. Estrogen levels returned to normal after treatment was discontinued.
5. Patients should be counseled on the possibility of the development or worsening of depression and the occurrence of memory disorders.
6. The induced hypoestrogenic state **also** results in a loss in bone density over the course of treatment, some of which may not be reversible. Clinical studies show that concurrent hormonal therapy with norethindrone acetate 5 mg daily is effective in reducing loss of bone mineral density that occurs with LUPRON. (All patients received calcium supplementation with 1000 mg elemental calcium.) (See *Changes in Bone Density* section).
7. If the symptoms of endometriosis recur after a course of therapy, retreatment with a six-month course of LUPRON DEPOT and norethindrone acetate 5 mg daily may be considered. Retreatment beyond this one six-month course cannot be recommended. It is recom-

mended that bone density be assessed before retreatment begins to ensure that values are within normal limits. Retreatment with LUPRON DEPOT alone is not recommended.
8. In patients with major risk factors for decreased bone mineral content such as chronic alcohol and/or tobacco use, strong family history of osteoporosis, or chronic use of drugs that can reduce bone mass such as anticonvulsants or corticosteroids, LUPRON DEPOT therapy may pose an additional risk. In these patients, the risks and benefits must be weighed carefully before therapy with LUPRON DEPOT alone is instituted, and concomitant treatment with norethindrone acetate 5 mg daily should be considered. Retreatment with gonadotropin-releasing hormone analogs, including LUPRON is not advisable in patients with major risk factors for loss of bone mineral content.
9. Because norethindrone acetate may cause some degree of fluid retention, conditions which might be influenced by this factor, such as epilepsy, migraine, asthma, cardiac or renal dysfunctions require careful observation during norethindrone acetate add-back therapy.
10. Patients who have a history of depression should be carefully observed during treatment with norethindrone acetate and norethindrone acetate should be discontinued if severe depression occurs.

Convulsions
There have been postmarketing reports of convulsions in patients on leuprolide acetate therapy. These included patients with and without concurrent medications and comorbid conditions.

Laboratory Tests
See **ADVERSE REACTIONS** section.

Drug Interactions
See **CLINICAL PHARMACOLOGY, Pharmacokinetics.**

Drug/Laboratory Test Interactions
Administration of LUPRON DEPOT in therapeutic doses results in suppression of the pituitary-gonadal system. Normal function is usually restored within three months after treatment is discontinued. Therefore, diagnostic tests of pituitary gonadotropic and gonadal functions conducted during treatment and for up to three months after discontinuation of LUPRON DEPOT may be misleading.

Carcinogenesis, Mutagenesis, Impairment of Fertility
A two-year carcinogenicity study was conducted in rats and mice. In rats, a dose-related increase of benign pituitary hyperplasia and benign pituitary adenomas was noted at 24 months when the drug was administered subcutaneously at high daily doses (0.6 to 4 mg/kg). There was a significant but not dose-related increase of pancreatic islet-cell adenomas in females and of testicular interstitial cell adenomas in males (highest incidence in the low dose group). In mice, no leuprolide acetate-induced tumors or pituitary abnormalities were observed at a dose as high as 60 mg/kg for two years. Patients have been treated with leuprolide acetate for up to three years with doses as high as 10 mg/day and for two years with doses as high as 20 mg/day without demonstrable pituitary abnormalities.

Mutagenicity studies have been performed with leuprolide acetate using bacterial and mammalian systems. These studies provided no evidence of a mutagenic potential.

Clinical and pharmacologic studies in adults (> 18 years) with leuprolide acetate and similar analogs have shown reversibility of fertility suppression when the drug is discontinued after continuous administration for periods of up to 24 weeks. Although no clinical studies have been completed in children to assess the full reversibility of fertility suppression, animal studies (prepubertal and adult rats and monkeys) with leuprolide acetate and other GnRH analogs have shown functional recovery.

Pregnancy
Teratogenic Effects
Pregnancy Category X (See **CONTRAINDICATIONS** section). When administered on day 6 of pregnancy at test dosages of 0.00024, 0.0024, and 0.024 mg/kg (1/300 to 1/3 of the human dose) to rabbits, LUPRON DEPOT produced a dose-related increase in major fetal abnormalities. Similar studies in rats failed to demonstrate an increase in fetal malformations. There was increased fetal mortality and decreased

Continued on next page

Information on the AbbVie, Inc. products listed on these pages is from the prescribing information in use as of July 31, 2016. For more information, please visit rxabbvie.com or call 1-800-633-9110.

fetal weights with the two higher doses of LUPRON DEPOT in rabbits and with the highest dose (0.024 mg/kg) in rats.

Nursing Mothers

It is not known whether LUPRON DEPOT is excreted in human milk. Because many drugs are excreted in human milk, and because the effects of LUPRON DEPOT on lactation and/or the breast-fed child have not been determined, LUPRON DEPOT should not be used by nursing mothers.

Pediatric Use

Safety and effectiveness of LUPRON DEPOT–3 Month 11.25 mg have not been established in pediatric patients. Experience with LUPRON DEPOT for treatment of endometriosis has been limited to women 18 years of age and older. See LUPRON DEPOT-PED® (leuprolide acetate for depot suspension) labeling for the safety and effectiveness in children with central precocious puberty.

Geriatric Use

This product has not been studied in women over 65 years of age and is not indicated in this population.

ADVERSE REACTIONS

Clinical Trials

The **monthly formulation of LUPRON DEPOT 3.75 mg** was utilized in controlled clinical trials that studied the drug in 166 endometriosis and 166 uterine fibroids patients. Adverse events reported in ≥ 5% of patients in either of these populations and thought to be potentially related to drug are noted in the following table.

[See table 2 below]

In one controlled clinical trial utilizing the monthly formulation of LUPRON DEPOT, patients diagnosed with uterine fibroids received a higher dose (7.5 mg) of LUPRON DEPOT. Events seen with this dose that were thought to be potentially related to drug and were not seen at the lower dose included glossitis, hypesthesia, lactation, pyelonephritis, and urinary disorders. Generally, a higher incidence of hypoestrogenic effects was observed at the higher dose.

In a pharmacokinetic trial involving 20 healthy female subjects receiving LUPRON DEPOT–3 Month 11.25 mg, a few

adverse events were reported with this formulation that were not reported previously. These included face edema, agitation, laryngitis, and ear pain.

In a Phase IV study involving endometriosis patients receiving LUPRON DEPOT 3.75 mg (N=20) or LUPRON DEPOT–3 Month 11.25 mg (N=21), similar adverse events were reported by the two groups of patients. In general the safety profiles of the two formulations were comparable in this study.

Table 3 lists the potentially drug-related adverse events observed in at least 5% of patients in any treatment group, during the first 6 months of treatment in the add-back clinical studies, in which patients were treated with monthly LUPRON DEPOT 3.75 mg with or without norethindrone acetate co-treatment.

[See table 3 at top of next page]

In the controlled clinical trial, 50 of 51 (98%) patients in the LD group (LUPRON DEPOT 3.75 mg) and 48 of 55 (87%) patients in the LD/N group (LUPRON DEPOT 3.75 mg plus norethindrone acetate 5 mg daily) reported experiencing hot flashes on one or more occasions during treatment. During Month 6 of treatment, 32 of 37 (86%) patients in the LD group and 22 of 38 (58%) patients in the LD/N group reported having experienced hot flashes. The mean number of days on which hot flashes were reported during this month of treatment was 19 and 7 in the LD and LD/N treatment groups, respectively. The mean maximum number of hot flashes in a day during this month of treatment was 5.8 and 1.9 in the LD and LD/N treatment groups, respectively.

Changes in Bone Density

In controlled clinical studies, patients with endometriosis (six months of therapy) or uterine fibroids (three months of therapy) were treated with LUPRON DEPOT 3.75 mg. In endometriosis patients, vertebral bone density as measured by dual energy x-ray absorptiometry (DEXA) decreased by an average of 3.2% at six months compared with the pretreatment value. Clinical studies demonstrate that concurrent hormonal therapy (norethindrone acetate 5 mg daily) and calcium supplementation is effective in significantly reducing the loss of bone mineral density that occurs with LUPRON treatment, without compromising the efficacy of

LUPRON in relieving symptoms of endometriosis. LUPRON DEPOT 3.75 mg plus norethindrone acetate 5 mg daily was evaluated in two clinical trials. The results from this regimen were similar in both studies. LUPRON DEPOT 3.75 mg was used as a control group in one study. The bone mineral density data of the lumbar spine from these two studies are presented in Table 4.

[See table 4 on page 728]

In the Phase IV, six-month pharmacokinetic/pharmacodynamic study in endometriosis patients who were treated with LUPRON DEPOT 3.75 mg or LUPRON DEPOT–3 Month 11.25 mg, vertebral bone density measured by DEXA decreased compared with baseline by an average of 3.0% and 2.8% at six months for the two groups, respectively. When LUPRON DEPOT 3.75 mg was administered for three months in uterine fibroid patients, vertebral trabecular bone mineral density as assessed by quantitative digital radiography (QDR) revealed a mean decrease of 2.7% compared with baseline. Six months after discontinuation of therapy, a trend toward recovery was observed. Use of LUPRON DEPOT for longer than three months (uterine fibroids) or six months (endometriosis) or in the presence of other known risk factors for decreased bone mineral content may cause additional bone loss and **is not recommended.**

Changes in Laboratory Values During Treatment

Liver Enzymes

Three percent of uterine fibroid patients treated with LUPRON DEPOT 3.75 mg, manifested posttreatment transaminase values that were at least twice the baseline value and above the upper limit of the normal range. None of the laboratory increases were associated with clinical symptoms.

In two other clinical trials, 6 of 191 patients receiving LUPRON DEPOT 3.75 mg plus norethindrone acetate 5 mg daily for up to 12 months developed an elevated (at least twice the upper limit of normal) SGPT or GGT. Five of the 6 increases were observed beyond 6 months of treatment. None were associated with an elevated bilirubin concentration.

Lipids

Triglycerides were increased above the upper limit of normal in 12% of the endometriosis patients who received LUPRON DEPOT 3.75 mg and in 32% of the subjects receiving LUPRON DEPOT–3 Month 11.25 mg.

Of those endometriosis and uterine fibroid patients whose pretreatment cholesterol values were in the normal range, mean change following therapy was +16 mg/dL to +17 mg/dL in endometriosis patients and +11 mg/dL to +29 mg/dL in uterine fibroid patients. In the endometriosis treated patients, increases from the pretreatment values were statistically significant ($p < 0.03$). There was essentially no increase in the LDL/HDL ratio in patients from either population receiving LUPRON DEPOT 3.75 mg.

In two other clinical trials, LUPRON DEPOT 3.75 mg plus norethindrone acetate 5 mg daily were evaluated for 12 months of treatment. LUPRON DEPOT 3.75 mg was used as a control group in one study. Percent changes from baseline for serum lipids and percentages of patients with serum lipid values outside of the normal range in the two studies are summarized in the tables below.

[See table 5 on page 728]

Changes from baseline tended to be greater at Week 52. After treatment, mean serum lipid levels from patients with follow up data returned to pretreatment values.

[See Table 6 on page 728]

Low HDL-cholesterol (<40 mg/dL) and elevated LDL-cholesterol (>160 mg/dL) are recognized risk factors for cardiovascular disease. The long-term significance of the observed treatment-related changes in serum lipids in women with endometriosis is unknown. Therefore assessment of cardiovascular risk factors should be considered prior to initiation of concurrent treatment with LUPRON and norethindrone acetate.

Chemistry

Slight to moderate mean increases were noted for glucose, uric acid, BUN, creatinine, total protein, albumin, bilirubin, alkaline phosphatase, LDH, calcium, and phosphorus. None of these increases were clinically significant. In the hormonal add-back studies LUPRON DEPOT in combination with norethindrone acetate was associated with elevations of GGT and SGPT in 6% to 7% of patients.

Postmarketing

The following adverse reactions have been identified during postapproval use of LUPRON DEPOT. Because these reactions are reported voluntarily from a population of uncertain size, it is not always possible to reliably estimate their frequency or establish a causal relationship to drug exposure.

Table 2 ADVERSE EVENTS REPORTED TO BE CAUSALLY RELATED TO DRUG IN ≥ 5% OF PATIENTS									
	Endometriosis (2 Studies)						**Uterine Fibroids (4 Studies)**		
	LUPRON DEPOT 3.75 mg N=166		Danazol N=136		Placebo N=31		LUPRON DEPOT 3.75 mg N=166		Placebo N=163
	N	(%)	N	(%)	N	(%)	N	(%)	N	(%)
Body as a Whole										
Asthenia	5	(3)	9	(7)	0	(0)	14	(8.4)	8	(4.9)
General pain	31	(19)	22	(16)	1	(3)	14	(8.4)	10	(6.1)
Headache*	53	(32)	30	(22)	2	(6)	43	(25.9)	29	(17.8)
Cardiovascular System										
Hot flashes/sweats*	139	(84)	77	(57)	9	(29)	121	(72.9)	29	(17.8)
Gastrointestinal System										
Nausea/vomiting	21	(13)	17	(13)	1	(3)	8	(4.8)	6	(3.7)
GI disturbances*	11	(7)	8	(6)	1	(3)	5	(3.0)	2	(1.2)
Metabolic and Nutritional Disorders										
Edema	12	(7)	17	(13)	1	(3)	9	(5.4)	2	(1.2)
Weight gain/loss	22	(13)	36	(26)	0	(0)	5	(3.0)	2	(1.2)
Endocrine System										
Acne	17	(10)	27	(20)	0	(0)	0	(0)	0	(0)
Hirsutism	2	(1)	9	(7)	1	(3)	1	(0.6)	0	(0)
Musculoskeletal System										
Joint disorder*	14	(8)	11	(8)	0	(0)	13	(7.8)	5	(3.1)
Myalgia*	1	(1)	7	(5)	0	(0)	1	(0.6)	0	(0)
Nervous System										
Decreased libido*	19	(11)	6	(4)	0	(0)	3	(1.8)	0	(0)
Depression/emotional lability*	36	(22)	27	(20)	1	(3)	18	(10.8)	7	(4.3)
Dizziness	19	(11)	4	(3)	0	(0)	3	(1.8)	6	(3.7)
Nervousness*	8	(5)	11	(8)	0	(0)	8	(4.8)	1	(0.6)
Neuromuscular disorders*	11	(7)	17	(13)	0	(0)	3	(1.8)	0	(0)
Paresthesias	12	(7)	11	(8)	0	(0)	2	(1.2)	1	(0.6)
Skin and Appendages										
Skin reactions	17	(10)	20	(15)	1	(3)	5	(3.0)	2	(1.2)
Urogenital System										
Breast changes/tenderness/pain*	10	(6)	12	(9)	0	(0)	3	(1.8)	7	(4.3)
Vaginitis*	46	(28)	23	(17)	0	(0)	19	(11.4)	3	(1.8)

In these same studies, symptoms reported in < 5% of patients included: *Body as a Whole* - Body odor, Flu syndrome, Injection site reactions; *Cardiovascular System* - Palpitations, Syncope, Tachycardia; *Digestive System* - Appetite changes, Dry mouth, Thirst; *Endocrine System* - Androgen-like effects; *Hemic and Lymphatic System* - Ecchymosis, Lymphadenopathy; *Nervous System* - Anxiety*, Insomnia/Sleep disorders*, Delusions, Memory disorder, Personality disorder; *Respiratory System* - Rhinitis; *Skin and Appendages* - Alopecia, Hair disorder, Nail disorder; *Special Senses* - Conjunctivitis, Ophthalmologic disorders*, Taste perversion; *Urogenital System* - Dysuria*, Lactation, Menstrual disorders.

* = Possible effect of decreased estrogen.

Table 3 TREATMENT-RELATED ADVERSE EVENTS OCCURRING IN ≥ 5% OF PATIENTS

	Controlled Study				Open Label Study	
	LD - Only* N=51		LD/N† N=55		LD/N† N=136	
Adverse Events	N	(%)	N	(%)	N	(%)
Any Adverse Event	50	(98)	53	(96)	126	(93)
Body as a Whole						
Asthenia	9	(18)	10	(18)	15	(11)
Headache/Migraine	33	(65)	28	(51)	63	(46)
Injection Site Reaction	1	(2)	5	(9)	4	(3)
Pain	12	(24)	16	(29)	29	(21)
Cardiovascular System						
Hot flashes/Sweats	50	(98)	48	(87)	78	(57)
Digestive System						
Altered Bowel Function	7	(14)	8	(15)	14	(10)
Changes in Appetite	2	(4)	0	(0)	8	(6)
GI Disturbance	2	(4)	4	(7)	6	(4)
Nausea/Vomiting	13	(25)	16	(29)	17	(13)
Metabolic and Nutritional Disorders						
Edema	0	(0)	5	(9)	9	(7)
Weight Changes	6	(12)	7	(13)	6	(4)
Nervous System						
Anxiety	3	(6)	0	(0)	11	(8)
Depression/Emotional Lability	16	(31)	15	(27)	46	(34)
Dizziness/Vertigo	8	(16)	6	(11)	10	(7)
Insomnia/Sleep Disorder	16	(31)	7	(13)	20	(15)
Libido Changes	5	(10)	2	(4)	10	(7)
Memory Disorder	3	(6)	1	(2)	6	(4)
Nervousness	4	(8)	2	(4)	15	(11)
Neuromuscular Disorder	1	(2)	5	(9)	4	(3)
Skin and Appendages						
Alopecia	0	(0)	5	(9)	4	(3)
Androgen-Like Effects	2	(4)	3	(5)	24	(18)
Skin/Mucous Membrane Reaction	2	(4)	5	(9)	15	(11)
Urogenital System						
Breast Changes/Pain/Tenderness	3	(6)	7	(13)	11	(8)
Menstrual Disorders	1	(2)	0	(0)	7	(5)
Vaginitis	10	(20)	8	(15)	11	(8)

* LD-Only = LUPRON DEPOT 3.75 mg
† LD/N = LUPRON DEPOT 3.75 mg plus norethindrone acetate 5 mg

During postmarketing surveillance with other dosage forms and in the same and/or different populations, the following adverse events were reported. Like other drugs in this class, mood swings, including depression, have been reported. There have been rare reports of suicidal ideation and attempt. Many, but not all, of these patients had a history of depression or other psychiatric illness. Patients should be counseled on the possibility of development or worsening of depression during treatment with LUPRON.

Symptoms consistent with an anaphylactoid or asthmatic process have been rarely reported. Rash, urticaria, and photosensitivity reactions have also been reported.

Localized reactions including induration and abscess have been reported at the site of injection.

Symptoms consistent with fibromyalgia (eg: joint and muscle pain, headaches, sleep disorders, gastrointestinal distress, and shortness of breath) have been reported individually and collectively.

Other events reported are:

Hepato-biliary disorder: Rarely reported serious liver injury

Injury, poisoning and procedural complications: Spinal fracture

Investigations: Decreased WBC

Musculoskeletal and Connective tissue disorder: Tenosynovitis-like symptoms

Nervous System Disorder: Convulsion, peripheral neuropathy, paralysis

Vascular Disorder: Hypotension

Cases of serious venous and arterial thromboembolism have been reported, including deep vein thrombosis, pulmonary embolism, myocardial infarction, stroke, and transient ischemic attack. Although a temporal relationship was reported in some cases, most cases were confounded by risk factors or concomitant medication use. It is unknown if there is a causal association between the use of GnRH analogs and these events.

Pituitary apoplexy

During post-marketing surveillance, rare cases of pituitary apoplexy (a clinical syndrome secondary to infarction of the pituitary gland) have been reported after the administration of gonadotropin-releasing hormone agonists. In a ma-

jority of these cases, a pituitary adenoma was diagnosed, with a majority of pituitary apoplexy cases occurring within 2 weeks of the first dose, and some within the first hour. In these cases, pituitary apoplexy has presented as sudden headache, vomiting, visual changes, ophthalmoplegia, altered mental status, and sometimes cardiovascular collapse. Immediate medical attention has been required.

See other LUPRON DEPOT and LUPRON Injection package inserts for other events reported in the same and different patient populations.

OVERDOSAGE

In clinical trials using daily subcutaneous leuprolide acetate in patients with prostate cancer, doses as high as 20 mg/day for up to two years caused no adverse effects differing from those observed with the 1 mg/day dose.

DOSAGE AND ADMINISTRATION

LUPRON DEPOT Must Be Administered Under the Supervision of a Physician.

Endometriosis

The recommended duration of treatment with LUPRON DEPOT–3 Month 11.25 mg alone or in combination with norethindrone acetate is six months. The choice of LUPRON DEPOT alone or LUPRON DEPOT plus norethindrone acetate therapy for initial management of the symptoms and signs of endometriosis should be made by the health care professional in consultation with the patient and should take into consideration the risks and benefits of the addition of norethindrone to LUPRON DEPOT alone.

If the symptoms of endometriosis recur after a course of therapy, retreatment with a six-month course of LUPRON DEPOT–3 Month 11.25 mg administered every three months and norethindrone acetate 5 mg daily may be considered. Retreatment beyond this one six-month course cannot be recommended. It is recommended that bone density be assessed before retreatment begins to ensure that values are within normal limits. LUPRON DEPOT alone is not recommended for retreatment. If norethindrone acetate is contraindicated for the individual patient, then retreatment is not recommended.

An assessment of cardiovascular risk and management of risk factors such as cigarette smoking is recommended before beginning treatment with LUPRON DEPOT and norethindrone acetate.

Uterine Leiomyomata (Fibroids)

The recommended dose of LUPRON DEPOT–3 Month 11.25 mg is one injection. The symptoms associated with uterine leiomyomata will recur following discontinuation of therapy. If additional treatment with LUPRON DEPOT–3 Month 11.25 mg is contemplated, bone density should be assessed prior to initiation of therapy to ensure that values are within normal limits.

Due to different release characteristics, a fractional dose of the 3-month depot formulation is not equivalent to the same dose of the monthly formulation and should not be given.

For optimal performance of the prefilled dual chamber syringe (PDS), read and follow the following instructions:
Reconstitution and Administration Instructions

• The lyophilized microspheres are to be reconstituted and administered as a single intramuscular injection.
• Since LUPRON DEPOT does not contain a preservative, the suspension should be injected immediately or discarded if not used within two hours.
• As with other drugs administered by injection, the injection site should be varied periodically.

1. The LUPRON DEPOT powder should be visually inspected and the syringe should NOT BE USED if clumping or caking is evident. A thin layer of powder on the wall of the syringe is considered normal prior to mixing with the diluent. The diluent should appear clear.

2. To prepare for injection, screw the white plunger into the end stopper until the stopper begins to turn.

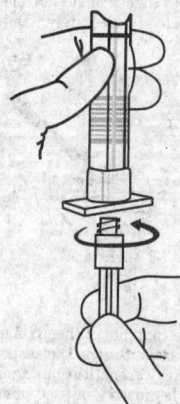

3. Hold the syringe UPRIGHT. Release the diluent by SLOWLY PUSHING (6 to 8 seconds) the plunger until the first stopper is at the blue line in the middle of the barrel.

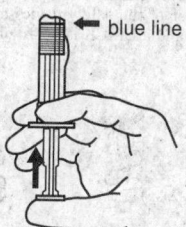

← blue line

4. Keep the syringe UPRIGHT. Mix the microspheres (powder) thoroughly by gently shaking the syringe until the powder forms a uniform suspension. The suspension will appear milky. If the powder adheres to the stopper or caking/clumping is present, tap the syringe with your finger to disperse. DO NOT USE if any of the powder has not gone into suspension.

5. Hold the syringe UPRIGHT. With the opposite hand pull the needle cap upward without twisting.

6. Keep the syringe UPRIGHT. Advance the plunger to expel the air from the syringe. Now the syringe is ready for injection.

7. After cleaning the injection site with an alcohol swab, the intramuscular injection should be performed by inserting the needle at a 90 degree angle into the gluteal area, an-

Continued on next page

Information on the AbbVie, Inc. products listed on these pages is from the prescribing information in use as of July 31, 2016. For more information, please visit rxabbvie.com or call 1-800-633-9110.

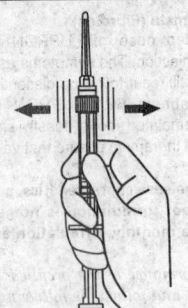

terior thigh, or deltoid; injection sites should be alternated.

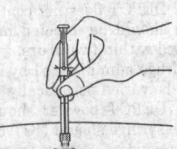

NOTE: Aspirated blood would be visible just below the luer lock connection if a blood vessel is accidentally penetrated. If present, blood can be seen through the transparent LuproLoc® safety device. If blood is present remove the needle immediately. Do not inject the medication.

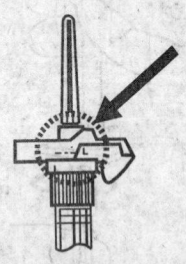

8. Inject the entire contents of the syringe intramuscularly at the time of reconstitution. The suspension settles very quickly following reconstitution; therefore, LUPRON DEPOT should be mixed and used immediately.

AFTER INJECTION

9. Withdraw the needle. Once the syringe has been withdrawn, activate immediately the LuproLoc® safety device by pushing the arrow on the lock upward towards the needle tip with the thumb or finger, as illustrated, until the needle cover of the safety device over the needle is fully extended and a CLICK is heard or felt.

CLICK

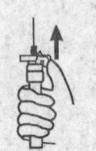 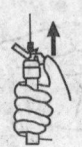 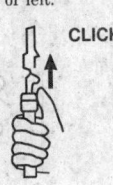

ADDITIONAL INFORMATION
• Dispose of the syringe according to local regulations/procedures.

HOW SUPPLIED

Each LUPRON DEPOT – 3 Month 11.25 mg kit (NDC 0074-3663-03) contains:
• one prefilled dual-chamber syringe
• one plunger
• two alcohol swabs
• a complete prescribing information enclosure

Each syringe contains sterile lyophilized microspheres which are leuprolide acetate incorporated in a biodegradable polymer of polylactic acid. When mixed with 1.5 mL of the diluent, LUPRON DEPOT–3 Month 11.25 mg is administered as a single IM injection **EVERY THREE MONTHS.**

Store at 25°C (77°F); excursions permitted to 15-30°C (59-86°F) [See USP Controlled Room Temperature]

REFERENCES

1. NIOSH Alert: Preventing occupational exposures to antineoplastic and other hazardous drugs in healthcare settings. 2004. U.S. Department of Health and Human Services, Public Health Service, Centers for Disease Control and Prevention, National Institute for Occupational Safety and Health, DHHS (NIOSH) Publication No. 2004-165.
2. OSHA Technical Manual, TED 1-0.15A, Section VI: Chapter 2. Controlling Occupational Exposure to Hazardous Drugs. OSHA, 1999. http://www.osha.gov/dts/osta/otm/otm_vi/otm_vi_2.html
3. American Society of Health-System Pharmacists. ASHP guidelines on handling hazardous drugs. *Am J Health-Syst Pharm.* 2006; 63; 1172-1193.
4. Polovich, M., White, J.M., & Kelleher, L.O. (eds.) 2005. Chemotherapy and biotherapy guidelines and recommendations for practice (2nd. Ed.) Pittsburgh, PA: Oncology Nursing Society.

Manufactured for
AbbVie Inc.
North Chicago, IL 60064
by Takeda Pharmaceutical Company Limited
Osaka, Japan 540-8645
™ - Trademark
® - Registered Trademark
(No. 3663)
Ref: 03-A892 - Revised October, 2013
© 2013, AbbVie Inc.
Shown in Product Identification Guide, page 505

Table 4 MEAN PERCENT CHANGE FROM BASELINE IN BONE MINERAL DENSITY OF LUMBAR SPINE

	LUPRON DEPOT 3.75 mg		LUPRON DEPOT 3.75 mg plus norethindrone acetate 5 mg daily			
	Controlled Study		Controlled Study		Open Label Study	
	N	Change (Mean, 95% CI)#	N	Change (Mean, 95% CI)#	N	Change (Mean, 95% CI)#
Week 24*	41	-3.2% (-3.8, -2.6)	42	-0.3% (-0.8, 0.3)	115	-0.2% (-0.6, 0.2)
Week 52†	29	-6.3% (-7.1, -5.4)	32	-1.0% (-1.9, -0.1)	84	-1.1% (-1.6, -0.5)

* Includes on-treatment measurements that fell within 2-252 days after the first day of treatment.
† Includes on-treatment measurements >252 days after the first day of treatment.
# 95% CI: 95% Confidence Interval

Table 5 SERUM LIPIDS: MEAN PERCENT CHANGES FROM BASELINE VALUES AT TREATMENT WEEK 24

	LUPRON DEPOT 3.75 mg		LUPRON DEPOT 3.75 mg plus norethindrone acetate 5 mg daily			
	Controlled Study (n=39)		Controlled Study (n=41)		Open Label Study (n=117)	
	Baseline Value*	Wk 24 % Change	Baseline Value*	Wk 24 % Change	Baseline Value*	Wk 24 % Change
Total Cholesterol	170.5	9.2%	179.3	0.2%	181.2	2.8%
HDL Cholesterol	52.4	7.4%	51.8	-18.8%	51.0	-14.6%
LDL Cholesterol	96.6	10.9%	101.5	14.1%	109.1	13.1%
LDL/HDL Ratio	2.0†	5.0%	2.1†	43.4%	2.3†	39.4%
Triglycerides	107.8	17.5%	130.2	9.5%	105.4	13.8%

* mg/dL
† ratio

Table 6 PERCENTAGE OF PATIENTS WITH SERUM LIPID VALUES OUTSIDE OF THE NORMAL RANGE

	LUPRON DEPOT 3.75 mg		LUPRON DEPOT 3.75 mg plus norethindrone acetate 5 mg daily			
	Controlled Study (n=39)		Controlled Study (n=41)		Open Label Study (n=117)	
	Wk 0	Wk 24*	Wk 0	Wk 24*	Wk 0	Wk 24*
Total Cholesterol (>240 mg/dL)	15%	23%	15%	20%	6%	7%
HDL Cholesterol (<40 mg/dL)	15%	10%	15%	44%	15%	41%
LDL Cholesterol (>160 mg/dL)	0%	8%	5%	7%	9%	11%
LDL/HDL Ratio (>4.0)	0%	3%	2%	15%	7%	21%
Triglycerides (>200 mg/dL)	13%	13%	12%	10%	5%	9%

* Includes all patients regardless of baseline value.

LUPRON DEPOT®   ℞
[lū-prŏn]
(leuprolide acetate for depot suspension)
7.5 mg for 1-Month Administration
22.5 mg for 3-Month Administration
30 mg for 4-Month Administration
45 mg for 6-Month Administration

HIGHLIGHTS OF PRESCRIBING INFORMATION
These highlights do not include all the information needed to use LUPRON DEPOT safely and effectively. See full prescribing information for LUPRON DEPOT.
LUPRON DEPOT (leuprolide acetate for depot suspension)
Initial U.S. Approval: 1989

——————RECENT MAJOR CHANGES——————

Dosage and Administration (2)   6/2016

——————INDICATIONS AND USAGE——————

LUPRON DEPOT is a gonadotropin releasing hormone (GnRH) agonist indicated for:
• palliative treatment of advanced prostatic cancer. (1)

——————DOSAGE AND ADMINISTRATION——————

LUPRON DEPOT must be administered under the supervision of a physician. Due to different release characteristics, the dosage strengths are not additive and must be selected based upon the desired dosing schedule. (2)
• LUPRON DEPOT 7.5 mg for 1-month administration, given as a single intramuscular injection every 4 weeks. (2.1)

- LUPRON DEPOT 22.5 mg for 3-month administration, given as a single intramuscular injection every 12 weeks. (2.2)
- LUPRON DEPOT 30 mg for 4-month administration, given as a single intramuscular injection every 16 weeks. (2.3)
- LUPRON DEPOT 45 mg for 6-month administration, given as a single intramuscular injection every 24 weeks. (2.4)

———DOSAGE FORMS AND STRENGTHS———

7.5 mg, 22.5 mg, 30 mg, and 45 mg injections in a kit with prefilled dual chamber syringe. (3)

———————CONTRAINDICATIONS———————

- Hypersensitivity to GnRH, GnRH agonist or any of the excipients in LUPRON DEPOT. (4)
- Pregnancy. (4, 8.1)

————WARNINGS AND PRECAUTIONS————

- Increased serum testosterone (~ 50% above baseline) during first week of treatment; monitor serum testosterone and PSA. (5.1, 5.6)
  ○ Isolated cases of transient worsening of symptoms, or additional signs and symptoms of prostate cancer during the first few weeks of treatment. (5.1)
  ○ A small number of patients may experience a temporary increase in bone pain which can be managed symptomatically. (5.1)
  ○ Isolated cases of ureteral obstruction and spinal cord compression have been reported with GnRH agonists, which may contribute to paralysis with or without fatal complications. (5.1)
- Hyperglycemia and Diabetes: Hyperglycemia and an increased risk of developing diabetes have been reported in men receiving GnRH analogs. Monitor blood glucose level and manage according to current clinical practice. (5.2)
- Cardiovascular Diseases: Increased risk of myocardial infarction, sudden cardiac death and stroke has been reported in association with use of GnRH analogs in men. Monitor for cardiovascular disease and manage according to current clinical practice. (5.3)
- Effect on QT/QTc Interval: Androgen deprivation therapy may prolong the QT interval. Consider risks and benefits. (5.4)
- Convulsions have been observed in patients with or without a history of predisposing factors. Manage convulsions according to the current clinical practice. (5.5)

———————ADVERSE REACTIONS———————

- LUPRON DEPOT 7.5 mg for 1-month administration: The most common adverse reactions (>10%) were general pain, hot flashes/sweats, GI disorders, edema, respiratory disorder, urinary disorder. (6.1)
- LUPRON DEPOT 22.5 mg for 3-month administration: The most common adverse reactions (>10%) were general pain, injection site reaction, hot flashes/sweats, GI disorders, joint disorders, testicular atrophy, urinary disorders. (6.2)
- LUPRON DEPOT 30 mg for 4-month administration: The most common adverse reactions (>10%) were asthenia, flu syndrome, general pain, headache, injection site reaction, hot flashes/sweats, GI disorders, edema, skin reaction, urinary disorders. (6.3)
- LUPRON DEPOT 45 mg for 6-month administration: The most common adverse reactions (>10%) were hot flush, injection site pain, upper respiratory infection, and fatigue. (6.4)

In postmarketing experience, mood swings, depression, rare reports of suicidal ideation and attempt, rare reports of pituitary apoplexy, and rare reports of serious drug-induced liver injury have been reported. (6.5)

To report SUSPECTED ADVERSE REACTIONS, contact AbbVie Inc. at 1-800-633-9110 or FDA at 1-800-FDA-1088 or www.fda.gov/medwatch

————USE IN SPECIFIC POPULATIONS————

- Pediatric: These LUPRON DEPOT formulations are not indicated for use in children. See the LUPRON DEPOT PED® package insert for the use of leuprolide acetate in children with central precocious puberty.
- Geriatric: This label reflects clinical trials for LUPRON DEPOT in prostate cancer in which the majority of the subjects studied were at least 65 years of age.

See 17 for PATIENT COUNSELING INFORMATION.

Revised: 6/2016

FULL PRESCRIBING INFORMATION: CONTENTS*

* Sections or subsections omitted from the full prescribing information are not listed.

FULL PRESCRIBING INFORMATION

1　INDICATIONS AND USAGE

LUPRON DEPOT 7.5 mg for 1-month administration, 22.5 mg for 3-month administration, 30 mg for 4-month administration, and 45 mg for 6-month administration (leuprolide acetate) are indicated in the palliative treatment of advanced prostatic cancer.

LUPRON DEPOT is a gonadotropin releasing hormone (GnRH) agonist.

2　DOSAGE AND ADMINISTRATION

LUPRON DEPOT must be administered under the supervision of a physician.

In patients treated with GnRH analogues for prostate cancer, treatment is usually continued upon development of metastatic castration-resistant prostate cancer.

[See table 1 above]

2.1　LUPRON DEPOT 7.5 mg for 1-Month Administration

The recommended dose of LUPRON DEPOT 7.5 mg for 1-month administration is one injection every 4 weeks. Do

Table 1. LUPRON DEPOT Recommended Dosing				
Dosage	7.5 mg for 1-Month Administration	22.5 mg for 3-Month Administration	30 mg for 4-Month Administration	45 mg for 6-Month Administration
Recommended dose	1 injection every 4 weeks	1 injection every 12 weeks	1 injection every 16 weeks	1 injection every 24 weeks

not use concurrently a fractional dose, or a combination of doses of this or any depot formulation due to different release characteristics.

Incorporated in a depot formulation, the lyophilized microspheres must be reconstituted and should be administered every 4 weeks as a single intramuscular injection.

For optimal performance of the prefilled dual chamber syringe (PDS), read and follow the instructions in Section 2.5.

2.2　LUPRON DEPOT 22.5 mg for 3-Month Administration

The recommended dose of LUPRON DEPOT 22.5 mg for 3-month administration is one injection every 12 weeks. Do not use concurrently a fractional dose, or a combination of doses of this or any depot formulation due to different release characteristics.

Incorporated in a depot formulation, the lyophilized microspheres must be reconstituted and should be administered every 12 weeks as a single intramuscular injection.

For optimal performance of the prefilled dual chamber syringe (PDS), read and follow the instructions in Section 2.5.

2.3　LUPRON DEPOT 30 mg for 4-Month Administration

The recommended dose of LUPRON DEPOT 30 mg for 4-month administration is one injection every 16 weeks. Do not use concurrently a fractional dose, or a combination of doses of this or any depot formulation due to different release characteristics.

Incorporated in a depot formulation, the lyophilized microspheres must be reconstituted and should be administered every 16 weeks as a single intramuscular injection.

For optimal performance of the prefilled dual chamber syringe (PDS), read and follow the instructions in Section 2.5.

2.4　LUPRON DEPOT 45 mg for 6-Month Administration

The recommended dose of LUPRON DEPOT 45 mg for 6-month administration is one injection every 24 weeks. Do not use concurrently a fractional dose, or a combination of doses of this or any depot formulation due to different release characteristics.

Incorporated in a depot formulation, the lyophilized microspheres must be reconstituted and should be administered every 24 weeks as a single intramuscular injection.

For optimal performance of the prefilled dual chamber syringe (PDS), read and follow the instructions in Section 2.5.

2.5　Reconstitution and Administration for Injection of LUPRON DEPOT

- Reconstitute and administer the lyophilized microspheres as a single intramuscular injection.
- Inject the suspension immediately or discard if not used within two hours, because LUPRON DEPOT does not contain a preservative.

1. Visually inspect the LUPRON DEPOT powder. DO NOT USE the syringe if clumping or caking is evident. A thin layer of powder on the wall of the syringe is considered normal prior to mixing with the diluent. The diluent should appear clear and colorless.

2. To prepare for injection, screw the white plunger into the end stopper until the stopper begins to turn (see Figure 1 and Figure 2).

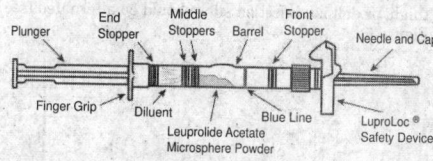

Figure 1

Continued on next page

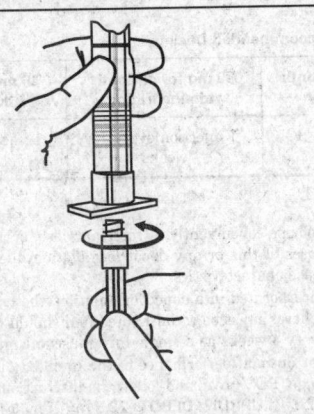

Figure 2

3. Hold the syringe UPRIGHT. Release the diluent by SLOWLY PUSHING (6 to 8 seconds) the plunger until the first middle stopper is at the blue line in the middle of the barrel (see Figure 3).

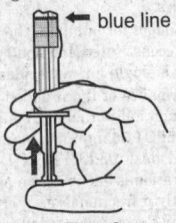

← blue line

Figure 3

4. Keep the syringe UPRIGHT. Mix the microspheres (powder) thoroughly by gently shaking the syringe until the powder forms a uniform suspension. The suspension will appear milky. If the powder adheres to the stopper or caking/clumping is present, tap the syringe with your finger to disperse. DO NOT USE if any of the powder has not gone into suspension (see Figure 4).

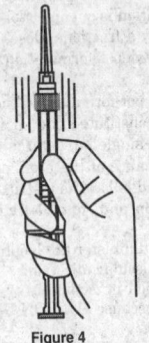

Figure 4

5. Keep the syringe UPRIGHT. With the opposite hand pull the needle cap upward without twisting.
6. Keep the syringe UPRIGHT. Advance the plunger to expel the air from the syringe. Now the syringe is ready for injection.
7. After cleaning the injection site with an alcohol swab, administer the intramuscular injection by inserting the needle at a 90 degree angle into the gluteal area, anterior thigh, or deltoid; injection sites should be alternated (see Figure 5).

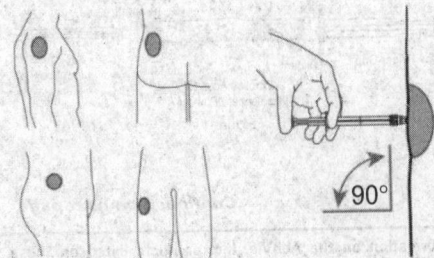

90°

Figure 5

NOTE: If a blood vessel is accidentally penetrated, aspi-

rated blood will be visible just below the luer lock (see Figure 6) and can be seen through the transparent LuproLoc® safety device. If blood is present, remove the needle immediately. Do not inject the medication. [See Figure 6 below]

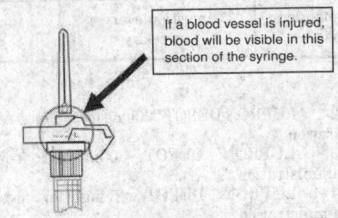

If a blood vessel is injured, blood will be visible in this section of the syringe.

Figure 6

8. Inject the entire contents of the syringe intramuscularly.
9. Withdraw the needle. Once the syringe has been withdrawn, immediately activate the LuproLoc® safety device by pushing the arrow on the lock upward towards the needle tip with the thumb or finger, as illustrated, until the needle cover of the safety device over the needle is fully extended and a CLICK is heard or felt (see Figure 7).

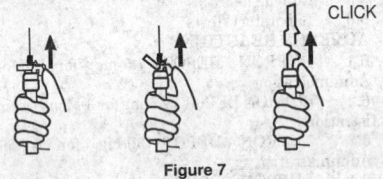

CLICK

Figure 7

10. Dispose of the syringe according to local regulations/procedures.

3   DOSAGE FORMS AND STRENGTHS

LUPRON DEPOT 7.5 mg for 1-month administration, 22.5 mg for 3-month administration, 30 mg for 4-month administration, and 45 mg for 6-month administration are each supplied as a kit with prefilled dual chamber syringe.

4   CONTRAINDICATIONS

LUPRON DEPOT is contraindicated in:

• **Hypersensitivity**
LUPRON DEPOT is contraindicated in individuals with known hypersensitivity to GnRH agonists or any of the excipients in LUPRON DEPOT. Reports of anaphylactic reactions to GnRH agonists have been reported in the medical literature.

• **Pregnancy**
LUPRON DEPOT may cause fetal harm when administered to a pregnant woman. Expected hormonal changes that occur with LUPRON DEPOT treatment increase the risk for pregnancy loss and fetal harm when administered to a pregnant woman. LUPRON DEPOT is contraindicated in women who are or may become pregnant. If this drug is used during pregnancy, or if the patient becomes pregnant while taking this drug, the patient should be apprised of the potential hazard to the fetus [see Use in Specific Populations (8.1)].

5   WARNINGS AND PRECAUTIONS

5.1   Tumor Flare
Initially, LUPRON DEPOT, like other GnRH agonists, causes increases in serum levels of testosterone to approximately 50% above baseline during the first weeks of treatment. Isolated cases of ureteral obstruction and spinal cord compression have been observed, which may contribute to paralysis with or without fatal complications. Transient worsening of symptoms may develop. A small number of patients may experience a temporary increase in bone pain, which can be managed symptomatically.
Patients with metastatic vertebral lesions and/or with urinary tract obstruction should be closely observed during the first few weeks of therapy.

5.2   Hyperglycemia and Diabetes
Hyperglycemia and an increased risk of developing diabetes have been reported in men receiving GnRH agonists. Hyperglycemia may represent development of diabetes mellitus or worsening of glycemic control in patients with diabetes. Monitor blood glucose and/or glycosylated hemoglobin (HbA1c) periodically in patients receiving a GnRH agonist and manage with current practice for treatment of hyperglycemia or diabetes.

5.3   Cardiovascular Diseases
Increased risk of developing myocardial infarction, sudden cardiac death and stroke has been reported in association

with use of GnRH agonists in men. The risk appears low based on the reported odds ratios, and should be evaluated carefully along with cardiovascular risk factors when determining a treatment for patients with prostate cancer. Patients receiving a GnRH agonist should be monitored for symptoms and signs suggestive of development of cardiovascular disease and be managed according to current clinical practice.

5.4   Effect on QT/QTc Interval
Androgen deprivation therapy may prolong the QT/QTc interval. Providers should consider whether the benefits of androgen deprivation therapy outweigh the potential risks in patients with congenital long QT syndrome, congestive heart failure, frequent electrolyte abnormalities, and in patients taking drugs known to prolong the QT interval. Electrolyte abnormalities should be corrected. Consider periodic monitoring of electrocardiograms and electrolytes.

5.5   Convulsions
Postmarketing reports of convulsions have been observed in patients on leuprolide acetate therapy. These included patients with a history of seizures, epilepsy, cerebrovascular disorders, central nervous system anomalies or tumors, and in patients on concomitant medications that have been associated with convulsions such as bupropion and SSRIs. Convulsions have also been reported in patients in the absence of any of the conditions mentioned above. Patients receiving a GnRH agonist who experience convulsion should be managed according to current clinical practice.

5.6   Laboratory Tests
Monitor serum levels of testosterone following injection of LUPRON DEPOT 7.5 mg for 1-month administration, 22.5 mg for 3-month administration, 30 mg for 4-month administration, or 45 mg for 6-month administration. In the majority of patients, testosterone levels increased above baseline, and then declined thereafter to castrate levels (< 50 ng/dL) within four weeks. [see Clinical Studies (14) and Adverse Reactions (6)].

6   ADVERSE REACTIONS

Because clinical trials are conducted under widely varying conditions, adverse reaction rates observed in the clinical trials of a drug cannot be directly compared to rates in the clinical trials of another drug and may not reflect the rates observed in practice.

6.1   LUPRON DEPOT 7.5 mg for 1-Month Administration
In the majority of patients testosterone levels increased above baseline during the first week, declining thereafter to baseline levels or below by the end of the second week of treatment.
Potential exacerbations of signs and symptoms during the first few weeks of treatment is a concern in patients with vertebral metastases and/or urinary obstruction or hematuria which, if aggravated, may lead to neurological problems such as temporary weakness and/or paresthesia of the lower limbs or worsening of urinary symptoms [see Warnings and Precautions (5.1)].
In a clinical trial of LUPRON DEPOT 7.5 mg for 1-month administration, the following adverse reactions were reported in 5% or more of the patients during the initial 24-week treatment period.

Table 2. Adverse Reactions Reported in ≥ 5% of Patients

LUPRON DEPOT 7.5 mg for 1-Month Administration (N=56)		
	N	(%)
Body As A Whole		
General pain	13	(23.2)
Infection	3	(5.4)
Cardiovascular System		
Hot flashes/sweats*	32	(57.1)
Digestive System		
GI disorders	8	(14.3)
Metabolic and Nutritional Disorders		
Edema	8	(14.3)
Nervous System		
Libido decreased*	3	(5.4)
Respiratory System		
Respiratory disorder	6	(10.7)
Urogenital System		
Urinary disorder	7	(12.5)
Impotence*	3	(5.4)
Testicular atrophy*	3	(5.4)
* Due to the expected physiologic effect of decreased testosterone levels.		

In this same study, the following adverse reactions were reported in less than 5% of the patients on LUPRON DEPOT 7.5 mg for 1-month administration.

Body As A Whole - Asthenia, Cellulitis, Fever, Headache, Injection site reaction, Neoplasm

Cardiovascular System - Angina, Congestive heart failure

Digestive System - Anorexia, Dysphagia, Eructation, Peptic ulcer

Hemic and Lymphatic System - Ecchymosis

Musculoskeletal System - Myalgia

Nervous System - Agitation, Insomnia/sleep disorders, Neuromuscular disorders

Respiratory System - Emphysema, Hemoptysis, Lung edema, Sputum increased

Skin and Appendages - Hair disorder, Skin reaction

Urogenital System - Balanitis, Breast enlargement, Urinary tract infection

Laboratory Abnormalities

Abnormalities of certain parameters were observed, but their relationship to drug treatment are difficult to assess in this population. The following were recorded in ≥5% of patients at final visit: Decreased albumin, decreased hemoglobin/hematocrit, decreased prostatic acid phosphatase, decreased total protein, decreased urine specific gravity, hyperglycemia, hyperuricemia, increased BUN, increased creatinine, increased liver function tests (AST, LDH), increased phosphorus, increased platelets, increased prostatic acid phosphatase, increased total cholesterol, increased urine specific gravity, leukopenia.

6.2 LUPRON DEPOT 22.5 mg for 3-Month Administration

In two clinical trials of LUPRON DEPOT 22.5 mg for 3-month administration, the following adverse reactions were reported to have a possible or probable relationship to drug as ascribed by the treating physician in 5% or more of the patients receiving the drug. **Often, causality is difficult to assess in patients with metastatic prostate cancer.** Reactions considered not drug-related are excluded.

Table 3. Adverse Reactions Reported in ≥ 5% of Patients

LUPRON DEPOT 22.5 mg for 3-Month Administration		
Body System/Reaction	N=94	(%)
Body As A Whole		
Asthenia	7	(7.4)
General Pain	25	(26.6)
Headache	6	(6.4)
Injection Site Reaction	13	(13.8)
Cardiovascular System		
Hot flashes/Sweats	55	(58.5)
Digestive System		
GI Disorders	15	(16.0)
Musculoskeletal System		
Joint Disorders	11	(11.7)
Central/Peripheral Nervous System		
Dizziness/Vertigo	6	(6.4)
Insomnia/Sleep Disorders	8	(8.5)
Neuromuscular Disorders	9	(9.6)
Respiratory System		
Respiratory Disorders	6	(6.4)
Skin and Appendages		
Skin Reaction	8	(8.5)
Urogenital System		
Testicular Atrophy	19	(20.2)
Urinary Disorders	14	(14.9)

In these same studies, the following adverse reactions were reported in less than 5% of the patients on LUPRON DEPOT 22.5 mg for 3-month administration.

Body As A Whole - Enlarged abdomen, Fever

Cardiovascular System - Arrhythmia, Bradycardia, Heart failure, Hypertension, Hypotension, Varicose vein

Digestive System - Anorexia, Duodenal ulcer, Increased appetite, Thirst/dry mouth

Hemic and Lymphatic System - Anemia, Lymphedema

Metabolic and Nutritional Disorders - Dehydration, Edema

Central/Peripheral Nervous System - Anxiety, Delusions, Depression, Hypesthesia, Libido decreased*, Nervousness, Paresthesia

Respiratory System - Epistaxis, Pharyngitis, Pleural effusion, Pneumonia

Special Senses - Abnormal vision, Amblyopia, Dry eyes, Tinnitus

Urogenital System - Gynecomastia, Impotence*, Penis disorders, Testis disorders.

*Physiologic effect of decreased testosterone.

Laboratory Abnormalities

Abnormalities of certain parameters were observed, but are difficult to assess in this population. The following were recorded in ≥5% of patients: Increased BUN, Hyperglycemia,

Hyperlipidemia (total cholesterol, LDL-cholesterol, triglycerides), Hyperphosphatemia, Abnormal liver function tests, Increased PT, Increased PTT. Additional laboratory abnormalities reported were: Decreased platelets, Decreased potassium and Increased WBC.

6.3 LUPRON DEPOT 30 mg for 4-Month Administration

The 4-month formulation of LUPRON DEPOT 30 mg was utilized in clinical trials that studied the drug in 49 nonorchiectomized prostate cancer patients for 32 weeks or longer and in 24 orchiectomized prostate cancer patients for 20 weeks.

In the above described clinical trials, the following adverse reactions were reported in ≥ 5% of the patients during the treatment period.

[See table 4 above]

In these same studies, the following adverse reactions were reported in less than 5% of the patients on LUPRON DEPOT 30 mg for 4-month administration.

Body As A Whole - Abscess, Accidental injury, Allergic reaction, Cyst, Fever, Generalized edema, Hernia, Neck pain, Neoplasm

Cardiovascular System - Atrial fibrillation, Deep thrombophlebitis, Hypertension

Digestive System - Anorexia, Eructation, Gastrointestinal hemorrhage, Gingivitis, Gum hemorrhage, Hepatomegaly, Increased appetite, Intestinal obstruction, Periodontal abscess

Hemic and Lymphatic System - Lymphadenopathy

Metabolic and Nutritional Disorders - Healing abnormal, Hypoxia, Weight loss

Musculoskeletal System - Leg cramps, Pathological fracture, Ptosis

Nervous System - Abnormal thinking, Amnesia, Confusion, Convulsion, Dementia, Depression, Insomnia/sleep disorders, Libido decreased*, Neuropathy, Paralysis

Respiratory System - Asthma, Bronchitis, Hiccup, Lung disorder, Sinusitis, Voice alteration

Skin and Appendages - Herpes zoster, Melanosis

Urogenital System - Bladder carcinoma, Epididymitis, Impotence*, Prostate disorder, Testicular atrophy*, Urinary incontinence, Urinary tract infection.

*Physiologic effect of decreased testosterone.

Laboratory Abnormalities

Abnormalities of certain parameters were observed, but their relationship to drug treatment is difficult to assess in this population. The following were recorded in ≥ 5% of patients: Decreased bicarbonate, Decreased hemoglobin/hematocrit/RBC, Hyperlipidemia (total cholesterol, LDL-cholesterol, triglycerides), Decreased HDL-cholesterol, Eosinophilia, Increased glucose, Increased liver function tests (ALT, AST, GGTP, LDH), Increased phosphorus. Additional laboratory abnormalities were reported: Increased BUN and PT, Leukopenia, Thrombocytopenia, Uricaciduria.

Table 4. Adverse Reactions Reported in ≥ 5% of Patients

Body System/Events	LUPRON DEPOT 30 mg for 4-Month Administration			
	Nonorchiectomized Study 013		Orchiectomized Study 012	
	N=49	(%)	N=24	(%)
Body As A Whole				
Asthenia	6	(12.2)	1	(4.2)
Flu Syndrome	6	(12.2)	0	(0.0)
General Pain	16	(32.7)	1	(4.2)
Headache	5	(10.2)	1	(4.2)
Injection Site Reaction	4	(8.2)	9	(37.5)
Cardiovascular System				
Hot flashes/Sweats	23	(46.9)	2	(8.3)
Digestive System				
GI Disorders	5	(10.2)	3	(12.5)
Metabolic and Nutritional Disorders				
Dehydration	4	(8.2)	0	(0.0)
Edema	4	(8.2)	5	(20.8)
Musculoskeletal System				
Joint Disorder	8	(16.3)	1	(4.2)
Myalgia	4	(8.2)	0	(0.0)
Nervous System				
Dizziness/Vertigo	3	(6.1)	2	(8.3)
Neuromuscular Disorders	3	(6.1)	1	(4.2)
Paresthesia	4	(8.2)	1	(4.2)
Respiratory System				
Respiratory Disorder	4	(8.2)	1	(4.2)
Skin and Appendages				
Skin Reaction	6	(12.2)	0	(0.0)
Urogenital System				
Urinary Disorders	5	(10.2)	4	(16.7)

6.4 LUPRON DEPOT 45 mg for 6-Month Administration

One open label, multicenter study was conducted with LUPRON DEPOT 45 mg for 6-month administration in 151 prostate cancer patients. Patients were treated for 48 weeks, with 139/151 receiving two injections 24 weeks apart.

In the above described clinical trial, the following adverse events were reported in ≥ 5% of the patients during the treatment period. The Table 5 includes all adverse events reported in ≥ 5% of patients as well as the incidences of these adverse events that were considered, by the treating physician, to have a definite or possible relationship to LUPRON.

[See table 5 on next page]

The following adverse events led to discontinuation; fatigue, hot flush, second primary neoplasm, asthenia, coronary artery disease, constipation, hyperkalemia, and sleep disorder. Serious adverse events in ≥ 2% of patients, regardless of causality, included chronic obstructive pulmonary disease, coronary artery disease/angina, cerebrovascular accident/transient ischemic attack, pneumonia, and second primary neoplasms.

Laboratory Abnormalities

At baseline, 13.9% of patients had a CTCAE v4.0 grade 1 or 2 decreased hemoglobin. During the study, 42.4% of subjects had grade 1 decreased hemoglobin (10 - <12·5 g/dL), 2.0% had grade 2 (8 - <10 g/dL) and 1.3% of subjects had grade 3 or 4 (<8 g/dL). Likewise, 28.5% of patients had a grade 1 or 2 increased cholesterol at baseline while 55.0% had grade 1 increased cholesterol (>199- 300 mg/dL), 3.3% had a grade 2 increase (>300-400 mg/dL), and 0.7% of subjects had grade 3 (>400 mg/dL) during the study.

6.5 Postmarketing

The following adverse reactions have been identified during post-approval use of LUPRON DEPOT. Because these reactions are reported voluntarily from a population of uncertain size, it is not always possible to reliably estimate their frequency or establish a causal relationship to drug exposure.

During postmarketing surveillance, which includes other dosage forms and other patient populations, the following adverse reactions were reported.

Like other drugs in this class, mood swings, including depression, have been reported. There have been very rare reports of suicidal ideation and attempt. Many, but not all, of

Continued on next page

Information on the AbbVie, Inc. products listed on these pages is from the prescribing information in use as of July 31, 2016. For more information, please visit rxabbvie.com or call 1-800-633-9110.

these patients had a history of depression or other psychiatric illness. Patients should be counseled on the possibility of development or worsening of depression during treatment with LUPRON.

Symptoms consistent with an anaphylactoid or asthmatic process have been rarely (incidence rate of about 0.002%) reported. Rash, urticaria, and photosensitivity reactions have also been reported.

Changes in Bone Density - Decreased bone density has been reported in the medical literature in men who have had orchiectomy or who have been treated with a GnRH agonist analog. In a clinical trial, 25 men with prostate cancer, 12 of whom had been treated previously with leuprolide acetate for at least six months, underwent bone density studies as a result of pain. The leuprolide-treated group had lower bone density scores than the nontreated control group. It can be anticipated that long periods of medical castration in men will have effects on bone density.

Pituitary apoplexy - During post-marketing surveillance, rare cases of pituitary apoplexy (a clinical syndrome secondary to infarction of the pituitary gland) have been reported after the administration of gonadotropin-releasing hormone agonists. In a majority of these cases, a pituitary adenoma was diagnosed, with a majority of pituitary apoplexy cases occurring within 2 weeks of the first dose, and some within the first hour. In these cases, pituitary apoplexy has presented as sudden headache, vomiting, visual changes, ophthalmoplegia, altered mental status, and sometimes cardiovascular collapse. Immediate medical attention has been required.

Localized reactions including induration and abscess have been reported at the site of injection.

Symptoms consistent with fibromyalgia (e.g., joint and muscle pain, headaches, sleep disorders, gastrointestinal distress, and shortness of breath) have been reported individually and collectively.

Cardiovascular System - Hypotension, Myocardial infarction, Pulmonary embolism

Respiratory, thoracic and mediastinal disorder - Interstitial lung disease

Hepato-biliary disorder - Serious drug-induced liver injury

Hemic and Lymphatic System - Decreased WBC

Central/Peripheral Nervous System - Convulsion, Peripheral neuropathy, Spinal fracture/paralysis

Endocrine System - Diabetes

Musculoskeletal System - Tenosynovitis-like symptoms

Urogenital System - Prostate pain

See other LUPRON DEPOT and LUPRON Injection package inserts for other reactions reported in women and pediatric populations.

7 DRUG INTERACTIONS

No pharmacokinetic-based drug-drug interaction studies have been conducted with LUPRON DEPOT.

7.1 Drug/Laboratory Test Interactions

Administration of LUPRON DEPOT in therapeutic doses results in suppression of the pituitary-gonadal system. Normal function is usually restored within three months after treatment is discontinued. Due to the suppression of the pituitary-gonadal system by LUPRON DEPOT, diagnostic tests of pituitary gonadotropic and gonadal functions conducted during treatment and up to three months after discontinuation of LUPRON DEPOT may be affected.

8 USE IN SPECIFIC POPULATIONS

8.1 Pregnancy

Pregnancy Category X *[see Contraindications (4)].*

Risk Summary

LUPRON DEPOT may cause fetal harm when administered to a pregnant woman. The monthly formulation of leuprolide acetate caused embryo-fetal toxicity in animals at doses less than the human dose based on body surface area using an estimated daily dose. Expected hormonal changes that occur with LUPRON DEPOT treatment increase the risk for pregnancy loss and fetal harm when administered to a pregnant woman. LUPRON DEPOT is con-

traindicated in women who are pregnant while receiving the drug. If this drug is used during pregnancy, or if the patient becomes pregnant while taking this drug, apprise the patient of the potential hazard to the fetus and the potential risk for pregnancy loss.

Animal Data

Major fetal abnormalities were observed in rabbits after a single administration of the monthly formulation of leuprolide acetate on day 6 of pregnancy at doses of 0.00024, 0.0024, and 0.024 mg/kg (approximately 1/1600 to 1/16 the human dose based on body surface area using an estimated daily dose in animals and humans). Since a depot formulation was utilized in the study, a sustained exposure to leuprolide was expected throughout the period of organogenesis and to the end of gestation. Similar studies in rats did not demonstrate an increase in fetal malformations, however, there was increased fetal mortality and decreased fetal weights with the two higher doses of the monthly formulation of leuprolide acetate in rabbits and with the highest dose (0.024 mg/kg) in rats.

8.3 Nursing Mothers

LUPRON DEPOT is not indicated for use in nursing mothers *[see Indications and Usage (1)].* It is not known whether leuprolide is excreted in human milk. Because many drugs are excreted in human milk and because of the potential for serious adverse reactions in nursing infants from LUPRON DEPOT, a decision should be made to discontinue nursing or discontinue the drug taking into account the importance of the drug to the mother.

8.4 Pediatric Use

See LUPRON DEPOT-PED® (leuprolide acetate for depot suspension) labeling for the safety and effectiveness in children with central precocious puberty.

8.5 Geriatric Use

In the clinical trials for LUPRON DEPOT in prostate cancer 80% of the subjects studied were at least 65 years of age. Therefore, the labeling reflects the efficacy and safety of LUPRON DEPOT in this population.

8.6 Males of Reproductive Potential

Infertility

LUPRON DEPOT may reduce fertility based on animal studies and its mechanism of action. There are no data in humans relating to male fertility following treatment with leuprolide acetate. In animal studies, administration of leuprolide acetate to rats as a monthly depot formulation caused atrophy of the reproductive organs and suppression of reproductive function. These changes were reversible upon cessation of treatment *[see Nonclinical Toxicology (13.1)].*

10 OVERDOSAGE

There is no experience of overdosage in clinical trials. In rats, a single subcutaneous dose of 100 mg/kg (approximately 4,000 times the estimated daily human dose based on body surface area), resulted in dyspnea, decreased activity, and excessive scratching. In early clinical trials with daily subcutaneous leuprolide acetate, doses as high as 20 mg/day for up to two years caused no adverse effects differing from those observed with the 1 mg/day dose.

11 DESCRIPTION

Leuprolide acetate is a synthetic nonapeptide analog of naturally occurring gonadotropin-releasing hormone (GnRH). The analog possesses greater potency than the natural hormone. The chemical name is 5-oxo-L-prolyl-L-histidyl-L-tryptophyl-L-seryl-L-tyrosyl-D-leucyl-L-leucyl-L-arginyl-N-ethyl-L-prolinamide acetate (salt) with the following structural formula:

[See structural formula below]

LUPRON DEPOT 7.5 mg for 1-month administration is available in a prefilled dual-chamber syringe containing sterile lyophilized microspheres which, when mixed with diluent, becomes a suspension intended as a monthly intramuscular injection.

The front chamber of LUPRON DEPOT 7.5 mg for 1-month administration prefilled dual-chamber syringe contains leuprolide acetate (7.5 mg), purified gelatin (1.3 mg), DL-lactic and glycolic acids copolymer (66.2 mg), and D-mannitol (13.2 mg). The second chamber of diluent contains carboxymethylcellulose sodium (5 mg), D-mannitol (50 mg), polysorbate 80 (1 mg), water for injection, USP, and glacial acetic acid, USP to control pH.

LUPRON DEPOT 22.5 mg for 3-month administration is available in a prefilled dual-chamber syringe containing sterile lyophilized microspheres which, when mixed with diluent, become a suspension intended as an intramuscular injection to be given ONCE EVERY 12 WEEKS.

The front chamber of LUPRON DEPOT 22.5 mg for 3-month administration prefilled dual-chamber syringe contains leuprolide acetate (22.5 mg), polylactic acid (198.6 mg) and D-mannitol (38.9 mg). The second chamber of diluent contains carboxymethylcellulose sodium (7.5 mg), D-mannitol (75.0 mg), polysorbate 80 (1.5 mg), water for injection, USP, and glacial acetic acid, USP to control pH.

Table 5. Adverse Events in ≥ 5% of Patients

LUPRON DEPOT 45 mg for 6-Month Administration

Adverse Event	Treatment Emergent N = 151	(%)	Treatment Related N = 151	(%)
Hot Flush/Flushing	89	58.9	88	58.3
Injection Site Pain/Discomfort	29	19.2	16	10.6
Upper Respiratory Tract Infection/Influenza-like Illness[1]	32	21.2	0	0
Fatigue/Lethargy	20	13.2	18	11.9
Constipation	15	9.9	5	3.3
Arthralgia	14	9.3	2	1.3
Insomnia/Sleep Disorder	13	8.6	5	3.3
Headache/Sinus Headache	12	7.9	3	2.0
Musculoskeletal Pain/ Myalgia	12	7.9	3	2.0
Second Primary Neoplasm[2]	11	7.3	0	0
Cough	10	6.6	2	1.3
Hematuria/Hemorrhagic Cystitis	10	6.6	0	0
Hypertension/BP Increased	10	6.6	3	2.0
Rash	9	6.0	3	2.0
Dysuria	9	6.0	1	0.7
Urinary Tract Infection/Cystitis	9	6.0	0	0
Anemia/Hemoglobin Decreased	10	6.6	2	1.3
Back Pain	8	5.3	0	0
COPD	8	5.3	0	0
Dizziness	8	5.3	3	2.0
Dyspnea/Dyspnea on Exertion	8	5.3	2	1.3
Nocturia	8	5.3	2	1.3
Peripheral/Pitting Edema	8	5.3	2	1.3
Coronary Artery Disease/Angina	8	5.3	1	0.7

[1]Includes influenza, nasal congestion, nasopharyngitis, rhinorrhea, upper respiratory tract infection, and viral upper respiratory tract infection

[2]Includes basal cell carcinoma, bladder transitional cell carcinoma, lung neoplasm, malignant melanoma, non-Hodgkin's lymphoma, and squamous cell carcinoma

LUPRON DEPOT 30 mg for 4-month administration is available in a prefilled dual-chamber syringe containing sterile lyophilized microspheres which, when mixed with diluent, become a suspension intended as an intramuscular injection to be given **ONCE EVERY 16 WEEKS**.

The front chamber of LUPRON DEPOT 30 mg for 4-month administration prefilled dual-chamber syringe contains leuprolide acetate (30 mg), polylactic acid (264.8 mg) and D-mannitol (51.9 mg). The second chamber of diluent contains carboxymethylcellulose sodium (7.5 mg), D-mannitol (75.0 mg), polysorbate 80 (1.5 mg), water for injection, USP, and glacial acetic acid, USP to control pH.

LUPRON DEPOT 45 mg for 6-month administration is available in a prefilled dual-chamber syringe containing sterile lyophilized microspheres which, when mixed with diluent, become a suspension intended as an intramuscular injection to be given **ONCE EVERY 24 WEEKS**.

The front chamber of LUPRON DEPOT 45 mg for 6-month administration prefilled dual-chamber syringe contains leuprolide acetate (45 mg), polylactic acid (169.9 mg), D-mannitol (39.7 mg), and stearic acid (10.1 mg). The second chamber of diluent contains carboxymethylcellulose sodium (7.5 mg), D-mannitol (75.0 mg), polysorbate 80 (1.5 mg), water for injection, USP, and glacial acetic acid, USP to control pH.

12 CLINICAL PHARMACOLOGY

12.1 Mechanism of Action

Leuprolide acetate, a GnRH agonist, acts as an inhibitor of gonadotropin secretion. Animal studies indicate that following an initial stimulation, continuous administration of leuprolide acetate results in suppression of ovarian and testicular steroidogenesis. This effect was reversible upon discontinuation of drug therapy.

Administration of leuprolide acetate has resulted in inhibition of the growth of certain hormone dependent tumors (prostatic tumors in Noble and Dunning male rats and DMBA-induced mammary tumors in female rats) as well as atrophy of the reproductive organs.

12.2 Pharmacodynamics

In humans, administration of leuprolide acetate results in an initial increase in circulating concentrations of luteinizing hormone (LH) and follicle stimulating hormone (FSH), leading to a transient increase in concentrations of the gonadal steroids (testosterone and dihydrotestosterone in males, and estrone and estradiol in premenopausal females). However, continuous administration of leuprolide acetate results in decreased concentrations of LH and FSH. In males, testosterone is reduced to castrate concentrations. In premenopausal females, estrogens are reduced to postmenopausal concentrations. These decreases occur within two to four weeks after initiation of treatment, and castrate concentrations of testosterone in prostatic cancer patients have been demonstrated for more than five years.

Leuprolide acetate is not active when given orally.

12.3 Pharmacokinetics

Absorption

LUPRON DEPOT 7.5 mg for 1-Month Administration

Following a single injection of LUPRON DEPOT 7.5 mg for 1-month administration to patients, mean plasma measured concentrations were 20 ng/mL at 4 hours and 0.36 ng/mL at 4 weeks. However, intact leuprolide and an inactive major metabolite could not be distinguished by the assay which was employed in the study.

LUPRON DEPOT 22.5 mg for 3-Month Administration

Following a single injection of LUPRON DEPOT 22.5 mg for 3-month administration in patients, mean peak plasma concentrations were 48.9 ng/mL at 4 hours and then declined to 0.67 ng/mL at 12 weeks. Leuprolide appeared to be released at a constant rate following the onset of steady-state concentrations during the third week after dosing, providing steady plasma concentrations through the 12-week dosing interval. However, intact leuprolide and an inactive major metabolite could not be distinguished by the assay which was employed in the study. The initial burst, followed by a decline to a steady-state concentration, was similar to the release pattern seen with the monthly formulation.

LUPRON DEPOT 30 mg for 4-Month Administration

Following a single injection of LUPRON DEPOT 30 mg for 4-month administration in sixteen orchiectomized prostate cancer patients, mean plasma concentrations were 59.3 ng/mL at 4 hours and then declined to 0.30 ng/mL at 16 weeks. Mean plasma concentrations from weeks 3.5 to 16 was 0.44 ± 0.20 ng/mL (range: 0.20-1.06). Leuprolide appeared to be released at a constant rate following the onset of steady-state concentrations during the fourth week after dosing, providing steady plasma concentrations throughout the 16-week dosing interval. However, intact leuprolide and an inactive major metabolite could not be distinguished by the assay which was employed in the study. The initial burst, followed by a decline to a steady-state concentration, was similar to the release pattern seen with the other depot formulations.

LUPRON DEPOT 45 mg for 6-Month Administration

Following a single injection of LUPRON DEPOT 45 mg for 6-month administration in 26 prostate cancer patients, mean peak plasma concentration of 6.7 ng/mL was observed at 2 hours and then declined to 0.07 ng/mL at 24 weeks. Leuprolide appeared to be released continuously following the onset of steady-state concentrations during the third week after dosing providing steady plasma concentrations through the 24-week dosing interval. The initial burst, followed by a decline to a steady-state concentration, was similar to the release pattern seen with the other depot formulations. In this study, mean plasma concentration-time profiles were similar after the first and second dose.

Distribution

The mean steady-state volume of distribution of leuprolide following intravenous bolus administration to healthy male volunteers was 27 L. *In vitro* binding to human plasma proteins ranged from 43% to 49%.

Elimination

The mean systemic clearance of leuprolide following intravenous bolus administration to healthy male volunteers was 7.6 L/h, and terminal elimination half-life was approximately 3 hours based on a two compartment model.

Following administration of LUPRON DEPOT 3.75 mg to 3 patients, less than 5% of the dose was recovered as parent and M-I metabolite in the urine.

13 NONCLINICAL TOXICOLOGY

13.1 Carcinogenesis, Mutagenesis, Impairment of Fertility

Two-year carcinogenicity studies were conducted in rats and mice. In rats, a dose-related increase of benign pituitary hyperplasia and benign pituitary adenomas was noted at 24 months when the drug was administered subcutaneously at daily doses (0.6 to 4 mg/kg). There was a significant but not dose-related increase of pancreatic islet-cell adenomas in females and of testicular interstitial cell adenomas in males (highest incidence in the low dose group). In mice, no leuprolide acetate-induced tumors or pituitary abnormalities were observed at a dose as high as 60 mg/kg for two years. Patients have been treated with leuprolide acetate for up to three years with doses as high as 10 mg/day and for two years with doses as high as 20 mg/day without demonstrable pituitary abnormalities.

Genotoxicity studies were conducted with leuprolide acetate using bacterial and mammalian systems. These studies provided no evidence of mutagenic effects or chromosomal aberrations.

Leuprolide may reduce male and female fertility. Administration of leuprolide acetate to male and female rats at dose of 0.024, 0.24, and 2.4 mg/kg as monthly depot formulation for up to 3 months (approximately as low as 1/30 of the human dose based on body surface area using an estimated daily dose in animals and humans) caused atrophy of the reproductive organs, and suppression of reproductive function. These changes were reversible upon cessation of treatment.

14 CLINICAL STUDIES

14.1 LUPRON DEPOT 7.5 mg for 1-Month Administration

In an open-label, non-comparative, multicenter clinical study of LUPRON DEPOT 7.5 mg for 1-month administration, 56 patients with stage D_2 prostatic adenocarcinoma and no prior systemic treatment were enrolled. The objectives were to determine if a 7.5 mg depot formulation of leuprolide injected once every 4 weeks would reduce and maintain serum testosterone to castrate range (≤50 ng/dL), to evaluate objective clinical response, and to assess the safety of the formulation. During the initial 24 weeks, serum testosterone was measured weekly, biweekly, or every four weeks and objective tumor response assessments were performed at Weeks 12 and 24. Once the patient completed the initial 24-week treatment phase, treatment continued at the investigator's discretion. Data from the initial 24-week treatment phase are summarized in this section.

In the majority of patients, serum testosterone increased by 50% or more above baseline during the first week of treatment. Serum testosterone suppressed to the castrate range within 30 days of the initial depot injection in 94% (51/54) of patients for whom testosterone suppression was achieved (2 patients withdrew prior to onset of suppression) and within 66 days in all 54 patients. Mean serum testosterone suppressed to castrate level by Week 3. The median dosing interval between injections was 28 days. One escape from suppression (2 consecutive testosterone values greater than 50 ng/dL after achieving castrate level) was noted at Week 18, associated with a substantial dosing delay. In this patient, serum testosterone returned to the castrate range at the next monthly measurement. Serum testosterone was minimally above the castrate range on a single occasion for 4 other patients. No clinical significance was attributed to these rises in testosterone.

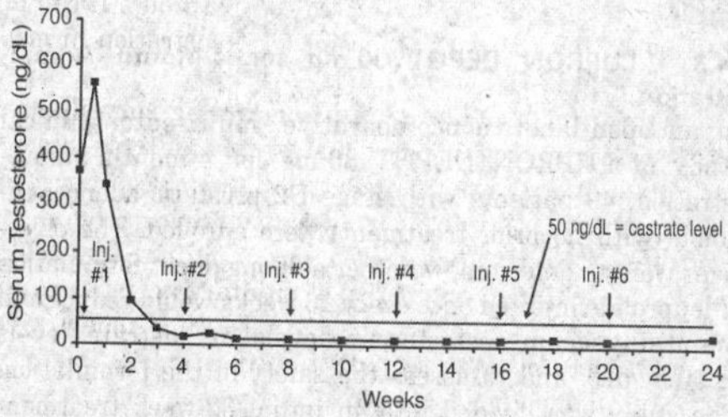

Figure 8. LUPRON DEPOT 7.5 mg for 1-Month Administration Mean Serum Testosterone Concentrations

Secondary efficacy endpoints evaluated included objective tumor response, assessed by clinical evaluations of tumor burden (complete response, partial response, objectively stable, and progression), as well as changes in local disease status, assessed by digital rectal examination, and changes in prostatic acid phosphatase (PAP). These evaluations were performed at Weeks 12 and 24. The objective tumor response analysis showed a "no progression" (ie. complete or partial response, or stable disease) in 77% (40/52) of patients at Week 12, and in 84% (42/50) of patients at Week 24. Local disease improved or remained stable in all (42) patients evaluated at Week 12 and in 98% (41/42) of patients elevated at Week 24. PAP normalized or decreased at Week 12 and/or 24 in the majority of patients with elevated baseline PAP.

Periodic monitoring of serum testosterone and PSA levels is recommended, especially if the anticipated clinical or biochemical response to treatment has not been achieved. It should be noted that results of testosterone determinations are dependent on assay methodology. It is advisable to be aware of the type and precision of the assay methodology to make appropriate clinical and therapeutic decisions.

14.2 LUPRON DEPOT 22.5 mg for 3-Month Administration

In clinical studies, serum testosterone was suppressed to castrate within 30 days in 87 of 92 (95%) patients and within an additional two weeks in three patients. Two patients did not suppress for 15 and 28 weeks, respectively. Suppression was maintained in all of these patients with the exception of transient minimal testosterone elevations in one of them, and in another an increase in serum testosterone to above the castrate range was recorded during the 12 hour observation period after a subsequent injection. This represents stimulation of gonadotropin secretion.

[See Figure 9 on top of next page]

An 85% rate of "no progression" was achieved during the initial 24 weeks of treatment. A decrease from baseline in serum PSA of ≥90% was reported in 71% of the patients and a change to within the normal range (≤3.99 ng/mL) in 63% of the patients.

Periodic monitoring of serum testosterone and PSA levels is recommended, especially if the anticipated clinical or biochemical response to treatment has not been achieved. It should be noted that results of testosterone determinations are dependent on assay methodology. It is advisable to be aware of the type and precision of the assay methodology to make appropriate clinical and therapeutic decisions.

Continued on next page

Information on the AbbVie, Inc. products listed on these pages is from the prescribing information in use as of July 31, 2016. For more information, please visit rxabbvie.com or call 1-800-633-9110.

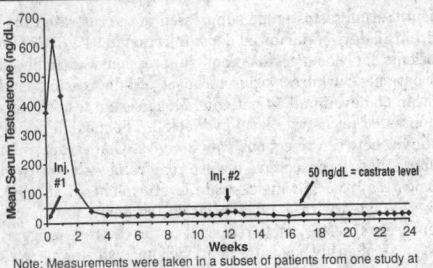

Note: Measurements were taken in a subset of patients from one study at Weeks 10.5, 11.5, 12.5, 22.5 and 23.5

Figure 9. LUPRON DEPOT 22.5 mg for 3-Month Administration Mean Serum Testosterone Concentrations

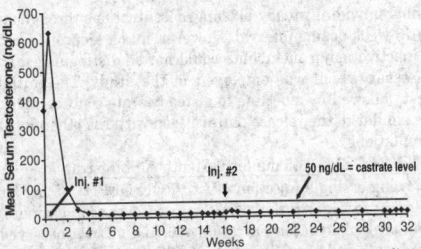

Note: Measurements were taken in a subset of patients from one study at Weeks 14.5, 15.5, 16.5, 30.5, 31 and 31.5

Figure 10. LUPRON DEPOT 30 mg for 4-Month Administration Mean Serum Testosterone Concentrations

14.3   LUPRON DEPOT 30 mg for 4-Month Administration

In an open-label, noncomparative, multicenter clinical study of LUPRON DEPOT 30 mg for 4-month administration, 49 patients with stage D2 prostatic adenocarcinoma (with no prior treatment) were enrolled. The objectives were to determine whether a 30 mg depot formulation of leuprolide injected once every 16 weeks would reduce and maintain serum testosterone levels at castrate levels (≤ 50 ng/dL), and to assess the safety of the formulation. The study was divided into an initial 32-week treatment phase and a long-term treatment phase. Serum testosterone levels were determined biweekly or weekly during the first 32 weeks of treatment. Once the patient completed the initial 32-week treatment period, treatment continued at the investigator's discretion with serum testosterone levels being done every 4 months prior to the injection.

In the majority of patients, testosterone levels increased 50% or more above the baseline during the first week of treatment. Mean serum testosterone subsequently suppressed to castrate levels within 30 days of the first injection in 94% of patients and within 43 days in all 49 patients during the initial 32-week treatment period. The median dosing interval between injections was 112 days. One escape from suppression (two consecutive testosterone values greater than 50 ng/dL after castrate levels achieved) was noted at Week 16. In this patient, serum testosterone increased to above the castrate range following the second depot injection (Week 16) but returned to the castrate level by Week 18. No adverse reactions were associated with this rise in serum testosterone. A second patient had a rise in testosterone at Week 17, then returned to the castrate level by Week 18 and remained there through Week 32. In the long-term treatment phase two patients experienced testosterone elevations, both at Week 48. Testosterone for one patient returned to the castrate range at Week 52, and one patient discontinued the study at Week 48 due to disease progression.

Secondary efficacy endpoints evaluated in the study were the objective tumor response as assessed by clinical evaluations of tumor burden (complete response, partial response, objectively stable and progression) and evaluations of changes in prostatic involvement and prostate-specific antigen (PSA). These evaluations were performed at Weeks 16 and 32 of the treatment phase. The long-term treatment phase monitored PSA at each visit (every 16 weeks). The objective tumor response analysis showed "no progression" (i.e. complete or partial response, or stable disease) in 86% (37/43) of patients at Week 16, and in 77% (37/48) of patients at Week 32. Local disease improved or remained stable in all patients evaluated at Week 16 and/or 32. For patients with elevated baseline PSA, 50% (23/46) had a normal PSA (less than 4.0 ng/mL) at Week 16, and 51% (19/37) had a normal PSA at Week 32.

Periodic monitoring of serum testosterone and PSA levels is recommended, especially if the anticipated clinical or biochemical response to treatment has not been achieved. It should be noted that results of testosterone determinations are dependent on assay methodology. It is advisable to be aware of the type and precision of the assay methodology to make appropriate clinical and therapeutic decisions.

Using historical comparisons, the safety and efficacy of LUPRON DEPOT 30 mg for 4-month administration appear similar to the other LUPRON DEPOT formulations. [See Figure 10 below]

14.4   LUPRON DEPOT 45 mg for 6-Month Administration

An open-label, non-comparative, multicenter clinical study of LUPRON DEPOT 45 mg for 6-month administration en-

rolled 151 patients with prostate cancer. The study drug was administered as two intramuscular injections of LUPRON DEPOT 45 mg at 24 week intervals (139/151 received 2 injections), and patients were followed for a total of 48 weeks.

Among 148 patients who had testosterone value at Week 4, serum testosterone was suppressed to castrate levels (< 50 ng/dL) from Week 4 through Week 48 in an estimated 93.4% (two-sided 95% CI: 89.2%, 97.6%) of patients. One patient failed to achieve testosterone suppression by Week 4, and eight patients had escapes from suppression (any testosterone value > 50 ng/dL after castrate levels were achieved). Mean testosterone levels increased to 608 ng/dL from a baseline of 435 ng/dL during the first week of treatment. By Week 4, the mean testosterone concentration had decreased to below castrate levels (16 ng/dL).

Periodic monitoring of serum testosterone levels is recommended, especially if the anticipated clinical or biochemical response to treatment has not been achieved. Testosterone determinations are dependent on assay methodology and it is advisable to be aware of the type and precision of the assay methodology to make appropriate clinical and therapeutic decisions.

Figure 11 below shows the mean testosterone concentration at various time points.

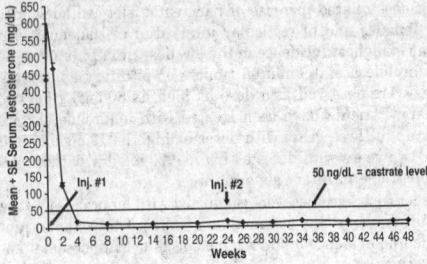

Figure 11. LUPRON DEPOT 45 mg for 6-Month Administration Serum Testosterone Concentrations (Mean + SE)

16   HOW SUPPLIED/STORAGE AND HANDLING

Each LUPRON DEPOT 7.5 mg for 1-month administration kit (NDC 0074-3642-03), 22.5 mg for 3-month administration kit (NDC 0074-3346-03), 30 mg for 4-month administration kit (NDC 0074-3683-03), 45 mg for 6-month administration kit (NDC 0074-3473-03) contains:

• one prefilled dual-chamber syringe containing needle with LuproLoc® safety device
• one plunger
• two alcohol swabs
• a complete prescribing information enclosure

The prefilled dual-chamber syringe of LUPRON DEPOT 7.5 mg for 1-month administration contains sterile lyophilized microspheres of leuprolide acetate incorporated in a biodegradable lactic acid/glycolic acid copolymer.

The prefilled dual-chamber syringe of LUPRON DEPOT 22.5 mg for 3-month administration, 30 mg for 4-month administration, 45 mg for 6-month administration contains sterile lyophilized microspheres of leuprolide acetate incorporated in a biodegradable lactic acid copolymer.

When mixed with 1 mL of accompanying diluent, LUPRON DEPOT 7.5 mg for 1-month administration is administered as a single monthly intramuscular injection.

When mixed with 1.5 mL of accompanying diluent, LUPRON DEPOT 22.5 mg for 3-month administration is administered as a single intramuscular injection EVERY **12 WEEKS**.

When mixed with 1.5 mL of accompanying diluent, LUPRON DEPOT 30 mg for 4-month administration is administered as a single intramuscular injection EVERY **16 WEEKS**.

When mixed with 1.5 mL of accompanying diluent, LUPRON DEPOT 45 mg for 6-month administration is administered as a single intramuscular injection EVERY **24 WEEKS**.

Store at 25°C (77°F); excursions permitted to 15°C–30°C (59°F–86°F) [See USP Controlled Room Temperature].

17   PATIENT COUNSELING INFORMATION

Information for Patients

Patients should be informed that:

• If they experience an allergic reaction to other drugs like LUPRON DEPOT, they should not use this drug.
• LUPRON DEPOT is usually continued, often with additional medication, after the development of metastatic castration-resistant prostate cancer.
• The most common side effects associated with LUPRON DEPOT are hot flashes, pain (especially joint pain and back pain), injection site pain and fatigue.
• LUPRON DEPOT may cause impotence.
• The increase in testosterone that occurs during the first weeks of therapy can cause an increase in urinary symptoms or pain.
• If they have metastatic cancer to the spine or urinary tract, they need close medical attention during the first weeks of therapy.
• They should notify their doctor if they develop new or worsened symptoms after beginning LUPRON DEPOT treatment.

Manufactured for
AbbVie Inc.
North Chicago, IL 60064
by Takeda Pharmaceutical Company Limited
Osaka, Japan 540-8645
™–Trademark
®–Registered Trademark
(No. 3346) (No. 3683) (No. 3473) (No. 3642)
03-B364-R7 June, 2016
©2016 AbbVie Inc.
Shown in Product Identification Guide, page 506

LUPRON DEPOT-PED®   ℞
(leuprolide acetate for depot suspension)
7.5 mg, 11.25 mg, 15 mg, and 30 mg

HIGHLIGHTS OF PRESCRIBING INFORMATION

These highlights do not include all the information needed to use LUPRON DEPOT-PED safely and effectively. See full prescribing information for LUPRON DEPOT-PED.

LUPRON DEPOT-PED (leuprolide acetate for depot suspension) Injection, Powder, Lyophilized, For Suspension

Initial U.S. Approval: 1993

————INDICATIONS AND USAGE————

LUPRON DEPOT-PED is a gonadotropin releasing hormone (GnRH) agonist indicated in the treatment of children with central precocious puberty. (1)

————DOSAGE AND ADMINISTRATION————

• LUPRON DEPOT-PED is administered as a single intramuscular injection. The starting dose 7.5 mg, 11.25 mg, or 15 mg for 1-month administration is based on the child's weight. (2)
• LUPRON DEPOT-PED is administered as a single intramuscular injection. The doses are either 11.25 mg or 30 mg for 3-month administration.(2)
• Hormonal and clinical parameters should be monitored during treatment to ensure adequate suppression. (2)
• The injection site should be varied periodically. (2)

————DOSAGE FORMS AND STRENGTHS————

LUPRON DEPOT-PED 7.5 mg, 11.25 mg, or 15 mg for 1-month administration and LUPRON DEPOT-PED 11.25 mg or 30 mg for 3-month administration are provided in a prefilled dual chamber syringe for intramuscular injection. (3)

————CONTRAINDICATIONS————

• Hypersensitivity reactions. (4)
• Pregnancy. (4,8.1)

————WARNINGS AND PRECAUTIONS————

• An increase in clinical signs and symptoms of puberty may be observed during the first 2-4 weeks of therapy since gonadotropins and sex steroids rise above baseline because of the initial stimulatory effect of the drug before being suppressed. (5.1)

- Convulsions have been observed in patients with or without a history of seizures, epilepsy, cerebrovascular disorders, central nervous system anomalies or tumors, and in patients on concomitant medications that have been associated with convulsions. (5.2)

ADVERSE REACTIONS

- Adverse events related to suppression of endogenous sex steroid secretion may occur with LUPRON DEPOT-PED 7.5 mg, 11.25 mg, or 15 mg for 1-month administration. (6.1, 6.3)
- In clinical studies for LUPRON DEPOT-PED 11.25 mg or 30 mg for 3-month administration, the most frequent (≥ 2 patients) adverse reactions were: injection site pain, weight increased, headache, mood altered, and injection site swelling. (6.2)

To report SUSPECTED ADVERSE REACTIONS, contact AbbVie Inc. at 1-800-633-9110 or FDA at 1-800-FDA-1088 or www.fda.gov/medwatch

USE IN SPECIFIC POPULATIONS

- The use of LUPRON DEPOT-PED in children under 2 years is not recommended. (8.4)

See 17 for PATIENT COUNSELING INFORMATION.

Revised: 4/2012

FULL PRESCRIBING INFORMATION: CONTENTS*

* Sections or subsections omitted from the full prescribing information are not listed.

FULL PRESCRIBING INFORMATION

1   INDICATIONS AND USAGE

LUPRON DEPOT-PED is indicated in the treatment of children with central precocious puberty (CPP).

CPP is defined as early onset of secondary sexual characteristics (generally earlier than 8 years of age in girls and 9 years of age in boys) associated with pubertal pituitary gonadotropin activation. It may show a significantly advanced bone age that can result in diminished adult height.

Prior to initiation of treatment a clinical diagnosis of CPP should be confirmed by measurement of blood concentra-

---

tions of luteinizing hormone (LH) (basal or stimulated with a GnRH analog), sex steroids, and assessment of bone age versus chronological age. Baseline evaluations should include height and weight measurements, diagnostic imaging of the brain (to rule out intracranial tumor), pelvic/testicular/adrenal ultrasound (to rule out steroid secreting tumors), human chorionic gonadotropin levels (to rule out a chorionic gonadotropin secreting tumor), and adrenal steroid measurements to exclude congenital adrenal hyperplasia.

2   DOSAGE AND ADMINISTRATION

2.1   Dose and Principles of Dosing 7.5 mg, 11.25 mg, or 15 mg for 1-month administration

LUPRON DEPOT-PED must be administered under the supervision of a physician.

LUPRON DEPOT-PED is administered as a single intramuscular injection once a month. The starting dose will be dictated by the child's weight, as indicated in the table below.

Table 1. Dosing Recommendations Based on Body Weight for LUPRON DEPOT-PED 1-month Formulations

Body Weight	Recommended Dose
≤ 25 kg	7.5 mg
> 25-37.5 kg	11.25 mg
> 37.5 kg	15 mg

The dose of LUPRON DEPOT-PED must be individualized for each child. If adequate hormonal and clinical suppression is not achieved with the starting dose, it should be increased to the next available higher dose (e.g. 11.25 mg or 15 mg at the next monthly injection). Similarly, the dose may be adjusted with changes in body weight. The injection site should be varied periodically.

The goal of therapy is to suppress pituitary gonadotropins and peripheral sex steroids, and to arrest progression of secondary sexual characteristics. Hormonal and clinical parameters should be monitored after 1–2 months of initiating therapy and with each dose change to ensure adequate pituitary gonadotropin suppression. Once a dose that results in adequate hormonal suppression is found, it can often be maintained for the duration of therapy in most children. It is recommended, however, that adequate hormonal suppression be verified in such patients as weight can increase significantly while on therapy.

Each LUPRON DEPOT-PED strength and formulation has different release characteristics. Do not use partial syringes or a combination of syringes to achieve a particular dose.

LUPRON DEPOT-PED should be discontinued at the appropriate age of onset of puberty at the discretion of the physician.

For optimal performance of the prefilled dual chamber syringe (PDS), read and follow the instructions in Section 2.3.

2.2   Dose and Principles of Dosing 11.25 mg or 30 mg for 3-month administration

LUPRON DEPOT-PED 11.25 mg or 30 mg for 3-month administration must be administered under the supervision of a physician.

LUPRON DEPOT-PED 11.25 mg or 30 mg for 3-month administration should be administered once every three months (12 weeks) as a single intramuscular injection. Regardless of the dose chosen, the goal of therapy is to suppress pituitary gonadotropins and peripheral sex steroids, and to arrest progression of secondary sexual characteristics. Hormonal and clinical parameters should be monitored during treatment, for instance at month 2-3, month 6 and further as judged clinically appropriate, to ensure adequate suppression. In case of inadequate suppression, other available GnRH agonists indicated for the treatment of CPP should be considered.

Each LUPRON DEPOT-PED 11.25 mg or 30 mg for 3-month administration strength and formulation has different release characteristics. Do not use partial syringes or a combination of syringes to achieve a particular dose.

LUPRON DEPOT-PED 11.25 mg or 30 mg for 3-month administration treatment should be discontinued at the appropriate age of onset of puberty at the discretion of the physician.

For optimal performance of the prefilled dual chamber syringe (PDS), read and follow the instructions in Section 2.3.

2.3   Reconstitution and Administration Instructions

- The lyophilized microspheres are to be reconstituted and administered as a single intramuscular injection.
- Since LUPRON DEPOT-PED does not contain a preservative, the suspension should be injected immediately or discarded if not used within two hours.
- As with other drugs administered by injection, the injection site should be varied periodically.

1. The LUPRON DEPOT-PED powder should be visually inspected and the syringe should NOT BE USED if clumping or caking is evident. A thin layer of powder on the wall of the syringe is considered normal prior to mixing with the diluent. The diluent should appear clear.
2. To prepare for injection, screw the white plunger into the end stopper until the stopper begins to turn.

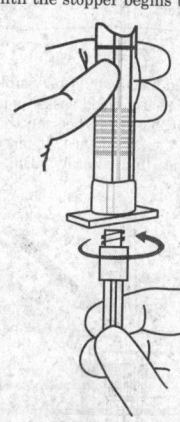

3. Hold the syringe UPRIGHT. Release the diluent by SLOWLY PUSHING (6 to 8 seconds) the plunger until the first stopper is <u>at the blue line</u> in the middle of the barrel.

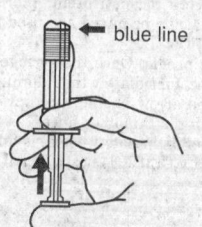

← blue line

4. Keep the syringe UPRIGHT. Mix the microspheres (powder) thoroughly by gently shaking the syringe until the powder forms a uniform suspension. The suspension will appear milky. If the powder adheres to the stopper or caking/clumping is present, tap the syringe with your finger to disperse. DO NOT USE if any of the powder has not gone into suspension.

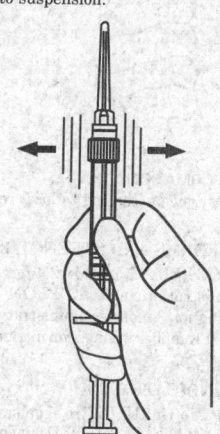

Continued on next page

5. Hold the syringe UPRIGHT. With the opposite hand pull the needle cap upward without twisting.
6. Keep the syringe UPRIGHT. Advance the plunger to expel the air from the syringe.
   Now the syringe is ready for injection.
7. After cleaning the injection site with an alcohol swab, the intramuscular injection should be performed by inserting the needle at a 90 degree angle into the gluteal area, anterior thigh, or shoulder; injection sites should be alternated.

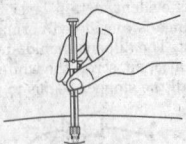

NOTE: Aspirated blood would be visible just below the luer lock connection if a blood vessel is accidentally penetrated. If present, blood can be seen through the transparent LuproLoc® safety device. If blood is present remove the needle immediately. Do not inject the medication.

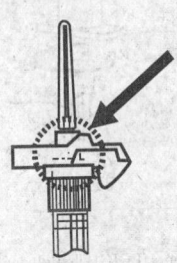

8. Inject the entire contents of the syringe intramuscularly at the time of reconstitution. The suspension settles very quickly following reconstitution; therefore, LUPRON DEPOT-PED should be mixed and used immediately.

AFTER INJECTION

9. Withdraw the needle. Once the syringe has been withdrawn, activate immediately the LuproLoc® safety device by pushing the arrow on the lock upward towards the needle tip with the thumb or finger, as illustrated, until the needle cover of the safety device is fully extended over the needle and a CLICK is heard or felt.

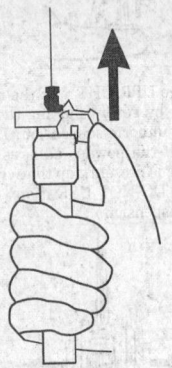

ADDITIONAL INFORMATION
• Dispose of the syringe according to local regulations/procedures.

3 DOSAGE FORMS AND STRENGTHS

LUPRON DEPOT-PED 7.5 mg, 11.25 mg, or 15 mg for 1-month administration and LUPRON DEPOT-PED 11.25 mg or 30 mg for 3-month administration is provided in a prefilled dual chamber syringe for intramuscular injection.

4 CONTRAINDICATIONS

• Hypersensitivity to GnRH, GnRH agonists or any of the excipients in LUPRON DEPOT-PED. Reports of anaphylactic reactions to GnRH agonists have been reported in the medical literature.
• All formulations of LUPRON DEPOT may cause fetal harm if administered to a pregnant woman. When LUPRON DEPOT was administered subcutaneously to rabbits it produced a dose related increase in major fetal abnormalities, and fetal mortality. The possibility exists that spontaneous abortion may occur if the drug is administered during pregnancy. LUPRON DEPOT-PED is con-

traindicated in women who are or may become pregnant. If this drug is inadvertently used during pregnancy, or if the patient becomes pregnant while taking this drug, the patient should be apprised of the potential hazard to the fetus.

5 WARNINGS AND PRECAUTIONS

5.1 Initial Rise of Gonadotropins and Sex Steroid Levels

During the early phase of therapy, gonadotropins and sex steroids rise above baseline because of the initial stimulatory effect of the drug. Therefore, an increase in clinical signs and symptoms of puberty may be observed *[see Clinical Pharmacology (12.3)]*.

5.2 Convulsions

Postmarketing reports of convulsions have been observed in patients on leuprolide acetate therapy. These included patients with a history of seizures, epilepsy, cerebrovascular disorders, central nervous system anomalies or tumors, and patients on concomitant medications that have been associated with convulsions such as bupropion and SSRIs. Convulsions have also been reported in patients in the absence of any of the conditions mentioned above.

5.3 Monitoring and Laboratory Tests

Response to LUPRON DEPOT-PED 7.5 mg, 11.25 mg, or 15 mg for 1-month administration should be monitored with a GnRHa stimulation test, basal LH or serum concentration of sex steroid levels beginning 1-2 months following initiation of therapy, with changing doses, or potentially during therapy in order to confirm maintenance of efficacy. Measurement of bone age for advancement should be done every 6-12 months.

Response to LUPRON DEPOT-PED 11.25 mg or 30 mg for 3-month administration should be monitored with a GnRHa stimulation test, basal LH or serum concentration of sex steroid levels at months 2-3, month 6 and further as judged clinically appropriate, to ensure adequate suppression. Additionally, height (for calculation of growth rate) and bone age should be assessed every 6-12 months.

Once a therapeutic dose has been established, gonadotropin and sex steroid levels will decline to prepubertal levels. Gonadotropins and/or sex steroids may increase or rise above prepubertal levels if the dose is inadequate. Noncompliance with drug regimen or inadequate dosing may result in inadequate control of the pubertal process with gonadotropins and/or sex steroids increasing above prepubertal levels *[see Clinical Studies (14) and Adverse Reactions (6)]*.

6 ADVERSE REACTIONS

The most common adverse reactions with GnRH agonists including LUPRON DEPOT-PED 7.5 mg, 11.25 mg, or 15 mg for 1-month administration and LUPRON DEPOT-PED 11.25 mg or 30 mg for 3-month administration are injection site reactions/pain including abscess, general pain, headache, emotional lability and hot flushes/sweating. During the early phase of therapy, gonadotropins and sex steroids rise above baseline because of the initial stimulatory effect of the drug (hormonal flare effect). Therefore, an increase in clinical signs and symptoms of puberty may be observed *[see Warnings and Precautions (5.1)]*.

6.1 LUPRON DEPOT-PED 7.5 mg, 11.25 mg, or 15 mg for 1-month administration - Clinical Trials Experience

Because clinical studies are conducted under widely varying conditions, adverse reaction rates observed in the clinical studies of a drug cannot be directly compared to rates in the clinical studies of another drug and may not reflect the rates observed in practice.

In two studies of children with central precocious puberty, in 2% or more of the patients receiving the drug, the following adverse reactions were reported to have a possible or probable relationship to drug as ascribed by the treating physician. Reactions which are not considered drug-related are excluded.

Table 2. Percentage of Patients with Treatment-Emergent Adverse Reactions Occurring in ≥ 2% of Pediatric Patients Receiving LUPRON DEPOT-PED 1-month

	Number of Patients (N = 421)	
	N	(%)
Body as a Whole		
Injection Site Reactions Including Abscess*	37	(9)
General Pain	12	(3)
Headache	11	(3)
Cardiovascular System		
Vasodilation	9	(2)
Integumentary System (Skin and Appendages)		
Acne/Seborrhea	13	(3)
Rash Including Erythema Multiforme	12	(3)
Nervous System		
Emotional Lability	19	(5)
Urogenital System		
Vaginitis/Vaginal Bleeding/ Vaginal Discharge	13	(3)

* Most events were mild or moderate in severity.

Less Common Adverse Reactions
The following treatment-emergent adverse reactions were reported in less than 2% of the patients and are listed below by body system.
Body as a Whole – aggravation of preexisting tumor and decreased vision, allergic reaction, body odor, fever, flu syndrome, hypertrophy, infection; *Cardiovascular System* – bradycardia, hypertension, peripheral vascular disorder, syncope; *Digestive System* – constipation, dyspepsia, dysphagia, gingivitis, increased appetite, nausea/vomiting; *Endocrine System* – accelerated sexual maturity, feminization, goiter; *Hemic and Lymphatic System* – purpura; *Metabolic and Nutritional Disorders* – growth retarded, peripheral edema, weight gain; *Musculoskeletal System* – arthralgia, joint disorder, myalgia, myopathy; *Nervous System* – depression, hyperkinesia, nervousness, somnolence; *Respiratory System* – asthma, epistaxis, pharyngitis, rhinitis, sinusitis; *Integumentary System (Skin and Appendages)* – alopecia, hair disorder, hirsutism, leukoderma, nail disorder, skin hypertrophy; *Urogenital System* – cervix disorder/neoplasm, dysmenorrhea, gynecomastia/breast disorders, menstrual disorder, urinary incontinence.
Laboratory: The following laboratory events were reported as adverse reactions: antinuclear antibody present and increased sedimentation rate.

6.2 LUPRON DEPOT-PED 11.25 mg or 30 mg for 3-month administration - Clinical Trials Experience

Because clinical studies are conducted under widely varying conditions, adverse reaction rates observed in the clinical studies of a drug cannot be directly compared to rates in the clinical studies of another drug and may not reflect the rates observed in practice.
[See table 3 at top of next page]
Less Common Adverse Reactions
The following treatment-emergent adverse reactions were reported in one patient and are listed below by system organ class:
Gastrointestinal Disorders – abdominal pain, nausea; *General Disorders and Administration Site Conditions* – asthenia, gait disturbance, injection site abscess sterile, injection site hematoma, injection site induration, injection site warmth, irritability; *Metabolic and Nutritional Disorders* – decreased appetite, obesity; *Musculoskeletal and Connective Tissue Disorders* - musculoskeletal pain, pain in extremity; *Nervous System Disorders* – crying, dizziness; *Psychiatric Disorders* – tearfulness; *Respiratory, Thoracic and Mediastinal Disorders* – cough; *Skin and Subcutaneous Tissue Disorders* – hyperhidrosis; *Vascular Disorders* – pallor.

6.3 Postmarketing

The following adverse events have been observed with this or other formulations of leuprolide acetate injection. As leuprolide has multiple indications, and therefore patient populations, some of these adverse events may not be applicable to every patient.
Allergic reactions (anaphylactic, rash, urticaria, and photosensitivity reactions) have also been reported.
Gastrointestinal Disorders: nausea, abdominal pain, vomiting;
General Disorders and Administration Site Conditions: chest pain, injection site reactions including induration and abscess have been reported;

Table 3. Percentage of Patients with Treatment-Emergent Adverse Reactions Occurring in ≥ 2 Pediatric Patients Receiving LUPRON DEPOT-PED 11.25 mg or 30 mg for 3-month administration.

	11.25 mg every 3 Months N=42		30 mg every 3 Months N=42		Overall N = 84	
	N	%	N	%	N	%
Injection site pain	8	(19)	9	(21)	17	(20)
Weight increased	3	(7)	3	(7)	6	(7)
Headache	1	(2)	3	(7)	4	(5)
Mood altered	2	(5)	2	(5)	4	(5)
Injection site swelling	1	(2)	1	(2)	2	(2)

Investigations: decreased WBC, weight increased;
Metabolism and Nutrition Disorders: diabetes mellitus;
Musculoskeletal and Connective Tissue Disorders: tenosynovitis-like symptoms;
Nervous System Disorders: neuropathy peripheral, convulsion, spinal fracture/paralysis;
Skin and Subcutaneous Tissue Disorders: hot flush, flushing, hyperhidrosis;
Reproductive System and Breast Disorders: prostate pain;
Vascular Disorders: hypertension, hypotension.
Pituitary apoplexy: During post-marketing surveillance, rare cases of pituitary apoplexy (a clinical syndrome secondary to infarction of the pituitary gland) have been reported after the administration of gonadotropin-releasing hormone agonists. In a majority of these cases, a pituitary adenoma was diagnosed, with a majority of pituitary apoplexy cases occurring within 2 weeks of the first dose, and some within the first hour. In these cases, pituitary apoplexy has presented as sudden headache, vomiting, visual changes, ophthalmoplegia, altered mental status, and sometimes cardiovascular collapse. Immediate medical attention has been required.
See other LUPRON DEPOT and LUPRON Injection package inserts for other events reported in different patient populations.

7 DRUG INTERACTIONS
No pharmacokinetic-based drug-drug interaction studies have been conducted; however, drug interactions are not expected to occur *[see Clinical Pharmacology (12.3)]*.

7.1 Drug/Laboratory Test Interactions
Administration of LUPRON DEPOT-PED in therapeutic doses results in suppression of the pituitary-gonadal system. Therefore, diagnostic tests of pituitary gonadotropic and gonadal functions conducted during treatment and up to six months after discontinuation of LUPRON DEPOT-PED may be affected. Normal pituitary-gonadal function is usually restored within six months after treatment with LUPRON DEPOT-PED is discontinued.

8 USE IN SPECIFIC POPULATIONS
8.1 Pregnancy
Pregnancy Category X
LUPRON DEPOT-PED is contraindicated in women who are or may become pregnant while receiving the drug *[see Contraindications (4)]*.
Safe use of leuprolide acetate in pregnancy has not been established in clinical studies. Before starting and during treatment with leuprolide acetate, it is advisable to establish whether the patient is pregnant. Leuprolide acetate is not a contraceptive. If contraception is required, a nonhormonal method of contraception should be used.
When LUPRON DEPOT was administered subcutaneously to groups of rabbits as one time dosing on day 6 of pregnancy at test dosages of 0.00024, 0.0024, and 0.024 mg/kg (1/1900 to 1/19 of the human pediatric dose) it produced a dose-related increase in major fetal abnormalities. Similar studies in rats failed to demonstrate an increase in fetal malformations. There was increased fetal mortality and decreased fetal weights with the two higher doses of LUPRON DEPOT in rabbits and with the highest dose in rats. No fetal malformations but increase in fetal resorptions and mortality were observed in rat and rabbit when the daily injection formulation of leuprolide acetate was dosed subcutaneously once daily at lower doses (0.1-1 mcg/kg/day in rabbit; 10 mcg/kg/day in rat) during the period of organogenesis. The effects on fetal mortality are logical consequences of the alterations in hormonal levels brought about

by this drug. Therefore, the possibility exists that spontaneous abortion may occur if the drug is administered during pregnancy.

8.3 Nursing Mothers
It is not known whether leuprolide acetate is excreted in human milk. LUPRON DEPOT-PED should not be used by nursing mothers.

8.4 Pediatric Use
Safety and effectiveness in pediatric patients below the age of 2 years have not been established. The use of LUPRON DEPOT-PED in children under 2 years is not recommended.

8.5 Geriatric Use
LUPRON DEPOT 1-month 7.5 mg and 4-month 30 mg are indicated for the palliative treatment of advanced prostate cancer. For LUPRON DEPOT-PED 11.25 mg or 15 mg for 1-month administration and LUPRON DEPOT-PED 11.25 mg or 30 mg for 3-month administration, no clinical information is available for persons aged 65 and over.

10 OVERDOSAGE
In early clinical trials using leuprolide acetate in adult patients, doses as high as 20 mg/day for up to two years caused no adverse effects differing from those observed with the 1 mg/day dose.
In rats, subcutaneous administration of leuprolide acetate as a single dose 225 times the recommended human pediatric dose, expressed on a per body weight basis, resulted in dyspnea, decreased activity, and local irritation at the injection site. There is no evidence at present that there is a clinical counterpart of this phenomenon.
In cases of overdosage, standard of care monitoring and management principles should be followed.

11 DESCRIPTION
Leuprolide acetate is a synthetic nonapeptide analog of naturally occurring gonadotropin-releasing hormone (GnRH or LH-RH). The analog possesses greater potency than the natural hormone. The chemical name is 5-oxo-L-prolyl-L-histidyl-L-tryptophyl-L-seryl-L-tyrosyl-D-leucyl-L-leucyl-L-arginyl-N-ethyl-L-prolinamide acetate (salt) with the following structural formula:
[See structural formula at top of next page]

LUPRON DEPOT-PED 7.5 mg, 11.25 mg, or 15 mg for 1-month administration
LUPRON DEPOT-PED is available in a prefilled dual-chamber syringe containing sterile lyophilized microspheres which, when mixed with diluent, become a suspension intended as a single intramuscular injection.
The front chamber of LUPRON DEPOT-PED 7.5 mg, 11.25 mg, and 15 mg prefilled dual-chamber syringe contains leuprolide acetate (7.5/11.25/15 mg), purified gelatin (1.3/1.95/2.6 mg), DL-lactic and glycolic acids copolymer (66.2/99.3/132.4 mg), and D-mannitol (13.2/19.8/26.4 mg). The second chamber of diluent contains carboxymethylcellulose sodium (5 mg), D-mannitol (50 mg), polysorbate 80 (1 mg), water for injection, USP, and glacial acetic acid, USP to control pH.

LUPRON DEPOT-PED 11.25 mg or 30 mg for 3-month administration
LUPRON DEPOT-PED 11.25 mg or 30 mg for 3-month administration is available in a prefilled dual-chamber syringe containing sterile lyophilized microspheres which, when mixed with diluent, become a suspension intended as an intramuscular injection to be given **ONCE EVERY THREE MONTHS**.
The front chamber of LUPRON DEPOT-PED 11.25 mg for 3-month administration prefilled dual-chamber syringe contains leuprolide acetate (11.25 mg), polylactic acid (99.3 mg)

and D-mannitol (19.45 mg). The second chamber of diluent contains carboxymethylcellulose sodium (7.5 mg), D-mannitol (75.0 mg), polysorbate 80 (1.5 mg), water for injection, USP, and glacial acetic acid, USP to control pH.
The front chamber of LUPRON DEPOT-PED 30 mg for 3-month administration prefilled dual-chamber syringe contains leuprolide acetate (30 mg), polylactic acid (264.8 mg) and D-mannitol (51.9 mg). The second chamber of diluent contains carboxymethylcellulose sodium (7.5 mg), D-mannitol (75.0 mg), polysorbate 80 (1.5 mg), water for injection, USP, and glacial acetic acid, USP to control pH.

12 CLINICAL PHARMACOLOGY
12.1 Mechanism of Action
Leuprolide acetate, a GnRH agonist, acts as a potent inhibitor of gonadotropin secretion when given continuously and in therapeutic doses. Human studies indicate that following an initial stimulation of gonadotropins, chronic stimulation with leuprolide acetate results in suppression or "downregulation" of these hormones and consequent suppression of ovarian and testicular steroidogenesis. These effects are reversible on discontinuation of drug therapy.
Leuprolide acetate is not active when given orally.

12.3 Pharmacokinetics
Absorption
LUPRON DEPOT-PED 7.5 mg, 11.25 mg, or 15 mg for 1-month administration
Following a single LUPRON DEPOT-PED 7.5 mg for 1-month administration to adult patients, mean peak leuprolide plasma concentration was almost 20 ng/mL at 4 hours and then declined to 0.36 ng/mL at 4 weeks. However, intact leuprolide and an inactive major metabolite could not be distinguished by the assay which was employed in the study. Nondetectable leuprolide plasma concentrations have been observed during chronic LUPRON DEPOT-PED 7.5 mg administration, but testosterone levels appear to be maintained at castrate levels.
In a study of 55 children with central precocious puberty, doses of 7.5 mg, 11.25 mg and 15.0 mg of LUPRON DEPOT-PED were given every 4 weeks and in a subset of 22 children, trough leuprolide plasma levels were determined according to weight categories as summarized below:

Patient Weight Range (kg)	Group Weight Average (kg)	Dose (mg)	Trough Plasma Leuprolide Level Mean ±SD (ng/mL)*
20.2 - 27.0	22.7	7.5	0.77±0.033
28.4 - 36.8	32.5	11.25	1.25±1.06
39.3 - 57.5	44.2	15.0	1.59±0.65

* Group average values determined at Week 4 immediately prior to leuprolide injection. Drug levels at 12 and 24 weeks were similar to respective 4 week levels.

LUPRON DEPOT-PED 11.25 mg or 30 mg for 3-month administration
Following a single LUPRON DEPOT-PED 11.25 mg or 30 mg for 3-month administration to children with CPP, leuprolide concentrations increased with increasing dose with mean peak leuprolide plasma concentration of 19.1 and 52.5 ng/mL at 1 hour for the 11.25 and 30 mg dose levels, respectively. The concentrations then declined to 0.08 and 0.25 ng/mL at 2 weeks after dosing for the 11.25 and 30 mg dose levels. Mean leuprolide plasma concentration remained constant from month 1 to month 3 for both 11.25 and 30 mg doses. The mean leuprolide concentrations 3 months after the first and second injections were similar indicating no accumulation of leuprolide from repeated administration.
Distribution
The mean steady-state volume of distribution of leuprolide following intravenous bolus administration to healthy male volunteers was 27 L. *In vitro* binding to human plasma proteins ranged from 43% to 49%.

Continued on next page

Information on the AbbVie, Inc. products listed on these pages is from the prescribing information in use as of July 31, 2016. For more information, please visit rxabbvie.com or call 1-800-633-9110.

Metabolism

In healthy male volunteers, a 1 mg bolus of leuprolide administered intravenously revealed that the mean systemic clearance was 7.6 L/h, with a terminal elimination half-life of approximately 3 hours based on a two compartment model.

In rats and dogs, administration of ^{14}C-labeled leuprolide was shown to be metabolized to smaller inactive peptides; a pentapeptide (Metabolite I), tripeptides (Metabolites II and III) and a dipeptide (Metabolite IV). These fragments may be further catabolized.

The major metabolite (M-I) plasma concentrations measured in 5 prostate cancer patients reached maximum concentration 2 to 6 hours after dosing and were approximately 6% of the peak parent drug concentration. One week after dosing, mean plasma M-I concentrations were approximately 20% of mean leuprolide concentrations.

Excretion

Following administration of LUPRON DEPOT 3.75 mg to 3 patients, less than 5% of the dose was recovered as parent and M-I metabolite in the urine.

Specific Populations

The pharmacokinetics of LUPRON DEPOT-PED has not been determined in patients with hepatic or renal impairment.

Drug-Drug Interactions

No pharmacokinetic-based drug-drug interaction studies have been conducted with LUPRON DEPOT-PED. However, because leuprolide acetate is a peptide that is primarily degraded by peptidase and not by cytochrome P-450 enzymes as noted in specific studies, and the drug is only about 46% bound to plasma proteins, drug interactions are not expected to occur.

13 NONCLINICAL TOXICOLOGY

13.1 Carcinogenesis, Mutagenesis, Impairment of Fertility

A two-year carcinogenicity study was conducted in rats and mice. In rats, a dose-related increase of benign pituitary hyperplasia and benign pituitary adenomas was noted at 24 months when the drug was administered subcutaneously at high daily doses (0.6 to 4 mg/kg). There was a significant but not dose-related increase of pancreatic islet-cell adenomas in females and of testicular interstitial cell adenomas in males (highest incidence in the low dose group). In mice, no leuprolide acetate-induced tumors or pituitary abnormalities were observed at a dose as high as 60 mg/kg for two years. Adult patients have been treated with leuprolide acetate for up to three years with doses as high as 10 mg/day and for two years with doses as high as 20 mg/day without demonstrable pituitary abnormalities. Following subcutaneous administration of LUPRON DEPOT to male and female rats before mating there was atrophy of the reproductive organs and suppression of reproductive performance.

Following a study with leuprolide acetate, immature male rats demonstrated tubular degeneration in the testes even after a recovery period. In spite of the failure to recover histologically, the treated males proved to be as fertile as the controls. Also, no histologic changes were observed in the female rats following the same protocol. In both sexes, the offspring of the treated animals appeared normal. The effect of the treatment of the parents on the reproductive performance of the F1 generation has been evaluated using LUPRON DEPOT formulation to groups of rats as one-time subcutaneous dose of 0.024 mg/kg (1/19 of the pediatric dose) on Day 15 of gestation or dosing on parturition day at doses up to 8 mg/kg (18 fold of the pediatric dose). There was no effect on growth, morphological development and reproductive performance of F1 generation.

14 CLINICAL STUDIES

14.1 LUPRON DEPOT-PED 7.5 mg, 11.25 mg, or 15 mg for 1-month administration

In children with central precocious puberty (CPP), therapeutic doses of LUPRON DEPOT-PED reduce stimulated and basal gonadotropins to prepubertal levels. Testosterone and estradiol are also reduced to prepubertal levels in males and females respectively. Reduction of gonadotropins and sex steroids allow a return to age-appropriate physical and psychological growth and development. The following effects have been noted with the chronic administration of leuprolide: cessation of menses (in girls), normalization and stabilization of linear growth and bone age advancement, stabilization of clinical signs and symptoms of puberty.

55 CPP subjects (49 females and 6 males, naïve to previous GnRHa treatment), were treated with LUPRON

DEPOT-PED 1-month formulations until age appropriate for entry into puberty (see treatment period data below) and a subset of 40 subjects were then followed post-treatment (see follow-up period data below).

Treatment Period Data:

During the treatment period, LUPRON DEPOT-PED suppressed gonadotropins and sex steroids to prepubertal levels. Suppression of peak stimulated LH concentrations to < 1.75 mIU/mL was achieved in 96% of subjects by month 1. Five subjects required increased doses of study drug to achieve or retain LH suppression. The number and percentage of subjects with suppression of peak stimulated LH < 1.75 mIU/mL and mean ± SD peak stimulated LH over time is shown in Table 4. The mean ± SD age at the start of treatment was 7 ± 2 years and the duration of treatment was 4 ± 2 years. Six months after the treatment period was finished, the mean peak stimulated LH was 20.6 ± SD 13.7 mIU/mL (n=30).

Table 4. The number and percentage of patients with peak stimulated LH < 1.75 mIU/mL and Mean (SD) peak LH at each clinic visit

Weeks on Study	n with peak stimulated LH < 1.75 mIU/mL/N with a LH measurement for that week		Mean (SD) peak LH
	n/N	%	
Baseline	0/55	0%	35.0 (21.32)
Week 4	53/55	96.4%	0.8 (0.57)
Week 12	48/54	88.9%	1.1 (1.77)
Week 24	48/53	90.6%	0.8 (0.79)
Week 36	51/54	94.4%	0.6 (0.43)
Week 48	51/54	94.4%	0.6 (0.47)
Week 72	52/52	100%	0.5 (0.30)
Week 96	46/46	100%	0.4 (0.33)
Week 120	40/40	100%	0.4 (0.27)
Week 144	36/36	100%	0.4 (0.24)
Week 168	27/28	96.4%	1.2 (4.58)
Week 216	18/19	94.7%	0.5 (0.90)
Week 240	16/17	94.1%	0.4 (0.62)
Week 264	14/15	95.3%	0.4 (0.41)
Week 288	11/11	100%	0.3 (0.22)
Week 312	9/9	100%	0.4 (0.20)
Week 336	6/6	100%	0.3 (0.10)
Week 360	6/6	100%	0.3 (0.13)
Week 384	5/5	100%	0.2 (0.10)
Week 408	3/3	100%	0.2 (0.09)
Week 432	2/2	100%	0.3 (0.04)
Week 456	2/2	100%	0.2 (0.04)
Week 480	1/1	100%	0.2 (NA)
Week 504	1/1	100%	0.2 (NA)

Suppression (defined as regression or no change) of the clinical/physical signs of puberty was achieved in most patients. In females, suppression of breast development ranged from 66.7 to 90.6% of subjects during the first 5 years of treatment. The mean stimulated estradiol was 15.1 pg/mL at baseline, decreased to the lower level of detection (5.0 pg/mL) by Week 4 and was maintained there during the first 5 years of treatment. In males, suppression of genitalia development ranged from 60% to 100% of subjects during the first 5 years of treatment. The mean stimulated testosterone was 347.7 ng/dL at baseline and was maintained at levels no greater than 25.3 ng/dL during the first 5 years of treatment.

A "flare effect" of transient bleeding or spotting during the first 4 weeks of treatment was observed in 19.4% (7/36) females who had not reached menarche at baseline. After the first 4 weeks and for the remainder of the treatment period, no subject reported menstrual-like bleeding, and only rare spotting was noted.

In many subjects, growth rate decreased on treatment, as did bone age: chronological age ratio. Through year 5, the mean growth rate ranged between 3.4 and 5.6 cm/yr. The mean ratio of bone age to chronological age decreased from 1.5 at baseline to 1.1 by end of treatment. The mean height standard deviation score changed from 1.6 at baseline to 0.7 at the end of the treatment phase.

Follow-up Period Data:

35 females and 5 males participated in a post-treatment follow-up period to assess reproductive function (in females) and final height. At 6 months post-treatment, most subjects reverted to pubertal levels of LH (87.9%) and clinical signs of resumption of pubertal progression were evident with increase in breast development in girls (66.7%) and increase in genitalia development in boys (80%).

Of the 40 patients evaluated in the follow-up, 33 were observed until they reached final or near-final adult height. These patients had a mean increase in final adult height compared to baseline predicted adult height. The mean final adult height standard deviation score was -0.2.

After stopping treatment, regular menses were reported for all female subjects who reached 12 years of age during follow-up; mean time to menses was approximately 1.5 years; mean age of onset of menstruation after stopping treatment was 12.9 years. Data to assess reproductive function was collected in a post-study survey of 20 girls who reached adulthood (ages 18-26): menstrual cycles were reported to be normal in 80% of women; 12 pregnancies were reported for a total of 7 of the 20 subjects, including multiple pregnancies for 4 subjects.

14.2 LUPRON DEPOT-PED 11.25 mg or 30 mg for 3-month administration

In a randomized, open-label clinical study of LUPRON DEPOT-PED 3-Month formulations, 84 subjects (76 female, 8 male) between 1 and 11 years of age received the LUPRON DEPOT-PED 11.25 mg or 30 mg for 3-month administration formulation. Each dose group had an equal number of treatment-naïve patients who had pubertal LH levels and patients previously treated with GnRHa therapies who had prepubertal LH levels at the time of study entry. The percentage of subjects with suppression of peak-stimulated LH to < 4.0 mIU/mL, as determined by assessments at months 2, 3 and 6 is 78.6% in the 11.25 mg dose and 95.2% in the 30 mg dose as shown in Table 5.

[See table 5 on next page]

The mean peak stimulated LH levels for all visits are shown by dose and subgroup (naïve vs. previously treated subjects) in Figures 1 and 2.

[See Figures 1 and 2 on next page]

For the LUPRON DEPOT-PED 11.25 mg dose for 3-month administration, 93% (39/42) of subjects and for LUPRON DEPOT-PED 30 mg dose for 3-month administration 100% (42/42) of subjects had sex steroid (estradiol or testosterone) suppressed to prepubertal levels at all visits. Clinical suppression of puberty in female patients was observed in 29 of 32 (90.6%) and 28 of 34 (82.4%) of patients in the 11.25 mg and 30 mg groups, respectively, at month 6. Clinical suppression of puberty in males was observed in 1 of 2 (50.0%) and 2 of 5 (40.0%) patients in the 11.25 mg and 30 mg groups, respectively, at month 6. In subjects with complete data for bone age, 29 of 33 (87.9 %) in the 11.25 mg group and 30 of 40 in the 30 mg group (75.0%) had a decrease in the ratio of bone age to chronological age at month 6 compared to screening.

16   HOW SUPPLIED/STORAGE AND HANDLING

LUPRON DEPOT-PED 7.5 mg, 11.25 mg, or 15 mg for 1-month administration is packaged as follows:

1-month Kit with prefilled dual-chamber syringe	7.5 mg	NDC 0074-2108-03
1-month Kit with prefilled dual-chamber syringe	11.25 mg	NDC 0074-2282-03
1-month Kit with prefilled dual-chamber syringe	15 mg	NDC 0074-2440-03

LUPRON DEPOT-PED 11.25 mg or 30 mg for 3-month administration is packaged as follows:

3-month Kit with prefilled dual-chamber syringe	11.25 mg	NDC 0074-3779-03
3-month Kit with prefilled dual-chamber syringe	30 mg	NDC 0074-9694-03

LUPRON DEPOT-PED prefilled syringe for 1-month administration contains sterile lyophilized microspheres of leuprolide acetate incorporated in a biodegradable lactic acid/glycolic acid copolymer.

LUPRON DEPOT-PED prefilled syringe for 3-month administration contains sterile lyophilized microspheres of leuprolide acetate incorporated in a biodegradable lactic acid polymer.

When mixed with 1 milliliter of accompanying diluent, LUPRON DEPOT-PED for 1-month administration is administered as a single intramuscular injection. When mixed with 1.5 milliliter of accompanying diluent, LUPRON DEPOT-PED for 3-month administration is administered as a single intramuscular injection.

Each kit contains:
• one prefilled dual-chamber syringe containing 1½ inch needle with LuproLoc® safety device
• one plunger
• two alcohol swabs
• population, dose and frequency confirmation insert
• a complete prescribing information enclosure
Store at 25°C (77°F); excursions permitted to 15-30°C (59-86°F) [See USP Controlled Room Temperature]

17   PATIENT COUNSELING INFORMATION

Information for Parents
Prior to starting therapy with LUPRON DEPOT-PED, patients should be informed that:
• All formulations are contraindicated in women who are or may become pregnant. If this drug is used during pregnancy, or if the patient becomes pregnant while taking the drug, the patient should be informed of the potential risk to the fetus.
• Continuous therapy is important and that adherence to the recommended drug administration schedule (monthly for LUPRON DEPOT-PED for 1-month administration and every three months for LUPRON DEPOT-PED for 3-month administration) must be accepted if therapy is to be successful. If the injection schedule is not followed, pubertal development may begin again.
• During the first weeks of treatment, signs of puberty, e.g., vaginal bleeding, may occur. This is a common initial effect of the drug. If these symptoms continue beyond the second month of treatment, the physician should be notified.
• The most common side effects related to treatment with LUPRON DEPOT-PED for 1-month or 3-month administration in clinical studies are: pain, acne/seborrhea, injection site reactions including pain, swelling and abscess, rash including erythema multiforme, vaginitis/bleeding/discharge, increased weight, headache, and altered mood.
• After injection, some pain and irritation is expected; however if more severe symptoms occur, the physician should

be contacted. Any unusual signs or symptoms should be reported to the physician.
• The parents should notify the physician if new or worsened symptoms develop after beginning treatment.
Manufactured for
AbbVie Inc.
North Chicago, IL 60064
by Takeda Pharmaceutical Company Limited
Osaka, Japan 540-8645
™ - Trademark
® - Registered Trademark
Ref: 03-A822-R23-Revised: June, 2013
©2013 AbbVie Inc.
Shown in Product Identification Guide, page 506

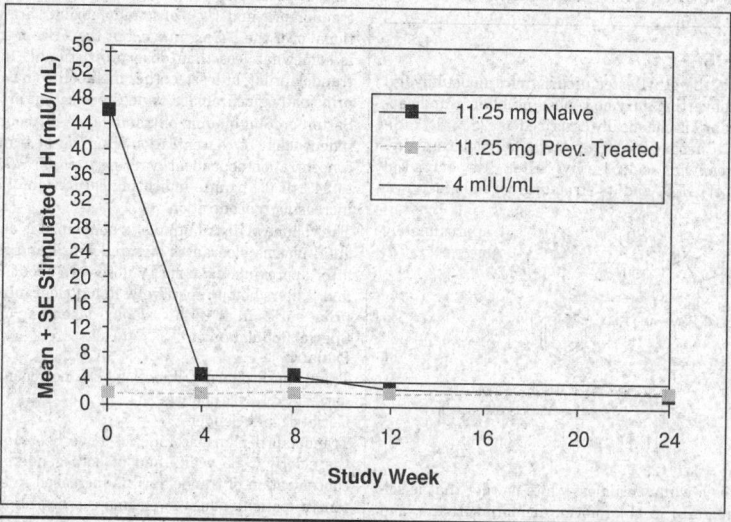

Figure 1. Mean Peak Stimulated LH for LUPRON DEPOT-PED 11.25 mg for 3-month administration

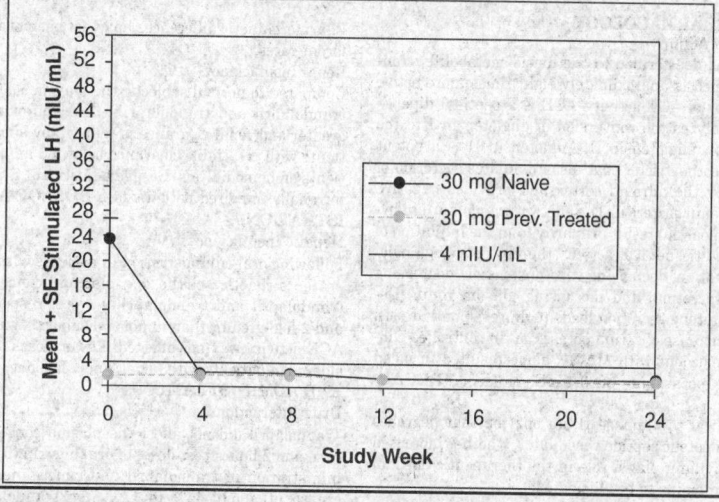

Figure 2. Mean Peak Stimulated LH for LUPRON DEPOT-PED 30 mg for 3-month administration

Table 5. Suppression of Peak-Stimulated LH from Month 2 Through Month 6

Parameter	LUPRON DEPOT-PED 11.25 mg every 3 Months			LUPRON DEPOT-PED 30 mg every 3 Months		
	Naïve N = 21	Prev Trt[a] N = 21	Total N = 42	Naïve N = 21	Prev Trt[a] N = 21	Total N = 42
Percent with Suppression	76.2	81.0	78.6	90.5	100	95.2
2-sided 95% CI	52.8, 91.8	58.1, 94.6	63.2, 89.7	69.6, 98.8	83.9, 100	83.8, 99.4

a. Previously treated with GnRHa for at least 6 months prior to enrollment in pivotal Study L-CP07-167.

MAVIK®
[*MAH-vic*]
(trandolapril tablets)   ℞

> **WARNING: FETAL TOXICITY**
> • When pregnancy is detected, discontinue MAVIK as soon as possible.

Continued on next page

Physicians' Desk Reference®, the trusted drug reference for over 70 years

- Drugs that act directly on the renin-angiotensin system can cause injury and death to the developing fetus (See **WARNINGS: Fetal Toxicity**).

DESCRIPTION

Trandolapril is the ethyl ester prodrug of a nonsulfhydryl angiotensin converting enzyme (ACE) inhibitor, trandolaprilat. Trandolapril is chemically described as (2S, 3aR, 7aS)-1-[(S)-N-[(S)-1-Carboxy-3-phenylpropyl]alanyl] hexahydro-2-indolinecarboxylic acid, 1-ethyl ester. Its empirical formula is $C_{24}H_{34}N_2O_5$ and its structural formula is

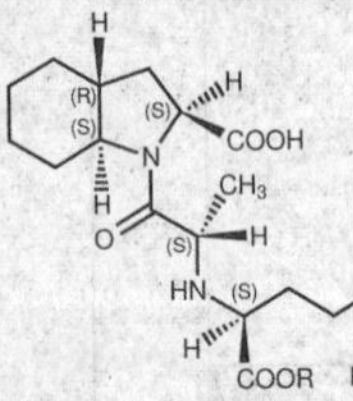

COOR   R = C_2H_5, Trandolapril
= H , Trandolaprilat (diacid)

M.W. = 430.54
Melting Point = 125°C
Trandolapril is a white or almost white powder that is soluble (> 100 mg/mL) in chloroform, dichloromethane, and methanol. MAVIK tablets contain 1 mg, 2 mg, or 4 mg of trandolapril for oral administration. Each tablet also contains corn starch, croscarmellose sodium, hypromellose, iron oxide, lactose monohydrate, povidone, sodium stearyl fumarate.

CLINICAL PHARMACOLOGY

Mechanism of Action

Trandolapril is deesterified to the diacid metabolite, trandolaprilat, which is approximately eight times more active as an inhibitor of ACE activity. ACE is a peptidyl dipeptidase that catalyzes the conversion of angiotensin I to the vasoconstrictor, angiotensin II. Angiotensin II is a potent peripheral vasoconstrictor that also stimulates secretion of aldosterone by the adrenal cortex and provides negative feedback for renin secretion. The effect of trandolapril in hypertension appears to result primarily from the inhibition of circulating and tissue ACE activity thereby reducing angiotensin II formation, decreasing vasoconstriction, decreasing aldosterone secretion, and increasing plasma renin. Decreased aldosterone secretion leads to diuresis, natriuresis, and a small increase of serum potassium. In controlled clinical trials, treatment with MAVIK alone resulted in mean increases in potassium of 0.1 mEq/L (see **PRECAUTIONS**.)

ACE is identical to kininase II, an enzyme that degrades bradykinin, a potent peptide vasodilator; whether increased levels of bradykinin play a role in the therapeutic effect of trandolapril remains to be elucidated.

While the principal mechanism of antihypertensive effect is thought to be through the renin-angiotensin-aldosterone system, trandolapril exerts antihypertensive actions even in patients with low-renin hypertension. MAVIK was an effective antihypertensive in all races studied. Both black patients (usually a predominantly low-renin group) and non-black patients responded to 2 to 4 mg of MAVIK.

Pharmacokinetics and Metabolism

Pharmacokinetics

Trandolapril's ACE-inhibiting activity is primarily due to its diacid metabolite, trandolaprilat. Cleavage of the ester group of trandolapril, primarily in the liver, is responsible for conversion. Absolute bioavailability after oral administration of trandolapril is about 10% as trandolapril and 70% as trandolaprilat. After oral trandolapril under fasting conditions, peak trandolapril levels occur at about one hour and peak trandolaprilat levels occur between 4 and 10 hours. The elimination half-life of trandolapril is about 6 hours. At steady state, the effective half-life of trandolaprilat is 22.5 hours. Like all ACE inhibitors, trandolaprilat also has a prolonged terminal elimination phase, involving a small fraction of administered drug, probably representing binding to plasma and tissue ACE. During multiple dosing of trandolapril, there is no significant accumulation of trandolaprilat. Food slows absorption of trandolapril, but does not affect AUC or C_{max} of trandolaprilat or C_{max} of trandolapril.

Metabolism and Excretion

After oral administration of trandolapril, about 33% of parent drug and metabolites are recovered in urine, mostly as trandolaprilat, with about 66% in feces. The extent of the absorbed dose which is biliary excreted has not been determined. Plasma concentrations (C_{max} and AUC of trandolapril and C_{max} of trandolaprilat) are dose proportional over the 1-4 mg range, but the AUC of trandolaprilat is somewhat less than dose proportional. In addition to trandolaprilat, at least 7 other metabolites have been found, principally glucuronides or deesterification products. Serum protein binding of trandolapril is about 80%, and is independent of concentration. Binding of trandolaprilat is concentration-dependent, varying from 65% at 1000 ng/mL to 94% at 0.1 ng/mL, indicating saturation of binding with increasing concentration.

The volume of distribution of trandolapril is about 18 liters. Total plasma clearances of trandolapril and trandolaprilat after approximately 2 mg IV doses are about 52 liters/hour and 7 liters/hour respectively. Renal clearance of trandolaprilat varies from 1-4 liters/hour, depending on dose.

Special Populations

Pediatric

Trandolapril pharmacokinetics have not been evaluated in patients < 18 years of age.

Geriatric and Gender

Trandolapril pharmacokinetics have been investigated in the elderly (> 65 years) and in both genders. The plasma concentration of trandolapril is increased in elderly hypertensive patients, but the plasma concentration of trandolaprilat and inhibition of ACE activity are similar in elderly and young hypertensive patients. The pharmacokinetics of trandolapril and trandolaprilat and inhibition of ACE activity are similar in male and female elderly hypertensive patients.

Race

Pharmacokinetic differences have not been evaluated in different races.

Renal Insufficiency

Compared to normal subjects, the plasma concentrations of trandolapril and trandolaprilat are approximately 2-fold greater and renal clearance is reduced by about 85% in patients with creatinine clearance below 30 ml/min and in patients on hemodialysis. Dosage adjustment is recommended in renally impaired patients (see **DOSAGE AND ADMINISTRATION**).

Hepatic Insufficiency

Following oral administration in patients with mild to moderate alcoholic cirrhosis, plasma concentrations of trandolapril and trandolaprilat were, respectively, 9-fold and 2-fold greater than in normal subjects, but inhibition of ACE activity was not affected. Lower doses should be considered in patients with hepatic insufficiency (see **DOSAGE AND ADMINISTRATION**).

Drug Interactions

Trandolapril did not affect the plasma concentration (pre-dose and 2 hours post-dose) of oral digoxin (0.25 mg). Coadministration of trandolapril and cimetidine led to an increase of about 44% in C_{max} for trandolapril, but no difference in the pharmacokinetics of trandolaprilat or in ACE inhibition. Coadministration of trandolapril and furosemide led to an increase of about 25% in the renal clearance of trandolaprilat, but no effect was seen on the pharmacokinetics of furosemide or trandolaprilat or on ACE inhibition.

Pharmacodynamics and Clinical Effects

A single 2-mg dose of MAVIK produces 70 to 85% inhibition of plasma ACE activity at 4 hours with about 10% decline at 24 hours and about half the effect manifest at 8 days. Maximum ACE inhibition is achieved with a plasma trandolaprilat concentration of 2 ng/mL. ACE inhibition is a function of trandolaprilat concentration, not trandolapril concentration. The effect of trandolapril on exogenous angiotensin I was not measured.

Hypertension

Four placebo-controlled dose response studies were conducted using once-daily oral dosing of MAVIK in doses from 0.25 to 16 mg per day in 827 black and non-black patients with mild to moderate hypertension. The minimal effective once-daily dose was 1 mg in non-black patients and 2 mg in black patients. Further decreases in trough supine diastolic blood pressure were obtained in non-black patients with higher doses, and no further response was seen with doses above 4 mg (up to 16 mg). The antihypertensive effect diminished somewhat at the end of the dosing interval, but trough/peak ratios are well above 50% for all effective doses. There was a slightly greater effect on the diastolic pressure, but no difference on systolic pressure with b.i.d. dosing.

During chronic therapy, the maximum reduction in blood pressure with any dose is achieved within one week. Following 6 weeks of monotherapy in placebo-controlled trials in patients with mild to moderate hypertension, once-daily doses of 2 to 4 mg lowered supine or standing systolic/diastolic blood pressure 24 hours after dosing by an average 7-10/4-5 mmHg below placebo responses in non-black patients. Once-daily doses of 2 to 4 mg lowered blood pressure 4-6/3-4 mmHg in black patients. Trough to peak ratios for effective doses ranged from 0.5 to 0.9. There were no differences in response between men and women, but responses were somewhat greater in patients under 60 than in patients over 60 years old. Abrupt withdrawal of MAVIK has not been associated with a rapid increase in blood pressure. Administration of MAVIK to patients with mild to moderate hypertension results in a reduction of supine, sitting and standing blood pressure to about the same extent without compensatory tachycardia.

Symptomatic hypotension is infrequent, although it can occur in patients who are salt- and/or volume-depleted (see **WARNINGS**). Use of MAVIK in combination with thiazide diuretics gives a blood pressure lowering effect greater than that seen with either agent alone, and the additional effect of trandolapril is similar to the effect of monotherapy.

Heart Failure Post Myocardial Infarction or Left Ventricular Dysfunction Post Myocardial Infarction

The Trandolapril Cardiac Evaluation (TRACE) Trial was a Danish, 27-center, double-blind, placebo controlled, parallel-group study of the effect of trandolapril on all-cause mortality in stable patients with echocardiographic evidence of left ventricular dysfunction 3 to 7 days after a myocardial infarction. Subjects with residual ischemia or overt heart failure were included. Patients tolerant of a test dose of 1 mg trandolapril were randomized to placebo (n=873) or trandolapril (n=876) and followed for 24 months. Among patients randomized to trandolapril, who began treatment on 1 mg, 62% were successfully titrated to a target dose of 4 mg once daily over a period of weeks. The use of trandolapril was associated with a 16% reduction in the risk of all-cause mortality (p=0.042), largely cardiovascular mortality. Trandolapril was also associated with a 20% reduction in the risk of progression of heart failure (p=0.047), defined by a time-to-first-event analysis of death attributed to heart failure, hospitalization for heart failure, or requirement for open-label ACE inhibitor for the treatment of heart failure. There was no significant effect of treatment on other endpoints: subsequent hospitalization, incidence of recurrent myocardial infarction, exercise tolerance, ventricular function, ventricular dimensions, or NYHA class.

The population in TRACE was entirely Caucasian and had less usage than would be typical in a U.S. population of other post-infarction interventions: 42% thrombolysis, 16% beta-adrenergic blockade, and 6.7% PTCA or CABG during the entire period of follow-up. Blood pressure control, especially in the placebo group, was poor: 47 to 53% of patients randomized to placebo and 32 to 40% of patients randomized to trandolapril had blood pressures > 140/95 at 90-day follow-up visits.

INDICATIONS AND USAGE

Hypertension

MAVIK is indicated for the treatment of hypertension. It may be used alone or in combination with other antihypertensive medication such as hydrochlorothiazide.

Heart Failure Post Myocardial Infarction or Left-Ventricular Dysfunction Post Myocardial Infarction

MAVIK is indicated in stable patients who have evidence of left-ventricular systolic dysfunction (identified by wall motion abnormalities) or who are symptomatic from congestive heart failure within the first few days after sustaining acute myocardial infarction. Administration of trandolapril to Caucasian patients has been shown to decrease the risk of death (principally cardiovascular death) and to decrease the risk of heart failure-related hospitalization (see **CLINICAL PHARMACOLOGY - Heart Failure or Left-Ventricular Dysfunction Post Myocardial Infarction** for details of the survival trial).

CONTRAINDICATIONS

MAVIK is contraindicated in patients who are hypersensitive to this product, in patients with hereditary/idiopathic angioedema and in patients with a history of angioedema related to previous treatment with an ACE inhibitor.

Do not co-administer aliskiren with MAVIK in patients with diabetes (see **PRECAUTIONS, Drug Interactions**).

WARNINGS

Anaphylactoid and Possibly Related Reactions

Presumably because angiotensin converting enzyme inhibitors affect the metabolism of eicosanoids and polypeptides, including endogenous bradykinin, patients receiving ACE inhibitors, including MAVIK, may be subject to a variety of adverse reactions, some of them serious.

Anaphylactoid Reactions During Desensitization

Two patients undergoing desensitizing treatment with hymenoptera venom while receiving ACE inhibitors sustained life-threatening anaphylactoid reactions. In the same patients, these reactions did not occur when ACE inhibitors were temporarily withheld, but they reappeared when the ACE inhibitors were inadvertently readministered.

Anaphylactoid Reactions During Membrane Exposure

Anaphylactoid reactions have been reported in patients dialyzed with high-flux membranes and treated concomitantly with an ACE inhibitor. Anaphylactoid reactions have also been reported in patients undergoing low-density lipoprotein apheresis with dextran sulfate absorption.

Head and Neck Angioedema

In controlled trials ACE inhibitors (for which adequate data are available) cause a higher rate of angioedema in black than in non-black patients.

Angioedema of the face, extremities, lips, tongue, glottis, and larynx has been reported in patients treated with ACE inhibitors including MAVIK. Symptoms suggestive of angioedema or facial edema occurred in 0.13% of MAVIK-treated patients. Two of the four cases were life-threatening and resolved without treatment or with medication (corticosteroids). Angioedema associated with laryngeal edema can be fatal. If laryngeal stridor or angioedema of the face, tongue or glottis occurs, treatment with MAVIK should be discontinued immediately, the patient treated in accordance with accepted medical care and carefully observed until the swelling disappears. In instances where swelling is confined to the face and lips, the condition generally resolves without treatment; antihistamines may be useful in relieving symptoms. **Where there is involvement of the tongue, glottis, or larynx, likely to cause airway obstruction, emergency therapy, including but not limited to subcutaneous epinephrine solution 1:1,000 (0.3 to 0.5 mL) should be promptly administered** (see **PRECAUTIONS - Information for Patients** and **ADVERSE REACTIONS**).

Intestinal Angioedema

Intestinal angioedema has been reported in patients treated with ACE inhibitors. These patients presented with abdominal pain (with or without nausea or vomiting); in some cases there was no prior history of facial angioedema and C-1 esterase levels were normal. The angioedema was diagnosed by procedures including abdominal CT scan or ultrasound, or at surgery, and symptoms resolved after stopping the ACE inhibitor. Intestinal angioedema should be included in the differential diagnosis of patients on ACE inhibitors presenting with abdominal pain.

Hypotension

MAVIK can cause symptomatic hypotension. Like other ACE inhibitors, MAVIK has only rarely been associated with symptomatic hypotension in uncomplicated hypertensive patients. Symptomatic hypotension is most likely to occur in patients who have been salt- or volume-depleted as a result of prolonged treatment with diuretics, dietary salt restriction, dialysis, diarrhea, or vomiting. Volume and/or salt depletion should be corrected before initiating treatment with MAVIK (see **PRECAUTIONS - Drug Interactions** and **ADVERSE REACTIONS**). In controlled and uncontrolled studies, hypotension was reported as an adverse event in 0.6% of patients and led to discontinuations in 0.1% of patients.

In patients with concomitant congestive heart failure, with or without associated renal insufficiency, ACE inhibitor therapy may cause excessive hypotension, which may be associated with oliguria or azotemia, and rarely, with acute renal failure and death. In such patients, MAVIK therapy should be started at the recommended dose under close medical supervision. These patients should be followed closely during the first 2 weeks of treatment and, thereafter, whenever the dosage of MAVIK or diuretic is increased (see **DOSAGE AND ADMINISTRATION**). Care in avoiding hypotension should also be taken in patients with ischemic heart disease, aortic stenosis, or cerebrovascular disease.

If symptomatic hypotension occurs, the patient should be placed in the supine position and, if necessary, normal saline may be administered intravenously. A transient hypotensive response is not a contraindication to further doses; however, lower doses of MAVIK or reduced concomitant diuretic therapy should be considered.

Neutropenia/Agranulocytosis

Another ACE inhibitor, captopril, has been shown to cause agranulocytosis and bone marrow depression rarely in patients with uncomplicated hypertension, but more frequently in patients with renal impairment, especially if they also have a collagen-vascular disease such as systemic lupus erythematosus or scleroderma. Available data from clinical trials of trandolapril are insufficient to show that trandolapril does not cause agranulocytosis at similar rates. As with other ACE inhibitors, periodic monitoring of white blood cell counts in patients with collagen-vascular disease and/or renal disease should be considered.

Hepatic Failure

ACE inhibitors rarely have been associated with a syndrome of cholestatic jaundice, fulminant hepatic necrosis, and death. The mechanism of this syndrome is not understood. Patients receiving ACE inhibitors who develop jaundice should discontinue the ACE inhibitor and receive appropriate medical follow-up.

Fetal Toxicity

Pregnancy Category D

Use of drugs that act on the renin-angiotensin system during the second and third trimesters of pregnancy reduces fetal renal function and increases fetal and neonatal morbidity and death. Resulting oligohydramnios can be associated with fetal lung hypoplasia and skeletal deformations. Potential neonatal adverse effects include skull hypoplasia, anuria, hypotension, renal failure, and death. When pregnancy is detected, discontinue MAVIK as soon as possible. These adverse outcomes are usually associated with use of these drugs in the second and third trimester of pregnancy. Most epidemiologic studies examining fetal abnormalities after exposure to antihypertensive use in the first trimester have not distinguished drugs affecting the renin-angiotensin system from other antihypertensive agents. Appropriate management of maternal hypertension during pregnancy is important to optimize outcomes for both mother and fetus.

In the unusual case that there is no appropriate alternative to therapy with drugs affecting the renin-angiotensin system for a particular patient, apprise the mother of the potential risk to the fetus. Perform serial ultrasound examinations to assess the intra-amniotic environment. If oligohydramnios is observed, discontinue MAVIK, unless it is considered lifesaving for the mother. Fetal testing may be appropriate, based on the week of pregnancy. Patients and physicians should be aware, however, that oligohydramnios may not appear until after the fetus has sustained irreversible injury. Closely observe infants with histories of *in utero* exposure to MAVIK for hypotension, oliguria, and hyperkalemia (See **PRECAUTIONS, Pediatric Use**).

Doses of 0.8 mg/kg/day (9.4 mg/m^2/day) in rabbits, 1000 mg/kg/day (7000 mg/m^2/day) in rats, and 25 mg/kg/day (295 mg/m^2/day) in cynomolgus monkeys did not produce teratogenic effects. These doses represent 10 and 3 times (rabbits), 1250 and 2564 times (rats), and 312 and 108 times (monkeys) the maximum projected human dose of 4 mg based on body-weight and body-surface-area, respectively assuming a 50 kg woman.

PRECAUTIONS
General

Impaired Renal Function

As a consequence of inhibiting the renin-angiotensin-aldosterone system, changes in renal function may be anticipated in susceptible individuals. In patients with severe heart failure whose renal function may depend on the activity of the renin-angiotensin-aldosterone system, treatment with ACE inhibitors, including MAVIK® (trandolapril), may be associated with oliguria and/or progressive azotemia and rarely with acute renal failure and/or death.

In hypertensive patients with unilateral or bilateral renal artery stenosis, increases in blood urea nitrogen and serum creatinine have been observed in some patients following ACE inhibitor therapy. These increases were almost always reversible upon discontinuation of the ACE inhibitor and/or diuretic therapy. In such patients, renal function should be monitored during the first few weeks of therapy.

Some hypertensive patients with no apparent preexisting renal vascular disease have developed increases in blood urea and serum creatinine, usually minor and transient, especially when ACE inhibitors have been given concomitantly with a diuretic. This is more likely to occur in patients with preexisting renal impairment. Dosage reduction and/or discontinuation of any diuretic and/or the ACE inhibitor may be required. Evaluation of hypertensive patients should always include assessment of renal function (see **DOSAGE AND ADMINISTRATION**).

Hyperkalemia and Potassium-sparing Diuretics

In clinical trials, hyperkalemia (serum potassium > 6.00 mEq/L) occurred in approximately 0.4% of hypertensive patients receiving MAVIK. In most cases, elevated serum potassium levels were isolated values, which resolved despite continued therapy. None of these patients were discontinued from the trials because of hyperkalemia. Risk factors for the development of hyperkalemia include renal insufficiency, diabetes mellitus, and the concomitant use of potassium-sparing diuretics, potassium supplements, and/or potassium-containing salt substitutes, which should be used cautiously, if at all, with MAVIK (see **PRECAUTIONS - Drug Interactions**).

Cough

Presumably due to the inhibition of the degradation of endogenous bradykinin, persistent nonproductive cough has been reported with all ACE inhibitors, always resolving after discontinuation of therapy. ACE inhibitor-induced cough should be considered in the differential diagnosis of cough. In controlled trials of trandolapril, cough was present in 2% of trandolapril patients and 0% of patients given placebo. There was no evidence of a relationship to dose.

Surgery/Anesthesia

In patients undergoing major surgery or during anesthesia with agents that produce hypotension, MAVIK will block angiotensin II formation secondary to compensatory renin release. If hypotension occurs and is considered to be due to this mechanism, it can be corrected by volume expansion.

Information for Patients

Angioedema

Angioedema, including laryngeal edema, may occur at any time during treatment with ACE inhibitors, including MAVIK. Patients should be so advised and told to report immediately any signs or symptoms suggesting angioedema (swelling of face, extremities, eyes, lips, tongue, difficulty in swallowing or breathing) and to stop taking the drug until they have consulted with their physician (see **WARNINGS** and **ADVERSE REACTIONS**).

Symptomatic Hypotension

Patients should be cautioned that light-headedness can occur, especially during the first days of MAVIK therapy, and should be reported to a physician. If actual syncope occurs, patients should be told to stop taking the drug until they have consulted with their physician (see **WARNINGS**).

All patients should be cautioned that inadequate fluid intake, excessive perspiration, diarrhea, or vomiting, resulting in reduced fluid volume, may precipitate an excessive fall in blood pressure with the same consequences of light-headedness and possible syncope.

Patients planning to undergo any surgery and/or anesthesia should be told to inform their physician that they are taking an ACE inhibitor that has a long duration of action.

Hyperkalemia

Patients should be told not to use potassium supplements or salt substitutes containing potassium without consulting their physician (see **PRECAUTIONS**).

Neutropenia

Patients should be told to report promptly any indication of infection (e.g., sore throat, fever) which could be a sign of neutropenia.

Pregnancy

Female patients of childbearing age should be told about the consequences of exposure to MAVIK during pregnancy. Discuss treatment options with women planning to become pregnant. Patients should be asked to report pregnancies to their physicians as soon as possible.

NOTE: As with many other drugs, certain advice to patients being treated with MAVIK is warranted. This information is intended to aid in the safe and effective use of this medication. It is not a disclosure of all possible adverse or intended effects.

Drug Interactions

Dual Blockade of the Renin-Angiotensin System (RAS)

Dual blockade of the RAS with angiotensin receptor blockers, ACE inhibitors, or aliskiren is associated with increased risks of hypotension, hyperkalemia, and changes in renal function (including acute renal failure) compared to

Continued on next page

Information on the AbbVie, Inc. products listed on these pages is from the prescribing information in use as of July 31, 2016. For more information, please visit rxabbvie.com or call 1-800-633-9110.

monotherapy. Closely monitor blood pressure, renal function and electrolytes in patients on MAVIK and other agents that affect the RAS.

Do not co-administer aliskiren with MAVIK in patients with diabetes. Avoid use of aliskiren with MAVIK in patients with renal impairment (GFR <60 ml/min).

Concomitant Diuretic Therapy

As with other ACE inhibitors, patients on diuretics, especially those on recently instituted diuretic therapy, may experience an excessive reduction of blood pressure after initiation of therapy with MAVIK. The possibility of exacerbation of hypotensive effects with MAVIK may be minimized by either discontinuing the diuretic or cautiously increasing salt intake prior to initiation of treatment with MAVIK. If it is not possible to discontinue the diuretic, the starting dose of trandolapril should be reduced (see **DOSAGE AND ADMINISTRATION**).

Agents Increasing Serum Potassium

Trandolapril can attenuate potassium loss caused by thiazide diuretics and increase serum potassium when used alone. Use of potassium-sparing diuretics (spironolactone, triamterene, or amiloride), potassium supplements, or potassium-containing salt substitutes concomitantly with ACE inhibitors can increase the risk of hyperkalemia. If concomitant use of such agents is indicated, they should be used with caution and with appropriate monitoring of serum potassium (see **PRECAUTIONS**).

Antidiabetic Agents

Concomitant use of ACE inhibitors and antidiabetic medicines (insulin or oral hypoglycemic agents) may cause an increased blood glucose lowering effect with greater risk of hypoglycemia.

Lithium

Increased serum lithium levels and symptoms of lithium toxicity have been reported in patients receiving concomitant lithium and ACE inhibitor therapy. These drugs should be coadministered with caution, and frequent monitoring of serum lithium levels is recommended. If a diuretic is also used, the risk of lithium toxicity may be increased.

Non-Steroidal Anti-Inflammatory Agents including Selective Cyclooxygenase-2 Inhibitors (COX-2 Inhibitors)

In patients who are elderly, volume-depleted (including those on diuretic therapy), or with compromised renal function, co-administration of NSAIDs, including selective COX-2 inhibitors, with ACE inhibitors, including trandolapril, may result in deterioration of renal function, including possible acute renal failure. These effects are usually reversible. Monitor renal function periodically in patients receiving trandolapril and NSAID therapy.

The antihypertensive effect of ACE inhibitors, including trandolapril may be attenuated by NSAIDs.

Gold

Nitritoid reactions (symptoms include facial flushing, nausea, vomiting and hypotension) have been reported rarely in patients on therapy with injectable gold (sodium aurothiomalate) and concomitant ACE inhibitor therapy including MAVIK.

Other

No clinically significant pharmacokinetic interaction has been found between trandolaprilat and food, cimetidine, digoxin, or furosemide.

The anticoagulant effect of warfarin was not significantly changed by trandolapril.

The hypotensive effect of certain inhalation anesthetics may be enhanced by ACE inhibitors including trandolapril (see **PRECAUTIONS**-Surgery/Anesthesia).

Carcinogenesis, Mutagenesis, Impairment of Fertility

Long-term studies were conducted with oral trandolapril administered by gavage to mice (78 weeks) and rats (104 and 106 weeks). No evidence of carcinogenic potential was seen in mice dosed up to 25 mg/kg/day (85 mg/m²/day) or rats dosed up to 8 mg/kg/day (60 mg/m²/day). These doses are 313 and 32 times (mice), and 100 and 23 times (rats) the maximum recommended human daily dose (MRHDD) of 4 mg based on body-weight and body-surface-area, respectively assuming a 50 kg individual. The genotoxic potential of trandolapril was evaluated in the microbial mutagenicity (Ames) test, the point mutation and chromosome aberration assays in Chinese hamster V79 cells, and the micronucleus test in mice. There was no evidence of mutagenic or clastogenic potential in these in vitro and in vivo assays.

Reproduction studies in rats did not show any impairment of fertility at doses up to 100 mg/kg/day (710 mg/m²/day) of trandolapril, or 1250 and 260 times the MRHDD on the basis of body-weight and body-surface-area, respectively.

Nursing Mothers

Radiolabeled trandolapril or its metabolites are secreted in rat milk. MAVIK should not be administered to nursing mothers.

Geriatric Use

In placebo-controlled studies of MAVIK, 31.1% of patients were 60 years and older, 20.1% were 65 years and older, and 2.3% were 75 years and older. No overall differences in effectiveness or safety were observed between these patients and younger patients. (Greater sensitivity of some older individual patients cannot be ruled out.)

Pediatric Use

Neonates with a history of in utero exposure to MAVIK:
If oliguria or hypotension occurs, direct attention toward support of blood pressure and renal perfusion. Exchange transfusions or dialysis may be required as a means of reversing hypotension and/or substituting for disordered renal function.

The safety and effectiveness of MAVIK in pediatric patients have not been established.

ADVERSE REACTIONS

The safety experience in U.S. placebo-controlled trials included 1069 hypertensive patients, of whom 832 received MAVIK. Nearly 200 hypertensive patients received MAVIK for over one year in open-label trials. In controlled trials, withdrawals for adverse events were 2.1% on placebo and 1.4% on MAVIK. Adverse events considered at least possibly related to treatment occurring in 1% of MAVIK-treated patients and more common on MAVIK than placebo, pooled for all doses, are shown below, together with the frequency of discontinuation of treatment because of these events.

ADVERSE EVENTS IN PLACEBO-CONTROLLED HYPERTENSION TRIALS

	Occurring at 1% or greater MAVIK (N=832) % Incidence (% Discontinuance)	PLACEBO (N=237) % Incidence (% Discontinuance)
Cough	1.9 (0.1)	0.4 (0.4)
Dizziness	1.3 (0.2)	0.4 (0.4)
Diarrhea	1.0 (0.0)	0.4 (0.0)

Headache and fatigue were all seen in more than 1% of MAVIK-treated patients but were more frequently seen on placebo. Adverse events were not usually persistent or difficult to manage.

Left Ventricular Dysfunction Post Myocardial Infarction

Adverse reactions related to MAVIK occurring at a rate greater than that observed in placebo-treated patients with left ventricular dysfunction, are shown below. The incidences represent the experiences from the TRACE study. The follow-up time was between 24 and 50 months for this study.

Percentage of Patients with Adverse Events Greater Than Placebo

Adverse Event	Placebo-Controlled (TRACE) Mortality Study Trandolapril N=876	Placebo N=873
Cough	35	22
Dizziness	23	17
Hypotension	11	6.8
Elevated serum uric acid	15	13
Elevated BUN	9.0	7.6
PICA or CABG	7.3	6.1
Dyspepsia	6.4	6.0
Syncope	5.9	3.3
Hyperkalemia	5.3	2.8
Bradycardia	4.7	4.4
Hypocalcemia	4.7	3.9
Myalgia	4.7	3.1
Elevated creatinine	4.7	2.4
Gastritis	4.2	3.6
Cardiogenic shock	3.8	< 2
Intermittent claudication	3.8	< 2
Stroke	3.3	3.2
Asthenia	3.3	2.6

Clinical adverse experiences possibly or probably related or of uncertain relationship to therapy occurring in 0.3% to 1.0% (except as noted) of the patients treated with MAVIK (with or without concomitant calcium ion antagonist or diuretic) in controlled or uncontrolled trials (N=1134) and less frequent, clinically significant events seen in clinical trials or post-marketing experience include (listed by body system):

General Body Function
Chest pain.
Cardiovascular
AV first degree block, bradycardia, edema, flushing, and palpitations.
Central Nervous System
Drowsiness, insomnia, paresthesia, vertigo.
Dermatologic
Pruritus, rash, pemphigus.
Eye, Ear, Nose, Throat
Epistaxis, throat inflammation, upper respiratory tract infection.
Emotional, Mental, Sexual States
Anxiety, impotence, decreased libido.
Gastrointestinal
Abdominal distention, abdominal pain/cramps, constipation, dyspepsia, diarrhea, vomiting, nausea.
Hemopoietic
Decreased leukocytes, decreased neutrophils.
Metabolism and Endocrine
Increased liver enzymes including SGPT (ALT).
Musculoskeletal System
Extremity pain, muscle cramps, gout.
Pulmonary
Dyspnea.

Postmarketing

The following adverse reactions were identified during post approval use of MAVIK. Because these reactions are reported voluntarily from a population of uncertain size, it is not always possible to reliably estimate their frequency or establish a causal relationship to drug exposure.

General Body Function
Malaise, fever.
Cardiovascular
Myocardial infarction, myocardial ischemia, angina pectoris, cardiac failure, ventricular tachycardia, tachycardia, transient ischemic attack, arrhythmia.
Central Nervous System
Cerebral hemorrhage.
Dermatologic
Alopecia, sweating, Stevens-Johnson syndrome and toxic epidermal necrolysis.
Emotional, Mental, Sexual States
Hallucination, depression.
Gastrointestinal
Dry mouth, pancreatitis, jaundice and hepatitis.
Hemopoietic
Agranulocytosis, pancytopenia.
Metabolism and Endocrine
Increased SGOT (AST).
Pulmonary
Bronchitis.
Renal and Urinary
Renal failure.
Clinical Laboratory Test Findings
Hematology
Thrombocytopenia.
Serum Electrolytes
Hyponatremia.
Creatinine and Blood Urea Nitrogen
Increases in creatinine levels occurred in 1.1% of patients receiving MAVIK alone and 7.3% of patients treated with MAVIK, a calcium ion antagonist and a diuretic. Increases in blood urea nitrogen levels occurred in 0.6% of patients receiving MAVIK alone and 1.4% of patients receiving MAVIK, a calcium ion antagonist, and a diuretic. None of these increases required discontinuation of treatment. Increases in these laboratory values are more likely to occur in patients with renal insufficiency or those pretreated with a diuretic and, based on experience with other ACE inhibitors, would be expected to be especially likely in patients with renal artery stenosis (see **PRECAUTIONS** and **WARNINGS**).

Liver Function Tests

Occasional elevation of transaminases at the rate of 3X upper normals occurred in 0.8% of patients and persistent increase in bilirubin occurred in 0.2% of patients. Discontinuation for elevated liver enzymes occurred in 0.2% of patients.

Other

Another potentially important adverse experience, eosinophilic pneumonitis, has been attributed to other ACE inhibitors.

OVERDOSAGE

No data are available with respect to overdosage in humans. The oral LD_{50} of trandolapril in mice was 4875 mg/Kg in males and 3990 mg/Kg in females. In rats, an oral dose of 5000 mg/Kg caused low mortality (1 male out of 5; 0 females). In dogs, an oral dose of 1000 mg/Kg did not cause mortality and abnormal clinical signs were not observed. In humans, the most likely clinical manifestation would be symptoms attributable to severe hypotension. Symptoms also expected with ACE inhibitors are hypotension, hyperkalemia, and renal failure.

Laboratory determinations of serum levels of trandolapril and its metabolites are not widely available, and such determinations have, in any event, no established role in the management of trandolapril overdose. No data are available to suggest that physiological maneuvers (e.g., maneuvers to change the pH of the urine) might accelerate elimination of trandolapril and its metabolites. Trandolaprilat is removed by hemodialysis. Angiotensin II could presumably serve as a specific antagonist antidote in the setting of trandolapril overdose, but angiotensin II is essentially unavailable outside of scattered research facilities. Because the hypotensive effect of trandolapril is achieved through vasodilation and effective hypovolemia, it is reasonable to treat trandolapril overdose by infusion of normal saline solution.

DOSAGE AND ADMINISTRATION

Hypertension

The recommended initial dosage of MAVIK for patients not receiving a diuretic is 1 mg once daily in non-black patients and 2 mg in black patients. Dosage should be adjusted according to the blood pressure response. Generally, dosage adjustments should be made at intervals of at least 1 week. Most patients have required dosages of 2 to 4 mg once daily. There is little clinical experience with doses above 8 mg.

Patients inadequately treated with once-daily dosing at 4 mg may be treated with twice-daily dosing. If blood pressure is not adequately controlled with MAVIK monotherapy, a diuretic may be added.

In patients who are currently being treated with a diuretic, symptomatic hypotension occasionally can occur following the initial dose of MAVIK. To reduce the likelihood of hypotension, the diuretic should, if possible, be discontinued two to three days prior to beginning therapy with MAVIK (see **WARNINGS**). Then, if blood pressure is not controlled with MAVIK alone, diuretic therapy should be resumed. If the diuretic cannot be discontinued, an initial dose of 0.5 mg MAVIK should be used with careful medical supervision for several hours until blood pressure has stabilized. The dosage should subsequently be titrated (as described above) to the optimal response (see **WARNINGS, PRECAUTIONS, and DRUG INTERACTIONS**).

Concomitant administration of MAVIK with potassium supplements, potassium salt substitutes, or potassium sparing diuretics can lead to increases of serum potassium (see **PRECAUTIONS**).

Heart Failure Post Myocardial Infarction or Left-Ventricular Dysfunction Post Myocardial Infarction

The recommended starting dose is 1 mg, once daily. Following the initial dose, all patients should be titrated (as tolerated) toward a target dose of 4 mg, once daily. If a 4 mg dose is not tolerated, patients can continue therapy with the greatest tolerated dose.

Dosage Adjustment in Renal Impairment or Hepatic Cirrhosis

For patients with a creatinine clearance < 30 mL/min. or with hepatic cirrhosis, the recommended starting dose, based on clinical and pharmacokinetic data, is 0.5 mg daily. Patients should subsequently have their dosage titrated (as described above) to the optimal response.

HOW SUPPLIED

MAVIK® (trandolapril tablets) are supplied as follows:

1 mg tablet - Salmon colored, round shaped, scored, compressed tablets, with the "a" logo on one side and code identification letters FT on the other side. NDC 0074-2278-13 - bottles of 100 NDC 0074-2278-11 - unit dose packs of 100

2 mg tablet - Yellow colored, round shaped, compressed tablets, with the "a" logo on one side and code identification letters FX on the other side. NDC 0074-2279-13 - bottles of 100 NDC 0074-2279-11 - unit dose packs of 100

4 mg tablet - Rose colored, round shaped, compressed tablets, with the "a" logo on one side and code identification letters FZ on the other side. NDC 0074-2280-13 - bottles of 100 NDC 0074-2280-11 - unit dose packs of 100

Dispense in well-closed container with safety closure.

Storage

Store at controlled room temperature: 20-25°C (68-77°F) see USP.

Manufactured by

Halo Pharmaceutical Inc.
Whippany, N.J. 07981, U.S.A.

for

AbbVie Inc.
North Chicago, IL 60064, U.S.A.

03-A670 December 2012

Shown in Product Identification Guide, page 506

MIVACRON® INJECTION
(mivacurium chloride)   ℞

This drug should be administered only by adequately trained individuals familiar with its actions, characteristics, and hazards.

DESCRIPTION

MIVACRON (mivacurium chloride) is a short-acting, nondepolarizing skeletal muscle relaxant for intravenous (IV) administration. Mivacurium chloride is [R-[R*,R*-(E)]]-2, 2'-[(1,8-dioxo-4-octene-1,8-diyl)bis(oxy-3,1-propanediyl)] bis[1,2,3,4-tetrahydro-6,7-dimethoxy-2-methyl-1-[(3,4,5-trimethoxyphenyl)methyl]isoquinolinium] dichloride. The molecular formula is $C_{58}H_{80}Cl_2N_2O_{14}$ and the molecular weight is 1100.18. The structural formula is:

The partition coefficient of the compound is 0.015 in a 1-octanol/distilled water system at 25°C.

Mivacurium chloride is a mixture of three stereoisomers: (1R,1'R, 2S, 2'S), the *trans-trans* diester; (1R,1'R, 2R, 2'S), the *cis-trans* diester; and (1R,1'R , 2R, 2'R), the *cis-cis* diester. The *trans-trans* and *cis-trans* stereoisomers comprise 92% to 96% of mivacurium chloride and their neuromuscular blocking potencies are not significantly different from each other or from mivacurium chloride. The *cis-cis* diester has been estimated from studies in cats to have one-tenth the neuromuscular blocking potency of the other two stereoisomers.

MIVACRON Injection is a sterile, non-pyrogenic solution (pH 3.5 to 5) containing mivacurium chloride equivalent to 2 mg/mL mivacurium in Water for Injection. Hydrochloric acid may have been added to adjust pH.

CLINICAL PHARMACOLOGY

MIVACRON (a mixture of three stereoisomers) binds competitively to cholinergic receptors on the motor end-plate to antagonize the action of acetylcholine, resulting in a block of neuromuscular transmission. This action is antagonized by acetylcholinesterase inhibitors, such as neostigmine.

Pharmacodynamics

The time to maximum neuromuscular block is similar for recommended doses of MIVACRON and intermediate-acting agents (e.g., atracurium), but longer than for the ultra-short-acting agent, succinylcholine. The clinically effective duration of action of MIVACRON (a mixture of three stereoisomers) is one-third to one-half that of intermediate-acting agents and 2 to 2.5 times that of succinylcholine.

The average ED_{95} (dose required to produce 95% suppression of the adductor pollicis muscle twitch response to ulnar nerve stimulation) of MIVACRON is 0.07 mg/kg (range: 0.05 mg/kg to 0.09 mg/kg) in adults receiving opioid/nitrous oxide/oxygen anesthesia. The pharmacodynamics of doses of MIVACRON greater than or equal to ED_{95} administered over 5 to 15 seconds during opioid/nitrous oxide/oxygen anesthesia are summarized in Table 1. The mean time for spontaneous recovery of the twitch response from 25% to 75% of control amplitude is about 6 minutes (range: 3 to 9 minutes, n = 32) following an initial dose of 0.15 mg/kg MIVACRON and 7 to 8 minutes (range: 4 to 24 minutes, n = 85) following initial doses of 0.2 or 0.25 mg/kg MIVACRON.

Volatile anesthetics may decrease the dosing requirement for MIVACRON and prolong the duration of action; the magnitude of these effects may be increased as the concentration of the volatile agent is increased. Isoflurane and enflurane (administered with nitrous oxide/oxygen to achieve 1.25 MAC [Minimum Alveolar Concentration]) may decrease the effective dose of MIVACRON by as much as 25%, and may prolong the clinically effective duration of action and decrease the average infusion requirement by as much as 35% to 40%. At equivalent MAC values, halothane has little or no effect on the ED_{50} of MIVACRON, but may prolong the duration of action and decrease the average infusion requirement by as much as 20% (see **CLINICAL PHARMACOLOGY - Individualization of Dosages** subsection and **PRECAUTIONS - Drug Interactions**).

[See table 1 above]

Administration of MIVACRON over 30 to 60 seconds does not alter the time to maximum neuromuscular block or the duration of action. The duration of action of MIVACRON may be prolonged in patients with reduced plasma cholinesterase (pseudocholinesterase) activity (see **PRECAUTIONS - Reduced Plasma Cholinesterase Activity** and **CLINICAL PHARMACOLOGY - Individualization of Dosages** subsection).

Continued on next page

Table 1. Pharmacodynamic Dose Response During Opioid/Nitrous Oxide/Oxygen Anesthesia

Initial Dose of MIVACRON* (mg/kg)		Time to Maximum Block[†] (min)	5% Recovery (min)	Time to Spontaneous Recovery[†]			T_4/T_1 Ratio ≥ 75%[§] (min)
				25% Recovery[‡] (min)	95% Recovery[§] (min)		
Adults							
0.07 to 0.1	[n = 47]	4.9 (2-7.6)	11 (7-19)	13 (8-24)	21 (10-36)		21 (10-36)
0.15	[n = 50]	3.3 (1.5-8.8)	13 (6-31)	16 (9-38)	26 (16-41)		26 (15-45)
0.2‖	[n = 50]	2.5 (1.2-6)	16 (10-29)	20 (10-36)	31 (15-51)		34 (19-56)
0.25‖	[n = 48]	2.3 (1-4.8)	19 (11-29)	23 (14-38)	34 (22-64)		43 (26-75)
Children 2 to 12 Years							
0.11 to 0.12	[n = 17]	2.8 (1.2-4.6)	5 (3-9)	7 (4-10)	–		–
0.2	[n = 18]	1.9 (1.3-3.3)	7 (3-12)	10 (6-15)	19 (14-26)		16 (12-23)
0.25	[n = 9]	1.6 (1-2.2)	7 (4-9)	9 (5-12)	–		–

* Doses administered over 5 to 15 seconds.
† Values shown are medians of means from individual studies (range of individual patient values).
‡ Clinically effective duration of neuromuscular block.
§ Data available for as few as 40% of adults in specific dose groups and for 22% of children in the 0.2 mg/kg dose group due to administration of reversal agents or additional doses of MIVACRON prior to 95% recovery or T_4/T_1 ratio recovery to greater than or equal to 75%.
‖ Rapid administration not recommended due to possibility of decreased blood pressure. Administer 0.2 mg/kg over 30 seconds; administer 0.25 mg/kg as divided dose (0.15 mg/kg followed 30 seconds later by 0.1 mg/kg). (See **DOSAGE AND ADMINISTRATION**.)

Interpatient variability in duration of action occurs with MIVACRON as with other neuromuscular blocking agents. However, analysis of data from 224 patients in clinical studies receiving various doses of MIVACRON during opioid/nitrous oxide/oxygen anesthesia with a variety of premedicants and varying lengths of surgery indicated that approximately 90% of the patients had clinically effective durations of block within 8 minutes of the median duration predicted from the dose-response data shown in Table 1. Variations in plasma cholinesterase activity, including values within the normal range and values as low as 20% below the lower limit of the normal range, were not associated with clinically significant effects on duration. The variability in duration, however, was greater in patients with plasma cholinesterase activity at or slightly below the lower limit of the normal range.

When administered during the induction of adequate anesthesia using thiopental or propofol, nitrous oxide/oxygen, and co-induction agents such as fentanyl and/or midazolam, doses of 0.15 mg/kg (2 × ED_{95}) MIVACRON administered over 5 to 15 seconds or 0.2 mg/kg MIVACRON administered over 30 seconds produced generally good-to-excellent tracheal intubation conditions in 2.5 to 3 and 2 to 2.5 minutes, respectively. A dose of 0.25 mg/kg MIVACRON administered as a divided dose (0.15 mg/kg followed 30 seconds later by 0.1 mg/kg) produced generally good-to-excellent intubation conditions in 1.5 to 2 minutes after initiating the dosing regimen.

Repeated administration of maintenance doses or continuous infusion of MIVACRON for up to 2.5 hours is not associated with development of tachyphylaxis or cumulative neuromuscular blocking effects in ASA Physical Status I-II patients. Based on pharmacokinetic studies in 82 adults receiving infusions of MIVACRON for longer than 2.5 hours, spontaneous recovery of neuromuscular function after infusion is independent of the duration of infusion and comparable to recovery reported for single doses (Table 1).

MIVACRON was administered as an infusion for as long as 4 to 6 hours in 20 adult patients and 19 geriatric patients. In most patients, after a brief period of adjustment, the rate of MIVACRON required to maintain 89% to 99% T_1 suppression remained relatively constant over time. There was a subset of patients in each group whose infusion rates did not stabilize quickly and decreased (by greater than or equal to 30%) over the period of infusion. The rate of spontaneous recovery in these patients was comparable with that of patients having stable infusion rates and not dependent on the duration of infusion. These patients, however, tended to have higher infusion requirements (i.e., greater than 8 mcg/kg/min) during the first 30 minutes of infusion than patients with stable infusion rates, although their final infusion rates were similar to those with stable infusion rates. There were no clinically important differences in infusion rate requirements between geriatric and young patients (see **Pharmacokinetics - Special Populations - Geriatric Patients**).

The neuromuscular block produced by MIVACRON is readily antagonized by anticholinesterase agents. As seen with other nondepolarizing neuromuscular blocking agents, the more profound the neuromuscular block at the time of reversal, the longer the time and the greater the dose of anticholinesterase agent required for recovery of neuromuscular function.

In children (2 to 12 years), MIVACRON has a higher ED_{95} (0.1 mg/kg), faster onset, and shorter duration of action than in adults. The mean time for spontaneous recovery of the twitch response from 25% to 75% of control amplitude is about 5 minutes (n = 4) following an initial dose of 0.2 mg/kg MIVACRON. Recovery following reversal is faster in children than in adults (Table 1).

Hemodynamics

Administration of MIVACRON in doses up to and including 0.15 mg/kg (2 × ED_{95}) over 5 to 15 seconds to ASA Physical Status I-II patients during opioid/nitrous oxide/oxygen anesthesia is associated with minimal changes in mean arterial blood pressure (MAP) or heart rate (HR) (Table 2).

Table 2. Cardiovascular Dose Response During Opioid/Nitrous Oxide/Oxygen Anesthesia

Initial Dose of MIVACRON* (mg/kg)		% of Patients With ≥ 30% Change: MAP Dec	MAP Inc	HR Dec	HR Inc
Adults					
0.07 to 0.1	[n = 49]	0%	2%	0%	0%
0.15	[n = 53]	4%	4%	4%	2%
0.2†	[n = 53]	30%	0%	0%	8%
0.25†	[n = 44]	39%	2%	0%	14%
Children 2 to 12 years					
0.11 to 0.12	[n = 17]	0%	6%	0%	0%
0.2	[n = 17]	0%	0%	0%	0%
0.25	[n = 8]	13%	0%	0%	0%

* Doses administered over 5 to 15 seconds.
† Rapid administration not recommended due to possibility of decreased blood pressure. Administer 0.2 mg/kg over 30 seconds; administer 0.25 mg/kg as divided dose (0.15 mg/kg followed 30 seconds later by 0.1 mg/kg). (See **DOSAGE AND ADMINISTRATION**.)

Higher doses of greater than or equal to 0.2 mg/kg (greater than or equal to 3 × ED_{95}) may be associated with transient decreases in MAP and increases in HR in some patients. These decreases in MAP are usually maximal within 1 to 3 minutes following the dose, typically resolve without treatment in an additional 1 to 3 minutes, and are usually associated with increases in plasma histamine concentration. Decreases in MAP can be minimized by administering MIVACRON over 30 to 60 seconds (see **CLINICAL PHARMACOLOGY - Individualization of Dosages** subsection and **PRECAUTIONS - General**).

Analysis of 426 patients in clinical studies receiving initial doses of MIVACRON up to and including 0.3 mg/kg during opioid/nitrous oxide/oxygen anesthesia showed that high initial doses and a rapid rate of injection contributed to a greater probability of experiencing a decrease of greater than or equal to 30% in MAP after administration of MIVACRON. Obese patients also had a greater probability of experiencing a decrease of greater than or equal to 30% in MAP when dosed on the basis of actual body weight, thereby receiving a larger dose than if dosed on the basis of ideal body weight (see **CLINICAL PHARMACOLOGY - Individualization of Dosages** subsection and **PRECAUTIONS - General**).

Children experience minimal changes in MAP or HR after administration of doses of MIVACRON up to and including 0.2 mg/kg over 5 to 15 seconds, but higher doses (greater than or equal to 0.25 mg/kg) may be associated with transient decreases in MAP (Table 2).

Following a dose of 0.15 mg/kg MIVACRON administered over 60 seconds, adult patients with significant cardiovascular disease undergoing coronary artery bypass grafting or valve replacement procedures showed no clinically important changes in MAP or HR. Transient decreases in MAP were observed in some patients after doses of 0.2 to 0.25 mg/kg MIVACRON administered over 60 seconds. The number of patients in whom these decreases in MAP required treatment was small.

Pharmacokinetics

MIVACRON is a mixture of isomers which do not interconvert *in vivo*. The *cis-trans* and *trans-trans* isomers (92% to 96% of the mixture) are equipotent. The steady-state concentrations of the *cis-trans* and *trans-trans* isomers doubled after the infusion rate was increased from 5 to 10 mcg/kg/min, indicating that their pharmacokinetics is dose-proportional.

Table 3. Stereoisomer Pharmacokinetic Parameters* of Mivacurium in ASA Physical Status I-II Adult Patients† [n = 18] During Opioid/Nitrous Oxide/Oxygen Anesthesia

Parameter	*trans-trans* isomer	*cis-trans* isomer
Elimination Half-life ($t_{1/2}$ min)	2 (1-3.6)	1.8 (0.8-4.8)
Volume of Distribution‡ (mL/kg)	147 (67-254)	276 (79-772)
Plasma Clearance (mL/min/kg)	53 (26-98)	99 (44-199)

* Values shown are mean (range).
† Ages 31 to 48 years.
‡ Volume of distribution during the terminal elimination phase.

The *cis-cis* isomer (6% of the mixture) has approximately one-tenth the neuromuscular blocking potency of the *trans-trans* and *cis-trans* isomers in cats. Neuromuscular blocking effects due to the *cis-cis* isomer cannot be ruled out in humans; however, modeling of clinical pharmacokinetic-pharmacodynamic data suggests that the *cis-cis* isomer produces minimal (less than 5%) neuromuscular block during a 2-hour infusion. In studies of ASA Physical Status I-II patients receiving infusions of MIVACRON lasting as long as 4 to 6 hours, the 5% to 25% and the 25% to 75% recovery indices were independent of the duration of infusion, suggesting that the *cis-cis* isomer does not affect the rate of post-infusion recovery.

Distribution

The volume of distribution of *cis-trans* and *trans-trans* isomers in healthy surgical patients is relatively small, reflecting limited tissue distribution (Table 3). The volume of distribution of *cis-cis* isomers is also small and averaged 335 mL/kg (range 192 to 523) in the 18 healthy surgical patients whose data are displayed in Table 3. The protein binding of mivacurium has not been determined due to its rapid hydrolysis by plasma cholinesterase.

Metabolism

Enzymatic hydrolysis by plasma cholinesterase is the primary mechanism for inactivation of mivacurium and yields a quaternary alcohol and a quaternary monoester metabolite. Tests in which these two metabolites were administered to cats and dogs suggest that each metabolite is unlikely to produce clinically significant neuromuscular, autonomic, or cardiovascular effects following administration of MIVACRON.

The mean ± S.D. *in vitro* $t_{1/2}$ values of the *trans-trans* and the *cis-trans* isomers were 1.3 ± 0.3 and 0.8 ± 0.2 minutes, respectively, in human plasma from healthy male (n = 5) and female (n = 5) volunteers. The mean *in vivo* $t_{1/2}$ values for the more potent *trans-trans* and *cis-trans* isomers in healthy surgical patients (Table 3) were similar to those found *in vitro*, suggesting that hydrolysis by plasma cholinesterase is the predominant elimination pathway for these isomers. The mean ± S.D. *in vitro* $t_{1/2}$ of the less potent *cis-cis* isomer was 276 ± 130 minutes, while the mean ± S.D. *in vivo* $t_{1/2}$ for the *cis-cis* isomer in healthy surgical patients was 53 ± 20 minutes. These data suggest that *in vivo*, pathways other than hydrolysis by plasma cholinesterase contribute to the elimination of the *cis-cis* isomer.

Elimination

The clearance (CL) values of the two more potent isomers, *cis-trans* and *trans-trans*, are very high and are dependent on plasma cholinesterase activity (Table 3). The combination of high CL and low distribution volume results in $t_{1/2}$ values of approximately 2 minutes for the two more potent isomers. The short $t_{1/2}$ and high CL of the more potent isomers are consistent with the short duration of action of MIVACRON.

The CL of the less potent *cis-cis* isomer is not dependent on plasma cholinesterase. The mean ± S.D. CL was 4.6 ± 1.1 mL/min/kg and $t_{1/2}$ was 53 ± 20 minutes in the 18 healthy surgical patients whose data are displayed in Table 3.

Renal and biliary excretion of unchanged mivacurium are minor elimination pathways; urine and bile are important elimination pathways for the two metabolites.

Special Populations

Geriatric Patients (greater than or equal to 60 years)

Two pharmacokinetic/pharmacodynamic studies of MIVACRON have been conducted in geriatric patients. The first study compared the pharmacokinetics and pharmacodynamics of mivacurium in 19 geriatric patients with those in 20 adult patients receiving infusions for as long as 4 to 6 hours. The average infusion rate required to produce 89% to 99% T_1 suppression was slightly (~ 14%) lower in geriatric patients. This difference is not regarded as clinically important, but is most likely secondary to differences in pharmacokinetics (i.e., a lower CL of the *cis-trans* and *trans-trans* isomers in geriatric patients) (Table 4). The rate of post-infusion spontaneous recovery was not dependent on duration of infusion and appeared to be comparable in these geriatric patients and adult patients. Two pharmacodynamic studies in which patients received infusions for a shorter duration (2 to 3 hours) have shown that the infusion rate requirements were lower (by 38%) in geriatric patients (64 to 86 years of age) than in younger patients (18 to 41 years of age).

Table 4. Stereoisomer Pharmacokinetic Parameters* of Mivacurium in ASA Physical Status I-II Adult Patients [18-58 Years] and Geriatric Patients [60-81 Years] During Opioid/Nitrous Oxide/Oxygen Anesthesia

Parameter	Isomer	Adult Patients (n = 12)	Geriatric Patients (n = 8)
Plasma Clearance (mL/min/kg)	trans-trans isomer	54 (34 - 129)	32 (18 - 55)
	cis-trans isomer	91 (27 - 825)	47 (24 - 93)

* Values shown are median (range).

The second pharmacokinetic/pharmacodynamic study showed no clinically important differences in the pharmacokinetics of the individual isomers nor the ED_{95} determined for 36 young adult patients (18 to 40 years) and 35 geriatric patients (greater than or equal to 65 years) during opioid/nitrous oxide/oxygen anesthesia. Following infusions for up to 3.5 hours in these patients, the rate of spontaneous recovery was slightly (~ 2 to 4 minutes, on average) slower in the geriatric patients than in young adult patients.

In a third study of the pharmacodynamics of 0.1 mg/kg MIVACRON administered to eight geriatric patients (68 to 77 years) and nine adult patients (18 to 49 years) during N_2O/O_2/isoflurane anesthesia, the time to onset was approximately 1.5 minutes slower in geriatric patients than in adult patients. In addition, the clinical duration was slightly (~ 3 minutes, on average) longer in geriatric patients than in adult patients; these differences are not considered clinically important.

Although these studies showed conflicting findings, in general, the clearances of the more potent isomers are most likely lower in geriatric patients. This difference does not lead to clinically important differences in the ED_{95} of MIVACRON or the infusion rate of MIVACRON required to produce 95% T_1 suppression in geriatric patients. However, the time to onset may be slower, the duration may be slightly longer, the rate of recovery may be slightly slower, therefore MIVACRON requirements may be lower in geriatric patients.

Patients with Renal Disease

An early clinical trial showed that the clinically effective duration of action of 0.15 mg/kg MIVACRON was about 1.5 times longer in kidney transplant patients than in healthy patients, presumably due to reduced clearance of one or more isomers. A second study was conducted in seven patients with mild to moderate renal impairment, eight patients with severe renal dysfunction (not undergoing transplantation), and 11 patients with normal renal function. This study showed that the pharmacokinetics of the more potent (cis-trans and trans-trans) isomers were not statistically significantly affected by renal impairment or failure (Table 5). However, the CL of the cis-cis isomer was lower and the $t_{1/2}$ values of the cis-cis isomer and metabolites were longer in patients with renal impairment or failure than in patients with normal renal function. The second study also showed that there were no differences in the average infusion rate required to produce 89% to 99% T_1 suppression, nor were there any differences in the post-infusion recovery profile among these populations (Table 5). A third study in a similar population showed that patients with renal dysfunction had a longer duration and a slower rate of recovery than patients with normal renal function. This study did, however, confirm that there were no differences in the average infusion rate required to produce 89% to 99% T_1 suppression in these patient populations. Therefore, although there were minor differences in the pharmacokinetics of the cis-cis isomer and metabolites, there were no clinically significant differences in the infusion rate requirements of MIVACRON in patients with mild, moderate, or severe renal dysfunction receiving infusions of MIVACRON for an average of 1 to 2 hours; however, the duration may be longer and the rate of recovery may be slower following administration of MIVACRON in some patients with renal dysfunction.

[See table 5 above]

Patients with Hepatic Disease

The clinically effective duration of action of 0.15 mg/kg MIVACRON was three times longer in eight patients with end-stage liver disease (undergoing liver transplantation) than in eight healthy patients and is likely related to the markedly decreased plasma cholinesterase activity (30% of healthy patient values) which could decrease the clearance of the trans-trans and cis-trans isomers (see **PRECAUTIONS - Reduced Plasma Cholinesterase Activity**).

Table 5. Stereoisomer Pharmacokinetic Parameters* of Mivacurium in ASA Physical Status I-II Adult Patients with Normal Renal Function [Serum Creatinine less than or equal to 1 mg/dL], Patients with Mild to Moderate Renal Dysfunction [Serum Creatinine 1.3 to 2.7 mg/dL] and Patients with Severe Renal Dysfunction [Serum Creatinine greater than 6.2 mg/dL] During Opioid/Nitrous Oxide/Oxygen Anesthesia

Parameter	Isomer	Normal Renal Function (n = 10)	Mild to Moderate Renal Dysfunction (n = 8)	Severe Renal Dysfunction (n = 7)
Plasma Clearance (mL/min/kg)	trans-trans isomer	54 (19 - 91)	49 (43 - 59)	53 (17 - 82)
	cis-trans isomer	97‡ (28 - 215)	93 (72 - 115)	110 (23 - 199)
	cis-cis isomer	4 (2.9 - 5.4)	2.5 (1.9 - 3.8)	2.8 (2.1 - 4.7)
Volume of Distribution† (mL/kg)	trans-trans isomer	179 (67 - 492)	243 (119 - 707)	238 (93 - 397)
	cis-trans isomer	303§ (97 - 776)	474 (284 - 908)	416‖ (64 - 802)
	cis-cis isomer	287 (169 - 424)	323 (254 - 473)	276 (213 - 351)
Half-life (min)	trans-trans isomer	2.6 (1 - 6.8)	3.6 (1.7 - 10.7)	3.2 (1.6 - 4.1)
	cis-trans isomer	2.3§ (0.7 - 5.2)	3.7 (2.2 - 6.9)	2.6‖ (1.2 - 5.1)
	cis-cis isomer	52 (28 - 80)	90 (66 - 103)	73 (34 - 111)
25% to 75% Recovery Index (min)		10.8¶ (7.3 - 19.9)	9.2 (5.2 - 13.8)	10.3§ (4.1 - 14.2)

* Values shown are mean (range).
† Volume of distribution during the terminal elimination phase.
‡ n = 9
§ n = 8
‖ n = 6
¶ n = 11

A separate study compared the pharmacokinetics and pharmacodynamics of mivacurium in patients with mild or moderate cirrhosis to healthy adults with normal hepatic function (Table 6). Although the number of patients in each group is small, the CL values of the more potent isomers, trans-trans and cis-trans, are lower in patients with mild to moderate cirrhosis as expected based on the marked decreases in plasma cholinesterase activity in this population (see **PRECAUTIONS - Reduced Plasma Cholinesterase Activity**).

[See table 6 on next page]

Individualization of Dosages

Doses of MIVACRON should be individualized and a peripheral nerve stimulator should be used to measure neuromuscular function during administration of MIVACRON in order to monitor drug effect, determine the need for additional doses, and confirm recovery from neuromuscular block.

Based on the known actions of MIVACRON (a mixture of three stereoisomers) and other neuromuscular blocking agents, the following factors should be considered when administering MIVACRON:

Renal or Hepatic Impairment

A dose of 0.15 mg/kg MIVACRON is recommended for facilitation of tracheal intubation in patients with renal or hepatic impairment. However, the clinically effective duration of block produced by this dose may be about 1.5 times longer in patients with end-stage kidney disease and about 3 times longer in patients with end-stage liver disease than in patients with normal renal and hepatic function. Infusion rates should be decreased by as much as 50% in patients with hepatic disease depending on the degree of hepatic impairment (see **PRECAUTIONS - Renal and Hepatic Disease**). No infusion rate adjustments are necessary in patients with renal impairment.

Reduced Plasma Cholinesterase Activity

The possibility of prolonged neuromuscular block following administration of MIVACRON must be considered in patients with reduced plasma cholinesterase (pseudocholinesterase) activity. MIVACRON should be used with great caution, if at all, in patients known or suspected of being homozygous for the atypical plasma cholinesterase gene (see **WARNINGS**). Doses of 0.03 mg/kg produced complete neuromuscular block for 26 to 128 minutes in three such patients; thus initial doses greater than 0.03 mg/kg are not recommended in homozygous patients. Infusions of MIVACRON are not recommended in homozygous patients. MIVACRON has been used safely in patients heterozygous for the atypical plasma cholinesterase gene and in genotypically normal patients with reduced plasma cholinesterase activity. After an initial dose of 0.15 mg/kg MIVACRON, the clinically effective duration of block in heterozygous patients may be approximately 10 minutes longer than in patients with normal genotype and normal plasma cholinesterase activity. Lower infusion rates of MIVACRON are recommended in these patients (see **PRECAUTIONS - Reduced Plasma Cholinesterase Activity**).

Drugs or Conditions Causing Potentiation of or Resistance to Neuromuscular Block

As with other neuromuscular blocking agents, MIVACRON may have profound neuromuscular blocking effects in cachectic or debilitated patients, patients with neuromuscular diseases, and patients with carcinomatosis. In these or other patients in whom potentiation of neuromuscular block or difficulty with reversal may be anticipated, the initial dose should be decreased. A test dose of not more than 0.015 to 0.02 mg/kg, which represents the lower end of the dose-response curve for MIVACRON, is recommended in such patients (see **PRECAUTIONS - General**).

The neuromuscular blocking action of MIVACRON is potentiated by isoflurane or enflurane anesthesia. Recommended initial doses of MIVACRON (see **DOSAGE AND ADMINISTRATION**) may be used for intubation prior to the administration of these agents. If MIVACRON is first administered after establishment of stable-state isoflurane or enflurane anesthesia (administered with nitrous oxide/oxygen to achieve 1.25 MAC), the initial dose of MIVACRON should be reduced by as much as 25%, and the infusion rate reduced by as much as 35% to 40%. A greater potentiation of the neuromuscular blocking action of MIVACRON may be expected with higher concentrations of enflurane or isoflurane. The use of halothane requires no adjustment of the initial dose of MIVACRON, but may prolong the duration of action and decrease the average infusion rate by as much as 20% (see **PRECAUTIONS - Drug Interactions**).

When MIVACRON is administered to patients receiving certain antibiotics, magnesium salts, lithium, local anesthetics, procainamide and quinidine, longer durations of neuromuscular block may be expected and infusion requirements may be lower (see **PRECAUTIONS - Drug Interactions**).

When MIVACRON is administered to patients chronically receiving phenytoin or carbamazepine, slightly shorter durations of neuromuscular block may be anticipated and infusion rate requirements may be higher (see **PRECAUTIONS - Drug Interactions**).

Severe acid-base and/or electrolyte abnormalities may potentiate or cause resistance to the neuromuscular blocking action of MIVACRON. No data are available in such patients and no dosing recommendations can be made (see **PRECAUTIONS - General**).

Burns

While patients with burns are known to develop resistance to nondepolarizing neuromuscular blocking agents, they may also have reduced plasma cholinesterase activity. Consequently, in these patients, a test dose of not more than 0.015 to 0.02 mg/kg MIVACRON is recommended, followed

Continued on next page

Information on the AbbVie, Inc. products listed on these pages is from the prescribing information in use as of July 31, 2016. For more information, please visit rxabbvie.com or call 1-800-633-9110.

by additional appropriate dosing guided by the use of a neuromuscular block monitor (see **PRECAUTIONS - General**).

Cardiovascular Disease

In patients with clinically significant cardiovascular disease, the initial dose of MIVACRON should be 0.15 mg/kg or less, administered over 60 seconds (see **CLINICAL PHARMACOLOGY - Hemodynamics** subsection and **PRECAUTIONS - General**).

Obesity

Obese patients (patients weighing greater than or equal to 30% more than their ideal body weight) dosed on the basis of actual body weight, thereby receiving a larger dose than if dosed on the basis of ideal body weight, had a greater probability of experiencing a decrease of greater than or equal to 30% in MAP effect (see **CLINICAL PHARMACOLOGY - Hemodynamics** subsection and **PRECAUTIONS - General**). Therefore, in obese patients, the initial dose should be determined using the patient's ideal body weight (IBW), according to the following formulae:

Men:	IBW in kg = (106 + [6 × inches in height above 5 feet])/2.2

Women:	IBW in kg = (100 + [5 × inches in height above 5 feet])/2.2

Allergy and Sensitivity

In patients with any history suggestive of a greater sensitivity to the release of histamine or related mediators (e.g., asthma), the initial dose of MIVACRON should be 0.15 mg/kg or less, administered over 60 seconds (see **PRECAUTIONS - General**).

INDICATIONS AND USAGE

MIVACRON is a short-acting neuromuscular blocking agent indicated for inpatients and outpatients, as an adjunct to general anesthesia, to facilitate tracheal intubation and to provide skeletal muscle relaxation during surgery or mechanical ventilation.

CONTRAINDICATIONS

MIVACRON is contraindicated in patients with known hypersensitivity to the product and its components.

WARNINGS

Anaphylaxis

Severe anaphylactic reactions to neuromuscular blocking agents, including MIVACRON, have been reported. These reactions have in some cases been life-threatening and fatal. Due to the potential severity of these reactions, the necessary precautions, such as the immediate availability of appropriate emergency treatment, should be taken. Precautions should also be taken in those individuals who have had previous anaphylactic reactions to other neuromuscular blocking agents since cross-reactivity between neuromuscular blocking agents, both depolarizing and non-depolarizing, has been reported in this class of drugs.

Administration

MIVACRON should be administered in carefully adjusted dosage by or under the supervision of experienced clinicians who are familiar with the drug's actions and the possible complications of its use. The drug should not be administered unless personnel and facilities for resuscitation and life support (tracheal intubation, artificial ventilation, oxygen therapy), and an antagonist of MIVACRON are immediately available. It is recommended that a peripheral nerve stimulator be used to measure neuromuscular function during the administration of MIVACRON in order to monitor drug effect, determine the need for additional drug, and confirm recovery from neuromuscular block. MIVACRON has no known effect on consciousness, pain threshold, or cerebration. To avoid distress to the patient, neuromuscular block should not be induced before unconsciousness.

MIVACRON is metabolized by plasma cholinesterase and should be used with great caution, if at all, in patients known to be or suspected of being homozygous for the atypical plasma cholinesterase gene.

MIVACRON Injection is acidic (pH 3.5 to 5) and may not be compatible with alkaline solutions having a pH greater than 8.5 (e.g., barbiturate solutions).

PRECAUTIONS

General

Although MIVACRON (a mixture of three stereoisomers) is not a potent histamine releaser, the possibility of substantial histamine release must be considered. Release of histamine is related to the dose and speed of injection.

Caution should be exercised in administering MIVACRON to patients with clinically significant cardiovascular disease and patients with any history suggesting a greater sensitivity to the release of histamine or related mediators (e.g., asthma). In such patients, the initial dose of MIVACRON should be 0.15 mg/kg or less, administered over 60 seconds; assurance of adequate hydration and careful monitoring of hemodynamic status are important (see **CLINICAL PHARMACOLOGY - Hemodynamics** and **Individualization of Dosages**).

Obese patients may be more likely to experience clinically significant transient decreases in MAP than non-obese patients when the dose of MIVACRON is based on actual rather than ideal body weight. Therefore, in obese patients, the initial dose should be determined using the patient's ideal body weight (see **CLINICAL PHARMACOLOGY - Hemodynamics and Individualization of Dosages**).

Recommended doses of MIVACRON have no clinically significant effects on heart rate; therefore, MIVACRON will not counteract the bradycardia produced by many anesthetic agents or by vagal stimulation.

Neuromuscular blocking agents may have a profound effect in patients with neuromuscular diseases (e.g., myasthenia gravis and the myasthenic syndrome). In these and other conditions in which prolonged neuromuscular block is a possibility (e.g., carcinomatosis), the use of a peripheral nerve stimulator and a dose of not more than 0.015 to 0.02 mg/kg MIVACRON is recommended to assess the level of neuromuscular block and to monitor dosage requirements (see **CLINICAL PHARMACOLOGY - Individualization of Dosages**).

MIVACRON has not been studied in patients with burns. Resistance to nondepolarizing neuromuscular blocking agents may develop in patients with burns, depending upon the time elapsed since the injury and the size of the burn. Patients with burns may have reduced plasma cholinesterase activity which may offset this resistance (see **CLINICAL PHARMACOLOGY - Individualization of Dosages**). Acid-base and/or serum electrolyte abnormalities may potentiate or antagonize the action of neuromuscular blocking agents. The action of neuromuscular blocking agents may be enhanced by magnesium salts administered for the management of toxemia of pregnancy (see **CLINICAL PHARMACOLOGY - Individualization of Dosages**).

No data are available to support the use of MIVACRON by intramuscular injection.

Allergic Reactions

Since allergic cross-reactivity has been reported in this class, request information from your patients about previous anaphylactic reactions to other neuromuscular blocking agents. In addition, inform your patients that severe anaphylactic reactions to neuromuscular blocking agents, including MIVACRON have been reported (see **CONTRAINDICATIONS**).

Renal and Hepatic Disease

The possibility of prolonged neuromuscular block must be considered when MIVACRON is used in patients with renal or hepatic disease (see **CLINICAL PHARMACOLOGY - Pharmacokinetics**). Most patients with chronic hepatic disease such as hepatitis, liver abscess, and cirrhosis of the liver exhibit a marked reduction in plasma cholinesterase activity. Patients with acute or chronic renal disease may also show a reduction in plasma cholinesterase activity (see **CLINICAL PHARMACOLOGY - Individualization of Dosages**).

Reduced Plasma Cholinesterase Activity

The possibility of prolonged neuromuscular block following administration of MIVACRON must be considered in patients with reduced plasma cholinesterase (pseudocholinesterase) activity.

Plasma cholinesterase activity may be diminished in the presence of genetic abnormalities of plasma cholinesterase (e.g., patients heterozygous or homozygous for the atypical plasma cholinesterase gene), pregnancy, liver or kidney disease, malignant tumors, infections, burns, anemia, decompensated heart disease, peptic ulcer, or myxedema. Plasma cholinesterase activity may also be diminished by chronic administration of oral contraceptives, glucocorticoids, or certain monoamine oxidase inhibitors and by irreversible inhibitors of plasma cholinesterase (e.g., organophosphate insecticides, echothiophate, and certain antineoplastic drugs).

MIVACRON has been used safely in patients heterozygous for the atypical plasma cholinesterase gene. At doses of 0.1 to 0.2 mg/kg MIVACRON, the clinically effective duration of action was 8 minutes to 11 minutes longer in patients heterozygous for the atypical gene than in genotypically normal patients.

As with succinylcholine, patients homozygous for the atypical plasma cholinesterase gene (one in 2500 patients) are extremely sensitive to the neuromuscular blocking effect of MIVACRON. In three such adult patients, a small dose of 0.03 mg/kg (approximately the ED_{10-20} in genotypically normal patients) produced complete neuromuscular block for 26 to 128 minutes. Once spontaneous recovery had begun, neuromuscular block in these patients was antagonized with conventional doses of neostigmine. One adult patient, who was homozygous for the atypical plasma cholinesterase gene, received a dose of 0.18 mg/kg MIVACRON and exhibited complete neuromuscular block for about 4 hours. Response to post-tetanic stimulation was present after 4 hours, all four responses to train-of-four stimulation were present after 6 hours, and the patient was extubated after 8 hours. Reversal was not attempted in this patient.

Malignant Hyperthermia (MH)

In a study of MH-susceptible pigs, MIVACRON did not trigger MH. MIVACRON has not been studied in MH-susceptible patients. Because MH can develop in the absence of established triggering agents, the clinician should be prepared to recognize and treat MH in any patient undergoing general anesthesia.

Long-Term Use in the Intensive Care Unit (ICU)

No data are available on the long-term use of MIVACRON in patients undergoing mechanical ventilation in the ICU.

Drug Interactions

Although MIVACRON (a mixture of three stereoisomers) has been administered safely following succinylcholine-

Table 6. Pharmacokinetic and Pharmacodynamic Parameters* of Mivacurium in ASA Physical Status I-II Patients and In Patients with Mild or Moderate Cirrhosis During Opioid/Nitrous Oxide/Oxygen Anesthesia

Parameter	Isomer	Normal Hepatic Function (n = 10)	Degree of Hepatic Failure	
			Mild Cirrhosis (n = 5)	Moderate Cirrhosis (n = 6)
Plasma Clearance (mL/min/kg)	*trans-trans* isomer	66 (34 - 99)	43 (22 - 64)	31 (11 - 66)
	cis-trans isomer	124‡ (57 - 218)	73 (34 - 111)	52 (18 - 128)
	cis-cis isomer	8.6 (4.5 - 13.3)	8.6 (4.5 - 16.7)	5.6 (3.5 - 9.7)
Volume of Distribution† (mL/kg)	*trans-trans* isomer	204‡ (94 - 269)	221 (118 - 457)	191 (74 - 273)
	cis-trans isomer	201‡ (89 - 411)	152 (102 - 256)	111 (56 - 164)
	cis-cis isomer§	–	–	–
Half-life (min)	*trans-trans* isomer	2.4‡ (1.3 - 3.9)	3.7 (1.7 - 5.1)	5.3 (1.7 - 8.5)
	cis-trans isomer	1.2‡ (0.6 - 2.1)	1.6 (1 - 2.1)	1.9 (0.9 - 3)
	cis-cis isomer§	–		
25% to 75% Recovery Index (min)		7.3 (4.7 - 9.6)	9.5 (5.7 - 12.3)	16.4 (6.3 - 26.2)

* Values shown are mean (range).
† Volume of distribution during the terminal elimination phase.
‡ n = 9
§ Not available.

facilitated tracheal intubation, the interaction between MIVACRON and succinylcholine has not been systematically studied. Prior administration of succinylcholine can potentiate the neuromuscular blocking effects of nondepolarizing agents. Evidence of spontaneous recovery from succinylcholine should be observed before the administration of MIVACRON.

The use of MIVACRON before succinylcholine to attenuate some of the side effects of succinylcholine has not been studied.

There are no clinical data on the use of MIVACRON with other nondepolarizing neuromuscular blocking agents.

Isoflurane and enflurane (administered with nitrous oxide/oxygen to achieve 1.25 MAC) decrease the ED_{50} of MIVACRON by as much as 25% (see **CLINICAL PHARMACOLOGY - Pharmacodynamics** and **Individualization of Dosages**). These agents may also prolong the clinically effective duration of action and decrease the average infusion requirement of MIVACRON by as much as 35% to 40%. A greater potentiation of the neuromuscular blocking effects of MIVACRON may be expected with higher concentrations of enflurane or isoflurane. Halothane has little or no effect on the ED_{50}, but may prolong the duration of action and decrease the average infusion requirement by as much as 20%.

Other drugs which may enhance the neuromuscular blocking action of nondepolarizing agents such as MIVACRON include certain antibiotics (e.g., aminoglycosides, tetracyclines, bacitracin, polymyxins, lincomycin, clindamycin, colistin, and sodium colistimethate), magnesium salts, lithium, local anesthetics, procainamide, and quinidine. The neuromuscular blocking effect of MIVACRON may be enhanced by drugs that reduce plasma cholinesterase activity (e.g., chronically administered oral contraceptives, glucocorticoids, or certain monoamine oxidase inhibitors) or by drugs that irreversibly inhibit plasma cholinesterase (see **PRECAUTIONS - Reduced Plasma Cholinesterase Activity** subsection).

Resistance to the neuromuscular blocking action of nondepolarizing neuromuscular blocking agents has been demonstrated in patients chronically administered phenytoin or carbamazepine. While the effects of chronic phenytoin or carbamazepine therapy on the action of MIVACRON are unknown, slightly shorter durations of neuromuscular block may be anticipated and infusion rate requirements may be higher.

Carcinogenesis, Mutagenesis, Impairment of Fertility

Carcinogenesis and fertility studies have not been performed. MIVACRON was evaluated in a battery of four short-term mutagenicity tests. It was non-mutagenic in the Ames Salmonella assay, the mouse lymphoma assay, the human lymphocyte assay, and the *in vivo* rat bone marrow cytogenetic assay.

Pregnancy

Teratogenic Effects

Pregnancy Category C

Teratology testing in nonventilated pregnant rats and mice treated subcutaneously with maximum subparalyzing doses of MIVACRON revealed no maternal or fetal toxicity or teratogenic effects. There are no adequate and well-controlled studies of MIVACRON in pregnant women. Because animal studies are not always predictive of human response, and the doses used were subparalyzing, MIVACRON should be used during pregnancy only if the potential benefit justifies the potential risk to the fetus.

Labor and Delivery

The use of MIVACRON during labor, vaginal delivery, or cesarean section has not been studied in humans and it is not known whether MIVACRON administered to the mother has effects on the fetus. Doses of 0.08 and 0.2 mg/kg MIVACRON given to female beagles undergoing cesarean section resulted in negligible levels of the stereoisomers in MIVACRON in umbilical vessel blood of neonates and no deleterious effects on the puppies.

Nursing Mothers

It is not known whether any of the stereoisomers of mivacurium are excreted in human milk. Because many drugs are excreted in human milk, caution should be exercised following administration of MIVACRON to a nursing woman.

Pediatric Use

MIVACRON has not been studied in pediatric patients below the age of 2 years (see **CLINICAL PHARMACOLOGY** and **DOSAGE AND ADMINISTRATION** for clinical experience and recommendations for use in children 2 to 12 years of age).

Geriatric Use

MIVACRON was safely administered during clinical trials to 64 geriatric (greater than or equal to 65 years) patients, including 31 patients with significant cardiovascular disease (see **PRECAUTIONS - General** subsection). In general, the clearances of MIVACRON are most likely lower, the duration may be longer, the rate of recovery may be slower, therefore, MIVACRON requirements may be lower in geriatric patients (see **CLINICAL PHARMACOLOGY - Special Populations - Geriatric Patients**).

ADVERSE REACTIONS
Observed in Clinical Trials

MIVACRON (a mixture of three stereoisomers) was well tolerated during extensive clinical trials in inpatients and outpatients. Prolonged neuromuscular block, which is an important adverse experience associated with neuromuscular blocking agents as a class, was reported as an adverse experience in three of 2074 patients administered MIVACRON. The most commonly reported adverse experience following the administration of MIVACRON was transient, dose-dependent cutaneous flushing about the face, neck, and/or chest. Flushing was most frequently noted after the initial dose of MIVACRON and was reported in about 25% of adult patients who received 0.15 mg/kg MIVACRON over 5 to 15 seconds. When present, flushing typically began within 1 to 2 minutes after the dose of MIVACRON and lasted for 3 to 5 minutes. Of 105 patients who experienced flushing after 0.15 mg/kg MIVACRON, two patients also experienced mild hypotension that was not treated, and one patient experienced moderate wheezing that was successfully treated.

Overall, hypotension was infrequently reported as an adverse experience in the clinical trials of MIVACRON. One of 332 (0.3%) healthy adults who received 0.15 mg/kg MIVACRON over 5 to 15 seconds and none of 37 cardiac surgery patients who received 0.15 mg/kg MIVACRON over 60 seconds were treated for a decrease in blood pressure in association with the administration of MIVACRON. One to two percent of healthy adults given greater than or equal to 0.2 mg/kg MIVACRON over 5 to 15 seconds, 2% to 3% of healthy adults given 0.2 mg/kg over 30 seconds, none of 100 healthy adults given 0.25 mg/kg as a divided dose (0.15 mg/kg followed in 30 seconds by 0.1 mg/kg), and 2% to 4% of cardiac surgery patients given greater than or equal to 0.2 mg/kg over 60 seconds were treated for a decrease in blood pressure. None of the 63 children who received the recommended dose of 0.2 mg/kg MIVACRON was treated for a decrease in blood pressure in association with the administration of MIVACRON.

The following adverse experiences were reported in patients administered MIVACRON (all events judged by investigators during the clinical trials to have a possible causal relationship):

Incidence Greater Than 1%

Cardiovascular

Flushing (16%)

Incidence Less Than 1%

Cardiovascular

Hypotension, tachycardia, bradycardia, cardiac arrhythmia, phlebitis

Respiratory

Bronchospasm, wheezing, hypoxemia

Dermatological

Rash, urticaria, erythema, injection site reaction

Nonspecific

Prolonged drug effect

Neurologic

Dizziness

Musculoskeletal

Muscle spasms

Observed in Clinical Practice

Based on initial clinical practice experience in patients who received MIVACRON, spontaneously reported adverse events are uncommon. Some of these events occurred at recommended doses and required treatment.

Anaphylaxis/Anaphylactoid Reactions: From postmarketing surveillance, MIVACRON has been associated with reports of anaphylactic/anaphylactoid reactions which in some cases have been life-threatening and fatal. Because these reactions were reported voluntarily from a population of uncertain size, it is not possible to reliably estimate their frequency (see **WARNINGS** and **PRECAUTIONS**). In some of these reports, sensitivity to MIVACRON was confirmed using skin test procedures.

Other adverse reaction data from clinical practice are insufficient to establish a causal relationship or to support an estimate of their incidence. These adverse events include:

Musculoskeletal

Diminished drug effect, prolonged drug effect

Cardiovascular

Hypotension (rarely severe), flushing

Respiratory

Bronchospasm

Integumentary

Rash

OVERDOSAGE

Overdosage with neuromuscular blocking agents may result in neuromuscular block beyond the time needed for surgery and anesthesia. The primary treatment is maintenance of a patent airway and controlled ventilation until recovery of normal neuromuscular function is assured. Once evidence of recovery from neuromuscular block is observed, further recovery may be facilitated by administration of an anticholinesterase agent (e.g., neostigmine, edrophonium) in conjunction with an appropriate anticholinergic agent (see Antagonism of Neuromuscular Block subsection below). Overdosage may increase the risk of hemodynamic side effects, especially decreases in blood pressure. If needed, cardiovascular support may be provided by proper positioning of the patient, fluid administration, and/or vasopressor agent administration.

Antagonism of Neuromuscular Block

Antagonists (such as neostigmine) should not be administered when complete neuromuscular block is evident or suspected. The use of a peripheral nerve stimulator to evaluate recovery and antagonism of neuromuscular block is recommended.

Administration of 0.03 to 0.064 mg/kg neostigmine or 0.5 mg/kg edrophonium at approximately 10% recovery from neuromuscular block (range: 1 to 15) produced 95% recovery of the muscle twitch response and a T_4/T_1 ratio greater than or equal to 75% in about 10 minutes. The times from 25% recovery of the muscle twitch response to T_4/T_1 ratio greater than or equal to 75% following these doses of antagonists averaged about 7 to 9 minutes. In comparison, average times for spontaneous recovery from 25% to T_4/T_1 greater than or equal to 75% were 12 to 13 minutes.

Patients administered antagonists should be evaluated for adequate clinical evidence of antagonism, e.g., 5-second head lift and grip strength. Ventilation must be supported until no longer required.

Antagonism may be delayed in the presence of debilitation, carcinomatosis, and the concomitant use of certain broad spectrum antibiotics, or anesthetic agents and other drugs which enhance neuromuscular block or separately cause respiratory depression (see **PRECAUTIONS - Drug Interactions**). Under such circumstances the management is the same as that of prolonged neuromuscular block (see **OVERDOSAGE**).

DOSAGE AND ADMINISTRATION

MIVACRON SHOULD ONLY BE ADMINISTERED INTRAVENOUSLY.

The dosage information provided below is intended as a guide only. Doses of MIVACRON should be individualized (see **CLINICAL PHARMACOLOGY - Individualization of Dosages**). Factors that may warrant dosage adjustment include but may not be limited to: the presence of significant kidney, liver, or cardiovascular disease, obesity (patients weighing greater than or equal to 30% more than ideal body weight for height), asthma, reduction in plasma cholinesterase activity, and the presence of inhalational anesthetic agents.

When using MIVACRON or other neuromuscular blocking agents to facilitate tracheal intubation, it is important to recognize that the most important factors affecting intubation are the depth of general anesthesia and the level of neuromuscular block. Satisfactory intubating conditions can usually be achieved before complete neuromuscular block is attained if there is adequate anesthesia.

Continued on next page

Information on the AbbVie, Inc. products listed on these pages is from the prescribing information in use as of July 31, 2016. For more information, please visit rxabbvie.com or call 1-800-633-9110.

The use of a peripheral nerve stimulator will permit the most advantageous use of MIVACRON, minimize the possibility of overdosage or underdosage, and assist in the evaluation of recovery. When using a stimulator to monitor onset of neuromuscular block, clinical studies have shown that all four twitches of the train-of-four response may be present, with little or no fade, at the times recommended for intubation. Therefore, as with other neuromuscular blocking agents, it is important to use other criteria, such as clinical evaluation of the status of relaxation of jaw muscles and vocal cords, in conjunction with peripheral muscle twitch monitoring, to guide the appropriate time of intubation.

The onset of conditions suitable for tracheal intubation occurs earlier after a conventional intubating dose of succinylcholine than after recommended doses of MIVACRON.

Adults

Initial Doses

Doses of 0.15 mg/kg administered over 5 to 15 seconds, 0.2 mg/kg administered over 30 seconds, or 0.25 mg/kg administered in divided doses (0.15 mg/kg followed in 30 seconds by 0.1 mg/kg) are recommended for facilitation of tracheal intubation for most patients (see Table 7).

Table 7. Recommended Initial Dosing Regimens for Adults

Dosing Paradigm*	Anesthetic Induction Technique Studied	Time to Generally Good-to-Excellent Intubating Conditions
0.15 mg/kg, intravenous (over 5 to 15 sec)	Thiopental/opioid/N₂O/O₂ or propofol/opioid	2.5 to 3 min after completion of dose
0.2 mg/kg, intravenous (over 30 sec)	Thiopental/opioid/N₂O/O₂ or propofol/opioid	2 to 2.5 min after completion of dose
0.25 mg/kg, intravenous (0.15 mg/kg followed in 30 sec by 0.1 mg/kg)	Propofol/opioid	1.5 to 2 min after completion of 0.15 mg/kg dose

*Dosing instituted after induction of adequate general anesthesia.

The purpose of slowed or divided dosing of MIVACRON at doses above 0.15 mg/kg is to minimize the transient decreases in blood pressure observed in some patients given these doses over 5 to 15 seconds (see **CLINICAL PHARMACOLOGY, PRECAUTIONS,** and **ADVERSE REACTIONS**). The quality of intubation conditions does not significantly differ for the times and doses of MIVACRON recommended in Table 7, but the onset of suitable intubation conditions may be reached earlier with higher doses. The choice of a particular dose and regimen should be based on individual circumstances and patient requirements (see **CLINICAL PHARMACOLOGY - Individualization of Dosages**).

In patients with clinically significant cardiovascular disease and in patients with any history suggesting a greater sensitivity to the release of histamine or other mediators (e.g., asthma), the dose of MIVACRON should be 0.15 mg/kg or less, administered over 60 seconds (see **PRECAUTIONS**). No data are available on the use of doses of MIVACRON above 0.15 mg/kg in patients with clinically significant kidney or liver disease.

Clinically effective neuromuscular block may be expected to last for 15 to 20 minutes (range: 9 to 38 minutes) and spontaneous recovery may be expected to be 95% complete in 25 to 30 minutes (range: 16 to 41 minutes) following 0.15 mg/kg MIVACRON administered to patients receiving opioid/nitrous oxide/oxygen anesthesia. The expected duration of clinically effective block and time to 95% spontaneous recovery following 0.2 mg/kg MIVACRON are approximately 20 and 30 minutes, respectively, and following 0.25 mg/kg MIVACRON are approximately 25 and 35 minutes. Initiation of maintenance dosing during opioid/nitrous oxide/oxygen anesthesia is generally required approximately 15, 20 and 25 minutes following initial doses of 0.15 mg/kg, 0.2 mg/kg, and 0.25 mg/kg MIVACRON, respectively (see Table 1). Maintenance doses of 0.1 mg/kg each provide approximately 15 minutes of additional clinically effective block. For shorter or longer durations of action, smaller or larger maintenance doses may be administered. The neuromuscular blocking action of MIVACRON is potentiated by isoflurane or enflurane anesthesia. Recommended initial doses of MIVACRON may be used to facilitate tracheal intubation prior to the administration of these agents; however, if MIVACRON is first administered after establishment of stable-state isoflurane or enflurane anesthesia (administered with nitrous oxide/oxygen to achieve 1.25 MAC), the initial dose of MIVACRON may be reduced by as much as 25%. Greater reductions in the dose of MIVACRON may be required with higher concentrations of enflurane or isoflurane. With halothane, which has only a minimal potentiating effect on MIVACRON, a smaller dosage reduction may be considered.

Continuous Infusion

Continuous infusion of MIVACRON may be used to maintain neuromuscular block. Upon early evidence of spontaneous recovery from an initial dose, an initial infusion rate of 9 to 10 mcg/kg/min is recommended. If continuous infusion is initiated simultaneously with the administration of an initial dose, a lower initial infusion rate should be used (e.g., 4 mcg/kg/min). In either case, the initial infusion rate should be adjusted according to the response to peripheral nerve stimulation and to clinical criteria. On average, an infusion rate of 5 to 7 mcg/kg/min (range: 1 to 15 mcg/kg/min) may be expected to maintain neuromuscular block within the range of 89% to 99% for extended periods in adults receiving opioid/nitrous oxide/oxygen anesthesia. In some patients, particularly those with higher infusion requirements (greater than 8 mcg/kg/min) during the first 30 minutes, the infusion rate required to maintain 89% to 99% T₁ suppression may decrease gradually (by greater than or equal to 30%) with time over a 4- to 6-hour period of infusion (see **CLINICAL PHARMACOLOGY - Pharmacodynamics**). Reduction of the infusion rate by up to 35% to 40% should be considered when MIVACRON is administered during stable-state conditions of isoflurane or enflurane anesthesia (administered with nitrous oxide/oxygen to achieve 1.25 MAC). Greater reductions in the infusion rate of MIVACRON may be required with greater concentrations of enflurane or isoflurane. With halothane, smaller reductions in infusion rate may be required.

Children

Initial Doses

Dosage requirements for MIVACRON on a mg/kg basis are higher in children than in adults. Onset and recovery of neuromuscular block occur more rapidly in children than in adults (see **CLINICAL PHARMACOLOGY**).

The recommended dose of MIVACRON for facilitating tracheal intubation in children 2 to 12 years of age is 0.2 mg/kg administered over 5 to 15 seconds. When administered during stable opioid/nitrous oxide/oxygen anesthesia, 0.2 mg/kg of MIVACRON produces maximum neuromuscular block in an average of 1.9 minutes (range: 1.3 to 3.3 minutes) and clinically effective block for 10 minutes (range: 6 to 15 minutes). Maintenance doses are generally required more frequently in children than in adults. Administration of doses of MIVACRON above the recommended range (greater than 0.2 mg/kg) is associated with transient decreases in MAP in some children (see **CLINICAL PHARMACOLOGY - Hemodynamics**). MIVACRON has not been studied in pediatric patients below the age of 2 years.

Continuous Infusion

Children require higher infusion rates of MIVACRON than adults. During opioid/nitrous oxide/oxygen anesthesia, the infusion rate required to maintain 89% to 99% neuromuscular block averages 14 mcg/kg/min (range: 5 to 31 mcg/kg/min). The principles for infusion of MIVACRON in adults are also applicable to children (see above).

Infusion Rate Tables

For adults and children the amount of infusion solution required per hour depends upon the clinical requirements of the patient, the concentration of MIVACRON in the infusion solution, and the patient's weight. The contribution of the infusion solution to the fluid requirements of the patient must be considered. Table 8 provides guidelines for delivery in mL/hr (equivalent to microdrops/min when 60 microdrops = 1 mL) of MIVACRON Injection (2 mg/mL).

[See table 8 below]

MIVACRON Injection Compatibility and Admixtures

Y-site Administration

MIVACRON Injection may not be compatible with alkaline solutions having a pH greater than 8.5 (e.g., barbiturate solutions).

Studies have shown that MIVACRON Injection is compatible with:

- 5% Dextrose Injection, USP
- 0.9% Sodium Chloride Injection, USP
- 5% Dextrose and 0.9% Sodium Chloride Injection, USP
- Lactated Ringer's Injection, USP
- 5% Dextrose in Lactated Ringer's Injection
- Sufenta® (sufentanil citrate) Injection, diluted as directed
- Alfenta® (alfentanil hydrochloride) Injection, diluted as directed
- Sublimaze® (fentanyl citrate) Injection, diluted as directed
- Versed® (midazolam hydrochloride) Injection, diluted as directed
- Inapsine® (droperidol) Injection, diluted as directed

Compatibility studies with other parenteral products have not been conducted.

Dilution Stability

MIVACRON Injection diluted to 0.5 mg mivacurium per mL in 5% Dextrose Injection, USP, 5% Dextrose and 0.9% Sodium Chloride Injection, USP, 0.9% Sodium Chloride Injection, USP, Lactated Ringer's Injection, USP, or 5% Dextrose in Lactated Ringer's Injection is physically and chemically stable when stored in PVC (polyvinylchloride) bags at 5° to 25°C (41° to 77°F) for up to 24 hours. Aseptic techniques should be used to prepare the diluted product. Admixtures of MIVACRON should be prepared for single patient use only and used within 24 hours of preparation. The unused portion of diluted MIVACRON should be discarded after each case.

NOTE: Parenteral drug products should be inspected visually for particulate matter and discoloration prior to administration whenever solution and container permit. Solutions which are not clear and colorless should not be used.

HOW SUPPLIED

MIVACRON Injection, 2 mg mivacurium in each mL.

List	Fill	Container	Quantity	NDC#
4365	5 mL	Single-Dose Fliptop Vial	10 per Carton	NDC 0074-4365-05
4365	10 mL	Single-Dose Fliptop Vial	10 per Carton	NDC 0074-4365-10

STORAGE

Store MIVACRON Injection at 25°C (77°F). Excursions permitted between 15°- 30°C (59°- 86°F). DO NOT FREEZE.

Table 8. Infusion Rates for Maintenance of Neuromuscular Block During Opioid/Nitrous Oxide/Oxygen Anesthesia Using MIVACRON Injection (2 mg/mL)

Patient Weight (kg)	Drug Delivery Rate (mcg/kg/min)									
	4	5	6	7	8	10	14	16	18	20
	Infusion Delivery Rate (mL/hr)									
10	1.2	1.5	1.8	2.1	2.4	3	4.2	4.8	5.4	6
15	1.8	2.3	2.7	3.2	3.6	4.5	6.3	7.2	8.1	9
20	2.4	3	3.6	4.2	4.8	6	8.4	9.6	10.8	12
25	3	3.8	4.5	5.3	6	7.5	10.5	12	13.5	15
35	4.2	5.3	6.3	7.4	8.4	10.5	14.7	16.8	18.9	21
50	6	7.5	9	10.5	12	15	21	24	27	30
60	7.2	9	10.8	12.6	14.4	18	25.2	28.8	32.4	36
70	8.4	10.5	12.6	14.7	16.8	21	29.4	33.6	37.8	42
80	9.6	12	14.4	16.8	19.2	24	33.6	38.4	43.2	48
90	10.8	13.5	16.2	18.9	21.6	27	37.8	43.2	48.6	54
100	12	15	18	21	24	30	42	48	54	60

MIVACRON is a registered trademark of GlaxoSmithKline, licensed for use by AbbVie Inc.

Sufenta, Alfenta, Sublimaze, Versed, and Inapsine are not trademarks of AbbVie Inc.

©AbbVie Inc. 2014
Manufactured for
AbbVie Inc.
North Chicago, IL 60064, USA
January 2015
10000000126431

MODERIBA™
[*Mah-duh-RYE-bah*]
(ribavirin, USP)
Tablets

℞

HIGHLIGHTS OF PRESCRIBING INFORMATION
These highlights do not include all the information needed to use Moderiba™ (ribavirin, USP) safely and effectively. See full prescribing information for Moderiba (ribavirin, USP).

Moderiba™ (ribavirin, USP) Tablets for oral use
Initial U.S. Approval: 2002

> **WARNING: RISK OF SERIOUS DISORDERS AND RIBAVIRIN-ASSOCIATED EFFECTS**
> *See full prescribing information for complete boxed warning.*
> - Ribavirin monotherapy, including Moderiba, is not effective for the treatment of chronic hepatitis C virus infection (Boxed Warning).
> - The hemolytic anemia associated with ribavirin therapy may result in worsening of cardiac disease and lead to fatal and nonfatal myocardial infarctions. Patients with a history of significant or unstable cardiac disease should not be treated with Moderiba (2.3, 5.2, 6.1).
> - Significant teratogenic and embryocidal effects have been demonstrated in all animal species exposed to ribavirin. Therefore, Moderiba is contraindicated in women who are pregnant and in the male partners of women who are pregnant. Extreme care must be taken to avoid pregnancy during therapy and for 6 months after completion of treatment in both female patients and in female partners of male patients who are taking Moderiba therapy (4, 5.1, 8.1).

INDICATIONS AND USAGE
Moderiba is a nucleoside analogue indicated for the treatment of chronic hepatitis C (CHC) virus infection in combination with peginterferon alfa-2a in patients 5 years of age and older with compensated liver disease not previously treated with interferon alpha, and in adult CHC patients coinfected with HIV (1)

DOSAGE AND ADMINISTRATION
- CHC: Moderiba is administered according to body weight and genotype (2.1)
- CHC with HIV coinfection: 800 mg by mouth daily for a total of 48 weeks, regardless of genotype (2.2)
- Dose reduction or discontinuation is recommended in patients experiencing certain adverse reactions or renal impairment (2.3, 2.4)

DOSAGE FORMS AND STRENGTHS
- Moderiba (ribavirin, USP) tablets 200 mg (3)
- Moderiba (ribavirin, USP) tablets 400 mg (3)
- Moderiba (ribavirin, USP) tablets 600 mg (3)

CONTRAINDICATIONS
- Pregnant women and men whose female partners are pregnant (4, 5.1, 8.1)
- Hemoglobinopathies (4)
- Coadministration with didanosine (4, 7.1)
Moderiba in combination with peginterferon alfa-2a is contraindicated in patients with:
- Autoimmune hepatitis (4)
- Hepatic decompensation in cirrhotic patients (4, 5.3)

WARNINGS AND PRECAUTIONS
- Birth defects and fetal death with ribavirin: Do not use in pregnancy and for 6 months after treatment. Patients must have a negative pregnancy test prior to therapy, use at least 2 forms of contraception and undergo monthly pregnancy tests (4, 5.1, 8.1)
Peginterferon alfa-2a/Moderiba: Patients exhibiting the following conditions should be closely monitored and may require dose reduction or discontinuation of therapy:
- Hemolytic anemia may occur with a significant initial drop in hemoglobin. This may result in worsening cardiac disease leading to fatal or nonfatal myocardial infarctions (5.2, 6.1)
- Risk of hepatic failure and death: Monitor hepatic function during treatment and discontinue treatment for hepatic decompensation (5.3)
- Severe hypersensitivity reactions including urticaria, angioedema, bronchoconstriction, and anaphylaxis, and serious skin reactions such as Stevens-Johnson Syndrome (5.4)
- Pulmonary disorders, including pulmonary function impairment and pneumonitis, including fatal cases of pneumonia (5.5)
- Severe depression and suicidal ideation, autoimmune and infectious disorders, suppression of bone marrow function, pancreatitis, and diabetes (5)
- Bone marrow suppression with azathioprine coadministration (5.6)
- Growth impairment with combination therapy in pediatric patients (5.8)

ADVERSE REACTIONS
The most common adverse reactions (frequency greater than 40%) in adults receiving combination therapy are fatigue/asthenia, pyrexia, myalgia, and headache. (6.1)
The most common adverse reactions in pediatric subjects were similar to those seen in adults. (6.1)

To report SUSPECTED ADVERSE REACTIONS, contact AbbVie Inc. at 1-800-633-9110 or FDA at 1-800-FDA-1088 or www.fda.gov/medwatch.

DRUG INTERACTIONS
- Nucleoside analogues: Closely monitor for toxicities. Discontinue nucleoside reverse transcriptase inhibitors or reduce dose or discontinue interferon, ribavirin or both with worsening toxicities (7.1)
- Azathioprine: Concomitant use of azathioprine with ribavirin has been reported to induce severe pancytopenia and may increase the risk of azathioprine-related myelotoxicity (7.3)

USE IN SPECIFIC POPULATIONS
- Ribavirin Pregnancy Registry (8.1)
- Pediatrics: Safety and efficacy in pediatric patients less than 5 years old have not been established (8.4)
- Renal Impairment: Dose should be reduced in patients with creatinine clearance less than or equal to 50 mL/min (8.7)
- Organ Transplant: Safety and efficacy have not been studied (8.10)

See 17 for PATIENT COUNSELING INFORMATION and Medication Guide.

Revised: 2/2015

FULL PRESCRIBING INFORMATION

> **WARNING: RISK OF SERIOUS DISORDERS AND RIBAVIRIN-ASSOCIATED EFFECTS**
> Moderiba monotherapy is not effective for the treatment of chronic hepatitis C virus infection and should not be used alone for this indication.
> The primary clinical toxicity of ribavirin is hemolytic anemia. The anemia associated with ribavirin therapy may result in worsening of cardiac disease and lead to fatal and nonfatal myocardial infarctions. Patients with a history of significant or unstable cardiac disease should not be treated with Moderiba [see Warnings and Precautions (5.2), Adverse Reactions (6.1), and Dosage and Administration (2.3)].
> Significant teratogenic and/or embryocidal effects have been demonstrated in all animal species exposed to ribavirin. In addition, ribavirin has a multiple dose half-life of 12 days, and it may persist in non-plasma compartments for as long as 6 months. Therefore, ribavirin, including Moderiba, is contraindicated in women who are pregnant and in the male partners of women who are pregnant. Extreme care must be taken to avoid pregnancy during therapy and for 6 months after completion of therapy in both female patients and in female partners of male patients who are taking ribavirin therapy. At least two reliable forms of effective contraception must be utilized during treatment and during the 6-month post treatment follow-up period [see Contraindications (4), Warnings and Precautions (5.1), and Use in Specific Populations (8.1)].

1 INDICATIONS AND USAGE
Moderiba (ribavirin, USP) in combination with peginterferon alfa-2a is indicated for the treatment of patients 5 years of age and older with chronic hepatitis C (CHC) virus infection who have compensated liver disease and have not been previously treated with interferon alpha.
The following points should be considered when initiating Moderiba combination therapy with peginterferon alfa-2a:
- This indication is based on clinical trials of combination therapy in patients with CHC and compensated liver disease, some of whom had histological evidence of cirrhosis (Child-Pugh class A), and in adult patients with clinically stable HIV disease and CD4 count greater than 100 cells/mm³.

Continued on next page

- This indication is based on achieving undetectable HCV-RNA after treatment for 24 or 48 weeks, based on HCV genotype, and maintaining a Sustained Virologic Response (SVR) 24 weeks after the last dose.
- Safety and efficacy data are not available for treatment longer than 48 weeks.
- The safety and efficacy of ribavirin and peginterferon alfa-2a therapy have not been established in liver or other organ transplant recipients, patients with decompensated liver disease, or previous non-responders to interferon therapy.
- The safety and efficacy of ribavirin therapy for the treatment of adenovirus, RSV, parainfluenza or influenza infections have not been established. Moderiba should not be used for these indications. Ribavirin for inhalation has a separate package insert, which should be consulted if ribavirin inhalation therapy is being considered.

2   DOSAGE AND ADMINISTRATION

Moderiba (ribavirin, USP) should be taken with food. Moderiba should be given in combination with peginterferon alfa-2a; it is important to note that Moderiba should never be given as monotherapy. See Peginterferon alfa-2a Package Insert for all instructions regarding peginterferon alfa-2a dosing and administration.

2.1   Chronic Hepatitis C Monoinfection

Adult Patients

The recommended dose of Moderiba tablets is provided in **Table 1**. The recommended duration of treatment for patients previously untreated with ribavirin and interferon is 24 to 48 weeks.

The daily dose of Moderiba is 800 mg to 1200 mg administered orally in two divided doses. The dose should be individualized to the patient depending on baseline disease characteristics (e.g., genotype), response to therapy, and tolerability of the regimen (see **Table 1**).

Table 1 Peginterferon alfa-2a and Moderiba Dosing Recommendations

Hepatitis C Virus (HCV) Genotype	Peginterferon alfa-2a Dose* (once weekly)	Moderiba Dose (daily)	Duration
Genotypes 1, 4	180 mcg	<75 kg = 1000 mg	48 weeks
		≥75 kg = 1200 mg	48 weeks
Genotypes 2, 3	180 mcg	800 mg	24 weeks

Genotypes 2 and 3 showed no increased response to treatment beyond 24 weeks (see **Table 10**).
Data on genotypes 5 and 6 are insufficient for dosing recommendations.
*See Peginterferon alfa-2a Package Insert for further details on peginterferon alfa-2a dosing and administration, including dose modification in patients with renal impairment.

Pediatric Patients

Peginterferon alfa-2a is administered as 180 mcg/1.73m^2 × BSA once weekly subcutaneously, to a maximum dose of 180 mcg, and should be given in combination with ribavirin. The recommended treatment duration for patients with genotype 2 or 3 is 24 weeks and for other genotypes is 48 weeks.

Moderiba should be given in combination with peginterferon alfa-2a. Moderiba is available as a 200 mg, 400 mg and 600 mg tablet and therefore the healthcare provider should determine if this sized tablet can be swallowed by the pediatric patient. The recommended doses for Moderiba are provided in **Table 2**. Patients who initiate treatment prior to their 18th birthday should maintain pediatric dosing through the completion of therapy.

Table 2 Moderiba Dosing Recommendations for Pediatric Patients

Body Weight in kilograms (kg)	Moderiba Daily Dose*	Moderiba Number of Tablets
23 – 33	400 mg/day	1 × 200 mg tablet A.M. 1 × 200 mg tablet P.M.
34 – 46	600 mg/day	1 × 200 mg tablet A.M. 2 × 200 mg tablets P.M.**
47 – 59	800 mg/day	2 × 200 mg tablets A.M.** 2 × 200 mg tablets P.M.**
60 – 74	1000 mg/day	2 × 200 mg tablets A.M.** 3 × 200 mg tablets P.M.***
≥75	1200 mg/day	3 × 200 mg tablets A.M.*** 3 × 200 mg tablets P.M.***

*approximately 15 mg/kg/day
**or 1 × 400 mg tablet
***or 1 × 600 mg tablet

2.2   Chronic Hepatitis C with HIV Coinfection

Adult Patients

The recommended dose for treatment of chronic hepatitis C in patients coinfected with HIV is peginterferon alfa-2a 180 mcg subcutaneous once weekly and Moderiba 800 mg by mouth daily for a total duration of 48 weeks, regardless of HCV genotype.

2.3   Dose Modifications

Adult and Pediatric Patients

If severe adverse reactions or laboratory abnormalities develop during combination Moderiba/peginterferon alfa-2a therapy, the dose should be modified or discontinued, if appropriate, until the adverse reactions abate or decrease in severity. If intolerance persists after dose adjustment, Moderiba/peginterferon alfa-2a therapy should be discontinued. **Table 3** provides guidelines for dose modifications and discontinuation based on the patient's hemoglobin concentration and cardiac status.

Moderiba should be administered with caution to patients with pre-existing cardiac disease. Patients should be assessed before commencement of therapy and should be appropriately monitored during therapy. If there is any deterioration of cardiovascular status, therapy should be stopped *[see Warnings and Precautions (5.2)].*

[See table 3 below]

The guidelines for Moderiba dose modifications outlined in this table apply to laboratory abnormalities or adverse reactions other than decreases in hemoglobin values.

Adult Patients

Once Moderiba has been withheld due to either a laboratory abnormality or clinical adverse reaction, an attempt may be made to restart Moderiba at 600 mg daily and further increase the dose to 800 mg daily. However, it is not recommended that Moderiba be increased to the original assigned dose (1000 mg to 1200 mg).

Pediatric Patients

Upon resolution of a laboratory abnormality or clinical adverse reaction, an increase in Moderiba dose to the original dose may be attempted depending upon the physician's judgment. If Moderiba has been withheld due to a laboratory abnormality or clinical adverse reaction, an attempt may be made to restart Moderiba at one-half the full dose.

2.4   Renal Impairment

The total daily dose of Moderiba should be reduced for patients with creatinine clearance less than or equal to 50 mL/min; and the weekly dose of peginterferon alfa-2a should be reduced for creatinine clearance less than 30 mL/min as follows in **Table 4** *[see Use in Specific Populations (8.7), Pharmacokinetics (12.3), and Peginterferon alfa-2a Package Insert].*

Table 4 Dosage Modification for Renal Impairment

Creatinine Clearance	Peginterferon alfa-2a Dose (once weekly)	Moderiba Dose (daily)
30 to 50 mL/min	180 mcg	Alternating doses, 200 mg and 400 mg every other day
Less than 30 mL/min	135 mcg	200 mg daily
Hemodialysis	135 mcg	200 mg daily

The dose of Moderiba should not be further modified in patients with renal impairment. If severe adverse reactions or laboratory abnormalities develop, Moderiba should be discontinued, if appropriate, until the adverse reactions abate or decrease in severity. If intolerance persists after restarting Moderiba, Moderiba/peginterferon alfa-2a therapy should be discontinued.

No data are available for pediatric subjects with renal impairment.

2.5   Discontinuation of Dosing

Discontinuation of peginterferon alfa-2a/Moderiba therapy should be considered if the patient has failed to demonstrate at least a 2 log$_{10}$ reduction from baseline in HCV RNA by 12 weeks of therapy, or undetectable HCV RNA levels after 24 weeks of therapy.

Peginterferon alfa-2a/Moderiba therapy should be discontinued in patients who develop hepatic decompensation during treatment *[see Warnings and Precautions (5.3)].*

3   DOSAGE FORMS AND STRENGTHS

Moderiba (ribavirin, USP) is available as tablets for oral administration.

Each Moderiba 200-mg tablet contains 200 mg of ribavirin, USP and is a capsule-shaped, light blue colored, film-coated tablet, debossed with "200" on one side and the logo "3RP" on the other side.

Each Moderiba 400-mg tablet contains 400 mg of ribavirin, USP and is a capsule-shaped, medium blue colored, film-coated tablet, debossed with "400" on one side and the logo "3RP" on the other side.

Each Moderiba 600-mg tablet contains 600 mg of ribavirin, USP and is a capsule-shaped, dark blue colored, film-coated tablet, debossed with "600" on one side and the logo "3RP" on the other side.

4   CONTRAINDICATIONS

Moderiba (ribavirin, USP) is contraindicated in:

- Women who are pregnant. Moderiba may cause fetal harm when administered to a pregnant woman. Moderiba is contraindicated in women who are or may become pregnant. If this drug is used during pregnancy, or if the patient becomes pregnant while taking this drug, the patient

Table 3 Moderiba Dose Modification Guidelines in Adults and Pediatrics

	Laboratory Values	
Body weight in kilograms (kg)	Hemoglobin <10 g/dL in patients with no cardiac disease, or Decrease in hemoglobin of ≥2 g/dL during any 4 week period in patients with history of stable cardiac disease	Hemoglobin <8.5 g/dL in patients with no cardiac disease, or Hemoglobin <12 g/dL despite 4 weeks at reduced dose in patients with history of stable cardiac disease
Adult Patients older than 18 years of age		
Any weight	1 × 200 mg tablet A.M. 2 × 200 mg tablets or 1 × 400 mg tablet P.M.	Discontinue Moderiba
Pediatric Patients 5 to 18 years of age		
23 – 33 kg	1 × 200 mg tablet A.M.	
34 – 46 kg	1 × 200 mg tablet A.M. 1 × 200 mg tablet P.M.	
47 – 59 kg	1 × 200 mg tablet A.M. 1 × 200 mg tablet P.M.	Discontinue Moderiba
60 – 74 kg	1 × 200 mg tablet A.M. 2 × 200 mg tablets P.M. or 1 × 400 mg tablet P.M.	
≥75 kg	1 × 200 mg tablet A.M. 2 × 200 mg tablets P.M. or 1 × 400 mg tablet P.M.	

should be apprised of the potential hazard to the fetus *[see Warnings and Precautions (5.1), Use in Specific Populations (8.1), and Patient Counseling Information (17)]*.

• Men whose female partners are pregnant.
• Patients with hemoglobinopathies (e.g., thalassemia major or sickle-cell anemia).
• In combination with didanosine. Reports of fatal hepatic failure, as well as peripheral neuropathy, pancreatitis, and symptomatic hyperlactatemia/lactic acidosis have been reported in clinical trials *[see Drug Interactions (7.1)]*.

Moderiba and peginterferon alfa-2a combination therapy is contraindicated in patients with:

• Autoimmune hepatitis.
• Hepatic decompensation (Child-Pugh score greater than 6; class B and C) in cirrhotic CHC monoinfected patients before treatment *[see Warnings and Precautions (5.3)]*.
• Hepatic decompensation (Child-Pugh score greater than or equal to 6) in cirrhotic CHC patients coinfected with HIV before treatment *[see Warnings and Precautions (5.3)]*.

5 WARNINGS AND PRECAUTIONS

Significant adverse reactions associated with Moderiba (ribavirin, USP)/peginterferon alfa-2a combination therapy include severe depression and suicidal ideation, hemolytic anemia, suppression of bone marrow function, autoimmune and infectious disorders, ophthalmologic disorders, cerebrovascular disorders, pulmonary dysfunction, colitis, pancreatitis, and diabetes.

The Peginterferon alfa-2a Package Insert should be reviewed in its entirety for additional safety information prior to initiation of combination treatment.

5.1 Pregnancy

Moderiba may cause birth defects and/or death of the exposed fetus. Ribavirin has demonstrated significant teratogenic and/or embryocidal effects in all animal species in which adequate studies have been conducted. These effects occurred at doses as low as one twentieth of the recommended human dose of ribavirin.

Moderiba therapy should not be started unless a report of a negative pregnancy test has been obtained immediately prior to planned initiation of therapy. Extreme care must be taken to avoid pregnancy in female patients and in female partners of male patients. Patients should be instructed to use at least two forms of effective contraception during treatment and for 6 months after treatment has been stopped. Pregnancy testing should occur monthly during Moderiba therapy and for 6 months after therapy has stopped *[see Boxed Warning, Contraindications (4), Use in Specific Populations (8.1), and Patient Counseling Information (17)]*.

5.2 Anemia

The primary toxicity of ribavirin is hemolytic anemia, which was observed in approximately 13% of all ribavirin/peginterferon alfa-2a-treated subjects in clinical trials. Anemia associated with ribavirin occurs within 1 to 2 weeks of initiation of therapy. Because the initial drop in hemoglobin may be significant, it is advised that hemoglobin or hematocrit be obtained pretreatment and at week 2 and week 4 of therapy or more frequently if clinically indicated. Patients should then be followed as clinically appropriate. Caution should be exercised in initiating treatment in any patient with baseline risk of severe anemia (e.g., spherocytosis, history of gastrointestinal bleeding) *[see Dosage and Administration (2.3)]*.

Fatal and nonfatal myocardial infarctions have been reported in patients with anemia caused by ribavirin. Patients should be assessed for underlying cardiac disease before initiation of ribavirin therapy. Patients with pre-existing cardiac disease should have electrocardiograms administered before treatment, and should be appropriately monitored during therapy. If there is any deterioration of cardiovascular status, therapy should be suspended or discontinued *[see Dosage and Administration (2.3)]*. Because cardiac disease may be worsened by drug-induced anemia, patients with a history of significant or unstable cardiac disease should not use Moderiba *[see Boxed Warning and Dosage and Administration (2.3)]*.

5.3 Hepatic Failure

Chronic hepatitis C (CHC) patients with cirrhosis may be at risk of hepatic decompensation and death when treated with alpha interferons, including peginterferon alfa-2a. Cirrhotic CHC patients coinfected with HIV receiving highly active antiretroviral therapy (HAART) and interferon alfa-2a with or without ribavirin appear to be at increased risk for the development of hepatic decompensation com-

pared to patients not receiving HAART. In Study NR15961 *[see Clinical Studies (14.3)]*, among 129 CHC/HIV cirrhotic patients receiving HAART, 14 (11%) of these patients across all treatment arms developed hepatic decompensation resulting in 6 deaths. All 14 patients were on NRTIs, including stavudine, didanosine, abacavir, zidovudine, and lamivudine. These small numbers of patients do not permit discrimination between specific NRTIs or the associated risk. During treatment, patients' clinical status and hepatic function should be closely monitored for signs and symptoms of hepatic decompensation. Treatment with peginterferon alfa-2a/Moderiba should be discontinued immediately in patients with hepatic decompensation *[see Contraindications (4)]*.

5.4 Hypersensitivity

Severe acute hypersensitivity reactions (e.g., urticaria, angioedema, bronchoconstriction, and anaphylaxis) have been observed during alpha interferon and ribavirin therapy. If such a reaction occurs, therapy with peginterferon alfa-2a and Moderiba should be discontinued immediately and appropriate medical therapy instituted. Serious skin reactions including vesiculobullous eruptions, reactions in the spectrum of Stevens-Johnson Syndrome (erythema multiforme major) with varying degrees of skin and mucosal involvement and exfoliative dermatitis (erythroderma) have been reported in patients receiving peginterferon alfa-2a with and without ribavirin. Patients developing signs or symptoms of severe skin reactions must discontinue therapy *[see Adverse Reactions (6.2)]*.

5.5 Pulmonary Disorders

Dyspnea, pulmonary infiltrates, pneumonitis, pulmonary hypertension, and pneumonia have been reported during therapy with ribavirin and interferon. Occasional cases of fatal pneumonia have occurred. In addition, sarcoidosis or the exacerbation of sarcoidosis has been reported. If there is evidence of pulmonary infiltrates or pulmonary function impairment, patients should be closely monitored and, if appropriate, combination Moderiba/Peginterferon alfa-2a treatment should be discontinued.

5.6 Bone Marrow Suppression

Pancytopenia (marked decreases in RBCs, neutrophils and platelets) and bone marrow suppression have been reported in the literature to occur within 3 to 7 weeks after the concomitant administration of pegylated interferon/ribavirin and azathioprine. In this limited number of patients (n=8), myelotoxicity was reversible within 4 to 6 weeks upon withdrawal of both HCV antiviral therapy and concomitant azathioprine and did not recur upon reintroduction of either treatment alone. Peginterferon alfa-2a, Moderiba, and azathioprine should be discontinued for pancytopenia, and pegylated interferon/ribavirin should not be re-introduced with concomitant azathioprine *[see Drug Interactions (7.3)]*.

5.7 Pancreatitis

Moderiba and peginterferon alfa-2a therapy should be suspended in patients with signs and symptoms of pancreatitis, and discontinued in patients with confirmed pancreatitis.

5.8 Impact on Growth in Pediatric Patients

Pediatric subjects treated with peginterferon alfa-2a plus ribavirin combination therapy showed a delay in weight and height increases after 48 weeks of therapy compared with baseline. Both weight and height for age z-scores as well as the percentiles of the normative population for subject weight and height decreased during treatment. At the end of 2 years follow-up after treatment, most subjects had returned to baseline normative growth curve percentiles for weight and height (mean weight for age percentile was 64% at baseline and 60% at 2 years post-treatment; mean height percentile was 54% at baseline and 56% at 2 years post-treatment). At the end of treatment, 43% of subjects experienced a weight percentile decrease of 15 percentiles or more, and 25% experienced a height percentile decrease of 15 percentiles or more on the normative growth curves. At 2 years post-treatment, 16% of subjects remained 15 percentiles or more below their baseline weight curve and 11% remained 15 percentiles or more below their baseline height curve.

5.9 Laboratory Tests

Before beginning peginterferon alfa-2a/Moderiba combination therapy, standard hematological and biochemical laboratory tests are recommended for all patients. Pregnancy screening for women of childbearing potential must be performed. Patients who have pre-existing cardiac abnormalities should have electrocardiograms administered before treatment with peginterferon alfa-2a/Moderiba.

After initiation of therapy, hematological tests should be performed at 2 weeks and 4 weeks and biochemical tests

should be performed at 4 weeks. Additional testing should be performed periodically during therapy. In adult clinical studies, the CBC (including hemoglobin level and white blood cell and platelet counts) and chemistries (including liver function tests and uric acid) were measured at 1, 2, 4, 6, and 8 weeks, and then every 4 to 6 weeks or more frequently if abnormalities were found. In the pediatric clinical trial, hematological and chemistry assessments were at 1, 3, 5, and 8 weeks, then every 4 weeks. Thyroid stimulating hormone (TSH) was measured every 12 weeks. Monthly pregnancy testing should be performed during combination therapy and for 6 months after discontinuing therapy.

The entrance criteria used for the clinical studies of ribavirin and peginterferon alfa-2a may be considered as a guideline to acceptable baseline values for initiation of treatment:

• Platelet count greater than or equal to 90,000 cells/mm^3 (as low as 75,000 cells/mm^3 in HCV patients with cirrhosis or 70,000 cells/mm^3 in patients with CHC and HIV)
• Absolute neutrophil count (ANC) greater than or equal to 1500 cells/mm^3
• TSH and T$_4$ within normal limits or adequately controlled thyroid function
• CD4+ cell count greater than or equal to 200 cells/mm^3 or CD4+ cell count greater than or equal to 100 cells/mm^3 but less than 200 cells/mm^3 and HIV-1 RNA less than 5,000 copies/mm^3 in patients coinfected with HIV
• Hemoglobin greater than or equal to 12 g/dL for women and greater than or equal to 13 g/dL for men in CHC monoinfected patients
• Hemoglobin greater than or equal to 11 g/dL for women and greater than or equal to 12 g/dL for men in patients with CHC and HIV

6 ADVERSE REACTIONS

Peginterferon alfa-2a in combination with ribavirin causes a broad variety of serious adverse reactions *[see Boxed Warning and Warnings and Precautions (5)]*. The most common serious or life-threatening adverse reactions induced or aggravated by ribavirin/peginterferon alfa-2a include depression, suicide, relapse of drug abuse/overdose, and bacterial infections each occurring at a frequency of less than 1%. Hepatic decompensation occurred in 2% (10/574) CHC/HIV patients *[see Warnings and Precautions (5.3)]*.

6.1 Clinical Studies Experience

Because clinical trials are conducted under widely varying conditions, adverse reaction rates observed in the clinical trials of a drug cannot be directly compared to rates in the clinical trials of another drug and may not reflect the rates observed in clinical practice.

Adult Patients

In the pivotal registration trials NV15801 and NV15942, 886 patients received ribavirin for 48 weeks at doses of 1000/1200 mg based on body weight. In these trials, one or more serious adverse reactions occurred in 10% of CHC monoinfected subjects and in 19% of CHC/HIV subjects receiving peginterferon alfa-2a alone or in combination with ribavirin. The most common serious adverse event (3% in CHC and 5% in CHC/HIV) was bacterial infection (e.g., sepsis, osteomyelitis, endocarditis, pyelonephritis, pneumonia). Other serious adverse reactions occurred at a frequency of less than 1% and included: suicide, suicidal ideation, psychosis, aggression, anxiety, drug abuse and drug overdose, angina, hepatic dysfunction, fatty liver, cholangitis, arrhythmia, diabetes mellitus, autoimmune phenomena (e.g., hyperthyroidism, hypothyroidism, sarcoidosis, systemic lupus erythematosus, rheumatoid arthritis), peripheral neuropathy, aplastic anemia, peptic ulcer, gastrointestinal bleeding, pancreatitis, colitis, corneal ulcer, pulmonary embolism, coma, myositis, cerebral hemorrhage, thrombotic thrombocytopenic purpura, psychotic disorder, and hallucination.

The percentage of patients in clinical trials who experienced one or more adverse events was 98%. The most commonly reported adverse reactions were psychiatric reactions, including depression, insomnia, irritability, anxiety, and flu-like symptoms such as fatigue, pyrexia, myalgia, headache and rigors. Other common reactions were anorexia, nausea and vomiting, diarrhea, arthralgias, injection site reactions,

Continued on next page

Information on the AbbVie, Inc. products listed on these pages is from the prescribing information in use as of July 31, 2016. For more information, please visit rxabbvie.com or call 1-800-633-9110.

Table 5 Adverse Reactions Occurring in greater than or equal to 5% of Patients in Chronic Hepatitis C Clinical Trials (Study NV15801)

Body System	CHC Combination Therapy Study NV15801	
	peginterferon alfa-2a 180 mcg + 1000 mg or 1200 mg ribavirin tablets 48 weeks	interferon alfa-2b + 1000 mg or 1200 mg ribavirin capsules 48 weeks
	N=451 %	N=443 %
Application Site Disorders		
Injection site reaction	23	16
Endocrine Disorders		
Hypothyroidism	4	5
Flu-like Symptoms and Signs		
Fatigue/Asthenia	65	68
Pyrexia	41	55
Rigors	25	37
Pain	10	9
Gastrointestinal		
Nausea/Vomiting	25	29
Diarrhea	11	10
Abdominal pain	8	9
Dry mouth	4	7
Dyspepsia	6	5
Hematologic*		
Lymphopenia	14	12
Anemia	11	11
Neutropenia	27	8
Thrombocytopenia	5	<1
Metabolic and Nutritional		
Anorexia	24	26
Weight decrease	10	10
Musculoskeletal, Connective Tissue and Bone		
Myalgia	40	49
Arthralgia	22	23
Back pain	5	5
Neurological		
Headache	43	49
Dizziness (excluding vertigo)	14	14
Memory impairment	6	5
Psychiatric		
Irritability/Anxiety/Nervousness	33	38
Insomnia	30	37
Depression	20	28
Concentration impairment	10	13
Mood alteration	5	6
Resistance Mechanism Disorders		
Overall	12	10
Respiratory, Thoracic and Mediastinal		
Dyspnea	13	14
Cough	10	7
Dyspnea exertional	4	7
Skin and Subcutaneous Tissue		
Alopecia	28	33
Pruritus	19	18
Dermatitis	16	13
Dry skin	10	13
Rash	8	5
Sweating increased	6	5
Eczema	5	4
Visual Disorders		
Vision blurred	5	2

*Severe hematologic abnormalities (lymphocyte less than 500 cells/mm^3; hemoglobin less than 10 g/dL; neutrophil less than 750 cells/mm^3; platelet less than 50,000 cells/mm^3).

alopecia, and pruritus. **Table 5** shows rates of adverse events occurring in greater than or equal to 5% subjects receiving pegylated interferon and ribavirin combination therapy in the CHC Clinical Trial, NV15801.

Ten percent of CHC monoinfected patients receiving 48 weeks of therapy with peginterferon alfa-2a in combination with ribavirin discontinued therapy; 16% of CHC/HIV coinfected patients discontinued therapy. The most common reasons for discontinuation of therapy were psychiatric, flu-like syndrome (e.g., lethargy, fatigue, headache), dermatologic and gastrointestinal disorders and laboratory abnormalities (thrombocytopenia, neutropenia, and anemia).

Overall 39% of patients with CHC or CHC/HIV required modification of peginterferon alfa-2a and/or ribavirin therapy. The most common reason for dose modification of peginterferon alfa-2a in CHC and CHC/HIV patients was for laboratory abnormalities; neutropenia (20% and 27%, re-

spectively) and thrombocytopenia (4% and 6%, respectively). The most common reason for dose modification of ribavirin in CHC and CHC/HIV patients was anemia (22% and 16%, respectively).

Peginterferon alfa-2a dose was reduced in 12% of patients receiving 1000 mg to 1200 mg ribavirin for 48 weeks and in 7% of patients receiving 800 mg ribavirin for 24 weeks. Ribavirin dose was reduced in 21% of patients receiving 1000 mg to 1200 mg ribavirin for 48 weeks and in 12% of patients receiving 800 mg ribavirin for 24 weeks.

Chronic hepatitis C monoinfected patients treated for 24 weeks with peginterferon alfa-2a and 800 mg ribavirin were observed to have lower incidence of serious adverse events (3% vs. 10%), hemoglobin less than 10 g/dL (3% vs. 15%), dose modification of peginterferon alfa-2a (30% vs. 36%) and ribavirin (19% vs. 38%), and of withdrawal from treatment (5% vs. 15%) compared to patients treated for 48 weeks with

peginterferon alfa-2a and 1000 mg or 1200 mg ribavirin. On the other hand, the overall incidence of adverse events appeared to be similar in the two treatment groups.
[See table 5]

Pediatric Subjects

In a clinical trial with 114 pediatric subjects (5 to 17 years of age) treated with peginterferon alfa-2a alone or in combination with ribavirin, dose modifications were required in approximately one-third of subjects, most commonly for neutropenia and anemia. In general, the safety profile observed in pediatric subjects was similar to that seen in adults. In the pediatric study, the most common adverse events in subjects treated with combination therapy peginterferon alfa-2a and ribavirin for up to 48 weeks were influenza-like illness (91%), upper respiratory tract infection (60%), headache (64%), gastrointestinal disorder (56%), skin disorder (47%), and injection-site reaction (45%). Seven subjects receiving combination peginterferon alfa-2a and ribavirin treatment for 48 weeks discontinued therapy for safety reasons (depression, psychiatric evaluation abnormal, transient blindness, retinal exudates, hyperglycemia, type 1 diabetes mellitus, and anemia). Severe adverse events were reported in 2 subjects in the peginterferon alfa-2a plus ribavirin combination therapy group (hyperglycemia and cholecystectomy).

Growth inhibition was observed in pediatric subjects. During combination therapy for up to 48 weeks with peginterferon alfa-2a and ribavirin, negative changes in weight for age z-score and height for age z-score after 48 weeks of therapy compared with baseline were observed [see Warnings and Precautions (5.8)].
[See table 6 on next page]

In pediatric subjects randomized to combination therapy, the incidence of most adverse reactions were similar for the entire treatment period (up to 48 weeks plus 24 weeks follow-up) in comparison to the first 24 weeks, and increased only slightly for headache, gastrointestinal disorder, irritability and rash. The majority of adverse reactions occurred in the first 24 weeks of treatment.

Common Adverse Reactions in CHC with HIV Coinfection (Adults)

The adverse event profile of coinfected patients treated with peginterferon alfa-2a/ribavirin in Study NR15961 was generally similar to that shown for monoinfected patients in Study NV15801 (**Table 5**). Events occurring more frequently in coinfected patients were neutropenia (40%), anemia (14%), thrombocytopenia (8%), weight decrease (16%), and mood alteration (9%).

Laboratory Test Abnormalities

Adult Patients

Anemia due to hemolysis is the most significant toxicity of ribavirin therapy. Anemia (hemoglobin less than 10 g/dL) was observed in 13% of all ribavirin and peginterferon alfa-2a combination-treated patients in clinical trials. The maximum drop in hemoglobin occurred during the first 8 weeks of initiation of ribavirin therapy [see Dosage and Administration (2.3)].

Table 7 Selected Laboratory Abnormalities During Treatment With Ribavirin in Combination With Either Peginterferon alfa-2a or Interferon alfa-2b

Laboratory Parameter	Peginterferon alfa-2a + Ribavirin 1000/ 1200 mg 48 wks (N=887)	Interferon alfa-2b + Ribavirin 1000/ 1200 mg 48 wks (N=443)
Neutrophils (cells/mm^3)		
1,000 <1,500	34%	38%
500 <1,000	49%	21%
<500	5%	1%
Platelets (cells/mm^3)		
50,000 – <75,000	11%	4%
20,000 – <50,000	5%	<1%
<20,000	0	0
Hemoglobin (g/dL)		
8.5 – 9.9	11%	11%
<8.5	2%	<1%

Pediatric Patients

Decreases in hemoglobin, neutrophils and platelets may require dose reduction or permanent discontinuation from treatment [see Dosage and Administration (2.4)]. Most lab-

Table 6 Percentage of Pediatric Subjects with Adverse Reactions* During First 24 Weeks of Treatment by Treatment Group and for 24 Weeks Post-treatment (in at Least 10% of Subjects)

System Organ Class	Study NV17424	
	peginterferon alfa-2a 180 mcg/1.73 m² × BSA + ribavirin tablets 15 mg/kg (N=55)	peginterferon alfa-2a 180 mcg/1.73 m² × BSA + Placebo** (N=59)
	%	%
General disorders and administration site conditions		
Influenza like illness	91	81
Injection site reaction	44	42
Fatigue	25	20
Irritability	24	14
Gastrointestinal disorders		
Gastrointestinal disorder	49	44
Nervous system disorders		
Headache	51	39
Skin and subcutaneous tissue disorders		
Rash	15	10
Pruritus	11	12
Musculoskeletal, connective tissue and bone disorders		
Musculoskeletal pain	35	29
Psychiatric disorders		
Insomnia	9	12
Metabolism and nutrition disorders		
Decreased appetite	11	14

*Displayed adverse drug reactions include all grades of reported adverse clinical events considered possibly, probably, or definitely related to study drug.

**Subjects in the peginterferon alfa-2a plus placebo arm who did not achieve undetectable viral load at week 24 switched to combination treatment thereafter. Therefore, only the first 24 weeks are presented for the comparison of combination therapy with monotherapy.

oratory abnormalities noted during the clinical trial returned to baseline levels shortly after discontinuation of treatment.

Table 8 Selected Hematologic Abnormalities During First 24 Weeks of Treatment by Treatment Group in Previously Untreated Pediatric Subjects

Laboratory Parameter	Peginterferon alfa-2a 180 mcg/1.73 m² × BSA + Ribavirin tablets 15 mg/kg (N=55)	Peginterferon alfa-2a 180 mcg/1.73 m² × BSA + Placebo* (N=59)
Neutrophils (cells/mm³)		
1,000 - <1,500	31%	39%
750 - <1,000	27%	17%
500 - <750	25%	15%
<500	7%	5%
Platelets (cells/mm³)		
75,000 - <100,000	4%	2%
50,000 - <75,000	0%	2%
<50,000	0%	0%
Hemoglobin (g/dL)		
8.5 – <10	7%	3%
<8.5	0%	0%

*Subjects in the peginterferon alfa-2a plus placebo arm who did not achieve undetectable viral load at week 24 switched to combination treatment thereafter. Therefore, only the first 24 weeks are presented for the comparison of combination therapy with monotherapy.

In patients randomized to combination therapy, the incidence of abnormalities during the entire treatment phase (up to 48 weeks plus 24 weeks follow-up) in comparison to the first 24 weeks increased slightly for neutrophils between 500 and 1,000 cells/mm³ and hemoglobin values between 8.5 and 10 g/dL. The majority of hematologic abnormalities occurred in the first 24 weeks of treatment.

6.2 Postmarketing Experience

The following adverse reactions have been identified and reported during post-approval use of peginterferon alfa-2a/ribavirin combination therapy. Because these reactions are reported voluntarily from a population of uncertain size, it is not always possible to reliably estimate their frequency or establish a causal relationship to drug exposure.

Blood and Lymphatic System disorders
Pure red cell aplasia
Ear and Labyrinth disorders
Hearing impairment, hearing loss

Eye disorders
Serous retinal detachment
Immune disorders
Liver and renal graft rejection
Metabolism and Nutrition disorders
Dehydration
Skin and Subcutaneous Tissue disorders
Stevens-Johnson Syndrome (SJS)
Toxic epidermal necrolysis (TEN)

7 DRUG INTERACTIONS

Results from a pharmacokinetic sub-study demonstrated no pharmacokinetic interaction between peginterferon alfa-2a and ribavirin.

7.1 Nucleoside Reverse Transcriptase Inhibitors (NRTIs)

In vitro data indicate ribavirin reduces phosphorylation of lamivudine, stavudine, and zidovudine. However, no pharmacokinetic (e.g., plasma concentrations or intracellular triphosphorylated active metabolite concentrations) or pharmacodynamic (e.g., loss of HIV/HCV virologic suppression) interaction was observed when ribavirin and lamivudine (n=18), stavudine (n=10), or zidovudine (n=6) were co-administered as part of a multi-drug regimen to HCV/HIV coinfected patients.

In Study NR15961 among the CHC/HIV coinfected cirrhotic patients receiving NRTIs cases of hepatic decompensation (some fatal) were observed [see *Warnings and Precautions (5.3)*].

Patients receiving peginterferon alfa-2a/Moderiba (ribavirin, USP) and NRTIs should be closely monitored for treatment associated toxicities. Physicians should refer to prescribing information for the respective NRTIs for guidance regarding toxicity management. In addition, dose reduction or discontinuation of peginterferon alfa-2a, Moderiba or both should also be considered if worsening toxicities are observed, including hepatic decompensation (e.g., Child-Pugh greater than or equal to 6) [see *Warnings and Precautions (5.3) and Dosage and Administration (2.3)*].

Didanosine

Co-administration of Moderiba and didanosine is contraindicated. Didanosine or its active metabolite (dideoxyadenosine 5'-triphosphate) concentrations are increased when didanosine is co-administered with ribavirin, which could cause or worsen clinical toxicities. Reports of fatal hepatic failure, as well as peripheral neuropathy, pancreatitis, and symptomatic hyperlactatemia/lactic acidosis have been reported in clinical trials [see *Contraindications (4)*].

Zidovudine

In Study NR15961, patients who were administered zidovudine in combination with peginterferon alfa-2a/ribavirin developed severe neutropenia (ANC less than 500) and severe anemia (hemoglobin less than 8 g/dL) more frequently than

similar patients not receiving zidovudine (neutropenia 15% vs. 9%) (anemia 5% vs. 1%). Discontinuation of zidovudine should be considered as medically appropriate.

7.2 Drugs Metabolized by Cytochrome P450

In vitro studies indicate that ribavirin does not inhibit CYP 2C9, CYP 2C19, CYP 2D6 or CYP 3A4.

7.3 Azathioprine

The use of ribavirin to treat chronic hepatitis C in patients receiving azathioprine has been reported to induce severe pancytopenia and may increase the risk of azathioprine-related myelotoxicity. Inosine monophosphate dehydrogenase (IMDH) is required for one of the metabolic pathways of azathioprine. Ribavirin is known to inhibit IMDH, thereby leading to accumulation of an azathioprine metabolite, 6-methylthioinosine monophosphate (6-MTITP), which is associated with myelotoxicity (neutropenia, thrombocytopenia, and anemia). Patients receiving azathioprine with ribavirin should have complete blood counts, including platelet counts, monitored weekly for the first month, twice monthly for the second and third months of treatment, then monthly or more frequently if dosage or other therapy changes are necessary [see *Warnings and Precautions (5.7)*].

8 USE IN SPECIFIC POPULATIONS

8.1 Pregnancy

Teratogenic Effects

Pregnancy: Category X [see *Contraindications (4)*].

Ribavirin produced significant embryocidal and/or teratogenic effects in all animal species in which adequate studies have been conducted. Malformations of the skull, palate, eye, jaw, limbs, skeleton, and gastrointestinal tract were noted. The incidence and severity of teratogenic effects increased with escalation of the drug dose. Survival of fetuses and offspring was reduced [see *Contraindications (4) and Warnings and Precautions (5.1)*].

In conventional embryotoxicity/teratogenicity studies in rats and rabbits, observed no-effect dose levels were well below those for proposed clinical use (0.3 mg/kg/day for both the rat and rabbit; approximately 0.06 times the recommended daily human dose of ribavirin). No maternal toxicity or effects on offspring were observed in a peri/postnatal toxicity study in rats dosed orally at up to 1 mg/kg/day (approximately 0.01 times the maximum recommended daily human dose of ribavirin).

Treatment and Post treatment: Potential Risk to the Fetus

Ribavirin is known to accumulate in intracellular components from where it is cleared very slowly. It is not known whether ribavirin is contained in sperm, and if so, will exert a potential teratogenic effect upon fertilization of the ova. However, because of the potential human teratogenic effects of ribavirin, male patients should be advised to take every precaution to avoid risk of pregnancy for their female partners.

Moderiba should not be used by pregnant women or by men whose female partners are pregnant. Female patients of childbearing potential and male patients with female partners of childbearing potential should not receive Moderiba unless the patient and his/her partner are using effective contraception (two reliable forms) during therapy and for 6 months post therapy [see *Contraindications (4)*].

Ribavirin Pregnancy Registry

A Ribavirin Pregnancy Registry has been established to monitor maternal-fetal outcomes of pregnancies of female patients and female partners of male patients exposed to ribavirin during treatment and for 6 months following cessation of treatment. Healthcare providers and patients are encouraged to report such cases by calling 1-800-593-2214.

8.3 Nursing Mothers

It is not known whether ribavirin is excreted in human milk. Because many drugs are excreted in human milk and to avoid any potential for serious adverse reactions in nursing infants from ribavirin, a decision should be made either to discontinue nursing or therapy with Moderiba, based on the importance of the therapy to the mother.

8.4 Pediatric Use

Pharmacokinetic evaluations in pediatric patients have not been performed.

Continued on next page

Information on the AbbVie, Inc. products listed on these pages is from the prescribing information in use as of July 31, 2016. For more information, please visit rxabbvie.com or call 1-800-633-9110.

Safety and effectiveness of Moderiba tablets have not been established in patients below the age of 5 years.

8.5 Geriatric Use

Clinical studies of ribavirin and peginterferon alfa-2a did not include sufficient numbers of subjects aged 65 or over to determine whether they respond differently from younger subjects. Specific pharmacokinetic evaluations for ribavirin in the elderly have not been performed. The risk of toxic reactions to this drug may be greater in patients with impaired renal function. The dose of Moderiba should be reduced in patients with creatinine clearance less than or equal to 50 mL/min; and the dose of peginterferon alfa-2a should be reduced in patients with creatinine clearance less than 30 mL/min *[see Dosage and Administration (2.5); Use in Specific Populations (8.7)]*.

8.6 Race

A pharmacokinetic study in 42 subjects demonstrated there is no clinically significant difference in ribavirin pharmacokinetics among Black (n=14), Hispanic (n=13) and Caucasian (n=15) subjects.

8.7 Renal Impairment

Renal function should be evaluated in all patients prior to initiation of Moderiba by estimating the patient's creatinine clearance.

A clinical trial evaluated treatment with ribavirin and peginterferon alfa-2a in 50 CHC subjects with moderate (creatinine clearance 30 – 50 mL/min) or severe (creatinine clearance less than 30 mL/min) renal impairment or end stage renal disease (ESRD) requiring chronic hemodialysis (HD). In 18 subjects with ESRD receiving chronic HD, ribavirin was administered at a dose of 200 mg daily with no apparent difference in the adverse event profile in comparison to subjects with normal renal function. Dose reductions and temporary interruptions of ribavirin (due to ribavirin-related adverse reactions, mainly anemia) were observed in up to one-third ESRD/HD subjects during treatment; and only one-third of these subjects received ribavirin for 48 weeks. Ribavirin plasma exposures were approximately 20% lower in subjects with ESRD on HD compared to subjects with normal renal function receiving the standard 1000/1200 mg ribavirin daily dose.

Subjects with moderate (n=17) or severe (n=14) renal impairment did not tolerate 600 mg or 400 mg daily doses of ribavirin, respectively, due to ribavirin-related adverse reactions, mainly anemia, and exhibited 20 to 30% higher ribavirin plasma exposures (despite frequent dose modifications) compared to subjects with normal renal function (creatinine clearance greater than 80 mL/min) receiving the standard dose of ribavirin. Discontinuation rates were higher in subjects with severe renal impairment compared to that observed in subjects with moderate renal impairment or normal renal function. Pharmacokinetic modeling and simulation indicates that a dose of 200 mg daily in patients with severe renal impairment and a dose of 200 mg daily alternating with 400 mg the following day in patients with moderate renal impairment will provide plasma ribavirin exposure similar to patients with normal renal function receiving the approved regimen of ribavirin. These doses have not been studied in patients *[see Dosage and Administration (2.4), Use in Specific Populations (8.7), and Clinical Pharmacology (12.3)]*.

Based on the pharmacokinetic and safety results from this trial, patients with creatinine clearance less than or equal to 50 mL/min should receive a reduced dose of ribavirin; and patients with creatinine clearance less than 30 mL/min should receive a reduced dose of peginterferon alfa-2a. The clinical and hematologic status of patients with creatinine clearance less than or equal to 50 mL/min receiving ribavirin should be carefully monitored. Patients with clinically significant laboratory abnormalities or adverse reactions which are persistently severe or worsening should have therapy withdrawn *[see Dosage and Administration (2.5), Clinical Pharmacology (12.3), and Peginterferon alfa-2a Package Insert]*.

8.8 Hepatic Impairment

The effect of hepatic impairment on the pharmacokinetics of ribavirin following administration of ribavirin has not been evaluated. The clinical trials of ribavirin were restricted to patients with Child-Pugh class A disease.

8.9 Gender

No clinically significant differences in the pharmacokinetics of ribavirin were observed between male and female subjects.

Ribavirin pharmacokinetics, when corrected for weight, are similar in male and female patients.

8.10 Organ Transplant Recipients

The safety and efficacy of peginterferon alfa-2a and ribavirin treatment have not been established in patients with liver and other transplantations. As with other alpha interferons, liver and renal graft rejections have been reported on peginterferon alfa-2a, alone or in combination with ribavirin *[see Adverse Reactions (6.2)]*.

10 OVERDOSAGE

No cases of overdose with ribavirin have been reported in clinical trials. Hypocalcemia and hypomagnesemia have been observed in persons administered greater than the recommended dosage of ribavirin. In most of these cases, ribavirin was administered intravenously at dosages up to and in some cases exceeding four times the recommended maximum oral daily dose.

11 DESCRIPTION

Moderiba (ribavirin, USP) is a nucleoside analogue with antiviral activity. The chemical name of ribavirin is 1-β-D-ribofuranosyl-1*H*-1,2,4-triazole-3-carboxamide and has the following structural formula:

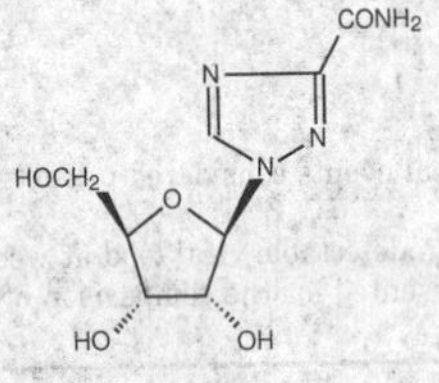

The molecular formula of ribavirin is $C_8H_{12}N_4O_5$ and the molecular weight is 244.2. Ribavirin is a white to off-white powder. It is freely soluble in water and slightly soluble in anhydrous alcohol.

Moderiba is available as a blue-colored (shade depending on strength), capsule-shaped, film-coated tablet for oral administration. Each tablet contains 200 mg, 400 mg, or 600 mg of ribavirin and the following inactive ingredients: microcrystalline cellulose, lactose monohydrate, croscarmellose sodium, povidone, magnesium stearate, and purified water. The coating of the 200 mg tablet contains partially hydrolyzed polyvinyl alcohol, titanium dioxide, polyethylene glycol 3350, talc, FD&C blue #2 [indigo carmine aluminum lake], and carnauba wax. The coating of the 400 mg and 600 mg tablet contains partially hydrolyzed polyvinyl alcohol, titanium dioxide, polyethylene glycol 3350, talc, FD&C blue #1 [brilliant blue FCF aluminum lake], and carnauba wax.

Moderiba complies with Organic Impurities: Procedure 1 of the current USP Monograph for Ribavirin Tablets.

12 CLINICAL PHARMACOLOGY

12.1 Mechanism of Action

Ribavirin is an antiviral drug *[see Microbiology (12.4)]*.

12.3 Pharmacokinetics

Multiple dose ribavirin pharmacokinetic data are available for HCV patients who received ribavirin in combination with peginterferon alfa-2a. Following administration of 1200 mg/day with food for 12 weeks mean±SD (n=39; body weight greater than 75 kg) $AUC_{0\text{-}12hr}$ was 25,361±7110 ng·hr/mL and C_{max} was 2748±818 ng/mL. The average time to reach C_{max} was 2 hours. Trough ribavirin plasma concentrations following 12 weeks of dosing with food were 1662±545 ng/mL in HCV infected patients who received 800 mg/day (n=89), and 2112±810 ng/mL in patients who received 1200 mg/day (n=75; body weight greater than 75 kg).

The terminal half-life of ribavirin following administration of a single oral dose of ribavirin is about 120 to 170 hours. The total apparent clearance following administration of a single oral dose of ribavirin is about 26 L/h. There is extensive accumulation of ribavirin after multiple dosing (twice daily) such that the C_{max} at steady state was four-fold higher than that of a single dose.

Effect of Food on Absorption of Ribavirin

Bioavailability of a single oral dose of ribavirin was increased by co-administration with a high-fat meal. The absorption was slowed (T_{max} was doubled) and the $AUC_{0\text{-}192h}$ and C_{max} increased by 42% and 66%, respectively, when ribavirin was taken with a high-fat meal compared with fasting conditions *[see Dosage and Administration (2.1) and Patient Counseling Information (17)]*.

Elimination and Metabolism

The contribution of renal and hepatic pathways to ribavirin elimination after administration of ribavirin is not known. *In vitro* studies indicate that ribavirin is not a substrate of CYP450 enzymes.

Renal Impairment

A clinical trial evaluated 50 CHC subjects with either moderate (creatinine clearance 30 to 50 mL/min) or severe (creatinine clearance less than 30 mL/min) renal impairment or end stage renal disease (ESRD) requiring chronic hemodialysis (HD). The apparent clearance of ribavirin was reduced in subjects with creatinine clearance less than or equal to 50 mL/min, including subjects with ESRD on HD, exhibiting approximately 30% of the value found in subjects with normal renal function. Pharmacokinetic modeling and simulation indicates that a dose of 200 mg daily in patients with severe renal impairment and a dose of 200 mg daily alternating with 400 mg the following day in patients with moderate renal impairment will provide plasma ribavirin exposures similar to that observed in patients with normal renal function receiving the standard 1000/1200 mg ribavirin daily dose. These doses have not been studied in patients.

In 18 subjects with ESRD receiving chronic HD, ribavirin was administered at a dose of 200 mg daily. Ribavirin plasma exposures in these subjects were approximately 20% lower compared to subjects with normal renal function receiving the standard 1000/1200 mg ribavirin daily dose *[see Dosage and Administration (2.4), Use in Specific Populations (8.7)]*.

Plasma ribavirin is removed by hemodialysis with an extraction ratio of approximately 50%; however, due to the large volume of distribution of ribavirin, plasma exposure is not expected to change with hemodialysis.

12.4 Microbiology

Mechanism of Action

The mechanism by which ribavirin contributes to its antiviral efficacy in the clinic is not fully understood. Ribavirin has direct antiviral activity in tissue culture against many RNA viruses. Ribavirin increases the mutation frequency in the genomes of several RNA viruses and ribavirin triphosphate inhibits HCV polymerase in a biochemical reaction.

Antiviral Activity in Cell Culture

In the stable HCV cell culture model system (HCV replicon), ribavirin inhibited autonomous HCV RNA replication with a 50% effective concentration (EC_{50}) value of 11-21 mcM. In the same model, PEG-IFN α-2a also inhibited HCV RNA replication, with an EC_{50} value of 0.1-3 ng/mL. The combination of PEG-IFN α-2a and ribavirin was more effective at inhibiting HCV RNA replication than either agent alone.

Resistance

Different HCV genotypes display considerable clinical variability in their response to PEG-IFN-α and ribavirin therapy. Viral genetic determinants associated with the variable response have not been definitively identified.

Cross-resistance

Cross-resistance between IFN α and ribavirin has not been observed.

13 NONCLINICAL TOXICOLOGY

13.1 Carcinogenesis, Mutagenesis, Impairment of Fertility

Carcinogenesis

In a p53 (+/-) mouse carcinogenicity study up to the maximum tolerated dose of 100 mg/kg/day, ribavirin was not oncogenic. Ribavirin was also not oncogenic in a rat 2-year carcinogenicity study at doses up to the maximum tolerated dose of 60 mg/kg/day. On a body surface area basis, these doses are approximately 0.5 and 0.6 times the maximum recommended daily human dose of ribavirin, respectively.

Mutagenesis

Ribavirin demonstrated mutagenic activity in the *in vitro* mouse lymphoma assay. No clastogenic activity was observed in an *in vivo* mouse micronucleus assay at doses up to 2000 mg/kg. However, results from studies published in the literature show clastogenic activity in the in vivo mouse micronucleus assay at oral doses up to 2000 mg/kg. A dominant lethal assay in rats was negative, indicating that if mutations occurred in rats they were not transmitted through male gametes.

Impairment of Fertility

In a fertility study in rats, ribavirin showed a marginal reduction in sperm counts at the dose of 100 mg/kg/day with no effect on fertility. Upon cessation of treatment, total recovery occurred after 1 spermatogenesis cycle. Abnormalities in sperm were observed in studies in mice designed to evaluate the time course and reversibility of ribavirin-induced testicular degeneration at doses of 15 to 150 mg/kg/day (approximately 0.1 to 0.8 times the maximum recommended daily human dose of ribavirin) administered for 3 to 6 months. Upon cessation of treatment, essentially total recovery from ribavirin-induced testicular toxicity was apparent within 1 or 2 spermatogenic cycles.

Female patients of childbearing potential and male patients with female partners of childbearing potential should not receive Moderiba unless the patient and his/her partner are using effective contraception (two reliable forms). Based on a multiple dose half-life ($t_{1/2}$) of ribavirin of 12 days, effective contraception must be utilized for 6 months post therapy (i.e., 15 half-lives of clearance for ribavirin).

No reproductive toxicology studies have been performed using peginterferon alfa-2a in combination with ribavirin. However, peginterferon alfa-2a and ribavirin when administered separately, each has adverse effects on reproduction. It should be assumed that the effects produced by either agent alone would also be caused by the combination of the two agents.

13.2 Animal Toxicology and/or Pharmacology

In a study in rats, it was concluded that dominant lethality was not induced by ribavirin at doses up to 200 mg/kg for 5 days (up to 1.7 times the maximum recommended human dose of ribavirin).

Long-term studies in the mouse and rat (18 to 24 months; dose 20 to 75, and 10 to 40 mg/kg/day, respectively, approximately 0.1 to 0.4 times the maximum daily human dose of ribavirin) have demonstrated a relationship between chronic ribavirin exposure and an increased incidence of vascular lesions (microscopic hemorrhages) in mice. In rats, retinal degeneration occurred in controls, but the incidence was increased in ribavirin-treated rats.

14 CLINICAL STUDIES

14.1 Chronic Hepatitis C Patients

Adult Patients

The safety and effectiveness of peginterferon alfa-2a in combination with ribavirin for the treatment of hepatitis C virus infection were assessed in two randomized controlled clinical trials. All patients were adults, had compensated liver disease, detectable hepatitis C virus, liver biopsy diagnosis of chronic hepatitis, and were previously untreated with interferon. Approximately 20% of patients in both studies had compensated cirrhosis (Child-Pugh class A). Patients coinfected with HIV were excluded from these studies.

In Study NV15801, patients were randomized to receive either peginterferon alfa-2a 180 mcg subcutaneous once weekly with an oral placebo, peginterferon alfa-2a 180 mcg once weekly with ribavirin 1000 mg by mouth (body weight less than 75 kg) or 1200 mg by mouth (body weight greater than or equal to 75 kg) or interferon alfa-2b 3 MIU subcutaneous three times a week plus ribavirin 1000 mg or 1200 mg by mouth. All patients received 48 weeks of therapy followed by 24 weeks of treatment-free follow-up. Ribavirin or placebo treatment assignment was blinded. Sustained virological response was defined as undetectable (less than 50 IU/mL) HCV RNA on or after study week 68. Peginterferon alfa-2a in combination with ribavirin resulted in a higher SVR compared to peginterferon alfa-2a alone or interferon alfa-2b and ribavirin (**Table 9**). In all treatment arms, patients with viral genotype 1, regardless of viral load, had a lower response rate to peginterferon alfa-2a in combination with ribavirin compared to patients with other viral genotypes.

[See table 9 above]

Table 9 Sustained Virologic Response (SVR) to Combination Therapy (Study NV15801)

	Interferon alfa-2b + Ribavirin 1000 mg or 1200 mg	Peginterferon alfa-2a + placebo	Peginterferon alfa-2a + Ribavirin Tablets 1000 mg or 1200 mg
All patients	197/444 (44%)	65/224 (29%)	241/453 (53%)
Genotype 1	103/285 (36%)	29/145 (20%)	132/298 (44%)
Genotypes 2–6	94/159 (59%)	36/79 (46%)	109/155 (70%)

Difference in overall treatment response (Peginterferon alfa-2a/ribavirin – Interferon alfa-2b/ribavirin) was 9% (95% CI 2.3, 15.3).

In Study NV15942, all patients received peginterferon alfa-2a 180 mcg subcutaneous once weekly and were randomized to treatment for either 24 or 48 weeks and to a ribavirin dose of either 800 mg or 1000 mg/1200 mg (for body weight less than 75 kg/greater than or equal to 75 kg). Assignment to the four treatment arms was stratified by viral genotype and baseline HCV viral titer. Patients with genotype 1 and high viral titer (defined as greater than 2×10^6 HCV RNA copies/mL serum) were preferentially assigned to treatment for 48 weeks.

Sustained Virologic Response (SVR) and HCV Genotype

HCV 1 and 4- Irrespective of baseline viral titer, treatment for 48 weeks with peginterferon alfa-2a and 1000 mg or 1200 mg of ribavirin resulted in higher SVR (defined as undetectable HCV RNA at the end of the 24-week treatment-free follow-up period) compared to shorter treatment (24 weeks) and/or 800 mg ribavirin.

HCV 2 and 3- Irrespective of baseline viral titer, treatment for 24 weeks with peginterferon alfa-2a and 800 mg of ribavirin resulted in a similar SVR compared to longer treatment (48 weeks) and/or 1000 mg or 1200 mg of ribavirin (see **Table 10**).

The numbers of patients with genotype 5 and 6 were too few to allow for meaningful assessment.

[See table 10 on next page]

Pediatric Patients

Previously untreated pediatric subjects 5 through 17 years of age (55% less than 12 years old) with chronic hepatitis C, compensated liver disease and detectable HCV RNA were treated with ribavirin approximately 15 mg/kg/day plus peginterferon alfa-2a 180 mcg/1.73 m^2 × body surface area once weekly for 48 weeks. All subjects were followed for 24 weeks post-treatment. Sustained virological response (SVR) was defined as undetectable (less than 50 IU/mL) HCV RNA on or after study week 68. A total of 114 subjects were randomized to receive either combination treatment of ribavirin plus peginterferon alfa-2a or peginterferon alfa-2a monotherapy; subjects failing peginterferon alfa-2a monotherapy at 24 weeks or later could receive open-label ribavirin plus peginterferon alfa-2a. The initial randomized arms were balanced for demographic factors; 55 subjects received initial combination treatment of ribavirin plus peginterferon alfa-2a and 59 received peginterferon alfa-2a plus placebo; in the overall intent-to-treat population, 45% were female, 80% were Caucasian, and 81% were infected with HCV genotype 1. The SVR results are summarized in **Table 11**.

[See table 11 on next page]

14.2 Other Treatment Response Predictors

Treatment response rates are lower in patients with poor prognostic factors receiving pegylated interferon alpha therapy. In studies NV15801 and NV15942, treatment response rates were lower in patients older than 40 years (50% vs. 66%), in patients with cirrhosis (47% vs. 59%), in patients weighing over 85 kg (49% vs. 60%), and in patients with genotype 1 with high vs. low viral load (43% vs. 56%). African-American patients had lower response rates compared to Caucasians.

In studies NV15801 and NV15942, lack of early virologic response by 12 weeks (defined as HCV RNA undetectable or greater than 2 $\log_{10}$ lower than baseline) was grounds for discontinuation of treatment. Of patients who lacked an early viral response by 12 weeks and completed a recommended course of therapy despite a protocol-defined option to discontinue therapy, 5/39 (13%) achieved an SVR. Of patients who lacked an early viral response by 24 weeks, 19 completed a full course of therapy and none achieved an SVR.

14.3 Chronic Hepatitis C/HIV Coinfected Patients

In Study NR15961, patients with CHC/HIV were randomized to receive either peginterferon alfa-2a 180 mcg subcutaneous once weekly plus an oral placebo, peginterferon alfa-2a 180 mcg once weekly plus ribavirin 800 mg by mouth daily or interferon alfa-2a, 3 MIU subcutaneous three times a week plus ribavirin 800 mg by mouth daily. All patients received 48 weeks of therapy and sustained virologic response (SVR) was assessed at 24 weeks of treatment-free follow-up. Ribavirin or placebo treatment assignment was blinded in the peginterferon alfa-2a treatment arms. All patients were adults, had compensated liver disease, detectable hepatitis C virus, liver biopsy diagnosis of chronic hepatitis C, and were previously untreated with interferon. Patients also had CD4+ cell count greater than or equal to 200 cells/mm^3 or CD4+ cell count greater than or equal to 100 cells/mm^3 but less than 200 cells/mm^3 and HIV-1 RNA less than 5000 copies/mL, and stable status of HIV. Approximately 15% of patients in the study had cirrhosis. Results are shown in **Table 12**.

[See table 12 on next page]

Treatment response rates were lower in CHC/HIV patients with poor prognostic factors (including HCV genotype 1, HCV RNA greater than 800,000 IU/mL, and cirrhosis) receiving pegylated interferon alpha therapy.

Of the patients who did not demonstrate either undetectable HCV RNA or at least a 2 $\log_{10}$ reduction from baseline in HCV RNA titer by 12 weeks of peginterferon alfa-2a and ribavirin combination therapy, 2% (2/85) achieved an SVR.

In CHC patients with HIV coinfection who received 48 weeks of peginterferon alfa-2a alone or in combination with ribavirin treatment, mean and median HIV RNA titers did not increase above baseline during treatment or 24 weeks post treatment.

16 HOW SUPPLIED/STORAGE AND HANDLING

Moderiba (ribavirin, USP) is available as tablets for oral administration.

Each Moderiba 200-mg tablet contains 200 mg of ribavirin, USP and is a capsule-shaped, light blue colored, film-coated tablet, debossed with "200" on one side and the logo "3RP" on the other side.

Each Moderiba 400-mg tablet contains 400 mg of ribavirin, USP and is a capsule-shaped, medium blue colored, film-coated tablet, debossed with "400" on one side and the logo "3RP" on the other side.

Each Moderiba 600-mg tablet contains 600 mg of ribavirin, USP and is a capsule-shaped, dark blue colored, film-coated tablet, debossed with "600" on one side and the logo "3RP" on the other side.

They are packaged as follows:

200 mg Bottles of 168 NDC 0074-3197-16

Moderiba™ is also available in blister packs as follows:

Moderiba™ 600 Dose Pack Carton contains a total of 28 - 200 mg Moderiba tablets and 28 - 400 mg Moderiba tablets. Each carton contains 4 individual Moderiba™ 600 Dose Packs. Each individual Moderiba™ 600 Dose Pack contains 7 (seven) - 200 mg Moderiba tablets and 7 (seven) - 400 mg Moderiba tablets.

Each 200 mg Moderiba tablet contains 200 mg of ribavirin and is a capsule-shaped, light blue colored, film-coated tablet, debossed with "200" on one side and the logo "3RP" on the other side. Each 400 mg Moderiba tablet contains 400 mg of ribavirin and is a capsule-shaped, medium blue colored, film-coated tablet, debossed with "400" on one side and the logo "3RP" on the other side.

Moderiba™ 600 Dose Pack Carton
NDC: 0074-3224-56
Moderiba™ 600 Dose Pack
NDC: 0074-3224-14

Moderiba™ 800 Dose Pack Carton contains a total of 56 - 400 mg Moderiba tablets. Each carton contains 4 individual Moderiba 800 Dose Packs. Each individual Moderiba 800 Dose Pack contains 14 (fourteen) - 400 mg Moderiba tablets. Each 400 mg Moderiba tablet contains 400 mg of ribavirin and is a capsule-shaped, medium blue colored, film-coated tablet, debossed with "400" on one side and the logo "3RP" on the other side.

Moderiba™ 800 Dose Pack Carton
NDC: 0074-3239-56
Moderiba™ 800 Dose Pack
NDC: 0074-3239-14

Moderiba™ 1000 Dose Pack Carton contains a total of 28 - 400 mg Moderiba tablets and 28 - 600 mg Moderiba tablets.

Continued on next page

Information on the AbbVie, Inc. products listed on these pages is from the prescribing information in use as of July 31, 2016. For more information, please visit rxabbvie.com or call 1-800-633-9110.

Each carton contains 4 individual Moderiba 1000 Dose Packs. Each individual Moderiba 1000 Dose Pack contains 7 (seven) - 400 mg Moderiba tablets and 7 (seven) - 600 mg Moderiba tablets.

Each 400 mg Moderiba tablet contains 400 mg of ribavirin and is a capsule-shaped, medium blue colored, film-coated tablet, debossed with "400" on one side and the logo "3RP" on the other side. Each 600 mg Moderiba tablet contains 600 mg of ribavirin and is a capsule-shaped, dark blue colored, film-coated tablet, debossed with "600" on one side and the logo "3RP" on the other side.

Moderiba™ 1000 Dose Pack Carton
NDC: 0074-3271-56
Moderiba™ 1000 Dose Pack
NDC: 0074-3271-14
Moderiba™ 1200 Dose Pack Carton contains a total of 56 - 600 mg Moderiba tablets. Each carton contains 4 individual Moderiba 1200 Dose Packs. Each individual Moderiba 1200 Dose Pack contains 14 (fourteen) - 600 mg Moderiba tablets.
Each 600 mg Moderiba tablet contains 600 mg of ribavirin and is a capsule-shaped, dark blue colored, film-coated tablet, debossed with "600" on one side and the logo "3RP" on the other side.
Moderiba™ 1200 Dose Pack Carton
NDC: 0074-3282-56
Moderiba™ 1200 mg Dose Pack
NDC: 0074-3282-14

Storage and Handling
Store the Moderiba™ Tablets bottle at 25°C (77°F); excursions are permitted between 15°C and 30°C (59°F and 86°F) [see USP Controlled Room Temperature]. Keep bottle tightly closed.

17 PATIENT COUNSELING INFORMATION
• "See FDA-approved patient labeling (Medication Guide)"

Pregnancy
Patients must be informed that ribavirin may cause birth defects and/or death of the exposed fetus. Moderiba therapy must not be used by women who are pregnant or by men whose female partners are pregnant. Extreme care must be taken to avoid pregnancy in female patients and in female partners of male patients taking Moderiba therapy and for 6 months post therapy. Patients should use two reliable methods of birth control while taking Moderiba therapy and for 6 months post therapy. Moderiba therapy should not be initiated until a report of a negative pregnancy test has been obtained immediately prior to initiation of therapy. Patients must perform a pregnancy test monthly during therapy and for 6 months post therapy.

Female patients of childbearing potential and male patients with female partners of childbearing potential must be advised of the teratogenic/embryocidal risks and must be instructed to practice effective contraception during Moderiba therapy and for 6 months post therapy. Patients should be advised to notify the healthcare provider immediately in the event of a pregnancy [see Contraindications (4) and Warnings and Precautions (5.1)].

Anemia
The most common adverse event associated with ribavirin is anemia, which may be severe [see Boxed Warning, Warnings and Precautions (5.2) and Adverse Reactions (6.1)]. Patients should be advised that laboratory evaluations are required prior to starting Moderiba therapy and periodically thereafter [see Warnings and Precautions (5.9)]. It is advised that patients be well hydrated, especially during the initial stages of treatment.

Patients who develop dizziness, confusion, somnolence, and fatigue should be cautioned to avoid driving or operating machinery.

Patients should be advised to take Moderiba with food.

Patients should be questioned about prior history of drug abuse before initiating Moderiba/peginterferon alfa-2a, as relapse of drug addiction and drug overdoses have been reported in patients treated with interferons.

Patients should be advised not to drink alcohol, as alcohol may exacerbate chronic hepatitis C infection.

Patients should be informed about what to do in the event they miss a dose of Moderiba. The missed doses should be taken as soon as possible during the same day. Patients should not double the next dose. Patients should be advised to call their healthcare provider if they have questions.

Patients should be informed that the effect of peginterferon alfa-2a/Moderiba treatment of hepatitis C infection on transmission is not known, and that appropriate precautions to prevent transmission of hepatitis C virus during treatment or in the event of treatment failure should be taken.

Patients should be informed regarding the potential benefits and risks attendant to the use of Moderiba. Instructions on appropriate use should be given, including review of the contents of the enclosed MEDICATION GUIDE, which is not a disclosure of all or possible adverse effects.

U.S. Patent No. 7,723,310
C139.00015
70010441

MEDICATION GUIDE
Moderiba™ (Mah-duh-RYE-bah)
(ribavirin, USP)
Tablets
Read this Medication Guide carefully before you start taking Moderiba and read the Medication Guide each time you get more Moderiba. There may be new information. This information does not take the place of talking to your healthcare provider about your medical condition or your treatment.
Also read the Medication Guide for PEGASYS[1] (peginterferon alfa-2a).

What is the most important information I should know about Moderiba?
1. **You should not take Moderiba alone to treat chronic hepatitis C infection.** Moderiba should be used with peginterferon alfa-2a to treat chronic hepatitis C infection.
2. **Moderiba may cause you to have a blood problem (hemolytic anemia) that can worsen any heart problems you have, and cause you to have a heart attack or die.** Tell your healthcare provider if you have ever had any heart problems. Moderiba may not be right for you. If you have chest pain while you take Moderiba, get emergency medical attention right away.
3. **Moderiba may cause birth defects or death of your unborn baby.** If you are pregnant or your sexual partner is pregnant, do not take Moderiba. You or your sexual partner should not become pregnant while you take Moderiba and for 6 months after treatment is over. You must use two forms of birth control when you take Moderiba and for the 6 months after treatment.
   • Females must have a pregnancy test before starting Moderiba, every month while treated with Moderiba, and every month for the 6 months after treatment with Moderiba.

• If you or your female sexual partner becomes pregnant while taking Moderiba or within 6 months after you stop taking Moderiba, tell your healthcare provider right away. You or your healthcare provider should contact the **Ribavirin Pregnancy Registry by calling 1-800-593-2214.** The Ribavirin Pregnancy Registry collects information about what happens to mothers and their babies if the mother takes Moderiba while she is pregnant.

What is Moderiba?
Moderiba is a prescription medicine used with another medicine called peginterferon alfa-2a to treat chronic (lasting a long time) hepatitis C infection in people 5 years and older whose liver still works normally, and who have not been treated before with a medicine called an interferon alpha. It is not known if Moderiba is safe and will work in children under 5 years of age.

Who should not take Moderiba?
See "What is the most important information I should know about Moderiba?"
Do not take Moderiba if you:
• **have certain types of hepatitis** caused by your immune system attacking your liver (autoimmune hepatitis)
• **have certain blood disorders,** such as thalassemia major or sickle-cell anemia (hemoglobinopathies)
• **take didanosine** (Videx[®2] or Videx EC[®2])
Talk to your healthcare provider before starting treatment with Moderiba if you have any of these medical conditions.

What should I tell my healthcare provider before taking Moderiba?
Before you take Moderiba, tell your healthcare provider if you have or have had:
• **treatment for hepatitis C that did not work for you**
• **serious allergic reactions to Moderiba or to any of the ingredients in Moderiba.** See the end of this Medication Guide for a list of ingredients.
• **breathing problems.** Moderiba may cause or worsen your breathing problems you already have.
• **vision problems.** Moderiba may cause eye problems or worsen eye problems you already have. You should have an eye exam before you start treatment with Moderiba.
• **certain blood disorders such as anemia**
• **high blood pressure, heart problems or have had a heart attack.** Your healthcare provider should test your blood and heart before you start treatment with Moderiba.
• **thyroid problems**

Table 10 Sustained Virologic Response as a Function of Genotype (Study NV15942)

	24 Weeks Treatment		48 Weeks Treatment	
	Peginterferon alfa-2a + Ribavirin 800 mg (N=207)	Peginterferon alfa-2a + Ribavirin 1000 mg or 1200 mg* (N=280)	Peginterferon alfa-2a + Ribavirin 800 mg (N=361)	Peginterferon alfa-2a + Ribavirin 1000 mg or 1200 mg* (N=436)
Genotype 1	29/101 (29%)	48/118 (41%)	99/250 (40%)	138/271 (51%)
Genotypes 2, 3	79/96 (82%)	116/144 (81%)	75/99 (76%)	117/153 (76%)
Genotype 4	0/5 (0%)	7/12 (58%)	5/8 (63%)	9/11 (82%)

*1000 mg for body weight less than 75 kg; 1200 mg for body weight greater than or equal to 75 kg.

Table 11 Sustained Virologic Response (Study NV17424)

	Peginterferon alfa-2a 180 mcg/1.73 m² × BSA + Ribavirin 15 mg/kg* (N=55)	Peginterferon alfa-2a 180 mcg/1.73 m² × BSA + Placebo* (N=59)
All HCV genotypes**	29 (53%)	12 (20%)
HCV genotype 1	21/45 (47%)	8/47 (17%)
HCV non-genotype 1***	8/10 (80%)	4/12 (33%)

*Results indicate undetectable HCV-RNA defined as HCV RNA less than 50 IU/mL at 24 weeks post-treatment using the AMPLICOR HCV test v2
**Scheduled treatment duration was 48 weeks regardless of the genotype
***Includes HCV genotypes 2, 3 and others

Table 12 Sustained Virologic Response in Patients With Chronic Hepatitis C Coinfected With HIV (Study NR15961)

	Interferon alfa-2a + Ribavirin 800 mg (N=289)	peginterferon alfa-2a + Placebo (N=289)	peginterferon alfa-2a + Ribavirin 800 mg (N=290)
All patients	33 (11%)	58 (20%)	116 (40%)
Genotype 1	12/171 (7%)	24/175 (14%)	51/176 (29%)
Genotypes 2, 3	18/89 (20%)	32/90 (36%)	59/95 (62%)

- diabetes. Moderiba and peginterferon alfa-2a combination therapy may make your diabetes worse or harder to treat.
- **liver problems** other than hepatitis C virus infection
- **human immunodeficiency virus (HIV)** or other immunity problems
- **mental health problems**, including depression or thoughts of suicide
- **kidney problems**
- **an organ transplant**
- **drug addiction or abuse**
- **infection with hepatitis B virus**
- **any other medical condition**
- **are breast feeding.** It is not known if Moderiba passes into your breast milk. You and your healthcare provider should decide if you will take Moderiba or breast-feed.

Tell your healthcare provider about all the medicines you take, including prescription and non-prescription medicines, vitamins and herbal supplements. Some medicines can cause serious side effects if taken while you also take Moderiba. Some medicines may affect how Moderiba works or Moderiba may affect how your other medicines work.

Especially tell your healthcare provider if you take any medicines to treat HIV, including didanosine (Videx[2] or Videx EC[2]), or if you take azathioprine (Imuran[3] or Azasan[4]).

Know the medicines you take. Keep a list of them to show your healthcare provider or pharmacist when you get a new medicine.

How should I take Moderiba?

- Take Moderiba exactly as your healthcare provider tells you. Your healthcare provider will tell you how much Moderiba to take and when to take it. For children 5 years of age and older your healthcare provider will prescribe the dose of Moderiba based on weight.
- Take Moderiba with food.
- If you miss a dose of Moderiba, take the missed dose as soon as possible during the same day. Do not double the next dose. If you have questions about what to do, call your healthcare provider.
- If you take too much Moderiba, call your healthcare provider or local Poison Control Center right away, or go to the nearest hospital emergency room right away.
- Your healthcare provider should do blood tests before you start treatment with Moderiba, at weeks 2 and 4 of treatment, and then as needed to see how well you are tolerating treatment and to check for side effects. Your healthcare provider may change your dose of Moderiba based on blood test results or side effects you may have.
- If you have heart problems, your healthcare provider should check your heart by doing an electrocardiogram before you start treatment with Moderiba, and if needed during treatment.

What should I avoid while taking Moderiba?

- Moderiba can make you feel tired, dizzy, or confused. You should not drive or operate machinery if you have any of these symptoms.
- Do not drink alcohol, including beer, wine, and liquor. This may make your liver disease worse.

What are the possible side effects of Moderiba?

Moderiba may cause serious side effects including:

See "What is the most important information I should know about Moderiba?"

- **Swelling and irritation of your pancreas (pancreatitis).** You may have stomach pain, nausea, vomiting or diarrhea.
- **Severe allergic reactions.** Symptoms may include hives, wheezing, trouble breathing, chest pain, swelling of your mouth, tongue, or lips, or severe rash.
- **Serious breathing problems.** Difficulty breathing may be a sign of a serious lung infection (pneumonia) that can lead to death.
- **Serious eye problems** that may lead to vision loss or blindness.
- **Liver problems.** Some people may get worsening of liver function. Tell your healthcare provider right away if you have any of these symptoms: stomach bloating, confusion, brown urine, and yellow eyes.
- **Severe depression**
- **Suicidal thoughts and attempts**
- **Effect on growth in children.** Children can experience a delay in weight gain and height increase while being treated with peginterferon alfa-2a and Moderiba. Catch-up in growth happens after treatment stops, but some children may not reach the height that they were expected to have before treatment. Talk to your healthcare provider if you are concerned about your child's growth during treatment with peginterferon alfa-2a and Moderiba.

Call your healthcare provider or get medical help right away if you have any of the symptoms listed above. These may be signs of a serious side effect of Moderiba treatment.

Common side effects of Moderiba taken with peginterferon alfa-2a include:

- flu-like symptoms-feeling tired, headache, shaking along with high temperature (fever), and muscle or joint aches
- mood changes, feeling irritable, anxiety, and difficulty sleeping
- loss of appetite, nausea, vomiting, and diarrhea
- hair loss
- itching

Tell your healthcare provider about any side effect that bothers you or that does not go away.

These are not all the possible side effects of Moderiba treatment. For more information, ask your healthcare provider or pharmacist.

Call your doctor for medical advice about side effects. You may report side effects to FDA at 1-800-FDA-1088.

You may also report side effects to AbbVie Inc. at 1-800-633-9110.

How should I store Moderiba?

- Store Moderiba tablets between 59°F and 86°F (15°C and 30°C).
- Keep the bottle tightly closed.

Keep Moderiba and all medicines out of the reach of children.

General information about the safe and effective use of Moderiba

It is not known if treatment with Moderiba in combination with peginterferon alfa-2a will prevent an infected person from spreading the hepatitis C virus to another person while on treatment.

Medicines are sometimes prescribed for purposes other than those listed in a Medication Guide. Do not use Moderiba for a condition for which it was not prescribed. Do not give Moderiba to other people, even if they have the same symptoms that you have. It may harm them.

This Medication Guide summarizes the most important information about Moderiba. If you would like more information, talk with your healthcare provider. You can ask your healthcare provider or pharmacist for information about Moderiba that is written for healthcare professionals.

What are the ingredients in Moderiba?

Active Ingredient: ribavirin

Inactive Ingredients: microcrystalline cellulose, lactose monohydrate, croscarmellose sodium, povidone, magnesium stearate, and purified water. The tablet is coated with partially hydrolyzed polyvinyl alcohol, polyethylene glycol 3350, talc, titanium dioxide, FD&C blue #2 [indigo carmine aluminum lake] (200 mg tablet only), FD&C blue #1 [brilliant blue FCF aluminum lake] (400 mg and 600 mg tablets only), and carnauba wax.

This Medication Guide has been approved by the U.S. Food and Drug Administration.

[1]PEGASYS is a trademark of Hoffmann-La Roche, Inc.
[2]Videx and Videx EC is a registered trademark of Bristol-Myers Squibb Company
[3]Imuran is a registered trademark of Prometheus Laboratories, Inc.
[4]Azasan is a registered trademark of Salix Pharmaceuticals, Inc.

Distributed by
AbbVie Inc.
North Chicago, IL 60064 USA
C139.00016 – Revised February, 2015
70010440
Printed in USA
U.S. Patent No. 7,723,310
Copyright © 2015 by Kadmon Pharmaceuticals, LLC. All rights reserved.

Shown in Product Identification Guide, page 506

NIASPAN®   ℞

[ny-a-span]
(niacin extended-release)
tablet, film coated, extended release for oral use.

HIGHLIGHTS OF PRESCRIBING INFORMATION
These highlights do not include all the information needed to use NIASPAN® safely and effectively. See full prescribing information for NIASPAN.

NIASPAN (niacin extended-release) tablet, film coated, extended release for oral use.
Initial U.S. Approval: 1997

RECENT MAJOR CHANGES

Indications and Usage, Combination With a Statin – removal (1)	4/2015
Dosage and Administration, Combination With a Statin – removal (2)	4/2015

INDICATIONS AND USAGE

NIASPAN contains extended-release niacin (nicotinic acid), and is indicated:

- To reduce elevated TC, LDL-C, Apo B and TG, and to increase HDL-C in patients with primary hyperlipidemia and mixed dyslipidemia. (1)
- To reduce the risk of recurrent nonfatal myocardial infarction in patients with a history of myocardial infarction and hyperlipidemia. (1)
- In combination with a bile acid binding resin:
  - Slows progression or promotes regression of atherosclerotic disease in patients with a history of coronary artery disease (CAD) and hyperlipidemia. (1)
  - As an adjunct to diet to reduce elevated TC and LDL-C in adult patients with primary hyperlipidemia. (1)
- To reduce TG in adult patients with severe hypertriglyceridemia. (1)

Limitations of use:
Addition of NIASPAN did not reduce cardiovascular morbidity or mortality among patients treated with simvastatin in a large, randomized controlled trial (5.1).

DOSAGE AND ADMINISTRATION

- NIASPAN should be taken at bedtime with a low-fat snack. (2)
- Dose range: 500 mg to 2000 mg once daily. (2)
- Therapy with NIASPAN must be initiated at 500 mg at bedtime in order to reduce the incidence and severity of side effects which may occur during early therapy and should not be increased by more than 500 mg in any four week period. (2)
- Maintenance dose: 1000 to 2000 mg once daily. (2)
- Doses greater than 2000 mg daily are not recommended. (2)

DOSAGE FORMS AND STRENGTHS

Unscored film-coated tablets for oral administration: 500, 750 and 1000 mg niacin extended-release. (3)

CONTRAINDICATIONS

- Active liver disease, which may include unexplained persistent elevations in hepatic transaminase levels. (4, 5.3)
- Active peptic ulcer disease. (4)
- Arterial bleeding. (4)
- Known hypersensitivity to product components. (4, 6.1)

WARNINGS AND PRECAUTIONS

- Severe hepatic toxicity has occurred in patients substituting sustained-release niacin for immediate-release niacin at equivalent doses. (5.3)
- Myopathy has been reported in patients taking NIASPAN. The risk for myopathy and rhabdomyolysis are increased among elderly patients; patients with diabetes, renal failure, or uncontrolled hypothyroidism; and patients being treated with a statin. (5.2)
- Liver enzyme abnormalities and monitoring: Persistent elevations in hepatic transaminase can occur. Monitor liver enzymes before and during treatment. (5.3)
- Use with caution in patients with unstable angina or in the acute phase of an MI. (5)
- NIASPAN can increase serum glucose levels. Glucose levels should be closely monitored in diabetic or potentially diabetic patients particularly during the first few months of use or dose adjustment. (5.4)

ADVERSE REACTIONS

Most common adverse reactions (incidence >5% and greater than placebo) are flushing, diarrhea, nausea, vomiting, increased cough, and pruritus. (6.1)

Flushing of the skin may be reduced in frequency or severity by pretreatment with aspirin (up to the recommended dose of 325 mg taken 30 minutes prior to NIASPAN dose). (2)

To report SUSPECTED ADVERSE REACTIONS, contact AbbVie Inc. at 1-800-633-9110 or FDA at 1-800-FDA-1088 or www.fda.gov/medwatch.

Continued on next page

Information on the AbbVie, Inc. products listed on these pages is from the prescribing information in use as of July 31, 2016. For more information, please visit rxabbvie.com or call 1-800-633-9110.

----------DRUG INTERACTIONS----------

- Statins: Caution should be used when prescribing niacin with statins as these agents can increase risk of myopathy/rhabdomyolysis. (5.2, 7.1)
- Bile Acid Sequestrants: Bile acid sequestrants have a high niacin-binding capacity and should be taken at least 4 - 6 hours before NIASPAN administration. (7.2)

----------USE IN SPECIFIC POPULATIONS----------

- Renal impairment: NIASPAN should be used with caution in patients with renal impairment. (5, 8.6)
- Hepatic impairment: NIASPAN is contraindicated in active liver disease or significant or unexplained hepatic dysfunction or unexplained elevations of serum transaminases. (4, 5, 5.3, 8.7)

See 17 for PATIENT COUNSELING INFORMATION and FDA-approved patient labeling.

Revised: 4/2015

FULL PRESCRIBING INFORMATION: CONTENTS*

* Sections or subsections omitted from the full prescribing information are not listed.

FULL PRESCRIBING INFORMATION

1   INDICATIONS AND USAGE

Therapy with lipid-altering agents should be only one component of multiple risk factor intervention in individuals at significantly increased risk for atherosclerotic vascular disease due to hyperlipidemia. Niacin therapy is indicated as an adjunct to diet when the response to a diet restricted in saturated fat and cholesterol and other nonpharmacologic measures alone has been inadequate.

1. NIASPAN is indicated to reduce elevated TC, LDL-C, Apo B and TG levels, and to increase HDL-C in patients with primary hyperlipidemia and mixed dyslipidemia.
2. In patients with a history of myocardial infarction and hyperlipidemia, niacin is indicated to reduce the risk of recurrent nonfatal myocardial infarction.
3. In patients with a history of coronary artery disease (CAD) and hyperlipidemia, niacin, in combination with a bile acid binding resin, is indicated to slow progression or promote regression of atherosclerotic disease.
4. NIASPAN in combination with a bile acid binding resin is indicated to reduce elevated TC and LDL-C levels in adult patients with primary hyperlipidemia.
5. Niacin is also indicated as adjunctive therapy for treatment of adult patients with severe hypertriglyceridemia who present a risk of pancreatitis and who do not respond adequately to a determined dietary effort to control them.

Limitations of Use

Addition of NIASPAN did not reduce cardiovascular morbidity or mortality among patients treated with simvastatin in a large, randomized controlled trial (AIM-HIGH) [see Warnings and Precautions (5.1)].

2   DOSAGE AND ADMINISTRATION

NIASPAN should be taken at bedtime, after a low-fat snack, and doses should be individualized according to patient response. Therapy with NIASPAN must be initiated at 500 mg at bedtime in order to reduce the incidence and severity of side effects which may occur during early therapy. The recommended dose escalation is shown in Table 1 below.

[See table 1 below]

Maintenance Dose

The daily dosage of NIASPAN should not be increased by more than 500 mg in any 4-week period. The recommended maintenance dose is 1000 mg (two 500 mg tablets or one 1000 mg tablet) to 2000 mg (two 1000 mg tablets or four 500 mg tablets) once daily at bedtime. Doses greater than 2000 mg daily are not recommended. Women may respond at lower NIASPAN doses than men [see Clinical Studies (14.2)].

Single-dose bioavailability studies have demonstrated that two of the 500 mg and one of the 1000 mg tablet strengths are interchangeable but three of the 500 mg and two of the 750 mg tablet strengths are not interchangeable.

Flushing of the skin [see Adverse Reactions (6.1)] may be reduced in frequency or severity by pretreatment with aspirin (up to the recommended dose of 325 mg taken 30 minutes prior to NIASPAN dose). Tolerance to this flushing develops rapidly over the course of several weeks. Flushing, pruritus, and gastrointestinal distress are also greatly reduced by slowly increasing the dose of niacin and avoiding administration on an empty stomach. Concomitant alcoholic, hot drinks or spicy foods may increase the side effects of flushing and pruritus and should be avoided around the time of NIASPAN ingestion.

Equivalent doses of NIASPAN should not be substituted for sustained-release (modified-release, timed-release) niacin preparations or immediate-release (crystalline) niacin [see Warnings and Precautions (5)]. Patients previously receiving other niacin products should be started with the recommended NIASPAN titration schedule (see Table 1), and the dose should subsequently be individualized based on patient response.

If NIASPAN therapy is discontinued for an extended period, reinstitution of therapy should include a titration phase (see Table 1).

NIASPAN tablets should be taken whole and should not be broken, crushed or chewed before swallowing.

Dosage in Patients with Renal or Hepatic Impairment

Use of NIASPAN in patients with renal or hepatic impairment has not been studied. NIASPAN is contraindicated in patients with significant or unexplained hepatic dysfunction. NIASPAN should be used with caution in patients with renal impairment [see Warnings and Precautions (5)].

3   DOSAGE FORMS AND STRENGTHS

- 500 mg unscored, medium-orange, film-coated, capsule-shaped tablets
- 750 mg unscored, medium-orange, film-coated, capsule-shaped tablets
- 1000 mg unscored, medium-orange, film-coated, capsule-shaped tablets

4   CONTRAINDICATIONS

NIASPAN is contraindicated in the following conditions:

- Active liver disease or unexplained persistent elevations in hepatic transaminases [see Warnings and Precautions (5.3)]
- Patients with active peptic ulcer disease
- Patients with arterial bleeding
- Hypersensitivity to niacin or any component of this medication [see Adverse Reactions (6.1)]

5   WARNINGS AND PRECAUTIONS

NIASPAN preparations should not be substituted for equivalent doses of immediate-release (crystalline) niacin. For patients switching from immediate-release niacin to NIASPAN, therapy with NIASPAN should be initiated with low doses (i.e., 500 mg at bedtime) and the NIASPAN dose should then be titrated to the desired therapeutic response [see Dosage and Administration (2)].

Caution should also be used when NIASPAN is used in patients with unstable angina or in the acute phase of an MI, particularly when such patients are also receiving vasoactive drugs such as nitrates, calcium channel blockers, or adrenergic blocking agents.

Niacin is rapidly metabolized by the liver, and excreted through the kidneys. NIASPAN is contraindicated in patients with significant or unexplained hepatic impairment [see Contraindications (4) and Warnings and Precautions (5.3)] and should be used with caution in patients with renal impairment. Patients with a past history of jaundice, hepatobiliary disease, or peptic ulcer should be observed closely during NIASPAN therapy.

5.1   Mortality and Coronary Heart Disease Morbidity

NIASPAN has not been shown to reduce cardiovascular morbidity or mortality among patients already treated with a statin.

The Atherothrombosis Intervention in Metabolic Syndrome with Low HDL/High Triglycerides: Impact on Global Health Outcomes (AIM-HIGH) trial was a randomized placebo-controlled trial of 3414 patients with stable, previously diagnosed cardiovascular disease. Mean baseline lipid levels were LDL-C 74 mg/dL, HDL-C 35 mg/dL, non-HDL-C 111 mg/dL and median triglyceride level of 163-177 mg/dL. Ninety-four percent of patients were on background statin therapy prior to entering the trial. All participants received simvastatin, 40 to 80 mg per day, plus ezetimibe 10 mg per day if needed, to maintain an LDL-C level of 40-80 mg/dL, and were randomized to receive NIASPAN 1500-2000 mg/day (n=1718) or matching placebo (IR Niacin, 100-150 mg, n=1696). On-treatment lipid changes at two years for LDL-C were -12.0% for the simvastatin plus NIASPAN group and -5.5% for the simvastatin plus placebo group. HDL-C increased by 25.0% to 42 mg/dL in the simvastatin plus NIASPAN group and by 9.8% to 38 mg/dL in the simvastatin plus placebo group (P<0.001). Triglyceride levels decreased by 28.6% in the simvastatin plus NIASPAN group and by 8.1% in the simvastatin plus placebo group. The primary outcome was an ITT composite of the first study occurrence of coronary heart disease death, nonfatal myocardial infarction, ischemic stroke, hospitalization for acute coronary syndrome or symptom-driven coronary or cerebral revascularization procedures. The trial was stopped after a mean follow-up period of 3 years owing to a lack of efficacy. The primary outcome occurred in 282 patients in the simvastatin plus NIASPAN group (16.4%) and in 274 patients in the simvastatin plus placebo group (16.2%) (HR 1.02 [95% CI, 0.87-1.21], P=0.79. In an ITT analysis, there were 42 cases of first occurrence of ischemic stroke reported, 27 (1.6%) in the simvastatin plus NIASPAN group and 15 (0.9%) in the simvastatin plus placebo group, a non-statistically significant result (HR 1.79, [95%CI =

Table 1. Recommended Dosing

	Week(s)	Daily dose	NIASPAN Dosage
INITIAL TITRATION SCHEDULE	1 to 4	500 mg	1 NIASPAN 500 mg tablet at bedtime
	5 to 8	1000 mg	1 NIASPAN 1000 mg tablet or 2 NIASPAN 500 mg tablets at bedtime
	*	1500 mg	2 NIASPAN 750 mg tablets or 3 NIASPAN 500 mg tablets at bedtime
	*	2000 mg	2 NIASPAN 1000 mg tablets or 4 NIASPAN 500 mg tablets at bedtime

* After Week 8, titrate to patient response and tolerance. If response to 1000 mg daily is inadequate, increase dose to 1500 mg daily; may subsequently increase dose to 2000 mg daily. Daily dose should not be increased more than 500 mg in a 4-week period, and doses above 2000 mg daily are not recommended. Women may respond at lower doses than men.

0.95-3.36], p=0.071). The on-treatment ischemic stroke events were 19 for the simvastatin plus NIASPAN group and 15 for the simvastatin plus placebo group [*see Adverse Reactions (6.1)*].

5.2 Skeletal Muscle

Cases of rhabdomyolysis have been associated with concomitant administration of lipid-altering doses (≥1 g/day) of niacin and statins. Elderly patients and patients with diabetes, renal failure, or uncontrolled hypothyroidism are particularly at risk. Monitor patients for any signs and symptoms of muscle pain, tenderness, or weakness, particularly during the initial months of therapy and during any periods of upward dosage titration. Periodic serum creatine phosphokinase (CPK) and potassium determinations should be considered in such situations, but there is no assurance that such monitoring will prevent the occurrence of severe myopathy.

5.3 Liver Dysfunction

Cases of severe hepatic toxicity, including fulminant hepatic necrosis, have occurred in patients who have substituted sustained-release (modified-release, timed-release) niacin products for immediate-release (crystalline) niacin at equivalent doses.

NIASPAN should be used with caution in patients who consume substantial quantities of alcohol and/or have a past history of liver disease. Active liver diseases or unexplained transaminase elevations are contraindications to the use of NIASPAN.

Niacin preparations have been associated with abnormal liver tests. In three placebo-controlled clinical trials involving titration to final daily NIASPAN doses ranging from 500 to 3000 mg, 245 patients received NIASPAN for a mean duration of 17 weeks. No patient with normal serum transaminase levels (AST, ALT) at baseline experienced elevations to more than 3 times the upper limit of normal (ULN) during treatment with NIASPAN. In these studies, fewer than 1% (2/245) of NIASPAN patients discontinued due to transaminase elevations greater than 2 times the ULN.

Liver-related tests should be performed on all patients during therapy with NIASPAN. Serum transaminase levels, including AST and ALT (SGOT and SGPT), should be monitored before treatment begins, every 6 to 12 weeks for the first year, and periodically thereafter (e.g., at approximately 6-month intervals). Special attention should be paid to patients who develop elevated serum transaminase levels, and in these patients, measurements should be repeated promptly and then performed more frequently. If the transaminase levels show evidence of progression, particularly if they rise to 3 times ULN and are persistent, or if they are associated with symptoms of nausea, fever, and/or malaise, the drug should be discontinued.

5.4 Laboratory Abnormalities

Increase in Blood Glucose: Niacin treatment can increase fasting blood glucose. Frequent monitoring of blood glucose should be performed to ascertain that the drug is producing no adverse effects. Diabetic patients may experience a dose-related increase in glucose intolerance. Diabetic or potentially diabetic patients should be observed closely during treatment with NIASPAN, particularly during the first few months of use or dose adjustment; adjustment of diet and/or hypoglycemic therapy may be necessary.

Reduction in platelet count: NIASPAN has been associated with small but statistically significant dose-related reductions in platelet count (mean of -11% with 2000 mg). Caution should be observed when NIASPAN is administered concomitantly with anticoagulants; platelet counts should be monitored closely in such patients.

Increase in Prothrombin Time (PT): NIASPAN has been associated with small but statistically significant increases in prothrombin time (mean of approximately +4%); accordingly, patients undergoing surgery should be carefully evaluated. Caution should be observed when NIASPAN is administered concomitantly with anticoagulants; prothrombin time should be monitored closely in such patients.

Increase in Uric Acid: Elevated uric acid levels have occurred with niacin therapy, therefore use with caution in patients predisposed to gout.

Decrease in Phosphorus: In placebo-controlled trials, NIASPAN has been associated with small but statistically significant, dose-related reductions in phosphorus levels (mean of -13% with 2000 mg). Although these reductions were transient, phosphorus levels should be monitored periodically in patients at risk for hypophosphatemia.

6 ADVERSE REACTIONS

Because clinical studies are conducted under widely varying conditions, adverse reaction rates observed in the clinical studies of a drug cannot be directly compared to rates in the clinical studies of another drug and may not reflect the rates observed in practice.

6.1 Clinical Studies Experience

In the placebo-controlled clinical trials database of 402 patients (age range 21-75 years, 33% women, 89% Caucasians, 7% Blacks, 3% Hispanics, 1% Asians) with a median treatment duration of 16 weeks, 16% of patients on NIASPAN and 4% of patients on placebo discontinued due to adverse reactions. The most common adverse reactions in the group of patients treated with NIASPAN that led to treatment discontinuation and occurred at a rate greater than placebo were flushing (6% vs. 0%), rash (2% vs. 0%), diarrhea (2% vs. 0%), nausea (1% vs. 0%), and vomiting (1% vs. 0%). The most commonly reported adverse reactions (incidence >5% and greater than placebo) in the NIASPAN controlled clinical trial database of 402 patients were flushing, diarrhea, nausea, vomiting, increased cough and pruritus.

In the placebo-controlled clinical trials, flushing episodes (i.e., warmth, redness, itching and/or tingling) were the most common treatment-emergent adverse reactions (reported by as many as 88% of patients) for NIASPAN. Spontaneous reports suggest that flushing may also be accompanied by symptoms of dizziness, tachycardia, palpitations, shortness of breath, sweating, burning sensation/skin burning sensation, chills, and/or edema, which in rare cases may lead to syncope. In pivotal studies, 6% (14/245) of NIASPAN patients discontinued due to flushing. In comparisons of immediate-release (IR) niacin and NIASPAN, although the proportion of patients who flushed was similar, fewer flushing episodes were reported by patients who received NIASPAN. Following 4 weeks of maintenance therapy at daily doses of 1500 mg, the incidence of flushing over the 4-week period averaged 8.6 events per patient for IR niacin versus 1.9 following NIASPAN.

Other adverse reactions occurring in ≥5% of patients treated with NIASPAN and at an incidence greater than placebo are shown in Table 2 below.

[See table 2 above]

In general, the incidence of adverse events was higher in women compared to men.

Atherothrombosis Intervention in Metabolic Syndrome with Low HDL/High Triglycerides: Impact on Global Health Outcomes (AIM-HIGH)

In AIM-HIGH involving 3414 patients (mean age of 64 years, 15% women, 92% Caucasians, 34% with diabetes mellitus) with stable, previously diagnosed cardiovascular disease, all patients received simvastatin, 40 to 80 mg per day, plus ezetimibe 10 mg per day if needed, to maintain an LDL-C level of 40-80 mg/dL, and were randomized to receive NIASPAN 1500-2000 mg/day (n=1718) or matching placebo (IR Niacin, 100-150 mg, n=1696). The incidence of the adverse reactions of "blood glucose increased" (6.4% vs. 4.5%) and "diabetes mellitus" (3.6% vs. 2.2%) was significantly higher in the simvastatin plus NIASPAN group as compared to the simvastatin plus placebo group. There were 5 cases of rhabdomyolysis reported, 4 (0.2%) in the simvastatin plus NIASPAN group and one (<0.1%) in the simvastatin plus placebo group [*see Warnings and Precautions (5.1)*].

6.2 Postmarketing Experience

Because the below reactions are reported voluntarily from a population of uncertain size, it is generally not possible to reliably estimate their frequency or establish a causal relationship to drug exposure.

The following additional adverse reactions have been identified during post-approval use of NIASPAN:

Hypersensitivity reactions, including anaphylaxis, angioedema, urticaria, flushing, dyspnea, tongue edema, larynx edema, face edema, peripheral edema, laryngismus, and vesiculobullous rash; maculopapular rash; dry skin; tachycardia; palpitations; atrial fibrillation; other cardiac arrhythmias; syncope; hypotension; postural hypotension; blurred vision; macular edema; peptic ulcers; eructation; flatulence; hepatitis; jaundice; decreased glucose tolerance; gout; myalgia; myopathy; dizziness; insomnia; asthenia; nervousness; paresthesia; dyspnea; sweating; burning sensation/skin burning sensation; skin discoloration, and migraine.

Clinical Laboratory Abnormalities

Chemistry: Elevations in serum transaminases [*see Warnings and Precautions (5.3)*], LDH, fasting glucose, uric acid, total bilirubin, amylase and creatine kinase, and reduction in phosphorus.

Hematology: Slight reductions in platelet counts and prolongation in prothrombin time [*see Warnings and Precautions (5.4)*].

7 DRUG INTERACTIONS

7.1 Statins

Caution should be used when prescribing niacin (≥1 gm/day) with statins as these drugs can increase risk of myopathy/rhabdomyolysis [*see Warnings and Precautions (5) and Clinical Pharmacology (12.3)*].

7.2 Bile Acid Sequestrants

An *in vitro* study results suggest that the bile acid-binding resins have high niacin binding capacity. Therefore, 4 to 6 hours, or as great an interval as possible, should elapse between the ingestion of bile acid-binding resins and the administration of NIASPAN [*see Clinical Pharmacology (12.3)*].

7.3 Aspirin

Concomitant aspirin may decrease the metabolic clearance of nicotinic acid. The clinical relevance of this finding is unclear.

Continued on next page

Information on the AbbVie, Inc. products listed on these pages is from the prescribing information in use as of July 31, 2016. For more information, please visit rxabbvie.com or call 1-800-633-9110.

Table 2. Treatment-Emergent Adverse Reactions by Dose Level in ≥ 5% of Patients and at an Incidence Greater than Placebo; Regardless of Causality Assessment in Placebo-Controlled Clinical Trials

	Placebo-Controlled Studies NIASPAN Treatment@				
			Recommended Daily Maintenance Doses [†]		
	Placebo (n = 157) %	500 mg‡ (n = 87) %	1000 mg (n = 110) %	1500 mg (n = 136) %	2000 mg (n = 95) %
Gastrointestinal Disorders					
Diarrhea	13	7	10	10	14
Nausea	7	5	6	4	11
Vomiting	4	0	2	4	9
Respiratory					
Cough, Increased	6	3	2	< 2	8
Skin and Subcutaneous Tissue Disorders					
Pruritus	2	8	0	3	0
Rash	0	5	5	5	0
Vascular Disorders					
Flushing&	19	68	69	63	55

Note: Percentages are calculated from the total number of patients in each column.
[†] Adverse reactions are reported at the initial dose where they occur.
@ Pooled results from placebo-controlled studies; for NIASPAN, n = 245 and median treatment duration = 16 weeks. Number of NIASPAN patients (n) are not additive across doses.
‡ The 500 mg/day dose is outside the recommended daily maintenance dosing range [*see Dosage and Administration (2)*].
& 10 patients discontinued before receiving 500 mg, therefore they were not included.

7.4 Antihypertensive Therapy

Niacin may potentiate the effects of ganglionic blocking agents and vasoactive drugs resulting in postural hypotension.

7.5 Other

Vitamins or other nutritional supplements containing large doses of niacin or related compounds such as nicotinamide may potentiate the adverse effects of NIASPAN.

7.6 Laboratory Test Interactions

Niacin may produce false elevations in some fluorometric determinations of plasma or urinary catecholamines. Niacin may also give false-positive reactions with cupric sulfate solution (Benedict's reagent) in urine glucose tests.

8 USE IN SPECIFIC POPULATIONS

8.1 Pregnancy

Pregnancy Category C.

Animal reproduction studies have not been conducted with niacin or with NIASPAN. It is also not known whether niacin at doses typically used for lipid disorders can cause fetal harm when administered to pregnant women or whether it can affect reproductive capacity. If a woman receiving niacin for primary hyperlipidemia becomes pregnant, the drug should be discontinued. If a woman being treated with niacin for hypertriglyceridemia conceives, the benefits and risks of continued therapy should be assessed on an individual basis.

8.3 Nursing Mothers

Niacin is excreted into human milk but the actual infant dose or infant dose as a percent of the maternal dose is not known. Because of the potential for serious adverse reactions in nursing infants from lipid-altering doses of nicotinic acid, a decision should be made whether to discontinue nursing or to discontinue the drug, taking into account the importance of the drug to the mother. No studies have been conducted with NIASPAN in nursing mothers.

8.4 Pediatric Use

Safety and effectiveness of niacin therapy in pediatric patients (≤16 years) have not been established.

8.5 Geriatric Use

Of 979 patients in clinical studies of NIASPAN, 21% of the patients were age 65 and over. No overall differences in safety and effectiveness were observed between these patients and younger patients, and other reported clinical experience has not identified differences in responses between the elderly and younger patients, but greater sensitivity of some older individuals cannot be ruled out.

8.6 Renal Impairment

No studies have been performed in this population. NIASPAN should be used with caution in patients with renal impairment *[see Warnings and Precautions (5)]*.

8.7 Hepatic Impairment

No studies have been performed in this population. NIASPAN should be used with caution in patients with a past history of liver disease and/or who consume substantial quantities of alcohol. Active liver disease, unexplained transaminase elevations and significant or unexplained hepatic dysfunction are contraindications to the use of NIASPAN *[see Contraindications (4.0) and Warnings and Precautions (5.3)]*.

8.8 Gender

Data from the clinical trials suggest that women have a greater hypolipidemic response than men at equivalent doses of NIASPAN.

10 OVERDOSAGE

Supportive measures should be undertaken in the event of an overdose.

11 DESCRIPTION

NIASPAN (niacin tablet, film-coated extended-release), contains niacin, which at therapeutic doses is an antihyperlipidemic agent. Niacin (nicotinic acid, or 3-pyridinecarboxylic acid) is a white, crystalline powder, very soluble in water, with the following structural formula:

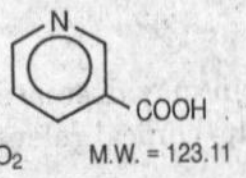

$C_6H_5NO_2$ M.W. = 123.11

NIASPAN is an unscored, medium-orange, film-coated tablet for oral administration and is available in three tablet strengths containing 500, 750, and 1000 mg niacin. NIASPAN tablets also contain the inactive ingredients hypromellose, povidone, stearic acid, and polyethylene glycol, and the following coloring agents: FD&C yellow #6/sunset yellow FCF Aluminum Lake, synthetic red and yellow iron oxides, and titanium dioxide.

12 CLINICAL PHARMACOLOGY

12.1 Mechanism of Action

The mechanism by which niacin alters lipid profiles has not been well defined. It may involve several actions including partial inhibition of release of free fatty acids from adipose tissue, and increased lipoprotein lipase activity, which may increase the rate of chylomicron triglyceride removal from plasma. Niacin decreases the rate of hepatic synthesis of VLDL and LDL, and does not appear to affect fecal excretion of fats, sterols, or bile acids.

12.3 Pharmacokinetics

Absorption

Due to extensive and saturable first-pass metabolism, niacin concentrations in the general circulation are dose dependent and highly variable. Time to reach the maximum niacin plasma concentrations was about 5 hours following NIASPAN. To reduce the risk of gastrointestinal (GI) upset, administration of NIASPAN with a low-fat meal or snack is recommended.

Single-dose bioavailability studies have demonstrated that the 500 mg and 1000 mg tablet strengths are dosage form equivalent but the 500 mg and 750 mg tablet strengths are not dosage form equivalent.

Metabolism

The pharmacokinetic profile of niacin is complicated due to extensive first-pass metabolism that is dose-rate specific and, at the doses used to treat dyslipidemia, saturable. In humans, one pathway is through a simple conjugation step with glycine to form nicotinuric acid (NUA). NUA is then excreted in the urine, although there may be a small amount of reversible metabolism back to niacin. The other pathway results in the formation of nicotinamide adenine dinucleotide (NAD). It is unclear whether nicotinamide is formed as a precursor to, or following the synthesis of, NAD. Nicotinamide is further metabolized to at least N-methylnicotinamide (MNA) and nicotinamide-N-oxide (NNO). MNA is further metabolized to two other compounds, N-methyl-2-pyridone-5-carboxamide (2PY) and N-methyl-4-pyridone-5-carboxamide (4PY). The formation of 2PY appears to predominate over 4PY in humans. At the doses used to treat hyperlipidemia, these metabolic pathways are saturable, which explains the nonlinear relationship between niacin dose and plasma concentrations following multiple-dose NIASPAN administration.

Nicotinamide does not have hypolipidemic activity; the activity of the other metabolites is unknown.

Elimination

Following single and multiple doses, approximately 60 to 76% of the niacin dose administered as NIASPAN was recovered in urine as niacin and metabolites; up to 12% was recovered as unchanged niacin after multiple dosing. The ratio of metabolites recovered in the urine was dependent on the dose administered.

Pediatric Use

No pharmacokinetic studies have been performed in this population (≤16 years) *[see Use in Specific Populations (8.4)]*.

Geriatric Use

No pharmacokinetic studies have been performed in this population (> 65 years) *[see Use in Specific Populations (8.5)]*.

Renal Impairment

No pharmacokinetic studies have been performed in this population. NIASPAN should be used with caution in patients with renal disease *[see Warnings and Precautions (5)]*.

Hepatic Impairment

No pharmacokinetic studies have been performed in this population. Active liver disease, unexplained transaminase elevations and significant or unexplained hepatic dysfunction are contraindications to the use of NIASPAN *[see Contraindications (4) and Warnings and Precautions (5.3)]*.

Gender

Steady-state plasma concentrations of niacin and metabolites after administration of NIASPAN are generally higher in women than in men, with the magnitude of the difference varying with dose and metabolite. This gender differences observed in plasma levels of niacin and its metabolites may be due to gender-specific differences in metabolic rate or volume of distribution. Recovery of niacin and metabolites in urine, however, is generally similar for men and women, indicating that absorption is similar for both genders *[see Gender (8.8)]*.

Drug interactions

Fluvastatin

Niacin did not affect fluvastatin pharmacokinetics *[see Drug Interactions (7.1)]*.

Lovastatin

When NIASPAN 2000 mg and lovastatin 40 mg were co-administered, NIASPAN increased lovastatin C_{max} and AUC by 2% and 14%, respectively, and decreased lovastatin acid C_{max} and AUC by 22% and 2%, respectively. Lovastatin reduced NIASPAN bioavailability by 2-3% *[see Drug Interactions (7.1)]*.

Simvastatin

When NIASPAN 2000 mg and simvastatin 40 mg were co-administered, NIASPAN increased simvastatin C_{max} and AUC by 1% and 9%, respectively, and simvastatin acid C_{max} and AUC by 2% and 18%, respectively. Simvastatin reduced NIASPAN bioavailability by 2% *[see Drug Interactions (7.1)]*.

Bile Acid Sequestrants

An *in vitro* study was carried out investigating the niacin-binding capacity of colestipol and cholestyramine. About 98% of available niacin was bound to colestipol, with 10 to 30% binding to cholestyramine *[see Drug Interactions (7.2)]*.

13 NONCLINICAL TOXICOLOGY

13.1 Carcinogenesis and Mutagenesis and Impairment of Fertility

Niacin administered to mice for a lifetime as a 1% solution in drinking water was not carcinogenic. The mice in this study received approximately 6 to 8 times a human dose of 3000 mg/day as determined on a mg/m^2 basis. Niacin was negative for mutagenicity in the Ames test. No studies on impairment of fertility have been performed. No studies have been conducted with NIASPAN regarding carcinogenesis, mutagenesis, or impairment of fertility.

14 CLINICAL STUDIES

14.1 Niacin Clinical Studies

Niacin's ability to reduce mortality and the risk of definite, nonfatal myocardial infarction (MI) has been assessed in long-term studies. The Coronary Drug Project, completed in 1975, was designed to assess the safety and efficacy of niacin and other lipid-altering drugs in men 30 to 64 years old with a history of MI. Over an observation period of 5 years, niacin treatment was associated with a statistically significant reduction in nonfatal, recurrent MI. The incidence of definite, nonfatal MI was 8.9% for the 1,119 patients randomized to nicotinic acid versus 12.2% for the 2,789 patients who received placebo (p<0.004). Total mortality was similar in the two groups at 5 years (24.4% with nicotinic acid versus 25.4% with placebo; p=N.S.). At the time of a 15-year follow-up, there were 11% (69) fewer deaths in the niacin group compared to the placebo cohort (52.0% versus 58.2%; p=0.0004). However, mortality at 15 years was not an original endpoint of the Coronary Drug Project. In addition, patients had not received niacin for approximately 9 years, and confounding variables such as concomitant medication use and medical or surgical treatments were not controlled.

The Cholesterol-Lowering Atherosclerosis Study (CLAS) was a randomized, placebo-controlled, angiographic trial testing combined colestipol and niacin therapy in 162 non-smoking males with previous coronary bypass surgery. The primary, per-subject cardiac endpoint was global coronary artery change score. After 2 years, 61% of patients in the placebo cohort showed disease progression by global change score (n=82), compared with only 38.8% of drug-treated subjects (n=80), when both native arteries and grafts were considered (p<0.005); disease regression also occurred more frequently in the drug-treated group (16.2% versus 2.4%; p=0.002). In a follow-up to this trial in a subgroup of 103 patients treated for 4 years, again, significantly fewer patients in the drug-treated group demonstrated progression than in the placebo cohort (48% versus 85%, respectively; p<0.0001).

The Familial Atherosclerosis Treatment Study (FATS) in 146 men ages 62 and younger with Apo B levels ≥125 mg/dL, established coronary artery disease, and family histories of vascular disease, assessed change in severity of disease in the proximal coronary arteries by quantitative arteriography. Patients were given dietary counseling and randomized to treatment with either conventional therapy with double placebo (or placebo plus colestipol if the LDL-C was elevated); lovastatin plus colestipol; or niacin plus colestipol. In the conventional therapy group, 46% of patients had disease progression (and no regression) in at least one of nine proximal coronary segments; regression was the only change in 11%. In contrast, progression (as the only change) was seen in only 25% in the niacin plus colestipol group, while regression was observed in 39%. Though not an original endpoint of the trial, clinical events (death, MI, or revascularization for worsening angina) occurred in 10 of 52 patients who received conventional therapy, compared with 2 of 48 who received niacin plus colestipol.

14.2 NIASPAN Clinical Studies

Placebo-Controlled Clinical Studies in Patients with Primary Hyperlipidemia and Mixed Dyslipidemia: In two randomized, double-blind, parallel, multi-center, placebo-controlled trials, NIASPAN dosed at 1000, 1500 or 2000 mg daily at bedtime with a low-fat snack for 16 weeks (including 4 weeks of dose escalation) favorably altered lipid profiles compared to placebo (Table 3). Women appeared to have a greater response than men at each NIASPAN dose level (see *Gender Effect,* below).

[See table 3 above]

In a double-blind, multi-center, forced dose-escalation study, monthly 500 mg increases in NIASPAN resulted in incremental reductions of approximately 5% in LDL-C and Apo B levels in the daily dose range of 500 mg through 2000 mg (Table 4). Women again tended to have a greater response to NIASPAN than men (see *Gender Effect,* below).

[See table 4 on next page]

Pooled results for major lipids from these three placebo-controlled studies are shown below (Table 5).

[See table 5 on next page]

Gender Effect: Combined data from the three placebo-controlled NIASPAN studies in patients with primary hyperlipidemia and mixed dyslipidemia suggest that, at each NIASPAN dose level studied, changes in lipid concentrations are greater for women than for men (Table 6).

[See table 6 on next page]

Other Patient Populations: In a double-blind, multi-center, 19-week study the lipid-altering effects of NIASPAN (forced titration to 2000 mg at bedtime) were compared to baseline in patients whose primary lipid abnormality was a low level of HDL-C (HDL-C ≤40 mg/dL, TG ≤400 mg/dL, and LDL-C ≤160, or <130 mg/dL in the presence of CHD). Results are shown below (Table 7).

[See table 7 on next page]

At NIASPAN 2000 mg/day, median changes from baseline (25th, 75th percentiles) for LDL-C, HDL-C, and TG were -3% (-14, +12%), +27% (+13, +38%), and -33% (-50, -19%), respectively.

16 HOW SUPPLIED/STORAGE AND HANDLING

NIASPAN tablets are supplied as unscored, medium-orange, film-coated, capsule-shaped (containing 500 or 750 mg of niacin) or oval shaped (containing 1000 mg of niacin) tablets, in an extended-release formulation. Tablets are printed with the "a" logo and the tablet strength (500, 750 or 1000). Tablets are supplied in bottles of 30 and 90 as shown below.

500 mg tablets: bottles of 30 - NDC# 0074-3074-30
500 mg tablets: bottles of 90 - NDC# 0074-3074-90
750 mg tablets: bottles of 30 - NDC# 0074-3079-30
750 mg tablets: bottles of 90 - NDC# 0074-3079-90
1000 mg tablets: bottles of 30 - NDC# 0074-3080-30
1000 mg tablets: bottles of 90 - NDC# 0074-3080-90

Storage: Store at room temperature 20° to 25°C (68° to 77°F).

17 PATIENT COUNSELING INFORMATION

17.1 Patient Counseling

Patients should be advised to adhere to their National Cholesterol Education Program (NCEP) recommended diet, a regular exercise program, and periodic testing of a fasting lipid panel.

Patients should be advised to inform other healthcare professionals prescribing a new medication that they are taking NIASPAN.

The patient should be informed of the following:

Dosing Time

NIASPAN tablets should be taken at bedtime, after a low-fat snack. Administration on an empty stomach is not recommended.

Tablet Integrity

NIASPAN tablets should not be broken, crushed or chewed, but should be swallowed whole.

Dosing Interruption

If dosing is interrupted for any length of time, their physician should be contacted prior to restarting therapy; re-titration is recommended.

Muscle Pain

Notify their physician of any unexplained muscle pain, tenderness, or weakness promptly. They should discuss all medication, both prescription and over the counter, with their physician.

Flushing

Flushing (warmth, redness, itching and/or tingling of the skin) is a common side effect of niacin therapy that may subside after several weeks of consistent NIASPAN use. Flushing may vary in severity and is more likely to occur with initiation of therapy, or during dose increases. By dosing at bedtime, flushing will most likely occur during sleep. However, if awakened by flushing at night, the patient should get up slowly, especially if feeling dizzy, feeling faint, or taking blood pressure medications. Advise patients of the symptoms of flushing and how they differ from the symptoms of a myocardial infarction.

Use of Aspirin Medication

Taking aspirin (up to the recommended dose of 325 mg) approximately 30 minutes before dosing can minimize flushing.

Diet

Avoid ingestion of alcohol, hot beverages and spicy foods around the time of taking NIASPAN to minimize flushing.

Supplements

Notify their physician if they are taking vitamins or other nutritional supplements containing niacin or nicotinamide.

Dizziness

Notify their physician if symptoms of dizziness occur.

Diabetics

If diabetic, to notify their physician of changes in blood glucose.

Pregnancy

Discuss future pregnancy plans with your patients, and discuss when to stop NIASPAN if they are trying to conceive. Patients should be advised that if they become pregnant, they should stop taking NIASPAN and call their healthcare professional.

Breastfeeding

Women who are breastfeeding should be advised to not use NIASPAN. Patients, who have a lipid disorder and are breastfeeding should be advised to discuss the options with their healthcare professional.

© AbbVie Inc. 2015
Manufactured by:
AbbVie LTD, Barceloneta, PR 00617
For AbbVie Inc.
North Chicago, IL 60064, USA
Ref. 03-B103-R10-Revised April, 2015

PATIENT INFORMATION

NIASPAN® (ny-a-span)
(niacin extended-release) tablets

Read this information carefully before you start taking NIASPAN and each time you get a refill. There may be new information. This information does not take the place of talking with your doctor about your medical condition or your treatment.

What is NIASPAN?

NIASPAN is a prescription medicine used with diet and exercise to increase the good cholesterol (HDL) and lower the bad cholesterol (LDL) and fats (triglycerides) in your blood.

- NIASPAN is also used to lower the risk of heart attack in people who have had a heart attack and have high cholesterol.
- In people with coronary artery disease and high cholesterol, NIASPAN, when used with a bile acid-binding resin (another cholesterol medicine) can slow down or lessen the build-up of plaque (fatty deposits) in your arteries.
- In people with heart problems and well-controlled cholesterol, taking NIASPAN with another cholesterol-lowering medicine (simvastatin) does not reduce heart attacks or strokes more than taking simvastatin alone.

It is not known if NIASPAN is safe and effective in children 16 years of age and under.

Who should not take NIASPAN?

Do not take NIASPAN if you have:

- liver problems
- a stomach ulcer
- bleeding problems
- an allergy to niacin or any of the ingredients in NIASPAN. See the end of this leaflet for a complete list of ingredients in NIASPAN.

What should I tell my doctor before taking NIASPAN?

Before you take NIASPAN, tell your doctor, if you:

- have diabetes. Tell your doctor if your blood sugar levels change after you take NIASPAN.
- have gout
- have kidney problems
- are pregnant or plan to become pregnant. It is not known if NIASPAN will harm your unborn baby. Talk to your doctor if you are pregnant or plan to become pregnant while taking NIASPAN.
- are breastfeeding or plan to breastfeed. NIASPAN can pass into your breast milk. You and your doctor should decide if you will take NIASPAN or breastfeed. You should not do both. Talk to your doctor about the best way to feed your baby if you take NIASPAN.

Tell your doctor about all the medicines you take, including prescription and non-prescription medicines, vitamins, herbal supplements or other nutritional supplements containing niacin or nicotinamide. NIASPAN and other medicines may affect each other causing side effects. NIASPAN may affect the way other medicines work, and other medicines may affect how NIASPAN works.

Especially tell your doctor if you take:

- other medicines to lower cholesterol or triglycerides
- aspirin
- blood pressure medicines
- blood thinner medicines
- large amounts of alcohol

Know the medicines you take. Keep a list of them to show your doctor and pharmacist when you get a new medicine.

How should I take NIASPAN?

- Take NIASPAN exactly as your doctor tells you to take it.
- Take NIASPAN tablets whole. Do not break, crush or chew NIASPAN tablets before swallowing.
- Take NIASPAN 1 time a day at bedtime after a low-fat snack. NIASPAN should not be taken on an empty stomach.
- All forms of niacin are not the same as NIASPAN. Do not switch between forms of niacin without first talking to your doctor as severe liver damage can occur.
- Do not change your dose or stop taking NIASPAN unless your doctor tells you to.
- If you need to stop taking NIASPAN, call your doctor before you start taking NIASPAN again. Your doctor may need to lower your dose of NIASPAN.
- If you forget to take a dose of NIASPAN, take it as soon as you remember.
- If you take too much NIASPAN, call your doctor right away.
- Medicines used to lower your cholesterol called bile acid resins, such as colestipol and cholestyramine, should not be taken at the same time of day as NIASPAN. You should take NIASPAN and the bile acid resin medicine at least 4 to 6 hours apart.
- Your doctor may do blood tests before you start taking NIASPAN and during your treatment. You should see your doctor regularly to check your cholesterol and triglyceride levels and to check for side effects.

Continued on next page

Information on the AbbVie, Inc. products listed on these pages is from the prescribing information in use as of July 31, 2016. For more information, please visit rxabbvie.com or call 1-800-633-9110.

Table 3. Lipid Response to NIASPAN Therapy

Treatment	n	Mean Percent Change from Baseline to Week 16*				
		TC	LDL-C	HDL-C	TG	Apo B
NIASPAN 1000 mg at bedtime	41	-3	-5	+18	-21	-6
NIASPAN 2000 mg at bedtime	41	-10	-14	+22	-28	-16
Placebo	40	0	-1	+4	0	+1
NIASPAN 1500 mg at bedtime	76	-8	-12	+20	-13	-12
Placebo	73	+2	+1	+2	+12	+1

n = number of patients at baseline;
* Mean percent change from baseline for all NIASPAN doses was significantly different ($p < 0.05$) from placebo.

What are the possible side effects of NIASPAN?
NIASPAN may cause serious side effects, including:
- **severe liver problems. Signs of liver problems include:**
  ◦ increased tiredness
  ◦ dark colored urine (tea-colored)
  ◦ loss of appetite
  ◦ light colored stools
  ◦ nausea
  ◦ right upper stomach (abdomen) pain
  ◦ yellowing of your skin or whites of your eye
  ◦ itchy skin
- **unexplained muscle pain, tenderness or weakness**
- **high blood sugar level (glucose)**

Call your doctor right away if you have any of the side effects listed above.
The most common side effects of NIASPAN include:
- flushing
- diarrhea
- nausea
- vomiting
- increased cough
- rash

Flushing is the most common side effect of NIASPAN.
Flushing happens when tiny blood vessels near the surface of the skin (especially on the face, neck, chest and/or back) open wider. Symptoms of flushing may include any or all of the following:
- warmth
- redness
- itching
- tingling of the skin

Flushing does not always happen. If it does, it is usually within 2 to 4 hours after taking a dose of NIASPAN. Flushing may last for a few hours. Flushing is more likely to happen when you first start taking NIASPAN or when your dose of NIASPAN is increased. Flushing may get better after several weeks.
If you wake up at night because of flushing, get up slowly, especially if you:
- feel dizzy or faint
- take blood pressure medicines

To lower your chance of flushing:
- Ask your doctor if you can take aspirin to help lower the flushing side effect from NIASPAN. You can take aspirin (up to the recommended dose of 325 mg) about 30 minutes before you take NIASPAN to help lower the flushing side effect.
- Do not drink hot beverages (including coffee), alcohol, or eat spicy foods around the time you take NIASPAN.
- Take NIASPAN with a low-fat snack to lessen upset stomach.

People with high cholesterol and heart disease are at risk for a heart attack. Symptoms of a heart attack may be different from a flushing reaction from NIASPAN. **The following may be symptoms of a heart attack due to heart disease and not a flushing reaction:**
- chest pain
- pain in other areas of your upper body such as one or both arms, back, neck, jaw or stomach
- shortness of breath
- sweating
- nausea
- lightheadedness

The chest pain you have with a heart attack may feel like uncomfortable pressure, squeezing, fullness or pain that lasts more than a few minutes, or that goes away and comes back. Heart attacks may be sudden and intense, but often start slowly, with mild pain or discomfort.
Call your doctor right away if you have any symptoms of a heart attack.
Tell your doctor if you have any side effect that bothers you or does not go away.
These are not all the possible side effects of NIASPAN. For more information, ask your doctor or pharmacist.
Call your doctor for medical advice about side effects. You may report side effects to FDA at 1-800-FDA-1088.
How should I store NIASPAN?
- Store NIASPAN at 68°F to 77°F (20°C to 25°C).
Keep NIASPAN and all medicines out of the reach of children.
General information about the safe and effective use of NIASPAN.
Medicines are sometimes prescribed for purposes other than those listed in a Patient Information leaflet. Do not use NIASPAN for a condition for which it was not prescribed. Do not give NIASPAN to other people, even if they have the same symptoms that you have. It may harm them.

This leaflet summarizes the most important information about NIASPAN. If you would like more information, talk with your doctor. You can ask your pharmacist or doctor for information about NIASPAN that is written for health professionals.
For more information, go to www.NIASPAN.com or call AbbVie Inc. Medical Information at 1-800-633-9110.
What are the ingredients in NIASPAN?
Active ingredient: niacin
Inactive Ingredients: hypromellose, povidone, stearic acid, and polyethylene glycol, and the following coloring agents: FD&C yellow #6/sunset yellow FCF Aluminum Lake, synthetic red and yellow iron oxides, and titanium dioxide
This Patient Information has been approved by the U.S. Food and Drug Administration.
Manufactured by: AbbVie LTD, Barceloneta, PR 00617
For AbbVie Inc.
North Chicago, IL 60064, USA

Table 4. Lipid Response in Dose-Escalation Study

Treatment	n	TC	LDL-C	HDL-C	TG	Apo B
			Mean Percent Change from Baseline*			
Placebo‡	44	-2	-1	+5	-6	-2
NIASPAN	87					
500 mg at bedtime		-2	-3	+10	-5	-2
1000 mg at bedtime		-5	-9	+15	-11	-7
1500 mg at bedtime		-11	-14	+22	-28	-15
2000 mg at bedtime		-12	-17	+26	-35	-16

n = number of patients enrolled;
‡ Placebo data shown are after 24 weeks of placebo treatment.
* For all NIASPAN doses except 500 mg, mean percent change from baseline was significantly different ($p < 0.05$) from placebo for all lipid parameters shown.

Table 5. Selected Lipid Response to NIASPAN in Placebo-Controlled Clinical Studies*

NIASPAN Dose	n	LDL-C	HDL-C	TG
		Mean Baseline and Median Percent Change from Baseline (25th, 75th Percentiles)		
1000 mg at bedtime	104			
Baseline (mg/dL)		218	45	172
Percent Change		-7 (-15, 0)	+14 (+7, +23)	-16 (-34, +3)
1500 mg at bedtime	120			
Baseline (mg/dL)		212	46	171
Percent Change		-13 (-21, -4)	+19 (+9, +31)	-25 (-45, -2)
2000 mg at bedtime	85			
Baseline (mg/dL)		220	44	160
Percent Change		-16 (-26, -7)	+22 (+15, +34)	-38 (-52, -14)

* Represents pooled analyses of results; minimum duration on therapy at each dose was 4 weeks.

Table 6. Effect of Gender on NIASPAN Dose Response

NIASPAN Dose	n (M/F)	LDL-C M	LDL-C F	HDL-C M	HDL-C F	TG M	TG F	Apo B M	Apo B F
		Mean Percent Change from Baseline							
500 mg at bedtime	50/37	-2	-5	+11	+8	-3	-9	-1	-5
1000 mg at bedtime	76/52	-6*	-11*	+14	+20	-10	-20	-5*	-10*
1500 mg at bedtime	104/59	-12	-16	+19	+24	-17	-28	-13	-15
2000 mg at bedtime	75/53	-15	-18	+23	+26	-30	-36	-16	-16

n = number of male/female patients enrolled.
* Percent change significantly different between genders ($p < 0.05$).

Table 7. Lipid Response to NIASPAN in Patients with Low HDL-C

	n	TC	LDL-C	HDL-C	TG	Apo B†
		Mean Baseline and Mean Percent Change from Baseline*				
Baseline (mg/dL)	88	190	120	31	194	106
Week 19 (% Change)	71	-3	0	+26	-30	-9

n = number of patients
* Mean percent change from baseline was significantly different ($p < 0.05$) for all lipid parameters shown except LDL-C.
† n = 72 at baseline and 69 at week 19.

Ref. 03-B103–R10–Revised April, 2015
Shown in Product Identification Guide, page 506

NIMBEX®   ℞
[nĭm-bĕks]
(cisatracurium besylate)
Injection

This drug should be administered only by adequately trained individuals familiar with its actions, characteristics, and hazards.
NOT FOR USE IN NEONATES
CONTAINS BENZYL ALCOHOL

DESCRIPTION
NIMBEX® (cisatracurium besylate) is a nondepolarizing skeletal muscle relaxant for intravenous administration.

Compared to other neuromuscular blocking agents, it is intermediate in its onset and duration of action. Cisatracurium besylate is one of 10 isomers of atracurium besylate and constitutes approximately 15% of that mixture. Cisatracurium besylate is [1R-[1α,2α(1′R*,2′R*)]]-2,2′- [1,5-pentanediylbis[oxy(3-oxo-3,1-propanediyl)]]bis[1-[(3,4-dimethoxyphenyl)methyl]-1,2,3,4-tetrahydro-6,7-dimethoxy-2-methylisoquinolinium] dibenzenesulfonate. The molecular formula of the cisatracurium parent biscation is $C_{53}H_{72}N_2O_{12}$ and the molecular weight is 929.2. The molecular formula of cisatracurium as the besylate salt is $C_{65}H_{82}N_2O_{18}S_2$ and the molecular weight is 1243.50. The structural formula of cisatracurium besylate is:

The log of the partition coefficient of cisatracurium besylate is -2.12 in a 1-octanol/distilled water system at 25°C.
NIMBEX Injection is a sterile, non-pyrogenic aqueous solution provided in 5 mL, 10 mL, and 20 mL vials. The pH is adjusted to 3.25 to 3.65 with benzenesulfonic acid. The 5 mL and 10 mL vials each contain cisatracurium besylate, equivalent to 2 mg/mL cisatracurium. The 20 mL vial, **intended for ICU use only**, contains cisatracurium besylate, equivalent to 10 mg/mL cisatracurium. The 10 mL vial, intended for multiple-dose use, contains 0.9% benzyl alcohol as a preservative. The 5 mL and 20 mL vials are single-use vials and do not contain benzyl alcohol.
Cisatracurium besylate slowly loses potency with time at a rate of approximately 5% per year under refrigeration (5°C). NIMBEX should be refrigerated at 2° to 8°C (36° to 46°F) in the carton to preserve potency. The rate of loss in potency increases to approximately 5% per *month* at 25°C (77°F). Upon removal from refrigeration to room temperature storage conditions (25°C/77°F), use NIMBEX within 21 days, even if rerefrigerated.

CLINICAL PHARMACOLOGY
NIMBEX binds competitively to cholinergic receptors on the motor end-plate to antagonize the action of acetylcholine, resulting in block of neuromuscular transmission. This action is antagonized by acetylcholinesterase inhibitors such as neostigmine.

Pharmacodynamics
The neuromuscular blocking potency of NIMBEX is approximately threefold that of atracurium besylate. The time to maximum block is up to 2 minutes longer for equipotent doses of NIMBEX compared to atracurium besylate. The clinically effective duration of action and rate of spontaneous recovery from equipotent doses of NIMBEX and atracurium besylate are similar.
The average ED_{95} (dose required to produce 95% suppression of the adductor pollicis muscle twitch response to ulnar nerve stimulation) of cisatracurium is 0.05 mg/kg (range: 0.048 to 0.053) in adults receiving opioid/nitrous oxide/oxygen anesthesia. For comparison, the average ED_{95} for atracurium when also expressed as the parent bis-cation is 0.17 mg/kg under similar anesthetic conditions.
The pharmacodynamics of $2 \times ED_{95}$ to $8 \times ED_{95}$ doses of cisatracurium administered over 5 to 10 seconds during opioid/nitrous oxide/oxygen anesthesia are summarized in Table 1. When the dose is doubled, the clinically effective duration of block increases by approximately 25 minutes. Once recovery begins, the rate of recovery is independent of dose. Isoflurane or enflurane administered with nitrous oxide/oxygen to achieve 1.25 MAC [Minimum Alveolar Concentration] may prolong the clinically effective duration of action of initial and maintenance doses, and decrease the average infusion rate requirement of NIMBEX. The magnitude of these effects may depend on the duration of administration of the volatile agents. Fifteen to 30 minutes of exposure to 1.25 MAC isoflurane or enflurane had minimal effects on the duration of action of initial doses of NIMBEX and therefore, no adjustment to the initial dose should be necessary when NIMBEX is administered shortly after initiation of volatile agents. In long surgical procedures during enflurane or isoflurane anesthesia, less frequent maintenance dosing, lower maintenance doses, or reduced infusion rates of NIMBEX may be necessary. The average infusion rate requirement may be decreased by as much as 30% to 40%.

Table 1. Pharmacodynamic Dose Response* of NIMBEX During Opioid/Nitrous Oxide/Oxygen Anesthesia

Initial Dose of NIMBEX (mg/kg)	Time to 90% Block (min)	Time to Maximum Block (min)	Time to Spontaneous Recovery				
			5% Recovery (min)	25% Recovery[†] (min)	95% Recovery (min)	T_4:T_1 Ratio[‡]≥70% (min)	25%-75% Recovery Index (min)
Adults							
0.1 (2 × ED$_{95}$) (n[§]=98)	3.3 (1.0-8.7)	5.0 (1.2-17.2)	33 (15-51)	42 (22-63)	64 (25-93)	64 (32-91)	13 (5-30)
0.15[∥] (3 × ED$_{95}$) (n=39)	2.6 (1.0-4.4)	3.5 (1.6-6.8)	46 (28-65)	55 (44-74)	76 (60-103)	75 (63-98)	13 (11-16)
0.2 (4 × ED$_{95}$) (n=30)	2.4 (1.5-4.5)	2.9 (1.9-5.2)	59 (31-103)	65 (43-103)	81 (53-114)	85 (55-114)	12 (2-30)
0.25 (5 × ED$_{95}$) (n=15)	1.6 (0.8-3.3)	2.0 (1.2-3.7)	70 (58-85)	78 (66-86)	91 (76-109)	97 (82-113)	8 (5-12)
0.4 (8 × ED$_{95}$) (n=15)	1.5 (1.3-1.8)	1.9 (1.4-2.3)	83 (37-103)	91 (59-107)	121 (110-134)	126 (115-137)	14 (10-18)
Infants (1-23 mos.)							
0.15** (n=18-26)	1.5 (0.7-3.2)	2.0 (1.3-4.3)	36 (28-50)	43 (34-58)	64 (54-84)	59 (49-76)	11.3 (7.3-18.3)
Children (2-12 yr)							
0.08¶ (2 × ED$_{95}$) (n=60)	2.2 (1.2-6.8)	3.3 (1.7-9.7)	22 (11-38)	29 (20-46)	52 (37-64)	50 (37-62)	11 (7-15)
0.1 (n=16)	1.7 (1.3-2.7)	2.8 (1.8-6.7)	21 (13-31)	28 (21-38)	46 (37-58)	44 (36-58)	10 (7-12)
0.15** (n=23-24)	2.1 (1.3-2.8)	3.0 (1.5-8.0)	29 (19-38)	36 (29-46)	55 (45-72)	54 (44-66)	10.6 (8.5-17.7)

* Values shown are medians of means from individual studies. Values in parentheses are ranges of individual patient values.
† Clinically effective duration of block.
‡ Train-of-four ratio.
§ n=the number of patients with Time to Maximum Block data.
∥ Propofol anesthesia.
¶ Halothane anesthesia.
** Thiopentone, alfentanil, N_2O/O_2 anesthesia

The onset, duration of action, and recovery profiles of NIMBEX during propofol/oxygen or propofol/nitrous oxide/oxygen anesthesia are similar to those during opioid/nitrous oxide/oxygen anesthesia.
[See table 1 above]
When administered during the induction of adequate anesthesia using propofol, nitrous oxide/oxygen, and co-induction agents (e.g., fentanyl and midazolam), GOOD or EXCELLENT conditions for tracheal intubation occurred in 96/102 (94%) patients in 1.5 to 2.0 minutes following 0.15 mg/kg cisatracurium and in 97/110 (88%) patients in 1.5 minutes following 0.2 mg/kg cisatracurium.
In one intubation study during thiopental anesthesia in which fentanyl and midazolam were administered two minutes prior to induction, intubation conditions were assessed at 120 seconds. Table 2 displays these results in this study of 51 patients.

Table 2. Study of Tracheal Intubation Comparing Two Doses of Cisatracurium (Thiopental Anesthesia)

Intubating Conditions at 120 seconds	3 × ED$_{95}$ 0.15 mg/kg n = 26	4 × ED$_{95}$ 0.20 mg/kg n = 25
Excellent and Good		
Proportion	23/26	24/25
Percent	88%	96%
95% CI	76,100	88,100
Excellent		
Proportion	8/26	15/26
Percent	31%	60%
Good		
Proportion	15/26	9/25
Percent	58%	36%

While GOOD or EXCELLENT intubation conditions were achieved in the majority of patients in this setting, EXCELLENT intubation conditions were more frequently achieved with the 0.2 mg/kg dose (60%) than the 0.15 mg/kg dose (31%) when intubation was attempted 2.0 minutes following cisatracurium.

A second study evaluated intubation conditions after 3 and 4 × ED$_{95}$ (0.15 mg/kg and 0.20 mg/kg) following induction with fentanyl and midazolam and either thiopental or propofol anesthesia. This study compared intubation conditions produced by these doses of cisatracurium after 1.5 minutes. Table 3 displays these results.
[See table 3 on page 766]
EXCELLENT intubation conditions were more frequently observed with the 0.2 mg/kg dose when intubation was attempted 1.5 minutes following cisatracurium.
A third study in pediatric patients (ages 1 month to 12 years) evaluated intubation conditions at 120 seconds after 0.15 mg/kg NIMBEX following induction with either halothane (with halothane/nitrous oxide/oxygen maintenance) or thiopentone and fentanyl (with thiopentone/fentanyl nitrous oxide/oxygen maintenance). The results are summarized in Table 4.
[See table 4 on page 766]
EXCELLENT or GOOD intubating conditions were produced 120 seconds following 0.15 mg/kg NIMBEX in 88/90 (98%) of patients induced with halothane and in 85/90 (94%) of patients induced with thiopentone and fentanyl. There were no patients for whom intubation was not possible, but there were 7/120 patients ages 1-12 years for whom intubating conditions were described as poor.
Repeated administration of maintenance doses or a continuous infusion of NIMBEX for up to 3 hours is not associated with development of tachyphylaxis or cumulative neuromuscular blocking effects. The time needed to recover from successive maintenance doses does not change with the number of doses administered as long as partial recovery is allowed to occur between doses. Maintenance doses can therefore be administered at relatively regular intervals

Continued on next page

Information on the AbbVie, Inc. products listed on these pages is from the prescribing information in use as of July 31, 2016. For more information, please visit rxabbvie.com or call 1-800-633-9110.

with predictable results. The rate of spontaneous recovery of neuromuscular function after infusion is independent of the duration of infusion and comparable to the rate of recovery following initial doses (Table 1).

Long-term infusion (up to 6 days) of NIMBEX during mechanical ventilation in the ICU has been evaluated in two studies. In a randomized, double-blind study using presence of a single twitch during train-of-four (TOF) monitoring to regulate dosage, patients treated with NIMBEX (n = 19) recovered neuromuscular function (T_4:T_1 ratio ≥ 70%) following termination of infusion in approximately 55 minutes (range: 20 to 270) whereas those treated with vecuronium (n = 12) recovered in 178 minutes (range: 40 minutes to 33 hours). In another study comparing NIMBEX and atracurium, patients recovered neuromuscular function in approximately 50 minutes for both NIMBEX (range: 20 to 175; n = 34) and atracurium (range: 35 to 85; n = 15).

The neuromuscular block produced by NIMBEX is readily antagonized by anticholinesterase agents once recovery has started. As with other nondepolarizing neuromuscular blocking agents, the more profound the neuromuscular block at the time of reversal, the longer the time required for recovery of neuromuscular function.

In children (2 to 12 years) cisatracurium has a lower ED_{95} than in adults (0.04 mg/kg, halothane/nitrous oxide/oxygen anesthesia). At 0.1 mg/kg during opioid anesthesia,

Figure 3. Heart Rate and MAP Change at 1 Minute After the Initial Dose, By Age Group Treatment Group: NIMBEX 0:3 x ED_{95} Opioid Intubation at 120 Sec.

1-11 Months

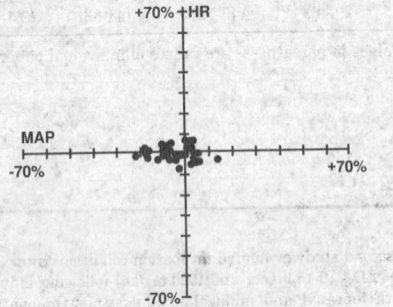

1-5 Years

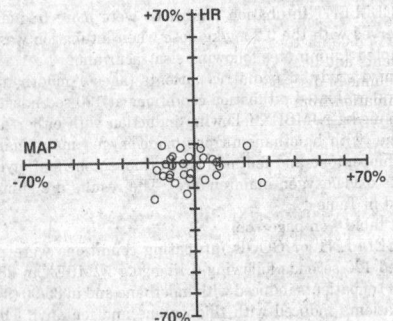

5-13 Years

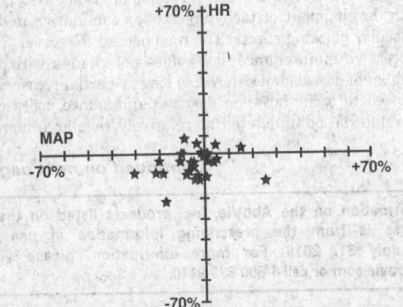

cisatracurium had a faster onset and shorter duration of action in children than in adults (Table 1). Recovery following reversal is faster in children than in adults.

At 0.15 mg/kg during opioid anesthesia, cisatracurium had a faster onset and longer clinically effective duration of action in infants aged 1-23 months compared to children aged 2-12 years (Table 1).

Studies were conducted during both opioid-based and halothane-based anesthesia in children aged 1-11 months, 1-4 years, and 5-12 years. Cisatracurium had a faster onset and longer duration of action in infants 1-11 months compared to children 1-4 years, who in turn have a faster onset and longer duration of action for cisatracurium compared to children 5-12 years.

The mean time to onset of maximum T_1 suppression was generally faster for pediatric patients induced with halothane compared to thiopentone/fentanyl and the clinically effective duration (time to 25% recovery) was longer (by up to 15%) for pediatric patients under halothane anesthesia.

Hemodynamics Profile

The cardiovascular profile of NIMBEX allows it to be administered by rapid bolus at higher multiples of the ED_{95} than atracurium. NIMBEX has no dose-related effects on mean arterial blood pressure (MAP) or heart rate (HR) following doses ranging from 2 to 8 × ED_{95} (> 0.1 to > 0.4 mg/kg), administered over 5 to 10 seconds, in healthy adult patients (Figure 1) or in patients with serious cardiovascular disease (Figure 2).

A total of 141 patients undergoing coronary artery bypass grafting (CABG) have been administered NIMBEX in three active controlled clinical trials and have received doses ranging from 2 to 8 × ED_{95}. While the hemodynamic profile was comparable in both the NIMBEX and active control groups, data for doses above 0.3 mg/kg in this population are limited.

Unlike atracurium, NIMBEX® (cisatracurium besylate), at therapeutic doses of 2 × ED_{95} to 8 × ED_{95} (0.1 to 0.4 mg/kg), administered over 5 to 10 seconds, does not cause dose-related elevations in mean plasma histamine concentration. [See Figure 2 in next column]

Figure 1. Maximum Percent Change from Preinjection in Heart Rate (HR) and Mean Arterial Pressure (MAP) During First 5 Minutes after Initial 4 x ED_{95} to 8 x ED_{95} Doses of NIMBEX in Healthy Adult Patients Receiving Opioid/Nitrous Oxide/Oxygen Anesthesia (n = 44)

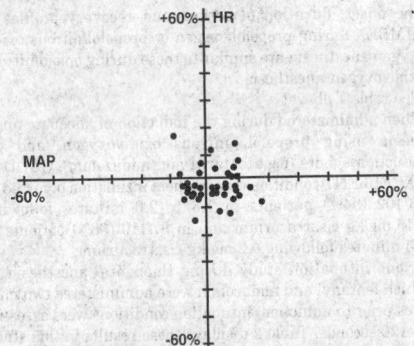

No clinically significant changes in MAP or HR were observed following administration of doses up to 0.1 mg/kg NIMBEX over 5 to 10 seconds in 2- to 12-year-old children receiving either halothane/nitrous oxide/oxygen or opioid/nitrous oxide/oxygen anesthesia. Doses of 0.15 mg/kg NIMBEX administered over 5 seconds were not consistently associated with changes in HR and MAP in pediatric patients aged 1 month to 12 years receiving opioid/nitrous oxide/oxygen or halothane/nitrous oxide/oxygen anesthesia. [See Figure 3 in previous column] [See Figure 4 on next page]

Pharmacokinetics

General

The neuromuscular blocking activity of NIMBEX is due to parent drug. Cisatracurium plasma concentration-time data following IV bolus administration are best described by a two-compartment open model (with elimination from both compartments) with an elimination half-life ($t_{1/2}\beta$) of 22 minutes, a plasma clearance (CL) of 4.57 mL/min/kg, and a volume of distribution at steady state (V_{ss}) of 145 mL/kg. Cisatracurium undergoes organ-independent Hofmann elimination (a chemical process dependent on pH and temperature) to form the monoquaternary acrylate metabolite

Figure 2. Percent Change from Preinjection in Heart Rate (HR) and Mean Arterial Pressure (MAP) 10 Minutes After an Initial 4 x ED_{95} to 8 x ED_{95} Dose of NIMBEX in Patients Undergoing CABG Surgery Receiving Oxygen/Fentanyl/Midazolam/ Anesthesia (n = 54)

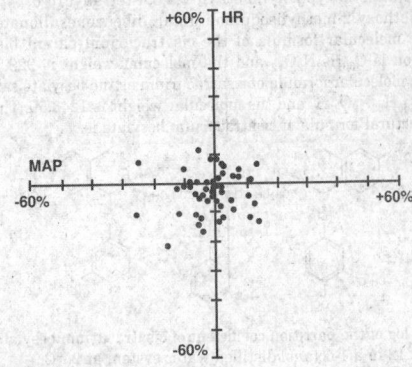

and laudanosine, neither of which has any neuromuscular blocking activity (see **Pharmacokinetics** -Metabolism section). Following administration of radiolabeled cisatracurium, 95% of the dose was recovered in the urine; less than 10% of the dose was excreted as unchanged parent drug. Laudanosine, a metabolite of cisatracurium (and atracurium) has been noted to cause transient hypotension and, in higher doses, cerebral excitatory effects when administered to several animal species. The relationship between CNS excitation and laudanosine concentrations in humans has not been established (see **PRECAUTIONS - Long-term Use in the Intensive Care Unit**). Because cisatracurium is three times more potent than atracurium and lower doses are required, the corresponding laudanosine concentrations following cisatracurium are one third of those that would be expected following an equipotent dose of atracurium (see **Pharmacokinetics** - Special Populations -*Intensive Care Unit Patients*).

Results from population pharmacokinetic/pharmacodynamic (PK/PD) analyses from 241 healthy surgical patients are summarized in Table 5.

Table 5. Key Population PK/PD Parameter Estimates for Cisatracurium in Healthy Surgical Patients* Following 0.1 (2 × ED_{95}) to 0.4 mg/kg (8 × ED_{95}) NIMBEX

Parameter	Estimate[†]	Magnitude of Interpatient Variability (CV)[‡]
CL (mL/min/kg)	4.57	16%
V_{ss} (mL/kg)[§]	145	27%
k_{eo} (min-1)[∥]	0.0575	61%
EC_{50} (ng/mL)[¶]	141	52%

* Healthy male non-obese patients 19-64 years of age with creatinine clearance values greater than 70 mL/min who received cisatracurium during opioid anesthesia and had venous samples collected.

† The percent standard error of the mean (%SEM) ranged from 3% to 12% indicating good precision for the PK/PD estimates.

‡ Expressed as a coefficient of variation; the %SEM ranged from 20% to 35% indicating adequate precision for the estimates of interpatient variability.

§ V_{ss} is the volume of distribution at steady state estimated using a two-compartment model with elimination from both compartments. V_{ss} is equal to the sum of the volume in the central compartment (V_c) and the volume in the peripheral compartment (Vp); interpatient variability could only be estimated for V_c.

∥ Rate constant describing the equilibration between plasma concentrations and neuromuscular block.

¶ Concentration required to produce 50% T_1 suppression; an index of patient sensitivity.

The magnitude of interpatient variability in CL was low (16%), as expected based on the importance of Hofmann elimination (see **Pharmacokinetics** -Elimination). The magnitudes of interpatient variability in CL and volume of distribution were low in comparison to those for k_{eo} and EC_{50}. This suggests that any alterations in the time course of

Figure 4. Heart Rate and MAP Change at 1 Minute After the Initial Dose, By Age Group Treatment Group: NIMBEX H:3 x ED₉₅ Halothane Intubation at 120 Sec.

1-11 Months

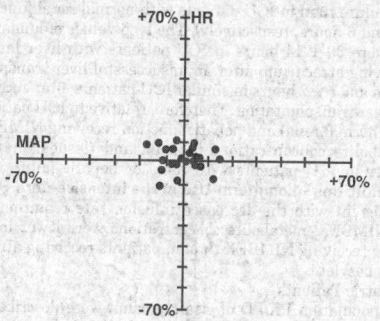

1-5 Years

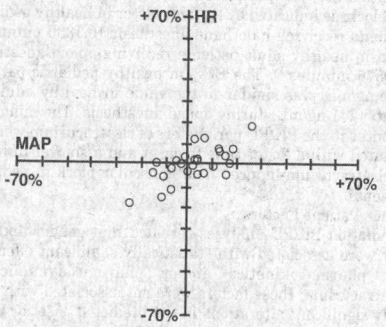

5-13 Years

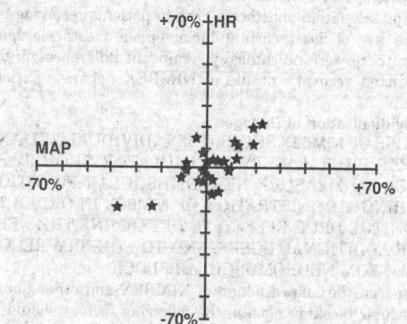

cisatracurium-induced block are more likely to be due to variability in the pharmacodynamic parameters than in the pharmacokinetic parameters. Parameter estimates from the population pharmacokinetic analyses were supported by noncompartmental pharmacokinetic analyses on data from healthy patients and from special patient populations. Conventional pharmacokinetic analyses have shown that the pharmacokinetics of cisatracurium are proportional to dose between 0.1 ($2 \times ED_{95}$) and 0.2 ($4 \times ED_{95}$) mg/kg cisatracurium. In addition, population pharmacokinetic analyses revealed no statistically significant effect of initial dose on CL for doses between 0.1 ($2 \times ED_{95}$) and 0.4 ($8 \times ED_{95}$) mg/kg cisatracurium.

Distribution

The volume of distribution of cisatracurium is limited by its large molecular weight and high polarity. The V_{ss} was equal to 145 mL/kg (Table 4) in healthy 19- to 64-year-old surgical patients receiving opioid anesthesia. The V_{ss} was 21% larger in similar patients receiving inhalation anesthesia (see **Pharmacokinetics** - Special Populations -*Other Patient Factors*).

Protein Binding

The binding of cisatracurium to plasma proteins has not been successfully studied due to its rapid degradation at physiologic pH. Inhibition of degradation requires non-physiological conditions of temperature and pH which are associated with changes in protein binding.

Metabolism

The degradation of cisatracurium is largely independent of liver metabolism. Results from *in vitro* experiments suggest that cisatracurium undergoes Hofmann elimination (a pH and temperature-dependent chemical process) to form laudanosine (see **PRECAUTIONS - Long-term Use in the Intensive Care Unit**) and the monoquaternary acrylate metabolite. The monoquaternary acrylate undergoes hydrolysis by non-specific plasma esterases to form the monoquaternary alcohol (MQA) metabolite. The MQA metabolite can also undergo Hofmann elimination but at a much slower rate than cisatracurium. Laudanosine is further metabolized to desmethyl metabolites which are conjugated with glucuronic acid and excreted in the urine.

Organ-independent Hofmann elimination is the predominant pathway for the elimination of cisatracurium. The liver and kidney play a minor role in the elimination of cisatracurium but are primary pathways for the elimination of metabolites. Therefore, the $t_{1/2}\beta$ values of metabolites (including laudanosine) are longer in patients with kidney or liver dysfunction and metabolite concentrations may be higher after long-term administration (see **PRECAUTIONS - Long-term Use in the Intensive Care Unit**). Most importantly, C_{max} values of laudanosine are significantly lower in healthy surgical patients receiving infusions of NIMBEX than in patients receiving infusions of atracurium (mean ± SD C_{max}: 60 ± 52 and 342 ± 93 ng/mL, respectively).

Elimination

Clearance and Half-life

Mean CL values for cisatracurium ranged from 4.5 to 5.7 mL/min/kg in studies of healthy surgical patients. Compartmental pharmacokinetic modeling suggests that approximately 80% of the CL is accounted for by Hofmann elimination and the remaining 20% by renal and hepatic elimination. These findings are consistent with the low magnitude of interpatient variability in CL (16%) estimated as part of the population PK/PD analyses and with the recovery of parent and metabolites in urine. Following ^{14}C-cisatracurium administration to 6 healthy male patients, 95% of the dose was recovered in the urine (mostly as conjugated metabolites) and 4% in the feces; less than 10% of the dose was excreted as unchanged parent drug in the urine. In 12 healthy surgical patients receiving non-radiolabeled cisatracurium who had Foley catheters placed for surgical management, approximately 15% of the dose was excreted unchanged in the urine.

In studies of healthy surgical patients, mean $t_{1/2}\beta$ values of cisatracurium ranged from 22 to 29 minutes and were consistent with the $t_{1/2}\beta$ of cisatracurium *in vitro* (29 minutes). The mean ± SD $t_{1/2}\beta$ values of laudanosine were 3.1 ± 0.4 and 3.3 ± 2.1 hours in healthy surgical patients receiving NIMBEX (n = 10) or atracurium (n = 10), respectively. During IV infusions of NIMBEX, peak plasma concentrations (C_{max}) of laudanosine and the MQA metabolite are approximately 6% and 11% of the parent compound, respectively.

Special Populations

Geriatric Patients (≥ 65 years)

The results of conventional pharmacokinetic analysis from a study of 12 healthy elderly patients and 12 healthy young adult patients receiving a single IV dose of 0.1 mg/kg NIMBEX are summarized in Table 6. Plasma clearances of cisatracurium were not affected by age; however, the volumes of distribution were slightly larger in elderly patients than in young patients resulting in slightly longer $t_{1/2}\beta$ values for cisatracurium. The rate of equilibration between plasma cisatracurium concentrations and neuromuscular block was slower in elderly patients than in young patients (mean ± SD k_{eo}: 0.071 ± 0.036 and 0.105 ± 0.021 minutes⁻¹, respectively); there was no difference in the patient sensitivity to cisatracurium-induced block, as indicated by EC_{50} values (mean ± SD EC_{50}: 91 ± 22 and 89 ± 23 ng/mL, respectively). These changes were consistent with the 1-minute slower times to maximum block in elderly patients receiving 0.1 mg/kg NIMBEX, when compared to young patients receiving the same dose. The minor differences in PK/PD parameters of cisatracurium between elderly patients and young patients were not associated with clinically significant differences in the recovery profile of NIMBEX® (cisatracurium besylate).

Table 6. Pharmacokinetic Parameters* of Cisatracurium in Healthy Elderly and Young Adult Patients Following 0.1 mg/kg (2 × ED₉₅) NIMBEX (Isoflurane/Nitrous Oxide/Oxygen Anesthesia)

Parameter	Healthy Elderly Patients	Healthy Young Adult Patients
Elimination Half-Life ($t_{1/2}\beta$, min)	25.8 ± 3.6[†]	22.1 ± 2.5
Volume of Distribution at Steady State[‡] (mL/kg)	156 ± 17[†]	133 ± 15
Plasma Clearance (mL/min/kg)	5.7 ± 1.0	5.3 ± 0.9

* Values presented are mean ± SD.
† P < 0.05 for comparisons between healthy elderly and healthy young adult patients.
‡ Volume of distribution is underestimated because elimination from the peripheral compartment is ignored.

Patients with Hepatic Disease

Table 7 summarizes the conventional pharmacokinetic analysis from a study of NIMBEX in 13 patients with end-stage liver disease undergoing liver transplantation and 11 healthy adult patients undergoing elective surgery. The slightly larger volumes of distribution in liver transplant patients were associated with slightly higher plasma clearances of cisatracurium. The parallel changes in these parameters resulted in no difference in $t_{1/2}\beta$ values. There were no differences in k_{eo} or EC_{50} between patient groups. The times to maximum block were approximately one minute faster in liver transplant patients than in healthy adult patients receiving 0.1 mg/kg NIMBEX. These minor differences in pharmacokinetics were not associated with clinically significant differences in the recovery profile of NIMBEX.

The $t_{1/2}\beta$ values of metabolites are longer in patients with hepatic disease and concentrations may be higher after long-term administration (see **Pharmacokinetics** - Special Populations - *Intensive Care Unit Patients*).

Table 7. Pharmacokinetic Parameters* of Cisatracurium in Healthy Adult Patients and in Patients Undergoing Liver Transplantation Following 0.1 mg/kg (2 × ED₉₅) NIMBEX (Isoflurane/Nitrous Oxide/Oxygen Anesthesia)

Parameter	Liver Transplant Patients	Healthy Adult Patients
Elimination Half-Life ($t_{1/2}\beta$, min)	24.4 ± 2.9	23.5 ± 3.5
Volume of Distribution at Steady State[‡] (mL/kg)	195 ± 38[†]	161 ± 23
Plasma Clearance (mL/min/kg)	6.6 ± 1.1[†]	5.7 ± 0.8

* Values presented are mean ± SD.
† P < 0.05 for comparisons between liver transplant patients and healthy adult patients.
‡ Volume of distribution is underestimated because elimination from the peripheral compartment is ignored.

Patients with Renal Dysfunction

Results from a conventional pharmacokinetic study of NIMBEX in 13 healthy adult patients and 15 patients with end-stage renal disease (ESRD) undergoing elective surgery are summarized in Table 8. The PK/PD parameters of cisatracurium were similar in healthy adult patients and ESRD patients. The times to 90% block were approximately one minute slower in ESRD patients following 0.1 mg/kg NIMBEX. There were no differences in the durations or rates of recovery of NIMBEX between ESRD and healthy adult patients.

The $t_{1/2}\beta$ values of metabolites are longer in patients with renal failure and concentrations may be higher after long-term administration (see **Pharmacokinetics** - Special Populations - *Intensive Care Unit Patients*).

Table 8. Pharmacokinetic Parameters* for Cisatracurium in Healthy Adult Patients and in Patients With End-Stage Renal Disease (ESRD) Receiving 0.1 mg/kg (2 × ED₉₅) NIMBEX (Opioid/Nitrous Oxide/Oxygen Anesthesia)

Continued on next page

Information on the AbbVie, Inc. products listed on these pages is from the prescribing information in use as of July 31, 2016. For more information, please visit rxabbvie.com or call 1-800-633-9110.

Table 3. Study of Tracheal Intubation Comparing Three Doses of Cisatracurium (Thiopental or Propofol Anesthesia)

Intubating Conditions at 90 seconds	3 × ED$_{95}$ 0.15 mg/kg Propofol n = 31	3 × ED$_{95}$ 0.15 mg/kg Thiopental n = 31	4 × ED$_{95}$ 0.20 mg/kg Propofol n = 30	4 × ED$_{95}$ 0.20 mg/kg Thiopental n = 28
Excellent and Good				
Proportion	29/31	28/31	28/30	27/28
Percent	94%	90%	93%	96%
95% CI	85,100	80,100	84,100	90,100
Excellent				
Proportion	18/31	17/31	22/30	16/28
Percent	58%	55%	70%	57%
Good				
Proportion	11/31	11/31	6/30	11/28
Percent	35%	35%	20%	39%

Table 4. Study of Tracheal Intubation for Pediatrics Stratified by Age Group (0.15 mg/kg NIMBEX with Halothane or Thiopentone/ Fentanyl Anesthesia)

Intubating Conditions at 120 seconds**	NIMBEX 0.15 mg/kg 1-11 mo. n = 30 Halothane Anesthesia	NIMBEX 0.15 mg/kg 1-11 mo. n = 30 Thiopentone/ Fentanyl Anesthesia	NIMBEX 0.15 mg/kg 1- 4 years n = 31 Halothane Anesthesia	NIMBEX 0.15 mg/kg 1- 4 years n = 31 Thiopentone/ Fentanyl Anesthesia	NIMBEX 0.15 mg/kg 5-12 years n = 30 Halothane Anesthesia	NIMBEX 0.15 mg/kg 5-12 years n = 30 Thiopentone/ Fentanyl Anesthesia
Excellent and Good						
Proportion	30/30	30/30	29/30	26/30	29/30	29/30
Percent	100%	100%	97%	87%	97%	97%
Excellent						
Proportion	30/30	25/30	27/30	19/30	22/30	21/30
Percent	100%	83%	90%	63%	73%	70%
Good						
Proportion	0	5/30	2/30	7/30	7/30	8/30
Percent	0%	17%	7%	23%	23%	27%
Poor						
Proportion	0/30	0/30	1/30	4/30	1/30	1/30
Percent	0%	0%	3%	13%	3%	3%

** **Excellent:** Easy passage of the tube without coughing. Vocal cords relaxed and abducted.
Good: Passage of tube with slight coughing and/or bucking. Vocal cords relaxed and abducted.
Poor: Passage of tube with moderate coughing and/or bucking. Vocal cords moderately adducted.
Response of patient requires adjustment of ventilation pressure and/or rate.

Parameter	Healthy Adult Patients	ESRD Patients
Elimination Half-Life ($t_{1/2}\beta$, min)	29.4 ± 4.1	32.3 ± 6.3
Volume of Distribution at Steady State† (mL/kg)	149 ± 35	160 ± 32
Plasma Clearance (mL/min/kg)	4.66 ± 0.86	4.26 ± 0.62

* Values presented are mean ± SD.
† Volume of distribution is underestimated because elimination from the peripheral compartment is ignored.

Population pharmacokinetic analyses revealed that patients with creatinine clearances ≤ 70 mL/min had a slower rate of equilibration between plasma concentrations and neuromuscular block than patients with normal renal function; this change was associated with a slightly slower (~ 40 seconds) predicted time to 90% T_1 suppression in patients with renal dysfunction following 0.1 mg/kg NIMBEX. There was no clinically significant alteration in the recovery profile of NIMBEX in patients with renal dysfunction. The recovery profile of NIMBEX is unchanged in the presence of renal or hepatic failure, which is consistent with predominantly organ-independent elimination.

Intensive Care Unit (ICU) Patients
The pharmacokinetics of cisatracurium, atracurium, and their metabolites were determined in six ICU patients receiving NIMBEX and in six ICU patients receiving atracurium and are presented in Table 9. The plasma clearances of cisatracurium and atracurium are similar. The volume of distribution was larger and the $t_{1/2}\beta$ was longer for cisatracurium than for atracurium. The relationships between plasma cisatracurium or atracurium concentrations and neuromuscular block have not been evaluated in ICU patients. The minor differences in pharmacokinetics were not associated with any differences in the recovery profiles of NIMBEX and atracurium in ICU patients.
[See table 9 below]
Plasma metabolite pharmacokinetics are listed in Table 9.
Limited pharmacokinetic data are available for patients with liver/kidney dysfunction receiving NIMBEX. Data from studies of atracurium demonstrate that renal/hepatic failure in ICU patients produces little to no effect on its pharmacokinetics, but decreases the biotransformation and elimination of the metabolites. Following atracurium, $t_{1/2}\beta$ values for laudanosine were longer in ICU patients with renal failure than in ICU patients with normal renal function (15 and 6 hours, respectively). The $t_{1/2}\beta$ values of laudanosine were 39 ± 14 hours in ICU patients with liver failure receiving atracurium after an unsuccessful liver transplantation and 5 ± 2 hours in similar ICU patients after successful liver transplantation. Therefore, relative to ICU patients with normal renal and hepatic function receiving NIMBEX, metabolite concentrations (plasma and tissues) may be higher in ICU patients with renal or hepatic failure (see **Precautions - Long-term Use in the Intensive Care Unit**). Consistent with the decreased infusion rate requirements for NIMBEX, metabolite concentrations were lower in patients receiving NIMBEX than in patients receiving atracurium besylate.
Pediatric Patients
The population PK/PD of cisatracurium were described in 20 healthy pediatric patients during halothane anesthesia, using the same model developed for healthy adult patients. The CL was higher in healthy pediatric patients (5.89 mL/min/kg) than in healthy adult patients (4.57 mL/min/kg) during opioid anesthesia. The rate of equilibration between plasma concentrations and neuromuscular block, as indicated by k_{eo}, was faster in healthy pediatric patients receiving halothane anesthesia (0.1330 minutes^{-1}) than in healthy adult patients receiving opioid anesthesia (0.0575 minutes^{-1}). The EC$_{50}$ in healthy pediatric patients (125 ng/mL) was similar to the value in healthy adult patients (141 ng/mL) during opioid anesthesia. The minor differences in the PK/PD parameters of cisatracurium were associated with a faster time to onset and a shorter duration of cisatracurium-induced neuromuscular block in pediatric patients.
Other Patient Factors
Population PK/PD analyses revealed that gender and obesity were associated with statistically significant effects on the pharmacokinetics and/or pharmacodynamics of cisatracurium; these factors were not associated with clinically significant alterations in the predicted onset or recovery profile of NIMBEX. The use of inhalation agents was associated with a 21% larger V_{ss}, a 78% larger k_{eo}, and a 15% lower EC$_{50}$ for cisatracurium. These changes resulted in a slightly faster (~45 seconds) predicted time to 90% T_1 suppression in patients receiving 0.1 mg/kg cisatracurium during inhalation anesthesia than in patients receiving the same dose of cisatracurium during opioid anesthesia; however, there were no clinically significant differences in the predicted recovery profile of NIMBEX between patient groups.

Individualization of Dosages
DOSES OF **NIMBEX** SHOULD BE INDIVIDUALIZED AND A PERIPHERAL NERVE STIMULATOR SHOULD BE USED TO MEASURE NEUROMUSCULAR FUNCTION DURING ADMINISTRATION OF **NIMBEX** IN ORDER TO MONITOR DRUG EFFECT, TO DETERMINE THE NEED FOR ADDITIONAL DOSES, AND TO CONFIRM RECOVERY FROM NEUROMUSCULAR BLOCK.
Based on the known action of NIMBEX and other neuromuscular blocking agents, the following factors should be considered when administering NIMBEX.
Renal and Hepatic Disease
See **PRECAUTIONS** section.
Long-Term Use in the Intensive Care Unit (ICU)
The long-term infusion (up to 6 days) of NIMBEX during mechanical ventilation in the ICU has been evaluated in two studies. Average infusion rates of approximately 3 mcg/kg/min (range: 0.5 to 10.2) were required to achieve adequate neuromuscular block. As with other neuromuscular blocking agents, these data indicate the presence of wide interpatient variability in dosage requirements. In addition, dosage requirements may increase or decrease with time (see **PRECAUTIONS**). Use of NIMBEX in the ICU for longer than 6 days has not been studied.
Drugs or Conditions Causing Potentiation of or Resistance to Neuromuscular Block
Persons with certain pre-existing conditions or receiving certain drugs may require individualization of dosing (see **PRECAUTIONS**).
Burns
Patients with burns have been shown to develop resistance to nondepolarizing neuromuscular blocking agents, and may require individualization of dosing (see **PRECAUTIONS**).

Table 9. Parameter Estimates* for Cisatracurium, Atracurium, and Metabolites in ICU Patients After Long-Term (24-48 Hour) Administration of NIMBEX or Atracurium Besylate

	Parameter	Cisatracurium (n = 6)	Atracurium (n = 6)
Parent Compound	CL (mL/min/kg)	7.45 ± 1.02	7.49 ± 0.66†
	$t_{1/2}\beta$ (min)	26.8 ± 11.1	16.5 ± 6.0†
	Vβ (mL/kg)‡	280 ± 103	178 ± 71†
Laudanosine	C$_{max}$ (ng/mL)	707 ± 360	2318 ± 1498
	$t_{1/2}\beta$ (hrs)	6.6 ± 4.1	8.4 ± 7.3
MQA metabolite	C$_{max}$ (ng/mL)	152-181§	943 ± 333‖
	$t_{1/2}\beta$ (min)	26-31§	21-58§

* Presented as mean ± standard deviation.
† n = 5.
‡ Volume of distribution during the terminal elimination phase, an underestimate because elimination from the peripheral compartment is ignored.
§ n = 2, range presented.
‖ n = 3.

INDICATIONS AND USAGE

NIMBEX is an intermediate-onset/intermediate-duration neuromuscular blocking agent indicated for inpatients and outpatients as an adjunct to general anesthesia, to facilitate tracheal intubation, and to provide skeletal muscle relaxation during surgery or mechanical ventilation in the ICU.

CONTRAINDICATIONS

NIMBEX is contraindicated in patients with known hypersensitivity to the product and its components. The 10 mL multiple-dose vials of Nimbex is contraindicated for use in premature infants because the formulation contains benzyl alcohol. (See WARNINGS and PRECAUTIONS – Pediatric Use).

WARNINGS

Anaphylaxis

Severe anaphylactic reactions to neuromuscular blocking agents, including NIMBEX, have been reported. These reactions have in some cases been life-threatening and fatal. Due to the potential severity of these reactions, the necessary precautions, such as the immediate availability of appropriate emergency treatment, should be taken. Precautions should also be taken in those individuals who have had previous anaphylactic reactions to other neuromuscular blocking agents since cross-reactivity between neuromuscular blocking agents, both depolarizing and non-depolarizing, has been reported in this class of drugs.

Administration

NIMBEX SHOULD BE ADMINISTERED IN CAREFULLY ADJUSTED DOSAGE BY OR UNDER THE SUPERVISION OF EXPERIENCED CLINICIANS WHO ARE FAMILIAR WITH THE DRUG'S ACTIONS AND THE POSSIBLE COMPLICATIONS OF ITS USE. THE DRUG SHOULD NOT BE ADMINISTERED UNLESS PERSONNEL AND FACILITIES FOR RESUSCITATION AND LIFE SUPPORT (TRACHEAL INTUBATION, ARTIFICIAL VENTILATION, OXYGEN THERAPY), AND AN ANTAGONIST OF NIMBEX ARE IMMEDIATELY AVAILABLE. IT IS RECOMMENDED THAT A PERIPHERAL NERVE STIMULATOR BE USED TO MEASURE NEUROMUSCULAR FUNCTION DURING THE ADMINISTRATION OF NIMBEX IN ORDER TO MONITOR DRUG EFFECT, DETERMINE THE NEED FOR ADDITIONAL DOSES, AND CONFIRM RECOVERY FROM NEUROMUSCULAR BLOCK.

NIMBEX HAS NO KNOWN EFFECT ON CONSCIOUSNESS, PAIN THRESHOLD, OR CEREBRATION. TO AVOID DISTRESS TO THE PATIENT, NEUROMUSCULAR BLOCK SHOULD NOT BE INDUCED BEFORE UNCONSCIOUSNESS.

NIMBEX Injection is acidic (pH 3.25 to 3.65) and may not be compatible with alkaline solutions having a pH greater than 8.5 (e.g., barbiturate solutions).

The 10 mL multiple-dose vials of NIMBEX contain benzyl alcohol, which is potentially toxic when administered locally to neural tissue. Exposure to excessive amounts of benzyl alcohol has been associated with toxicity (hypotension, metabolic acidosis), particularly in neonates, and an increased incidence of kernicterus, particularly in small preterm infants. There have been rare reports of deaths, primarily in preterm infants, associated with exposure to excessive amounts of benzyl alcohol. The amount of benzyl alcohol from medications is usually considered negligible compared to that received in flush solution containing benzyl alcohol. Administration of high dosages of medications containing this preservative must take into account the total amount of benzyl alcohol administered. The amount of benzyl alcohol at which toxicity may occur is not known. If the patient requires more than the recommended dosages or other medications containing this preservative, the practitioner must consider the daily metabolic load of benzyl alcohol from these combined sources. Single-use vials (5 mL and 20 mL) of NIMBEX do not contain benzyl alcohol (see WARNINGS and PRECAUTIONS - Pediatric Use).

PRECAUTIONS

Because of its intermediate onset of action, NIMBEX is not recommended for rapid sequence endotracheal intubation.
Recommended doses of NIMBEX® (cisatracurium besylate) have no clinically significant effects on heart rate; therefore, NIMBEX will not counteract the bradycardia produced by many anesthetic agents or by vagal stimulation.

Neuromuscular blocking agents may have a profound effect in patients with neuromuscular diseases (e.g., myasthenia gravis and the myasthenic syndrome). In these and other conditions in which prolonged neuromuscular block is a possibility (e.g., carcinomatosis), the use of a peripheral nerve stimulator and a dose of not more than 0.02 mg/kg NIMBEX is recommended to assess the level of neuromuscular block and to monitor dosage requirements.

Patients with burns have been shown to develop resistance to nondepolarizing neuromuscular blocking agents, including atracurium. The extent of altered response depends upon the size of the burn and the time elapsed since the burn injury. NIMBEX has not been studied in patients with burns; however, based on its structural similarity to atracurium, the possibility of increased dosing requirements and shortened duration of action must be considered if NIMBEX is administered to burn patients.

Patients with hemiparesis or paraparesis also may demonstrate resistance to nondepolarizing muscle relaxants in the affected limbs. To avoid inaccurate dosing, neuromuscular monitoring should be performed on a non-paretic limb.

Acid-base and/or serum electrolyte abnormalities may potentiate or antagonize the action of neuromuscular blocking agents. No data are available to support the use of NIMBEX by intramuscular injection.

Allergic Reactions

Since allergic cross-reactivity has been reported in this class, request information from your patients about previous anaphylactic reactions to other neuromuscular blocking agents. In addition, inform your patients that severe anaphylactic reactions to neuromuscular blocking agents, including NIMBEX have been reported (see CONTRAINDICATIONS).

Renal and Hepatic Disease

No clinically significant alterations in the recovery profile were observed in patients with renal dysfunction or in patients with end-stage liver disease following a 0.1 mg/kg dose of cisatracurium. The onset time was approximately 1 minute faster in patients with end-stage liver disease and approximately 1 minute slower in patients with renal dysfunction than in healthy adult control patients.

Malignant Hyperthermia (MH)

In a study of MH-susceptible pigs, cisatracurium besylate (highest dose 2000 mcg/kg equivalent to $3 \times ED_{95}$ in pigs and $40 \times ED_{95}$ in humans) did not trigger MH. Cisatracurium besylate has not been studied in MH-susceptible patients. Because MH can develop in the absence of established triggering agents, the clinician should be prepared to recognize and treat MH in any patient undergoing general anesthesia.

Long-Term Use in the Intensive Care Unit (ICU)

Long-term infusion (up to 6 days) of NIMBEX during mechanical ventilation in the ICU has been safely used in two studies. Dosage requirements may increase or decrease with time (see CLINICAL PHARMACOLOGY - Individualization of Doses).

Little information is available on the plasma levels and clinical consequences of cisatracurium metabolites that may accumulate during days to weeks of cisatracurium administration in ICU patients. Laudanosine, a major, biologically active metabolite of atracurium and cisatracurium without neuromuscular blocking activity, produces transient hypotension and, in higher doses, cerebral excitatory effects (generalized muscle twitching and seizures) when administered to several species of animals. There have been rare spontaneous reports of seizures in ICU patients who have received atracurium or other agents. These patients usually had predisposing causes (such as cranial trauma, cerebral edema, hypoxic encephalopathy, viral encephalitis, uremia). There are insufficient data to determine whether or not laudanosine contributes to seizures in ICU patients. Consistent with the decreased infusion rate requirements for NIMBEX, laudanosine concentrations were lower in patients receiving NIMBEX than in patients receiving atracurium for up to 48 hours (see Pharmacokinetics -Special Populations - Intensive Care Unit Patients).

In a randomized, double-blind study using train-of-four nerve stimulator monitoring to maintain at least one visible twitch, evaluable patients treated with NIMBEX (n = 19) recovered neuromuscular function ($T_4:T_1$ ratio ≥ 70%) following termination of infusion in approximately 55 minutes (range: 20 to 270) whereas evaluable vecuronium-treated patients (n = 12) recovered in 178 minutes (range: 40 minutes to 33 hours). In another study comparing NIMBEX and atracurium, patients recovered neuromuscular function in approximately 50 minutes for both NIMBEX (range: 20 to 175; n = 34) and atracurium (range: 35 to 85; n = 15).

WHENEVER THE USE OF NIMBEX OR ANY OTHER NEUROMUSCULAR BLOCKING AGENT IN THE ICU IS CONTEMPLATED, IT IS RECOMMENDED THAT NEUROMUSCULAR FUNCTION BE MONITORED DURING ADMINISTRATION WITH A NERVE STIMULATOR. ADDITIONAL DOSES OF NIMBEX OR ANY OTHER NEUROMUSCULAR BLOCKING AGENT SHOULD NOT BE GIVEN BEFORE THERE IS A DEFINITE RESPONSE TO NERVE STIMULATION. IF NO RESPONSE IS ELICITED, INFUSION ADMINISTRATION SHOULD BE DISCONTINUED UNTIL A RESPONSE RETURNS.

The effects of hemofiltration, hemodialysis, and hemoperfusion on plasma levels of NIMBEX and its metabolites are unknown.

Drug Interactions

NIMBEX has been used safely following varying degrees of recovery from succinylcholine-induced neuromuscular block. Administration of 0.1 mg/kg ($2 \times ED_{95}$) NIMBEX at 10% or 95% recovery following an intubating dose of succinylcholine (1 mg/kg) produced ≥ 95% neuromuscular block. The time to onset of maximum block following NIMBEX is approximately 2 minutes faster with prior administration of succinylcholine. Prior administration of succinylcholine had no effect on the duration of neuromuscular block following initial or maintenance bolus doses of NIMBEX. Infusion requirements of NIMBEX in patients administered succinylcholine prior to infusions of NIMBEX were comparable to or slightly greater than when succinylcholine was not administered.

The use of NIMBEX before succinylcholine to attenuate some of the side effects of succinylcholine has not been studied.

Although not studied systematically in clinical trials, no drug interactions were observed when vecuronium, pancuronium, or atracurium were administered following varying degrees of recovery from single doses or infusions of NIMBEX.

Isoflurane or enflurane administered with nitrous oxide/oxygen to achieve 1.25 MAC [Minimum Alveolar Concentration] may prolong the clinically effective duration of action of initial and maintenance doses of NIMBEX and decrease the required infusion rate of NIMBEX. The magnitude of these effects may depend on the duration of administration of the volatile agents. Fifteen to 30 minutes of exposure to 1.25 MAC isoflurane or enflurane had minimal effects on the duration of action of initial doses of NIMBEX and therefore, no adjustment to the initial dose should be necessary when NIMBEX is administered shortly after initiation of volatile agents. In long surgical procedures during enflurane or isoflurane anesthesia, less frequent maintenance dosing, lower maintenance doses, or reduced infusion rates of NIMBEX may be necessary. The average infusion rate requirement may be decreased by as much as 30% to 40%.

In clinical studies propofol had no effect on the duration of action or dosing requirements for NIMBEX.

Other drugs which may enhance the neuromuscular blocking action of nondepolarizing agents such as NIMBEX include certain antibiotics (e.g., aminoglycosides, tetracyclines, bacitracin, polymyxins, lincomycin, clindamycin, colistin, and sodium colistemethate), magnesium salts, lithium, local anesthetics, procainamide, and quinidine.

Resistance to the neuromuscular blocking action of nondepolarizing neuromuscular blocking agents has been demonstrated in patients chronically administered phenytoin or carbamazepine. While the effects of chronic phenytoin or carbamazepine therapy on the action of NIMBEX are unknown, slightly shorter durations of neuromuscular block may be anticipated and infusion rate requirements may be higher.

Drug/Laboratory Test Interactions

None known.

Carcinogenesis, Mutagenesis, Impairment of Fertility

Carcinogenesis and fertility studies have not been performed. Cisatracurium besylate was evaluated in a battery of four short-term mutagenicity tests. It was non-mutagenic in the Ames Salmonella assay, a rat bone marrow cytogenetic assay, and an in vitro human lymphocyte cytogenetics assay. As was the case with atracurium, the mouse lymphoma assay was positive both in the presence and absence

Continued on next page

Information on the AbbVie, Inc. products listed on these pages is from the prescribing information in use as of July 31, 2016. For more information, please visit rxabbvie.com or call 1-800-633-9110.

of exogenous metabolic activation (rat liver S-9). In the absence of S-9, cisatracurium besylate was positive at *in vitro* cisatracurium concentrations of 40 mcg/mL and higher. The highest non-mutagenic concentration (30 mcg/mL) and incubation time (4 hours) resulted in an AUC approximately 120 times that noted in clinical studies and approximately 8.5 times the mean peak clinical concentration noted. In the presence of S-9, cisatracurium besylate was positive at a cisatracurium concentration of 300 mcg/mL but not at lower or higher concentrations.

Pregnancy
Teratogenic Effects
Pregnancy Category B
Teratology testing in nonventilated pregnant rats treated subcutaneously with maximum subparalyzing doses (4 mg/kg daily; equivalent to 8 × the human ED_{95} following a bolus dose of 0.2 mg/kg IV) and in ventilated rats treated intravenously with paralyzing doses of NIMBEX at 0.5 and 1.0 mg/kg; equivalent to 10 × and 20 × the human ED_{95} dose, respectively, revealed no maternal or fetal toxicity or teratogenic effects. There are no adequate and well-controlled studies of NIMBEX in pregnant women. Because animal studies are not always predictive of human response, NIMBEX should be used during pregnancy only if clearly needed.

Labor and Delivery
The use of NIMBEX during labor, vaginal delivery, or cesarean section has not been studied in humans and it is not known whether NIMBEX administered to the mother has effects on the fetus. Doses of 0.2 or 0.4 mg/kg cisatracurium given to female beagles undergoing cesarean section resulted in negligible levels of cisatracurium in umbilical vessel blood of neonates and no deleterious effects on the puppies. The action of neuromuscular blocking agents may be enhanced by magnesium salts administered for the management of toxemia of pregnancy.

Nursing Mothers
It is not known whether cisatracurium besylate is excreted in human milk. Because many drugs are excreted in human milk, caution should be exercised following administration of NIMBEX to a nursing woman.

Pediatric Use
NIMBEX has not been studied in pediatric patients below the age of 1 month (see **CLINICAL PHARMACOLOGY** and **DOSAGE AND ADMINISTRATION** for clinical experience and recommendations for use in children 1 month to 12 years of age). Intubation of the trachea in patients 1-4 years old was facilitated more reliably when NIMBEX was used in combination with Halothane than when opioids and nitrous oxide were used for induction of anesthesia.

The 10 mL multiple-dose vials of NIMBEX contain benzyl alcohol as a preservative. Benzyl alcohol, a component of this product, has been associated with serious adverse events and death, particularly in pediatric patients. The "gasping syndrome", (characterized by central nervous system depression, metabolic acidosis, gasping respirations, and high levels of benzyl alcohol and its metabolites found in the blood and urine) has been associated with benzyl alcohol dosages >99 mg/kg/day in neonates and low-birth-weight neonates. Additional symptoms may include gradual neurological deterioration, seizures, intracranial hemorrhage, hematologic abnormalities, skin breakdown, hepatic and renal failure, hypotension, bradycardia, and cardiovascular collapse. Although normal therapeutic doses of this product deliver amounts of benzyl alcohol that are substantially lower than those reported in association with the "gasping syndrome", the minimum amount of benzyl alcohol at which toxicity may occur is not known. Premature and low-birth-weight infants, as well as patients receiving high dosages, may be more likely to develop toxicity. Practitioners administering this and other medications containing benzyl alcohol should consider the combined daily metabolic load of benzyl alcohol from all sources.

Geriatric Use
Of the total number of subjects in clinical studies of NIMBEX, 57 were 65 and over, 63 were 70 and over, and 15 were 80 and over. The geriatric population included a subset of patients with significant cardiovascular disease (see **CLINICAL PHARMACOLOGY - Hemodynamics Profile** and Special Populations - *Geriatric Patients* subsections). No overall differences in safety or effectiveness were observed between these subjects and younger subjects, and other reported clinical experience has not identified differences in responses between elderly and younger subjects, but greater sensitivity of some older individuals to NIMBEX cannot be ruled out.

Minor differences in the pharmacokinetics of cisatracurium between elderly and young adult patients are not associated with clinically significant differences in the recovery profile of NIMBEX following a single 0.1 mg/kg dose; the time to maximum block is approximately 1 minute slower in elderly patients (see **CLINICAL PHARMACOLOGY - Pharmacokinetics**).

ADVERSE REACTIONS
Observed in Clinical Trials of Surgical Patients
Adverse experiences were uncommon among the 945 surgical patients who received NIMBEX in conjunction with other drugs in US and European clinical studies in the course of a wide variety of procedures in patients receiving opioid, propofol, or inhalation anesthesia. The following adverse experiences were judged by investigators during the clinical trials to have a possible causal relationship to administration of NIMBEX:
Incidence Greater than 1%
None.
Incidence Less than 1%
Cardiovascular
bradycardia (0.4%)
hypotension (0.2%)
flushing (0.2%).
Respiratory
bronchospasm (0.2%).
Dermatological
rash (0.1%).

Observed in Clinical Trials of Intensive Care Unit Patients
Adverse experiences were uncommon among the 68 ICU patients who received NIMBEX in conjunction with other drugs in US and European clinical studies. One patient experienced bronchospasm. In one of the two ICU studies, a randomized and double-blind study of ICU patients using TOF neuromuscular monitoring, there were two reports of prolonged recovery (167 and 270 minutes) among 28 patients administered NIMBEX and 13 reports of prolonged recovery (range: 90 minutes to 33 hours) among 30 patients administered vecuronium.

Observed During Clinical Practice
In addition to adverse events reported from clinical trials, the following events have been identified during post-approval use of cisatracurium besylate in conjunction with one or more anesthetic agents in clinical practice. Because they are reported voluntarily from a population of unknown size, estimates of frequency cannot be made. These events have been chosen for inclusion due to a combination of their seriousness, frequency of reporting, or potential causal connection to cisatracurium besylate.
General
Histamine release, hypersensitivity reactions including anaphylactic or anaphylactoid reactions which in some cases have been life threatening and fatal. Because these reactions were reported voluntarily from a population of uncertain size, it is not possible to reliably estimate their frequency (see **WARNINGS** and **PRECAUTIONS**). There are rare reports of wheezing, laryngospasm, bronchospasm, rash and itching following administration of NIMBEX in children. These reported adverse events were not serious and their etiology could not be established with certainty.
Musculoskeletal
Prolonged neuromuscular block, inadequate neuromuscular block, muscle weakness, and myopathy.

OVERDOSAGE
Overdosage with neuromuscular blocking agents may result in neuromuscular block beyond the time needed for surgery and anesthesia. The primary treatment is maintenance of a patent airway and controlled ventilation until recovery of normal neuromuscular function is assured. Once recovery from neuromuscular block begins, further recovery may be facilitated by administration of an anticholinesterase agent (e.g., neostigmine, edrophonium) in conjunction with an appropriate anticholinergic agent (see Antagonism of Neuromuscular Block below).

Antagonism of Neuromuscular Block
ANTAGONISTS (SUCH AS NEOSTIGMINE AND EDROPHONIUM) SHOULD NOT BE ADMINISTERED WHEN COMPLETE NEUROMUSCULAR BLOCK IS EVIDENT OR SUSPECTED. THE USE OF A PERIPHERAL NERVE STIMULATOR TO EVALUATE RECOVERY AND ANTAGONISM OF NEUROMUSCULAR BLOCK IS RECOMMENDED.
Administration of 0.04 to 0.07 mg/kg neostigmine at approximately 10% recovery from neuromuscular block (range: 0 to

15%) produced 95% recovery of the muscle twitch response and a $T_4:T_1$ ratio ≥ 70% in an average of 9 to 10 minutes. The times from 25% recovery of the muscle twitch response to a $T_4:T_1$ ratio ≥ 70% following these doses of neostigmine averaged 7 minutes. The mean 25% to 75% recovery index following reversal was 3 to 4 minutes.
Administration of 1.0 mg/kg edrophonium at approximately 25% recovery from neuromuscular block (range: 16% to 30%) produced 95% recovery and a $T_4:T_1$ ratio ≥ 70% in an average of 3 to 5 minutes.
Patients administered antagonists should be evaluated for evidence of adequate clinical recovery (e.g., 5-second head lift and grip strength). Ventilation must be supported until no longer required.
The onset of antagonism may be delayed in the presence of debilitation, cachexia, carcinomatosis, and the concomitant use of certain broad spectrum antibiotics, or anesthetic agents and other drugs which enhance neuromuscular block or separately cause respiratory depression (see **PRECAUTIONS - Drug Interactions**). Under such circumstances the management is the same as that of prolonged neuromuscular block (see **OVERDOSAGE**).

DOSAGE AND ADMINISTRATION
NOTE: CONTAINS BENZYL ALCOHOL (see **WARNINGS** and **PRECAUTIONS – Pediatric Use**)
NIMBEX SHOULD ONLY BE ADMINISTERED INTRAVENOUSLY.
The dosage information provided below is intended as a guide only. Doses of NIMBEX should be individualized (see CLINICAL PHARMACOLOGY - Individualization of Dosages). The use of a peripheral nerve stimulator will permit the most advantageous use of NIMBEX, minimize the possibility of overdosage or underdosage, and assist in the evaluation of recovery.
Adults
Initial Doses
One of two intubating doses of NIMBEX may be chosen, based on the desired time to tracheal intubation and the anticipated length of surgery. In addition to the dose of neuromuscular blocking agent, the presence of co-induction agents (e.g., fentanyl and midazolam) and the depth of anesthesia are factors that can influence intubation conditions. Doses of 0.15 (3 × ED_{95}) and 0.20 (4 × ED_{95}) mg/kg NIMBEX, as components of a propofol/nitrous oxide/oxygen induction-intubation technique, may produce generally GOOD or EXCELLENT conditions for intubation in 2.0 and 1.5 minutes, respectively. Similar intubation conditions may be expected when these doses of NIMBEX are administered as components of a thiopental/nitrous oxide/oxygen induction-intubation technique. In two intubation studies using thiopental or propofol and midazolam and fentanyl as co-induction agents, EXCELLENT intubation conditions were most frequently achieved with the 0.2 mg/kg compared to 0.15 mg/kg dose of cisatracurium. The clinically effective durations of action for 0.15 and 0.20 mg/kg NIMBEX during propofol anesthesia are 55 minutes (range: 44 to 74 minutes) and 61 minutes (range: 41 to 81 minutes), respectively. Lower doses may result in a longer time for the development of satisfactory intubation conditions. Doses up to 8 × ED_{95} NIMBEX have been safely administered to healthy adult patients and patients with serious cardiovascular disease. These larger doses are associated with longer clinically effective durations of action (see **CLINICAL PHARMACOLOGY**).
Because slower times to onset of complete neuromuscular block were observed in elderly patients and patients with renal dysfunction, extending the interval between administration of NIMBEX and the intubation attempt for these patients may be required to achieve adequate intubation conditions.
A dose of 0.03 mg/kg NIMBEX is recommended for maintenance of neuromuscular block during prolonged surgical procedures. Maintenance doses of 0.03 mg/kg each sustain neuromuscular block for approximately 20 minutes. Maintenance dosing is generally required 40 to 50 minutes following an initial dose of 0.15 mg/kg NIMBEX and 50 to 60 minutes following an initial dose of 0.20 mg/kg NIMBEX, but the need for maintenance doses should be determined by clinical criteria. For shorter or longer durations of action, smaller or larger maintenance doses may be administered. Isoflurane or enflurane administered with nitrous oxide/oxygen to achieve 1.25 MAC (Minimum Alveolar Concentration) may prolong the clinically effective duration of action of initial and maintenance doses. The magnitude of these

effects may depend on the duration of administration of the volatile agents. Fifteen to 30 minutes of exposure to 1.25 MAC isoflurane or enflurane had minimal effects on the duration of action of initial doses of NIMBEX and therefore, no adjustment to the initial dose should be necessary when NIMBEX is administered shortly after initiation of volatile agents. In long surgical procedures during enflurane or isoflurane anesthesia, less frequent maintenance dosing or lower maintenance doses of NIMBEX may be necessary. No adjustments to the initial dose of NIMBEX are required when used in patients receiving propofol anesthesia.

Children
Initial Doses
The recommended dose of NIMBEX for children 2 to 12 years of age is 0.10-0.15 mg/kg administered over 5 to 10 seconds during either halothane or opioid anesthesia. When administered during stable opioid/nitrous oxide/oxygen anesthesia, 0.10 mg/kg NIMBEX produces maximum neuromuscular block in an average of 2.8 minutes (range: 1.8 to 6.7 minutes) and clinically effective block for 28 minutes (range: 21 to 38 minutes). When administered during stable opioid/nitrous oxide/oxygen anesthesia, 0.15 mg/kg NIMBEX produces maximum neuromuscular block in about 3.0 minutes (range: 1.5 to 8.0 minutes) and clinically effective block (time to 25% recovery) for 36 minutes (range: 29 to 46 minutes).

Infants
Initial Doses
The recommended dose of NIMBEX for intubation of infants 1 month to 23 months is 0.15 mg/kg administered over 5 to 10 seconds during either halothane or opioid anesthesia. When administered during stable opioid/nitrous oxide/oxygen anesthesia, 0.15 mg/kg NIMBEX produces maximum neuromuscular block in about 2.0 minutes (range: 1.3 to 3.4 minutes) and clinically effective block (time to 25% recovery) for about 43 minutes (range: 34 to 58 minutes).

Use by Continuous Infusion
Infusion in the Operating Room (OR)
After administration of an initial bolus dose of NIMBEX, a diluted solution of NIMBEX can be administered by continuous infusion to adults and children age 2 or more years for maintenance of neuromuscular block during extended surgical procedures. Infusion of NIMBEX should be individualized for each patient. The rate of administration should be adjusted according to the patient's response as determined by peripheral nerve stimulation. Accurate dosing is best achieved using a precision infusion device.
Infusion of NIMBEX should be initiated only after early evidence of spontaneous recovery from the initial bolus dose. An initial infusion rate of 3 mcg/kg/min may be required to rapidly counteract the spontaneous recovery of neuromuscular function. Thereafter, a rate of 1 to 2 mcg/kg/min should be adequate to maintain continuous neuromuscular block in the range of 89% to 99% in most pediatric and adult patients under opioid/nitrous oxide/oxygen anesthesia.
Reduction of the infusion rate by up to 30% to 40% should be considered when NIMBEX is administered during stable isoflurane or enflurane anesthesia (administered with nitrous oxide/oxygen at the 1.25 MAC level). Greater reductions in the infusion rate of NIMBEX may be required with longer durations of administration of isoflurane or enflurane.
The rate of infusion of atracurium required to maintain adequate surgical relaxation in patients undergoing coronary artery bypass surgery with induced hypothermia (25° to 28°C) is approximately half the rate required during normothermia. Based on the structural similarity between NIMBEX and atracurium, a similar effect on the infusion rate of NIMBEX may be expected.
Spontaneous recovery from neuromuscular block following discontinuation of infusion of NIMBEX may be expected to proceed at a rate comparable to that following administration of a single bolus dose.
Infusion in the Intensive Care Unit (ICU)
The principles for infusion of NIMBEX in the OR are also applicable to use in the ICU. An infusion rate of approximately 3 mcg/kg/min (range: 0.5 to 10.2 mcg/kg/min) should provide adequate neuromuscular block in adult patients in the ICU. There may be wide interpatient variability in dosage requirements and these may increase or decrease with time (see **PRECAUTIONS - Long-Term Use in the Intensive Care Unit [ICU]**). Following recovery from neuromuscular block, readministration of a bolus dose may be necessary to quickly re-establish neuromuscular block prior to reinstitution of the infusion.

Infusion Rate Tables
The amount of infusion solution required per minute will depend upon the concentration of NIMBEX in the infusion solution, the desired dose of NIMBEX, and the patient's weight. The contribution of the infusion solution to the fluid requirements of the patient also must be considered. Tables 10 and 11 provide guidelines for delivery, in mL/hr (equivalent to microdrops/minute when 60 microdrops = 1 mL), of NIMBEX solutions in concentrations of 0.1 mg/mL (10 mg/100 mL) or 0.4 mg/mL (40 mg/100 mL).

Table 10. Infusion Rates of NIMBEX for Maintenance of Neuromuscular Block During Opioid/Nitrous Oxide/Oxygen Anesthesia for a Concentration of 0.1 mg/mL

Patient Weight (kg)	Drug Delivery Rate (mcg/kg/min)				
	1.0	1.5	2.0	3.0	5.0
	Infusion Delivery Rate (mL/hr)				
10	6	9	12	18	30
45	27	41	54	81	135
70	42	63	84	126	210
100	60	90	120	180	300

Table 11. Infusion Rates of NIMBEX for Maintenance of Neuromuscular Block During Opioid/Nitrous Oxide/Oxygen Anesthesia for a Concentration of 0.4 mg/mL

Patient Weight (kg)	Drug Delivery Rate (mcg/kg/min)				
	1.0	1.5	2.0	3.0	5.0
	Infusion Delivery Rate (mL/hr)				
10	1.5	2.3	3.0	4.5	7.5
45	6.8	10.1	13.5	20.3	33.8
70	10.5	15.8	21.0	31.5	52.5
100	15.0	22.5	30.0	45.0	75.0

NIMBEX Injection Compatibility and Admixtures
Y-site Administration
NIMBEX Injection is acidic (pH = 3.25 to 3.65) and may not be compatible with alkaline solution having a pH greater than 8.5 (e.g., barbiturate solutions).
Studies have shown that NIMBEX Injection is compatible with:
- 5% Dextrose Injection, USP
- 0.9% Sodium Chloride Injection, USP
- 5% Dextrose and 0.9% Sodium Chloride Injection, USP
- SUFENTA® (sufentanil citrate) Injection, diluted as directed
- ALFENTA® (alfentanil hydrochloride) Injection, diluted as directed
- SUBLIMAZE® (fentanyl citrate) Injection, diluted as directed
- VERSED® (midazolam hydrochloride) Injection, diluted as directed
- Droperidol Injection, diluted as directed
NIMBEX Injection is not compatible with DIPRIVAN® (propofol) Injection or TORADOL® (ketorolac) Injection for Y-site administration. Studies of other parenteral products have not been conducted.
Dilution Stability
NIMBEX Injection diluted in 5% Dextrose Injection, USP; 0.9% Sodium Chloride Injection, USP; or 5% Dextrose and 0.9% Sodium Chloride Injection, USP to 0.1 mg/mL may be stored either under refrigeration or at room temperature for 24 hours without significant loss of potency. Dilutions to 0.1 mg/mL or 0.2 mg/mL in 5% Dextrose and Lactated Ringer's Injection may be stored under refrigeration for 24 hours.
NIMBEX Injection should not be diluted in Lactated Ringer's Injection, USP due to chemical instability.
NOTE: Parenteral drug products should be inspected visually for particulate matter and discoloration prior to administration whenever solution and container permit. Solutions which are not clear, or contain visible particulates, should not be used. NIMBEX Injection is a colorless to slightly yellow or greenish-yellow solution.

HOW SUPPLIED
NIMBEX Injection, 2 mg cisatracurium per mL, is supplied in the following:

List No.	Container	Size

| 4378 | Single-dose Vial | 5 mL |
| 4380 | Multiple-dose Vial | 10 mL |

NOTE: 10 mL Multiple-dose Vials contain 0.9% w/v benzyl alcohol as a preservative (see **WARNINGS** concerning newborn infants).
NIMBEX Injection, 10 mg cisatracurium per mL is supplied in the following:

| 4382 | Single-dose Vial | 20 mL |

Intended only for use in the ICU.
STORAGE
NIMBEX Injection should be refrigerated at 2° to 8°C (36° to 46°F) in the carton to preserve potency. Protect from light. DO NOT FREEZE. Upon removal from refrigeration to room temperature storage conditions (25°C/77°F), use NIMBEX Injection within 21 days even if rerefrigerated.
Nimbex® is a registered trademark of GlaxoSmithKline, licensed for use by AbbVie Inc.
©2013 AbbVie Inc.
Mfd By: Hospira, Inc.
Lake Forest, IL 60045 USA
For: AbbVie Inc.
North Chicago, IL 60064 USA
EN-3172 Revised January, 2013
Shown in Product Identification Guide, page 506

NORVIR®
[*NOR-VEER*]
(ritonavir)
tablet, for oral use
NORVIR
(ritonavir)
solution, for oral use

HIGHLIGHTS OF PRESCRIBING INFORMATION
These highlights do not include all the information needed to use NORVIR safely and effectively. See full prescribing information for NORVIR.
NORVIR (ritonavir) tablet, for oral use
NORVIR (ritonavir) solution, for oral use
Initial U.S. Approval: 1996

> **WARNING: DRUG-DRUG INTERACTIONS LEADING TO POTENTIALLY SERIOUS AND/OR LIFE THREATENING REACTIONS**
> *See full prescribing information for complete boxed warning*
> Co-administration of NORVIR with several classes of drugs including sedative hypnotics, antiarrhythmics, or ergot alkaloid preparations may result in potentially serious and/or life-threatening adverse events due to possible effects of NORVIR on the hepatic metabolism of certain drugs. Review medications taken by patients prior to prescribing NORVIR or when prescribing other medications to patients already taking NORVIR [*see Contraindications (4), Warnings and Precautions (5.1), Drug Interactions (7), and Clinical Pharmacology (12.3)*].

RECENT MAJOR CHANGES
Warnings and Precautions
 Risk of Serious Adverse Reactions Due to
 Drug Interactions (5.1)   03/2015

INDICATIONS AND USAGE
NORVIR is an HIV protease inhibitor indicated in combination with other antiretroviral agents for the treatment of HIV-1 infection (1)

DOSAGE AND ADMINISTRATION
- Dose modification for NORVIR is necessary when used with other protease inhibitors (2)

Continued on next page

- Adult patients: 600 mg twice-day with meals (2.1)
- Pediatrics patients: The recommended twice daily dose for children greater than one month of age is based on body surface area and should not exceed 600 mg twice daily with meals (2.2)
- NORVIR oral solution should not be administered to neonates before a postmenstrual age (first day of the mother's last menstrual period to birth plus the time elapsed after birth) of 44 weeks has been attained (2.2, 5.2)

DOSAGE FORMS AND STRENGTHS

- Tablet: 100 mg ritonavir (3)
- Oral solution: 80 mg ritonavir per milliliter (3)

CONTRAINDICATIONS

- NORVIR is contraindicated in patients with known hypersensitivity to ritonavir (e.g., toxic epidermal necrolysis, Stevens-Johnson syndrome) or any of its ingredients (4)
- Co-administration with drugs highly dependent on CYP3A for clearance and for which elevated plasma concentrations may be associated with serious and/or life-threatening events (4)
- Co-administration with drugs that significantly reduce ritonavir (4)

WARNINGS AND PRECAUTIONS

The following have been observed in patients receiving NORVIR:

- The concomitant use of NORVIR and certain other drugs may result in known or potentially significant drug interactions. Consult the full prescribing information prior to and during treatment for potential drug interactions. (5.1, 7.2)
- Toxicity in preterm neonates: NORVIR oral solution should not be used in preterm neonates in the immediate postnatal period because of possible toxicities. A safe and effective dose of NORVIR oral solution in this patient population has not been established (2.2, 5.2)
- Hepatic Reactions: Fatalities have occurred. Monitor liver function before and during therapy, especially in patients with underlying hepatic disease, including hepatitis B and hepatitis C, or marked transaminase elevations (5.3, 8.6)
- Pancreatitis: Fatalities have occurred; suspend therapy as clinically appropriate (5.4)
- Allergic Reactions/Hypersensitivity: Allergic reactions have been reported and include anaphylaxis, toxic epidermal necrolysis, Stevens-Johnson syndrome, bronchospasm and angioedema. Discontinue treatment if severe reactions develop (5.5, 6.2)
- PR interval prolongation may occur in some patients. Cases of second and third degree heart block have been reported. Use with caution with patients with preexisting conduction system disease, ischemic heart disease, cardiomyopathy, underlying structural heart disease or when administering with other drugs that may prolong the PR interval (5.6, 12.3)
- Total cholesterol and triglycerides elevations: Monitor prior to therapy and periodically thereafter (5.7)
- Patients may develop new onset or exacerbations of diabetes mellitus, hyperglycemia (5.8)
- Patients may develop immune reconstitution syndrome (5.9)
- Patients may develop redistribution/accumulation of body fat (5.10)
- Hemophilia: Spontaneous bleeding may occur, and additional factor VIII may be required (5.11)

ADVERSE REACTIONS

The most frequently reported adverse drug reactions among patients receiving NORVIR alone or in combination with other antiretroviral drugs were gastrointestinal (including diarrhea, nausea, vomiting, abdominal pain (upper and lower)), neurological disturbances (including paresthesia and oral paresthesia), rash, and fatigue/asthenia (6.1)

To report SUSPECTED ADVERSE REACTIONS, contact AbbVie Inc. at 1-800-633-9110 or FDA at 1-800-FDA-1088 or www.fda.gov/medwatch.

DRUG INTERACTIONS

- Co-administration of NORVIR can alter the concentrations of other drugs. The potential for drug-drug interactions must be considered prior to and during therapy (4, 5.1, 7, 12.3)

USE IN SPECIFIC POPULATIONS

- Nursing Mothers: Because of both the potential for HIV transmission and the potential for serious adverse reactions in nursing infants, mothers should be instructed not to breastfeed if they are receiving NORVIR (8.3)

See 17 for PATIENT COUNSELING INFORMATION and FDA-approved patient labeling.
Revised: 11/2015

FULL PRESCRIBING INFORMATION

> **WARNING: DRUG-DRUG INTERACTIONS LEADING TO POTENTIALLY SERIOUS AND/OR LIFE THREATENING REACTIONS**
>
> Co-administration of NORVIR with several classes of drugs including sedative hypnotics, antiarrhythmics, or ergot alkaloid preparations may result in potentially serious and/or life-threatening adverse events due to possible effects of NORVIR on the hepatic metabolism of certain drugs. Review medications taken by patients prior to prescribing NORVIR or when prescribing other medications to patients already taking NORVIR *[see Contraindications (4), Warnings and Precautions (5.1), Drug Interactions (7), and Clinical Pharmacology (12.3)].*

1   INDICATIONS AND USAGE

NORVIR is indicated in combination with other antiretroviral agents for the treatment of HIV-1 infection.

2   DOSAGE AND ADMINISTRATION

NORVIR® (ritonavir) is administered orally. NORVIR tablets should be swallowed whole, and not chewed, broken or crushed. Take NORVIR with meals. Patients may improve the taste of NORVIR oral solution by mixing with chocolate milk, Ensure®, or Advera® within one hour of dosing.

General Dosing Guidelines

Patients who take the 600 mg twice daily soft gel capsule NORVIR dose may experience more gastrointestinal side effects such as nausea, vomiting, abdominal pain or diarrhea when switching from the soft gel capsule to the tablet formulation because of greater maximum plasma concentration (C_{max}) achieved with the tablet formulation relative to the soft gel capsule *[see Clinical Pharmacology (12.3)].* Patients should also be aware that these adverse events (gastrointestinal or paresthesias) may diminish as therapy is continued.

Dose Modification for NORVIR

Dose reduction of NORVIR is necessary when used with other protease inhibitors: atazanavir, darunavir, fosamprenavir, saquinavir, and tipranavir.

Prescribers should consult the full prescribing information and clinical study information of these protease inhibitors if they are co-administered with a reduced dose of ritonavir *[see Warnings and Precautions (5), and Drug Interactions (7)].*

2.1   Adult Patients

Recommended Dosage for Treatment of HIV-1:

The recommended dosage of ritonavir is 600 mg twice daily by mouth to be taken with meals. Use of a dose titration schedule may help to reduce treatment-emergent adverse events while maintaining appropriate ritonavir plasma levels. Ritonavir should be started at no less than 300 mg twice daily and increased at 2 to 3 day intervals by 100 mg twice daily. The maximum dose of 600 mg twice daily should not be exceeded upon completion of the titration.

2.2   Pediatric Patients

Ritonavir should be used in combination with other antiretroviral agents *[see Dosage and Administration (2)].* The recommended dosage of ritonavir in children greater than 1 month is 350 to 400 mg per m^2 twice daily by mouth to be taken with meals and should not exceed 600 mg twice daily. Ritonavir should be started at 250 mg per m^2 twice daily and increased at 2 to 3 day intervals by 50 mg per m^2 twice daily. If patients do not tolerate 400 mg per m^2 twice daily due to adverse events, the highest tolerated dose may be used for maintenance therapy in combination with other antiretroviral agents, however, alternative therapy should be considered. When possible, dose should be administered using a calibrated dosing syringe.

NORVIR oral solution should not be administered to neonates before a postmenstrual age (first day of the mother's last menstrual period to birth plus the time elapsed after birth) of 44 weeks has been attained *[see Warnings and Precautions (5.2)].*

NORVIR oral solution contains 43.2% (v/v) alcohol and 26.57% (w/v) propylene glycol. Special attention should be given to accurate calculation of the dose of NORVIR, transcription of the medication order, dispensing information and dosing instructions to minimize the risk for medication errors, and overdose. This is especially important for young children. Total amounts of alcohol and propylene glycol from all medicines that are to be given to pediatric patients 1 to 6 months of age should be taken into account in order to avoid toxicity from these excipients *[see Warnings and Precautions (5.2) and Overdosage (10)].*

[See table 1 on next page]

Body surface area (BSA) can be calculated as follows[1]:

$$BSA\ (m^2) = \sqrt{\frac{Ht\ (Cm) \times Wt\ (kg)}{3600}}$$

3   DOSAGE FORMS AND STRENGTHS

- NORVIR Tablets
  White film-coated ovaloid tablets debossed with the "a" logo and the code NK providing 100 mg ritonavir.
- NORVIR Oral Solution
  Orange-colored liquid containing 600 mg ritonavir per 7.5 mL marked dosage cup (80 mg per mL).

4   CONTRAINDICATIONS

- When co-administering NORVIR with other protease inhibitors, see the full prescribing information for that protease inhibitor including contraindication information.

Table 1. Pediatric Dosage Guidelines

Body Surface Area (m^2)	Twice Daily Dose 250 mg per m^2	Twice Daily Dose 300 mg per m^2	Twice Daily Dose 350 mg per m^2	Twice Daily Dose 400 mg per m^2
0.20	0.6 mL (50 mg)	0.75 mL (60 mg)	0.9 mL (70 mg)	1.0 mL (80 mg)
0.25	0.8 mL (62.5 mg)	0.9 mL (75 mg)	1.1 mL (87.5 mg)	1.25 mL (100 mg)
0.50	1.6 mL (125 mg)	1.9 mL (150 mg)	2.2 mL (175 mg)	2.5 mL (200 mg)
0.75	2.3 mL (187.5 mg)	2.8 mL (225 mg)	3.3 mL (262.5 mg)	3.75 mL (300 mg)
1.00	3.1 mL (250 mg)	3.75 mL (300 mg)	4.4 mL (350 mg)	5 mL (400 mg)
1.25	3.9 mL (312.5 mg)	4.7 mL (375 mg)	5.5 mL (437.5 mg)	6.25 mL (500 mg)
1.50	4.7 mL (375 mg)	5.6 mL (450 mg)	6.6 mL (525 mg)	7.5 mL (600 mg)

- NORVIR is contraindicated in patients with known hypersensitivity (e.g., toxic epidermal necrolysis (TEN) or Stevens-Johnson syndrome) to ritonavir or any of its ingredients.
- Co-administration of NORVIR with several classes of drugs (including sedative hypnotics, antiarrhythmics, or ergot alkaloid preparations) is contraindicated and may result in potentially serious and/or life-threatening adverse events due to possible effects of NORVIR on the hepatic metabolism of these drugs (see Table 2). Voriconazole and St. John's Wort are exceptions in that co-administration of NORVIR and voriconazole results in a significant decrease in plasma concentrations of voriconazole, and co-administration of NORVIR with St. John's Wort may result in decreased ritonavir plasma concentrations.

[See table 2 on next page]

5 WARNINGS AND PRECAUTIONS

When co-administering NORVIR with other protease inhibitors, see the full prescribing information for that protease inhibitor including important Warnings and Precautions.

5.1 Risk of Serious Adverse Reactions Due to Drug Interactions

Initiation of NORVIR, a CYP3A inhibitor, in patients receiving medications metabolized by CYP3A or initiation of medications metabolized by CYP3A in patients already receiving NORVIR, may increase plasma concentrations of medications metabolized by CYP3A. Initiation of medications that inhibit or induce CYP3A may increase or decrease concentrations of NORVIR, respectively. These interactions may lead to:

- Clinically significant adverse reactions, potentially leading to severe, life-threatening, or fatal events from greater exposures of concomitant medications.
- Clinically significant adverse reactions from greater exposures of NORVIR.
- Loss of therapeutic effect of NORVIR and possible development of resistance.

See Table 5 for steps to prevent or manage these possible and known significant drug interactions, including dosing recommendations *[see Drug Interactions (7)]*. Consider the potential for drug interactions prior to and during NORVIR therapy; review concomitant medications during NORVIR therapy, and monitor for the adverse reactions associated with the concomitant medications *[see Contraindications(4) and Drug Interactions (7)]*.

5.2 Toxicity in Preterm Neonates

NORVIR oral solution contains the excipients alcohol (43.2% v/v) and propylene glycol (26.57% w/v). When administered concomitantly with propylene glycol, ethanol competitively inhibits the metabolism of propylene glycol, which may lead to elevated concentrations. Preterm neonates may be at an increased risk of propylene glycol-associated adverse events due to diminished ability to metabolize propylene glycol, thereby leading to accumulation and potential adverse events. Postmarketing life-threatening cases of cardiac toxicity (including complete AV block, bradycardia, and cardiomyopathy), lactic acidosis, acute renal failure, CNS depression and respiratory complications leading to death have been reported, predominantly in preterm neonates receiving lopinavir/ritonavir oral solution which also contains the excipients alcohol and propylene glycol.

NORVIR oral solution should not be used in preterm neonates in the immediate postnatal period because of possible toxicities. However, if the benefit of using NORVIR oral solution to treat HIV infection in infants immediately after birth outweighs the potential risks, infants should be monitored closely for increases in serum osmolality and serum creatinine, and for toxicity related to NORVIR oral solution including: hyperosmolality, with or without lactic acidosis, renal toxicity, CNS depression (including stupor, coma, and apnea), seizures, hypotonia, cardiac arrhythmias and ECG changes, and hemolysis. Total amounts of alcohol and propylene glycol from all medicines that are to be given to infants should be taken into account in order to avoid toxicity from these excipients *[see Dosage and Administration (2.2) and Overdosage (10)]*.

5.3 Hepatic Reactions

Hepatic transaminase elevations exceeding 5 times the upper limit of normal, clinical hepatitis, and jaundice have occurred in patients receiving NORVIR alone or in combination with other antiretroviral drugs (see Table 4). There may be an increased risk for transaminase elevations in patients with underlying hepatitis B or C. Therefore, caution should be exercised when administering NORVIR to patients with pre-existing liver diseases, liver enzyme abnormalities, or hepatitis. Increased AST/ALT monitoring should be considered in these patients, especially during the first three months of NORVIR treatment *[see Use in Specific Populations (8.6)]*.

There have been postmarketing reports of hepatic dysfunction, including some fatalities. These have generally occurred in patients taking multiple concomitant medications and/or with advanced AIDS.

5.4 Pancreatitis

Pancreatitis has been observed in patients receiving NORVIR therapy, including those who developed hypertriglyceridemia. In some cases fatalities have been observed. Patients with advanced HIV disease may be at increased risk of elevated triglycerides and pancreatitis *[see Warnings and Precautions (5.7)]*. Pancreatitis should be considered if clinical symptoms (nausea, vomiting, abdominal pain) or abnormalities in laboratory values (such as increased serum lipase or amylase values) suggestive of pancreatitis should occur. Patients who exhibit these signs or symptoms should be evaluated and NORVIR therapy should be discontinued if a diagnosis of pancreatitis is made.

5.5 Allergic Reactions/Hypersensitivity

Allergic reactions including urticaria, mild skin eruptions, bronchospasm, and angioedema have been reported. Cases of anaphylaxis, toxic epidermal necrolysis (TEN), and Stevens-Johnson syndrome have also been reported. Discontinue treatment if severe reactions develop.

5.6 PR Interval Prolongation

Ritonavir prolongs the PR interval in some patients. Post marketing cases of second or third degree atrioventricular block have been reported in patients.

NORVIR should be used with caution in patients with underlying structural heart disease, preexisting conduction system abnormalities, ischemic heart disease, cardiomyopathies, as these patients may be at increased risk for developing cardiac conduction abnormalities.

The impact on the PR interval of co-administration of ritonavir with other drugs that prolong the PR interval (including calcium channel blockers, beta-adrenergic blockers, digoxin and atazanavir) has not been evaluated. As a result, co-administration of ritonavir with these drugs should be undertaken with caution, particularly with those drugs metabolized by CYP3A. Clinical monitoring is recommended *[see Drug Interactions (7), and Clinical Pharmacology (12.3)]*.

5.7 Lipid Disorders

Treatment with NORVIR therapy alone or in combination with saquinavir has resulted in substantial increases in the concentration of total cholesterol and triglycerides *[see Adverse Reactions (6.1)]*. Triglyceride and cholesterol testing should be performed prior to initiating NORVIR therapy and at periodic intervals during therapy. Lipid disorders should be managed as clinically appropriate, taking into account any potential drug-drug interactions with NORVIR and HMG CoA reductase inhibitors *[see Contraindications (4) and Drug Interactions (7)]*.

5.8 Diabetes Mellitus/Hyperglycemia

New onset diabetes mellitus, exacerbation of pre-existing diabetes mellitus, and hyperglycemia have been reported during postmarketing surveillance in HIV-infected patients receiving protease inhibitor therapy. Some patients required either initiation or dose adjustments of insulin or oral hypoglycemic agents for treatment of these events. In some cases, diabetic ketoacidosis has occurred. In those patients who discontinued protease inhibitor therapy, hyperglycemia persisted in some cases. Because these events have been reported voluntarily during clinical practice, estimates of frequency cannot be made and a causal relationship between protease inhibitor therapy and these events has not been established.

5.9 Immune Reconstitution Syndrome

Immune reconstitution syndrome has been reported in HIV-infected patients treated with combination antiretroviral therapy, including NORVIR. During the initial phase of combination antiretroviral treatment, patients whose immune system responds may develop an inflammatory response to indolent or residual opportunistic infections (such as *Mycobacterium avium* infection, cytomegalovirus, *Pneumocystis jiroveci* pneumonia, or tuberculosis), which may necessitate further evaluation and treatment.

Autoimmune disorders (such as Graves' disease, polymyositis, and Guillain-Barré syndrome) have also been reported to occur in the setting of immune reconstitution, however, the time to onset is more variable, and can occur many months after initiation of treatment.

5.10 Fat Redistribution

Redistribution/accumulation of body fat including central obesity, dorsocervical fat enlargement (buffalo hump), peripheral wasting, facial wasting, breast enlargement, and "cushingoid appearance" have been observed in patients receiving antiretroviral therapy. The mechanism and long-term consequences of these events are currently unknown. A causal relationship has not been established.

5.11 Patients with Hemophilia

There have been reports of increased bleeding, including spontaneous skin hematomas and hemarthrosis, in patients with hemophilia type A and B treated with protease inhibitors. In some patients additional factor VIII was given. In more than half of the reported cases, treatment with protease inhibitors was continued or reintroduced. A causal relationship between protease inhibitor therapy and these events has not been established.

5.12 Resistance/Cross-resistance

Varying degrees of cross-resistance among protease inhibitors have been observed. Continued administration of ritonavir 600 mg twice daily following loss of viral suppression may increase the likelihood of cross-resistance to other protease inhibitors *[see Microbiology (12.4)]*.

5.13 Laboratory Tests

Ritonavir has been shown to increase triglycerides, cholesterol, SGOT (AST), SGPT (ALT), GGT, CPK, and uric acid. Appropriate laboratory testing should be performed prior to initiating NORVIR therapy and at periodic intervals or if any clinical signs or symptoms occur during therapy.

6 ADVERSE REACTIONS

The following adverse reactions are discussed in greater detail in other sections of the labeling.

- Drug Interactions *[see Warnings and Precautions (5.1)]*
- Hepatotoxicity *[see Warnings and Precautions (5.3)]*
- Pancreatitis *[see Warnings and Precautions (5.4)]*
- Allergic Reactions/Hypersensitivity *[see Warnings and Precautions (5.5)]*

When co-administering NORVIR with other protease inhibitors, see the full prescribing information for that protease inhibitor including adverse reactions.

6.1 Clinical Trial Experience

Because clinical trials are conducted under widely varying conditions, adverse reactions rates observed in the clinical

Continued on next page

Information on the AbbVie, Inc. products listed on these pages is from the prescribing information in use as of July 31, 2016. For more information, please visit rxabbvie.com or call 1-800-633-9110.

trials of a drug cannot be directly compared to rates in the clinical trials of another drug and may not reflect the rates observed in practice.

Adverse Reactions in Adults

The safety of NORVIR alone and in combination with other antiretroviral agents was studied in 1,755 adult patients. Table 3 lists treatment-emergent Adverse Reactions (with possible or probable relationship to study drug) occurring in greater than or equal to 1% of adult patients receiving NORVIR in combined Phase II/IV studies.

The most frequently reported adverse drug reactions among patients receiving NORVIR alone or in combination with other antiretroviral drugs were gastrointestinal (including diarrhea, nausea, vomiting, abdominal pain (upper and lower)), neurological disturbances (including paresthesia and oral paresthesia), rash, and fatigue/asthenia.

Table 3. Treatment-Emergent Adverse Reactions (With Possible or Probable Relationship to Study Drug) Occurring in greater than or equal to 1% of Adult Patients Receiving NORVIR in Combined Phase II/IV Studies (N = 1,755)

Adverse Reactions	n	%
Eye disorders		
Blurred vision	113	6.4
Gastrointestinal disorders		
Abdominal Pain (upper and lower)*	464	26.4
Diarrhea including severe with electrolyte imbalance*	1,192	67.9
Dyspepsia	201	11.5
Flatulence	142	8.1
Gastrointestinal hemorrhage*	41	2.3
Gastroesophageal reflux disease (GERD)	19	1.1
Nausea	1,007	57.4
Vomiting*	559	31.9
General disorders and administration site conditions		
Fatigue including asthenia*	811	46.2
Hepatobiliary disorders		
Blood bilirubin increased (including jaundice)*	25	1.4
Hepatitis (including increased AST, ALT, GGT)*	153	8.7
Immune system disorders		
Hypersensivity including urticatria and face edema*	114	8.2
Metabolism and nutrition disorders		
Edema and peripheral edema*	110	6.3
Gout*	24	1.4
Hypercholesterolemia*	52	3.0
Hypertriglyceridemia*	158	9.0
Lipodystrophy acquired*	51	2.9
Musculoskeletal and connective tissue disorders		
Arthralgia and back pain*	326	18.6
Myopathy/creatine phosphokinase increased*	66	3.8
Myalgia	156	8.9
Nervous system disorders		
Dizziness*	274	15.6
Dysgeusia*	285	16.2
Paresthesia (including oral paresthesia)*	889	50.7
Peripheral neuropathy	178	10.1
Syncope*	58	3.3
Psychiatric disorders		
Confusion*	52	3.0
Disturbance in attention	44	2.5
Renal and urinary disorders		
Increased urination*	74	4.2
Respiratory, thoracic and mediastinal disorders		
Coughing*	380	21.7
Oropharyngeal Pain*	279	15.9
Skin and subcutaneous tissue disorders		
Acne*	67	3.8
Pruritus*	214	12.2
Rash (includes erythematous and maculopapular)*	475	27.1
Vascular disorders		
Flushing, feeling hot*	232	13.2
Hypertension*	58	3.3
Hypotension including orthostatic hypotension*	30	1.7
Peripheral coldness*	21	1.2

Table 2. Drugs that are Contraindicated with NORVIR

Drug Class	Drugs Within Class That Are Contraindicated With NORVIR**	Clinical Comments
Alpha₁-adrenoreceptor antagonist	Alfuzosin HCL	Potential for hypotension.
Antiarrhythmics	Amiodarone, flecainide, propafenone, quinidine	Potential for cardiac arrhythmias.
Antifungal	Voriconazole	Co-administration of voriconazole with ritonavir 400 mg every 12 hours significantly decreases voriconazole plasma concentrations and may lead to loss of antifungal response. Voriconazole is contraindicated with ritonavir doses of 400 mg every 12 hours or greater *[see Drug Interactions (7.2)]*.
Ergot Derivatives	Dihydroergotamine, ergotamine, methylergonovine	Potential for acute ergot toxicity characterized by vasospasm and ischemia of the extremities and other tissues including the central nervous system.
GI Motility Agent	Cisapride	Potential for cardiac arrhythmias.
Herbal Products	St. John's Wort (hypericum perforatum)	Co-administration of NORVIR with St. John's Wort may result in decreased ritonavir plasma concentrations and may lead to loss of virologic response and possible resistance to NORVIR or to the class of protease inhibitors.
HMG-CoA Reductase Inhibitors:	Lovastatin, simvastatin	Potential for myopathy including rhabdomyolysis.
Neuroleptic	Pimozide	Potential for cardiac arrhythmias.
PDE5 enzyme inhibitor	Sildenafil* (Revatio®) only when used for the treatment of pulmonary arterial hypertension (PAH)	A safe and effective dose has not been established when used with ritonavir. There is an increased potential for sildenafil-associated adverse events, including visual abnormalities, hypotension, prolonged erection, and syncope *[see Drug Interactions (7.2)]*.
Sedative/hypnotics	Oral midazolam, triazolam	Prolonged or increased sedation or respiratory depression *[see Drug Interactions (7.2)]*.

* see *Drug Interactions (7)* for co-administration of sildenafil in patients with erectile dysfunction.
** For additional information for these contraindicated drugs, *see also Drug Interactions (7)*.

* Represents a medical concept including several similar MedDRA PTs

Laboratory Abnormalities in Adults
Table 4 shows the percentage of adult patients who developed marked laboratory abnormalities.
[See table 4 on next page]
Adverse Reactions in Pediatric Patients
NORVIR has been studied in 265 pediatric patients greater than 1 month to 21 years of age. The adverse event profile observed during pediatric clinical trials was similar to that for adult patients.
Vomiting, diarrhea, and skin rash/allergy were the only drug-related clinical adverse events of moderate to severe intensity observed in greater than or equal to 2% of pediatric patients enrolled in NORVIR clinical trials.
Laboratory Abnormalities in Pediatric Patients
The following Grade 3-4 laboratory abnormalities occurred in greater than 3% of pediatric patients who received treatment with NORVIR® (ritonavir) either alone or in combination with reverse transcriptase inhibitors: neutropenia (9%), hyperamylasemia (7%), thrombocytopenia (5%), anemia (4%), and elevated AST (3%).

6.2   Postmarketing Experience
The following adverse events (not previously mentioned in the labeling) have been reported during post-marketing use of NORVIR. Because these reactions are reported voluntarily from a population of unknown size, it is not possible to reliably estimate their frequency or establish a causal relationship to NORVIR exposure.
Body as a Whole
Dehydration, usually associated with gastrointestinal symptoms, and sometimes resulting in hypotension, syncope, or renal insufficiency has been reported. Syncope, orthostatic hypotension, and renal insufficiency have also been reported without known dehydration.
Co-administration of ritonavir with ergotamine or dihydroergotamine has been associated with acute ergot toxicity characterized by vasospasm and ischemia of the extremities and other tissues including the central nervous system.

Table 4. Percentage of Adult Patients, by Study and Treatment Group, with Chemistry and Hematology Abnormalities Occurring in greater than 3% of Patients Receiving NORVIR

Variable	Limit	Study 245 Naive Patients			Study 247 Advanced Patients		Study 462 PI-Naive Patients
		NORVIR plus ZDV	NORVIR	ZDV	NORVIR	Placebo	NORVIR plus Saquinavir
Chemistry	**High**						
Cholesterol	> 240 mg/dL	30.7	44.8	9.3	36.5	8.0	65.2
CPK	> 1000 IU/L	9.6	12.1	11.0	9.1	6.3	9.9
GGT	> 300 IU/L	1.8	5.2	1.7	19.6	11.3	9.2
SGOT (AST)	> 180 IU/L	5.3	9.5	2.5	6.4	7.0	7.8
SGPT (ALT)	> 215 IU/L	5.3	7.8	3.4	8.5	4.4	9.2
Triglycerides	> 800 mg/dL	9.6	17.2	3.4	33.6	9.4	23.4
Triglycerides	> 1500 mg/dL	1.8	2.6	-	12.6	0.4	11.3
Triglycerides Fasting	> 1500 mg/dL	1.5	1.3	-	9.9	0.3	-
Uric Acid	> 12 mg/dL	-	-	-	3.8	0.2	1.4
Hematology	**Low**						
Hematocrit	< 30%	2.6	-	0.8	17.3	22.0	0.7
Hemoglobin	< 8.0 g/dL	0.9	-	-	3.8	3.9	-
Neutrophils	≤ 0.5 × 10^9/L	-	-	-	6.0	8.3	-
RBC	< 3.0 × 10^{12}/L	1.8	-	5.9	18.6	24.4	-
WBC	< 2.5 × 10^9/L	-	0.9	6.8	36.9	59.4	3.5

- Indicates no events reported.

Cardiovascular System
First-degree AV block, second-degree AV block, third-degree AV block, right bundle branch block have been reported [see Warnings and Precautions (5.6)].
Cardiac and neurologic events have been reported when ritonavir has been co-administered with disopyramide, mexiletine, nefazodone, fluoxetine, and beta blockers. The possibility of drug interaction cannot be excluded.

Endocrine System
Cushing's syndrome and adrenal suppression have been reported when ritonavir has been co-administered with fluticasone propionate or budesonide.

Nervous System
There have been postmarketing reports of seizure. Also, see Cardiovascular System.

Skin and subcutaneous tissue disorders
Toxic epidermal necrolysis (TEN) has been reported.

7 DRUG INTERACTIONS

See also Contraindications (4), Warnings and Precautions (5.1), and Clinical Pharmacology (12.3)
When co-administering NORVIR® (ritonavir) with other protease inhibitors (atazanavir, darunavir, fosamprenavir, saquinavir, and tipranavir), see the full prescribing information for that protease inhibitor including important information for drug interactions.

7.1 Potential for NORVIR to Affect Other Drugs
Ritonavir has been found to be an inhibitor of cytochrome P450 3A (CYP3A) and may increase plasma concentrations of agents that are primarily metabolized by CYP3A. Agents that are extensively metabolized by CYP3A and have high first pass metabolism appear to be the most susceptible to large increases in AUC (greater than 3-fold) when co-administered with ritonavir. Thus, co-administration of NORVIR with drugs highly dependent on CYP3A for clearance and for which elevated plasma concentrations are associated with serious and/or life-threatening events is contraindicated. Co-administration with other CYP3A substrates may require a dose adjustment or additional monitoring as shown in Table 5.
Ritonavir also inhibits CYP2D6 to a lesser extent. Co-administration of substrates of CYP2D6 with ritonavir could result in increases (up to 2-fold) in the AUC of the other agent, possibly requiring a proportional dosage reduction. Ritonavir also appears to induce CYP3A, CYP1A2, CYP2C9, CYP2C19, and CYP2B6 as well as other enzymes, including glucuronosyl transferase.

7.2 Established and Other Potentially Significant Drug Interactions
Table 5 provides a list of established or potentially clinically significant drug interactions. Alteration in dose or regimen may be recommended based on drug interaction studies or predicted interaction [see Clinical Pharmacology (12.3) for magnitude of interaction].
[See table 5 on pages 774 to 778]

8 USE IN SPECIFIC POPULATIONS

When co-administering NORVIR® (ritonavir) with other protease inhibitors, see the full prescribing information for the co-administered protease inhibitor including important information for use in special populations.

8.1 Pregnancy
Pregnancy Category B
Antiretroviral Pregnancy Registry: To monitor maternal-fetal outcomes of pregnant women exposed to NORVIR, an Antiretroviral Pregnancy Registry has been established. Physicians are encouraged to register patients by calling 1–800–258–4263.

Human Data
There are no adequate and well-controlled studies in pregnant women. NORVIR should be used during pregnancy only if the potential benefit justifies the potential risk to the fetus.

Antiretroviral Pregnancy Registry:
As of January 2012, the Antiretroviral Pregnancy Registry (APR) has received prospective reports of 3860 exposures to ritonavir containing regimens (1567 exposed in the first trimester and 2293 exposed in the second and third trimester). Birth defects occurred in 35 of the 1567 (2.2%) live births (first trimester exposure) and 59 of the 2293 (2.6%) live births (second/third trimester exposure).
Among pregnant women in the U.S. reference population, the background rate of birth defects is 2.7%. There was no association between ritonavir and overall birth defects observed in the APR.

Animal Data
No treatment related malformations were observed when ritonavir was administered to pregnant rats or rabbits. De-velopmental toxicity observed in rats (early resorptions, decreased fetal body weight and ossification delays and developmental variations) occurred at a maternally toxic dosage at an exposure equivalent to approximately 30% of that achieved with the proposed therapeutic dose. A slight increase in the incidence of cryptorchidism was also noted in rats at an exposure approximately 22% of that achieved with the proposed therapeutic dose.
Developmental toxicity observed in rabbits (resorptions, decreased litter size and decreased fetal weights) also occurred at a maternally toxic dosage equivalent to 1.8 times the proposed therapeutic dose based on a body surface area conversion factor.

8.3 Nursing Mothers
The Centers for Disease Control and Prevention recommend that HIV-infected mothers not breastfeed their infants to avoid risking postnatal transmission of HIV. It is not known whether ritonavir is secreted in human milk. Because of both the potential for HIV transmission and the potential for serious adverse reactions in nursing infants, mothers should be instructed not to breastfeed if they are receiving NORVIR.

8.4 Pediatric Use
In HIV-infected patients age greater than 1 month to 21 years, the antiviral activity and adverse event profile seen during clinical trials and through postmarketing experience were similar to that for adult patients.

8.5 Geriatric Use
Clinical studies of NORVIR did not include sufficient numbers of subjects aged 65 and over to determine whether they respond differently from younger subjects. In general, dose selection for an elderly patient should be cautious, usually starting at the low end of the dosing range, reflecting the greater frequency of decreased hepatic, renal or cardiac function, and of concomitant disease or other drug therapy.

8.6 Hepatic Impairment
No dose adjustment of ritonavir is necessary for patients with either mild (Child-Pugh Class A) or moderate (Child-Pugh Class B) hepatic impairment. No pharmacokinetic or safety data are available regarding the use of ritonavir in subjects with severe hepatic impairment (Child-Pugh Class C); therefore, ritonavir is not recommended for use in patients with severe hepatic impairment [see Warnings and Precautions (5.3), Clinical Pharmacology (12.3)].

10 OVERDOSAGE

10.1 Acute Overdosage - Human Overdose Experience
Human experience of acute overdose with NORVIR® (ritonavir) is limited. One patient in clinical trials took NORVIR 1500 mg per day for two days. The patient reported paresthesias which resolved after the dose was decreased. A post-marketing case of renal failure with eosinophilia has been reported with ritonavir overdose.
The approximate lethal dose was found to be greater than 20 times the related human dose in rats and 10 times the related human dose in mice.

10.2 Management of Overdosage
NORVIR oral solution contains 43.2% (v/v) alcohol and 26.57% (w/v) propylene glycol. Ingestion of the product over the recommended dose by a young child could result in significant toxicity and could potentially be lethal.
Treatment of overdose with NORVIR consists of general supportive measures including monitoring of vital signs and observation of the clinical status of the patient. There is no specific antidote for overdose with NORVIR. If indicated, elimination of unabsorbed drug should be achieved by gastric lavage; usual precautions should be observed to maintain the airway. Administration of activated charcoal may also be used to aid in removal of unabsorbed drug. Since ritonavir is extensively metabolized by the liver and is highly protein bound, dialysis is unlikely to be beneficial in significant removal of the drug. However, dialysis can remove both alcohol and propylene glycol in the case of overdose with ritonavir oral solution. A Certified Poison Control Center should be consulted for up-to-date information on the management of overdose with NORVIR.

11 DESCRIPTION

NORVIR (ritonavir) is an inhibitor of HIV protease with activity against the Human Immunodeficiency Virus (HIV).

Continued on next page

Information on the AbbVie, Inc. products listed on these pages is from the prescribing information in use as of July 31, 2016. For more information, please visit rxabbvie.com or call 1-800-633-9110.

Ritonavir is chemically designated as 10-Hydroxy-2-methyl-5-(1-methylethyl)-1- [2-(1-methylethyl)-4-thiazolyl]-3,6-dioxo-8,11-bis(phenylmethyl)-2,4,7,12- tetraazatridecan-13-oic acid, 5-thiazolylmethyl ester, [5S-(5R*,8R*,10R*,11R*)]. Its molecular formula is $C_{37}H_{48}N_6O_5S_2$, and its molecular weight is 720.95. Ritonavir has the following structural formula:

[See structural formula on page 778]

Ritonavir is a white-to-light-tan powder. Ritonavir has a bitter metallic taste. It is freely soluble in methanol and ethanol, soluble in isopropanol and practically insoluble in water.

NORVIR tablets are available for oral administration in a strength of 100 mg ritonavir with the following inactive ingredients: copovidone, anhydrous dibasic calcium phosphate, sorbitan monolaurate, colloidal silicon dioxide, and sodium stearyl fumarate. The following are the ingredients in the film coating: hypromellose, titanium dioxide, polyethylene glycol 400, hydroxypropyl cellulose, talc, polyethylene glycol 3350, colloidal silicon dioxide, and polysorbate 80.

NORVIR oral solution is available for oral administration as 80 mg per mL of ritonavir in a peppermint and caramel flavored vehicle. Each 8-ounce bottle contains 19.2 grams of ritonavir. NORVIR oral solution also contains ethanol, water, polyoxyl 35 castor oil, propylene glycol, anhydrous citric acid to adjust pH, saccharin sodium, peppermint oil, creamy caramel flavoring, and FD&C Yellow No. 6.

12   CLINICAL PHARMACOLOGY
12.1   Mechanism of Action
Ritonavir is an antiviral drug *[see Microbiology (12.4)].*

12.3   Pharmacokinetics
The pharmacokinetics of ritonavir have been studied in healthy volunteers and HIV-infected patients (CD_4 greater than or equal to 50 cells per μL). See Table 6 for ritonavir pharmacokinetic characteristics.

Absorption
The absolute bioavailability of ritonavir has not been determined. After a 600 mg dose of oral solution, peak concentrations of ritonavir were achieved approximately 2 hours and 4 hours after dosing under fasting and non-fasting (514 KCal; 9% fat, 12% protein, and 79% carbohydrate) conditions, respectively.

NORVIR tablets are not bioequivalent to NORVIR capsules. Under moderate fat conditions (857 kcal; 31% fat, 13% protein, 56% carbohydrates), when a single 100 mg NORVIR dose was administered as a tablet compared with a capsule, $AUC_{(0-\infty)}$ met equivalence criteria but mean C_{max} was increased by 26% (92.8% confidence intervals: ↑15 -↑39%). No information is available comparing NORVIR tablets to NORVIR capsules under fasting conditions.

Effect of Food on Oral Absorption
When the oral solution was given under non-fasting conditions, peak ritonavir concentrations decreased 23% and the extent of absorption decreased 7% relative to fasting conditions. Dilution of the oral solution, within one hour of administration, with 240 mL of chocolate milk, Advera® or Ensure® did not significantly affect the extent and rate of ritonavir absorption. Administration of a single 600 mg dose oral solution under non-fasting conditions yielded mean ± SD areas under the plasma concentration-time curve (AUCs) of 129.0 ± 39.3 mg•h per mL.

A food effect is observed for NORVIR tablets. Food decreased the bioavailability of the ritonavir tablets when a single 100 mg dose of NORVIR was administered. Under high fat conditions (907 kcal; 52% fat, 15% protein, 33% carbohydrates), a 23% decrease in mean $AUC_{(0-\infty)}$ [90% confidence intervals: ↓30%-↓15%], and a 23% decrease in mean C_{max} [90% confidence intervals: ↓34%-↓11%]) was observed relative to fasting conditions. Under moderate fat conditions, a 21% decrease in mean $AUC_{(0-\infty)}$ [90% confidence intervals: ↓28%-↓13%], and a 22% decrease in mean C_{max} [90% confidence intervals: ↓33%-↓9%]) was observed relative to fasting conditions.

However, the type of meal administered did not change ritonavir tablet bioavailability when high fat was compared to moderate fat meals.

Metabolism
Nearly all of the plasma radioactivity after a single oral 600 mg dose of ^{14}C-ritonavir oral solution (n = 5) was attributed to unchanged ritonavir. Five ritonavir metabolites have been identified in human urine and feces. The isopropylthiazole oxidation metabolite (M-2) is the major metabo-

Table 5. Established and Other Potentially Significant Drug Interactions

Concomitant Drug Class: Drug Name	Effect on Concentration of Ritonavir or Concomitant Drug	Clinical Comment
HIV-Antiviral Agents		
HIV-1 Protease Inhibitor: atazanavir	When co-administered with reduced doses of atazanavir and ritonavir ↑ atazanavir (↑ AUC, ↑ C_{max}, ↑ C_{min})	Atazanavir plasma concentrations achieved with atazanavir 300 mg once daily and ritonavir 100 mg once daily are higher than those achieved with atazanavir 400 mg once daily. See the complete prescribing information for Reyataz® (atazanavir) for details on co-administration of atazanavir 300 mg once daily with ritonavir 100 mg once daily.
HIV-1 Protease Inhibitor: darunavir	When co-administered with reduced doses of ritonavir ↑ darunavir (↑ AUC, ↑ C_{max}, ↑ C_{min})	See the complete prescribing information for Prezista® (darunavir) for details on co-administration of darunavir 600 mg twice daily with ritonavir 100 mg twice daily or darunavir 800 mg once daily with ritonavir 100 mg once daily.
HIV-1 Protease Inhibitor: fosamprenavir	When co-administered with reduced doses of ritonavir ↑ amprenavir (↑ AUC, ↑ C_{max}, ↑ C_{min})	See the complete prescribing information for Lexiva® (fosamprenavir) for details on co-administration of fosamprenavir 700 mg twice daily with ritonavir 100 mg twice daily, fosamprenavir 1400 mg once daily with ritonavir 200 mg once daily or fosamprenavir 1400 mg once daily with ritonavir 100 mg once daily.
HIV-1 Protease Inhibitor: indinavir	When co-administered with reduced doses of indinavir and ritonavir ↑ indinavir (↔ AUC, ↓ C_{max}, ↑ C_{min})	Alterations in concentrations are noted when reduced doses of indinavir are co-administered with NORVIR. Appropriate doses for this combination, with respect to efficacy and safety, have not been established.
HIV-1 Protease Inhibitor: saquinavir	When co-administered with reduced doses of ritonavir ↑ saquinavir (↑ AUC, ↑ C_{max}, ↑ C_{min})	See the complete prescribing information for Invirase® (saquinavir) for details on co-administration of saquinavir 1000 mg twice daily with ritonavir 100 mg twice daily. Saquinavir/ritonavir should not be given together with rifampin, due to the risk of severe hepatotoxicity (presenting as increased hepatic transaminases) if the three drugs are given together.
HIV-1 Protease Inhibitor: tipranavir	When co-administered with reduced doses of ritonavir ↑ tipranavir (↑ AUC, ↑ C_{max}, ↑ C_{min})	See the complete prescribing information for Aptivus® (tipranavir) for details on co-administration of tipranavir 500 mg twice daily with ritonavir 200 mg twice daily. There have been reports of clinical hepatitis and hepatic decompensation including some fatalities. All patients should be followed closely with clinical and laboratory monitoring, especially those with chronic hepatitis B or C co-infection, as these patients have an increased risk of hepatotoxicity. Liver function tests should be performed prior to initiating therapy with tipranavir/ritonavir, and frequently throughout the duration of treatment.
Non-Nucleoside Reverse Transcriptase Inhibitor: delavirdine	↑ ritonavir (↑ AUC, ↑ C_{max}, ↑ C_{min})	Appropriate doses of this combination with respect to safety and efficacy have not been established.
HIV-1 CCR5 – antagonist: maraviroc	↑ maraviroc	Concurrent administration of maraviroc with ritonavir will increase plasma levels of maraviroc. For specific dosage adjustment recommendations, please refer to the complete prescribing information for Selzentry® (maraviroc).
Integrase Inhibitor: Raltegravir	↓ raltegravir	The effects of ritonavir on raltegravir with ritonavir dosage regimens greater than 100 mg twice daily have not been evaluated, however raltegravir concentrations may be decreased with ritonavir coadministration.
Other Agents		
Analgesics, Narcotic: tramadol, propoxyphene		A dose decrease may be needed for these drugs when co-administered with ritonavir.
Anesthetic: meperidine	↓ meperidine/ ↑ normeperidine (metabolite)	Dosage increase and long-term use of meperidine with ritonavir are not recommended due to the increased concentrations of the metabolite normeperidine which has both analgesic activity and CNS stimulant activity (e.g., seizures).
Antialcoholics: disulfiram/ metronidazole		Ritonavir formulations contain alcohol, which can produce disulfiram-like reactions when co-administered with disulfiram or other drugs that produce this reaction (e.g., metronidazole).
Antiarrhythmics: disopyramide, lidocaine, mexiletine	↑ antiarrhythmics	Caution is warranted and therapeutic concentration monitoring is recommended for antiarrhythmics when co-administered with ritonavir, if available.

This table is continued on the next page

Table 5 *(Cont.)* **Established and Other Potentially Significant Drug Interactions**

Concomitant Drug Class: Drug Name	Effect on Concentration of Ritonavir or Concomitant Drug	Clinical Comment
Anticancer Agents: dasatinib, nilotinib, vincristine, vinblastine	↑ anticancer agents	Concentrations of these drugs may be increased when co-administered with ritonavir resulting in the potential for increased adverse events usually associated with these anticancer agents. For vincristine and vinblastine, consideration should be given to temporarily withholding the ritonavir containing antiretroviral regimen in patients who develop significant hematologic or gastrointestinal side effects when ritonavir is administered concurrently with vincristine or vinblastine. Clinicians should be aware that if the ritonavir containing regimen is withheld for a prolonged period, consideration should be given to altering the regimen to not include a CYP3A or P-gp inhibitor in order to control HIV-1 viral load. A decrease in the dosage or an adjustment of the dosing interval of nilotinib and dasatinib may be necessary for patients requiring co-administration with strong CYP3A inhibitors such as NORVIR. Please refer to the nilotinib and dasatinib prescribing information for dosing instructions.
Anticoagulant: warfarin	↓ R-warfarin ↓↑ S-warfarin	Initial frequent monitoring of the INR during ritonavir and warfarin co-administration is indicated.
Anticoagulant: rivaroxaban	↑ rivaroxaban	Avoid concomitant use of rivaroxaban and ritonavir. Co-administration of ritonavir and rivaroxaban is expected to result in increased exposure of rivaroxaban which may lead to risk of increased bleeding.
Anticonvulsants: carbamazepine, clonazepam, ethosuximide	↑ anticonvulsants	Use with caution. A dose decrease may be needed for these drugs when co-administered with ritonavir and therapeutic concentration monitoring is recommended for these anticonvulsants, if available.
Anticonvulsants: divalproex, lamotrigine, phenytoin	↓ anticonvulsants	Use with caution. A dose increase may be needed for these drugs when co-administered with ritonavir and therapeutic concentration monitoring is recommended for these anticonvulsants, if available.
Antidepressants: nefazodone, selective serotonin reuptake inhibitors (SSRIs): e.g. fluoxetine, paroxetine, tricyclics: e.g. amitriptyline, nortriptyline	↑ antidepressants	A dose decrease may be needed for these drugs when co-administered with ritonavir.
Antidepressant: bupropion	↓ bupropion ↓ active metabolite, hydroxybupropion	Concurrent administration of bupropion with ritonavir may decrease plasma levels of both bupropion and its active metabolite (hydroxybupropion). Patients receiving ritonavir and bupropion concurrently should be monitored for an adequate clinical response to bupropion.
Antidepressant: desipramine	↑ desipramine	Dosage reduction and concentration monitoring of desipramine is recommended.
Antidepressant: trazodone	↑ trazodone	Concomitant use of trazodone and NORVIR increases plasma concentrations of trazodone. Adverse events of nausea, dizziness, hypotension and syncope have been observed following co-administration of trazodone and NORVIR. If trazodone is used with a CYP3A4 inhibitor such as ritonavir, the combination should be used with caution and a lower dose of trazodone should be considered.
Antiemetic: dronabinol	↑ dronabinol	A dose decrease of dronabinol may be needed when co-administered with ritonavir.
Antifungal: ketoconazole itraconazole voriconazole	↑ ketoconazole ↑ itraconazole ↓ voriconazole	High doses of ketoconazole or itraconazole (greater than 200 mg per day) are not recommended. Co-administration of voriconazole and ritonavir doses of 400 mg every 12 hours or greater is contraindicated. Co-administration of voriconazole and ritonavir 100 mg should be avoided, unless an assessment of the benefit/risk to the patient justifies the use of voriconazole.

This table is continued on the next page

excreted as unchanged parent drug. Upon multiple dosing, ritonavir accumulation is less than predicted from a single dose possibly due to a time and dose-related increase in clearance.

Table 6. Ritonavir Pharmacokinetic Characteristics

Parameter	N	Values (Mean ± SD)
$V_\beta/F^\ddagger$	91	0.41 ± 0.25 L/kg
$t_{1/2}$		3 - 5 h
CL/F SS†	10	8.8 ± 3.2 L/h
CL/F‡	91	4.6 ± 1.6 L/h
CL_R	62	< 0.1 L/h
RBC/Plasma Ratio		0.14
Percent Bound*		98 to 99%

† SS = steady state; patients taking ritonavir 600 mg q12h.
‡ Single ritonavir 600 mg dose.
* Primarily bound to human serum albumin and alpha-1 acid glycoprotein over the ritonavir concentration range of 0.01 to 30 µg/mL.

Effects on Electrocardiogram

QTcF interval was evaluated in a randomized, placebo and active (moxifloxacin 400 mg once-daily) controlled crossover study in 45 healthy adults, with 10 measurements over 12 hours on Day 3. The maximum mean (95% upper confidence bound) time-matched difference in QTcF from placebo after baseline correction was 5.5 (7.6) milliseconds (msec) for 400 mg twice-daily ritonavir. Ritonavir 400 mg twice daily resulted in Day 3 ritonavir exposure that was approximately 1.5 fold higher than observed with ritonavir 600 mg twice-daily dose at steady state.

PR interval prolongation was also noted in subjects receiving ritonavir in the same study on Day 3. The maximum mean (95% confidence interval) difference from placebo in the PR interval after baseline correction was 22 (25) msec for 400 mg twice-daily ritonavir *[see Warnings and Precautions (5.6)]*.

Special Populations

Gender, Race and Age

No age-related pharmacokinetic differences have been observed in adult patients (18 to 63 years). Ritonavir pharmacokinetics have not been studied in older patients.

A study of ritonavir pharmacokinetics in healthy males and females showed no statistically significant differences in the pharmacokinetics of ritonavir. Pharmacokinetic differences due to race have not been identified.

Pediatric Patients

Steady-state pharmacokinetics were evaluated in 37 HIV-infected patients ages 2 to 14 years receiving doses ranging from 250 mg per m² twice-daily to 400 mg per m² twice-daily in PACTG Study 310, and in 41 HIV-infected patients ages 1 month to 2 years at doses of 350 and 450 mg per m² twice-daily in PACTG Study 345. Across dose groups, ritonavir steady-state oral clearance (CL/F/m²) was approximately 1.5 to 1.7 times faster in pediatric patients than in adult subjects. Ritonavir concentrations obtained after 350 to 400 mg per m² twice-daily in pediatric patients greater than 2 years were comparable to those obtained in adults receiving 600 mg (approximately 330 mg per m²) twice-daily. The following observations were seen regarding ritonavir concentrations after administration with 350 or 450 mg per m² twice-daily in children less than 2 years of age. Higher ritonavir exposures were not evident with 450 mg per m² twice-daily compared to the 350 mg per m² twice-daily. Ritonavir trough concentrations were somewhat lower than those obtained in adults receiving 600 mg twice-daily. The area under the ritonavir plasma concentration time curve and trough concentrations obtained after administration with 350 or 450 mg per m² twice-daily in children

lite and has antiviral activity similar to that of parent drug; however, the concentrations of this metabolite in plasma are low. *In vitro* studies utilizing human liver microsomes have demonstrated that cytochrome P450 3A (CYP3A) is the major isoform involved in ritonavir metabolism, although CYP2D6 also contributes to the formation of M–2.

Elimination

In a study of five subjects receiving a 600 mg dose of ¹⁴C-ritonavir oral solution, 11.3 ± 2.8% of the dose was excreted into the urine, with 3.5 ± 1.8% of the dose excreted as unchanged parent drug. In that study, 86.4 ± 2.9% of the dose was excreted in the feces with 33.8 ± 10.8% of the dose

Continued on next page

Information on the AbbVie, Inc. products listed on these pages is from the prescribing information in use as of July 31, 2016. For more information, please visit rxabbvie.com or call 1-800-633-9110.

less than 2 years were approximately 16% and 60% lower, respectively, than that obtained in adults receiving 600 mg twice daily.

Renal Impairment

Ritonavir pharmacokinetics have not been studied in patients with renal impairment, however, since renal clearance is negligible, a decrease in total body clearance is not expected in patients with renal impairment.

Hepatic Impairment

Dose-normalized steady-state ritonavir concentrations in subjects with mild hepatic impairment (400 mg twice-daily, n = 6) were similar to those in control subjects dosed with 500 mg twice-daily. Dose-normalized steady-state ritonavir exposures in subjects with moderate hepatic impairment (400 mg twice-daily, n= 6) were about 40% lower than those in subjects with normal hepatic function (500 mg twice-daily, n = 6). Protein binding of ritonavir was not statistically significantly affected by mild or moderately impaired hepatic function. No dose adjustment is recommended in patients with mild or moderate hepatic impairment. However, health care providers should be aware of the potential for lower ritonavir concentrations in patients with moderate hepatic impairment and should monitor patient response carefully. Ritonavir has not been studied in patients with severe hepatic impairment.

Drug Interactions

[see also *Contraindications (4), Warnings and Precautions (5.1)*, and *Drug Interactions (7)*]

Table 7 and Table 8 summarize the effects on AUC and C_{max}, with 95% confidence intervals (95% CI), of co-administration of ritonavir with a variety of drugs. For information about clinical recommendations see Table 5 in *Drug Interactions (7)*.

[See table 7 on page 779]

[See table 8 on pages 780 and 781]

12.4   Microbiology

Mechanism of Action

Ritonavir is a peptidomimetic inhibitor of the HIV-1 protease. Inhibition of HIV protease renders the enzyme incapable of processing the *gag-pol* polyprotein precursor which leads to production of non-infectious immature HIV particles.

Antiviral Activity in Cell Culture

The activity of ritonavir was assessed in acutely infected lymphoblastoid cell lines and in peripheral blood lymphocytes. The concentration of drug that inhibits 50% (EC_{50}) value of viral replication ranged from 3.8 to 153 nM depending upon the HIV-1 isolate and the cells employed. The average EC_{50} value for low passage clinical isolates was 22 nM (n = 13). In MT$_4$ cells, ritonavir demonstrated additive effects against HIV-1 in combination with either didanosine (ddI) or zidovudine (ZDV). Studies which measured cytotoxicity of ritonavir on several cell lines showed that greater than 20 μM was required to inhibit cellular growth by 50% resulting in a cell culture therapeutic index of at least 1000.

Resistance

HIV-1 isolates with reduced susceptibility to ritonavir have been selected in cell culture. Genotypic analysis of these isolates showed mutations in the HIV-1 protease gene leading to amino acid substitutions I84V, V82F, A71V, and M46I. Phenotypic (n = 18) and genotypic (n = 48) changes in HIV-1 isolates from selected patients treated with ritonavir were monitored in phase I/II trials over a period of 3 to 32 weeks. Substitutions associated with the HIV-1 viral protease in isolates obtained from 43 patients appeared to occur in a stepwise and ordered fashion at positions V82A/F/T/S, I54V, A71V/T, and I36L, followed by combinations of substitutions at an additional 5 specific amino acid positions (M46I/L, K20R, I84V, L33F and L90M). Of 18 patients for whom both phenotypic and genotypic analysis were performed on free virus isolated from plasma, 12 showed reduced susceptibility to ritonavir in cell culture. All 18 patients possessed one or more substitutions in the viral protease gene. The V82A/F substitution appeared to be necessary but not sufficient to confer phenotypic resistance. Phenotypic resistance was defined as a greater than or equal to 5-fold decrease in viral sensitivity in cell culture from baseline.

Cross-Resistance to Other Antiretrovirals

Among protease inhibitors variable cross-resistance has been recognized. Serial HIV-1 isolates obtained from six patients during ritonavir therapy showed a decrease in ritonavir susceptibility in cell culture but did not demonstrate a concordant decrease in susceptibility to saquinavir in cell culture when compared to matched baseline isolates. However, isolates from two of these patients demonstrated

decreased susceptibility to indinavir in cell culture (8-fold). Isolates from 5 patients were also tested for cross-resistance to amprenavir and nelfinavir; isolates from 3 patients had a decrease in susceptibility to nelfinavir (6- to 14-fold), and none to amprenavir. Cross-resistance between ritonavir and reverse transcriptase inhibitors is unlikely because of the different enzyme targets involved. One ZDV-resistant HIV-1 isolate tested in cell culture retained full susceptibility to ritonavir.

13   NONCLINICAL TOXICOLOGY

13.1   Carcinogenesis, Mutagenesis, Impairment of Fertility

Carcinogenesis

Carcinogenicity studies in mice and rats have been carried out on ritonavir. In male mice, at levels of 50, 100 or 200 mg per kg per day, there was a dose dependent increase in the incidence of both adenomas and combined adenomas and carcinomas in the liver. Based on AUC measurements, the exposure at the high dose was approximately 0.3-fold for males that of the exposure in humans with the recommended therapeutic dose (600 mg twice-daily). There were no carcinogenic effects seen in females at the dosages tested. The exposure at the high dose was approximately 0.6-fold for the females that of the exposure in humans. In rats dosed at levels of 7, 15 or 30 mg per kg per day there were no carcinogenic effects. In this study, the exposure at

Table 5 *(Cont.)* Established and Other Potentially Significant Drug Interactions

Concomitant Drug Class: Drug Name	Effect on Concentration of Ritonavir or Concomitant Drug	Clinical Comment
Anti-gout: colchicine	↑ colchicine	Patients with renal or hepatic impairment should not be given colchicine with ritonavir. <u>Treatment of gout flares-co-administration of colchicine in patients on ritonavir:</u> 0.6 mg (one tablet) for one dose, followed by 0.3 mg (half tablet) one hour later. Dose to be repeated no earlier than three days. <u>Prophylaxis of gout flares-co-administration of colchicine in patients on ritonavir:</u> If the original colchicine regimen was 0.6 mg twice a day, the regimen should be adjusted to 0.3 mg once a day. If the original colchicine regimen was 0.6 mg once a day, the regimen should be adjusted to 0.3 mg once every other day. <u>Treatment of familial Mediterranean fever (FMF)-co-administration of colchicine in patients on ritonavir:</u> Maximum daily dose of 0.6 mg (may be given as 0.3 mg twice a day).
Anti-infective: clarithromycin	↑ clarithromycin	For patients with renal impairment the following dosage adjustments should be considered: <ul><li>For patients with CL_{CR} 30 to 60 mL per min the dose of clarithromycin should be reduced by 50%.</li><li>For patients with CL_{CR} less than 30 mL per min the dose of clarithromycin should be decreased by 75%.</li></ul> No dose adjustment for patients with normal renal function is necessary.
Antimycobacterial: bedaquiline	↑ bedaquiline	Bedaquiline should only be used with ritonavir if the benefit of co-administration outweighs the risk.
Antimycobacterial: rifabutin	↑ rifabutin and rifabutin metabolite	Dosage reduction of rifabutin by at least three-quarters of the usual dose of 300 mg per day is recommended (e.g., 150 mg every other day or three times a week). Further dosage reduction may be necessary.
Antimycobacterial: rifampin	↓ ritonavir	May lead to loss of virologic response. Alternate antimycobacterial agents such as rifabutin should be considered (see Antimycobacterial: rifabutin, for dose reduction recommendations).
Antiparasitic: atovaquone	↓ atovaquone	Clinical significance is unknown; however, increase in atovaquone dose may be needed.
Antiparasitic: quinine	↑ quinine	A dose decrease of quinine may be needed when co-administered with ritonavir.
Antipsychotics: quetiapine	↑ quetiapine	<u>Initiation of NORVIR in patients taking quetiapine:</u> Consider alternative antiretroviral therapy to avoid increases in quetiapine exposures. If coadministration is necessary, reduce the quetiapine dose to 1/6 of the current dose and monitor for quetiapine-associated adverse reactions. Refer to the quetiapine prescribing information for recommendations on adverse reaction monitoring. <u>Initiation of quetiapine in patients taking NORVIR:</u> Refer to the quetiapine prescribing information for initial dosing and titration of quetiapine.
β-Blockers: metoprolol, timolol	↑ Beta-Blockers	Caution is warranted and clinical monitoring of patients is recommended. A dose decrease may be needed for these drugs when co-administered with ritonavir.
Bronchodilator: theophylline	↓ theophylline	Increased dosage of theophylline may be required; therapeutic monitoring should be considered.
Calcium channel blockers: diltiazem, nifedipine, verapamil	↑ calcium channel blockers	Caution is warranted and clinical monitoring of patients is recommended. A dose decrease may be needed for these drugs when co-administered with ritonavir.

This table is continued on the next page

Table 5 (Cont.) Established and Other Potentially Significant Drug Interactions

Concomitant Drug Class: Drug Name	Effect on Concentration of Ritonavir or Concomitant Drug	Clinical Comment
Digoxin	↑ digoxin	Concomitant administration of ritonavir with digoxin may increase digoxin levels. Caution should be exercised when co-administering ritonavir with digoxin, with appropriate monitoring of serum digoxin levels.
Endothelin receptor antagonists: bosentan	↑ bosentan	Co-administration of bosentan in patients on ritonavir: In patients who have been receiving ritonavir for at least 10 days, start bosentan at 62.5 mg once daily or every other day based upon individual tolerability. Co-administration of ritonavir in patients on bosentan: Discontinue use of bosentan at least 36 hours prior to initiation of ritonavir. After at least 10 days following the initiation of ritonavir, resume bosentan at 62.5 mg once daily or every other day based upon individual tolerability.
HCV-Protease Inhibitor: simeprevir	↑simeprevir	It is not recommended to co-administer ritonavir with simeprevir.
HMG-CoA Reductase Inhibitor: atorvastatin rosuvastatin	↑ atorvastatin ↑ rosuvastatin	Titrate atorvastatin and rosuvastatin dose carefully and use the lowest necessary dose. If NORVIR is used with another protease inhibitor, see the complete prescribing information for the concomitant protease inhibitor for details on co-administration with atorvastatin and rosuvastatin.
Immunosuppressants: cyclosporine, tacrolimus, sirolimus (rapamycin)	↑ immunosuppressants	Therapeutic concentration monitoring is recommended for immunosuppressant agents when co-administered with ritonavir.
Inhaled or Intranasal Steroid: e.g. fluticasone budesonide	↑ glucocorticoids	Concomitant use of ritonavir and fluticasone or other glucocorticoids that are metabolized by CYP3A is not recommended unless the potential benefit of treatment outweighs the risk of systemic corticosteroid effects. Concomitant use may result in increased steroid concentrations and reduced serum cortisol concentrations. Systemic corticosteroid effects including Cushing's syndrome and adrenal suppression have been reported during postmarketing use in patients when ritonavir has been coadministered with fluticasone propionate or budesonide.
Long-acting beta-adrenoceptor agonist: salmeterol	↑ salmeterol	Concurrent administration of salmeterol and ritonavir is not recommended. The combination may result in increased risk of cardiovascular adverse events associated with salmeterol, including QT prolongation, palpitations and sinus tachycardia.
Narcotic Analgesic: methadone fentanyl	↓ methadone ↑ fentanyl	Dosage increase of methadone may be considered. Concentrations of fentanyl are expected to increase. Careful monitoring of therapeutic and adverse effects (including potentially fatal respiratory depression) is recommended when fentanyl is concomitantly administered with NORVIR.
Neuroleptics: perphenazine, risperidone, thioridazine	↑ neuroleptics	A dose decrease may be needed for these drugs when co-administered with ritonavir.
Oral Contraceptives or Patch Contraceptives: ethinyl estradiol	↓ ethinyl estradiol	Alternate methods of contraception should be considered.

This table is continued on the next page

the high dose was approximately 6% that of the exposure in humans with the recommended therapeutic dose. Based on the exposures achieved in the animal studies, the significance of the observed effects is not known.

Mutagenesis

However, ritonavir was found to be negative for mutagenic or clastogenic activity in a battery of *in vitro* and *in vivo* assays including the Ames bacterial reverse mutation assay using *S. typhimurium* and *E. coli*, the mouse lymphoma assay, the mouse micronucleus test and chromosomal aberration assays in human lymphocytes.

Impairment of Fertility

Ritonavir produced no effects on fertility in rats at drug exposures approximately 40% (male) and 60% (female) of that achieved with the proposed therapeutic dose. Higher dosages were not feasible due to hepatic toxicity.

14 CLINICAL STUDIES

The activity of NORVIR® (ritonavir) as monotherapy or in combination with nucleoside reverse transcriptase inhibitors has been evaluated in 1446 patients enrolled in two double-blind, randomized trials.

14.1 Advanced Patients with Prior Antiretroviral Therapy

Study 247 was a randomized, double-blind trial (with open-label follow-up) conducted in HIV-infected patients with at least nine months of prior antiretroviral therapy and baseline CD_4 cell counts less than or equal to 100 cells per µL. NORVIR 600 mg twice-daily or placebo was added to each patient's baseline antiretroviral therapy regimen, which could have consisted of up to two approved antiretroviral agents. The study accrued 1,090 patients, with mean baseline CD_4 cell count at study entry of 32 cells per µL. After the clinical benefit of NORVIR® (ritonavir) therapy was

demonstrated, all patients were eligible to switch to open-label NORVIR for the duration of the follow-up period. Median duration of double-blind therapy with NORVIR and placebo was 6 months. The median duration of follow-up through the end of the open-label phase was 13.5 months for patients randomized to NORVIR and 14 months for patients randomized to placebo.

The cumulative incidence of clinical disease progression or death during the double-blind phase of Study 247 was 26% for patients initially randomized to NORVIR compared to 42% for patients initially randomized to placebo. This difference in rates was statistically significant.

Cumulative mortality through the end of the open-label follow-up phase for patients enrolled in Study 247 was 18% (99/543) for patients initially randomized to NORVIR compared to 26% (142/547) for patients initially randomized to placebo. This difference in rates was statistically significant. However, since the analysis at the end of the open-label phase includes patients in the placebo arm who were switched from placebo to NORVIR therapy, the survival benefit of NORVIR cannot be precisely estimated.

During the double-blind phase of Study 247, CD_4 cell counts increases from baseline for patients randomized to NORVIR at Week 2 and Week 4 were observed. From Week 4 and through Week 24, mean CD_4 cell counts for patients randomized to NORVIR appeared to plateau. In contrast, there was no apparent change in mean CD_4 cell counts for patients randomized to placebo at any visit between baseline and Week 24 of the double-blind phase of Study 247.

14.2 Patients without Prior Antiretroviral Therapy

In Study 245, 356 antiretroviral-naive HIV-infected patients (mean baseline CD_4 = 364 cells per µL) were randomized to receive either NORVIR 600 mg twice-daily, zidovudine 200 mg three-times-daily, or a combination of these drugs.

During the double-blind phase of study 245, greater mean CD_4 cell count increases were observed from baseline to Week 12 in the NORVIR-containing arms compared to the zidovudine arms. Mean CD_4 cell count changes subsequently appeared to plateau through Week 24 in the NORVIR arm, whereas mean CD_4 cell counts gradually diminished through Week 24 in the zidovudine and NORVIR plus zidovudine arms.

Greater mean reductions in plasma HIV-1 RNA levels were observed from baseline to Week 2 for the NORVIR-containing arms compared to the zidovudine arm. After Week 2 and through Week 24, mean plasma HIV-1 RNA levels either remained stable in the NORVIR and zidovudine arms or gradually rebounded toward baseline in the NORVIR plus zidovudine arm.

15 REFERENCES

1. Sewester CS. Calculations. In: Drug Facts and Comparisons. St. Louis, MO: J.B. Lippincott Co; January, 1997:xix.

16 HOW SUPPLIED/STORAGE AND HANDLING

NORVIR (ritonavir) tablets and NORVIR (ritonavir) oral solution are available in the following strengths and package sizes:

16.1 NORVIR Tablets, 100 mg Ritonavir

NORVIR (ritonavir) tablets are white film-coated ovaloid tablets debossed with the "a" logo and the code NK.
Bottles of 30 tablets each (NDC 0074-3333-30).

Recommended Storage

Store at or below 30°C (86°F). Exposure to temperatures up to 50°C (122°F) for seven days permitted. Dispense in original container or USP equivalent tight container (60 mL or less). For patient use: exposure of this product to high humidity outside the original or USP equivalent tight container (60 mL or less) for longer than 2 weeks is not recommended.

16.2 NORVIR Oral Solution, 80 mg per mL Ritonavir

NORVIR (ritonavir) oral solution is an orange-colored liquid, supplied in amber-colored, multi-dose bottles containing 600 mg ritonavir per 7.5 mL marked dosage cup (80 mg per mL).
240 mL bottles (NDC 0074-1940-63).

Continued on next page

Information on the AbbVie, Inc. products listed on these pages is from the prescribing information in use as of July 31, 2016. For more information, please visit rxabbvie.com or call 1-800-633-9110.

Recommended Storage

Store NORVIR oral solution at room temperature 20°-25°C (68°-77°F). Do not refrigerate. Shake well before each use. Use by product expiration date.

Product should be stored and dispensed in the original container.

Avoid exposure to excessive heat. Keep cap tightly closed.

17 PATIENT COUNSELING INFORMATION

Advise the patient to read the FDA-approved patient labeling (Patient Information)

Patients or parents of patients should be informed that:

General Information

❑ They should pay special attention to accurate administration of their dose to minimize the risk of accidental overdose or underdose of NORVIR.

❑ They should inform their healthcare provider if their children's weight changes in order to make sure that the child's NORVIR dose is the correct one.

❑ Take NORVIR with meals.

❑ For adult patients taking NORVIR tablets, the maximum dose of 600 mg twice daily by mouth with meals should not be exceeded.

❑ Patients should remain under the care of a physician while using NORVIR. Patients should be advised to take NORVIR and other concomitant antiretroviral therapy every day as prescribed. NORVIR must always be used in combination with other antiretroviral drugs. Patients should not alter the dose or discontinue therapy without consulting with their doctor. If a dose of NORVIR is missed patients should take the dose as soon as possible and then return to their normal schedule. However, if a dose is skipped the patient should not double the next dose.

❑ NORVIR is not a cure for HIV-1 infection and patients may continue to experience illnesses associated with HIV-1 infection, including opportunistic infections. Patients should remain under the care of a physician when using NORVIR.

Patients should be advised to avoid doing things that can spread HIV-1 infection to others.

• **Do not share needles or other injection equipment.**

• **Do not share personal items that can have blood or body fluids on them, like toothbrushes and razor blades.**

• **Do not have any kind of sex without protection.** Always practice safe sex by using a latex or polyurethane condom to lower the chance of sexual contact with semen, vaginal secretions, or blood.

• **Do not breastfeed.** We do not know if NORVIR can be passed to the baby through breast milk and whether it could harm the baby. Also, mothers with HIV-1 should not breastfeed because HIV-1 can be passed to the baby in the breast milk.

❑ Sustained decreases in plasma HIV-1 RNA have been associated with a reduced risk of progression to AIDS and death.

Drug Interactions

❑ NORVIR may interact with some drugs; therefore, patients should be advised to report to their doctor the use of any other prescription, non-prescription medication or herbal products, particularly St. John's Wort.

❑ If they are receiving estrogen-based hormonal contraceptives, additional or alternate contraceptive measures should be used during therapy with NORVIR.

Potential Adverse Effects

❑ Pre-existing liver disease including Hepatitis B or C can worsen with use of NORVIR. This can be seen as worsening of transaminase elevations or hepatic decompensation. Patients should be advised that their liver function tests will need to be monitored closely especially during the first several months of NORVIR treatment and that they should notify their healthcare provider if they develop the signs and symptoms of worsening liver disease including loss of appetite, abdominal pain, jaundice, and itchy skin.

❑ Pancreatitis, including some fatalities, has been observed in patients receiving NORVIR therapy. Your patients should let you know of signs and symptoms (nausea, vomiting, and abdominal pain) that might be suggestive of pancreatitis.

❑ Skin rashes ranging in severity from mild to Stevens-Johnson syndrome have been reported in patients receiving NORVIR. Patients should be advised to contact their healthcare provider if they develop a rash while taking

NORVIR. The healthcare provider will determine if treatment should be continued or an alternative antiretroviral regimen used.

❑ NORVIR may produce changes in the electrocardiogram (e.g., PR prolongation). Patients should consult their physician if they experience symptoms such as dizziness, lightheadedness, abnormal heart rhythm or loss of consciousness.

❑ Treatment with NORVIR therapy can result in substantial increases in the concentration of total cholesterol and triglycerides.

❑ New onset of diabetes or exacerbation of pre-existing diabetes mellitus, and hyperglycemia have been reported. Patients should be advised to notify their healthcare provider if they develop the signs and symptoms of diabetes mellitus including frequent urination, excessive thirst, extreme hunger or unusual weight loss and/or an increased blood sugar while on NORVIR as they may require a change in their diabetes treatment or new treatment.

❑ Immune reconstitution syndrome has been reported in HIV-infected patients treated with combination antiretroviral therapy, including NORVIR.

❑ Redistribution or accumulation of body fat may occur in patients receiving antiretroviral therapy and that the cause and long term health effects of these conditions are not known at this time.

❑ Patients with hemophilia may experience increased bleeding when treated with protease inhibitors such as NORVIR.

❑ If they are receiving avanafil, sildenafil, tadalafil, or vardenafil for the treatment of erectile dysfunction, they may be at an increased risk of associated adverse reactions including hypotension, visual changes, and sustained erection, and should promptly report any symptoms to their doctor. They should seek medical assistance

Table 5 *(Cont.)* Established and Other Potentially Significant Drug Interactions		
Concomitant Drug Class: Drug Name	**Effect on Concentration of Ritonavir or Concomitant Drug**	**Clinical Comment**
PDE5 Inhibitors: avanafil sildenafil, tadalafil, vardenafil	↑ avanafil ↑ sildenafil ↑ tadalafil ↑ vardenafil	Do not use ritonavir with avanafil because a safe and effective avanafil dosage regimen has not been established. Particular caution should be used when prescribing sildenafil, tadalafil or vardenafil in patients receiving ritonavir. Coadministration of ritonavir with these drugs is expected to substantially increase their concentrations and may result in an increase in PDE5 inhibitor associated adverse events, including hypotension, syncope, visual changes, and prolonged erection. Use of PDE5 inhibitors for pulmonary arterial hypertension (PAH): Sildenafil (Revatio®) is contraindicated when used for the treatment of pulmonary arterial hypertension (PAH) because a safe and effective dose has not been established when used with ritonavir *[see Contraindications (4)]*. The following dose adjustments are recommended for use of tadalafil (Adcirca™) with ritonavir: Co-administration of ADCIRCA in patients on ritonavir: In patients receiving ritonavir for at least one week, start ADCIRCA at 20 mg once daily. Increase to 40 mg once daily based upon individual tolerability. Co-administration of ritonavir in patients on ADCIRCA: Avoid use of ADCIRCA during the initiation of ritonavir. Stop ADCIRCA at least 24 hours prior to starting ritonavir. After at least one week following the initiation of ritonavir, resume ADCIRCA at 20 mg once daily. Increase to 40 mg once daily based upon individual tolerability. Use of PDE5 inhibitors for the treatment of erectile dysfunction: It is recommended not to exceed the following doses: • Sildenafil: 25 mg every 48 hours • Tadalafil: 10 mg every 72 hours • Vardenafil: 2.5 mg every 72 hours Use with increased monitoring for adverse events.
Sedative/hypnotics: buspirone, clorazepate, diazepam, estazolam, flurazepam, zolpidem	↑ sedative/hypnotics	A dose decrease may be needed for these drugs when co-administered with ritonavir.
Sedative/hypnotics: Parenteral midazolam	↑ midazolam	Co-administration of oral midazolam with NORVIR is CONTRAINDICATED. Concomitant use of parenteral midazolam with NORVIR may increase plasma concentrations of midazolam. Co-administration should be done in a setting which ensures close clinical monitoring and appropriate medical management in case of respiratory depression and/or prolonged sedation. Dosage reduction for midazolam should be considered, especially if more than a single dose of midazolam is administered.
Steroids (systemic): e.g. budesonide, dexamethasone, prednisone	↑ glucocorticoids	Concomitant use of glucocorticoids that are metabolized by CYP3A is not recommended unless the potential benefit of treatment outweighs the risk of systemic corticosteroid effects. Concomitant use may result in increased steroid concentrations and reduced serum cortisol concentrations. This may increase the risk for development of systemic corticosteroid effects including Cushing's syndrome and adrenal suppression.
Stimulant: methamphetamine	↑ methamphetamine	Use with caution. A dose decrease of methamphetamine may be needed when co-administered with ritonavir.

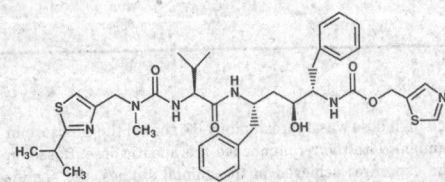

Table 7. Drug Interactions - Pharmacokinetic Parameters for Ritonavir in the Presence of the Co-administered Drug

Co-administered Drug	Dose of Co-administered Drug (mg)	Dose of NORVIR (mg)	N	AUC % (95% CI)	C_{max} (95% CI)	C_{min} (95% CI)
Clarithromycin	500 q12h, 4 d	200 q8h, 4 d	22	↑ 12% (2, 23%)	↑ 15% (2, 28%)	↑ 14% (-3, 36%)
Didanosine	200 q12h, 4 d	600 q12h, 4 d	12	↔	↔	↔
Fluconazole	400 single dose, day 1; 200 daily, 4 d	200 q6h, 4 d	8	↑ 12% (5, 20%)	↑ 15% (7, 22%)	↑ 14% (0, 26%)
Fluoxetine	30 q12h, 8 d	600 single dose, 1 d	16	↑ 19% (7, 34%)	↔	ND
Ketoconazole	200 daily, 7 d	500 q12h, 10 d	12	↑ 18% (-3, 52%)	↑ 10% (-11, 36%)	ND
Rifampin	600 or 300 daily, 10 d	500 q12h, 20 d	7, 9*	↓ 35% (7, 55%)	↓ 25% (-5, 46%)	↓ 49% (-14, 91%)
Voriconazole	400 q12h, 1 d; then 200 q12h, 8 d	400 q12h, 9 d		↔	↔	ND
Zidovudine	200 q8h, 4 d	300 q6h, 4 d	10	↔	↔	↔

immediately if they develop a sustained penile erection lasting more than 4 hours while taking NORVIR and a PDE 5 Inhibitor such as Stendra®, Viagra®, Cialis® or Levitra®. If they are currently using or planning to use avanafil or tadalafil (for the treatment of pulmonary arterial hypertension) they should ask their doctor about potential adverse reactions these medications may cause when taken with NORVIR. The doctor may choose not to keep them on avanafil, or may adjust the dose of tadalafil while initiating treatment with NORVIR. Concomitant use of Revatio® (sildenafil) with NORVIR is contraindicated in patients with pulmonary arterial hypertension (PAH).

❑ Continued NORVIR therapy at a dose of 600 mg twice daily following loss of viral suppression may increase the likelihood of cross-resistance to other protease inhibitors.
NORVIR tablets and oral solution are manufactured by:
AbbVie Inc.
North Chicago, IL 60064 USA
© 2015 AbbVie Inc. All rights reserved.
03-B235

Patient Information
NORVIR® (NOR-VEER)
(ritonavir) Tablet
NORVIR® (NOR-VEER)
(ritonavir) Oral Solution
Read this Patient Information before you start taking NORVIR and each time you get a refill. There may be new information. This information does not take the place of talking to your doctor about your medical condition or your treatment.

What is the most important information I should know about NORVIR?
• NORVIR can interact with other medicines and cause serious side effects. It is important to know the medicines that should not be taken with NORVIR. See the section "Who should not take NORVIR?"

What is NORVIR?
NORVIR is a prescription anti-HIV medicine used with other anti-HIV medicines to treat people with human immunodeficiency virus (HIV) infection. NORVIR is a type of anti-HIV medicine called a protease inhibitor. HIV is the virus that causes AIDS (Acquired Immune Deficiency Syndrome).

When used with other HIV medicines, NORVIR may reduce the amount of HIV in your blood (called "viral load"). NORVIR may also help to increase the number of CD_4 (T) cells in your blood which help fight off other infections. Reducing the amount of HIV and increasing the CD_4 (T) cell count may improve your immune system. This may reduce your risk of death or infections that can happen when your immune system is weak (opportunistic infections). Patients who took NORVIR in clinical studies had significant reductions in both death and AIDS defining diseases; however NORVIR may not have these effects in all patients.
NORVIR does not cure HIV infection or AIDS and you may continue to experience illnesses associated with HIV-1 infection, including opportunistic infections. You should remain under the care of a doctor when using NORVIR.

Avoid doing things that can spread HIV-1 infection.
• **Do not share needles or other injection equipment.**
• **Do not share personal items that can have blood or body fluids on them, like toothbrushes and razor blades.**
• **Do not have any kind of sex without protection.** Always practice safe sex by using a latex or polyurethane condom to lower the chance of sexual contact with semen, vaginal secretions, or blood.

Who should not take NORVIR?
Do not take NORVIR if you are allergic to ritonavir or any of the ingredients in NORVIR. See the end of this leaflet for a complete list of ingredients in NORVIR.
Do not take NORVIR with any of the following medicines:
• alfuzosin (Uroxatral)
• amiodarone (Cordarone, Nexterone, Pacerone), flecainide (Tambocor), propafenone (Rythmol) or quinidine (Nuedext, Quinaglute, Cardioquin, Quinidex, and others)
• voriconazole (VFend) if NORVIR dose is 400 mg every 12 hours or greater
• dihydroergotamine (D.H.E. 45, Embolex, Migranal), ergotamine (Cafergot, Ergomar) methylergonovine (Methergine)
• cisapride (Propulsid)
• St. John's Wort (Hypericum perforatum)
• the cholesterol lowering medicines lovastatin (Mevacor, Altoprev, Advicor) or simvastatin (Zocor, Simcor, Vytorin)
• pimozide (Orap)
• sildenafil (Revatio) only when used for the treatment of pulmonary arterial hypertension
• oral midazolam or triazolam (Halcion)
Serious problems can happen if you or your child takes any of these medicines with NORVIR.

What should I tell my doctor before taking NORVIR?
Before taking NORVIR, tell your doctor if you:
• have liver problems, including Hepatitis B or Hepatitis C.
• have heart problems.
• have high blood sugar (diabetes).
• have bleeding problems or hemophilia.
• are pregnant or plan to become pregnant. It is not known if NORVIR can harm your unborn baby.
  Pregnancy Registry: There is a pregnancy registry for women who take antiviral medicines during pregnancy. The purpose of the registry is to collect information about the health of you and your baby. Talk to your doctor about how you can take part in this registry.
• are breastfeeding. **Do not breastfeed if you take NORVIR**
  • You should not breastfeed if you have HIV-1 because of the risk of passing HIV-1 to your baby.
  • It is not known if NORVIR passes into your breast milk.
  • Talk to your doctor about the best way to feed your baby.
Tell your doctor about all the medicines you take including prescription and nonprescription medicines, vitamins, and herbal supplements. Taking NORVIR and certain other medicines may affect each other causing serious side effects. NORVIR may affect the way other medicines work and other medicines may affect how NORVIR works.
Especially tell your doctor if you take:
• medicine to treat HIV
• estrogen-based contraceptives (birth control). NORVIR might reduce the effectiveness of estrogen-based contraceptives. You must take additional precautions for birth control such as a condom.

• medicine for pain such as tramadol (Ryzolt, Ultracet, Conzip, Ultram), propoxyphene, or meperidine (Demerol)
• medicine to treat alcohol abuse such as disulfiram (Antabuse)
• medicine for your heart such as disopyramide (Norpace), lidocaine (Xylocaine Viscous), mexiletine, digoxin (Lanoxin), nifedipine (Procardia, Adalat, Afeditab CR), diltiazem (Cardizem, Dilacor, Cartia, Diltzac, Dilt, Taztia, Tiazac) or verapamil (Calan, Covera, Isoptin, Tarka, Verelan)
• medicines for panic disorder or anxiety such as buspirone, clorazepate, diazepam, estazolam, flurazepam, and zolpidem
• medicine for cancer such as dasatinib (Sprycel), nilotinib (Tasigna) vincristine, or vinblastine
• warfarin (Coumadin, Jantoven), rivaroxaban (Xarelto)
• medicine for seizures such as carbamazepine (Carbatrol, Equetro, Tegretol, Epitol), clonazepam (Klonopin), ethosuximide (Zarontin, Ethosuximide), divalproex (Depakote, Divalproex Sodium), lamotrigine (Lamictal) or phenytoin (Dilantin, Phenytek)
• medicine for depression such as nefazodone, bupropion (Wellbutrin, Aplenzin, Zyban), desipramine (Norpramin) or trazadone, fluoxetine (Prozac), paroxetine (Paxil), amitriptyline, or nortriptyline
• medicine for nausea and vomiting such as dronabinol (Marinol) or perphenazine
• medicine for fungal infections such as ketoconazole (Nizoral), itraconazole (Sporanox, Onmel) or voriconazole (VFend)
• colchicine (Colcrys, Col-Probenecid, Probenecid and Colchine)
• medicine for infections such as clarithromycin (Prevpac, Biaxin), rifabutin (Mycobutin), rifampin (Rimactane, Rifadin, Rifater, Rifamate), atovaquone (Mepron, Malarone), bedaquiline (Sirturo), quinine (Qualaquin) or metronidazole (Flagyl, Helidac, Metrocream)
• medicine used to treat blood pressure, a heart attack, heart failure, or to lower pressure in the eye such as metoprolol (Lopressor, Toprol-XL), timolol (Cosopt, Betimol, Timoptic, Isatolol, Combigan)
• medicine for lung disease such as theophylline and salmeterol (Serevent)
• bosentan (Tracleer)
• medicine to treat Hepatitis C such as simeprevir (Olysio)
• medicine to prevent organ transplant failure such as cyclosporine (Gengraf, Sandimmune, Neoral), tacrolimus (Prograf,) sirolimus (Rapamune)
• steroids such as dexamethasone, fluticasone (Advair Diskus, Veramyst, Flovent, Flonase), budesonide (Entocort EC, Pulmicort, Rhinocort), or prednisone
• a narcotic medicine such as methadone (Methadose, Dolophine Hydrochloride) or fentanyl (Abstral, Actiq, Fentora, Lazanda, Onsolis, Duragesic)
• medicine to treat schizophrenia such as risperidone (Risperdal) or thioridazine
• medicine to treat psychosis such as quetiapine (Seroquel)
• medicine to treat erectile dysfunction or pulmonary hypertension such as avanafil (Stendra), sildenafil (Viagra, Revatio), vardenafil (Levitra, Staxyn), tadalafil (Cialis, Adcirca). If you are taking avanafil (Stendra), your doctor may need to change it to a different medicine.
• midazolam by injection
• methamphetamine (Desoxyn)
• cholesterol lowering medicine such as atorvastatin (Lipitor) or rosuvastatin (Crestor)
This is not a complete list of medicines that you should tell your doctor that you are taking. Ask your doctor, provider or pharmacist if you are not sure if your medicine is one that is listed above.

Know the medicines you take. Keep a list of them to show your doctor or pharmacist when you get a new medicine. Do not start any new medicines while you are taking NORVIR without first talking with your doctor.

How should I take NORVIR?
• Take NORVIR exactly as prescribed by your doctor.
• You should stay under a doctor's care when taking NORVIR. Do not change your dose of NORVIR or stop your treatment without talking with your doctor first.
• If your child is taking NORVIR, your child's doctor will decide the right dose based on your child's height and weight. Tell your doctor if your child's weight changes.

Continued on next page

Table 8. Drug Interactions - Pharmacokinetic Parameters for Co-administered Drug in the Presence of NORVIR

Co-administered Drug	Dose of Co-administered Drug (mg)	Dose of NORVIR (mg)	N	AUC % (95% CI)	C_{max} (95% CI)	C_{min} (95% CI)
Alprazolam	1, single dose	500 q12h, 10 d	12	↓ 12% (-5, 30%)	↓ 16% (5, 27%)	ND
Avanafil	50, single dose	600 q12h	14[6]	↑ 13-fold	↑ 2.4-fold	ND
Clarithromycin 14-OH clarithromycin metabolite	500 q12h, 4 d	200 q8h, 4 d	22	↑ 77% (56, 103%) ↓ 100%	↑ 31% (15, 51%) ↓ 99%	↑ 2.8-fold (2.4, 3.3×) ↓ 100%
Desipramine 2-OH desipramine metabolite	100, single dose	500 q12h, 12 d	14	↑ 145% (103, 211%) ↓ 15% (3, 26%)	↑ 22% (12, 35%) ↓ 67% (62, 72%)	ND ND
Didanosine	200 q12h, 4 d	600 q12h, 4 d	12	↓ 13% (0, 23%)	↓ 16% (5, 26%)	↔
Ethinyl estradiol	50 µg single dose	500 q12h, 16 d	23	↓ 40% (31, 49%)	↓ 32% (24, 39%)	ND
Fluticasone propionate aqueous nasal spray	200 mcg qd, 7 d	100 mg q12h, 7 d	18	↑ approximately 350-fold[5]	↑ approximately 25-fold[5]	
Indinavir[1] Day 14 Day 15	400 q12h, 15 d	400 q12h, 15 d	10	↑ 6% (-14, 29%) ↓ 7% (-22, 28%)	↓ 51% (40, 61%) ↓ 62% (52, 70%)	↑ 4-fold (2.8, 6.8×) ↑ 4-fold (2.5, 6.5×)
Ketoconazole	200 daily, 7 d	500 q12h, 10 d	12	↑ 3.4-fold (2.8, 4.3×)	↑ 55% (40, 72%)	ND
Meperidine Normeperidine metabolite	50 oral single dose	500 q12h, 10 d	8 6	↓ 62% (59, 65%) ↑ 47% (-24, 345%)	↓ 59% (42, 72%) ↑ 87% (42, 147%)	ND ND
Methadone[2]	5, single dose	500 q12h, 15 d	11	↓ 36% (16, 52%)	↓ 38% (28, 46%)	ND
Raltegravir	400, single dose	100 q12h, 16 d	10	↓ 16% (-30, 1%)	↓ 24% (-45, 4%)	↓ 1% (-30, 40%)
Rivaroxaban	10, single dose (days 0 and 7)	600 q12h (days 2 to 7)	12	↑ 150% (130-170%)[7]	↑ 60% (40-70%)[7]	ND
Rifabutin 25-O-desacetyl rifabutin metabolite	150 daily, 16 d	500 q12h, 10 d	5, 11*	↑ 4-fold (2.8, 6.1×) ↑ 38-fold (28, 56×)	↑ 2.5-fold (1.9, 3.4×) ↑ 16-fold (13, 20×)	↑ 6-fold (3.5, 18.3×) ↑ 181-fold (ND)

This table is continued on the next page

Your child should take NORVIR with food. If your child does not tolerate NORVIR Oral Solution, ask your child's doctor for advice.

- Swallow NORVIR tablets whole. Do not chew, break, or crush tablets before swallowing. If you cannot swallow NORVIR tablets whole, tell your doctor. You may need a different medicine.
- Take NORVIR with meals.
- NORVIR Oral Solution is peppermint or caramel flavored. You can take it alone, or may improve the taste by mixing it with 8 ounces of chocolate milk, Ensure®, or Advera® NORVIR Oral Solution should be taken within 1 hour if mixed with these fluids. Ask your doctor, nurse or pharmacist about other ways to improve the taste of NORVIR Oral Solution.
- Do not run out of NORVIR. Get your NORVIR prescription refilled from you doctor or pharmacy before you run out.
- If you miss a dose of NORVIR, take it as soon as possible and then take your next scheduled dose at its regular time. If it is almost time for your next dose, wait and take the next dose at the regular time. Do not double the next dose.
- If you take too much NORVIR, call your local poison control center or go to the nearest hospital emergency room right away.

What are the possible side effects of NORVIR?
NORVIR can cause serious side effects including:
- See "What is the most important information I should know about NORVIR?"
- **Liver disease.** Some people taking NORVIR in combination with other anti-HIV medicines have developed liver problems which may be life-threatening. Your doctor should do regular blood tests during your combination

treatment with NORVIR. If you have chronic hepatitis B or C infection, your doctor should check your blood tests more often because you have an increased chance of developing liver problems. Tell your doctor if you have any of the below signs and symptoms of liver problems:
- loss of appetite
- pain or tenderness on your right side below your ribs
- yellowing of your skin or whites of your eyes
- itchy skin
- **Swelling of your pancreas (Pancreatitis).** NORVIR can cause serious pancreas problems, which may lead to death. Tell your doctor right away if you have signs or symptoms of pancreatitis such as:
- nausea
- vomiting
- stomach (abdomen) pain
- **Allergic Reactions.** Sometimes these allergic reactions can become severe and require treatment in a hospital. You should call your doctor right away if you develop a rash. Stop taking NORVIR and get medical help right away if you have any of the following symptoms of a severe allergic reaction:
- trouble breathing
- wheezing
- dizziness or fainting
- throat tightness or hoarseness
- fast heartbeat or pounding in your chest (tachycardia)
- sweating
- swelling of your face, lips or tongue
- muscle or joint pain
- blisters or skin lesions
- mouth sores or ulcers

- **Changes in the electrical activity of your heart called PR prolongation.** PR prolongation can cause irregular heartbeats. Tell your doctor right away if you have symptoms such as:
- dizziness
- lightheadedness
- feel faint or pass out
- abnormal heart beat
- **Increase in cholesterol and triglyceride levels.** Treatment with NORVIR® (ritonavir) may increase your blood levels of cholesterol and triglycerides. Your doctor should do blood tests before you start your treatment with NORVIR and regularly to check for an increase in your cholesterol and triglycerides levels.
- **Diabetes and high blood sugar (hyperglycemia).** Some people who take protease inhibitors including NORVIR can get high blood sugar, develop diabetes, or your diabetes can get worse. Tell your doctor if you notice an increase in thirst or urinate often while taking NORVIR.
- **Changes in your immune system (Immune reconstitution syndrome)** can happen when you start taking HIV medicines. Your immune system may get stronger and begin to fight infections that have been hidden in your body for a long time. Call your doctor right away if you start having new symptoms after starting your HIV medicine.
- **Change in body fat.** These changes can happen in people who take antiretroviral therapy. The changes may include an increase amount of fat in the upper back and neck ("buffalo hump"), breast, and around the back and stomach area. Loss of fat from the legs, arms, and face may also happen. The exact cause and long-term health effects of these conditions are not known.
- **Increased bleeding for hemophiliacs.** Some people with hemophilia have increased bleeding with protease inhibitors including NORVIR.

The most common side effects of NORVIR include:
- diarrhea
- nausea
- vomiting
- upper and lower stomach (abdomen) pain
- tingling feeling or numbness in hands or feet or around the lips
- rash
- feeling weak or tired

NORVIR liquid contains a large amount of alcohol. If a toddler or young child accidentally drinks more than the recommended dose of NORVIR, it could make him/her sick from too much alcohol. Contact your local poison control center or emergency room immediately if this happens.

Tell your doctor if you have any side effect that bothers you or that does not go away.

These are not all of the possible side effects of NORVIR. For more information, ask your doctor or pharmacist.

Call your doctor for medical advice about side effects. You may report side effects to FDA at 1-800-FDA-1088.

How should I store NORVIR?
- Store NORVIR Oral Solution at room temperature between 68°F to 77°F (20°C to 25°C).
- Store NORVIR tablets below 30°C (86°F). Exposure to temperatures up to 50°C (122°F) for seven days permitted.
- Do not refrigerate NORVIR Oral Solution.
- Shake NORVIR Oral Solution well before each use.
- Keep NORVIR Oral Solution away from heat.
- Store NORVIR tablets and NORVIR oral solution in the original container given to you by the pharmacist.
- Exposure of NORVIR tablets to high humidity outside the original container for longer than 2 weeks is not recommended.
- Use NORVIR tablets and NORVIR Oral Solution by the expiration date on the bottle.

Keep NORVIR and all medicines out of the reach of children.

General information about NORVIR

Medicines are sometimes prescribed for purposes other than those listed in a Patient Information Leaflet. Do not use this medicine for a condition for which it was not prescribed. Do not share this medicine with other people.

This leaflet summarizes the most important information about NORVIR. If you would like more information, talk to your doctor. You can ask your doctor or pharmacist for information about NORVIR that is written for healthcare professionals.

Information on the AbbVie, Inc. products listed on these pages is from the prescribing information in use as of July 31, 2016. For more information, please visit rxabbvie.com or call 1-800-633-9110.

Table 8 (cont.) Drug Interactions - Pharmacokinetic Parameters for Co-administered Drug in the Presence of NORVIR

Co-administered Drug	Dose of Co-administered Drug (mg)	Dose of NORVIR (mg)	N	AUC % (95% CI)	C_{max} (95% CI)	C_{min} (95% CI) Sildenafil
Simeprevir	200 mg qd, 7 d	100 mg bid, 15 d	12	↑ 618% (463%-815%)[8]	↑370% (284%-476%)[8]	↑1335% (929%-1901%)[8]
Sulfamethoxazole[3]	800, single dose	500 q12h, 12 d	15	↓ 20% (16, 23%)	↔	ND
Tadalafil	20 mg, single dose	200 mg q12h		↑ 124%	↔	ND
Theophylline	3 mg/kg q8h, 15 d	500 q12h, 10 d	13, 11*	↓ 43% (42, 45%)	↓ 32% (29, 34%)	↓ 57% (55, 59%)
Trazodone	50 mg, single dose	200 mg q12h, 4 doses	10	↑ 2.4-fold	↑ 34%	
Trimethoprim[3]	160, single dose	500 q12h, 12 d	15	↑ 20% (3, 43%)	↔	ND
Vardenafil	5 mg	600 q12h		↑ 49-fold	↑ 13-fold	ND
Voriconazole	400 q12h, 1 d; then 200 q12h, 8 d	400 q12h, 9 d		↓ 82%	↓ 66%	
	400 q12h, 1 d; then 200 q12h, 8 d	100 q12h, 9 d		↓ 39%	↓ 24%	
Warfarin S-Warfarin R-Warfarin	5, single dose	400 q12h, 12d	12	↑ 9% (-17, 44%)[4] ↓ 33% (-38, -27%)[4]	↓ 9% (-16, -2%)[4] ↔	ND ND
Zidovudine	200 q8h, 4 d	300 q6h, 4 d	9	↓ 25% (15, 34%)	↓ 27% (4, 45%)	ND

1 Ritonavir and indinavir were co-administered for 15 days; Day 14 doses were administered after a 15%-fat breakfast (757 Kcal) and 9%-fat evening snack (236 Kcal), and Day 15 doses were administered after a 15%-fat breakfast (757 Kcal) and 32%-fat dinner (815 Kcal). Indinavir C_{min} was also increased 4-fold. Effects were assessed relative to an indinavir 800 mg q8h regimen under fasting conditions.
2 Effects were assessed on a dose-normalized comparison to a methadone 20 mg single dose.
3 Sulfamethoxazole and trimethoprim taken as single combination tablet.
4 90% CI presented for R- and S-warfarin AUC and C_{max} ratios.
5 This significant increase in plasma fluticasone propionate exposure resulted in a significant decrease (86%) in plasma cortisol AUC.
6 For the reference arm: N=14 for C_{max} and $AUC_{(0-inf)}$, and for the test arm: N=13 for C_{max} and N=4 for $AUC_{(0-inf)}$.
7 90% CI presented for rivaroxaban
8 90% CI presented for simeprevir (change in exposure presented as percentage increase)
↑ Indicates increase.
↓ Indicates decrease.
↔ Indicates no change.
* Parallel group design; entries are subjects receiving combination and control regimens, respectively.

For more information, call 1-800-633-9110.
What are the ingredients in NORVIR?
Active ingredient: ritonavir
Inactive ingredients:
NORVIR Tablet: copovidone, anhydrous dibasic calcium phosphate, sorbitan monolaurate, colloidal silicon dioxide, and sodium stearyl fumarate. The film coating contains: hypromellose, titanium dioxide, polyethylene glycol 400, hydroxypropyl cellulose, talc, polyethylene glycol 3350, colloidal silicon dioxide, and polysorbate 80.
NORVIR Oral Solution: ethanol, water, polyoxyl 35 castor oil, propylene glycol, anhydrous citric acid to adjust pH, saccharin sodium, peppermint oil, creamy caramel flavoring, and FD&C Yellow No. 6.
This Patient Information has been approved by the U.S. Food and Drug Administration.

NORVIR tablets and oral solution are manufactured by: AbbVie Inc.
North Chicago, IL 60064 USA
Revised: November 2015
The brands listed are trademarks of their respective owners and are not trademarks of AbbVie Inc. The makers of these brands are not affiliated with and do not endorse AbbVie Inc. or its products.

Shown in Product Identification Guide, page 506

PROMETRIUM®   ℞
[pro-mē-trē-um]
(progesterone, USP)
Capsules 100 mg
Capsules 200 mg

WARNING: CARDIOVASCULAR DISORDERS, BREAST CANCER AND PROBABLE DEMENTIA FOR ESTROGEN PLUS PROGESTIN THERAPY

Cardiovascular Disorders and Probable Dementia
Estrogens plus progestin therapy should not be used for the prevention of cardiovascular disease or dementia. (See **CLINICAL STUDIES** and **WARNINGS, Cardiovascular disorders and Probable dementia.**)
The Women's Health Initiative (WHI) estrogen plus progestin substudy reported increased risks of deep vein thrombosis, pulmonary embolism, stroke and myocardial infarction in postmenopausal women (50 to 79 years of age) during 5.6 years of treatment with daily oral conjugated estrogens (CE) [0.625 mg] combined with medroxyprogesterone acetate (MPA) [2.5 mg], relative to placebo. (See **CLINICAL STUDIES** and **WARNINGS, Cardiovascular disorders.**)
The WHI Memory Study (WHIMS) estrogen plus progestin ancillary study of the WHI reported an increased risk of developing probable dementia in postmenopausal women 65 years of age or older during 4 years of treatment with daily CE (0.625 mg) combined with MPA (2.5 mg), relative to placebo. It is unknown whether this finding applies to younger postmeno-

---

pausal women. (See **CLINICAL STUDIES** and **WARNINGS, Probable dementia** and **PRECAUTIONS, Geriatric Use.**)
Breast Cancer
The WHI estrogen plus progestin substudy also demonstrated an increased risk of invasive breast cancer. (See **CLINICAL STUDIES** and **WARNINGS, Malignant neoplasms, Breast Cancer.**)
In the absence of comparable data, these risks should be assumed to be similar for other doses of CE and MPA, and other combinations and dosage forms of estrogens and progestins.
Progestins with estrogens should be prescribed at the lowest effective doses and for the shortest duration consistent with treatment goals and risks for the individual woman.

DESCRIPTION

PROMETRIUM® (progesterone, USP) Capsules contain micronized progesterone for oral administration. Progesterone has a molecular weight of 314.47 and a molecular formula of $C_{21}H_{30}O_2$. Progesterone (pregn-4-ene-3, 20-dione) is a white or creamy white, odorless, crystalline powder practically insoluble in water, soluble in alcohol, acetone and dioxane and sparingly soluble in vegetable oils, stable in air, melting between 126° and 131°C. The structural formula is:

Progesterone is synthesized from a starting material from a plant source and is chemically identical to progesterone of human ovarian origin. PROMETRIUM Capsules are available in multiple strengths to afford dosage flexibility for optimum management. PROMETRIUM Capsules contain 100 mg or 200 mg micronized progesterone.
The inactive ingredients for PROMETRIUM Capsules 100 mg include: peanut oil NF, gelatin NF, glycerin USP, lecithin NF, titanium dioxide USP, FD&C Red No. 40, and D&C Yellow No. 10.
The inactive ingredients for PROMETRIUM Capsules 200 mg include: peanut oil NF, gelatin NF, glycerin USP, lecithin NF, titanium dioxide USP, D&C Yellow No. 10, and FD&C Yellow No. 6.

CLINICAL PHARMACOLOGY

PROMETRIUM Capsules are an oral dosage form of micronized progesterone which is chemically identical to progesterone of ovarian origin. The oral bioavailability of progesterone is increased through micronization.
Pharmacokinetics
A. Absorption
After oral administration of progesterone as a micronized soft-gelatin capsule formulation, maximum serum concentrations were attained within 3 hours. The absolute bioavailability of micronized progesterone is not known. Table 1 summarizes the mean pharmacokinetic parameters in postmenopausal women after five oral daily doses of PROMETRIUM Capsules 100 mg as a micronized soft-gelatin capsule formulation.

TABLE 1. Pharmacokinetic Parameters of PROMETRIUM Capsules

Parameter	PROMETRIUM Capsules Daily Dose		
	100 mg	200 mg	300 mg
C_{max} (ng/mL)	17.3 ± 21.9ª	38.1 ± 37.8	60.6 ± 72.5
T_{max} (hr)	1.5 ± 0.8	2.3 ± 1.4	1.7 ± 0.6

Continued on next page

Information on the AbbVie, Inc. products listed on these pages is from the prescribing information in use as of July 31, 2016. For more information, please visit rxabbvie.com or call 1-800-633-9110.

AUC$_{(0-10)}$ (ng × hr/mL)	43.3 ± 30.8	101.2 ± 66.0	175.7 ± 170.3

ª Mean ± S.D.

Serum progesterone concentrations appeared linear and dose proportional following multiple dose administration of PROMETRIUM® (progesterone, USP) Capsules 100 mg over the dose range 100 mg per day to 300 mg per day in postmenopausal women. Although doses greater than 300 mg per day were not studied in females, serum concentrations from a study in male volunteers appeared linear and dose proportional between 100 mg per day and 400 mg per day. The pharmacokinetic parameters in male volunteers were generally consistent with those seen in postmenopausal women.

B. Distribution
Progesterone is approximately 96 percent to 99 percent bound to serum proteins, primarily to serum albumin (50 to 54 percent) and transcortin (43 to 48 percent).

C. Metabolism
Progesterone is metabolized primarily by the liver largely to pregnanediols and pregnanolones. Pregnanediols and pregnanolones are conjugated in the liver to glucuronide and sulfate metabolites. Progesterone metabolites which are excreted in the bile may be deconjugated and may be further metabolized in the intestine via reduction, dehydroxylation, and epimerization.

D. Excretion
The glucuronide and sulfate conjugates of pregnanediol and pregnanolone are excreted in the bile and urine. Progesterone metabolites are eliminated mainly by the kidneys. Progesterone metabolites which are excreted in the bile may undergo enterohepatic recycling or may be excreted in the feces.

E. Special Populations
The pharmacokinetics of PROMETRIUM Capsules have not been assessed in low body weight or obese patients.

Hepatic Insufficiency: The effect of hepatic impairment on the pharmacokinetics of PROMETRIUM Capsules has not been studied.

Renal Insufficiency: The effect of renal impairment on the pharmacokinetics of PROMETRIUM Capsules has not been studied.

F. Food–Drug Interaction
Concomitant food ingestion increased the bioavailability of PROMETRIUM Capsules relative to a fasting state when administered to postmenopausal women at a dose of 200 mg.

G. Drug Interactions
The metabolism of progesterone by human liver microsomes was inhibited by ketoconazole (IC$_{50}$ < 0.1 µM). Ketoconazole is a known inhibitor of cytochrome P450 3A4, hence these data suggest that ketoconazole or other known inhibitors of this enzyme may increase the bioavailability of progesterone. The clinical relevance of the *in vitro* findings is unknown.

Coadministration of conjugated estrogens and PROMETRIUM Capsules to 29 postmenopausal women over a 12-day period resulted in an increase in total estrone concentrations (C$_{max}$ 3.68 ng/mL to 4.93 ng/mL) and total equilin concentrations (C$_{max}$ 2.27 ng/mL to 3.22 ng/mL) and a decrease in circulating 17β estradiol concentrations (C$_{max}$ 0.037 ng/mL to 0.030 ng/mL). The half-life of the conjugated estrogens was similar with coadministration of PROMETRIUM Capsules. Table 2 summarizes the pharmacokinetic parameters.
[See table 2 on next page]

CLINICAL STUDIES
Effects on the endometrium
In a randomized, double-blind clinical trial, 358 postmenopausal women, each with an intact uterus, received treatment for up to 36 months. The treatment groups were: PROMETRIUM® (progesterone, USP) Capsules at the dose of 200 mg per day for 12 days per 28-day cycle in combination with conjugated estrogens 0.625 mg per day (n=120); conjugated estrogens 0.625 mg per day only (n=119); or placebo (n=119). The subjects in all three treatment groups were primarily Caucasian women (87 percent or more of each group). The results for the incidence of endometrial hyperplasia in women receiving up to 3 years of treatment are shown in Table 3. A comparison of the PROMETRIUM Capsules plus conjugated estrogens treatment group to the conjugated estrogens only group showed a significantly lower

rate of hyperplasia (6 percent combination product versus 64 percent estrogen alone) in the PROMETRIUM Capsules plus conjugated estrogens treatment group throughout 36 months of treatment.
[See table 3 on page 784]
The times to diagnosis of endometrial hyperplasia over 36 months of treatment are shown in Figure 1. This figure illustrates graphically that the proportion of patients with hyperplasia was significantly greater for the conjugated estrogens group (64 percent) compared to the conjugated estrogens plus PROMETRIUM Capsules group (6 percent).

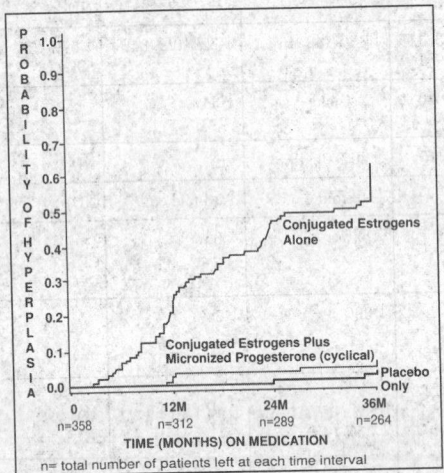

Figure 1. Time to Hyperplasia in Women Receiving up to 36 Months of Treatment

The discontinuation rates due to hyperplasia over the 36 months of treatment are as shown in Table 4. For any degree of hyperplasia, the discontinuation rate for patients who received conjugated estrogens plus PROMETRIUM Capsules was similar to that of the placebo only group, while the discontinuation rate for patients who received conjugated estrogens alone was significantly higher. Women who permanently discontinued treatment due to hyperplasia were similar in demographics to the overall study population.
[See table 4 on page 784]

Effects on secondary amenorrhea
In a single-center, randomized, double-blind clinical study that included premenopausal women with secondary amenorrhea for at least 90 days, administration of 10 days of PROMETRIUM® (progesterone, USP) Capsules therapy resulted in 80 percent of women experiencing withdrawal bleeding within 7 days of the last dose of PROMETRIUM Capsules, 300 mg per day (n=20), compared to 10 percent of women experiencing withdrawal bleeding in the placebo group (n=21).

In a multicenter, parallel-group, open label, postmarketing dosing study that included premenopausal women with secondary amenorrhea for at least 90 days, administration of 10 days of PROMETRIUM Capsules during two 28-day treatment cycles, 300 mg per day (n=107) or 400 mg per day (n=99), resulted in 73.8 percent and 76.8 percent of women, respectively, experiencing withdrawal bleeding.

The rate of secretory transformation was evaluated in a multicenter, randomized, double-blind clinical study in estrogen-primed postmenopausal women. PROMETRIUM Capsules administered orally for 10 days at 400 mg per day (n=22) induced complete secretory changes in the endometrium in 45 percent of women compared to 0 percent in the placebo group (n=23).

A second multicenter, parallel-group, open label postmarketing dosing study in premenopausal women with secondary amenorrhea for at least 90 days also evaluated the rate of secretory transformation. All subjects received daily oral conjugated estrogens over 3 consecutive 28-day treatment cycles and PROMETRIUM Capsules, 300 mg per day (n=107) or 400 mg per day (n=99) for 10 days of each treatment cycle. The rate of complete secretory transformation was 21.5 percent and 28.3 percent, respectively.

Women's Health Initiative Studies
The Women's Health Initiative (WHI) enrolled approximately 27,000 predominantly healthy postmenopausal women in two substudies to assess the risks and benefits of

daily oral conjugated estrogens (CE) [0.625 mg]-alone or in combination with medroxyprogesterone acetate (MPA) [2.5 mg] compared to placebo in the prevention of certain chronic diseases. The primary endpoint was the incidence of coronary heart disease [(CHD) defined as nonfatal myocardial infarction (MI), silent MI and CHD death], with invasive breast cancer as the primary adverse outcome. A "global index" included the earliest occurrence of CHD, invasive breast cancer, stroke, pulmonary embolism (PE), endometrial cancer (only in the CE plus MPA substudy), colorectal cancer, hip fracture, or death due to other cause. These sub studies did not evaluate the effects of CE–alone or CE plus MPA on menopausal symptoms.

WHI Estrogen Plus Progestin Substudy
The WHI estrogen plus progestin substudy was stopped early. According to the predefined stopping rule, after an average follow-up of 5.6 years of treatment, the increased risk of breast cancer and cardiovascular events exceeded the specified benefits included in the "global index." The absolute excess risk of events in the "global index" was 19 per 10,000 women-years.
For those outcomes included in the WHI "global index" that reached statistical significance after 5.6 years of follow-up, the absolute excess risks per 10,000 women-years in the group treated with CE plus MPA were 7 more CHD events, 8 more strokes, 10 more PEs, and 8 more invasive breast cancers, while the absolute risk reductions per 10,000 women-years were 6 fewer colorectal cancers and 5 fewer hip fractures.
Results of the estrogen plus progestin substudy, which included 16,608 women (average 63 years of age, range 50 to 79; 83.9 percent White, 6.8 percent Black, 5.4 percent Hispanic, 3.9 percent Other) are presented in Table 5. These results reflect centrally adjudicated data after an average follow-up of 5.6 years.
[See table 5 on page 785]
Timing of the initiation of estrogen plus progestin therapy relative to the start of menopause may affect the overall risk benefit profile. The WHI estrogen plus progestin substudy stratified for age showed in women 50 to 59 years of age a non-significant trend toward reducing risk of overall mortality [hazard ratio (HR) 0.69 (95 percent CI, 0.44-1.07)].

Women's Health Initiative Memory Study
The estrogen plus progestin Women's Health Initiative Memory Study (WHIMS), an ancillary study of WHI, enrolled 4,532 predominantly healthy postmenopausal women 65 years of age and older (47 percent were 65 to 69 years of age; 35 percent were 70 to 74 years of age; and 18 percent were 75 years of age and older) to evaluate the effects of daily CE (0.625 mg) plus MPA (2.5 mg) on the incidence of probable dementia (primary outcome) compared to placebo. After an average follow-up of 4 years, the relative risk of probable dementia for CE plus MPA versus placebo was 2.05 (95 percent CI, 1.21 – 3.48). The absolute risk of probable dementia for CE plus MPA versus placebo was 45 versus 22 per 10,000 women-years. Probable dementia as defined in this study included Alzheimer's disease (AD), vascular dementia (VaD) and mixed type (having features of both AD and VaD). The most common classification of probable dementia in the treatment group and the placebo group was AD. Since the ancillary study was conducted in women 65 to 79 years of age, it is unknown whether these findings apply to younger postmenopausal women. (See **WARNINGS, Probable dementia** and **PRECAUTIONS, Geriatric Use.**)

INDICATIONS AND USAGE
PROMETRIUM® (progesterone, USP) Capsules are indicated for use in the prevention of endometrial hyperplasia in nonhysterectomized postmenopausal women who are receiving conjugated estrogens tablets. They are also indicated for use in secondary amenorrhea.

CONTRAINDICATIONS
PROMETRIUM Capsules should not be used in women with any of the following conditions:
1. **PROMETRIUM Capsules should not be used in patients with known hypersensitivity to its ingredients. PROMETRIUM Capsules contain peanut oil and should never be used by patients allergic to peanuts.**
2. Undiagnosed abnormal genital bleeding.
3. Known, suspected, or history of breast cancer.
4. Active deep vein thrombosis, pulmonary embolism or history of these conditions.
5. Active arterial thromboembolic disease (for example, stroke and myocardial infarction), or a history of these conditions.

6. Known liver dysfunction or disease.
7. Known or suspected pregnancy.

WARNINGS
See **BOXED WARNING**.

1. Cardiovascular disorders
An increased risk of pulmonary embolism, deep vein thrombosis (DVT), stroke, and myocardial infarction has been reported with estrogen plus progestin therapy. Should any of these occur or be suspected, estrogen with progestin therapy should be discontinued immediately.

Risk factors for arterial vascular disease (for example, hypertension, diabetes mellitus, tobacco use, hypercholesterolemia, and obesity) and/or venous thromboembolism (for example, personal history or family history of venous thromboembolism [VTE], obesity, and systemic lupus erythematosus) should be managed appropriately.

a. Stroke
In the Women's Health Initiative (WHI) estrogen plus progestin substudy, a statistically significant increased risk of stroke was reported in women 50 to 79 years of age receiving daily CE (0.625 mg) plus MPA (2.5 mg) compared to women in the same age group receiving placebo (33 versus 25 per 10,000 women-years). The increase in risk was demonstrated after the first year and persisted. (See **CLINICAL STUDIES**.) Should a stroke occur or be suspected, estrogen plus progestin therapy should be discontinued immediately.

b. Coronary Heart Disease
In the WHI estrogen plus progestin substudy, there was a statistically non-significant increased risk of coronary heart disease (CHD) events (defined as nonfatal myocardial infarction [MI], silent MI, or CHD death) reported in women receiving daily CE (0.625 mg) plus MPA (2.5 mg) compared to women receiving placebo (41 versus 34 per 10,000 women-years). An increase in relative risk was demonstrated in year 1 and a trend toward decreasing relative risk was reported in years 2 through 5. (See **CLINICAL STUDIES**.)

In postmenopausal women with documented heart disease (n = 2,763, average age 66.7 years), in a controlled clinical trial of secondary prevention of cardiovascular disease (Heart and Estrogen/Progestin Replacement Study [HERS]), treatment with daily CE (0.625 mg) plus MPA (2.5 mg) demonstrated no cardiovascular benefit. During an average follow-up of 4.1 years, treatment with CE plus MPA did not reduce the overall rate of CHD events in postmenopausal women with established coronary heart disease. There were more CHD events in the CE plus MPA-treated group than in the placebo group in year 1, but not during the subsequent years. Two thousand, three hundred and twenty-one (2,321) women from the original HERS trial agreed to participate in an open-label extension of HERS, HERS II. Average follow-up in HERS II was an additional 2.7 years, for a total of 6.8 years overall. Rates of CHD events were comparable among women in the CE plus MPA group and the placebo group in HERS, HERS II, and overall.

c. Venous Thromboembolism
In the WHI estrogen plus progestin substudy, a statistically significant 2-fold greater rate of VTE (DVT and pulmonary embolism [PE]) was reported in women receiving daily CE (0.625 mg) plus MPA (2.5 mg) compared to women receiving placebo (35 versus 17 per 10,000 women-years). Statistically significant increases in risk for both DVT (26 versus 13 per 10,000 women-years) and PE (18 versus 8 per 10,000 women-years) were also demonstrated. The increase in VTE risk was demonstrated during the first year and persisted. (See **CLINICAL STUDIES**.) Should a VTE occur or be suspected, estrogen plus progestin therapy should be discontinued immediately.

If feasible, estrogens with progestins should be discontinued at least 4 to 6 weeks before surgery of the type associated with an increased risk of thromboembolism, or during periods of prolonged immobilization.

2. Malignant neoplasms
a. Breast Cancer
The most important randomized clinical trial providing information about breast cancer in estrogen plus progestin users is the Women's Health Initiative (WHI) substudy of daily CE (0.625 mg) plus MPA (2.5 mg). After a mean follow-up of 5.6 years, the estrogen plus progestin substudy reported an increased risk of invasive breast cancer in women who took daily CE plus MPA. In this substudy, prior use of estrogen-alone or estrogen plus progestin therapy was reported by 26 percent of the women. The relative risk

TABLE 2. Mean (± S.D.) Pharmacokinetic Parameters for Estradiol, Estrone, and Equilin Following Coadministration of Conjugated Estrogens 0.625 mg and PROMETRIUM Capsules 200 mg for 12 Days to Postmenopausal Women

Drug	Conjugated Estrogens			Conjugated Estrogens plus PROMETRIUM Capsules		
	C_{max} (ng/mL)	T_{max} (hr)	$AUC_{(0-24h)}$ (ng × h/mL)	C_{max} (ng/mL)	T_{max} (hr)	$AUC_{(0-24h)}$ (ng × h/mL)
Estradiol	0.037 ± 0.048	12.7 ± 9.1	0.676 ± 0.737	0.030 ± 0.032	17.32 ± 1.21	0.561 ± 0.572
Estrone Total[a]	3.68 ± 1.55	10.6 ± 6.8	61.3 ± 26.36	4.93 ± 2.07	7.5 ± 3.8	85.9 ± 41.2
Equilin Total[a]	2.27 ± 0.95	6.0 ± 4.0	28.8 ± 13.0	3.22 ± 1.13	5.3 ± 2.6	38.1 ± 20.2

[a] Total estrogens is the sum of conjugated and unconjugated estrogen.

of invasive breast cancer was 1.24 (95 percent nCI, 1.01-1.54), and the absolute risk was 41 versus 33 cases per 10,000 women-years, for CE plus MPA compared with placebo.

Among women who reported prior use of hormone therapy, the relative risk of invasive breast cancer was 1.86, and the absolute risk was 46 versus 25 cases per 10,000 women-years, for estrogen plus progestin compared with placebo. Among women who reported no prior use of hormone therapy, the relative risk of invasive breast cancer was 1.09, and the absolute risk was 40 versus 36 cases per 10,000 women-years for CE plus MPA compared with placebo. In the same substudy, invasive breast cancers were larger, were more likely to be node positive, and were diagnosed at a more advanced stage in the CE (0.625 mg) plus MPA (2.5 mg) group compared with the placebo group. Metastatic disease was rare, with no apparent difference between the two groups. Other prognostic factors such as histologic subtype, grade and hormone receptor status did not differ between the groups. (See **CLINICAL STUDIES**.)

Consistent with the WHI clinical trials, observational studies have also reported an increased risk of breast cancer for estrogen plus progestin therapy, and a smaller increased risk for estrogen-alone therapy, after several years of use. The risk increased with duration of use, and appeared to return to baseline over about 5 years after stopping treatment (only the observational studies have substantial data on risk after stopping). Observational studies also suggest that the risk of breast cancer was greater, and became apparent earlier, with estrogen plus progestin therapy as compared to estrogen-alone therapy. However, these studies have not generally found significant variation in the risk of breast cancer among different estrogen plus progestin combinations, doses, or routes of administration.

The use of estrogen plus progestin has been reported to result in an increase in abnormal mammograms requiring further evaluation. All women should receive yearly breast examinations by a healthcare provider and perform monthly breast self-examinations. In addition, mammography examinations should be scheduled based on patient age, risk factors, and prior mammogram results.

b. Endometrial Cancer
An increased risk of endometrial cancer has been reported with the use of unopposed estrogen therapy in a woman with a uterus. The reported endometrial cancer risk among unopposed estrogen users is about 2 to 12 times greater than in non-users, and appears dependent on duration of treatment and on estrogen dose. Most studies show no significant increased risk associated with the use of estrogens for less than 1 year. The greatest risk appears associated with prolonged use, with increased risks of 15- to 24-fold for 5 to 10 years or more and this risk has been shown to persist for at least 8 to 15 years after estrogen therapy is discontinued.

Clinical surveillance of all women using estrogen plus progestin therapy is important. Adequate diagnostic measures, including directed or random endometrial sampling when indicated, should be undertaken to rule out malignancy in all cases of undiagnosed persistent or recurring abnormal genital bleeding. There is no evidence that the use of natural estrogens results in a different endometrial risk profile than synthetic estrogens of equivalent estrogen dose. Adding a progestin to estrogen therapy in postmenopausal women has been shown to reduce the risk of endometrial hyperplasia, which may be a precursor to endometrial cancer.

c. Ovarian Cancer
The WHI estrogen plus progestin substudy reported a statistically non-significant increased risk of ovarian cancer. After an average follow-up of 5.6 years, the relative risk for ovarian cancer for CE plus MPA versus placebo was 1.58 (95 percent nCI, 0.77 – 3.24). The absolute risk for CE plus MPA versus placebo was 4 versus 3 cases per 10,000 women-years. In some epidemiologic studies, the use of estrogen plus progestin and estrogen-only products, in particular for 5 or more years, has been associated with an increased risk of ovarian cancer. However, the duration of exposure associated with increased risk is not consistent across all epidemiologic studies and some report no association.

3. Probable dementia
In the estrogen plus progestin Women's Health Initiative Memory Study (WHIMS), an ancillary study of WHI, a population of 4,532 postmenopausal women 65 to 79 years of age was randomized to daily CE (0.625 mg) plus MPA (2.5 mg) or placebo.

In the WHIMS estrogen plus progestin ancillary study, after an average follow-up of 4 years, 40 women in the CE plus MPA group and 21 women in the placebo group were diagnosed with probable dementia. The relative risk of probable dementia for estrogen plus progestin versus placebo was 2.05 (95 percent CI, 1.21-3.48). The absolute risk of probable dementia for CE plus MPA versus placebo was 45 versus 22 cases per 10,000 women-years. It is unknown whether these findings apply to younger postmenopausal women. (See **CLINICAL STUDIES** and **PRECAUTIONS, Geriatric Use**.)

4. Vision abnormalities
Retinal vascular thrombosis has been reported in patients receiving estrogen. Discontinue estrogen plus progestin therapy pending examination if there is sudden partial or complete loss of vision, or if there is a sudden onset of proptosis, diplopia or migraine. If examination reveals papilledema or retinal vascular lesions, estrogen plus progestin therapy should be permanently discontinued.

PRECAUTIONS
A. General
1. Addition of a progestin when a woman has not had a hysterectomy
Studies of the addition of a progestin for 10 or more days of a cycle of estrogen administration, or daily with estrogen in a continuous regimen, have reported a lowered incidence of endometrial hyperplasia than would be induced by estrogen treatment alone. Endometrial hyperplasia may be a precursor to endometrial cancer.

There are, however, possible risks that may be associated with the use of progestins with estrogens compared with estrogen-alone regimens. These include an increased risk of breast cancer.

2. Fluid Retention
Progesterone may cause some degree of fluid retention. Women with conditions that might be influenced by this factor, such as cardiac or renal dysfunction, warrant careful observation.

Continued on next page

3. Dizziness and Drowsiness
PROMETRIUM® (progesterone, USP) Capsules may cause transient dizziness and drowsiness and should be used with caution when driving a motor vehicle or operating machinery. PROMETRIUM Capsules should be taken as a single daily dose at bedtime.

B. Patient Information
General: **This product contains peanut oil and should not be used if you are allergic to peanuts.**
Physicians are advised to discuss the contents of the Patient Information leaflet with patients for whom they prescribe PROMETRIUM Capsules.

C. Drug-Laboratory Test Interactions
The following laboratory results may be altered by the use of estrogen plus progestin therapy:
• Increased sulfobromophthalein retention and other hepatic function tests.
• Coagulation tests: increase in prothrombin factors VII, VIII, IX and X.
• Pregnanediol determination.
• Thyroid function: increase in PBI, and butanol extractable protein bound iodine and decrease in T3 uptake values.

D. Carcinogenesis, Mutagenesis, Impairment of Fertility
Progesterone has not been tested for carcinogenicity in animals by the oral route of administration. When implanted into female mice, progesterone produced mammary carcinomas, ovarian granulosa cell tumors and endometrial stromal sarcomas. In dogs, long-term intramuscular injections produced nodular hyperplasia and benign and malignant mammary tumors. Subcutaneous or intramuscular injections of progesterone decreased the latency period and increased the incidence of mammary tumors in rats previously treated with a chemical carcinogen.
Progesterone did not show evidence of genotoxicity in *in vitro* studies for point mutations or for chromosomal damage. *In vivo* studies for chromosome damage have yielded positive results in mice at oral doses of 1000 mg/kg and 2000 mg/kg. Exogenously administered progesterone has been shown to inhibit ovulation in a number of species and it is expected that high doses given for an extended duration would impair fertility until the cessation of treatment.

E. Pregnancy
PROMETRIUM Capsules should not be used during pregnancy. (See **CONTRAINDICATIONS**).
Pregnancy Category B: Reproductive studies have been performed in mice at doses up to 9 times the human oral dose, in rats at doses up to 44 times the human oral dose, in rabbits at a dose of 10 mcg/day delivered locally within the uterus by an implanted device, in guinea pigs at doses of approximately one-half the human oral dose and in rhesus monkeys at doses approximately the human dose, all based on body surface area, and have revealed little or no evidence of impaired fertility or harm to the fetus due to progesterone.

F. Nursing Women
Detectable amounts of progestin have been identified in the milk of nursing women receiving progestins. Caution should be exercised when PROMETRIUM Capsules are administered to a nursing woman.

G. Pediatric Use
PROMETRIUM Capsules are not indicated in children. Clinical studies have not been conducted in the pediatric population.

H. Geriatric Use
There have not been sufficient numbers of geriatric women involved in clinical studies utilizing PROMETRIUM Capsules to determine whether those over 65 years of age differ from younger subjects in their response to PROMETRIUM Capsules.

The Women's Health Initiative Study
In the Women's Health Initiative (WHI) estrogen plus progestin substudy (daily CE [0.625 mg] plus MPA [2.5 mg] versus placebo), there was a higher relative risk of nonfatal stroke and invasive breast cancer in women greater than 65 years of age. (See **CLINICAL STUDIES** and **WARNINGS**, **Cardiovascular disorders** and **Malignant neoplasms**.)
The Women's Health Initiative Memory Study
In the Women's Health Initiative Memory Study (WHIMS) of postmenopausal women 65 to 79 years of age, there was an increased risk of developing probable dementia in the estrogen plus progestin ancillary study when compared to placebo. (See **CLINICAL STUDIES** and **WARNINGS, Probable dementia**.)

ADVERSE REACTIONS
See **BOXED WARNING**, **WARNINGS** and **PRECAUTIONS**.
Because clinical trials are conducted under widely varying conditions, adverse reaction rates observed in the clinical trials of a drug cannot be directly compared to rates in the clinical trials of another drug and may not reflect the rates observed in practice.
In a multicenter, randomized, double-blind, placebo-controlled clinical trial, the effects of PROMETRIUM Capsules on the endometrium was studied in a total of 875 postmenopausal women. Table 6 lists adverse reactions greater than or equal to 2 percent of women who received cyclic PROMETRIUM Capsules 200 mg daily (12 days per calendar month cycle) with 0.625 mg conjugated estrogens or placebo.

TABLE 3. Incidence of Endometrial Hyperplasia in Women Receiving 3 Years of Treatment

Endometrial Diagnosis	Treatment Group					
	Conjugated Estrogens 0.625 mg + PROMETRIUM Capsules 200 mg (cyclical)		Conjugated Estrogens 0.625 mg (alone)		Placebo	
	Number of patients	% of patients	Number of patients	% of patients	Number of patients	% of patients
	n=117		n=115		n=116	
HYPERPLASIA [a]	7	6	74	64	3	3
Adenocarcinoma	0	0	0	0	1	1
Atypical hyperplasia	1	1	14	12	0	0
Complex hyperplasia	0	0	27	23	1	1
Simple hyperplasia	6	5	33	29	1	1

[a] Most advanced result to least advanced result:
Adenocarcinoma > atypical hyperplasia > complex hyperplasia > simple hyperplasia

TABLE 4. Discontinuation Rate Due to Hyperplasia Over 36 Months of Treatment

Most Advanced Biopsy Result Through 36 Months of Treatment	Treatment Group					
	Conjugated Estrogens + PROMETRIUM Capsules (cyclical)		Conjugated Estrogens (alone)		Placebo	
	n=120		n=119		n=119	
	Number of patients	% of patients	Number of patients	% of patients	Number of patients	% of patients
Adenocarcinoma	0	0	0	0	1	1
Atypical hyperplasia	1	1	10	8	0	0
Complex hyperplasia	0	0	21	18	1	1
Simple hyperplasia	1	1	13	11	0	0

TABLE 6. Adverse Reactions (≥ 2%) Reported in an 875 Patient Placebo-Controlled Trial in Postmenopausal Women Over a 3-Year Period [Percentage (%) of Patients Reporting]

	PROMETRIUM Capsules 200 mg with Conjugated Estrogens 0.625 mg	Placebo
	(n=178)	(n=174)
Headache	31	27
Breast Tenderness	27	6
Joint Pain	20	29
Depression	19	12
Dizziness	15	9
Abdominal Bloating	12	5
Hot Flashes	11	35
Urinary Problems	11	9
Abdominal Pain	10	10
Vaginal Discharge	10	3
Nausea / Vomiting	8	7
Worry	8	4
Chest Pain	7	5
Diarrhea	7	4
Night Sweats	7	17
Breast Pain	6	2
Swelling of Hands and Feet	6	9
Vaginal Dryness	6	10

TABLE 5. Relative and Absolute Risk Seen in the Estrogen Plus Progestin Substudy of WHI at an Average of 5.6 Years[a, b]

Event	Relative Risk CE/MPA versus Placebo (95% nCI [c])	CE/MPA n = 8,506	Placebo n = 8,102
		Absolute Risk per 10,000 Women-Years	
CHD events	1.23 (0.99-1.53)	41	34
Non-fatal MI	*1.28 (1.00-1.63)*	*31*	*25*
CHD death	*1.10 (0.70-1.75)*	*8*	*8*
All stroke	1.31 (1.03-1.88)	33	25
Ischemic Stroke	*1.44 (1.09-1.90)*	*26*	*18*
Deep vein thrombosis [d]	1.95 (1.43-2.67)	26	13
Pulmonary embolism	2.13 (1.45-3.11)	18	8
Invasive breast cancer [e]	1.24 (1.01-1.54)	41	33
Colorectal cancer	0.61 (0.42-0.87)	10	16
Endometrial cancer [d]	0.81 (0.48-1.36)	6	7
Cervical cancer [d]	1.44 (0.47-4.42)	2	1
Hip fracture	0.67 (0.47-0.96)	11	16
Vertebral fractures [d]	0.65 (0.46-0.92)	11	17
Lower arm/wrist fractures [d]	0.71 (0.59-0.85)	44	62
Total fractures [d]	0.76 (0.69-0.83)	152	199
Overall mortality [f]	1.00 (0.83-1.19)	52	52
Global Index [g]	1.13 (1.02-1.25)	184	165

[a] Adapted from numerous WHI publications. WHI publications can be viewed at www.nhlbi.nih.gov/whi.
[b] Results are based on centrally adjudicated data.
[c] Nominal confidence intervals unadjusted for multiple looks and multiple comparisons.
[d] Not included in Global Index.
[e] Includes metastatic and non-metastatic breast cancer with the exception of *in situ* breast cancer.
[f] All deaths, except from breast or colorectal cancer, definite or probable CHD, PE or cerebrovascular disease.
[g] A subset of the events was combined in a "global index" defined as the earliest occurrence of CHD events, invasive breast cancer, stroke, pulmonary embolism, endometrial cancer, colorectal cancer, hip fracture, or death due to other causes.

Constipation	3	2		Abdominal Pain (Cramping)	20	13
Breast Carcinoma	2	<1		Diarrhea	8	4
Breast Excisional Biopsy	2	<1		Nausea	8	0
Cholecystectomy	2	<1		Back Pain	8	8
				Musculoskeletal Pain	12	4
				Irritability	8	4
				Breast Pain	16	8
				Infection Viral	12	0
				Coughing	8	0

Effects on Secondary Amenorrhea

In a multicenter, randomized, double-blind, placebo-controlled clinical trial, the effects of PROMETRIUM® (progesterone, USP) Capsules on secondary amenorrhea was studied in 49 estrogen-primed postmenopausal women. Table 7 lists adverse reactions greater than or equal to 5 percent of women who received PROMETRIUM Capsules or placebo.

TABLE 7. Adverse Reactions (≥ 5%) Reported in Patients Using 400 mg/day in a Placebo-Controlled Trial in Estrogen-Primed Postmenopausal Women

Adverse Experience	PROMETRIUM Capsules 400 mg	Placebo
	n=25	n=24
	Percentage (%) of Patients	
Fatigue	8	4
Headache	16	8
Dizziness	24	4
Abdominal Distension (Bloating)	8	8

In a multicenter, parallel-group, open label postmarketing dosing study consisting of three consecutive 28-day treatment cycles, 220 premenopausal women with secondary amenorrhea were randomized to receive daily conjugated estrogens therapy (0.625 mg conjugated estrogens) and PROMETRIUM Capsules, 300 mg per day (n=113) or PROMETRIUM Capsules, 400 mg per /day (n=107) for 10 days of each treatment cycle. Overall, the most frequently reported treatment-emergent adverse reactions, reported in greater than or equal to 5 percent of subjects, were nausea, fatigue, vaginal mycosis, nasopharyngitis, upper respiratory tract infection, headache, dizziness, breast tenderness, abdominal distension, acne, dysmenorrhea, mood swing, and urinary tract infection.

Postmarketing Experience:
The following additional adverse reactions have been reported with PROMETRIUM Capsules. Because these reactions are reported voluntarily from a population of uncertain size, it is not always possible to reliably estimate the frequency or establish a causal relationship to drug exposure.

Genitourinary System: endometrial carcinoma, hypospadia, intra-uterine death, menorrhagia, menstrual disorder, metrorrhagia, ovarian cyst, spontaneous abortion.
Cardiovascular: circulatory collapse, congenital heart disease (including ventricular septal defect and patent ductus arteriosus), hypertension, hypotension, tachycardia.
Gastrointestinal: acute pancreatitis, cholestasis, cholestatic hepatitis, dysphagia, hepatic failure, hepatic necrosis, hepatitis, increased liver function tests (including alanine aminotransferase increased, aspartate aminotransferase increased, gamma-glutamyl transferase increased), jaundice, swollen tongue.
Skin: alopecia, pruritus, urticaria.
Eyes: blurred vision, diplopia, visual disturbance.
Central Nervous System: aggression, convulsion, depersonalization, depressed consciousness, disorientation, dysarthria, loss of consciousness, paresthesia, sedation, stupor, syncope (with and without hypotension), transient ischemic attack, suicidal ideation.
During initial therapy, a few women have experienced a constellation of many or all of the following symptoms: extreme dizziness and/or drowsiness, blurred vision, slurred speech, difficulty walking, loss of consciousness, vertigo, confusion, disorientation, feeling drunk, and shortness of breath.
Miscellaneous: abnormal gait, anaphylactic reaction, arthralgia, blood glucose increased, choking, cleft lip, cleft palate, difficulty walking, dyspnea, face edema, feeling abnormal, feeling drunk, hypersensitivity, asthma, muscle cramp, throat tightness, tinnitus, vertigo, weight decreased, weight increased.

OVERDOSAGE

No studies on overdosage have been conducted in humans. In the case of overdosage, PROMETRIUM® (progesterone, USP) Capsules should be discontinued and the patient should be treated symptomatically.

DOSAGE AND ADMINISTRATION

Prevention of Endometrial Hyperplasia
PROMETRIUM Capsules should be given as a single daily dose at bedtime, 200 mg orally for 12 days sequentially per 28-day cycle, to a postmenopausal woman with a uterus who is receiving daily conjugated estrogens tablets.

Treatment of Secondary Amenorrhea
PROMETRIUM Capsules may be given as a single daily dose of 400 mg at bedtime for 10 days.
Some women may experience difficulty swallowing PROMETRIUM Capsules. For these women, PROMETRIUM Capsules should be taken with a glass of water while in the standing position.

HOW SUPPLIED

PROMETRIUM (progesterone, USP) Capsules 100 mg are round, peach-colored capsules branded with black imprint "SV."
NDC 0032-1708-01 (Bottle of 100)
PROMETRIUM (progesterone, USP) Capsules 200 mg are oval, pale yellow-colored capsules branded with black imprint "SV2."
NDC 0032-1711-01 (Bottle of 100)
Store at 25°C (77°F); excursions permitted to 15° to 30°C (59° to 86°F) [See USP Controlled Room Temperature].
Protect from excessive moisture.
Dispense in tight, light-resistant container as defined in USP/NF, accompanied by a Patient Insert.
Keep out of reach of children.
Manufactured by:
Catalent Pharma Solutions
St. Petersburg, FL 33716
Marketed by:
AbbVie Inc.
North Chicago, IL 60064, USA
© AbbVie Inc. 2013
Ref: 500032 Rev 09/13 - Revised: September, 2013

Continued on next page

Information on the AbbVie, Inc. products listed on these pages is from the prescribing information in use as of July 31, 2016. For more information, please visit rxabbvie.com or call 1-800-633-9110.

PATIENT INFORMATION

PROMETRIUM® (progesterone, USP)

Capsules 100 mg

Capsules 200 mg

Read this PATIENT INFORMATION before you start taking PROMETRIUM® (progesterone, USP) Capsules and read what you get each time you refill your PROMETRIUM Capsules prescription. There may be new information. This information does not take the place of talking to your healthcare provider about your medical condition or your treatment.

WHAT IS THE MOST IMPORTANT INFORMATION I SHOULD KNOW ABOUT PROMETRIUM CAPSULES (A Progesterone Hormone)?

- Progestins with estrogens should not be used to prevent heart disease, heart attacks, strokes, or dementia.
- Using progestins with estrogens may increase your chance of getting heart attacks, strokes, breast cancer, and blood clots.
- Using progestins with estrogens may increase your chance of getting dementia, based on a study of women age 65 and older.
- You and your healthcare provider should talk regularly about whether you still need treatment with PROMETRIUM Capsules.

THIS PRODUCT CONTAINS PEANUT OIL AND SHOULD NOT BE USED IF YOU ARE ALLERGIC TO PEANUTS.

What is PROMETRIUM Capsules?

PROMETRIUM Capsules contain the female hormone called progesterone.

What is PROMETRIUM Capsules used for?

Treatment of Menstrual Irregularities

PROMETRIUM Capsules are used for the treatment of secondary amenorrhea (absence of menstrual periods in women who have previously had a menstrual period) due to a decrease in progesterone. When you do not produce enough progesterone, menstrual irregularities can occur. If your healthcare provider has determined your body does not produce enough progesterone on its own, PROMETRIUM Capsules may be prescribed to provide the progesterone you need.

Protection of the Endometrium (Lining of the Uterus)

PROMETRIUM Capsules are used in combination with estrogen-containing medications in a postmenopausal woman with a uterus (womb). Taking estrogen-alone increases the chance of developing a condition called endometrial hyperplasia that may lead to cancer of the lining of the uterus (womb). The addition of a progestin is generally recommended for a woman with a uterus to reduce the chance of getting cancer of the uterus (womb).

Who should not take PROMETRIUM Capsules?

Do not start taking PROMETRIUM Capsules if you:

- Are allergic to peanuts
- Have unusual vaginal bleeding
- Currently have or have had certain cancers

   Estrogen plus progestin treatment may increase the chance of getting certain types of cancers, including cancer of the breast or uterus. If you have or have had cancer, talk with your healthcare provider about whether you should take PROMETRIUM Capsules.

- Had a stroke or heart attack
- Currently have or have had blood clots
- Currently have or have had liver problems
- Are allergic to PROMETRIUM Capsules or any of its ingredients

   See the list of ingredients in PROMETRIUM Capsules at the end of this leaflet.

- Think you may be pregnant

Tell your healthcare provider:

- If you are breastfeeding. The hormone in PROMETRIUM Capsules can pass into your breast milk.
- About all of your medical problems. Your healthcare provider may need to check you more carefully if you have certain conditions, such as asthma (wheezing), epilepsy (seizures), diabetes, migraine, endometriosis, lupus, problems with your heart, liver, thyroid, or kidneys, or have high calcium levels in your blood.
- About all the medicines you take. This includes prescription and nonprescription medicines, vitamins, and herbal supplements. Some medicines may affect how PROMETRIUM Capsules work. PROMETRIUM Capsules may also affect how your other medicines work.

How should I take PROMETRIUM Capsules?

1. Prevention of Endometrial Hyperplasia: A postmenopausal woman with a uterus who is taking estrogens should take a single daily dose of 200 mg PROMETRIUM Capsules at bedtime for 12 continuous days per 28-day cycle.

2. Secondary Amenorrhea: PROMETRIUM Capsules may be given as a single daily dose of 400 mg at bedtime for 10 days.

3. PROMETRIUM Capsules are to be taken at bedtime as some women become very drowsy and/or dizzy after taking PROMETRIUM Capsules. In a few cases, symptoms may include blurred vision, difficulty speaking, difficulty with walking, and feeling abnormal. If you experience these symptoms, discuss them with your healthcare provider right away.

4. If you experience difficulty in swallowing PROMETRIUM Capsules, it is recommended that you take your daily dose at bedtime with a glass of water while in the standing position.

What are the possible side effects of PROMETRIUM Capsules?

Side effects are grouped by how serious they are and how often they happen when you are treated:

Serious, but less common side effects include:

- *Risk to the Fetus:* Cases of cleft palate, cleft lip, hypospadias, ventricular septal defect, patent ductus arteriosus, and other congenital heart defects.
- *Abnormal Blood Clotting:* Stroke, heart attack, pulmonary embolus, visual loss or blindness.

Some of the warning signs of serious side effects include:

- Changes in vision or speech
- Sudden new severe headaches
- Severe pains in your chest or legs with or without shortness of breath, weakness and fatigue
- Dizziness and faintness
- Vomiting

Call your healthcare provider right away if you get any of these warning signs, or any other unusual symptoms that concern you.

Less serious, but common side effects include:

- Headaches
- Breast pain
- Irregular vaginal bleeding or spotting
- Stomach or abdominal cramps, bloating
- Nausea and vomiting
- Hair loss
- Fluid retention
- Vaginal yeast infection

These are not all the possible side effects of PROMETRIUM Capsules. For more information, ask your healthcare provider or pharmacist for advice about side effects. You may report side effects to AbbVie Inc. at 1-800-633-9110 or to FDA at 1-800-FDA-1088.

What can I do to lower my chances of getting a serious side effect with PROMETRIUM Capsules?

- Talk with your healthcare provider regularly about whether you should continue taking PROMETRIUM Capsules.
- See your healthcare provider right away if you get unusual vaginal bleeding while taking PROMETRIUM Capsules.
- Have a pelvic exam, breast exam, and mammogram (breast X-ray) every year unless your healthcare provider tells you something else. If members of your family have had breast cancer or if you have ever had breast lumps or an abnormal mammogram, you may need to have breast exams more often.
- If you have high blood pressure, high cholesterol (fat in the blood), diabetes, are overweight, or if you use tobacco, you may have higher chances for getting heart disease. Ask your healthcare provider for ways to lower your chances for getting heart disease.

General information about safe and effective use of PROMETRIUM Capsules

- Medicines are sometimes prescribed for conditions that are not mentioned in patient information leaflets. Do not take PROMETRIUM Capsules for conditions for which it was not prescribed.
- Your healthcare provider has prescribed this drug for you and you alone. Do not give PROMETRIUM Capsules to other people, even if they have the same symptoms you have. It may harm them.
- PROMETRIUM Capsules should be taken as a single daily dose at bedtime. Some women may experience extreme dizziness and/or drowsiness during initial therapy. In a few cases, symptoms may include blurred vision, difficulty speaking, difficulty with walking, and feeling abnormal. If you experience these symptoms, discuss them with your healthcare provider right away.

- Use caution when driving a motor vehicle or operating machinery as dizziness or drowsiness may occur.

Keep PROMETRIUM Capsules out of the reach of children.

This leaflet provides a summary of the most important information about PROMETRIUM Capsules. If you would like more information, talk with your healthcare provider or pharmacist. You can ask for information about PROMETRIUM Capsules that is written for health professionals. You can get more information by calling the toll free number 1-800-633-9110.

What are the ingredients in PROMETRIUM Capsules?

Active ingredient: 100 mg or 200 mg micronized progesterone

The inactive ingredients for PROMETRIUM Capsules 100 mg include: peanut oil NF, gelatin NF, glycerin USP, lecithin NF, titanium dioxide USP, FD&C Red No. 40, and D&C Yellow No. 10.

The inactive ingredients for PROMETRIUM Capsules 200 mg include: peanut oil NF, gelatin NF, glycerin USP, lecithin NF, titanium dioxide USP, D&C Yellow No. 10, and FD&C Yellow No. 6.

HOW SUPPLIED

PROMETRIUM Capsules 100 mg are round, peach-colored capsules branded with black imprint "SV."

PROMETRIUM Capsules 200 mg are oval, pale yellow-colored capsules branded with black imprint "SV2."

Store at 25°C (77°F); excursions permitted to 15° to 30°C (59° to 86°F) [See USP Controlled Room Temperature].

Protect from excessive moisture.

Manufactured by:

Catalent Pharma Solutions

St. Petersburg, FL 33716

Marketed by:

AbbVie Inc.

North Chicago, IL 60064, USA

© AbbVie Inc. 2013

Ref: 500033 Rev 09/13 - Revised: September, 2013

SURVANTA®   ℞

(beractant)

intratracheal suspension

Sterile Suspension

For Intratracheal Administration Only

DESCRIPTION

SURVANTA® (beractant) Intratracheal Suspension is a sterile, non-pyrogenic pulmonary surfactant intended for intratracheal use only. It is a natural bovine lung extract containing phospholipids, neutral lipids, fatty acids, and surfactant-associated proteins to which colfosceril palmitate (dipalmitoylphosphatidylcholine), palmitic acid, and tripalmitin are added to standardize the composition and to mimic surface-tension lowering properties of natural lung surfactant. The resulting composition provides 25 mg/mL phospholipids (including 11.0-15.5 mg/mL disaturated phosphatidylcholine), 0.5-1.75 mg/mL triglycerides, 1.4-3.5 mg/mL free fatty acids, and less than 1.0 mg/mL protein. It is suspended in 0.9% sodium chloride solution, and heat-sterilized. SURVANTA contains no preservatives. Its protein content consists of two hydrophobic, low molecular weight, surfactant-associated proteins commonly known as SP-B and SP-C. It does not contain the hydrophilic, large molecular weight surfactant-associated protein known as SP-A.

Each mL of SURVANTA contains 25 mg of phospholipids. It is an off-white to light brown liquid supplied in single-use glass vials containing 4 mL (100 mg phospholipids) or 8 mL (200 mg phospholipids).

CLINICAL PHARMACOLOGY

Endogenous pulmonary surfactant lowers surface tension on alveolar surfaces during respiration and stabilizes the alveoli against collapse at resting transpulmonary pressures. Deficiency of pulmonary surfactant causes Respiratory Distress Syndrome (RDS) in premature infants. SURVANTA replenishes surfactant and restores surface activity to the lungs of these infants.

Activity

In vitro, SURVANTA reproducibly lowers minimum surface tension to less than 8 dynes/cm as measured by the pulsating bubble surfactometer and Wilhelmy Surface Balance. *In situ*, SURVANTA restores pulmonary compliance to excised rat lungs artificially made surfactant-deficient.

In vivo, single SURVANTA doses improve lung pressure-volume measurements, lung compliance, and oxygenation in premature rabbits and sheep.

Animal Metabolism

SURVANTA is administered directly to the target organ, the lungs, where biophysical effects occur at the alveolar surface. In surfactant-deficient premature rabbits and lambs, alveolar clearance of radio-labelled lipid components of SURVANTA is rapid. Most of the dose becomes lung-associated within hours of administration, and the lipids enter endogenous surfactant pathways of reutilization and recycling. In surfactant-sufficient adult animals, SURVANTA clearance is more rapid than in premature and young animals. There is less reutilization and recycling of surfactant in adult animals.

Limited animal experiments have not found effects of SURVANTA on endogenous surfactant metabolism. Precursor incorporation and subsequent secretion of saturated phosphatidylcholine in premature sheep are not changed by SURVANTA treatments.

No information is available about the metabolic fate of the surfactant-associated proteins in SURVANTA. The metabolic disposition in humans has not been studied.

Clinical Studies

Clinical effects of SURVANTA were demonstrated in six single-dose and four multiple-dose randomized, multicenter, controlled clinical trials involving approximately 1700 infants. Three open trials, including a Treatment IND, involved more than 8500 infants. Each dose of SURVANTA in all studies was 100 mg phospholipids/kg birth weight and was based on published experience with Surfactant TA, a lyophilized powder dosage form of SURVANTA having the same composition.

Prevention Studies

Infants of 600-1250 g birth weight and 23 to 29 weeks estimated gestational age were enrolled in two *multiple-dose* studies. A dose of SURVANTA was given within 15 minutes of birth to prevent the development of RDS. Up to three additional doses in the first 48 hours, as often as every 6 hours, were given if RDS subsequently developed and infants required mechanical ventilation with an $FiO_2 \geq 0.30$. Results of the studies at 28 days of age are shown in Table 1.

TABLE 1

Study 1

	SURVANTA	Control	P-Value
Number infants studied	119	124	
Incidence of RDS (%)	27.6	63.5	< 0.001
Death due to RDS (%)	2.5	19.5	< 0.001
Death or BPD due to RDS (%)	48.7	52.8	0.536
Death due to any cause (%)	7.6	22.8	0.001
Air Leaks[a] (%)	5.9	21.7	0.001
Pulmonary interstitial emphysema (%)	20.8	40.0	0.001

Study 2[b]

	SURVANTA	Control	P-Value
Number infants studied	91	96	
Incidence of RDS (%)	28.6	48.3	0.007
Death due to RDS (%)	1.1	10.5	0.006
Death or BPD due to RDS (%)	27.5	44.2	0.018
Death due to any cause [c](%)	16.5	13.7	0.633
Air Leaks [a](%)	14.5	19.6	0.374
Pulmonary interstitial emphysema (%)	26.5	33.2	0.298

[a]Pneumothorax or pneumopericardium
[b]Study discontinued when Treatment IND initiated
[c]No cause of death in the SURVANTA group was significantly increased; the higher number of deaths in this group was due to the sum of all causes.

Rescue Studies

Infants of 600-1750 g birth weight with RDS requiring mechanical ventilation and an $FiO_2 \geq 0.40$ were enrolled in two *multiple-dose* rescue studies. The initial dose of SURVANTA was given after RDS developed and before 8 hours of age.

Infants could receive up to three additional doses in the first 48 hours, as often as every 6 hours, if they required mechanical ventilation and an $FiO_2 \geq 0.30$. Results of the studies at 28 days of age are shown in Table 2.

TABLE 2

Study 3[a]

	SURVANTA	Control	P-Value
Number infants studied	198	193	
Death due to RDS (%)	11.6	18.1	0.071
Death or BPD due to RDS (%)	59.1	66.8	0.102
Death due to any cause (%)	21.7	26.4	0.285
Air Leaks[b] (%)	11.8	29.5	<0.001
Pulmonary interstitial emphysema (%)	16.3	34.0	<0.001

Study 4

	SURVANTA	Control	P-Value
Number infants studied	204	203	
Death due to RDS (%)	6.4	22.3	< 0.001
Death or BPD due to RDS (%)	43.6	63.4	< 0.001
Death due to any cause (%)	15.2	28.2	0.001
Air Leaks[b] (%)	11.2	22.2	0.005
Pulmonary interstitial emphysema (%)	20.8	44.4	< 0.001

[a]Study discontinued when Treatment IND initiated
[b]Pneumothorax or pneumopericardium

Acute Clinical Effects

Marked improvements in oxygenation may occur within minutes of administration of SURVANTA.

All controlled clinical studies with SURVANTA provided information regarding the acute effects of SURVANTA on the arterial-alveolar oxygen ratio (a/APO₂), FiO_2, and mean airway pressure (MAP) during the first 48 to 72 hours of life. Significant improvements in these variables were sustained for 48-72 hours in SURVANTA-treated infants in four single-dose and two multiple-dose rescue studies and in two multiple-dose prevention studies. In the single-dose prevention studies, the FiO_2 improved significantly.

Indications and Usage

SURVANTA is indicated for prevention and treatment ("rescue") of Respiratory Distress Syndrome (RDS) (hyaline membrane disease) in premature infants. SURVANTA significantly reduces the incidence of RDS, mortality due to RDS and air leak complications.

Prevention

In premature infants less than 1250 g birth weight or with evidence of surfactant deficiency, give SURVANTA as soon as possible, preferably within 15 minutes of birth.

Rescue

To treat infants with RDS confirmed by x-ray and requiring mechanical ventilation, give SURVANTA as soon as possible, preferably by 8 hours of age.

Contraindications

None known.

Warnings

SURVANTA is intended for intratracheal use only.
SURVANTA CAN RAPIDLY AFFECT OXYGENATION AND LUNG COMPLIANCE. Therefore, its use should be restricted to a highly supervised clinical setting with immediate availability of clinicians experienced with intubation, ventilator management, and general care of premature infants. Infants receiving SURVANTA should be frequently monitored with arterial or transcutaneous measurement of systemic oxygen and carbon dioxide.
DURING THE DOSING PROCEDURE, TRANSIENT EPISODES OF BRADYCARDIA AND DECREASED OXYGEN SATURATION HAVE BEEN REPORTED. If these occur, stop the dosing procedure and initiate appropriate measures to alleviate the condition. After stabilization, resume the dosing procedure.

Precautions
General

Rales and moist breath sounds can occur transiently after administration. Endotracheal suctioning or other remedial action is not necessary unless clear-cut signs of airway obstruction are present.

Increased probability of post-treatment nosocomial sepsis in SURVANTA-treated infants was observed in the controlled clinical trials (Table 3). The increased risk for sepsis among SURVANTA-treated infants was not associated with increased mortality among these infants. The causative organisms were similar in treated and control infants. There was no significant difference between groups in the rate of post-treatment infections other than sepsis.

Use of SURVANTA in infants less than 600 g birth weight or greater than 1750 g birth weight has not been evaluated in controlled trials. There is no controlled experience with use of SURVANTA in conjunction with experimental therapies for RDS (eg, high-frequency ventilation or extracorporeal membrane oxygenation).

No information is available on the effects of doses other than 100 mg phospholipids/kg, more than four doses, dosing more frequently than every 6 hours, or administration after 48 hours of age.

Carcinogenesis, Mutagenesis, Impairment of Fertility

Carcinogenicity studies have not been performed with SURVANTA. SURVANTA was negative when tested in the Ames test for mutagenicity. Using the maximum feasible dose volume, SURVANTA up to 500 mg phospholipids/kg/day (approximately one-third the premature infant dose based on mg/m²/day) was administered subcutaneously to newborn rats for 5 days. The rats reproduced normally and there were no observable adverse effects in their offspring.

Adverse Reactions

The most commonly reported adverse experiences were associated with the dosing procedure. In the multiple-dose controlled clinical trials, each dose of SURVANTA was divided into four quarter-doses which were instilled through a catheter inserted into the endotracheal tube by briefly disconnecting the endotracheal tube from the ventilator. Transient bradycardia occurred with 11.9% of *doses.* Oxygen desaturation occurred with 9.8% of *doses.*

Other reactions during the dosing procedure occurred with fewer than 1% of doses and included endotracheal tube reflux, pallor, vasoconstriction, hypotension, endotracheal tube blockage, hypertension, hypocarbia, hypercarbia, and apnea. No deaths occurred during the dosing procedure, and all reactions resolved with symptomatic treatment.

The occurrence of concurrent illnesses common in premature infants was evaluated in the controlled trials. The rates in all controlled studies are in Table 3.

TABLE 3

| Concurrent Event | All Controlled Studies | | |
	SURVANTA (%)	Control (%)	P-Value[a]
Patent ductus arteriosus	46.9	47.1	0.814
Intracranial hemorrhage	48.1	45.2	0.241
Severe intracranial hemorrhage	24.1	23.3	0.693
Pulmonary air leaks	10.9	24.7	< 0.001
Pulmonary interstitial emphysema	20.2	38.4	< 0.001
Necrotizing enterocolitis	6.1	5.3	0.427
Apnea	65.4	59.6	0.283
Severe apnea	46.1	42.5	0.114
Post-treatment sepsis	20.7	16.1	0.019
Post-treatment infection	10.2	9.1	0.345
Pulmonary hemorrhage	7.2	5.3	0.166

[a]P-value comparing groups in controlled studies

When all controlled studies were pooled, there was no difference in intracranial hemorrhage. However, in one of the single-dose rescue studies and one of the multiple-dose prevention studies, the rate of intracranial hemorrhage was significantly higher in SURVANTA patients than control patients (63.3% *v* 30.8%, P = 0.001; and 48.8% *v* 34.2%, P = 0.047, respectively). The rate in a Treatment IND involving approximately 8100 infants was lower than in the controlled trials.

Continued on next page

Information on the AbbVie, Inc. products listed on these pages is from the prescribing information in use as of July 31, 2016. For more information, please visit rxabbvie.com or call 1-800-633-9110.

In the controlled clinical trials, there was no effect of SURVANTA on results of common laboratory tests: white blood cell count and serum sodium, potassium, bilirubin, and creatinine.

More than 4300 pretreatment and post-treatment serum samples from approximately 1500 patients were tested by Western Blot Immunoassay for antibodies to surfactant-associated proteins SP-B and SP-C. No IgG or IgM antibodies were detected.

Several other complications are known to occur in premature infants. The following conditions were reported in the controlled clinical studies. The rates of the complications were not different in treated and control infants, and none of the complications were attributed to SURVANTA.

Respiratory
lung consolidation, blood from the endotracheal tube, deterioration after weaning, respiratory decompensation, subglottic stenosis, paralyzed diaphragm, respiratory failure.

Cardiovascular
hypotension, hypertension, tachycardia, ventricular tachycardia, aortic thrombosis, cardiac failure, cardio-respiratory arrest, increased apical pulse, persistent fetal circulation, air embolism, total anomalous pulmonary venous return.

Gastrointestinal
abdominal distention, hemorrhage, intestinal perforations, volvulus, bowel infarct, feeding intolerance, hepatic failure, stress ulcer.

Renal
renal failure, hematuria.

Hematologic
coagulopathy, thrombocytopenia, disseminated intravascular coagulation.

Central Nervous System
seizures.

Endocrine/Metabolic
adrenal hemorrhage, inappropriate ADH secretion, hyperphosphatemia.

Musculoskeletal
inguinal hernia.

Systemic
fever, deterioration.

Follow-Up Evaluations
To date, no long-term complications or sequelae of SURVANTA therapy have been found.

Single-Dose Studies
Six-month adjusted-age follow-up evaluations of 232 infants (115 treated) demonstrated no clinically important differences between treatment groups in pulmonary and neurologic sequelae, incidence or severity of retinopathy of prematurity, rehospitalizations, growth, or allergic manifestations.

Multiple-Dose Studies
Six-month adjusted age follow-up evaluations have been completed in 631 (345 treated) of 916 surviving infants. There were significantly less cerebral palsy and need for supplemental oxygen in SURVANTA infants than controls. Wheezing at the time of examination was significantly more frequent among SURVANTA infants, although there was no difference in bronchodilator therapy.

Final twelve-month follow-up data from the multiple-dose studies are available from 521 (272 treated) of 909 surviving infants. There was significantly less wheezing in SURVANTA infants than controls, in contrast to the six-month results. There was no difference in the incidence of cerebral palsy at twelve months.

Twenty-four month adjusted age evaluations were completed in 429 (226 treated) of 906 surviving infants. There were significantly fewer SURVANTA infants with rhonchi, wheezing, and tachypnea at the time of examination. No other differences were found.

Overdosage
Overdosage with SURVANTA has not been reported. Based on animal data, overdosage might result in acute airway obstruction. Treatment should be symptomatic and supportive.

Rales and moist breath sounds can transiently occur after SURVANTA is given, and do not indicate overdosage. Endotracheal suctioning or other remedial action is not required unless clear-cut signs of airway obstruction are present.

Dosage and Administration
FOR INTRATRACHEAL ADMINISTRATION ONLY.
SURVANTA should be administered by or under the supervision of clinicians experienced in intubation, ventilator management, and general care of premature infants.

Marked improvements in oxygenation may occur within minutes of administration of SURVANTA. Therefore, frequent and careful clinical observation and monitoring of systemic oxygenation are essential to avoid hyperoxia.

Review of audiovisual instructional materials describing dosage and administration procedures is recommended before using SURVANTA. Materials are available upon request from AbbVie Inc.

Dosage
Each dose of SURVANTA is 100 mg of phospholipids/kg birth weight (4 mL/kg). The SURVANTA DOSING CHART shows the total dosage for a range of birth weights.

SURVANTA DOSING CHART			
Weight (grams)	Total Dose (mL)	Weight (grams)	Total Dose (mL)
600-650	2.6	1301-1350	5.4
651-700	2.8	1351-1400	5.6
701-750	3.0	1401-1450	5.8
751-800	3.2	1451-1500	6.0
801-850	3.4	1501-1550	6.2
851-900	3.6	1551-1600	6.4
901-950	3.8	1601-1650	6.6
951-1000	4.0	1651-1700	6.8
1001-1050	4.2	1701-1750	7.0
1051-1100	4.4	1751-1800	7.2
1101-1150	4.6	1801-1850	7.4
1151-1200	4.8	1851-1900	7.6
1201-1250	5.0	1901-1950	7.8
1251-1300	5.2	1951-2000	8.0

Four doses of SURVANTA can be administered in the first 48 hours of life. Doses should be given no more frequently than every 6 hours.

Directions for Use
SURVANTA should be inspected visually for discoloration prior to administration. The color of SURVANTA is off-white to light brown. If settling occurs during storage, swirl the vial gently (DO NOT SHAKE) to redisperse. Some foaming at the surface may occur during handling and is inherent in the nature of the product.

SURVANTA is stored refrigerated (2-8°C). Date and time need to be recorded in the box on front of the carton or vial, whenever SURVANTA is removed from the refrigerator. Before administration, SURVANTA should be warmed by standing at room temperature for at least 20 minutes or warmed in the hand for at least 8 minutes. ARTIFICIAL WARMING METHODS SHOULD NOT BE USED. If a prevention dose is to be given, preparation of SURVANTA should begin before the infant's birth.

Unopened, unused vials of SURVANTA that have been warmed to room temperature may be returned to the refrigerator within 24 hours of warming, and stored for future use. SURVANTA SHOULD NOT BE REMOVED FROM THE REFRIGERATOR FOR MORE THAN 24 HOURS. SURVANTA SHOULD NOT BE WARMED AND RETURNED TO THE REFRIGERATOR MORE THAN ONCE. Each single-use vial of SURVANTA should be entered only once. Used vials with residual drug should be discarded. SURVANTA DOES NOT REQUIRE RECONSTITUTION OR SONICATION BEFORE USE.

Dosing Procedures
General
SURVANTA is administered intratracheally by instillation through a 5 French end-hole catheter. The catheter can be inserted into the infant's endotracheal tube without interrupting ventilation by passing the catheter through a neonatal suction valve attached to the endotracheal tube. Alternatively, SURVANTA can be instilled through the catheter by briefly disconnecting the endotracheal tube from the ventilator.

The neonatal suction valve used for administering SURVANTA should be a type that allows entry of the catheter into the endotracheal tube without interrupting ventilation and also maintains a closed airway circuit system by sealing the valve around the catheter.

If the neonatal suction valve is used, the catheter should be rigid enough to pass easily into the endotracheal tube. A very soft and pliable catheter may twist or curl within the neonatal suction valve. The length of the catheter should be shortened so that the tip of the catheter protrudes just beyond the end of the endotracheal tube above the infant's carina. SURVANTA should not be instilled into a mainstem bronchus.

To ensure homogenous distribution of SURVANTA throughout the lungs, each dose is divided into *four quarter-doses*. Each quarter-dose is administered with the infant in a different position. The recommended positions are:
• Head and body inclined 5-10° down, head turned to the right
• Head and body inclined 5-10° down, head turned to the left
• Head and body inclined 5-10° up, head turned to the right
• Head and body inclined 5-10° up, head turned to the left
The dosing procedure is facilitated if one person administers the dose while another person positions and monitors the infant.

First Dose
Determine the total dose of SURVANTA from the SURVANTA DOSING CHART based on the infant's birth weight. Slowly withdraw the entire contents of the vial into a plastic syringe through a large-gauge needle (eg, at least 20 gauge). DO NOT FILTER SURVANTA AND AVOID SHAKING.

Attach the premeasured 5 French end-hole catheter to the syringe. Fill the catheter with SURVANTA. Discard excess SURVANTA through the catheter so that only the total dose to be given remains in the syringe.

BEFORE ADMINISTERING SURVANTA, assure proper placement and patency of the endotracheal tube. At the discretion of the clinician, the endotracheal tube may be suctioned before administering SURVANTA. The infant should be allowed to stabilize before proceeding with dosing.

In the prevention strategy, weigh, intubate and stabilize the infant. Administer the dose as soon as possible after birth, preferably within 15 minutes. Position the infant appropriately and gently inject the first quarter-dose through the catheter over 2-3 seconds.

After administration of the first quarter-dose, remove the catheter from the endotracheal tube. Manually ventilate with a hand-bag with sufficient oxygen to prevent cyanosis, at a rate of 60 breaths/minute, and sufficient positive pressure to provide adequate air exchange and chest wall excursion.

In the rescue strategy, the first dose should be given as soon as possible after the infant is placed on a ventilator for management of RDS. In the clinical trials, immediately before instilling the first quarter-dose, the infant's ventilator settings were changed to rate 60/minute, inspiratory time 0.5 second, and FiO_2 1.0.

Position the infant appropriately and gently inject the first quarter-dose through the catheter over 2-3 seconds. After administration of the first quarter-dose, remove the catheter from the endotracheal tube and continue mechanical ventilation.

In both strategies, ventilate the infant for at least 30 seconds or until stable. Reposition the infant for instillation of the next quarter-dose.

Instill the remaining quarter-doses using the same procedures. After instillation of each quarter-dose, remove the catheter and ventilate for at least 30 seconds or until the infant is stabilized. After instillation of the final quarter-dose, remove the catheter without flushing it. Do not suction the infant for 1 hour after dosing unless signs of significant airway obstruction occur.

AFTER COMPLETION OF THE DOSING PROCEDURE, RESUME USUAL VENTILATOR MANAGEMENT AND CLINICAL CARE.

Repeat Doses
The dosage of SURVANTA for repeat doses is also 100 mg phospholipids/kg and is based on the infant's birth weight. The infant should not be reweighed for determination of the SURVANTA dosage. Use the SURVANTA DOSING CHART to determine the total dosage.

The need for additional doses of SURVANTA is determined by evidence of continuing respiratory distress. Using the following criteria for redosing, significant reductions in mortality due to RDS were observed in the multiple-dose clinical trials with SURVANTA.

Dose no sooner than 6 hours after the preceding dose if the infant remains intubated and requires at least 30% inspired oxygen to maintain a PaO_2 less than or equal to 80 torr.

Radiographic confirmation of RDS should be obtained before administering additional doses to those who received a prevention dose.

Prepare SURVANTA and position the infant for administration of each quarter-dose as previously described. After instillation of each quarter-dose, remove the dosing catheter from the endotracheal tube and ventilate the infant for at least 30 seconds or until stable.

In the clinical studies, ventilator settings used to administer repeat doses were different than those used for the first dose. For repeat doses, the FiO_2 was increased by 0.20 or an amount sufficient to prevent cyanosis. The ventilator delivered a rate of 30/minute with an inspiratory time less than 1.0 second. If the infant's pretreatment rate was 30 or greater, it was left unchanged during SURVANTA instillation.

Manual hand-bag ventilation should not be used to administer repeat doses. DURING THE DOSING PROCEDURE, VENTILATOR SETTINGS MAY BE ADJUSTED AT THE DISCRETION OF THE CLINICIAN TO MAINTAIN APPROPRIATE OXYGENATION AND VENTILATION. AFTER COMPLETION OF THE DOSING PROCEDURE, RESUME USUAL VENTILATOR MANAGEMENT AND CLINICAL CARE.

Dosing Precautions

If an infant experiences bradycardia or oxygen desaturation during the dosing procedure, stop the dosing procedure and initiate appropriate measures to alleviate the condition. After the infant has stabilized, resume the dosing procedure. Rales and moist breath sounds can occur transiently after administration of SURVANTA. Endotracheal suctioning or other remedial action is unnecessary unless clear-cut signs of airway obstruction are present.

How Supplied

SURVANTA (beractant) Intratracheal Suspension is supplied in single-use glass vials containing 4 mL (NDC 0074-1040-04) or 8 mL of SURVANTA (NDC 0074-1040-08). Each milliliter contains 25 mg of phospholipids suspended in 0.9% sodium chloride solution. The color is off-white to light brown.

Store unopened vials at refrigeration temperature (2-8°C). Protect from light. Store vials in carton until ready for use. Vials are for single use only. Upon opening, discard unused drug.

LITHO IN USA

AbbVie Inc.

North Chicago, IL 60064, U.S.A.

03-A683 December, 2012

Shown in Product Identification Guide, page 506

SYNTHROID®   ℞

[sĭn-thrŏĭd]

(levothyroxine sodium tablets, USP)

DESCRIPTION

SYNTHROID (levothyroxine sodium tablets, USP) contain synthetic crystalline L-3,3′,5,5′-tetraiodothyronine sodium salt [levothyroxine (T_4) sodium]. Synthetic T_4 is identical to that produced in the human thyroid gland. Levothyroxine (T_4) sodium has an empirical formula of $C_{15}H_{10}I_4N\ NaO_4 \bullet H_2O$, molecular weight of 798.86 g/mol (anhydrous), and structural formula as shown:

[See structural formula in column 3]

Inactive Ingredients

Acacia, confectioner's sugar (contains corn starch), lactose monohydrate, magnesium stearate, povidone, and talc. The following are the color additives by tablet strength:

Strength (mcg)	Color additive(s)
25	FD&C Yellow No. 6 Aluminum Lake*
50	None
75	FD&C Red No. 40 Aluminum Lake, FD&C Blue No. 2 Aluminum Lake
88	FD&C Blue No. 1 Aluminum Lake, FD&C Yellow No. 6 Aluminum Lake*, D&C Yellow No. 10 Aluminum Lake
100	D&C Yellow No. 10 Aluminum Lake, FD&C Yellow No. 6 Aluminum Lake*
112	D&C Red No. 27 & 30 Aluminum Lake
125	FD&C Yellow No. 6 Aluminum Lake*, FD&C Red No. 40 Aluminum Lake, FD&C Blue No. 1 Aluminum Lake
137	FD&C Blue No. 1 Aluminum Lake
150	FD&C Blue No. 2 Aluminum Lake
175	FD&C Blue No. 1 Aluminum Lake, D&C Red No. 27 & 30 Aluminum Lake
200	FD&C Red No. 40 Aluminum Lake
300	D&C Yellow No. 10 Aluminum Lake, FD&C Yellow No. 6 Aluminum Lake*, FD&C Blue No. 1 Aluminum Lake

*Note – FD&C Yellow No. 6 is orange in color.

Meets USP Dissolution Test 3

CLINICAL PHARMACOLOGY

Thyroid hormone synthesis and secretion is regulated by the hypothalamic-pituitary-thyroid axis. Thyrotropin-releasing hormone (TRH) released from the hypothalamus stimulates secretion of thyrotropin-stimulating hormone, TSH, from the anterior pituitary. TSH, in turn, is the physiologic stimulus for the synthesis and secretion of thyroid hormones, L-thyroxine (T_4) and L-triiodothyronine (T_3), by the thyroid gland. Circulating serum T_3 and T_4 levels exert a feedback effect on both TRH and TSH secretion. When serum T_3 and T_4 levels increase, TRH and TSH secretion decrease. When thyroid hormone levels decrease, TRH and TSH secretion increase.

The mechanisms by which thyroid hormones exert their physiologic actions are not completely understood, but it is thought that their principal effects are exerted through control of DNA transcription and protein synthesis. T_3 and T_4 diffuse into the cell nucleus and bind to thyroid receptor proteins attached to DNA. This hormone nuclear receptor complex activates gene transcription and synthesis of messenger RNA and cytoplasmic proteins.

Thyroid hormones regulate multiple metabolic processes and play an essential role in normal growth and development, and normal maturation of the central nervous system and bone. The metabolic actions of thyroid hormones include augmentation of cellular respiration and thermogenesis, as well as metabolism of proteins, carbohydrates and lipids. The protein anabolic effects of thyroid hormones are essential to normal growth and development.

The physiological actions of thyroid hormones are produced predominantly by T_3, the majority of which (approximately 80%) is derived from T_4 by deiodination in peripheral tissues.

Levothyroxine, at doses individualized according to patient response, is effective as replacement or supplemental therapy in hypothyroidism of any etiology, except transient hypothyroidism during the recovery phase of subacute thyroiditis.

Levothyroxine is also effective in the suppression of pituitary TSH secretion in the treatment or prevention of various types of euthyroid goiters, including thyroid nodules, Hashimoto's thyroiditis, multinodular goiter and, as adjunctive therapy in the management of thyrotropin-dependent well-differentiated thyroid cancer (see INDICATIONS AND USAGE, PRECAUTIONS, and DOSAGE AND ADMINISTRATION).

Pharmacokinetics

Absorption

Absorption of orally administered T_4 from the gastrointestinal (GI) tract ranges from 40% to 80%. The majority of the levothyroxine dose is absorbed from the jejunum and upper ileum. The relative bioavailability of SYNTHROID tablets, compared to an equal nominal dose of oral levothyroxine sodium solution, is approximately 93%. T_4 absorption is increased by fasting, and decreased in malabsorption syndromes and by certain foods such as soybean infant formula. Dietary fiber decreases bioavailability of T_4. Absorption may also decrease with age. In addition, many drugs and foods affect T_4 absorption (see PRECAUTIONS - Drug Interactions and Drug-Food Interactions).

Distribution

Circulating thyroid hormones are greater than 99% bound to plasma proteins, including thyroxine-binding globulin (TBG), thyroxine-binding prealbumin (TBPA), and albumin (TBA), whose capacities and affinities vary for each hormone. The higher affinity of both TBG and TBPA for T_4 partially explains the higher serum levels, slower metabolic

clearance, and longer half-life of T_4 compared to T_3. Protein-bound thyroid hormones exist in reverse equilibrium with small amounts of free hormone. Only unbound hormone is metabolically active. Many drugs and physiologic conditions affect the binding of thyroid hormones to serum proteins (see PRECAUTIONS - Drug Interactions and Drug-Laboratory Test Interactions). Thyroid hormones do not readily cross the placental barrier (see PRECAUTIONS - Pregnancy).

Metabolism

T_4 is slowly eliminated (see Table 1). The major pathway of thyroid hormone metabolism is through sequential deiodination. Approximately eighty-percent of circulating T_3 is derived from peripheral T_4 by monodeiodination. The liver is the major site of degradation for both T_4 and T_3, with T_4 deiodination also occurring at a number of additional sites, including the kidney and other tissues. Approximately 80% of the daily dose of T_4 is deiodinated to yield equal amounts of T_3 and reverse T_3 (rT_3). T_3 and rT_3 are further deiodinated to diiodothyronine. Thyroid hormones are also metabolized via conjugation with glucuronides and sulfates and excreted directly into the bile and gut where they undergo enterohepatic recirculation.

Elimination

Thyroid hormones are primarily eliminated by the kidneys. A portion of the conjugated hormone reaches the colon unchanged and is eliminated in the feces. Approximately 20% of T_4 is eliminated in the stool. Urinary excretion of T_4 decreases with age.

[See table 1 on next page]

INDICATIONS AND USAGE

Levothyroxine sodium is used for the following indications:

Hypothyroidism

As replacement or supplemental therapy in congenital or acquired hypothyroidism of any etiology, except transient hypothyroidism during the recovery phase of subacute thyroiditis. Specific indications include: primary (thyroidal), secondary (pituitary), and tertiary (hypothalamic) hypothyroidism and subclinical hypothyroidism. Primary hypothyroidism may result from functional deficiency, primary atrophy, partial or total congenital absence of the thyroid gland, or from the effects of surgery, radiation, or drugs, with or without the presence of goiter.

Pituitary TSH Suppression

In the treatment or prevention of various types of euthyroid goiters (see WARNINGS and PRECAUTIONS), including thyroid nodules (see WARNINGS and PRECAUTIONS), subacute or chronic lymphocytic thyroiditis (Hashimoto's thyroiditis), multinodular goiter (see WARNINGS and PRECAUTIONS) and, as an adjunct to surgery and radioiodine therapy in the management of thyrotropin-dependent well-differentiated thyroid cancer.

CONTRAINDICATIONS

Levothyroxine is contraindicated in patients with untreated subclinical (suppressed serum TSH level with normal T_3 and T_4 levels) or overt thyrotoxicosis of any etiology and in patients with acute myocardial infarction. Levothyroxine is contraindicated in patients with uncorrected adrenal insufficiency since thyroid hormones may precipitate an acute adrenal crisis by increasing the metabolic clearance of glucocorticoids (see PRECAUTIONS). SYNTHROID is contraindicated in patients with hypersensitivity to any of the inactive ingredients in SYNTHROID tablets (See DESCRIPTION - Inactive Ingredients).

Continued on next page

WARNINGS

> **Boxed Warning**
>
> WARNING: Thyroid hormones, including SYNTHROID, either alone or with other therapeutic agents, should not be used for the treatment of obesity or for weight loss. In euthyroid patients, doses within the range of daily hormonal requirements are ineffective for weight reduction. Larger doses may produce serious or even life threatening manifestations of toxicity, particularly when given in association with sympathomimetic amines such as those used for their anorectic effects.

Levothyroxine sodium should not be used in the treatment of male or female infertility unless this condition is associated with hypothyroidism.

In patients with nontoxic diffuse goiter or nodular thyroid disease, particularly the elderly or those with underlying cardiovascular disease, levothyroxine sodium therapy is contraindicated if the serum TSH level is already suppressed due to the risk of precipitating overt thyrotoxicosis (see **CONTRAINDICATIONS**). If the serum TSH level is not suppressed, SYNTHROID should be used with caution in conjunction with careful monitoring of thyroid function for evidence of hyperthyroidism and clinical monitoring for potential associated adverse cardiovascular signs and symptoms of hyperthyroidism.

PRECAUTIONS

General
Levothyroxine has a narrow therapeutic index. Regardless of the indication for use, careful dosage titration is necessary to avoid the consequences of over- or under-treatment. These consequences include, among others, effects on growth and development, cardiovascular function, bone metabolism, reproductive function, cognitive function, emotional state, gastrointestinal function, and on glucose and lipid metabolism. Many drugs interact with levothyroxine sodium necessitating adjustments in dosing to maintain therapeutic response (see **Drug Interactions**).

Effects on Bone Mineral Density
In women, long-term levothyroxine sodium therapy has been associated with increased bone resorption, thereby decreasing bone mineral density, especially in postmenopausal women on greater than replacement doses or in women who are receiving suppressive doses of levothyroxine sodium. The increased bone resorption may be associated with increased serum levels and urinary excretion of calcium and phosphorous, elevations in bone alkaline phosphatase and suppressed serum parathyroid hormone levels. Therefore, it is recommended that patients receiving levothyroxine sodium be given the minimum dose necessary to achieve the desired clinical and biochemical response.

Patients with Underlying Cardiovascular Disease
Exercise caution when administering levothyroxine to patients with cardiovascular disorders and to the elderly in whom there is an increased risk of occult cardiac disease. In these patients, levothyroxine therapy should be initiated at lower doses than those recommended in younger individuals or in patients without cardiac disease (see **WARNINGS, PRECAUTIONS - Geriatric Use**, and **DOSAGE AND ADMINISTRATION**). If cardiac symptoms develop or worsen, the levothyroxine dose should be reduced or withheld for one week and then cautiously restarted at a lower dose. Overtreatment with levothyroxine sodium may have adverse cardiovascular effects such as an increase in heart rate, cardiac wall thickness, and cardiac contractility and may precipitate angina or arrhythmias. Patients with coronary artery disease who are receiving levothyroxine therapy should be monitored closely during surgical procedures, since the possibility of precipitating cardiac arrhythmias may be greater in those treated with levothyroxine. Concomitant administration of levothyroxine and sympathomimetic agents to patients with coronary artery disease may precipitate coronary insufficiency.

Patients with Nontoxic Diffuse Goiter or Nodular Thyroid Disease
Exercise caution when administering levothyroxine to patients with nontoxic diffuse goiter or nodular thyroid disease in order to prevent precipitation of thyrotoxicosis (see **WARNINGS**). If the serum TSH is already suppressed, levothyroxine sodium should not be administered (see **CONTRAINDICATIONS**).

Table 1. Pharmacokinetic Parameters of Thyroid Hormones in Euthyroid Patients

Hormone	Ratio in Thyroglobulin	Biologic Potency	$t_{1/2}$ (days)	Protein Binding (%)[2]
Levothyroxine (T$_4$)	10 - 20	1	6-7[1]	99.96
Liothyronine (T$_3$)	1	4	≤ 2	99.5

[1] 3 to 4 days in hyperthyroidism, 9 to 10 days in hypothyroidism
[2] Includes TBG, TBPA, and TBA

Table 2. Drug-Thyroidal Axis Interactions

Drug or Drug Class	Effect
Drugs that may reduce TSH secretion – the reduction is not sustained; therefore, hypothyroidism does not occur	
Dopamine/Dopamine Agonists Glucocorticoids Octreotide	Use of these agents may result in a transient reduction in TSH secretion when administered at the following doses: Dopamine (≥ 1 mcg/kg/min); Glucocorticoids (hydrocortisone ≥ 100 mg/day or equivalent); Octreotide (> 100 mcg/day).
Drugs that alter thyroid hormone secretion	
Drugs that may decrease thyroid hormone secretion, which may result in hypothyroidism	
Aminoglutethimide Amiodarone Iodide (including iodine-containing radiographic contrast agents) Lithium Methimazole Propylthiouracil (PTU) Sulfonamides Tolbutamide	Long-term lithium therapy can result in goiter in up to 50% of patients, and either subclinical or overt hypothyroidism, each in up to 20% of patients. The fetus, neonate, elderly and euthyroid patients with underlying thyroid disease (e.g., Hashimoto's thyroiditis or with Grave's disease previously treated with radioiodine or surgery) are among those individuals who are particularly susceptible to iodine-induced hypothyroidism. Oral cholecystographic agents and amiodarone are slowly excreted, producing more prolonged hypothyroidism than parenterally administered iodinated contrast agents. Long-term aminoglutethimide therapy may minimally decrease T$_4$ and T$_3$ levels and increase TSH, although all values remain within normal limits in most patients.
Drugs that may increase thyroid hormone secretion, which may result in hyperthyroidism	
Amiodarone Iodide (including iodine-containing radiographic contrast agents)	Iodide and drugs that contain pharmacologic amounts of iodide may cause hyperthyroidism in euthyroid patients with Grave's disease previously treated with antithyroid drugs or in euthyroid patients with thyroid autonomy (e.g., multinodular goiter or hyperfunctioning thyroid adenoma). Hyperthyroidism may develop over several weeks and may persist for several months after therapy discontinuation. Amiodarone may induce hyperthyroidism by causing thyroiditis.
Drugs that may decrease T$_4$ absorption, which may result in hypothyroidism	
Antacids - Aluminum & Magnesium Hydroxides - Simethicone Bile Acid Sequestrants - Cholestyramine - Colestipol Calcium Carbonate Cation Exchange Resins - Kayexalate Ferrous Sulfate Orlistat Sucralfate	Concurrent use may reduce the efficacy of levothyroxine by binding and delaying or preventing absorption, potentially resulting in hypothyroidism. Calcium carbonate may form an insoluble chelate with levothyroxine, and ferrous sulfate likely forms a ferric-thyroxine complex. Administer levothyroxine at least 4 hours apart from these agents. Patients treated concomitantly with orlistat and levothyroxine should be monitored for changes in thyroid function.

This table is continued on the next page

Associated Endocrine Disorders

Hypothalamic/pituitary hormone deficiencies

In patients with secondary or tertiary hypothyroidism, additional hypothalamic/pituitary hormone deficiencies should be considered, and, if diagnosed, treated (see **PRECAUTIONS - Autoimmune polyglandular syndrome** for adrenal insufficiency).

Autoimmune polyglandular syndrome

Occasionally, chronic autoimmune thyroiditis may occur in association with other autoimmune disorders such as adrenal insufficiency, pernicious anemia, and insulin-dependent diabetes mellitus. Patients with concomitant adrenal insufficiency should be treated with replacement glucocorticoids prior to initiation of treatment with levothyroxine sodium. Failure to do so may precipitate an acute adrenal crisis when thyroid hormone therapy is initiated, due to increased metabolic clearance of glucocorticoids by thyroid hormone. Patients with diabetes mellitus may require upward adjustments of their antidiabetic therapeutic regimens when treated with levothyroxine (see **PRECAUTIONS - Drug Interactions**).

Other associated medical conditions

Infants with congenital hypothyroidism appear to be at increased risk for other congenital anomalies, with cardiovascular anomalies (pulmonary stenosis, atrial septal defect, and ventricular septal defect) being the most common association.

Information for Patients

Patients should be informed of the following information to aid in the safe and effective use of SYNTHROID:

1. Notify your physician if you are allergic to any foods or medicines, are pregnant or intend to become pregnant, are breast-feeding or are taking any other medications, including prescription and over-the-counter preparations.
2. Notify your physician of any other medical conditions you may have, particularly heart disease, diabetes, clotting disorders, and adrenal or pituitary gland problems. Your dose of medications used to control these other conditions may need to be adjusted while you are taking SYNTHROID. If you have diabetes, monitor your blood and/or urinary glucose levels as directed by your physician and immediately report any changes to your physician. If you are taking anticoagulants (blood thinners), your clotting status should be checked frequently.
3. Use SYNTHROID only as prescribed by your physician. Do not discontinue or change the amount you take or how often you take it, unless directed to do so by your physician.
4. The levothyroxine in SYNTHROID is intended to replace a hormone that is normally produced by your thyroid gland. Generally, replacement therapy is to be taken for life, except in cases of transient hypothyroidism, which is usually associated with an inflammation of the thyroid gland (thyroiditis).
5. Take SYNTHROID as a single dose, preferably on an empty stomach, one-half to one hour before breakfast. Levothyroxine absorption is increased on an empty stomach.
6. It may take several weeks before you notice an improvement in your symptoms.
7. Notify your physician if you experience any of the following symptoms: rapid or irregular heartbeat, chest pain, shortness of breath, leg cramps, headache, nervousness, irritability, sleeplessness, tremors, change in appetite, weight gain or loss, vomiting, diarrhea, excessive sweating, heat intolerance, fever, changes in menstrual periods, hives or skin rash, or any other unusual medical event.
8. Notify your physician if you become pregnant while taking SYNTHROID. It is likely that your dose of SYNTHROID will need to be increased while you are pregnant.
9. Notify your physician or dentist that you are taking SYNTHROID prior to any surgery.
10. Partial hair loss may occur rarely during the first few months of SYNTHROID therapy, but this is usually temporary.
11. SYNTHROID should not be used as a primary or adjunctive therapy in a weight control program.
12. Keep SYNTHROID out of the reach of children. Store SYNTHROID away from heat, moisture, and light.
13. Agents such as iron and calcium supplements and antacids can decrease the absorption of levothyroxine sodium tablets. Therefore, levothyroxine sodium tablets should not be administered within 4 hours of these agents.

Laboratory Tests

General

The diagnosis of hypothyroidism is confirmed by measuring TSH levels using a sensitive assay (second generation assay sensitivity ≤ 0.1 mIU/L or third generation assay sensitivity ≤ 0.01 mIU/L) and measurement of free-T_4.

The adequacy of therapy is determined by periodic assessment of appropriate laboratory tests and clinical evaluation. The choice of laboratory tests depends on various factors including the etiology of the underlying thyroid disease, the presence of concomitant medical conditions, including pregnancy, and the use of concomitant medications (see **PRECAUTIONS - Drug Interactions** and **Drug-Laboratory Test Interactions**). Persistent clinical and laboratory evidence of hypothyroidism despite an apparent adequate replacement dose of SYNTHROID may be evidence of inadequate absorption, poor compliance, drug interactions, or decreased T_4 potency of the drug product.

Adults

In adult patients with primary (thyroidal) hypothyroidism, serum TSH levels (using a sensitive assay) alone may be used to monitor therapy. The frequency of TSH monitoring during levothyroxine dose titration depends on the clinical situation but it is generally recommended at 6-8 week intervals until normalization. For patients who have recently initiated levothyroxine therapy and whose serum TSH has normalized or in patients who have had their dosage or brand of levothyroxine changed, the serum TSH concentration should be measured after 8-12 weeks. When the optimum replacement dose has been attained, clinical (physical examination) and biochemical monitoring may be performed every 6-12 months, depending on the clinical situation, and whenever there is a change in the patient's status. It is recommended that a physical examination and a serum

Continued on next page

Information on the AbbVie, Inc. products listed on these pages is from the prescribing information in use as of July 31, 2016. For more information, please visit rxabbvie.com or call 1-800-633-9110.

Table 2 (Cont.) Drug-Thyroidal Axis Interactions

Drug or Drug Class	Effect
Drugs that may alter T_4 and T_3 serum transport - but FT_4 concentration remains normal; and therefore, the patient remains euthyroid	

Drugs that may increase serum TBG concentration	Drugs that may decrease serum TBG concentration
Clofibrate Estrogen-containing oral contraceptives Estrogens (oral) Heroin / Methadone 5-Fluorouracil Mitotane Tamoxifen	Androgens / Anabolic Steroids Asparaginase Glucocorticoids Slow-Release Nicotinic Acid

Drugs that may cause protein-binding site displacement	
Furosemide (> 80 mg IV) Heparin Hydantoins Non Steroidal Anti-Inflammatory Drugs - Fenamates - Phenylbutazone Salicylates (> 2 g/day)	Administration of these agents with levothyroxine results in an initial transient increase in FT_4. Continued administration results in a decrease in serum T_4 and normal FT_4 and TSH concentrations and, therefore, patients are clinically euthyroid. Salicylates inhibit binding of T_4 and T_3 to TBG and transthyretin. An initial increase in serum FT_4 is followed by return of FT_4 to normal levels with sustained therapeutic serum salicylate concentrations, although total-T_4 levels may decrease by as much as 30%.

Drugs that may alter T_4 and T_3 metabolism	

Drugs that may increase hepatic metabolism, which may result in hypothyroidism	
Carbamazepine Hydantoins Phenobarbital Rifampin	Stimulation of hepatic microsomal drug-metabolizing enzyme activity may cause increased hepatic degradation of levothyroxine, resulting in increased levothyroxine requirements. Phenytoin and carbamazepine reduce serum protein binding of levothyroxine, and total- and free- T_4 may be reduced by 20% to 40%, but most patients have normal serum TSH levels and are clinically euthyroid.

Drugs that may decrease T_4 5'-deiodinase activity	
Amiodarone Beta-adrenergic antagonists - (e.g., Propranolol > 160 mg/day) Glucocorticoids - (e.g., Dexamethasone ≥ 4 mg/day) Propylthiouracil (PTU)	Administration of these enzyme inhibitors decreases the peripheral conversion of T_4 to T_3, leading to decreased T_3 levels. However, serum T_4 levels are usually normal but may occasionally be slightly increased. In patients treated with large doses of propranolol (> 160 mg/day), T_3 and T_4 levels change slightly, TSH levels remain normal, and patients are clinically euthyroid. It should be noted that actions of particular beta-adrenergic antagonists may be impaired when the hypothyroid patient is converted to the euthyroid state. Short-term administration of large doses of glucocorticoids may decrease serum T_3 concentrations by 30% with minimal change in serum T_4 levels. However, long-term glucocorticoid therapy may result in slightly decreased T_3 and T_4 levels due to decreased TBG production (see above).

This table is continued on the next page

Table 2 *(Cont.)* Drug-Thyroidal Axis Interactions

Drug or Drug Class	Effect
Miscellaneous	
Anticoagulants (oral) - Coumarin Derivatives - Indandione Derivatives	Thyroid hormones appear to increase the catabolism of vitamin K-dependent clotting factors, thereby increasing the anticoagulant activity of oral anticoagulants. Concomitant use of these agents impairs the compensatory increases in clotting factor synthesis. Prothrombin time should be carefully monitored in patients taking levothyroxine and oral anticoagulants and the dose of anticoagulant therapy adjusted accordingly.
Antidepressants - Tricyclics (e.g., Amitriptyline) - Tetracyclics (e.g., Maprotiline) - Selective Serotonin Reuptake Inhibitors (SSRIs; e.g., Sertraline)	Concurrent use of tri/tetracyclic antidepressants and levothyroxine may increase the therapeutic and toxic effects of both drugs, possibly due to increased receptor sensitivity to catecholamines. Toxic effects may include increased risk of cardiac arrhythmias and CNS stimulation; onset of action of tricyclics may be accelerated. Administration of sertraline in patients stabilized on levothyroxine may result in increased levothyroxine requirements.
Antidiabetic Agents - Biguanides - Meglitinides - Sulfonylureas - Thiazolidinediones - Insulin	Addition of levothyroxine to antidiabetic or insulin therapy may result in increased antidiabetic agent or insulin requirements. Careful monitoring of diabetic control is recommended, especially when thyroid therapy is started, changed, or discontinued.
Cardiac Glycosides	Serum digitalis glycoside levels may be reduced in hyperthyroidism or when the hypothyroid patient is converted to the euthyroid state. Therapeutic effect of digitalis glycosides may be reduced.

This table is continued on the next page

TSH measurement be performed at least annually in patients receiving SYNTHROID (see **WARNINGS, PRECAUTIONS,** and **DOSAGE AND ADMINISTRATION**).
Pediatrics
In patients with congenital hypothyroidism, the adequacy of replacement therapy should be assessed by measuring both serum TSH (using a sensitive assay) and total- or free- T_4. During the first three years of life, the serum total- or free- T_4 should be maintained at all times in the upper half of the normal range. While the aim of therapy is to also normalize the serum TSH level, this is not always possible in a small percentage of patients, particularly in the first few months of therapy. TSH may not normalize due to a resetting of the pituitary-thyroid feedback threshold as a result of *in utero* hypothyroidism. Failure of the serum T_4 to increase into the upper half of the normal range within 2 weeks of initiation of SYNTHROID therapy and/or of the serum TSH to decrease below 20 mU/L within 4 weeks should alert the physician to the possibility that the child is not receiving adequate therapy. Careful inquiry should then be made regarding compliance, dose of medication administered, and method of administration prior to raising the dose of SYNTHROID.
The recommended frequency of monitoring of TSH and total or free T_4 in children is as follows: at 2 and 4 weeks after the initiation of treatment; every 1-2 months during the first year of life; every 2-3 months between 1 and 3 years of age; and every 3 to 12 months thereafter until growth is completed. More frequent intervals of monitoring may be necessary if poor compliance is suspected or abnormal values are obtained. It is recommended that TSH and T_4 levels, and a physical examination, if indicated, be performed 2 weeks after any change in SYNTHROID dosage. Routine clinical examination, including assessment of mental and physical growth and development, and bone maturation, should be performed at regular intervals (see **PRECAUTIONS - Pediatric Use** and **DOSAGE AND ADMINISTRATION**).

Secondary (Pituitary) and Tertiary (Hypothalamic) Hypothyroidism
Adequacy of therapy should be assessed by measuring serum free-T_4 levels, which should be maintained in the upper half of the normal range in these patients.
Drug Interactions
Many drugs affect thyroid hormone pharmacokinetics and metabolism (e.g., absorption, synthesis, secretion, catabolism, protein binding, and target tissue response) and may alter the therapeutic response to SYNTHROID. In addition, thyroid hormones and thyroid status have varied effects on the pharmacokinetics and actions of other drugs. A listing of drug-thyroidal axis interactions is contained in Table 2.
The list of drug-thyroidal axis interactions in Table 2 may not be comprehensive due to the introduction of new drugs that interact with the thyroidal axis or the discovery of previously unknown interactions. The prescriber should be aware of this fact and should consult appropriate reference sources (e.g., package inserts of newly approved drugs, medical literature) for additional information if a drug-drug interaction with levothyroxine is suspected.
[See table 2 on pages 790 through 793]
Oral anticoagulants
Levothyroxine increases the response to oral anticoagulant therapy. Therefore, a decrease in the dose of anticoagulant may be warranted with correction of the hypothyroid state or when the SYNTHROID dose is increased. Prothrombin time should be closely monitored to permit appropriate and timely dosage adjustments (see **Table 2**).
Digitalis glycosides
The therapeutic effects of digitalis glycosides may be reduced by levothyroxine. Serum digitalis glycoside levels may be decreased when a hypothyroid patient becomes euthyroid, necessitating an increase in the dose of digitalis glycosides (see **Table 2**).
Drug-Food Interactions
Consumption of certain foods may affect levothyroxine absorption thereby necessitating adjustments in dosing. Soy-

bean flour (infant formula), cotton seed meal, walnuts, and dietary fiber may bind and decrease the absorption of levothyroxine sodium from the GI tract.
Drug-Laboratory Test Interactions
Changes in TBG concentration must be considered when interpreting T_4 and T_3 values, which necessitates measurement and evaluation of unbound (free) hormone and/or determination of the free T_4 index (FT$_4$I). Pregnancy, infectious hepatitis, estrogens, estrogen-containing oral contraceptives, and acute intermittent porphyria increase TBG concentrations. Decreases in TBG concentrations are observed in nephrosis, severe hypoproteinemia, severe liver disease, acromegaly, and after androgen or corticosteroid therapy (see also **Table 2**). Familial hyper- or hypo-thyroxine binding globulinemias have been described, with the incidence of TBG deficiency approximating 1 in 9000.
Carcinogenesis, Mutagenesis, and Impairment of Fertility
Animal studies have not been performed to evaluate the carcinogenic potential, mutagenic potential or effects on fertility of levothyroxine. The synthetic T_4 in SYNTHROID is identical to that produced naturally by the human thyroid gland. Although there has been a reported association between prolonged thyroid hormone therapy and breast cancer, this has not been confirmed. Patients receiving SYNTHROID for appropriate clinical indications should be titrated to the lowest effective replacement dose.
Pregnancy
Category A
Studies in women taking levothyroxine sodium during pregnancy have not shown an increased risk of congenital abnormalities. Therefore, the possibility of fetal harm appears remote. SYNTHROID should not be discontinued during pregnancy and hypothyroidism diagnosed during pregnancy should be promptly treated.
Hypothyroidism during pregnancy is associated with a higher rate of complications, including spontaneous abortion, pre-eclampsia, stillbirth and premature delivery. Maternal hypothyroidism may have an adverse effect on fetal and childhood growth and development. During pregnancy, serum T_4 levels may decrease and serum TSH levels increase to values outside the normal range. Since elevations in serum TSH may occur as early as 4 weeks gestation, pregnant women taking SYNTHROID should have their TSH measured during each trimester. An elevated serum TSH level should be corrected by an increase in the dose of SYNTHROID. Since postpartum TSH levels are similar to preconception values, the SYNTHROID dosage should return to the pre-pregnancy dose immediately after delivery. A serum TSH level should be obtained 6-8 weeks postpartum.
Thyroid hormones cross the placental barrier to some extent as evidenced by levels in cord blood of athyreotic fetuses being approximately one-third maternal levels. Transfer of thyroid hormone from the mother to the fetus, however, may not be adequate to prevent *in utero* hypothyroidism.
Nursing Mothers
Although thyroid hormones are excreted only minimally in human milk, caution should be exercised when SYNTHROID is administered to a nursing woman. However, adequate replacement doses of levothyroxine are generally needed to maintain normal lactation.
Pediatric Use
General
The goal of treatment in pediatric patients with hypothyroidism is to achieve and maintain normal intellectual and physical growth and development.
The initial dose of levothyroxine varies with age and body weight (see **DOSAGE AND ADMINISTRATION - Table 3**). Dosing adjustments are based on an assessment of the individual patient's clinical and laboratory parameters (see **PRECAUTIONS - Laboratory Tests**).
In children in whom a diagnosis of permanent hypothyroidism has not been established, it is recommended that levothyroxine administration be discontinued for a 30-day trial period, but only after the child is at least 3 years of age. Serum T_4 and TSH levels should then be obtained. If the T_4 is low and the TSH high, the diagnosis of permanent hypothyroidism is established, and levothyroxine therapy should be reinstituted. If the T_4 and TSH levels are normal, euthyroidism may be assumed and, therefore, the hypothyroidism can be considered to have been transient. In this instance, however, the physician should carefully monitor the child and repeat the thyroid function tests if any signs or symptoms of hypothyroidism develop. In this setting, the clinician should have a high index of suspicion of relapse. If the

Table 2 *(Cont.)* **Drug-Thyroidal Axis Interactions**

Drug or Drug Class	Effect
Cytokines - Interferon-α - Interleukin-2	Therapy with interferon-α has been associated with the development of antithyroid microsomal antibodies in 20% of patients and some have transient hypothyroidism, hyperthyroidism, or both. Patients who have antithyroid antibodies before treatment are at higher risk for thyroid dysfunction during treatment. Interleukin-2 has been associated with transient painless thyroiditis in 20% of patients. Interferon-β and -γ have not been reported to cause thyroid dysfunction.
Growth Hormones - Somatrem - Somatropin	Excessive use of thyroid hormones with growth hormones may accelerate epiphyseal closure. However, untreated hypothyroidism may interfere with growth response to growth hormone.
Ketamine	Concurrent use may produce marked hypertension and tachycardia; cautious administration to patients receiving thyroid hormone therapy is recommended.
Methylxanthine Bronchodilators - (e.g., Theophylline)	Decreased theophylline clearance may occur in hypothyroid patients; clearance returns to normal when the euthyroid state is achieved.
Radiographic Agents	Thyroid hormones may reduce the uptake of ^{123}I, ^{131}I, and ^{99m}Tc.
Sympathomimetics	Concurrent use may increase the effects of sympathomimetics or thyroid hormone. Thyroid hormones may increase the risk of coronary insufficiency when sympathomimetic agents are administered to patients with coronary artery disease.
Chloral Hydrate Diazepam Ethionamide Lovastatin Metoclopramide 6-Mercaptopurine Nitroprusside Para-aminosalicylate sodium Perphenazine Resorcinol (excessive topical use) Thiazide Diuretics	These agents have been associated with thyroid hormone and/or TSH level alterations by various mechanisms.

Strength (mcg)	Color	NDC# for bottles of 90	NDC # for bottles of 100	NDC # for bottles of 1000	NDC # for unit dose cartons of 100
25	orange	0074-4341-90	0074-4341-13	0074-4341-19	--
50	white	0074-4552-90	0074-4552-13	0074-4552-19	0074-4552-11
75	violet	0074-5182-90	0074-5182-13	0074-5182-19	0074-5182-11
88	olive	0074-6594-90	0074-6594-13	0074-6594-19	--
100	yellow	0074-6624-90	0074-6624-13	0074-6624-19	0074-6624-11
112	rose	0074-9296-90	0074-9296-13	0074-9296-19	--
125	brown	0074-7068-90	0074-7068-13	0074-7068-19	0074-7068-11
137	turquoise	0074-3727-90	0074-3727-13	0074-3727-19	--
150	blue	0074-7069-90	0074-7069-13	0074-7069-19	0074-7069-11
175	lilac	0074-7070-90	0074-7070-13	0074-7070-19	--
200	pink	0074-7148-90	0074-7148-13	0074-7148-19	0074-7148-11
300	green	0074-7149-90	0074-7149-13	0074-7149-19	--

results of the levothyroxine withdrawal test are inconclusive, careful follow-up and subsequent testing will be necessary.

Since some more severely affected children may become clinically hypothyroid when treatment is discontinued for 30 days, an alternate approach is to reduce the replacement dose of levothyroxine by half during the 30-day trial period. If, after 30 days, the serum TSH is elevated above 20 mU/L, the diagnosis of permanent hypothyroidism is confirmed, and full replacement therapy should be resumed. However, if the serum TSH has not risen to greater than 20 mU/L, levothyroxine treatment should be discontinued for another 30-day trial period followed by repeat serum T_4 and TSH testing.

The presence of concomitant medical conditions should be considered in certain clinical circumstances and, if present, appropriately treated (see **PRECAUTIONS**).

Congenital Hypothyroidism

(see **PRECAUTIONS - Laboratory Tests and DOSAGE AND ADMINISTRATION**)

Rapid restoration of normal serum T_4 concentrations is essential for preventing the adverse effects of congenital hypothyroidism on intellectual development as well as on overall physical growth and maturation. Therefore, SYNTHROID therapy should be initiated immediately upon diagnosis and is generally continued for life.

During the first 2 weeks of SYNTHROID therapy, infants should be closely monitored for cardiac overload, arrhythmias, and aspiration from avid suckling.

The patient should be monitored closely to avoid undertreatment or overtreatment. Undertreatment may have deleterious effects on intellectual development and linear growth. Overtreatment has been associated with craniosynostosis in infants, and may adversely affect the tempo of brain maturation and accelerate the bone age with resultant premature closure of the epiphyses and compromised adult stature.

Acquired Hypothyroidism in Pediatric Patients

The patient should be monitored closely to avoid undertreatment and overtreatment. Undertreatment may result in poor school performance due to impaired concentration and slowed mentation and in reduced adult height. Overtreatment may accelerate the bone age and result in premature epiphyseal closure and compromised adult stature.

Treated children may manifest a period of catch-up growth, which may be adequate in some cases to normalize adult height. In children with severe or prolonged hypothyroidism, catch-up growth may not be adequate to normalize adult height.

Geriatric Use

Because of the increased prevalence of cardiovascular disease among the elderly, levothyroxine therapy should not be initiated at the full replacement dose (see **WARNINGS, PRECAUTIONS,** and **DOSAGE AND ADMINISTRATION**).

ADVERSE REACTIONS

Adverse reactions associated with levothyroxine therapy are primarily those of hyperthyroidism due to therapeutic overdosage (see **PRECAUTIONS** and **OVERDOSAGE**). They include the following:

General

fatigue, increased appetite, weight loss, heat intolerance, fever, excessive sweating;

Central nervous system

headache, hyperactivity, nervousness, anxiety, irritability, emotional lability, insomnia;

Musculoskeletal

tremors, muscle weakness;

Cardiovascular

palpitations, tachycardia, arrhythmias, increased pulse and blood pressure, heart failure, angina, myocardial infarction, cardiac arrest;

Respiratory

dyspnea;

Gastrointestinal

diarrhea, vomiting, abdominal cramps and elevations in liver function tests;

Continued on next page

Information on the AbbVie, Inc. products listed on these pages is from the prescribing information in use as of July 31, 2016. For more information, please visit rxabbvie.com or call 1-800-633-9110.

Dermatologic
hair loss, flushing;
Endocrine
decreased bone mineral density;
Reproductive
menstrual irregularities, impaired fertility.
Pseudotumor cerebri and slipped capital femoral epiphysis have been reported in children receiving levothyroxine therapy. Overtreatment may result in craniosynostosis in infants and premature closure of the epiphyses in children with resultant compromised adult height.
Seizures have been reported rarely with the institution of levothyroxine therapy.
Inadequate levothyroxine dosage will produce or fail to ameliorate the signs and symptoms of hypothyroidism.
Hypersensitivity reactions to inactive ingredients have occurred in patients treated with thyroid hormone products. These include urticaria, pruritus, skin rash, flushing, angioedema, various GI symptoms (abdominal pain, nausea, vomiting and diarrhea), fever, arthralgia, serum sickness and wheezing. Hypersensitivity to levothyroxine itself is not known to occur.

Overdosage
The signs and symptoms of overdosage are those of hyperthyroidism (see **PRECAUTIONS** and **ADVERSE REACTIONS**). In addition, confusion and disorientation may occur. Cerebral embolism, shock, coma, and death have been reported. Seizures have occurred in a child ingesting 18 mg of levothyroxine. Symptoms may not necessarily be evident or may not appear until several days after ingestion of levothyroxine sodium.

Treatment of Overdosage
Levothyroxine sodium should be reduced in dose or temporarily discontinued if signs or symptoms of overdosage occur.

Acute Massive Overdosage
This may be a life-threatening emergency, therefore, symptomatic and supportive therapy should be instituted immediately. If not contraindicated (e.g., by seizures, coma, or loss of the gag reflex), the stomach should be emptied by emesis or gastric lavage to decrease gastrointestinal absorption. Activated charcoal or cholestyramine may also be used to decrease absorption. Central and peripheral increased sympathetic activity may be treated by administering β-receptor antagonists, e.g., propranolol, provided there are no medical contraindications to their use. Provide respiratory support as needed; control congestive heart failure and arrhythmia; control fever, hypoglycemia, and fluid loss as necessary. Large doses of antithyroid drugs (e.g., methimazole or propylthiouracil) followed in one to two hours by large doses of iodine may be given to inhibit synthesis and release of thyroid hormones. Glucocorticoids may be given to inhibit the conversion of T_4 to T_3. Plasmapheresis, charcoal hemoperfusion and exchange transfusion have been reserved for cases in which continued clinical deterioration occurs despite conventional therapy. Because T_4 is highly protein bound, very little drug will be removed by dialysis.

DOSAGE AND ADMINISTRATION
General Principles
The goal of replacement therapy is to achieve and maintain a clinical and biochemical euthyroid state. The goal of suppressive therapy is to inhibit growth and/or function of abnormal thyroid tissue. The dose of SYNTHROID that is adequate to achieve these goals depends on a variety of factors including the patient's age, body weight, cardiovascular status, concomitant medical conditions, including pregnancy, concomitant medications, and the specific nature of the condition being treated (see **WARNINGS** and **PRECAUTIONS**). Hence, the following recommendations serve only as dosing guidelines. Dosing must be individualized and adjustments made based on periodic assessment of the patient's clinical response and laboratory parameters (see **PRECAUTIONS** - Laboratory Tests).
SYNTHROID is administered as a single daily dose, preferably one-half to one-hour before breakfast. SYNTHROID should be taken at least 4 hours apart from drugs that are known to interfere with its absorption (see **PRECAUTIONS** - Drug Interactions).
Due to the long half-life of levothyroxine, the peak therapeutic effect at a given dose of levothyroxine sodium may not be attained for 4-6 weeks.

Caution should be exercised when administering SYNTHROID to patients with underlying cardiovascular disease, to the elderly, and to those with concomitant adrenal insufficiency (see **PRECAUTIONS**).
Specific Patient Populations
Hypothyroidism in Adults and in Children in Whom Growth and Puberty are Complete
(see **WARNINGS** and **PRECAUTIONS** - Laboratory Tests)
Therapy may begin at full replacement doses in otherwise healthy individuals less than 50 years old and in those older than 50 years who have been recently treated for hyperthyroidism or who have been hypothyroid for only a short time (such as a few months). The average full replacement dose of levothyroxine sodium is approximately 1.7 mcg/kg/day (e.g., **100-125 mcg/day** for a 70 kg adult). Older patients may require less than 1 mcg/kg/day. Levothyroxine sodium doses greater than 200 mcg/day are seldom required. An inadequate response to daily doses ≥ 300 mcg/day is rare and may indicate poor compliance, malabsorption, and/or drug interactions.
For most patients older than 50 years or for patients under 50 years of age with underlying cardiac disease, an initial starting dose of **25-50 mcg/day** of levothyroxine sodium is recommended, with gradual increments in dose at 6-8 week intervals, as needed. The recommended starting dose of levothyroxine sodium in elderly patients with cardiac disease is **12.5-25 mcg/day**, with gradual dose increments at 4-6 week intervals. The levothyroxine sodium dose is generally adjusted in 12.5-25 mcg increments until the patient with primary hypothyroidism is clinically euthyroid and the serum TSH has normalized.
In patients with severe hypothyroidism, the recommended initial levothyroxine sodium dose is **12.5-25 mcg/day** with increases of 25 mcg/day every 2-4 weeks, accompanied by clinical and laboratory assessment, until the TSH level is normalized.
In patients with secondary (pituitary) or tertiary (hypothalamic) hypothyroidism, the levothyroxine sodium dose should be titrated until the patient is clinically euthyroid and the serum free- T_4 level is restored to the upper half of the normal range.
Pediatric Dosage - Congenital or Acquired Hypothyroidism (see **PRECAUTIONS** - Laboratory Tests)
General Principles
In general, levothyroxine therapy should be instituted at full replacement doses as soon as possible. Delays in diagnosis and institution of therapy may have deleterious effects on the child's intellectual and physical growth and development.
Undertreatment and overtreatment should be avoided (see **PRECAUTIONS** - Pediatric Use). SYNTHROID may be administered to infants and children who cannot swallow intact tablets by crushing the tablet and suspending the freshly crushed tablet in a small amount (5-10 mL or 1-2 teaspoons) of water. This suspension can be administered by spoon or by dropper. **DO NOT STORE THE SUSPENSION**. Foods that decrease absorption of levothyroxine, such as soybean infant formula, should not be used for administering levothyroxine sodium tablets (see **PRECAUTIONS** - Drug-Food Interactions).
Newborns
The recommended starting dose of levothyroxine sodium in newborn infants is **10-15 mcg/kg/day** . A lower starting dose (e.g., 25 mcg/day) should be considered in infants at risk for cardiac failure, and the dose should be increased in 4-6 weeks as needed based on clinical and laboratory response to treatment. In infants with very low (< 5 mcg/dL) or undetectable serum T_4 concentrations, the recommended initial starting dose is **50 mcg/day** of levothyroxine sodium.
Infants and Children
Levothyroxine therapy is usually initiated at full replacement doses, with the recommended dose per body weight decreasing with age (see **Table 3**). However, in children with chronic or severe hypothyroidism, an initial dose of **25 mcg/day** of levothyroxine sodium is recommended with increments of 25 mcg every 2-4 weeks until the desired effect is achieved.
Hyperactivity in an older child can be minimized if the starting dose is one-fourth of the recommended full replacement dose, and the dose is then increased on a weekly basis by an amount equal to one-fourth the full-recommended replacement dose until the full recommended replacement dose is reached.

Table 3. Levothyroxine Sodium Dosing Guidelines for Pediatric Hypothyroidism

AGE	Daily Dose Per Kg Body Weight[a]
0-3 months	10-15 mcg/kg/day
3-6 months	8-10 mcg/kg/day
6-12 months	6-8 mcg/kg/day
1-5 years	5-6 mcg/kg/day
6-12 years	4-5 mcg/kg/day
> 12 years but growth and puberty incomplete	2-3 mcg/kg/day
Growth and puberty complete	1.7 mcg/kg/day

[a] The dose should be adjusted based on clinical response and laboratory parameters (see **PRECAUTIONS** - Laboratory Tests and Pediatric Use).

Pregnancy
Pregnancy may increase levothyroxine requirements (see **PREGNANCY**).

Subclinical Hypothyroidism
If this condition is treated, a lower levothyroxine sodium dose (e.g., **1 mcg/kg/day**) than that used for full replacement may be adequate to normalize the serum TSH level. Patients who are not treated should be monitored yearly for changes in clinical status and thyroid laboratory parameters.
TSH Suppression in Well-differentiated Thyroid Cancer and Thyroid Nodules
The target level for TSH suppression in these conditions has not been established with controlled studies. In addition, the efficacy of TSH suppression for benign nodular disease is controversial. Therefore, the dose of SYNTHROID used for TSH suppression should be individualized based on the specific disease and the patient being treated.
In the treatment of well-differentiated (papillary and follicular) thyroid cancer, levothyroxine is used as an adjunct to surgery and radioiodine therapy. Generally, TSH is suppressed to < 0.1 mU/L, and this usually requires a levothyroxine sodium dose of **greater than 2 mcg/kg/day**. However, in patients with high-risk tumors, the target level for TSH suppression may be < 0.01 mU/L.
In the treatment of benign nodules and nontoxic multinodular goiter, TSH is generally suppressed to a higher target (e.g., 0.1 to either 0.5 or 1.0 mU/L) than that used for the treatment of thyroid cancer. Levothyroxine sodium is contraindicated if the serum TSH is already suppressed due to the risk of precipitating overt thyrotoxicosis (see **CONTRAINDICATIONS, WARNINGS** and **PRECAUTIONS**).

Myxedema Coma
Myxedema coma is a life-threatening emergency characterized by poor circulation and hypometabolism, and may result in unpredictable absorption of levothyroxine sodium from the gastrointestinal tract. Therefore, oral thyroid hormone drug products are not recommended to treat this condition. Thyroid hormone products formulated for intravenous administration should be administered.

HOW SUPPLIED

SYNTHROID® (levothyroxine sodium tablets, USP) are round, color coded, scored and debossed with "SYNTHROID" on one side and potency on the other side. They are supplied as follows:
[See table at bottom of page 793]

Storage Conditions
Store at 25°C (77°F); excursions permitted to 15-30°C (59-86°F) [see USP Controlled Room Temperature]. SYNTHROID tablets should be protected from light and moisture.
(Nos. 4341, 4552, 5182, 6594, 9296, 7068, 3727, 7069, 7070, 7148, 7149)
03-A663-R7-Rev. September, 2012
AbbVie Inc.
North Chicago, IL 60064, U.S.A.

TARKA® ℞

(trandolapril/verapamil hydrochloride ER tablets)

> **WARNING: FETAL TOXICITY**
> - **When pregnancy is detected, discontinue TARKA as soon as possible.**
> - **Drugs that act directly on the renin-angiotensin system can cause injury and death to the developing fetus (see WARNINGS: Fetal Toxicity).**

DESCRIPTION

TARKA (trandolapril/verapamil hydrochloride ER) combines a slow release formulation of a calcium channel blocker, verapamil hydrochloride, and an immediate release formulation of an angiotensin converting enzyme inhibitor, trandolapril.

Verapamil Component

Verapamil hydrochloride is chemically described as benzeneacetonitrile, α[3-[[2-(3,4-dimethoxyphenyl)ethyl] methylamino]propyl]-3, 4-dimethoxy-α-(1-methylethyl) hydrochloride. Its empirical formula is $C_{27}H_{38}N_2O_4$ HCl and its structural formula is:

[See structural formula in column 3]

Verapamil hydrochloride is an almost white crystalline powder, with a molecular weight of 491.08. It is soluble in water, chloroform, and methanol. It is practically free of odor, with a bitter taste.

Trandolapril Component

Trandolapril is the ethyl ester prodrug of a nonsulfhydryl angiotensin converting enzyme (ACE) inhibitor, trandolaprilat. It is chemically described as (2S,3aR,7aS)-1-[(S)-N-[(S)-1-Carboxy-3-phenylpropyl]alanyl] hexahydro-2-indolinecarboxylic acid, 1-ethyl ester. Its empirical formula is C_{24} H_{34} N_2O_5 and its structural formula is:

[See structural formula on next page]

Trandolapril is a white or almost white powder with a molecular weight of 430.54. It is soluble (>100 mg/mL) in chloroform, dichloromethane, and methanol.

TARKA tablets are formulated for oral administration, containing verapamil hydrochloride as a controlled release formulation and trandolapril as an immediate release formulation. The tablet strengths are trandolapril 2 mg/verapamil hydrochloride ER 180 mg, trandolapril 1 mg/verapamil hydrochloride ER 240 mg, trandolapril 2 mg/verapamil hydrochloride ER 240 mg, and trandolapril 4 mg/verapamil hydrochloride ER 240 mg. The tablets also contain the following ingredients: corn starch, dioctyl sodium sulfosuccinate, ethanol, hydroxypropyl cellulose, hypromellose, lactose monohydrate, magnesium stearate, microcrystalline cellulose, polyethylene glycol, povidone, purified water, silicon dioxide, sodium alginate, sodium stearyl fumarate, synthetic iron oxides, talc, and titanium dioxide.

CLINICAL PHARMACOLOGY

Verapamil hydrochloride and trandolapril have been used individually and in combination for the treatment of hypertension. For the four dosing strengths, the antihypertensive effect of the combination is approximately additive to the individual components.

Verapamil Component

Verapamil is a calcium channel blocker that exerts its pharmacologic effects by modulating the influx of ionic calcium across the cell membrane of the arterial smooth muscle as well as in conductile and contractile myocardial cells. Verapamil exerts antihypertensive effects by decreasing systemic vascular resistance, usually without orthostatic decreases in blood pressure or reflex tachycardia. During isometric or dynamic exercise, verapamil does not alter systolic cardiac function in patients with normal ventricular function. Verapamil does not alter total serum calcium levels.

Trandolapril Component

Trandolapril is de-esterified to its diacid metabolite, trandolaprilat. Both inhibit angiotensin-converting enzyme (ACE) in human subjects and in animals. Trandolaprilat is about 8 times more potent than trandolapril. ACE is a peptidyl dipeptidase that catalyzes the conversion of angiotensin I to the vasoconstrictor, angiotensin II. Angiotensin II also stimulates aldosterone secretion by the adrenal cortex. Inhibition of ACE results in decreased plasma angiotensin II, which leads to decreased vasopressor activity and to decreased aldosterone secretion. The latter decrease may result in a small increase of serum potassium. In controlled clinical trials, treatment with TARKA resulted in mean increases in potassium of 0.1 mEq/L (see **PRECAUTIONS**). Removal of angiotensin II negative feedback on renin secretion leads to increased plasma renin activity (PRA). ACE is identical to kininase II, an enzyme that degrades bradykinin. Whether increased levels of bradykinin, a potent vasodepressor peptide, play a role in the therapeutic effect of TARKA remains to be elucidated.

While the mechanism through which trandolapril lowers blood pressure is believed to be primarily suppression of the renin-angiotensin-aldosterone system, trandolapril has an antihypertensive effect even in patients with low renin hypertension. Trandolapril is an effective antihypertensive in all races studied. Both black patients (usually a predominantly low renin group) and non-black patients respond to 2 to 4 mg of trandolapril.

Pharmacokinetics and Metabolism

TARKA

Following a single oral dose of TARKA in healthy subjects, peak plasma concentrations are reached within 0.5-2 hours for trandolapril and within 4-15 hours for verapamil. Peak plasma concentrations of the active desmethyl metabolite of verapamil, norverapamil, are reached within 5-15 hours. Cleavage of the ester group converts trandolapril to its active diacid metabolite, trandolaprilat, which reaches peak plasma concentrations within 2-12 hours. The pharmacokinetics of trandolapril and trandolaprilat are not altered when trandolapril is administered in combination with verapamil, compared to monotherapy.

The AUC and C_{max} for both verapamil and norverapamil are increased when 240 mg of controlled release verapamil is administered concomitantly with 4 mg trandolapril. The increase in C_{max} is 54 and 30% and the AUC is increased by 65 and 32% for verapamil and norverapamil, respectively. Administration of TARKA 4/240 (4 mg trandolapril and 240 mg verapamil hydrochloride ER) with a high-fat meal does not alter the bioavailability of trandolapril whereas verapamil peak concentrations and area under the curve (AUC) decrease 37% and 28%, respectively. Food thus decreases verapamil bioavailability and the time to peak plasma concentration for both verapamil and norverapamil are delayed by approximately 7 hours. Both optical isomers of verapamil are similarly affected.

The elimination half life of trandolapril is about 6 hours. At steady state, the effective half-life of trandolaprilat is 22.5 hours. Like all ACE inhibitors, trandolaprilat also has a prolonged terminal elimination phase, involving a small fraction of administered drug, probably representing binding to plasma and tissue ACE.

The terminal half-life of verapamil is 6-11 hours. Steady-state plasma concentrations of the two components are achieved after about a week of once-daily dosing of TARKA. At steady-state, plasma concentrations of verapamil and trandolaprilat are up to two-fold higher than those observed after a single oral TARKA dose.

The pharmacokinetics of verapamil and trandolaprilat are significantly different in the elderly (≥65 years) than in younger subjects. The bioavailability of verapamil and norverapamil are increased by 87% and 77%, respectively, and that of trandolapril by approximately 35% in the elderly. AUCs are approximately 80% and 35% higher, respectively.

Verapamil Component

With the immediate release formulation, more than 90% of the orally administered dose is absorbed with peak plasma concentrations of verapamil observed 1 to 2 hours after dosing. A delayed rate but similar extent of absorption is observed for the sustained release formulation when compared to the immediate release formulation. Because of the rapid biotransformation of verapamil during its first pass through the portal circulation, absolute bioavailability ranges from 20% to 35%. A nonlinear correlation exists between verapamil dose and plasma concentrations.

In early dose titration with verapamil, a relationship exists between plasma concentrations of verapamil and prolongation of the PR interval. However, during chronic administration, this relationship may disappear. No relationship has been established between the plasma concentration of verapamil and reduction in blood pressure.

In healthy subjects, orally administered verapamil undergoes extensive metabolism in the liver. Twelve metabolites have been identified in plasma; all except norverapamil are present in trace amounts only. Approximately 70% of an administered dose is excreted as metabolites in the urine and 16% or more in the feces within 5 days. Urinary excretion of unchanged drug is about 3% to 4% of the dose. Verapamil is approximately 90% bound to plasma proteins.

In patients with hepatic insufficiency, verapamil clearance is decreased about 30% and the elimination half-life is prolonged up to 14 to 16 hours (see **PRECAUTIONS**). In pa-

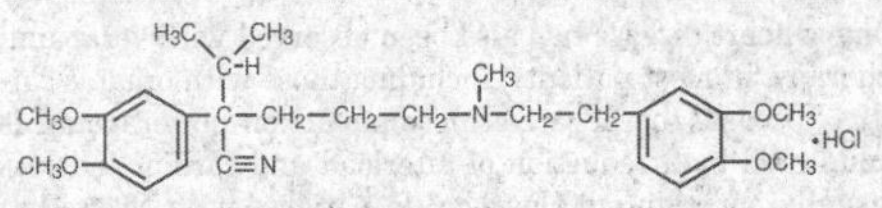

tients with liver dysfunction, a dosage adjustment may be required. In the elderly (≥65 years), verapamil clearance is reduced resulting in increases in elimination half-life.

Trandolapril Component

Following oral administration of trandolapril, the absolute bioavailability of trandolapril is approximately 10% as trandolapril and 70% as trandolaprilat. Plasma concentrations of trandolaprilat but not trandolapril increase in proportion with dose. Plasma concentrations of trandolaprilat decline in a triphasic manner. The more prolonged terminal elimination phase probably represents a small fraction of dose saturably bound to ACE.

After an oral radiolabeled dose of trandolapril, excretion of trandolapril and metabolites account for 33% of the dose in the urine and about 66% in the feces. Less than 1% of the dose is excreted in the urine as unchanged drug. Serum protein binding of trandolapril is about 80%, and is independent of concentration. Binding of trandolaprilat is concentration-dependent, varying from 65% at 1000 ng/mL to 94% at 0.1 ng/mL, indicating saturation of binding with increasing concentration.

Compared to normal subjects, the plasma concentrations of trandolapril and trandolaprilat are approximately 2-fold greater and renal clearance is reduced by about 85% in patients with creatinine clearance below 30 mL/min and in patients on hemodialysis. Dosage adjustment is recommended in renally impaired patients (see **DOSAGE AND ADMINISTRATION**).

Following oral administration in patients with mild to moderate alcoholic cirrhosis, plasma concentrations of trandolapril and trandolaprilat were, respectively, 9-fold and 2-fold greater than in normal subjects, but inhibition of ACE activity was not affected. Lower doses should be considered in patients with hepatic insufficiency (see **DOSAGE AND ADMINISTRATION**).

Pharmacodynamics

TARKA

Verapamil does not interfere with ACE inhibition by trandolapril. Trandolapril does not alter the effect of verapamil on intra-cardiac conduction.

Verapamil Component

Verapamil dilates the main coronary arteries and coronary arterioles, both in normal and ischemic regions, and is a potent inhibitor of coronary artery spasm. This property increases myocardial oxygen delivery in patients with coronary artery spasm, and is responsible for the effectiveness of verapamil in vasospastic (Prinzmetal's or variant) as well as unstable angina at rest.

Verapamil regularly reduces the total systemic resistance (afterload) by dilating peripheral arterioles. By decreasing the influx of calcium, verapamil prolongs the effective refractory period within the AV node and slows AV conduction in a rate-related manner.

Normal sinus rhythm is usually not affected, but in patients with sick sinus syndrome, verapamil may interfere with sinus node impulse generation and may induce sinus arrest or sinoatrial block. Atrioventricular block can occur in patients without preexisting conduction defects (see **WARNINGS**).

Verapamil does not alter the normal atrial action potential or intraventricular conduction time, but depresses amplitude, velocity of depolarization and conduction in depressed atrial fibers. Verapamil may shorten the antegrade effective refractory period of accessory bypass tracts. Acceleration of ventricular rate and/or ventricular fibrillation has been reported in patients with atrial flutter or atrial fibrillation and a coexisting accessory AV pathway following administration of verapamil (see **WARNINGS**).

Hemodynamics and Myocardial Metabolism: Verapamil reduces afterload and myocardial contractility. Improved left ventricular diastolic function in patients with idiopathic hypertrophic subaortic stenosis (IHSS) and those with cor-

Continued on next page

Information on the AbbVie, Inc. products listed on these pages is from the prescribing information in use as of July 31, 2016. For more information, please visit rxabbvie.com or call 1-800-633-9110.

onary heart disease has also been observed with verapamil therapy. In most patients, including those with organic cardiac disease, the negative inotropic action of verapamil is countered by a reduction of afterload and cardiac index is usually not reduced. However, in patients with severe left ventricular dysfunction (e.g., pulmonary wedge pressure about 20 mmHg or ejection fraction less than 30%), or in patients taking beta-adrenergic blocking agents or other cardio-depressant drugs, deterioration of ventricular function may occur (see **PRECAUTIONS - Drug Interactions**).
Pulmonary Function: Verapamil does not induce bronchoconstriction and hence, does not impair ventilatory function.

Trandolapril Component

After a single 2 mg dose of trandolapril, inhibition of ACE activity reaches a maximum (70-85%) at 4 hours with about 10% decline at 24 hours. Eight days after dosing, ACE inhibition is still 40%.

Four placebo-controlled dose response studies were conducted using once daily oral dosing of trandolapril in doses from 0.25 to 16 mg per day in 827 black and non-black patients with mild to moderate hypertension. The minimal effective once daily dose was 1.0 mg in non-black patients and 2.0 mg in black patients. Further decreases in trough supine diastolic blood pressure were obtained in non-black patients with higher doses, and no further response was seen with doses above 4 mg (up to 16 mg). The antihypertensive effect diminished somewhat at the end of the dosing interval.

During chronic therapy, the maximum reduction in blood pressure with any dose is achieved within one week. Following 6 weeks of monotherapy in placebo-controlled trials in patients with mild to moderate hypertension, once daily doses of 2 to 4 mg lowered supine or standing systolic/diastolic blood pressure 24 hours after dosing by an average 7-10/4-5 mmHg below placebo responses in non-black patients. Once daily doses of 2 to 4 mg lowered blood pressures 4-6/3-4 mmHg below placebo responses in black patients.

CLINICAL STUDIES

In controlled clinical trials, once daily doses of TARKA, trandolapril 4 mg/verapamil HCl ER 240 mg or trandolapril 2 mg/verapamil HCl ER 180 mg, decreased placebo-corrected seated pressure (systolic/diastolic) 24 hours after dosing by about 7-12/6-8 mmHg. Each of the components of TARKA added to the antihypertensive effect. Treatment effects were consistent across age groups (<65, ≥65 years), and gender (male, female).

Blood pressure reductions were significantly greater for the TARKA 4/240 combination than for either of the components used alone.

The antihypertensive effects of TARKA have continued during therapy for at least 1 year.

INDICATIONS AND USAGE

TARKA is indicated for the treatment of hypertension.

This fixed combination drug is not indicated for the initial therapy of hypertension (see DOSAGE AND ADMINISTRATION).

In using TARKA, consideration should be given to the fact that an angiotensin converting enzyme inhibitor, captopril, has caused agranulocytosis, particularly in patients with renal impairment or collagen vascular disease, and that available data are insufficient to show that trandolapril does not have similar risk (see **WARNINGS - Neutropenia/Agranulocytosis**).

CONTRAINDICATIONS

TARKA is contraindicated in patients who are hypersensitive to any ACE inhibitor or verapamil.

Because of the verapamil component, TARKA is contraindicated in:

1. Severe left ventricular dysfunction (see **WARNINGS**).
2. Hypotension (systolic pressure less than 90 mmHg) or cardiogenic shock.
3. Sick sinus syndrome (except in patients with a functioning artificial ventricular pacemaker).
4. Second- or third-degree AV block (except in patients with a functioning artificial ventricular pacemaker).
5. Patients with atrial flutter or atrial fibrillation and an accessory bypass tract (e.g. Wolff-Parkinson-White, Lown-Ganong-Levine syndromes) (see **WARNINGS**).

Because of the trandolapril component, TARKA is contraindicated in patients with a history of angioedema related to previous treatment with an angiotensin converting enzyme (ACE) inhibitor.

Do not co-administer aliskiren with TARKA in patients with diabetes (see **PRECAUTIONS, Drug Interactions**).

WARNINGS

Heart Failure

Verapamil Component

Verapamil has a negative inotropic effect which, in most patients, is compensated by its afterload reduction (decreased systemic vascular resistance) properties without a net impairment of ventricular performance. In clinical experience with 4,954 patients, 87 (1.8%) developed congestive heart failure or pulmonary edema. Verapamil should be avoided in patients with severe left ventricular dysfunction (e.g., ejection fraction less than 30%, pulmonary wedge pressure above 20 mmHg, or severe symptoms of cardiac failure) and in patients with any degree of ventricular dysfunction if they are receiving a beta adrenergic blocker (see **PRECAUTIONS - Drug Interactions**). Patients with milder ventricular dysfunction should, if possible, be controlled with optimum doses of digitalis and/or diuretics before verapamil treatment (Note interactions with digoxin under: **PRECAUTIONS**).

Trandolapril Component

Trandolapril, as an ACE inhibitor, may cause excessive hypotension in patients with congestive heart failure (see **WARNINGS - Hypotension**).

Hypotension

Verapamil Component

Occasionally, the pharmacologic action of verapamil may produce a decrease in blood pressure below normal levels which may result in dizziness or symptomatic hypotension.

Trandolapril Component

Trandolapril can cause symptomatic hypotension. Like other ACE inhibitors, trandolapril has only rarely been associated with symptomatic hypotension in uncomplicated hypertensive patients. Symptomatic hypotension is most likely to occur in patients who are salt- or volume-depleted as a result of prolonged treatment with diuretics, dietary salt restriction, dialysis, diarrhea, or vomiting. Volume and/or salt depletion should be corrected before initiating treatment with trandolapril (see **PRECAUTIONS - Drug Interactions** and **ADVERSE REACTIONS**).

In controlled studies, hypotension was observed in 0.6% of patients receiving any combination of trandolapril and verapamil HCl ER.

In patients with concomitant congestive heart failure, with or without associated renal insufficiency, ACE inhibitor therapy may cause excessive hypotension, which may be associated with oliguria or azotemia, and, rarely, with acute renal failure and death (see **DOSAGE AND ADMINISTRATION**).

If symptomatic hypotension occurs, the patient should be placed in the supine position and, if necessary, normal saline may be administered intravenously. A transient hypotensive response is not a contraindication to further doses; however, lower doses of verapamil HCl ER and/or trandolapril or reduced concomitant diuretic therapy should be considered.

Elevated Liver Enzymes/Hepatic Failure

Verapamil Component

Elevations of transaminases with and without concomitant elevations in alkaline phosphatase and bilirubin have been reported. Such elevations have sometimes been transient and may disappear even in the face of continued verapamil treatment. Several cases of hepatocellular injury related to verapamil have been proven by rechallenge; half of these had clinical symptoms (malaise, fever, and/or right upper quadrant pain) in addition to elevations of SGOT, SGPT, and alkaline phosphatase.

Trandolapril Component

ACE inhibitors rarely have been associated with a syndrome of cholestatic jaundice, fulminant hepatic necrosis, and death. The mechanism of this syndrome is not understood. Patients receiving ACE inhibitors who develop jaundice should discontinue the ACE inhibitor and receive appropriate medical follow-up.

Liver abnormalities were noted in 3.2% of patients taking any of several combinations of trandolapril/verapamil doses. Periodic monitoring of liver function in patients taking TARKA is therefore prudent.

Accessory Bypass Tract (Wolff-Parkinson-White or Lown-Ganong-Levine Syndromes)

Verapamil Component

Some patients with paroxysmal and/or chronic atrial fibrillation or atrial flutter and a coexisting accessory AV pathway have developed increased antegrade conduction across the accessory pathway bypassing the AV node, producing a very rapid ventricular response or ventricular fibrillation after receiving intravenous verapamil (or digitalis). Although a risk of this occurring with oral verapamil has not been established, such patients receiving oral verapamil may be at risk and its use in these patients is contraindicated (see **CONTRAINDICATIONS**).

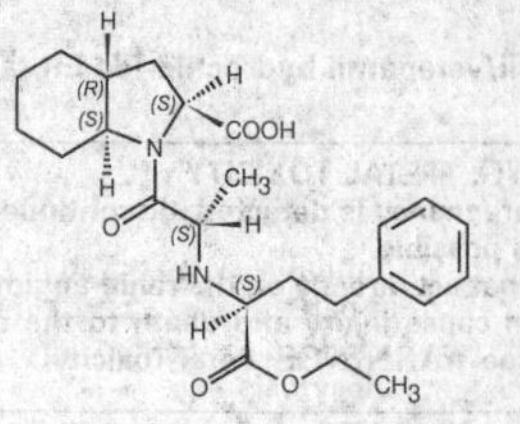

Treatment is usually DC-cardioversion. Cardioversion has been used safely and effectively after oral verapamil.

Atrioventricular Block

Verapamil Component

The effect of verapamil on AV conduction and the SA node may lead to asymptomatic first-degree AV block and transient bradycardia, sometimes accompanied by nodal escape rhythms. PR interval prolongation is correlated with verapamil plasma concentrations, especially during the early titration phases of therapy. Higher degrees of AV block, however, were infrequently (0.8%) observed. Marked first-degree block or progressive development to second- or third-degree AV block requires a reduction in dosage or, in rare instances, discontinuation of verapamil HCl and institution of appropriate therapy depending upon the clinical situation.

Patients with Hypertrophic Cardiomyopathy (IHSS)

Verapamil Component

In 120 patients with hypertrophic cardiomyopathy (most of them refractory or intolerant to propranolol) who received therapy with verapamil at doses up to 720 mg/day, a variety of serious adverse effects were seen. Three patients died in pulmonary edema; all had severe left ventricular outflow obstruction and a past history of left ventricular dysfunction. Eight other patients had pulmonary edema and/or severe hypotension; abnormally high (over 20 mmHg) capillary wedge pressure and a marked left ventricular outflow obstruction were present in most of these patients. Sinus bradycardia occurred in 11% of the patients, second-degree AV block in 4% and sinus arrest in 2%. It must be appreciated that this group of patients had a serious disease with a high mortality rate. Most adverse effects responded well to dose reduction and only rarely did verapamil have to be discontinued.

Anaphylactoid and Possibly Related Reactions

Presumably because angiotensin-converting enzyme inhibitors affect the metabolism of eicosanoids and polypeptides, including endogenous bradykinin, patients receiving ACE inhibitors, including trandolapril may be subject to a variety of adverse reactions, some of them serious.

Angioedema

Angioedema of the face, extremities, lips, tongue, glottis, and larynx has been reported in patients treated with ACE inhibitors including trandolapril. Symptoms suggestive of angioedema or facial edema occurred in 0.13% of trandolapril-treated patients. Two of the four cases were life-threatening and resolved without treatment or with medication (corticosteroids). Angioedema associated with laryngeal edema can be fatal. If laryngeal stridor or angioedema of the face, tongue or glottis occurs, treatment with TARKA should be discontinued immediately, the patient treated in accordance with accepted medical care and carefully observed until the swelling disappears. In instances where swelling is confined to the face and lips, the condition generally resolves without treatment; antihistamines may be useful in relieving symptoms. **Where there is involvement of the tongue, glottis, or larynx, likely to cause airway obstruction, emergency therapy, including but not limited to subcutaneous epinephrine solution 1:1,000 (0.3 to 0.5 mL) should be promptly administered** (see **PRECAUTIONS** and **ADVERSE REACTIONS**).

Patients receiving coadministration of an ACE inhibitor with an mTOR (mammalian target of rapamycin) inhibitor (e.g., temsirolimus, sirolimus, everolimus) may be at increased risk for angioedema.

Anaphylactoid Reactions During Desensitization

Two patients undergoing desensitizing treatment with hymenoptera venom while receiving ACE inhibitors sustained life-threatening anaphylactoid reactions. In the same patients, these reactions did not occur when ACE inhibitors were temporarily withheld, but they reappeared when the ACE inhibitors were inadvertently readministered.

Anaphylactoid Reactions During Membrane Exposure
Anaphylactoid reactions have been reported in patients dialyzed with high-flux membranes and treated concomitantly with an ACE inhibitor. Anaphylactoid reactions have also been reported in patients undergoing low-density lipoprotein apheresis with dextran sulfate absorption.

Neutropenia/Agranulocytosis
Trandolapril Component
Another ACE inhibitor, captopril, has been shown to cause agranulocytosis and bone marrow depression rarely in patients with uncomplicated hypertension, but more frequently in patients with renal impairment, especially if they also have a collagen-vascular disease such as systemic lupus erythematosus or scleroderma. Available data from clinical trials of trandolapril or TARKA are insufficient to show that trandolapril does not cause agranulocytosis at similar rates. As with other ACE inhibitors, periodic monitoring of white blood cell counts in patients with collagen-vascular disease and/or renal disease should be considered.

Fetal Toxicity
Pregnancy Category D
Trandolapril Component
Use of drugs that act on the renin-angiotensin system during the second and third trimesters of pregnancy reduces fetal renal function and increases fetal and neonatal morbidity and death. Resulting oligohydramnios can be associated with fetal lung hypoplasia and skeletal deformations. Potential neonatal adverse effects include skull hypoplasia, anuria, hypotension, renal failure, and death. When pregnancy is detected, discontinue TARKA as soon as possible. These adverse outcomes are usually associated with use of these drugs in the second and third trimester of pregnancy. Most epidemiologic studies examining fetal abnormalities after exposure to antihypertensive use in the first trimester have not distinguished drugs affecting the renin-angiotensin system from other antihypertensive agents. Appropriate management of maternal hypertension during pregnancy is important to optimize outcomes for both mother and fetus.
In the unusual case that there is no appropriate alternative to therapy with drugs affecting the renin-angiotensin system for a particular patient, apprise the mother of the potential risk to the fetus. Perform serial ultrasound examinations to assess the intra-amniotic environment. If oligohydramnios is observed, discontinue TARKA, unless it is considered lifesaving for the mother. Fetal testing may be appropriate, based on the week of pregnancy. Patients and physicians should be aware, however, that oligohydramnios may not appear until after the fetus has sustained irreversible injury. Closely observe infants with histories of *in utero* exposure to TARKA for hypotension, oliguria, and hyperkalemia (see **PRECAUTIONS - Pediatric Use**).
Doses of 0.8 mg/kg/day (9.4 mg/m2/day) in rabbits, 1000 mg/kg/day (7000 mg/m2/day) in rats, and 25 mg/kg/day (295 mg/m2/day) in cynomolgus monkeys did not produce teratogenic effects. These doses represent 10 and 3 times (rabbits), 1250 and 2564 times (rats), and 312 and 108 times (monkeys) the maximum projected human dose of 4 mg based on body-weight and body-surface-area, respectively assuming a 50 kg woman.
Trandolapril in doses of 0.8 mg/kg/day in rabbits, 100.0 mg/kg/day in rats, and 25 mg/kg/day in cynomolgus monkeys (10, 1250, and 312 times the maximum projected human dose, respectively, assuming a 50 kg woman) did not produce teratogenic effects.

PRECAUTIONS

Use in Patients with Impaired Hepatic Function
TARKA has not been evaluated in subjects with impaired hepatic function.
Verapamil Component
Since verapamil is highly metabolized by the liver, it should be administered cautiously to patients with impaired hepatic function. Severe liver dysfunction prolongs the elimination half-life of immediate release verapamil to about 14 to 16 hours; hence, approximately 30% of the dose given to patients with normal liver function should be administered to these patients.
Careful monitoring for abnormal prolongation of the PR interval or other signs of excessive pharmacologic effects (see **OVERDOSAGE**) should be carried out.
Trandolapril Component
Trandolapril and trandolaprilat concentrations increase in patients with impaired liver function.

Use in Patients with Impaired Renal Function
TARKA has not been evaluated in patients with impaired renal function.
Verapamil Component
About 70% of an administered dose of verapamil is excreted as metabolites in the urine. Verapamil is not removed by hemodialysis. Until further data are available, verapamil should be administered cautiously to patients with impaired renal function. These patients should be carefully monitored for abnormal prolongation of the PR interval or other signs of overdosage (see **OVERDOSAGE**).
Trandolapril Component
As a consequence of inhibiting the renin-angiotensin-aldosterone system, changes in renal function may be anticipated in susceptible individuals. In patients with severe heart failure whose renal function may depend on the activity of the renin-angiotensin-aldosterone system, treatment with ACE inhibitors, including trandolapril, may be associated with oliguria and/or progressive azotemia and rarely with acute renal failure and/or death.
In hypertensive patients with unilateral or bilateral renal artery stenosis, increases in blood urea nitrogen and serum creatinine have been observed in some patients following ACE inhibitor therapy. These increases were almost always reversible upon discontinuation of the ACE inhibitor and/or diuretic therapy. In such patients, renal function should be monitored during the first few weeks of therapy.
Some hypertensive patients with no apparent pre-existing renal vascular disease have developed increases in blood urea and serum creatinine, usually minor and transient, especially when ACE inhibitors have been given concomitantly with a diuretic. This is more likely to occur in patients with pre-existing renal impairment. Dosage reduction and/or discontinuation of any diuretic and/or the ACE inhibitor may be required.
Evaluation of hypertensive patients should always include assessment of renal function (see **DOSAGE AND ADMINISTRATION**).

Use in Patients with Attenuated (Decreased) Neuromuscular Transmission
Verapamil Component
It has been reported that verapamil decreases neuromuscular transmission in patients with Duchenne's muscular dystrophy, and that verapamil prolongs recovery from the neuromuscular blocking agent vecuronium. It may be necessary to decrease the dosage of verapamil when it is administered to patients with attenuated neuromuscular transmission (see **PRECAUTIONS - Surgery/Anesthesia**).

Hyperkalemia and Potassium-sparing Diuretics
Trandolapril Component
In clinical trials, hyperkalemia (serum potassium > 6.00 mEq/L) occurred in approximately 0.4 percent of hypertensive patients receiving trandolapril and in 0.8% of patients receiving a dose of trandolapril (0.5-8 mg) in combination with a dose of verapamil SR (120-240 mg). In most cases, elevated serum potassium levels were isolated values, which resolved despite continued therapy. None of these patients were discontinued from the trials because of hyperkalemia. Risk factors for the development of hyperkalemia include renal insufficiency, diabetes mellitus, and the concomitant use of potassium-sparing diuretics, potassium supplements, and/or potassium-containing salt substitutes, which should be used cautiously, if at all, with trandolapril (see **PRECAUTIONS - Drug Interactions**).

Cough
Presumably due to the inhibition of the degradation of endogenous bradykinin, persistent nonproductive cough has been reported with all ACE inhibitors, always resolving after discontinuation of therapy. ACE inhibitor-induced cough should be considered in the differential diagnosis of cough. In controlled trials of trandolapril, cough was present in 2% of trandolapril patients and 0% of patients given placebo. There was no evidence of a relationship to dose.

Surgery/anesthesia
Trandolapril Component
In patients undergoing major surgery or during anesthesia with agents that produce hypotension, trandolapril will block angiotensin II formation secondary to compensatory renin release. If hypotension occurs and is considered to be due to this mechanism, it can be corrected by volume expansion (see **PRECAUTIONS - Use in Patients with Attenuated (Decreased) Neuromuscular Transmission**).

Drug Interactions
In vitro metabolic studies indicate that verapamil is metabolized by cytochrome P450 including CYP3A4, CYP1A2, CYP2C8, CYP2C9 and CYP2C18. Verapamil has been shown to be an inhibitor of CYP3A4 enzymes and P-glycoprotein (P-gp).
Clinically significant interactions have been reported with inhibitors of CYP3A4 (e.g. erythromycin, ritonavir) causing elevation of plasma levels of verapamil while inducers of CYP3A4 (e.g. rifampin) have caused a lowering of plasma levels of verapamil. Therefore, patients receiving inhibitors or inducers of the cytochrome P450 system should be monitored for drug interactions.

Digitalis
Clinical use of verapamil in digitalized patients has shown the combination to be well tolerated if digoxin doses are properly adjusted. Chronic verapamil treatment can increase serum digoxin levels by 50 to 75% during the first week of therapy, and this can result in digoxin toxicity. In patients with hepatic cirrhosis, the influence of verapamil on digoxin kinetics is magnified. Verapamil may reduce total body clearance and extrarenal clearance of digitoxin by 27% and 29%, respectively. Maintenance digoxin doses should be reduced when verapamil is administered, and the patient should be carefully monitored to avoid over- or under-digitalization. Whenever overdigitalization is suspected, the daily dose of digoxin should be reduced or temporarily discontinued. Upon discontinuation of any verapamil-containing regime including TARKA (trandolapril/verapamil hydrochloride ER), the patient should be reassessed to avoid underdigitalization. No clinically significant pharmacokinetic interaction has been found between trandolapril (or its metabolites) and digoxin.

Lithium
Verapamil Component
Increased sensitivity to the effects of lithium (neurotoxicity) has been reported during concomitant verapamil-lithium therapy with either no change or an increase in serum lithium levels. Increased serum lithium levels and symptoms of lithium toxicity have been reported in patients receiving concomitant lithium and ACE inhibitor therapy. TARKA and lithium should be coadministered with caution, and frequent monitoring of serum lithium levels is recommended. If a diuretic is also used, the risk of lithium toxicity may be increased.

Clarithromycin
Hypotension, bradyarrhythmias, and lactic acidosis have been observed in patients receiving concurrent clarithromycin.

Erythromycin
Hypotension, bradyarrhythmias, and lactic acidosis have been observed in patients receiving concurrent erythromycin ethylsuccinate.

Cimetidine
The interaction between cimetidine and chronically administered verapamil has not been studied. Variable results on clearance have been obtained in acute studies of healthy volunteers; clearance of verapamil was either reduced or unchanged. No clinically significant pharmacokinetic interaction has been found between trandolapril (or its metabolites) and cimetidine.

Antiarrhythmic Agents
Verapamil Component
Disopyramide Phosphate
Data on possible interactions between verapamil and disopyramide phosphate are not available. Therefore, disopyramide should not be administered within 48 hours before or 24 hours after verapamil administration.

Flecainide
A study of healthy volunteers showed that the concomitant administration of flecainide and verapamil may have additive effects on myocardial contractility, AV conduction, and repolarization. Concomitant therapy with flecainide and verapamil may result in additive negative inotropic effect and prolongation of atrioventricular conduction.

Quinidine
In a small number of patients with hypertrophic cardiomyopathy (IHSS), concomitant use of verapamil and quinidine resulted in significant hypotension. Until further data are obtained, combined therapy of verapamil and quinidine in patients with hypertrophic cardiomyopathy should probably be avoided.

Continued on next page

Information on the AbbVie, Inc. products listed on these pages is from the prescribing information in use as of July 31, 2016. For more information, please visit rxabbvie.com or call 1-800-633-9110.

The electrophysiological effects of quinidine and verapamil on AV conduction were studied in 8 patients. Verapamil significantly counteracted the effects of quinidine on AV conduction. There has been a report of increased quinidine levels during verapamil therapy.

Antihypertensive Agents

Concomitant use of TARKA with other antihypertensive agents including diuretics, vasodilators, beta-adrenergic blockers, and alpha-antagonists may result in additive hypotensive effects. There are reports that verapamil may result in higher concentrations of the alpha-agonists prazosin and terazosin.

Dual Blockade of the Renin-Angiotensin System (RAS)
Trandolapril Component

Dual blockade of the RAS with angiotensin receptor blockers, ACE inhibitors, or aliskiren is associated with increased risks of hypotension, hyperkalemia, and changes in renal function (including acute renal failure) compared to monotherapy. Most patients receiving the combination of two RAS inhibitors do not obtain any additional benefit compared to monotherapy. In general, avoid combined use of RAS inhibitors. Closely monitor blood pressure, renal function and electrolytes in patients on TARKA and other agents that affect the RAS.

Do not co-administer aliskiren with TARKA in patients with diabetes. Avoid use of aliskiren with TARKA in patients with renal impairment (GFR <60 ml/min).

Beta Blockers
Verapamil Component

Concomitant therapy with beta-adrenergic blockers and verapamil may result in additive negative effects on heart rate, atrioventricular conduction, and/or cardiac contractility. Drug interaction studies have indicated that the maximum concentrations of metoprolol and propanolol are increased after the administration of verapamil. The use of verapamil in combination with a beta-adrenergic blocker should be used only with caution, and close monitoring. Asymptomatic bradycardia (36 beats/min) with a wandering atrial pacemaker has been observed in a patient receiving concomitant timolol (a beta-adrenergic blocker) eyedrops and oral verapamil.

Concomitant Diuretic Therapy
Trandolapril Component

As with other ACE inhibitors, patients on diuretics, especially those on recently instituted diuretic therapy, may occasionally experience an excessive reduction of blood pressure after initiation of therapy with TARKA. The possibility of exacerbation of hypotensive effects with TARKA may be minimized by either discontinuing the diuretic or cautiously increasing salt intake prior to initiation of treatment with TARKA. If it is not possible to discontinue the diuretic, the starting dose of TARKA should be reduced (see **DOSAGE AND ADMINISTRATION**). No clinically significant pharmacokinetic interaction has been found between trandolapril (or its metabolites) and furosemide.

Agents Increasing Serum Potassium
Trandolapril Component

Trandolapril can attenuate potassium loss caused by thiazide diuretics and increase serum potassium when used alone. Use of potassium-sparing diuretics (spironolactone, triamterene, or amiloride), potassium supplements, or potassium-containing salt substitutes concomitantly with ACE inhibitors can increase the risk of hyperkalemia. If concomitant use of such agents is indicated, they should be used with caution and with appropriate monitoring of serum potassium (see **PRECAUTIONS**).

HMG-CoA Reductase Inhibitors ("Statins")
Verapamil component

The use of HMG-CoA reductase inhibitors that are CYP3A4 substrates in combination with verapamil has been associated with reports of myopathy/rhabdomyolysis.

Co-administration of multiple doses of 10 mg of verapamil with 80 mg simvastatin resulted in exposure to simvastatin 2.5-fold that following simvastatin alone. Limit the dose of simvastatin in patients on verapamil to 10 mg daily. Limit the daily dose of lovastatin to 40 mg. Lower starting and maintenance doses of other CYP3A4 substrates (e.g., atorvastatin) may be required as verapamil may increase the plasma concentration of these drugs.

Non-Steroidal Anti-Inflammatory Agents including Selective Cyclooxygenase-2 Inhibitors (COX-2 Inhibitors)
Trandolapril component

In patients who are elderly, volume-depleted (including those on diuretic therapy), or with compromised renal function, co-administration of NSAIDs, including selective COX-2 inhibitors, with ACE inhibitors, including trandolapril, may result in deterioration of renal function, including possible acute renal failure. These effects are usually reversible. Monitor renal function periodically in patients receiving trandolapril and NSAID therapy.

The antihypertensive effect of ACE inhibitors, including trandolapril may be attenuated by NSAIDs.

Other (Verapamil Component)
Nitrates

Verapamil has been given concomitantly with short- and long-acting nitrates without any undesirable drug interactions. The pharmacologic profile of both drugs and the clinical experience suggest beneficial interactions.

Carbamazepine

Verapamil may increase carbamazepine concentrations during combined therapy. This may produce carbamazepine side effects such as diplopia, headache, ataxia, or dizziness.

Anti-infective Agents

Therapy with rifampin may markedly reduce oral verapamil bioavailability. There have been reports that erythromycin and telithromycin may increase concentrations of verapamil.

Barbiturates

Phenobarbital therapy may increase verapamil clearance.

Immunosuppressive Agents

Verapamil therapy may increase serum levels of cyclosporin, sirolimus and tacrolimus.

Theophylline

Verapamil therapy may inhibit the clearance and increase the plasma levels of theophylline.

Tranquilizers/ Anti-depressants

Due to metabolism via the CYP enzyme system, there have been reports that verapamil may increase the concentrations of buspirone, midazolam, almotriptan and imipramine.

Colchicine

Colchicine is a substrate for both CYP3A and the efflux transporter, P-gp. Verapamil is known to inhibit CYP3A and P-gp. When verapamil and colchicine are administered together, the potential inhibition of P-gp and/or CYP3A by verapamil may lead to increased exposure to colchicine (see **PRECAUTIONS - Drug Interactions**).

Other

Concentrations of verapamil may be increased by the concomitant administration of protease inhibitors such as ritonavir, and reduced by the concomitant administration of sulfinpyrazone, or St John's Wort.

Concentrations of doxorubicin may be increased by the administration of verapamil.

There have been reports that verapamil may elevate the concentrations of the oral anti-diabetic glyburide.

Inhalation Anesthetics

Animal experiments have shown that inhalation anesthetics depress cardiovascular activity by decreasing the inward movement of calcium ions. When used concomitantly, inhalation anesthetics and calcium antagonists, such as verapamil, should be titrated carefully to avoid excessive cardiovascular depression.

Neuromuscular Blocking Agents

Clinical data and animal studies suggest that verapamil may potentiate the activity of neuromuscular blocking agents (curare-like and depolarizing). It may be necessary to decrease the dose of verapamil and/or the dose of the neuromuscular blocking agent when the drugs are used concomitantly.

Gold

Nitritoid reactions (symptoms include facial flushing, nausea, vomiting and hypotension) have been reported rarely in patients on therapy with injectable gold (sodium aurothiomalate) and concomitant ACE inhibitor therapy including TARKA.

Other (Trandolapril Component)

No clinically significant pharmacokinetic interaction has been found between trandolapril (or its metabolites) and nifedipine.

The anticoagulant effect of warfarin was not significantly changed by trandolapril.

Mammalian Target of Rapamycin (mTOR) Inhibitors

Patients taking concomitant mTOR inhibitor (e.g., temsirolimus, sirolimus, everolimus) therapy may be at increased risk for angioedema (see **WARNINGS - Angioedema**).

Anti-diabetic Agents

The concomitant use of ACE inhibitors such as trandolapril with antidiabetic medications (insulin or oral hypoglycemic agents) may result in increased blood glucose lowering effects.

Carcinogenesis, Mutagenesis, Impairment of Fertility
Verapamil Component

An 18-month toxicity study in rats, at a low multiple (6 fold) of the maximum recommended human dose, and not the maximum tolerated dose, did not suggest a tumorigenic potential. There was no evidence of a carcinogenic potential of verapamil administered in the diet of rats for two years at doses of 10, 35, and 120 mg/kg per day or approximately 1×, 3.5×, and 12×, respectively, the maximum recommended human daily dose (480 mg per day or 9.6 mg/kg/day).

Verapamil was not mutagenic in the Ames test in 5 test strains at 3 mg per plate, with or without metabolic activation.

Studies in female rats at daily dietary doses up to 5.5 times (55 mg/kg/day) the maximum recommended human dose did not show impaired fertility. Effects on male fertility have not been determined.

Trandolapril Component

Long-term studies were conducted with oral trandolapril administered by gavage to mice (78 weeks) and rats (104 and 106 weeks). No evidence of carcinogenic potential was seen in mice dosed up to 25 mg/kg/day (85 mg/m^2/day) or rats dosed up to 8 mg/kg/day (60 mg/m^2/day). These doses are 313 and 32 times (mice), and 100 and 23 times (rats) the maximum recommended human daily dose (MRHDD) of 4 mg based on body-weight and body-surface-area, respectively assuming a 50 kg individual. The genotoxic potential of trandolapril was evaluated in the microbial mutagenicity (Ames) test, the point mutation and chromosome aberration assays in Chinese hamster V79 cells, and the micronucleus test in mice. There was no evidence of mutagenic or clastogenic potential in these *in vitro* and *in vivo* assays.

Reproduction studies in rats did not show any impairment of fertility at doses up to 100 mg/kg/day (710 mg/m^2/day) of trandolapril, or 1250 and 260 times the MRHDD on the basis of body-weight and body-surface-area, respectively.

Pregnancy

Female patients of childbearing age should be told about the consequences of exposure to TARKA during pregnancy. Discuss treatment options with women planning to become pregnant. Patients should be asked to report pregnancies to their physicians as soon as possible.

Nursing Mothers

Verapamil is excreted in human milk. Radiolabeled trandolapril or its metabolites are secreted in rat milk. TARKA should not be administered to nursing mothers.

Geriatric Use

In placebo-controlled studies, where 23% of patients receiving TARKA were 65 years and older, and 2.4% were 75 years and older, no overall differences in effectiveness or safety were observed between these patients and younger patients. However, greater sensitivity of some older individual patients cannot be ruled out.

Pediatric Use

Neonates with a history of *in utero* exposure to TARKA: If oliguria or hypotension occurs, direct attention toward support of blood pressure and renal perfusion. Exchange transfusions or dialysis may be required as a means of reversing hypotension and/or substituting for disordered renal function.

The safety and effectiveness of TARKA in children below the age of 18 have not been established.

Animal Pharmacology and/or Animal Toxicology

In chronic animal toxicology studies, verapamil caused lenticular and/or suture line changes at 30 mg/kg/day or greater and frank cataracts at 62.5 mg/kg/day or greater in the beagle dog but not the rat. Development of cataracts due to verapamil has not been reported in man.

ADVERSE REACTIONS

TARKA has been evaluated in over 1,957 subjects and patients. Of these, 541 patients, including 23% elderly patients, participated in U.S. controlled clinical trials, and 251 were studied in foreign controlled clinical trials. In clinical trials with TARKA, no adverse experiences peculiar to this combination drug have been observed. Adverse experiences that have occurred have been limited to those that have been previously reported with verapamil or trandolapril. TARKA has been evaluated for long-term safety in 272 patients treated for 1 year or more. Adverse experiences were usually mild and transient.

Discontinuation of therapy because of adverse events in U.S. placebo-controlled hypertension studies was required in 2.6% and 1.9% of patients treated with TARKA and placebo, respectively.

Adverse experiences occurring in 1% or more of the 541 patients in placebo-controlled hypertension trials who were treated with a range of trandolapril (0.5-8 mg) and verapamil (120-240 mg) combinations are shown below. [See table above]

Other clinical adverse experiences possibly, probably, or definitely related to drug treatment occurring in 0.3% or more of patients treated with trandolapril/verapamil combinations with or without concomitant diuretic in controlled or uncontrolled trials (N = 990) and less frequent, clinically significant events (in italics) include the following:

Cardiovascular
Angina, AV block second degree, bundle branch block, edema, flushing, hypotension, myocardial infarction , palpitations, premature ventricular contractions, nonspecific ST-T changes, near syncope, tachycardia.

Central Nervous System
Drowsiness, hypesthesia, insomnia, loss of balance, paresthesia, vertigo.

Dermatologic
Pruritus, rash.

Emotional, Mental, Sexual States
Anxiety, impotence, abnormal mentation.

Eye, Ear, Nose, Throat
Epistaxis, tinnitus, upper respiratory tract infection, blurred vision.

Gastrointestinal
Diarrhea, dyspepsia, dry mouth, nausea.

General Body Function
Chest pain, malaise, weakness.

Genitourinary
Endometriosis, hematuria, nocturia, polyuria, proteinuria.

Hemopoietic
Decreased leukocytes, decreased neutrophils.

Musculoskeletal System
Arthralgias/myalgias, gout (increased uric acid).

Pulmonary
Dyspnea.

Angioedema
Angioedema has been reported in 3 (0.15%) patients receiving TARKA in U.S. and foreign studies (N = 1,957). Angioedema associated with laryngeal edema may be fatal. If angioedema of the face, extremities, lips, tongue, glottis, and/or larynx occurs, treatment with TARKA should be discontinued and appropriate therapy instituted immediately (see **WARNINGS**).

Hypotension
(See **WARNINGS**). In hypertensive patients, hypotension occurred in 0.6% and near syncope occurred in 0.1%. Hypotension or syncope was a cause for discontinuation of therapy in 0.4% of hypertensive patients.

Treatment of Acute Cardiovascular Adverse Reactions
The frequency of cardiovascular adverse reactions which require therapy is rare, hence, experience with their treatment is limited. Whenever severe hypotension or complete AV block occur following oral administration of TARKA (verapamil component), the appropriate emergency measures should be applied immediately, e.g., intravenously administered isoproterenol HCl, levarterenol bitartrate, atropine (all in the usual doses), or calcium gluconate (10% solution). In patients with hypertrophic cardiomyopathy (IHSS), alpha-adrenergic agents (phenylephrine, metaraminol bitartrate or methoxamine) should be used to maintain blood pressure, and isoproterenol and levarterenol should be avoided. If further support is necessary, inotropic agents (dopamine or dobutamine) may be administered. Actual treatment and dosage should depend on the severity of the clinical situation and the judgment and experience of the treating physician.

Other
Other adverse experiences (in addition to those in table and listed above) that have been reported with the individual components are listed below.

Verapamil Component
Cardiovascular
(See **WARNINGS**). CHF/pulmonary edema, AV block 3°, atrioventricular dissociation, claudication, purpura (vasculitis), syncope.

Digestive System
Gingival hyperplasia. Reversible, (upon discontinuation of verapamil) nonobstructive, paralytic ileus has been infrequently reported in association with the use of verapamil.

Hemic and Lymphatic
Ecchymosis or bruising.

Nervous System
Cerebrovascular accident, confusion, psychotic symptoms, shakiness, somnolence.

Skin
Exanthema, hair loss, hyperkeratosis, maculae, sweating, urticaria, Stevens-Johnson syndrome, erythema multiform.

Urogenital
Gynecomastia, galactorrhea/hyperprolactinemia, increased urination, spotty menstruation.

Trandolapril Component
Emotional, Mental, Sexual States
Decreased libido.

Gastrointestinal
Pancreatitis.

Clinical Laboratory Test Findings
Hematology
(See **WARNINGS**). Low white blood cells, low neutrophils, low lymphocytes, low platelets.

Serum Electrolytes
Hyperkalemia (see **PRECAUTIONS**), hyponatremia.

Renal Function Tests
Increases in creatinine and blood urea nitrogen levels occurred in 1.1 percent and 0.3 percent, respectively, of patients receiving TARKA with or without hydrochlorothiazide therapy. None of these increases required discontinuation of treatment. Increases in these laboratory values are more likely to occur in patients with renal insufficiency or those pretreated with a diuretic and, based on experience with other ACE inhibitors, would be expected to be especially likely in patients with renal artery stenosis (see **PRECAUTIONS** and **WARNINGS**).

Liver Function Tests
Elevations of liver enzymes (SGOT, SGPT, LDH, and alkaline phosphatase) and/or serum bilirubin occurred. Discontinuation for elevated liver enzymes occurred in 0.9 percent of patients (see **WARNINGS**).

Post Marketing Experience
There has been a single postmarketing report of paralysis (tetraparesis) associated with the combined use of verapamil and colchicine. This may have been caused by colchicine crossing the blood-brain barrier due to CYP3A4 and P-gp inhibition by verapamil. Combined use of verapamil and colchicine is not recommended (see **PRECAUTIONS - Drug Interactions**).

OVERDOSAGE
No specific information is available on the treatment of overdosage with TARKA.

Verapamil Component
Overdose with verapamil may lead to pronounced hypotension, bradycardia, and conduction system abnormalities (e.g., junctional rhythm with AV dissociation and high degree AV block, including asystole). Other symptoms secondary to hypoperfusion (e.g., metabolic acidosis, hyperglycemia, hyperkalemia, renal dysfunction, and convulsions) may be evident.

Treat all verapamil overdoses as serious and maintain observation for at least 48 hours, preferably under continuous hospital care. Delayed pharmacodynamic consequences may occur with the sustained release formulation. Verapamil is known to decrease gastrointestinal transit time. In cases of overdose, tablets of ISOPTIN SR have occasionally been reported to form concretions within the stomach or intestines. These concretions have not been visible on plain radiographs of the abdomen, and no medical means of gastrointestinal emptying is of proven efficacy in removing them. Endoscopy might reasonably be considered in cases of overdose when symptoms are unusually prolonged. Verapamil cannot be removed by hemodialysis.

Treatment of overdosage should be supportive. Beta adrenergic stimulation or parenteral administration of calcium solutions may increase calcium ion flux across the slow channel, and have been used effectively in treatment of deliberate overdosage with verapamil. The following measures may be considered:

Bradycardia and Conduction System Abnormalities
Atropine, isoproterenol, and cardiac pacing.

Hypotension
Intravenous fluids, vasopressors (e.g., dopamine, dobutamine), calcium solutions (e.g., 10% calcium chloride solution).

Cardiac Failures
Inotropic agents (e.g., isoproterenol, dopamine, dobutamine), diuretics. Asystole should be handled by the usual measures including cardiopulmonary resuscitation.

Trandolapril Component
The oral LD$_{50}$ of trandolapril in mice was 4875 mg/kg in males and 3990 mg/kg in females. In rats, an oral dose of 5000 mg/kg caused low mortality (1 male out of 5; 0 females). In dogs, an oral dose of 1000 mg/kg did not cause mortality and abnormal clinical signs were not observed.

In humans, the most likely clinical manifestation would be symptoms attributable to severe hypotension. Laboratory determinations of serum levels of trandolapril and its metabolites are not widely available, and such determinations have, in any event, no established role in the management of trandolapril overdose. No data are available to suggest that physiological maneuvers (e.g., maneuvers to change pH of the urine) might accelerate elimination of trandolapril

Continued on next page

ADVERSE EVENTS OCCURRING in ≥ 1% of TARKA PATIENTS IN U.S. PLACEBO-CONTROLLED TRIALS		
	TARKA **(N = 541)** % Incidence (% Discontinuance)	**PLACEBO** **(N = 206)** % Incidence (% Discontinuance)
AV Block First Degree	3.9 (0.2)	0.5 (0.0)
Bradycardia	1.8 (0.0)	0.0 (0.0)
Bronchitis	1.5 (0.0)	0.5 (0.0)
Chest Pain	2.2 (0.0)	1.0 (0.0)
Constipation	3.3 (0.0)	1.0 (0.0)
Cough	4.6 (0.0)	2.4 (0.0)
Diarrhea	1.5 (0.2)	1.0 (0.0)
Dizziness	3.1 (0.0)	1.9 (0.5)
Dyspnea	1.3 (0.0)	0.0 (0.0)
Edema	1.3 (0.0)	2.4 (0.0)
Fatigue	2.8 (0.4)	2.4 (0.0)
Headache(s)+	8.9 (0.0)	9.7 (0.5)
Increased Liver Enzymes*	2.8 (0.2)	1.0 (0.0)
Nausea	1.5 (0.0)	0.5 (0.0)
Pain Extremity(ies)	1.1 (0.2)	0.5 (0.0)
Pain Back+	2.2 (0.0)	2.4 (0.0)
Pain Joint(s)	1.7 (0.0)	1.0 (0.0)
Upper Respiratory Tract Infection(s)+	5.4 (0.0)	7.8 (0.0)
Upper Respiratory Tract Congestion+	2.4 (0.0)	3.4 (0.0)

* Also includes increase in SGPT, SGOT, Alkaline Phosphatase
+ Incidence of adverse events is higher in Placebo group than TARKA patients

Information on the AbbVie, Inc. products listed on these pages is from the prescribing information in use as of July 31, 2016. For more information, please visit rxabbvie.com or call 1-800-633-9110.

and its metabolites. It is not known if trandolapril or trandolaprilat can be usefully removed from the body by hemodialysis.

Angiotensin II could presumably serve as a specific antagonist antidote in the setting of trandolapril overdose, but angiotensin II is essentially unavailable outside of scattered research facilities. Because the hypotensive effect of trandolapril is achieved through vasodilation and effective hypovolemia, it is reasonable to treat trandolapril overdose by infusion of normal saline solution.

DOSAGE AND ADMINISTRATION

The recommended usual dosage range of trandolapril for hypertension is 1 to 4 mg per day administered in a single dose or two divided doses. The recommended usual dosage range of Isoptin-SR for hypertension is 120 to 480 mg per day administered in a single dose or two divided doses.

The hazards (see **WARNINGS**) of trandolapril are generally independent of dose; those of verapamil are a mixture of dose-dependent phenomena (primarily dizziness, AV block, constipation) and dose-independent phenomena, the former much more common than the latter. Therapy with any combination of trandolapril and verapamil will thus be associated with both sets of dose-independent hazards. The dose-dependent side effects of verapamil have not been shown to be decreased by the addition of trandolapril nor vice versa. Rarely, the dose-independent hazards of trandolapril are serious. To minimize dose-independent hazards, it is usually appropriate to begin therapy with TARKA only after a patient has either (a) failed to achieve the desired antihypertensive effect with one or the other monotherapy at its respective maximally recommended dose and shortest dosing interval, or (b) the dose of one or the other monotherapy cannot be increased further because of dose-limiting side effects.

Clinical trials with TARKA have explored only once-a-day doses. The antihypertensive effect and or adverse effects of adding 4 mg of trandolapril once-a-day to a dose of 240 mg Isoptin-SR administered twice-a-day has not been studied, nor have the effects of adding as little of 180 mg Isoptin-SR to 2 mg trandolapril administered twice-a-day been evaluated. Over the dose range of Isoptin-SR 120 to 240 mg once-a-day and trandolapril 0.5 to 8 mg once-a-day, the effects of the combination increase with increasing doses of either component.

Replacement Therapy

For convenience, patients receiving trandolapril (up to 8 mg) and verapamil (up to 240 mg) in separate tablets, administered once-a-day, may instead wish to receive tablets of TARKA containing the same component doses.

TARKA should be administered with food.

HOW SUPPLIED

TARKA 2/180 mg tablets are supplied as pink, oval, film-coated tablets containing 2 mg trandolapril in an immediate release form and 180 mg verapamil hydrochloride in a sustained release form. The tablet is debossed with a triangle and 182 on one side and plain on the other side.

NDC 0074-3287-13 - bottles of 100

TARKA 1/240 mg tablets are supplied as white, oval, film-coated tablets containing 1 mg trandolapril in an immediate release form and 240 mg verapamil hydrochloride in a sustained release form. The tablet is debossed with a triangle and 241 on one side and plain on the other side.

NDC 0074-3288-13 - bottles of 100

TARKA 2/240 mg tablets are supplied as gold, oval, film-coated tablets containing 2 mg trandolapril in an immediate release form and 240 mg verapamil hydrochloride in a sustained release form. The tablet is debossed with a triangle and 242 on one side and plain on the other side.

NDC 0074-3289-13 - bottles of 100

TARKA 4/240 mg tablets are supplied as reddish-brown, oval, film-coated tablets containing 4 mg trandolapril in an immediate release form and 240 mg verapamil hydrochloride in a sustained release form. The tablet is debossed with a triangle and 244 on one side and plain on the other side.

NDC 0074-3290-13 - bottles of 100

Dispense in well-closed container with safety closure.

Storage

Store at 15°-25°C (59°-77°F) see USP.

AbbVie Inc.

North Chicago, IL 60064, U.S.A.

03-B298 January 2016

Shown in Product Identification Guide, page 506

TECHNIVIE™   ℞
[TEK-ni-vee]
(ombitasvir, paritaprevir and ritonavir) tablets

HIGHLIGHTS OF PRESCRIBING INFORMATION
These highlights do not include all the information needed to use TECHNIVIE safely and effectively. See full prescribing information for TECHNIVIE.
TECHNIVIE™ (ombitasvir, paritaprevir and ritonavir) tablets, for oral use
Initial U.S. Approval: 2015

—————————— **INDICATIONS AND USAGE** ——————————

TECHNIVIE is a fixed-dose combination of ombitasvir, a hepatitis C virus NS5A inhibitor, paritaprevir, a hepatitis C virus NS3/4A protease inhibitor, and ritonavir, a CYP3A inhibitor and is indicated in combination with ribavirin for the treatment of patients with genotype 4 chronic hepatitis C virus (HCV) infection without cirrhosis. (1)

————————— **DOSAGE AND ADMINISTRATION** —————————

• Testing Prior to Initiation: Assess baseline hepatic laboratory and clinical parameters. (2.1)
• Recommended dosage: Two tablets taken orally once daily (in the morning) with a meal without regard to fat or calorie content. TECHNIVIE is recommended to be used in combination with ribavirin. (2.2)

Patient Population	Treatment	Duration
Genotype 4 without cirrhosis	TECHNIVIE + ribavirin*	12 weeks

*TECHNIVIE administered without ribavirin for 12 weeks may be considered for treatment-naïve patients who cannot take or tolerate ribavirin *[see Microbiology (12.4) and Clinical Studies (14)]*.

————————— **DOSAGE FORMS AND STRENGTHS** —————————

Tablets: 12.5 mg ombitasvir, 75 mg paritaprevir, 50 mg ritonavir. (3)

—————————— **CONTRAINDICATIONS** ——————————

• The contraindications to ribavirin also apply to this combination regimen. (4)
• Patients with moderate to severe hepatic impairment. (4, 5.1, 8.6, 12.3)
• Co-administration with drugs that are: highly dependent on CYP3A for clearance; moderate and strong inducers of CYP3A. (4)
• Known hypersensitivity to ritonavir (e.g. toxic epidermal necrolysis, Stevens-Johnson syndrome). (4)

————————— **WARNINGS AND PRECAUTIONS** —————————

• Hepatic Decompensation and Hepatic Failure in Patient with Cirrhosis: Hepatic decompensation and hepatic failure, including liver transplantation or fatal outcomes, have been reported mostly in patients with advanced cirrhosis. Discontinue treatment in patients who develop evidence of hepatic decompensation. (5.1)
• ALT Elevations: Discontinue ethinyl estradiol-containing medications prior to starting TECHNIVIE (alternative contraceptive methods are recommended). Perform hepatic laboratory testing on all patients during the first 4 weeks of treatment. For ALT elevations on TECHNIVIE, monitor closely and follow recommendations in full prescribing information. (5.2)
• Risks Associated With Ribavirin Combination Treatment: The warnings and precautions for ribavirin also apply to this combination regimen. (5.3)
• Drug Interactions: The concomitant use of TECHNIVIE and certain other drugs may result in known or potentially significant drug interactions, some of which may lead to loss of therapeutic effect of TECHNIVIE. (5.4)

——————————— **ADVERSE REACTIONS** ———————————

The most commonly reported adverse reactions (incidence greater than 10% of subjects, all grades) observed with treatment with ombitasvir, paritaprevir and ritonavir with ribavirin for 12 weeks were asthenia, fatigue, nausea and insomnia. (6.1)

To report SUSPECTED ADVERSE REACTIONS, contact AbbVie Inc. at 1-800-633-9110 or FDA at 1-800-FDA-1088 or www.fda.gov/medwatch.

——————————— **DRUG INTERACTIONS** ———————————

Co-administration of TECHNIVIE can alter the plasma concentrations of some drugs and some drugs may alter the plasma concentrations of TECHNIVIE. The potential for drug-drug interactions must be considered before and during treatment. Consult the full prescribing information. prior to and during treatment for potential drug interactions. (4, 5.4, 7, 12.3)

See 17 for PATIENT COUNSELING INFORMATION and Medication Guide.

Revised: 6/2016

Table 2. Drugs that are Contraindicated with TECHNIVIE

Drug Class	Drug(s) within Class that are Contraindicated	Clinical Comments
Alpha1-adrenoreceptor antagonist	Alfuzosin HCl	Potential for hypotension.
Anti-gout	Colchicine	Potential for serious and/or life-threatening reactions in patients with renal and/or hepatic impairment.
Anti-anginal	Ranolazine	Potential for serious and/or life-threatening reactions.
Antiarrhythmic	Dronedarone	Potential for serious and/or life-threatening reactions such as cardiac arrhythmias.
Anticonvulsants	Carbamazepine, phenytoin, phenobarbital	Ombitasvir, paritaprevir and ritonavir exposures may decrease leading to a potential loss of therapeutic activity of TECHNIVIE.
Antimycobacterial	Rifampin	Ombitasvir, paritaprevir and ritonavir exposures may decrease leading to a potential loss of therapeutic activity of TECHNIVIE.
Antipsychotic	Lurasidone Pimozide	Potential for serious and/or life-threatening reactions. Potential for serious and/or life-threatening reactions such as cardiac arrhythmias.
Ergot derivatives	Ergotamine, dihydroergotamine, methylergonovine	Acute ergot toxicity characterized by vasospasm and tissue ischemia has been associated with co-administration of ritonavir and ergonovine, ergotamine, dihydroergotamine, or methylergonovine.
Ethinyl estradiol-containing products	Ethinyl estradiol-containing medications such as combined oral contraceptives	Potential for ALT elevations *[see Warnings and Precautions (5.2)]*.
GI Motility Agent	Cisapride	Potential for serious and/or life threatening reactions such as cardiac arrhythmias
Herbal Product	St. John's Wort (*Hypericum perforatum*)	Ombitasvir, paritaprevir and ritonavir exposures may decrease leading to a potential loss of therapeutic activity of TECHNIVIE.
HMG-CoA Reductase Inhibitors	Lovastatin, simvastatin	Potential for myopathy including rhabdomyolysis.
Non-nucleoside reverse transcriptase inhibitor	Efavirenz	Co-administration of efavirenz based regimens with paritaprevir, ritonavir was poorly tolerated and resulted in liver enzyme elevations.
Phosphodiesterase-5 (PDE5) inhibitor	Sildenafil when dosed as Revatio for the treatment of pulmonary arterial hypertension (PAH)	There is increased potential for sildenafil-associated adverse events such as visual disturbances, hypotension, priapism, and syncope.
Sedatives/hypnotics	Triazolam Orally administered midazolam	Triazolam and orally administered midazolam are extensively metabolized by CYP3A4. Coadministration of triazolam or orally administered midazolam with TECHNIVIE may cause large increases in the concentration of these benzodiazepines. The potential exists for serious and/or life threatening events such as prolonged or increased sedation or respiratory depression.

FULL PRESCRIBING INFORMATION

1 INDICATIONS AND USAGE

TECHNIVIE is indicated in combination with ribavirin for the treatment of patients with genotype 4 chronic hepatitis C virus (HCV) infection without cirrhosis.

2 DOSAGE AND ADMINISTRATION

2.1 Testing Prior to Initiation of TECHNIVIE
Prior to initiation of TECHNIVIE, assess baseline hepatic laboratory and clinical parameters *[see Contraindications (4) and Warnings and Precautions (5.1 and 5.2)]*.

2.2 Recommended Dosage in Adults
TECHNIVIE is ombitasvir, paritaprevir and ritonavir fixed dose combination tablets.
The recommended dosage of TECHNIVIE is two tablets taken orally once daily (in the morning). Take TECHNIVIE with a meal without regard to fat or calorie content *[see Clinical Pharmacology (12.3)]*.
TECHNIVIE is used in combination with ribavirin (RBV). When administered with TECHNIVIE, the recommended dosage of RBV is based on weight: 1000 mg per day for subjects less than 75 kg and 1200 mg per day for those weighing at least 75 kg, divided and administered twice-daily with food. For ribavirin dosage modifications, refer to the ribavirin prescribing information.
Table 1 shows the recommended TECHNIVIE treatment regimen and duration for HCV genotype 4 patients without cirrhosis.

Table 1. Treatment Regimen and Duration for Patients with HCV Genotype 4 without Cirrhosis

Patient Population	Treatment	Duration
Genotype 4 without cirrhosis	TECHNIVIE + ribavirin*	12 weeks

*TECHNIVIE administered without RBV for 12 weeks may be considered for treatment-naïve patients who cannot take or tolerate ribavirin *[see Microbiology (12.4) and Clinical Studies (14)]*.

2.3 Dosage in Patients with Hepatic Impairment
TECHNIVIE is contraindicated in patients with moderate to severe hepatic impairment (Child-Pugh B and C) *[see Contraindications (4), Warnings and Precautions (5.1), Use in Specific Populations (8.6), and Clinical Pharmacology (12.3)]*.

3 DOSAGE FORMS AND STRENGTHS

TECHNIVIE is a pink-colored, film-coated, oblong, biconvex-shaped tablet debossed "AV1" on one side. Each tablet contains 12.5 mg ombitasvir, 75 mg paritaprevir and 50 mg ritonavir.

4 CONTRAINDICATIONS

- The contraindications to ribavirin also apply to this combination regimen. Refer to the ribavirin prescribing information for a list of contraindications for ribavirin.
- TECHNIVIE is contraindicated:
  - In patients with moderate to severe hepatic impairment (Child-Pugh B and C) due to risk of potential toxicity *[see Warnings and Precautions (5.1), Use in Specific Populations (8.6) and Clinical Pharmacology (12.3)]*.
  - With drugs that are highly dependent on CYP3A for clearance and for which elevated plasma concentrations are associated with serious and/or life-threatening events.
  - With drugs that are moderate or strong inducers of CYP3A and may lead to reduced efficacy of TECHNIVIE.
  - In patients with known hypersensitivity to ritonavir (e.g. toxic epidermal necrolysis (TEN) or Stevens-Johnson syndrome).

Continued on next page

Information on the AbbVie, Inc. products listed on these pages is from the prescribing information in use as of July 31, 2016. For more information, please visit rxabbvie.com or call 1-800-633-9110.

Table 2 lists drugs that are contraindicated with TECHNIVIE [see Drug Interactions (7)].
[See table on previous page]

5   WARNINGS AND PRECAUTIONS

5.1   Risk of Hepatic Decompensation and Hepatic Failure in Patients with Cirrhosis

TECHNIVIE is not indicated in patients with cirrhosis. Hepatic decompensation and hepatic failure, including liver transplantation or fatal outcomes, have been reported post-marketing in patients treated with ombitasvir, paritaprevir, ritonavir with and without dasabuvir and with and without ribavirin. Most patients with these severe outcomes had evidence of advanced cirrhosis prior to initiating therapy. Reported cases typically occurred within one to four weeks of initiating therapy and were characterized by the acute onset of rising direct serum bilirubin levels without ALT elevations in association with clinical signs and symptoms of hepatic decompensation. Because these events are reported voluntarily from a population of uncertain size, it is not always possible to reliably estimate their frequency or establish a causal relationship to drug exposure. Discontinue treatment in patients who develop evidence of hepatic decompensation.

TECHNIVIE is contraindicated in patients with moderate to severe hepatic impairment (Child-Pugh B and C) [see Contraindications (4), Adverse Reactions (6.2), Use in Specific Populations (8.6), and Clinical Pharmacology (12.3)].

5.2   Increased Risk of ALT Elevations

During clinical trials with ombitasvir, paritaprevir and ritonavir with or without dasabuvir and with or without ribavirin, elevations of ALT to greater than 5 times the upper limit of normal (ULN) occurred in approximately 1% of subjects [see Adverse Reactions (6.1)]. ALT elevations were typically asymptomatic, occurred during the first 4 weeks of treatment, and declined within two to eight weeks of onset with continued dosing.

These ALT elevations were significantly more frequent in female subjects who were using ethinyl estradiol-containing medications such as combined oral contraceptives, contraceptive patches or contraceptive vaginal rings. Ethinyl estradiol-containing medications must be discontinued prior to starting therapy with TECHNIVIE [see Contraindications (4)]. Alternative methods of contraception (e.g., progestin only contraception or non-hormonal methods) are recommended during TECHNIVIE therapy. Ethinyl estradiol-containing medications can be restarted approximately 2 weeks following completion of treatment with TECHNIVIE.

Women using estrogens other than ethinyl estradiol, such as estradiol and conjugated estrogens used in hormone replacement therapy had a rate of ALT elevation similar to those not receiving any estrogens. Due to the limited number of subjects taking these other estrogens in clinical studies, caution is warranted for co-administration with TECHNIVIE [see Adverse Reactions (6.1)].

Hepatic laboratory testing should be performed during the first 4 weeks of starting treatment and as clinically indicated thereafter. If ALT is found to be elevated above baseline levels, it should be repeated and monitored closely:

- Patients should be instructed to consult their health care professional without delay if they have onset of fatigue, weakness, lack of appetite, nausea and vomiting, jaundice or discolored feces.
- Consider discontinuing TECHNIVIE if ALT levels remain persistently greater than 10 times the ULN.
- Discontinue TECHNIVIE if ALT elevation is accompanied by signs or symptoms of liver inflammation or increasing direct bilirubin, alkaline phosphatase, or INR.

5.3   Risks Associated With Ribavirin Combination Treatment

The warnings and precautions for ribavirin, in particular the pregnancy avoidance warning, apply to this combination regimen. Refer to the ribavirin prescribing information for a full list of the warnings and precautions for ribavirin.

5.4   Risk of Adverse Reactions or Reduced Therapeutic Effect Due to Drug Interactions

The concomitant use of TECHNIVIE and certain other drugs may result in known or potentially significant drug interactions, some of which may lead to:

- Loss of therapeutic effect of TECHNIVIE and possible development of resistance
- Possible clinically significant adverse reactions from greater exposures of concomitant drugs or components of TECHNIVIE.

See Table 4 for steps to prevent or manage these possible and known significant drug interactions [see Drug Interactions (7)]. Consider the potential for drug interactions prior to and during TECHNIVIE therapy; review concomitant medications during TECHNIVIE therapy; and monitor for the adverse reactions associated with the concomitant drugs [see Contraindications (4) and Drug Interactions (7)].

5.5   Risk of HIV-1 Protease Inhibitor Drug Resistance in HCV/HIV-1 Co-infected Patients

The ritonavir component of TECHNIVIE is also an HIV-1 protease inhibitor and can select for HIV-1 protease inhibitor resistance-associated substitutions. Any HCV/HIV-1 coinfected patients treated with TECHNIVIE should also be on a suppressive antiretroviral drug regimen to reduce the risk of HIV-1 protease inhibitor drug resistance.

6   ADVERSE REACTIONS

TECHNIVIE should be administered with ribavirin (RBV). Refer to the prescribing information for ribavirin for a list of ribavirin-associated adverse reactions.

The following adverse reaction is described below and elsewhere in the labeling:

- Risk of Hepatic Decompensation and Hepatic Failure in Patients with Cirrhosis [see Warnings and Precautions (5.1)]
- Increased Risk of ALT Elevations [see Warnings and Precautions (5.2)]

6.1   Clinical Trials Experience

Because clinical trials are conducted under widely varying conditions, adverse reaction rates observed in clinical trials of ombitasvir, paritaprevir and ritonavir cannot be directly compared to rates in the clinical trials of another drug and may not reflect the rates observed in practice.

The safety assessment of TECHNIVIE is based on data from a clinical study that included 135 HCV genotype 4-infected subjects without cirrhosis, 91 who received ombitasvir 25 mg, paritaprevir 150 mg and ritonavir 100 mg (administered as one ombitasvir 25 mg tablet, three paritaprevir 50 mg tablets and one ritonavir 100 mg capsule) once daily with ribavirin for 12 weeks and 44 subjects without cirrhosis who received ombitasvir 25 mg, paritaprevir 150 mg, and ritonavir 100 mg (administered as one ombitasvir 25 mg tablet, three paritaprevir 50 mg tablets and one ritonavir 100 mg capsule) once daily without ribavirin for 12 weeks (PEARL-I).

Adverse reactions that occurred in subjects treated with ombitasvir, paritaprevir and ritonavir with or without ribavirin for 12 weeks are listed in Table 3. The majority of adverse reactions in PEARL-I were mild in severity. None of the subjects who received ombitasvir, paritaprevir and ritonavir with ribavirin experienced a serious adverse reaction. None of the subjects receiving ombitasvir, paritaprevir and ritonavir with or without ribavirin discontinued treatment due to an adverse reaction.

[See table 3 below]

Laboratory Abnormalities

Serum ALT Elevations

None of the 135 HCV GT4 infected subjects treated with TECHNIVIE experienced post-baseline serum ALT levels greater than 5 times the upper limit of normal (ULN) after starting treatment [see Warnings and Precautions (5.2)].

Serum Bilirubin Elevations

Post-baseline elevations in bilirubin at least 2 times ULN were observed in 5% (7/134) of subjects receiving TECHNIVIE; all of whom were also receiving RBV. These bilirubin increases were predominately indirect and related to the inhibition of the bilirubin transporters OATP1B1/1B3 by paritaprevir and possibly ribavirin-induced hemolysis. Bilirubin elevations occurred early after initiation of treatment, peaked by study Week 1, and generally resolved with ongoing therapy. Bilirubin elevations were generally not associated with serum ALT elevations.

Anemia / Decreased Hemoglobin

The mean change from baseline in hemoglobin levels in subjects treated with TECHNIVIE in combination with ribavirin was -2.1 g/dL and the mean change in subjects treated with TECHNIVIE alone was -0.4 g/dL. Decreases in hemoglobin levels occurred early in treatment (Week 1-2) with further reductions through Week 3. Hemoglobin values remained low during the remainder of treatment and returned towards baseline levels by post-treatment Week 4. One subject treated with TECHNIVIE with ribavirin had a single hemoglobin level decrease to less than 8 g/dL during treatment. Four percent (4/91) of subjects treated with TECHNIVIE with ribavirin underwent ribavirin dose reductions to manage anemia/decreased hemoglobin levels; none received a blood transfusion or erythropoietin. No subjects treated with TECHNIVIE alone had a hemoglobin level less than 8 g/dL.

6.2   Post-Marketing Experience

The following adverse reactions have been identified during post approval use of TECHNIVIE. Because these reactions are reported voluntarily from a population of uncertain size, it is not always possible to reliably estimate their frequency or establish a causal relationship to drug exposure.

Immune System Disorders: Hypersensitivity reactions (including angioedema).

Hepatobiliary Disorders: Hepatic decompensation, hepatic failure [see Warnings and Precautions (5.1)].

7   DRUG INTERACTIONS

7.1   Potential for TECHNIVIE to Affect Other Drugs

Paritaprevir is an inhibitor of OATP1B1 and OATP1B3 and paritaprevir and ritonavir are inhibitors of BCRP and P-gp.

Table 3. Selected Adverse Reactions (All Grades) with ≥5% Frequency Reported in Subjects Treated with Ombitasvir, Paritaprevir and Ritonavir with or without Ribavirin for 12 Weeks

Adverse Reaction	PEARL-I	
	Ombitasvir, paritaprevir, ritonavir + RBV 12 Weeks N = 91 %	Ombitasvir, paritaprevir, ritonavir 12 Weeks N = 44 %
Asthenia	29	25
Fatigue	15	7
Nausea	14	9
Insomnia	13	5
Pruritus*	7	5
Skin reactions$,#	7	5

*Grouped term 'pruritus' includes the preferred terms pruritus and pruritus generalized.
$Grouped term 'skin reactions' includes the preferred terms rash, erythema, eczema, rash maculo-papular, rash macular, dermatitis, rash papular, skin exfoliation, rash pruritic, rash erythematous, rash generalized, dermatitis allergic, dermatitis contact, exfoliative rash, photosensitivity reaction, psoriasis, skin reaction, ulcer and urticaria.
#The majority of events were graded as mild in severity. There were no serious events or severe cutaneous reactions, such as Stevens Johnson Syndrome (SJS), toxic epidermal necrolysis (TEN), erythema multiforme (EM) or drug rash with eosinophilia and systemic symptoms (DRESS).

Table 4. Established Drug Interactions Based on Drug Interaction Trials

Concomitant Drug Class: Drug Name	Effect on Concentration	Clinical Comments
ANGIOTENSIN RECEPTOR BLOCKERS e.g.		
valsartan*, losartan*, candesartan*	↑ angiotensin receptor blockers	Decrease the dose of the angiotensin receptor blockers and monitor patients for signs and symptoms of hypotension and/or worsening renal function. If such events occur, consider further dose reduction of the angiotensin receptor blocker or switching to an alternative to the angiotensin receptor blocker.
ANTIARRHYTHMICS		
digoxin	↑ digoxin	Decrease digoxin dose by 30-50%. Appropriate monitoring of serum digoxin levels is recommended.
amiodarone*, bepridil*, disopyramide*, flecainide*, lidocaine (systemic)*, mexiletine*, propafenone*, quinidine*	↑ antiarrhythmics	Therapeutic monitoring (if available) is recommended for antiarrhythmics when co-administered with TECHNIVIE.
ANTIDIABETIC DRUGS		
metformin	↔ metformin	Monitor for signs of onset of lactic acidosis such as respiratory distress, somnolence, and non-specific abdominal distress or worsening renal function. Concomitant metformin use in patients with renal insufficiency or hepatic impairment is not recommended. Refer to the prescribing information of metformin for further guidance.
ANTIFUNGALS		
ketoconazole	↑ ketoconazole	When TECHNIVIE is co-administered with ketoconazole, the maximum daily dose of ketoconazole should be limited to 200 mg per day.
voriconazole*	↓ voriconazole	Co-administration of TECHNIVIE with voriconazole is not recommended unless an assessment of the benefit-to-risk ratio justifies the use of voriconazole.
ANTIPSYCHOTICS		
quetiapine*	↑ quetiapine	• Initiation of TECHNIVIE in patients taking quetiapine: Consider alternative anti-HCV therapy to avoid increases in quetiapine exposures. If coadministration is necessary, reduce the quetiapine dose to 1/6th of the current dose and monitor for quetiapine-associated adverse reactions. Refer to the quetiapine prescribing information for recommendations on adverse reaction monitoring. • Initiation of quetiapine in patients taking TECHNIVIE: Refer to the quetiapine prescribing information for initial dosing and titration of quetiapine.
CALCIUM CHANNEL BLOCKERS		
amlodipine, nifedipine*, diltiazem*, verapamil*	↑ calcium channel blockers	Decrease the dose of the calcium channel blocker. The dose of amlodipine should be decreased by at least 50%. Clinical monitoring of patients is recommended for edema and/or signs and symptoms of hypotension. If such events occur, consider further dose reduction of the calcium channel blocker or switching to an alternative to the calcium channel blocker.

This table is continued on the next page

Ritonavir is an inhibitor of CYP3A4. Co-administration of TECHNIVIE with drugs that are substrates of CYP3A, P-gp, BCRP, OATP1B1 or OATP1B3 may result in increased plasma concentrations of such drugs [see also *Contraindications (4), Warnings and Precautions (5.4), and Clinical Pharmacology (12.3)*].

7.2   Potential for Other Drugs to Affect One or More Components of TECHNIVIE

Paritaprevir and ritonavir are primarily metabolized by CYP3A enzymes. Co-administration of TECHNIVIE with strong inhibitors of CYP3A may increase paritaprevir and ritonavir concentrations. Ombitasvir is primarily metabolized via amide hydrolysis while CYP enzymes play a minor role in its metabolism. Ombitasvir, paritaprevir and ritonavir are substrates of P-gp. Paritaprevir is a substrate of BCRP, OATP1B1 and OATP1B3. Inhibition of P-gp, BCRP, OATP1B1 or OATP1B3 may increase the plasma concentrations of the various components of TECHNIVIE.

7.3   Established and Other Potential Drug Interactions

If dosage adjustments of concomitant medications are made due to treatment with TECHNIVIE, dosages should be readjusted after administration of TECHNIVIE is completed. Dosage adjustment is not required for TECHNIVIE. Table 4 provides the effect of co-administration of TECHNIVIE™ (ombitasvir, paritaprevir and ritonavir) tablets on concentrations of concomitant drugs and the effect of concomitant drugs on the various components of TECHNIVIE. See *Contraindications (4)* for drugs that are contraindicated with TECHNIVIE. Refer to the ritonavir prescribing information for other potentially significant drug interactions with ritonavir.

[See table 4 above]

7.4   Drugs without Clinically Significant Interactions with TECHNIVIE

No dosage adjustments are recommended when TECHNIVIE is co-administered with the following medications: abacavir, dolutegravir, duloxetine, emtricitabine/tenofovir disoproxil fumarate, escitalopram, gemfibrozil, lamivudine, methadone, progestin only contraceptives, raltegravir, sofosbuvir, sulfamethoxazole, trimethoprim, rosuvastatin, warfarin and zolpidem.

8   USE IN SPECIFIC POPULATIONS

8.1   Pregnancy

Pregnancy Category B

Risk Summary

Adequate and well controlled studies with TECHNIVIE have not been conducted in pregnant women. In animal reproduction studies, no evidence of teratogenicity was observed with the administration of ombitasvir (mice and rabbits), paritaprevir or ritonavir (mice and rats) at exposures higher than the recommended clinical dose [see Data]. Because animal reproduction studies are not always predictive of human response, TECHNIVIE should be used during pregnancy only if clearly needed.

When TECHNIVIE is administered with ribavirin, the combination regimen is contraindicated in pregnant women and in men whose female partners are pregnant. Refer to the ribavirin prescribing information for more information on use of ribavirin in males and females of child-bearing potential.

Data

Animal data

In animal reproduction studies, there was no evidence of teratogenicity in offspring born to animals treated throughout pregnancy with ombitasvir and its major inactive human metabolites (M29, M36), paritaprevir or ritonavir. For ombitasvir, the highest dose tested produced exposures approximately 29-fold (mouse) or 4-fold (rabbit) the exposures in humans at the recommended clinical dose. The highest doses of the major, inactive human metabolites similarly tested produced exposures approximately 26-fold the exposures in humans at the recommended clinical dose. For

Continued on next page

paritaprevir, ritonavir, the highest doses tested produced exposures approximately 143-fold (mouse) or 12-fold (rat) the exposures of paritaprevir in humans at the recommended clinical dose.

8.3 Nursing Mothers

It is not known whether any of the components of TECHNIVIE or their metabolites are present in human milk. Unchanged ombitasvir, paritaprevir and its hydrolysis product M13 were the predominant components observed in the milk of lactating rats, without effect on nursing pups. The developmental and health benefits of breastfeeding should be considered along with the mother's clinical need for TECHNIVIE and any potential adverse effects on the breastfed child from TECHNIVIE or from the underlying maternal condition.

When TECHNIVIE is administered with ribavirin, the nursing mother's information for ribavirin also applies to this combination regimen (see prescribing information for ribavirin).

8.4 Pediatric Use

Safety and effectiveness of TECHNIVIE in pediatric patients less than 18 years of age have not been established.

8.5 Geriatric Use

No dosage adjustment of TECHNIVIE is warranted in geriatric patients. Clinical study PEARL-I did not include sufficient numbers of patients older than 65 years of age to assess safety or efficacy, or to determine if they responded differently than younger patients.

8.6 Hepatic Impairment

No dosage adjustment of TECHNIVIE is required in patients with mild hepatic impairment (Child-Pugh A). TECHNIVIE is contraindicated in patients with moderate to severe hepatic impairment (Child-Pugh B and C) *[see Dosage and Administration (2.3), Contraindications (4), Warnings and Precautions (5.1) and Clinical Pharmacology (12.3)]*.

8.7 Renal Impairment

No dosage adjustment of TECHNIVIE is required in patients with mild, moderate or severe renal impairment. TECHNIVIE has not been studied in patients on dialysis. For patients that require ribavirin, refer to the ribavirin prescribing information for information regarding use in patients with renal impairment *[see Clinical Pharmacology (12.3)]*.

10   OVERDOSAGE

In case of overdose, it is recommended that the patient be monitored for any signs or symptoms of adverse reactions and appropriate symptomatic treatment be instituted immediately.

11   DESCRIPTION

TECHNIVIE is a fixed-dose combination tablet containing ombitasvir, paritaprevir, and ritonavir for oral administration.

Ombitasvir, paritaprevir, ritonavir fixed dose combination tablet includes a hepatitis C virus NS5A inhibitor (ombitasvir), a hepatitis C virus NS3/4A protease inhibitor (paritaprevir), and a CYP3A inhibitor (ritonavir) that inhibits CYP3A mediated metabolism of paritaprevir, thereby providing increased plasma concentration of paritaprevir.

Ombitasvir

The chemical name of ombitasvir is Dimethyl ([(2S,5S)-1-(4-*tert*-butylphenyl) pyrrolidine-2,5-diyl]bis{benzene-4,1-diylcarbamoyl(2S)pyrrolidine-2,1-diyl[(2S)-3-methyl-1-oxobutane-1,2-diyl]})biscarbamate hydrate. The molecular formula is $C_{50}H_{67}N_7O_8 \cdot 4.5H_2O$ (hydrate) and the molecular weight for the drug substance is 975.20 (hydrate). The drug substance is white to light yellow to light pink powder, and is practically insoluble in aqueous buffers but is soluble in ethanol. Ombitasvir has the following molecular structure: [See first structural formula on next page]

Paritaprevir

The chemical name of paritaprevir is (2R,6S,12Z,13aS,14aR,16aS)-N-(cyclopropylsulfonyl)-6-[[(5-methylpyrazin-2-yl)carbonyl]amino]-5,16-dioxo-2-(phenanthridin-6-yloxy)-1,2,3,6,7,8,9,10,11,13a,14,15,16,16a-tetradecahydrocyclopropa[e]pyrrolo[1,2-*a*][1,4] diazacyclopentadecine-14a(5H)-carboxamide dihydrate. The molecular formula is $C_{40}H_{43}N_7O_7S \cdot 2H_2O$ (dihydrate) and the molecular weight for the drug substance is 801.91 (dihydrate). The drug sub-

---

Table 4 *(Cont.)* Established Drug Interactions Based on Drug Interaction Trials

Concomitant Drug Class: Drug Name	Effect on Concentration	Clinical Comments
CORTICOSTEROIDS (INHALED/NASAL)		
fluticasone*	↑ fluticasone	Concomitant use of TECHNIVIE with inhaled or nasal fluticasone may reduce serum cortisol concentrations. Alternative corticosteroids should be considered, particularly for long term use.
DIURETICS		
furosemide	↑ furosemide (C_{max})	Clinical monitoring of patients is recommended and therapy should be individualized based on patient's response.
HIV-ANTIVIRAL AGENTS		
atazanavir or atazanavir/ritonavir	↑ paritaprevir	Co-administration of TECHNIVIE with atazanavir or atazanavir/ritonavir is not recommended.
darunavir/ritonavir	↓ darunavir (C_{trough})	When co-administered with TECHNIVIE, darunavir 800 mg (without ritonavir) should be taken at the same time as TECHNIVIE.
lopinavir/ritonavir	↑ paritaprevir	Co-administration of TECHNIVIE with lopinavir/ritonavir is not recommended.
rilpivirine	↑ rilpivirine	Co-administration of TECHNIVIE with rilpivirine once daily is not recommended due to potential for QT interval prolongation with higher concentrations of rilpivirine.
HMG CoA REDUCTASE INHIBITORS		
pravastatin	↑ pravastatin	When TECHNIVIE is co-administered with pravastatin, the dose of pravastatin should not exceed 40 mg per day.
IMMUNOSUPPRESSANTS		
cyclosporine	↑ cyclosporine	When initiating therapy with TECHNIVIE, reduce cyclosporine dose to 1/5th of the patient's current cyclosporine dose. Measure cyclosporine blood concentrations to determine subsequent dose modifications. Upon completion of TECHNIVIE therapy, the appropriate time to resume pre-TECHNIVIE dose of cyclosporine should be guided by assessment of cyclosporine blood concentrations. Frequent assessment of renal function and cyclosporine-related side effects is recommended.
tacrolimus	↑ tacrolimus	When initiating therapy with TECHNIVIE, the dose of tacrolimus needs to be reduced. Do not administer tacrolimus on the day TECHNIVIE is initiated. Beginning the day after TECHNIVIE is initiated; reinitiate tacrolimus at a reduced dose based on tacrolimus blood concentrations. Typical tacrolimus dosing is 0.5 mg every 7 days. Measure tacrolimus blood concentrations and adjust dose or dosing frequency to determine subsequent dose modifications. Upon completion of TECHNIVIE therapy, the appropriate time to resume pre-TECHNIVIE dose of tacrolimus should be guided by assessment of tacrolimus blood concentrations. Frequent assessment of renal function and tacrolimus related side effects is recommended.

This table is continued on the next page

Table 4 (Cont.) Established Drug Interactions Based on Drug Interaction Trials

Concomitant Drug Class: Drug Name	Effect on Concentration	Clinical Comments
LONG ACTING BETA-ADRENOCEPTOR AGONIST		
salmeterol*	↑ salmeterol	Concurrent administration of TECHNIVIE and salmeterol is not recommended. The combination may result in increased risk of cardiovascular adverse events associated with salmeterol, including QT prolongation, palpitations and sinus tachycardia.
MUSCLE RELAXANTS		
carisoprodol	↓ carisoprodol ↔ mepobramate (metabolite of carisoprodol)	Increase dose if clinically indicated.
cyclobenzaprine	↓ cyclobenzaprine ↓ norcyclobenzaprine (metabolite of cyclobenzaprine)	Increase dose if clinically indicated.
NARCOTIC ANALGESICS		
buprenorphine/naloxone	↑ buprenorphine ↑ norbuprenorphine (metabolite of buprenorphine)	Patients should be closely monitored for sedation and cognitive effects.
Hydrocodone/acetaminophen	↑ hydrocodone ↔ acetaminophen	Reduce the dose of hydrocodone by 50% and monitor patients for respiratory depression and sedation at frequent intervals. Upon completion of TECHNIVIE therapy, adjust the hydrocodone dose and monitor for signs of opioid withdrawal.
PROTON PUMP INHIBITORS		
omeprazole	↓ omeprazole	Monitor patients for decreased efficacy of omeprazole. Consider increasing the omeprazole dose in patients whose symptoms are not well controlled; avoid use of more than 40 mg per day of omeprazole.
SEDATIVES/HYPNOTICS		
alprazolam	↑ alprazolam	Clinical monitoring of patients is recommended. A decrease in alprazolam dose can be considered based on clinical response.
diazepam	↓ diazepam ↓ nordiazepam (metabolite of diazepam)	Increase dose if clinically indicated.

*Not studied.
See Clinical Pharmacology, Tables 7 and 8.
The direction of the arrow indicates the direction of the change in exposures (C_{max} and AUC) (↑ = increase of more than 20%, ↓ = decrease of more than 20%).

stance is white to off-white powder with very low water solubility. Paritaprevir has the following molecular structure:

Ritonavir
The chemical name of ritonavir is [5S-(5R*,8R*,10R*, 11R*)]10-Hydroxy-2-methyl-5-(1-methyethyl)-1-[2-(1-methylethyl)-4-thiazolyl]-3,6-dioxo-8,11-bis(phenylmethyl)-2,4,7,12-tetraazatridecan-13-oic acid,5-thiazolylmethyl ester. The molecular formula is $C_{37}H_{48}N_6O_5S_2$ and the molecular weight for the drug substance is 720.95. The drug substance is white to off white to light tan powder practically insoluble in water and freely soluble in methanol and ethanol. Ritonavir has the following molecular structure:

Ombitasvir, Paritaprevir, Ritonavir Fixed-Dose Combination Tablets
Ombitasvir, paritaprevir and ritonavir film-coated tablets are co-formulated immediate release tablets. The tablet contains copovidone, K value 28, vitamin E polyethylene glycol succinate, propylene glycol monolaurate Type I, sorbitan monolaurate, colloidal silicon dioxide/colloidal anhydrous silica, sodium stearyl fumarate, polyvinyl alcohol, polyethylene glycol 3350/macrogol 3350, talc, titanium dioxide, and iron oxide red. The strength for the tablet is 12.5 mg ombitasvir, 75 mg paritaprevir, 50 mg ritonavir.

12   CLINICAL PHARMACOLOGY
12.1   Mechanism of Action
TECHNIVIE combines two direct-acting hepatitis C virus antiviral agents with distinct mechanisms of action *[see Microbiology (12.4)]*.
Ritonavir is not active against HCV. Ritonavir is a potent CYP3A inhibitor that increases peak and trough plasma drug concentrations of paritaprevir and overall drug exposure (i.e., area under the curve).
12.2   Pharmacodynamics
Cardiac Electrophysiology
The effect of a combination of ombitasvir, paritaprevir and ritonavir plus dasabuvir on QTc interval was evaluated in a randomized, double blind, placebo and active-controlled

Continued on next page

Information on the AbbVie, Inc. products listed on these pages is from the prescribing information in use as of July 31, 2016. For more information, please visit rxabbvie.com or call 1-800-633-9110.

Table 5. Pharmacokinetic Properties of the Components of TECHNIVIE

	Ombitasvir	Paritaprevir	Ritonavir
Absorption			
T_{max} (hr)	~ 5	~ 4-5	~ 4-5
Absolute bioavailability (%)	48	53	NA
Effect of moderate fat meal (relative to fasting)[a]	1.82 (1.61-2.05)	3.11 (2.16-4.46)	1.49 (1.23-1.79)
Effect of high fat meal (relative to fasting)[a]	1.76 (1.56-1.99)	2.80 (1.95-4.02)	1.44 (1.19-1.73)
Accumulation[b]	0.90- to 1.03-fold	1.5- to 2-fold	
Distribution			
% Bound to human plasma proteins	99.9	97-98.6	>99
Blood-to-plasma ratio	0.49	0.7	0.6
Volume of distribution at steady state (Vss) (L)	173	103	21.5[c]
Metabolism			
Metabolism	amide hydrolysis followed by oxidative metabolism	CYP3A4 (major), CYP3A5	CYP3A (major), CYP2D6
Elimination[d]			
Major route of elimination	biliary excretion	metabolism	metabolism
$t_{1/2}$ (hr)[e]	21-25	5.5	4
% of dose excreted in feces[f]	90.2	88	86.4
% of dose excreted unchanged in feces[f]	87.8	1.1	33.8
% of dose excreted in urine[f]	1.91	8.8	11.3
% of dose excreted unchanged in urine[f]	0.03	0.05	3.5

NA - data not available
a. Values refer to mean non-fasting/fasting ratios (90% Confidence Interval) in systemic exposure (AUC). Moderate fat meal ~600 Kcal, 20-30% calories from fat. High fat meal ~900 Kcal, 60% calories from fat.
b. Steady state exposures are achieved after approximately 12 days of dosing.
c. It is apparent volume of distribution (V/F) for ritonavir.
d. Ombitasvir, paritaprevir, and ritonavir do not inhibit organic anion transporter (OAT1) *in vivo* and based on *in vitro* data, are not expected to inhibit organic cation transporter (OCT2), organic anion transporter (OAT3), or multidrug and toxin extrusion proteins (MATE1 and MATE2K) at clinically relevant concentrations.
e. $t_{1/2}$ values refer to the mean elimination half-life.
f. Dosing in mass balance studies: single dose administration of [^{14}C]ombitasvir; single dose administration of [^{14}C]paritaprevir co-dosed with 100 mg ritonavir.

(moxifloxacin 400 mg) 4-way crossover thorough QT study in 60 healthy subjects. At concentrations approximately 6 and 1.8 times the therapeutic concentrations of paritaprevir and ombitasvir, the combination did not prolong QTc to any clinically relevant extent.

12.3   Pharmacokinetics
The pharmacokinetic properties of the components of TECHNIVIE are provided in Table 5. Based on the population pharmacokinetic analysis, the median steady-state pharmacokinetic parameters of ombitasvir, paritaprevir, and ritonavir in HCV-infected subjects are provided in Table 6.
[See table 5 above]
[See table 6 on next page]
Specific Populations
Hepatic Impairment
The single dose pharmacokinetics of ombitasvir, paritaprevir, ritonavir and another antiviral drug were evaluated in non-HCV infected subjects with mild hepatic impairment (Child-Pugh A; score of 5-6), moderate hepatic impairment (Child-Pugh B, score of 7-9) and severe hepatic impairment (Child-Pugh C, score of 10-15).
Relative to subjects with normal hepatic function, ombitasvir, paritaprevir and ritonavir mean AUC values decreased by 8%, 29% and 34%, respectively, in subjects with mild hepatic impairment.
Relative to subjects with normal hepatic function, ombitasvir and ritonavir mean AUC values decreased by 30% and 30%, respectively and paritaprevir mean AUC values increased by 62% in subjects with moderate hepatic impairment.
Relative to subjects with normal hepatic function, paritaprevir and ritonavir mean AUC values increased by 945% and 13% respectively and ombitasvir mean AUC values decreased by 54% in subjects with severe hepatic impairment *[see Dosage and Administration (2.3), Contraindications (4), Warnings and Precautions (5.1) and Use in Specific Populations (8.6)]*.
Renal Impairment
The single dose pharmacokinetics of ombitasvir, paritaprevir and ritonavir were evaluated in non-HCV infected subjects with mild (CL_{cr}: 60 to 89 mL/min), moderate (CL_{cr}: 30 to 59 mL/min), and severe (CL_{cr}: 15 to 29 mL/min) renal impairment.
Overall, changes in exposure of ombitasvir, paritaprevir, and ritonavir in non-HCV infected subjects with mild-, moderate- and severe renal impairment are not expected to be clinically relevant. Pharmacokinetic data are not available on the use of TECHNIVIE™ (ombitasvir, paritaprevir and ritonavir) tablets in non-HCV infected subjects with End Stage Renal Disease (ESRD).
Relative to subjects with normal renal function, ritonavir AUC values increased by 40%, while ombitasvir and paritaprevir AUC values were unchanged in subjects with mild renal impairment.
Relative to subjects with normal renal function, ritonavir AUC values increased by 76%, while ombitasvir and paritaprevir AUC values were unchanged in subjects with moderate renal impairment.
Relative to subjects with normal renal function, paritaprevir and ritonavir AUC values increased by 25% and 108%, respectively, while ombitasvir AUC values were unchanged in subjects with severe renal impairment.
Pediatric Population
The pharmacokinetics of TECHNIVIE in pediatric patients less than 18 years of age has not been established *[see Use in Specific Populations (8.4)]*.
Sex
No dosage adjustment is recommended based on sex or body weight.
Race/Ethnicity
No dosage adjustment is recommended based on race or ethnicity.
Age
No dosage adjustment is recommended in geriatric patients *[see Use in Specific Populations (8.5)]*.
Drug Interactions
See also Contraindications (4), Warnings and Precautions (5.4), Drug Interactions (7)
The effects of drugs discussed in Table 4 on the exposures of the individual components of TECHNIVIE are shown in Table 7. For information regarding clinical recommendations, see *Drug Interactions (7)*.
[See table 7 on pages 807 through 809]

Table 6. Steady-State Pharmacokinetic Parameters of Ombitasvir, Paritaprevir, and Ritonavir Following Oral Administration of TECHNIVIE in HCV-Infected Subjects

Pharmacokinetic Parameter[a]	Ombitasvir	Paritaprevir	Ritonavir
C_{max} (ng/mL)	82	194	543
AUC_{0-24} (ng*h/mL)	1239	2276	6072

a. Median values reported based on the population PK analysis.

Table 7. Drug Interactions: Change in Pharmacokinetic Parameters of the Individual Components of TECHNIVIE in the Presence of Co-administered Drug

Co-administered Drug	Dose of Co-administered Drug (mg)	n	DAA	Ratio (with/without co-administered drug) of DAA Pharmacokinetic Parameters (90% CI); No Effect = 1.00		
				C_{max}	AUC	C_{min}
Alprazolam[a]	0.5 single dose	12	ombitasvir	0.98 (0.93, 1.04)	1.00 (0.96, 1.04)	0.98 (0.93, 1.04)
			paritaprevir	0.91 (0.64, 1.31)	0.96 (0.73, 1.27)	1.12 (1.02, 1.23)
			ritonavir	0.92 (0.84, 1.02)	0.96 (0.89, 1.03)	1.01 (0.94, 1.09)
Amlodipine[a]	5 single dose	14	ombitasvir	1.00 (0.95, 1.06)	1.00 (0.97, 1.04)	1.00 (0.97, 1.04)
			paritaprevir	0.77 (0.64, 0.94)	0.78 (0.68, 0.88)	0.88 (0.80, 0.95)XXXX
			ritonavir	0.96 (0.87, 1.06)	0.93 (0.89, 0.98)	0.95 (0.89, 1.01)
Atazanavir[b]	300 once daily	10	ombitasvir	0.83 (0.74, 0.94)	0.91 (0.81, 1.02)	0.98 (0.87, 1.11)
			paritaprevir	2.74 (1.76, 4.27)	2.87 (2.08, 3.97)	3.71 (2.87, 4.79)
			ritonavir	0.85 (0.72, 0.99)	0.97 (0.84, 1.13)	1.45 (1.29, 1.64)
Carbamazepine[a]	200 once daily followed by 200 twice daily	12	ombitasvir	0.69 (0.61, 0.78)	0.69 (0.64, 0.74)	NA
			paritaprevir	0.34 (0.25, 0.48)	0.30 (0.23, 0.38)	NA
			ritonavir	0.17 (0.12, 0.24)	0.13 (0.09, 0.17)	NA
Carisoprodol[a]	250 single dose	14	ombitasvir	0.98 (0.92, 1.04)	0.95 (0.92, 0.97)	0.96 (0.92, 0.99)
			paritaprevir	0.88 (0.75, 1.03)	0.96 (0.85, 1.08)	1.14 (1.02, 1.27)
			ritonavir	0.94 (0.87, 1.02)	0.94 (0.88, 0.99)	0.95 (0.89, 1.03)
Cyclobenzaprine[a]	5 single dose	14	ombitasvir	0.98 (0.92, 1.04)	1.00 (0.97, 1.03)	1.01 (0.98, 1.04)
			paritaprevir	1.14 (0.99, 1.32)	1.13 (1.00, 1.28)	1.13 (1.01, 1.25)
			ritonavir	0.93 (0.87, 0.99)	1.00 (0.95, 1.06)	1.13 (1.05, 1.21)
Cyclosporine	10 single dose[c]	12	ombitasvir	1.06 (1.02, 1.11)	1.10 (1.07, 1.12)	1.10 (1.06, 1.14)
			paritaprevir	1.39 (1.10, 1.75)	1.46 (1.29, 1.64)	1.18 (1.08, 1.30)
			ritonavir	1.13 (0.94, 1.35)	1.20 (1.10, 1.30)	1.11 (0.89, 1.37)

This table is continued on the next page

Table 8 summarizes the effects of TECHNIVIE on the pharmacokinetics of co-administered drugs which showed clinically relevant changes. For information regarding clinical recommendations, see *Drug Interactions (7)*.
[See table 8 on pages 810 and 811]

12.4 Microbiology

Mechanism of Action

TECHNIVIE combines two direct-acting antiviral agents with distinct mechanisms of action and non-overlapping resistance profiles to target HCV at multiple steps in the viral lifecycle.

Ombitasvir

Ombitasvir is an inhibitor of HCV NS5A, which is essential for viral RNA replication and virion assembly. The mechanism of action of ombitasvir has been characterized based on cell culture antiviral activity and drug resistance mapping studies.

Paritaprevir

Paritaprevir is an inhibitor of HCV NS3/4A protease which is necessary for the proteolytic cleavage of the HCV encoded polyprotein (into mature forms of the NS3, NS4A, NS4B, NS5A, and NS5B proteins) and is essential for viral replication. In a biochemical assay, paritaprevir inhibited the proteolytic activity of a recombinant HCV genotype 4a NS3/4A protease enzyme with an IC_{50} value of 0.16 nM.

Antiviral Activity

Ombitasvir

The EC_{50} values of ombitasvir against HCV replicons containing NS5A from a single isolate each of genotype 4a and genotype 4d were 1.7 pM and 0.38 pM, respectively. Ombitasvir had a median EC_{50} value of 0.21 pM (range 0.10 pM to 0.36 pM; n=9) against transient HCV replicons containing NS5A genes from a panel of genotype 4a isolates from treatment-naïve subjects.

Paritaprevir

The EC_{50} values of paritaprevir against HCV replicons containing NS3 from a single isolate each of genotype 4a and genotype 4d were 0.09 nM and 0.015 nM, respectively.

Ritonavir

In HCV replicon cell culture assays, ritonavir did not exhibit a direct antiviral effect and the presence of ritonavir did not affect the antiviral activity of paritaprevir.

Resistance

In Cell Culture

Exposure of HCV genotype 4a replicons to ombitasvir or paritaprevir resulted in the emergence of drug resistant replicons carrying amino acid substitutions in NS5A or NS3, respectively. Amino acid substitutions in NS5A or NS3 selected in cell culture or identified in clinical study PEARL-I were phenotypically characterized in genotype 4 replicons.

For ombitasvir, in an HCV genotype 4a replicon, NS5A substitution L28V reduced ombitasvir antiviral activity by 21-fold. In an HCV genotype 4d replicon, substitutions L28V alone and L28V in combination with T58S reduced ombitasvir antiviral activity by 310- and 760-fold, respectively. Ombitasvir activity against an HCV genotype 4d replicon was not reduced by a T58P polymorphism, which represents the consensus sequence observed at this position for HCV genotype 4a and 4d subjects in PEARL-I.

For paritaprevir, in an HCV genotype 4a replicon, NS3 substitutions R155C, A156T/V, and D168H/V reduced paritaprevir antiviral activity by 40- to 323-fold. In an HCV genotype 4d replicon, NS3 substitutions Y56H and D168V reduced paritaprevir antiviral activity by 8- and 313-fold, respectively, while a combination of Y56H and D168V reduced the activity of paritaprevir by 12,533-fold.

In Clinical Studies

In the clinical study PEARL-I, three subjects with HCV genotype 4 infection experienced virologic failure (2 post-treatment relapse, 1 on-treatment failure). All 3 virologic failures were observed in a regimen containing paritaprevir/ritonavir and ombitasvir without ribavirin. Treatment-emergent, resistance-associated substitutions were detected

Continued on next page

Table 7 *(Cont.)* **Drug Interactions: Change in Pharmacokinetic Parameters of the Individual Components of TECHNIVIE in the Presence of Co-administered Drug**

Co-administered Drug	Dose of Co-administered Drug (mg)	n	DAA	Ratio (with/without co-administered drug) of DAA Pharmacokinetic Parameters (90% CI); No Effect = 1.00		
				C_{max}	AUC	C_{min}
Darunavir[b]	800 once daily	9	ombitasvir	1.01 (0.87, 1.17)	1.01 (0.91, 1.11)	1.06 (0.99, 1.13)
			paritaprevir	2.09 (1.35, 3.24)	1.94 (1.36, 2.75)	1.85 (1.41, 2.42)
			ritonavir	0.83 (0.68, 1.01)	0.80 (0.73, 0.87)	0.91 (0.78, 1.06)
Diazepam[a]	2 single dose	13	ombitasvir	1.00 (0.93, 1.08)	0.98 (0.93, 1.03)	0.93 (0.88, 0.98)
			paritaprevir	0.95 (0.77, 1.18)	0.91 (0.78, 1.07)	0.92 (0.82, 1.03)
			ritonavir	1.10 (1.02, 1.19)	1.06 (0.98, 1.14)	0.98 (0.92, 1.03)
Digoxin	0.5 single dose	11	ombitasvir	0.99 (0.95-1.04)	1.02 (0.98-1.06)	1.01 (0.98-1.05)
			paritaprevir	1.15 (0.97-1.36)	1.12 (1.00-1.25)	0.97 (0.84-1.13)
			ritonavir	1.06 (0.99-1.13)	1.01 (0.98-1.05)	0.95 (0.86-1.04)
Ethinyl estradiol/ Norgestimate	Ethinyl estradiol 0.035 and Norgestimate 0.25 once daily	7[d]	ombitasvir	1.05 (0.81, 1.35)	0.97 (0.81, 1.15)	0.96 (0.88, 1.12)
			paritaprevir	0.70 (0.40, 1.21)	0.66 (0.42, 1.04)	0.87 (0.67, 1.14)
			ritonavir	0.80 (0.53, 1.21)	0.71 (0.54, 0.94)	0.79 (0.68, 0.93)
Furosemide[a]	20 single dose	12	ombitasvir	1.14 (1.03, 1.26)	1.07 (1.01, 1.12)	1.12 (1.08, 1.16)
			paritaprevir	0.93 (0.63, 1.36)	0.92 (0.70, 1.21)	1.26 (1.16, 1.38)
			ritonavir	1.10 (0.96, 1.27)	1.04 (0.92, 1.18)	1.07 (0.99, 1.17)
Hydrocodone/ Acetaminophen[a]	5/300 single dose	15	ombitasvir	1.01 (0.93, 1.10)	0.97 (0.93, 1.02)	0.93 (0.90, 0.97)
			paritaprevir	1.01 (0.80, 1.27)	1.03 (0.89, 1.18)	1.10 (0.97, 1.26)
			ritonavir	1.01 (0.90, 1.13)	1.03 (0.96, 1.09)	1.01 (0.93, 1.10)

This table is continued on the next page

at the time of failure in all 3 subjects and included D168V (with or without Y56H) in NS3, and L28S and L28V (with or without M31I or T58S) in NS5A.

Persistence of Resistance-Associated Substitutions

The persistence of ombitasvir or paritaprevir resistance-associated amino acid substitutions in NS5A or NS3, respectively, in HCV genotype 4 has not been studied. In HCV genotype 1, persistence of ombitasvir and paritaprevir resistance-associated substitutions through 24 or 48 weeks post-treatment has been observed in subjects who experienced virologic failure with ombitasvir- and paritaprevir-containing regimens. The long-term clinical impact of the emergence or persistence of virus containing ombitasvir or paritaprevir resistance-associated substitutions is unknown.

Effect of Baseline HCV Polymorphisms on Treatment Response

Phylogenetic analysis of HCV sequences from genotype 4-infected subjects in the clinical study PEARL-I, identified 7 HCV genotype 4 subtypes (4a, 4b, 4c, 4d, 4f, 4g/4k, 4o). Most subjects were infected with either subtype 4a (38%) or 4d (52%); 1 to 7 subjects were infected with each of the other genotype 4 subtypes. Among subjects enrolled at U.S. study sites, 16/18 (89%) were infected with HCV subtype 4a; one subject each was infected with subtype 4c or 4d. Three subjects who experienced virologic failure with the regimen containing paritaprevir/ritonavir and ombitasvir without ribavirin were infected with HCV subtype 4d.

Baseline HCV polymorphisms are not expected to impact the likelihood of achieving SVR when TECHNIVIE™ (ombitasvir, paritaprevir and ritonavir) tablets is used as recommended to treat HCV genotype 4 infected patients, based on the low virologic failure rate observed in PEARL-I.

Cross-resistance

Cross-resistance may occur among NS5A inhibitors and among NS3/4A protease inhibitors within each individual class. The impact of prior ombitasvir or paritaprevir treatment experience on the efficacy of other NS5A inhibitors or NS3/4A protease inhibitors has not been studied. Similarly, the efficacy of TECHNIVIE has not been studied in subjects who have failed prior treatment with another NS5A inhibitor, NS3/4A protease inhibitor, or NS5B inhibitor.

13 NONCLINICAL TOXICOLOGY

13.1 Carcinogenesis, Mutagenesis, Impairment of Fertility

Carcinogenesis and Mutagenesis

Ombitasvir

Ombitasvir was not carcinogenic in a 6-month transgenic mouse study up to the highest dose tested (150 mg per kg per day).

Similarly, ombitasvir was not carcinogenic in a 2-year rat study up to the highest dose tested (30 mg per kg per day), resulting in ombitasvir exposures approximately 16-fold higher than those in humans at 25 mg.

Ombitasvir and its major inactive human metabolites (M29, M36) were not genotoxic in a battery of *in vitro* or *in vivo* assays, including bacterial mutagenicity, chromosome aberration using human peripheral blood lymphocytes and *in vivo* mouse micronucleus assays.

Paritaprevir, ritonavir

Paritaprevir, ritonavir was not carcinogenic in a 6-month transgenic mouse study up to the highest dose tested (300/30 mg per kg per day). Similarly, paritaprevir, ritonavir was not carcinogenic in a 2-year rat study up to the highest dose tested (300/30 mg per kg per day), resulting in paritaprevir exposures approximately 11-fold higher than those in humans at 150 mg.

Paritaprevir was positive in an *in vitro* chromosome aberration test using human lymphocytes. Paritaprevir was negative in a bacterial mutation assay, and in two *in vivo* genetic toxicology assays (rat bone marrow micronucleus and rat liver Comet tests).

TECHNIVIE is administered with ribavirin. Refer to the prescribing information for ribavirin for information on carcinogenesis and mutagenesis.

Impairment of Fertility

Ombitasvir

Ombitasvir had no effects on embryo-fetal viability or on fertility when evaluated in mice up to the highest dose of 200 mg per kg per day. Ombitasvir exposures at this dose were approximately 26-fold the exposure in humans at the recommended clinical dose.

Paritaprevir, ritonavir

Table 7 *(Cont.)* Drug Interactions: Change in Pharmacokinetic Parameters of the Individual Components of TECHNIVIE in the Presence of Co-administered Drug

Co-administered Drug	Dose of Co-administered Drug (mg)	n	DAA	Ratio (with/without co-administered drug) of DAA Pharmacokinetic Parameters (90% CI); No Effect = 1.00		
				C_{max}	AUC	C_{min}
Ketoconazole	400 once daily	12	ombitasvir	0.98 (0.92, 1.04)	1.26 (1.20, 1.32)	NA
			paritaprevir	1.72 (1.32, 2.26)	2.16 (1.76, 2.66)	NA
			ritonavir	1.27 (1.11, 1.45)	1.51 (1.36, 1.68)	NA
Lopinavir/ ritonavir	400/100 twice daily	18	ombitasvir	1.07 (1.01, 1.13)	1.25 (1.19, 1.32)	1.48 (1.39, 1.57)
			paritaprevir	4.76 (3.54, 6.39)	6.10 (4.30, 8.67)	12.33 (7.30, 20.84)
			ritonavir	1.74 (1.39, 2.17)	2.78 (2.42, 3.20)	10.02 (7.66, 13.11)
Lopinavir/ ritonavir[e]	800/200 once daily	11	ombitasvir	0.97 (0.87, 1.08)	1.09 (1.00, 1.19)	1.24 (1.13, 1.35)
			paritaprevir	1.78 (1.26, 2.52)	3.55 (2.37, 5.32)	14.78 (9.41, 23.23)
			ritonavir	1.80 (1.30, 2.48)	3.09 (2.36, 4.06)	23.16 (15.55, 34.51)
Omeprazole	40 once daily	12	ombitasvir	0.96 (0.81, 1.14)	1.00 (0.88, 1.12)	0.97 (0.89, 1.107)
			paritaprevir	1.02 (0.64, 1.62)	0.93 (0.64, 1.34)	0.83 (0.67, 1.04)
			ritonavir	1.06 (0.95, 1.18)	1.07 (0.96, 1.21)	1.07 (0.97, 1.18)
Pravastatin	10 once daily	10	ombitasvir	0.98 (0.90, 1.06)	0.94 (0.88, 1.02)	0.97 (0.90, 1.03)
			paritaprevir	1.44 (1.15, 1.81)	1.33 (1.09, 1.62)	1.28 (0.83, 1.96)
			ritonavir	1.10 (0.98, 1.24)	1.08 (0.93, 1.27)	0.97 (0.91, 1.04)
Rilpivirine[a]	25 once daily (morning)[f]	10	ombitasvir	1.11 (1.02, 1.20)	1.09 (1.04, 1.14)	1.05 (1.01, 1.08)
			paritaprevir	1.30 (0.94, 1.81)	1.23 (0.93, 1.64)	0.95 (0.84, 1.07)
			ritonavir	1.10 (0.98, 1.24)	1.08 (0.93, 1.27)	0.97 (0.91, 1.04)
Tacrolimus	0.5 single dose[g]	11	ombitasvir	0.94 (0.89, 1.00)	0.95 (0.91, 1.00)	0.95 (0.92, 0.99)
			paritaprevir	0.71 (0.55, 0.91)	0.79 (0.69, 0.92)	0.84 (0.74, 0.97)
			ritonavir	0.884 (0.76, 0.93)	0.89 (0.85, 0.93)	1.04 (0.96, 1.13)

a. Study evaluated interaction with ombitasvir/paritaprevir/ritonavir plus dasabuvir; results extrapolated to ombitasvir/ paritaprevir/ritonavir.
b. Atazanavir or darunavir administered with ombitasvir/paritaprevir/ritonavir in the morning was compared to atazanavir or darunavir administered with 100 mg ritonavir in the morning.
c. 10 mg cyclosporine was administered with ombitasvir/paritaprevir/ritonavir in the test arm and 100 mg cyclosporine was administered in the reference arm without ombitasvir/paritaprevir/ritonavir.
d. Data shown is combined data for ombitasvir/paritaprevir/ritonavir with (N=3) and without (N=4) dasabuvir.
e. Lopinavir/ritonavir administered in the evening, 12 hours after morning dose of ombitasvir/paritaprevir/ritonavir.
f. Similar changes were observed when rilpivirine was dosed in the evening with food or 4 hours after food.
g. 0.5 mg tacrolimus was administered with ombitasvir/paritaprevir/ritonavir in the test arm and 2 mg tacrolimus was administered in the reference arm without ombitasvir/paritaprevir/ritonavir.

NA: not available/not applicable; DAA: Direct-acting antiviral agent; CI: Confidence interval
Doses of ombitasvir, paritaprevir, ritonavir were 25 mg, 150 mg and 100 mg, respectively.
For studies conducted with ombitasvir/paritaprevir/ritonavir plus dasabuvir, doses of dasabuvir were 250 mg or 400 mg (both doses showed similar exposures).

Ombitasvir, paritaprevir and ritonavir were dosed once daily (and where applicable, dasabuvir was dosed twice daily) in all the above studies except studies with ketoconazole and carbamazepine that used single doses.

Paritaprevir, ritonavir had no effects on embryo-fetal viability or on fertility when evaluated in rats up to the highest dose of 300/30 mg per kg per day. Paritaprevir exposures at this dose were approximately 3- to 8-fold the exposure in humans at the recommended clinical dose.
TECHNIVIE is administered with ribavirin. Refer to the prescribing information for ribavirin for information on Impairment of Fertility.

14 CLINICAL STUDIES
14.1 Clinical Trial Results in Adults with Chronic GT4 HCV Infection without Cirrhosis
The efficacy and safety of TECHNIVIE was evaluated in a single clinical trial in subjects with genotype 4 (GT4) chronic hepatitis virus (HCV) infection. PEARL-I was a randomized, global, multicenter, open-label trial that enrolled 135 adults with HCV GT4 infection without cirrhosis who were either treatment-naïve or did not achieve a virologic response with prior treatment with pegylated interferon/ribavirin (pegIFN/RBV). Previous exposure to HCV direct-acting antivirals was prohibited. Treatment-naïve subjects were randomized in a 1:1 ratio to receive one ombitasvir 25 mg tablet, three paritaprevir 50 mg tablets and one ritonavir 100 mg capsule once-daily with food with or without ribavirin for 12 weeks. PegIFN/RBV treatment-experienced subjects received one ombitasvir 25 mg tablet, three paritaprevir 50 mg tablets and one ritonavir 100 mg capsule once-daily with food in combination with ribavirin for 12 weeks. The ribavirin dosage was 1000 mg per day for subjects weighing less than 75 kg or 1200 mg per day for subjects weighing greater than or equal to 75 kg. The primary endpoint was sustained virologic response defined as HCV RNA below the lower limit of quantification (<LLOQ) 12 weeks after the end of treatment (SVR12) using the CO-BAS TaqMan HCV test (version 2.0), for use with the High Pure System, which has an LLOQ of 25 IU per mL.
HCV GT4-infected subjects had a median age of 51 years (range: 19 to 70); 64% were treatment-naïve, 17% were prior pegIFN/RBV null responders; 7% were prior pegIFN/RBV partial responders, 13% were prior pegIFN/RBV relapsers; 65% were male; 9% were Black; 14% had a body mass index at least 30 kg/m[2]; 70% had baseline HCV RNA levels at least 800,000 IU/mL; 79% had IL28B (rs12979860) non-CC genotype; 7% had bridging fibrosis (F3).
Table 9 presents the SVR12 rates.
[See table 9 on page 812]
Among 131 HCV GT4 infected subjects in PEARL-I who achieved SVR12, virologic response data at post-treatment week 24 were available from 129 subjects, and 129/129 (100%) subjects maintained their response through 24 weeks post-treatment (SVR24).

16 HOW SUPPLIED/STORAGE AND HANDLING
TECHNIVIE is dispensed in a monthly carton for a total of 28 days of therapy. Each monthly carton contains four weekly cartons. Each weekly carton contains seven daily dose packs.
Each child resistant daily dose pack contains two TECHNIVIE tablets. The NDC number is 0074-3082-28.
TECHNIVIE is a pink-colored, film-coated, oblong, biconvex-shaped tablet debossed with "AV1" on one side. Each tablet contains 12.5 mg ombitasvir, 75 mg paritaprevir and 50 mg ritonavir.
Store at or below 30°C (86°F).

17 PATIENT COUNSELING INFORMATION
Advise the patient to read the FDA-approved patient labeling (Medication Guide).
Inform patients to review the Medication Guide for ribavirin *[see Warnings and Precautions (5.3)]*.
Risk of ALT Elevations or Hepatic Decompensation and Failure
Inform patients to watch for early warning signs of liver inflammation or failure, such as fatigue, weakness, lack of appetite, nausea and vomiting, as well as later signs such as jaundice, onset of confusion, abdominal swelling, and discolored feces, and to consult their health care professional without delay if such symptoms occur *[see Warnings and Precautions (5.1 and 5.2) and Adverse Reactions (6.1)]*.

Continued on next page

Information on the AbbVie, Inc. products listed on these pages is from the prescribing information in use as of July 31, 2016. For more information, please visit rxabbvie.com or call 1-800-633-9110.

Table 8. Drug Interactions: Change in Pharmacokinetic Parameters for Co-administered Drug in the Presence of TECHNIVIE

Co-administered Drug	Dose of Co-administered Drug (mg)	n	Ratio (with/without TECHNIVIE) of Co-administered Drug Pharmacokinetic Parameters (90% CI); No Effect = 1.00		
			C_{max}	AUC	C_{min}
Alprazolam[a]	0.5 single dose	12	1.09 (1.03, 1.15)	1.34 (1.15, 1.55)	NA
Amlodipine[a]	5 single dose	14	1.26 (1.11, 1.44)	2.57 (2.31, 2.86)	NA
Atazanavir[b]	300 once daily	11	0.90 (0.83, 0.97)	0.93 (0.85, 1.02)	0.81 (0.72, 0.91)
Buprenorphine	Buprenorphine: 4 to 24 once daily and Naloxone: 1 to 6 once daily	11	1.19 (1.01, 1.40)[c]	1.51 (1.27, 1.78)[c]	1.65 (1.30, 2.08)[c]
Norbuprenorphine			1.82 (1.41, 2.36)[c]	2.11 (1.65, 2.70)[c]	1.87 (1.48, 2.36)[c]
Naloxone			0.99 (0.84, 1.16)[c]	1.11 (0.91, 1.37)[c]	NA
Carbamazepine[a]	200 once daily followed by 200 twice daily	12	1.10 (1.07, 1.14)	1.17 (1.13, 1.22)	1.35 (1.27, 1.45)
Carbamazepine's metabolite, carbamazepine-10,11-epoxide (CBZE)			0.84 (0.82, 0.87)	0.75 (0.73, 0.77)	0.57 (0.54, 0.61)
Carisoprodol[a]	250 single dose	14	0.54 (0.47, 0.63)	0.62 (0.55, 0.70)	NA
Carisoprodol's metabolite, meprobamate			1.17 (1.10, 1.25)	1.09 (1.03, 1.16)	NA
Cyclobenzaprine[a]	5 single dose	14	0.68 (0.61, 0.75)	0.60 (0.53, 0.68)	NA
Cyclobenzaprine's metabolite norcyclobenzaprine			1.03 (0.87, 1.23)	0.74 (0.64, 0.85)	NA
Cyclosporine	10 single dose[d]	12	0.83 (0.72, 0.94)[c]	4.28 (3.66, 5.01)[c]	12.85 (10.61, 15.55)[c]
Darunavir[b]	800 once daily	9	0.99 (0.92, 1.08)	0.92 (0.84, 1.00)	0.74 (0.63, 0.88)
Diazepam[a]	2 single dose	13	1.18 (1.07, 1.30)	0.78 (0.73, 0.82)	NA
Diazepam's metabolite nordiazepam			1.10 (1.03, 1.19)	0.56 (0.45, 0.70)	NA
Digoxin	0.5 single dose	11	1.58 (1.43-1.73)	1.36 (1.21-1.53)	1.24 (1.07-1.43)

This table is continued on the next page

Pregnancy
Advise patients to avoid pregnancy during treatment and within 6 months of stopping treatment with TECHNIVIE with ribavirin. Inform patients to notify their health care provider immediately in the event of a pregnancy *[see Use in Specific Populations (8.1)]*.

Drug Interactions
Inform patients that TECHNIVIE may interact with some drugs; therefore, patients should be advised to report to their healthcare provider the use of any prescription, non-prescription medication or herbal products *[see Contraindications (4), Warnings and Precautions (5.4) and Drug Interactions (7)]*.
Inform patients that contraceptives containing ethinyl estradiol are contraindicated with TECHNIVIE *[see Contraindications (4) and Warnings and Precautions (5.2)]*.

Administration
Advise patients to take TECHNIVIE every day at the regularly scheduled time with a meal without regard to fat or calorie content *[see Dosage and Administration (2.1)]*.
Inform patients that it is important not to miss or skip doses and to take TECHNIVIE for the duration that is recommended by the healthcare provider.
TECHNIVIE is manufactured by AbbVie Inc., North Chicago, IL 60064.
TECHNIVIE and NORVIR are trademarks of AbbVie Inc. All other brands listed are trademarks of their respective owners and are not trademarks of AbbVie Inc. The makers of these brands are not affiliated with and do not endorse AbbVie Inc. or its products.

MEDICATION GUIDE
TECHNIVIE™ (TEK-ni-vee)
(ombitasvir, paritaprevir and ritonavir tablets)

Important: TECHNIVIE is taken in combination with ribavirin. You should also read the Medication Guide that comes with ribavirin.

What is the most important information I should know about TECHNIVIE?
TECHNIVIE may cause severe liver problems, especially in people with certain types of cirrhosis. These severe liver problems can lead to the need for a liver transplant, or can lead to death.
TECHNIVIE can cause increases in your liver function blood test results, especially if you use ethinyl estradiol-containing medicines (such as some birth control products).

- You must stop using ethinyl estradiol-containing medicines before you start treatment with TECHNIVIE. See the section **"Who should not take TECHNIVIE?"** for a list of these medicines.
- If you use these medicines as a method of birth control, you must use another method of birth control during treatment with TECHNIVIE, and for about 2 weeks after you finish treatment with TECHNIVIE. Your healthcare provider will tell you when you may begin taking ethinyl estradiol-containing medicines.
- Your healthcare provider should do blood tests to check your liver function during the first 4 weeks and then as needed, during treatment with TECHNIVIE.
- Your healthcare provider may tell you to stop taking TECHNIVIE if you develop signs or symptoms of liver problems.
- Tell your healthcare provider right away if you develop any of the following symptoms, or if they worsen during treatment with TECHNIVIE:
  ○ tiredness
  ○ weakness
  ○ loss of appetite
  ○ nausea and vomiting
  ○ yellowing of your skin or eyes
  ○ color changes in your stools
  ○ confusion
  ○ swelling of the stomach area

What is TECHNIVIE?
- TECHNIVIE is a prescription medicine used with ribavirin to treat people with genotype 4 chronic (lasting a long time) hepatitis C virus (HCV) infection without cirrhosis. You should also read the Medication Guide for ribavirin.
- TECHNIVIE is not for people with certain types of liver problems.
- Each TECHNIVIE tablet contains the medicines ombitasvir, paritaprevir and ritonavir.
It is not known if TECHNIVIE is safe and effective in children under 18 years of age.

Who should not take TECHNIVIE?
Do not take TECHNIVIE if you:
- **have severe liver problems**
- **take any of the following medicines:**
  ○ alfuzosin hydrochloride (Uroxatral®)
  ○ carbamazepine (Carbatrol®, Epitol®, Equetro®, Tegretol®, TEGRETOL-XR®, TERIL®)
  ○ cisapride (Propulsid®)
  ○ colchicine (Colcrys®) in patients who have certain kidney or liver problems
  ○ dronedarone (Multaq®)
  ○ efavirenz (Atripla®, Sustiva®)
  ○ ergot containing medicines including:
    • ergotamine tartrate (Cafergot®, Ergomar®, Ergostat®, Medihaler®, Migergot®, Wigraine®, Wigrettes®)
    • dihydroergotamine mesylate (D.H.E. 45®, Migranal®)
    • methylergonovine (Ergotrate®, Methergine®)
  ○ ethinyl estradiol-containing medicines:
    • combination birth control pills or patches, such as Lo Loestrin® FE, Norinyl®, Ortho Tri-Cyclen Lo®, Ortho Evra®
    • hormonal vaginal rings such as NuvaRing®
    • the hormone replacement therapy medicine, Fem HRT®
  ○ lovastatin (Advicor®, Altoprev®, Mevacor®)
  ○ lurasidone (Latuda®)
  ○ midazolam, when taken by mouth
  ○ phenytoin, (Dilantin®, Phenytek®)
  ○ phenobarbital (Luminal®)
  ○ pimozide (Orap®)
  ○ ranolazine (Ranexa®)
  ○ rifampin (Rifadin®, Rifamate®, Rifater® Rimactane®)
  ○ sildenafil citrate (Revatio®), when taken for pulmonary artery hypertension (PAH)
  ○ simvastatin (Simcor®, Vytorin®, Zocor®)
  ○ St. John's wort (Hypericum perforatum) or a product that contains St. John's wort
  ○ triazolam (Halcion®)
- **have had a severe skin rash after taking ritonavir (Norvir®)**

What should I tell my healthcare provider before taking TECHNIVIE?
Before taking TECHNIVIE tell your healthcare provider about all your medical conditions, including if you:
- have liver problems other than hepatitis C infection. See **"Who should not take TECHNIVIE?"**
- have HIV infection

Table 8 *(Cont.)* Drug Interactions: Change in Pharmacokinetic Parameters for Co-administered Drug in the Presence of TECHNIVIE

Co-administered Drug	Dose of Co-administered Drug (mg)	n	Ratio (with/without TECHNIVIE) of Co-administered Drug Pharmacokinetic Parameters (90% CI); No Effect = 1.00		
			C_{max}	AUC	C_{min}
Ethinyl Estradiol[e]	Ethinyl estradiol 0.035 and Norgestimate 0.25 once daily	8	1.16 (0.90, 1.50)	1.06 (0.96, 1.17)	1.12 (0.94, 1.33)
Norelgestromin[e]		9	2.01 (1.77, 2.29)	2.60 (2.30, 2.95)	3.11 (2.51, 3.85)
Norgestrel[e]		9	2.26 (1.91, 2.67)	2.54 (2.09, 3.09)	2.93 (2.39, 3.57)
Furosemide[a]	20 single dose	12	1.42 (1.17, 1.72)	1.08 (1.00, 1.17)	NA
Hydrocodone[a]	5 single dose	15	1.27 (1.14, 1.40)	1.90 (1.72, 2.10)	NA
Ketoconazole	400 once daily	12	1.10 (1.05, 1.16)	2.05 (1.93, 2.18)	NA
Lopinavir/ritonavir[f]	400/100 twice daily	18	1.06 (0.99, 1.14)	1.13 (1.09, 1.17)	1.34 (1.26, 1.42)
Lopinavir/ritonavir[f,g]	800/200 once daily	12	1.05 (0.95, 1.17)	1.17 (1.09, 1.26)	3.50 (2.69, 4.56)
Omeprazole	40 once daily	12	0.48 (0.29, 0.78)	0.46 (0.27, 0.77)	NA
Pravastatin	10 once daily	10	1.43 (1.09, 1.88)	1.76 (1.46, 2.13)	NA
Rilpivirine[a]	25 once daily (morning)[h]	8	2.55 (2.08, 3.12)	3.25 (2.80, 3.77)	3.62 (3.12, 4.21)
Tacrolimus	0.5 single dose[i]	11	4.27 (3.49, 5.22)[c]	85.81 (67.88, 108.49)[c]	24.61 (19.69, 30.77)[c]

a. Study evaluated interaction with ombitasvir/paritaprevir/ritonavir plus dasabuvir; results extrapolated to ombitasvir/paritaprevir/ritonavir.
b. Atazanavir or darunavir administered with ombitasvir/paritaprevir/ritonavir in the morning was compared to atazanavir or darunavir administered with 100 mg ritonavir in the morning.
c. Dose normalized parameters reported.
d. 10 mg cyclosporine was administered with ombitasvir/paritaprevir/ritonavir in the test arm and 100 mg cyclosporine was administered in the reference arm without ombitasvir/paritaprevir/ritonavir.
e. Data shown is combined data for ombitasvir/paritaprevir/ritonavir with (N=3) and without (N=6) dasabuvir.
f. Lopinavir parameters are reported.
g. Lopinavir/ritonavir administered in the evening, 12 hours after morning dose of ombitasvir/paritaprevir/ritonavir.
h. Similar increases were observed when rilpivirine was dosed in the evening with food or 4 hours after food.
i. 0.5 mg tacrolimus was administered with ombitasvir/paritaprevir/ritonavir in the test arm and 2 mg tacrolimus was administered in the reference arm without ombitasvir/paritaprevir/ritonavir.
NA: not available/not applicable; CI: Confidence interval.
Doses of ombitasvir, paritaprevir and ritonavir were 25 mg, 150 mg and 100 mg, respectively.
For studies conducted with ombitasvir/paritaprevir/ritonavir plus dasabuvir, doses of dasabuvir were 250 mg or 400 mg (both doses showed similar exposures).
Ombitasvir, paritaprevir and ritonavir were dosed once daily (and where applicable, dasabuvir was dosed twice daily) in all the above studies except studies with ketoconazole and carbamazepine that used single doses.

• have had a liver transplant. If you take the medicines tacrolimus (Prograf®) or cyclosporine (Gengraf®, Neoral®, Sandimmune®) to help prevent rejection of your transplanted liver, the amount of these medicines in your blood may increase during treatment with TECHNIVIE.
  ○ Your healthcare provider should check the level of tacrolimus or cyclosporine in your blood, and if needed may change your dose of these medicines or how often you take them.
  ○ When you finish taking TECHNIVIE or if you have to stop TECHNIVIE for any reason, your healthcare provider should tell you what dose of tacrolimus or cyclosporine to take and how often you should take it.
• are pregnant or plan to become pregnant. It is not known if TECHNIVIE will harm your unborn baby. **When taking TECHNIVIE in combination with ribavirin you should also read the ribavirin Medication Guide for important pregnancy information.**
• are breastfeeding or plan to breastfeed. It is not known if TECHNIVIE passes into your breast milk. Talk to your healthcare provider about the best way to feed your baby if you take TECHNIVIE.
Tell your healthcare provider about all the medicines you take, including prescription and over-the-counter medicines, vitamins, and herbal supplements. Some medicines interact with TECHNIVIE. **Keep a list of your medicines to show your healthcare provider and pharmacist.**
• You can ask your healthcare provider or pharmacist for a list of medicines that interact with TECHNIVIE.
• **Do not start taking a new medicine without telling your healthcare provider.** Your healthcare provider can tell you if it is safe to take TECHNIVIE with other medicines.
• When you finish treatment with TECHNIVIE:
  ○ If your healthcare provider changed the dose of one of your usual medicines during treatment with TECHNIVIE: Ask your healthcare provider about when you should change back to your original dose after you finish treatment with TECHNIVIE.
  ○ If your healthcare provider told you to stop taking one of your usual medicines during treatment with TECHNIVIE: Ask your healthcare provider if you should start taking these medicines again after you finished treatment with TECHNIVIE.

How should I take TECHNIVIE?
• Take TECHNIVIE exactly as your healthcare provider tells you to take it. Do not change your dose unless your healthcare provider tells you to.

• Do not stop taking TECHNIVIE without first talking with your healthcare provider.
• Take 2 TECHNIVIE tablets every day in the morning, with a meal.
• If you take too much TECHNIVIE, call your healthcare provider or go to the nearest emergency room right away.
• TECHNIVIE comes in **monthly cartons that contain enough medicine for 28 days**.
  ○ Each monthly carton of TECHNIVIE contains **4 smaller cartons.**
  ○ Each of the 4 smaller cartons contains enough child resistant **daily dose packs** of medicine to last for **7 days (1 week).**
  ○ Each **daily dose pack** contains all of your TECHNIVIE medicine for **1 day** (2 tablets).
  ○ Follow the instructions on each daily dose pack about how to remove the tablets.
  ○ It is important that you do not miss or skip doses of TECHNIVIE during treatment.
  ○ If you take too much TECHNIVIE, call your healthcare provider or go to the nearest hospital emergency room right away.

What are the possible side effects of TECHNIVIE?
TECHNIVIE can cause serious side effects. See "What is the most important information I should know about TECHNIVIE?"
Common side effects of TECHNIVIE when used with ribavirin include:
• feeling weak   • nausea
• tiredness   • sleep problems
These are not all the possible side effects of TECHNIVIE. Call your doctor for medical advice about side effects. You may report side effects to FDA at 1-800-FDA-1088.

How should I store TECHNIVIE?
• Store TECHNIVIE at or below 86°F (30°C).
Keep TECHNIVIE and all medicines out of the reach of children.

General information about the safe and effective use of TECHNIVIE
Medicines are sometimes prescribed for purposes other than those listed in a Medication Guide. Do not use TECHNIVIE for a condition for which it was not prescribed. Do not give TECHNIVIE to other people, even if they have the same symptoms that you have. It may harm them. You can ask your pharmacist or healthcare provider for information about TECHNIVIE that is written for health professionals.

What are the ingredients in TECHNIVIE?
Active ingredients: ombitasvir, paritaprevir, and ritonavir
Inactive ingredients: copovidone, K value 28, vitamin E polyethylene glycol succinate, propylene glycol monolaurate Type I, sorbitan monolaurate, colloidal silicon dioxide/colloidal anhydrous silica, sodium stearyl fumarate, polyvinyl alcohol, polyethylene glycol 3350/macrogol 3350, talc, titanium dioxide, and red iron oxide.
Manufactured by AbbVie Inc., North Chicago, IL 60064.
TECHNIVIE and NORVIR are trademarks of AbbVie Inc. All other brands listed are trademarks of their respective owners and are not trademarks of AbbVie Inc. The makers of these brands are not affiliated with and do not endorse AbbVie Inc. or its products.
For more information go to www.technivie.com or call 1-844-283-2464.

This Medication Guide has been approved by the U.S. Food and Drug Administration.   Issued: June 2016
03-B365

Continued on next page

Information on the AbbVie, Inc. products listed on these pages is from the prescribing information in use as of July 31, 2016. For more information, please visit rxabbvie.com or call 1-800-633-9110.

Table 9. SVR12 for HCV Genotype 4-Infected Subjects without Cirrhosis

Treatment outcome	Ombitasvir + Paritaprevir + Ritonavir with RBV for 12 weeks		Ombitasvir + Paritaprevir + Ritonavir for 12 weeks
	Treatment-naïve	Treatment-experienced	Treatment-naïve
	% (n/N)	% (n/N)	% (n/N)
Overall SVR12	100 % (42/42)	100% (49/49)	91% (40/44)
Outcome for subjects without SVR12			
On-treatment VF[a]	0% (0/42)	0% (0/49)	2% (1/44)
Relapse[b]	0% (0/42)	0% (0/49)	5% (2/42)
Other[c]	0% (0/42)	0% (0/49)	2% (1/44)

VF = virologic failure

a. On-treatment VF was defined as confirmed HCV ≥ 25 IU/mL after HCV RNA < 25 IU/mL during treatment, confirmed increase from nadir in HCV RNA > 1 $\log_{10}$ IU/mL during treatment, or HCV RNA ≥ 25 IU/mL persistently during treatment with at least 6 weeks of treatment.

b. Relapse was defined as confirmed HCV RNA ≥ 25 IU/mL post-treatment before or during SVR12 window among subjects with HCV RNA less than 25 IU/mL at last observation during at least 11 weeks of treatment.

c. Other includes subjects not achieving SVR12 but not experiencing on-treatment VF or relapse (e.g. lost to follow-up).

TRICOR®
Ŗ

[tri cŏr]
(fenofibrate)
Tablet for oral use

HIGHLIGHTS OF PRESCRIBING INFORMATION
These highlights do not include all the information needed to use TRICOR safely and effectively. See full prescribing information for TRICOR.
TRICOR (fenofibrate) Tablet for oral use
Initial U.S. Approval: 1993

────────INDICATIONS AND USAGE────────

TRICOR is a peroxisome proliferator receptor alpha (PPARα) activator indicated as an adjunct to diet:
• To reduce elevated LDL-C, Total-C, TG and Apo B, and to increase HDL-C in adult patients with primary hypercholesterolemia or mixed dyslipidemia (1.1).
• For treatment of adult patients with severe hypertriglyceridemia (1.2).
Important Limitations of Use: Fenofibrate was not shown to reduce coronary heart disease morbidity and mortality in patients with type 2 diabetes mellitus (5.1).

────────DOSAGE AND ADMINISTRATION────────

• Primary hypercholesterolemia or mixed dyslipidemia: Initial dose of 145 mg once daily (2.2).
• Severe hypertriglyceridemia: Initial dose of 48 to 145 mg once daily. Maximum dose is 145 mg (2.3).
• Renally impaired patients: Initial dose of 48 mg once daily (2.4).
• Geriatric patients: Select the dose on the basis of renal function (2.5).
• Maybe taken without regard to meals (2.1).

────────DOSAGE FORMS AND STRENGTHS────────

Oral Tablets: 48 mg and 145 mg (3).

────────CONTRAINDICATIONS────────

• Severe renal dysfunction, including patients receiving dialysis (4, 8.6, 12.3).
• Active liver disease (4, 5.3).
• Gallbladder disease (4, 5.5).
• Known hypersensitivity to fenofibrate (4).
• Nursing mothers (4, 8.3).

────────WARNINGS AND PRECAUTIONS────────

• Myopathy and rhabdomyolysis have been reported in patients taking fenofibrate. The risks for myopathy and rhabdomyolysis are increased when fibrates are co-administered with a statin (with a significantly higher rate observed for gemfibrozil), particularly in elderly patients and patients with diabetes, renal failure, or hypothyroidism (5.2).
• TRICOR can increase serum transaminases. Monitor liver tests, including ALT, periodically during therapy (5.3).
• TRICOR can reversibly increase serum creatinine levels (5.4). Monitor renal function periodically in patients with renal impairment (8.6).
• TRICOR increases cholesterol excretion into the bile, leading to risk of cholelithiasis. If cholelithiasis is suspected, gallbladder studies are indicated (5.5).

• Exercise caution in concomitant treatment with oral coumarin anticoagulants. Adjust the dosage of coumarin anticoagulant to maintain the prothrombin time/INR at the desired level to prevent bleeding complications (5.6).

────────ADVERSE REACTIONS────────

The most common adverse reactions (> 2% and at least 1% greater than placebo) are abnormal liver tests, increased AST, increased ALT, increased CPK, and rhinitis (6).
To report SUSPECTED ADVERSE REACTIONS, contact AbbVie Inc. at 1-800-633-9110 or FDA at 1-800-FDA-1088 or www.fda.gov/medwatch

────────DRUG INTERACTIONS────────

• Coumarin anticoagulants: (7.1).
• Immunosuppressants: (7.2).
• Bile acid resins: (7.3).

────────USE IN SPECIFIC POPULATIONS────────

• Geriatric Use: Determine dose selection based on renal function (8.5).
• Renal Impairment: Avoid use in patients with severe renal impairment. Dose reduction is required in patients with mild to moderate renal impairment (8.6).
See 17 for PATIENT COUNSELING INFORMATION.
Revised: 2/2016

FULL PRESCRIBING INFORMATION

1 INDICATIONS AND USAGE
1.1 Primary Hypercholesterolemia or Mixed Dyslipidemia
TRICOR is indicated as adjunctive therapy to diet to reduce elevated low-density lipoprotein cholesterol (LDL-C), total cholesterol (Total-C), Triglycerides and apolipoprotein B (Apo B), and to increase high-density lipoprotein cholesterol (HDL-C) in adult patients with primary hypercholesterolemia or mixed dyslipidemia.
1.2 Severe Hypertriglyceridemia
TRICOR is also indicated as adjunctive therapy to diet for treatment of adult patients with severe hypertriglyceridemia. Improving glycemic control in diabetic patients showing fasting chylomicronemia will usually obviate the need for pharmacologic intervention.
Markedly elevated levels of serum triglycerides (e.g. > 2,000 mg/dL) may increase the risk of developing pancreatitis. The effect of fenofibrate therapy on reducing this risk has not been adequately studied.
1.3 Important Limitations of Use
Fenofibrate at a dose equivalent to 145 mg of TRICOR was not shown to reduce coronary heart disease morbidity and mortality in a large, randomized controlled trial of patients with type 2 diabetes mellitus *[see Warnings and Precautions (5.1)]*.

2 DOSAGE AND ADMINISTRATION
2.1 General Considerations
Patients should be placed on an appropriate lipid-lowering diet before receiving TRICOR, and should continue this diet during treatment with TRICOR. TRICOR tablets can be given without regard to meals.
The initial treatment for dyslipidemia is dietary therapy specific for the type of lipoprotein abnormality. Excess body weight and excess alcoholic intake may be important factors in hypertriglyceridemia and should be addressed prior to any drug therapy. Physical exercise can be an important ancillary measure. Diseases contributory to hyperlipidemia, such as hypothyroidism or diabetes mellitus should be looked for and adequately treated. Estrogen therapy, thiazide diuretics and beta-blockers, are sometimes associated with massive rises in plasma triglycerides, especially in subjects with familial hypertriglyceridemia. In such cases, discontinuation of the specific etiologic agent may obviate the need for specific drug therapy of hypertriglyceridemia. Lipid levels should be monitored periodically and consideration should be given to reducing the dosage of TRICOR® (fenofibrate tablets) if lipid levels fall significantly below the targeted range.
Therapy should be withdrawn in patients who do not have an adequate response after two months of treatment with the maximum recommended dose of 145 mg once daily.
2.2 Primary Hypercholesterolemia or Mixed Dyslipidemia
The initial dose of TRICOR is 145 mg once daily.
2.3 Severe Hypertriglyceridemia
The initial dose is 48 to 145 mg per day. Dosage should be individualized according to patient response, and should be

adjusted if necessary following repeat lipid determinations at 4 to 8 week intervals. The maximum dose is 145 mg once daily.

2.4 Impaired Renal Function

Treatment with TRICOR should be initiated at a dose of 48 mg per day in patients having mild to moderately impaired renal function, and increased only after evaluation of the effects on renal function and lipid levels at this dose. The use of TRICOR should be avoided in patients with severe renal impairment *[see Use in Specific Populations (8.6) and Clinical Pharmacology (12.3)]*.

2.5 Geriatric Patients

Dose selection for the elderly should be made on the basis of renal function *[see Use in Specific Populations (8.5)]*.

3 DOSAGE FORMS AND STRENGTHS

- 48 mg yellow tablets, imprinted with the code identification letters "FI".
- 48 mg yellow tablets, imprinted with the "a" logo and code identification letters "FI".
- 145 mg white tablets, imprinted with the code identification letters "FO".
- 145 mg white tablets, imprinted with the "a" logo and code identification letters "FO".

4 CONTRAINDICATIONS

TRICOR is contraindicated in:
- patients with severe renal impairment, including those receiving dialysis *[see Clinical Pharmacology (12.3)]*.
- patients with active liver disease, including those with primary biliary cirrhosis and unexplained persistent liver function abnormalities *[see Warnings and Precautions (5.3)]*.
- patients with preexisting gallbladder disease *[see Warnings and Precautions (5.5)]*.
- nursing mothers *[see Use in Specific Populations (8.3)]*.
- patients with known hypersensitivity to fenofibrate or fenofibric acid *[see Warnings and Precautions (5.9)]*.

5 WARNINGS AND PRECAUTIONS

5.1 Mortality and Coronary Heart Disease Morbidity

The effect of TRICOR on coronary heart disease morbidity and mortality and non-cardiovascular mortality has not been established.

The Action to Control Cardiovascular Risk in Diabetes Lipid (ACCORD Lipid) trial was a randomized placebo-controlled study of 5518 patients with type 2 diabetes mellitus on background statin therapy treated with fenofibrate. The mean duration of follow-up was 4.7 years. Fenofibrate plus statin combination therapy showed a non-significant 8% relative risk reduction in the primary outcome of major adverse cardiovascular events (MACE), a composite of non-fatal myocardial infarction, non-fatal stroke, and cardiovascular disease death (hazard ratio [HR] 0.92, 95% CI 0.79-1.08) (p=0.32) as compared to statin monotherapy. In a gender subgroup analysis, the hazard ratio for MACE in men receiving combination therapy versus statin monotherapy was 0.82 (95% CI 0.69-0.99), and the hazard ratio for MACE in women receiving combination therapy versus statin monotherapy was 1.38 (95% CI 0.98-1.94) (interaction p=0.01). The clinical significance of this subgroup finding is unclear.

The Fenofibrate Intervention and Event Lowering in Diabetes (FIELD) study was a 5-year randomized, placebo-controlled study of 9795 patients with type 2 diabetes mellitus treated with fenofibrate. Fenofibrate demonstrated a non-significant 11% relative reduction in the primary outcome of coronary heart disease events (hazard ratio [HR] 0.89, 95% CI 0.75-1.05, p=0.16) and a significant 11% reduction in the secondary outcome of total cardiovascular disease events (HR 0.89 [0.80-0.99], p=0.04). There was a non-significant 11% (HR 1.11 [0.95, 1.29], p=0.18) and 19% (HR 1.19 [0.90, 1.57], p=0.22) increase in total and coronary heart disease mortality, respectively, with fenofibrate as compared to placebo.

Because of chemical, pharmacological, and clinical similarities between TRICOR (fenofibrate tablets), clofibrate, and gemfibrozil, the adverse findings in 4 large randomized, placebo-controlled clinical studies with these other fibrate drugs may also apply to TRICOR.

In the Coronary Drug Project, a large study of post myocardial infarction of patients treated for 5 years with clofibrate, there was no difference in mortality seen between the clofibrate group and the placebo group. There was however, a difference in the rate of cholelithiasis and cholecystitis requiring surgery between the two groups (3.0% vs. 1.8%).

In a study conducted by the World Health Organization (WHO), 5000 subjects without known coronary artery disease were treated with placebo or clofibrate for 5 years and followed for an additional one year. There was a statistically significant, higher age - adjusted all-cause mortality in the clofibrate group compared with the placebo group (5.70% vs. 3.96%, p = < 0.01). Excess mortality was due to a 33% increase in non-cardiovascular causes, including malignancy, post-cholecystectomy complications, and pancreatitis. This appeared to confirm the higher risk of gallbladder disease seen in clofibrate-treated patients studied in the Coronary Drug Project.

The Helsinki Heart Study was a large (n=4081) study of middle-aged men without a history of coronary artery disease. Subjects received either placebo or gemfibrozil for 5 years, with a 3.5 year open extension afterward. Total mortality was numerically higher in the gemfibrozil randomization group but did not achieve statistical significance (p = 0.19, 95% confidence interval for relative risk G:P = .91-1.64). Although cancer deaths trended higher in the gemfibrozil group (p = 0.11), cancers (excluding basal cell carcinoma) were diagnosed with equal frequency in both study groups. Due to the limited size of the study, the relative risk of death from any cause was not shown to be different than that seen in the 9 year follow-up data from World Health Organization study (RR=1.29).

A secondary prevention component of the Helsinki Heart Study enrolled middle-aged men excluded from the primary prevention study because of known or suspected coronary heart disease. Subjects received gemfibrozil or placebo for 5 years. Although cardiac deaths trended higher in the gemfibrozil group, this was not statistically significant (hazard ratio 2.2, 95% confidence interval: 0.94-5.05). The rate of gallbladder surgery was not statistically significant between study groups, but did trend higher in the gemfibrozil group, (1.9% vs. 0.3%, p = 0.07).

5.2 Skeletal Muscle

Fibrates increase the risk for myopathy and have been associated with rhabdomyolysis. The risk for serious muscle toxicity appears to be increased in elderly patients and in patients with diabetes, renal insufficiency, or hypothyroidism.

Myopathy should be considered in any patient with diffuse myalgias, muscle tenderness or weakness, and/or marked elevations of creatine phosphokinase (CPK) levels.

Patients should be advised to report promptly unexplained muscle pain, tenderness or weakness, particularly if accompanied by malaise or fever. CPK levels should be assessed in patients reporting these symptoms, and TRICOR therapy should be discontinued if markedly elevated CPK levels occur or myopathy/myositis is suspected or diagnosed.

Data from observational studies indicate that the risk for rhabdomyolysis is increased when fibrates, in particular gemfibrozil, are co-administered with an HMG-CoA reductase inhibitor (statin). The combination should be avoided unless the benefit of further alterations in lipid levels is likely to outweigh the increased risk of this drug combination *[see Clinical Pharmacology (12.3)]*.

Cases of myopathy, including rhabdomyolysis, have been reported with fenofibrates co-administered with colchicine, and caution should be exercised when prescribing fenofibrate with colchicine *[see Drug Interactions (7.4)]*.

5.3 Liver Function

Fenofibrate at doses equivalent to 96 mg to 145 mg TRICOR per day has been associated with increases in serum transaminases [AST (SGOT) or ALT (SGPT)]. In a pooled analysis of 10 placebo-controlled trials, increases to > 3 times the upper limit of normal occurred in 5.3% of patients taking fenofibrate versus 1.1% of patients treated with placebo.

When transaminase determinations were followed either after discontinuation of treatment or during continued treatment, a return to normal limits was usually observed. The incidence of increases in transaminases related to fenofibrate therapy appear to be dose related. In an 8-week dose-ranging study, the incidence of ALT or AST elevations to at least three times the upper limit of normal was 13% in patients receiving dosages equivalent to 96 mg to 145 mg TRICOR per day and was 0% in those receiving dosages equivalent to 48 mg or less TRICOR per day, or placebo. Hepatocellular, chronic active and cholestatic hepatitis associated with fenofibrate therapy have been reported after exposures of weeks to several years. In extremely rare cases, cirrhosis has been reported in association with chronic active hepatitis.

Baseline and regular periodic monitoring of liver function, including serum ALT (SGPT) should be performed for the duration of therapy with TRICOR, and therapy discontinued if enzyme levels persist above three times the normal limit.

5.4 Serum Creatinine

Elevations in serum creatinine have been reported in patients on fenofibrate. These elevations tend to return to baseline following discontinuation of fenofibrate. The clinical significance of these observations is unknown. Monitor renal function in patients with renal impairment taking TRICOR. Renal monitoring should also be considered for patients taking TRICOR at risk for renal insufficiency such as the elderly and patients with diabetes.

5.5 Cholelithiasis

Fenofibrate, like clofibrate and gemfibrozil, may increase cholesterol excretion into the bile, leading to cholelithiasis. If cholelithiasis is suspected, gallbladder studies are indicated. TRICOR therapy should be discontinued if gallstones are found.

5.6 Coumarin Anticoagulants

Caution should be exercised when coumarin anticoagulants are given in conjunction with TRICOR because of the potentiation of coumarin-type anticoagulant effects in prolonging the Prothrombin Time/International Normalized Ratio (PT/INR). To prevent bleeding complications, frequent monitoring of PT/INR and dose adjustment of the anticoagulant are recommended until PT/INR has stabilized *[see Drug Interactions (7.1)]*.

5.7 Pancreatitis

Pancreatitis has been reported in patients taking fenofibrate, gemfibrozil, and clofibrate. This occurrence may represent a failure of efficacy in patients with severe hypertriglyceridemia, a direct drug effect, or a secondary phenomenon mediated through biliary tract stone or sludge formation with obstruction of the common bile duct.

5.8 Hematologic Changes

Mild to moderate hemoglobin, hematocrit, and white blood cell decreases have been observed in patients following initiation of fenofibrate therapy. However, these levels stabilize during long-term administration. Thrombocytopenia and agranulocytosis have been reported in individuals treated with fenofibrate. Periodic monitoring of red and white blood cell counts are recommended during the first 12 months of TRICOR administration.

5.9 Hypersensitivity Reactions

Acute hypersensitivity reactions such as Stevens-Johnson syndrome and toxic epidermal necrolysis requiring patient hospitalization and treatment with steroids have been reported in individuals treated with fenofibrates. Urticaria was seen in 1.1 vs. 0%, and rash in 1.4 vs. 0.8% of fenofibrate and placebo patients respectively in controlled trials.

5.10 Venothromboembolic Disease

In the FIELD trial, pulmonary embolus (PE) and deep vein thrombosis (DVT) were observed at higher rates in the fenofibrate- than the placebo-treated group. Of 9,795 patients enrolled in FIELD, there were 4,900 in the placebo group and 4,895 in the fenofibrate group. For DVT, there were 48 events (1%) in the placebo group and 67 (1%) in the fenofibrate group (p = 0.074); and for PE, there were 32 (0.7%) events in the placebo group and 53 (1%) in the fenofibrate group (p = 0.022).

In the Coronary Drug Project, a higher proportion of the clofibrate group experienced definite or suspected fatal or nonfatal pulmonary embolism or thrombophlebitis than the placebo group (5.2% vs. 3.3% at five years; p < 0.01).

5.11 Paradoxical Decreases in HDL Cholesterol Levels

There have been postmarketing and clinical trial reports of severe decreases in HDL cholesterol levels (as low as 2 mg/dL) occurring in diabetic and non-diabetic patients initiated on fibrate therapy. The decrease in HDL-C is mirrored by a decrease in apolipoprotein A1. This decrease has been reported to occur within 2 weeks to years after initiation of fibrate therapy. The HDL-C levels remain depressed until fibrate therapy has been withdrawn; the response to withdrawal of fibrate therapy is rapid and sustained. The clinical significance of this decrease in HDL-C is unknown. It is recommended that HDL-C levels be checked within the first few months after initiation of fibrate therapy. If a severely depressed HDL-C level is detected, fibrate therapy should be withdrawn, and the HDL-C level monitored until it has returned to baseline, and fibrate therapy should not be re-initiated.

Continued on next page

Information on the AbbVie, Inc. products listed on these pages is from the prescribing information in use as of July 31, 2016. For more information, please visit rxabbvie.com or call 1-800-633-9110.

6 ADVERSE REACTIONS

6.1 Clinical Trials Experience

Because clinical studies are conducted under widely varying conditions, adverse reaction rates observed in the clinical studies of a drug cannot be directly compared to rates in the clinical studies of another drug and may not reflect the rates observed in practice.

Adverse events reported by 2% or more of patients treated with fenofibrate (and greater than placebo) during the double-blind, placebo-controlled trials, regardless of causality, are listed in Table 1 below. Adverse events led to discontinuation of treatment in 5.0% of patients treated with fenofibrate and in 3.0% treated with placebo. Increases in liver function tests were the most frequent events, causing discontinuation of fenofibrate treatment in 1.6% of patients in double-blind trials.

Table 1. Adverse Reactions Reported by 2% or More of Patients Treated with Fenofibrate and Greater than Placebo During the Double-Blind, Placebo-Controlled Trials

BODY SYSTEM	Fenofibrate*	Placebo
Adverse Reaction	(N=439)	(N=365)
BODY AS A WHOLE		
Abdominal Pain	4.6%	4.4%
Back Pain	3.4%	2.5%
Headache	3.2%	2.7%
DIGESTIVE		
Nausea	2.3%	1.9%
Constipation	2.1%	1.4%
METABOLIC AND NUTRITIONAL DISORDERS		
Abnormal Liver Function Tests	7.5%**	1.4%
Increased ALT	3.0%	1.6%
Increased CPK	3.0%	1.4%
Increased AST	3.4%**	0.5%
RESPIRATORY		
Respiratory Disorder	6.2%	5.5%
Rhinitis	2.3%	1.1%

* Dosage equivalent to 145 mg TRICOR.
** Significantly different from Placebo.

6.2 Postmarketing Experience

The following adverse reactions have been identified during postapproval use of fenofibrate: myalgia, rhabdomyolysis, pancreatitis, acute renal failure, muscle spasm, hepatitis, cirrhosis, anemia, arthralgia, decreases in hemoglobin, decreases in hematocrit, white blood cell decreases, asthenia, and severely depressed HDL-cholesterol levels. Because these reactions are reported voluntarily from a population of uncertain size, it is not always possible to reliably estimate their frequency or establish a causal relationship to drug exposure.

7 DRUG INTERACTIONS

7.1 Coumarin Anticoagulants

Potentiation of coumarin-type anticoagulant effects has been observed with prolongation of the PT/INR.

Caution should be exercised when coumarin anticoagulants are given in conjunction with TRICOR® (fenofibrate tablets). The dosage of the anticoagulants should be reduced to maintain the PT/INR at the desired level to prevent bleeding complications. Frequent PT/INR determinations are advisable until it has been definitely determined that the PT/INR has stabilized [see Warnings and Precautions (5.6)].

7.2 Immunosuppressants

Immunosuppressants such as cyclosporine and tacrolimus can produce nephrotoxicity with decreases in creatinine clearance and rises in serum creatinine, and because renal excretion is the primary elimination route of fibrate drugs including TRICOR, there is a risk that an interaction will lead to deterioration of renal function. The benefits and risks of using TRICOR (fenofibrate tablets) with immunosuppressants and other potentially nephrotoxic agents should be carefully considered, and the lowest effective dose employed and renal function monitored.

7.3 Bile Acid Binding Resins

Since bile acid binding resins may bind other drugs given concurrently, patients should take TRICOR at least 1 hour before or 4 to 6 hours after a bile acid binding resin to avoid impeding its absorption.

7.4 Colchicine

Cases of myopathy, including rhabdomyolysis, have been reported with fenofibrates co-administered with colchicine, and caution should be exercised when prescribing fenofibrate with colchicine.

8 USE IN SPECIFIC POPULATIONS

8.1 Pregnancy

Pregnancy Category C

Safety in pregnant women has not been established. There are no adequate and well controlled studies of fenofibrate in pregnant women. Fenofibrate should be used during pregnancy only if the potential benefit justifies the potential risk to the fetus.

In female rats given oral dietary doses of 15, 75, and 300 mg/kg/day of fenofibrate from 15 days prior to mating through weaning, maternal toxicity was observed at 0.3 times the MRHD, based on body surface area comparisons; mg/m².

In pregnant rats given oral dietary doses of 14, 127, and 361 mg/kg/day from gestation day 6-15 during the period of organogenesis, adverse developmental findings were not observed at 14 mg/kg/day (less than 1 times the MRHD, based on body surface area comparisons; mg/m²). At higher multiples of human doses evidence of maternal toxicity was observed.

In pregnant rabbits given oral gavage doses of 15, 150, and 300 mg/kg/day from gestation day 6-18 during the period of organogenesis and allowed to deliver, aborted litters were observed at 150 mg/kg/day (10 times the MRHD, based on body surface area comparisons: mg/m²). No developmental findings were observed at 15 mg/kg/day (at less than 1 times the MRHD, based on body surface area comparisons; mg/m²).

In pregnant rats given oral dietary doses of 15, 75, and 300 mg/kg/day from gestation day 15 through lactation day 21 (weaning), maternal toxicity was observed at less than 1 times the maximum recommended human dose (MRHD), based on body surface area comparisons; mg/m².

8.3 Nursing Mothers

Fenofibrate should not be used in nursing mothers. A decision should be made whether to discontinue nursing or to discontinue the drug, taking into account the importance of the drug to the mother.

8.4 Pediatric Use

Safety and effectiveness have not been established in pediatric patients.

8.5 Geriatric Use

Fenofibric acid is known to be substantially excreted by the kidney, and the risk of adverse reactions to this drug may be greater in patients with impaired renal function. Fenofibric acid exposure is not influenced by age. Since elderly patients have a higher incidence of renal impairment, dose selection for the elderly should be made on the basis of renal function [see Dosage and Administration (2.5) and Clinical Pharmacology (12.3)]. Elderly patients with normal renal function should require no dose modifications. Consider monitoring renal function in elderly patients taking TRICOR.

8.6 Renal Impairment

The use of TRICOR should be avoided in patients who have severe renal impairment [see Contraindications (4)]. Dose reduction is required in patients with mild to moderate renal impairment [see Dosage and Administration (2.4) and Clinical Pharmacology (12.3)]. Monitoring renal function in patients with renal impairment is recommended.

8.7 Hepatic Impairment

The use of TRICOR has not been evaluated in subjects with hepatic impairment [see Contraindications (4) and Clinical Pharmacology (12.3)].

10 OVERDOSAGE

There is no specific treatment for overdose with TRICOR. General supportive care of the patient is indicated, including monitoring of vital signs and observation of clinical status, should an overdose occur. If indicated, elimination of unabsorbed drug should be achieved by emesis or gastric lavage; usual precautions should be observed to maintain the airway. Because fenofibric acid is highly bound to plasma proteins, hemodialysis should not be considered.

11 DESCRIPTION

TRICOR® (fenofibrate tablets), is a lipid regulating agent available as tablets for oral administration. Each tablet contains 48 mg or 145 mg of fenofibrate. The chemical name for fenofibrate is 2-[4-(4-chlorobenzoyl) phenoxy]-2-methyl-propanoic acid, 1-methylethyl ester with the following structural formula:

The empirical formula is $C_{20}H_{21}O_4Cl$ and the molecular weight is 360.83; fenofibrate is insoluble in water. The melting point is 79-82°C. Fenofibrate is a white solid which is stable under ordinary conditions.

Inactive Ingredients

Each tablet contains hypromellose 2910 (3 cps), docusate sodium, sucrose, sodium lauryl sulfate, lactose monohydrate, silicified microcrystalline cellulose, crospovidone, and magnesium stearate.

In addition, individual tablets contain:

48 mg tablets

polyvinyl alcohol, titanium dioxide, talc, soybean lecithin, xanthan gum, D&C Yellow #10 aluminum lake, FD&C Yellow #6 /sunset yellow FCF aluminum lake, FD&C Blue #2 /indigo carmine aluminum lake.

145 mg tablets

polyvinyl alcohol, titanium dioxide, talc, soybean lecithin, xanthan gum.

12 CLINICAL PHARMACOLOGY

12.1 Mechanism of Action

The active moiety of TRICOR is fenofibric acid. The pharmacological effects of fenofibric acid in both animals and humans have been extensively studied through oral administration of fenofibrate.

The lipid-modifying effects of fenofibric acid seen in clinical practice have been explained *in vivo* in transgenic mice and *in vitro* in human hepatocyte cultures by the activation of peroxisome proliferator activated receptor α (PPARα). Through this mechanism, fenofibrate increases lipolysis and elimination of triglyceride-rich particles from plasma by activating lipoprotein lipase and reducing production of apoprotein C-III (an inhibitor of lipoprotein lipase activity).

The resulting decrease in TG produces an alteration in the size and composition of LDL from small, dense particles (which are thought to be atherogenic due to their susceptibility to oxidation), to large buoyant particles. These larger particles have a greater affinity for cholesterol receptors and are catabolized rapidly. Activation of PPARα also induces an increase in the synthesis of apolipoproteins A-I, A-II and HDL-cholesterol.

Fenofibrate also reduces serum uric acid levels in hyperuricemic and normal individuals by increasing the urinary excretion of uric acid.

12.2 Pharmacodynamics

A variety of clinical studies have demonstrated that elevated levels of total-C, LDL-C, and apo B, an LDL membrane complex, are associated with human atherosclerosis. Similarly, decreased levels of HDL-C and its transport complex, apolipoprotein A (apo AI and apo AII) are associated with the development of atherosclerosis. Epidemiologic investigations have established that cardiovascular morbidity and mortality vary directly with the level of total-C, LDL-C, and TG, and inversely with the level of HDL-C. The independent effect of raising HDL-C or lowering triglycerides (TG) on the risk of cardiovascular morbidity and mortality has not been determined.

Fenofibric acid, the active metabolite of fenofibrate, produces reductions in total cholesterol, LDL cholesterol, apolipoprotein B, total triglycerides and triglyceride rich lipoprotein (VLDL) in treated patients. In addition, treatment with fenofibrate results in increases in high density lipoprotein (HDL) and apolipoproteins apoAI and apoAII.

12.3 Pharmacokinetics

Plasma concentrations of fenofibric acid after administration of three 48 mg or one 145 mg tablets are equivalent under fed conditions to one 200 mg micronized fenofibrate capsule.

Fenofibrate is a pro-drug of the active chemical moiety fenofibric acid. Fenofibrate is converted by ester hydrolysis in the body to fenofibric acid which is the active constituent measurable in the circulation.

Absorption

The absolute bioavailability of fenofibrate cannot be determined as the compound is virtually insoluble in aqueous media suitable for injection. However, fenofibrate is well absorbed from the gastrointestinal tract. Following oral administration in healthy volunteers, approximately 60% of a single dose of radiolabelled fenofibrate appeared in urine, primarily as fenofibric acid and its glucuronate conjugate, and 25% was excreted in the feces. Peak plasma levels of fenofibric acid occur within 6 to 8 hours after administration.

Exposure to fenofibric acid in plasma, as measured by C_{max} and AUC, is not significantly different when a single 145 mg dose of fenofibrate is administered under fasting or nonfasting conditions.

Distribution

Upon multiple dosing of fenofibrate, fenofibric acid steady state is achieved within 9 days. Plasma concentrations of fenofibric acid at steady state are approximately double of those following a single dose. Serum protein binding was approximately 99% in normal and hyperlipidemic subjects.

Metabolism

Following oral administration, fenofibrate is rapidly hydrolyzed by esterases to the active metabolite, fenofibric acid; no unchanged fenofibrate is detected in plasma.

Fenofibric acid is primarily conjugated with glucuronic acid and then excreted in urine. A small amount of fenofibric acid is reduced at the carbonyl moiety to a benzhydrol metabolite which is, in turn, conjugated with glucuronic acid and excreted in urine.

In vivo metabolism data indicate that neither fenofibrate nor fenofibric acid undergo oxidative metabolism (e.g., cytochrome P450) to a significant extent.

Elimination

After absorption, fenofibrate is mainly excreted in the urine in the form of metabolites, primarily fenofibric acid and fenofibric acid glucuronide. After administration of radiolabelled fenofibrate, approximately 60% of the dose appeared in the urine and 25% was excreted in the feces.

Fenofibric acid is eliminated with a half-life of 20 hours, allowing once daily dosing.

Special Populations

Geriatrics

In elderly volunteers 77 to 87 years of age, the oral clearance of fenofibric acid following a single oral dose of fenofibrate was 1.2 L/h, which compares to 1.1 L/h in young adults. This indicates that a similar dosage regimen can be used in elderly with normal renal function, without increasing accumulation of the drug or metabolites *[see Dosage and Administration (2.5) and Use in Specific Populations (8.5)]*.

Pediatrics

The pharmacokinetics of TRICOR® (fenofibrate tablets) has not been studied in pediatric populations.

Gender

No pharmacokinetic difference between males and females has been observed for fenofibrate.

Race

The influence of race on the pharmacokinetics of fenofibrate has not been studied, however fenofibrate is not metabolized by enzymes known for exhibiting inter-ethnic variability.

Renal Impairment

The pharmacokinetics of fenofibric acid was examined in patients with mild, moderate, and severe renal impairment. Patients with severe renal impairment (estimated glomerular filtration rate [eGFR] < 30 mL/min/1.73m^2) showed 2.7-fold increase in exposure for fenofibric acid and increased accumulation of fenofibric acid during chronic dosing compared to that of healthy subjects. Patients with mild to moderate renal impairment (eGFR 30-59 mL/min/1.73m^2) had similar exposure but an increase in the half-life for fenofibric acid compared to that of healthy subjects. Based on these findings, the use of TRICOR should be avoided in patients who have severe renal impairment and dose reduction is required in patients having mild to moderate renal impairment *[see Dosage and Administration (2.4)]*.

Hepatic Impairment

No pharmacokinetic studies have been conducted in patients with hepatic impairment.

Drug-drug Interactions

In vitro studies using human liver microsomes indicate that fenofibrate and fenofibric acid are not inhibitors of cytochrome (CYP) P450 isoforms CYP3A4, CYP2D6, CYP2E1, or CYP1A2. They are weak inhibitors of CYP2C8, CYP2C19 and CYP2A6, and mild-to-moderate inhibitors of CYP2C9 at therapeutic concentrations.

Table 2 describes the effects of co-administered drugs on fenofibric acid systemic exposure. Table 3 describes the effects of co-administered fenofibrate or fenofibric acid on other drugs.

[See table 2 above]
[See table 3 above]

13 NONCLINICAL TOXICOLOGY

13.1 Carcinogenesis and Mutagenesis and Impairment of Fertility

Two dietary carcinogenicity studies have been conducted in rats with fenofibrate. In the first 24-month study, Wistar rats were dosed with fenofibrate at 10, 45, and 200 mg/kg/day, approximately 0.3, 1, and 6 times the maximum recommended human dose (MRHD), based on body surface area comparisons (mg/m^2). At a dose of 200 mg/kg/

day (at 6 times the MRHD), the incidence of liver carcinomas was significantly increased in both sexes. A statistically significant increase in pancreatic carcinomas was observed in males at 1 and 6 times the MRHD; an increase in pancreatic adenomas and benign testicular interstitial cell tumors was observed at 6 times the MRHD in males. In a second 24-month rat carcinogenicity study in a different strain of rats (Sprague-Dawley), doses of 10 and 60 mg/kg/day (0.3 and 2 times the MRHD) produced significant increases in the incidence of pancreatic acinar adenomas in both sexes and increases in testicular interstitial cell tumors in males at 2 times the MRHD.

A 117-week carcinogenicity study was conducted in rats comparing three drugs: fenofibrate 10 and 60 mg/kg/day (0.3 and 2 times the MRHD), clofibrate (400 mg/kg/day; 2 times the human dose), and gemfibrozil (250 mg/kg/day; 2 times the human dose, based on mg/m^2 surface area). Fenofibrate increased pancreatic acinar adenomas in both sexes. Clofibrate increased hepatocellular carcinoma and pancreatic acinar adenomas in males and hepatic neoplastic

nodules in females. Gemfibrozil increased hepatic neoplastic nodules in males and females, while all three drugs increased testicular interstitial cell tumors in males.

In a 21-month study in CF-1 mice, fenofibrate 10, 45, and 200 mg/kg/day (approximately 0.2, 1, and 3 times the MRHD on the basis of mg/m^2 surface area) significantly increased the liver carcinomas in both sexes at 3 times the MRHD. In a second 18-month study at 10, 60, and 200 mg/kg/day, fenofibrate significantly increased the liver carcinomas in male mice and liver adenomas in female mice at 3 times the MRHD.

Electron microscopy studies have demonstrated peroxisomal proliferation following fenofibrate administration to

Continued on next page

Information on the AbbVie, Inc. products listed on these pages is from the prescribing information in use as of July 31, 2016. For more information, please visit rxabbvie.com or call 1-800-633-9110.

Table 2. Effects of Co-Administered Drugs on Fenofibric Acid Systemic Exposure from Fenofibrate Administration

Co-Administered Drug	Dosage Regimen of Co-Administered Drug	Dosage Regimen of Fenofibrate	Changes in Fenofibric Acid Exposure	
			AUC	C_{max}
Lipid-lowering agents				
Atorvastatin	20 mg once daily for 10 days	Fenofibrate 160 mg[1] once daily for 10 days	↓2%	↓4%
Pravastatin	40 mg as a single dose	Fenofibrate 3 × 67 mg[2] as a single dose	↓1%	↓2%
Fluvastatin	40 mg as a single dose	Fenofibrate 160 mg[1] as a single dose	↓2%	↓10%
Anti-diabetic agents				
Glimepiride	1 mg as a single dose	Fenofibrate 145 mg[1] once daily for 10 days	↑1%	↓1%
Metformin	850 mg three times daily for 10 days	Fenofibrate 54 mg[1] three times daily for 10 days	↓9%	↓6%
Rosiglitazone	8 mg once daily for 5 days	Fenofibrate 145 mg[1] once daily for 14 days	↑10%	↑3%

[1] TriCor (fenofibrate) oral tablet
[2] TriCor (fenofibrate) oral micronized capsule

Table 3. Effects of Fenofibrate Co-Administration on Systemic Exposure of Other Drugs

Dosage Regimen of Fenofibrate	Dosage Regimen of Co-Administered Drug	Change in Co-Administered Drug Exposure		
		Analyte	AUC	C_{max}
Lipid-lowering agents				
Fenofibrate 160 mg[1] once daily for 10 days	Atorvastatin, 20 mg once daily for 10 days	Atorvastatin	↓17%	0%
Fenofibrate 3 × 67 mg[2] as a single dose	Pravastatin, 40 mg as a single dose	Pravastatin	↑13%	↑13%
		3α-Hydroxyl-iso-pravastatin	↑26%	↑29%
Fenofibrate 160 mg[1] as a single dose	Fluvastatin, 40 mg as a single dose	(+)-3R, 5S-Fluvastatin	↑15%	↑16%
Anti-diabetic agents				
Fenofibrate 145 mg[1] once daily for 10 days	Glimepiride, 1 mg as a single dose	Glimepiride	↑35%	↑18%
Fenofibrate 54 mg[1] three times daily for 10 days	Metformin, 850 mg three times daily for 10 days	Metformin	↑3%	↑6%
Fenofibrate 145 mg[1] once daily for 14 days	Rosiglitazone, 8 mg once daily for 5 days	Rosiglitazone	↑6%	↓1%

[1] TriCor (fenofibrate) oral tablet
[2] TriCor (fenofibrate) oral micronized capsule

Table 4. Mean Percent Change in Lipid Parameters at End of Treatment[†]

Treatment Group	Total-C	LDL-C	HDL-C	TG
Pooled Cohort				
Mean baseline lipid values (n=646)	306.9 mg/dL	213.8 mg/dL	52.3 mg/dL	191.0 mg/dL
All FEN (n=361)	-18.7%*	-20.6%*	+11.0%*	-28.9%*
Placebo (n=285)	-0.4%	-2.2%	+0.7%	+7.7%
Baseline LDL-C > 160 mg/dL and TG < 150 mg/dL				
Mean baseline lipid values (n=334)	307.7 mg/dL	227.7 mg/dL	58.1 mg/dL	101.7 mg/dL
All FEN (n=193)	-22.4%*	-31.4%*	+9.8%*	-23.5%*
Placebo (n=141)	+0.2%	-2.2%	+2.6%	+11.7%
Baseline LDL-C >160 mg/dL and TG ≥ 150 mg/dL				
Mean baseline lipid values (n=242)	312.8 mg/dL	219.8 mg/dL	46.7 mg/dL	231.9 mg/dL
All FEN (n=126)	-16.8%*	-20.1%*	+14.6%*	-35.9%*
Placebo (n=116)	-3.0%	-6.6%	+2.3%	+0.9%

† Duration of study treatment was 3 to 6 months.
* p = < 0.05 vs. Placebo

Table 5. Effects of TRICOR in Patients With Severe Hypertriglyceridemia

Study 1

Baseline TG levels 350 to 499 mg/dL	Placebo				TRICOR			
	N	Baseline (Mean)	Endpoint (Mean)	% Change (Mean)	N	Baseline (Mean)	Endpoint (Mean)	% Change (Mean)
Triglycerides	28	449	450	-0.5	27	432	223	-46.2*
VLDL Triglycerides	19	367	350	2.7	19	350	178	-44.1*
Total Cholesterol	28	255	261	2.8	27	252	227	-9.1*
HDL Cholesterol	28	35	36	4	27	34	40	19.6*
LDL Cholesterol	28	120	129	12	27	128	137	14.5
VLDL Cholesterol	27	99	99	5.8	27	92	46	-44.7*

Study 2

Baseline TG levels 500 to 1500 mg/dL	Placebo				TRICOR			
	N	Baseline (Mean)	Endpoint (Mean)	% Change (Mean)	N	Baseline (Mean)	Endpoint (Mean)	% Change (Mean)
Triglycerides	44	710	750	7.2	48	726	308	-54.5*
VLDL Triglycerides	29	537	571	18.7	33	543	205	-50.6*
Total Cholesterol	44	272	271	0.4	48	261	223	-13.8*
HDL Cholesterol	44	27	28	5.0	48	30	36	22.9*
LDL Cholesterol	42	100	90	-4.2	45	103	131	45.0*
VLDL Cholesterol	42	137	142	11.0	45	126	54	-49.4*

* =p < 0.05 vs. Placebo

the rat. An adequate study to test for peroxisome proliferation in humans has not been done, but changes in peroxisome morphology and numbers have been observed in humans after treatment with other members of the fibrate class when liver biopsies were compared before and after treatment in the same individual.

Mutagenesis: Fenofibrate has been demonstrated to be devoid of mutagenic potential in the following tests: Ames, mouse lymphoma, chromosomal aberration and unscheduled DNA synthesis in primary rat hepatocytes.

Impairment of Fertility: In fertility studies rats were given oral dietary doses of fenofibrate, males received 61 days prior to mating and females 15 days prior to mating through weaning which resulted in no adverse effect on fertility at doses up to 300 mg/kg/day (~10 times the MRHD, based on mg/m² surface area comparisons).

14 CLINICAL STUDIES

14.1 Primary Hypercholesterolemia (Heterozygous Familial and Nonfamilial) and Mixed Dyslipidemia

The effects of fenofibrate at a dose equivalent to 145 mg TRICOR® (fenofibrate tablets) per day were assessed from four randomized, placebo-controlled, double-blind, parallel-group studies including patients with the following mean baseline lipid values: total-C 306.9 mg/dL; LDL-C 213.8 mg/dL; HDL-C 52.3 mg/dL; and triglycerides 191.0 mg/dL. TRICOR therapy lowered LDL-C, Total-C, and the LDL-C/HDL-C ratio. TRICOR therapy also lowered triglycerides and raised HDL-C (see Table 4 above).

[See table 4 above]

In a subset of the subjects, measurements of apo B were conducted. TRICOR treatment significantly reduced apo B from baseline to endpoint as compared with placebo (-25.1% vs. 2.4%, p < 0.0001, n=213 and 143 respectively).

14.2 Severe Hypertriglyceridemia

The effects of fenofibrate on serum triglycerides were studied in two randomized, double-blind, placebo-controlled clinical trials of 147 hypertriglyceridemic patients. Patients were treated for eight weeks under protocols that differed only in that one entered patients with baseline TG levels of 500 to 1500 mg/dL, and the other TG levels of 350 to 500 mg/dL. In patients with hypertriglyceridemia and normal cholesterolemia with or without hyperchylomicronemia, treatment with fenofibrate at dosages equivalent to TRICOR 145 mg per day decreased primarily very low density lipoprotein (VLDL) triglycerides and VLDL cholesterol. Treatment of patients with elevated triglycerides often results in an increase of LDL-C (see Table 5).

[See table 5 above]

The effect of TRICOR on cardiovascular morbidity and mortality has not been determined.

16 HOW SUPPLIED/STORAGE AND HANDLING

TRICOR® (fenofibrate tablets) is available in two strengths:

48 mg

Yellow tablets, imprinted with the code identification letters "FI", available in bottles of 90 (NDC 0074-3173-90).

Yellow tablets, imprinted with the "a" logo and code identification letters "FI", available in bottles of 90 (NDC 0074-6122-90).

145 mg

White tablets, imprinted with the code identification letters "FO", available in bottles of 90 (NDC 0074-3189-90).

White tablets, imprinted with the "a" logo and code identification letters "FO", available in bottles of 90 (NDC 0074-6123-90).

Storage

Store at 25°C (77°F); excursions permitted to 15-30°C (59-86°F).

[See USP Controlled Room Temperature]. Keep out of the reach of children. Protect from moisture.

17 PATIENT COUNSELING INFORMATION

Patients should be advised:
• of the potential benefits and risks of TRICOR.
• not to use TRICOR if there is a known hypersensitivity to fenofibrate or fenofibric acid.
• of medications that should not be taken in combination with TRICOR.
• that if they are taking coumarin anticoagulants, TRICOR may increase their anti-coagulant effect, and increased monitoring may be necessary.
• to continue to follow an appropriate lipid-modifying diet while taking TRICOR.
• to take TRICOR once daily, without regard to food, at the prescribed dose, swallowing each tablet whole.
• to return for routine monitoring.
• to inform their physician of all medications, supplements, and herbal preparations they are taking and any change to their medical condition. Patients should also be advised to inform their physicians prescribing a new medication that they are taking TRICOR.
• to inform their physician of any muscle pain, tenderness, or weakness; onset of abdominal pain; or any other new symptoms.

Manufactured for AbbVie Inc., North Chicago, IL 60064, U.S.A.

by Fournier Laboratories Ireland Limited, Anngrove, Carrigtwohill Co. Cork, Ireland.

03-B251 February, 2016

Shown in Product Identification Guide, page 506

TRILIPIX® ℞
[try-lip-iks]
(fenofibric acid)
capsule, delayed release for oral use

HIGHLIGHTS OF PRESCRIBING INFORMATION

These highlights do not include all the information needed to use TRILIPIX safely and effectively. See full prescribing information for TRILIPIX.

TRILIPIX® (fenofibric acid) capsule, delayed release for oral use

Initial U.S. Approval: 2008

RECENT MAJOR CHANGES

Indications and Usage, Combination With a Statin – removal (1)	4/2015
Dosage and Administration, Combination With a Statin – removal (2)	4/2015

INDICATIONS AND USAGE

Trilipix is a peroxisome proliferator-activated receptor (PPAR) alpha agonist indicated as adjunctive therapy to diet to:
• Reduce TG in patients with severe hypertriglyceridemia (1.1).
• Reduce elevated LDL-C, Total-C, TG and Apo B, and to increase HDL-C in patients with primary hypercholesterolemia or mixed dyslipidemia (1.2).

Limitations of Use: Fenofibrate at a dose equivalent to 135 mg of Trilipix did not reduce coronary heart disease morbidity and mortality in patients with type 2 diabetes mellitus (5.1).

DOSAGE AND ADMINISTRATION

• Hypertriglyceridemia: 45 to 135 mg once daily (2.2).
• Primary hypercholesterolemia or mixed dyslipidemia: 135 mg once daily (2.3).
• Renally impaired patients: 45 mg once daily (2.4).
• Maximum dose: 135 mg once daily (2.1).
• May be taken without regard to food (2.1).

DOSAGE FORMS AND STRENGTHS

Oral Delayed Release Capsules: 45 mg and 135 mg (3).

CONTRAINDICATIONS

• Severe renal dysfunction, including patients receiving dialysis (4, 12.3).
• Active liver disease (4, 5.3).
• Gallbladder disease (4, 5.5).
• Nursing mothers (4, 8.3).
• Known hypersensitivity to fenofibric acid or fenofibrate (4, 5.9).

WARNINGS AND PRECAUTIONS

• Myopathy and rhabdomyolysis have been reported in patients taking fenofibrate. The risks for myopathy and rhabdomyolysis are increased in elderly patients; patients with diabetes, renal failure, or hypothyroidism; and patients being treated with a statin (5.2).
• Trilipix can increase serum transaminases. Liver tests should be monitored periodically (5.3).
• Trilipix can reversibly increase serum creatinine levels (5.4). Renal function should be monitored periodically in patients with renal insufficiency (8.6).

- Trilipix increases cholesterol excretion into the bile, leading to risk of cholelithiasis. If cholelithiasis is suspected, gallbladder studies are indicated (5.5).
- Exercise caution in concomitant treatment with oral coumarin anticoagulants. Adjust the dosage of coumarin anticoagulant to maintain the prothrombin time/INR at the desired level to prevent bleeding complications (5.6).

ADVERSE REACTIONS

The most common adverse events reported during clinical trials with fenofibrate (≥ 2% and at least 1% greater than placebo) were abnormal liver tests, increased AST, increased ALT, increased CPK, and rhinitis (6.1).

To report SUSPECTED ADVERSE REACTIONS, contact AbbVie Inc. at 1-800-633-9110 or FDA at 1-800-FDA-1088 or www.fda.gov/medwatch

DRUG INTERACTIONS

- Coumarin Anticoagulants: (7.1).
- Bile Acid Binding Resins: (7.2).
- Immunosuppressants: (7.3).

USE IN SPECIFIC POPULATIONS

- Geriatric Use: Dose selection for the elderly should be made on the basis of renal function (8.5).
- Renal Impairment: Trilipix should be avoided in patients with severe renal impairment. Dose adjustment is required in patients with mild to moderate renal impairment (8.6).

See 17 for PATIENT COUNSELING INFORMATION and Medication Guide.

Revised: 4/2015

FULL PRESCRIBING INFORMATION

1 INDICATIONS AND USAGE

1.1 Treatment of Severe Hypertriglyceridemia

Trilipix is indicated as adjunctive therapy to diet to reduce triglycerides (TG) in patients with severe hypertriglyceridemia. Improving glycemic control in diabetic patients showing fasting chylomicronemia will usually obviate the need for pharmacological intervention. Markedly elevated levels of serum triglycerides (e.g. > 2,000 mg/dL) may increase the risk of developing pancreatitis. The effect of Trilipix therapy on reducing this risk has not been adequately studied.

1.2 Treatment of Primary Hypercholesterolemia or Mixed Dyslipidemia

Trilipix is indicated as adjunctive therapy to diet to reduce elevated low-density lipoprotein cholesterol (LDL-C), total cholesterol (Total-C), triglycerides (TG), and apolipoprotein B (Apo B), and to increase high-density lipoprotein cholesterol (HDL-C) in patients with primary hypercholesterolemia or mixed dyslipidemia.

1.3 Limitations of Use

Fenofibrate at a dose equivalent to 135 mg of Trilipix did not reduce coronary heart disease morbidity and mortality in 2 large, randomized controlled trials of patients with type 2 diabetes mellitus [see Warnings and Precautions (5.1)].

1.4 General Considerations for Treatment

Laboratory studies should be performed to establish that lipid levels are abnormal before instituting Trilipix therapy. Every reasonable attempt should be made to control serum lipids with non-drug methods including appropriate diet, exercise, weight loss in obese patients, and control of any medical problems such as diabetes mellitus and hypothyroidism that may be contributing to the lipid abnormalities. Medications known to exacerbate hypertriglyceridemia (beta-blockers, thiazides, estrogens) should be discontinued or changed if possible, and excessive alcohol intake should be addressed before triglyceride-lowering drug therapy is considered. If the decision is made to use lipid-altering drugs, the patient should be instructed that this does not reduce the importance of adhering to diet.

Drug therapy is not indicated for patients who have elevations of chylomicrons and plasma triglycerides, but who have normal levels of VLDL.

2 DOSAGE AND ADMINISTRATION

2.1 General Considerations

Patients should be placed on an appropriate lipid-lowering diet before receiving Trilipix and should continue this diet during treatment. Trilipix delayed release capsules can be taken without regard to meals. Patients should be advised to swallow Trilipix capsules whole. Do not open, crush, dissolve, or chew capsules. Serum lipids should be monitored periodically.

2.2 Severe Hypertriglyceridemia

The initial dose of Trilipix is 45 to 135 mg once daily. Dosage should be individualized according to patient response, and should be adjusted if necessary following repeat lipid determinations at 4 to 8 week intervals. The maximum dose is 135 mg once daily.

2.3 Primary Hypercholesterolemia or Mixed Dyslipidemia

The dose of Trilipix is 135 mg once daily.

2.4 Impaired Renal Function

Treatment with Trilipix should be initiated at a dose of 45 mg once daily in patients with mild to moderate renal impairment and should only be increased after evaluation of the effects on renal function and lipid levels at this dose. The use of Trilipix should be avoided in patients with severely impaired renal function [see Use in Specific Populations (8.6) and Clinical Pharmacology (12.3)].

2.5 Geriatric Patients

Dose selection for the elderly should be made on the basis of renal function [see Use in Specific Populations (8.5)].

3 DOSAGE FORMS AND STRENGTHS

- 45 mg capsules with a reddish-brown cap imprinted in white ink the "a" logo and a yellow body imprinted in black ink the number "45".
- 135 mg capsules with a blue cap imprinted in white ink the "a" logo and a yellow body imprinted in black ink the number "135".

4 CONTRAINDICATIONS

Trilipix is contraindicated in:

- patients with severe renal impairment, including those receiving dialysis [see Clinical Pharmacology (12.3)].
- patients with active liver disease, including those with primary biliary cirrhosis and unexplained persistent liver function abnormalities [see Warnings and Precautions (5.3)].
- patients with preexisting gallbladder disease [see Warnings and Precautions (5.5)].
- nursing mothers [see Use in Specific Populations (8.3)].
- patients with hypersensitivity to fenofibric acid or fenofibrate [see Warnings and Precautions (5.9)].

5 WARNINGS AND PRECAUTIONS

5.1 Mortality and Coronary Heart Disease Morbidity

The effect of Trilipix on coronary heart disease morbidity and mortality and non-cardiovascular mortality has not been established. Because of similarities between Trilipix and fenofibrate, clofibrate, and gemfibrozil, the findings in the following large randomized, placebo-controlled clinical studies with these fibrate drugs may also apply to Trilipix.

The Action to Control Cardiovascular Risk in Diabetes Lipid (ACCORD Lipid) trial was a randomized placebo-controlled study of 5518 patients with type 2 diabetes mellitus on background statin therapy treated with fenofibrate. The mean duration of follow-up was 4.7 years. Fenofibrate plus statin combination therapy showed a non-significant 8% relative risk reduction in the primary outcome of major adverse cardiovascular events (MACE), a composite of non-fatal myocardial infarction, non-fatal stroke, and cardiovascular disease death [HR] 0.92, 95% CI 0.79-1.08) (p=0.32) as compared to statin monotherapy. In a gender subgroup analysis, the hazard ratio for MACE in men receiving combination therapy versus statin monotherapy was 0.82 (95% CI 0.69-0.99), and the hazard ratio for MACE in women receiving combination therapy versus statin monotherapy was 1.38 (95% CI 0.98-1.94) (interaction p=0.01). The clinical significance of this subgroup finding is unclear.

The Fenofibrate Intervention and Event Lowering in Diabetes (FIELD) study was a 5-year randomized, placebo-controlled study of 9795 patients with type 2 diabetes mellitus treated with fenofibrate. Fenofibrate demonstrated a non-significant 11% relative reduction in the primary outcome of coronary heart disease events (hazard ratio [HR] 0.89, 95% CI 0.75-1.05, p = 0.16) and a significant 11% reduction in the secondary outcome of total cardiovascular disease events (HR 0.89 [0.80-0.99], p = 0.04). There was a non-significant 11% (HR 1.11 [0.95, 1.29], p = 0.18) and 19% (HR 1.19 [0.90, 1.57], p = 0.22) increase in total and coronary heart disease mortality, respectively, with fenofibrate as compared to placebo.

In the Coronary Drug Project, a large study of post-myocardial infarction patients treated for 5 years with clofibrate, there was no difference in mortality seen between the clofibrate group and the placebo group. There was, however, a difference in the rate of cholelithiasis and cholecystitis requiring surgery between the two groups (3.0% vs. 1.8%).

In a study conducted by the World Health Organization (WHO), 5000 subjects without known coronary artery disease were treated with placebo or clofibrate for 5 years and followed for an additional one year. There was a statistically significant, higher age-adjusted all-cause mortality in the clofibrate group compared with the placebo group (5.70% vs. 3.96%, p = < 0.01). Excess mortality was due to a 33% increase in non-cardiovascular causes, including malignancy, post-cholecystectomy complications, and pancreatitis. This appeared to confirm the higher risk of gallbladder disease seen in clofibrate-treated patients studied in the Coronary Drug Project.

The Helsinki Heart Study was a large (N = 4081) study of middle-aged men without a history of coronary artery disease. Subjects received either placebo or gemfibrozil for 5 years, with a 3.5 year open extension afterward. Total mortality was numerically higher in the gemfibrozil randomization group but did not achieve statistical significance

Continued on next page

Information on the AbbVie, Inc. products listed on these pages is from the prescribing information in use as of July 31, 2016. For more information, please visit rxabbvie.com or call 1-800-633-9110.

(p = 0.19, 95% confidence interval for relative risk G:P = 0.91-1.64). Although cancer deaths trended higher in the gemfibrozil group (p = 0.11), cancers (excluding basal cell carcinoma) were diagnosed with equal frequency in both study groups. Due to the limited size of the study, the relative risk of death from any cause was not shown to be different than that seen in the 9 year follow-up data from WHO study (RR = 1.29). A secondary prevention component of the Helsinki Heart Study enrolled middle-aged men excluded from the primary prevention study because of known or suspected coronary heart disease. Subjects received gemfibrozil or placebo for 5 years. Although cardiac deaths trended higher in the gemfibrozil group, this was not statistically significant (hazard ratio 2.2, 95% confidence interval: 0.94-5.05).

5.2 Skeletal Muscle
Fibrates increase the risk of myositis or myopathy and have been associated with rhabdomyolysis. The risk for serious muscle toxicity appears to be increased in elderly patients and in patients with diabetes, renal failure, or hypothyroidism.

Myopathy should be considered in any patient with diffuse myalgias, muscle tenderness or weakness, and/or marked elevations of CPK levels. Patients should promptly report unexplained muscle pain, tenderness or weakness, particularly if accompanied by malaise or fever. CPK levels should be assessed in patients reporting these symptoms, and Trilipix should be discontinued if markedly elevated CPK levels occur or myopathy or myositis is suspected or diagnosed.

Data from observational studies suggest that the risk for rhabdomyolysis is increased when fibrates are co-administered with a statin.

Cases of myopathy, including rhabdomyolysis, have been reported with fenofibrates co-administered with colchicine, and caution should be exercised when prescribing fenofibrate with colchicine *[see Drug Interactions (7.4)]*.

5.3 Liver Function
Trilipix at a dose of 135 mg once daily has been associated with increases in serum transaminases [AST (SGOT) or ALT (SGPT)]. In a pooled analysis of three 12-week, double-blind, controlled studies of Trilipix, increases in ALT and AST to >3 times the upper limit of normal on two consecutive occasions occurred in 1.9% and 0.2%, respectively, of patients receiving Trilipix without other lipid-altering drugs. Increases in ALT and/or AST were not accompanied by increases in bilirubin or clinically significant increases in alkaline phosphatase.

In a pooled analysis of 10 placebo-controlled trials of fenofibrate, increases to > 3 times the upper limit of normal in ALT occurred in 5.3% of patients taking fenofibrate versus 1.1% of patients treated with placebo. The incidence of increases in transaminases observed with fenofibrate therapy may be dose related. In an 8-week dose-ranging study of fenofibrate in hypertriglyceridemia, the incidence of ALT or AST elevations ≥ 3 times the upper limit of normal was 13% in patients receiving dosages equivalent to 90 mg to 135 mg Trilipix once daily and was 0% in those receiving dosages equivalent to 45 mg Trilipix once daily or less, or placebo. Hepatocellular, chronic active, and cholestatic hepatitis observed with fenofibrate therapy have been reported after exposures of weeks to several years. In extremely rare cases, cirrhosis has been reported in association with chronic active hepatitis.

Baseline and regular monitoring of liver function, including serum ALT (SGPT) should be performed for the duration of therapy with Trilipix, and therapy discontinued if enzyme levels persist above 3 times the upper limit of normal.

5.4 Serum Creatinine
Reversible elevations in serum creatinine have been reported in patients receiving Trilipix as well as patients receiving fenofibrate. In the pooled analysis of three 12-week, double-blind, controlled studies of Trilipix, increases in creatinine to > 2 mg/dL occurred in 0.8% of patients treated with Trilipix without other lipid-altering drugs. Elevations in serum creatinine were generally stable over time with no evidence for continued increases in serum creatinine with long-term therapy and tended to return to baseline following discontinuation of treatment. The clinical significance of these observations is unknown. Monitoring renal function in patients with renal impairment taking Trilipix is suggested. Renal monitoring should be considered for patients at risk for renal insufficiency, such as the elderly and those with diabetes.

5.5 Cholelithiasis
Trilipix, like fenofibrate, clofibrate, and gemfibrozil, may increase cholesterol excretion into the bile, potentially leading to cholelithiasis. If cholelithiasis is suspected, gallbladder studies are indicated. Trilipix therapy should be discontinued if gallstones are found.

5.6 Coumarin Anticoagulants
Caution should be exercised when Trilipix is given in conjunction with oral coumarin anticoagulants. Trilipix may potentiate the anticoagulant effects of these agents resulting in prolongation of the prothrombin time/International Normalized Ratio (PT/INR). Frequent monitoring of PT/INR and dose adjustment of the oral anticoagulant are recommended until the PT/INR has stabilized in order to prevent bleeding complications *[see Drug Interactions (7.1)]*.

5.7 Pancreatitis
Pancreatitis has been reported in patients taking drugs of the fibrate class, including Trilipix. This occurrence may represent a failure of efficacy in patients with severe hypertriglyceridemia, a direct drug effect, or a secondary phenomenon mediated through biliary tract stone or sludge formation with obstruction of the common bile duct.

5.8 Hematological Changes
Mild to moderate hemoglobin, hematocrit, and white blood cell decreases have been observed in patients following initiation of Trilipix and fenofibrate therapy. However, these levels stabilize during long-term administration. Thrombocytopenia and agranulocytosis have been reported in individuals treated with fenofibrates. Periodic monitoring of red and white blood cell counts are recommended during the first 12 months of Trilipix administration.

5.9 Hypersensitivity Reactions
Acute hypersensitivity reactions such as Stevens-Johnson syndrome and toxic necrolysis requiring patient hospitalization and treatment with steroids have been reported in individuals treated with fenofibrates.

5.10 Venothromboembolic Disease
In the FIELD trial, pulmonary embolus (PE) and deep vein thrombosis (DVT) were observed at higher rates in the fenofibrate- than the placebo-treated group. Of 9,795 patients enrolled in FIELD, there were 4,900 in the placebo group and 4,895 in the fenofibrate group. For DVT, there were 48 events (1%) in the placebo group and 67 (1%) in the fenofibrate group (p = 0.074); and for PE, there were 32 (0.7%) events in the placebo group and 53 (1%) in the fenofibrate group (p = 0.022).

In the Coronary Drug Project, a higher proportion of the clofibrate group experienced definite or suspected fatal or nonfatal PE or thrombophlebitis than the placebo group (5.2% vs. 3.3% at five years; p < 0.01).

5.11 Paradoxical Decreases in HDL Cholesterol Levels
There have been postmarketing and clinical trial reports of severe decreases in HDL cholesterol levels (as low as 2 mg/dL) occurring in diabetic and non-diabetic patients initiated on fibrate therapy. The decrease in HDL-C is mirrored by a decrease in apolipoprotein A1. This decrease has been reported to occur within 2 weeks to years after initiation of fibrate therapy. The HDL-C levels remain depressed until fibrate therapy has been withdrawn; the response to withdrawal of fibrate therapy is rapid and sustained. The clinical significance of this decrease in HDL-C is unknown. It is recommended that HDL-C levels be checked within the first few months after initiation of fibrate therapy. If a severely depressed HDL-C level is detected, fibrate therapy should be withdrawn, and the HDL-C level monitored until it has returned to baseline, and fibrate therapy should not be re-initiated.

6 ADVERSE REACTIONS
6.1 Clinical Trials Experience
Because clinical studies are conducted under widely varying conditions, adverse reaction rates observed in the clinical studies of a drug cannot be directly compared to rates in the clinical studies of another drug and may not reflect the rates observed in practice.

Fenofibric acid is the active metabolite of fenofibrate. Adverse events reported by 2% or more of patients treated with fenofibrate and greater than placebo during double-blind, placebo-controlled trials are listed in Table 1. Adverse events led to discontinuation of treatment in 5.0% of patients treated with fenofibrate and in 3.0% treated with placebo. Increases in liver tests were the most frequent events, causing discontinuation of fenofibrate treatment in 1.6% of patients in double-blind trials.

Table 1. Adverse Events Reported by 2% or More of Patients Treated with Fenofibrate and Greater than Placebo During the Double-Blind, Placebo-Controlled Trials

BODY SYSTEM Adverse Event	Fenofibrate* (N = 439)	Placebo (N = 365)
BODY AS A WHOLE		
Abdominal Pain	4.6%	4.4%
Back Pain	3.4%	2.5%
Headache	3.2%	2.7%
DIGESTIVE		
Nausea	2.3%	1.9%
Constipation	2.1%	1.4%
INVESTIGATIONS		
Abnormal Liver Tests	7.5%	1.4%
Increased AST	3.4%	0.5%
Increased ALT	3.0%	1.6%
Increased Creatine Phosphokinase	3.0%	1.4%
RESPIRATORY		
Respiratory Disorder	6.2%	5.5%
Rhinitis	2.3%	1.1%

* Dosage equivalent to 135 mg Trilipix

Clinical trials with Trilipix did not include a placebo-control arm. However, the adverse event profile of Trilipix was generally consistent with that of fenofibrate. The following adverse events not listed above were reported in ≥ 3% of patients taking Trilipix alone:

Gastrointestinal Disorders: Diarrhea, dyspepsia
General Disorders and Administration Site Conditions: Pain
Infections and Infestations: Nasopharyngitis, sinusitis, upper respiratory tract infection
Musculoskeletal and Connective Tissue Disorders: Arthralgia, myalgia, pain in extremity
Nervous System Disorders: Dizziness

6.2 Postmarketing Experience
The following adverse events have been identified during postapproval use of fenofibrate: rhabdomyolysis, pancreatitis, renal failure, muscle spasms, acute renal failure, hepatitis, cirrhosis, anemia, asthenia, and severely depressed HDL-cholesterol levels.

Because these events are reported voluntarily from a population of uncertain size, it is not always possible to reliably estimate their frequency or establish a causal relationship to drug exposure.

7 DRUG INTERACTIONS
7.1 Coumarin Anticoagulants
Potentiation of coumarin-type anticoagulant effect has been observed with prolongation of the PT/INR.

Caution should be exercised when oral coumarin anticoagulants are given in conjunction with Trilipix. The dosage of the anticoagulant should be reduced to maintain the PT/INR at the desired level to prevent bleeding complications. Frequent PT/INR determinations are advisable until it has been definitely determined that the PT/INR has stabilized *[see Warnings and Precautions (5.6)]*.

7.2 Bile Acid Binding Resins
Since bile acid binding resins may bind other drugs given concurrently, patients should take Trilipix at least 1 hour before or 4 to 6 hours after a bile acid resin to avoid impeding its absorption.

7.3 Immunosuppressants
Immunosuppressants such as cyclosporine and tacrolimus can produce nephrotoxicity with decreases in creatinine clearance and rises in serum creatinine, and because renal excretion is the primary elimination route of drugs of the fibrate class including Trilipix, there is a risk that an interaction will lead to deterioration of renal function. The benefits and risks of using Trilipix with immunosuppressants and other potentially nephrotoxic agents should be carefully considered, and the lowest effective dose employed.

7.4 Colchicine
Cases of myopathy, including rhabdomyolysis, have been reported with fenofibrates co-administered with colchicine, and caution should be exercised when prescribing fenofibrate with colchicine.

8 USE IN SPECIFIC POPULATIONS
8.1 Pregnancy
Pregnancy Category: C

The safety of Trilipix in pregnant women has not been established. There are no adequate and well controlled studies of Trilipix in pregnant women. Trilipix should be used during pregnancy only if the potential benefit justifies the potential risk to the fetus.

In pregnant rats given oral dietary doses of 14, 127, and 361 mg/kg/day from gestation day 6-15 during the period of organogenesis, adverse developmental findings were not observed at 14 mg/kg/day (less than 1 times the maximum recommended human dose [MRHD], based on body surface area comparisons; mg/m^2). At higher multiples of human doses evidence of maternal toxicity was observed.

In pregnant rabbits given oral gavage doses of 15, 150, and 300 mg/kg/day from gestation day 6-18 during the period of organogenesis and allowed to deliver, aborted litters were observed at 150 mg/kg/day (10 times the MRHD, based on body surface area comparisons; mg/m^2). No developmental findings were observed at 15 mg/kg/day (at less than 1 times the MRHD, based on body surface area comparisons; mg/m^2).

In pregnant rats given oral dietary doses of 15, 75, and 300 mg/kg/day from gestation day 15 through lactation day 21 (weaning), maternal toxicity was observed at less than 1 times the MRHD, based on body surface area comparisons; mg/m^2.

8.3 Nursing Mothers

Trilipix should not be used in nursing mothers. A decision should be made whether to discontinue nursing or to discontinue the drug taking into account the importance of the drug to the mother.

8.4 Pediatric Use

The safety and effectiveness of Trilipix in pediatric patients have not been established.

8.5 Geriatric Use

Trilipix is substantially excreted by the kidney as fenofibric acid and fenofibric acid glucuronide, and the risk of adverse reactions to this drug may be greater in patients with impaired renal function. Fenofibric acid exposure is not influenced by age. Since elderly patients have a higher incidence of renal impairment, dose selection for the elderly should be made on the basis of renal function *[see Dosage and Administration (2.5) and Clinical Pharmacology (12.3)]*. Elderly patients with normal renal function should require no dose modifications. Consider monitoring renal function in elderly patients taking Trilipix.

8.6 Renal Impairment

The use of Trilipix should be avoided in patients who have severe renal impairment *[see Contraindications (4)]*. Dose reduction is required in patients with mild to moderate renal impairment *[see Dosage and Administration (2.4) and Clinical Pharmacology (12.3)]*. Monitoring renal function in patients with renal impairment is recommended.

8.7 Hepatic Impairment

The use of Trilipix has not been evaluated in subjects with hepatic impairment *[see Contraindications (4) and Clinical Pharmacology (12.3)]*.

10 OVERDOSAGE

There is no specific treatment for overdose with Trilipix. General supportive care of the patient is indicated, including monitoring of vital signs and observation of clinical status, should an overdose occur. If indicated, elimination of unabsorbed drug should be achieved by emesis or gastric lavage; usual precautions should be observed to maintain the airway. Because Trilipix is highly bound to plasma proteins, hemodialysis should not be considered.

11 DESCRIPTION

Trilipix (fenofibric acid) is a lipid regulating agent available as delayed release capsules for oral administration. Each delayed release capsule contains choline fenofibrate, equivalent to 45 mg or 135 mg of fenofibric acid. The chemical name for choline fenofibrate is ethanaminium, 2-hydroxy-N,N,N-trimethyl, 2-{4-(4-chlorobenzoyl)phenoxy] -2-methylpropanoate (1:1) with the following structural formula:

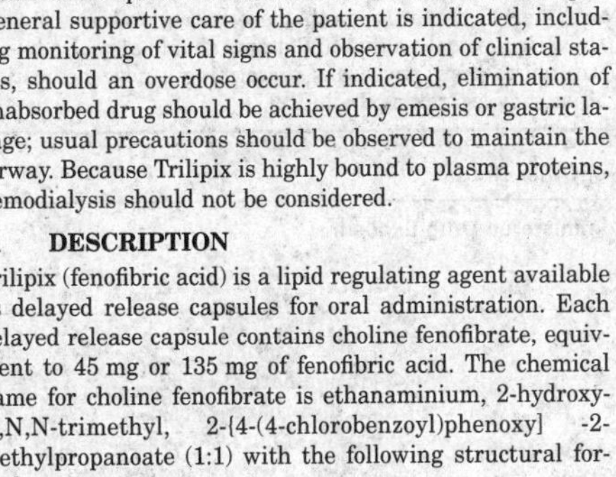

The empirical formula is $C_{22}H_{28}ClNO_5$ and the molecular weight is 421.91. Choline fenofibrate is freely soluble in water. The melting point is approximately 210°C. Choline fenofibrate is a white to yellow powder, which is stable under ordinary conditions.

Each delayed release capsule contains enteric coated minitablets comprised of choline fenofibrate and the following inactive ingredients: hypromellose, povidone, water, hydroxylpropyl cellulose, colloidal silicon dioxide, sodium stearyl fumarate, methacrylic acid copolymer, talc, triethyl citrate. The capsule shell of the 45 mg capsule contains the following inactive ingredients: gelatin, titanium dioxide, yellow iron oxide, black iron oxide, and red iron oxide. The capsule shell of the 135 mg capsule contains the following inactive ingredients: gelatin, titanium dioxide, yellow iron oxide, and FD&C Blue #2.

12 CLINICAL PHARMACOLOGY

12.1 Mechanism of Action

The active moiety of Trilipix is fenofibric acid. The pharmacological effects of fenofibric acid in both animals and humans have been extensively studied through oral administration of fenofibrate.

The lipid-modifying effects of fenofibric acid seen in clinical practice have been explained *in vivo* in transgenic mice and *in vitro* in human hepatocyte cultures by the activation of peroxisome proliferator activated receptor α (PPARα). Through this mechanism, fenofibric acid increases lipolysis and elimination of triglyceride-rich particles from plasma by activating lipoprotein lipase and reducing production of Apo CIII (an inhibitor of lipoprotein lipase activity).

Activation of PPARα also induces an increase in the synthesis of HDL-C and Apo AI and AII.

12.3 Pharmacokinetics

Trilipix contains fenofibric acid, which is the only circulating pharmacologically active moiety in plasma after oral administration of Trilipix. Fenofibric acid is also the circulating pharmacologically active moiety in plasma after oral administration of fenofibrate, the ester of fenofibric acid.

Plasma concentrations of fenofibric acid after administration of one 135 mg Trilipix delayed release capsule are equivalent to those after one 200 mg capsule of micronized fenofibrate administered under fed conditions.

Absorption

Fenofibric acid is well absorbed throughout the gastrointestinal tract. The absolute bioavailability of fenofibric acid is approximately 81%.

Peak plasma levels of fenofibric acid occur within 4 to 5 hours after a single dose administration of Trilipix capsule under fasting conditions.

Fenofibric acid exposure in plasma, as measured by C_{max} and AUC, is not significantly different when a single 135 mg dose of Trilipix is administered under fasting or nonfasting conditions.

Distribution

Upon multiple dosing of Trilipix, fenofibric acid levels reach steady state within 8 days. Plasma concentrations of fenofibric acid at steady state are approximately slightly more than double those following a single dose. Serum protein binding is approximately 99% in normal and dyslipidemic subjects.

Metabolism

Fenofibric acid is primarily conjugated with glucuronic acid and then excreted in urine. A small amount of fenofibric acid is reduced at the carbonyl moiety to a benzhydrol metabolite which is, in turn, conjugated with glucuronic acid and excreted in urine.

In vivo metabolism data after fenofibrate administration indicate that fenofibric acid does not undergo oxidative metabolism (e.g., cytochrome P450) to a significant extent.

Elimination

After absorption, Trilipix is primarily excreted in the urine in the form of fenofibric acid and fenofibric acid glucuronide. Fenofibric acid is eliminated with a half-life of approximately 20 hours, allowing once daily administration of Trilipix.

Specific Populations

Geriatrics

In five elderly volunteers 77 to 87 years of age, the oral clearance of fenofibric acid following a single oral dose of fenofibrate was 1.2 L/h, which compares to 1.1 L/h in young adults. This indicates that an equivalent dose of Trilipix can be used in elderly subjects with normal renal function, without increasing accumulation of the drug or metabolites *[see Use in Specific Populations (8.5)]*.

Pediatrics

The pharmacokinetics of Trilipix has not been studied in pediatric populations.

Gender

No pharmacokinetic difference between males and females has been observed for Trilipix.

Race

The influence of race on the pharmacokinetics of Trilipix has not been studied; however, fenofibric acid is not metabolized by enzymes known for exhibiting inter-ethnic variability.

Renal Impairment

The pharmacokinetics of fenofibric acid was examined in patients with mild, moderate, and severe renal impairment. Patients with severe renal impairment (estimated glomerular filtration rate [eGFR] <30 mL/min/1.73m^2) showed a 2.7-fold increase in exposure for fenofibric acid and increased accumulation of fenofibric acid during chronic dosing compared to that of healthy subjects. Patients with mild to moderate renal impairment (eGFR 30-59 mL/min/1.73m^2) had similar exposure but an increase in the half-life for fenofibric acid compared to that of healthy subjects. Based on these findings, the use of Trilipix should be avoided in patients who have severe renal impairment and dose reduction is required in patients having mild to moderate renal impairment *[see Dosage and Administration (2.4)]*.

Hepatic Impairment

No pharmacokinetic studies have been conducted in patients with hepatic impairment.

Drug-drug Interactions

In vitro studies using human liver microsomes indicate that fenofibric acid is not an inhibitor of cytochrome (CYP) P450 isoforms CYP3A4, CYP2D6, CYP2E1, or CYP1A2. It is a weak inhibitor of CYP2C8, CYP2C19, and CYP2A6, and mild-to-moderate inhibitor of CYP2C9 at therapeutic concentrations.

Comparison of atorvastatin exposures when atorvastatin (80 mg once daily for 10 days) is given in combination with fenofibric acid (Trilipix 135 mg once daily for 10 days) and ezetimibe (10 mg once daily for 10 days) versus when atorvastatin is given in combination with ezetimibe only (ezetimibe 10 mg once daily and atorvastatin, 80 mg once daily for 10 days): The C_{max} decreased by 1% for atorvastatin and ortho-hydroxy-atorvastatin and increased by 2% for parahydroxy-atorvastatin. The AUC decreased 6% and 9% for atorvastatin and orthohydroxy-atorvastatin, respectively, and did not change for para-hydroxy-atorvastatin.

Comparison of ezetimibe exposures when ezetimibe (10 mg once daily for 10 days) is given in combination with fenofibric acid (Trilipix 135 mg once daily for 10 days) and atorvastatin (80 mg once daily for 10 days) versus when ezetimibe is given in combination with atorvastatin only (ezetimibe 10 mg once daily and atorvastatin, 80 mg once daily for 10 days): The C_{max} increased by 26% and 7% for total and free ezetimibe, respectively. The AUC increased by 27% and 12% for total and free ezetimibe, respectively.

Table 2 describes the effects of co-administered drugs on fenofibric acid systemic exposure. Table 3 describes the effects of co-administered fenofibric acid on other drugs.

[See table 2 at top of next page]

[See table 3 at bottom of next page]

13 NONCLINICAL TOXICOLOGY

13.1 Carcinogenesis, Mutagenesis, Impairment of Fertility

Trilipix (fenofibric acid)

No carcinogenicity and fertility studies have been conducted with choline fenofibrate or fenofibric acid. However, because fenofibrate is rapidly converted to its active metabolite, fenofibric acid, either during or immediately following absorption both in animals and humans, studies conducted with fenofibrate are relevant for the assessment of the toxicity profile of fenofibric acid. A similar toxicity spectrum is expected after treatment with either Trilipix or fenofibrate.

Fenofibrate

Two dietary carcinogenicity studies have been conducted in rats with fenofibrate. In the first 24-month study, Wistar rats were dosed with fenofibrate at 10, 45, and 200 mg/kg/day, approximately 0.3, 1, and 6 times the maximum recommended human dose (MRHD), based on body surface area comparisons (mg/m^2). At a dose of 200 mg/kg/day (6 times the MRHD), the incidence of liver

Continued on next page

carcinomas was significantly increased in both sexes. A statistically significant increase in pancreatic carcinomas was observed in males at 1 and 6 times the MRHD; an increase in pancreatic adenomas and benign testicular interstitial cell tumors was observed at 6 times the MRHD in males. In a second 24-month rat carcinogenicity study in a different strain of rats (Sprague-Dawley), (doses of 10 and 60 mg/kg/day (0.3 and 2 times the MRHD), produced significant increases in the incidence of pancreatic acinar adenomas in both sexes and increases in interstitial cell tumors of the testes at 2 times the MRHD.

A 117-week carcinogenicity study was conducted in rats comparing three drugs: fenofibrate 10 and 60 mg/kg/day (0.3 and 2 times the MRHD), clofibrate (400 mg/kg/day; 2 times the human dose), and gemfibrozil (250 mg/kg/day; 2 times the MRHD). Fenofibrate increased pancreatic acinar adenomas in both sexes. Clofibrate increased hepatocellular carcinoma and pancreatic acinar adenomas in males and hepatic neoplastic nodules in females. Gemfibrozil increased hepatic neoplastic nodules in males and females, while all three drugs increased testicular interstitial tumors in males.

In a 21-month study in CF-1 mice, fenofibrate 10, 45, and 200 mg/kg/day (approximately 0.2, 1, and 3 times the MRHD on the basis of mg/m² surface area) significantly increased the liver carcinomas in both sexes at 3 times the MRHD. In a second 18-month study at 10, 60, and 200 mg/kg/day, fenofibrate significantly increased the liver carcinomas in male and female mice at 3 times the MRHD. Electron microscopy studies have demonstrated peroxisomal proliferation following fenofibrate administration to the rat. An adequate study to test for peroxisome proliferation in humans has not been done, but changes in peroxisome morphology and numbers have been observed in humans after treatment with other members of the fibrate class when liver biopsies were compared before and after treatment in the same individual.

Mutagenesis:
Fenofibrate has been demonstrated to be devoid of mutagenic potential in the following tests: Ames, and micronucleus *in vivo*/rat. In addition, fenofibric acid, has been demonstrated to be devoid of mutagenic potential in the following tests: Ames, mouse lymphoma, chromosomal aberration and sister chromatid exchange in human lymphocytes, and unscheduled DNA synthesis in primary rat hepatocytes.

Impairment of Fertility:
In a fertility study, rats were given oral dietary doses of fenofibrate. Males received doses for 61 days prior to mating and females for 15 days prior to mating through weaning, which resulted in no adverse effect on fertility at doses up to 300 mg/kg/day (~10 times the MRHD, based on mg/m² surface area comparisons).

14 CLINICAL STUDIES
14.1 Severe Hypertriglyceridemia
The effects of fenofibrate on serum triglycerides were studied in two randomized, double-blind, placebo-controlled clinical trials of 147 hypertriglyceridemic patients. Patients were treated for eight weeks under protocols that differed only in that one entered patients with baseline TG levels of 500 to 1500 mg/dL, and the other TG levels of 350 to 500 mg/dL. In patients with hypertriglyceridemia and nor-

mal cholesterolemia with or without hyperchylomicronemia, treatment with fenofibrate at dosages equivalent to 135 mg once daily of Trilipix decreased primarily VLDL-TG and VLDL-C. Treatment of patients with elevated TG often results in an increase of LDL-C (Table 4).
[See table 4 on next page]
14.2 Primary Hypercholesterolemia (Heterozygous Familial and Nonfamilial) and Mixed Dyslipidemia
The effects of fenofibrate at a dose equivalent to Trilipix 135 mg once daily were assessed from four randomized, placebo-controlled, double-blind, parallel-group studies including patients with the following mean baseline lipid values: Total-C 306.9 mg/dL; LDL-C 213.8 mg/dL; HDL-C 52.3 mg/dL; and triglycerides 191.0 mg/dL. Fenofibrate therapy lowered LDL-C, Total-C, and the LDL-C/HDL-C ratio. Fenofibrate therapy also lowered triglycerides and raised HDL-C (Table 5).
[See table 5 on next page]
In a subset of the subjects, measurements of Apo B were conducted. Fenofibrate treatment significantly reduced Apo B from baseline to endpoint as compared with placebo (-25.1% vs. 2.4%, p < 0.0001, n = 213 and 143, respectively).

16 HOW SUPPLIED/STORAGE AND HANDLING
Trilipix (fenofibric acid) delayed release capsules 45 mg have a reddish-brown cap imprinted in white ink the "a" logo and a yellow body imprinted in black ink the number "45".

Bottles of 90 (NDC 0074-9642-90).
Trilipix (fenofibric acid) delayed release capsules 135 mg have a blue cap imprinted in white ink the "a" logo and a yellow body imprinted in black ink the number "135".
Bottles of 90 (NDC 0074-9189-90).
Store at 25°C (77°F); excursions permitted to 15°-30°C (59° to 86°F) [See USP controlled room temperature]. Keep out of the reach of children. Protect from moisture.

17 PATIENT COUNSELING INFORMATION
See Medication Guide
17.1 Patient Counseling
Patients should be advised:
• of the potential benefits and risks of Trilipix.
• to read the Medication Guide before starting Trilipix therapy and to reread it each time the prescription is renewed.
• of medications that should not be taken in combination with Trilipix.
• to continue to follow an appropriate lipid-modifying diet while taking Trilipix.
• to take Trilipix once daily, without regard to food, at the prescribed dose, swallowing each capsule whole.
• to return for routine monitoring.
• to inform their physician of all medications, supplements, and herbal preparations they are taking and any change to their medical condition. Patients should also be advised to inform their physicians prescribing a new medication that they are taking Trilipix.

Table 2. Effects of Co-Administered Drugs on Fenofibric Acid Systemic Exposure from Trilipix or Fenofibrate Administration

Co-Administered Drug	Dosage Regimen of Co-Administered Drug	Dosage Regimen of Trilipix or Fenofibrate	Changes in Fenofibric Acid Exposure AUC	Cmax
Lipid-lowering agents				
Rosuvastatin	40 mg once daily for 10 days	Trilipix 135 mg once daily for 10 days	↓2%	↓2%
Atorvastatin	20 mg once daily for 10 days	Fenofibrate 160 mg[1] once daily for 10 days	↓2%	↓4%
Atorvastatin + ezetimibe	Atorvastatin, 80 mg once daily and ezetimibe, 10 mg once daily for 10 days	Trilipix 135 mg once daily for 10 days	↑5%	↑5%
Pravastatin	40 mg as a single dose	Fenofibrate 3 × 67 mg[2] as a single dose	↓1%	↓2%
Fluvastatin	40 mg as a single dose	Fenofibrate 160 mg[1] as a single dose	↓2%	↓10%
Simvastatin	80 mg once daily for 7 days	Fenofibrate 160 mg[1] once daily for 7 days	↓5%	↓11%
Anti-diabetic agents				
Glimepiride	1 mg as a single dose	Fenofibrate 145 mg[1] once daily for 10 days	↑1%	↓1%
Metformin	850 mg 3 times daily for 10 days	Fenofibrate 54 mg[1] 3 times daily for 10 days	↓9%	↓6%
Rosiglitazone	8 mg once daily for 5 days	Fenofibrate 145 mg[1] once daily for 14 days	↑10%	↑3%
Gastrointestinal agents				
Omeprazole	40 mg once daily for 5 days	Trilipix 135 mg as a single dose fasting	↑6%	↑17%
Omeprazole	40 mg once daily for 5 days	Trilipix 135 mg as a single dose with food	↑4%	↓2%

[1] TriCor (fenofibrate) oral tablet
[2] TriCor (fenofibrate) oral micronized capsule

Table 3. Effects of Trilipix or Fenofibrate Co-Administration on Systemic Exposure of Other Drugs

Dosage Regimen of Trilipix or Fenofibrate	Dosage Regimen of Co-Administered Drug	Change in Co-Administered Drug Exposure Analyte	AUC	Cmax
Lipid-lowering agents				
Trilipix 135 mg once daily for 10 days	Rosuvastatin, 40 mg once daily for 10 days	Rosuvastatin	↑6%	↑20%
Fenofibrate 160 mg[1] once daily for 10 days	Atorvastatin, 20 mg once daily for 10 days	Atorvastatin	↓17%	0%
Fenofibrate 3 × 67 mg[2] as a single dose	Pravastatin, 40 mg as a single dose	Pravastatin	↑13%	↑13%
		3α-Hydroxyl-iso-pravastatin	↑26%	↑29%
Fenofibrate 160 mg[1] as a single dose	Fluvastatin, 40 mg as a single dose	(+)-3R, 5S-Fluvastatin	↑15%	↑16%
Fenofibrate 160 mg[1] once daily for 7 days	Simvastatin, 80 mg once daily for 7 days	Simvastatin acid	↓36%	↓11%
		Simvastatin	↓11%	↓17%
		Active HMG-CoA Inhibitors	↓12%	↓1%
		Total HMG-CoA Inhibitors	↓8%	↓10%
Anti-diabetic agents				
Fenofibrate 145 mg[1] once daily for 10 days	Glimepiride, 1 mg as a single dose	Glimepiride	↑35%	↑18%
Fenofibrate 54 mg[1] 3 times daily for 10 days	Metformin, 850 mg 3 times daily for 10 days	Metformin	↑3%	↑6%
Fenofibrate 145 mg[1] once daily for 14 days	Rosiglitazone, 8 mg once daily for 5 days	Rosiglitazone	↑6%	↓1%

[1] TriCor (fenofibrate) oral tablet
[2] TriCor (fenofibrate) oral micronized capsule

Table 4. Effects of Fenofibrate in Patients With Severe Hypertriglyceridemia

Study 1 Baseline TG levels 350 to 499 mg/dL	Placebo N	Baseline Mean (mg/dL)	Endpoint Mean (mg/dL)	Mean % Change	Fenofibrate N	Baseline Mean (mg/dL)	Endpoint Mean (mg/dL)	Mean % Change
Triglycerides	28	449	450	-0.5	27	432	223	-46.2*
VLDL Triglycerides	19	367	350	2.7	19	350	178	-44.1*
Total Cholesterol	28	255	261	2.8	27	252	227	-9.1*
HDL Cholesterol	28	35	36	4	27	34	40	19.6*
LDL Cholesterol	28	120	129	12	27	128	137	14.5
VLDL Cholesterol	27	99	99	5.8	27	92	46	-44.7*
Study 2 Baseline TG levels 500 to 1500 mg/dL	**Placebo N**	**Baseline Mean (mg/dL)**	**Endpoint Mean (mg/dL)**	**Mean % Change**	**Fenofibrate N**	**Baseline Mean (mg/dL)**	**Endpoint Mean (mg/dL)**	**Mean % Change**
Triglycerides	44	710	750	7.2	48	726	308	-54.5*
VLDL Triglycerides	29	537	571	18.7	33	543	205	-50.6*
Total Cholesterol	44	272	271	0.4	48	261	223	-13.8*
HDL Cholesterol	44	27	28	5.0	48	30	36	22.9*
LDL Cholesterol	42	100	90	-4.2	45	103	131	45.0*
VLDL Cholesterol	42	137	142	11.0	45	126	54	-49.4*

* = p < 0.05 vs. Placebo

Table 5. Mean Percent Change in Lipid Parameters at End of Treatment[†]

Treatment Group	Total-C (mg/dL)	LDL-C (mg/dL)	HDL-C (mg/dL)	TG (mg/dL)
Pooled Cohort				
Mean baseline lipid values (n = 646)	306.9	213.8	52.3	191.0
All Fenofibrate (n = 361)	-18.7%*	-20.6%*	+11.0%*	-28.9%*
Placebo (n = 285)	-0.4%	-2.2%	+0.7%	+7.7%
Baseline LDL-C > 160 mg/dL and TG < 150 mg/dL				
Mean baseline lipid values (n = 334)	307.7	227.7	58.1	101.7
All Fenofibrate (n = 193)	-22.4%*	-31.4%*	+9.8%*	-23.5%*
Placebo (n = 141)	+0.2%	-2.2%	+2.6%	+11.7%
Baseline LDL-C > 160 mg/dL and TG ≥ 150 mg/dL				
Mean baseline lipid values (n = 242)	312.8	219.8	46.7	231.9
All Fenofibrate (n = 126)	-16.8%*	-20.1%*	+14.6%*	-35.9%*
Placebo (n = 116)	-3.0%	-6.6%	+2.3%	+0.9%

† Duration of study treatment was 3 to 6 months
* p = < 0.05 vs. Placebo

- to inform their physician of any muscle pain, tenderness, or weakness; onset of abdominal pain; or any other new symptoms.

©AbbVie Inc. 2015

Manufactured for AbbVie Inc., North Chicago, IL 60064, U.S.A. by Fournier Laboratories Ireland Limited, Anngrove, Carrigtwohill Co. Cork, Ireland, or AbbVie LTD, Barceloneta, PR 00617.

Ref: 03-B105-R8-April, 2015

MEDICATION GUIDE

Trilipix®

(try-lip-iks)

(fenofibric acid, delayed release capsules)

Read this Medication Guide before you start taking Trilipix and each time you get a refill. There may be new information. This information does not take the place of talking to your healthcare provider about your medical condition or your treatment.

What is the most important information I should know about Trilipix?

Trilipix can cause muscle pain, tenderness or weakness, which may be symptoms of a rare but serious muscle condition called rhabdomyolysis. In some cases rhabdomyolysis can cause kidney damage and death. The risk of rhabdomyolysis may be higher when Trilipix is given with statins. If you take a statin, tell your healthcare provider.

What is Trilipix?

Trilipix is a prescription medicine used to treat cholesterol in the blood by lowering the total amount of triglycerides and LDL (bad) cholesterol, and increasing the HDL (good) cholesterol. **Trilipix has not been shown to lower your risk of having heart problems or a stroke.** You should be on a low fat and low cholesterol diet while you take Trilipix.

The safety and effectiveness of Trilipix in children is not known.

Who should not take Trilipix?

Do not take Trilipix if you:

- are allergic to fenofibric acid, or any of the ingredients in Trilipix. See the end of this Medication Guide for a list of all the ingredients in Trilipix.
- have severe kidney disease.
- have liver disease.
- have gallbladder disease.
- are a nursing mother.

Talk to your healthcare provider before you take Trilipix if you have any of these conditions.

What should I tell my healthcare provider before taking Trilipix?

Before taking Trilipix, tell your healthcare provider about all your medical conditions, including if you:

- are allergic to any medicines.
- have ever had kidney problems.
- have ever had liver problems.
- have ever had gallbladder problems.
- are pregnant or if you plan to become pregnant. It is not known if Trilipix will harm your unborn baby.
- are breastfeeding or plan to breastfeed. It is not known if Trilipix passes into your breast milk. You and your healthcare provider should decide if you will take Trilipix or breastfeed. You should not do both.

Tell your healthcare provider about all the medicines you take, including prescription and non-prescription medicines, vitamins and herbal supplements.

Using Trilipix with certain other medicines can affect the way these medicines work and other medicines may affect how Trilipix works. In some cases, using Trilipix with other medicines can cause serious side effects.

Know all the medicines you take. Keep a list of them and show it to your healthcare provider when you get a new medicine.

It is especially important to tell your healthcare provider if you take any of the medicines listed below:

- **anticoagulants**, also known as blood thinners (warfarin, Coumadin)
- **bile acid resins**
- **cyclosporine**

Ask your healthcare provider if you are not sure if your medicine is one of these.

How should I take Trilipix?

- You should be on a low fat and low cholesterol diet while you take Trilipix.
- Take Trilipix one time each day as prescribed by your healthcare provider.
- Take Trilipix with or without food.
- Swallow Trilipix capsules whole. Do not break, crush, dissolve, or chew Trilipix capsules before swallowing. If you cannot swallow Trilipix capsules whole, tell your healthcare provider, you may need a different medicine.
- If you miss a dose of Trilipix, take it as soon as you remember. If it is almost time for your next dose, just skip the missed dose. Take the next dose at your regular time. If you are not sure about your dosing, call your healthcare provider. **Do not take more than one dose of Trilipix a day unless your healthcare provider tells you to.**
- If you take too much Trilipix, contact your healthcare provider or your local emergency department.
- Do not change your dose or stop Trilipix unless your healthcare provider tells you to.
- Your healthcare provider may do blood tests before you start taking Trilipix and during treatment. See your healthcare provider regularly to check your cholesterol and triglyceride levels and to check for side effects.

What are the possible side effects with Trilipix?

Trilipix may cause serious side effects, including:

- **muscle pain, tenderness, or weakness.** See "What is the most important information that I should know about Trilipix?"
- **tiredness and fever.**
- **abdominal pain, nausea, or vomiting.** These may be signs of inflammation (swelling) of the gallbladder or pancreas.

Call your healthcare provider right away if you have any of these serious side effects.

The most common side effects with Trilipix include:

- headache
- heartburn (indigestion)
- nausea
- muscle aches
- increases in muscle or liver enzymes that are measured by blood tests

Tell your healthcare provider if you have any side effect that bothers you or that does not go away. These are not all the possible side effects of Trilipix. For more information, ask your healthcare provider or pharmacist.

Call your doctor for medical advice about side effects. You may report side effects to FDA at 1-800-FDA-1088.

How do I store Trilipix?

- Store Trilipix between 59° to 86° F (15° to 30° C).
- Protect Trilipix from moisture.

Keep Trilipix and all medicines out of the reach of children.

General information about the safe and effective use of Trilipix

Medicines are sometimes prescribed for conditions that are not mentioned in the Medication Guide. Do not use Trilipix for a condition for which it was not prescribed. Do not give Trilipix to other people, even if they have the same condition you have. It may harm them.

This Medication Guide summarizes the most important information about Trilipix. If you would like more information, talk to your healthcare provider. You can also ask your pharmacist or healthcare provider for information that is written for health professionals.

For more information go to www.Trilipix.com or call 1-800-633-9110.

What are the ingredients in Trilipix?

Active Ingredient: Fenofibric acid

Inactive Ingredients: Hypromellose, povidone, water, hydroxylpropyl cellulose, colloidal silicon dioxide, sodium stearyl fumarate, methacrylic acid copolymer, talc, triethyl citrate, gelatin, titanium dioxide, and yellow iron oxide. Additionally, the 45 mg capsule shell contains black iron oxide and red iron oxide, and the 135 mg capsule shell contains FD&C Blue #2.

© AbbVie Inc. 2015

Manufactured for AbbVie Inc., North Chicago, IL 60064, U.S.A. by Fournier Laboratories Ireland Limited, Anngrove, Carrigtwohill Co. Cork, Ireland, or AbbVie LTD, Barceloneta, PR 00617.

Continued on next page

Ref: 03-B105-R8 April, 2015
This Medication Guide has been approved by the U.S. Food and Drug Administration.
Shown in Product Identification Guide, page 506

ULTANE®   ℞
[ul-tān]
(sevoflurane)
volatile liquid for inhalation

DESCRIPTION
ULTANE (sevoflurane), volatile liquid for inhalation, a nonflammable and nonexplosive liquid administered by vaporization, is a halogenated general inhalation anesthetic drug. Sevoflurane is fluoromethyl 2,2,2,-trifluoro-1-(trifluoromethyl) ethyl ether and its structural formula is:

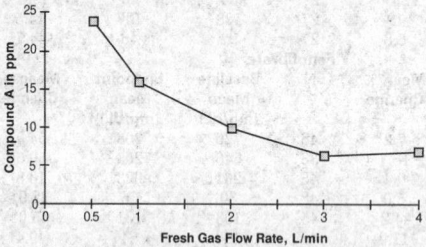

Sevoflurane, Physical Constants are:

Molecular weight	200.05
Boiling point at 760 mm Hg	58.6°C
Specific gravity at 20°C	1.520 - 1.525
Vapor pressure in mm Hg	157 mm Hg at 20°C
	197 mm Hg at 25°C
	317 mm Hg at 36°C

Distribution Partition Coefficients at 37°C:

Blood/Gas	0.63 - 0.69
Water/Gas	0.36
Olive Oil/Gas	47 - 54
Brain/Gas	1.15

Mean Component/Gas Partition Coefficients at 25°C for Polymers Used Commonly in Medical Applications:

Conductive rubber	14.0
Butyl rubber	7.7
Polyvinylchloride	17.4
Polyethylene	1.3

Sevoflurane is nonflammable and nonexplosive as defined by the requirements of International Electrotechnical Commission 601-2-13.

Sevoflurane is a clear, colorless, liquid containing no additives. Sevoflurane is not corrosive to stainless steel, brass, aluminum, nickel-plated brass, chrome-plated brass or copper beryllium. Sevoflurane is nonpungent. It is miscible with ethanol, ether, chloroform, and benzene, and it is slightly soluble in water. Sevoflurane is stable when stored under normal room lighting conditions according to instructions. No discernible degradation of sevoflurane occurs in the presence of strong acids or heat. When in contact with alkaline CO_2 absorbents (e.g Baralyme® and to a lesser extent soda lime) within the anesthesia machine, sevoflurane can undergo degradation under certain conditions. Degradation of sevoflurane is minimal, and degradants are either undetectable or present in non-toxic amounts when used as directed with fresh absorbents. Sevoflurane degradation and subsequent degradant formation are enhanced by increasing absorbent temperature increased sevoflurane concentration, decreased fresh gas flow and desiccated CO_2 absorbents (especially with potassium hydroxide containing absorbents e.g. Baralyme).

Sevoflurane alkaline degradation occurs by two pathways. The first results from the loss of hydrogen fluoride with the formation of pentafluoroisopropenyl fluoromethyl ether, (PIFE, $C_4H_2F_6O$), also known as Compound A, and trace amounts of pentafluoromethoxy isopropyl fluoromethyl ether, (PMFE, $C_5H_6F_6O$), also known as Compound B. The second pathway for degradation of sevoflurane, which occurs primarily in the presence of desiccated CO_2 absorbents, is discussed later.

In the first pathway, the defluorination pathway, the production of degradants in the anesthesia circuit results from

the extraction of the acidic proton in the presence of a strong base (KOH and/or NaOH) forming an alkene (Compound A) from sevoflurane similar to formation of 2-bromo-2-chloro-1,1-difluoro ethylene (BCDFE) from halothane. Laboratory simulations have shown that the concentration of these degradants is inversely correlated with the fresh gas flow rate (See Figure 1).

Figure 1. Fresh Gas Flow Rate versus Compound A Levels in a Circle Absorber System

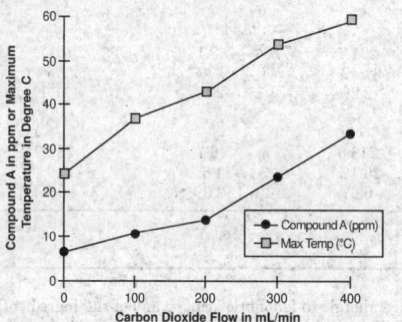

Since the reaction of carbon dioxide with absorbents is exothermic, the temperature increase will be determined by quantities of CO_2 absorbed, which in turn will depend on fresh gas flow in the anesthesia circle system, metabolic status of the patient, and ventilation. The relationship of temperature produced by varying levels of CO_2 and Compound A production is illustrated in the following *in vitro* simulation where CO_2 was added to a circle absorber system.

Figure 2. Carbon Dioxide Flow versus Compound A and Maximum Temperature

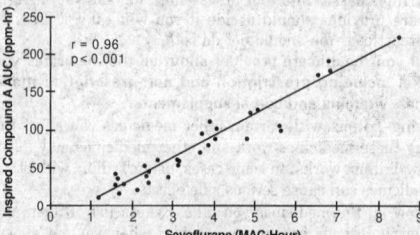

Compound A concentration in a circle absorber system increases as a function of increasing CO_2 absorbent temperature and composition (Baralyme producing higher levels than soda lime), increased body temperature, and increased minute ventilation, and decreasing fresh gas flow rates. It has been reported that the concentration of Compound A increases significantly with prolonged dehydration of Baralyme. Compound A exposure in patients also has been shown to rise with increased sevoflurane concentrations and duration of anesthesia. In a clinical study in which sevoflurane was administered to patients under low flow conditions for ≥ 2 hours at flow rates of 1 Liter/minute, Compound A levels were measured in an effort to determine the relationship between MAC hours and Compound A levels produced. The relationship between Compound A levels and sevoflurane exposure are shown in Figure 2a.

Figure 2a. ppm·hr versus MAC·hr at Flow Rate of 1 L/min

r = 0.96
p < 0.001

Compound A has been shown to be nephrotoxic in rats after exposures that have varied in duration from one to three hours. No histopathologic change was seen at a concentration of up to 270 ppm for one hour. Sporadic single cell necrosis of proximal tubule cells has been reported at a concentration of 114 ppm after a 3-hour exposure to

Compound A in rats. The LC_{50} reported at 1 hour is 1050-1090 ppm (male-female) and, at 3 hours, 350-490 ppm (male-female).

An experiment was performed comparing sevoflurane plus 75 or 100 ppm Compound A with an active control to evaluate the potential nephrotoxicity of Compound A in non-human primates. A single 8-hour exposure of Sevoflurane in the presence of Compound A produced single-cell renal tubular degeneration and single-cell necrosis in cynomolgus monkeys. These changes are consistent with the increased urinary protein, glucose level and enzymic activity noted on days one and three on the clinical pathology evaluation. This nephrotoxicity produced by Compound A is dose and duration of exposure dependent.

At a fresh gas flow rate of 1 L/min, mean maximum concentrations of Compound A in the anesthesia circuit in clinical settings are approximately 20 ppm (0.002%) with soda lime and 30 ppm (0.003%) with Baralyme in adult patients; mean maximum concentrations in pediatric patients with soda lime are about half those found in adults. The highest concentration observed in a single patient with Baralyme was 61 ppm (0.0061%) and 32 ppm (0.0032%) with soda lime. The levels of Compound A at which toxicity occurs in humans is not known.

The second pathway for degradation of sevoflurane occurs primarily in the presence of desiccated CO_2 absorbents and leads to the dissociation of sevoflurane into hexafluoroisopropanol (HFIP) and formaldehyde. HFIP is inactive, non-genotoxic, rapidly glucuronidated and cleared by the liver. Formaldehyde is present during normal metabolic processes. Upon exposure to a highly desiccated absorbent, formaldehyde can further degrade into methanol and formate. Formate can contribute to the formation of carbon monoxide in the presence of high temperature that can be associated with desiccated Baralyme®. Methanol can react with Compound A to form the methoxy addition product Compound B. Compound B can undergo further HF elimination to form Compounds C, D, and E.

Sevoflurane degradants were observed in the respiratory circuit of an experimental anesthesia machine using desiccated CO_2 absorbents and maximum sevoflurane concentrations (8%) for extended periods of time (> 2 hours). Concentrations of formaldehyde observed with desiccated soda lime in this experimental anesthesia respiratory circuit were consistent with levels that could potentially result in respiratory irritation. Although KOH containing CO_2 absorbents are no longer commercially available, in the laboratory experiments, exposure of sevoflurane to the desiccated KOH containing CO_2 absorbent, Baralyme, resulted in the detection of substantially greater degradant levels.

CLINICAL PHARMACOLOGY
Sevoflurane is an inhalational anesthetic agent for use in induction and maintenance of general anesthesia. Minimum alveolar concentration (MAC) of sevoflurane in oxygen for a 40-year-old adult is 2.1%. The MAC of sevoflurane decreases with age (see **DOSAGE AND ADMINISTRATION** for details).

Pharmacokinetics
Uptake and Distribution
Solubility
Because of the low solubility of sevoflurane in blood (blood/gas partition coefficient @ 37°C = 0.63-0.69), a minimal amount of sevoflurane is required to be dissolved in the blood before the alveolar partial pressure is in equilibrium with the arterial partial pressure. Therefore there is a rapid rate of increase in the alveolar (end-tidal) concentration (F_A) toward the inspired concentration (F_I) during induction.

Induction of Anesthesia
In a study in which seven healthy male volunteers were administered 70% $N_2O/30\%O_2$ for 30 minutes followed by 1.0% sevoflurane and 0.6% isoflurane for another 30 minutes the F_A/F_I ratio was greater for sevoflurane than isoflurane at all time points. The time for the concentration in the alveoli to reach 50% of the inspired concentration was 4-8 minutes for isoflurane and approximately 1 minute for sevoflurane.

F_A/F_I data from this study were compared with F_A/F_I data of other halogenated anesthetic agents from another study. When all data were normalized to isoflurane, the uptake and distribution of sevoflurane was shown to be faster than isoflurane and halothane, but slower than desflurane. The results are depicted in Figure 3.

Recovery from Anesthesia
The low solubility of sevoflurane facilitates rapid elimination via the lungs. The rate of elimination is quantified as the rate of change of the alveolar (end-tidal) concentration following termination of anesthesia (F_A), relative to the last

alveolar concentration (Fa_O) measured immediately before discontinuance of the anesthetic. In the healthy volunteer study described above, rate of elimination of sevoflurane was similar compared with desflurane, but faster compared with either halothane or isoflurane. These results are depicted in Figure 4.

Figure 3. Ratio of Concentration of Anesthetic in Alveolar Gas to Inspired Gas

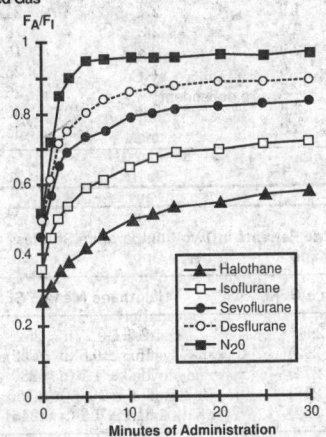

Figure 4. Concentration of Anesthetic in Alveolar Gas Following Termination of Anesthesia

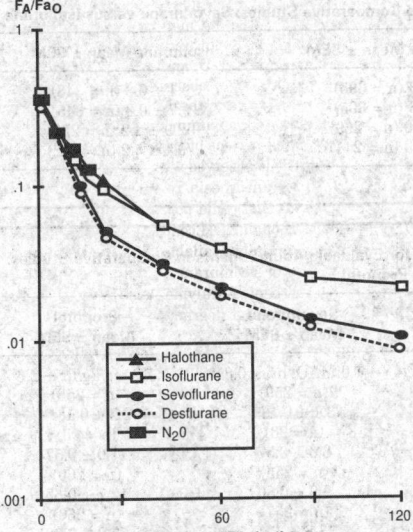

Yasuda N, Lockhart S, Eger EI II, et al: Comparison of kinetics of sevoflurane and isoflurane in humans. Anesth Analg 72:316, 1991.

Protein Binding

The effects of sevoflurane on the displacement of drugs from serum and tissue proteins have not been investigated. Other fluorinated volatile anesthetics have been shown to displace drugs from serum and tissue proteins *in vitro*. The clinical significance of this is unknown. Clinical studies have shown no untoward effects when sevoflurane is administered to patients taking drugs that are highly bound and have a small volume of distribution (e.g., phenytoin).

Metabolism

Sevoflurane is metabolized by cytochrome P450 2E1, to hexafluoroisopropanol (HFIP) with release of inorganic fluoride and CO_2. Once formed HFIP is rapidly conjugated with glucuronic acid and eliminated as a urinary metabolite. No other metabolic pathways for sevoflurane have been identified. *In vivo* metabolism studies suggest that approximately 5% of the sevoflurane dose may be metabolized. Cytochrome P450 2E1 is the principal isoform identified for sevoflurane metabolism and this may be induced by chronic exposure to isoniazid and ethanol. This is similar to the metabolism of isoflurane and enflurane and is distinct from that of methoxyflurane which is metabolized via a variety of cytochrome P450 isoforms. The metabolism of sevoflurane is not inducible by barbiturates. As shown in Figure 5, inor-

ganic fluoride concentrations peak within 2 hours of the end of sevoflurane anesthesia and return to baseline concentrations within 48 hours post-anesthesia in the majority of cases (67%). The rapid and extensive pulmonary elimination of sevoflurane minimizes the amount of anesthetic available for metabolism.

Figure 5. Serum Inorganic Fluoride Concentrations for Sevoflurane and Other Volatile Anesthetics

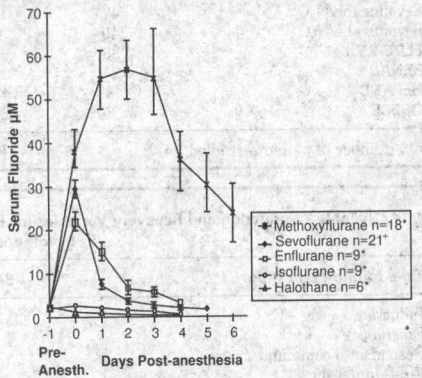

Cousins M.J., Greenstein L.R., Hitt B.A., et al: Metabolism and renal effects of enflurane in man. Anesthesiology 44:44; 1976[*] and Sevo-93-044[+].

Legend:

Pre-Anesth. = Pre-anesthesia

Elimination

Up to 3.5% of the sevoflurane dose appears in the urine as inorganic fluoride. Studies on fluoride indicate that up to 50% of fluoride clearance is nonrenal (via fluoride being taken up into bone).

Pharmacokinetics of Fluoride Ion

Fluoride ion concentrations are influenced by the duration of anesthesia, the concentration of sevoflurane administered, and the composition of the anesthetic gas mixture. In studies where anesthesia was maintained purely with sevoflurane for periods ranging from 1 to 6 hours, peak fluoride concentrations ranged between 12 µM and 90 µM. As shown in Figure 6, peak concentrations occur within 2 hours of the end of anesthesia and are less than 25 µM (475 ng/mL) for the majority of the population after 10 hours. The half-life is in the range of 15-23 hours.

It has been reported that following administration of methoxyflurane, serum inorganic fluoride concentrations > 50 µM were correlated with the development of vasopressin-resistant, polyuric, renal failure. In clinical trials with sevoflurane, there were no reports of toxicity associated with elevated fluoride ion levels.

Figure 6. Fluoride Ion Concentrations Following Administration of Sevoflurane (mean MAC = 1.27, mean duration = 2.06 hr) Mean Fluoride Ion Concentrations (n = 48)

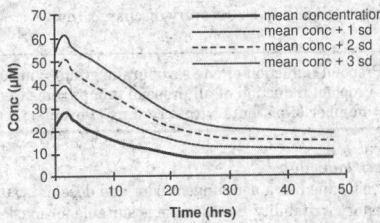

Fluoride Concentrations After Repeat Exposure and in Special Populations

Fluoride concentrations have been measured after single, extended, and repeat exposure to sevoflurane in normal surgical and special patient populations, and pharmacokinetic parameters were determined.

Compared with healthy individuals, the fluoride ion half-life was prolonged in patients with renal impairment, but not in the elderly. A study in 8 patients with hepatic impairment suggests a slight prolongation of the half-life. The mean half-life in patients with renal impairment averaged approximately 33 hours (range 21-61 hours) as compared to a mean of approximately 21 hours (range 10-48 hours) in normal healthy individuals. The mean half-life in the elderly (greater than 65 years) approximated 24 hours (range 18-72 hours). The mean half-life in individuals with hepatic

impairment was 23 hours (range 16-47 hours). Mean maximal fluoride values (C_{max}) determined in individual studies of special populations are displayed below.

[See table 1 on next page]

Pharmacodynamics

Changes in the depth of sevoflurane anesthesia rapidly follow changes in the inspired concentration.

In the sevoflurane clinical program, the following recovery variables were evaluated:

1. **Time to events measured from the end of study drug:**
   - Time to removal of the endotracheal tube (extubation time)
   - Time required for the patient to open his/her eyes on verbal command (emergence time)
   - Time to respond to simple command (e.g., squeeze my hand) or demonstrates purposeful movement (response to command time, orientation time)

2. **Recovery of cognitive function and motor coordination was evaluated based on:**
   - psychomotor performance tests (Digit Symbol Substitution Test [DSST], Treiger Dot Test)
   - the results of subjective (Visual Analog Scale [VAS]) and objective (objective pain-discomfort scale [OPDS]) measurements
   - time to administration of the first post-anesthesia analgesic medication
   - assessments of post-anesthesia patient status

3. **Other recovery times were:**
   - time to achieve an Aldrete Score of ≥ 8
   - time required for the patient to be eligible for discharge from the recovery area, per standard criteria at site
   - time when the patient was eligible for discharge from the hospital
   - time when the patient was able to sit up or stand without dizziness

Some of these variables are summarized as follows:

[See table 2 on next page]
[See table 3 on next page]
[See table 4 on next page]

Cardiovascular Effects

Sevoflurane was studied in 14 healthy volunteers (18-35 years old) comparing sevoflurane-O_2 (Sevo/O_2) to sevoflurane-N_2O/O_2 (Sevo/N_2O/O_2) during 7 hours of anesthesia. During controlled ventilation, hemodynamic parameters measured are shown in Figures 7-10:

Figure 7. Heart Rate

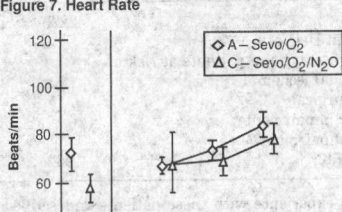

Figure 8. Mean Arterial Pressure

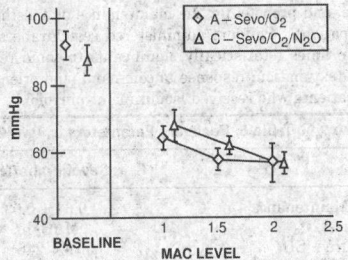

Continued on next page

Information on the AbbVie, Inc. products listed on these pages is from the prescribing information in use as of July 31, 2016. For more information, please visit rxabbvie.com or call 1-800-633-9110.

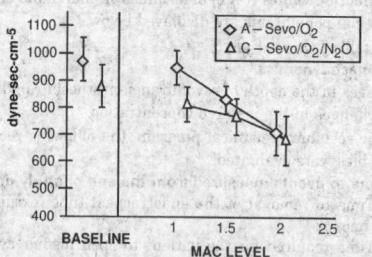

Figure 9. Systemic Vascular Resistance

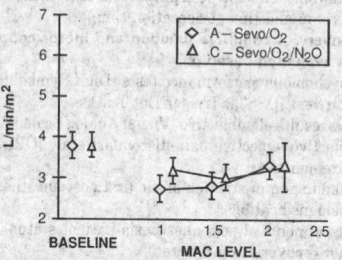

Figure 10. Cardiac Index

Sevoflurane is a dose-related cardiac depressant. Sevoflurane does not produce increases in heart rate at doses less than 2 MAC.

A study investigating the epinephrine induced arrhythmogenic effect of sevoflurane versus isoflurane in adult patients undergoing transsphenoidal hypophysectomy demonstrated that the threshold dose of epinephrine (i.e., the dose at which the first sign of arrhythmia was observed) producing multiple ventricular arrhythmias was 5 mcg/kg with both sevoflurane and isoflurane. Consequently, the interaction of sevoflurane with epinephrine appears to be equal to that seen with isoflurane.

Clinical Trials

Sevoflurane was administered to a total of 3185 patients prior to sevoflurane NDA submission. The types of patients are summarized as follows:

Table 5. Patients Receiving Sevoflurane in Clinical Trials

Type of Patients	Number	Studied
ADULT	2223	
Cesarean Delivery		29
Cardiovascular and patients at risk of myocardial ischemia		246
Neurosurgical		22
Hepatic impairment		8
Renal impairment		35
PEDIATRIC	962	

Clinical experience with these patients is described below.

Adult Anesthesia

The efficacy of sevoflurane in comparison to isoflurane, enflurane, and propofol was investigated in 3 outpatient and 25 inpatient studies involving 3591 adult patients. Sevoflurane was found to be comparable to isoflurane, enflurane, and propofol for the maintenance of anesthesia in adult patients. Patients administered sevoflurane showed shorter times (statistically significant) to some recovery events (extubation, response to command, and orientation) than patients who received isoflurane or propofol.

Table 1. Fluoride Ion Estimates in Special Populations Following Administration of Sevoflurane

	n	Age (yr)	Duration (hr)	Dose (MAC·hr)	C_{max} (μM)
PEDIATRIC PATIENTS					
Anesthetic					
Sevoflurane-O_2	76	0-11	0.8	1.1	12.6
Sevoflurane-O_2	40	1-11	2.2	3.0	16.0
Sevoflurane/N_2O	25	5-13	1.9	2.4	21.3
Sevoflurane/N_2O	42	0-18	2.4	2.2	18.4
Sevoflurane/N_2O	40	1-11	2.0	2.6	15.5
ELDERLY	33	65-93	2.6	1.4	25.6
RENAL	21	29-83	2.5	1.0	26.1
HEPATIC	8	42-79	3.6	2.2	30.6
OBESE	35	24-73	3.0	1.7	38.0

n = number of patients studied.

Table 2. Induction and Recovery Variables for Evaluable Pediatric Patients in Two Comparative Studies: Sevoflurane versus Halothane

Time to End-Point (min)	Sevoflurane Mean ± SEM	Halothane Mean ± SEM
Induction	2.0 ± 0.2 (n = 294)	2.7 ± 0.2 (n = 252)
Emergence	11.3 ± 0.7 (n = 293)	15.8 ± 0.8 (n = 252)
Response to command	13.7 ± 1.0 (n = 271)	19.3 ± 1.1 (n = 230)
First analgesia	52.2 ± 8.5 (n = 216)	67.6 ± 10.6 (n = 150)
Eligible for recovery discharge	76.5 ± 2.0 (n = 292)	81.1 ± 1.9 (n = 246)

n = number of patients with recording of events.

Table 3. Recovery Variables for Evaluable Adult Patients in Two Comparative Studies: Sevoflurane versus Isoflurane

Time to Parameter: (min)	Sevoflurane Mean ± SEM	Isoflurane Mean ± SEM
Emergence	7.7 ± 0.3 (n = 395)	9.1 ± 0.3 (n = 348)
Response to command	8.1 ± 0.3 (n = 395)	9.7 ± 0.3 (n = 345)
First analgesia	42.7 ± 3.0 (n = 269)	52.9 ± 4.2 (n = 228)
Eligible for recovery discharge	87.6 ± 5.3 (n = 244)	79.1 ± 5.2 (n = 252)

n = number of patients with recording of recovery events.

Table 4. Meta-Analyses for Induction and Emergence Variables for Evaluable Adult Patients in Comparative Studies: Sevoflurane versus Propofol

Parameter	No. of Studies	Sevoflurane Mean ± SEM	Propofol Mean ± SEM
Mean maintenance anesthesia exposure	3	1.0 MAC·hr. ± 0.8 (n = 259)	7.2 mg/kg/hr ± 2.6 (n = 258)
Time to induction: (min)	1	3.1 ± 0.18* (n = 93)	2.2 ± 0.18** (n = 93)
Time to emergence: (min)	3	8.6 ± 0.57 (n = 255)	11.0 ± 0.57 (n = 260)
Time to respond to command: (min)	3	9.9 ± 0.60 (n = 257)	12.1 ± 0.60 (n = 260)
Time to first analgesia: (min)	3	43.8 ± 3.79 (n = 177)	57.9 ± 3.68 (n = 179)
Time to eligibility for recovery discharge: (min)	3	116.0 ± 4.15 (n = 257)	115.6 ± 3.98 (n = 261)

* Propofol induction of one sevoflurane group = mean of 178.8 mg ± 72.5 SD (n = 165)
** Propofol induction of all propofol groups = mean of 170.2 mg ± 60.6 SD (n = 245)
n = number of patients with recording of events.

Mask Induction

Sevoflurane has a nonpungent odor and does not cause respiratory irritation. Sevoflurane is suitable for mask induction in adults. In 196 patients, mask induction was smooth and rapid, with complications occurring with the following frequencies: cough, 6%; breathholding, 6%; agitation, 6%; laryngospasm, 5%.

Ambulatory Surgery

Sevoflurane was compared to isoflurane and propofol for maintenance of anesthesia supplemented with N_2O in two studies involving 786 adult (18-84 years of age) ASA Class I, II, or III patients. Shorter times to emergence and response to commands (statistically significant) were observed with sevoflurane compared to isoflurane and propofol.

[See table 6 below]

Inpatient Surgery

Sevoflurane was compared to isoflurane and propofol for maintenance of anesthesia supplemented with N_2O in two multicenter studies involving 741 adult ASA Class I, II or III (18-92 years of age) patients. Shorter times to emergence, command response, and first post-anesthesia analgesia (statistically significant) were observed with sevoflurane compared to isoflurane and propofol.

Table 6. Recovery Parameters in Two Outpatient Surgery Studies: Least Squares Mean ± SEM

	Sevoflurane/N_2O	Isoflurane/N_2O	Sevoflurane/N_2O	Propofol/N_2O
Mean Maintenance Anesthesia Exposure ± SD	0.64 ± 0.03 MAC·hr. (n = 245)	0.66 ± 0.03 MAC·hr. (n = 249)	0.8 ± 0.5 MAC·hr. (n = 166)	7.3 ± 2.3 mg/kg/hr. (n = 166)
Time to Emergence (min)	8.2 ± 0.4 (n = 246)	9.3 ± 0.3 (n = 251)	8.3 ± 0.7 (n = 137)	10.4 ± 0.7 (n = 142)
Time to Respond to Commands (min)	8.5 ± 0.4 (n = 246)	9.8 ± 0.4 (n = 248)	9.1 ± 0.7 (n = 139)	11.5 ± 0.7 (n = 143)
Time to First Analgesia (min)	45.9 ± 4.7 (n = 160)	59.1 ± 6.0 (n = 252)	46.1 ± 5.4 (n = 83)	60.0 ± 4.7 (n = 88)
Time to Eligibility for Discharge from Recovery Area (min)	87.6 ± 5.3 (n = 244)	79.1 ± 5.2 (n = 252)	103.1 ± 3.8 (n = 139)	105.1 ± 3.7 (n = 143)

n = number of patients with recording of recovery events.

[See table 7 above]

Pediatric Anesthesia

The concentration of sevoflurane required for maintenance of general anesthesia is age-dependent (see **DOSAGE AND ADMINISTRATION**). Sevoflurane or halothane was used to anesthetize 1620 pediatric patients aged 1 day to 18 years, and ASA physical status I or II (948 sevoflurane, 672 halothane). In one study involving 90 infants and children, there were no clinically significant decreases in heart rate compared to awake values at 1 MAC. Systolic blood pressure decreased 15-20% in comparison to awake values following administration of 1 MAC sevoflurane; however, clinically significant hypotension requiring immediate intervention did not occur. Overall incidences of bradycardia [more than 20 beats/min lower than normal (80 beats/min)] in comparative studies was 3% for sevoflurane and 7% for halothane. Patients who received sevoflurane had slightly faster emergence times (12 vs. 19 minutes), and a higher incidence of post-anesthesia agitation (14% vs. 10%). Sevoflurane (n = 91) was compared to halothane (n = 89) in a single-center study for elective repair or palliation of congenital heart disease. The patients ranged in age from 9 days to 11.8 years with an ASA physical status of II, III, and IV (18%, 68%, and 13% respectively). No significant differences were demonstrated between treatment groups with respect to the primary outcome measures: cardiovascular decompensation and severe arterial desaturation. Adverse event data was limited to the study outcome variables collected during surgery and before institution of cardiopulmonary bypass.

Mask Induction

Sevoflurane has a nonpungent odor and is suitable for mask induction in pediatric patients. In controlled pediatric studies in which mask induction was performed, the incidence of induction events is shown below (see **ADVERSE REACTIONS**).

Table 8. Incidence of Pediatric Induction Events

	Sevoflurane (n = 836)	Halothane (n = 660)
Agitation	14%	11%
Cough	6%	10%
Breathholding	5%	6%
Secretions	3%	3%
Laryngospasm	2%	2%
Bronchospasm	< 1%	0%

n = number of patients.

Ambulatory Surgery

Sevoflurane (n = 518) was compared to halothane (n = 382) for the maintenance of anesthesia in pediatric outpatients. All patients received N_2O and many received fentanyl, midazolam, bupivacaine, or lidocaine. The time to eligibility for discharge from post-anesthesia care units was similar between agents (see **CLINICAL PHARMACOLOGY** and **ADVERSE REACTIONS**).

Cardiovascular Surgery

Coronary Artery Bypass Graft (CABG) Surgery

Sevoflurane was compared to isoflurane as an adjunct with opioids in a multicenter study of 273 patients undergoing CABG surgery. Anesthesia was induced with midazolam (0.1-0.3 mg/kg); vecuronium (0.1-0.2 mg/kg), and fentanyl (5-15 mcg/kg). Both isoflurane and sevoflurane were administered at loss of consciousness in doses of 1.0 MAC and titrated until the beginning of cardiopulmonary bypass to a maximum of 2.0 MAC. The total dose of fentanyl did not exceed 25 mcg/kg. The average MAC dose was 0.49 for sevoflurane and 0.53 for isoflurane. There were no significant differences in hemodynamics, cardioactive drug use, or ischemia incidence between the two groups. Outcome was also equivalent. In this small multicenter study, sevoflurane appears to be as effective and as safe as isoflurane for supplementation of opioid anesthesia for coronary bypass grafting.

Non-Cardiac Surgery Patients at Risk for Myocardial Ischemia

Sevoflurane-N_2O was compared to isoflurane-N_2O for maintenance of anesthesia in a multicenter study in 214 patients, age 40-87 years who were at mild-to-moderate risk for myocardial ischemia and were undergoing elective noncardiac surgery. Forty-six percent (46%) of the operations were cardiovascular, with the remainder evenly divided between gastrointestinal and musculoskeletal and small num-

bers of other surgical procedures. The average duration of surgery was less than 2 hours. Anesthesia induction usually was performed with thiopental (2-5 mg/kg) and fentanyl (1-5 mcg/kg). Vecuronium (0.1-0.2 mg/kg) was also administered to facilitate intubation, muscle relaxation or immobility during surgery. The average MAC dose was 0.49 for both anesthetics. There was no significant difference between the anesthetic regimens for intraoperative hemodynamics, cardioactive drug use, or ischemic incidents, although only 83 patients in the sevoflurane group and 85 patients in the isoflurane group were successfully monitored for ischemia. The outcome was also equivalent in terms of adverse events, death, and postoperative myocardial infarction. Within the limits of this small multicenter study in patients at mild-to-moderate risk for myocardial ischemia, sevoflurane was a satisfactory equivalent to isoflurane in providing supplemental inhalation anesthesia to intravenous drugs.

Cesarean Section

Sevoflurane (n = 29) was compared to isoflurane (n = 27) in ASA Class I or II patients for the maintenance of anesthesia during cesarean section. Newborn evaluations and recovery events were recorded. With both anesthetics, Apgar scores averaged 8 and 9 at 1 and 5 minutes, respectively.

Use of sevoflurane as part of general anesthesia for elective cesarean section produced no untoward effects in mother or neonate. Sevoflurane and isoflurane demonstrated equivalent recovery characteristics. There was no difference between sevoflurane and isoflurane with regard to the effect on the newborn, as assessed by Apgar Score and Neurological and Adaptive Capacity Score (average = 29.5). The safety of sevoflurane in labor and vaginal delivery has not been evaluated.

Neurosurgery

Three studies compared sevoflurane to isoflurane for maintenance of anesthesia during neurosurgical procedures. In a study of 20 patients, there was no difference between sevoflurane and isoflurane with regard to recovery from anesthesia. In 2 studies, a total of 22 patients with intracranial pressure (ICP) monitors received either sevoflurane or isoflurane. There was no difference between sevoflurane and isoflurane with regard to ICP response to inhalation of 0.5, 1.0, and 1.5 MAC inspired concentrations of volatile agent during N_2O-O_2-fentanyl anesthesia. During progressive hyperventilation from $PaCO_2$ = 40 to $PaCO_2$ = 30, ICP response to hypocarbia was preserved with sevoflurane at both 0.5 and 1.0 MAC concentrations. In patients at risk for elevations of ICP, sevoflurane should be administered cautiously in conjunction with ICP-reducing maneuvers such as hyperventilation.

Hepatic Impairment

A multicenter study (2 sites) compared the safety of sevoflurane and isoflurane in 16 patients with mild-to-moderate hepatic impairment utilizing the lidocaine MEGX assay for assessment of hepatocellular function. All patients received intravenous propofol (1-3 mg/kg) or thiopental (2-7 mg/kg) for induction and succinylcholine, vecuronium, or atracurium for intubation. Sevoflurane or isoflurane was administered in either 100% O_2 or up to 70% N_2O/O_2. Neither drug adversely affected hepatic function. No serum inorganic fluoride level exceeded 45 μM/L, but sevoflurane patients had prolonged terminal disposition of fluoride, as evidenced by longer inorganic fluoride half-life than patients with normal hepatic function (23 hours vs. 10-48 hours).

Renal Impairment

Sevoflurane was evaluated in renally impaired patients with baseline serum creatinine > 1.5 mg/dL. Fourteen pa-

tients who received sevoflurane were compared with 12 patients who received isoflurane. In another study, 21 patients who received sevoflurane were compared with 20 patients who received enflurane. Creatinine levels increased in 7% of patients who received sevoflurane, 8% of patients who received isoflurane, and 10% of patients who received enflurane. Because of the small number of patients with renal insufficiency (baseline serum creatinine greater than 1.5 mg/dL) studied, the safety of sevoflurane administration in this group has not yet been fully established. Therefore, sevoflurane should be used with caution in patients with renal insufficiency (see **WARNINGS**).

INDICATIONS AND USAGE

Sevoflurane is indicated for induction and maintenance of general anesthesia in adult and pediatric patients for inpatient and outpatient surgery.

Sevoflurane should be administered only by persons trained in the administration of general anesthesia. Facilities for maintenance of a patent airway, artificial ventilation, oxygen enrichment, and circulatory resuscitation must be immediately available. Since level of anesthesia may be altered rapidly, only vaporizers producing predictable concentrations of sevoflurane should be used.

CONTRAINDICATIONS

Sevoflurane can cause malignant hyperthermia. It should not be used in patients with known sensitivity to sevoflurane or to other halogenated agents nor in patients with known or suspected susceptibility to malignant hyperthermia.

WARNINGS

Although data from controlled clinical studies at low flow rates are limited, findings taken from patient and animal studies suggest that there is a potential for renal injury which is presumed due to Compound A. Animal and human studies demonstrate that sevoflurane administered for more than 2 MAC•hours and at fresh gas flow rates of < 2 L/min may be associated with proteinuria and glycosuria.

While a level of Compound A exposure at which clinical nephrotoxicity might be expected to occur has not been established, it is prudent to consider all of the factors leading to Compound A exposure in humans, especially duration of exposure, fresh gas flow rate, and concentration of sevoflurane. During sevoflurane anesthesia the clinician should adjust inspired concentration and fresh gas flow rate to minimize exposure to Compound A. To minimize exposure to Compound A, sevoflurane exposure should not exceed 2 MAC•hours at flow rates of 1 to < 2 L/min. Fresh gas flow rates < 1 L/min are not recommended.

Because clinical experience in administering sevoflurane to patients with renal insufficiency (creatinine > 1.5 mg/dL) is limited, its safety in these patients has not been established.

Sevoflurane may be associated with glycosuria and proteinuria when used for long procedures at low flow rates. The safety of low flow sevoflurane on renal function was evaluated in patients with normal preoperative renal function. One study compared sevoflurane (N = 98) to an active con-

Continued on next page

Table 7. Recovery Parameters in Two Inpatient Surgery Studies: Least Squares Mean ± SEM

	Sevoflurane/N2O	Isoflurane/N2O	Sevoflurane/N2O	Propofol/N2O
Mean Maintenance Anesthesia Exposure ± SD	1.27 MAC•hr. ± 0.05 (n = 271)	1.58 MAC•hr. ± 0.06 (n = 282)	1.43 MAC•hr. ± 0.94 (n = 93)	7.0 mg/kg/hr ± 2.9 (n = 92)
Time to Emergence (min)	11.0 ± 0.6 (n = 270)	16.4 ± 0.6 (n = 281)	8.8 ± 1.2 (n = 92)	13.2 ± 1.2 (n = 92)
Time to Respond to Commands (min)	12.8 ± 0.7 (n = 270)	18.4 ± 0.7 (n = 281)	11.0 ± 1.20 (n = 92)	14.4 ± 1.21 (n = 91)
Time to First Analgesia (min)	46.1 ± 3.0 (n = 233)	55.4 ± 3.2 (n = 242)	37.8 ± 3.3 (n = 82)	49.2 ± 3.3 (n = 79)
Time to Eligibility for Discharge from Recovery Area (min)	139.2 ± 15.6 (n = 268)	165.9 ± 16.3 (n = 282)	148.4 ± 8.9 (n = 92)	141.4 ± 8.9 (n = 92)

n = number of patients with recording of recovery events.

trol (N = 90) administered for ≥ 2 hours at a fresh gas flow rate of ≤ 1 Liter/minute. Per study defined criteria (Hou et al.) one patient in the sevoflurane group developed elevations of creatinine, in addition to glycosuria and proteinuria. This patient received sevoflurane at fresh gas flow rates of ≤ 800 mL/minute. Using these same criteria, there were no patients in the active control group who developed treatment emergent elevations in serum creatinine.

Sevoflurane may present an increased risk in patients with known sensitivity to volatile halogenated anesthetic agents. KOH containing CO_2 absorbents are not recommended for use with sevoflurane.

Reports of QT prolongation, associated with torsade de pointes (in exceptional cases, fatal), have been received. Caution should be exercised when administering sevoflurane to susceptible patients (e.g. patients with congenital Long QT Syndrome or patients taking drugs that can prolong the QT interval).

Malignant Hyperthermia

In susceptible individuals, potent inhalation anesthetic agents, including sevoflurane, may trigger a skeletal muscle hypermetabolic state leading to high oxygen demand and the clinical syndrome known as malignant hyperthermia. Sevoflurane can induce malignant hyperthermia in genetically susceptible individuals, such as those with certain inherited ryanodine receptor mutations. The clinical syndrome is signaled by hypercapnia, and may include muscle rigidity, tachycardia, tachypnea, cyanosis, arrhythmias, and/or unstable blood pressure. Some of these nonspecific signs may also appear during light anesthesia, acute hypoxia, hypercapnia, and hypovolemia.

In clinical trials, one case of malignant hyperthermia was reported. In addition, there have been postmarketing reports of malignant hyperthermia. Some of these cases have been fatal.

Treatment of malignant hyperthermia includes discontinuation of triggering agents (e.g., sevoflurane), administration of intravenous dantrolene sodium (consult prescribing information for intravenous dantrolene sodium for additional information on patient management), and application of supportive therapy. Supportive therapy may include efforts to restore body temperature, respiratory and circulatory support as indicated, and management of electrolyte-fluid-acid-base abnormalities. Renal failure may appear later, and urine flow should be monitored and sustained if possible.

Perioperative Hyperkalemia

Use of inhaled anesthetic agents has been associated with rare increases in serum potassium levels that have resulted in cardiac arrhythmias and death in pediatric patients during the postoperative period. Patients with latent as well as overt neuromuscular disease, particularly Duchenne muscular dystrophy, appear to be most vulnerable. Concomitant use of succinylcholine has been associated with most, but not all, of these cases. These patients also experienced significant elevations in serum creatine kinase levels and, in some cases, changes in urine consistent with myoglobinuria. Despite the similarity in presentation to malignant hyperthermia, none of these patients exhibited signs or symptoms of muscle rigidity or hypermetabolic state. Early and aggressive intervention to treat the hyperkalemia and resistant arrhythmias is recommended; as is subsequent evaluation for latent neuromuscular disease.

PRECAUTIONS

During the maintenance of anesthesia, increasing the concentration of sevoflurane produces dose-dependent decreases in blood pressure. Due to sevoflurane's insolubility in blood, these hemodynamic changes may occur more rapidly than with other volatile anesthetics. Excessive decreases in blood pressure or respiratory depression may be related to depth of anesthesia and may be corrected by decreasing the inspired concentration of sevoflurane.

Rare cases of seizures have been reported in association with sevoflurane use (see **PRECAUTIONS - Pediatric Use** and **ADVERSE REACTIONS**).

The recovery from general anesthesia should be assessed carefully before a patient is discharged from the post-anesthesia care unit.

Drug Interactions

In clinical trials, no significant adverse reactions occurred with other drugs commonly used in the perioperative period, including: central nervous system depressants, autonomic drugs, skeletal muscle relaxants, anti-infective agents, hormones and synthetic substitutes, blood derivatives, and cardiovascular drugs.

Intravenous Anesthetics

Sevoflurane administration is compatible with barbiturates, propofol, and other commonly used intravenous anesthetics.

Benzodiazepines and Opioids

Benzodiazepines and opioids would be expected to decrease the MAC of sevoflurane in the same manner as with other inhalational anesthetics. Sevoflurane administration is compatible with benzodiazepines and opioids as commonly used in surgical practice.

Nitrous Oxide

As with other halogenated volatile anesthetics, the anesthetic requirement for sevoflurane is decreased when administered in combination with nitrous oxide. Using 50% N_2O, the MAC equivalent dose requirement is reduced approximately 50% in adults, and approximately 25% in pediatric patients (see **DOSAGE AND ADMINISTRATION**).

Neuromuscular Blocking Agents

As is the case with other volatile anesthetics, sevoflurane increases both the intensity and duration of neuromuscular blockade induced by nondepolarizing muscle relaxants. When used to supplement alfentanil-N_2O anesthesia, sevoflurane and isoflurane equally potentiate neuromuscular block induced with pancuronium, vecuronium or atracurium. Therefore, during sevoflurane anesthesia, the dosage adjustments for these muscle relaxants are similar to those required with isoflurane.

Potentiation of neuromuscular blocking agents requires equilibration of muscle with delivered partial pressure of sevoflurane. Reduced doses of neuromuscular blocking agents during induction of anesthesia may result in delayed onset of conditions suitable for endotracheal intubation or inadequate muscle relaxation.

Among available nondepolarizing agents, only vecuronium, pancuronium and atracurium interactions have been studied during sevoflurane anesthesia. In the absence of specific guidelines:

1. For endotracheal intubation, do not reduce the dose of nondepolarizing muscle relaxants.
2. During maintenance of anesthesia, the required dose of nondepolarizing muscle relaxants is likely to be reduced compared to that during N_2O/opioid anesthesia. Administration of supplemental doses of muscle relaxants should be guided by the response to nerve stimulation.

The effect of sevoflurane on the duration of depolarizing neuromuscular blockade induced by succinylcholine has not been studied.

Hepatic Function

Results of evaluations of laboratory parameters (e.g., ALT, AST, alkaline phosphatase, and total bilirubin, etc.), as well as investigator-reported incidence of adverse events relating to liver function, demonstrate that sevoflurane can be administered to patients with normal or mild-to-moderately impaired hepatic function. However, patients with severe hepatic dysfunction were not investigated.

Occasional cases of transient changes in postoperative hepatic function tests were reported with both sevoflurane and reference agents. Sevoflurane was found to be comparable to isoflurane with regard to these changes in hepatic function.

Very rare cases of mild, moderate and severe post-operative hepatic dysfunction or hepatitis with or without jaundice have been reported from postmarketing experiences. Clinical judgement should be exercised when sevoflurane is used in patients with underlying hepatic conditions or under treatment with drugs known to cause hepatic dysfunction (see **ADVERSE REACTIONS**).

It has been reported that previous exposure to halogenated hydrocarbon anesthetics may increase the potential for hepatic injury.

Desiccated CO_2 Absorbents

An exothermic reaction occurs when sevoflurane is exposed to CO_2 absorbents. This reaction is increased when the CO_2 absorbent becomes desiccated, such as after an extended period of dry gas flow through the CO_2 absorbent canisters. Rare cases of extreme heat, smoke, and/or spontaneous fire in the anesthesia breathing circuit have been reported during sevoflurane use in conjunction with the use of desiccated CO_2 absorbent, specifically those containing potassium hydroxide (e.g. Baralyme). KOH containing CO_2 absorbents are not recommended for use with sevoflurane. An unusually delayed rise or unexpected decline of inspired sevoflurane concentration compared to the vaporizer setting may be associated with excessive heating of the CO_2 absorbent and chemical breakdown of sevoflurane.

As with other inhalational anesthetics, degradation and production of degradation products can occur when sevoflurane is exposed to desiccated absorbents. When a clinician suspects that the CO_2 absorbent may be desiccated, it should be replaced. The color indicator of most CO_2 absorbents may not change upon desiccation. Therefore, the lack of significant color change should not be taken as an assurance of adequate hydration. CO_2 absorbents should be replaced routinely regardless of the state of the color indicator.

Carcinogenesis, Mutagenesis, Impairment of Fertility

Studies on carcinogenesis have not been performed for either sevoflurane or Compound A. No mutagenic effect of sevoflurane was noted in the Ames test, mouse micronucleus test, mouse lymphoma mutagenicity assay, human lymphocyte culture assay, mammalian cell transformation assay, ^{32}P DNA adduct assay, and no chromosomal aberrations were induced in cultured mammalian cells.

Similarly, no mutagenic effect of Compound A was noted in the Ames test, the Chinese hamster chromosomal aberration assay and the *in vivo* mouse micronucleus assay. However, positive responses were observed in the human lymphocyte chromosome aberration assay. These responses were seen only at high concentrations and in the absence of metabolic activation (human S-9).

Pregnancy Category B

Reproduction studies have been performed in rats and rabbits at doses up to 1 MAC (minimum alveolar concentration) without CO_2 absorbent and have revealed no evidence of impaired fertility or harm to the fetus due to sevoflurane at 0.3 MAC, the highest nontoxic dose. Developmental and reproductive toxicity studies of sevoflurane in animals in the presence of strong alkalies (i.e., degradation of sevoflurane and production of Compound A) have not been conducted. There are no adequate and well-controlled studies in pregnant women. Because animal reproduction studies are not always predictive of human response, sevoflurane should be used during pregnancy only if clearly needed.

Labor and Delivery

Sevoflurane has been used as part of general anesthesia for elective cesarean section in 29 women. There were no untoward effects in mother or neonate (see **PHARMACODYNAMICS - Clinical Trials**). The safety of sevoflurane in labor and delivery has not been demonstrated.

Nursing Mothers

The concentrations of sevoflurane in milk are probably of no clinical importance 24 hours after anesthesia. Because of rapid washout, sevoflurane concentrations in milk are predicted to be below those found with many other volatile anesthetics.

Geriatric Use

MAC decreases with increasing age. The average concentration of sevoflurane to achieve MAC in an 80 year old is approximately 50% of that required in a 20 year old.

Pediatric Use

Induction and maintenance of general anesthesia with sevoflurane have been established in controlled clinical trials in pediatric patients aged 1 to 18 years (see **PHARMACODYNAMICS - Clinical Trials** and **ADVERSE REACTIONS**). Sevoflurane has a nonpungent odor and is suitable for mask induction in pediatric patients.

The concentration of sevoflurane required for maintenance of general anesthesia is age dependent. When used in combination with nitrous oxide, the MAC equivalent dose of sevoflurane should be reduced in pediatric patients. MAC in premature infants has not been determined (see **PRECAUTIONS - Drug Interactions** and **DOSAGE AND ADMINISTRATION** for recommendations in pediatric patients 1 day of age and older).

The use of sevoflurane has been associated with seizures (see **PRECAUTIONS** and **ADVERSE REACTIONS**). The majority of these have occurred in children and young adults starting from 2 months of age, most of whom had no predisposing risk factors. Clinical judgement should be exercised when using sevoflurane in patients who may be at risk for seizures.

ADVERSE REACTIONS

Adverse events are derived from controlled clinical trials conducted in the United States, Canada, and Europe. The reference drugs were isoflurane, enflurane, and propofol in adults and halothane in pediatric patients. The studies were conducted using a variety of premedications, other anesthetics, and surgical procedures of varying length. Most adverse events reported were mild and transient, and may reflect the surgical procedures, patient characteristics (including disease) and/or medications administered.

Of the 5182 patients enrolled in the clinical trials, 2906 were exposed to sevoflurane, including 118 adults and 507 pediatric patients who underwent mask induction. Each patient was counted once for each type of adverse event. Adverse events reported in patients in clinical trials and considered to be possibly or probably related to sevoflurane are presented within each body system in order of decreasing frequency in the following listings. One case of malignant hyperthermia was reported in pre-registration clinical trials.

Adverse Events During the Induction Period (from Onset of Anesthesia by Mask Induction to Surgical Incision) Incidence > 1%

Adult Patients (N = 118)

Cardiovascular

Bradycardia 5%, Hypotension 4%, Tachycardia 2%

Nervous System

Agitation 7%

Respiratory System

Laryngospasm 8%, Airway obstruction 8%, Breathholding 5%, Cough Increased 5%

Pediatric Patients (N = 507)

Cardiovascular

Tachycardia 6%, Hypotension 4%

Nervous System

Agitation 15%

Respiratory System

Breathholding 5%, Cough Increased 5%, Laryngospasm 3%, Apnea 2%

Digestive System

Increased salivation 2%

Adverse Events During Maintenance and Emergence Periods, Incidence > 1% (N = 2906)

Body as a whole

Fever 1%, Shivering 6%, Hypothermia 1%, Movement 1%, Headache 1%

Cardiovascular

Hypotension 11%, Hypertension 2%, Bradycardia 5%, Tachycardia 2%

Nervous System

Somnolence 9%, Agitation 9%, Dizziness 4%, Increased salivation 4%

Digestive System

Nausea 25%, Vomiting 18%

Respiratory System

Cough increased 11%, Breathholding 2%, Laryngospasm 2%

Adverse Events, All Patients in Clinical Trials (N = 2906), All Anesthetic Periods, Incidence < 1% (Reported in 3 or More Patients)

Body as a whole

Asthenia, Pain

Cardiovascular

Arrhythmia, Ventricular Extrasystoles, Supraventricular Extrasystoles, Complete AV Block, Bigeminy, Hemorrhage, Inverted T Wave, Atrial Fibrillation, Atrial Arrhythmia, Second Degree AV Block, Syncope, S-T Depressed

Nervous System

Crying, Nervousness, Confusion, Hypertonia, Dry Mouth, Insomnia

Respiratory System

Sputum Increased, Apnea, Hypoxia, Wheezing, Bronchospasm, Hyperventilation, Pharyngitis, Hiccup, Hypoventilation, Dyspnea, Stridor

Metabolism and Nutrition

Increases in LDH, AST, ALT, BUN, Alkaline Phosphatase, Creatinine, Bilirubinemia, Glycosuria, Fluorosis, Albuminuria, Hypophosphatemia, Acidosis, Hyperglycemia

Hemic and Lymphatic System

Leucocytosis, Thrombocytopenia

Skin and Special Senses

Amblyopia, Pruritus, Taste Perversion, Rash, Conjunctivitis

Urogenital

Urination Impaired, Urine Abnormality, Urinary Retention, Oliguria

See **WARNINGS** for information regarding malignant hyperthermia.

Post-Marketing Adverse Events

The following adverse events have been identified during post-approval use of Ultane (sevoflurane USP). Due to the spontaneous nature of these reports, the actual incidence and relationship of Ultane to these events cannot be established with certainty.

CNS

Seizures — Post-marketing reports indicate that sevoflurane use has been associated with seizures. The ma-

jority of cases were in children and young adults, most of whom had no medical history of seizures. Several cases reported no concomitant medications, and at least one case was confirmed by EEG. Although many cases were single seizures that resolved spontaneously or after treatment, cases of multiple seizures have also been reported. Seizures have occurred during, or soon after sevoflurane induction, during emergence, and during post-operative recovery up to a day following anesthesia.

Cardiac

Cardiac arrest

Hepatic

• Cases of mild, moderate and severe post-operative hepatic dysfunction or hepatitis with or without jaundice have been reported. Histological evidence was not provided for any of the reported hepatitis cases. In most of these cases, patients had underlying hepatic conditions or were under treatment with drugs known to cause hepatic dysfunction. Most of the reported events were transient and resolved spontaneously (see **PRECAUTIONS**).

• Hepatic necrosis

• Hepatic failure

Other

• Malignant hyperthermia (see **CONTRAINDICATIONS** and **WARNINGS**)

• Allergic reactions, such as rash, urticaria, pruritus, bronchospasm, anaphylactic or anaphylactoid reactions (see **CONTRAINDICATIONS**)

• Reports of hypersensitivity (including contact dermatitis, rash, dyspnea, wheezing, chest discomfort, swelling face, or anaphylactic reaction) have been received, particularly in association with long-term occupational exposure to inhaled anesthetic agents, including sevoflurane (see **OCCUPATIONAL CAUTION**).

Laboratory Findings

• Transient elevations in glucose, liver function tests, and white blood cell count may occur as with use of other anesthetic agents.

OVERDOSAGE

In the event of overdosage, or what may appear to be overdosage, the following action should be taken: discontinue administration of sevoflurane, maintain a patent airway, initiate assisted or controlled ventilation with oxygen, and maintain adequate cardiovascular function.

DOSAGE AND ADMINISTRATION

The concentration of sevoflurane being delivered from a vaporizer during anesthesia should be known. This may be accomplished by using a vaporizer calibrated specifically for sevoflurane. The administration of general anesthesia must be individualized based on the patient's response.

Replacement of Desiccated CO_2 Absorbents

When a clinician suspects that the CO_2 absorbent may be desiccated, it should be replaced. The exothermic reaction that occurs with sevoflurane and CO_2 absorbents is increased when the CO_2 absorbent becomes desiccated, such as after an extended period of dry gas flow through the CO_2 absorbent canisters (see **PRECAUTIONS**).

Pre-anesthetic Medication

No specific premedication is either indicated or contraindicated with sevoflurane. The decision as to whether or not to premedicate and the choice of premedication is left to the discretion of the anesthesiologist.

Induction

Sevoflurane has a nonpungent odor and does not cause respiratory irritation; it is suitable for mask induction in pediatrics and adults.

Maintenance

Surgical levels of anesthesia can usually be achieved with concentrations of 0.5 - 3% sevoflurane with or without the concomitant use of nitrous oxide. Sevoflurane can be administered with any type of anesthesia circuit.

Table 9. MAC Values for Adults and Pediatric Patients According to Age

Age of Patient (years)	Sevoflurane in Oxygen	Sevoflurane in 65% N₂O/35% O₂
0 - 1 months #	3.3%	
1 - < 6 months	3.0%	
6 months - < 3 years	2.8%	2.0%@
3 - 12	2.5%	
25	2.6%	1.4%
40	2.1%	1.1%
60	1.7%	0.9%
80	1.4%	0.7%

\# Neonates are full-term gestational age. MAC in premature infants has not been determined.

@ In 1 - < 3 year old pediatric patients, 60% N₂O/40% O₂ was used.

HOW SUPPLIED

ULTANE (sevoflurane), Volatile Liquid for Inhalation, is packaged in amber colored bottles containing 250 mL sevoflurane, List 4456, NDC # 0074-4456-04 (plastic).

SAFETY AND HANDLING

Occupational Caution

There is no specific work exposure limit established for sevoflurane. However, the National Institute for Occupational Safety and Health has recommended an 8 hour time-weighted average limit of 2 ppm for halogenated anesthetic agents in general (0.5 ppm when coupled with exposure to N₂O) (see **ADVERSE REACTIONS**).

Storage

Store at controlled room temperature, 15° - 30°C (59° - 86°F). See USP.

Product of Japan

Product inquiries should be directed to AbbVie Inc., North Chicago, IL 60064, USA

Manufactured by:

AbbVie Inc., North Chicago, IL 60064, USA under license from Maruishi Pharmaceutical Company LTD. 2-3-5, Fushimi-machi, Chuo-Ku, Osaka, Japan.

©AbbVie Inc. 2014

03-A903 March 2014

Shown in Product Identification Guide, page 506

VENCLEXTA™   ℞

[*ven-KLEKS-tuh*]

(venetoclax)

tablets

HIGHLIGHTS OF PRESCRIBING INFORMATION

These highlights do not include all the information needed to use VENCLEXTA safely and effectively. See full prescribing information for VENCLEXTA.

VENCLEXTA™ (venetoclax) tablets, for oral use

Initial U.S. Approval: 2016

—————INDICATIONS AND USAGE—————

VENCLEXTA is a BCL-2 inhibitor indicated for the treatment of patients with chronic lymphocytic leukemia (CLL) with 17p deletion, as detected by an FDA approved test, who have received at least one prior therapy.

This indication is approved under accelerated approval based on overall response rate. Continued approval for this indication may be contingent upon verification and description of clinical benefit in a confirmatory trial. (1)

————DOSAGE AND ADMINISTRATION————

• Initiate therapy with VENCLEXTA at 20 mg once daily for 7 days, followed by a weekly ramp-up dosing schedule to the recommended daily dose of 400 mg. (2.2)

• VENCLEXTA tablets should be taken orally once daily with a meal and water. Do not chew, crush, or break tablets. (2.2)

• Perform prophylaxis for tumor lysis syndrome. (2.3)

————DOSAGE FORMS AND STRENGTHS————

Tablets: 10 mg, 50 mg, 100 mg (3)

—————CONTRAINDICATIONS—————

Concomitant use of VENCLEXTA with strong inhibitors of CYP3A at initiation and during ramp-up phase is contraindicated. (2.5, 4, 7.1)

————WARNINGS AND PRECAUTIONS————

• Tumor Lysis Syndrome (TLS): Anticipate TLS; assess risk in all patients. Premedicate with anti-hyperuricemics and ensure adequate hydration. Employ more intensive measures (intravenous hydration, frequent monitoring, hospitalization) as overall risk increases. (2.3, 5.1)

• Neutropenia: Monitor blood counts and for signs of infection; manage as medically appropriate. (2.4, 5.2)

Continued on next page

- Immunization: Do not administer live attenuated vaccines prior to, during, or after VENCLEXTA treatment. (5.3)
- Embryo-Fetal Toxicity: May cause embryo-fetal harm. Advise females of reproductive potential of the potential risk to a fetus and to use effective contraception during treatment. (5.4)

————————ADVERSE REACTIONS————————

The most common adverse reactions (≥20%) were neutropenia, diarrhea, nausea, anemia, upper respiratory tract infection, thrombocytopenia, and fatigue. (6.1)
To report SUSPECTED ADVERSE REACTIONS, contact AbbVie Inc. at 1-800-633-9110 or FDA at 1-800-FDA-1088 or www.fda.gov/medwatch.

————————DRUG INTERACTIONS————————

Avoid concomitant use of VENCLEXTA with moderate CYP3A inhibitors, strong or moderate CYP3A inducers, P-gp inhibitors, or narrow therapeutic index P-gp substrates. (2.5, 7.1, 7.2)

- If a moderate CYP3A inhibitor or a P-gp inhibitor must be used, reduce the VENCLEXTA dose by at least 50%. (2.5, 7.1)
- If a strong CYP3A inhibitor must be used after the ramp-up phase, reduce the VENCLEXTA dose by at least 75%. (2.5, 7.1)
- If a narrow therapeutic index P-gp substrate must be used, it should be taken at least 6 hours before VENCLEXTA. (7.2)

————————USE IN SPECIFIC POPULATIONS————————

- Lactation: Discontinue breastfeeding. (8.2)

See 17 for PATIENT COUNSELING INFORMATION and Medication Guide.

Revised: 4/2016

FULL PRESCRIBING INFORMATION: CONTENTS*

* Sections or subsections omitted from the full prescribing information are not listed.

FULL PRESCRIBING INFORMATION

1   INDICATIONS AND USAGE

VENCLEXTA is indicated for the treatment of patients with chronic lymphocytic leukemia (CLL) with 17p deletion, as detected by an FDA approved test, who have received at least one prior therapy.

This indication is approved under accelerated approval based on overall response rate [see Clinical Studies (14)]. Continued approval for this indication may be contingent upon verification and description of clinical benefit in a confirmatory trial.

2   DOSAGE AND ADMINISTRATION
2.1   Patient Selection
Select patients for the treatment of relapsed or refractory CLL with VENCLEXTA based on the presence of 17p deletions in blood specimens [see Indications and Usage (1) and Clinical Studies (14)]. Patients without 17p deletion at diagnosis should be retested at relapse because acquisition of 17p deletion can occur. Information on FDA-approved tests for the detection of 17p deletions in CLL is available at: http://www.fda.gov/CompanionDiagnostics.
2.2   Recommended Dosage
Assess patient-specific factors for level of risk of tumor lysis syndrome (TLS) and provide prophylactic hydration and anti-hyperuricemics to patients prior to first dose of VENCLEXTA to reduce risk of TLS [see Dosage and Administration (2.3) and Warnings and Precautions (5.1)]. Administer the VENCLEXTA dose according to a weekly ramp-up schedule over 5 weeks to the recommended daily dose of 400 mg as shown in Table 1. The 5-week ramp-up dosing schedule is designed to gradually reduce tumor burden (debulk) and decrease the risk of TLS.
Instruct patients to take VENCLEXTA tablets with a meal and water at approximately the same time each day. VENCLEXTA tablets should be swallowed whole and not chewed, crushed, or broken prior to swallowing.

Table 1. Dosing Schedule for Ramp-Up Phase

Week	VENCLEXTA Daily Dose
1	20 mg
2	50 mg
3	100 mg
4	200 mg
5 and beyond	400 mg

The Starting Pack provides the first 4 weeks of VENCLEXTA according to the ramp-up schedule. Once the ramp-up phase is completed, the 400 mg dose is achieved using 100 mg tablets supplied in bottles [see How Supplied/Storage and Handling (16)].
VENCLEXTA should be taken orally once daily until disease progression or unacceptable toxicity is observed.
2.3   Risk Assessment and Prophylaxis for Tumor Lysis Syndrome
VENCLEXTA can cause rapid reduction in tumor and thus poses a risk for TLS in the initial 5-week ramp-up phase. Changes in blood chemistries consistent with TLS that require prompt management can occur as early as 6 to 8 hours following the first dose of VENCLEXTA and at each dose increase.
The risk of TLS is a continuum based on multiple factors, including tumor burden and comorbidities. Perform tumor burden assessments, including radiographic evaluation (e.g., CT scan), assess blood chemistry (potassium, uric acid, phosphorus, calcium, and creatinine) in all patients and correct pre-existing abnormalities prior to initiation of treatment with VENCLEXTA. Reduced renal function (creatinine clearance [CrCl] <80 mL/min) further increases the risk. The risk may decrease as tumor burden decreases [see Warnings and Precautions (5.1) and Use in Specific Populations (8.6)].
Table 2 below describes the recommended TLS prophylaxis and monitoring during VENCLEXTA treatment based on tumor burden determination from clinical trial data.
[See table 2 below]
2.4   Dose Modifications Based on Toxicities
Interrupt dosing or reduce dose for toxicities. See Table 3 for dose modifications for hematologic and other toxicities related to VENCLEXTA, and Table 4 for dose. For patients who have had a dosing interruption greater than 1 week during the first 5 weeks of ramp-up phase or greater than 2 weeks when at the daily dose of 400 mg, reassess for risk of TLS to determine if reinitiation with a reduced dose is necessary (e.g., all or some levels of the dose ramp-up schedule) [see Dosage and Administration (2.2, 2.3)].

Table 2. Recommended TLS Prophylaxis Based on Tumor Burden From Clinical Trial Data (consider all patient co-morbidities before final determination of prophylaxis and monitoring schedule)

Tumor Burden		Prophylaxis		Blood Chemistry Monitoring[c,d]
		Hydration[a]	Anti-hyperuricemics	Setting and Frequency of Assessments
Low	All LN <5 cm AND ALC <25 ×10⁹/L	Oral (1.5-2 L)	Allopurinol[b]	Outpatient • Pre-dose, 6 to 8 hours, 24 hours at first dose of 20 mg and 50 mg • Pre-dose at subsequent ramp-up doses
Medium	Any LN 5 cm to <10 cm OR ALC ≥25 ×10⁹/L	Oral (1.5-2 L) and consider additional intravenous	Allopurinol	Outpatient • Pre-dose, 6 to 8 hours, 24 hours at first dose of 20 mg and 50 mg • Pre-dose at subsequent ramp-up doses • Consider hospitalization for patients with CrCl <80ml/min at first dose of 20 mg and 50 mg; see below for monitoring in hospital
High	Any LN ≥10 cm OR ALC ≥25 ×10⁹/L AND any LN ≥5 cm	Oral (1.5-2L) and intravenous (150-200 mL/hr as tolerated)	Allopurinol; consider rasburicase if baseline uric acid is elevated	In hospital at first dose of 20 mg and 50 mg • Pre-dose, 4, 8,12 and 24 hours Outpatient at subsequent ramp-up doses • Pre-dose, 6 to 8 hours, 24 hours

ALC = absolute lymphocyte count; LN = lymph node.
[a]Administer intravenous hydration for any patient who cannot tolerate oral hydration.
[b]Start allopurinol or xanthine oxidase inhibitor 2 to 3 days prior to initiation of VENCLEXTA.
[c]Evaluate blood chemistries (potassium, uric acid, phosphorus, calcium, and creatinine); review in real time.
[d]For patients at risk of TLS, monitor blood chemistries at 6 to 8 hours and at 24 hours at each subsequent ramp-up dose.

Table 3. Recommended Dose Modifications for Toxicities[a]

Event	Occurrence	Action
Tumor Lysis Syndrome		
Blood chemistry changes or symptoms suggestive of TLS	Any	Withhold the next day's dose. If resolved within 24 to 48 hours of last dose, resume at the same dose.
		For any blood chemistry changes requiring more than 48 hours to resolve, resume at a reduced dose (see Table 4) *[see Dosage and Administration (2.3)].*
		For any events of clinical TLS,[b] resume at a reduced dose following resolution (see Table 4) *[see Dosage and Administration (2.3)].*
Non-Hematologic Toxicities		
Grade 3 or 4 non-hematologic toxicities	1st occurrence	Interrupt VENCLEXTA. Once the toxicity has resolved to Grade 1 or baseline level, VENCLEXTA therapy may be resumed at the same dose. No dose modification is required.
	2nd and subsequent occurrences	Interrupt VENCLEXTA. Follow dose reduction guidelines in Table 4 when resuming treatment with VENCLEXTA after resolution. A larger dose reduction may occur at the discretion of the physician.
Hematologic Toxicities		
Grade 3 or 4 neutropenia with infection or fever; or Grade 4 hematologic toxicities (except lymphopenia) *[see Warnings and Precautions (5.2)]*	1st occurrence	Interrupt VENCLEXTA. To reduce the infection risks associated with neutropenia, granulocyte-colony stimulating factor (G-CSF) may be administered with VENCLEXTA if clinically indicated. Once the toxicity has resolved to Grade 1 or baseline level, VENCLEXTA therapy may be resumed at the same dose.
	2nd and subsequent occurrences	Interrupt VENCLEXTA. Consider using G-CSF as clinically indicated. Follow dose reduction guidelines in Table 4 when resuming treatment with VENCLEXTA after resolution. A larger dose reduction may occur at the discretion of the physician.

Consider discontinuing VENCLEXTA for patients who require dose reductions to less than 100 mg for more than 2 weeks.
[a]Adverse reactions were graded using NCI CTCAE version 4.0.
[b]Clinical TLS was defined as laboratory TLS with clinical consequences such as acute renal failure, cardiac arrhythmias, or sudden death and/or seizures.

Table 4. Dose Modification for Toxicity During VENCLEXTA Treatment

Dose at Interruption, mg	Restart Dose, mg[a]
400	300
300	200
200	100
100	50
50	20
20	10

[a]During the ramp-up phase, continue the reduced dose for 1 week before increasing the dose.

2.5 Dose Modifications for Use with CYP3A and P-gp Inhibitors

Concomitant use of VENCLEXTA with *strong* CYP3A inhibitors at initiation and during ramp-up phase is contraindicated. Concomitant use of VENCLEXTA with strong CYP3A inhibitors increases venetoclax exposure (i.e., C_{max} and AUC) and may increase the risk for TLS at initiation and during ramp-up phase *[see Contraindications (4)].* For patients who have completed the ramp-up phase and are on a steady daily dose of VENCLEXTA, reduce the VENCLEXTA dose by at least 75% when *strong* CYP3A inhibitors must be used concomitantly.
Avoid concomitant use of VENCLEXTA with *moderate* CYP3A inhibitors or P-gp inhibitors. Consider alternative treatments. If a moderate CYP3A inhibitor or a P-gp inhibitor must be used, reduce the VENCLEXTA dose by at least 50%. Monitor these patients more closely for signs of toxicities *[see Dosage and Administration (2.4)].*
Resume the VENCLEXTA dose that was used prior to initiating the CYP3A inhibitor or P-gp inhibitor 2 to 3 days after discontinuation of the inhibitor *[see Dosage and Administration (2.4) and Drug Interactions (7.1)].*
The recommendations for managing drug-drug interactions are summarized in Table 5.

Table 5. Management of Potential VENCLEXTA Interactions with CYP3A and P-gp Inhibitors

Inhibitors	Initiation and Ramp-Up Phase	Steady Daily Dose (After Ramp-Up Phase)
Strong CYP3A inhibitor	Contraindicated	Avoid inhibitor use or reduce the VENCLEXTA dose by at least 75%
Moderate CYP3A inhibitor	Avoid inhibitor use or reduce the VENCLEXTA dose by at least 50%	
P-gp inhibitor		

2.6 Missed Dose

If the patient misses a dose of VENCLEXTA within 8 hours of the time it is usually taken, the patient should take the missed dose as soon as possible and resume the normal daily dosing schedule. If a patient misses a dose by more than 8 hours, the patient should not take the missed dose and should resume the usual dosing schedule the next day. If the patient vomits following dosing, no additional dose should be taken that day. The next prescribed dose should be taken at the usual time.

3 DOSAGE FORMS AND STRENGTHS

Table 6. VENCLEXTA Tablet Strength and Description

Tablet Strength	Description of Tablet
10 mg	Round, biconvex shaped, pale yellow film-coated tablet debossed with "V" on one side and "10" on the other side
50 mg	Oblong, biconvex shaped, beige film-coated tablet debossed with "V" on one side and "50" on the other side
100 mg	Oblong, biconvex shaped, pale yellow film-coated tablet debossed with "V" on one side and "100" on the other side

4 CONTRAINDICATIONS

Concomitant use of VENCLEXTA with *strong* CYP3A inhibitors at initiation and during ramp-up phase is contraindicated *[see Dosage and Administration (2.5) and Drug Interactions (7.1)].*

5 WARNINGS AND PRECAUTIONS

5.1 Tumor Lysis Syndrome

Tumor lysis syndrome, including fatal events and renal failure requiring dialysis, has occurred in previously treated CLL patients with high tumor burden when treated with VENCLEXTA *[see Adverse Reactions (6.1)].*
VENCLEXTA can cause rapid reduction in tumor and thus poses a risk for TLS in the initial 5-week ramp-up phase. Changes in blood chemistries consistent with TLS that require prompt management can occur as early as 6 to 8 hours following the first dose of VENCLEXTA and at each dose increase.
The risk of TLS is a continuum based on multiple factors, including tumor burden (see Table 2) and comorbidities. Reduced renal function (CrCl <80 mL/min) further increases the risk. Patients should be assessed for risk and should receive appropriate prophylaxis for TLS, including hydration and anti-hyperuricemics. Monitor blood chemistries and manage abnormalities promptly. Interrupt dosing if needed. Employ more intensive measures (intravenous hydration, frequent monitoring, hospitalization) as overall risk increases *[see Dosage and Administration (2.3, 2.4) and Use in Specific Populations (8.6)].*
Concomitant use of VENCLEXTA with strong or moderate CYP3A inhibitors and P-gp inhibitors increases venetoclax exposure, may increase the risk of TLS at initiation and during ramp-up phase and may require VENCLEXTA dose adjustment *[see Dosage and Administration (2.5) and Drug Interactions (7.1)].*

5.2 Neutropenia

Grade 3 or 4 neutropenia occurred in 41% (98/240) of patients treated with VENCLEXTA *[see Adverse Reactions (6.1)].* Monitor complete blood counts throughout the treatment period. Interrupt dosing or reduce dose for severe neutropenia. Consider supportive measures including antimicrobials for signs of infection and use of growth factors (e.g., G-CSF) *[see Dosage and Administration (2.4)].*

5.3 Immunization

Do not administer live attenuated vaccines prior to, during, or after treatment with VENCLEXTA until B-cell recovery occurs. The safety and efficacy of immunization with live attenuated vaccines during or following VENCLEXTA therapy have not been studied. Advise patients that vaccinations may be less effective.

5.4 Embryo-Fetal Toxicity

Based on its mechanism of action and findings in animals, VENCLEXTA may cause embryo-fetal harm when administered to a pregnant woman. In an embryo-fetal study conducted in mice, administration of venetoclax to pregnant animals at exposures equivalent to that observed in patients at the recommended dose of 400 mg daily resulted in post-implantation loss and decreased fetal weight. There are no adequate and well-controlled studies in pregnant woman using VENCLEXTA. Advise females of reproductive potential to avoid pregnancy during treatment. If VENCLEXTA is used during pregnancy or if the patient becomes pregnant while taking VENCLEXTA, the patient should be apprised of the potential hazard to the fetus *[see Use in Specific Populations (8.1)].*

6 ADVERSE REACTIONS

The following serious adverse events are discussed in greater detail in other sections of the labeling:
• Tumor Lysis Syndrome *[see Warnings and Precautions (5.1)]*
• Neutropenia *[see Warnings and Precautions (5.2)]*
Because clinical trials are conducted under widely variable conditions, adverse event rates observed in clinical trials of a drug cannot be directly compared with rates of clinical trials of another drug and may not reflect the rates observed in practice.

6.1 Clinical Trial Experience

The safety of single agent VENCLEXTA at the 400 mg recommended daily dose following a dose ramp-up schedule is based on pooled data of 240 patients with previously treated CLL from two phase 2 trials and one phase 1 trial. In the pooled dataset, the median age was 66 years (range: 29 to 85 years), 95% were white, and 69% were male. The median

Continued on next page

number of prior therapies was 3 (range: 1 to 12). The median duration of treatment with VENCLEXTA at the time of data analysis was approximately 10.3 months (range: 0 to 34.1 months). Approximately 46% of patients received VENCLEXTA for more than 48 weeks.

The most common adverse reactions (≥20%) of any grade were neutropenia, diarrhea, nausea, anemia, upper respiratory tract infection, thrombocytopenia, and fatigue.

Serious adverse reactions were reported in 43.8% of patients. The most frequent serious adverse reactions (≥2%) were pneumonia, febrile neutropenia, pyrexia, autoimmune hemolytic anemia (AIHA), anemia, and TLS.

Discontinuations due to adverse reactions occurred in 8.3% of patients. The most frequent adverse reactions leading to drug discontinuation were thrombocytopenia and AIHA.

Dosage adjustments due to adverse reactions occurred in 9.6% of patients. The most frequent adverse reactions leading to dose adjustments were neutropenia, febrile neutropenia, and thrombocytopenia.

Adverse reactions reported in 3 trials of patients with previously treated CLL using single agent VENCLEXTA are presented in Table 7.

[See table 7 below]

Tumor Lysis Syndrome

Tumor lysis syndrome is an important identified risk when initiating VENCLEXTA. In the initial Phase 1 dose-finding trials, which had shorter (2-3 week) ramp-up phase and higher starting dose, the incidence of TLS was 12% (9/77; 4 laboratory TLS, 5 clinical TLS), including 2 fatal events and 3 events of acute renal failure, 1 requiring dialysis.

The risk of TLS was reduced after revision of the dosing regimen and modification to prophylaxis and monitoring measures *[see Dosage and Administration (2.2, 2.3)]*. In venetoclax clinical trials, patients with any measurable lymph node ≥10 cm or those with both an ALC ≥25 × 10⁹/L and any measurable lymph node ≥5 cm were hospitalized to enable more intensive hydration and monitoring for the first day of dosing at 20 mg and 50 mg during the ramp-up phase.

In 66 patients with CLL starting with a daily dose of 20 mg and increasing over 5 weeks to a daily dose of 400 mg, the rate of TLS was 6%. All events either met laboratory TLS criteria (laboratory abnormalities that met ≥2 of the follow-ing within 24 hours of each other: potassium >6 mmol/L, uric acid >476 µmol/L, calcium <1.75 mmol/L, or phosphorus >1.5 mmol/L); or were reported as TLS events. The events occurred in patients who had a lymph node(s) ≥5 cm or ALC ≥25 × 10⁹/L. No TLS with clinical consequences such as acute renal failure, cardiac arrhythmias or sudden death and/or seizures was observed in these patients. All patients had CrCl ≥50 mL/min.

Laboratory abnormalities relevant to TLS observed in 66 patients with CLL who followed the dose ramp-up schedule and TLS prophylaxis measures are presented in Table 8.

Table 8. Adverse Reactions of TLS and Relevant Laboratory Abnormalities Reported in Patients with CLL

Parameter	All Grades (%) N=66	Grade ≥3 (%) N=66
Laboratory TLS[a]	6	6
Hyperkalemia[b]	20	2
Hyperphosphatemia[c]	15	3
Hypocalcemia[d]	9	3
Hyperuricemia[e]	6	2

[a]Laboratory abnormalities that met ≥2 of the following criteria within 24 hours of each other: potassium >6 mmol/L, uric acid >476 µmol/L, calcium <1.75 mmol/L, or phosphorus >1.5 mmol/L; or were reported as TLS events.
[b]Hyperkalemia/blood potassium increased.
[c]Hyperphosphatemia/blood phosphorus increased.
[d]Hypocalcemia/blood calcium decreased.
[e]Hyperuricemia/blood uric acid increased.

7 DRUG INTERACTIONS
7.1 Effects of Other Drugs on VENCLEXTA
Venetoclax is predominantly metabolized by CYP3A4/5.
Strong CYP3A Inhibitors
Concomitant use of VENCLEXTA with strong CYP3A inhibitors (e.g., ketoconazole, conivaptan, clarithromycin, indinavir, itraconazole, lopinavir, ritonavir, telaprevir, posa-conazole and voriconazole) at initiation and during ramp-up phase is contraindicated *[see Contraindications (4) and Clinical Pharmacology (12.3)]*.

For patients who have completed the ramp-up phase and are on a steady daily dose of VENCLEXTA, reduce the VENCLEXTA dose by at least 75% when used concomitantly with strong CYP3A inhibitors. Resume the VENCLEXTA dose that was used prior to initiating the CYP3A inhibitor 2 to 3 days after discontinuation of the inhibitor *[see Dosage and Administration (2.4, 2.5) and Clinical Pharmacology (12.3)]*.

Co-administration of ketoconazole increased venetoclax C_{max} by 2.3-fold and AUC_∞ by 6.4-fold.

Moderate CYP3A Inhibitors and P-gp Inhibitors
Avoid concomitant use of moderate CYP3A inhibitors (e.g., erythromycin, ciprofloxacin, diltiazem, dronedarone, fluconazole, verapamil) or P-gp inhibitors (e.g., amiodarone, azithromycin, captopril, carvedilol, cyclosporine, felodipine, quercetin, quinidine, ranolazine, ticagrelor) with VENCLEXTA. Consider alternative treatments. If a moderate CYP3A inhibitor or a P-gp inhibitor must be used, reduce the VENCLEXTA dose by at least 50%. Monitor patients more closely for signs of VENCLEXTA toxicities *[see Dosage and Administration (2.4, 2.5) and Clinical Pharmacology (12.3)]*.

Resume the VENCLEXTA dose that was used prior to initiating the CYP3A inhibitor or P-gp inhibitor 2 to 3 days after discontinuation of the inhibitor *[see Dosage and Administration (2.5) and Clinical Pharmacology (12.3)]*.

Avoid grapefruit products, Seville oranges, and starfruit during treatment with VENCLEXTA, as they contain inhibitors of CYP3A.

Co-administration of a single dose of rifampin, a P-gp inhibitor, increased venetoclax C_{max} by 106% and AUC_∞ by 78%.

CYP3A Inducers
Avoid concomitant use of VENCLEXTA with strong CYP3A inducers (e.g., carbamazepine, phenytoin, rifampin, St. John's wort) or moderate CYP3A inducers (e.g., bosentan, efavirenz, etravirine, modafinil, nafcillin). Consider alternative treatments with less CYP3A induction *[see Clinical Pharmacology (12.3)]*.

Co-administration of multiple doses of rifampin, a strong CYP3A inducer, decreased venetoclax C_{max} by 42% and AUC_∞ by 71%.

7.2 Effects of VENCLEXTA on Other Drugs
Warfarin
In a drug-drug interaction study in healthy subjects, administration of a single dose of venetoclax with warfarin resulted in an 18% to 28% increase in C_{max} and AUC_∞ of R-warfarin and S-warfarin. Because venetoclax was not dosed to steady state, it is recommended that the international normalized ratio (INR) be monitored closely in patients receiving warfarin.

P-gp substrates
In vitro data suggest venetoclax has inhibition potential on P-gp substrates at therapeutic dose levels in the gut. Therefore, co-administration of narrow therapeutic index P-gp substrates (e.g., digoxin, everolimus, and sirolimus) with VENCLEXTA should be avoided. If a narrow therapeutic index P-gp substrate must be used, it should be taken at least 6 hours before VENCLEXTA.

8 USE IN SPECIFIC POPULATIONS
8.1 Pregnancy
Risk Summary
There are no available human data on the use of VENCLEXTA in pregnant women. Based on toxicity observed in mice, VENCLEXTA may cause fetal harm when administered to pregnant women. In mice, venetoclax was fetotoxic at exposures 1.2 times the human clinical exposure based on AUC at the recommended human dose of 400 mg daily. If VENCLEXTA is used during pregnancy or if the patient becomes pregnant while taking VENCLEXTA, the patient should be apprised of the potential risk to a fetus.

The background risk in the U.S. general population of major birth defects is 2% to 4% and of miscarriage is 15% to 20% of clinically recognized pregnancies.

Data
Animal data
In embryo-fetal development studies, venetoclax was administered to pregnant mice and rabbits during the period of organogenesis. In mice, venetoclax was associated with increased post-implantation loss and decreased fetal body weight at 150 mg/kg/day (maternal exposures approxi-

Table 7. Adverse Reactions Reported in ≥10% (Any Grade) or ≥5% (Grade 3 or 4) of Patients with CLL

Body System	Adverse Reaction	Any Grade (%) N=240	Grade 3 or 4 (%) N=240
Blood and lymphatic system disorders	Neutropenia[a]	45	41
	Anemia[b]	29	18
	Thrombocytopenia[c]	22	15
	Febrile neutropenia	5	5
Gastrointestinal disorders	Diarrhea	35	<1
	Nausea	33	<1
	Vomiting	15	<1
	Constipation	14	0
General disorders and administration site conditions	Fatigue	21	2
	Pyrexia	16	<1
	Peripheral edema	11	<1
Infections and infestations	Upper respiratory tract infection	22	1
	Pneumonia	8	5
Metabolic and nutrition disorders	Hypokalemia	12	4
Musculoskeletal and connective tissue disorders	Back pain	10	<1
Nervous system disorders	Headache	15	<1
Respiratory, thoracic, and mediastinal disorders	Cough	13	0

Adverse Reactions graded using NCI Common Terminology Criteria for Adverse Events version 4.0.
[a]Neutropenia/neutrophil count decreased.
[b]Anemia/hemoglobin decreased.
[c]Thrombocytopenia/platelet count decreased.

mately 1.2 times the human AUC exposure at the recommended dose of 400 mg daily). No teratogenicity was observed in either the mouse or the rabbit.

8.2 Lactation
Risk Summary
There are no data on the presence of VENCLEXTA in human milk, the effects of VENCLEXTA on the breastfed child, or the effects of VENCLEXTA on milk production. Because many drugs are excreted in human milk and because the potential for serious adverse reactions in breastfed infants from VENCLEXTA is unknown, advise nursing women to discontinue breastfeeding during treatment with VENCLEXTA.

8.3 Females and Males of Reproductive Potential
VENCLEXTA may cause fetal harm *[see Warnings and Precautions (5.4) and Use in Specific Populations (8.1)]*.
Pregnancy Testing
Females of reproductive potential should undergo pregnancy testing before initiation of VENCLEXTA *[see Use in Specific Populations (8.1)]*.
Contraception
Advise females of reproductive potential to use effective contraception during treatment with VENCLEXTA and for at least 30 days after the last dose *[see Use in Specific Populations (8.1)]*.
Infertility
Based on findings in animals, male fertility may be compromised by treatment with VENCLEXTA *[see Nonclinical Toxicology (13.1)]*.

8.4 Pediatric Use
Safety and effectiveness have not been established in pediatric patients.

8.5 Geriatric Use
Of the 106 patients with previously treated CLL with 17p deletion who were evaluated for efficacy, 57% were ≥65 years of age and 17% were ≥75 years of age.
Of the 240 patients with previously treated CLL evaluated for safety from 3 open-label trials, 58% were ≥65 years of age and 17% were ≥75 years of age.
No overall differences in safety and effectiveness were observed between older and younger patients.

8.6 Renal Impairment
Patients with reduced renal function (CrCl <80 mL/min) are at increased risk of TLS. These patients may require more intensive prophylaxis and monitoring to reduce the risk of TLS when initiating treatment with VENCLEXTA *[see Dosage and Administration (2.3, 2.4)]*.
No specific clinical trials have been conducted in subjects with renal impairment. Less than 0.1% of radioactive VENCLEXTA dose was detected in urine. No dose adjustment is needed for patients with mild or moderate renal impairment (CrCl ≥30 mL/min) based on results of the population pharmacokinetic analysis *[see Clinical Pharmacology (12.3)]*. A recommended dose has not been determined for patients with severe renal impairment (CrCl <30 mL/min) or patients on dialysis.

8.7 Hepatic Impairment
No specific clinical trials have been conducted in subjects with hepatic impairment, however human mass balance study showed that venetoclax undergoes hepatic elimination. Although no dose adjustment is recommended in patients with mild or moderate hepatic impairment based on results of the population pharmacokinetic analysis *[see Clinical Pharmacology (12.3)]*, a trend for increased adverse events was observed in patients with moderate hepatic impairment; monitor these patients more closely for signs of toxicity during the initiation and dose ramp-up phase. A recommended dose has not been determined for patients with severe hepatic impairment.

10 OVERDOSAGE
There is no specific antidote for VENCLEXTA. For patients who experience overdose, closely monitor and provide appropriate supportive treatment; during ramp-up phase interrupt VENCLEXTA and monitor carefully for signs and symptoms of TLS along with other toxicities *[see Dosage and Administration (2.3, 2.4)]*. Based on venetoclax large volume of distribution and extensive protein binding, dialysis is unlikely to result in significant removal of venetoclax.

11 DESCRIPTION
Venetoclax is a selective inhibitor of BCL-2 protein. It is a light yellow to dark yellow solid with the empirical formula $C_{45}H_{50}ClN_7O_7S$ and a molecular weight of 868.44. Venetoclax has very low aqueous solubility. Venetoclax is described chemically as 4-(4-{[2-(4-chlorophenyl)-4,4-di-

methylcyclohex-1-en-1-yl]methyl}piperazin-1-yl)-N-({3-nitro-4-[(tetrahydro-2H-pyran-4-ylmethyl)amino]phenyl}sulfonyl)-2-(1H-pyrrolo[2,3-b]pyridin-5-yloxy)benzamide) and has the following chemical structure:

VENCLEXTA tablets for oral administration are supplied as pale yellow or beige tablets that contain 10, 50, or 100 mg venetoclax as the active ingredient. Each tablet also contains the following inactive ingredients: copovidone, colloidal silicon dioxide, polysorbate 80, sodium stearyl fumarate, and calcium phosphate dibasic. In addition, the 10 mg and 100 mg coated tablets include the following: iron oxide yellow, polyvinyl alcohol, polyethylene glycol, talc, and titanium dioxide. The 50 mg coated tablets also include the following: iron oxide yellow, iron oxide red, iron oxide black, polyvinyl alcohol, talc, polyethylene glycol and titanium dioxide. Each tablet is debossed with "V" on one side and "10", "50" or "100" corresponding to the tablet strength on the other side.

12 CLINICAL PHARMACOLOGY
12.1 Mechanism of Action
Venetoclax is a selective and orally bioavailable small-molecule inhibitor of BCL-2, an anti-apoptotic protein. Overexpression of BCL-2 has been demonstrated in CLL cells where it mediates tumor cell survival and has been associated with resistance to chemotherapeutics. Venetoclax helps restore the process of apoptosis by binding directly to the BCL-2 protein, displacing pro-apoptotic proteins like BIM, triggering mitochondrial outer membrane permeabilization and the activation of caspases. In nonclinical studies, venetoclax has demonstrated cytotoxic activity in tumor cells that overexpress BCL-2.

12.2 Pharmacodynamics
Cardiac Electrophysiology
The effect of multiple doses of VENCLEXTA up to 1200 mg once daily on the QTc interval was evaluated in an open-label, single-arm study in 176 patients with previously treated hematologic malignancies. VENCLEXTA had no large effect on QTc interval (i.e., > 20 ms) and there was no relationship between venetoclax exposure and change in QTc interval.

12.3 Pharmacokinetics
Absorption
Following multiple oral administrations under fed conditions, maximum plasma concentration of venetoclax was reached 5-8 hours after dose. Venetoclax steady state AUC increased proportionally over the dose range of 150-800 mg. Under low-fat meal conditions, venetoclax mean (± standard deviation) steady state C_{max} was 2.1 ± 1.1 µg/mL and AUC_{0-24} was 32.8 ± 16.9 µg•h/mL at the 400 mg once daily dose.
Food Effect
Administration with a low-fat meal increased venetoclax exposure by approximately 3.4-fold and administration with a high-fat meal increased venetoclax exposure by 5.1- to 5.3-fold compared to fasting conditions. Venetoclax should be administered with a meal *[see Dosage and Administration (2.2)]*.
Distribution
Venetoclax is highly bound to human plasma protein with unbound fraction in plasma <0.01 across a concentration range of 1-30 µM (0.87-26 µg/mL). The mean blood-to-

plasma ratio was 0.57. The population estimate for apparent volume of distribution (Vd_{ss}/F) of venetoclax ranged from 256-321 L in patients.
Elimination
The population estimate for the terminal elimination half-life of venetoclax was approximately 26 hours. The pharmacokinetics of venetoclax does not change over time.
Metabolism
In vitro studies demonstrated that venetoclax is predominantly metabolized by CYP3A4/5. M27 was identified as a major metabolite in plasma with an inhibitory activity against BCL-2 that is at least 58-fold lower than venetoclax *in vitro*.
Excretion
After single oral administration of 200 mg radiolabeled [^{14}C]-venetoclax dose to healthy subjects, >99.9% of the dose was recovered in feces and <0.1% of the dose was excreted in urine within 9 days, indicating that hepatic elimination is responsible for the clearance of venetoclax from the systemic circulation. Unchanged venetoclax accounted for 20.8% of the administered radioactive dose excreted in feces.

Special Populations
Age, Race, Sex, and Weight
Based on population pharmacokinetic analyses, age, race, sex, and weight do not have a clinically meaningful effect on venetoclax clearance.
Renal Impairment
Based on a population pharmacokinetic analysis that included 211 subjects with mild renal impairment (CrCl ≥60 and <90 mL/min, calculated by Cockcroft-Gault equation), 83 subjects with moderate renal impairment (CrCl ≥30 and <60 mL/min) and 210 subjects with normal renal function (CrCl ≥90 mL/min), venetoclax exposures in subjects with mild or moderate renal impairment are similar to those with normal renal function. The pharmacokinetics of venetoclax has not been studied in subjects with severe renal impairment (CrCl <30 mL/min) or subjects on dialysis *[see Use in Specific Populations (8.6)]*.
Hepatic Impairment
Based on a population pharmacokinetic analysis that included 69 subjects with mild hepatic impairment, 7 subjects with moderate hepatic impairment and 429 subjects with normal hepatic function, venetoclax exposures are similar in subjects with mild and moderate hepatic impairment and normal hepatic function. The NCI Organ Dysfunction Working Group criteria for hepatic impairment were used in the analysis. Mild hepatic impairment was defined as normal total bilirubin and aspartate transaminase (AST) > upper limit of normal (ULN) or total bilirubin >1.0 to 1.5 times ULN, moderate hepatic impairment as total bilirubin >1.5 to 3.0 times ULN, and severe hepatic impairment as total bilirubin >3.0 times ULN. The pharmacokinetics of venetoclax has not been studied in subjects with severe hepatic impairment *[see Use in Specific Populations (8.7)]*.
Drug Interactions
Ketoconazole
Co-administration of 400 mg once daily ketoconazole, a strong CYP3A, P-gp and BCRP inhibitor, for 7 days in 11 previously treated NHL patients increased venetoclax C_{max} by 2.3-fold and AUC_{∞} by 6.4-fold *[see Drug Interactions (7.1)]*.
Rifampin multiple doses
Co-administration of 600 mg once daily rifampin, a strong CYP3A inducer, for 13 days in 10 healthy subjects decreased venetoclax C_{max} by 42% and AUC_{∞} by 71% *[see Drug Interactions (7.1)]*.
Rifampin single dose
Co-administration of a 600 mg single dose of rifampin, an OATP1B1/1B3 and P-gp inhibitor, in 11 healthy subjects increased venetoclax C_{max} by 106% and AUC_{∞} by 78% *[see Drug Interactions (7.1)]*.
Gastric Acid Reducing Agents
Based on population pharmacokinetic analysis, gastric acid reducing agents (e.g., proton pump inhibitors, H2-receptor antagonists, antacids) do not affect venetoclax bioavailability.

Continued on next page

Information on the AbbVie, Inc. products listed on these pages is from the prescribing information in use as of July 31, 2016. For more information, please visit rxabbvie.com or call 1-800-633-9110.

Warfarin

In a drug-drug interaction study in three healthy subjects, administration of a single 400 mg dose of venetoclax with 5 mg warfarin resulted in 18% to 28% increase in C_{max} and AUC_∞ of R-warfarin and S-warfarin *[see Drug Interactions (7.2)]*.

In vitro Studies

In vitro studies indicated that venetoclax is not an inhibitor or inducer of CYP1A2, CYP2B6, CYP2C19, CYP2D6, or CYP3A4 at clinically relevant concentrations. Venetoclax is a weak inhibitor of CYP2C8, CYP2C9, and UGT1A1 *in vitro*, but it is not predicted to cause clinically relevant inhibition due to high plasma protein binding. Venetoclax is not an inhibitor of UGT1A4, UGT1A6, UGT1A9, or UGT2B7. Venetoclax is a P-gp and BCRP substrate as well as a P-gp and BCRP inhibitor and weak OATP1B1 inhibitor *in vitro*. To avoid a potential interaction in the gastrointestinal tract, co-administration of narrow therapeutic index P-gp substrates such as digoxin with VENCLEXTA should be avoided. If a narrow therapeutic index P-gp substrate must be used, it should be taken at least 6 hours before VENCLEXTA. Venetoclax is not expected to inhibit OATP1B3, OCT1, OCT2, OAT1, OAT3, MATE1, or MATE2K at clinically relevant concentrations.

13 NONCLINICAL TOXICOLOGY

13.1 Carcinogenesis, Mutagenesis, Impairment of Fertility

Carcinogenicity studies have not been conducted with venetoclax.

Venetoclax was not mutagenic in an *in vitro* bacterial mutagenicity (Ames) assay, did not induce numerical or structural aberrations in an *in vitro* chromosome aberration assay using human peripheral blood lymphocytes, and was not clastogenic in an *in vivo* mouse bone marrow micronucleus assay at doses up to 835 mg/kg. The M27 metabolite was negative for genotoxic activity in *in vitro* Ames and chromosome aberration assays.

Fertility and early embryonic development studies were conducted in male and female mice. These studies evaluate mating, fertilization, and embryonic development through implantation. There were no effects of venetoclax on estrus cycles, mating, fertility, corpora lutea, uterine implants or live embryos per litter at dosages up to 600 mg/kg/day. However, a risk to human male fertility exists based on testicular toxicity (germ cell loss) observed in dogs at exposures as low as 0.5 times the human AUC exposure at the recommend dose.

13.2 Animal Toxicology and/or Pharmacology

In dogs, venetoclax caused single-cell necrosis in various tissues, including the gallbladder, exocrine pancreas, and stomach with no evidence of disruption of tissue integrity or organ dysfunction; these findings were minimal to mild in magnitude. Following a 4-week dosing period and subsequent 4-week recovery period, minimal single-cell necrosis was still present in some tissues and reversibility has not been assessed following longer periods of dosing or recovery. In addition, after approximately 3 months of daily dosing in dogs, venetoclax caused progressive white discoloration of the hair coat, due to loss of melanin pigment.

14 CLINICAL STUDIES

The efficacy of VENCLEXTA was established in an open-label, single-arm, multicenter clinical trial of 106 patients with CLL with 17p deletion who had received at least one prior therapy. In the study, 17p deletion was confirmed in peripheral blood specimens from patients using Vysis CLL FISH Probe Kit, which is FDA approved for selection of patients for VENCLEXTA treatment. Patients received VENCLEXTA via a weekly ramp-up schedule starting at 20 mg and ramping to 50 mg, 100 mg, 200 mg and finally 400 mg once daily. Patients continued to receive 400 mg of VENCLEXTA orally once daily until disease progression or unacceptable toxicity.

The efficacy of VENCLEXTA was evaluated by overall response rate (ORR) as assessed by an Independent Review Committee (IRC) using the International Workshop for Chronic Lymphocytic Leukemia (IWCLL) updated National Cancer Institute-sponsored Working Group (NCI-WG) guidelines (2008).

Table 9 summarizes the baseline demographic and disease characteristics of the study population.

Table 9. Baseline Patient Characteristics

Characteristics	N = 106
Age, years; median (range)	67 (37-83)
White; %	97.1
Male; %	65.1
ECOG performance status; % 0	39.6
1	51.9
2	8.5
Tumor burden; % Absolute lymphocyte count $\geq 25 \times 10^9$/L	50.0
One or more nodes ≥ 5 cm	52.8
Number of prior therapies; median (range)	2.5 (1-10)
Time since diagnosis, months; median (range)[a]	79.4 (1.2-385.6)

[a]N=105.

The median time on treatment at the time of evaluation was 12.1 months (range: 0 to 21.5 months). Efficacy results are shown in Table 10.

Table 10. Efficacy Results for Patients with Previously Treated CLL with 17p Deletion by IRC

	VENCLEXTA N=106
ORR, n (%) (95% CI)	85 (80.2) (71.3, 87.3)
CR + CRi, n (%) CR, n (%) CRi, n (%)	8 (7.5) 6 (5.7) 2 (1.9)
nPR, n (%)	3 (2.8)
PR, n (%)	74 (69.8)

CI = confidence interval; CR = complete remission; CRi = complete remission with incomplete marrow recovery; IRC = independent review committee; nPR = nodular partial remission; ORR = overall response rate (CR + CRi + nPR + PR); PR = partial remission.

The median time to first response was 0.8 months (range: 0.1 to 8.1 months). Median duration of response (DOR) has not been reached with approximately 12 months median follow-up. The DOR ranged from 2.9 to 19.0+ months.

Minimal residual disease (MRD) was evaluated in peripheral blood and bone marrow for patients who achieved CR or CRi, following treatment with VENCLEXTA. Three percent (3/106) were MRD negative in the peripheral blood and bone marrow (less than one CLL cell per 10^4 leukocytes).

16 HOW SUPPLIED/STORAGE AND HANDLING

VENCLEXTA is dispensed as follows:

Packaging Presentation	Number of Tablets	National Drug Code (NDC)
Starting Pack	Each pack contains four weekly wallet blister packs: • Week 1 (14 × 10 mg tablets) • Week 2 (7 × 50 mg tablets) • Week 3 (7 × 100 mg tablets) • Week 4 (14 × 100 mg tablets)	0074-0579-28
10 mg Wallet	14 × 10 mg tablets	0074-0561-14
50 mg Wallet	7 × 50 mg tablets	0074-0566-07
10 mg Unit Dose	2 × 10 mg tablets	0074-0561-11
50 mg Unit Dose	1 × 50 mg tablet	0074-0566-11
100 mg Unit Dose	1 × 100 mg tablet	0074-0576-11
100 mg Bottle	120 × 100 mg tablets	0074-0576-22

VENCLEXTA 10 mg film-coated tablets are round, biconvex shaped, pale yellow debossed with "V" on one side and "10" on the other side.

VENCLEXTA 50 mg film-coated tablets are oblong, biconvex shaped, beige debossed with "V" on one side and "50" on the other side.

VENCLEXTA 100 mg film-coated tablets are oblong, biconvex shaped, pale yellow debossed with "V" on one side and "100" on the other side.

Store at or below 86°F (30°C).

17 PATIENT COUNSELING INFORMATION

Advise the patient to read the FDA-approved patient labeling (Medication Guide).

• **Tumor Lysis Syndrome**

Advise patients of the potential risk of TLS, particularly at treatment initiation and during ramp-up phase, and to immediately report any signs and symptoms associated with this event (fever, chills, nausea, vomiting, confusion, shortness of breath, seizure, irregular heartbeat, dark or cloudy urine, unusual tiredness, muscle pain, and/or joint discomfort) to their doctor for evaluation *[see Warnings and Precautions (5.1)]*.

Advise patients to be adequately hydrated every day when taking VENCLEXTA to reduce the risk of TLS. The recommended volume is 6 to 8 glasses (approximately 56 ounces total) of water each day. Patients should drink water starting 2 days before and on the day of the first dose, and every time the dose is increased *[see Dosage and Administration (2.3)]*.

Advise patients of the importance of keeping scheduled appointments for blood work or other laboratory tests *[see Dosage and Administration (2.3)]*.

Advise patients that it may be necessary to take VENCLEXTA in the presence of a doctor to allow monitoring for TLS.

• **Neutropenia**

Advise patients to contact their doctor immediately if they develop a fever or any signs of infection. Advise patients of the need for periodic monitoring of blood counts *[see Warnings and Precautions (5.2)]*.

• **Drug Interactions**

Advise patients to avoid consuming grapefruit products, Seville oranges, or starfruit during treatment with VENCLEXTA. Advise patients that VENCLEXTA may interact with some drugs; therefore, advise patients to inform their doctor of the use of any prescription medication, over-the-counter drugs, vitamins and herbal products *[see Contraindications (4) and Drug Interactions (7.1)]*.

• **Immunizations**

Advise patients to avoid vaccination with live vaccines because they may not be safe or effective during treatment with VENCLEXTA *[see Warnings and Precautions (5.3)]*.

• **Pregnancy and Lactation**

Advise women of the potential risk to the fetus and to avoid pregnancy during treatment with VENCLEXTA. Advise female patients of reproductive potential to use effective contraception during therapy and for at least 30 days after completing of therapy. Advise females to contact their doctor if they become pregnant, or if pregnancy is suspected, during treatment with VENCLEXTA. Also advise patients not to breastfeed while taking VENCLEXTA *[see Warnings and Precautions (5.4), and Use in Specific Populations (8.1, 8.2, and 8.3)]*.

• **Male Infertility**

Advise patients of the possibility of infertility and possible use of sperm banking for males of reproductive potential *[see Use in Specific Populations (8.3)]*.

Instructions for Taking VENCLEXTA

Advise patients to take VENCLEXTA exactly as prescribed and not to change their dose or to stop taking VENCLEXTA unless they are told to do so by their doctor. Advise patients to take VENCLEXTA orally once daily, at approximately the same time each day, according to their doctor's instructions and that the tablets should be swallowed whole with a meal and water without being chewed, crushed, or broken *[see Dosage and Administration (2.2)]*.

Advise patients to keep VENCLEXTA in the original packaging during the first 4 weeks of treatment, and not to transfer the tablets to a different container.

Advise patients that if a dose of VENCLEXTA is missed by less than 8 hours, to take the missed dose right away and take the next dose as usual. If a dose of VENCLEXTA is missed by more than 8 hours, advise patients to wait and take the next dose at the usual time *[see Dosage and Administration (2.6)]*.

Advise patients not to take any additional dose that day if they vomit after taking VENCLEXTA, and to take the next dose at the usual time the following day.

Manufactured and Marketed by:
AbbVie Inc.
North Chicago, IL 60064
and
Marketed by:
Genentech USA, Inc.
A Member of the Roche Group
South San Francisco, CA 94080-4990
© 2016 AbbVie Inc.
© 2016 Genentech, Inc.
03-B232 April 2016

MEDICATION GUIDE
VENCLEXTA™ (ven-KLEKS-tuh)
(venetoclax)
tablets

What is the most important information I should know about VENCLEXTA?
VENCLEXTA can cause serious side effects, including:
Tumor lysis syndrome (TLS). TLS is caused by the fast breakdown of cancer cells. TLS can cause kidney failure, the need for dialysis treatment, and may lead to death. Your doctor will do tests to check your risk of getting TLS before you start taking VENCLEXTA. You will receive other medicines before starting and during treatment with VENCLEXTA to help reduce your risk of TLS. You may also need to receive intravenous (IV) fluids into your vein. Your doctor will do blood tests in your first 5 weeks of treatment to check you for TLS during treatment with VENCLEXTA. It is important to keep your appointments for blood tests. Tell your doctor right away if you have any symptoms of TLS during treatment with VENCLEXTA, including:

- fever
- chills
- nausea
- vomiting
- confusion
- shortness of breath
- seizures
- irregular heartbeat
- dark or cloudy urine
- unusual tiredness
- muscle or joint pain

Drink plenty of water when taking VENCLEXTA to help reduce your risk of getting TLS. Drink 6 to 8 glasses (about 56 ounces total) of water each day, starting 2 days before your first dose, on the day of your first dose of VENCLEXTA, and each time your dose is increased. Your doctor may delay, decrease your dose, or stop treatment with VENCLEXTA if you have side effects. See "What are the possible side effects of VENCLEXTA?" for more information about side effects.

What is VENCLEXTA?
VENCLEXTA is a prescription medicine used to treat people with chronic lymphocytic leukemia (CLL) with 17p deletion, who have received at least one prior treatment. It is not known if VENCLEXTA is safe and effective in children.

Who should not take VENCLEXTA? Certain medicines must not be taken when you first start taking VENCLEXTA and while your dose is being slowly increased.
- Tell your doctor about all the medicines you take, including prescription and over-the-counter medicines, vitamins, and herbal supplements. VENCLEXTA and other medicines may affect each other causing serious side effects.
- Do not start new medicines during treatment with VENCLEXTA without first talking with your doctor.

What should I tell my doctor before taking VENCLEXTA?
Before taking VENCLEXTA, tell your doctor about all of your medical conditions, including if you:
- have kidney or liver problems
- have problems with your body salts or electrolytes, such as potassium, phosphorus, or calcium
- have a history of high uric acid levels in your blood or gout
- are scheduled to receive a vaccine. You should not receive a "live vaccine" before, during, or after treatment with VENCLEXTA, until your doctor tells you it is okay. If you are not sure about the type of immunization or vaccine, ask your doctor. These vaccines may not be safe or may not work as well during treatment with VENCLEXTA.
- are pregnant or plan to become pregnant. VENCLEXTA may harm your unborn baby. If you are able to become pregnant, your doctor should do a pregnancy test before you start treatment with VENCLEXTA. Females who are able to become pregnant should use effective birth control during treatment and for 30 days after the last dose of VENCLEXTA. If you become pregnant or think you are pregnant, tell your doctor right away.
- are breastfeeding or plan to breastfeed. It is not known if VENCLEXTA passes into your breast milk. Do not breastfeed during treatment with VENCLEXTA.

Tell your doctor about all the medicines you take, including prescription and over-the-counter medicines, vitamins, and herbal supplements. VENCLEXTA and other medicines may affect each other causing serious side effects. See "Who should not take VENCLEXTA?"

How should I take VENCLEXTA?
- Take VENCLEXTA exactly as your doctor tells you to take it. Do not change your dose of VENCLEXTA or stop taking VENCLEXTA unless your doctor tells you to.
- When you first take VENCLEXTA:
  - You may need to take VENCLEXTA at the hospital or clinic to monitor for TLS.
  - Your doctor will start VENCLEXTA at a low dose. Your dose will be slowly increased weekly over 5 weeks up to the full dose. Read the Quick Start Guide that comes with VENCLEXTA before your first dose.
- Follow the instructions about drinking water described in the section of this Medication Guide about TLS called "What is the most important information I should know about VENCLEXTA?" and also in the Quick Start Guide.
- Take VENCLEXTA 1 time a day with a meal and water at about the same time each day.
- Swallow VENCLEXTA tablets whole. Do not chew, crush, or break the tablets.
- If you miss a dose of VENCLEXTA and it has been less than 8 hours, take your dose as soon as possible. If you miss a dose of VENCLEXTA and it has been more than 8 hours, skip the missed dose and take the next dose at your usual time.
- If you vomit after taking VENCLEXTA, do not take an extra dose. Take the next dose at your usual time the next day.

What should I avoid while taking VENCLEXTA?
- You should not drink grapefruit juice, eat grapefruit, Seville oranges (often used in marmalades), or starfruit while you are taking VENCLEXTA. These products may increase the amount of VENCLEXTA in your blood.

What are the possible side effects of VENCLEXTA?
VENCLEXTA can cause serious side effects, including:
- See "What is the most important information I should know about VENCLEXTA?"
- **Low white blood cell count (neutropenia).** Low white blood cell counts are common with VENCLEXTA, but can also be severe. Your doctor will do blood tests to check your blood counts during treatment with VENCLEXTA. Tell your doctor right away if you have a fever or any signs of an infection while taking VENCLEXTA.

The most common side effects of VENCLEXTA include:
- diarrhea
- nausea
- low red blood cell count
- upper respiratory tract infection
- low platelet count
- feeling tired

VENCLEXTA may cause fertility problems in males. This may affect your ability to father a child. Talk to your doctor if you have concerns about fertility.

Tell your doctor if you have any side effect that bothers you or that does not go away.

These are not all the possible side effects of VENCLEXTA. For more information, ask your doctor or pharmacist.

Call your doctor for medical advice about side effects. You may report side effects to FDA at 1-800-FDA-1088.

How should I store VENCLEXTA?
- Store VENCLEXTA at or below 86°F (30°C).
- Keep VENCLEXTA tablets in the original package during the first 4 weeks of treatment. **Do not** transfer the tablets to a pillbox or other container.

Keep VENCLEXTA and all medicines out of reach of children.

General information about the safe and effective use of VENCLEXTA.
Medicines are sometimes prescribed for purposes other than those listed in a Medication Guide. Do not use VENCLEXTA for a condition for which it was not prescribed. Do not give VENCLEXTA to other people, even if they have the same symptoms that you have. It may harm them. You can ask your doctor or pharmacist for information about VENCLEXTA that is written for health professionals.

What are the ingredients in VENCLEXTA?
Active ingredient: venetoclax
Inactive ingredients: copovidone, colloidal silicon dioxide, polysorbate 80, sodium stearyl fumarate, and calcium phosphate dibasic.
The 10 mg and 100 mg coated tablets also include the following: iron oxide yellow, polyvinyl alcohol, polyethylene glycol, talc, titanium dioxide. The 50 mg coated tablets also include the following: iron oxide yellow, iron oxide red, iron oxide black, polyvinyl alcohol, talc, polyethylene glycol, and titanium dioxide.

Manufactured and Marketed by:
AbbVie Inc.
North Chicago, IL 60064
© 2016 AbbVie Inc.
03-B232

Marketed by:
Genentech USA, Inc.
A Member of the Roche Group
South San Francisco, CA 94080-4990
© 2016 Genentech, Inc.

This Medication Guide has been approved by the U.S. Food and Drug Administration.   Issued: 04/2016

Shown in Product Identification Guide, page 506

Continued on next page

VICODIN®
VICODIN ES®
VICODIN HP®
(hydrocodone bitartrate and acetaminophen)
TABLETS, USP

WARNING

> **HEPATOTOXICITY**
> ACETAMINOPHEN HAS BEEN ASSOCIATED WITH CASES OF ACUTE LIVER FAILURE, AT TIMES RESULTING IN LIVER TRANSPLANT AND DEATH. MOST OF THE CASES OF LIVER INJURY ARE ASSOCIATED WITH THE USE OF ACETAMINOPHEN AT DOSES THAT EXCEED 4000 MILLIGRAMS PER DAY, AND OFTEN INVOLVE MORE THAN ONE ACETAMINOPHEN-CONTAINING PRODUCT.

DESCRIPTION
Hydrocodone bitartrate and acetaminophen is supplied in tablet form for oral administration.
WARNING: May be habit-forming (see **PRECAUTIONS, Information for Patients/Caregivers,** and **DRUG ABUSE AND DEPENDENCE**).
Hydrocodone bitartrate is an opioid analgesic and antitussive and occurs as fine, white crystals or as a crystalline powder. It is affected by light. The chemical name is 4,5α-epoxy-3-methoxy-17-methylmorphinan-6-one tartrate (1:1) hydrate (2:5). It has the following structural formula:
Acetaminophen, 4'-hydroxyacetanilide, a slightly bitter, white, odorless, crystalline powder, is a non-opiate, non-salicylate analgesic and antipyretic. It has the following structural formula:

$C_{18}H_{21}NO_3 \cdot C_4H_6O_6 \cdot 2\frac{1}{2}H_2O$ M.W. = 494.490

$C_8H_9NO_2$ M.W. = 151.16

Hydrocodone Bitartrate and Acetaminophen Tablets, USP is available in the following strengths:

VICODIN®: Hydrocodone Bitartrate.................. 5 mg
WARNING: May be habit-forming.
Acetaminophen............................. 300 mg
VICODIN ES®: Hydrocodone Bitartrate............... 7.5 mg
WARNING: May be habit-forming.
Acetaminophen............................. 300 mg
VICODIN HP®: Hydrocodone Bitartrate.................. 10 mg
WARNING: May be habit-forming.
Acetaminophen............................. 300 mg

In addition each tablet contains the following inactive ingredients: colloidal silicon dioxide, crospovidone, magnesium stearate, microcrystalline cellulose, povidone, pregelatinized starch, and stearic acid.

This product complies with USP dissolution test 2.

CLINICAL PHARMACOLOGY

Hydrocodone is a semisynthetic narcotic analgesic and antitussive with multiple actions qualitatively similar to those of codeine. Most of these involve the central nervous system and smooth muscle. The precise mechanism of action of hydrocodone and other opiates is not known, although it is believed to relate to the existence of opiate receptors in the central nervous system. In addition to analgesia, narcotics may produce drowsiness, changes in mood and mental clouding.

The analgesic action of acetaminophen involves peripheral influences, but the specific mechanism is as yet undetermined. Antipyretic activity is mediated through hypothalamic heat regulating centers. Acetaminophen inhibits prostaglandin synthetase. Therapeutic doses of acetaminophen have negligible effects on the cardiovascular or respiratory systems; however, toxic doses may cause circulatory failure and rapid, shallow breathing.

Pharmacokinetics

The behavior of the individual components is described below.

Hydrocodone

Following a 10 mg oral dose of hydrocodone administered to five adult male subjects, the mean peak concentration was 23.6 ± 5.2 ng/mL. Maximum serum levels were achieved at 1.3 ± 0.3 hours and the half-life was determined to be 3.8 ± 0.3 hours. Hydrocodone exhibits a complex pattern of metabolism including O-demethylation, N-demethylation and 6-keto reduction to the corresponding 6-α- and 6-β-hydroxy- metabolites. See **OVERDOSAGE** for toxicity information.

Acetaminophen

Acetaminophen is rapidly absorbed from the gastrointestinal tract and is distributed throughout most body tissues. The plasma half-life is 1.25 to 3 hours, but may be increased by liver damage and following overdosage. Elimination of acetaminophen is principally by liver metabolism (conjugation) and subsequent renal excretion of metabolites. Approximately 85% of an oral dose appears in the urine within 24 hours of administration, most as the glucuronide conjugate, with small amounts of other conjugates and unchanged drug. See **OVERDOSAGE** for toxicity information.

INDICATIONS AND USAGE

Hydrocodone bitartrate and acetaminophen tablets are indicated for the relief of moderate to moderately severe pain.

CONTRAINDICATIONS

This product should not be administered to patients who have previously exhibited hypersensitivity to hydrocodone or acetaminophen.

Patients known to be hypersensitive to other opioids may exhibit cross sensitivity to hydrocodone.

WARNINGS

Hepatotoxicity

Acetaminophen has been associated with cases of acute liver failure, at times resulting in liver transplant and death. Most of the cases of liver injury are associated with the use of acetaminophen at doses that exceed 4000 milligrams per day, and often involve more than one acetaminophen-containing product. The excessive intake of acetaminophen may be intentional to cause self-harm or unintentional as patients attempt to obtain more pain relief or unknowingly take other acetaminophen-containing products.

The risk of acute liver failure is higher in individuals with underlying liver disease and in individuals who ingest alcohol while taking acetaminophen.

Instruct patients to look for acetaminophen or APAP on package labels and not to use more than one product that contains acetaminophen. Instruct patients to seek medical attention immediately upon ingestion of more than 4000 milligrams of acetaminophen per day, even if they feel well.

Serious skin reactions

Rarely, acetaminophen may cause serious skin reactions such as acute generalized exanthematous pustulosis (AGEP), Stevens-Johnson Syndrome (SJS), and toxic epidermal necrolysis (TEN), which can be fatal. Patients should be informed about the signs of serious skin reactions, and use of the drug should be discontinued at the first appearance of skin rash or any other sign of hypersensitivity.

Hypersensitivity/anaphylaxis

There have been post-marketing reports of hypersensitivity and anaphylaxis associated with use of acetaminophen. Clinical signs included swelling of the face, mouth and throat, respiratory distress, urticaria, rash, pruritus, and vomiting. There were infrequent reports of life-threatening anaphylaxis requiring emergency medical attention. Instruct patients to discontinue hydrocodone bitartrate and acetaminophen tablets immediately and seek medical care if they experience these symptoms. Do not prescribe hydrocodone bitartrate and acetaminophen tablets for patients with acetaminophen allergy.

Respiratory Depression

At high doses or in sensitive patients, hydrocodone may produce dose-related respiratory depression by acting directly on the brain stem respiratory center. Hydrocodone also affects the center that controls respiratory rhythm, and may produce irregular and periodic breathing.

Head Injury and Increased Intracranial Pressure

The respiratory depressant effects of narcotics and their capacity to elevate cerebrospinal fluid pressure may be markedly exaggerated in the presence of head injury, other intracranial lesions or a preexisting increase in intracranial pressure. Furthermore, narcotics produce adverse reactions which may obscure the clinical course of patients with head injuries.

Acute Abdominal Conditions

The administration of narcotics may obscure the diagnosis or clinical course of patients with acute abdominal conditions.

PRECAUTIONS

General

Special Risk Patients

As with any narcotic analgesic agent, hydrocodone bitartrate and acetaminophen tablets should be used with caution in elderly or debilitated patients and those with severe impairment of hepatic or renal function, hypothyroidism, Addison's disease, prostatic hypertrophy or urethral stricture. The usual precautions should be observed and the possibility of respiratory depression should be kept in mind.

Cough Reflex

Hydrocodone suppresses the cough reflex; as with all narcotics, caution should be exercised when hydrocodone bitartrate and acetaminophen tablets are used postoperatively and in patients with pulmonary disease.

Information for Patients/Caregivers

- Do not take hydrocodone bitartrate and acetaminophen tablets if you are allergic to any of its ingredients.
- If you develop signs of allergy such as a rash or difficulty breathing stop taking hydrocodone bitartrate and acetaminophen tablets and contact your healthcare provider immediately.
- Do not take more than 4000 milligrams of acetaminophen per day. Call your doctor if you took more than the recommended dose.

Hydrocodone, like all narcotics, may impair the mental and/or physical abilities required for the performance of potentially hazardous tasks such as driving a car or operating machinery; patients should be cautioned accordingly.

Alcohol and other CNS depressants may produce an additive CNS depression, when taken with this combination product, and should be avoided.

Hydrocodone may be habit forming. Patients should take the drug only for as long as it is prescribed, in the amounts prescribed, and no more frequently than prescribed.

Laboratory Tests

In patients with severe hepatic or renal disease, effects of therapy should be monitored with serial liver and/or renal function tests.

Drug Interactions

Patients receiving other narcotics, antihistamines, antipsychotics, antianxiety agents, or other CNS depressants (including alcohol) concomitantly with hydrocodone bitartrate and acetaminophen tablets may exhibit an additive CNS depression. When combined therapy is contemplated, the dose of one or both agents should be reduced.

The use of MAO inhibitors or tricyclic antidepressants with hydrocodone preparations may increase the effect of either the antidepressant or hydrocodone.

Drug/Laboratory Test Interactions

Acetaminophen may produce false-positive test results for urinary 5-hydroxyindoleacetic acid.

Carcinogenesis, Mutagenesis, Impairment of Fertility

No adequate studies have been conducted in animals to determine whether hydrocodone or acetaminophen have a potential for carcinogenesis, mutagenesis, or impairment of fertility.

Pregnancy

Teratogenic Effects

Pregnancy Category C

There are no adequate and well-controlled studies in pregnant women. Hydrocodone bitartrate and acetaminophen tablets should be used during pregnancy only if the potential benefit justifies the potential risk to the fetus.

Nonteratogenic Effects

Babies born to mothers who have been taking opioids regularly prior to delivery will be physically dependent. The withdrawal signs include irritability and excessive crying, tremors, hyperactive reflexes, increased respiratory rate, increased stools, sneezing, yawning, vomiting, and fever. The intensity of the syndrome does not always correlate with the duration of maternal opioid use or dose. There is no consensus on the best method of managing withdrawal.

Labor and Delivery

As with all narcotics, administration of this product to the mother shortly before delivery may result in some degree of respiratory depression in the newborn, especially if higher doses are used.

Nursing Mothers

Acetaminophen is excreted in breast milk in small amounts, but the significance of its effects on nursing infants is not known. It is not known whether hydrocodone is excreted in human milk. Because many drugs are excreted in human milk and because of the potential for serious adverse reactions in nursing infants from hydrocodone and acetaminophen, a decision should be made whether to discontinue nursing or to discontinue the drug, taking into account the importance of the drug to the mother.

Pediatric Use

Safety and effectiveness in pediatric patients have not been established.

Geriatric Use

Clinical studies of hydrocodone bitartrate and acetaminophen tablets did not include sufficient numbers of subjects aged 65 and over to determine whether they respond differently from younger subjects. Other reported clinical experience has not identified differences in responses between the elderly and younger patients. In general, dose selection for an elderly patient should be cautious, usually starting at the low end of the dosing range, reflecting the greater frequency of decreased hepatic, renal, or cardiac function, and of concomitant disease or other drug therapy.

Hydrocodone and the major metabolites of acetaminophen are known to be substantially excreted by the kidney. Thus the risk of toxic reactions may be greater in patients with impaired renal function due to accumulation of the parent compound and/or metabolites in the plasma. Because elderly patients are more likely to have decreased renal function, care should be taken in dose selection, and it may be useful to monitor renal function.

Hydrocodone may cause confusion and over-sedation in the elderly; elderly patients generally should be started on low doses of hydrocodone bitartrate and acetaminophen tablets and observed closely.

ADVERSE REACTIONS

The most frequently reported adverse reactions are light-headedness, dizziness, sedation, nausea and vomiting. These effects seem to be more prominent in ambulatory than in nonambulatory patients, and some of these adverse reactions may be alleviated if the patient lies down.
Other adverse reactions include:

Central Nervous System
Drowsiness, mental clouding, lethargy, impairment of mental and physical performance, anxiety, fear, dysphoria, psychic dependence, mood changes.

Gastrointestinal System
Prolonged administration of hydrocodone bitartrate and acetaminophen tablets may produce constipation.

Genitourinary System
Ureteral spasm, spasm of vesical sphincters and urinary retention have been reported with opiates.

Respiratory Depression
Hydrocodone bitartrate may produce dose-related respiratory depression by acting directly on the brain stem respiratory centers (see **OVERDOSAGE**).

Special Senses
Cases of hearing impairment or permanent loss have been reported predominantly in patients with chronic overdose.

Dermatological
Skin rash, pruritus.
The following adverse drug events may be borne in mind as potential effects of acetaminophen: allergic reactions, rash, thrombocytopenia, agranulocytosis.
Potential effects of high dosage are listed in the **OVERDOSAGE** section.

DRUG ABUSE AND DEPENDENCE

Controlled Substance
Hydrocone bitartrate and acetaminophen tablets is classified as a Schedule III controlled substance.

Abuse and Dependence
Psychic dependence, physical dependence, and tolerance may develop upon repeated administration of narcotics; therefore, this product should be prescribed and administered with caution. However, psychic dependence is unlikely to develop when hydrocodone bitartrate and acetaminophen tablets are used for a short time for the treatment of pain. Physical dependence, the condition in which continued administration of the drug is required to prevent the appearance of a withdrawal syndrome, assumes clinically significant proportions only after several weeks of continued narcotic use, although some mild degree of physical dependence may develop after a few days of narcotic therapy. Tolerance, in which increasingly large doses are required in order to produce the same degree of analgesia, is manifested initially by a shortened duration of analgesic effect, and subsequently by decreases in the intensity of analgesia. The rate of development of tolerance varies among patients.

OVERDOSAGE

Following an acute overdosage, toxicity may result from hydrocodone or acetaminophen.

Signs and Symptoms
Hydrocodone: Serious overdose with hydrocodone is characterized by respiratory depression (a decrease in respiratory rate and/or tidal volume, Cheyne-Stokes respiration, cyanosis), extreme somnolence progressing to stupor or coma, skeletal muscle flaccidity, cold and clammy skin, and sometimes bradycardia and hypotension. In severe overdosage, apnea, circulatory collapse, cardiac arrest and death may occur.

Acetaminophen: In acetaminophen overdosage: dose-dependent, potentially fatal hepatic necrosis is the most serious adverse effect. Renal tubular necrosis, hypoglycemic coma, and coagulation defects may also occur.
Early symptoms following a potentially hepatotoxic overdose may include: nausea, vomiting, diaphoresis and general malaise. Clinical and laboratory evidence of hepatic toxicity may not be apparent until 48 to 72 hours post-ingestion.

Treatment
A single or multiple drug overdose with hydrocodone and acetaminophen is a potentially lethal polydrug overdose, and consultation with a regional poison control center is recommended.

Immediate treatment includes support of cardiorespiratory function and measures to reduce drug absorption.
Oxygen, intravenous fluids, vasopressors, and other supportive measures should be employed as indicated. Assisted or controlled ventilation should also be considered.
For hydrocodone overdose, primary attention should be given to the reestablishment of adequate respiratory exchange through provision of a patent airway and the institution of assisted or controlled ventilation. The narcotic antagonist naloxone hydrochloride is a specific antidote against respiratory depression which may result from overdosage or unusual sensitivity to narcotics, including hydrocodone. Since the duration of action of hydrocodone may exceed that of the antagonist, the patient should be kept under continued surveillance, and repeated doses of the antagonist should be administered as needed to maintain adequate respiration. A narcotic antagonist should not be administered in the absence of clinically significant respiratory or cardiovascular depression.
Gastric decontamination with activated charcoal should be administered just prior to N-acetylcysteine (NAC) to decrease systemic absorption if acetaminophen ingestion is known or suspected to have occurred within a few hours of presentation. Serum acetaminophen levels should be obtained immediately if the patient presents 4 hours or more after ingestion to assess potential risk of hepatotoxicity; acetaminophen levels drawn less than 4 hours post-ingestion may be misleading. To obtain the best possible outcome, NAC should be administered as soon as possible where impending or evolving liver injury is suspected. Intravenous NAC may be administered when circumstances preclude oral administration.
Vigorous supportive therapy is required in severe intoxication. Procedures to limit the continuing absorption of the drug must be readily performed since the hepatic injury is dose dependent and occurs early in the course of intoxication.

DOSAGE AND ADMINISTRATION

Dosage should be adjusted according to the severity of the pain and the response of the patient. However, it should be kept in mind that tolerance to hydrocodone can develop with continued use and that the incidence of untoward effects is dose related.

VICODIN® (Hydrocodone Bitartrate and Acetaminophen Tablets, USP 5 mg/300 mg): The usual adult dosage is one or two tablets every four to six hours as needed for pain. The total daily dosage should not exceed 8 tablets.

VICODIN ES® (Hydrocodone Bitartrate and Acetaminophen Tablets, USP 7.5 mg/300 mg): The usual adult dosage is one tablet every four to six hours as needed for pain. The total daily dosage should not exceed 6 tablets.

VICODIN HP® (Hydrocodone Bitartrate and Acetaminophen Tablets, USP 10 mg/300 mg): The usual adult dosage is one tablet every four to six hours as needed for pain. The total daily dosage should not exceed 6 tablets.

HOW SUPPLIED

VICODIN®, VICODIN ES® and VICODIN HP® (Hydrocodone Bitartrate and Acetaminophen) Tablets, USP are supplied as follows:

VICODIN® 5 mg/300 mg
White, capsule-shaped, bisected tablets, debossed "5" score "300" on one side and "VICODIN" on the other side in bottles of 100 and 500 tablets:
Bottles of 100 - NDC 0074-3041-13
Bottles of 500 - NDC 0074-3041-53

VICODIN ES® 7.5 mg/300 mg
White, capsule-shaped, bisected tablets, debossed "7.5" score "300" on one side and "VICODIN ES" on the other side in bottles of 100 and 500 tablets:
Bottles of 100 - NDC 0074-3043-13
Bottles of 500 - NDC 0074-3043-53

VICODIN HP® 10 mg/300 mg
White, capsule-shaped, bisected tablets, debossed "10" score "300" on one side and "VICODIN HP" on the other side in bottles of 100 and 500 tablets:
Bottles of 100 - NDC 0074-3054-13
Bottles of 500 - NDC 0074-3054-53

STORAGE

Store at 20° to 25°C (68° to 77°F), [See USP Controlled Room Temperature].

PHARMACIST: Dispense in a tight, light-resistant container with a child-resistant closure.
A Schedule III Narcotic

© AbbVie Inc. 2014
Manufactured for
AbbVie Inc.
North Chicago, IL 60064 U.S.A.
Manufactured by:
Mikart, Inc.
Atlanta, GA 30318
Ref. 1122F00 Rev. 08/14 - Rev. August, 2014
Shown in Product Identification Guide, page 506

VICOPROFEN®   ℂℹ ℞
(hydrocodone bitartrate and ibuprofen tablets)
7.5 mg/200 mg

DESCRIPTION

Each VICOPROFEN tablet contains:
Hydrocodone Bitartrate, USP 7.5 mg
Ibuprofen, USP 200 mg
VICOPROFEN is supplied in a fixed combination tablet form for oral administration. VICOPROFEN combines the opioid analgesic agent, hydrocodone bitartrate, with the nonsteroidal anti-inflammatory (NSAID) agent, ibuprofen. Hydrocodone bitartrate is a semisynthetic and centrally acting opioid analgesic. Its chemical name is: 4,5 α-epoxy-3-methoxy-17-methylmorphinan-6-one tartrate (1:1) hydrate (2:5). Its chemical formula is: $C_{18}H_{21}NO_3 \cdot C_4H_6O_6 \cdot 2\frac{1}{2}H_2O$, and the molecular weight is 494.50. Its structural formula is:

Ibuprofen is a nonsteroidal anti-inflammatory agent [nonselective COX inhibitor] with analgesic and antipyretic properties. Its chemical name is: (±)-2-(*p*-isobutylphenyl) propionic acid. Its chemical formula is: $C_{13}H_{18}O_2$, and the molecular weight is: 206.29. Its structural formula is:

Inactive ingredients in VICOPROFEN tablets include: colloidal silicon dioxide, corn starch, croscarmellose sodium, hypromellose, magnesium stearate, microcrystalline cellulose, polyethylene glycol, polysorbate 80, propylene glycol and titanium dioxide.

CLINICAL PHARMACOLOGY

Hydrocodone Component
Hydrocodone is a semisynthetic opioid analgesic and antitussive with multiple actions qualitatively similar to those of codeine. Most of these involve the central nervous system and smooth muscle. The precise mechanism of action of hydrocodone and other opioids is not known, although it is believed to relate to the existence of opiate receptors in the central nervous system. In addition to analgesia, opioids may produce drowsiness, changes in mood, and mental clouding.

Ibuprofen Component
Ibuprofen is a non-steroidal anti-inflammatory agent that possesses analgesic and antipyretic activities. Its mode of action, like that of other NSAIDs, is not completely understood, but may be related to inhibition of cyclooxygenase ac-

Continued on next page

tivity and prostaglandin synthesis. Ibuprofen is a peripherally acting analgesic. Ibuprofen does not have any known effects on opiate receptors.

Pharmacokinetics

Absorption

After oral dosing with the VICOPROFEN tablet, a peak hydrocodone plasma level of 27 ng/mL is achieved at 1.7 hours, and a peak ibuprofen plasma level of 30 mcg/mL is achieved at 1.8 hours. The effect of food on the absorption of either component from the VICOPROFEN tablet has not been established.

Distribution

Ibuprofen is highly protein-bound (99%) like most other non-steroidal anti-inflammatory agents. Although the extent of protein binding of hydrocodone in human plasma has not been definitely determined, structural similarities to related opioid analgesics suggest that hydrocodone is not extensively protein bound. As most agents in the 5-ring morphinan group of semi-synthetic opioids bind plasma protein to a similar degree (range 19% [hydromorphone] to 45% [oxycodone]), hydrocodone is expected to fall within this range.

Metabolism

Hydrocodone exhibits a complex pattern of metabolism, including *O*-demethylation, *N*-demethylation, and 6-keto reduction to the corresponding 6-α-and 6-β-hydroxy metabolites. Hydromorphone, a potent opioid, is formed from the *O*-demethylation of hydrocodone and contributes to the total analgesic effect of hydrocodone. The *O*- and *N*- demethylation processes are mediated by separate P-450 isoenzymes: CYP2D6 and CYP3A4, respectively.

Ibuprofen is present in this product as a racemate, and following absorption it undergoes interconversion in the plasma from the R-isomer to the S-isomer. Both the R- and S- isomers are metabolized to two primary metabolites: (+)-2-4′-(2hydroxy-2-methyl-propyl) phenyl propionic acid and (+)-2-4′-(2carboxypropyl) phenyl propionic acid, both of which circulate in the plasma at low levels relative to the parent.

Elimination

Hydrocodone and its metabolites are eliminated primarily in the kidneys, with a mean plasma half-life of 4.5 hours. Ibuprofen is excreted in the urine, 50% to 60% as metabolites and approximately 15% as unchanged drug and conjugate. The plasma half-life is 2.2 hours.

Special Populations

No significant pharmacokinetic differences based on age or gender have been demonstrated. The pharmacokinetics of hydrocodone and ibuprofen from VICOPROFEN has not been evaluated in children.

Renal Impairment

The effect of renal insufficiency on the pharmacokinetics of the VICOPROFEN dosage form has not been determined.

CLINICAL STUDIES

In single-dose studies of post surgical pain (abdominal, gynecological, orthopedic), 940 patients were studied at doses of one or two tablets. VICOPROFEN produced greater efficacy than placebo and each of its individual components given at the same dose. No advantage was demonstrated for the two-tablet dose.

INDICATIONS AND USAGE

Carefully consider the potential benefits and risks of VICOPROFEN and other treatment options before deciding to use VICOPROFEN. Use the lowest effective dose for the shortest duration consistent with individual patient treatment goals (see **WARNINGS**).

VICOPROFEN tablets are indicated for the short-term (generally less than 10 days) management of acute pain. VICOPROFEN is not indicated for the treatment of such conditions as osteoarthritis or rheumatoid arthritis.

CONTRAINDICATIONS

VICOPROFEN is contraindicated in patients with known hypersensitivity to hydrocodone or ibuprofen. Patients known to be hypersensitive to other opioids may exhibit cross-sensitivity to hydrocodone.

VICOPROFEN should not be given to patients who have experienced asthma, urticaria, or allergic-type reactions after taking aspirin or other NSAIDs. Severe, rarely fatal, anaphylactic-like reactions to NSAIDs have been reported in such patients (see **WARNINGS – Anaphylactoid Reactions**, and **PRECAUTIONS - Preexisting Asthma**).

VICOPROFEN is contraindicated for the treatment of perioperative pain in the setting of coronary artery bypass graft (CABG) surgery (see **WARNINGS**).

WARNINGS

CARDIOVASCULAR EFFECTS

Cardiovascular Thrombotic Events

Clinical trials of several COX-2 selective and nonselective NSAIDs of up to three years duration have shown an increased risk of serious cardiovascular (CV) thrombotic events, myocardial infarction, and stroke, which can be fatal. All NSAIDs, both COX-2 selective and nonselective, may have a similar risk. Patients with known CV disease or risk factors for CV disease may be at greater risk. To minimize the potential risk for an adverse CV event in patients treated with an NSAID, the lowest effective dose should be used for the shortest duration possible. Physicians and patients should remain alert for the development of such events, even in the absence of previous CV symptoms. Patients should be informed about the signs and/or symptoms of serious CV events and the steps to take if they occur.

There is no consistent evidence that concurrent use of aspirin mitigates the increased risk of serious CV thrombotic events associated with NSAID use. The concurrent use of aspirin and an NSAID does increase the risk of serious GI events (see **GI WARNINGS**).

Two large, controlled, clinical trials of a COX-2 selective NSAID for the treatment of pain in the first 10-14 days following CABG surgery found an increased incidence of myocardial infarction and stroke (see **CONTRAINDICATIONS**).

Hypertension

NSAID-containing products, including VICOPROFEN, can lead to onset of new hypertension or worsening of preexisting hypertension, either of which may contribute to the increased incidence of CV events. Patients taking thiazides or loop diuretics may have impaired response to these therapies when taking NSAIDs. NSAID-containing products, including VICOPROFEN, should be used with caution in patients with hypertension. Blood pressure (BP) should be monitored closely during the initiation of NSAID treatment and throughout the course of therapy.

Congestive Heart Failure and Edema

Fluid retention and edema have been observed in some patients taking NSAIDs. VICOPROFEN should be used with caution in patients with fluid retention or heart failure.

Misuse Abuse and Diversion of Opioids

VICOPROFEN contains hydrocodone an opioid agonist, and is a Schedule II controlled substance. Opioid agonists have the potential for being abused and are sought by abusers and people with addiction disorders, and are subject to diversion.

VICOPROFEN can be abused in a manner similar to other opioid agonists, legal or illicit. This should be considered when prescribing or dispensing VICOPROFEN in situations where the physician or pharmacist is concerned about an increased risk of misuse, abuse or diversion (see **DRUG ABUSE AND DEPENDENCE**).

Respiratory Depression

At high doses or in opioid-sensitive patients, hydrocodone may produce dose-related respiratory depression by acting directly on the brain stem respiratory centers. Hydrocodone also affects the center that controls respiratory rhythm, and may produce irregular and periodic breathing.

Head Injury and Increased Intracranial Pressure

The respiratory depressant effects of opioids and their capacity to elevate cerebrospinal fluid pressure may be markedly exaggerated in the presence of head injury, intracranial lesions or a pre-existing increase in intracranial pressure. Furthermore, opioids produce adverse reactions, which may obscure the clinical course of patients with head injuries.

Acute Abdominal Conditions

The administration of opioids may obscure the diagnosis or clinical course of patients with acute abdominal conditions.

Gastrointestinal (GI) Effects - Risk of GI Ulceration, Bleeding and Perforation

NSAIDs, including VICOPROFEN, can cause serious gastrointestinal (GI) adverse events including inflammation, bleeding, ulceration, and perforation of the stomach, small intestine, or large intestine, which can be fatal. These serious adverse events can occur at any time, with or without warning symptoms, in patients treated with NSAIDs. Only one in five patients who develops a serious upper GI adverse event on NSAID therapy, is symptomatic. Upper GI ulcers, gross bleeding, or perforation caused by NSAIDs occur in approximately 1% of patients treated for 3-6 months, and in about 2-4% of patients treated for one year. These trends continue with longer duration of use, increasing the likelihood of developing a serious GI event at some time during the course of therapy. However, even short-term therapy is not without risk.

NSAIDs should be prescribed with extreme caution in those with a prior history of ulcer disease or gastrointestinal bleeding. Patients with a *prior history of peptic ulcer disease and/or gastrointestinal bleeding who* use NSAIDs have a greater than 10-fold increased risk for developing a GI bleed compared to patients with neither of these risk factors. Other factors that increase the risk for GI bleeding in patients treated with NSAIDs include concomitant use of oral corticosteroids or anticoagulants, longer duration of NSAID therapy, smoking, use of alcohol, older age, and poor general health status. Most spontaneous reports of fatal GI events are in elderly or debilitated patients and therefore, special care should be taken in treating this population.

To minimize the potential risk for an adverse GI event in patients treated with an NSAID, the lowest effective dose should be used for the shortest possible duration. Patients and physicians should remain alert for signs and symptoms of GI ulceration and bleeding during NSAID therapy and promptly initiate additional evaluation and treatment if a serious GI adverse event is suspected. This should include discontinuation of the NSAID until a serious GI adverse event is ruled out. For high-risk patients, alternate therapies that do not involve NSAIDs should be considered.

Renal Effects

Long-term administration of NSAIDs has resulted in renal papillary necrosis and other renal injury. Renal toxicity has also been seen in patients in whom renal prostaglandins have a compensatory role in the maintenance of renal perfusion. In these patients, administration of a nonsteroidal anti-inflammatory drug may cause a dose-dependent reduction in prostaglandin formation and, secondarily, in renal blood flow, which may precipitate overt renal decompensation. Patients at greatest risk of this reaction are those with impaired renal function, heart failure, liver dysfunction, those taking diuretics and ACE inhibitors, and the elderly. Discontinuation of NSAID therapy is usually followed by recovery to the pretreatment state.

Advanced Renal Disease

No information is available from controlled clinical studies regarding the use of VICOPROFEN in patients with advanced renal disease. Therefore, treatment with VICOPROFEN is not recommended in patients with advanced renal disease. If VICOPROFEN therapy must be initiated, close monitoring of the patient's renal function is advisable.

Anaphylactoid Reactions

As with other NSAID-containing products, anaphylactoid reactions may occur in patients without known prior exposure to VICOPROFEN. VICOPROFEN should not be given to patients with the aspirin triad. This symptom complex typically occurs in asthmatic patients who experience rhinitis with or without nasal polyps, or who exhibit severe, potentially fatal bronchospasm after taking aspirin or other NSAIDs. Fatal reactions to NSAIDs have been reported in such patients (see **CONTRAINDICATIONS** and **PRECAUTIONS** - Pre-existing Asthma). Emergency help should be sought in cases where an anaphylactoid reaction occurs.

Skin Reactions

Products containing NSAIDs, including VICOPROFEN, can cause serious skin adverse events such as exfoliative dermatitis, Stevens-Johnson Syndrome (SJS), and toxic epidermal necrolysis (TEN), which can be fatal. These serious events may occur without warning. Patients should be informed about the signs and symptoms of serious skin manifestations and use of the drug should be discontinued at the first appearance of skin rash or any other sign of hypersensitivity.

Pregnancy

As with other NSAID-containing products, VICOPROFEN should be avoided in late pregnancy because it may cause premature closure of the ductus arteriosus.

PRECAUTIONS

General

VICOPROFEN cannot be expected to substitute for corticosteroids or to treat corticosteroid insufficiency. Abrupt discontinuation of corticosteroids may lead to disease exacerbation. Patients on prolonged corticosteroid therapy should have their therapy tapered slowly if a decision is made to discontinue corticosteroids.

The pharmacological activity of VICOPROFEN in reducing fever and inflammation may diminish the utility of these diagnostic signs in detecting complications of presumed noninfectious, painful conditions.

Special Risk Patients

As with any opioid analgesic agent, VICOPROFEN tablets should be used with caution in elderly or debilitated patients, and those with severe impairment of hepatic or renal function, hypothyroidism, Addison's disease, prostatic hypertrophy or urethral stricture. The usual precautions should be observed and the possibility of respiratory depression should be kept in mind.

Cough Reflex

Hydrocodone suppresses the cough reflex; as with opioids, caution should be exercised when VICOPROFEN is used postoperatively and in patients with pulmonary disease.

Hepatic Effects

Borderline elevations of one or more liver enzymes may occur in up to 15% of patients taking NSAIDs including ibuprofen as found in VICOPROFEN. These laboratory abnormalities may progress, may remain essentially unchanged, or may be transient with continued therapy. Notable elevations of SGPT (ALT) or SGOT (AST) (approximately three or more times the upper limit of normal) have been reported in approximately 1% of patients in clinical trials with NSAIDS. In addition, rare cases of severe hepatic reactions, including jaundice and fatal fulminant hepatitis, liver necrosis and hepatic failure, some of them with fatal outcomes have been reported.

A patient with symptoms and/or signs suggesting liver dysfunction, or in whom an abnormal liver test has occurred, should be evaluated for evidence of the development of more severe hepatic reactions while on VICOPROFEN therapy. If clinical signs and symptoms consistent with liver disease develop, or if systemic manifestations occur (e.g., eosinophilia, rash, etc.), VICOPROFEN should be discontinued.

Hematological Effects

Anemia is sometimes seen in patients receiving NSAIDs including ibuprofen as found in VICOPROFEN. This may be due to fluid retention, occult or gross GI blood loss, or an incompletely described effect upon erythropoiesis. Patients on long-term treatment with NSAIDs including ibuprofen, should have their hemoglobin or hematocrit checked if they exhibit any signs or symptoms of anemia.

NSAIDs inhibit platelet aggregation and have been shown to prolong bleeding time in some patients. Unlike aspirin, their effect on platelet function is quantitatively less, of shorter duration, and reversible. Patients receiving VICOPROFEN who may be adversely affected by alterations in platelet function, such as those with coagulation disorders or patients receiving anticoagulants, should be carefully monitored.

Pre-existing Asthma

Patients with asthma may have aspirin-sensitive asthma. The use of aspirin in patients with aspirin-sensitive asthma has been associated with severe bronchospasm, which may be fatal. Since cross-reactivity between aspirin and other NSAIDs has been reported in such aspirin-sensitive patients, VICOPROFEN should not be administered to patients with this form of aspirin sensitivity and should be used with caution in patients with pre-existing asthma.

Aseptic Meningitis

Aseptic meningitis with fever and coma has been observed on rare occasions in patients on ibuprofen therapy as found in VICOPROFEN. Although it is probably more likely to occur in patients with systemic lupus erythematosus and related connective tissue diseases, it has been reported in patients who do not have an underlying chronic disease. If signs or symptoms of meningitis develop in a patient on VICOPROFEN, the possibility of its being related to ibuprofen should be considered.

Information for Patients

Patients should be informed of the following information before initiating therapy with an NSAID and periodically during the course of ongoing therapy. Patients should also be encouraged to read the NSAID Medication Guide that accompanies each prescription dispensed.

1. VICOPROFEN® (hydrocodone bitartrate 7.5 mg and ibuprofen 200 mg), like other opioid-containing analgesics, may impair mental and/or physical abilities required for the performance of potentially hazardous tasks such as driving a car or operating machinery; patients should be cautioned accordingly.
2. Alcohol and other CNS depressants may produce an additive CNS depression, when taken with this combination product, and should be avoided.
3. VICOPROFEN can be abused in a manner similar to other opioid agonists, legal or illicit. VICOPROFEN may be habit-forming. Patients should take the drug only for as long as it is prescribed, in the amounts prescribed, and no more frequently than prescribed.
4. VICOPROFEN, like other NSAID-containing products, may cause serious CV side effects, such as MI or stroke, which may result in hospitalization and even death. Although serious CV events can occur without warning symptoms, patients should be alert for the signs and symptoms of chest pain, shortness of breath, weakness, slurring of speech, and should ask for medical advice when observing any indicative sign or symptoms. Patients should be apprised of the importance of this follow-up (see **WARNINGS, Cardiovascular Effects**).
5. VICOPROFEN, like other NSAID-containing products, can cause GI discomfort and serious GI side effects, such as ulcers and bleeding, which may result in hospitalization and even death. Although serious GI tract ulcerations and bleeding can occur without warning symptoms, patients should be alert for the signs and symptoms of ulcerations and bleeding, and should ask for medical advice when observing any indicative sign or symptoms including epigastric pain, dyspepsia, melena, and hematemesis. Patients should be apprised of the importance of this follow-up (see **WARNINGS, Gastrointestinal Effects: Risk of Ulceration, Bleeding, and Perforation**).
6. VICOPROFEN, like other NSAID-containing products, can cause serious skin side effects such as exfoliative dermatitis, SJS, and TEN, which may result in hospitalizations and even death. Although serious skin reactions may occur without warning, patients should be alert for the signs and symptoms of skin rash and blisters, fever, or other signs of hypersensitivity such as itching, and should ask for medical advice when observing any indicative signs or symptoms. Patients should be advised to stop the drug immediately if they develop any type of rash and contact their physicians as soon as possible.
7. Patients should promptly report signs or symptoms of unexplained weight gain or edema to their physicians.
8. Patients should be informed of the warning signs and symptoms of hepatotoxicity (e.g., nausea, fatigue, lethargy, pruritus, jaundice, right upper quadrant tenderness, and "flu-like" symptoms). If these occur, patients should be instructed to stop therapy and seek immediate medical therapy.
9. Patients should be informed of the signs of an anaphylactoid reaction (e.g., difficulty breathing, swelling of the face or throat). If these occur, patients should be instructed to seek immediate emergency help (see **WARNINGS**).
10. In late pregnancy, as with other NSAIDs, VICOPROFEN should be avoided because it may cause premature closure of the ductus arteriosus.
11. Patients should be instructed to report any signs of blurred vision or other eye symptoms.

Laboratory Tests

Because serious GI tract ulcerations and bleeding can occur without warning symptoms, physicians should monitor for signs or symptoms of GI bleeding. Patients on long-term treatment with NSAIDs should have their CBC and a chemistry profile checked periodically. If clinical signs and symptoms consistent with liver or renal disease develop, systemic manifestations occur (e.g., eosinophilia, rash, etc.) or if abnormal liver tests persist or worsen, VICOPROFEN should be discontinued.

Drug Interactions

ACE-inhibitors

Reports suggest that NSAIDs may diminish the antihypertensive effect of ACE-inhibitors. This interaction should be given consideration in patients taking VICOPROFEN concomitantly with ACE-inhibitors.

Anticholinergics

The concurrent use of anticholinergics with hydrocodone preparations may produce paralytic ileus.

Antidepressants

The use of Monoamine Oxidase Inhibitors (MAOIs) or tricyclic antidepressants with VICOPROFEN may increase the effect of either the antidepressant or hydrocodone.

MAOIs have been reported to intensify the effects of at least one opioid drug causing anxiety, confusion and significant depression of respiration or coma. The use of hydrocodone is not recommended for patients taking MAOIs or within 14 days of stopping such treatment.

Aspirin

When VICOPROFEN is administered with aspirin, the protein binding of aspirin is reduced, although the clearance of free VICOPROFEN is not altered. The clinical significance of this interaction is not known; however, as with other NSAID-containing products, concomitant administration of VICOPROFEN and aspirin is not generally recommended because of the potential of increased adverse effects.

CNS Depressants

Patients receiving other opioids, antihistamines, antipsychotics, antianxiety agents, or other CNS depressants (including alcohol) concomitantly with VICOPROFEN may exhibit an additive CNS depression. When combined therapy is contemplated, the dose of one or both agents should be reduced.

Diuretics

Ibuprofen has been shown to reduce the natriuretic effect of furosemide and thiazides in some patients. This response has been attributed to inhibition of renal prostaglandin synthesis. During concomitant therapy with VICOPROFEN the patient should be observed closely for signs of renal failure (see **WARNINGS** - Renal Effects), as well as diuretic efficacy.

Lithium

Ibuprofen has been shown to elevate plasma lithium concentration and reduce renal lithium clearance. The mean minimum lithium concentration increased 15% and the renal clearance was decreased by approximately 20%. This effect has been attributed to inhibition of renal prostaglandin synthesis by ibuprofen. Thus, when VICOPROFEN and lithium are administered concurrently, patients should be observed for signs of lithium toxicity.

Methotrexate

Ibuprofen, as well as other NSAIDs, has been reported to competitively inhibit methotrexate accumulation in rabbit kidney slices. This may indicate that ibuprofen could enhance the toxicity of methotrexate. Caution should be used when VICOPROFEN is administered concomitantly with methotrexate.

Mixed Agonist/Antagonist Opioid Analgesics

Agonist/antagonist analgesics (i.e., pentazocine, nalbuphine, butorphanol and buprenorphine) should be administered with caution to patients who have received or are receiving a course of therapy with a pure opioid agonist analgesic such as hydrocodone. In this situation, mixed agonist/antagonist analgesics may reduce the analgesic effect of hydrocodone and/or may precipitate withdrawal symptoms in these patients.

Neuromuscular Blocking Agents

Hydrocodone, as well as other opioid analgesics, may enhance the neuromuscular blocking action of skeletal muscle relaxants and produce an increased degree of respiratory depression.

Warfarin

The effects of warfarin and NSAIDs on GI bleeding are synergistic, such that users of both drugs together have a risk of serious GI bleeding higher than users of either drug alone.

Carcinogenicity, Mutagenicity, and Impairment of Fertility

The carcinogenic and mutagenic potential of VICOPROFEN has not been investigated. The ability of VICOPROFEN to impair fertility has not been assessed.

Pregnancy

Pregnancy Category C.

Teratogenic Effects

Reproductive studies conducted in rats and rabbits have not demonstrated evidence of developmental abnormalities.

VICOPROFEN, administered to rabbits at 95 mg/kg (5.72 and 1.9 times the maximum clinical dose based on body weight and surface area, respectively), a maternally toxic dose, resulted in an increase in the percentage of litters and fetuses with any major abnormality and an increase in the number of litters and fetuses with one or more nonossified metacarpals (a minor abnormality). VICOPROFEN, administered to rats at 166 mg/kg (10.0 and 1.66 times the maximum clinical dose based on body weight and surface area, respectively), a maternally toxic dose, did not result in any reproductive toxicity. However, animal reproduction studies are not always predictive of human response. There are no adequate and well-controlled studies in pregnant women. VICOPROFEN should be used during pregnancy only if the potential benefit justifies the potential risk to the fetus.

Nonteratogenic Effects

Because of the known effects of nonsteroidal antiinflammatory drugs on the fetal cardiovascular system (closure of the ductus arteriosus), use during pregnancy (par-

Continued on next page

Information on the AbbVie, Inc. products listed on these pages is from the prescribing information in use as of July 31, 2016. For more information, please visit rxabbvie.com or call 1-800-633-9110.

ticularly late pregnancy) should be avoided. Babies born to mothers who have been taking opioids regularly prior to delivery will be physically dependent. The withdrawal signs include irritability and excessive crying, tremors, hyperactive reflexes, increased respiratory rate, increased stools, sneezing, yawning, vomiting, and fever. The intensity of the syndrome does not always correlate with the duration of maternal opioid use or dose. There is no consensus on the best method of managing withdrawal.

Labor and Delivery
As with other drugs known to inhibit prostaglandin synthesis, an increased incidence of dystocia and delayed parturition occurred in rats. Administration of VICOPROFEN is not recommended during labor and delivery. The effects of VICOPROFEN on labor and delivery in pregnant women are unknown.

Nursing Mothers
It is not known whether hydrocodone is excreted in human milk. In limited studies, an assay capable of detecting 1 mcg/mL did not demonstrate ibuprofen in the milk of lactating mothers. However, because of the limited nature of the studies, and because of the potential for serious adverse reactions in nursing infants from VICOPROFEN, a decision should be made whether to discontinue nursing or to discontinue the drug, taking into account the importance of the drug to the mother.

Pediatric Use
The safety and effectiveness of VICOPROFEN in pediatric patients below the age of 16 have not been established.

Geriatric Use
In controlled clinical trials there was no difference in tolerability between patients < 65 years of age and those ≥ 65, apart from an increased tendency of the elderly to develop constipation. However, because the elderly may be more sensitive to the renal and gastrointestinal effects of nonsteroidal anti-inflammatory agents as well as possible increased risk of respiratory depression with opioids, extra caution and reduced dosages should be used when treating the elderly with VICOPROFEN.

ADVERSE REACTIONS
VICOPROFEN was administered to approximately 300 pain patients in a safety study that employed dosages and a duration of treatment sufficient to encompass the recommended usage (see **DOSAGE AND ADMINISTRATION**). Adverse event rates generally increased with increasing daily dose. The event rates reported below are from approximately 150 patients who were in a group that received one tablet of VICOPROFEN an average of three to four times daily. The overall incidence rates of adverse experiences in the trials were fairly similar for this patient group and those who received the comparison treatment, acetaminophen 600 mg with codeine 60 mg.

The following lists adverse events that occurred with an incidence of 1% or greater in clinical trials of VICOPROFEN, without regard to the causal relationship of the events to the drug. To distinguish different rates of occurrence in clinical studies, the adverse events are listed as follows:
name of adverse event = less than 3%
*adverse events marked with an asterisk * = 3% to 9%*
adverse event rates over 9% are in parentheses.

Body as a Whole
Abdominal pain*; Asthenia*; Fever; Flu syndrome; Headache (27%); Infection*; Pain.

Cardiovascular
Palpitations; Vasodilation.

Central Nervous System
Anxiety*; Confusion; Dizziness (14%); Hypertonia; Insomnia*; Nervousness*; Paresthesia; Somnolence (22%); Thinking abnormalities.

Digestive
Anorexia; Constipation (22%); Diarrhea*; Dry mouth*; Dyspepsia (12%); Flatulence*; Gastritis; Melena; Mouth ulcers; Nausea (21%); Thirst; Vomiting*.

Metabolic and Nutritional Disorders
Edema*.

Respiratory
Dyspnea; Hiccups; Pharyngitis; Rhinitis.

Skin and Appendages
Pruritus*; Sweating*.

Special Senses
Tinnitus.

Urogenital
Urinary frequency.

Incidence less than 1%
Body as a Whole
Allergic reaction.

Cardiovascular
Arrhythmia; Hypotension; Tachycardia.

Central Nervous System
Agitation; Abnormal dreams; Decreased libido; Depression; Euphoria; Mood changes; Neuralgia; Slurred speech; Tremor, Vertigo.

Digestive
Chalky stool; "Clenching teeth"; Dysphagia; Esophageal spasm; Esophagitis; Gastroenteritis; Glossitis; Liver enzyme elevation.

Metabolic and Nutritional
Weight decrease.

Musculoskeletal
Arthralgia; Myalgia.

Respiratory
Asthma; Bronchitis; Hoarseness; Increased cough; Pulmonary congestion; Pneumonia; Shallow breathing; Sinusitis.

Skin and Appendages
Rash; Urticaria.

Special Senses
Altered vision; Bad taste; Dry eyes.

Urogenital
Cystitis; Glycosuria; Impotence; Urinary incontinence; Urinary retention.

DRUG ABUSE AND DEPENDENCE
Misuse Abuse and Diversion of Opioids
VICOPROFEN contains hydrocodone, an opioid agonist, and is a Schedule II controlled substance. VICOPROFEN, and other opioids used in analgesia can be abused and are subject to criminal diversion.

Addiction is a primary, chronic, neurobiologic disease, with genetic, psychosocial, and environmental factors influencing its development and manifestations. It is characterized by behaviors that include one or more of the following: impaired control over drug use, compulsive use, continued use despite harm, and craving. Drug addiction is a treatable disease utilizing a multidisciplinary approach, but relapse is common.

"Drug seeking" behavior is very common in addicts and drug abusers. Drug-seeking tactics include emergency calls or visits near the end of office hours, refusal to undergo appropriate examination, testing or referral, repeated "loss" of prescriptions, tampering with prescriptions and reluctance to provide prior medical records or contact information for other treating physician(s). "Doctor shopping" to obtain additional prescriptions is common among drug abusers and people suffering from untreated addiction.

Abuse and addiction are separate and distinct from physical dependence and tolerance. Physical dependence usually assumes clinically significant dimensions only after several weeks of continued opioid use, although a mild degree of physical dependence may develop after a few days of opioid therapy. Tolerance, in which increasingly large doses are required in order to produce the same degree of analgesia, is manifested initially by a shortened duration of analgesic effect, and subsequently by decreases in the intensity of analgesia. The rate of development of tolerance varies among patients. Physicians should be aware that abuse of opioids can occur in the absence of true addiction and is characterized by misuse for non-medical purposes, often in combination with other psychoactive substances. VICOPROFEN, like other opioids, may be diverted for non-medical use. Record-keeping of prescribing information, including quantity, frequency, and renewal requests is strongly advised. Proper assessment of the patient, proper prescribing practices, periodic re-evaluation of therapy, and proper dispensing and storage are appropriate measures that help to limit abuse of opioid drugs.

OVERDOSAGE
Following an acute overdosage, toxicity may result from hydrocodone and/or ibuprofen.

Signs and Symptoms
Hydrocodone Component
Serious overdose with hydrocodone is characterized by respiratory depression (a decrease in respiratory rate and/or tidal volume, Cheyne-Stokes respiration, cyanosis) extreme somnolence progressing to stupor or coma, skeletal muscle flaccidity, cold and clammy skin, and sometimes bradycardia and hypotension. In severe overdosage, apnea, circulatory collapse, cardiac arrest and death may occur.

Ibuprofen Component
Symptoms include gastrointestinal irritation with erosion and hemorrhage or perforation, kidney damage, liver damage, heart damage, hemolytic anemia, agranulocytosis, thrombocytopenia, aplastic anemia, and meningitis. Other symptoms may include headache, dizziness, tinnitus, confusion, blurred vision, mental disturbances, skin rash, stomatitis, edema, reduced retinal sensitivity, corneal deposits, and hyperkalemia.

Treatment
Primary attention should be given to the re-establishment of adequate respiratory exchange through provision of a patent airway and the institution of assisted or controlled ventilation. Naloxone, a narcotic antagonist, can reverse respiratory depression and coma associated with opioid overdose or unusual sensitivity to opioids, including hydrocodone. Therefore, an appropriate dose of naloxone hydrochloride should be administered intravenously with simultaneous efforts at respiratory resuscitation. Since the duration of action of hydrocodone may exceed that of the naloxone, the patient should be kept under continuous surveillance and repeated doses of the antagonist should be administered as needed to maintain adequate respiration. Supportive measures should be employed as indicated. Gastric emptying may be useful in removing unabsorbed drug. In cases where consciousness is impaired it may be inadvisable to perform gastric lavage. If gastric lavage is performed, little drug will likely be recovered if more than an hour has elapsed since ingestion. Ibuprofen is acidic and is excreted in the urine; therefore, it may be beneficial to administer alkali and induce diuresis. In addition to supportive measures the use of oral activated charcoal may help to reduce the absorption and reabsorption of ibuprofen. Dialysis is not likely to be effective for removal of ibuprofen because it is very highly bound to plasma proteins.

DOSAGE AND ADMINISTRATION
Carefully consider the potential benefits and risks of VICOPROFEN and other treatment options before deciding to use VICOPROFEN. Use the lowest effective dose for the shortest duration consistent with individual patient treatment goals (see **WARNINGS**).

After observing the response to initial therapy with VICOPROFEN, the dose and frequency should be adjusted to suit an individual patient's needs.

For the short-term (generally less than 10 days) management of acute pain, the recommended dose of VICOPROFEN is one tablet every 4 to 6 hours, as necessary. Dosage should not exceed 5 tablets in a 24-hour period. It should be kept in mind that tolerance to hydrocodone can develop with continued use and that the incidence of untoward effects is dose related.

The lowest effective dose or the longest dosing interval should be sought for each patient (see **WARNINGS**), especially in the elderly. After observing the initial response to therapy with VICOPROFEN, the dose and frequency of dosing should be adjusted to suit the individual patient's need, without exceeding the total daily dose recommended.

HOW SUPPLIED
VICOPROFEN tablets are available as:
White film-coated round convex tablets, engraved with "VP" over "a" logo on one side and plain on the other side.
Bottles of 100-NDC 0074-2277-14
Bottles of 500-NDC 0074-2277-54
Hospital Unit Dosage Package-100 tablets
(4 × 25 tablets)-NDC 0074-2277-12

Storage
Store at 25°C (77°F); excursions permitted to 15°-30°C (59°-86°F). [See USP Controlled Room Temperature].
Dispense in a tight, light-resistant container.
A Schedule II Controlled Substance.
© AbbVie Inc. 2014

Medication Guide
for
Non-Steroidal Anti-Inflammatory Drugs (NSAIDs)
(See the end of this Medication Guide for a list of prescription NSAID medicines.)

What is the most important information I should know about medicines called Non-Steroidal Anti-Inflammatory Drugs (NSAIDs)?
NSAID medicines may increase the chance of a heart attack or stroke that can lead to death.
This chance increases:
• with longer use of NSAID medicines
• in people who have heart disease
NSAID medicines should never be used right before or after a heart surgery called a "coronary artery bypass graft (CABG)."

NSAID medicines can cause ulcers and bleeding in the stomach and intestines at any time during treatment. Ulcers and bleeding:
• can happen without warning symptoms
• may cause death
The chance of a person getting an ulcer or bleeding increases with:
• taking medicines called "corticosteroids" and "anticoagulants"
• longer use
• smoking
• drinking alcohol
• older age
• having poor health
NSAID medicines should only be used:
• exactly as prescribed
• at the lowest dose possible for your treatment
• for the shortest time needed
What are Non-Steroidal Anti-Inflammatory Drugs (NSAIDs)?
NSAID medicines are used to treat pain and redness, swelling, and heat (inflammation) from medical conditions such as:
• different types of arthritis
• menstrual cramps and other types of short-term pain
Who should not take a Non-Steroidal Anti-Inflammatory Drug (NSAID)?
Do not take an NSAID medicine:
• if you had an asthma attack, hives, or other allergic reaction with aspirin or any other NSAID medicine
• for pain right before or after heart bypass surgery
Tell your healthcare provider:
• about all your medical conditions.
• about all of the medicines you take. NSAIDs and some other medicines can interact with each other and cause serious side effects. **Keep a list of your medicines to show to your healthcare provider and pharmacist.**
• if you are pregnant. **NSAID medicines should not be used by pregnant women late in their pregnancy.**
• if you are breastfeeding. **Talk to your doctor.**
What are the possible side effects of Non-Steroidal Anti-Inflammatory Drugs (NSAIDs)?

Serious side effects include:	Other side effects include:
• heart attack	• stomach pain
• stroke	• constipation
• high blood pressure	• diarrhea
• heart failure from body swelling (fluid retention)	• gas
• kidney problems including kidney failure	• heartburn
	• nausea
• bleeding and ulcers in the stomach and intestine	• vomiting
	• dizziness
• low red blood cells (anemia)	
• life-threatening skin reactions	
• life-threatening allergic reactions	
• liver problems including liver failure	
• asthma attacks in people who have asthma	

Get emergency help right away if you have any of the following symptoms:
• shortness of breath or trouble breathing
• chest pain
• weakness in one part or side of your body
• slurred speech
• swelling of the face or throat
Stop your NSAID medicine and call your healthcare provider right away if you have any of the following symptoms:
• nausea
• more tired or weaker than usual
• itching
• your skin or eyes look yellow
• stomach pain
• flu-like symptoms
• vomit blood
• there is blood in your bowel movement or it is black and sticky like tar
• unusual weight gain
• skin rash or blisters with fever
• swelling of the arms and legs, hands and feet
These are not all the side effects with NSAID medicines. Talk to your healthcare provider or pharmacist for more information about NSAID medicines. Call your doctor for medical advice about side effects. You may report side effects to FDA at 1-800-FDA-1088.

Other information about Non-Steroidal Anti-Inflammatory Drugs (NSAIDs)
• Aspirin is an NSAID medicine but it does not increase the chance of a heart attack. Aspirin can cause bleeding in the brain, stomach, and intestines. Aspirin can also cause ulcers in the stomach and intestines.
• Some of these NSAID medicines are sold in lower doses without a prescription (over the counter). Talk to your healthcare provider before using over the counter NSAIDs for more than 10 days.

NSAID medicines that need a prescription

Generic Name	Tradename
Celecoxib	Celebrex
Diclofenac	Cataflam, Voltaren, Arthrotec (combined with misoprostol)
Diflunisal	Dolobid
Etodolac	Lodine, Lodine XL
Fenoprofen	Nalfon, Nalfon 200
Flurbirofen	Ansaid
Ibuprofen	Motrin, Tab-Profen, Vicoprofen* (combined with hydrocodone), Combunox (combined with oxycodone)
Indomethacin	Indocin, Indocin SR, Indo-Lemmon, Indomethagan
Ketoprofen	Oruvail
Ketorolac	Toradol
Mefenamic Acid	Ponstel
Meloxicam	Mobic
Nabumetone	Relafen
Naproxen	Naprosyn, Anaprox, Anaprox DS, EC-Naproxyn, Naprelan, Naprapac (copackaged with lansoprazole)
Oxaprozin	Daypro
Piroxicam	Feldene
Sulindac	Clinoril
Tolmetin	Tolectin, Tolectin DS, Tolectin 600

* Vicoprofen contains the same dose of ibuprofen as over-the-counter (OTC) NSAIDs, and is usually used for less than 10 days to treat pain. The OTC NSAID label warns that long term continuous use may increase the risk of heart attack or stroke.

Manufactured by Halo Pharmaceutical Inc.
Whippany, NJ 07981 U.S.A.
for AbbVie Inc.
North Chicago, IL 60064 U.S.A.
This Medication Guide has been approved by the U.S. Food and Drug Administration.
Ref. 03-B024-R6-Rev. August, 2014
Shown in Product Identification Guide, page 507

VIEKIRA PAK™
[vee-KEE-rah-pak]
(ombitasvir, paritaprevir, and ritonavir tablets; dasabuvir tablets), co-packaged for oral use

℞

HIGHLIGHTS OF PRESCRIBING INFORMATION
These highlights do not include all the information needed to use VIEKIRA PAK safely and effectively. See full prescribing information for VIEKIRA PAK.
VIEKIRA PAK™ (ombitasvir, paritaprevir, and ritonavir tablets; dasabuvir tablets), co-packaged for oral use

Initial U.S. Approval: 2014

——INDICATIONS AND USAGE——
VIEKIRA PAK is indicated for the treatment of adult patients with chronic hepatitis C virus (HCV):
• genotype 1b without cirrhosis or with compensated cirrhosis
• genotype 1a without cirrhosis or with compensated cirrhosis for use in combination with ribavirin.
VIEKIRA PAK includes ombitasvir, a hepatitis C virus NS5A inhibitor, paritaprevir, a hepatitis C virus NS3/4A protease inhibitor, ritonavir, a CYP3A inhibitor and dasabuvir, a hepatitis C virus non-nucleoside NS5B palm polymerase inhibitor. (1)

——DOSAGE AND ADMINISTRATION——
Testing Prior to Initiation - Assess for laboratory and clinical evidence of hepatic decompensation. (2.1)
Recommended dosage: Two ombitasvir, paritaprevir, ritonavir 12.5/75/50 mg tablets once daily (in the morning) and one dasabuvir 250 mg tablet twice daily (morning and evening) with a meal without regard to fat or calorie content. (2.1)

Treatment Regimen and Duration by Patient Population

Patient Population	Treatment*	Duration
Genotype 1a, without cirrhosis	VIEKIRA PAK + ribavirin	12 weeks
Genotype 1a, with compensated cirrhosis	VIEKIRA PAK + ribavirin	24 weeks**
Genotype 1b, with or without compensated cirrhosis	VIEKIRA PAK	12 weeks

*Note: Follow the genotype 1a dosing recommendations in patients with an unknown genotype 1 subtype or with mixed genotype 1 infection.
**VIEKIRA PAK administered with ribavirin for 12 weeks may be considered for some patients based on prior treatment history [See Clinical Studies (14.3)].

• HCV/HIV-1 co-infection: For patients with HCV/HIV-1 co-infection, follow the dosage recommendations in the table above. (2.1)
• Liver Transplant Recipients: In liver transplant recipients with normal hepatic function and mild fibrosis (Metavir fibrosis score ≤2), the recommended duration of VIEKIRA PAK with ribavirin is 24 weeks. (2.3)

——DOSAGE FORMS AND STRENGTHS——
Tablets:
• Ombitasvir, paritaprevir, ritonavir: 12.5/75/50 mg (3)
• Dasabuvir: 250 mg (3)

——CONTRAINDICATIONS——
• Patients with moderate to severe hepatic impairment. (4, 5.1, 8.6, 12.3)
• If VIEKIRA PAK is administered with ribavirin, the contraindications to ribavirin also apply to this combination regimen. (4)
• Co-administration with drugs that are: highly dependent on CYP3A for clearance; moderate or strong inducers of CYP3A and strong inducers of CYP2C8; and strong inhibitors of CYP2C8. (4)

Continued on next page

Information on the AbbVie, Inc. products listed on these pages is from the prescribing information in use as of July 31, 2016. For more information, please visit rxabbvie.com or call 1-800-633-9110.

• Known hypersensitivity to ritonavir (e.g. toxic epidermal necrolysis, Stevens-Johnson syndrome). (4)

WARNINGS AND PRECAUTIONS

• **Hepatic Decompensation and Hepatic Failure in Patient with Cirrhosis:** Hepatic decompensation and hepatic failure, including liver transplantation or fatal outcomes, have been reported mostly in patients with advanced cirrhosis. Monitor for clinical signs and symptoms of hepatic decompensation. (5.1)
• **ALT Elevations:** Discontinue ethinyl estradiol-containing medications prior to starting VIEKIRA PAK (alternative contraceptive methods are recommended). Perform hepatic laboratory testing on all patients during the first 4 weeks of treatment. For ALT elevations on VIEKIRA PAK, monitor closely and follow recommendations in full prescribing information. (5.2)
• **Risks Associated With Ribavirin Combination Treatment:** If VIEKIRA PAK is administered with ribavirin, the warnings and precautions for ribavirin also apply to this combination regimen. (5.3)
• **Drug Interactions:** The concomitant use of VIEKIRA PAK and certain other drugs may result in known or potentially significant drug interactions, some of which may lead to loss of therapeutic effect of VIEKIRA PAK. (5.4)

ADVERSE REACTIONS

In subjects receiving VIEKIRA PAK with ribavirin, the most commonly reported adverse reactions (greater than 10% of subjects) were fatigue, nausea, pruritus, other skin reactions, insomnia and asthenia. In subjects receiving VIEKIRA PAK without ribavirin, the most commonly reported adverse reactions (greater than or equal to 5% of subjects) were nausea, pruritus and insomnia. (6.1)

To report SUSPECTED ADVERSE REACTIONS, contact AbbVie Inc. at 1-800-633-9110 or FDA at 1-800-FDA-1088 or www.fda.gov/medwatch.

DRUG INTERACTIONS

Co-administration of VIEKIRA PAK can alter the plasma concentrations of some drugs and some drugs may alter the plasma concentrations of VIEKIRA PAK. The potential for drug interactions must be considered before and during treatment. Consult the full prescribing information prior to and during treatment for potential drug interactions. (4, 5.4, 7, 12.3)

See 17 for PATIENT COUNSELING INFORMATION and Medication Guide.

Revised: 6/2016

FULL PRESCRIBING INFORMATION: CONTENTS*

* Sections or subsections omitted from the full prescribing information are not listed.

FULL PRESCRIBING INFORMATION

1   INDICATIONS AND USAGE

VIEKIRA PAK is indicated for the treatment of adult patients with chronic hepatitis C virus (HCV) [see Dosage and Administration (2.2) and Clinical Studies (14)]:
• genotype 1b without cirrhosis or with compensated cirrhosis
• genotype 1a without cirrhosis or with compensated cirrhosis for use in combination with ribavirin

2   DOSAGE AND ADMINISTRATION

2.1   Testing Prior to Initiation of VIEKIRA PAK

Prior to initiation of VIEKIRA PAK, assess for laboratory and clinical evidence of hepatic decompensation [see Warnings and Precautions (5.1 and 5.2)].

2.2   Recommended Dosage in Adults

VIEKIRA PAK is ombitasvir, paritaprevir, ritonavir fixed dose combination tablets copackaged with dasabuvir tablets.

The recommended oral dosage of VIEKIRA PAK is two ombitasvir, paritaprevir, ritonavir tablets once daily (in the morning) and one dasabuvir tablet twice daily (morning and evening). Take VIEKIRA PAK with a meal without regard to fat or calorie content [see Clinical Pharmacology (12.3)]. VIEKIRA PAK is used in combination with ribavirin (RBV) in certain patient populations (see Table 1). When administered with VIEKIRA PAK, the recommended dosage of RBV is based on weight: 1000 mg/day for subjects <75 kg and 1200 mg/day for those ≥75 kg, divided and administered twice-daily with food. For ribavirin dosage modifications, refer to the ribavirin prescribing information.

For patients with HCV/HIV-1 co-infection, follow the dosage recommendations in Table 1. Refer to Drug Interactions (7) for dosage recommendations for concomitant HIV-1 antiviral drugs.

Table 1 shows the recommended VIEKIRA PAK treatment regimen and duration based on patient population.

Table 1. Treatment Regimen and Duration by Patient Population (Treatment-Naïve or Interferon-Experienced)

Patient Population	Treatment*	Duration
Genotype 1a, without cirrhosis	VIEKIRA PAK + ribavirin	12 weeks
Genotype 1a, with compensated cirrhosis (Child-Pugh A)	VIEKIRA PAK + ribavirin	24 weeks**
Genotype 1b, with or without compensated cirrhosis (Child-Pugh A)	VIEKIRA PAK	12 weeks

*Note: Follow the genotype 1a dosing recommendations in patients with an unknown genotype 1 subtype or with mixed genotype 1 infection.

**VIEKIRA PAK administered with ribavirin for 12 weeks may be considered for some patients based on prior treatment history [see Clinical Studies (14.3)].

2.3   Use in Liver Transplant Recipients

In liver transplant recipients with normal hepatic function and mild fibrosis (Metavir fibrosis score 2 or lower), the recommended duration of VIEKIRA PAK with ribavirin is 24 weeks, irrespective of HCV genotype 1 subtype [see Clinical Studies (14.6)]. When VIEKIRA PAK is administered with calcineurin inhibitors in liver transplant recipients, dosage adjustment of calcineurin inhibitors is needed [see Drug Interactions (7)].

2.4   Hepatic Impairment

VIEKIRA PAK is contraindicated in patients with moderate to severe hepatic impairment (Child-Pugh B and C) [see Contraindications (4), Warnings and Precautions (5.1), Use in Specific Populations (8.6), and Clinical Pharmacology (12.3)].

3   DOSAGE FORMS AND STRENGTHS

VIEKIRA PAK is ombitasvir, paritaprevir, ritonavir fixed dose combination tablets copackaged with dasabuvir tablets.
• Ombitasvir, paritaprevir, ritonavir 12.5/75/50 mg tablets are pink-colored, film-coated, oblong biconvex shaped, debossed with "AV1" on one side.
• Dasabuvir 250 mg tablets are beige-colored, film-coated, oval-shaped, debossed with "AV2" on one side. Each tablet contains 270.3 mg dasabuvir sodium monohydrate equivalent to 250 mg dasabuvir.

4   CONTRAINDICATIONS

• VIEKIRA PAK is contraindicated in patients with moderate to severe hepatic impairment (Child-Pugh B and C) due to risk of potential toxicity [see Warnings and Precautions (5.1), Use in Specific Populations (8.6) and Clinical Pharmacology (12.3)].
• If VIEKIRA PAK is administered with ribavirin, the contraindications to ribavirin also apply to this combination regimen. Refer to the ribavirin prescribing information for a list of contraindications for ribavirin.
• VIEKIRA PAK is contraindicated:
  ○ With drugs that are highly dependent on CYP3A for clearance and for which elevated plasma concentrations are associated with serious and/or life-threatening events.
  ○ With drugs that are moderate or strong inducers of CYP3A and strong inducers of CYP2C8 and may lead to reduced efficacy of VIEKIRA PAK.
  ○ With drugs that are strong inhibitors of CYP2C8 and may increase dasabuvir plasma concentrations and the risk of QT prolongation.
  ○ In patients with known hypersensitivity to ritonavir (e.g. toxic epidermal necrolysis (TEN) or Stevens-Johnson syndrome).

Table 2 lists drugs that are contraindicated with VIEKIRA PAK [see Drug Interactions (7)].

[See table 2 on next page]

5   WARNINGS AND PRECAUTIONS

5.1   Risk of Hepatic Decompensation and Hepatic Failure in Patients with Cirrhosis

Hepatic decompensation and hepatic failure, including liver transplantation or fatal outcomes, have been reported post-marketing in patients treated with VIEKIRA PAK. Most patients with these severe outcomes had evidence of advanced cirrhosis prior to initiating therapy with VIEKIRA PAK. Reported cases typically occurred within one to four weeks of initiating therapy and were characterized by the acute onset of rising direct serum bilirubin levels without ALT elevations in association with clinical signs and symptoms of hepatic decompensation. Because these events are reported voluntarily from a population of uncertain size, it is not always possible to reliably estimate their frequency or establish a causal relationship to drug exposure.

VIEKIRA PAK is contraindicated in patients with moderate to severe hepatic impairment (Child-Pugh B and C) [see Contraindications (4), Adverse Reactions (6.2), Use in Specific Populations (8.6), and Clinical Pharmacology (12.3)].

For patients with cirrhosis:
• Monitor for clinical signs and symptoms of hepatic decompensation (such as ascites, hepatic encephalopathy, variceal hemorrhage).
• Hepatic laboratory testing including direct bilirubin levels should be performed at baseline and during the first 4 weeks of starting treatment and as clinically indicated.
• Discontinue VIEKIRA PAK in patients who develop evidence of hepatic decompensation.

5.2   Increased Risk of ALT Elevations

During clinical trials with VIEKIRA PAK with or without ribavirin, elevations of ALT to greater than 5 times the upper limit of normal (ULN) occurred in approximately 1% of

Table 2. Drugs that are Contraindicated with VIEKIRA PAK

Drug Class	Drug(s) within Class that are Contraindicated	Clinical Comments
Alpha1-adrenoreceptor antagonist	Alfuzosin HCL	Potential for hypotension.
Anti-anginal	Ranolazine	Potential for serious and/or life-threatening reactions.
Antiarrhythmic	Dronedarone	Potential for serious and/or life-threatening reactions such as cardiac arrhythmias.
Anticonvulsants	Carbamazepine, phenytoin, phenobarbital	Ombitasvir, paritaprevir, ritonavir and dasabuvir exposures may decrease leading to a potential loss of therapeutic activity of VIEKIRA PAK.
Anti-gout	Colchicine	Potential for serious and/or life-threatening reactions in patients with renal and/or hepatic impairment.
Antihyperlipidemic agent	Gemfibrozil	Increase in dasabuvir exposures by 10-fold which may increase the risk of QT prolongation.
Antimycobacterial	Rifampin	Ombitasvir, paritaprevir, ritonavir and dasabuvir exposures may decrease leading to a potential loss of therapeutic activity of VIEKIRA PAK.
Antipsychotic	Lurasidone Pimozide	Potential for serious and/or life-threatening reactions. Potential for serious and/or life-threatening reactions such as cardiac arrhythmias.
Ergot derivatives	Ergotamine, dihydroergotamine, methylergonovine	Acute ergot toxicity characterized by vasospasm and tissue ischemia has been associated with co-administration of ritonavir and ergotamine, dihydroergotamine, or methylergonovine.
Ethinyl estradiol-containing products	Ethinyl estradiol-containing medications such as combined oral contraceptives	Potential for ALT elevations [see Warnings and Precautions (5.2)].
GI Motility Agent	Cisapride	Potential for serious and/or life threatening reactions such as cardiac arrhythmias
Herbal Product	St. John's Wort (Hypericum perforatum)	Ombitasvir, paritaprevir, ritonavir and dasabuvir exposures may decrease leading to a potential loss of therapeutic activity of VIEKIRA PAK.
HMG-CoA Reductase Inhibitors	Lovastatin, simvastatin	Potential for myopathy including rhabdomyolysis.
Non-nucleoside reverse transcriptase inhibitor	Efavirenz	Co-administration of efavirenz based regimens with paritaprevir, ritonavir plus dasabuvir was poorly tolerated and resulted in liver enzyme elevations.
Phosphodiesterase-5 (PDE5) inhibitor	Sildenafil when dosed as Revatio for the treatment of pulmonary arterial hypertension (PAH)	There is increased potential for sildenafil-associated adverse events such as visual disturbances, hypotension, priapism, and syncope.
Sedatives/hypnotics	Triazolam Orally administered midazolam	Triazolam and orally administered midazolam are extensively metabolized by CYP3A4. Coadministration of triazolam or orally administered midazolam with VIEKIRA PAK may cause large increases in the concentration of these benzodiazepines. The potential exists for serious and/or life threatening events such as prolonged or increased sedation or respiratory depression.

all subjects [see Adverse Reactions (6.1)]. ALT elevations were typically asymptomatic, occurred during the first 4 weeks of treatment, and declined within two to eight weeks of onset with continued dosing of VIEKIRA PAK with or without ribavirin.

These ALT elevations were significantly more frequent in female subjects who were using ethinyl estradiol-containing medications such as combined oral contraceptives, contraceptive patches or contraceptive vaginal rings. Ethinyl estradiol-containing medications must be discontinued prior to starting therapy with VIEKIRA PAK [see Contraindications (4)]. Alternative methods of contraception (e.g, progestin only contraception or non-hormonal methods) are recommended during VIEKIRA PAK therapy. Ethinyl estradiol-containing medications can be restarted approximately 2 weeks following completion of treatment with VIEKIRA PAK.

Women using estrogens other than ethinyl estradiol, such as estradiol and conjugated estrogens used in hormone replacement therapy had a rate of ALT elevation similar to those not receiving any estrogens; however, due to the lim-

ited number of subjects taking these other estrogens, caution is warranted for co-administration with VIEKIRA PAK [see Adverse Reactions (6.1)].

Hepatic laboratory testing should be performed during the first 4 weeks of starting treatment and as clinically indicated thereafter. If ALT is found to be elevated above baseline levels, it should be repeated and monitored closely:

- Patients should be instructed to consult their health care professional without delay if they have onset of fatigue, weakness, lack of appetite, nausea and vomiting, jaundice or discolored feces.
- Consider discontinuing VIEKIRA PAK if ALT levels remain persistently greater than 10 times the ULN.
- Discontinue VIEKIRA PAK if ALT elevation is accompanied by signs or symptoms of liver inflammation or increasing direct bilirubin, alkaline phosphatase, or INR.

5.3   Risks Associated With Ribavirin Combination Treatment

If VIEKIRA PAK is administered with ribavirin, the warnings and precautions for ribavirin, in particular the pregnancy avoidance warning, apply to this combination regimen. Refer to the ribavirin prescribing information for a full list of the warnings and precautions for ribavirin.

5.4   Risk of Adverse Reactions or Reduced Therapeutic Effect Due to Drug Interactions

The concomitant use of VIEKIRA PAK and certain other drugs may result in known or potentially significant drug interactions, some of which may lead to:

- Loss of therapeutic effect of VIEKIRA PAK and possible development of resistance
- Possible clinically significant adverse reactions from greater exposures of concomitant drugs or components of VIEKIRA PAK.

See Table 5 for steps to prevent or manage these possible and known significant drug interactions, including dosing recommendations [see Drug Interactions (7)]. Consider the potential for drug interactions prior to and during VIEKIRA PAK therapy; review concomitant medications during VIEKIRA PAK therapy; and monitor for the adverse reactions associated with the concomitant drugs [see Contraindications (4) and Drug Interactions (7)].

5.5   Risk of HIV-1 Protease Inhibitor Drug Resistance in HCV/HIV-1 Co-infected Patients

The ritonavir component of VIEKIRA PAK is also an HIV-1 protease inhibitor and can select for HIV-1 protease inhibitor resistance-associated substitutions. Any HCV/HIV-1 co-infected patients treated with VIEKIRA PAK should also be on a suppressive antiretroviral drug regimen to reduce the risk of HIV-1 protease inhibitor drug resistance.

6   ADVERSE REACTIONS

If VIEKIRA PAK is administered with ribavirin (RBV), refer to the prescribing information for ribavirin for a list of ribavirin-associated adverse reactions.

The following adverse reaction is described below and elsewhere in the labeling:

- Risk of Hepatic Decompensation and Hepatic Failure in Patients with Cirrhosis [see Warnings and Precautions (5.1)]
- Increased Risk of ALT Elevations [see Warnings and Precautions (5.2)]

6.1   Clinical Trials Experience

Because clinical trials are conducted under widely varying conditions, adverse reaction rates observed in clinical trials of VIEKIRA PAK cannot be directly compared to rates in the clinical trials of another drug and may not reflect the rates observed in practice.

The safety assessment was based on data from seven clinical trials in more than 2,000 subjects who received VIEKIRA PAK with or without ribavirin for 12 or 24 weeks.

VIEKIRA PAK with Ribavirin in Placebo-Controlled Trials

The safety of VIEKIRA PAK™ (ombitasvir, paritaprevir, and ritonavir tablets; dasabuvir tablets) in combination with ribavirin was assessed in 770 subjects with chronic HCV genotype 1 (GT1) infection in two placebo-controlled trials (SAPPHIRE-I and -II) [see Clinical Studies (14.1, 14.2)]. Adverse reactions that occurred more often in subjects treated with VIEKIRA PAK in combination with ribavirin compared to placebo were fatigue, nausea, pruritus, other skin reactions, insomnia, and asthenia (see Table 3). The majority of the adverse reactions were mild in severity. Two percent of subjects experienced a serious adverse event (SAE). The proportion of subjects who permanently discontinued treatment due to adverse reactions was less than 1%.

Table 3. Adverse Reactions with ≥5% Greater Frequency Reported in Subjects with Chronic HCV GT1 Infection Treated with VIEKIRA PAK in Combination with Ribavirin Compared to Placebo for 12 Weeks

	SAPPHIRE-I and -II	
	VIEKIRA PAK + RBV 12 Weeks N = 770 %	Placebo 12 Weeks N = 255 %
Fatigue	34	26
Nausea	22	15
Pruritus*	18	7

Continued on next page

Information on the AbbVie, Inc. products listed on these pages is from the prescribing information in use as of July 31, 2016. For more information, please visit rxabbvie.com or call 1-800-633-9110.

Table 5. Established Drug Interactions Based on Drug Interaction Trials

Concomitant Drug Class: Drug Name	Effect on Concentration	Clinical Comments
ANGIOTENSIN RECEPTOR BLOCKERS e.g.		
valsartan[*] losartan[*] candesartan[*]	↑ angiotensin receptor blockers	Decrease the dose of the angiotensin receptor blockers and monitor patients for signs and symptoms of hypotension and/or worsening renal function. If such events occur, consider further dose reduction of the angiotensin receptor blocker or switching to an alternative to the angiotensin receptor blocker.
ANTIARRHYTHMICS		
amiodarone[*], bepridil[*], disopyramide[*], flecainide[*], lidocaine (systemic)[*], mexiletine[*], propafenone[*], quinidine[*]	↑ antiarrhythmics	Therapeutic concentration monitoring (if available) is recommended for antiarrhythmics when co-administered with VIEKIRA PAK.
ANTIDIABETIC DRUGS		
metformin	↔ metformin	Monitor for signs of onset of lactic acidosis such as respiratory distress, somnolence, and non-specific abdominal distress or worsening renal function. Concomitant metformin use in patients with renal insufficiency or hepatic impairment is not recommended. Refer to the prescribing information of metformin for further guidance.
ANTIFUNGALS		
ketoconazole	↑ ketoconazole	When VIEKIRA PAK is co-administered with ketoconazole, the maximum daily dose of ketoconazole should be limited to 200 mg per day.
voriconazole[*]	↓ voriconazole	Co-administration of VIEKIRA PAK with voriconazole is not recommended unless an assessment of the benefit-to-risk ratio justifies the use of voriconazole.
ANTIPSYCHOTICS		
quetiapine[*]	↑ quetiapine	• Initiation of VIEKIRA PAK in patients taking quetiapine: Consider alternative anti-HCV therapy to avoid increases in quetiapine exposures. If coadministration is necessary, reduce the quetiapine dose to 1/6th of the current dose and monitor for quetiapine-associated adverse reactions. Refer to the quetiapine prescribing information for the recommendations on adverse reaction monitoring. • Initiation of quetiapine in patients taking VIEKIRA PAK: Refer to the quetiapine prescribing information for initial dosing and titration of quetiapine.
CALCIUM CHANNEL BLOCKERS		
amlodipine[*] nifedipine[*] diltiazem[*] verapamil[*]	↑ calcium channel blockers	Decrease the dose of the calcium channel blocker. The dose of amlodipine should be decreased by at least 50%. Clinical monitoring of patients is recommended for edema and/or signs and symptoms of hypotension. If such events occur, consider further dose reduction of the calcium channel blocker or switching to an alternative to the calcium channel blocker.
CORTICOSTEROIDS (INHALED/NASAL)		
fluticasone[*]	↑ fluticasone	Concomitant use of VIEKIRA PAK with inhaled or nasal fluticasone may reduce serum cortisol concentrations. Alternative corticosteroids should be considered, particularly for long term use.
DIURETICS		
furosemide	↑ furosemide (C_{max})	Clinical monitoring of patients is recommended and therapy should be individualized based on patient's response.

This table is continued on the next page

Skin reactions[§]	16	9
Insomnia	14	8
Asthenia	14	7

*Grouped term 'pruritus' included the preferred terms pruritus and pruritus generalized.
§Grouped terms: rash, erythema, eczema, rash maculo-papular, rash macular, dermatitis, rash papular, skin exfoliation, rash pruritic, rash erythematous, rash generalized, dermatitis allergic, dermatitis contact, exfoliative rash, photosensitivity reaction, psoriasis, skin reaction, ulcer, urticaria.

VIEKIRA PAK with and without Ribavirin in Regimen-Controlled Trials
VIEKIRA PAK with and without ribavirin was assessed in 401 and 509 subjects with chronic HCV infection, respectively, in three clinical trials (PEARL-II, PEARL-III and PEARL-IV) *[see Clinical Studies (14.1, 14.2)]*. Pruritus, nausea, insomnia, and asthenia were identified as adverse events occurring more often in subjects treated with VIEKIRA PAK in combination with ribavirin (see Table 4). The majority of adverse events were mild to moderate in severity. The proportion of subjects who permanently discontinued treatment due to adverse events was less than 1% for both VIEKIRA PAK in combination with ribavirin and VIEKIRA PAK alone.

Table 4. Adverse Events with ≥5% Greater Frequency Reported in Subjects with Chronic HCV GT1 Infection Treated with VIEKIRA PAK in Combination with Ribavirin Compared to VIEKIRA PAK for 12 Weeks

	PEARL-II, -III and -IV	
	VIEKIRA PAK + RBV 12 Weeks N = 401 %	VIEKIRA PAK 12 Weeks N = 509 %
Nausea	16	8
Pruritus*	13	7
Insomnia	12	5
Asthenia	9	4

*Grouped term 'pruritus' included the preferred terms pruritus and pruritus generalized.

VIEKIRA PAK with Ribavirin in GT1-infected Subjects with Compensated Cirrhosis
VIEKIRA PAK with ribavirin was assessed in 380 subjects with genotype 1 infection and compensated cirrhosis who were treated with VIEKIRA PAK plus ribavirin for 12 (n=208) or 24 (n=172) weeks duration (TURQUOISE-II) *[see Clinical Studies (14.1, 14.3)]*. The type and severity of adverse events in subjects with compensated cirrhosis was comparable to non-cirrhotic subjects in other phase 3 trials. Fatigue, skin reactions and dyspnea occurred at least 5% more often in subjects treated for 24 weeks. The majority of adverse events occurred during the first 12 weeks of dosing in both treatment arms. Most of the adverse events were mild to moderate in severity. The proportion of subjects treated with VIEKIRA PAK for 12 and 24 weeks with SAEs was 6% and 5%, respectively and 2% of subjects permanently discontinued treatment due to adverse events in each treatment arm.
VIEKIRA PAK without Ribavirin in GT1b-infected Subjects with Compensated Cirrhosis
VIEKIRA PAK without ribavirin for 12 weeks was assessed in 60 subjects with genotype 1b infection and compensated cirrhosis (TURQUOISE-III) *[see Clinical Studies (14.1, 14.3)]*. The type and severity of adverse events and laboratory abnormalities in genotype 1b-infected subjects with compensated cirrhosis were comparable to subjects in other trials without ribavirin.
Skin Reactions
In PEARL-II, -III and -IV, 7% of subjects receiving VIEKIRA PAK alone and 10% of subjects receiving VIEKIRA PAK with ribavirin reported rash-related events. In SAPPHIRE-I and -II 16% of subjects receiving VIEKIRA PAK with ribavirin and 9% of subjects receiving placebo re-

Table 5 *(Cont.)* Established Drug Interactions Based on Drug Interaction Trials

Concomitant Drug Class: Drug Name	Effect on Concentration	Clinical Comments
HIV-ANTIVIRAL AGENTS		
atazanavir/ritonavir once daily	↑ paritaprevir	When coadministered with VIEKIRA PAK, atazanavir 300 mg (without ritonavir) should only be given in the morning.
darunavir/ritonavir	↓ darunavir (C_{trough})	Co-administration of VIEKIRA PAK with darunavir/ritonavir is not recommended.
lopinavir/ritonavir	↑ paritaprevir	Co-administration of VIEKIRA PAK with lopinavir/ritonavir is not recommended.
rilpivirine	↑ rilpivirine	Co-administration of VIEKIRA PAK with rilpivirine once daily is not recommended due to potential for QT interval prolongation with higher concentrations of rilpivirine.
HMG CoA REDUCTASE INHIBITORS		
rosuvastatin	↑ rosuvastatin	When VIEKIRA PAK is co-administered with rosuvastatin, the dose of rosuvastatin should not exceed 10 mg per day.
pravastatin	↑ pravastatin	When VIEKIRA PAK is co-administered with pravastatin, the dose of pravastatin should not exceed 40 mg per day.
IMMUNOSUPPRESSANTS		
cyclosporine	↑ cyclosporine	When initiating therapy with VIEKIRA PAK, reduce cyclosporine dose to 1/5th of the patient's current cyclosporine dose. Measure cyclosporine blood concentrations to determine subsequent dose modifications. Upon completion of VIEKIRA PAK therapy, the appropriate time to resume pre-VIEKIRA PAK dose of cyclosporine should be guided by assessment of cyclosporine blood concentrations. Frequent assessment of renal function and cyclosporine-related side effects is recommended.
tacrolimus	↑ tacrolimus	When initiating therapy with VIEKIRA PAK, the dose of tacrolimus needs to be reduced. Do not administer tacrolimus on the day VIEKIRA PAK is initiated. Beginning the day after VIEKIRA PAK is initiated; reinitiate tacrolimus at a reduced dose based on tacrolimus blood concentrations. Typical tacrolimus dosing is 0.5 mg every 7 days. Measure tacrolimus blood concentrations and adjust dose or dosing frequency to determine subsequent dose modifications. Upon completion of VIEKIRA PAK therapy, the appropriate time to resume pre-VIEKIRA PAK dose of tacrolimus should be guided by assessment of tacrolimus blood concentrations. Frequent assessment of renal function and tacrolimus related side effects is recommended.
LONG ACTING BETA-ADRENOCEPTOR AGONIST		
salmeterol⁺	↑ salmeterol	Concurrent administration of VIEKIRA PAK and salmeterol is not recommended. The combination may result in increased risk of cardiovascular adverse events associated with salmeterol, including QT prolongation, palpitations and sinus tachycardia.
MUSCLE RELAXANTS		
carisoprodol	↑ carisoprodol ↔ mepobramate (metabolite of carisoprodol)	Increase dose if clinically indicated.
cyclobenzaprine	↓ cyclobenzaprine ↓ norcyclobenzaprine (metabolite ofcyclobenzaprine)	Increase dose if clinically indicated.

This table is continued on the next page

ported skin reactions. In TURQUOISE-II, 18% and 24% of subjects receiving VIEKIRA PAK with ribavirin for 12 or 24 weeks reported skin reactions. The majority of events were graded as mild in severity. There were no serious events or severe cutaneous reactions, such as Stevens Johnson Syndrome (SJS), toxic epidermal necrolysis (TEN), erythema multiforme (EM) or drug rash with eosinophilia and systemic symptoms (DRESS).

Laboratory Abnormalities

Serum ALT Elevations

Approximately 1% of subjects treated with VIEKIRA PAK experienced post-baseline serum ALT levels greater than 5 times the upper limit of normal (ULN) after starting treatment. The incidence increased to 25% (4/16) among women taking a concomitant ethinyl estradiol containing medication *[see Contraindications (4) and Warnings and Precautions (5.2)]*. The incidence of clinically relevant ALT elevations among women using estrogens other than ethinyl estradiol, such as estradiol and conjugated estrogens used in hormone replacement therapy was 3% (2/59).

ALT elevations were typically asymptomatic, generally occurred during the first 4 weeks of treatment (mean time 20 days, range 8-57 days) and most resolved with ongoing therapy. The majority of these ALT elevations were assessed as drug-related liver injury. Elevations in ALT were generally not associated with bilirubin elevations. Cirrhosis was not a risk factor for elevated ALT *[see Warnings and Precautions (5.2)]*.

Serum Bilirubin Elevations

Post-baseline elevations in bilirubin at least $2 \times$ ULN were observed in 15% of subjects receiving VIEKIRA PAK with ribavirin compared to 2% in those receiving VIEKIRA PAK alone. These bilirubin increases were predominantly indirect and related to the inhibition of the bilirubin transporters OATP1B1/1B3 by paritaprevir and ribavirin-induced hemolysis. Bilirubin elevations occurred after initiation of treatment, peaked by study Week 1, and generally resolved with ongoing therapy. Bilirubin elevations were not associated with serum ALT elevations.

Anemia / Decreased Hemoglobin

Across all Phase 3 studies, the mean change from baseline in hemoglobin levels in subjects treated with VIEKIRA PAK in combination with ribavirin was -2.4 g/dL and the mean change in subjects treated with VIEKIRA PAK alone was -0.5 g/dL. Decreases in hemoglobin levels occurred early in treatment (Week 1-2) with further reductions through Week 3. Hemoglobin values remained low during the remainder of treatment and returned towards baseline levels by post-treatment Week 4. Less than 1% of subjects treated with VIEKIRA PAK with ribavirin had hemoglobin levels decrease to less than 8.0 g/dL during treatment. Seven percent of subjects treated with VIEKIRA PAK in combination with ribavirin underwent a ribavirin dose reduction due to a decrease in hemoglobin levels; three subjects received a blood transfusion and five required erythropoietin. One patient discontinued therapy due to anemia. No subjects treated with VIEKIRA PAK alone had a hemoglobin level less than 10 g/dL.

VIEKIRA PAK in HCV/HIV-1 Co-infected Subjects

VIEKIRA PAK with ribavirin was assessed in 63 subjects with HCV/HIV-1 co-infection who were on stable antiretroviral therapy. The most common adverse events occurring in at least 10% of subjects were fatigue (48%), insomnia (19%), nausea (17%), headache (16%), pruritus (13%), cough (11%), irritability (10%), and ocular icterus (10%).

Elevations in total bilirubin greater than 2 x ULN (mostly indirect) occurred in 34 (54%) subjects. Fifteen of these subjects were also receiving atazanavir at the time of bilirubin elevation and nine also had adverse events of ocular icterus, jaundice or hyperbilirubinemia. None of the subjects with hyperbilirubinemia had concomitant elevations of aminotransferases *[see Warnings and Precautions (5.5), Adverse Reactions (6.1) and Clinical Studies (14.6)]*. No subject experienced a grade 3 ALT elevation.

Seven subjects (11%) had at least one post-baseline hemoglobin value of less than 10 g/dL, and six of these subjects had a ribavirin dose modification; no subject in this small cohort required a blood transfusion or erythropoietin.

Continued on next page

Information on the AbbVie, Inc. products listed on these pages is from the prescribing information in use as of July 31, 2016. For more information, please visit rxabbvie.com or call 1-800-633-9110.

Table 5 *(Cont.)* **Established Drug Interactions Based on Drug Interaction Trials**

Concomitant Drug Class: Drug Name	Effect on Concentration	Clinical Comment
NARCOTIC ANALGESICS		
buprenorphine/naloxone	↑ buprenorphine ↑ norbuprenorphine (metabolite of buprenorphine)	Patients should be closely monitored for sedation and cognitive effects.
Acetaminophen/hydrocodone	↑ hydrocodone ↔ acetaminophen	Reduce the dose of hydrocodone by 50% and monitor patients for respiratory depression and sedation at frequent intervals. Upon completion of VIEKIRA PAK therapy, adjust the hydrocodone dose and monitor for signs of opioid withdrawal.
PROTON PUMP INHIBITORS		
omeprazole	↓ omeprazole	Monitor patients for decreased efficacy of omeprazole. Consider increasing the omeprazole dose in patients whose symptoms are not well controlled; avoid use of more than 40 mg per day of omeprazole.
SEDATIVES/HYPNOTICS		
alprazolam	↑ alprazolam	Clinical monitoring of patients is recommended. A decrease in alprazolam dose can be considered based on clinical response.
diazepam	↓ diazepam ↓ nordiazepam (metabolite of diazepam)	Increase dose if clinically indicated.

See Clinical Pharmacology, Tables 8 and 9.
The direction of the arrow indicates the direction of the change in exposures (C_{max} and AUC) (↑ = increase of more than 20%, ↓ = decrease of more than 20%, ↔ = no change or change less than 20%).
*not studied.

Median declines in CD4+ T-cell counts of 47 cells/mm^3 and 62 cells/mm^3 were observed at the end of 12 and 24 weeks of treatment, respectively, and most returned to baseline levels post-treatment. Two subjects had CD4+ T-cell counts decrease to less than 200 cells/mm^3 during treatment without a decrease in CD4%. No subject experienced an AIDS-related opportunistic infection.

VIEKIRA PAK in Selected Liver Transplant Recipients
VIEKIRA PAK with ribavirin was assessed in 34 post-liver transplant subjects with recurrent HCV infection. Adverse events occurring in more than 20% of subjects included fatigue 50%, headache 44%, cough 32%, diarrhea 26%, insomnia 26%, asthenia 24%, nausea 24%, muscle spasms 21% and rash 21%. Ten subjects (29%) had at least one post-baseline hemoglobin value of less than 10 g/dL. Ten subjects underwent a ribavirin dose modification due to decrease in hemoglobin and 3% (1/34) had an interruption of ribavirin. Five subjects received erythropoietin, all of whom initiated ribavirin at the starting dose of 1000 to 1200 mg daily. No subject received a blood transfusion *[see Clinical Studies (14.5)]*.

6.2   Post-Marketing Adverse Reactions
The following adverse reactions have been identified during post approval use of VIEKIRA PAK. Because these reactions are reported voluntarily from a population of uncertain size, it is not always possible to reliably estimate their frequency or establish a causal relationship to drug exposure.
Immune System Disorders: Hypersensitivity reactions (including angioedema).
Hepatobiliary Disorders: Hepatic decompensation, hepatic failure *[see Warnings and Precautions (5.1)]*.

7   DRUG INTERACTIONS
7.1   Potential for VIEKIRA PAK to Affect Other Drugs
Ombitasvir, paritaprevir, and dasabuvir are inhibitors of UGT1A1, and ritonavir is an inhibitor of CYP3A4. Paritaprevir is an inhibitor of OATP1B1 and OATP1B3 and paritaprevir, ritonavir and dasabuvir are inhibitors of BCRP. Co-administration of VIEKIRA PAK with drugs that are substrates of CYP3A, UGT1A1, BCRP, OATP1B1 or OATP1B3 may result in increased plasma concentrations of such drugs *[see Contraindications (4), Warnings and Precautions (5.4), and Clinical Pharmacology (12.3)]*.

7.2   Potential for Other Drugs to Affect One or More Components of VIEKIRA PAK
Paritaprevir and ritonavir are primarily metabolized by CYP3A enzymes. Co-administration of VIEKIRA PAK with strong inhibitors of CYP3A may increase paritaprevir and ritonavir concentrations. Dasabuvir is primarily metabolized by CYP2C8 enzymes. Co-administration of VIEKIRA PAK with drugs that inhibit CYP2C8 may increase dasabuvir plasma concentrations. Ombitasvir is primarily metabolized via amide hydrolysis while CYP enzymes play a minor role in its metabolism. Ombitasvir, paritaprevir, dasabuvir and ritonavir are substrates of P-gp. Ombitasvir, paritaprevir and dasabuvir are substrates of BCRP. Paritaprevir is a substrate of OATP1B1 and OATP1B3. Inhibition of P-gp, BCRP, OATP1B1 or OATP1B3 may increase the plasma concentrations of the various components of VIEKIRA PAK.

7.3   Established and Other Potential Drug Interactions
If dose adjustments of concomitant medications are made due to treatment with VIEKIRA PAK, doses should be re-adjusted after administration of VIEKIRA PAK is completed. Dose adjustment is not required for VIEKIRA PAK. Table 5 provides the effect of co-administration of VIEKIRA PAK on concentrations of concomitant drugs and the effect of concomitant drugs on the various components of VIEKIRA PAK. See *Contraindications (4)* for drugs that are contraindicated with VIEKIRA PAK. Refer to the ritonavir prescribing information for other potentially significant drug interactions with ritonavir.
[See table 5 on pages 842-844]

7.4   Drugs without Clinically Significant Interactions with VIEKIRA PAK
No dose adjustments are recommended when VIEKIRA PAK is co-administered with the following medications: abacavir, dolutegravir, digoxin, duloxetine, emtricitabine/tenofovir disoproxil fumarate, escitalopram, lamivudine, methadone, progestin only contraceptives, raltegravir, sofosbuvir, sulfamethoxazole, trimethoprim, warfarin and zolpidem.

8   USE IN SPECIFIC POPULATIONS
8.1   Pregnancy
Risk Summary
If VIEKIRA PAK is administered with ribavirin, the combination regimen is contraindicated in pregnant women and in men whose female partners are pregnant. Refer to the ribavirin prescribing information for more information on use in pregnancy.
No adequate human data are available to establish whether or not VIEKIRA PAK poses a risk to pregnancy outcomes. In animal reproduction studies, no adverse developmental effects were observed when the components of VIEKIRA PAK were administered separately during organogenesis and lactation. During organogenesis, the exposures were up to 28 and 4 times (mice and rabbits, respectively; ombitasvir), 8 and 98 times (mice and rats, respectively; paritaprevir, ritonavir), and 24 and 6 times (rats and rabbits, respectively; dasabuvir) exposures at the recommended clinical dose of VIEKIRA PAK. In rodent pre/postnatal developmental studies, maternal systemic exposures (AUC) to ombitasvir, paritaprevir and dasabuvir were approximately 25, 17 and 44 times, respectively, the exposure in humans at the recommended clinical dose *[see Data]*.
The background risk of major birth defects and miscarriage for the indicated population is unknown. In the U.S. general population, the estimated background risk of major birth defects and miscarriage in clinically recognized pregnancies is 2% to 4% and 15% to 20%, respectively.
Data
Animal data
Ombitasvir
Ombitasvir was administered orally to pregnant mice (0, 15, 50, or 150 mg/kg/day) and rabbits (0, 10 or 60 mg/kg/day) during the period of organogenesis (on gestation days (GD) 6 to 15, and GD 7 to 19, respectively). There were no ombitasvir-related embryofetal effects (malformations or fetal toxicity) at any dose level in either species. The systemic exposures at the highest doses were 28-times higher (mice) and 4-times higher (rabbits) than the exposures in humans at the recommended clinical dose.
In a pre- and postnatal developmental study in mice, ombitasvir was administered orally at 0, 10, 40, or 200 mg/kg/day from GD 6 to lactation day 20. There were no ombitasvir-related effects at maternal exposures 25-times higher than exposures in humans at the recommended clinical dose.
The major human metabolites of ombitasvir, M29 and M36, were tested in pregnant mice during the period of organogenesis from GD 6 to 15. M29 was administered orally at doses of 0, 1, 2.5 or 4.5 mg/kg/day. M36 was dosed orally at doses 1.5, 3, or 6 mg/kg/day. In both cases, there were no treatment related embryofetal effects (malformations or fetal toxicity) at any dose level. The highest doses produced exposures approximately 26-times higher than the exposures in humans at the recommended clinical dose.
Paritaprevir/ritonavir
Paritaprevir/ritonavir was administered orally to pregnant rats (0/0, 30/15, 100/15, 450/45 mg/kg/day) and mice (0/0, 30/30, 100/30, or 300/30 mg/kg/day) during the period of organogenesis (on GD 6 to 17, and GD 6 to 15, respectively). There were no test article-related embryofetal effects (malformations or fetal toxicity) at any dose level in either species. The highest systemic exposure of paritaprevir was 8-times higher (rats) and 98-times higher (mice) than the exposures in humans at the recommended clinical dose.
In a pre- and postnatal developmental study in rats, paritaprevir/ritonavir were administered orally at 0/0, 6/30, 30/30, or 300/30 mg/kg/day from GD 7 to lactation day 20. There were no treatment related effects at maternal exposures 17-times higher than exposures in humans at the recommended clinical dose.
Dasabuvir
Dasabuvir was administered orally to pregnant rats (0, 60, 300 and 800 mg/kg/day) and rabbits (0, 100, 200 or 400 mg/kg/day) during the period of organogenesis (on GD 6 to 17 and GD 7 to 20, respectively). There were no test article-related embryofetal effects (malformations or fetal toxicity) at any dose level in either species. The highest systemic exposure of dasabuvir was 24-times higher (rats) and 6-times higher (rabbits) than the exposures in humans at the recommended clinical dose.
In a pre- and postnatal developmental study in rats, dasabuvir was administered orally at 0, 50, 200, or 800 mg/kg/day from GD 7 to lactation day 21. There were no

Table 6. Pharmacokinetic Properties of the Components of VIEKIRA PAK

	Ombitasvir	Paritaprevir	Ritonavir	Dasabuvir
Absorption				
T_{max} (hr)	~ 5	~ 4-5	~ 4-5	~ 4
Absolute bioavailability (%)	48	53	NA	70
Effect of moderate fat meal (relative to fasting)[a]	1.82 (1.61-2.05)	3.11 (2.16-4.46)	1.49 (1.23-1.79)	1.30 (1.08-1.55)
Effect of high fat meal (relative to fasting)[a]	1.76 (1.56-1.99)	2.80 (1.95-4.02)	1.44 (1.19-1.73)	1.22 (1.01-1.46)
Accumulation[b]	0.90- to 1.03-fold	1.5- to 2-fold		0.96-fold
Distribution				
% Bound to human plasma proteins	99.9	97-98.6	>99	>99.5
Blood-to-plasma ratio	0.49	0.7	0.6	0.7
Volume of distribution at steady state (Vss) (L)	173	103	21.5[c]	149
Metabolism				
Metabolism	amide hydrolysis followed by oxidative metabolism	CYP3A4 (major), CYP3A5	CYP3A (major), CYP2D6	CYP2C8 (major), CYP3A
Elimination[d]				
Major route of elimination	biliary excretion	metabolism	metabolism	metabolism
$t_{1/2}$ (hr)[e]	21-25	5.5	4	5.5-6
% of dose excreted in feces[f]	90.2	88	86.4	94.4
% of dose excreted unchanged in feces[f]	87.8	1.1	33.8	26.2
% of dose excreted in urine[f]	1.91	8.8	11.3	~ 2
% of dose excreted unchanged in urine[f]	0.03	0.05	3.5	0.03

NA - data not available
a. Values refer to mean non-fasting/fasting ratios (90% CI) in systemic exposure (AUC). Moderate fat meal ~600 Kcal, 20-30% calories from fat. High fat meal ~900 Kcal, 60% calories from fat.
b. Steady state exposures are achieved after approximately 12 days of dosing.
c. It is apparent volume of distribution (V/F) for ritonavir.
d. Ombitasvir, paritaprevir, ritonavir, and dasabuvir do not inhibit organic anion transporter (OAT1) *in vivo* and based on *in vitro* data, are not expected to inhibit organic cation transporter (OCT2), organic anion transporter (OAT3), or multidrug and toxin extrusion proteins (MATE1 and MATE2K) at clinically relevant concentrations.
e. $t_{1/2}$ values refer to the mean elimination half-life.
f. Dosing in mass balance studies: single dose administration of [^{14}C]ombitasvir; single dose administration of [^{14}C]paritaprevir co-dosed with 100 mg ritonavir; single dose administration of [^{14}C]dasabuvir.

Table 7. Steady-State Pharmacokinetic Parameters of Ombitasvir, Paritaprevir, Ritonavir and Dasabuvir Following Oral Administration of VIEKIRA PAK in HCV-Infected Subjects

Pharmacokinetic Parameter[a]	Ombitasvir	Paritaprevir	Ritonavir	Dasabuvir
C_{max} (ng/mL)	68	262	682	667
AUC_{tau} (ng*h/mL)[b]	1000	2220	6180	3240

a. Median values reported based on the population PK analysis.
b. AUC_{0-24} for ombitasvir, paritaprevir, ritonavir and AUC_{0-12} for dasabuvir.

treatment-related effects at maternal exposures 44-times higher than exposures in humans at the recommended clinical dose.

8.2 Lactation
Risk Summary
It is not known whether VIEKIRA PAK and its metabolites are present in human breast milk, affect human milk production or have effects on the breastfed infant. Unchanged ombitasvir, paritaprevir and its hydrolysis product M13, and dasabuvir were the predominant components observed in the milk of lactating rats, without effect on nursing pups [see Data].

The developmental and health benefits of breastfeeding should be considered along with the mother's clinical need for VIEKIRA PAK and any potential adverse effects on the breastfed child from VIEKIRA PAK or from the underlying maternal condition.
If VIEKIRA PAK is administered with ribavirin, the nursing mother's information for ribavirin also applies to this combination regimen. Refer to the ribavirin prescribing information for more information on use during lactation.
Data
Animal Data
Ombitasvir

No effects of ombitasvir on growth and postnatal development were observed in nursing pups at the highest dose tested (200 mg/kg/day) in mice. Maternal systemic exposure (AUC) to ombitasvir was approximately 25 times the exposure in humans at the recommended clinical dose. Although not measured directly, ombitasvir was likely present in the milk of lactating mice in this study, since systemic exposure was observed in nursing pups on post-natal day 21 (approximately 16% of maternal exposure).
When ombitasvir was administered to lactating rats (5 mg/kg on post-partum day 10 to 11), milk exposure (AUC) was 4 times higher than that in plasma, with unchanged parent drug (91%) accounting for the majority of drug-related material in milk.
Paritaprevir/ritonavir
No effects of paritaprevir/ritonavir on growth and postnatal development were observed in nursing pups at the highest dose tested (300/30 mg/kg/day) in rats. Maternal systemic exposure (AUC) to paritaprevir was approximately 17 times the exposure in humans at the recommended clinical dose. Although not measured directly, paritaprevir was likely present in the milk of lactating rats at the high dose in this study, since systemic exposure was observed in nursing pups on post-natal day 15 (approximately 0.3 % of maternal exposure).
When paritaprevir/ritonavir was administered to lactating rats (30/15 mg/kg on post-partum day 10 to 11), milk exposure (AUC) was half that in plasma, with the hydrolysis product M13 (84%) and unchanged parent drug (16%) accounting for all paritaprevir-related material in milk.
Dasabuvir
No effects of dasabuvir on growth and postnatal development were observed in nursing pups at the highest dose tested (800 mg/kg/day) in rats. Maternal systemic exposure (AUC) to dasabuvir was approximately 44 times the exposure in humans at the recommended clinical dose. Although not measured directly, dasabuvir was likely present in the milk of lactating rats in this study, since systemic exposure was observed in nursing pups on post-natal day 14 (approximately 14% of maternal exposure).
When dasabuvir was administered to lactating rats (5 mg/kg on post-partum day 10 to 11), milk exposure (AUC) was 2 times higher than that in plasma, with unchanged parent drug (78%) accounting for the majority of drug-related material in milk.

8.3 Females and Males of Reproductive Potential
If VIEKIRA PAK™ (ombitasvir, paritaprevir, and ritonavir tablets; dasabuvir tablets) is administered with ribavirin, the information for ribavirin with regard to pregnancy testing, contraception, and infertility also applies to this combination regimen. Refer to ribavirin prescribing information for additional information.

8.4 Pediatric Use
Safety and effectiveness of VIEKIRA PAK in pediatric patients less than 18 years of age have not been established.

8.5 Geriatric Use
No dosage adjustment of VIEKIRA PAK is warranted in geriatric patients. Of the total number of subjects in clinical studies of VIEKIRA PAK, 8.5% (174/2053) were 65 and over. No overall differences in safety or effectiveness were observed between these subjects and younger subjects, and other reported clinical experience has not identified differences in responses between the elderly and younger subjects, but greater sensitivity of some older individuals cannot be ruled out.

8.6 Hepatic Impairment
No dosage adjustment of VIEKIRA PAK is required in patients with mild hepatic impairment (Child-Pugh A). VIEKIRA PAK is contraindicated in patients with moderate to severe (Child-Pugh B and C) hepatic impairment [see Contraindications (4), Warnings and Precautions (5.1) and Clinical Pharmacology (12.3)].

8.7 Renal Impairment
No dosage adjustment of VIEKIRA PAK is required in patients with mild, moderate or severe renal impairment, including those on dialysis. For patients that require ribavi-

Continued on next page

Information on the AbbVie, Inc. products listed on these pages is from the prescribing information in use as of July 31, 2016. For more information, please visit rxabbvie.com or call 1-800-633-9110.

rin, refer to the ribavirin prescribing information for information regarding use in patients with renal impairment [see Clinical Pharmacology (12.3)].

10 OVERDOSAGE

In case of overdose, it is recommended that the patient be monitored for any signs or symptoms of adverse reactions and appropriate symptomatic treatment instituted immediately.

11 DESCRIPTION

VIEKIRA PAK is ombitasvir, paritaprevir, ritonavir fixed dose combination tablets copackaged with dasabuvir tablets.

Ombitasvir, paritaprevir, ritonavir fixed dose combination tablet includes a hepatitis C virus NS5A inhibitor (ombitasvir), a hepatitis C virus NS3/4A protease inhibitor (paritaprevir), and a CYP3A inhibitor (ritonavir) that inhibits CYP3A mediated metabolism of paritaprevir, thereby providing increased plasma concentration of paritaprevir. Dasabuvir is a hepatitis C virus non-nucleoside NS5B palm polymerase inhibitor, which is supplied as separate tablets in the copackage. Both tablets are for oral administration.
Ombitasvir
The chemical name of ombitasvir is Dimethyl ([(2S,5S)-1-(4-tert-butylphenyl) pyrrolidine-2,5-diyl]bis{benzene-4, 1-diylcarbamoyl(2S)pyrrolidine-2,1-diyl[(2S)-3-methyl-1-oxobutane-1,2-diyl]})biscarbamate hydrate. The molecular formula is $C_{50}H_{67}N_7O_8 \cdot 4.5H_2O$ (hydrate) and the molecular weight for the drug substance is 975.20 (hydrate). The drug substance is white to light yellow to light pink powder, and is practically insoluble in aqueous buffers but is soluble in ethanol. Ombitasvir has the following molecular structure:

Paritaprevir
The chemical name of paritaprevir is (2R,6S,12Z,13aS, 14aR,16aS)-N-(cyclopropylsulfonyl)-6-[[(5-methylpyrazin-2-yl)carbonyl]amino]-5,16-dioxo-2-(phenanthridin-6-yloxy)-1,2,3,6,7,8,9,10,11,13a,14,15,16,16a-tetradecahydrocyclo-propa[e]pyrrolo[1,2-a][1,4] diazacyclopentadecine-14a(5H)-carboxamide dihydrate. The molecular formula is $C_{40}H_{43}N_7O_7S \cdot 2H_2O$ (dihydrate) and the molecular weight for the drug substance is 801.91 (dihydrate). The drug substance is white to off-white powder with very low water solubility. Paritaprevir has the following molecular structure:

Ritonavir
The chemical name of ritonavir is [5S-(5R*,8R*,10R*,11R*)]10-Hydroxy-2-methyl-5-(1-methyethyl)-1-[2-(1-methylethyl)-4-thiazolyl]-3,6-dioxo-8,11-bis(phenylmethyl)-2,4,7,12-tetraazatridecan-13-oic acid,5-thiazolylmethyl ester. The molecular formula is $C_{37}H_{48}N_6O_5S_2$ and the molecular weight for the drug substance is 720.95. The drug substance is white to off white to light tan powder practically insoluble in water and freely soluble in methanol and ethanol. Ritonavir has the following molecular structure:
[See molecular structure on next page]
Ombitasvir, Paritaprevir, Ritonavir Fixed-Dose Combination Tablets

Table 8. Drug Interactions: Change in Pharmacokinetic Parameters of the Individual Components of VIEKIRA PAK in the Presence of Co-administered Drug

Co-administered Drug	Dose of Co-administered Drug (mg)	n	DAA	Ratio (with/without co-administered drug) of DAA Pharmacokinetic Parameters (90% CI); No Effect = 1.00		
				C_{max}	AUC	C_{min}
Alprazolam	0.5 single dose	12	ombitasvir	0.98 (0.93, 1.04)	1.00 (0.96, 1.04)	0.98 (0.93, 1.04)
			paritaprevir	0.91 (0.64, 1.31)	0.96 (0.73, 1.27)	1.12 (1.02, 1.23)
			ritonavir	0.92 (0.84, 1.02)	0.96 (0.89, 1.03)	1.01 (0.94, 1.09)
			dasabuvir	0.93 (0.83, 1.04)	0.98 (0.87, 1.11)	1.00 (0.87, 1.15)
Amlodipine	5 single dose	14	ombitasvir	1.00 (0.95, 1.06)	1.00 (0.97, 1.04)	1.00 (0.97, 1.04)
			paritaprevir	0.77 (0.64, 0.94)	0.78 (0.68, 0.88)	0.88 (0.80, 0.95)
			ritonavir	0.96 (0.87, 1.06)	0.93 (0.89, 0.98)	0.95 (0.89, 1.01)
			dasabuvir	1.05 (0.97, 1.14)	1.01 (0.96, 1.06)	0.95 (0.89, 1.01)
Atazanavir/ ritonavir[a]	Atazanavir 300 and ritonavir 100 once daily in the evening	11	ombitasvir	0.83 (0.72, 0.96)	0.90 (0.78, 1.02)	1.00 (0.89, 1.13)
			paritaprevir	2.19 (1.61, 2.98)	3.16 (2.40, 4.17)	11.95 (8.94, 15.98)
			ritonavir	1.60 (1.38, 1.86)	3.18 (2.74, 3.69)	24.65 (18.64, 32.60)
			dasabuvir	0.81 (0.73, 0.91)	0.81 (0.71, 0.92)	0.80 (0.65, 0.98)
Carbamazepine	200 once daily followed by 200 twice daily	12	ombitasvir	0.69 (0.61, 0.78)	0.69 (0.64, 0.74)	NA
			paritaprevir	0.34 (0.25, 0.48)	0.30 (0.23, 0.38)	NA
			ritonavir	0.17 (0.12, 0.24)	0.13 (0.09, 0.17)	NA
			dasabuvir	0.45 (0.41, 0.50)	0.30 (0.28, 0.33)	NA
Carisoprodol	250 single dose	14	ombitasvir	0.98 (0.92, 1.04)	0.95 (0.92, 0.97)	0.96 (0.92, 0.99)
			paritaprevir	0.88 (0.75, 1.03)	0.96 (0.85, 1.08)	1.14 (1.02, 1.27)
			ritonavir	0.94 (0.87, 1.02)	0.94 (0.88, 0.99)	0.95 (0.89, 1.03)
			dasabuvir	0.96 (0.91, 1.01)	1.02 (0.97, 1.07)	1.00 (0.92, 1.10)
Cyclobenzaprine	5 single dose	14	ombitasvir	0.98 (0.92, 1.04)	1.00 (0.97, 1.03)	1.01 (0.98, 1.04)
			paritaprevir	1.14 (0.99, 1.32)	1.13 (1.00, 1.28)	1.13 (1.01, 1.25)
			ritonavir	0.93 (0.87, 0.99)	1.00 (0.95, 1.06)	1.13 (1.05, 1.21)
			dasabuvir	0.98 (0.90, 1.07)	1.01 (0.96, 1.06)	1.13 (1.07, 1.18)

This table is continued on the next page

Table 8 *(Cont.)* Drug Interactions: Change in Pharmacokinetic Parameters of the Individual Components of VIEKIRA PAK in the Presence of Co-administered Drug

Co-administered Drug	Dose of Co-administered Drug (mg)	n	DAA	Ratio (with/without co-administered drug) of DAA Pharmacokinetic Parameters (90% CI); No Effect = 1.00		
				C_{max}	AUC	C_{min}
Cyclosporine	30 single dose[b]	10	ombitasvir	0.99 (0.92, 1.07)	1.08 (1.05, 1.11)	1.15 (1.08, 1.23)
			paritaprevir	1.44 (1.16, 1.78)	1.72 (1.49, 1.99)	1.85 (1.58, 2.18)
			ritonavir	0.90 (0.78, 1.04)	1.11 (1.04, 1.19)	1.49 (1.28, 1.74)
			dasabuvir	0.66 (0.58, 0.75)	0.70 (0.65, 0.76)	0.76 (0.71, 0.82)
Darunavir[c]	800 once daily	9	ombitasvir	0.86 (0.77, 0.95)	0.86 (0.79, 0.94)	0.87 (0.82, 0.92)
			paritaprevir	1.54 (1.14, 2.09)	1.29 (1.04, 1.61)	1.30 (1.09, 1.54)
			ritonavir	0.84 (0.72, 0.98)	0.85 (0.78, 0.93)	1.07 (0.93, 1.23)
			dasabuvir	1.10 (0.88, 1.37)	0.94 (0.78, 1.14)	0.90 (0.76, 1.06)
Darunavir/ ritonavir[d]	Darunavir 600 twice daily and ritonavir 100 once daily in the evening	7	ombitasvir	0.76 (0.65, 0.88)	0.73 (0.66, 0.80)	0.73 (0.64, 0.83)
			paritaprevir	0.70 (0.43, 1.12)	0.59 (0.44, 0.79)	0.83 (0.69, 1.01)
			ritonavir	1.61 (1.30, 2.00)	1.28 (1.12, 1.45)	0.88 (0.79, 0.99)
			dasabuvir	0.84 (0.67, 1.05)	0.73 (0.62, 0.86)	0.54 (0.49, 0.61)
Darunavir/ ritonavir[e]	Darunavir 800 and ritonavir 100 once daily in the evening	12	ombitasvir	0.87 (0.82, 0.93)	0.87 (0.81, 0.93)	0.87 (0.80, 0.95)
			paritaprevir	0.70 (0.50, 0.99)	0.81 (0.60, 1.09)	1.59 (1.23, 2.05)
			ritonavir	1.19 (1.06, 1.33)	1.70 (1.54, 1.88)	14.15 (11.66, 17.18)
			dasabuvir	0.75 (0.64, 0.88)	0.72 (0.64, 0.82)	0.65 (0.58, 0.72)
Diazepam	2 single dose	13	ombitasvir	1.00 (0.93, 1.08)	0.98 (0.93, 1.03)	0.93 (0.88, 0.98)
			paritaprevir	0.95 (0.77, 1.18)	0.91 (0.78, 1.07)	0.92 (0.82, 1.03)
			ritonavir	1.10 (1.02, 1.19)	1.06 (0.98, 1.14)	0.98 (0.92, 1.03)
			dasabuvir	1.05 (0.98, 1.13)	1.01 (0.94, 1.08)	1.05 (0.98, 1.12)

Ombitasvir, paritaprevir, and ritonavir film-coated tablets are co-formulated immediate release tablets. The tablet contains copovidone, K value 28, vitamin E polyethylene glycol succinate, propylene glycol monolaurate Type I, sorbitan monolaurate, colloidal silicon dioxide/colloidal anhydrous silica, sodium stearyl fumarate, polyvinyl alcohol, polyethylene glycol 3350/macrogol 3350, talc, titanium dioxide, and iron oxide red. The strength for the tablet is 12.5 mg ombitasvir, 75 mg paritaprevir, 50 mg ritonavir.
Dasabuvir
The chemical name of dasabuvir is Sodium 3-(3-*tert*-butyl-4-methoxy-5-{6-[(methylsulfonyl)amino]naphthalene-2-yl}phenyl)-2,6-dioxo-3,6-dihydro-2H-pyrimidin-1-ide hydrate (1:1:1). The molecular formula is $C_{26}H_{26}N_3O_5S \cdot Na \cdot H_2O$ (salt, hydrate) and the molecular weight of the drug substance is 533.57 (salt, hydrate). The drug substance is white to pale yellow to pink powder, slightly soluble in water and very slightly soluble in methanol and isopropyl alcohol. Dasabuvir has the following molecular structure:

Dasabuvir is formulated as a 250 mg film-coated, immediate release tablet containing microcrystalline cellulose (D50-100 um), microcrystalline cellulose (D50-50 um); lactose monohydrate, copovidone, croscarmellose sodium, colloidal silicon dioxide/anhydrous colloidal silica, magnesium stearate, polyvinyl alcohol, titanium dioxide, polyethylene glycol 3350/macrogol 3350, talc, and iron oxide yellow, iron oxide red and iron oxide black. Each tablet contains 270.3 mg dasabuvir sodium monohydrate equivalent to 250 mg dasabuvir.

12   CLINICAL PHARMACOLOGY
12.1   Mechanism of Action
VIEKIRA PAK combines three direct-acting hepatitis C virus antiviral agents with distinct mechanisms of action *[see Microbiology (12.4)]*.
Ritonavir is not active against HCV. Ritonavir is a potent CYP3A inhibitor that increases peak and trough plasma drug concentrations of paritaprevir and overall drug exposure (i.e., area under the curve).
12.2   Pharmacodynamics
Cardiac Electrophysiology
The effect of a combination of ombitasvir, paritaprevir, ritonavir, and dasabuvir on QTc interval was evaluated in a randomized, double blind, placebo and active-controlled (moxifloxacin 400 mg) 4-way crossover thorough QT study in 60 healthy subjects. At concentrations approximately 6, 1.8 and 2 times the therapeutic concentrations of paritaprevir, ombitasvir, and dasabuvir, the combination did not prolong QTc to any clinically relevant extent.
12.3   Pharmacokinetics
The pharmacokinetic properties of the components of VIEKIRA PAK are provided in Table 6. Based on the population pharmacokinetic analysis, the median steady-state

Continued on next page

This table is continued on the next page

Table 8 *(Cont.)* Drug Interactions: Change in Pharmacokinetic Parameters of the Individual Components of VIEKIRA PAK in the Presence of Co-administered Drug

Co-administered Drug	Dose of Co-administered Drug (mg)	n	DAA	Ratio (with/without co-administered drug) of DAA Pharmacokinetic Parameters (90% CI); No Effect = 1.00		
				C_{max}	AUC	C_{min}
Ethinyl estradiol/ Norgestimate	Ethinyl estradiol 0.035 and Norgestimate 0.25 once daily	7[f]	ombitasvir	1.05 (0.81, 1.35)	0.97 (0.81, 1.15)	1.00 (0.88, 1.12)
			paritaprevir	0.70 (0.40, 1.21)	0.66 (0.42, 1.04)	0.87 (0.67, 1.14)
			ritonavir	0.80 (0.53, 1.21)	0.71 (0.54, 0.94)	0.79 (0.68, 0.93)
			dasabuvir	0.51 (0.22, 1.18)	0.48 (0.23, 1.02)	0.53 (0.30, 0.95)
Furosemide	20 single dose	12	ombitasvir	1.14 (1.03, 1.26)	1.07 (1.01, 1.12)	1.12 (1.08, 1.16)
			paritaprevir	0.93 (0.63, 1.36)	0.92 (0.70, 1.21)	1.26 (1.16, 1.38)
			ritonavir	1.10 (0.96, 1.27)	1.04 (0.92, 1.18)	1.07 (0.99, 1.17)
			dasabuvir	1.12 (0.96, 1.31)	1.09 (0.96, 1.23)	1.06
Gemfibrozil[g]	600 twice daily	11	ombitasvir	NA	NA	NA
			paritaprevir	1.21 (0.94, 1.57)	1.38 (1.18, 1.61)	NA
			ritonavir	0.84 (0.69, 1.03)	0.90 (0.78, 1.04)	NA
			dasabuvir	2.01 (1.71, 2.38)	11.25 (9.05, 13.99)	NA
Hydrocodone/ Acetaminophen	5/300 single dose	15	ombitasvir	1.01 (0.93, 1.10)	0.97 (0.93, 1.02)	0.93 (0.90, 0.97)
			paritaprevir	1.01 (0.80, 1.27)	1.03 (0.89, 1.18)	1.10 (0.97, 1.26)
			ritonavir	1.01 (0.90, 1.13)	1.03 (0.96, 1.09)	1.01 (0.93, 1.10)
			dasabuvir	1.13 (1.01, 1.26)	1.12 (1.05, 1.19)	1.16
Ketoconazole	400 once daily	12	ombitasvir	0.98 (0.90, 1.06)	1.17 (1.11, 1.24)	NA
			paritaprevir	1.37 (1.11, 1.69)	1.98 (1.63, 2.42)	NA
			ritonavir	1.27 (1.04, 1.56)	1.57 (1.36, 1.81)	NA
			dasabuvir	1.16 (1.03, 1.32)	1.42 (1.26, 1.59)	NA
Lopinavir/ ritonavir	400/100 twice daily	6	ombitasvir	1.14 (1.01, 1.28)	1.17 (1.07, 1.28)	1.24 (1.14, 1.34)
			paritaprevir	2.04 (1.30, 3.20)	2.17 (1.63, 2.89)	2.36 (1.00, 5.55)
			ritonavir	1.55 (1.16, 2.09)	2.05 (1.49, 2.81)	5.25 (3.33, 8.28)
			dasabuvir	0.99 (0.75, 1.31)	0.93 (0.75, 1.15)	0.68 (0.57, 0.80)

This table is continued on the next page

pharmacokinetic parameters of ombitasvir, paritaprevir, ritonavir and dasabuvir in HCV–infected subjects are provided in Table 7.

[See table 6 on top of page 845]

[See table 7 on bottom of page 845]

Specific Populations

Hepatic Impairment

The single dose pharmacokinetics of ombitasvir, paritaprevir, ritonavir and dasabuvir were evaluated in non-HCV infected subjects with mild hepatic impairment (Child-Pugh Category A; score of 5-6), moderate hepatic impairment (Child-Pugh Category B, score of 7-9) and severe hepatic impairment (Child-Pugh Category C, score of 10-15).

Relative to subjects with normal hepatic function, ombitasvir, paritaprevir and ritonavir AUC values decreased by 8%, 29% and 34%, respectively, and dasabuvir AUC values increased by 17% in subjects with mild hepatic impairment.

Relative to subjects with normal hepatic function, ombitasvir, ritonavir and dasabuvir AUC values decreased by 30%, 30% and 16%, respectively, and paritaprevir AUC values increased by 62% in subjects with moderate hepatic impairment.

Relative to subjects with normal hepatic function, paritaprevir, ritonavir and dasabuvir AUC values increased by 945%, 13%, and 325% respectively, and ombitasvir AUC values decreased by 54% in subjects with severe hepatic impairment *[see Dosage and Administration (2.4), Contraindications (4), Warnings and Precautions (5.1) and Use in Specific Populations (8.6)]*.

Renal Impairment

The single dose pharmacokinetics of ombitasvir, paritaprevir, ritonavir and dasabuvir were evaluated in non-HCV infected subjects with mild (CL_{cr}: 60 to 89 mL/min), moderate (CL_{cr}: 30 to 59 mL/min), and severe (CL_{cr}: 15 to 29 mL/min) renal impairment.

Overall, changes in exposure of ombitasvir, paritaprevir, ritonavir and dasabuvir in non-HCV infected subjects with mild-, moderate- and severe renal impairment are not expected to be clinically relevant. Pharmacokinetic data are not available on the use of VIEKIRA PAK in non-HCV infected subjects with End Stage Renal Disease (ESRD).

Relative to subjects with normal renal function, paritaprevir, ritonavir and dasabuvir AUC values increased by 19%, 42% and 21%, respectively, while ombitasvir AUC values were unchanged in subjects with mild renal impairment.

Relative to subjects with normal renal function, paritaprevir, ritonavir and dasabuvir AUC values increased by 33%, 80% and 37%, respectively, while ombitasvir AUC values were unchanged in subjects with moderate renal impairment.

Relative to subjects with normal renal function, paritaprevir, ritonavir and dasabuvir AUC values increased by 45%, 114% and 50%, respectively, while ombitasvir AUC values were unchanged in subjects with severe renal impairment *[see Use in Specific Populations (8.7)]*.

Pediatric Population

The pharmacokinetics of VIEKIRA PAK in pediatric patients less than 18 years of age has not been established *[see Use in Specific Populations (8.4)]*.

Sex

No dose adjustment is recommended based on sex or body weight.

Race / Ethnicity

No dose adjustment is recommended based on race or ethnicity.

Age

No dose adjustment is recommended in geriatric patients *[see Use in Specific Populations (8.5)]*.

Drug Interaction Studies

See also Contraindications (4), Warnings and Precautions (5.4), Drug Interactions (7)

The effects of drugs discussed in Table 5 on the exposures of the individual components of VIEKIRA PAK are shown in Table 8. For information regarding clinical recommendations, see *Drug Interactions (7)*.

[See table 8 on pages 846 through 850]

Table 9 summarizes the effects of VIEKIRA PAK™ (ombitasvir, paritaprevir, and ritonavir tablets; dasabuvir tablets) on the pharmacokinetics of co-administered drugs

Table 8 *(Cont.)* Drug Interactions: Change in Pharmacokinetic Parameters of the Individual Components of VIEKIRA PAK in the Presence of Co-administered Drug

Co-administered Drug	Dose of Co-administered Drug (mg)	n	DAA	Ratio (with/without co-administered drug) of DAA Pharmacokinetic Parameters (90% CI); No Effect = 1.00		
				C_{max}	AUC	C_{min}
Lopinavir/ ritonavir[h]	800/200 once daily	12	ombitasvir	0.87 (0.83, 0.92)	0.97 (0.94, 1.02)	1.11 (1.06, 1.16)
			paritaprevir	0.99 (0.79, 1.25)	1.87 (1.40, 2.52)	8.23 (5.18, 13.07)
			ritonavir	1.57 (1.34, 1.83)	2.62 (2.32, 2.97)	19.46 (15.93, 23.77)
			dasabuvir	0.56 (0.47, 0.66)	0.54 (0.46, 0.65)	0.47 (0.39, 0.58)
Omeprazole	40 once daily	11	ombitasvir	1.02 (0.95, 1.09)	1.05 (0.98, 1.12)	1.04 (0.98, 1.11)
			paritaprevir	1.19 (1.04, 1.36)	1.18 (1.03, 1.37)	0.92 (0.76, 1.12)
			ritonavir	1.04 (0.96, 1.12)	1.02 (0.97, 1.08)	0.97 (0.89, 1.05)
			dasabuvir	1.13 (1.03, 1.25)	1.08 (0.98, 1.20)	1.05 (0.93, 1.19)
Pravastatin	10 once daily	12	ombitasvir	0.95 (0.89, 1.02)	0.94 (0.89, 0.99)	0.94 (0.89, 0.99)
			paritaprevir	0.96 (0.69, 1.32)	1.13 (0.92, 1.38)	1.39 (1.21, 1.59)
			ritonavir	0.89 (0.73, 1.09)	0.95 (0.86, 1.05)	1.08 (0.98, 1.19)
			dasabuvir	1.00 (0.87, 1.14)	0.96 (0.85, 1.09)	1.03 (0.91, 1.15)
Rosuvastatin	5 once daily	11	ombitasvir	0.92 (0.82, 1.04)	0.89 (0.83, 0.95)	0.88 (0.83, 0.94)
			paritaprevir	1.59 (1.13, 2.23)	1.52 (1.23, 1.90)	1.43 (1.22, 1.68)
			ritonavir	0.98 (0.84, 1.15)	1.02 (0.93, 1.12)	1.00 (0.90, 1.12)
			dasabuvir	1.07 (0.92, 1.24)	1.08 (0.92, 1.26)	1.15 (1.05, 1.25)

This table is continued on the next page

which showed clinically relevant changes. For information regarding clinical recommendations, see *Drug Interactions (7).*

[See table 9 on pages 851 and 852]

12.4   Microbiology
Mechanism of Action
VIEKIRA PAK combines three direct-acting antiviral agents with distinct mechanisms of action and non-overlapping resistance profiles to target HCV at multiple steps in the viral lifecycle.
Ombitasvir
Ombitasvir is an inhibitor of HCV NS5A, which is essential for viral RNA replication and virion assembly. The mechanism of action of ombitasvir has been characterized based on cell culture antiviral activity and drug resistance mapping studies.
Paritaprevir
Paritaprevir is an inhibitor of the HCV NS3/4A protease which is necessary for the proteolytic cleavage of the HCV encoded polyprotein (into mature forms of the NS3, NS4A, NS4B, NS5A, and NS5B proteins) and is essential for viral replication. In a biochemical assay, paritaprevir inhibited the proteolytic activity of recombinant HCV genotype 1a and 1b NS3/4A protease enzymes with IC_{50} values of 0.18 nM and 0.43 nM, respectively.
Dasabuvir
Dasabuvir is a non-nucleoside inhibitor of the HCV RNA-dependent RNA polymerase encoded by the NS5B gene, which is essential for replication of the viral genome. In a biochemical assay, dasabuvir inhibited a panel of genotype 1a and 1b NS5B polymerases with median IC_{50} values of 2.8 nM (range 2.4 nM to 4.2 nM; n = 3) and 3.7 nM (range 2.2 nM to 10.7 nM; n = 4), respectively. Based on drug resistance mapping studies of HCV genotypes 1a and 1b, dasabuvir targets the palm domain of the NS5B polymerase, and is therefore referred to as a non-nucleoside NS5B-palm polymerase inhibitor.
Antiviral Activity
Ombitasvir
The EC_{50} values of ombitasvir against genotype 1a-H77 and 1b-Con1 strains in HCV replicon cell culture assays were 14.1 pM and 5 pM, respectively. The median EC_{50} values of ombitasvir against HCV replicons containing NS5A genes from a panel of genotype 1a and 1b isolates from treatment-naïve subjects were 0.68 pM (range 0.35 to 0.88 pM; n = 11) and 0.94 pM (range 0.74 to 1.5 pM; n = 11), respectively.
Paritaprevir
The EC_{50} values of paritaprevir against genotype 1a-H77 and 1b-Con1 strains in HCV replicon cell culture assay were 1.0 nM and 0.21 nM, respectively. The median EC_{50} values of paritaprevir against HCV replicons containing NS3 genes from a panel of genotype 1a and 1b isolates from treatment-naïve subjects were 0.68 nM (range 0.43 nM to 1.87 nM; n = 11) and 0.06 nM (range 0.03 nM to 0.09 nM; n = 9), respectively.
Ritonavir
In HCV replicon cell culture assays, ritonavir did not exhibit a direct antiviral effect and the presence of ritonavir did not affect the antiviral activity of paritaprevir.
Dasabuvir
The EC_{50} values of dasabuvir against genotype 1a-H77 and 1b-Con1 strains in HCV replicon cell culture assays were 7.7 nM and 1.8 nM, respectively. The median EC_{50} values of dasabuvir against HCV replicons containing NS5B genes from a panel of genotype 1a and 1b isolates from treatment-naïve subjects were 0.6 nM (range 0.4 nM to 2.1 nM; n = 11) and 0.3 nM (range 0.2 nM to 2 nM; n = 10), respectively.
Combination Antiviral Activity
Evaluation of pairwise combinations of ombitasvir, paritaprevir, dasabuvir and ribavirin in HCV genotype 1 replicon cell culture assays showed no evidence of antagonism in antiviral activity.
Resistance
In Cell Culture
Exposure of HCV genotype 1a and 1b replicons to ombitasvir, paritaprevir or dasabuvir resulted in the emergence of drug resistant replicons carrying amino acid sub-

Continued on next page

Information on the AbbVie, Inc. products listed on these pages is from the prescribing information in use as of July 31, 2016. For more information, please visit rxabbvie.com or call 1-800-633-9110.

Table 8 *(Cont.)* Drug Interactions: Change in Pharmacokinetic Parameters of the Individual Components of VIEKIRA PAK in the Presence of Co-administered Drug

Co-administered Drug	Dose of Co-administered Drug (mg)	n	DAA	Ratio (with/without co-administered drug) of DAA Pharmacokinetic Parameters (90% CI); No Effect = 1.00		
				C_{max}	AUC	C_{min}
Rilpivirine	25 once daily (morning)[i]	10	ombitasvir	1.11 (1.02, 1.20)	1.09 (1.04, 1.14)	1.05 (1.01, 1.08)
			paritaprevir	1.30 (0.94, 1.81)	1.23 (0.93, 1.64)	0.95 (0.84, 1.07)
			ritonavir	1.10 (0.98, 1.24)	1.08 (0.93, 1.27)	0.97 (0.91, 1.04)
			dasabuvir	1.18 (1.02, 1.37)	1.17 (0.99, 1.38)	1.10 (0.89, 1.37)
Tacrolimus	2 single dose	12	ombitasvir	0.93 (0.88, 0.99)	0.94 (0.89, 0.98)	0.94 (0.91, 0.96)
			paritaprevir	0.57 (0.42, 0.78)	0.66 (0.54, 0.81)	0.73 (0.66, 0.80)
			ritonavir	0.76 (0.63, 0.91)	0.87 (0.79, 0.97)	1.03 (0.89, 1.19)
			dasabuvir	0.85 (0.73, 0.98)	0.90 (0.80, 1.02)	1.01 (0.91, 1.11)

a. Atazanavir plus 100 mg ritonavir administered in the evening, 12 hours after morning dose of VIEKIRA PAK.
b. 30 mg cyclosporine was administered with VIEKIRA PAK in the test arm and 100 mg cyclosporine was administered in the reference arm without VIEKIRA PAK.
c. Darunavir administered with VIEKIRA PAK in the morning was compared to darunavir administered with 100 mg ritonavir in the morning.
d. Darunavir administered with VIEKIRA PAK in the morning and with 100 mg ritonavir in the evening was compared to darunavir administered with 100 mg ritonavir in the morning and evening.
e. Darunavir plus 100 mg ritonavir administered in the evening, 12 hours after the morning dose of VIEKIRA PAK compared to darunavir administered with 100 mg ritonavir in the evening.
f. N=3 for dasabuvir.
g. Study was conducted with paritaprevir, ritonavir and dasabuvir.
h. Lopinavir/ritonavir administered in the evening, 12 hours after morning dose of VIEKIRA PAK.
i. Similar increases were observed when rilpivirine was dosed in the evening with food or 4 hours after food.
NA: not available/not applicable; DAA: Direct-acting antiviral agent; CI: Confidence interval
Doses of ombitasvir, paritaprevir, and ritonavir were 25 mg, 150 mg and 100 mg. Doses of dasabuvir were 250 mg or 400 mg (both doses showed similar exposures).
Ombitasvir, paritaprevir and ritonavir were dosed once daily and dasabuvir was dosed twice daily in all the above studies except studies with gemfibrozil, ketoconazole and carbamazepine that used single doses.

stitutions in NS5A, NS3, or NS5B, respectively. Amino acid substitutions in NS5A, NS3, or NS5B selected in cell culture or identified in Phase 2b and 3 clinical trials were phenotypically characterized in genotype 1a or 1b replicons.
For ombitasvir, in HCV genotype 1a replicons single NS5A substitutions M28T/V, Q30E/R, L31V, H58D, and Y93C/H/L/N reduced ombitasvir antiviral activity by 58- to 67,000-fold. In genotype 1b replicons, single NS5A substitutions L28T, L31F/V, and Y93H reduced ombitasvir antiviral activity by 8- to 661-fold. In general, combinations of ombitasvir resistance-associated substitutions in HCV genotype 1a or 1b replicons further reduced ombitasvir antiviral activity.
For paritaprevir, in HCV genotype 1a replicons single NS3 substitutions F43L, R155G/K/S, A156T, and D168A/E/F/H/N/V/Y reduced paritaprevir antiviral activity by 7- to 219-fold. An NS3 Q80K substitution in a genotype 1a replicon reduced paritaprevir antiviral activity by 3-fold. Combinations of V36M, Y56H, or E357K with R155K or D168 substitutions reduced the activity of paritaprevir by an additional 2- to 7-fold relative to the single R155K or D168 substitutions in genotype 1a replicons. In genotype 1b replicons single NS3 substitutions A156T and D168A/H/V reduced paritaprevir antiviral activity by 7- to 159-fold. The combination of Y56H with D168 substitutions reduced the activity of paritaprevir by an additional 16- to 26-fold relative to the single D168 substitutions in genotype 1b replicons.
For dasabuvir, in HCV genotype 1a replicons single NS5B substitutions C316Y, M414I/T, E446K/Q, Y448C/H, A553T, G554S, S556G/R, and Y561H reduced dasabuvir antiviral activity by 8- to 1,472-fold. In genotype 1b replicons, single NS5B substitutions C316H/N/Y, S368T, N411S, M414I/T, Y448C/H, A553V, S556G and D559G reduced dasabuvir antiviral activity by 5- to 1,569-fold.
In Clinical Studies
In a pooled analysis of subjects treated with regimens containing ombitasvir, paritaprevir, and dasabuvir with or without ribavirin (for 12 or 24 weeks) in Phase 2b and Phase 3 clinical trials, resistance analyses were conducted for 64 subjects who experienced virologic failure (20 with on-treatment virologic failure, 44 with post-treatment relapse). Treatment-emergent substitutions observed in the viral populations of these subjects are shown in Table 10. Treatment-emergent substitutions were detected in all 3 HCV drug targets in 30/57 (53%) HCV genotype 1a infected subjects, and 1/6 (17%) HCV genotype 1b infected subjects.
[See table 10 on page 853]
Persistence of Resistance-Associated Substitutions
The persistence of ombitasvir, paritaprevir, and dasabuvir treatment-emergent amino acid substitutions in NS5A, NS3, and NS5B, respectively, was assessed in HCV genotype 1a-infected subjects in Phase 2 trials whose virus had at least 1 treatment-emergent resistance-associated substitution in the drug target, and with available data through at least 24 weeks post-treatment. Population and clonal nucleotide sequence analyses (assay sensitivity approximately 5-10%) were conducted to detect the persistence of viral populations with treatment-emergent substitutions.
For ombitasvir, viral populations with 1 or more resistance-associated treatment-emergent substitutions in NS5A persisted at detectable levels through at least Post-Treatment Week 24 in 24/24 (100%) subjects, and through Post-Treatment Week 48 in 18/18 (100%) subjects with available data.
For paritaprevir, viral populations with 1 or more treatment-emergent substitutions in NS3 persisted at detectable levels through at least Post-Treatment Week 24 in 17/29 (59%) subjects, and through Post-Treatment Week 48 in 5/22 (23%) subjects with available data. Resistance-associated variant R155K remained detectable in 5/8 (63%) subjects through Post-Treatment Week 24, and in 1/5 (20%) subjects through Post-Treatment Week 48. Resistance-associated D168 substitutions remained detectable in 6/22 (27%) subjects through Post-Treatment Week 24, and were no longer detectable through Post-Treatment Week 48.
For dasabuvir, viral populations with 1 or more treatment-emergent substitutions in NS5B persisted at detectable levels through at least Post-Treatment Week 24 in 11/16 (69%) subjects, and through Post-Treatment Week 48 in 8/15 (53%) subjects with available data. Treatment-emergent S556G persisted through Post-Treatment Week 48 in 6/9 (67%) subjects.
Among HCV genotype 1b infected subjects who experienced virologic failure with a regimen including ombitasvir and

Table 9. Drug Interactions: Change in Pharmacokinetic Parameters for Co-administered Drug in the Presence of VIEKIRA PAK

Co-administered Drug	Dose of Co-administered Drug (mg)	n	Ratio (with/without VIEKIRA PAK) of Co-administered Drug Pharmacokinetic Parameters (90% CI); No Effect = 1.00		
			C_{max}	AUC	C_{min}
Alprazolam	0.5 single dose	12	1.09 (1.03, 1.15)	1.34 (1.15, 1.55)	NA
Amlodipine	5 single dose	14	1.26 (1.11, 1.44)	2.57 (2.31, 2.86)	NA
Atazanavir/ ritonavir[a]	Atazanavir 300 and ritonavir 100 once daily in the evening	12	1.02 (0.92, 1.13)[b]	1.19 (1.11, 1.28)[b]	1.68 (1.44, 1.95)[b]
Buprenorphine	Buprenorphine: 4 to 24 once daily and Naloxone 1 to 6 once daily	10	2.18 (1.78, 2.68)[c]	2.07 (1.78, 2.40)[c]	3.12 (2.29, 4.27)[c]
Norbuprenorphine			2.07 (1.42, 3.01)[c]	1.84 (1.30, 2.60)[c]	2.10 (1.49, 2.97)[c]
Naloxone			1.18 (0.81, 1.73)	1.28 (0.92, 1.79)[c]	NA
Carbamazepine	200 once daily followed by 200 twice daily	12	1.10 (1.07, 1.14)	1.17 (1.13, 1.22)	1.35 (1.27, 1.45)
Carbamazepine's metabolite, carbamazepine-10,11-epoxide (CBZE)			0.84 (0.82, 0.87)	0.75 (0.73, 0.77)	0.57 (0.54, 0.61)
Carisoprodol	250 single dose	14	0.54 (0.47, 0.63)	0.62 (0.55, 0.70)	NA
Carisoprodol's metabolite, mepobramate			1.17 (1.10, 1.25)	1.09 (1.03, 1.16)	NA
Cyclobenzaprine	5 single dose	14	0.68 (0.61, 0.75)	0.60 (0.53, 0.68)	NA
Cyclobenzaprine's metabolite norcyclobenzaprine			1.03 (0.87, 1.23)	0.74 (0.64, 0.85)	NA
Cyclosporine	30 single dose[d]	10	1.01 (0.85, 1.20)[c]	5.82 (4.73, 7.14)[c]	15.80 (13.81, 18.09)[c]
Darunavir[e]	800 once daily	8	0.92 (0.87, 0.98)[b]	0.76 (0.71, 0.82)[b]	0.52 (0.47, 0.58)[b]
Darunavir/ ritonavir[f]	Darunavir 600 twice daily and ritonavir 100 once daily in the evening	7	0.87 (0.79, 0.96)[b]	0.80 (0.74, 0.86)[b]	0.57 (0.48, 0.67)[b]
Darunavir/ ritonavir[g]	Darunavir 800 and ritonavir 100 once daily in the evening	10	0.79 (0.70, 0.90)[b]	1.34 (1.25, 1.43)[b]	0.54 (0.48, 0.62)[b]

This table is continued on the next page

paritaprevir, a treatment-emergent NS5A Y93H substitution persisted through at least Post-Treatment Week 48 in 2/2 subjects, and a NS3 D168V treatment-emergent substitution persisted through Post-Treatment Week 24 in 2/4 subjects, but was no longer detectable through Post-Treatment Week 48 (0/4 subjects).

The lack of detection of virus containing a resistance-associated substitution does not indicate that the resistant virus is no longer present at clinically significant levels. The long-term clinical impact of the emergence or persistence of virus containing VIEKIRA PAK-resistance-associated substitutions is unknown.

Effect of Baseline HCV Polymorphisms on Treatment Response

A pooled analysis of subjects in the Phase 3 clinical trials of ombitasvir, paritaprevir, and dasabuvir with or without ribavirin was conducted to explore the association between baseline HCV NS5A, NS3, or NS5B resistance-associated polymorphisms and treatment outcome. Baseline samples from HCV genotype 1a infected subjects who experienced virologic failure (n=47), as well as samples from a subset of demographically matched subjects who achieved SVR (n=94), were analyzed to compare the frequencies of resistance-associated polymorphisms in these two populations. The NS3 Q80K polymorphism was detected in approximately 38% of subjects in this analysis and was enriched approximately 2-fold in virologic failure subjects compared to SVR-achieving subjects. Ombitasvir resistance-associated polymorphisms in NS5A (pooling data from all resistance-associated amino acid positions) were detected in approximately 22% of subjects in this analysis and similarly were enriched approximately 2-fold in virologic failure subjects. Dasabuvir resistance-associated polymorphisms in NS5B were detected in approximately 5% of subjects in this analysis and were not enriched in virologic failure subjects.

In contrast to the Phase 3 subset analysis, no association of NS3 or NS5A polymorphisms and treatment outcome was seen in an analysis of noncirrhotic HCV genotype 1a-infected subjects (n=174 for NS3 and n=183 for NS5A) who received ombitasvir, paritaprevir, and dasabuvir with or without ribavirin (for 12 or 24 weeks) in a Phase 2b trial.

Baseline HCV polymorphisms are not expected to have a substantial impact on the likelihood of achieving SVR when VIEKIRA PAK is used as recommended for HCV genotype 1a and 1b infected patients, based on the low virologic failure rates observed in clinical trials.

Cross-resistance

Cross-resistance is expected among NS5A inhibitors, NS3/4A protease inhibitors, and non-nucleoside NS5B-palm inhibitors by class. Dasabuvir retained full activity against HCV replicons containing a single NS5B L159F, S282T, or V321A substitution, which are associated with resistance or prior exposure to nucleos(t)ide analogue NS5B polymerase inhibitors. In clinical trials of VIEKIRA PAK™ (ombitasvir, paritaprevir, and ritonavir tablets; dasabuvir tablets), no subjects who experienced virologic failure had treatment-emergent substitutions potentially associated with resistance to nucleos(t)ide analogue NS5B polymerase inhibitors.

The impact of prior ombitasvir, paritaprevir, or dasabuvir treatment experience on the efficacy of other NS5A inhibitors, NS3/4A protease inhibitors, or NS5B inhibitors has not been studied. Similarly, the efficacy of VIEKIRA PAK has not been studied in subjects who have failed prior treatment with another NS5A inhibitor, NS3/4A protease inhibitor, or NS5B inhibitor.

13   NONCLINICAL TOXICOLOGY
13.1   Carcinogenesis, Mutagenesis, Impairment of Fertility
Carcinogenesis and Mutagenesis
Ombitasvir
Ombitasvir was not carcinogenic in a 6-month transgenic mouse study up to the highest dose tested (150 mg per kg per day). Similarly, ombitasvir was not carcinogenic in a 2-year rat study up to the highest dose tested (30 mg per kg per day), resulting in ombitasvir exposures approximately 16-fold higher than those in humans at 25 mg.

Continued on next page

Information on the AbbVie, Inc. products listed on these pages is from the prescribing information in use as of July 31, 2016. For more information, please visit rxabbvie.com or call 1-800-633-9110.

Table 9 *(Cont.)* Drug Interactions: Change in Pharmacokinetic Parameters for Co-administered Drug in the Presence of VIEKIRA PAK

Co-administered Drug	Dose of Co-administered Drug (mg)	n	Ratio (with/without VIEKIRA PAK) of Co-administered Drug Pharmacokinetic Parameters (90% CI); No Effect = 1.00		
			C_{max}	AUC	C_{min}
Diazepam	2 single dose	13	1.18 (1.07, 1.30)	0.78 (0.73, 0.82)	NA
Diazepam's metabolite nordiazepam			1.10 (1.03, 1.19)	0.56 (0.45, 0.70)	NA
Ethinyl Estradiol	Ethinyl estradiol 0.035 and Norgestimate 0.25 once daily	8	1.16 (0.90, 1.50)	1.06 (0.96, 1.17)	1.12 (0.94, 1.33)
Norelgestromin		9	2.01 (1.77, 2.29)	2.60 (2.30, 2.95)	3.11 (2.51, 3.85)
Norgestrel		9	2.26 (1.91, 2.67)	2.54 (2.09, 3.09)	2.93 (2.39, 3.57)
Furosemide	20 single dose	12	1.42 (1.17, 1.72)	1.08 (1.00, 1.17)	NA
Ketoconazole	400 once daily	12	1.15 (1.09, 1.21)	2.17 (2.05, 2.29)	NA
Hydrocodone	5 single dose	15	1.27 (1.14, 1.40)	1.90 (1.72, 2.10)	NA
Lopinavir/ ritonavir	400/100 twice daily	6	0.87 (0.76, 0.99)[b]	0.94 (0.81, 1.10)[b]	1.15 (0.93, 1.42)[b]
Lopinavir/ ritonavir[h]	800/200 once daily	12	0.86 (0.80, 0.93)[b]	0.94 (0.87, 1.01)[b]	3.18 (2.49, 4.06)[b]
Omeprazole	40 once daily	11	0.62 (0.48, 0.80)	0.62 (0.51, 0.75)	NA
Pravastatin	10 once daily	12	1.37 (1.11, 1.69)	1.82 (1.60, 2.08)	NA
Rosuvastatin	5 once daily	11	7.13 (5.11, 9.96)	2.59 (2.09, 3.21)	0.59 (0.51, 0.69)
Rilpivirine	25 once daily (morning)[i]	8	2.55 (2.08, 3.12)	3.25 (2.80, 3.77)	3.62 (3.12, 4.21)
Tacrolimus	2 single dose	12	3.99 (3.21, 4.97)[c]	57.13 (45.53, 71.69)[c]	16.56 (12.97, 21.16)[c]

a. Atazanavir plus 100 mg ritonavir administered in the evening, 12 hours after morning dose of VIEKIRA PAK.
b. Atazanavir or darunavir or lopinavir parameters are reported.
c. Dose normalized parameters reported.
d. 30 mg cyclosporine was administered with VIEKIRA PAK in the test arm and 100 mg cyclosporine was administered in the reference arm without VIEKIRA PAK.
e. Darunavir administered with VIEKIRA PAK in the morning was compared to darunavir administered with 100 mg ritonavir in the morning.
f. Darunavir administered with VIEKIRA PAK in the morning and with 100 mg ritonavir in the evening was compared to darunavir administered with 100 mg ritonavir in the morning and evening.
g. Darunavir plus 100 mg ritonavir administered in the evening, 12 hours after morning dose of VIEKIRA PAK compared to darunavir administered with 100 mg ritonavir in the evening.
h. Lopinavir/ritonavir administered in the evening, 12 hours after morning dose of VIEKIRA PAK.
i. Similar increases were observed when rilpivirine was dosed in the evening with food or 4 hours after food.
NA: not available/not applicable; CI: Confidence interval
Doses of ombitasvir, paritaprevir, and ritonavir were 25 mg, 150 mg and 100 mg. Doses of dasabuvir were 250 mg or 400 mg (both doses showed similar exposures).
Ombitasvir, paritaprevir and ritonavir were dosed once daily and dasabuvir was dosed twice daily in all the above studies except studies with ketoconazole and carbamazepine that used single doses.

Ombitasvir and its major inactive human metabolites (M29, M36) were not genotoxic in a battery of *in vitro* or *in vivo* assays, including bacterial mutagenicity, chromosome aberration using human peripheral blood lymphocytes and *in vivo* mouse micronucleus assays.

Paritaprevir, ritonavir
Paritaprevir, ritonavir was not carcinogenic in a 6-month transgenic mouse study up to the highest dose tested (300/30 mg per kg per day). Similarly, paritaprevir, ritonavir was not carcinogenic in a 2-year rat study up to the highest dose tested (300/30 mg per kg per day), resulting in paritaprevir exposures approximately 9-fold higher than those in humans at 150 mg.
Paritaprevir was positive in an *in vitro* chromosome aberration test using human lymphocytes. Paritaprevir was negative in a bacterial mutation assay, and in two *in vivo* genetic toxicology assays (rat bone marrow micronucleus and rat liver Comet tests).

Dasabuvir
Dasabuvir was not carcinogenic in a 6-month transgenic mouse study up to the highest dose tested (2000 mg per kg per day). Similarly, dasabuvir was not carcinogenic in a 2-year rat study up to the highest dose tested (800 mg per kg per day), resulting in dasabuvir exposures approximately 19-fold higher than those in humans at 500 mg.
Dasabuvir was not genotoxic in a battery of *in vitro* or *in vivo* assays, including bacterial mutagenicity, chromosome aberration using human peripheral blood lymphocytes and *in vivo* rat micronucleus assays.
If VIEKIRA PAK is administered with ribavirin, refer to the prescribing information for ribavirin for information on carcinogenesis, and mutagenesis.

Impairment of Fertility
Ombitasvir
Ombitasvir had no effects on embryo-fetal viability or on fertility when evaluated in mice up to the highest dose of 200 mg per kg per day. Ombitasvir exposures at this dose were approximately 25-fold the exposure in humans at the recommended clinical dose.

Paritaprevir, ritonavir
Paritaprevir, ritonavir had no effects on embryo-fetal viability or on fertility when evaluated in rats up to the highest dose of 300/30 mg per kg per day. Paritaprevir exposures at this dose were approximately 2- to 5-fold the exposure in humans at the recommended clinical dose.

Dasabuvir
Dasabuvir had no effects on embryo-fetal viability or on fertility when evaluated in rats up to the highest dose of 800 mg per kg per day. Dasabuvir exposures at this dose were approximately 16-fold the exposure in humans at the recommended clinical dose.
If VIEKIRA PAK is administered with ribavirin, refer to the prescribing information for ribavirin for information on Impairment of Fertility.

14 CLINICAL STUDIES
14.1 Description of Clinical Trials
Table 11 presents the clinical trial design including different treatment arms that were conducted with VIEKIRA PAK with or without ribavirin in subjects with chronic hepatitis C (HCV) genotype 1 (GT1) infection. For detailed description of trial design and recommended regimen and duration *[see Dosage and Administration (2) and Clinical Studies (14)]*.
[See table 11 on page 854]
VIEKIRA PAK with RBV was also evaluated in the following two studies:
• HCV GT1-infected liver transplant recipients (CORAL-I) *[see Clinical Studies (14.5)]*.
• Subjects with HCV GT1 co-infected with HIV-1 (TURQUOISE-I) *[see Clinical Studies (14.6)]*.
In all clinical trials, the ombitasvir, paritaprevir, ritonavir dose was 25/150/100 mg once daily and the dasabuvir dose was 250 mg twice daily. Doses of drugs in VIEKIRA PAK were not adjusted. For subjects who received RBV, the RBV dose was 1000 mg per day for subjects weighing less than 75 kg or 1200 mg per day for subjects weighing greater than or equal to 75 kg. RBV dose adjustments were performed according to the RBV labeling.
In all clinical trials, sustained virologic response was defined as HCV RNA below the lower limit of quantification (<LLOQ) 12 weeks after the end of treatment (SVR12). Plasma HCV RNA levels were measured using the COBAS TaqMan HCV test (version 2.0), for use with the High Pure System, which has an LLOQ of 25 IU per mL. Outcomes for

Table 10. Treatment-Emergent Amino Acid Substitutions in the Pooled Analysis of VIEKIRA PAK with and without Ribavirin Regimens (12- or 24-week durations) in Phase 2b and Phase 3 Clinical Trials

Target	Emergent Amino Acid Substitutions	Genotype 1a N = 58[a] % (n)	Genotype 1b N = 6 % (n)
NS3	Any of the following NS3 substitutions: V36A/M/T, F43L, V55I, Y56H, Q80L, I132V, R155K, A156G, D168(any), P334S, S342P, E357K, V406A/I, T449I, P470S, V23A (NS4A)	88 (51)	67 (4)
	V36A/M/T[b]	7 (4)	--
	V55I[b]	7 (4)	--
	Y56H[b]	10 (6)	50 (3)
	I132V[b]	7 (4)	--
	R155K	16 (9)	--
	D168 (any)[d]	72 (42)	67 (4)
	D168V	59 (34)	50 (3)
	P334S[b,c]	7 (4)	--
	E357K[b,c]	5 (3)	17 (1)
	V406A/I[b,c]	5 (3)	--
	T449I[b,c]	5 (3)	--
	P470S[b,c]	5 (3)	--
	NS4A V23A[b]	--	17 (1)
	F43L[b], Q80L[b], A156G, S342P[b,c]	<5%	--
NS5A	Any of the following NS5A substitutions: K24R, M28A/T/V, Q30E/K/R, H/Q54Y, H58D/P/R, Y93C/H/N	78 (45)	33 (2)
	K24R	5 (3)	--
	M28A/T/V	33 (19)	--
	Q30E/K/R	47 (27)	--
	H/Q54Y	--	17 (1)
	H58D/P/R	7 (4)	--
	Y93C/N	5 (3)	--
	Y93H	--	33 (2)
NS5B	Any of the following NS5B substitutions: G307R, C316Y, M414I/T, E446K/Q, A450V, A553I/T/V, G554S, S556G/R, G558R, D559G/I/N/V, Y561H	67 (38)	33 (2)
	C316Y	4 (2)	17 (1)
	M414I	--	17 (1)
	M414T	5 (3)	17 (1)
	A553I/T/V	7 (4)	--
	S556G/R	39 (22)	17 (1)
	D559G/I/N/V	7 (4)	--
	Y561H	5 (3)	--
	G307R, E446K/Q, A450V, G554S, G558R	<5%	--

a. N = 57 for the NS5B target.
b. Substitutions were observed in combination with other emergent substitutions at NS3 position R155 or D168.
c. Position located in NS3 helicase domain.
d. D168A/F/H/I/L/N/T/V/Y.

subjects not achieving an SVR12 were recorded as on-treatment virologic failure (VF), post-treatment virologic relapse through post-treatment Week 12 or failure due to other non-virologic reasons (e.g., premature discontinuation, adverse event, lost to follow-up, consent withdrawn).

14.2   Clinical Trial Results in Adults with Chronic HCV Genotype 1a and 1b Infection without Cirrhosis
Subjects with Chronic HCV GT1a Infection without Cirrhosis

Subjects with HCV GT1a infection without cirrhosis treated with VIEKIRA PAK with RBV for 12 weeks in SAPPHIRE-I and -II and in PEARL-IV [see Clinical Studies (14.1)] had a median age of 53 years (range: 18 to 70); 63% of the subjects were male; 90% were White; 7% were Black/African American; 8% were Hispanic or Latino; 19% had a body mass index of at least 30 kg per m², 55% of patients were enrolled in

US sites; 72% had IL28B (rs12979860) non-CC genotype; 85% had baseline HCV RNA levels of at least 800,000 IU per mL.

Table 12 presents treatment outcomes for HCV GT1a treatment-naïve and treatment-experienced subjects treated with VIEKIRA PAK with RBV for 12 weeks in SAPPHIRE-I, PEARL-IV and SAPPHIRE-II.

Treatment-naïve, HCV GT1a-infected subjects without cirrhosis treated with VIEKIRA PAK in combination with RBV for 12 weeks in PEARL-IV had a significantly higher SVR12 rate than subjects treated with VIEKIRA PAK alone (97% and 90% respectively; difference +7% with 95% confidence interval, +1% to +12%). VIEKIRA PAK alone was not studied in treatment-experienced subjects with GT1a infection. In SAPPHIRE-I and SAPPHIRE-II, no placebo subject achieved a HCV RNA <25 IU/mL during treatment.

Table 12. SVR12 for HCV Genotype 1a-Infected Subjects without Cirrhosis Who Were Treatment-Naïve or Previously Treated with PegIFN/RBV

	VIEKIRA PAK with RBV for 12 Weeks % (n/N)
GT1a treatment-naïve	
SAPPHIRE-I SVR12	96% (308/322)
Outcome for subjects without SVR12	
On-treatment VF	<1% (1/322)
Relapse	2% (6/314)
Other	2% (7/322)
PEARL-IV SVR12	97% (97/100)
Outcome for subjects without SVR12	
On-treatment VF	1% (1/100)
Relapse	1% (1/98)
Other	1% (1/100)
GT1a treatment-experienced	
SAPPHIRE-II SVR12	96% (166/173)
Outcome for subjects without SVR12	
On-treatment VF	0% (0/173)
Relapse	3% (5/172)
Other	1% (2/173)
SVR12 by Prior pegIFN Experience	
Null Responder	95% (83/87)
Partial Responder	100% (36/36)
Relapser	94% (47/50)

Subjects with Chronic HCV GT1b Infection without Cirrhosis
Subjects with HCV GT1b infection without cirrhosis were treated with VIEKIRA PAK with or without RBV for 12 weeks in PEARL-II and -III [see Clinical Studies (14.1)]. Subjects had a median age of 52 years (range: 22 to 70); 47% of the subjects were male; 93% were White; 5% were Black/African American; 2% were Hispanic or Latino; 21% had a body mass index of at least 30 kg per m²; 21% of patients

Continued on next page

Information on the AbbVie, Inc. products listed on these pages is from the prescribing information in use as of July 31, 2016. For more information, please visit rxabbvie.com or call 1-800-633-9110.

were enrolled in US sites; 83% had IL28B (rs12979860) non-CC genotype; 77% had baseline HCV RNA levels of at least 800,000 IU per mL.

The SVR rate for HCV GT1b-infected subjects without cirrhosis treated with VIEKIRA PAK without RBV for 12 weeks in PEARL-II (treatment-experienced: null responder, n=32; partial responder, n=26; relapser, n=33) and PEARL-III (treatment-naïve, n=209) was 100%.

14.3   Clinical Trial Results in Adults with Chronic HCV Genotype 1a and 1b Infection and Compensated Cirrhosis

VIEKIRA PAK with and without ribavirin was evaluated in two clinical trials in patients with compensated cirrhosis. TURQUOISE-II was an open-label trial that enrolled 380 HCV GT1-infected subjects with cirrhosis and mild hepatic impairment (Child-Pugh A) who were either treatment-naïve or did not achieve SVR with prior treatment with pegIFN/RBV. Subjects were randomized to receive VIEKIRA PAK in combination with RBV for either 12 or 24 weeks of treatment. Treated subjects had a median age of 58 years (range: 21 to 71); 70% of the subjects were male; 95% were White; 3% were Black/African American; 12% were Hispanic or Latino; 28% had a body mass index of at least 30 kg per m², 43% of patients were enrolled in US sites; 82% had IL28B (rs12979860) non-CC genotype; 86% had baseline HCV RNA levels of at least 800,000 IU per mL; 69% had HCV GT1a infection, 31% had HCV GT1b infection; 42% were treatment-naïve, 36% were prior pegIFN/RBV null responders, 8% were prior pegIFN/RBV partial responders, 14% were prior pegIFN/RBV relapsers; 15% had platelet counts of less than 90×10^9 per L; 50% had albumin less than 4.0 mg per dL.

TURQUOISE-III was an open-label trial that enrolled 60 HCV GT1b-infected subjects with cirrhosis and mild hepatic impairment (Child-Pugh A) who were either treatment-naïve or did not achieve SVR with prior treatment with pegIFN/RBV. Subjects received VIEKIRA PAK without RBV for 12 weeks. Treated subjects had a median age of 61 years (range: 26 to 78); including 45% treatment-naïve and 55% pegIFN/RBV treatment-experienced; 25% were ≥65 years; 62% were male; 12% were Black; 5% were Hispanic or Latino; 28% had a body mass index of at least 30 kg per m², 40% of patients were enrolled in US sites; 22% had platelet counts of less than 90×10^9 per L; 17% had albumin less than 35 g/L; 92% had baseline HCV RNA levels of at least 800,000 IU per mL; 83% had IL28B (rs12979860) non-CC genotype.

Table 13 presents treatment outcomes for GT1a- and GT1b-infected treatment-naïve and treatment-experienced subjects. In GT1a infected subjects, the overall SVR12 rate difference between 24 and 12 weeks of treatment with VIEKIRA PAK with RBV was +6% with 95% confidence interval, -0.1% to +13% with differences varying by pretreatment history.

[See table 13 on next page]

14.4   Effect of Ribavirin Dose Reductions on SVR12

Seven percent of subjects (101/1551) treated with VIEKIRA PAK with RBV had a RBV dose adjustment due to a decrease in hemoglobin level; of these, 98% (98/100) achieved an SVR12.

14.5   Clinical Trial of Selected Liver Transplant Recipients (CORAL-I)

VIEKIRA PAK with RBV was administered for 24 weeks to 34 HCV GT1-infected liver transplant recipients who were at least 12 months post transplantation at enrollment with normal hepatic function and mild fibrosis (Metavir fibrosis score F2 or lower). The initial dose of RBV was left to the discretion of the investigator with 600 to 800 mg per day being the most frequently selected dose range at initiation of VIEKIRA PAK and at the end of treatment.

Of the 34 subjects (29 with HCV GT1a infection and 5 with HCV GT1b infection) enrolled, (97%) achieved SVR12 (97% in subjects with GT1a infection and 100% of subjects with GT1b infection). One subject with HCV GT1a infection relapsed post-treatment.

14.6   Clinical Trial in Subjects with HCV/HIV-1 Co-infection (TURQUOISE-I)

In an open-label clinical trial 63 subjects with HCV GT1 infection co-infected with HIV-1 were treated for 12 or 24 weeks with VIEKIRA PAK in combination with RBV. Subjects were on a stable HIV-1 antiretroviral therapy (ART) regimen that included tenofovir disoproxil fumarate plus emtricitabine or lamivudine, administered with ritonavir boosted atazanavir or raltegravir. Subjects on atazanavir stopped the ritonavir component of their HIV-1 ART regimen upon initiating treatment with VIEKIRA PAK in com-

Table 11. Clinical Trials Conducted with VIEKIRA PAK With or Without Ribavirin (RBV) in Subjects with Chronic HCV GT1 Infection

Trial	Population	Study Arms and Duration (Number of Subjects Treated)
SAPPHIRE-I (double-blind)	GT1 (a and b) TN[a] without cirrhosis	• VIEKIRA PAK + RBV for 12 weeks (473) • Placebo for 12 weeks (158)
SAPPHIRE-II (double-blind)	GT1 (a and b) TE[b] without cirrhosis	• VIEKIRA PAK + RBV for 12 weeks (297) • Placebo for 12 weeks (97)
PEARL-II (open-label)	GT1b TE without cirrhosis	• VIEKIRA PAK + RBV for 12 weeks (88) • VIEKIRA PAK for 12 weeks (91)
PEARL-III (double-blind)	GT1b TN without cirrhosis	• VIEKIRA PAK + RBV for 12 weeks (210) • VIEKIRA PAK for 12 weeks (209)
PEARL-IV (double-blind)	GT1a TN without cirrhosis	• VIEKIRA PAK + RBV for 12 weeks (100) • VIEKIRA PAK for 12 weeks (205)
TURQUOISE-II (open-label)	GT1 (a and b) TN & TE with compensated cirrhosis	• VIEKIRA PAK + RBV for 12 weeks (208) • VIEKIRA PAK + RBV for 24 weeks (172)
TURQUOISE-III (open-label)	GT1b TN & TE with compensated cirrhosis	• VIEKIRA PAK for 12 weeks (60)

a. TN, treatment-naïve was defined as not having received any prior therapy for HCV infection.
b. TE, treatment-experienced subjects were defined as having failed to respond to prior treatment with pegIFN/RBV.

bination with RBV. Atazanavir was taken with the morning dose of VIEKIRA PAK. The ritonavir component of the HIV-1 ART regimen was restarted after completion of treatment with VIEKIRA PAK and RBV.

Treated subjects had a median age of 51 years (range: 31 to 69); 24% of subjects were black; 81% of subjects had IL28B (rs12979860) non-CC genotype; 19% of subjects had compensated cirrhosis; 67% of subjects were HCV treatment-naïve; 33% of subjects had failed prior treatment with pegIFN/RBV; 89% of subjects had HCV genotype 1a infection. The SVR12 rates were 91% (51/56) for subjects with HCV GT1a infection and 100% (7/7) for those with HCV GT1b infection. Of the 5 subjects who were non-responders, 1 experienced virologic breakthrough, 1 discontinued treatment, 1 experienced relapse and 2 subjects had evidence of HCV reinfection post-treatment.

One subject had confirmed HIV-1 RNA >400 copies/mL during the post-treatment period. This subject had no evidence of resistance to the ART regimen. No subjects switched their ART regimen due to loss of plasma HIV-1 RNA suppression.

14.7   Durability of Response

In an open-label clinical trial, 92% of subjects (526/571) who received various combinations of the direct acting antivirals included in VIEKIRA PAK with or without RBV achieved SVR12, and 99% of those who achieved SVR12 maintained their response through 48 weeks post-treatment (SVR48).

16   HOW SUPPLIED/STORAGE AND HANDLING

VIEKIRA PAK™ (ombitasvir, paritaprevir, and ritonavir tablets; dasabuvir tablets) is dispensed in a monthly carton for a total of 28 days of therapy. Each monthly carton contains four weekly cartons. Each weekly carton contains seven daily dose packs.

Each child resistant daily dose pack contains four tablets: two 12.5/75/50 mg ombitasvir, paritaprevir, ritonavir tablets and two 250 mg dasabuvir tablets, and indicates which tablets need to be taken in the morning and evening. The NDC number is 0074-3093-28.

Ombitasvir, paritaprevir, ritonavir 12.5/75/50 mg tablets are pink-colored, film-coated, oblong biconvex shaped, debossed with "AV1" on one side. Dasabuvir 250 mg tablets are beige-colored, film-coated, oval-shaped, debossed with "AV2" on one side.

Store at or below 30°C (86°F).

17   PATIENT COUNSELING INFORMATION

Advise the patient to read the FDA-approved patient labeling (Medication Guide).

Inform patients to review the Medication Guide for ribavirin *[see Warnings and Precautions (5.3)]*.

Risk of ALT Elevations or Hepatic Decompensation and Failure

Inform patients to watch for early warning signs of liver inflammation or failure, such as fatigue, weakness, lack of appetite, nausea and vomiting, as well as later signs such as jaundice, onset of confusion, abdominal swelling, and discol-

ored feces, and to consult their health care professional without delay if such symptoms occur *[see Warnings and Precautions (5.1 and 5.2) and Adverse Reactions (6)]*.

Pregnancy

Advise patients taking VIEKIRA PAK with ribavirin to avoid pregnancy during treatment and within 6 months of stopping ribavirin. Inform patients to notify their health care provider immediately in the event of a pregnancy *[see Use in Specific Populations (8.1)]*.

Drug Interactions

Inform patients that VIEKIRA PAK may interact with some drugs; therefore, patients should be advised to report to their healthcare provider the use of any prescription, nonprescription medication or herbal products *[see Contraindications (4), Warnings and Precautions (5.4) and Drug Interactions (7)]*.

Inform patients that contraceptives containing ethinyl estradiol are contraindicated with VIEKIRA PAK *[see Contraindications (4) and Warnings and Precautions (5.2)]*.

Administration

Advise patients to take VIEKIRA PAK every day at the regularly scheduled time with a meal without regard to fat or calorie content *[see Dosage and Administration (2.1)]*.

Inform patients that it is important not to miss or skip doses and to take VIEKIRA PAK for the duration that is recommended by the healthcare provider.

Manufactured by AbbVie Inc., North Chicago, IL 60064.

VIEKIRA PAK and NORVIR are trademarks of AbbVie Inc. All other brands listed are trademarks of their respective owners and are not trademarks of AbbVie Inc. The makers of these brands are not affiliated with and do not endorse AbbVie Inc. or its products.

© 2016 AbbVie Inc. All rights reserved.

03-B366

Table 13. TURQUOISE-II and TURQUOISE III: SVR12 for Chronic HCV Genotype 1-Infected Subjects with Compensated Cirrhosis Who Were Treatment-Naïve or Previously Treated with pegIFN/RBV

| | GT1a (TURQUOISE-II) | | GT1b (TURQUOISE-III) |
	VIEKIRA PAK with RBV for 24 Weeks % (n/N)	VIEKIRA PAK with RBV for 12 Weeks % (n/N)	VIEKIRA PAK without RBV for 12 Weeks % (n/N)
SVR12	95% (115/121)	89% (124/140)	100% (60/60)
Outcome for subjects without SVR12			
On-treatment VF	2% (3/121)	<1% (1/140)	0
Relapse	1% (1/116)	8% (11/135)	0
Other	2% (2/121)	3% (4/140)	0
SVR12 for Naïve	95% (53/56)	92% (59/64)	100% (27/27)
SVR12 by Prior pegIFN Experience			100% (33/33)
Null Responder	93% (39/42)	80% (40/50)	100% (7/7)
Partial Responder	100% (10/10)	100% (11/11)	100% (5/5)
Relapser	100% (13/13)	93% (14/15)	100% (3/3)

MEDICATION GUIDE
VIEKIRA PAK™ (vee-KEE-rah-pak)
(ombitasvir, paritaprevir, and ritonavir tablets; dasabuvir tablets)
co-packaged for oral use

Important: When taking VIEKIRA PAK in combination with ribavirin, you should also read the Medication Guide that comes with ribavirin.

What is the most important information I should know about VIEKIRA PAK?
VIEKIRA PAK may cause severe liver problems, especially in people with certain types of cirrhosis. These severe liver problems can lead to the need for a liver transplant, or can lead to death.
VIEKIRA PAK can cause increases in your liver function blood test results, especially if you use ethinyl estradiol-containing medicines (such as some birth control products).
- You must stop using ethinyl estradiol-containing medicines before you start treatment with VIEKIRA PAK. See the section **"Who should not take VIEKIRA PAK?"** for a list of these medicines.
- If you use these medicines as a method of birth control, you must use another method of birth control during treatment with VIEKIRA PAK, and for about **2** weeks after you finish treatment with VIEKIRA PAK. Your healthcare provider will tell you when you may begin taking ethinyl estradiol-containing medicines.
- Your healthcare provider should do blood tests to check your liver function during the first 4 weeks and then as needed, during treatment with VIEKIRA PAK.

- Your healthcare provider may tell you to stop taking VIEKIRA PAK if you develop signs or symptoms of liver problems.
- Tell your healthcare provider right away if you develop any of the following symptoms, or if they worsen during treatment with VIEKIRA PAK:
  - tiredness
  - weakness
  - loss of appetite
  - nausea and vomiting
  - yellowing of your skin or eyes
  - color changes in your stools
  - confusion
  - swelling of the stomach area

What is VIEKIRA PAK?
- VIEKIRA PAK is a prescription medicine used with or without ribavirin to treat genotype 1 chronic (lasting a long time) hepatitis C virus (HCV) infection.
- VIEKIRA PAK can be used in people who have compensated cirrhosis.
- VIEKIRA PAK is not for people with advanced cirrhosis (decompensated). If you have cirrhosis, talk to your healthcare provider before taking VIEKIRA PAK. VIEKIRA PAK is not for people with certain types of liver problems.

- VIEKIRA PAK contains 2 different types of tablets:
  - The pink tablet contains the medicines ombitasvir, paritaprevir, and ritonavir
  - The beige tablet contains dasabuvir
It is not known if VIEKIRA PAK is safe and effective in children under 18 years of age.

Who should not take VIEKIRA PAK?
Do not take VIEKIRA PAK if you:
- **have certain liver problems**
- **take any of the following medicines:**
  - alfuzosin hydrochloride (Uroxatral®)
  - carbamazepine (Carbatrol®, Epitol®, Equetro®, Tegretol®, TEGRETOL-XR®, TERIL®)
  - cisapride (Propulsid®)
  - colchicine (Colcrys®) in patients who have certain kidney or liver problems
  - dronedarone (Multaq®)
  - efavirenz (Atripla®, Sustiva®)
  - ergot containing medicines including:
    - ergotamine tartrate (Cafergot®, Ergomar®, Ergostat®, Medihaler®, Migergot®, Wigraine®, Wigrettes®)
    - dihydroergotamine mesylate (D.H.E. 45®, Migranal®)
    - methylergonovine (Ergotrate® Methergine®)
  - ethinyl estradiol-containing medicines:
    - combination birth control pills or patches, such as Lo Loestrin® FE, Norinyl®, Ortho Tri-Cyclen Lo®, Ortho Evra®
    - hormonal vaginal rings such as NuvaRing®
    - the hormone replacement therapy medicine, Fem HRT®
  - gemfibrozil (Lopid®)
  - lovastatin (Advicor®, Altoprev®, Mevacor®)
  - lurasidone (Latuda®)
  - midazolam, when taken by mouth
  - phenytoin (Dilantin®, Phenytek®)
  - phenobarbital (Luminal®)
  - pimozide (Orap®)
  - ranolazine (Ranexa®)
  - rifampin (Rifadin®, Rifamate®, Rifater®, Rimactane®)
  - sildenafil citrate (Revatio®), when taken for pulmonary artery hypertension (PAH)
  - simvastatin (Simcor®, Vytorin®, Zocor®)
  - St. John's wort (Hypericum perforatum) or a product that contains St. John's wort
  - triazolam (Halcion®)
- **have had a severe skin rash after taking ritonavir (Norvir®)**

What should I tell my healthcare provider before taking VIEKIRA PAK?
Before taking VIEKIRA PAK tell your healthcare provider about all your medical conditions, including if you:
- have liver problems other than hepatitis C infection. See **"Who should not take VIEKIRA PAK?"**
- have HIV infection
- have had a liver transplant. If you take the medicines tacrolimus (Prograf®) or cyclosporine (Gengraf®, Neoral®, Sandimmune®) to help prevent rejection of your transplanted liver, the amount of these medicines in your blood may increase during treatment with VIEKIRA PAK.

  - Your healthcare provider should check the level of tacrolimus or cyclosporine in your blood, and if needed may change your dose of these medicines or how often you take them.
  - When you finish taking VIEKIRA PAK or if you have to stop VIEKIRA PAK for any reason, your healthcare provider should tell you what dose of tacrolimus or cyclosporine to take and how often you should take it.
- are pregnant or plan to become pregnant. It is not known if VIEKIRA PAK will harm your unborn baby. **When taking VIEKIRA PAK in combination with ribavirin you should also read the ribavirin Medication Guide for important pregnancy information.**
- are breastfeeding or plan to breastfeed. It is not known if VIEKIRA PAK passes into your breast milk. Talk to your healthcare provider about the best way to feed your baby if you take VIEKIRA PAK.

Tell your healthcare provider about all the medicines you take, including prescription and over-the-counter medicines, vitamins, and herbal supplements. Some medicines interact with VIEKIRA PAK. **Keep a list of your medicines to show your healthcare provider and pharmacist.**
- You can ask your healthcare provider or pharmacist for a list of medicines that interact with VIEKIRA PAK.
- **Do not start taking a new medicine without telling your healthcare provider.** Your healthcare provider can tell you if it is safe to take VIEKIRA PAK with other medicines.
- When you finish treatment with VIEKIRA PAK:
  - If your healthcare provider changed the dose of one of your usual medicines during treatment with VIEKIRA PAK: Ask your healthcare provider about when you should change back to your original dose after you finish treatment with VIEKIRA PAK.
  - If your healthcare provider told you to stop taking one of your usual medicines during treatment with VIEKIRA PAK: Ask your healthcare provider if you should start taking these medicines again after you finished treatment with VIEKIRA PAK.

How should I take VIEKIRA PAK?
- Take VIEKIRA PAK™ (ombitasvir, paritaprevir, and ritonavir tablets; dasabuvir tablets) exactly as your healthcare provider tells you to take it. Do not change your dose.
- Do not stop taking VIEKIRA PAK without first talking with your healthcare provider.
- Take VIEKIRA PAK tablets every day, with a meal.
- VIEKIRA PAK comes in **monthly cartons that contain enough medicine for 28 days.**
- Each monthly carton of VIEKIRA PAK contains **4 smaller cartons.**
- Each of the 4 smaller cartons contains enough child resistant **daily dose packs** of medicine to last for **7 days (1 week).**
- Each **daily dose pack** contains all of your VIEKIRA PAK medicine for **1 day** (4 tablets). Follow the instructions on each daily dose pack about how to remove the tablets.

- Take VIEKIRA PAK tablets with a meal as follows:
  - Take the **2** pink tablets (ombitasvir, paritaprevir, and ritonavir), with **1** of the beige tablets (dasabuvir), at about the same time every morning.
  - Take the **second** beige tablet (dasabuvir), at about the same time every evening.
- It is important that you do not miss or skip doses of VIEKIRA PAK during treatment.
- If you take too much VIEKIRA PAK, call your healthcare provider or go to the nearest hospital emergency room right away.

What are the possible side effects of VIEKIRA PAK?
VIEKIRA PAK can cause serious side effects. See "What is the most important information I should know about VIEKIRA PAK?"
Common side effects of VIEKIRA PAK when used with ribavirin include:
- tiredness
- nausea
- itching
- skin reactions such as redness or rash
- sleep problems
- feeling weak
Common side effects of VIEKIRA PAK when used without ribavirin include:

Continued on next page

Information on the AbbVie, Inc. products listed on these pages is from the prescribing information in use as of July 31, 2016. For more information, please visit rxabbvie.com or call 1-800-633-9110.

• nausea
• itching
• sleep problems

These are not all the possible side effects of VIEKIRA PAK. Call your doctor for medical advice about side effects. You may report side effects to FDA at 1-800-FDA-1088.

How should I store VIEKIRA PAK?
• Store VIEKIRA PAK at or below 86°F (30°C).Keep VIEKIRA PAK and all medicines out of the reach of children.

General information about the safe and effective use of VIEKIRA PAK
Medicines are sometimes prescribed for purposes other than those listed in a Medication Guide. Do not use VIEKIRA PAK for a condition for which it was not prescribed. Do not give VIEKIRA PAK to other people, even if they have the same symptoms that you have. It may harm them. You can ask your pharmacist or healthcare provider for information about VIEKIRA PAK that is written for health professionals.

What are the ingredients in VIEKIRA PAK?
Ombitasvir, paritaprevir, and ritonavir tablets:
Active ingredients: ombitasvir, paritaprevir, and ritonavir
Inactive ingredients: copovidone, K value 28, vitamin E polyethylene glycol succinate, propylene glycol monolaurate Type I, sorbitan monolaurate, colloidal silicon dioxide/colloidal anhydrous silica, sodium stearyl fumarate, polyvinyl alcohol, polyethylene glycol 3350/macrogol 3350, talc, titanium dioxide, and red iron oxide.
Dasabuvir tablets:
Active ingredients: dasabuvir
Inactive ingredients: microcrystalline cellulose (D50-100 um), microcrystalline cellulose (D50-50 um), lactose monohydrate, copovidone, croscarmellose sodium, colloidal silicon dioxide/anhydrous colloidal silica, magnesium stearate, polyvinyl alcohol, titanium dioxide, polyethylene glycol 3350/macrogol 3350, talc and iron oxide yellow, iron oxide red and iron oxide black.
Manufactured by AbbVie Inc., North Chicago, IL 60064. VIEKIRA PAK and NORVIR are trademarks of AbbVie Inc. All other brands listed are trademarks of their respective owners and are not trademarks of AbbVie Inc. The makers of these brands are not affiliated with and do not endorse AbbVie Inc. or its products.
For more information go to www.viekira.com or call 1-844-484-3547.

This Medication Guide has been approved by the U.S. Food and Drug Administration.
Revised: June 2016
03-B366
Shown in Product Identification Guide, page 507

VIEKIRA XR™ ℞
[*vee-KEE-rah-XR*]
(dasabuvir, ombitasvir, paritaprevir, and ritonavir) extended-release tablets, for oral use

HIGHLIGHTS OF PRESCRIBING INFORMATION
These highlights do not include all the information needed to use VIEKIRA XR safely and effectively. See full prescribing information for VIEKIRA XR.
VIEKIRA XR™ (dasabuvir, ombitasvir, paritaprevir, and ritonavir) extended-release tablets, for oral use
Initial U.S. Approval: 2014

---INDICATIONS AND USAGE---
VIEKIRA XR includes dasabuvir, a hepatitis C virus nonnucleoside NS5B palm polymerase inhibitor, ombitasvir, a hepatitis C virus NS5A inhibitor, paritaprevir, a hepatitis C virus NS3/4A protease inhibitor, and ritonavir, a CYP3A inhibitor and is indicated for the treatment of adult patients with chronic hepatitis C virus (HCV):
• genotype 1b infection without cirrhosis or with compensated cirrhosis
• genotype 1a infection without cirrhosis or with compensated cirrhosis for use in combination with ribavirin. (1)

---DOSAGE AND ADMINISTRATION---
Testing Prior to Initiation - Assess for laboratory and clinical evidence of hepatic decompensation. (2.1)
Recommended dosage: Three tablets taken once daily. VIEKIRA XR must be taken with a meal because administration under fasting conditions may result in reduced virologic response and possible development of resistance. (2.2)

Treatment Regimen and Duration by Patient Population

Patient Population	Treatment*	Duration
Genotype 1a, without cirrhosis	VIEKIRA XR + ribavirin	12 weeks
Genotype 1a, with compensated cirrhosis	VIEKIRA XR + ribavirin	24 weeks**
Genotype 1b, with or without compensated cirrhosis	VIEKIRA XR	12 weeks

*Note: Follow the genotype 1a dosing recommendations in patients with an unknown genotype 1 subtype or with mixed genotype 1 infection.
**VIEKIRA XR administered with ribavirin for 12 weeks may be considered for some patients based on prior treatment history [See Clinical Studies (14.3)].

• HCV/HIV-1 co-infection: For patients with HCV/HIV-1 co-infection, follow the dosage recommendations in the table above. (2.2)
• Liver Transplant Recipients: In liver transplant recipients with normal hepatic function and mild fibrosis (Metavir fibrosis score ≤2), the recommended duration of VIEKIRA XR with ribavirin is 24 weeks. (2.4)

---DOSAGE FORMS AND STRENGTHS---
Extended-release tablets: 200 mg dasabuvir, 8.33 mg ombitasvir, 50 mg paritaprevir, and 33.33 mg ritonavir (3)

---CONTRAINDICATIONS---
• Patients with moderate to severe hepatic impairment. (4, 5.1, 8.6, 12.3)
• If VIEKIRA XR is administered with ribavirin, the contraindications to ribavirin also apply to this combination regimen. (4)
• Co-administration with drugs that are: highly dependent on CYP3A for clearance; moderate or strong inducers of CYP3A or strong inducers of CYP2C8; and strong inhibitors of CYP2C8. (4)
• Known hypersensitivity to ritonavir (e.g. toxic epidermal necrolysis, Stevens-Johnson syndrome). (4)

---WARNINGS AND PRECAUTIONS---
• Hepatic Decompensation and Hepatic Failure in Patient with Cirrhosis: Hepatic decompensation and hepatic failure, including liver transplantation or fatal outcomes, have been reported mostly in patients with advanced cirrhosis. Monitor for clinical signs and symptoms of hepatic decompensation. (5.1)
• ALT Elevations: Discontinue ethinyl estradiol-containing medications prior to starting VIEKIRA XR (alternative contraceptive methods are recommended). Perform hepatic laboratory testing on all patients during the first 4 weeks of treatment. For ALT elevations on VIEKIRA XR, monitor closely and follow recommendations in full prescribing information. (5.2)
• Risks Associated With Ribavirin Combination Treatment: If VIEKIRA XR is administered with ribavirin, the warnings and precautions for ribavirin also apply to this combination regimen. (5.3)
• Drug Interactions: The concomitant use of VIEKIRA XR and certain other drugs may result in known or potentially significant drug interactions, some of which may lead to loss of therapeutic effect of VIEKIRA XR. (5.4)

---ADVERSE REACTIONS---
In subjects receiving the combination of dasabuvir with ombitasvir, paritaprevir, ritonavir with ribavirin, the most commonly reported adverse reactions (greater than 10% of subjects) were fatigue, nausea, pruritus, other skin reactions, insomnia and asthenia. In subjects receiving the combination of dasabuvir with ombitasvir, paritaprevir, ritonavir without ribavirin, the most commonly reported adverse reactions (greater than or equal to 5% of subjects) were nausea, pruritus and insomnia. (6.1)

To report SUSPECTED ADVERSE REACTIONS, contact AbbVie Inc. at 1-800-633-9110 or FDA at 1-800-FDA-1088 or www.fda.gov/medwatch.

---DRUG INTERACTIONS---
Co-administration of VIEKIRA XR can alter the plasma concentrations of some drugs and some drugs may alter the plasma concentrations of VIEKIRA XR. The potential for drug interactions must be considered before and during treatment. Consult the full prescribing information prior to and during treatment for potential drug interactions. (4, 5.4, 7, 12.3)
See 17 for PATIENT COUNSELING INFORMATION and Medication Guide.

Revised: 7/2016

FULL PRESCRIBING INFORMATION: CONTENTS*
* Sections or subsections omitted from the full prescribing information are not listed.

FULL PRESCRIBING INFORMATION

1   INDICATIONS AND USAGE
VIEKIRA XR is indicated for the treatment of adult patients with chronic hepatitis C virus (HCV) [see Dosage and Administration (2.2) and Clinical Studies (14)]:
• genotype 1b infection without cirrhosis or with compensated cirrhosis
• genotype 1a infection without cirrhosis or with compensated cirrhosis for use in combination with ribavirin.

2   DOSAGE AND ADMINISTRATION
2.1   Testing Prior to Initiation of VIEKIRA XR
Prior to initiation of VIEKIRA XR, assess for laboratory and clinical evidence of hepatic decompensation [see Warnings and Precautions (5.1 and 5.2)].

Table 2. Drugs that are Contraindicated with VIEKIRA XR

Drug Class	Drug(s) within Class that are Contraindicated	Clinical Comments
Alpha1-adrenoreceptor antagonist	Alfuzosin HCL	Potential for hypotension.
Anti-anginal	Ranolazine	Potential for serious and/or life-threatening reactions.
Antiarrhythmic	Dronedarone	Potential for serious and/or life-threatening reactions such as cardiac arrhythmias.
Anticonvulsants	Carbamazepine, phenytoin, phenobarbital	VIEKIRA XR exposures may decrease leading to a potential loss of therapeutic activity of VIEKIRA XR.
Anti-gout	Colchicine	Potential for serious and/or life-threatening reactions in patients with renal and/or hepatic impairment.
Antihyperlipidemic agent	Gemfibrozil	Increase in dasabuvir exposures by 10-fold which may increase the risk of QT prolongation.
Antimycobacterial	Rifampin	VIEKIRA XR exposures may decrease leading to a potential loss of therapeutic activity of VIEKIRA XR.
Antipsychotic	Lurasidone Pimozide	Potential for serious and/or life-threatening reactions. Potential for serious and/or life-threatening reactions such as cardiac arrhythmias.
Ergot derivatives	Ergotamine, dihydroergotamine, methylergonovine	Acute ergot toxicity characterized by vasospasm and tissue ischemia has been associated with co-administration of ritonavir and ergonovine, ergotamine, dihydroergotamine, or methylergonovine.
Ethinyl estradiol-containing products	Ethinyl estradiol-containing medications such as combined oral contraceptives	Potential for ALT elevations *[see Warnings and Precautions (5.2)]*.
GI Motility Agent	Cisapride	Potential for serious and/or life threatening reactions such as cardiac arrhythmias.
Herbal Product	St. John's Wort (*Hypericum perforatum*)	VIEKIRA XR exposures may decrease leading to a potential loss of therapeutic activity of VIEKIRA XR.
HMG-CoA Reductase Inhibitors	Lovastatin, simvastatin	Potential for myopathy including rhabdomyolysis.
Non-nucleoside reverse transcriptase inhibitor	Efavirenz	Co-administration of efavirenz based regimens with paritaprevir, ritonavir plus dasabuvir was poorly tolerated and resulted in liver enzyme elevations.
Phosphodiesterase-5 (PDE5) inhibitor	Sildenafil when dosed as Revatio for the treatment of pulmonary arterial hypertension (PAH)	There is increased potential for sildenafil-associated adverse events such as visual disturbances, hypotension, priapism, and syncope.
Sedatives/hypnotics	Triazolam Orally administered midazolam	Triazolam and orally administered midazolam are extensively metabolized by CYP3A4. Coadministration of triazolam or orally administered midazolam with VIEKIRA XR may cause large increases in the concentration of these benzodiazepines. The potential exists for serious and/or life threatening events such as prolonged or increased sedation or respiratory depression.

2.2   Recommended Dosage in Adults
VIEKIRA XR is a 4-drug fixed-dose combination, extended-release tablet containing 200 mg of dasabuvir, 8.33 mg of ombitasvir, 50 mg of paritaprevir, and 33.33 mg of ritonavir. The recommended dosage of VIEKIRA XR is three tablets taken orally once daily.
• VIEKIRA XR must be taken with a meal because administration under fasting conditions may result in reduced virologic response and possible development of resistance *[see Clinical Pharmacology (12.3)]*.
• Swallow tablets whole. Splitting, crushing, or chewing tablets may compromise the extended-release performance, efficacy, and/or safety of VIEKIRA XR.
• For optimal release of dasabuvir, alcohol should not be consumed within 4 hours of taking VIEKIRA XR.
VIEKIRA XR is used in combination with ribavirin (RBV) in certain patient populations (see Table 1). When administered with VIEKIRA XR, the recommended dosage of RBV is based on weight: 1000 mg/day for subjects <75 kg and 1200 mg/day for those ≥75 kg, divided and administered twice-daily with food. The starting dosage and on-treatment dosage of RBV can be decreased based on changes in hemoglobin levels and/or creatinine clearance. For ribavirin dosage modifications, refer to the ribavirin prescribing information.
For patients with HCV/HIV-1 co-infection, follow the dosage recommendations in Table 1. Refer to *Drug Interactions (7)* for dosage recommendations for concomitant HIV-1 antiviral drugs.
Table 1 shows the recommended VIEKIRA XR treatment regimen and duration based on patient population.

Table 1. Treatment Regimen and Duration by Patient Population (Treatment-Naïve or Interferon-Experienced)

Patient Population	Treatment*	Duration
Genotype 1a, without cirrhosis	VIEKIRA XR + ribavirin	12 weeks
Genotype 1a, with compensated cirrhosis (Child-Pugh A)	VIEKIRA XR + ribavirin	24 weeks**
Genotype 1b, with or without compensated cirrhosis (Child-Pugh A)	VIEKIRA XR	12 weeks

*Note: Follow the genotype 1a dosing recommendations in patients with an unknown genotype 1 subtype or with mixed genotype 1 infection.
**VIEKIRA XR administered with ribavirin for 12 weeks may be considered for some patients based on prior treatment history *[see Clinical Studies (14.3)]*.

2.3   Use in Liver Transplant Recipients
In liver transplant recipients with normal hepatic function and mild fibrosis (Metavir fibrosis score 2 or lower), the recommended duration of VIEKIRA XR with ribavirin is 24 weeks, irrespective of HCV genotype 1 subtype *[see Clinical Studies (14.6)]*. When VIEKIRA XR is administered with calcineurin inhibitors in liver transplant recipients, dosage adjustment of calcineurin inhibitors is needed *[see Drug Interactions (7)]*.
2.4   Hepatic Impairment
VIEKIRA XR is contraindicated in patients with moderate to severe hepatic impairment (Child-Pugh B and C) *[see Contraindications (4), Warnings and Precautions (5.1), Use in Specific Populations (8.6), and Clinical Pharmacology (12.3)]*.
3   DOSAGE FORMS AND STRENGTHS
Extended-release tablet: 200 mg of dasabuvir (equivalent to 216.2 mg of dasabuvir sodium monohydrate), 8.33 mg of ombitasvir, 50 mg of paritaprevir, and 33.33 mg of ritonavir. The tablets are pale yellow-colored, film-coated, oblong shaped, debossed with "3QD" on one side.
4   CONTRAINDICATIONS
• VIEKIRA XR is contraindicated in patients with moderate to severe hepatic impairment (Child-Pugh B and C) due to

Continued on next page

Information on the AbbVie, Inc. products listed on these pages is from the prescribing information in use as of July 31, 2016. For more information, please visit rxabbvie.com or call 1-800-633-9110.

risk of potential toxicity [see Warnings and Precautions (5.1), Use in Specific Populations (8.6) and Clinical Pharmacology (12.3)].

- If VIEKIRA XR is administered with ribavirin, the contraindications to ribavirin also apply to this combination regimen. Refer to the ribavirin prescribing information for a list of contraindications for ribavirin.
- VIEKIRA XR is contraindicated:
  - With drugs that are highly dependent on CYP3A for clearance and for which elevated plasma concentrations are associated with serious and/or life-threatening events.
  - With drugs that are moderate or strong inducers of CYP3A and strong inducers of CYP2C8 and may lead to reduced efficacy of VIEKIRA XR.
  - With drugs that are strong inhibitors of CYP2C8 and may increase dasabuvir plasma concentrations and the risk of QT prolongation.
  - In patients with known hypersensitivity to ritonavir (e.g. toxic epidermal necrolysis (TEN) or Stevens-Johnson syndrome).

Table 2 lists drugs that are contraindicated with VIEKIRA XR [see Drug Interactions (7)].
[See table 2 on previous page]

5   WARNINGS AND PRECAUTIONS

5.1   Risk of Hepatic Decompensation and Hepatic Failure in Patients with Cirrhosis

Hepatic decompensation and hepatic failure, including liver transplantation or fatal outcomes, have been reported postmarketing in patients treated with the components of VIEKIRA XR. Most patients with these severe outcomes had evidence of advanced cirrhosis prior to initiating therapy. Reported cases typically occurred within one to four weeks of initiating therapy and were characterized by the acute onset of rising direct serum bilirubin levels without ALT elevations in association with clinical signs and symptoms of hepatic decompensation. Because these events are reported voluntarily from a population of uncertain size, it is not always possible to reliably estimate their frequency or establish a causal relationship to drug exposure.

VIEKIRA XR is contraindicated in patients with moderate to severe hepatic impairment (Child-Pugh B and C) [see Contraindications (4), Adverse Reactions (6.2), Use in Specific Populations (8.6), and Clinical Pharmacology (12.3)].

For patients with cirrhosis:

- Monitor for clinical signs and symptoms of hepatic decompensation (such as ascites, hepatic encephalopathy, variceal hemorrhage).
- Hepatic laboratory testing including direct bilirubin levels should be performed at baseline and during the first 4 weeks of starting treatment and as clinically indicated.
- Discontinue VIEKIRA XR in patients who develop evidence of hepatic decompensation.

5.2   Increased Risk of ALT Elevations

During clinical trials with the combination of dasabuvir tablets and ombitasvir, paritaprevir, and ritonavir tablets (components of VIEKIRA XR) with or without ribavirin, elevations of ALT to greater than 5 times the upper limit of normal (ULN) occurred in approximately 1% of all subjects [see Adverse Reactions (6.1)]. ALT elevations were typically asymptomatic, occurred during the first 4 weeks of treatment, and declined within two to eight weeks of onset with continued dosing.

These ALT elevations were significantly more frequent in female subjects who were using ethinyl estradiol-containing medications such as combined oral contraceptives, contraceptive patches or contraceptive vaginal rings. Ethinyl estradiol-containing medications must be discontinued prior to starting therapy with VIEKIRA XR [see Contraindications (4)]. Alternative methods of contraception (e.g., progestin only contraception or non-hormonal methods) are recommended during VIEKIRA XR therapy. Ethinyl estradiol-containing medications can be restarted approximately 2 weeks following completion of treatment with VIEKIRA XR.

Women using estrogens other than ethinyl estradiol, such as estradiol and conjugated estrogens used in hormone replacement therapy had a rate of ALT elevation similar to those not receiving any estrogens; however, due to the limited number of subjects taking these other estrogens, caution is warranted for co-administration with VIEKIRA XR [see Adverse Reactions (6.1)].

Hepatic laboratory testing should be performed during the first 4 weeks of starting treatment and as clinically indicated thereafter. If ALT is found to be elevated above baseline levels, it should be repeated and monitored closely:

Table 5. Established Drug Interactions Based on Drug Interaction Trials

Concomitant Drug Class: Drug Name	Effect on Concentration	Clinical Comments
ANGIOTENSIN RECEPTOR BLOCKERS		
valsartan* losartan* candesartan*	↑ angiotensin receptor blockers	Decrease the dose of the angiotensin receptor blockers and monitor patients for signs and symptoms of hypotension and/or worsening renal function. If such events occur, consider further dose reduction of the angiotensin receptor blocker or switching to an alternative to the angiotensin receptor blocker.
ANTIARRHYTHMICS		
amiodarone*, bepridil*, disopyramide*, flecainide*, lidocaine (systemic)*, mexiletine*, propafenone*, quinidine*	↑ antiarrhythmics	Contraindicated antiarrhythmics [see Contraindications (4)]. Therapeutic concentration monitoring (if available) is recommended for antiarrhythmics when co-administered with VIEKIRA XR.
ANTIDIABETIC DRUGS		
metformin	↔ metformin	Monitor for signs of onset of lactic acidosis such as respiratory distress, somnolence, and non-specific abdominal distress or worsening renal function. Concomitant metformin use in patients with renal insufficiency or hepatic impairment is not recommended. Refer to the prescribing information of metformin for further guidance.
ANTIFUNGALS		
ketoconazole	↑ ketoconazole	When VIEKIRA XR is co-administered with ketoconazole, the maximum daily dose of ketoconazole should be limited to 200 mg per day.
voriconazole*	↓ voriconazole	Co-administration of VIEKIRA XR with voriconazole is not recommended unless an assessment of the benefit-to-risk ratio justifies the use of voriconazole.
ANTIPSYCHOTIC		
quetiapine*	↑ quetiapine	Contraindicated antipsychotics [see Contraindications (4)]. Quetiapine: • Initiation of VIEKIRA XR in patients taking quetiapine: Consider alternative anti-HCV therapy to avoid increases in quetiapine exposures. If coadministration is necessary, reduce the quetiapine dose to 1/6th of the current dose and monitor for quetiapine-associated adverse reactions. Refer to the quetiapine prescribing information for the recommendations on adverse reaction monitoring. • Initiation of quetiapine in patients taking VIEKIRA XR: Refer to the quetiapine prescribing information for initial dosing and titration of quetiapine.
CALCIUM CHANNEL BLOCKERS		
amlodipine nifedipine* diltiazem* verapamil*	↑ calcium channel blockers	Decrease the dose of the calcium channel blocker. The dose of amlodipine should be decreased by at least 50%. Clinical monitoring of patients is recommended for edema and/or signs and symptoms of hypotension. If such events occur, consider further dose reduction of the calcium channel blocker or switching to an alternative to the calcium channel blocker.
CORTICOSTEROIDS (INHALED/NASAL)		
fluticasone*	↑ fluticasone	Concomitant use of VIEKIRA XR with inhaled or nasal fluticasone may reduce serum cortisol concentrations. Alternative corticosteroids should be considered, particularly for long term use.
DIURETICS		
furosemide	↑ furosemide (C_{max})	Clinical monitoring of patients is recommended and therapy should be individualized based on patient's response.

This table is continued on the next page

Table 5 (Cont.) Established Drug Interactions Based on Drug Interaction Trials

Concomitant Drug Class: Drug Name	Effect on Concentration	Clinical Comments
ANTIRETROVIRAL AGENTS: PROTEASE INHIBITORS		
atazanavir/ritonavir once daily	↑ paritaprevir	When coadministered with VIEKIRA XR, atazanavir 300 mg (without ritonavir) should only be given in the morning.
darunavir/ritonavir	↓ darunavir (C_{trough})	Co-administration of VIEKIRA XR with darunavir/ritonavir is not recommended.
lopinavir/ritonavir	↑ paritaprevir	Co-administration of VIEKIRA XR with lopinavir/ritonavir is not recommended.
ANTIRETROVIRAL AGENTS: NON-NUCLEOSIDE REVERSE TRANSCRIPTASE INHIBITORS		
rilpivirine	↑ rilpivirine	Contraindicated non-nucleoside reverse transcriptase inhibitors [see Contraindications (4)]. Rilpivirine: Co-administration of VIEKIRA XR with rilpivirine once daily is not recommended due to potential for QT interval prolongation with higher concentrations of rilpivirine.
HMG CoA REDUCTASE INHIBITORS:		
pravastatin rosuvastatin	↑ pravastatin ↑ rosuvastatin	Contraindicated HMG CoA Reductase Inhibitors [see Contraindications (4)]. Rosuvastatin: Dose of rosuvastatin should not exceed 10 mg per day. Pravastatin: Dose of pravastatin should not exceed 40 mg per day.
IMMUNOSUPPRESSANTS		
cyclosporine	↑ cyclosporine	When initiating therapy with VIEKIRA XR, reduce cyclosporine dose to 1/5th of the patient's current cyclosporine dose. Measure cyclosporine blood concentrations to determine subsequent dose modifications. Upon completion of VIEKIRA XR therapy, the appropriate time to resume pre-VIEKIRA XR dose of cyclosporine should be guided by assessment of cyclosporine blood concentrations. Frequent assessment of renal function and cyclosporine-related side effects is recommended.
tacrolimus	↑ tacrolimus	When initiating therapy with VIEKIRA XR, the dose of tacrolimus needs to be reduced. Do not administer tacrolimus on the day VIEKIRA XR is initiated. Beginning the day after VIEKIRA XR is initiated; reinitiate tacrolimus at a reduced dose based on tacrolimus blood concentrations. Typical tacrolimus dosing is 0.5 mg every 7 days. Measure tacrolimus blood concentrations and adjust dose or dosing frequency to determine subsequent dose modifications. Upon completion of VIEKIRA XR therapy, the appropriate time to resume pre-VIEKIRA XR dose of tacrolimus should be guided by assessment of tacrolimus blood concentrations. Frequent assessment of renal function and tacrolimus related side effects is recommended.
LONG ACTING BETA-ADRENOCEPTOR AGONIST		
salmeterol*	↑ salmeterol	Concurrent administration of VIEKIRA XR and salmeterol is not recommended. The combination may result in increased risk of cardiovascular adverse events associated with salmeterol, including QT prolongation, palpitations and sinus tachycardia.
MUSCLE RELAXANTS		
carisoprodol	↓ carisoprodol ↔ mepobramate (metabolite of carisoprodol)	Increase dose if clinically indicated.
cyclobenzaprine	↓ cyclobenzaprine ↓ norcyclobenzaprine (metabolite of cyclobenzaprine)	Increase dose if clinically indicated.

This table is continued on the next page

- Patients should be instructed to consult their health care professional without delay if they have onset of fatigue, weakness, lack of appetite, nausea and vomiting, jaundice or discolored feces.
- Consider discontinuing VIEKIRA XR if ALT levels remain persistently greater than 10 times the ULN.
- Discontinue VIEKIRA XR if ALT elevation is accompanied by signs or symptoms of liver inflammation or increasing direct bilirubin, alkaline phosphatase, or INR.

5.3   Risks Associated With Ribavirin Combination Treatment

If VIEKIRA XR is administered with ribavirin, the warnings and precautions for ribavirin, in particular the pregnancy avoidance warning, apply to this combination regimen. Refer to the ribavirin prescribing information for a full list of the warnings and precautions for ribavirin.

5.4   Risk of Adverse Reactions or Reduced Therapeutic Effect Due to Drug Interactions

The concomitant use of VIEKIRA XR and certain other drugs may result in known or potentially significant drug interactions, some of which may lead to:

- Loss of therapeutic effect of VIEKIRA XR and possible development of resistance
- Possible clinically significant adverse reactions from greater exposures of concomitant drugs or components of VIEKIRA XR.

See Table 5 for steps to prevent or manage these possible and known significant drug interactions, including dosing recommendations [see Drug Interactions (7)]. Consider the potential for drug interactions prior to and during VIEKIRA XR therapy; review concomitant medications during VIEKIRA XR therapy; and monitor for the adverse reactions associated with the concomitant drugs [see Contraindications (4) and Drug Interactions (7)].

5.5   Risk of HIV-1 Protease Inhibitor Drug Resistance in HCV/HIV-1 Co-infected Patients

The ritonavir component of VIEKIRA XR is also an HIV-1 protease inhibitor and can select for HIV-1 protease inhibitor resistance-associated substitutions. Any HCV/HIV-1 co-infected patients treated with VIEKIRA XR should also be on a suppressive antiretroviral drug regimen to reduce the risk of HIV-1 protease inhibitor drug resistance.

6   ADVERSE REACTIONS

The following adverse reaction is described below and elsewhere in the labeling:

- Risk of Hepatic Decompensation and Hepatic Failure in Patients with Cirrhosis [see Warnings and Precautions (5.1)]
- Increased Risk of ALT Elevations [see Warnings and Precautions (5.2)]

6.1   Clinical Trials Experience

Because clinical trials are conducted under widely varying conditions, adverse reaction rates observed in clinical trials of VIEKIRA XR cannot be directly compared to rates in the clinical trials of another drug and may not reflect the rates observed in practice.

If VIEKIRA XR™ (dasabuvir, ombitasvir, paritaprevir, and ritonavir) is administered with ribavirin (RBV), refer to the prescribing information for ribavirin for a list of ribavirin-associated adverse reactions.

The safety assessment was based on data from seven clinical trials in more than 2,000 subjects who received the components of VIEKIRA XR with or without ribavirin for 12 or 24 weeks.

Components of VIEKIRA XR with Ribavirin in GT 1-Infected Subjects without Cirrhosis

The safety of the components of VIEKIRA XR with ribavirin were assessed in 770 subjects with chronic HCV genotype 1 (GT1) infection without cirrhosis in two placebo-controlled trials (SAPPHIRE-I and -II) [see Clinical Studies (14.1, 14.2)]. Adverse reactions that occurred more often in subjects treated with the components of VIEKIRA XR with ribavirin compared to placebo were fatigue, nausea, pruritus, other skin reactions, insomnia, and asthenia (see Table 3). The majority of the adverse reactions were mild in severity. Two percent of subjects experienced a serious adverse event (SAE). The proportion of subjects who permanently discontinued treatment due to adverse reactions was less than 1%.

Continued on next page

Table 5 *(Cont.)* Established Drug Interactions Based on Drug Interaction Trials

Concomitant Drug Class: Drug Name	Effect on Concentration	Clinical Comments
NARCOTIC ANALGESICS		
acetaminophen/hydrocodone	↑ hydrocodone ↔ acetaminophen	Reduce the dose of hydrocodone by 50% and monitor patients for respiratory depression and sedation at frequent intervals. Upon completion of VIEKIRA XR therapy, adjust the hydrocodone dose and monitor for signs of opioid withdrawal.
buprenorphine/naloxone	↑ buprenorphine ↑ norbuprenorphine (metabolite of buprenorphine)	Patients should be closely monitored for sedation and cognitive effects.
PROTON PUMP INHIBITORS		
omeprazole	↓ omeprazole	Monitor patients for decreased efficacy of omeprazole. Consider increasing the omeprazole dose in patients whose symptoms are not well controlled; avoid use of more than 40 mg per day of omeprazole.
SEDATIVES/HYPNOTICS		
alprazolam	↑ alprazolam	Contraindicated Sedatives/Hypnotics *[see Contraindications (4)].* Alprazolam: Clinical monitoring of patients is recommended. A decrease in alprazolam dose can be considered based on clinical response.
diazepam	↓ diazepam ↓ nordiazepam (metabolite of diazepam)	Increase dose if clinically indicated.

See Clinical Pharmacology, Tables 7 and 8.
The direction of the arrow indicates the direction of the change in exposures (C_{max} and AUC) (↑ = *increase of more than 20%,* ↓ = *decrease of more than 20%,* ↔ = *no change or change less than 20%*).
˙not studied.

Table 3. Adverse Reactions with ≥5% Greater Frequency Reported in Subjects with Chronic HCV GT1 Infection without Cirrhosis Treated with the Components of VIEKIRA XR with Ribavirin Compared to Placebo for 12 Weeks

	SAPPHIRE-I and -II	
	Components of VIEKIRA XR + RBV 12 Weeks N = 770 %	Placebo 12 Weeks N = 255 %
Fatigue	34	26
Nausea	22	15
Pruritus*	18	7
Skin reactions[§]	16	9
Insomnia	14	8
Asthenia	14	7

*Grouped term 'pruritus' included the preferred terms pruritus and pruritus generalized.
[§]Grouped terms: rash, erythema, eczema, rash maculo-papular, rash macular, dermatitis, rash papular, skin exfoliation, rash pruritic, rash erythematous, rash generalized, dermatitis allergic, dermatitis contact, exfoliative rash, photosensitivity reaction, psoriasis, skin reaction, ulcer, urticaria.

Components of VIEKIRA XR with and without Ribavirin in GT1-Infected Subjects without Cirrhosis
The components of VIEKIRA XR with and without ribavirin were assessed in 401 and 509 subjects with chronic HCV infection GT1 infection without cirrhosis, respectively, in three clinical trials (PEARL-II, PEARL-III and PEARL-IV) *[see Clinical Studies (14.1, 14.2)].* Pruritus, nausea, insomnia, and asthenia were identified as adverse events occurring more often in subjects treated with the components of VIEKIRA XR with ribavirin (see Table 4). The majority of adverse events were mild to moderate in severity. The proportion of subjects who permanently discontinued treatment due to adverse events was less than 1% for the components of VIEKIRA XR with or without ribavirin.

Table 4. Adverse Events with ≥5% Greater Frequency Reported in Subjects with Chronic HCV GT1 Infection without Cirrhosis Treated with the Components of VIEKIRA XR with or without Ribavirin for 12 Weeks

	PEARL-II, -III and -IV	
	Components of VIEKIRA XR + RBV 12 Weeks N = 401 %	Components of VIEKIRA XR without RBV 12 Weeks N = 509 %
Nausea	16	8
Pruritus*	13	7
Insomnia	12	5
Asthenia	9	4

*Grouped term 'pruritus' included the preferred terms pruritus and pruritus generalized.

Components of VIEKIRA XR with Ribavirin in GT1-Infected Subjects with Compensated Cirrhosis
The components of VIEKIRA XR with ribavirin were assessed in 380 subjects with genotype 1 infection and compensated cirrhosis who were treated with the components of VIEKIRA XR plus ribavirin for 12 (n=208) or 24 (n=172) weeks duration (TURQUOISE-II) *[see Clinical Studies (14.1, 14.3)].* The type and severity of adverse events in subjects with compensated cirrhosis was comparable to non-cirrhotic subjects in other phase 3 trials. Fatigue, skin reactions and dyspnea occurred at least 5% more often in subjects treated for 24 weeks. The majority of adverse events occurred during the first 12 weeks of dosing in both treatment arms. Most of the adverse events were mild to moderate in severity. The proportion of subjects treated with the components of VIEKIRA XR for 12 and 24 weeks who experienced SAEs were 6% and 5%, respectively and 2% of subjects permanently discontinued treatment due to adverse events in each treatment arm.
Components of VIEKIRA XR without Ribavirin in GT1b-Infected Subjects with Compensated Cirrhosis
The components of VIEKIRA XR without ribavirin for 12 weeks was assessed in 60 subjects with genotype 1b infection and compensated cirrhosis (TURQUOISE-III) *[see Clinical Studies (14.1, 14.3)].* The type and severity of adverse events and laboratory abnormalities in genotype 1b-infected subjects with compensated cirrhosis were comparable to subjects in other trials without ribavirin.
Skin Reactions
In PEARL-II, -III and -IV, 7% of subjects receiving the components of VIEKIRA XR alone and 10% of subjects receiving the components of VIEKIRA XR with ribavirin reported rash-related events. In SAPPHIRE-I and -II 16% of subjects receiving the components of VIEKIRA XR with ribavirin and 9% of subjects receiving placebo reported skin reactions. In TURQUOISE-II, 18% and 24% of subjects receiving the components of VIEKIRA XR with ribavirin for 12 or 24 weeks reported skin reactions. The majority of events were graded as mild in severity. There were no serious events or severe cutaneous reactions, such as Stevens Johnson Syndrome (SJS), toxic epidermal necrolysis (TEN), erythema multiforme (EM) or drug rash with eosinophilia and systemic symptoms (DRESS).

PDR® Pharmacy Discount Card is available to help reduce the cost of prescriptions for cash-paying patients. Print a card at PDR.net/printcard or download now on iTunes® or Google Play™.

Table 6. Pharmacokinetic Properties of the Components of VIEKIRA XR

	Ombitasvir	Paritaprevir	Ritonavir	Dasabuvir
Absorption				
T_{max} (hr) median values	5	5	4	8
Absolute bioavailability (%)	48	53	NA	70
Effect of high fat meal relative to fasting[a,b]	1.96 (1.83-2.15)	4.60 (3.8-5.57)	2.13 (1.86-2.43)	5.92 (5.06-6.92)
Accumulation[c]	0.90- to 1.03-fold	1.5- to 2-fold		0.96-fold
Distribution				
% Bound to human plasma proteins	99.9	97-98.6	>99	>99.5
Blood-to-plasma ratio	0.49	0.7	0.6	0.7
Volume of distribution at steady state (Vss) (L)	173	103	21.5[d]	149
Metabolism				
Metabolism	amide hydrolysis followed by oxidative metabolism	CYP3A4 (major), CYP3A5	CYP3A (major), CYP2D6	CYP2C8 (major), CYP3A
Elimination[e]				
Major route of elimination	biliary excretion	metabolism	metabolism	metabolism
$t_{1/2}$ (hr)[f]	21-25	5.5	4	5.5-6
% of dose excreted in feces[g]	90.2	88	86.4	94.4
% of dose excreted unchanged in feces[g]	87.8	1.1	33.8	26.2
% of dose excreted in urine[g]	1.91	8.8	11.3	~ 2
% of dose excreted unchanged in urine[g]	0.03	0.05	3.5	0.03

NA - data not available
a. High fat meal of 753 Kcal; 55.3% calories from fat, 27.8% calories from carbohydrates, and 16.9% calories from protein.
b. Similar results are expected for ombitasvir, paritaprevir and dasabuvir under moderate fat meal conditions.
c. Steady state exposures are achieved after approximately 12 days of dosing.
d. It is apparent volume of distribution (V/F) for ritonavir.
e. Ombitasvir, paritaprevir, ritonavir, and dasabuvir do not inhibit organic anion transporter (OAT1) *in vivo* and based on *in vitro* data, are not expected to inhibit organic cation transporter (OCT2), organic anion transporter (OAT3), or multidrug and toxin extrusion proteins (MATE1 and MATE2K) at clinically relevant concentrations.
f. $t_{1/2}$ values refer to the mean elimination half-life.
g. Dosing in mass balance studies: single dose administration of [14C] ombitasvir; single dose administration of [14C] paritaprevir co-dosed with 100 mg ritonavir; single dose administration of [14C] dasabuvir.

Laboratory Abnormalities
Serum ALT Elevations
Approximately 1% of subjects treated with the components of VIEKIRA XR experienced post-baseline serum ALT levels greater than 5 times the upper limit of normal (ULN) after starting treatment. The incidence increased to 25% (4/16) among women taking a concomitant ethinyl estradiol containing medication [see Contraindications (4) and Warnings and Precautions (5.2)]. The incidence of clinically relevant ALT elevations among women using estrogens other than ethinyl estradiol, such as estradiol and conjugated estrogens used in hormone replacement therapy was 3% (2/59). ALT elevations were typically asymptomatic, generally occurred during the first 4 weeks of treatment (mean time 20 days, range 8-57 days) and most resolved with ongoing therapy. The majority of these ALT elevations were assessed as drug-related liver injury. Elevations in ALT were generally not associated with bilirubin elevations. Cirrhosis was not a risk factor for elevated ALT [see Warnings and Precautions (5.2)].
Serum Bilirubin Elevations

Post-baseline elevations in bilirubin at least 2 × ULN were observed in 15% of subjects receiving the components of VIEKIRA XR with ribavirin compared to 2% in those receiving the components of VIEKIRA XR without ribavirin. These bilirubin increases were predominately indirect and related to the inhibition of the bilirubin transporters OATP1B1/1B3 by paritaprevir and ribavirin-induced hemolysis. Bilirubin elevations occurred after initiation of treatment, peaked by study Week 1, and generally resolved with ongoing therapy. Bilirubin elevations were not associated with serum ALT elevations.
Anemia/Decreased Hemoglobin
Across all Phase 3 studies, the mean change from baseline in hemoglobin levels in subjects treated with the components of VIEKIRA XR with ribavirin was -2.4 g/dL and the mean change in subjects treated with the components of VIEKIRA XR without ribavirin was -0.5 g/dL. Decreases in hemoglobin levels occurred early in treatment (Week 1-2) with further reductions through Week 3. Hemoglobin values remained low during the remainder of treatment and returned towards baseline levels by post-treatment Week 4.

Less than 1% of subjects treated with the components of VIEKIRA XR with ribavirin had hemoglobin levels decrease to less than 8.0 g/dL during treatment. Seven percent of subjects treated with the components of VIEKIRA XR with ribavirin underwent a ribavirin dose reduction due to a decrease in hemoglobin levels; three subjects received a blood transfusion and five required erythropoietin. One patient discontinued therapy due to anemia. No subjects treated with the components of VIEKIRA XR without ribavirin had a hemoglobin level less than 10 g/dL.
Components of VIEKIRA XR with Ribavirin in HCV/HIV-1 Co-infected Subjects
The components of VIEKIRA XR with ribavirin were assessed in 63 subjects with HCV/HIV-1 co-infection who were on stable antiretroviral therapy. The most common adverse events occurring in at least 10% of subjects were fatigue (48%), insomnia (19%), nausea (17%), headache (16%), pruritus (13%), cough (11%), irritability (10%), and ocular icterus (10%).
Elevations in total bilirubin greater than 2 x ULN (mostly indirect) occurred in 34 (54%) subjects. Fifteen of these subjects were also receiving atazanavir at the time of bilirubin elevation and nine also had adverse events of ocular icterus, jaundice or hyperbilirubinemia. None of the subjects with hyperbilirubinemia had concomitant elevations of aminotransferases [see Warnings and Precautions (5.5), Adverse Reactions (6.1) and Clinical Studies (14.6)]. No subject experienced a grade 3 ALT elevation.
Seven subjects (11%) had at least one post-baseline hemoglobin value of less than 10 g/dL, and six of these subjects had a ribavirin dose modification; no subject in this small cohort required a blood transfusion or erythropoietin.
Median declines in CD4+ T-cell counts of 47 cells/mm³ and 62 cells/mm³ were observed at the end of 12 and 24 weeks of treatment, respectively, and most returned to baseline levels post-treatment. Two subjects had CD4+ T-cell counts decrease to less than 200 cells/mm³ during treatment without a decrease in CD4%. No subject experienced an AIDS-related opportunistic infection.
Components of VIEKIRA XR with Ribavirin in Selected Liver Transplant Recipients
The components of VIEKIRA XR with ribavirin were assessed in 34 post-liver transplant subjects with recurrent HCV infection. Adverse events occurring in more than 20% of subjects included fatigue 50%, headache 44%, cough 32%, diarrhea 26%, insomnia 26%, asthenia 24%, nausea 24%, muscle spasms 21% and rash 21%. Ten subjects (29%) had at least one post-baseline hemoglobin value of less than 10 g/dL. Ten subjects underwent a ribavirin dose modification due to decrease in hemoglobin and 3% (1/34) had an interruption of ribavirin. Five subjects received erythropoietin, all of whom initiated ribavirin at the starting dose of 1000 to 1200 mg daily. No subject received a blood transfusion [see Clinical Studies (14.5)].

6.2   Postmarketing Experience
The following adverse reactions have been identified during post approval use of the components of VIEKIRA XR. Because these reactions are reported voluntarily from a population of uncertain size, it is not always possible to reliably estimate their frequency or establish a causal relationship to drug exposure.
Immune System Disorders: Hypersensitivity reactions (including angioedema).
Hepatobiliary Disorders: Hepatic decompensation, hepatic failure [see Warnings and Precautions (5.1)].

7   DRUG INTERACTIONS
7.1   Potential for VIEKIRA XR to Affect Other Drugs
Dasabuvir, ombitasvir, and paritaprevir are inhibitors of UGT1A1, and ritonavir is an inhibitor of CYP3A4. Paritaprevir is an inhibitor of OATP1B1 and OATP1B3 and dasabuvir, paritaprevir, and ritonavir are inhibitors of BCRP. Co-administration of VIEKIRA XR with drugs that are substrates of CYP3A, UGT1A1, BCRP, OATP1B1 or OATP1B3 may result in increased plasma concentrations of such drugs [see also Contraindications (4), Warnings and Precautions (5.4), and Clinical Pharmacology (12.3)].

Continued on next page

7.2 Potential for Other Drugs to Affect One or More Components of VIEKIRA XR

Paritaprevir and ritonavir are primarily metabolized by CYP3A enzymes. Co-administration of VIEKIRA XR with strong inhibitors of CYP3A may increase paritaprevir and ritonavir concentrations. Dasabuvir is primarily metabolized by CYP2C8 enzymes. Co-administration of VIEKIRA XR with drugs that inhibit CYP2C8 may increase dasabuvir plasma concentrations. Ombitasvir is primarily metabolized via amide hydrolysis while CYP enzymes play a minor role in its metabolism. Ombitasvir, paritaprevir, dasabuvir and ritonavir are substrates of P-gp. Ombitasvir, paritaprevir and dasabuvir are substrates of BCRP. Paritaprevir is a substrate of OATP1B1 and OATP1B3. Inhibition of P-gp, BCRP, OATP1B1 or OATP1B3 may increase the plasma concentrations of the various components of VIEKIRA XR.

7.3 Established and Other Potential Drug Interactions

If dose adjustments of concomitant medications are made due to treatment with VIEKIRA XR, doses should be re-adjusted after administration of VIEKIRA XR is completed. Table 5 provides the effect of co-administration of VIEKIRA XR on concentrations of concomitant drugs and the effect of concomitant drugs on the various components of VIEKIRA XR. Refer to Contraindications for drugs that are contraindicated with VIEKIRA XR *[see Contraindications (4)].* Refer to the ritonavir prescribing information for other potentially significant drug interactions with ritonavir.

[See table 5 on pages 858 through 860]

7.4 Drugs without Clinically Significant Interactions with VIEKIRA XR

No dosage adjustments are recommended when VIEKIRA XR™ (dasabuvir, ombitasvir, paritaprevir, and ritonavir) is co-administered with the following medications: abacavir, dolutegravir, digoxin, duloxetine, emtricitabine/tenofovir disoproxil fumarate, escitalopram, lamivudine, methadone, progestin only contraceptives, raltegravir, sofosbuvir, sulfamethoxazole, trimethoprim, warfarin and zolpidem.

8 USE IN SPECIFIC POPULATIONS

8.1 Pregnancy

Risk Summary

If VIEKIRA XR is administered with ribavirin, the combination regimen is contraindicated in pregnant women and in men whose female partners are pregnant. Refer to the ribavirin prescribing information for more information on use in pregnancy.

No adequate human data are available to establish whether or not VIEKIRA XR poses a risk to pregnancy outcomes. In animal reproduction studies, no adverse developmental effects were observed when the components of VIEKIRA XR were administered separately during organogenesis and lactation. During organogenesis, the exposures were up to 28 and 4 times (mice and rabbits, respectively; ombitasvir), 8 and 98 times (mice and rats, respectively; paritaprevir, ritonavir), and 24 and 6 times (rats and rabbits, respectively; dasabuvir) exposures at the recommended clinical dose of VIEKIRA XR. In rodent pre/postnatal developmental studies, maternal systemic exposures (AUC) to ombitasvir, paritaprevir and dasabuvir were approximately 25, 17 and 44 times, respectively, the exposure in humans at the recommended clinical dose *[see Data].*

The background risk of major birth defects and miscarriage for the indicated population is unknown. In the U.S. general population, the estimated background risk of major birth defects and miscarriage in clinically recognized pregnancies is 2% to 4% and 15% to 20%, respectively.

Data

Animal data

Dasabuvir

Dasabuvir was administered orally to pregnant rats (0, 60, 300 and 800 mg/kg/day) and rabbits (0, 100, 200 or 400 mg/kg/day) during the period of organogenesis (on GD 6 to 17 and GD 7 to 20, respectively). There were no test article-related embryofetal effects (malformations or fetal toxicity) at any dose level in either species. The highest systemic exposure of dasabuvir was 24-times higher (rats) and 6-times higher (rabbits) than the exposures in humans at the recommended clinical dose.

In a pre- and postnatal developmental study in rats, dasabuvir was administered orally at 0, 50, 200, or 800 mg/kg/day from GD 7 to lactation day 21. There were no treatment-related effects at maternal exposures 44-times higher than exposures in humans at the recommended clinical dose.

Ombitasvir

Ombitasvir was administered orally to pregnant mice (0, 15, 50, or 150 mg/kg/day) and rabbits (0, 10 or 60 mg/kg/day) during the period of organogenesis (on gestation days (GD) 6 to 15, and GD 7 to 19, respectively). There were no ombitasvir-related embryofetal effects (malformations or fetal toxicity) at any dose level in either species. The systemic exposures at the highest doses were 28-times higher (mice) and 4-times higher (rabbits) than the exposures in humans at the recommended clinical dose.

In a pre- and postnatal developmental study in mice, ombitasvir was administered orally at 0, 10, 40, or 200 mg/kg/day from GD 6 to lactation day 20. There were no ombitasvir-related effects at maternal exposures 25-times higher than exposures in humans at the recommended clinical dose.

The major human metabolites of ombitasvir, M29 and M36, were tested in pregnant mice during the period of organogenesis from GD 6 to 15. M29 was administered orally at doses of 0, 1, 2.5 or 4.5 mg/kg/day. M36 was dosed orally at doses 1.5, 3, or 6 mg/kg/day. In both cases, there were no treatment related embryofetal effects (malformations or fetal toxicity) at any dose level. The highest doses produced exposures approximately 26-times higher than the exposures in humans at the recommended clinical dose.

Paritaprevir/ritonavir

Paritaprevir/ritonavir was administered orally to pregnant rats (0/0, 30/15, 100/15, 450/45 mg/kg/day) and mice (0/0, 30/30, 100/30, or 300/30 mg/kg/day) during the period of organogenesis (on GD 6 to 17, and GD 6 to 15, respectively). There were no test article-related embryofetal effects (malformations or fetal toxicity) at any dose level in either species. The highest systemic exposure of paritaprevir was 8-times higher (rats) and 98-times higher (mice) than the exposures in humans at the recommended clinical dose.

In a pre- and postnatal developmental study in rats, paritaprevir/ritonavir were administered orally at 0/0, 6/30, 30/30, or 300/30 mg/kg/day from GD 7 to lactation day 20. There were no treatment related effects at maternal exposures 17-times higher than exposures in humans at the recommended clinical dose.

8.2 Lactation

Risk Summary

It is not known whether VIEKIRA XR and its metabolites are present in human breast milk, affect human milk production or have effects on the breastfed infant. Unchanged ombitasvir, paritaprevir and its hydrolysis product M13, and dasabuvir were the predominant components observed in the milk of lactating rats, without effect on nursing pups *[see Data].*

The developmental and health benefits of breastfeeding should be considered along with the mother's clinical need for VIEKIRA XR and any potential adverse effects on the breastfed child from VIEKIRA XR or from the underlying maternal condition.

If VIEKIRA XR is administered with ribavirin, the nursing mother's information for ribavirin also applies to this combination regimen. Refer to the ribavirin prescribing information for more information on use during lactation.

Data

Animal Data

Dasabuvir

No effects of dasabuvir on growth and postnatal development were observed in nursing pups at the highest dose tested (800 mg/kg/day) in rats. Maternal systemic exposure (AUC) to dasabuvir was approximately 44 times the exposure in humans at the recommended clinical dose. Although not measured directly, dasabuvir was likely present in the milk of lactating rats in this study, since systemic exposure was observed in nursing pups on post-natal day 14 (approximately 14% of maternal exposure).

When dasabuvir was administered to lactating rats (5 mg/kg on post-partum day 10 to 11), milk exposure (AUC) was 2 times higher than that in plasma, with unchanged parent drug (78%) accounting for the majority of drug-related material in milk.

Ombitasvir

No effects of ombitasvir on growth and postnatal development were observed in nursing pups at the highest dose tested (200 mg/kg/day) in mice. Maternal systemic exposure (AUC) to ombitasvir was approximately 25 times the exposure in humans at the recommended clinical dose. Although not measured directly, ombitasvir was likely present in the milk of lactating mice in this study, since systemic exposure was observed in nursing pups on post-natal day 21 (approximately 16% of maternal exposure).

When ombitasvir was administered to lactating rats (5 mg/kg on post-partum day 10 to 11), milk exposure (AUC) was 4 times higher than that in plasma, with unchanged parent drug (91%) accounting for the majority of drug-related material in milk.

Paritaprevir/ritonavir

No effects of paritaprevir/ritonavir on growth and postnatal development were observed in nursing pups at the highest dose tested (300/30 mg/kg/day) in rats. Maternal systemic exposure (AUC) to paritaprevir was approximately 17 times the exposure in humans at the recommended clinical dose. Although not measured directly, paritaprevir was likely present in the milk of lactating rats at the high dose in this study, since systemic exposure was observed in nursing pups on post-natal day 15 (approximately 0.3 % of maternal exposure).

When paritaprevir/ritonavir was administered to lactating rats (30/15 mg/kg on post-partum day 10 to 11), milk exposure (AUC) was half that in plasma, with the hydrolysis product M13 (84%) and unchanged parent drug (16%) accounting for all paritaprevir-related material in milk.

8.3 Females and Males of Reproductive Potential

If VIEKIRA XR is administered with ribavirin, the information for ribavirin with regard to pregnancy testing, contraception, and infertility also applies to this combination regimen. Refer to ribavirin prescribing information for additional information.

8.4 Pediatric Use

Safety and effectiveness of VIEKIRA XR in pediatric patients less than 18 years of age have not been established.

8.5 Geriatric Use

No dosage adjustment of VIEKIRA XR is warranted in geriatric patients. Of the total number of subjects in clinical studies of the components of VIEKIRA XR, 8.5% (174/2053) were 65 and over. No overall differences in safety or effectiveness were observed between these subjects and younger subjects, and other reported clinical experience has not identified differences in responses between the elderly and younger subjects, but greater sensitivity of some older individuals cannot be ruled out.

8.6 Hepatic Impairment

No dosage adjustment of VIEKIRA XR is required in patients with mild hepatic impairment (Child-Pugh A). VIEKIRA XR is contraindicated in patients with moderate to severe (Child-Pugh B and C) hepatic impairment *[see Contraindications (4), Warnings and Precautions (5.1) and Clinical Pharmacology (12.3)].*

8.7 Renal Impairment

No dosage adjustment of VIEKIRA XR is required in patients with mild, moderate or severe renal impairment, including those on dialysis. For patients that require ribavirin, refer to the ribavirin prescribing information for information regarding use in patients with renal impairment *[see Clinical Pharmacology (12.3)].*

10 OVERDOSAGE

In case of overdose, it is recommended that the patient be monitored for any signs or symptoms of adverse reactions and appropriate symptomatic treatment instituted immediately.

11 DESCRIPTION

VIEKIRA XR fixed dose combination, extended-release tablet includes a hepatitis C virus non-nucleoside NS5B palm polymerase inhibitor (dasabuvir), a hepatitis C virus NS5A inhibitor (ombitasvir), a hepatitis C virus NS3/4A protease inhibitor (paritaprevir), and a CYP3A inhibitor (ritonavir) that inhibits CYP3A mediated metabolism of paritaprevir, thereby providing increased plasma concentration of paritaprevir. The tablets are for oral administration.

Dasabuvir

The chemical name of dasabuvir is Sodium 3-(3-*tert*-butyl-4-methoxy-5-[6-[(methylsulfonyl)amino]naphthalene-2-yl]phenyl)-2,6-dioxo-3,6-dihydro-2H-pyrimidin-1-ide hydrate (1:1:1). The molecular formula is $C_{26}H_{26}N_3O_5S \bullet Na \bullet H_2O$ (salt, hydrate) and the molecular weight of the drug substance is 533.57 (salt, hydrate). The drug substance is white to pale yellow to pink powder, slightly soluble in water and very slightly soluble in methanol and isopropyl alcohol. Dasabuvir has the following molecular structure:[See molecular structure on next page]

Ombitasvir

The chemical name of ombitasvir is Dimethyl ([(2S,5S)-1-(4-*tert*-butylphenyl) pyrrolidine-2,5-diyl]bis(benzene-4,1-diylcarbamoyl(2S)pyrrolidine-2,1-diyl[(2S)-3-methyl-1-oxobutane-1,2-diyl]))biscarbamate hydrate. The molecular

Table 7. Drug Interactions: Change in Pharmacokinetic Parameters of Dasabuvir, Ombitasvir, Paritaprevir, and Ritonavir in the Presence of Co-administered Drug

Co-administered Drug	Dose of Co-administered Drug (mg)	n	DAA	Ratio (with/without co-administered drug) of DAA Pharmacokinetic Parameters (90% CI); No Effect = 1.00		
				C_{max}	AUC	C_{min}
Alprazolam	0.5 single dose	12	dasabuvir	0.93 (0.83, 1.04)	0.98 (0.87, 1.11)	1.00 (0.87, 1.15)
			ombitasvir	0.98 (0.93, 1.04)	1.00 (0.96, 1.04)	0.98 (0.93, 1.04)
			paritaprevir	0.91 (0.64, 1.31)	0.96 (0.73, 1.27)	1.12 (1.02, 1.23)
			ritonavir	0.92 (0.84, 1.02)	0.96 (0.89, 1.03)	1.01 (0.94, 1.09)
Amlodipine	5 single dose	14	dasabuvir	1.05 (0.97, 1.14)	1.01 (0.96, 1.06)	0.95 (0.89, 1.01)
			ombitasvir	1.00 (0.95, 1.06)	1.00 (0.97, 1.04)	1.00 (0.97, 1.04)
			paritaprevir	0.77 (0.64, 0.94)	0.78 (0.68, 0.88)	0.88 (0.80, 0.95)
			ritonavir	0.96 (0.87, 1.06)	0.93 (0.89, 0.98)	0.95 (0.89, 1.01)
Atazanavir/ritonavir[a]	Atazanavir 300 and ritonavir 100 once daily in the evening	11	dasabuvir	0.81 (0.73, 0.91)	0.81 (0.71, 0.92)	0.80 (0.65, 0.98)
			ombitasvir	0.83 (0.72, 0.96)	0.90 (0.78, 1.02)	1.00 (0.89, 1.13)
			paritaprevir	2.19 (1.61, 2.98)	3.16 (2.40, 4.17)	11.95 (8.94, 15.98)
			ritonavir	1.60 (1.38, 1.86)	3.18 (2.74, 3.69)	24.65 (18.64, 32.60)
Carbamazepine	200 once daily followed by 200 twice daily	12	dasabuvir	0.45 (0.41, 0.50)	0.30 (0.28, 0.33)	NA
			ombitasvir	0.69 (0.61, 0.78)	0.69 (0.64, 0.74)	NA
			paritaprevir	0.34 (0.25, 0.48)	0.30 (0.23, 0.38)	NA
			ritonavir	0.17 (0.12, 0.24)	0.13 (0.09, 0.17)	NA
Carisoprodol	250 single dose	14	dasabuvir	0.96 (0.91, 1.01)	1.02 (0.97, 1.07)	1.00 (0.92, 1.10)
			ombitasvir	0.98 (0.92, 1.04)	0.95 (0.92, 0.97)	0.96 (0.92, 0.99)
			paritaprevir	0.88 (0.75, 1.03)	0.96 (0.85, 1.08)	1.14 (1.02, 1.27)
			ritonavir	0.94 (0.87, 1.02)	0.94 (0.88, 0.99)	0.95 (0.89, 1.03)
Cyclobenzaprine	5 single dose	14	dasabuvir	0.98 (0.90, 1.07)	1.01 (0.96, 1.06)	1.13 (1.07, 1.18)
			ombitasvir	0.98 (0.92, 1.04)	1.00 (0.97, 1.03)	1.01 (0.98, 1.04)
			paritaprevir	1.14 (0.99, 1.32)	1.13 (1.00, 1.28)	1.13 (1.01, 1.25)
			ritonavir	0.93 (0.87, 0.99)	1.00 (0.95, 1.06)	1.13 (1.05, 1.21)

This table is continued on the next page

formula is $C_{50}H_{67}N_7O_8 \bullet 4.5H_2O$ (hydrate) and the molecular weight for the drug substance is 975.20 (hydrate). The drug substance is white to light yellow to light pink powder, and is practically insoluble in aqueous buffers but is soluble in ethanol. Ombitasvir has the following molecular structure:

Paritaprevir
The chemical name of paritaprevir is (2R,6S,12Z,13aS, 14aR,16aS)-N-(cyclopropylsulfonyl)-6-{[(5-methylpyrazin-2-yl)carbonyl]amino}-5,16-dioxo-2-(phenanthridin-6-yloxy)-1,2,3,6,7,8,9,10,11,13a,14,15,16,16a-tetradecahydrocy-clopropa[e]pyrrolo[1,2-a][1,4] diazacyclopentadecine-14a (5H)-carboxamide dihydrate. The molecular formula is $C_{40}H_{43}N_7O_7S \bullet 2H_2O$ (dihydrate) and the molecular weight for the drug substance is 801.91 (dihydrate). The drug substance is white to off-white powder with very low water solubility. Paritaprevir has the following molecular structure:

Ritonavir
The chemical name of ritonavir is [5S-(5R*,8R*,10R*, 11R*)]10-Hydroxy-2-methyl-5-(1-methyethyl)-1-[2-(1-me-thylethyl)-4-thiazolyl]-3,6-dioxo-8,11-bis(phenylmethyl)-2,4,7,12-tetraazatridecan-13-oic acid,5-thiazolylmethyl ester. The molecular formula is $C_{37}H_{48}N_6O_5S_2$ and the molecular weight for the drug substance is 720.95. The drug substance is white to off white to light tan powder practically insoluble in water and freely soluble in methanol and ethanol. Ritonavir has the following molecular structure:

Continued on next page

Table 7 *(Cont.)* Drug Interactions: Change in Pharmacokinetic Parameters of Dasabuvir, Ombitasvir, Paritaprevir, and Ritonavir in the Presence of Co-administered Drug

Co-administered Drug	Dose of Co-administered Drug (mg)	n	DAA	Ratio (with/without co-administered drug) of DAA Pharmacokinetic Parameters (90% CI); No Effect = 1.00		
				C_{max}	AUC	C_{min} C_{min}
Cyclosporine	30 single dose[b]	10	dasabuvir	0.66 (0.58, 0.75)	0.70 (0.5, 0.76)	0.76 (0.71, 0.82)
			ombitasvir	0.99 (0.92, 1.07)	1.08 (1.05, 1.11)	1.15 (1.08, 1.23)
			paritaprevir	1.44 (1.16, 1.78)	1.72 (1.49, 1.99)	1.85 (1.58, 2.18)
			ritonavir	0.90 (0.78, 1.04)	1.11 (1.04, 1.19)	1.49 (1.28, 1.74)
Darunavir[c]	800 once daily	9	dasabuvir	1.10 (0.88, 1.37)	0.94 (0.78, 1.14)	0.90 (0.76, 1.06)
			ombitasvir	0.86 (0.77, 0.95)	0.86 (0.79, 0.94)	0.87 (0.82, 0.92)
			paritaprevir	1.54 (1.14, 2.09)	1.29 (1.04, 1.61)	1.30 (1.09, 1.54)
			ritonavir	0.84 (0.72, 0.98)	0.85 (0.78, 0.93)	1.07 (0.93, 1.23)
Darunavir/ ritonavir[d]	Darunavir 600 twice daily and ritonavir 100 once daily in the evening	7	dasabuvir	0.84 (0.67, 1.05)	0.73 (0.62, 0.86)	0.54 (0.49, 0.61)
			ombitasvir	0.76 (0.65, 0.88)	0.73 (0.66, 0.80)	0.73 (0.64, 0.83)
			paritaprevir	0.70 (0.43, 1.12)	0.59 (0.44, 0.79)	0.83 (0.69, 1.01)
			ritonavir	1.61 (1.30, 2.00)	1.28 (1.12, 1.45)	0.88 (0.79, 0.99)
Darunavir/ ritonavir[e]	Darunavir 800 and ritonavir 100 once daily in the evening	12	dasabuvir	0.75 (0.64, 0.88)	0.72 (0.64, 0.82)	0.65 (0.58, 0.72)
			ombitasvir	0.87 (0.82, 0.93)	0.87 (0.81, 0.93)	0.87 (0.80, 0.95)
			paritaprevir	0.70 (0.50, 0.99)	0.81 (0.60, 1.09)	1.59 (1.23, 2.05)
			ritonavir	1.19 (1.06, 1.33)	1.70 (1.54, 1.88)	14.15 (11.66, 17.18)
Diazepam	2 single dose	13	dasabuvir	1.05 (0.98, 1.13)	1.01 (0.94, 1.08)	1.05 (0.98, 1.12)
			ombitasvir	1.00 (0.93, 1.08)	0.98 (0.93, 1.03)	0.93 (0.88, 0.98)
			paritaprevir	0.95 (0.77, 1.18)	0.91 (0.78, 1.07)	0.92 (0.82, 1.03)
			ritonavir	1.10 (1.02, 1.19)	1.06 (0.98, 1.14)	0.98 (0.92, 1.03)

This table is continued on the next page

Dasabuvir, Ombitasvir, Paritaprevir, Ritonavir Film-Coated Bilayer Tablets

Dasabuvir, ombitasvir, paritaprevir, and ritonavir film-coated bilayer tablets consist of an extended release (ER) layer and an immediate release (IR) layer. The ER layer contains 200 mg dasabuvir (equivalent to 216.2 mg of dasabuvir sodium monohydrate). The ER layer of the tablet also contains copovidone, K value 28, hypromellose 2208, 17,700 (mPa*s), colloidal silicon dioxide/colloidal anhydrous silica and magnesium stearate. The IR layer contains 8.33 mg ombitasvir, 50 mg paritaprevir and 33.33 mg ritonavir. Strength of ombitasvir and paritaprevir in the drug product are expressed on the anhydrous basis. The IR layer of the tablet also contains copovidone, K value 28, vitamin E polyethylene glycol succinate, propylene glycol monolaurate, sorbitan monolaurate, colloidal silicon dioxide/colloidal anhydrous silica. The tablet coating contains hypromellose (6 mPa*s), hypromellose (15 mPa*s), polyethylene glycol 400, hydroxypropyl cellulose, polysorbate 80, polyethylene glycol 3350/macrogol 4000, talc, titanium dioxide, colloidal silicon dioxide/colloidal anhydrous silica and iron oxide yellow.

12 CLINICAL PHARMACOLOGY

12.1 Mechanism of Action

VIEKIRA XR combines three direct-acting hepatitis C virus antiviral agents with distinct mechanisms of action *[see Microbiology (12.4)]*.

Ritonavir is not active against HCV. Ritonavir is a potent CYP3A inhibitor that increases peak and trough plasma drug concentrations of paritaprevir and overall drug exposure (i.e., area under the curve).

12.2 Pharmacodynamics

Cardiac Electrophysiology

The effect of a combination of ombitasvir, paritaprevir, ritonavir, and dasabuvir on QTc interval was evaluated in a randomized, double blind, placebo and active-controlled (moxifloxacin 400 mg) 4-way crossover thorough QT study in 60 healthy subjects. At concentrations approximately 6, 1.8 and 2 times the therapeutic concentrations of paritaprevir, ombitasvir, and dasabuvir, the combination did not prolong QTc to any clinically relevant extent.

12.3 Pharmacokinetics

Dasabuvir, ombitasvir, paritaprevir, and ritonavir film-coated bilayer tablets consist of an extended-release (ER) layer of dasabuvir and an immediate-release (IR) layer of ombitasvir, paritaprevir and ritonavir.

The pharmacokinetic properties of the components of VIEKIRA XR are provided in Table 6.

[See table 6 on page 861]

Specific Populations

There are no clinically relevant changes in the pharmacokinetics of the components of VIEKIRA XR in relation to sex, race/ethnicity, or geriatric age *[see Use in Specific Populations (8.5)]*. The pharmacokinetics of VIEKIRA XR in pediatric patients less than 18 years of age have not been established *[see Use in Specific Populations (8.4)]*.

Hepatic Impairment

The single dose pharmacokinetics of the combination of dasabuvir, ombitasvir, paritaprevir, and ritonavir were evaluated in non-HCV infected subjects with mild hepatic impairment (Child-Pugh Category A; score of 5-6), moderate hepatic impairment (Child-Pugh Category B, score of 7-9) and severe hepatic impairment (Child-Pugh Category C, score of 10-15).

Relative to subjects with normal hepatic function, dasabuvir AUC values increased by 17%, and ombitasvir, paritaprevir and ritonavir AUC values decreased by 8%, 29% and 34%, respectively, in subjects with mild hepatic impairment.

Relative to subjects with normal hepatic function, dasabuvir, ombitasvir, and ritonavir AUC values decreased by 16%, 30%, and 30% respectively, and paritaprevir AUC values increased by 62% in subjects with moderate hepatic impairment.

Relative to subjects with normal hepatic function, dasabuvir, paritaprevir, and ritonavir AUC values increased by 325%, 945%, and 13%, respectively, and ombitasvir AUC values decreased by 54% in subjects with severe hepatic impairment.

Renal Impairment

The single dose pharmacokinetics of the combination of dasabuvir, ombitasvir, paritaprevir, and ritonavir were evaluated in non-HCV infected subjects with mild (CL_{cr}: 60 to 89 mL/min), moderate (CL_{cr}: 30 to 59 mL/min), and severe (CL_{cr}: 15 to 29 mL/min) renal impairment.

Table 7 *(Cont.)* **Drug Interactions: Change in Pharmacokinetic Parameters of Dasabuvir, Ombitasvir, Paritaprevir, and Ritonavir in the Presence of Co-administered Drug**

Co-administered Drug	Dose of Co-administered Drug (mg)	n	DAA	Ratio (with/without co-administered drug) of DAA Pharmacokinetic Parameters (90% CI); No Effect = 1.00		
				C_{max}	AUC	C_{min}
Ethinyl estradiol/ Norgestimate	Ethinyl estradiol 0.035 and Norgestimate 0.25 once daily	7[f]	dasabuvir	0.51 (0.22, 1.18)	0.48 (0.23, 1.02)	0.53 (0.30, 0.95)
			ombitasvir	1.05 (0.81, 1.35)	0.97 (0.81, 1.15)	1.00 (0.88, 1.12)
			paritaprevir	0.70 (0.40, 1.21)	0.66 (0.42, 1.04)	0.87 (0.67, 1.14)
			ritonavir	0.80 (0.53, 1.21)	0.71 (0.54, 0.94)	0.79 (0.68, 0.93)
Furosemide	20 single dose	12	dasabuvir	1.12 (0.96, 1.31)	1.09 (0.96, 1.23)	1.06 (0.98, 1.14)
			ombitasvir	1.14 (1.03, 1.26)	1.07 (1.01, 1.12)	1.12 (1.08, 1.16)
			paritaprevir	0.93 (0.63, 1.36)	0.92 (0.70, 1.21)	1.26 (1.16, 1.38)
			ritonavir	1.10 (0.96, 1.27)	1.04 (0.92, 1.18)	1.07 (0.99, 1.17)
Gemfibrozil[g]	600 twice daily	11	dasabuvir	2.01 (1.71, 2.38)	11.25 (9.05, 13.99)	NA
			ombitasvir	NA	NA	NA
			paritaprevir	1.21 (0.94, 1.57)	1.38 (1.18, 1.61)	NA
			ritonavir	0.84 (0.69, 1.03)	0.90 (0.78, 1.04)	NA
Hydrocodone/ Acetaminophen	5/300 single dose	15	dasabuvir	1.13 (1.01, 1.26)	1.12 (1.05, 1.19)	1.16 (1.08, 1.25)
			ombitasvir	1.01 (0.93, 1.10)	0.97 (0.93, 1.02)	0.93 (0.90, 0.97)
			paritaprevir	1.01 (0.80, 1.27)	1.03 (0.89, 1.18)	1.10 (0.97, 1.26)
			ritonavir	1.01 (0.90, 1.13)	1.03 (0.96, 1.09)	1.01 (0.93, 1.10)
Ketoconazole	400 once daily	12	dasabuvir	1.16 (1.03, 1.32)	1.42 (1.26, 1.59)	NA
			ombitasvir	0.98 (0.90, 1.06)	1.17 (1.11, 1.24)	NA
			paritaprevir	1.37 (1.11, 1.69)	1.98 (1.63, 2.42)	NA
			ritonavir	1.27 (1.04, 1.56)	1.57 (1.36, 1.81)	NA
Lopinavir/ ritonavir	400/100 twice daily	6	dasabuvir	0.99 (0.75, 1.31)	0.93 (0.75, 1.15)	0.68 (0.57, 0.80)
			ombitasvir	1.14 (1.01, 1.28)	1.17 (1.07, 1.28)	1.24 (1.14, 1.34)
			paritaprevir	2.04 (1.30, 3.20)	2.17 (1.63, 2.89)	2.36 (1.00, 5.55)
			ritonavir	1.55 (1.16, 2.09)	2.05 (1.49, 2.81)	5.25 (3.33, 8.28)

This table is continued on the next page

Pharmacokinetic data are not available on the use of VIEKIRA XR™ (dasabuvir, ombitasvir, paritaprevir, and ritonavir) in non-HCV infected subjects with End Stage Renal Disease (ESRD).

Relative to subjects with normal renal function, dasabuvir, paritaprevir, and ritonavir AUC values increased by 21%, 19%, and 42% respectively, while ombitasvir AUC values were unchanged in subjects with mild renal impairment.

Relative to subjects with normal renal function, dasabuvir, paritaprevir, and ritonavir AUC values increased by 37%, 33%, and 80% respectively, while ombitasvir AUC values were unchanged in subjects with moderate renal impairment.

Relative to subjects with normal renal function, dasabuvir, paritaprevir, and ritonavir AUC values increased by 50%, 45%, and 114% respectively, while ombitasvir AUC values were unchanged in subjects with severe renal impairment *[see Use in Specific Populations (8.7)]*.

Drug Interaction Studies
See also Contraindications (4), Warnings and Precautions (5.4), Drug Interactions (7)
All drug-drug interaction trials were conducted with VIEKIRA PAK. The effects of some drugs discussed in Table 5 on the exposures of dasabuvir, ombitasvir, paritaprevir, and ritonavir are shown in Table 7. For information regarding clinical recommendations, see *Drug Interactions (7)*.
[See table 7 on pages 863 through 867]
Table 8 summarizes the effects of dasabuvir, ombitasvir, paritaprevir, and ritonavir on the pharmacokinetics of co-administered drugs which showed clinically relevant changes. For information regarding clinical recommendations, see *Drug Interactions (7)*.
[See table 8 on page 868 and 869]

12.4   Microbiology
Mechanism of Action
VIEKIRA XR™ (dasabuvir, ombitasvir, paritaprevir, and ritonavir) combines three direct-acting antiviral agents with distinct mechanisms of action and non-overlapping resistance profiles to target HCV at multiple steps in the viral lifecycle.
Dasabuvir
Dasabuvir is a non-nucleoside inhibitor of the HCV RNA-dependent RNA polymerase encoded by the NS5B gene, which is essential for replication of the viral genome. In a biochemical assay, dasabuvir inhibited a panel of genotype 1a and 1b NS5B polymerases with median IC_{50} values of 2.8 nM (range 2.4 nM to 4.2 nM; n = 3) and 3.7 nM (range 2.2 nM to 10.7 nM; n = 4), respectively. Based on drug resistance mapping studies of HCV genotypes 1a and 1b, dasabuvir targets the palm domain of the NS5B polymerase, and is therefore referred to as a non-nucleoside NS5B-palm polymerase inhibitor.
Ombitasvir
Ombitasvir is an inhibitor of HCV NS5A, which is essential for viral RNA replication and virion assembly. The mechanism of action of ombitasvir has been characterized based on cell culture antiviral activity and drug resistance mapping studies.
Paritaprevir
Paritaprevir is an inhibitor of the HCV NS3/4A protease which is necessary for the proteolytic cleavage of the HCV encoded polyprotein (into mature forms of the NS3, NS4A, NS4B, NS5A, and NS5B proteins) and is essential for viral replication. In a biochemical assay, paritaprevir inhibited the proteolytic activity of recombinant HCV genotype 1a and 1b NS3/4A protease enzymes with IC_{50} values of 0.18 nM and 0.43 nM, respectively.
Antiviral Activity
Dasabuvir
The EC_{50} values of dasabuvir against genotype 1a-H77 and 1b-Con1 strains in HCV replicon cell culture assays were 7.7 nM and 1.8 nM, respectively. The median EC_{50} values of dasabuvir against HCV replicons containing NS5B genes from a panel of genotype 1a and 1b isolates from treatment-naïve subjects were 0.6 nM (range 0.4 nM to 2.1 nM; n = 11) and 0.3 nM (range 0.2 nM to 2 nM; n = 10), respectively.
Ombitasvir

Continued on next page

The EC_{50} values of ombitasvir against genotype 1a-H77 and 1b-Con1 strains in HCV replicon cell culture assays were 14.1 pM and 5 pM, respectively. The median EC_{50} values of ombitasvir against HCV replicons containing NS5A genes from a panel of genotype 1a and 1b isolates from treatment-naïve subjects were 0.68 pM (range 0.35 to 0.88 pM; n = 11) and 0.94 pM (range 0.74 to 1.5 pM; n = 11), respectively.

Paritaprevir
The EC_{50} values of paritaprevir against genotype 1a-H77 and 1b-Con1 strains in the HCV replicon cell culture assay were 1.0 nM and 0.21 nM, respectively. The median EC_{50} values of paritaprevir against HCV replicons containing NS3 genes from a panel of genotype 1a and 1b isolates from treatment-naïve subjects were 0.68 nM (range 0.43 nM to 1.87 nM; n = 11) and 0.06 nM (range 0.03 nM to 0.09 nM; n = 9), respectively.

Ritonavir
In HCV replicon cell culture assays, ritonavir did not exhibit a direct antiviral effect and the presence of ritonavir did not affect the antiviral activity of paritaprevir.

Combination Antiviral Activity
Evaluation of pairwise combinations of ombitasvir, paritaprevir, dasabuvir and ribavirin in HCV genotype 1 replicon cell culture assays showed no evidence of antagonism in antiviral activity.

Resistance
In Cell Culture
Exposure of HCV genotype 1a and 1b replicons to ombitasvir, paritaprevir or dasabuvir resulted in the emergence of drug resistant replicons carrying amino acid substitutions in NS5A, NS3, or NS5B, respectively. Amino acid substitutions in NS5A, NS3, or NS5B selected in cell culture or identified in Phase 2b and 3 clinical trials were phenotypically characterized in genotype 1a or 1b replicons.
For dasabuvir, in HCV genotype 1a replicons single NS5B substitutions C316Y, M414I/T, E446K/Q, Y448C/H, A553T, G554S, S556G/R, and Y561H reduced dasabuvir antiviral activity by 8- to 1,472-fold. In genotype 1b replicons, single NS5B substitutions C316H/N/Y, S368T, N411S, M414I/T, Y448C/H, A553V, S556G and D559G reduced dasabuvir antiviral activity by 5- to 1,569-fold.
For ombitasvir, in HCV genotype 1a replicons single NS5A substitutions M28T/V, Q30E/R, L31V, H58D, and Y93C/H/L/N reduced ombitasvir antiviral activity by 58- to 67,000-fold. In genotype 1b replicons, single NS5A substitutions L28T, L31F/V, and Y93H reduced ombitasvir antiviral activity by 8- to 661-fold. In general, combinations of ombitasvir resistance-associated substitutions in HCV genotype 1a or 1b replicons further reduced ombitasvir antiviral activity.
For paritaprevir, in HCV genotype 1a replicons single NS3 substitutions F43L, R155G/K/S, A156T, and D168A/E/F/H/N/V/Y reduced paritaprevir antiviral activity by 7- to 219-fold. An NS3 Q80K substitution in a genotype 1a replicon reduced paritaprevir antiviral activity by 3-fold. Combinations of V36M, Y56H, or E357K with R155K or D168 substitutions reduced the activity of paritaprevir by an additional 2- to 7-fold relative to the single R155K or D168 substitutions in genotype 1a replicons. In genotype 1b replicons single NS3 substitutions A156T and D168A/H/V reduced paritaprevir antiviral activity by 7- to 159-fold. The combination of Y56H with D168 substitutions reduced the activity of paritaprevir by an additional 16- to 26-fold relative to the single D168 substitutions in genotype 1b replicons.

In Clinical Studies
In a pooled analysis of subjects treated with regimens containing dasabuvir, ombitasvir, paritaprevir, and ritonavir with or without ribavirin (for 12 or 24 weeks) in Phase 2b and Phase 3 clinical trials, resistance analyses were conducted for 64 subjects who experienced virologic failure (20 with on-treatment virologic failure, 44 with post-treatment relapse). Treatment-emergent substitutions observed in the viral populations of these subjects are shown in Table 9. Treatment-emergent substitutions were detected in all 3 HCV drug targets in 30/57 (53%) HCV genotype 1a infected subjects, and 1/6 (17%) HCV genotype 1b infected subjects. [See Table 9 on page 870]

Persistence of Resistance-Associated Substitutions
The persistence of dasabuvir, ombitasvir, and paritaprevir treatment-emergent amino acid substitutions in NS5B, NS5A, and NS3, respectively, was assessed in HCV genotype 1a-infected subjects in Phase 2 trials whose virus had at least 1 treatment-emergent resistance-associated substitution in the drug target, and with available data through at least 24 weeks post-treatment. Population and clonal nu-

cleotide sequence analyses (assay sensitivity approximately 5-10%) were conducted to detect the persistence of viral populations with treatment-emergent substitutions.
For dasabuvir, viral populations with 1 or more treatment-emergent substitutions in NS5B persisted at detectable levels through at least Post-Treatment Week 24 in 11/16 (69%) subjects, and through Post-Treatment Week 48 in 8/15 (53%) subjects with available data. Treatment-emergent S556G persisted through Post-Treatment Week 48 in 6/9 (67%) subjects.
For ombitasvir, viral populations with 1 or more resistance-associated treatment-emergent substitutions in NS5A persisted at detectable levels through at least Post-Treatment Week 24 in 24/24 (100%) subjects, and through Post-Treatment Week 48 in 18/18 (100%) subjects with available data.
For paritaprevir, viral populations with 1 or more treatment-emergent substitutions in NS3 persisted at detectable levels through at least Post-Treatment Week 24 in

17/29 (59%) subjects, and through Post-Treatment Week 48 in 5/22 (23%) subjects with available data. Resistance-associated variant R155K remained detectable in 5/8 (63%) subjects through Post-Treatment Week 24, and in 1/5 (20%) subjects through Post-Treatment Week 48. Resistance-associated D168 substitutions remained detectable in 6/22 (27%) subjects through Post-Treatment Week 24, and were no longer detectable through Post-Treatment Week 48.
Among HCV genotype 1b infected subjects who experienced virologic failure with a regimen including ombitasvir and paritaprevir, a treatment-emergent NS5A Y93H substitution persisted through at least Post-Treatment Week 48 in 2/2 subjects, and a NS3 D168V treatment-emergent substitution persisted through Post-Treatment Week 24 in 2/4 subjects, but was no longer detectable through Post-Treatment Week 48 (0/4 subjects).
The lack of detection of virus containing a resistance-associated substitution does not indicate that the resistant virus is no longer present at clinically significant levels. The

Table 7 *(Cont.)* Drug Interactions: Change in Pharmacokinetic Parameters of Dasabuvir, Ombitasvir, Paritaprevir, and Ritonavir in the Presence of Co-administered Drug

Co-administered Drug	Dose of Co-administered Drug (mg)	n	DAA	Ratio (with/without co-administered drug) of DAA Pharmacokinetic Parameters (90% CI); No Effect = 1.00		
				C_{max}	AUC	C_{min}
Lopinavir/ ritonavir[h]	800/200 once daily	12	dasabuvir	0.56 (0.47, 0.66)	0.54 (0.46, 0.65)	0.47 (0.39, 0.58)
			ombitasvir	0.87 (0.83, 0.92)	0.97 (0.94, 1.02)	1.11 (1.06, 1.16)
			paritaprevir	0.99 (0.79, 1.25)	1.87 (1.40, 2.52)	8.23 (5.18, 13.07)
			ritonavir	1.57 (1.34, 1.83)	2.62 (2.32, 2.97)	19.46 (15.93, 23.77)
Omeprazole	40 once daily	11	dasabuvir	1.13 (1.03, 1.25)	1.08 (0.98, 1.20)	1.05 (0.93, 1.19)
			ombitasvir	1.02 (0.95, 1.09)	1.05 (0.98, 1.12)	1.04 (0.98, 1.11)
			paritaprevir	1.19 (1.04, 1.36)	1.18 (1.03, 1.37)	0.92 (0.76, 1.12)
			ritonavir	1.04 (0.96, 1.12)	1.02 (0.97, 1.08)	0.97 (0.89, 1.05)
Pravastatin	10 once daily	12	dasabuvir	1.00 (0.87, 1.14)	0.96 (0.85, 1.09)	1.03 (0.91, 1.15)
			ombitasvir	0.95 (0.89, 1.02)	0.94 (0.89, 0.99)	0.94 (0.89, 0.99)
			paritaprevir	0.96 (0.69, 1.32)	1.13 (0.92, 1.38)	1.39 (1.21, 1.59)
			ritonavir	0.89 (0.73, 1.09)	0.95 (0.86, 1.05)	1.08 (0.98, 1.19)
Rilpivirine	25 once daily (morning)[i]	10	dasabuvir	1.18 (1.02, 1.37)	1.17 (0.99, 1.38)	1.10 (0.89, 1.37)
			ombitasvir	1.11 (1.02, 1.20)	1.09 (1.04, 1.14)	1.05 (1.01, 1.08)
			paritaprevir	1.30 (0.94, 1.81)	1.23 (0.93, 1.64)	0.95 (0.84, 1.07)
			ritonavir	1.10 (0.98, 1.24)	1.08 (0.93, 1.27)	0.97 (0.91, 1.04)

This table is continued on the next page

Table 7 *(Cont.)* Drug Interactions: Change in Pharmacokinetic Parameters of Dasabuvir, Ombitasvir, Paritaprevir, and Ritonavir in the Presence of Co-administered Drug

Co-administered Drug	Dose of Co-administered Drug (mg)	n	DAA	Ratio (with/without co-administered drug) of DAA Pharmacokinetic Parameters (90% CI); No Effect = 1.00		
				C_{max}	AUC	C_{min}
Rosuvastatin	5 once daily	11	dasabuvir	1.07 (0.92, 1.24)	1.08 (0.92, 1.26)	1.15 (1.05, 1.25)
			ombitasvir	0.92 (0.82, 1.04)	0.89 (0.83, 0.95)	0.88 (0.83, 0.94)
			paritaprevir	1.59 (1.13, 2.23)	1.52 (1.23, 1.90)	1.43 (1.22, 1.68)
			ritonavir	0.98 (0.84, 1.15)	1.02 (0.93, 1.12)	1.00 (0.90, 1.12)
Tacrolimus	2 single dose	12	dasabuvir	0.85 (0.73, 0.98)	0.90 (0.80, 1.02)	1.01 (0.91, 1.11)
			ombitasvir	0.93 (0.88, 0.99)	0.94 (0.89, 0.98)	0.94 (0.91, 0.96)
			paritaprevir	0.57 (0.42, 0.78)	0.66 (0.54, 0.81)	0.73 (0.66, 0.80)
			ritonavir	0.76 (0.63, 0.91)	0.87 (0.79, 0.97)	1.03 (0.89, 1.19)

a. Atazanavir plus 100 mg ritonavir administered in the evening, 12 hours after morning dose of the components of VIEKIRA XR.
b. 30 mg cyclosporine was administered with the components of VIEKIRA XR in the test arm and 100 mg cyclosporine was administered in the reference arm without the components of VIEKIRA XR.
c. Darunavir administered with the components of VIEKIRA XR in the morning was compared to darunavir administered with 100 mg ritonavir in the morning.
d. Darunavir administered with the components of VIEKIRA XR in the morning and with 100 mg ritonavir in the evening was compared to darunavir administered with 100 mg ritonavir in the morning and evening.
e. Darunavir plus 100 mg ritonavir administered in the evening, 12 hours after the morning dose of the components of VIEKIRA XR compared to darunavir administered with 100 mg ritonavir in the evening.
f. N=3 for dasabuvir.
g. Study was conducted with paritaprevir, ritonavir and dasabuvir.
h. Lopinavir/ritonavir administered in the evening, 12 hours after morning dose of the components of VIEKIRA XR.
i. Similar increases were observed when rilpivirine was dosed in the evening with food or 4 hours after food.
NA: not available/not applicable; DAA: Direct-acting antiviral agent; CI: Confidence interval
Doses of dasabuvir were 250 mg or 400 mg (both doses showed similar exposures). Doses of ombitasvir, paritaprevir, and ritonavir were 25 mg, 150 mg and 100 mg.
Dasabuvir was dosed twice daily and ombitasvir, paritaprevir and ritonavir were dosed once daily in all the above studies except studies with gemfibrozil, ketoconazole and carbamazepine that used single doses.

long-term clinical impact of the emergence or persistence of virus containing VIEKIRA XR-resistance-associated substitutions is unknown.
Effect of Baseline HCV Polymorphisms on Treatment Response
A pooled analysis of subjects in the Phase 3 clinical trials of dasabuvir, ombitasvir, and paritaprevir with or without ribavirin was conducted to explore the association between baseline HCV NS5B, NS5A, or NS3 resistance-associated polymorphisms and treatment outcome. Baseline samples from HCV genotype 1a infected subjects who experienced virologic failure (n=47), as well as samples from a subset of demographically matched subjects who achieved SVR (n=94), were analyzed to compare the frequencies of resistance-associated polymorphisms in these two populations. The NS3 Q80K polymorphism was detected in approximately 38% of subjects in this analysis and was enriched approximately 2-fold in virologic failure subjects compared to SVR-achieving subjects. Ombitasvir resistance-associated polymorphisms in NS5A (pooling data from all resistance-associated amino acid positions) were detected in approximately 22% of subjects in this analysis and similarly were enriched approximately 2-fold in viro-

logic failure subjects. Dasabuvir resistance-associated polymorphisms in NS5B were detected in approximately 5% of subjects in this analysis and were not enriched in virologic failure subjects.
In contrast to the Phase 3 subset analysis, no association of NS3 or NS5A polymorphisms and treatment outcome was seen in an analysis of noncirrhotic HCV genotype 1a-infected subjects (n=174 for NS3 and n=183 for NS5A) who received dasabuvir, ombitasvir, and paritaprevir with or without ribavirin (for 12 or 24 weeks) in a Phase 2b trial. Baseline HCV polymorphisms are not expected to have a substantial impact on the likelihood of achieving SVR when VIEKIRA XR is used as recommended for HCV genotype 1a and 1b infected patients, based on the low virologic failure rates observed in clinical trials.
Cross-resistance
Cross-resistance is expected among NS5A inhibitors, NS3/4A protease inhibitors, and non-nucleoside NS5B-palm inhibitors by class. Dasabuvir retained full activity against HCV replicons containing a single NS5B L159F, S282T, or V321A substitution, which are associated with resistance or prior exposure to nucleot(s)ide analogue NS5B polymerase inhibitors. In clinical trials of the components of VIEKIRA

XR, no subjects who experienced virologic failure had treatment-emergent substitutions potentially associated with resistance to nucleot(s)ide analogue NS5B polymerase inhibitors.
The impact of prior dasabuvir, ombitasvir, or paritaprevir treatment experience on the efficacy of other NS5B inhibitors, NS5A inhibitors, or NS3/4A protease inhibitors has not been studied. Similarly, the efficacy of VIEKIRA XR has not been studied in subjects who have failed prior treatment with another NS5B inhibitor, NS5A inhibitor, or NS3/4A protease inhibitor.

13 NONCLINICAL TOXICOLOGY
13.1 Carcinogenesis, Mutagenesis, Impairment of Fertility
Carcinogenesis and Mutagenesis
Dasabuvir
Dasabuvir was not carcinogenic in a 6-month transgenic mouse study up to the highest dose tested (2000 mg per kg per day). Similarly, dasabuvir was not carcinogenic in a 2-year rat study up to the highest dose tested (800 mg per kg per day), resulting in dasabuvir exposures approximately 19-fold higher than those in humans at 500 mg.
Dasabuvir was not genotoxic in a battery of *in vitro* or *in vivo* assays, including bacterial mutagenicity, chromosome aberration using human peripheral blood lymphocytes and *in vivo* rat micronucleus assays.
Ombitasvir
Ombitasvir was not carcinogenic in a 6-month transgenic mouse study up to the highest dose tested (150 mg per kg per day). Similarly, ombitasvir was not carcinogenic in a 2-year rat study up to the highest dose tested (30 mg per kg per day), resulting in ombitasvir exposures approximately 16-fold higher than those in humans at 25 mg.
Ombitasvir and its major inactive human metabolites (M29, M36) were not genotoxic in a battery of *in vitro* or *in vivo* assays, including bacterial mutagenicity, chromosome aberration using human peripheral blood lymphocytes and *in vivo* mouse micronucleus assays.
Paritaprevir, ritonavir
Paritaprevir, ritonavir was not carcinogenic in a 6-month transgenic mouse study up to the highest dose tested (300/30 mg per kg per day). Similarly, paritaprevir, ritonavir was not carcinogenic in a 2-year rat study up to the highest dose tested (300/30 mg per kg per day), resulting in paritaprevir exposures approximately 9-fold higher than those in humans at 150 mg.
Paritaprevir was positive in an *in vitro* chromosome aberration test using human lymphocytes. Paritaprevir was negative in a bacterial mutation assay, and in two *in vivo* genetic toxicology assays (rat bone marrow micronucleus and rat liver Comet tests).
If VIEKIRA XR is administered with ribavirin, refer to the prescribing information for ribavirin for information on carcinogenesis, and mutagenesis.
Impairment of Fertility
Dasabuvir
Dasabuvir had no effects on embryo-fetal viability or on fertility when evaluated in rats up to the highest dose of 800 mg per kg per day. Dasabuvir exposures at this dose were approximately 16-fold the exposure in humans at the recommended clinical dose.

Continued on next page

Information on the AbbVie, Inc. products listed on these pages is from the prescribing information in use as of July 31, 2016. For more information, please visit rxabbvie.com or call 1-800-633-9110.

Ombitasvir

Ombitasvir had no effects on embryo-fetal viability or on fertility when evaluated in mice up to the highest dose of 200 mg per kg per day. Ombitasvir exposures at this dose were approximately 25-fold the exposure in humans at the recommended clinical dose.

Paritaprevir, ritonavir

Paritaprevir, ritonavir had no effects on embryo-fetal viability or on fertility when evaluated in rats up to the highest dose of 300/30 mg per kg per day. Paritaprevir exposures at this dose were approximately 2- to 5-fold the exposure in humans at the recommended clinical dose.

If VIEKIRA XR is administered with ribavirin, refer to the prescribing information for ribavirin for information on Impairment of Fertility.

14   CLINICAL STUDIES
14.1   Description of Clinical Trials

Table 10 presents the clinical trial design including different treatment arms that were conducted with the components of VIEKIRA XR™ (dasabuvir, ombitasvir, paritaprevir, and ritonavir) with or without ribavirin in subjects with chronic hepatitis C (HCV) genotype 1 (GT1) infection. For detailed description of trial design and recommended regimen and duration *[see Dosage and Administration (2) and Clinical Studies (14)].*

[See table 10 on page 871]

The components of VIEKIRA XR with RBV were also evaluated in the following two studies:

• HCV GT1-infected liver transplant recipients (CORAL-I) *[see Clinical Studies (14.5)].*
• Subjects with HCV GT1 co-infected with HIV-1 (TURQUOISE-I) *[see Clinical Studies (14.6)].*

In all clinical trials, the ombitasvir, paritaprevir, ritonavir dose was 25/150/100 mg once daily and the dasabuvir dose was 250 mg twice daily and doses were not adjusted. For subjects who received RBV, the RBV dose was 1000 mg per day for subjects weighing less than 75 kg or 1200 mg per day for subjects weighing greater than or equal to 75 kg. RBV dose adjustments were performed according to the RBV labeling.

In all clinical trials, sustained virologic response was defined as HCV RNA below the lower limit of quantification (<LLOQ) 12 weeks after the end of treatment (SVR12). Plasma HCV RNA levels were measured using the COBAS TaqMan HCV test (version 2.0), for use with the High Pure System, which has an LLOQ of 25 IU per mL. Outcomes for subjects not achieving an SVR12 were recorded as on-treatment virologic failure (VF), post-treatment virologic relapse through post-treatment Week 12 or failure due to other non-virologic reasons (e.g., premature discontinuation, adverse event, lost to follow-up, consent withdrawn).

14.2   Clinical Trial Results in Adults with Chronic HCV Genotype 1a and 1b Infection without Cirrhosis

Subjects with Chronic HCV GT1a Infection without Cirrhosis

Subjects with HCV GT1a infection without cirrhosis treated with the components of VIEKIRA XR with RBV for 12 weeks in SAPPHIRE-I and -II and in PEARL-IV *[see Clinical Studies (14.1)]* had a median age of 53 years (range: 18 to 70); 63% of the subjects were male; 90% were White; 7% were Black/African American; 8% were Hispanic or Latino; 19% had a body mass index of at least 30 kg per m², 55% of patients were enrolled in US sites; 72% had IL28B (rs12979860) non-CC genotype; 85% had baseline HCV RNA levels of at least 800,000 IU per mL.

Table 11 presents treatment outcomes for HCV GT1a treatment-naïve and treatment-experienced subjects treated with the components of VIEKIRA XR with RBV for 12 weeks in SAPPHIRE-I, PEARL-IV and SAPPHIRE-II. Treatment-naïve, HCV GT1a-infected subjects without cirrhosis treated with the components of VIEKIRA XR with RBV for 12 weeks in PEARL-IV had a significantly higher SVR12 rate than subjects treated with the components of VIEKIRA XR without RBV (97% and 90% respectively; difference +7% with 95% confidence interval, +1% to +12%). The components of VIEKIRA XR without RBV were not studied in treatment-experienced subjects with GT1a infection.

In SAPPHIRE-I and SAPPHIRE-II, no placebo subject achieved a HCV RNA <25 IU/mL during treatment.

Table 8. Drug Interactions: Change in Pharmacokinetic Parameters for Co-administered Drug in the Presence of VIEKIRA XR

Co-administered Drug	Dose of Co-administered Drug (mg)	n	Ratio (with/without the Components of VIEKIRA XR) of Co-administered Drug Pharmacokinetic Parameters (90% CI); No Effect = 1.00		
			C_{max}	AUC	C_{min}
Alprazolam	0.5 single dose	12	1.09 (1.03, 1.15)	1.34 (1.15, 1.55)	NA
Amlodipine	5 single dose	14	1.26 (1.11, 1.44)	2.57 (2.31, 2.86)	NA
Atazanavir/ ritonavir[a]	Atazanavir 300 and ritonavir 100 once daily in the evening	12	1.02 (0.92, 1.13)[b]	1.19 (1.11, 1.28)[b]	1.68 (1.44, 1.95)[b]
Buprenorphine	Buprenorphine: 4 to 24 once daily and Naloxone 1 to 6 once daily	10	2.18 (1.78, 2.68)[c]	2.07 (1.78, 2.40)[c]	3.12 (2.29, 4.27)[c]
Norbuprenorphine			2.07 (1.42, 3.01)[c]	1.84 (1.30, 2.60)[c]	2.10 (1.49, 2.97)[c]
Naloxone			1.18 (0.81, 1.73)	1.28 (0.92, 1.79)[c]	NA
Carbamazepine	200 once daily followed by 200 twice daily	12	1.10 (1.07, 1.14)	1.17 (1.13, 1.22)	1.35 (1.27, 1.45)
Carbamazepine's metabolite, carbamazepine-10,11-epoxide (CBZE)			0.84 (0.82, 0.87)	0.75 (0.73, 0.77)	0.57 (0.54, 0.61)
Carisoprodol	250 single dose	14	0.54 (0.47, 0.63)	0.62 (0.55, 0.70)	NA
Carisoprodol's metabolite, mepobramate			1.17 (1.10, 1.25)	1.09 (1.03, 1.16)	NA
Cyclobenzaprine	5 single dose	14	0.68 (0.61, 0.75)	0.60 (0.53, 0.68)	NA
Cyclobenzaprine's metabolite, norcyclobenzaprine			1.03 (0.87, 1.23)	0.74 (0.64, 0.85)	NA
Cyclosporine	30 single dose[d]	10	1.01 (0.85, 1.20)[c]	5.82 (4.73, 7.14)[c]	15.80 (13.81, 18.09)[c]
Darunavir[e]	800 once daily	8	0.92 (0.87, 0.98)[b]	0.76 (0.71, 0.82)[b]	0.52 (0.47, 0.58)[b]
Darunavir/ ritonavir[f]	Darunavir 600 twice daily and ritonavir 100 once daily in the evening	7	0.87 (0.79, 0.96)[b]	0.80 (0.74, 0.86)[b]	0.57 (0.48, 0.67)[b]
Darunavir/ ritonavir[g]	Darunavir 800 and ritonavir 100 once daily in the evening	10	0.79 (0.70, 0.90)[b]	1.34 (1.25, 1.43)[b]	0.54 (0.48, 0.62)[b]
Diazepam	2 single dose	13	1.18 (1.07, 1.30)	0.78 (0.73, 0.82)	NA
Diazepam's metabolite, nordiazepam			1.10 (1.03, 1.19)	0.56 (0.45, 0.70)	NA

This table is continued on the next page

Table 8 (Cont.) Drug Interactions: Change in Pharmacokinetic Parameters for Co-administered Drug in the Presence of VIEKIRA XR

Co-administered Drug	Dose of Co-administered Drug (mg)	n	Ratio (with/without the Components of VIEKIRA XR) of Co-administered Drug Pharmacokinetic Parameters (90% CI); No Effect = 1.00		
			C_{max}	AUC m	C_{min}
Ethinyl Estradiol	Ethinyl estradiol 0.035 and Norgestimate 0.25 once daily	8	1.16 (0.90, 1.50)	1.06 (0.96, 1.17)	1.12 (0.94, 1.33)
Norelgestromin		9	2.01 (1.77, 2.29)	2.60 (2.30, 2.95)	3.11 (2.51, 3.85)
Norgestrel		9	2.26 (1.91, 2.67)	2.54 (2.09, 3.09)	2.93 (2.39, 3.57)
Furosemide	20 single dose	12	1.42 (1.17, 1.72)	1.08 (1.00, 1.17)	NA
Hydrocodone	5 single dose	15	1.27 (1.14, 1.40)	1.90 (1.72, 2.10)	NA
Ketoconazole	400 once daily	12	1.15 (1.09, 1.21)	2.17 (2.05, 2.29)	NA
Lopinavir/ ritonavir	400/100 twice daily	6	0.87 (0.76, 0.99)[b]	0.94 (0.81, 1.10)[b]	1.15 (0.93, 1.42)[b]
Lopinavir/ ritonavir[h]	800/200 once daily	12	0.86 (0.80, 0.93)[b]	0.94 (0.87, 1.01)[b]	3.18 (2.49, 4.06)[b]
Omeprazole	40 once daily	11	0.62 (0.48, 0.80)	0.62 (0.51, 0.75)	NA
Pravastatin	10 once daily	12	1.37 (1.11, 1.69)	1.82 (1.60, 2.08)	NA
Rilpivirine	25 once daily (morning)[i]	8	2.55 (2.08, 3.12)	3.25 (2.80, 3.77)	3.62 (3.12, 4.21)
Rosuvastatin	5 once daily	11	7.13 (5.11, 9.96)	2.59 (2.09, 3.21)	0.59 (0.51, 0.69)
Tacrolimus	2 single dose	12	3.99 (3.21, 4.97)[c]	57.13 (45.53, 71.69)[c]	16.56 (12.97, 21.16)[c]

a. Atazanavir plus 100 mg ritonavir administered in the evening, 12 hours after morning dose of the components of VIEKIRA XR.
b. Atazanavir or darunavir or lopinavir parameters are reported.
c. Dose normalized parameters reported.
d. 30 mg cyclosporine was administered with the components of VIEKIRA XR in the test arm and 100 mg cyclosporine was administered in the reference arm without the components of VIEKIRA XR.
e. Darunavir administered with the components of VIEKIRA XR in the morning was compared to darunavir administered with 100 mg ritonavir in the morning.
f. Darunavir administered with the components of VIEKIRA XR in the morning and with 100 mg ritonavir in the evening was compared to darunavir administered with 100 mg ritonavir in the morning and evening.
g. Darunavir plus 100 mg ritonavir administered in the evening, 12 hours after morning dose of the components of VIEKIRA XR compared to darunavir administered with 100 mg ritonavir in the evening.
h. Lopinavir/ritonavir administered in the evening, 12 hours after morning dose of the components of VIEKIRA XR.
i. Similar increases were observed when rilpivirine was dosed in the evening with food or 4 hours after food.
NA: not available/not applicable; CI: Confidence interval
Doses of dasabuvir were 250 mg or 400 mg (both doses showed similar exposures). Doses of ombitasvir, paritaprevir, and ritonavir were 25 mg, 150 mg and 100 mg.
Dasabuvir was dosed twice daily and ombitasvir, paritaprevir and ritonavir were dosed once daily in all the above studies except studies with ketoconazole and carbamazepine that used single doses.

Table 11. SVR12 for HCV Genotype 1a-Infected Subjects without Cirrhosis Who Were Treatment-Naïve or Previously Treated with PegIFN/RBV

	Components of VIEKIRA XR + RBV for 12 Weeks % (n/N)
GT1a treatment-naïve	
SAPPHIRE-I SVR12	96% (308/322)
Outcome for subjects without SVR12	
On-treatment VF	<1% (1/322)
Relapse	2% (6/314)
Other	2% (7/322)
PEARL-IV SVR12	97% (97/100)
Outcome for subjects without SVR12	
On-treatment VF	1% (1/100)
Relapse	1% (1/98)
Other	1% (1/100)
GT1a treatment-experienced	
SAPPHIRE-II SVR12	96% (166/173)
Outcome for subjects without SVR12	
On-treatment VF	0% (0/173)
Relapse	3% (5/172)
Other	1% (2/173)
SVR12 by Prior pegIFN Experience	
Null Responder	95% (83/87)
Partial Responder	100% (36/36)
Relapser	94% (47/50)

Subjects with Chronic HCV GT1b Infection without Cirrhosis
Subjects with HCV GT1b infection without cirrhosis were treated with the components of VIEKIRA XR with or without RBV for 12 weeks in PEARL-II and -III [see Clinical Studies (14.1)]. Subjects had a median age of 52 years (range: 22 to 70); 47% of the subjects were male; 93% were White; 5% were Black/African American; 2% were Hispanic or Latino; 21% had a body mass index of at least 30 kg per m², 21% of patients were enrolled in US sites; 83% had IL28B (rs12979860) non-CC genotype; 77% had baseline HCV RNA levels of at least 800,000 IU per mL.
The SVR rate for HCV GT1b-infected subjects without cirrhosis treated with the components of VIEKIRA XR without RBV for 12 weeks in PEARL-II (treatment-experienced: null responder, n=32; partial responder, n=26; relapser, n=33) and PEARL-III (treatment-naïve, n=209) was 100%.
14.3 Clinical Trial Results in Adults with Chronic HCV Genotype 1a and 1b Infection and Compensated Cirrhosis
The components of VIEKIRA XR with and without ribavirin were evaluated in two clinical trials in patients with compensated cirrhosis.
TURQUOISE-II was an open-label trial that enrolled 380 HCV GT1 subjects with cirrhosis and mild hepatic impairment (Child-Pugh A) who were either treatment-naïve or did not achieve SVR with prior treatment with pegIFN/

Continued on next page

Information on the AbbVie, Inc. products listed on these pages is from the prescribing information in use as of July 31, 2016. For more information, please visit rxabbvie.com or call 1-800-633-9110.

RBV. Subjects were randomized to receive the components of VIEKIRA XR with RBV for either 12 or 24 weeks of treatment.

Treated subjects had a median age of 58 years (range: 21 to 71); 70% of the subjects were male; 95% were White; 3% were Black/African American; 12% were Hispanic or Latino; 28% had a body mass index of at least 30 kg per m²; 43% of patients were enrolled in US sites; 82% had IL28B (rs12979860) non-CC genotype; 86% had baseline HCV RNA levels of at least 800,000 IU per mL; 69% had HCV GT1a infection, 31% had HCV GT1b infection; 42% were treatment-naïve, 36% were prior pegIFN/RBV null responders; 8% were prior pegIFN/RBV partial responders, 14% were prior pegIFN/RBV relapsers; 15% had platelet counts of less than 90×10^9 per L; 50% had albumin less than 4.0 mg per dL.

TURQUOISE-III was an open-label trial that enrolled 60 HCV GT1b-infected subjects with cirrhosis and mild hepatic impairment (Child-Pugh A) who were either treatment-naïve or did not achieve SVR with prior treatment with pegIFN/RBV. Subjects received the components of VIEKIRA XR without RBV for 12 weeks. Treated subjects had a median age of 61 years (range: 26 to 78); including 45% treatment-naïve and 55% pegIFN/RBV treatment-experienced; 25% were ≥65 years; 62% were male; 12% were Black; 5% were Hispanic or Latino; 28% had a body mass index of at least 30 kg per m²; 40% of patients were enrolled in US sites; 22% had platelet counts of less than 90×10^9 per L; 17% had albumin less than 35 g/L; 92% had baseline HCV RNA levels of at least 800,000 IU per mL; 83% had IL28B (rs12979860) non-CC genotype.

Table 12 presents treatment outcomes for GT1a- and GT1b-infected treatment-naïve and treatment-experienced subjects.

In GT1a infected subjects, the overall SVR12 rate difference between 24 and 12 weeks of treatment with the components of VIEKIRA XR with RBV was +6% with 95% confidence interval (-0.1% to +13% with differences varying by pretreatment history).

[See table 12 on next page]

14.4 Effect of Ribavirin Dose Reductions on SVR12

Seven percent of subjects (101/1551) treated with the components of VIEKIRA XR with RBV had a RBV dose adjustment due to a decrease in hemoglobin level; of these, 98% (98/100) achieved an SVR12.

14.5 Clinical Trial of Selected Liver Transplant Recipients (CORAL-I)

The components of VIEKIRA XR with RBV were administered for 24 weeks to 34 HCV GT1-infected liver transplant recipients who were at least 12 months post transplantation at enrollment with normal hepatic function and mild fibrosis (Metavir fibrosis score F2 or lower). The initial dose of RBV was left to the discretion of the investigator with 600 to 800 mg per day being the most frequently selected dose range at initiation of the components of VIEKIRA XR and at the end of treatment.

Of the 34 subjects (29 with HCV GT1a infection and 5 with HCV GT1b infection) enrolled, (97%) achieved SVR12 (97% in subjects with GT1a infection and 100% of subjects with GT1b infection). One subject with HCV GT1a infection relapsed post-treatment.

14.6 Clinical Trial in Subjects with HCV/HIV-1 Co-infection (TURQUOISE-I)

In an open-label clinical trial 63 subjects with HCV GT1 infection co-infected with HIV-1 were treated for 12 or 24 weeks with the components of VIEKIRA XR with RBV. Subjects were on a stable HIV-1 antiretroviral therapy (ART) regimen that included tenofovir disoproxil fumarate plus emtricitabine or lamivudine, administered with ritonavir boosted atazanavir or raltegravir. Subjects on atazanavir stopped the ritonavir component of their HIV-1 ART regimen upon initiating treatment with the components of VIEKIRA XR with RBV. Atazanavir was taken with the morning dose. The ritonavir component of the HIV-1 ART regimen was restarted after completion of treatment.

Treated subjects had a median age of 51 years (range: 31 to 69); 24% of subjects were black; 81% of subjects had IL28B (rs12979860) non-CC genotype; 19% of subjects had compensated cirrhosis; 67% of subjects were HCV treatment-naïve; 33% of subjects had failed prior treatment with pegIFN/RBV; 89% of subjects had HCV genotype 1a infection. The SVR12 rates were 91% (51/56) for subjects with HCV GT1a infection and 100% (7/7) for those with HCV GT1b infection. Of the 5 subjects who were non-responders, 1 experienced virologic breakthrough, 1 discontinued treatment, 1 experienced relapse and 2 subjects had evidence of HCV re-infection post-treatment.

Table 9. Treatment-Emergent Amino Acid Substitutions in the Pooled Analysis of the Components of VIEKIRA XR with and without Ribavirin Regimens (12- or 24-week durations) in Phase 2b and Phase 3 Clinical Trials

Target	Emergent Amino Acid Substitutions	Genotype 1a N = 58[a] % (n)	Genotype 1b N = 6 % (n)
NS3	Any of the following NS3 substitutions: V36A/M/T, F43L, V55I, Y56H, Q80L, I132V, R155K, A156G, D168(any), P334S, S342P, E357K, V406A/I, T449I, P470S, V23A (NS4A)	88 (51)	67 (4)
	V36A/M/T[b]	7 (4)	--
	V55I[b]	7 (4)	--
	Y56H[b]	10 (6)	50 (3)
	I132V[b]	7 (4)	--
	R155K	16 (9)	--
	D168 (any)[d]	72 (42)	67 (4)
	D168V	59 (34)	50 (3)
	P334S[b,c]	7 (4)	--
	E357K[b,c]	5 (3)	17 (1)
	V406A/I[b,c]	5 (3)	--
	T449I[b,c]	5 (3)	--
	P470S[b,c]	5 (3)	--
	NS4A V23A[b]	--	17 (1)
	F43L[b], Q80L[b], A156G, S342P[b,c]	<5%	
NS5A	Any of the following NS5A substitutions: K24R, M28A/T/V, Q30E/K/R, H/Q54Y, H58D/P/R, Y93C/H/N	78 (45)	33 (2)
	K24R	5 (3)	--
	M28A/T/V	33 (19)	--
	Q30E/K/R	47 (27)	--
	H/Q54Y	--	17 (1)
	H58D/P/R	7 (4)	--
	Y93C/N	5 (3)	--
	Y93H	--	33 (2)
NS5B	Any of the following NS5B substitutions: G307R, C316Y, M414I/T, E446K/Q, A450V, A553I/T/V, G554S, S556G/R, G558R, D559G/I/N/V, Y561H	67 (38)	33 (2)
	C316Y	4 (2)	17 (1)
	M414I	--	17 (1)
	M414T	5 (3)	17 (1)
	A553I/T/V	7 (4)	--
	S556G/R	39 (22)	17 (1)
	D559G/I/N/V	7 (4)	--
	Y561H	5 (3)	--
	G307R, E446K/Q, A450V, G554S, G558R	<5%	

a. N = 57 for the NS5B target.
b. Substitutions were observed in combination with other emergent substitutions at NS3 position R155 or D168.
c. Position located in NS3 helicase domain.
d. D168A/F/H/I/L/N/T/V/Y.

Table 10. Clinical Trials Conducted with the Components of VIEKIRA XR With or Without Ribavirin (RBV) in Subjects with Chronic HCV GT1 Infection

Trial	Population	Study Arms and Duration (Number of Subjects Treated)
SAPPHIRE-I (double-blind)	GT1 (a and b) TN[a] without cirrhosis	• Components of VIEKIRA XR + RBV for 12 weeks (473) • Placebo for 12 weeks (158)
SAPPHIRE-II (double-blind)	GT1 (a and b) TE[b] without cirrhosis	• Components of VIEKIRA XR + RBV for 12 weeks (297) • Placebo for 12 weeks (97)
PEARL-II (open-label)	GT1b TE without cirrhosis	• Components of VIEKIRA XR + RBV for 12 weeks (88) • Components of VIEKIRA XR for 12 weeks (91)
PEARL-III (double-blind)	GT1b TN without cirrhosis	• Components of VIEKIRA XR + RBV for 12 weeks (210) • Components of VIEKIRA XR for 12 weeks (209)
PEARL-IV (double-blind)	GT1a TN without cirrhosis	• Components of VIEKIRA XR + RBV for 12 weeks (100) • Components of VIEKIRA XR for 12 weeks (205)
TURQUOISE-II (open-label)	GT1 (a and b) TN & TE with compensated cirrhosis	• Components of VIEKIRA XR + RBV for 12 weeks (208) • Components of VIEKIRA XR + RBV for 24 weeks (172)
TURQUOISE-III (open-label)	GT1b TN & TE with compensated cirrhosis	• Components of VIEKIRA XR for 12 weeks (60)

a. TN, treatment-naïve was defined as not having received any prior therapy for HCV infection.
b. TE, treatment-experienced subjects were defined as having failed to respond to prior treatment with pegIFN/RBV.

Table 12. TURQUOISE-II: SVR12 for Chronic HCV Genotype 1-Infected Subjects with Cirrhosis Who Were Treatment-Naïve or Previously Treated with pegIFN/RBV

	GT1a (TURQUOISE-II)		GT1b (TURQUOISE-III)
	Components of VIEKIRA XR + RBV for 24 Weeks % (n/N)	Components of VIEKIRA XR + RBV for 12 Weeks % (n/N)	Components of VIEKIRA XR without RBV for 12 Weeks % (n/N)
SVR12	95% (115/121)	89% (124/140)	100% (60/60)
Outcome for subjects without SVR12			
On-treatment VF	2% (3/121)	<1% (1/140)	0
Relapse	1% (1/116)	8% (11/135)	0
Other	2% (2/121)	3% (4/140)	0
SVR12 for Naïve	95% (53/56)	92% (59/64)	100% (27/27)
SVR12 by Prior pegIFN Experience			100% (33/33)
Null Responder	93% (39/42)	80% (40/50)	100% (7/7)
Partial Responder	100% (10/10)	100% (11/11)	100% (5/5)
Relapser	100% (13/13)	93% (14/15)	100% (3/3)

One subject had confirmed HIV-1 RNA >400 copies/mL during the post-treatment period. This subject had no evidence of resistance to the ART regimen. No subjects switched their ART regimen due to loss of plasma HIV-1 RNA suppression.

14.7 Durability of Response

In an open-label clinical trial, 92% of subjects (526/571) who received various combinations of the direct acting antivirals included in VIEKIRA XR with or without RBV achieved SVR12, and 99% of those who achieved SVR12 maintained their response through 48 weeks post-treatment (SVR48).

16 HOW SUPPLIED/STORAGE AND HANDLING

VIEKIRA XR is dispensed in a monthly carton for a total of 28 days of therapy. Each monthly carton contains four weekly cartons. Each weekly carton contains seven daily dose packs.

Each child-resistant daily dose pack contains three tablets. The NDC number is 0074-0063-28.

Dasabuvir, ombitasvir, paritaprevir, and ritonavir 200 mg/8.33 mg/50 mg/33.33 mg tablets are pale yellow-colored, film-coated, oblong shaped, debossed with "3QD" on one side.

Store at or below 30°C (86°F).

17 PATIENT COUNSELING INFORMATION

Advise the patient to read the FDA-approved patient labeling (Medication Guide).

Inform patients to review the Medication Guide for ribavirin [see Warnings and Precautions (5.3)].

Risk of ALT Elevations or Hepatic Decompensation and Failure

Inform patients to watch for early warning signs of liver inflammation or failure, such as fatigue, weakness, lack of appetite, nausea and vomiting, as well as later signs such as jaundice, onset of confusion, abdominal swelling, and discolored feces, and to consult their health care professional without delay if such symptoms occur [see Warnings and Precautions (5.1 and 5.2) and Adverse Reactions (6)].

Pregnancy

Advise patients taking VIEKIRA XR with ribavirin to avoid pregnancy during treatment and within 6 months of stopping ribavirin. Inform patients to notify their health care provider immediately in the event of a pregnancy [see Use in Specific Populations (8.1)].

Drug Interactions

Inform patients that VIEKIRA XR may interact with some drugs; therefore, patients should be advised to report to their healthcare provider the use of any prescription, nonprescription medication or herbal products [see Contraindications (4), Warnings and Precautions (5.4) and Drug Interactions (7)].

Inform patients that contraceptives containing ethinyl estradiol are contraindicated with VIEKIRA XR [see Contraindications (4) and Warnings and Precautions (5.2)].

Administration

Advise patients to take VIEKIRA XR every day at the regularly scheduled time and that VIEKIRA XR must be taken with a meal because taking it under fasting conditions may result in reduced virologic response and possible development of resistance. Inform patients to swallow tablets whole and not to consume alcohol within 4 hours of taking VIEKIRA XR [see Dosage and Administration (2.2)].

Inform patients that it is important not to miss or skip doses and to take VIEKIRA XR for the duration that is recommended by the healthcare provider.

Manufactured by AbbVie Inc., North Chicago, IL 60064.

VIEKIRA XR and NORVIR are trademarks of AbbVie Inc. All other brands listed are trademarks of their respective owners and are not trademarks of AbbVie Inc. The makers of these brands are not affiliated with and do not endorse AbbVie Inc. or its products.

© 2016 AbbVie Inc. All rights reserved.

03-B193

Continued on next page

MEDICATION GUIDE
VIEKIRA XR™ (vee-KEE-rah-XR)
(dasabuvir, ombitasvir, paritaprevir, and ritonavir)
extended-release tablets
for oral use

Important: When taking VIEKIRA XR in combination with ribavirin, you should also read the Medication Guide that comes with ribavirin.

What is the most important information I should know about VIEKIRA XR?

VIEKIRA XR may cause severe liver problems, especially in people with certain types of cirrhosis. These severe liver problems can lead to the need for a liver transplant, or can lead to death.

VIEKIRA XR can cause increases in your liver function blood test results, especially if you use ethinyl estradiol-containing medicines (such as some birth control products).

- You must stop using ethinyl estradiol-containing medicines before you start treatment with VIEKIRA XR. See the section **"Who should not take VIEKIRA XR?"** for a list of these medicines.
- If you use these medicines as a method of birth control, you must use another method of birth control during treatment with VIEKIRA XR, and for about **2** weeks after you finish treatment with VIEKIRA XR. Your healthcare provider will tell you when you may begin taking ethinyl estradiol-containing medicines.
- Your healthcare provider should do blood tests to check your liver function during the first 4 weeks and then as needed, during treatment with VIEKIRA XR.
- Your healthcare provider may tell you to stop taking VIEKIRA XR if you develop signs or symptoms of liver problems.
- Tell your healthcare provider right away if you develop any of the following symptoms, or if they worsen during treatment with VIEKIRA XR:
  - tiredness
  - weakness
  - loss of appetite
  - nausea and vomiting
  - yellowing of your skin or eyes
  - color changes in your stools
  - confusion
  - swelling of the stomach area

What is VIEKIRA XR?

- VIEKIRA XR is a prescription medicine used with or without ribavirin to treat people with genotype 1 chronic (lasting a long time) hepatitis C virus (HCV) infection.
- VIEKIRA XR can be used in people who have compensated cirrhosis.
- VIEKIRA XR is not for people with advanced cirrhosis (decompensated). If you have cirrhosis, talk to your healthcare provider before taking VIEKIRA XR. VIEKIRA XR is not for people with certain types of liver problems.

It is not known if VIEKIRA XR is safe and effective in children under 18 years of age.

Who should not take VIEKIRA XR?
Do not take VIEKIRA XR if you:
- **have certain liver problems**
- **take any of the following medicines:**
  - alfuzosin hydrochloride (Uroxatral®)
  - carbamazepine (Carbatrol®, Epitol®, Equetro®, Tegretol®, TEGRETOL-XR®, TERIL®)
  - cisapride (Propulsid®)
  - colchicine (Colcrys®) in patients who have certain kidney or liver problems
  - dronedarone (Multaq®)
  - efavirenz (Atripla®, Sustiva®)
  - ergot containing medicines including:
    - ergotamine tartrate (Cafergot®, Ergomar®, Ergostat®, Medihaler®, Migergot®, Wigraine®, Wigrettes®)
    - dihydroergotamine mesylate (D.H.E. 45®, Migranal®)
    - methylergonovine (Ergotrate®, Methergine®)
  - ethinyl estradiol-containing medicines:
    - combination birth control pills or patches, such as Lo Loestrin® FE, Norinyl®, Ortho Tri-Cyclen Lo®, Ortho Evra®
    - hormonal vaginal rings such as NuvaRing®
    - the hormone replacement therapy medicine, Fem HRT®

- gemfibrozil (Lopid®)
- lovastatin (Advicor®, Altoprev®, Mevacor®)
- lurasidone (Latuda®)
- midazolam, when taken by mouth
- phenytoin (Dilantin®, Phenytek®)
- phenobarbital (Luminal®)
- pimozide (Orap®)
- ranolazine (Ranexa®)
- rifampin (Rifadin®, Rifamate®, Rifater®, Rimactane)
- sildenafil citrate (Revatio®), when taking for pulmonary artery hypertension (PAH)
- simvastatin (Simcor®, Vytorin®, Zocor®)
- St. John's wort (Hypericum perforatum) or a product that contains St. John's wort
- Triazolam (Halcion®)
- **have had a severe skin rash after taking ritonavir (Norvir®)**

What should I tell my healthcare provider before taking VIEKIRA XR?
Before taking VIEKIRA XR tell your healthcare provider about all your medical conditions, including if you:
- have liver problems other than hepatitis C infection. See **"Who should not take VIEKIRA XR?"**
- have HIV infection
- have had a liver transplant. If you take the medicines tacrolimus (Prograf®) or cyclosporine (Gengraf®, Neoral®, Sandimmune®) to help prevent rejection of your transplanted liver, the amount of these medicines in your blood may increase during treatment with VIEKIRA XR.
  - Your healthcare provider should check the level of tacrolimus or cyclosporine in your blood, and if needed may change your dose of these medicines or how often you take them.
  - When you finish taking VIEKIRA XR or if you have to stop VIEKIRA XR for any reason, your healthcare provider should tell you what dose of tacrolimus or cyclosporine to take and how often you should take it.
- are pregnant or plan to become pregnant. It is not known if VIEKIRA XR will harm your unborn baby. **When taking VIEKIRA XR in combination with ribavirin you should also read the ribavirin Medication Guide for important pregnancy information.**
- are breastfeeding or plan to breastfeed. It is not known if VIEKIRA XR passes into your breast milk. Talk to your healthcare provider about the best way to feed your baby if you take VIEKIRA XR.

Tell your healthcare provider about all the medicines you take, including prescription and over-the-counter medicines, vitamins, and herbal supplements. Some medicines interact with VIEKIRA XR. **Keep a list of your medicines to show your healthcare provider and pharmacist.**
- You can ask your healthcare provider or pharmacist for a list of medicines that interact with VIEKIRA XR.
- **Do not start taking a new medicine without telling your healthcare provider.** Your healthcare provider can tell you if it is safe to take VIEKIRA XR with other medicines.
- When you finish treatment with VIEKIRA XR:
  - If your healthcare provider changed the dose of one of your usual medicines during treatment with VIEKIRA XR: Ask your healthcare provider about when you should change back to your original dose after you finish treatment with VIEKIRA XR.
  - If your healthcare provider told you to stop taking one of your usual medicines during treatment with VIEKIRA XR: Ask your healthcare provider if you should start taking these medicines again after you finished treatment with VIEKIRA XR.

How should I take VIEKIRA XR?
- Take VIEKIRA XR™ (dasabuvir, ombitasvir, paritaprevir, and ritonavir) exactly as your healthcare provider tells you to take it. Do not change your dose.
- Do not stop taking VIEKIRA XR without first talking with your healthcare provider.
- Take VIEKIRA XR tablets one time each day.
- **VIEKIRA XR tablets must be taken with a meal.**
- Swallow VIEKIRA XR tablets whole. Do not split, crush, or chew the tablets.
- Do not drink alcohol within 4 hours of taking VIEKIRA XR.
- VIEKIRA XR comes in **monthly cartons that contain enough medicine for 28 days.**
  - Each monthly carton of VIEKIRA XR contains **4 smaller cartons.**
  - Each of the 4 smaller cartons contains enough child resistant **daily dose packs** of medicine to last for **7 days (1 week).**

- Each **daily dose pack** contains all of your VIEKIRA XR medicine for **1 day** (3 tablets). Follow the instructions on each daily dose pack about how to remove the tablets.
- It is important that you do not miss or skip doses of VIEKIRA XR during treatment.
- If you take too much VIEKIRA XR, call your healthcare provider or go to the nearest hospital emergency room right away.

What are the possible side effects of VIEKIRA XR?
VIEKIRA XR can cause serious side effects. See "What is the most important information I should know about VIEKIRA XR?"

Common side effects of VIEKIRA XR when used with ribavirin include:

- tiredness
- nausea
- itching
- skin reactions such as redness or rash
- sleep problems
- feeling weak

Common side effects of VIEKIRA XR when used without ribavirin include:
- nausea
- itching
- sleep problems

These are not all the possible side effects of VIEKIRA XR. Call your doctor for medical advice about side effects. You may report side effects to FDA at 1-800-FDA-1088.

How should I store VIEKIRA XR?
- Store VIEKIRA XR at or below 86°F (30°C).

Keep VIEKIRA XR and all medicines out of the reach of children.

General information about the safe and effective use of VIEKIRA XR

Medicines are sometimes prescribed for purposes other than those listed in a Medication Guide. Do not use VIEKIRA XR for a condition for which it was not prescribed. Do not give VIEKIRA XR to other people, even if they have the same symptoms that you have. It may harm them. You can ask your pharmacist or healthcare provider for information about VIEKIRA XR that is written for health professionals.

What are the ingredients in VIEKIRA XR?
Active ingredients: dasabuvir, ombitasvir, paritaprevir, and ritonavir
Inactive ingredients:
- The extended release layer contains: copovidone, K value 28, hypromellose 2208, 17,700 (mPa*s), colloidal silicon dioxide/colloidal anhydrous silica, and magnesium stearate.
- The immediate release layer contains: copovidone, K value 28, vitamin E polyethylene glycol succinate, propylene glycol monolaurate, sorbitan monolaurate, colloidal silicon dioxide/colloidal anhydrous silica.
- The tablet coating contains: hypromellose (6 mPa*s), hypromellose (15 mPa*s), polyethylene glycol 400, hydroxypropyl cellulose, polysorbate 80, polyethylene glycol 3350/macrogol 4000, talc, titanium dioxide, colloidal silicon dioxide/colloidal anhydrous silica and iron oxide yellow.

Manufactured by AbbVie Inc., North Chicago, IL 60064. VIEKIRA XR and NORVIR are trademarks of AbbVie Inc. All other brands listed are trademarks of their respective owners and are not trademarks of AbbVie Inc. The makers of these brands are not affiliated with and do not endorse AbbVie Inc. or its products.

For more information go to www.viekira.com or call 1-844-843-5472.

This Medication Guide has been approved by the U.S. Food and Drug Administration.   Issued: July 2016

03-B193

Shown in Product Identification Guide, page 507

ZEMPLAR® ℞
[zĕm-plər]
(paricalcitol) capsules

HIGHLIGHTS OF PRESCRIBING INFORMATION
**These highlights do not include all the information needed to use ZEMPLAR safely and effectively.
See full prescribing information for ZEMPLAR.
ZEMPLAR (paricalcitol) capsules
Initial U.S. Approval: 1998**

───────INDICATIONS AND USAGE───────
Zemplar is a vitamin D analog indicated for the prevention and treatment of secondary hyperparathyroidism associated with

• Chronic kidney disease (CKD) Stages 3 and 4 (1.1).
• CKD Stage 5 in patients on hemodialysis (HD) or peritoneal dialysis (PD) (1.2).

───────DOSAGE AND ADMINISTRATION───────
• CKD Stages 3 and 4: Zemplar Capsules may be administered once daily or every other day, three times a week (2.1).
• CKD Stage 5: Zemplar Capsules are dosed every other day, three times a week (2.2). To minimize the risk of hypercalcemia patients should be treated only after their baseline serum calcium has been reduced to 9.5 mg/dL or lower.
[See first table above]
[See second table above]

───────DOSAGE FORMS AND STRENGTHS───────
Capsules: 1 mcg and 2 mcg (3).

───────CONTRAINDICATIONS───────
Evidence of hypercalcemia or vitamin D toxicity (4).

───────WARNINGS AND PRECAUTIONS───────
• Hypercalcemia: Excessive administration of Zemplar Capsules can cause over suppression of PTH, hypercalcemia, hypercalciuria, hyperphosphatemia, and adynamic bone disease. Prescription-based doses of vitamin D and its derivatives should be withheld during Zemplar treatment (5.1).
• Digitalis toxicity: Potentiated by hypercalcemia of any cause. Use caution when Zemplar Capsules are prescribed concomitantly with digitalis compounds (5.2).
• Laboratory tests: Monitor serum calcium, serum phosphorus, and serum or plasma iPTH during initial dosing or following any dose adjustment. Zemplar Capsules may increase serum creatinine and therefore decrease the estimated GFR (eGFR) (5.3).
• Aluminum overload and toxicity: Avoid excessive use of aluminum containing compounds (5.4).

───────ADVERSE REACTIONS───────
The most common adverse reactions (> 5% and more frequent than placebo) include diarrhea, hypertension, dizziness and vomiting.

To report SUSPECTED ADVERSE REACTIONS, contact AbbVie Inc. at 1-800-633-9110 or FDA at 1-800-FDA-1088 or www.fda.gov/medwatch

───────DRUG INTERACTIONS───────
• Strong CYP3A inhibitors (e.g. ketoconazole) will increase the exposure of paricalcitol. Use with caution (7.1).
• Cholestyramine, Mineral Oil: Intestinal absorption of Zemplar may be reduced if administered simultaneously with mineral oil or cholestyramine (7.2,7.3).
See 17 for PATIENT COUNSELING INFORMATION.
Revised: 10/2015

FULL PRESCRIBING INFORMATION

1   INDICATIONS AND USAGE
1.1   Chronic Kidney Disease Stages 3 and 4
Zemplar Capsules are indicated for the prevention and treatment of secondary hyperparathyroidism associated with Chronic Kidney Disease (CKD) Stages 3 and 4.
1.2   Chronic Kidney Disease Stage 5
Zemplar Capsules are indicated for the prevention and treatment of secondary hyperparathyroidism associated with CKD Stage 5 in patients on hemodialysis (HD) or peritoneal dialysis (PD).

2   DOSAGE AND ADMINISTRATION
2.1   Chronic Kidney Disease Stages 3 and 4
Zemplar Capsules may be administered daily or three times a week. When dosing three times weekly, the dose should be administered not more frequently than every other day. The total weekly doses for both daily and three times a week dosage regimens are similar [see *Clinical Studies (14.1)*].
Zemplar Capsules may be taken without regard to food. No dosing adjustment is required in patients with mild and moderate hepatic impairment.
Initial Dose

Initial Dosage

	CKD Stages 3, 4		CKD Stage 5
Baseline intact parathyroid (iPTH) Level	Starting Dose		Dose in micrograms is based on baseline iPTH level (pg/mL)/80. Dose three times a week (e.g. every other day).
≤ 500 pg/mL	1 mcg daily or 2 mcg three times a week (e.g. every other day)		
> 500 pg/mL	2 mcg daily or 4 mcg three times a week (e.g. every other day)		

Dose Titration

	CKD Stages 3, 4		CKD Stage 5
iPTH Level Relative to Baseline	Dosing Recommendation		Dose in micrograms is based on most recent iPTH level (pg/mL)/80 with adjustments based on serum calcium and phosphorous levels. Dose three times a week (e.g. every other day).
Decreased by < 30%	Increase dose by 1 mcg daily or 2 mcg three times a week (e.g. every other day)		
Decreased by ≥ 30% and ≤ 60%	Maintain dose		
Decreased by > 60% or iPTH < 60 pg/mL	Decrease dose by 1 mcg daily or 2 mcg three times a week (e.g. every other day)		

The initial dose of Zemplar Capsules for CKD Stages 3 and 4 patients is based on baseline intact parathyroid hormone (iPTH) levels.

Baseline iPTH Level	Daily Dose	Three Times a Week Dose*
≤ 500 pg/mL	1 mcg	2 mcg
> 500 pg/mL	2 mcg	4 mcg

* To be administered not more often than every other day

Dose Titration
Dosing must be individualized and based on serum or plasma iPTH levels, with monitoring of serum calcium and serum phosphorus. The following is a suggested approach to dose titration.

iPTH Level Relative to Baseline	Zemplar Capsule Dose	Dose Adjustment at 2 to 4 Week Intervals	
		Daily Dosage	Three Times a Week Dosage*
The same, increased or decreased by < 30%	Increase dose by	1 mcg	2 mcg
Decreased by ≥ 30% and ≤ 60%	Maintain dose	-	-
Decreased by > 60% or iPTH < 60 pg/mL	Decrease dose by	1 mcg	2 mcg

* To be administered not more often than every other day

Continued on next page

Information on the AbbVie, Inc. products listed on these pages is from the prescribing information in use as of July 31, 2016. For more information, please visit rxabbvie.com or call 1-800-633-9110.

If a patient is taking the lowest dose, 1 mcg, on the daily regimen and a dose reduction is needed, the dose can be decreased to 1 mcg three times a week. If a further dose reduction is required, the drug should be withheld as needed and restarted at a lower dosing frequency. If a patient is on a calcium-based phosphate binder, the phosphate-binder dose may be decreased or withheld, or the patient may be switched to a non-calcium-based phosphate binder. If hypercalcemia is observed, the dose of Zemplar should be reduced or withheld until these parameters are normalized.

Serum calcium and phosphorus levels should be closely monitored after initiation of Zemplar Capsules, during dose titration periods and during co-administration with strong CYP3A inhibitors [see *Warnings and Precautions (5.3)*, *Drug Interactions (7)* and *Clinical Pharmacology (12.3)*].

2.2　Chronic Kidney Disease Stage 5
Zemplar Capsules are to be administered three times a week, not more frequently than every other day.

Zemplar Capsules may be taken without regard to food. No dosing adjustment is required in patients with mild and moderate hepatic impairment.

Initial Dose
The initial dose of Zemplar Capsules in micrograms is based on a baseline iPTH level (pg/mL)/80. To minimize the risk of hypercalcemia patients should be treated only after their baseline serum calcium has been adjusted to 9.5 mg/dL or lower [see *Clinical Pharmacology (12.2)* and *Clinical Studies (14.2)*].

Dose Titration
Subsequent dosing should be individualized and based on iPTH, serum calcium and phosphorus levels. A suggested dose titration of Zemplar Capsules is based on the following formula:

Titration dose (micrograms) = most recent iPTH level (pg/ml)/80

Serum calcium and phosphorus levels should be closely monitored after initiation, during dose titration periods, and with co-administration of strong P450 3A inhibitors. If an elevated serum calcium is observed and the patient is on a calcium-based phosphate binder, the binder dose may be decreased or withheld, or the patient may be switched to a non-calcium-based phosphate binder. If serum calcium is elevated, the dose should be decreased by 2 to 4 micrograms lower than that calculated by the most recent iPTH/80. If further adjustment is required, the dose of paricalcitol capsules should be reduced or withheld until these parameters are normalized.

As iPTH approaches the target range, small, individualized dose adjustments may be necessary in order to achieve a stable iPTH. In situations where monitoring of iPTH, Ca or P occurs less frequently than once per week, a more modest initial and dose titration ratio (e.g., iPTH/100) may be warranted.

3　DOSAGE FORMS AND STRENGTHS
Zemplar Capsules are available as 1 mcg and 2 mcg soft gelatin capsules.
• 1 mcg:　oval, gray capsule imprinted with the "a" logo and "ZA"
• 2 mcg:　oval, orange-brown capsule imprinted with the "a" logo and "ZF"

4　CONTRAINDICATIONS
Zemplar Capsules should not be given to patients with evidence of
• hypercalcemia or
• vitamin D toxicity [see *Warnings and Precautions (5.1)*].

5　WARNINGS AND PRECAUTIONS
Excessive administration of vitamin D compounds, including Zemplar Capsules, can cause over suppression of PTH, hypercalcemia, hypercalciuria, hyperphosphatemia, and adynamic bone disease.

5.1　Hypercalcemia
Progressive hypercalcemia due to overdosage of vitamin D and its metabolites may be so severe as to require emergency attention [see *Overdosage (10)*]. Acute hypercalcemia may exacerbate tendencies for cardiac arrhythmias and seizures and may potentiate the action of digitalis. Chronic hypercalcemia can lead to generalized vascular calcification and other soft-tissue calcification. Concomitant administration of high doses of calcium-containing preparations or thiazide diuretics with Zemplar may increase the risk of hypercalcemia. High intake of calcium and phosphate concomitant with vitamin D compounds may lead to serum abnormalities requiring more frequent patient monitoring and individualized dose titration. Patients also should be in-

formed about the symptoms of elevated calcium, which include feeling tired, difficulty thinking clearly, loss of appetite, nausea, vomiting, constipation, increased thirst, increased urination and weight loss.

Prescription-based doses of vitamin D and its derivatives should be withheld during Zemplar treatment to avoid hypercalcemia.

5.2　Digitalis Toxicity
Digitalis toxicity is potentiated by hypercalcemia of any cause. Use caution when Zemplar Capsules are prescribed concomitantly with digitalis compounds.

5.3　Laboratory Tests
During the initial dosing or following any dose adjustment of medication, serum calcium, serum phosphorus, and serum or plasma iPTH should be monitored at least every two weeks for 3 months, then monthly for 3 months, and every 3 months thereafter.

In pre-dialysis patients, Zemplar Capsules may increase serum creatinine and therefore decrease the estimated GFR (eGFR). Similar effects have also been seen with calcitriol.

5.4　Aluminum Overload and Toxicity
Aluminum-containing preparations (e.g., antacids, phosphate binders) should not be administered chronically with Zemplar, as increased blood levels of aluminum and aluminum bone toxicity may occur.

6　ADVERSE REACTIONS
Because clinical studies are conducted under widely varying conditions, adverse reaction rates observed in the clinical studies of a drug cannot be directly compared to rates in the clinical studies of another drug and may not reflect the rates observed in practice.

6.1　Clinical Trials Experience
CKD Stages 3 and 4
The safety of Zemplar Capsules has been evaluated in three 24-week (approximately six-month), double-blind, placebo-controlled, multicenter clinical studies involving 220 CKD Stages 3 and 4 patients. Six percent (6%) of Zemplar Capsules treated patients and 4% of placebo treated patients discontinued from clinical studies due to an adverse event. Adverse events occurring in the Zemplar Capsules group at a frequency of 2% or greater and more frequently than in the placebo group are presented in Table 1:

Table 1. Treatment-Emergent Adverse Events by Body System Occurring in ≥ 2% of Subjects in the Zemplar-Treated Group of Three, Double-Blind, Placebo-Controlled, Phase 3, CKD Stages 3 and 4 Studies; All Treated Patients

Adverse Event[a]	Number (%) of Subjects			
	Zemplar Capsules (n = 107)		Placebo (n = 113)	
Overall	88	(82%)	86	(76%)
Ear and Labyrinth Disorders				
Vertigo	5	(4.7%)	0	(0.0%)
Gastrointestinal Disorders				
Abdominal Discomfort	4	(3.7%)	1	(0.9%)
Constipation	4	(3.7%)	4	(3.5%)
Diarrhea	7	(6.5%)	5	(4.4%)
Nausea	6	(5.6%)	4	(3.5%)
Vomiting	5	(4.7%)	5	(4.4%)
General Disorders and Administration Site Conditions				
Chest Pain	3	(2.8%)	1	(0.9%)
Edema	6	(5.6%)	5	(4.4%)
Pain	4	(3.7%)	4	(3.5%)
Immune System Disorders				
Hypersensitivity	6	(5.6%)	2	(1.8%)
Infections and Infestations				
Fungal Infection	3	(2.8%)	0	(0.0%)
Gastroenteritis	3	(2.8%)	3	(2.7%)
Infection	3	(2.8%)	3	(2.7%)
Sinusitis	3	(2.8%)	1	(0.9%)
Urinary Tract Infection	3	(2.8%)	1	(0.9%)
Viral Infection	8	(7.5%)	8	(7.1%)
Metabolism and Nutrition Disorders				
Dehydration	3	(2.8%)	1	(0.9%)
Musculoskeletal and Connective Tissue Disorders				
Arthritis	5	(4.7%)	0	(0.0%)
Back Pain	3	(2.8%)	1	(0.9%)
Muscle Spasms	3	(2.8%)	0	(0.0%)
Nervous System Disorders				
Dizziness	5	(4.7%)	5	(4.4%)
Headache	5	(4.7%)	5	(4.4%)
Syncope	3	(2.8%)	1	(0.9%)
Psychiatric Disorders				
Depression	3	(2.8%)	0	(0.0%)
Respiratory, Thoracic and Mediastinal Disorders				
Cough	3	(2.8%)	2	(1.8%)
Oropharyngeal Pain	4	(3.7%)	0	(0.0%)
Skin and Subcutaneous Tissue Disorders				
Pruritus	3	(2.8%)	3	(2.7%)
Rash	4	(3.7%)	1	(0.9%)
Skin Ulcer	3	(2.8%)	0	(0.0%)
Vascular Disorders				
Hypertension	7	(6.5%)	4	(3.5%)
Hypotension	5	(4.7%)	3	(2.7%)

a. Includes only events more common in the Zemplar treatment group.

The following adverse reactions, with a causal relationship to Zemplar, occurred in <2% of the Zemplar treated patients in the above double-blind, placebo-controlled clinical trial data set.
Gastrointestinal Disorders:　Dry mouth
Investigations:　Hepatic enzyme abnormal
Nervous System Disorders:　Dysgeusia
Skin and Subcutaneous Tissue Disorders:　Urticaria
CKD Stage 5
The safety of Zemplar Capsules has been evaluated in one 12-week, double-blind, placebo-controlled, multicenter clinical study involving 88 CKD Stage 5 patients. Sixty-one patients received Zemplar Capsules and 27 patients received placebo.

The proportion of patients who terminated prematurely from the study due to adverse events was 7% for Zemplar Capsules treated patients and 7% for placebo patients.

Adverse events occurring in the Zemplar Capsules group at a frequency of 2% or greater and more frequently than in the placebo group are as follows:

Table 2. Treatment-Emergent Adverse Events by Body System Occurring in ≥ 2% of Subjects in the Zemplar-Treated Group, Double-Blind, Placebo-Controlled, Phase 3, CKD Stage 5 Study; All Treated Patients

Adverse Events[a]	Number (%) of Subjects			
	Zemplar Capsules (n=61)		Placebo (n = 27)	
Overall	43	(70%)	19	(70%)
Gastrointestinal Disorders				
Constipation	3	(4.9%)	0	(0.0%)
Diarrhea	7	(11.5%)	3	(11.1%)
Vomiting	4	(6.6%)	0	(0.0%)
General Disorders and Administration Site Conditions				
Fatigue	2	(3.3%)	0	(0.0%)
Edema Peripheral	2	(3.3%)	0	(0.0%)
Infections and Infestations				
Nasopharyngitis	5	(8.2%)	2	(7.4%)
Peritonitis	3	(4.9%)	0	(0.0%)
Sinusitis	2	(3.3%)	0	(0.0%)
Urinary Tract Infection	2	(3.3%)	0	(0.0%)
Metabolism and Nutrition Disorders				
Fluid Overload	3	(4.9%)	0	(0.0%)
Hypoglycemia	2	(3.3%)	0	(0.0%)
Nervous System Disorders				
Dizziness	4	(6.6%)	0	(0.0%)
Headache	2	(3.3%)	0	(0.0%)
Psychiatric Disorders				
Anxiety	2	(3.3%)	0	(0.0%)
Insomnia	3	(4.9%)	0	(0.0%)
Renal and Urinary Disorders				
Renal Failure Chronic	2	(3.3%)	0	(0.0%)

a. Includes only events more common in the Zemplar treatment group.

The following adverse reactions, with a causal relationship to Zemplar, occurred in <2% of the Zemplar treated patients in the above double-blind, placebo-controlled clinical trial data set.

Gastrointestinal Disorders: Gastroesophageal reflux disease

Metabolism and Nutrition Disorders: Decreased appetite, hypercalcemia, hypocalcemia

Reproductive System and Breast Disorders: Breast tenderness

Skin and Subcutaneous Tissue Disorders: Acne

6.2 Postmarketing Experience

The following additional adverse reactions have been reported during post-approval use and post-approval clinical trials with the active ingredient in Zemplar capsules:

Immune System Disorders: Angioedema (including laryngeal edema)

Metabolism and Nutrition Disorders: Hypercalcemia
Investigations: Blood creatinine increased

7 DRUG INTERACTIONS
7.1 CYP3A Inhibitors

Since paricalcitol is partially metabolized by CYP3A, exposure of paricalcitol will be increased while paricalcitol is co-administered with strong CYP3A inhibitors including the following drugs but not limited to: ketoconazole, atazanavir, clarithromycin, indinavir, itraconazole, nefazodone, nelfinavir, ritonavir, saquinavir, telithromycin or voriconazole. Dose adjustment of Zemplar Capsules may be required, and iPTH and serum calcium concentrations should be closely monitored if a patient initiates or discontinues therapy with a strong CYP3A4 inhibitor [see *Clinical Pharmacology (12.3)*].

7.2 Cholestyramine

Drugs that impair intestinal absorption of fat-soluble vitamins, such as cholestyramine, may interfere with the absorption of Zemplar Capsules.

7.3 Mineral Oil

The use of mineral oil or other substances that may affect absorption of fat may influence the absorption of Zemplar Capsules.

8 USE IN SPECIFIC POPULATIONS
8.1 Pregnancy
Pregnancy Category C.

Paricalcitol has been shown to cause minimal decreases in fetal viability (5%) when administered daily to rabbits at a dose 0.5 times a human dose of 14 mcg or 0.24 mcg/kg (based on body surface area, mcg/m²), and when administered to rats at a dose two times the 0.24 mcg/kg human dose (based on body surface area, mcg/m²). At the highest dose tested, 20 mcg/kg administered three times per week in rats (13 times the 14 mcg human dose based on surface area, mcg/m²), there was a significant increase in the mortality of newborn rats at doses that were maternally toxic and are known to produce hypercalcemia in rats. No other effects on offspring development were observed.

Paricalcitol was not teratogenic at the doses tested.
Paricalcitol (20 mcg/kg) has been shown to cross the placental barrier in rats. There are no adequate and well-controlled clinical studies in pregnant women. Zemplar Capsules should be used during pregnancy only if the potential benefit to the mother justifies the potential risk to the fetus.

8.3 Nursing Mothers

Studies in rats have shown that paricalcitol is present in the milk. It is not known whether paricalcitol is excreted in human milk. In the nursing patient, a decision should be made whether to discontinue nursing or to discontinue the drug, taking into account the importance of the drug to the mother.

8.4 Pediatric Use

Safety and efficacy of Zemplar Capsules in pediatric patients have not been established.

8.5 Geriatric Use

Of the total number (n = 220) of CKD Stages 3 and 4 patients in clinical studies of Zemplar Capsules, 49% were age 65 and over, while 17% were age 75 and over. Of the total number (n = 88) of CKD Stage 5 patients in the pivotal study of Zemplar Capsules, 28% were age 65 and over, while 6% were age 75 and over. No overall differences in safety and effectiveness were observed between these patients and younger patients, and other reported clinical experience has not identified differences in responses between the elderly and younger patients, but greater sensitivity of some older individuals cannot be ruled out.

10 OVERDOSAGE

Excessive administration of Zemplar Capsules can cause hypercalcemia, hypercalciuria, and hyperphosphatemia, and over suppression of PTH [see *Warnings and Precautions (5.1)*].

Treatment of Overdosage

The treatment of acute overdosage of Zemplar Capsules should consist of general supportive measures. If drug ingestion is discovered within a relatively short time, induction of emesis or gastric lavage may be of benefit in preventing further absorption. If the drug has passed through the stomach, the administration of mineral oil may promote its fecal elimination. Serial serum electrolyte determinations (especially calcium), rate of urinary calcium excretion, and assessment of electrocardiographic abnormalities due to hypercalcemia should be obtained. Such monitoring is critical in patients receiving digitalis. Discontinuation of supple-

mental calcium and institution of a low-calcium diet are also indicated in accidental overdosage. Due to the relatively short duration of the pharmacological action of paricalcitol, further measures are probably unnecessary. If persistent and markedly elevated serum calcium levels occur, there are a variety of therapeutic alternatives that may be considered depending on the patient's underlying condition. These include the use of drugs such as phosphates and corticosteroids, as well as measures to induce an appropriate forced diuresis.

Zemplar is not significantly removed by dialysis.

11 DESCRIPTION

Paricalcitol, USP, the active ingredient in Zemplar Capsules, is a synthetically manufactured, metabolically active vitamin D analog of calcitriol with modifications to the side chain (D₂) and the A (19-nor) ring. Zemplar is indicated for the prevention and treatment of secondary hyperparathyroidism in chronic kidney disease. Zemplar is available as soft gelatin capsules for oral administration containing 1 microgram or 2 micrograms of paricalcitol. Each capsule also contains medium chain triglycerides, alcohol, and butylated hydroxytoluene. The medium chain triglycerides are fractionated from coconut oil or palm kernel oil. The capsule shell is composed of gelatin, glycerin, titanium dioxide, iron oxide red (2 microgram capsules only), iron oxide yellow (2 microgram capsules only), iron oxide black (1 microgram capsules only), and water.

Paricalcitol is a white, crystalline powder with the empirical formula of $C_{27}H_{44}O_3$, which corresponds to a molecular weight of 416.64. Paricalcitol is chemically designated as 19-nor-1α,3β,25-trihydroxy-9,10-secoergosta-5(Z),7(E),22 (E)-triene and has the following structural formula:

12 CLINICAL PHARMACOLOGY

Secondary hyperparathyroidism is characterized by an elevation in parathyroid hormone (PTH) associated with inadequate levels of active vitamin D hormone. The source of vitamin D in the body is from synthesis in the skin as vitamin D₃ and from dietary intake as either vitamin D₂ or D₃. Both vitamin D₂ and D₃ require two sequential hydroxylations in the liver and the kidney to bind to and to activate the vitamin D receptor (VDR). The endogenous VDR activator, calcitriol [1,25(OH)₂D₃], is a hormone that binds to VDRs that are present in the parathyroid gland, intestine, kidney, and bone to maintain parathyroid function and calcium and phosphorus homeostasis, and to VDRs found in many other tissues, including prostate, endothelium and immune cells. VDR activation is essential for the proper formation and maintenance of normal bone. In the diseased kidney, the activation of vitamin D is diminished, resulting in a rise of PTH, subsequently leading to secondary hyperparathyroidism and disturbances in the calcium and phosphorus homeostasis. Decreased levels of 1,25(OH)₂D₃ have been observed in early stages of chronic kidney disease. The decreased levels of 1,25(OH)₂D₃ and resultant elevated PTH levels, both of which often precede abnormalities in serum calcium and phosphorus, affect bone turnover rate and may result in renal osteodystrophy.

12.1 Mechanism of Action

Paricalcitol is a synthetic, biologically active vitamin D₂ analog of calcitriol. Preclinical and *in vitro* studies have demonstrated that paricalcitol's biological actions are mediated through binding of the VDR, which results in the selective activation of vitamin D responsive pathways. Vitamin D and paricalcitol have been shown to reduce parathyroid hormone levels by inhibiting PTH synthesis and secretion.

Continued on next page

Information on the AbbVie, Inc. products listed on these pages is from the prescribing information in use as of July 31, 2016. For more information, please visit rxabbvie.com or call 1-800-633-9110.

12.2 Pharmacodynamics

Paricalcitol decreases serum intact parathyroid hormone (iPTH) and increases serum calcium and serum phosphorous in both HD and PD patients. This observed relationship was quantified using a mathematical model for HD and PD patient populations separately. Computer-based simulations of 100 trials in HD or PD patients (N = 100) using these relationships predict slightly lower efficacy (at least two consecutive ≥ 30% reductions from baseline iPTH) with lower hypercalcemia rates (at least two consecutive serum calcium ≥ 10.5 mg/dL) for lower iPTH-based dosing regimens. Further lowering of hypercalcemia rates was predicted if the treatment with paricalcitol is initiated in patients with lower serum calcium levels at screening.

Based on these simulations, a dosing regimen of iPTH/80 with a screening serum calcium ≤ 9.5 mg/dL, approximately 76.5% (95% CI: 75.6% – 77.3%) of HD patients are predicted to achieve at least two consecutive weekly ≥ 30% reductions from baseline iPTH over a duration of 12 weeks. The predicted incidence of hypercalcemia is 0.8% (95% CI: 0.7% – 1.0%). In PD patients, with this dosing regimen, approximately 83.3% (95% CI: 82.6% – 84.0%) of patients are predicted to achieve at least two consecutive weekly ≥ 30% reductions from baseline iPTH. The predicted incidence of hypercalcemia is 12.4% (95% CI: 11.7% - 13.0%) [*see Clinical Studies (14.2) and Dosage and Administration (2.2)*].

12.3 Pharmacokinetics

Absorption

The mean absolute bioavailability of Zemplar Capsules under low-fat fed condition ranged from 72% to 86% in healthy subjects, CKD Stage 5 patients on HD, and CKD Stage 5 patients on PD. A food effect study in healthy subjects indicated that the C_{max} and $AUC_{0-\infty}$ were unchanged when paricalcitol was administered with a high fat meal compared to fasting. Food delayed T_{max} by about 2 hours. The $AUC_{0-\infty}$ of paricalcitol increased proportionally over the dose range of 0.06 to 0.48 mcg/kg in healthy subjects.

Distribution

Paricalcitol is extensively bound to plasma proteins (≥ 99.8%). The mean apparent volume of distribution following a 0.24 mcg/kg dose of paricalcitol in healthy subjects was 34 L. The mean apparent volume of distribution following a 4 mcg dose of paricalcitol in CKD Stage 3 and a 3 mcg dose in CKD Stage 4 patients is between 44 and 46 L.

Metabolism

After oral administration of a 0.48 mcg/kg dose of ^{3}H-paricalcitol, parent drug was extensively metabolized, with only about 2% of the dose eliminated unchanged in the feces, and no parent drug was found in the urine. Several metabolites were detected in both the urine and feces. Most of the systemic exposure was from the parent drug. Two minor metabolites, relative to paricalcitol, were detected in human plasma. One metabolite was identified as 24(R)-hydroxy paricalcitol, while the other metabolite was unidentified. The 24(R)-hydroxy paricalcitol is less active than paricalcitol in an *in vivo* rat model of PTH suppression.

In vitro data suggest that paricalcitol is metabolized by multiple hepatic and non-hepatic enzymes, including mitochondrial CYP24, as well as CYP3A4 and UGT1A4. The identified metabolites include the product of 24(R)-hydroxylation, 24,26- and 24,28-dihydroxylation and direct glucuronidation.

Elimination

Paricalcitol is eliminated primarily via hepatobiliary excretion; approximately 70% of the radiolabeled dose is recovered in the feces and 18% is recovered in the urine. While the mean elimination half-life of paricalcitol is 4 to 6 hours in healthy subjects, the mean elimination half-life of paricalcitol in CKD Stages 3, 4, and 5 (on HD and PD) patients ranged from 14 to 20 hours.

[See table 3 below]

Specific Populations

Geriatric

The pharmacokinetics of paricalcitol has not been investigated in geriatric patients greater than 65 years [*see Use in Specific Populations (8.5)*].

Pediatric

The pharmacokinetics of paricalcitol has not been investigated in patients less than 18 years of age.

Gender

The pharmacokinetics of paricalcitol following single doses over the 0.06 to 0.48 mcg/kg dose range was gender independent.

Hepatic Impairment

The disposition of paricalcitol (0.24 mcg/kg) was compared in patients with mild (n = 5) and moderate (n = 5) hepatic impairment (as indicated by the Child-Pugh method) and subjects with normal hepatic function (n = 10). The pharmacokinetics of unbound paricalcitol was similar across the range of hepatic function evaluated in this study. No dose adjustment is required in patients with mild and moderate hepatic impairment. The influence of severe hepatic impairment on the pharmacokinetics of paricalcitol has not been evaluated.

Renal Impairment

Following administration of Zemplar Capsules, the pharmacokinetic profile of paricalcitol for CKD Stage 5 on HD or PD was comparable to that in CKD 3 or 4 patients. Therefore, no special dose adjustments are required other than those recommended in the Dosage and Administration section [*see Dosage and Administration (2)*].

Drug Interactions

An *in vitro* study indicates that paricalcitol is neither an inhibitor of CYP1A2, CYP2A6, CYP2B6, CYP2C8, CYP2C9, CYP2C19, CYP2D6, CYP2E1 or CYP3A nor an inducer of CYP2B6, CYP2C9 or CYP3A. Hence, paricalcitol is neither expected to inhibit nor induce the clearance of drugs metabolized by these enzymes.

Omeprazole

The effect of omeprazole (40 mg capsule), a strong inhibitor of CYP2C19, on paricalcitol (four 4 mcg capsules) pharmacokinetics was investigated in a single dose, crossover study in healthy subjects. The pharmacokinetics of paricalcitol was not affected when omeprazole was administered approximately 2 hours prior to the paricalcitol dose.

Ketoconazole

The effect of multiple doses of ketoconazole, a strong inhibitor of CYP3A, administered as 200 mg BID for 5 days on the pharmacokinetics of paricalcitol (4 mcg capsule) has been studied in healthy subjects. The C_{max} of paricalcitol was minimally affected, but $AUC_{0-\infty}$ approximately doubled in the presence of ketoconazole. The mean half-life of paricalcitol was 17.0 hours in the presence of ketoconazole as compared to 9.8 hours, when paricalcitol was administered alone [*see Drug Interactions (7)*].

13 NONCLINICAL TOXICOLOGY

13.1 Carcinogenesis, Mutagenesis and Impairment of Fertility

In a 104-week carcinogenicity study in CD-1 mice, an increased incidence of uterine leiomyoma and leiomyosarcoma was observed at subcutaneous doses of 1, 3, 10 mcg/kg given three times weekly (2 to 15 times the AUC at a human dose of 14 mcg, equivalent to 0.24 mcg/kg based on AUC). The incidence rate of uterine leiomyoma was significantly different than the control group at the highest dose of 10 mcg/kg. In a 104-week carcinogenicity study in rats, there was an increased incidence of benign adrenal pheochromocytoma at subcutaneous doses of 0.15, 0.5, 1.5 mcg/kg (< 1 to 7 times the exposure following a human dose of 14 mcg, equivalent to 0.24 mcg/kg based on AUC). The increased incidence of pheochromocytomas in rats may be related to the alteration of calcium homeostasis by paricalcitol. Paricalcitol did not exhibit genetic toxicity *in vitro* with or without metabolic activation in the microbial mutagenesis assay (Ames Assay), mouse lymphoma mutagenesis assay (L5178Y), or a human lymphocyte cell chromosomal aberration assay. There was also no evidence of genetic toxicity in an *in vivo* mouse micronucleus assay. Paricalcitol had no effect on fertility (male or female) in rats at intravenous doses up to 20 mcg/kg/dose (equivalent to 13 times a human dose of 14 mcg based on surface area, mcg/m^2).

14 CLINICAL STUDIES

14.1 Chronic Kidney Disease Stages 3 and 4

The safety and efficacy of Zemplar Capsules were evaluated in three, 24-week, double blind, placebo-controlled, randomized, multicenter, Phase 3 clinical studies in CKD Stages 3 and 4 patients. Two studies used an identical three times a week dosing design, and one study used a daily dosing design. A total of 107 patients received Zemplar Capsules and 113 patients received placebo. The mean age of the patients was 63 years, 68% were male, 71% were Caucasian, and 26% were African-American. The average baseline iPTH was 274 pg/mL (range: 145-856 pg/mL). The average duration of CKD prior to study entry was 5.7 years. At study entry 22% were receiving calcium based phosphate binders and/or calcium supplements. Baseline 25-hydroxyvitamin D levels were not measured.

The initial dose of Zemplar Capsules was based on baseline iPTH. If iPTH was ≤ 500 pg/mL, Zemplar Capsules were administered 1 mcg daily or 2 mcg three times a week, not more than every other day. If iPTH was > 500 pg/mL, Zemplar Capsules were administered 2 mcg daily or 4 mcg three times a week, not more than every other day. The dose was increased by 1 mcg daily or 2 mcg three times a week every 2 to 4 weeks until iPTH levels were reduced by at least 30% from baseline. The overall average weekly dose of Zemplar Capsules was 9.6 mcg/week in the daily regimen and 9.5 mcg/week in the three times a week regimen.

In the clinical studies, doses were titrated for any of the following reasons: if iPTH fell to < 60 pg/mL, or decreased > 60% from baseline, the dose was reduced or temporarily withheld; if iPTH decreased < 30% from baseline and serum calcium was ≤ 10.3 mg/dL and serum phosphorus was ≤ 5.5 mg/dL, the dose was increased; and if iPTH decreased between 30 to 60% from baseline and serum calcium and phosphorus were ≤ 10.3 mg/dL and ≤ 5.5 mg/dL, respectively, the dose was maintained. Additionally, if serum calcium was between 10.4 to 11.0 mg/dL, the dose was reduced irrespective of iPTH, and the dose was withheld if serum calcium was > 11.0 mg/dL. If serum phosphorus was > 5.5 mg/dL, dietary counseling was provided, and phosphate binders could have been initiated or increased. If the elevation persisted, the Zemplar Capsules dose was decreased. Seventy-seven percent (77%) of the Zemplar Capsules treated patients and 82% of the placebo treated patients completed the 24-week treatment. The primary efficacy endpoint of at least two consecutive ≥ 30% reductions from baseline iPTH was achieved by 91% of Zemplar Capsules treated patients and 13% of the placebo treated patients (p < 0.001). The proportion of Zemplar Capsules treated patients achieving two consecutive ≥ 30% reductions was similar between the daily and the three times a week regimens (daily: 30/33, 91%; three times a week: 62/68, 91%).

The incidence of hypercalcemia (defined as two consecutive serum calcium values > 10.5 mg/dL), and hyperphosphatemia in Zemplar Capsules treated patients was similar to placebo. There were no treatment related adverse events associated with hypercalcemia or hyperphosphatemia in the Zemplar Capsules group. No increases in urinary calcium or phosphorous were detected in Zemplar Capsules treated patients compared to placebo.

The pattern of change in the mean values for serum iPTH during the studies is shown in Figure 1.

The mean changes from baseline to final treatment visit in serum iPTH, calcium, phosphorus, calcium-phosphorus product, and bone-specific alkaline phosphatase are shown in Table 4.

Table 3. Paricalcitol Capsule Pharmacokinetic Characteristics in CKD Stages 3, 4, and 5 Patients

Pharmacokinetic Parameters	CKD Stage 3 n = 15*	CKD Stage 4 n = 14*	CKD Stage 5 HD** n = 14	CKD Stage 5 PD** n = 8
C_{max} (ng/mL)	0.11 ± 0.04	0.06 ± 0.01	0.575 ± 0.17	0.413 ± 0.06
$AUC_{0-\infty}$ (ng•h/mL)	2.42 ± 0.61	2.13 ± 0.73	11.67 ± 3.23	13.41 ± 5.48
CL/F (L/h)	1.77 ± 0.50	1.52 ± 0.36	1.82 ± 0.75	1.76 ± 0.77
V/F (L)	43.7 ± 14.4	46.4 ± 12.4	38 ± 16.4	48.7 ± 15.6
$t_{1/2}$	16.8 ± 2.65	19.7 ± 7.2	13.9 ± 5.1	17.7 ± 9.6

* Four mcg paricalcitol capsules were given to CKD Stage 3 patients; three mcg paricalcitol capsules were given to CKD Stage 4 patients.

** CKD Stage 5 HD and PD patients received a 0.24 mcg/kg dose of paricalcitol as capsules.

Figure 1. Mean Values for Serum iPTH Over Time in the Three Double-Blind, Placebo-Controlled, Phase 3, CKD Stages 3 and 4 Studies Combined

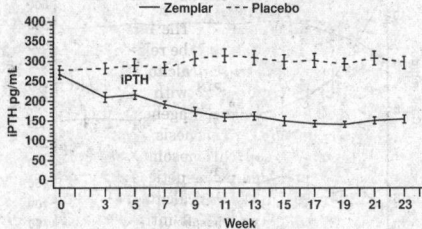

Table 4. Mean Changes from Baseline to Final Treatment Visit in Serum iPTH, Bone Specific Alkaline Phosphatase, Calcium, Phosphorus, and Calcium × Phosphorus Product in Three Combined Double-Blind, Placebo-Controlled, Phase 3, CKD Stages 3 and 4 Studies

	Zemplar Capsules	Placebo
iPTH (pg/mL)	n = 104	n = 110
Mean Baseline Value	266	279
Mean Final Treatment Value	162	315
Mean Change from Baseline (SE)	-104 (9.2)	+35 (9.0)
Bone Specific Alkaline Phosphatase (mcg/L)	n = 101	n = 107
Mean Baseline	17.1	18.8
Mean Final Treatment Value	9.2	17.4
Mean Change from Baseline (SE)	-7.9 (0.76)	-1.4 (0.74)
Calcium (mg/dL)	n = 104	n = 110
Mean Baseline	9.3	9.4
Mean Final Treatment Value	9.5	9.3
Mean Change from Baseline (SE)	+0.2 (0.04)	-0.1 (0.04)
Phosphorus (mg/dL)	n = 104	n = 110
Mean Baseline	4.0	4.0
Mean Final Treatment Value	4.3	4.3
Mean Change from Baseline (SE)	+0.3 (0.08)	+0.3 (0.08)
Calcium × Phosphorus Product (mg²/dL²)	n = 104	n = 110
Mean Baseline	36.7	36.9
Mean Final Treatment Value	40.7	39.7
Mean Change from Baseline (SE)	+4.0 (0.74)	+2.9 (0.72)

14.2 Chronic Kidney Disease Stage 5

The safety and efficacy of Zemplar Capsules were evaluated in a Phase 3, 12-week, double blind, placebo-controlled, randomized, multicenter study in patients with CKD Stage 5 on HD or PD. The study used a three times a week dosing design. A total of 61 patients received Zemplar Capsules and 27 patients received placebo. The mean age of the patients was 57 years, 67% were male, 50% were Caucasian, 45% were African- American, and 53% were diabetic. The average baseline iPTH was 701 pg/mL (range: 216-1933 pg/mL). The average time since first dialysis across all subjects was 3.3 years.

The initial dose of Zemplar Capsules was based on baseline iPTH/60. Subsequent dose adjustments were based on

iPTH/60 as well as primary chemistry results that were measured once a week. Starting at Treatment Week 2, study drug was maintained, increased or decreased weekly based on the results of the previous week's calculation of iPTH/60. Zemplar Capsules were administered three times a week, not more than every other day.

The proportion of patients achieving at least two consecutive weekly ≥ 30% reductions from baseline iPTH was 88% of Zemplar Capsules treated patients and 13% of the placebo treated patients. The proportion of patients achieving at least two consecutive weekly ≥ 30% reductions from baseline iPTH was similar for HD and PD patients.

The incidence of hypercalcemia (defined as two consecutive serum calcium values > 10.5 mg/dL) in patients treated with Zemplar Capsules was 6.6% as compared to 0% for patients given placebo. In PD patients the incidence of hypercalcemia in patients treated with Zemplar Capsules was 21% as compared to 0% for patients given placebo. The patterns of change in the mean values for serum iPTH are shown in Figure 2. The rate of hypercalcemia with Zemplar Capsules may be reduced with a lower dosing regimen based on the iPTH/80 formula as shown by computer simulations. The hypercalcemia rate can be further predicted to decrease, if the treatment is initiated in only those with baseline serum calcium ≤ 9.5 mg/dL [*see Clinical Pharmacology (12.2) and Dosage and Administration (2.2)*].

Figure 2. Mean Values for Serum iPTH Over Time in a Phase 3, Double-Blind, Placebo-Controlled CKD Stage 5 Study

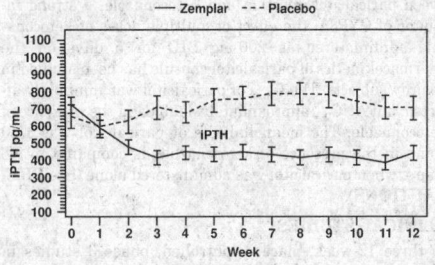

16 HOW SUPPLIED/STORAGE AND HANDLING

Zemplar Capsules are available as 1 mcg and 2 mcg capsules.

The 1 mcg capsule is an oval, gray, soft gelatin capsule imprinted with the "a" logo and ZA, and is available in the following package size:
Bottles of 30 (NDC 0074-4317-30)

The 2 mcg capsule is an oval, orange-brown, soft gelatin capsule imprinted with the "a" logo and ZF, and is available in the following package size:
Bottles of 30 (NDC 0074-4314-30)

Storage

Store Zemplar Capsules at 25°C (77°F). Excursions permitted between 15°- 30°C (59°- 86°F). See USP Controlled Room Temperature.

17 PATIENT COUNSELING INFORMATION

Patients should be advised:
• of the most common adverse reactions with use of Zemplar Capsules, which include diarrhea, hypertension, dizziness and vomiting.
• to adhere to instructions regarding diet and phosphorus restriction.
• to contact a health care provider if you develop symptoms of elevated calcium, (e.g. feeling tired, difficulty thinking clearly, loss of appetite, nausea, vomiting, constipation, increased thirst, increased urination and weight loss).
• to return to the physician's office for routine monitoring. More frequent monitoring is necessary during the initiation of therapy, following dose changes or when potentially interacting medications are started or discontinued.
• to inform their physician of all medications, including prescription and nonprescription drugs, supplements, and herbal preparations they are taking and any change to their medical condition. Patients should also be advised to inform their physicians prescribing a new medication that they are taking Zemplar Capsules.

© 2015 AbbVie Inc.
Manufactured for
AbbVie Inc.
North Chicago, IL 60064, U.S.A.
03-B217 October, 2015
Shown in Product Identification Guide, page 507

ZEMPLAR® ℞
[*zĕm-plar*]
(paricalcitol) Injection
Fliptop Vial

DESCRIPTION

Paricalcitol, USP, the active ingredient in Zemplar Injection, is a synthetically manufactured analog of calcitriol, the metabolically active form of vitamin D indicated for the prevention and treatment of secondary hyperparathyroidism associated with chronic kidney disease (CKD) Stage 5. Zemplar is available as a sterile, clear, colorless, aqueous solution for intravenous injection. Each mL contains paricalcitol, 2 mcg or 5 mcg and the following inactive ingredients: alcohol, 20% (v/v) and propylene glycol, 30% (v/v).

Paricalcitol is a white powder chemically designated as 19-nor-1α,3β,25-trihydroxy-9,10-secoergosta-5(Z),7(E),22(E)-triene and has the following structural formula:

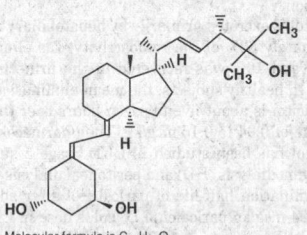

Molecular formula is $C_{27}H_{44}O_3$.
Molecular weight is 416.64.

CLINICAL PHARMACOLOGY

Secondary hyperparathyroidism is characterized by an elevation in parathyroid hormone (PTH) associated with inadequate levels of active vitamin D hormone. The source of vitamin D in the body is from synthesis in the skin and from dietary intake. Vitamin D requires two sequential hydroxylations in the liver and the kidney to bind to and to activate the vitamin D receptor (VDR). The endogenous VDR activator, calcitriol [1,25(OH)$_2$ D$_3$], is a hormone that binds to VDRs that are present in the parathyroid gland, intestine, kidney, and bone to maintain parathyroid function and calcium and phosphorus homeostasis, and to VDRs found in many other tissues, including prostate, endothelium and immune cells. VDR activation is essential for the proper formation and maintenance of normal bone. In the diseased kidney, the activation of vitamin D is diminished, resulting in a rise of PTH, subsequently leading to secondary hyperparathyroidism, and disturbances in the calcium and phosphorus homeostasis. The decreased levels of 1,25(OH)$_2$ D$_3$ and resultant elevated PTH levels, both of which often precede abnormalities in serum calcium and phosphorus, affect bone turnover rate and may result in renal osteodystrophy.

Mechanism of Action

Paricalcitol is a synthetic, biologically active vitamin D analog of calcitriol with modifications to the side chain (D$_2$) and the A (19-nor) ring. Preclinical and *in vitro* studies have demonstrated that paricalcitol's biological actions are mediated through binding of the VDR, which results in the selective activation of vitamin D responsive pathways. Vitamin D and paricalcitol have been shown to reduce parathyroid hormone levels by inhibiting PTH synthesis and secretion.

Pharmacokinetics

Within two hours after administering Zemplar intravenous doses ranging from 0.04 to 0.24 mcg/kg, concentrations of paricalcitol decreased rapidly; thereafter, concentrations of paricalcitol declined log-linearly. No accumulation of paricalcitol was observed with three times a week dosing.

Distribution

Paricalcitol is extensively bound to plasma proteins (≥99.8%). In healthy subjects, the steady state volume of distribution is approximately 23.8 L. The mean volume of distribution following a 0.24 mcg/kg dose of paricalcitol in CKD Stage 5 subjects requiring hemodialysis (HD) and peritoneal dialysis (PD) is between 31 and 35 L.

Continued on next page

Metabolism

After IV administration of a 0.48 mcg/kg dose of ^{3}H-paricalcitol, parent drug was extensively metabolized, with only about 2% of the dose eliminated unchanged in the feces and no parent drug found in the urine. Several metabolites were detected in both the urine and feces. Most of the systemic exposure was from the parent drug. Two minor metabolites, relative to paricalcitol, were detected in human plasma. One metabolite was identified as 24(R)-hydroxy paricalcitol, while the other metabolite was unidentified. The 24(R)-hydroxy paricalcitol is less active than paricalcitol in an *in vivo* rat model of PTH suppression.

In vitro data suggest that paricalcitol is metabolized by multiple hepatic and non-hepatic enzymes, including mitochondrial CYP24, as well as CYP3A4 and UGT1A4. The identified metabolites include the product of 24(R)-hydroxylation (present at low levels in plasma), as well as 24,26- and 24,28-dihydroxylation and direct glucuronidation.

Elimination

Paricalcitol is excreted primarily by hepatobiliary excretion. Approximately 63% of the radioactivity was eliminated in the feces and 19% was recovered in the urine in healthy subjects. In healthy subjects, the mean elimination half-life of paricalcitol is about five to seven hours over the studied dose range of 0.04 to 0.16 mcg/kg. The pharmacokinetics of paricalcitol has been studied in CKD Stage 5 subjects requiring hemodialysis (HD) and peritoneal dialysis (PD). The mean elimination half-life of paricalcitol after administration of 0.24 mcg/kg paricalcitol IV bolus dose in CKD Stage 5 HD and PD patients is 13.9 and 15.4 hours, respectively (Table 1).

Table 1 Mean ± SD Paricalcitol Pharmacokinetic Parameters in CKD Stage 5 Subjects Following Single 0.24 mcg/kg IV Bolus Dose

	CKD Stage 5-HD (n=14)	CKD Stage 5-PD (n=8)
C_{max} (ng/mL)	1.680 ± 0.511	1.832 ± 0.315
$AUC_{0-\infty}$ (ng•h/mL)	14.51 ± 4.12	16.01 ± 5.98
β (1/h)	0.050 ± 0.023	0.045 ± 0.026
$t_{1/2}$ (h)†	13.9 ± 7.3	15.4 ± 10.5
CL (L/h)	1.49 ± 0.60	1.54 ± 0.95
Vd_β (L)	30.8 ± 7.5	34.9 ± 9.5

† harmonic mean ± pseudo standard deviation, HD: hemodialysis, PD: peritoneal dialysis

No accumulation of paricalcitol was observed with three times a week dosing which is consistent with the observed half-life.

Special Populations

Geriatric
The pharmacokinetics of paricalcitol have not been investigated in geriatric patients greater than 65 years.

Pediatrics
The pharmacokinetics of paricalcitol have not been investigated in patients less than 18 years of age.

Gender
The pharmacokinetics of paricalcitol were gender independent.

Hepatic Impairment
The disposition of paricalcitol (0.24 mcg/kg) was compared in patients with mild (n=5) and moderate (n=5) hepatic impairment (as indicated by the Child-Pugh method) and subjects with normal hepatic function (n=10). The pharmacokinetics of unbound paricalcitol were similar across the range of hepatic function evaluated in this study. No dose adjustment is required in patients with mild and moderate hepatic impairment. The influence of severe hepatic impairment on the pharmacokinetics of paricalcitol has not been evaluated.

Renal Impairment
The pharmacokinetics of paricalcitol have been studied in CKD Stage 5 subjects requiring hemodialysis (HD) and peritoneal dialysis (PD). Hemodialysis procedure has essentially no effect on paricalcitol elimination. However, compared to healthy subjects, CKD Stage 5 subjects showed a decreased CL and increased half-life (see **Pharmacokinetics -Elimination**).

Drug Interactions
An *in vitro* study indicates that paricalcitol is not an inhibitor of CYP1A2, CYP2A6, CYP2B6, CYP2C8, CYP2C9, CYP2C19, CYP2D6, CYP2E1, or CYP3A at concentrations up to 50 nM (21 ng/mL) (approximately 20-fold greater than that obtained after highest tested dose). In fresh primary cultured hepatocytes, the induction observed at paricalcitol concentrations up to 50 nM was less than two-fold for CYP2B6, CYP2C9 or CYP3A, where the positive controls rendered a six- to nineteen-fold induction. Hence, paricalcitol is not expected to inhibit or induce the clearance of drugs metabolized by these enzymes.

Drug interactions with paricalcitol injection have not been studied.

Omeprazole
The pharmacokinetic interaction between paricalcitol capsule (16 mcg) and omeprazole (40 mg; oral), a strong inhibitor of CYP2C19, was investigated in a single dose, crossover study in healthy subjects. The pharmacokinetics of paricalcitol were unaffected when omeprazole was administrated approximately 2 hours prior to the paricalcitol dose.

Ketoconazole
Although no data are available for the drug interaction between paricalcitol injection and ketoconazole, a strong inhibitor of CYP3A, the effect of multiple doses of ketoconazole administered as 200 mg BID for 5 days on the pharmacokinetics of paricalcitol capsule has been studied in healthy subjects. The C_{max} of paricalcitol was minimally affected, but $AUC_{0-\infty}$ approximately doubled in the presence of ketoconazole. The mean half-life of paricalcitol was 17.0 hours in the presence of ketoconazole as compared to 9.8 hours, when paricalcitol was administered alone (See **PRE-CAUTIONS**).

CLINICAL STUDIES

In three 12-week, placebo-controlled, phase 3 studies in chronic kidney disease Stage 5 patients on dialysis, the dose of Zemplar was started at 0.04 mcg/kg 3 times per week. The dose was increased by 0.04 mcg/kg every 2 weeks until intact parathyroid hormone (iPTH) levels were decreased at least 30% from baseline or a fifth escalation brought the dose to 0.24 mcg/kg, or iPTH fell to less than 100 pg/mL, or the Ca × P product was greater than 75 within any 2 week period, or serum calcium became greater than 11.5 mg/dL at any time.

Patients treated with Zemplar achieved a mean iPTH reduction of 30% within 6 weeks. In these studies, there was no significant difference in the incidence of hypercalcemia or hyperphosphatemia between Zemplar and placebo-treated patients. The results from these studies are as follows:
[See table below]

A long-term, open-label safety study of 164 CKD Stage 5 patients (mean dose of 7.5 mcg three times per week), demonstrated that mean serum Ca, P, and Ca × P remained within clinically appropriate ranges with PTH reduction (mean decrease of 319 pg/mL at 13 months).

INDICATIONS AND USAGE

Zemplar is indicated for the prevention and treatment of secondary hyperparathyroidism associated with chronic kidney disease Stage 5.

CONTRAINDICATIONS

Zemplar should not be given to patients with evidence of vitamin D toxicity, hypercalcemia, or hypersensitivity to any ingredient in this product (see **WARNINGS**).

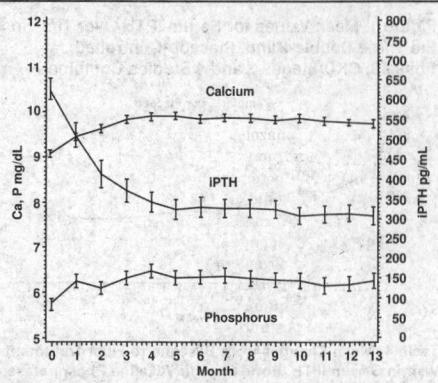

WARNINGS

Acute overdose of Zemplar may cause hypercalcemia, and require emergency attention (see **OVERDOSAGE**). During dose adjustment, serum calcium and phosphorus levels should be monitored closely (e.g., twice weekly). If clinically significant hypercalcemia develops, the dose should be reduced or interrupted. Chronic administration of Zemplar may place patients at risk of hypercalcemia, elevated Ca × P product, and metastatic calcification. Chronic hypercalcemia can lead to generalized vascular calcification and other soft-tissue calcification.

Concomitant administration of high doses of calcium-containing preparations or thiazide diueretics with Zemplar may increase the risk of hypercalcemia. High intake of calcium and phosphate concomitant with vitamin D compounds may lead to serum abnormalities requiring more frequent patient monitoring and individualized dose titration. Patients also should be informed about the symptoms of elevated calcium, which include feeling tired, difficulty thinking clearly, loss of appetite, nausea, vomiting, constipation, increased thirst, increased urination and weight loss.

Prescription-based doses of vitamin D and its derivatives should be withheld during Zemplar treatment to avoid hypercalcemia.

Aluminum-containing preparations (e.g., antacids, phosphate binders) should not be administered chronically with Zemplar, as increased blood levels of aluminum and aluminum bone toxicity may occur.

PRECAUTIONS

General
Digitalis toxicity is potentiated by hypercalcemia of any cause, so caution should be applied when digitalis compounds are prescribed concomitantly with Zemplar. Adynamic bone lesions may develop if PTH levels are suppressed to abnormal levels.

Information for the Patient
The patient should be instructed that, to ensure effectiveness of Zemplar therapy, it is important to adhere to a dietary regimen of calcium supplementation and phosphorus restriction. Appropriate types of phosphate-binding compounds may be needed to control serum phosphorus levels in patients with chronic kidney disease (CKD) Stage 5, but excessive use of aluminum containing compounds should be avoided (see **WARNINGS**). Patients should also be carefully informed about the symptoms of elevated calcium (see **WARNINGS**).

Laboratory Tests
During the initial phase of medication, serum calcium and phosphorus should be determined frequently (e.g., twice weekly). Once dosage has been established, serum calcium and phosphorus should be measured at least monthly. Measurements of serum or plasma PTH are recommended every 3 months. During dose adjustment of Zemplar, laboratory tests may be required more frequently.

Drug Interactions
Specific interaction studies were not performed with Zemplar Injection. Paricalcitol is not expected to inhibit the clearance of drugs metabolized by cytochrome P450 enzymes CYP1A2, CYP2A6, CYP2B6, CYP2C8, CYP2C9, CYP2C19, CYP2D6, CYP2E1, or CYP3A nor induce the clearance of drug metabolized by CYP2B6, CYP2C9 or CYP3A.

A multiple dose drug-drug interaction study with ketoconazole and paricalcitol capsule demonstrated that ketoconazole approximately doubled paricalcitol $AUC_{0-\infty}$ (see **CLINICAL PHARMACOLOGY**). Since paricalcitol is partially

Group (No. of Pts.)		Baseline Mean (Range)	Mean (SE) Change From Baseline to Final Evaluation
PTH (pg/mL)	Zemplar (n = 40)	783 (291 – 2076)	-379 (43.7)
	placebo (n = 38)	745 (320 –1671)	-69.6 (44.8)
Alkaline Phosphatase (U/L)	Zemplar (n = 31)	150 (40 – 600)	-41.5 (10.6)
	placebo (n = 34)	169 (56 – 911)	+2.6 (10.1)
Calcium (mg/dL)	Zemplar (n = 40)	9.3 (7.2 – 10.4)	+0.47 (0.1)
	placebo (n = 38)	9.1 (7.8 – 10.7)	+0.02 (0.1)
Phosphorus (mg/dL)	Zemplar (n = 40)	5.8 (3.7 – 10.2)	+0.47 (0.3)
	placebo (n = 38)	6.0 (2.8 – 8.8)	-0.47 (0.3)
Calcium × Phosphorus Product	Zemplar (n = 40)	54 (32 – 106)	+7.9 (2.2)
	placebo (n = 38)	54 (26 – 77)	-3.9 (2.3)

metabolized by CYP3A and ketoconazole is known to be a strong inhibitor of cytochrome P450 3A enzyme, care should be taken while paricalcitol is co-administered with ketoconazole and other strong P450 3A inhibitors including the following drugs but not limited to: atazanavir, clarithromycin, indinavir, itraconazole, nefazodone, nelfinavir, ritonavir, saquinavir, telithromycin or voriconazole.

Digitalis toxicity is potentiated by hypercalcemia of any cause, so caution should be applied when digitalis compounds are prescribed concomitantly with Zemplar.

Carcinogenesis, Mutagenesis, Impairment of Fertility

In a 104-week carcinogenicity study in CD-1 mice, an increased incidence of uterine leiomyoma and leiomyosarcoma was observed at subcutaneous doses of 1, 3, 10 mcg/kg (2 to 15 times the AUC at a human dose of 14 mcg, equivalent to 0.24 mcg/kg based on AUC). The incidence rate of uterine leiomyoma was significantly different than the control group at the highest dose of 10 mcg/kg.

In a 104-week carcinogenicity study in rats, there was an increased incidence of benign adrenal pheochromocytoma at subcutaneous doses of 0.15, 0.5, 1.5 mcg/kg (< 1 to 7 times the exposure following a human dose of 14 mcg, equivalent to 0.24 mcg/kg based on AUC). The increased incidence of pheochromocytomas in rats may be related to the alteration of calcium homeostasis by paricalcitol.

Paricalcitol did not exhibit genetic toxicity *in vitro* with or without metabolic activation in the microbial mutagenesis assay (Ames Assay), mouse lymphoma mutagenesis assay (L5178Y), or a human lymphocyte cell chromosomal aberration assay. There was also no evidence of genetic toxicity in an *in vivo* mouse micronucleus assay. Zemplar had no effect on fertility (male or female) in rats at intravenous doses up to 20 mcg/kg/dose [equivalent to 13 times the highest recommended human dose (0.24 mcg/kg) based on surface area, mg/m^2].

Pregnancy

Pregnancy Category C

Paricalcitol has been shown to cause minimal decreases in fetal viability (5%) when administered daily to rabbits at a dose 0.5 times the 0.24 mcg/kg human dose (based on surface area, mg/m^2) and when administered to rats at a dose 2 times the 0.24 mcg/kg human dose (based on plasma levels of exposure). At the highest dose tested (20 mcg/kg 3 times per week in rats, 13 times the 0.24 mcg/kg human dose based on surface area), there was a significant increase of the mortality of newborn rats at doses that were maternally toxic (hypercalcemia). No other effects on offspring development were observed. Paricalcitol was not teratogenic at the doses tested.

There are no adequate and well-controlled studies in pregnant women. Zemplar should be used during pregnancy only if the potential benefit to the mother justifies the potential risk to the fetus.

Nursing Mothers

Studies in rats have shown that paricalcitol is present in the milk. It is not known whether paricalcitol is excreted in human milk. In the nursing patient, a decision should be made whether to discontinue nursing or to discontinue the drug, taking into account the importance of the drug to the mother.

Pediatric Use

The safety and effectiveness of Zemplar were examined in a 12-week randomized, double-blind, placebo-controlled study of 29 pediatric patients, aged 5-19 years, with end-stage renal disease on hemodialysis and nearly all had received some form of vitamin D prior to the study. Seventy-six percent of the patients were male, 52% were Caucasian and 45% were African-American. The initial dose of Zemplar was 0.04 mcg/kg 3 times per week based on baseline iPTH level of less than 500 pg/mL, or 0.08 mcg/kg 3 times a week, based on baseline iPTH level of ≥ 500 pg/mL, respectively. The dose of Zemplar was adjusted in 0.04 mcg/kg increments based on the levels of serum iPTH, calcium and Ca × P. The mean baseline levels of iPTH were 841 pg/mL for the 15 Zemplar-treated patients and 740 pg/mL for the 14 placebo-treated subjects. The mean dose of Zemplar administered was 4.6 mcg (range: 0.8 mcg – 9.6 mcg). Ten of the 15 (67%) Zemplar-treated patients and 2 of the 14 (14%) placebo-treated patients completed the trial. Ten of the placebo patients (71%) were discontinued due to excessive elevations in iPTH levels as defined by 2 consecutive iPTH levels > 700 pg/mL and greater than baseline after 4 weeks of treatment.

In the primary efficacy analysis, 9 of 15 (60%) subjects in the Zemplar group had 2 consecutive 30% decreases from baseline iPTH compared with 3 of 14 (21%) patients in the placebo group (95% CI for the difference between groups −1%, 63%). Twenty-three percent of Zemplar vs. 31% of placebo patients had at least one serum calcium level > 10.3 mg/dL, and 40% vs. 14% of Zemplar vs. placebo subjects had at least one Ca × P ion product > 72 (mg/dL)^2. The overall percentage of serum calcium measurements > 10.3 mg/dL was 7% in the Zemplar group and 7% in the placebo group; the overall percentage of patients with Ca × P product > 72 (mg/dL)^2 was 8% in the Zemplar group and 7% in the placebo group. No subjects in either the Zemplar group or placebo group developed hypercalcemia (defined as at least one calcium value > 11.2 mg/dL) during the study.

Geriatric Use

Of the 40 patients receiving Zemplar in the three phase 3 placebo-controlled CKD Stage 5 studies, 10 patients were 65 years or over. In these studies, no overall differences in efficacy or safety were observed between patients 65 years or older and younger patients.

ADVERSE REACTIONS

Zemplar has been evaluated for safety in clinical studies in 609 CKD Stage 5 patients. In four, placebo-controlled, double-blind, multicenter studies, discontinuation of therapy due to any adverse event occurred in 6.5% of 62 patients treated with Zemplar (dosage titrated as tolerated, see **CLINICAL PHARMACOLOGY - Clinical Studies**) and 2.0% of 51 patients treated with placebo for 1 to 3 months. Adverse events occurring in the Zemplar group at a frequency of 2% or greater and with an incidence greater than that in the placebo group, regardless of causality, are presented in the following table:

Adverse Event Incidence Rates for All Treated Patients In All Placebo-Controlled Studies

Adverse Event	Zemplar (n = 62) %	Placebo (n = 51) %
Overall	71	78
Cardiac Disorders		
Palpitations	3.2	0.0
Gastrointestinal Disorders		
Dry Mouth	3.2	2.0
Gastrointestinal Hemorrhage	4.8	2.0
Nausea	12.9	7.8
Vomiting	8.1	5.9
General Disorders and Administration Site Conditions		
Chills	4.8	2.0
Edema	6.5	0.0
Malaise	3.2	0.0
Pyrexia	4.8	2.0
Infections and Infestations		
Influenza	4.8	3.9
Pneumonia	4.8	0.0
Sepsis	4.8	2.0
Musculoskeletal and Connective Tissue Disorders		
Arthralgia	4.8	3.9

A patient who reported the same medical term more than once was counted only once for that medical term.

Safety parameters (changes in mean Ca, P, Ca × P) in an open-label safety study up to 13 months in duration support the long-term safety of Zemplar in this patient population (see **CLINICAL STUDIES**).

Other Adverse Reactions Observed During Clinical Evaluation of Zemplar Injection

The following adverse reactions, with a causal relationship to Zemplar, occurred in <2% of the Zemplar treated patients in the above double-blind, placebo-controlled clinical trial data set. In addition, the following also includes adverse reactions reported in Zemplar-treated patients who participated in other studies (non placebo-controlled), including double-blind, active-controlled and open-label studies:

Blood and Lymphatic System Disorders:
Anemia, lymphadenopathy

Cardiac Disorders:
Arrhythmia, atrial flutter, cardiac arrest

Ear and Labyrinth Disorders:
Ear discomfort

Endocrine Disorders:
Hyperparathyroidism, hypoparathyroidism

Eye Disorders:
Conjunctivitis, glaucoma, ocular hyperemia

Gastrointestinal Disorders:

Abdominal discomfort, constipation, diarrhea, dysphagia, gastritis, intestinal ischemia, rectal hemorrhage

General Disorders and Administration Site Conditions:
Asthenia, chest discomfort, chest pain, condition aggravated, edema peripheral, fatigue, feeling abnormal, gait disturbance, injection site extravasation, injection site pain, pain, swelling, thirst

Infections and Infestations:
Nasopharyngitis, upper respiratory tract infection, vaginal infection

Investigations:
Aspartate aminotransferase increased, bleeding time prolonged, heart rate irregular, laboratory test abnormal, weight decreased

Metabolism and Nutrition Disorders:
Decreased appetite, hypercalcemia, hyperkalemia, hyperphosphatemia, hypocalcemia

Musculoskeletal and Connective Tissue Disorders:
Joint stiffness, muscle twitching, myalgia

Neoplasms Benign, Malignant and Unspecified:
Breast cancer

Nervous System Disorders:
Cerebrovascular accident, dizziness, dysgeusia, headache, hypoesthesia, myoclonus, paresthesia, syncope, unresponsive to stimuli

Psychiatric Disorders:
Agitation, confusional state, delirium, insomnia, nervousness, restlessness

Reproductive System and Breast Disorders:
Breast pain, erectile dysfunction

Respiratory, Thoracic and Mediastinal Disorders:
Cough, dyspnea, orthopnea, pulmonary edema, wheezing

Skin and Subcutaneous Tissue Disorders:
Alopecia, blister, hirsutism, night sweats, rash pruritic, pruritus, skin burning sensation

Vascular Disorders:
Hypertension, hypotension

Additional Adverse Events Reported During Postmarketing Experience

Allergic reactions, such as rash, urticaria, and angioedema (including laryngeal edema) have been reported.

OVERDOSAGE

Overdosage of Zemplar may lead to hypercalcemia, hypercalciuria, hyperphosphatemia, and over suppression of PTH. (see **WARNINGS**).

Treatment of Overdosage and Hypercalcemia

The treatment of acute overdosage should consist of general supportive measures. Serial serum electrolyte determinations (especially calcium), rate of urinary calcium excretion, and assessment of electrocardiographic abnormalities due to hypercalcemia should be obtained. Such monitoring is critical in patients receiving digitalis. Discontinuation of supplemental calcium and institution of a low calcium diet are also indicated in acute overdosage.

General treatment of hypercalcemia due to overdosage consists of immediate dose reduction or suspension of Zemplar therapy, institution of a low calcium diet, withdrawal of calcium supplements, patient mobilization, and attention to fluid and electrolyte imbalances. Serum calcium levels should be determined at least weekly until normocalcemia ensues. When serum calcium levels have returned to within normal limits, Zemplar may be reinitiated at a lower dose. If persistent and markedly elevated serum calcium levels occur, there are a variety of therapeutic alternatives that may be considered. These include the use of drugs such as phosphates and corticosteroids as well as measures to induce diuresis. Also, one may consider dialysis against a calcium-free dialysate.

Zemplar is not significantly removed by dialysis.

DOSAGE AND ADMINISTRATION

The currently accepted target range for iPTH levels in CKD Stage 5 patients is no more than 1.5 to 3 times the nonuremic upper limit of normal.

Continued on next page

List No.	Volume/Container	Concentration	Total Content	Vial Type
4637-01	1 mL/Fliptop Vial	2 mcg/mL	2 mcg	Single-dose
1658-01	1 mL/Fliptop Vial	5 mcg/mL	5 mcg	Single-dose
1658-05	2 mL/Fliptop Vial	5 mcg/mL	10 mcg	Multi-dose

The recommended initial dose of Zemplar is 0.04 mcg/kg to 0.1 mcg/kg (2.8 – 7 mcg) administered as a bolus dose no more frequently than every other day at any time during dialysis.

If a satisfactory response is not observed, the dose may be increased by 2 to 4 mcg at 2- to 4-week intervals. During any dose adjustment period, serum calcium and phosphorus levels should be monitored more frequently, and if an elevated calcium level or a Ca × P product greater than 75 is noted, the drug dosage should be immediately reduced or interrupted until these parameters are normalized. Then, Zemplar should be reinitiated at a lower dose. If a patient is on a calcium-based phosphate binder, the dose may be decreased or withheld, or the patient may be switched to a non-calcium-based phosphate binder. Zemplar doses may need to be decreased as the PTH levels decrease in response to therapy. Thus, incremental dosing must be individualized.

The following table is a suggested approach in dose titration:

Suggested Dosing Guidelines

PTH Level	Zemplar Dose
the same or increasing	increase
decreasing by < 30%	increase
decreasing by > 30%, < 60%	maintain
decreasing by > 60%	decrease
one and one-half to three times upper limit of normal	maintain

The influence of mild to moderately impaired hepatic function on paricalcitol pharmacokinetics is sufficiently small that no dosing adjustment is required.

Parenteral drug products should be inspected visually for particulate matter and discoloration prior to administration whenever solution and container permit.

After initial vial use, the contents of the multi-dose vial remain stable up to seven days when stored at controlled room temperature (see **HOW SUPPLIED**). Discard unused portion of the single-dose vial.

HOW SUPPLIED

Zemplar Injection is available as 2 mcg/mL (**NDC** 0074-4637-01) and 5 mcg/mL (**NDC** 0074-1658-01 and **NDC** 0074-1658-05) in trays of 25 vials.

[See table above]

Store at 25°C (77°F). Excursions permitted between 15° - 30°C (59° - 86°F).

© AbbVie Inc.

Manufactured for
AbbVie Inc.
North Chicago, IL 60064, U.S.A.
Ref. EN-2945-Rev. January, 2013

Amgen
ONE AMGEN CENTER DRIVE
THOUSAND OAKS, CA 91320-1799

For Product Inquiries and
Adverse Event Reporting Contact:
Amgen Medical Information
(800) 772-6436
FAX: (866) 292-6436
Sales and Ordering:
Amgen Trade Operations
(800) 282-6436
FAX: (866) 292-6436

IMLYGIC   ℞
[imm-LY-jik]
(talimogene laherparepvec)
Suspension for intralesional injection

HIGHLIGHTS OF PRESCRIBING INFORMATION
These highlights do not include all the information needed to use IMLYGIC™ safely and effectively. See full prescribing information for IMLYGIC.
IMLYGIC (talimogene laherparepvec)
Suspension for intralesional injection
Initial U.S. Approval: 2015

INDICATIONS AND USAGE
IMLYGIC is a genetically modified oncolytic viral therapy indicated for the local treatment of unresectable cutaneous, subcutaneous, and nodal lesions in patients with melanoma recurrent after initial surgery.
Limitations of use: IMLYGIC has not been shown to improve overall survival or have an effect on visceral metastases. (1)

DOSAGE AND ADMINISTRATION
• Administer IMLYGIC by injection into cutaneous, subcutaneous, and/or nodal lesions. (2)
• Recommended starting dose is up to a maximum of 4 mL of IMLYGIC at a concentration of 10^6 (1 million) plaque-forming units (PFU) per mL. Subsequent doses should be administered up to 4 mL of IMLYGIC at a concentration of 10^8 (100 million) PFU per mL. (2)

DOSAGE FORMS AND STRENGTHS
• Injection: 10^6 (1 million) PFU per mL, 10^8 (100 million) PFU per mL in single-use vials (3)

CONTRAINDICATIONS
• Immunocompromised Patients (4.1)
• Pregnant Patients (4.2)

WARNINGS AND PRECAUTIONS
• Accidental Exposure to IMLYGIC: Accidental exposure may lead to transmission of IMLYGIC and herpetic infection. Healthcare providers and close contacts should avoid direct contact with injected lesions, dressings, or body fluids of treated patients. Healthcare providers who are immunocompromised or pregnant should not prepare or administer IMLYGIC. If accidental exposure occurs, exposed individuals should clean the affected area. (5.1)
• Herpetic Infection: Patients who develop herpetic infections should be advised to follow standard hygienic practices to prevent viral transmission. (5.2)
• Injection Site Complications: Consider the risks and benefits before continuing IMLYGIC treatment if persistent infection or delayed healing develops. (5.3)
• Immune-Mediated Events: Consider the risks and benefits of IMLYGIC before initiating treatment in patients who have underlying autoimmune disease or before continuing treatment in patients who develop immune-mediated events. (5.4)
• Plasmacytoma at Injection Site: Consider the risks and benefits in patients with multiple myeloma or in whom plasmacytoma develops during treatment. (5.5)

ADVERSE REACTIONS
• The most commonly reported adverse drug reactions (≥ 25%) in IMLYGIC-treated patients were fatigue, chills, pyrexia, nausea, influenza-like illness, and injection site pain. (6)
To report SUSPECTED ADVERSE REACTIONS, contact Amgen at 1-855-IMLYGIC (1-855-465-9442) or FDA at 1-800-FDA-1088 or www.fda.gov/medwatch.

USE IN SPECIFIC POPULATIONS
• Pregnancy: Women of childbearing potential should be advised to use an effective method of contraception to prevent pregnancy during treatment with IMLYGIC. (8.1)
• Lactation: Discontinue drug or nursing. (8.2)
See 17 for PATIENT COUNSELING INFORMATION and Medication Guide.

Revised: 10/2015

FULL PRESCRIBING INFORMATION

1   INDICATIONS AND USAGE
IMLYGIC is a genetically modified oncolytic viral therapy indicated for the local treatment of unresectable cutaneous, subcutaneous, and nodal lesions in patients with melanoma recurrent after initial surgery.
Limitations of use: IMLYGIC has not been shown to improve overall survival or have an effect on visceral metastases.

2   DOSAGE AND ADMINISTRATION
For intralesional injection only. Do not administer intravenously.
2.1   Dose
Administer IMLYGIC by injection into cutaneous, subcutaneous, and/or nodal lesions that are visible, palpable, or detectable by ultrasound guidance.
IMLYGIC is provided in single-use vials of 1 mL each in two different dose strengths:
• 10^6 (1 million) plaque-forming units (PFU) per mL (light green cap) – for initial dose only
• 10^8 (100 million) PFU per mL (royal blue cap) – for all subsequent doses
Recommended Dose and Schedule
The total injection volume for each treatment visit should not exceed 4 mL for all injected lesions combined. It may not be possible to inject all lesions at each treatment visit or over the full course of treatment. Previously injected and/or

uninjected lesion(s) may be injected at subsequent treatment visits. The initial recommended dose is up to 4 mL of IMLYGIC at a concentration of 10^6 (1 million) PFU per mL. The recommended dose for subsequent administrations is up to 4 mL of IMLYGIC at a concentration of 10^8 (100 million) PFU per mL. The recommended dosing schedule for IMLYGIC is shown in Table 1.
[See table above]

Dose Volume Determination (per Lesion)
Use Table 2 to determine the volume of IMLYGIC injection for each lesion.

Table 2. Determination of IMLYGIC Injection Volume Based on Lesion Size

Lesion Size (longest dimension)	Injection Volume
> 5 cm	up to 4 mL
> 2.5 cm to 5 cm	up to 2 mL
> 1.5 cm to 2.5 cm	up to 1 mL
> 0.5 cm to 1.5 cm	up to 0.5 mL
≤ 0.5 cm	up to 0.1 mL

When lesions are clustered together, inject them as a single lesion according to Table 2.
Continue IMLYGIC treatment for at least 6 months unless other treatment is required or until there are no injectable lesions to treat.
Reinitiate IMLYGIC treatment if new unresectable cutaneous, subcutaneous, or nodal lesions appear after a complete response.

2.2 Preparation and Handling
Healthcare providers who are immunocompromised or pregnant should not prepare or administer IMLYGIC and should not come into direct contact with the IMLYGIC injection sites, dressings, or body fluids of treated patients [see Warnings and Precautions (5.1)].
Avoid accidental exposure to IMLYGIC and follow universal biohazard precautions for preparation, administration, and handling of IMLYGIC:
• Wear personal protective equipment (protective gown or laboratory coat, safety glasses or face shield, and gloves) while preparing or administering IMLYGIC.
• Avoid accidental exposure to IMLYGIC, especially contact with skin, eyes, and mucous membranes.
  ○ Cover any exposed wounds before handling.
  ○ In the event of an accidental occupational exposure (e.g., through a splash to the eyes or mucous membranes), flush with clean water for at least 15 minutes.
  ○ In the event of exposure to broken skin or needle stick, clean the affected area thoroughly with soap and water and/or a disinfectant.
• Treat all IMLYGIC spills with a virucidal agent such as 1% sodium hypochlorite and blot using absorbent materials.
• Dispose of all materials that may have come in contact with IMLYGIC (e.g., vial, syringe, needle, cotton gauze, gloves, masks, or dressings) in accordance with universal biohazard precautions.
• Advise patients to place used dressings and cleaning materials into a sealed plastic bag and dispose in household waste.

Thawing IMLYGIC Vials
1. Determine the total volume required for injection, up to 4 ml [see Dosage and Administration (2.1)].
2. Thaw frozen IMLYGIC vials at room temperature [20° to 25°C (68° to 77°F)] until IMLYGIC is liquid (approximately 30 minutes). Do not expose the vial to higher temperatures. Keep the vial in original carton during thawing.
3. Swirl gently. Do NOT shake.
4. After thawing, administer IMLYGIC immediately or store in its original vial and carton, protected from light in a refrigerator [2° to 8°C (36° to 46°F)] for no longer than the specified duration in Table 3. Do not refreeze IMLYGIC after thawing. Discard any IMLYGIC vial left in the refrigerator longer than the specified times in Table 3.

Table 3. Storage Times for Thawed IMLYGIC Vial at 2° to 8°C (36° to 46°F)

10^6 (1 million) PFU per mL	10^8 (100 million) PFU per mL
12 hours	48 hours

Table 1. Recommended Dose and Schedule for IMLYGIC

Treatment	Treatment Interval	Maximum Injection Volume per Treatment Visit (all lesions combined)	Dose Strength	Prioritization of Lesions to be Injected
Initial	–	4 mL	10^6 (1 million) PFU per mL	• Inject largest lesion(s) first. • Prioritize injection of remaining lesion(s) based on lesion size until maximum injection volume is reached or until all injectable lesion(s) have been treated.
Second	3 weeks after initial treatment	4 mL	10^8 (100 million) PFU per mL	• Inject any new lesion(s) (lesions that have developed since initial treatment) first. • Prioritize injection of remaining lesion(s) based on lesion size until maximum injection volume is reached or until all injectable lesion(s) have been treated.
All subsequent treatments (including reinitiation)	2 weeks after previous treatment	4 mL	10^8 (100 million) PFU per mL	• Inject any new lesion(s) (lesions that have developed since previous treatment) first. • Prioritize injection of remaining lesion(s) based on lesion size until maximum injection volume is reached or until all injectable lesion(s) have been treated.

5. Prepare sterile syringes and needles. A detachable needle of 18–26G may be used for IMLYGIC withdrawal and a detachable needle of 22–26G may be used for injection. Small unit syringes (e.g., 0.5 mL insulin syringes) are recommended for better injection control.
6. Using aseptic technique, remove the vial cap and withdraw the product from the vial into the syringe(s), noting the total volume. Avoid generating aerosols when loading syringes with product, and use a biologic safety cabinet if available.

2.3 Administration
Follow the steps below to administer IMLYGIC to patients:
Pre-Injection
1. Clean the lesion and surrounding areas with an alcohol swab and let dry.
2. Treat the injection site with a topical or local anesthetic agent, if necessary. Do not inject anesthetic agent directly into the lesion. Inject anesthetic agent around the periphery of the lesion.
Injection
1. Inject IMLYGIC intralesionally into cutaneous, subcutaneous, and/or nodal lesions that are visible, palpable, or detectable by ultrasound guidance. Using a single insertion point, inject IMLYGIC along multiple tracks as far as the radial reach of the needle allows within the lesion to achieve even and complete dispersion. Multiple insertion points may be used if a lesion is larger than the radial reach of the needle.

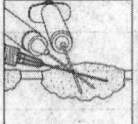 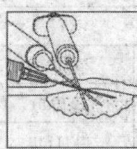 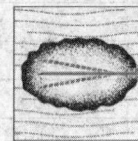

Figure 1: Injection administration for cutaneous lesions

Figure 2: Injection administration for subcutaneous lesions

Figure 3: Injection administration for nodal lesions

2. Inject IMLYGIC evenly and completely within the lesion by pulling the needle back without exiting the lesion. Redirect the needle as many times as necessary while injecting the remainder of the dose of IMLYGIC. Continue until the full dose is evenly and completely dispersed.
3. When removing the needle, withdraw it from the lesion slowly to avoid leakage of IMLYGIC at the insertion point.
4. Repeat steps 1-2 under pre-injection and steps 1-3 under injection for other lesions to be injected.
5. Use a new needle any time the needle is completely removed from a lesion and each time a different lesion is injected.
Post-Injection
1. Apply pressure to the injection site(s) with sterile gauze for at least 30 seconds.
2. Swab the injection site(s) and surrounding area with alcohol.
3. Change gloves and cover the injected lesion(s) with an absorbent pad and dry occlusive dressing.
4. Wipe the exterior of occlusive dressing with alcohol.
5. Advise patients to:

• Keep the injection site(s) covered for at least the first week after each treatment visit or longer if the injection site is weeping or oozing.
• Replace the dressing if it falls off.

3 DOSAGE FORMS AND STRENGTHS
• Initial dose only: 10^6 (1 million) PFU per mL solution in 1 mL single-use vial (light green cap)
• Subsequent doses: 10^8 (100 million) PFU per mL solution in 1 mL single-use vial (royal blue cap)

4 CONTRAINDICATIONS
4.1 Immunocompromised Patients
IMLYGIC is a live, attenuated herpes simplex virus and may cause life-threatening disseminated herpetic infection in patients who are immunocompromised. Do not administer IMLYGIC to immunocompromised patients, including those with a history of primary or acquired immunodeficient states, leukemia, lymphoma, AIDS or other clinical manifestations of infection with human immunodeficiency viruses, and those on immunosuppressive therapy [see Nonclinical Toxicology (13.2)].
4.2 Pregnant Patients
Do not administer IMLYGIC to pregnant patients.

5 WARNINGS AND PRECAUTIONS
5.1 Accidental Exposure to IMLYGIC
Accidental exposure may lead to transmission of IMLYGIC and herpetic infection. Accidental needle stick and splashback to the eyes have been reported in healthcare providers during preparation and administration of IMLYGIC.
Healthcare providers, close contacts (household members, caregivers, sex partners, or persons sharing the same bed), pregnant women, and newborns should avoid direct contact with injected lesions, dressings, or body fluids of treated patients [see Dosage and Administration (2.2)]. Healthcare providers who are immunocompromised or pregnant should not prepare or administer IMLYGIC.
Caregivers should wear protective gloves when assisting patients in applying or changing occlusive dressings and observe safety precautions for disposal of used dressings, gloves, and cleaning materials [see Dosage and Administration (2.2)].
In the event of an accidental exposure to IMLYGIC, exposed individuals should clean the affected area thoroughly with soap and water and/or a disinfectant. If signs or symptoms of herpetic infection develop, the exposed individuals should contact their healthcare provider for appropriate treatment [see Warnings and Precautions (5.2)].
Patients should avoid touching or scratching injection sites or their occlusive dressings, as doing so could lead to inadvertent transfer of IMLYGIC to other areas of the body.
5.2 Herpetic Infection
In clinical studies, herpetic infections (including cold sores and herpetic keratitis) have been reported in patients treated with IMLYGIC. Disseminated herpetic infection may also occur in immunocompromised patients [see Contraindications (4.1)].

Continued on next page

Patients who develop suspicious herpes-like lesions should follow standard hygienic practices to prevent viral transmission. Patients or close contacts with suspected herpetic infections should also contact their healthcare provider to evaluate the lesions. Suspected herpetic lesions should be reported to Amgen at 1-855-IMLYGIC (1-855-465-9442); patients or close contacts have the option of follow-up testing for further characterization of the infection.

IMLYGIC is sensitive to acyclovir. Acyclovir or other antiviral agents may interfere with the effectiveness of IMLYGIC. Therefore, consider the risks and benefits of IMLYGIC treatment before administering antiviral agents to manage herpetic infection.

5.3 Injection Site Complications

Necrosis or ulceration of tumor tissue may occur during IMLYGIC treatment. Cellulitis and systemic bacterial infection have been reported in clinical studies. Careful wound care and infection precautions are recommended, particularly if tissue necrosis results in open wounds.

In clinical studies, impaired healing at the injection site has been reported. IMLYGIC may increase the risk of impaired healing in patients with underlying risk factors (e.g., previous radiation at the injection site or lesions in poorly vascularized areas). One patient had an amputation of a lower extremity 6 months after IMLYGIC injection due to an infected non-healing wound. This wound area had been treated with surgery and radiation prior to IMLYGIC treatment and had previous wound complications.

If there is persistent infection or delayed healing of the injection site(s), consider the risks and benefits of IMLYGIC before continuing treatment with IMLYGIC.

5.4 Immune-Mediated Events

IMLYGIC may result in immune-mediated events. In clinical studies, immune-mediated events, including glomerulo-

nephritis, vasculitis, pneumonitis, worsening psoriasis, and vitiligo have been reported in patients treated with IMLYGIC.

Consider the risks and benefits of IMLYGIC before initiating treatment in patients who have underlying autoimmune disease or before continuing treatment in patients who develop immune-mediated events.

5.5 Plasmacytoma at Injection Site

In a clinical study, a plasmacytoma has been reported in proximity to the injection site after administration of IMLYGIC in a patient with smoldering multiple myeloma. Consider the risks and benefits of IMLYGIC in patients with multiple myeloma or in whom plasmacytoma develops during treatment.

6 ADVERSE REACTIONS

The most commonly reported adverse drug reactions (≥ 25%) in IMLYGIC-treated patients were fatigue, chills, pyrexia, nausea, influenza-like illness, and injection site pain.

The following adverse reactions are discussed in greater detail in another section of the label:

- Herpetic Infection *[see Warnings and Precautions (5.2)]*
- Injection Site Complications *[see Warnings and Precautions (5.3)]*

6.1 Clinical Trials Experience

Because clinical trials are conducted under widely varying conditions, adverse reaction rates observed in the clinical trials of a drug cannot be directly compared to rates in the clinical trials of another drug and may not reflect the rates observed in practice.

The safety of IMLYGIC was evaluated in 419 patients who received at least 1 dose of either IMLYGIC (n = 292) or subcutaneously administered granulocyte-macrophage colony-

stimulating factor (GM-CSF) (n = 127) in an open-label, randomized clinical study of patients with stage IIIB, IIIC, and IV melanoma that was not considered to be surgically resectable *[see Clinical Studies (14)]*. The median duration of exposure to IMLYGIC was 23 weeks (5.3 months). Twenty-six patients were exposed to IMLYGIC for at least 1 year.

Most adverse reactions reported were mild or moderate in severity and generally resolved within 72 hours. The most common grade 3 or higher adverse reaction was cellulitis *[see Warnings and Precautions (5.3)]*.

Pyrexia, chills, and influenza-like illness can occur any time during IMLYGIC treatment but were more frequent during the first 3 months of treatment.

Table 4 below lists adverse reactions with a 5% or greater incidence in the IMLYGIC arm compared to the GM-CSF arm in the clinical study *[see Clinical Studies (14)]*.

[See table 4 below]

Other adverse reactions associated with IMLYGIC in the open-label, randomized study include glomerulonephritis, vitiligo, cellulitis, and oral herpes.

7 DRUG INTERACTIONS

IMLYGIC is sensitive to acyclovir. Acyclovir or other antiherpetic viral agents may interfere with the effectiveness of IMLYGIC. No drug interaction studies have been conducted with IMLYGIC.

8 USE IN SPECIFIC POPULATIONS

8.1 Pregnancy

Risk Summary

Adequate and well-controlled studies with IMLYGIC have not been conducted in pregnant women. No effects on embryo-fetal development have been observed in a study conducted in pregnant mice. The design of the study limits application of the animal data to humans *[see Data]*.

In the U.S. general population, the estimated background risk of major birth defects and miscarriage in clinically recognized pregnancies is 2-4% and 15-20%, respectively.

Clinical Considerations

If the patient becomes pregnant while taking IMLYGIC, the patient should be apprised of the potential hazards to the fetus and neonate. Women of childbearing potential should be advised to use an effective method of contraception to prevent pregnancy during treatment with IMLYGIC.

If a pregnant woman has an infection with wild-type Herpes Simplex Virus Type 1 (HSV-1) (primary or reactivation), there is potential for the virus to cross the placental barrier and also a risk of transmission during birth due to viral shedding. Infections with wild-type HSV-1 have been associated with serious adverse effects, including multi-organ failure and death, if a fetus or neonate contracts the wild-type herpes infection. While there are no clinical data to date on IMLYGIC infections in pregnant women, there could be a risk to the fetus or neonate if IMLYGIC were to act in the same manner.

Data

Animal Data

No effects on embryo-fetal development were observed when IMLYGIC was intravenously administered during organogenesis to immunocompetent pregnant mice at doses up to 4 × 10⁸ (400 million) PFU per kg (60-fold higher, on a PFU per kg basis, compared to the maximum clinical dose). Levels of IMLYGIC DNA in pooled fetal blood were at or below the assay detection level. Study design limitations included: 1) administration of IMLYGIC expressing human granulocyte-macrophage colony-stimulating factor (huGM-CSF), which is not biologically active in mice; 2) unknown transplacental kinetics of IMLYGIC following intravenous administration in pregnant mice; and 3) unknown significance of IMLYGIC dose extrapolation from animal to human based on body weight.

8.2 Lactation

Risk Summary

There is no information regarding the presence of IMLYGIC in human milk, the effects on the breastfed infant, or the effects on milk production. The developmental and health benefits of breastfeeding should be considered along with the mother's clinical need for IMLYGIC and any potential adverse effects on the breastfed infant from IMLYGIC or from the underlying maternal condition.

Clinical Considerations

Because medicinal products can be found in human milk, a decision should be made whether to discontinue nursing or to discontinue IMLYGIC while nursing.

Table 4. Adverse Reactions Reported with At Least a 5% Greater Incidence in Patients Treated with IMLYGIC Compared to GM-CSF

Adverse Reactions	IMLYGIC (n = 292)		GM-CSF (n = 127)	
	Any Grade n (%)	Grade 3 n (%)	Any Grade n (%)	Grade 3 n (%)
General disorders and administration site conditions				
Fatigue	147 (50.3)	6 (2.1)	46 (36.2)	1 (< 1)
Chills	142 (48.6)		11 (8.7)	
Pyrexia	125 (42.8)		11 (8.7)	
Influenza-like illness	89 (30.5)	2 (< 1)	19 (15.0)	
Injection site pain	81 (27.7)	2 (< 1)	8 (6.3)	
Gastrointestinal disorders				
Nausea	104 (35.6)	1 (< 1)	25 (19.7)	
Vomiting	62 (21.2)	5 (1.7)	12 (9.5)	
Diarrhea	55 (18.8)	1 (< 1)	14 (11.0)	
Constipation	34 (11.6)		8 (6.3)	1 (< 1)
Abdominal pain	26 (8.9)	2 (< 1)	3 (2.4)	
Musculoskeletal and connective tissue disorders				
Myalgia	51 (17.5)	1 (< 1)	7 (5.5)	
Arthralgia	50 (17.1)	2 (< 1)	11 (8.7)	
Pain in extremity	48 (16.4)	4 (1.4)	12 (9.5)	1 (< 1)
Nervous system disorders				
Headache	55 (18.8)	2 (< 1)	12 (9.5)	
Dizziness	28 (9.6)		4 (3.2)	
Respiratory, thoracic, and mediastinal disorders				
Oropharyngeal pain	17 (5.8)		1 (< 1)	
Investigations				
Weight decreased	17 (5.8)	1 (< 1)	1 (< 1)	

8.3   Females and Males of Reproductive Potential

No nonclinical or clinical studies were performed to evaluate the effect of IMLYGIC on fertility.

8.4   Pediatric Use

Safety and effectiveness of IMLYGIC have not been established in pediatric patients.

8.5   Geriatric Use

In clinical studies, no overall differences in safety or efficacy were observed between geriatric patients ($\geq$ 65 years old) and younger patients.

8.6   Renal Impairment

No clinical studies have been conducted to evaluate the effect of renal impairment on the pharmacokinetics of IMLYGIC.

8.7   Hepatic Impairment

No clinical studies have been conducted to evaluate the effect of hepatic impairment on the pharmacokinetics of IMLYGIC.

10   OVERDOSAGE

There is no clinical experience with an overdose with IMLYGIC. Doses up to 4 mL at dose strength of 10^8 (100 million) PFU per mL every 2 weeks (maximum cumulative dose of 222.5 $\times$ 10^8 PFU) have been administered in clinical studies, with no evidence of dose-limiting toxicity. The maximum dose of IMLYGIC that can be safely administered has not been determined. In the event of a suspected overdose, the patient should be treated symptomatically and supportive measures instituted as required *[see Warnings and Precautions (5)]*.

11   DESCRIPTION

IMLYGIC (talimogene laherparepvec) is a sterile suspension for intralesional injection. IMLYGIC is a live, attenuated HSV-1 that has been genetically modified to express huGM-CSF. The parental virus for IMLYGIC was a primary isolate, which was subsequently altered using recombinant methods to result in gene deletions and insertions.

Each vial contains 1 mL deliverable volume of IMLYGIC at either 1×10^6 (1 million) PFU per mL or 1×10^8 (100 million) PFU per mL concentrations and the following excipients: disodium hydrogen phosphate dihydrate (15.4 mg), sodium dihydrogen phosphate dihydrate (2.44 mg), sodium chloride (8.5 mg), myo-inositol (40 mg), sorbitol (20 mg), and water for injection.

The 10^6 (1 million) PFU per mL vial of IMLYGIC contains a clear to semi-translucent liquid following thaw from its frozen state. The 10^8 (100 million) PFU per mL vial of IMLYGIC contains a semi-translucent to opaque liquid following thaw from its frozen state. The liquid in each vial may contain white, visible, variously shaped, virus-containing particles.

Each vial of IMLYGIC may also contain residual components of VERO cells including DNA and protein and trace quantities of fetal bovine serum.

The product contains no preservative.

12   CLINICAL PHARMACOLOGY

12.1   Mechanism of Action

IMLYGIC has been genetically modified to replicate within tumors and to produce the immune stimulatory protein GM-CSF. IMLYGIC causes lysis of tumors, followed by release of tumor-derived antigens, which together with virally derived GM-CSF may promote an antitumor immune response. However, the exact mechanism of action is unknown.

12.3   Pharmacokinetics

Biodistribution (within the body) and Viral Shedding (excretion/secretion)

IMLYGIC viral DNA levels in various tissues and secretions were determined using a quantitative polymerase chain reaction (qPCR) assay. Infectious IMLYGIC at the injection sites and at some potential herpetic lesions was also quantified using viral infectivity assays.

Nonclinical data

Following repeat intratumoral administration in mice, IMLYGIC DNA was primarily detected in the tumor, blood, spleen, lymph node, liver, heart, and kidney. IMLYGIC DNA was not detected in bone marrow, eyes, lachrymal glands, nasal mucosa, or feces. The highest level of IMLYGIC DNA was found in the injected tumor. IMLYGIC DNA was found in the injected tumor through 84 days and in blood samples through 14 days after the last administration of IMLYGIC.

Clinical data

The biodistribution and shedding of intralesionally administered IMLYGIC are being investigated in an ongoing study measuring IMLYGIC DNA and virus in blood, oral mucosa, urine, injection site, and occlusive dressings. In the initial 20 patients with melanoma who received IMLYGIC intralesional injection at a dose and schedule similar to that of the clinical study *[see Clinical Studies (14)]*, available data indicate that IMLYGIC DNA was present in the blood in 17 (85%) patients and in urine of 4 (20%) patients during the study. The peak levels of IMLYGIC DNA in the urine were detected on the day of treatment. Infectious IMLYGIC virus was detected at the site of injection in 3 (15%) patients at a single time point each, and all within the first week after the initial injection. The exterior of the occlusive dressings was positive for IMLYGIC DNA in 14 (70%) patients during the study; however, no infectious virus was detected on the exterior of the occlusive dressing. The number of patients with measurable levels of IMLYGIC DNA on the exterior of occlusive dressings declined over time with no measurable DNA by the third treatment in 13 patients tested.

13   NONCLINICAL TOXICOLOGY

13.2   Animal Toxicology and/or Pharmacology

Repeated intratumoral administration at 2 x 10^8 (200 million) PFU per kg (30-fold maximum proposed clinical dose, extrapolated based on body weight) did not demonstrate any adverse effects in immunocompetent mice. Severe combined immunodeficient (SCID) mice administered repeat intratumoral injections of IMLYGIC at a dose of 30-fold maximum proposed clinical dose developed systemic viral infection (viral inclusion bodies or necrosis in enteric neurons in the gastrointestinal tract, adrenal gland, skin, pancreatic islet cells, eye, pineal gland, and brain).

14   CLINICAL STUDIES

The safety and efficacy of intralesional injections of IMLYGIC compared with subcutaneously administered GM-CSF was evaluated in a multicenter, open-label, randomized clinical study in patients with stage IIIB, IIIC, and IV melanoma that was considered to be not surgically resectable. IMLYGIC was injected into cutaneous, subcutaneous, or nodal melanoma lesions and was not injected into visceral lesions. Previous systemic treatment for melanoma was allowed. Patients with active cerebral metastases, bony metastases, extensive visceral disease, primary ocular or mucosal melanoma, evidence of immunosuppression, or receiving treatment with a systemic antiherpetic agent were excluded from the study.

The study included 250 (57%) men and 186 (43%) women. The mean age was 63 (range: 22 to 94) years. Most patients (98%) were white. Seventy percent (70%) of patients had baseline Eastern Cooperative Oncology Group (ECOG) performance status of zero. Seventy percent (70%) of patients had stage IV disease (27% M1a; 21% M1b; and 22% M1c), and 30% had stage III disease. Fifty-three percent (53%) of patients had received prior therapy for melanoma (other than or in addition to surgery, adjuvant therapy, or radiation), and 58% were seropositive for wild-type HSV-1 at baseline.

A total of 436 patients were randomized to receive either IMLYGIC (n = 295) or GM-CSF (n = 141). IMLYGIC was administered by intralesional injection at an initial concentration of 10^6 (1 million) PFU per mL on Day 1, followed by a concentration of 10^8 (100 million) PFU per mL on Day 21 and every 2 weeks thereafter, at a dose of up to 4 mL per visit. GM-CSF was administered subcutaneously in 28-day cycles, i.e., 125 μg/m^2 daily for 14 days followed by 14 days without GM-CSF administration.

Patients were to be treated for at least 6 months or until there were no injectable lesions. During this period, treatment could continue despite an increase in size in existing lesion(s) and/or development of new lesion(s), unless the patient developed intolerable toxicity or the investigator believed that it was in the best interest of the patient to stop treatment or to be given other therapy for melanoma. After 6 months of treatment, patients were to continue treatment until clinically relevant disease progression (i.e., disease progression associated with a decline in performance status and/or alternative therapy was required in the opinion of the investigator), up to 12 months. Patients experiencing a response at 12 months after the start of treatment could continue treatment for up to an additional 6 months, unless there were no remaining injectable lesions or disease progression. All patients were to be followed for survival status for at least 36 months.

The major efficacy outcome was durable response rate (DRR), defined as the percent of patients with complete response (CR) or partial response (PR) maintained continuously for a minimum of 6 months. Tumor responses were determined according to World Health Organization (WHO) response criteria modified to allow patients who developed new lesions or disease progression of existing lesions to continue the treatment and be evaluated later for tumor response.

The DRR was 16.3% in the IMLYGIC arm and 2.1% in the GM-CSF arm in the overall study population. The unadjusted relative risk was 7.6 (95% CI: 2.4, 24.1), with a p-value < 0.0001. The median time to response was 4.1 (range: 1.2 to 16.7) months in the IMLYGIC arm.

There was no statistically significant difference in overall survival (OS) between the IMLYGIC and the GM-CSF arms. The median OS in the overall study population was 22.9 months in the IMLYGIC arm and 19.0 months in the GM-CSF arm (p = 0.116).

16   HOW SUPPLIED/STORAGE AND HANDLING

How Supplied

- IMLYGIC is provided as a sterile frozen suspension in a single-use, cyclic olefin polymer (COP) plastic resin vial with a chlorobutyl elastomer stopper, aluminum seal, and polypropylene cap. Each vial contains a retrievable minimal volume of 1 mL.
- The vial cap is color coded:
  - 10^6 (1 million) PFU per mL is light green (NDC 55513-078-01).
  - 10^8 (100 million) PFU per mL is royal blue (NDC 55513-079-01).

Storage and Handling

- Store and transport IMLYGIC at –90°C to –70°C (–130°F to –94°F).
- Protect IMLYGIC from light.
- Store IMLYGIC in the carton until use.
- Thaw IMLYGIC immediately prior to administration *[see Dosage and Administration (2.2)]*.
- Do not draw IMLYGIC into a syringe until immediately prior to administration *[see Dosage and Administration (2.2)]*.

17   PATIENT COUNSELING INFORMATION

Advise patients and/or close contacts to:

- **Read the FDA-approved patient labeling (Medication Guide).**
- Follow instructions below to prevent viral transmission *[see Warnings and Precautions (5.1)]*:
  ○ Avoid direct contact with injection sites, dressings, or body fluids of patients.
  ○ Wear gloves when changing dressing.
  ○ Avoid touching or scratching injection sites.
  ○ Keep injection sites covered for at least the first week after each treatment visit or longer if the injection site is weeping or oozing. Replace dressing if it falls off.
  ○ Dispose of used dressings and cleaning materials in household waste in a sealed plastic bag.
- Female patients of childbearing potential should use an effective method of contraception to prevent pregnancy during treatment with IMLYGIC *[see Contraindications (4.2) and Use in Specific Populations (8.1)]*.
- Close contacts who are pregnant or immunocompromised should not change dressings or clean injection sites *[see Warnings and Precautions (5.1)]*.
- In case of accidental exposure to IMLYGIC, clean the exposed area with soap and water and/or a disinfectant. Patients or close contacts with suspected herpetic infections should contact their healthcare provider to evaluate the lesions. Suspected herpetic lesions should be reported to Amgen at 1-855-IMLYGIC (1-855-465-9442); patients or close contacts have the option of follow-up testing for further characterization of the infection *[see Warnings and Precautions (5.1) and (5.2)]*.

IMLYGIC™ (talimogene laherparepvec)

Manufactured by:
BioVex, Inc., a subsidiary of Amgen Inc.
One Amgen Center Drive
Thousand Oaks, California 91320-1799
Patent: http://pat.amgen.com/Imlygic/
© 2015 Amgen Inc. All rights reserved.
v1

Medication Guide

IMLYGIC™ (imm-LY-jik)
(talimogene laherparepvec)

Read the Medication Guide before you start treatment with IMLYGIC and before each IMLYGIC treatment. There may be new information. This Medication Guide does not tell you everything about IMLYGIC. Talk with your healthcare provider if you have any questions about treatment with IMLYGIC.

Continued on next page

What is IMLYGIC?

IMLYGIC is a prescription medicine used to treat a type of cancer called melanoma when it is on your skin or in your lymph glands. IMLYGIC is a weakened form of Herpes Simplex Virus Type 1, which is commonly called the cold sore virus. Your healthcare provider will inject IMLYGIC directly into your tumor(s).

IMLYGIC may not help you live longer and may not shrink cancer in your organs (for example, lung or liver).

Who should not get IMLYGIC?

You should not get IMLYGIC if you are pregnant or have a weakened immune system (for example, an immune deficiency, blood or bone marrow cancer, steroid use, or HIV/AIDS).

What should I tell my healthcare provider before I get IMLYGIC?

Before getting IMLYGIC, tell your healthcare provider if you:
- Are taking steroids or other medicines that suppress your immune system.
- Are taking antiviral medicines to treat or prevent herpes, such as acyclovir.
- Have or ever had medical conditions such as:
  ○ HIV infection or AIDS.
  ○ Blood or bone marrow cancer.
  ○ Autoimmune disease.
  ○ Other medical conditions that can weaken your immune system.
- Have close contact with someone who has a weakened immune system or is pregnant.
- Are pregnant or plan to become pregnant.
  ○ IMLYGIC may harm your unborn baby.
  ○ You should not become pregnant during treatment with IMLYGIC.
  ○ Talk to your healthcare provider about effective birth control methods.
- Are breastfeeding or plan to breastfeed.

Tell your healthcare provider about all the medicines you take, including prescription and over-the-counter medicines, vitamins, and herbal supplements. IMLYGIC may affect the way other medicines work and other medicines may affect how IMLYGIC works.

How is IMLYGIC given?

Your healthcare provider will inject IMLYGIC directly into your tumor(s) with a needle and syringe. You will get a second treatment 3 weeks after the first treatment. After that, you will get treatments every 2 weeks for as long as you have tumor(s). You can get treated for 6 months or longer. Your healthcare provider will decide which tumor(s) to inject and may not inject every one.

It is important to care for the treatment sites properly so that IMLYGIC does not spread to other people. Your healthcare provider will show you how to do this.

What should I avoid while getting IMLYGIC?

IMLYGIC virus can spread to other areas of your body or to your close contacts (household members, caregivers, sex partners, or persons sharing the same bed).

Do the following to avoid spreading IMLYGIC to other areas of your body or to your close contacts:
- Avoid direct contact between your treatment sites, dressings, or body fluids and close contacts (for example, use condoms when engaging in sexual activity, avoid kissing close contacts if either has an open mouth sore).
- Wear gloves while putting on or changing your dressings.
- Keep treatment sites covered with airtight and watertight dressings for at least 1 week after each treatment (or longer if the treatment site is weeping or oozing).
- If the dressing comes loose or falls off, replace it right away with a clean dressing.
- Place all used dressings and cleaning materials in a sealed plastic bag and throw them away in the garbage.
- Do not touch or scratch the treatment sites.

What are possible side effects of IMLYGIC?

The most common side effects of IMLYGIC include:
- Tiredness
- Chills
- Fever
- Nausea
- Flu-like symptoms
- Pain at treatment site

Tell your doctor right away if you get any of these signs and symptoms of herpes infection:
- Pain, burning, or tingling in a blister around the mouth or genitals or on the fingers or ears
- Eye pain, light sensitivity, discharge from the eyes, or blurry vision
- Weakness in arms or legs
- Extreme drowsiness (feeling sleepy)

- Mental confusion

If you think you have a herpes infection, inform your healthcare provider. You or your healthcare provider should call Amgen at 1-855-IMLYGIC (1-855-465-9442) for follow-up testing if needed.

These are not all the possible side effects of IMLYGIC. Your healthcare provider can give you more detailed information. Tell your healthcare provider if you have any side effects that bother you or that do not go away. You may report side effects to FDA at 1-800-FDA-1088.

What are the ingredients in IMLYGIC?

Active ingredient: talimogene laherparepvec

Inactive ingredients: di-sodium hydrogen phosphate dihydrate, sodium dihydrogen phosphate dihydrate, sodium chloride, myo-inositol, sorbitol, and water for injection

This Medication Guide summarizes the most important information about IMLYGIC. If you would like more information, talk with your healthcare provider. You can ask your healthcare provider for information about IMLYGIC that was written for healthcare professionals.

This Medication Guide has been approved by the U.S. Food and Drug Administration.

IMLYGIC™ (talimogene laherparepvec)

Manufactured by:
BioVex, Inc., a subsidiary of Amgen Inc.
One Amgen Center Drive
Thousand Oaks, California 91320-1799
Patent: http://pat.amgen.com/Imlygic/
©2015 Amgen Inc. All rights reserved.
Revised:10/2015
v1

Shown in Product Identification Guide, page 507

Concordia Pharmaceuticals Inc.
**5 CANEWOOD INDUSTRIAL PARK
ST. MICHAEL, BARBADOS
BB11005**

Phone:
1 (246) 621-1861
Fax: 1 (246) 621-1860
Email: info@concordiarx.com

DIBENZYLINE®   ℞
(phenoxybenzamine hydrochloride capsules, USP)
10 mg adrenergic, *alpha*-receptor-blocking agent

DESCRIPTION

Each Dibenzyline capsule, with red cap and body, is imprinted WPC 001 and 10 mg, and contains 10 mg of Phenoxybenzamine Hydrochloride USP. Inactive ingredients consist of D&C Red No. 33, FD&C Red No. 3, FD&C Yellow No. 6, Gelatin NF, and Lactose NF.

Dibenzyline is *N*-(2-Chloroethyl)-*N*-(1-methyl-2-phenoxyethyl)benzylamine hydrochloride:

Phenoxybenzamine hydrochloride is a colorless, crystalline powder with a molecular weight of 340.3, which melts between 136° and 141°C. It is soluble in water, alcohol and chloroform; insoluble in ether.

CLINICAL PHARMACOLOGY

Dibenzyline (phenoxybenzamine hydrochloride) is a long-acting, adrenergic, *alpha*-receptor-blocking agent, which can produce and maintain "chemical sympathectomy" by oral administration. It increases blood flow to the skin, mucosa and abdominal viscera, and lowers both supine and erect blood pressures. It has no effect on the parasympathetic system.

Twenty to 30 percent of orally administered phenoxybenzamine appears to be absorbed in the active form.[1]

The half-life of orally administered phenoxybenzamine hydrochloride is not known; however, the half-life of intravenously administered drug is approximately 24 hours. De-

monstrable effects with intravenous administration persist for at least 3 to 4 days, and the effects of daily administration are cumulative for nearly a week.[1]

INDICATION AND USAGE

Dibenzyline is indicated in the treatment of pheochromocytoma, to control episodes of hypertension and sweating. If tachycardia is excessive, it may be necessary to use a *beta*-blocking agent concomitantly.

CONTRAINDICATIONS

Conditions where a fall in blood pressure may be undesirable; hypersensitivity to the drug or any of its components.

WARNING

Dibenzyline-induced *alpha*-adrenergic blockade leaves *beta*-adrenergic receptors unopposed. Compounds that stimulate both types of receptors may, therefore, produce an exaggerated hypotensive response and tachycardia.

PRECAUTIONS

General – Administer with caution in patients with marked cerebral or coronary arteriosclerosis or renal damage. Adrenergic blocking effect may aggravate symptoms of respiratory infections.

Drug Interactions [2]

Dibenzyline (phenoxybenzamine hydrochloride) may interact with compounds that stimulate both *alpha*- and *beta*-adrenergic receptors (i.e., epinephrine) to produce an exaggerated hypotensive response and tachycardia. (See WARNING)

Dibenzyline blocks hyperthermia production by levarterenol, and blocks hypothermia production by reserpine.

Carcinogenesis and Mutagenesis

Case reports of carcinoma in humans after long-term treatment with phenoxybenzamine have been reported. Hence long-term use of phenoxybenzamine is not recommended.[3,4] Carefully weigh the benefits and risks before prescribing this drug.

Phenoxybenzamine hydrochloride showed *in vitro* mutagenic activity in the Ames test and mouse lymphoma assay; it did not show mutagenic activity *in vivo* in the micronucleus test in mice. In rats and mice, repeated intraperitoneal administration of phenoxybenzamine hydrochloride (three times per week for up to 52 weeks) resulted in peritoneal sarcomas. Chronic oral dosing in rats (for up to 2 years) produced malignant tumors of the small intestine and non-glandular stomach, as well as ulcerative and/or erosive gastritis of the glandular stomach. Whereas squamous cell carcinomas of the non-glandular stomach were observed at all tested doses of phenoxybenzamine hydrochloride, there was a no-observed-effect-level of 10 mg/kg for tumors (carcinomas and sarcomas) of the small intestine. This dose is, on a body surface area basis, about twice the maximum recommended human dosage of 20 mg b.i.d.

Pregnancy

Teratogenic Effects

Adequate reproductive studies in animals have not been performed with Dibenzyline (phenoxybenzamine hydrochloride). It is also not known whether Dibenzyline can cause fetal harm when administered to a pregnant woman. Dibenzyline should be given to a pregnant woman only if clearly needed.

Nursing Mothers

It is not known whether this drug is excreted in human milk. Because many drugs are excreted in human milk, and because of the potential for serious adverse reactions from phenoxybenzamine hydrochloride, a decision should be made whether to discontinue nursing or to discontinue the drug, taking into account the importance of the drug to the mother.

Pediatric Use

Safety and effectiveness in pediatric patients have not been established.

ADVERSE REACTIONS

The following adverse reactions have been observed, but there are insufficient data to support an estimate of their frequency.

Autonomic Nervous System*: Postural hypotension, tachycardia, inhibition of ejaculation, nasal congestion, miosis.

*These so-called "side effects" are actually evidence of adrenergic blockade and vary according to the degree of blockade.

Miscellaneous: Gastrointestinal irritation, drowsiness, fatigue.

To report SUSPECTED ADVERSE REACTIONS, contact Concordia Pharmaceuticals Inc. at 1-877-370-1142 or FDA at 1-800-FDA-1088 or www.fda.gov/medwatch.

OVERDOSAGE

SYMPTOMS – These are largely the result of blocking of the sympathetic nervous system and of the circulating epinephrine. They may include postural hypotension, resulting in dizziness or fainting; tachycardia, particularly postural; vomiting; lethargy; shock.

TREATMENT

When symptoms and signs of overdosage exist, discontinue the drug. Treatment of circulatory failure, if present, is a prime consideration. In cases of mild overdosage, recumbent position with legs elevated usually restores cerebral circulation. In the more severe cases, the usual measures to combat shock should be instituted. Usual pressor agents are *not* effective. Epinephrine is contraindicated because it stimulates both *alpha-* and *beta-* receptors; since *alpha-* receptors are blocked, the net effect of epinephrine administration is vasodilation and a further drop in blood pressure (epinephrine reversal).

The patient may have to be kept flat for 24 hours or more in the case of overdose, as the effect of the drug is prolonged. Leg bandages and an abdominal binder may shorten the period of disability.

I.V. Infusion of levarterenol bitartrate** may be used to combat severe hypotensive reactions, because it stimulates *alpha*-receptors primarily. Although Dibenzyline (phenoxybenzamine hydrochloride) is an *alpha*-adrenergic blocking agent, a sufficient dose of levarterenol bitartrate will overcome this effect.

The oral LD$_{50}$ for phenoxybenzamine hydrochloride is approximately 2000 mg/kg in rats and approximately 500 mg/kg in guinea pigs.

DOSAGE AND ADMINISTRATION

The dosage should be adjusted to fit the needs of each patient. Small initial doses should be *slowly* increased until the desired effect is obtained or the side effects from blockade become troublesome. *After each increase, the patient should be observed on that level before instituting another increase.* The dosage should be carried to a point where symptomatic relief and/or objective improvement are obtained, but not so high that the side effects from blockade become troublesome.

Initially, 10 mg of Dibenzyline (phenoxybenzamine hydrochloride) twice a day. Dosage should be increased every other day, usually to 20 to 40 mg 2 or 3 times a day, until an optimal dosage is obtained, as judged by blood pressure control.

Long-term use of phenoxybenzamine is not recommended (see PRECAUTIONS Carcinogenesis and Mutagenesis).

STORAGE

Store at 25°C (77°F); excursions permitted to 15°- 30°C (59°- 86°F) [See USP Controlled Room Temperature]. Dispense in a tight container.

HOW SUPPLIED

Dibenzyline (phenoxybenzamine hydrochloride) capsules, 10 mg, in bottles of 100 (NDC 59212-001-01).

REFERENCES

1. Weiner, N.: Drugs That Inhibit Adrenergic Nerves and Block Adrenergic Receptors, in Goodman, L., and Gilman, A., *The Pharmacological Basis of Therapeutics*, ed. 6, New York, Macmillan Publishing Co., 1980, p. 179; p. 182.
2. Martin, E.W.: *Drug Interactions Index 1978/1979*, Philadelphia, J.B. Lippincott Co., 1978, pp. 209-210.
3. Nettesheim O, Hoffken G, Gahr M, Breidert M: Haematemesis and dysphagia in a 20-year-old woman with congenital spine malformation and situs inversus partialis [German]. Zeitschrift fur Gastroenterologie. 2003; 41(4):319-24.
4. Vaidyanathan S, Mansour P, Soni BM, Hughes PL, Singh G: Chronic lymphocytic leukaemia, synchronous small cell carcinoma and squamous neoplasia of the urinary bladder in a paraplegic man following long-term phenoxybenzamine therapy. Spinal Cord. 2006;44(3):188-91.
**Available as Levophed® (brand of norepinephrine bitartrate) from Hospira Inc.
Made in Canada
©2015 Concordia Pharmaceuticals Inc.

Manufactured for
Concordia Pharmaceuticals Inc.
St. Michael, Barbados BB11005
Rev. 2_06/2016 N0702J DIB_PI
Shown in Product Identification Guide, page 507

DONNATAL®   R

(Phenobarbital, Hyoscyamine Sulfate, Atropine Sulfate, Scopolamine Hydrobromide)
Elixir
Rx Only
Revised: 08/2016

DESCRIPTION

Donnatal® Elixir - Grape
Each 5 mL (teaspoonful) of elixir (alcohol not more than 23.8%) contains:

Phenobarbital, USP ....16.2 mg
Hyoscyamine Sulfate, USP ....0.1037 mg
Atropine Sulfate, USP ....0.0194 mg
Scopolamine Hydrobromide, USP ....0.0065 mg
Inactive Ingredients
Purified Water, Glycerin, Sorbitol, Ethyl Alcohol, Sucrose, Saccharin Sodium, Artificial and Natural Grape Flavor, FD&C Red #3, and FD&C Blue #1.
Donnatal® Elixir - Mint
Each 5 mL (teaspoonful) of elixir (alcohol not more than 23.8%) contains:

Phenobarbital, USP ....16.2 mg
Hyoscyamine Sulfate, USP ....0.1037 mg
Atropine Sulfate, USP ....0.0194 mg
Scopolamine Hydrobromide, USP ....0.0065 mg
Inactive Ingredients
Purified Water, Glycerin, Sorbitol, Ethyl Alcohol, Sucrose, Saccharin Sodium, Natural Mint Flavor, FD&C Yellow #5, and FD&C Blue #1.

CLINICAL PHARMACOLOGY

This drug combination provides natural belladonna alkaloids in a specific, fixed ratio combined with phenobarbital to provide peripheral anticholinergic/antispasmodic action and mild sedation.

INDICATIONS AND USAGE

Based on a review of this drug by the National Academy of Sciences–National Research Council and/or other information, FDA has classified the indications as follows: "Possibly" effective: For use as adjunctive therapy in the treatment of irritable bowel syndrome (irritable colon, spastic colon, mucous colitis) and acute enterocolitis.
May also be useful as adjunctive therapy in the treatment of duodenal ulcer.
Final classification of the less-than-effective indications requires further investigation.
IT HAS NOT BEEN SHOWN CONCLUSIVELY WHETHER ANTICHOLINERGIC/ANTISPASMODIC DRUGS AID IN THE HEALING OF A DUODENAL ULCER, DECREASE THE RATE OF RECURRENCES OR PREVENT COMPLICATIONS.

CONTRAINDICATIONS

- glaucoma;
- obstructive uropathy (for example, bladder neck obstruction due to prostatic hypertrophy);
- obstructive disease of the gastrointestinal tract (as in achalasia, pyloroduodenal stenosis, etc.);
- paralytic ileus, intestinal atony of the elderly or debilitated patient;
- unstable cardiovascular status in acute hemorrhage;
- severe ulcerative colitis especially if complicated by toxic megacolon;
- myasthenia gravis;
- hiatal hernia associated with reflux esophagitis;
- in patients with known hypersensitivity to any of the ingredients.

Phenobarbital is contraindicated in acute intermittent porphyria and in those patients in whom phenobarbital produces restlessness and/or excitement.

WARNINGS

Donnatal® Elixir can cause fetal harm when administered to a pregnant woman. Animal reproduction studies have not been conducted with Donnatal® Elixir. If this drug is used during pregnancy, or if the patient becomes pregnant while taking this drug, the patient should be apprised of the potential hazard to the fetus.

In the presence of a high environmental temperature, heat prostration can occur with belladonna alkaloids (fever and heatstroke due to decreased sweating).
Diarrhea may be an early symptom of incomplete intestinal obstruction, especially in patients with ileostomy or colostomy. In this instance, treatment with this drug would be inappropriate and possibly harmful.
Donnatal® Elixir may produce drowsiness or blurred vision. The patient should be warned, not to engage in activities requiring mental alertness, such as operating a motor vehicle or other machinery, and not to perform hazardous work.
Phenobarbital may decrease the effect of anticoagulants, and necessitate larger doses of the anticoagulant for optimal effect. When the phenobarbital is discontinued, the dose of the anticoagulant may have to be decreased.
Phenobarbital may be habit forming and should not be administered to individuals known to be addiction prone or to those with a history of physical and/or psychological dependence upon drugs.
Since barbiturates are metabolized in the liver, they should be used with caution and initial doses should be small in patients with hepatic dysfunction.

PRECAUTIONS
General
Use with caution in patients with:
- autonomic neuropathy
- hepatic or renal disease
- hyperthyroidism
- coronary heart disease
- congestive heart failure
- cardiac arrhythmias
- tachycardia
- hypertension

Belladonna alkaloids may produce a delay in gastric emptying (antral stasis) which would complicate the management of gastric ulcer.
Do not rely on the use of the drug in the presence of complication of biliary tract disease.
Theoretically, with overdosage, a curare-like action may occur.
Donnatal® Elixir – Mint contains FD&C Yellow No. 5 (tartrazine) which may cause allergic-type reactions (including bronchial asthma) in certain susceptible persons. Although the overall incidence of FD&C Yellow No. 5 (tartrazine) sensitivity in the general population is low, it is frequently seen in patients who also have aspirin hypersensitivity.
Information for Patients
Donnatal® Elixir may produce drowsiness or blurred vision. The patient should be warned, should these occur, not to engage in activities requiring mental alertness, such as operating a motor vehicle or other machinery, and not to perform hazardous work.
Drug Interactions
Phenobarbital may decrease the effect of anticoagulants, and necessitate larger doses of the anticoagulant for optimal effect. When the phenobarbital is discontinued, the dose of the anticoagulant may have to be decreased.
Carcinogenesis, Mutagenesis, Impairment of Fertility
Long-term studies in animals have not been performed to evaluate carcinogenic potential.
Pregnancy
Pregnancy Category D
Animal reproduction studies have not been conducted with Donnatal® Elixir. There is positive evidence of human fetal risk based on adverse reaction data from investigational or marketing experience or studies in humans, but potential benefits may warrant use of the drug in pregnant women despite potential risks (*see WARNINGS*).
Nursing Mothers
It is not known whether this drug is excreted in human milk. Because many drugs are excreted in human milk, caution should be exercised when Donnatal® Elixir is administered to a nursing woman.
Geriatric Use
Elderly patients may react with symptoms of excitement, agitation, drowsiness, and other untoward manifestations to even small doses of the drug.

ADVERSE REACTIONS

Adverse reactions may include xerostomia; urinary hesitancy and retention; blurred vision; tachycardia; palpitation; mydriasis; cycloplegia; increased ocular tension; loss of taste sense; headache; nervousness; drowsiness; weakness;

Continued on next page

dizziness; insomnia; nausea; vomiting; impotence; suppression of lactation; constipation; bloated feeling; musculoskeletal pain; severe allergic reaction or drug idiosyncrasies, including anaphylaxis, urticaria, and other dermal manifestations; and decreased sweating.

Acquired hypersensitivity to barbiturates consists chiefly in allergic reactions that occur especially in persons who tend to have asthma, urticaria, angioedema, and similar conditions. Hypersensitivity reactions in this category include localized swelling, particularly of the eyelids, cheeks, or lips, and erythematous dermatitis. Rarely, exfoliative dermatitis (e.g. Stevens-Johnson syndrome and toxic epidermal necrolysis) may be caused by phenobarbital and can prove fatal. The skin eruption may be associated with fever, delirium, and marked degenerative changes in the liver and other parenchymatous organs. In a few cases, megaloblastic anemia has been associated with the chronic use of phenobarbital.

Phenobarbital may produce excitement in some patients, rather than a sedative effect.

To report SUSPECTED ADVERSE REACTIONS, contact Concordia Pharmaceuticals Inc. at 1-877-370-1142 or the FDA at 1-800-FDA-1088 or www.fda.gov/medwatch.

DRUG ABUSE AND DEPENDENCE
Abuse

Phenobarbital may be habit forming and should not be administered to individuals known to be addiction prone or to those with a history of physical and/or psychological dependence upon drugs (*see WARNINGS*).
Dependence

In patients habituated to barbiturates, abrupt withdrawal may produce delirium or convulsions.

OVERDOSAGE

The signs and symptoms of overdose are headache, nausea, vomiting, blurred vision, dilated pupils, hot and dry skin, dizziness, dryness of the mouth, difficulty in swallowing, and CNS stimulation. Treatment should consist of gastric lavage, emetics, and activated charcoal. If indicated, parenteral cholinergic agents such as physostigmine or bethanechol chloride should be used.

DOSAGE AND ADMINISTRATION

The dosage of Donnatal® Elixir should be adjusted to the needs of the individual patient to assure symptomatic control with a minimum of adverse effects.
Donnatal® Elixir. Adults: One or two teaspoonfuls of elixir three or four times a day according to conditions and severity of symptoms.
Pediatric patients: may be dosed every 4 to 6 hours. Use a pediatric dosing device or oral syringe to measure the dose.

Starting Dosage

Body weight	Every 4 hours	Every 6 hours
10 lb. (4.5 kg)	0.5 mL	0.75 mL
20 lb. (9.1 kg)	1 mL	1.5 mL
30 lb. (13.6 kg)	1.5 mL	2 mL
50 lb. (22.7 kg)	2.5 mL	3.75 mL
75 lb. (34 kg)	3.75 mL	5 mL
100 lb. (45.4 kg)	5 mL	7.5 mL

HOW SUPPLIED

Donnatal® Elixir - Grape is a purple colored, grape flavored liquid.
• 4 fl oz (118 mL) bottles- NDC 59212-423-04.
• 1 Pint (473 mL) bottles- NDC 59212-423-16.
Donnatal® Elixir - Mint is a green colored, mint flavored liquid.
• 4 fl oz (118 mL) bottles- NDC 59212-422-04.
• 1 Pint (473 mL) bottles- NDC 59212-422-16.
Avoid Freezing
Store Donnatal® Elixir at 20°- 25ºC (68º - 77ºF) [see USP Controlled Room Temperature]. Protect from light and moisture.
Dispense in a tight, light-resistant container as defined in the USP using a child-resistant closure.
Manufactured For:
Concordia Pharmaceuticals Inc.
St. Michael, Barbados BB11005
www.donnatal.com
Manufactured By:
IriSys, LLC
San Diego, CA 92121
Revised: 6_08/2016
Shown in Product Identification Guide, page 507

DONNATAL® TABLETS   ℞
(phenobarbital, hyoscyamine sulfate, atropine sulfate, scopolamine hydrobromide)
tablets
Rx Only
Revised: 3/2015

DESCRIPTION
Donnatal® Tablets
Each Donnatal® Tablet contains:
Phenobarbital, USP ....16.2 mg
Hyoscyamine Sulfate, USP ....0.1037 mg
Atropine Sulfate, USP ....0.0194 mg
Scopolamine Hydrobromide, USP ....0.0065 mg

Inactive Ingredients
Dibasic Calcium Phosphate Dihydrate, Compressible Sugar, Microcrystalline Cellulose, Sodium Starch Glycolate, Stearic Acid, Silicon Dioxide Colloidal, Magnesium Stearate.

CLINICAL PHARMACOLOGY
This drug combination provides natural belladonna alkaloids in a specific, fixed ratio combined with phenobarbital to provide peripheral anticholinergic/antispasmodic action and mild sedation.

INDICATIONS AND USAGE
Based on a review of this drug by the National Academy of Sciences–National Research Council and/or other information, FDA has classified the indications as follows: "Possibly" effective: For use as adjunctive therapy in the treatment of irritable bowel syndrome (irritable colon, spastic colon, mucous colitis) and acute enterocolitis.
May also be useful as adjunctive therapy in the treatment of duodenal ulcer.
Final classification of the less-than-effective indications requires further investigation.
IT HAS NOT BEEN SHOWN CONCLUSIVELY WHETHER ANTICHOLINERGIC/ANTISPASMODIC DRUGS AID IN THE HEALING OF A DUODENAL ULCER, DECREASE THE RATE OF RECURRENCES OR PREVENT COMPLICATIONS.

CONTRAINDICATIONS
• glaucoma;
• obstructive uropathy (for example, bladder neck obstruction due to prostatic hypertrophy);
• obstructive disease of the gastrointestinal tract (as in achalasia, pyloroduodenal stenosis, etc.);
• paralytic ileus, intestinal atony of the elderly or debilitated patient;
• unstable cardiovascular status in acute hemorrhage;
• severe ulcerative colitis especially if complicated by toxic megacolon;
• myasthenia gravis;
• hiatal hernia associated with reflux esophagitis;
• in patients with known hypersensitivity to any of the ingredients.
Phenobarbital is contraindicated in acute intermittent porphyria and in those patients in whom phenobarbital produces restlessness and/or excitement.

WARNINGS
Donnatal® Tablets can cause fetal harm when administered to a pregnant woman. Animal reproduction studies have not been conducted with Donnatal® Tablets. If this drug is used during pregnancy, or if the patient becomes pregnant while taking this drug, the patient should be apprised of the potential hazard to the fetus.
In the presence of a high environmental temperature, heat prostration can occur with belladonna alkaloids (fever and heatstroke due to decreased sweating).
Diarrhea may be an early symptom of incomplete intestinal obstruction, especially in patients with ileostomy or colostomy. In this instance, treatment with this drug would be inappropriate and possibly harmful.
Donnatal® Tablets may produce drowsiness or blurred vision. The patient should be warned, should these occur, not to engage in activities requiring mental alertness, such as operating a motor vehicle or other machinery, and not to perform hazardous work.
Phenobarbital may decrease the effect of anticoagulants, and necessitate larger doses of the anticoagulant for optimal effect. When the phenobarbital is discontinued, the dose of the anticoagulant may have to be decreased.

Phenobarbital may be habit forming and should not be administered to individuals known to be addiction prone or to those with a history of physical and/or psychological dependence upon drugs.
Since barbiturates are metabolized in the liver, they should be used with caution and initial doses should be small in patients with hepatic dysfunction.

PRECAUTIONS
General
Use with caution in patients with:
• autonomic neuropathy
• hepatic or renal disease
• hyperthyroidism
• coronary heart disease
• congestive heart failure
• cardiac arrhythmias
• tachycardia
• hypertension
Belladonna alkaloids may produce a delay in gastric emptying (antral stasis) which would complicate the management of gastric ulcer.
Do not rely on the use of the drug in the presence of complication of biliary tract disease.
Theoretically, with overdosage, a curare-like action may occur.
Information for Patients
Donnatal® Tablets may produce drowsiness or blurred vision. The patient should be warned, should these occur, not to engage in activities requiring mental alertness, such as operating a motor vehicle or other machinery, and not to perform hazardous work.
Drug Interactions
Phenobarbital may decrease the effect of anticoagulants, and necessitate larger doses of the anticoagulant for optimal effect. When the phenobarbital is discontinued, the dose of the anticoagulant may have to be decreased.
Carcinogenesis, Mutagenesis, Impairment of Fertility
Long-term studies in animals have not been performed to evaluate carcinogenic potential.
Pregnancy
Pregnancy Category D
Animal reproduction studies have not been conducted with Donnatal® Tablets. There is positive evidence of human fetal risk based on adverse reaction data from investigational or marketing experience or studies in humans, but potential benefits may warrant use of the drug in pregnant women despite potential risks (*see WARNINGS*).
Nursing Mothers
It is not known whether this drug is excreted in human milk. Because many drugs are excreted in human milk, caution should be exercised when Donnatal® Tablets are administered to a nursing woman.
Geriatric Use
Elderly patients may react with symptoms of excitement, agitation, drowsiness, and other untoward manifestations to even small doses of the drug.

ADVERSE REACTIONS
Adverse reactions may include xerostomia; urinary hesitancy and retention; blurred vision; tachycardia; palpitation; mydriasis; cycloplegia; increased ocular tension; loss of taste sense; headache; nervousness; drowsiness; weakness; dizziness; insomnia; nausea; vomiting; impotence; suppression of lactation; constipation; bloated feeling; musculoskeletal pain; severe allergic reaction or drug idiosyncrasies, including anaphylaxis, urticaria, and other dermal manifestations; and decreased sweating.

Acquired hypersensitivity to barbiturates consists chiefly in allergic reactions that occur especially in persons who tend to have asthma, urticaria, angioedema, and similar conditions. Hypersensitivity reactions in this category include localized swelling, particularly of the eyelids, cheeks, or lips, and erythematous dermatitis. Rarely, exfoliative dermatitis (e.g. Stevens-Johnson syndrome and toxic epidermal necrolysis) may be caused by phenobarbital and can prove fatal. The skin eruption may be associated with fever, delirium, and marked degenerative changes in the liver and other parenchymatous organs. In a few cases, megaloblastic anemia has been associated with the chronic use of phenobarbital.

Phenobarbital may produce excitement in some patients, rather than a sedative effect.

To report SUSPECTED ADVERSE REACTIONS, contact Concordia Pharmaceuticals Inc. at 1-877-370-1142 or the FDA at 1-800-FDA-1088 or www.fda.gov/medwatch.

DRUG ABUSE AND DEPENDENCE

Abuse

Phenobarbital may be habit forming and should not be administered to individuals known to be addiction prone or to those with a history of physical and/or psychological dependence upon drugs (*see WARNINGS*).

Dependence

In patients habituated to barbiturates, abrupt withdrawal may produce delirium or convulsions.

OVERDOSAGE

The signs and symptoms of overdose are headache, nausea, vomiting, blurred vision, dilated pupils, hot and dry skin, dizziness, dryness of the mouth, difficulty in swallowing, and CNS stimulation. Treatment should consist of gastric lavage, emetics, and activated charcoal. If indicated, parenteral cholinergic agents such as physostigmine or bethanechol chloride should be used.

DOSAGE AND ADMINISTRATION

The dosage of Donnatal® Tablets should be adjusted to the needs of the individual patient to assure symptomatic control with a minimum of adverse effects.

Donnatal® Tablets - Adults: One or two Donnatal® Tablets three or four times a day according to condition and severity of symptoms.

HOW SUPPLIED

Donnatal® Tablets are supplied as: white, D-shaped, flat faced beveled edge tablets debossed "D" on one side and "Donnatal" on the other side.

- Bottles of 100 tablets - NDC 59212-425-10.
- Bottles of 1000 tablets - NDC 59212-425-11.
- Bottles of 4 tablets - NDC 59212-425-04.

Store at 20°-25°C (68°-77°F) [See USP Controlled Room Temperature]. Protect from light and moisture.

Dispense in a tight, light-resistant container as defined in the USP using a child-resistant closure.

Manufactured For:
Concordia Pharmaceuticals Inc.
St. Michael, Barbados BB11005
www.donnatal.com
Manufactured By:
IriSys, LLC
San Diego, CA 92121
Revised: 3/15

Shown in Product Identification Guide, page 507

DUTOPROL   ℞
(metoprolol succinate extended release/hydrochlorothiazide) tablets, for oral use

HIGHLIGHTS OF PRESCRIBING INFORMATION

These highlights do not include all the information needed to use DUTOPROL safely and effectively. See full prescribing information for DUTOPROL.

DUTOPROL® (metoprolol succinate extended release/hydrochlorothiazide) tablets, for oral use
Initial U.S. Approval: 2006

WARNING: CARDIAC ISCHEMIA AFTER ABRUPT DISCONTINUATION

See full prescribing information for complete boxed warning.

Following abrupt cessation of therapy with beta-blockers, exacerbations of angina pectoris and myocardial infarction have occurred. Warn patients against interruption or discontinuation of therapy without the physician's advice (5.1)

————INDICATIONS AND USAGE————

DUTOPROL is the combination tablet of metoprolol succinate, a beta adrenoceptor blocker and hydrochlorothiazide (HCTZ), a thiazide diuretic, indicated for the treatment of hypertension, to lower blood pressure. Lowering blood pressure reduces the risk of fatal and nonfatal cardiovascular events, primarily strokes and myocardial infarctions. (1)

————DOSAGE AND ADMINISTRATION————

- Usual dose range: Hydrochlorothiazide 12.5 to 25 mg and metoprolol succinate 25 to 200 mg dosed once daily. (2.1)

————DOSAGE FORMS AND STRENGTHS————

Tablets (metoprolol succinate/HCTZ mg): 25/12.5 mg, 50/12.5 mg, 100/12.5 mg. (3)

————CONTRAINDICATIONS————

- Hypersensitivity to metoprolol succinate or hydrochlorothiazide or other sulfonamide-derived drugs. (4)
- Cardiogenic shock or decompensated heart failure. (4)
- Sinus bradycardia, sick sinus syndrome, and greater than first-degree block unless a permanent pacemaker is in place. (4)
- Anuria. (4)

————WARNINGS AND PRECAUTIONS————

- May worsen congestive heart failure. (5.2)
- Bronchospasm: Avoid beta-blockers. (5.3)
- Bradycardia. (5.4)
- Avoid discontinuing therapy prior to major surgery. (5.5)
- May mask symptoms of hypoglycemia. (5.6)
- Monitor serum electrolytes and creatinine periodically. (5.7)
- Peripheral vascular disease: Can aggravate symptoms of arterial insufficiency. (5.9)

————ADVERSE REACTIONS————

Adverse events which occurred greater than 1% more frequently in patients treated with DUTOPROL than placebo were: nasopharyngitis and fatigue. (6.1)

To report SUSPECTED ADVERSE REACTIONS, contact Concordia Pharmaceuticals Inc. at 1-877-370-1142 or FDA at 1-800-FDA-1088 or www.fda.gov/medwatch.

————DRUG INTERACTIONS————

- Catecholamine-depleting drugs (e.g., MAO inhibitors): Hypotension, bradycardia. (7.1)
- CYP2D6 inhibitors: Increased metoprolol concentration. (12.3)
- Digitalis glycosides, clonidine, diltiazem and verapamil: Bradycardia. (5.4, 7.1)
- Clonidine: Rebound hypertension following clonidine withdrawal. (7.1)
- Antidiabetic drugs: Dosage adjustment may be required. (7.2)
- Cholestyramine and colestipol: Reduced absorption of thiazides. (7.2)
- Lithium: Risk of lithium toxicity. (7.2)
- Non-Steroidal Anti-Inflammatory Drugs (NSAIDs): Reduced diuretic, natriuretic, and antihypertensive effects of diuretics. (7.2)

————USE IN SPECIFIC POPULATIONS————

- Nursing Mothers: Consider possible infant exposure. (8.3)

See 17 for PATIENT COUNSELING INFORMATION.

Revised: 6/2015

FULL PRESCRIBING INFORMATION: CONTENTS*

WARNING: CARDIAC ISCHEMIA AFTER ABRUPT DISCONTINUATION

FULL PRESCRIBING INFORMATION

WARNING: CARDIAC ISCHEMIA AFTER ABRUPT DISCONTINUATION

Following abrupt discontinuation of therapy with beta adrenergic blockers, exacerbations of angina pectoris and myocardial infarction have occurred.

When discontinuing chronically administered DUTOPROL, particularly in patients with ischemic heart disease, gradually reduce the dose over a period of 1–2 weeks and monitor the patient. If angina markedly worsens or acute coronary insufficiency develops, promptly resume therapy, at least temporarily, and take other measures appropriate for the management of unstable angina. Warn patients against interruption or discontinuation of therapy without the physician's advice.

Because coronary artery disease is common and may be unrecognized, avoid abrupt discontinuation of DUTOPROL therapy even in patients treated only for hypertension [see Warnings and Precautions (5.1)].

---

1   INDICATIONS AND USAGE

DUTOPROL (metoprolol succinate extended release and hydrochlorothiazide) is a combination tablet of metoprolol succinate, a beta adrenoceptor blocking agent and hydrochlorothiazide, a diuretic. DUTOPROL is indicated for the treatment of hypertension, to lower blood pressure. Lowering blood pressure lowers the risk of fatal and non-fatal cardiovascular (CV) events, primarily strokes and myocardial infarction. These benefits have been seen in controlled trials of antihypertensive drugs from a wide variety of pharmacologic classes including metoprolol and hydrochlorothiazide. Control of high blood pressure should be part of comprehensive cardiovascular risk management, including, as appropriate, lipid control, diabetes management, antithrombotic therapy, smoking cessation, exercise, and limited sodium intake. Many patients will require more than 1 drug to achieve blood pressure goals. For specific advice on goals and management, see published guidelines, such as those of the National High Blood Pressure Education Program's Joint National Committee on Prevention, Detection, Evaluation, and Treatment of High Blood Pressure (JNC).

Numerous antihypertensive drugs, from a variety of pharmacologic classes and with different mechanisms of action, have been shown in randomized controlled trials to reduce cardiovascular morbidity and mortality, and it can be concluded that it is blood pressure reduction, and not some other pharmacologic property of the drugs, that is largely responsible for those benefits. The largest and most consistent cardiovascular outcome benefit has been a reduction in the risk of stroke, but reductions in myocardial infarction and cardiovascular mortality also have been seen regularly.

Elevated systolic or diastolic pressure causes increased cardiovascular risk, and the absolute risk increase per mmHg

Continued on next page

is greater at higher blood pressures, so that even modest reductions of severe hypertension can provide substantial benefit. Relative risk reduction from blood pressure reduction is similar across populations with varying absolute risk, so the absolute benefit is greater in patients who are at higher risk independent of their hypertension (for example, patients with diabetes or hyperlipidemia), and such patients would be expected to benefit from more aggressive treatment to a lower blood pressure goal.

Some antihypertensive drugs have smaller blood pressure effects (as monotherapy) in black patients, and many antihypertensive drugs have additional approved indications and effects (e.g., on angina, heart failure, or diabetic kidney disease). These considerations may guide selection of therapy.

DUTOPROL may be administered with other antihypertensive agents.

2   DOSAGE AND ADMINISTRATION
2.1   Dosing Information
The recommended starting dose of DUTOPROL (metoprolol succinate extended release and hydrochlorothiazide) is 25 mg/12.5 mg taken orally once daily with or without food. Depending on the blood pressure response, the dose may be titrated at intervals of 2 weeks to a maximum recommended dose of 200 mg/25 mg (two DUTOPROL 100 mg/12.5 mg tablets) once daily *[see Clinical Studies (14).]*

For specific advice on blood pressure goals, see published guidelines, such as those of the National High Blood Pressure Education Program's Joint National Committee on Prevention, Detection, Evaluation, and Treatment of High Blood Pressure (JNC).

2.2   Use with and Switching from other Anti-Hypertensive Drugs
DUTOPROL may be administered with other antihypertensive drugs. Patients titrated to the individual components (metoprolol succinate and hydrochlorothiazide) may instead receive the corresponding dose of DUTOPROL.

A patient whose blood pressure is inadequately controlled by metoprolol succinate alone or hydrochlorothiazide alone may be switched to DUTOPROL.

3   DOSAGE FORMS AND STRENGTHS
25/12.5 mg tablets: Yellow, circular, biconvex, film-coated tablet engraved with "A" above "IH" on one side.

50/12.5 mg tablets: Light orange, circular, biconvex, film-coated tablet engraved with "A" above "IK" on one side.

100/12.5 mg tablets: Yellow, circular, biconvex, film-coated tablet engraved with "A" above "IL" on one side and scored on the other side.

4   CONTRAINDICATIONS
DUTOPROL is contraindicated in patients with:
• Cardiogenic shock or decompensated heart failure.
• Sinus bradycardia, sick sinus syndrome, and greater than first-degree block unless a permanent pacemaker is in place.
• Anuria
• Hypersensitivity to metoprolol succinate or hydrochlorothiazide or to other sulfonamide-derived drugs.

5   WARNINGS AND PRECAUTIONS
5.1   Cardiac Ischemia after Abrupt Discontinuation
Following abrupt cessation of therapy with beta adrenergic blockers, exacerbations of angina pectoris and myocardial infarction may occur. When discontinuing chronically administered DUTOPROL, particularly in patients with ischemic heart disease, gradually reduce the dosage over a period of 1–2 weeks and monitor the patient. If angina markedly worsens or acute coronary ischemia develops, promptly resume therapy and take measures appropriate for the management of unstable angina. Warn patients not to interrupt therapy without their physician's advice. Because coronary artery disease is common and may be unrecognized, avoid abrupt discontinuation of DUTOPROL in patients treated only for hypertension.

5.2   Heart Failure
Worsening cardiac failure may occur during up-titration of beta-blockers. If such symptoms occur, increase diuretics and restore clinical stability (compensated heart failure) before advancing the dose of DUTOPROL *[see Dosage and Administration (2)]*. It may be necessary to lower the dose of DUTOPROL or temporarily discontinue it *[see Boxed Warning.]* Such episodes do not preclude subsequent successful titration of DUTOPROL.

5.3   Bronchospasm
Beta adrenergic blockers can cause bronchospasm. Patients with bronchospastic disease should, in general, not receive beta adrenergic blockers. Because of its relative beta$_1$ cardio-selectivity, however, metoprolol-containing products including DUTOPROL may be used in patients with bronchospastic disease who do not respond to or cannot tolerate other antihypertensive treatment. Because beta$_1$-selectivity is not absolute, in such patients use the lowest possible DUTOPROL dose and have bronchodilators (e.g., beta$_2$-agonists) readily available or administer concomitantly.

5.4   Bradycardia
Bradycardia, including sinus pause, heart block, and cardiac arrest have occurred with the use of Dutoprol. Patients with first-degree atrioventricular block, sinus node dysfunction, or conduction disorders (including Wolff-Parkinson-White) may be at increased risk. The concomitant use of beta adrenergic blockers and non-dihydropyridine calcium channel blockers (e.g., verapamil and diltiazem), digoxin or clonidine increases the risk of significant bradycardia. Monitor heart rate and rhythm in patients receiving Dutoprol. If severe bradycardia develops, reduce or stop Dutoprol.

5.5   Risks of Use in Major Surgery
Avoid initiation of high-dose regimen of DUTOPROL in patients with cardiovascular risk factors undergoing non-cardiac surgery, since use in such patients has been associated with bradycardia, hypotension, stroke and death. Chronically administered beta adrenergic blockers should not be routinely withdrawn prior to major surgery; however, the impaired ability of the heart to respond to reflex adrenergic stimuli may augment the risks of general anesthesia and surgical procedures *[see Warnings and Precautions (5.1)]*.

5.6   Masked Signs of Hypoglycemia
Beta adrenergic blockers may mask tachycardia occurring with hypoglycemia, but other manifestations such as dizziness and sweating may not be significantly affected.

5.7   Electrolyte and Metabolic Effects
DUTOPROL contains hydrochlorothiazide which can cause hypokalemia and hyponatremia. Hypomagnesemia can result in hypokalemia which may be difficult to treat despite potassium repletion. Monitor serum electrolytes periodically.

Hydrochlorothiazide may alter glucose tolerance and raise serum levels of cholesterol and triglycerides.

Hydrochlorothiazide reduces clearance of uric acid and may cause or exacerbate hyperuricemia and precipitate gout in susceptible patients.

Hydrochlorothiazide decreases urinary calcium excretion and may cause elevations of serum calcium. Monitor calcium levels.

5.8   Renal Impairment
Patients with chronic kidney disease, severe heart failure, or volume depletion may be at increased risk for developing acute renal failure on drugs containing hydrochlorothiazide, including DUTOPROL.

5.9   Exacerbated Symptoms of Peripheral Vascular Disease
Beta adrenergic blockers can precipitate or aggravate symptoms of arterial insufficiency in patients with peripheral vascular disease.

5.10   Increased Blood Pressure in Patients with Pheochromocytoma
Administration of beta adrenergic blockers alone in patients with pheochromocytoma has been associated with a paradoxical increase in blood pressure because of the attenuation of beta-mediated vasodilatation in skeletal muscle. If DUTOPROL is used in patients with pheochromocytoma, first initiate an alpha-blocker.

5.11   Thyrotoxicosis after Discontinuation in Patients with Hyperthyroidism
Beta adrenergic blockers may mask certain clinical signs of hyperthyroidism, such as tachycardia. Abrupt withdrawal of a beta adrenergic blocker may precipitate a thyroid storm. Therefore, in patients with hyperthyroidism discontinue DUTOPROL gradually.

5.12   Reduced Effectiveness of Epinephrine in Treating Anaphylaxis
Beta adrenergic blocker- treated patients treated with epinephrine for a severe anaphylactic reaction may be less responsive to the typical doses of epinephrine. In these patients, consider other medications.

5.13   Acute Myopia and Secondary Angle-Closure Glaucoma
Hydrochlorothiazide, a sulfonamide, can cause acute transient myopia and acute angle-closure glaucoma (idiosyncratic reactions). Symptoms include acute onset of decreased visual acuity or ocular pain and typically occur within hours to weeks of hydrochlorothiazide initiation.

Risk factors for developing acute angle-closure glaucoma may include a history of sulfonamide or penicillin allergy.

Untreated acute angle-closure glaucoma can lead to permanent vision loss. Given that DUTOPROL contains hydrochlorothiazide, if these symptoms occur, discontinue DUTOPROL. Consider prompt medical or surgical treatment if the intraocular pressure remains uncontrolled.

5.14   Exacerbation of Systemic Lupus Erythematosus
Hydrochlorothiazide can exacerbate or activate systemic lupus erythematosus.

6   ADVERSE REACTIONS
6.1   Clinical Trials Experience
Because clinical trials are conducted under widely varying conditions, adverse reaction rates observed in the clinical trials of a drug cannot be directly compared to rates in the clinical trials of another drug and may not reflect the rates observed in practice. The adverse reaction information from clinical trials does, however, provide a basis for identifying the adverse events that appear to be related to drug use and for approximating rates.

Metoprolol   succinate   extended   release/ hydrochlorothiazide

The metoprolol succinate extended release and hydrochlorothiazide combination was evaluated for safety in 891 patients with hypertension in clinical trials. In a randomized, double-blind, placebo-controlled, factorial trial (Study 1), 843 patients were treated with various combinations of metoprolol succinate (doses of 25 to 200 mg) and hydrochlorothiazide (doses of 6.25 to 25 mg) *[see Clinical Studies (14)]*. Adverse events which occurred more than 1% more frequently in patients treated with DUTOPROL than placebo were: nasopharyngitis (3.4% vs 1.3%) and fatigue (2.6% vs 0.7%).

The adverse reactions of metoprolol succinate extended release are a mixture of dose-dependent phenomena (primarily bradycardia and fatigue) and those of hydrochlorothiazide are a mixture of dose-dependent (primarily hypokalemia) and dose independent phenomena (e.g., pancreatitis), the former much more common than the latter. Therapy with DUTOPROL will be associated with both sets of dose independent reactions.

Laboratory Abnormalities
Liver Enzyme Tests—Increases in liver enzymes or serum bilirubin.

6.2   Post-Marketing Experience
The following adverse reactions have been identified during post-approval use of DUTOPROL, metoprolol succinate extended release, and/or hydrochlorothiazide. Because these reactions are reported voluntarily from a population of uncertain size, it is not always possible to estimate their frequency reliably or establish a causal relationship to drug exposure.

Metoprolol
The following adverse reactions have been reported for immediate release metoprolol tartrate. Most adverse reactions have been mild and transient.

Central Nervous System: Confusion, short-term memory loss, headache, somnolence, nightmares, insomnia, anxiety/nervousness, hallucinations, paresthesia, dizziness

Cardiovascular: Shortness of breath, bradycardia, cold extremities; arterial insufficiency (usually of the Raynaud type), palpitations, peripheral edema, syncope, chest pain

Respiratory: Dyspnea

Gastrointestinal: Diarrhea, nausea, dry mouth, gastric pain, constipation, flatulence, heartburn, hepatitis, vomiting.

Hypersensitivity Reactions: Pruritus, rash

Miscellaneous: Musculoskeletal pain, arthralgia, blurred vision, decreased libido, male impotence, tinnitus, reversible alopecia, dry eyes, worsening of psoriasis, Peyronie's disease, sweating, photosensitivity, taste disturbance, depression

Other Beta-Adrenergic Blockers
In addition, adverse reactions not listed above, that have been reported with other beta-adrenoceptor blockers and should be considered potential adverse reactions to DUTOPROL.

Central Nervous System: Reversible mental depression progressing to catatonia; an acute reversible syndrome characterized by disorientation for time and place, emotional lability, clouded sensorium, and decreased performance on neuropsychometrics.

Hematologic: Non-thrombocytopenic purpura, thrombocytopenic purpura

Hypersensitivity Reactions: Laryngospasm, and respiratory distress

Hydrochlorothiazide

Adverse reactions that have been reported with hydrochlorothiazide are listed below:

Body as a Whole: Weakness

Cardiovascular: Orthostatic hypotension

Digestive: Pancreatitis, jaundice (intrahepatic cholestatic jaundice), sialadenitis, cramping, gastric irritation, anorexia

Hematologic: Aplastic anemia, agranulocytosis, leukopenia, hemolytic anemia, thrombocytopenia

Hypersensitivity Reactions: Anaphylactic reactions, necrotizing angiitis (vasculitis and cutaneous vasculitis), respiratory distress including pneumonitis and pulmonary edema, photosensitivity, fever, urticaria

Metabolic: Glycosuria

Musculoskeletal: Muscle spasm

Nervous System/Psychiatric: Vertigo, paresthesias, restlessness

Renal: Interstitial nephritis

Skin: Erythema multiforme including Stevens-Johnson syndrome, exfoliative dermatitis including toxic epidermal necrolysis

Special Senses: Transient blurred vision, xanthopsia

7 DRUG INTERACTIONS

7.1 Drug Interactions with Metoprolol

Reserpine, monoamine oxidase (MAO) inhibitors: The concomitant use of catecholamine-depleting drugs (e.g., reserpine, monoamine oxidase (MAO) inhibitors) with beta adrenergic blockers may have an additive affect and increase the risk of hypotension or bradycardia. Observe patients treated with DUTOPROL plus a catecholamine depletor for evidence of hypotension or marked bradycardia, which may produce vertigo, syncope, or postural hypotension.

CYP2D6 Inhibitors: Drugs that inhibit CYP2D6 such as quinidine, fluoxetine, paroxetine, and propafenone are likely to increase metoprolol concentration *[see Clinical Pharmacology (12.3)].*

Nondihydropyridine Calcium Channel Blockers: *[See Warnings and Precautions (5.4)].*

Digoxin: Digitalis glycosides slow atrioventricular conduction and decrease heart rate. Concomitant use of digoxin with beta adrenergic blockers increases the risk of bradycardia.

Clonidine: Clonidine slows conduction and decrease heart rate. Concomitant use with beta adrenergic blockers increases the risk of bradycardia. If clonidine and DUTOPROL are to both be discontinued, withdraw DUTOPROL several days before the gradual withdrawal of clonidine to reduce the risk of rebound hypertension following the clonidine withdrawal. If a patient is to switch from clonidine to DUTOPROL, delay the introduction of DUTOPROL for several days after discontinuation of clonidine.

Epinephrine: *[See Warnings and Precautions (5.12)].*

7.2 Drug Interactions with Hydrochlorothiazide

Antidiabetic drugs (oral agents and insulin): Dosage adjustment of the antidiabetic drug may be required.

Ion exchange resins: Absorption of hydrochlorothiazide is impaired in the presence of anionic exchange resins. Single doses of either cholestyramine or colestipol resins bind the hydrochlorothiazide and reduce its absorption from the gastrointestinal tract by up to 85% and 43%, respectively. Stagger the dosage of hydrochlorothiazide and ion exchange resins (e.g., cholestyramine and colestipol resins) such that hydrochlorothiazide is administered at least 4 hours before or 4-6 hours after the administration of resins to minimize the interaction.

Lithium: Diuretics reduce the renal clearance of lithium and increase the risk of lithium toxicity. Monitor serum lithium concentrations during concurrent use.

Non-Steroidal Anti-Inflammatory Drugs: NSAIDs can reduce the diuretic, natriuretic, and antihypertensive effects of thiazide diuretics.

8 USE IN SPECIFIC POPULATIONS

8.1 Pregnancy

Pregnancy Category C

Metoprolol/Hydrochlorothiazide

Oral administration of metoprolol tartrate/hydrochlorothiazide combinations to pregnant rats during organogenesis at doses up to 200/50 mg/kg/day (10 and 20 times the MRHD for metoprolol and hydrochlorothiazide, respectively) or to pregnant rabbits at doses up to 25/6.25 mg/kg/day (about 2.5 and 5 times the MRHD for metoprolol and hydrochlorothiazide, respectively) produced no teratogenic effects. A 200/50 mg/kg/day metoprolol tartrate/hydrochlorothiazide combination administered to rats from mid-late gestation through lactation produced increased post-implantation loss and decreased neonatal survival.

Metoprolol

There are no adequate and well-controlled studies of metoprolol in pregnant women. Metoprolol tartrate has been shown to increase post-implantation loss and decrease neonatal survival in rats at doses up to 22 times, on a mg/m^2 basis, the daily dose of 200 mg in a 60-kg patient. Distribution studies in mice confirm exposure of the fetus when metoprolol tartrate is administered to the pregnant animal. These studies have revealed no evidence of impaired fertility or teratogenicity. Because animal reproduction studies are not always predictive of human response, use this drug during pregnancy only if clearly needed.

Hydrochlorothiazide

The use of thiazide diuretics in pregnant women requires that the anticipated benefit be weighed against possible hazards to the fetus. These hazards include fetal or neonatal jaundice, pancreatitis, thrombocytopenia, and possibly other adverse reactions, which have occurred in the adult. Hydrochlorothiazide administered to pregnant mice and rats during organogenesis at doses up to 3000 and 1000 mg/kg/day (600 and 400 times the MRHD), respectively, produced no harm to the fetus. Thiazides cross the placental barrier and appear in the cord blood.

8.3 Nursing Mothers

Metoprolol is excreted in breast milk in very small quantities. An infant consuming 1 liter of breast milk daily would receive a dose of less than 1 mg of metoprolol. Thiazide diurectics appear in human milk. Consider possible infant exposure when DUTOPROL is administered to a nursing woman.

8.4 Pediatric Use

Safety and effectiveness in pediatric patients have not been established.

8.5 Geriatric Use

Of the 849 subjects randomized to treatment with both metoprolol succinate extended release and hydrochlorothiazide in a factorial clinical study, 129 (15%) were 65 and over, while 16 (2%) were 75 and over. No overall differences in safety or effectiveness were observed between these subjects and younger subjects. Greater sensitivity of some older individuals cannot be ruled out. In addition, patients 70 to 84 years of age were studied in two clinical outcome trials (n=3025), which included a treatment regimen of a thiazide diuretic or beta adrenergic blocker (metoprolol succinate extended release, atenolol or pindolol) or their combination have not identified differences in responses between the elderly and younger patients.

Hydrochlorothiazide is known to be substantially excreted by the kidney, and the risk of toxic reactions to this drug may be greater in patients with impaired renal function.

8.6 Use in Patients with Hepatic Impairment

Hydrochlorothiazide

Minor alterations of fluid and electrolyte balance may precipitate hepatic coma in patients with impaired hepatic function or progressive liver disease.

8.7 Use in Patients with Renal Impairment

Safety and effectiveness of DUTOPROL in patients with severe renal impairment (CrCL≤30 ml/min) have not been established. No dose adjustment is required in patients with moderate renal impairment (CrCL 30-60 ml/min).

10 OVERDOSAGE

10.1 Signs and Symptoms

The most frequently observed signs expected with overdosage of a beta adrenergic blocker are bradycardia and bradyarrhythmia, hypotension, heart failure, cardiac conduction disturbances and bronchospasm.

With thiazide diuretics, acute intoxication is rare. The most prominent feature of overdose is acute loss of fluid, electrolytes and magnesium. Signs and symptoms of overdose may include hypotension, dizziness, muscle cramps, renal impairment or failure, and sedation/impairment of consciousness. Altered laboratory findings can also occur (e.g. hypokalemia, hypomagnesaemia, hyponatremia, hypochloremia, alkalosis, increased BUN).

10.2 Management

Care should be provided at a facility that can provide appropriate supporting measures, monitoring and supervision as treatment is symptomatic and supportive and there is no specific antidote. Limited data suggest that neither metoprolol nor hydrochlorothiazide is dialyzable. If justified, gastric lavage and/or activated charcoal can be administered.

Based on the expected pharmacologic actions and recommendations for other beta adrenergic blockers and hydrochlorothiazide, the following measures should be considered when clinically warranted.

Bradycardia and conduction disturbances: Use atropine, adrenergic-stimulating drugs or pacemaker.

Hypotension, acute heart failure, and shock: Treat with suitable volume expansion, injection of glucagon (if necessary, followed by an intravenous infusion of glucagon), intravenous administration of adrenergic drugs such as dobutamine, with α_1 receptor agonist drugs added in the presence of vasodilation.

Bronchospasm: Can usually be reversed by bronchodilators.

11 DESCRIPTION

DUTOPROL® (metoprolol succinate extended release/hydrochlorothiazide) combines a beta adrenoceptor blocker and a thiazide diuretic.

Metoprolol succinate is chemically described as (±)1-(isopropylamino)-3-[p-(2-methoxyethyl) phenoxy]-2-propanol succinate (2:1) (salt). Its structural formula is:

Metoprolol succinate is a white crystalline powder with a molecular weight of 652.8. It is freely soluble in water, soluble in methanol, sparingly soluble in ethanol, slightly soluble in dichloromethane and 2-propanol, and practically insoluble in ethyl-acetate, acetone, diethylether and heptane. Hydrochlorothiazide is 6-chloro-3,4-dihydro-2H-1,2,4-benzothiadiazine-7-sulfonamide 1,1-dioxide. Its empirical formula is $C_7H_8ClN_3O_4S_2$ and its structural formula is:

Hydrochlorothiazide is a white, or practically white, crystalline powder with a molecular weight of 297.74, which is slightly soluble in water, but freely soluble in sodium hydroxide solution.

DUTOPROL is for oral administration supplied in 3 tablet strengths of metoprolol succinate extended release and hydrochlorothiazide.

DUTOPROL 25/12.5 contains 23.75 mg of metoprolol succinate extended release, equivalent to 25 mg of metoprolol tartrate and 12.5 mg of hydrochlorothiazide. DUTOPROL 50/12.5 contains 47.5 mg of metoprolol succinate extended release, equivalent to 50 mg of metoprolol tartrate, and 12.5 mg of hydrochlorothiazide. DUTOPROL 100/12.5 contains 95 mg of metoprolol succinate extended release, equivalent to 100 mg of metoprolol tartrate, and 12.5 mg of hydrochlorothiazide. The inactive ingredients of the tablets are silicon dioxide, ethylcellulose, hydroxypropyl cellulose, cornstarch, microcrystalline cellulose, polyvinyl pyrrolidone, sodium stearyl fumarate, hydroxypropyl methylcellulose, polyethylene glycol 6000, titanium dioxide, iron oxide (yellow), iron oxide (red) and paraffin.

12 CLINICAL PHARMACOLOGY

12.1 Mechanism of Action

The mechanism of the antihypertensive effects of beta adrenergic blockers has not been elucidated. However, several possible mechanisms have been proposed: (1) competitive antagonism of catecholamines at peripheral (especially cardiac) adrenergic neuron sites, leading to decreased cardiac output; (2) a central effect leading to reduced sympathetic outflow to the periphery; and (3) suppression of renin activity.

The mechanism of the antihypertensive effect of thiazide diurectics is unknown.

Continued on next page

12.2 Pharmacodynamics

Metoprolol

Clinical pharmacology studies have confirmed the beta adrenergic blocker activity of metoprolol, as shown by (1) reduction in heart rate and cardiac output at rest and upon exercise, (2) reduction of systolic blood pressure upon exercise, (3) inhibition of isoproterenol-induced tachycardia, and (4) reduction of reflex orthostatic tachycardia.

Metoprolol is a $beta_1$-selective (cardioselective) adrenergic receptor blocker. This preferential effect is not absolute, however, and at higher plasma concentrations, metoprolol also inhibits $beta_2$-adrenoreceptors, chiefly located in the bronchial and vascular musculature. Metoprolol has no intrinsic sympathomimetic activity, and membrane-stabilizing activity is detectable only at plasma concentrations much greater than required for beta-blockade. Animal and human experiments indicate that metoprolol slows the sinus rate and decreases AV nodal conduction.

The relative $beta_1$-selectivity of metoprolol is demonstrated by the following: (1) In healthy subjects, metoprolol is unable to reverse the $beta_2$-mediated vasodilating effects of epinephrine. This contrasts with the effect of nonselective beta-blockers, which completely reverse the vasodilating effects of epinephrine. (2) In asthmatic patients, metoprolol reduces FEV_1 and FVC significantly less than a nonselective beta-blocker, propranolol, at equivalent $beta_1$-receptor blocking doses.

The relationship between plasma metoprolol levels and reduction in exercise heart rate is independent of the pharmaceutical formulation. Using an E_{max} model, the maximum effect is a 30% reduction in exercise heart rate, which is attributed to $beta_1$-blockade. $Beta_1$-blocking effects in the range of 30–80% of the maximal effect (approximately 8–23% reduction in exercise heart rate) correspond to metoprolol plasma concentrations from 30-540 nmol/L. The relative $beta_1$-selectivity of metoprolol diminishes and blockade of $beta_2$-adrenoceptors increases at higher plasma concentrations above 300 nmol/L.

Although beta-adrenergic receptor blockade is useful in the treatment of hypertension there are situations in which sympathetic stimulation is vital. In patients with severely damaged hearts, adequate ventricular function may depend on sympathetic drive. In the presence of AV block, beta-blockade may prevent the necessary facilitating effect of sympathetic activity on conduction. $Beta_2$-adrenergic blockade results in passive bronchial constriction by interfering with endogenous adrenergic bronchodilator activity in patients subject to bronchospasm and may also interfere with exogenous bronchodilators in such patients.

Hydrochlorothiazide

Hydrochlorothiazide is a thiazide diuretic. Thiazides affect the renal tubular mechanisms of electrolyte reabsorption, directly increasing excretion of sodium and chloride in approximately equimolar amounts. Indirectly, the diuretic action of hydrochlorothiazide reduces plasma volume, with consequent increases in plasma renin activity, increases in aldosterone secretion, increases in urinary potassium loss, and decreases in serum potassium.

After oral administration of hydrochlorothiazide, diuresis begins within 2 hours, peaks in about 4 hours and lasts about 6 to 12 hours.

The following pharmacodynamic drug interactions may occur with hydrochlorothiazide:

Alcohol, barbiturates, or narcotics: Orthostatic hypotension.

Skeletal muscle relaxants, nondepolarizing (e.g., tubocurarine): Possible increased responsiveness to the muscle relaxant.

Corticosteroids, ACTH: Intensified electrolyte depletion, particularly hypokalemia.

12.3 Pharmacokinetics

Metoprolol/hydrochlorothiazide

After single oral doses of DUTOPROL, plasma levels of metoprolol and of hydrochlorothiazide are similar to levels obtained after single doses of TOPROL XL and hydrochlorothiazide. Peak plasma concentrations (C_{max}) of metoprolol and hydrochlorothiazide occur within 10-12 hours and 2 hours of dose intake, respectively.

The rate and extent of absorption of metoprolol/ hydrochlorothiazide are similar in the fasting state and after a high-fat meal after administration of DUTOPROL.

Metoprolol

Absorption of metoprolol is complete following oral administration. The absolute bioavailability of metoprolol after oral administration of immediate release metoprolol is estimated to be about 50% because of pre-systemic metabolism. Plasma levels achieved are highly variable after oral administration of immediate release metoprolol.

Metoprolol is known to cross the blood brain barrier following oral administration and CSF concentrations close to that observed in plasma have been reported. About 12% of the drug is bound to human serum albumin.

Metoprolol is primarily metabolized by CYP2D6. Metoprolol is a racemic mixture of R- and S- enantiomers, and when administered orally, it exhibits stereoselective metabolism that is dependent on oxidation phenotype. CYP2D6 is absent (poor metabolizers) in about 8% of Caucasians and about 2% of most other populations. CYP2D6 can be inhibited by a number of drugs. Concomitant use with CYP2D6 inhibitors or administration of metoprolol in poor metabolizers will increase blood levels of metoprolol several-fold, decreasing metoprolol's cardioselectivity *[see Drug Interactions (7.2)]*.

Elimination is mainly by biotransformation in the liver, and the plasma half-life ranges from approximately 3 to 7 hours. Less than 5% of an oral dose and 10% of an intravenous dose of metoprolol is recovered unchanged in the urine; the rest is excreted by the kidneys as metabolites that appear to have no beta blocking activity.

The systemic availability and half-life of metoprolol in patients with renal failure do not differ to a clinically significant degree from those in healthy subjects.

Metoprolol succinate extended release

The metoprolol component of DUTOPROL is bioequivalent to TOPROL-XL. In comparison to immediate release metoprolol, the plasma metoprolol levels following administration of TOPROL-XL are characterized by lower peaks, longer time to peak and significantly lower peak to trough variation (PTT ratio). The peak plasma levels following once-daily administration of TOPROL-XL average one-fourth to one-half the peak plasma levels obtained following a corresponding dose of immediate release metoprolol, administered once daily or in divided doses. At steady state the average bioavailability of metoprolol following administration of TOPROL-XL, across the dosage range of 50 to 400 mg once daily, was 77% relative to the corresponding single or divided doses of immediate release metoprolol. Nevertheless, over the 24-hour dosing interval, β_1-blockade is similar and dose-related *[see Clinical Pharmacology (12)]*.

Pharmacokinetic drug interactions: In healthy subjects with CYP2D6 extensive metabolizer phenotype, coadministration of quinidine 100 mg and immediate-release metoprolol 200 mg tripled the concentration of S-metoprolol and doubled the metoprolol elimination half-life. Coadministration of propafenone 150 mg t.i.d. with immediate-release metoprolol 50 mg t.i.d. resulted in two- to five-fold increases in the steady-state concentration of metoprolol. These increases in plasma concentration would decrease the cardioselectivity of metoprolol.

Hydrochlorothiazide

The pharmacokinetics of hydrochlorothiazide is dose proportional in the range of 12.5 to 75 mg.

The estimated absolute bioavailability of hydrochlorothiazide after oral administration is about 70%. Peak plasma hydrochlorothiazide concentrations (C_{max}) are reached within 2 to 5 hours after oral administration. There is no clinically significant effect of food on the bioavailability of hydrochlorothiazide.

Hydrochlorothiazide binds to albumin (40 to 70%) and distributes into erythrocytes. Following oral administration, plasma hydrochlorothiazide concentrations decline bi-exponentially, with a mean distribution half-life of about 2 hours and an elimination half-life of about 10 hours.

About 70% of an orally administered dose of hydrochlorothiazide is eliminated in the urine as unchanged drug.

Pharmacokinetic drug interactions: Absorption of hydrochlorothiazide is impaired in the presence of ionic exchange resins. Single doses of either cholestyramine or colestipol resins bind the hydrochlorothiazide and reduce its absorption from the gastrointestinal tract by up to 85% and 43%, respectively.

13 NONCLINICAL TOXICOLOGY

13.1 Carcinogenesis, Mutagenesis, Impairment of Fertility

Metoprolol/hydrochlorothiazide

Carcinogenicity and mutagenicity studies have not been conducted with combinations of metoprolol and hydrochlorothiazide.

A combination of metoprolol tartrate and hydrochlorothiazide produced no adverse effects on the fertility and reproductive performance of male and female rats at doses of up to 200/50 mg/kg/day [about 10 and 20 times the maximum recommended human dose (MRHD) of metoprolol and hydrochlorothiazide, respectively, on a mg/m^2 basis].

Metoprolol

Long-term studies in animals have been conducted to evaluate the carcinogenic potential of metoprolol tartrate. In 2-year studies in rats at oral dosage levels of up to 800 mg/kg/day (41 times, on a mg/m^2 basis, the daily dose of 200 mg for a 60-kg patient), there was no increase in the development of spontaneously occurring benign or malignant neoplasms of any type. The only histologic changes that appeared to be drug related were an increased incidence of generally mild focal accumulation of foamy macrophages in pulmonary alveoli and a slight increase in biliary hyperplasia. In a 21-month study in Swiss albino mice at three oral dosage levels of up to 750 mg/kg/day (about 18 times, on a mg/m^2 basis, the daily dose of 200 mg for a 60-kg patient), benign lung tumors (small adenomas) occurred more frequently in female mice receiving the highest dose than in untreated control animals. There was no increase in malignant or total (benign plus malignant) lung tumors, nor in the overall incidence of tumors or malignant tumors. This 21-month study was repeated in CD-1 mice, and no statistically or biologically significant differences were observed between treated and control mice of either sex for any type of tumor.

All genotoxicity tests performed with metoprolol tartrate (a dominant lethal study in mice, chromosomal studies in somatic cells, a *Salmonella*/mammalian-microsome mutagenicity test, and a nucleus anomaly test in somatic interphase nuclei) and metoprolol succinate (a *Salmonella*/mammalian-microsome mutagenicity test) were negative.

No evidence of impaired fertility was observed in a study of metoprolol tartrate performed in rats at doses up to 22 times, on a mg/m^2 basis, the daily dose of 200 mg in a 60 kg patient.

Hydrochlorothiazide

Two-year feeding studies in mice and rats uncovered no evidence of a carcinogenic potential of hydrochlorothiazide in female mice at doses of up to 600 mg/kg/day (about 120 times the MRHD of 25 mg/day) or in male and female rats at doses of up to 100 mg/kg/day (about 40 times the MRHD). However, there was equivocal evidence of hepatocarcinogenicity in male mice.

Hydrochlorothiazide was not genotoxic in the Ames bacterial mutagenicity test or the *in vitro* Chinese Hamster Ovary (CHO) test for chromosomal aberrations. Nor was it genotoxic *in vivo* in assays using mouse germinal cell chromosomes, Chinese hamster bone marrow chromosomes, and the Drosophila sex-linked recessive lethal trait gene. Positive results were obtained in the *in vitro* CHO Sister Chromatid Exchange (clastogenicity) test, the Mouse Lymphoma Cell (mutagenicity) assay and the *Aspergillus* nidulans nondisjunction assay.

Hydrochlorothiazide had no adverse effects on the fertility of mice and rats of either sex in studies wherein these species were exposed, via their diet, to doses of up to 100 and 4 mg/kg/day (about 20 and 1.6 times the MRHD, on a mg/m^2 basis), respectively, prior to mating and throughout gestation.

14 CLINICAL STUDIES

A randomized, double-blind, placebo-controlled, 8-week, factorial study (Study 1) (N=1571) evaluated the antihypertensive effects of various doses (given once daily) of metoprolol succinate extended release (25, 50, 100 and 200 mg) and hydrochlorothiazide (6.25, 12.5 and 25 mg), and 9 of their combinations. The trial established that metoprolol succinate extended release and hydrochlorothiazide both contributed to the antihypertensive effect, as measured by the change from baseline to week 8 in sitting diastolic (p= 0.0015) and systolic (p=0.0006) blood pressure. The predicted values for the drugs' effects are shown in Table 1.

[See table 1 on next page]

Blood pressure declines were apparent within 2 weeks and were maintained throughout the 8-week study. The blood pressure lowering effect 24 hours post-dosing retained approximately 96% of the peak effect (6 hours post-dosing). The antihypertensive effect was similar regardless of age or gender, and the blood pressure response to the metoprolol

Table 1. Placebo-corrected Change from Baseline* in SBP/DBP at Week 8 in Study 1

		Metoprolol				
		0 mg	25 mg	50 mg	100 mg	200 mg
HCTZ	0 mg	0/0	-2.0/-1.4	-3.7/-2.6	-6.1/-4.5	-7.0/-6.1
	6.25 mg	-3.5/-1.9	-5.5/-3.3	-7.2/-4.5	-9.6/-6.4	-10.5/-8.0†
	12.5 mg	-5.9/-3.3	-7.9/-4.7	-9.6/-5.9	-12.0/-7.8	-12.9/-9.3
	25 mg	-7.7/-4.3	-9.7/-5.7†	-11.4/-6.9†	-13.8/-8.8	-14.7/-10.4

* Predicted values from a least-squares quadratic regression model.
† These doses were not studied.
SBP = systolic blood pressure; DBP = diastolic blood pressure

succinate extended release and hydrochlorothiazide combination appears similar in black and non-black patients.

16   HOW SUPPLIED/STORAGE AND HANDLING

DUTOPROL is supplied as circular, biconvex, film-coated tablets engraved on one side.

Metoprolol/ Hydrochloro- thiazide	Engraving	Scored	NDC 59212-xxxx-xx Bottle/30
25/12.5 mg	A IH	No	087-30
50/12.5 mg	A IK	No	095-30
100/12.5 mg	A IL	Yes	097-30

Store at 25°C (77°F). Excursions permitted to 15-30°C (59-86°F). (See USP Controlled Room Temperature.)

17   PATIENT COUNSELING INFORMATION

Avoid Abrupt Discontinuation
Advise patients to take DUTOPROL regularly and continuously, as directed. If a dose is missed, instruct the patient to take only the next scheduled dose (without doubling the dose). Instruct patients not to interrupt or discontinue DUTOPROL without consulting a healthcare provider. *[See Boxed Warning and Warnings and Precautions (5.1)].*

Bronchospasm
Inform patients that beta adrenergic blockers can cause bronchospasm and to inform their healthcare providers if they start to wheeze or have difficulty breathing. *[See Warnings and Precautions (5.3)]*

Electrolyte Changes
Inform patients that they may need blood tests to monitor their serum electrolytes. *[See Warnings and Precautions (5.7)].*

Acute Myopia and Secondary Angle-Closure Glaucoma
Inform patients to report decreased visual acuity or ocular pain and to stop DUTOPROL and contact their healthcare provider right away if these symptoms occur. *[See Warnings and Precautions (5.13)].*

Hypersensitivity Reaction
Instruct patients that hypersensitivity reactions to DUTOPROL may occur. *[See Contraindications (4)].*

Lithium Toxicity
Instruct patients to inform other doctors that they are taking a diuretic. *[See Drug Interactions (7.2)].*

All trademarks are the property of Concordia Pharmaceuticals Inc.
Revised 1_06/2015
Manufactured for:
Concordia Pharmaceuticals Inc.
St. Michael, Barbados BB11005
© 2015, Concordia Pharmaceuticals Inc.
DUT_PI
Shown in Product Identification Guide, page 508

DYRENIUM®   ℞
(triamterene USP)
Capsules 50 mg and 100 mg potassium-sparing diuretic

> **Warnings**
> Abnormal elevation of serum potassium levels (greater than or equal to 5.5 mEq/liter) can occur with all potassium-sparing agents, including Dyrenium. Hyperkalemia is more likely to occur in patients with renal impairment and diabetes (even without evidence of renal impairment), and in the elderly or severely ill. Since uncorrected hyperkalemia may be fatal, serum potassium levels must be monitored at frequent intervals especially in patients receiving Dyrenium, when dosages are changed or with any illness that may influence renal function.

DESCRIPTION

Each capsule for oral use, with opaque red cap and body, contains Triamterene USP, 50 or 100 mg, and is imprinted with the product name, DYRENIUM, strength (50 mg or 100 mg) and WPC 002 (for the 50-mg strength) and WPC 003 (for the 100-mg strength). Inactive ingredients consist of D&C Red No. 33, FD&C Yellow No. 6, Gelatin NF, Lactose NF, Magnesium Stearate NF, and Titanium Dioxide USP. Triamterene is 2,4,7-triamino-6-phenyl-pteridine:

Its molecular weight is 253.27. At 50°C, triamterene is slightly soluble in water. It is soluble in dilute ammonia, dilute aqueous sodium hydroxide and dimethylformamide. It is sparingly soluble in methanol.

CLINICAL PHARMACOLOGY

Triamterene has a unique mode of action; it inhibits the reabsorption of sodium ions in exchange for potassium and hydrogen ions at that segment of the distal tubule under the control of adrenal mineralocorticoids (especially aldosterone). This activity is not directly related to aldosterone secretion or antagonism; it is a result of a direct effect on the renal tubule.
The fraction of filtered sodium reaching this distal tubular exchange site is relatively small, and the amount which is exchanged depends on the level of mineralocorticoid activity. Thus, the degree of natriuresis and diuresis produced by inhibition of the exchange mechanism is necessarily limited. Increasing the amount of available sodium and the level of mineralocorticoid activity by the use of more proximally acting diuretics will increase the degree of diuresis and potassium conservation.
Triamterene occasionally causes increases in serum potassium which can result in hyperkalemia. It does not produce alkalosis, because it does not cause excessive excretion of titratable acid and ammonium.
Triamterene has been shown to cross the placental barrier and appear in the cord blood of animals.

Pharmacokinetics

Onset of action is 2 to 4 hours after ingestion. In normal volunteers the mean peak serum levels were 30 ng/mL at 3

---

hours. The average percent of drug recovered in the urine (0 to 48 hours) was 21%. Triamterene is primarily metabolized to the sulfate conjugate of hydroxytriamterene. Both the plasma and urine levels of this metabolite greatly exceed triamterene levels. Triamterene is rapidly absorbed, with somewhat less than 50% of the oral dose reaching the urine. Most patients will respond to Dyrenium (triamterene) during the first day of treatment. Maximum therapeutic effect, however, may not be seen for several days. Duration of diuresis depends on several factors, especially renal function, but it generally tapers off 7 to 9 hours after administration.

INDICATIONS AND USAGE

Dyrenium (triamterene) is indicated in the treatment of edema associated with congestive heart failure, cirrhosis of the liver and the nephrotic syndrome; steroid-induced edema, idiopathic edema and edema due to secondary hyperaldosteronism.
Dyrenium may be used alone or with other diuretics, either for its added diuretic effect or its potassium-sparing potential. It also promotes increased diuresis when patients prove resistant or only partially responsive to thiazides or other diuretics because of secondary hyperaldosteronism.
Usage in Pregnancy. The routine use of diuretics in an otherwise healthy woman is inappropriate and exposes mother and fetus to unnecessary hazard. Diuretics do not prevent development of toxemia of pregnancy, and there is no satisfactory evidence that they are useful in the treatment of developed toxemia.
Edema during pregnancy may arise from pathological causes or from the physiologic and mechanical consequences of pregnancy. Diuretics are indicated in pregnancy (however, see PRECAUTIONS below) when edema is due to pathologic causes, just as they are in the absence of pregnancy. Dependent edema in pregnancy, resulting from restriction of venous return by the expanded uterus, is properly treated through elevation of the lower extremities and use of support hose; use of diuretics to lower intravascular volume in this case is illogical and unnecessary. There is hypervolemia during normal pregnancy which is harmful to neither the fetus nor the mother (in the absence of cardiovascular disease), but which is associated with edema, including generalized edema, in the majority of pregnant women. If this edema produces discomfort, increased recumbency will often provide relief. In rare instances, this edema may cause extreme discomfort which is not relieved by rest. In these cases, a short course of diuretics may provide relief and may be appropriate.

CONTRAINDICATIONS

Anuria. Severe or progressive kidney disease or dysfunction, with the possible exception of nephrosis. Severe hepatic disease. Hypersensitivity to the drug or any of its components.
Dyrenium (triamterene) should not be used in patients with pre-existing elevated serum potassium, as is sometimes seen in patients with impaired renal function or azotemia, or in patients who develop hyperkalemia while on the drug. Patients should not be placed on dietary potassium supplements, potassium salts or potassium-containing salt substitutes in conjunction with Dyrenium.
Dyrenium should not be given to patients receiving other potassium-sparing agents, such as spironolactone, amiloride hydrochloride, or other formulations containing triamterene. Two deaths have been reported in patients receiving concomitant spironolactone and Dyrenium or Dyazide®. Although dosage recommendations were exceeded in one case and in the other serum electrolytes were not properly monitored, these two drugs should not be given concomitantly.

> **WARNINGS**
> Abnormal elevation of serum potassium levels (greater than or equal to 5.5 mEq/liter) can occur with all potassium-sparing agents, including Dyrenium. Hyperkalemia is more likely to occur in patients with renal impairment and diabetes (even without evidence of renal impairment), and in the elderly or severely ill. Since uncorrected hyperkalemia may be fatal, serum potassium levels must be monitored at frequent intervals especially in patients receiving Dyrenium, when dosages are changed or with any illness that may influence renal function.

Continued on next page

There have been isolated reports of hypersensitivity reactions; therefore, patients should be observed regularly for the possible occurrence of blood dyscrasias, liver damage or other idiosyncratic reactions.

Periodic BUN and serum potassium determinations should be made to check kidney function, especially in patients with suspected or confirmed renal insufficiency. It is particularly important to make serum potassium determinations in elderly or diabetic patients receiving the drug; these patients should be observed carefully for possible serum potassium increases.

If hyperkalemia is present or suspected, an electrocardiogram should be obtained. If the ECG shows no widening of the QRS or arrhythmia in the presence of hyperkalemia, it is usually sufficient to discontinue Dyrenium (triamterene) and any potassium supplementation, and substitute a thiazide alone. Sodium polystyrene sulfonate (Kayexalate®, Concordia Pharmaceuticals Inc.) may be administered to enhance the excretion of excess potassium. **The presence of a widened QRS complex or arrhythmia in association with hyperkalemia requires prompt additional therapy.** For tachyarrhythmia, infuse 44 mEq of sodium bicarbonate or 10 mL of 10% calcium gluconate or calcium chloride over several minutes. For asystole, bradycardia or A-V block transvenous pacing is also recommended.

The effect of calcium and sodium bicarbonate is transient and repeated administration may be required. When indicated by the clinical situation, excess K+ may be removed by dialysis or oral or rectal administration of Kayexalate®. Infusion of glucose and insulin has also been used to treat hyperkalemia.

PRECAUTIONS

General

Dyrenium (triamterene) tends to conserve potassium rather than to promote the excretion as do many diuretics and, occasionally, can cause increases in serum potassium which, in some instances, can result in hyperkalemia. In rare instances, hyperkalemia has been associated with cardiac irregularities.

Electrolyte imbalance often encountered in such diseases as congestive heart failure, renal disease or cirrhosis may be aggravated or caused independently by any effective diuretic agent including Dyrenium. The use of full doses of a diuretic when salt intake is restricted can result in a low-salt syndrome.

Triamterene can cause mild nitrogen retention, which is reversible upon withdrawal of the drug, and is seldom observed with intermittent (every-other-day) therapy.

Triamterene may cause a decreasing alkali reserve, with the possibility of metabolic acidosis.

By the very nature of their illness, cirrhotics with splenomegaly sometimes have marked variations in their blood. Since triamterene is a weak folic acid antagonist, it may contribute to the appearance of megaloblastosis in cases where folic acid stores have been depleted. Therefore, periodic blood studies in these patients are recommended. They should also be observed for exacerbations of underlying liver disease.

Triamterene has elevated uric acid, especially in persons predisposed to gouty arthritis.

Triamterene has been reported in renal stones in association with other calculus components. Dyrenium should be used with caution in patients with histories of renal stones.

Information for Patients

To help avoid stomach upset, it is recommended that the drug be taken after meals.

If a single daily dose is prescribed, it may be preferable to take it in the morning to minimize the effect of increased frequency of urination on nighttime sleep.

If a dose is missed, the patient should not take more than the prescribed dose at the next dosing interval.

Laboratory Tests

Hyperkalemia will rarely occur in patients with adequate urinary output, but it is a possibility if large doses are used for considerable periods of time. If hyperkalemia is observed, Dyrenium (triamterene) should be withdrawn. The normal adult range of serum potassium is 3.5 to 5.0 mEq per liter, with 4.5 mEq often being used for a reference point. Potassium levels persistently above 6 mEq per liter require careful observation and treatment. Normal potassium levels tend to be higher in neonates (7.7 mEq per liter) than in adults.

Serum potassium levels do not necessarily indicate true body potassium concentration. A rise in plasma pH may cause a decrease in plasma potassium concentration and an increase in the intracellular potassium concentration. Because Dyrenium conserves potassium, it has been theorized that in patients who have received intensive therapy or been given the drug for prolonged periods, a rebound kaliuresis could occur upon abrupt withdrawal. In such patients, withdrawal of Dyrenium should be gradual.

Drug Interactions

Caution should be used when lithium and diuretics are used concomitantly because diuretic-induced sodium loss may reduce the renal clearance of lithium and increase serum lithium levels with risk of lithium toxicity. Patients receiving such combined therapy should have serum lithium levels monitored closely and the lithium dosage adjusted if necessary.

A possible interaction resulting in acute renal failure has been reported in a few subjects when indomethacin, a nonsteroidal anti-inflammatory agent, was given with triamterene. Caution is advised in administering nonsteroidal anti-inflammatory agents with triamterene.

The effects of the following drugs may be potentiated when given together with triamterene: antihypertensive medication, other diuretics, preanesthetic and anesthetic agents, skeletal muscle relaxants (non-depolarizing).

Potassium-sparing agents should be used with caution in conjunction with angiotensin-converting enzyme (ACE) inhibitors due to an increased risk of hyperkalemia.

The following agents, given together with triamterene, may promote serum potassium accumulation and possibly result in hyperkalemia because of the potassium-sparing nature of triamterene, especially in patients with renal insufficiency: blood from blood bank (may contain up to 30 mEq of potassium per liter of plasma or up to 65 mEq per liter of whole blood when stored for more than 10 days); low-salt milk (may contain up to 60 mEq of potassium per liter); potassium-containing medications (such as parenteral penicillin G potassium); salt substitutes (most contain substantial amounts of potassium).

Dyrenium (triamterene) may raise blood glucose levels; for adult-onset diabetes, dosage adjustments of hypoglycemic agents may be necessary during and/or after therapy; concurrent use with chlorpropamide may increase the risk of severe hyponatremia.

Drug/Laboratory Test Interactions

Triamterene and quinidine have similar fluorescence spectra; thus, triamterene will interfere with the fluorescent measurement of quinidine.

Carcinogenesis, Mutagenesis, Impairment of Fertility

Carcinogenesis: In studies conducted under the auspices of the National Toxicology Program, groups of rats were fed diets containing 0, 150, 300 or 600 ppm of triamterene, and groups of mice were fed diets containing 0, 100, 200 or 400 ppm triamterene. Male and female rats exposed to the highest tested concentration received triamterene at about 25 and 30 mg/kg/day, respectively. Male and female mice exposed to the highest tested concentration received triamterene at about 45 and 60 mg/kg/day, respectively.

There was an increased incidence of hepatocellular neoplasia (primarily adenomas) in male and female mice at the highest dosage level. These doses represent 7.5X and 10X the Maximum Recommended Human Dose (MRHD) of 300 mg/kg/day (or 6 mg/day based on a 50 kg patient) for male and female mice, respectively, when based on body weight and 0.7X and 0.9X the MRHD when based on body-surface area.

Although hepatocellular neoplasia (exclusively adenomas) in the rat study was limited to triamterene-exposed males, incidence was not dose dependent and there was no statistically significant difference from control incidence at any dose level.

Mutagenesis: Triamterene was not mutagenic in bacteria (Salmonella typhimurium strains TA98, TA100, TA1535 or TA1537) with or without metabolic activation. It did not induce chromosomal aberrations in Chinese hamster ovary (CHO) cells in vitro with or without metabolic activation, but it did induce sister chromatid exchanges in CHO cells in vitro with and without metabolic activation.

Impairment of Fertility: Studies of the effects of triamterene on animal reproductive function have not been conducted.

Pregnancy

Teratogenic Effects: Reproduction studies have been performed in rats at doses as high as 20 times the Maximum Recommended Human Dose (MRHD) on the basis of body weight, and 6 times the MRHD on the basis of body-surface area, without evidence of harm to the fetus due to triamterene. Because animal reproduction studies are not always predictive of human response, this drug should be used during pregnancy only if clearly needed.

Nonteratogenic Effects: Triamterene has been shown to cross the placental barrier and appear in cord blood. The use of triamterene in pregnant women requires that the anticipated benefits be weighed against possible hazards to the fetus. These possible hazards include adverse reactions which have occurred in the adult.

Nursing Mothers:

Triamterene has not been studied in nursing mothers. Triamterene appears in animal milk and is likely present in human milk. If use of the drug product is deemed essential, the patient should stop nursing.

Pediatric Use:

Safety and effectiveness in pediatric patients have not been established.

ADVERSE REACTIONS

Adverse effects are listed in decreasing order of frequency; however, the most serious adverse effects are listed first, regardless of frequency. All adverse effects occur rarely (that is, 1 in 1000, or less).

Hypersensitivity: anaphylaxis, rash, photosensitivity.

Metabolic: hyperkalemia, hypokalemia.

Renal: azotemia, elevated BUN and creatinine, renal stones, acute interstitial nephritis (rare), acute renal failure (one case of irreversible renal failure has been reported).

Gastrointestinal: jaundice and/or liver enzyme abnormalities, nausea and vomiting, diarrhea.

Hematologic: thrombocytopenia, megaloblastic anemia.

Central Nervous System: weakness, fatigue, dizziness, headache, dry mouth.

To report SUSPECTED ADVERSE REACTIONS, contact Concordia Pharmaceuticals Inc. at 1-877-370-1142 or FDA at 1-800-FDA-1088 or www.fda.gov/medwatch.

OVERDOSAGE

In the event of overdosage, it can be theorized that electrolyte imbalance would be the major concern, with particular attention to possible hyperkalemia. Other symptoms that might be seen would be nausea and vomiting, other G.I. disturbances and weakness. It is conceivable that some hypotension could occur. As with an overdose of any drug, immediate evacuation of the stomach should be induced through emesis and gastric lavage. Careful evaluation of the electrolyte pattern and fluid balance should be made. There is no specific antidote.

Reversible acute renal failure following ingestion of 50 tablets of a product containing a combination of 50 mg triamterene and 25 mg hydrochlorothiazide has been reported.

The oral LD50 in mice is 380 mg/kg. The amount of drug in a single dose ordinarily associated with symptoms of overdose or likely to be life-threatening is not known.

Although triamterene is 67% protein bound, there may be some benefit to dialysis in cases of overdosage.

DOSAGE AND ADMINISTRATION

Adult Dosage

Dosage should be titrated to the needs of the individual patient. When used alone, the usual starting dose is 100 mg twice daily after meals. When combined with another diuretic or antihypertensive agent, the total daily dosage of each agent should usually be lowered initially and then adjusted to the patient's needs. The total daily dosage should not exceed 300 mg. Please refer to PRECAUTIONS–General.

When Dyrenium (triamterene) is added to other diuretic therapy or when patients are switched to Dyrenium from other diuretics, all potassium supplementation should be discontinued.

HOW SUPPLIED

Capsules: 50 mg in bottles of 100, and 100 mg in bottles of 100.

STORAGE

Store at 25°C (77°F); excursions permitted to 15°-30°C (59°-86°F) [See USP Controlled Room Temperature]. Dispense in a tight, light resistant container.

50 mg 100s: NDC 59212-002-01

100 mg 100s: NDC 59212-003-01

©2015 Concordia Pharmaceuticals Inc.

Manufactured for

Concordia Pharmaceuticals Inc.

St. Michael, Barbados BB11005

Made in Canada

Rev. 2_06/2016 N0170E DYR_PI

Shown in Product Identification Guide, page 508

KAPVAY   ℞

[*KAP-vay*]

(clonidine hydrochloride)

extended-release tablets, for oral use

HIGHLIGHTS OF PRESCRIBING INFORMATION

These highlights do not include all the information needed to use KAPVAY safely and effectively. See full prescribing information for KAPVAY.

KAPVAY (clonidine hydrochloride) extended-release tablets, for oral use

Initial U.S. Approval: 1974

INDICATIONS AND USAGE

KAPVAY® is a centrally acting alpha$_2$-adrenergic agonist indicated for the treatment of attention deficit hyperactivity disorder (ADHD) as monotherapy or as adjunctive therapy to stimulant medications. (1)

DOSAGE AND ADMINISTRATION

• Start with one 0.1 mg tablet at bedtime for one week. Increase daily dosage in increments of 0.1 mg/day at weekly intervals until the desired response is achieved. Take twice a day, with either an equal or higher split dosage being given at bedtime, as depicted below (2.2)

Total Daily Dose	Morning Dose	Bedtime Dose
0.1 mg/day		0.1 mg
0.2 mg/day	0.1 mg	0.1 mg
0.3 mg/day	0.1 mg	0.2 mg
0.4 mg/day	0.2 mg	0.2 mg

• Do not crush, chew or break tablet before swallowing. (2.1)
• Do not substitute for other clonidine products on a mg-per-mg basis, because of differing pharmacokinetic profiles. (2.1)
• When discontinuing, taper the dose in decrements of no more than 0.1 mg every 3 to 7 days to avoid rebound hypertension. (2.3)

DOSAGE FORMS AND STRENGTHS

Extended-release tablets: 0.1 mg and 0.2 mg, not scored. (3)

CONTRAINDICATIONS

History of a hypersensitivity reaction to clonidine. Reactions have included generalized rash, urticaria, angioedema. (4)

WARNINGS AND PRECAUTIONS

• Hypotension/bradycardia/syncope: Titrate slowly and monitor vital signs frequently in patients at risk for hypotension, heart block, bradycardia, syncope, cardiovascular disease, vascular disease, cerebrovascular disease or chronic renal failure. Measure heart rate and blood pressure prior to initiation of therapy, following dose increases, and periodically while on therapy. Avoid concomitant use of drugs with additive effects unless clinically indicated. Advise patients to avoid becoming dehydrated or overheated. (5.1)
• Somnolence/Sedation: Has been observed with KAPVAY. Consider the potential for additive sedative effects with CNS depressant drugs. Caution patients against operating heavy equipment or driving until they know how they respond to KAPVAY. (5.2)
• Cardiac Conduction Abnormalities: May worsen sinus node dysfunction and atrioventricular (AV) block, especially in patients taking other sympatholytic drugs. Titrate slowly and monitor vital signs frequently. (5.5)

ADVERSE REACTIONS

Most common adverse reactions (incidence at least 5% and twice the rate of placebo) as monotherapy in ADHD: somnolence, fatigue, irritability, nightmare, insomnia, constipation, dry mouth. (6.1)

Most common adverse reactions (incidence at least 5% and twice the rate of placebo) as adjunct therapy to psychostimulant in ADHD: somnolence, fatigue, decreased appetite, dizziness. (6.1)

To report SUSPECTED ADVERSE REACTIONS, contact Concordia Pharmaceuticals Inc. at 1-877-370-1142 or FDA at 1-800-FDA-1088 or *www.fda.gov/medwatch*.

DRUG INTERACTIONS

• Sedating Drugs: Clonidine may potentiate the CNS-depressive effects of alcohol, barbiturates or other sedating drugs. (7)
• Tricyclic Antidepressants: May reduce the hypotensive effect of clonidine. (7)
• Drugs Known to Affect Sinus Node Function or AV Nodal Conduction: Caution is warranted in patients receiving clonidine concomitantly with agents known to affect sinus node function or AV nodal conduction (e.g., digitalis, calcium channel blockers and beta-blockers) due to a potential for additive effects such as bradycardia and AV block. (7)
• Antihypertensive drugs: Use caution when coadministered with KAPVAY. (7)

USE IN SPECIFIC POPULATIONS

• Based on animal data, KAPVAY may cause fetal harm. (8.1)
• Renal Impairment: The dosage of KAPVAY must be adjusted according to the degree of impairment, and patients should be carefully monitored. (8.6, 12.3)

See 17 for PATIENT COUNSELING INFORMATION and FDA-approved patient labeling.

Revised: 8/2016

FULL PRESCRIBING INFORMATION: CONTENTS*

FULL PRESCRIBING INFORMATION

1   INDICATIONS AND USAGE

KAPVAY® (clonidine hydrochloride) extended-release is indicated for the treatment of attention deficit hyperactivity disorder (ADHD) as monotherapy and as adjunctive therapy to stimulant medications [see Clinical Studies (14)].

2   DOSAGE AND ADMINISTRATION

2.1   General Dosing Information

KAPVAY is an extended-release tablet to be taken orally with or without food. Swallow tablets whole. Do not crush, chew, or break tablets because this will increase the rate of clonidine release.

Due to the lack of controlled clinical trial data and differing pharmacokinetic profiles, substitution of KAPVAY for other clonidine products on a mg-per-mg basis is not recommended [see Clinical Pharmacology (12.3)].

2.2   Dose Selection

The dose of KAPVAY, administered either as monotherapy or as adjunctive therapy to a psychostimulant, should be individualized according to the therapeutic needs and response of the patient. Dosing should be initiated with one 0.1 mg tablet at bedtime, and the daily dosage should be adjusted in increments of 0.1 mg/day at weekly intervals until the desired response is achieved. Doses should be taken twice a day, with either an equal or higher split dosage being given at bedtime (see Table 1).

Table 1 KAPVAY Dosing Guidance

Total Daily Dose	Morning Dose	Bedtime Dose
0.1 mg/day		0.1 mg
0.2 mg/day	0.1 mg	0.1 mg
0.3 mg/day	0.1 mg	0.2 mg
0.4 mg/day	0.2 mg	0.2 mg

Doses of KAPVAY higher than 0.4 mg/day (0.2 mg twice daily) were not evaluated in clinical trials for ADHD and are not recommended.

When KAPVAY is being added-on to a psychostimulant, the dose of the psychostimulant can be adjusted depending on the patient's response to KAPVAY.

2.3   Discontinuation

When discontinuing KAPVAY, the total daily dose should be tapered in decrements of no more than 0.1 mg every 3 to 7 days to avoid rebound hypertension [see Warnings and Precautions (5.3)].

2.4   Missed Doses

If patients miss a dose of KAPVAY, they should skip that dose and take the next dose as scheduled. Do not take more than the prescribed total daily amount of KAPVAY in any 24-hour period.

3   DOSAGE FORMS AND STRENGTHS

KAPVAY tablets are available in two strengths, 0.1 mg and 0.2 mg as an extended-release formulation. Both the 0.1 mg and 0.2 mg tablets are white, non-scored, standard convex with debossing on one side. The 0.1 mg tablets are round and the 0.2 mg tablets are oval. KAPVAY tablets must be swallowed whole and never crushed, cut or chewed.

4   CONTRAINDICATIONS

KAPVAY is contraindicated in patients with a history of a hypersensitivity reaction to clonidine. Reactions have included generalized rash, urticaria, and angioedema [see Adverse Reactions (6)].

5   WARNINGS AND PRECAUTIONS

5.1   Hypotension/Bradycardia

Treatment with KAPVAY can cause dose-related decreases in blood pressure and heart rate [see Adverse Reactions (6.1)]. Measure heart rate and blood pressure prior to initiation of therapy, following dose increases, and periodically while on therapy. Titrate KAPVAY slowly in patients with a history of hypotension, and those with underlying conditions that may be worsened by hypotension and bradycardia; e.g., heart block, bradycardia, cardiovascular disease, vascular disease, cerebrovascular disease, or chronic renal failure. In patients who have a history of syncope or may have a condition that predisposes them to syncope, such as hypotension, orthostatic hypotension, bradycardia, or dehydration, advise patients to avoid becoming dehydrated or overheated. Monitor blood pressure and heart rate, and adjust dosages accordingly in patients treated concomitantly with antihypertensives or other drugs that can reduce blood pressure or heart rate or increase the risk of syncope.

5.2   Sedation and Somnolence

Somnolence and sedation were commonly reported adverse reactions in clinical studies. In patients that completed 5 weeks of therapy in a controlled, fixed dose pediatric monotherapy study, 31% of patients treated with 0.4 mg/day and 38% treated with 0.2 mg/day versus 4% of placebo treated patients reported somnolence as an adverse event. In patients that completed 5 weeks of therapy in a controlled flexible dose pediatric adjunctive to stimulants study, 19%

Continued on next page

of patients treated with KAPVAY+stimulant versus 7% treated with placebo+stimulant reported somnolence. Before using KAPVAY with other centrally active depressants (such as phenothiazines, barbiturates, or benzodiazepines), consider the potential for additive sedative effects. Caution patients against operating heavy equipment or driving until they know how they respond to treatment with KAPVAY. Advise patients to avoid use with alcohol.

5.3 Rebound Hypertension
Abrupt discontinuation of KAPVAY can cause rebound hypertension. In adults with hypertension, sudden cessation of clonidine hydrochloride extended-release formulation treatment in the 0.2 to 0.6 mg/day range resulted in reports of headache, tachycardia, nausea, flushing, warm feeling, brief lightheadedness, tightness in chest, and anxiety. In adults with hypertension, sudden cessation of treatment with immediate-release clonidine has, in some cases, resulted in symptoms such as nervousness, agitation, headache, and tremor accompanied or followed by a rapid rise in blood pressure and elevated catecholamine concentrations in the plasma.

No studies evaluating abrupt discontinuation of KAPVAY in children with ADHD have been conducted; however, to minimize the risk of rebound hypertension, gradually reduce the dose of KAPVAY in decrements of no more than 0.1 mg every 3 to 7 days. Patients should be instructed not to discontinue KAPVAY therapy without consulting their physician due to the potential risk of withdrawal effects.

5.4 Allergic Reactions
In patients who have developed localized contact sensitization to clonidine transdermal system, continuation of clonidine transdermal system or substitution of oral KAPVAY therapy may be associated with the development of a generalized skin rash.

In patients who develop an allergic reaction from clonidine transdermal system, substitution of oral KAPVAY may also elicit an allergic reaction (including generalized rash, urticaria, or angioedema).

5.5 Cardiac Conduction Abnormalities
The sympatholytic action of clonidine may worsen sinus node dysfunction and atrioventricular (AV) block, especially in patients taking other sympatholytic drugs. There have been post-marketing reports of patients with conduction abnormalities and/or taking other sympatholytic drugs who developed severe bradycardia requiring IV atropine, IV isoproterenol, and temporary cardiac pacing while taking clonidine. Titrate KAPVAY slowly and monitor vital signs frequently in patients with cardiac conduction abnormalities or patients concomitantly treated with other sympatholytic drugs.

6 ADVERSE REACTIONS
The following serious adverse reactions are described in greater detail elsewhere in labeling:
• Hypotension/bradycardia *[see Warnings and Precautions (5.1)]*
• Sedation and somnolence *[see Warnings and Precautions (5.2)]*
• Rebound hypertension *[see Warnings and Precautions (5.3)]*
• Allergic reactions *[see Warnings and Precautions (5.4)]*
• Cardiac Conduction Abnormalities *[see Warnings and Precautions (5.5)]*

6.1 Clinical Trial Experience
Because clinical trials are conducted under widely varying conditions, adverse reaction rates observed in the clinical trials of a drug cannot be directly compared to rates in the clinical trials of another drug and may not reflect the rates observed in practice.

Two KAPVAY ADHD clinical studies (Study 1, CLON-301 and Study 2, CLON-302) evaluated 256 patients in two 8-week placebo-controlled studies.

A third KAPVAY ADHD clinical study (Study 3, SHN-KAP-401) evaluated 135 children and adolescents in a 40-week placebo-controlled randomized-withdrawal study.

Study 1: Fixed-dose KAPVAY Monotherapy
Study 1 (CLON-301) was a short-term, multi-center, randomized, double-blind, placebo-controlled study of two fixed doses (0.2 mg/day or 0.4 mg/day) of KAPVAY in children and adolescents (6 to 17 years of age) who met DSM-IV criteria for ADHD hyperactive or combined inattentive/hyperactive subtypes.

Most Common Adverse Reactions (incidence of ≥ 5% and at least twice the rate of placebo): somnolence, fatigue, irritability, insomnia, nightmare, constipation, dry mouth.

Adverse Events Leading to Discontinuation of KAPVAY –Five patients (7%) in the low dose group (0.2 mg), 15 patients (20%) in the high dose group (0.4 mg), and 1 patient in the placebo group (1%) reported adverse reactions that led to discontinuation. The most common adverse reactions that led to discontinuation were somnolence and fatigue. Commonly observed adverse reactions (incidence of ≥2% in either active treatment group and greater than the rate on placebo) during the treatment period are listed in Table 2. [See table 2 below]

Commonly observed adverse reactions (incidence of >2% in either active treatment group and greater than the rate on placebo) during the taper period are listed in Table 3.

Table 3 Common Adverse Reactions in the Fixed-Dose Monotherapy Trial -Taper Period* (Study 1)

Preferred Term	Percentage of Patients Reporting Event		
	KAPVAY 0.2 mg/day N=76	KAPVAY 0.4 mg/day N=78	Placebo (N=76)
Abdominal Pain Upper	0%	6%	3%
Headache	5%	2%	3%
Gastrointestinal Viral	0%	5%	0%
Somnolence	2%	3%	0%
Heart Rate Increased	0%	3%	0%
Otitis Media Acute	3%	0%	0%

* Taper Period: 0.2 mg dose, week 8; 0.4 mg dose, weeks 6-8; Placebo dose, weeks 6-8

Study 2: Flexible-dose KAPVAY as Adjunctive Therapy to Psychostimulants
Study 2 (CLON-302) was a short-term, randomized, double-blind, placebo-controlled study of a flexible dose of KAPVAY as adjunctive therapy to a psychostimulant in children and adolescents (6 to 17 years) who met DSM-IV criteria for ADHD hyperactive or combined inattentive/hyperactive subtypes during which KAPVAY was initiated at 0.1 mg/day and titrated up to 0.4 mg/day over a 3-week period. Most KAPVAY treated patients (75.5%) were escalated to the maximum dose of 0.4 mg/day.

Most Common Adverse Reactions (incidence of ≥ 5% and at least twice the rate of placebo): somnolence, fatigue, decreased appetite, dizziness.

Adverse Events Leading to Discontinuation – There was one patient in the CLON+STM group (1%) who discontinued because of an adverse event (severe bradyphrenia, with severe fatigue).

Commonly observed adverse reactions (incidence of ≥2% in the treatment group and greater than the rate on placebo) during the treatment period are listed in Table 4. [See table 4 on next page]

Commonly observed adverse reactions (incidence of ≥2% in the treatment group and greater than the rate on placebo) during the taper period are listed in Table 5.

Table 5 Common Adverse Reactions in the Flexible-Dose Adjunctive to Stimulant Therapy Trial - Taper Period* (Study 2)

Preferred Term	Percentage of Patients Reporting Event	
	KAPVAY+STM (N=102)	PBO+STM (N=96)
Nasal Congestion	4%	2%
Headache	3%	1%
Irritability	3%	2%
Throat Pain	3%	1%
Gastroenteritis Viral	2%	0%

Table 2 Common Adverse Reactions in the Fixed-Dose Monotherapy Trial-Treatment Period (Study 1)

Preferred Term	Percentage of Patients Reporting Event		
	KAPVAY 0.2 mg/day N=76	KAPVAY 0.4 mg/day N=78	Placebo (N=76)
PSYCHIATRIC DISORDERS			
Somnolence*	38%	31%	4%
Nightmare	4%	9%	0%
Emotional Disorder	4%	4%	1%
Aggression*	3%	1%	0%
Tearfulness	1%	3%	0%
Enuresis	0%	4%	0%
Sleep Terror	3%	0%	0%
Poor Quality Sleep	0%	3%	1%
NERVOUS SYSTEM DISORDERS			
Headache	20%	13%	16%
Insomnia	5%	6%	1%
Tremor	1%	4%	0%
Abnormal Sleep-Related Event	3%	1%	0%
GASTROINTESTINAL DISORDERS	15%	10%	12%
Upper Abdominal Pain	4%	5%	3%
Nausea	1%	6%	0%
Constipation	0%	5%	1%
Dry Mouth			
GENERAL DISORDERS			
Fatigue†	16%	13%	1%
Irritability	9%	5%	4%
CARDIAC DISORDERS			
Dizziness	7%	3%	5%
Bradycardia	0%	4%	0%
INVESTIGATIONS			
Increased Heart Rate	0%	3%	0%
METABOLISM AND NUTRITION DISORDERS			
Decreased Appetite	3%	4%	4%

* Somnolence includes the terms "somnolence" and "sedation".
† Fatigue includes the terms "fatigue" and "lethargy".

Rash	2%	0%

* Taper Period: weeks 6-8

Adverse Reactions Leading to Discontinuation

Thirteen percent (13%) of patients receiving KAPVAY discontinued from the pediatric monotherapy study due to adverse events, compared to 1% in the placebo group. The most common adverse reactions leading to discontinuation of KAPVAY monotherapy treated patients were from somnolence/sedation (5%) and fatigue (4%).

Effect on Blood Pressure and Heart Rate

In patients that completed 5 weeks of treatment in a controlled, fixed-dose monotherapy study in pediatric patients, during the treatment period the maximum placebo-subtracted mean change in systolic blood pressure was -4.0 mmHg on KAPVAY 0.2 mg/day and -8.8 mmHg on KAPVAY 0.4 mg/day. The maximum placebo-subtracted mean change in diastolic blood pressure was -4.0 mmHg on KAPVAY 0.2 mg/day and -7.3 mmHg on KAPVAY 0.4 mg/day. The maximum placebo-subtracted mean change in heart rate was -4.0 beats per minute on KAPVAY 0.2 mg/day and -7.7 beats per minute on KAPVAY 0.4 mg/day.

During the taper period of the fixed-dose monotherapy study the maximum placebo-subtracted mean change in systolic blood pressure was +3.4 mmHg on KAPVAY 0.2 mg/day and -5.6 mmHg on KAPVAY 0.4 mg/day. The maximum placebo-subtracted mean change in diastolic blood pressure was +3.3 mmHg on KAPVAY 0.2 mg/day and -5.4 mmHg on KAPVAY 0.4 mg/day. The maximum placebo-subtracted mean change in heart rate was -0.6 beats per minute on KAPVAY 0.2 mg/day and -3.0 beats per minute on KAPVAY 0.4 mg/day.

6.2 Postmarketing Experience

The following adverse reactions have been identified during post-approval use of KAPVAY. Because these reactions are reported voluntarily from a population of uncertain size, it is not always possible to reliably estimate their frequency or establish a causal relationship to drug exposure. These events exclude those already mentioned in 6.1:

Psychiatric: hallucinations
Cardiovascular: Q-T prolongation

7 DRUG INTERACTIONS

The following have been reported with other oral immediate release formulations of clonidine:
[See table 6 above]

Table 6 Clinically Important Drug Interactions

Concomitant Drug Name or Drug Class	Clinical Rationale	Clinical Recommendation
Tricyclic antidepressants	Increase blood pressure and may counteract clonidine's hypotensive effects	Monitor blood pressure and adjust as needed
Antihypertensive drugs	Potentiate clonidine's hypotensive effects	Monitor blood pressure and adjust as needed
CNS depressants	Potentiate sedating effects	Avoid use
Drugs that affect sinus node function or AV node conduction (e.g., digitalis, calcium channel blockers, beta blockers)	Potentiate bradycardia and risk of AV block	Avoid use

---

8 USE IN SPECIFIC POPULATIONS

8.1 Pregnancy

Pregnancy Category C:

Risk Summary

There are no adequate or well-controlled studies with KAPVAY in pregnant women. In animal embryofetal studies, increased resorptions were seen in rats and mice administered oral clonidine hydrochloride from implantation through organogenesis at 10 and 5 times, respectively, the maximum recommended human dose (MRHD). No embryotoxic or teratogenic effects were seen in rabbits administered oral clonidine hydrochloride during organogenesis at doses up to 3 times the MRHD. KAPVAY should be used during pregnancy only if the potential benefit justifies the potential risk to the fetus.

Animal Data

Oral administration of clonidine hydrochloride to pregnant rabbits during the period of embryo/fetal organogenesis at doses of up to 80 mcg/kg/day (approximately 3 times the oral maximum recommended daily dose [MRHD] of 0.4 mg/day on a mg/m^2 basis) produced no evidence of teratogenic or embryotoxic potential. In pregnant rats, however, doses as low as 15 mcg/kg/day (1/3 the MRHD on a mg/m^2 basis) were associated with increased resorptions in a study in which dams were treated continuously from 2 months prior to mating and throughout gestation. Increased resorptions were not associated with treatment at the same or at higher dose levels (up to 3 times the MRHD) when treatment of the dams was restricted to gestation days 6-15. Increases in resorptions were observed in both rats and mice at 500 mcg/kg/day (10 and 5 times the MRHD in rats and mice, respectively) or higher when the animals were treated on gestation days 1-14; 500 mcg/kg/day was the lowest dose employed in this study.

8.3 Nursing Mothers

Clonidine hydrochloride is present in human milk. The developmental and health benefits of breastfeeding should be considered along with the mother's clinical need for KAPVAY and any potential adverse effects on the breastfed child from KAPVAY or from the underlying maternal condition. Exercise caution when KAPVAY is administered to a nursing woman.

8.4 Pediatric Use

The safety and efficacy of KAPVAY in the treatment of ADHD have been established in pediatric patients 6 to 17 years of age. Use of KAPVAY in pediatric patients 6 to 17 years of age is supported by three adequate and well-controlled studies; a short-term, placebo-controlled monotherapy trial, a short-term adjunctive therapy trial and a longer-term randomized monotherapy trial *[see Clinical Studies (14)]*. Safety and efficacy in pediatric patients below the age of 6 years has not been established.

Juvenile Animal Data

In studies in juvenile rats, clonidine hydrochloride alone or in combination with methylphenidate had an effect on bone growth at clinically relevant doses and produced a slight delay in sexual maturation in males at 3 times the maximum recommended human dose (MRHD) for clonidine and methylphenidate.

In a study where juvenile rats were treated orally with clonidine hydrochloride from day 21 of age to adulthood, a slight delay in onset of preputial separation (delayed sexual maturation) was seen in males treated with 300 mcg/kg/day, which is approximately 3 times the MRHD of 0.4 mg/day on a mg/m^2 basis. The no-effect dose was 100 mcg/kg/day, which is approximately equal to the MRHD. There was no drug effects on fertility or on other measures of sexual or neurobehavioral development.

In a study where juvenile rats were treated with clonidine alone (300 mcg/kg/day) or in combination with methylphenidate (10 mg/kg/day in females and 50/30 mg/kg/day in males; the dose was lowered from 50 to 30 mg/kg/day in males due to self-injurious behavior during the first week of treatment) from day 21 of age to adulthood, decreases in bone mineral density and mineral content were observed in males treated with 300 mcg/kg/day clonidine alone and in combination with 50/30 mg/kg/day methylphenidate and a decrease in femur length was observed in males treated with the combination at the end of the treatment period. These doses are approximately 3 times the MRHD of 0.4 mg/day clonidine and 54 mg/day methylphenidate on a mg/m^2 basis. All these effects in male were not reversed at the end of a 4-week recovery period. In addition, similar findings were seen in males treated with a lower dose of clonidine (30 mcg/kg/day) in combination with 50 mg/kg/day of methylphenidate and a decrease in femur length was observed in females treated with clonidine alone at the end of the recovery period. These effects were accompanied by a decrease in body weight gain in treated animals during the treatment period but the effect was reversed at the end of the recovery period. A delay in preputial separation (sexual maturation) was observed in males treated with the combination treatment of 300 mcg/kg/day clonidine and 50/30 mg/kg/day methylphenidate. There was no effect on reproduction or sperm analysis in these males.

8.6 Renal Impairment

The impact of renal impairment on the pharmacokinetics of clonidine in children has not been assessed. The initial dos-

---

Table 4 Common Adverse Reactions in the Flexible-Dose Adjunctive to Stimulant Therapy Trial - Treatment Period (Study 2)

Preferred Term	Percentage of Patients Reporting Event	
	KAPVAY+STM (N=102)	PBO+STM (N=96)
PSYCHIATRIC DISORDERS		
Somnolence*	19%	7%
Aggression	2%	1%
Affect Lability	2%	1%
Emotional Disorder	2%	0%
GENERAL DISORDERS		
Fatigue†	14%	4%
Irritability	2%	7%
NERVOUS SYSTEM DISORDERS		
Headache	7%	12%
Insomnia	4%	3%
GASTROINTESTINAL DISORDERS		
Upper Abdominal Pain	7%	4%
RESPIRATORY DISORDERS		
Nasal Congestion	2%	2%
METABOLISM AND NUTRITION DISORDERS		
Decreased Appetite	6%	3%
CARDIAC DISORDERS		
Dizziness	5%	1%

* Somnolence includes the terms: "somnolence" and "sedation".
† Fatigue includes the terms "fatigue" and "lethargy".

Continued on next page

age of KAPVAY should be based on degree of impairment. Monitor patients carefully for hypotension and bradycardia, and titrate to higher doses cautiously. Since only a minimal amount of clonidine is removed during routine hemodialysis, there is no need to give supplemental KAPVAY following dialysis.

9 DRUG ABUSE AND DEPENDENCE
9.1 Controlled Substance
KAPVAY is not a controlled substance and has no known potential for abuse or dependence.

10 OVERDOSAGE
Symptoms
Clonidine overdose: hypertension may develop early and may be followed by hypotension, bradycardia, respiratory depression, hypothermia, drowsiness, decreased or absent reflexes, weakness, irritability and miosis. The frequency of CNS depression may be higher in children than adults. Large overdoses may result in reversible cardiac conduction defects or dysrhythmias, apnea, coma and seizures. Signs and symptoms of overdose generally occur within 30 minutes to two hours after exposure.

Treatment
Consult with a Certified Poison Control Center (1-800-222-1222) for up-to-date guidance and advice.

11 DESCRIPTION
KAPVAY (clonidine hydrochloride) extended-release is a centrally acting alpha$_2$-adrenergic agonist available as 0.1 mg or 0.2 mg extended-release tablets for oral administration. Each 0.1 mg and 0.2 mg tablet is equivalent to 0.087 mg and 0.174 mg, respectively, of the free base.

The inactive ingredients are sodium lauryl sulfate, lactose monohydrate, hypromellose type 2208, partially pregelatinized starch, colloidal silicon dioxide, and magnesium stearate. The formulation is designed to delay the absorption of active drug in order to decrease peak to trough plasma concentration differences. Clonidine hydrochloride is an imidazoline derivative and exists as a mesomeric compound. The chemical name is 2-(2,6-dichlorophenylamino)-2-imidazoline hydrochloride. The following is the structural formula:

$C_9H_9Cl_2N_3 \cdot HCl$ Mol. Wt. 266.56

Clonidine hydrochloride is an odorless, bitter, white, crystalline substance soluble in water and alcohol.

12 CLINICAL PHARMACOLOGY
12.1 Mechanism of Action
Clonidine stimulates alpha$_2$-adrenergic receptors in the brain. Clonidine is not a central nervous system stimulant. The mechanism of action of clonidine in ADHD is not known.

12.2 Pharmacodynamics
Clonidine is a known antihypertensive agent. By stimulating alpha$_2$-adrenergic receptors in the brain stem, clonidine reduces sympathetic outflow from the central nervous system and decreases peripheral resistance, renal vascular resistance, heart rate, and blood pressure.

12.3 Pharmacokinetics
Single-dose Pharmacokinetics in Adults
Immediate-release clonidine hydrochloride and KAPVAY have different pharmacokinetic characteristics; dose substitution on a milligram for milligram basis will result in dif-

ferences in exposure. A comparison across studies suggests that the Cmax is 50% lower for KAPVAY compared to immediate-release clonidine hydrochloride.

Following oral administration of an immediate release formulation, plasma clonidine concentration peaks in approximately 3 to 5 hours and the plasma half-life ranges from 12 to 16 hours. The half-life increases up to 41 hours in patients with severe impairment of renal function. Following oral administration about 40-60% of the absorbed dose is recovered in the urine as unchanged drug in 24 hours.

About 50% of the absorbed dose is metabolized in the liver. Although studies of the effect of renal impairment and studies of clonidine excretion have not been performed with KAPVAY, results are likely to be similar to those of the immediate release formulation.

The pharmacokinetic profile of KAPVAY administration was evaluated in an open-label, three-period, randomized, crossover study of 15 healthy adult subjects who received three single-dose regimens of clonidine: 0.1 mg of KAPVAY under fasted conditions, 0.1 mg of KAPVAY following a high fat meal, and 0.1 mg of clonidine immediate-release (Catapres®) under fasted conditions. Treatments were separated by one-week washout periods.

Mean concentration-time data from the 3 treatments are shown in Table 7 and Figure 1. After administration of KAPVAY, maximum clonidine concentrations were approximately 50% of the Catapres maximum concentrations and occurred approximately 5 hours later relative to Catapres. Similar elimination half-lives were observed and total systemic bioavailability following KAPVAY was approximately 89% of that following Catapres.

Food had no effect on plasma concentrations, bioavailability, or elimination half-life.

[See table 7 below]

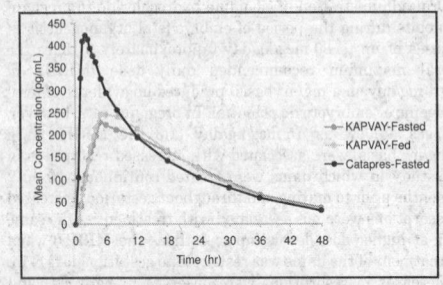

Figure 1 Mean Clonidine Concentration-Time Profiles after Single Dose Administration

Multiple-dose Pharmacokinetics in Children and Adolescents
Plasma clonidine concentrations in children and adolescents (0.1 mg bid and 0.2 mg bid) with ADHD are greater than those of adults with hypertension with children and adolescents receiving higher doses on a mg/kg basis. Body weight normalized clearance (CL/F) in children and adolescents was higher than CL/F observed in adults with hypertension. Clonidine concentrations in plasma increased with increases in dose over the dose range of 0.2 to 0.4 mg/day. Clonidine CL/F was independent of dose administered over the 0.2 to 0.4 mg/day dose range. Clonidine CL/F appeared to decrease slightly with increases in age over the range of 6 to 17 years, and females had a 23% lower CL/F than males. The incidence of "sedation-like" AEs (somnolence and fatigue) appeared to be independent of clonidine dose or concentration within the studied dose range in the titration study. Results from the add-on study showed that clonidine

CL/F was 11% higher in patients who were receiving methylphenidate and 44% lower in those receiving amphetamine compared to subjects not on adjunctive therapy.

13 NONCLINICAL TOXICOLOGY
13.1 Carcinogenesis, Mutagenesis and Impairment of Fertility
Clonidine HCl was not carcinogenic when administered in the diet of rats (for up to 132 weeks) or mice (for up to 78 weeks) at doses of up to 1620 (male rats), 2040 (female rats), or 2500 (mice) mcg/kg/day. These doses are approximately 20, 25, and 15 times, respectively, the maximum recommended human dose (MRHD) of 0.4 mg/day on a mg/m^2 basis.

There was no evidence of genotoxicity in the Ames test for mutagenicity or mouse micronucleus test for clastogenicity. Fertility of male or female rats was unaffected by clonidine HCl doses as high as 150 mcg/kg/day (approximately 3 times the MRHD on a mg/m^2 basis). In a separate experiment, fertility of female rats appeared to be adversely affected at dose levels of 500 and 2000 mcg/kg/day (10 and 40 times the MRHD on a mg/m^2 basis).

14 CLINICAL STUDIES
Efficacy of KAPVAY in the treatment of ADHD was established in children and adolescents (6 to 17 years) in:
- One short-term, placebo-controlled monotherapy trial (Study 1)
- One short-term adjunctive therapy to psychostimulants trial (Study 2)
- One randomized withdrawal trial as monotherapy (Study 3)

Short-term Monotherapy and Adjunctive Therapy to Psychostimulant Studies for ADHD
The efficacy of KAPVAY in the treatment of ADHD was established in 2 (one monotherapy and one adjunctive therapy) placebo-controlled trials in pediatric patients aged 6 to 17, who met DSM-IV criteria of ADHD hyperactive or combined hyperactive/inattentive subtypes. Signs and symptoms of ADHD were evaluated using the investigator administered and scored ADHD Rating Scale-IV-Parent Version (ADHDRS-IV) total score including hyperactive/impulsivity and inattentive subscales.

Study 1 (CLON-301), was an 8-week randomized, double-blind, placebo-controlled, fixed dose study of children and adolescents aged 6 to 17 (N=236) with a 5-week primary efficacy endpoint. Patients were randomly assigned to one of the following three treatment groups: KAPVAY (CLON) 0.2 mg/day (N=78), KAPVAY 0.4 mg/day (N=80), or placebo (N=78). Dosing for the KAPVAY groups started at 0.1 mg/day and was titrated in increments of 0.1 mg/week to their respective dose (as divided doses). Patients were maintained at their dose for a minimum of 2 weeks before being gradually tapered down to 0.1 mg/day at the last week of treatment. At both doses, improvements in ADHD symptoms were statistically significantly superior in KAPVAY-treated patients compared with placebo-treated patients at the end of 5 weeks as measured by the ADHDRS-IV total score (Table 8).

Study 2 (CLON-302) was an 8-week randomized, double-blind, placebo-controlled, flexible dose study in children and adolescents aged 6 to 17 (N=198) with a 5-week primary efficacy end point. Patients had been treated with a psychostimulant (methylphenidate or amphetamine) for four weeks with inadequate response. Patients were randomly assigned to one of two treatment groups: KAPVAY adjunct to a psychostimulant (N=102) or psychostimulant alone (N=96). The KAPVAY dose was initiated at 0.1 mg/day and doses were titrated in increments of 0.1 mg/week up to 0.4 mg/day, as divided doses, over a 3-week period based on tolerability and clinical response. The dose was maintained for a minimum of 2 weeks before being gradually tapered to 0.1 mg/day at the last week of treatment. ADHD symptoms were statistically significantly improved in KAPVAY plus stimulant group compared with the stimulant alone group at the end of 5 weeks as measured by the ADHDRS-IV total score (Table 8).

[See table 8 on next page]

Maintenance Monotherapy for ADHD
Study 3 (SHN-KAP-401), was a double-blind, placebo-controlled, randomized-withdrawal study in children and adolescents aged 6 to 17 years (n=253) with DSM-IV-TR diagnosis of ADHD. The study consisted of a 10-week, open-label phase (4 weeks of dose optimization and 6 weeks of dose maintenance), a 26-week double-blind phase, and a 4-week taper-down and follow-up phase. All patients were

Table 7 Pharmacokinetic Parameters of Clonidine in Healthy Adult Volunteers

Parameter	CATAPRES-Fasted n=15 Mean	CATAPRES-Fasted n=15 SD	KAPVAY-Fed n=15 Mean	KAPVAY-Fed n=15 SD	KAPVAY-Fasted n=14 MEAN	KAPVAY-Fasted n=14 SD
C$_{max}$ (pg/mL)	443	59.6	235	34.7	258	33.3
AUC$_{inf}$ (hr*pg/mL)	7313	1812	6505	1728	6729	1650
hT$_{max}$ (hr)	2.07	0.5	6.80	3.61	6.50	1.23
T$_{1/2}$ (hr)	12.57	3.11	12.67	3.76	12.65	3.56

initiated at 0.1 mg/day and increased at weekly intervals in increments of 0.1 mg/day until reaching personalized optimal dose (0.1, 0.2, 0.3 or 0.4 mg/day, as divided doses). Eligible patients had to demonstrate treatment response as defined by ≥ 30% reduction in ADHD-RS-IV total score and a Clinical Global Impression-Improvement score of 1 or 2 during the open label phase. Patients who sustained treatment response (n=135) until the end of the open label phase were randomly assigned to one of the two treatment groups, KAPVAY (N=68) and Placebo (N=67), to evaluate the long-term efficacy of maintenance dose of KAPVAY in the double-blind phase. The primary efficacy endpoint was the percentage of patients with treatment failure defined as a ≥ 30% increase (worsening) in ADHD-RS-IV total score and ≥ 2 points increase (worsening) in Clinical Global Impression – Severity Scale in 2 consecutive visits or early termination for any reason. A total of 73 patients experienced treatment failure in the double-blind phase: 31 patients (45.6%) in the KAPVAY group and 42 patients (62.7%) in the placebo group, with a statistically significant difference in the primary endpoint favoring KAPVAY (Table 9). The cumulative proportion of patients with treatment failure over time during the double-blind phase is displayed in Figure 2.

Table 9 Treatment Failure: Double-Blind Full Analysis Set (Study 3)

Study 3	Double-Blind Full Analysis Set	
	Kapvay®	Placebo
Number of subjects	68	67
Number of treatment failures	31 (45.6%)	42 (62.7%)
Basis of Treatment Failure		
Clinical criteria[a,b]	11 (16.2%)	9 (13.4%)
Lack of efficacy[c]	1 (1.5%)	3 (4.5%)
Withdrawal of informed assent/ consent	4 (5.9%)	20 (29.9%)
Other early terminations	15 (22.1%)	10 (14.9%)

ADHD-RS-IV = Attention Deficit Hyperactivity Disorder-Rating Scale-4th edition; CGI-S = Clinical Global Impression-Severity
[a] At the same 2 consecutive visits a (1) 30% or greater reduction in ADHD-RS-IV, and (2) 2-point or more increase in CGI-S.
[b] Two subjects (1 placebo and 1 KAPVAY) withdrew consent, but met the clinical criteria for treatment failure.
[c] Three subjects (all placebo) discontinued the study due to treatment failure, but met only the criterion for ADHD-RS-IV.

[See Figure 2 at top of next column]

16 HOW SUPPLIED/STORAGE AND HANDLING

KAPVAY extended-release tablets are white, non-scored, standard convex with debossing ("651" for 0.1 mg and "652" for 0.2 mg) on one side.
NDC 59212-658-60 – 0.1 mg round tablets supplied in bottles containing 60 tablets.
NDC 59212-659-60 – 0.2 mg oval tablets supplied in bottles containing 60 tablets.

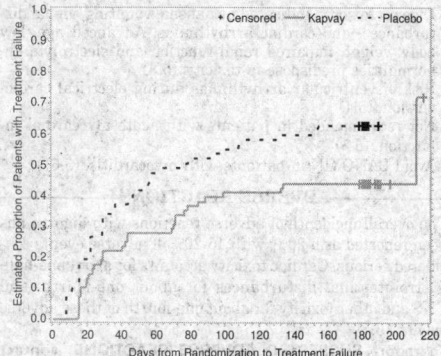

Figure 2: Kaplan-Meier Estimation of Cumulative Proportion of Patients with Treatment Failure (Study 3)

Store at 20°-25°C (68°-77°F) [see USP Controlled Room Temperature].
Dispense in a tight container.

17 PATIENT COUNSELING INFORMATION

Advise the patient to read the FDA-approved Patient Labeling (Patient Information)
Dosage and Administration
Advise patients that KAPVAY must be swallowed whole, never crushed, cut, or chewed, and may be taken with or without food. When initiating treatment, provide dosage escalation instructions [see Dosage and Administration (2.1)].
Missed Dose
If patients miss a dose of KAPVAY, advise them to skip the dose and take the next dose as scheduled and not to take more than the prescribed total daily amount of KAPVAY in any 24-hour period [see Dosage and Administration (2.4)].
Hypotension/Bradycardia
Advise patients who have a history of syncope or may have a condition that predisposes them to syncope, such as hypotension, orthostatic hypotension, bradycardia, or dehydration, to avoid becoming dehydrated or overheated [see Warnings and Precautions (5.1)].
Sedation and Somnolence
Instruct patients to use caution when driving a car or operating hazardous machinery until they know how they will respond to treatment with KAPVAY. Also advise patients to avoid the use of KAPVAY with other centrally active depressants and with alcohol [see Warnings and Precautions (5.2)].
Rebound Hypertension
Advise patients not to discontinue KAPVAY abruptly [see Warnings and Precautions (5.3)].
Allergic Reactions
Advise patients to discontinue KAPVAY and seek immediate medical attention if any signs or symptoms of a hypersensitivity reaction occur, such as generalized rash, urticaria, or angioedema [see Warnings and Precautions (5.4)].
Patient Information
KAPVAY® (KAP-vay)
(clonidine hydrochloride) Extended-Release Tablets
Read the Patient Information that comes with KAPVAY before you start taking it and each time you get a refill. There may be new information. This Patient Information leaflet does not take the place of talking to your doctor about your medical condition or treatment.

What is KAPVAY?
KAPVAY is a prescription medicine used for the treatment of Attention-Deficit Hyperactivity Disorder (ADHD). Your doctor may prescribe KAPVAY alone or together with certain other ADHD medicines.
• KAPVAY is not a central nervous system (CNS) stimulant.
• KAPVAY should be used as part of a total treatment program for ADHD that may include counseling or other therapies.
Who should not take KAPVAY?
• Do not take KAPVAY if you are allergic to clonidine in KAPVAY. See the end of this leaflet for a complete list of ingredients in KAPVAY.
What should I tell my doctor before taking KAPVAY?
Before you take KAPVAY, tell your doctor if you:
• have kidney problems
• have low or high blood pressure
• have a history of passing out (syncope)
• have heart problems, including history of heart attack
• have had a stroke or have stroke symptoms
• had a skin reaction (such as a rash) after taking clonidine in a transdermal form (skin patch)
• have any other medical conditions
• are pregnant or plan to become pregnant. It is not known if KAPVAY will harm your unborn baby. Talk to your doctor if you are pregnant or plan to become pregnant.
• are breastfeeding or plan to breastfeed. KAPVAY can pass into your breast milk. Talk to your doctor about the best way to feed your baby if you take KAPVAY.
Tell your doctor about all of the medicines that you take, including prescription and non-prescription medicines, vitamins, and herbal supplements.
KAPVAY and certain other medicines may affect each other causing serious side effects. Sometimes the doses of other medicines may need to be changed while taking KAPVAY.
Especially tell your doctor if you take:
• anti-depression medicines
• heart or blood pressure medicine
• other medicines that contain clonidine
• a medicine that makes you sleepy (sedation)
Ask your doctor or pharmacist for a list of these medicines, if you are not sure if your medicine is listed above.
Know the medicines that you take. Keep a list of your medicines with you to show your doctor and pharmacist when you get a new medicine.
How should I take KAPVAY?
• Take KAPVAY exactly as your doctor tells you to take it.
• Your doctor will tell you how many KAPVAY tablets to take and when to take them. Your doctor may change your dose of KAPVAY. Do not change your dose of KAPVAY without talking to your doctor.
• Do not stop taking KAPVAY without talking to your doctor.
• KAPVAY can be taken with or without food.
• KAPVAY should be taken 2 times a day (in the morning and at bedtime).
• If you miss a dose of KAPVAY, skip the missed dose. Just take the next dose at your regular time. Do not take two doses at the same time.
• Take KAPVAY tablets whole. Do not chew, crush or break KAPVAY tablets. Tell your doctor if you cannot swallow KAPVAY tablets whole. You may need a different medicine.
• If you take too much KAPVAY, call your Poison Control Center or go to the nearest hospital emergency room right away.
What should I avoid while taking KAPVAY?
• Do not drink alcohol or take other medicines that make you sleepy or dizzy while taking KAPVAY until you talk with your doctor. KAPVAY taken with alcohol or medicines that cause sleepiness or dizziness may make your sleepiness or dizziness worse.
• Do not drive, operate heavy machinery or do other dangerous activities until you know how KAPVAY will affect you.
• Avoid becoming dehydrated or overheated.
What are possible side effects of KAPVAY?
KAPVAY may cause serious side effects, including:
• **Low blood pressure and low heart rate**. Your doctor should check your heart rate and blood pressure before starting treatment and regularly during treatment with KAPVAY.
• Sleepiness.
• Withdrawal symptoms. Suddenly stopping KAPVAY may cause withdrawal symptoms including: increased blood pressure, headache, increased heart rate, lightheadedness, tightness in your chest and nervousness.
The most common side effects of KAPVAY include:
• sleepiness

Table 8 Short-Term Trials

Study Number	Treatment Group	Primary Efficacy Measure: ADHDRS-IV Total Score		
		Mean Baseline Score (SD)	LS Mean Change from Baseline (SE)	Placebo-subtracted Difference[a] (95% CI)
Study 1	KAPVAY (0.2 mg/day)	43.8 (7.47)	-15.0 (1.38)	-8.5 (-12.2, - 4.8)
	KAPVAY (0.4 mg/day)	44.6 (7.73)	-15.6 (1.33)	-9.1 (-12.8, - 5.5)
	Placebo	45.0 (8.53)	-6.5 (1.35)	--
Study 2	KAPVAY (0.4 mg/day) + Psychostimulant	38.9 (6.95)	-15.8 (1.18)	-4.5 (-7.8, -1.1)
	Psychostimulant alone	39.0 (7.68)	-11.3 (1.24)	--

SD: standard deviation; SE: standard error; LS Mean: least-squares mean; CI: unadjusted confidence interval.
[a] Difference (drug minus placebo) in least-squares mean change from baseline.

Continued on next page

- tiredness
- irritability
- trouble sleeping (insomnia)
- nightmare
- constipation
- dry mouth
- decreased appetite
- dizziness

Tell your doctor if you have any side effects that bother you or that does not go away.

These are not all of the possible side effects of KAPVAY. For more information, ask your doctor or pharmacist.

Call your doctor for medical advice about side effects. You may report side effects to FDA at 1-800-FDA-1088.

How should I store KAPVAY?

- Store KAPVAY between 68°-77°F (20°-25°C).
- Keep KAPVAY in a tightly closed container.

Keep KAPVAY and all medicines out of the reach of children.

General information about the safe and effective use of KAPVAY

Medicines are sometimes prescribed for purposes other than those listed in a Patient Information leaflet. Do not use KAPVAY for a condition for which it was not prescribed.

Do not give KAPVAY to other people, even if they have the same symptoms that you have. It may harm them.

This Patient Information leaflet summarizes the most important information about KAPVAY. If you would like more information, talk with your doctor. You can also ask your doctor or pharmacist for information about KAPVAY that is written for healthcare professionals.

For more information about KAPVAY, go to www.KAPVAY.com or call 1-877-370-1142.

What are the ingredients in KAPVAY?

- Active Ingredient: clonidine hydrochloride
- Inactive Ingredients: sodium lauryl sulfate, lactose monohydrate, hypromellose type 2208, partially pregelatinized starch, colloidal silicon dioxide, and magnesium stearate

Revised: 8/2016
Manufactured for:
Concordia Pharmaceuticals Inc.
St. Michael, Barbados BB11005
Kapvay® is a registered trademark of Concordia Pharmaceuticals Inc.

Shown in Product Identification Guide, page 508

LANOXIN® ℞
(digoxin)
tablets, for oral use

HIGHLIGHTS OF PRESCRIBING INFORMATION
These highlights do not include all the information needed to use LANOXIN safely and effectively. See full prescribing information for LANOXIN.
LANOXIN® (digoxin) tablets, for oral use
Initial U.S. Approval: 1954

————INDICATIONS AND USAGE————
LANOXIN is a cardiac glycoside indicated for:
- Treatment of mild to moderate heart failure in adults. (1.1)
- Increasing myocardial contractility in pediatric patients with heart failure. (1.2)
- Control of resting ventricular rate in patients with chronic atrial fibrillation in adults. (1.3)

————DOSAGE AND ADMINISTRATION————
LANOXIN dose is based on patient-specific factors (age, lean body weight, renal function, etc.). See full prescribing information. Monitor for toxicity and therapeutic effect. (2)

————DOSAGE FORMS AND STRENGTHS————
Unscored Tablets: 62.5 and 187.5 mcg.
Scored Tablets: 125 and 250 mcg. (3)

————CONTRAINDICATIONS————
- Ventricular fibrillation. (4)
- Known hypersensitivity to digoxin or other forms of digitalis. (4)

————WARNINGS AND PRECAUTIONS————
- Risk of rapid ventricular response leading to ventricular fibrillation in patients with AV accessory pathway. (5.1)
- Risk of advanced or complete heart block in patients with sinus node disease and AV block. (5.2)

- Digoxin toxicity: Indicated by nausea, vomiting, visual disturbances, and cardiac arrhythmias. Advanced age, low body weight, impaired renal function and electrolyte abnormalities predispose to toxicity. (5.3)
- Risk of ventricular arrhythmias during electrical cardioversion. (5.4)
- Not recommended in patients with acute myocardial infarction. (5.5)
- Avoid LANOXIN in patients with myocarditis. (5.6)

————ADVERSE REACTIONS————
The overall incidence of adverse reactions with digoxin has been reported as 5-20%, with 15-20% of adverse events considered serious. Cardiac toxicity accounts for about one-half, gastrointestinal disturbances for about one-fourth, and CNS and other toxicity for about one-fourth of these adverse events. (6.1)

To report SUSPECTED ADVERSE REACTIONS, contact Concordia Pharmaceuticals Inc. at 1-877-370-1142 or FDA at 1-800-FDA-1088 or www.fda.gov/medwatch.

————DRUG INTERACTIONS————
- PGP Inducers/Inhibitors: Drugs that induce or inhibit PGP have the potential to alter digoxin pharmacokinetics. (7.1)
- The potential for drug-drug interactions must be considered prior to and during drug therapy. See full prescribing information. (7.2, 7.3, 12.3)

————USE IN SPECIFIC POPULATIONS————
- Pregnant patients: It is unknown whether use during pregnancy can cause fetal harm. (8.1)
- Pediatric patients: Newborn infants display variability in tolerance to LANOXIN. (8.4)
- Geriatric patients: Consider renal function in dosage selection, and carefully monitor for side effects. (8.5)
- Renal impairment: LANOXIN is excreted by the kidneys. Consider renal function during dosage selection. (8.6)

See 17 for PATIENT COUNSELING INFORMATION.

Revised: 7/2015

FULL PRESCRIBING INFORMATION

1   INDICATIONS AND USAGE
1.1   Heart Failure in Adults
LANOXIN is indicated for the treatment of mild to moderate heart failure in adults. LANOXIN increases left ventricular ejection fraction and improves heart failure symptoms as evidenced by improved exercise capacity and decreased heart failure-related hospitalizations and emergency care, while having no effect on mortality. Where possible, LANOXIN should be used in combination with a diuretic and an angiotensin-converting enzyme (ACE) inhibitor.

1.2   Heart Failure in Pediatric Patients
LANOXIN increases myocardial contractility in pediatric patients with heart failure.

1.3   Atrial Fibrillation in Adults
LANOXIN is indicated for the control of ventricular response rate in adult patients with chronic atrial fibrillation.

2   DOSAGE AND ADMINISTRATION
2.1   Important Dosing and Administration Information
In selecting a LANOXIN dosing regimen, it is important to consider factors that affect digoxin blood levels (e.g., body weight, age, renal function, concomitant drugs) since toxic levels of digoxin are only slightly higher than therapeutic levels. Dosing can be either initiated with a loading dose followed by maintenance dosing if rapid titration is desired or initiated with maintenance dosing without a loading dose.

Consider interruption or reduction in LANOXIN dose prior to electrical cardioversion *[see Warnings and Precautions (5.4)]*.

Use digoxin solution to obtain the appropriate dose in infants, young pediatric patients, or patients with very low body weight.

2.2   Loading Dosing Regimen in Adults and Pediatric Patients
For adults and pediatric patients if a loading dosage is to be given, administer half the total loading dose initially, then ¼ the loading dose every 6-8 hours twice, with careful assessment of clinical response and toxicity before each dose. The recommended loading dose is displayed in Table 1.

Table 1. Recommended LANOXIN Oral Loading Dose

Age	Total Oral Loading Dose (mcg/kg) Administer half the total loading dose initially, then ¼ the loading dose every 6 to 8 hours twice
5 to 10 years	20-45
Adults and pediatric patients over 10 years	10-15

mcg = microgram

2.3   Maintenance Dosing in Adults and Pediatric Patients Over 10 Years Old
The maintenance dose is based on lean body weight, renal function, age, and concomitant products *[see Clinical Pharmacology (12.3)]*.

The recommended **starting** maintenance dose in adults and pediatric patients over 10 years old with normal renal function is given in Table 2. Doses may be increased every 2 weeks according to clinical response, serum drug levels, and toxicity.

Table 2. Recommended Starting LANOXIN Maintenance Dosage in Adults and Pediatric Patients Over 10 Years Old

Age	Total Oral Maintenance Dose, mcg/kg/day (given once daily)
Adults and pediatric patients over 10 years	3.4-5.1

mcg = microgram

Table 3 provides the recommended (once daily) maintenance dose for adults and pediatric patients over 10 years old (to be given once daily) according to lean body weight and renal function. The doses are based on studies in adult patients with heart failure. Alternatively, the maintenance dose may be estimated by the following formula (peak body stores lost each day through elimination):

Total Maintenance Dose = Loading Dose (i.e., Peak Body Stores) × % Daily Loss/100

(% Daily Loss = 14 + Creatinine clearance/5)

Reduce the dose of LANOXIN in patients whose lean weight is an abnormally small fraction of their total body mass because of obesity or edema.

[See table 3 above]

2.4 Maintenance Dosing in Pediatric Patients Less Than 10 Years Old

The starting maintenance dose for heart failure in pediatric patients less than 10 years old is based on lean body weight, renal function, age, and concomitant products *[see Clinical Pharmacology (12.3)]*. The recommended **starting** maintenance dose for pediatric patients between 5 years and 10 years old is given in Table 4. These recommendations assume the presence of normal renal function.

Table 4. Recommended Starting LANOXIN Oral Maintenance Dosage in Pediatric Patients between 5 and 10 Years Old

Age	Oral Maintenance Dose, mcg/kg/dose
5 years to 10 years	3.2-6.4 **Twice daily**

Table 5 provides average daily maintenance dose requirements for pediatric patients between 5 and 10 years old (to be given twice daily) with heart failure based on age, lean body weight, and renal function.

[See table 5 above]

2.5 Monitoring to Assess Safety, Efficacy, and Therapeutic Blood Levels

Monitor for signs and symptoms of digoxin toxicity and clinical response. Adjust dose based on toxicity, efficacy, and blood levels.

Serum digoxin levels less than 0.5 ng/mL have been associated with diminished efficacy, while levels above 2 ng/mL have been associated with increased toxicity without increased benefit.

Interpret the serum digoxin concentration in the overall clinical context, and do not use an isolated measurement of serum digoxin concentration as the basis for increasing or decreasing the LANOXIN dose. Serum digoxin concentrations may be falsely elevated by endogenous digoxin-like substances *[see Drug Interactions (7.4)]*. If the assay is sensitive to these substances, consider obtaining a baseline digoxin level before starting LANOXIN and correct post-treatment values by the reported baseline level.

Obtain serum digoxin concentrations just before the next scheduled LANOXIN dose or at least 6 hours after the last dose. The digoxin concentration is likely to be 10-25% lower when sampled right before the next dose (24 hours after dosing) compared to sampling 8 hours after dosing (using once-daily dosing). However, there will be only minor differences in digoxin concentrations using twice daily dosing whether sampling is done at 8 or 12 hours after a dose.

2.6 Switching from Intravenous Digoxin to Oral Digoxin

When switching from intravenous to oral digoxin formulations, make allowances for differences in bioavailability when calculating maintenance dosages (see Table 6).

[See table 6 on next page]

Table 3. Recommended Maintenance Dose (in micrograms given once daily) of LANOXIN in Pediatric Patients Over 10 Years Old and Adults by Lean Body Weight and by Renal Function[a]

Corrected Creatinine Clearance[b]	Lean Body Weight[d]								Number of Days Before Steady State Achieved[c]
	kg	40	50	60	70	80	90	100	
10 mL/min		62.5*	125	125	187.5	187.5	187.5	250	19
20 mL/min		125	125	125	187.5	187.5	250	250	16
30 mL/min		125	125	187.5	187.5	250	250	312.5	14
40 mL/min		125	187.5	187.5	250	250	312.5	312.5	13
50 mL/min		125	187.5	187.5	250	250	312.5	312.5	12
60 mL/min		125	187.5	250	250	312.5	312.5	375	11
70 mL/min		187.5	187.5	250	250	312.5	375	375	10
80 mL/min		187.5	187.5	250	312.5	312.5	375	437.5	9
90 mL/min		187.5	250	250	312.5	375	437.5	437.5	8
100 mL/min		187.5	250	312.5	312.5	375	437.5	500	7

[a] Doses are rounded to the nearest dose possible using whole LANOXIN tablets. Recommended doses approximately 30 percent lower than the calculated dose are designated with an *. Monitor digoxin levels in patients receiving these initial doses and increase dose if needed.

[b] *For adults*, creatinine clearance was corrected to 70-kg body weight or 1.73 m²body surface area. If only serum creatinine concentrations (Scr) are available, a corrected Ccr may be estimated in men as (140 – Age)/Scr. For women, this result should be multiplied by 0.85.

For *pediatric* patients, the modified Schwartz equation may be used. The formula is based on height in cm and Scr in mg/dL where k is a constant. Ccr is corrected to 1.73 m²body surface area. During the first year of life, the value of k is 0.33 for pre-term babies and 0.45 for term infants. The k is 0.55 for pediatric patients and adolescent girls and 0.7 for adolescent boys.

GFR (mL/min/1.73 m²) = (k × Height)/Scr

[c] If no loading dose administered.

[d] The doses listed assume average body composition.

Table 5. Recommended Maintenance Dose (in micrograms given TWICE daily) of LANOXIN in Pediatric Patients between 5 and 10 Years of Age[a] Based upon Lean Body Weight and Renal Function[a,b]

Corrected Creatinine Clearance[c]	Lean Body Weight					Number of Days Before Steady State Achieved[d]
	kg	20	30	40	50	60	
10 mL/min		-	62.5	62.5*	125	125	19
20 mL/min		62.5	62.5	125	125	125	16
30 mL/min		62.5	62.5*	125	125	187.5	14
40 mL/min		62.5	62.5*	125	187.5	187.5	13
50 mL/min		62.5	125	125	187.5	187.5	12
60 mL/min		62.5	125	125	187.5	250	11
70 mL/min		62.5	125	187.5	187.5	250	10
80 mL/min		62.5*	125	187.5	187.5	250	9
90 mL/min		62.5*	125	187.5	250	250	8
100 mL/min		62.5*	125	187.5	250	312.5	7

[a] Recommended are doses to be given twice daily.

[b] The doses are rounded to the nearest dose possible using whole LANOXIN tablets. Recommended doses approximately 30 percent lower than the calculated dose are designated with an *. Monitor digoxin levels in patients receiving these initial doses and increase dose if needed.

[c] The modified Schwartz equation may be used to estimate creatinine clearance. See footnote b under Table 3.

[d] If no loading dose administered.

3 DOSAGE FORMS AND STRENGTHS

Unscored Tablets: 62.5 mcg are peach, round with "U3A" imprinted on one side.

Scored Tablets: 125 mcg are yellow, round, scored tablets with "Y3B" imprinted on one side.

Unscored Tablets: 187.5 mcg are blue, round with "F3F" imprinted on one side.

Scored Tablets: 250 mcg are white, round, scored tablets with "X3A" imprinted on one side.

4 CONTRAINDICATIONS

LANOXIN is contraindicated in patients with:
• Ventricular fibrillation *[see Warnings and Precautions (5.1)]*

• Known hypersensitivity to digoxin (reactions seen include unexplained rash, swelling of the mouth, lips or throat or a difficulty in breathing). A hypersensitivity reaction to other digitalis preparations usually constitutes a contraindication to digoxin.

5 WARNINGS AND PRECAUTIONS

5.1 Ventricular Fibrillation in Patients With Accessory AV Pathway (Wolff-Parkinson-White Syndrome)

Patients with Wolff-Parkinson-White syndrome who develop atrial fibrillation are at high risk of ventricular fibrillation. Treatment of these patients with digoxin leads to greater slowing of conduction in the atrioventricular node

Continued on next page

than in accessory pathways, and the risks of rapid ventricular response leading to ventricular fibrillation are thereby increased.

5.2 Sinus Bradycardia and Sino-atrial Block

LANOXIN may cause severe sinus bradycardia or sinoatrial block particularly in patients with pre-existing sinus node disease and may cause advanced or complete heart block in patients with pre-existing incomplete AV block. Consider insertion of a pacemaker before treatment with digoxin.

5.3 Digoxin Toxicity

Signs and symptoms of digoxin toxicity include anorexia, nausea, vomiting, visual changes and cardiac arrhythmias [first-degree, second-degree (Wenckebach), or third-degree heart block (including asystole); atrial tachycardia with block; AV dissociation; accelerated junctional (nodal) rhythm; unifocal or multiform ventricular premature contractions (especially bigeminy or trigeminy); ventricular tachycardia; and ventricular fibrillation]. Toxicity is usually associated with digoxin levels greater than 2 ng/mL although symptoms may also occur at lower levels. Low body weight, advanced age or impaired renal function, hypokalemia, hypercalcemia, or hypomagnesemia may predispose to digoxin toxicity. Obtain serum digoxin levels in patients with signs or symptoms of digoxin therapy and interrupt or adjust dose if necessary *[see Adverse Reactions (6) and Overdosage (10)]*. Assess serum electrolytes and renal function periodically.

The earliest and most frequent manifestation of digoxin toxicity in infants and children is the appearance of cardiac arrhythmias, including sinus bradycardia. In children, the use of digoxin may produce any arrhythmia. The most common are conduction disturbances or supraventricular tachyarrhythmias, such as atrial tachycardia (with or without block) and junctional (nodal) tachycardia. Ventricular arrhythmias are less common. Sinus bradycardia may be a sign of impending digoxin intoxication, especially in infants, even in the absence of first-degree heart block. Any arrhythmias or alteration in cardiac conduction that develops in a child taking digoxin should initially be assumed to be a consequence of digoxin intoxication.

Given that adult patients with heart failure have some symptoms in common with digoxin toxicity, it may be difficult to distinguish digoxin toxicity from heart failure. Misidentification of their etiology might lead the clinician to continue or increase LANOXIN dosing, when dosing should actually be suspended. When the etiology of these signs and symptoms is not clear, measure serum digoxin levels.

5.4 Risk of Ventricular Arrhythmias During Electrical Cardioversion

It may be desirable to reduce the dose of or discontinue LANOXIN for 1 to 2 days prior to electrical cardioversion of atrial fibrillation to avoid the induction of ventricular arrhythmias, but physicians must consider the consequences of increasing the ventricular response if digoxin is decreased or withdrawn. If digitalis toxicity is suspected, elective cardioversion should be delayed. If it is not prudent to delay cardioversion, the lowest possible energy level should be selected to avoid provoking ventricular arrhythmias.

5.5 Risk of Ischemia in Patients With Acute Myocardial Infarction

LANOXIN is not recommended in patients with acute myocardial infarction because digoxin may increase myocardial oxygen demand and lead to ischemia.

5.6 Vasoconstriction In Patients With Myocarditis

LANOXIN can precipitate vasoconstriction and may promote production of pro-inflammatory cytokines; therefore, avoid use in patients with myocarditis.

5.7 Decreased Cardiac Output in Patients With Preserved Left Ventricular Systolic Function

Patients with heart failure associated with preserved left ventricular ejection fraction may experience decreased cardiac output with use of LANOXIN. Such disorders include restrictive cardiomyopathy, constrictive pericarditis, amyloid heart disease, and acute cor pulmonale. Patients with idiopathic hypertrophic subaortic stenosis may have worsening of the outflow obstruction due to the inotropic effects of digoxin. Patients with amyloid heart disease may be more susceptible to digoxin toxicity at therapeutic levels because of an increased binding of digoxin to extracellular amyloid fibrils.

LANOXIN should generally be avoided in these patients, although it has been used for ventricular rate control in the subgroup of patients with atrial fibrillation.

5.8 Reduced Efficacy In Patients With Hypocalcemia

Hypocalcemia can nullify the effects of digoxin in humans; thus, digoxin may be ineffective until serum calcium is restored to normal. These interactions are related to the fact that digoxin affects contractility and excitability of the heart in a manner similar to that of calcium.

Table 6. Comparison of the Systemic Availability and Equivalent Doses of Oral and Intravenous LANOXIN

	Absolute Bioavailability	Equivalent Doses (mcg)			
LANOXIN Tablets	60-80%	62.5	125	250	500
LANOXIN Intravenous Injection	100%	50	100	200	400

5.9 Altered Response in Thyroid Disorders and Hypermetabolic States

Hypothyroidism may reduce the requirements for digoxin.

Heart failure and/or atrial arrhythmias resulting from hypermetabolic or hyperdynamic states (e.g., hyperthyroidism, hypoxia, or arteriovenous shunt) are best treated by addressing the underlying condition. Atrial arrhythmias associated with hypermetabolic states are particularly resistant to digoxin treatment. Patients with beri beri heart disease may fail to respond adequately to digoxin if the underlying thiamine deficiency is not treated concomitantly.

6 ADVERSE REACTIONS

The following adverse reactions are included in more detail in the Warnings and Precautions section of the label:

- Cardiac arrhythmias *[see Warnings and Precautions (5.1, 5.2)]*
- Digoxin Toxicity *[see Warnings and Precautions (5.3)]*

6.1 Clinical Trials Experience

Because clinical trials are conducted under widely varying conditions, adverse reaction rates observed in the clinical trials of a drug cannot be directly compared to rates in the clinical trials of another drug and may not reflect the rates observed in clinical practice.

In general, the adverse reactions of LANOXIN are dose-dependent and occur at doses higher than those needed to achieve a therapeutic effect. Hence, adverse reactions are less common when LANOXIN is used within the recommended dose range, is maintained within the therapeutic serum concentration range, and when there is careful attention to concurrent medications and conditions.

In the DIG trial (a trial investigating the effect of digoxin on mortality and morbidity in patients with heart failure), the incidence of hospitalization for suspected digoxin toxicity was 2% in patients taking LANOXIN compared to 0.9% in patients taking placebo *[see Clinical Studies (14.1)]*.

The overall incidence of adverse reactions with digoxin has been reported as 5-20%, with 15-20% of adverse events considered serious. Cardiac toxicity accounts for about one-half, gastrointestinal disturbances for about one-fourth, and CNS and other toxicity for about one-fourth of these adverse events.

Gastrointestinal: In addition to nausea and vomiting, the use of digoxin has been associated with abdominal pain, intestinal ischemia, and hemorrhagic necrosis of the intestines.

CNS: Digoxin can cause headache, weakness, dizziness, apathy, confusion, and mental disturbances (such as anxiety, depression, delirium, and hallucination).

Other: Gynecomastia has been occasionally observed following the prolonged use of digoxin. Thrombocytopenia and maculopapular rash and other skin reactions have been rarely observed.

7 DRUG INTERACTIONS

Digoxin has a narrow therapeutic index, increased monitoring of serum digoxin concentrations and for potential signs and symptoms of clinical toxicity is necessary when initiating, adjusting, or discontinuing drugs that may interact with digoxin. Prescribers should consult the prescribing information of any drug which is co-prescribed with digoxin for potential drug interaction information.

7.1 P-Glycoprotein (PGP) Inducers/Inhibitors

Digoxin is a substrate of P-glycoprotein, at the level of intestinal absorption, renal tubular section and biliary-intestinal secretion. Therefore, drugs that induce/inhibit P-glycoprotein have the potential to alter digoxin pharmacokinetics.

7.2 Pharmacokinetic Drug Interactions

[See table on next page]

7.3 Potentially Significant Pharmacodynamic Drug Interactions

Because of considerable variability of pharmacodynamic interactions, the dosage of digoxin should be individualized when patients receive these medications concurrently.

[See table on page 902]

7.4 Drug/Laboratory Test Interactions

Endogenous substances of unknown composition (digoxin-like immunoreactive substances [DLIS]) can interfere with standard radioimmunoassays for digoxin. The interference most often causes results to be falsely positive or falsely elevated, but sometimes it causes results to be falsely reduced. Some assays are more subject to these failings than others. Several LC/MS/MS methods are available that may provide less susceptibility to DLIS interference. DLIS are present in up to half of all neonates and in varying percentages of pregnant women, patients with hypertrophic cardiomyopathy, patients with renal or hepatic dysfunction, and other patients who are volume-expanded for any reason. The measured levels of DLIS (as digoxin equivalents) are usually low (0.2-0.4 ng/mL), but sometimes they reach levels that would be considered therapeutic or even toxic.

In some assays, spironolactone, canrenone, and potassium canrenoate may be falsely detected as digoxin, at levels up to 0.5 ng/mL. Some traditional Chinese and Ayurvedic medicine substances like Chan Su, Siberian Ginseng, Asian Ginseng, Ashwagandha or Dashen can cause similar interference.

Spironolactone and DLIS are much more extensively protein-bound than digoxin. As a result, assays of free digoxin levels in protein-free ultrafiltrate (which tend to be about 25% less than total levels, consistent with the usual extent of protein binding) are less affected by spironolactone or DLIS. It should be noted that ultrafiltration does not solve all interference problems with alternative medicines. The use of an LC/MS/MS method may be the better option according to the good results it provides, especially in terms of specificity and limit of quantization.

8 USE IN SPECIFIC POPULATIONS

8.1 Pregnancy

Pregnancy Category C

LANOXIN should be given to a pregnant woman only if clearly needed. It is also not known whether digoxin can cause fetal harm when administered to a pregnant woman or can affect reproductive capacity. Animal reproduction studies have not been conducted with digoxin.

8.2 Labor and Delivery

There are not enough data from clinical trials to determine the safety and efficacy of digoxin during labor and delivery.

8.3 Nursing Mothers

Studies have shown that digoxin distributes into breast milk, and that the milk-to-serum concentration ratio is approximately 0.6-0.9. However, the estimated exposure of a nursing infant to digoxin via breastfeeding is far below the usual infant maintenance dose. Therefore, this amount should have no pharmacologic effect upon the infant.

8.4 Pediatric Use

The safety and effectiveness of LANOXIN in the control of ventricular rate in children with atrial fibrillation have not been established.

The safety and effectiveness of LANOXIN in the treatment of heart failure in children have not been established in adequate and well-controlled studies. However, in published literature of children with heart failure of various etiologies (e.g., ventricular septal defects, anthracycline toxicity, patent ductus arteriosus), treatment with digoxin has been associated with improvements in hemodynamic parameters and in clinical signs and symptoms.

Newborn infants display considerable variability in their tolerance to digoxin. Premature and immature infants are particularly sensitive to the effects of digoxin, and the dosage of the drug must not only be reduced but must be individualized according to their degree of maturity.

8.5 Geriatric Use

The majority of clinical experience gained with digoxin has been in the elderly population. This experience has not identified differences in response or adverse effects between the elderly and younger patients. However, this drug is known to be substantially excreted by the kidney, and the risk of toxic reactions to this drug may be greater in pa-

Digoxin concentrations increased greater than 50%

	Digoxin Serum Concentration Increase	Digoxin AUC Increase	Recommendations
Amiodarone	70%	NA	Measure serum digoxin concentrations before initiating concomitant drugs. Reduce digoxin concentrations by decreasing dose by approximately 30-50% or by modifying the dosing frequency and continue monitoring.
Captopril	58%	39%	
Clarithromycin	NA	70%	
Dronedarone	NA	150%	
Gentamicin	129-212%	NA	
Erythromycin	100%	NA	
Itraconazole	80%	NA	
Lapatinib	NA	180%	
Nitrendipine	57%	15%	
Propafenone	NA	60-270%	
Quinidine	100%	NA	
Ranolazine	50%	NA	
Ritonavir	NA	86%	
Telaprevir	50%	85%	
Tetracycline	100%	NA	
Verapamil	50-75%	NA	

Digoxin concentrations increased less than 50%

	Digoxin Serum Concentration Increase	Digoxin AUC Increase	Recommendations
Atorvastatin	22%	15%	Measure serum digoxin concentrations before initiating concomitant drugs. Reduce digoxin concentrations by decreasing the dose by approximately 15-30% or by modifying the dosing frequency and continue monitoring.
Carvedilol	16%	14%	
Conivaptan	33%	43%	
Diltiazem	20%	NA	
Indomethacin	40%	NA	
Nefazodone	27%	15%	
Nifedipine	45%	NA	
Propantheline	24%	24%	
Quinine	NA	33%	
Rabeprazole	29%	19%	
Saquinavir	27%	49%	
Spironolactone	25%	NA	
Telmisartan	20-49%	NA	
Ticagrelor	31%	28%	
Tolvaptan	30%	20%	
Trimethoprim	22-28%	NA	

Digoxin concentrations increased, but magnitude is unclear

Alprazolam, azithromycin, cyclosporine, diclofenac, diphenoxylate, epoprostenol, esomeprazole, ibuprofen, ketoconazole, lansoprazole, metformin, omeprazole	Measure serum digoxin concentrations before initiating concomitant drugs. Continue monitoring and reduce digoxin dose as necessary.

Digoxin concentrations decreased

Acarbose, activated charcoal, albuterol, antacids, certain cancer chemotherapy or radiation therapy, cholestyramine, colestipol, extenatide, kaolin-pectin, meals high in bran, metoclopramide, miglitol, neomycin, penicillamine, phenytoin, rifampin, St. John's Wort, sucralfate, and sulfasalazine	Measure serum digoxin concentrations before initiating concomitant drugs. Continue monitoring and increase digoxin dose by approximately 20-40% as necessary.

NA = Not available/reported

tients with impaired renal function. Because elderly patients are more likely to have decreased renal function, care should be taken in dose selection, which should be based on renal function, and it may be useful to monitor renal function *[see Dosage and Administration (2.1)]*.

8.6 Renal Impairment

The clearance of digoxin can be primarily correlated with the renal function as indicated by creatinine clearance. Tables 3 and 5 provide the usual daily maintenance dose requirements for digoxin based on creatinine clearance *[see Dosage and Administration (2.3)]*.

Digoxin is primarily excreted by the kidneys; therefore, patients with impaired renal function require smaller than usual maintenance doses of digoxin *[see Dosage and Administration (2.3)]*. Because of the prolonged elimination half-life, a longer period of time is required to achieve an initial or new steady-state serum concentration in patients with renal impairment than in patients with normal renal function. If appropriate care is not taken to reduce the dose of digoxin, such patients are at high risk for toxicity, and toxic effects will last longer in such patients than in patients with normal renal function.

8.7 Hepatic Impairment

Plasma digoxin concentrations in patients with acute hepatitis generally fall within the range of profiles in a group of healthy subjects.

8.8 Malabsorption

The absorption of digoxin is reduced in some malabsorption conditions such as chronic diarrhea.

10 OVERDOSAGE

10.1 Signs and Symptoms in Adults and Children

The signs and symptoms of toxicity are generally similar to those described in the Adverse Reactions (6.1) but may be more frequent and can be more severe. Signs and symptoms of digoxin toxicity become more frequent with levels above 2 ng/mL. However, in deciding whether a patient's symptoms are due to digoxin, the clinical state together with serum electrolyte levels and thyroid function are important factors *[see Dosage and Administration (2)]*.

Adults: The most common signs and symptoms of digoxin toxicity are nausea, vomiting, anorexia, and fatigue that occur in 30-70% of patients who are overdosed. Extremely high serum concentrations produce hyperkalemia especially in patients with impaired renal function. Almost every type of cardiac arrhythmia has been associated with digoxin overdose and multiple rhythm disturbances in the same patient are common. Peak cardiac effects occur 3-6 hours following ingestion and may persist for 24 hours or longer. Arrhythmias that are considered more characteristic of digoxin toxicity are new-onset Mobitz type 1 A-V block, accelerated junctional rhythms, non-paroxysmal atrial tachycardia with A-V block, and bi-directional ventricular tachycardia. Cardiac arrest from asystole or ventricular fibrillation is usually fatal.

Digoxin toxicity is related to serum concentration. As digoxin serum levels increase above 1.2 ng/mL, there is a potential for increase in adverse reactions. Furthermore, lower potassium levels increases the risk for adverse reactions. In adults with heart disease, clinical observations suggest that an overdose of digoxin of 10-15 mg results in death of half of patients. A dose above 25 mg ingested by an adult without heart disease appeared to be uniformly fatal if no Digoxin Immune Fab (DIGIBIND®, DIGIFAB®) was administered.

Among the extra-cardiac manifestations, gastrointestinal symptoms (e.g., nausea, vomiting, anorexia) are very common (up to 80% incidence) and precede cardiac manifestations in approximately half of the patients in most literature reports. Neurologic manifestations (e.g., dizziness, various CNS disturbances), fatigue, and malaise are very common. Visual manifestations may also occur with aberration in color vision (predominance of yellow green) the most frequent. Neurological and visual symptoms may persist after other signs of toxicity have resolved. In chronic toxicity, non-specific extra-cardiac symptoms, such as malaise and weakness, may predominate.

Children: In pediatric patients, signs and symptoms of toxicity can occur during or shortly after the dose of digoxin. Frequent non-cardiac effects are similar to those observed in adults although nausea and vomiting are not seen frequently in infants and small pediatric patients. Other reported manifestations of overdose are weight loss in older age groups, failure to thrive in infants, abdominal pain

Continued on next page

caused by mesenteric artery ischemia, drowsiness, and behavioral disturbances including psychotic episodes. Arrhythmias and combinations of arrhythmias that occur in adult patients can also occur in pediatric patients although sinus tachycardia, supraventricular tachycardia, and rapid atrial fibrillation are seen less frequently in pediatric patients. Pediatric patients are more likely to develop A-V conduction disturbances, or sinus bradycardia. Any arrhythmia in a child treated with digoxin should be considered related to digoxin until otherwise ruled out. In pediatric patients aged 1-3 years without heart disease, clinical observations suggest that an overdose of digoxin of 6-10 mg would result in death of half of the patients. In the same population, a dose above 10 mg resulted in death if no Digoxin Immune Fab were administered.

10.2 Treatment

Chronic Overdose

If there is suspicion of toxicity, discontinue LANOXIN and place the patient on a cardiac monitor. Correct factors such as electrolyte abnormalities, thyroid dysfunction, and concomitant medications *[see Dosage and Administration (2.5)]*. Correct hypokalemia by administering potassium so that serum potassium is maintained between 4.0 and 5.5 mmol/L. Potassium is usually administered orally, but when correction of the arrhythmia is urgent and serum potassium concentration is low, potassium may be administered by the intravenous route. Monitor electrocardiogram for any evidence of potassium toxicity (e.g., peaking of T waves) and to observe the effect on the arrhythmia. Avoid potassium salts in patients with bradycardia or heart block. Symptomatic arrhythmias may be treated with Digoxin Immune Fab.

Acute Overdose

Patients who have intentionally or accidently ingested massive doses of digoxin should receive activated charcoal orally or by nasogastric tube regardless of the time since ingestion since digoxin recirculates to the intestine by enterohepatic circulation. In addition to cardiac monitoring, temporarily discontinue LANOXIN until the adverse reaction resolves. Correct factors that may be contributing to the adverse reactions *[see Warnings and Precautions (5)]*. In particular, correct hypokalemia and hypomagnesemia. Digoxin is not effectively removed from the body by dialysis because of its large extravascular volume of distribution. Life threatening arrhythmias (ventricular tachycardia, ventricular fibrillation, high degree A-V block, bradyarrhythma, sinus arrest) or hyperkalemia requires administration of Digoxin Immune Fab. Digoxin Immune Fab has been shown to be 80-90% effective in reversing signs and symptoms of digoxin toxicity. Bradycardia and heart block caused by digoxin are parasympathetically mediated and respond to atropine. A temporary cardiac pacemaker may also be used. Ventricular arrhythmias may respond to lidocaine or phenytoin. When a large amount of digoxin has been ingested, especially in patients with impaired renal function, hyperkalemia may be present due to release of potassium from skeletal muscle. In this case, treatment with Digoxin Immune Fab is indicated; an initial treatment with glucose and insulin may be needed if the hyperkalemia is life-threatening. Once the adverse reaction has resolved, therapy with LANOXIN may be reinstituted following a careful reassessment of dose.

11 DESCRIPTION

LANOXIN (digoxin) is one of the cardiac (or digitalis) glycosides, a closely related group of drugs having in common specific effects on the myocardium. These drugs are found in a number of plants. Digoxin is extracted from the leaves of *Digitalis lanata*. The term "digitalis" is used to designate the whole group of glycosides. The glycosides are composed of 2 portions: a sugar and a cardenolide (hence "glycosides"). Digoxin is described chemically as (3β,5β,12β)-3-[(*O*-2,6-dideoxy-β-*D-ribo*-hexopyranosyl-(1→4)-*O*-2,6-dideoxy-β-*D-ribo*-hexopyranosyl-(1→4)-2,6-dideoxy-β-*D-ribo*-hexopyr-

anosyl)oxy]-12,14-dihydroxy-card-20(22)-enolide. Its molecular formula is $C_{41}H_{64}O_{14}$, its molecular weight is 780.95, and its structural formula is:

Digoxin exists as odorless white crystals that melt with decomposition above 230°C. The drug is practically insoluble in water and in ether; slightly soluble in diluted (50%) alcohol and in chloroform; and freely soluble in pyridine.

LANOXIN is supplied as 62.5 mcg (unscored), 125 mcg (scored), 187.5 mcg (unscored), and 250 mcg (scored) tablets for oral administration. Each tablet contains the labeled amount of digoxin USP and the following inactive ingredients: corn and potato starches, lactose and magnesium stearate. The 125 mcg tablets contain D&C Yellow No. 10 and FD&C Yellow No. 6, the 62.5 mcg tablets contain FD&C Yellow No. 6 and the 187.5 mcg tablets contain D&C Green Dye No. 5.

Drugs that Affect Renal Function		A decline in GFR or tubular secretion, as from ACE inhibitors, angiotensin receptor blockers, nonsteroidal anti-inflammatory drugs [NSAIDS], COX-2 inhibitors may impair the excretion of digoxin.
Antiarrhythmics	Dofetilide	Concomitant administration with digoxin was associated with a higher rate of torsades de pointes
	Sotalol	Proarrhythmic events were more common in patients receiving sotalol and digoxin than on either alone; it is not clear whether this represents an interaction or is related to the presence of CHF, a known risk factor for proarrhythmia, in patients receiving digoxin.
	Dronedarone	Sudden death was more common in patients receiving digoxin with dronedarone than on either alone; it is not clear whether this represents an interaction or is related to the presence of advanced heart disease, a known risk factor for sudden death in patients receiving digoxin.
Parathyroid Hormone Analog	Teriparatide	Sporadic case reports have suggested that hypercalcemia may predispose patients to digitalis toxicity. Teriparatide transiently increases serum calcium.
Thyroid supplement	Thyroid	Treatment of hypothyroidism in patients taking digoxin may increase the dose requirements of digoxin.
Sympathomimetics	Epinephrine Norepinephrine Dopamine	Can increase the risk of cardiac arrhythmias
Neuromuscular Blocking Agents	Succinylcholine	May cause sudden extrusion of potassium from muscle cells causing arrhythmias in patients taking digoxin.
Supplements	Calcium	If administered rapidly by intravenous route, can produce serious arrhythmias in digitalized patients.
Beta-adrenergic blockers and calcium channel blockers		Additive effects on AV node conduction can result in bradycardia and advanced or complete heart block.

12 CLINICAL PHARMACOLOGY

12.1 Mechanism of Action

All of digoxin's actions are mediated through its effects on Na-K ATPase. This enzyme, the "sodium pump," is responsible for maintaining the intracellular milieu throughout the body by moving sodium ions out of and potassium ions into cells. By inhibiting Na-K ATPase, digoxin

- causes increased availability of intracellular calcium in the myocardium and conduction system, with consequent increased inotropy, increased automaticity, and reduced conduction velocity
- indirectly causes parasympathetic stimulation of the autonomic nervous system, with consequent effects on the sino-atrial (SA) and atrioventricular (AV) nodes
- reduces catecholamine reuptake at nerve terminals, rendering blood vessels more sensitive to endogenous or exogenous catecholamines
- increases baroreceptor sensitization, with consequent increased carotid sinus nerve activity and enhanced sympathetic withdrawal for any given increment in mean arterial pressure
- increases (at higher concentrations) sympathetic outflow from the central nervous system (CNS) to both cardiac and peripheral sympathetic nerves
- allows (at higher concentrations) progressive efflux of intracellular potassium, with consequent increase in serum potassium levels

The cardiologic consequences of these direct and indirect effects are an increase in the force and velocity of myocardial systolic contraction (positive inotropic action), a slowing of the heart rate (negative chronotropic effect), decreased conduction velocity through the AV node, and a decrease in the degree of activation of the sympathetic nervous system and renin-angiotensin system (neurohormonal deactivating effect).

12.2 Pharmacodynamics

The times to onset of pharmacologic effect and to peak effect of preparations of LANOXIN are shown in Table 7.

[See table 7 below]

Hemodynamic Effects: Short- and long-term therapy with the drug increases cardiac output and lowers pulmonary artery pressure, pulmonary capillary wedge pressure, and systemic vascular resistance in patients with heart failure. These hemodynamic effects are accompanied by an increase in the left ventricular ejection fraction and a decrease in end-systolic and end-diastolic dimensions.

ECG Changes: The use of therapeutic doses of LANOXIN may cause prolongation of the PR interval and depression of

Table 7. Times to Onset of Pharmacologic Effect and to Peak Effect of Preparations of LANOXIN

Product	Time to Onset of Effect[a]	Time to Peak Effect[a]
LANOXIN Tablets	0.5-2 hours	2-6 hours
LANOXIN Injection/IV	5-30 minutes[b]	1-4 hours

[a] Documented for ventricular response rate in atrial fibrillation, inotropic effects and electrocardiographic changes.
[b] Depending upon rate of infusion.

Mcg	Scored	Color	Imprint	NDC 59212-xxx-xx		
				Bottle/100	Bottle/1000	Unit dose/100
62.5	No	Peach	U3A	240-55	240-75	Not applicable
125	Yes	Yellow	Y3B	242-55 242-57	242-75 242-76	242-56
187.5	No	Blue	F3F	245-55	245-75	Not applicable
250	Yes	White	X3A	249-55 249-57	249-75 249-76	249-56

the ST segment on the electrocardiogram. LANOXIN may produce false positive ST-T changes on the electrocardiogram during exercise testing. These electrophysiologic effects are not indicative of toxicity. LANOXIN does not significantly reduce heart rate during exercise.

12.3 Pharmacokinetics

Note: The following data are from studies performed in adults, unless otherwise stated.

Absorption: Following oral administration, peak serum concentrations of digoxin occur at 1 to 3 hours. Absorption of digoxin from LANOXIN Tablets has been demonstrated to be 60-80% complete compared to an identical intravenous dose of digoxin (absolute bioavailability). When LANOXIN Tablets are taken after meals, the rate of absorption is slowed, but the total amount of digoxin absorbed is usually unchanged. When taken with meals high in bran fiber, however, the amount absorbed from an oral dose may be reduced. Comparisons of the systemic availability and equivalent doses for oral preparations of LANOXIN are shown in Dosage and Administration (2.6).

Digoxin is a substrate for P-glycoprotein. As an efflux protein on the apical membrane of enterocytes, P-glycoprotein may limit the absorption of digoxin.

In some patients, orally administered digoxin is converted to inactive reduction products (e.g., dihydrodigoxin) by colonic bacteria in the gut. Data suggest that 1 in 10 patients treated with digoxin tablets, colonic bacteria will degrade 40% or more of the ingested dose. As a result, certain antibiotics may increase the absorption of digoxin in such patients. Although inactivation of these bacteria by antibiotics is rapid, the serum digoxin concentration will rise at a rate consistent with the elimination half-life of digoxin. Serum digoxin concentration relates to the extent of bacterial inactivation, and may be as much as doubled in some cases *[see Drug Interactions (7.2)]*.

Patients with malabsorption syndromes (e.g., short bowel syndrome, celiac sprue, jejunoileal bypass) may have a reduced ability to absorb orally administered digoxin.

Distribution: Following drug administration, a 6-8 hour tissue distribution phase is observed. This is followed by a much more gradual decline in the serum concentration of the drug, which is dependent on the elimination of digoxin from the body. The peak height and slope of the early portion (absorption/distribution phases) of the serum concentration-time curve are dependent upon the route of administration and the absorption characteristics of the formulation. Clinical evidence indicates that the early high serum concentrations do not reflect the concentration of digoxin at its site of action, but that with chronic use, the steady-state post-distribution serum concentrations are in equilibrium with tissue concentrations and correlate with pharmacologic effects. In individual patients, these post-distribution serum concentrations may be useful in evaluating therapeutic and toxic effects *[see Dosage and Administration (2.1)]*.

Digoxin is concentrated in tissues and therefore has a large apparent volume of distribution (approximately 475-500 L). Digoxin crosses both the blood-brain barrier and the placenta. At delivery, the serum digoxin concentration in the newborn is similar to the serum concentration in the mother. Approximately 25% of digoxin in the plasma is bound to protein. Serum digoxin concentrations are not significantly altered by large changes in fat tissue weight, so that its distribution space correlates best with lean (i.e., ideal) body weight, not total body weight.

Metabolism: Only a small percentage (13%) of a dose of digoxin is metabolized in healthy volunteers. The urinary metabolites, which include dihydrodigoxin, digoxigenin bis-digitoxoside, and their glucuronide and sulfate conjugates, are polar in nature and are postulated to be formed via hydrolysis, oxidation, and conjugation. The metabolism of

digoxin is not dependent upon the cytochrome P-450 system, and digoxin is not known to induce or inhibit the cytochrome P-450 system.

Excretion: Elimination of digoxin follows first-order kinetics (that is, the quantity of digoxin eliminated at any time is proportional to the total body content). Following intravenous administration to healthy volunteers, 50-70% of a digoxin dose is excreted unchanged in the urine. Renal excretion of digoxin is proportional to creatinine clearance and is largely independent of urine flow. In healthy volunteers with normal renal function, digoxin has a half-life of 1.5-2 days. The half-life in anuric patients is prolonged to 3.5-5 days. Digoxin is not effectively removed from the body by dialysis, exchange transfusion, or during cardiopulmonary bypass because most of the drug is bound to extravascular tissues.

Special Populations: *Geriatrics:* Because of age-related declines in renal function, elderly patients would be expected to eliminate digoxin more slowly than younger subjects. Elderly patients may also exhibit a lower volume of distribution of digoxin due to age-related loss of lean muscle mass. Thus, the dosage of digoxin should be carefully selected and monitored in elderly patients *[see Use in Specific Populations (8.5)]*.

Gender: In a study of 184 patients, the clearance of digoxin was 12% lower in female than in male patients. This difference is not likely to be clinically important.

Hepatic Impairment: Because only a small percentage (approximately 13%) of a dose of digoxin undergoes metabolism, hepatic impairment would not be expected to significantly alter the pharmacokinetics of digoxin. In a small study, plasma digoxin concentration profiles in patients with acute hepatitis generally fell within the range of profiles in a group of healthy subjects. No dosage adjustments are recommended for patients with hepatic impairment; however, serum digoxin concentrations should be used as appropriate to help guide dosing in these patients.

Renal Impairment: Since the clearance of digoxin correlates with creatinine clearance, patients with renal impairment generally demonstrate prolonged digoxin elimination half-lives and greater exposures to digoxin. Therefore, titrate carefully in these patients based on clinical response and based on monitoring of serum digoxin concentrations, as appropriate.

Race: The impact of race differences on digoxin pharmacokinetics have not been formally studied. Because digoxin is primarily eliminated as unchanged drug via the kidney and because there are no important differences in creatinine clearance among races, pharmacokinetic differences due to race are not expected.

13 NONCLINICAL TOXICOLOGY

13.1 Carcinogenesis, Mutagenesis, Impairment of Fertility

Digoxin showed no genotoxic potential in *in vitro* studies (Ames test and mouse lymphoma). No data are available on the carcinogenic potential of digoxin, nor have studies been conducted to assess its potential to affect fertility.

14 CLINICAL STUDIES

14.1 Chronic Heart Failure

Two 12-week, double-blind, placebo-controlled studies enrolled 178 (RADIANCE trial) and 88 (PROVED trial) adult patients with NYHA Class II or III heart failure previously treated with oral digoxin, a diuretic, and an ACE inhibitor (RADIANCE only) and randomized them to placebo or treatment with LANOXIN Tablets. Both trials demonstrated better preservation of exercise capacity in patients randomized to LANOXIN. Continued treatment with LANOXIN reduced the risk of developing worsening heart failure, as evidenced by heart failure-related hospitalizations and emergency care and the need for concomitant heart failure therapy.

DIG Trial of LANOXIN in Patients with Heart Failure
The Digitalis Investigation Group (DIG) main trial was a 37-week, multicenter, randomized, double-blind mortality study comparing digoxin to placebo in 6800 adult patients with heart failure and left ventricular ejection fraction less than or equal to 0.45. At randomization, 67% were NYHA class I or II, 71% had heart failure of ischemic etiology, 44% had been receiving digoxin, and most were receiving a concomitant ACE inhibitor (94%) and diuretics (82%). As in the smaller trials described above, patients who had been receiving open-label digoxin were withdrawn from this treatment before randomization. Randomization to digoxin was again associated with a significant reduction in the incidence of hospitalization, whether scored as number of hospitalizations for heart failure (relative risk 75%), risk of having at least one such hospitalization during the trial (RR 72%), or number of hospitalizations for any cause (RR 94%). On the other hand, randomization to digoxin had no apparent effect on mortality (RR 99%, with confidence limits of 91-107%).

14.2 Chronic Atrial Fibrillation

Digoxin has also been studied as a means of controlling the ventricular response to chronic atrial fibrillation in adults. Digoxin reduced the resting heart rate, but not the heart rate during exercise.

In 3 different randomized, double-blind trials that included a total of 315 adult patients, digoxin was compared to placebo for the conversion of recent-onset atrial fibrillation to sinus rhythm. Conversion was equally likely, and equally rapid, in the digoxin and placebo groups. In a randomized 120-patient trial comparing digoxin, sotalol, and amiodarone, patients randomized to digoxin had the lowest incidence of conversion to sinus rhythm, and the least satisfactory rate control when conversion did not occur.

In at least one study, digoxin was studied as a means of delaying reversion to atrial fibrillation in adult patients with frequent recurrence of this arrhythmia. This was a randomized, double-blind, 43-patient crossover study. Digoxin increased the mean time between symptomatic recurrent episodes by 54%, but had no effect on the frequency of fibrillatory episodes seen during continuous electrocardiographic monitoring.

16 HOW SUPPLIED/STORAGE AND HANDLING

LANOXIN Tablets have "LANOXIN" on one side and are supplied as follows:
[See table above]

Store at 25°C (77°F); excursions permitted to 15 to 30°C (59 to 86°F) [See USP Controlled Room Temperature] in a dry place and protect from light. Keep out of reach of children.

Dispense in tight, light-resistant container.

17 PATIENT COUNSELING INFORMATION

• Advise patients that digoxin is used to treat heart failure and heart arrhythmias.
• Instruct patients to take this medication as directed.
• Advise patients that many drugs can interact with LANOXIN. Instruct patients to inform their doctor and pharmacist if they are taking any over the counter medications, including herbal medication, or are started on a new prescription.
• Advise patient that blood tests will be necessary to ensure that their LANOXIN dose is appropriate for them.
• Advise patients to contact their doctor or a health care professional if they experience nausea, vomiting, persistent diarrhea, confusion, weakness, or visual disturbances (including blurred vision, green-yellow color disturbances, halo effect) as these could be signs that the dose of LANOXIN may be too high.
• Advise parents or caregivers that the symptoms of having too high LANOXIN doses may be difficult to recognize in infants and pediatric patients. Symptoms such as weight loss, failure to thrive in infants, abdominal pain, and behavioral disturbances may be indications of digoxin toxicity.
• Instruct the patient to monitor and record their heart rate and blood pressure daily.
• Instruct women of childbearing potential who become or are planning to become pregnant to consult a physician prior to initiation or continuing therapy with LANOXIN.

LANOXIN is a registered trademark of GlaxoSmithKline
Manufactured for:
Concordia Pharmaceuticals Inc.
St. Michael, Barbados BB11005
©2015, Concordia Pharmaceuticals Inc. All rights reserved.
Shown in Product Identification Guide, page 508

Continued on next page

NILANDRON
(nilutamide)
Tablets

℞

DESCRIPTION

NILANDRON® tablets contain nilutamide, a nonsteroidal, orally active antiandrogen having the chemical name 5,5-dimethyl-3-[4-nitro-3-(trifluoromethyl)phenyl]-2,4-imidazolidinedione with the following structural formula:

Nilutamide is a microcrystalline, white to practically white powder with a molecular weight of 317.25. Its molecular formula is $C_{12}H_{10}F_3N_3O_4$.

It is freely soluble in ethyl acetate, acetone, chloroform, ethyl alcohol, dichloromethane, and methanol. It is slightly soluble in water [<0.1% W/V at 25°C (77°F)]. It melts between 153°C and 156°C (307.4°F and 312.8°F).

Each NILANDRON tablet contains 150 mg of nilutamide. Other ingredients in NILANDRON tablets are corn starch, lactose, povidone, docusate sodium, magnesium stearate, and talc.

CLINICAL PHARMACOLOGY

Mechanism of Action

Prostate cancer is known to be androgen sensitive and responds to androgen ablation. In animal studies, nilutamide has demonstrated antiandrogenic activity without other hormonal (estrogen, progesterone, mineralocorticoid, and glucocorticoid) effects. In vitro, nilutamide blocks the effects of testosterone at the androgen receptor level. In vivo, nilutamide interacts with the androgen receptor and prevents the normal androgenic response.

Pharmacokinetics

Absorption:

Analysis of blood, urine, and feces samples following a single oral 150-mg dose of [^{14}C]-nilutamide in patients with metastatic prostate cancer showed that the drug is rapidly and completely absorbed and that it yields high and persistent plasma concentrations.

Distribution:

After absorption of the drug, there is a detectable distribution phase. There is moderate binding of the drug to plasma proteins and low binding to erythrocytes. The binding is nonsaturable except in the case of alpha-1-glycoprotein, which makes a minor contribution to the total concentration of proteins in the plasma. The results of binding studies do not indicate any effects that would cause nonlinear pharmacokinetics.

Metabolism:

The results of a human metabolism study using ^{14}C-radiolabelled tablets show that nilutamide is extensively metabolized and less than 2% of the drug is excreted unchanged in urine after 5 days. Five metabolites have been isolated from human urine. Two metabolites display an asymmetric center, due to oxidation of a methyl group, resulting in the formation of D- and L-isomers. One of the metabolites was shown, in vitro, to possess 25 to 50% of the pharmacological activity of the parent drug, and the D-isomer of the active metabolite showed equal or greater potency compared to the L-isomer. However, the pharmacokinetics and the pharmacodynamics of the metabolites have not been fully investigated.

Elimination:

The majority (62%) of orally administered [^{14}C]-nilutamide is eliminated in the urine during the first 120 hours after a single 150-mg dose. Fecal elimination is negligible, ranging from 1.4% to 7% of the dose after 4 to 5 days. Excretion of radioactivity in urine likely continues beyond 5 days. The mean elimination half-life of nilutamide determined in studies in which subjects received a single dose of 100–300 mg ranged from 38.0 to 59.1 hours with most values between 41 and 49 hours. The elimination of at least one metabolite is generally longer than that of unchanged nilutamide (59–126 hours). During multiple dosing of 150 mg nilutamide (given as 3×50 mg) twice a day, steady state was reached within 2 to 4 weeks for most patients, and mean steady state AUC_{0-12} was 110% higher than the $AUC_{0-\infty}$ obtained from the first 150 mg dose. These data and in vitro metabolism data suggest that, upon multiple dosing, metabolic enzyme inhibition may occur for this drug.

Clinical Studies

Nilutamide through its antiandrogenic activity can complement surgical castration, which suppresses only testicular androgens. The effects of the combined therapy were studied in patients with previously untreated metastatic prostate cancer.

In a double-blind, randomized, multicenter study that enrolled 457 patients (225 treated with orchiectomy and NILANDRON, 232 treated with orchiectomy and placebo), the NILANDRON group showed a statistically significant benefit in time to progression and time to death. The results are summarized below.

	NILANDRON	PLACEBO
Median Survival (months)	27.3	23.6
Progression-Free Survival (months)	21.1	14.9
Complete or Partial Regression	41%	24%
Improvement in Bone Pain	54%	37%

INDICATIONS AND USAGE

Metastatic Prostate Cancer

NILANDRON tablets are indicated for use in combination with surgical castration for the treatment of metastatic prostate cancer (Stage D₂).

For maximum benefit, NILANDRON treatment must begin on the same day as or on the day after surgical castration.

CONTRAINDICATIONS

NILANDRON tablets are contraindicated:
• in patients with severe hepatic impairment (baseline hepatic enzymes should be evaluated prior to treatment)
• in patients with severe respiratory insufficiency
• in patients with hypersensitivity to nilutamide or any component of this preparation.

WARNINGS

> **Interstitial Pneumonitis**
>
> Interstitial pneumonitis has been reported in 2% of patients in controlled clinical trials in patients exposed to nilutamide. A small study in Japanese subjects showed that 8 of 47 patients (17%) developed interstitial pneumonitis. Reports of interstitial changes including pulmonary fibrosis that led to hospitalization and death have been reported rarely postmarketing. Symptoms included exertional dyspnea, cough, chest pain, and fever. X-rays showed interstitial or alveolo-interstitial changes, and pulmonary function tests revealed a restrictive pattern with decreased DLco. Most cases occurred within the first 3 months of treatment with NILANDRON, and most reversed with discontinuation of therapy. A routine chest X-ray should be performed prior to initiating treatment with NILANDRON. Baseline pulmonary function tests may be considered. Patients should be instructed to report any new or worsening shortness of breath that they experience while on NILANDRON. **If symptoms occur, NILANDRON should be immediately discontinued until it can be determined if the symptoms are drug related.**

Hepatitis

Rare cases of death or hospitalization due to severe liver injury have been reported post-marketing in association with the use of NILANDRON. Hepatotoxicity in these reports generally occurred within the first 3 to 4 months of treatment. Hepatitis or marked increases in liver enzymes leading to drug discontinuation occurred in 1% of NILANDRON patients in controlled clinical trials.

Serum transaminase levels should be measured prior to starting treatment with NILANDRON, at regular intervals for the first 4 months of treatment, and periodically thereafter. Liver function tests should also be obtained at the first sign or symptom suggestive of liver dysfunction, e.g. nausea, vomiting, abdominal pain, fatigue, anorexia, "flu-like" symptoms, dark urine, jaundice, or right upper quadrant tenderness. If at any time, a patient has jaundice, or their ALT rises above 2 times the upper limit of normal, NILANDRON should be immediately discontinued with close followup of liver function tests until resolution.

Use in Women

NILANDRON has no indication for women, and should not be used in this population, particularly for non-serious or non-life threatening conditions.

Other

Foreign postmarketing surveillance has revealed isolated cases of aplastic anemia in which a causal relationship with NILANDRON could not be ascertained.

PRECAUTIONS

General

Antiandrogen Withdrawal Syndrome

Patients whose disease progresses while being treated with an antiandrogen may experience clinical improvement with discontinuation of the antiandrogen.

Information For Patients

Patients should be informed that NILANDRON tablets should be started on the day of, or on the day after, surgical castration. They should also be informed that they should not interrupt their dosing of NILANDRON or stop taking this medication without consulting their physician.

Because of the possibility of interstitial pneumonitis, patients should also be told to report immediately any dyspnea or aggravation of pre-existing dyspnea.

Because of the possibility of hepatitis, patients should be told to consult with their physician should nausea, vomiting, abdominal pain, or jaundice occur.

Because of the possibility of an intolerance to alcohol (facial flushes, malaise, hypotension) following ingestion of NILANDRON, it is recommended that intake of alcoholic beverages be avoided by patients who experience this reaction. This effect has been reported in about 5% of patients treated with NILANDRON.

In clinical trials, 13% to 57% of patients receiving NILANDRON reported a delay in adaptation to dark, ranging from seconds to a few minutes, when passing from a lighted area to a dark area. This effect sometimes does not abate as drug treatment is continued. Patients who experience this effect should be cautioned about driving at night or through tunnels. This effect can be alleviated by the wearing of tinted glasses.

Drug Interactions

In vitro, nilutamide has been shown to inhibit the activity of liver cytochrome P-450 isoenzymes and, therefore, may reduce the metabolism of compounds requiring these systems. Consequently, drugs with a low therapeutic margin, such as vitamin K antagonists, phenytoin, and theophylline, could have a delayed elimination and increases in their serum half-life leading to a toxic level. The dosage of these drugs or others with a similar metabolism may need to be modified if they are administered concomitantly with nilutamide. For example, when vitamin K antagonists are administered concomitantly with nilutamide, prothrombin time should be carefully monitored and, if necessary, the dosage of vitamin K antagonists should be reduced.

Carcinogenesis, Mutagenesis, Impairment Of Fertility

Administration of nilutamide to rats for 18 months at doses of 0, 5, 15, or 45 mg/kg/day produced benign Leydig cell tumors in 35% of the high-dose male rats (AUC exposures in high-dose rats were approximately 1–2 times human AUC exposures with therapeutic doses). The increased incidence of Leydig cell tumors is secondary to elevated luteinizing hormone (LH) concentrations resulting from loss of feedback inhibition at the pituitary. Elevated LH and testosterone concentrations are not observed in castrated men receiving NILANDRON. Nilutamide had no effect on the incidence, size, or time of onset of any spontaneous tumor in rats.

Nilutamide displayed no mutagenic effects in a variety of in vitro and in vivo tests (Ames test, mouse micronucleus test, and two chromosomal aberration tests).

In reproduction studies in rats, nilutamide had no effect on the reproductive function of males and females, and no lethal, teratogenic, or growth-suppressive effects on fetuses were found. The maximal dose at which nilutamide did not affect reproductive function in either sex or have an effect on fetuses was estimated to be 45 mg/kg orally (AUC exposures in rats approximately 1–2 times human therapeutic AUC exposures).

Pregnancy

Animal reproduction studies have not been conducted with nilutamide. It is also not known whether nilutamide can cause fetal harm when administered to a pregnant woman or can affect reproductive capacity. Nilutamide should be given to a pregnant woman only if clearly needed.

Pediatric Use

Safety and effectiveness in pediatric patients have not been determined.

Animal Pharmacology and Toxicology

Administration of NILANDRON to beagle dogs resulted in drug-related deaths at dose levels that produce AUC exposures in dogs much lower than the AUC exposures of men receiving the therapeutic doses of 150 and 300 mg/day. Nilutamide-induced toxicity in dogs was cumulative with progressively lower doses producing death when given for longer durations. Nilutamide given to dogs at 60 mg/kg/day (1–2 times human AUC exposure) for 1 month produced 100% mortality. Administration of 20 and 30 mg/kg/day nilutamide (1/2–1 times human AUC exposure) for 6 months resulted in 20% and 70% mortality in treated dogs. Administration to dogs of 3, 6, and 12 mg/kg/day nilutamide (1/10–1/2 human AUC exposure) for 1 year resulted in 8%, 33%, and 50% mortality, respectively. **A "no-effect level" for nilutamide-induced mortality in dogs was not identified.** Pathology data from the one-year oral toxicity study suggest that the deaths in dogs were secondary to liver toxicity. Marked-to-massive hepatocellular swelling and vacuolization were observed in affected dogs. Liver toxicity in dogs was not consistently associated with elevations of liver enzymes.

Administration of nilutamide to rats at a dose level of 45 mg/kg/day (AUC exposure in rats 1–2 times human therapeutic AUC exposures) for 18 months increased the incidence of lung pathology (granulomatous inflammation and chronic alveolitis).

The hepatic and pulmonary adverse effects observed in nilutamide-treated animals and men are similar to effects observed with another nitroaromatic compound, nitrofurantoin. Nilutamide and nitrofurantoin are both metabolized in vitro to nitroanion free-radicals by microsomal NADPH-cytochrome P450 reductase in the lungs and liver of rats and humans.

ADVERSE REACTIONS

The following adverse experiences were reported during a multicenter clinical trial comparing NILANDRON + surgical castration versus placebo + surgical castration. The most frequently reported (greater than 5%) adverse experiences during treatment with NILANDRON tablets in combination with surgical castration are listed below. For comparison, adverse experiences seen with surgical castration and placebo are also listed.

Adverse Experience	NILANDRON + surgical castration (N=225) % All	Placebo + surgical castration (N=232) % All
Cardiovascular System		
Hypertension	5.3	2.6
Digestive System		
Nausea	9.8	6.0
Constipation	7.1	3.9
Endocrine System		
Hot flushes	28.4	22.4
Metabolic and Nutritional System		
Increased AST	8.0	3.9
Increased ALT	7.6	4.3
Nervous System		
Dizziness	7.1	3.4
Respiratory System		
Dyspnea	6.2	7.3
Special Senses		
Impaired adaptation to dark	12.9	1.3
Abnormal vision	6.7	1.7
Urogenital System		
Urinary tract infection	8.0	9.1

The overall incidence of adverse experiences was 86% (194/225) for the NILANDRON group and 81% (188/232) for the placebo group.

The following adverse experiences were reported during a multicenter clinical trial comparing NILANDRON + leuprolide versus placebo + leuprolide. The most frequently reported (greater than 5%) adverse experiences during treatment with NILANDRON tablets in combination with leuprolide are listed below. For comparison, adverse experiences seen with leuprolide and placebo are also listed.

Adverse Experience	NILANDRON + leuprolide (N=209) % All	Placebo + leuprolide (N=202) % All
Body as a Whole		
Pain	26.8	27.7
Headache	13.9	10.4
Asthenia	19.1	20.8
Back pain	11.5	16.8
Abdominal pain	10.0	5.4
Chest pain	7.2	4.5
Flu syndrome	7.2	3.0
Fever	5.3	6.4
Cardiovascular System		
Hypertension	9.1	9.9
Digestive System		
Nausea	23.9	8.4
Constipation	19.6	16.8
Anorexia	11.0	6.4
Dyspepsia	6.7	4.5
Vomiting	5.7	4.0
Endocrine System		
Hot flushes	66.5	59.4
Impotence	11.0	12.9
Libido decreased	11.0	4.5
Hemic and Lymphatic System		
Anemia	7.2	6.4
Metabolic and Nutritional System		
Increased AST	12.9	13.9
Peripheral edema	12.4	17.3
Increased ALT	9.1	8.9
Musculoskeletal System		
Bone Pain	6.2	5.0
Nervous System		
Insomnia	16.3	15.8
Dizziness	10.0	11.4
Depression	8.6	7.4
Hypesthesia	5.3	2.0
Respiratory System		
Dyspnea	10.5	7.4
Upper respiratory infection	8.1	10.9
Pneumonia	5.3	3.5
Skin and Appendages		
Sweating	6.2	3.0
Body hair loss	5.7	0.5
Dry skin	5.3	2.5
Rash	5.3	4.0
Special Senses		
Impaired adaptation to dark	56.9	5.4
Chromatopsia	8.6	0.0
Impaired adaptation to light	7.7	1.0
Abnormal vision	6.2	4.5
Urogenital System		
Testicular atrophy	16.3	12.4
Gynecomastia	10.5	11.9
Urinary tract infection	8.6	21.3
Hematuria	8.1	7.9
Urinary tract disorder	7.2	10.4
Nocturia	6.7	6.4

The overall incidence of adverse experiences is 99.5% (208/209) for the NILANDRON group and 98.5% (199/202) for the placebo group.

Some frequently occurring adverse experiences, for example hot flushes, impotence, and decreased libido, are known to be associated with low serum androgen levels and known to occur with medical or surgical castration alone. Notable was the higher incidence of visual disturbances (variously described as impaired adaptation to darkness, abnormal vision, and colored vision), which led to treatment discontinuation in 1% to 2% of patients.

Interstitial pneumonitis occurred in one (<1%) patient receiving NILANDRON in combination with surgical castration and in seven patients (3%) receiving NILANDRON in combination with leuprolide and one patient receiving placebo in combination with leuprolide. Overall, it has been reported in 2% of patients receiving NILANDRON. This included a report of interstitial pneumonitis in 8 of 47 patients (17%) in a small study performed in Japan.

In addition, the following adverse experiences were reported in 2 to 5% of patients treated with NILANDRON in combination with leuprolide or orchiectomy.

Body as a Whole: Malaise (2%).

Cardiovascular System: Angina (2%), heart failure (3%), syncope (2%).

Digestive System: Diarrhea (2%), gastrointestinal disorder (2%), gastrointestinal hemorrhage (2%), melena (2%).

Metabolic and Nutritional System: Alcohol intolerance (5%), edema (2%), weight loss (2%).

Musculoskeletal System: Arthritis (2%).

Nervous System: Dry mouth (2%), nervousness (2%), paresthesia (3%).

Respiratory System: Cough increased (2%), interstitial lung disease (2%), lung disorder (4%), rhinitis (2%).

Skin and Appendages: Pruritus (2%).

Special Senses: Cataract (2%), photophobia (2%).

Laboratory Values: Haptoglobin increased (2%), leukopenia (3%), alkaline phosphatase increased (3%), BUN increased (2%), creatinine increased (2%), hyperglycemia (4%).

To report SUSPECTED ADVERSE REACTIONS, contact Concordia Pharmaceuticals Inc. at 1-877-370-1142 or FDA at 1-800-FDA-1088 or www.fda.gov/medwatch.

OVERDOSAGE

One case of massive overdosage has been published. A 79-year-old man attempted suicide by ingesting 13 g of nilutamide (i.e., 43 times the maximum recommended dose). Despite immediate gastric lavage and oral administration of activated charcoal, plasma nilutamide levels peaked at 6 times the normal range 2 hours after ingestion. There were no clinical signs or symptoms or changes in parameters such as transaminases or chest X-ray. Maintenance treatment (150 mg/day) was resumed 30 days later. In repeated-dose tolerance studies, doses of 600 mg/day and 900 mg/day were administered to 9 and 4 patients, respectively. The ingestion of these doses was associated with gastrointestinal disorders, including nausea and vomiting, malaise, headache, and dizziness. In addition, a transient elevation in hepatic enzyme levels was noted in one patient. Since nilutamide is protein bound, dialysis may not be useful as treatment for overdose. As in the management of overdosage with any drug, it should be borne in mind that multiple agents may have been taken. If vomiting does not occur spontaneously, it should be induced if the patient is alert. General supportive care, including frequent monitoring of the vital signs and close observation of the patient, is indicated.

DOSAGE AND ADMINISTRATION

The recommended dosage is 300 mg once a day for 30 days, followed thereafter by 150 mg once a day. NILANDRON tablets can be taken with or without food.

HOW SUPPLIED

NILANDRON 150 mg tablets are supplied in boxes of 30 tablets. Each box contains 3 child-resistant, PVC, aluminum foil-backed blisters of 10 tablets (NDC 59212-111-14). Each white, biconvex, cylindrical (10 mm in diameter) tablet has a triangular logo on one side and an internal reference number (168D) on the other.

Store at 25°C (77°F); excursions permitted between 15–30°C (59–86°F) [see USP Controlled Room Temperature]. Protect from light. Keep out of reach of children.

Revised 1_11/2015

Manufactured for:
Concordia Pharmaceuticals Inc.
St. Michael, Barbados BB11005
Made in France
© 2015 Concordia Pharmaceuticals Inc.
All rights reserved.

Shown in Product Identification Guide, page 508

Continued on next page

ORAPRED ODT℞
(prednisolone sodium phosphate)
orally disintegrating tablets

HIGHLIGHTS OF PRESCRIBING INFORMATION
These highlights do not include all the information needed to use Orapred ODT® safely and effectively. See full prescribing information for Orapred ODT.

Orapred ODT® (prednisolone sodium phosphate orally disintegrating tablets)
Initial U.S. Approval: 1955

INDICATIONS AND USAGE
Orapred ODT is a corticosteroid indicated
- as an anti-inflammatory or immunosuppressive agent for certain allergic, dermatologic, gastrointestinal, hematologic, ophthalmologic, nervous system, renal, respiratory, rheumatologic, specific infectious diseases or conditions and organ transplantation (1)
- for the treatment of certain endocrine conditions (1)
- for palliation of certain neoplastic conditions (1)

DOSAGE AND ADMINISTRATION
Individualize dosing based on disease severity and patient response (2):
- Initial Dose: 10 mg to 60 mg of prednisolone (as 13.4 mg to 80.6 mg of prednisolone sodium phosphate)
- Maintenance Dose: Use lowest dosage that will maintain an adequate clinical response
- Discontinuation: Withdraw gradually if discontinuing long-term or high-dose therapy
- Take with food to avoid gastrointestinal (GI) irritation
DO NOT BREAK OR USE PARTIAL ORAPRED ODT TABLETS. USE AN APPROPRIATE FORMULATION OF PREDNISOLONE IF INDICATED DOSE CANNOT BE OBTAINED USING ORAPRED ODT.

DOSAGE FORMS AND STRENGTHS
Orally Disintegrating Tablets:
- 10 mg Tablets (as 13.4 mg prednisolone sodium phosphate) (3)
- 15 mg Tablets (as 20.2 mg prednisolone sodium phosphate) (3)
- 30 mg Tablets (as 40.3 mg prednisolone sodium phosphate) (3)

CONTRAINDICATIONS
- Hypersensitivity to prednisolone or any components of this product. (4)

WARNINGS AND PRECAUTIONS
- Hypothalamic-pituitary-adrenal (HPA) axis suppression, Cushing's syndrome and hyperglycemia: Monitor patients for these conditions with chronic use. Taper doses gradually for withdrawal after chronic use. (5.1)
- Infections: Increased susceptibility to new infection and increased risk of exacerbation, dissemination, or reactivation of latent infection. Signs and symptoms of infection may be masked. (5.2)
- Elevated blood pressure, salt and water retention and hypokalemia:
  Monitor blood pressure and sodium, potassium serum levels. (5.3)
- GI perforation: increased risk in patients with certain GI disorders. Signs and symptoms may be masked. (5.4)
- Behavioral and mood disturbances: May include euphoria, insomnia, mood swings, personality changes, severe depression, and psychosis.
  Existing conditions may be aggravated. (5.5)
- Decreases in bone density: Monitor bone density in patients receiving long term corticosteroid therapy. (5.6)
- Ophthalmic effects: May include cataracts, infections and glaucoma.
  Monitor intraocular pressure if corticosteroid therapy is continued for more than 6 weeks. (5.7)
- Live or live attenuated vaccines: Do not administer to patients receiving immunosuppressive doses of corticosteroids. (5.8)
- Negative effects on growth and development: Monitor pediatric patients on long-term corticosteroid therapy. (5.9)
- Use in pregnancy: Fetal harm can occur with first trimester use. Apprise women of potential harm to the fetus. (5.10)

ADVERSE REACTIONS
Common adverse reactions for corticosteroids include fluid retention, alteration in glucose tolerance, elevation in blood pressure, behavioral and mood changes, increased appetite and weight gain. (6)

To report SUSPECTED ADVERSE REACTIONS, contact Concordia Pharmaceuticals Inc. at 1-877-370-1142 or FDA at 1-800-FDA-1088 or www.fda.gov/medwatch.

DRUG INTERACTIONS
- Anticoagulant Agents: May enhance or diminish anticoagulant effects. Monitor coagulation indices. (7)
- Antidiabetic Agents: May increase blood glucose concentrations. Dose adjustments of antidiabetic agents may be required. (7)
- CYP 3A4 inducers and inhibitors: May, respectively, increase or decrease clearance of corticosteroids, necessitating dose adjustment. (7)
- Cyclosporine: Increase in activity of both, cyclosporine and corticosteroid when administered concurrently. Convulsions have been reported with concurrent use. (7)
- NSAIDS including aspirin and salicylates: Increased risk of gastrointestinal side effects. (7)

See 17 for PATIENT COUNSELING INFORMATION.
Revised: 7/2015

FULL PRESCRIBING INFORMATION: CONTENTS*

FULL PRESCRIBING INFORMATION

1   INDICATIONS AND USAGE
Orapred ODT (prednisolone sodium phosphate orally disintegrating tablet) is indicated in the treatment of the following diseases or conditions:

1.1   Allergic Conditions
Control of severe or incapacitating allergic conditions intractable to adequate trials of conventional treatment in adult and pediatric populations with:
- Atopic dermatitis
- Drug hypersensitivity reactions
- Seasonal or perennial allergic rhinitis

- Serum sickness

1.2   Dermatologic Diseases
- Bullous dermatitis herpetiformis
- Contact dermatitis
- Exfoliative erythroderma
- Mycosis fungoides
- Pemphigus
- Severe erythema multiforme (Stevens-Johnson syndrome)

1.3   Endocrine Conditions
- Congenital adrenal hyperplasia
- Hypercalcemia of malignancy
- Nonsuppurative thyroiditis
- Primary or secondary adrenocortical insufficiency: hydrocortisone or cortisone is the first choice; synthetic analogs may be used in conjunction with mineralocorticoids where applicable.

1.4   Gastrointestinal Diseases
During acute episodes in:
- Crohn's Disease
- Ulcerative colitis

1.5   Hematologic Diseases
- Acquired (autoimmune) hemolytic anemia
- Diamond-Blackfan anemia
- Idiopathic thrombocytopenic purpura in adults
- Pure red cell aplasia
- Secondary thrombocytopenia in adults

1.6   Neoplastic Conditions
For the treatment of:
- Acute leukemia
- Aggressive lymphomas

1.7   Nervous System Conditions
- Acute exacerbations of multiple sclerosis
- Cerebral edema associated with primary or metastatic brain tumor, craniotomy or head injury

1.8   Ophthalmic Conditions
- Sympathetic ophthalmia
- Uveitis and ocular inflammatory conditions unresponsive to topical corticosteroids

1.9   Conditions Related to Organ Transplantation
- Acute or chronic solid organ rejection

1.10   Pulmonary Diseases
- Acute exacerbations of chronic obstructive pulmonary disease (COPD)
- Allergic bronchopulmonary aspergillosis
- Aspiration pneumonitis
- Asthma
- Fulminating or disseminated pulmonary tuberculosis when used concurrently with appropriate chemotherapy
- Hypersensitivity pneumonitis
- Idiopathic bronchiolitis obliterans with organizing pneumonia
- Idiopathic eosinophilic pneumonias
- Idiopathic pulmonary fibrosis Pneumocystis carinii pneumonia (PCP) associated with hypoxemia occurring in an HIV (+) individual who is also under treatment with appropriate anti-PCP antibiotics
- Symptomatic sarcoidosis

1.11   Renal Conditions
To induce a diuresis or remission of proteinuria in nephrotic syndrome, without uremia, of the idiopathic type or that due to lupus erythematosus

1.12   Rheumatologic Conditions
As adjunctive therapy for short term administration (to tide the patient over an acute episode or exacerbation) in:
- Acute gouty arthritis
During an exacerbation or as maintenance therapy in selected cases of:
- Ankylosing spondylitis
- Dermatomyositis /polymyositis
- Polymyalgia rheumatica/temporal arteritis
- Psoriatic arthritis
- Relapsing polychondritis
- Rheumatoid arthritis, including juvenile rheumatoid arthritis (selected cases may require low dose maintenance therapy)
- Sjogren's syndrome
- Systemic lupus erythematosus
- Vasculitis

1.13   Specific Infectious Diseases
- Trichinosis with neurologic or myocardial involvement
- Tuberculous meningitis with subarachnoid block or impending block, (used concurrently with appropriate anti-tuberculous chemotherapy

2   DOSAGE AND ADMINISTRATION
2.1   Recommended Dosing
Dosage of Orapred ODT should be individualized according to the severity of the disease and the response of the patient. For pediatric patients, the recommended dosage should be governed by the same considerations rather than strict adherence to the ratio indicated by age or body weight.

Do not break or use partial Orapred ODT tablets. Use an appropriate formulation of prednisolone if indicated dose cannot be obtained using Orapred ODT. This may become important in the treatment of conditions that require tapering doses that cannot be adequately accommodated by Orapred ODT, e.g., tapering the dose below 10 mg.

The initial dose of Orapred ODT may vary from 10 to 60 mg (prednisolone base) per day, depending on the specific disease entity being treated. In situations of less severity, lower doses will generally suffice while in selected patients higher initial doses may be required. The initial dosage should be maintained or adjusted until a satisfactory response is noted. If after a reasonable period of time, there is a lack of satisfactory clinical response, Orapred should be discontinued and the patient placed on other appropriate therapy. IT SHOULD BE EMPHASIZED THAT DOSAGE REQUIREMENTS ARE VARIABLE AND MUST BE INDIVIDUALIZED ON THE BASIS OF THE DISEASE UNDER TREATMENT AND THE RESPONSE OF THE PATIENT. After a favorable response is noted, the proper maintenance dosage should be determined by decreasing the initial drug dosage in small decrements at appropriate time intervals until the lowest dosage that will maintain an adequate clinical response is reached. It should be kept in mind that constant monitoring is needed in regard to drug dosage. Included in the situations which may make dosage adjustments necessary are changes in clinical status secondary to remissions or exacerbations in the disease process, the patient's individual drug responsiveness, and the effect of patient exposure to stressful situations not directly related to the disease entity under treatment; in this latter situation it may be necessary to increase the dosage of Orapred ODT for a period of time consistent with the patient's condition. If after long term therapy the drug is to be stopped, it is recommended that it be withdrawn gradually rather than abruptly.

Orapred ODT are packaged in a blister. Patients should be instructed not to remove the tablet from the blister until just prior to dosing. The blister pack should then be peeled open, and the orally disintegrating tablet placed on the tongue, where tablets may be swallowed whole as any conventional tablet, or allowed to dissolve in the mouth, with or without the assistance of water. Orally disintegrating tablet dosage forms are friable and are not intended to be cut, split, or broken.

Multiple Sclerosis
In the treatment of acute exacerbations of multiple sclerosis, daily doses of 200 mg of prednisolone for a week followed by 80 mg every other day for one month have been shown to be effective.

Pediatric
In pediatric patients, the initial dose of Orapred may vary depending on the specific disease entity being treated. The range of initial doses is 0.14 to 2 mg/kg/day in three or four divided doses (4 to 60 mg/m²bsa/day).

Nephrotic Syndrome
The standard regimen used to treat nephrotic syndrome in pediatric patients is 60 mg/m²/day given in three divided doses for 4 weeks, followed by 4 weeks of single dose alternate-day therapy at 40 mg/m²/day.

Asthma
The National Heart, Lung, and Blood Institute (NHLBI) recommended dosing for systemic *prednisone, prednisolone or methylprednisolone* in children whose asthma is uncontrolled by inhaled corticosteroids and long-acting bronchodilators is 1-2 mg/kg/day in single or divided doses.

It is further recommended that short course, or "burst" therapy, be continued until a child achieves a peak expiratory flow rate of 80% of his or her personal best or symptoms resolve. This usually requires 3 to 10 days of treatment, although it can take longer. There is no evidence that tapering the dose after improvement will prevent a relapse.

2.2   Recommended Monitoring
Blood pressure, body weight, routine laboratory studies, including serum potassium and fasting blood glucose, should be obtained at regular intervals during prolonged therapy. Appropriate diagnostic studies should be performed in patients with known or suspected peptic ulcer disease and in patients at risk for reactivation of latent tuberculosis infections.

2.3   Corticosteroid Comparison Chart
For the purpose of comparison, one 10 mg Orapred ODT tablet (13.4 mg prednisolone sodium phosphate) is equivalent to the following milligram dosage of the various glucocorticoids:

Betamethasone 1.75 mg	Paramethasone 4 mg
Cortisone 50 mg	Prednisolone 10 mg
Dexamethasone 1.75 mg	Prednisone 10 mg
Hydrocortisone 40 mg	Triamcinolone 8 mg
Methylprednisolone 8 mg	

These dose relationships apply only to oral or intravenous administration of these compounds. When these substances or their derivatives are injected intramuscularly or into joint spaces, their relative properties may be greatly altered.

3   DOSAGE FORMS AND STRENGTHS
Orally disintegrating tablets:
• 10 mg prednisolone (as 13.4 mg prednisolone sodium phosphate)
• 15 mg prednisolone (as 20.2 mg prednisolone sodium phosphate)
• 30 mg prednisolone (as 40.3 mg prednisolone sodium phosphate)

4   CONTRAINDICATIONS
Orapred ODT is contraindicated in patients who are hypersensitive to corticosteroids such as prednisolone or any components of this product. Rare instances of anaphylactoid reactions have occurred in patients receiving corticosteroid therapy.

5   WARNINGS AND PRECAUTIONS
5.1   Alterations in Endocrine Function
Hypothalamic-pituitary-adrenal (HPA) axis suppression, Cushing's syndrome, and hyperglycemia. Monitor patients for these conditions with chronic use.

Corticosteroids can produce reversible HPA axis suppression with the potential for glucocorticosteroid insufficiency after withdrawal of treatment. Drug induced secondary adrenocortical insufficiency may be minimized by gradual reduction of dosage. This type of relative insufficiency may persist for months after discontinuation of therapy; therefore, in any situation of stress occurring during that period, hormone therapy should be reinstituted.

Since mineralocorticoid secretion may be impaired, salt and/or a mineralocorticoid should be administered concurrently. Mineralocorticoid supplementation is of particular importance in infancy.

Metabolic clearance of corticosteroids is decreased in hypothyroid patients and increased in hyperthyroid patients. Changes in thyroid status of the patient may necessitate adjustment in dosage.

5.2   Increased Risks Related to Infections
Corticosteroids may increase the risks related to infections with any pathogen, including viral, bacterial, fungal, protozoan, or helminthic infections. The degree to which the dose, route and duration of corticosteroid administration correlates with the specific risks of infection is not well characterized, however, with increasing doses of corticosteroids, the rate of occurrence of infectious complications increases. Corticosteroids may mask some signs of infection and may reduce resistance to new infections.

Corticosteroids may exacerbate infections and increase risk of disseminated infection.

The use of Orapred in active tuberculosis should be restricted to those cases of fulminating or disseminated tuberculosis in which the corticosteroid is used for the management of the disease in conjunction with an appropriate antituberculous regimen.

Chickenpox and measles can have a more serious or even fatal course in non-immune children or adults on corticosteroids. In children or adults who have not had these diseases, particular care should be taken to avoid exposure. If a patient is exposed to chickenpox, prophylaxis with varicella zoster immune globulin (VZIG) may be indicated. If patient is exposed to measles, prophylaxis with pooled intramuscular immunoglobulin (IG) may be indicated. If chickenpox develops, treatment with antiviral agents may be considered.

Corticosteroids should be used with great care in patients with known or suspected Strongyloides (threadworm) infestation. In such patients, corticosteroid-induced immunosuppression may lead to Strongyloides hyperinfection and dissemination with widespread larval migration, often accompanied by severe enterocolitis and potentially fatal gram-negative septicemia.

Corticosteroids may exacerbate systemic fungal infections and therefore should not be used in the presence of such infections unless they are needed to control drug reactions. *Corticosteroids may increase risk of reactivation or exacerbation of latent infection.*

If corticosteroids are indicated in patients with latent tuberculosis or tuberculin reactivity, close observation is necessary as reactivation of the disease may occur. During prolonged corticosteroid therapy, these patients should receive chemoprophylaxis.

Corticosteroids may activate latent amebiasis. Therefore, it is recommended that latent or active amebiasis be ruled out before initiating corticosteroid therapy in any patient who has spent time in the tropics or in any patient with unexplained diarrhea.

Corticosteroids should not be used in cerebral malaria.

5.3   Alterations in Cardiovascular/Renal Function
Corticosteroids can cause elevation of blood pressure, salt and water retention, and increased excretion of potassium and calcium. These effects are less likely to occur with the synthetic derivatives except when used in large doses. Dietary salt restriction and potassium supplementation may be necessary. These agents should be used with caution in patients with hypertension, congestive heart failure, or renal insufficiency.

Literature reports suggest an association between use of corticosteroids and left ventricular free wall rupture after a recent myocardial infarction; therefore, therapy with corticosteroids should be used with caution in these patients.

5.4   Use in Patients with Gastrointestinal Disorders
There is an increased risk of gastrointestinal (GI) perforation in patients with certain GI disorders. Signs of GI perforation, such as peritoneal irritation, may be masked in patients receiving corticosteroids.

Corticosteroids should be used with caution if there is a probability of impending perforation, abscess or other pyogenic infections; diverticulitis; fresh intestinal anastomoses; and active or latent peptic ulcer.

5.5   Behavioral and Mood Disturbances
Corticosteroid use may be associated with central nervous system effects ranging from euphoria, insomnia, mood swings, personality changes, and severe depression, to frank psychotic manifestations. Also, existing emotional instability or psychotic tendencies may be aggravated by corticosteroids.

5.6   Decrease in Bone Density
Corticosteroids decrease bone formation and increase bone resorption both through their effect on calcium regulation (i.e., decreasing absorption and increasing excretion) and inhibition of osteoblast function. This, together with a decrease in the protein matrix of the bone secondary to an increase in protein catabolism, and reduced sex hormone production, may lead to inhibition of bone growth in children and adolescents and the development of osteoporosis at any age. Special consideration should be given to patients at increased risk of osteoporosis (e.g., postmenopausal women) before initiating corticosteroid therapy and bone density should be monitored in patients on long term corticosteroid therapy.

5.7   Ophthalmic Effects
Prolonged use of corticosteroids may produce posterior subcapsular cataracts, glaucoma with possible damage to the optic nerves, and may enhance the establishment of secondary ocular infections due to fungi or viruses.

The use of oral corticosteroids is not recommended in the treatment of optic neuritis and may lead to an increase in the risk of new episodes.

Intraocular pressure may become elevated in some individuals. If steroid therapy is continued for more than 6 weeks, intraocular pressure should be monitored.

Patients with Ocular Herpes Simplex
Corticosteroids should be used cautiously in patients with ocular herpes simplex because of possible corneal perforation. Corticosteroids **should not be used** in active ocular herpes simplex.

5.8   Vaccination
Administration of live or live attenuated vaccines is contraindicated in patients receiving immunosuppressive doses of corticosteroids. Killed or inactivated vaccines may be administered; however, the response to such vaccines cannot be predicted. Immunization procedures may be undertaken in patients who are receiving corticosteroids as replacement therapy, e.g., for Addison's disease.

Continued on next page

While on corticosteroid therapy, patients should not be vaccinated against smallpox. Other immunization procedures should not be undertaken in patients who are on corticosteroids, especially on high dose, because of possible hazards of neurological complications and a lack of antibody response.

5.9 Effect on Growth and Development

Long-term use of corticosteroids can have negative effects on growth and development in children. Growth and development of pediatric patients on prolonged corticosteroid therapy should be carefully monitored.

5.10 Use in Pregnancy

Prednisolone can cause fetal harm when administered to a pregnant woman. Human and animal studies suggest that use of corticosteroids during the first trimester of pregnancy is associated with an increased risk of orofacial clefts, intrauterine growth restriction and decreased birth weight. If this drug is used during pregnancy, or if the patient becomes pregnant while using this drug, the patient should be apprised of the potential hazard to the fetus. [see *Use in Specific Populations (8.1)*].

5.11 Neuromuscular Effects

Although controlled clinical trials have shown corticosteroids to be effective in speeding the resolution of acute exacerbations of multiple sclerosis, they do not show that they affect the ultimate outcome or natural history of the disease. The studies do show that relatively high doses of corticosteroids are necessary to demonstrate a significant effect. [see *Dosage and Administration (3)*].

An acute myopathy has been observed with the use of high doses of corticosteroids, most often occurring in patients with disorders of neuromuscular transmission (e.g., myasthenia gravis), or in patients receiving concomitant therapy with neuromuscular blocking drugs (e.g., pancuronium). This acute myopathy is generalized, may involve ocular and respiratory muscles, and may result in quadriparesis. Elevation of creatinine kinase may occur. Clinical improvement or recovery after stopping corticosteroids may require weeks to years.

5.12 Kaposi's Sarcoma

Kaposi's sarcoma has been reported to occur in patients receiving corticosteroid therapy, most often for chronic conditions. Discontinuation of corticosteroids may result in clinical improvement.

6 ADVERSE REACTIONS

Common adverse reactions for corticosteroids include fluid retention, alteration in glucose tolerance, elevation in blood pressure, behavioral and mood changes, increased appetite and weight gain.

Allergic Reactions: Anaphylactoid reaction, anaphylaxis, angioedema

Cardiovascular: Bradycardia, cardiac arrest, cardiac arrhythmias, cardiac enlargement, circulatory collapse, congestive heart failure, fat embolism, hypertension, hypertrophic cardiomyopathy in premature infants, myocardial rupture following recent myocardial infarction, pulmonary edema, syncope, tachycardia, thromboembolism, thrombophlebitis, vasculitis

Dermatologic: Acne, allergic dermatitis, cutaneous and subcutaneous atrophy, dry scalp, edema, facial erythema, hyper or hypo-pigmentation, impaired wound healing, increased sweating, petechiae and ecchymoses, rash, sterile abscess, striae, suppressed reactions to skin tests, thin fragile skin, thinning scalp hair, urticaria

Endocrine: Abnormal fat deposits, decreased carbohydrate tolerance, development of Cushingoid state, hirsutism, manifestations of latent diabetes mellitus and increased requirements for insulin or oral hypoglycemic agents in diabetics, menstrual irregularities, moon facies, secondary adrenocortical and pituitary unresponsiveness (particularly in times of stress, as in trauma, surgery or illness), suppression of growth in children

Fluid and Electrolyte Disturbances: Fluid retention, potassium loss, hypertension, hypokalemic alkalosis, sodium retention

Gastrointestinal: Abdominal distention; elevation in serum liver enzyme levels (usually reversible upon discontinuation); hepatomegaly, hiccups, malaise, nausea, pancreatitis; peptic ulcer with possible perforation and hemorrhage; ulcerative esophagitis

General: Increased appetite and weight gain

Metabolic: Negative nitrogen balance due to protein catabolism

Musculoskeletal: Aseptic necrosis of femoral and humeral heads; charcot-like arthropathy, loss of muscle mass; muscle weakness; osteoporosis; pathologic fracture of long bones; steroid myopathy; tendon rupture; vertebral compression fractures

Neurological: Arachnoiditis, convulsions; depression, emotional instability, euphoria, headache; increased intracranial pressure with papilledema (pseudotumor cerebri) usually following discontinuation of treatment; insomnia, meningitis, mood swings, neuritis, neuropathy, paraparesis/paraplegia, paresthesia, personality changes, sensory disturbances, vertigo

Ophthalmic: Exophthalmos; glaucoma; increased intraocular pressure; posterior subcapsular cataracts

Reproductive: Alteration in motility and number of spermatozoa

7 DRUG INTERACTIONS

- **Aminoglutethimide:** Aminoglutethimide may lead to loss of corticosteroid-induced adrenal suppression.
- **Amphotericin B:** There have been cases reported in which concomitant use of Amphotericin B and hydrocortisone was followed by cardiac enlargement and congestive heart failure (see also Potassium depleting agents).
- **Anticholinesterase agents:** Concomitant use of anticholinesterase agents and corticosteroids may produce severe weakness in patients with myasthenia gravis. If possible, anticholinesterase agents should be withdrawn at least 24 hours before initiating corticosteroid therapy.
- **Anticoagulant agents:** Co-administration of corticosteroids and warfarin usually results in inhibition of response to warfarin, although there have been some conflicting reports. Therefore, coagulation indices should be monitored frequently to maintain the desired anticoagulant effect.
- **Antidiabetic Agents:** Because corticosteroids may increase blood glucose concentrations, dosage adjustments of antidiabetic agents may be required.
- **Antitubercular drugs:** Serum concentrations of isoniazid may be decreased.
- **CYP 3A4 inducers (e.g. barbiturates, phenytoin, carbamazepine, and rifampin):** Drugs such as barbiturates, phenytoin, ephedrine, and rifampin, which induce hepatic microsomal drug metabolizing enzyme activity may enhance metabolism of prednisolone and require that the dosage of Orapred be increased.
- **CYP 3A4 inhibitors (e.g., ketoconazole, macrolide antibiotics):** Ketoconazole has been reported to decrease the metabolism of certain corticosteroids by up to 60% leading to an increased risk of corticosteroid side effects.
- **Cholestyramine:** Cholestyramine may increase the clearance of corticosteroids.
- **Cyclosporine:** Increased activity of both cyclosporine and corticosteroids may occur when the two are used concurrently. Convulsions have been reported with this concurrent use.
- **Digitalis:** Patients on digitalis glycosides may be at increased risk of arrhythmias due to hypokalemia.
- **Estrogens, including oral contraceptives:** Estrogens may decrease the hepatic metabolism of certain corticosteroids thereby increasing their effect.
- **NSAIDS, including aspirin and salicylates:** Concomitant use of aspirin or other non-steroidal anti-inflammatory agents and corticosteroids increases the risk of gastrointestinal side effects. Aspirin should be used cautiously in conjunction with corticosteroids in hypoprothrombinemia. The clearance of salicylates may be increased with concurrent use of corticosteroids.
- **Potassium-depleting agents (e.g., diuretics, Amphotericin B):** When corticosteroids are administered concomitantly with potassium-depleting agents, patients should be observed closely for development of hypokalemia.
- **Skin Tests:** Corticosteroids may suppress reactions to skin tests.
- **Toxoids and live or inactivated Vaccines:** Due to inhibition of antibody response, patients on prolonged corticosteroid therapy may exhibit a diminished response to toxoids and live or inactivated vaccines. Corticosteroids may also potentiate the replication of some organisms contained in live attenuated vaccines.

8 USE IN SPECIFIC POPULATIONS

8.1 Pregnancy

Pregnancy Category D [see *Warnings and Precautions (5.10)*]

Orapred has not been formally evaluated in clinical or nonclinical studies for effects on pregnancy and fetal development. Multiple cohort and case controlled studies in humans suggest that maternal corticosteroid use during the first trimester increases the incidence of cleft lip with or without cleft palate from about 1/1000 infants to 3-5/1000 infants. Two prospective case control studies showed decreased birth weight in infants exposed to maternal corticosteroids in utero. In humans, the risk of decreased birth weight appears to be dose related and may be minimized by administering lower corticosteroid doses. It is likely that underlying maternal conditions contribute to intrauterine growth restriction and decreased birth weight, but it is unclear to what extent these maternal conditions contribute to the increased risk of orofacial clefts.

Thus, prednisolone can cause fetal harm when used during pregnancy. Orapred should be used during pregnancy only if the potential benefit justifies the potential risk to the fetus. If this drug is used during pregnancy, or if the patient becomes pregnant while using this drug, the patient should be apprised of the potential hazard to the fetus. Infants born to mothers who have received corticosteroids during pregnancy should be carefully observed for signs of hypoadrenalism.

Published literature indicates prednisolone has been shown to be teratogenic in rats, rabbits, hamsters, and mice with increased incidence of cleft palate in offspring, supportive of the clinical data. In teratogenicity studies, cleft palate along with an elevation of fetal lethality (or increase in resorptions) and reductions in fetal body weight was seen in rats at maternal doses of 30 mg/kg (equivalent to 290 mg in a 60 kg individual based on mg/m^2 body surface comparison) and higher. Cleft palate was observed in mice at a maternal dose of 20 mg/kg (equivalent to 100 mg in a 60 kg individual based on mg/m^2 comparison). Additionally, constriction of the ductus arteriosus was observed in fetuses of pregnant rats exposed to prednisolone.

8.3 Nursing Mothers

Prednisolone is secreted in human milk. Reports suggest that prednisolone concentrations in human milk are 5 to 25% of maternal serum levels, and that total infant daily doses are small, about 0.14% of the maternal daily dose. Therefore, caution should be exercised when prednisolone is administered to a nursing woman. High doses of corticosteroids for long periods could potentially produce problems in infant growth and development and interfere with endogenous corticosteroid production. The risk of infant exposure to prednisolone through breast milk should be weighed against the known benefits of breastfeeding for both the mother and baby. If prednisolone must be prescribed to a breastfeeding mother, the lowest dose should be prescribed to achieve the desired clinical effect.

8.4 Pediatric Use

The efficacy and safety of prednisolone in the pediatric population are based on the well-established course of effect of corticosteroids, which is similar in pediatric and adult populations. Published studies provide evidence of efficacy and safety in pediatric patients for the treatment of nephrotic syndrome (>2 years of age), and aggressive lymphomas and leukemias (>1 month of age). However, some of these conclusions and other indications for pediatric use of corticosteroid, e.g., severe asthma and wheezing, are based on adequate and well-controlled trials conducted in adults, on the premises that the course of the diseases and their pathophysiology are considered to be substantially similar in both populations.

The adverse effects of prednisolone in pediatric patients are similar to those in adults [see *Adverse Reactions (6)*]. Like adults, pediatric patients should be carefully observed with frequent measurements of blood pressure, weight, height, intraocular pressure, and clinical evaluation for the presence of infection, psychosocial disturbances, thromboembolism, peptic ulcers, cataracts, and osteoporosis. Children, who are treated with corticosteroids by any route, including systemically administered corticosteroids, may experience a decrease in their growth velocity. This negative impact of corticosteroids on growth has been observed at low systemic doses and in the absence of laboratory evidence of HPA axis suppression (i.e., cosyntropin stimulation and basal cortisol plasma levels).

Growth velocity may therefore be a more sensitive indicator of systemic corticosteroid exposure in children than some commonly used tests of HPA axis function. The linear growth of children treated with corticosteroids by any route should be monitored, and the potential growth effects of prolonged treatment should be weighed against clinical benefits obtained and the availability of other treatment alternatives. In order to minimize the potential growth effects of corticosteroids, children should be titrated to the lowest effective dose.

8.5 Geriatric Use

No overall differences in safety or effectiveness were observed between elderly subjects and younger subjects, and other reported clinical experience with prednisolone has not identified differences in responses between the elderly and younger patients. However, the incidence of corticosteroid-induced side effects may be increased in geriatric patients and appear to be dose-related. Osteoporosis is the most frequently encountered complication, which occurs at a higher incidence rate in corticosteroid-treated geriatric patients as compared to younger populations and in age-matched controls. Losses of bone mineral density appear to be greatest early on in the course of treatment and may recover over time after steroid withdrawal or use of lower doses (i.e., ≤5 mg/day). Prednisolone doses of 7.5 mg/day or higher, have been associated with an increased relative risk of both vertebral and nonvertebral fractures, even in the presence of higher bone density compared to patients with involutional osteoporosis.

Routine screening of geriatric patients, including regular assessments of bone mineral density and institution of fracture prevention strategies, along with regular review of Orapred indication should be undertaken to minimize complications and keep the Orapred dose at the lowest acceptable level. Co-administration of bisphosphonates has been shown to retard the rate of bone loss in corticosteroid-treated males and postmenopausal females, and these agents are recommended in the prevention and treatment of corticosteroid-induced osteoporosis.

It has been reported that equivalent weight-based doses yield higher total and unbound prednisolone plasma concentrations and reduced renal and non-renal clearance in elderly patients compared to younger populations. However, it is not clear whether dosing reductions would be necessary in elderly patients, since these pharmacokinetic alterations may be offset by age-related differences in responsiveness of target organs and/or less pronounced suppression of adrenal release of cortisol. Dose selection for an elderly patient should be cautious, usually starting at the low end of the dosing range, reflecting the greater frequency of decreased hepatic, renal, or cardiac function, and of concomitant disease or other drug therapy.

This drug is known to be substantially excreted by the kidney, and the risk of toxic reactions to this drug may be greater in patients with impaired renal function. Because elderly patients are more likely to have decreased renal function, care should be taken in dose selection, and it may be useful to monitor renal function.

10 OVERDOSAGE

The effects of accidental ingestion of large quantities of prednisolone over a very short period of time have not been reported, but prolonged use of the drug can produce mental symptoms, moon face, abnormal fat deposits, fluid retention, excessive appetite, weight gain, hypertrichosis, acne, striae, ecchymosis, increased sweating, pigmentation, dry scaly skin, thinning scalp hair, increased blood pressure, tachycardia, thrombophlebitis, decreased resistance to infection, negative nitrogen balance with delayed bone and wound healing, headache, weakness, menstrual disorders, accentuated menopausal symptoms, neuropathy, fractures, osteoporosis, peptic ulcer, decreased glucose tolerance, hypokalemia, and adrenal insufficiency. Hepatomegaly and abdominal distention have been observed in children.

Treatment of acute overdosage is by immediate gastric lavage or emesis followed by supportive and symptomatic therapy. For chronic overdosage in the face of severe disease requiring continuous steroid therapy, the dosage of prednisolone may be reduced only temporarily, or alternate day treatment may be introduced.

11 DESCRIPTION

Orapred ODT (prednisolone sodium phosphate disintegrating tablets) is a sodium salt of the phosphoester of the glucocorticoid prednisolone. Glucocorticoids are adrenocortical steroids, both naturally occurring and synthetic, which are readily absorbed from the gastrointestinal tract.

Prednisolone sodium phosphate occurs as white or slightly yellow, friable granules or powder. It is freely soluble in water; soluble in methanol; slightly soluble in alcohol and in chloroform; and very slightly soluble in acetone and in dioxane.

The chemical name of prednisolone sodium phosphate is pregna-1, 4-diene-3, 20-dione, 11, 17-dihydroxy-21-(phosphonooxy)-, disodium salt, (11ß)-. The empirical formula is $C_{21}H_{27}Na_2O_8P$; the molecular weight is 484.39. Its chemical structure is:

[See structural formula at top of next column]

Each orally disintegrating tablet also contains the following inactive ingredients: citric acid, colloidal silicon dioxide,

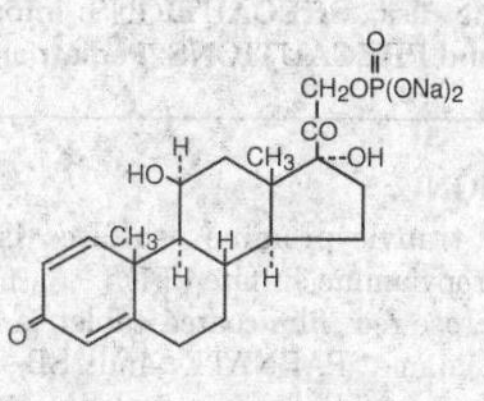

crospovidone, grape flavor, hypromellose, magnesium stearate, mannitol, methacrylate copolymer, microcrystalline cellulose, sodium bicarbonate, sucralose, and sucrose.

12 CLINICAL PHARMACOLOGY

12.1 Mechanism of Action

Prednisolone is a synthetic adrenocortical steroid drug with predominantly glucocorticoid properties. Some of these properties reproduce the physiological actions of endogenous glucocorticosteroids, but others do not necessarily reflect any of the adrenal hormones' normal functions; they are seen only after administration of large therapeutic doses of the drug. The pharmacological effects of prednisolone which are due to its glucocorticoid properties include: promotion of gluconeogenesis; increased deposition of glycogen in the liver; inhibition of the utilization of glucose; anti-insulin activity; increased catabolism of protein; increased lipolysis; stimulation of fat synthesis and storage; increased glomerular filtration rate and resulting increase in urinary excretion of urate (creatinine excretion remains unchanged); and increased calcium excretion. Depressed production of eosinophils and lymphocytes occurs, but erythropoiesis and production of polymorphonuclear leukocytes are stimulated. Inflammatory processes (edema, fibrin deposition, capillary dilatation, migration of leukocytes and phagocytosis) and the later stages of wound healing (capillary proliferation, deposition of collagen, cicatrization) are inhibited. Prednisolone can stimulate secretion of various components of gastric juice. Suppression of the production of corticotropin may lead to suppression of endogenous corticosteroids. Prednisolone has slight mineralocorticoid activity, whereby entry of sodium into cells and loss of intracellular potassium is stimulated. This is particularly evident in the kidney, where rapid ion exchange leads to sodium retention and hypertension.

12.3 Pharmacokinetics

Absorption:

Oral administration of single doses of 30 mg prednisolone base equivalent of Orapred ODT, and Pediapred Solution to 21 adult volunteers yielded comparable pharmacokinetic data:

Table 1. Comparison of Mean Pharmacokinetic Parameters (%CV) in Healthy Volunteers Following a Single Dose of 30 mg Orapred ODT and Pediapred Solution,

Dose*	$AUC_{0-\infty}$ (ng·hr/mL)	C_{max} (ng·hr/mL)†
(30 mg prednisolone base equivalent)	(± S.D.)	(± S.D.)
Pediapred Solution	2426.1 (360.0)	461.33 (77.94)
Orapred ODT	2408.1 (361.5)	420.91 (78.28)

*Administered under fasting conditions.
†Mean values of 21 normal volunteers

Distribution:

Prednisolone is 70-90% protein-bound in the plasma and the volume of distribution is reported as 0.22 - 0.7 L/kg.

Metabolism:

Prednisolone is reported to be metabolized mainly in the liver and excreted in the urine as sulfate and glucuronide conjugates.

Excretion:

Prednisolone is eliminated from the plasma with a mean (± SD) half-life of 2.6 (± 0.27) hours.

Special Populations

The systemic availability, metabolism and elimination of prednisolone after administration of single weight-based doses (0.8 mg/kg) of intravenous (IV) prednisolone and oral prednisone were reported in a small study of 19 younger (23 to 34 years) and 12 geriatric (65 to 89 years) subjects. Results showed that the systemic availability of total and unbound prednisolone, as well as interconversion between prednisolone and prednisone were independent of age. The mean unbound fraction of prednisolone was higher, and the steady-state volume of distribution (V_{ss}) of unbound prednisolone was reduced in elderly patients. Plasma prednisolone concentrations were higher in elderly subjects, and the higher AUCs of total and unbound prednisolone were most likely reflective of an impaired metabolic clearance, evidenced by reduced fractional urinary clearance of 6b-hydroxyprednisolone. Despite these findings of higher total and unbound prednisolone concentrations, elderly subjects had higher AUCs of cortisol, suggesting that the elderly population is less sensitive to suppression of endogenous cortisol or their capacity for hepatic inactivation of cortisol is diminished.

13 NONCLINICAL TOXICOLOGY

13.1 Carcinogenesis, Mutagenesis, Impairment of Fertility

Orapred was not formally evaluated in carcinogenicity studies. Review of the published literature identified the potential for malignancy at doses within the therapeutic range. In a 2-year study, male Sprague-Dawley rats administered prednisolone in drinking water at an estimated continuous daily prednisolone consumption of 368 mcg/kg/day (equivalent to 3.5 mg/day in a 60 kg individual based on an mg/m^2 body surface area comparison) developed increased incidences of hepatic adenomas. However infrequent administration of prednisolone did not result in malignancy. In an 18-month study, intermittent (1, 2, 4.5 or 9 times per month) oral gavage of 3 mg/kg prednisolone did not induce tumors in female Sprague-Dawley rats (equivalent to 29 mg in a 60 kg individual based on a mg/m^2 body surface area comparison).

Orapred was not formally evaluated for genotoxicity. However, in published studies prednisolone was not mutagenic with or without metabolic activation in the Ames bacterial reverse mutation assay using *Salmonella typhimurium* and *Escherichia coli*, or in a mammalian cell gene mutation assay using mouse lymphoma L5178Y cells, according to current evaluation standards. In a published chromosomal aberration study in Chinese Hamster Lung (CHL) cells, a slight increase was seen in the incidence of structural chromosomal aberrations with metabolic activation at the highest concentration tested, however, the effect appears to be equivocal.

Orapred was not formally evaluated in fertility studies. However, alterations in motility and numbers of spermatozoa, and menstrual irregularities have been described with clinical use [see *Adverse Reactions (6)*].

16 HOW SUPPLIED/STORAGE AND HANDLING

Orapred ODT (prednisolone sodium phosphate orally disintegrating tablets) 13.4 mg prednisolone sodium phosphate (equivalent to 10 mg prednisolone base) is a white, flat faced, bevelled tablet, debossed with ORA on one side and 10 on the other. Supplied as:

- NDC 59212-700-48: 48 tablets per carton. Each carton has 8 cards containing 6 tablets.

Orapred ODT (prednisolone sodium phosphate orally disintegrating tablets) 20.2 mg prednisolone sodium phosphate (equivalent to 15 mg prednisolone base) is a white, flat faced, bevelled tablet, debossed with ORA on one side and 15 on the other. Supplied as:

- NDC 59212-701-48: 48 tablets per carton. Each carton has 8 cards containing 6 tablets.

Orapred ODT: (prednisolone sodium phosphate orally disintegrating tablets) 40.3 mg prednisolone sodium phosphate (equivalent to 30 mg prednisolone base) is a white, flat faced, beveled tablets, debossed with ORA on one side and 30 on the other. Supplied as:

- NDC 59212-702-48: 48 tablets per carton. Each carton has 8 cards containing 6 tablets.

Store at 20 to 25°C (68 to 77°F); excursions permitted to 15 to 30°C (59 to 86°F). [See USP controlled Room Temperature]. Protect from moisture.

Do not break or use partial Orapred ODT tablets. Keep out of the reach of children.

17 PATIENT COUNSELING INFORMATION

Advise patients not to discontinue the use of Orapred abruptly or without medical supervision, to advise any healthcare provider that they are taking it, and to seek medical advice at once should they develop fever or other

Continued on next page

signs of infection. Inform patients to take Orapred exactly as prescribed, follow the instructions on the prescription label, and not stop taking Orapred without first checking with their health-care providers, as there may be a need for gradual dose reduction.

Patients should discuss with their physician if they have had recent or ongoing infections or if they have recently received a vaccine.

Warn patients who are on immunosuppressant doses of corticosteroids to avoid exposure to chickenpox or measles. Advise patients that if they are exposed, to seek medical advice without delay.

There are a number of medicines that can interact with Orapred. Patients should inform their healthcare provider of all the medicines they are taking, including over-the counter and prescription medicines (such as phenytoin, diuretics, digitalis or digoxin, rifampin, amphotericin B, cyclosporine, insulin or diabetes medicines, ketoconazole, estrogens including birth control pills and hormone replacement therapy, blood thinners such as warfarin, aspirin or other NSAIDS, barbiturates), dietary supplements, and herbal products. If patients are taking any of these drugs, alternate therapy, dosage adjustment, and/or a special test may be needed during the treatment.

For missed doses, inform patients to take the missed dose as soon as they remember. If it is almost time for the next dose, the missed dose should be skipped and the medicine taken at the next regularly scheduled time. Advise patients not to take an extra dose to make up for the missed dose.

Inform patients to take Orapred with food to avoid GI irritation.

Advise patients of common adverse reactions that could occur with Orapred use to include fluid retention, alteration in glucose tolerance, elevation in blood pressure, behavioral and mood changes, increased appetite and weight gain.

Orapred ODT tablets are packaged in a blister. Patients should be instructed not to remove the tablet from the blister until just prior to dosing. The blister pack should then be peeled open, and the orally disintegrating tablet placed on the tongue, where the tablets may be swallowed whole as any conventional tablet, or allowed to dissolve in the mouth, with or without the assistance of water. Orally disintegrating tablet dosage forms are friable and are not intended to be cut, split, or broken.

Revised 07/2015

Manufactured for:

Concordia Pharmaceuticals Inc.

St. Michael, Barbados BB11005

U.S. Patent No. 6,740,341

Orapred ODT® is a registered trademark of Concordia Pharmaceuticals Inc.

For inquiries call 1-877-370-1142

Shown in Product Identification Guide, page 508

PARNATE ℞

[*PAR-nate*]

(tranylcypromine sulfate)

Tablets

Suicidality and Antidepressant Drugs

Antidepressants increased the risk compared to placebo of suicidal thinking and behavior (suicidality) in children, adolescents, and young adults in short-term studies of major depressive disorder (MDD) and other psychiatric disorders. Anyone considering the use of PARNATE or any other antidepressant in a child, adolescent, or young adult must balance this risk with the clinical need. Short-term studies did not show an increase in the risk of suicidality with antidepressants compared to placebo in adults beyond age 24; there was a reduction in risk with antidepressants compared to placebo in adults aged 65 and older. Depression and certain other psychiatric disorders are themselves associated with increases in the risk of suicide. Patients of all ages who are started on antidepressant therapy should be monitored appropriately and observed closely for clinical worsening, suicidality, or unusual changes in behavior. Families and caregivers should be advised of the need for close observation and communication with the prescriber. PARNATE is not approved for use in pediatric patients. (See

WARNINGS TO PHYSICIANS: Clinical Worsening and Suicide Risk, PRECAUTIONS: Information for Patients, and PRECAUTIONS: Pediatric Use.)

DESCRIPTION

Chemically, tranylcypromine sulfate is (±)-*trans*-2-phenylcyclopropylamine sulfate (2:1).

Each round, rose-red, film-coated tablet is debossed with the product name PARNATE and SB and contains tranylcypromine sulfate equivalent to 10 mg of tranylcypromine. Inactive ingredients consist of microcrystalline cellulose NF, citric acid anhydrous USP, croscarmellose sodium NF, D&C Red No. 7, FD&C Blue No. 2, FD&C Yellow No. 6, gelatin NF, lactose NF, magnesium stearate NF, talc USP, titanium dioxide USP, carnauba wax NF, polyethylene glycol 400 and 8000 NF, and hypromellose USP.

ACTION

Tranylcypromine is a non-hydrazine monoamine oxidase inhibitor with a rapid onset of activity. It increases the concentration of epinephrine, norepinephrine, and serotonin in storage sites throughout the nervous system and, in theory, this increased concentration of monoamines in the brain stem is the basis for its antidepressant activity. When tranylcypromine is withdrawn, monoamine oxidase activity is recovered in 3 to 5 days, although the drug is excreted in 24 hours.

INDICATIONS

For the treatment of Major Depressive Episode Without Melancholia.

PARNATE should be used in adult patients who can be closely supervised. It should rarely be the first antidepressant drug given. Rather, the drug is suited for patients who have failed to respond to the drugs more commonly administered for depression.

The effectiveness of PARNATE has been established in adult outpatients, most of whom had a depressive illness which would correspond to a diagnosis of Major Depressive Episode Without Melancholia. As described in the American Psychiatric Association's Diagnostic and Statistical Manual, third edition (DSM III), Major Depressive Episode implies a prominent and relatively persistent (nearly every day for at least 2 weeks) depressed or dysphoric mood that usually interferes with daily functioning and includes at least 4 of the following 8 symptoms: change in appetite, change in sleep, psychomotor agitation or retardation, loss of interest in usual activities or decrease in sexual drive, increased fatigability, feelings of guilt or worthlessness, slowed thinking or impaired concentration, and suicidal ideation or attempts.

The effectiveness of PARNATE in patients who meet the criteria for Major Depressive Episode with Melancholia (endogenous features) has not been established.

SUMMARY OF CONTRAINDICATIONS

PARNATE should not be administered in combination with any of the following: MAO inhibitors or dibenzazepine derivatives; sympathomimetics (including amphetamines); some central nervous system depressants (including narcotics and alcohol); antihypertensive, diuretic, antihistaminic, sedative, or anesthetic drugs; bupropion HCl; buspirone HCl; dextromethorphan; cheese or other foods with a high tyramine content; or excessive quantities of caffeine.

PARNATE should not be administered to any patient with a confirmed or suspected cerebrovascular defect or to any patient with cardiovascular disease, hypertension, or history of headache.

(For complete discussion of contraindications and warnings, see below.)

CONTRAINDICATIONS

PARNATE is contraindicated:

1. In patients with cerebrovascular defects or cardiovascular disorders

PARNATE should not be administered to any patient with a confirmed or suspected cerebrovascular defect or to any patient with cardiovascular disease or hypertension.

2. In the presence of pheochromocytoma

PARNATE should not be used in the presence of pheochromocytoma since such tumors secrete pressor substances.

3. In combination with MAO inhibitors or with dibenzazepine-related entities

PARNATE should not be administered together or in rapid succession with other MAO inhibitors or with

dibenzazepine-related entities. Hypertensive crises or severe convulsive seizures may occur in patients receiving such combinations.

In patients being transferred to PARNATE from another MAO inhibitor or from a dibenzazepine-related entity, allow a medication-free interval of at least a week, then initiate PARNATE using half the normal starting dosage for at least the first week of therapy. Similarly, at least a week should elapse between the discontinuance of PARNATE and the administration of another MAO inhibitor or a dibenzazepine-related entity, or the readministration of PARNATE.

The following list includes some other MAO inhibitors, dibenzazepine-related entities and tricyclic antidepressants.

Other MAO Inhibitors

Generic Name

Furazolidone

Isocarboxazid

Pargyline HCl

Pargyline HCl and methylclothiazide

Phenelzine sulfate

Procarbazine HCl

Dibenzazepine-Related and Other Tricyclics

Generic Name

Amitriptyline HCl

Perphenazine and amitriptyline HCl

Clomipramine hydrochloride

Desipramine HCl

Imipramine HCl

Nortriptyline HCl

Protriptyline HCl

Doxepin HCl

Carbamazepine

Cyclobenzaprine HCl

Amoxapine

Maprotiline HCl

Trimipramine maleate

4. In combination with bupropion

The concurrent administration of an MAO inhibitor and bupropion hydrochloride is contraindicated. At least 14 days should elapse between discontinuation of an MAO inhibitor and initiation of treatment with bupropion hydrochloride.

5. In combination with selective serotonin reuptake inhibitors (SSRIs) or selective norepinephrine reuptake inhibitors (SNRIs)

As a general rule, PARNATE should not be administered in combination with any SSRI or SNRI. There have been reports of serious, sometimes fatal, reactions (including hyperthermia, rigidity, myoclonus, autonomic instability with possible rapid fluctuations of vital signs, and mental status changes that include extreme agitation progressing to delirium and coma) in patients receiving a SSRI (e.g., fluoxetine) or a SNRI (e.g., venlafaxine) in combination with a monoamine oxidase inhibitor (MAOI), and in patients who have recently discontinued a SSRI or SNRI and are then started on an MAOI. Some cases presented with features resembling neuroleptic malignant syndrome. Therefore SSRIs and SNRIs should not be used in combination with an MAOI, or within 14 days of discontinuing therapy with an MAOI.

Since fluoxetine and its major metabolite have very long elimination half-lives, at least 5 weeks should be allowed after stopping fluoxetine before starting an MAOI.

At least 2 weeks should be allowed after stopping sertraline or paroxetine before starting an MAOI.

At least one week should be allowed after stopping a SNRI (e.g., venlafaxine) before starting a MAOI.

6. In combination with buspirone

PARNATE should not be used in combination with buspirone HCl, since several cases of elevated blood pressure have been reported in patients taking MAO inhibitors who were then given buspirone HCl. At least 10 days should elapse between the discontinuation of PARNATE and the institution of buspirone HCl.

7. In combination with sympathomimetics

PARNATE should not be administered in combination with sympathomimetics, including amphetamines which may be found in many herbal preparations as well as over-the-counter drugs such as cold, hay fever or weight-reducing preparations that contain vasoconstrictors.

During therapy with PARNATE, it appears that certain patients are particularly vulnerable to the effects of sympathomimetics when the activity of certain enzymes is inhibited. Use of sympathomimetics and compounds such as guanethidine, methyldopa, reserpine, dopamine, levodopa, and tryptophan with PARNATE may precipitate hypertension, headache, and related symptoms. Cerebral hemorrhage may also occur. The combination of MAOIs and tryptophan has been reported to cause behavioral and neurologic syndromes including disorientation, confusion, amnesia, delirium, agitation, hypomanic signs, ataxia, myoclonus, hyperreflexia, shivering, ocular oscillations, and Babinski's signs.

8. In combination with meperidine
Do not use meperidine concomitantly with MAO inhibitors or within 2 or 3 weeks following MAOI therapy. Serious reactions have been precipitated with concomitant use, including coma, severe hypertension or hypotension, severe respiratory depression, convulsions, malignant hyperpyrexia, excitation, peripheral vascular collapse, and death. It is thought that these reactions may be mediated by accumulation of 5-HT (serotonin) consequent to MAO inhibition.

9. In combination with dextromethorphan
The combination of MAO inhibitors and dextromethorphan has been reported to cause brief episodes of psychosis or bizarre behavior.

10. In combination with cheese or other foods with a high tyramine content
When excessive amounts of tyramine are consumed in conjunction with tranylcypromine, or within 2 weeks of stopping treatment, a serious and sometimes fatal hypertensive reaction may occur.

Tyramine occurs naturally in some foods or may occur from the bacterial breakdown of protein in foods which are fermented, aged, or spoiled. Foods that have reliably been shown to contain a high tyramine content and may also have been reported to induce a serious hypertensive reaction when consumed with tranylcypromine are:

- all matured or aged cheeses (note: all cheeses are considered matured or aged except fresh cottage cheese, cream cheese, ricotta, and processed cheese. All non-cheese dairy products can be consumed providing they are fresh)
- all aged, cured or fermented meat, fish, or poultry (note: meat, fish, or poultry that has not undergone aging, curing or fermenting and that is bought fresh, stored correctly and eaten fresh is not contraindicated)
- all fermented soybean products (e.g., soy sauce, miso, fermented tofu)
- sauerkraut
- fava or broad bean pods
- banana peel (but not the pulp)
- concentrated yeast extracts (e.g., Marmite or Vegemite spread)
- all tap/draught beers (note: some bottled beers, including non-alcoholic beer, may also pose a risk).

Patients should be advised to minimize or avoid use of all alcoholic beverages while taking PARNATE. Patients should be advised to adhere to the following dietary guidance about eating fresh foods:

Foods may be deliberately aged as part of their processing and these are contraindicated (see list above). Foods may also naturally age over time, even if they are refrigerated. It is therefore extremely important that patients are instructed to buy and eat only fresh foods or those which have been properly frozen. They should avoid eating foods if they are unsure of their storage conditions or freshness and they should be cautious of foods of unknown age or composition even if refrigerated.

The longer food is left to deteriorate and the larger the quantity of food eaten, the greater the potential quantity of tyramine ingested. Where there is any doubt, patients should be advised to either avoid the food or consume it in strict moderation if it is not otherwise contraindicated.

Patients should also be warned that tyramine levels may vary by brand or even batch and a person may absorb different amounts of tyramine from a particular food at different times. Therefore, if they have accidentally consumed a prohibited food on one occasion and not had a reaction, this does not mean that they will not have a serious hypertensive reaction if they consume the same food on a different occasion.

11. In patients undergoing elective surgery
Patients taking PARNATE should not undergo elective surgery requiring general anesthesia. Also, they should not be given cocaine or local anesthesia containing sympathomimetic vasoconstrictors. The possible combined hypotensive effects of PARNATE and spinal anesthesia should be kept in mind. PARNATE should be discontinued at least 10 days prior to elective surgery.

ADDITIONAL CONTRAINDICATIONS
In general, the physician should bear in mind the possibility of a lowered margin of safety when PARNATE is administered in combination with potent drugs.

1. PARNATE should not be used in combination with some central nervous system depressants such as narcotics and alcohol, or with hypotensive agents. A marked potentiating effect on these classes of drugs has been reported.
2. Anti-parkinsonism drugs should be used with caution in patients receiving PARNATE since severe reactions have been reported.
3. PARNATE should not be used in patients with a history of liver disease or in those with abnormal liver function tests.
4. Excessive use of caffeine in any form should be avoided in patients receiving PARNATE.

WARNINGS TO PHYSICIANS
Clinical Worsening and Suicide Risk: Patients with major depressive disorder (MDD), both adult and pediatric, may experience worsening of their depression and/or the emergence of suicidal ideation and behavior (suicidality) or unusual changes in behavior, whether or not they are taking antidepressant medications, and this risk may persist until significant remission occurs. Suicide is a known risk of depression and certain other psychiatric disorders, and these disorders themselves are the strongest predictors of suicide. There has been a long-standing concern, however, that antidepressants may have a role in inducing worsening of depression and the emergence of suicidality in certain patients during the early phases of treatment. Pooled analyses of short-term placebo-controlled trials of antidepressant drugs (SSRIs and others) showed that these drugs increase the risk of suicidal thinking and behavior (suicidality) in children, adolescents, and young adults (ages 18-24) with major depressive disorder (MDD) and other psychiatric disorders. Short-term studies did not show an increase in the risk of suicidality with antidepressants compared to placebo in adults beyond age 24; there was a reduction with antidepressants compared to placebo in adults aged 65 and older. The pooled analyses of placebo-controlled trials in children and adolescents with MDD, obsessive compulsive disorder (OCD), or other psychiatric disorders included a total of 24 short-term trials of 9 antidepressant drugs in over 4,400 patients. The pooled analyses of placebo-controlled trials in adults with MDD or other psychiatric disorders included a total of 295 short-term trials (median duration of 2 months) of 11 antidepressant drugs in over 77,000 patients. There was considerable variation in risk of suicidality among drugs, but a tendency toward an increase in the younger patients for almost all drugs studied. There were differences in absolute risk of suicidality across the different indications, with the highest incidence in MDD. The risk differences (drug vs placebo), however, were relatively stable within age strata and across indications. These risk differences (drug-placebo difference in the number of cases of suicidality per 1,000 patients treated) are provided in Table 1.

Table 1.

Age Range	Drug-Placebo Difference in Number of Cases of Suicidality per 1,000 Patients Treated
Increases Compared to Placebo	
<18	14 additional cases
18-24	5 additional cases
Decreases Compared to Placebo	
25-64	1 fewer case
≥65	6 fewer cases

No suicides occurred in any of the pediatric trials. There were suicides in the adult trials, but the number was not sufficient to reach any conclusion about drug effect on suicide.

It is unknown whether the suicidality risk extends to longer-term use, i.e., beyond several months. However, there is substantial evidence from placebo-controlled maintenance trials in adults with depression that the use of antidepressants can delay the recurrence of depression.

All patients being treated with antidepressants for any indication should be monitored appropriately and observed closely for clinical worsening, suicidality, and unusual changes in behavior, especially during the initial few months of a course of drug therapy, or at times of dose changes, either increases or decreases.

The following symptoms, anxiety, agitation, panic attacks, insomnia, irritability, hostility, aggressiveness, impulsivity, akathisia (psychomotor restlessness), hypomania, and mania, have been reported in adult and pediatric patients being treated with antidepressants for major depressive disorder as well as for other indications, both psychiatric and nonpsychiatric. Although a causal link between the emergence of such symptoms and either the worsening of depression and/or the emergence of suicidal impulses has not been established, there is concern that such symptoms may represent precursors to emerging suicidality.

Consideration should be given to changing the therapeutic regimen, including possibly discontinuing the medication, in patients whose depression is persistently worse, or who are experiencing emergent suicidality or symptoms that might be precursors to worsening depression or suicidality, especially if these symptoms are severe, abrupt in onset, or were not part of the patient's presenting symptoms.

Families and caregivers of patients being treated with antidepressants for major depressive disorder or other indications, both psychiatric and nonpsychiatric, should be alerted about the need to monitor patients for the emergence of agitation, irritability, unusual changes in behavior, and the other symptoms described above, as well as the emergence of suicidality, and to report such symptoms immediately to healthcare providers. Such monitoring should include daily observation by families and caregivers.

Prescriptions for PARNATE should be written for the smallest quantity of tablets consistent with good patient management, in order to reduce the risk of overdose.

Screening Patients for Bipolar Disorder: A major depressive episode may be the initial presentation of bipolar disorder. It is generally believed (though not established in controlled trials) that treating such an episode with an antidepressant alone may increase the likelihood of precipitation of a mixed/manic episode in patients at risk for bipolar disorder. Whether any of the symptoms described above represent such a conversion is unknown. However, prior to initiating treatment with an antidepressant, patients with depressive symptoms should be adequately screened to determine if they are at risk for bipolar disorder; such screening should include a detailed psychiatric history, including a family history of suicide, bipolar disorder, and depression. It should be noted that PARNATE is not approved for use in treating bipolar depression.

PARNATE is a potent agent with the capability of producing serious side effects. PARNATE is not recommended in those depressive reactions where other antidepressant drugs may be effective. **It should be reserved for patients who can be closely supervised and who have not responded satisfactorily to the drugs more commonly administered for depression.**

Before prescribing, the physician should be completely familiar with the full material on dosage, side effects, and contraindications on these pages, with the principles of MAO inhibitor therapy and the side effects of this class of drugs. Also, the physician should be familiar with the symptomatology of mental depressions and alternate methods of treatment to aid in the careful selection of patients for therapy with PARNATE.

Pregnancy Warning: Use of any drug in pregnancy, during lactation or in women of childbearing age requires that the potential benefits of the drug be weighed against its possible hazards to mother and child.

Animal reproductive studies show that PARNATE passes through the placental barrier into the fetus of the rat, and into the milk of the lactating dog. The absence of a harmful action of PARNATE on fertility or on postnatal development by either prenatal treatment or from the milk of treated animals has not been demonstrated. Tranylcypromine is excreted in human milk.

WARNING TO THE PATIENT
Patients should be instructed to report promptly the occurrence of headache or other unusual symptoms, i.e., palpitation and/or tachycardia, a sense of constriction in the throat or chest, sweating, dizziness, neck stiffness, nausea, or vomiting.

Patients should be warned against eating the foods listed in Section 11 under Contraindications while on therapy with PARNATE. Also, they should be told not to drink alcoholic beverages. The patient should also be warned about the possibility of hypotension and faintness, as well as drowsiness sufficient to impair performance of potentially hazardous tasks such as driving a car or operating machinery.

Continued on next page

Patients should also be cautioned not to take concomitant medications, whether prescription or over-the-counter drugs such as cold, hay fever, or weight-reducing preparations, without the advice of a physician. They should be advised not to consume excessive amounts of caffeine in any form. Likewise, they should inform other physicians, and their dentist, about their use of PARNATE.

See PRECAUTIONS—Information for Patients for information regarding clinical worsening and suicide risk.

WARNINGS

Hypertensive Crisis: The most important reaction associated with PARNATE is the occurrence of hypertensive crises which have sometimes been fatal.

These crises are characterized by some or all of the following symptoms: occipital headache which may radiate frontally, palpitation, neck stiffness or soreness, nausea or vomiting, sweating (sometimes with fever and sometimes with cold, clammy skin), and photophobia. Either tachycardia or bradycardia may be present, and associated constricting chest pain and dilated pupils may occur. **Intracranial bleeding, sometimes fatal in outcome, has been reported in association with the paradoxical increase in blood pressure.** In all patients taking PARNATE, blood pressure should be followed closely to detect evidence of any pressor response. It is emphasized that full reliance should not be placed on blood pressure readings, but that the patient should also be observed frequently.

Therapy should be discontinued immediately upon the occurrence of palpitation or frequent headaches during therapy with PARNATE. These signs may be prodromal of a hypertensive crisis.

Important:

Recommended treatment in hypertensive crises

If a hypertensive crisis occurs, PARNATE should be discontinued and therapy to lower blood pressure should be instituted immediately. Headache tends to abate as blood pressure is lowered. On the basis of present evidence, phentolamine is recommended. (The dosage reported for phentolamine is 5 mg I.V.) Care should be taken to administer this drug slowly in order to avoid producing an excessive hypotensive effect. Fever should be managed by means of external cooling. Other symptomatic and supportive measures may be desirable in particular cases. Do not use parenteral reserpine.

PRECAUTIONS

Hypotension: Hypotension has been observed during therapy with PARNATE. Symptoms of postural hypotension are seen most commonly but not exclusively in patients with pre-existent hypertension; blood pressure usually returns rapidly to pretreatment levels upon discontinuation of the drug. At doses above 30 mg daily, postural hypotension is a major side effect and may result in syncope. Dosage increases should be made more gradually in patients showing a tendency toward hypotension at the beginning of therapy. Postural hypotension may be relieved by having the patient lie down until blood pressure returns to normal.

Also, when PARNATE is combined with those phenothiazine derivatives or other compounds known to cause hypotension, the possibility of additive hypotensive effects should be considered.

There have been reports of drug dependency in patients using doses of tranylcypromine significantly in excess of the therapeutic range. Some of these patients had a history of previous substance abuse. The following withdrawal symptoms have been reported: restlessness, anxiety, depression, confusion, hallucinations, headache, weakness, and diarrhea.

Drugs which lower the seizure threshold, including MAO inhibitors, should not be used with contrasting agents used before myelography. As with other MAO inhibitors, PARNATE should be discontinued at least 48 hours before myelography and should not be resumed for at least 24 hours postprocedure.

MAO inhibitors may have the capacity to suppress anginal pain that would otherwise serve as a warning of myocardial ischemia.

The usual precautions should be observed in patients with impaired renal function since there is a possibility of cumulative effects in such patients.

Older patients may suffer more morbidity than younger patients during and following an episode of hypertension or malignant hyperthermia. Older patients have less compensatory reserve to cope with any serious adverse reaction. Therefore, PARNATE should be used with caution in the elderly population.

Although excretion of PARNATE is rapid, inhibition of MAO may persist up to 10 days following discontinuation.

Because the influence of PARNATE on the convulsive threshold is variable in animal experiments, suitable precautions should be taken if epileptic patients are treated.

Some MAO inhibitors have contributed to hypoglycemic episodes in diabetic patients receiving insulin or oral hypoglycemic agents. Therefore, PARNATE should be used with caution in diabetics using these drugs.

PARNATE may aggravate coexisting symptoms in depression, such as anxiety and agitation.

Use PARNATE with caution in hyperthyroid patients because of their increased sensitivity to pressor amines.

PARNATE should be administered with caution to patients receiving disulfiram tablets. In a single study, rats given high intraperitoneal doses of d or l isomers of tranylcypromine sulfate plus disulfiram experienced severe toxicity including convulsions and death. Additional studies in rats given high oral doses of racemic tranylcypromine sulfate (PARNATE) and disulfiram produced no adverse interaction.

Information for Patients: Prescribers or other health professionals should inform patients, their families, and their caregivers about the benefits and risks associated with treatment with PARNATE and should counsel them in its appropriate use. A patient Medication Guide about "Antidepressant Medicines, Depression and Other Serious Mental Illnesses, and Suicidal Thoughts or Actions" is available for PARNATE. The prescriber or health professional should instruct patients, their families, and their caregivers to read the Medication Guide and should assist them in understanding its contents. Patients should be given the opportunity to discuss the contents of the Medication Guide and to obtain answers to any questions they may have. The complete text of the Medication Guide is reprinted at the end of this document.

Patients should be advised of the following issues and asked to alert their prescriber if these occur while taking PARNATE.

Clinical Worsening and Suicide Risk: Patients, their families, and their caregivers should be encouraged to be alert to the emergence of anxiety, agitation, panic attacks, insomnia, irritability, hostility, aggressiveness, impulsivity, akathisia (psychomotor restlessness), hypomania, mania, other unusual changes in behavior, worsening of depression, and suicidal ideation, especially early during antidepressant treatment and when the dose is adjusted up or down. Families and caregivers of patients should be advised to look for the emergence of such symptoms on a day-to-day basis, since changes may be abrupt. Such symptoms should be reported to the patient's prescriber or health professional, especially if they are severe, abrupt in onset, or were not part of the patient's presenting symptoms. Symptoms such as these may be associated with an increased risk for suicidal thinking and behavior and indicate a need for very close monitoring and possibly changes in the medication.

Pediatric Use: Safety and effectiveness in the pediatric population have not been established (see BOX WARNING and WARNINGS—Clinical Worsening and Suicide Risk). Anyone considering the use of PARNATE in a child or adolescent must balance the potential risks with the clinical need.

ADVERSE REACTIONS

Overstimulation which may include increased anxiety, agitation, and manic symptoms is usually evidence of excessive therapeutic action. Dosage should be reduced, or a phenothiazine tranquilizer should be administered concomitantly. Patients may experience restlessness or insomnia; may notice some weakness, drowsiness, episodes of dizziness or dry mouth; or may report nausea, diarrhea, abdominal pain, or constipation. Most of these effects can be relieved by lowering the dosage or by giving suitable concomitant medication.

Tachycardia, significant anorexia, edema, palpitation, blurred vision, chills, and impotence have each been reported.

Headaches without blood pressure elevation have occurred. Rare instances of hepatitis, skin rash, and alopecia have been reported.

Impaired water excretion compatible with the syndrome of inappropriate secretion of antidiuretic hormone (SIADH) has been reported.

Tinnitus, muscle spasm, tremors, myoclonic jerks, numbness, paresthesia, urinary retention, and retarded ejaculation have been reported.

Hematologic disorders including anemia, leukopenia, agranulocytosis, and thrombocytopenia have been reported.

Post-Introduction Reports: The following are spontaneously reported adverse events temporally associated with use of PARNATE. No clear relationship between PARNATE and these events has been established. Localized scleroderma, flare-up of cystic acne, ataxia, confusion, disorientation, memory loss, urinary frequency, urinary incontinence, urticaria, fissuring in corner of mouth, akinesia.

To report SUSPECTED ADVERSE REACTIONS, contact Concordia Pharmaceuticals Inc. at 1-877-370-1142 or FDA at 1-800-FDA-1088 or *www.fda.gov/medwatch*.

DOSAGE AND ADMINISTRATION

Dosage should be adjusted to the requirements of the individual patient. Improvement should be seen within 48 hours to 3 weeks after starting therapy.

The usual effective dosage is 30 mg per day, usually given in divided doses. If there are no signs of improvement after a reasonable period (up to 2 weeks), then the dosage may be increased in 10 mg per day increments at intervals of 1 to 3 weeks; the dosage range may be extended to a maximum of 60 mg per day from the usual 30 mg per day.

OVERDOSAGE

Symptoms: The characteristic symptoms that may be caused by overdosage are usually those described above. However, an intensification of these symptoms and sometimes severe additional manifestations may be seen, depending on the degree of overdosage and on individual susceptibility. Some patients exhibit insomnia, restlessness and anxiety, progressing in severe cases to agitation, mental confusion, and incoherence. Hypotension, dizziness, weakness, and drowsiness may occur, progressing in severe cases to extreme dizziness and shock. A few patients have displayed hypertension with severe headache and other symptoms. Rare instances have been reported in which hypertension was accompanied by twitching or myoclonic fibrillation of skeletal muscles with hyperpyrexia, sometimes progressing to generalized rigidity and coma.

Treatment: Because strategies for the management of overdose are continually evolving, it is advisable to contact a Poison Control Center to determine the latest recommendations for the management of an overdose of any drug. Telephone numbers for the certified Poison Control Centers are listed in the *Physicians' Desk Reference* (PDR).

Treatment should normally consist of general supportive measures, close observation of vital signs and steps to counteract specific symptoms as they occur, since MAO inhibition may persist. The management of hypertensive crises is described under WARNINGS in the HYPERTENSIVE CRISES section.

External cooling is recommended if hyperpyrexia occurs. Barbiturates have been reported to help relieve myoclonic reactions, but frequency of administration should be controlled carefully because PARNATE may prolong barbiturate activity. When hypotension requires treatment, the standard measures for managing circulatory shock should be initiated. If pressor agents are used, the rate of infusion should be regulated by careful observation of the patient because an exaggerated pressor response sometimes occurs in the presence of MAO inhibition. Remember that the toxic effect of PARNATE may be delayed or prolonged following the last dose of the drug. Therefore, the patient should be closely observed for at least a week. It is not known if tranylcypromine is dialyzable.

HOW SUPPLIED

PARNATE is supplied as round, rose-red, film-coated tablets debossed with the product name PARNATE and SB and contains tranylcypromine sulfate equivalent to 10 mg of tranylcypromine, in bottles of 100 with a desiccant.

10 mg 100's: NDC 59212-447-10

Store between 15° and 30°C (59° and 86°F). Dispense in a tight, light-resistant container.

Medication Guide

Antidepressant Medicines, Depression and Other Serious Mental Illnesses, and Suicidal Thoughts or Actions

PARNATE® (PAR-nate) (tranylcypromine sulfate) Tablets

Read the Medication Guide that comes with you or your family member's antidepressant medicine. This Medication Guide is only about the risk of suicidal thoughts and actions with antidepressant medicines. **Talk to your, or your family member's, healthcare provider about:**

• All risks and benefits of treatment with antidepressant medicines

- All treatment choices for depression or other serious mental illness

What is the most important information I should know about antidepressant medicines, depression and other serious mental illnesses, and suicidal thoughts or actions?
1. **Antidepressant medicines may increase suicidal thoughts or actions in some children, teenagers, and young adults within the first few months of treatment.**
2. **Depression and other serious mental illnesses are the most important causes of suicidal thoughts and actions.** Some people may have a particularly high risk of having suicidal thoughts or actions. These include people who have (or have a family history of) bipolar illness (also called manic-depressive illness) or suicidal thoughts or actions.
3. **How can I watch for and try to prevent suicidal thoughts and actions in myself or a family member?**
- Pay close attention to any changes, especially sudden changes, in mood, behaviors, thoughts, or feelings. This is very important when an antidepressant medicine is started or when the dose is changed.
- Call the healthcare provider right away to report new or sudden changes in mood, behavior, thoughts, or feelings.
- Keep all follow-up visits with the healthcare provider as scheduled. Call the healthcare provider between visits as needed, especially if you have concerns about symptoms.

Call a healthcare provider right away if you or your family member has any of the following symptoms, especially if they are new, worse, or worry you:
- Thoughts about suicide or dying
- Attempts to commit suicide
- New or worse depression
- New or worse anxiety
- Feeling very agitated or restless
- Panic attacks
- Trouble sleeping (insomnia)
- New or worse irritability
- Acting aggressive, being angry, or violent
- Acting on dangerous impulses
- An extreme increase in activity and talking (mania)
- Other unusual changes in behavior or mood

What else do I need to know about antidepressant medicines?
- **Never stop an antidepressant medicine without first talking to a healthcare provider.** Stopping an antidepressant medicine suddenly can cause other symptoms.
- **Antidepressants are medicines used to treat depression and other illnesses.** It is important to discuss all the risks of treating depression and also the risks of not treating it. Patients and their families or other caregivers should discuss all treatment choices with the healthcare provider, not just the use of antidepressants.
- **Antidepressant medicines have other side effects.** Call your doctor for medical advice about side effects. You may report side effects to FDA at 1-800-FDA-1088.
- **Antidepressant medicines can interact with other medicines.** Know all of the medicines that you or your family member takes. Keep a list of all medicines to show the healthcare provider. Do not start new medicines without first checking with your healthcare provider.
- **Not all antidepressant medicines prescribed for children are FDA approved for use in children.** Talk to your child's healthcare provider for more information.

This Medication Guide has been approved by the U.S. Food and Drug Administration for all antidepressants.
06/2016
Manufactured for:
Concordia Pharmaceuticals Inc.
St. Michael, Barbados BB11005
©2015 Concordia Pharmaceuticals Inc. All rights reserved.
Shown in Product Identification Guide, page 508

PLAQUENIL®   ℞
Hydroxychloroquine Sulfate
Tablets, USP

WARNING
PHYSICIANS SHOULD COMPLETELY FAMILIARIZE THEMSELVES WITH THE COMPLETE CONTENTS OF THIS LEAFLET BEFORE PRESCRIBING HYDROXYCHLOROQUINE.

DESCRIPTION
Hydroxychloroquine sulfate is a colorless crystalline solid, soluble in water to at least 20 percent; chemically the drug is 2-[[4-[(7-Chloro-4-quinolyl)amino]pentyl]ethylamino] ethanol sulfate (1:1).

PLAQUENIL (hydroxychloroquine sulfate) tablets contain 200 mg hydroxychloroquine sulfate, equivalent to 155 mg base, and are for oral administration.
Inactive Ingredients: Dibasic Calcium Phosphate, Hydroxypropyl Methylcellulose, Magnesium Stearate, Polyethylene glycol 400, Polysorbate 80, Corn Starch, Titanium Dioxide.

ACTIONS
The drug possesses antimalarial actions and also exerts a beneficial effect in lupus erythematosus (chronic discoid or systemic) and acute or chronic rheumatoid arthritis. The precise mechanism of action is not known.

INDICATIONS
PLAQUENIL is indicated for the suppressive treatment and treatment of acute attacks of malaria due to *Plasmodium vivax*, *P. malariae*, *P. ovale*, and susceptible strains of *P. falciparum*. It is also indicated for the treatment of discoid and systemic lupus erythematosus, and rheumatoid arthritis.

CONTRAINDICATIONS
Use of this drug is contraindicated (1) in the presence of retinal or visual field changes attributable to any 4-aminoquinoline compound, (2) in patients with known hypersensitivity to 4-aminoquinoline compounds, and (3) for long-term therapy in children.

WARNINGS, General
PLAQUENIL is not effective against chloroquine-resistant strains of *P. falciparum*.
Before starting a long-term treatment, both eyes should be carefully examined for visual acuity, central visual field, and color vision. Examination should also include fundoscopy. These examinations should be repeated at least annually. Retinal toxicity is largely dose-related.
The risk of retinal damage is small with daily doses of up to 6.5 mg/kg body weight. Exceeding the recommended daily dose sharply increases the risk of retinal toxicity. This examination should be more frequent and adapted to the patient in the following situations:
- daily dosage exceeding 6.5 mg/kg ideal body weight. Absolute body weight used as a guide to dosage could result in an overdosage in the obese;
- renal insufficiency;
- cumulative dose more than 200 g;
- elderly;
- impaired visual acuity.
If any visual disturbance occurs (visual acuity, color vision), the drug should be immediately discontinued and the patient closely observed for possible progression of the abnormality. Retinal changes (and visual disturbances) may progress even after cessation of the therapy. (see ADVERSE REACTIONS).
Suicidal behavior has been reported in very rare cases in patients treated with hydroxychloroquine.
Children are especially sensitive to the 4-aminoquinoline compounds. A number of fatalities have been reported following the accidental ingestion of chloroquine, sometimes in relatively small doses (0.75 g or 1 g in one 3-year-old child). Patients should be strongly warned to keep these drugs out of the reach of children.
Use of PLAQUENIL in patients with psoriasis may precipitate a severe attack of psoriasis. When used in patients with porphyria the condition may be exacerbated. The preparation should not be used in these conditions unless in the judgment of the physician the benefit to the patient outweighs the possible hazard.

Usage in Pregnancy
Usage of this drug during pregnancy should be avoided except in the suppression or treatment of malaria when in the judgment of the physician the benefit outweighs the possible hazard. It should be noted that radioactively-tagged chloroquine administered intravenously to pregnant, pigmented CBA mice passed rapidly across the placenta. It accumulated selectively in the melanin structures of the fetal eyes and was retained in the ocular tissues for five months after the drug had been eliminated from the rest of the body.

PRECAUTIONS, General
Antimalarial compounds should be used with caution in patients with hepatic disease or alcoholism or in conjunction with known hepatotoxic drugs.
Periodic blood cell counts should be made if patients are given prolonged therapy. If any severe blood disorder appears which is not attributable to the disease under treatment, discontinuation of the drug should be considered. The

drug should be administered with caution in patients having G-6-PD (glucose-6-phosphate dehydrogenase) deficiency.

ADVERSE REACTIONS
Psychiatric disorders: Nervousness, emotional lability, psychosis, suicidal behavior.
Nervous system disorders: Dizziness, headache, and convulsions have been reported with this class of drugs.
Eye disorders: Retinopathy with changes in pigmentation and visual field defects have been reported. In its early form, it appears reversible on discontinuation of hydroxychloroquine. If allowed to develop, there may be a risk of progression even after treatment withdrawal. Cases of maculopathies and macular degeneration have been reported and may be irreversible.
Skin and subcutaneous tissue disorders: Bullous eruptions including very rare cases of Erythema multiforme, Stevens-Johnson syndrome, toxic epidermal necrolysis, photosensitivity, and exfoliative dermatitis have been reported.

OVERDOSAGE
The 4-aminoquinoline compounds are very rapidly and completely absorbed after ingestion, and in accidental overdosage, or rarely with lower doses in hypersensitive patients, toxic symptoms may occur within 30 minutes. The symptoms of overdosage may include headache, drowsiness, visual disturbances, cardiovascular collapse, convulsions, hypokalemia, rhythm and conduction disorders including QT prolongation, torsade de pointe, ventricular tachycardia and ventricular fibrillation, followed by sudden potentially fatal respiratory and cardiac arrest. Immediate medical attention is required, as these effects may appear shortly after the overdose. Treatment is symptomatic and must be prompt with immediate evacuation of the stomach by emesis (at home, before transportation to the hospital) or gastric lavage until the stomach is completely emptied. If finely powdered, activated charcoal is introduced by the stomach tube, after lavage, and within 30 minutes after ingestion of the tablets, it may inhibit further intestinal absorption of the drug. To be effective, the dose of activated charcoal should be at least five times the estimated dose of hydroxychloroquine ingested. Convulsions, if present, should be controlled before attempting gastric lavage. If due to cerebral stimulation, cautious administration of an ultrashort-acting barbiturate may be tried but, if due to anoxia, it should be corrected by oxygen administration, artificial respiration or, in shock with hypotension, by vasopressor therapy. Because of the importance of supporting respiration, tracheal intubation or tracheostomy, followed by gastric lavage, may also be necessary. Exchange transfusions have been used to reduce the level of 4-aminoquinoline drug in the blood.
A patient who survives the acute phase and is asymptomatic should be closely observed for at least six hours. Fluids may be forced, and sufficient ammonium chloride (8 g daily in divided doses for adults) may be administered for a few days to acidify the urine to help promote urinary excretion in cases of both overdosage and sensitivity.

MALARIA
Actions
Like chloroquine phosphate, USP, PLAQUENIL is highly active against the erythrocytic forms of *P. vivax* and *P. malariae* and most strains of *P. falciparum* (but not the gametocytes of *P. falciparum*).
PLAQUENIL does not prevent relapses in patients with *P. vivax* or *P. malariae* malaria because it is not effective against exo-erythrocytic forms of the parasite, nor will it prevent *P. vivax* or *P. malariae* infection when administered as a prophylactic. It is highly effective as a suppressive agent in patients with *P. vivax* or *P. malariae* malaria, in terminating acute attacks, and significantly lengthening the interval between treatment and relapse. In patients with *P. falciparum* malaria, it abolishes the acute attack and effects complete cure of the infection, unless due to a resistant strain of *P. falciparum*.
Indications
PLAQUENIL is indicated for the treatment of acute attacks and suppression of malaria.
Warnings
In recent years, it has been found that certain strains of *P. falciparum* have become resistant to 4-aminoquinoline compounds (including hydroxychloroquine) as shown by the fact that normally adequate doses have failed to prevent or cure

Continued on next page

clinical malaria or parasitemia. Treatment with quinine or other specific forms of therapy is therefore advised for patients infected with a resistant strain of parasites.

Before starting a long-term treatment, both eyes should be carefully examined for visual acuity, central visual field and color vision. Examination should also include fundoscopy. These examinations should be repeated at least annually. Retinal toxicity is largely dose-related.

The risk of retinal damages is small with daily doses of up to 6.5 mg/kg body weight. Exceeding the recommended daily dose sharply increases the risk of retinal toxicity. This examination should be more frequent and adapted to the patient in the following situations:

• daily dosage exceeding 6.5 mg/kg ideal body weight. Absolute body weight used as a guide to dosage could result in an overdosage in the obese;
• renal insufficiency;
• cumulative dose more than 200 g;
• elderly;
• impaired visual acuity.

If any visual disturbance occurs (visual acuity, color vision), the drug should be immediately discontinued and the patient closely observed for possible progression of the abnormality. Retinal changes (and visual disturbances) may progress even after cessation of the therapy. (see ADVERSE REACTIONS).

Suicidal behavior has been reported in very rare cases in patients treated with hydroxychloroquine.

Adverse Reactions

Following the administration in doses adequate for the treatment of an acute malarial attack, mild and transient headache, dizziness, and gastrointestinal complaints (diarrhea, anorexia, nausea, abdominal cramps and, on rare occasions, vomiting) may occur. Cardiomyopathy has been rarely reported with high daily dosages of hydroxychloroquine.

Psychiatric disorders: Nervousness, emotional lability, psychosis, suicidal behavior.

Nervous system disorders: Dizziness, headache, and convulsions have been reported with this class of drugs.

Eye disorders: Retinopathy with changes in pigmentation and visual field defects have been reported. In its early form, it appears reversible on discontinuation of hydroxychloroquine. If allowed to develop, there may be a risk of progression even after treatment withdrawal. Cases of maculopathies and macular degeneration have been reported and may be irreversible.

Skin and subcutaneous tissue disorders: Bullous eruptions including very rare cases of Erythema multiforme, Stevens-Johnson syndrome, toxic epidermal necrolysis, photosensitivity and exfoliative dermatitis have been reported.

Dosage and Administration

One tablet of 200 mg of hydroxychloroquine sulfate is equivalent to 155 mg base.

Malaria

Suppression

In adults, 400 mg (=310 mg base) on exactly the same day of each week. *In infants and children,* the weekly suppressive dosage is 5 mg, calculated as base, per kg of body weight, but should not exceed the adult dose regardless of weight. If circumstances permit, suppressive therapy should begin two weeks prior to exposure. However, failing this, in adults an initial double (loading) dose of 800 mg (=620 mg base), or in children 10 mg base/kg may be taken in two divided doses, six hours apart. The suppressive therapy should be continued for eight weeks after leaving the endemic area.

Treatment of the acute attack

In adults, an initial dose of 800 mg (= 620 mg base) followed by 400 mg (=310 mg base) in six to eight hours and 400 mg (=310 mg base) on each of two consecutive days (total 2 g hydroxychloroquine sulfate or 1.55 g base). An alternative method, employing a single dose of 800 mg (=620 mg base), has also proved effective.

The dosage for adults may also be calculated on the basis of body weight; this method is preferred for infants and children. A total dose representing 25 mg of base per kg of body weight is administered in three days, as follows:

First dose: 10 mg base per kg (but not exceeding a single dose of 620 mg base).

Second dose: 5 mg base per kg (but not exceeding a single dose of 310 mg base) 6 hours after first dose.

Third dose: 5 mg base per kg 18 hours after second dose.

Fourth dose: 5 mg base per kg 24 hours after third dose.

For radical cure of *vivax* and *malariae* malaria concomitant therapy with an 8-aminoquinoline compound is necessary.

LUPUS ERYTHEMATOSUS AND RHEUMATOID ARTHRITIS

Indications

PLAQUENIL is useful in patients with the following disorders who have not responded satisfactorily to drugs with less potential for serious side effects: lupus erythematosus (chronic discoid and systemic) and acute or chronic rheumatoid arthritis.

Warnings

PHYSICIANS SHOULD COMPLETELY FAMILIARIZE THEMSELVES WITH THE COMPLETE CONTENTS OF THIS LEAFLET BEFORE PRESCRIBING PLAQUENIL.

Irreversible retinal damage has been observed in some patients who had received long-term or high-dosage 4-aminoquinoline therapy for discoid and systemic lupus erythematosus, or rheumatoid arthritis.

When prolonged therapy with any Antimalarial compound is contemplated, initial (base line) and periodic (every three months) ophthalmologic examinations (including visual acuity, expert slit-lamp, funduscopic, and visual field tests) should be performed.

If there is any indication of abnormality in the visual acuity, visual field, color vision, or retinal macular areas (such as pigmentary changes, loss of foveal reflex), or any visual symptoms (such as light flashes and streaks) which are not fully explainable by difficulties of accommodation or corneal opacities, the drug should be discontinued immediately and the patient closely observed for possible progression. Retinal changes (and visual disturbances) may progress even after cessation of therapy (see ADVERSE REACTIONS).

Retinal toxicity is largely dose-related. The risk of retinal damages is small with daily doses of up to 6.5 mg/kg body weight. Exceeding the recommended daily dose sharply increases the risk of retinal toxicity. This examination should be more frequent and adapted to the patient in the following situations:

• daily dosage exceeding 6.5 mg/kg ideal body weight. Absolute body weight used as a guide to dosage could result in an overdosage in the obese;
• renal insufficiency;
• cumulative dose more than 200 g;
• elderly;
• impaired visual acuity.

All patients on long-term therapy with this preparation should be questioned and examined periodically, including the testing of knee and ankle reflexes, to detect any evidence of muscular weakness. If weakness occurs, discontinue the drug.

In the treatment of rheumatoid arthritis, if objective improvement (such as reduced joint swelling, increased mobility) does not occur within six months, the drug should be discontinued. Safe use of the drug in the treatment of juvenile arthritis has not been established.

Suicidal behavior has been reported in very rare cases in patients treated with hydroxychloroquine.

Precautions

Dermatologic reactions to PLAQUENIL may occur and, therefore, proper care should be exercised when it is administered to any patient receiving a drug with a significant tendency to produce dermatitis.

The methods recommended for early diagnosis of "chloroquine retinopathy" consist of (1) funduscopic examination of the macula for fine pigmentary disturbances or loss of the foveal reflex and (2) examination of the central visual field with a small red test object for pericentral or paracentral scotoma or determination of retinal thresholds to red. Any unexplained visual symptoms, such as light flashes or streaks, should also be regarded with suspicion as possible manifestations of retinopathy.

If serious toxic symptoms occur from overdosage or sensitivity, it has been suggested that ammonium chloride (8 g daily in divided doses for adults) be administered orally three or four days a week for several months after therapy has been stopped, as acidification of the urine increases renal excretion of the 4-aminoquinoline compounds by 20 to 90 percent. However, caution must be exercised in patients with impaired renal function and/or metabolic acidosis.

Adverse Reactions

Not all of the following reactions have been observed with every 4-aminoquinoline compound during long-term therapy, but they have been reported with one or more and should be borne in mind when drugs of this class are administered. Adverse effects with different compounds vary in type and frequency.

CNS Reactions: Irritability, nervousness, emotional changes, nightmares, psychosis, headache, dizziness, vertigo, tinnitus, nystagmus, nerve deafness, convulsions, ataxia and suicidal behavior.

Neuromuscular Reactions: Skeletal muscle palsies or skeletal muscle myopathy or neuromyopathy leading to progressive weakness and atrophy of proximal muscle groups which may be associated with mild sensory changes, depression of tendon reflexes and abnormal nerve conduction.

Ocular Reactions:

A. *Ciliary body:* Disturbance of accommodation with symptoms of blurred vision. This reaction is dose-related and reversible with cessation of therapy.

B. *Cornea:* Transient edema, punctate to lineal opacities, decreased corneal sensitivity. The corneal changes, with or without accompanying symptoms (blurred vision, halos around lights, photophobia), are fairly common, but reversible. Corneal deposits may appear as early as three weeks following initiation of therapy.

The incidence of corneal changes and visual side effects appears to be considerably lower with hydroxychloroquine than with chloroquine.

C. *Retina:* Macula: Edema, atrophy, abnormal pigmentation (mild pigment stippling to a "bull's-eye" appearance), loss of foveal reflex, increased macular recovery time following exposure to a bright light (photo-stress test), elevated retinal threshold to red light in macular, paramacular, and peripheral retinal areas. **Cases of maculopathies and macular degeneration have been reported and may be irreversible.**

Other fundus changes include optic disc pallor and atrophy, attenuation of retinal arterioles, fine granular pigmentary disturbances in the peripheral retina and prominent choroidal patterns in advanced stage.

D. *Visual field defects:* Pericentral or paracentral scotoma, central scotoma with decreased visual acuity, rarely field constriction, abnormal color vision.

The most common visual symptoms attributed to the retinopathy are: reading and seeing difficulties (words, letters, or parts of objects missing), photophobia, blurred distance vision, missing or blacked out areas in the central or peripheral visual field, light flashes and streaks.

Retinopathy appears to be dose related and has occurred within several months (rarely) to several years of daily therapy; a small number of cases have been reported several years after antimalarial drug therapy was discontinued. It has not been noted during prolonged use of weekly doses of the 4-aminoquinoline compounds for suppression of malaria.

Patients with retinal changes may have visual symptoms or may be asymptomatic (with or without visual field changes). Rarely scotomatous vision or field defects may occur without obvious retinal change.

Retinopathy may progress even after the drug is discontinued. In a number of patients, early retinopathy (macular pigmentation sometimes with central field defects) diminished or regressed completely after therapy was discontinued. If allowed to develop, there may be a risk of progression even after treatment withdrawal. Paracentral scotoma to red targets (sometimes called "premaculopathy") is indicative of early retinal dysfunction which is usually reversible with cessation of therapy.

A small number of cases of retinal changes have been reported as occurring in patients who received only hydroxychloroquine. These usually consisted of alteration in retinal pigmentation which was detected on periodic ophthalmologic examination; visual field defects were also present in some instances. A case of delayed retinopathy has been reported with loss of vision starting one year after administration of hydroxychloroquine had been discontinued.

Dermatologic Reactions: Bleaching of hair, alopecia, pruritus, skin and mucosal pigmentation, photosensitivity, and skin eruptions (urticarial, morbilliform, lichenoid, maculopapular, purpuric, erythema multiforme, erythema annulare centrifugum, Stevens-Johnson syndrome, toxic epidermal necrolysis, acute generalized exanthematous pustulosis, and exfoliative dermatitis).

Hematologic Reactions: Various blood dyscrasias such as aplastic anemia, agranulocytosis, leukopenia, anemia, thrombocytopenia (hemolysis in individuals with glucose-6-phosphate dehydrogenase (G-6-PD) deficiency).

Gastrointestinal Reactions: Anorexia, nausea, vomiting, diarrhea, and abdominal cramps. Isolated cases of abnormal liver function and fulminant hepatic failure.

Allergic Reactions: Urticaria, angioedema and bronchospasm have been reported.

Miscellaneous Reactions: Weight loss, lassitude, exacerbation or precipitation of porphyria and nonlight-sensitive psoriasis.

Cardiomyopathy has been rarely reported with high daily dosages of hydroxychloroquine.

To report SUSPECTED ADVERSE REACTIONS, contact Concordia Pharmaceuticals Inc. at 1-877-370-1142 or FDA at 1-800-FDA-1088 or *www.fda.gov/medwatch*.

Dosage and Administration

One tablet of hydroxychloroquine sulfate, 200 mg, is equivalent to 155 mg base.

Lupus erythematosus

Initially, the average *adult* dose is 400 mg (=310 mg base) once or twice daily. This may be continued for several weeks or months, depending on the response of the patient. For prolonged maintenance therapy, a smaller dose, from 200 mg to 400 mg (=155 mg to 310 mg base) daily will frequently suffice.

The incidence of retinopathy has been reported to be higher when this maintenance dose is exceeded.

Rheumatoid arthritis

The compound is cumulative in action and will require several weeks to exert its beneficial therapeutic effects, whereas minor side effects may occur relatively early. Several months of therapy may be required before maximum effects can be obtained. If objective improvement (such as reduced joint swelling, increased mobility) does not occur within six months, the drug should be discontinued. Safe use of the drug in the treatment of juvenile rheumatoid arthritis has not been established.

Initial dosage

In **adults**, from 400 mg to 600 mg (=310 mg to 465 mg base) daily, each dose to be taken with a meal or a glass of milk. In a small percentage of patients, troublesome side effects may require temporary reduction of the initial dosage. Later (usually from five to ten days), the dose may gradually be increased to the optimum response level, often without return of side effects.

Maintenance dosage

When a good response is obtained (usually in four to twelve weeks), the dosage is reduced by 50 percent and continued at a usual maintenance level of 200 mg to 400 mg (=155 mg to 310 mg base) daily, each dose to be taken with a meal or a glass of milk. The incidence of retinopathy has been reported to be higher when this maintenance dose is exceeded. Should a relapse occur after medication is withdrawn, therapy may be resumed or continued on an intermittent schedule if there are no ocular contraindications.

Corticosteroids and salicylates may be used in conjunction with this compound, and they can generally be decreased gradually in dosage or eliminated after the drug has been used for several weeks. When gradual reduction of steroid dosage is indicated, it may be done by reducing every four to five days the dose of cortisone by no more than from 5 mg to 15 mg; of hydrocortisone from 5 mg to 10 mg; of prednisolone and prednisone from 1 mg to 2.5 mg; of methylprednisolone and triamcinolone from 1 mg to 2 mg; and of dexamethasone from 0.25 mg to 0.5 mg.

HOW SUPPLIED

PLAQUENIL tablets are white, to off-white, film coated tablets imprinted "PLAQUENIL" on one face in black ink. Each tablet contains 200 mg hydroxychloroquine sulfate (equivalent to 155 mg base). Bottles of 100 tablets (NDC 59212-562-10 & 59212-562-20).

Dispense in a tight, light-resistant container as defined in the USP/NF. Keep out of the reach of children.

Store at room temperature up to 30° C (86° F).

Manufactured for:

Concordia Pharmaceuticals Inc.
St. Michael, Barbados BB11005
Revised 08/2015
©2015 Concordia Pharmaceuticals Inc. All rights reserved.
PLA_PI

Shown in Product Identification Guide, page 508

UROXATRAL® ℞
[yoo-ROX-uh-trahl]
(alfuzosin HCl)
extended-release tablets

HIGHLIGHTS OF PRESCRIBING INFORMATION
These highlights do not include all the information needed to use UROXATRAL safely and effectively. See full prescribing information for UROXATRAL.
UROXATRAL® (alfuzosin HCl) extended-release tablets
Initial U.S. Approval: 2003

---INDICATIONS AND USAGE---
UROXATRAL is an alpha adrenergic antagonist, indicated for the treatment of signs and symptoms of benign prostatic hyperplasia. (1)
Important Limitations of Use:
UROXATRAL is not indicated for treatment of hypertension. (1.1)
UROXATRAL is not indicated for use in the pediatric population. (1.1, 8.4, 12.3)

---DOSAGE AND ADMINISTRATION---
10 mg once daily with food and with the same meal each day. (2)
Tablets should not be chewed or crushed (2, 12.3)

---DOSAGE FORMS AND STRENGTHS---
Extended-release tablet: 10 mg (3)

---CONTRAINDICATIONS---
• Moderate or severe hepatic impairment (4, 8.7, 12.3)
• Co-administration with potent CYP3A4 inhibitors (e.g. ketoconazole, itraconazole, ritonavir) (4, 5.4, 7.1, 12.3)
• Known hypersensitivity (e.g., urticaria or angioedema) to alfuzosin or any of the ingredients (4, 6.2)

---WARNINGS AND PRECAUTIONS---
• Postural hypotension/syncope: Care should be taken in patients with symptomatic hypotension or who have had a hypotensive response to other medications or are concomitantly treated with antihypertensive medication or nitrates (5.1)
• Use with caution in patients with severe renal impairment (creatinine clearance <30 mL/min) (5.2, 8.6, 12.3)
• Use with caution in patients with mild hepatic impairment (5.3, 8.7, 12.3)
• Should not be used in combination with other alpha adrenergic antagonists (5.4, 7.2)
• Prostate carcinoma should be ruled out prior to treatment (5.5)
• Intraoperative Floppy Iris Syndrome (IFIS) during cataract surgery may require modifications to the surgical technique (5.6)
• Discontinue UROXATRAL if symptoms of angina pectoris appear or worsen (5.8)
• Use with caution in patients with a history of QT prolongation or who are taking medications which prolong the QT interval (5.9, 12.2)

---ADVERSE REACTIONS---
Most common adverse reactions in clinical studies (incidence ≥2% and at a higher incidence than placebo): dizziness, upper respiratory tract infection, headache, fatigue. (6.1)

To report SUSPECTED ADVERSE REACTIONS, contact Concordia Pharmaceuticals Inc. at 1-877-370-1142 or FDA at 1-800-FDA-1088 or *www.fda.gov/medwatch*.

---DRUG INTERACTIONS---
• Concomitant use of PDE5 inhibitors with alpha adrenergic antagonists, including UROXATRAL, can potentially cause symptomatic hypotension (5.4, 7.4)

See 17 for PATIENT COUNSELING INFORMATION and FDA-approved patient labeling.

Revised: 8/2015

FULL PRESCRIBING INFORMATION: CONTENTS*

FULL PRESCRIBING INFORMATION

1   INDICATIONS AND USAGE

UROXATRAL is indicated for the treatment of signs and symptoms of benign prostatic hyperplasia.

1.1   Important Limitations of Use

UROXATRAL is not indicated for the treatment of hypertension.

UROXATRAL is not indicated for use in the pediatric population.

2   DOSAGE AND ADMINISTRATION

The recommended dosage is one 10 mg UROXATRAL (alfuzosin HCl) extended-release tablet once daily. The extent of absorption of alfuzosin is 50% lower under fasting conditions. Therefore, Uroxatral should be taken with food and with the same meal each day. The tablets should not be chewed or crushed.

3   DOSAGE FORMS AND STRENGTHS

UROXATRAL (alfuzosin HCl) extended-release tablet 10 mg is available as a round, three-layer tablet: one white layer between two yellow layers, debossed with X10.

4   CONTRAINDICATIONS

UROXATRAL is contraindicated for use:

• in patients with moderate or severe hepatic impairment (Childs-Pugh categories B and C), since alfuzosin blood levels are increased in these patients *[see Use in Specific Populations (8.7) and Clinical Pharmacology (12.3)]*.

• with potent CYP3A4 inhibitors such as ketoconazole, itraconazole, and ritonavir, since alfuzosin blood levels are increased *[see Drug Interactions (7.1) and Clinical Pharmacology (12.3)]*.

• in patients with known hypersensitivity, such as urticaria and angioedema, to alfuzosin hydrochloride or any component of UROXATRAL tablets *[see Adverse Reactions (6.2)]*

5   WARNINGS AND PRECAUTIONS

5.1   Postural Hypotension

Postural hypotension with or without symptoms (e.g., dizziness) may develop within a few hours following administration of UROXATRAL. As with other alpha adrenergic antagonists, there is a potential for syncope. Patients should be warned of the possible occurrence of such events and should avoid situations where injury could result should syncope occur. There may be an increased risk of hypotension/postural hypotension and syncope when taking UROXATRAL concomitantly with anti-hypertensive medication and nitrates. Care should be taken when UROXATRAL is administered to patients with symptomatic hypotension or patients who have had a hypotensive response to other medications.

5.2   Patients with Renal Impairment

Caution should be exercised when UROXATRAL is administered in patients with severe renal impairment (*creatinine clearance < 30 mL/min*) *[see Use in Specific Populations (8.6) and Clinical Pharmacology (12.3)]*.

5.3   Patients with Hepatic Impairment

UROXATRAL is contraindicated for use in patients with moderate or severe hepatic impairment *[see Contraindica-*

Continued on next page

tions (4), Use in Specific Populations (8.7) and Clinical Pharmacology (12.3)]. Although the pharmacokinetics of UROXATRAL have not been studied in patients with mild hepatic impairment, caution should be exercised when UROXATRAL is administered to such patients *[see Use in Specific Populations (8.7) and Clinical Pharmacology (12.3)].*

5.4 Drug-Drug Interactions

Potent CYP3A4 Inhibitors: UROXATRAL is contraindicated for use with potent CYP3A4 inhibitors (e.g. ketoconazole, itraconazole, ritonavir) since alfuzosin blood levels are increased *[see Contraindications (4), Drug Interactions (7.1) and Clinical Pharmacology (12.3)].*

Other alpha adrenergic antagonists: UROXATRAL is an alpha adrenergic antagonist and should not be used in combination with other alpha adrenergic antagonist *[see Drug Interactions (7.2)].*

Phosphodiesterase-5 (PDE5) Inhibitors: PDE5-inhibitors are also vasodilators. Caution is advised for concomitant use of PDE5-inhibitors and UROXATRAL, as this combination can potentially cause symptomatic hypotension *[see Drug Interactions (7.4)].*

5.5 Prostatic Carcinoma

Carcinoma of the prostate and benign prostatic hyperplasia (BPH) cause many of the same symptoms. These two diseases frequently coexist. Therefore, patients thought to have BPH should be examined to rule out the presence of carcinoma of the prostate prior to starting treatment with UROXATRAL.

5.6 Intraoperative Floppy Iris Syndrome (IFIS)

IFIS has been observed during cataract surgery in some patients on or previously treated with alpha adrenergic antagonists. This variant of small pupil syndrome is characterized by the combination of a flaccid iris that billows in response to intraoperative irrigation currents, progressive intraoperative miosis despite preoperative dilation with standard mydriatic drugs, and potential prolapse of the iris toward the phacoemulsification incisions. The patient's ophthalmologist should be prepared for possible modifications to their surgical technique, such as the utilization of iris hooks, iris dilator rings, or viscoelastic substances.

There does not appear to be a benefit of stopping alpha adrenergic antagonist therapy prior to cataract surgery.

5.7 Priapism

Rarely (probably less than 1 in 50,000), alfuzosin, like other alpha adrenergic antagonists, has been associated with priapism (persistent painful penile erection unrelated to sexual activity). Because this condition can lead to permanent impotence if not properly treated, patients should be advised about the seriousness of the condition *[see Adverse Reactions (6.2) and Patient Counseling Information [17.3]).*

5.8 Coronary Insufficiency

If symptoms of angina pectoris should appear or worsen, UROXATRAL should be discontinued.

5.9 Patients with Congenital or Acquired QT Prolongation

Use with caution in patients with acquired or congenital QT prolongation or who are taking medications that prolong the QT interval *[see Clinical Pharmacology (12.2)].*

6 ADVERSE REACTIONS

6.1 Clinical Trials Experience

Because clinical trials are conducted under widely varying conditions, adverse reaction rates observed in the clinical trials of a drug cannot be directly compared to rates in the clinical trials of another drug and may not reflect the rates observed in clinical practice.

The incidence of adverse reactions has been ascertained from 3 placebo-controlled clinical trials involving 1,608 men where daily doses of 10 and 15 mg alfuzosin were evaluated. In these 3 trials, 473 men received UROXATRAL (alfuzosin HCl) 10 mg extended-release tablets. In these trials, 4% of patients taking UROXATRAL (alfuzosin HCl) 10 mg extended-release tablets withdrew from the trial due to adverse reactions, compared with 3% in the placebo group.

Table 1 summarizes adverse reactions that occurred in ≥2% of patients receiving UROXATRAL, and at a higher incidence than that of the placebo group. In general, the adverse reactions seen in long-term use were similar in type and frequency to the events described below for the 3-month trials.

Table 1 — Adverse Reactions Occurring in ≥2% of UROXATRAL-Treated Patients and More Frequently than with Placebo in 3-Month Placebo-Controlled Clinical Trials

Adverse Reaction	Placebo (n=678)	UROXATRAL (n=473)
Dizziness	19 (2.8%)	27 (5.7%)
Upper respiratory tract infection	4 (0.6%)	14 (3.0%)
Headache	12 (1.8%)	14 (3.0%)
Fatigue	12 (1.8%)	13 (2.7%)

The following adverse reactions, reported by between 1% and 2% of patients receiving UROXATRAL and occurring more frequently than with placebo, are listed alphabetically by body system and by decreasing frequency within body system:

Body as a whole: pain

Gastrointestinal system: abdominal pain, dyspepsia, constipation, nausea

Reproductive system: impotence

Respiratory system: bronchitis, sinusitis, pharyngitis

Signs and Symptoms of Orthostasis in Clinical Trials: The adverse reactions related to orthostasis that occurred in the double-blind phase 3 trials with alfuzosin 10 mg are summarized in Table 2. Approximately 20% to 30% of patients in these trials were taking antihypertensive medication.

Table 2— Number (%) of Patients with Symptoms Possibly Associated with Orthostasis in 3-Month Placebo-Controlled Clinical Trials

Symptoms	Placebo (n=678)	UROXATRAL (n=473)
Dizziness	19 (2.8%)	27 (5.7%)
Hypotension or postural hypotension	0	2 (0.4%)
Syncope	0	1 (0.2%)

Testing for blood pressure changes or orthostatic hypotension was conducted in three controlled studies. Decreased systolic blood pressure (≤90 mm Hg, with a decrease ≥20 mm Hg from baseline) was observed in none of the 674 placebo patients and 1 (0.2%) of the 469 UROXATRAL patients. Decreased diastolic blood pressure (≤50 mm Hg, with a decrease ≥15 mm Hg from baseline) was observed in 3 (0.4%) of the placebo patients and in 4 (0.9%) of the UROXATRAL patients. A positive orthostatic test (decrease in systolic blood pressure of ≥20 mm Hg upon standing from the supine position) was seen in 52 (7.7%) of placebo patients and in 31 (6.6%) of the UROXATRAL patients.

6.2 Post-Marketing Experience

The following adverse reactions have been identified during post approval use of UROXATRAL. Because these reactions are reported voluntarily from a population of uncertain size, it is not always possible to reliably estimate their frequency or establish a causal relationship to drug exposure.

General disorders: edema

Cardiac disorders: tachycardia, chest pain, angina pectoris in patients with pre-existing coronary artery disease, atrial fibrillation

Gastrointestinal disorders: diarrhea

Hepatobiliary disorders: hepatocellular and cholestatic liver injury (including cases with jaundice leading to drug discontinuation)

Respiratory system disorders: rhinitis

Reproductive system disorders: priapism

Skin and subcutaneous tissue disorders: rash, pruritis, urticaria, angioedema, toxic epidermal necrolysis

Vascular disorders: flushing

Blood and lymphatic system disorders: thrombocytopenia

During cataract surgery, a variant of small pupil syndrome known as Intraoperative Floppy Iris Syndrome (IFIS) has been reported in some patients on or previously treated with alpha adrenergic antagonists *[see Warnings and Precautions (5.6)].*

7 DRUG INTERACTIONS

7.1 CYP3A4 Inhibitors

UROXATRAL is contraindicated for use with potent CYP3A4 inhibitors such as ketoconazole, itraconazole, or ritonavir, since alfuzosin blood levels are increased *[see Contraindications (4), Warnings and Precautions (5.4) and Clinical Pharmacology (12.3)].*

7.2 Alpha Adrenergic Antagonists

The pharmacokinetic and pharmacodynamic interactions between UROXATRAL and other alpha adrenergic antagonists have not been determined. However, interactions may be expected, and UROXATRAL should not be used in combination with other alpha adrenergic antagonists *[see Warnings and Precautions (5.4)].*

7.3 Antihypertensive Medication and Nitrates

There may be an increased risk of hypotension/postural hypotension and syncope when taking UROXATRAL concomitantly with anti-hypertensive medication and nitrates *[see Warnings and Precautions (5.1)].*

7.4 PDE5 Inhibitors

Caution is advised when alpha adrenergic antagonists, including UROXATRAL, are co-administered with PDE5 inhibitors. Alpha adrenergic antagonists and PDE5 inhibitors are both vasodilators that can lower blood pressure. Concomitant use of these two drug classes can potentially cause symptomatic hypotension *[see Warnings and Precautions (5.4)].*

8 USE IN SPECIFIC POPULATIONS

8.1 Pregnancy

Pregnancy Category B. UROXATRAL is not indicated for use in women, and there are no studies of alfuzosin in pregnant women

Alfuzosin was not teratogenic, embryotoxic or fetotoxic in rats at plasma exposure levels (based on AUC of unbound drug) up to 1200 times (maternal oral dose of 250 mg/kg/day) the maximum recommended human dose (MRHD) of 10 mg. In rabbits administered up to 3 times the MRHD (based on body surface area) (maternal oral dose of 100 mg/kg/day) no embryofetal toxicity or teratogenicity was observed. Gestation was slightly prolonged in rats at exposure levels (based on AUC of unbound drug) approximately 12 times (greater than 5 mg/kg/day oral maternal dose) the MRHD, but difficulties with parturition were not observed.

8.4 Pediatric Use

UROXATRAL is not indicated for use in the pediatric population.

Efficacy of alfuzosin hydrochloride was not demonstrated in a randomized, double-blind, placebo-controlled, efficacy and safety trial conducted in 172 patients ages 2 to 16 years with elevated detrusor leak point pressure (LPP≥40 cm H_2O) of neurologic origin treated with alfuzosin hydrochloride using pediatric formulations. The trial included a 12-week efficacy phase followed by a 40-week safety extension period. No statistically significant difference in the proportion of patients achieving a detrusor leak point pressure of <40 cm H_20 was observed between the alfuzosin and placebo groups.

During the placebo-controlled trial, the adverse reactions reported in ≥2% of patients treated with alfuzosin and at a higher incidence than in the placebo group were: pyrexia, headache, respiratory tract infection, cough, epistaxis and diarrhea. The adverse reactions reported for the whole 12-month trial period, which included the open-label extension, were similar in type and frequency to the reactions observed during the 12-week period.

Alfuzosin hydrochloride was not studied in patients below the age of 2.

8.5 Geriatric Use

Of the total number of subjects in clinical studies of UROXATRAL, 48% were 65 years of age and over, whereas 11% were 75 and over. No overall differences in safety or effectiveness were observed between these subjects and younger subjects, but greater sensitivity of some older individuals cannot be ruled out *[see Clinical Pharmacology (12.3)]*

8.6 Renal Impairment

Systemic exposure was increased by approximately 50% in pharmacokinetic studies of patients with mild, moderate, and severe renal impairment *[see Clinical Pharmacology (12.3)].* In phase 3 studies, the safety profile of patients with mild (n=172) or moderate (n=56) renal impairment was similar to the patients with normal renal function in those studies. Safety data are available in only a limited number of patients (n=6) with creatinine clearance below 30 mL/min; therefore, caution should be exercised when UROXATRAL is administered in patients with severe renal impairment *[see Warnings and Precautions (5.2)].*

8.7 Hepatic Impairment

The pharmacokinetics of UROXATRAL have not been studied in patients with mild hepatic impairment. UROXATRAL is contraindicated for use in patients with moderate or severe hepatic impairment *[see Contraindications (4), Warnings and Precautions (5.3) and Clinical Pharmacology (12.3)].*

10   OVERDOSAGE

Should overdose of UROXATRAL lead to hypotension, support of the cardiovascular system is of first importance. Restoration of blood pressure and normalization of heart rate may be accomplished by keeping the patient in the supine position. If this measure is inadequate, then the administration of intravenous fluids should be considered. If necessary, vasopressors should then be used, and the renal function should be monitored and supported as needed. Alfuzosin is 82% to 90% protein bound; therefore, dialysis may not be of benefit.

11   DESCRIPTION

Each UROXATRAL extended-release tablet contains 10 mg alfuzosin hydrochloride as the active ingredient. Alfuzosin hydrochloride is a white to off-white crystalline powder that melts at approximately 240°C. It is freely soluble in water, sparingly soluble in alcohol, and practically insoluble in dichloromethane.

Alfuzosin hydrochloride is (R,S)-N-[3-[(4-amino-6,7-dimethoxy-2-quinazolinyl) methylamino] propyl] tetrahydro-2-furancarboxamide hydrochloride. The empirical formula of alfuzosin hydrochloride is $C_{19}H_{27}N_5O_4 \bullet HCl$. The molecular weight of alfuzosin hydrochloride is 425.9. Its structural formula is:

The tablet also contains the following inactive ingredients: colloidal silicon dioxide (NF), ethylcellulose (NF), hydrogenated castor oil (NF), hydroxypropyl methylcellulose (USP), magnesium stearate (NF), mannitol (USP), microcrystalline cellulose (NF), povidone (USP), and yellow ferric oxide (NF).

12   CLINICAL PHARMACOLOGY

12.1   Mechanism of Action

Alfuzosin is a selective antagonist of post-synaptic alpha$_1$-adrenoreceptors, which are located in the prostate, bladder base, bladder neck, prostatic capsule, and prostatic urethra.

12.2   Pharmacodynamics

Alfuzosin exhibits selectivity for alpha adrenergic receptors in the lower urinary tract. Blockade of these adrenoreceptors can cause smooth muscle in the bladder neck and prostate to relax, resulting in an improvement in urine flow and a reduction in symptoms of BPH.

Cardiac Electrophysiology

The effect of 10 mg and 40 mg alfuzosin on QT interval was evaluated in a double-blind, randomized, placebo and active-controlled (moxifloxacin 400 mg), 4-way crossover single dose study in 45 healthy white male subjects aged 19 to 45 years. The QT interval was measured at the time of peak alfuzosin plasma concentrations. The 40 mg dose of alfuzosin was chosen because this dose achieves higher blood levels than those achieved with the co-administration of UROXATRAL and ketoconazole 400 mg. Table 3 summarizes the effect on uncorrected QT and mean corrected QT interval (QTc) with different methods of correction (Fridericia, population-specific and subject-specific correction methods) at the time of peak alfuzosin plasma concentrations. No single one of these correction methodologies is known to be more valid. The mean change of heart rate associated with a 10 mg dose of alfuzosin in this study was 5.2 beats/minute and 5.8 beats/minute with 40 mg alfuzosin. The change in heart rate with moxifloxacin was 2.8 beats/minute.

[See table 3 above]

The QT effect appeared greater for 40 mg compared to 10 mg alfuzosin. The effect of the highest alfuzosin dose (four times the therapeutic dose) studied did not appear as large as that of the active control moxifloxacin at its therapeutic dose. This study, however, was not designed to make direct statistical comparisons between the drugs or the dose levels. There has been no signal of Torsade de Pointes in the extensive post-marketing experience with alfuzosin outside the United States.

A separate post-marketing QT study evaluated the effect of the co-administration of 10 mg alfuzosin with a drug of similar QT effect size. In this study, the mean placebo-subtracted QTcF increase of alfuzosin 10 mg alone was 1.9 msec (upperbound 95% CI, 5.5 msec). The concomitant administration of the two drugs showed an increased QT ef-

Table 3. Mean QT and QTc changes in msec (95% CI) from baseline at T_{max} (relative to placebo) with different methodologies to correct for effect of heart rate.

Drug/Dose	QT	Fridericia method	Population-specific method	Subject-specific method
Alfuzosin 10 mg	-5.8 (-10.2, -1.4)	4.9 (0.9, 8.8)	1.8 (-1.4, 5.0)	1.8 (-1.3, 5.0)
Alfuzosin 40 mg	-4.2 (-8.5, 0.2)	7.7 (1.9, 13.5)	4.2 (-0.6, 9.0)	4.3 (-0.5, 9.2)
Moxifloxacin *400 mg	6.9 (2.3, 11.5)	12.7 (8.6, 16.8)	11.0 (7.0, 15.0)	11.1 (7.2, 15.0)

* Active control

fect when compared with either drug alone. This QTcF increase [5.9 msec (UB 95% CI, 9.4 msec)] was not more than additive. Although this study was not designed to make direct statistical comparisons between drugs, the QT increase with both drugs given together appeared to be lower than the QTcF increase seen with the positive control moxifloxacin 400 mg [10.2 msec (UB 95% CI, 13.8 msec)]. The clinical impact of these QTc changes is unknown.

12.3   Pharmacokinetics

The pharmacokinetics of UROXATRAL have been evaluated in adult healthy male volunteers after single and/or multiple administration with daily doses ranging from 7.5 mg to 30 mg, and in patients with BPH at doses from 7.5 mg to 15 mg.

Absorption

The absolute bioavailability of UROXATRAL 10 mg tablets under fed conditions is 49%. Following multiple dosing of 10 mg UROXATRAL under fed conditions, the time to maximum concentration is 8 hours. C_{max} and AUC_{0-24} are 13.6 (SD = 5.6) ng/mL and 194 (SD = 75) ng•h/mL, respectively. UROXATRAL exhibits linear kinetics following single and multiple dosing up to 30 mg. Steady-state plasma levels are reached with the second dose of UROXATRAL administration. Steady-state alfuzosin plasma concentrations are 1.2- to 1.6-fold higher than those observed after a single administration.

Effect of Food

As illustrated in Figure 1, the extent of absorption is 50% lower under fasting conditions. Therefore, UROXATRAL should be taken with food and with the same meal each day [see Dosage and Administration (2)].

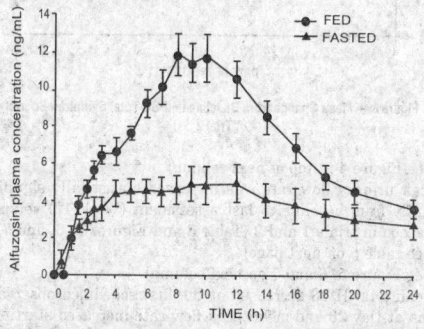

Figure 1 – Mean (SEM) Alfuzosin Plasma Concentration-Time Profiles after a Single Administration of UROXATRAL 10 mg tablets to 8 Healthy Middle-Aged Male Volunteers in Fed and Fasted States

Distribution

The volume of distribution following intravenous administration in healthy male middle-aged volunteers was 3.2 L/kg. Results of *in vitro* studies indicate that alfuzosin is moderately bound to human plasma proteins (82% to 90%), with linear binding over a wide concentration range (5 to 5,000 ng/mL).

Metabolism

Alfuzosin undergoes extensive metabolism by the liver, with only 11% of the administered dose excreted unchanged in the urine. Alfuzosin is metabolized by three metabolic pathways: oxidation, O-demethylation, and N-dealkylation. The metabolites are not pharmacologically active. CYP3A4 is the principal hepatic enzyme isoform involved in its metabolism.

Excretion

Following oral administration of ^{14}C-labeled alfuzosin solu-

tion, the recovery of radioactivity after 7 days (expressed as a percentage of the administered dose) was 69% in feces and 24% in urine. Following oral administration of UROXATRAL 10 mg tablets, the apparent elimination half-life is 10 hours.

Specific Populations

Geriatric Use: In a pharmacokinetic assessment during phase 3 clinical studies in patients with BPH, there was no relationship between peak plasma concentrations of alfuzosin and age. However, trough levels were positively correlated with age. The concentrations in subjects ≥75 years of age were approximately 35% greater than in those below 65 years of age.

Renal Impairment: The Pharmacokinetic profiles of UROXATRAL 10 mg tablets in subjects with normal renal function (CL_{CR} >80 mL/min), mild impairment (CL_{CR} 60 to 80 mL/min), moderate impairment (CL_{CR} 30 to 59 mL/min), and severe impairment (CL_{CR} <30 mL/min) were compared. These clearances were calculated by the Cockcroft-Gault formula. Relative to subjects with normal renal function, the mean C_{max} and AUC values were increased by approximately 50% in patients with mild, moderate, or severe renal impairment [see Warnings and Precautions (5.2) and Use in Specific Populations (8.6)].

Hepatic Impairment: The pharmacokinetics of UROXATRAL have not been studied in patients with mild hepatic impairment. In patients with moderate and severe hepatic insufficiency (Child-Pugh categories B and C), the plasma apparent clearance (CL/F) was reduced to approximately one-third to one-fourth that observed in healthy subjects. This reduction in clearance results in three to four-fold higher plasma concentrations of alfuzosin in these patients compared to healthy subjects. Therefore, UROXATRAL is contraindicated in patients with moderate to severe hepatic impairment [see Contraindications (4), Warnings and Precautions (5.3) and Use in Specific Populations (8.7)].

Pediatric Use: UROXATRAL tablets are not indicated for use in the pediatric population [see Indications and Usage (1.1) and Use in Specific Populations (8.4)].

Drug-Drug Interactions

Metabolic Interactions

CYP3A4 is the principal hepatic enzyme isoform involved in the metabolism of alfuzosin.

Potent CYP3A4 Inhibitors

Repeated oral administration of 400 mg/day of ketoconazole, a potent inhibitor of CYP3A4, increased alfuzosin C_{max} by 2.3-fold and AUC_{last} by 3.2-fold, following a single 10 mg dose of alfuzosin.

In another study, repeated oral administration of a lower (200 mg/day) dose of ketoconazole increased alfuzosin C_{max} by 2.1-fold and AUC_{last} by 2.5-fold, following a single 10 mg dose of alfuzosin.

Therefore, UROXATRAL is contraindicated for co-administration with potent inhibitors of CYP3A4 (e.g., ketoconazole, itraconazole, or ritonavir) because of increased alfuzosin exposure[see Contraindications (4), Warnings and Precautions (5.4) and Drug Interactions (7.1)].

Moderate CYP3A4 Inhibitors

Diltiazem: Repeated co-administration of 240 mg/day of diltiazem, a moderately-potent inhibitor of CYP3A4, with 7.5 mg/day (2.5 mg three times daily) alfuzosin (equivalent to the exposure with UROXATRAL) increased the C_{max} and AUC_{0-24} of alfuzosin 1.5- and 1.3-fold, respectively. Alfuzosin increased the C_{max} and AUC_{0-12} of diltiazem 1.4-fold. Although no changes in blood pressure were observed in this

Continued on next page

study, diltiazem is an antihypertensive medication and the combination of UROXATRAL and antihypertensive medications has the potential to cause hypotension in some patients *[see Warnings and Precautions (5.1)]*.

In human liver microsomes, at concentrations that are achieved at the therapeutic dose, alfuzosin did not inhibit CYP1A2, 2A6, 2C9, 2C19, 2D6 or 3A4 isoenzymes. In primary culture of human hepatocytes, alfuzosin did not induce CYP1A, 2A6 or 3A4 isoenzymes.

Other Interactions

Warfarin: Multiple dose administration of an immediate release tablet formulation of alfuzosin 5 mg twice daily for six days to six healthy male volunteers did not affect the pharmacological response to a single 25 mg oral dose of warfarin.

Digoxin: Repeated co-administration of UROXATRAL 10 mg tablets and digoxin 0.25 mg/day for 7 days did not influence the steady-state pharmacokinetics of either drug.

Cimetidine: Repeated administration of 1 g/day cimetidine increased both alfuzosin C_{max} and AUC values by 20%.

Atenolol: Single administration of 100 mg atenolol with a single dose of 2.5 mg of an immediate release alfuzosin tablet in eight healthy young male volunteers increased alfuzosin C_{max} and AUC values by 28% and 21%, respectively. Alfuzosin increased atenolol C_{max} and AUC values by 26% and 14%, respectively. In this study, the combination of alfuzosin with atenolol caused significant reductions in mean blood pressure and in mean heart rate. *[see Warnings and Precautions (5.1)]*.

Hydrochlorothiazide: Single administration of 25 mg hydrochlorothiazide did not modify the pharmacokinetic parameters of alfuzosin. There was no evidence of pharmacodynamic interaction between alfuzosin and hydrochlorothiazide in the 8 patients in this study.

13   NONCLINICAL TOXICOLOGY

13.1   Carcinogenesis, Mutagenesis, Impairment of Fertility

There was no evidence of a drug-related increase in the incidence of tumors in mice following dietary administration of 100 mg/kg/day alfuzosin for 98 weeks (13 and 15 times the maximum recommended human dose [MRHD] of 10 mg based on AUC of unbound drug), in females and males, respectively. The highest dose tested in female mice may not have constituted a maximally tolerated dose. Likewise, there was no evidence of a drug-related increase in the incidence of tumors in rats following dietary administration of 100 mg/kg/day alfuzosin for 104 weeks (53 and 37 times the MRHD in females and males, respectively).

Alfuzosin showed no evidence of mutagenic effect in the Ames and mouse lymphoma assays, and was free of any clastogenic effects in the Chinese hamster ovary cell and *in vivo* mouse micronucleus assays. Alfuzosin treatment did not induce DNA repair in a human cell line.

There was no evidence of reproductive organ toxicity when male rats were administered oral doses of several hundred times (250 mg/kg/day for 26 weeks) the MRHD of alfuzosin. No impairment of fertility was observed following oral (gavage) administration to male rats at doses of up to 125 mg/kg/day for 70 days. Estrous cycling was inhibited in rats and dogs at approximately 12 and 18 times the MRHD respectively (doses of 25 mg/kg and 20 mg/kg, respectively), but did not result in impaired fertility in female rats.

14   CLINICAL STUDIES

Three randomized placebo-controlled, double-blind, parallel-arm, 12-week trials were conducted with the 10 mg daily dose of alfuzosin. In these three trials, 1,608 patients [mean age 64.2 years, range 49–92 years; Caucasian (96.1%), Black (1.6%), Asian (1.1%), Other (1.2%)] were randomized and 473 patients received UROXATRAL 10 mg daily. Table 4 provides the results of the three trials that evaluated the 10 mg dose.

There were two primary efficacy variables in these three studies. The International Prostate Symptom Score (IPSS, or AUA Symptom Score) consists of seven questions that assess the severity of both irritative (frequency, urgency, nocturia) and obstructive (incomplete emptying, stopping and starting, weak stream, and pushing or straining) symptoms, with possible scores ranging from 0 to 35 with higher numerical scores on the IPSS total symptom score representing greater severity of symptoms. The second efficacy variable was peak urinary flow rate. The peak flow rate was measured just prior to the next dose in study 2 and on average at 16 hours post-dosing in trials 1 and 3.

There was a statistically significant reduction from baseline to last assessment (Week 12) in the IPSS total symptom score versus placebo in all three studies, indicating a reduction in symptom severity (Table 5 and Figures 2, 3, and 4). [See table 4 below]

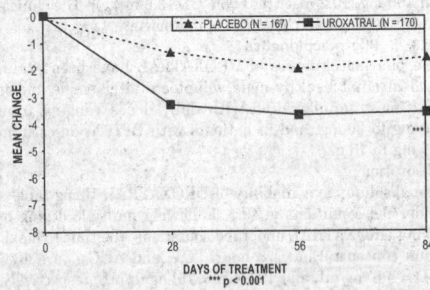

Figure 2 — Mean Change from Baseline in IPSS Total Symptom Score: Trial 1

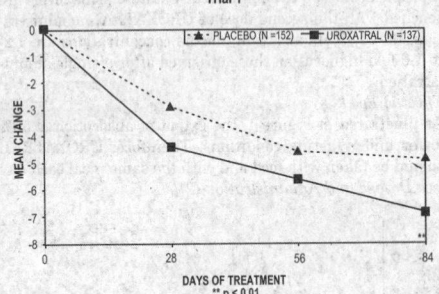

Figure 3 — Mean Change from Baseline in IPSS Total Symptom Score: Trial 2

[See Figure 4 at top of next column]

Peak urinary flow rate was increased statistically significantly from baseline to last assessment (Week 12) versus placebo in trials 1 and 2 (Table 5 and Figures 5, 6, and 7).
[See table 5 on next page]
[See Figure 5, 6 and 7 on next column]

Mean total IPSS decreased at the first scheduled observation at Day 28 and mean peak flow rate increased starting at the first scheduled observation at Day 14 in trials 2 and 3 and Day 28 in trial 1.

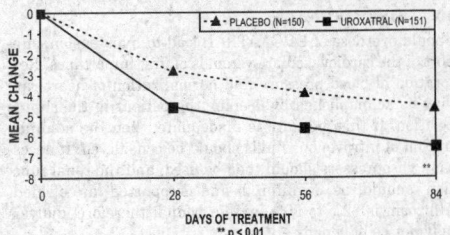

Figure 4 — Mean Change from Baseline in IPSS Total Symptom Score: Trial 3

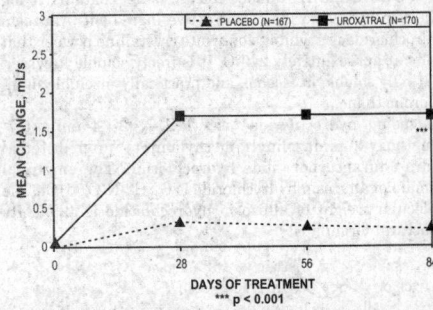

Figure 5 — Mean Change from Baseline in Peak Urine Flow Rate (mL/s): Trial 1

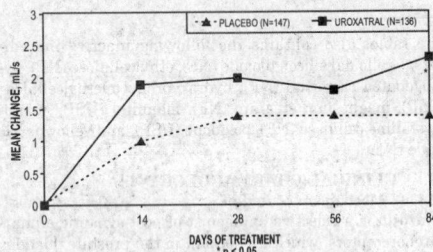

Figure 6 — Mean Change from Baseline in Peak Urine Flow Rate (mL/s): Trial 2

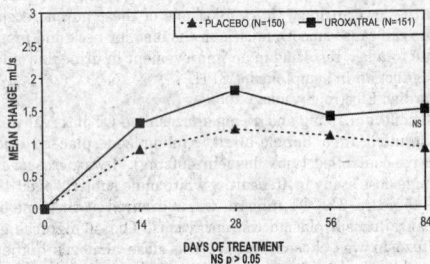

Figure 7 — Mean Change from Baseline in Peak Urine Flow Rate (mL/s): Trial 3

16   HOW SUPPLIED/STORAGE AND HANDLING

UROXATRAL is supplied as follows:

Package	NDC Number
Bottles of 100	59212-200-10 & 59212-200-20

UROXATRAL (alfuzosin HCl) extended-release tablet 10 mg is available as a round, three-layer tablet: one white layer between two yellow layers, debossed with X10.
Store at 25°C (77°F); excursions permitted to 15° to 30°C (59° to 86°F) [see USP Controlled Room Temperature]. Dispense in a tight, light-resistant container as described in the USP.
Protect from light and moisture.
Keep UROXATRAL out of reach of children.

17   PATIENT COUNSELING INFORMATION

See FDA-approved patient labeling.

17.1   Hypotension/Syncope

Patients should be told about the possible occurrence of symptoms related to postural hypotension, such as dizziness, when beginning UROXATRAL, and they should be cautioned about driving, operating machinery, or performing hazardous tasks during this period. This is important

Table 4 — Mean Change (SD) from Baseline to week 12 in International Prostate Symptom Score in Three Randomized, Controlled, Double Blind Trials

Symptom Score	Trial 1		Trial 2		Trial 3	
	Placebo (n=167)	UROXATRAL 10 mg (n=170)	Placebo (n=152)	UROXATRAL 10 mg (n=137)	Placebo (n=150)	UROXATRAL 10 mg (n=151)
Total symptom score						
Baseline	18.2 (6.4)	18.2 (6.3)	17.7 (4.1)	17.3 (3.5)	17.7 (5.0)	18.0 (5.4)
Change*	-1.6 (5.8)	-3.6 (4.8)	-4.9 (5.9)	-6.9 (4.9)	-4.6 (5.8)	-6.5 (5.2)
p-value	0.001		0.002		0.007	

* Difference between baseline and week 12.

Table 5 — Mean (SD) Change from Baseline to Week 12 in Peak Urine Flow Rate (mL/sec) in Three Randomized, Controlled, Double-Blind Trials

	Trial 1		Trial 2		Trial 3	
	Placebo (n=167)	UROXATRAL 10 mg (n=170)	Placebo (n=147)	UROXATRAL 10 mg (n=136)	Placebo (n=150)	UROXATRAL 10 mg (n=151)
Mean Peak flow rate						
Baseline	10.2 (4.0)	9.9 (3.9)	9.2 (2.0)	9.4 (1.9)	9.3 (2.6)	9.5 (3.0)
Change*	0.2 (3.5)	1.7 (4.2)	1.4 (3.2)	2.3 (3.6)	0.9 (3.0)	1.5 (3.3)
p-value	0.0004		0.03		0.22	

* Difference between baseline and week 12.

for those with low blood pressure or who are taking antihypertensive medications or nitrates *[see Warnings and Precautions (5.1)]*.

17.2   Intraoperative Floppy Iris Syndrome
Patients should be instructed to tell their ophthalmologist about their use of UROXATRAL before cataract surgery or other procedures involving the eyes, even if the patient is no longer taking UROXATRAL *[see Warnings and Precautions (5.6)]*.

17.3   Priapism
Patients should be advised about the possibility of priapism resulting from treatment with UROXATRAL and medications in the same class. Although this reaction is extremely rare, but if not brought to immediate medical attention, can lead to permanent erectile dysfunction (impotence) *[see Warnings and Precautions (5.7)]*.

17.4   Instructions of Use
UROXATRAL should be taken with food and with the same meal each day.
Patients should be advised not to crush or chew UROXATRAL tablets.
Manufactured for:
Concordia Pharmaceuticals Inc.
St. Michael, Barbados BB11005
©2015 Concordia Pharmaceuticals Inc. All rights reserved.
URO_PI

PATIENT INFORMATION
UROXATRAL®(yoo-ROX-uh-trahl)
(Alfuzosin hydrochloride extended-release tablets)
Read the Patient Information that comes with UROXATRAL before you start using it and each time you get a refill. There may be new information. This leaflet does not take the place of talking with your doctor about your condition or your treatment. You and your doctor should talk about all your medicines, including UROXATRAL, now and at your regular checkups.
What is the most important information I should know about UROXATRAL?
UROXATRAL **can cause serious side effects, including a sudden drop in blood pressure, especially when you start treatment.** This may cause you to faint, or to feel dizzy or lightheaded.
• Your risk of having this problem may be increased if you take UROXATRAL with certain other medicine that lowers blood pressure:
  ◦ medicines for high blood pressure
  ◦ a nitrate medicine for angina Ask your doctor if you are not sure if you are taking one of these medicines.
• **Do not drive, operate machinery, or do any dangerous activities until you know how UROXATRAL affects you.** This is especially important if you already have a problem with low blood pressure or take medicines to treat high blood pressure.
• If you begin to feel dizzy or lightheaded, lie down with your legs and feet up. If your symptoms do not improve call your doctor.
See the section "What are the possible side effects of UROXATRAL?" for more information about side effects.
What is UROXATRAL?
UROXATRAL is a prescription medicine that is called an "alpha-blocker". UROXATRAL is used in adult men to treat the symptoms of benign prostatic hyperplasia (BPH). UROXATRAL may help to relax the muscles in the prostate and the bladder which may lessen the symptoms of BPH and improve urine flow.

Before prescribing UROXATRAL, your doctor may examine your prostate gland and do a blood test called a prostate specific antigen (PSA) test to check for prostate cancer. Prostate cancer and BPH can cause the same symptoms. Prostate cancer needs a different treatment.
UROXATRAL is not for use in women or children.
Some medicines called "alpha-blockers" are used to treat high blood pressure. UROXATRAL is not for the treatment of high blood pressure.
Who should not take UROXATRAL?
Do not take UROXATRAL if you:
• have certain liver problems
• take antifungal medicines like ketoconazole or itraconazole (Sporanox)
• take anti-HIV medicines like ritonavir (Norvir, Kaletra)
• are allergic to alfuzosin hydrochloride or any of the ingredients in UROXATRAL.
  See the end of this leaflet for a complete list of ingredients in UROXATRAL.
Before taking UROXATRAL, tell your doctor if you:
• have liver problems
• have kidney problems
• have had low blood pressure, especially after taking another medicine. Signs of low blood pressure are fainting, dizziness, and lightheadedness.
• have a heart problem called angina
• or any family members have a rare heart condition known as congenital prolongation of the QT interval.
Tell your doctor about all the medicines you take, including prescription and non-prescription medicines, vitamins and herbal supplements. Some of your other medicines may affect the way UROXATRAL works and cause serious side effects. See "What is the most important information I should know about UROXATRAL?"
Especially tell your doctor if you take:
• another alpha blocker medicine
• a medicine to treat high blood pressure
• a medicine to treat angina
• a medicine to treat erectile dysfunction (ED)
• the antifungal medicines like ketoconazole or itraconazole (Sporanox)
• the anti-HIV medicine like, ritonavir (Norvir, Kaletra)
Ask your doctor or pharmacist if you are not sure if your medicine is one of those listed above.
What you need to know while taking UROXATRAL (alfuzosin HCl) tablets
• If you have an eye surgery for cataract (clouding of the eye) planned, tell your ophthalmologist that you are using UROXATRAL or have previously been treated with an alpha-blocker.
How do I take UROXATRAL?
• Take UROXATRAL exactly as your doctor prescribes it.
• Take UROXATRAL after the same meal each day. Do not take it on an empty stomach.
• Swallow the UROXATRAL tablet whole. Do not crush, split, or chew UROXATRAL tablets.
• If you take too much UROXATRAL call your local poison control center or emergency room right away.
What are the possible side effects of UROXATRAL?
UROXATRAL can cause serious side effects, including:
• **See "What is the most important information I should know about UROXATRAL?"**
• **A painful erection that will not go away.** UROXATRAL can cause a painful erection (priapism), which cannot be relieved by having sex. If this happens, get medical help right away. If priapism is not treated, you may not be able to get an erection in the future.

The most common side effects with UROXATRAL are:
• dizziness
• headache
• tiredness
Call your doctor if you get any side effect that bothers you. These are not all the side effects of UROXATRAL. For more information ask your doctor or pharmacist.
Call your doctor for medical advice about side effects. You may report side effects to FDA at 1-800-FDA-1088.
How do I store UROXATRAL?
• Store UROXATRAL between 59°F and 86°F (15°C and 30°C).
• Protect from light and moisture.
Keep UROXATRAL and all medicines out of the reach of children.
General information about UROXATRAL:
Medicines are sometimes prescribed for conditions that are not mentioned in patient information leaflets. Do not use UROXATRAL for a condition for which it was not prescribed. Do not give UROXATRAL to other people, even if they have the same symptoms you have. It may harm them. This leaflet summarizes the most important information about UROXATRAL. If you would like more information, talk with your doctor. You can ask your doctor or pharmacist for information about UROXATRAL that is written for health professionals.
You may also visit our website at www.concordiarx.com.
What are the ingredients of UROXATRAL?
Active Ingredient: alfuzosin hydrochloride
Inactive Ingredients: colloidal silicon dioxide (NF), ethylcellulose (NF), hydrogenated castor oil (NF), hydroxypropyl methylcellulose (USP), magnesium stearate (NF), mannitol (USP), microcrystalline cellulose (NF), povidone (USP), and yellow ferric oxide (NF).
Manufactured for:
Concordia Pharmaceuticals Inc.
St. Michael, Barbados BB11005
©2015 Concordia Pharmaceuticals Inc. All rights reserved.
URO_PI
Shown in Product Identification Guide, page 508

ZONEGRAN®   ℞
(zonisamide)
capsules, for oral administration
Rx Only

DESCRIPTION
ZONEGRAN® (zonisamide) is an antiseizure drug chemically classified as a sulfonamide and unrelated to other antiseizure agents. The active ingredient is zonisamide, 1,2-benzisoxazole-3-methanesulfonamide. The empirical formula is $C_8H_8N_2O_3S$ with a molecular weight of 212.23. Zonisamide is a white powder, pKa = 10.2, and is moderately soluble in water (0.80 mg/mL) and 0.1 N HCl (0.50 mg/mL).
The chemical structure is:

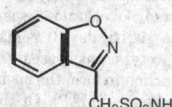

ZONEGRAN is supplied for oral administration as capsules containing 25 mg or 100 mg zonisamide.
Each 25 mg capsule contains the labeled amount of zonisamide plus the following inactive ingredients: microcrystalline cellulose, hydrogenated vegetable oil, sodium lauryl sulfate, gelatin, and titanium dioxide.
Each 100 mg capsule contains the labeled amount of zonisamide plus the following inactive ingredients: microcrystalline cellulose, hydrogenated vegetable oil, sodium lauryl sulfate, gelatin, titanium dioxide, FD&C Red No. 40 and FD&C Yellow No. 6.

CLINICAL PHARMACOLOGY
Mechanism of Action:
The precise mechanism(s) by which zonisamide exerts its antiseizure effect is unknown. Zonisamide demonstrated anticonvulsant activity in several experimental models. In animals, zonisamide was effective against tonic extension seizures induced by maximal electroshock but ineffective against clonic seizures induced by subcutaneous pentylenetetrazol. Zonisamide raised the threshold for generalized

Continued on next page

seizures in the kindled rat model and reduced the duration of cortical focal seizures induced by electrical stimulation of the visual cortex in cats. Furthermore, zonisamide suppressed both interictal spikes and the secondarily generalized seizures produced by cortical application of tungstic acid gel in rats or by cortical freezing in cats. The relevance of these models to human epilepsy is unknown.

Zonisamide may produce these effects through action at sodium and calcium channels. In vitro pharmacological studies suggest that zonisamide blocks sodium channels and reduces voltage-dependent, transient inward currents (T-type Ca^{2+} currents), consequently stabilizing neuronal membranes and suppressing neuronal hypersynchronization. In vitro binding studies have demonstrated that zonisamide binds to the GABA/benzodiazepine receptor ionophore complex in an allosteric fashion which does not produce changes in chloride flux. Other in vitro studies have demonstrated that zonisamide (10–30 µg/mL) suppresses synaptically-driven electrical activity without affecting postsynaptic GABA or glutamate responses (cultured mouse spinal cord neurons) or neuronal or glial uptake of [^{3}H]-GABA (rat hippocampal slices). Thus, zonisamide does not appear to potentiate the synaptic activity of GABA. In vivo microdialysis studies demonstrated that zonisamide facilitates both dopaminergic and serotonergic neurotransmission.

Zonisamide is a carbonic anhydrase inhibitor. The contribution of this pharmacological action to the therapeutic effects of zonisamide is unknown. However, as a carbonic anhydrase inhibitor, zonisamide may cause metabolic acidosis (see WARNINGS, Metabolic Acidosis subsection).

Pharmacokinetics:

Absorption

Following a 200–400 mg oral zonisamide dose, peak plasma concentrations (range: 2–5 µg/mL) in normal volunteers occur within 2–6 hours. In the presence of food, the time to maximum concentration is delayed, occurring at 4–6 hours, but food has no effect on the bioavailability of zonisamide. Zonisamide absorption is dose-proportional in the range of 200-400 mg. Cmax and AUC, however, increase disproportionately at 800 mg, possibly due to saturable binding of zonisamide to red blood cells. Once a stable dose is reached, steady state is achieved within 14 days.

Distribution

The apparent volume of distribution (V/F) of zonisamide is about 1.45 L/kg following a 400 mg oral dose. Zonisamide, at concentrations of 1.0–7.0 µg/mL, is approximately 40% bound to human plasma proteins. Zonisamide extensively binds to erythrocytes, resulting in an eight-fold higher concentration of zonisamide in red blood cells than in plasma. Protein binding of zonisamide is unaffected in the presence of therapeutic concentrations of phenytoin, phenobarbital or carbamazepine.

Metabolism and Elimination

Following oral administration of ^{14}C-zonisamide to healthy volunteers, only zonisamide was detected in plasma. Zonisamide is excreted primarily in urine as parent drug and as the glucuronide of a metabolite. Following multiple dosing, 62% of the radiolabeled dose was recovered in the urine, with 3% in the feces by day 10. Zonisamide undergoes acetylation by N-acetyl-transferases to form N-acetyl zonisamide and reduction to form the open ring metabolite, 2–sulfamoylacetyl phenol (SMAP). Of the excreted dose, 35% was recovered as zonisamide, 15% as N-acetyl zonisamide, and 50% as the glucuronide of SMAP. Reduction of zonisamide to SMAP is mediated by cytochrome P450 isozyme 3A4 (CYP3A4). Zonisamide does not induce its own metabolism. The plasma clearance of oral zonisamide is approximately 0.30–0.35 mL/min/kg in patients not receiving enzyme-inducing antiepilepsy drugs (AEDs). The clearance of zonisamide is increased to 0.5 mL/min/kg in patients concurrently on enzyme-inducing AEDs.

After a single-dose administration, renal clearance of zonisamide is approximately 3.5 mL/min. The clearance of an oral dose of zonisamide from red blood cells is 2 mL/min. The elimination half-life of zonisamide in plasma is approximately 63 hours. The elimination half-life of zonisamide in red blood cells is approximately 105 hours.

Specific Populations:

Renal Impairment: Single 300 mg zonisamide doses were administered to three groups of volunteers. Group 1 was a healthy group with a creatinine clearance ranging from 70–152 mL/min. Group 2 and Group 3 had creatinine clearances ranging from 14.5–59 mL/min and 10–20 mL/min, respectively. Zonisamide renal clearance decreased with

decreasing renal function (3.42, 2.50, 2.23 mL/min, respectively). Marked renal impairment (creatinine clearance < 20 mL/min) was associated with an increase in zonisamide AUC of 35% (see DOSAGE AND ADMINISTRATION section).

Hepatic Impairment: The pharmacokinetics of zonisamide in patients with impaired liver function have not been studied (see DOSAGE AND ADMINISTRATION section).

Age: The pharmacokinetics of a 300 mg single dose of zonisamide was similar in young (mean age 28 years) and elderly subjects (mean age 69 years).

Gender and Race: Information on the effect of gender and race on the pharmacokinetics of zonisamide is not available.

Effects of ZONEGRAN on cytochrome P450 enzymes

In vitro studies using human liver microsomes show insignificant (<25%) inhibition of cytochrome P450 isozymes 1A2, 2A6, 2C9, 2C19, 2D6, 2E1, 3A4, 2B6 or 2C8 at zonisamide levels approximately two-fold or greater than clinically relevant unbound serum concentrations. Therefore ZONEGRAN is not expected to affect the pharmacokinetics of other drugs via cytochrome P450-mediated mechanisms.

Potential for ZONEGRAN to affect other drugs

Anti-epileptic drugs

In epileptic patients, steady state dosing with ZONEGRAN resulted in no clinically relevant pharmacokinetic effects on carbamazepine, lamotrigine, phenytoin, or sodium valproate.

Oral contraceptives

In healthy subjects, steady state dosing with ZONEGRAN did not affect serum concentrations of ethinylestradiol or norethisterone in a combined oral contraceptive.

CYP2D6 substrates

Coadministration of multiple dosing of zonisamide up to 400 mg/day with single 50-mg doses of desipramine did not significantly affect the pharmacokinetic parameters of desipramine, a probe drug for CYP2D6 activity.

P-gp substrate

An in vitro study showed that zonisamide is a weak inhibitor of P-gp (MDR1) with an IC_{50} of 267 µmol/L. There is a theoretical potential for zonisamide to affect the pharmacokinetics of drugs which are P-gp substrates.

Caution is advised when starting or stopping ZONEGRAN or changing the ZONEGRAN dose in patients who are also receiving drugs which are P-gp substrates (e.g., digoxin, quinidine)

Potential for Medicinal Product to Affect ZONEGRAN

Concomitant medications that can induce or inhibit CYP3A4 or N-acetyl-transferases may affect the pharmacokinetics of zonisamide. Drugs which inhibit or induce glucuronide conjugation are not expected to influence the pharmacokinetics of zonisamide.

The absence of a clinically significant pharmacokinetic interaction between zonisamide and lamotrigine indicates a low potential for zonisamide to interact with substances which are metabolized by UDP-GT.

CYP3A4 Induction: Drugs that induce liver enzymes increase the metabolism and clearance of zonisamide and decrease its half-life. The half-life of zonisamide following a 400 mg dose in patients concurrently on enzyme-inducing AEDs such as phenytoin, carbamazepine, or phenobarbital was between 27-38 hours; the half-life of zonisamide in patients concurrently on the non-enzyme inducing AED, valproate, was 46 hours.

These effects are unlikely to be of clinical significance when ZONEGRAN is added to existing therapy; however, changes in zonisamide concentrations may occur if concomitant CYP3A4 inducing anti-epileptic or other drugs are withdrawn, dose adjusted or introduced, an adjustment of the ZONEGRAN dose may be required. If co-administration with a potent CYP3A4 inducer (e.g., rifampicin) is necessary, the patient should be closely monitored and the dose of ZONEGRAN and other drugs that are CYP3A4 substrate may need to be adjusted.

CYP3A4 Inhibition: Steady-state dosing of either ketoconazole (400 mg/day) or cimetidine (1200 mg/day) had no clinically relevant effects on the single dose pharmacokinetics of zonisamide given to healthy subjects. Therefore, modification of ZONEGRAN dosing is not necessary when co-administered with known CYP3A4 inhibitors.

Interactions of Zonisamide with Other Carbonic Anhydrase Inhibitors:

Concomitant use of ZONEGRAN, a carbonic anhydrase inhibitor, with any other carbonic anhydrase inhibitor (e.g., topiramate, acetazolamide or dichlorphenamide), may in-

crease the severity of metabolic acidosis and may also increase the risk of kidney stone formation. Therefore, if ZONEGRAN is given concomitantly with another carbonic anhydrase inhibitor, the patient should be monitored for the appearance or worsening of metabolic acidosis (see PRECAUTIONS, Drug Interactions subsection).

Clinical Studies:

The effectiveness of ZONEGRAN as adjunctive therapy (added to other antiepilepsy drugs) has been established in three multicenter, placebo-controlled, double blind, 3-month clinical trials (two domestic, one European) in 499 patients with refractory partial onset seizures with or without secondary generalization. Each patient had a history of at least four partial onset seizures per month in spite of receiving one or two antiepilepsy drugs at therapeutic concentrations. The 499 patients (209 women, 290 men) ranged in age from 13–68 years with a mean age of about 35 years. In the two US studies, over 80% of patients were Caucasian; 100% of patients in the European study were Caucasian. ZONEGRAN or placebo was added to the existing therapy. The primary measure of effectiveness was median percent reduction from baseline in partial seizure frequency. The secondary measure was proportion of patients achieving a 50% or greater seizure reduction from baseline (responders). The results described below are for all partial seizures in the intent-to-treat populations.

In the first study (n = 203), all patients had a 1-month baseline observation period, then received placebo or ZONEGRAN in one of two dose escalation regimens; either 1) 100 mg/day for five weeks, 200 mg/day for one week, 300 mg/day for one week, and then 400 mg/day for five weeks; or 2) 100 mg/day for one week, followed by 200 mg/day for five weeks, then 300 mg/day for one week, then 400 mg/day for five weeks. This design allowed a 100 mg vs. placebo comparison over weeks 1–5, and a 200 mg vs. placebo comparison over weeks 2–6; the primary comparison was 400 mg (both escalation groups combined) vs. placebo over weeks 8–12. The total daily dose was given as twice a day dosing. Statistically significant treatment differences favoring ZONEGRAN were seen for doses of 100, 200, and 400 mg/day.

In the second (n = 152) and third (n = 138) studies, patients had a 2–3 month baseline, then were randomly assigned to placebo or ZONEGRAN for three months. ZONEGRAN was introduced by administering 100 mg/day for the first week, 200 mg/day the second week, then 400 mg/day for two weeks, after which the dose (ZONEGRAN or placebo) could be adjusted as necessary to a maximum dose of 20 mg/kg/day or a maximum plasma level of 40 µg/mL. In the second study, the total daily dose was given as twice a day dosing; in the third study, it was given as a single daily dose. The average final maintenance doses received in the studies were 530 and 430 mg/day in the second and third studies, respectively. Both studies demonstrated statistically significant differences favoring ZONEGRAN for doses of 400–600 mg/day, and there was no apparent difference between once daily and twice daily dosing (in different studies). Analysis of the data (first 4 weeks) during titration demonstrated statistically significant differences favoring ZONEGRAN at doses between 100 and 400 mg/day. The primary comparison in both trials was for any dose over Weeks 5–12.

[See table 1 on next page]

[See table 2 on next page]

Figure 1 presents the proportion of patients (X-axis) whose percentage reduction from baseline in the all partial seizure rate was at least as great as that indicated on the Y-axis in the second and third placebo-controlled trials. A positive value on the Y-axis indicates an improvement from baseline (i.e., a decrease in seizure rate), while a negative value indicates a worsening from baseline (i.e., an increase in seizure rate). Thus, in a display of this type, the curve for an effective treatment is shifted to the left of the curve for placebo. The proportion of patients achieving any particular level of reduction in seizure rate was consistently higher for the ZONEGRAN groups compared to the placebo groups. For example, Figure 1 indicates that approximately 27% of patients treated with ZONEGRAN experienced a 75% or greater reduction, compared to approximately 12% in the placebo groups.

[See Figure 1 in next column]

No differences in efficacy based on age, sex or race, as measured by a change in seizure frequency from baseline, were detected.

INDICATIONS AND USAGE

ZONEGRAN is indicated as adjunctive therapy in the treatment of partial seizures in adults with epilepsy.

Table 1. Median % Reduction in All Partial Seizures and % Responders in Primary Efficacy Analyses: Intent-To-Treat Analysis

Study	Median % reduction in partial seizures		% Responders	
	ZONEGRAN	Placebo	ZONEGRAN	Placebo
Study 1: Weeks 8-12:	n=98 40.5%*	n=72 9.0%	n=98 41.8%*	n=72 22.2%
Study 2: Weeks 5-12:	n=69 29.6%*	n=72 -3.2%	n=69 29.0%	n=72 15.0%
Study 3: Weeks 5-12:	n=67 27.2%*	n=66 -1.1%	n=67 28.0%*	n=66 12.0%

* p<0.05 compared to placebo

Table 2. Median % Reduction in All Partial Seizures and % Responders for Dose Analyses in Study 1: Intent-To-Treat Analysis

Dose Group	Median % reduction in partial seizures		% Responders	
	ZONEGRAN	Placebo	ZONEGRAN	Placebo
100-400 mg/day: Weeks 1-12:	n=112 32.3%*	n=83 5.6%	n=112 32.1%*	n=83 9.6%
100 mg/day: Weeks 1-5:	n=56 24.7%*	n=80 8.3%	n=56 25.0%*	n=80 11.3%
200 mg/day: Weeks 2-6:	n=55 20.4%*	n=82 4.0%	n=55 25.5%*	n=82 9.8%

* p<0.05 compared to placebo

Figure 1 Proportion of Patients Achieving Differing Levels of Seizure Reduction in ZONEGRAN and Placebo Groups in Studies 2 and 3

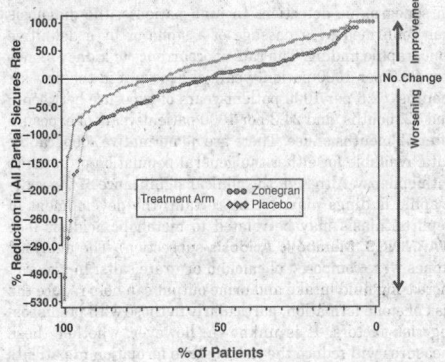

CONTRAINDICATIONS

ZONEGRAN is contraindicated in patients who have demonstrated hypersensitivity to sulfonamides or zonisamide.

WARNINGS

Potentially Fatal Reactions to Sulfonamides: Fatalities have occurred, although rarely, as a result of severe reactions to sulfonamides (zonisamide is a sulfonamide) including Stevens-Johnson syndrome, toxic epidermal necrolysis, fulminant hepatic necrosis, agranulocytosis, aplastic anemia, and other blood dyscrasias. Such reactions may occur when a sulfonamide is readministered irrespective of the route of administration. If signs of hypersensitivity or other serious reactions occur, discontinue zonisamide immediately. Specific experience with sulfonamide-type adverse reaction to zonisamide is described below.

Serious Skin Reactions: Consideration should be given to discontinuing ZONEGRAN in patients who develop an otherwise unexplained rash. If the drug is not discontinued, patients should be observed frequently. Seven deaths from severe rash [i.e. Stevens-Johnson syndrome (SJS) and toxic epidermal necrolysis (TEN)] were reported in the first 11 years of marketing in Japan. All of the patients were receiving other drugs in addition to zonisamide. In postmarketing experience from Japan, a total of 49 cases of SJS or TEN have been reported, a reporting rate of 46 per million patient-years of exposure. Although this rate is greater than background, it is probably an underestimate of the true incidence because of under-reporting. There were no confirmed cases of SJS or TEN in the US, European, or Japanese development programs.

In the US and European randomized controlled trials, 6 of 269 (2.2%) zonisamide patients discontinued treatment because of rash compared to none on placebo. Across all trials during the US and European development, rash that led to discontinuation of zonisamide was reported in 1.4% of patients (12.0 events per 1000 patient-years of exposure). During Japanese development, serious rash or rash that led to study drug discontinuation was reported in 2.0% of patients (27.8 events per 1000 patient-years). Rash usually occurred early in treatment, with 85% reported within 16 weeks in the US and European studies and 90% reported within two weeks in the Japanese studies. There was no apparent relationship of dose to the occurrence of rash.

Serious Hematologic Events: Two confirmed cases of aplastic anemia and one confirmed case of agranulocytosis were reported in the first 11 years of marketing in Japan, rates greater than generally accepted background rates. There were no cases of aplastic anemia and two confirmed cases of agranulocytosis in the US, European, or Japanese development programs. There is inadequate information to assess the relationship, if any, between dose and duration of treatment and these events.

Drug Reaction with Eosinophilia and Systemic Symptoms (DRESS)/Multi-Organ Hypersensitivity: Drug Reaction with Eosinophilia and Systemic Symptoms (DRESS), also known as multi-organ hypersensitivity, has occurred with ZONEGRAN. Some of these events have been fatal or life-threatening. DRESS typically, although not exclusively, presents with fever, rash, lymphadenopathy and/or facial swelling, in association with other organ system involvement, such as hepatitis, nephritis, hematologic abnormalities, myocarditis, or myositis, sometimes resembling an acute viral infection. Eosinophilia is often present. This disorder is variable in its expression, and other organ systems not noted here may be involved. It is important to note that early manifestations of hypersensitivity (e.g., fever, lymphadenopathy) may be present even though rash is not evident. If such signs or symptoms are present, the patient should be evaluated immediately. ZONEGRAN should be discontinued if an alternative etiology for the signs or symptoms cannot be established.

Oligohidrosis and Hyperthermia in Pediatric Patients: Oligohidrosis, sometimes resulting in heat stroke and hospitalization, is seen in association with zonisamide in pediatric patients.

During the pre-approval development program in Japan, one case of oligohidrosis was reported in 403 pediatric patients, an incidence of 1 case per 285 patient-years of exposure. While there were no cases reported in the US or European development programs, fewer than 100 pediatric patients participated in these trials.

In the first 11 years of marketing in Japan, 38 cases were reported, an estimated reporting rate of about 1 case per 10,000 patient-years of exposure. In the first year of marketing in the US, 2 cases were reported, an estimated reporting rate of about 12 cases per 10,000 patient-years of exposure. These rates are underestimates of the true incidence because of under-reporting. There has also been one report of heat stroke in an 18-year-old patient in the US. Decreased sweating and an elevation in body temperature above normal characterized these cases. Many cases were reported after exposure to elevated environmental temperatures. Heat stroke, requiring hospitalization, was diagnosed in some cases. There have been no reported deaths.

Pediatric patients appear to be at an increased risk for zonisamide-associated oligohidrosis and hyperthermia. Patients, especially pediatric patients, treated with ZONEGRAN should be monitored closely for evidence of decreased sweating and increased body temperature, especially in warm or hot weather. Caution should be used when zonisamide is prescribed with other drugs that predispose patients to heat-related disorders; these drugs include, but are not limited to, carbonic anhydrase inhibitors and drugs with anticholinergic activity.

The practitioner should be aware that the safety and effectiveness of zonisamide in pediatric patients have not been established, and that zonisamide is not approved for use in pediatric patients.

Suicidal Behavior and Ideation

Antiepileptic drugs (AEDs), including ZONEGRAN, increase the risk of suicidal thoughts or behavior in patients taking these drugs for any indication. Patients treated with any AED for any indication should be monitored for the emergence or worsening of depression, suicidal thoughts or behavior, and/or any unusual changes in mood or behavior. Pooled analyses of 199 placebo-controlled clinical trials (mono- and adjunctive therapy) of 11 different AEDs showed that patients randomized to one of the AEDs had approximately twice the risk (adjusted Relative Risk 1.8, 95% CI: 1.2, 2.7) of suicidal thinking or behavior compared to patients randomized to placebo. In these trials, which had a median treatment duration of 12 weeks, the estimated incidence rate of suicidal behavior or ideation among 27,863 AED-treated patients was 0.43%, compared to 0.24% among 16,029 placebo-treated patients, representing an increase of approximately one case of suicidal thinking or behavior for every 530 patients treated. There were four suicides in drug-treated patients in the trials and none in placebo-treated patients, but the number is too small to allow any conclusion about drug effect on suicide.

The increased risk of suicidal thoughts or behavior with AEDs was observed as early as one week after starting drug treatment with AEDs and persisted for the duration of treatment assessed. Because most trials included in the analysis did not extend beyond 24 weeks, the risk of suicidal thoughts or behavior beyond 24 weeks could not be assessed.

The risk of suicidal thoughts or behavior was generally consistent among drugs in the data analyzed. The finding of increased risk with AEDs of varying mechanisms of action and across a range of indications suggests that the risk applies to all AEDs used for any indication. The risk did not vary substantially by age (5-100 years) in the clinical trials analyzed.

Continued on next page

Table 3 shows absolute and relative risk by indication for all evaluated AEDs.

Table 3. Risk by Indication for Antiepileptic Drugs in the Pooled Analysis

Indication	Placebo Patients with Events Per 1000 Patients	Drug Patients with Events Per 1000 Patients	Relative Risk: Incidence of Events in Drug Patients/Incidence in Placebo Patients	Risk Difference: Additional Drug Patients with Events Per 1000 Patients
Epilepsy	1.0	3.4	3.5	2.4
Psychiatric	5.7	8.5	1.5	2.9
Other	1.0	1.8	1.9	0.9
Total	2.4	4.3	1.8	1.9

The relative risk for suicidal thoughts or behavior was higher in clinical trials for epilepsy than in clinical trials for psychiatric or other conditions, but the absolute risk differences were similar for the epilepsy and psychiatric indications.

Anyone considering prescribing ZONEGRAN or any other AED must balance the risk of suicidal thoughts or behavior with the risk of untreated illness. Epilepsy and many other illnesses for which AEDs are prescribed are themselves associated with morbidity and mortality and an increased risk of suicidal thoughts and behavior. Should suicidal thoughts and behavior emerge during treatment, the prescriber needs to consider whether the emergence of these symptoms in any given patient may be related to the illness being treated.

Patients, their caregivers, and families should be informed that AEDs increase the risk of suicidal thoughts and behavior and should be advised of the need to be alert for the emergence or worsening of the signs and symptoms of depression, any unusual changes in mood or behavior, or the emergence of suicidal thoughts, behavior, or thoughts about self-harm. Behaviors of concern should be reported immediately to healthcare providers (see **WARNINGS, Cognitive/ Neuropsychiatric Adverse Events** subsection below).

Metabolic Acidosis:

Zonisamide causes hyperchloremic, non-anion gap, metabolic acidosis (i.e., decreased serum bicarbonate below the normal reference range in the absence of chronic respiratory alkalosis) (see **PRECAUTIONS, Laboratory Tests** subsection). This metabolic acidosis is caused by renal bicarbonate loss due to the inhibitory effect of zonisamide on carbonic anhydrase. Generally, zonisamide-induced metabolic acidosis occurs early in treatment, but it can develop at any time during treatment. Metabolic acidosis generally appears to be dose-dependent and can occur at doses as low as 25 mg daily.

Conditions or therapies that predispose to acidosis (such as renal disease, severe respiratory disorders, status epilepticus, diarrhea, ketogenic diet, or specific drugs) may be additive to the bicarbonate lowering effects of zonisamide.

Some manifestations of acute or chronic metabolic acidosis include hyperventilation, nonspecific symptoms such as fatigue and anorexia, or more severe sequelae including cardiac arrhythmias or stupor. Chronic, untreated, metabolic acidosis may increase the risk for nephrolithiasis or nephrocalcinosis. Nephrolithiasis has been observed in the clinical development program in 4% of adults treated with ZONEGRAN, has also been detected by renal ultrasound in 8% of pediatric treated patients who had at least one ultrasound prospectively collected, and was reported as an adverse event in 3% (4/133) of pediatric patients (see **PRECAUTIONS, Kidney Stones** subsection).

Chronic, untreated metabolic acidosis may result in osteomalacia (referred to as rickets in pediatric patients) and/or osteoporosis with an increased risk for fracture. Of potential relevance, zonisamide treatment was associated with reductions in serum phosphorus and increases in serum alkaline phosphatase, changes that may be related to metabolic acidosis and osteomalacia (see **PRECAUTIONS, Laboratory Tests** subsection).

Chronic, untreated metabolic acidosis in pediatric patients may reduce growth rates. A reduction in growth rate may eventually decrease the maximal height achieved. The effect of zonisamide on growth and bone-related sequelae has not been systematically investigated.

Measurement of baseline and periodic serum bicarbonate during treatment is recommended. If metabolic acidosis develops and persists, consideration should be given to reducing the dose or discontinuing zonisamide (using dose tapering). If the decision is made to continue patients on zonisamide in the face of persistent acidosis, alkali treatment should be considered.

Serum bicarbonate was not measured in the adjunctive controlled trials of adults with epilepsy. However, serum bicarbonate was studied in three clinical trials for indications which have not been approved: a placebo-controlled trial for migraine prophylaxis in adults, a controlled trial for monotherapy in epilepsy in adults, and an open label trial for adjunctive treatment of epilepsy in pediatric patients (3-16 years). In adults, mean serum bicarbonate reductions ranged from approximately 2 mEq/L at daily doses of 100 mg to nearly 4 mEq/L at daily doses of 300 mg. In pediatric patients, mean serum bicarbonate reductions ranged from approximately 2 mEq/L at daily doses from above 100 mg up to 300 mg, to nearly 4 mEq/L at daily doses from above 400 mg up to 600 mg.

In two controlled studies in adults, the incidence of a persistent treatment-emergent decrease in serum bicarbonate to less than 20 mEq/L (observed at 2 or more consecutive visits or the final visit) was dose-related at relatively low zonisamide doses. In the monotherapy trial of epilepsy, the incidence of a persistent treatment-emergent decrease in serum bicarbonate was 21% for daily zonisamide doses of 25 mg or 100 mg, and was 43% at a daily dose of 300 mg. In a placebo-controlled trial for prophylaxis of migraine, the incidence of a persistent treatment-emergent decrease in serum bicarbonate was 7% for placebo, 29% for 150 mg daily, and 34% for 300 mg daily. The incidence of persistent markedly abnormally low serum bicarbonate (decrease to less than 17 mEq/L and more than 5 mEq/L from a pretreatment value of at least 20 mEq/L) in these controlled trials was 2% or less.

In the pediatric study, the incidence of persistent, treatment-emergent decreases in serum bicarbonate to levels less than 20 mEq/L was 52% at doses up to 100 mg daily, was 90% for a wide range of doses up to 600 mg daily, and generally appeared to increase with higher doses. The incidence of a persistent markedly abnormally low serum bicarbonate value was 4% at doses up to 100 mg daily, was 18% for a wide range of doses up to 600 mg daily, and generally appeared to increase with higher doses. Some patients experienced moderately severe serum bicarbonate decrements down to a level as low as 10 mEq/L.

The relatively high frequencies of varying severities of metabolic acidosis observed in this study of pediatric patients (compared to the frequency and severity observed in various clinical trial development programs in adults) suggest that pediatric patients may be more likely to develop metabolic acidosis than adults.

Seizures on Withdrawal:

As with other AEDs, abrupt withdrawal of ZONEGRAN in patients with epilepsy may precipitate increased seizure frequency or status epilepticus. Dose reduction or discontinuation of zonisamide should be done gradually.

Teratogenicity:

Women of child bearing potential who are given zonisamide should be advised to use effective contraception. Zonisamide was teratogenic in mice, rats, and dogs and embryolethal in monkeys when administered during the period of organogenesis. A variety of fetal abnormalities, including cardiovascular defects, and embryo-fetal deaths occurred at maternal plasma levels similar to or lower than therapeutic levels in humans. These findings suggest that the use of ZONEGRAN during pregnancy in humans may present a significant risk to the fetus (see **PRECAUTIONS, Pregnancy** subsection). Zonisamide should be used during pregnancy only if the potential benefit justifies the potential risk to the fetus.

Cognitive/Neuropsychiatric Adverse Events:

Use of ZONEGRAN was frequently associated with central nervous system-related adverse events. The most significant of these can be classified into three general categories: 1) psychiatric symptoms, including depression and psychosis, 2) psychomotor slowing, difficulty with concentration, and speech or language problems, in particular, word-finding difficulties, and 3) somnolence or fatigue.

In placebo-controlled trials, 2.2% of patients discontinued ZONEGRAN or were hospitalized for depression compared to 0.4% of placebo patients. Among all epilepsy patients treated with ZONEGRAN, 1.4% were discontinued and

1.0% were hospitalized because of reported depression or suicide attempts. In placebo-controlled trials, 2.2% of patients discontinued ZONEGRAN or were hospitalized due to psychosis or psychosis-related symptoms compared to none of the placebo patients. Among all epilepsy patients treated with ZONEGRAN, 0.9% were discontinued and 1.4% were hospitalized because of reported psychosis or related symptoms.

Psychomotor slowing and difficulty with concentration occurred in the first month of treatment and were associated with doses above 300 mg/day. Speech and language problems tended to occur after 6–10 weeks of treatment and at doses above 300 mg/day. Although in most cases these events were of mild to moderate severity, they at times led to withdrawal from treatment.

Somnolence and fatigue were frequently reported CNS adverse events during clinical trials with ZONEGRAN. Although in most cases these events were of mild to moderate severity, they led to withdrawal from treatment in 0.2% of the patients enrolled in controlled trials. Somnolence and fatigue tended to occur within the first month of treatment. Somnolence and fatigue occurred most frequently at doses of 300–500 mg/day. **Patients should be cautioned about this possibility and special care should be taken by patients if they drive, operate machinery, or perform any hazardous task.**

PRECAUTIONS

General:

Somnolence is commonly reported, especially at higher doses of ZONEGRAN (see **WARNINGS: Cognitive/ Neuropsychiatric Adverse Events** subsection). Zonisamide is metabolized by the liver and eliminated by the kidneys; caution should therefore be exercised when administering ZONEGRAN to patients with hepatic and renal dysfunction (see **CLINICAL PHARMACOLOGY, Specific Populations** subsection).

Kidney Stones:

Among 991 patients treated during the development of ZONEGRAN, 40 patients (4.0%) with epilepsy receiving ZONEGRAN developed clinically possible or confirmed kidney stones (e.g., clinical symptomatology, sonography, etc.), a rate of 34 per 1000 patient-years of exposure (40 patients with 1168 years of exposure). Of these, 12 were symptomatic, and 28 were described as possible kidney stones based on sonographic detection. In nine patients, the diagnosis was confirmed by a passage of a stone or by a definitive sonographic finding. The rate of occurrence of kidney stones was 28.7 per 1000 patient-years of exposure in the first six months, 62.6 per 1000 patient-years of exposure between 6 and 12 months, and 24.3 per 1000 patient-years of exposure after 12 months of use. There are no normative sonographic data available for either the general population or patients with epilepsy. Although the clinical significance of the sonographic findings may not be certain, the development of nephrolithiasis may be related to metabolic acidosis (see **WARNINGS, Metabolic Acidosis** subsection). The analyzed stones were composed of calcium or urate salts. In general, increasing fluid intake and urine output can help reduce the risk of stone formation, particularly in those with predisposing risk factors. It is unknown, however, whether these measures will reduce the risk of stone formation in patients treated with ZONEGRAN.

Although not approved in pediatric patients, sonographic findings consistent with nephrolithiasis were also detected in 8% of a subset of ZONEGRAN treated pediatric patients who had at least one renal ultrasound prospectively performed in a clinical development program investigating open-label treatment. The incidence of kidney stone as an adverse event was 3% (see **WARNINGS, Metabolic Acidosis** subsection).

Effect on Renal Function:

In several clinical studies, zonisamide was associated with a statistically significant 8% mean increase from baseline of serum creatinine and blood urea nitrogen (BUN) compared to essentially no change in the placebo patients. The increase appeared to persist over time but was not progressive; this has been interpreted as an effect on glomerular filtration rate (GFR). There were no episodes of unexplained acute renal failure in clinical development in the US, Europe, or Japan. The decrease in GFR appeared within the first 4 weeks of treatment. In a 30-day study, the GFR returned to baseline within 2–3 weeks of drug discontinuation. There is no information about reversibility, after drug discontinuation, of the effects on GFR after long-term use.

ZONEGRAN should be discontinued in patients who develop acute renal failure or a clinically significant sustained increase in the creatinine/BUN concentration. ZONEGRAN should not be used in patients with renal failure (estimated GFR < 50 mL/min) as there has been insufficient experience concerning drug dosing and toxicity.

Status Epilepticus:
Estimates of the incidence of treatment emergent status epilepticus in ZONEGRAN treated patients are difficult because a standard definition was not employed. Nonetheless, in controlled trials, 1.1% of patients treated with ZONEGRAN had an event labeled as status epilepticus compared to none of the patients treated with placebo. Among patients treated with ZONEGRAN across all epilepsy studies (controlled and uncontrolled), 1.0% of patients had an event reported as status epilepticus.

Information for Patients:
Patients should be informed of the availability of a Medication Guide, and they should be instructed to read the Medication Guide prior to taking ZONEGRAN. Patients should be instructed to take ZONEGRAN only as prescribed.
Patients should be advised as follows: (See Medication Guide)

1. **ZONEGRAN may produce drowsiness, especially at higher doses. Patients should be advised not to drive a car or operate other complex machinery until they have gained experience on ZONEGRAN sufficient to determine whether it affects their performance. Because of the potential of zonisamide to cause CNS depression, as well as other cognitive and/or neuropsychiatric adverse events, zonisamide should be used with caution if used in combination with alcohol or other CNS depressants.**
2. Patients should contact their physician immediately if a skin rash develops or seizures worsen.
3. Patients should contact their physician immediately if they develop signs or symptoms, such as sudden back pain, abdominal pain, and/or blood in the urine that could indicate a kidney stone. Increasing fluid intake and urine output may reduce the risk of stone formation, particularly in those with predisposing risk factors for stones.
4. Patients should contact their physician immediately if a child has been taking ZONEGRAN and is not sweating as usual with or without a fever.
5. Because zonisamide can cause hematological complications, patients should contact their physician immediately if they develop a fever, sore throat, oral ulcers, or easy bruising.
6. **Suicidal Thinking and Behavior** - Patients, their caregivers, and families should be counseled that AEDs, including ZONEGRAN, may increase the risk of suicidal thoughts and behavior and should be advised of the need to be alert for the emergence or worsening of symptoms of depression, any unusual changes in mood or behavior, or the emergence of suicidal thoughts, behavior, or thoughts about self-harm. Behaviors of concern should be reported immediately to healthcare providers.
7. Patients should contact their physician immediately if they develop fast breathing, fatigue/tiredness, loss of appetite, or irregular heart beat or palpitations (possible manifestations of metabolic acidosis).
8. As with other AEDs, patients should contact their physician if they intend to become pregnant or are pregnant during ZONEGRAN therapy. Patients should notify their physician if they intend to breast-feed or are breast-feeding an infant.
   Patients should be encouraged to enroll in the North American Antiepileptic Drug (NAAED) Pregnancy Registry if they become pregnant. This registry is collecting information about the safety of antiepileptic drugs during pregnancy. To enroll, patients can call the toll free number 1-888-233-2334 (see **PRECAUTIONS, Pregnancy** subsection).

Laboratory Tests:
In several clinical studies, zonisamide was associated with a mean increase in the concentration of serum creatinine and blood urea nitrogen (BUN) of approximately 8% over the baseline measurement. Consideration should be given to monitoring renal function periodically (see **PRECAUTIONS, Effect on Renal Function** subsection).
Zonisamide increases serum chloride and alkaline phosphatase and decreases serum bicarbonate (see **WARNINGS, Metabolic Acidosis** subsection), phosphorus, calcium, and albumin.
Drug Interactions with CNS Depressants: Concomitant administration of ZONEGRAN and alcohol or other CNS depressant drugs has not been evaluated in clinical studies. Because of the potential of zonisamide to cause CNS depression, as well as other cognitive and/or neuropsychiatric ad-

verse events, zonisamide should be used with caution if used in combination with alcohol or other CNS depressants.
Other Carbonic Anhydrase Inhibitors: Concomitant use of ZONEGRAN, a carbonic anhydrase inhibitor, with any other carbonic anhydrase inhibitor (e.g., topiramate, acetazolamide or dichlorphenamide), may increase the severity of metabolic acidosis and may also increase the risk of kidney stone formation. Therefore, if ZONEGRAN is given concomitantly with another carbonic anhydrase inhibitor, the patient should be monitored for the appearance or worsening of metabolic acidosis (see **CLINICAL PHARMACOLOGY, Interactions of Zonisamide with Other Carbonic Anhydrase Inhibitors** subsection).

Carcinogenicity, Mutagenesis, Impairment of Fertility:
No evidence of carcinogenicity was found in mice or rats following dietary administration of zonisamide for two years at doses of up to 80 mg/kg/day. In mice, this dose is approximately equivalent to the maximum recommended human dose (MRHD) of 400 mg/day on a mg/m² basis. In rats, this dose is 1–2 times the MRHD on a mg/m² basis.
Zonisamide was mutagenic in an in vitro chromosomal aberration assay in CHL cells. Zonisamide was not mutagenic or clastogenic in other in vitro assays (Ames, mouse lymphoma tk assay, chromosomal aberration in human lymphocytes) or in the in vivo rat bone marrow cytogenetics assay. Rats treated with zonisamide (20, 60, or 200 mg/kg) before mating and during the initial gestation phase showed signs of reproductive toxicity (decreased corpora lutea, implantations, and live fetuses) at all doses. The low dose in this study is approximately 0.5 times the maximum recommended human dose (MRHD) on a mg/m² basis.
Pregnancy: (see **WARNINGS, Teratogenicity** subsection):
Zonisamide may cause serious adverse fetal effects, based on clinical and nonclinical data. Zonisamide was teratogenic in multiple animal species.
Zonisamide treatment causes metabolic acidosis in humans. The effect of zonisamide-induced metabolic acidosis has not been studied in pregnancy; however, metabolic acidosis in pregnancy (due to other causes) may be associated with decreased fetal growth, decreased fetal oxygenation, and fetal death, and may affect the fetus's ability to tolerate labor. Pregnant patients should be monitored for metabolic acidosis and treated as in the non-pregnant state. (See **WARNINGS, Metabolic Acidosis** subsection.)
Newborns of mothers treated with zonisamide should be monitored for metabolic acidosis because of transfer of zonisamide to the fetus and possible occurrence of transient metabolic acidosis following birth. Transient metabolic acidosis has been reported in neonates born to mothers treated during pregnancy with a different carbonic anhydrase inhibitor.
Zonisamide was teratogenic in mice, rats, and dogs and embryolethal in monkeys when administered during the period of organogenesis. Fetal abnormalities or embryo-fetal deaths occurred in these species at zonisamide dosage and maternal plasma levels similar to or lower than therapeutic levels in humans, indicating that use of this drug in pregnancy entails a significant risk to the fetus. A variety of external, visceral, and skeletal malformations was produced in animals by prenatal exposure to zonisamide. Cardiovascular defects were prominent in both rats and dogs.
Following administration of zonisamide (10, 30, or 60 mg/kg/day) to pregnant dogs during organogenesis, increased incidences of fetal cardiovascular malformations (ventricular septal defects, cardiomegaly, various valvular and arterial anomalies) were found at doses of 30 mg/kg/day or greater. The low effect dose for malformations produced peak maternal plasma zonisamide levels (25 µg/mL) about 0.5 times the highest plasma levels measured in patients receiving the maximum recommended human dose (MRHD) of 400 mg/day. In dogs, cardiovascular malformations were found in approximately 50% of all fetuses exposed to the high dose, which was associated with maternal plasma levels (44 µg/mL) approximately equal to the highest levels measured in humans receiving the MRHD. Incidences of skeletal malformations were also increased at the high dose, and fetal growth retardation and increased frequencies of skeletal variations were seen at all doses in this study. The low dose produced maternal plasma levels (12 µg/mL) about 0.25 times the highest human levels.
In cynomolgus monkeys, administration of zonisamide (10 or 20 mg/kg/day) to pregnant animals during organogenesis resulted in embryo-fetal deaths at both doses. The possibility that these deaths were due to malformations cannot be ruled out. The lowest embryolethal dose in monkeys was as-

sociated with peak maternal plasma zonisamide levels (5 µg/mL) approximately 0.1 times the highest levels measured in patients at the MRHD.
In a mouse embryo-fetal development study, treatment of pregnant animals with zonisamide (125, 250, or 500 mg/kg/day) during the period of organogenesis resulted in increased incidences of fetal malformations (skeletal and/or craniofacial defects) at all doses tested. The low dose in this study is approximately 1.5 times the MRHD on a mg/m² basis. In rats, increased frequencies of malformations (cardiovascular defects) and variations (persistent cords of thymic tissue, decreased skeletal ossification) were observed among the offspring of dams treated with zonisamide (20, 60, or 200 mg/kg/day) throughout organogenesis at all doses. The low effect dose is approximately 0.5 times the MRHD on a mg/m² basis.
Perinatal death was increased among the offspring of rats treated with zonisamide (10, 30, or 60 mg/kg/day) from the latter part of gestation up to weaning at the high dose, or approximately 1.4 times the MRHD on a mg/m² basis. The no effect level of 30 mg/kg/day is approximately 0.7 times the MRHD on a mg/m² basis.
There are no adequate and well-controlled studies in pregnant women. ZONEGRAN should be used during pregnancy only if the potential benefit justifies the potential risk to the fetus.
To provide information regarding the effects of in utero exposure to ZONEGRAN, physicians are advised to recommend that pregnant patients taking ZONEGRAN enroll in the NAAED Pregnancy Registry. This can be done by calling the toll free number 1-888-233-2334, and must be done by patients themselves. Information on the registry can also be found at the website http://www.aedpregnancyregistry.org/.
Labor and Delivery:
The effects of ZONEGRAN on labor and delivery in humans are unknown.
Use in Nursing Mothers:
Zonisamide is excreted in human milk. Because of the potential for serious adverse reactions in nursing infants from ZONEGRAN, a decision should be made whether to discontinue nursing or to discontinue drug, taking into account the importance of the drug to the mother.
Pediatric Use:
The safety and effectiveness of ZONEGRAN in children under age 16 have not been established. Cases of oligohidrosis and hyperpyrexia have been reported (see **WARNINGS, Oligohidrosis and Hyperthermia in Pediatric Patients** subsection). Zonisamide commonly causes metabolic acidosis in pediatric patients (see **WARNINGS, Metabolic Acidosis** subsection). Chronic untreated metabolic acidosis in pediatric patients may cause nephrolithiasis and/or nephrocalcinosis, osteoporosis and/or osteomalacia (potentially resulting in rickets), and may reduce growth rates. A reduction in growth rate may eventually decrease the maximal height achieved. The effect of zonisamide on growth and bone-related sequelae has not been systematically investigated.
Geriatric Use:
Single dose pharmacokinetic parameters are similar in elderly and young healthy volunteers (see **CLINICAL PHARMACOLOGY, Specific Populations** subsection). Clinical studies of zonisamide did not include sufficient numbers of subjects aged 65 and over to determine whether they respond differently from younger subjects. Other reported clinical experience has not identified differences in responses between the elderly and younger patients. In general, dose selection for an elderly patient should be cautious, usually starting at the low end of the dosing range, reflecting the greater frequency of decreased hepatic, renal, or cardiac function, and of concomitant disease or other drug therapy.

ADVERSE REACTIONS

The most common adverse reactions with ZONEGRAN (an incidence at least 4% greater than placebo) in controlled clinical trials and shown in descending order of frequency were somnolence, anorexia, dizziness, ataxia, agitation/irritability, and difficulty with memory and/or concentration.
In controlled clinical trials, 12% of patients receiving ZONEGRAN as adjunctive therapy discontinued due to an adverse reaction compared to 6% receiving placebo. Approximately 21% of the 1,336 patients with epilepsy who received ZONEGRAN in clinical studies discontinued treatment because of an adverse reaction. The most common

Continued on next page

adverse reactions leading to discontinuation were somnolence, fatigue and/or ataxia (6%), anorexia (3%), difficulty concentrating (2%), difficulty with memory, mental slowing, nausea/vomiting (2%), and weight loss (1%). Many of these adverse reactions were dose-related (see **WARNINGS** and **PRECAUTIONS**).

Adverse Reaction Incidence in Controlled Clinical Trials:
Table 4 lists adverse reactions that occurred in at least 2% of patients treated with ZONEGRAN in controlled clinical trials that were numerically more common in the ZONEGRAN group. In these studies, either ZONEGRAN or placebo was added to the patient's current AED therapy.

Table 4. Adverse Reactions in Placebo-Controlled, Add-On Trials (Events that occurred in at least 2% of ZONEGRAN-treated patients and occurred more frequently in ZONEGRAN-treated than placebo-treated patients)

BODY SYSTEM/PREFERRED TERM	ZONEGRAN (n=269) %	PLACEBO (n=230) %
BODY AS A WHOLE		
Headache	10	8
Abdominal Pain	6	3
Flu Syndrome	4	3
DIGESTIVE		
Anorexia	13	6
Nausea	9	6
Diarrhea	5	2
Dyspepsia	3	1
Constipation	2	1
Dry Mouth	2	1
HEMATOLOGIC AND LYMPHATIC		
Ecchymosis	2	1
METABOLIC AND NUTRITIONAL		
Weight Loss	3	2
NERVOUS SYSTEM		
Dizziness	13	7
Ataxia	6	1
Nystagmus	4	2
Paresthesia	4	1
NEUROPSYCHIATRIC AND COGNITIVE DYSFUNCTION-ALTERED COGNITIVE FUNCTION		
Confusion	6	3
Difficulty Concentrating	6	2
Difficulty with Memory	6	2
Mental Slowing	4	2
NEUROPSYCHIATRIC AND COGNITIVE DYSFUNCTION-BEHAVIORAL ABNORMALITIES (NON-PSYCHOSIS-RELATED)		
Agitation/Irritability	9	4
Depression	6	3
Insomnia	6	3
Anxiety	3	2
Nervousness	2	1
NEUROPSYCHIATRIC AND COGNITIVE DYSFUNCTION-BEHAVIORAL ABNORMALITIES (PSYCHOSIS-RELATED)		
Schizophrenic/Schizophreniform Behavior	2	0
NEUROPSYCHIATRIC AND COGNITIVE DYSFUNCTION-CNS DEPRESSION		
Somnolence	17	7
Fatigue	8	6
Tiredness	7	5
NEUROPSYCHIATRIC AND COGNITIVE DYSFUNCTION-SPEECH AND LANGUAGE ABNORMALITIES		
Speech Abnormalities	5	2
Difficulties in Verbal Expression	2	<1
RESPIRATORY		
Rhinitis	2	1
SKIN AND APPENDAGES		
Rash	3	2
SPECIAL SENSES		
Diplopia	6	3
Taste Perversion	2	0

Other Adverse Reactions in Clinical Trials:
ZONEGRAN has been administered to 1,598 individuals during all clinical trials, only some of which were placebo-controlled. The frequencies represent the proportion of the 1,598 individuals exposed to ZONEGRAN who experienced an event on at least one occasion. All events are included except those already listed in the previous table or discussed in **WARNINGS** or **PRECAUTIONS**, trivial events, those too general to be informative, and those not reasonably associated with ZONEGRAN.

Events are further classified within each category and listed in order of decreasing frequency as follows: <u>frequent</u> occurring in at least 1:100 patients; <u>infrequent</u> occurring in 1:100 to 1:1000 patients; <u>rare</u> occurring in fewer than 1:1000 patients.

Body as a Whole: *Frequent:* Accidental injury, asthenia. *Infrequent:* Chest pain, flank pain, malaise, allergic reaction, face edema, neck rigidity. *Rare:* Lupus erythematosus.

Cardiovascular: *Infrequent:* Palpitation, tachycardia, vascular insufficiency, hypotension, hypertension, thrombophlebitis, syncope, bradycardia. *Rare:* Atrial fibrillation, heart failure, pulmonary embolus, ventricular extrasystoles.

Digestive: *Frequent:* Vomiting. *Infrequent:* Flatulence, gingivitis, gum hyperplasia, gastritis, gastroenteritis, stomatitis, cholelithiasis, glossitis, melena, rectal hemorrhage, ulcerative stomatitis, gastro-duodenal ulcer, dysphagia, gum hemorrhage. *Rare:* Cholangitis, hematemesis, cholecystitis, cholestatic jaundice, colitis, duodenitis, esophagitis, fecal incontinence, mouth ulceration.

Hematologic and Lymphatic: *Infrequent:* Leukopenia, anemia, immunodeficiency, lymphadenopathy. *Rare:* Thrombocytopenia, microcytic anemia, petechia.

Metabolic and Nutritional: *Infrequent:* Peripheral edema, weight gain, edema, thirst, dehydration. *Rare:* Hypoglycemia, hyponatremia, lactic dehydrogenase increased, SGOT increased, SGPT increased.

Musculoskeletal: *Infrequent:* Leg cramps, myalgia, myasthenia, arthralgia, arthritis.

Nervous System: *Frequent:* Tremor, convulsion, abnormal gait, hyperesthesia, incoordination. *Infrequent:* Hypertonia, twitching, abnormal dreams, vertigo, libido decreased, neuropathy, hyperkinesia, movement disorder, dysarthria, cerebrovascular accident, hypotonia, peripheral neuritis, reflexes increased. *Rare:* Dyskinesia, dystonia, encephalopathy, facial paralysis, hypokinesia, hyperesthesia, myoclonus, oculogyric crisis.

Behavioral Abnormalities –Non-Psychosis-Related: *Infrequent:* Euphoria.

Respiratory: *Frequent:* Pharyngitis, cough increased. *Infrequent:* Dyspnea. *Rare:* Apnea, hemoptysis.

Skin and Appendages: *Frequent:* Pruritus. *Infrequent:* Maculopapular rash, acne, alopecia, dry skin, sweating, eczema, urticaria, hirsutism, pustular rash, vesiculobullous rash.

Special Senses: *Frequent:* Amblyopia, tinnitus. *Infrequent:* Conjunctivitis, parosmia, deafness, visual field defect, glaucoma. *Rare:* Photophobia, iritis.

Urogenital: *Infrequent:* Urinary frequency, dysuria, urinary incontinence, hematuria, impotence, urinary retention, urinary urgency, amenorrhea, polyuria, nocturia. *Rare:* Albuminuria, enuresis, bladder pain, bladder calculus, gynecomastia, mastitis, menorrhagia.

POST MARKETING EXPERIENCE

The following serious adverse reactions have been reported since approval and use of ZONEGRAN worldwide. These reactions are reported voluntarily from a population of uncertain size; therefore, it is not possible to estimate their frequency or establish a causal relationship to drug exposure. Acute pancreatitis, rhabdomyolysis, increased creatine phosphokinase, and drug reaction with eosinophilia and systemic symptoms (DRESS) (see **WARNINGS**).

To report SUSPECTED ADVERSE REACTIONS, contact Concordia Pharmaceuticals Inc. at 1-877-370-1142 or the FDA at 1-800-FDA-1088 or www.fda.gov/medwatch.

DRUG ABUSE AND DEPENDENCE

The abuse and dependence potential of ZONEGRAN has not been evaluated in human studies (see **WARNINGS, Cognitive/Neuropsychiatric Adverse Events** subsection). In a series of animal studies, zonisamide did not demonstrate abuse liability and dependence potential. Monkeys did not self-administer zonisamide in a standard reinforcing paradigm. Rats exposed to zonisamide did not exhibit signs of physical dependence of the CNS-depressant type. Rats did not generalize the effects of diazepam to zonisamide in a standard discrimination paradigm after training, suggesting that zonisamide does not have abuse potential of the benzodiazepine-CNS depressant type.

OVERDOSAGE

Human Experience:
Experience with ZONEGRAN daily doses over 800 mg/day is limited. During ZONEGRAN clinical development, three patients ingested unknown amounts of ZONEGRAN as suicide attempts, and all three were hospitalized with CNS symptoms. One patient became comatose and developed bradycardia, hypotension, and respiratory depression; the zonisamide plasma level was 100.1 μg/mL measured 31 hours post-ingestion. Zonisamide plasma levels fell with a half-life of 57 hours, and the patient became alert five days later.

Management:
No specific antidotes for ZONEGRAN overdosage are available. Following a suspected recent overdose, emesis should be induced or gastric lavage performed with the usual precautions to protect the airway. General supportive care is indicated, including frequent monitoring of vital signs and close observation.

Zonisamide has a long half-life (see **CLINICAL PHARMACOLOGY** section). Due to the low protein binding of zonisamide (40%), renal dialysis may be effective. The effectiveness of renal dialysis as a treatment of overdose has not been formally studied. A poison control center should be contacted for information on the management of ZONEGRAN overdosage.

DOSAGE AND ADMINISTRATION

ZONEGRAN (zonisamide) is recommended as adjunctive therapy for the treatment of partial seizures in adults. Safety and efficacy in pediatric patients below the age of 16 have not been established. ZONEGRAN should be administered once or twice daily, using 25 mg or 100 mg capsules. ZONEGRAN is given orally and can be taken with or without food. Capsules should be swallowed whole.

Adults over Age 16:
The prescriber should be aware that, because of the long half-life of zonisamide, up to two weeks may be required to achieve steady state levels upon reaching a stable dose or following dosage adjustment. Although the regimen described below is one that has been shown to be tolerated, the prescriber may wish to prolong the duration of treatment at the lower doses in order to fully assess the effects of zonisamide at steady state, noting that many of the side effects of zonisamide are more frequent at doses of 300 mg per day and above. Although there is some evidence of greater response at doses above 100–200 mg/day, the increase appears small and formal dose-response studies have not been conducted.

The initial dose of ZONEGRAN should be 100 mg daily. After two weeks, the dose may be increased to 200 mg/day for at least two weeks. It can be increased to 300 mg/day and 400 mg/day, with the dose stable for at least two weeks to achieve steady state at each level. Evidence from controlled trials suggests that ZONEGRAN doses of 100–600 mg/day are effective, but there is no suggestion of increasing response above 400 mg/day (see **CLINICAL PHARMACOLOGY, Clinical Studies** subsection). There is little experience with doses greater than 600 mg/day.

Patients with Renal or Hepatic Disease:
Because zonisamide is metabolized in the liver and excreted by the kidneys, patients with renal or hepatic disease should be treated with caution, and might require slower titration and more frequent monitoring (see **CLINICAL PHARMACOLOGY** and **PRECAUTIONS**).

HOW SUPPLIED

ZONEGRAN is available as 25 mg and 100 mg two-piece hard gelatin capsules. The capsules are printed in black with "ZONEGRAN 25" or "ZONEGRAN 100," respectively. ZONEGRAN is available in bottles of 100 with strengths and colors as follows:

Dosage Strength	Capsule Colors	NDC #
25 mg	White opaque body with white opaque cap.	59212-681-10
100 mg	White opaque body with red opaque cap.	59212-680-10

Store at 25°C (77°F), excursions permitted to 15–30°C (59–86°F) [see USP Controlled Room Temperature], in a dry place and protected from light.

Manufactured for:
Concordia Pharmaceuticals Inc.
St. Michael, Barbados BB11005
ZONEGRAN® is a registered trademark of Dainippon Pharmaceutical Co., Ltd. and licensed exclusively to Concordia Pharmaceuticals Inc.
© 2015 Concordia Pharmaceuticals Inc.
Revised: 04/2016

Medication Guide
ZONEGRAN® (ZO-nuh-gran)
(zonisamide) capsules
What is the most important information I should know about ZONEGRAN?
ZONEGRAN may cause serious side effects, including:
1. Serious skin rash that can cause death.
2. Serious allergic reactions that may affect different parts of the body.
3. Less sweating and increase in your body temperature (fever).
4. Suicidal thoughts or actions in some people.
5. Increased level of acid in your blood (metabolic acidosis).
6. Problems with your concentration, attention, memory, thinking, speech, or language.
7. Blood cell changes such as reduced red and white blood cell counts.
These serious side effects are described below.
1. ZONEGRAN may cause a serious skin rash that can cause death. These serious skin reactions are more likely to happen when you begin taking ZONEGRAN within the first 4 months of treatment but may occur at later times.
2. ZONEGRAN can cause other types of allergic reactions or serious problems that may affect different parts of the body such as your liver, kidneys, heart, or blood cells. You may or may not have a rash with these types of reactions. These reactions can be very serious and can cause death. Call your health care provider right away if you have:
   ◦ fever
   ◦ severe muscle pain
   ◦ rash
   ◦ swollen lymph glands
   ◦ swelling of your face
   ◦ unusual bruising or bleeding
   ◦ weakness, fatigue
   ◦ yellowing of your skin or the white part of your eyes
3. ZONEGRAN may cause you to sweat less and to increase your body temperature (fever). You may need to be hospitalized for this. You should watch for decreased sweating and fever, especially when it is hot and especially in children taking ZONEGRAN.
   Call your health care provider right away if you have:
   ◦ high fever, recurring fever, or long lasting fever
   ◦ less sweat than normal
4. Like other antiepileptic drugs, ZONEGRAN may cause suicidal thoughts or actions in a very small number of people, about 1 in 500.
   Call a healthcare provider right away if you have any of these symptoms, especially if they are new, worse, or worry you:
   ◦ thoughts about suicide or dying
   ◦ attempt to commit suicide
   ◦ new or worse depression
   ◦ new or worse anxiety
   ◦ feeling agitated or restless
   ◦ panic attacks
   ◦ trouble sleeping (insomnia)
   ◦ new or worse irritability
   ◦ acting aggressive, being angry, or violent
   ◦ acting on dangerous impulses
   ◦ an extreme increase in activity and talking (mania)
   ◦ other unusual changes in behavior or mood
   ◦ Suicidal thoughts or actions can be caused by things other than medicines. If you have suicidal thoughts or actions, your healthcare provider may check for other causes.
   How can I watch for early symptoms of suicidal thoughts and actions?
   ◦ Pay attention to any changes, especially sudden changes, in mood, behaviors, thoughts, or feelings.
   ◦ Keep all follow-up visits with your healthcare provider as scheduled.
   Call your healthcare provider between visits as needed, especially if you are worried about symptoms.
   Do not stop ZONEGRAN without first talking to a healthcare provider.
   Stopping ZONEGRAN suddenly can cause serious problems. Stopping a seizure medicine suddenly in a patient who has epilepsy can cause seizures that will not stop (status epilepticus).

5. ZONEGRAN can increase the level of acid in your blood (metabolic acidosis). If left untreated, metabolic acidosis can cause brittle or soft bones (osteoporosis, osteomalacia, osteopenia), kidney stones and can slow the rate of growth in children. Metabolic acidosis can happen with or without symptoms.
   Sometimes people with metabolic acidosis will:
   ◦ feel tired
   ◦ not feel hungry (loss of appetite)
   ◦ feel changes in heartbeat
   ◦ have trouble thinking clearly
   Your healthcare provider should do a blood test to measure the level of acid in your blood before and during your treatment with ZONEGRAN.
6. ZONEGRAN may cause problems with your concentration, attention, memory, thinking, speech, or language.
7. ZONEGRAN can cause blood cell changes such as reduced red and white blood cell counts. Call your healthcare provider if you develop fever, sore throat, sores in your mouth, or unusual bruising.
ZONEGRAN can have other serious side effects. For more information ask your healthcare provider or pharmacist. Tell your healthcare provider if you have any side effect that bothers you. Be sure to read the section titled "What are the possible side effects of ZONEGRAN?"
What is ZONEGRAN?
ZONEGRAN is a prescription medicine that is used with other medicines to treat partial seizures in adults.
It is not known if ZONEGRAN is safe or effective in children under 16 years of age.
Do not take ZONEGRAN:
Do not take ZONEGRAN if you are allergic to medicines that contain sulfa.
Before taking ZONEGRAN, tell your healthcare provider about all your medical conditions, including if you:
• have or have had depression, mood problems or suicidal thoughts or behavior
• have kidney problems
• have liver problems
• have a history of metabolic acidosis (too much acid in your blood)
• have weak, brittle bones or soft bones (osteomalacia, osteopenia or osteoporosis)
• have a growth problem
• are on a diet high in fat called a ketogenic diet
• have diarrhea
Tell your healthcare provider if you:
• are pregnant or plan to become pregnant. ZONEGRAN may harm your unborn baby. Women who can become pregnant should use effective birth control. Tell your healthcare provider right away if you become pregnant while taking ZONEGRAN.
You and your healthcare provider should decide if you should take ZONEGRAN while you are pregnant.
If you become pregnant while taking ZONEGRAN, talk to your healthcare provider about registering with the North American Antiepileptic Drug Pregnancy Registry. You can enroll in this registry by calling 1-888-233-2334. The purpose of this registry is to collect information about the safety of antiepileptic drugs during pregnancy.
• are breastfeeding or plan to breastfeed. ZONEGRAN can pass into your breast milk. It is not known if ZONEGRAN in your breast milk can harm your baby. Talk to your healthcare provider about the best way to feed your baby if you take ZONEGRAN.
Tell your healthcare provider about all the medicines you take, including prescription and over-the-counter medicines, vitamins and herbal supplements.
How should I take ZONEGRAN?
• Take ZONEGRAN exactly as prescribed. Your healthcare prescriber may change your dose. Your healthcare provider will tell you how much ZONEGRAN to take.
• Take ZONEGRAN with or without food.
• Swallow the capsules whole.
• If you take too much ZONEGRAN, call your local Poison Control Center or go to the nearest emergency room right away.
• Do not stop taking ZONEGRAN without talking to your healthcare provider. Stopping ZONEGRAN suddenly can cause serious problems, including seizures that will not stop (status epilepticus).
What should I avoid while taking ZONEGRAN?
• Do not drink alcohol or take other drugs that make you sleepy or dizzy while taking ZONEGRAN until you talk to your health care provider. ZONEGRAN taken with alcohol or drugs that cause sleepiness or dizziness may make your sleepiness or dizziness worse.
• Do not drive, operate heavy machinery, or do other dangerous activities until you know how ZONEGRAN affects you. ZONEGRAN can slow your thinking and motor skills.

What are the possible side effects of ZONEGRAN?
ZONEGRAN can cause serious side effects. See "What is the most important information I should know about ZONEGRAN?"
Other serious side effects include:
• **kidney stones**. Back pain, stomach pain, or blood in your urine may mean you have kidney stones. Drink plenty of fluids while you take ZONEGRAN to lower your chance of getting kidney stones.
• **problems with mood or thinking** (new or worse depression; sudden changes in mood, behavior, or loss of contact with reality, sometimes associated with hearing voices or seeing things that are not really there; feeling sleepy or tired; trouble concentrating; speech and language problems). Call your healthcare provider right away if you have any of the symptoms listed above.
The most common side effects of ZONEGRAN include:
• drowsiness
• loss of appetite
• dizziness
• problems with concentration or memory
• trouble with walking and coordination
• agitation or irritability
Side effects can happen at any time, but are more likely to happen during the first several weeks after starting ZONEGRAN.
These are not all of the possible side effects of ZONEGRAN. Call your doctor for medical advice about side effects. You may report side effects to FDA at 1-800-FDA-1088.
How should I store ZONEGRAN?
• Store ZONEGRAN between 59°F to 86°F (15°C to 30°C)
• Keep ZONEGRAN dry and away from light
Keep ZONEGRAN and all medicines out of the reach of children.
General Information about the safe and effective use of ZONEGRAN
Medicines are sometimes prescribed for purposes other than those listed in a Medication Guide. Do not use ZONEGRAN for a condition for which it was not prescribed. Do not give ZONEGRAN to other people, even if they have the same symptoms that you have. It may harm them. You can ask your pharmacist or healthcare provider for information about ZONEGRAN that is written for health professionals.
What are the ingredients in ZONEGRAN?
Active ingredient: zonisamide
Inactive ingredients in ZONEGRAN 25 mg capsules: microcrystalline cellulose, hydrogenated vegetable oil, sodium lauryl sulfate, gelatin, and titanium dioxide
Inactive ingredients in ZONEGRAN 100 mg capsules: microcrystalline cellulose, hydrogenated vegetable oil, sodium lauryl sulfate, gelatin, and titanium dioxide, FD&C Red No. 40 and FD&C Yellow No. 6
Manufactured for:
Concordia Pharmaceuticals Inc.
St. Michael, Barbados BB11005
ZONEGRAN® is a registered trademark of Dainippon Pharmaceutical Co., Ltd. and licensed exclusively to Concordia Pharmaceuticals Inc.
This Medication Guide has been approved by the U.S. Food and Drug Administration. Revised: April 2016
Shown in Product Identification Guide, page 508

CSL BEHRING
1020 First Avenue
PO Box 61501
King of Prussia, PA 19406-0901

Direct Inquiries to:
Phone: (610) 878-4000
www.CslBehring-us.com

BERINERT®
C1 Esterase Inhibitor (Human)
Freeze-Dried Powder for Reconstitution

HIGHLIGHTS OF PRESCRIBING INFORMATION
These highlights do not include all the information needed to use Berinert safely and effectively. See full prescribing information for Berinert.
Berinert [C1 Esterase Inhibitor (Human)]

℞

Continued on next page

For intravenous use. Freeze-Dried Powder for Reconstitution.
Initial U.S. Approval: 2009

---RECENT MAJOR CHANGES---

Indications and Usage (1)   07/2016

---INDICATIONS AND USAGE---

Berinert is a plasma-derived C1 Esterase Inhibitor (Human) indicated for the treatment of acute abdominal, facial, or laryngeal hereditary angioedema (HAE) attacks in adult and pediatric patients. (1)
The safety and efficacy of Berinert for prophylactic therapy have not been established. (1)

---DOSAGE AND ADMINISTRATION---

For intravenous use only.
• Store the vial in the original carton in order to protect from light. Store at 2-25°C (36-77°F). Do not freeze. (2)
• Administer 20 International Units per kg body weight. (2)
• Reconstitute Berinert prior to use using the Sterile Water for Injection, USP provided. (2.1)
• Use a silicone-free syringe for reconstitution and administration. (2.1)
• Administer at room temperature within 8 hours of reconstitution. (2.1)
• Inject at a rate of approximately 4 mL per minute. (2.2)
• Do not mix Berinert with other medicinal products or solutions. (2.2)
• Appropriately trained patients may self-administer upon recognition of an HAE attack. (2.2)

---DOSAGE FORMS AND STRENGTHS---

• 500 International Units lyophilized concentrate in a single-use vial for reconstitution with 10 mL of Sterile Water for Injection, USP. (3)

---CONTRAINDICATIONS---

• Do not use in patients with a history of life-threatening immediate hypersensitivity reactions, including anaphylaxis, to C1 esterase inhibitor preparations. (4)

---WARNINGS AND PRECAUTIONS---

• Hypersensitivity reactions may occur. Epinephrine should be immediately available to treat any acute severe hypersensitivity reactions following discontinuation of administration. (5.1)
• Serious arterial and venous thromboembolic (TE) events have been reported at the recommended dose of C1 Esterase Inhibitor (Human) products, including Berinert, following administration in patients with HAE. Risk factors may include the presence of an indwelling venous catheter/access device, prior history of thrombosis, underlying atherosclerosis, use of oral contraceptives or certain androgens, morbid obesity, and immobility. Benefits of treatment of HAE attacks should be weighed against the risks of TE events in patients with underlying risk factors. Monitor patients with known risk factors for TE events during and after Berinert administration.
TE events have also been reported following administration of a C1 Esterase Inhibitor (Human) product when used for unapproved indications at higher than recommended doses.[1] (5.2)
• Berinert is made from human plasma and may contain infectious agents, eg, viruses and, theoretically, the Creutzfeldt-Jakob disease (CJD) agent. (5.3)
• Laryngeal attacks: Following self-administration of Berinert for laryngeal attacks, advise patients to immediately seek medical attention. (5.4)

---ADVERSE REACTIONS---

• The most serious adverse reaction reported in subjects who received Berinert was an increase in the severity of pain associated with HAE. (6.1)
• The most common adverse reaction reported in greater than 4% of the subjects and greater than placebo among subjects who received Berinert in the placebo-controlled clinical trial was dysgeusia. (6.1)
To report SUSPECTED ADVERSE REACTIONS, contact the CSL Behring Pharmacovigilance Department at 1-866-915-6958 or to the FDA at 1-800-FDA-1088 or www.fda.gov/medwatch.

---USE IN SPECIFIC POPULATIONS---

• Pregnancy: Use only if clearly needed. (8.1)
• Compared to adults, when adjusted for baseline, the half-life of Berinert was shorter and clearance (on per kg basis) was faster in children. The clinical implication of this difference is not known. (12.3)

See 17 for PATIENT COUNSELING INFORMATION and FDA-approved patient labeling.

       Revised: 7/2016

FULL PRESCRIBING INFORMATION
Berinert® [C1 Esterase Inhibitor (Human)]
Freeze-dried powder

1   INDICATIONS AND USAGE

Berinert is a plasma-derived concentrate of C1 Esterase Inhibitor (Human) indicated for the treatment of acute abdominal, facial, or laryngeal hereditary angioedema (HAE) attacks in adult and pediatric patients.
The safety and efficacy of Berinert for prophylactic therapy have not been established.

2   DOSAGE AND ADMINISTRATION

For Intravenous Use Only.
Administer Berinert at a dose of 20 International Units (IU) per kg body weight by intravenous injection. Doses lower than 20 IU/kg body weight should not be administered.
Berinert is provided as a freeze-dried powder for reconstitution with the Sterile Water for Injection, USP provided. Store the vial in the original carton in order to protect from light. Do not freeze.

2.1   Preparation and Handling
• Check the expiration date on the product vial label. Do not use beyond the expiration date.
• Prepare and administer using aseptic techniques [see Dosage and Administration (2.2)].
• Use a silicone-free syringe for reconstitution and administration of Berinert.
• After reconstitution and prior to administration, inspect Berinert visually for particulate matter and discoloration. The reconstituted solution should be colorless, clear, and free from visible particles. Do not use if the solution is cloudy, discolored, or contains particulates.
• The Berinert vial is for single use only. Berinert contains no preservative. Any product that has been reconstituted should be used promptly. The reconstituted solution must be used within 8 hours. Discard partially used vials.
• Do not freeze the reconstituted solution.

2.2   Reconstitution and Administration
Each Berinert vial containing 500 IU of C1 esterase inhibitor as a lyophilized concentrate for reconstitution with 10 mL of Sterile Water for Injection, USP provided.
Use either the Mix2Vial® transfer set provided with Berinert [see How Supplied/Storage and Handling (16.1)] or a commercially available double-ended needle and vented filter spike.

Reconstitution
The procedures below are provided as general guidelines for the reconstitution and administration of Berinert.
[See table on pages 927 through 929]
Administration
• Do not mix Berinert with other medicinal products. Administer Berinert by a separate infusion line.
• Use aseptic technique when administering Berinert.
• Use a silicone-free syringe.
• Follow recommended venipuncture guidelines for initiating intravenous therapy.
• Administer Berinert by slow intravenous injection at a rate of approximately 4 mL per minute. Please refer to the illustration in step 6 of the self-administration section in the Patient Product Information (PPI) section.
• For self-administration, provide the patient with instructions and training for intravenous injection outside of a clinic setting so patients may self-administer Berinert upon recognition of symptoms of an HAE attack [see Patient Counseling Information (17)].
• After administration, immediately discard any unused product and all used disposable supplies in accordance with local requirements.

3   DOSAGE FORMS AND STRENGTHS

• Berinert is available in a single-use vial that contains 500 IU of C1 esterase inhibitor as a lyophilized concentrate.
• Each vial must be reconstituted with 10 mL of Sterile Water for Injection, USP provided.

4   CONTRAINDICATIONS

Berinert is contraindicated in individuals who have experienced life-threatening hypersensitivity reactions, including anaphylaxis, to C1 esterase inhibitor preparations.

5.1   WARNINGS AND PRECAUTIONS
5.1   Hypersensitivity
Severe hypersensitivity reactions may occur. Epinephrine should be immediately available for treatment of acute severe hypersensitivity reaction [see Patient Counseling Information (17)]. The signs and symptoms of hypersensitivity reactions may include hives, generalized urticaria, tightness of the chest, wheezing, hypotension, and/or anaphylaxis during or after injection of Berinert.
Because hypersensitivity reactions may have symptoms similar to HAE attacks, treatment methods should be carefully considered. In case of suspected hypersensitivity, immediately discontinue administration of Berinert and institute appropriate treatment.
5.2   Thromboembolic Events
Serious arterial and venous thromboembolic (TE) events have been reported at the recommended dose of C1 Esterase Inhibitor (Human) products, including Berinert, following administration in patients with HAE. Risk factors may include the presence of an indwelling venous catheter/access device, prior history of thrombosis, underlying atherosclerosis, use of oral contraceptives or certain androgens, morbid obesity, and immobility. Benefits of treatment of HAE attacks should be weighed against the risks of TE events in patients with underlying risk factors. Monitor patients with known risk factors for TE events during and after Berinert administration.
TE events have also been reported following administration of a C1 Esterase Inhibitor (Human) product when used for unapproved indications at higher than recommended doses[1,2] [see Overdosage (10) and Nonclinical Toxicology (13.2)].
5.3   Transmission of Infectious Agents
Because Berinert is made from human blood, it may contain infectious agents (eg, viruses and, theoretically, the Creutzfeldt-Jakob disease [CJD] agent) that can cause disease. The risk that such products will transmit an infectious agent has been reduced by screening plasma donors for prior exposure to certain viruses, by testing for the presence of certain current virus infections, and by processes demonstrated to inactivate and/or remove certain viruses during manufacturing [see Description (11) and Patient Counseling Information (17)].
Despite these measures, such products may still potentially transmit disease. There is also the possibility that unknown infectious agents may be present in such products.
Since 1979, a few suspected cases of viral transmission have been reported with the use of Berinert outside the US, including cases of acute hepatitis C. From the incomplete information available from these cases, it was not possible to determine with certainty if the infections were or were not related to prior administration of Berinert. With the introduction of the pasteurization step (heat treatment in aque-

1. Ensure that the Berinert vial and diluent vial are at room temperature.

2. Place the Berinert vial, diluent vial and Mix2Vial transfer set on a flat surface.

3. Remove the flip caps from the Berinert and diluent vials. Wipe the vial stoppers with the alcohol swab provided. Allow to dry prior to opening the Mix2Vial transfer set package.

4. Open the Mix2Vial transfer set package by peeling away the lid (Figure 1). Leave the Mix2Vial transfer set in the clear package.

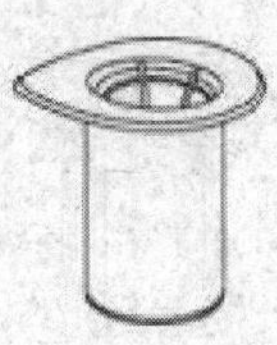

Figure 1

5. Place the diluent vial on a flat surface and hold the vial tightly. Grip the Mix2Vial transfer set together with the clear package and push the plastic spike at the blue end of the Mix2Vial transfer set firmly through the center of the stopper of the diluent vial (Figure 2).

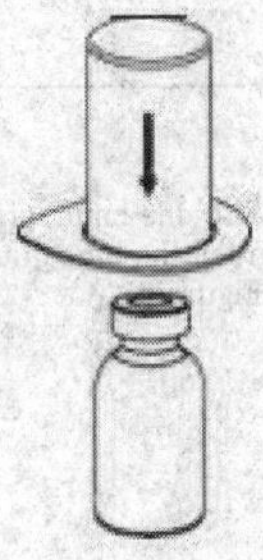

Figure 2

6. Carefully remove the clear package from the Mix2Vial transfer set. Make sure that you pull up only the clear package, and not the Mix2Vial transfer set (Figure 3).

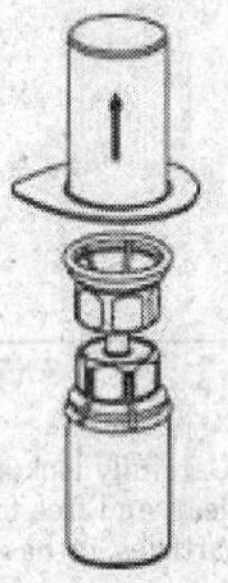

Figure 3

7. With the Berinert vial placed firmly on a flat surface, invert the diluent vial with the Mix2Vial transfer set attached and push the plastic spike of the transparent adapter firmly through the center of the stopper of the Berinert vial (Figure 4). The diluent will automatically transfer into the Berinert vial.

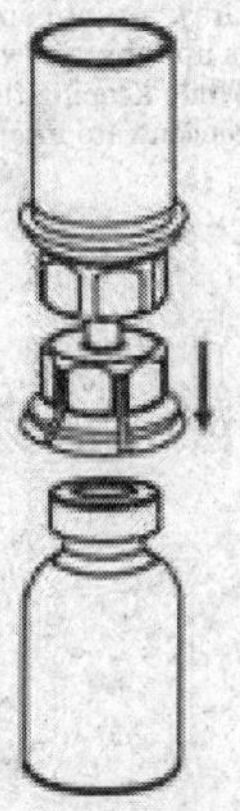

Figure 4

ous solution at 60°C for 10 hours) in 1985, case reports on suspected transmission of viruses have not demonstrated a causal relationship to the administration of Berinert.

The physician should discuss the risks and benefits of this product with the patient before prescribing or administering it to the patient [see *Patient Counseling Information (17)*].

All infections thought by a physician possibly to have been transmitted by Berinert should be reported by lot number, by the physician, or other healthcare provider to the CSL Behring Pharmacovigilance Department at 1-866-915-6958.

5.4 Laryngeal Attacks

Given the potential for airway obstruction during acute laryngeal HAE attacks, patients self-administering Berinert should be advised to immediately seek medical attention in an appropriate healthcare facility after treatment with Berinert.

6 ADVERSE REACTIONS

The most serious adverse reaction reported in subjects enrolled in clinical studies who received Berinert was an increase in the severity of pain associated with HAE.

The most common adverse reaction reported in greater than 4% of the subjects and greater than placebo among subjects who received Berinert in the placebo-controlled clinical trial was dysgeusia.

6.1 Clinical Trials Experience

Because clinical studies are conducted under widely varying conditions, adverse reaction rates observed in the clinical trials of a drug cannot be directly compared to rates in the clinical trials of another drug and may not reflect the rates observed in practice.

Placebo-controlled Clinical Study

In the placebo-controlled clinical study, referred to as the randomized clinical trial (RCT) [see *Clinical Studies (14)*], 124 subjects experiencing an acute moderate to severe abdominal or facial HAE attack were treated with Berinert (either a 10 IU per kg body weight or a 20 IU per kg body weight dose), or placebo (physiological saline solution).

The treatment-emergent serious adverse reactions/events that occurred in 5 subjects in the RCT were laryngeal edema, facial attack with laryngeal edema, swelling (shoulder and chest), exacerbation of hereditary angioedema, and laryngospasm.

Table 1: Adverse Reactions* Occurring up to 4 hours After Initial Infusion in More Than 4% of subjects[†]

Adverse Reactions	Number (%) of subjects Reporting Adverse Reactions Berinert 20 IU/kg (n=43)	Number (%) of subjects Reporting Adverse Reactions Placebo Group (n=42)
Nausea[†]	3 (7%)	5 (11.9%)
Dysgeusia	2 (4.7%)	0 (0)
Abdominal Pain[†]	2 (4.7%)	3 (7.1%)
Vomiting[†]	1 (2.3%)	3 (7.1%)
Diarrhea[†]	0 (0)	4 (9.5%)
Headache	0 (0)	2 (4.8%)

* Comprises adverse events that began within 4 hours of infusion; these events were considered adverse reactions irrespective of reported causality.
† The following abdominal symptoms were identified in the protocol as associated with HAE abdominal attacks: abdominal pain, bloating, cramps, nausea, vomiting, and diarrhea.

Table 2: Adverse Reactions* Occurring in More Than 4% of subjects up to 72 hours After Infusion of Initial or Rescue Medication[†] by Intent-to-Treat

Adverse Reactions	Number (%) of subjects Reporting Adverse Reactions[†‡] Berinert 20 IU/kg (n=43)	Number (%) of subjects Reporting Adverse Reactions[†‡] Placebo Group (n=42)
Nausea	3 (7%)	11 (26.2%)

This table is continued on the next page

Continued on next page

Headache	3 (7%)	5 (11.9%)
Abdominal Pain	3 (7%)	5 (11.9%)
Dysgeusia	2 (4.7%)	1 (2.4%)
Vomiting	1 (2.3%)	7 (16.7%)
Pain	1 (2.3%)	4 (9.5%)
Muscle spasms	1 (2.3%)	4 (9.5%)
Diarrhea	0 (0)	8 (19%)
Back pain	0 (0)	2 (4.8%)
Facial pain	0 (0)	2 (4.8%)

* Comprises adverse events that began within 72 hours of infusion; these events were considered adverse reactions irrespective of reported causality.

† If a subject experienced no relief or insufficient relief of symptoms within 4 hours after infusion, investigators had the option to administer a blinded second infusion ("rescue" treatment) of Berinert (20 IU/kg for the placebo group or 10 IU/kg for the 10 IU/kg group), or placebo (for the 20 IU/kg group).

‡ Adverse reactions following either initial treatment and/or blinded "rescue" treatment. Because more subjects in the placebo randomization group than in the Berinert randomization group received rescue treatment, the median observation period in this analysis for subjects randomized to placebo was slightly longer than for subjects randomized to receive Berinert.

Subjects were tested at baseline and after 3 months for possible exposure to Parvovirus B19, hepatitis B, hepatitis C, and HIV-1 and HIV-2. No subject who underwent testing evidenced seroconversion or treatment-emergent positive polymerase chain reaction testing for these pathogens.

Open-Label Extension Study

In the safety analysis of the open-label extension study, 57 subjects with 1085 acute moderate to severe abdominal, facial, peripheral, and laryngeal attacks received a 20 IU/kg body weight dose of Berinert *[see Clinical Studies (14)]*. This study provides additional safety data in subjects who received multiple infusions of the product for sequential HAE attacks (one infusion per attack).

Table 3 lists the adverse reactions that occurred in the safety analysis of the open-label extension study in ≥2 subjects or associated with ≥5 attacks during infusion or within 24 hours or 72 hours after the end of a Berinert infusion.

[See table 3 on page 932]
[See table 4 on next page]

The incidence and type of adverse reactions with Berinert when administered for treatment of multiple consecutive acute HAE attacks of any type was similar to those previously observed. As in the placebo-controlled study, no proven cases of infections due to HIV-1/2, HAV, HBV, HCV or Parvovirus B19 were observed during the study.

6.2 Postmarketing Experience

Because postmarketing reporting of adverse reactions is voluntary and from a population of uncertain size, it is not always possible to reliably estimate the frequency of these reactions or establish a causal relationship to product exposure.

Adverse reactions reported in Europe since 1979 in patients receiving Berinert for treatment of HAE include hypersensitivity/anaphylactic reactions, injection-site pain, injection-site redness, chills, and fever.

TE Events Associated with HAE Treatment

TE events including basilar artery thrombosis, multiple pulmonary microemboli, and thrombosis have been reported with the use of Berinert at the recommended dose following treatment of HAE.

TE Events Associated with Use in Unapproved Indications

TE events have also been reported with the use of Berinert in patients receiving higher than recommended doses during cardiac surgery (unapproved indication) include carotid artery thrombosis, cerebral thrombosis, myocardial infarction, pulmonary embolism, renal vein thrombosis, sagittal sinus thrombosis, inferior vena cava thrombosis, superior vena cava thrombosis, internal jugular vein thrombosis, and peripheral venous thrombosis.[1]

8. With the diluent and Berinert vial still attached to the Mix2Vial transfer set, gently swirl the Berinert vial to ensure that the Berinert is fully dissolved (Figure 5). Do not shake the vial.

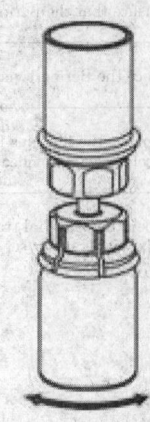

Figure 5

9. With one hand, grasp the Berinert-side of the Mix2Vial transfer set and with the other hand grasp the blue diluent-side of the Mix2Vial transfer set and unscrew the set into two pieces (Figure 6).

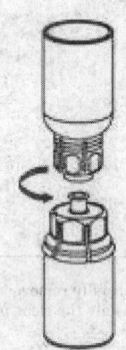

Figure 6

10. Carefully look at reconstituted solution in each vial of Berinert. It should be colorless, clear, and free from visible particles. **Do not use the vial if** the liquid looks cloudy, contains particles, or has changed color. Do not use if the expiration date on the label has expired.

11. Draw air into an empty, sterile syringe. Use a silicone-free syringe. While the Berinert vial is upright, screw the syringe to the Mix2Vial transfer set. Inject air into the Berinert vial. While keeping the syringe plunger pressed, invert the system upside down and draw the concentrate into the syringe by pulling the plunger back slowly (Figure 7).

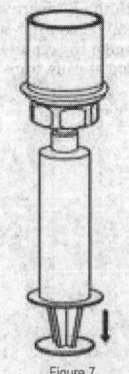

Figure 7

This table is continued on the next page

The following adverse reactions, identified by system organ class, have been attributed to Berinert during post-approval use outside the US.

- *Immune System Disorder: Hypersensitivity / anaphylactic reactions, and shock*
- *General / Body as a Whole: Pain on injection, redness at injection site, chills, and fever*

7 DRUG INTERACTIONS

No drug interaction studies have been conducted.

8 USE IN SPECIFIC POPULATIONS

8.1 Pregnancy

Risk Summary

Background risk (general population)

A review of available data suggests that major birth defects occur in 2-4% of the U.S. general population and that miscarriage occurs in 15-20% of clinically recognized pregnancies, regardless of drug exposure.

Data

Risk in Berinert patients

In a retrospective case collection study, 20 pregnant women ranging in age from 20 to 35 years received Berinert with repeated doses up to 3,500 IU per attack; these women reported no complications during delivery and no harmful effects on their 34 neonates. Berinert should be given to a pregnant woman only if clearly needed.

8.2 Lactation

Risk Summary

It is not known whether Berinert is excreted in human milk. Because many drugs are excreted in human milk, caution should be exercised when Berinert is administered to a nursing woman.

8.4 Pediatric Use

Safety and efficacy of Berinert have been evaluated in 12 pediatric patients with HAE (age range 10 to 16 years) in the placebo controlled and open-label extension studies. Berinert was also evaluated in 18 pediatric patients with HAE (age range 5 to 11 years) in a Registry Study conducted in the US and Europe. The safety profile observed in the pediatric population was similar to that observed in adults. The pharmacokinetics of Berinert were evaluated in 5 pediatric subjects (ages 6 through 13) *[see Clinical Pharmacology (12.3), Table 7]*.

8.5 Geriatric Use

The safety and efficacy of Berinert in the geriatric population have not been evaluated in controlled clinical studies. Berinert was evaluated in 27 geriatric subjects (age range 65 to 83 years) with HAE in a Registry Study conducted in the US and Europe. The safety profile observed in the geriatric population was similar to that observed in the younger populations studied.

10 OVERDOSAGE

The development of thrombosis has been reported after doses exceeding 20 IU/kg body weight of Berinert when used for unapproved indications in newborns and young children with congenital heart anomalies during or after cardiac surgery under extracorporeal circulation.[1]

The maximum dose administered in clinical studies in hereditary angioedema was 20 IU/kg body weight.

11 DESCRIPTION

Berinert is a human plasma-derived, purified, pasteurized, lyophilized concentrate of C1 esterase inhibitor to be reconstituted for intravenous administration. Berinert is prepared from large pools of human plasma from US donors. The potency of C1 esterase inhibitor is expressed in Inter-national Units (IU), which is related to the current WHO Standard for C1 esterase inhibitor products.

C1 esterase inhibitor is a soluble, single-chain glycoprotein containing 478 amino acid residues organized into three beta-sheets and eight or nine alpha-helices.[3] The heavily glycosylated molecule has an apparent molecular weight of 105 kD, of which the carbohydrate chains comprise 26% to 35%.[4]

Each 500 IU vial of reconstituted Berinert contains 400-625 IU C1 esterase inhibitor, 50 to 80 mg total protein, 85 to 115 mg glycine, 70 to 100 mg sodium chloride, and 25 to 35 mg sodium citrate.

All plasma used in the manufacture of Berinert is obtained from US donors and is tested using serological assays for hepatitis B surface antigen and antibodies to HIV-1/2 and HCV. Additionally, the plasma is tested with Nucleic Acid Testing (NAT) for HBV, HCV, HIV-1 and HAV and found to be non-reactive (negative). In addition, the plasma is also tested by NAT for Human Parvovirus B19. Only plasma that has passed virus screening is used for production, and the limit for Parvovirus B19 in the fractionation pool is set not to exceed 10^4 IU of Parvovirus B19 DNA per mL.

The manufacturing process for Berinert includes multiple steps that reduce the risk of virus transmission. The virus inactivation/reduction capacity consists of three steps:

- Pasteurization in aqueous solution at 60°C for 10 hours
- Hydrophobic interaction chromatography
- Virus filtration (also called nanofiltration) by two filters, 20 nm and 15 nm, in series

This was evaluated in a series of in vitro spiking experiments. The total mean cumulative virus inactivation/reduction is shown in Table 5.

[See table 5 on page 933]

12 CLINICAL PHARMACOLOGY

12.1 Mechanism of Action

C1 esterase inhibitor is a normal constituent of human plasma and belongs to the group of serine protease inhibitors (serpins) that includes antithrombin III, $alpha_1$-protease inhibitor, $alpha_2$-antiplasmin, and heparin cofactor II. As with the other inhibitors in this group, C1 esterase inhibitor has an important inhibiting potential on several of the major cascade systems of the human body, including the complement system, the intrinsic coagulation (contact) system, the fibrinolytic system, and the coagulation cascade. Regulation of these systems is performed through the formation of complexes between the proteinase and the inhibitor, resulting in inactivation of both and consumption of the C1 esterase inhibitor.

C1 esterase inhibitor, which is usually activated during the inflammatory process, inactivates its substrate by covalently binding to the reactive site. C1 esterase inhibitor is the only known inhibitor for the subcomponent of the com-

---

12. Now that the concentrate has been transferred into the syringe, firmly grasp the barrel of the syringe (keeping the plunger facing down) and unscrew the syringe from the Mix2Vial transfer set (Figure 8). Attach the syringe to a suitable intravenous administration set.

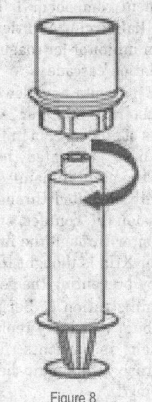

Figure 8

13. If patient requires more than one vial, pool the contents of multiple vials into one syringe. A new unused Mix2Vial transfer set should be used for each Berinert vial.

14. Do not refrigerate after reconstitution. When reconstitution is carried out using aseptic technique, administration may begin within 8 hours, provided the solution has been stored at up to 25°C (77°F). Do not refrigerate or freeze the reconstituted solution. Only store the reconstituted product in the vial.

Table 4: Summary of Adverse Reactions* by Type of Attack (Safety subject Population)

Overall ARs	Abdominal (n=51)	Peripheral (n=30)	Laryngeal (n=16)	Facial (n=21)	Other (n=3)
Subjects with ARs	17 (33.3%)	7 (23.3%)	2 (12.5%)	0 (0)	0 (0)
Subjects with serious ARs	1 (2.0%)	0 (0)	0 (0)	0 (0)	0 (0)
Study medication permanently discontinued due to ARs	1 (2.0%)	0 (0)	0 (0)	0 (0)	0 (0)
Most frequent ARs (≥3 subjects overall)					
Headache	5 (9.8%)	0 (0)	0 (0)	0 (0)	0 (0)
Nasopharyngitis	1 (2.0%)	2 (6.7%)	0 (0)	0 (0)	0 (0)
Other ARs (<3 subjects overall)					
Abdominal discomfort	0 (0)	1 (3.3%)	0 (0)	0 (0)	0 (0)
Dizziness	1 (2.0%)	0 (0)	0 (0)	0 (0)	0 (0)
Dry mouth	0 (0)	1 (3.3%)	0 (0)	0 (0)	0 (0)
Erythema infectiosum	1 (2.0%)	0 (0)	0 (0)	0 (0)	0 (0)
Headache	1 (2.0%)	0 (0)	0 (0)	0 (0)	0 (0)
Infusion-related reaction	1 (2.0%)	0 (0)	0 (0)	0 (0)	0 (0)
Influenza like illness	1 (2.0%)	0 (0)	1 (6.3%)	0 (0)	0 (0)
Pruritus	0 (0)	1 (3.3%)	0 (0)	0 (0)	0 (0)
Rash	0 (0)	1 (3.3%)	0 (0)	0 (0)	0 (0)

N = number of subjects

Only ARs associated with attacks of the respective subgroups were included in the analysis.

* Because of the allowance of rescue medication in both study arms, all listed adverse events were considered to be at least potentially related to study medication (eg, adverse reactions), regardless of the investigator's opinion concerning causality.

Continued on next page

plement component 1 (C1r), C1s, coagulation factor XIIa, and kallikrein. Additionally, C1 esterase inhibitor is the main inhibitor for coagulation factor XIa of the intrinsic coagulation cascade.

HAE patients have low levels of endogenous or functional C1 esterase inhibitor. Although the events that induce attacks of angioedema in HAE patients are not well defined, it has been postulated that increased vascular permeability and the clinical manifestation of HAE attacks may be primarily mediated through contact system activation. Suppression of contact system activation by C1 esterase inhibitor through the inactivation of plasma kallikrein and factor XIIa is thought to modulate this vascular permeability by preventing the generation of bradykinin.[5]

Administration of Berinert to patients with C1 esterase inhibitor deficiency replaces the missing or malfunctioning protein in patients. The plasma concentration of C1 esterase inhibitor in healthy volunteers is approximately 270 mg/L.[6]

12.3 Pharmacokinetics

The pharmacokinetics of Berinert were evaluated in an open-label, uncontrolled, single-center study in 40 subjects (35 adults and 5 children under 16 years of age) with either mild or severe HAE. All subjects received a single intravenous injection of Berinert ranging from 500 IU to 1500 IU. Blood samples were taken during an attack-free period at baseline and for up to 72 hours after drug administration. Pharmacokinetic parameters were estimated using non-compartmental analysis (with or without baseline adjustment). Table 6 summarizes the pharmacokinetic parameters in 35 adult subjects with HAE.

Table 6: Pharmacokinetic Parameters of Berinert in Adult subjects with HAE by Non-compartmental Analysis (n=35)

Parameters	Unadjusted for baseline	Adjusted for baseline
$AUC_{(0-t)}$ (hr × IU/mL)*	27.5 ± 8.5 (15.7-44.7)	12.8 ± 6.7 (3.9-34.7)
CL (mL/hr/kg)	0.60 ± 0.17 (0.34-0.96)	1.44 ± 0.67 (0.43-3.85)
V_{ss} (mL/kg)	18.6 ± 4.9 (11.1-27.6)	35.4 ± 10.5 (14.1-56.1)
Half-life (hrs)	21.9 ± 1.7 (16.5-24.4)	18.4 ± 3.5 (7.4-22.8)
MRT (hrs)	31.5 ± 2.4 (23.7-35.2)	26.4 ± 5.0 (10.7-33.0)

AUC: Area under the curve
CL: Clearance
V_{ss}: Volume steady state
MRT: Mean residence time
* Based on a 15 IU/kg dose. Numbers in parenthesis are the range.

Table 7 summarizes the pharmacokinetic parameters in 5 pediatric subjects (ages 6 through 13) with HAE. When adjusted for baseline, compared to adults, the half-life of Berinert was shorter and clearance (on per kg basis) was faster in this limited cohort of children. However, the clinical implication of this difference is not known.

Table 7: Pharmacokinetic Parameters of Berinert in Pediatric subjects (n=5)* with HAE by Non-compartmental Analysis

Parameters	Unadjusted for baseline	Adjusted for baseline
$AUC_{(0-t)}$ (hr × IU/mL)†	25.45 ± 5.8 (16.8-31.7)	9.78 ± 4.37 (4.1-15.2)
CL (mL/hr/kg)	0.62 ± 0.17 (0.47-0.89)	1.9 ± 1.1 (0.98-3.69)
V_{ss} (mL/kg)	19.8 ± 4.0 (16.7-26.1)	38.8 ± 8.9 (31.9-54.0)
Half-life (hrs)	22.4 ± 1.6 (20.3-24.4)	16.7 ± 5.8 (7.4-22.5)
MRT (hrs)	32.3 ± 2.3 (29.3-35.2)	24.0 ± 8.3 (10.7-32.4)

AUC: Area under the curve
CL: Clearance
V_{ss}: Volume steady state
MRT: Mean residence time
* Age Range: 6-13 years
† Based on a 15 IU/kg dose. Numbers in parenthesis are the range.

1. Ensure that the BERINERT vial and diluent vial are at room temperature.

2. Place the BERINERT vial, diluent vial and Mix2Vial transfer set on a flat surface.

3. Remove the flip caps from the BERINERT and diluent vials. Wipe the vial stoppers with the alcohol swab provided. Allow to dry prior to opening the Mix2Vial transfer set package.

4. Open the Mix2Vial transfer set package by peeling away the lid (Figure 1). Leave the Mix2Vial transfer set in the clear package.

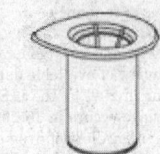
Figure 1

5. Place the diluent vial on a flat surface and hold the vial tightly. Grip the Mix2Vial transfer set together with the clear package and push the plastic spike at the blue end of the Mix2Vial transfer set firmly through the center of the stopper of the diluent vial (Figure 2).

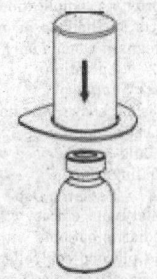
Figure 2

6. Carefully remove the clear package from the Mix2Vial transfer set. Make sure that you pull up only the clear package, and not the Mix2Vial transfer set (Figure 3).

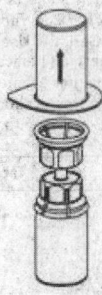
Figure 3

7. With the BERINERT vial placed firmly on a flat surface, invert the diluent vial with the Mix2Vial transfer set attached and push the plastic spike of the transparent adapter firmly through the center of the stopper of the BERINERT vial (Figure 4). The diluent will automatically transfer into the BERINERT vial.

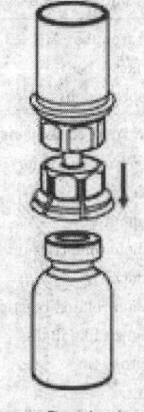
Figure 4

This table is continued on the next page

8. With the diluent and BERINERT vial still attached to the Mix2Vial transfer set, gently swirl the BERINERT vial to ensure that the BERINERT is fully dissolved (Figure 5). Do not shake the vial.

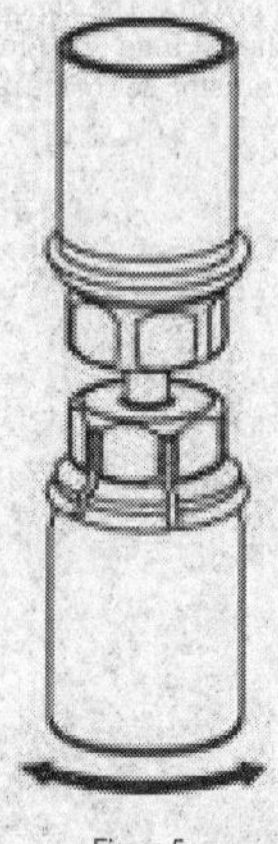

Figure 5

9. With one hand, grasp the BERINERT-side of the Mix2Vial transfer set and with the other hand grasp the blue diluent-side of the Mix2Vial transfer set and unscrew the set into two pieces (Figure 6).

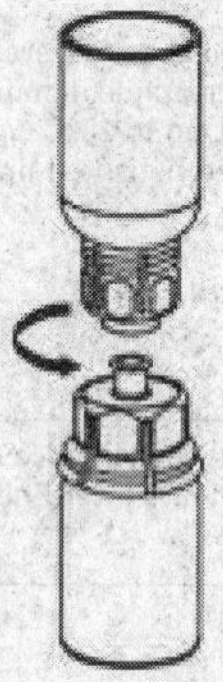

Figure 6

10. Carefully look at reconstituted solution in each vial of BERINERT. It should be colorless, clear, and free from visible particles. **Do not use the vial if** the liquid looks cloudy, contains particles, or has changed color. Do not use if the expiration date on the label has expired.

11. Draw air into an empty, sterile syringe. Use a silicone-free syringe. While the BERINERT vial is upright, screw the syringe to the Mix2Vial transfer set. Inject air into the BERINERT vial. While keeping the syringe plunger pressed, invert the system upside down and draw the concentrate into the syringe by pulling the plunger back slowly (Figure 7).

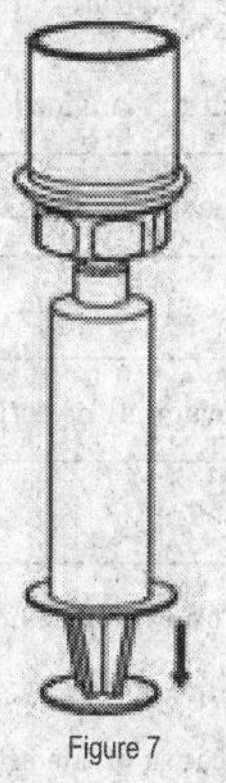

Figure 7

This table is continued on the next page

Studies have not been conducted to evaluate the pharmacokinetics of Berinert in special patient populations identified by gender, race, geriatric age, or the presence of renal or hepatic impairment.

13 NONCLINICAL TOXICOLOGY

13.1 Carcinogenesis, Mutagenesis, Impairment of Fertility

No animal studies have been completed to evaluate the effects of Berinert on carcinogenesis, mutagenesis, and impairment of fertility.

13.2 Animal Toxicology and/or Pharmacology

Acute intravenous toxicity of Berinert was performed in mice at 1500, 3000, and 6000 IU/kg and in rats at 1000, 2000, and 3000 IU/kg. Berinert was well tolerated and no signs of toxicity were observed up to the highest dose administered.

Repeat intravenous dose toxicity was studied in a 14-day repeat dose study in rats at doses of 20, 60, and 200 IU/kg/day. Berinert was well tolerated and no toxicity was observed up to the highest dose administered. No antibody response against C1 esterase inhibitor could be demonstrated in this study after multiple dosing with Berinert.

In a safety pharmacology study, Berinert was administered to beagle dogs intravenously at a cumulative dose of 3500 IU/kg. No adverse effects were seen on the cardiovascular and respiratory system. There was a drop in body temperature, reduced coagulation time, and a decrease in thrombocyte aggregation.

Local intravenous tolerance of Berinert was evaluated in rabbits at 1500 IU. No pathological changes were noted at the time of injection or during the following 24 hours. No pathological signs were noted during necropsy.

A study in pigs investigating cardioprotective effects of C1 esterase inhibitor suggests a risk of thrombosis from intravenous administration of C1 esterase inhibitor products at doses of 200 IU/kg; however, in this model, cardioprotective effects were observed at a dose of 40 IU/kg.[2]

14 CLINICAL STUDIES

The safety and efficacy of Berinert in the treatment of acute abdominal or facial attacks in subjects with hereditary angioedema were demonstrated in a placebo-controlled, double-blind, prospective, multinational, randomized, parallel-group, dose-finding, three-arm, clinical study, referred to as the randomized clinical trial (RCT). The RCT assessed the efficacy and safety of Berinert in 124 adult and pediatric subjects with C1 esterase inhibitor deficiency who were experiencing an acute moderate to severe attack of abdominal or facial HAE. Subjects ranged in age from six to 72 years of age; 67.7% were female and 32.3% were male; and approximately 90% were Caucasian.

The study objectives were to evaluate whether Berinert shortens the time to onset of relief of symptoms of an abdominal or facial attack compared to placebo and to compare the efficacy of two different doses of Berinert. The time to onset of relief of symptoms was determined by the subject's response to a standard question posed at appropriate time intervals for as long as 24 hours after start of treatment, taking into account all single HAE symptoms. In addition the severity of individual HAE symptoms was assessed over time.

Subjects were randomized to receive a single 10 IU/kg body weight dose of Berinert (39 subjects), a single 20 IU/kg dose of Berinert (43 subjects), or a single dose of placebo (42 subjects) by slow intravenous infusion (recommended to be given at a rate of approximately 4 mL per minute) within 5 hours of an HAE attack. At least 70% of the subjects in each treatment group were required to be experiencing an abdominal attack.

If a subject experienced no relief or insufficient relief of symptoms by 4 hours after infusion, investigators had the option to administer a second infusion of Berinert (20 IU/kg for the placebo group, 10 IU/kg for the 10 IU/kg group), or placebo (for the 20 IU/kg group). This masked (blinded) "rescue study medication" was administered to subjects and they were then followed until complete resolution of symptoms was achieved. Adverse events were collected for up to 7 to 9 days following the initial administration of Berinert or placebo.

In the rare case that a subject developed life-threatening laryngeal edema after inclusion into the study, immediate start of open-label treatment with a 20 IU/kg body weight dose of Berinert was allowed.

Continued on next page

All subjects who received confounding medication (rescue medication) before symptom relief were regarded as "non-responders". Therefore, time to onset of symptom relief was set at 24 hours if a subject received any rescue medication (ie, rescue study medication, narcotic analgesics, non-narcotic analgesics, anti-emetics, open-label C1 inhibitor, androgens at increased dose, or fresh frozen plasma) between 5 hours before administration of blinded study medication until time to onset of relief.

For the trial to be considered successful, the study protocol specified the following criteria for the differences between the Berinert 20 IU/kg and the placebo group:

• The time to onset of relief of symptoms of the HAE attack had to achieve a one-sided p-value of less than 0.0249 for the final analysis, and at least one of the following criteria had to demonstrate a trend in favor of Berinert with a one-sided p-value of less than 0.1:
  ◦ The proportion of subjects with increased intensity of clinical HAE symptoms between 2 and 4 hours after start of treatment with study medication compared to baseline, or
  ◦ The number of vomiting episodes within 4 hours after start of study treatment.

Subjects treated with 20 IU/kg body weight of Berinert experienced a significant reduction (p=0.0016; "Wilcoxon Rank Sum test") in time to onset of relief from symptoms of an HAE attack as compared to placebo (median of 48 minutes for Berinert 20 IU/kg body weight, as compared to a median of >4 hours for placebo). The time to onset of relief from symptoms of an HAE attack for subjects in the 10 IU/kg dose of Berinert was not statistically significantly different from that of subjects in the placebo group.

Figure 9 is a Kaplan-Meier curve showing the percentage of subjects reporting onset of relief of HAE attack symptoms as a function of time. Individual time points beyond 4 hours are not presented on the graph, because the protocol permitted blinded rescue medication, analgesics, and/or anti-emetics to be administered starting 4 hours after randomized blinded study medication had been administered.

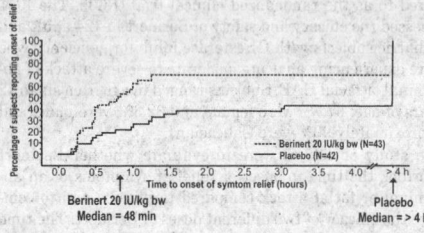

Figure 9: Time to Onset of Symptom Relief with Imputation to >4 hours for subjects Who Received any Rescue Medication* or Non-narcotic Analgesics Before Start of Relief

* Included rescue study medication (as blinded C1 inhibitor or placebo given as rescue medication), open-label C1 inhibitor, narcotic and non-narcotic analgesics, anti-emetics, androgens at increased dose, or fresh frozen plasma.

In addition, the efficacy of Berinert 20 IU/kg body weight could be confirmed by observing a reduction in the intensity of single HAE symptoms at an earlier time compared to placebo. For abdominal attacks Figure 10 shows the time to start of relief of the *last* symptom to improve that was already present at baseline. Pre-defined abdominal HAE symptoms included pain, nausea, vomiting, cramps and diarrhea. Figure 11 shows the respective time to start of relief of the *first* symptom to improve that was already present at baseline.

[See Figures 10 and 11 on next page]

For facial attacks, single HAE symptoms were recorded. In addition, photos were taken at pre-determined time points and assessed by the members of an independent Data Safety Monitoring Board (DSMB), who were blinded as to treatment, center and other outcome measures. The change in the severity of the edema when compared to baseline was assessed on a scale with outcomes "no change", "better", "worse" and "resolved". Figure 12 shows the time to start of relief from serial facial photographs by DSMB assessment.

[See Figure 12 on next page]

Table 8 compares additional endpoints, including changes in HAE symptoms and use of rescue medication in subjects receiving Berinert at 20 IU/kg body weight and placebo.

12. Now that the concentrate has been transferred into the syringe, firmly grasp the barrel of the syringe (keeping the plunger facing down) and unscrew the syringe from the Mix2Vial transfer set (Figure 8). Attach the syringe to a suitable intravenous administration set.

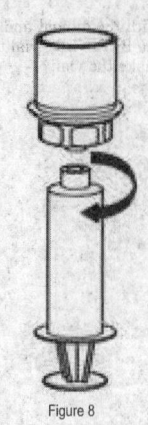

Figure 8

13. If patient is to receive more than one vial, pool the contents of multiple vials into one syringe. A new unused Mix2Vial transfer set should be used for each BERINERT vial.

14. Do not refrigerate after reconstitution. When reconstitution is carried out using aseptic technique, administration may begin within 8 hours, provided the solution has been stored at up to 25°C (77°F). Do not refrigerate or freeze the reconstituted solution. Only store the reconstituted product in the vial.

Table 3: Incidence of subjects and Attacks with Adverse Reactions (ARs)* Starting during Infusion or Within 24 hours or 72 hours after End of an Infusion (Experienced by ≥2 subjects or Associated with ≥5 Attacks Overall) by Preferred Term (Safety subject and Attack Populations)

Preferred term	Number (%) of subjects (n=57)		Number (%) of Attacks (n=1085)	
	ARs within 24 hours	ARs within 72 hours	ARs within 24 hours	ARs within 72 hours
Any preferred term	**13 (22.8%)**	**20 (35.1%)**	**27 (2.5%)**	**41 (3.8%)**
Headache	2 (3.5%)	4 (7.0%)	3 (0.3%)	6 (0.6%)
Nasopharyngitis	1 (1.8%)	2 (3.5%)	1 (<0.1%)	2 (0.2%)
Abdominal pain or discomfort	1 (1.8%)	3 (5.3%)	2 (0.2%)	6 (0.6%)
Upper respiratory tract infection	0 (0)	1 (1.8%)	0 (0)	1 (<0.1%)
Hereditary angioedema†	1 (1.8%)	1 (1.8%)	1 (<0.1%)	1 (<0.1%)
Influenza like illness	1 (1.8%)	2 (3.5%)	1 (<0.1%)	2 (0.2%)
Rash	2 (3.5%)	2 (3.5%)	2 (0.2%)	2 (0.2%)
Vulvovaginal mycotic infection	0 (0)	2 (3.5%)	0 (0)	2 (0.2%)
Nausea	1 (1.8%)	1 (1.8%)	4 (0.4%)	5 (0.5%)

N = total number of subjects/attacks

Data are sorted by decreasing frequency by number of subjects.

* Because of the allowance of rescue medication in both study arms, all listed adverse events were considered to be at least potentially related to study medication (eg, adverse reactions), regardless of the investigator's opinion concerning causality.

† Hereditary angioedema attacks were only to be reported as adverse reaction if it was a worsening of symptoms during a treated attack. New attacks were not to be reported as adverse reactions. Although the adverse reaction of hereditary angioedema in subject 22301 was a new attack that started after the previous attack had completely resolved, this attack was reported as an adverse reaction, because the attack was not included in the study and treated outside study site with medication other than the study medication.

Step 1: Assemble supplies
Gather the BERINERT syringe, the following disposable supplies (not provided with BERINERT), and other items (sharps or other container, treatment diary or log book):
- Standard butterfly catheter infusion set (IV administration set with winged adapter and needle)
- Sterile syringe (Use a silicone-free syringe).
- Tourniquet
- Sterile gauze and tape, or transparent dressing
- Bandage (adhesive dressing)
- Gloves (if recommended by your healthcare provider)
- Alcohol wipe for cleaning the skin

Step 2: Wash hands
- Thoroughly wash and dry your hands.
- If you have been told to wear gloves when preparing your infusion, put the gloves on.

Step 3: Clean surface
Thoroughly clean a table or other flat surface using one or more of the alcohol wipes.

Step 4: Prime the infusion set
As instructed by your healthcare provider:
- To prime (fill) the infusion tubing, connect the syringe filled with BERINERT to the infusion set tubing and gently push on the syringe plunger to fill the tubing with BERINERT (Figure 9).

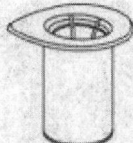

Figure 1

Step 5: Prepare the infusion site
- Apply a tourniquet above the site of the infusion.
- Prepare the infusion site by wiping the skin well with an alcohol swab and allow it to dry (Figure 10).

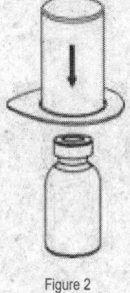

Figure 2

This table is continued on the next page

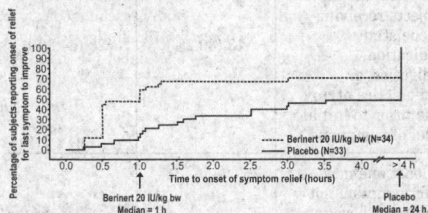

Figure 10: Time to Start of Relief of the *Last* Symptom to Improve (Abdominal Attacks) with Imputation to >4 hours for subjects Who Received any Rescue Medication* Before Start of Relief

* Included rescue study medication (as blinded C1 inhibitor or placebo given as rescue medication), open-label C1 inhibitor, narcotic and non-narcotic analgesics, anti-emetics, androgens at increased dose, or fresh frozen plasma.

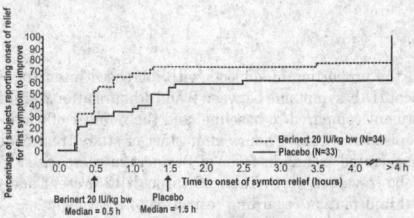

Figure 11: Time to Start of Relief of the *First* Symptom to Improve (Abdominal Attacks) with Imputation to >4 hours for subjects Who Received Any Rescue Medication* Before Start of Relief

* Included rescue study medication (as blinded C1 inhibitor or placebo given as rescue medication), open-label C1 inhibitor, narcotic and non-narcotic analgesics, anti-emetics, androgens at increased dose, or fresh frozen plasma.

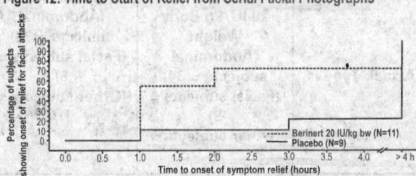

Figure 12: Time to Start of Relief from Serial Facial Photographs*

* Includes facial attacks in subjects with concomitant abdominal attacks.

Table 5: Mean Virus Inactivation/Reductions in Berinert

Virus Studied	Pasteurization [$\log_{10}$]	Hydrophobic Interaction Chromatography [$\log_{10}$]	Virus Filtration [$\log_{10}$]	Total Cumulative [$\log_{10}$]
Enveloped Viruses				
HIV-1	≥6.6	≥4.5	≥5.1	≥16.2
BVDV	≥9.2	≥4.7	≥5.3	≥19.2
PRV	6.3	≥6.5	≥7.1	≥19.9
WNV	≥7.0	ND	≥8.0	≥15.0
Non-Enveloped Viruses				
HAV	≥6.4	2.8	≥5.3	≥14.5
CPV	1.4	6.4	≥7.2	≥15.0
B19V	3.9	ND	ND	NA

HIV-1, Human immunodeficiency virus type 1, a model for HIV-1 and HIV-2
BVDV, Bovine viral diarrhea virus, a model for HCV
PRV, Pseudorabies virus, a model for large enveloped DNA viruses
WNV, West Nile virus
HAV, Hepatitis A virus
CPV, Canine parvovirus
B19V, Human Parvovirus B19
ND, Not determined
NA, Not applicable

Table 8: Changes in HAE Symptoms and Use of Rescue Medication in subjects Receiving Berinert 20 IU/kg Body Weight vs. Placebo

Additional Endpoints	Number (%) of subjects Berinert 20 IU/kg Body Weight Group (n=43)	Number (%) of subjects Placebo Group (n=42)
Onset of symptom relief within 60 minutes after administration of study medication *(post-hoc)*	27 (62.8%)	11 (26.2%)
Onset of symptom relief within 4 hours after administration of study medication	30 (69.8%)	18 (42.9%)
Number of vomiting episodes within 4 hours after start of study treatment*	6 episodes	35 episodes
Worsened intensity of clinical HAE symptoms between 2 and 4 hours after administration of study medication compared to baseline†	0 (0%)	12 (28.6%)

Continued on next page

	Berinert 20 IU/kg	Placebo
Number (percent) of combined abdominal and facial attack subjects receiving rescue study medication, analgesics, or anti-emetics at any time prior to initial relief of symptoms	13 (30.2%)	23 (54.8%)
At least one new HAE symptom not present at baseline and starting within 4 hours after administration of study medication	2 (4.6%)	6 (14.3%)

* p-value = 0.033
† p-value = 0.00008

Both the proportion of subjects with increased intensity of clinical HAE symptoms between 2 and 4 hours after start of treatment compared to baseline, and the number of vomiting episodes within 4 hours after start of study treatment demonstrated trends in favor of Berinert in comparison to placebo (p-values <0.1). Tables 9 through 12 present additional information regarding responses to treatment.

Table 9: Proportion of subjects Experiencing Start of Self-Reported Relief of Symptoms by 4 hours by Attack Type

Attack Type	Berinert 20 IU/kg Body Weight (Abdominal subjects = 34) (Facial subjects = 9) (Other subjects = 0)	Placebo Group (Abdominal subjects = 33) (Facial subjects = 8) (Other subjects = 1)*
Abdominal	24 (70.6%)	15 (45.5%)
Facial	6 (66.7%)	3 (37.5%)

* Laryngeal edema initially classified as facial edema.

Table 10: Proportion of subjects Experiencing Reduction in Severity of at Least One Individual HAE Attack Symptom by 4 hours

Attack Type	Berinert 20 IU/kg Body Weight (Abdominal subjects = 34) (Facial subjects = 9)	Placebo Group (Abdominal subjects = 33) (Facial subjects = 8)
Abdominal	33 (97.1%)	29 (87.9%)
Facial	6 (66.7%)	4 (50%)

Table 11: Proportion of subjects with Facial Attacks Demonstrating Improvement in Serial Facial Photographs by 4 hours*

Attack Type	Berinert 20 IU/kg Body Weight (Subjects = 9)	Placebo Group (Subjects = 8)
Facial	7 (77.8%)	2 (25%)

* Based on masked (blinded) evaluation by data safety monitoring board.

Table 12: Proportion of subjects with Abdominal and Facial Attacks Receiving Rescue Study Medication at any Time Prior to Complete Relief of Symptoms

Attack Type	Berinert 20 IU/kg Body Weight (Abdominal subjects = 34) (Facial subjects = 9)	Placebo Group (Abdominal subjects = 33) (Facial subjects = 8)
Abdominal	7 (20.6%)	17 (51.5%)
Facial	1 (11.1%)	6 (75%)

No subjects treated with Berinert at 20 IU/kg body weight reported worsening of symptoms at 4 hours after administration of study medication compared to baseline.

Step 6: Infusion
As instructed by your healthcare provider:
• Insert the butterfly needle of the infusion set tubing into your vein (Figure 11).
• If necessary, use sterile gauze and tape or transparent dressing to hold the needle in place.
• To make sure that the needle is in a vein, gently pull back on the syringe plunger and check to see if blood is in the tubing (Figure 12). If there is blood present, then the needle is in a vein. If there is no blood present, remove the needle and repeat this step using a new needle, new administration tubing, and a different injection site.
• Remove the tourniquet.
• Inject the BERINERT solution slowly at a rate of approximately 4 mL per minute (Figure 13).

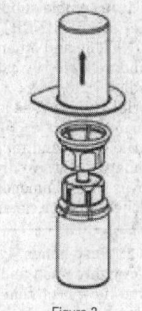

Figure 3

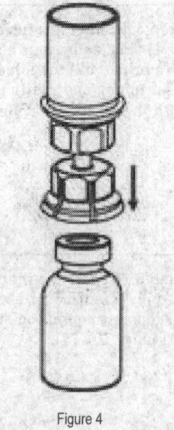

Figure 4

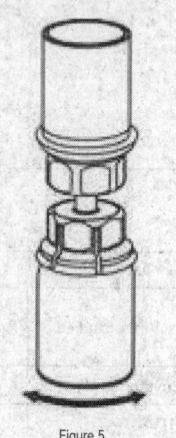

Figure 5

This table is continued on the next page

The study demonstrated that the Berinert 20 IU/kg body weight dose was significantly more efficacious than the Berinert 10 IU/kg body weight dose or placebo.
Open-Label Extension Study
Berinert was evaluated in a prospective, open-label, uncontrolled, multicenter extension study conducted at 15 centers in the US and Canada in subjects who had participated in the RCT study for the treatment of acute abdominal or facial attacks in subjects with hereditary angioedema.
The purpose of this extension study was to provide Berinert to subjects who had participated in the RCT study and who experienced any type of subsequent HAE attack (ie, abdominal, facial, peripheral, or laryngeal).
The safety analysis of the open-label extension study included a total of 57 subjects (19 males and 38 females, age range: 10 to 53 years) with 1085 HAE attacks treated with 20 IU/kg body weight dose of Berinert per attack, who were observed at the study site until onset of relief of HAE symptoms, and were followed up for adverse reactions for 7 to 9

days following treatment of each HAE attack *[see Adverse Reactions (6.1)].* During the extension study, 51 subjects experienced 747 abdominal attacks, 21 subjects experienced 51 facial attacks, 30 subjects experienced 235 peripheral attacks, and 16 subjects experienced 48 laryngeal attacks. Some study subjects may have experienced HAE attacks in more than one location.

An analysis of laryngeal HAE attacks showed that the median time to initial onset of symptom relief and median time to complete resolution in the per-attack analysis were 0.25 hours and 8.4 hours, respectively (Table 13), which were the shortest times among the various attack locations.

Table 13: Time to Initial Onset of Symptom Relief and Time to Complete Resolution of HAE Symptoms for Laryngeal Attacks

Statistic	Laryngeal (n=48)
Time to initial onset of symptom relief [hours]	
Median (range)	0.25 (0.10 - 1.25)
95% CI for median	[0.23; 0.42]
Time to complete resolution of HAE symptoms [hours]	
Median (range)	8.4 (0.6 - 61.8*)
95% CI for median	[6.2; 21.5]

CI = confidence interval
HAE = hereditary angioedema
N = number of attacks
* The maximum time to complete resolution of 61.8 hours was an imputed value. subject 29301 had 2 laryngeal attacks with missing times to complete resolution of HAE symptoms, which were imputed with the maximum time to complete resolution of HAE symptoms observed for an abdominal attack in this subject.

There were no clinically relevant or consistent data suggesting that gender, age group, race/ethnic group, type of HAE, routine use of androgens, or presence of detectable anti-C1 Esterase Inhibitor antibodies had an effect on the time to initial or complete relief of symptoms following Berinert.

The prospective open-label extension study demonstrated that, in comparison to untreated historical control data retrospectively collected at a study center in Germany over a 20 year period[7], the Berinert 20 IU/kg body weight dose appeared to be effective in ameliorating laryngeal HAE attacks by achieving complete resolution of HAE symptoms within 24 hours from attack onset in the majority of subjects. The treatment effects observed with Berinert in the extension study are consistent with the findings from the placebo-controlled efficacy trial.

15 REFERENCES

1. German Medical Profession's Drugs Committee. Severe thrombus formation of Berinert® HS. *Deutsches Ärzteblatt.* 2000;97:B-864.
2. Horstick, G *et al.* Application of C1-Esterase Inhibitor During Reperfusion of Ischemic Myocardium: Dose-Related Beneficial Versus Detrimental Effects. *Circulation.* 2001;104:3125-3131.
3. Carrell RW, Boswell DR. Serpins: the superfamily of plasma serine proteinase inhibitors. In: Barrett A, Salvesen G, eds. *Proteinase Inhibitors.* Amsterdam: Elsevier. 1986;12:403-420.
4. Harrison RA. Human C1 inhibitor: Improved isolation and preliminary structural characterization. *Biochemistry* 1983;22:5001-5007.
5. Davis AE, The pathophysiology of hereditary angioedema. *Clin Immunol.* 2005;114:3-9.
6. Nuijens JH, Eerenberg-Belmer AJM, Huijbregts CCM, et al. Proteolytic inactivation of plasma C1 inhibitor in sepsis. *J Clin Invest.* 1989;84:443-450.
7. Bork K, Barnstedt SE. Treatment of 193 Episodes of Laryngeal Edema with C1 Inhibitor Concentrate in Patients with Hereditary Angioedema. *Arch Intern Med.* 2001;161:714-718.

16 HOW SUPPLIED/STORAGE AND HANDLING

16.1 How Supplied

- Berinert is supplied in a single-use vial.
- 500 IU vial of Berinert for reconstitution with 10 mL of Sterile Water for Injection, USP.
- The components used in the packaging for Berinert are latex-free.

Each product presentation includes a package insert and the following components:

[See table at top of next page]

Step 7: Clean up

- After infusing the entire amount of BERINERT, remove the infusion set (Figure 14) and cover the infusion site with a bandage (Figure 15), holding pressure on the site for a few minutes.
- Dispose of all unused solution, the empty vials, and the used needles and syringe in an appropriate container used for throwing away waste that might hurt others if not handled properly.

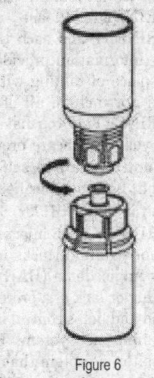

Figure 6

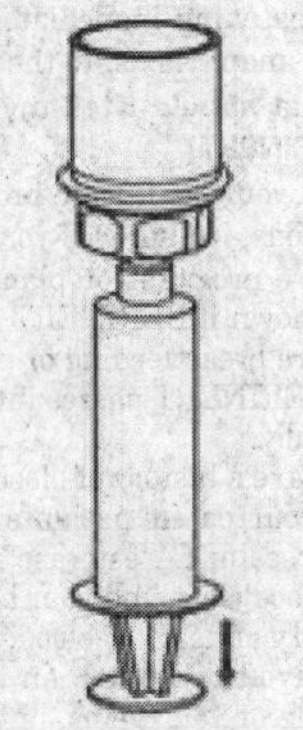

Figure 7

Step 8: Record treatment

- Record the lot number from the BERINERT vial label in your treatment diary or log book with the date and time of infusion every time you use BERINERT.

16.2 Storage and Handling

- When stored at temperatures of 2-25°C (36-77°F), Berinert is stable for the period indicated by the expiration date on the carton and vial label (up to 30 months).
- Keep Berinert in its original carton until ready to use.
- Do not freeze.
- Protect from light.

17 PATIENT COUNSELING INFORMATION

See FDA-approved patient labeling (Patient Product Information).

Inform patients to immediately report the following to their physician:

- Signs and symptoms of allergic hypersensitivity reactions, such as hives, urticaria, tightness of the chest, wheezing, hypotension and/or anaphylaxis experienced during or after injection of Berinert *[see Warnings and Precautions (5.1)]*
- Signs and symptoms of a thromboembolic event including pain and/or swelling of an arm or leg with warmth over the affected area, discoloration of an arm or leg, unexplained shortness of breath, chest pain or discomfort that worsens on deep breathing, unexplained rapid pulse, numbness or weakness on one side of the body. Advise patients with known risk factors for thromboembolic events that they are at an increased risk for these events *[see Warnings and Precautions (5.2)].*
- Advise female patients to notify their physician if they become pregnant or intend to become pregnant during the treatment of acute abdominal or facial attacks of HAE with Berinert.
- Advise patients to notify their physician if they are breastfeeding or plan to breastfeed.
- Advise patients to consult with their healthcare professional prior to travel.
- Advise patients/caregivers to bring an adequate supply of Berinert when traveling.
- Advise patients to bring Berinert with them when they visit a healthcare provider/facility for an acute HAE attack.
- Advise patients that, because Berinert is made from human blood, it may carry a risk of transmitting infectious agents, eg, viruses, and, theoretically, the Creutzfeldt-Jakob (CJD) agent *[see Warnings and Precautions (5.3) and Description (11)].* Inform patients of the risks and benefits of Berinert before prescribing or administering it to the patient.

Self-administration — Ensure that the patient (or caregiver) is an appropriate candidate for self-administration, this includes, but not limited to a determination that:

- The patient (or caregiver) is reliably able to recognize the signs and symptoms of their HAE attacks.
- The patient (or caregiver) has the necessary dexterity and comprehension to be trained to self-administer.

If self-administration is deemed appropriate, ensure that the patient/caregiver receives clear instructions and training on intravenous administration in the home or other appropriate setting and has demonstrated the ability to perform intravenous infusions.

- Ensure the patients/caregivers understand the importance of not starting self-administration if the attack (regardless of type) has progressed to a point that the patient/caregiver would be unable to successfully prepare or administer Berinert.
- Given the potential for airway obstruction during acute laryngeal HAE attacks, patients self-administering Berinert should be advised to immediately seek medical attention in an appropriate healthcare facility in addition to treatment with Berinert.
- To help exclude the possibility that another potentially serious medical cause may be responsible for their symptoms, advise patients self-administering Berinert to contact their healthcare provider after treating suspected abdominal HAE attacks.
- Instruct patients/caregivers to record the lot number from the Berinert vial label every time they use Berinert.

The attached BERINERT "Patient Product Information (PPI)" contains more detailed instructions for patients/caregivers who will be self-administering BERINERT.

FDA-Approved Patient Labeling – Patient Product Information (PPI)

BERINERT (BEAR-i-nert)

C1 Esterase Inhibitor (Human)

Freeze-Dried Powder for Reconstitution

Continued on next page

This leaflet summarizes important information about BERINERT. Please read it carefully before using BERINERT and each time you get a refill. There may be new information provided. This information does not take the place of talking with your healthcare provider, and it does not include all of the important information about BERINERT. If you have any questions after reading this, ask your healthcare provider.

Do not attempt to self-administer unless you have been taught how by your healthcare provider.

What is BERINERT?

BERINERT is an injectable medicine used to treat swelling and/or painful attacks in adults and children with Hereditary Angioedema (HAE). HAE is caused by the poor functioning or lack of a protein called C1 that is present in your blood and helps control inflammation (swelling) and parts of the immune system. BERINERT contains C1 esterase inhibitor, a protein that helps control C1.

Who should not use BERINERT?

You should not use BERINERT if you have experienced life-threatening immediate hypersensitivity reactions, including anaphylaxis, to the product.

What should I tell my healthcare provider before using BERINERT?

Tell your healthcare provider about all of your medical conditions, including if you:
- Are pregnant or planning to become pregnant. It is not known if BERINERT can harm your unborn baby.
- Are breastfeeding or plan to breastfeed. It is not known if BERINERT passes into your milk and if it can harm your baby.
- Have a history of blood clotting problems. Blood clots have occurred in patients receiving BERINERT. Very high doses of C1 esterase inhibitor could increase the risk of blood clots. Tell your healthcare provider if you have a history of heart or blood vessel disease, stroke, blood clots, or have thick blood, an indwelling catheter/access device in one of your veins, or have been immobile for some time. These things may increase your risk of having a blood clot after using BERINERT. Also, tell your healthcare provider what drugs you are using, as some drugs, such as birth control pills or certain androgens, may increase your risk of developing a blood clot.

Tell your healthcare provider and pharmacist about all of the medicines you take, including all prescription and non-prescription medicines such as over-the-counter medicines, supplements, or herbal remedies.

What are the possible side effects of BERINERT?

Allergic reactions may occur with BERINERT. Call your healthcare provider or seek emergency support services right away if you have any of the following symptoms after using BERINERT:
- **wheezing**
- **difficulty breathing**
- **chest tightness**
- **turning blue (look at lips and gums)**
- **fast heartbeat**
- **swelling of the face**
- **faintness**
- **rash**
- **hives**

Signs of a blood clot include:
- pain and/or swelling of an arm or leg with warmth over the affected area
- discoloration of an arm or leg
- unexplained shortness of breath
- chest pain or discomfort that worsens on deep breathing
- unexplained rapid pulse
- numbness or weakness on one side of the body

In clinical studies, the most serious adverse reaction reported in subjects who received BERINERT was an increase in the severity of pain associated with HAE.

In clinical studies, the most common adverse reaction reported among subjects who received BERINERT in the placebo-controlled clinical trial was dysgeusia (bad taste in mouth).

Because BERINERT is made from human blood, it may carry a risk of transmitting infectious agents, eg, viruses, and, theoretically, the Creutzfeldt-Jakob (CJD) agent.

These are not all the possible side effects of BERINERT.

Tell your healthcare provider about any side effect that bothers you or that does not go away. You can also report side effects to the FDA at 1-800-FDA-1088.

How should I store BERINERT?
- Keep BERINERT in its original carton to protect from light until ready to use.

Presentation	Carton NDC Number	Components
500 IU	63833-825-02	• Berinert in a single-use vial [NDC 63833-835-01] • 10 mL vial of Sterile Water for Injection, USP [NDC 63833-765-15] • Mix2Vial filter transfer set • Alcohol swab

- When stored at temperatures of 2-25°C (36-77°F), BERINERT is stable for the period indicated by the expiration date on the carton and vial label.
- Do not freeze.

What else should I know about BERINERT?

Medicines are sometimes prescribed for purposes other than those listed here. Do not use BERINERT for a condition for which it is not prescribed. Do not share BERINERT with other people, even if they have the same symptoms that you have.

This leaflet summarizes the most important information about BERINERT. If you would like more information, talk to your healthcare provider. You can ask your healthcare provider or pharmacist for information about BERINERT that was written for healthcare professionals. For more information, go to www.BERINERT.com or call 1-877-236-4423.

What are the symptoms of a facial, abdominal or laryngeal Hereditary Angioedema (HAE) attack?

Early HAE symptoms appear anywhere from minutes to one to two days before the attack worsens. HAE attacks can last hours to several days, and range in severity. Itching is not a typical feature of HAE attacks.

Facial attacks — These attacks can occur in areas around the eyes and mouth, and result from local edema of tissue beneath the skin (subcutaneous).

Abdominal attacks — These attacks appear as pain (colic), nausea, vomiting, and/or diarrhea. These symptoms result from the swelling of walls of the gastrointestinal tract.

Laryngeal attacks — Swelling of the voice box (laryngeal edema) can occur by itself, or with swelling of the lips, tongue, uvula (the piece of mouth tissue that hangs down from the top of the mouth over the back of the tongue), and soft palate (the soft tissue at the back of the mouth). Removing a tooth and oral surgery can trigger a laryngeal attack. Laryngeal swelling can develop in minutes or hours.

Many HAE attacks involve only one location of the body at a time, although combination attacks, such as cutaneous attacks that spread to involve the larynx (the voice box), can occur.

What other diseases or symptoms could resemble a HAE attack?

Some abdominal-related causes that can appear as an HAE attack include:
- Appendicitis
- Heartburn
- Gall bladder attack
- Diverticulitis
- Pancreatitis
- Stomach ulcer
- General abdominal distress

Other symptoms that can appear as an HAE attack include:
- Allergic reactions (eg, insect bites and rash)

What should I know about self-administration?
- At the first symptoms of an attack, you should immediately prepare the prescribed dose of BERINERT for self-administration.
- You should not start self-administration if the attack (regardless of type) has progressed to a point where you are unable to successfully dissolve BERINERT or to administer BERINERT.

Instructions for Use
- **Do not attempt to self-administer unless you have been taught how by your healthcare provider.**
- **See the step-by-step instructions for injecting BERINERT at the end of this leaflet.** You should always follow the specific instructions given by your healthcare provider. The steps listed below are general guidelines for using BERINERT. If you are unsure of the steps, please contact your healthcare provider or pharmacist before using.
- Your healthcare provider will prescribe the dose that you should administer, which is based on your body weight.
- After self-administering BERINERT for an acute laryngeal HAE attack, immediately seek medical attention in an appropriate healthcare facility after treatment with BERINERT.

- Contact your healthcare provider after treating suspected abdominal HAE attacks to help exclude the possibility that another potentially serious medical cause may be responsible for your symptoms.
- **Call your healthcare provider right away if swelling is not controlled after using BERINERT.**
- Bring BERINERT with you when you visit a healthcare provider/facility for an acute HAE attack.
- Talk to your healthcare provider before traveling to make sure you have an adequate supply of BERINERT.

Reconstitution and Administration
- Each BERINERT vial contains 500 IU of C1 esterase inhibitor as a lyophilized concentrate for reconstitution with 10 mL of Sterile Water for Injection, USP provided.
- Check the expiration date on the product vial label. Do not use beyond the expiration date.
- Use either the Mix2Vial transfer set provided with BERINERT or a commercially available double-ended needle and vented filter spike.
- Prepare and administer using aseptic techniques.
- After reconstitution and prior to administration inspect BERINERT. The reconstituted solution should be colorless, clear, and free from visible particles. Do not use if the solution is cloudy, discolored, or contains particulates.

Reconstitution

The procedures below are provided as general guidelines for the reconstitution of BERINERT.
[See table on pages 930 through 932]

SELF-ADMINISTRATION (Intravenous Infusion)

Your healthcare provider will teach you how to safely administer BERINERT. It is important that BERINERT is injected directly into a visible vein. Do not inject into surrounding tissues or into an artery. Once you learn how to self-administer, follow the instructions provided below.
[See table on pages 933 thought 935]

This Patient Package Insert has been approved by the US Food and Drug Administration.

Manufactured by:
CSL Behring GmbH
35041 Marburg, Germany
US License No. 1765
Distributed by:
CSL Behring LLC
Kankakee, IL 60901 USA
Mix2Vial® is a registered trademark of Medimop Medical Projects, Ltd., a subsidiary of West Pharmaceuticals Services, Inc.
Shown in Product Identification Guide, page 508

HIZENTRA® ℞
Immune Globulin Subcutaneous (Human)
20% Liquid

HIGHLIGHTS OF PRESCRIBING INFORMATION
These highlights do not include all the information needed to use HIZENTRA safely and effectively. See full prescribing information for HIZENTRA.
HIZENTRA, Immune Globulin Subcutaneous (Human), 20% Liquid
Initial U.S. Approval: 2010

WARNING: THROMBOSIS
See full prescribing information for complete boxed warning.
- **Thrombosis may occur with immune globulin products, including Hizentra. Risk factors may include: advanced age, prolonged immobilization, hypercoagulable conditions, history of venous or arterial thrombosis, use of estrogens, indwelling vascular catheters, hyperviscosity, and cardiovascular risk factors.**
- **For patients at risk of thrombosis, administer Hizentra at the minimum dose and infusion rate practicable. Ensure adequate hydration in patients before administration. Monitor for signs and symptoms of thrombosis and assess blood viscosity in patients at risk for hyperviscosity.**

RECENT MAJOR CHANGES

Dosage and Administration (2.2, 2.3)	01/2015
Warnings and Precautions (5.4, 5.5, 5.7)	01/2015

INDICATIONS AND USAGE

Hizentra is an Immune Globulin Subcutaneous (Human) (IGSC), 20% Liquid indicated for the treatment of primary immunodeficiency (PI) in adults and pediatric patients 2 years of age and older (1).

DOSAGE AND ADMINISTRATION

For subcutaneous infusion only. Do not inject into a blood vessel.
Administer at regular intervals from daily up to every two weeks (biweekly).
Dosage (2.2)
Before switching to Hizentra, obtain the patient's serum IgG trough level to guide subsequent dose adjustments.
• **Weekly:** Start Hizentra 1 week after last IGIV infusion

$$\text{Initial weekly dose} = \frac{\text{Previous IGIV dose (in grams)} \times 1.37}{\text{No. of weeks between IGIV doses}}$$

• **Biweekly:** Start Hizentra 1 or 2 weeks after the last IGIV infusion or 1 week after the last weekly Hizentra/IGSC infusion. Administer twice the calculated weekly dose.
• **Frequent dosing (2 to 7 times per week):** Start Hizentra 1 week after the last IGIV or Hizentra/IGSC infusion. Divide the calculated weekly dose by the desired number of times per week.
• Adjust the dose based on clinical response and serum IgG trough levels (*see Dose Adjustment*).
Administration (2.3)
• Infusion sites – 1 to 4 injection sites simultaneously, with at least 2 inches between sites.

Infusion Parameters*	Infusion Number			
	1st	2nd to 4th	5th	6th and above
Volume (mL/site)	≤ 15	≤ 20		≤ 25
Rate (mL/hr/site)	15			≤ 25

* As tolerated

DOSAGE FORMS AND STRENGTHS

0.2 g per mL (20%) protein solution for subcutaneous injection (3)

CONTRAINDICATIONS

• Anaphylactic or severe systemic reaction to human immune globulin or components of Hizentra, such as polysorbate 80 (4)
• Hyperprolinemia (type I or II) (Hizentra contains the stabilizer L-proline) (4)
• IgA-deficient patients with antibodies against IgA and a history of hypersensitivity (4)

WARNINGS AND PRECAUTIONS

• IgA-deficient patients with anti-IgA antibodies are at greater risk of severe hypersensitivity and anaphylactic reactions (5.1).
• Thrombosis may occur following treatment with immune globulin products, including Hizentra (5.2).
• Aseptic meningitis syndrome has been reported with IGIV or IGSC treatment (5.3).
• Monitor renal function, including blood urea nitrogen, serum creatinine, and urine output in patients at risk of acute renal failure (5.4).
• Monitor for clinical signs and symptoms of hemolysis (5.5).
• Monitor for pulmonary adverse reactions (transfusion-related acute lung injury [TRALI]) (5.6).
• Hizentra is made from human plasma and may contain infectious agents, e.g., viruses, the variant Creutzfeldt-Jakob disease (vCJD) agent and, theoretically, the Creutzfeldt-Jakob disease (CJD) agent (5.7).

ADVERSE REACTIONS

The most common adverse reactions observed in ≥5% of study subjects were local reactions (i.e., swelling, redness, heat, pain, and itching at the injection site), headache, diarrhea, fatigue, back pain, nausea, pain in extremity, cough, rash, pruritus, vomiting, abdominal pain (upper), migraine, and pain (6).
To report SUSPECTED ADVERSE REACTIONS, contact CSL Behring Pharmacovigilance at 1-866-915-6958 or FDA at 1-800-FDA-1088 or *www.fda.gov/medwatch*.

DRUG INTERACTIONS

The passive transfer of antibodies may interfere with the response to live virus vaccines (7.1), and lead to misinterpretation of the results of serological testing (5.8, 7.2).

USE IN SPECIFIC POPULATIONS

• Pregnancy: No human or animal data. Use only if clearly needed (8.1).
• Pediatric: No specific dose requirements are necessary to achieve the desired serum IgG levels (8.4).
See 17 for PATIENT COUNSELING INFORMATION and FDA-approved patient labeling.

Revised: 1/2015

FULL PRESCRIBING INFORMATION: CONTENTS*
WARNING: THROMBOSIS
1 INDICATIONS AND USAGE
2 DOSAGE AND ADMINISTRATION
  2.1 Preparation and Handling
  2.2 Dosage
  2.3 Administration
3 DOSAGE FORMS AND STRENGTHS
4 CONTRAINDICATIONS
5 WARNINGS AND PRECAUTIONS
  5.1 Hypersensitivity
  5.2 Thrombosis
  5.3 Aseptic Meningitis Syndrome (AMS)
  5.4 Renal Dysfunction/Failure
  5.5 Hemolysis
  5.6 Transfusion-Related Acute Lung Injury (TRALI)
  5.7 Transmissible Infectious Agents
  5.8 Laboratory Tests
6 ADVERSE REACTIONS
  6.1 Clinical Trials Experience
  6.2 Postmarketing Experience
7 DRUG INTERACTIONS
  7.1 Live Virus Vaccines
  7.2 Serological Testing
8 USE IN SPECIFIC POPULATIONS
  8.1 Pregnancy
  8.3 Nursing Mothers
  8.4 Pediatric Use
  8.5 Geriatric Use
11 DESCRIPTION
12 CLINICAL PHARMACOLOGY
  12.1 Mechanism of Action
  12.3 Pharmacokinetics
13 NONCLINICAL TOXICOLOGY
  13.2 Animal Toxicology and/or Pharmacology
14 CLINICAL STUDIES
  14.1 US Study
  14.2 European Study
15 REFERENCES
16 HOW SUPPLIED/STORAGE AND HANDLING
  16.1 How Supplied
  16.2 Storage and Handling
17 PATIENT COUNSELING INFORMATION
* Sections or subsections omitted from the full prescribing information are not listed.

FULL PRESCRIBING INFORMATION

WARNING: THROMBOSIS
• **Thrombosis may occur with immune globulin products**[1-3]**, including Hizentra. Risk factors may include: advanced age, prolonged immobilization, hypercoagulable conditions, history of venous or arterial thrombosis, use of estrogens, indwelling central vascular catheters, hyperviscosity, and cardiovascular risk factors. Thrombosis may occur in the absence of known risk factors *(see Warnings and Precautions [5.2], Patient Counseling Information [17])*.**
• **For patients at risk of thrombosis, administer Hizentra at the minimum dose and infusion rate practicable. Ensure adequate hydration in patients before administration. Monitor for signs and symptoms of thrombosis and assess blood viscosity in patients at risk for hyperviscosity *(see Warnings and Precautions [5.2])*.**

---

1 INDICATIONS AND USAGE
Hizentra is an Immune Globulin Subcutaneous (Human) (IGSC), 20% Liquid indicated as replacement therapy for primary humoral immunodeficiency (PI) in adults and pediatric patients 2 years of age and older. This includes, but is not limited to, the humoral immune defect in congenital agammaglobulinemia, common variable immunodeficiency, X-linked agammaglobulinemia, Wiskott-Aldrich syndrome, and severe combined immunodeficiencies.

2 DOSAGE AND ADMINISTRATION
For subcutaneous infusion only. Do not inject into a blood vessel.
2.1 Preparation and Handling
Hizentra is a clear and pale yellow to light brown solution. Do not use if the solution is cloudy or contains particulates.
• Prior to administration, visually inspect each vial of Hizentra for particulate matter or discoloration, whenever the solution and container permit.
• Do not freeze. Do not use any solution that has been frozen.
• Check the product expiration date on the vial label. Do not use beyond the expiration date.
• Do not mix Hizentra with other products.
• Do not shake the Hizentra vial.
• Use aseptic technique when preparing and administering Hizentra.
• The Hizentra vial is for single-use only. Discard all used administration supplies and any unused product immediately after each infusion in accordance with local requirements.
2.2 Dosage
• Hizentra can be administered at regular intervals from daily up to every two weeks (biweekly).
• Individualize the dose based on the patient's clinical response to Hizentra therapy and serum immunoglobulin G (IgG) trough levels.
• Before receiving treatment with Hizentra:
  ○ Ensure that patients have received Immune Globulin Intravenous (Human) (IGIV) treatment at regular intervals for at least 3 months.
  ○ Obtain the patient's serum IgG trough level to guide subsequent dose adjustments (*see below under Dose Adjustment*).
Dosage for patients switching to Hizentra from Immune Globulin Intravenous (Human) (IGIV)
• Establish the initial weekly dose of Hizentra by converting the monthly IGIV dose into a weekly equivalent and increasing it using a dose adjustment factor. The goal is to achieve a systemic serum IgG exposure (area under the concentration-time curve [AUC]) not inferior to that of the previous IGIV treatment.
  ○ To calculate the initial weekly dose of Hizentra, divide the previous IGIV dose in grams by the number of weeks between doses during the patient's IGIV treatment (e.g., 3 or 4); then multiply this by the dose adjustment factor of 1.37. [see *Pharmacokinetics (12.3, Table 8)*]

$$\text{Initial Hizentra dose} = \frac{\text{Previous IGIV dose (in grams)} \times 1.37}{\text{Number of weeks between IGIV doses}}$$

  ○ To convert the Hizentra dose (in grams) to milliliters (mL), multiply the calculated dose (in grams) by 5.
• Provided the total weekly dose is maintained, any dosing interval from daily up to biweekly can be used and will result in systemic serum IgG exposure that is comparable to the previous IGIV or weekly Hizentra treatment [see *Pharmacokinetics (12.3)*].
• For biweekly dosing, multiply the calculated Hizentra weekly dose by 2.
• For frequent dosing (2 to 7 times per week), divide the calculated weekly dose by the desired number of times per week (e.g., for 3 times per week dosing, divide weekly dose by 3).
Dosage for patients switching to Hizentra from IGSC
• The previous weekly IGSC dose should be maintained.
• For biweekly dosing, multiply the previous weekly dose by 2.
• For frequent dosing (2 to 7 times per week), divide the previous weekly dose by the desired number of times per week (e.g., for 3 times per week dosing, divide weekly dose by 3).
Start Hizentra treatment:
• For weekly or frequent dosing, start treatment with Hizentra 1 week after the patient's last IGIV infusion or Hizentra/IGSC infusion.

Continued on next page

• For biweekly dosing, start treatment 1 or 2 weeks after the last IGIV infusion or 1 week after the last weekly Hizentra/IGSC infusion.

Dose Adjustment

Over time, the dose may need to be adjusted to achieve the desired clinical response and serum IgG trough level, irrespective of the frequency of administration. To determine if a dose adjustment should be considered, measure the patient's serum IgG trough level 2 to 3 months after switching to Hizentra.

Weekly dosing: When switching from IGIV to weekly Hizentra dosing, the target serum IgG trough level is projected to be approximately 16% higher than the last trough level during prior IGIV therapy *[see Pharmacokinetics (12.3)]*.

Biweekly dosing: When switching from IGIV to biweekly Hizentra dosing, the target serum IgG trough level is projected to be approximately 10% higher than the last IGIV trough level. When switching from weekly to biweekly Hizentra dosing, the target trough is projected to be approximately 5% lower than the last trough level on weekly therapy *[see Pharmacokinetics (12.3)]*.

Frequent dosing: When switching from weekly dosing to more frequent Hizentra dosing, the target serum IgG trough level is projected to be approximately 3 to 4% higher than the last trough level on weekly therapy *[see Pharmacokinetics (12.3)]*.

To adjust the dose based on trough levels, calculate the difference (in mg/dL) between the patient's serum IgG trough level and the target IgG trough level for weekly or biweekly dosing. Then find this difference in Table 1 (Column 1) and, based on the Hizentra dosing frequency (for weekly or biweekly) and the patient's body weight, locate the corresponding adjustment amount (in mL) by which to increase (or decrease) the dose. For frequent dosing, add the weekly increment from Table 1 to the weekly-equivalent dose and then divide by the number of days of dosing.

Use the patient's clinical response as the primary consideration in dose adjustment. Additional dosage increments may be indicated based on the patient's clinical response (infection frequency and severity).

[See table 1 below]

For example, if a patient with a body weight of 70 kg has an actual IgG trough level of 900 mg/dL and the target trough level is 1000 mg/dL, this results in a difference of 100 mg/dL. Therefore, increase the weekly dose of Hizentra by 10 mL. For biweekly dosing, increase the biweekly dose by 20 mL. For 2 times per week dosing, increase the dose by 5 mL.

Monitor the patient's clinical response, and repeat the dose adjustment as needed.

Dosage requirements for patients switching to Hizentra from another IGSC product: If a patient on Hizentra does not maintain an adequate clinical response or a serum IgG trough level equivalent to that of the previous IGSC treatment, the physician may want to adjust the dose. For such patients, Table 1 also provides guidance for dose adjustment if their desired IGSC trough level is known.

Measles Exposure

Administer a minimum total weekly Hizentra dose of 200 mg/kg body weight for two consecutive weeks if a patient is at risk of measles exposure (i.e., due to an outbreak in the US or travel to endemic areas outside of the US. For biweekly dosing, one infusion of a minimum of 400 mg/kg is recommended. If a patient has been exposed to measles, ensure this minimum dose is administered as soon as possible after exposure.

2.3   Administration

Hizentra is for subcutaneous infusion only. Do not inject into a blood vessel.

Hizentra is intended for subcutaneous administration using an infusion pump. Infuse Hizentra in the abdomen, thigh, upper arm, and/or lateral hip.

• Injection sites – A Hizentra dose may be infused into multiple injection sites. Use up to 4 sites simultaneously or up to 12 sites consecutively per infusion. Injection sites should be at least 2 inches apart. Change the actual site of injection with each administration.

• Volume – For the first infusion of Hizentra, do not exceed a volume of 15 mL per injection site. The volume may be increased to 20 mL per site for the fifth infusion and then to 25 mL per site as tolerated.

• Rate – For the first infusion of Hizentra, the recommended flow rate is 15 mL per hour per site. For subsequent infusions, the flow rate may be increased to 25 mL per hour per site as tolerated.

Follow the steps below and use aseptic technique to administer Hizentra.

[See table on next page]

For self-administration, provide the patient with instructions and training for subcutaneous infusion in the home or other appropriate setting.

3   DOSAGE FORMS AND STRENGTHS

Hizentra is a 0.2 g/mL (20%) protein solution for subcutaneous injection.

4   CONTRAINDICATIONS

Hizentra is contraindicated in patients who have had an anaphylactic or severe systemic reaction to the administration of human immune globulin or to components of Hizentra, such as polysorbate 80.

Hizentra is contraindicated in patients with hyperprolinemia (type I or II) because it contains the stabilizer L-proline *[see Description (11)]*.

Hizentra is contraindicated in IgA-deficient patients with antibodies against IgA and a history of hypersensitivity *[see Description (11)]*.

5   WARNINGS AND PRECAUTIONS

5.1   Hypersensitivity

Severe hypersensitivity reactions may occur to human immune globulin or components of Hizentra, such as polysorbate 80. If a hypersensitivity reaction occurs, discontinue the Hizentra infusion immediately and institute appropriate treatment.

Individuals with IgA deficiency can develop anti-IgA antibodies and anaphylactic reactions (including anaphylaxis and shock) after administration of blood components containing IgA. Patients with known antibodies to IgA may

have a greater risk of developing potentially severe hypersensitivity and anaphylactic reactions with administration of Hizentra. Hizentra contains ≤50 mcg/mL IgA *[see Description (11)]*.

5.2   Thrombosis

Thrombosis may occur following treatment with immune globulin products[1-3], including Hizentra. Risk factors may include: advanced age, prolonged immobilization, hypercoagulable conditions, history of venous or arterial thrombosis, use of estrogens, indwelling central vascular catheters, hyperviscosity, and cardiovascular risk factors. Thrombosis may occur in the absence of known risk factors.

Consider baseline assessment of blood viscosity in patients at risk for hyperviscosity, including those with cryoglobulins, fasting chylomicronemia/markedly high triacylglycerols (triglycerides), or monoclonal gammopathies. For patients at risk of thrombosis, administer Hizentra at the minimum dose and infusion rate practicable. Ensure adequate hydration in patients before administration. Monitor for signs and symptoms of thrombosis and assess blood viscosity in patients at risk for hyperviscosity *[see Boxed Warning, Patient Counseling Information (17)]*.

5.3   Aseptic Meningitis Syndrome (AMS)

AMS has been reported with use of IGIV[4] or IGSC. The syndrome usually begins within several hours to 2 days following immune globulin treatment. AMS is characterized by the following signs and symptoms: severe headache, nuchal rigidity, drowsiness, fever, photophobia, painful eye movements, nausea, and vomiting. Cerebrospinal fluid (CSF) studies frequently show pleocytosis up to several thousand cells per cubic millimeter, predominantly from the granulocytic series, and elevated protein levels up to several hundred mg/dL. AMS may occur more frequently in association with high doses (≥2 g/kg) and/or rapid infusion of immune globulin product.

Patients exhibiting such signs and symptoms should receive a thorough neurological examination, including CSF studies, to rule out other causes of meningitis. Discontinuation of immune globulin treatment has resulted in remission of AMS within several days without sequelae.

5.4   Renal Dysfunction/Failure

Acute renal dysfunction/failure, acute tubular necrosis, proximal tubular nephropathy, osmotic nephrosis and death may occur with use of human immune globulin products, especially those containing sucrose.[5] Hizentra does not contain sucrose. Ensure that patients are not volume depleted before administering Hizentra.

For patients judged to be at risk for developing renal dysfunction, including patients with any degree of pre-existing renal insufficiency, diabetes mellitus, age greater than 65, volume depletion, sepsis, paraproteinemia, or patients receiving known nephrotoxic drugs, monitor renal function and consider lower, more frequent dosing *[see Dosing and Administration (2.3)]*.

Periodic monitoring of renal function and urine output is particularly important in patients judged to have a potential increased risk of developing acute renal failure.[6] Assess renal function, including measurement of blood urea nitrogen (BUN) and serum creatinine, before the initial infusion of Hizentra and at appropriate intervals thereafter. If renal function deteriorates, consider discontinuing Hizentra.

5.5   Hemolysis

Hizentra can contain blood group antibodies that may act as hemolysins and induce *in vivo* coating of red blood cells (RBCs) with immunoglobulin, causing a positive direct antiglobulin (Coombs') test result and hemolysis.[7-9] Delayed hemolytic anemia can develop subsequent to immune globulin therapy due to enhanced RBC sequestration, and acute hemolysis, consistent with intravascular hemolysis, has been reported.[10]

Monitor recipients of Hizentra for clinical signs and symptoms of hemolysis. If signs and/or symptoms of hemolysis are present after Hizentra infusion, perform appropriate confirmatory laboratory testing.

5.6   Transfusion-Related Acute Lung Injury (TRALI)

Noncardiogenic pulmonary edema may occur in patients administered human immune globulin products.[11] TRALI is characterized by severe respiratory distress, pulmonary edema, hypoxemia, normal left ventricular function, and fever. Typically, it occurs within 1 to 6 hours following transfusion. Patients with TRALI may be managed using oxygen therapy with adequate ventilatory support.

Monitor Hizentra recipients for pulmonary adverse reactions. If TRALI is suspected, perform appropriate tests for the presence of anti-neutrophil antibodies in both the product and patient's serum.

Table 1: Incremental Adjustment (mL)* of the Hizentra Dose† Based on the Difference (±mg/dL) from the Target Serum IgG Trough Level

Difference From Target Serum IgG Trough Level (mg/dL)	Dosing Frequency	Weight Adjusted Dose Increment (mL)*				
		Weight Group				
		>10 to 30 kg	>30 to 50 kg	>50 to 70 kg	>70 to 90 kg	>90 kg
50	Weekly‡	n/a	2.5	5	5	10
	Biweekly	5	5	10	10	20
100	Weekly	2.5	5	10	10	15
	Biweekly	5	10	20	20	30
200	Weekly	5	10	15	20	30
	Biweekly	10	20	30	40	60

n/a, not applicable.

* Incremental adjustments based on slopes of the pharmacometric model-predicted relationship between serum IgG trough level and Hizentra dose increments of 1 mg/kg per week.

† Includes biweekly, weekly or frequent dosing.

‡ To determine the dose increment for frequent dosing, add the weekly increment to the weekly-equivalent dose and then divide by the number of days of dosing.

5.7 Transmissible Infectious Agents

Because Hizentra is made from human plasma, it may carry a risk of transmitting infectious agents, e.g., viruses, the variant Creutzfeldt-Jakob disease (vCJD) agent and, theoretically, the Creutzfeldt-Jakob disease (CJD) agent. This also applies to unknown or emerging viruses and other pathogens. No cases of transmission of viral diseases or CJD have been associated with the use of Hizentra. All infections suspected by a physician possibly to have been transmitted by Hizentra should be reported to CSL Behring Pharmacovigilance at 1-866-915-6958.

5.8 Laboratory Tests

Various passively transferred antibodies in immunoglobulin preparations may lead to misinterpretation of the results of serological testing.

6 ADVERSE REACTIONS

The most common adverse reactions (ARs), observed in ≥5% of study subjects receiving Hizentra, were local reactions (e.g., swelling, redness, heat, pain, and itching at the injection site), headache, diarrhea, fatigue, back pain, nausea, pain in extremity, cough, rash, pruritus, vomiting, abdominal pain (upper), migraine, and pain.

6.1 Clinical Trials Experience

Because clinical studies are conducted under widely varying conditions, AR rates observed in clinical studies of a product cannot be directly compared to rates in the clinical studies of another product and may not reflect the rates observed in clinical practice.

US Study

The safety of Hizentra was evaluated in a clinical study in the US for 15 months (3-month wash-in/wash-out period followed by a 12-month efficacy period) in subjects with PI who had been treated previously with IGIV every 3 or 4 weeks.

The safety analyses included 49 subjects in the intention-to-treat (ITT) population. The ITT population consisted of all subjects who received at least one dose of Hizentra [see *Clinical Studies (14)*].

Subjects were treated with Hizentra at weekly median doses ranging from 66 to 331 mg/kg body weight (mean: 181.4 mg/kg) during the wash-in/wash-out period and from 72 to 379 mg/kg (mean: 213.2 mg/kg) during the efficacy period. The 49 subjects received a total of 2264 weekly infusions of Hizentra.

Table 2 summarizes the most frequent adverse reactions (ARs) (experienced by at least 2 subjects) occurring during or within 72 hours after the end of an infusion. Local reactions were assessed by the investigators 15 to 45 minutes post-infusion and by the subjects 24 hours post-infusion. The investigators then evaluated the ARs arising from the subject assessments. Local reactions were the most frequent ARs observed, with injection-site reactions (e.g., swelling, redness, heat, pain, and itching at the site of injection) comprising 98% of local reactions.

Table 2: Incidence of Subjects with Adverse Reactions (ARs) (Experienced by 2 or More Subjects) and Rate per Infusion (ITT Population), US Study

AR (≥2 Subjects)	ARs* Occurring During or Within 72 Hours of Infusion	
	Number (%) of Subjects (n=49)	Number (Rate†) of ARs (n=2264 Infusions)
Local reactions‡	49 (100)	1322 (0.584)
Other ARs:		
Headache	12 (24.5)	32 (0.014)
Diarrhea	5 (10.2)	6 (0.003)
Fatigue	4 (8.2)	4 (0.002)
Back pain	4 (8.2)	5 (0.002)
Nausea	4 (8.2)	4 (0.002)
Pain in extremity	4 (8.2)	6 (0.003)
Cough	4 (8.2)	4 (0.002)
Vomiting	3 (6.1)	3 (0.001)
Abdominal pain, upper	3 (6.1)	3 (0.001)
Migraine	3 (6.1)	4 (0.002)
Pain	3 (6.1)	4 (0.002)
Arthralgia	2 (4.1)	3 (0.001)
Contusion	2 (4.1)	3 (0.001)
Rash	2 (4.1)	3 (0.001)
Urticaria	2 (4.1)	2 (< 0.001)

* Excluding infections.
† Rate of ARs per infusion.
‡ Includes injection-site reactions as well as bruising, scabbing, pain, irritation, cysts, eczema, and nodules at the injection site.

The ratio of infusions with ARs, including local reactions, to all infusions was 1303 to 2264 (57.6%). Excluding local reactions, the corresponding ratio was 56 to 2264 (2.5%).

Table 3 summarizes injection-site reactions based on investigator assessments 15 to 45 minutes after the end of the 683 infusions administered during regularly scheduled visits (every 4 weeks).

Table 3: Investigator Assessments* of Injection-Site Reactions by Infusion, US Study

Injection-Site Reaction	Number† (Rate‡) of Reactions (n=683 Infusions§)
Edema/induration	467 (0.68)
Erythema	346 (0.51)
Local heat	108 (0.16)
Local pain	88 (0.13)
Itching	64 (0.09)

* 15 to 45 minutes after the end of infusions administered at regularly scheduled visits (every 4 weeks).
† For multiple injection sites, every site was judged, but only the site with the strongest reaction was recorded.
‡ Rate of injection-site reactions per infusion.
§ Number of infusions administered during regularly scheduled visits.

Most local reactions were either mild (93.4%) or moderate (6.3%) in intensity.

No deaths or serious ARs occurred during the study. Two subjects withdrew from the study due to ARs. One subject experienced a severe injection-site reaction one day after the third weekly infusion, and the other subject experienced moderate myositis. Both reactions were judged to be "at least possibly related" to the administration of Hizentra.

European Study

In a clinical study conducted in Europe, the safety of Hizentra was evaluated for 10 months (3-month wash-in/wash-out period followed by a 7-month efficacy period) in 51 subjects with PI who had been treated previously with IGIV every 3 or 4 weeks or with IGSC weekly.

Subjects were treated with Hizentra at weekly median doses ranging from 59 to 267 mg/kg body weight (mean: 118.8 mg/kg) during the wash-in/wash-out period and from 59 to 243 mg/kg (mean: 120.1 mg/kg) during the efficacy period. The 51 subjects received a total of 1831 weekly infusions of Hizentra.

Table 4 summarizes the most frequent ARs (experienced by at least 2 subjects) occurring during or within 72 hours after the end of an infusion. Local reactions were assessed by the subjects between 24 and 72 hours post-infusion. The investigators then evaluated the ARs arising from the subject assessments.

1. **Assemble supplies** – Gather the Hizentra vial(s), disposable supplies (not provided with Hizentra), and other items (infusion pump, sharps or other container, patient's treatment diary/log book) needed for the infusion.
2. **Clean surface** – Thoroughly clean a flat surface using an alcohol wipe.
3. **Wash hands** – Thoroughly wash and dry hands. The use of gloves when preparing and administering Hizentra is optional.
4. **Check vials** – Carefully inspect each vial of Hizentra. Do not use the vial if the liquid looks cloudy, contains particles, or has changed color, if the protective cap is missing, or if the expiration date on the label has passed.
5. **Transfer Hizentra from vial(s) to syringe**
   - Remove the protective cap from the vial to expose the central portion of the rubber stopper of the Hizentra vial.
   - Clean the stopper with an alcohol wipe and allow it to dry.
     - If using a transfer device, follow the instructions provided by the device manufacturer.
     - If using a needle and a syringe to transfer Hizentra, follow the instructions below.
     - Attach a sterile transfer needle to a sterile syringe. Pull back on the plunger of the syringe to draw air into the syringe that is equal to the amount of Hizentra to be withdrawn.
     - Insert the transfer needle into the center of the vial stopper and, to avoid foaming, inject the air into headspace of the vial (not into the liquid).
     - Withdraw the desired volume of Hizentra.
   - When using multiple vials to achieve the desired dose, repeat this step.

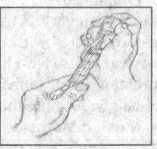

6. **Prepare infusion pump and tubing** – Follow the manufacturer's instructions for preparing the pump, using subcutaneous administration sets and tubing, as needed. Be sure to prime the tubing with Hizentra to ensure that no air is left in the tubing.
7. **Prepare injection site(s)**
   - The number and location of injection sites depends on the volume of the total dose. Infuse Hizentra into a maximum of 4 sites simultaneously; or up to 12 consecutively per infusion. Injection sites should be at least 2 inches apart.
   - Using an antiseptic skin preparation, clean each site beginning at the center and working outward in a circular motion. Allow each site to dry before proceeding.

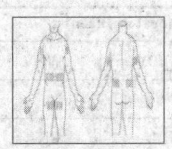

8. **Insert needle(s)**
   - Grasp the skin between 2 fingers and insert the needle into the subcutaneous tissue.
   - If necessary, use sterile gauze and tape or transparent dressing to hold the needle in place.
   - Before starting the infusion, attach a sterile syringe to the end of the primed administration tubing and gently pull back on the plunger to make sure no blood is flowing back into the tubing. If blood is present, remove and discard the needle and tubing. Repeat the process beginning with step 6 (priming) using a new needle, new infusion tubing, and a different injection site.

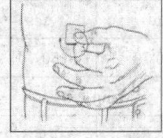

9. **Start infusion** – Follow the manufacturer's instructions to turn on the infusion pump.
10. **Record treatment** – Remove the peel-off portion of the label from each vial used, and affix it to the patient's treatment diary/log book or scan the vial if recording the infusion electronically.
11. **Clean up** – After administration is complete, turn off the infusion pump. Take off the tape or dressing and remove the needle set from the infusion site(s). Disconnect the tubing from the pump. Immediately discard any unused product and all used disposable supplies in accordance with local requirements. Clean and store the pump according to the manufacturer's instructions.

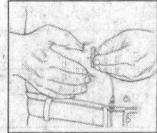

Continued on next page

Table 4: Incidence of Subjects with Adverse Reactions (ARs)* (Experienced by 2 or More Subjects) and Rate per Infusion, European Study

AR (≥2 Subjects)	ARs* Occurring During or Within 72 Hours of Infusion	
	Number (%) of Subjects (n=51)	Number (Rate†) of ARs (n=1831 Infusions)
Local reactions‡	24 (47.1)	105 (0.057)
Other ARs:		
Headache	9 (17.6)	20 (0.011)
Rash	4 (7.8)	4 (0.002)
Pruritus	4 (7.8)	13 (0.007)
Fatigue	3 (5.9)	5 (0.003)
Abdominal pain, upper	2 (3.9)	3 (0.002)
Arthralgia	2 (3.9)	2 (0.001)
Erythema	2 (3.9)	4 (0.002)
Abdominal discomfort	2 (3.9)	3 (0.002)
Back pain	2 (3.9)	2 (0.001)
Hematoma	2 (3.9)	3 (0.002)
Hypersensitivity	2 (3.9)	4 (0.002)

* Excluding infections.
† Rate of ARs per infusion.
‡ Includes infusion-related reaction; infusion-site mass; infusion/injection-site erythema, hematoma, induration, inflammation, edema, pain, pruritus, rash, reaction, swelling; injection-site extravasation, nodule; puncture-site reaction.

The proportion of subjects reporting local reactions decreased over time from approximately 20% following the first infusion to <5% by the end of the study.
Three subjects withdrew from the study due to ARs of mild to moderate intensity. One subject experienced injection-site pain and injection-site pruritus; the second subject experienced injection-site reaction, fatigue, and feeling cold; and the third subject experienced injection-site reaction and hypersensitivity. All reactions were judged by the investigator to be "at least possibly related" to the administration of Hizentra.

Biweekly (Every Two Weeks) or Frequent (2 To 7 Times per Week) Dosing
No data regarding ARs are available for these alternative Hizentra dosing regimens because no clinical trials using these regimens were conducted; however, it is unlikely that the safety profile is qualitatively different from that of weekly dosing.

6.2   Postmarketing Experience
Because postmarketing reporting of adverse reactions is voluntary and from a population of uncertain size, it is not al-ways possible to reliably estimate the frequency of these reactions or establish a causal relationship to product exposure.
Hizentra
The following adverse reactions have been identified during postmarketing use of Hizentra. This list does not include reactions already reported in clinical studies with Hizentra *[see Adverse Reactions (6.1)]*.
• *Infusion reactions:* Allergic-anaphylactic reactions such as swollen face or tongue and pharyngeal edema, pyrexia, chills, dizziness, hypertension/changes in blood pressure, malaise.
• *Cardiovascular:* Chest discomfort (including chest pain)
• *Respiratory:* Dyspnea
• *Neurological:* Tremor, burning sensation
The following adverse reactions have been reported during postmarketing use of immune globulin products[5]:
• *Infusion reactions:* Tachycardia, flushing, wheezing, rigors, myalgia
• *Renal:* Osmotic nephropathy
• *Respiratory:* Apnea, Acute Respiratory Distress Syndrome (ARDS), cyanosis, hypoxemia, pulmonary edema, bronchospasm
• *Cardiovascular:* Cardiac arrest, vascular collapse, hypotension
• *Neurological:* Coma, loss of consciousness, seizures, aseptic meningitis syndrome
• *Integumentary:* Stevens-Johnson syndrome, epidermolysis, erythema multiforme, dermatitis (e.g., bullous dermatitis)
• *Hematologic:* Pancytopenia, leukopenia, hemolysis, positive direct antiglobulin (Coombs') test
• *Gastrointestinal:* Hepatic dysfunction
To report SUSPECTED ADVERSE REACTIONS, contact CSL Behring Pharmacovigilance at 1-866-915-6958 or FDA at 1-800-FDA-1088 or *www.fda.gov/medwatch.*

7   DRUG INTERACTIONS
7.1   Live Virus Vaccines
The passive transfer of antibodies with immunoglobulin administration may interfere with the response to live virus vaccines such as measles, mumps, rubella, and varicella *[see Patient Counseling Information (17)]*.
7.2   Serological Testing
Various passively transferred antibodies in immunoglobulin preparations may lead to misinterpretation of the results of serological testing.

8   USE IN SPECIFIC POPULATIONS
8.1   Pregnancy
Pregnancy Category C. Animal reproduction studies have not been conducted with Hizentra. It is not known whether Hizentra can cause fetal harm when administered to a pregnant woman or can affect reproduction capacity. Hizentra should be given to pregnant women only if clearly needed.
8.3   Nursing Mothers
Hizentra has not been evaluated in nursing mothers.
8.4   Pediatric Use
Clinical Studies (Weekly Dosing)

The safety and effectiveness of weekly Hizentra have been established in the pediatric age groups 2 to 16. Hizentra was evaluated in 10 pediatric subjects with PI (3 children and 7 adolescents) in a study conducted in the US *[see Clinical Studies (14)]* and in 23 pediatric subjects with PI (18 children and 5 adolescents) in Europe. There were no differences in the pharmacokinetics, safety and efficacy profiles as compared with adult subjects. No pediatric-specific dose requirements were necessary to achieve the desired serum IgG levels.
Pharmacokinetic Modeling and Simulation (Biweekly or more Frequent Dosing)
The biweekly (every two weeks) or more frequent dosing (2 to 7 times per week) regimens, developed from population PK-based modeling and simulation, included 57 pediatric subjects (32 from Hizentra clinical studies) *[see Pharmacokinetics (12.3)]*. Hizentra dosing is adjusted to body weight. No pediatric-specific dose requirements are necessary for these regimens.
Safety and effectiveness of Hizentra in pediatric patients below the age of 2 have not been established.
8.5   Geriatric Use
Of the 49 subjects evaluated in the US clinical study of Hizentra, 6 subjects were 65 years of age or older. No overall differences in safety or efficacy were observed between these subjects and younger subjects. The clinical study of Hizentra in Europe did not include subjects over the age of 65.

11   DESCRIPTION
Hizentra, Immune Globulin Subcutaneous (Human), 20% Liquid, is a ready-to-use, sterile 20% (0.2 g/mL) protein liquid preparation of polyvalent human immunoglobulin G (IgG) for subcutaneous administration. Hizentra is manufactured from large pools of human plasma by a combination of cold alcohol fractionation, octanoic acid fractionation, and anion exchange chromatography. The IgG proteins are not subjected to heating or to chemical or enzymatic modification. The Fc and Fab functions of the IgG molecule are retained. Fab functions tested include antigen binding capacities, and Fc functions tested include complement activation and Fc-receptor-mediated leukocyte activation (determined with complexed IgG).
Hizentra has a purity of ≥98% IgG and a pH of 4.6 to 5.2. Hizentra contains approximately 250 mmol/L (range: 210 to 290 mmol/L) L-proline (a nonessential amino acid) as a stabilizer, 8 to 30 mg/L polysorbate 80, and trace amounts of sodium. Hizentra contains ≤50 mcg/mL IgA. Hizentra contains no carbohydrate stabilizers (e.g., sucrose, maltose) and no preservative.
Plasma units used in the manufacture of Hizentra are tested using FDA-licensed serological assays for hepatitis B surface antigen and antibodies to human immunodeficiency virus (HIV)-1/2 and hepatitis C virus (HCV) as well as FDA-licensed Nucleic Acid Testing (NAT) for HBV, HCV and HIV-1. All plasma units have been found to be nonreactive (negative) in these tests. In addition, the plasma has been tested for B19 virus (B19V) DNA by NAT. Only plasma that passes virus screening is used for production, and the limit for B19V in the fractionation pool is set not to exceed 10^4 IU of B19V DNA per mL.
The manufacturing process for Hizentra includes three steps to reduce the risk of virus transmission. Two of these are dedicated virus clearance steps: pH 4 incubation to inactivate enveloped viruses; and virus filtration to remove, by size exclusion, both enveloped and non-enveloped viruses as small as approximately 20 nanometers. In addition, a depth filtration step contributes to the virus reduction capacity.[12]
These steps have been independently validated in a series of *in vitro* experiments for their capacity to inactivate and/or remove both enveloped and non-enveloped viruses. Table 5 shows the virus clearance during the manufacturing process for Hizentra, expressed as the mean $\log_{10}$ reduction factor (LRF).
[See table 5 below]
The manufacturing process was also investigated for its capacity to decrease the infectivity of an experimental agent of transmissible spongiform encephalopathy (TSE), considered a model for CJD and its variant (vCJD).[12] Several of the production steps have been shown to decrease infectivity of an experimental TSE model agent. TSE reduction steps include octanoic acid fractionation (≥6.4 $\log_{10}$), depth filtration (2.6 $\log_{10}$), and virus filtration (≥5.8 $\log_{10}$). These studies

Table 5: Virus Inactivation/Removal in Hizentra*

	HIV-1	PRV	BVDV	WNV	EMCV	MVM
Virus Property						
Genome	RNA	DNA	RNA	RNA	RNA	DNA
Envelope	Yes	Yes	Yes	Yes	No	No
Size (nm)	80-100	120-200	50-70	50-70	25-30	18-24
Manufacturing Step	**Mean LRF**					
pH 4 incubation	≥5.4	≥5.9	4.6	≥7.8	nt	nt
Depth filtration	≥5.3	≥6.3	2.1	3.0	4.2	2.3
Virus filtration	≥5.3	≥5.5	≥5.1	≥5.9	≥5.4	≥5.5
Overall Reduction (Log₁₀ Units)	≥16.0	≥17.7	≥11.8	≥16.7	≥9.6	≥7.8

HIV-1, human immunodeficiency virus type 1, a model for HIV-1 and HIV-2; PRV, pseudorabies virus, a nonspecific model for large enveloped DNA viruses (e.g., herpes virus); BVDV, bovine viral diarrhea virus, a model for hepatitis C virus; WNV, West Nile virus; EMCV, encephalomyocarditis virus, a model for hepatitis A virus; MVM, minute virus of mice, a model for a small highly resistant non-enveloped DNA virus (e.g., parvovirus); LRF, $\log_{10}$ reduction factor; nt, not tested; na, not applicable.

* The virus clearance of human parvovirus B19 was investigated experimentally at the pH 4 incubation step. The estimated LRF obtained was ≥5.3.

provide reasonable assurance that low levels of vCJD/CJD agent infectivity, if present in the starting material, would be removed.

12 CLINICAL PHARMACOLOGY
12.1 Mechanism of Action
Hizentra supplies a broad spectrum of opsonizing and neutralizing IgG antibodies against a wide variety of bacterial and viral agents. The mechanism of action in PI has not been fully elucidated.

12.3 Pharmacokinetics
Clinical Studies
The pharmacokinetics (PK) of Hizentra was evaluated in a PK substudy of subjects (14 adults, 1 pediatric subject 6 to <12 years, and 3 adolescent subjects 12 to <16 years) with PI participating in the 15-month efficacy and safety study *[see Clinical Studies (14)]*. All PK subjects were treated previously with Privigen®, Immune Globulin Intravenous (Human), 10% Liquid and were switched to weekly subcutaneous treatment with Hizentra. After a 3-month wash-in/wash-out period, doses were adjusted individually with the goal of providing a systemic serum IgG exposure (area under the IgG serum concentration vs time curve; AUC) not inferior to that of the previous weekly-equivalent IGIV dose. Table 6 summarizes PK parameters for subjects in the substudy following treatment with Hizentra and IGIV.

Table 6: Pharmacokinetics Parameters of Hizentra and IGIV, US Study

	Hizentra	IGIV* (Privigen®)
Number of subjects	18	18
Dose* (mg/kg)		
Mean	228	152
Range	141-381	86-254
IgG peak levels (mg/dL)		
Mean	1616	2564
Range	1090-2825	2046-3456
IgG trough levels (mg/dL)		
Mean	1448	1127
Range	952-2623	702-1810
AUC† (day × mg/dL)		
Mean	10560	10320
Range	7210-18670	8051-15530
CL‡ (mL/day/kg)		
Mean	2.2	1.3§
Range	1.2-3.7	0.9-2.1

AUC, area under the curve; CL, clearance.
* For IGIV: weekly-equivalent dose.
† Standardized to a 7-day period.
‡ Apparent clearance (CL/F) for Hizentra (F = bioavailability)
§ Based on n=25 from the US Privigen PI study.

For the 19 subjects completing the wash-in/wash-out period, the average dose adjustment for Hizentra was 153% (range: 126% to 187%) of the previous weekly-equivalent IGIV dose. After 12 weeks of treatment with Hizentra at this individually adjusted dose, the final steady-state AUC determinations were made in 18 of the 19 subjects. The geometric mean ratio of the steady-state AUCs, standardized to a weekly treatment period, for Hizentra vs IGIV treatment was 1.002 (range: 0.77 to 1.20) with a 90% confidence limit of 0.951 to 1.055 for the 18 subjects.

With Hizentra, peak serum levels are lower (1616 vs 2564 mg/dL) than those achieved with IGIV while trough levels are generally higher (1448 vs 1127 mg/dL). In contrast to IGIV administered every 3 to 4 weeks, weekly subcutaneous administration results in relatively stable steady-state serum IgG levels.[13,14] After the subjects had reached steady-state with weekly administration of Hizentra, peak serum IgG levels were observed after a mean of 2.9 days (range: 0 to 7 days) in 18 subjects.

Table 7 summarizes PK parameters at steady state for pediatric subjects (age groups: 6 to <12 and 12 to <16 years) and adults subjects (>16 years) in the European Hizentra study following weekly treatment *[see Clinical Studies*

Table 7: Pediatric Pharmacokinetics Parameters of Hizentra, European Study

	Age Group			Total (n=23)
	6 to <12 years (n=9)	12 to <16 years (n=3)	16 to <65 years (n=11)	
Dose (mg/kg)				
Mean	120	115	117	118
Range	71-170	72-150	87-156	71-170
IgG trough levels (mg/dL)				
Mean	731	764	754	746
Range	531-915	615-957	505-898	505-957
AUC_{0-7d} (day × mg/dL)				
Mean	5230	5491	5452	5370
Range	3890-6950	4480-6750	3860-6810	3860-6950
CL (mL/day/kg)				
Mean	2.19	2.17	2.30	2.23
Range	1.57-3.05	1.38-3.34	1.82-3.01	1.38-3.34

AUC_{0-7d}, area under the curve for the 7-day dosing interval; CL, apparent clearance (CL/F) (F = bioavailability).

(14.2)]. Pediatric PK parameters are similar to those of adult subjects; thus no pediatric specific dose requirements are needed for Hizentra dosing.
[See table 7 above]

Pharmacokinetic Modeling and Simulation
Biweekly (Every Two Weeks) or more Frequent Dosing
Pharmacokinetic characterization of biweekly or more frequent dosing of Hizentra was undertaken using population PK-based modeling and simulation. Serum IgG concentration data consisted of 3837 samples from 151 unique pediatric and adult subjects with PI from four clinical studies of IGIV (Privigen®) and/or Hizentra. Of the 151 subjects, 94 were adult subjects (63 from Hizentra clinical studies) and 57 were pediatric subjects (32 from Hizentra clinical studies). Compared with weekly administration, PK modeling and simulation predicted that administration of Hizentra on a biweekly basis at double the weekly dose results in comparable IgG exposure [equivalent AUCs, with a slightly higher IgG peak (C_{max}) and slightly lower trough (C_{min})]. In addition, PK modeling and simulation predicted that for the same total weekly dose, Hizentra infusions given 2, 3, 5, or 7 times per week (frequent dosing) produce IgG exposures comparable to weekly dosing [equivalent AUCs, with a slightly lower IgG peak (C_{max}) and slightly higher trough (C_{min})]. Frequent dosing reduces the peak-to-trough variation in Hizentra exposure, thus resulting in more sustained IgG exposures. See Table 8 (columns for AUC, C_{max} and C_{min}).

Dose Adjustment Factor
Using data from four clinical studies, results of model-based simulations demonstrated that weekly or biweekly Hizentra dosing regimens with an IGIV:IGSC dose adjustment factor of 1:1.37 adequately maintain median $AUC_{0-28days}$ and C_{min} ratios at ≥90% of values observed with 4-weekly IGIV dosing. See Table 8 (top two rows).

Prediction of Trough Levels Following Regimen Changes
PK modeling and simulation also predicted changes in trough levels after switching from (a) monthly IGIV to weekly or biweekly Hizentra dosing, (b) weekly to biweekly Hizentra dosing, or (c) weekly to more frequent dosing. Table 8 (last column) shows the predicted changes in steady-state IgG trough levels after switching between the various dosing regimens.
[See table 8 on next page]

Pediatric Pharmacokinetics
PK-based modeling and simulation results indicate that, similar to observations from the clinical study with weekly Hizentra dosing (Table 7), body weight-adjusted biweekly dosing accounted for age-related (>3 years) differences in clearance of Hizentra, thereby maintaining systemic IgG exposure (AUC values) in the therapeutic range.

13 NONCLINICAL TOXICOLOGY
13.2 Animal Toxicology and/or Pharmacology
Long- and short-term memory loss was seen in juvenile rats in a study modeling hyperprolinemia. In this study, rats received daily subcutaneous injections with L-proline from day 6 to day 28 of life.[15] The daily amounts of L-proline used in this study were more than 60 times higher than the L-proline dose that would result from the administration of 400 mg/kg body weight of Hizentra once weekly. In unpublished studies using the same animal model (i.e., rats) dosed

with the same amount of L-proline with a dosing interval relevant to IGSC treatment (i.e., on 5 consecutive days on days 9 to 13, or once weekly on days 9, 16, and 23), no effects on learning and memory were observed. The clinical relevance of these studies is not known.

14 CLINICAL STUDIES
14.1 US Study
A prospective, open-label, multicenter, single-arm, clinical study conducted in the US evaluated the efficacy, tolerability, and safety of Hizentra in 49 adult and pediatric subjects with PI. Subjects previously receiving monthly treatment with IGIV were switched to weekly subcutaneous administration of Hizentra for 15 months. Following a 3-month wash-in/wash-out period, subjects received a dose adjustment to achieve an equivalent AUC to their previous IGIV dose *[see Pharmacokinetics (12.3)]* and continued treatment for a 12-month efficacy period. The efficacy analyses included 38 subjects in the modified intention-to-treat (MITT) population. The MITT population consisted of subjects who completed the wash-in/wash-out period and received at least one infusion of Hizentra during the efficacy period.

Although 5% of the administered doses could not be verified, the weekly median doses of Hizentra ranged from 72 to 379 mg/kg body weight during the efficacy period. The mean dose was 213.2 mg/kg, which was 149% of the previous IGIV dose.

In the study, the number of injection sites per infusion ranged from 1 to 12. In 73% of infusions, the number of injection sites was 4 or fewer. Up to 4 simultaneous injection sites were permitted using 2 pumps; however, more than 4 sites could be used consecutively during one infusion. The infusion flow rate did not exceed 50 mL per hour for all injection sites combined. During the efficacy period, the median duration of a weekly infusion ranged from 1.6 to 2.0 hours.

The study evaluated the annual rate of serious bacterial infections (SBIs), defined as bacterial pneumonia, bacteremia/septicemia, osteomyelitis/septic arthritis, bacterial meningitis, and visceral abscess. The study also evaluated the annual rate of any infections, the use of antibiotics for infection (prophylaxis or treatment), the days out of work/school/kindergarten/day care or unable to perform normal activities due to infections, hospitalizations due to infections, and serum IgG trough levels.

Table 9 summarizes the efficacy results for subjects in the efficacy period (MITT population) of the study. No subjects experienced an SBI in this study.

Table 9: Summary of Efficacy Results (MITT Population)

Number of subjects (efficacy period)	38
Total number of subject days	12,697
Infections	
Annual rate of SBIs*	0 SBIs per subject year†
Annual rate of any infections	2.76 infections/subject year‡

Continued on next page

Antibiotic use for infection (prophylaxis or treatment)	
Number of subjects (%)	27 (71.1)
Annual rate	48.5 days/subject year
Total number of subject days	12,605
Days out of work/school/ kindergarten/day care or unable to perform normal activities due to infections	
Number of days (%)	71 (0.56)
Annual rate	2.06 days/subject year
Hospitalizations due to infections	
Number of days (%)	7 (0.06)§
Annual rate	0.2 days/subject year

* Defined as bacterial pneumonia, bacteremia/septicemia, osteomyelitis/septic arthritis, bacterial meningitis, and visceral abscess.
† Upper 99% confidence limit: 0.132.
‡ 95% confidence limits: 2.235; 3.370.
§ Based on 1 subject.

The mean IgG trough levels increased by 24.2%, from 1009 mg/dL prior to the study to 1253 mg/dL during the efficacy period.

14.2 European Study

In a prospective, open-label, multicenter, single-arm, clinical study conducted in Europe, 51 adult and pediatric subjects with PI switched from monthly IGIV (31 subjects) or weekly IGSC (20 subjects) to weekly treatment with Hizentra. For the 46 subjects in the efficacy analysis, the weekly mean dose in the efficacy period was 120.1 mg/kg (range 59 to 243 mg/kg), which was 104% of the previous weekly equivalent IGIV or weekly IGSC dose.

None of the subjects had an SBI during the efficacy period, resulting in an annualized rate of 0 (upper one-sided 99% confidence limit of 0.192) SBIs per subject. The annualized rate of any infections was 5.18 infections per subject for the efficacy period.

15 REFERENCES

1. Dalakas MC. High-dose intravenous immunoglobulin and serum viscosity: risk of precipitating thromboembolic events. *Neurology* 1994;44:223-226.
2. Woodruff RK, Grigg AP, Firkin FC, Smith IL. Fatal thrombotic events during treatment of autoimmune thrombocytopenia with intravenous immunoglobulin in elderly patients. *Lancet* 1986;2:217-218.
3. Wolberg AS, Kon RH, Monroe DM, Hoffman M. Coagulation factor XI is a contaminant in intravenous immunoglobulin preparations. *Am J Hematol* 2000;65:30-34.
4. Gabor EP, Meningitis and skin reaction after intravenous immune globulin therapy. *Ann Intern Med* 1997;127:1130.
5. Pierce LR, Jain N. Risks associated with the use of intravenous immunoglobulin. *Trans Med Rev* 2003;17:241-251.
6. Cayco AV, Perazella MA, Hayslett JP. Renal insufficiency after intravenous immune globulin therapy: a report of two cases and an analysis of the literature. *J Am Soc Nephrol* 1997;8:1788-1793.
7. Copelan EA, Strohm PL, Kennedy MS, Tutschka PJ. Hemolysis following intravenous immune globulin therapy. *Transfusion* 1986;26:410-412.
8. Thomas MJ, Misbah SA, Chapel HM, Jones M, Elrington G, Newsom-Davis J. Hemolysis after high-dose intravenous Ig. *Blood* 1993;15:3789.
9. Wilson JR, Bhoopalam N, Fisher M. Hemolytic anemia associated with intravenous immunoglobulin. *Muscle Nerve* 1997;20:1142-1145.
10. Kessary-Shoham H, Levy Y, Shoenfeld Y, Lorber M, Gershon H. *In vivo* administration of intravenous immunoglobulin (IVIg) can lead to enhanced erythrocyte sequestration. *J Autoimmun* 1999;13:129-135.
11. Rizk A, Gorson KC, Kenney L, Weinstein R. Transfusion-related acute lung injury after the infusion of IVIG. *Transfusion* 2001;41:264-268.
12. Stucki M, Boschetti N, Schäfer W, et al. Investigations of prion and virus safety of a new liquid IVIG product. *Biologicals* 2008;36:239-247.
13. Smith GN, Griffiths B, Mollison D, Mollison PL. Uptake of IgG after intramuscular and subcutaneous injection. *Lancet* 1972;1:1208-1212.
14. Waniewski I, Gardulf A, Hammarström L. Bioavailability of γ-globulin after subcutaneous infusions in patients with common variable immunodeficiency. *J Clin Immunol* 1994;14:90-97.
15. Bavaresco CS, Streck EL, Netto CA, et al. Chronic hyperprolinemia provokes a memory deficit in the Morris Water Maze Task. *Metabolic Brain Disease* 2005;20:73-80.

Table 8: Predicted Ratios* [Median (5th, 95th percentiles)] of AUC, C_{max} and C_{min} and Changes in IgG Trough Levels after Switching Between IgG Dosing Regimens

IgG Dosing Regimen Switch		AUC	C_{max}	C_{min}	Predicted Change in Trough†
From:	To:				
IGIV	Weekly Hizentra‡	0.97 (0.90-1.04)	0.68 (0.60-0.76)	1.16 (1.07-1.26)	16% increase
IGIV	Biweekly Hizentra§	0.97 (0.91-1.04)	0.71 (0.63-0.78)	1.10 (1.02-1.18)	10% increase
Weekly Hizentra	Biweekly Hizentra§	1.00 (0.98-1.03)	1.06 (1.02-1.09)	0.95 (0.92-0.98)	5% decrease
Weekly Hizentra	2 times per week Hizentra	1.01 (0.98-1.03)	0.99 (0.96-1.02)	1.03 (1.00-1.06)	3% increase
Weekly Hizentra	3 times per week Hizentra	1.01 (0.98-1.03)	0.99 (0.96-1.02)	1.04 (1.01-1.07)	4% increase
Weekly Hizentra	5 times per week Hizentra (daily for 5 days)	1.01 (0.98-1.03)	0.99 (0.97-1.01)	1.04 (1.01-1.06)	4% increase
Weekly Hizentra	Daily Hizentra (7 times per week)	1.00 (0.98-1.03)	0.98 (0.95-1.01)	1.04 (1.02-1.08)	4% increase

AUC, area under the curve, calculated as $AUC_{0-28days}$ for the IGIV to Hizentra switches, $AUC_{0-14days}$ for the weekly to biweekly Hizentra switch, and $AUC_{0-7days}$ for weekly to more frequent Hizentra switches; C_{max}, maximum IgG concentration; C_{min}, minimum IgG concentration during a 28-day period (for the IGIV to Hizentra switches), a 14-day period (for the weekly to biweekly Hizentra switch), or a 7-day period (for the weekly to more frequent Hizentra switches).
* Ratios are based on comparison of second regimen vs. first regimen.
† Approximate change in trough based on predicted median C_{min} ratio.
‡ Weekly dose based on dose adjustment factor of 1.37 when switching from IGIV.
§ Biweekly dose = 2× weekly dose, based on dose adjustment factor of 1.37 when switching from IGIV.

16 HOW SUPPLIED/STORAGE AND HANDLING

16.1 How Supplied

• Hizentra is supplied in a single-use, tamper-evident vial containing 0.2 grams of protein per mL of preservative-free liquid.

Each product presentation includes a package insert and the following components:

Presentation	Carton NDC Number	Components
5 mL	44206-451-01	Vial containing 1 gram of protein (NDC 44206-451-90)
10 mL	44206-452-02	Vial containing 2 grams of protein (NDC 44206-452-91)
20 mL	44206-454-04	Vial containing 4 grams of protein (NDC 44206-454-92)
50 mL	44206-455-10	Vial containing 10 grams of protein (NDC 44206-455-93)

16.2 Storage and Handling

• Keep Hizentra in its original carton to protect it from light.
• Each vial label contains a peel-off strip with the vial size and product lot number for use in recording doses in a patient treatment record.
• When stored at room temperature (up to 25°C [77°F]), Hizentra is stable for up to 30 months, as indicated by the expiration date printed on the outer carton and vial label.
• Do not shake.
• Do not freeze. Do not use product that has been frozen.
• The components used in the packaging for Hizentra contain no latex.

17 PATIENT COUNSELING INFORMATION

Advise the patient to read the FDA-approved patient labeling (Patient Information).
Inform patients to immediately report the following signs and symptoms to their healthcare provider:

• Hypersensitivity reactions to Hizentra (including hives, generalized urticaria, tightness of the chest, wheezing, hypotension, and anaphylaxis) *(see Warnings and Precautions [5.1])*.
• Pain and/or swelling of an arm or leg with warmth over the affected area, discoloration of an arm or leg, unexplained shortness of breath, chest pain or discomfort that worsens on deep breathing, unexplained rapid pulse, or numbness or weakness on one side of the body *(see Warnings and Precautions [5.2])*.
• Severe headache, neck stiffness, drowsiness, fever, sensitivity to light, painful eye movements, nausea, and vomiting *(see Warnings and Precautions [5.3])*.
• Decreased urine output, sudden weight gain, fluid retention/edema, and/or shortness of breath *(see Warnings and Precautions [5.4])*.
• Fatigue, increased heart rate, yellowing of the skin or eyes, and dark-colored urine *(see Warnings and Precautions [5.5])*.
• Severe breathing problems, lightheadedness, drops in blood pressure, and fever *(see Warnings and Precautions [5.6])*.

Inform patients that because Hizentra is made from human blood, it may carry a risk of transmitting infectious agents, e.g., viruses, the variant Creutzfeldt-Jakob disease (vCJD) agent and, theoretically, the Creutzfeldt-Jakob disease (CJD) agent *(see Warnings and Precautions [5.7] and Description [11])*.

Inform patients that Hizentra may interfere with the response to live virus vaccines (e.g., measles, mumps, rubella, and varicella) and to notify their immunizing physician of recent therapy with Hizentra *(see Drug Interactions [7])*.

Home Treatment for Primary Humoral Immunodeficiency with Subcutaneous Administration

• If self-administration is deemed to be appropriate, ensure that the patient receives clear instructions and training on subcutaneous administration in the home or other appropriate setting and has demonstrated the ability to independently administer subcutaneous infusions.
• Ensure the patient understands the importance of adhering to their prescribed administration schedule to maintain appropriate steady IgG levels.
• Instruct patients to scan the vial if recording the infusion electronically and keep a diary/log book that includes information about each infusion such as, the time, date, dose, lot number(s) and any reactions.
• Inform the patient that mild to moderate local injection-site reactions (e.g., swelling and redness) are a common side effect of subcutaneous therapy, but to contact their healthcare professional if a local reaction increases in severity or persists for more than a few days.

Step 1: Assemble supplies
Gather the Hizentra vial(s), the following disposable supplies (not provided with Hizentra), and other items (infusion pump, sharps or other container, treatment diary or log book):

   Infusion administration tubing
   Needle or catheter sets (for subcutaneous infusion)
   Y-site connectors (if needed)
   Alcohol wipes
   Antiseptic skin preps
   Syringes
   Transfer device or needle(s)
   Gauze and tape, or transparent dressing
   Gloves (if recommended by your doctor)

Step 2: Clean surface
Thoroughly clean a table or other flat surface using one of the alcohol wipes.

Step 3: Wash hands

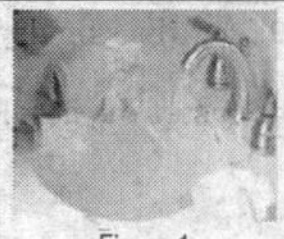

- Thoroughly wash and dry your hands (Figure 1).
- If you have been told to wear gloves when preparing your infusion, put the gloves on.

Step 4: Check vials
Carefully look at the liquid in each vial of Hizentra (Figure 2). Hizentra is a pale yellow to light brown solution. Check for particles or color changes. **Do not use the vial if:**

- The liquid looks cloudy, contains particles, or has changed color.
- The protective cap is missing.
- The expiration date on the label has passed.

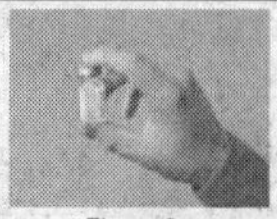

Step 5: Transfer Hizentra from vial(s) to syringe
- Take the protective cap off the vial (Figure 3).

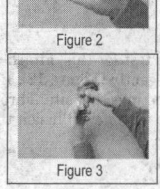

Figure 1

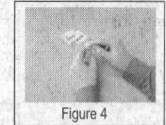

Figure 2

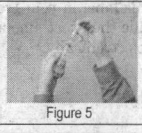

Figure 3

Clean the vial stopper with an alcohol wipe (Figure 4). Let the stopper dry.

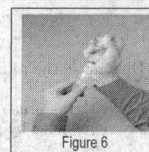

Figure 4

- Attach a needle or transfer device to a syringe tip, using aseptic technique. If using a transfer device, follow the instructions provided by the device manufacturer. If using a needle and a syringe to transfer Hizentra, follow the instructions below.
  - Attach a sterile transfer needle to a sterile syringe (Figure 5).
  - Pull out the plunger of the syringe to fill the syringe with air. Make sure the amount of air is the same as the amount of Hizentra you will transfer from the vial.
  - Put the Hizentra vial on a flat surface. Keeping the vial upright, insert the transfer needle into the center of the rubber stopper.
  - Check that the tip of the needle is not in the liquid. Then, push the plunger of the syringe down. This will inject the air from the syringe into the airspace of the vial.
  - Leaving the needle in the stopper, carefully turn the vial upside down (Figure 6).
  - Slowly pull back on the plunger of the syringe to fill the syringe with Hizentra.
  - Take the filled syringe and needle out of the stopper. Take off the needle and throw it away in the sharps container.

Figure 5

Figure 6

This table is continued on the next page

- Inform patients of the importance of having an infusion needle long enough to reach the subcutaneous tissue and of changing the actual site of injection with each infusion. Explain that Hizentra is for subcutaneous infusion only, and must not be injected into a blood vessel. Make sure patients know how to avoid blood vessels and check if the needle has entered a blood vessel.
- Inform patients to consider adjusting the injection-site location, volume per site, and rate of infusion based on how infusions are tolerated.
- Inform patient to interrupt or terminate the Hizentra infusion if a hypersensitivity reaction occurs.
- Inform patients that they should be tested regularly to make sure they have the correct levels of Hizentra (IgG) in their blood. These tests may result in adjustments to the Hizentra dose.

Hizentra
Immune Globulin Subcutaneous (Human), 20% Liquid
Information for Patients
This patient package insert summarizes important information about Hizentra. Please read it carefully before using this medicine. This information does not take the place of talking with your healthcare professional, and it does not include all of the important information about Hizentra. If you have any questions after reading this, ask your healthcare professional.

What is the most important information I should know about Hizentra?
Hizentra is supposed to be infused under your skin only. DO NOT inject Hizentra into a blood vessel (vein or artery).

What is Hizentra?
Hizentra (Hi – ZEN – tra) is a prescription medicine used to treat primary immune deficiency (PI). Hizentra is made from human plasma. It contains antibodies, called immunoglobulin G (IgG), that healthy people have to fight germs (bacteria and viruses).
People with PI get a lot of infections. Hizentra helps lower the number of infections you will get.

Who should <u>NOT</u> take Hizentra?
Do not take Hizentra if you have too much proline in your blood (called "hyperprolinemia") or if you have had reactions to polysorbate 80.

Tell your doctor if you have had a serious reaction to other immune globulin medicines or if you have been told that you also have a deficiency of the immunoglobulin called IgA. Tell your doctor if you have a history of heart or blood vessel disease or blood clots, have thick blood, or have been immobile for some time. These things may increase your risk of having a blood clot after using Hizentra. Also tell your doctor what drugs you are using, as some drugs, such as those that contain the hormone estrogen (for example, birth control pills), may increase your risk of developing a blood clot.

How should I take Hizentra?
You will take Hizentra through an infusion, only under your skin. Make sure that the infusion is not into a blood vessel. You will place up to 4 needles into different areas of your body each time you use Hizentra. The needles are attached to a pump with an infusion tube. You can have infusions as often as every day up to every two weeks. For weekly infusions, it can take about 1 to 2 hours to complete an infusion; however, this time may be shorter or longer depending on the dose and frequency your doctor has prescribed for you. Instructions for using Hizentra are at the end of this patient package insert (see "How do I use Hizentra?"). Do not use Hizentra by yourself until you have been taught how by your doctor or healthcare professional.

What should I avoid while taking Hizentra?
Vaccines may not work well for you while you are taking Hizentra. Tell your doctor or healthcare professional that you are taking Hizentra before you get a vaccine.
Tell your doctor or healthcare professional if you are pregnant or plan to become pregnant, or if you are nursing.

What are possible side effects of Hizentra?
The most common side effects with Hizentra are:
- Redness, swelling, itching, and/or bruising at the injection site
- Headache/migraine
- Nausea and/or vomiting
- Pain (including pain in the chest, back, joints, arms, legs)
- Fatigue
- Diarrhea
- Stomach ache/bloating
- Cough
- Rash (including hives)
- Itching
- Fever and/or chills
- Shortness of breath
- Dizziness

Tell your doctor right away or go to the emergency room if you have hives, trouble breathing, wheezing, dizziness, or fainting. These could be signs of a bad allergic reaction.
Tell your doctor right away if you have any of the following symptoms. They could be signs of a serious problem.
- Reduced urination, sudden weight gain, or swelling in your legs. These could be signs of a kidney problem.
- Pain and/or swelling of an arm or leg with warmth over the affected area, discoloration of an arm or leg, unexplained shortness of breath, chest pain or discomfort that worsens on deep breathing, unexplained rapid pulse, or numbness or weakness on one side of the body. These could be signs of a blood clot.
- Bad headache with nausea, vomiting, stiff neck, fever, and sensitivity to light. These could be signs of a brain swelling called meningitis.
- Brown or red urine, fast heart rate, yellow skin or eyes. These could be signs of a blood problem.
- Chest pains or trouble breathing.
- Fever over 100°F. This could be a sign of an infection.

Tell your doctor about any side effects that concern you. You can ask your doctor to give you more information that is available to healthcare professionals.

How do I use Hizentra?
Infuse Hizentra only after you have been trained by your doctor or healthcare professional. Below are step-by-step instructions to help you remember how to use Hizentra. Ask your doctor or healthcare professional about any instructions you do not understand.

Instructions for use
Hizentra comes in single-use vials.
Keep Hizentra in the storage box at room temperature.
Manufactured by:
CSL Behring AG
Bern, Switzerland
US License No. 1766
Distributed by:
CSL Behring LLC
Kankakee, IL 60901 USA
Shown in Product Identification Guide, page 508

When using multiple vials to achieve the desired dose, repeat this step.

Step 6: Prepare infusion pump and tubing
Prepare the infusion pump (following the manufacturer's instructions) and prime (fill) the infusion tubing. To prime the tubing, connect the syringe filled with Hizentra to the infusion tubing and gently push on the syringe plunger to fill the tubing with Hizentra (Figure 7).

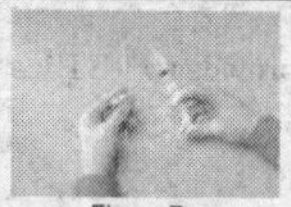

Step 7: Prepare injection site(s)
• Select an area on your abdomen, thigh, upper arm, or side of upper leg/hip for the infusion (Figure 8).
• Use a different site from the last time you infused Hizentra. New sites should be at least 1 inch from a previous site.
• Never infuse into areas where the skin is tender, bruised, red, or hard. Avoid infusing into scars or stretch marks.
• If you are using more than one injection site, be sure the injection sites are at least 2 inches apart.
• During an infusion, do not use more than 4 injection sites at the same time.
• Clean the skin at each site with an antiseptic skin prep (Figure 9). Let the skin dry.

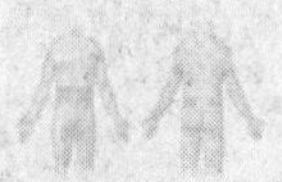

Step 8: Insert needle(s)
• With two fingers, pinch together the skin around the injection site. Insert the needle under the skin (Figure 10).

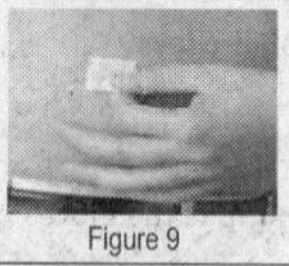

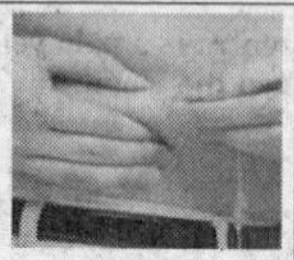

• Put sterile gauze and tape or a transparent dressing over the injection site (Figure 11). This will keep the needle from coming out.

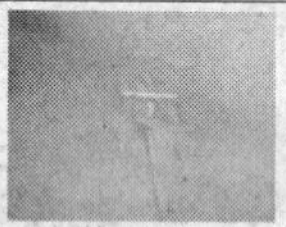

• Make sure you are not injecting Hizentra into a blood vessel. To test for this, attach a sterile syringe to the end of the infusion tubing. Pull the plunger back gently (Figure 12). If you see any blood flowing back into the tubing, take the needle out of the injection site. Throw away the tubing and needle. Start the infusion over at a different site with new infusion tubing and a new needle.

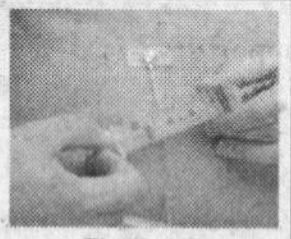

Step 9: Start infusion
Follow the manufacturer's instructions to turn on the infusion pump (Figure 13).

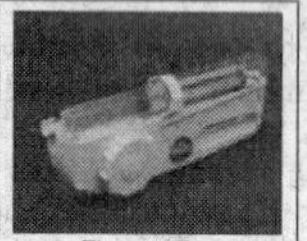

Step 10: Record treatment (Figure 14)
Peel off the removable part of the label of the Hizentra vial. Put this label in your treatment diary or log book with the date and time of the infusion. Also include the exact amount of Hizentra that you infused. Scan the vial if recording the infusion electronically.

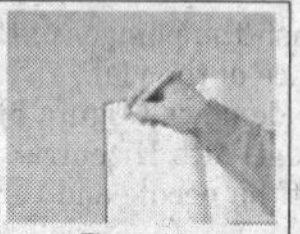

Step 11: Clean up
• When all the Hizentra has been infused, turn off the pump.
• Take off the dressing and take the needle out of the injection site. Disconnect the tubing from the pump.
• Throw away any Hizentra that is leftover in the single-use vial, along with the used disposable supplies, in the sharps or other container (Figure 15) as recommended by your healthcare professional.
• Clean and store the infusion pump, following the manufacturer's instructions.

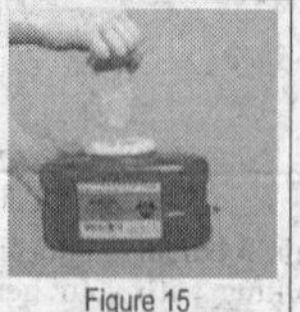

Be sure to tell your doctor about any problems you have doing your infusions. Your doctor may ask to see your treatment diary or log book, so be sure to take it with you each time you visit the doctor's office.

Call your doctor for medical advice about side effects. You can also report side effects to FDA at 1-800-FDA-1088 or *www.fda.gov/medwatch*.

Figure 7

Figure 8

Figure 9

Figure 10

Figure 11

Figure 12

Figure 13

Figure 14

Figure 15

• Kcentra was not studied in subjects who had a thromboembolic event, myocardial infarction, disseminated intravascular coagulation, cerebral vascular accident, transient ischemic attack, unstable angina pectoris, or severe peripheral vascular disease within the prior 3 months. Kcentra may not be suitable in patients with thromboembolic events in the prior 3 months. (5.2)

RECENT MAJOR CHANGES

Indications and Usage (1)	12/2013
Dosage and Administration (2.1)	11/2013
Warnings and Precautions (5.2)	12/2013

INDICATIONS AND USAGE

Kcentra, Prothrombin Complex Concentrate (Human), is a blood coagulation factor replacement product indicated for the urgent reversal of acquired coagulation factor deficiency induced by Vitamin K antagonist (VKA, e.g., warfarin) therapy in adult patients with:
• acute major bleeding or
• need for an urgent surgery/invasive procedure. (1)

DOSAGE AND ADMINISTRATION

For intravenous use only.
• Kcentra dosing should be individualized based on the patient's baseline International Normalized Ratio (INR) value, and body weight. (2.1)
• Administer Vitamin K concurrently to patients receiving Kcentra to maintain factor levels once the effects of Kcentra have diminished.
• The safety and effectiveness of repeat dosing have not been established and it is not recommended. (2.1)
• Administer reconstituted Kcentra at a rate of 0.12 mL/kg/min (~3 units/kg/min) up to a maximum rate of 8.4 mL/min (~210 units/min). (2.3)

Pre-treatment INR	2–< 4	4–6	> 6
Dose* of Kcentra (units† of Factor IX) / kg body weight	25	35	50
Maximum dose‡ (units of Factor IX)	Not to exceed 2500	Not to exceed 3500	Not to exceed 5000

* Dosing is based on body weight. Dose based on actual potency as stated on the carton, which will vary from 20--31 Factor IX units/mL after reconstitution. Nominal potency is 500 or 1000 units per vial, approximately 25 units per mL after reconstitution.
† Units refer to International Units.
‡ Dose is based on body weight up to but not exceeding 100 kg. For patients weighing more than 100 kg, maximum dose should not be exceeded.

DOSAGE FORMS AND STRENGTHS

• Kcentra is available as a single-use vial containing coagulation Factors II, VII, IX and X, and antithrombotic Proteins C and S as a lyophilized concentrate. (3)

CONTRAINDICATIONS

Kcentra is contraindicated in patients with:
• Known anaphylactic or severe systemic reactions to Kcentra or any components in Kcentra including heparin, Factors II, VII, IX, X, Proteins C and S, Antithrombin III and human albumin. (4)
• Disseminated intravascular coagulation. (4)
• Known heparin-induced thrombocytopenia. Kcentra contains heparin. (4)

WARNINGS AND PRECAUTIONS

• Hypersensitivity reactions may occur. If necessary, discontinue administration and institute appropriate treatment. (5.1)
• Arterial and venous thromboembolic complications have been reported in patients receiving Kcentra. Monitor patients receiving Kcentra for signs and symptoms of thromboembolic events. Kcentra was not studied in subjects who had a thrombotic or thromboembolic (TE) event within the prior 3 months. Kcentra may not be suitable in patients with thromboembolic events in the prior 3 months. (5.2)
• Kcentra is made from human blood and may carry a risk of transmitting infectious agents, e.g., viruses, the variant Creutzfeldt-Jakob disease (vCJD) agent, and theoretically,

---

KCENTRA® ℞
Prothrombin Complex Concentrate (Human)
For Intravenous Use, Lyophilized Powder for Reconstitution

HIGHLIGHTS OF PRESCRIBING INFORMATION
These highlights do not include all the information needed to use KCENTRA safely and effectively. See full prescribing information for KCENTRA.
KCENTRA (Prothrombin Complex Concentrate (Human))
For Intravenous Use, Lyophilized Powder for Reconstitution
Initial U.S. Approval: 2013

WARNING: ARTERIAL AND VENOUS THROMBOEMBOLIC COMPLICATIONS

Patients being treated with Vitamin K antagonists (VKA) therapy have underlying disease states that predispose them to thromboembolic events. Potential benefits of reversing VKA should be weighed against the potential risks of thromboembolic events, especially in patients with the history of a thromboembolic event. Resumption of anticoagulation should be carefully considered as soon as the risk of thromboembolic events outweighs the risk of acute bleeding.
• Both fatal and non-fatal arterial and venous thromboembolic complications have been reported with Kcentra in clinical trials and post marketing surveillance. Monitor patients receiving Kcentra for signs and symptoms of thromboembolic events.

ADVERSE REACTIONS

- The most common adverse reactions (ARs) (frequency ≥ 2.8%) observed in subjects receiving Kcentra were headache, nausea/vomiting, hypotension, and anemia. (6)
- The most serious ARs were thromboembolic events including stroke, pulmonary embolism, and deep vein thrombosis. (6)

To report SUSPECTED ADVERSE REACTIONS, contact CSL Behring at 1-866-915-6958 or FDA at 1-800-FDA-1088 or *www.fda.gov/medwatch*.

USE IN SPECIFIC POPULATIONS

Pregnancy: No human or animal data. Use only if clearly needed. (8.1)

See 17 for PATIENT COUNSELING INFORMATION.

Revised: 9/2014

FULL PRESCRIBING INFORMATION: CONTENTS*
WARNING: ARTERIAL AND VENOUS THROMBOEM-BOLIC COMPLICATIONS

FULL PRESCRIBING INFORMATION

> **WARNING: ARTERIAL AND VENOUS THROMBO-EMBOLIC COMPLICATIONS**
>
> **Patients being treated with Vitamin K antagonists (VKA) therapy have underlying disease states that predispose them to thromboembolic events. Potential benefits of reversing VKA should be weighed against the potential risks of thromboembolic events (TE), especially in patients with the history of a thromboembolic event. Resumption of anticoagulation should be carefully considered as soon as the risk of thromboembolic events outweighs the risk of acute bleeding.**
>
> - **Both fatal and non-fatal arterial and venous thromboembolic complications have been reported with Kcentra in clinical trials and post marketing surveillance. Monitor patients receiving Kcentra for signs and symptoms of thromboembolic events. (5.2)**
> - **Kcentra was not studied in subjects who had a thromboembolic event, myocardial infarction, disseminated intravascular coagulation, cerebral vascular accident, transient ischemic attack, unstable angina pectoris, or severe peripheral vascular disease within the prior 3 months. Kcentra may not be suitable in patients with thromboembolic events in the prior 3 months. (5.2)**

1   INDICATIONS AND USAGE

Kcentra, (Prothrombin Complex Concentrate (Human)), is a blood coagulation factor replacement product indicated for the urgent reversal of acquired coagulation factor deficiency induced by Vitamin K antagonist (VKA, e.g., warfarin) therapy in adult patients with:

- acute major bleeding or
- need for an urgent surgery/invasive procedure.

2   DOSAGE AND ADMINISTRATION

For intravenous use only.

2.1   Dosage

- Measurement of INR prior to treatment and close to the time of dosing is important because coagulation factors may be unstable in patients with acute major bleeding or an urgent need for surgery and other invasive procedures.
- Individualize Kcentra dosing based on the patient's current pre-dose International Normalized Ratio (INR) value, and body weight (*see Table 1*).
- The actual potency per vial of Factors II, VII, IX and X, Proteins C and S is stated on the carton.
- Administer Vitamin K concurrently to patients receiving Kcentra. Vitamin K is administered to maintain Vitamin K-dependent clotting factor levels once the effects of Kcentra have diminished.
- The safety and effectiveness of repeat dosing have not been established and it is not recommended.
- Dose ranging within pre-treatment INR groups has not been studied in randomized clinical trials of Kcentra.

Table 1: Dosage Required for Reversal of VKA Anticoagulation in Patients with acute major bleeding or need for an urgent surgery/invasive procedure

Pre-treatment INR	2–< 4	4–6	> 6
Dose* of Kcentra (units† of Factor IX) / kg body weight	25	35	50
Maximum dose‡ (units of Factor IX)	Not to exceed 2500	Not to exceed 3500	Not to exceed 5000

* Dosing is based on body weight. Dose based on actual potency as stated on the carton, which will vary from 20–31 Factor IX units/mL after reconstitution. Nominal potency is 500 or 1000 units per vial, approximately 25 units per mL after reconstitution.
† Units refer to International Units.
‡ Dose is based on body weight up to but not exceeding 100 kg. For patients weighing more than 100 kg, maximum dose should not be exceeded.

Example dosing calculation for 80 kg patient

For example, an 80 kg patient with a baseline of INR of 5.0, the dose would be 2,800 Factor IX units of Kcentra, calculated as follows based on INR range of 4–6, see *Table 1*:

$$35 \text{ units of Factor IX/kg} \times 80 \text{ kg} = 2{,}800 \text{ units of Factor IX required*}$$

* For a vial with an actual potency of 30 units/mL Factor IX, 93 mL would be given (2,800 U/30 U per mL = 93 mL).

Monitor INR and clinical response during and after treatment. In clinical trials, Kcentra decreased the INR to ≤ 1.3 within 30 minutes in most subjects. The relationship between this or other INR values and clinical hemostasis in patients has not been established *[see Clinical Studies (14)]*.

2.2   Preparation and Reconstitution

- Reconstitute using aseptic technique with 20 mL (500 U kit) or 40 mL (1000 U kit) of diluent provided with the kit.
- Visually inspect parenteral drug products for particulate matter and discoloration prior to administration whenever solution and container permit. Reconstituted Kcentra solution should be colorless, clear to slightly opalescent, and free from visible particles. Do not use solutions that are cloudy or have deposits.
- Kcentra is for single use only. Contains no preservatives. Discard partially used vials.

The procedures provided in *Table 2* are general guidelines for the preparation and reconstitution of Kcentra.

Reconstitute at room temperature as follows:

[See table 2 on pages 946 through 948]

2.3   Administration

- Do not mix Kcentra with other medicinal products; administer through a separate infusion line.
- Use aseptic technique when administering Kcentra.
- Administer at room temperature.
- Administer by intravenous infusion at a rate of 0.12 mL/kg/min (~3 units/kg/min), up to a maximum rate of 8.4 mL/min (~210 units/min).

- No blood should enter the syringe, as there is a possibility of fibrin clot formation.

3   DOSAGE FORMS AND STRENGTHS

- Kcentra is available as a single use vial containing coagulation Factors II, VII, IX and X, antithrombotic Proteins C and S as a lyophilized concentrate.
- Kcentra potency (units) is defined by Factor IX content. The range of Factor IX units per vial is 400–620 units for the 500 U kit and 800–1240 units for the 1000 U kit. When reconstituted, the final concentration of drug product in Factor IX units will be in a range from 20–31 units/mL.
- The actual content of Factor IX as measured in units of potency is stated on the vial.
- The actual units of potency for each coagulation factor (Factors II, VII, IX and X), and Proteins C and S are stated on the carton.

4   CONTRAINDICATIONS

Kcentra is contraindicated in:

- Patients with known anaphylactic or severe systemic reactions to Kcentra or any components in Kcentra including heparin, Factors II, VII, IX, X, Proteins C and S, Antithrombin III and human albumin.
- Patients with disseminated intravascular coagulation (DIC).
- Patients with known heparin-induced thrombocytopenia (HIT). Kcentra contains heparin *[see Description (11)]*.

5   WARNINGS AND PRECAUTIONS

5.1   Hypersensitivity Reactions

Hypersensitivity reactions including flushing, urticaria, tachycardia, anxiety, angioedema, wheezing, nausea, vomiting, hypotension, tachypnea, dyspnea, pulmonary edema, and bronchospasm have been observed with Kcentra.

If severe allergic reaction or anaphylactic type reactions occur, immediately discontinue administration, and institute appropriate treatment.

5.2   Thromboembolic Risk/Complications

Both fatal and non-fatal arterial thromboembolic events (including acute myocardial infarction and arterial thrombosis), and venous thromboembolic events (including pulmonary embolism and venous thrombosis) and disseminated intravascular coagulation have been reported with Kcentra in clinical trials and post marketing surveillance *[see Adverse Reactions (6) and Clinical Studies (14)]*. Patients being treated with VKA therapy have underlying disease states that predispose them to thromboembolic events. Reversing VKA therapy exposes patients to the thromboembolic risk of their underlying disease. Resumption of anticoagulation should be carefully considered following administration of Kcentra and Vitamin K once the risk of thromboembolic events outweighs the risk of bleeding.

Thromboembolic events occurred more frequently following Kcentra compared to plasma in a randomized, plasma controlled trial in subjects requiring urgent reversal of VKA anticoagulation due to acute major bleeding, and the excess in thromboembolic events was more pronounced among subjects who had a history of prior thromboembolic event, although these differences were not statistically significant *[see Adverse Reactions (6.1), Clinical Studies (14)]*. Potential benefits of treatment with Kcentra should be weighed against the potential risks of thromboembolic events *[see Adverse Reactions (6)]*. Patients with a history of thrombotic events, myocardial infarction, cerebral vascular accident, transient ischemic attack, unstable angina pectoris, severe peripheral vascular disease, or disseminated intravascular coagulation, within the previous 3 months were excluded from participating in the plasma-controlled RCT. Kcentra may not be suitable in patients with thromboembolic events in the prior 3 months. Because of the risk of thromboembolism associated with reversal of VKA, closely monitor patients for signs and symptoms of thromboembolism during and after administration of Kcentra. *[see 17 Patient Counseling Information]*

5.3   Transmissible Infectious Agents

Because Kcentra is made from human blood, it may carry a risk of transmitting infectious agents, e.g., viruses, the variant Creutzfeldt-Jakob disease (vCJD) agent, and, theoretically, the Creutzfeldt-Jakob disease agent. There is also the possibility that unknown infectious agents may be present in such products. Despite the use of two dedicated virus reduction steps in manufacturing to reduce risks, such products may still potentially transmit disease.

Reports of suspected virus transmission of hepatitis A, B, C, and HIV were generally confounded by concomitant admin-

Continued on next page

Table 2: Kcentra Reconstitution Instructions

1. Ensure that the Kcentra vial and diluent vial are at room temperature. Prepare and administer using aseptic technique.	
2. Place the Kcentra vial, diluent vial, and Mix2Vial® transfer set on a flat surface.	
3. Remove Kcentra and diluent vial flip caps. Wipe the stoppers with the alcohol swab provided and allow to dry prior to opening the Mix2Vial transfer set package.	
4. Open the Mix2Vial transfer set package by peeling away the lid. [*Fig. 1*] Leave the Mix2Vial transfer set in the clear package.	Fig. 1
5. Place the diluent vial on a flat surface and hold the vial tightly. Grip the Mix2Vial transfer set together with the clear package and push the plastic spike at the blue end of the Mix2Vial transfer set firmly through the center of the stopper of the diluent vial. [*Fig. 2*]	Fig. 2
6. Carefully remove the clear package from the Mix2Vial transfer set. Make sure that you pull up only the clear package, not the Mix2Vial transfer set. [*Fig. 3*]	Fig. 3
7. With the Kcentra vial placed firmly on a flat surface, invert the diluent vial with the Mix2Vial transfer set attached and push the plastic spike of the transparent adapter firmly through the center of the stopper of the Kcentra vial. [*Fig. 4*] The diluent will automatically transfer into the Kcentra vial.	Fig. 4

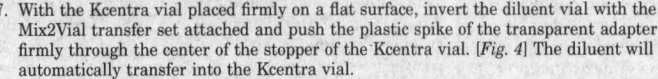

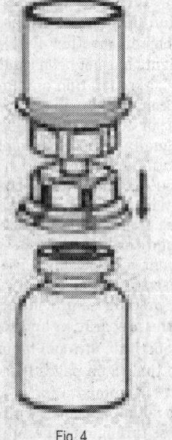

This table is continued on the next page

istration of blood/blood components and/or other plasma-derived products. No causal relationship to Kcentra administration was established for any of these reports since introduction of a virus filtration step in 1996.

All infections thought by a physician to have been possibly transmitted by Kcentra should be reported by the physician or other healthcare provider to the CSL Behring Pharmacovigilance Department at 1-866-915-6958 or FDA at 1-800-FDA-1088 or *www.fda.gov/medwatch*.

6 ADVERSE REACTIONS

The most common adverse reactions (ARs) (frequency ≥ 2.8%) observed in subjects receiving Kcentra were headache, nausea/vomiting, hypotension, and anemia.

The most serious ARs were thromboembolic events including stroke, pulmonary embolism, and deep vein thrombosis. The following serious adverse reactions are described below and/or elsewhere in the labeling:

- Hypersensitivity Reactions *[see Warnings and Precautions (5.1)]*
- Arterial and venous thromboembolic complications *[see Boxed Warning and Warnings and Precautions (5.2)]*
- Possible transmission of infectious agents *[see Warnings and Precautions (5.3)]*

6.1 Clinical Trials Experience

Because clinical studies are conducted under widely varying conditions, adverse reaction rates observed in the clinical trials of a drug cannot be directly compared to rates in the clinical trials of another drug and may not reflect the rates observed in practice.

Randomized, Plasma-Controlled Trial in Acute Major Bleeding

In a prospective, randomized, open-label, active-controlled multicenter non-inferiority trial, 212 subjects who required urgent reversal of VKA therapy due to acute major bleeding were enrolled and randomized to treatment; 103 were treated with Kcentra and 109 with plasma. Subjects with a history of a thrombotic event, myocardial infarction, cerebral vascular accident, transient ischemic attack, unstable angina pectoris, severe peripheral vascular disease, or disseminated intravascular coagulation, within the previous 3 months were excluded from participating. Subjects ranged in age from 26 years to 96 years.

Randomized, Plasma-Controlled Trial in Urgent Surgery/Invasive Procedures

In a prospective, randomized, open-label, active-controlled, multicenter non-inferiority trial, 176 subjects who required urgent reversal of VKA therapy due to the need for an urgent surgical or urgent invasive procedure were enrolled; 88 were treated with Kcentra and 88 with plasma. Subjects ranged in age from 27 years to 94 years.

Adverse reactions are summarized for Kcentra and plasma in the Acute Major Bleeding and Urgent Surgery/Invasive Procedures RCTs (*see Table 3*).

Adverse Reactions are defined as adverse events that began during or within 72 hours of test product infusion plus adverse events considered possibly/probably related or related to study treatment according to the investigator, sponsor, or the blinded safety adjudication board (SAB), and with at least a 1.3-fold difference between treatments.

Table 3: Adverse Reactions Reported in more than 5 Subjects (≥ 2.8%) Following Kcentra or Plasma Administration in RCTs

	No. (%) of subjects	
	Kcentra (N = 191)	Plasma (N = 197)
Nervous system disorders		
Headache	14 (7.3%)	7 (3.6%)
Respiratory, thoracic, and mediastinal disorders		
Pleural effusion	8 (4.2%)	3 (1.5%)
Respiratory distress/dyspnea/ hypoxia	7 (3.7%)	10 (5.1%)
Pulmonary edema	3 (1.6%)	10 (5.1%)
Gastrointestinal disorders		
Nausea/vomiting	12 (6.3%)	8 (4.1%)
Diarrhea	4 (2.1%)	7 (3.6%)
Cardiac disorders		
Tachycardia	9 (4.7%)	2 (1.0%)
Atrial fibrillation	8 (4.2%)	6 (3.0%)
Metabolism and nutrition disorders		
Fluid overload*	5 (2.6%)	16 (8.1%)
Hypokalemia	9 (4.7%)	14 (7.1%)

8. With the diluent and Kcentra vial still attached to the Mix2Vial transfer set, gently swirl the Kcentra vial to ensure that the Kcentra is fully dissolved. [*Fig. 5*] Do not shake the vial.

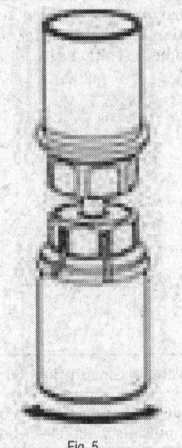

Fig. 5

9. With one hand, grasp the Kcentra side of the Mix2Vial transfer set and with the other hand grasp the blue diluent-side of the Mix2Vial transfer set, and unscrew the set into two pieces. [*Fig. 6*]

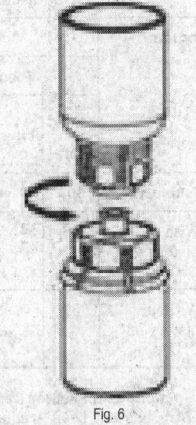

Fig. 6

10. Draw air into an empty, sterile syringe. While the Kcentra vial is upright, screw the syringe to the Mix2Vial transfer set. Inject air into the Kcentra vial. While keeping the syringe plunger pressed, invert the system upside down and draw the concentrate into the syringe by pulling the plunger back slowly. [*Fig. 7*]

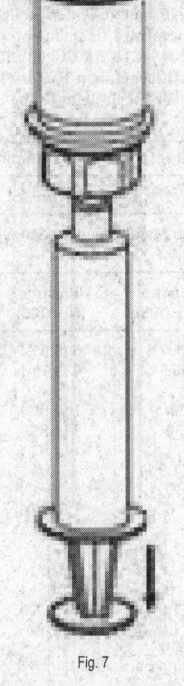

Fig. 7

This table is continued on the next page

Psychiatric disorders		
Insomnia	9 (4.7%)	6 (3.0%)
Vascular disorders		
Hypotension[†]	14 (7.3%)	10 (5.1%)
Injury, poisoning, and procedural complications		
Skin laceration/contusion/ subcutaneous hematoma	8 (4.2%)	5 (2.5%)
Blood and lymphatic disorders		
Anemia[‡]	11 (5.8%)	16 (8.1%)

* Includes fluid overload and cardiac failure congestive
† Includes orthostatic hypotension, hypotension, and hemorrhagic shock
‡ Includes anemia, hemoglobin decreased, and hematocrit decreased

Serious adverse reactions in subjects receiving Kcentra in both RCTs included ischemic cerebrovascular accident (stroke), DVT, thrombosis, and venous insufficiency. Serious adverse reactions in both RCTs for plasma included myocardial ischemia, myocardial infarction, fluid overload, embolic cerebral infarction, pulmonary edema, respiratory failure, and DVT.

There were a total of 10 subjects (9.7%) who died in the Kcentra group (1 additional death occurred on day 46 just after completion of the study reporting period) and 5 (4.6%) who died in the plasma group in the plasma-controlled RCT in acute major bleeding. The 95% confidence interval for the Kcentra minus plasma between-group difference in deaths ranged from -2.7% to 13.5%. From the plasma-controlled RCT in urgent surgery/invasive procedures, there were a total of 3 subjects (3.4%) who died in the Kcentra group (1 additional death occurred on day 48 after completion of the study reporting period) and 8 (9.1%) who died in the Plasma group. The 95% confidence interval for the Kcentra minus plasma between-group difference in deaths in this trial ranged from -14.6% to 2.7%. One death in the Kcentra group in the RCT in Acute Major Bleeding and one death in the plasma group in the RCT in urgent surgery/invasive procedures were considered possibly related to study treatment according to an assessment of masked data by an independent safety adjudication board. No factors common to all deaths were identified, except for the frequent findings of a high comorbidity burden, advanced age, and death after being placed on comfort care. Although, a greater proportion of subjects in the RCT in acute major bleeding than in the RCT in surgery/invasive procedure received the highest two recommended doses of Kcentra because more subjects in the trial in acute major bleeding had a baseline INR in the ranges of 4–6 and > 6.0, an analysis of deaths and factor levels in subjects with major bleeding revealed that subjects who died had similar median factor levels to subjects that did not die. Additionally, outliers with supraphysiologic factor levels did not have a mortality rate out of proportion to the overall population.

Fluid Overload
There were 9 subjects (4.7%, all non-related by investigator assessment) in the Kcentra group who experienced fluid overload in the plasma-controlled RCTs in acute major bleeding and urgent surgery/invasive procedures and 25 (12.7%, 13 events related by investigator assessment) who had fluid overload in the plasma group. The 95% confidence interval for the Kcentra minus Plasma between-group difference in fluid overload event incidence ranged from -14.1% to -2.0%.

Subgroup analyses of the RCTs in acute major bleeding and urgent surgery/invasive procedures according to whether subjects with fluid overload events had a prior history of congestive heart failure are presented in Table 4.
[See table 4 on next page]

Thromboembolic Events
In RCTs, there were 13 subjects (6.8%) in the Kcentra group who experienced possible thromboembolic events (TEEs) and 14 (7.1%) who had TEEs in the plasma group. The incidence of thromboembolic (TE) adverse reactions assessed as at least possibly related to study treatment by the Investigator or, in the case of serious thromboembolic events, the blinded safety adjudication board (SAB) was 9 (4.7%) in the Kcentra group and 7 (3.6%) in the plasma group. When also considering the events which began during or within 72 hours of test product infusion, the incidence was 9 (4.7%) in the Kcentra group and 8 (4.1%) in the plasma group.

Continued on next page

TE events observed in the acute major bleeding and the urgent surgery/invasive procedures RCTs are shown in Table 5.

[See table 5 below]

Subgroup analyses of the RCTs according to whether subjects with thromboembolic events had a prior history of a thromboembolic event are presented in Table 6.

[See table 6 on next page]

The European Bleeding and Surgical Study: In a prospective, open label, single-arm, multicenter safety and efficacy trial, 17 subjects who required urgent reversal of VKA due to acute bleeding were enrolled and 26 subjects who required urgent reversal of Vitamin K antagonist due to the need for an urgent surgical/invasive procedure were enrolled, all were treated with Kcentra. Subjects ranged in age from 22 years to 85 years. Serious adverse reactions considered possibly related to Kcentra included a suspected pulmonary embolism which occurred in one subject following a second dose of Kcentra. A single non-fatal TE event occurred in another Kcentra-treated subject in that trial.

6.2 Postmarketing Experience

No adverse reactions other than those addressed in Warnings And Precautions (5) and Adverse Reactions (6) have been observed in the postmarketing use of Kcentra outside the US since 1996.

8 USE IN SPECIFIC POPULATIONS

8.1 Pregnancy

Pregnancy Category C. Animal reproduction studies have not been conducted with Kcentra. It is also not known whether Kcentra can cause fetal harm when administered to a pregnant woman or can affect reproduction capacity. Kcentra should be prescribed for a pregnant woman only if clearly needed.

8.2 Labor and Delivery

Kcentra has not been studied for use during labor and delivery. Safety and effectiveness in labor and delivery have not been established.

8.3 Nursing Mothers

It is not known whether Kcentra is excreted in human milk. Because many drugs are excreted in human milk, use Kcentra only if clearly needed when treating a nursing woman.

8.4 Pediatric Use

The safety and efficacy of Kcentra in the pediatric population has not been studied.

8.5 Geriatric Use

Of the total number of subjects (431) with acute major bleeding or with the need for an urgent surgery/invasive procedure treated to reverse VKA anticoagulation in three clinical studies, 66% were 65 years old or greater and 39% were 75 years old or greater. There were no clinically significant differences between the safety profile of Kcentra and plasma in any age group.

11. Now that the concentrate has been transferred into the syringe, firmly grasp the barrel of the syringe (keeping the plunger facing down) and unscrew the syringe from the Mix2Vial transfer set. [*Fig. 8*] Attach the syringe to a suitable intravenous administration set.

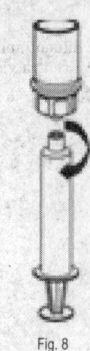

Fig. 8

12. After reconstitution, administration should begin promptly or within 4 hours.

13. If the same patient is to receive more than one vial, you may pool the contents of multiple vials. Use a separate unused Mix2Vial transfer set for each product vial.

Table 4: Subjects with Fluid Overload Events by Prior History of Congestive Heart Failure in RCTs

Subgroup	Acute Major Bleeding Study				Urgent Surgery/Invasive Procedures Study			
	Kcentra		Plasma		Kcentra		Plasma	
	N	Fluid Overload N (%)	N	Fluid Overload N (%)	N	Fluid Overload N (%)	N	Fluid Overload N (%)
All subjects	103	6 (5.8)	109	14 (12.8)	88	3 (3.4)	88	11 (12.5)
With history of CHF	46	4 (8.7)	44	11 (25.0)	24	1 (4.2)	36	6 (16.7)
Without history of CHF	57	2 (3.5)	65	3 (4.6)	64	2 (3.1)	52	5 (9.6)

8.6 Congenital Factor Deficiencies

Kcentra has not been studied in patients with congenital factor deficiencies.

11 DESCRIPTION

Kcentra is a purified, heat-treated, nanofiltered and lyophilized non-activated four-factor Prothrombin Complex Concentrate (Human) prepared from human U.S. Source Plasma (21 CFR 640.60). It contains the Vitamin K dependent Coagulation Factors II, VII, IX and X, and the antithrombotic Proteins C and S. Factor IX is the lead factor for

the potency of the preparation as stated on the vial label. The excipients are human antithrombin III, heparin, human albumin, sodium chloride, and sodium citrate. Kcentra is sterile, pyrogen-free, and does not contain preservatives.

The product contents are shown in Table 7 and listed as ranges for the blood coagulation factors.

Table 7: Composition per Vial of Kcentra *

Ingredient	Kcentra 500 units	Kcentra 1000 units
Total protein	120–280 mg	240–560 mg
Factor II	380–800 units	760–1600 units
Factor VII	200–500 units	400–1000 units
Factor IX	400–620 units	800–1240 units
Factor X	500–1020 units	1000–2040 units
Protein C	420–820 units	840–1640 units
Protein S	240–680 units	480–1360 units
Heparin	8–40 units	16–80 units
Antithrombin III	4–30 units	8–60 units
Human albumin	40–80 mg	80–160 mg
Sodium chloride	60–120 mg	120–240 mg
Sodium citrate	40–80 mg	80–160 mg
HCl	Small amounts	Small amounts
NaOH	Small amounts	Small amounts

* Exact potency of coagulant and antithrombotic proteins are listed on the carton

All plasma used in the manufacture of Kcentra is obtained from US donors and is tested using serological assays for

Table 5: Adverse Reactions (TEEs only) Following Kcentra or Plasma Administration in RCTs

System Organ Class	No. (%) of subjects			
	Acute Major Bleeding Study		Urgent Surgery/Invasive Procedures Study	
	Kcentra (N = 103)	Plasma (N = 109)	Kcentra (N = 88)	Plasma (N = 88)
Any possible TEE*	9 (8.7%)	6 (5.5%)	4 (4.5)	8 (9.1)
TEE Adverse reactions	6 (5.5%)	4 (3.7%)	4 (4.5)	4 (4.5)
Cardiac disorders				
Myocardial infarction	0	1 (0.9%)	0	2 (2.3)
Myocardial ischemia	0	2 (1.8%)	0	0
Nervous system disorders				
Ischemic cerebrovascular accident (stroke)	2 (1.9%)	0	1 (1.1)	0
Embolic cerebral infarction	0	0	0	1 (1.1)
Cerebrovascular disorder	0	1 (0.9%)	0	0
Vascular disorders				
Venous thrombosis calf	1 (1.0%)	0	0	0
Venous thrombosis radial vein	0	0	1 (1.1)	0
Thrombosis (microthrombosis of toes)	0	0	1 (1.1)	0
Deep vein thrombosis (DVT)	1 (1.0%)	0	1 (1.1)	1 (1.1)
Fistula Clot	1 (1.0%)	0	0	0
Unknown Cause of Death (not confirmed TEE)				
Sudden death	1 (1.0%)	0	0	0

* The tabulation of possible TEEs includes subjects with confirmed TEEs as well as 3 subjects in the Acute Major Bleeding RCT Kcentra group that died of unknown causes on days 7, 31, and 38 and 1 subject in the Urgent Surgery/ Invasive Procedures RCT plasma group that died of unknown causes on day 18. The death on day 7 was considered possibly related to study product by the SAB and is tabulated as an adverse reaction.

hepatitis B surface antigen and antibodies to HIV-1/2 and HCV. The plasma is tested with Nucleic Acid Testing (NAT) for HCV, HIV-1, HAV, and HBV, and found to be non-reactive (negative), and the plasma is also tested by NAT for human parvovirus B19 (B19V) in order to exclude donations with high titers. The limit for B19V in the fractionation pool is set not to exceed 10^4 units of B19V DNA per mL. Only plasma that passed virus screening is used for production. The Kcentra manufacturing process includes various steps, which contribute towards the reduction/ inactivation of viruses. Kcentra is manufactured from cryo-depleted plasma that is adsorbed via ion exchange chromatography, heat treated in aqueous solution for 10 hours at 60°C, precipitated, adsorbed to calcium phosphate, virus filtered, and lyophilized.

Manufacturing steps were independently validated in a series of in-vitro experiments for their virus inactivation / reduction capacity for both enveloped and non-enveloped viruses. Table 8 shows the virus clearance during the manufacturing process for Kcentra, expressed as the mean $\log_{10}$ reduction factor.

[See table 8 above]

Table 8: Mean Virus Reduction Factors [$\log_{10}$] of Kcentra

Virus Studied	Manufacturing Steps			Overall Virus Reduction [$\log_{10}$]
	Heat treatment ("Pasteurization")	Ammonium sulphate precipitation followed by Ca Phosphate adsorption	2 × 20nm Virus Filtration	
Enveloped Viruses				
HIV	≥ 5.9	≥ 5.9	≥ 6.6	≥ 18.4
BVDV	≥ 8.5	2.2	≥ 6.0	≥ 16.7
PRV	3.8	7.2	≥ 6.6	≥ 17.6
WNV	≥ 7.4	n.d.	≥ 8.1	≥ 15.5
Non-Enveloped Viruses				
HAV	4.0	1.8	≥ 6.1	≥ 11.9
CPV	[0.5]*	1.5	6.5	8.0

HIV Human immunodeficiency virus, a model for HIV-1 and HIV-2

BVDV Bovine viral diarrhea virus, model for HCV

PRV Pseudorabies virus, a model for large enveloped DNA viruses

WNV West Nile virus

HAV Hepatitis A virus

CPV Canine parvovirus, model for B19V

n.d. not determined

* Reduction factor below 1 $\log_{10}$ was not considered in calculating the overall virus reduction. Studies using human parvovirus B19, which are considered experimental in nature, have demonstrated a virus reduction factor of 3.5 $\log_{10}$ by heat treatment.

12 CLINICAL PHARMACOLOGY

12.1 Mechanism of Action

Kcentra contains the Vitamin K-dependent coagulation Factors II (FII), VII (FVII), IX (FIX), and X (FX), together known as the Prothrombin Complex, and the antithrombotic Protein C and Protein S.

A dose-dependent acquired deficiency of the Vitamin K-dependent coagulation factors occurs during Vitamin K antagonist treatment. Vitamin K antagonists exert anticoagulant effects by blocking carboxylation of glutamic acid residues of the Vitamin K-dependent coagulation factors during hepatic synthesis, lowering both factor synthesis and function. The administration of Kcentra rapidly increases plasma levels of the Vitamin K-dependent coagulation Factors II, VII, IX, and X as well as the antithrombotic Proteins C and S.

Coagulation Factor II

Factor II (prothrombin) is converted to thrombin by activated FX (FXa) in the presence of Ca^{2+}, FV, and phospholipids.

Coagulation Factor VII

Factor VII (proconvertin) is converted to the activated form (FVIIa) by splitting of an internal peptide link. The FVIIa-TF complex activates Factor IX and initiates the primary coagulation pathway by activating FX in the presence of phospholipids and calcium ions.

Coagulation Factor IX

Factor IX (antihemophilic globulin B, or Christmas factor) is activated by the FVIIa-TF complex and by FXIa. Factor IXa in the presence of FVIIIa activates FX to FXa.

Coagulation Factor X

Factor X (Stuart-Prower factor) activation involves the cleavage of a peptide bond by the FVIIIa-Factor IXa complex or the TF-FVIIa complex. Factor Xa forms a complex with activated FV (FVa) that converts prothrombin to thrombin in the presence of phospholipids and calcium ions.

Protein C

Protein C, when activated by thrombin, exerts an antithrombotic effect by inhibiting FVa and FVIIIa leading to a decrease in thrombin formation, and has indirect profibrinolytic activity by inhibiting plasminogen activator inhibitor-1.

Protein S

Protein S exists in a free form (40%) and in a complex with C4b-binding protein (60%). Protein S (free form) functions as a cofactor for activated Protein C in the inactivation of FVa and FVIIIa, leading to antithrombotic activity.

12.2 Pharmacodynamics

International Normalized Ratio (INR)

In the plasma-controlled RCT in acute major bleeding, the INR was determined at varying time points after the start or end of infusion, depending upon study design. The median INR was above 3.0 prior to the infusion and dropped to a median value of 1.20 by the 30 minute time point after start of Kcentra infusion. By contrast, the median value for plasma was 2.4 at 30 minutes after the start of infusion. The INR differences between Kcentra and plasma were statistically significant in randomized plasma-controlled trial in bleeding up to 12 hours after start of infusion [see Table 9].

The relationship between these or other INR values and clinical hemostasis in patients has not been established [see Clinical Studies (14)].

[See table 9 on next page]

12.3 Pharmacokinetics

Fifteen healthy subjects received 50 units/kg of Kcentra. No subjects were receiving VKA therapy or were experiencing acute bleeding. A single intravenous Kcentra infusion produced a rapid and sustained increase in plasma concentration of Factors II, VII, IX and X as well as Proteins C and S. The PK analysis [see Table 10] shows that factor II had the longest half-life (59.7 hours) and factor VII the shortest (4.2 hours) in healthy subjects. PK parameters obtained from data derived from the study of healthy subjects may not be directly applicable to patients with INR elevation due to VKA anticoagulation therapy.

[See table 10 on next page]

The mean in vivo recovery (IVR) of infused factors was calculated in subjects who received Kcentra. The IVR is the increase in measurable factor levels in plasma (units/dL) that may be expected following an infusion of factors (units/kg) administered as a dose of Kcentra. The in vivo recovery ranged from 1.15 (Factor IX) to 2.81 (Protein S) [see Table 11].

[See table 11 on next page]

13 NONCLINICAL TOXICOLOGY

13.1 Carcinogenesis, Mutagenesis, Impairment of Fertility

Long-term studies in animals to evaluate the carcinogenic potential of Kcentra, or studies to determine the effects of Kcentra on genotoxicity or fertility have not been performed. An assessment of the carcinogenic potential of Kcentra was completed and suggests minimal carcinogenic risk from product use.

14 CLINICAL STUDIES

Acute Major Bleeding RCT: The efficacy of Kcentra has been evaluated in a prospective, open-label, (blinded assessor), active-controlled, non-inferiority, multicenter RCT in subjects who had been treated with VKA therapy and who required urgent replacement of their Vitamin K-dependent clotting factors to treat acute major bleeding. A total of 216 subjects with acquired coagulation factor deficiency due to oral Vitamin K antagonist therapy were randomized to a single dose of Kcentra or plasma. Two hundred twelve (212) subjects received Kcentra or plasma for acute major bleeding in the setting of a baseline INR ≥ 2.0 and recent use of a VKA anticoagulant. The doses of Kcentra (25 units/kg, 35 units/kg, or 50 units/kg) based on nominal Factor IX content and plasma (10 mL/kg, 12 mL/kg, or 15 mL/kg) were

Table 6: Subjects with Thromboembolic Events by Prior History of TE Event in RCTs

	Acute Major Bleeding Study				Urgent Surgery/Invasive Procedures Study			
	Kcentra		Plasma		Kcentra		Plasma	
	N	TE Events* N (%)	N	TE Events N (%)	N	TE Events* N (%)	N	TE Events N (%)
All subjects	103	9 (8.7)	109	6 (5.5)	88	4 (4.5)	88	8 (9.1)
With history of TE event†	69	8 (11.6)	79	3 (3.8)	55	3 (5.5)	62	5 (8.1)
Without history of TE event	34	1 (2.9)	30	3 (10.0)	33	1 (3.0)	26	3 (11.5)

* One additional subject in the Acute Major Bleeding RCT who had received Kcentra, not listed in the table, had an upper extremity venous thrombosis in association with an indwelling catheter. Two additional subjects in the Urgent Surgery/Invasive Procedures RCT who had received Kcentra, not listed in the table, had non-intravascular events (catheter-related/IVC filter insertion).

† History of prior TE event greater than 3 months from study entry (TE event within 3 months not studied).

Continued on next page

calculated according to the subject's baseline INR (2–< 4, 4–6, > 6, respectively). The observation period lasted for 90 days after the infusion of Kcentra or plasma. The modified efficacy (ITT-E) population for Kcentra included 98 subjects and for plasma included 104 subjects. Additionally, intravenous Vitamin K was administered.

The efficacy endpoint was hemostatic efficacy for the time period from the start of infusion of Kcentra or plasma until 24 hours. Efficacy was adjudicated as "effective" or "not effective" by a blinded, independent Endpoint Adjudication Board for all subjects who received study product. Criteria for effective hemostasis were based upon standard clinical assessments including vital signs, hemoglobin measurements, and CT assessments at pre-defined time points, as relevant to the type of bleeding (i.e., gastrointestinal, intracranial hemorrhage, visible, musculoskeletal, etc.). The proportion of subjects with effective hemostasis was 72.4% in the Kcentra group and 65.4% in the plasma group. The lower limit of the 95% confidence interval (CI) for the difference in proportions of Kcentra minus plasma was -5.8%, which exceeded -10% and thereby demonstrated the non-inferiority of Kcentra versus plasma (the study's primary objective) *[see Table 12]*. Because the lower limit of the CI was not greater than zero, the prospectively defined criterion for superiority of Kcentra for hemostatic efficacy (a secondary objective) was not met.

Table 12: Rating of Hemostatic Efficacy in Subjects with Acute Major Bleeding

Rating	No. (%) of subjects [95% CI]		Difference Kcentra – Plasma (%) [95% CI]*
	Kcentra (N = 98)	Plasma (N = 104)	
"Effective" hemostasis	71 (72.4%) [62.3; 82.6]	68 (65.4%) [54.9; 75.8]	(7.1%) [-5.8; 19.9]

CI = confidence interval; N = number of subjects
* Kcentra non-inferior to plasma if lower limit of 95% CI > –10%; Kcentra superior to plasma if lower limit of 95% CI > 0.

Results of a post-hoc analysis of hemostatic efficacy stratified by actual dose of Kcentra or plasma administered in the acute major bleeding RCT are presented in Table 13.

Table 13: Rating of Hemostatic Efficacy Stratified by Actual Dose of Kcentra or Plasma (Number and % of Subjects rated "Effective" in Acute Major Bleeding RCT

	Low Dose	Mid Dose	High Dose
	N = 49 (K)	N = 22 (K)	N = 26 (K)
	N = 55 (P)	N = 18 (P)	N = 31 (P)
Kcentra	36 (74.5%)	16 (72.7%)	18 (69.2%)
Plasma	38 (69.1%)	11 (61.1%)	19 (61.3%)
Difference*	(4.4%)	(11.6%)	(7.9%)
95% CI K– P	-13.2–21.9	-17.4–40.6	-17.0–32.9

* Kcentra minus Plasma

An additional endpoint was the reduction of INR to ≤ 1.3 at 30 minutes after the end of infusion of Kcentra or plasma for all subjects that received study product. The proportion of subjects with this decrease in INR was 62.2% in the Kcentra group and 9.6% in the plasma group. The 95% confidence interval for the difference in proportions of Kcentra minus plasma was 39.4% to 65.9%. The lower limit of the 95% CI of 39.4% demonstrated superiority of Kcentra versus plasma for this endpoint *[see Table 14]*.

Table 14: Decrease of INR (1.3 or Less at 30 Minutes after End of Infusion) in Acute Major Bleeding RCT

Rating	No. (%) of subjects [95% CI]		Difference Kcentra – Plasma (%) [95% CI]*
	Kcentra (N = 98)	Plasma (N = 104)	
Decrease of INR to ≤ 1.3 at 30 min	61 (62.2%) [52.6; 71.8]	10 (9.6%) [3.9; 15.3]	(52.6%) [39.4; 65.9]

Table 9: Median INR (Min-Max) after Start of Infusion in RCTs

Study	Treatment	Baseline	30 min	1 hr	2-3 hr	6-8 hr	12 hr	24 hr
Acute Major Bleeding Study	Kcentra (N = 98)	3.90 (1.8–20.0)	1.20* (0.9–6.7)	1.30* (0.9–5.4)	1.30* (0.9–2.5)	1.30* (0.9–2.1)	1.20* (0.9–2.2)	1.20 (0.9–3.8)
	Plasma (N = 104)	3.60 (1.9–38.9)	2.4 (1.4–11.4)	2.1 (1.0–11.4)	1.7 (1.1–4.1)	1.5 (1.0–3.0)	1.4 (1.0–3.0)	1.3 (1.0–2.9)
Urgent Surgery/ Invasive Procedures Study	Kcentra (N = 87)	2.90 (2.0–17.0)	1.30* (0.9–7.0)	1.20* (0.9–2.5)	1.30* (0.9–39.2)	1.30* (1.0–10.3)	NC	1.20 (0.9–2.7)
	Plasma (N = 81)	2.90 (2.0–26.7)	2.15 (1.4–5.4)	1.90 (1.3–5.7)	1.70 (1.1–3.7)	1.60 (1.0–5.8)	NC	1.30 (1.0–2.7)

INR = international normalized ratio; NC = not collected.

* Statistically significant difference compared to plasma by 2-sided Wilcoxon test

Table 10: Vitamin K-Dependent Coagulation Factor Pharmacokinetics after a Single Kcentra Infusion in Healthy Subjects (n=15) Mean (SD)*

Parameter	Factor IX	Factor II	Factor VII	Factor X	Protein C	Protein S
Terminal half-life (h)	42.4 (41.6)	60.4 (25.5)	5.0 (1.9)	31.8 (8.7)	49.6 (32.7)	50.4 (13.4)
IVR (%/units/kg bw)*	1.6 (0.4)	2.2 (0.3)	2.5 (0.4)	2.2 (0.4)	2.9 (0.3)	2.0 (0.3)
AUC (IU/dL × h)	1850.8 (1001.4)	7282.2 (2324.9)	512.9 (250.1)	6921.5 (1730.5)	5397.5 (2613.9)	3651.6 (916.3)
Clearance (mL/ kg × h)	3.7 (1.6)	1.0 (0.3)	7.4 (4.1)	1.3 (0.3)	1.5 (0.9)	1.2 (0.3)
MRT (h)†	47.3 (49.5)	82.0 (34.2)	7.1 (2.7)	45.9 (12.6)	62.4 (42.1)	70.3 (18.3)
Vd$_{ss}$ (mL/kg)‡	114.3 (54.6)	71.4 (13.7)	45.0 (10.7)	55.5 (6.7)	62.2 (17.4)	78.8 (11.6)

* IVR: In Vivo Recovery

† MRT: Mean Residence Time

‡ Vd$_{ss}$: Volume of Distribution at steady state

Table 11: In vivo Recovery in RCTs*

Parameter	Incremental (units/dL per units/kg b.w.)			
	Acute Major Bleeding Study (N = 98)		Urgent Surgery/Invasive Procedures Study (N = 87)	
	Mean (SD)	95% CI†	Mean (SD)	95% CI†
Factor IX	1.29 (0.71)	(1.14–1.43)	1.15 (0.57)	(1.03–1.28)
Factor II	2.00 (0.88)	(1.82–2.18)	2.14 (0.74)	(1.98–2.31)
Factor VII	2.15 (2.96)	(1.55–2.75)	1.90 (4.50)	(0.92–2.88)
Factor X	1.96 (0.87)	(1.79–2.14)	1.94 (0.69)	(1.79–2.09)
Protein C	2.04 (0.96)	(1.85–2.23)	1.88 (0.68)	(1.73–2.02)
Protein S	2.17 (1.66)	(1.83–2.50)	2.81 (1.95)	(2.38–3.23)

* ITT-E: Intention to Treat – Efficacy Population
† CI: Confidence Interval

CI = confidence interval; INR = international normalized ratio; N = total subjects
* Kcentra non-inferior to plasma if lower limit of 95% CI > –10%; Kcentra superior to plasma if lower limit of 95% CI > 0.

Urgent Surgery/Invasive Procedure RCT: The efficacy of Kcentra has been evaluated in a prospective, open-label, active-controlled, non-inferiority, multicenter RCT in subjects who had been treated with VKA therapy and who required urgent replacement of their Vitamin K-dependent clotting factors because of their need for an urgent surgery/ invasive procedure. A total of 181 subjects with acquired coagulation factor deficiency due to oral Vitamin K antagonist therapy were randomized to a single dose of Kcentra or plasma. One hundred seventy-six (176) subjects received Kcentra or plasma because of their need for an urgent surgery/ invasive procedure in the setting of a baseline INR ≥ 2.0 and recent use of a VKA anticoagulant. The doses of Kcentra (25 units/kg, 35 units/kg, or 50 units/kg) based on nominal Factor IX content and plasma (10 mL/kg, 12 mL/kg, or 15 mL/kg) were calculated according to the subject's baseline INR (2–< 4, 4–6, > 6, respectively). The observation period lasted for 90 days after the infusion of Kcentra or plasma. The modified efficacy (ITT-E) population for Kcentra included 87 subjects and for plasma included 81 subjects. Additionally, oral or intravenous Vitamin K was administered.

The efficacy endpoint was hemostatic efficacy for the time period from the start of infusion of Kcentra or plasma until the end of the urgent surgery/invasive procedure. Criteria for effective hemostasis were based upon the difference between predicted and actual blood losses, subjective hemostasis rating, and the need for additional blood products containing coagulation factors. The proportion of subjects with effective hemostasis was 89.7% in the Kcentra group and 75.3% in the plasma group. The lower limit of the 95% confidence interval (CI) for the difference in proportions of Kcentra minus plasma was 2.8%, which exceeded -10% and thereby demonstrated the non-inferiority of Kcentra versus plasma (the study's primary objective) *[see Table 15]*. Because the lower limit of the CI was greater than 0, the prospectively defined criterion for superiority of Kcentra for hemostatic efficacy (a secondary objective) was also met.

Table 15: Rating of Hemostatic Efficacy in Urgent Surgery/Invasive Procedure RCT

Rating	No. (%) of subjects [95% CI]		Difference Kcentra – Plasma (%)
	Kcentra (N = 87)	Plasma (N = 81)	[95% CI]*
"Effective" hemostasis	78 (89.7%) [83.3; 96.1]	61 (75.3%) [65.9; 84.7]	(14.3%) [2.8; 25.8]

CI = confidence interval; N = number of subjects
* Kcentra non-inferior to plasma if lower limit of 95% CI > –10%; Kcentra superior to plasma if lower limit of 95% CI > 0.

Results of a post-hoc analysis of hemostatic efficacy stratified by actual dose of Kcentra or plasma administered in the urgent surgery/invasive procedure RCT are presented in Table 16.

Table 16: Rating of Hemostatic Efficacy Stratified by Actual Dose of Kcentra or Plasma (Number and % of Subjects rated "Effective" in Urgent Surgery/ Invasive Procedure RCT

	Low Dose	Mid Dose	High Dose
	N = 69 (K)	N = 10 (K)	N = 8 (K)
	N = 62 (P)	N = 10 (P)	N = 9 (P)
Kcentra	63 (91.3%)	8 (80.0%)	7 (87.5%)
Plasma	48 (77.4%)	7 (70.0%)	6 (66.7%)
Difference*	(13.9%)	(10.0%)	(20.8%)
95% CI K–P	1.4–26.6	-26.5–43.5	-19.8–53.7

* Kcentra minus Plasma

An additional endpoint was the reduction of INR to ≤ 1.3 at 30 minutes after the end of infusion of Kcentra or plasma for all subjects that received study product. The proportion of subjects with this decrease in INR was 55.2% in the Kcentra group and 9.9% in the plasma group. The 95% confidence interval for the difference in proportions of Kcentra minus plasma was 31.9% to 56.4%. The lower limit of the 95% CI of 31.9% demonstrated superiority of Kcentra versus plasma for this endpoint *[see Table 17]*. The relationship between a decrease in INR to less than or equal to 1.3 and clinical hemostatic efficacy has not been established.

Table 17: Decrease of INR (1.3 or Less at 30 Minutes after End of Infusion) in Urgent Surgery/Invasive Procedure RCT

Rating	No. (%) of subjects [95% CI]		Difference Kcentra – Plasma (%)
	Kcentra (N = 87)	Plasma (N = 81)	[95% CI]*
Decrease of INR to ≤ 1.3 at 30 min	48 (55.2%) [44.7; 65.6]	8 (9.9%) [3.4; 16.4]	(45.3%) [31.9; 56.4]

CI = confidence interval; INR = international normalized ratio; N = total subjects
* Kcentra non-inferior to plasma if lower limit of 95% CI > -10%; Kcentra superior to plasma if lower limit of 95% CI > 0.

The European Bleeding and Surgical Study was an open-label, single-arm, multicenter study.[1] Forty-three (43) subjects who were receiving VKA were treated with Kcentra, because they either (1) required a surgical or an invasive diagnostic intervention (26 subjects), or (2) experienced an acute bleeding event (17 subjects). The dose of Kcentra (25 units/kg, 35 units/kg, or 50 units/kg) based on nominal Factor IX content was calculated according to the subject's baseline INR value (2–< 4, 4–6, > 6). The endpoint was the decrease of the INR to ≤ 1.3 within 30 minutes after end of Kcentra infusion in subjects who received any portion of study product.

Of the 17 evaluable subjects receiving Kcentra for acute bleeding, 16 subjects (94%) experienced a decrease in INR to ≤ 1.3 within 30 minutes after the end of the Kcentra infusion.

In RCTs, levels of Coagulation Factors II, VII, IX, X, and Antithrombotic Proteins C and S were measured after the infusion of Kcentra or plasma and the results were similar for subjects with acute major bleeding or subjects requiring an urgent surgery or invasive procedure. In the plasma-controlled RCT in acute major bleeding, the mean duration of Kcentra infusion was 24 minutes (± 32 minutes) and the mean duration of infusion for plasma was 169 minutes (± 143 minutes). The mean infusion volume of Kcentra was 105 mL ± 37 mL and the mean infusion volume of plasma was 865 mL ± 269 mL. In the plasma-controlled RCT for patients needing urgent surgery/invasive procedures, the mean duration of Kcentra infusion was 21 minutes (± 14 minutes) and the mean duration of infusion for plasma was 141 minutes (± 113 minutes). The mean infusion volume of Kcentra was 90 mL ± 32 mL and the mean infusion volume of plasma was 819 mL ± 231 mL.

The increase in mean factor levels over time following Kcentra and plasma administration in the plasma-controlled RCT in acute major bleeding is shown in *Figure 9* below (the mean factor levels over time following Kcentra and plasma administration in the plasma-controlled RCT for patients needing urgent surgery/invasive procedures are not shown, but showed similar profiles). Levels of some factors continued to increase at later time points, consistent with the effect of concomitant Vitamin K treatment. Formal pharmacokinetic parameters were not derived because of the effect of Vitamin K on factor levels at time points required for pharmacokinetic profiling.
[See figure 9 above]

15 REFERENCES

1. Pabinger I, Brenner B, Kalina U, *et al*. Prothrombin complex concentrate (Beriplex P/N) for emergency anticoagulation reversal: a prospective multinational clinical trial. *Journal of Thrombosis and Haemostasis* 2008; 6: 622-631.

16 HOW SUPPLIED/STORAGE AND HANDLING

16.1 How Supplied

• Kcentra is supplied in a single-use vial.
• The actual units of potency of all coagulation factors (Factors II, VII, IX and X), Proteins C and S in units are stated on each Kcentra carton.
• The Kcentra packaging components are not made with natural rubber latex.

Each kit consists of the following:

Carton NDC Number	Components
63833-386-02	• 500 units Kcentra in a single-use vial [NDC 63833-396-01] • 20 mL vial of Sterile Water for Injection, USP [NDC 63833-761-20] • Mix2Vial filter transfer set • Alcohol swab
63833-387-02	• 1000 units Kcentra in a single-use vial [NDC 63833-397-01] • 40 mL vial of Sterile Water for Injection, USP [NDC 63833-761-40] • Mix2Vial filter transfer set • Alcohol swab

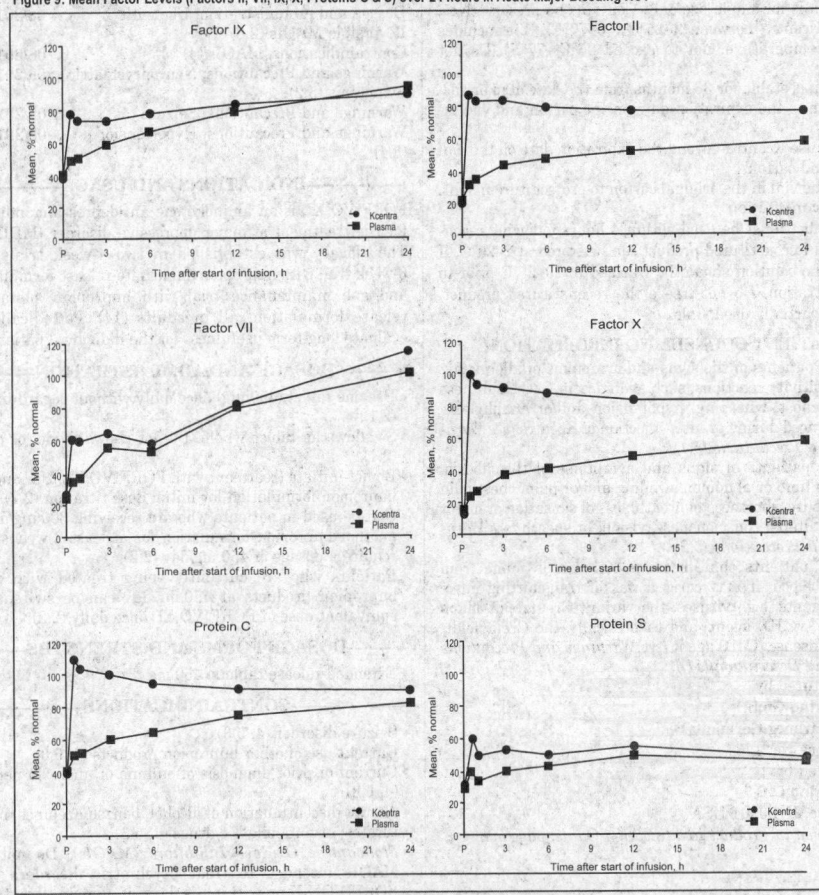

Figure 9: Mean Factor Levels (Factors II, VII, IX, X, Proteins C & S) over 24 hours in Acute Major Bleeding RCT

Time axis is scheduled measuring time: hours after start of infusion (P=pre-infusion)

16.2　Storage and Handling

Prior to Reconstitution

- Kcentra is for single use only. Contains no preservatives.
- Store Kcentra between 2–25°C (36–77°F), this includes room temperature, not to exceed 25°C (77°F). Do not freeze.
- Kcentra is stable for 36 months from the date of manufacture, up to the expiration date on the carton and vial labels.
- Do not use Kcentra beyond the expiration date on the vial label and carton.
- Store the vial in the original carton to protect it from light.

After Reconstitution

The product must be used within 4 hours following reconstitution. Reconstituted product can be stored at 2–25°C. If cooled, the solution should be warmed to 20–25°C prior to administration. Do not freeze the reconstituted product. Discard partially used vials.

17　PATIENT COUNSELING INFORMATION

- Inform patients of the signs and symptoms of allergic hypersensitivity reactions, such as urticaria, rash, tightness of the chest, wheezing, hypotension and/or anaphylaxis experienced during or after injection of Kcentra *[see Warnings and Precautions (5.1)]*.
- Inform patients of signs and symptoms of thrombosis, such as limb or abdomen swelling and/or pain, chest pain or pressure, shortness of breath, loss of sensation or motor power, altered consciousness, vision, or speech *[see Warnings and Precautions (5.2)]*.
- Inform patients that, because Kcentra is made from human blood, it may carry a risk of transmitting infectious agents, e.g., viruses, the variant Creutzfeldt-Jakob disease (vCJD) agent, and theoretically, the Creutzfeldt-Jakob disease (CJD) agent *[see Warnings and Precautions (5.3) and Description (11)]*.

Manufactured by:

CSL Behring GmbH

35041 Marburg Germany

US License No. 1765

Distributed by:

CSL Behring LLC

Kankakee, IL 60901 USA

Shown in Product Identification Guide, page 508

Edgemont Pharmaceuticals, LLC

1250 Capital of Texas Hwy South,
Building 3, Suite 400
Austin, TX 78746

Toll Free: (888) 594-4332

Fax: (512) 329-2094

customerservice@edgemontpharma.com

FORFIVO XL　　　　　　　　　　℞

[Fore fye' voe Eks el]

(bupropion hydrochloride extended-release tablets)
for oral use

HIGHLIGHTS OF PRESCRIBING INFORMATION

These highlights do not include all the information needed to use FORFIVO XL® safely and effectively. See full prescribing information for FORFIVO XL.

FORFIVO XL (bupropion hydrochloride extended-release tablets), for oral use

Initial U.S. Approval: 1985

WARNING: SUICIDAL THOUGHTS AND BEHAVIORS; AND NEUROPSYCHIATRIC REACTIONS

See full prescribing information for complete boxed warning

- **Increased risk of suicidal thinking and behavior in children, adolescents, and young adults taking antidepressants (5.1).**
- **Monitor for worsening and emergence of suicidal thoughts and behaviors (5.1).**
- **Serious neuropsychiatric events have been reported in patients taking bupropion for smoking cessation. (5.2).**

——————RECENT MAJOR CHANGES——————

Dosage and Administration, Discontinuation　08/2016
(2.4)

Dosage and Administration, Switching　　08/2016
To/From MAOIs (2.7)

Dosage and Administration, Use with　　08/2016
Reversible MAOIs (2.8)

Contraindications, MAOIs (4)　　　　08/2016

Warnings and Precautions, Neuropsychiatric　08/2016
Symptoms (5.2)

Warnings and Precautions, Seizure (5.3)　08/2016

Warnings and Precautions, Hypertension　08/2016
(5.4)

——————INDICATIONS AND USAGE——————

FORFIVO XL is an aminoketone antidepressant indicated for the treatment of major depressive disorder (MDD) (1). The efficacy was established in two 4-week trials, one 6-week trial with bupropion immediate-release formulation, and one maintenance trial with bupropion sustained-release formulation, all in adults (14). Periodically re-evaluate long-term usefulness for the individual patient (1).

——————DOSAGE AND ADMINISTRATION——————

- Use one tablet (450 mg) once daily without regard to food (2.1).
- Swallow the tablet whole. Do not chew, divide, or crush (2.1).
- Do not initiate treatment with FORFIVO XL. Use another bupropion formulation for initial dose titration (2.2).
- Can be used in patients who are receiving 300 mg/day of another bupropion formulation for at least 2 weeks, and require a dosage of 450 mg/day (2.2).
- Patients who are currently being treated with other bupropion products at 450 mg/day can be switched to equivalent dose of FORFIVO XL once daily (2.2).

——————DOSAGE FORMS AND STRENGTHS——————

- Extended-release tablets: 450 mg (3)

——————CONTRAINDICATIONS——————

- Seizure disorder (4, 5.3)
- Current use of other bupropion products (4, 5.3)
- Current or prior diagnosis of bulimia or anorexia nervosa (4, 5.3)
- Abrupt discontinuation of alcohol, benzodiazepines, barbiturates, or antiepileptic drugs (4, 5.3)
- *Monoamine Oxidase Inhibitors (MAOIs):* Do not use MAOIs intended to treat psychiatric disorders with FORFIVO XL or within 14 days of stopping treatment with FORFIVO XL. Do not use FORFIVO XL within 14 days of stopping an MAOI intended to treat psychiatric disorders. In addition, do not start FORFIVO XL in a patient who is being treated with linezolid or intravenous methylene blue. (4, 7.6)
- Known hypersensitivity to bupropion or other ingredients of FORFIVO XL (4, 5.8)

——————WARNINGS AND PRECAUTIONS——————

- *Seizure Risk:* The risk is dose dependent. Discontinue if seizure occurs (4, 5.3, 7.3).
- *Hypertension:* FORFIVO XL can increase blood pressure. Monitor blood pressure before initiating treatment and periodically during treatment (5.4).
- *Activation of Mania/Hypomania:* Screen patients for bipolar disorder and monitor for these symptoms (5.5).
- *Psychosis and Other Neuropsychiatric Reactions:* Discontinue if such reactions occur (5.6).
- *Angle-closure Glaucoma:* Angle-closure glaucoma has occurred in patients with untreated anatomically narrow angles treated with antidepressants (5.7).

——————ADVERSE REACTIONS——————

Most common adverse reactions are (incidence ≥ 5%; ≥ 2 times placebo rate): dry mouth, nausea, insomnia, dizziness, pharyngitis, abdominal pain, agitation, anxiety, tremor, palpitation, sweating, tinnitus, myalgia, anorexia, urinary frequency, rash (6.1)

To report SUSPECTED ADVERSE REACTIONS, contact Edgemont Pharmaceuticals, LLC at 1-888- 594-4332 or FDA at 1-800-FDA-1088 or *www.fda.gov/medwatch*.

——————DRUG INTERACTIONS——————

- *CYP2B6 Inhibitors:* Ticlopidine or clopidogrel may increase bupropion exposure. Coadministration of FORFIVO XL with ticlopidine or clopidogrel is not recommended (7.1).
- *CYP2B6 Inducers:* Dose increase may be necessary if coadministered with CYP2B6 inducers (eg, ritonavir, lopinavir, efavirenz, carbamazepine, phenobarbital, and phenytoin) based on clinical exposure, but should not exceed the maximum recommended dose (7.1).

- *Drugs Metabolized by CYP2D6:* Bupropion inhibits CYP2D6 and can increase concentrations of: antidepressants (eg, venlafaxine, nortriptyline, imipramine, desipramine, paroxetine, fluoxetine, sertraline), antipsychotics (eg, haloperidol, risperidone, thioridazine), beta blockers (eg, metoprolol), and Type 1C antiarrhythmics (eg, propafenone, flecainide). Consider dose reduction when using with bupropion (7.2).
- *Drugs That Lower Seizure Threshold:* Dose FORFIVO XL with extreme caution (5.3, 7.3).
- *Dopaminergic Drugs (levodopa and amantadine):* CNS toxicity can occur when used concomitantly with FORFIVO XL (7.4).
- *MAOIs:* Increased risk of hypertensive reactions can occur when used concomitantly with FORFIVO XL (7.6).
- *Drug-Laboratory Test Interactions:* FORFIVO XL can cause false-positive urine test results for amphetamines (7.7).

——————USE IN SPECIFIC POPULATIONS——————

- *Pregnancy:* Use only if benefit outweighs potential risk to the fetus (8.1).
- *Renal Impairment:* Because there is no lower dose strength for FORFIVO XL, FORFIVO XL is not recommended in patients with renal impairment (8.6).
- *Hepatic Impairment:* Because there is no lower dose strength for FORFIVO XL, FORFIVO XL is not recommended in patients with hepatic impairment (8.7).

See 17 for PATIENT COUNSELING INFORMATION and Medication Guide.

Revised: 8/2016

FULL PRESCRIBING INFORMATION: CONTENTS*

WARNING: SUICIDAL THOUGHTS AND BEHAVIORS; AND NEUROPSYCHIATRIC REACTIONS

13   NONCLINICAL TOXICOLOGY
    13.1   Carcinogenesis, Mutagenesis, Impairment of Fertility
14   CLINICAL STUDIES
16   HOW SUPPLIED/STORAGE AND HANDLING
17   PATIENT COUNSELING INFORMATION
MEDICATION GUIDE

* Sections or subsections omitted from the full prescribing information are not listed.

FULL PRESCRIBING INFORMATION

WARNING: SUICIDAL THOUGHTS AND BE-HAVIORS; AND NEUROPSYCHIATRIC REAC-TIONS

SUICIDALITY AND ANTIDEPRESSANT DRUGS
Antidepressants increased the risk of suicidal thoughts and behavior in children, adolescents, and young adults in short-term trials. These trials did not show an increase in the risk of suicidal thoughts and behavior with antidepressant use in subjects aged 65 and older [see *Warnings and Precautions (5.1)*].
In patients of all ages who are started on antidepressant therapy, monitor closely for worsening and for emergence of suicidal thoughts and behaviors. Advise families and caregivers of the need for close observation and communication with the prescriber. FORFIVO XL is not approved for use in pediatric patients [see *Warnings and Precautions (5.1)*].
NEUROPSYCHIATRIC REACTIONS IN PATIENTS TAK-ING BUPROPION FOR SMOKING CESSATION
Serious neuropsychiatric reactions have occurred in patients taking bupropion for smoking cessation [see *Warnings and Precautions (5.2)*]. The majority of these reactions occurred during bupropion treatment, but some occurred in the context of discontinuing treatment. In many cases, a causal relationship to bupropion treatment is not certain, because depressed mood may be a symptom of nicotine withdrawal. However, some of the cases occurred in patients taking bupropion who continued to smoke. Although FORFIVO XL is not approved for smoking cessation, observe all patients for neuropsychiatric reactions. Instruct the patient to contact a healthcare provider if such reactions occur [see *Warnings and Precautions (5.2)*].

---

1   INDICATIONS AND USAGE
FORFIVO XL (bupropion hydrochloride extended-release tablets) is indicated for the treatment of major depressive disorder (MDD), as defined by the Diagnostic and Statistical Manual (DSM).
The efficacy of the immediate-release formulation of bupropion was established in two 4-week controlled inpatient trials and one 6-week controlled outpatient trial of adult patients with MDD. The efficacy of the sustained-release formulation of bupropion in the maintenance treatment of MDD was established in a long-term (up to 44 weeks), placebo-controlled trial in patients who had responded to bupropion in an 8-week study of acute treatment [see *Clinical Studies (14)*].
The physician who elects to use FORFIVO XL for extended periods should periodically reevaluate the long-term usefulness of the drug for the individual patient.

2   DOSAGE AND ADMINISTRATION
2.1   General Instructions for Use
One tablet (450 mg) of FORFIVO XL should be taken once daily without regard to meals. FORFIVO XL should be swallowed whole and not crushed, divided, or chewed.
2.2   Initial Treatment with FORFIVO XL
Do not initiate treatment with FORFIVO XL because the 450-mg tablet is the only available dose formulation. Use another bupropion formulation for initial dose titration (referring to prescribing information of other bupropion products).
FORFIVO XL can be used in patients who are receiving 300 mg/day of another bupropion formulation for at least 2 weeks, and require a dosage of 450 mg/day.
Patients who are currently being treated with other bupropion products at 450 mg/day can be switched to an equivalent dose of FORFIVO XL once daily.
2.3   Maintenance Treatment with FORFIVO XL
It is generally agreed that acute episodes of depression require several months or longer of sustained antidepressant

treatment beyond the response in the acute episode. It is unknown whether the 450-mg dose needed for maintenance treatment is identical to the dose that provided an initial response. Periodically reassess the need for maintenance treatment and the appropriate dose for such treatment.
2.4   To Discontinue FORFIVO XL, Taper the Dose
Because the 450-mg tablet is the only available dose formulation, use another bupropion formulation for tapering the dose prior to discontinuation (referring to prescribing information of other bupropion products).
2.5   Patients with Impaired Hepatic Function
Because there is no lower dose strength for FORFIVO XL, FORFIVO XL is not recommended in patients with hepatic impairment [see *Use in Specific Populations (8.7)* and *Clinical Pharmacology (12.3)*].
2.6   Patients with Impaired Renal Function
Because there is no lower dose strength for FORFIVO XL, FORFIVO XL is not recommended in patients with renal impairment [see *Use in Specific Populations (8.6)* and *Clinical Pharmacology (12.3)*].
2.7   Switching a Patient To or From a Monoamine Oxidase Inhibitor (MAOI) Antidepressant
At least 14 days should elapse between discontinuation of an MAOI intended to treat depression and initiation of therapy with FORFIVO XL. Conversely, at least 14 days should be allowed after stopping FORFIVO XL before starting an MAOI antidepressant [see *Contraindications (4)* and *Drug Interactions (7.6)*].
2.8   Use of FORFIVO XL with Reversible MAOIs Such as Linezolid or Methylene Blue
Do not start FORFIVO XL in a patient who is being treated with a reversible MAOI such as linezolid or intravenous methylene blue. Drug interactions can increase the risk of hypertensive reactions. In a patient who requires more urgent treatment of a psychiatric condition, nonpharmacological interventions, including hospitalization, should be considered [see *Contraindications (4)*].
In some cases, a patient already receiving therapy with FORFIVO XL may require urgent treatment with linezolid or intravenous methylene blue. If acceptable alternatives to linezolid or intravenous methylene blue treatment are not available and the potential benefits of linezolid or intravenous methylene blue treatment are judged to outweigh the risks of hypertensive reactions in a particular patient, FORFIVO XL should be stopped promptly, and linezolid or intravenous methylene blue can be administered. The patient should be monitored for 2 weeks or until 24 hours after the last dose of linezolid or intravenous methylene blue, whichever comes first. Therapy with FORFIVO XL may be resumed 24 hours after the last dose of linezolid or intravenous methylene blue.
The risk of administering methylene blue by nonintravenous routes (such as oral tablets or by local injection) or in intravenous doses much lower than 1 mg/kg with FORFIVO XL is unclear. The clinician should, nevertheless, be aware of the possibility of a drug interaction with such use [see *Contraindications (4)* and *Drug Interactions (7.6)*].

3   DOSAGE FORMS AND STRENGTHS
FORFIVO XL Extended-Release Tablets, 450 mg of bupropion hydrochloride, are white to off-white, oval tablets with the logo "Forfivo" printed on one side.

4   CONTRAINDICATIONS
• FORFIVO XL is contraindicated in patients with a seizure disorder [see *Warnings and Precautions (5.3)*].
• FORFIVO XL is contraindicated in patients treated currently with other bupropion products because the incidence of seizure is dose dependent [see *Warnings and Precautions (5.3)*].
• FORFIVO XL is contraindicated in patients with a current or prior diagnosis of bulimia or anorexia nervosa because a higher incidence of seizures was observed in such patients treated with bupropion [see *Warnings and Precautions (5.3)*].
• FORFIVO XL is contraindicated in patients undergoing abrupt discontinuation of alcohol, benzodiazepines, barbiturates, and antiepileptic drugs [see *Warnings and Precautions (5.3)* and *Drug Interactions (7.3)*].
• The use of MAOIs (intended to treat psychiatric disorders) concomitantly with FORFIVO XL or within 14 days of discontinuing treatment with FORFIVO XL is contraindicated. There is an increased risk of hypertensive reactions when FORFIVO XL is used concomitantly with MAOIs. The use of FORFIVO XL within 14 days of discontinuing treatment with an MAOI is also contraindicated. Starting FORFIVO XL in a patient treated with reversible MAOIs

such as linezolid or intravenous methylene blue is contraindicated [see *Dosage and Administration (2.8)*, *Warnings and Precautions (5.4)*, and *Drug Interactions (7.6)*].
• FORFIVO XL is contraindicated in patients with known hypersensitivity to bupropion or the other ingredients of FORFIVO XL tablets. Anaphylactoid/anaphylactic reactions and Stevens-Johnson syndrome have been reported [see *Warnings and Precautions (5.8)*].

5   WARNINGS AND PRECAUTIONS
5.1   Suicidal Thoughts and Behaviors in Children, Adolescents, and Young Adults
Patients with MDD, both adult and pediatric, may experience worsening of their depression and/or the emergence of suicidal ideation and behavior (suicidality) or unusual changes in behavior, whether or not they are taking antidepressant medications, and this risk may persist until significant remission occurs. Suicide is a known risk of depression and certain other psychiatric disorders, and these disorders themselves are the strongest predictors of suicide. There has been a long-standing concern that antidepressants may have a role in inducing worsening of depression and the emergence of suicidality in certain patients during the early phases of treatment.
Pooled analyses of short-term, placebo-controlled trials of antidepressant drugs (SSRIs and others) show that these drugs increase the risk of suicidal thinking and behavior (suicidality) in children, adolescents, and young adults (ages 18 to 24) with MDD and other psychiatric disorders. Short-term studies did not show an increase in the risk of suicidality with antidepressants compared to placebo in adults beyond age 24; there was a reduction with antidepressants compared to placebo in adults aged 65 and older. The pooled analyses of placebo-controlled trials in children and adolescents with MDD, obsessive compulsive disorder (OCD), or other psychiatric disorders included a total of 24 short-term trials of 9 antidepressant drugs in over 4400 patients. The pooled analyses of placebo-controlled trials in adults with MDD or other psychiatric disorders included a total of 295 short-term trials (median duration of 2 months) of 11 antidepressant drugs in over 77,000 patients. There was considerable variation in risk of suicidality among drugs, but a tendency toward an increase in the younger patients for almost all drugs studied. There were differences in absolute risk of suicidality across the different indications, with the highest incidence in MDD. The risk differences (drug vs placebo), however, were relatively stable within age strata and across indications. These risk differences (drug-placebo difference in the number of cases of suicidality per 1000 patients treated) are provided in Table 1.

Table 1. Risk Differences in the Number of Suicidality Cases by Age Group in the Pooled Placebo-controlled Trials of Antidepressants in Pediatric and Adult Patients

Age Range (Years)	Drug-Placebo Difference in Number of Cases of Suicidality per 1000 Patients Treated
	Increases Compared to Placebo
< 18	14 additional cases
18-24	5 additional cases
	Decreases Compared to Placebo
25-64	1 fewer case
≥ 65	6 fewer cases

No suicides occurred in any of the pediatric trials. There were suicides in the adult trials, but the number was not sufficient to reach any conclusion about drug effect on suicide.
It is unknown whether the suicidality risk extends to longer-term use, ie, beyond several months. However, there is substantial evidence from placebo-controlled maintenance trials in adults with depression that the use of antidepressants can delay the recurrence of depression.
All patients being treated with antidepressants for any indication should be monitored appropriately and observed closely for clinical worsening, suicidality, and unusual changes in behavior, especially during the initial few months of a course of drug therapy, or at times of dose changes, either increases or decreases [see *Boxed Warning* and *Use in Specific Populations (8.4)*].
The following symptoms, anxiety, agitation, panic attacks, insomnia, irritability, hostility, aggressiveness, impulsivity, akathisia (psychomotor restlessness), hypomania, and ma-

Continued on next page

nia have been reported in adult and pediatric patients being treated with antidepressants for MDD as well as for other indications, both psychiatric and nonpsychiatric. Although a causal link between the emergence of such symptoms and either the worsening of depression and/or the emergence of suicidal impulses has not been established, there is concern that such symptoms may represent precursors to emerging suicidality.

Consideration should be given to changing the therapeutic regimen, including possibly discontinuing the medication, in patients whose depression is persistently worse, or who are experiencing emergent suicidality or symptoms that might be precursors to worsening depression or suicidality, especially if these symptoms are severe, abrupt in onset, or were not part of the patient's presenting symptoms.

Families and caregivers of patients being treated with antidepressants for MDD or other indications, both psychiatric and nonpsychiatric, should be alerted about the need to monitor patients for the emergence of agitation, irritability, unusual changes in behavior, and the other symptoms described above, as well as the emergence of suicidality, and to report such symptoms immediately to healthcare providers. Such monitoring should include daily observation by families and caregivers [see *Patient Counseling Information (17)*]. Prescriptions for FORFIVO XL should be written for the smallest quantity of tablets consistent with good patient management, in order to reduce the risk of overdose.

5.2 Neuropsychiatric Symptoms and Suicide Risk in Smoking Cessation Treatment

FORFIVO XL is not approved for smoking cessation treatment, but bupropion hydrochloride sustained-release is approved for this use. Serious neuropsychiatric symptoms have been reported in patients taking bupropion for smoking cessation. These have included changes in mood (including depression and mania), psychosis, hallucinations, paranoia, delusions, homicidal ideation, hostility, agitation, aggression, anxiety, and panic, as well as suicidal ideation, suicide attempt, and completed suicide [see *Boxed Warning* and *Adverse Reactions (6.2)*]. Observe patients for the occurrence of neuropsychiatric reactions. Instruct patients to contact a healthcare professional if such reactions occur.

In many of these cases, a causal relationship to bupropion treatment is not certain, because depressed mood can be a symptom of nicotine withdrawal. However, some of the cases occurred in patients taking bupropion who continued to smoke.

5.3 Seizure

Bupropion can cause seizure. The risk of seizure is dose related. FORFIVO XL should be discontinued and not restarted in patients who experience a seizure while on treatment.

The risk of seizures is also related to patient factors, clinical situations, and concomitant medications that lower the seizure threshold. Consider these risks before initiating treatment with FORFIVO XL. FORFIVO XL is contraindicated in patients with a seizure disorder or conditions that increase the risk of seizure (eg, severe head injury, arteriovenous malformation, central nervous system [CNS] tumor or CNS infection, severe stroke, anorexia nervosa or bulimia, or abrupt discontinuation of alcohol, benzodiazepines, barbiturates, and antiepileptic drugs) [see *Contraindications (4)*]. The following conditions can also increase the risk of seizure: concomitant use of other medications that lower the seizure threshold (eg, other bupropion products, antipsychotics, tricyclic antidepressants, theophylline, and systemic corticosteroids); metabolic disorders (eg, hypoglycemia, hyponatremia, severe hepatic impairment, and hypoxia), or use of illicit drugs (eg, cocaine) or abuse or misuse of prescription drugs such as CNS stimulants. Additional predisposing conditions include diabetes mellitus treated with oral hypoglycemic drugs or insulin, use of anorectic drugs, excessive use of alcohol, use of benzodiazepines, sedatives/hypnotics, or opiates.

Incidence of Seizure with Bupropion Use

The incidence of seizure with bupropion extended-release has not been formally evaluated in clinical trials. In studies using bupropion hydrochloride sustained-release up to 300 mg/day, the incidence of seizure was approximately 0.1% (1/1000 patients). In a large prospective, follow-up study, the seizure incidence was approximately 0.4% (13/3200 patients) with bupropion hydrochloride immediate-release in the range of 300 to 450 mg/day.

Additional data accumulated for bupropion immediate-release suggests that the estimated seizure incidence in-

creases almost tenfold between 450 and 600 mg/day. The 600-mg dose is twice the usual adult dose and one and one-third the maximum recommended daily dose (450 mg) of FORFIVO XL. This disproportionate increase in seizure incidence with dose incrementation calls for caution in dosing.

5.4 Hypertension

Treatment with FORFIVO XL can result in elevated blood pressure and hypertension. Assess blood pressure before initiating treatment with FORFIVO XL, and monitor periodically during treatment. The risk of hypertension is increased if FORFIVO XL is used concomitantly with MAOIs or other drugs that increase dopaminergic or noradrenergic activity [see *Contraindications (4)*].

Data from a comparative trial of the sustained-release formulation of bupropion hydrochloride, nicotine transdermal system (NTS), the combination of sustained-release bupropion hydrochloride plus NTS, and placebo as an aid to smoking cessation suggest a higher incidence of treatment-emergent hypertension in patients treated with the combination of sustained-release bupropion hydrochloride and NTS. In this trial, 6.1% of subjects treated with the combination of sustained-release bupropion and NTS had treatment-emergent hypertension compared to 2.5%, 1.6%, and 3.1% of subjects treated with sustained-release bupropion, NTS, and placebo, respectively. The majority of these subjects had evidence of pre-existing hypertension. Three subjects (1.2%) treated with the combination of sustained-release bupropion and NTS and 1 subject (0.4%) treated with NTS had study medication discontinued due to hypertension compared with none of the subjects treated with sustained-release bupropion or placebo. Monitoring of blood pressure is recommended in patients who receive the combination of bupropion and nicotine replacement.

In a clinical trial of bupropion immediate-release in MDD subjects with stable congestive heart failure (N = 36), bupropion was associated with an exacerbation of pre-existing hypertension in 2 patients, leading to discontinuation of bupropion treatment. There are no controlled studies assessing the safety of bupropion in patients with a recent history of myocardial infarction or unstable cardiac disease.

5.5 Activation of Mania/Hypomania

Antidepressant treatment can precipitate a manic, mixed, or hypomanic manic episode. The risk appears to be increased in patients with bipolar disorder or who have risk factors for bipolar disorder. Prior to initiating FORFIVO XL, screen patients for a history of bipolar disorder and the presence of risk factors for bipolar disorder (eg, family history of bipolar disorder, suicide, or depression). FORFIVO XL is not approved for the treatment of bipolar depression.

5.6 Psychosis and Other Neuropsychiatric Reactions

Depressed patients treated with bupropion have had a variety of neuropsychiatric signs and symptoms, including delusions, hallucinations, psychosis, concentration disturbance, paranoia, and confusion. Some of these patients had a diagnosis of bipolar disorder. In some cases, these symptoms abated upon dose reduction and/or withdrawal of treatment. Discontinue FORFIVO XL if these reactions occur.

5.7 Angle-closure Glaucoma

Angle-closure Glaucoma: The pupillary dilation that occurs following use of many antidepressant drugs including FORFIVO XL may trigger an angle closure attack in a patient with anatomically narrow angles who does not have a patent iridectomy.

5.8 Hypersensitivity Reactions

Anaphylactoid/anaphylactic reactions have occurred during clinical trials with bupropion. Reactions have been characterized by symptoms such as pruritus, urticaria, angioedema, and dyspnea, requiring medical treatment. In addition, there have been rare, spontaneous postmarketing reports of erythema multiforme, Stevens-Johnson syndrome, and anaphylactic shock associated with bupropion. Instruct patients to discontinue FORFIVO XL and consult a healthcare provider if they develop an allergic or anaphylactoid/anaphylactic reaction (eg, skin rash, pruritus, hives, chest pain, edema, and shortness of breath) during treatment.

There are reports of arthralgia, myalgia, fever with rash, and other symptoms of serum sickness suggestive of delayed hypersensitivity.

6   ADVERSE REACTIONS

The following adverse reactions are discussed in greater detail in other sections of the labeling:
- Suicidal thoughts and behaviors in children, adolescents, and young adults [see *Warnings and Precautions (5.1)*]

- Neuropsychiatric symptoms and suicide risk in smoking cessation treatment [see *Warnings and Precautions (5.2)*]
- Seizure [see *Warnings and Precautions (5.3)*]
- Hypertension [see *Warnings and Precautions (5.4)*]
- Activation of mania or hypomania [see *Warnings and Precautions (5.5)*]
- Psychosis and other neuropsychiatric events [see *Warnings and Precautions (5.6)*]
- Angle-closure Glaucoma [see *Warnings and Precautions (5.7)*]
- Hypersensitivity reactions [see *Warnings and Precautions (5.8)*]

6.1   Clinical Trials Experience

Because clinical trials are conducted under widely varying conditions, adverse reaction rates observed in the clinical trials of a drug cannot be directly compared to rates in the clinical trials of another drug and may not reflect the rates observed in clinical practice.

Commonly Observed Adverse Reactions in Controlled Clinical Trials of Sustained-release Bupropion Hydrochloride

Adverse reactions that occurred in at least 5% of patients treated with bupropion hydrochloride sustained-release (300 and 400 mg/day) and at a rate at least twice the placebo rate are listed below.

300 mg/day of bupropion hydrochloride sustained-release: anorexia, dry mouth, rash, sweating, tinnitus, and tremor.

400 mg/day of bupropion hydrochloride sustained-release: abdominal pain, agitation, anxiety, dizziness, dry mouth, insomnia, myalgia, nausea, palpitation, pharyngitis, sweating, tinnitus, and urinary frequency.

FORFIVO XL is bioequivalent to three 150-mg tablets of WELLBUTRIN XL®, which has been demonstrated to have similar bioavailability both to the immediate-release and the sustained-release formulations of bupropion. The information included under this subsection and under subsection 6.2 is based primarily on data from controlled clinical trials with the sustained-release and extended-release formulations of bupropion hydrochloride.

Major Depressive Disorder

Adverse Reactions Leading to Discontinuation of Treatment with Bupropion Hydrochloride Immediate-release, Bupropion Hydrochloride Sustained-release, and Bupropion Hydrochloride Extended-release Formulations in Major Depressive Disorder Trials

In placebo-controlled clinical trials with bupropion hydrochloride sustained-release, 4%, 9%, and 11% of the placebo, 300 mg/day, and 400 mg/day groups, respectively, discontinued treatment because of adverse reactions. The specific adverse reactions leading to discontinuation in at least 1% of the 300-mg/day or 400-mg/day groups and at a rate at least twice the placebo rate are listed in Table 2.

Table 2. Treatment Discontinuation Due to Adverse Reactions in Placebo-controlled Trials in Major Depressive Disorder

Adverse Reaction Term	Placebo (N = 385)	Bupropion Hydrochloride Sustained-release 300 mg/day (N = 376)	Bupropion Hydrochloride Sustained-release 400 mg/day (N = 114)
Rash	0.0%	2.4%	0.9%
Nausea	0.3%	0.8%	1.8%
Agitation	0.3%	0.3%	1.8%
Migraine	0.3%	0.0%	1.8%

In clinical trials with bupropion hydrochloride immediate-release, 10% of patients and volunteers discontinued due to an adverse reaction. Reactions resulting in discontinuation (in addition to those listed above for the sustained-release formulation) included vomiting, seizures, and sleep disturbances.

Adverse Reactions Occurring at an Incidence of > 1% in Patients Treated With Bupropion Hydrochloride Immediate-release or Bupropion Hydrochloride Sustained-release Formulations in Major Depressive Disorder Trials

Table 3 summarizes the adverse reactions that occurred in placebo-controlled trials in patients treated with bupropion hydrochloride sustained-release at 300 mg/day and 400 mg/day. These include reactions that occurred in either the 300-mg/day or 400-mg/day group at an incidence of 1% or more and were more frequent than in the placebo group.

[See table 3 on next page]

The following additional adverse reactions occurred in controlled trials of bupropion hydrochloride immediate-release

(300 to 600 mg/day) at an incidence of at least 1% more frequently than in the placebo group: cardiac arrhythmia (5% vs 4%), hypertension (4% vs 2%), hypotension (3% vs 2%), menstrual complaints (5% vs 1%), akathisia (2% vs 1%), impaired sleep quality (4% vs 2%), sensory disturbance (4% vs 3%), confusion (8% vs 5%), decreased libido (3% vs 2%), hostility (6% vs 4%), auditory disturbance (5% vs 3%), and gustatory disturbance (3% vs 1%).

Changes in Body Weight

Table 4 presents the incidence of body weight changes (≥ 5 lbs) in the short-term MDD trials using bupropion hydrochloride sustained-release. There was a dose-related decrease in body weight.

Table 4. Incidence of Weight Gain or Weight Loss (≥ 5 lbs) in Placebo-controlled Trials of Bupropion Hydrochloride Sustained-release Tablets for Major Depressive Disorder

Weight Change	Placebo (N = 347)	Bupropion Hydrochloride Sustained-release 300 mg/day (N = 339)	Bupropion Hydrochloride Sustained-release 400 mg/day (N = 112)
Gained > 5 lbs	4%	3%	2%
Lost > 5 lbs	6%	14%	19%

6.2 Postmarketing Experience

The following adverse reactions have been identified during postapproval use of bupropion hydrochloride. Because these reactions are reported voluntarily from a population of uncertain size, it is not always possible to reliably estimate their frequency or establish a causal relationship to drug exposure.

Body (General)—chills, facial edema, edema, peripheral edema, musculoskeletal chest pain, photosensitivity, and malaise.

Cardiovascular—postural hypotension, hypertension, stroke, vasodilation, syncope, complete atrioventricular block, extrasystoles, myocardial infarction, phlebitis, and pulmonary embolism.

Digestive—abnormal liver function, bruxism, gastric reflux, gingivitis, glossitis, increased salivation, jaundice, mouth ulcers, stomatitis, thirst, edema of tongue, colitis, esophagitis, gastrointestinal hemorrhage, gum hemorrhage, hepatitis, intestinal perforation, liver damage, pancreatitis, and stomach ulcer.

Endocrine—hyperglycemia, hypoglycemia, and syndrome of inappropriate antidiuretic hormone secretion.

Hemic and Lymphatic—ecchymosis, anemia, leukocytosis, leukopenia, lymphadenopathy, pancytopenia, and thrombocytopenia. Altered PT and/or INR, associated with hemorrhagic or thrombotic complications, were observed when bupropion was coadministered with warfarin.

Metabolic and Nutritional—glycosuria.

Musculoskeletal—leg cramps, fever/rhabdomyolysis, and muscle weakness.

Nervous System—abnormal coordination, depersonalization, emotional lability, hyperkinesia, hypertonia, hypesthesia, vertigo, amnesia, ataxia, derealization, abnormal electroencephalogram (EEG), aggression, akinesia, aphasia, coma, dysarthria, dyskinesia, dystonia, euphoria, extrapyramidal syndrome, hypokinesia, increased libido, neuralgia, neuropathy, paranoid ideation, restlessness, suicide attempt, and unmasking tardive dyskinesia.

Respiratory—bronchospasm and pneumonia.

Skin—maculopapular rash, alopecia, angioedema, exfoliative dermatitis, and hirsutism.

Special Senses—accommodation abnormality, dry eye, deafness, increased intraocular pressure, angle-closure glaucoma, and mydriasis.

Urogenital—impotence, polyuria, prostate disorder, abnormal ejaculation, cystitis, dyspareunia, dysuria, gynecomastia, menopause, painful erection, salpingitis, urinary incontinence, urinary retention, and vaginitis.

7 DRUG INTERACTIONS

7.1 Potential for Other Drugs to Affect FORFIVO XL

Bupropion is primarily metabolized to hydroxybupropion by CYP2B6. Therefore, the potential exists for drug interactions between FORFIVO XL and drugs that are inhibitors or inducers of CYP2B6.

Table 3. Adverse Reactions in Placebo-controlled Trials for Major Depressive Disorder

Body System/Adverse Reaction	Placebo (n = 385)	Bupropion Hydrochloride Sustained-release 300 mg/day (N = 376)	Bupropion Hydrochloride Sustained-release 400 mg/day (N = 114)
Body (General)			
Headache	23%	26%	25%
Infection	6%	8%	9%
Abdominal pain	2%	3%	9%
Asthenia	2%	2%	4%
Chest pain	1%	3%	4%
Pain	2%	2%	3%
Fever	—	1%	2%
Cardiovascular			
Palpitation	2%	2%	6%
Flushing	—	1%	4%
Migraine	1%	1%	4%
Hot flashes	1%	1%	3%
Digestive			
Dry mouth	7%	17%	24%
Nausea	8%	13%	18%
Constipation	7%	10%	5%
Diarrhea	6%	5%	7%
Anorexia	2%	5%	3%
Vomiting	2%	4%	2%
Dysphagia	0%	0%	2%
Musculoskeletal			
Myalgia	3%	2%	6%
Arthralgia	1%	1%	4%
Arthritis	0%	0%	2%
Twitch	—	1%	2%
Nervous System			
Insomnia	6%	11%	16%
Dizziness	5%	7%	11%
Agitation	2%	3%	9%
Anxiety	3%	5%	6%
Tremor	1%	6%	3%
Nervousness	3%	5%	3%
Somnolence	2%	2%	3%
Irritability	2%	3%	2%
Memory decreased	1%	—	3%
Paresthesia	1%	1%	2%
Central nervous system stimulation	1%	2%	1%
Respiratory			
Pharyngitis	2%	3%	11%
Sinusitis	2%	3%	1%
Increased cough	1%	1%	2%
Skin			
Sweating	2%	6%	5%
Rash	1%	5%	4%
Pruritus	2%	2%	4%
Urticaria	0%	2%	1%
Special Senses			
Tinnitus	2%	6%	6%
Taste perversion	—	2%	4%
Blurred vision or diplopia	2%	3%	2%
Urogenital			
Urinary frequency	2%	2%	5%
Urinary urgency	0%	—	2%
Vaginal hemorrhage[a]	—	0%	2%
Urinary tract infection	—	1%	0%

[a] = Incidence based on the number of female patients.
— = Denotes adverse reactions occurring in greater than 0 but less than 0.5% of patients.

Inhibitors of CYP2B6

Ticlopidine and Clopidogrel: Concomitant treatment with these drugs can increase bupropion exposures but decrease hydroxybupropion exposure. Coadministration of FORFIVO XL with ticlopidine or clopidogrel is not recommended [see *Clinical Pharmacology (12.3)*].

Inducers of CYP2B6

Ritonavir, Lopinavir, and Efavirenz: Concomitant treatment with these drugs can decrease bupropion and hydroxybupropion exposure. Patients receiving any of these drugs with bupropion may need increased doses of bupropion, but the maximum recommended dose of bupropion should not be exceeded [see *Clinical Pharmacology (12.3)*].

Carbamazepine, Phenobarbital, and Phenytoin: Although not systematically studied, these drugs may induce metabolism of bupropion and may decrease bupropion exposure [see *Clinical Pharmacology (12.3)*]. If bupropion is used concomitantly with a CYP inducer, it may be necessary to increase the dose of bupropion but the maximum recommended dose should not be exceeded.

7.2 Potential for FORFIVO XL to Affect Other Drugs Drugs Metabolized by CYP2D6

Bupropion and its metabolites (erythrohydrobupropion, threohydrobupropion, and hydroxybupropion) are CYP2D6 inhibitors. Therefore, coadministration of bupropion with drugs that are metabolized by CYP2D6 can increase the exposures of drugs that are substrates of CYP2D6. Such drugs include antidepressants (eg, venlafaxine, nortriptyline, imipramine, desipramine, paroxetine, fluoxetine, and sertraline), antipsychotics (eg, haloperidol, risperidone, and thioridazine), beta-blockers (eg, metoprolol), and Type 1C antiarrhythmics (eg, propafenone, and flecainide). When used concomitantly with bupropion, it may be necessary to decrease the dose of these CYP2D6 substrates, particularly for drugs with a narrow therapeutic index.

Continued on next page

Drugs that require metabolic activation by CYP2D6 to be effective (eg, tamoxifen) theoretically could have reduced efficacy when administered concomitantly with inhibitors of CYP2D6 such as bupropion. Patients treated concomitantly with FORFIVO XL and such drugs may require increased doses of the drug [see *Clinical Pharmacology (12.3)*].

7.3   Drugs that Lower Seizure Threshold

Because there is no lower strength for FORFIVO XL, concurrent administration of FORFIVO XL tablets and agents that lower the seizure threshold (eg, other bupropion products, antipsychotics, antidepressants, theophylline, or systemic corticosteroids) should be undertaken only with extreme caution [see *Warnings and Precautions (5.3)*].

7.4   Dopaminergic Drugs (Levodopa and Amantadine)

Bupropion, levodopa, and amantadine have dopamine agonist effects. CNS toxicity has been reported when bupropion was coadministered with levodopa or amantadine. Adverse reactions have included restlessness, agitation, tremor, ataxia, gait disturbance, vertigo, and dizziness. It is presumed that the toxicity results from cumulative dopamine agonist effects. Because there is no lower strength for FORFIVO XL, administration of FORFIVO XL tablets to patients receiving either levodopa or amantadine concurrently should be undertaken with caution.

7.5   Use with Alcohol

In postmarketing experience, there have been rare reports of adverse neuropsychiatric events or reduced alcohol tolerance in patients who were drinking alcohol during treatment with bupropion. Alcohol increased the release rate of FORFIVO XL in vitro. The consumption of alcohol during treatment with FORFIVO XL should be avoided.

7.6   Monoamine Oxidase Inhibitors (MAOIs)

Bupropion inhibits the reuptake of dopamine and norepinephrine. Concomitant use of MAOIs and bupropion is contraindicated because there is an increased risk of hypertensive reactions if bupropion is used concomitantly with MAOIs. Studies in animals demonstrate that the acute toxicity of bupropion is enhanced by the MAOI phenelzine. At least 14 days should elapse between discontinuation of an MAOI intended to treat depression and initiation of treatment with FORFIVO XL. Conversely, at least 14 days should be allowed after stopping FORFIVO XL before starting an MAOI antidepressant [see *Dosage and Administration (2.7, 2.8)* and *Contraindications (4)*].

7.7   Drug-Laboratory Test Interactions

False-positive urine immunoassay screening tests for amphetamines have been reported in patients taking bupropion. This is due to lack of specificity of some screening tests. False-positive test results may result even following discontinuation of bupropion therapy. Confirmatory tests such as gas chromatography/mass spectrometry, will distinguish bupropion from amphetamines.

8   USE IN SPECIFIC POPULATIONS

8.1   Pregnancy

Pregnancy Category C

Risk Summary

Data from epidemiological studies including pregnant women exposed to bupropion in the first trimester indicate no increased risk of congenital malformations. All pregnancies regardless of drug exposure have a background rate of 2% to 4% for major malformations and 15% to 20% for pregnancy loss. No clear evidence of teratogenic activity was found in reproductive developmental studies conducted in rats and rabbits. However, in rabbits, slightly increased incidences of fetal malformations and skeletal variations were observed at doses approximately equal to the maximum recommended human dose (MRHD) and greater and decreased fetal weights were seen at doses twice the MRHD and greater. FORFIVO XL should be used during pregnancy only if the potential benefit justifies the potential risk to the fetus.

Clinical Considerations

Consider the risk of untreated depression when discontinuing or changing treatment with antidepressant medications during pregnancy and postpartum.

Human Data

Data from the international bupropion Pregnancy Registry (675 first-trimester exposures) and a retrospective cohort study using the United Healthcare database (1213 first-trimester exposures) did not show an increased risk for malformations overall.

No increased risk for cardiovascular malformations overall has been observed after bupropion exposure during the first trimester. The prospectively observed rate of cardiovascular malformations in pregnancies with exposure to bupropion

in the first trimester from the international Pregnancy Registry was 1.3% (9 cardiovascular malformations/675 first-trimester maternal bupropion exposures), which is similar to the background rate of cardiovascular malformations (approximately 1%). Data from the United Healthcare database and a case-control study (6853 infants with cardiovascular malformations and 5753 with non-cardiovascular malformations) from the National Birth Defects Prevention Study (NBDPS) did not show an increased risk for cardiovascular malformations overall after bupropion exposure during the first trimester.

Study findings on bupropion exposure during the first trimester and risk for left ventricular outflow tract obstruction (LVOTO) are inconsistent and do not allow conclusions regarding possible association. The United Healthcare database lacked sufficient power to evaluate this association; the NBDPS found increased risk for LVOTO (N = 10; adjusted OR = 2.6; 95% CI: 1.2, 5.7) and the Slone Epidemiology case-control study did not find increased risk for LVOTO.

Study findings on bupropion exposure during the first trimester and risk for ventricular septal defect (VSD) are inconsistent and do not allow conclusions regarding a possible association. The Slone Epidemiology study found an increased risk for VSD following first-trimester maternal bupropion exposure (N = 17; adjusted OR = 2.5; 95% CI: 1.3, 5.0) but did not find an increased risk for any other cardiovascular malformations studied (including LVOTO, as above). The NBDPS and United Healthcare database study did not find an association between first-trimester maternal bupropion exposure and VSD.

For the findings of LVOTO and VSD, the studies were limited by the small number of exposed cases, inconsistent findings among studies, and the potential for chance findings from multiple comparisons in case-control studies.

Animal Data

In studies conducted in rats and rabbits, bupropion was administered orally at doses of up to 450 and 150 mg/kg/day, respectively (approximately 11 and 7 times the MRHD, respectively, on a mg/m^2 basis), during the period of organogenesis. No clear evidence of teratogenic activity was found in either species; however, in rabbits, slightly increased incidences of fetal malformations and skeletal variations were observed at the lowest dose tested (25 mg/kg/day, approximately equal to the MRHD on a mg/m^2 basis) and greater. Decreased fetal weights were observed at 50 mg/kg and greater. When rats were administered bupropion at oral doses of up to 300 mg/kg/day (approximately 7 times the MRHD on a mg/m^2 basis) prior to mating and throughout pregnancy and lactation, there were no apparent adverse effects on offspring development.

8.3   Nursing Mothers

Bupropion and its metabolites are present in human milk. In a lactation study of 10 women, levels of orally dosed bupropion and its active metabolites were measured in expressed milk. The average daily infant exposure (assuming 150 mL/kg daily consumption) to bupropion and its active metabolites was 2% of the maternal weight-adjusted dose. Exercise caution when FORFIVO XL is administered to a nursing woman.

8.4   Pediatric Use

Safety and effectiveness in the pediatric population have not been established. When considering the use of FORFIVO XL in a child or adolescent, balance the potential risks with the clinical need [see *Boxed Warning*, and *Warnings and Precautions (5.1)*].

8.5   Geriatric Use

Of the approximately 6000 patients who participated in clinical trials with bupropion hydrochloride sustained-release tablets (depression and smoking cessation studies), 275 were ≥ 65 years of age and 47 were ≥ 75 years of age. In addition, several hundred patients ≥ 65 years of age participated in clinical trials using the immediate-release formulation of bupropion hydrochloride (depression studies). No overall differences in safety or effectiveness were observed between these subjects and younger subjects. Reported clinical experience has not identified differences in responses between the elderly and younger patients, but greater sensitivity of some older individuals cannot be ruled out.

Bupropion is extensively metabolized in the liver to active metabolites, which are further metabolized and excreted by the kidneys. The risk of adverse reactions may be greater in patients with impaired renal function. Because elderly patients are more likely to have decreased renal function, it may be necessary to consider this factor in dose selection; it may be useful to monitor renal function [see *Dosage and Administration (2.6)*, *Use in Specific Populations (8.6)*, and *Clinical Pharmacology (12.3)*].

8.6   Renal Impairment

Because there is no lower strength for FORFIVO XL, FORFIVO XL is not recommended in patients with renal impairment [see *Clinical Pharmacology (12.3)*].

8.7   Hepatic Impairment

Because there is no lower strength for FORFIVO XL, FORFIVO XL is not recommended in patients with hepatic impairment [see *Clinical Pharmacology (12.3)*].

9   DRUG ABUSE AND DEPENDENCE

9.1   Controlled Substance

Bupropion is not a controlled substance.

9.2   Abuse

Humans

Controlled clinical studies of bupropion hydrochloride (immediate-release formulation) conducted in normal volunteers, in subjects with a history of multiple drug abuse, and in depressed patients demonstrated an increase in motor activity and agitation/excitement.

In a population of individuals experienced with drugs of abuse, a single dose of 400 mg of bupropion hydrochloride produced mild amphetamine-like activity as compared to placebo on the Morphine-Benzedrine Subscale of the Addiction Research Center Inventories (ARCI), and a score intermediate between placebo and amphetamine on the Liking Scale of the ARCI. These scales measure general feelings of euphoria and drug desirability.

Findings in clinical trials, however, are not known to reliably predict the abuse potential of drugs. Nonetheless, evidence from single-dose studies does suggest that the recommended daily dosage of bupropion when administered in divided doses is not likely to be significantly reinforcing to amphetamine or CNS-stimulant abusers. However, higher doses (that could not be tested because of the risk of seizure) might be modestly attractive to those who abuse CNS-stimulant drugs.

Bupropion hydrochloride extended-release tablets are intended for oral use only. The inhalation of crushed tablets or injection of dissolved bupropion has been reported. Seizures and/or cases of death have been reported when bupropion has been administered intranasally or by parenteral injection.

Animals

Studies in rodents and primates demonstrated that bupropion exhibits some pharmacologic actions common to psychostimulants. In rodents, it has been shown to increase locomotor activity, elicit a mild stereotyped behavioral response, and increase rates of responding in several schedule-controlled behavior paradigms. In primate models assessing the positive reinforcing effects of psychoactive drugs, bupropion was self-administered intravenously. In rats, bupropion produced amphetamine-like and cocaine-like discriminative stimulus effects in drug discrimination paradigms used to characterize the subjective effects of psychoactive drugs.

10   OVERDOSAGE

10.1   Human Overdose Experience

Overdoses of up to 30 g or more of bupropion have been reported. Seizure was reported in approximately one third of all cases. Other serious reactions reported with overdoses of bupropion alone included hallucinations, loss of consciousness, sinus tachycardia, and ECG changes such as conduction disturbances or arrhythmias. Fever, muscle rigidity, rhabdomyolysis, hypotension, stupor, coma, and respiratory failure have been reported mainly when bupropion was part of multiple drug overdoses.

Although most patients recovered without sequelae, deaths associated with overdoses of bupropion alone have been reported in patients ingesting large doses of the drug. Multiple uncontrolled seizures, bradycardia, cardiac failure, and cardiac arrest prior to death were reported in these patients.

10.2   Overdosage Management

Consult a Certified Poison Control Center for up-to-date guidance and advice. Telephone numbers for certified poison control centers are listed in the *Physicians' Desk Reference* (PDR). Call 1-800-222-1222 or refer to www.poison.org.

There are no known antidotes for bupropion. In case of an overdose, provide supportive care, including close medical supervision and monitoring. Consider the possibility of multiple drug overdose.

11   DESCRIPTION

FORFIVO XL (bupropion hydrochloride), an antidepressant of the aminoketone class, is chemically unrelated to tricyclic, tetracyclic, selective serotonin re-uptake inhibitor, or other known antidepressant agents. Its structure closely resembles that of diethylpropion; it is related to phenylethylamines. It is designated as (±)-2-(tert-Butylamino)-3'-chloropropiophenone hydrochloride. The molecular weight is 276.2. The empirical formula is $C_{13}H_{18}ClNO \bullet HCl$. Bupropion hydrochloride powder is white or almost white, crystalline, and soluble in water. It has a bitter taste and produces the sensation of local anesthesia on the oral mucosa. The structural formula is:

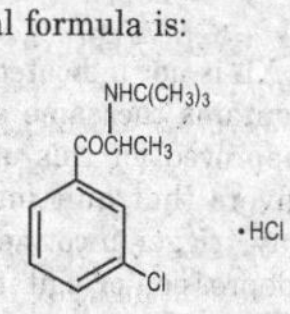

FORFIVO XL tablets are supplied for oral administration of 450 mg of bupropion hydrochloride as white to off-white extended-release tablets. Each film-coated tablet contains the labeled amount of bupropion hydrochloride and the inactive ingredients: hydroxypropyl cellulose, hydrochloric acid, polyvinyl pyrrolidone and polyvinyl acetate blend, polyethylene oxide, stearic acid, colloidal silicon dioxide, magnesium stearate, hydroxypropylmethyl cellulose, triacetin, talc, methacrylic acid copolymer, polyethylene glycol 8000, titanium dioxide and carboxymethyl cellulose sodium. The logo "Forfivo" is printed on one side of the tablet with edible black ink.

12 CLINICAL PHARMACOLOGY

12.1 Mechanism of Action

The mechanism of action of bupropion is unknown, as is the case with other antidepressants. However, it is presumed that this action is mediated by noradrenergic and/or dopaminergic mechanisms. Bupropion is a relatively weak inhibitor of the neuronal uptake of norepinephrine and dopamine, and does not inhibit monoamine oxidase or the reuptake of serotonin.

12.3 Pharmacokinetics

Bupropion is a racemic mixture. The pharmacologic activity and pharmacokinetics of the individual enantiomers have not been studied.

Following single dosing under fasted conditions of FORFIVO XL tablets, the maximum peak plasma concentration (C_{max}), and the area under the plasma concentration versus time curve of bupropion from zero to infinity (AUC_{inf}), were 207.46 (± 59.40) ng/mL, and 2147.53 (± 664.12) ng•hr/mL, respectively. The elimination half-life (± SD) of bupropion after a single dose was 14.44 (± 5.00) hours.

In a single-dose study under fasting conditions, one FORFIVO XL tablet given once daily and three WELLBUTRIN XL 150 mg tablets once daily were evaluated. Equivalence was demonstrated for peak concentration and area under the curve for bupropion and the 3 metabolites (hydroxybupropion, erythrohydrobupropion, and threohydrobupropion).

Absorption

Following single oral administration of FORFIVO XL tablets to healthy volunteers, the median time to peak plasma concentrations for bupropion was approximately 5 hours under fasted conditions, and 12 hours under fed conditions. The presence of food did not affect the maximum peak plasma concentration for bupropion, however, mean systemic exposure to bupropion was increased by 25% when FORFIVO XL tablets were taken with food. The food effect is not considered clinically significant and FORFIVO XL can be taken with or without food.

Distribution

In vitro tests show that bupropion is 84% bound to human plasma proteins at concentrations up to 200 mcg/mL. The extent of protein binding of the hydroxybupropion metabolite is similar to that for bupropion, whereas the extent of protein binding of the threohydrobupropion metabolite is about half that of bupropion.

Metabolism

Bupropion is extensively metabolized in humans. Three metabolites are active: hydroxybupropion, which is formed via hydroxylation of the *tert*-butyl group of bupropion, and the amino-alcohol isomers threohydrobupropion and erythrohydrobupropion, which are formed via reduction of the carbonyl group. In vitro findings suggest that CYP2B6 is the principal isoenzyme involved in the formation of hydroxybupropion, while cytochrome P450 isoenzymes are not involved in the formation of threohydrobupropion. Oxidation of the bupropion side chain results in the formation of a glycine conjugate of meta-chlorobenzoic acid, which is then excreted as the major urinary metabolite. The potency and toxicity of the metabolites relative to bupropion have not been fully characterized. However, it has been demonstrated in an antidepressant screening test in mice that hydroxybupropion is one half as potent as bupropion, while threohydrobupropion and erythrohydrobupropion are 5-fold less potent than bupropion. This may be of clinical importance because the plasma concentrations of the metabolites are as high or higher than those of bupropion.

In humans, peak plasma concentrations of hydroxybupropion occur approximately 10 hours after administration of a single dose of FORFIVO XL under fasted conditions and 16 hours under fed conditions. Following administration of WELLBUTRIN XL, peak plasma concentrations of hydroxybupropion are approximately 7 times the peak level of the parent drug at steady state. The elimination half-life of hydroxybupropion is approximately 20 (± 5) hours, and its AUC at steady state is about 13 times that of bupropion. The times to peak concentrations for the erythrohydrobupropion and threohydrobupropion metabolites are similar to that of the hydroxybupropion metabolite. However, the elimination half-lives of erythrohydrobupropion and threohydrobupropion are longer, approximately 33 (± 10) and 37 (± 13) hours, respectively, and steady-state AUCs are 1.4 and 7 times that of bupropion, respectively.

Bupropion and its metabolites exhibit linear kinetics following chronic administration of 300 to 450 mg/day of bupropion hydrochloride.

Elimination

Following oral administration of 200 mg of ^{14}C-bupropion in humans, 87% and 10% of the radioactive dose were recovered in the urine and feces, respectively. Only 0.5% of the oral dose was excreted as unchanged bupropion.

Population Subgroups

Factors or conditions altering metabolic capacity (eg, liver disease, congestive heart failure [CHF], age, concomitant medications, etc) or elimination may be expected to influence the degree and extent of accumulation of the active metabolites of bupropion. The elimination of the major metabolites of bupropion may be affected by reduced renal or hepatic function because they are moderately polar compounds and are likely to undergo further metabolism or conjugation in the liver prior to urinary excretion.

Renal Impairment

There is limited information on the pharmacokinetics of bupropion in patients with renal impairment. An intertrial comparison between normal subjects and patients with end-stage renal failure demonstrated that the parent drug C_{max} and AUC values were comparable in the 2 groups, whereas the hydroxybupropion and threohydrobupropion metabolites had a 2.3- and 2.8-fold increase, respectively, in AUC for subjects with end-stage renal failure. A second study, comparing normal subjects and subjects with moderate to severe renal impairment (GFR 30.9 ± 10.8 mL/min) showed that after a single 150-mg dose of sustained-release bupropion, exposure to bupropion was approximately 2-fold higher in subjects with impaired renal function while levels of the hydroxybupropion and threo/erythrohydrobupropion (combined) metabolites were similar in the 2 groups. Bupropion is extensively metabolized in the liver to active metabolites, which are further metabolized and subsequently excreted by the kidneys. The elimination of the major metabolites of bupropion may be reduced by impaired renal function [see *Dosage and Administration (2.6)* and *Use in Specific Populations (8.6)*].

Hepatic Impairment

The effect of hepatic impairment on the pharmacokinetics of bupropion was characterized in 2 single-dose studies, one in subjects with alcoholic liver disease and one in subjects with mild to severe cirrhosis. The first trial demonstrated that the half-life of hydroxybupropion was significantly longer in 8 subjects with alcoholic liver disease than in 8 healthy volunteers (32 ± 14 hours versus 21 ± 5 hours, respectively). Although not statistically significant, the AUCs for bupropion and hydroxybupropion were more variable and tended to be greater (by 53% to 57%) in patients with alcoholic liver disease. The differences in half-life for bupropion and the other metabolites in the 2 groups were minimal.

The second trial demonstrated no statistically significant differences in the pharmacokinetics of bupropion and its active metabolites in 9 subjects with mild to moderate hepatic cirrhosis compared to 8 healthy volunteers. However, more variability was observed in some of the pharmacokinetic parameters for bupropion (AUC, C_{max}, and T_{max}) and its active metabolites ($t_{½}$) in subjects with mild to moderate hepatic cirrhosis. In addition, in patients with severe hepatic cirrhosis, the bupropion C_{max} and AUC were substantially increased (mean difference: by approximately 70% and 3-fold, respectively) and more variable when compared to values in healthy volunteers; the mean bupropion half-life was also longer (29 hours in subjects with severe hepatic cirrhosis vs 19 hours in healthy subjects). For the metabolite hydroxybupropion, the mean C_{max} was approximately 69% lower. For the combined amino-alcohol isomers threohydrobupropion and erythrohydrobupropion, the mean C_{max} was approximately 31% lower. The mean AUC increased by about 1.5-fold for hydroxybupropion and about 2.5-fold for threo/erythrohydrobupropion. The median T_{max} was observed 19 hours later for hydroxybupropion and 31 hours later for threo/erythrohydrobupropion. The mean half-lives for hydroxybupropion and threo/erythrohydrobupropion were increased 5- and 2-fold, respectively, in patients with severe hepatic cirrhosis compared to healthy volunteers [see *Dosage and Administration (2.5)* and *Use in Specific Populations (8.7)*].

Left Ventricular Dysfunction

During a chronic dosing study with bupropion in 14 depressed patients with left ventricular dysfunction (history of CHF or an enlarged heart on x-ray), there was no apparent effect on the pharmacokinetics of bupropion or its metabolites, compared to healthy volunteers.

Age

The effects of age on the pharmacokinetics of bupropion and its metabolites have not been fully characterized, but an exploration of steady-state bupropion concentrations from several depression efficacy studies involving patients dosed in a range of 300 to 750 mg/day, on a 3 times daily schedule, revealed no relationship between age (18 to 83 years) and plasma concentration of bupropion. A single-dose pharmacokinetic study demonstrated that the disposition of bupropion and its metabolites in elderly subjects was similar to that in younger subjects. These data suggest that there is no prominent effect of age on bupropion concentration; however, another single- and multiple-dose pharmacokinetic study suggested that the elderly are at increased risk for accumulation of bupropion and its metabolites [see *Use in Specific Populations (8.5)*].

Gender

A single-dose study involving 12 healthy male and 12 healthy female volunteers revealed no sex-related differences in the pharmacokinetic parameters of bupropion. In addition, pooled analysis of bupropion pharmacokinetic data from 90 healthy male and 90 healthy female volunteers revealed no sex-related differences in the peak plasma concentrations of bupropion. The mean systemic exposure (AUC) was approximately 13% higher in male volunteers compared to female volunteers.

Smokers

The effects of cigarette smoking on the pharmacokinetics of bupropion hydrochloride were studied in 34 healthy male and female volunteers; 17 were chronic cigarette smokers and 17 were nonsmokers. Following oral administration of a single 150-mg dose of bupropion, there was no statistically significant difference in C_{max}, half-life, T_{max}, AUC, or clearance of bupropion or its active metabolites between smokers and nonsmokers.

Drug Interactions

Potential for Other Drugs to Affect FORFIVO XL

In vitro studies indicate that bupropion is primarily metabolized to hydroxybupropion by CYP2B6. Therefore, the potential exists for drug interactions between FORFIVO XL and drugs that are inhibitors or inducers of CYP2B6. In addition, in vitro studies suggest that paroxetine, sertraline, norfluoxetine, fluvoxamine, and nelfinavir, inhibit the hydroxylation of bupropion.

Inhibitors of CYP2B6

Ticlopidine, Clopidogrel: In a study in healthy male volunteers, clopidogrel 75 mg once daily or ticlopidine 250 mg twice daily increased exposures (C_{max} and AUC) of bupropion by 40% and 60% for clopidogrel and by 38% and 85% for ticlopidine, respectively. The exposures of hydroxybupropion were decreased.

Prasugrel: In healthy subjects, prasugrel increased bupropion C_{max} and AUC values by 14% and 18%, respectively, and decreased C_{max} and AUC values of hydroxybupropion by 32% and 24%, respectively.

Continued on next page

Cimetidine: Following oral administration of bupropion 300 mg with and without cimetidine 800 mg in 24 healthy young male volunteers, the pharmacokinetics of bupropion and hydroxybupropion were unaffected. However, there were 16% and 32% increases in the AUC and C_{max}, respectively, of the combined moieties of threohydrobupropion and erythrohydrobupropion.

Citalopram: Citalopram did not affect the pharmacokinetics of bupropion and its 3 metabolites.

Inducers of CYP2B6

Ritonavir and Lopinavir: In a healthy volunteer study, ritonavir 100 mg twice daily reduced the AUC and C_{max} of bupropion by 22% and 21%, respectively. The exposure of the hydroxybupropion metabolite was decreased by 23%, threohydrobupropion decreased by 38%, and erythrohydrobupropion decreased by 48%. In a second healthy volunteer study, ritonavir 600 mg twice daily decreased the AUC and the C_{max} of bupropion by 66% and 62%, respectively. The exposure of the hydroxybupropion metabolite was decreased by 78%, threohydrobupropion decreased by 50%, and erythrohydrobupropion decreased by 68%.

In another healthy volunteer study, lopinavir 400 mg/ritonavir 100 mg twice daily decreased bupropion AUC and C_{max} by 57%. The AUC and C_{max} of the hydroxybupropion metabolite were decreased by 50% and 31%, respectively.

Efavirenz: In a study of healthy volunteers, efavirenz 600 mg once daily for 2 weeks reduced the AUC and C_{max} of bupropion by approximately 55% and 34%, respectively. The AUC of hydroxybupropion was unchanged, whereas C_{max} of hydroxybupropion was increased by 50%.

Carbamazepine, Phenobarbital, Phenytoin: Although not systematically studied, these drugs may induce the metabolism of bupropion.

Potential for FORFIVO XL to Affect Other Drugs

Animal data indicated that bupropion may be an inducer of drug-metabolizing enzymes in humans. In a study of 8 healthy male volunteers, following a 14-day administration of bupropion 100 mg 3 times daily, there was no evidence of induction of its own metabolism. Nevertheless, there may be the potential for clinically important alterations of blood levels of coadministered drugs.

Drugs Metabolized by CYP2D6

In vitro, bupropion and hydroxybupropion are CYP2D6 inhibitors. In a clinical study of 15 male subjects (19 to 35 years of age) who were extensive metabolizers of CYP2D6, bupropion given as 150 mg twice daily followed by a single dose of 50 mg desipramine increased the C_{max}, AUC, and $t_{1/2}$ of desipramine by an average of approximately 2-, 5-, and 2-fold, respectively. The effect was present for at least 7 days after the last dose of bupropion. Concomitant use of bupropion with other drugs metabolized by CYP2D6 has not been formally studied.

Citalopram: Although citalopram is not primarily metabolized by CYP2D6, in one study bupropion increased the C_{max} and AUC of citalopram by 30% and 40%, respectively.

Lamotrigine: Multiple oral doses of bupropion had no statistically significant effects on the single-dose pharmacokinetics of lamotrigine in 12 healthy volunteers.

13   NONCLINICAL TOXICOLOGY

13.1   Carcinogenesis, Mutagenesis, Impairment of Fertility

Lifetime carcinogenicity studies were performed in rats and mice at doses up to 300 and 150 mg/kg/day bupropion hydrochloride, respectively. These doses are approximately 7 and 2 times the MRHD, respectively, on a mg/m² basis. In the rat study there was an increase in nodular proliferative lesions of the liver at doses of 100 to 300 mg/kg/day of bupropion hydrochloride (approximately 2 to 7 times the MRHD on a mg/m² basis); lower doses were not tested. The question of whether or not such lesions may be precursors of neoplasms of the liver is currently unresolved. Similar liver lesions were not seen in the mouse study, and no increase in malignant tumors of the liver and other organs was seen in either study.

Bupropion produced a positive response (2 to 3 times control mutation rate) in 2 of 5 strains in one Ames bacterial mutagenicity assay, but was negative in another. Bupropion produced an increase in chromosomal aberrations in 1 of 3 in vivo rat bone marrow cytogenetic studies.

A fertility study in rats at doses up to 300 mg/kg/day revealed no evidence of impaired fertility.

14   CLINICAL STUDIES

The efficacy of bupropion in the treatment of MDD was established with the immediate-release formulation of bupropion hydrochloride in two 4-week, placebo-controlled trials in adult inpatients with MDD and in one 6-week, placebo-controlled trial in adult outpatients with MDD. In the first study, the bupropion dose range was 300 to 600 mg/day administered in 3 divided doses; 78% of patients were treated with doses of 300 to 450 mg/day. The trial demonstrated the efficacy of bupropion as measured by the Hamilton Depression Rating Scale (HDRS) total score, the HDRS depressed mood item (item 1), and the Clinical Global Impressions-Severity Scale (CGI-S). The second study included 2 fixed doses of bupropion (300 and 450 mg/day) and placebo. This trial demonstrated the efficacy of bupropion for only the 450-mg dose. The efficacy results were significant for the HDRS total score and the CGI-S score, but not for HDRS item 1. In the third study, outpatients were treated with bupropion at 300 mg/day. This study demonstrated the efficacy of bupropion as measured by the HDRS total score, the HDRS item 1, the Montgomery-Asberg Depression Rating Scale (MADRS), the CGI-S score, and the CGI-Improvement Scale (CGI-I) score. A longer-term, placebo-controlled, randomized withdrawal trial demonstrated the efficacy of bupropion hydrochloride sustained-release in the maintenance treatment of MDD. The trial included adult outpatients meeting DSM-IV criteria for MDD, recurrent type, who had responded during an 8-week open-label trial of bupropion 300 mg/day. Responders were randomized to continuation of bupropion at 300 mg/day or placebo, for up to 44 weeks of observation for relapse. Response during the open-label phase was defined as a CGI-I score of 1 (very much improved) or 2 (much improved) for each of the final 3 weeks. Relapse during the double-blind phase was defined as the investigator's judgment that drug treatment was needed for worsening depressive symptoms. Patients in the bupropion group experienced significantly lower relapse rates over the subsequent 44 weeks compared to those in the placebo group.

Although there are no independent trials demonstrating the efficacy of bupropion extended-release in the acute treatment of MDD, studies have demonstrated similar bioavailability between the immediate-, sustained-, and extended-release formulations of bupropion hydrochloride under steady-state conditions (ie, the exposures [C_{max} and AUC] for bupropion and its metabolites are similar among the 3 formulations). Further, it has been demonstrated that FORFIVO XL is bioequivalent to WELLBUTRIN XL.

16   HOW SUPPLIED/STORAGE AND HANDLING

FORFIVO XL Extended-Release Tablets, 450 mg of bupropion hydrochloride, are white to off-white, oblong-shaped tablets printed with the "Forfivo" logo on one side supplied in bottles of 30 tablets
(NDC 49909-010-30). °

Store at 20°C to 25°C (68°F to 77°F) [see USP Controlled Room Temperature].

17   PATIENT COUNSELING INFORMATION

Advise the patient to read the FDA-approved patient labeling (Medication Guide).

Inform patients, their families, and their caregivers about the benefits and risks associated with treatment with FORFIVO XL and counsel them in its appropriate use.

A patient Medication Guide about "Antidepressant Medicines, Depression and Other Serious Mental Illnesses, and Suicidal Thoughts or Actions", "Quitting Smoking, Quit-smoking Medications, Changes in Thinking and Behavior, Depression, and Suicidal Thoughts or Actions" and "What Other Important Information Should I Know about FORFIVO XL" is available for FORFIVO XL. Instruct patients, their families, and their caregivers to read the Medication Guide and assist them in understanding its contents. Patients should be given the opportunity to discuss the contents of the Medication Guide and to obtain answers to any questions they may have. The complete text of the Medication Guide is reprinted at the end of this document. Advise patients regarding the following issues and to alert their prescriber if these occur while taking FORFIVO XL.

Suicidal Thoughts and Behaviors

Instruct patients, their families, and/or their caregivers to be alert to the emergence of anxiety, agitation, panic attacks, insomnia, irritability, hostility, aggressiveness, impulsivity, akathisia (psychomotor restlessness), hypomania, mania, other unusual changes in behavior, worsening of depression, and suicidal ideation, especially early during antidepressant treatment and when the dose is adjusted up or down. Advise families and caregivers of patients to observe for the emergence of such symptoms on a day-to-day basis,

since changes may be abrupt. Such symptoms should be reported to the patient's prescriber or health professional, especially if they are severe, abrupt in onset, or were not part of the patient's presenting symptoms. Symptoms such as these may be associated with an increased risk for suicidal thinking and behavior and indicate a need for very close monitoring and possibly changes in the medication.

Neuropsychiatric Symptoms and Suicide Risk in Smoking Cessation Treatment

Although FORFIVO XL is not indicated for smoking cessation treatment, it contains the same active ingredient as ZYBAN® which is approved for this use. Advise patients, families, and caregivers that quitting smoking, with or without ZYBAN, may trigger nicotine withdrawal symptoms (eg, including depression or agitation), or worsen pre-existing psychiatric illness. Some patients have experienced changes in mood (including depression and mania), psychosis, hallucinations, paranoia, delusions, homicidal ideation, aggression, anxiety, and panic, as well as suicidal ideation, suicide attempt, and completed suicide when attempting to quit smoking while taking ZYBAN. If patients develop agitation, hostility, depressed mood, or changes in thinking or behavior that are not typical for them, or if patients develop suicidal ideation or behavior, they should be urged to report these symptoms to their healthcare provider immediately.

Severe Allergic Reactions

Educate patients on the symptoms of hypersensitivity and to discontinue FORFIVO XL if they have a severe allergic reaction.

Seizure

Instruct patients to discontinue and not restart FORFIVO XL if they experience a seizure while on treatment. Advise patients that the excessive use or the abrupt discontinuation of alcohol, benzodiazepines, antiepileptic drugs, or sedatives/hypnotics can increase the risk of seizure. Advise patients to avoid the use of alcohol.

Angle-closure Glaucoma

Patients should be advised that taking FORFIVO XL can cause mild pupillary dilation, which in susceptible individuals, can lead to an episode of angle-closure glaucoma. Pre-existing glaucoma is almost always open-angle glaucoma because angle-closure glaucoma, when diagnosed, can be treated definitively with iridectomy. Open-angle glaucoma is not a risk factor for angle-closure glaucoma. Patients may wish to be examined to determine whether they are susceptible to angle closure, and have a prophylactic procedure (eg, iridectomy), if they are susceptible [see *Warnings and Precautions (5.7)*].

Bupropion-containing Products

Educate patients that FORFIVO XL contains the same active ingredient (bupropion) found in ZYBAN, which is used as an aid to smoking cessation treatment, and that FORFIVO XL should not be used in combination with ZYBAN or any other medications that contain bupropion hydrochloride (such as WELLBUTRIN XL, the extended-release formulation; WELLBUTRIN SR®, the sustained-release formulation; WELLBUTRIN®, the immediate-release formulation; and APLENZIN®, a bupropion hydrobromide formulation). In addition, there are a number of generic bupropion hydrochloride products for the immediate-, sustained-, and extended-release formulations.

Potential for Cognitive and Motor Impairment

Advise patients that any CNS-active drug like FORFIVO XL tablets may impair their ability to perform tasks requiring judgment or motor and cognitive skills. Advise patients that until they are reasonably certain that FORFIVO XL tablets do not adversely affect their performance, they should refrain from driving an automobile or operating complex, hazardous machinery. FORFIVO XL treatment may lead to decreased alcohol tolerance.

Concomitant Medications

Counsel patients to notify their healthcare provider if they are taking or plan to take any prescription or over-the-counter drugs, because FORFIVO XL tablets and other drugs may affect each other's metabolism.

Pregnancy

Advise patients to notify their healthcare provider if they become pregnant or intend to become pregnant during therapy.

Precautions for Nursing Mothers

Communicate with the patient and pediatric healthcare provider regarding the infant's exposure to bupropion through human milk. Instruct patients to immediately contact the infant's healthcare provider if they note any side effect in the infant that concerns them or is persistent.

Administration Information

Instruct patients to swallow FORFIVO XL tablets whole so that the release rate is not altered. Instruct patients that FORFIVO XL tablets should not be chewed, divided, or crushed. FORFIVO XL may be taken with or without food. FORFIVO XL is a registered trademark of IntelGenx Corporation. All other products/brand names are trademarks of their respective owners.

Manufactured by:
Pillar5 Pharma, Inc.
Arnprior, Ontario, K7S 0C9
Canada
For:
Edgemont Pharmaceuticals, LLC
Austin, TX 78746
FFO_V5

MEDICATION GUIDE

FORFIVO XL®

Fore fye' voe Eks el

(bupropion hydrochloride extended-release tablets)

Read this Medication Guide carefully before you start using FORFIVO XL and each time you get a refill. There may be new information. This information does not take the place of talking to your healthcare provider about your medical condition or your treatment. If you have any questions about FORFIVO XL, ask your healthcare provider or pharmacist.

IMPORTANT: Be sure to read the three sections of this Medication Guide. The first section is about the risk of suicidal thoughts and actions with antidepressant medicines; the second section is about the risk of changes in thinking and behavior, depression and suicidal thoughts or actions with medicines used to quit smoking; and the third section is entitled "What Other Important Information Should I Know About FORFIVO XL?"

Antidepressant Medicines, Depression and Other Serious Mental Illnesses, and Suicidal Thoughts or Actions

This section of the Medication Guide is only about the risk of suicidal thoughts and actions with antidepressant medicines. **Talk to your healthcare provider or your family member's healthcare provider about:**

• all risks and benefits of treatment with antidepressant medicines
• all treatment choices for depression or other serious mental illness

What is the most important information I should know about antidepressant medicines, depression and other serious mental illnesses, and suicidal thoughts or actions?

• **Antidepressant medicines may increase suicidal thoughts or actions in some children, teenagers, or young adults within the first few months of treatment.**
• **Depression or other serious mental illnesses are the most important causes of suicidal thoughts or actions. Some** people may have a particularly high risk of having suicidal thoughts or actions. These include people who have (or have a family history of) bipolar illness (also called manic-depressive illness) or suicidal thoughts or actions.
• **How can I watch for and try to prevent suicidal thoughts and actions in myself or a family member?**
  ○ Pay close attention to any changes, especially sudden changes in mood, behaviors, thoughts, or feelings. This is very important when an antidepressant medicine is started or when the dose is changed.
  ○ Call your healthcare provider right away to report new or sudden changes in mood, behavior, thoughts, or feelings.
  ○ Keep all follow-up visits with your healthcare provider as scheduled. Call the healthcare provider between visits as needed, especially if you have concerns about symptoms.

Call your healthcare provider right away if you or your family member has any of the following symptoms, especially if they are new, worse, or worry you:

• thoughts about suicide or dying
• attempts to commit suicide
• new or worse depression
• new or worse anxiety
• feeling very agitated or restless
• panic attacks
• trouble sleeping (insomnia)
• new or worse irritability
• acting aggressive, being angry, or violent
• acting on dangerous impulses
• an extreme increase in activity and talking (mania)
• other unusual changes in behavior or mood

What else do I need to know about antidepressant medicines?

• **Never stop an antidepressant medicine without first talking to a healthcare provider.** Stopping an antidepressant medicine suddenly can cause other symptoms.
• **Antidepressants are medicines used to treat depression and other illnesses.** It is important to discuss all the risks of treating depression and also the risks of not treating it. Patients and their families or other caregivers should discuss all treatment choices with the healthcare provider, not just the use of antidepressants.
• **Antidepressant medicines have other side effects.** Talk to the healthcare provider about the side effects of the medicine prescribed for you or your family member.
• **Antidepressant medicines can interact with other medicines.** Know all of the medicines that you or your family member takes. Keep a list of all medicines to show the healthcare provider. Do not start new medicines without first checking with your healthcare provider.
• It is not known if FORFIVO XL is safe and effective in children under the age of 18.

Quitting Smoking, Quit-smoking Medications, Changes in Thinking and Behavior, Depression, and Suicidal Thoughts or Actions

This section of the Medication Guide is only about the risk of changes in thinking andbehavior, depression and suicidal thoughts or actions with drugs used to quit smoking.

Although FORFIVO XL is not a treatment for quitting smoking, it contains thesame active ingredient (bupropion hydrochloride) as ZYBAN® which is used to help patients quit smoking.

Some people have had changes in behavior, hostility, agitation, depression, suicidal thoughts or actions while taking bupropion to help them quit smoking. These symptoms can develop during treatment with bupropion or after stopping treatment with bupropion.

If you, your family member, or your caregiver notice agitation, hostility, depression or changes in thinking or behavior that are not typical for you, or you have any of the following symptoms, stop taking bupropion and call your healthcare provider right away:

• thoughts about suicide or dying
• attempts to commit suicide
• new or worse depression
• new or worse anxiety
• panic attacks
• feeling very agitated or restless
• acting aggressive, being angry, or violent
• acting on dangerous impulses
• an extreme increase in activity and talking (mania)
• abnormal thoughts or sensations
• seeing or hearing things that are not there (hallucinations)
• feeling people are against you (paranoia)
• feeling confused
• other unusual changes in behavior or mood

When you try to quit smoking, with or without bupropion, you may have symptoms that may be due to nicotine withdrawal, including urge to smoke, depressed mood, trouble sleeping, irritability, frustration, anger, feeling anxious, difficulty concentrating, restlessness, decreased heart rate, and increased appetite or weight gain. Some people have even experienced suicidal thoughts when trying to quit smoking without medication. Sometimes quitting smoking can lead to worsening of mental health problems that you already have, such as depression.

Before taking bupropion, tell your healthcare provider if you have ever had depression or other mental illness. You should also tell your healthcare provider about any symptoms you had during other times you tried to quit smoking, with or without bupropion.

What Other Important Information Should I Know About FORFIVO XL?

• **Seizures: There is a chance of having a seizure (convulsion, fit) with FORFIVO XL, especially in people:**
  ○ with certain medical problems
  ○ who take certain medicines

The chance of having seizures increases with higher doses of bupropion. For more information, see the sections **"Who should not take FORFIVO XL?"** and **"What should I tell my healthcare provider before using FORFIVO XL?"** Tell your healthcare provider about all of your medical conditions and all the medicines you take. **Do not take any other medicines while you are taking FORFIVO XL unless your healthcare provider has said it is okay to take them.**

If you have a seizure while taking FORFIVO XL, stop taking the tablets and call your healthcare provider right away. Do not take FORFIVO XL again if you have a seizure.

• **High blood pressure (hypertension): Some people get high blood pressure that can be severe, while taking FORFIVO XL.** The chance of high blood pressure may be higher if you also use nicotine replacement therapy (such as a nicotine patch) to help you stop smoking.
• **Manic episodes:** Some people may have periods of mania while taking FORFIVO XL, including:
  ○ greatly increased energy
  ○ severe trouble sleeping
  ○ racing thoughts
  ○ reckless behavior
  ○ unusually grand ideas
  ○ excessive happiness or irritability
  ○ talking more or faster than usual If you have any of the above symptoms of mania, call your healthcare provider.
• **Unusual thoughts or behaviors:** Some people may have unusual thoughts or behaviors while taking FORFIVO XL, including delusions (believing you are someone else), hallucinations (seeing or hearing things that are not there), paranoia (feeling that people are against you), or feeling confused. If this happens to you, call your healthcare provider.
• **Visual problems:**
  ○ eye pain
  ○ changes in vision
  ○ swelling or redness in or around the eye Only some people are at risk for these problems. You may want to undergo an eye examination to see if you are at risk and receive preventative treatment if you are.
• **Severe allergic reactions: Some people have severe allergic reactions to FORFIVO XL. Stop taking FORFIVO XL and call your healthcare provider right away** if you get a rash, itching, hives, fever, swollen lymph glands, painful sores in the mouth or around the eyes, swelling of the lips or tongue, chest pain, or have trouble breathing. These could be signs of a serious allergic reaction.

What is FORFIVO XL?

FORFIVO XL is a prescription medicine used to treat adults with a certain type of depression called major depressive disorder.

Who should not take FORFIVO XL?

Do not take FORFIVO XL if you:

• have or had a seizure disorder or epilepsy.
• have or had an eating disorder such as anorexia nervosa or bulimia.
• **are taking any other medicines that contain bupropion, including ZYBAN (used to help people stop smoking), APLENZIN®, WELLBUTRIN®, WELLBUTRIN SR®, or WELLBUTRIN XL®.** Bupropion is the same active ingredient that is in FORFIVO XL.
• abruptly stop drinking alcohol, or use medicines called sedatives (these make you sleepy) or benzodiazepines, or antiseizure medications, and you stop using them all of a sudden.
• take a monoamine oxidase inhibitor (MAOI). Ask your healthcare provider or pharmacist if you are not sure if you take an MAOI, including the antibiotic linezolid.
  ○ do not take an MAOI within 2 weeks of stopping FORFIVO XL unless directed to do so by your healthcare provider.
  ○ do not start FORFIVO XL if you stopped taking an MAOI in the last 2 weeks unless directed to do so by your healthcare provider.
• are allergic to the active ingredient in FORFIVO XL, bupropion hydrochloride, or to any of the inactive ingredients. See the end of this Medication Guide for a complete list of ingredients in FORFIVO XL.

What should I tell my healthcare provider before using FORFIVO XL?

• Tell your healthcare provider if you have ever had depression, suicidal thoughts or actions, or other mental health problems. See "Antidepressant Medicines, Depression and Other Serious Mental Illnesses, and Suicidal Thoughts or Actions."

Tell your healthcare provider about your other medical conditions including if you:

1. have liver problems, especially cirrhosis of the liver
2. have kidney problems
3. have, or have had, an eating disorder such as anorexia nervosa or bulimia
4. have had a head injury
5. have had a seizure (convulsion, fit)
6. have a tumor in your nervous system (brain or spine)
7. have had a heart attack, heart problems, or high blood pressure
8. are a diabetic taking insulin or other medications to control your blood sugar
9. drink alcohol

Continued on next page

10. abuse prescription medicines or street drugs
11. are pregnant or plan to become pregnant
12. are breastfeeding. FORFIVO XL passes into your milk in small amounts.

Tell your healthcare provider about all the medicines you take, including prescription and over-the-counter medicines, vitamins, and herbal supplements. Many medicines increase your chances of having seizures or cause other serious side effects if you take them while you are using FORFIVO XL.

How should I take FORFIVO XL?

• Take FORFIVO XL exactly as prescribed by your healthcare provider.
• **Do not chew, cut, or crush FORFIVO XL tablets.**
• You may take FORFIVO XL with or without food.
• If you take too much FORFIVO XL, or overdose, call your local emergency room or poison control center right away.
• **Do not take any other medicines while using FORFIVO XL unless your healthcare provider has told you it is okay.**
• If you are taking FORFIVO XL for the treatment of major depressive disorder, it may take several weeks for you to feel that FORFIVO XL is working. Once you feel better, it is important to keep taking FORFIVO XL exactly as directed by your healthcare provider. Call your healthcare provider if you do not feel FORFIVO XL is working for you.
• Do not change your dose or stop taking FORFIVO XL without talking with your healthcare provider first.

What should I avoid while taking FORFIVO XL?

• Do not drink alcohol while taking FORFIVO XL.
• Do not drive a car or use heavy machinery until you know how FORFIVO XL affects you. FORFIVO XL can impair your ability to do these things safely.

What are the possible side effects of FORFIVO XL?

FORFIVO XL may cause serious side effects.

• See "What Other Important Information Should I Know About FORFIVO XL?"

The most common side effects of FORFIVO XL include:

• dry mouth
• nervousness
• constipation
• headache
• nausea and vomiting
• trouble sleeping
• dizziness
• shakiness (tremor)
• fast heartbeat
• heavy sweating

If you have nausea, take your medicine with food. If you have trouble sleeping, do not take your medicine too close to bedtime.

Tell your healthcare provider right away about any side effects that bother you.

These are not all the possible side effects of FORFIVO XL. For more information, ask your healthcare provider or pharmacist.

Call your doctor for medical advice about side effects. You may report side effects to FDA at 1-800-FDA-1088.

You may also report side effects to Edgemont Pharmaceuticals, LLC at **1-888-594-4332.**

How should I store FORFIVO XL?

Store FORFIVO XL between 68°F to 77°F (20°C to 25°C).

Keep FORFIVO XL and all medicines out of the reach of children.

General information about FORFIVO XL

• Medicines are sometimes prescribed for purposes other than those listed in a Medication Guide. Do not use FORFIVO XL for a condition for which it was not prescribed. Do not give FORFIVO XL to other people, even if they have the same symptoms you have. It may harm them.
• If you take a urine drug screening test, FORFIVO XL may make the test result positive for amphetamines. If you tell the person giving you the drug screening test that you are taking FORFIVO XL, they can do a more specific drug screening test that should not have this problem.

This Medication Guide summarizes the most important information about FORFIVO XL. If you would like more information, talk with your healthcare provider. You may ask your healthcare provider or pharmacist for information about FORFIVO XL that is written for healthcare professionals.

For more information about FORFIVO XL, go to *www.forfivoxl.com* or call **1-888-594-4332.**

What are the ingredients in FORFIVO XL?

Active ingredient: bupropion hydrochloride.

Inactive ingredients: hydroxypropyl cellulose, hydrochloric acid, polyvinyl pyrrolidone and polyvinyl acetate blend, polyethylene oxide, stearic acid, colloidal silicon dioxide, magnesium stearate, hydroxypropylmethyl cellulose, triacetin, talc, methacrylic acid copolymer, polyethylene glycol 8000, titanium dioxide and carboxymethyl cellulose sodium. The tablets are printed with edible black ink.

FORFIVO XL is a registered trademark of IntelGenx Corporation. All other product/brand names are trademarks of their respective owners.

Rx only

This Medication Guide has been approved by the U.S. Food and Drug Administration.

Manufactured by:
Pillar5 Pharma, Inc.
Arnprior, Ontario, K7S 0C9
Canada

For:
**Edgemont Pharmaceuticals, LLC
Austin, TX 78746**
Revised August 2016
FFO_V5

Shown in Product Identification Guide, page 508

Egalet US Inc.
**600 Lee Road, Suite 100
WAYNE, PA 19087**

Tel: 1-800-518-1084

OXAYDO™   Ⓒ Ⓡ
**(oxycodone HCl, USP)
Tablets for oral use only**

HIGHLIGHTS OF PRESCRIBING INFORMATION
These highlights do not include all the information needed to use OXAYDO safely and effectively. See full prescribing information for OXAYDO.

OXAYDO™ (oxycodone HCl, USP) Tablets for oral use only – CII

Initial U.S. Approval: 1982

————INDICATIONS AND USAGE————
• OXAYDO (oxycodone HCl) is an opioid agonist indicated for the management of acute and chronic moderate to severe pain where the use of an opioid analgesic is appropriate. (1)

————DOSAGE AND ADMINISTRATION————
• Opioid naïve - start dosing with 5 mg to 15 mg every 4 to 6 hours as needed for pain. (2.2)
• Take each tablet, with enough water to ensure complete swallowing immediately after placing it in the mouth. (2, 17)
• Must be swallowed whole and is not amenable to crushing and dissolution. Do not use OXAYDO for administration via nasogastric, gastric or other feeding tubes as it may cause obstruction of feeding tubes. (2, 17)

————DOSAGE FORMS AND STRENGTHS————
Tablets: 5 mg and 7.5 mg (oxycodone HCl) (3)

————CONTRAINDICATIONS————
• Known hypersensitivity to oxycodone, oxycodone salts, any components of the product, or in any situation where opioids are contraindicated (4)
• Respiratory depression (4)
• Paralytic ileus (4)
• Acute or severe bronchial asthma or hypercarbia (4)

————WARNINGS AND PRECAUTIONS————
• Respiratory depression: Increased risk in elderly, debilitated patients, those suffering from conditions accompanied by hypoxia, hypercapnia, or upper airway obstruction. (5.1)
• Controlled substance: Oxycodone HCl is a Schedule II controlled substance with an abuse liability similar to other opioids. (5.2)
• CNS effects: Additive CNS depressive effects when used in conjunction with alcohol, other opioids, or illicit drugs. (5.3)
• Elevation of intracranial pressure: May be markedly exaggerated in the presence of head injury, or other intracranial lesions. (5.4)
• Hypotensive effect: Increased risk with compromised ability to maintain blood pressure. (5.5)

• Prolonged gastric obstruction: In patients with gastrointestinal obstruction, especially paralytic ileus. (5.6)
• Sphincter of Oddi spasm and diminished biliary/pancreatic secretions. Increased risk with biliary tract disease. (5.7)
• Special Risk Groups: Use with caution and in reduced dosages in patients with severe renal or hepatic impairment, Addison's disease, hypothyroidism, prostatic hypertrophy, or urethral stricture, or in elderly or debilitated patients. (5.8)
• Impaired mental/physical abilities: Must use caution with potentially hazardous activities. (5.9)
• Concomitant use of CYP3A4 inhibitors may increase opioid effects. (5.10)

————ADVERSE REACTIONS————
The most common adverse reactions are nausea, constipation, vomiting, headache, pruritus, insomnia, dizziness, asthenia, and somnolence. (6.1)

To report SUSPECTED ADVERSE REACTIONS, contact Egalet US Inc. at 1-800-518-1084 or FDA at 1-800-FDA-1088 or www.fda.gov/medwatch.

————DRUG INTERACTIONS————
• CNS Depressants: Increased risk of respiratory depression, hypotension, profound sedation, or coma. Possible additive central nervous system depression with central nervous system depressants. (7.1)
• Muscle relaxants: Enhances the neuromuscular blocking action of skeletal muscle relaxants and produces an increased degree of respiratory depression. (7.2)
• Mixed agonist/antagonist analgesics (i.e., pentazocine, nalbuphine, butorphanol, and buprenorphine): May reduce the analgesic effects and/or may precipitate withdrawal symptoms. (7.3)
• Monoamine Oxidase Inhibitors (MAOIs): Use not recommended with or within 14 days of stopping MAOIs. (7.4)
• The CYP3A4 enzyme plays a major role in the metabolism of oxycodone: drugs that inhibit CYP3A4 activity may cause decreased clearance of oxycodone which could lead to an increase in oxycodone plasma concentrations. (7.5)
• Anticholinergics: Increased risk for urinary retention and severe constipation. (7.6)

————USE IN SPECIFIC POPULATIONS————
• Geriatric patients: Use caution during dose selection, starting at the low end of the dosing range while carefully monitoring for adverse reactions. (8.5)
• Patients with hepatic impairment (8.6) or renal impairment (8.7): Dose initiation should follow a conservative approach, monitor patients closely and adjust the dose based on clinical response.
• Use in pregnancy only if potential benefit justifies the risk to the fetus (8.1). Women in labor (8.2) and nursing mothers (8.3) should not use OXAYDO.
• Safety and effectiveness in pediatric patients (< 18 years) have not been established. (8.4)

See 17 for PATIENT COUNSELING INFORMATION.
Revised: 4/2015

FULL PRESCRIBING INFORMATION

1 INDICATIONS AND USAGE

OXAYDO is an immediate-release oral formulation of oxycodone HCl indicated for the management of acute and chronic moderate to severe pain where the use of an opioid analgesic is appropriate.

2 DOSAGE AND ADMINISTRATION

Selection of patients for treatment with OXAYDO should be governed by the same principles that apply to the use of other potent opioid analgesics. Opioid analgesics given on a fixed-dosage schedule have a narrow therapeutic index in certain patient populations, especially when combined with other drugs, and should be reserved for cases where the benefits of opioid analgesia outweigh the known risks of respiratory depression, altered mental state, and postural hypotension. Healthcare providers should individualize treatment in every case, using non-opioid analgesics, opioids and/or combination products when necessary, and chronic opioid therapy with drugs such as OXAYDO in a progressive plan of pain management such as outlined by the World Health Organization, the Agency for Health Care Policy and Research, and the American Pain Society.

OXAYDO must be swallowed whole. Take each tablet with enough water to ensure complete swallowing immediately after placing in the mouth [see Patient Counseling Information (17)]. OXAYDO is not amenable to crushing and dissolution. Do not administer OXAYDO via nasogastric, gastric or other feeding tubes as it may cause obstruction of feeding tubes.

2.1 Individualization of Dose

The dose of OXAYDO should be individually adjusted according to severity of pain, and the patient's response, weight, age, and prior analgesic treatment experience. Although it is not possible to list every condition that is important to the selection of the initial dose of OXAYDO, attention must be given to:
1. the daily dose, potency and characteristics of a pure agonist or mixed agonist/antagonist the patient has been taking previously
2. the reliability of the relative potency estimate to calculate the dose of oxycodone HCl needed
3. the degree of opioid tolerance
4. the general condition and medical status of the patient
5. the balance between pain management and adverse reactions
6. the type and severity of the patient's pain
7. risk factors for abuse or addiction, including a prior history of abuse or addiction

2.2 Initiation of Therapy

Patients who have not been receiving opioid analgesics should be started on OXAYDO in a dosing range of 5 mg to 15 mg every 4 to 6 hours as needed for pain. The dose should be titrated based upon the individual patient's response to their initial dose of OXAYDO.

Patients with chronic pain may need to be dosed at the lowest dosage level that will achieve acceptable analgesia and tolerable adverse reactions, on an around-the-clock basis rather than on an as needed basis.

Hepatic Impairment

Since oxycodone is extensively metabolized in the liver, its clearance may decrease in patients with hepatic impairment. Dose initiation in such patients should follow a conservative approach. Dosages should be adjusted according to the clinical situation [see Use in Specific Populations (8.6)].

Renal Impairment

Published data reported that elimination of oxycodone was impaired in patients with end-stage renal failure. The mean elimination half-life was prolonged in uremic patients due to increased volume of distribution and reduced clearance. Dose initiation in such patients should follow a conservative approach. Dosages should be adjusted according to the clinical situation [see Use in Specific Populations (8.7)].

2.3 Conversion to OXAYDO

Conversion from Fixed-Ratio Oral Opioid/Non-Opioid Combinations

When converting patients from fixed-ratio opioid/non-opioid drug regimens to OXAYDO, determine whether or not to continue the non-opioid analgesic. Titrate the dose of OXAYDO in response to the level of analgesia and adverse reactions afforded by the dosing regimen regardless of whether the non-opioid is continued.

Conversion from Other Oral Opioid Therapy to OXAYDO

If a patient has been receiving opioid-containing medications prior to taking OXAYDO, factor the potency of the prior opioid relative to oxycodone into the selection of the total daily dose of oxycodone.

In converting patients from other opioids to OXAYDO, close observation and adjustment of dosage based upon the patient's response to OXAYDO is imperative.

2.4 Maintenance of Therapy

Continual re-evaluation of the patient receiving OXAYDO is important, with special attention to the maintenance of pain management and the relative incidence of adverse reactions associated with therapy. If the level of pain increases, effort should be made to identify the source of the increased pain, while adjusting the dose as described above to decrease the level of pain.

During chronic therapy, especially for non-cancer-related pain (or pain associated with other terminal illnesses), the continued need for the use of opioid analgesics must be reassessed as appropriate.

2.5 Cessation of Therapy

When a patient no longer requires therapy with OXAYDO after chronic use, it is important that therapy be gradually tapered over time to prevent the development of an opioid abstinence syndrome (narcotic withdrawal). In general, therapy can be decreased by 25% to 50% per day with careful monitoring for signs and symptoms of withdrawal [see Drug Abuse and Dependence (9.3) for a description of the signs and symptoms of withdrawal]. If the patient develops these signs or symptoms, the dose should be raised to the previous level and tapered more slowly, either by increasing the interval between decreases, decreasing the amount of change in dose, or both. It is not known at what dose of OXAYDO that treatment may be discontinued without risk of the opioid abstinence syndrome occurring.

3 DOSAGE FORMS AND STRENGTHS

OXAYDO is supplied as white, debossed tablets in two strengths, 5 mg and 7.5 mg of oxycodone HCl, USP, as noted below.

Strength	Description
5 mg	Round, convex, white tablet, debossed "5" on one side, letter "O" on other side.
7.5 mg	Round, convex, white tablet, debossed "7.5" on one side, letter "O" on other side.

4 CONTRAINDICATIONS

OXAYDO is contraindicated in patients with respiratory depression in unmonitored settings and in the absence of resuscitative equipment.

OXAYDO is contraindicated in any patient who has or is suspected of having paralytic ileus.

OXAYDO is contraindicated in patients with acute or severe bronchial asthma or hypercarbia.

OXAYDO is contraindicated in patients with known hypersensitivity to oxycodone, oxycodone salts, or any components of the product.

5 WARNINGS AND PRECAUTIONS

5.1 Respiratory Depression

Respiratory depression is the primary risk of OXAYDO. Respiratory depression occurs more frequently in elderly or debilitated patients, in those suffering from conditions accompanied by hypoxia, hypercapnia, or upper airway obstruction, or following large initial doses of opioids given to non-tolerant patients, or when opioids are given in conjunction with other agents that depress respiration (e.g., benzodiazepines, tricyclic antidepressants, and sedative-hypnotics).

OXAYDO must be used with extreme caution in patients with chronic obstructive pulmonary disease or cor pulmonale, and in patients having substantially decreased respiratory reserve (e.g., severe kyphoscoliosis), hypoxia, hypercapnia, or pre-existing respiratory depression. In such patients, even usual therapeutic doses of OXAYDO may decrease respiratory drive to the point of apnea. In these patients, alternative non-opioid analgesics should be considered, and opioids must be employed only under careful medical supervision at the lowest effective dose.

5.2 Misuse and Abuse of Opioids

OXAYDO contains oxycodone HCl, an opioid agonist and a Schedule II controlled substance. Such drugs are sought by drug abusers and people with addiction disorders.

OXAYDO can be abused in a manner similar to other opioid agonists, legal or illicit. This should be considered when prescribing or dispensing oxycodone HCl in situations where the physician or pharmacist is concerned about an increased risk of misuse or abuse.

OXAYDO may be abused by crushing, chewing, snorting or injecting the product. These practices pose a significant risk to the abuser that could result in overdose and death [see Drug Abuse and Dependence (9)].

Concerns about abuse and addiction should not prevent the proper management of pain. Healthcare professionals should contact their State Professional Licensing Board or State Controlled Substances Authority for information on how to prevent and detect abuse or misuse of this product.

5.3 Central Nervous System Depressants

Patients receiving narcotic analgesics, general anesthetics, phenothiazines, benzodiazepines, other tranquilizers, sedative-hypnotics, or other central nervous system depressants concomitantly with OXAYDO may exhibit an additive central nervous system depression. Interactive effects resulting in respiratory depression, hypotension, profound sedation, or coma may result if these drugs are taken in combination with the usual dosage of OXAYDO. When such combined therapy is contemplated, the dose of one or both agents should be reduced.

Patients should not consume alcoholic beverages, or any medications containing alcohol while taking OXAYDO.

5.4 Head Injury and Increased Intracranial Pressure

In the presence of head injury, intracranial lesions or a pre-existing increase in intracranial pressure, the possible respiratory depressant effects of OXAYDO and its potential to elevate cerebrospinal fluid pressure (resulting from vasodilation following CO_2 retention) may be markedly exaggerated. Furthermore, OXAYDO can produce effects on pupillary response and consciousness, which may obscure neurologic signs of further increases in intracranial pressure in patients with head injuries.

5.5 Hypotensive Effect

OXAYDO may cause severe hypotension in patients whose ability to maintain blood pressure has been compromised by a depleted intravascular volume, or after concurrent administration with drugs such as phenothiazines, general anesthetics or other agents which compromise vasomotor tone. OXAYDO may produce orthostatic hypotension in ambulatory patients. OXAYDO must be administered with caution to patients in circulatory shock, since vasodilation produced by the drug may further reduce cardiac output and blood pressure.

5.6 Gastrointestinal Effects

Do not administer OXAYDO to patients with gastrointestinal obstruction, especially paralytic ileus because oxycodone HCl diminishes propulsive peristaltic waves in the gastrointestinal tract and may prolong the obstruction.

The administration of OXAYDO may obscure the diagnosis or clinical course in patients with acute abdominal condition.

5.7 Use in Pancreatic/Biliary Tract Disease

Use OXAYDO with caution in patients with biliary tract disease, including acute pancreatitis, as oxycodone HCl may cause spasm of the sphincter of Oddi and diminish biliary and pancreatic secretions.

Continued on next page

5.8 Special Risk Groups

Use OXAYDO with caution and in reduced dosages in patients with severe renal or hepatic impairment, Addison's disease, hypothyroidism, prostatic hypertrophy, or urethral stricture, and in elderly or debilitated patients [see Use in Specific Populations (8)].

Exercise caution in the administration of OXAYDO to patients with CNS depression, toxic psychosis, acute alcoholism and delirium tremens. All opioids may aggravate convulsions in patients with convulsive disorders, and all opioids may induce or aggravate seizures in some clinical settings.

Keep OXAYDO out of the reach of children. In case of accidental ingestion, seek emergency medical help immediately.

5.9 Driving and Operating Machinery

OXAYDO may impair the mental and/or physical abilities required for the performance of potentially hazardous tasks such as driving a car or operating heavy machinery. The patient using OXAYDO must be cautioned accordingly [see Drug Interactions (7)].

5.10 Cytochrome P450 3A4 Inhibitors and Inducers

Since the CYP3A4 isoenzyme plays a major role in the metabolism of oxycodone, drugs that alter CYP3A4 activity may cause changes in clearance of oxycodone which could lead to changes in oxycodone plasma concentrations. The expected clinical results with CYP3A4 inhibitors would be an increase in oxycodone plasma concentrations and possibly increased or prolonged opioid effects. The expected clinical results with CYP3A4 inducers would be a decrease in oxycodone plasma concentrations, lack of efficacy or, possibly, development of an abstinence syndrome in a patient who had developed physical dependence to oxycodone.

If co-administration is necessary, caution is advised when initiating oxycodone treatment in patients currently taking, or discontinuing, CYP3A4 inhibitors or inducers. Evaluate these patients at frequent intervals and consider dose adjustments until stable drug effects are achieved [see Drug Interactions (7.5) and Clinical Pharmacology (12.3)].

6 ADVERSE REACTIONS

6.1 Clinical Studies

Because clinical trials are conducted under widely varying conditions, the adverse reaction rates observed in clinical trials of a drug cannot be directly compared to rates in the clinical trials of another drug and may not reflect the rates observed in clinical practice.

Serious adverse reactions that may be associated with OXAYDO include: respiratory depression, respiratory arrest, circulatory depression, cardiac arrest, hypotension, and/or shock [see Warnings and Precautions (5) and Overdosage (10)].

The common adverse reactions seen on initiation of therapy with OXAYDO are dose-dependent, and their frequency depends on the clinical setting, the patient's level of opioid tolerance, and host factors specific to the individual. They should be expected and managed as a part of opioid therapy. The most frequent of the adverse reactions include nausea, constipation, vomiting, headache, and pruritus.

The frequency of adverse reactions during initiation of opioid therapy may be minimized by careful individualization of starting dosage, slow titration and the avoidance of large rapid swings in plasma concentration of the opioid. Many of these adverse reactions will abate as therapy is continued and some degree of tolerance is developed, but others may be expected to remain throughout therapy.

In all patients for whom dosing information was available (n=191) from open-label and double-blind studies involving oxycodone, the following adverse reactions were recorded in oxycodone-treated patients with an incidence of ≥3%. In descending order of frequency they were: nausea, constipation, vomiting, headache, pruritus, insomnia, dizziness, asthenia, and somnolence.

The following adverse reactions occurred in less than 3% of patients involved in clinical trials with oxycodone:

Body as a Whole: abdominal pain, accidental injury, allergic reaction, back pain, chills and fever, fever, flu syndrome, infection, neck pain, pain, photosensitivity reaction, and sepsis.

Cardiovascular: deep vein thrombophlebitis, heart failure, hemorrhage, hypotension, migraine, palpitation, and tachycardia.

Digestive: anorexia, diarrhea, dyspepsia, dysphagia, gingivitis, glossitis, and nausea and vomiting.

Hematopoietic and Lymphatic: anemia and leukopenia.

Metabolism and Nutrition: edema, gout, hyperglycemia, iron deficiency anemia, and peripheral edema.

Musculoskeletal: arthralgia, arthritis, bone pain, myalgia, and pathological fracture.

Nervous System: agitation, anxiety, confusion, dry mouth, hypertonia, hypesthesia, nervousness, neuralgia, personality disorder, tremor, and vasodilation.

Respiratory: bronchitis, cough increased, dyspnea, epistaxis, laryngismus, lung disorder, pharyngitis, rhinitis, and sinusitis.

Skin and Appendages: herpes simplex, rash, sweating, and urticaria.

Special Senses: amblyopia.

Urogenital: urinary tract infection.

7 DRUG INTERACTIONS

7.1 Central Nervous System Depressants

Other central nervous system (CNS) depressants including sedatives, hypnotics, general anesthetics, antiemetics, phenothiazines, other tranquilizers, and alcohol increase the risk of respiratory depression, hypotension, profound sedation, or coma. Use OXAYDO with caution and in reduced dosages in patients taking these agents.

Patients should not consume alcoholic beverages, or any medications containing alcohol while taking OXAYDO.

7.2 Muscle Relaxants

OXAYDO may enhance the neuromuscular blocking action of skeletal muscle relaxants and produce an increased degree of respiratory depression.

7.3 Mixed Agonist/Antagonist Opioid Analgesics

Do not administer mixed agonist/antagonist analgesics (i.e., pentazocine, nalbuphine, butorphanol and buprenorphine) to patients who have received or are receiving a course of therapy with a pure opioid agonist analgesic such as oxycodone HCl. In these patients, mixed agonist/antagonist analgesics may reduce the analgesic effect of oxycodone HCl and/or may precipitate withdrawal symptoms.

7.4 Monoamine Oxidase Inhibitors (MAOIs)

Monoamine oxidase inhibitors have been reported to intensify the effects of at least one opioid drug causing anxiety, confusion, and significant depression of respiration or coma. The use of OXAYDO is not recommended for patients taking MAOIs or within 14 days of stopping such treatment.

7.5 Agents Affecting Cytochrome P450 Enzymes

CYP3A4 Inhibitors

A published study showed that the co-administration with voriconazole, a CYP3A4 inhibitor, significantly increased the plasma concentrations of oxycodone. Inhibition of CYP3A4 activity by its inhibitors, such as macrolide antibiotics (e.g., erythromycin), azole-antifungal agents (e.g., ketoconazole), and protease inhibitors (e.g., ritonavir), may prolong opioid effects. If co-administration is necessary, caution is advised when initiating therapy with, currently taking, or discontinuing CYP3A4 inhibitors. Evaluate these patients at frequent intervals and consider dose adjustments until stable drug effects are achieved [see Clinical Pharmacology (12.3)].

CYP3A4 Inducers

A published study showed that the co-administration of rifampin, a drug metabolizing enzyme inducer, significantly decreased plasma oxycodone concentrations. Induction of CYP3A4 activity by its inducers, such as rifampin, carbamazepine, and phenytoin, may lead to a lack of efficacy or, possibly, development of an abstinence syndrome in a patient who had developed physical dependence to oxycodone. If co-administration is necessary, caution is advised when initiating therapy with, currently taking, or discontinuing CYP3A4 inducers. Evaluate these patients at frequent intervals and consider dose adjustments until stable drug effects are achieved [see Clinical Pharmacology (12.3)].

CYP2D6 Inhibitors

Oxycodone is metabolized in part to oxymorphone via the cytochrome p450 isoenzyme CYP2D6. While this pathway may be blocked by a variety of drugs (e.g., certain cardiovascular drugs, including amiodarone and quinidine, and antidepressants), such blockade has not yet been shown to be of clinical significance with this agent. However, clinicians should be aware of this possible interaction.

7.6 Anticholinergics

Anticholinergics or other medications with anticholinergic activity when used concurrently with opioid analgesics may result in increased risk of urinary retention and/or severe constipation, which may lead to paralytic ileus.

8 USE IN SPECIFIC POPULATIONS

8.1 Pregnancy

Teratogenic Effects: Pregnancy Category B: There are no adequate and well-controlled studies of oxycodone use during pregnancy. Based on limited human data in the literature, oxycodone does not appear to increase the risk of congenital malformations. Animal reproduction studies have not revealed evidence of teratogenicity or fetal harm. Because animal reproduction studies are not always predictive of human response, OXAYDO should be used during pregnancy only if clearly needed.

Reproduction studies in Sprague-Dawley rats and New Zealand rabbits revealed that when oxycodone was administered orally at doses up to 16 mg/kg and 25 mg/kg (approximately 2 and 5 times the daily oral dose of 90 mg on a mg/m^2 basis) respectively, it was not teratogenic or embryofetal toxic.

Non-teratogenic Effects

Neonates whose mothers have taken oxycodone chronically may exhibit respiratory depression and/or withdrawal symptoms, either at birth and/or in the nursery.

8.2 Labor and Delivery

Opioids cross the placenta and may produce respiratory depression and psycho-physiologic effects in neonates. OXAYDO is not recommended for use in women during or immediately prior to labor. Occasionally, opioid analgesics may prolong labor through actions which temporarily reduce the strength, duration, and frequency of uterine contractions. Neonates, whose mothers received opioid analgesics during labor, must be observed closely for signs of respiratory depression. A specific narcotic antagonist, naloxone, must be available for reversal of narcotic-induced respiratory depression in the neonate.

8.3 Nursing Mothers

Low levels of oxycodone have been detected in maternal milk. The amount of oxycodone delivered to the infant depends on the plasma concentration of the mother, the amount of milk ingested by the infant, and the extent of first-pass metabolism. There is potential for serious adverse reactions in nursing infants from oxycodone that includes respiratory depression, sedation and potentially withdrawal symptoms when the mother stops taking oxycodone HCl. As such, one should consider either discontinuing nursing or discontinuing the drug, while taking into account the importance of the drug to the mother.

8.4 Pediatric Use

The safety, effectiveness, and pharmacokinetics of OXAYDO in pediatric patients below the age of 18 have not been established.

8.5 Geriatric Use

Elderly patients (aged 65 years or older) may have increased sensitivity to OXAYDO. Use caution when selecting a dose for an elderly patient, usually starting at the low end of the dosing range, reflecting the greater frequency of decreased hepatic, renal, or cardiac function, concomitant disease, and use of other drug therapy.

8.6 Hepatic Impairment

Since oxycodone is extensively metabolized in the liver, its clearance may decrease in patients with hepatic impairment. Follow a conservative approach to initiate dosing in patients with hepatic impairment. Monitor patients closely and adjust the dose based on clinical response [see Dosage and Administration (2.2)].

8.7 Renal Impairment

Information from oxycodone HCl indicates that patients with renal impairment (defined as a creatinine clearance <60 mL/min) had higher plasma concentrations of oxycodone than subjects with normal renal function. Use a conservative approach to initiate dosing in patients with renal impairment. Monitor patients closely and adjust the dose based on clinical response [see Dosage and Administration (2.2)].

9 DRUG ABUSE AND DEPENDENCE

9.1 Controlled Substance

OXAYDO contains oxycodone HCl, a mu-agonist opioid of the morphine type and a Schedule II controlled substance. OXAYDO, like other opioids used in analgesia, can be abused and is subject to criminal diversion.

9.2 Abuse

Abuse of OXAYDO poses a hazard of overdose and death. This risk is increased with concurrent abuse of alcohol or other substances.

"Drug-seeking" behavior is very common in persons with substance abuse disorders. Drug-seeking tactics include emergency calls or visits near the end of office hours, refusal to undergo appropriate examination, testing or referral, repeated "loss" of prescriptions, tampering with prescriptions and reluctance to provide prior medical records or contact information for other treating healthcare provider(s). "Doctor shopping" to obtain additional prescriptions is common among drug abusers and people suffering from untreated addiction.

Abuse and addiction are separate and distinct from physical dependence and tolerance. Drug addiction is characterized by compulsive use, use for non-medical purposes, and continued use despite harm or risk of harm. Drug addiction is a treatable disease, utilizing a multi-disciplinary approach, but relapse is common. Healthcare providers should be aware that addiction may not be accompanied by concurrent tolerance and symptoms of physical dependence. The converse is also true. In addition, abuse of opioids can occur in the absence of true addiction and is characterized by intentional non-therapeutic use of a drug for its rewarding psychological or physiological effects, often in combination with other psychoactive substances. Misuse includes use of a drug in ways other than prescribed or directed by a healthcare provider. Careful record-keeping of prescribing information, including quantity, frequency, and renewal requests is strongly advised.

OXAYDO is intended for oral use only. Abuse of OXAYDO poses a risk of overdose and death. The risk of overdose and death is increased with concurrent abuse of alcohol or other central nervous system depressants. Parenteral drug abuse is commonly associated with transmission of infectious diseases such as hepatitis and HIV.

In a double-blind, active-comparator, crossover study in 40 non-dependent recreational opioid users, "drug liking" responses and single-dose safety of crushed OXAYDO tablets were compared with crushed immediate-release Oxycodone tablets when subjects self-administered the drug intranasally. The presence of sequence effects resulted in questionable reliability of the second period data. First period data demonstrated small numeric differences in the median and mean drug liking scores, lower in response to OXAYDO than immediate-release oxycodone. Thirty percent of subjects exposed to OXAYDO responded that they would not take the drug again compared to 5% of subjects exposed to immediate-release oxycodone. Study subjects self-administering OXAYDO reported a higher incidence of nasopharyngeal and facial adverse events and a decreased ability to completely insufflate two crushed tablets within a fixed time period (21 of 40 subjects). The clinical significance of the difference in drug liking and difference in response to taking the drug again reported in this study has not yet been established. There is no evidence that OXAYDO has a reduced abuse liability compared to immediate-release oxycodone.

Proper assessment of the patient, proper prescribing practices, periodic re-evaluation of therapy, and proper dispensing and storage are appropriate measures that help to limit abuse of opioid drugs.

Infants born to mothers physically dependent on opioids will also be physically dependent and may exhibit respiratory difficulties and withdrawal symptoms.

9.3 Dependence

Tolerance is the need for increasing doses of opioids to maintain a defined effect such as analgesia (in the absence of disease progression or other external factors). Physical dependence is manifested by withdrawal symptoms after abrupt discontinuation of a drug or upon administration of an antagonist. Physical dependence and tolerance are not unusual during chronic opioid therapy.

The opioid abstinence or withdrawal syndrome is characterized by some or all of the following: restlessness, lacrimation, rhinorrhea, yawning, perspiration, chills, myalgia, and mydriasis. Other symptoms also may develop, including irritability, anxiety, backache, joint pain, weakness, abdominal cramps, insomnia, nausea, anorexia, vomiting, diarrhea, or increased blood pressure, respiratory rate, or heart rate. In general, opioids should not be abruptly discontinued.

10 OVERDOSAGE

10.1 Signs and Symptoms

Acute overdose with OXAYDO can be manifested by respiratory depression (a decrease in respiratory rate and/or tidal volume, Cheyne-Stokes respiration, cyanosis), extreme somnolence progressing to stupor or coma, skeletal muscle flaccidity, cold and clammy skin, constricted pupils, and in some cases, pulmonary edema, bradycardia, hypotension, cardiac arrest and death.

Oxycodone HCl may cause miosis, even in total darkness. Pinpoint pupils are a sign of opioid overdose but are not pathognomonic (e.g., pontine lesions of hemorrhagic or ischemic origin may produce similar findings). Marked mydriasis rather than miosis may be seen with hypoxia in overdose situations.

10.2 Treatment

To treat OXAYDO overdose, primary attention must be given to the re-establishment of a patent airway and institution of assisted or controlled ventilation. Supportive measures (including oxygen and vasopressors) must be employed in the management of circulatory shock and pulmonary edema accompanying overdose as indicated. Cardiac arrest or arrhythmias may require cardiac massage or defibrillation.

The pure opioid antagonist naloxone is a specific antidote to respiratory depression resulting from opioid overdose. Opioid antagonists should not be administered in the absence of clinically significant respiratory or circulatory depression secondary to OXAYDO overdose. If needed, the appropriate dose of naloxone HCl should be administered simultaneously with efforts at respiratory resuscitation (see prescribing information for naloxone HCl for the details).

Since the duration of action of OXAYDO is expected to exceed that of the antagonist, the patient must be kept under continued surveillance and repeated doses of the antagonist should be administered as needed to maintain adequate respiration. Opioid antagonists must be administered cautiously to persons who are suspected to be physically dependent on any opioid agonist, including oxycodone (see Opioid-Tolerant Individuals).

Opioid-Tolerant Individuals: In an individual physically dependent on opioids, administration of a usual dose of antagonist will precipitate an acute withdrawal. The severity of the withdrawal syndrome produced will depend on the degree of physical dependence and the dose of the antagonist administered. Reserve use of an opioid antagonist for cases where such treatment is clearly needed. If it is necessary to treat serious respiratory depression in the physically dependent patient, initiate administration of the antagonist with care and by titration with smaller than usual doses.

11 DESCRIPTION

OXAYDO (oxycodone HCl, USP) tablets are an immediate-release opioid analgesic intended for oral administration only. OXAYDO contains oxycodone HCl, USP as the active analgesic ingredient. The tablets are round, convex, white and debossed with the strength (5 or 7.5) on one side and the letter "O" on the other side. OXAYDO also contains colloidal silicon dioxide NF; crospovidone NF; magnesium stearate NF; microcrystalline cellulose NF; polyethylene oxide NF; and sodium lauryl sulfate NF.

Chemically, oxycodone HCl is 4,5α-epoxy-14-hydroxy-3-methoxy-17-methylmorphinan-6-one HCl, a white, odorless crystalline powder. Oxycodone HCl is soluble in water (1 g in 6 to 7 mL). The molecular weight of oxycodone HCl is 351.82. The molecular formula for oxycodone HCl is $C_{18}H_{21}NO_4 \cdot HCl$, and the structure is:

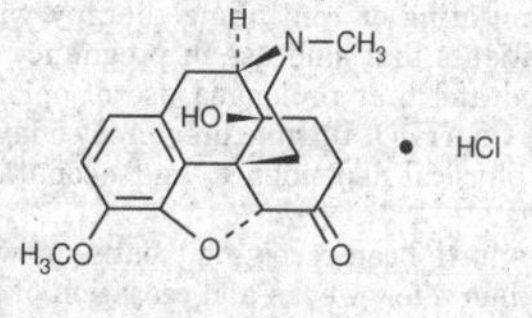

12 CLINICAL PHARMACOLOGY

12.1 Mechanism of Action

Oxycodone HCl is a pure opioid agonist and is relatively selective for the mu receptor, although it can interact with other opioid receptors at higher doses. The principal therapeutic action of oxycodone is analgesia. Like all pure opioid agonists, there is no ceiling effect to analgesia.

12.2 Pharmacodynamics

The relationship between the plasma level of oxycodone and the analgesic response will depend on the patient's age, state of health, medical condition, and extent of previous opioid treatment.

The minimum effective plasma concentration of oxycodone to achieve analgesia will vary widely among patients, especially among patients who have been previously treated with potent agonist opioids. Thus, patients need to be treated with individualized titration of dosage to the desired effect. The minimum effective analgesic concentration of oxycodone for any individual patient may increase over time with repeated dosing due to an increase in pain and/or development of tolerance.

Effects on Central Nervous System

Oxycodone produces respiratory depression by direct action on brainstem respiratory centers. The respiratory depression involves both a reduction in the responsiveness of the brain stem respiratory centers to increases in carbon dioxide tension and to electrical stimulation.

Oxycodone depresses the cough reflex by direct effect on the cough center in the medulla. Oxycodone causes miosis, even in total darkness. Pinpoint pupils are a sign of opioid overdose but are not pathognomonic (e.g., pontine lesions of hemorrhagic or ischemic origins may produce similar findings). Marked mydriasis rather than miosis may be seen due to hypoxia in overdose situations.

Effects on Gastrointestinal Tract and Other Smooth Muscle

Gastric, biliary, and pancreatic secretions are decreased by oxycodone HCl. Oxycodone, like other opioid analgesics, produces some degree of nausea and vomiting which is caused by direct stimulation of the chemoreceptor trigger zone located in the medulla. The frequency and severity of emesis gradually diminishes with time.

Oxycodone may cause a decrease in the secretion of hydrochloric acid in the stomach that reduces motility while increasing the tone of the antrum of the stomach and duodenum. Digestion of food in the small intestine is delayed and propulsive contractions are decreased. Propulsive peristaltic waves in the colon are decreased, while tone may be increased to the point of spasm resulting in constipation. Other opioid-induced effects may include a reduction in biliary and pancreatic secretions, spasm of sphincter of Oddi, and transient elevations in serum amylase.

Effects on Cardiovascular System

Oxycodone, in therapeutic doses, produces peripheral vasodilation (arterial and venous), decreased peripheral resistance, and inhibits baroreceptor reflexes. Manifestations of histamine release and/or peripheral vasodilation may include pruritus, flushing, red eyes, sweating, and/or orthostatic hypotension.

Caution must be used in hypovolemic patients, such as those suffering acute myocardial infarction, because oxycodone may cause or further aggravate their hypotension. Caution must also be used in patients with cor pulmonale who have received therapeutic doses of opioids.

Endocrine System

Opioid agonists have been shown to have a variety of effects on the secretion of hormones. Opioids inhibit the secretion of ACTH, cortisol, and luteinizing hormone (LH) in humans. They also stimulate prolactin, growth hormone (GH) secretion, and pancreatic secretion of insulin and glucagon in humans and other species, rats, and dogs. Thyroid stimulating hormone (TSH) has been shown to be both inhibited and stimulated by opioids.

Chronic use of opioids may influence the hypothalamic-pituitary-gonadal axis, leading to hormonal changes that may manifest as symptoms of hypogonadism.

Immune System

Opioids have been shown to have a variety of effects on components of the immune system in *in vitro* and animal models. The clinical significance of these findings is unknown.

12.3 Pharmacokinetics

The analgesic activity of OXAYDO is primarily due to the parent drug oxycodone.

The pharmacokinetics of oxycodone after OXAYDO administration are characterized by peak plasma concentrations occurring on average within 1.2 to 1.4 hours of the first dose under fasted conditions. Thereafter, oxycodone concentrations fall with an average terminal half-life ranging between 3-4 hours. OXAYDO is bioequivalent with Oxycodone immediate-release tablets in the fasted state, with no differences identified in the time to peak exposure (T_{max}) and terminal elimination half-life ($T_{½}$) of oxycodone between administration of OXAYDO and Oxycodone immediate-release tablets. Dose proportionality was established for OXAYDO at doses of 5 mg, 10 mg, and 15 mg (oxycodone HCl) based on proportional increases in oxycodone C_{max} and AUC exposure levels.

Food Effect

When administered with a high fat meal, mean AUC values are increased by 21% and peak concentrations are decreased by 14%. Food causes a delay in T_{max} from 1.25 to 3.00 hours. These changes in oxycodone pharmacokinetics are not considered clinically relevant; therefore, OXAYDO can be taken without regard to food.

Absorption

Continued on next page

The oral bioavailability of oxycodone is 60% to 87%. The high oral bioavailability of oxycodone (compared to other oral opioids) is due to lower pre-systemic and/or first-pass metabolism of oxycodone compared to other oral opioids.

Distribution

Following intravenous administration, the volume of distribution for oxycodone was 2.6 L/kg. Plasma protein binding of oxycodone at 37°C and a pH of 7.4 was approximately 45%. Oxycodone has been found in breast milk [*see Use in Specific Populations (8.3)*].

Metabolism

Oxycodone HCl is extensively metabolized by multiple metabolic pathways to noroxycodone, oxymorphone, and noroxymorphone, which are subsequently glucuronidated. CYP3A4 mediated N-demethylation to noroxycodone is the primary metabolic pathway of oxycodone with less contribution from CYP2D6 mediated O-demethylation to oxymorphone. Therefore, the formation of these and related metabolites can, in theory, be affected by other drugs. The major circulating metabolite is noroxycodone with an AUC ratio of 0.6 relative to that of oxycodone. Noroxycodone is reported to be a considerably weaker analgesic than oxycodone. Oxymorphone, although possessing analgesic activity, is present in the plasma only in low concentrations. The correlation between oxymorphone concentrations and opioid effects was much less than that seen with oxycodone plasma concentrations. The analgesic activity profile of other metabolites is not known.

Excretion

Oxycodone and its metabolites are excreted primarily via the kidney. The amounts measured in the urine have been reported as follows: free oxycodone up to 19%; conjugated oxycodone up to 50%; free oxymorphone 0%; and conjugated oxymorphone ≤14%. Both free and conjugated noroxycodone have been found in urine but not quantified. The total plasma clearance was 0.8 L/min for adults. Apparent elimination half-life of oxycodone following the administration of oxycodone was 3.5 to 4 hours.

Special Populations

Elderly: Information obtained from oxycodone indicate that the plasma concentrations of oxycodone did not appear to be increased in patients over the age of 65.

Gender: Information obtained from oxycodone support the lack of gender effect on the pharmacokinetics of oxycodone.

Renal Insufficiency: Information obtained from oxycodone indicate that patients with renal impairment (defined as creatinine clearance <60 mL/min) had higher plasma concentrations of oxycodone than subjects with normal renal function [*see Dosage and Administration (2.2)*].

Hepatic Failure: Since oxycodone is extensively metabolized, its clearance may decrease in patients with hepatic impairment [*see Dosage and Administration (2.2)*].

Drug-Drug Interactions

CYP3A4 Inhibitors

CYP3A4 is the major enzyme involved in noroxycodone formation. A published study showed that the coadministration of voriconazole, a CYP3A4 inhibitor, increased oxycodone AUC and C_{max} by 3.6 and 1.7 fold, respectively [*see Warnings and Precautions (5.10) and Drug Interactions (7.5)*].

CYP3A4 Inducers

A published study showed that the co-administration of rifampin, a drug metabolizing enzyme inducer, decreased oxycodone AUC and C_{max} values by 86% and 63%, respectively [*see Warnings and Precautions (5.10) and Drug Interactions (7.5)*].

CYP2D6 Inhibitors

Oxycodone is metabolized in part to oxymorphone via the cytochrome p450 isoenzyme CYP2D6. While this pathway may be blocked by a variety of drugs (e.g., certain cardiovascular drugs and antidepressants), such blockade has not yet been shown to be of clinical significance with this agent.

13 NONCLINICAL TOXICOLOGY

13.1 Carcinogenesis, Mutagenesis, Impairment of Fertility

Carcinogenesis

Studies of oxycodone HCl to evaluate its carcinogenic potential have not been conducted.

Mutagenesis

Oxycodone HCl was genotoxic in an *in vitro* mouse lymphoma assay in the presence of metabolic activation. There was no evidence of genotoxic potential in an *in vitro* bacterial reverse mutation assay (*Salmonella typhimurium* and *Escherichia coli*) and in an assay for chromosomal aberrations (*in vivo* mouse bone marrow micronucleus assay).

Impairment of Fertility

The potential effects of oxycodone on male and female fertility have not been evaluated.

16 HOW SUPPLIED/STORAGE AND HANDLING

OXAYDO (oxycodone HCl, USP) is supplied as round, convex, white tablets as follows:

5 mg tablets debossed with the strength "5" on one side and the letter "O" on the other side.

NDC 69344-113-11 Bottles of 100 tablets

7.5 mg tablets debossed with the strength "7.5" on one side and the letter "O" on the other side.

NDC 69344-213-11 Bottles of 100 tablets

Dispense in tight container as defined in the USP, with a child-resistant closure.

Store at 25°C (77°F); with excursions permitted to 15°-30°C (59°-86°F) [See USP Controlled Room Temperature].

Protect from moisture.

Handling

All opioids, including OXAYDO, are liable to diversion and misuse both by the general public and healthcare workers and must be handled accordingly.

DEA Schedule II Order Form Required

Prescribing Information as of April 2015

Distributed by Egalet US Inc., Wayne, PA 19087

17 PATIENT COUNSELING INFORMATION

Provide the following information to patients receiving OXAYDO or their caregivers:

- Advise patients that OXAYDO is a narcotic pain reliever and must be taken only as directed.
- Advise patients to take each tablet with enough water to ensure complete swallowing immediately after placing in the mouth. Advise patients that OXAYDO tablets must be swallowed whole. Do not crush or dissolve. Do not use OXAYDO for administration via nasogastric, gastric or other feeding tubes as it may cause obstruction of feeding tubes.
- Advise patients not to pre-soak, lick or otherwise wet the tablet prior to placing in the mouth.
- Advise patients to take OXAYDO only as directed.
- Advise patients not to adjust the dose of OXAYDO without consulting with a physician or other healthcare professional.
- Advise patients that OXAYDO may cause drowsiness, dizziness, or lightheadedness and may impair mental and/or physical ability required for the performance of potentially hazardous tasks (e.g., driving, operating heavy machinery). Advise patients started on OXAYDO or patients whose dose has been adjusted to refrain from any potentially dangerous activity until it is established that they are not adversely affected.
- Instruct patients not to combine OXAYDO with central nervous system depressants (sleep aids, tranquilizers) except by the orders of the prescribing physician, and not to combine with alcohol because dangerous additive effects may occur, resulting in serious injury or death.
- Instruct women of childbearing potential who become or are planning to become pregnant to consult a physician prior to initiating or continuing therapy with OXAYDO. Advise patients that safe use in pregnancy has not been established and that prolonged use of opioid analgesics, including OXAYDO, during pregnancy may cause fetal-neonatal physical dependence, and neonatal withdrawal may occur.
- If patients have been receiving treatment with OXAYDO for more than a few weeks and cessation of therapy is indicated, counsel them on the importance of safely tapering the dose and that abruptly discontinuing the medication could precipitate withdrawal symptoms. Provide a dose schedule to help patients gradually discontinue the medication.
- Advise patients that sharing this OXAYDO can result in fatal overdose and death.
- Advise patients that OXAYDO is a potential drug of abuse. They must protect it from theft. Patients should keep OXAYDO in a locked cabinet, drawer, or medicine safe. It must never be given to anyone other than the individual for whom it was prescribed.
- Instruct patients to keep OXAYDO in a secure place out of the reach of children. When OXAYDO is no longer needed, the unused tablets should be destroyed by flushing them down the toilet.
- Advise patients taking OXAYDO of the potential for severe constipation; appropriate laxatives and/or stool softeners as well as other appropriate treatments should be initiated from the onset of opioid therapy.
- Advise patients of the most common adverse reactions that may occur while taking OXAYDO: nausea, constipation, vomiting, headache, pruritus, insomnia, dizziness, asthenia, and somnolence.
- Advise patients to call 911 or the local Poison Control center and get emergency help immediately if they take more OXAYDO than prescribed.
- Advise patients that if they miss a dose to take it as soon as possible. If it is almost time for the next dose, skip the missed dose and take the next dose at the regularly scheduled time. Do not take 2 doses at once unless instructed by their healthcare provider. If they are not sure about their dosing, call their healthcare provider.

Rx Only

Distributed by:

Egalet US Inc., Wayne, PA 19087

Revised: 4/2015

LBL #: 201.00

Shown in Product Identification Guide, page 508

SPRIX®

℞

[spriks]

(ketorolac tromethamine)

Nasal Spray

HIGHLIGHTS OF PRESCRIBING INFORMATION

These highlights do not include all the information needed to use SPRIX® safely and effectively. See full prescribing information for SPRIX®.

SPRIX® (ketorolac tromethamine) Nasal Spray

Initial U.S. Approval: 1989

WARNING: RISK OF SERIOUS CARDIOVASCULAR AND GASTROINTESTINAL EVENTS

See full prescribing information for complete boxed warning.

- Nonsteroidal anti-inflammatory drugs (NSAIDS) cause an increased risk of serious cardiovascular thrombotic events, including myocardial infarction and stroke, which can be fatal. This risk may occur early in treatment and may increase with duration of use (5.1)
- SPRIX® is contraindicated in the setting of coronary artery bypass graft (CABG) surgery (4, 5.1)
- NSAIDS cause an increased risk of serious gastrointestinal (GI) adverse events including bleeding, ulceration, and perforation of the stomach or intestines, which can be fatal. These events can occur at any time during use and without warning symptoms. Elderly patients and patients with a prior history of peptic ulcer disease and/or GI bleeding are at greater risk for serious GI events (5.2)

RECENT MAJOR CHANGES

Boxed Warning	5/2016
Warnings and Precautions, Cardiovascular Thrombotic Events (5.1)	5/2016
Warnings and Precautions, Heart Failure and Edema (5.5)	5/2016

INDICATIONS AND USAGE

SPRIX is a nonsteroidal anti-inflammatory drug indicated in adult patients for the short term (up to 5 days) management of moderate to moderately severe pain that requires analgesia at the opioid level. (1)

DOSAGE AND ADMINISTRATION

- Use the lowest effective dosage for shortest duration consistent with individual patient treatment goals. (2.1)
- SPRIX is not an inhaled product. For adult patients < 65 years of age: 31.5 mg (one 15.75 mg spray in each nostril) every 6 to 8 hours. The maximum daily dose is 126 mg. (2.2, 2.3)
- For patients ≥ 65 years of age, renally impaired patients, and patients less than 50 kg (110 lbs): 15.75 mg (one 15.75 mg spray in only one nostril) every 6 to 8 hours. The maximum daily dose is 63 mg. (2.4)
- SPRIX nasal spray should be discarded within 24 hours of taking the first dose, even if the bottle still contains some medication. (2.5)

DOSAGE FORMS AND STRENGTHS

SPRIX (ketorolac tromethamine) Nasal Spray: 15.75 mg of ketorolac tromethamine in each 100 μL spray. Each 1.7 g bottle contains 8 sprays. (3)

CONTRAINDICATIONS

- Known hypersensitivity to ketorolac or any components of the drug product (4)

- History of asthma, urticaria, or other allergic-type reactions after taking aspirin or other NSAIDs (4)
- In the setting of CABG surgery (4)
- Use in patients with active peptic ulcer disease or with recent GI bleeding or perforation (4)
- Use as a prophylactic analgesic before any major surgery (4)
- Use in patients with advanced renal disease or patients at risk for renal failure due to volume depletion (4)
- Use in patients with suspected or confirmed cerebrovascular bleeding, patients with hemorrhagic diathesis, incomplete hemostasis, and those at high risk of bleeding (4)
- Use in labor and delivery (4)

————WARNINGS AND PRECAUTIONS————

- Hepatotoxicity: Inform patients of warning signs and symptoms of hepatotoxicity. Discontinue if abnormal liver tests persist or worsen or if clinical signs and symptoms of liver disease develop. (5.3)
- Hypertension: Patients taking some antihypertensive medications may have impaired response to these therapies when taking NSAIDs. Monitor blood pressure. (5.4, 7)
- Heart Failure and Edema: Avoid use of SPRIX in patients with severe heart failure unless benefits are expected to outweigh risk of worsening heart failure. (5.5)
- Renal Toxicity: Monitor renal function in patients with renal or hepatic impairment, heart failure, dehydration, or hypovolemia. Avoid use of SPRIX in patients with advanced renal disease unless benefits are expected to outweigh risk of worsening renal function. (5.6)
- Anaphylactic Reactions: Seek emergency help if an anaphylactic reaction occurs. (5.7)
- Exacerbation of Asthma Related to Aspirin Sensitivity: SPRIX is contraindicated in patients with aspirin-sensitive asthma. Monitor patients with preexisting asthma (without aspirin sensitivity). (5.8)
- Serious Skin Reactions: Discontinue SPRIX at first appearance of skin rash or other signs of hypersensitivity. (5.9)
- Premature Closure of Fetal Ductus Arteriosus: Avoid use in pregnant women starting at 30 weeks gestation. (5.10, 8.1)
- Hematologic Toxicity: Monitor hemoglobin or hematocrit in patients with any signs or symptoms of anemia. Do not use SPRIX in patients for whom hemostasis is critical. (5.11, 7)
- Limitations of Use: SPRIX should not be used concomitantly with IM/IV or oral ketorolac, aspirin, or other NSAIDs. (5.15)

————ADVERSE REACTIONS————

Most common adverse reactions (incidence ≥2%) in patients treated with SPRIX and occurring at a rate at least twice that of placebo are nasal discomfort, rhinalgia, increased lacrimation, throat irritation, oliguria, rash, bradycardia, decreased urine output, increased ALT and/or AST, hypertension, and rhinitis. (6.1)

To report SUSPECTED ADVERSE REACTIONS, contact Egalet US Inc. at 1-800-518-1084 or FDA at 1-800-FDA-1088 or www.fda.gov/medwatch.

————DRUG INTERACTIONS————

- Drugs that Interfere with Hemostasis (e.g. warfarin, aspirin, SSRIs/SNRIs): Monitor patients for bleeding who are concomitantly taking SPRIX with drugs that interfere with hemostasis. Concomitant use of SPRIX and analgesic doses of aspirin is not generally recommended. (7)
- ACE Inhibitors, Angiotensin Receptor Blockers (ARB), or Beta-Blockers: Concomitant use with SPRIX may diminish the antihypertensive effect of these drugs. Monitor blood pressure. (7)
- ACE Inhibitors and ARBs: Concomitant use with SPRIX in elderly, volume depleted, or those with renal impairment may result in deterioration of renal function. In such high risk patients, monitor for signs of worsening renal function. (7)
- Diuretics: NSAIDs can reduce natriuretic effect of furosemide and thiazide diuretics. Monitor patients to assure diuretic efficacy including antihypertensive effects. (7)
- Digoxin: Concomitant use with SPRIX can increase serum concentration and prolong half-life of digoxin. Monitor serum digoxin levels. (7)

————USE IN SPECIFIC POPULATIONS————

Pregnancy: Use of NSAIDs during the third trimester of pregnancy increases the risk of premature closure of the fetal ductus arteriosus. Avoid use of NSAIDs in pregnant women starting at 30 weeks gestation. (5.10, 8.1)

Infertility: NSAIDs are associated with reversible infertility. Consider withdrawal of SPRIX in women who have difficulties conceiving. (8.3)

See 17 for PATIENT COUNSELING INFORMATION and Medication Guide.

Revised: 7/2016

FULL PRESCRIBING INFORMATION: CONTENTS*
WARNING: RISK OF SERIOUS CARDIOVASCULAR AND GASTROINTESTINAL EVENTS

* Sections or subsections omitted from the full prescribing information are not listed.

FULL PRESCRIBING INFORMATION

> **WARNING: RISK OF SERIOUS CARDIOVASCULAR AND GASTROINTESTINAL EVENTS**
> **Cardiovascular Thrombotic Events**
> - **Nonsteroidal anti-inflammatory drugs (NSAIDs) cause an increased risk of serious cardiovascular thrombotic events, including myocardial infarction and stroke, which can be fatal. This risk may occur early in treatment and may increase with duration of use [see Warnings and Precautions (5.1)].**
> - **SPRIX® is contraindicated in the setting of coronary artery bypass graft (CABG) surgery [see Contraindications (4) and Warnings and Precautions (5.1)].**
>
> **Gastrointestinal Bleeding, Ulceration, and Perforation**
> - **NSAIDS cause an increased risk of serious gastrointestinal (GI) adverse events including bleeding, ulceration, and perforation of the stomach or intestines, which can be fatal. These events can occur at any time during use and without warning symptoms. Elderly patients and patients with a prior history of peptic ulcer disease and/or GI bleeding are at greater risk for serious GI events [see Warnings and Precautions (5.2)].**

1   INDICATIONS AND USAGE

SPRIX is indicated in adult patients for the short term (up to 5 days) management of moderate to moderately severe pain that requires analgesia at the opioid level.

---

2   DOSAGE AND ADMINISTRATION

2.1   General Dosing Instructions

Use the lowest effective dosage for the shortest duration consistent with individual patient treatment goals [see *Warnings and Precautions (5)*].

The total duration of use of SPRIX alone or sequentially with other formulations of ketorolac (IM/IV or oral) must not exceed 5 days because of the potential for increasing the frequency and severity of adverse reactions associated with the recommended doses [see *Warnings and Precautions (5.15)*].

Do not use SPRIX concomitantly with other formulations of ketorolac or other NSAIDs [see *Warnings and Precautions (5.15)*].

2.2   Administration

SPRIX is not an inhaled product. Do not inhale when administering this product.

Instruct patients to administer as follows:

1. First hold the finger flange with fingers, and remove the clear plastic cover with opposite hand; then remove the blue plastic safety clip. Keep the clear plastic cover; and throw away the blue plastic safety clip.
2. Before using the bottle for the **FIRST** time, activate the pump. To activate the pump, hold the bottle at arm's length away from the body with index finger and middle finger resting on the top of the finger flange and thumb supporting the base. **Press down evenly and release the pump 5 times.** Patient may not see a spray the first few times he/she presses down.
   The bottle is now ready to use. There is no need to activate the pump again if more doses are used from the bottle.
3. It's important to get the medication to the correct place in the nose so it will be most effective.
   - Blow nose gently to clear nostrils.
   - Sit up straight or stand. Tilt head slightly forward.
   - Insert the tip of the container into your right nostril.
   - Point the container away from the center of your nose.
   - Hold your breath and spray once into your right nostril, pressing down evenly on both sides.
   - Immediately after administration, resume breathing through mouth to reduce expelling the product. Also pinch the nose to help retain the spray if it starts to drip.
   If only one spray per dose is prescribed, administration is complete; skip to Step 5 below.
4. If a dose of 2 sprays is prescribed, repeat the process in Step 3 for the left nostril. Again, be sure to point the spray away from the center of nose. Spray once into the left nostril.
5. Replace the clear plastic cover and place the bottle in a cool, dry location out of direct sunlight, such as inside a medication cabinet. Keep out of reach of children.

2.3   Adult Patients < 65 Years of Age

The recommended dose is 31.5 mg SPRIX (one 15.75 mg spray in each nostril) every 6 to 8 hours. The maximum daily dose is 126 mg (four doses).

2.4   Reduced Doses for Special Populations

For patients ≥ 65 years of age, renally impaired patients, and adult patients less than 50 kg (110 lbs), the recommended dose is 15.75 mg SPRIX (one 15.75 mg spray in only one nostril) every 6 to 8 hours. The maximum daily dose is 63 mg (four doses) [see *Warnings and Precautions (5.2, 5.6)*].

2.5   Discard Used SPRIX Bottle after 24 Hours

Do not use any single SPRIX bottle for more than one day as it will not deliver the intended dose after 24 hours. Therefore, the bottle must be discarded no more than 24 hours after taking the first dose, even if the bottle still contains some liquid.

3   DOSAGE FORMS AND STRENGTHS

SPRIX (ketorolac tromethamine) Nasal spray: 15.75 mg of ketorolac tromethamine in each 100 µL spray. Each 1.7 g bottle contains 8 sprays.

4   CONTRAINDICATIONS

SPRIX is contraindicated in the following patients:
- Known hypersensitivity (e.g., anaphylactic reactions and serious skin reactions) to ketorolac or any components of the drug product [see *Warning and Precautions (5.7, 5.9)*].
- History of asthma, urticaria, or other allergic-type reactions after taking aspirin or other NSAIDs. Severe, sometimes fatal, anaphylactic reactions to NSAIDs have been reported in such patients [see *Warning and Precautions (5.7, 5.8)*]

Continued on next page

- In the setting of coronary artery bypass graft (CABG) surgery [see *Warnings and Precautions (5.1)*]
- Use in patients with active peptic ulcer disease and in patients with recent gastrointestinal bleeding or perforation [see *Warnings and Precautions (5.2)*]
- Use as a prophylactic analgesic before any major surgery [see *Warnings and Precautions (5.11)*]
- Use in patients with advanced renal disease or patients at risk for renal failure due to volume depletion [see *Warnings and Precautions (5.6)*]
- Use in labor and delivery. Through its prostaglandin synthesis inhibitory effect, ketorolac may adversely affect fetal circulation and inhibit uterine contractions, thus increasing the risk of uterine hemorrhage [see *Use in Specific Populations (8.1)*]
- Use in patients with suspected or confirmed cerebrovascular bleeding, hemorrhagic diathesis, incomplete hemostasis, or those for whom hemostasis is critical [see *Warnings and Precautions (5.11), Drug Interactions (7)*]
- Concomitant use with probenecid [see *Drug Interactions (7)*]
- Concomitant use with pentoxifylline [see *Drug Interactions (7)*]

5 WARNINGS AND PRECAUTIONS

5.1 Cardiovascular Thrombotic Events

Clinical trials of several COX-2 selective and nonselective NSAIDs of up to three years duration have shown an increased risk of serious cardiovascular (CV) thrombotic events, including myocardial infarction (MI) and stroke, which can be fatal. Based on available data, it is unclear that the risk for CV thrombotic events is similar for all NSAIDs. The relative increase in serious CV thrombotic events over baseline conferred by NSAID use appears to be similar in those with and without known CV disease or risk factors for CV disease. However, patients with known CV disease or risk factors had a higher absolute incidence of excess serious CV thrombotic events, due to their increased baseline rate. Some observational studies found that this increased risk of serious CV thrombotic events began as early as the first weeks of treatment. The increase in CV thrombotic risk has been observed most consistently at higher doses.

To minimize the potential risk for an adverse CV event in NSAID-treated patients, use the lowest effective dose for the shortest duration possible. Physicians and patients should remain alert for the development of such events, throughout the entire treatment course, even in the absence of previous CV symptoms. Patients should be informed about the symptoms of serious CV events and the steps to take if they occur.

There is no consistent evidence that concurrent use of aspirin mitigates the increased risk of serious CV thrombotic events associated with NSAID use. The concurrent use of aspirin and an NSAID, such as ketorolac, increases the risk of serious gastrointestinal (GI) events [see *Warnings and Precautions (5.2)*].

Status Post Coronary Artery Bypass Graft (CABG) Surgery
Two large, controlled clinical trials of a COX-2 selective NSAID for the treatment of pain in the first 10–14 days following CABG surgery found an increased incidence of myocardial infarction and stroke. NSAIDs are contraindicated in the setting of CABG [see *Contraindications (4)*].

Post-MI Patients
Observational studies conducted in the Danish National Registry have demonstrated that patients treated with NSAIDs in the post-MI period were at increased risk of reinfarction, CV-related death, and all-cause mortality beginning in the first week of treatment. In this same cohort, the incidence of death in the first year post-MI was 20 per 100 person years in NSAID-treated patients compared to 12 per 100 person years in non-NSAID exposed patients. Although the absolute rate of death declined somewhat after the first year post-MI, the increased relative risk of death in NSAID users persisted over at least the next four years of follow-up. Avoid the use of SPRIX in patients with a recent MI unless the benefits are expected to outweigh the risk of recurrent CV thrombotic events. If SPRIX is used in patients with a recent MI, monitor patients for signs of cardiac ischemia.

5.2 Gastrointestinal Bleeding, Ulceration, and Perforation

SPRIX is contraindicated in patients with active peptic ulcers and/or GI bleeding and in patients with recent gastrointestinal bleeding or perforation [see *Contraindications (4)*].

NSAIDs, including ketorolac, cause serious gastrointestinal (GI) adverse events including inflammation, bleeding, ulcer-

ation, and perforation of the esophagus, stomach, small intestine, or large intestine, which can be fatal. These serious adverse events can occur at any time, with or without warning symptoms, in patients treated with NSAIDs. Only one in five patients who develop a serious upper GI adverse event on NSAID therapy is symptomatic. Upper GI ulcers, gross bleeding, or perforation caused by NSAIDs occurred in approximately 1% of patients treated for 3-6 months, and in about 2%-4% of patients treated for one year. However, even short-term NSAID therapy is not without risk.

Risk Factors for GI Bleeding, Ulceration, and Perforation
Patients with a prior history of peptic ulcer disease and/or GI bleeding who used NSAIDs had a greater than 10-fold increased risk for developing a GI bleed compared to patients without these risk factors. Other factors that increase the risk of GI bleeding in patients treated with NSAIDs include longer duration of NSAID therapy; concomitant use of oral corticosteroids, aspirin, anticoagulants, or selective serotonin reuptake inhibitors (SSRIs); smoking; use of alcohol; older age; and poor general health status. Most postmarketing reports of fatal GI events occurred in elderly or debilitated patients. Additionally, patients with advanced liver disease and/or coagulopathy are at increased risk for GI bleeding.

Strategies to Minimize the GI Risks in NSAID-treated patients:
- Use the lowest effective dosage for the shortest possible duration.
- Avoid administration of more than one NSAID at a time.
- Avoid use in patients at higher risk unless benefits are expected to outweigh the increased risk of bleeding. For such patients, consider alternate therapies other than NSAIDs. Do not use Sprix in those with active GI bleeding.
- Remain alert for signs and symptoms of GI ulceration and bleeding during NSAID therapy.
- If a serious GI adverse event is suspected, promptly initiate evaluation and treatment, and discontinue SPRIX until a serious GI adverse event is ruled out.
- In the setting of concomitant use of low-dose aspirin for cardiac prophylaxis, monitor patients more closely for evidence of GI bleeding [see *Drug Interactions (7)*].
- Use great care when giving SPRIX to patients with a history of inflammatory bowel disease (ulcerative colitis, Crohn's disease) as their condition may be exacerbated.

5.3 Hepatotoxicity

Elevations of ALT or AST (three or more times the upper limit of normal [ULN]) have been reported in approximately 1% of NSAID-treated patients in clinical trials. In addition, rare, sometimes fatal, cases of severe hepatic injury, including fulminant hepatitis, liver necrosis, and hepatic failure have been reported.

Elevations of ALT or AST (less than three times ULN) may occur in up to 15% of patients treated with NSAIDs including ketorolac.

Inform patients of the warning signs and symptoms of hepatotoxicity (e.g., nausea, fatigue, lethargy, diarrhea, pruritus, jaundice, right upper quadrant tenderness, and "flu-like" symptoms). If clinical signs and symptoms consistent with liver disease develop, or if systemic manifestations occur (e.g., eosinophilia, rash, etc.), discontinue SPRIX immediately, and perform a clinical evaluation of the patient.

5.4 Hypertension

NSAIDs, including SPRIX, can lead to new onset of hypertension or worsening of preexisting hypertension, either of which may contribute to the increased incidence of CV events. Patients taking angiotensin converting enzyme (ACE) inhibitors, thiazide diuretics, or loop diuretics may have impaired response to these therapies when taking NSAIDs [see *Drug Interactions (7)*].

Monitor blood pressure (BP) during the initiation of NSAID treatment and throughout the course of therapy.

5.5 Heart Failure and Edema

The Coxib and traditional NSAID Trialists' Collaboration meta-analysis of randomized controlled trials demonstrated an approximately two-fold increase in hospitalizations for heart failure in COX-2 selective-treated patients and nonselective NSAID-treated patients compared to placebo-treated patients. In a Danish National Registry study of patients with heart failure, NSAID use increased the risk of MI, hospitalization for heart failure, and death.

Additionally, fluid retention and edema have been observed in some patients treated with NSAIDs. Use of ketorolac may blunt the CV effects of several therapeutic agents used to treat these medical conditions (e.g., diuretics, ACE inhibitors, or angiotensin receptor blockers [ARBs]) [see *Drug Interactions (7)*].

Avoid the use of SPRIX in patients with severe heart failure unless the benefits are expected to outweigh the risk of worsening heart failure. If SPRIX is used in patients with severe heart failure, monitor patients for signs of worsening heart failure.

5.6 Renal Toxicity and Hyperkalemia

Ketorolac and its metabolites are eliminated primarily by the kidneys. Patients with reduced creatinine clearance will have diminished clearance of the drug [see *Clinical Pharmacology (12.3)*]. SPRIX is contraindicated in patients with advanced renal impairment [see *Contraindications (4)*].

Renal Toxicity
Long-term administration of NSAIDs has resulted in renal papillary necrosis and other renal injury. Renal toxicity has also been seen in patients in whom renal prostaglandins have a compensatory role in the maintenance of renal perfusion. In these patients, administration of an NSAID may cause a dose-dependent reduction in prostaglandin formation and, secondarily, in renal blood flow, which may precipitate overt renal decompensation. Patients at greatest risk of this reaction are those with impaired renal function, dehydration, hypovolemia, heart failure, liver dysfunction, those taking diuretics and ACE inhibitors or ARBs, and the elderly. Discontinuation of NSAID therapy is usually followed by recovery to the pretreatment state.

No information is available from controlled clinical studies regarding the use of SPRIX in patients with advanced renal disease. The renal effects of SPRIX may hasten the progression of renal dysfunction in patients with preexisting renal disease.

Correct volume status in dehydrated or hypovolemic patients prior to initiating SPRIX. Monitor renal function in patients with renal or hepatic impairment, heart failure, dehydration, or hypovolemia during use of SPRIX [see *Drug Interactions (7)*]. Avoid the use of SPRIX in patients with advanced renal disease unless the benefits are expected to outweigh the risk of worsening renal function. If SPRIX is used in patients with advanced renal disease, monitor patients for signs of worsening renal function.

Hyperkalemia
Increases in serum potassium concentration, including hyperkalemia, have been reported with use of NSAIDs, even in some patients without renal impairment. In patients with normal renal function, these effects have been attributed to a hyporeninemic-hypoaldosteronism state.

5.7 Anaphylactic Reactions

Ketorolac has been associated with anaphylactic reactions in patients with and without known hypersensitivity to ketorolac and in patients with aspirin-sensitive asthma [see *Contraindications (4) and Warnings and Precautions (5.8)*]. Seek emergency help if an anaphylactic reaction occurs.

5.8 Exacerbation of Asthma Related to Aspirin Sensitivity

A subpopulation of patients with asthma may have aspirin-sensitive asthma which may include chronic rhinosinusitis complicated by nasal polyps; severe, potentially fatal bronchospasm; and/or intolerance to aspirin and other NSAIDs. Because cross-reactivity between aspirin and other NSAIDs has been reported in such aspirin-sensitive patients, SPRIX is contraindicated in patients with this form of aspirin sensitivity [see *Contraindications (4)*]. When SPRIX is used in patients with preexisting asthma (without known aspirin sensitivity), monitor patients for changes in the signs and symptoms of asthma.

5.9 Serious Skin Reactions

NSAIDs, including ketorolac, can cause serious skin adverse reactions such as exfoliative dermatitis, Stevens-Johnson Syndrome (SJS), and toxic epidermal necrolysis (TEN), which can be fatal. These serious events may occur without warning. Inform patients about the signs and symptoms of serious skin reactions, and to discontinue the use of SPRIX at the first appearance of skin rash or any other sign of hypersensitivity. SPRIX is contraindicated in patients with previous serious skin reactions to NSAIDs [see *Contraindications (4)*].

5.10 Premature Closure of Fetal Ductus Arteriosus

Ketorolac may cause premature closure of the fetal ductus arteriosus. Avoid use of NSAIDs, including SPRIX, in pregnant women starting at 30 weeks of gestation (third trimester) [see *Use in Specific Populations (8.1)*].

5.11 Hematologic Toxicity

Anemia has occurred in NSAID-treated patients. This may be due to occult or gross blood loss, fluid retention, or an incompletely described effect upon erythropoiesis. If a patient treated with SPRIX has any signs or symptoms of anemia, monitor hemoglobin or hematocrit. Do not use SPRIX in patients for whom hemostasis is critical [see *Contraindications (4), Drug Interactions (7)*].

NSAIDs, including SPRIX, may increase the risk of bleeding events. Co-morbid conditions such as coagulation disorders or concomitant use of warfarin, other anticoagulants, antiplatelet agents (e.g., aspirin), serotonin reuptake inhibitors (SSRIs) and serotonin norepinephrine reuptake inhibitors (SNRIs) may increase this risk. Monitor these patients for signs of bleeding [see *Drug Interactions (7)*].

The concurrent use of ketorolac and therapy that affects hemostasis, including prophylactic low dose heparin (2500 to 5000 units q12h), warfarin and dextrans, has not been studied extensively, but may also be associated with an increased risk of bleeding. Until data from such studies are available, carefully weigh the benefits against the risks and use such concomitant therapy in these patients only with extreme caution. Monitor patients receiving therapy that affects hemostasis closely.

In clinical trials, serious adverse events related to bleeding were more common in patients treated with SPRIX than placebo. In clinical trials and in postmarketing experience with ketorolac IV and IM dosing, postoperative hematomas and other signs of wound bleeding have been reported in association with peri-operative use. Therefore, use SPRIX with caution in the postoperative setting when hemostasis is critical.

5.12 Masking of Inflammation and Fever
The pharmacological activity of SPRIX in reducing inflammation, and possibly fever, may diminish the utility of diagnostic signs in detecting infections.

5.13 Laboratory Monitoring
Because serious GI bleeding, hepatotoxicity, and renal injury can occur without warning symptoms or signs, consider monitoring patients on long-term NSAID treatment with a CBC and a chemistry profile periodically [see *Warnings and Precautions (5.2, 5.3, 5.6)*].

5.14 Eye Exposure
Avoid contact of SPRIX with the eyes. If eye contact occurs, wash out the eye with water or saline, and consult a physician if irritation persists for more than an hour.

5.15 Limitations of Use
The total duration of use of SPRIX alone or sequentially with other forms of ketorolac is not to exceed 5 days. SPRIX must not be used concomitantly with other forms of ketorolac or other NSAIDs [see *Dosage and Administration (2.1)*].

6 ADVERSE REACTIONS
The following adverse reactions are discussed in greater detail in other sections of the labeling:

- Cardiovascular Thrombotic Events [see *Warnings and Precautions (5.1)*]
- GI Bleeding, Ulceration and Perforation [see *Warnings and Precautions (5.2)*]
- Hepatotoxicity [see *Warnings and Precautions (5.3)*]
- Hypertension [see *Warnings and Precautions (5.4)*]
- Heart Failure and Edema [see *Warnings and Precautions (5.5)*]
- Renal Toxicity and Hyperkalemia [see *Warnings and Precautions (5.6)*]
- Anaphylactic Reactions [see *Warnings and Precautions (5.7)*]
- Serious Skin Reactions [see *Warnings and Precautions (5.9)*]
- Hematologic Toxicity [see *Warnings and Precautions (5.11)*]

6.1 Clinical Trials Experience
Because clinical trials are conducted under widely varying conditions, adverse reaction rates observed in the clinical trials of a drug cannot be directly compared to rates in the clinical trials of another drug and may not reflect the rates observed in practice.

The data described below reflect exposure to SPRIX in patients enrolled in placebo-controlled efficacy studies of acute pain following major surgery. The studies enrolled 828 patients (183 men, 645 women) ranging from 18 years to over 75 years of age.

The patients in the postoperative pain studies had undergone major abdominal, orthopedic, gynecologic, or other surgery; 455 patients received SPRIX (31.5 mg) three or four times a day for up to 5 days, and 245 patients received placebo. Most patients were receiving concomitant opioids, primarily PCA morphine.

The most frequently reported adverse reactions were related to local symptoms, i.e., nasal discomfort or irritation. These reactions were generally mild and transient in nature.

The most common drug-related adverse events leading to premature discontinuation were nasal discomfort or nasal pain (rhinalgia).

Table 1: Post-Operative Patients with Adverse Reactions Observed at a Rate of 2% or More and at Least Twice the Incidence of the Placebo Group.

	SPRIX (N = 455)	Placebo (N = 245)
Nasal discomfort	15%	2%
Rhinalgia	13%	<1%
Lacrimation increased	5%	0%
Throat irritation	4%	<1%
Oliguria	3%	1%
Rash	3%	<1%
Bradycardia	2%	<1%
Urine output decreased	2%	<1%
ALT and/or AST increased	2%	1%
Hypertension	2%	1%
Rhinitis	2%	<1%

In controlled clinical trials in major surgery, primarily knee and hip replacements and abdominal hysterectomies, seven patients (N=455, 1.5%) treated with SPRIX experienced serious adverse events of bleeding (4 patients) or hematoma (3 patients) at the operative site versus one patient (N=245, 0.4%) treated with placebo (hematoma). Six of the seven patients treated with SPRIX underwent a surgical procedure and/or blood transfusion and the placebo patient subsequently required a blood transfusion.

Adverse Reactions Reported in Clinical Trials with Other Dosage Forms of Ketorolac or Other NSAIDs

Adverse reaction rates increase with higher doses of ketorolac. It is necessary to remain alert for the severe complications of treatment with ketorolac, such as GI ulceration, bleeding, and perforation, postoperative bleeding, acute renal failure, anaphylactic and anaphylactoid reactions, and liver failure. These complications can be serious in certain patients for whom ketorolac is indicated, especially when the drug is used inappropriately.

In patients taking ketorolac or other NSAIDs in clinical trials, the most frequently reported adverse experiences in approximately 1% to 10% of patients are:

Gastrointestinal (GI) experiences including:

abdominal pain	constipation/	dyspepsia
flatulence	diarrhea	GI ulcers (gastric/
gross bleeding/	GI fullness	duodenal)
perforation	heartburn	nausea*
stomatitis	vomiting	

Other experiences:

abnormal renal	anemia	dizziness
function	edema	elevated liver
drowsiness	hypertension	enzymes
headache*	pruritus	increased bleeding
injection site pain	tinnitus	time
rash		purpura
		sweating

Incidence greater than 10%

Additional adverse experiences reported occasionally (<1% in patients taking ketorolac or other NSAIDs in clinical trials) include:
Body as a Whole: fever, infection, sepsis
Cardiovascular System: congestive heart failure, palpitation, pallor, tachycardia, syncope
Digestive System: anorexia, dry mouth, eructation, esophagitis, excessive thirst, gastritis, glossitis, hematemesis, hepatitis, increased appetite, jaundice, melena, rectal bleeding
Hemic and Lymphatic: ecchymosis, eosinophilia, epistaxis, leukopenia, thrombocytopenia

Metabolic and Nutritional: weight change
Nervous System: abnormal dreams, abnormal thinking, anxiety, asthenia, confusion, depression, euphoria, extrapyramidal symptoms, hallucinations, hyperkinesis, inability to concentrate, insomnia, nervousness, paresthesia, somnolence, stupor, tremors, vertigo, malaise
Respiratory: asthma, dyspnea, pulmonary edema, rhinitis
Special Senses: abnormal taste, abnormal vision, blurred vision, hearing loss
Urogenital: cystitis, dysuria, hematuria, increased urinary frequency, interstitial nephritis, oliguria/polyuria, proteinuria, renal failure, urinary retention

6.2 Postmarketing Experience
The following adverse reactions have been identified during post approval use of ketorolac or other NSAIDs. Because these reactions are reported voluntarily from a population of uncertain size, it is not always possible to reliably estimate their frequency or establish a causal relationship to drug exposure.

Other observed reactions (reported from postmarketing experience in patients taking ketorolac or other NSAIDs) are:
Body as a Whole: angioedema, death, hypersensitivity reactions such as anaphylaxis, anaphylactoid reaction, laryngeal edema, tongue edema, myalgia
Cardiovascular: arrhythmia, bradycardia, chest pain, flushing, hypotension, myocardial infarction, vasculitis
Dermatologic: exfoliative dermatitis, erythema multiforme, Lyell's syndrome, bullous reactions including Stevens-Johnson syndrome and toxic epidermal necrolysis
Gastrointestinal: acute pancreatitis, liver failure, ulcerative stomatitis, exacerbation of inflammatory bowel disease (ulcerative colitis, Crohn's disease)
Hemic and Lymphatic: agranulocytosis, aplastic anemia, hemolytic anemia, lymphadenopathy, pancytopenia, postoperative wound hemorrhage (rarely requiring blood transfusion)
Metabolic and Nutritional: hyperglycemia, hyperkalemia, hyponatremia
Nervous System: aseptic meningitis, convulsions, coma, psychosis
Respiratory: bronchospasm, respiratory depression, pneumonia
Special Senses: conjunctivitis
Urogenital: flank pain with or without hematuria and/or azotemia, hemolytic uremic syndrome

7 DRUG INTERACTIONS
See Table 2 for clinically significant drug interactions with ketorolac.

Table 2: Clinically Significant Drug Interactions with Ketorolac

Drugs that Interfere with Hemostasis

Clinical Impact:	• Ketorolac and anticoagulants such as warfarin have a synergistic effect on bleeding. The concomitant use of ketorolac and anticoagulants have an increased risk of serious bleeding compared to the use of either drug alone [see *Clinical Pharmacology (12.3)*]. • Serotonin release by platelets plays an important role in hemostasis. Case-control and cohort epidemiological studies showed that concomitant use of drugs that interfere with serotonin reuptake and an NSAID may potentiate the risk of bleeding more than an NSAID alone. • When ketorolac is administered concurrently with pentoxifylline, there is an increased risk of bleeding.
Intervention:	Monitor patients with concomitant use of SPRIX with anticoagulants (e.g., warfarin), antiplatelet agents (e.g., aspirin), selective serotonin reuptake inhibitors (SSRIs), and serotonin norepinephrine reuptake inhibitors (SNRIs) for signs of bleeding [see *Warnings and Precautions (5.11)*]. Concomitant use of SPRIX and pentoxifylline is contraindicated [see *Contraindications (4) and Warnings and Precautions (5.11)*].

Continued on next page

Aspirin

Clinical Impact:	Controlled clinical studies showed that the concomitant use of NSAIDs and analgesic doses of aspirin does not produce any greater therapeutic effect than the use of NSAIDs alone. In a clinical study, the concomitant use of an NSAID and aspirin was associated with a significantly increased incidence of GI adverse reactions as compared to use of the NSAID alone [see *Warnings and Precautions (5.2)*].
Intervention:	Concomitant use of SPRIX and analgesic doses of aspirin is not generally recommended because of the increased risk of bleeding [see *Warnings and Precautions (5.11)*]. SPRIX is not a substitute for low dose aspirin for cardiovascular protection.

ACE Inhibitors, Angiotensin Receptor Blockers, and Beta-blockers

Clinical Impact:	• NSAIDs may diminish the antihypertensive effect of angiotensin converting enzyme (ACE) inhibitors, angiotensin receptor blockers (ARBs), or beta-blockers (including propranolol). • In patients who are elderly, volume-depleted (including those on diuretic therapy), or have renal impairment, co-administration of an NSAID with ACE inhibitors or ARBs may result in deterioration of renal function, including possible acute renal failure. These effects are usually reversible.
Intervention:	• During concomitant use of SPRIX and ACE-inhibitors, ARBs, or beta-blockers, monitor blood pressure to ensure that the desired blood pressure is obtained. • During concomitant use of SPRIX and ACE-inhibitors or ARBs in patients who are elderly, volume-depleted, or have impaired renal function, monitor for signs of worsening renal function [see *Warnings and Precautions (5.6)*]. • When these drugs are administered concomitantly, patients should be adequately hydrated. Assess renal function at the beginning of the concomitant treatment and periodically thereafter.

Diuretics

Clinical Impact:	Clinical studies, as well as post-marketing observations, showed that NSAIDs reduced the natriuretic effect of loop diuretics (e.g., furosemide) and thiazide diuretics in some patients. This effect has been attributed to the NSAID inhibition of renal prostaglandin synthesis
Intervention:	During concomitant use of SPRIX with diuretics, observe patients for signs of worsening renal function, in addition to assuring diuretic efficacy including antihypertensive effects [see *Warnings and Precautions (5.6)*].

Digoxin

Clinical Impact:	The concomitant use of ketorolac with digoxin has been reported to increase the serum concentration and prolong the half-life of digoxin.
Intervention:	During concomitant use of SPRIX and digoxin, monitor serum digoxin levels.

Lithium

Clinical Impact:	NSAIDs have produced elevations in plasma lithium levels and reductions in renal lithium clearance. The mean minimum lithium concentration increased

15%, and the renal clearance decreased by approximately 20%. This effect has been attributed to NSAID inhibition of renal prostaglandin synthesis.

Intervention:	During concomitant use of SPRIX and lithium, monitor patients for signs of lithium toxicity.

Methotrexate

Clinical Impact:	Concomitant use of NSAIDs and methotrexate may increase the risk for methotrexate toxicity (e.g., neutropenia, thrombocytopenia, renal dysfunction).
Intervention:	During concomitant use of SPRIX and methotrexate, monitor patients for methotrexate toxicity.

Cyclosporine

Clinical Impact:	Concomitant use of SPRIX and cyclosporine may increase cyclosporine's nephrotoxicity.
Intervention:	During concomitant use of SPRIX and cyclosporine, monitor patients for signs of worsening renal function.

NSAIDs and Salicylates

Clinical Impact:	Concomitant use of ketorolac with other NSAIDs or salicylates (e.g., diflunisal, salsalate) increases the risk of GI toxicity, with little or no increase in efficacy [see *Warnings and Precautions (5.2)* and *Clinical Pharmacology (12.3)*].
Intervention:	The concomitant use of ketorolac with other NSAIDs or salicylates is not recommended.

Pemetrexed

Clinical Impact:	Concomitant use of SPRIX and pemetrexed may increase the risk of pemetrexed-associated myelosuppression, renal, and GI toxicity (see the pemetrexed prescribing information).
Intervention:	During concomitant use of SPRIX and pemetrexed, in patients with renal impairment whose creatinine clearance ranges from 45 to 79 mL/min, monitor for myelosuppression, renal and GI toxicity. NSAIDs with short elimination half-lives (e.g., diclofenac, indomethacin) should be avoided for a period of two days before, the day of, and two days following administration of pemetrexed. In the absence of data regarding potential interaction between pemetrexed and NSAIDs with longer half-lives (e.g., meloxicam, nabumetone), patients taking these NSAIDs should interrupt dosing for at least five days before, the day of, and two days following pemetrexed administration.

Probenecid

Clinical Impact:	Concomitant administration of oral ketorolac and probenecid results in increased half-life and systemic exposure. [see *Clinical Pharmacology (12.3)*].
Intervention:	Concomitant use of SPRIX and probenecid is contraindicated.

Antiepileptic Drugs

Clinical Impact:	Sporadic cases of seizures have been reported during concomitant use of ketorolac and antiepileptic drugs (phenytoin, carbamazepine).
Intervention:	During concomitant use of SPRIX and antiepileptic drugs, monitor patients for seizures.

Psychoactive Drugs

Clinical Impact:	Hallucinations have been reported when ketorolac was used in patients taking psychoactive drugs (fluoxetine, thiothixene, alprazolam).
Intervention:	During concomitant use of SPRIX and psychoactive drugs, monitor patients for hallucinations.

Nondepolarizing Muscle Relaxants

Clinical Impact:	In postmarketing experience there have been reports of a possible interaction between ketorolac and nondepolarizing muscle relaxants that resulted in apnea. The concurrent use of ketorolac with muscle relaxants has not been formally studied.
Intervention:	During concomitant use of SPRIX and nondepolarizing muscle relaxants, monitor patients for apnea.

8   USE IN SPECIFIC POPULATIONS

8.1   Pregnancy

Pregnancy Category C prior to 30 weeks gestation; Category D starting at 30 weeks gestation.

Risk Summary

Use of NSAIDs, including SPRIX, during the third trimester of pregnancy increases the risk of premature closure of the fetal ductus arteriosus. Avoid use of NSAIDs, including SPRIX, in pregnant women starting at 30 weeks of gestation (third trimester).

There are no adequate and well-controlled studies of SPRIX in pregnant women. Data from observational studies regarding potential embryofetal risks of NSAID use in women in the first or second trimesters of pregnancy are inconclusive. In the general U.S. population, all clinically recognized pregnancies, regardless of drug exposure, have a background rate of 2-4% for major malformations, and 15-20% for pregnancy loss. In animal reproduction studies in rabbits and rats tested at 0.6 and 1.5 times the human systemic exposure, respectively, at the recommended maximum IN dose of 31.5 mg four times a day, there was no evidence of teratogenicity or other adverse developmental outcomes (see Data). Based on animal data, prostaglandins have been shown to have an important role in endometrial vascular permeability, blastocyst implantation, and decidualization. In animal studies, administration of prostaglandin synthesis inhibitors such as ketorolac, resulted in increased pre- and post-implantation loss.

Clinical Considerations

Labor or Delivery

There are no studies on the effects of SPRIX during labor or delivery. In animal studies, NSAIDs, including ketorolac, inhibit prostaglandin synthesis, cause delayed parturition, and increase the incidence of stillbirth.

Data

Human Data

There are no adequate and well-controlled studies of SPRIX in pregnant women.

Animal Data

Reproduction studies have been performed during organogenesis using daily oral doses of ketorolac tromethamine at 3.6 mg/kg (0.6 times the human systemic exposure at the recommended maximum IN dose of 31.5 mg qid, based on area-under-the-plasma-concentration curve [AUC]) in rabbits and at 10 mg/kg (1.5 times the human AUC) in rats. These studies did not reveal evidence of teratogenicity or other adverse developmental outcomes. However, because animal dosing was limited by maternal toxicity, these studies do not adequately assess ketorolac's potential to cause adverse developmental outcomes in humans.

8.2   Lactation

Risk Summary

Ketorolac is excreted in human milk. The developmental and health benefits of breastfeeding should be considered along with the mother's clinical need for SPRIX and any potential adverse effects on the breastfed infant from the SPRIX or from the underlying maternal condition.

Clinical Considerations

Exercise caution when administering SPRIX to a nursing woman. Available information has not shown any specific adverse events in nursing infants; however, instruct patients to contact their infant's health care provider if they note any adverse events.

Data

Limited data from one published study involving ten nursing mothers 2-6 days postpartum showed low levels of ketorolac in breast milk. Levels were undetectable (less than 5 ng/mL) in 4 of the patients. After a single administration of 10 mg ketorolac, the maximum milk concentration observed was 7.3 ng/mL, and the maximum milk to plasma ratio was 0.037. After 1 day of dosing (10 mg every 6 hours), the maximum milk concentration was 7.9 ng/mL, and the maximum milk-to-plasma ratio was 0.025. Assuming a daily intake of 400-1000 mL of human milk per day and a maternal body weight of 60 kg, the calculated maximum daily infant exposure was 0.00263 mg/kg/day, which is 0.4% of the maternal weight adjusted dose.

8.3 Females and Males of Reproductive Potential

Infertility

Females

Based on the mechanism of action, the use of prostaglandin-mediated NSAIDs, including SPRIX, may delay or prevent rupture of ovarian follicles, which has been associated with reversible infertility in some women. Published animal studies have shown that administration of prostaglandin synthesis inhibitors has the potential to disrupt prostaglandin-mediated follicular rupture required for ovulation. Small studies in women treated with NSAIDs have also shown a reversible delay in ovulation. Consider withdrawal of NSAIDs, including SPRIX, in women who have difficulties conceiving or who are undergoing investigation of infertility.

8.4 Pediatric Use

The safety and effectiveness of ketorolac in pediatric patients 17 years of age and younger have not been established.

8.5 Geriatric Use

Exercise caution when treating the elderly (65 years and older) with SPRIX. Elderly patients, compared to younger patients, are at greater risk for NSAID-associated serious cardiovascular, gastrointestinal, and/or renal adverse reactions. If the anticipated benefit for the elderly patient outweighs these potential risks, start dosing at the low end of the dosing range, and monitor patients for adverse effects [*see Dosage and Administration (2.4), Warnings and Precautions (5.1, 5.2, 5.3, 5.6, 5.13), Clinical Pharmacology (12.3)*].

After observing the response to initial therapy with SPRIX, adjust the dose and frequency to suit an individual patient's needs.

Ketorolac and its metabolites are known to be substantially excreted by the kidneys, and the risk of adverse reactions to this drug may be greater in patients with impaired renal function. Because elderly patients are more likely to have decreased renal function, use caution in this patient population, and it may be useful to monitor renal function [*see Clinical Pharmacology (12.3)*].

10 OVERDOSAGE

Symptoms following acute NSAID overdosages have been typically limited to lethargy, drowsiness, nausea, vomiting, and epigastric pain, which have been generally reversible with supportive care. Gastrointestinal bleeding has occurred. Hypertension, acute renal failure, respiratory depression, and coma have occurred, but were rare [*see Warnings and Precautions (5.1, 5.2, 5.4, 5.6)*].

There has been no experience with overdosage of SPRIX. In controlled overdosage studies with IM ketorolac injection, daily doses of 360 mg given for five days (approximately 3 times the maximum daily dose of SPRIX) caused abdominal pain and peptic ulcers, which healed after discontinuation of dosing. Single overdoses of ketorolac tromethamine have been variously associated with abdominal pain, nausea, vomiting, hyperventilation, peptic ulcers and/or erosive gastritis, and renal dysfunction.

Manage patients with symptomatic and supportive care following an NSAID overdosage. There are no specific antidotes. Consider emesis and/or activated charcoal (60 to 100 grams in adults, 1 to 2 grams per kg of body weight in pediatric patients) and/or osmotic cathartic in symptomatic patients seen within four hours of ingestion or in patients with a large overdosage (5 to 10 times the recommended dosage). Forced diuresis, alkalinization of urine, hemodialysis, or hemoperfusion may not be useful due to high protein binding.

For additional information about overdosage treatment contact a poison control center (1-800-222-1222).

11 DESCRIPTION

SPRIX (ketorolac tromethamine) Nasal Spray is a member of the pyrrolo-pyrrole group of nonsteroidal anti-inflammatory drugs, available as a clear, colorless to yellow solution packaged in a glass vial with a snap on spray pump that delivers 15.75 mg ketorolac tromethamine per spray and is intended for intranasal administration. The chemical name is (±)-5-benzoyl-2,3-dihydro-1H-pyrrolizine-1-carboxylic acid, compound with 2-amino-2-(hydroxymethyl)-1,3-propanediol (1:1). The molecular weight is 376.41.

Its molecular formula is $C_{19}H_{24}N_2O_6(C_{15}H_{13}NO_3 \bullet C_4H_{11}NO_3)$, and it has the following chemical structure.

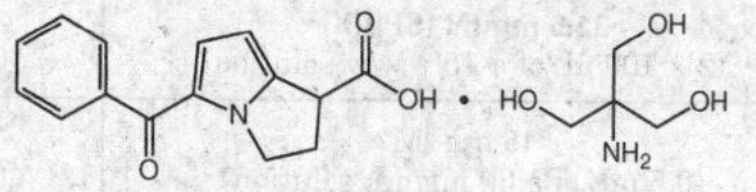

Ketorolac tromethamine is highly water-soluble, allowing its formulation in an aqueous nasal spray product at pH 7.2. The inactive ingredients in SPRIX include: edetate disodium (EDTA), monobasic potassium phosphate, sodium hydroxide, and water for injection.

12 CLINICAL PHARMACOLOGY

12.1 Mechanism of Action

Ketorolac has analgesic, anti-inflammatory, and antipyretic properties.

The mechanism of action of SPRIX, like that of other NSAIDs, is not completely understood but involves inhibition of cyclooxygenase (COX-1 and COX-2), an early component of the arachidonic acid cascade, resulting in the reduced synthesis of prostaglandins, thromboxanes, and prostacyclin.

Ketorolac is a potent inhibitor of prostaglandin synthesis *in vitro*. Ketorolac concentrations reached during therapy have produced *in vivo* effects. Prostaglandins sensitize afferent nerves and potentiate the action of bradykinin in inducing pain in animal models. Prostaglandins are mediators of inflammation. Because ketorolac is an inhibitor of prostaglandin synthesis, its mode of action may be due to a decrease of prostaglandins in peripheral tissues.

12.3 Pharmacokinetics

The half-lives of ketorolac by the IN and IM routes were similar. The bioavailability of ketorolac by the IN route of administration of a 31.5 mg dose was approximately 60% compared to IM administration. (See Table 3).

[See table 3 on next page]

Absorption

In a study in which SPRIX (31.5 mg) was administered to healthy volunteers four times daily for 5 days, the C_{max}, t_{max}, and AUC values following the final dose were comparable to those obtained in the single-dose study. Accumulation of ketorolac has not been studied in special populations, geriatric, pediatric, renal failure or hepatic disease patients.

Distribution

Scintigraphic assessment of drug disposition of ketorolac following SPRIX intranasal dosing demonstrated that most of the ketorolac was deposited in the nasal cavity and pharynx, with less than 20% deposited in the esophagus and stomach, and zero or negligible deposition in the lungs (<0.5%).

The mean apparent volume (Vβ) of ketorolac tromethamine following complete distribution was approximately 13 liters. This parameter was determined from single-dose data. The ketorolac tromethamine racemate has been shown to be highly protein bound (99.2%). Nevertheless, plasma concentrations as high as 10 mcg/mL will only occupy approximately 5% of the albumin binding sites. Thus, the unbound fraction for each enantiomer will be constant over the therapeutic range. A decrease in serum albumin, however, will result in increased free drug concentrations. Therapeutic concentrations of digoxin, warfarin, ibuprofen, naproxen, piroxicam, acetaminophen, phenytoin, and tolbutamide did not alter ketorolac protein binding. *In vitro* studies indicate that, at therapeutic concentrations of salicylate (300 mcg/mL), the binding of ketorolac was reduced from approximately 99.2% to 97.5%, representing a potential twofold increase in unbound ketorolac plasma levels.

The mean apparent volume (Vβ) of ketorolac tromethamine following complete distribution was approximately 13 liters. This parameter was determined from single-dose data. The ketorolac tromethamine racemate has been shown to be highly protein bound (99.2%). Nevertheless, plasma concentrations as high as 10 mcg/mL will only occupy approximately 5% of the albumin binding sites. Thus, the unbound fraction for each enantiomer will be constant over the therapeutic range. A decrease in serum albumin, however, will result in increased free drug concentrations. Therapeutic concentrations of digoxin, warfarin, ibuprofen, naproxen, piroxicam, acetaminophen, phenytoin, and tolbutamide did not alter ketorolac protein binding. *In vitro* studies indicate that, at therapeutic concentrations of salicylate (300 mcg/mL), the binding of ketorolac was reduced from approximately 99.2% to 97.5%, representing a potential twofold increase in unbound ketorolac plasma levels.

The *in vitro* binding of warfarin to plasma proteins is only slightly reduced by ketorolac (99.5% control vs. 99.3%) when ketorolac plasma concentrations reach 5 to 10 mcg/mL.

Ketorolac tromethamine is excreted in human milk.

Elimination

Metabolism

Ketorolac tromethamine is largely metabolized in the liver. The metabolic products are hydroxylated and conjugated forms of the parent drug. The products of metabolism, and some unchanged drug, are excreted in the urine. There is no evidence in animal or human studies that ketorolac induces or inhibits hepatic enzymes capable of metabolizing itself or other drugs.

Excretion

The principal route of elimination of ketorolac and its metabolites is renal. About 92% of a given dose is found in the urine, approximately 40% as metabolites and 60% as unchanged ketorolac. Approximately 6% of a dose is excreted in the feces. A single-dose study with 10 mg ketorolac tromethamine (n = 9) demonstrated that the S-enantiomer is cleared approximately two times faster than the R-enantiomer and that the clearance was independent of the route of administration. This means that the ratio of S/R plasma concentrations decreases with time after each dose. There is little or no inversion of the R- to S- form in humans. The half-life of the ketorolac tromethamine S-enantiomer was approximately 2.5 hours (SD ± 0.4) compared with 5 hours (SD ± 1.7) for the R-enantiomer. In other studies, the half-life for the racemate has been reported to lie within the range of 5 to 6 hours.

Specific Populations

Geriatric: A single-dose study was conducted to compare the pharmacokinetics of SPRIX (31.5 mg) in subjects ≥ age 65 to the pharmacokinetics in subjects < age 65. Exposure to ketorolac was increased by 23% for the ≥ 65 population as compared to subjects < 65. Peak concentrations of 2028 and 1840 ng/mL were observed for the elderly and nonelderly adult populations, respectively, at 0.75 h after dosing. In the elderly population a longer terminal half-life was observed as compared to the nonelderly adults (4.5 h vs. 3.3 h, respectively).

Race: Pharmacokinetic differences due to race have not been identified.

Hepatic Impairment: There was no significant difference in estimates of half-life, AUC_∞ and C_{max} in 7 patients with liver disease compared to healthy volunteers.

Renal Impairment: Based on single-dose data only, the mean half-life of ketorolac tromethamine in renally impaired patients is between 6 and 19 hours, and is dependent on the extent of the impairment. There is poor correlation between creatinine clearance and total ketorolac tromethamine clearance in the elderly and populations with renal impairment (r = 0.5).

In patients with renal disease, the AUC_∞ of each enantiomer increased by approximately 100% compared with healthy volunteers. The volume of distribution doubles for the S-enantiomer and increases by 1/5th for the R-enantiomer. The increase in volume of distribution of ketorolac tromethamine implies an increase in unbound fraction. The AUC_∞-ratio of the ketorolac tromethamine enantiomers in healthy subjects and patients remained similar, indicating there was no selective excretion of either enantiomer in patients compared to healthy subjects.

Allergic Rhinitis: Comparison of the pharmacokinetics of SPRIX in subjects with allergic rhinitis to data from a previous study in healthy subjects showed no differences that would be of clinical consequence for the efficacy or safety of SPRIX.

Drug Interaction Studies

Aspirin: When NSAIDs were administered with aspirin, the protein binding of NSAIDs were reduced, although the clearance of free NSAID was not altered. The clinical significance of this interaction is not known. See Table 2 for clinically significant drug interactions of NSAIDs with aspirin [*see Drug Interactions (7)*].

Continued on next page

Other Nasal Spray Products: A study was conducted in subjects with symptomatic allergic rhinitis to assess the effects of the commonly used nasal spray products oxymetazoline hydrochloride and fluticasone propionate on the pharmacokinetics of SPRIX. Subjects received a single dose of oxymetazoline nasal spray followed by a single dose (31.5 mg) of SPRIX 30 min later. Subjects also received fluticasone nasal spray (200 mcg as 2 × 50 mcg in each nostril) for seven days, with a single dose (31.5 mg) of SPRIX on the 7th day. Administration of these common intranasal products had no effect of clinical significance on the rate or extent of ketorolac absorption.

Probenecid: Concomitant administration of oral ketorolac and probenecid resulted in decreased clearance and volume of distribution of ketorolac and significant increases in ketorolac plasma levels (total AUC increased approximately threefold from 5.4 to 17.8 mcg/h/mL), and terminal half-life increased approximately twofold from 6.6 to 15.1 hours [*see Drug Interactions (7)*].

13 NONCLINICAL TOXICOLOGY

13.1 Carcinogenesis, Mutagenesis, Impairment of Fertility

Carcinogenesis

An 18-month study in mice with oral doses of ketorolac at 2 mg/kg/day (approximately 1.3 times the human systemic exposure at the recommended maximum IN dose of 31.5 mg four times a day, based on area-under-the-plasma-concentration curve [AUC]), and a 24-month study in rats at 5 mg/kg/day (approximately 0.8 times the human AUC) showed no evidence of tumorigenicity.

Mutagenesis

Ketorolac was not mutagenic in the Ames test, unscheduled DNA synthesis and repair, or in forward mutation assays. Ketorolac did not cause chromosome breakage in the *in vivo* mouse micronucleus assay. At 1590 µg/mL and at higher concentrations, ketorolac increased the incidence of chromosomal aberrations in Chinese hamster ovarian cells.

Impairment of fertility

Impairment of fertility did not occur in male or female rats at oral doses of 9 mg/kg (approximately 1.3 times the human AUC) and 16 mg/kg (approximately 2.4 times the human AUC) of ketorolac, respectively.

14 CLINICAL STUDIES

14.1 Postoperative Pain

The effect of SPRIX on acute pain was evaluated in two multi-center, randomized, double-blind, placebo-controlled studies.

In a study of adults who had undergone elective abdominal or orthopedic surgery, 300 patients were randomized and treated with SPRIX or placebo administered every 8 hours and morphine administered via patient controlled analgesia on an as needed basis. Efficacy was demonstrated as a statistically significant greater reduction in the summed pain intensity difference over 48 hours in patients who received SPRIX as compared to those receiving placebo. The clinical relevance of this is reflected in the finding that patients treated with SPRIX required 36% less morphine over 48 hours than patients treated with placebo.

In a study of adults who had undergone elective abdominal surgery, 321 patients were randomized and treated with SPRIX or placebo administered every 6 hours and morphine administered via patient controlled analgesia on an as needed basis. Efficacy was demonstrated as a statistically significant greater reduction in the summed pain intensity difference over 48 hours in patients who received SPRIX as compared to those receiving placebo. The clinical relevance of this is reflected in the finding that patients treated with SPRIX required 26% less morphine over 48 hours than patients treated with placebo.

16 HOW SUPPLIED/STORAGE AND HANDLING

SPRIX (ketorolac tromethamine) Nasal Spray, 15.75 mg/spray, are single-day preservative-free spray bottles, supplied as:

NDC 69344-144-43 Carton containing 5 single-day nasal spray bottles

NDC 69344-144-53 Carton containing 1 single-day nasal spray bottle

Each single-day nasal spray bottle contains a sufficient quantity of solution to deliver 8 sprays for a total of 126 mg of ketorolac tromethamine. Each spray delivers 15.75 mg of ketorolac tromethamine. The delivery system is designed to administer precisely metered doses of 100 µL per spray.

Table 3: Pharmacokinetic Parameters of Ketorolac Tromethamine after Intramuscular (IM) and Intranasal (IN) Administration

Ketorolac Tromethamine	C_{max} (SD) ng/mL	t_{max} (range) hours	$AUC_{0-\infty}$ (SD) ng·h/mL	$T_{1/2}$ (SD) hours
30 mg IM (1.0 mL of a 30 mg/mL solution)	2382.2 (432.7)	0.75 (0.25-1.03)	11152.8 (4260.1)	4.80 (1.18)
31.5 mg IN (SPRIX) (2 × 100 µL of a 15% w/w solution)	1805.8 (882.8)	0.75 (0.50-2.00)	7477.3 (3654.4)	5.24 (1.33)
15 mg IM (0.5 mL of a 30 mg/mL solution)	1163.4 (279.9)	0.75 (0.25-1.50)	5196.3 (2076.7)	5.00 (1.72)

C_{max} = maximum plasma concentration; t_{max} = time of C_{max}; $AUC_{0-\infty}$ = complete area under the concentration-time curve; $T_{1/2}$ = half-life; SD = standard deviation. All values are means, except t_{max}, for which medians are reported.

Storage

Protect from light and freezing. Store unopened SPRIX between 2°C to 8°C (36°F to 46°F). During use, keep containers of SPRIX Nasal Spray at controlled room temperature, between 15°C to 30°C (59°F to 86°F), out of direct sunlight. Bottles of SPRIX should be discarded within 24 hours of priming.

17 PATIENT COUNSELING INFORMATION

Advise the patient to read the FDA-approved patient labeling (Medication Guide and Instructions for Use) that accompanies each prescription dispensed. Instruct all patients to read and closely follow the FDA-approved SPRIX Patient Instructions to ensure proper administration of SPRIX. When prescribing SPRIX, inform patients or their caregivers of the potential risks of ketorolac treatment, instruct patients to seek medical advice if they develop treatment-related adverse events, advise patients not to give SPRIX to other family members, and advise patients to discard any unused drug. Inform patients, families, or their caregivers of the following information before initiating therapy with SPRIX and periodically during the course of ongoing therapy.

Cardiovascular Thrombotic Events

Advise patients to be alert for the symptoms of cardiovascular thrombotic events, including chest pain, shortness of breath, weakness, or slurring of speech, and to report any of these symptoms to their health care provider immediately [*see Warnings and Precautions (5.1)*].

Gastrointestinal Bleeding, Ulceration, and Perforation

Advise patients to report symptoms of ulcerations and bleeding, including epigastric pain, dyspepsia, melena, and hematemesis to their health care provider. In the setting of concomitant use of low-dose aspirin for cardiac prophylaxis, inform patients of the increased risk for and the signs and symptoms of GI bleeding [*see Contraindications (4), Warnings and Precautions (5.2)*].

Hepatotoxicity

Inform patients of the warning signs and symptoms of hepatotoxicity (e.g., nausea, fatigue, lethargy, pruritus, diarrhea, jaundice, right upper quadrant tenderness, and "flu-like" symptoms). If these occur, instruct patients to stop SPRIX and seek immediate medical therapy [*see Warnings and Precautions (5.3)*].

Heart Failure and Edema

Advise patients to be alert for the symptoms of congestive heart failure including shortness of breath, unexplained weight gain, or edema and to contact their healthcare provider if such symptoms occur [*see Warnings and Precautions (5.5)*].

Anaphylactic Reactions

Inform patients of the signs of an anaphylactic reaction (e.g., difficulty breathing, swelling of the face or throat). Instruct patients to seek immediate emergency help if these occur [*see Contraindications (4) and Warnings and Precautions (5.7)*].

Serious Skin Reactions

Advise patients to stop SPRIX immediately if they develop any type of rash and to contact their healthcare provider as soon as possible [*see Warnings and Precautions (5.9)*].

Female Fertility

Advise females of reproductive potential who desire pregnancy that NSAIDs, including SPRIX, may be associated with a reversible delay in ovulation [*see Use in Specific Populations (8.3)*].

Fetal Toxicity

Inform pregnant women to avoid use of SPRIX and other NSAIDs starting at 30 weeks gestation because of the risk of the premature closing of the fetal ductus arteriosus [*see Warnings and Precautions (5.10) and Use in Specific Populations (8.1)*].

Avoid Concomitant Use of NSAIDs

Inform patients that the concomitant use of SPRIX with other NSAIDs or salicylates (e.g., diflunisal, salsalate) is not recommended due to the increased risk of gastrointestinal toxicity, and little or no increase in efficacy [*see Warnings and Precautions (5.2) and Drug Interactions (7)*]. Alert patients that NSAIDs may be present in "over the counter" medications for treatment of colds, fever, or insomnia.

Use of NSAIDS and Low-Dose Aspirin

Inform patients not to use low-dose aspirin concomitantly with SPRIX until they talk to their healthcare provider [*see Drug Interactions (7)*].

Renal Effects

SPRIX is eliminated by the kidneys. Advise patients to maintain adequate fluid intake and request medical advice if urine output decreases significantly [*see Contraindications (4), Warnings and Precautions (5.6)*].

Limitations of Use

Instruct patients not to use SPRIX for more than 5 days. Use of SPRIX alone or in combination with any other ketorolac product for more than 5 days increases the risk for serious complications including GI bleeding and renal injury [*see Dosage and Administration (2)*].

Single-Day Container

Instruct patients not to use any single bottle of SPRIX for more than one day [*see Dosage and Administration (2.5)*].

Nasal Discomfort

Advise patients that they may experience transient, mild to moderate nasal irritation or discomfort upon dosing.

Manufactured for and Distributed by:

Egalet US Inc.
Wayne, PA 19087

Issued: May/2016   LBL # 101.01

Medication Guide for Nonsteroidal Anti-inflammatory Drugs (NSAIDs)

What is the most important information I should know about medicines called Nonsteroidal Anti-inflammatory Drugs (NSAIDs)?

NSAIDs can cause serious side effects, including:

- **Increased risk of a heart attack or stroke that can lead to death.** This risk may happen early in treatment and may increase:
  - with increasing doses of NSAIDs
  - with longer use of NSAIDs

Do not take NSAIDs right before or after a heart surgery called a "coronary artery bypass graft (CABG)."

Avoid taking NSAIDs after a recent heart attack, unless your healthcare provider tells you to. You may have an increased risk of another heart attack if you take NSAIDs after a recent heart attack.

- **Increased risk of bleeding, ulcers, and tears (perforation) of the esophagus (tube leading from the mouth to the stomach), stomach and intestines:**
  - anytime during use
  - without warning symptoms
  - that may cause death

The risk of getting an ulcer or bleeding increases with:
- past history of stomach ulcers, or stomach or intestinal bleeding with use of NSAIDs
- taking medicines called "corticosteroids", "anticoagulants", "SSRIs", or "SNRIs"
- increasing doses of older age

NSAIDs
○ longer use of NSAIDs
○ smoking
○ drinking alcohol
○ poor health
○ advanced liver disease
○ bleeding problems

NSAIDs should only be used:
○ exactly as prescribed
○ at the lowest dose possible for your treatment
○ for the shortest time needed

What are NSAIDs?
NSAIDs are used to treat pain and redness, swelling, and heat (inflammation) from medical conditions such as different types of arthritis, menstrual cramps, and other types of short-term pain.

Who should not take NSAIDs?
Do not take NSAIDs:
• if you have had an asthma attack, hives, or other allergic reaction with aspirin or any other NSAIDs.
• right before or after heart bypass surgery.

Before taking NSAIDs, tell your healthcare provider about all of your medical conditions, including if you:
• have liver or kidney problems
• have high blood pressure
• have asthma
• are pregnant or plan to become pregnant. Talk to your healthcare provider if you are considering taking NSAIDs during pregnancy.
  You should not take NSAIDs after 29 weeks of pregnancy.
• are breastfeeding or plan to breast feed.
Tell your healthcare provider about all of the medicines you take, including prescription or over-the-counter medicines, vitamins or herbal supplements. NSAIDs and some other medicines can interact with each other and cause serious side effects. Do not start taking any new medicine without talking to your healthcare provider first.

What are the possible side effects of NSAIDs?
NSAIDs can cause serious side effects, including:
See "What is the most important information I should know about medicines called Nonsteroidal Anti-inflammatory Drugs (NSAIDs)?"
• new or worse high blood pressure
• heart failure
• liver problems including liver failure
• kidney problems including kidney failure
• low red blood cells (anemia)
• life-threatening skin reactions
• life-threatening allergic reactions
• **Other side effects of NSAIDs include:** stomach pain, constipation, diarrhea, gas, heartburn, nausea, vomiting, and dizziness.
Get emergency help right away if you get any of the following symptoms:
• shortness of breath or trouble breathing
• chest pain
• weakness in one part or side of your body
• slurred speech
• swelling of the face or throat

Stop taking your NSAID and call your healthcare provider right away if you get any of the following symptoms:
• nausea
• more tired or weaker than usual
• diarrhea
• itching
• your skin or eyes look yellow
• indigestion or stomach pain
• flu-like symptoms
• vomit blood
• there is blood in your bowel movement or it is black and sticky like tar
• unusual weight gain
• skin rash or blisters with fever
• swelling of the arms, legs, hands and feet

If you take too much of your NSAID, call your healthcare provider or get medical help right away.
These are not all the possible side effects of NSAIDs. For more information, ask your healthcare provider or pharmacist about NSAIDs.
Call your doctor for medical advice about side effects. You may report side effects to FDA at 1-800-FDA-1088.

Other information about NSAIDs
• Aspirin is an NSAID but it does not increase the chance of a heart attack. Aspirin can cause bleeding in the brain, stomach, and intestines. Aspirin can also cause ulcers in the stomach and intestines.
• Some NSAIDs are sold in lower doses without a prescription (over-the-counter). Talk to your healthcare provider before using over-the-counter NSAIDs for more than 10 days.

General information about the safe and effective use of NSAIDs
Medicines are sometimes prescribed for purposes other than those listed in a Medication Guide. Do not use NSAIDs for a condition for which it was not prescribed. Do not give NSAIDs to other people, even if they have the same symptoms that you have. It may harm them.
If you would like more information about NSAIDs, talk with your healthcare provider. You can ask your pharmacist or healthcare provider for information about NSAIDs that is written for health professionals.

Manufactured for: Egalet US Inc., Wayne, PA 19087
Distributed by: Egalet US Inc., Wayne, PA 19087
For more information, go to www.sprix.com or call 1-800-518-1084.

This Medication Guide has been approved by the U.S. Food and Drug Administration.

Instructions for Use
SPRIX® (spriks)
(ketorolac tromethamine)
Nasal Spray
Read this Instructions for Use before you start using SPRIX and each time you get a refill. There may be new information. This information does not take the place of talking to your healthcare provider about your medical condition or your treatment.
Important information:
• **SPRIX is for use in your nose only. Do not breathe in (inhale) SPRIX.**
• Each SPRIX bottle has enough pain medicine for 1 day.
• Throw away each SPRIX bottle within 24 hours of taking your first dose, even if the bottle still contains unused medicine.
Your healthcare provider has prescribed SPRIX to treat moderate to severe pain.
• Use SPRIX exactly as your healthcare provider tells you to use it.
• Your healthcare provider will tell you how many sprays you should use each time you use SPRIX.
• Do not use SPRIX for more than 5 days. If you still have pain after 5 days, contact your healthcare provider.
• Do not use SPRIX more than every 6 hours.
• It is important that you drink plenty of fluids while you are using SPRIX. Tell your healthcare provider if you urinate less while using SPRIX.
You may have discomfort or irritation in your nose when using SPRIX. This usually lasts for a short time. Do not breathe in (inhale) SPRIX while spraying.
Using SPRIX Nasal Spray
Parts of your SPRIX bottle

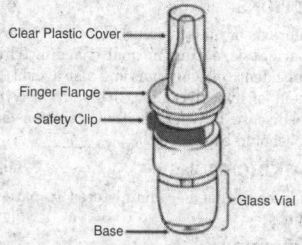

Clear Plastic Cover
Finger Flange
Safety Clip
Glass Vial
Base

Follow the instructions below to use SPRIX.
Before you use SPRIX for the first time, you will need to prime the bottle.
Priming SPRIX:
Step 1. Hold the finger flange with your fingers (**see Figure A**), and remove the clear plastic cover with your opposite hand. Keep the clear plastic cover for later. Remove and throw away the blue plastic safety clip.
[See Figure A on next column]
If the clear plastic cover is improperly removed, the tip of the bottle may be pulled off of the glass vial. If this happens, place the tip back onto the glass vial by lining it up carefully and gently pushing it back on until it is back in the correct position (**see Figure B**). The SPRIX bottle should work properly again.
See Figure B on next column]
Step 2. Hold the SPRIX bottle upright at arm's length away from you with your index finger and middle finger resting on the top of the finger flange and your thumb supporting the base (**see Figure C**).

Figure A

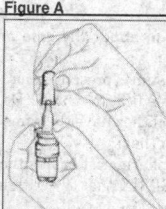

Figure B

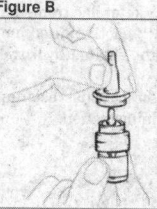

Press down on the finger flange and release the pump 5 times. You may not see a spray the first few times you press down.
Now the pump is primed and ready to use. You do not need to prime the pump again if you use more doses from this bottle.

Figure C

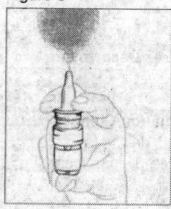

Step 3. Blow your nose to clear your nostrils.
Step 4. Sit up straight or stand.
Step 5. Keep your head tilted downward toward your toes.
Step 6. Place the tip of the SPRIX bottle into your right nostril.
Step 7. Hold the SPRIX bottle upright and aim the tip toward the back of your nose (**see Figure D**).

Figure D

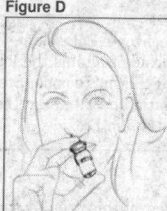

Step 8. Hold your breath and spray 1 time into your right nostril, pressing down on both sides of the finger flange (**see Figure D**).
Step 9. Breathe in gently through your mouth after you use SPRIX. You may also pinch your nose to help keep the medicine in your nose.
Step 10. If your healthcare provider has prescribed only 1 spray per dose for you, you have now finished your dose, skip to Step 12 below.
Step 11. If your healthcare provider has prescribed 2 sprays for you, repeat steps 3 - 9 above for your left nostril. Be sure to point the spray away from the center of your nose. Spray 1 time into your left nostril.
Step 12. When you are finished using SPRIX, put the clear plastic cover back on the SPRIX bottle.
How should I store SPRIX?
• Store unopened SPRIX bottles between 36°F to 46°F (2°C to 8°C).
• Keep opened bottles of SPRIX at room temperature.
• Keep SPRIX out of direct sunlight.
• Do not freeze SPRIX.
• SPRIX does not contain a preservative. Throw away each SPRIX bottle within 24 hours of taking your first dose, even if the bottle still contains unused medicine.
Keep SPRIX and all medicines out of the reach of children.

Continued on next page

General information about the safe and effective use of SPRIX.

Medicines are sometimes prescribed for purposes other than those listed in a Medication Guide. Do not give SPRIX to other people, even if they have the same symptoms that you have. It may harm them.

You can ask your pharmacist or healthcare provider for information about SPRIX that is written for health professionals.

What are the ingredients in SPRIX?
Active ingredient: ketorolac tromethamine
Inactive ingredient: edetate disodium (EDTA), monobasic potassium phosphate, sodium hydroxide, and water for injection
This Instructions for Use has been approved by the U.S. Food and Drug Administration.
Distributed by:
Egalet US Inc.
Wayne, PA 19087

LBL # 102.01   Revised: 5/2016
Shown in Product Identification Guide, page 508

Glenwood
111 CEDAR LANE
ENGLEWOOD, NJ 07631

Direct Inquiries to:
Professional Services Department
201 569-0050
800 542-0772
For Medical Information Contact:
In Emergencies:
Professional Services Department
201 569-0050
800 542-0772

POTABA®   ℞
Aminobenzoate Potassium, USP
Systemic ANTIFIBROSIS THERAPY

FORMULA: POTABA® is chemically pure potassium p-aminobenzoate.

DESCRIPTION
POTABA® (Aminobenzoate Potassium, USP) is available in Capsules. Each Capsule contains the following inactive ingredients: Colloidal Silicon Dioxide, Stearic Acid. Capsule Shell contains: Gelatin and Titanium Dioxide. The imprinting ink contains Titanium Dioxide.

INDICATIONS
Based on a review of this drug by the National Academy of Sciences-National Research Council and/or other information, FDA has classified the indications as follows:
"Possibly" effective: Potassium aminobenzoate is possibly effective in the treatment of scleroderma, dermatomyositis, morphea, linear scleroderma, pemphigus, and Peyronie's disease.
Final classification of the less-than-effective indications requires further investigation.

ADVANTAGES: POTABA® offers a means of treatment of serious and often chronic entities involving fibrosis and non-suppurative inflammation.

PHARMACOLOGY
p-Aminobenzoate is considered a member of the vitamin B complex. Small amounts are found in cereal, eggs, milk and meats. Detectable amounts are normally present in human blood, spinal fluid, urine, and sweat. PABA is a component of several biologically important systems, and it participates in a number of fundamental biological processes.
It has been suggested that the antifibrosis action of POTABA® is due to its mediation of increased oxygen uptake at the tissue level. Fibrosis is believed to occur from either too much serotonin or too little monoamine oxidase (MAO) activity over a period of time. Monoamine oxidase requires an adequate supply of oxygen to function properly.

By increasing oxygen supply at the tissue level POTABA® may enhance MAO activity and prevent or bring about regression of fibrosis.[3]

CLINICAL USES
PEYRONIE'S DISEASE: 21 patients with Peyronie's disease were placed on POTABA® therapy for periods ranging from 3 months to 2 years. Pain disappeared from 16 of 16 cases in which it had been present. There was objective improvement in penile deformity in 10 of 17 patients, and decrease in plaque size in 16 of 21. The authors suggest that this medication offers no hazard of further local injury as may result from other therapy. There were no significant untoward effects encountered on long-term POTABA® therapy.[5,10]
SCLERODERMA: Of 135 patients with diffuse systemic sclerosis treated with POTABA® every patient but one has shown softening of the involved skin if treatment has been continued for 3 months or longer. The responses have been reported in a number of publications.[9] The treatment program consists of systemic antifibrosis therapy with POTABA®, physical therapy, including deep breathing exercises and dynamic traction splints where indicated, and bethanechol chloride for relief of dysphagia as well as small doses of reserpine for amelioration of Raynaud's phenomena.[1,3]
DERMATOMYOSITIS: Five patients with scleroderma and 2 with dermatomyositis were treated with POTABA®. There was striking clinical improvement in each patient. Doses of 15-20 grams per day were well tolerated, and patients were easily able to take these doses.[6]
MORPHEA and LINEAR SCLERODERMA: All 14 patients with localized forms of scleroderma placed on long-term POTABA® treatment showed softening of the sclerotic component of their disorder. Treatment is particularly indicated in patients where persistent compressive sclerosis may contribute even greater disfigurement or functional embarrassment from secondary pressure atrophy.[8,9]

DOSAGE & ADMINISTRATION
The average adult daily dose of POTABA® is 12 grams, usually given in four to six divided doses. Capsules 0.5 gram are given at the rate of 4 capsules 6 times daily, or 6 given four times daily, usually with meals, and at bedtime with a snack.
Children are given 1 gram of POTABA® daily in divided doses for each 10 lbs. of body weight.
SIDE EFFECTS: Anorexia, nausea, fever and rash have occurred infrequently and subside with omission of the drug. Desensitization can be accomplished and treatment resumed.
USAGE IN PREGNANCY: Safety for use in pregnancy or during lactation has not been established.

PRECAUTIONS
Should anorexia or nausea occur, therapy is interrupted until the patient is eating normally again. This permits prompt subsidence of symptoms and also avoids the possible development of hypoglycemia. Give cautiously to patients with renal disease. If hypersensitivity reaction should occur, POTABA® should be stopped.

CONTRAINDICATIONS
POTABA® should not be administered to patients taking sulfonamides.

HOW SUPPLIED
POTABA® (Aminobenzoate Potassium, USP) Capsules 0.5 grams are supplied as No. 0 White/White Opaque Hard Gelatin Capsule Printed "POTABA 51" in black ink.
NDC-0516-0051-10 bottle of 1000
Rx only.

REFERENCES
1. From: Inflammation and Diseases of Connective Tissue, Edited by Drs. Lewis C. Mills and John H. Moyer, Published by W. B. Saunders Company, Phila. 1961.
3. Zarafonetis, Chris J. D.: Treatment of Scleroderma, Annals of Int. Med. 50:343-365 (1959).
5. Zarafonetis, C. J. D., and Horrax, T.M.: Treatment of Peyronie's Disease with POTABA, Journ. of Urology 81:770-772 (June 1959).
6. Grace. William J., Kennedy, Richard J., Formato, Anthony: Therapy of Scleroderma and Dermatomyositis, N.Y. State J. of Med. 63:140-144, 1963.
8. Zarafonetis, C. J. D.: Treatment of Localized Forms of Scleroderma, Am. J. Med. Sci. 243:147-158. 1962.
9. Zarafonetis, Chris J. D.: Antifibrotic Therapy With POTABA, Amer. Jrnl. of Med. Sci. 248: No. 5/551-561 (Nov. 1964).
10. Horrax, Trudeau M.: Peyronie's Disease, Scientific Exhibit, Amer. Urological Assn. Annl. Meet., New Orleans, May 1965.
GLENWOOD, LLC
111 Cedar Lane
Englewood, NJ 07631
REV. 11/10
Shown in Product Identification Guide, page 508

Gordon Laboratories
6801 LUDLOW STREET
UPPER DARBY, PA 19082

Direct inquiries to:
Customer Service
(610) 734-2011
Fax (610) 734-2049
Website: http://www.gordonlabs.net
E-mail: gordonlabs@att.net
For medical emergencies contact:
David Dercher   (610) 734-2011
                                 Fax (610) 734-2049

FORMADON   ℞

INDICATIONS
Used as a drying agent for pre and postsurgical removal of warts; and as an antiperspirant in the treatment of severe conditions of hyperhidrosis and bromidrosis.
ACTIVE INGREDIENT: Formaldehyde (10% of U.S.P. strength).

DESCRIPTION
Formadon provides a preferable vehicle for the topical application of formalin solution (10% U.S.P. strength formaldehyde). It is formulated with an aqueous perfumed base which helps minimize the characteristic pungent odor.

PHARMACOLOGY
Formalin, a solution of formaldehyde, has been extensively used as a drying agent as well as a disinfectant. Direct topical application of formalin solution has been an extremely useful way of dealing with odor-causing bacteria on the surface of the skin. The elimination of hyperhidrosis is of paramount importance in reducing bacteria associated with odor and wetness. Formalin, in drying the skin surface, reduces bacteria flora which can thrive in moisture.

CONTRAINDICATIONS/WARNINGS
Avoid frequent use. Avoid contact with eyes or mucous membranes. Do not apply to open wounds. Should signs of irritation develop, medication should be discontinued. Irritates eyes, nose, and throat. Avoid breathing vapors. Use with adequate ventilation. In the event of eye contact, flush copiously with water and get medical attention. **Keep out of reach of children. For external use only.** Harmful if swallowed. Contact a local Poison Control Center immediately. **Do not induce vomiting.** If conscious, give eight ounces (240 mL) of milk, water or water with activated charcoal. Keep well closed in a cool place. **Federal law prohibits dispensing without a prescription.**

DIRECTIONS
Apply to feet twice weekly or as prescribed by a Physician.

HOW SUPPLIED
2 oz. sponge tip bottle NDC 10481-1050-05
4 oz. plastic bottle NDC 10481-1050-2
Shown in Product Identification Guide, page 509

GORDOCHOM™ Solution   OTC
[gördö'kŏm]

DESCRIPTION
Gordochom is an antifungal solution for topical use containing 25% Undecylenic Acid and Chloroxylenol as its active ingredients in a penetrating oil base. Undecylenic Acid is

chemically 10 hendecenoic acid having the empirical formula $C_{11}H_{20}O_2$ and the chemical bond structure $CH_2=CH$ $(CH_2)8\ CO_2H$.

Undecylenic Acid is a colorless to pale yellow liquid. It is insoluble in water and soluble in alcohol, chloroform and ether.

Chloroxylenol is chemically 2-chloro-5-hydroxy-1,3-dimethylbenzene having the empirical formula C_8H_9ClO.

CLINICAL PHARMACOLOGY

Undecylenic Acid is a fungistatic agent employed in the treatment of tinea pedis, ringworm and dermatophytosis. Chloroxylenol is a topical antiseptic, germicide and antifungal agent effective against a wide variety of causative fungi and yeast organisms. Among those affected by Chloroxylenol are candida albicans, aspergillus niger, aspergillus flavus, trichophyton rubrum, trichophyton mentagrophytes, penicillum luteum and epidermophyton floccosum.

The penetrating oil base vehicle serves as a delivery system, enhancing the impregnation of Undecylenic Acid and Chloroxylenol as antimicrobial agents.

INDICATIONS

Cures athlete's foot (tinea pedis), and ringworm (tinea corporis).

CONTRAINDICATIONS

Gordochom is contraindicated in patients who are sensitive to Undecylenic Acid or Chloroxylenol.

WARNINGS

For external use only. Not for opthalmic or optic use. Avoid inhaling and contact with eyes or other mucous membranes. Not to be applied over blistered, raw or oozing areas of skin or over deep puncture wounds.

PRECAUTIONS

If a reaction suggesting sensitivity or chemical irritation should occur with the use of Gordochom, treatment should be discontinued. Use of Gordochom in pregnancy has not been established. **Keep out of reach of children.**

ADVERSE REACTIONS

No significant adverse reactions have been reported. However, attention should be paid to localized hypersensitivity.

DOSAGE AND ADMINISTRATION

Cleanse and dry affected areas. Apply a thin application twice a day (morning and night) to the affected area, or as recommended by your physician. For athlete's foot, pay special attention to the spaces between the toes; wear well-fitting, ventilated shoes, and change shoes and socks at least once daily. For athlete's foot and ringworm, use daily for 4 weeks. If condition persists longer, consult a physician. This product has not been proven effective on the scalp or nails.

HOW SUPPLIED

Gordochom is available in 1 oz. bottles with special brush applicator. (NDC 10481-8010-2)

Store at controlled room temperatures (59°–86°F).

Shown in Product Identification Guide, page 509

Incyte Corporation
1801 AUGUSTINE CUT-OFF
WILMINGTON, DE 19803

Direct Inquiries;
Tel: 1-855-4-INCYTE (1-855-446-2983)
Tel: 302.498.6700
Medical Information Contact
1-855-4-MEDINFO (1-855-463-3463)
medinfo@incyte.com
Normal business hours: 8am to 8pm ET, Mon-Fri

JAKAFI®
(ruxolitinib)
tablets, for oral use

℞

HIGHLIGHTS OF PRESCRIBING INFORMATION
These highlights do not include all the information needed to use JAKAFI safely and effectively. See full prescribing information for JAKAFI.
JAKAFI® (ruxolitinib) tablets, for oral use

Initial U.S. Approval: 2011

---——RECENT MAJOR CHANGES——---
Warnings and Precautions (5.2), (5.5)   03/2016

---——INDICATIONS AND USAGE——---
Jakafi is a kinase inhibitor indicated for treatment of patients with:
• intermediate or high-risk myelofibrosis, including primary myelofibrosis, post-polycythemia vera myelofibrosis and post-essential thrombocythemia myelofibrosis. (1.1)
• polycythemia vera who have had an inadequate response to or are intolerant of hydroxyurea. (1.2)

---——DOSAGE AND ADMINISTRATION——---
Doses should be individualized based on safety and efficacy. Starting doses per indication are noted below.
Myelofibrosis (2.1)
• The starting dose of Jakafi is based on patient's baseline platelet count:
  • Greater than 200×10^9/L: 20 mg given orally twice daily
  • 100×10^9/L to 200×10^9/L: 15 mg given orally twice daily
  • 50×10^9/L to less than 100×10^9/L: 5 mg given orally twice daily
• Monitor complete blood counts every 2 to 4 weeks until doses are stabilized, and then as clinically indicated. Modify or interrupt dosing for thrombocytopenia.
Polycythemia Vera (2.2)
• The starting dose of Jakafi is 10 mg given orally twice daily.

---——DOSAGE FORMS AND STRENGTHS——---
Tablets: 5 mg, 10 mg, 15 mg, 20 mg and 25 mg. (3)

---——CONTRAINDICATIONS——---
None. (4)

---——WARNINGS AND PRECAUTIONS——---
• Thrombocytopenia, Anemia and Neutropenia: Manage by dose reduction, or interruption, or transfusion. (5.1)
• Risk of Infection: Assess patients for signs and symptoms of infection and initiate appropriate treatment promptly. Serious infections should have resolved before starting therapy with Jakafi. (5.2)
• Symptom Exacerbation Following Interruption or Discontinuation: Manage with supportive care and consider resuming treatment with Jakafi. (5.3)
• Risk of Non-Melanoma Skin Cancer: Perform periodic skin examinations. (5.4)
• Lipid Elevations: Assess lipid levels 8-12 weeks from start of therapy and treat as needed. (5.5)

---——ADVERSE REACTIONS——---
The most common hematologic adverse reactions (incidence > 20%) are thrombocytopenia and anemia. The most common non-hematologic adverse reactions (incidence >10%) are bruising, dizziness and headache. (6.1)
To report SUSPECTED ADVERSE REACTIONS, contact Incyte Corporation at 1-855-463-3463 or FDA at 1-800-FDA-1088 or *www.fda.gov/medwatch*

---——DRUG INTERACTIONS——---
• Strong CYP3A4 Inhibitors or Fluconazole: Reduce, interrupt, or discontinue Jakafi doses as recommended. (2.3) (7.1) Avoid use of Jakafi with fluconazole doses greater than 200 mg.

---——USE IN SPECIFIC POPULATIONS——---
• Renal Impairment: Reduce Jakafi starting dose or avoid treatment as recommended. (2.4) (8.6)
• Hepatic Impairment: Reduce Jakafi starting dose or avoid treatment as recommended. (2.4) (8.7)
• Nursing Mothers: Discontinue nursing or discontinue the drug taking into account the importance of the drug to the mother. (8.3)
See 17 for PATIENT COUNSELING INFORMATION and FDA-approved patient labeling.

Revised: 3/2016

FULL PRESCRIBING INFORMATION

1.   INDICATIONS AND USAGE
1.1   Myelofibrosis
Jakafi is indicated for treatment of patients with intermediate or high-risk myelofibrosis, including primary myelofibrosis, post-polycythemia vera myelofibrosis and post-essential thrombocythemia myelofibrosis.
1.2   Polycythemia Vera
Jakafi is indicated for treatment of patients with polycythemia vera who have had an inadequate response to or are intolerant of hydroxyurea.

2.   DOSAGE AND ADMINISTRATION
2.1   Myelofibrosis
The recommended starting dose of Jakafi is based on platelet count (Table 1). A complete blood count (CBC) and platelet count must be performed before initiating therapy, every 2 to 4 weeks until doses are stabilized, and then as clinically indicated [*see Warnings and Precautions (5.1)*]. Doses may be titrated based on safety and efficacy.

Table 1: Jakafi Starting Doses for Myelofibrosis

Platelet Count	Starting Dose
Greater than 200×10^9/L	20 mg orally twice daily
100×10^9/L to 200×10^9/L	15 mg orally twice daily
50×10^9/L to less than 100×10^9/L	5 mg orally twice daily

2.1.1 Dose Modification Guidelines for Hematologic Toxicity for Patients with Myelofibrosis Starting Treatment with a Platelet Count of 100×10^9/L or Greater
Treatment Interruption and Restarting Dosing
Interrupt treatment for platelet counts less than 50×10^9/L or absolute neutrophil count (ANC) less than 0.5×10^9/L. After recovery of platelet counts above 50×10^9/L and ANC above 0.75×10^9/L, dosing may be restarted. Table 2 illustrates the maximum allowable dose that may be used in restarting Jakafi after a previous interruption.

Continued on next page

Table 2: Myelofibrosis: Maximum Restarting Doses for Jakafi after Safety Interruption for Thrombocytopenia for Patients Starting Treatment with a Platelet Count of 100 × 10⁹/L or Greater

Current Platelet Count	Maximum Dose When Restarting Jakafi Treatment*
Greater than or equal to 125×10^9/L	20 mg twice daily
100 to less than 125×10^9/L	15 mg twice daily
75 to less than 100×10^9/L	10 mg twice daily for at least 2 weeks; if stable, may increase to 15 mg twice daily
50 to less than 75×10^9/L	5 mg twice daily for at least 2 weeks; if stable, may increase to 10 mg twice daily
Less than 50×10^9/L	Continue hold

* Maximum doses are displayed. When restarting, begin with a dose at least 5 mg twice daily below the dose at interruption.

Following treatment interruption for ANC below 0.5×10^9/L, after ANC recovers to 0.75×10^9/L or greater, restart dosing at the higher of 5 mg once daily or 5 mg twice daily below the largest dose in the week prior to the treatment interruption.

Dose Reductions

Dose reductions should be considered if the platelet counts decrease as outlined in Table 3 with the goal of avoiding dose interruptions for thrombocytopenia.

[See table 3 below]

2.1.2 Dose Modification Based on Insufficient Response for Patients with Myelofibrosis Starting Treatment with a Platelet Count of 100 × 10⁹/L or Greater

If the response is insufficient and platelet and neutrophil counts are adequate, doses may be increased in 5 mg twice daily increments to a maximum of 25 mg twice daily. Doses should not be increased during the first 4 weeks of therapy and not more frequently than every 2 weeks.

Consider dose increases in patients who meet all of the following conditions:

a. Failure to achieve a reduction from pretreatment baseline in either palpable spleen length of 50% or a 35% reduction in spleen volume as measured by computed tomography (CT) or magnetic resonance imaging (MRI);

b. Platelet count greater than 125×10^9/L at 4 weeks and platelet count never below 100×10^9/L;

c. ANC Levels greater than 0.75×10^9/L.

Based on limited clinical data, long-term maintenance at a 5 mg twice daily dose has not shown responses and continued use at this dose should be limited to patients in whom the benefits outweigh the potential risks. Discontinue Jakafi if there is no spleen size reduction or symptom improvement after 6 months of therapy.

2.1.3 Dose Modifications for Hematologic Toxicity for Patients with Myelofibrosis Starting Treatment with Platelet Counts of 50 × 10⁹/L to Less Than 100 × 10⁹/L

This section applies only to patients with platelet counts of 50×10^9/L to less than 100×10^9/L prior to any treatment with ruxolitinib. See Section 2.1.1 for dose modifications for

hematological toxicity in patients whose platelet counts were 100×10^9/L or more prior to starting treatment with ruxolitinib.

Treatment Interruption and Restarting Dosing

Interrupt treatment for platelet counts less than 25×10^9/L or ANC less than 0.5×10^9/L.

After recovery of platelet counts above 35×10^9/L and ANC above 0.75×10^9/L, dosing may be restarted. Restart dosing at the higher of 5 mg once daily or 5 mg twice daily below the largest dose in the week prior to the decrease in platelet count below 25×10^9/L or ANC below 0.5×10^9/L that led to dose interruption.

Dose Reductions

Reduce the dose of ruxolitinib for platelet counts less than 35×10^9/L as described in Table 4.

Table 4: Myelofibrosis: Dosing Modifications for Thrombocytopenia for Patients with Starting Platelet Count of 50 × 10⁹/L to Less Than 100 × 10⁹/L

Platelet Count	Dosing Recommendations
Less than 25×10^9/L	• Interrupt dosing.
25×10^9/L to less than 35×10^9/L AND the platelet count decline is less than 20% during the prior four weeks	• Decrease dose by 5 mg once daily. • For patients on 5 mg once daily, maintain dose at 5 mg once daily.
25×10^9/L to less than 35×10^9/L AND the platelet count decline is 20% or greater during the prior four weeks	• Decrease dose by 5 mg twice daily. • For patients on 5 mg twice daily, decrease the dose to 5 mg once daily. • For patients on 5 mg once daily, maintain dose at 5 mg once daily.

2.1.4 Dose Modifications Based on Insufficient Response for Patients with Myelofibrosis and Starting Platelet Count of 50 × 10⁹/L to Less Than 100 × 10⁹/L

Do not increase doses during the first 4 weeks of therapy, and do not increase the dose more frequently than every 2 weeks.

If the response is insufficient as defined in Section 2.1.2, doses may be increased by increments of 5 mg daily to a maximum of 10 mg twice daily if:

a. the platelet count has remained at least 40×10^9/L, and

b. the platelet count has not fallen by more than 20% in the prior 4 weeks, and

c. the ANC is more than 1×10^9/L, and

d. the dose has not been reduced or interrupted for an adverse event or hematological toxicity in the prior 4 weeks.

Continuation of treatment for more than 6 months should be limited to patients in whom the benefits outweigh the potential risks. Discontinue Jakafi if there is no spleen size reduction or symptom improvement after 6 months of therapy.

2.1.5 Dose Modification for Bleeding

Interrupt treatment for bleeding requiring intervention regardless of current platelet count. Once the bleeding event has resolved, consider resuming treatment at the prior dose if the underlying cause of bleeding has been controlled. If the bleeding event has resolved but the underlying cause persists, consider resuming treatment with Jakafi at a lower dose.

2.2 Polycythemia Vera

The recommended starting dose of Jakafi is 10 mg twice daily. Doses may be titrated based on safety and efficacy.

2.2.1 Dose Modification Guidelines for Patients with Polycythemia Vera

A complete blood count (CBC) and platelet count must be performed before initiating therapy, every 2 to 4 weeks until doses are stabilized, and then as clinically indicated [see *Warnings and Precautions (5.1)*].

Dose Reductions

Dose reductions should be considered for hemoglobin and platelet count decreases as described in Table 5.

Table 5: Polycythemia Vera: Dose Reductions

Hemoglobin and/or Platelet Count	Dosing Recommendations
Hemoglobin greater than or equal to 12 g/dL AND platelet count greater than or equal to 100×10^9/L	• No change required.
Hemoglobin 10 to less than 12 g/dL AND platelet count 75 to less than 100×10^9/L	• Dose reductions should be considered with the goal of avoiding dose interruptions for anemia and thrombocytopenia.
Hemoglobin 8 to less than 10 g/dL OR platelet count 50 to less than 75×10^9/L	• Reduce dose by 5 mg twice daily. • For patients on 5 mg twice daily, decrease the dose to 5 mg once daily.
Hemoglobin less than 8 g/dL OR platelet count less than 50×10^9/L	• Interrupt dosing.

Treatment Interruption and Restarting Dosing

Interrupt treatment for hemoglobin less than 8 g/dL, platelet counts less than 50×10^9/L or ANC less than 1.0×10^9/L. After recovery of the hematologic parameter(s) to acceptable levels, dosing may be restarted.

Table 6 illustrates the dose that may be used in restarting Jakafi after a previous interruption.

Table 6: Polycythemia Vera: Restarting Doses for Jakafi after Safety Interruption for Hematologic Parameter(s)

Use the **most severe category** of a patient's hemoglobin, platelet count, or ANC abnormality to determine the corresponding maximum restarting dose.

Hemoglobin, Platelet Count, or ANC	Maximum Restarting Dose
Hemoglobin less than 8 g/dL OR platelet count less than 50×10^9/L OR ANC less than 1×10^9/L	Continue hold
Hemoglobin 8 to less than 10 g/dL OR platelet count 50 to less than 75×10^9/L OR ANC 1 to less than 1.5×10^9/L	5 mg twice daily* or no more than 5 mg twice daily less than the dose which resulted in dose interruption
Hemoglobin 10 to less than 12 g/dL OR platelet count 75 to less than 100×10^9/L OR ANC 1.5 to less than 2×10^9/L	10 mg twice daily* or no more than 5 mg twice daily less than the dose which resulted in dose interruption
Hemoglobin greater than or equal to 12 g/dL OR platelet count greater than or equal to 100×10^9/L OR ANC greater than or equal to 2×10^9/L	15 mg twice daily* or no more than 5 mg twice daily less than the dose which resulted in dose interruption

* Continue treatment for at least 2 weeks; if stable, may increase dose by 5 mg twice daily.

Patients who had required dose interruption while receiving a dose of 5 mg twice daily, may restart at a dose of 5 mg twice daily or 5 mg once daily, but not higher, once hemo-

Table 3: Myelofibrosis: Dosing Recommendations for Thrombocytopenia for Patients Starting Treatment with a Platelet Count of 100 × 10⁹/L or Greater

Platelet Count	25 mg twice daily — New Dose	20 mg twice daily — New Dose	15 mg twice daily — New Dose	10 mg twice daily — New Dose	5 mg twice daily — New Dose
	Dose at Time of Platelet Decline				
100 to less than 125×10^9/L	20 mg twice daily	15 mg twice daily	No Change	No Change	No Change
75 to less than 100×10^9/L	10 mg twice daily	10 mg twice daily	10 mg twice daily	No Change	No Change
50 to less than 75×10^9/L	5 mg twice daily	5 mg twice daily	5 mg twice daily	5 mg twice daily	No Change
Less than 50×10^9/L	Hold	Hold	Hold	Hold	Hold

globin is greater than or equal to 10 g/dL, platelet count is greater than or equal to 75×10^9/L, and ANC is greater than or equal to 1.5×10^9/L.

Dose Management after Restarting Treatment

After restarting Jakafi following treatment interruption, doses may be titrated, but the maximum total daily dose should not exceed 5 mg less than the dose that resulted in the dose interruption. An exception to this is dose interruption following phlebotomy-associated anemia, in which case the maximal total daily dose allowed after restarting Jakafi would not be limited.

2.2.2 Dose Modifications Based on Insufficient Response for Patients with Polycythemia Vera

If the response is insufficient and platelet, hemoglobin, and neutrophil counts are adequate, doses may be increased in 5 mg twice daily increments to a maximum of 25 mg twice daily. Doses should not be increased during the first 4 weeks of therapy and not more frequently than every two weeks. Consider dose increases in patients who meet all of the following conditions:

1. Inadequate efficacy as demonstrated by one or more of the following:
   a. Continued need for phlebotomy
   b. WBC greater than the upper limit of normal range
   c. Platelet count greater than the upper limit of normal range
   d. Palpable spleen that is reduced by less than 25% from Baseline
2. Platelet count greater than or equal to 140×10^9/L
3. Hemoglobin greater than or equal to 12 g/dL
4. ANC greater than or equal to 1.5×10^9/L

2.3 Dose Modification for Drug Interactions Concomitant Use with Strong CYP3A4 Inhibitors or Fluconazole

Modify the dose of Jakafi when given concomitantly with strong CYP3A4 inhibitors (such as but not limited to boceprevir, clarithromycin, conivaptan, grapefruit juice, indinavir, itraconazole, ketoconazole, lopinavir/ritonavir, mibefradil, nefazodone, nelfinavir, posaconazole, ritonavir, saquinavir, telaprevir, telithromycin, voriconazole) and fluconazole doses of less than or equal to 200 mg as follows [*see Drug Interactions (7.1)*], according to Table 7.

Table 7: Dose Modification for Drug Interactions

Patients on concomitant strong CYP3A4 inhibitors or fluconazole doses of less than or equal to 200 mg	Recommended Dose Modification
Starting Dose for Patients with Myelofibrosis with a platelet count:	
• Greater than or equal to 100×10^9/L	10 mg twice daily
• 50×10^9/L to less than 100 $\times 10^9$/L	5 mg once daily
Starting Dose for Patients with Polycythemia Vera	5 mg twice daily
All Patients on a Stable Dose of:	
• Greater than or equal to 10 mg twice daily	Decrease dose by 50% (round up to the closest available tablet strength)
• 5 mg twice daily	5 mg once daily
• 5 mg once daily	Avoid strong CYP3A4 inhibitor or fluconazole treatment or interrupt Jakafi treatment for the duration of strong CYP3A4 inhibitor or fluconazole use

Avoid the use of fluconazole doses of greater than 200 mg daily concomitantly with Jakafi.

Additional dose modifications should be made with careful monitoring of safety and efficacy.

2.4 Organ Impairment

Renal Impairment

Modify the dose of Jakafi accordingly in patients with moderate or severe renal impairment.

[See table 8 below]

Table 8: Dosing for Renal Impairment

Renal Impairment Status	Platelet Count	Recommended Starting Dosage
Patients with Myelofibrosis Moderate (CrCl 30–59 mL/min) or Severe (CrCl 15–29 mL/min)	Greater than 150×10^9/L	No dose modification needed
	100×10^9/L - 150×10^9/L	10 mg twice daily
	50 - less than 100×10^9/L	5 mg daily
	Less than 50×10^9/L	Avoid use [*see Use in Specific Populations (8.6)*]
Patients with Polycythemia Vera Moderate (CrCl 30-59 mL/min) or Severe (CrCl 15-29 mL/min)	Any	5 mg twice daily

Patients on Dialysis

The recommended starting dose for patients with myelofibrosis with end stage renal disease on dialysis is 15 mg once after a dialysis session for patients with a platelet count between 100×10^9/L and 200×10^9/L or 20 mg for patients with a platelet count of greater than 200×10^9/L. The recommended starting dose for patients with polycythemia vera with end stage renal disease on dialysis is 10 mg. Additional dose modifications should be made with frequent monitoring of safety and efficacy. Avoid use of Jakafi in patients with end stage renal disease (CrCl less than 15 mL/min) not requiring dialysis [*see Use in Specific Populations (8.6)*].

Hepatic Impairment

The dose of Jakafi should be reduced in patients with hepatic impairment.

[See table 9 on next page]

2.5 Method of Administration

Jakafi is dosed orally and can be administered with or without food.

If a dose is missed, the patient should not take an additional dose, but should take the next usual prescribed dose.

When discontinuing Jakafi therapy for reasons other than thrombocytopenia, gradual tapering of the dose of Jakafi may be considered, for example by 5 mg twice daily each week.

For patients unable to ingest tablets, Jakafi can be administered through a nasogastric tube (8 French or greater) as follows:

• Suspend one tablet in approximately 40 mL of water with stirring for approximately 10 minutes.

• Within 6 hours after the tablet has dispersed, the suspension can be administered through a nasogastric tube using an appropriate syringe.

The tube should be rinsed with approximately 75 mL of water. The effect of tube feeding preparations on Jakafi exposure during administration through a nasogastric tube has not been evaluated.

3. DOSAGE FORMS AND STRENGTHS

5 mg tablets - round and white with "INCY" on one side and "5" on the other.
10 mg tablets - round and white with "INCY" on one side and "10" on the other.
15 mg tablets - oval and white with "INCY" on one side and "15" on the other.
20 mg tablets - capsule-shaped and white with "INCY" on one side and "20" on the other.
25 mg tablets - oval and white with "INCY" on one side and "25" on the other.

4. CONTRAINDICATIONS

None.

5. WARNINGS AND PRECAUTIONS

5.1 Thrombocytopenia, Anemia and Neutropenia

Treatment with Jakafi can cause thrombocytopenia, anemia and neutropenia. [*see Dosage and Administration (2.1)*].

Manage thrombocytopenia by reducing the dose or temporarily interrupting Jakafi. Platelet transfusions may be necessary [*see Dosage and Administration (2.1.1), and Adverse Reactions (6.1)*].

Patients developing anemia may require blood transfusions and/or dose modifications of Jakafi.

Severe neutropenia (ANC less than 0.5×10^9/L) was generally reversible by withholding Jakafi until recovery [*see Adverse Reactions (6.1)*].

Perform a pre-treatment complete blood count (CBC) and monitor CBCs every 2 to 4 weeks until doses are stabilized, and then as clinically indicated. [*see Dosage and Administration (2.1.1), and Adverse Reactions (6.1)*].

5.2 Risk of Infection

Serious bacterial, mycobacterial, fungal and viral infections have occurred. Delay starting therapy with Jakafi until active serious infections have resolved. Observe patients receiving Jakafi for signs and symptoms of infection and manage promptly.

Tuberculosis

Tuberculosis infection has been reported in patients receiving Jakafi. Observe patients receiving Jakafi for signs and symptoms of active tuberculosis and manage promptly.

Prior to initiating Jakafi, patients should be evaluated for tuberculosis risk factors, and those at higher risk should be tested for latent infection. Risk factors include, but are not limited to, prior residence in or travel to countries with a high prevalence of tuberculosis, close contact with a person with active tuberculosis, and a history of active or latent tuberculosis where an adequate course of treatment cannot be confirmed.

For patients with evidence of active or latent tuberculosis, consult a physician with expertise in the treatment of tuberculosis before starting Jakafi. The decision to continue Jakafi during treatment of active tuberculosis should be based on the overall risk-benefit determination.

PML

Progressive multifocal leukoencephalopathy (PML) has occurred with ruxolitinib treatment for myelofibrosis. If PML is suspected, stop Jakafi and evaluate.

Herpes Zoster

Advise patients about early signs and symptoms of herpes zoster and to seek treatment as early as possible if suspected [*see Adverse Reactions (6.1)*].

Hepatitis B

Hepatitis B viral load (HBV-DNA titer) increases, with or without associated elevations in alanine aminotransferase and aspartate aminotransferase, have been reported in patients with chronic HBV infections taking Jakafi. The effect of Jakafi on viral replication in patients with chronic HBV infection is unknown. Patients with chronic HBV infection should be treated and monitored according to clinical guidelines.

5.3 Symptom Exacerbation Following Interruption or Discontinuation of Treatment with Jakafi

Following discontinuation of Jakafi, symptoms from myeloproliferative neoplasms may return to pretreatment levels over a period of approximately one week. Some patients with myelofibrosis have experienced one or more of the following adverse events after discontinuing Jakafi: fever, respiratory distress, hypotension, DIC, or multi-organ failure. If one or more of these occur after discontinuation of, or while tapering the dose of Jakafi, evaluate for and treat any intercurrent illness and consider restarting or increasing the dose of Jakafi. Instruct patients not to interrupt or discontinue Jakafi therapy without consulting their physician. When discontinuing or interrupting therapy with Jakafi for reasons other than thrombocytopenia or neutropenia [*see Dosage and Administration (2.5)*], consider tapering the dose of Jakafi gradually rather than discontinuing abruptly.

5.4 Non-Melanoma Skin Cancer

Non-melanoma skin cancers including basal cell, squamous cell, and Merkel cell carcinoma have occurred in patients treated with Jakafi. Perform periodic skin examinations.

5.5 Lipid Elevations

Treatment with Jakafi has been associated with increases in lipid parameters including total cholesterol, low-density lipoprotein (LDL) cholesterol, and triglycerides. The effect of these lipid parameter elevations on cardiovascular morbidity and mortality has not been determined in patients

Continued on next page

treated with Jakafi. Assess lipid parameters approximately 8-12 weeks following initiation of Jakafi therapy. Monitor and treat according to clinical guidelines for the management of hyperlipidemia.

6. ADVERSE REACTIONS

The following serious adverse reactions are discussed in greater detail in other sections of the labeling:

- Thrombocytopenia, Anemia and Neutropenia [see *Warnings and Precautions (5.1)*]
- Risk of Infection [see *Warnings and Precautions (5.2)*]
- Symptom Exacerbation Following Interruption or Discontinuation of Treatment with Jakafi [see *Warnings and Precautions (5.3)*]
- Non-Melanoma Skin Cancer [see *Warnings and Precautions (5.4)*]

Because clinical trials are conducted under widely varying conditions, adverse reaction rates observed in the clinical trials of a drug cannot be directly compared to rates in the clinical trials of another drug and may not reflect the rates observed in practice.

6.1 Clinical Trials Experience in Myelofibrosis

The safety of Jakafi was assessed in 617 patients in six clinical studies with a median duration of follow-up of 10.9 months, including 301 patients with myelofibrosis in two Phase 3 studies.

In these two Phase 3 studies, patients had a median duration of exposure to Jakafi of 9.5 months (range 0.5 to 17 months), with 89% of patients treated for more than 6 months and 25% treated for more than 12 months. One hundred and eleven (111) patients started treatment at 15 mg twice daily and 190 patients started at 20 mg twice daily. In patients starting treatment with 15 mg twice daily (pre-treatment platelet counts of 100 to 200×10^9/L) and 20 mg twice daily (pretreatment platelet counts greater than 200×10^9/L), 65% and 25% of patients, respectively, required a dose reduction below the starting dose within the first 8 weeks of therapy.

In a double-blind, randomized, placebo-controlled study of Jakafi, among the 155 patients treated with Jakafi, the most frequent adverse drug reactions were thrombocytopenia and anemia [see *Table 11*]. Thrombocytopenia, anemia and neutropenia are dose related effects. The three most frequent non-hematologic adverse reactions were bruising, dizziness and headache [see *Table 10*].

Discontinuation for adverse events, regardless of causality, was observed in 11% of patients treated with Jakafi and 11% of patients treated with placebo.

Table 10 presents the most common adverse reactions occurring in patients who received Jakafi in the double-blind, placebo-controlled study during randomized treatment.

[See table 10 below]

Description of Selected Adverse Drug Reactions

Anemia

In the two Phase 3 clinical studies, median time to onset of first CTCAE Grade 2 or higher anemia was approximately 6 weeks. One patient (<1%) discontinued treatment because

of anemia. In patients receiving Jakafi, mean decreases in hemoglobin reached a nadir of approximately 1.5 to 2.0 g/dL below baseline after 8 to 12 weeks of therapy and then gradually recovered to reach a new steady state that was approximately 1.0 g/dL below baseline. This pattern was observed in patients regardless of whether they had received transfusions during therapy.

In the randomized, placebo-controlled study, 60% of patients treated with Jakafi and 38% of patients receiving placebo received red blood cell transfusions during randomized treatment. Among transfused patients, the median number of units transfused per month was 1.2 in patients treated with Jakafi and 1.7 in placebo treated patients.

Thrombocytopenia

In the two Phase 3 clinical studies, in patients who developed Grade 3 or 4 thrombocytopenia, the median time to onset was approximately 8 weeks. Thrombocytopenia was generally reversible with dose reduction or dose interruption. The median time to recovery of platelet counts above 50×10^9/L was 14 days. Platelet transfusions were administered to 5% of patients receiving Jakafi and to 4% of patients receiving control regimens. Discontinuation of treatment because of thrombocytopenia occurred in <1% of patients receiving Jakafi and <1% of patients receiving control regimens. Patients with a platelet count of 100×10^9/L to 200×10^9/L before starting Jakafi had a higher frequency of Grade 3 or 4 thrombocytopenia compared to patients with a platelet count greater than 200×10^9/L (17% versus 7%).

Neutropenia

In the two Phase 3 clinical studies, 1% of patients reduced or stopped Jakafi because of neutropenia.

Table 11 provides the frequency and severity of clinical hematology abnormalities reported for patients receiving treatment with Jakafi or placebo in the placebo-controlled study.

[See table on next page]

Additional Data from the Placebo-controlled Study

25% of patients treated with Jakafi and 7% of patients treated with placebo developed newly occurring or worsening Grade 1 abnormalities in alanine transaminase (ALT).

The incidence of greater than or equal to Grade 2 elevations was 2% for Jakafi with 1% Grade 3 and no Grade 4 ALT elevations.

17% of patients treated with Jakafi and 6% of patients treated with placebo developed newly occurring or worsening Grade 1 abnormalities in aspartate transaminase (AST). The incidence of Grade 2 AST elevations was <1% for Jakafi with no Grade 3 or 4 AST elevations.

17% of patients treated with Jakafi and <1% of patients treated with placebo developed newly occurring or worsening Grade 1 elevations in cholesterol. The incidence of Grade 2 cholesterol elevations was <1% for Jakafi with no Grade 3 or 4 cholesterol elevations.

6.2 Clinical Trial Experience in Polycythemia Vera

In a randomized, open-label, active-controlled study, 110 patients with polycythemia vera resistant to or intolerant of hydroxyurea received Jakafi and 111 patients received best available therapy [see *Clinical Studies (14.2)*]. The most frequent adverse drug reaction was anemia. Table 12 presents the most frequent non-hematologic treatment emergent adverse events occurring up to Week 32.

Discontinuation for adverse events, regardless of causality, was observed in 4% of patients treated with Jakafi.

[See table 12 on next page]

Other clinically important treatment emergent adverse events observed in less than 6% of patients treated with Jakafi were:

Weight gain, hypertension, and urinary tract infections

Clinically relevant laboratory abnormalities are shown in Table 13.

[See table 13 on page 978]

7. DRUG INTERACTIONS

7.1 Drugs That Inhibit or Induce Cytochrome P450 Enzymes

Ruxolitinib is metabolized by CYP3A4 and to a lesser extent by CYP2C9.

CYP3A4 inhibitors: The C_{max} and AUC of ruxolitinib increased 33% and 91%, respectively following concomitant administration with the strong CYP3A4 inhibitor ketoconazole in healthy subjects. Concomitant administration with mild or moderate CYP3A4 inhibitors did not result in an exposure change requiring intervention [see *Pharmacokinetics (12.3)*].

When administering Jakafi with strong CYP3A4 inhibitors, consider dose reduction [see *Dosage and Administration (2.3)*].

Fluconazole: The AUC of ruxolitinib is predicted to increase by approximately 100% to 300% following concomitant administration with the combined CYP3A4 and CYP2C9 inhibitor fluconazole at doses of 100 mg to 400 mg once daily, respectively [see *Pharmacokinetics (12.3)*].

Avoid the concomitant use of Jakafi with fluconazole doses of greater than 200 mg daily [see *Dosage and Administration (2.3)*].

CYP3A4 inducers: The C_{max} and AUC of ruxolitinib decreased 32% and 61%, respectively, following concomitant administration with the strong CYP3A4 inducer rifampin in healthy subjects. No dose adjustment is recommended; however, monitor patients frequently and adjust the Jakafi dose based on safety and efficacy [see *Pharmacokinetics (12.3)*].

8. USE IN SPECIFIC POPULATIONS

8.1 Pregnancy

Pregnancy Category C

Risk Summary

There are no adequate and well-controlled studies of Jakafi in pregnant women. In embryofetal toxicity studies, treatment with ruxolitinib resulted in an increase in late resorp-

Table 9: Dosing for Hepatic Impairment

Hepatic Impairment Status	Platelet Count	Recommended Starting Dosage
Patients with Myelofibrosis Mild, Moderate, or Severe (Child-Pugh categories A, B, C)	Greater than 150×10^9/L	No dose modification needed
	100×10^9/L - 150×10^9/L	10 mg twice daily
	50 - less than 100×10^9/L	5 mg daily
	Less than 50×10^9/L	Avoid use [see *Use in Specific Populations (8.7)*]
Patients with Polycythemia Vera Mild, Moderate, or Severe (Child-Pugh categories A, B, C)	Any	5 mg twice daily

Table 10: Myelofibrosis: Adverse Reactions Occurring in Patients on Jakafi in the Double-blind, Placebo-controlled Study During Randomized Treatment

Adverse Reactions	Jakafi (N=155)			Placebo (N=151)		
	All Grades* (%)	Grade 3 (%)	Grade 4 (%)	All Grades* (%)	Grade 3 (%)	Grade 4 (%)
Bruising[†]	23	<1	0	15	0	0
Dizziness[‡]	18	<1	0	7	0	0
Headache	15	0	0	5	0	0
Urinary Tract Infections[§]	9	0	0	5	<1	<1
Weight Gain[¶]	7	<1	0	1	<1	0
Flatulence	5	0	0	<1	0	0
Herpes Zoster[#]	2	0	0	<1	0	0

* National Cancer Institute Common Terminology Criteria for Adverse Events (CTCAE), version 3.0
† includes contusion, ecchymosis, hematoma, injection site hematoma, periorbital hematoma, vessel puncture site hematoma, increased tendency to bruise, petechiae, purpura
‡ includes dizziness, postural dizziness, vertigo, balance disorder, Meniere's Disease, labyrinthitis
§ includes urinary tract infection, cystitis, urosepsis, urinary tract infection bacterial, kidney infection, pyuria, bacteria urine, bacteria urine identified, nitrite urine present
¶ includes weight increased, abnormal weight gain
# includes herpes zoster and post-herpetic neuralgia

tions and reduced fetal weights at maternally toxic doses. Jakafi should be used during pregnancy only if the potential benefit justifies the potential risk to the fetus.

Animal Data

Ruxolitinib was administered orally to pregnant rats or rabbits during the period of organogenesis, at doses of 15, 30 or 60 mg/kg/day in rats and 10, 30 or 60 mg/kg/day in rabbits. There was no evidence of teratogenicity. However, decreases of approximately 9% in fetal weights were noted in rats at the highest and maternally toxic dose of 60 mg/kg/day. This dose results in an exposure (AUC) that is approximately 2 times the clinical exposure at the maximum recommended dose of 25 mg twice daily. In rabbits, lower fetal weights of approximately 8% and increased late resorptions were noted at the highest and maternally toxic dose of 60 mg/kg/day. This dose is approximately 7% the clinical exposure at the maximum recommended dose.

In a pre- and post-natal development study in rats, pregnant animals were dosed with ruxolitinib from implantation through lactation at doses up to 30 mg/kg/day. There were no drug-related adverse findings in pups for fertility indices or for maternal or embryofetal survival, growth and devel-

opment parameters at the highest dose evaluated (34% the clinical exposure at the maximum recommended dose of 25 mg twice daily).

8.3   Nursing Mothers

It is not known whether ruxolitinib is excreted in human milk. Ruxolitinib and/or its metabolites were excreted in the milk of lactating rats with a concentration that was 13-fold the maternal plasma. Because many drugs are excreted in human milk and because of the potential for serious adverse reactions in nursing infants from Jakafi, a decision should be made to discontinue nursing or to discontinue the drug, taking into account the importance of the drug to the mother.

8.4   Pediatric Use

The safety and effectiveness of Jakafi in pediatric patients have not been established.

8.5   Geriatric Use

Of the total number of patients with myelofibrosis in clinical studies with Jakafi, 52% were 65 years and older, while 15% were 75 years and older. No overall differences in safety or effectiveness of Jakafi were observed between these patients and younger patients.

8.6   Renal Impairment

The safety and pharmacokinetics of single dose Jakafi (25 mg) were evaluated in a study in healthy subjects [CrCl 72-164 mL/min (N=8)] and in subjects with mild [CrCl 53-83 mL/min (N=8)], moderate [CrCl 38-57 mL/min (N=8)], or severe renal impairment [CrCl 15-51 mL/min (N=8)]. Eight (8) additional subjects with end stage renal disease requiring hemodialysis were also enrolled.

The pharmacokinetics of ruxolitinib was similar in subjects with various degrees of renal impairment and in those with normal renal function. However, plasma AUC values of ruxolitinib metabolites increased with increasing severity of renal impairment. This was most marked in the subjects with end stage renal disease requiring hemodialysis. The change in the pharmacodynamic marker, pSTAT3 inhibition, was consistent with the corresponding increase in metabolite exposure. Ruxolitinib is not removed by dialysis; however, the removal of some active metabolites by dialysis cannot be ruled out.

When administering Jakafi to patients with myelofibrosis and moderate (CrCl 30-59 mL/min) or severe renal impairment (CrCl 15-29 mL/min) with a platelet count between 50×10^9/L and 150×10^9/L, a dose reduction is recommended. A dose reduction is also recommended for patients with polycythemia vera and moderate (CrCl 30-59 mL/min) or severe renal impairment (CrCl 15-29 mL/min). In all patients with end stage renal disease on dialysis, a dose reduction is recommended [*see Dosage and Administration (2.4)*].

8.7   Hepatic Impairment

The safety and pharmacokinetics of single dose Jakafi (25 mg) were evaluated in a study in healthy subjects (N=8) and in subjects with mild [Child-Pugh A (N=8)], moderate [Child-Pugh B (N=8)], or severe hepatic impairment [Child-Pugh C (N=8)]. The mean AUC for ruxolitinib was increased by 87%, 28% and 65%, respectively, in patients with mild, moderate and severe hepatic impairment compared to patients with normal hepatic function. The terminal elimination half-life was prolonged in patients with hepatic impairment compared to healthy controls (4.1-5.0 hours versus 2.8 hours). The change in the pharmacodynamic marker, pSTAT3 inhibition, was consistent with the corresponding increase in ruxolitinib exposure except in the severe (Child-Pugh C) hepatic impairment cohort where the pharmacodynamic activity was more prolonged in some subjects than expected based on plasma concentrations of ruxolitinib.

When administering Jakafi to patients with myelofibrosis and any degree of hepatic impairment and with a platelet count between 50×10^9/L and 150×10^9/L, a dose reduction is recommended. A dose reduction is also recommended for patients with polycythemia vera and hepatic impairment [*see Dosage and Administration (2.4)*].

10.   OVERDOSAGE

There is no known antidote for overdoses with Jakafi. Single doses up to 200 mg have been given with acceptable acute tolerability. Higher than recommended repeat doses are associated with increased myelosuppression including leukopenia, anemia and thrombocytopenia. Appropriate supportive treatment should be given.

Hemodialysis is not expected to enhance the elimination of ruxolitinib.

11.   DESCRIPTION

Ruxolitinib phosphate is a kinase inhibitor with the chemical name (*R*)-3-(4-(7*H*-pyrrolo[2,3-*d*]pyrimidin-4-yl)-1*H*-pyrazol-1-yl)-3-cyclopentylpropanenitrile phosphate and a molecular weight of 404.36. Ruxolitinib phosphate has the following structural formula:

Table 11: Myelofibrosis: Worst Hematology Laboratory Abnormalities in the Placebo-Controlled Study*

Laboratory Parameter	Jakafi (N=155)			Placebo (N=151)		
	All Grades[†] (%)	Grade 3 (%)	Grade 4 (%)	All Grades (%)	Grade 3 (%)	Grade 4 (%)
Thrombocytopenia	70	9	4	31	1	0
Anemia	96	34	11	87	16	3
Neutropenia	19	5	2	4	<1	1

* Presented values are worst Grade values regardless of baseline
† National Cancer Institute Common Terminology Criteria for Adverse Events, version 3.0

Table 12: Polycythemia Vera: Treatment Emergent Adverse Events Occurring in ≥ 6% of Patients on Jakafi in the Open-Label, Active-controlled Study up to Week 32 of Randomized Treatment

Adverse Events	Jakafi (N=110)		Best Available Therapy (N=111)	
	All Grades* (%)	Grade 3-4 (%)	All Grades (%)	Grade 3-4 (%)
Headache	16	<1	19	<1
Abdominal Pain[†]	15	<1	15	<1
Diarrhea	15	0	7	<1
Dizziness[‡]	15	0	13	0
Fatigue	15	0	15	3
Pruritus	14	<1	23	4
Dyspnea[§]	13	3	4	0
Muscle Spasms	12	<1	5	0
Nasopharyngitis	9	0	8	0
Constipation	8	0	3	0
Cough	8	0	5	0
Edema[¶]	8	0	7	0
Arthralgia	7	0	6	<1
Asthenia	7	0	11	2
Epistaxis	6	0	3	0
Herpes Zoster[#]	6	<1	0	0
Nausea	6	0	4	0

* National Cancer Institute Common Terminology Criteria for Adverse Events (CTCAE), version 3.0
† includes abdominal pain, abdominal pain lower, and abdominal pain upper
‡ includes dizziness and vertigo
§ includes dyspnea and dyspnea exertional
¶ includes edema and peripheral edema
# includes herpes zoster and post-herpetic neuralgia

Continued on next page

Ruxolitinib phosphate is a white to off-white to light pink powder and is soluble in aqueous buffers across a pH range of 1 to 8.

Jakafi (ruxolitinib) Tablets are for oral administration. Each tablet contains ruxolitinib phosphate equivalent to 5 mg, 10 mg, 15 mg, 20 mg and 25 mg of ruxolitinib free base together with microcrystalline cellulose, lactose monohydrate, magnesium stearate, colloidal silicon dioxide, sodium starch glycolate, povidone and hydroxypropyl cellulose.

12. CLINICAL PHARMACOLOGY

12.1 Mechanism of Action

Ruxolitinib, a kinase inhibitor, inhibits Janus Associated Kinases (JAKs) JAK1 and JAK2 which mediate the signaling of a number of cytokines and growth factors that are important for hematopoiesis and immune function. JAK signaling involves recruitment of STATs (signal transducers and activators of transcription) to cytokine receptors, activation and subsequent localization of STATs to the nucleus leading to modulation of gene expression.

Myelofibrosis (MF) and polycythemia vera (PV) are myeloproliferative neoplasms (MPN) known to be associated with dysregulated JAK1 and JAK2 signaling. In a mouse model of JAK2V617F-positive MPN, oral administration of ruxolitinib prevented splenomegaly, preferentially decreased JAK2V617F mutant cells in the spleen and decreased circulating inflammatory cytokines (eg, TNF-α, IL-6).

12.2 Pharmacodynamics

Ruxolitinib inhibits cytokine induced STAT3 phosphorylation in whole blood from healthy subjects and patients with MF and PV. Jakafi administration resulted in maximal inhibition of STAT3 phosphorylation 2 hours after dosing which returned to near baseline by 10 hours in both healthy subjects and patients with MF and PV.

12.3 Pharmacokinetics

Absorption

In clinical studies, ruxolitinib is rapidly absorbed after oral Jakafi administration with maximal plasma concentration (C_{max}) achieved within 1 to 2 hours post-dose. Based on a mass balance study in humans, oral absorption of ruxolitinib was estimated to be at least 95%. Mean ruxolitinib C_{max} and total exposure (AUC) increased proportionally over a single dose range of 5 to 200 mg. There were no clinically relevant changes in the pharmacokinetics of ruxolitinib upon administration of Jakafi with a high-fat meal, with the mean C_{max} moderately decreased (24%) and the mean AUC nearly unchanged (4% increase).

Distribution

The mean volume of distribution at steady-state is 72 L in patients with MF with an associated inter-subject variability of 29% and 75 L in patients with PV with an associated inter-subject variability of 23%. Binding to plasma proteins *in vitro* is approximately 97%, mostly with albumin.

Metabolism

In vitro studies suggest that ruxolitinib is metabolized by CYP3A4 and to a lesser extent by CYP2C9.

Elimination

Following a single oral dose of [^{14}C]-labeled ruxolitinib in healthy adult subjects, elimination was predominately through metabolism with 74% of radioactivity excreted in urine and 22% excretion via feces. Unchanged drug accounted for less than 1% of the excreted total radioactivity. The mean elimination half-life of ruxolitinib is approximately 3 hours and the mean half-life of ruxolitinib + metabolites is approximately 5.8 hours.

Effects of Age, Gender, or Race

In healthy subjects, no significant differences in ruxolitinib pharmacokinetics were observed with regard to gender and race. In a population pharmacokinetic evaluation in patients with MF, no relationship was apparent between oral clearance and patient age or race, and in women, clearance was 17.7 L/h and in men, 22.1 L/h with 39% inter-subject variability. Clearance was 12.7 L/h in patients with PV, with a 42% inter-subject variability, and no relationship was apparent between oral clearance and gender, patient age or race in this patient population.

Drug Interactions

Strong CYP3A4 inhibitors : In a trial of 16 healthy volunteers, a single dose of 10 mg of Jakafi was administered alone on Day 1 and a single dose of 10 mg of Jakafi was administered on Day 5 in combination with 200 mg of ketoconazole (a strong CYP3A4 inhibitor, given twice daily on Days 2 to 5). Ketoconazole increased ruxolitinib C_{max} and

AUC by 33% and 91%, respectively. Ketoconazole also prolonged ruxolitinib half-life from 3.7 to 6.0 hours [*see Dosage and Administration (2.3) and Drug Interactions (7.1)*].

Fluconazole : Simulations using physiologically-based pharmacokinetic (PBPK) models suggested that fluconazole (a dual CYP3A4 and CYP2C9 inhibitor) increases steady state ruxolitinib AUC by approximately 100% to 300% following concomitant administration of 10 mg of Jakafi twice daily with 100 mg to 400 mg of fluconazole once daily, respectively [*see Dosage and Administration (2.3) and Drug Interactions (7.1)*].

Mild or moderate CYP3A4 inhibitors : In a trial of 15 healthy volunteers, a single dose of 10 mg of Jakafi was administered alone on Day 1 and a single dose of 10 mg of Jakafi was administered on Day 5 in combination with 500 mg of erythromycin (a moderate CYP3A4 inhibitor, given twice daily on Days 2 to 5). Erythromycin increased ruxolitinib C_{max} and AUC by 8% and 27%, respectively [*see Drug Interactions (7.1)*].

CYP3A4 inducers : In a trial of 12 healthy volunteers, a single dose of 50 mg of Jakafi was administered alone on Day 1 and a single dose of 50 mg of Jakafi was administered on Day 13 in combination with 600 mg of rifampin (a strong CYP3A4 inducer, given once daily on Days 3 to 13). Rifampin decreased ruxolitinib C_{max} and AUC by 32% and 61%, respectively. In addition, the relative exposure to ruxolitinib's active metabolites increased approximately 100% [*see Drug Interactions (7.1)*].

In vitro studies : *In vitro*, ruxolitinib and its M18 metabolite do not inhibit CYP1A2, CYP2B6, CYP2C8, CYP2C9, CYP2C19, CYP2D6 or CYP3A4. Ruxolitinib is not an inducer of CYP1A2, CYP2B6 or CYP3A4 at clinically relevant concentrations.

In vitro, ruxolitinib and its M18 metabolite do not inhibit the P-gp, BCRP, OATP1B1, OATP1B3, OCT1, OCT2, OAT1 or OAT3 transport systems at clinically relevant concentrations. Ruxolitinib is not a substrate for the P-gp transporter.

12.4 Thorough QT Study

The effect of single dose ruxolitinib 25 mg and 200 mg on QTc interval was evaluated in a randomized, placebo-, and active-controlled (moxifloxacin 400 mg) four-period crossover thorough QT study in 47 healthy subjects. In a study with demonstrated ability to detect small effects, the upper bound of the one-sided 95% confidence interval for the largest placebo adjusted, baseline-corrected QTc based on Fridericia correction method (QTcF) was below 10 ms, the threshold for regulatory concern. The dose of 200 mg is adequate to represent the high exposure clinical scenario.

13. NONCLINICAL TOXICOLOGY

13.1 Carcinogenesis, Mutagenesis, Impairment of Fertility

Ruxolitinib was not carcinogenic in the 6-month Tg.rasH2 transgenic mouse model or in a 2-year carcinogenicity study in the rat.

Ruxolitinib was not mutagenic in a bacterial mutagenicity assay (Ames test) or clastogenic in *in vitro* chromosomal aberration assay (cultured human peripheral blood lymphocytes) or *in vivo* in a rat bone marrow micronucleus assay. In a fertility study, ruxolitinib was administered to male rats prior to and throughout mating and to female rats prior to mating and up to the implantation day (gestation day 7). Ruxolitinib had no effect on fertility or reproductive function in male or female rats at doses of 10, 30 or 60 mg/kg/day. However, in female rats doses of greater than or equal to 30 mg/kg/day resulted in increased post-implantation loss. The exposure (AUC) at the dose of 30 mg/kg/day is approximately 34% the clinical exposure at the maximum recommended dose of 25 mg twice daily.

14. CLINICAL STUDIES

14.1 Myelofibrosis

Two randomized Phase 3 studies (Studies 1 and 2) were conducted in patients with myelofibrosis (either primary myelofibrosis, post-polycythemia vera myelofibrosis or post-essential thrombocythemia-myelofibrosis). In both studies, patients had palpable splenomegaly at least 5 cm below the costal margin and risk category of intermediate 2 (2 prognostic factors) or high risk (3 or more prognostic factors) based on the International Working Group Consensus Criteria (IWG).

The starting dose of Jakafi was based on platelet count. Patients with a platelet count between 100 and 200 × 10^9/L were started on Jakafi 15 mg twice daily and patients with a platelet count greater than 200 × 10^9/L were started on Jakafi 20 mg twice daily. Doses were then individualized based upon tolerability and efficacy with maximum doses of 20 mg twice daily for patients with platelet counts between 100 to less than or equal to 125 × 10^9/L, of 10 mg twice daily for patients with platelet counts between 75 to less than or equal to 100 × 10^9/L, and of 5 mg twice daily for patients with platelet counts between 50 to less than or equal to 75 × 10^9/L.

Study 1

Study 1 was a double-blind, randomized, placebo-controlled study in 309 patients who were refractory to or were not candidates for available therapy. The median age was 68 years (range 40 to 91 years) with 61% of patients older than 65 years and 54% were male. Fifty percent (50%) of patients had primary myelofibrosis, 31% had post-polycythemia vera myelofibrosis and 18% had post-essential thrombocythemia myelofibrosis. Twenty-one percent (21%) of patients had red blood cell transfusions within 8 weeks of enrollment in the study. The median hemoglobin count was 10.5 g/dL and the median platelet count was 251 × 10^9/L. Patients had a median palpable spleen length of 16 cm below the costal margin, with 81% having a spleen length 10 cm or greater below the costal margin. Patients had a median spleen volume as measured by magnetic resonance imaging (MRI) or computed tomography (CT) of 2595 cm^3 (range 478 cm^3 to 8881 cm^3). (The upper limit of normal is approximately 300 cm^3).

Patients were dosed with Jakafi or matching placebo. The primary efficacy endpoint was the proportion of patients

Table 13: Polycythemia Vera: Selected Laboratory Abnormalities in the Open-Label, Active-controlled Study up to Week 32 of Randomized Treatment*

Laboratory Parameter	Jakafi (N=110)			Best Available Therapy (N=111)		
	All Grades[†] (%)	Grade 3 (%)	Grade 4 (%)	All Grades (%)	Grade 3 (%)	Grade 4 (%)
Hematology						
Anemia	72	<1	<1	58	0	0
Thrombocytopenia	27	5	<1	24	3	<1
Neutropenia	3	0	<1	10	<1	0
Chemistry						
Hypercholesterolemia	35	0	0	8	0	0
Elevated ALT	25	<1	0	16	0	0
Elevated AST	23	0	0	23	<1	0
Hypertriglyceridemia	15	0	0	13	0	0

* Presented values are worst Grade values regardless of baseline
† National Cancer Institute Common Terminology Criteria for Adverse Events, version 3.0

achieving greater than or equal to a 35% reduction from baseline in spleen volume at Week 24 as measured by MRI or CT.

Secondary endpoints included duration of a 35% or greater reduction in spleen volume and proportion of patients with a 50% or greater reduction in Total Symptom Score from baseline to Week 24 as measured by the modified Myelofibrosis Symptom Assessment Form (MFSAF) v2.0 diary.

Study 2

Study 2 was an open-label, randomized study in 219 patients. Patients were randomized 2:1-to Jakafi versus best available therapy. Best available therapy was selected by the investigator on a patient-by-patient basis. In the best available therapy arm, the medications received by more than 10% of patients were hydroxyurea (47%) and glucocorticoids (16%). The median age was 66 years (range 35 to 85 years) with 52% of patients older than 65 years and 57% were male. Fifty-three percent (53%) of patients had primary myelofibrosis, 31% had post-polycythemia vera myelofibrosis and 16% had post-essential thrombocythemia myelofibrosis. Twenty-one percent (21%) of patients had red blood cell transfusions within 8 weeks of enrollment in the study. The median hemoglobin count was 10.4 g/dL and the median platelet count was 236×10^9/L. Patients had a median palpable spleen length of 15 cm below the costal margin, with 70% having a spleen length 10 cm or greater below the costal margin. Patients had a median spleen volume as measured by MRI or CT of 2381 cm^3 (range 451 cm^3 to 7765 cm^3).

The primary efficacy endpoint was the proportion of patients achieving 35% or greater reduction from baseline in spleen volume at Week 48 as measured by MRI or CT.

A secondary endpoint in Study 2 was the proportion of patients achieving a 35% or greater reduction of spleen volume as measured by MRI or CT from baseline to Week 24.

Study 1 and 2 Efficacy Results

Efficacy analyses of the primary endpoint in Studies 1 and 2 are presented in Table 14 below. A significantly larger proportion of patients in the Jakafi group achieved a 35% or greater reduction in spleen volume from baseline in both studies compared to placebo in Study 1 and best available therapy in Study 2. A similar proportion of patients in the Jakafi group achieved a 50% or greater reduction in palpable spleen length.

[See table 14 above]

Figure 1 shows the percent change from baseline in spleen volume for each patient at Week 24 (Jakafi N=139, placebo N=106) or the last evaluation prior to Week 24 for patients who did not complete 24 weeks of randomized treatment (Jakafi N=16, placebo N=47). One (1) patient (placebo) with a missing baseline spleen volume is not included.

[See Figure 1 on next page]

In Study 1, myelofibrosis symptoms were a secondary endpoint and were measured using the modified Myelofibrosis Symptom Assessment Form (MFSAF) v2.0 diary. The modified MFSAF is a daily diary capturing the core symptoms of myelofibrosis (abdominal discomfort, pain under left ribs, night sweats, itching, bone/muscle pain and early satiety). Symptom scores ranged from 0 to 10 with 0 representing symptoms "absent" and 10 representing "worst imaginable" symptoms. These scores were added to create the daily total score, which has a maximum of 60.

Table 15 presents assessments of Total Symptom Score from baseline to Week 24 in Study 1 including the proportion of patients with at least a 50% reduction (ie, improvement in symptoms). At baseline, the mean Total Symptom Score was 18.0 in the Jakafi group and 16.5 in the placebo group. A higher proportion of patients in the Jakafi group had a 50% or greater reduction in Total Symptom Score than in the placebo group, with a median time to response of less than 4 weeks.

Table 15: Improvement in Total Symptom Score in Patients with Myelofibrosis

	Jakafi (N=148)	Placebo (N=152)
Number (%) of Patients with 50% or Greater Reduction in Total Symptom Score by Week 24	68 (46)	8 (5)
P-value	< 0.0001	

Figure 2 shows the percent change from baseline in Total Symptom Score for each patient at Week 24 (Jakafi N=129, placebo N=103) or the last evaluation on randomized ther-

apy prior to Week 24 for patients who did not complete 24 weeks of randomized treatment (Jakafi N=16, placebo N=42). Results are excluded for 5 patients with a baseline Total Symptom Score of zero, 8 patients with missing baseline and 6 patients with insufficient post-baseline data.

[See Figure 2 on next page]

Figure 3 displays the proportion of patients with at least a 50% improvement in each of the individual symptoms that comprise the Total Symptom Score indicating that all 6 of the symptoms contributed to the higher Total Symptom Score response rate in the group treated with Jakafi.

[See Figure 3 on next page]

Overall survival was a secondary endpoint in both Study 1 and Study 2. Patients in the control groups were eligible for crossover in both studies, and the median times to crossover were 9 months in Study 1 and 17 months in Study 2.

Figure 4 and Figure 5 show Kaplan-Meier curves of overall survival at prospectively planned analyses after all patients remaining on study had completed 144 weeks on study.

[See Figures 4 and 5 on page 981]

14.2 Polycythemia Vera

Study 3 was a randomized, open-label, active-controlled Phase 3 study conducted in 222 patients with polycythemia vera. Patients had been diagnosed with polycythemia vera for at least 24 weeks, had an inadequate response to or were intolerant of hydroxyurea, required phlebotomy and exhibited splenomegaly. All patients were required to demonstrate hematocrit control between 40-45% prior to randomization. The age ranged from 33 to 90 years with 30% of patients over 65 years of age and 66% were male. Patients had a median spleen volume as measured by MRI or CT of 1272 cm^3 (range 254 cm^3 to 5147 cm^3) and median palpable spleen length below the costal margin was 7 cm.

Patients were randomized to Jakafi or best available therapy. The starting dose of Jakafi was 10 mg twice daily. Doses were then individualized based upon tolerability and efficacy with a maximum dose of 25 mg twice daily. At Week 32, 98 patients were still on Jakafi with 8% receiving greater than 20 mg twice daily, 15% receiving 20 mg twice daily, 33% receiving 15 mg twice daily, 34% receiving 10 mg twice daily, and 10% receiving less than 10 mg twice daily. Best available therapy (BAT) was selected by the investigator on a patient-by-patient basis and included hydroxyurea (60%), interferon/pegylated interferon (12%), anagrelide (7%), pipobroman (2%), lenalidomide/thalidomide (5%), and observation (15%).

The primary endpoint was the proportion of subjects achieving a response at Week 32, with response defined as having achieved both hematocrit control (the absence of phlebotomy eligibility beginning at the Week 8 visit and continuing through Week 32) and spleen volume reduction (a greater than or equal to 35% reduction from baseline in spleen volume at Week 32). Phlebotomy eligibility was defined as a confirmed hematocrit greater than 45% that is at least 3 percentage points higher than the hematocrit obtained at baseline or a confirmed hematocrit greater than 48%, whichever was lower. Secondary endpoints included the proportion of all randomized subjects who achieved the primary endpoint and who maintained their response 48 weeks after randomization, and the proportion of subjects achieving complete hematological remission at Week 32 with complete hematological remission defined as achieving hematocrit control, platelet count less than or equal to 400×10^9/L, and white blood cell count less than or equal to 10×10^9/L.

Results of the primary and secondary endpoints are presented in Table 16. A significantly larger proportion of patients on the Jakafi arm achieved a response for the primary endpoint compared to best available therapy at Week 32 and maintained their response 48 weeks after random-

ization. A significantly larger proportion of patients on the Jakafi arm compared to best available therapy also achieved complete hematological remission at Week 32.

Table 16: Percent of Patients with Polycythemia Vera Achieving the Primary and Key Secondary Endpoints in Study 3 (Intent to Treat)

	Jakafi (N=110)	Best Available Therapy (N=112)
Number (%) of Patients Achieving a Primary Response at Week 32	25 (23%)	1 (<1%)
95% CI of the response rate (%)	(15%, 32%)	(0%, 5%)
P-value	< 0.0001	
Number (%) of Patients Achieving a Durable Primary Response at Week 48	22 (20%)	1 (<1%)
95% CI of the response rate (%)	(13%, 29%)	(0%, 5%)
P-value	< 0.0001	
Number (%) of Patients Achieving Complete Hematological Remission at Week 32	26 (24%)	9 (8%)
95% CI of the response rate (%)	(16%, 33%)	(4%, 15%)
P-value	0.0016	

Primary Response defined as having achieved both the absence of phlebotomy eligibility beginning at the Week 8 visit and continuing through Week 32 and a greater than or equal to 35% reduction from baseline in spleen volume at Week 32.

Additional analyses for Study 3 to assess durability of response were conducted at Week 80 only in the Jakafi arm. On this arm, 91 (83%) patients were still on treatment at the time of the Week 80 data cut-off. Of the 25 patients who achieved a primary response at Week 32, 19 (76% of the responders) maintained their response through Week 80, and of the 26 patients who achieved complete hematological remission at Week 32, 15 (58% of the responders) maintained their response through Week 80.

In an assessment of the individual components that make up the primary endpoint, there were 66 (60%) patients with hematocrit control on the Jakafi arm vs. 21 (19%) patients on best available therapy at Week 32; 51 (77% of hematocrit responders) patients on the Jakafi arm maintained hematocrit control through Week 80. There were 44 (40%) patients with spleen volume reduction from baseline greater than or equal to 35% on the Jakafi arm vs. 1 (<1%) patient on best available therapy at Week 32; 43 (98% of spleen volume reduction responders) patients on the Jakafi arm maintained spleen volume reduction through Week 80.

Table 14: Percent of Patients with Myelofibrosis Achieving 35% or Greater Reduction from Baseline in Spleen Volume at Week 24 in Study 1 and at Week 48 in Study 2 (Intent to Treat)

	Study 1		Study 2	
	Jakafi (N=155)	Placebo (N=154)	Jakafi (N=146)	Best Available Therapy (N=73)
Time Points	Week 24		Week 48	
Number (%) of Patients with Spleen Volume Reduction by 35% or More	65 (42)	1 (<1)	41 (29)	0
P-value	< 0.0001		< 0.0001	

Continued on next page

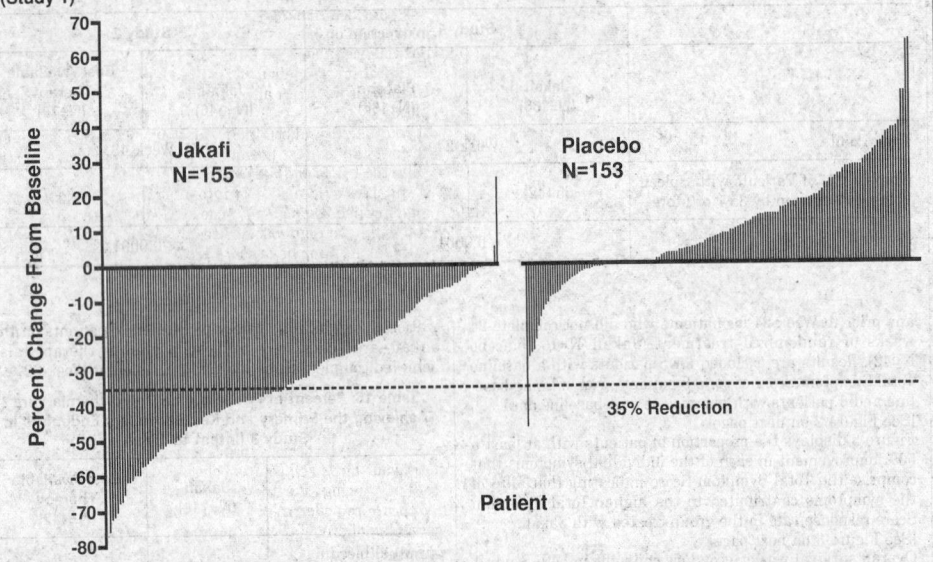

Figure 1: Percent Change from Baseline in Spleen Volume at Week 24 or Last Observation for Each Patient (Study 1)

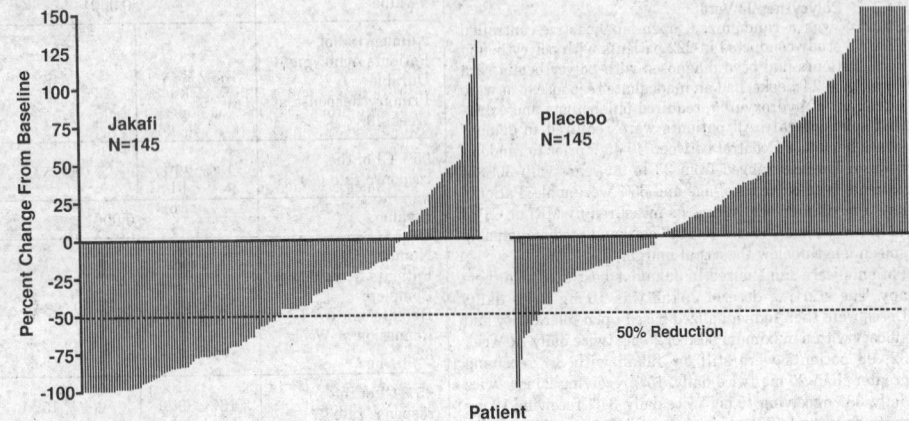

Figure 2: Percent Change from Baseline in Total Symptom Score at Week 24 or Last Observation for Each Patient (Study 1)

Worsening of Total Symptom Score is truncated at 150%.

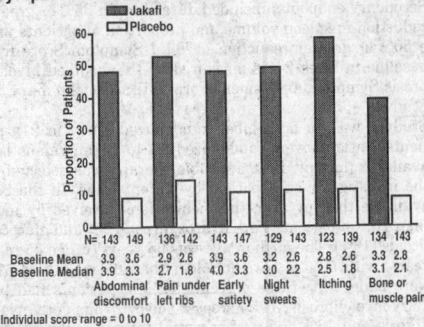

Figure 3: Proportion of Patients With Myelofibrosis Achieving 50% or Greater Reduction in Individual Symptom Scores at Week 24

Individual score range = 0 to 10

**Patient Information
JAKAFI® (JAK-ah-fye)
(ruxolitinib)
tablets**

Read this Patient Information before you start taking Jakafi and each time you get a refill. There may be new information. This information does not take the place of talking to your healthcare provider about your medical condition or treatment.

What is Jakafi?
Jakafi is a prescription medicine used to treat certain types of myelofibrosis.
Jakafi is also used to treat people with polycythemia vera who have already taken a medicine called hydroxyurea and it did not work well enough or they could not tolerate it.
It is not known if Jakafi is safe or effective in children.

What should I tell my healthcare provider before taking Jakafi?
Before taking Jakafi, tell your healthcare provider if you:
• have an infection
• have or had tuberculosis (TB), or have been in close contact with someone who has TB
• have or had hepatitis B
• have or have had liver problems
• have or have had kidney problems or are on dialysis. If you are on dialysis, Jakafi should be taken after your dialysis
• have had skin cancer in the past
• have any other medical conditions
• are pregnant or plan to become pregnant. It is not known if Jakafi will harm your unborn baby.
• are breastfeeding or plan to breastfeed. It is not known if Jakafi passes into your breast milk. You and your healthcare provider should decide if you will take Jakafi or breastfeed. You should not do both.
Tell your healthcare provider about all the medicines you take, including prescription and over-the-counter medicines, vitamins and herbal supplements. Taking Jakafi with certain other medicines may affect how Jakafi works. Especially tell your healthcare provider if you take medicine for:
• Fungal infections
• Bacterial infections
• HIV-AIDS
Ask your healthcare provider or pharmacist if you are not sure if your medicine is one listed above.
Know the medicines you take. Keep a list of them to show your healthcare provider and pharmacist when you get a new medicine.

How should I take Jakafi?
• Take Jakafi exactly as your healthcare provider tells you.
• Do not change your dose or stop taking Jakafi without first talking to your healthcare provider.
• You can take Jakafi with or without food.
• Jakafi may also be given through certain nasogastric tubes.
○ Tell your healthcare provider if you cannot take Jakafi

---

16. HOW SUPPLIED/STORAGE AND HANDLING
Jakafi (ruxolitinib) Tablets are available as follows:
[See table on bottom of next page]

17. PATIENT COUNSELING INFORMATION
See FDA-approved patient labeling (Patient Information). Discuss the following with patients prior to and during treatment with Jakafi:
Thrombocytopenia, Anemia and Neutropenia
Inform patients that Jakafi is associated with thrombocytopenia, anemia and neutropenia, and of the need to monitor complete blood counts before and during treatment. Advise patients to observe for and report bleeding.
Infections
Inform patients of the signs and symptoms of infection and to report any such signs and symptoms promptly.
Inform patients regarding the early signs and symptoms of herpes zoster and of progressive multifocal leukoencephalopathy, and advise patients to seek advice of a clinician if such symptoms are observed.
Symptom Exacerbation Following Interruption or Discontinuation of Treatment with Jakafi
Inform patients that after discontinuation of treatment, signs and symptoms from myeloproliferative neoplasms are expected to return. Instruct patients not to interrupt or discontinue Jakafi therapy without consulting their physician.

Non-Melanoma Skin Cancer
Inform patients that Jakafi may increase their risk of certain non-melanoma skin cancers. Advise patients to inform their healthcare provider if they have ever had any type of skin cancer or if they observe any new or changing skin lesions.
Lipid Elevations
Inform patients that Jakafi may increase blood cholesterol, and of the need to monitor blood cholesterol levels.
Drug-drug Interactions
Advise patients to inform their healthcare providers of all medications they are taking, including over-the-counter medications, herbal products and dietary supplements.
Dialysis
Inform patients on dialysis that their dose should not be taken before dialysis but only following dialysis.
Compliance
Advise patients to continue taking Jakafi every day for as long as their physician tells them and that this is a long-term treatment. Patients should not change dose or stop taking Jakafi without first consulting their physician. Patients should be aware that after discontinuation of treatment, signs and symptoms from myeloproliferative neoplasms are expected to return.
Manufactured for:
Incyte Corporation
Wilmington, DE 19803

Figure 4: Overall Survival - Kaplan-Meier Curves by Treatment Group in Study 1

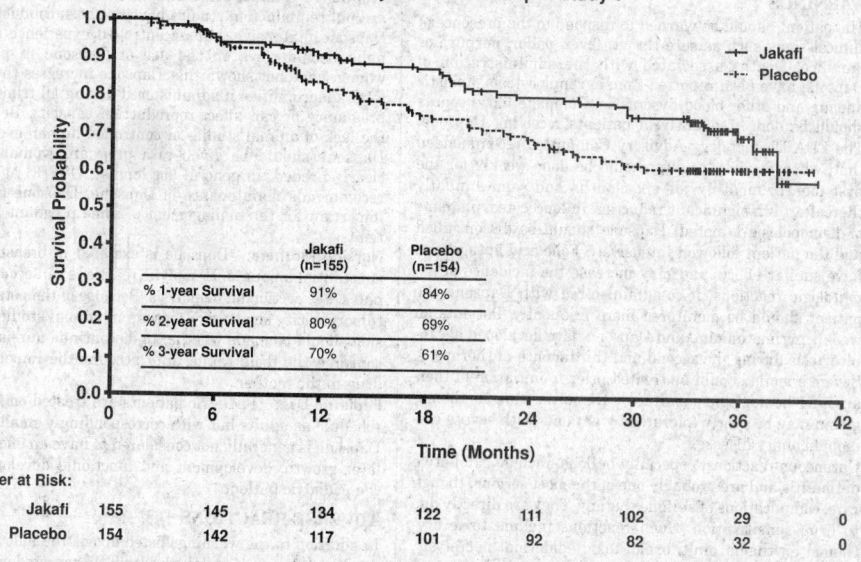

	Jakafi (n=155)	Placebo (n=154)
% 1-year Survival	91%	84%
% 2-year Survival	80%	69%
% 3-year Survival	70%	61%

Number at Risk:

Jakafi	155	145	134	122	111	102	29	0
Placebo	154	142	117	101	92	82	32	0

Figure 5: Overall Survival - Kaplan-Meier Curves by Treatment Group in Study 2

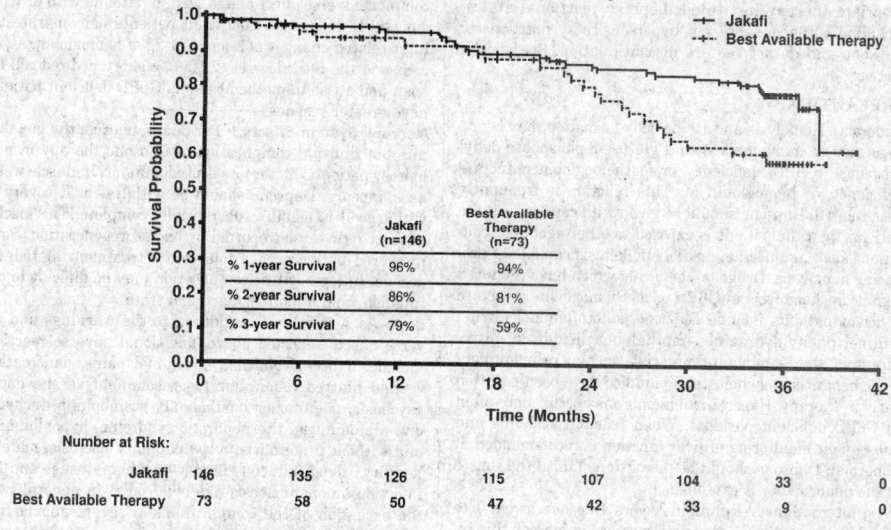

	Jakafi (n=146)	Best Available Therapy (n=73)
% 1-year Survival	96%	94%
% 2-year Survival	86%	81%
% 3-year Survival	79%	59%

Number at Risk:

Jakafi	146	135	126	115	107	104	33	0
Best Available Therapy	73	58	50	47	42	33	9	0

Jakafi Trade Presentations

NDC Number	Strength	Description	Tablets per Bottle
50881-005-60	5 mg	Round tablet with "INCY" on one side and "5" on the other	60
50881-010-60	10 mg	Round tablet with "INCY" on one side and "10" on the other	60
50881-015-60	15 mg	Oval tablet with "INCY" on one side and "15" on the other	60
50881-020-60	20 mg	Capsule shaped tablet with "INCY" on one side and "20" on the other	60
50881-025-60	25 mg	Oval tablet with "INCY" on one side and "25" on the other	60

Store at room temperature 20°C to 25°C (68°F to 77°F); excursions permitted between 15°C and 30°C (59°F and 86°F) [see USP Controlled Room Temperature].

by mouth. Your healthcare provider will decide if you can take Jakafi through a nasogastric tube.

○ Ask your healthcare provider to give you specific instruction on how to properly take Jakafi through a nasogastric tube.

• Do not drink grapefruit juice while taking Jakafi. Grapefruit juice can affect the amount of Jakafi in your blood.

• If you take too much Jakafi call your healthcare provider or go to the nearest hospital emergency room right away. Take the bottle of Jakafi with you.

• If you miss a dose of Jakafi, take your next dose at your regular time. Do not take 2 doses at the same time.

• You will have regular blood tests during your treatment with Jakafi. Your healthcare provider may change your dose of Jakafi or stop your treatment based on the results of your blood tests.

What are the possible side effects of Jakafi?
Jakafi can cause serious side effects including:
Low blood cell counts. Jakafi may cause low platelet counts (thrombocytopenia), low red blood cell counts (anemia), and low white blood cell counts (neutropenia). If you develop bleeding, stop Jakafi and call your healthcare provider. Your healthcare provider will do a blood test to check your blood cell counts before you start Jakafi and regularly during your treatment with Jakafi. Tell your healthcare provider right away if you develop or have worsening of any of these symptoms:

• unusual bleeding	• shortness of breath
• bruising	• fever
• tiredness	

Infection. You may be at risk for developing a serious infection during treatment with Jakafi. Tell your healthcare provider if you develop any of the following symptoms of infection:

• chills	• vomiting
• aches	• weakness
• fever	• painful skin rash or
• nausea	blisters

Skin cancers. Some people who take Jakafi have developed certain types of non-melanoma skin cancers. Tell your healthcare provider if you develop any new or changing skin lesions during treatment with Jakafi.

Cholesterol increases. You may have changes in your blood cholesterol levels. Your healthcare provider will do blood tests to check your cholesterol levels during treatment with Jakafi.

The most common side effects of Jakafi include:

• low platelet count (thrombocytopenia)	• dizziness
	• headache
• low red blood cell counts (anemia)	
• bruising	

Tell your healthcare provider about any side effect that bothers you or that does not go away.

These are not all the possible side effects of Jakafi. Ask your healthcare provider or pharmacist for more information.

Call your doctor for medical advice about side effects. You may report side effects to FDA at 1-800-FDA-1088. You may also report side effects to Incyte Corporation at 1-855-463-3463.

How should I store Jakafi?
• Store Jakafi at room temperature from 68°F to 77°F (20°C to 25°C).
Keep Jakafi and all medicines out of the reach of children.

General information about the safe and effective use of Jakafi.
Medicines are sometimes prescribed for purposes other than those listed in Patient Information. Do not use Jakafi for a condition for which it is not prescribed. Do not give Jakafi to other people, even if they have the same symptoms you have. It may harm them.

This Patient Information leaflet summarizes the most important information about Jakafi. If you would like more information, talk with your healthcare provider. You can ask your pharmacist or healthcare provider for information that is written for healthcare professionals. For more information call 1-855-463-3463 or go to www.jakafi.com.

Continued on next page

What are the ingredients in Jakafi?
Active ingredient: ruxolitinib phosphate
Inactive ingredients: microcrystalline cellulose, lactose monohydrate, magnesium stearate, colloidal silicon dioxide, sodium starch glycolate, povidone and hydroxypropyl cellulose

Manufactured for:
Incyte Corporation
Wilmington, DE 19803
Jakafi is a registered trademark of Incyte. All rights reserved.
U.S. Patent Nos. 7598257; 8415362; 8722693; 8822481; 8829013; 9079912
© 2011-2016 Incyte Corporation. All rights reserved.

This Patient Information has been approved by the U.S. Food and Drug Administration.
Revised: March 2016

Jacobus Pharmaceutical Co., Inc.

37 CLEVELAND LANE
P.O. BOX 5290
PRINCETON, NJ 08540

Direct All Inquiries to:
(609) 921-7447
FAX: (609) 799-1176

DAPSONE   ℞
[*dap´sŏne*]
Tablets, USP
25 mg & 100 mg

DESCRIPTION
Dapsone-USP, 4,4′-diaminodiphenylsulfone (DDS), is a primary treatment for Dermatitis herpetiformis. It is an antibacterial drug for susceptible cases of leprosy. It is a white, odorless crystalline powder, practically insoluble in water and insoluble in fixed and vegetable oils.
Dapsone is issued on prescription in tablets of 25 and 100 mg for oral use.

$$NH_2-\!\!\langle\ \rangle\!\!-SO_2-\!\!\langle\ \rangle\!\!-NH_2$$

Inactive Ingredients: Colloidal silicone dioxide, magnesium stearate, microcrystalline cellulose and corn starch.
Contains no ingredient made from a gluten-containing grain (wheat, barley, or rye).

CLINICAL PHARMACOLOGY
Actions: The mechanism of action in Dermatitis herpetiformis has not been established. By the kinetic method in mice, Dapsone is bactericidal as well as bacteriostatic against *Mycobacterium leprae*.
Absorption and Excretion: Dapsone, when given orally, is rapidly and almost completely absorbed. About 85 percent of the daily intake is recoverable from the urine mainly in the form of water-soluble metabolites. Excretion of the drug is slow and a constant blood level can be maintained with the usual dosage.
Blood Levels: Detected a few minutes after ingestion, the drug reaches peak concentration in 4-8 hours. Daily administration for at least eight days is necessary to achieve a plateau level. With doses of 200 mg daily, this level averaged 2.3 μg/ml with a range of 0.1-7.0 μg/ml. The half-life in the plasma in different individuals varies from ten hours to fifty hours and averages twenty-eight hours. Repeat tests in the same individual are constant. Daily administration (50-100 mg) in leprosy patients will provide blood levels in excess of the usual minimum inhibitory concentration even for patients with a short Dapsone half-life.

INDICATIONS AND USAGE
Dermatitis herpetiformis: (D.H.)
Leprosy: All forms of leprosy except for cases of proven Dapsone resistance.

CONTRAINDICATION
Hypersensitivity to Dapsone and/or its derivatives.

WARNINGS
The patient should be warned to respond to the presence of clinical signs such as sore throat, fever, pallor, purpura or jaundice. Deaths associated with the administration of Dapsone have been reported from agranulocytosis, aplastic anemia and other blood dyscrasias. Complete blood counts should be done frequently in patients receiving Dapsone. The FDA Dermatology Advisory Committee recommended that, when feasible, counts should be done weekly for the first month, monthly for six months and semi-annually thereafter. If a significant reduction in leucocytes, platelets or hemopoiesis is noted, Dapsone should be discontinued and the patient followed intensively. Folic acid antagonists have similar effects and may increase the incidence of hematologic reactions; if co-administered with Dapsone the patient should be monitored more frequently. Patients on weekly pyrimethamine and Dapsone have developed agranulocytosis during the second and third month of therapy. Severe anemia should be treated prior to initiation of therapy and hemoglobin monitored. Hemolysis and methemoglobin may be poorly tolerated by patients with severe cardiopulmonary disease.
Cutaneous reactions, especially bullous, include exfoliative dermatitis and are probably one of the most serious, though rare, complications of sulfone therapy. They are directly due to drug sensitization. Such reactions include toxic erythema, erythema multiforme, toxic epidermal necrolysis, morbilliform and scarlatiniform reactions, urticaria and erythema nodosum. If new or toxic dermatologic reactions occur, sulfone therapy must be promptly discontinued and appropriate therapy instituted. Leprosy reactional states, including cutaneous, are not hypersensitivity reactions to Dapsone and do not require discontinuation. See special section.

PRECAUTIONS
General: Hemolysis and Heinz body formation may be exaggerated in individuals with a glucose-6-phosphate dehydrogenase (G6PD) deficiency, or methemoglobin reductase deficiency, or hemoglobin M. This reaction is frequently dose-related. Dapsone should be given with caution to these patients or if the patient is exposed to other agents or conditions such as infection or diabetic ketosis capable of producing hemolysis. Drugs or chemicals which have produced significant hemolysis in G6PD or methemoglobin reductase deficient patients include Dapsone, sulfanilamide, nitrite, aniline, phenylhydrazine, napthalene, niridazole, nitrofurantoin and 8-amino-antimalarials such as primaquine. Toxic hepatitis and cholestatic jaundice have been reported early in therapy. Hyperbilirubinemia may occur more often in G6PD deficient patients. When feasible, baseline and subsequent monitoring of liver function is recommended; if abnormal, Dapsone should be discontinued until the source of the abnormality is established.
Drug Interactions: Rifampin lowers Dapsone levels 7 to 10-fold by accelerating plasma clearance; in leprosy this reduction has not required a change in dosage. Folic acid antagonists such as pyrimethamine may increase the likelihood of hematological reactions.
A modest interaction has been reported for patients receiving 100 mg Dapsone daily in combination with trimethoprim 5 mg/kg q6h. On Day 7, the serum Dapsone levels averaged 2.1 ± 1.0 μg/mL in comparison to 1.5 ± 0.5 μg/mL for Dapsone alone. On Day 7, trimethoprim levels averaged 18.4 ± 5.2 μg/mL in comparison to 12.4 ± 4.5 μg/mL for patients not receiving Dapsone. Thus, there is a mutual interaction between Dapsone and trimethoprim in which each raises the level of the other about 1.5 times.
A crossover study[1] designed to assess the potential of a drug interaction between Dapsone, 100 mg/day and trimethoprim, 200 mg every 12 hours, in eight asymptomatic HIV positive volunteers (average CD4 count 524 cells/mm³) demonstrated that there was not a significant drug interreaction between Dapsone and trimethoprim. However, an earlier report[2] also by Lee et al, in 78 HIV infected patients with acute *Pneumocystis carinii* pneumonia, receiving Dapsone, 100 mg/day and higher trimethoprim dose, 20 mg/kg/day, demonstrated that the serum levels of Dapsone were increased by 40% and trimethoprim levels were increased by 48% when the drugs were administered concurrently.
Carcinogenesis, mutagenesis: Dapsone has been found carcinogenic (sarcomagenic) for male rats and female mice causing mesenchymal tumors in the spleen and peritoneum, and thyroid carcinoma in female rats. Dapsone is not mutagenic with or without microsomal activation in *S. typhimurium* tester strains 1535, 1537, 1538, 98, or 100.

Pregnancy: Teratogenic Effects. Pregnancy Category C: Animal reproduction studies have not been conducted with Dapsone. Extensive, but uncontrolled experience and two published surveys on the use of Dapsone in pregnant women have not shown that Dapsone increases the risk of fetal abnormalities if administered during all trimesters of pregnancy or can affect reproduction capacity. Because of the lack of animal studies or controlled human experience, Dapsone should be given to a pregnant woman only if clearly needed. In general, for leprosy, USPHS at Carville recommends maintenance of Dapsone. Dapsone has been important for the management of some pregnant D.H. patients.
Nursing Mothers: Dapsone is excreted in breast milk in substantial amounts. Hemolytic reactions can occur in neonates. See section on hemolysis. Because of the potential for tumorgenicity shown for Dapsone in animal studies a decision should be made whether to discontinue nursing or discontinue the drug taking into account the importance of drug to the mother.
Pediatric Use: Pediatric patients are treated on the same schedule as adults but with correspondingly smaller doses. Dapsone is generally not considered to have an effect on the later growth, development and functional development of the pediatric patient.

ADVERSE REACTIONS
In addition to the warnings listed above, the following syndromes and serious reactions have been reported in patients on Dapsone.
Hematologic Effects: Dose-related hemolysis is the most common adverse effect and is seen in patients with or without G6PD deficiency. Almost all patients demonstrate the inter-related changes of a loss of 1-2g of hemoglobin, an increase in the reticulocytes (2-12%), a shortened red cell life span and a rise in methemoglobin. G6PD deficient patients have greater responses.
Nervous System Effects: Peripheral neuropathy is a definite but unusual complication of Dapsone therapy in non-leprosy patients. Motor loss is predominant. If muscle weakness appears, Dapsone should be withdrawn. Recovery on withdrawal is usually substantially complete. The mechanism of recovery is reported by axonal regeneration. Some recovered patients have tolerated retreatment at reduced dosage. In leprosy this complication may be difficult to distinguish from a leprosy reactional state.
Body As A Whole: In addition to the warnings and adverse effects reported above, additional adverse reactions include: nausea, vomiting, abdominal pains, pancreatitis, vertigo, blurred vision, tinnitus, insomnia, fever, headache, psychosis, phototoxicity, pulmonary eosinophilia, tachycardia, albuminuria, the nephrotic syndrome, hypoalbuminemia without proteinuria, renal papillary necrosis, male infertility, drug-induced Lupus erythematosus and an infectious mononucleosis-like syndrome. In general, with the exception of the complications of severe anoxia from overdosage (retinal and optic nerve damage, etc.) these adverse reactions have regressed off drug.

OVERDOSAGE
Nausea, vomiting, hyperexcitability can appear a few minutes up to 24 hours after ingestion of an overdosage. Methemoglobin induced depression, convulsions or severe cyanosis requires prompt treatment. In normal and methemoglobin reductase deficient patients, methylene blue, 1-2 mg/kg of body weight, given slowly intravenously, is the treatment of choice. The effect is complete in 30 minutes, but may have to be repeated if methemoglobin reaccumulates. For non-emergencies, if treatment is needed, methylene blue may be given orally in doses of 3-5 mg/kg every 4-6 hours. Methylene blue reduction depends on G6PD and should not be given to fully expressed G6PD deficient patients.

DOSAGE AND ADMINISTRATION
Dermatitis herpetiformis: The dosage should be individually titrated starting in adults with 50 mg daily and correspondingly smaller doses in children. If full control is not achieved within the range of 50-300 mg daily, higher doses may be tried. Dosage should be reduced to a minimum maintenance level as soon as possible. In responsive patients there is a prompt reduction in pruritus followed by clearance of skin lesions. There is no effect on the gastrointestinal component of the disease. Dapsone levels are influenced by acetylation rates. Patients with high acetylation rates, or who are receiving treatment affecting acetylation may require an adjustment in dosage.

A strict gluten free diet is an option for the patient to elect, permitting many to reduce or eliminate the need for Dapsone; the average time for dosage reduction is 8 months with a range of 4 months to 2 1/2 years and for dosage elimination 29 months with a range of 6 months to 9 years.

Leprosy: In order to reduce secondary Dapsone resistance, the WHO Expert Committee on Leprosy and the USPHS at Carville, LA, recommended that Dapsone should be commenced in combination with one or more anti-leprosy drugs. In the multidrug program Dapsone should be maintained at the full dosage of 100 mg daily without interruption (with corresponding smaller doses for children) and provided to all patients who have sensitive organisms with new or recrudescent disease or who have not yet completed a two year course of Dapsone monotherapy. For advice and other drugs, the USPHS at Carville, LA (1-800-642-2477) should be contacted. Before using other drugs consult appropriate product labeling.

In bacteriologically negative tuberculoid and indeterminate disease, the recommendation is the coadministration of Dapsone 100 mg daily with six months of Rifampin 600 mg daily. Under WHO, daily Rifampin may be replaced by 600 mg Rifampin monthly, if supervised. The Dapsone is continued until all signs of clinical activity are controlled - usually after an additional six months. Then Dapsone should be continued for an additional three years for tuberculoid and indeterminate patients and for five years for borderline tuberculoid patients.

In lepromatous and borderline lepromatous patients, the recommendation is the co-administration of Dapsone 100 mg daily with two years of Rifampin 600 mg daily. Under WHO daily Rifampin may be replaced by 600 mg Rifampin monthly, if supervised. One may elect the concurrent administration of a third anti-leprosy drug, usually either Clofazamine 50-100 mg daily or Ethionamide 250-500 mg daily. Dapsone 100 mg daily is continued 3-10 years until all signs of clinical activity are controlled with skin scrapings and biopsies negative for one year. Dapsone should then be continued for an additional 10 years for borderline patients and for life for lepromatous patients.

Secondary Dapsone resistance should be suspected whenever a lepromatous or borderline lepromatous patient receiving Dapsone treatment relapses clinically and bacteriologically, solid staining bacilli being found in the smears taken from the new active lesions. If such cases show no response to regular and supervised Dapsone therapy within three to six months or good compliance for the past 3-6 months can be assured, Dapsone resistance should be considered confirmed clinically. Determination of drug sensitivity using the mouse footpad method is recommended and, after prior arrangement, is available without charge from the USPHS, Carville, LA. Patients with proven Dapsone resistance should be treated with other drugs.

LEPROSY REACTIONAL STATES

Abrupt changes in clinical activity occur in leprosy with any effective treatment and are known as reactional states. The majority can be classified into two groups. The "Reversal" reaction (Type 1) may occur in borderline or tuberculoid leprosy patients often soon after chemotherapy is started. The mechanism is presumed to result from a reduction in the antigenic load: the patient is able to mount an enhanced delayed hypersensitivity response to residual infection leading to swelling ("Reversal") of existing skin and nerve lesions. If severe, or if neuritis is present, large doses of steroids should always be used. If severe, the patient should be hospitalized. In general anti-leprosy treatment is continued and therapy to suppress the reaction is indicated such as analgesics, steroids, or surgical decompression of swollen nerve trunks. USPHS at Carville, LA should be contacted for advice in management.

Erythema nodosum leprosum (ENL) (lepromatous reaction) (Type 2 reaction) occurs mainly in lepromatous patients and small numbers of borderline patients. Approximately 50% of treated patients show this reaction in the first year. The principal clinical features are fever and tender erythematous skin nodules sometimes associated with malaise, neuritis, orchitis, albuminuria, joint swelling, iritis, epistaxis or depression. Skin lesions can become pustular and/or ulcerate. Histologically there is a vasculitis with an intense polymorphonuclear infiltrate. Elevated circulating immune complexes are considered to be the mechanism of reaction. If severe, patients should be hospitalized. In general, anti-leprosy treatment is continued. Analgesics, steroids, and other agents available from USPHS, Carville, LA, are used to suppress the reaction.

HOW SUPPLIED

Dapsone Tablets USP, 25 mg are available as round white scored tablets, debossed "25" above and "102" below the score and on the obverse "JACOBUS" in a Unit of Use carton of 30 tablets (2 × 15). The blisters are light and child-resistant. NDC 49938-102-30.

Dapsone Tablets USP, 100 mg are available as round white scored tablets, debossed "100" above and "101" below the score and on the obverse "JACOBUS" in a Unit of Use carton of 30 tablets (2 × 15). The blisters are light and child-resistant. NDC 49938-101-30.

Dapsone Tablets USP, 25 mg are available as round white scored tablets, debossed "25" above and "102" below the score and on the obverse "JACOBUS" in a Unit of Use carton of 28 tablets (2 × 14). The blisters are light and child-resistant. NDC 49938-102-28.

Dapsone Tablets USP, 100 mg are available as round white scored tablets, debossed "100" above and "101" below the score and on the obverse "JACOBUS" in a Unit of Use carton of 28 tablets (2 × 14). The blisters are light and child-resistant. NDC 49938-101-28.

Dapsone Tablets USP, 25 mg are available as round white scored tablets, debossed "25" above and "102" below the score and on the obverse "JACOBUS" in light and child-resistant bottles of 100. NDC 49938-102-01.

Dapsone Tablets USP, 100 mg are available as round white scored tablets, debossed "100" above and "101" below the score and on the obverse "JACOBUS" in light and child-resistant bottles of 100. NDC 49938-101-01.

REFERENCES

1. Lee, B., et al., Zidovudine, Trimethoprim, and Dapsone Pharmacokinetic Interactions in Patients with HIV Infection. *Antimicrobial Agents and Chemotherapy*, May 1996; 1231-1236.
2. Lee, B., et al., Dapsone, Trimethoprim, and Sulfamethoxazole Plasma Levels During Treatment of Pneumocystis Carinii Pneumonia in Patients with AIDS, *Annals of Internal Medicine*, 1989; 110:606-611.

Store at 20° -25° C (68°-77°F). [see USP Controlled Room Temperature]. Protect from light.

Rx only. Keep this and all medication out of the reach of children.

JACOBUS PHARMACEUTICAL CO., INC.
P.O. Box 5290
Princeton, NJ 08540
Revised August 2016
PDR082016

PASER® GRANULES ℞

[Pa - ser]

(4 grams aminosalicylic acid delayed-release granules)

DESCRIPTION

PASER granules are a delayed release granule preparation of aminosalicylic acid (p-aminosalicylic acid; 4-aminosalicylic acid) for use with other anti-tuberculosis drugs for the treatment of all forms of active tuberculosis due to susceptible strains of tubercle bacilli. The granules are designed for gradual release to avoid high peak levels not useful (and perhaps toxic) with bacteriostatic drugs. Aminosalicylic acid is rapidly degraded in acid media; the protective acid-resistant outer coating is rapidly dissolved in neutral media so a mildly acidic food such as orange, apple or tomato juice, yogurt or apple sauce should be used.

Aminosalicylic acid (p-aminosalicylic acid) is 4-Amino-2-hydroxybenzoic acid. PASER granules are the free base of aminosalicylic acid and do NOT contain sodium or a sugar. The molecular formula is $C_7H_7NO_3$ with a molecular weight of 153.14. With heat p-aminosalicylic acid is decarboxylated to produce CO_2 and m-aminophenol. If the airtight packets are swollen, storage has been improper. DO NOT USE if packets are swollen or the granules have lost their tan color and are dark brown or purple.

The structural formula is:

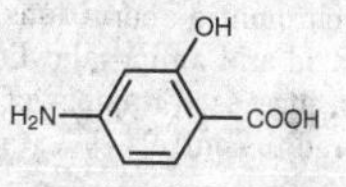

PASER granules are supplied as off-white tan colored granules with an average diameter of 1.5 mm and an average content of 60% aminosalicylic acid by weight. The acid resistant outer coating will be completely removed by a few minutes at a neutral pH. The inert ingredients are:

- colloidal silicon dioxide
- dibutyl sebacate
- hydroxypropyl methyl cellulose
- methacrylic acid copolymer
- microcrystalline cellulose
- talc

The packets contain 4 grams of aminosalicylic acid for oral administration three times a day by sprinkling on apple sauce or yogurt to be eaten without chewing. Suspension in an acidic fruit drink such as orange juice or tomato juice will protect the coating for at least 2 hours. Swirling the juice in the glass will help resuspend the granules if they sink.

CLINICAL PHARMACOLOGY

Mechanism of Action: Aminosalicylic acid is bacteriostatic against Mycobacterium tuberculosis. It inhibits the onset of bacterial resistance to streptomycin and isoniazid. The mechanism of action has been postulated to be inhibition of folic acid synthesis (but without potentiation with antifolic compounds) and/or inhibition of synthesis of the cell wall component, mycobactin, thus reducing iron uptake by M. tuberculosis.

Characteristics: The two major considerations in the clinical pharmacology of aminosalicylic acid are the prompt production of a toxic inactive metabolite under acid conditions and the short serum half life of one hour for the free drug. Both are discussed below.

After two hours in simulated gastric fluid, 10% of unprotected aminosalicylic acid is decarboxylated to form meta-aminophenol, a known hepatotoxin. The acid-resistant coating of the PASER granules protects against degradation in the stomach. The small granules are designed to escape the usual restriction on gastric emptying of large particles. Under neutral conditions such as are found in the small intestine or in neutral foods, the acid-resistant coating is dissolved within one minute. Care must be taken in the administration of these granules to protect the acid-resistant coating by maintaining the granules in an acidic food during dosage administration. Patients who have neutralized gastric acid with antacids will not need to protect the acid resistant coating with an acidic food since no acid is present to spoil the drug. Antacids may influence the absorption of other medications and are not necessary for PASER consumed with an acidic food.

Because PASER granules are protected by an enteric coating absorption does not commence until they leave the stomach; the soft skeletons of the granules remain and may be seen in the stool.

Absorption and excretion: In a single 4 gram pharmacokinetic study with food in normal volunteers the initial time to a 2µg/mL serum level of aminosalicylic acid was 2 hours with a range of 45 minutes to 24 hours; the median time to peak was 6 hours with a range of 1.5 to 24 hours; the mean peak level was 20 µg/mL with a range of 9 to 35 µg/mL; a level of 2 µg/mL was maintained for an average of 7.9 hours with a range of 5 to 9; a level of 1 µg/mL was maintained for an average of 8.8 hours with a range of 6 to 11.5 hours. The recommended schedule is 4 grams every 8 hours.

80% of aminosalicylic acid is excreted in the urine, with 50% or more of the dosage excreted in acetylated form. The acetylation process is not genetically determined as is the case for isoniazid. Aminosalicylic acid is excreted by glomerular filtration; although previously reported otherwise, probenecid, a tubular blocking agent, does not enhance plasma concentration. In a 1954 study thyroxine synthesis but not iodide uptake was reported reduced about 40% when the sodium salt (not PASER granules) of aminosalicylic acid was administered one hour before radio-iodine; the sodium salt typically produces a serum level over 120 µg/mL at one hour lasting one hour. Occasional goiter development can be prevented by the administration of thyroxine but not iodide. Penetration into the cerebrospinal fluid occurs only if the meminges are inflamed.

Approximately 50-60% of aminosalicylic acid is protein bound; binding is reported to be reduced 50% in kwashiorkor.

Microbiology: The aminosalicylic acid MIC for M. tuberculosis in 7H11 agar was less than 1.0 µg/mL for nine strains including three multidrug resistant strains, but 4 and 8 µg/mL for two other multidrug resistant strains. The 90% inhibition in 7H12 broth (Bactec) showed little dose response but was interpreted as being less than or equal to 0.12-0.25 µg/mL for eight strains of which three were multi-

Continued on next page

resistant, 0.50 µg/mL for one resistant strain, questionable for four non-resistant strains and greater than 1µg/mL for one non-resistant and three resistant strains. Aminosalicylic acid is not active in vitro against M. avium.

INDICATIONS AND USAGE

PASER is indicated for the treatment of tuberculosis in combination with other active agents. It is most commonly used in patients with Multi-drug Resistant TB (MDR-TB) or in situations when therapy with isoniazid and rifampin is not possible due to a combination of resistance and/or intolerance. When PASER is added to the treatment regimen in patients proven or suspected drug resistance, it should be accompanied by at least one and preferably two other new agents to which the patient's organism is known or expected to be susceptible.

CONTRAINDICATIONS

Hypersensitivity to any component of this medication. Severe renal disease.

Patients with severe renal disease will accumulate aminosalicylic acid and its acetyl metabolite but will continue to acetylate, thus leading exclusively to the inactive acetylated form; deacetylation, if any, is not significant.

The half life of free aminosalicylic acid in renal disease is 30.8 minutes in comparison to 26.4 minutes in normal volunteers. but the half life of the inactive metabolite is 309 minutes in uremic patients in comparison to 51 minutes in normal volunteers. Although aminosalicylic acid passes dialysis membranes, the frequency of dialysis usually is not comparable to the half-life of 50 minutes for the free acid. Patients with end stage renal disease should not receive aminosalicylic acid.

WARNINGS

Liver Function

In one retrospective study of 7492 patients on rapidly absorbed aminosalicylic acid preparations, drug-induced hepatitis occurred in 38 patients (0.5%); in these 38 the first symptom usually appeared within three months of the start of therapy with a rash as the most common event followed by fever and much less frequently by GI disturbances of anorexia, nausea or diarrhea. Only one patient was diagnosed on routine biochemistry.

Premonitory symptoms in 90% of these 38 patients preceded jaundice by a few days to several weeks with the mean time of onset 33 days with a range of 7-90 days. Half of the adverse reactions occurred during the third, fourth or fifth weeks. When aminosalicylic acid-induced hepatitis was diagnosed, hepatomegaly was invariably present with lymphadenopathy in 46%, leucocytosis in 79%, and eosinophilia in 55%. Prompt recognition with discontinuation led to the recovery of all 38 patients. If recognized in the premonitory stage, the reaction is reported to "settle" in 24 hours and no jaundice ensues. From other reported studies failure to recognize the reaction can result in a mortality of up to 21%. The patient must be monitored carefully during the first three months of therapy and treatment must be discontinued immediately at the first sign of a rash, fever or other premonitory signs of intolerance.

PRECAUTIONS

(1) General:

All drugs should be stopped at the first sign suggesting a hypersensitivity reaction. They may be restarted one at a time in very small but gradually increasing doses to determine whether the manifestations are drug-induced and, if so, which drug is responsible.

Desensitization has been accomplished successfully in 15 of 17 patients starting with 10 mg aminosalicylic acid given as a single dose. The dosage is doubled every 2 days until reaching a total of 1 gram after which the dosage is divided to follow the regular schedule of administration. If a mild temperature rise or skin reaction develops, the increment is to be dropped back one level or the progression held for one cycle. Reactions are rare after a total dosage of 1.5 grams. Patients with hepatic disease may not tolerate aminosalicylic acid as well as normal patients, even though the metabolism in patients with hepatic disease has been reported to be comparable to that in normal volunteers.

(2) Information for Patients:

The patient should be advised that the first signs of hypersensitivity include a rash, often followed by fever, and much less frequently, GI disturbances of anorexia, nausea or diarrhea. If such symptoms develop, the patient should immediately cease taking the medication and arrange for a prompt clinical visit.

Patients should be advised that poor compliance in taking anti-TB medication often leads to treatment failure, and, not infrequently, to the development of resistance of the organisms in the individual patient.

Patients should be advised that the skeleton of the granules may be seen in the stool.

The coating to protect the PASER granules dissolves promptly under neutral conditions; the granules therefore should be administered by sprinkling on acidic foods such as apple sauce or yogurt or by suspension in a fruit drink which will protect the coating, but the granules sink and will have to be swirled. The coating will last at least 2 hours in either system. All juices tested to date have been satisfactory; tested are: tomato, orange, grapefruit, grape, cranberry, apple, "fruit punch".

Patients should be advised to store PASER in a refrigerator or freezer. PASER packets may be stored at room temperature for short periods of time.

Patients should be advised NOT to use if the packets are swollen or the granules have lost their tan color and are dark brown or purple. The patient should inform the pharmacist or physician immediately and return the medication.

(3) Laboratory Tests:

Aminosalicylic acid has been reported to interfere technically with the serum determinations of albumin by dye-binding, SGOT by the azoene dye method and with qualitative urine tests for ketones, bilirubin, urobilinogen or porphobilinogen.

(4) Drug Interactions:

Aminosalicylic acid at a dosage of 12 grams in a rapidly available form has been reported to produce a 20 percent reduction in the acetylation of isoniazid, especially in patients who are rapid acetylators; INH serum levels, half lives and excretions in fast acetylators still remain half of the levels seen in slow acetylators with or without p-aminosalicylic acid. The effect is dose related and, while it has not been studied with the current delayed release preparation, the lower serum levels with this preparation will result in a reduced effect on the acetylation of INH.

Aminosalicylic acid has previously been reported to block the absorption of rifampin. A subsequent report has shown that this blockade was due to an excipient not included in PASER granules. Oral administration of a solution containing both aminosalicylic acid and rifampin showed full absorption of each product.

As a result of competition, Vitamin B_{12} absorption has been reduced 55% by 5 grams of aminosalicylic acid with clinically significant erythrocyte abnormalities developing after depletion; patients on therapy of more than one month should be considered for maintenance B_{12}.

A malabsorption syndrome can develop in patients on aminosalicylic acid but is usually not complete. The complete syndrome includes steatorrhea, an abnormal small bowel pattern on x-ray, villus atrophy, depressed cholesterol, reduced D-xylose and iron absorption. Triglyceride absorption always is normal.

In one literature report 8 hours after the last dosage of aminosalicylic acid at 2 gm qid serum digoxin levels were reduced 40% in two of ten patients but not changed in the remaining eight.

(5) Carcinogenesis, mutagenesis, impairment of fertility:

Sodium aminosalicylate produced an occipital bone defect, probably with a dose response, when administered to ten pregnant Wistar rats at five doses from 3.85 to 385 mg/kg from days 6 to 14. There were no significant changes from controls in any group in corpora lutea, early resorptions, total resorptions, fetal death, litter size, or hematomas. For all except the 77 mg/kg group, fetal weights were significantly greater than controls. Chinchilla rabbits on 5 mg/kg from days 7 to 14 did not show any significant differences as compared to controls for the same parameters studied.

Sodium aminosalicylic acid was not mutagenic in Ames tester strain TA 100. In human lymphocyte cultures in-vitro clastogenic effects of achromatic, chromatid, isochromatic breaks or chromatid translocations were not seen at 153 or 600 µg/mL. At 1500 and 3000 µg/mL there was a dose related increase in chromatid aberrations.

Patients on isoniazid and aminosalicylic acid have been reported to have an increased number of chromosomal aberrations as compared to controls.

(6) Pregnancy: Pregnancy Category C:

Aminosalicylic acid has been reported to produce occipital malformations in rats when given at doses within the human dose range. Although there probably is a dose response, the frequency of abnormalities was comparable to

controls at the highest level tested (two times the human dosage). When administered to rabbits at 5 mg/kg, throughout all three trimesters, no teratologic or embryocidal effects were seen. Literature reports on aminosalicylic acid in pregnant women always report coadministration of other medications. Because there are no adequate and well controlled studies of aminosalicylic acid in humans, PASER granules should be given to a pregnant woman only if clearly needed.

(8) Nursing mothers:

After administration of a different preparation of aminosalicylic acid to one patient, the maximum concentration in the milk was 1 µg/mL at 3 hours with a half-life of 2.5 hours; the maximum maternal plasma concentration was 70 µg/mL at two hours.

ADVERSE EFFECTS

The most common side effect is gastrointestinal intolerance manifested by nausea, vomiting, diarrhea, and abdominal pain.

Hypersensitivity reactions: Fever, skin eruptions of various types, including exfoliative dermatitis, infectious mononucleosis-like, or lymphoma-like syndrome, leucopenia, agranulocytosis, thrombocytopenia, Coombs' positive hemolytic anemia, jaundice, hepatitis, pericarditis, hypoglycemia, optic neuritis, encephalopathy, Leoffler's syndrome, vasculitis and a reduction in prothrombin.

Crystalluria may be prevented by the maintenance of urine at a neutral or an alkaline pH.

OVERDOSAGE

Overdosage has not been reported.

DOSAGE AND ADMINISTRATION

PASER granules should be administered with other drugs to which the organism is known or expected to be susceptible. It is most commonly administered to patients with Multi-drug Resistant TB (MDR-TB) or in other situations in which therapy with isoniazid or rifampin is not possible due to a combination of resistance and/or intolerance. The adult dosage of four grams (one packet) three times per day or correspondingly smaller doses in children should be given by sprinkling on apple sauce or yogurt or by swirling in the glass to suspend the granules in an acidic drink such as tomato or orange juice.

DO NOT USE if packet is swollen or the granules have lost their tan color, turning dark brown or purple.

HOW SUPPLIED

Carton of 30 PASER packets (NDC 49938-107-04).

Each packet contains four grams aminosalicylic acid.

PASER granules are supplied in packets containing 4 grams of aminosalicylic acid for administration three times a day by suspension in an acidic drink or food with a pH less than 5. Examples include apple sauce, yogurt, tomato or orange juice.

Distributors and Pharmacists: Store below 59°F (15°C) (in a refrigerator or freezer).

Patients are urged to store PASER in a refrigerator or freezer. PASER packets may be stored at room temperature for short periods of time.

AVOID EXCESSIVE HEAT. DO NOT USE if packet is swollen or the granules have lost their tan color, turning dark brown or purple.

JACOBUS PHARMACEUTICAL CO. INC.

P.O. Box 5290

Princeton, NJ 08540

2A JULY, 1996

Kowa Pharmaceuticals America, Inc.

530 INDUSTRIAL PARK BOULEVARD
MONTGOMERY, AL 36117

Tel: 334.288.1288
Fax: 334.288.2788
info@KowaPharma.com

LIVALO®　　　　　　　　　　℞
(pitavastatin)
Tablet, Film Coated for Oral use

HIGHLIGHTS OF PRESCRIBING INFORMATION
These highlights do not include all the information needed to use LIVALO® safely and effectively. See full prescribing information for LIVALO.

LIVALO (pitavastatin) Tablet, Film Coated for Oral use
Initial U.S. Approval: 2009

──────RECENT MAJOR CHANGES──────

None

──────INDICATIONS AND USAGE──────

LIVALO is a HMG-CoA reductase inhibitor indicated for:
• Patients with primary hyperlipidemia or mixed dyslipidemia as an adjunctive therapy to diet to reduce elevated total cholesterol (TC), low-density lipoprotein cholesterol (LDL-C), apolipoprotein B (Apo B), triglycerides (TG), and to increase high-density lipoprotein cholesterol (HDL-C) (1.1)

Limitations of Use (1.2):
• Doses of LIVALO greater than 4 mg once daily were associated with an increased risk for severe myopathy in pre-marketing clinical studies. Do not exceed 4 mg once daily dosing of LIVALO.
• The effect of LIVALO on cardiovascular morbidity and mortality has not been determined.
• LIVALO has not been studied in Fredrickson Type I, III, and V dyslipidemias.

──────DOSAGE AND ADMINISTRATION──────

• LIVALO can be taken with or without food, at any time of day (2.1) Dose Range: 1 mg to 4 mg once daily (2.1)
• Primary hyperlipidemia and mixed dyslipidemia: Starting dose 2 mg. When lowering of LDL-C is insufficient, the dosage may be increased to a maximum of 4 mg per day. (2.1)
• Moderate and severe renal impairment (glomerular filtration rate 30 – 59 and 15 - 29 mL/min/1.73 m², respectively) as well as end-stage renal disease on hemodialysis: Starting dose of 1 mg once daily and maximum dose of 2 mg once daily (2.2)

──────DOSAGE FORMS AND STRENGTHS──────

• Tablets: 1 mg, 2 mg, and 4 mg (3)

──────CONTRAINDICATIONS──────

• Known hypersensitivity to product components (4)
• Active liver disease, which may include unexplained persistent elevations in hepatic transaminase levels (4)
• Women who are pregnant or may become pregnant (4, 8.1)
• Nursing mothers (4, 8.3)
• Co-administration with cyclosporine (4, 7.1, 12.3)

──────WARNINGS AND PRECAUTIONS──────

• Skeletal muscle effects (e.g., myopathy and rhabdomyolysis): Risks increase in a dose-dependent manner, with advanced age (≥65), renal impairment, and inadequately treated hypothyroidism. Advise patients to promptly report unexplained and/or persistent muscle pain, tenderness, or weakness, and discontinue LIVALO (5.1)
• Liver enzyme abnormalities: Persistent elevations in hepatic transaminases can occur. Check liver enzyme tests before initiating therapy and as clinically indicated thereafter (5.2)

──────ADVERSE REACTIONS──────

The most frequent adverse reactions (rate ≥2.0% in at least one marketed dose) were myalgia, back pain, diarrhea, constipation and pain in extremity. (6)

To report SUSPECTED ADVERSE REACTIONS, contact Kowa Pharmaceuticals, Inc. at 1-877-334-3464 or FDA at 1-800-FDA-1088 or www.fda.gov/medwatch.

──────DRUG INTERACTIONS──────

• Erythromycin: Combination increases pitavastatin exposure. Limit LIVALO to 1 mg once daily (2.3, 7.2)
• Rifampin: Combination increases pitavastatin exposure. Limit LIVALO to 2 mg once daily (2.4, 7.3)
• Concomitant lipid-lowering therapies: Use with fibrates or lipid-modifying doses (≥1 g/day) of niacin increases the risk of adverse skeletal muscle effects. Caution should be used when prescribing with LIVALO. (5.1, 7.4, 7.5)

──────USE IN SPECIFIC POPULATIONS──────

• Pediatric use: Safety and effectiveness have not been established. (8.4)
• Renal impairment: Limitation of a starting dose of LIVALO 1 mg once daily and a maximum dose of LIVALO 2 mg once daily for patients with moderate and severe renal impairment as well as patients receiving hemodialysis (2.2, 8.6)

See 17 for PATIENT COUNSELING INFORMATION.
　　　　　　　　　　　　　　　　Revised: 2/2012

FULL PRESCRIBING INFORMATION

1　INDICATIONS AND USAGE

Drug therapy should be one component of multiple-risk-factor intervention in individuals who require modifications of their lipid profile. Lipid-altering agents should be used in addition to a diet restricted in saturated fat and cholesterol only when the response to diet and other nonpharmacological measures has been inadequate.

1.1　Primary Hyperlipidemia and Mixed Dyslipidemia
LIVALO® is indicated as an adjunctive therapy to diet to reduce elevated total cholesterol (TC), low-density lipopro-

tein cholesterol (LDL-C), apolipoprotein B (Apo B), triglycerides (TG), and to increase HDL-C in adult patients with primary hyperlipidemia or mixed dyslipidemia.

1.2　Limitations of Use
Doses of LIVALO greater than 4 mg once daily were associated with an increased risk for severe myopathy in premarketing clinical studies. Do not exceed 4 mg once daily dosing of LIVALO.
The effect of LIVALO on cardiovascular morbidity and mortality has not been determined.
LIVALO has not been studied in Fredrickson Type I, III, and V dyslipidemias.

2　DOSAGE AND ADMINISTRATION
2.1　General Dosing Information
The dose range for LIVALO is 1 to 4 mg orally once daily at any time of the day with or without food. The recommended starting dose is 2 mg and the maximum dose is 4 mg. The starting dose and maintenance doses of LIVALO should be individualized according to patient characteristics, such as goal of therapy and response.
After initiation or upon titration of LIVALO, lipid levels should be analyzed after 4 weeks and the dosage adjusted accordingly.
2.2　Dosage in Patients with Renal Impairment
Patients with moderate and severe renal impairment (glomerular filtration rate 30 – 59 mL/min/1.73 m² and 15 – 29 mL/min/1.73 m² not receiving hemodialysis, respectively) as well as end-stage renal disease receiving hemodialysis should receive a starting dose of LIVALO 1 mg once daily and a maximum dose of LIVALO 2 mg once daily.
2.3　Use with Erythromycin
In patients taking erythromycin, a dose of LIVALO 1 mg once daily should not be exceeded [see Drug Interactions (7.2)].
2.4　Use with Rifampin
In patients taking rifampin, a dose of LIVALO 2 mg once daily should not be exceeded [see Drug Interactions (7.3)].

3　DOSAGE FORMS AND STRENGTHS

1 mg: Round white film-coated tablet. Debossed "KC" on one side and "1" on the other side of the tablet.

2 mg: Round white film-coated tablet. Debossed "KC" on one side and "2" on the other side of the tablet.

4 mg: Round white film-coated tablet. Debossed "KC" on one side and "4" on the other side of the tablet.

4　CONTRAINDICATIONS

The use of LIVALO is contraindicated in the following conditions:
• Patients with a known hypersensitivity to any component of this product. Hypersensitivity reactions including rash, pruritus, and urticaria have been reported with LIVALO [see Adverse Reactions (6.1)].
• Patients with active liver disease which may include unexplained persistent elevations of hepatic transaminase levels [see Warnings and Precautions (5.2), Use in Specific Populations (8.7)].
• Women who are pregnant or may become pregnant. Because HMG-CoA reductase inhibitors decrease cholesterol synthesis and possibly the synthesis of other biologically active substances derived from cholesterol, LIVALO may cause fetal harm when administered to pregnant women. Additionally, there is no apparent benefit to therapy during pregnancy, and safety in pregnant women has not been established. If the patient becomes pregnant while taking this drug, the patient should be apprised of the potential hazard to the fetus and the lack of known clinical benefit with continued use during pregnancy [see Use in Specific Populations (8.1) and Nonclinical Toxicology (13.2)].
• Nursing mothers. Animal studies have shown that LIVALO passes into breast milk. Since HMG-CoA reductase inhibitors have the potential to cause serious adverse reactions in nursing infants, LIVALO, like other HMG-CoA reductase inhibitors, is contraindicated in pregnant or nursing mothers [see Use in Specific Populations (8.3) and Nonclinical Toxicology (13.2)].
• Co-administration with cyclosporine [see Drug Interactions (7.1) and Clinical Pharmacology (12.3)].

5　WARNINGS AND PRECAUTIONS
5.1　Skeletal Muscle Effects
Cases of myopathy and rhabdomyolysis with acute renal failure secondary to myoglobinuria have been reported with HMG-CoA reductase inhibitors, including LIVALO. These risks can occur at any dose level, but increase in a dose-dependent manner.

Continued on next page

LIVALO should be prescribed with caution in patients with predisposing factors for myopathy. These factors include advanced age (≥65 years), renal impairment, and inadequately treated hypothyroidism. The risk of myopathy may also be increased with concurrent administration of fibrates or lipid-modifying doses of niacin. LIVALO should be administered with caution in patients with impaired renal function, in elderly patients, or when used concomitantly with fibrates or lipid-modifying doses of niacin [see Drug Interactions (7.6), Use in Specific Populations (8.5, 8.6) and Clinical Pharmacology (12.3)].

Cases of myopathy, including rhabdomyolysis, have been reported with HMG-CoA reductase inhibitors coadministered with colchicine, and caution should be exercised when prescribing LIVALO with colchicine [see Drug Interactions (7.7)].

There have been rare reports of immune-mediated necrotizing myopathy (IMNM), an autoimmune myopathy, associated with statin use. IMNM is characterized by: proximal muscle weakness and elevated serum creatine kinase, which persist despite discontinuation of statin treatment; muscle biopsy showing necrotizing myopathy without significant inflammation; improvement with immunosuppressive agents.

LIVALO therapy should be discontinued if markedly elevated creatine kinase (CK) levels occur or myopathy is diagnosed or suspected. LIVALO therapy should also be temporarily withheld in any patient with an acute, serious condition suggestive of myopathy or predisposing to the development of renal failure secondary to rhabdomyolysis (e.g., sepsis, hypotension, dehydration, major surgery, trauma, severe metabolic, endocrine, and electrolyte disorders, or uncontrolled seizures). All patients should be advised to promptly report unexplained muscle pain, tenderness, or weakness, particularly if accompanied by malaise or fever or if muscle signs and symptoms persist after discontinuing LIVALO.

5.2 Liver Enzyme Abnormalities

Increases in serum transaminases (aspartate aminotransferase [AST]/serum glutamic-oxaloacetic transaminase, or alanine aminotransferase [ALT]/serum glutamic-pyruvic transaminase) have been reported with HMG-CoA reductase inhibitors, including LIVALO. In most cases, the elevations were transient and resolved or improved on continued therapy or after a brief interruption in therapy.

In placebo-controlled Phase 2 studies, ALT >3 times the upper limit of normal was not observed in the placebo, LIVALO 1 mg, or LIVALO 2 mg groups. One out of 202 patients (0.5%) administered LIVALO 4 mg had ALT >3 times the upper limit of normal.

It is recommended that liver enzyme tests be performed before the initiation of LIVALO and if signs or symptoms of liver injury occur.

There have been rare postmarketing reports of fatal and non-fatal hepatic failure in patients taking statins, including pitavastatin. If serious liver injury with clinical symptoms and/or hyperbilirubinemia or jaundice occurs during treatment with LIVALO, promptly interrupt therapy. If an alternate etiology is not found do not restart LIVALO.

As with other HMG-CoA reductase inhibitors, LIVALO should be used with caution in patients who consume substantial quantities of alcohol. Active liver disease, which may include unexplained persistent transaminase elevations, is a contraindication to the use of LIVALO [see Contraindications (4)].

5.3 Endocrine Function

Increases in HbA1c and fasting serum glucose levels have been reported with HMG-CoA reductase inhibitors, including LIVALO.

6 ADVERSE REACTIONS

The following serious adverse reactions are discussed in greater detail in other sections of the label:
- Rhabdomyolysis with myoglobinuria and acute renal failure and myopathy (including myositis) [see Warnings and Precautions (5.1)].
- Liver Enzyme Abnormalities [see Warning and Precautions (5.2)].

Of 4,798 patients enrolled in 10 controlled clinical studies and 4 subsequent open-label extension studies, 3,291 patients were administered pitavastatin 1 mg to 4 mg daily. The mean continuous exposure of pitavastatin (1 mg to 4 mg) was 36.7 weeks (median 51.1 weeks). The mean age of the patients was 60.9 years (range; 18 years – 89 years) and the gender distribution was 48% males and 52% females.

Table 1. Adverse Reactions* Reported by ≥2.0% of Patients Treated with LIVALO and > Placebo in Short-Term Controlled Studies

Adverse Reactions*	Placebo N= 208	LIVALO 1 mg N=309	LIVALO 2 mg N=951	LIVALO 4 mg N=1540
Back Pain	2.9%	3.9%	1.8%	1.4%
Constipation	1.9%	3.6%	1.5%	2.2%
Diarrhea	1.9%	2.6%	1.5%	1.9%
Myalgia	1.4%	1.9%	2.8%	3.1%
Pain in extremity	1.9%	2.3%	0.6%	0.9%

* Adverse reactions by MedDRA preferred term.

Table 2. Effect of Co-Administered Drugs on Pitavastatin Systemic Exposure

Co-administered drug	Dose regimen	Change in AUC*	Change in C_{max}*
Cyclosporine	Pitavastatin 2 mg QD for 6 days + cyclosporine 2 mg/kg on Day 6	↑ 4.6 fold†	↑ 6.6 fold †
Erythromycin	Pitavastatin 4 mg single dose on Day 4 + erythromycin 500 mg 4 times daily for 6 days	↑ 2.8 fold †	↑ 3.6 fold †
Rifampin	Pitavastatin 4 mg QD + rifampin 600 mg QD for 5 days	↑ 29%	↑ 2.0 fold
Atazanavir	Pitavastatin 4 mg QD + atazanavir 300 mg daily for 5 days	↑ 31%	↑ 60%
Darunavir/Ritonavir	Pitavastatin 4mg QD on Days 1-5 and 12-16 + darunavir/ritonavir 800mg/100 mg QD on Days 6-16	↓ 26%	↓ 4%
Lopinavir/Ritonavir	Pitavastatin 4 mg QD on Days 1-5 and 20-24 + lopinavir/ritonavir 400 mg/100 mg BID on Days 9 – 24	↓ 20%	↓4 %
Gemfibrozil	Pitavastatin 4 mg QD + gemfibrozil 600 mg BID for 7 days	↑ 45%	↑ 31%
Fenofibrate	Pitavastatin 4 mg QD + fenofibrate 160 mg QD for 7 days	↑18%	↑ 11%
Ezetimibe	Pitavastatin 2 mg QD + ezetimibe 10 mg for 7 days	↓ 2%	↓0.2%
Enalapril	Pitavastatin 4 mg QD + enalapril 20 mg daily for 5 days	↑ 6%	↓ 7%
Digoxin	Pitavastatin 4 mg QD + digoxin 0.25 mg for 7 days	↑ 4%	↓ 9%
Diltiazem LA	Pitavastatin 4 mg QD on Days 1-5 and 11-15 and diltiazem LA 240 mg on Days 6-15	↑10%	↑15%
Grapefruit Juice	Pitavastatin 2 mg single dose on Day 3 + grapefruit juice for 4 days	↑ 15%	↓ 12%
Itraconazole	Pitavastatin 4 mg single dose on Day 4 + itraconazole 200 mg daily for 5 days	↓ 23%	↓ 22%

*Data presented as x-fold change represent the ratio between co-administration and pitavastatin alone (i.e., 1-fold = no change). Data presented as % change represent % difference relative to pitavastatin alone (i.e., 0% = no change).
† Considered clinically significant [see Dosage and Administration (2) and Drug Interactions (7)]
BID = twice daily; QD = once daily; LA = Long Acting

Approximately 93% of the patients were Caucasian, 7% were Asian/Indian, 0.2% were African American and 0.3% were Hispanic and other.

6.1 Clinical Studies Experience

Because clinical studies on LIVALO are conducted in varying study populations and study designs, the frequency of adverse reactions observed in the clinical studies of LIVALO cannot be directly compared with that in the clinical studies of other HMG-CoA reductase inhibitors and may not reflect the frequency of adverse reactions observed in clinical practice.

Adverse reactions reported in ≥ 2% of patients in controlled clinical studies and at a rate greater than or equal to placebo are shown in Table 1. These studies had treatment duration of up to 12 weeks.

[See table above]

Other adverse reactions reported from clinical studies were arthralgia, headache, influenza, and nasopharyngitis.

The following laboratory abnormalities have also been reported: elevated creatine phosphokinase, transaminases, alkaline phosphatase, bilirubin, and glucose.

In controlled clinical studies and their open-label extensions, 3.9% (1 mg), 3.3% (2 mg), and 3.7% (4 mg) of pitavastatin-treated patients were discontinued due to adverse reactions. The most common adverse reactions that led to treatment discontinuation were: elevated creatine phosphokinase (0.6% on 4 mg) and myalgia (0.5% on 4 mg). Hypersensitivity reactions including rash, pruritus, and urticaria have been reported with LIVALO.

6.2 Postmarketing Experience

The following adverse reactions have been identified during postapproval use of LIVALO. Because these reactions are reported voluntarily from a population of uncertain size, it is not always possible to reliably estimate their frequency or establish a causal relationship to drug exposure.

Adverse reactions associated with LIVALO therapy reported since market introduction, regardless of causality assessment, include the following: abdominal discomfort, abdominal pain, dyspepsia, nausea, asthenia, fatigue, malaise, hepatitis, jaundice, fatal and non-fatal hepatic failure, dizziness, hypoesthesia, insomnia, depression, interstitial lung disease, erectile dysfunction and muscle spasms.

There have been rare postmarketing reports of cognitive impairment (e.g., memory loss, forgetfulness, amnesia, memory impairment, confusion) associated with statin use. These cognitive issues have been reported for all statins. The reports are generally nonserious, and reversible upon statin discontinuation, with variable times to symptom onset (1 day to years) and symptom resolution (median of 3 weeks).

There have been rare reports of immune-mediated necrotizing myopathy associated with statin use [see *Warnings and Precautions (5.1)*].

7 DRUG INTERACTIONS

7.1 Cyclosporine
Cyclosporine significantly increased pitavastatin exposure. Co-administration of cyclosporine with LIVALO is contraindicated [see *Contraindications (4) and Clinical Pharmacology (12.3)*].

7.2 Erythromycin
Erythromycin significantly increased pitavastatin exposure. In patients taking erythromycin, a dose of LIVALO 1 mg once daily should not be exceeded [see *Dosage and Administration (2.3) and Clinical Pharmacology (12.3)*].

7.3 Rifampin
Rifampin significantly increased pitavastatin exposure. In patients taking rifampin, a dose of LIVALO 2 mg once daily should not be exceeded [see *Dosage and Administration (2.4) and Clinical Pharmacology (12.3)*].

7.4 Gemfibrozil
Due to an increased risk of myopathy/rhabdomyolysis when HMG-CoA reductase inhibitors are coadministered with gemfibrozil, concomitant administration of LIVALO with gemfibrozil should be avoided.

7.5 Other Fibrates
Because it is known that the risk of myopathy during treatment with HMG-CoA reductase inhibitors is increased with concurrent administration of other fibrates, LIVALO should be administered with caution when used concomitantly with other fibrates [see *Warnings and Precautions (5.1), and Clinical Pharmacology (12.3)*].

7.6 Niacin
The risk of skeletal muscle effects may be enhanced when LIVALO is used in combination with niacin; a reduction in LIVALO dosage should be considered in this setting [see *Warnings and Precautions (5.1)*].

7.7 Colchicine
Cases of myopathy, including rhabdomyolysis, have been reported with HMG-CoA reductase inhibitors coadministered with colchicine, and caution should be exercised when prescribing LIVALO with colchicine.

7.8 Warfarin
LIVALO had no significant pharmacokinetic interaction with R- and S- warfarin. LIVALO had no significant effect on prothrombin time (PT) and international normalized ratio (INR) when administered to patients receiving chronic warfarin treatment [see *Clinical Pharmacology (12.3)*]. However, patients receiving warfarin should have their PT and INR monitored when pitavastatin is added to their therapy.

8 USE IN SPECIFIC POPULATIONS

8.1 Pregnancy
Teratogenic effects: Pregnancy Category X
LIVALO is contraindicated in women who are or may become pregnant. Serum cholesterol and TG increase during normal pregnancy, and cholesterol products are essential for fetal development. Atherosclerosis is a chronic process and discontinuation of lipid-lowering drugs during pregnancy should have little impact on long-term outcomes of primary hyperlipidemia therapy [see *Contraindications (4)*].

There are no adequate and well-controlled studies of LIVALO in pregnant women, although, there have been rare reports of congenital anomalies following intrauterine exposure to HMG-CoA reductase inhibitors. In a review of about 100 prospectively followed pregnancies in women exposed to other HMG-CoA reductase inhibitors, the incidences of congenital anomalies, spontaneous abortions, and fetal deaths/stillbirths did not exceed the rate expected in the general population. However, this study was only able to exclude a three-to-four-fold increased risk of congenital anomalies over background incidence. In 89% of these cases, drug treatment started before pregnancy and stopped during the first trimester when pregnancy was identified.

Reproductive toxicity studies have shown that pitavastatin crosses the placenta in rats and is found in fetal tissues at ≤36% of maternal plasma concentrations following a single dose of 1 mg/kg/day during gestation.

Table 3. Effect of Pitavastatin Co-Administration on Systemic Exposure to Other Drugs

Co-administered drug	Dose regimen		Change in AUC*	Change in C_{max}*
Atazanavir	Pitavastatin 4 mg QD + atazanavir 300 mg daily for 5 days		↑ 6%	↑ 13%
Darunavir	Pitavastatin 4mg QD on Days 1-5 and 12-16 + darunavir/ritonavir 800mg/100 mg QD on Days 6-16		↑ 3%	↑ 6%
Lopinavir	Pitavastatin 4 mg QD on Days 1-5 and 20-24 + lopinavir/ritonavir 400 mg/100 mg BID on Days 9 – 24		↓ 9%	↓ 7%
Ritonavir	Pitavastatin 4 mg QD on Days 1-5 and 20-24 + lopinavir/ritonavir 400 mg/100 mg BID on Days 9 – 24		↓ 11%	↓ 11%
Ritonavir	Pitavastatin 4mg QD on Days 1-5 and 12-16 + darunavir/ritonavir 800mg/100 mg QD on Days 6-16		↑ 8%	↑ 2%
Enalapril	Pitavastatin 4 mg QD + enalapril 20 mg daily for 5 days	Enalapril	↑ 12%	↑ 12%
		Enalaprilat	↓ 1%	↓ 1%
Warfarin	Individualized maintenance dose of warfarin (2 - 7 mg) for 8 days + pitavastatin 4 mg QD for 9 days	R-warfarin	↑ 7%	↑ 3%
		S-warfarin	↑ 6%	↑ 3%
Ezetimibe	Pitavastatin 2 mg QD + ezetimibe 10 mg for 7 days		↑ 9%	↑ 2%
Digoxin	Pitavastatin 4 mg QD + digoxin 0.25 mg for 7 days		↓ 3%	↓ 4%
Diltiazem LA	Pitavastatin 4 mg QD on Days 1-5 and 11-15 and diltiazem LA 240 mg on Days 6-15		↓ 2%	↓ 7%
Rifampin	Pitavastatin 4 mg QD + rifampin 600 mg QD for 5 days		↓ 15%	↓ 18%

*Data presented as % change represent % difference relative to the investigated drug alone (i.e., 0% = no change).
BID = twice daily; QD = once daily; LA = Long Acting

Table 4. Dose-Response in Patients with Primary Hypercholesterolemia (Adjusted Mean % Change from Baseline at Week 12)

Treatment	N	LDL-C	Apo-B	TC	TG	HDL-C
Placebo	53	-3	-2	-2	1	0
LIVALO 1mg	52	-32	-25	-23	-15	8
LIVALO 2mg	49	-36	-30	-26	-19	7
LIVALO 4mg	51#	-43	-35	-31	-18	5

The number of subjects for Apo-B was 49

Table 5. Response by Dose of LIVALO and Atorvastatin in Patients with Primary Hyperlipidemia or Mixed Dyslipidemia (Mean % Change from Baseline at Week 12)

Treatment	N	LDL-C	Apo-B	TC	TG	HDL-C	non-HDL-C
LIVALO 2 mg daily	315	-38	-30	-28	-14	4	-35
LIVALO 4 mg daily	298	-45	-35	-32	-19	5	-41
Atorvastatin 10 mg daily	102	-38	-29	-28	-18	3	-35
Atorvastatin 20 mg daily	102	-44	-36	-33	-22	2	-41
Atorvastatin 40 mg daily		----------------------Not Studied----------------------					
Atorvastatin 80 mg daily		----------------------Not Studied----------------------					

Embryo-fetal developmental studies were conducted in pregnant rats treated with 3, 10, 30 mg/kg/day pitavastatin by oral gavage during organogenesis. No adverse effects were observed at 3 mg/kg/day, systemic exposures 22 times human systemic exposure at 4 mg/day dose based on AUC.

Embryo-fetal developmental studies were conducted in pregnant rabbits treated with 0.1, 0.3, 1 mg/kg/day pitavastatin by oral gavage during the period of fetal organogenesis. Maternal toxicity consisting of reduced body weight and abortion was observed at all doses tested (4 times human systemic exposure at 4 mg/day based on AUC).

In perinatal/postnatal studies in pregnant rats given oral gavage doses of pitavastatin at 0.1, 0.3, 1, 3, 10, 30 mg/kg/day from organogenesis through weaning, maternal toxicity consisting of mortality at ≥0.3 mg/kg/day and impaired lactation at all doses contributed to the decreased survival of neonates in all dose groups (0.1 mg/kg/day represents approximately 1 time human systemic exposure at 4 mg/day dose based on AUC).

LIVALO may cause fetal harm when administered to a pregnant woman. If the patient becomes pregnant while taking LIVALO, the patient should be apprised of the potential risks to the fetus and the lack of known clinical benefit with continued use during pregnancy.

8.3 Nursing Mothers
It is not known whether pitavastatin is excreted in human milk, however, it has been shown that a small amount of

Continued on next page

Table 6. Response by Dose of LIVALO and Simvastatin in Patients with Primary Hyperlipidemia or Mixed Dyslipidemia (Mean % Change from Baseline at Week 12)

Treatment	N	LDL-C	Apo-B	TC	TG	HDL-C	non-HDL-C
LIVALO 2 mg daily	307	-39	-30	-28	-16	6	-36
LIVALO 4 mg daily	319	-44	-35	-32	-17	6	-41
Simvastatin 20 mg daily	107	-35	-27	-25	-16	6	-32
Simvastatin 40 mg daily	110	-43	-34	-31	-16	7	-39
Simvastatin 80 mg	--------------------------------Not Studied--------------------------------						

Table 7. Response by Dose of LIVALO and Pravastatin in Patients with Primary Hyperlipidemia or Mixed Dyslipidemia (Mean % Change from Baseline at Week 12)

Treatment	N	LDL-C	Apo-B	TC	TG	HDL-C	non-HDL-C
LIVALO 1 mg daily	207	-31	-25	-22	-13	1	-29
LIVALO 2 mg daily	224	-39	-31	-27	-15	2	-36
LIVALO 4 mg daily	210	-44	-37	-31	-22	4	-41
Pravastatin 10 mg daily	103	-22	-17	-15	-13	0	-20
Pravastatin 20 mg daily	96	-29	-22	-21	-11	-1	-27
Pravastatin 40 mg daily	102	-34	-28	-24	-15	1	-32
Pravastatin 80 mg daily	--------------------------------Not Studied--------------------------------						

another drug in this class passes into human milk. Rat studies have shown that pitavastatin is excreted into breast milk. Because another drug in this class passes into human milk and HMG-CoA reductase inhibitors have a potential to cause serious adverse reactions in nursing infants, women who require LIVALO treatment should be advised not to nurse their infants or to discontinue LIVALO [see Contraindications (4)].

8.4 Pediatric Use
Safety and effectiveness of LIVALO in pediatric patients have not been established.

8.5 Geriatric Use
Of the 2,800 patients randomized to LIVALO 1 mg to 4 mg in controlled clinical studies, 1,209 (43%) were 65 years and older. No significant differences in efficacy or safety were observed between elderly patients and younger patients. However, greater sensitivity of some older individuals cannot be ruled out.

8.6 Renal Impairment
Patients with moderate and severe renal impairment (glomerular filtration rate 30 – 59 mL/min/1.73 m^2 and 15 – 29 mL/min/1.73 m^2 not receiving hemodialysis, respectively) as well as end-stage renal disease receiving hemodialysis should receive a starting dose of LIVALO 1 mg once daily and a maximum dose of LIVALO 2 mg once daily [see Dosage and Administration (2.2) and Clinical Pharmacology (12.3)].

8.7 Hepatic Impairment
LIVALO is contraindicated in patients with active liver disease which may include unexplained persistent elevations of hepatic transaminase levels.

10 OVERDOSAGE
There is no known specific treatment in the event of overdose of pitavastatin. In the event of overdose, the patient should be treated symptomatically and supportive measures instituted as required. Hemodialysis is unlikely to be of benefit due to high protein binding ratio of pitavastatin.

11 DESCRIPTION
LIVALO (pitavastatin) is an inhibitor of HMG-CoA reductase. It is a synthetic lipid-lowering agent for oral administration.
The chemical name for pitavastatin is (+)monocalcium bis[(3R, 5S, 6E)-7-[2-cyclopropyl-4-(4-fluorophenyl)-3-quinolyl]-3,5-dihydroxy-6-heptenoate]. The structural formula is:
[See structural formula at top of next colmn]
The empirical formula for pitavastatin is $C_{50}H_{46}CaF_2N_2O_8$ and the molecular weight is 880.98. Pitavastatin is odorless

and occurs as white to pale-yellow powder. It is freely soluble in pyridine, chloroform, dilute hydrochloric acid, and tetrahydrofuran, soluble in ethylene glycol, sparingly soluble in octanol, slightly soluble in methanol, very slightly soluble in water or ethanol, and practically insoluble in acetonitrile or diethyl ether. Pitavastatin is hygroscopic and slightly unstable in light.
Each film-coated tablet of LIVALO contains 1.045 mg, 2.09 mg, or 4.18 mg of pitavastatin calcium, which is equivalent to 1 mg, 2 mg, or 4 mg, respectively of free base and the following inactive ingredients: lactose monohydrate, low substituted hydroxypropylcellulose, hypromellose, magnesium aluminometasilicate, magnesium stearate, and film coating containing the following inactive ingredients: hypromellose, titanium dioxide, triethyl citrate, and colloidal anhydrous silica.

12 CLINICAL PHARMACOLOGY
12.1 Mechanism of Action
Pitavastatin competitively inhibits HMG-CoA reductase, which is a rate-determining enzyme involved with biosynthesis of cholesterol, in a manner of competition with the substrate so that it inhibits cholesterol synthesis in the liver. As a result, the expression of LDL-receptors followed by the uptake of LDL from blood to liver is accelerated and then the plasma TC decreases. Further, the sustained inhibition of cholesterol synthesis in the liver decreases levels of very low density lipoproteins.

12.2 Pharmacodynamics
In a randomized, double-blind, placebo-controlled, 4-way parallel, active-comparator study with moxifloxacin in 174 healthy participants, LIVALO was not associated with clinically meaningful prolongation of the QTc interval or heart rate at daily doses up to 16 mg (4 times the recommended maximum daily dose).

12.3 Pharmacokinetics
Absorption: Pitavastatin peak plasma concentrations are achieved about 1 hour after oral administration. Both C_{max} and AUC_{0-inf} increased in an approximately dose-proportional manner for single LIVALO doses from 1 to 24 mg once daily. The absolute bioavailability of pitavastatin oral solution is 51%. Administration of LIVALO with a high fat meal (50% fat content) decreases pitavastatin C_{max} by 43% but does not significantly reduce pitavastatin AUC. The C_{max} and AUC of pitavastatin did not differ following evening or morning drug administration. In healthy volunteers receiving 4 mg pitavastatin, the percent change from baseline for LDL-C following evening dosing was slightly greater than that following morning dosing. Pitavastatin was absorbed in the small intestine but very little in the colon.
Distribution: Pitavastatin is more than 99% protein bound in human plasma, mainly to albumin and alpha 1-acid glycoprotein, and the mean volume of distribution is approximately 148 L. Association of pitavastatin and/or its metabolites with the blood cells is minimal.
Metabolism: Pitavastatin is marginally metabolized by CYP2C9 and to a lesser extent by CYP2C8. The major metabolite in human plasma is the lactone which is formed via an ester-type pitavastatin glucuronide conjugate by uridine 5'-diphosphate (UDP) glucuronosyltransferase (UGT1A3 and UGT2B7).
Excretion: A mean of 15% of radioactivity of orally administered, single 32 mg ^{14}C-labeled pitavastatin dose was excreted in urine, whereas a mean of 79% of the dose was excreted in feces within 7 days. The mean plasma elimination half-life is approximately 12 hours.
Race: In pharmacokinetic studies pitavastatin C_{max} and AUC were 21 and 5% lower, respectively in Black or African American healthy volunteers compared with those of Caucasian healthy volunteers. In pharmacokinetic comparison between Caucasian volunteers and Japanese volunteers, there were no significant differences in C_{max} and AUC.
Gender: In a pharmacokinetic study which compared healthy male and female volunteers, pitavastatin C_{max} and AUC were 60 and 54% higher, respectively in females. This had no effect on the efficacy or safety of LIVALO in women in clinical studies.
Geriatric: In a pharmacokinetic study which compared healthy young and elderly (≥65 years) volunteers, pitavastatin C_{max} and AUC were 10 and 30% higher, respectively, in the elderly. This had no effect on the efficacy or safety of LIVALO in elderly subjects in clinical studies.
Renal Impairment: In patients with moderate renal impairment (glomerular filtration rate of 30 – 59 mL/min/1.73 m^2) and end stage renal disease receiving hemodialysis, pitavastatin AUC_{0-inf} is 102 and 86% higher than those of healthy volunteers, respectively, while pitavastatin C_{max} is 60 and 40% higher than those of healthy volunteers, respectively. Patients received hemodialysis immediately before pitavastatin dosing and did not undergo hemodialysis during the pharmacokinetic study. Hemodialysis patients have 33 and 36% increases in the mean unbound fraction of pitavastatin as compared to healthy volunteers and patients with moderate renal impairment, respectively.
In another pharmacokinetic study, patients with severe renal impairment (glomerular filtration rate 15 – 29 mL/min/1.73 m^2) not receiving hemodialysis were administered a single dose of LIVALO 4 mg. The AUC_{0-inf} and the C_{max} were 36 and 18% higher, respectively, compared with those of healthy volunteers. For both patients with severe renal impairment and healthy volunteers, the mean percentage of protein-unbound pitavastatin was approximately 0.6%.
The effect of mild renal impairment on pitavastatin exposure has not been studied.
Hepatic Impairment: The disposition of pitavastatin was compared in healthy volunteers and patients with various degrees of hepatic impairment. The ratio of pitavastatin C_{max} between patients with moderate hepatic impairment (Child-Pugh B disease) and healthy volunteers was 2.7. The ratio of pitavastatin AUC_{inf} between patients with moderate hepatic impairment and healthy volunteers was 3.8. The ratio of pitavastatin C_{max} between patients with mild hepatic impairment (Child-Pugh A disease) and healthy volunteers was 1.3. The ratio of pitavastatin AUC_{inf} between patients with mild hepatic impairment and healthy volunteers was 1.6. Mean pitavastatin $t_{1/2}$ for moderate hepatic impairment, mild hepatic impairment, and healthy were 15, 10, and 8 hours, respectively.

Drug-Drug Interactions: The principal route of pitavastatin metabolism is glucuronidation via liver UGTs with subsequent formation of pitavastatin lactone. There is only minimal metabolism by the cytochrome P450 system. **Warfarin:** The steady-state pharmacodynamics (international normalized ratio [INR] and prothrombin time [PT]) and pharmacokinetics of warfarin in healthy volunteers were unaffected by the co-administration of LIVALO 4 mg daily. However, patients receiving warfarin should have their PT time or INR monitored when pitavastatin is added to their therapy.

[See table 2 on page 986]

[See table 3 on page 987]

13 NONCLINICAL TOXICOLOGY

13.1 Carcinogenesis, Mutagenesis, Impairment of Fertility

In a 92-week carcinogenicity study in mice given pitavastatin, at the maximum tolerated dose of 75 mg/kg/day with systemic maximum exposures (AUC) 26 times the clinical maximum exposure at 4 mg/day, there was an absence of drug-related tumors.

In a 92-week carcinogenicity study in rats given pitavastatin at 1, 5, 25 mg/kg/day by oral gavage there was a significant increase in the incidence of thyroid follicular cell tumors at 25 mg/kg/day, which represents 295 times human systemic exposures based on AUC at the 4 mg/day maximum human dose.

In a 26-week transgenic mouse (Tg rasH2) carcinogenicity study where animals were given pitavastatin at 30, 75, and 150 mg/kg/day by oral gavage, no clinically significant tumors were observed.

Pitavastatin was not mutagenic in the Ames test with *Salmonella typhimurium* and *Escherichia coli* with and without metabolic activation, the micronucleus test following a single administration in mice and multiple administrations in rats, the unscheduled DNA synthesis test in rats, and a Comet assay in mice. In the chromosomal aberration test, clastogenicity was observed at the highest doses tested which also elicited high levels of cytotoxicity.

Pitavastatin had no adverse effects on male and female rat fertility at oral doses of 10 and 30 mg/kg/day, respectively, at systemic exposures 56- and 354-times clinical exposure at 4 mg/day based on AUC.

Pitavastatin treatment in rabbits resulted in mortality in males and females given 1 mg/kg/day (30-times clinical systemic exposure at 4 mg/day based on AUC) and higher during a fertility study. Although the cause of death was not determined, rabbits had gross signs of renal toxicity (kidneys whitened) indicative of possible ischemia. Lower doses (15-times human systemic exposure) did not show significant toxicity in adult males and females. However, decreased implantations, increased resorptions, and decreased viability of fetuses were observed.

13.2 Animal Toxicology and/or Pharmacology

Central Nervous System Toxicity

CNS vascular lesions, characterized by perivascular hemorrhages, edema, and mononuclear cell infiltration of perivascular spaces, have been observed in dogs treated with several other members of this drug class. A chemically similar drug in this class produced dose-dependent optic nerve degeneration (Wallerian degeneration of retinogeniculate fibers) in dogs, at a dose that produced plasma drug levels about 30 times higher than the mean drug level in humans taking the highest recommended dose. Wallerian degeneration has not been observed with pitavastatin. Cataracts and lens opacities were seen in dogs treated for 52 weeks at a dose level of 1 mg/kg/day (9 times clinical exposure at the maximum human dose of 4 mg/day based on AUC comparisons.

14 CLINICAL STUDIES

14.1 Primary Hyperlipidemia or Mixed Dyslipidemia

Dose-ranging study: A multicenter, randomized, double-blind, placebo-controlled, dose-ranging study was performed to evaluate the efficacy of LIVALO compared with placebo in 251 patients with primary hyperlipidemia (Table 4). LIVALO given as a single daily dose for 12 weeks significantly reduced plasma LDL-C, TC, TG, and Apo-B compared to placebo and was associated with variable increases in HDL-C across the dose range.

[See table 4 on page 987]

Active-controlled study with atorvastatin (NK-104-301): LIVALO was compared with the HMG-CoA reductase inhibitor atorvastatin in a randomized, multicenter, double-blind, double-dummy, active-controlled, non-inferiority Phase 3 study of 817 patients with primary hyperlipidemia or mixed dyslipidemia. Patients entered a 6- to 8-week wash-out/dietary lead-in period and then were randomized to a 12-week treatment with either LIVALO or atorvastatin (Table 5). Non-inferiority of pitavastatin to a given dose of atorvastatin was considered to be demonstrated if the lower bound of the 95% CI for the mean treatment difference was greater than -6% for the mean percent change in LDL-C.

Lipid results are shown in Table 5. For the percent change from baseline to endpoint in LDL-C, LIVALO was non-inferior to atorvastatin for the two pairwise comparisons: LIVALO 2 mg vs. atorvastatin 10 mg and LIVALO 4 mg vs. atorvastatin 20 mg. Mean treatment differences (95% CI) were 0% (-3%, 3%) and 1% (-2%, 4%), respectively.

[See table 5 on page 987]

Active-controlled study with simvastatin (NK-104-302): LIVALO was compared with the HMG-CoA reductase inhibitor simvastatin in a randomized, multicenter, double-blind, double-dummy, active-controlled, non-inferiority Phase 3 study of 843 patients with primary hyperlipidemia or mixed dyslipidemia. Patients entered a 6- to 8-week wash-out/dietary lead-in period and then were randomized to a 12 week treatment with either LIVALO or simvastatin (Table 6). Non-inferiority of pitavastatin to a given dose of simvastatin was considered to be demonstrated if the lower bound of the 95% CI for the mean treatment difference was greater than -6% for the mean percent change in LDL-C.

Lipid results are shown in Table 6. For the percent change from baseline to endpoint in LDL-C, LIVALO was non-inferior to simvastatin for the two pairwise comparisons: LIVALO 2 mg vs. simvastatin 20 mg and LIVALO 4 mg vs. simvastatin 40 mg. Mean treatment differences (95% CI) were 4% (1%, 7%) and 1% (-2%, 4%), respectively.

[See table 6 on previous page]

Active-controlled study with pravastatin in elderly (NK-104-306): LIVALO was compared with the HMG-CoA reductase inhibitor pravastatin in a randomized, multicenter, double-blind, double-dummy, parallel group, active-controlled non-inferiority Phase 3 study of 942 elderly patients (≥65 years) with primary hyperlipidemia or mixed dyslipidemia. Patients entered a 6- to 8-week wash-out/dietary lead-in period, and then were randomized to a once daily dose of LIVALO or pravastatin for 12 weeks (Table 7). Non-inferiority of LIVALO to a given dose of pravastatin was assumed if the lower bound of the 95% CI for the treatment difference was greater than -6% for the mean percent change in LDL-C.

Lipid results are shown in Table 7. LIVALO significantly reduced LDL-C compared to pravastatin as demonstrated by the following pairwise dose comparisons: LIVALO 1 mg vs. pravastatin 10 mg, LIVALO 2 mg vs. pravastatin 20 mg and LIVALO 4 mg vs. pravastatin 40 mg. Mean treatment differences (95% CI) were 9% (6%, 12%), 10% (7%, 13%) and 10% (7%, 13%), respectively.

[See table 7 on previous page]

Active-controlled study with simvastatin in patients with ≥2 risk factors for coronary heart disease (NK-104-304): LIVALO was compared with the HMG-CoA reductase inhibitor simvastatin in a randomized, multicenter, double-blind, double-dummy, active-controlled, non-inferiority Phase 3 study of 351 patients with primary hyperlipidemia or mixed dyslipidemia with ≥2 risk factors for coronary heart disease. After a 6- to 8-week wash-out/dietary lead-in period, patients were randomized to a 12-week treatment with either LIVALO or simvastatin (Table 8). Non-inferiority of LIVALO to simvastatin was considered to be demonstrated if the lower bound of the 95% CI for the mean treatment difference was greater than -6% for the mean percent change in LDL-C.

Lipid results are shown in Table 8. LIVALO 4 mg was non-inferior to simvastatin 40 mg for percent change from baseline to endpoint in LDL-C. The mean treatment difference (95% CI) was 0% (-2%, 3%).

[See table 8 below]

Active-controlled study with atorvastatin in patients with type II diabetes mellitus (NK-104-305): LIVALO was compared with the HMG-CoA reductase inhibitor atorvastatin in a randomized, multicenter, double-blind, double-dummy, parallel group, active-controlled, non-inferiority Phase 3 study of 410 subjects with type II diabetes mellitus and combined dyslipidemia. Patients entered a 6- to 8-week washout/dietary lead-in period and were randomized to a once daily dose of LIVALO or atorvastatin for 12 weeks. Non-inferiority of LIVALO was considered to be demonstrated if the lower bound of the 95% CI for the mean treatment difference was greater than -6% for the mean percent change in LDL-C.

Lipid results are shown in Table 9. The treatment difference (95% CI) for LDL-C percent change from baseline was -2% (-6.2%, 1.5%). The two treatment groups were not statistically different on LDL-C. However, the lower limit of the CI was -6.2%, slightly exceeding the -6% non-inferiority limit so that the non-inferiority objective was not achieved.

[See table 9 above]

The treatment differences in efficacy in LDL-C change from baseline between LIVALO and active controls in the Phase 3 studies are summarized in Figure 1.

[See Figure 1 on next page]

16 HOW SUPPLIED/STORAGE AND HANDLING

LIVALO tablets for oral administration are provided as white, film-coated tablets that contain 1 mg, 2 mg, or 4 mg of pitavastatin. Each tablet has "KC" debossed on one side and a code number specific to the tablet strength on the other.

Packaging

LIVALO (pitavastatin) Tablets are supplied as;

- NDC 66869-104-90 : 1 mg. Round white film-coated tablet debossed "KC" on one face and "1" on the reverse; HDPE bottles of 90 tablets
- NDC 66869-204-90 : 2 mg. Round white film-coated tablet debossed "KC" on one face and "2" on the reverse; HDPE bottles of 90 tablets

Table 9. Response by Dose of LIVALO and Atorvastatin in Patients with Type II Diabetes Mellitus and Combined Dyslipidemia (Mean % Change from Baseline at Week 12)

Treatment	N	LDL-C	Apo-B	TC	TG	HDL-C	non-HDL-C
LIVALO 4 mg daily	274	-41	-32	-28	-20	7	-36
Atorvastatin 20 mg daily	136	-43	-34	-32	-27	8	-40
Atorvastatin 40 mg daily	----------------------------------Not Studied----------------------------------						
Atorvastatin 80 mg daily	----------------------------------Not Studied----------------------------------						

Table 8. Response by Dose of LIVALO and Simvastatin in Patients with Primary Hyperlipidemia or Mixed Dyslipidemia with ≥2 Risk Factors for Coronary Heart Disease (Mean % Change from Baseline at Week 12)

Treatment	N	LDL-C	Apo-B	TC	TG	HDL-C	non-HDL-C
LIVALO 4 mg daily	233	-44	-34	-31	-20	7	-40
Simvastatin 40 mg daily	118	-44	-34	-31	-15	5	-39
Simvastatin 80 mg daily	----------------------------------Not Studied----------------------------------						

Continued on next page

Figure 1. Treatment Difference in Adjusted Mean Percent Change in LDL-C

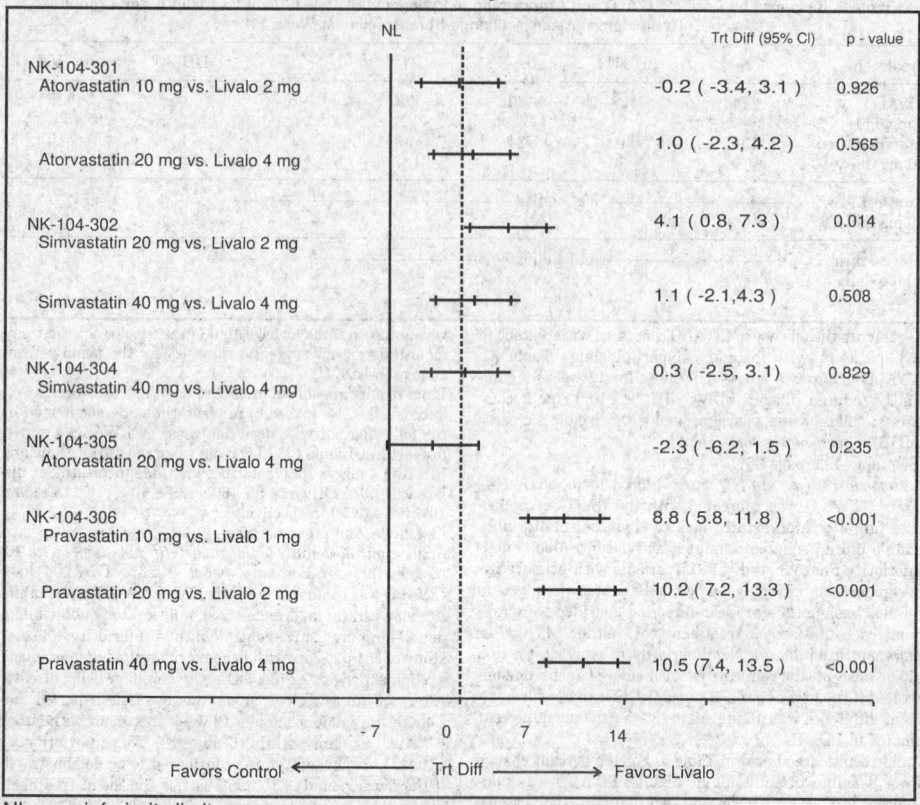

	Trt Diff (95% CI)	p - value
NK-104-301 Atorvastatin 10 mg vs. Livalo 2 mg	-0.2 (-3.4, 3.1)	0.926
Atorvastatin 20 mg vs. Livalo 4 mg	1.0 (-2.3, 4.2)	0.565
NK-104-302 Simvastatin 20 mg vs. Livalo 2 mg	4.1 (0.8, 7.3)	0.014
Simvastatin 40 mg vs. Livalo 4 mg	1.1 (-2.1, 4.3)	0.508
NK-104-304 Simvastatin 40 mg vs. Livalo 4 mg	0.3 (-2.5, 3.1)	0.829
NK-104-305 Atorvastatin 20 mg vs. Livalo 4 mg	-2.3 (-6.2, 1.5)	0.235
NK-104-306 Pravastatin 10 mg vs. Livalo 1 mg	8.8 (5.8, 11.8)	<0.001
Pravastatin 20 mg vs. Livalo 2 mg	10.2 (7.2, 13.3)	<0.001
Pravastatin 40 mg vs. Livalo 4 mg	10.5 (7.4, 13.5)	<0.001

Favors Control ← Trt Diff → Favors Livalo

NL=non-inferiority limit.

• NDC 66869-404-90 : 4 mg. Round white film-coated tablet debossed "KC" on one face and "4" on the reverse; HDPE bottles of 90 tablets

Storage

Store at room temperature between 15°C and 30°C (59° to 86° F) [see USP]. Protect from light.

17   PATIENT COUNSELING INFORMATION

The patient should be informed of the following:

17.1   Dosing Time

LIVALO can be taken at any time of the day with or without food.

17.2   Muscle Pain

Patients should be advised to promptly notify their physician of any unexplained muscle pain, tenderness, or weakness particularly if accompanied by malaise or fever, or if these muscle signs or symptoms persist after discontinuing LIVALO. They should discuss all medication, both prescription and over the counter, with their physician.

17.3   Pregnancy

Women of childbearing age should use an effective method of birth control to prevent pregnancy while using LIVALO. Discuss future pregnancy plans with your healthcare professional, and discuss when to stop LIVALO if you are trying to conceive. If you are pregnant, stop taking LIVALO and call your healthcare professional.

17.4   Breastfeeding

Women who are breastfeeding should not use LIVALO. If you have a lipid disorder and are breastfeeding, stop taking LIVALO and consult with your healthcare professional.

17.5   Liver Enzymes

It is recommended that liver enzyme tests be checked before the initiation of LIVALO and if signs or symptoms of liver injury occur. All patients treated with LIVALO should be advised to report promptly any symptoms that may indicate liver injury, including fatigue, anorexia, right upper abdominal discomfort, dark urine or jaundice.

LIVALO is a trademark of the Kowa group of companies.

© Kowa Pharmaceuticals America, Inc. (2009)

Manufactured under license from: Kowa Company, Limited Tokyo 103-8433 Japan

Product of Japan

Manufactured into tablets by: Patheon, Inc. Cincinnati, OH 45237 USA or by Kowa Company, LTD Nagoya, 462-0024

Japan

Marketed by: Kowa Pharmaceuticals America, Inc. Montgomery, AL 36117 USA

To request additional information or if you have questions concerning LIVALO please phone Kowa Pharmaceuticals America, Inc. at 877-8-LIVALO (877-854-8256) or fax your inquiry to 800-689-0244

Shown in Product Identification Guide, page 509

OREXIGEN THERAPEUTICS, INC.

**3344 N. Torrey Pines Court, Suite 200
La Jolla, CA 92037**

Direct Inquiries to:
Phone: (858) 875-8600
Fax: (858) 875-8650

CONTRAVE   ℞
[CON-trayv]
**(naltrexone HCl and bupropion HCl)
Extended-Release Tablets**

HIGHLIGHTS OF PRESCRIBING INFORMATION

These highlights do not include all the information needed to use CONTRAVE® safely and effectively. See full prescribing information for CONTRAVE.

CONTRAVE (naltrexone HCl and bupropion HCl) Extended-Release Tablets

Initial U.S. Approval: 2014

WARNING: SUICIDAL THOUGHTS AND BEHAV-IORS; AND NEUROPSYCHIATRIC REACTIONS

See full prescribing information for complete boxed warning

• **Increased risk of suicidal thinking and behavior in children, adolescents, and young adults taking antidepressants for major depressive disorder and other psychiatric disorders. (5.1)**

• **Monitor for worsening and emergence of suicidal thoughts and behaviors. (5.1)**
• **Serious neuropsychiatric events have been reported in patients taking bupropion for smoking cessation. (5.2)**
• **CONTRAVE has not been studied in pediatric patients. (5.1)**

INDICATIONS AND USAGE

CONTRAVE is a combination of naltrexone, an opioid antagonist, and bupropion, an aminoketone antidepressant, indicated as an adjunct to a reduced-calorie diet and increased physical activity for chronic weight management in adults with an initial body mass index (BMI) of:
• 30 kg/m² or greater (obese) or
• 27 kg/m² or greater (overweight) in the presence of at least one weight-related comorbidity (e.g., hypertension, type 2 diabetes mellitus, or dyslipidemia). (1)

Limitations of Use:
• The effect of CONTRAVE on cardiovascular morbidity and mortality has not been established. (1)
• The safety and effectiveness of CONTRAVE in combination with other products intended for weight loss, including prescription and over-the-counter drugs, and herbal preparations, have not been established. (1)

DOSAGE AND ADMINISTRATION

CONTRAVE dose escalation schedule (2.1):

	Morning Dose	Evening Dose
Week 1	1 tablet	None
Week 2	1 tablet	1 tablet
Week 3	2 tablets	1 tablet
Week 4 – Onward	2 tablets	2 tablets

DOSAGE FORMS AND STRENGTHS

Extended-Release Tablets: 8 mg naltrexone HCl /90 mg bupropion HCl (3)

CONTRAINDICATIONS

• Uncontrolled hypertension (4)
• Seizure disorders, anorexia nervosa or bulimia, or undergoing abrupt discontinuation of alcohol, benzodiazepines, barbiturates, and antiepileptic drugs (4)
• Use of other bupropion-containing products (4)
• Chronic opioid use (4)
• During or within 14 days of taking monoamine oxidase inhibitors (MAOI) (4)
• Known allergy to any of the ingredients in CONTRAVE (4)
• Pregnancy (4)

WARNINGS AND PRECAUTIONS

• Suicidal Behavior and Ideation: Monitor for depression or suicidal thoughts. Discontinue CONTRAVE if symptoms develop. (5.1)
• Risk of seizure may be minimized by adhering to the recommended dosing schedule and avoiding coadministration with high-fat meal. (5.3)
• Increase in Blood Pressure and Heart Rate: Monitor blood pressure and heart rate in all patients, especially those with cardiac or cerebrovascular disease. (5.5)
• Hepatotoxicity: Cases of hepatitis and clinically significant liver dysfunction observed with naltrexone exposure. (5.7)
• Angle-closure glaucoma: Angle-closure glaucoma has occurred in patients with untreated anatomically narrow angles treated with antidepressants. (5.9)
• Use of Antidiabetic Medications: Weight loss may cause hypoglycemia. Monitor blood glucose. (5.10)

ADVERSE REACTIONS

• Most common adverse reactions (greater than or equal to 5%): nausea, constipation, headache, vomiting, dizziness, insomnia, dry mouth and diarrhea. (6.1)

To report SUSPECTED ADVERSE REACTIONS, contact Orexigen Therapeutics, Inc. at 1-877-298-8340 or FDA at 1-800-FDA-1088 or *www.fda.gov/medwatch*.

DRUG INTERACTIONS

• MAOIs: Increased risk of hypertensive reactions can occur when used concomitantly. (7.1)
• Drugs Metabolized by CYP2D6: Bupropion inhibits CYP2D6 and can increase concentrations of: antidepressants, (e.g., selective serotonin reuptake inhibitors and many tricyclics), antipsychotics (e.g., haloperidol, risperi-

done and thioridazine), beta-blockers (e.g., metoprolol) and Type 1C antiarrhythmics (e.g., propafenone and flecainide): Consider dose reduction when using with CONTRAVE. (7.3)
- Concomitant Treatment with CYP2B6 Inhibitors (e.g., ticlopidine or clopidogrel) can increase bupropion exposure. Do not exceed one tablet twice daily when taken with CYP2B6 inhibitors. (2.5, 7.4)
- CYP2B6 Inducers (e.g., ritonavir, lopinavir, efavirenz, carbamazepine, phenobarbital, and phenytoin) may reduce efficacy by reducing bupropion exposure, avoid concomitant use. (7.4)
- Drugs that Lower Seizure Threshold: Dose CONTRAVE with caution. (5.3, 7.5)
- Dopaminergic Drugs (levodopa and amantadine): CNS toxicity can occur when used concomitantly with CONTRAVE. (7.6)
- Drug-Laboratory Test Interactions: CONTRAVE can cause false-positive urine test results for amphetamines. (7.8)

————USE IN SPECIFIC POPULATIONS————
- Nursing Mothers: Discontinue drug or nursing. (8.3)
- Pediatric Use: Safety and effectiveness not established and use not recommended. (8.4)

See 17 for PATIENT COUNSELING INFORMATION and Medication Guide.

Revised: 9/2016

FULL PRESCRIBING INFORMATION: CONTENTS*
WARNING: SUICIDAL THOUGHTS AND BEHAVIORS; AND NEUROPSYCHIATRIC REACTIONS

Table 1. BMI Conversion Chart

Weight (lb)		125	130	135	140	145	150	155	160	165	170	175	180	185	190	195	200	205	210	215	220	225
(kg)		56.8	59.1	61.4	63.6	65.9	68.2	70.5	72.7	75.0	77.3	79.5	81.8	84.1	86.4	88.6	90.9	93.2	95.5	97.7	100.0	102.3
Height (in)	(cm)																					
58	147.3	26	27	28	29	30	31	32	34	35	36	37	38	39	40	41	42	43	44	45	46	47
59	149.9	25	26	27	28	29	30	31	32	33	34	35	36	37	38	39	40	41	43	44	45	46
60	152.4	24	25	26	27	28	29	30	31	32	33	34	35	36	37	38	39	40	41	42	43	44
61	154.9	24	25	26	27	28	28	29	30	31	32	33	34	35	36	37	38	39	40	41	42	43
62	157.5	23	24	25	26	27	27	28	29	30	31	32	33	34	35	36	37	38	38	39	40	41
63	160.0	22	23	24	25	26	27	27	28	29	30	31	32	33	34	35	36	36	37	38	39	40
64	162.6	22	22	23	24	25	26	27	28	28	29	30	31	32	33	34	34	35	36	37	38	39
65	165.1	21	22	23	23	24	25	26	27	28	28	29	30	31	32	33	33	34	35	36	37	38
66	167.6	20	21	22	23	23	24	25	26	27	27	28	29	30	31	31	32	33	34	35	36	36
67	170.2	20	20	21	22	23	23	24	24	25	26	27	27	28	29	30	31	31	32	33	34	35
68	172.7	19	20	21	21	22	23	24	24	25	26	26	27	28	29	30	30	31	32	33	34	34
69	175.3	18	19	20	21	21	22	23	24	24	25	26	27	27	28	29	30	31	31	32	33	33
70	177.8	18	19	19	20	21	22	22	23	24	24	25	26	27	27	28	29	29	30	31	32	32
71	180.3	17	18	19	20	20	21	22	22	23	24	24	25	26	27	27	28	29	29	30	31	31
72	182.9	17	18	18	19	20	20	21	22	22	23	24	24	25	26	27	27	28	29	29	30	31
73	185.4	17	17	18	19	19	20	20	21	22	22	23	24	24	25	26	26	27	28	28	29	30
74	188.0	16	17	17	18	19	19	20	21	21	22	23	23	24	24	25	26	26	27	28	28	29
75	190.5	16	16	17	18	18	19	19	20	21	21	22	23	23	24	24	25	26	26	27	28	28
76	193.0	15	16	16	17	18	18	19	19	20	21	21	22	23	23	24	24	25	26	26	27	27

FULL PRESCRIBING INFORMATION

> **WARNING: SUICIDAL THOUGHTS AND BEHAVIORS; AND NEUROPSYCHIATRIC REACTIONS**
>
> **SUICIDALITY AND ANTIDEPRESSANT DRUGS**
> CONTRAVE® is not approved for use in the treatment of major depressive disorder or other psychiatric disorders. CONTRAVE contains bupropion, the same active ingredient as some other antidepressant medications (including, but not limited to, WELLBUTRIN, WELLBUTRIN SR, WELLBUTRIN XL and APLENZIN). Antidepressants increased the risk of suicidal thoughts and behavior in children, adolescents, and young adults in short-term trials. These trials did not show an increase in the risk of suicidal thoughts and behavior with antidepressant use in subjects over age 24; there was a reduction in risk with antidepressant use in subjects aged 65 and older. In patients of all ages who are started on CONTRAVE, monitor closely for worsening, and for the emergence of suicidal thoughts and behaviors. Advise families and caregivers of the need for close observation and communication with the prescriber. CONTRAVE is not approved for use in pediatric patients *[see Warnings and Precautions (5.1), Use in Specific Populations (8.4)]*.
>
> **NEUROPSYCHIATRIC REACTIONS IN PATIENTS TAKING BUPROPION FOR SMOKING CESSATION**
> Serious neuropsychiatric reactions have occurred in patients taking bupropion for smoking cessation *[see Warnings and Precautions (5.2)]*. The majority of these reactions occurred during bupropion treatment, but some occurred in the context of discontinuing treatment. In many cases, a causal relationship to bupropion treatment is not certain, because depressed mood may be a symptom of nicotine withdrawal. However, some of the cases occurred in patients taking bupropion who continued to smoke. Although CONTRAVE is not approved for smoking cessation, observe all patients for neuropsychiatric reactions. Instruct the patient to contact a healthcare provider if such reactions occur *[see Warnings and Precautions (5.2)]*.

---

1   INDICATIONS AND USAGE

CONTRAVE is indicated as an adjunct to a reduced-calorie diet and increased physical activity for chronic weight management in adults with an initial body mass index (BMI) of:

- 30 kg/m² or greater (obese) or
- 27 kg/m² or greater (overweight) in the presence of at least one weight-related comorbid condition (e.g., hypertension, type 2 diabetes mellitus, or dyslipidemia).

Limitations of Use:
- The effect of CONTRAVE on cardiovascular morbidity and mortality has not been established.
- The safety and effectiveness of CONTRAVE in combination with other products intended for weight loss, including prescription drugs, over-the-counter drugs, and herbal preparations, have not been established.

2   DOSAGE AND ADMINISTRATION
2.1   Recommended Dosing
CONTRAVE dosing should be escalated according to the following schedule:

	Morning Dose	Evening Dose
Week 1	1 tablet	None
Week 2	1 tablet	1 tablet
Week 3	2 tablets	1 tablet
Week 4 – Onward	2 tablets	2 tablets

A total daily dosage of two CONTRAVE 8 mg/90 mg tablets twice daily (32 mg/360 mg) is reached at the start of Week 4. CONTRAVE should be taken by mouth in the morning and in the evening. The tablets should not be cut, chewed, or crushed. Total daily doses greater than 32 mg/360 mg per day (two tablets twice daily) are not recommended. In clinical trials, CONTRAVE was administered with meals. However, CONTRAVE should not be taken with a high-fat meal because of a resulting significant increase in bupropion and naltrexone systemic exposure *[see Warnings and Precautions (5.3) and Clinical Pharmacology (12.3)]*.
Patients may develop elevated blood pressure or heart rate during CONTRAVE treatment; the risk may be greater during the initial three months of therapy *[see Warnings and Precautions (5.6)]*. Because patients with hypertension may be at increased risk for developing blood pressure elevations, such patients should be monitored for this potential effect when initiating treatment with CONTRAVE.
Response to therapy should be evaluated after 12 weeks at the maintenance dosage. If a patient has not lost at least 5% of baseline body weight, discontinue CONTRAVE, as it is unlikely that the patient will achieve and sustain clinically meaningful weight loss with continued treatment.
BMI is calculated by dividing weight (in kg) by height (in meters) squared. A BMI chart for determining BMI based on height and weight is provided in *Table 1*.
[See table above]

2.2   Dose Adjustment in Patients with Renal Impairment
In patients with moderate or severe renal impairment, the maximum recommended daily dose for CONTRAVE is two

Continued on next page

tablets (one tablet each morning and evening). CONTRAVE is not recommended for use in patients with end-stage renal disease. There is a lack of adequate information to guide dosing in patients with mild renal impairment *[see Use in Specific Population (8.6) and Clinical Pharmacology (12.3)]*.

2.3 Dose Adjustment in Patients with Hepatic Impairment

In patients with hepatic impairment, the maximum recommended daily dose of CONTRAVE is one tablet in the morning *[see Use in Specific Population (8.7) and Clinical Pharmacology (12.3)]*.

2.4 Switching a Patient To or From a Monoamine Oxidase Inhibitor (MAOI) Antidepressant

At least 14 days should elapse between discontinuation of an MAOI intended to treat depression and initiation of therapy with CONTRAVE. Conversely, at least 14 days should be allowed after stopping CONTRAVE before starting an MAOI antidepressant *[see Contraindications (4) and Drug Interactions (7.1)]*.

2.5 Concomitant Use with CYP2B6 Inhibitors

During concomitant use with CYP2B6 inhibitors (e.g., ticlopidine or clopidogrel), the maximum recommended daily dose of CONTRAVE is two tablets (one tablet each morning and evening) *[see Drug Interactions (7.4) and Clinical Pharmacology (12.3)]*.

3 DOSAGE FORMS AND STRENGTHS

CONTRAVE extended-release tri-layer tablets, 8 mg/90 mg, are blue, round, bi-convex, film-coated, and debossed with "NB-890" on one side.

4 CONTRAINDICATIONS

CONTRAVE is contraindicated in
- Uncontrolled hypertension *[see Warnings and Precautions (5.5)]*
- Seizure disorder or a history of seizures *[see Warnings and Precautions (5.3)]*
- Use of other bupropion-containing products (including, but not limited to, WELLBUTRIN, WELLBUTRIN SR, WELLBUTRIN XL, and APLENZIN)
- Bulimia or anorexia nervosa, which increase the risk for seizure *[see Warnings and Precautions (5.3)]*
- Chronic opioid or opiate agonist (e.g., methadone) or partial agonists (e.g., buprenorphine) use, or acute opiate withdrawal *[see Warnings and Precautions (5.4) and Drug Interactions (7.2)]*
- Patients undergoing an abrupt discontinuation of alcohol, benzodiazepines, barbiturates, and antiepileptic drugs *[see Warnings and Precautions (5.3) and Drug Interactions (7.7)]*
- Concomitant administration of monoamine oxidase inhibitors (MAOI). At least 14 days should elapse between discontinuation of MAOI and initiation of treatment with CONTRAVE. There is an increased risk of hypertensive reactions when CONTRAVE is used concomitantly with MAOIs. Starting CONTRAVE in a patient treated with reversible MAOIs such as linezolid or intravenous methylene blue is also contraindicated *[see Dosage and Administration (2.4), Drug Interactions (7.1)]*
- Known allergy to bupropion, naltrexone or any other component of CONTRAVE.
Anaphylactoid/anaphylactic reactions and Stevens-Johnson syndrome have been reported with bupropion *[see Warnings and Precautions (5.6)]*
- Pregnancy *[see Use in Specific Populations (8.1)]*

5 WARNINGS AND PRECAUTIONS

5.1 Suicidal Behavior and Ideation

CONTRAVE contains bupropion, a dopamine and norepinephrine re-uptake inhibitor that is similar to some drugs used for the treatment of depression; therefore, the following precautions pertaining to these products should be considered when treating patients with CONTRAVE.

Patients with major depressive disorder, both adult and pediatric, may experience worsening of their depression and/or the emergence of suicidal ideation and behavior (suicidality) or unusual changes in behavior, whether or not they are taking antidepressant medications, and this risk may persist until significant remission occurs. Suicide is a known risk of depression and certain other psychiatric disorders, and these disorders themselves are the strongest predictors of suicide. There has been a long-standing concern that antidepressants may have a role in inducing worsening of depression and the emergence of suicidality in certain patients during the early phases of treatment.

In placebo-controlled clinical trials with CONTRAVE for the treatment of obesity in adult patients, no suicides or suicide attempts were reported in studies up to 56 weeks duration with CONTRAVE (equivalent to bupropion doses of 360 mg/day). In these same studies, suicidal ideation was reported by 3 (0.20%) of 1,515 patients treated with placebo compared with 1 (0.03%) of 3,239 treated with CONTRAVE. Pooled analyses of short-term placebo-controlled trials of antidepressant drugs (selective serotonin re-uptake inhibitors [SSRIs] and others) show that these drugs increase the risk of suicidal thinking and behavior (suicidality) in children, adolescents, and young adults (ages 18 to 24) with major depressive disorder (MDD) and other psychiatric disorders. Short-term clinical trials did not show an increase in the risk of suicidality with antidepressants compared with placebo in adults beyond age 24; there was a reduction with antidepressants compared with placebo in adults aged 65 and older.

The pooled analyses of placebo-controlled trials of antidepressant drugs in children and adolescents with MDD, obsessive compulsive disorder (OCD), or other psychiatric disorders included a total of 24 short-term trials of nine antidepressant drugs in over 4,400 patients. The pooled analyses of placebo-controlled trials in adults with MDD or other psychiatric disorders included a total of 295 short-term trials (median duration of two months) of 11 antidepressant drugs in over 77,000 patients. There was considerable variation in risk of suicidality among drugs, but a tendency toward an increase in the younger patients for almost all drugs studied. There were differences in absolute risk of suicidality across the different indications, with the highest incidence in MDD. The risk differences (drug vs placebo), however, were relatively stable within age strata and across indications. These risk differences (drug-placebo difference in the number of cases of suicidality per 1,000 patients treated) are provided in *Table 2*.

Table 2. Risk Differences in the Number of Suicidality Cases by Age Group in the Pooled Placebo-Controlled Trials of Antidepressants in Pediatric and Adult Subjects

Age Range	Drug-Placebo Difference in Number of Cases of Suicidality per 1,000 Patients Treated
	Increases Compared to Placebo
<18	14 additional cases
18 to 24	5 additional cases
	Decreases Compared to Placebo
25 to 64	1 fewer case
≥65	6 fewer cases

No suicides occurred in any of the antidepressant pediatric trials. There were suicides in the adult antidepressant trials, but the number was not sufficient to reach any conclusion about drug effect on suicide.

It is unknown whether the suicidality risk extends to longer-term use, i.e., beyond several months. However, there is substantial evidence from placebo-controlled trials in adults with depression that the use of antidepressants can delay the recurrence of depression.

All patients being treated with antidepressants for any indication should be monitored appropriately and observed closely for clinical worsening, suicidality, and unusual changes in behavior, especially during the initial few months of a course of drug therapy, or at times of dose changes, either increases or decreases. This warning applies to CONTRAVE because one of its components, bupropion, is a member of an antidepressant class.

The following symptoms, anxiety, agitation, panic attacks, insomnia, irritability, hostility, aggressiveness, impulsivity, akathisia (psychomotor restlessness), hypomania, and mania, have been reported in adult and pediatric patients being treated with antidepressants for major depressive disorder as well as for other indications, both psychiatric and nonpsychiatric. Although a causal link between the emergence of such symptoms and either the worsening of depression and/or the emergence of suicidal impulses has not been established, there is concern that such symptoms may represent precursors to emerging suicidality.

Consideration should be given to changing the therapeutic regimen, including possibly discontinuing the medication, in patients whose depression is persistently worse, or who are experiencing emergent suicidality or symptoms that might be precursors to worsening depression or suicidality, especially if these symptoms are severe, abrupt in onset, or were not part of the patient's presenting symptoms.

Families and caregivers of patients being treated with antidepressants for major depressive disorder or other indications, both psychiatric and nonpsychiatric, should be alerted about the need to monitor patients for the emergence of anxiety, agitation, irritability, unusual changes in behavior, and the other symptoms described above, as well as the emergence of suicidality, and to report such symptoms immediately to healthcare providers. Such monitoring should include daily observation by families and caregivers. Prescriptions for CONTRAVE should be written for the smallest quantity of tablets consistent with good patient management, in order to reduce the risk of overdose.

5.2 Neuropsychiatric Symptoms and Suicide Risk in Smoking Cessation Treatment

CONTRAVE is not approved for smoking cessation treatment, but serious neuropsychiatric symptoms have been reported in patients taking bupropion for smoking cessation. These have included changes in mood (including depression and mania), psychosis, hallucinations, paranoia, delusions, homicidal ideation, hostility, agitation, aggression, anxiety, and panic, as well as suicidal ideation, suicide attempt, and completed suicide *[see Warnings and Precautions (5.1)]*. Observe patients for the occurrence of neuropsychiatric reactions. Instruct patients to contact a healthcare professional if such reactions occur.

In many of these cases, a causal relationship to bupropion treatment is not certain, because depressed mood can be a symptom of nicotine withdrawal. However, some of the cases occurred in patients taking bupropion who continued to smoke.

Depression, suicide, attempted suicide and suicidal ideation have been reported in the postmarketing experience with naltrexone used in the treatment of opioid dependence. No causal relationship has been demonstrated.

5.3 Seizures

Bupropion, a component of CONTRAVE, can cause seizures. The risk of seizure is dose-related. The incidence of seizure in patients receiving CONTRAVE in clinical trials was approximately 0.1% vs 0% on placebo. CONTRAVE should be discontinued and not restarted in patients who experience a seizure while being treated with CONTRAVE.

The risk of seizures is also related to patient factors, clinical situations, and concomitant medications that lower the seizure threshold. Consider these risks before initiating treatment with CONTRAVE. CONTRAVE is contraindicated in patients with a seizure disorder, current or prior diagnosis of anorexia nervosa or bulimia, or undergoing abrupt discontinuation of alcohol, benzodiazepines, barbiturates, and antiepileptic drugs. Caution should be used when prescribing CONTRAVE to patients with predisposing factors that may increase the risk of seizure including:
- history of head trauma or prior seizure, severe stroke, arteriovenous malformation, central nervous system tumor or infection, or metabolic disorders (e.g., hypoglycemia, hyponatremia, severe hepatic impairment, and hypoxia)
- excessive use of alcohol or sedatives, addiction to cocaine or stimulants, or withdrawal from sedatives
- patients with diabetes treated with insulin and/or oral diabetic medications (sulfonylureas and meglitinides) that may cause hypoglycemia
- concomitant administration of medications that may lower the seizure threshold, including other bupropion products, antipsychotics, tricyclic antidepressants, theophylline, systemic steroids

Recommendations for Reducing the Risk of Seizure: Clinical experience with bupropion suggests that the risk of seizure may be minimized by adhering to the recommended dosing recommendations *[see Dosage and Administration (2)]*, in particular:
- the total daily dose of CONTRAVE does not exceed 360 mg of the bupropion component (i.e., four tablets per day)
- the daily dose is administered in divided doses (twice daily)
- the dose is escalated gradually
- no more than two tablets are taken at one time
- coadministration of CONTRAVE with high-fat meals is avoided *[see Dosage and Administration (2.1) and Clinical Pharmacology (12.3)]*
- if a dose is missed, a patient should wait until the next scheduled dose to resume the regular dosing schedule

5.4 Patients Receiving Opioid Analgesics

Vulnerability to Opioid Overdose: CONTRAVE should not be administered to patients receiving chronic opioids, due to the naltrexone component, which is an opioid receptor antagonist *[see Contraindications (4)]*. If chronic opiate therapy is required, CONTRAVE treatment should be stopped. In patients requiring intermittent opiate treatment, CONTRAVE therapy should be temporarily discontinued and lower doses of opioids may be needed. Patients should be alerted that they may be more sensitive to opioids, even at lower doses, after CONTRAVE treatment is discontinued. An attempt by a patient to overcome any naltrexone opioid blockade by administering large amounts of exogenous opioids is especially dangerous and may lead to a fatal overdose or life-threatening opioid intoxication (e.g., respiratory arrest, circulatory collapse). Patients should be told of the serious consequences of trying to overcome the opioid blockade.

Precipitated Opioid Withdrawal: The symptoms of spontaneous opioid withdrawal, which are associated with the discontinuation of opioid in a dependent individual, are uncomfortable, but they are not generally believed to be severe or necessitate hospitalization. However, when withdrawal is precipitated abruptly, the resulting withdrawal syndrome can be severe enough to require hospitalization. To prevent occurrence of either precipitated withdrawal in patients dependent on opioids or exacerbation of a pre-existing subclinical withdrawal symptoms, opioid-dependent patients, including those being treated for alcohol dependence, should be opioid-free (including tramadol) before starting CONTRAVE treatment. An opioid-free interval of a minimum of 7 to 10 days is recommended for patients previously dependent on short-acting opioids, and those patients transitioning from buprenorphine or methadone may need as long as two weeks. Patients should be made aware of the risks associated with precipitated withdrawal and encouraged to give an accurate account of last opioid use.

5.5 Increase in Blood Pressure and Heart Rate

CONTRAVE can cause an increase in systolic and/or diastolic blood pressure as well as an increase in resting heart rate. In clinical practice with other bupropion-containing products, hypertension, in some cases severe and requiring acute treatment, has been reported. The clinical significance of the increases in blood pressure and heart rate observed with CONTRAVE treatment is unclear, especially for patients with cardiac and cerebrovascular disease, since patients with a history of myocardial infarction or stroke in the previous 6 months, life-threatening arrhythmias, or congestive heart failure were excluded from CONTRAVE clinical trials. Blood pressure and pulse should be measured prior to starting therapy with CONTRAVE and should be monitored at regular intervals consistent with usual clinical practice, particularly among patients with controlled hypertension prior to treatment *[see Dosage and Administration (2.1)]*. CONTRAVE should not be given to patients with uncontrolled hypertension *[see Contraindications (4)]*.

Among patients treated with CONTRAVE in placebo-controlled clinical trials, mean systolic and diastolic blood pressure was approximately 1 mmHg higher than baseline at Weeks 4 and 8, similar to baseline at Week 12, and approximately 1 mmHg below baseline between Weeks 24 and 56. In contrast, among patients treated with placebo, mean blood pressure was approximately 2 to 3 mmHg below baseline throughout the same time points, yielding statistically significant differences between the groups at every assessment during this period. The largest mean differences between the groups were observed during the first 12 weeks (treatment difference +1.8 to +2.4 mmHg systolic, all $p<0.001$; +1.7 to +2.1 mmHg diastolic, all $p<0.001$).

For heart rate, at both Weeks 4 and 8, mean heart rate was statistically significantly higher (2.1 bpm) in the CONTRAVE group compared with the placebo group; at Week 52, the difference between groups was +1.7 bpm ($p<0.001$).

In an ambulatory blood pressure monitoring substudy of 182 patients, the mean change from baseline in systolic blood pressure after 52 weeks of treatment was -0.2 mmHg for the CONTRAVE group and -2.8 mmHg for the placebo group (treatment difference, +2.6 mmHg, $p=0.08$); the mean change in diastolic blood pressure was +0.8 mmHg for the CONTRAVE group and -2.1 mmHg for the placebo group (treatment difference, +2.9 mmHg, $p=0.004$).

A greater percentage of subjects had adverse reactions related to blood pressure or heart rate in the CONTRAVE group compared to the placebo group (6.3% vs 4.2%, respectively), primarily attributable to adverse reactions of Hypertension/Blood Pressure Increased (5.9% vs 4.0%, respectively). These events were observed in both patients with and without evidence of preexisting hypertension. In a trial that enrolled individuals with diabetes, 12.0% of patients in the CONTRAVE group and 6.5% in the placebo group had a blood pressure-related adverse reaction.

5.6 Allergic Reactions

Anaphylactoid/anaphylactic reactions characterized by symptoms such as pruritus, urticaria, angioedema, and dyspnea requiring medical treatment have been reported in clinical trials with bupropion. In addition, there have been rare spontaneous postmarketing reports of erythema multiforme, Stevens-Johnson syndrome, and anaphylactic shock associated with bupropion. Instruct patients to discontinue CONTRAVE and consult a healthcare provider if they develop an allergic or anaphylactoid/anaphylactic reaction (e.g., skin rash, pruritus, hives, chest pain, edema, or shortness of breath) during treatment.

Arthralgia, myalgia, fever with rash, and other symptoms suggestive of delayed hypersensitivity have been reported in association with bupropion. These symptoms may resemble serum sickness.

5.7 Hepatotoxicity

Cases of hepatitis and clinically significant liver dysfunction were observed in association with naltrexone exposure during naltrexone clinical trials and in postmarketing reports for patients using naltrexone. Transient, asymptomatic hepatic transaminase elevations were also observed. When patients presented with elevated transaminases, there were often other potential causative or contributory etiologies identified, including pre-existing alcoholic liver disease, hepatitis B and/or C infection, and concomitant usage of other potentially hepatotoxic drugs. Although clinically significant liver dysfunction is not typically recognized as a manifestation of opioid withdrawal, opioid withdrawal that is precipitated abruptly may lead to systemic sequelae, including acute liver injury.

Patients should be warned of the risk of hepatic injury and advised to seek medical attention if they experience symptoms of acute hepatitis. Use of CONTRAVE should be discontinued in the event of symptoms and/or signs of acute hepatitis.

In CONTRAVE clinical trials, there were no cases of elevated transaminases greater than three times the upper limit of normal (ULN) in conjunction with an increase in bilirubin greater than two times ULN.

5.8 Activation of Mania

Bupropion, a component of CONTRAVE, is a drug used for the treatment of depression. Antidepressant treatment can precipitate a manic, mixed, or hypomanic episode. The risk appears to be increased in patients with bipolar disorder or who have risk factors for bipolar disorder. Prior to initiating CONTRAVE, screen patients for a history of bipolar disorder and the presence of risk factors for bipolar disorder (e.g., family history of bipolar disorder, suicide, or depression). CONTRAVE is not approved for use in treating bipolar depression. No activation of mania or hypomania was reported in the clinical trials evaluating effects of CONTRAVE in obese patients; however, patients receiving antidepressant medications and patients with a history of bipolar disorder or recent hospitalization because of psychiatric illness were excluded from CONTRAVE clinical trials.

5.9 Angle-Closure Glaucoma

The pupillary dilation that occurs following use of many antidepressant drugs including bupropion, a component of CONTRAVE, may trigger an angle-closure attack in a patient with anatomically narrow angles who does not have a patent iridectomy.

5.10 Potential Risk of Hypoglycemia in Patients with Type 2 Diabetes Mellitus on Antidiabetic Therapy

Weight loss may increase the risk of hypoglycemia in patients with type 2 diabetes mellitus treated with insulin and/or insulin secretagogues (e.g., sulfonylureas). Measurement of blood glucose levels prior to starting CONTRAVE and during CONTRAVE treatment is recommended in patients with type 2 diabetes. Decreases in medication doses for antidiabetic medications which are non-glucose-dependent should be considered to mitigate the risk of hypoglycemia. If a patient develops hypoglycemia after starting CONTRAVE, appropriate changes should be made to the antidiabetic drug regimen.

6 ADVERSE REACTIONS

The following adverse reactions are discussed in other sections of the labeling:

- Suicidal Behavior and Ideation *[see Warnings and Precautions (5.1)]*
- Neuropsychiatric Symptoms *[see Warnings and Precautions (5.2)]*
- Seizures *[see Contraindications (4), Warnings and Precautions (5.3)]*
- Increase in Blood Pressure and Heart Rate *[see Warnings and Precautions (5.5)]*
- Allergic Reactions *[see Warnings and Precautions (5.6)]*
- Angle-Closure Glaucoma *[see Warnings and Precautions (5.9)]*

6.1 Clinical Trials Experience

Because clinical trials are conducted under widely varying conditions, the adverse reaction rates observed in the clinical trials of a drug cannot be directly compared to rates in the clinical trials of another drug and may not reflect the rates observed in practice.

CONTRAVE was evaluated for safety in five double-blind placebo controlled trials in 4,754 overweight or obese patients (3,239 patients treated with CONTRAVE and 1,515 patients treated with placebo) for a treatment period up to 56 weeks. The majority of patients were treated with CONTRAVE 32 mg/360 mg total daily dose. In addition, some patients were treated with other combination daily doses including naltrexone up to 50 mg and bupropion up to 400 mg. All subjects received study drug in addition to diet and exercise counseling. One trial (N=793) evaluated patients participating in an intensive behavioral modification program and another trial (N= 505) evaluated patients with type 2 diabetes. In these randomized, placebo-controlled trials, 2,545 patients received CONTRAVE 32 mg/360 mg for a mean treatment duration of 36 weeks (median, 56 weeks). Baseline patient characteristics included a mean age of 46 years, 82% women, 78% white, 25% with hypertension, 13% with type 2 diabetes, 56% with dyslipidemia, 25% with BMI greater than 40 kg/m^2, and less than 2% with coronary artery disease. Dosing was initiated and increased weekly to reach the maintenance dose within 4 weeks.

In CONTRAVE clinical trials, 24% of subjects receiving CONTRAVE and 12% of subjects receiving placebo discontinued treatment because of an adverse event. The most frequent adverse reactions leading to discontinuation with CONTRAVE were nausea (6.3%), headache (1.7%) and vomiting (1.1%).

Common Adverse Reactions

Adverse reactions that were reported by greater than or equal to 2% of patients, and were more frequently reported by patients treated with CONTRAVE compared to placebo, are summarized in *Table 3*.

Table 3. Adverse Reactions Reported by Obese or Overweight Patients With an Incidence (%) of at Least 2% Among Patients Treated with CONTRAVE and More Common than with Placebo

Adverse Reaction	CONTRAVE 32 mg/360 mg N=2545 %	Placebo N=1515 %
Nausea	32.5	6.7
Constipation	19.2	7.2
Headache	17.6	10.4
Vomiting	10.7	2.9
Dizziness	9.9	3.4
Insomnia	9.2	5.9
Dry mouth	8.1	2.3
Diarrhea	7.1	5.2
Anxiety	4.2	2.8
Hot flush	4.2	1.2
Fatigue	4.0	3.4
Tremor	4.0	0.7
Upper abdominal pain	3.5	1.3
Viral gastroenteritis	3.5	2.6
Influenza	3.4	3.2
Tinnitus	3.3	0.6
Urinary tract infection	3.3	2.8

Continued on next page

Hypertension	3.2	2.2
Abdominal pain	2.8	1.4
Hyperhidrosis	2.6	0.6
Irritability	2.6	1.8
Blood pressure increased	2.4	1.5
Dysgeusia	2.4	0.7
Rash	2.4	2.0
Muscle strain	2.2	1.7
Palpitations	2.1	0.9

Other Adverse Reactions

The following additional adverse reactions were reported in less than 2% of patients treated with CONTRAVE but with an incidence at least twice that of placebo:

Cardiac Disorders: tachycardia, myocardial infarction
Ear and Labyrinth Disorders: vertigo, motion sickness
Gastrointestinal Disorders: lower abdominal pain, eructation, lip swelling, hematochezia, hernia
General Disorders and Administration Site Conditions: feeling jittery, feeling abnormal, asthenia, thirst, feeling hot
Hepatobiliary Disorders: cholecystitis
Infections and Infestations: pneumonia, staphylococcal infection, kidney infection
Investigations: increased blood creatinine, increased hepatic enzymes, decreased hematocrit
Metabolism and Nutrition Disorders: dehydration
Musculoskeletal and Connective Tissue Disorders: intervertebral disc protrusion, jaw pain
Nervous System Disorders: disturbance in attention, lethargy, intention tremor, balance disorder, memory impairment, amnesia, mental impairment, presyncope
Psychiatric Disorders: abnormal dreams, nervousness, dissociation (feeling spacey), tension, agitation, mood swings
Renal and Urinary Disorders: micturition urgency
Reproductive System and Breast Disorders: vaginal hemorrhage, irregular menstruation, erectile dysfunction, vulvovaginal dryness
Skin and Subcutaneous Tissue Disorders: alopecia

Psychiatric and Sleep Disorders

In the one-year controlled trials of CONTRAVE, the proportion of patients reporting one or more adverse reactions related to psychiatric and sleep disorders was higher in the CONTRAVE 32/360 mg group than the placebo group (22.2% and 15.5%, respectively). These events were further categorized into sleep disorders (13.8% CONTRAVE, 8.4% placebo), depression (6.3% CONTRAVE, 5.9% placebo), and anxiety (6.1% CONTRAVE, 4.4% placebo). Patients who were 65 years or older experienced more psychiatric and sleep disorder adverse reactions in the CONTRAVE group (28.6%) compared to placebo (6.3%), although the sample size in this subgroup was small (56 CONTRAVE, 32 placebo); the majority of these events were insomnia (10.7% CONTRAVE, 3.1% placebo) and depression (7.1% CONTRAVE, 3.1% placebo).

Neurocognitive Adverse Reactions

Adverse reactions involving attention, dizziness, and syncope occurred more often in individuals randomized to CONTRAVE 32/360 mg group compared to placebo (15.0% and 5.5%, respectively). The most common cognitive-related adverse reactions were attention disorders (2.5% CONTRAVE, 0.6% placebo). Adverse reactions involving dizziness and syncope were more common in patients treated with CONTRAVE (10.6%) than in placebo-treated patients (3.6%); dizziness accounted for almost all of these reported events (10.4% CONTRAVE, 3.4% placebo). Dizziness was the primary reason for discontinuation for 0.9% and 0.3% of patients in the CONTRAVE and placebo groups, respectively.

Increases in Serum Creatinine

In the one-year controlled trials of CONTRAVE, larger mean increases in serum creatinine from baseline to trial endpoint were observed in the CONTRAVE group compared with the placebo group (0.07 mg/dL and 0.01 mg/dL, respectively) as well as from baseline to the maximum value during follow-up (0.15 mg/dL and 0.07 mg/dL, respectively). Increases in serum creatinine that exceeded the upper limit of

normal and were also greater than or equal to 50% higher than baseline occurred in 0.6% of subjects receiving CONTRAVE compared to 0.1% receiving placebo. An *in vitro* drug-drug interaction study demonstrated that bupropion and its metabolites inhibit organic cation transporter 2 (OCT2), which is involved in the tubular secretion of creatinine, suggesting that the observed increase in serum creatinine may be the result of OCT2 inhibition.

Based on *in vitro* results and FDA guidance for Drug Interaction Studies, the ratios of the free (unbound) C_{max} and IC50 value of bupropion and hydroxybupropion were well below 0.1 suggesting a drug-drug interaction between CONTRAVE and OCT2 substrate due to bupropion and hydroxybupropion is unlikely. The ratio for the threohydrobupropion and erythrohydrobupropion metabolite mixture was 0.29, suggesting a drug-drug interaction between CONTRAVE and OCT2 due to threohydrobupropion and erythrohydrobupropion is possible.

7 DRUG INTERACTIONS

7.1 Monoamine Oxidase Inhibitors (MAOI)

Concomitant use of MAOIs and bupropion is contraindicated. Bupropion inhibits the re-uptake of dopamine and norepinephrine and can increase the risk for hypertensive reactions when used concomitantly with drugs that also inhibit the re-uptake of dopamine or norepinephrine, including MAOIs. Studies in animals demonstrate that the acute toxicity of bupropion is enhanced by the MAOI phenelzine. At least 14 days should elapse between discontinuation of an MAOI and initiation of treatment with CONTRAVE. Conversely, at least 14 days should be allowed after stopping CONTRAVE before starting an MAOI *[see Contraindications (4)]*.

7.2 Opioid Analgesics

Patients taking CONTRAVE may not fully benefit from treatment with opioid-containing medicines, such as cough and cold remedies, antidiarrheal preparations, and opioid analgesics. In patients requiring intermittent opiate treatment, CONTRAVE therapy should be temporarily discontinued and opiate dose should not be increased above the standard dose. CONTRAVE may be used with caution after chronic opioid use has been stopped for 7 to 10 days in order to prevent precipitation of withdrawal *[see Contraindications (4) and Warnings and Precautions (5.4)]*.

During CONTRAVE clinical studies, the use of concomitant opioid or opioid-like medications, including analgesics or antitussives, were excluded.

7.3 Potential for CONTRAVE to Affect Other Drugs Metabolized by CYP2D6

In a clinical study, CONTRAVE (32 mg naltrexone/360 mg bupropion) daily was coadministered with a 50 mg dose of metoprolol (a CYP2D6 substrate). CONTRAVE increased metoprolol AUC and C_{max} by approximately 4- and 2-fold, respectively, relative to metoprolol alone. Similar clinical drug interactions resulting in increased pharmacokinetic exposure of CYP2D6 substrates have also been observed with bupropion as a single agent with desipramine or venlafaxine.

Coadministration of CONTRAVE with drugs that are metabolized by CYP2D6 isozyme including certain antidepressants (SSRIs and many tricyclics), antipsychotics (e.g., haloperidol, risperidone and thioridazine), beta-blockers (e.g., metoprolol) and Type 1C antiarrhythmics (e.g., propafenone and flecainide), should be approached with caution and should be initiated at the lower end of the dose range of the concomitant medication. If CONTRAVE is added to the treatment regimen of a patient already receiving a drug metabolized by CYP2D6, the need to decrease the dose of the original medication should be considered, particularly for those concomitant medications with a narrow therapeutic index *[see Clinical Pharmacology (12.3)]*.

7.4 Potential for Other Drugs to Affect CONTRAVE

Bupropion is primarily metabolized to hydroxybupropion by CYP2B6. Therefore, the potential exists for drug interactions between CONTRAVE and drugs that are inhibitors or inducers of CYP2B6.

Inhibitors of CYP2B6: Ticlopidine and Clopidogrel: Concomitant treatment with these drugs can increase bupropion exposure but decrease hydroxybupropion exposure. During concomitant use with CYP2B6 inhibitors (e.g., ticlopidine or clopidogrel), the CONTRAVE daily dose should not exceed two tablets (one tablet each morning and evening) *[see Dosage and Administration (2.5) and Clinical Pharmacology (12.3)]*.

Inducers of CYP2B6: Ritonavir, Lopinavir, and Efavirenz: Concomitant treatment with these drugs can decrease

bupropion and hydroxybupropion exposure and may reduce efficacy. Avoiding concomitant use with ritonavir, lopinavir, or efavirenz is recommended *[see Clinical Pharmacology (12.3)]*.

7.5 Drugs That Lower Seizure Threshold

Use extreme caution when coadministering CONTRAVE with other drugs that lower seizure threshold (e.g., antipsychotics, antidepressants, theophylline, or systemic corticosteroids). Use low initial doses and increase the dose gradually. Concomitant use of other bupropion-containing products is contraindicated *[see Contraindications (4) and Warnings and Precautions (5.3)]*.

7.6 Dopaminergic Drugs (Levodopa and Amantadine)

Bupropion, levodopa, and amantadine have dopamine agonist effects. CNS toxicity has been reported when bupropion was coadministered with levodopa or amantadine. Adverse reactions have included restlessness, agitation, tremor, ataxia, gait disturbance, vertigo, and dizziness. It is presumed that the toxicity results from cumulative dopamine agonist effects. Use caution and monitor for such adverse reactions when administering CONTRAVE concomitantly with these drugs.

7.7 Use with Alcohol

In postmarketing experience, there have been rare reports of adverse neuropsychiatric events or reduced alcohol tolerance in patients who were drinking alcohol during treatment with bupropion. The consumption of alcohol during treatment with CONTRAVE should be minimized or avoided.

7.8 Drug-Laboratory Test Interactions

False-positive urine immunoassay screening tests for amphetamines have been reported in patients taking bupropion. This is due to lack of specificity of some screening tests. False-positive test results may result even following discontinuation of bupropion therapy. Confirmatory tests, such as gas chromatography/mass spectrometry, will distinguish bupropion from amphetamines.

7.9 Drug-Transporter Interactions

In vitro, CONTRAVE constituents inhibited the renal organic cation transporter OCT2 to a clinically relevant level. The systemic concentrations of substrate drugs transported by OCT2 (such as amantadine, amiloride, cimetidine, dopamine, famotidine, memantine, metformin, pindolol, procainamide, ranitidine, varenicline, oxaliplatin) are likely to increase as a result of reduced renal clearance when coadministered with CONTRAVE. Coadministration of CONTRAVE with such drugs should be approached with caution and patients should be monitored for adverse effects.

8 USE IN SPECIFIC POPULATIONS

8.1 Pregnancy

Pregnancy Category X

Risk Summary

CONTRAVE is contraindicated during pregnancy, because weight loss offers no potential benefit to a pregnant woman and may result in fetal harm. If this drug is used during pregnancy, or if the patient becomes pregnant while taking this drug, the patient should be apprised of the potential hazard of maternal weight loss to the fetus.

Clinical Considerations

A minimum weight gain, and no weight loss, is currently recommended for all pregnant women, including those who are already overweight or obese, due to the obligatory weight gain that occurs in maternal tissues during pregnancy.

Human Data

There are no adequate and well-controlled studies of CONTRAVE in pregnant women. In clinical studies, 21 (0.7%) of 3,024 women became pregnant while taking CONTRAVE: 11 carried to term and gave birth to a healthy infant, three had elective abortions, four had spontaneous abortions, and the outcome of three pregnancies were unknown.

Data from the international bupropion Pregnancy Registry (675 first trimester exposures) and a retrospective cohort study using the United Healthcare database (1,213 first trimester exposures) did not show an increased risk for malformations overall.

No increased risk for cardiovascular malformations overall has been observed after bupropion exposure during the first trimester. The prospectively observed rate of cardiovascular malformations in pregnancies with exposure to bupropion in the first trimester from the international Pregnancy Registry was 1.3% (9 cardiovascular malformations out of 675 first-trimester maternal bupropion exposures), which is similar to the background rate of cardiovascular malformations (approximately 1%). Data from the United Healthcare database and a case-control study (6,853 infants with cardiovascular malformations and 5,763 with non-cardiovascular malformations) from the National Birth Defects Prevention Study (NBDPS) did not show an increased risk for cardiovascular malformations overall after bupropion exposure during the first trimester.

Study findings on bupropion exposure during the first trimester and risk for left ventricular outflow tract obstruction (LVOTO) are inconsistent and do not allow conclusions regarding a possible association. The United Healthcare database lacked sufficient power to evaluate this association; the NBDPS found increased risk for LVOTO (n = 10; adjusted odds ratio [OR] = 2.6; 95% CI: 1.2, 5.7), and the Slone Epidemiology case control study did not find increased risk for LVOTO.

Study findings on bupropion exposure during the first trimester and risk for ventricular septal defect (VSD) are inconsistent and do not allow conclusions regarding a possible association. The Slone Epidemiology Study found an increased risk for VSD following first trimester maternal bupropion exposure (n = 17; adjusted OR = 2.5; 95% CI: 1.3, 5.0) but did not find increased risk for any other cardiovascular malformations studied (including LVOTO as above). The NBDPS and United Healthcare database study did not find an association between first trimester maternal bupropion exposure and VSD.

For the findings of LVOTO and VSD, the studies were limited by the small number of exposed cases, inconsistent findings among studies, and the potential for chance findings from multiple comparisons in case control studies.

Animal Data

Reproduction and developmental studies have not been conducted for the combined products naltrexone and bupropion in CONTRAVE. Safety margins were estimated using body surface area exposure (mg/m^2) based on a body weight of 100 kg.

Separate studies with bupropion and naltrexone have been conducted in pregnant rats and rabbits.

Naltrexone administered orally has been shown to increase the incidence of early fetal loss in rats administered ≥30 mg/kg/day (180 mg/m^2/day) and rabbits administered ≥60 mg/kg/day (720 mg/m^2/day), doses at least 15 and 60 times, respectively, the maximum recommended human dose [MRHD] of the naltrexone component in CONTRAVE on a mg/m^2 basis. There was no evidence of teratogenicity when naltrexone was administered orally to rats and rabbits during the period of major organogenesis at doses up to 200 mg/kg/day (approximately 100 and 200 times the recommended therapeutic dose, respectively, on a mg/m^2 basis). Rats do not form appreciable quantities of the major human metabolite, 6-beta-naltrexol; therefore, the potential reproductive toxicity of the metabolite in rats is not known.

Bupropion was administered orally in studies conducted in rats and rabbits at doses up to 450 and 150 mg/kg/day, respectively (approximately 20 and 15 times the MRHD, respectively, of the bupropion component in CONTRAVE on a mg/m^2 basis), during the period of organogenesis. No clear evidence of teratogenic activity was found in either species; however, in rabbits, slightly increased incidences of fetal malformations and skeletal variations were observed at the lowest dose tested (25 mg/kg/day, approximately 2 times the MRHD on a mg/m^2 basis) and greater. Decreased fetal weights were seen at 50 mg/kg and greater (approximately 5 times the MRHD of the bupropion component in CONTRAVE on a mg/m^2 basis). When rats were administered bupropion at oral doses of up to 300 mg/kg/day (approximately 15 times the MRHD of the bupropion component in CONTRAVE on a mg/m^2 basis) prior to mating and throughout pregnancy and lactation, there were no apparent adverse effects on offspring development.

8.3 Nursing Mothers

The constituents and metabolites of CONTRAVE have been shown to be secreted in human milk. Transfer of naltrexone and 6-beta-naltrexol into human milk has been reported with oral naltrexone. Bupropion and its metabolites are also secreted in human milk. CONTRAVE is not recommended for nursing mothers.

8.4 Pediatric Use

The safety and effectiveness of CONTRAVE in pediatric patients below the age of 18 have not been established and the use of CONTRAVE is not recommended in pediatric patients.

8.5 Geriatric Use

Of the 3,239 subjects who participated in clinical trials with CONTRAVE, 62 (2%) were 65 years and older and none were 75 years and older. Clinical studies of CONTRAVE did not include sufficient numbers of subjects aged 65 and over to determine whether they respond differently from younger subjects. Older individuals may be more sensitive to the central nervous system adverse effects of CONTRAVE. Naltrexone and bupropion are known to be substantially excreted by the kidney, and the risk of adverse reactions to CONTRAVE may be greater in patients with impaired renal function. Because elderly patients are more likely to have decreased renal function, care should be taken in dose selection, and it may be useful to monitor renal function. CONTRAVE should be used with caution in patients over 65 years of age.

8.6 Renal Impairment

A dedicated pharmacokinetic study has not been conducted for CONTRAVE in subjects with renal impairment. Based on information available for the individual constituents, systemic exposure is significantly higher for bupropion and metabolites (two- to three-fold), and naltrexone and their metabolites in subjects with moderate-to-severe renal impairment. Therefore, the maximum recommended daily maintenance dose for CONTRAVE is two tablets (one tablet each morning and evening) in patients with moderate or severe renal impairment. CONTRAVE is not recommended for use in patients with end-stage renal disease. There is a lack of adequate information to guide CONTRAVE dosing in patients with mild renal impairment *[see Dosage and Administration (2.2) and Clinical Pharmacology (12.3)]*.

8.7 Hepatic Impairment

CONTRAVE has not been evaluated in subjects with hepatic impairment. Based on information available for the individual constituents, systemic exposure is significantly higher for bupropion and metabolites (two- to three-fold), and naltrexone and their metabolites (up to 10-fold higher) in subjects with moderate-to-severe hepatic impairment. Therefore, the maximum recommended daily dose of CONTRAVE is one tablet in the morning in patients with hepatic impairment *[see Dosage and Administration (2.3) and Clinical Pharmacology (12.3)]*.

9 DRUG ABUSE AND DEPENDENCE

9.2 Abuse

Humans

CONTRAVE (naltrexone HCl and bupropion HCl) has not been systematically studied in humans for its potential for abuse, tolerance, or physical dependence. However, in outpatient clinical studies of up to 56 weeks in duration, there was no evidence of euphoric drug intoxication, physical dependence, diversion, or abuse. There was no evidence of an abstinence syndrome following abrupt or tapered drug discontinuation after 56 weeks of double-blind, placebo-controlled, randomized treatment.

Naltrexone is a pure opioid antagonist. It does not lead to physical or psychological dependence. Tolerance to the opioid antagonistic effect is not known to occur.

Controlled clinical trials of bupropion (immediate-release formulation) conducted in normal volunteers, in subjects with a history of multiple drug abuse, and in depressed subjects showed some increase in motor activity and agitation/excitement. In a population of individuals experienced with drugs of abuse, a single dose of 400 mg of bupropion produced mild amphetamine-like activity as compared with placebo on the Morphine-Benzedrine Subscale of the Addiction Research Center Inventories (ARCI) and a score intermediate between placebo and amphetamine on the Liking Scale of the ARCI. These scales measure general feelings of euphoria and drug desirability.

Findings in clinical trials, however, are not known to reliably predict the abuse potential of drugs. Nonetheless, evidence from single-dose studies does suggest that the recommended daily dosage of bupropion when administered in divided doses is not likely to be significantly reinforcing to amphetamine or CNS stimulant abusers.

The inhalation of crushed tablets or injection of dissolved bupropion has been reported. Seizures and/or cases of death have been reported when bupropion has been administered intranasally or by parenteral injection. CONTRAVE (naltrexone HCl and bupropion HCl) extended-release tablets are intended for oral use only.

Animals

Studies in rodents and primates have shown that bupropion exhibits some pharmacologic actions common to psychostimulants. In rodents, it has been shown to increase locomotor activity, elicit a mild stereotyped behavioral response, and increased rates of responding in several schedule-controlled behavior paradigms. In primate models assessing the positive reinforcing effects of psychoactive drugs, bupropion was self-administered intravenously. In rats, bupropion produced amphetamine-like and cocaine-like discriminative stimulus effects in drug discrimination paradigms used to characterize the subjective effects of psychoactive drugs.

10 OVERDOSAGE

Human Experience

There is no clinical experience with overdosage with CONTRAVE. The maximum daily dose of CONTRAVE administered in clinical trials contained 50 mg naltrexone and 400 mg bupropion. The most serious clinical implications of CONTRAVE overdose are likely those related to overdose of bupropion.

Overdoses of up to 30 grams or more of bupropion (equivalent of up to 83 times the recommended daily dose of CONTRAVE 32 mg/360 mg) have been reported. Seizure was reported in approximately one third of all cases. Other serious reactions reported with overdoses of bupropion alone included hallucinations, loss of consciousness, sinus tachycardia, and ECG changes such as conduction disturbances (including QRS prolongation) or arrhythmias. Fever, muscle rigidity, rhabdomyolysis, hypotension, stupor, coma, and respiratory failure have been reported mainly when bupropion was part of multiple drug overdoses.

Although most patients recovered without sequelae, deaths associated with overdoses of bupropion alone have been reported in patients ingesting large doses of the drug. Multiple uncontrolled seizures, bradycardia, cardiac failure, and cardiac arrest prior to death were reported in these patients.

There is limited experience with overdose of naltrexone monotherapy in humans. In one study, subjects who received 800 mg naltrexone daily (equivalent to 25 times the recommended daily dose of CONTRAVE 32 mg/360 mg) for up to one week showed no evidence of toxicity.

Animal Experience

In the mouse, rat, and guinea pig, the oral LD50s for naltrexone were 1,100 to 1,550 mg/kg; 1,450 mg/kg; and 1,490 mg/kg; respectively. High doses of naltrexone (generally greater than or equal to 1,000 mg/kg) produced salivation, depression/reduced activity, tremors, and convulsions. Mortality in animals due to high-dose naltrexone administration usually was due to clonic-tonic convulsions and/or respiratory failure.

Overdosage Management

If over-exposure occurs, call your poison control center at 1-800-222-1222. There are no known antidotes for CONTRAVE. In case of an overdose, provide supportive care, including close medical supervision and monitoring. Consider the possibility of multiple drug overdose. Ensure an adequate airway, oxygenation, and ventilation. Monitor cardiac rhythm and vital signs. Induction of emesis is not recommended.

11 DESCRIPTION

CONTRAVE extended-release tablets contain naltrexone hydrochloride and bupropion hydrochloride.

Naltrexone hydrochloride, USP, an opioid antagonist, is a synthetic congener of oxymorphone with no opioid agonist properties. Naltrexone differs in structure from oxymorphone in that the methyl group on the nitrogen atom is replaced by a cyclopropylmethyl group. Naltrexone hydrochloride is also related to the potent opioid antagonist, naloxone, or n-allylnoroxymorphone.

Naltrexone hydrochloride has the chemical name of morphinan-6-one, 17-(cyclopropylmethyl)-4,5-epoxy-3,14-dihydroxy-, hydrochloride, (5α)-. The empirical formula is $C_{20}H_{23}NO_4 \cdot HCl$ and the molecular weight is 377.86. The structural formula is:

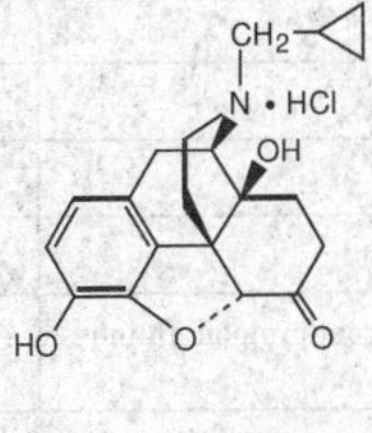

Continued on next page

Naltrexone hydrochloride is a white to yellowish, crystalline compound. It is soluble in water to the extent of about 100 mg/mL.

Bupropion hydrochloride is an antidepressant of the aminoketone class. Bupropion hydrochloride closely resembles the structure of diethylpropion. It is designated as (±)-1-(3 chlorophenyl)-2-[(1,1-dimethylethyl)amino]-1-propranone hydrochloride. It is related to phenylethylamines. The empirical formula is $C_{13}H_{18}ClNO•HCl$ and the molecular weight is 276.2. The structural formula is:

Bupropion hydrochloride powder is white, crystalline, and highly soluble in water.

CONTRAVE is available for oral administration as a round, bi-convex, film-coated, extended-release tablet. Each tablet has a trilayer core composed of two drug layers, containing the drug and excipients, separated by a more rapidly dissolving inert layer. Each tablet contains 8 mg of naltrexone hydrochloride and 90 mg of bupropion hydrochloride. Tablets are blue and are debossed with NB-890 on one side. Each tablet contains the following inactive ingredients: microcrystalline cellulose, hydroxypropyl cellulose, lactose anhydrous, L-cysteine hydrochloride, crospovidone, magnesium stearate, hypromellose, edetate disodium, lactose monohydrate, colloidal silicon dioxide, Opadry II Blue and FD&C Blue #2 aluminum lake.

12 CLINICAL PHARMACOLOGY

12.1 Mechanism of Action

CONTRAVE has two components: naltrexone, an opioid antagonist, and bupropion, a relatively weak inhibitor of the neuronal reuptake of dopamine and norepinephrine. Nonclinical studies suggest that naltrexone and bupropion have effects on two separate areas of the brain involved in the regulation of food intake: the hypothalamus (appetite regulatory center) and the mesolimbic dopamine circuit (reward system). The exact neurochemical effects of CONTRAVE leading to weight loss are not fully understood.

12.2 Pharmacodynamics

Combined, bupropion and naltrexone increased the firing rate of hypothalamic pro-opiomelanocortin (POMC) neurons *in vitro*, which are associated with regulation of appetite. The combination of bupropion and naltrexone also reduced food intake when injected directly into the ventral tegmental area of the mesolimbic circuit in mice, an area associated with regulation of reward pathways.

12.3 Pharmacokinetics

Absorption

Naltrexone

Following single oral administration of CONTRAVE (two 8 mg naltrexone/90 mg bupropion tablets) to healthy subjects, mean peak naltrexone concentration (C_{max}) was 1.4 ng/mL, time to peak concentration (T_{max}) was 2 hours, and extent of exposure (AUC_{0-inf}) was 8.4 ng·hr/mL.

Bupropion

Following single oral administration of CONTRAVE (two 8 mg naltrexone/90 mg bupropion tablets) to healthy subjects, mean peak bupropion concentration (C_{max}) was 168 ng/mL, time to peak concentration (T_{max}) was three hours, and extent of exposure (AUC_{0-inf}) was 1,607 ng·hr/mL.

Food Effect on Absorption

When CONTRAVE was administered with a high-fat meal, the AUC and C_{max} for naltrexone increased 2.1-fold and 3.7-fold, respectively, and the AUC and C_{max} for bupropion increased 1.4-fold and 1.8-fold, respectively. At steady state, the food effect increased AUC and C_{max} for naltrexone by 1.7-fold and 1.9-fold, respectively, and increased AUC and

C_{max} for bupropion by 1.1-fold and 1.3-fold, respectively. Thus, CONTRAVE should not be taken with high-fat meals because of the resulting significant increases in bupropion and naltrexone systemic exposure.

Distribution

Naltrexone

Naltrexone is 21% plasma protein bound. The mean apparent volume of distribution at steady state for naltrexone (V_{ss}/F) is 5,697 liters.

Bupropion

Bupropion is 84% plasma protein bound. The mean apparent volume of distribution at steady state for bupropion (V_{ss}/F) is 880 liters.

Metabolism and Excretion

Naltrexone

The major metabolite of naltrexone is 6-beta-naltrexol. The activity of naltrexone is believed to be the result of both the parent and the 6-beta-naltrexol metabolite. Though less potent, 6-beta-naltrexol is eliminated more slowly and thus circulates at much higher concentrations than naltrexone. Naltrexone and 6-beta-naltrexol are not metabolized by cytochrome P450 enzymes and *in vitro* studies indicate that there is no potential for inhibition or induction of important isozymes.

Naltrexone and its metabolites are excreted primarily by the kidney (53% to 79% of the dose). Urinary excretion of unchanged naltrexone accounts for less than 2% of an oral dose. Urinary excretion of unchanged and conjugated 6-beta-naltrexol accounts for 43% of an oral dose. The renal clearance for naltrexone ranges from 30 to 127 mL/min, suggesting that renal elimination is primarily by glomerular filtration. The renal clearance for 6-beta-naltrexol ranges from 230 to 369 mL/min suggesting an additional renal tubular secretory mechanism. Fecal excretion is a minor elimination pathway.

Following single oral administration of CONTRAVE tablets to healthy subjects, mean elimination half-life ($T_{1/2}$) was approximately 5 hours for naltrexone. Following twice daily administration of CONTRAVE, naltrexone did not accumulate and its kinetics appeared linear. However, in comparison to naltrexone, 6-beta-naltrexol accumulates to a larger extent (accumulation ratio ~3).

Bupropion

Bupropion is extensively metabolized with three active metabolites: hydroxybupropion, threohydrobupropion and erythrohydrobupropion. The metabolites have longer elimination half-lives than bupropion and accumulate to a greater extent. Following bupropion administration, more than 90% of the exposure is a result of metabolites. *In vitro* findings suggest that CYP2B6 is the principal isozyme involved in the formation of hydroxybupropion whereas cytochrome P450 isozymes are not involved in the formation of the other active metabolites. Bupropion and its metabolites inhibit CYP2D6. Plasma protein binding of hydroxybupropion is similar to that of bupropion (84%) whereas the other two metabolites have approximately half the binding.

Following oral administration of 200 mg of ^{14}C-bupropion in humans, 87% and 10% of the radioactive dose were recovered in the urine and feces, respectively. The fraction of the oral dose of bupropion excreted unchanged was 0.5%, a finding consistent with the extensive metabolism of bupropion.

Following single oral administration of CONTRAVE tablets to healthy subjects, mean elimination half-life ($T_{1/2}$) was approximately 21 hours for bupropion. Following twice daily administration of CONTRAVE, metabolites of bupropion, and to a lesser extent unchanged bupropion, accumulate and reach steady-state concentrations in approximately one week.

Specific Populations

Gender

Pooled analysis of CONTRAVE data suggested no clinically meaningful differences in the pharmacokinetic parameters of bupropion or naltrexone based on gender.

Race

Pooled analysis of CONTRAVE data suggested no clinically meaningful differences in the pharmacokinetic parameters of bupropion or naltrexone based on race.

Elderly

The pharmacokinetics of CONTRAVE have not been evaluated in the geriatric population. The effects of age on the pharmacokinetics of naltrexone or bupropion and their metabolites have not been fully characterized. An exploration of steady-state bupropion concentrations from several depression efficacy studies involving patients dosed in a range of 300 to 750 mg/day, on a three times daily schedule, revealed no relationship between age (18 to 83 years) and plasma concentration of bupropion. A single-dose pharmacokinetic study demonstrated that the disposition of bupropion and its metabolites in elderly subjects was similar to that of younger subjects. These data suggest there is no prominent effect of age on bupropion concentration; however, another pharmacokinetic study, single and multiple dose, has suggested that the elderly are at increased risk for accumulation of bupropion and its metabolites *[see Use in Specific Populations (8.5)]*.

Smokers

Pooled analysis of CONTRAVE data revealed no meaningful differences in the plasma concentrations of bupropion or naltrexone in smokers compared with nonsmokers. The effects of cigarette smoking on the pharmacokinetics of bupropion were studied in 34 healthy male and female volunteers; 17 were chronic cigarette smokers and 17 were nonsmokers. Following oral administration of a single 150 mg dose of bupropion, there was no statistically significant difference in C_{max}, half-life, T_{max}, AUC, or clearance of bupropion or its active metabolites between smokers and nonsmokers.

Hepatic Impairment

Pharmacokinetic data are not available with CONTRAVE in patients with hepatic impairment. The following information is available for individual constituents:

Naltrexone

An increase in naltrexone AUC of approximately 5- and 10-fold in patients with compensated and decompensated liver cirrhosis, respectively, compared with subjects with normal liver function, has been reported. These data also suggest that alterations in naltrexone bioavailability are related to liver disease severity.

Bupropion

The effect of hepatic impairment on the pharmacokinetics of bupropion was characterized in two single-dose trials, one trial in patients with alcoholic liver disease and a second trial in patients with mild-to-severe cirrhosis.

The first trial showed that the half-life of hydroxybupropion was significantly longer in eight patients with alcoholic liver disease than in eight healthy volunteers (32±14 hours vs 21±5 hours, respectively). Although not statistically significant, the AUCs for bupropion and hydroxybupropion were more variable and tended to be greater (by 53% to 57%) in patients with alcoholic liver disease. The differences in half-life for bupropion and the other metabolites in the two patient groups were minimal.

The second trial demonstrated no statistically significant differences in the pharmacokinetics of bupropion and its active metabolites in nine subjects with mild-to-moderate hepatic cirrhosis compared with eight healthy volunteers. However, more variability was observed in some of the pharmacokinetic parameters for bupropion (AUC, C_{max}, and T_{max}) and its active metabolites ($t_{1/2}$) in subjects with mild-to-moderate hepatic cirrhosis. In subjects with severe hepatic cirrhosis, significant alterations in the pharmacokinetics of bupropion and its metabolites were seen *(Table 4)*. [See table 4 below]

The dose of CONTRAVE should be reduced in patients with hepatic impairment *[see Dosage and Administration (2.3) and Use in Specific Populations (8.7)]*.

Renal Impairment

A dedicated pharmacokinetic study has not been conducted for CONTRAVE in subjects with renal impairment. The following information is available for the individual constituents:

Naltrexone

Limited information is available for naltrexone in patients with moderate to severe renal impairment. In a study of

Table 4. Pharmacokinetics of Bupropion and Metabolites in Patients With Severe Hepatic Cirrhosis: Ratio Relative to Healthy Matched Controls

	C_{max}	AUC	$t_{1/2}$	T_{max}*
Bupropion	1.69	3.12	1.43	0.5 h
Hydroxybupropion	0.31	1.28	3.88	19 h
Threo/erythrohydrobupropion amino alcohol	0.69	2.48	1.96	20 h

* = Difference

seven patients with end-stage renal disease requiring dialysis, peak plasma concentrations of naltrexone were elevated at least 6-fold compared to healthy subjects.

Bupropion

Limited information is available for bupropion in patients with moderate to severe renal impairment. An inter-trial comparison between normal subjects and patients with end-stage renal failure demonstrated that the bupropion C_{max} and AUC values were comparable in the two groups, whereas the hydroxybupropion and threohydrobupropion metabolites had a 2.3- and 2.8-fold increase, respectively, in AUC for patients with end-stage renal failure. A second trial, comparing normal subjects and patients with moderate-to-severe renal impairment (GFR 30.9 ± 10.8 mL/min) showed that exposure after a single 150 mg dose of sustained-release bupropion was approximately 2-fold higher in patients with impaired renal function while levels of the hydroxybupropion and threo/erythrohydrobupropion (combined) metabolites were similar in the two groups. The elimination of bupropion and/or the major metabolites of bupropion may be reduced by impaired renal function.

The dose of CONTRAVE should be reduced in patients with moderate or severe renal impairment. CONTRAVE is not recommended for use in patients with end-stage renal disease [see Dosage and Administration (2.2) and Use in Specific Populations (8.6)].

Drug Interactions

In Vitro Assessment of Drug Interactions

At therapeutically relevant concentrations, naltrexone and 6-beta-naltrexol are not major inhibitors of CYP isoforms CYP1A2, CYP2B6, CYP2C8, CYP2E1, CYP2C9, CYP2C19, CYP2D6 or CYP3A4. Both naltrexone and 6-beta-naltrexol are not major inducers of CYP isoforms CYP1A2, CYP2B6, or CYP3A4.

Bupropion and its metabolites (hydroxybupropion, erythrohydrobupropion, threohydrobupropion) are inhibitors of CYP2D6.

In vitro studies suggest that paroxetine, sertraline, norfluoxetine, fluvoxamine, and nelfinavir inhibit the hydroxylation of bupropion.

Bupropion (IC_{50} 9.3 mcM) and its metabolites, hydroxybupropion (IC_{50} 82 mcM) and threohydrobupropion and erythrohydrobupropion (1:1 mixture; IC_{50} 7.8 mcM), inhibited the renal organic transporter OCT2 to a clinically relevant level. The systemic concentrations of substrate drugs transported by OCT2 are likely to increase as a result of reduced renal clearance when coadministered with CONTRAVE.

Effects of Naltrexone/Bupropion on the Pharmacokinetics of Other Drugs

Drug interaction between CONTRAVE and CYP2D6 substrates (metoprolol) or other drugs (atorvastatin, glyburide, lisinopril, nifedipine, valsartan) has been evaluated. In addition, drug interaction between bupropion, a component of CONTRAVE, and CYP2D6 substrates (desipramine) or other drugs (citalopram, lamotrigine) has also been evaluated.

[See table 5 above]

Effects of Other Drugs on the Pharmacokinetics of Naltrexone/Bupropion

Drug interactions between CYP2B6 inhibitors (ticlopidine, clopidogrel, prasugrel), CYP2B6 inducers (ritonavir, lopinavir) and bupropion (one of the CONTRAVE components), or between other drugs (atorvastatin, glyburide, metoprolol, lisinopril, nifedipine, valsartan) and CONTRAVE have been evaluated. While not systematically studied, carbamazepine, phenobarbital, or phenytoin may induce the metabolism of bupropion.

[See table 6 on next page]

13   NONCLINICAL TOXICOLOGY

13.1   Carcinogenesis, Mutagenesis, Impairment of Fertility

Studies to evaluate carcinogenesis, mutagenesis, or impairment of fertility with the combined products in CONTRAVE have not been conducted. The following findings are from studies performed individually with naltrexone and bupropion. The potential carcinogenic, mutagenic and fertility effects of the metabolite 6-beta-naltrexol are unknown. Safety margins were estimated using body surface area exposure (mg/m^2) based on a body weight of 100 kg.

In a two-year carcinogenicity study in rats with naltrexone, there were small increases in the numbers of testicular mesotheliomas in males and tumors of vascular origin in males and females. The incidence of mesothelioma in males given naltrexone at a dietary dose of 100 mg/kg/day (approxi-

Table 5. Effect of Naltrexone/Bupropion Coadministration on Systemic Exposure of Other Drugs

Naltrexone/Bupropion Dosage	Coadministered Drug	
	Name and Dose Regimens	**Change in Systemic Exposure**
Initiate the following drugs at the lower end of the dose range during concomitant use with CONTRAVE [see Drug Interactions 7]:		
Bupropion 150 mg twice daily for 10 days	Desipramine 50 mg single dose	↑5-fold AUC, ↑2-fold C_{max}
Bupropion 300 mg (as XL) once daily for 14 days	Citalopram 40 mg once daily for 14 days	↑40% AUC, ↑30% C_{max}
Naltrexone/Bupropion 16 mg/180 mg twice daily for 7 days	Metoprolol 50 mg single dose	↑4-fold AUC, ↑2-fold C_{max}
No dose adjustment needed for the following drugs during concomitant use with CONTRAVE:		
Naltrexone/Bupropion 16 mg/180 mg single dose	Atorvastatin 80 mg single dose	No Effect
Naltrexone/Bupropion 16 mg/180 mg single dose	Glyburide 6 mg single dose	No Effect
Naltrexone/Bupropion 16 mg/180 mg single dose	Lisinopril 40 mg single dose	No Effect
Naltrexone/Bupropion 16 mg/180 mg single dose	Nifedipine 90 mg single dose	No Effect
Naltrexone/Bupropion 16 mg/180 mg single dose	Valsartan 320 mg single dose	No Effect
Bupropion 150 mg twice daily for 12 days	Lamotrigine 100 mg single dose	No Effect

mately 50 times the recommended therapeutic dose on a mg/m^2 basis for the naltrexone maintenance dose for CONTRAVE) was 6%, compared with a maximum historical incidence of 4%. The incidence of vascular tumors in males and females given dietary doses of 100 mg/kg/day was 4%, but only the incidence in females was increased compared with a maximum historical control incidence of 2%. There was no evidence of carcinogenicity in a two-year dietary study with naltrexone in male and female mice.

Lifetime carcinogenicity studies of bupropion were performed in rats and mice at doses up to 300 and 150 mg/kg/day, respectively. These doses are approximately 15 and 3 times the maximum recommended human dose (MRHD) of the bupropion component in CONTRAVE, respectively, on a mg/m^2 basis. In the rat study there was an increase in nodular proliferative lesions of the liver at doses of 100 to 300 mg/kg/day (approximately 5 to 15 times the MRHD of the bupropion component in CONTRAVE on a mg/m^2 basis); lower doses were not tested. The question of whether or not such lesions may be precursors of neoplasms of the liver is currently unresolved. Similar liver lesions were not seen in the mouse study, and no increase in malignant tumors of the liver and other organs was seen in either study.

There was limited evidence of a weak genotoxic effect of naltrexone in one gene mutation assay in a mammalian cell line, in the Drosophila recessive lethal assay, and in non-specific DNA repair tests with *E. coli*. However, no evidence of genotoxic potential was observed in a range of other *in vitro* tests, including assays for gene mutation in bacteria, yeast, or in a second mammalian cell line, a chromosomal aberration assay, and an assay for DNA damage in human cells. Naltrexone did not exhibit clastogenicity in an *in vivo* mouse micronucleus assay.

Bupropion produced a positive response (two to three times control mutation rate) in two of five strains in the Ames bacterial mutagenicity test and an increase in chromosomal aberrations in one of three *in vivo* rat bone marrow cytogenetic studies.

Naltrexone administered orally to rats caused a significant increase in pseudopregnancy and a decrease in pregnancy rates in rats at 100 mg/kg/day (approximately 50 times the MRHD of the naltrexone component in CONTRAVE on a mg/m^2 basis). There was no effect on male fertility at this dose level. The relevance of these observations to human fertility is not known.

A fertility study of bupropion in rats at doses up to 300 mg/kg/day (approximately 15 times the MRHD of the bupropion component in CONTRAVE on a mg/m^2 basis) revealed no evidence of impaired fertility.

14   CLINICAL STUDIES

The effects of CONTRAVE on weight loss in conjunction with reduced caloric intake and increased physical activity was studied in double-blind, placebo-controlled trials (BMI range 27 to 45 kg/m^2) with study durations of 16 to 56 weeks randomized to naltrexone (16 to 50 mg/day) and/or bupropion (300 to 400 mg/day) or placebo.

Effect on Weight Loss and Weight Maintenance

Four 56-week multicenter, double-blind, placebo-controlled obesity trials (CONTRAVE Obesity Research, or COR-I, COR-II, COR-BMOD, and COR-Diabetes) were conducted to evaluate the effect of CONTRAVE in conjunction with lifestyle modification in 4,536 patients randomized to CONTRAVE or placebo. The COR-I, COR-II, and COR-BMOD trials enrolled patients with obesity (BMI 30 kg/m^2 or greater) or overweight (BMI 27 kg/m^2 or greater) and at least one comorbidity (hypertension or dyslipidemia). The COR-Diabetes trial enrolled patients with BMI greater than 27 kg/m^2 with type 2 diabetes with or without hypertension and/or dyslipidemia.

Treatment was initiated with a three-week dose-escalation period followed by approximately 1 year of continued therapy. Patients were instructed to take CONTRAVE with food. COR-I and COR-II included a program consisting of a reduced-calorie diet resulting in an approximate 500 kcal/day decrease in caloric intake, behavioral counseling, and increased physical activity. COR-BMOD included an intensive behavioral modification program consisting of 28 group counseling sessions over 56 weeks as well as a prescribed diet and exercise regimen. COR-Diabetes evaluated patients with type 2 diabetes not achieving glycemic goal of a HbA1c less than 7% either with oral antidiabetic agents or with diet and exercise alone. Of the overall population from these four trials, 24% had hypertension, 54% had dyslipidemia at study entry, and 10% had type 2 diabetes.

Apart from COR-Diabetes, which only enrolled patients with type 2 diabetes, the demographic characteristics of patients were similar across all four trials. For the four trial populations combined, the mean age was 46 years, 83% were female, 77% were Caucasian, 18% were black, and 5% were other races. At baseline, mean BMI was 36 kg/m^2 and mean waist circumference was 110 cm.

A substantial percentage of randomized patients withdrew from the trials prior to Week 56: 45% for the placebo group and 46% for the CONTRAVE group. The majority of these patients discontinued within the first 12 weeks of treatment. Approximately 24% of patients treated with

Continued on next page

CONTRAVE and 12% of patients treated with placebo discontinued treatment because of an adverse reaction [see Adverse Reactions (6.1)].

The co-primary endpoints were percent change from baseline body weight and the proportion of patients achieving at least a 5% reduction in body weight. In the 56-week COR-I trial, the mean change in body weight was -5.4% among patients assigned to CONTRAVE 32 mg/360 mg compared with -1.3% among patients assigned to placebo (Intent-To-Treat [ITT] population), as shown in Table 7 and Figure 1. In this trial, the achievement of at least a 5% reduction in body weight from baseline occurred more frequently for patients treated with CONTRAVE 32 mg/360 mg compared with placebo (42% vs 17%; *Table 7*). Results from COR-BMOD and COR-Diabetes are shown in Table 7 and Figures 2 and 3.

[See table 7 on next page]

[See Figures 1, 2 and 3 on page 1001]

Effect on Cardiovascular and Metabolic Parameters

Changes in cardiovascular and metabolic parameters associated with obesity are presented for COR-I and COR-BMOD (*Table 8*). Changes in mean blood pressure and heart rate are further described elsewhere [see Warnings and Precautions (5.5)].

[See table 8 on page 1000]

Effect of CONTRAVE on Cardiometabolic Parameters and Anthropometry in Patients with Type 2 Diabetes Mellitus

Changes in glycemic control observed from baseline to Week 56 among patients with type 2 diabetes and obesity assigned to either CONTRAVE 32 mg/360 mg or placebo are shown in *Table 9*.

[See table 9 on page 1001]

Effect on Body Composition

In a subset of 124 patients (79 CONTRAVE, 45 placebo), body composition was measured using dual energy X-ray absorptiometry (DEXA). The DEXA assessment showed that mean total body fat mass decreased by 4.7 kg (11.7%) in the CONTRAVE group vs 1.4 kg (4.3%) in the placebo group at Week 52/LOCF (treatment difference, -3.3 kg [-7.4%], p<0.01).

16 HOW SUPPLIED/STORAGE AND HANDLING

CONTRAVE 8 mg/90 mg (naltrexone HCl 8 mg and bupropion HCl 90 mg) extended-release, tri-layer tablets are blue, round, bi-convex, film-coated tablets debossed with "NB-890" on one side. CONTRAVE tablets are available as follows:

NDC 51267-890-99   Bottles of 120 tablets

Storage

Store at 25°C (77°F); excursions permitted to 15° to 30°C (59° to 86°F) [see USP Controlled Room Temperature].

17 PATIENT COUNSELING INFORMATION

See FDA-Approved Patient Labeling (Medication Guide)

Patient information is printed at the end of this insert. This information and the instructions provided in the Medication Guide should be discussed with patients.

Patients should be advised to take CONTRAVE exactly as prescribed. Patients should be instructed to follow the dose escalation schedule and not to take more than the recommended dose of CONTRAVE.

Patients should be made aware that CONTRAVE contains the same active ingredient (bupropion) found in certain antidepressants and smoking cessation products (including, but not limited to, WELLBUTRIN, WELLBUTRIN SR, WELLBUTRIN XL, and APLENZIN) and that CONTRAVE should not be used in combination with any other medications that contain bupropion.

Patients should be advised that some patients have experienced changes in mood (including depression and mania), psychosis, hallucinations, paranoia, delusions, homicidal ideation, aggression, anxiety, and panic, as well as suicidal ideation, suicide attempt, and completed suicide when attempting to quit smoking while taking bupropion. If patients develop agitation, hostility, depressed mood, or changes in thinking or behavior that are not typical for them, or if patients develop suicidal ideation or behavior, they should be urged to report these symptoms to their healthcare provider immediately.

Patients should be advised of the potential serious risks associated with the use of CONTRAVE, including suicidality, seizures, and increases in blood pressure or heart rate.

Table 6. Effect of Coadministered Drugs on Systemic Exposure of Naltrexone/Bupropion

Name and Dose Regimens	Coadministered Drug	
	CONTRAVE Components	Change in Systemic Exposure
Do not exceed one tablet twice daily dose of CONTRAVE with the following drugs:		
Ticlopidine 250 mg twice daily for 4 days	Bupropion Hydroxybupropion	↑85% AUC, ↑38% C_{max} ↓84% AUC, ↓78% C_{max}
Clopidogrel 75 mg once daily for 4 days	Bupropion Hydroxybupropion	↑60% AUC, ↑40% C_{max} ↓52% AUC, ↓50% C_{max}
No dose adjustment needed for CONTRAVE with the following drugs:		
Atorvastatin 80 mg single dose	Naltrexone 6-beta naltrexol Bupropion Hydroxybupropion Threohydrobupropion Erythrohydrobupropion	No Effect No Effect No Effect No Effect No Effect No Effect
Lisinopril 40 mg single dose	Naltrexone 6-beta naltrexol Bupropion Hydroxybupropion Threohydrobupropion Erythrohydrobupropion	No Effect No Effect No Effect No Effect No Effect No Effect
Valsartan 320 mg single dose	Naltrexone 6-beta naltrexol Bupropion Hydroxybupropion Threohydrobupropion Erythrohydrobupropion	No Effect No Effect No Effect ↓14% AUC, No Effect on C_{max} No Effect No Effect
Cimetidine 800 mg single dose	Bupropion Hydroxybupropion Threo/Erythrohydrobupropion	No Effect No Effect ↑16% AUC, ↑32% C_{max}
Citalopram 40 mg once daily for 14 days	Bupropion Hydroxybupropion Threohydrobupropion Erythrohydrobupropion	No Effect No Effect No Effect No Effect
Metoprolol 50 mg single dose	Naltrexone 6-beta naltrexol Bupropion Hydroxybupropion Threohydrobupropion Erythrohydrobupropion	↓25% AUC, ↓29% C_{max} No Effect No Effect No Effect No Effect No Effect
Nifedipine 90 mg single dose	Naltrexone 6-beta naltrexol Bupropion Hydroxybupropion Threohydrobupropion Erythrohydrobupropion	↑24% AUC, ↑58% C_{max} No Effect No Effect on AUC, ↑22% C_{max} No Effect No Effect No Effect
Prasugrel 10 mg once daily for 6 days	Bupropion Hydroxybupropion	↑18% AUC, ↑14% C_{max} ↓24% AUC, ↓32% C_{max}
Use CONTRAVE with caution with the following drugs:		
Glyburide 6 mg single dose*	Naltrexone 6-beta naltrexol Bupropion Hydroxybupropion Threohydrobupropion Erythrohydrobupropion	↑2-fold AUC, ↑2-fold C_{max} No Effect ↑36% AUC, ↑18% C_{max} ↑22% AUC, ↑21% C_{max} No Effect on AUC, ↑15% C_{max} No Effect
Avoid concomitant use of CONTRAVE with following drugs:		
Ritonavir 100 mg twice daily for 17 days	Bupropion Hydroxybupropion Threohydrobupropion Erythrohydrobupropion	↓22% AUC, ↓21 % C_{max} ↓23% AUC, No Effect on C_{max} ↓38% AUC, ↓39 % C_{max} ↓48% AUC, ↓28 % C_{max}
600 mg twice daily for 8 days	Bupropion Hydroxybupropion Threohydrobupropion Erythrohydrobupropion	↓66% AUC, ↓62% C_{max} ↓78% AUC, ↓42 % C_{max} ↓50% AUC, ↓58% C_{max} ↓68% AUC, ↓48 % C_{max}
Lopinavir/Ritonavir 400 mg/100 mg twice daily for 14 days	Bupropion Hydroxybupropion	↓57% AUC, ↓57% C_{max} ↓50% AUC, ↓31% C_{max}
Efavirenz 600 mg once daily for 2 weeks	Bupropion Hydroxybupropion	↓55% AUC, ↓34% C_{max} No Effect on AUC, ↑50% C_{max}

*Results were confounded by the food-effect due to oral glucose coadministered with the treatment.

Patients should be advised to call their healthcare provider to report new or sudden changes in mood, behavior, thoughts, or feelings.

Patients should be advised that taking CONTRAVE can cause mild pupillary dilation, which in susceptible individuals, can lead to an episode of angle-closure glaucoma. Pre-existing glaucoma is almost always open-angle glaucoma because angle-closure glaucoma, when diagnosed, can be treated definitively with iridectomy. Open-angle glaucoma is not a risk factor for angle-closure glaucoma. Patients may wish to be examined to determine whether they are susceptible to angle closure, and have a prophylactic procedure (e.g., iridectomy), if they are susceptible.

Patients should be educated on the symptoms of hypersensitivity and to discontinue CONTRAVE if they have a severe allergic reaction to CONTRAVE.

Patients should be told that CONTRAVE should be discontinued and not restarted if they experience a seizure while on treatment.

Patients should be advised that the excessive use or abrupt discontinuation of alcohol, benzodiazepines, antiepileptic drugs, or sedatives/hypnotics can increase the risk of seizure. Patients should be advised to minimize or avoid use of alcohol.

Patients should be advised that if they previously used opioids, they may be more sensitive to lower doses of opioids and at risk of accidental overdose should they use opioids after CONTRAVE treatment is discontinued or temporarily interrupted.

Patients should be advised that because naltrexone, a component of CONTRAVE, can block the effects of opioids, they will not perceive any effect if they attempt to self-administer any opioid drug in small doses while on CONTRAVE. Further advise patients that the attempt to administer large doses of any opioid or to bypass the blockade while on CONTRAVE may lead to serious injury, coma, or death.

Patients should be off all opioids for a minimum of 7 to 10 days before starting CONTRAVE in order to avoid precipitation of withdrawal. Advise patients they should not take CONTRAVE if they have any symptoms of opioid withdrawal.

Patients should be advised to call their healthcare provider if they experience increased blood pressure or heart rate.

Patients should be advised to notify their healthcare provider if they are taking, or plan to take, any prescription or over-the-counter drugs. Concern is warranted because CONTRAVE and other drugs may affect each other's metabolism.

Patients should be advised to notify their healthcare provider if they become pregnant, intend to become pregnant, or are breastfeeding during therapy.

Patients with type 2 diabetes mellitus on antidiabetic therapy should be advised to monitor their blood glucose levels and report symptoms of hypoglycemia to their healthcare provider(s).

Patients should be advised to swallow CONTRAVE tablets whole so that the release rate is not altered. Do not chew, divide, or crush tablets.

Distributed by:

Orexigen Therapeutics, Inc.
La Jolla, CA 92037
CONTRAVE® is a registered trademark of Orexigen Therapeutics, Inc.
All other trademarks are the property of their respective owners.
©2016 Orexigen Therapeutics, Inc.
LBL-00022

Medication Guide
CONTRAVE® (CON-trayv)
(naltrexone HCl and bupropion HCl)
Extended-Release Tablets
Read this Medication Guide before you start taking CONTRAVE and each time you get a refill. There may be new information. This information does not take the place of talking with your healthcare provider about your medical problems or treatment.

What is the most important information I should know about CONTRAVE?

CONTRAVE can cause serious side effects, including:

• **Suicidal thoughts or actions.** One of the ingredients in CONTRAVE is bupropion. Bupropion has caused some people to have suicidal thoughts or actions or unusual changes in behavior, whether or not they are taking medicines used to treat depression.

Bupropion may increase suicidal thoughts or actions in some children, teenagers, and young adults within the first few months of treatment.

If you already have depression or other mental illnesses, taking bupropion may cause it to get worse, especially within the first few months of treatment.

Stop taking CONTRAVE and call a healthcare provider right away if you, or your family member, have any of the following symptoms, especially if they are new, worse, or worry you:

- ○ thoughts about suicide or dying
- ○ attempts to commit suicide
- ○ new or worse depression
- ○ new or worse anxiety
- ○ feeling very agitated or restless
- ○ panic attacks
- ○ trouble sleeping (insomnia)
- ○ new or worse irritability
- ○ acting aggressive, being angry, or violent
- ○ acting on dangerous impulses
- ○ an extreme increase in activity and talking (mania)
- ○ other unusual changes in behavior or mood

While taking CONTRAVE, you or your family members should:

- ○ Pay close attention to any changes, especially sudden changes, in mood, behaviors, thoughts, or feelings. This is very important when you start taking CONTRAVE or when your dose changes.
- ○ Keep all follow-up visits with your healthcare provider as scheduled. Call your healthcare provider between visits as needed, especially if you have concerns about symptoms.

CONTRAVE has not been studied in and is not approved for use in children under the age of 18.

What is CONTRAVE?

CONTRAVE is a prescription medicine which contains 2 medicines (naltrexone and bupropion) that may help some obese or overweight adults, who also have weight related medical problems, lose weight and keep the weight off.

• CONTRAVE should be used with a reduced calorie diet and increased physical activity.
• It is not known if CONTRAVE changes your risk of heart problems or stroke or of death due to heart problems or stroke.
• It is not known if CONTRAVE is safe and effective when taken with other prescription, over-the-counter, or herbal weight loss products.
• It is not known if CONTRAVE is safe and effective in children under 18 years of age.
• CONTRAVE is not approved to treat depression or other mental illnesses, or to help people quit smoking (smoking cessation). One of the ingredients in CONTRAVE, bupropion, is the same ingredient in some other medicines used to treat depression and to help people quit smoking.

Who should not take CONTRAVE?

Do not take CONTRAVE if you:

• have uncontrolled hypertension
• have or have had seizures
• use other medicines that contain bupropion such as WELLBUTRIN, WELLBUTRIN SR, WELLBUTRIN XL and APLENZIN
• have or have had an eating disorder called anorexia (eating very little) or bulimia (eating too much and vomiting to avoid gaining weight)
• are dependent on opioid pain medicines or use medicines to help stop taking opioids such as methadone or buprenorphine, or are in opiate withdrawal
• drink a lot of alcohol and abruptly stop drinking, or use medicines called sedatives (these make you sleepy), benzodiazepines, or anti-seizure medicines and you stop using them all of a sudden
• are taking medicines called monoamine oxidase inhibitors (MAOIs). Ask your healthcare provider or pharmacist if you are not sure if you take an MAOI, including linezolid. **Do not** start CONTRAVE until you have stopped taking your MAOI for at least 14 days.
• are allergic to naltrexone or bupropion or any of the ingredients in CONTRAVE. See the end of this Medication Guide for a complete list of ingredients in CONTRAVE.
• are pregnant or planning to become pregnant. Tell your healthcare provider right away if you become pregnant while taking CONTRAVE.

What should I tell my healthcare provider before taking CONTRAVE?

Before you take CONTRAVE, tell your healthcare provider if you:

• have or have had depression or other mental illnesses (such as bipolar disorder)

Table 7. Changes in Weight in 56-Week Trials with CONTRAVE (ITT/LOCF*)

	COR-I		COR-BMOD		COR-Diabetes	
	CONTRAVE 32 mg/ 360 mg	Placebo	CONTRAVE 32 mg/ 360 mg	Placebo	CONTRAVE 32 mg/ 360 mg	Placebo
N	538	536	565	196	321	166
Weight (kg)						
Baseline mean (SD)	99.8 (16.1)	99.5 (14.4)	100.3 (15.5)	101.8 (15.0)	104.2 (19.1)	105.3 (16.9)
LS Mean % Change From Baseline (SE)	-5.4 (0.3)	-1.3 (0.3)	-8.1 (0.4)	-4.9 (0.6)	-3.7 (0.3)	-1.7 (0.4)
Difference from placebo (95% CI)	-4.1† (-4.9, -3.3)		-3.2† (-4.5, -1.8)		-2.0† (-3.0, -1.0)	
Percentage of patients losing greater than or equal to 5% body weight	42	17	57	43	36	18
Risk difference vs placebo (95% CI)	25† (19, 30)		14† (6, 22)		18† (9, 25)	
Percentage of patients losing greater than or equal to 10% body weight	21	7	35	21	15	5
Risk difference vs placebo (95% CI)	14† (10, 18)		14† (7, 21)		10‡ (4, 15)	

Type 1 error was controlled across all 3 endpoints
*Based on last observation carried forward (LOCF) in all randomized subjects who had a baseline body weight measurement and at least one post baseline body weight measurement during the defined treatment phase. All available body weight data during the double-blind treatment phase are included in the analysis, including data collected from subjects who discontinued study drug.
†Difference from placebo, p<0.001
‡Difference from placebo, p<0.01
The percentages of patients who achieved at least 5% or at least 10% body weight loss from baseline were greater among those assigned to CONTRAVE, compared with placebo, in all four obesity trials (Table 7).

Continued on next page

Table 8. Change in Markers of Cardiovascular and Metabolic Parameters from Baseline in 56 Week Trials with CONTRAVE 32 mg/360 mg (COR-I and COR-BMOD)*

Parameter	COR-I			COR-BMOD		
	CONTRAVE 32 mg/360 mg N=471	Placebo N=511	CONTRAVE minus Placebo (LS Mean)	CONTRAVE 32 mg/360 mg N=482	Placebo N=193	CONTRAVE minus Placebo (LS Mean)
Triglycerides, mg/dL						
Baseline median (Q1, Q3)	113 (86, 158)	112 (78, 157)	-10.7†	110 (78, 162)	103 (76, 144)	-9.9†
Median % change	-11.6	1.7		-17.8	-7.4	
HDL-C, mg/dL						
Baseline mean (SD)	51.9 (13.6)	52.0 (13.6)	7.2	53.6 (13.5)	55.3 (12.9)	6.6
LS Mean % change (SE)	8.0 (0.9)	0.8 (0.9)		9.4 (1.0)	2.8 (1.6)	
LDL-C, mg/dL						
Baseline mean (SD)	118.8 (32.6)	119.7 (34.8)	-1.5	109.5 (27.5)	109.2 (27.3)	-2.9
LS Mean % change (SE)	-2.0 (1.0)	-0.5 (1.1)		7.1 (1.4)	10.0 (2.2)	
Waist circumference, cm						
Baseline mean (SD)	108.8 (11.3)	110.0 (12.2)	-3.8‡	109.3 (11.4)	109.0 (11.8)	-3.2‡
LS Mean change (SE)	-6.2 (0.4)	-2.5 (0.4)		-10.0 (0.5)	-6.8 (0.8)	
Heart rate, bpm						
Baseline mean (SD)	72.1 (8.7)	71.8 (8.0)	1.2	70.7 (8.3)	70.4 (9.0)	0.9
LS Mean change (SE)	1.0 (0.3)	-0.2 (0.3)		1.1 (0.4)	0.2 (0.5)	
Systolic blood pressure, mmHg						
Baseline mean (SD)	118.9 (9.8)	119.0 (9.8)	1.8	116.9 (9.9)	116.7 (10.9)	2.6
LS Mean change (SE)	-0.1 (0.4)	-1.9 (0.4)		-1.3 (0.5)	-3.9 (0.7)	
Diastolic blood pressure, mmHg						
Baseline mean (SD)	77.1 (7.2)	77.3 (6.6)	0.9	78.2 (7.2)	77.2 (7.4)	1.4
LS Mean change (SE)	0.0 (0.3)	-0.9 (0.3)		-1.4 (0.3)	-2.8 (0.5)	

Q1: first quartile; Q3: third quartile

*Based on last observation carried forward (LOCF) while on study drug

†Hodges-Lehmann estimate of treatment difference

‡Statistically significant vs placebo (p<0.001) based on the pre-specified closed testing procedure method for controlling Type I error

- have attempted suicide in the past
- have or have had seizures
- have had a head injury
- have had a tumor or infection of your brain or spine (central nervous system)
- have had a problem with low blood sugar (hypoglycemia) or low levels of sodium in your blood (hyponatremia)
- have or have had liver problems
- have high blood pressure
- have or have had a heart attack, heart problems, or have had a stroke
- have kidney problems
- are diabetic taking insulin or other medicines to control your blood sugar
- have or have had an eating disorder
- drink a lot of alcohol

- abuse prescription medicines or street drugs
- are over the age of 65
- have any other medical conditions
- are breastfeeding or plan to breastfeed. CONTRAVE can pass into your breast milk and may harm your baby. You and your healthcare provider should decide if you should take CONTRAVE or breastfeed. You should not do both.
- **Tell your healthcare provider about all the medicines you take** including prescription and over-the-counter medicines, vitamins, and herbal supplements.
CONTRAVE may affect the way other medicines work and other medicines may affect the way CONTRAVE works causing side effects.
Ask your healthcare provider for a list of these medicines if you are not sure.

Know the medicines you take. Keep a list of them to show your healthcare provider or pharmacist when you get a new medicine.
How should I take CONTRAVE?

How to take CONTRAVE

	Morning Dose	Evening Dose
Starting: Week 1	1 tablet	None
Week 2	1 tablet	1 tablet
Week 3	2 tablets	1 tablet
Week 4 Onward	2 tablets	2 tablets

- Take CONTRAVE exactly as your healthcare provider tells you to.
- **Do not** change your CONTRAVE dose without talking with your healthcare provider.
- Your healthcare provider will change your dose if needed.
- Your healthcare provider should tell you to stop taking CONTRAVE if you have not lost a certain amount of weight after 16 weeks of treatment.
- **Swallow CONTRAVE tablets whole. Do not cut, chew, or crush CONTRAVE tablets.** Tell your healthcare provider if you cannot swallow CONTRAVE tablets whole.
- **Do not** take more than 2 tablets in the morning and 2 tablets in the evening.
- **Do not** take more than 2 tablets at the same time or more than 4 tablets in 1 day.
- **Do not** take CONTRAVE with high-fat meals. It may increase your risk of seizures.
- If you miss a dose of CONTRAVE, wait until your next regular time to take it. **Do not** take more than 1 dose of CONTRAVE at a time.
- If you take too much CONTRAVE, call your healthcare provider or go to the nearest emergency room right away.

What should I avoid while taking CONTRAVE?
- **Do not** drink a lot of alcohol while taking CONTRAVE. If you drink a lot of alcohol, talk with your healthcare provider before suddenly stopping. If you suddenly stop drinking alcohol, you may increase your chance of having a seizure.

What are the possible side effects of CONTRAVE?
CONTRAVE may cause serious side effects, including:
- See "What is the most important information I should know about CONTRAVE?"
- **Seizures.** There is a risk of having a seizure when you take CONTRAVE. The risk of seizure is higher in people who:
  ○ take higher doses of CONTRAVE
  ○ have certain medical conditions
  ○ take CONTRAVE with certain other medicines
Do not take any other medicines while you are taking CONTRAVE unless your healthcare provider has said it is okay to take them.
If you have a seizure while taking CONTRAVE, stop taking CONTRAVE and call your healthcare provider right away. You should not take CONTRAVE again if you have a seizure.
- **Risk of opioid overdose.** One of the ingredients in CONTRAVE (naltrexone) can increase your chance of having an opioid overdose if you take opioid medicines while taking CONTRAVE.
You can accidentally overdose in 2 ways:
  ○ Naltrexone blocks the effects of opioids, such as heroin, methadone or opioid pain medicines. **Do not** take large amounts of opioids, including opioid-containing medicines, such as heroin or prescription pain pills, to try to overcome the opioid-blocking effects of naltrexone. This can lead to serious injury, coma, or death.
  ○ After you take naltrexone, its blocking effect slowly decreases and completely goes away over time. If you have used opioid street drugs or opioid-containing medicines in the past, using opioids in amounts that you used before treatment with naltrexone can lead to overdose and death. You may also be more sensitive to the effects of lower amounts of opioids:
    » after you have gone through detoxification
    » when your next dose of CONTRAVE is due
    » if you miss a dose of CONTRAVE
    » after you stop CONTRAVE treatment
It is important that you tell your family and the people closest to you of this increased sensitivity to opioids and the risk of overdose.
You or someone close to you should get emergency medical help right away if you:
  ○ have trouble breathing

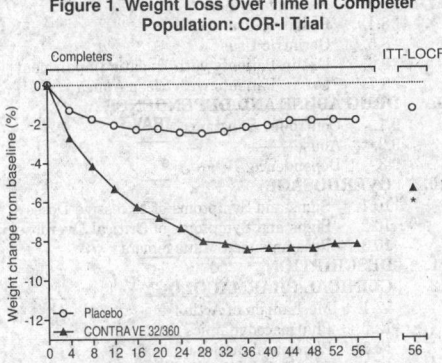

Figure 1. Weight Loss Over Time in Completer Population: COR-I Trial

*p<0.001 vs placebo
COR-I trial: 50.1% in the placebo group and 49.2% in the CONTRAVE group discontinued study drug.

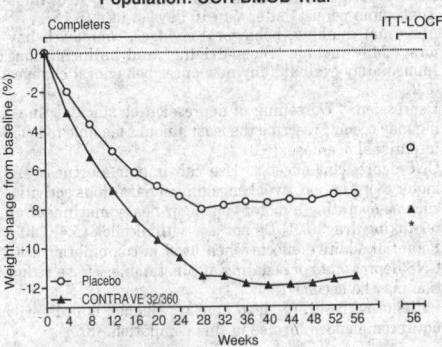

Figure 2. Weight Loss Over Time in Completer Population: COR-BMOD Trial

*p<0.001 vs placebo
COR-BMOD trial: 41.6% in the placebo group and 42.1% in the CONTRAVE group discontinued study drug.

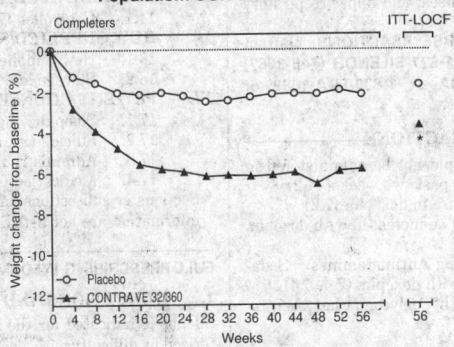

Figure 3. Weight Loss Over Time in Completer Population: COR-Diabetes Trial

*p<0.001 vs placebo
COR-Diabetes trial: 41.2% in the placebo group and 47.8% in the CONTRAVE group discontinued study drug.

Table 9. Changes in Cardiometabolic Parameters and Waist Circumference in Patients with Type 2 Diabetes Mellitus in a 56 Week Trial with CONTRAVE 32 mg/360 mg (COR-Diabetes)

	CONTRAVE 32 mg/360 mg N=265		Placebo N=159		
	Baseline	Change from Baseline (LS Mean)	Baseline	Change from Baseline (LS Mean)	CONTRAVE minus Placebo (LS Mean)
HbA1c (%)	8.0	-0.6	8.0	-0.1	-0.5*
Fasting Glucose (mg/dL)	160.0	-11.9	163.9	-4.0	-7.9
Waist Circumference (cm)	115.6	-5.0	114.3	-2.9	-2.1
Systolic blood pressure (mmHg)	125.0	0.0	124.5	-1.1	1.2
Diastolic blood pressure (mmHg)	77.5	-1.1	77.4	-1.5	0.4
Heart rate (bpm)	72.9	0.7	73.1	-0.2	0.9
	Baseline	% Change from Baseline (LS Mean)	Baseline	% Change from Baseline (LS Mean)	CONTRAVE minus Placebo (LS Mean)
Triglycerides (mg/dL)[†]	147 (98, 200)	-7.7	168 (114, 236)	-8.6	-3.3
HDL Cholesterol (mg/dL)	46.2	7.4	46.1	-0.2	7.6
LDL Cholesterol (mg/dL)	100.2	2.4	101.0	4.2	-1.9

Based on last observation carried forward (LOCF) while on study drug

*Statistically significant vs placebo (p<0.001) based on the pre-specified closed testing procedure method for controlling Type I error

[†]Values are baseline median (first and third quartiles), median % change, and the Hodges-Lehmann estimate of the median treatment difference

- become very drowsy with slowed breathing
- have slow, shallow breathing (little chest movement with breathing)
- feel faint, very dizzy, confused, or have unusual symptoms
- **Sudden opioid withdrawal.** People who take CONTRAVE must not use any type of opioid (must be opioid-free) including street drugs, prescription pain medicines (including tramadol), cough, cold, or diarrhea medicines that contain opioids, or opioid dependence treatments, buprenorphine or methadone, **for at least 7 to 10 days before starting CONTRAVE.** Using opioids in the 7 to 10 days before you start taking CONTRAVE may cause you to suddenly have symptoms of opioid withdrawal when you take it. Sudden opioid withdrawal can be severe, and you may need to go to the hospital. Tell your healthcare provider you are taking CONTRAVE before a medical procedure or surgery.
- **Severe allergic reactions.** Some people have had a severe allergic reaction to bupropion, one of the ingredients in CONTRAVE. **Stop taking CONTRAVE and call your healthcare provider or go to the nearest hospital emergency room right away** if you have any of the following signs and symptoms of an allergic reaction:
  - rash
  - itching
  - hives
  - fever
  - swollen lymph glands
  - painful sores in your mouth or around your eyes
  - swelling of your lips or tongue
  - chest pain
  - trouble breathing
- **Increases in blood pressure or heart rate.** Some people may get high blood pressure or have a higher heart rate when taking CONTRAVE. Your healthcare provider should check your blood pressure and heart rate before you start taking, and while you take CONTRAVE.
- **Liver damage or hepatitis.** One of the ingredients in CONTRAVE, naltrexone can cause liver damage or hepatitis. Stop taking CONTRAVE and tell your healthcare provider if you have any of the following symptoms of liver problems:
  - stomach area pain lasting more than a few days
  - dark urine
  - yellowing of the whites of your eyes
  - tiredness
  Your healthcare provider may need to stop treating you with CONTRAVE if you get signs or symptoms of a serious liver problem.
- **Manic episodes.** One of the ingredients in CONTRAVE, bupropion can cause some people who were manic or depressed in the past to become manic or depressed again.
- **Visual problems (angle-closure glaucoma).** One of the ingredients in CONTRAVE, bupropion, can cause some people to have visual problems (angle-closure glaucoma). Signs and symptoms of angle-closure glaucoma may include:
  - eye pain
  - changes in vision
  - swelling or redness in or around the eye
  Talk with your healthcare provider to find out if you are at risk for angle-closure glaucoma and to get treatment to prevent it if you are at risk.
- **Increased risk of low blood sugar (hypoglycemia) in people with type 2 diabetes mellitus who also take medicines to treat their diabetes.** Weight loss can cause low blood sugar in people with type 2 diabetes mellitus who also take medicines used to treat type 2 diabetes mellitus (such as insulin or sulfonylureas). You should check your blood sugar before you start taking CONTRAVE and while you take CONTRAVE.

The most common side effects of CONTRAVE include:
- nausea
- constipation
- headache
- vomiting
- dizziness
- trouble sleeping
- dry mouth
- diarrhea

Tell your healthcare provider about any side effect that bothers you or does not go away. These are not all the possible side effects of CONTRAVE. For more information, ask your healthcare provider or pharmacist.

Call your doctor for medical advice about side effects. You may report side effects to FDA at 1-800-FDA-1088.

How should I store CONTRAVE?

Store CONTRAVE at room temperature between 59°F to 86°F (15°C to 30°C).

Keep CONTRAVE and all medicines out of the reach of children.

General information about the safe and effective use of CONTRAVE.

Continued on next page

Medicines are sometimes prescribed for purposes other than those listed in a Medication Guide. Do not use CONTRAVE for a condition for which it was not prescribed. Do not give CONTRAVE to other people, even if they have the same symptoms or condition that you have. It may harm them. If you take a urine drug screening test, CONTRAVE may make the test result positive for amphetamines. If you tell the person giving you the drug screening test that you are taking CONTRAVE, they can do a more specific drug screening test that should not have this problem.

This Medication Guide summarizes the most important information about CONTRAVE. If you would like more information, talk with your healthcare provider. You can ask your pharmacist or healthcare provider for information about CONTRAVE that is written for health professionals. For more information, go to www.contrave.com or call 1-877-298-8340.

What are the ingredients in CONTRAVE?
Active ingredients: naltrexone hydrochloride and bupropion hydrochloride
Inactive ingredients: microcrystalline cellulose, hydroxypropyl cellulose, lactose anhydrous, L-cysteine hydrochloride, crospovidone, magnesium stearate, hypromellose, edetate disodium, lactose monohydrate, colloidal silicon dioxide, Opadry II Blue and FD&C Blue #2 aluminum lake
This Medication Guide has been approved by the U.S. Food and Drug Administration.
Distributed by:
Orexigen Therapeutics, Inc.
La Jolla, CA 92037
CONTRAVE® is a registered trademark of Orexigen Therapeutics, Inc.
All other trademarks are the property of their respective owners.
©2016 Orexigen Therapeutics, Inc.
Revised: September 2016
LBL-00022

Shown in Product Identification Guide, page 509

Pernix Therapeutics, LLC
10 North Park Place, Suite 201
Morristown, NJ 07960

Telephone: 800-793-2145
Fax: 862-260-8752

SILENOR®   ℞
[SI-leh-nor]
(doxepin)
tablets for oral administration

HIGHLIGHTS OF PRESCRIBING INFORMATION
These highlights do not include all the information needed to use Silenor safely and effectively. See full prescribing information for Silenor.
Silenor® (doxepin) tablets for oral administration
Initial U.S. Approval: 1969

————INDICATIONS AND USAGE————
Silenor (doxepin) tablets are indicated for the treatment of insomnia characterized by difficulties with sleep maintenance. (1, 14)

————DOSAGE AND ADMINISTRATION————
• Initial dose: 6 mg, once daily for adults (2.1) and 3 mg, once daily for the elderly. (2.1, 2.2)
• Take within 30 minutes of bedtime. Total daily dose should not exceed 6 mg. (2.3)
• Should not be taken within 3 hours of a meal. (2.3, 12.3)

————DOSAGE FORMS AND STRENGTHS————
• 3 mg and 6 mg tablets. Tablets not scored. (3)

————CONTRAINDICATIONS————
• Hypersensitivity to doxepin hydrochloride, inactive ingredients, or other dibenzoxepines. (4.1)
• Co-administration with Monoamine Oxidase Inhibitors (MAOIs): Do not administer if patient is taking MAOIs or has used MAOIs within the past two weeks. (4.2)
• Untreated narrow angle glaucoma or severe urinary retention. (4.3)

————WARNINGS AND PRECAUTIONS————
• Need to Evaluate for Co-morbid Diagnoses: Reevaluate if insomnia persists after 7 to 10 days of use. (5.1)
• Abnormal thinking, behavioral changes, complex behaviors: May include "Sleep-driving" and hallucinations. Immediately evaluate any new onset behavioral changes. (5.2)
• Depression: Worsening of depression or suicidal thinking may occur. Prescribe the least amount feasible to avoid intentional overdose. (5.3)
• CNS-depressant effects: Use can impair alertness and motor coordination. Avoid engaging in hazardous activities such as operating a motor vehicle or heavy machinery after taking drug. (5.4) Do not use with alcohol. (5.4, 7.3)
• Potential additive effects when used in combination with CNS depressants or sedating antihistamines. Dose reduction may be needed. (5.4, 7.4)
• Patients with severe sleep apnea: Silenor is ordinarily not recommended for use in this population. (8.7)

————ADVERSE REACTIONS————
• The most common treatment-emergent adverse reactions, reported in ≥ 2% of patients treated with Silenor, and more commonly than in patients treated with placebo, were somnolence/sedation, nausea, and upper respiratory tract infection. (6.1)

To report SUSPECTED ADVERSE REACTIONS, contact Pernix Therapeutics, LLC. at 1-877-SILENOR (745-3667) and www.silenor.com or FDA at 1-800-FDA-1088 or www.fda.gov/medwatch

————DRUG INTERACTIONS————
• MAO inhibitors: Silenor should not be administered in patients on MAOIs within the past two weeks. (4.2)
• Cimetidine: Increases exposure to doxepin. (7.2)
• Alcohol: Sedative effects may be increased with doxepin. (7.3, 5.4)
• CNS Depressants and Sedating Antihistamines: Sedative effects may be increased with doxepin. (7.4, 5.4)
• Tolazamide: A case of severe hypoglycemia has been reported. (7.5)

————USE IN SPECIFIC POPULATIONS————
• Pregnancy: Based on animal data, may cause fetal harm. (8.1)
• Nursing Mothers: Infant exposure via human milk. (8.3)
• Pediatric Use: Safety and effectiveness have not been evaluated. (8.4)
• Geriatric Use: The recommended starting dose is 3 mg. Monitor prior to considering dose escalation. (2.2, 8.5)
• Use in Patients with Comorbid Illness: Initiate treatment with 3 mg in patients with hepatic impairment or tendency to urinary retention. (8.6, 4.3)
See 17 for PATIENT COUNSELING INFORMATION and Medication Guide.

Revised: 3/2010

FULL PRESCRIBING INFORMATION: CONTENTS*

FULL PRESCRIBING INFORMATION

1.   INDICATIONS AND USAGE
Silenor is indicated for the treatment of insomnia characterized by difficulty with sleep maintenance. The clinical trials performed in support of efficacy were up to 3 months in duration [see *Clinical Studies (14)*].

2.   DOSAGE AND ADMINISTRATION
The dose of Silenor should be individualized.
2.1.   Dosing in Adults
The recommended dose of Silenor for adults is 6 mg once daily. A 3 mg once daily dose may be appropriate for some patients, if clinically indicated.
2.2.   Dosing in the Elderly
The recommended starting dose of Silenor in elderly patients (≥ 65 years old) is 3 mg once daily. The daily dose can be increased to 6 mg, if clinically indicated.
2.3.   Administration
Silenor should be taken within 30 minutes of bedtime. To minimize the potential for next day effects, Silenor should not be taken within 3 hours of a meal [see *Clinical Pharmacology (12.3)*].
The total Silenor dose should not exceed 6 mg per day.

3.   DOSAGE FORMS AND STRENGTHS
Silenor is an immediate-release, oval-shaped, tablet for oral administration available in strengths of 3 mg and 6 mg. The tablets are blue (3 mg) or green (6 mg) and are debossed with 3 or 6, respectively, on one side and SP on the other. Silenor tablets are not scored.

4.   CONTRAINDICATIONS
4.1.   Hypersensitivity
Silenor is contraindicated in individuals who have shown hypersensitivity to doxepin HCl, any of its inactive ingredients, or other dibenzoxepines.
4.2.   Co-administration with Monoamine Oxidase Inhibitors (MAOIs)
Serious side effects and even death have been reported following the concomitant use of certain drugs with MAO inhibitors. Do not administer Silenor if patient is currently on MAOIs or has used MAOIs within the past two weeks. The exact length of time may vary depending on the particular MAOI dosage and duration of treatment.
4.3.   Glaucoma and Urinary Retention
Silenor is contraindicated in individuals with untreated narrow angle glaucoma or severe urinary retention.

5.   WARNINGS AND PRECAUTIONS
5.1.   Need to Evaluate for Comorbid Diagnoses
Because sleep disturbances may be the presenting manifestation of a physical and/or psychiatric disorder, symptom-

atic treatment of insomnia should be initiated only after careful evaluation of the patient. **The failure of insomnia to remit after 7 to 10 days of treatment may indicate the presence of a primary psychiatric and/or medical illness that should be evaluated.** Exacerbation of insomnia or the emergence of new cognitive or behavioral abnormalities may be the consequence of an unrecognized psychiatric or physical disorder. Such findings have emerged during the course of treatment with hypnotic drugs.

5.2. Abnormal Thinking and Behavioral Changes

Complex behaviors such as "sleep-driving" (i.e., driving while not fully awake after ingestion of a hypnotic, with amnesia for the event) have been reported with hypnotics. These events can occur in hypnotic-naive as well as in hypnotic-experienced persons. Although behaviors such as "sleep-driving" may occur with hypnotics alone at therapeutic doses, the use of alcohol and other CNS depressants with hypnotics appears to increase the risk of such behaviors, as does the use of hypnotics at doses exceeding the maximum recommended dose. Due to the risk to the patient and the community, discontinuation of Silenor should be strongly considered for patients who report a "sleep-driving" episode. Other complex behaviors (e.g., preparing and eating food, making phone calls, or having sex) have been reported in patients who are not fully awake after taking a hypnotic. As with "sleep-driving", patients usually do not remember these events. Amnesia, anxiety and other neuro-psychiatric symptoms may occur unpredictably.

5.3. Suicide Risk and Worsening of Depression

In primarily depressed patients, worsening of depression, including suicidal thoughts and actions (including completed suicides), has been reported in association with the use of hypnotics.

Doxepin, the active ingredient in Silenor, is an antidepressant at doses 10- to 100-fold higher than in Silenor. Antidepressants increased the risk compared to placebo of suicidal thinking and behavior (suicidality) in children, adolescents, and young adults in short-term studies of major depressive disorder (MDD) and other psychiatric disorders. Risk from the lower dose of doxepin in Silenor can not be excluded.

It can rarely be determined with certainty whether a particular instance of the abnormal behaviors listed above is drug induced, spontaneous in origin, or a result of an underlying psychiatric or physical disorder. Nonetheless, the emergence of any new behavioral sign or symptom of concern requires careful and immediate evaluation.

5.4. CNS Depressant Effects

After taking Silenor, patients should confine their activities to those necessary to prepare for bed. Patients should avoid engaging in hazardous activities, such as operating a motor vehicle or heavy machinery, at night after taking Silenor, and should be cautioned about potential impairment in the performance of such activities that may occur the day following ingestion.

When taken with Silenor, the sedative effects of alcoholic beverages, sedating antihistamines, and other CNS depressants may be potentiated [*see Warnings and Precautions (5.2) and Drug Interactions (7.3, 7.4)*]. Patients should not consume alcohol with Silenor [*see Warnings and Precautions (5.2) and Drug Interactions (7.3)*]. Patients should be cautioned about potential additive effects of Silenor used in combination with CNS depressants or sedating antihistamines [*see Warnings and Precautions (5.2) and Drug Interactions (7.4)*].

6. ADVERSE REACTIONS

The following serious adverse reactions are discussed in greater detail in other sections of labeling:

- Abnormal thinking and behavioral changes [*see Warnings and Precautions (5.2)*].
- Suicide risk and worsening of depression [*see Warnings and Precautions (5.3)*].
- CNS Depressant effects [*see Warnings and Precautions (5.4)*].

6.1. Clinical Trials Experience

The pre-marketing development program for Silenor included doxepin HCl exposures in 1017 subjects (580 insomnia patients and 437 healthy subjects) from 12 studies conducted in the United States. 863 of these subjects (580 insomnia patients and 283 healthy subjects) participated in six randomized, placebo-controlled efficacy studies with Silenor doses of 1 mg, 3 mg, and 6 mg for up to 3-months in duration.

Because clinical studies are conducted under widely varying conditions, adverse reaction rates observed in the clinical studies of a drug cannot be directly compared to rates in the clinical studies of another drug and may not reflect the rates observed in practice. However, data from the Silenor studies provide the physician with a basis for estimating the relative contributions of drug and non-drug factors to adverse reaction incidence rates in the populations studied.

Associated with Discontinuation of Treatment

The percentage of subjects discontinuing Phase 1, 2, and 3 trials for an adverse reaction was 0.6% in the placebo group compared to 0.4%, 1.0%, and 0.7% in the Silenor 1 mg, 3 mg, and 6 mg groups, respectively. No reaction that resulted in discontinuation occurred at a rate greater than 0.5%.

Adverse Reactions Observed at an Incidence of ≥ 2% in Controlled Trials

Table 1 shows the incidence of treatment-emergent adverse reactions from three long-term (28 to 85 days) placebo-controlled studies of Silenor in adult (N=221) and elderly (N=494) subjects with chronic insomnia.

Reactions reported by Investigators were classified using a modified MedDRA dictionary of preferred terms for purposes of establishing incidence. The table includes only reactions that occurred in 2% or more of subjects who received Silenor 3 mg or 6 mg in which the incidence in subjects treated with Silenor was greater than the incidence in placebo-treated subjects.

Table 1 Incidence (%) of Treatment-Emergent Adverse Reactions in Long-term Placebo-Controlled Clinical Trials

System Organ Class Preferred Term*	Placebo (N=278)	Silenor 3 mg (N=157)	Silenor 6 mg (N=203)
Nervous System Disorders			
Somnolence/ Sedation	4	6	9
Infections and Infestations			
Upper Respiratory Tract Infection/ Nasopharyngitis	2	4	2
Gastroenteritis	0	2	0
Gastrointestinal Disorders			
Nausea	1	2	2
Vascular Disorders			
Hypertension	0	3	< 1

* Includes reactions that occurred at a rate of ≥ 2% in any Silenor-treated group and at a higher rate than placebo.

The most common treatment-emergent adverse reaction in the placebo and each of the Silenor dose groups was somnolence/sedation.

6.2. Studies Pertinent to Safety Concerns for Sleep-promoting Drugs

Residual Pharmacological Effect in Insomnia Trials

Five randomized, placebo-controlled studies in adults and the elderly assessed next-day psychomotor function within 1 hour of awakening utilizing the digit-symbol substitution test (DSST), symbol copying test (SCT), and visual analog scale (VAS) for sleepiness, following night time administration of Silenor.

In a one-night, double-blind study conducted in 565 healthy adult subjects experiencing transient insomnia, Silenor 6 mg showed modest negative changes in SCT and VAS.

In a 35-day, double-blind, placebo-controlled, parallel group study of Silenor 3 and 6 mg in 221 adults with chronic insomnia, small decreases in the DSST and SCT occurred in the 6 mg group.

In a 3-month, double-blind, placebo-controlled, parallel group study in 240 elderly subjects with chronic insomnia, Silenor 1 mg and 3 mg was comparable to placebo on DSST, SCT, and VAS.

6.3. Other Reactions Observed During the Premarketing Evaluation of Silenor

Silenor was administered to 1017 subjects in clinical trials in the United States. Treatment-emergent adverse reactions recorded by clinical investigators were standardized using a modified MedDRA dictionary of preferred terms.

The following is a list of MedDRA terms that reflect treatment-emergent adverse reactions reported by subjects treated with Silenor.

Adverse reactions are further categorized by body system and listed in order of decreasing frequency according to the following definitions: **Frequent** adverse reactions are those that occurred on one or more occasions in at least 1/100 subjects; **Infrequent** adverse reactions are those that occurred in fewer than 1/100 subjects and more than 1/1000 subjects. **Rare** adverse reactions are those that occurred in fewer than 1/1000 subjects. Adverse reactions that are listed in Table 1 are not included in the following listing of frequent, infrequent, and rare AEs.

Blood and Lymphatic System Disorders: Infrequent: anemia; Rare: thrombocythemia.

Cardiac Disorders: Rare: atrioventricular block, palpitations, tachycardia, ventricular extrasystoles.

Ear and Labyrinth Disorders: Rare: ear pain, hypoacusis, motion sickness, tinnitus, tympanic membrane perforation.

Eye Disorders: Infrequent: eye redness, vision blurred; Rare: blepharospasm, diplopia, eye pain, lacrimation decreased.

Gastrointestinal Disorders: Infrequent: abdominal pain, dry mouth, gastroesophageal reflux disease, vomiting; Rare: dyspepsia, constipation, gingival recession, haematochezia, lip blister.

General Disorders and Administration Site Conditions: Infrequent: asthenia, chest pain, fatigue; Rare: chills, gait abnormal, edema peripheral.

Hepatobiliary Disorders: Rare: hyperbilirubinemia.

Immune System Disorders: Rare: hypersensitivity.

Infections and Infestations: Infrequent: bronchitis, fungal infection, laryngitis, sinusitis, tooth infection, urinary tract infection, viral infection; Rare: cellulitis staphylococcal, eye infection, folliculitis, gastroenteritis viral, herpes zoster, infective tenosynovitis, influenza, lower respiratory tract infection, onychomycosis, pharyngitis, pneumonia.

Injury, Poisoning and Procedural Complications: Infrequent: back injury, fall, joint sprain; Rare: bone fracture, skin laceration.

Investigations: Infrequent: blood glucose increased; Rare: alanine aminotransferase increased, blood pressure decreased, blood pressure increased, electrocardiogram ST-T segment abnormal, electrocardiogram QRS complex abnormal, heart rate decreased, neutrophil count decreased, QRS axis abnormal, transaminases increased.

Metabolism and Nutrition Disorders: Infrequent: anorexia, decreased appetite, hyperkalemia, hypermagnesemia, increased appetite; Rare: hypokalemia.

Musculoskeletal and Connective Tissue Disorders: Infrequent: arthralgia, back pain, myalgia, neck pain, pain in extremity; Rare: joint range of motion decreased, muscle cramp, sensation of heaviness.

Neoplasms Benign, Malignant and Unspecified (Including Cysts and Polyps): Rare: lung adenocarcinoma stage I, malignant melanoma.

Nervous System Disorders: Frequent: dizziness; Infrequent: dysgeusia, lethargy, parasthesia, syncope; Rare: ageusia, ataxia, cerebrovascular accident, disturbance in attention, migraine, sleep paralysis, syncope vasovagal, tremor.

Psychiatric Disorders: Infrequent: abnormal dreams, adjustment disorder, anxiety, depression; Rare: confusional state, elevated mood, insomnia, libido decreased, nightmare.

Reproductive System and Breast Disorders: Rare: breast cyst, dysmenorrhea.

Renal and Urinary Disorders: Rare: dysuria, enuresis, hemoglobinuria, nocturia.

Respiratory, Thoracic and Mediastinal Disorders: Infrequent: nasal congestion, pharyngolaryngeal pain, sinus congestion, wheezing; Rare: cough, crackles lung, nasopharyngeal disorder, rhinorrhea, dyspnea.

Skin and Subcutaneous Tissue Disorders: Infrequent: skin irritation; Rare: cold sweat, dermatitis, erythema, hyperhidrosis, pruritis, rash, rosacea.

Surgical and Medical Procedures: Rare: arthrodesis.

Vascular Disorders: Infrequent: pallor; Rare: blood pressure inadequately controlled, hematoma, hot flush.

In addition, the reactions below have been reported for other tricyclics and may be idiosyncratic (not related to dose).

Continued on next page

Allergic: photosensitization, skin rash.
Hematologic: agranulocytosis, eosinophilia, leukopenia, purpura, thrombocytopenia.

7. DRUG INTERACTIONS

7.1. Cytochrome P450 Isozymes

Silenor is primarily metabolized by hepatic cytochrome P450 isozymes CYP2C19 and CYP2D6, and to a lesser extent, by CYP1A2 and CYP2C9. Inhibitors of these isozymes may increase the exposure of doxepin. Silenor is not an inhibitor of any CYP isozymes at therapeutically relevant concentrations. The ability of Silenor to induce CYP isozymes is not known.

7.2. Cimetidine

Silenor exposure is doubled with concomitant administration of cimetidine, a nonspecific inhibitor of CYP isozymes. A maximum dose of 3 mg is recommended in adults and elderly when cimetidine is co-administered with Silenor *[see Clinical Pharmacology (12.4)]*

7.3. Alcohol

When taken with Silenor, the sedative effects of alcohol may be potentiated [*see Warnings and Precautions (5.2, 5.4)*].

7.4. CNS Depressants and Sedating Antihistamines

When taken with Silenor, the sedative effects of sedating antihistamines and CNS depressants may be potentiated [*see Warnings and Precautions (5.2, 5.4)*].

7.5. Tolazamide

A case of severe hypoglycemia has been reported in a type II diabetic patient maintained on tolazamide (1 g/day) 11 days after the addition of oral doxepin (75 mg/day).

8. USE IN SPECIFIC POPULATIONS

8.1. Pregnancy

Pregnancy Category C

There are no adequate and well-controlled studies of Silenor in pregnant women. Silenor should be used during pregnancy only if the potential benefit justifies the potential risk to the fetus. Administration of doxepin to pregnant animals resulted in adverse effects on offspring development at doses greater than the maximum recommended human dose (MRHD) of 6 mg/day.

When doxepin (30, 100 and 150 mg/kg/day) was administered orally to pregnant rats during the period of organogenesis, developmental toxicity (increased incidences of fetal structural abnormalities and decreased fetal body weights) was noted at ≥100 mg/kg/day. The plasma exposures (AUC) at the no-effect dose for embryo-fetal developmental toxicity in rats (30 mg/kg/day) are approximately 6 and 3 times the plasma AUCs for doxepin and nordoxepin (the primary metabolite in humans), respectively, at the MRHD. When administered orally to pregnant rabbits (10, 30 and 60 mg/kg/day) during the period of organogenesis, fetal body weights were reduced at the highest dose in the absence of maternal toxicity. The plasma exposures (AUC) at the no-effect dose for developmental effects (30 mg/kg/day) are approximately 6 and 18 times the plasma AUCs for doxepin and nordoxepin, respectively, at the MRHD. Oral administration of doxepin (10, 30 and 100 mg/kg/day) to rats throughout the pregnancy and lactation periods resulted in decreased pup survival and transient growth delay at the highest dose. The plasma exposures (AUC) at the no-effect dose for adverse effects on pre- and postnatal development in rats (30 mg/kg/day) are approximately 3 and 2 times the plasma AUCs for doxepin and nordoxepin, respectively, at the MRHD.

8.2. Labor and Delivery

The effects of Silenor on labor and delivery in pregnant women are unknown.

8.3. Nursing Mothers

Doxepin is excreted in human milk after oral administration. There has been a report of apnea and drowsiness occurring in a nursing infant whose mother was taking the higher dose of doxepin used to treat depression. Caution should be exercised when Silenor is administered to nursing women.

8.4. Pediatric Use

The safety and effectiveness of Silenor in pediatric patients have not been evaluated.

8.5. Geriatric Use

A total of 362 subjects who were ≥ 65 years and 86 subjects who were ≥ 75 years received Silenor in controlled clinical studies. No overall differences in safety or effectiveness were observed between these subjects and younger adult subjects. Greater sensitivity of some older individuals cannot be ruled out.

Sleep-promoting drugs may cause confusion and over-sedation in the elderly. A starting dose of 3 mg is recommended in this population and evaluation prior to considering dose escalation is recommended *[see Dosage and Administration (2.2)]*.

8.6. Use in Patients with Hepatic Impairment

Patients with hepatic impairment may display higher doxepin concentrations than healthy individuals. Initiate Silenor treatment with 3 mg in patients with hepatic impairment and monitor closely for adverse daytime effects. *[see Clinical Pharmacology (12.5)]*

8.7. Use in Patients with Sleep Apnea

Silenor has not been studied in patients with obstructive sleep apnea. Since hypnotics have the capacity to depress respiratory drive, precautions should be taken if Silenor is prescribed to patients with compromised respiratory function. In patients with severe sleep apnea, Silenor is ordinarily not recommended for use.

9. DRUG ABUSE AND DEPENDENCE

9.1. Controlled Substance

Doxepin is not a controlled substance.

9.2. Abuse

Doxepin is not associated with abuse potential in animals or in humans. Physicians should carefully evaluate patients for history of drug abuse and follow such patients closely, observing them for signs of misuse or abuse of doxepin (e.g., incrementation of dose, drug-seeking behavior).

9.3. Dependence

In a brief assessment of adverse events observed during discontinuation of doxepin following chronic administration, no symptoms indicative of a withdrawal syndrome were observed. Thus, doxepin does not appear to produce physical dependence.

10. OVERDOSAGE

Doxepin is routinely administered for indications other than insomnia at doses 10- to 50-fold higher than the highest recommended dose of Silenor.

The signs and symptoms associated with doxepin use at doses several-fold higher than the maximum recommended dose (Excessive dose) of Silenor for the treatment of insomnia are described *[see Overdosage (10.1)]*, as are signs and symptoms associated with higher multiples of the maximum recommended dose (Critical overdose) *[see Overdosage (10.2)]*.

10.1. Signs and Symptoms of Excessive Doses

The following adverse effects have been associated with use of doxepin at doses higher than 6 mg.

Anticholinergic Effects: constipation and urinary retention.

Central Nervous System: disorientation, hallucinations, numbness, paresthesias, extrapyramidal symptoms, seizures, tardive dyskinesia.

Cardiovascular: hypotension.

Gastrointestinal: aphthous stomatitis, indigestion.

Endocrine: raised libido, testicular swelling, gynecomastia in males, enlargement of breasts and galactorrhea in the female, raising or lowering of blood sugar levels, and syndrome of inappropriate antidiuretic hormone secretion.

Other: tinnitus, weight gain, sweating, flushing, jaundice, alopecia, exacerbation of asthma, and hyperpyrexia (in association with chlorpromazine).

10.2. Signs and Symptoms of Critical Overdose

Manifestations of doxepin critical overdose include: cardiac dysrhythmias, severe hypotension, convulsions, and CNS depression including coma. Electrocardiogram changes, particularly in QRS axis or width, are clinically significant indicators of tricyclic compound toxicity. Other signs of overdose may include, but are not limited to: confusion, disturbed concentration, transient visual hallucinations, dilated pupils, agitation, hyperactive reflexes, stupor, drowsiness, muscle rigidity, vomiting, hypothermia, hyperpyrexia.

10.3. Recommended Management

As management of overdose is complex and changing, it is recommended that the physician contact a poison control center for current information on treatment. In addition, the possibility of a multiple drug ingestion should be considered.

If an overdose is suspected, an ECG should be obtained and cardiac monitoring should be initiated immediately. The patient's airway should be protected, an intravenous line should be established, and gastric decontamination should be initiated. A minimum of six hours of observation with cardiac monitoring and observation for signs of CNS or respiratory depression, hypotension, cardiac dysrhythmias and/or conduction blocks, and seizures is strongly advised. If signs of toxicity occur at any time during this period, extended monitoring is recommended. There are case reports of patients succumbing to fatal dysrhythmias late after overdose; these patients had clinical evidence of significant poisoning prior to death and most received inadequate gastrointestinal decontamination. Monitoring of plasma drug levels should not guide management of the patient.

Gastrointestinal Decontamination

All patients suspected of overdose should receive gastrointestinal decontamination. This should include large volume gastric lavage followed by administration of activated charcoal. If consciousness is impaired, the airway should be secured prior to lavage. Emesis is contraindicated.

Cardiovascular

A maximal limb-lead QRS duration of ≥0.10 seconds may be the best indication of the severity of an overdose. Serum alkalinization, using intravenous sodium bicarbonate should be used to maintain the serum pH in the range of 7.45 to 7.55 for patients with dysrhythmias and/or QRS widening. If the pH response is inadequate, hyperventilation may also be used. Concomitant use of hyperventilation and sodium bicarbonate should be done with extreme caution, with frequent pH monitoring. A pH >7.60 or a pCO_2 <20 mm Hg is undesirable. Dysrhythmias unresponsive to sodium bicarbonate therapy/hyperventilation may respond to lidocaine or phenytoin. Type 1A and 1C antiarrhythmics are generally contraindicated (e.g., quinidine, disopyramide, and procainamide).

In rare instances, hemoperfusion may be beneficial in acute refractory cardiovascular instability in patients with acute toxicity. However, hemodialysis, peritoneal dialysis, exchange transfusions, and forced diuresis generally have been reported as ineffective in treatment of tricyclic compound poisoning.

Central Nervous System

In patients with central nervous system depression, early intubation is advised because of the potential for abrupt deterioration. Seizures should be controlled with benzodiazepines, or, if these are ineffective, other anticonvulsants (e.g., phenobarbital or phenytoin). Physostigmine is not recommended except to treat life-threatening symptoms that have been unresponsive to other therapies, and then only in consultation with a poison control center.

Psychiatric Follow-up

Since overdose often is deliberate, patients may attempt suicide by other means during the recovery phase. Psychiatric referral may be appropriate.

Pediatric Management

The principles of management of child and adult overdoses are similar. It is strongly recommended that the physician contact the local poison control center for specific pediatric treatment.

11. DESCRIPTION

Silenor (doxepin) is available in 3 mg and 6 mg strength tablets for oral administration. Each tablet contains 3.39 mg or 6.78 mg doxepin hydrochloride, equivalent to 3 mg and 6mg of doxepin, respectively.

Chemically, doxepin hydrochloride is an (E) and (Z) geometric, isomeric mixture of 1 propanamine, 3-dibenz[*b,e*]oxepin-11(6*H*)ylidene-*N,N*-dimethyl-hydrochloride. It has the following structure:

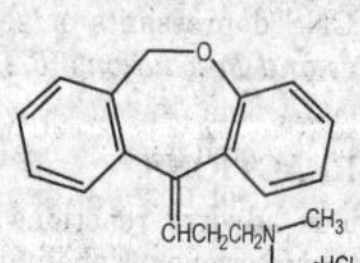

Doxepin hydrochloride is a white crystalline powder, with a slight amine-like odor, that is readily soluble in water. It has a molecular weight of 315.84 and molecular formula of $C_{19}H_{21}NO \cdot HCl$.

Each Silenor tablet includes the following inactive ingredients: microcrystalline cellulose, colloidal silicon dioxide, and magnesium stearate. The 3 mg tablet also contains FD&C Blue No.1. The 6 mg tablet also contains D&C Yellow No. 10 and FD&C Blue No. 1.

12. CLINICAL PHARMACOLOGY

12.1. Mechanism of Action

Doxepin binds with high affinity to the histamine H_1 receptor (Ki < 1 nM) where it functions as an antagonist. The exact mechanism by which doxepin exerts its sleep maintenance effect is unknown but is believed due to its antagonism of the H_1 receptor.

12.2. Pharmacodynamics
Cardiac Safety
In a thorough QTc prolongation clinical study in healthy subjects, doxepin had no effect on QT intervals or other electrocardiographic parameters after multiple daily doses up to 50 mg.

12.3. Pharmacokinetics
Absorption
The median time to peak concentrations (Tmax) of doxepin occurred at 3.5 hours postdose after oral administration of a 6 mg dose to fasted healthy subjects. Peak plasma concentrations (Cmax) of Silenor increased in approximately a dose-proportional manner for 3 mg and 6 mg doses. The AUC was increased by 41% and C_{max} by 15% when 6 mg Silenor was administered with a high fat meal. Additionally, compared to the fasted state, T_{max} was delayed by approximately 3 hours. Therefore, for faster onset and to minimize the potential for next day effects, it is recommended that Silenor not be taken within 3 hours of a meal [*see Dosage and Administration (2.3)*].

Distribution
Silenor is widely distributed throughout the body tissues. The mean apparent volume of distribution following a single 6 mg oral dose of Silenor to healthy subjects was 11,930 liters. Silenor is approximately 80% bound to plasma proteins.

Metabolism
Following oral administration, Silenor is extensively metabolized by oxidation and demethylation. The primary metabolite is N-desmethyldoxepin (nordoxepin).

The primary metabolite undergoes further biotransformation to glucuronide conjugates.

In vitro studies have shown that CYP2C19 and CYP2D6 are the major enzymes involved in doxepin metabolism, and that CYP1A2 and CYP2C9 are involved to a lesser extent.

Doxepin appears not to have inhibitory effects on human CYP enzymes at therapeutic concentrations. The potential of doxepin to induce metabolizing enzymes is not known. Doxepin is not a Pgp substrate.

Excretion
Doxepin is excreted in the urine mainly in the form of glucuronide conjugates.

Less than 3% of a doxepin dose is excreted in the urine as parent compound or nordoxepin. The apparent terminal half-life (t ½) of doxepin was 15.3 hours and for nordoxepin was 31 hours.

12.4. Drug Interactions
Since doxepin is metabolized by CYP2C19 and CYP2D6, inhibitors of these CYP isozymes may increase the exposure of doxepin.

Cimetidine:
The effect of cimetidine, a non-specific inhibitor of CYP1A2, 2C19, 2D6, and 3A4, on Silenor plasma concentrations was evaluated in healthy subjects. When cimetidine 300 mg BID was co-administered with a single dose of Silenor 6 mg, there was approximately a 2-fold increase in Silenor Cmax and AUC compared to Silenor given alone. A maximum dose of doxepin in adults and elderly should be 3 mg, when doxepin is co-administered with cimetidine.

Sertraline:
The effect of sertraline HCl, a selective serotonin reuptake inhibitor, on doxepin plasma concentrations was evaluated in a daytime study conducted with 24 healthy subjects. Following co-administration of doxepin 6 mg with sertraline 50 mg (at steady-state), the doxepin mean AUC and Cmax estimates were approximately 21% and 32% higher, respectively, than those obtained following administration of doxepin alone. Psychomotor function as measured by the digit symbol substitution test and symbol copy test performance was decreased more at 2-4 hours post dosing for the combination of sertraline and doxepin as compared to doxepin alone, but subjective measures of alertness were comparable for the two treatments.

12.5. Special Populations
Renal Impairment
The effects of renal impairment on doxepin pharmacokinetics have not been studied. Because only small amounts of doxepin and nordoxepin are eliminated in the urine, renal impairment would not be expected to result in significantly altered doxepin concentrations.

Hepatic Impairment
The effects of Silenor in patients with hepatic impairment have not been studied. Because doxepin is extensively metabolized by hepatic enzymes, patients with hepatic impairment may display higher doxepin concentrations than healthy individuals.

Poor Metabolizers of CYPs
Poor metabolizers of CYP2C19 and CYP2D6 may have higher doxepin plasma levels than normal subjects.

13. NONCLINICAL TOXICOLOGY
13.1. Carcinogenesis, Mutagenesis, Impairment of Fertility
Carcinogenesis
No evidence of carcinogenic potential was observed when doxepin was administered orally to hemizygous Tg.rasH2 mice for 26 weeks at doses of 25, 50, 75 and 100 mg/kg/day.

Mutagenesis
Doxepin was negative in *in vitro* (bacterial reverse mutation, chromosomal aberration in human lymphocytes) and *in vivo* (rat micronucleus) assays.

Impairment of Fertility
When doxepin (10, 30 and 100 mg/kg/day) was orally administered to male and female rats prior to, during and after mating, adverse effects on fertility (increased copulatory interval and decreased corpora lutea, implantation, viable embryos and litter size) and sperm parameters (increased percentages of abnormal sperm and decreased sperm motility) were observed. The plasma exposures (AUC) for doxepin and nordoxepin at the no-effect dose for adverse effects on reproductive performance and fertility in rats (10 mg/kg/day) are less than those in humans at the maximum recommended human dose of 6 mg/day.

14. CLINICAL STUDIES
14.1. Controlled Clinical Trials
The efficacy of Silenor for improving sleep maintenance was supported by six randomized, double-blind studies up to 3 months in duration that included 1,423 subjects, 18 to 93 years of age, with chronic (N=858) or transient (N=565) insomnia. Silenor was evaluated at doses of 1 mg, 3 mg, and 6 mg relative to placebo in inpatient (sleep laboratory) and outpatient settings.

The primary efficacy measures for assessment of sleep maintenance were the objective and subjective time spent awake after sleep onset (respectively, objective Wake After Sleep Onset [WASO] and subjective WASO).

Subjects in studies of chronic insomnia were required to have at least a 3-month history of insomnia.

Chronic Insomnia
Adults
A randomized, double-blind, parallel-group study was conducted in adults (N = 221) with chronic insomnia. Silenor 3 mg and 6 mg was compared to placebo out to 30 days.

Silenor 3 mg and 6 mg were superior to placebo on objective WASO. Silenor 3 mg was superior to placebo on subjective WASO at night 1 only. Silenor 6 mg was superior to placebo on subjective WASO at night 1, and nominally superior at some later time points out to Day 30.

Elderly
Elderly subjects with chronic insomnia were assessed in two parallel-group studies.

The first randomized, double-blind study assessed Silenor 1 mg and 3 mg relative to placebo for 3 months in inpatient and outpatient settings in elderly subjects (N=240) with chronic insomnia. Silenor 3 mg was superior to placebo on objective WASO.

The second randomized, double-blind study assessed Silenor 6 mg relative to placebo for 4 weeks in an outpatient setting in elderly subjects (N=254) with chronic insomnia. On subjective WASO, Silenor 6 mg was superior to placebo.

Transient Insomnia
Healthy adult subjects (N=565) experiencing transient insomnia during the first night in a sleep laboratory were evaluated in a randomized, double-blind, parallel-group, single-dose study of Silenor 6 mg relative to placebo. Silenor 6 mg was superior to placebo on objective WASO and subjective WASO.

Withdrawal Effects
Potential withdrawal effects were assessed in a 35-day double blind study of adults with chronic insomnia who were randomized to placebo, Silenor 3 mg, or Silenor 6 mg. There was no indication of a withdrawal syndrome after discontinuation of Silenor treatment (3 mg or 6 mg), as measured by the Tyrer's Symptom Checklist. Discontinuation-period emergent nausea and vomiting occurred in 5% of subjects treated with 6 mg Silenor, versus 0% in 3 mg and placebo subjects.

Rebound Insomnia Effects
Rebound insomnia, defined as a worsening in WASO compared with baseline following discontinuation of treatment, was assessed in a double-blind, 35-day study in adults with chronic insomnia. Silenor 3 mg and 6 mg showed no evidence of rebound insomnia.

16. HOW SUPPLIED/STORAGE AND HANDLING
16.1. How Supplied
Silenor 3 mg tablets are oval shaped, blue, identified with debossed markings of "3" on one side and "SP" on the other, and are supplied as:

NDC 42847-103-30	Bottle of 30
NDC 42847-103-10	Bottle of 100
NDC 42847-103-50	Bottle of 500
NDC 42847-103-03	Blister trade pack of 30

Silenor 6 mg tablets are oval shaped, green, identified with debossed markings of "6" on one side and "SP" on the other, and are supplied as:

NDC 42847-106-30	Bottle of 30
NDC 42847-106-10	Bottle of 100
NDC 42847-106-50	Bottle of 500
NDC 42847-106-03	Blister trade pack of 30

16.2. Storage and Handling
Store at controlled room temperature 20° - 25°C (68° - 77°F), protected from light.

17. PATIENT COUNSELING INFORMATION
Prescribers or other healthcare professionals should inform patients, their families, and their caregivers about the benefits and risks associated with treatment with hypnotics, should counsel them in appropriate use, and should instruct them to read the accompanying Medication Guide [*see Medication Guide (17.4)*].

17.1. Sleep-driving and Other Complex Behaviors
There have been reports of people getting out of bed after taking a hypnotic and driving their cars while not fully awake, often with no memory of the event. If a patient experiences such an episode, it should be reported to his or her doctor immediately, since "sleep-driving" can be dangerous. This behavior is more likely to occur when a hypnotic is taken with alcohol or other central nervous system depressants [*see Warnings and Precautions (5.2, 5.4) and Drug Interactions (7.3, 7.4)*]. Other complex behaviors (e.g., preparing and eating food, making phone calls, or having sex) have been reported in patients who are not fully awake after taking a hypnotic. As with "sleep-driving", patients usually do not remember these events.

In addition, patients should be advised to report all concomitant medications to the prescriber. Patients should be instructed to report events such as "sleep-driving" and other complex behaviors immediately to the prescriber.

17.2. Suicide risk and Worsening of Depression:
Patients, their families, and their caregivers should be encouraged to be alert to worsening of depression, including suicidal thoughts and actions. Such symptoms should be reported to the patient's prescriber or health professional.

17.3. Administration Instructions
Patients should be counseled to take Silenor within 30 minutes of bedtime and should confine their activities to those necessary to prepare for bed. Silenor tablets should not be taken with or immediately after a meal [*see Dosage and Administration (2.3)*]. Advise patients NOT to take Silenor when drinking alcohol [*see Warnings and Precautions (5.2, 5.4) and Drug Interactions (7.3)*].

17.4. Medication Guide
MEDICATION GUIDE
SILENOR® (SI-leh-nor) Tablets
(doxepin)

Read this Medication Guide before you start taking SILENOR and each time you get a refill. There may be new information. This information does not take the place of talking to your healthcare provider about your medical condition or treatment.

What is the most important information I should know about SILENOR?
After taking SILENOR, you may get up out of bed while not being fully awake and do an activity that you do not know you are doing. The next morning, you may not remember

Continued on next page

that you did anything during the night. You have a higher chance for doing these activities if you drink alcohol or take other medicines that make you sleepy with SILENOR. Reported activities include:

• driving a car ("sleep-driving")
• making and eating food
• talking on the phone
• having sex
• sleep-walking

Call your healthcare provider right away if you find out that you have done any of the above activities after taking SILENOR.

Important:

1. **Take SILENOR exactly as prescribed**
   • Do not take more SILENOR than prescribed.
   • Take SILENOR 30 minutes before bedtime. After taking SILENOR, you should only do activities needed to get ready for bed.
2. **Do not take SILENOR:**
   • with alcohol
   • if you take other medicines that can make you sleepy. Talk to your healthcare provider about all of your medicines. Your healthcare provider will tell you if you can take SILENOR with your other medicines
   • if you cannot get a full night of sleep before you must be active again

What is SILENOR?

SILENOR is a hypnotic (sleep) medicine that is used to treat people who have trouble staying asleep.

Who should not take SILENOR?

Do not take SILENOR if you:

• take a monoamine oxidase inhibitor (MAOI) medicine or have taken an MAOI in the last 14 days (2 weeks). Ask your healthcare provider if you are not sure if your medicine is an MAOI.
• have an eye problem called narrow angle glaucoma that is not being treated
• have trouble urinating
• are allergic to any of the ingredients in SILENOR. See the end of this Medication Guide for a complete list of ingredients in SILENOR.

Talk to your healthcare provider before taking this medicine if you have any of these conditions.

It is not known if SILENOR is safe and effective in children.

What should I tell my healthcare provider before taking SILENOR?

Before you take SILENOR, tell your healthcare provider if you:

• See "Who should not take Silenor?"
• have a history of depression, mental illness, or suicidal thoughts
• have severe sleep apnea
• have kidney or liver problems
• have a history of drug or alcohol abuse or addiction
• have a history of glaucoma or urinary retention
• have any other medical conditions
• are pregnant or plan to become pregnant. It is not known if SILENOR will harm your unborn baby. Talk to your healthcare provider if you are pregnant or plan to become pregnant.
• are breast-feeding or plan to breast-feed. SILENOR can pass into your milk and may harm your baby. Talk to your healthcare provider about the best way to feed your baby if you take SILENOR. You should not breast-feed while taking SILENOR.

Tell your doctor about all of the medicines you take including prescription and nonprescription medicines, vitamins and herbal supplements.

SILENOR and other medicines may affect each other causing side effects. SILENOR may affect the way other medicines work, and other medicines may affects how SILENOR works. Especially tell your healthcare provider if you take:

• a monoamine oxidase inhibitor (MAOI). See "Who should not take SILENOR?"
• cimetidine (Tagamet) or other medicines that can affect certain liver enzymes
• certain allergy medicines (antihistamines) or other medicines that can make you sleepy or affect your breathing
• the diabetes medicine tolazamide

Ask your doctor or pharmacist if you are not sure if your medicine is one that is listed above.

Know the medicines you take. Keep a list of your medicines with you to show your doctor and pharmacist each time you get a new medicine.

How should I take SILENOR?

• Take SILENOR exactly as your healthcare provider tells you to take it.

• Your doctor will tell you how many SILENOR to take and when to take them.
• Your doctor may change your dose if needed.
• **Take SILENOR within 30 minutes of bedtime.** After taking SILENOR, you should confine your activities to those necessary to prepare for bed.
• Do not take SILENOR within 3 hours of a meal. Silenor may not work as well, or may make you sleepy the next day if taken with or right after a meal.
• Do not take SILENOR unless you are able to get a full night of sleep before you must be active again.
• Call your doctor if your sleep problems get worse or do not get better within 7 to 10 days. This may mean that there is another condition causing your sleep problem.
• If you take too much SILENOR, call your doctor or get medical help right away.

What should I avoid while taking SILENOR?

• You should not drink alcohol while taking SILENOR. Alcohol can increase your chances of getting serious side effects with SILENOR.
• You should not drive, operate heavy machinery, or do other dangerous activities after SILENOR.

You may still feel drowsy the next day after taking SILENOR. Do not drive or do other dangerous activities after taking SILENOR until you feel fully awake.

What are the possible side effects of SILENOR?

SILENOR can cause serious side effects including:

• See "What is the most important information I should know about SILENOR?"

The most common side effect of SILENOR is drowsiness or tiredness.

Tell your healthcare provider if you have any side effect that bothers you or that does not go away.

These are not all the possible side effects of SILENOR. For more information ask your healthcare provider or pharmacist. **Call your doctor for medical advice about side effects. You may report side effects to the FDA at 1-800-FDA-1088.**

How should I store SILENOR?

• Store SILENOR between 68° and 77° F (20° to 25°C).
• Keep SILENOR in a tightly closed container, and away from light. Safely throw away medicine that is out of date or no longer needed.
• **Keep SILENOR and all medicines out of the reach of children.**

General Information about SILENOR

Medicines are sometimes prescribed for purposes other than those listed in a Medication Guide. Do not use SILENOR for a condition for which it was not prescribed. Do not share SILENOR with other people, even if you think they have the same symptoms that you have. It may harm them.

This Medication Guide summarizes the most important information about SILENOR. If you would like more information, talk with your healthcare provider. You can ask your healthcare provider or pharmacist for information about SILENOR that is written for healthcare professionals.

For more information, contact Pernix Therapeutics, LLC. at 1-877-SILENOR (745-3667) or visit http://www.silenor.com.

What are the ingredients in SILENOR?

Active Ingredient: doxepin hydrochloride

Inactive Ingredients: Microcrystalline cellulose, colloidal silicon dioxide, and magnesium stearate. The 3 mg tablet also contains FD&C Blue No. 1. The 6 mg tablet also contains FD&C Yellow No. 10 and FD&C Blue No. 1.

Manufactured by:
Pernix Therapeutics, LLC
Morristown, NJ 07960 USA

This Medication Guide has been approved by the U.S. Food and Drug Administration.

SIL-0030.03.P1A 09/14

Shown in Product Identification Guide, page 509

TREXIMET   ℞

[trex' i-met]
(sumatriptan and naproxen sodium) tablets, for oral use

HIGHLIGHTS OF PRESCRIBING INFORMATION

These highlights do not include all the information needed to use TREXIMET safely and effectively. See full prescribing information for TREXIMET.

TREXIMET (sumatriptan and naproxen sodium) tablets, for oral use

Initial U.S. Approval: 2008

WARNING: RISK OF SERIOUS CARDIOVASCULAR AND GASTROINTESTINAL EVENTS

See full prescribing information for complete boxed warning.

• Nonsteroidal anti-inflammatory drugs (NSAIDs) cause an increased risk of serious cardiovascular thrombotic events, including myocardial infarction and stroke, which can be fatal. This risk may occur early in treatment and may increase with duration of use. (5.1)
• TREXIMET is contraindicated in the setting of coronary artery bypass graft (CABG) surgery (4, 5.1)
• NSAIDs cause an increased risk of serious gastrointestinal (GI) adverse events including bleeding, ulceration, and perforation of the stomach or intestines, which can be fatal. These events can occur at any time during use and without warning symptoms. Elderly patients and patients with a prior history of peptic ulcer disease and/or GI bleeding are at greater risk for serious GI events. (5.2)

RECENT MAJOR CHANGES

Boxed Warning	05/2016
Contraindications (4)	05/2016
Warnings and Precautions (5.1, 5.2, 5.8, 5.9, 5.12, 5.13, 5.14, 5.16, 5.17, 5.19, 5.20)	05/2016

INDICATIONS AND USAGE

TREXIMET is a combination of sumatriptan, a serotonin (5-HT) 1b/1d receptor agonist (triptan), and naproxen sodium, a non-steroidal anti-inflammatory drug, indicated for the acute treatment of migraine with or without aura in adults and pediatric patients 12 years of age and older. (1)

Limitations of Use:
• Use only if a clear diagnosis of migraine headache has been established. (1)
• Not indicated for the prophylactic therapy of migraine attacks. (1)
• Not indicated for the treatment of cluster headache. (1)

DOSAGE AND ADMINISTRATION

Adults
• Recommended dosage: 1 tablet of 85/500 mg. (2.1)
• Maximum dosage in a 24-hour period: 2 tablets of 85/500 mg; separate doses by at least 2 hours. (2.1)

Pediatric Patients 12 to 17 years of Age
• Recommended dosage: 1 tablet of 10/60 mg. (2.2)
• Maximum dosage in a 24-hour period: 1 tablet of 85/500 mg.

Mild to Moderate Hepatic Impairment
• Recommended dosage: 1 tablet of 10/60 mg. (2.3, 8.7)

DOSAGE FORMS AND STRENGTHS

Tablets: 85 mg sumatriptan / 500 mg naproxen sodium (3)
            10 mg sumatriptan / 60 mg naproxen sodium (3)

CONTRAINDICATIONS

• History of coronary artery disease or coronary vasospasm. (4)
• In the setting of CABG surgery. (4)
• Wolff-Parkinson-White syndrome or other cardiac accessory conduction pathway disorders. (4)
• History of stroke, transient ischemic attack, or hemiplegic or basilar migraine. (4)
• Peripheral vascular disease. (4)
• Ischemic bowel disease. (4)
• Uncontrolled hypertension. (4)
• Recent (within 24 hours) use of another 5-HT$_1$ agonist (e.g., another triptan) or of ergotamine-containing medication. (4)
• Concurrent or recent (past 2 weeks) use of monoamine oxidase-A inhibitor. (4)
• History of asthma, urticaria, other allergic type reactions, rhinitis, or nasal polyps syndrome after taking aspirin or other NSAID/analgesic drugs. (4)
• Known hypersensitivity to sumatriptan, naproxen, or any components of TREXIMET (angioedema and anaphylaxis seen). (4)
• Third trimester of pregnancy. (4)
• Severe hepatic impairment. (4)

WARNINGS AND PRECAUTIONS

• Cardiovascular Thrombotic Events: Perform cardiac evaluation in patients with cardiovascular risk factors. (5.1)
• Arrhythmias: Discontinue TREXIMET if occurs. (5.3)
• Chest, Throat, Neck, and/or Jaw Pain/Tightness/Pressure: Generally not associated with myocardial ischemia; evaluate for coronary artery disease in patients at high risk. (5.4)
• Cerebrovascular Events: Discontinue TREXIMET if occurs. (5.5)

- Other Vasospasm Reactions: Discontinue TREXIMET if non-coronary vasospastic reaction occurs. (5.6)
- Hepatotoxicity: Inform patients of warning signs and symptoms of hepatotoxicity. Discontinue if abnormal liver tests persist or worsen or if clinical signs and symptoms of liver disease develop. (5.7)
- Hypertension: Patients taking some antihypertensive medications may have impaired response to these therapies when taking NSAIDs. Monitor blood pressure. (5.8)
- Heart Failure and Edema: Avoid use of TREXIMET in patients with severe heart failure unless benefits are expected to outweigh risk of worsening heart failure. (5.9)
- Medication Overuse Headache: Detoxification may be necessary. (5.10)
- Serotonin Syndrome: Discontinue TREXIMET if occurs. (5.11)
- Renal Toxicity and Hyperkalemia: Monitor renal function in patients with renal or hepatic impairment, heart failure, dehydration, or hypovolemia. Avoid use of TREXIMET in patients with advanced renal disease. (5.12)
- Anaphylactic Reactions: TREXIMET should not be given to patients with the aspirin triad. Seep emergency help if an anaphylactic reaction occurs.(5.13)
- Serious Skin Reactions: Discontinue TREXIMET at first sign of rash or other signs of hypersensitivity. (5.14)
- Hematologic Toxicity: Monitor hemoglobin or hematocrit in patients with any signs or symptoms of anemia. (5.16)
- Exacerbation of Asthma Related to Aspirin Sensitivity: TREXIMET is contraindicated in patients with aspirin-sensitive asthma. Monitor patients with preexisting asthma (without aspirin sensitivity). (5.17)

―――――――ADVERSE REACTIONS―――――――

The most common adverse reactions (incidence ≥2%) were:
- Adults: Dizziness, somnolence, nausea, chest discomfort/chest pain, neck/throat/jaw pain/tightness/pressure, paresthesia, dyspepsia, dry mouth. (6.1)
- Pediatrics: Hot flush (i.e., hot flash[es]) and muscle tightness. (6.1)

To report SUSPECTED ADVERSE REACTIONS, contact Pernix Therapeutics at 1-800-793-2145 or FDA at 1-800-FDA-1088 or www.fda.gov/medwatch.

―――――――DRUG INTERACTIONS―――――――

- Drugs that Interfere with Hemostasis (e.g. warfarin, aspirin, SSRIs/SNRIs): Monitor patients for bleeding who are concomitantly taking TREXIMET with drugs that interfere with hemostasis. Concomitant use of TREXIMET and analgesic doses of aspirin is not generally recommended. (7.1)
- ACE Inhibitors and ARBs: Concomitant use with TREXIMET in elderly, volume depleted, or those with renal impairment may result in deterioration of renal function. In such high risk patients, monitor for signs of worsening renal function. (7.1)
- Diuretics: NSAIDs can reduce natriuretic effect of loop and thiazide diuretics. Monitor patients to assure diuretic efficacy including antihypertensive effects. (7.1)
- Digoxin: Concomitant use with TREXIMET can increase serum concentration and prolong half-life of digoxin. Monitor serum digoxin levels. (7.1)
- Lithium: Increases lithium plasma levels. (7.1)
- Methotrexate: Increases methotrexate plasma levels. (7.1)

―――――USE IN SPECIFIC POPULATIONS―――――

- Pregnancy: Based on animal data, may cause fetal harm. (8.1)

See 17 for PATIENT COUNSELING INFORMATION and Medication Guide.

Revised: 5/2016

FULL PRESCRIBING INFORMATION: CONTENTS*
WARNING: RISK OF SERIOUS CARDIOVASCULAR AND GASTROINTESTINAL EVENTS
1   **INDICATIONS AND USAGE**
2   **DOSAGE AND ADMINISTRATION**
    2.1   Dosage in Adults
    2.2   Dosage in Pediatric Patients 12 to 17 Years of Age
    2.3   Dosing in Patients with Hepatic Impairment
    2.4   Administration Information
3   **DOSAGE FORMS AND STRENGTHS**
4   **CONTRAINDICATIONS**
5   **WARNINGS AND PRECAUTIONS**
    5.1   Cardiovascular Thrombotic Events
    5.2   Gastrointestinal Bleeding, Ulceration, and Perforation

    5.3   Arrhythmias
    5.4   Chest, Throat, Neck, and/or Jaw Pain/Tightness/Pressure
    5.5   Cerebrovascular Events
    5.6   Other Vasospasm Reactions
    5.7   Hepatotoxicity
    5.8   Hypertension
    5.9   Heart Failure and Edema
    5.10   Medication Overuse Headache
    5.11   Serotonin Syndrome
    5.12   Renal Toxicity and Hyperkalemia
    5.13   Anaphylactic Reactions
    5.14   Serious Skin Reactions
    5.15   Premature Closure of the Ductus Arteriosus
    5.16   Hematologic Toxicity
    5.17   Exacerbation of Asthma Related to Aspirin Sensitivity
    5.18   Seizures
    5.19   Masking of Inflammation and Fever
    5.20   Laboratory Monitoring
6   **ADVERSE REACTIONS**
    6.1   Clinical Trials Experience
7   **DRUG INTERACTIONS**
    7.1   Clinically Significant Drug Interactions with TREXIMET
    7.2   Drug/Laboratory Test Interactions
8   **USE IN SPECIFIC POPULATIONS**
    8.1   Pregnancy
    8.2   Labor and Delivery
    8.3   Nursing Mothers
    8.4   Pediatric Use
    8.5   Geriatric Use
    8.6   Renal Impairment
    8.7   Hepatic Impairment
10   **OVERDOSAGE**
11   **DESCRIPTION**
12   **CLINICAL PHARMACOLOGY**
    12.1   Mechanism of Action
    12.2   Pharmacodynamics
    12.3   Pharmacokinetics
13   **NONCLINICAL TOXICOLOGY**
    13.1   Carcinogenesis, Mutagenesis, Impairment of Fertility
    13.2   Animal Toxicology and/or Pharmacology
14   **CLINICAL STUDIES**
    14.1   Adults
    14.2   Pediatric Patients 12 to 17 Years of Age
16   **HOW SUPPLIED/STORAGE AND HANDLING**
17   **PATIENT COUNSELING INFORMATION**
* Sections or subsections omitted from the full prescribing information are not listed.

FULL PRESCRIBING INFORMATION
WARNING: RISK OF SERIOUS CARDIOVASCULAR AND GASTROINTESTINAL EVENTS

Cardiovascular Thrombotic Events
- **Nonsteroidal anti-inflammatory drugs (NSAIDs) cause an increased risk of serious cardiovascular thrombotic events, including myocardial infarction and stroke, which can be fatal. This risk may occur early in treatment and may increase with duration of use [see Warnings and Precautions (5.1)].**
- **TREXIMET is contraindicated in the setting of coronary artery bypass graft (CABG) surgery [see Contraindications (4) Warnings and Precautions (5.1)].**

Gastrointestinal Bleeding, Ulceration, and Perforation
- **NSAIDs cause an increased risk of serious gastrointestinal (GI) adverse events including bleeding, ulceration, and perforation of the stomach or intestines, which can be fatal. These events can occur at any time during use and without warning symptoms. Elderly patients and patients with a prior history of peptic ulcer disease and/or GI bleeding are at greater risk for serious GI events [see Warnings and Precautions (5.2)].**

1   INDICATIONS AND USAGE

TREXIMET is indicated for the acute treatment of migraine with or without aura in adults and pediatric patients 12 years of age and older.

Limitations of Use:
- Use only if a clear diagnosis of migraine headache has been established. If a patient has no response to the first migraine attack treated with TREXIMET, reconsider the diagnosis of migraine before TREXIMET is administered to treat any subsequent attacks.

- TREXIMET is not indicated for the prevention of migraine attacks.
- Safety and effectiveness of TREXIMET have not been established for cluster headache.

2   DOSAGE AND ADMINISTRATION
2.1   Dosage in Adults
The recommended dosage for adults is 1 tablet of TREXIMET 85/500 mg. TREXIMET 85/500 mg contains a dose of sumatriptan higher than the lowest effective dose. The choice of the dose of sumatriptan, and of the use of a fixed combination such as in TREXIMET 85/500 mg should be made on an individual basis, weighing the possible benefit of a higher dose of sumatriptan with the potential for a greater risk of adverse reactions.

The maximum recommended dosage in a 24-hour period is 2 tablets, taken at least 2 hours apart.

The safety of treating an average of more than 5 migraine headaches in adults in a 30-day period has not been established.

Use the lowest effective dosage for the shortest duration consistent with individual patient treatment goals [see Warnings and Precautions (5)].

2.2   Dosage in Pediatric Patients 12 to 17 Years of Age
The recommended dosage for pediatric patients 12 to 17 years of age is 1 tablet of TREXIMET 10/60 mg.

The maximum recommended dosage in a 24-hour period is 1 tablet of TREXIMET 85/500 mg.

The safety of treating an average of more than 2 migraine headaches in pediatric patients in a 30-day period has not been established.

Use the lowest effective dosage for the shortest duration consistent with individual patient treatment goals [see Warnings and Precautions (5)].

2.3   Dosing in Patients with Hepatic Impairment
TREXIMET is contraindicated in patients with severe hepatic impairment [see Contraindications (4), Use in Specific Populations (8.7), Clinical Pharmacology (12.3)].

In patients with mild to moderate hepatic impairment, the recommended dosage in a 24-hour period is 1 tablet of TREXIMET 10/60 mg [see Use in Specific Populations (8.7), Clinical Pharmacology (12.3)].

Use the lowest effective dosage for the shortest duration consistent with individual patient treatment goals [see Warnings and Precautions (5)].

2.4   Administration Information
TREXIMET may be administered with or without food. Tablets should not be split, crushed, or chewed.

3   DOSAGE FORMS AND STRENGTHS
10 mg sumatriptan/60 mg naproxen sodium, light-blue film-coated tablets, debossed on one side with "TREXIMET" and the other side with "10-60".

85 mg sumatriptan/500 mg naproxen sodium, blue film-coated tablets, debossed on one side with "TREXIMET".

4   CONTRAINDICATIONS
TREXIMET is contraindicated in the following patients:
- Ischemic coronary artery disease (CAD) (angina pectoris, history of myocardial infarction, or documented silent ischemia) or coronary artery vasospasm, including Prinzmetal's angina [see Warnings and Precautions (5.1)].
- In the setting of coronary artery bypass graft (CABG) surgery [see Warnings and Precautions (5.1)].
- Wolff-Parkinson-White syndrome or arrhythmias associated with other cardiac accessory conduction pathway disorders [see Warnings and Precautions (5.3)].
- History of stroke or transient ischemic attack (TIA) or history of hemiplegic or basilar migraine because these patients are at a higher risk of stroke [see Warnings and Precautions (5.5)].
- Peripheral vascular disease [see Warnings and Precautions (5.6)].
- Ischemic bowel disease [see Warnings and Precautions (5.6)].
- Uncontrolled hypertension [see Warnings and Precautions (5.8)].
- Recent use (i.e., within 24 hours) of ergotamine-containing medication, ergot-type medication (such as dihydroergotamine or methysergide), or another 5-hydroxytryptamine₁ (5-HT₁) agonist [see Drug Interactions (7)].
- Concurrent administration of a monoamine oxidase (MAO)-A inhibitor or recent (within 2 weeks) use of an MAO-A inhibitor [see Drug Interactions (7), Clinical Pharmacology (12.3)].
- History of asthma, urticaria, or allergic-type reactions after taking aspirin or other NSAIDs. Severe, sometimes fa-

Continued on next page

tal, anaphylactic reactions to NSAIDs have been reported in such patients *[see Warnings and Precautions (5.13, 5.14, 5.17)]*.

• Known hypersensitivity (e.g., anaphylactic reactions, angioedema, and serious skin reactions) to sumatriptan, naproxen, or any components of TREXIMET *[see Warnings and Precautions (5.14)]*.

• Third trimester of pregnancy *[see Warnings and Precautions (5.15), Use in Specific Populations (8.1)]*.

• Severe hepatic impairment *[see Warnings and Precautions (5.7), Use in Specific Populations (8.7), Clinical Pharmacology (12.3)]*.

5 WARNINGS AND PRECAUTIONS
5.1 Cardiovascular Thrombotic Events
The use of TREXIMET is contraindicated in patients with ischemic or vasospastic coronary artery disease (CAD) and in the setting of coronary artery bypass graft (CABG) surgery due to increased risk of serious cardiovascular events with sumatriptan and NSAIDS *[see Contraindications (4)]*.

Cardiovascular Events with Sumatriptan

There have been rare reports of serious cardiac adverse reactions, including acute myocardial infarction, occurring within a few hours following administration of sumatriptan. Some of these reactions occurred in patients without known CAD. TREXIMET may cause coronary artery vasospasm (Prinzmetal's angina), even in patients without a history of CAD.

Cardiovascular Thrombotic Events with Nonsteroidal Anti-inflammatory Drugs

Clinical trials of several COX-2 selective and nonselective NSAIDs of up to three years duration have shown an increased risk of serious cardiovascular (CV) thrombotic events, including myocardial infarction (MI) and stroke, which can be fatal. Based on available data, it is unclear that the risk for CV thrombotic events is similar for all NSAIDs. The relative increase in serious CV thrombotic events over baseline conferred by NSAID use appears to be similar in those with and without known CV disease or risk factors for CV disease. However, patients with known CV disease or risk factors had a higher absolute incidence of excess serious CV thrombotic events, due to their increased baseline rate. Some observational studies found that this increased risk of serious CV thrombotic events began as early as the first weeks of treatment. The increase in CV thrombotic risk has been observed most consistently at higher doses.

To minimize the potential risk for an adverse CV event in NSAID-treated patients, use the lowest effective dose for the shortest duration possible. Physicians and patients should remain alert for the development of such events, throughout the entire treatment course, even in the absence of previous CV symptoms. Patients should be informed about the symptoms of serious CV events and the steps to take if they occur.

There is no consistent evidence that concurrent use of aspirin mitigates the increased risk of serious CV thrombotic events associated with NSAID use. The concurrent use of aspirin and an NSAID, such as naproxen, increases the risk of serious gastrointestinal (GI) events *[see Warnings and Precautions (5.2)]*.

Status Post Coronary Artery Bypass Graft (CABG) Surgery

Two large, controlled clinical trials of a COX-2 selective NSAID for the treatment of pain in the first 10–14 days following CABG surgery found an increased incidence of myocardial infarction and stroke. NSAIDs are contraindicated in the setting of CABG *[see Contraindications (4)]*.

Post-MI Patients

Observational studies conducted in the Danish National Registry have demonstrated that patients treated with NSAIDs in the post-MI period were at increased risk of re-infarction, CV-related death, and all-cause mortality beginning in the first week of treatment. In this same cohort, the incidence of death in the first year post-MI was 20 per 100 person years in NSAID-treated patients compared to 12 per 100 person years in non-NSAID exposed patients. Although the absolute rate of death declined somewhat after the first year post-MI, the increased relative risk of death in NSAID users persisted over at least the next four years of follow-up.

Perform a cardiovascular evaluation in patients who have multiple cardiovascular risk factors (e.g., increased age, diabetes, hypertension, smoking, obesity, strong family history of CAD) prior to receiving TREXIMET. If there is evidence of CAD or coronary artery vasospasm, TREXIMET is contraindicated. For patients with multiple cardiovascular risk factors who have a negative cardiovascular evaluation,

consider administering the first dose of TREXIMET in a medically supervised setting and performing an electrocardiogram (ECG) immediately following administration of TREXIMET. For such patients, consider periodic cardiovascular evaluation in intermittent long-term users of TREXIMET.

Physicians and patients should remain alert for the development of cardiovascular events, even in the absence of previous cardiovascular symptoms. Patients should be informed about the signs and/or symptoms of serious cardiovascular events and the steps to take if they occur.

5.2 Gastrointestinal Bleeding, Ulceration, and Perforation
NSAIDs, including naproxen, a component of TREXIMET, cause serious gastrointestinal adverse events including inflammation, bleeding, ulceration, and perforation of the stomach, small intestine, or large intestine, which can be fatal. These serious adverse events can occur at any time, with or without warning symptoms, in patients treated with NSAIDs. Only 1 in 5 patients who develop a serious upper gastrointestinal adverse event on NSAID therapy is symptomatic. Upper gastrointestinal ulcers, gross bleeding, or perforation caused by NSAIDs appear to occur in approximately 1% of patients treated daily for 3 to 6 months and in about 2% to 4% of patients treated for 1 year. However, even short-term therapy is not without risk.

Among 3,302 adult patients with migraine who received TREXIMET in controlled and uncontrolled clinical trials, 1 patient experienced a recurrence of gastric ulcer after taking 8 doses over 3 weeks, and 1 patient developed a gastric ulcer after treating an average of 8 attacks per month over 7 months.

Risk Factors for GI Bleeding, Ulceration, and Perforation

Patients with a prior history of peptic ulcer disease and/or gastrointestinal bleeding who use NSAIDs have a greater than 10-fold increased risk for developing gastrointestinal bleeding compared with patients with neither of these risk factors. Other factors that increase the risk for gastrointestinal bleeding in patients treated with NSAIDs include longer duration of NSAID therapy; concomitant use of oral corticosteroids, aspirin, anticoagulants, or selective serotonin reuptake inhibitors (SSRIs); smoking; use of alcohol; older age; and poor general health status. Most postmarketing reports of fatal gastrointestinal events occurred in elderly or debilitated patients, and therefore special care should be taken in treating this population. Additionally, patients with advanced liver disease and/or coagulopathy are at increased risk for GI bleeding.

Strategies to Minimize the GI Risks in NSAID-treated patients:

• Use the lowest effective dosage for the shortest possible duration.
• Avoid administration of more than one NSAID at a time.
• Avoid use in patients at higher risk unless benefits are expected to outweigh the increased risk of bleeding. For high risk patients, as well as those with active GI bleeding, consider alternate therapies other than NSAIDs.
• Remain alert for signs and symptoms of GI ulceration and bleeding during NSAID therapy.
• If a serious GI adverse event is suspected, promptly initiate evaluation and treatment, and discontinue TREXIMET until a serious GI adverse event is ruled out.
• In the setting of concomitant use of low-dose aspirin for cardiac prophylaxis, monitor patients more closely for evidence of GI bleeding *[see Drug Interactions (7)]*.

5.3 Arrhythmias
Life-threatening disturbances of cardiac rhythm, including ventricular tachycardia and ventricular fibrillation leading to death, have been reported within a few hours following the administration of 5-HT$_1$ agonists. Discontinue TREXIMET if these disturbances occur. TREXIMET is contraindicated in patients with Wolff-Parkinson-White syndrome or arrhythmias associated with other cardiac accessory conduction pathway disorders.

5.4 Chest, Throat, Neck, and/or Jaw Pain/Tightness/Pressure
Sensations of tightness, pain, pressure, and heaviness in the precordium, throat, neck, and jaw commonly occur after treatment with sumatriptan and are usually non-cardiac in origin. However, perform a cardiac evaluation if these patients are at high cardiac risk. The use of TREXIMET is contraindicated in patients with CAD and those with Prinzmetal's variant angina.

5.5 Cerebrovascular Events
Cerebral hemorrhage, subarachnoid hemorrhage, and stroke have occurred in patients treated with 5-HT$_1$ ago-

nists, and some have resulted in fatalities. In a number of cases, it appears possible that the cerebrovascular events were primary, the 5-HT$_1$ agonist having been administered in the incorrect belief that the symptoms experienced were a consequence of migraine when they were not. Also, patients with migraine may be at increased risk of certain cerebrovascular events (e.g., stroke, hemorrhage, TIA). Discontinue TREXIMET if a cerebrovascular event occurs.

Before treating headaches in patients not previously diagnosed as migraineurs, and in migraineurs who present with atypical symptoms, exclude other potentially serious neurological conditions. TREXIMET is contraindicated in patients with a history of stroke or TIA *[see Contraindications (4)]*.

5.6 Other Vasospasm Reactions
Sumatriptan may cause non-coronary vasospastic reactions, such as peripheral vascular ischemia, gastrointestinal vascular ischemia and infarction (presenting with abdominal pain and bloody diarrhea), splenic infarction, and Raynaud's syndrome. In patients who experience symptoms or signs suggestive of non-coronary vasospasm reaction following the use of any 5-HT$_1$ agonist, rule out a vasospastic reaction before receiving additional TREXIMET.

Reports of transient and permanent blindness and significant partial vision loss have been reported with the use of 5-HT$_1$ agonists. Since visual disorders may be part of a migraine attack, a causal relationship between these events and the use of 5-HT$_1$ agonists have not been clearly established.

5.7 Hepatotoxicity
Borderline elevations of 1 or more liver tests may occur in up to 15% of patients who take NSAIDs including naproxen, a component of TREXIMET. Hepatic abnormalities may be the result of hypersensitivity rather than direct toxicity. These abnormalities may progress, may remain essentially unchanged, or may be transient with continued therapy. Notable (3 times the upper limit of normal) elevations of SGPT (ALT) or SGOT (AST) have been reported in approximately 1% of patients in clinical trials with NSAIDs. In addition, rare, sometimes fatal cases of severe hepatic injury, including jaundice and fatal fulminant hepatitis, liver necrosis, and hepatic failure have been reported with NSAIDs.

TREXIMET is contraindicated in patients with severe hepatic impairment *[see Use in Specific Populations (8.7), Clinical Pharmacology (12.3)]*. A patient with symptoms and/or signs suggesting liver dysfunction, or in whom an abnormal liver test has occurred, should be evaluated for evidence of the development of a more severe hepatic reaction while on therapy with TREXIMET. TREXIMET should be discontinued if clinical signs and symptoms consistent with liver disease develop, if systemic manifestations occur (e.g., eosinophilia, rash), or if abnormal liver tests persist or worsen.

Inform patients of the warning signs and symptoms of hepatotoxicity (e.g., nausea, fatigue, lethargy, diarrhea, pruritus, jaundice, right upper quadrant tenderness, and "flulike" symptoms). If clinical signs and symptoms consistent with liver disease develop, or if systemic manifestations occur (e.g., eosinophilia, rash, etc.), discontinue TREXIMET immediately, and perform a clinical evaluation of the patient.

5.8 Hypertension
Significant elevation in blood pressure, including hypertensive crisis with acute impairment of organ systems, has been reported on rare occasions in patients treated with 5-HT$_1$ agonists, including sumatriptan, a component of TREXIMET. This occurrence has included patients without a history of hypertension.

NSAIDs, including naproxen, a component of TREXIMET, can also lead to onset of new hypertension or worsening of preexisting hypertension, either of which may contribute to the increased incidence of cardiovascular events. Patients taking angiotensin converting enzyme (ACE) inhibitors, angiotensin receptor blockers (ARBs), beta-blockers, thiazide diuretics, or loop diuretics may have impaired response to these therapies when taking NSAIDs *[see Drug Interactions (7)]*.

Monitor blood pressure in patients treated with TREXIMET. TREXIMET is contraindicated in patients with uncontrolled hypertension *[see Contraindications (4)]*.

5.9 Heart Failure and Edema
The Coxib and traditional NSAID Trialists' Collaboration meta-analysis of randomized controlled trials demonstrated an approximately two-fold increase in hospitalizations for heart failure in COX-2 selective-treated patients and non-

selective NSAID-treated patients compared to placebo-treated patients. In a Danish National Registry study of patients with heart failure, NSAID use increased the risk of MI, hospitalization for heart failure, and death.

Additionally, fluid retention and edema have been observed in some patients treated with NSAIDs. Use of naproxen may blunt the CV effects of several therapeutic agents used to treat these medical conditions (e.g., diuretics, ACE inhibitors, or angiotensin receptor blockers [ARBs] *[see Drug Interactions (7)]*.

Avoid the use of TREXIMET in patients with severe heart failure unless the benefits are expected to outweigh the risk of worsening heart failure. If TREXIMET is used in patients with severe heart failure, monitor patients for signs of worsening heart failure.

Since each TREXIMET 85/500 mg tablet contains approximately 60 mg of sodium and each TREXIMET 10/60 mg tablet contains approximately 20 mg of sodium, this should be considered in patients whose overall intake of sodium must be severely restricted.

5.10 Medication Overuse Headache

Overuse of acute migraine drugs (e.g., ergotamine, triptans, opioids, or a combination of these drugs for 10 or more days per month) may lead to exacerbation of headache (medication overuse headache). Medication overuse headache may present as migraine-like daily headaches, or as a marked increase in frequency of migraine attacks. Detoxification of patients, including withdrawal of the overused drugs, and treatment of withdrawal symptoms (which often includes a transient worsening of headache) may be necessary.

5.11 Serotonin Syndrome

Serotonin syndrome may occur with TREXIMET, particularly during coadministration with selective serotonin reuptake inhibitors (SSRIs), serotonin norepinephrine reuptake inhibitors (SNRIs), tricyclic antidepressants (TCAs), and MAO inhibitors *[see Contraindications (4) and Drug Interactions (7.1)]*. Serotonin syndrome symptoms may include mental status changes (e.g., agitation, hallucinations, coma), autonomic instability (e.g., tachycardia, labile blood pressure, hyperthermia), neuromuscular aberrations (e.g., hyperreflexia, incoordination), and/or gastrointestinal symptoms (e.g., nausea, vomiting, diarrhea). The onset of symptoms usually occurs within minutes to hours of receiving a new or a greater dose of a serotonergic medication. Discontinue TREXIMET if serotonin syndrome is suspected.

5.12 Renal Toxicity and Hyperkalemia

Renal Toxicity

Long-term administration of NSAIDs has resulted in renal papillary necrosis and other renal injury. Renal toxicity has also been seen in patients in whom renal prostaglandins have a compensatory role in the maintenance of renal perfusion. In these patients administration of an NSAID may cause a dose-dependent reduction in prostaglandin formation and, secondarily, in renal blood flow, which may precipitate overt renal decompensation. Patients at greatest risk of this reaction are those with impaired renal function, dehydration, hypovolemia, heart failure, liver dysfunction, salt depletion, those taking diuretics and angiotensin-converting enzyme (ACE) inhibitors or ARBs, and the elderly. Discontinuation of NSAID therapy is usually followed by recovery to the pretreatment state.

TREXIMET should be discontinued if clinical signs and symptoms consistent with renal disease develop or if systemic manifestations occur.

TREXIMET is not recommended for use in patients with severe renal impairment (creatinine clearance [CrCl] <30 mL/min) unless the benefits are expected to outweigh the risk of worsening renal function *[see Use in Specific Populations (8.6), Clinical Pharmacology (12.3)]*. If TREXIMET is used in patients with advanced renal disease, monitor patients for signs of worsening renal function. Monitor renal function in patients with mild (CrCl = 60 to 89 mL/min) or moderate (CrCl = 30 to 59 mL/min) renal impairment, pre-existing kidney disease, or dehydration.

The renal effects of TREXIMET may hasten the progression of renal dysfunction in patients with pre-existing renal disease.

Correct volume status in dehydrated or hypovolemic patients prior to initiating TREXIMET. Monitor renal function in patients with renal or hepatic impairment, heart failure, dehydration, or hypovolemia during use of TREXIMET *[see Drug Interactions (7)]*. Avoid the use of TREXIMET in patients with advanced renal disease unless the benefits are expected to outweigh the risk of worsening renal function. If

TREXIMET is used in patients with advanced renal disease, monitor patients for signs of worsening renal function.

Hyperkalemia

Increases in serum potassium concentration, including hyperkalemia, have been reported with the use of NSAIDs, even in some patients without renal impairment. In patients with normal renal function, these effects have been attributed to a hyporeninemic-hypoaldosteronism state.

5.13 Anaphylactic Reactions

Anaphylactic reactions may occur in patients without known prior exposure to either component of TREXIMET. Such reactions can be life-threatening or fatal. In general, anaphylactic reactions to drugs are more likely to occur in individuals with a history of sensitivity to multiple allergens although anaphylactic reactions with naproxen have occurred in patient without known hypersensitivity to naproxen or to patients with aspirin sensitive asthma *[see Contraindications (4) and Warnings and Precautions (5.17)]*. TREXIMET should not be given to patients with the aspirin triad. This symptom complex typically occurs in patients with asthma who experience rhinitis with or without nasal polyps, or who exhibit severe, potentially fatal bronchospasm after taking aspirin or other NSAIDs *[see Contraindications (4)]*.

TREXIMET is contraindicated in patients with a history of hypersensitivity reaction to sumatriptan, naproxen, or any other component of TREXIMET. Naproxen has been associated with anaphylactic reactions in patients without known hypersensitivity to naproxen and in patients with aspirin-sensitive asthma *[see Contraindications (4) and Warnings and Precautions (5.17)]*. Seek emergency help if an anaphylactic reaction occurs.

5.14 Serious Skin Reactions

NSAID-containing products can cause serious skin adverse reactions such as exfoliative dermatitis, Stevens-Johnson syndrome (SJS), and toxic epidermal necrolysis (TEN), which can be fatal. These serious events may occur without warning. Inform patients about the signs and symptoms of serious skin reactions and to discontinue the use of TREXIMET at the first appearance of skin rash or any other sign of hypersensitivity. TREXIMET is contraindicated in patients with previous serious skin reactions to NSAIDs *[see Contraindications (4)]*.

5.15 Premature Closure of the Ductus Arteriosus

TREXIMET may cause premature closure of the ductus arteriosus. Avoid use of NSAIDs, including TREXIMET, in pregnant women starting at 30 weeks of gestation (third trimester) *[see Contraindications (4), Use in Specific Populations (8.1)]*.

5.16 Hematologic Toxicity

Anemia has occurred in patients receiving NSAIDs. This may be due to fluid retention, occult or gross gastrointestinal blood loss, or an incompletely described effect upon erythropoiesis. If a patient treated with TREXIMET has signs or symptoms of anemia, monitor hemoglobin or hematocrit.

NSAIDs, including TREXIMET, may increase the risk of bleeding events. Co-morbid conditions such as coagulation disorders or concomitant use of warfarin, other anticoagulants, antiplatelet agents (e.g., aspirin), serotonin reuptake inhibitors (SSRIs), and serotonin norepinephrine reuptake inhibitors (SNRIs) may increase this risk. Monitor these patients for signs of bleeding *[see Drug Interactions (7)]*.

5.17 Exacerbation of Asthma Related to Aspirin Sensitivity

A subpopulation of patients with asthma may have aspirin-sensitive asthma which may include chronic rhinosinusitis complicated by nasal polyps; severe, potentially fatal bronchospasm; and/or intolerance to aspirin and other NSAIDs. Because cross-reactivity between aspirin and other NSAIDs has been reported in such aspirin-sensitive patients, TREXIMET is contraindicated in patients with this form of aspirin sensitivity and should be used with caution in patients with preexisting asthma *[see Contraindications (4)]*. When TREXIMET is used in patients with preexisting asthma (without known aspirin sensitivity), monitor patients for changes in the signs and symptoms of asthma.

5.18 Seizures

Seizures have been reported following administration of sumatriptan. Some have occurred in patients with either a history of seizures or concurrent conditions predisposing to seizures. There are also reports in patients where no such predisposing factors are apparent. TREXIMET should be used with caution in patients with a history of epilepsy or conditions associated with a lowered seizure threshold.

5.19 Masking of Inflammation and Fever

The pharmacological activity of TREXIMET in reducing inflammation, and possibly fever, may diminish the utility of diagnostic signs in detecting infections.

5.20 Laboratory Monitoring

Because serious GI bleeding, hepatotoxicity, and renal injury can occur without warning symptoms or signs, consider monitoring patients on long-term NSAID treatment with a CBC and a chemistry profile periodically *[see Warnings and Precautions (5.2, 5.7, 5.12)]*.

6 ADVERSE REACTIONS

The following serious adverse reactions are described below and elsewhere in labeling:

- Cardiovascular Thrombotic Events *[see Warnings and Precautions (5.1)]*
- GI Bleeding, Ulceration and Perforation *[see Warnings and Precautions (5.2)]*
- Arrhythmias *[see Warnings and Precautions (5.3)]*
- Chest, Throat, Neck, and/or Jaw Pain/Tightness/Pressure *[see Warnings and Precautions (5.4)]*
- Cerebrovascular Events *[see Warnings and Precautions (5.5)]*
- Other Vasospasm Reactions *[see Warnings and Precautions (5.6)]*
- Hepatotoxicity *[see Warnings and Precautions (5.7)]*
- Hypertension *[see Warnings and Precautions (5.8)]*
- Heart Failure and Edema *[see Warnings and Precautions (5.9)]*
- Medication Overuse Headache *[see Warnings and Precautions (5.10)]*
- Serotonin Syndrome *[see Warnings and Precautions (5.11)]*
- Renal Toxicity and Hyperkalemia *[see Warnings and Precautions (5.12)]*
- Anaphylactic Reactions *[see Warnings and Precautions (5.13)]*
- Serious Skin Reactions *[see Warnings and Precautions (5.14)]*
- Hematological Toxicity *[see Warnings and Precautions (5.16)]*
- Exacerbation Asthma Related to Aspirin Sensitivity *[see Warnings and Precautions (5.17)]*
- Seizures *[see Warnings and Precautions (5.18)]*

6.1 Clinical Trials Experience

Because clinical trials are conducted under widely varying conditions, adverse reaction rates observed in the clinical trials of a drug cannot be directly compared with rates in the clinical trials of another drug and may not reflect the rates observed in practice.

Adults

The adverse reactions reported below are specific to the clinical trials with TREXIMET 85/500 mg. See also the full prescribing information for naproxen and sumatriptan products.

Table 1 lists adverse reactions that occurred in 2 placebo-controlled clinical trials (Study 1 and 2) in adult patients who received 1 dose of study drug. Only adverse reactions that occurred at a frequency of 2% or more in any group treated with TREXIMET 85/500 mg and that occurred at a frequency greater than the placebo group are included in Table 1.

[See table 1 on next page]

The incidence of adverse reactions in controlled clinical trials was not affected by gender or age of the patients. There were insufficient data to assess the impact of race on the incidence of adverse reactions.

Pediatric Patients 12 to 17 Years of Age

In a placebo-controlled clinical trial that evaluated pediatric patients 12 to 17 years of age who received 1 dose of TREXIMET 10/60 mg, 30/180 mg, or 85/500 mg, adverse reactions occurred in 13% of patients who received 10/60 mg, 9% of patients who received 30/180 mg, 13% who received 85/500 mg, and 8% who received placebo. No patients who received TREXIMET experienced adverse reactions leading to withdrawal from the trial. The incidence of adverse reactions in pediatric patients 12 to 17 years of age was comparable across all 3 doses compared with placebo. Table 2 lists adverse reactions that occurred in a placebo-controlled trial in pediatric patients 12 to 17 years of age at a frequency of 2% or more with TREXIMET and were more frequent than the placebo group.

[See table 2 on next page]

7 DRUG INTERACTIONS

7.1 Clinically Significant Drug Interactions with TREXIMET

See Table 3 for clinically significant drug interactions with NSAIDs or Sumatriptan

[See table 3 on pages 1011 and 1012]

Continued on next page

7.2 Drug/Laboratory Test Interactions

Blood Tests

Naproxen may decrease platelet aggregation and prolong bleeding time. This effect should be kept in mind when bleeding times are determined.

Urine Tests

The administration of naproxen sodium may result in increased urinary values for 17-ketogenic steroids because of an interaction between the drug and/or its metabolites with m-di-nitrobenzene used in this assay. Although 17-hydroxy-corticosteroid measurements (Porter-Silber test) do not appear to be artificially altered, it is suggested that therapy with naproxen be temporarily discontinued 72 hours before adrenal function tests are performed if the Porter-Silber test is to be used.

Naproxen may interfere with some urinary assays of 5-hydroxy indoleacetic acid (5HIAA).

8 USE IN SPECIFIC POPULATIONS

8.1 Pregnancy

Pregnancy Category C during the first two trimesters of pregnancy; Category X during the third trimester of pregnancy. There are no adequate and well-controlled studies in pregnant women. TREXIMET (sumatriptan and naproxen) should be used during the first and second trimester of pregnancy only if the potential benefit justifies the potential risk to the fetus. TREXIMET should not be used during the third trimester of pregnancy because inhibitors of prostaglandin synthesis (including naproxen) are known to cause premature closure of the ductus arteriosus in humans. In animal studies, administration of sumatriptan and naproxen, alone or in combination, during pregnancy resulted in developmental toxicity (increased incidences of fetal malformations, embryofetal and pup mortality, decreased embryofetal growth) at clinically relevant doses. Oral administration of sumatriptan combined with naproxen sodium (5/9, 25/45, or 50/90 mg/kg/day sumatriptan/naproxen sodium) or each drug alone (50/0 or 0/90 mg/kg/day sumatriptan/naproxen sodium) to pregnant rabbits during the period of organogenesis resulted in increased total incidences of fetal abnormalities at all doses and increased incidences of specific malformations (cardiac interventricular septal defect in the 50/90 mg/kg/day group, fused caudal vertebrae in the 50/0 and 0/90 mg/kg/day groups) and variations (absent intermediate lobe of the lung, irregular ossification of the skull, incompletely ossified sternal centra) at the highest dose of sumatriptan and naproxen alone and in combination. A no-effect dose for developmental toxicity in rabbits was not established. The lowest effect dose was 5/9 mg/kg/day sumatriptan/naproxen sodium, which was associated with plasma exposures (AUC) to sumatriptan and naproxen that were less than those attained at the maximum human daily dose (MHDD) of 170 mg sumatriptan and 1000 mg naproxen sodium (two tablets of TREXIMET 85/500 mg in a 24-hour period).

In previous developmental toxicity studies of sumatriptan, oral administration to pregnant rats during the period of organogenesis resulted in an increased incidence of fetal blood vessel abnormalities and decreased pup survival at doses of 250 mg/kg/day or higher. The highest no-effect dose was 60 mg/kg/day, which is approximately 3 times the MHDD of 170 mg sumatriptan on a mg/m² basis. Oral administration of sumatriptan to pregnant rabbits during the period of organogenesis resulted in increased incidences of vascular and skeletal abnormalities at a dose of 50 mg/kg/day and embryolethality at 100 mg/kg/day. The highest no-effect dose of sumatriptan for developmental toxicity in rabbits was 15 mg/kg/day, or approximately 2 times the MHDD of 170 mg sumatriptan on a mg/m² basis.

8.2 Labor and Delivery

Naproxen-containing products are not recommended in labor and delivery because, through its prostaglandin synthesis inhibitory effect, naproxen may adversely affect fetal circulation and inhibit uterine contractions, thus increasing the risk of uterine hemorrhage. In rat studies with NSAIDs, as with other drugs known to inhibit prostaglandin synthesis, an increased incidence of dystocia, delayed parturition, and decreased pup survival occurred.

8.3 Nursing Mothers

Both active components of TREXIMET, sumatriptan and naproxen, have been reported to be secreted in human milk. Because of the potential for serious adverse reactions in nursing infants from TREXIMET, a decision should be made whether to discontinue nursing or to discontinue the drug, taking into account the importance of the drug to the mother.

8.4 Pediatric Use

Safety and effectiveness of TREXIMET in pediatric patients under 12 years of age have not been established.

The safety and efficacy of TREXIMET for the acute treatment of migraine in pediatric patients 12 to 17 years of age was established in a double-blind, placebo-controlled trial [see Adverse Reactions (6.1) and Clinical Studies (14.2)].

8.5 Geriatric Use

Elderly patients, compared to younger patients, are at greater risk for NSAID-associated serious cardiovascular, gastrointestinal, and/or renal adverse reactions. TREXIMET is not recommended for use in elderly patients who have decreased renal function, higher risk for unrecognized CAD, and increases in blood pressure that may be more pronounced in the elderly [see Warnings and Precautions (5.1, 5.2, 5.3, 5.8,5.12) and Clinical Pharmacology (12.3)].

A cardiovascular evaluation is recommended for geriatric patients who have other cardiovascular risk factors (e.g., diabetes, hypertension, smoking, obesity, strong family history of CAD) prior to receiving TREXIMET [see Warnings and Precautions (5.1)].

8.6 Renal Impairment

TREXIMET is not recommended for use in patients with creatinine clearance less than 30 mL/min. Monitor the serum creatinine or creatinine clearance in patients with mild (CrCl = 60 to 89 mL/min) or moderate (CrCL = 30 to 59 mL/min) renal impairment, preexisting kidney disease, or dehydration [see Warnings and Precautions (5.12) and Clinical Pharmacology (12.3)].

8.7 Hepatic Impairment

TREXIMET is contraindicated in patients with severe hepatic impairment. For patients with mild or moderate hepatic impairment, the TREXIMET dose should be reduced. [see Contraindications (4), Warnings and Precautions (5.7), and Clinical Pharmacology (12.3)].

10 OVERDOSAGE

Patients (N = 670) have received single oral doses of 140 to 300 mg of sumatriptan without significant adverse effects. Volunteers (N = 174) have received single oral doses of 140 to 400 mg without serious adverse events.

Overdose of sumatriptan in animals has been fatal and has been heralded by convulsions, tremor, paralysis, inactivity, ptosis, erythema of the extremities, abnormal respiration, cyanosis, ataxia, mydriasis, salivation, and lacrimation.

Symptoms following acute NSAID overdosages have been typically limited to lethargy, drowsiness, nausea, vomiting and epigastric pain. Gastrointestinal bleeding has occurred. Hypertension, acute renal failure, respiratory depression, and coma have occurred, but were rare [see Warnings and Precautions (5.1, 5.2)].

Manage patients with symptomatic and supportive care following an NSAID overdosage. There are no specific antidotes. Consider emesis and/or activated charcoal (60 to 100 grams in adults, 1 to 2 grams per kg of body weight in pediatric patients) and/or osmotic cathartic in symptomatic patients seen within four hours of ingestion or in patients with a large overdosage (5 to 10 times the recommended dosage). Hemodialysis does not decrease the plasma concentration of naproxen because of the high degree of its protein binding. It is unknown what effect hemodialysis or peritoneal dialysis has on the serum concentrations of sumatriptan. Forced diuresis, alkalinization of urine, hemodialysis, or hemoperfusion may not be useful due to high protein binding.

For additional information about overdosage treatment contact a poison control center (1-800-222-1222).

11 DESCRIPTION

TREXIMET contains sumatriptan (as the succinate), a selective 5-hydroxytryptamine$_1$ (5-HT$_1$) receptor subtype agonist, and naproxen sodium, a member of the arylacetic acid group of NSAIDs.

Sumatriptan succinate is chemically designated as 3-[2-(dimethylamino)ethyl]-N-methyl-indole-5-methanesulfonamide succinate (1:1), and it has the following structure:

The empirical formula is $C_{14}H_{21}N_3O_2S \cdot C_4H_6O_4$, representing a molecular weight of 413.5. Sumatriptan succinate is a white to off-white powder that is readily soluble in water and in saline.

Naproxen sodium is chemically designated as (S)-6-methoxy-α-methyl-2-naphthaleneacetic acid, sodium salt, and it has the following structure:

Table 1. Adverse Reactions in Pooled Placebo-Controlled Trials in Adult Patients with Migraine

Adverse Reactions	TREXIMET 85/500 mg % (n = 737)	Placebo % (n = 752)	Sumatriptan 85 mg % (n = 735)	Naproxen Sodium 500 mg % (n = 732)
Nervous system disorders				
Dizziness	4	2	2	2
Somnolence	3	2	2	2
Paresthesia	2	<1	2	<1
Gastrointestinal disorders				
Nausea	3	1	3	<1
Dyspepsia	2	1	2	1
Dry mouth	2	1	2	<1
Pain and other pressure sensations				
Chest discomfort/chest pain	3	<1	2	1
Neck/throat/jaw pain/tightness/pressure	3	1	3	1

Table 2. Adverse Reactions in a Placebo-Controlled Trial in Pediatric Patients 12 to 17 Years of Age with Migraine

Adverse Reactions	TREXIMET 10/60 mg % (n = 96)	TREXIMET 30/180 mg % (n = 97)	TREXIMET 85/500 mg % (n = 152)	Placebo % (n = 145)
Vascular				
Hot flush (i.e., hot flash[es])	0	2	<1	0
Musculoskeletal				
Muscle tightness	0	0	2	0

Table 3. Clinically Significant Drug Interactions with naproxen or sumatriptan

Ergot-Containing Drugs

Clinical Impact:	Ergot-containing drugs have been reported to cause prolonged vasospastic reactions.
Intervention:	Because these effects may be additive, coadministration of TREXIMET and ergotamine-containing or ergot-type medications (like dihydroergotamine or methysergide) within 24 hours of each other is contraindicated.

Monoamine Oxidase-A Inhibitors

Clinical Impact:	MAO-A inhibitors increase systemic exposure of orally administered sumatriptan by 7-fold.
Intervention:	The use of TREXIMET in patients receiving MAO-A inhibitors is contraindicated.

Other 5-HT$_1$ Agonists

Clinical Impact:	5-HT$_1$ agonist drugs can cause vasospastic effects.
Intervention:	Because these effects may be additive, coadministration of TREXIMET and other 5 HT$_1$ agonists (e.g., triptans) within 24 hours of each other is contraindicated.

Drugs That Interfere with Hemostasis

Clinical Impact:	• Naproxen and anticoagulants such as warfarin have a synergistic effect on bleeding. The concomitant use of naproxen and anticoagulants have an increased risk of serious bleeding compared to the use of either drug alone. • Serotonin release by platelets plays an important role in hemostasis. Case-control and cohort epidemiological studies showed that concomitant use of drugs that interfere with serotonin reuptake and an NSAID may potentiate the risk of bleeding more than an NSAID alone.
Intervention:	Monitor patients with concomitant use of TREXIMET with anticoagulants (e.g., warfarin), antiplatelet agents (e.g., aspirin), selective serotonin reuptake inhibitors (SSRIs), and serotonin norepinephrine reuptake inhibitors (SNRIs) for signs of bleeding [see Warnings and Precautions (5.16)].

Aspirin

Clinical Impact:	Controlled clinical studies showed that the concomitant use of NSAIDs and analgesic doses of aspirin does not produce any greater therapeutic effect than the use of NSAIDs alone. In a clinical study, the concomitant use of an NSAID and aspirin was associated with a significantly increased incidence of GI adverse reactions as compared to use of the NSAID alone [see Warnings and Precautions (5.2) and Clinical Pharmacology (12.3)].
Intervention:	Concomitant use of TREXIMET and analgesic doses of aspirin is not generally recommended because of the increased risk of bleeding [see Warnings and Precautions (5.16)].

Selective Serotonin Reuptake Inhibitors/Serotonin Norepinephrine Reuptake Inhibitors and Serotonin Syndrome

Clinical Impact:	Cases of serotonin syndrome have been reported during coadministration of triptans and SSRIs, SNRIs, TCAs, and MAO inhibitors [see Warnings and Precautions (5.11)].
Intervention:	Discontinue TREXIMET if serotonin syndrome is suspected.

ACE Inhibitors, Angiotensin Receptor Blockers, and Beta-blockers

Clinical Impact:	• NSAIDs may diminish the antihypertensive effect of angiotensin converting enzyme (ACE) inhibitors, angiotensin receptor blockers (ARBs), or beta-blockers (including propranolol). • In patients who are elderly, volume-depleted (including those on diuretic therapy), or have renal impairment, co-administration of an NSAID with ACE inhibitors or ARBs may result in deterioration of renal function, including possible acute renal failure. These effects are usually reversible.
Intervention:	• During concomitant use of TREXIMET and ACE-inhibitors, ARBs, or beta-blockers, monitor blood pressure to ensure that the desired blood pressure is obtained [see Warnings and Precautions (5.8)]. • During concomitant use of TREXIMET and ACE-inhibitors or ARBs in patients who are elderly, volume-depleted, or have impaired renal function, monitor for signs of worsening renal function [see Warnings and Precautions (5.8)].

Diuretics

Clinical Impact:	Clinical studies, as well as post-marketing observations, showed that NSAIDs reduced the natriuretic effect of loop diuretics (e.g., furosemide) and thiazide diuretics in some patients. This effect has been attributed to the NSAID inhibition of renal prostaglandin synthesis.
Intervention:	During concomitant use of TREXIMET with diuretics, observe patients for signs of worsening renal function, in addition to assuring diuretic efficacy including antihypertensive effects [see Warnings and Precautions (5.8, 5.12)].

This table is continued on the next page.

The empirical formula is $C_{14}H_{13}NaO_3$, representing a molecular weight of 252.23. Naproxen sodium is a white-to-creamy white crystalline solid, freely soluble in water at neutral pH.

Each TREXIMET 85/500 mg tablet for oral administration contains 119 mg of sumatriptan succinate equivalent to 85 mg of sumatriptan and 500 mg of naproxen sodium. Each tablet also contains the inactive ingredients croscarmellose sodium, dibasic calcium phosphate, FD&C Blue No. 2, hypromellose, magnesium stearate, microcrystalline cellulose, povidone, sodium bicarbonate, talc, titanium dioxide, and triacetin.

Each TREXIMET 10/60 mg tablet for oral administration contains 14 mg of sumatriptan succinate equivalent to 10 mg of sumatriptan and 60 mg of naproxen sodium. Each tablet also contains the inactive ingredients croscarmellose sodium, dibasic calcium phosphate, FD&C Blue No. 2, magnesium stearate, microcrystalline cellulose, polyethylene glycol, polyvinyl alcohol, povidone, sodium bicarbonate, talc, and titanium dioxide.

12   CLINICAL PHARMACOLOGY

12.1   Mechanism of Action

TREXIMET contains sumatriptan and naproxen.

Sumatriptan binds with high affinity to cloned 5-HT$_{1B/1D}$ receptors. Sumatriptan presumably exerts its therapeutic effects in the treatment of migraine headache through agonist effects at the 5-HT$_{1B/1D}$ receptors on intracranial blood vessels and sensory nerves of the trigeminal system, which result in cranial vessel constriction and inhibition of neuropeptide release.

TREXIMET has analgesic, anti-inflammatory, and antipyretic properties. The mechanism of action of TREXIMET, like that of other NSAIDs, is not completely understood but involves inhibition of cyclooxygenase (COX-1 and COX-2). Naproxen is a potent inhibitor of prostaglandin synthesis in vitro. Naproxen concentrations reached during therapy have produced in vivo effects. Prostaglandins sensitize afferent nerves and potentiate the action of bradykinin in inducing pain in animal models. Prostaglandins are mediators of inflammation. Because naproxen is an inhibitor of prostaglandin synthesis, its mode of action may be due to a decrease of prostaglandins in peripheral tissues.

12.2   Pharmacodynamics

Blood Pressure

In a randomized, double-blind, parallel group, active control trial, TREXIMET 85/500 mg administered intermittently over 6 months did not increase blood pressure in a normotensive adult population (n = 122). However, significant elevation in blood pressure has been reported with 5-HT$_1$ agonists and NSAIDs in patients with and without a history of hypertension.

12.3   Pharmacokinetics

Absorption and Bioavailability

Sumatriptan, when given as TREXIMET 85/500 mg, has a mean C_{max} similar to that of sumatriptan succinate 100 mg tablets alone. The median T_{max} of sumatriptan, when given as TREXIMET 85/500 mg, was 1 hour (range: 0.3 to 4.0 hours), which is slightly different compared with sumatriptan succinate 100 mg tablets (median T_{max} of 1.5 hours). Naproxen, when given as TREXIMET 85/500 mg, has a C_{max} which is approximately 36% lower than naproxen sodium 550 mg tablets and a median T_{max} of 5 hours (range: 0.3 to 12 hours), which is approximately 4 hours later than from naproxen sodium tablets 550 mg. AUC values for sumatriptan and for naproxen are similar for TREXIMET 85/500 mg compared with sumatriptan succinate 100 mg tablets or naproxen sodium 550 mg tablets, respectively. In a crossover trial in 16 subjects, the pharmacokinetics of both components administered as TREXIMET 85/500 mg were similar during a migraine attack and during a migraine-free period.

Bioavailability of sumatriptan is approximately 15%, primarily due to presystemic (first-pass) metabolism and partly due to incomplete absorption.

Naproxen is absorbed from the gastrointestinal tract with an in vivo bioavailability of 95%.

Continued on next page

Food had no significant effect on the bioavailability of sumatriptan or naproxen administered as TREXIMET, but slightly delayed the T_{max} of sumatriptan by about 0.6 hour [see Dosage and Administration (2.3)].

Distribution
Plasma protein binding is 14% to 21%. The effect of sumatriptan on the protein binding of other drugs has not been evaluated. The volume of distribution of sumatriptan is 2.7 L/kg.

The volume of distribution of naproxen is 0.16 L/kg. At therapeutic levels naproxen is greater than 99% albumin bound. At doses of naproxen greater than 500 mg/day, there is a less-than-proportional increase in plasma levels due to an increase in clearance caused by saturation of plasma protein binding at higher doses (average trough C_{ss} = 36.5, 49.2, and 56.4 mg/L with 500-; 1,000-; and 1,500-mg daily doses of naproxen, respectively). However, the concentration of unbound naproxen continues to increase proportionally to dose.

Metabolism
In vitro studies with human microsomes suggest that sumatriptan is metabolized by monoamine oxidase (MAO), predominantly the A isoenzyme. No significant effect was seen with an MAO-B inhibitor.

Naproxen is extensively metabolized to 6-0-desmethyl naproxen, and both parent and metabolites do not induce metabolizing enzymes.

Elimination
The elimination half-life of sumatriptan is approximately 2 hours. Radiolabeled ^{14}C-sumatriptan administered orally is largely renally excreted (about 60%), with about 40% found in the feces. Most of a radiolabeled dose of sumatriptan excreted in the urine is the major metabolite indole acetic acid (IAA) or the IAA glucuronide, both of which are inactive. Three percent of the dose can be recovered as unchanged sumatriptan.

The clearance of naproxen is 0.13 mL/min/kg. Approximately 95% of the naproxen from any dose is excreted in the urine, primarily as naproxen (less than 1%), 6-0-desmethyl naproxen (less than 1%), or their conjugates (66% to 92%). The plasma half-life of the naproxen anion in humans is approximately 19 hours. The corresponding half-lives of both metabolites and conjugates of naproxen are shorter than 12 hours, and their rates of excretion have been found to coincide closely with the rate of naproxen disappearance from the plasma. In patients with renal failure, metabolites may accumulate.

Specific Populations
Geriatrics
The pharmacokinetics of TREXIMET in geriatric patients have not been studied. Elderly patients are more likely to have decreased hepatic function and decreased renal function [see Specific Populations (8.5)].

The pharmacokinetics of oral sumatriptan in the elderly (mean age: 72 years, 2 males and 4 females) and in patients with migraine (mean age: 38 years, 25 males and 155 females) were similar to that in healthy male subjects (mean age: 30 years).

Studies indicate that although total plasma concentration of naproxen is unchanged, the unbound plasma fraction, which represents <1% of the total concentration, increased in the elderly (range of unbound trough naproxen from 0.12% to 0.19% in elderly subjects versus 0.05% to 0.075% in younger subjects).

Pediatrics
A pharmacokinetic study compared 3 doses of TREXIMET in pediatric patients 12 to 17 years of age (n=24) with adults (n=26). The AUC and C_{max} of sumatriptan were 50-60% higher following a single dose of TREXIMET 10/60 mg in pediatric patients 12 to 17 years of age (n=7) compared with adult subjects (n=8), and were 6-26% higher following a single dose of TREXIMET 30/180 mg or 85/500 mg in pediatrics than adults. Naproxen pharmacokinetic parameters were similar between pediatrics and adults.

Renal Impairment
The effect of renal impairment on the pharmacokinetics of TREXIMET has not been studied. Since naproxen and its metabolites and conjugates are primarily excreted by the kidney, the potential exists for naproxen metabolites to accumulate in the presence of renal insufficiency. Elimination of naproxen is decreased in patients with severe renal impairment. [see Warnings and Precautions (5.12), Use in Specific Populations (8.6)].

Hepatic Impairment

The effect of hepatic impairment on the pharmacokinetics of TREXIMET has not been studied. In a study in patients with moderate hepatic impairment (n = 8) matched for sex, age, and weight with healthy subjects (n = 8), patients with hepatic impairment had an approximately 70% increase in AUC and C_{max} of sumatriptan and a T_{max} 40 minutes earlier compared to healthy subjects. The pharmacokinetics of sumatriptan in patients with severe hepatic impairment has not been studied.

Gender
In a pooled analysis of 5 pharmacokinetic trials, there was no effect of gender on the systemic exposure of TREXIMET.

Race
The effect of race on the pharmacokinetics of TREXIMET has not been studied. The systemic clearance and C_{max} of sumatriptan were similar in black (n = 34) and white (n = 38) healthy male subjects.

Drug Interaction Studies
Aspirin
When naproxen was administered with aspirin (>1 gram/day), the protein binding of naproxen was reduced, although the clearance of free naproxen was not altered. See Table 3 for clinically significant drug interactions of naproxen, an NSAID, with aspirin [see Drug Interactions (7)].

Propranolol
Propranolol 80 mg given twice daily had no significant effect on sumatriptan pharmacokinetics. See Table 3 for clinically significant drug interactions of propranolol, a beta-blocker, with TREXIMET [see Drug Interactions (7)].

13   NONCLINICAL TOXICOLOGY
13.1   Carcinogenesis, Mutagenesis, Impairment of Fertility
Carcinogenesis

Table 3 (Cont.) Clinically Significant Drug Interactions with naproxen or sumatriptan

Digoxin	
Clinical Impact:	The concomitant use of naproxen with digoxin has been reported to increase the serum concentration and prolong the half-life of digoxin.
Intervention:	During concomitant use of TREXIMET and digoxin, monitor serum digoxin levels.

Lithium	
Clinical Impact:	NSAIDs have produced elevations in plasma lithium levels and reductions in renal lithium clearance. The mean minimum lithium concentration increased 15%, and the renal clearance decreased by approximately 20%. This effect has been attributed to NSAID inhibition of renal prostaglandin synthesis.
Intervention:	During concomitant use of TREXIMET and lithium, monitor patients for signs of lithium toxicity.

Methotrexate	
Clinical Impact:	Concomitant administration of some NSAIDs with high-dose methotrexate therapy has been reported to elevate and prolong serum methotrexate levels, resulting in deaths from severe hematologic and gastrointestinal toxicity. Concomitant use of NSAIDs and methotrexate may increase the risk for methotrexate toxicity (e.g., neutropenia, thrombocytopenia, renal dysfunction).
Intervention:	During concomitant use of TREXIMET and methotrexate, monitor patients for methotrexate toxicity.

Cyclosporine	
Clinical Impact:	Concomitant use of NSAIDs and cyclosporine may increase cyclosporine's nephrotoxicity.
Intervention:	During concomitant use of TREXIMET and cyclosporine, monitor patients for signs of worsening renal function.

NSAIDs and Salicylates	
Clinical Impact:	Concomitant use of naproxen with other NSAIDs or salicylates (e.g., diflunisal, salsalate) increases the risk of GI toxicity, with little or no increase in efficacy [see Warnings and Precautions (5.2)].
Intervention:	The concomitant use of naproxen with other NSAIDs or salicylates is not recommended.

Pemetrexed	
Clinical Impact:	Concomitant use of NSAIDs and pemetrexed may increase the risk of pemetrexed-associated myelosuppression, renal, and GI toxicity (see the pemetrexed prescribing information).
Intervention:	During concomitant use of TREXIMET and pemetrexed, in patients with renal impairment whose creatinine clearance ranges from 45 to 79 mL/min, monitor for myelosuppression, renal and GI toxicity. NSAIDs with short elimination half-lives (e.g., diclofenac, indomethacin) should be avoided for a period of two days before, the day of, and two days following administration of pemetrexed. In the absence of data regarding potential interaction between pemetrexed and NSAIDs with longer half-lives (e.g., meloxicam, nabumetone), patients taking these NSAIDs should interrupt dosing for at least five days before, the day of, and two days following pemetrexed administration.

Probenecid	
Clinical Impact:	Probenecid given concurrently increases naproxen anion plasma levels and extends its plasma half-life significantly. The clinical significance of this is unknown. with probenecid.
Intervention:	Reduce the frequency of administration of Treximet when given concurrently

The carcinogenic potential of TREXIMET has not been studied.

In carcinogenicity studies in mouse and rat, sumatriptan was administered orally for 78 and 104 weeks, respectively, at doses up to 160 mg/kg/day. The highest doses tested are approximately 5 (mouse) and 9 (rat) times the maximum human daily dose (MHDD) of 170 mg sumatriptan on a mg/m^2 basis (two tablets of TREXIMET 85/500 mg in a 24-hour period).

The carcinogenic potential of naproxen was evaluated in a 2-year oral carcinogenicity study in rats at doses of 8, 16, and 24 mg/kg/day, and in another 2-year oral carcinogenicity study in rats at a dose of 8 mg/kg/day. No evidence of tumorigenicity was found in either study. The highest dose tested is less than the MHDD (1000 mg) of naproxen, on a mg/m^2 basis.

Mutagenesis

Sumatriptan and naproxen sodium tested alone and in combination were negative in an in vitro bacterial reverse mutation assay, and in an in vivo micronucleus assay in mice. The combination of sumatriptan and naproxen sodium was negative in an in vitro mouse lymphoma tk assay in the presence and absence of metabolic activation. However, in separate in vitro mouse lymphoma tk assays, naproxen sodium alone was reproducibly positive in the presence of metabolic activation.

Naproxen sodium alone and in combination with sumatriptan was positive in an in vitro clastogenicity assay in mammalian cells in the presence and absence of metabolic activation. The clastogenic effect for the combination was reproducible within this assay and was greater than observed with naproxen sodium alone. Sumatriptan alone was negative in these assays.

Chromosomal aberrations were not induced in peripheral blood lymphocytes following 7 days of twice-daily dosing with TREXIMET in human volunteers.

In previous studies, sumatriptan alone was negative in in vitro (bacterial reverse mutation [Ames], gene cell mutation in Chinese hamster V79/HGPRT, chromosomal aberration in human lymphocytes) and in vivo (rat micronucleus) assays.

Impairment of Fertility

The effect of TREXIMET on fertility in animals has not been studied.

When sumatriptan (5, 50, 500 mg/kg/day) was administered orally to male and female rats prior to and throughout the mating period, there was a drug-related decrease in fertility secondary to a decrease in mating in animals treated with doses greater than 5 mg/kg/day (less than the MHDD of 170 mg on a mg/m^2 basis). It is not clear whether this finding was due to an effect on males or females or both.

13.2 Animal Toxicology and/or Pharmacology

Corneal Opacities

Dogs receiving oral sumatriptan developed corneal opacities and defects in the corneal epithelium. Corneal opacities were seen at the lowest dosage tested, 2 mg/kg/day, and were present after 1 month of treatment. Defects in the corneal epithelium were noted in a 60-week study. Earlier examinations for these toxicities were not conducted and no-effect doses were not established. The lowest dose tested is less than the MHDD (170 mg) of sumatriptan on a mg/m^2 basis.

14 CLINICAL STUDIES

14.1 Adults

The efficacy of TREXIMET in the acute treatment of migraine with or without aura in adults was demonstrated in 2 randomized, double-blind, multicenter, parallel-group trials utilizing placebo and each individual active component of TREXIMET 85/500 mg (sumatriptan and naproxen sodium) as comparison treatments (Study 1 and Study 2). Patients enrolled in these 2 trials were predominately female (87%) and white (88%), with a mean age of 40 years (range: 18 to 65 years). Patients were instructed to treat a migraine of moderate to severe pain with 1 tablet. No rescue medication was allowed within 2 hours postdose. Patients evaluated their headache pain 2 hours after taking 1 dose of study medication; headache relief was defined as a reduction in headache severity from moderate or severe pain to mild or no pain. Associated symptoms of nausea, photophobia, and phonophobia were also evaluated. Sustained pain free was defined as a reduction in headache severity from moderate or severe pain to no pain at 2 hours postdose without a return of mild, moderate, or severe pain and no use of rescue medication for 24 hours postdose. The results from

MEDICATION GUIDE
TREXIMET® [trex' i-met] Tablets
(sumatriptan and naproxen sodium)

Read this Medication Guide before you start taking TREXIMET and each time you get a refill. There may be new information. This Medication Guide does not take the place of talking with your healthcare provider about your medical condition or treatment.

What is the most important information I should know about TREXIMET?
TREXIMET may increase your chance of a heart attack or stroke that can lead to death. TREXIMET contains 2 medicines: sumatriptan and naproxen sodium (a nonsteroidal anti-inflammatory drug [NSAID]).
• This risk may happen early in treatment and may increase:
  ○ with increasing doses of NSAIDs
  ○ with longer use of NSAIDs
Do not take TREXIMET right before or after a heart surgery called a "coronary artery bypass graft (CABG)."
Avoid taking TREXIMET after a recent heart attack, unless your healthcare provider tells you to. You may have an increased risk of another heart attack if you take NSAIDs after a recent heart attack.
Stop taking TREXIMET and get emergency help right away if you have any of the following symptoms of a heart attack or stroke:
• discomfort in the center of your chest that lasts for more than a few minutes, or that goes away and comes back
• severe tightness, pain, pressure, or heaviness in your chest, throat, neck, or jaw
• pain or discomfort in your arms, back, neck, jaw, or stomach
• shortness of breath with or without chest discomfort
• breaking out in a cold sweat
• nausea or vomiting
• feeling lightheaded
• weakness in one part or on one side of your body
• slurred speech
TREXIMET is not for people with risk factors for heart disease unless a heart exam is done and shows no problem. You have a higher risk for heart disease if you:
• have high blood pressure
• smoke
• have diabetes
• have high cholesterol levels
• are overweight
• have a family history of heart disease
TREXIMET can cause ulcers and bleeding in the stomach and intestines at any time during your treatment. Ulcers and bleeding can happen without warning symptoms and may cause death.
Your chance of getting an ulcer or bleeding increases with:
• past history of stomach ulcers, or stomach or intestinal bleeding with use of NSAIDs
• the use of medicines called "corticosteroids," "anticoagulants," and antidepressant medicines called "SSRIs" or "SNRIs"
• more frequent use
• drinking alcohol
• having poor health
• advanced liver disease
• bleeding problems
• longer use
• smoking
• older age
TREXIMET may cause serious allergic reactions or serious skin reactions that can be life-threatening. Stop taking TREXIMET and get emergency help right away if you develop:
• sudden wheezing
• rash
• problems breathing or swallowing
• blisters or bleeding of your lips, eye lids, mouth, nose, or genitals
• swelling of your lips, tongue, throat or body
• fainting
• reddening of your skin with blisters or peeling
TREXIMET should only be used exactly as prescribed, at the lowest dose possible for your treatment, and for the shortest time needed.
TREXIMET already contains an NSAID (naproxen). Do not use TREXIMET with other medicines to lessen pain or fever or with other medicines for colds or sleeping problems without talking to your healthcare provider first, because they may contain an NSAID also.

What is TREXIMET?
TREXIMET is a prescription medicine that contains sumatriptan and naproxen sodium (an NSAID). TREXIMET is used to treat acute migraine headaches with or without aura in patients 12 years of age and older.
TREXIMET is not used to treat other types of headaches such as hemiplegic (that make you unable to move on one side of your body) or basilar (rare form of migraine with aura) migraines.
TREXIMET is not used to prevent or decrease the number of migraine headaches you have.
It is not known if TREXIMET is safe and effective to treat cluster headaches.

Who should not take TREXIMET?
Do not take TREXIMET if you have:
• heart problems, history of heart problems, or right before or after heart bypass surgery
• had a stroke, transient ischemic attack (TIAs), or problems with your blood circulation
• hemiplegic migraines or basilar migraines. If you are not sure if you have these types of migraines, ask your healthcare provider.
• narrowing of blood vessels to your legs and arms (peripheral vascular disease), stomach (ischemic bowel disease), or kidneys
• uncontrolled high blood pressure
• taken any medicines in the last 24 hours that are called 5-HT$_1$ agonists that are triptans or contain ergotamine. Ask your healthcare provider for a list of these medicines if you are not sure.
• taken an antidepressant medicine called a monoamine oxidase (MAO) inhibitor within the last 2 weeks. Ask your healthcare provider for a list if you are not sure.
• had an asthma attack, hives, or other allergic reaction with aspirin or any other NSAID medicine
• an allergy to sumatriptan, naproxen, or any of the ingredients in TREXIMET. See "What are the ingredients in TREXIMET?" below for a complete list of ingredients.
• third trimester of pregnancy
• liver problems

What should I tell my healthcare provider before taking TREXIMET?
Before you take TREXIMET, tell your healthcare provider about all of your medical conditions, including if you:
• have high blood pressure
• have asthma
• have high cholesterol
• have diabetes

Study 1 and 2 are summarized in Table 4. In both trials, the percentage of patients achieving headache pain relief 2 hours after treatment was significantly greater among patients receiving TREXIMET 85/500 mg (65% and 57%) compared with those who received placebo (28% and 29%). Further, the percentage of patients who remained pain free without use of other medications through 24 hours postdose was significantly greater among patients receiving a single dose of TREXIMET 85/500 mg (25% and 23%) compared with those who received placebo (8% and 7%) or either sumatriptan (16% and 14%) or naproxen sodium (10%) alone.

[See table 4 on next page]

The percentage of patients achieving initial headache pain relief within 2 hours following treatment with TREXIMET 85/500 mg is shown in Figure 1.

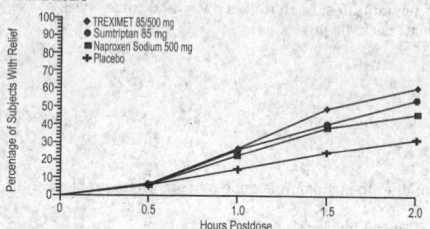

Figure 1. Percentage of Adult Patients with Initial Headache Pain Relief within 2 Hours

Compared with placebo, there was a decreased incidence of photophobia, phonophobia, and nausea 2 hours after the administration of TREXIMET 85/500 mg. The estimated probability of taking a rescue medication over the first 24 hours is shown in Figure 2.

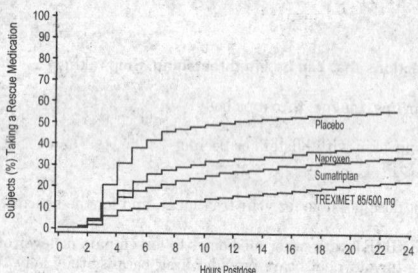

Figure 2. Estimated Probability of Adults Taking a Rescue Medication over the 24 Hours following the First Dose*

*Kaplan-Meier plot based on data obtained in the 2 clinical controlled trials providing evidence of efficacy with patients not using additional treatments censored to 24 hours. Plot also includes patients who had no response to the initial dose. No rescue medication was allowed within 2 hours postdose.

TREXIMET 85/500 mg was more effective than placebo regardless of the presence of aura; duration of headache prior to treatment; gender, age, or weight of the subject; or concomitant use of oral contraceptives or common migraine prophylactic drugs (e.g., beta-blockers, anti-epileptic drugs, tricyclic antidepressants).

14.2   Pediatric Patients 12 to 17 Years of Age

The efficacy of TREXIMET in the acute treatment of migraine with or without aura in pediatric patients 12 to 17 years of age was demonstrated in a randomized, double-blind, multicenter, parallel-group, placebo-controlled, multicenter trial comparing 3 doses of TREXIMET and placebo (Study 3). Patients enrolled in this trial were mostly female (59%) and white (81%), with a mean age of 15 years. Patients were required to have at least a 6-month history of migraine attacks with or without aura usually lasting 3 hours or more when untreated. Following a single-blind, placebo run-in phase, placebo nonresponders were randomized to receive a single dose of either TREXIMET 10/60 mg, 30/180 mg, 85/500 mg, or placebo. Patients were instructed to treat a single migraine attack with headache pain of moderate to severe intensity. No rescue medication was allowed within 2 hours postdose. Patients evaluated their headache pain 2 hours after taking 1 dose of study medication. Two-hour pain free was defined as a reduction in headache severity from moderate or severe pain to no pain at 2 hours postdose.

- smoke
- are overweight
- have heart problems or a family history of heart problems or stroke
- have kidney problems
- have liver problems
- have had epilepsy or seizures
- are not using effective birth control
- are pregnant, think you might be pregnant, or are trying to become pregnant. **TREXIMET should not be used by pregnant women during the third trimester of their pregnancy.**
- are breastfeeding or plan to breastfeed. The components of TREXIMET pass into your breast milk and may harm your baby. Talk with your healthcare provider about the best way to feed your baby if you take TREXIMET.

Tell your healthcare provider about all the medicines you take, including prescription and over-the-counter medicines, vitamins, and herbal supplements.

TREXIMET and certain other medicines can affect each other, causing serious side effects.

How should I take TREXIMET?

- Certain people should take their first dose of TREXIMET in their healthcare provider's office or in another medical setting. Ask your healthcare provider if you should take your first dose in a medical setting.
- Take TREXIMET exactly as your healthcare provider tells you to take it.
- Take TREXIMET tablets whole with water or other liquids.
- TREXIMET can be taken with or without food.
- If you do not get any relief after your first dose, do not take a second dose without first talking with your healthcare provider.
- If your headache comes back or you only get some relief from your headache:
  - For adults: a second dose may be taken 2 hours after the first dose. Do not take more than 2 doses of TREXIMET 85/500 mg in a 24-hour period.
  - For children 12 to 17 years of age: it is not known if taking more than 1 dose of TREXIMET in 24 hours is safe and effective. Talk to your healthcare provider about what to do if your headache does not go away or comes back.
- If you take too much TREXIMET, call your healthcare provider or go to the nearest hospital emergency room right away.
- You should write down when you have headaches and when you take TREXIMET so you can talk with your healthcare provider about how TREXIMET is working for you.

What should I avoid while taking TREXIMET?

TREXIMET can cause dizziness, weakness, or drowsiness. If you have these symptoms, do not drive a car, use machinery, or do anything where you need to be alert.

What are the possible side effects of TREXIMET?

TREXIMET may cause serious side effects. See "What is the most important information I should know about TREXIMET?"

These serious side effects include:

- changes in color or sensation in your fingers and toes (Raynaud's syndrome)
- new or worse high blood pressure
- heart failure from body swelling (fluid retention)
- kidney problems including kidney failure
- low red blood cells (anemia)
- liver problems including liver failure
- asthma attacks in people who have asthma
- stomach and intestinal problems (gastrointestinal and colonic ischemic events). Symptoms of gastrointestinal and colonic ischemic events include:
  - sudden or severe stomach pain
  - weight loss
  - constipation or diarrhea
  - fever
  - stomach pain after meals
  - nausea or vomiting
  - bloody diarrhea
- problems with blood circulation to your legs and feet (peripheral vascular ischemia). Symptoms of peripheral vascular ischemia include:
  - cramping and pain in your legs or hips
  - feeling of heaviness or tightness in your leg muscles
  - burning or aching pain in your feet or toes while resting
  - numbness, tingling, or weakness in your legs
  - cold feeling or color changes in 1 or both legs or feet
- medication overuse headaches. Some people who use too many TREXIMET tablets may have worse headaches (medication overuse headache). If your headaches get worse, your healthcare provider may decide to stop your treatment with TREXIMET.
- serotonin syndrome. Serotonin syndrome is a rare but serious problem that can happen in people using TREXIMET, especially if TREXIMET is used with antidepressant medicines called SSRIs or SNRIs.

Stop taking TREXIMET and call your healthcare provider right away if you have any of the following symptoms of serotonin syndrome:

- changes in blood pressure
- tight muscles
- mental changes such as seeing things that are not there (hallucinations), agitation, or coma
- fast heartbeat
- high body temperature
- trouble walking

- seizures. Seizures have happened in people taking sumatriptan, one of the ingredients in TREXIMET, who have never had seizures before. Talk with your healthcare provider about your chance of having seizures while you take TREXIMET.

The most common side effects of TREXIMET include:

- dizziness
- pain, discomfort, or stiffness in your neck, throat, jaw, or chest
- tingling or numbness in your fingers or toes
- dry mouth
- heartbeat problems
- feeling weak, drowsy, or tired
- nausea
- heartburn
- feeling hot
- muscle tightness

Stop TREXIMET and call your healthcare provider right away if you have any of the following symptoms:

- nausea that seems out of proportion to your migraine
- vomit blood
- yellow skin or eyes
- more tired or weaker than usual
- itching
- sudden or severe stomach pain
- blood in your bowel movement or it is black and sticky like tar
- unusual weight gain
- flu-like symptoms
- diarrhea
- tenderness in your upper right side

Results are summarized in Table 5. The percentage of patients who were pain free at 2 hours postdose was significantly greater among patients who received any of the 3 doses of TREXIMET compared with placebo.
[See table 5 below]
The percentage of pediatric patients who remained pain free without use of other medications 2 through 24 hours postdose was significantly greater after administration of a single dose of TREXIMET 85/500 mg compared with placebo. A greater percentage of pediatric patients who received a single dose of 10/60 mg or 30/180 mg remained pain free 2 through 24 hours postdose compared with placebo. Compared with placebo, the incidence of photophobia and phonophobia was significantly decreased 2 hours after the administration of a single dose of 85/500 mg, whereas, the incidence of nausea was comparable. There was a decreased incidence of photophobia, phonophobia, and nausea 2 hours after single-dose administration of 10/60 mg or 30/180 mg compared with placebo.

16   HOW SUPPLIED/STORAGE AND HANDLING

TREXIMET 85/500 mg contains 119 mg of sumatriptan succinate equivalent to 85 mg of sumatriptan and 500 mg of naproxen sodium and is supplied as blue film-coated tablets debossed on one side with *TREXIMET* in bottles of 9 tablets with desiccant (NDC 65224-850-09).
TREXIMET 10/60 mg contains 14 mg of sumatriptan succinate equivalent to 10 mg of sumatriptan and 60 mg of naproxen sodium and is supplied as light-blue film-coated tablets debossed on one side with *TREXIMET* and the other side with *10-60* in bottles of 9 tablets with desiccant (NDC 65224-860-09).
Store at 25°C (77°F); excursions permitted to 15°-30°C (59°-86°F) [see USP Controlled Room Temperature]. Do not repackage; dispense and store in original container with desiccant.

17   PATIENT COUNSELING INFORMATION

Advise the patient to read the FDA-approved patient labeling (Medication Guide) that accompanies each prescription dispensed. Inform patients, families, or their caregivers of the following information before initiating therapy with TREXIMET and periodically during the course of ongoing therapy.
Cardiovascular Thrombotic Events, Prinzmetal's Angina, Other Vasospasm-Related Events, Arrhythmias and Cerebrovascular Events
Advise patients to be alert for the symptoms of cardiovascular thrombotic effects such as myocardial infarction or stroke, which may result in hospitalization and even death.

• swelling of the arms, legs, hands, and feet
Tell your healthcare provider if you have any side effects that bother you or do not go away.
These are not all of the side effects of TREXIMET. For more information, ask your healthcare provider or pharmacist. Call your doctor for medical advice about side effects. You may report side effects to FDA at 1-800-FDA-1088.

How should I store TREXIMET?
Store TREXIMET at room temperature between 68°F to 77°F (20°C to 25°C).
Keep TREXIMET and all medicines out of the reach of children.

General information about the safe and effective use of TREXIMET
Medicines are sometimes prescribed for purposes other than those listed in a Medication Guide. Do not use TREXIMET for a condition for which it was not prescribed. Do not give TREXIMET to other people, even if they have the same problem you have. It may harm them.
This Medication Guide summarizes the most important information about TREXIMET. If you would like more information, talk with your healthcare provider. You can ask your healthcare provider or pharmacist for information about TREXIMET that is written for healthcare professionals.
For more information call 1-800-793-2145 or visit www.TREXIMET.com.

What are the ingredients in TREXIMET?
Active ingredients: sumatriptan succinate and naproxen sodium.
Inactive ingredients in all strengths: croscarmellose sodium, dibasic calcium phosphate, FD&C Blue No. 2, magnesium stearate, microcrystalline cellulose, povidone, sodium bicarbonate, talc, and titanium dioxide.
85/500-mg tablets also contain: hypromellose and triacetin.
10/60-mg tablets also contain: polyethylene glycol and polyvinyl alcohol.
TREXIMET is a registered trademark of Pernix Ireland Limited. The other brands listed are trademarks of their respective owners and are not trademarks of Pernix Ireland Limited. The makers of these brands are not affiliated with and do not endorse Pernix Ireland Limited or its products.
Pernix Ireland Limited, distributed by Pernix Therapeutics, LLC; Morristown, NJ 07960; ©2016, Pernix Ireland Limited. All rights reserved.

This Medication Guide has been approved by the U.S. Food and Drug Administration.

TRE-LC006.03 05/2016

Although serious cardiovascular events can occur without warning symptoms, patients should be alert for signs and symptoms of chest pain, shortness of breath, weakness, irregular heartbeat, significant rise in blood pressure, weakness and slurring of speech, and should be advised to report any of these symptoms to their health care provider immediately. Apprise patients of the importance of this follow-up [see Warnings and Precautions (5.1, 5.3, 5.5, 5.6, 5.8)].
Gastrointestinal Bleeding, Ulceration, and Perforation
Advise patients to report symptoms of ulcerations and bleeding, including epigastric pain, dyspepsia, melena, and hematemesis to their health care provider. In the setting of concomitant use of low-dose aspirin for cardiac prophylaxis, inform patients of the increased risk for and the signs and symptoms of GI bleeding [see Warnings and Precautions (5.2)].
Hepatotoxicity

Inform patients of the warning signs and symptoms of hepatotoxicity (e.g., nausea, fatigue, lethargy, pruritus, diarrhea, jaundice, right upper quadrant tenderness, and "flu-like" symptoms). If these occur, instruct patients to stop TREXIMET and seek immediate medical therapy [see Warnings and Precautions (5.7)].
Anaphylactic Reactions
Inform patients that anaphylactic reactions have occurred in patients receiving the components of TREXIMET. Such reactions can be life-threatening or fatal. In general, anaphylactic reactions to drugs are more likely to occur in individuals with a history of sensitivity to multiple allergens. Inform patients of the signs of an anaphylactic reaction (e.g., difficulty breathing, swelling of the face or throat). If these occur, patients should be instructed to seek immediate emergency help [see Contraindications (4), Warnings and Precautions (5.13)].
Serious Skin Reactions
Inform patients that TREXIMET, like other NSAID-containing products, may increase the risk of serious skin side effects such as exfoliative dermatitis, Stevens-Johnson syndrome, and toxic epidermal necrolysis, which may result in hospitalizations and even death. Although serious skin reactions may occur without warning, patients should be alert for the signs and symptoms of skin rash and blisters, fever, or other signs of hypersensitivity such as itching and should ask for medical advice when observing any indicative signs or symptoms. Advise patients to stop the drug immediately if they develop any type of rash and contact their healthcare providers as soon as possible [see Warnings and Precautions (5.14)].
Fetal Toxicity
Inform patients that TREXIMET should not be used during the third trimester of pregnancy because NSAID-containing products have been shown to cause premature closure of the ductus arteriosus. Inform patients that TREXIMET should be used during the first and second trimester of pregnancy only if the potential benefit justifies the potential risk to the fetus [see Contraindications (4), Warnings and Precautions (5.15), Use in Specific Populations (8.1)].
Nursing Mothers
Advise patients to notify their healthcare provider if they are breastfeeding or plan to breastfeed [see Use in Specific Populations (8.3)].
Heart Failure and Edema
Advise patients to be alert for the symptoms of congestive heart failure including shortness of breath, unexplained weight gain, or edema and to contact their healthcare provider if such symptoms occur [see Warnings and Precautions (5.9)].

Table 5. Percentage of Pediatric Patients 12 to 17 Years of Age with 2-Hour Pain-Free Response Following Treatment in Study 3*

Endpoint	TREXIMET 10/60 mg (n = 96)	TREXIMET 30/180 mg (n = 97)	TREXIMET 85/500 mg (n = 152)	Placebo (n = 145)
2-Hour Pain Free	29%[†]	27%[†]	24%[†]	10%

* P values provided only for prespecified comparisons.
† P<0.01 versus placebo.

Table 4. Percentage of Adult Patients with 2-Hour Pain Relief and Sustained Pain Free Following Treatment*

	TREXIMET 85/500 mg	Sumatriptan 85 mg	Naproxen Sodium 500 mg	Placebo
2-Hour Pain Relief				
Study 1	65%[†] n = 364	55% n = 361	44% n = 356	28% n = 360
Study 2	57%[†] n = 362	50% n = 362	43% n = 364	29% n = 382
Sustained Pain Free (2-24 Hours)				
Study 1	25%[‡] n = 364	16% n = 361	10% n = 356	8% n = 360
Study 2	23%[‡] n = 362	14% n = 362	10% n = 364	7% n = 382

* P values provided only for prespecified comparisons.
† P<0.05 versus placebo and sumatriptan.
‡ P <0.01 versus placebo, sumatriptan, and naproxen sodium.

Continued on next page

Concomitant Use with Other Triptans or Ergot Medications

Inform patients that use of TREXIMET within 24 hours of another triptan or an ergot-type medication (including dihydroergotamine or methysergide) is contraindicated *[see Contraindications (4), Drug Interactions (7.1)]*.

Serotonin Syndrome

Caution patients about the risk of serotonin syndrome with the use of TREXIMET or other triptans, particularly during concomitant use with SSRIs, SNRIs, TCAs, and MAO inhibitors *[see Warnings and Precautions (5.11), Drug Interactions (7.1)]*.

Medication Overuse Headache

Inform patients that use of acute migraine drugs for 10 or more days per month may lead to an exacerbation of headache and encourage patients to record headache frequency and drug use (e.g., by keeping a headache diary) *[see Warnings and Precautions (5.10)]*.

Ability to Perform Complex Tasks

Treatment with TREXIMET may cause somnolence and dizziness; instruct patients to evaluate their ability to perform complex tasks after administration of TREXIMET *[see Adverse Reactions (6.1)]*.

Asthma

Advise patients with preexisting asthma to seek immediate medical attention if their asthma worsens after taking TREXIMET. Patients with a history of aspirin-sensitive asthma should not take TREXIMET *[see Contraindications (4), Warnings and Precautions (5.17)]*.

Avoid Concomitant Use of NSAIDs

Inform patients that the concomitant use of TREXIMET with other NSAIDs or salicylates (e.g., diflunisal, salsalate) is not recommended due to the increased risk of gastrointestinal toxicity, and little or no increase in efficacy *[see Warnings and Precautions (5.2) and Drug Interactions (7)]*. Alert patients that NSAIDs may be present in "over the counter" medications for treatment of colds, fever, or insomnia.

Use of NSAIDS and Low-Dose Aspirin

Inform patients not to use low-dose aspirin concomitantly with TREXIMET until they talk to their healthcare provider *[see Drug Interactions (7)]*.

TREXIMET is a registered trademark of Pernix Ireland Limited. The other brands listed are trademarks of their respective owners and are not trademarks of Pernix Ireland Limited. The makers of these brands are not affiliated with and do not endorse Pernix Ireland Limited or its products. Pernix Ireland Limited, distributed by Pernix Therapeutics, LLC

Morristown, NJ 07960

©2016, Pernix Ireland Limited. All rights reserved.

May 2016

TRE-LC003.04

[See table on pages 1013 to 1015]

Shown in Product Identification Guide, page 509

Pfizer Inc.

235 EAST 42ND STREET
NEW YORK, NY 10017–5755

For updates to the product information listed below, please check the Pfizer Web site, http://www.pfizerpro.com, or call (800) 438-1985. For complete product listing, please see the Manufacturers' Index.

For Medical Information, Contact:
(800) 438-1985
24 hours a day, 7 days a week

Distribution:
1855 Shelby Oaks Drive North
Memphis, TN 38134
(901) 387-5200

Customer Service:
(800) 533-4535

Pfizer Companies Include:
Agouron Pharmaceuticals
King Pharmaceuticals Inc.
Pharmaceuticals Inc.
Parke-Davis
Pharmacia & Upjohn
G.D. Searle & Co.
Wyeth Pharmaceuticals – see Wyeth Pharmaceuticals

VIAGRA®

[vi-AG-rah]
(sildenafil citrate)
tablets, for oral use

℞

HIGHLIGHTS OF PRESCRIBING INFORMATION

These highlights do not include all the information needed to use VIAGRA safely and effectively. See full prescribing information for VIAGRA.

VIAGRA® (sildenafil citrate) tablets, for oral use
Initial U.S. Approval: 1998

RECENT MAJOR CHANGES

Contraindications, Concomitant Guanylate Cyclase (GC) Stimulators (4.3)

INDICATIONS AND USAGE

VIAGRA is a phosphodiesterase-5 (PDE5) inhibitor indicated for the treatment of erectile dysfunction (ED) (1)

DOSAGE AND ADMINISTRATION

- For most patients, the recommended dose is 50 mg taken, as needed, approximately 1 hour before sexual activity. However, VIAGRA may be taken anywhere from 30 minutes to 4 hours before sexual activity (2.1)
- Based on effectiveness and toleration, may increase to a maximum of 100 mg or decrease to 25 mg (2.1)
- Maximum recommended dosing frequency is once per day (2.1)

DOSAGE FORMS AND STRENGTHS

Tablets: 25 mg, 50 mg, 100 mg (3)

CONTRAINDICATIONS

- Administration of VIAGRA to patients using nitric oxide donors, such as organic nitrates or organic nitrites in any form. VIAGRA was shown to potentiate the hypotensive effect of nitrates (4.1, 7.1, 12.2)
- Known hypersensitivity to sildenafil or any component of tablet (4.2)
- Administration with guanylate cyclase (GC) stimulators, such as riociguat (4.3)

WARNINGS AND PRECAUTIONS

- Patients should not use VIAGRA if sexual activity is inadvisable due to cardiovascular status (5.1)
- Patients should seek emergency treatment if an erection lasts >4 hours. Use VIAGRA with caution in patients predisposed to priapism (5.2)
- Patients should stop VIAGRA and seek medical care if a sudden loss of vision occurs in one or both eyes, which could be a sign of non arteritic anterior ischemic optic neuropathy (NAION). VIAGRA should be used with caution, and only when the anticipated benefits outweigh the risks, in patients with a history of NAION. Patients with a "crowded" optic disc may also be at an increased risk of NAION. (5.3)
- Patients should stop VIAGRA and seek prompt medical attention in the event of sudden decrease or loss of hearing (5.4)
- Caution is advised when VIAGRA is co-administered with alpha-blockers or anti-hypertensives. Concomitant use may lead to hypotension (5.5)
- Decreased blood pressure, syncope, and prolonged erection may occur at higher sildenafil exposures. In patients taking strong CYP inhibitors, such as ritonavir, sildenafil exposure is increased. Decrease in VIAGRA dosage is recommended (2.4, 5.6)

ADVERSE REACTIONS

Most common adverse reactions (≥ 2%) include headache, flushing, dyspepsia, abnormal vision, nasal congestion, back pain, myalgia, nausea, dizziness and rash (6.1)

To report SUSPECTED ADVERSE REACTIONS, contact Pfizer at 1-800-438-1985 or FDA at 1-800-FDA-1088 or *www.fda.gov/medwatch.*

DRUG INTERACTIONS

- VIAGRA can potentiate the hypotensive effects of nitrates, alpha blockers, and anti-hypertensives (4.1, 5.5, 7.1, 7.2, 7.3, 12.2)
- With concomitant use of alpha blockers, initiate VIAGRA at 25 mg dose (2.3)
- CYP3A4 inhibitors (e.g., ritonavir, ketoconazole, itraconazole, erythromycin): Increase VIAGRA exposure (2.4, 7.4, 12.3)
- Ritonavir: Do not exceed a maximum single dose of 25 mg in a 48 hour period (2.4, 5.6)
- Erythromycin or strong CYP3A4 inhibitors (e.g., ketoconazole, itraconazole, saquinavir): Consider a starting dose of 25 mg (2.4, 7.4)

USE IN SPECIFIC POPULATIONS

- Geriatric use: Consider a starting dose of 25 mg (2.5, 8.5)
- Severe renal impairment: Consider a starting dose of 25 mg (2.5, 8.6)
- Hepatic impairment: Consider a starting dose of 25 mg (2.5, 8.7)

See 17 for PATIENT COUNSELING INFORMATION and FDA-approved patient labeling.

Revised: 11/2015

FULL PRESCRIBING INFORMATION

1   INDICATIONS AND USAGE

VIAGRA is indicated for the treatment of erectile dysfunction.

2   DOSAGE AND ADMINISTRATION

2.1   Dosage Information

For most patients, the recommended dose is 50 mg taken, as needed, approximately 1 hour before sexual activity. However, VIAGRA may be taken anywhere from 30 minutes to 4 hours before sexual activity.

The maximum recommended dosing frequency is once per day.

Based on effectiveness and toleration, the dose may be increased to a maximum recommended dose of 100 mg or decreased to 25 mg.

2.2   Use with Food

VIAGRA may be taken with or without food.

2.3 Dosage Adjustments in Specific Situations

VIAGRA was shown to potentiate the hypotensive effects of nitrates and its administration in patients who use nitric oxide donors such as organic nitrates or organic nitrites in any form is therefore contraindicated [see *Contraindications (4.1), Drug Interactions (7.1), and Clinical Pharmacology (12.2)*].

When VIAGRA is co-administered with an alpha-blocker, patients should be stable on alpha-blocker therapy prior to initiating VIAGRA treatment and VIAGRA should be initiated at 25 mg [see *Warnings and Precautions (5.5), Drug Interactions (7.2), and Clinical Pharmacology (12.2)*].

2.4 Dosage Adjustments Due to Drug Interactions

Ritonavir

The recommended dose for ritonavir-treated patients is 25 mg prior to sexual activity and the recommended maximum dose is 25 mg within a 48 hour period because concomitant administration increased the blood levels of sildenafil by 11-fold [see *Warnings and Precautions (5.6), Drug Interactions (7.4), and Clinical Pharmacology (12.3)*].

CYP3A4 Inhibitors

Consider a starting dose of 25 mg in patients treated with strong CYP3A4 inhibitors (e.g., ketoconazole, itraconazole, or saquinavir) or erythromycin. Clinical data have shown that co-administration with saquinavir or erythromycin increased plasma levels of sildenafil by about 3 fold [see *Drug Interactions (7.4) and Clinical Pharmacology (12.3)*].

2.5 Dosage Adjustments in Special Populations

Consider a starting dose of 25 mg in patients > 65 years, patients with hepatic impairment (e.g., cirrhosis), and patients with severe renal impairment (creatinine clearance <30 mL/minute) because administration of VIAGRA in these patients resulted in higher plasma levels of sildenafil [see *Use in Specific Populations (8.5, 8.6, 8.7) and Clinical Pharmacology (12.3)*].

3 DOSAGE FORMS AND STRENGTHS

VIAGRA is supplied as blue, film-coated, rounded-diamond-shaped tablets containing sildenafil citrate equivalent to 25 mg, 50 mg, or 100 mg of sildenafil. Tablets are debossed with PFIZER on one side and VGR25, VGR50 or VGR100 on the other to indicate the dosage strengths.

4 CONTRAINDICATIONS

4.1 Nitrates

Consistent with its known effects on the nitric oxide/cGMP pathway [see *Clinical Pharmacology (12.1, 12.2)*], VIAGRA was shown to potentiate the hypotensive effects of nitrates, and its administration to patients who are using nitric oxide donors such as organic nitrates or organic nitrites in any form either regularly and/or intermittently is therefore contraindicated.

After patients have taken VIAGRA, it is unknown when nitrates, if necessary, can be safely administered. Although plasma levels of sildenafil at 24 hours post dose are much lower than at peak concentration, it is unknown whether nitrates can be safely co-administered at this time point [see *Dosage and Administration (2.3), Drug Interactions (7.1), and Clinical Pharmacology (12.2)*].

4.2 Hypersensitivity Reactions

VIAGRA is contraindicated in patients with a known hypersensitivity to sildenafil, as contained in VIAGRA and REVATIO, or any component of the tablet. Hypersensitivity reactions have been reported, including rash and urticaria [see *Adverse Reactions (6.1)*].

4.3 Concomitant Guanylate Cyclase (GC) Stimulators

Do not use VIAGRA in patients who are using a GC stimulator, such as riociguat. PDE5 inhibitors, including VIAGRA, may potentiate the hypotensive effects of GC stimulators.

5 WARNINGS AND PRECAUTIONS

5.1 Cardiovascular

There is a potential for cardiac risk of sexual activity in patients with preexisting cardiovascular disease. Therefore, treatments for erectile dysfunction, including VIAGRA, should not be generally used in men for whom sexual activity is inadvisable because of their underlying cardiovascular status. The evaluation of erectile dysfunction should include a determination of potential underlying causes and the identification of appropriate treatment following a complete medical assessment.

VIAGRA has systemic vasodilatory properties that resulted in transient decreases in supine blood pressure in healthy volunteers (mean maximum decrease of 8.4/5.5 mmHg), [see *Clinical Pharmacology (12.2)*]. While this normally would be expected to be of little consequence in most patients, prior to prescribing VIAGRA, physicians should carefully consider whether their patients with underlying cardiovascular disease could be affected adversely by such vasodilatory effects, especially in combination with sexual activity. Use with caution in patients with the following underlying conditions which can be particularly sensitive to the actions of vasodilators including VIAGRA – those with left ventricular outflow obstruction (e.g., aortic stenosis, idiopathic hypertrophic subaortic stenosis) and those with severely impaired autonomic control of blood pressure.

There are no controlled clinical data on the safety or efficacy of VIAGRA in the following groups; if prescribed, this should be done with caution.

• Patients who have suffered a myocardial infarction, stroke, or life-threatening arrhythmia within the last 6 months;
• Patients with resting hypotension (BP <90/50 mmHg) or hypertension (BP >170/110 mmHg);
• Patients with cardiac failure or coronary artery disease causing unstable angina.

5.2 Prolonged Erection and Priapism

Prolonged erection greater than 4 hours and priapism (painful erections greater than 6 hours in duration) have been reported infrequently since market approval of VIAGRA. In the event of an erection that persists longer than 4 hours, the patient should seek immediate medical assistance. If priapism is not treated immediately, penile tissue damage and permanent loss of potency could result.

VIAGRA should be used with caution in patients with anatomical deformation of the penis (such as angulation, cavernosal fibrosis or Peyronie's disease), or in patients who have conditions which may predispose them to priapism (such as sickle cell anemia, multiple myeloma, or leukemia). However, there are no controlled clinical data on the safety or efficacy of VIAGRA in patients with sickle cell or related anemias.

5.3 Effects on the Eye

Physicians should advise patients to stop use of all phosphodiesterase type 5 (PDE5) inhibitors, including VIAGRA, and seek medical attention in the event of a sudden loss of vision in one or both eyes. Such an event may be a sign of non-arteritic anterior ischemic optic neuropathy (NAION), a rare condition and a cause of decreased vision including permanent loss of vision, that has been reported rarely postmarketing in temporal association with the use of all PDE5 inhibitors. Based on published literature, the annual incidence of NAION is 2.5–11.8 cases per 100,000 in males aged ≥ 50. An observational study evaluated whether recent use of PDE5 inhibitors, as a class, was associated with acute onset of NAION. The results suggest an approximate 2 fold increase in the risk of NAION within 5 half-lives of PDE5 inhibitor use. From this information, it is not possible to determine whether these events are related directly to the use of PDE5 inhibitors or to other factors [see *Adverse Reactions (6.2)*].

Physicians should consider whether their patients with underlying NAION risk factors could be adversely affected by use of PDE5 inhibitors. Individuals who have already experienced NAION are at increased risk of NAION recurrence. Therefore, PDE5 inhibitors, including VIAGRA, should be used with caution in these patients and only when the anticipated benefits outweigh the risks. Individuals with "crowded" optic disc are also considered at greater risk for NAION compared to the general population, however, evidence is insufficient to support screening of prospective users of PDE5 inhibitors, including VIAGRA, for this uncommon condition.

There are no controlled clinical data on the safety or efficacy of VIAGRA in patients with retinitis pigmentosa (a minority of these patients have genetic disorders of retinal phosphodiesterases); if prescribed, this should be done with caution.

5.4 Hearing Loss

Physicians should advise patients to stop taking PDE5 inhibitors, including VIAGRA, and seek prompt medical attention in the event of sudden decrease or loss of hearing. These events, which may be accompanied by tinnitus and dizziness, have been reported in temporal association to the intake of PDE5 inhibitors, including VIAGRA. It is not possible to determine whether these events are related directly to the use of PDE5 inhibitors or to other factors [see *Adverse Reactions (6.1, 6.2)*].

5.5 Hypotension when Co-administered with Alpha-blockers or Anti-hypertensives

Alpha-blockers

Caution is advised when PDE5 inhibitors are co-administered with alpha-blockers. PDE5 inhibitors, including VIAGRA, and alpha-adrenergic blocking agents are both vasodilators with blood pressure lowering effects. When vasodilators are used in combination, an additive effect on blood pressure may occur. In some patients, concomitant use of these two drug classes can lower blood pressure significantly [see *Drug Interactions (7.2) and Clinical Pharmacology (12.2)*] leading to symptomatic hypotension (e.g., dizziness, lightheadedness, fainting).

Consideration should be given to the following:

• Patients who demonstrate hemodynamic instability on alpha-blocker therapy alone are at increased risk of symptomatic hypotension with concomitant use of PDE5 inhibitors. Patients should be stable on alpha-blocker therapy prior to initiating a PDE5 inhibitor.
• In those patients who are stable on alpha-blocker therapy, PDE5 inhibitors should be initiated at the lowest dose [see *Dosage and Administration (2.3)*].
• In those patients already taking an optimized dose of a PDE5 inhibitor, alpha-blocker therapy should be initiated at the lowest dose. Stepwise increase in alpha-blocker dose may be associated with further lowering of blood pressure when taking a PDE5 inhibitor.
• Safety of combined use of PDE5 inhibitors and alpha-blockers may be affected by other variables, including intravascular volume depletion and other anti-hypertensive drugs.

Anti-hypertensives

VIAGRA has systemic vasodilatory properties and may further lower blood pressure in patients taking anti-hypertensive medications.

In a separate drug interaction study, when amlodipine, 5 mg or 10 mg, and VIAGRA, 100 mg were orally administered concomitantly to hypertensive patients mean additional blood pressure reduction of 8 mmHg systolic and 7 mmHg diastolic were noted [see *Drug Interactions (7.3) and Clinical Pharmacology (12.2)*].

5.6 Adverse Reactions with the Concomitant Use of Ritonavir

The concomitant administration of the protease inhibitor ritonavir substantially increases serum concentrations of sildenafil (11-fold increase in AUC). If VIAGRA is prescribed to patients taking ritonavir, caution should be used. Data from subjects exposed to high systemic levels of sildenafil are limited. Decreased blood pressure, syncope, and prolonged erection were reported in some healthy volunteers exposed to high doses of sildenafil (200–800 mg). To decrease the chance of adverse reactions in patients taking ritonavir, a decrease in sildenafil dosage is recommended [see *Dosage and Administration (2.4), Drug Interactions (7.4), and Clinical Pharmacology (12.3)*].

5.7 Combination with other PDE5 Inhibitors or Other Erectile Dysfunction Therapies

The safety and efficacy of combinations of VIAGRA with other PDE5 Inhibitors, including REVATIO or other pulmonary arterial hypertension (PAH) treatments containing sildenafil, or other treatments for erectile dysfunction have not been studied. Such combinations may further lower blood pressure. Therefore, the use of such combinations is not recommended.

5.8 Effects on Bleeding

There have been postmarketing reports of bleeding events in patients who have taken VIAGRA. A causal relationship between VIAGRA and these events has not been established. In humans, VIAGRA has no effect on bleeding time when taken alone or with aspirin. However, *in vitro* studies with human platelets indicate that sildenafil potentiates the antiaggregatory effect of sodium nitroprusside (a nitric oxide donor). In addition, the combination of heparin and VIAGRA had an additive effect on bleeding time in the anesthetized rabbit, but this interaction has not been studied in humans.

The safety of VIAGRA is unknown in patients with bleeding disorders and patients with active peptic ulceration.

5.9 Counseling Patients About Sexually Transmitted Diseases

The use of VIAGRA offers no protection against sexually transmitted diseases. Counseling of patients about the protective measures necessary to guard against sexually transmitted diseases, including the Human Immunodeficiency Virus (HIV), may be considered.

Continued on next page

6 ADVERSE REACTIONS

The following are discussed in more detail in other sections of the labeling:

- Cardiovascular [*see Warnings and Precautions (5.1)*]
- Prolonged Erection and Priapism [*see Warnings and Precautions (5.2)*]
- Effects on the Eye [*see Warnings and Precautions (5.3)*]
- Hearing Loss [*see Warnings and Precautions (5.4)*]
- Hypotension when Co-administered with Alpha-blockers or Anti-hypertensives [*see Warnings and Precautions (5.5)*]
- Adverse Reactions with the Concomitant Use of Ritonavir [*see Warnings and Precautions (5.6)*]
- Combination with other PDE5 Inhibitors or Other Erectile Dysfunction Therapies [*see Warnings and Precautions (5.7)*]
- Effects on Bleeding [*see Warnings and Precautions (5.8)*]
- Counseling Patients About Sexually Transmitted Diseases [*see Warnings and Precautions (5.9)*]

The most common adverse reactions reported in clinical trials (≥ 2%) are headache, flushing, dyspepsia, abnormal vision, nasal congestion, back pain, myalgia, nausea, dizziness, and rash.

6.1 Clinical Trials Experience

Because clinical trials are conducted under widely varying conditions, adverse reaction rates observed in the clinical trials of a drug cannot be directly compared to rates in the clinical trials of another drug and may not reflect the rates observed in clinical practice.

VIAGRA was administered to over 3700 patients (aged 19–87 years) during pre-marketing clinical trials worldwide. Over 550 patients were treated for longer than one year.

In placebo-controlled clinical studies, the discontinuation rate due to adverse reactions for VIAGRA (2.5%) was not significantly different from placebo (2.3%).

In fixed-dose studies, the incidence of some adverse reactions increased with dose. The type of adverse reactions in flexible-dose studies, which reflect the recommended dosage regimen, was similar to that for fixed-dose studies. At doses above the recommended dose range, adverse reactions were similar to those detailed in Table 1 below but generally were reported more frequently.

[See table 1 below]

When VIAGRA was taken as recommended (on an as-needed basis) in flexible-dose, placebo-controlled clinical trials of two to twenty-six weeks duration, patients took VIAGRA at least once weekly, and the following adverse reactions were reported:

Table 2. Adverse Reactions Reported by ≥2% of Patients Treated with VIAGRA and More Frequent than Placebo in Flexible-Dose Phase II/III Studies

Adverse Reaction	VIAGRA	PLACEBO
	N=734	N=725
Headache	16%	4%
Flushing	10%	1%
Dyspepsia	7%	2%
Nasal Congestion	4%	2%
Abnormal Vision*	3%	0%
Back pain	2%	2%
Dizziness	2%	1%
Rash	2%	1%

* Abnormal Vision: Mild and transient, predominantly color tinge to vision, but also increased sensitivity to light or blurred vision. In these studies, only one patient discontinued due to abnormal vision.

The following events occurred in <2% of patients in controlled clinical trials; a causal relationship to VIAGRA is uncertain. Reported events include those with a plausible relation to drug use; omitted are minor events and reports too imprecise to be meaningful:

Body as a Whole: face edema, photosensitivity reaction, shock, asthenia, pain, chills, accidental fall, abdominal pain, allergic reaction, chest pain, accidental injury.

Cardiovascular: angina pectoris, AV block, migraine, syncope, tachycardia, palpitation, hypotension, postural hypotension, myocardial ischemia, cerebral thrombosis, cardiac arrest, heart failure, abnormal electrocardiogram, cardiomyopathy.

Digestive: vomiting, glossitis, colitis, dysphagia, gastritis, gastroenteritis, esophagitis, stomatitis, dry mouth, liver function tests abnormal, rectal hemorrhage, gingivitis.

Hemic and Lymphatic: anemia and leukopenia.

Metabolic and Nutritional: thirst, edema, gout, unstable diabetes, hyperglycemia, peripheral edema, hyperuricemia, hypoglycemic reaction, hypernatremia.

Musculoskeletal: arthritis, arthrosis, myalgia, tendon rupture, tenosynovitis, bone pain, myasthenia, synovitis.

Nervous: ataxia, hypertonia, neuralgia, neuropathy, paresthesia, tremor, vertigo, depression, insomnia, somnolence, abnormal dreams, reflexes decreased, hypesthesia.

Respiratory: asthma, dyspnea, laryngitis, pharyngitis, sinusitis, bronchitis, sputum increased, cough increased.

Skin and Appendages: urticaria, herpes simplex, pruritus, sweating, skin ulcer, contact dermatitis, exfoliative dermatitis.

Special Senses: sudden decrease or loss of hearing, mydriasis, conjunctivitis, photophobia, tinnitus, eye pain, ear pain, eye hemorrhage, cataract, dry eyes.

Urogenital: cystitis, nocturia, urinary frequency, breast enlargement, urinary incontinence, abnormal ejaculation, genital edema and anorgasmia.

Analysis of the safety database from controlled clinical trials showed no apparent difference in adverse reactions in patients taking VIAGRA with and without anti-hypertensive medication. This analysis was performed retrospectively, and was not powered to detect any pre-specified difference in adverse reactions.

6.2 Postmarketing Experience

The following adverse reactions have been identified during post approval use of VIAGRA. Because these reactions are reported voluntarily from a population of uncertain size, it is not always possible to reliably estimate their frequency or establish a causal relationship to drug exposure. These events have been chosen for inclusion either due to their seriousness, reporting frequency, lack of clear alternative causation, or a combination of these factors.

Cardiovascular and cerebrovascular

Serious cardiovascular, cerebrovascular, and vascular events, including myocardial infarction, sudden cardiac death, ventricular arrhythmia, cerebrovascular hemorrhage, transient ischemic attack, hypertension, subarachnoid and intracerebral hemorrhages, and pulmonary hemorrhage have been reported post-marketing in temporal association with the use of VIAGRA. Most, but not all, of these patients had preexisting cardiovascular risk factors. Many of these events were reported to occur during or shortly after sexual activity, and a few were reported to occur shortly after the use of VIAGRA without sexual activity. Others were reported to have occurred hours to days after the use of VIAGRA and sexual activity. It is not possible to determine whether these events are related directly to VIAGRA, to sexual activity, to the patient's underlying cardiovascular disease, to a combination of these factors, or to other factors [*see Warnings and Precautions (5.1) and Patient Counseling Information (17)*].

Hemic and Lymphatic: vaso-occlusive crisis: In a small, prematurely terminated study of REVATIO (sildenafil) in patients with pulmonary arterial hypertension (PAH) secondary to sickle cell disease, vaso-occlusive crises requiring hospitalization were more commonly reported in patients who received sildenafil than in those randomized to placebo. The clinical relevance of this finding to men treated with VIAGRA for ED is not known.

Nervous: seizure, seizure recurrence, anxiety, and transient global amnesia.

Respiratory: epistaxis

Special senses:

Hearing: Cases of sudden decrease or loss of hearing have been reported postmarketing in temporal association with the use of PDE5 inhibitors, including VIAGRA. In some of the cases, medical conditions and other factors were reported that may have also played a role in the otologic adverse events. In many cases, medical follow-up information was limited. It is not possible to determine whether these reported events are related directly to the use of VIAGRA, to the patient's underlying risk factors for hearing loss, a combination of these factors, or to other factors [*see Warnings and Precautions (5.4) and Patient Counseling Information (17)*].

Ocular: diplopia, temporary vision loss/decreased vision, ocular redness or bloodshot appearance, ocular burning, ocular swelling/pressure, increased intraocular pressure, retinal edema, retinal vascular disease or bleeding, and vitreous traction/detachment.

Non-arteritic anterior ischemic optic neuropathy (NAION), a cause of decreased vision including permanent loss of vision, has been reported rarely post-marketing in temporal association with the use of phosphodiesterase type 5 (PDE5) inhibitors, including VIAGRA. Most, but not all, of these patients had underlying anatomic or vascular risk factors for developing NAION, including but not necessarily limited to: low cup to disc ratio ("crowded disc"), age over 50, diabetes, hypertension, coronary artery disease, hyperlipidemia and smoking. It is not possible to determine whether these events are related directly to the use of PDE5 inhibitors, to the patient's underlying vascular risk factors or anatomical defects, to a combination of these factors, or to other factors [*see Warnings and Precautions (5.3) and Patient Counseling Information (17)*].

Urogenital: prolonged erection, priapism [*see Warnings and Precautions (5.2) and Patient Counseling Information (17)*], and hematuria.

7 DRUG INTERACTIONS

7.1 Nitrates

Administration of VIAGRA with nitric oxide donors such as organic nitrates or organic nitrites in any form is contraindicated. Consistent with its known effects on the nitric oxide/cGMP pathway, VIAGRA was shown to potentiate the hypotensive effects of nitrates [*see Dosage and Administration (2.3), Contraindications (4.1), Clinical Pharmacology (12.2)*].

Table 1: Adverse Reactions Reported by ≥2% of Patients Treated with VIAGRA and More Frequent than Placebo in Fixed-Dose Phase II/III Studies

Adverse Reaction	25 mg (n=312)	50 mg (n=511)	100 mg (n=506)	Placebo (n=607)
Headache	16%	21%	28%	7%
Flushing	10%	19%	18%	2%
Dyspepsia	3%	9%	17%	2%
Abnormal vision*	1%	2%	11%	1%
Nasal congestion	4%	4%	9%	2%
Back pain	3%	4%	4%	2%
Myalgia	2%	2%	4%	1%
Nausea	2%	3%	3%	1%
Dizziness	3%	4%	3%	2%
Rash	1%	2%	3%	1%

* Abnormal Vision: Mild to moderate in severity and transient, predominantly color tinge to vision, but also increased sensitivity to light, or blurred vision.

7.2 Alpha-blockers

Use caution when co-administering alpha-blockers with VIAGRA because of potential additive blood pressure-lowering effects. When VIAGRA is co-administered with an alpha-blocker, patients should be stable on alpha-blocker therapy prior to initiating VIAGRA treatment and VIAGRA should be initiated at the lowest dose [*see Dosage and Administration (2.3),Warnings and Precautions (5.5), Clinical Pharmacology (12.2)*].

7.3 Amlodipine

When VIAGRA 100 mg was co-administered with amlodipine (5 mg or 10 mg) to hypertensive patients, the mean additional reduction on supine blood pressure was 8 mmHg systolic and 7 mmHg diastolic [*see Warnings and Precautions (5.5), Clinical Pharmacology (12.2)*].

7.4 Ritonavir and other CYP3A4 inhibitors

Co-administration of ritonavir, a strong CYP3A4 inhibitor, greatly increased the systemic exposure of sildenafil (11-fold increase in AUC). It is therefore recommended not to exceed a maximum single dose of 25 mg of VIAGRA in a 48 hour period [*see Dosage and Administration (2.4), Warnings and Precautions (5.6), Clinical Pharmacology (12.3)*].

Co-administration of erythromycin, a moderate CYP3A4 inhibitor, resulted in a 160% and 182% increases in sildenafil C_{max} and AUC, respectively. Co-administration of saquinavir, a strong CYP3A4 inhibitor, resulted in 140% and 210% increases in sildenafil C_{max} and AUC, respectively. Stronger CYP3A4 inhibitors such as ketoconazole or itraconazole could be expected to have greater effects than seen with saquinavir. A starting dose of 25 mg of VIAGRA should be considered in patients taking erythromycin or strong CYP3A4 inhibitors (such as saquinavir, ketoconazole, itraconazole) [*see Dosage and Administration (2.4), Clinical Pharmacology (12.3)*].

7.5 Alcohol

In a drug-drug interaction study sildenafil 50 mg given with alcohol 0.5 g/kg in which mean maximum blood alcohol levels of 0.08% was achieved, sildenafil did not potentiate the hypotensive effect of alcohol in healthy volunteers [*see Clinical Pharmacology (12.2)*].

8 USE IN SPECIFIC POPULATIONS

8.1 Pregnancy

Pregnancy Category B.
VIAGRA is not indicated for use in women. There are no adequate and well-controlled studies of sildenafil in pregnant women.

Risk Summary
Based on animal data, VIAGRA is not predicted to increase the risk of adverse developmental outcomes in humans.

Animal Data
No evidence of teratogenicity, embryotoxicity or fetotoxicity was observed in rats and rabbits which received up to 200 mg/kg/day during organogenesis. These doses represent, respectively, about 20 and 40 times the Maximum Recommended Human Dose (MRHD) on a mg/m² basis in a 50 kg subject. In the rat pre- and postnatal development study, the no observed adverse effect dose was 30 mg/kg/day given for 36 days. In the nonpregnant rat the AUC at this dose was about 20 times human AUC.

8.4 Pediatric Use

VIAGRA is not indicated for use in pediatric patients. Safety and effectiveness have not been established in pediatric patients.

8.5 Geriatric Use

Healthy elderly volunteers (65 years or over) had a reduced clearance of sildenafil resulting in approximately 84% and 107% higher plasma AUC values of sildenafil and its active N-desmethyl metabolite, respectively, compared to those seen in healthy young volunteers (18–45 years) [*see Clinical Pharmacology (12.3)*]. Due to age-differences in plasma protein binding, the corresponding increase in the AUC of free (unbound) sildenafil and its active N-desmethyl metabolite were 45% and 57%, respectively [*see Clinical Pharmacology (12.3)*].

Of the total number of subjects in clinical studies of Viagra, 18% were 65 years and older, while 2% were 75 years and older. No overall differences in safety or efficacy were observed between older (≥ 65 years of age) and younger (< 65 years of age) subjects.

However, since higher plasma levels may increase the incidence of adverse reactions, a starting dose of 25 mg should be considered in older subjects due to the higher systemic exposure [*see Dosage and Administration (2.5)*].

8.6 Renal Impairment

No dose adjustment is required for mild (CLcr=50–80 mL/min) and moderate (CLcr=30–49 mL/min) renal impairment. In volunteers with severe renal impairment (Clcr<30 mL/min), sildenafil clearance was reduced, resulting in higher plasma exposure of sildenafil (~2 fold), approximately doubling of C_{max} and AUC. A starting dose of 25 mg should be considered in patients with severe renal impairment [*see Dosage and Administration (2.5) and Clinical Pharmacology (12.3)*].

8.7 Hepatic Impairment

In volunteers with hepatic impairment (Child-Pugh Class A and B), sildenafil clearance was reduced, resulting in higher plasma exposure of sildenafil (47% for C_{max} and 85% for AUC). The pharmacokinetics of sildenafil in patients with severely impaired hepatic function (Child-Pugh Class C) have not been studied. A starting dose of 25 mg should be considered in patients with any degree of hepatic impairment [*see Dosage and Administration (2.5) and Clinical Pharmacology (12.3)*].

10 OVERDOSAGE

In studies with healthy volunteers of single doses up to 800 mg, adverse reactions were similar to those seen at lower doses but incidence rates and severities were increased.

In cases of overdose, standard supportive measures should be adopted as required. Renal dialysis is not expected to accelerate clearance as sildenafil is highly bound to plasma proteins and it is not eliminated in the urine.

11 DESCRIPTION

VIAGRA (sildenafil citrate), an oral therapy for erectile dysfunction, is the citrate salt of sildenafil, a selective inhibitor of cyclic guanosine monophosphate (cGMP)-specific phosphodiesterase type 5 (PDE5).

Sildenafil citrate is designated chemically as 1-[[3-(6,7-dihydro-1-methyl-7-oxo-3-propyl-1*H*-pyrazolo[4,3-*d*]pyrimidin-5-yl)-4-ethoxyphenyl]sulfonyl]-4-methylpiperazine citrate and has the following structural formula:

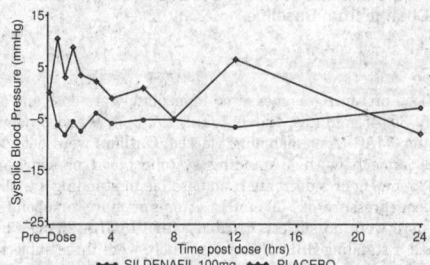

Sildenafil citrate is a white to off-white crystalline powder with a solubility of 3.5 mg/mL in water and a molecular weight of 666.7.

VIAGRA is formulated as blue, film-coated rounded-diamond-shaped tablets equivalent to 25 mg, 50 mg and 100 mg of sildenafil for oral administration. In addition to the active ingredient, sildenafil citrate, each tablet contains the following inactive ingredients: microcrystalline cellulose, anhydrous dibasic calcium phosphate, croscarmellose sodium, magnesium stearate, hypromellose, titanium dioxide, lactose, triacetin, and FD & C Blue #2 aluminum lake.

12 CLINICAL PHARMACOLOGY

12.1 Mechanism of Action

The physiologic mechanism of erection of the penis involves release of nitric oxide (NO) in the corpus cavernosum during sexual stimulation. NO then activates the enzyme guanylate cyclase, which results in increased levels of cyclic guanosine monophosphate (cGMP), producing smooth muscle relaxation in the corpus cavernosum and allowing inflow of blood.

Sildenafil enhances the effect of NO by inhibiting phosphodiesterase type 5 (PDE5), which is responsible for degradation of cGMP in the corpus cavernosum. Sildenafil has no direct relaxant effect on isolated human corpus cavernosum. When sexual stimulation causes local release of NO, inhibition of PDE5 by sildenafil causes increased levels of cGMP in the corpus cavernosum, resulting in smooth muscle relaxation and inflow of blood to the corpus cavernosum. Sildenafil at recommended doses has no effect in the absence of sexual stimulation.

Binding Characteristics

Studies *in vitro* have shown that sildenafil is selective for PDE5. Its effect is more potent on PDE5 than on other known phosphodiesterases (10-fold for PDE6, >80-fold for PDE1, >700-fold for PDE2, PDE3, PDE4, PDE7, PDE8, PDE9, PDE10, and PDE11). Sildenafil is approximately 4,000-fold more selective for PDE5 compared to PDE3.

PDE3 is involved in control of cardiac contractility. Sildenafil is only about 10-fold as potent for PDE5 compared to PDE6, an enzyme found in the retina which is involved in the phototransduction pathway of the retina. This lower selectivity is thought to be the basis for abnormalities related to color vision [*see Clinical Pharmacology (12.2)*].

In addition to human corpus cavernosum smooth muscle, PDE5 is also found in other tissues including platelets, vascular and visceral smooth muscle, and skeletal muscle, brain, heart, liver, kidney, lung, pancreas, prostate, bladder, testis, and seminal vesicle. The inhibition of PDE5 in some of these tissues by sildenafil may be the basis for the enhanced platelet antiaggregatory activity of NO observed *in vitro*, an inhibition of platelet thrombus formation *in vivo* and peripheral arterial-venous dilatation *in vivo*.

12.2 Pharmacodynamics

Effects of VIAGRA on Erectile Response: In eight double-blind, placebo-controlled crossover studies of patients with either organic or psychogenic erectile dysfunction, sexual stimulation resulted in improved erections, as assessed by an objective measurement of hardness and duration of erections (RigiScan®), after VIAGRA administration compared with placebo. Most studies assessed the efficacy of VIAGRA approximately 60 minutes post dose. The erectile response, as assessed by RigiScan®, generally increased with increasing sildenafil dose and plasma concentration. The time course of effect was examined in one study, showing an effect for up to 4 hours but the response was diminished compared to 2 hours.

Effects of VIAGRA on Blood Pressure: Single oral doses of sildenafil (100 mg) administered to healthy volunteers produced decreases in sitting blood pressure (mean maximum decrease in systolic/diastolic blood pressure of 8.3/5.3 mmHg). The decrease in sitting blood pressure was most notable approximately 1–2 hours after dosing, and was not different than placebo at 8 hours. Similar effects on blood pressure were noted with 25 mg, 50 mg and 100 mg of VIAGRA, therefore the effects are not related to dose or plasma levels within this dosage range. Larger effects were recorded among patients receiving concomitant nitrates [*see Contraindications (4.1)*].

Figure 1: Mean Change from Baseline in Sitting Systolic Blood Pressure, Healthy Volunteers.

Effects of VIAGRA on Blood Pressure When Nitroglycerin is Subsequently Administered: Based on the pharmacokinetic profile of a single 100 mg oral dose given to healthy normal volunteers, the plasma levels of sildenafil at 24 hours post dose are approximately 2 ng/mL (compared to peak plasma levels of approximately 440 ng/mL). In the following patients: age >65 years, hepatic impairment (e.g., cirrhosis), severe renal impairment (e.g., creatinine clearance <30 mL/min), and concomitant use of erythromycin or strong CYP3A4 inhibitors, plasma levels of sildenafil at 24 hours post dose have been found to be 3 to 8 times higher than those seen in healthy volunteers. Although plasma levels of sildenafil at 24 hours post dose are much lower than at peak concentration, it is unknown whether nitrates can be safely co-administered at this time point [*see Contraindications (4.1)*].

Effects of VIAGRA on Blood Pressure When Co-administered with Alpha-Blockers: Three double-blind, placebo-controlled, randomized, two-way crossover studies were conducted to assess the interaction of VIAGRA with doxazosin, an alpha-adrenergic blocking agent.

Study 1: VIAGRA with Doxazosin

In the first study, a single oral dose of VIAGRA 100 mg or matching placebo was administered in a 2-period crossover design to 4 generally healthy males with benign prostatic hyperplasia (BPH). Following at least 14 consecutive daily

Continued on next page

doses of doxazosin, VIAGRA 100 mg or matching placebo was administered simultaneously with doxazosin. Following a review of the data from these first 4 subjects (details provided below), the VIAGRA dose was reduced to 25 mg. Thereafter, 17 subjects were treated with VIAGRA 25 mg or matching placebo in combination with doxazosin 4 mg (15 subjects) or doxazosin 8 mg (2 subjects). The mean subject age was 66.5 years.

For the 17 subjects who received VIAGRA 25 mg and matching placebo, the placebo-subtracted mean maximum decreases from baseline (95% CI) in systolic blood pressure were as follows:

Placebo-subtracted mean maximum decrease in systolic blood pressure (mm Hg)	VIAGRA 25 mg
Supine	7.4 (-0.9, 15.7)
Standing	6.0 (-0.8, 12.8)

The mean profiles of the change from baseline in standing systolic blood pressure in subjects treated with doxazosin in combination with 25 mg VIAGRA or matching placebo are shown in Figure 2.

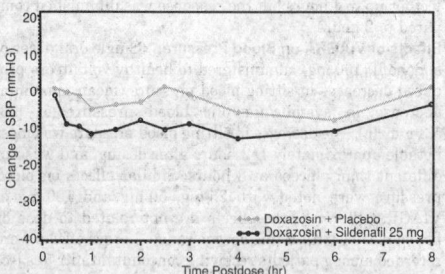

Figure 2: Mean Standing Systolic Blood Pressure Change from Baseline

Blood pressure was measured immediately pre-dose and at 15, 30, 45 minutes, and 1, 1.5, 2, 2.5, 3, 4, 6 and 8 hours after VIAGRA or matching placebo. Outliers were defined as subjects with a standing systolic blood pressure of <85 mmHg or a decrease from baseline in standing systolic blood pressure of >30 mmHg at one or more timepoints. There were no subjects treated with VIAGRA 25 mg who had a standing SBP < 85mmHg. There were three subjects with a decrease from baseline in standing systolic BP >30mmHg following VIAGRA 25 mg, one subject with a decrease from baseline in standing systolic BP > 30 mmHg following placebo and two subjects with a decrease from baseline in standing systolic BP > 30 mmHg following VIAGRA and placebo. No severe adverse events potentially related to blood pressure effects were reported in this group. Of the four subjects who received VIAGRA 100 mg in the first part of this study, a severe adverse event related to blood pressure effect was reported in one patient (postural hypotension that began 35 minutes after dosing with VIAGRA with symptoms lasting for 8 hours), and mild adverse events potentially related to blood pressure effects were reported in two others (dizziness, headache and fatigue at 1 hour after dosing; and dizziness, lightheadedness and nausea at 4 hours after dosing). There were no reports of syncope among these patients. For these four subjects, the placebo-subtracted mean maximum decreases from baseline in supine and standing systolic blood pressures were 14.8 mmHg and 21.5 mmHg, respectively. Two of these subjects had a standing SBP < 85mmHg. Both of these subjects were protocol violators, one due to a low baseline standing SBP, and the other due to baseline orthostatic hypotension.

Study 2: VIAGRA with Doxazosin
In the second study, a single oral dose of VIAGRA 50 mg or matching placebo was administered in a 2-period crossover design to 20 generally healthy males with BPH. Following at least 14 consecutive days of doxazosin, VIAGRA 50 mg or matching placebo was administered simultaneously with doxazosin 4 mg (17 subjects) or doxazosin 8 mg (3 subjects). The mean subject age in this study was 63.9 years.

Twenty subjects received VIAGRA 50 mg, but only 19 subjects received matching placebo. One patient discontinued the study prematurely due to an adverse event of hypotension following dosing with VIAGRA 50 mg. This patient had been taking minoxidil, a potent vasodilator, during the study.

For the 19 subjects who received both VIAGRA and matching placebo, the placebo-subtracted mean maximum decreases from baseline (95% CI) in systolic blood pressure were as follows:

Placebo-subtracted mean maximum decrease in systolic blood pressure (mm Hg)	VIAGRA 50 mg (95% CI)
Supine	9.08 (5.48, 12.68)
Standing	11.62 (7.34, 15.90)

The mean profiles of the change from baseline in standing systolic blood pressure in subjects treated with doxazosin in combination with 50 mg VIAGRA or matching placebo are shown in Figure 3.

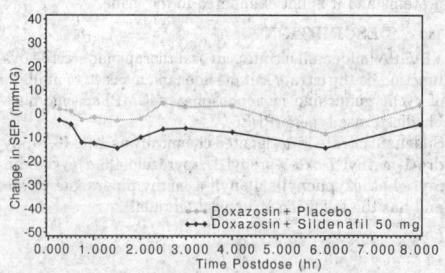

Figure 3: Mean Standing Systolic Blood Pressure Change from Baseline

Blood pressure was measured after administration of VIAGRA at the same times as those specified for the first doxazosin study. There were two subjects who had a standing SBP of < 85 mmHg. In these two subjects, hypotension was reported as a moderately severe adverse event, beginning at approximately 1 hour after administration of VIAGRA 50 mg and resolving after approximately 7.5 hours. There was one subject with a decrease from baseline in standing systolic BP >30mmHg following VIAGRA 50 mg and one subject with a decrease from baseline in standing systolic BP > 30 mmHg following both VIAGRA 50 mg and placebo. There were no severe adverse events potentially related to blood pressure and no episodes of syncope reported in this study.

Study 3: VIAGRA with Doxazosin
In the third study, a single oral dose of VIAGRA 100 mg or matching placebo was administered in a 3-period crossover design to 20 generally healthy males with BPH. In dose period 1, subjects were administered open-label doxazosin and a single dose of VIAGRA 50 mg simultaneously, after at least 14 consecutive days of doxazosin. If a subject did not successfully complete this first dosing period, he was discontinued from the study. Subjects who had successfully completed the previous doxazosin interaction study (using VIAGRA 50 mg), including no significant hemodynamic adverse events, were allowed to skip dose period 1. Treatment with doxazosin continued for at least 7 days after dose period 1. Thereafter, VIAGRA 100 mg or matching placebo was administered simultaneously with doxazosin 4 mg (14 subjects) or doxazosin 8 mg (6 subjects) in standard crossover fashion. The mean subject age in this study was 66.4 years.

Twenty-five subjects were screened. Two were discontinued after study period 1: one failed to meet pre-dose screening qualifications and the other experienced symptomatic hypotension as a moderately severe adverse event 30 minutes after dosing with open-label VIAGRA 50 mg. Of the twenty subjects who were ultimately assigned to treatment, a total of 13 subjects successfully completed dose period 1, and seven had successfully completed the previous doxazosin study (using VIAGRA 50 mg).

For the 20 subjects who received VIAGRA 100 mg and matching placebo, the placebo-subtracted mean maximum decreases from baseline (95% CI) in systolic blood pressure were as follows:

Placebo-subtracted mean maximum decrease in systolic blood pressure (mm Hg)	VIAGRA 100 mg
Supine	7.9 (4.6, 11.1)
Standing	4.3 (-1.8,10.3)

The mean profiles of the change from baseline in standing systolic blood pressure in subjects treated with doxazosin in combination with 100 mg VIAGRA or matching placebo are shown in Figure 4.

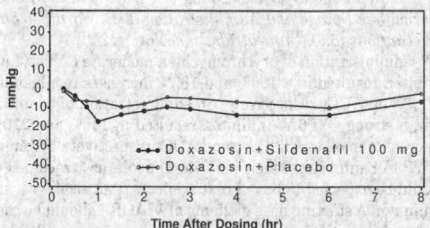

Figure 4: Mean Standing Systolic Blood Pressure Change from Baseline

Blood pressure was measured after administration of VIAGRA at the same times as those specified for the previous doxazosin studies. There were three subjects who had a standing SBP of < 85 mmHg. All three were taking VIAGRA 100 mg, and all three reported mild adverse events at the time of reductions in standing SBP, including vasodilation and lightheadedness. There were four subjects with a decrease from baseline in standing systolic BP > 30 mmHg following VIAGRA 100 mg, one subject with a decrease from baseline in standing systolic BP > 30 mmHg following placebo and one subject with a decrease from baseline in standing systolic BP > 30 mmHg following both VIAGRA and placebo. While there were no severe adverse events potentially related to blood pressure reported in this study, one subject reported moderate vasodilatation after both VIAGRA 50 mg and 100 mg. There were no episodes of syncope reported in this study.

Effect of VIAGRA on Blood Pressure When Co-administered with Anti-hypertensives: When VIAGRA 100 mg oral was co-administered with amlodipine, 5 mg or 10 mg oral, to hypertensive patients, the mean additional reduction on supine blood pressure was 8 mmHg systolic and 7 mmHg diastolic.

Effect of VIAGRA on Blood Pressure When Co-administered with Alcohol: VIAGRA (50 mg) did not potentiate the hypotensive effect of alcohol (0.5 g/kg) in healthy volunteers with mean maximum blood alcohol levels of 0.08%. The maximum observed decrease in systolic blood pressure was -18.5 mmHg when sildenafil was co-administered with alcohol versus -17.4 mmHg when alcohol was administered alone. The maximum observed decrease in diastolic blood pressure was -17.2 mmHg when sildenafil was co-administered with alcohol versus -11.1 mmHg when alcohol was administered alone. There were no reports of postural dizziness or orthostatic hypotension. The maximum recommended dose of 100 mg sildenafil was not evaluated in this study [see *Drug Interactions (7.5)*].

Effects of VIAGRA on Cardiac Parameters: Single oral doses of sildenafil up to 100 mg produced no clinically relevant changes in the ECGs of normal male volunteers.

Studies have produced relevant data on the effects of VIAGRA on cardiac output. In one small, open-label, uncontrolled, pilot study, eight patients with stable ischemic heart disease underwent Swan-Ganz catheterization. A total dose of 40 mg sildenafil was administered by four intravenous infusions.

The results from this pilot study are shown in Table 3; the mean resting systolic and diastolic blood pressures decreased by 7% and 10% compared to baseline in these patients. Mean resting values for right atrial pressure, pulmonary artery pressure, pulmonary artery occluded pressure and cardiac output decreased by 28%, 28%, 20% and 7% respectively. Even though this total dosage produced plasma sildenafil concentrations which were approximately 2 to 5 times higher than the mean maximum plasma concentrations following a single oral dose of 100 mg in healthy male volunteers, the hemodynamic response to exercise was preserved in these patients.

[See table 3 above]

In a double-blind study, 144 patients with erectile dysfunction and chronic stable angina limited by exercise, not receiving chronic oral nitrates, were randomized to a single dose of placebo or VIAGRA 100 mg 1 hour prior to exercise testing. The primary endpoint was time to limiting angina in the evaluable cohort. The mean times (adjusted for baseline) to onset of limiting angina were 423.6 and 403.7 seconds for sildenafil (N=70) and placebo, respectively. These results demonstrated that the effect of VIAGRA on the primary endpoint was statistically non-inferior to placebo.

Effects of VIAGRA on Vision: At single oral doses of 100 mg and 200 mg, transient dose-related impairment of color discrimination was detected using the Farnsworth-Munsell 100-hue test, with peak effects near the time of peak plasma levels. This finding is consistent with the inhibition of PDE6, which is involved in phototransduction in the retina. Subjects in the study reported this finding as difficulties in discriminating blue/green. An evaluation of visual function at doses up to twice the maximum recommended dose revealed no effects of VIAGRA on visual acuity, intraocular pressure, or pupillometry.

Effects of VIAGRA on Sperm: There was no effect on sperm motility or morphology after single 100 mg oral doses of VIAGRA in healthy volunteers.

12.3   Pharmacokinetics

VIAGRA is rapidly absorbed after oral administration, with a mean absolute bioavailability of 41% (range 25–63%). The pharmacokinetics of sildenafil are dose-proportional over the recommended dose range. It is eliminated predominantly by hepatic metabolism (mainly CYP3A4) and is converted to an active metabolite with properties similar to the parent, sildenafil. Both sildenafil and the metabolite have terminal half lives of about 4 hours.

Mean sildenafil plasma concentrations measured after the administration of a single oral dose of 100 mg to healthy male volunteers is depicted below:

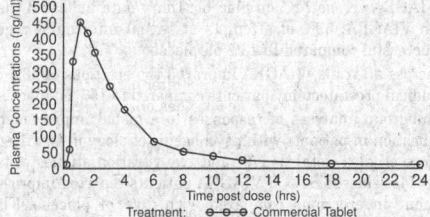

Treatment: ⊖–⊖–⊖ Commercial Tablet

Figure 5: Mean Sildenafil Plasma Concentrations in Healthy Male Volunteers.

Absorption and Distribution: VIAGRA is rapidly absorbed. Maximum observed plasma concentrations are reached within 30 to 120 minutes (median 60 minutes) of oral dosing in the fasted state. When VIAGRA is taken with a high fat meal, the rate of absorption is reduced, with a mean delay in T_{max} of 60 minutes and a mean reduction in C_{max} of 29%. The mean steady state volume of distribution (Vss) for sildenafil is 105 L, indicating distribution into the tissues. Sildenafil and its major circulating N-desmethyl metabolite are both approximately 96% bound to plasma proteins. Protein binding is independent of total drug concentrations.

Based upon measurements of sildenafil in semen of healthy volunteers 90 minutes after dosing, less than 0.001% of the administered dose may appear in the semen of patients.

Metabolism and Excretion: Sildenafil is cleared predominantly by the CYP3A4 (major route) and CYP2C9 (minor route) hepatic microsomal isoenzymes. The major circulating metabolite results from N-desmethylation of sildenafil, and is itself further metabolized. This metabolite has a PDE selectivity profile similar to sildenafil and an *in vitro* potency for PDE5 approximately 50% of the parent drug. Plasma concentrations of this metabolite are approximately 40% of those seen for sildenafil, so that the metabolite accounts for about 20% of sildenafil's pharmacologic effects.

After either oral or intravenous administration, sildenafil is excreted as metabolites predominantly in the feces (approximately 80% of administered oral dose) and to a lesser extent in the urine (approximately 13% of the administered oral dose). Similar values for pharmacokinetic parameters were seen in normal volunteers and in the patient population, using a population pharmacokinetic approach.

Pharmacokinetics in Special Populations

Geriatrics: Healthy elderly volunteers (65 years or over) had a reduced clearance of sildenafil, resulting in approximately 84% and 107% higher plasma AUC values of sildenafil and its active N-desmethyl metabolite, respectively, compared to those seen in healthy younger volunteers (18–45 years). Due to age-differences in plasma protein binding, the corresponding increase in the AUC of free (unbound) sildenafil and its active N-desmethyl metabolite were 45% and 57%, respectively [*see Dosage and Administration (2.5), and Use in Specific Populations (8.5)*]

Renal Impairment: In volunteers with mild (CLcr=50–80 mL/min) and moderate (CLcr=30–49 mL/min) renal impairment, the pharmacokinetics of a single oral dose of VIAGRA (50 mg) were not altered. In volunteers with severe (CLcr <30 mL/min) renal impairment, sildenafil clearance was reduced, resulting in approximately doubling of AUC and C_{max} compared to age-matched volunteers with no renal impairment [*see Dosage and Administration (2.5), and Use in Specific Populations (8.6)*].

In addition, N-desmethyl metabolite AUC and C_{max} values significantly increased by 200% and 79%, respectively in subjects with severe renal impairment compared to subjects with normal renal function.

Hepatic Impairment: In volunteers with hepatic impairment (Child-Pugh Class A and B), sildenafil clearance was reduced, resulting in increases in AUC (85%) and C_{max} (47%) compared to age-matched volunteers with no hepatic impairment. The pharmacokinetics of sildenafil in patients with severely impaired hepatic function (Child-Pugh Class C) have not been studied [*see Dosage and Administration (2.5), and Use in Specific Populations (8.7)*].

Therefore, age >65, hepatic impairment and severe renal impairment are associated with increased plasma levels of sildenafil. A starting oral dose of 25 mg should be considered in those patients [*see Dosage and Administration (2.5)*].

Drug Interaction Studies

Effects of Other Drugs on VIAGRA

Sildenafil metabolism is principally mediated by CYP3A4 (major route) and CYP2C9 (minor route). Therefore, inhibitors of these isoenzymes may reduce sildenafil clearance and inducers of these isoenzymes may increase sildenafil clearance. The concomitant use of erythromycin or strong CYP3A4 inhibitors (e.g., saquinavir, ketoconazole, itraconazole) as well as the nonspecific CYP inhibitor, cimetidine, is associated with increased plasma levels of sildenafil [*see Dosage and Administration (2.4)*].

In vivo studies:

Cimetidine (800 mg), a nonspecific CYP inhibitor, caused a 56% increase in plasma sildenafil concentrations when co-administered with VIAGRA (50 mg) to healthy volunteers. When a single 100 mg dose of VIAGRA was administered with erythromycin, a moderate CYP3A4 inhibitor, at steady state (500 mg bid for 5 days), there was a 160% increase in sildenafil C_{max} and a 182% increase in sildenafil AUC. In addition, in a study performed in healthy male volunteers, co-administration of the HIV protease inhibitor saquinavir, also a CYP3A4 inhibitor, at steady state (1200 mg tid) with Viagra (100 mg single dose) resulted in a 140% increase in sildenafil C_{max} and a 210% increase in sildenafil AUC. Viagra had no effect on saquinavir pharmacokinetics. A stronger CYP3A4 inhibitor such as ketoconazole or itraconazole could be expected to have greater effect than that seen with saquinavir. Population pharmacokinetic data from patients in clinical trials also indicated a reduction in sildenafil clearance when it was co-administered with CYP3A4 inhibitors (such as ketoconazole, erythromycin, or cimetidine) [*see Dosage and Administration (2.4) and Drug Interactions (7.4)*].

In another study in healthy male volunteers, co-administration with the HIV protease inhibitor ritonavir, which is a highly potent P450 inhibitor, at steady state (500 mg bid) with VIAGRA (100 mg single dose) resulted in a 300% (4-fold) increase in sildenafil C_{max} and a 1000% (11-fold) increase in sildenafil plasma AUC. At 24 hours the plasma levels of sildenafil were still approximately 200 ng/mL, compared to approximately 5 ng/mL when sildenafil was dosed alone. This is consistent with ritonavir's marked effects on a broad range of P450 substrates. VIAGRA had no effect on ritonavir pharmacokinetics [*see Dosage and Administration (2.4) and Drug Interactions (7.4)*].

Although the interaction between other protease inhibitors and sildenafil has not been studied, their concomitant use is expected to increase sildenafil levels.

In a study of healthy male volunteers, co-administration of sildenafil at steady state (80 mg t.i.d.) with endothelin receptor antagonist bosentan (a moderate inducer of CYP3A4, CYP2C9 and possibly of CYP2C19) at steady state (125 mg b.i.d.) resulted in a 63% decrease of sildenafil AUC and a 55% decrease in sildenafil C_{max}. Concomitant administration of strong CYP3A4 inducers, such as rifampin, is expected to cause greater decreases in plasma levels of sildenafil.

Single doses of antacid (magnesium hydroxide/aluminum hydroxide) did not affect the bioavailability of VIAGRA.

In healthy male volunteers, there was no evidence of a clinically significant effect of azithromycin (500 mg daily for 3 days) on the systemic exposure of sildenafil or its major circulating metabolite.

Pharmacokinetic data from patients in clinical trials showed no effect on sildenafil pharmacokinetics of CYP2C9 inhibitors (such as tolbutamide, warfarin), CYP2D6 inhibitors (such as selective serotonin reuptake inhibitors, tricyclic antidepressants), thiazide and related diuretics, ACE inhibitors, and calcium channel blockers. The AUC of the active metabolite, N-desmethyl sildenafil, was increased 62% by loop and potassium-sparing diuretics and 102% by nonspecific beta-blockers. These effects on the metabolite are not expected to be of clinical consequence.

Effects of VIAGRA on Other Drugs

In vitro studies:

Sildenafil is a weak inhibitor of the CYP isoforms 1A2, 2C9, 2C19, 2D6, 2E1 and 3A4 (IC50 >150 µM). Given sildenafil

Continued on next page

Table 3. Hemodynamic Data in Patients with Stable Ischemic Heart Disease after Intravenous Administration of 40 mg of Sildenafil

Means ± SD	At rest				After 4 minutes of exercise			
	N	Baseline (B2)	n	Sildenafil (D1)	n	Baseline	n	Sildenafil
PAOP (mmHg)	8	8.1 ± 5.1	8	6.5 ± 4.3	8	36.0 ± 13.7	8	27.8 ± 15.3
Mean PAP (mmHg)	8	16.7 ± 4	8	12.1 ± 3.9	8	39.4 ± 12.9	8	31.7 ± 13.2
Mean RAP (mmHg)	7	5.7 ± 3.7	8	4.1 ± 3.7	-	-	-	-
Systolic SAP (mmHg)	8	150.4 ± 12.4	8	140.6 ± 16.5	8	199.5 ± 37.4	8	187.8 ± 30.0
Diastolic SAP (mmHg)	8	73.6 ± 7.8	8	65.9 ± 10	8	84.6 ± 9.7	8	79.5 ± 9.4
Cardiac output (L/min)	8	5.6 ± 0.9	8	5.2 ± 1.1	8	11.5 ± 2.4	8	10.2 ± 3.5
Heart rate (bpm)	8	67 ± 11.1	8	66.9 ± 12	8	101.9 ± 11.6	8	99.0 ± 20.4

peak plasma concentrations of approximately 1 μM after recommended doses, it is unlikely that VIAGRA will alter the clearance of substrates of these isoenzymes.

***In vivo* studies:**

No significant interactions were shown with tolbutamide (250 mg) or warfarin (40 mg), both of which are metabolized by CYP2C9.

In a study of healthy male volunteers, sildenafil (100 mg) did not affect the steady state pharmacokinetics of the HIV protease inhibitors, saquinavir and ritonavir, both of which are CYP3A4 substrates.

VIAGRA (50 mg) did not potentiate the increase in bleeding time caused by aspirin (150 mg).

Sildenafil at steady state, at a dose not approved for the treatment of erectile dysfunction (80 mg t.i.d.) resulted in a 50% increase in AUC and a 42% increase in C_{max} of bosentan (125 mg b.i.d.).

13 NONCLINICAL TOXICOLOGY

13.1 Carcinogenesis, Mutagenesis, Impairment of Fertility

Carcinogenesis

Sildenafil was not carcinogenic when administered to rats for 24 months at a dose resulting in total systemic drug exposure (AUCs) for unbound sildenafil and its major metabolite of 29- and 42- times, for male and female rats, respectively, the exposures observed in human males given the Maximum Recommended Human Dose (MRHD) of 100 mg. Sildenafil was not carcinogenic when administered to mice for 18–21 months at dosages up to the Maximum Tolerated Dose (MTD) of 10 mg/kg/day, approximately 0.6 times the MRHD on a mg/m² basis.

Mutagenesis

Sildenafil was negative in *in vitro* bacterial and Chinese hamster ovary cell assays to detect mutagenicity, and *in vitro* human lymphocytes and *in vivo* mouse micronucleus assays to detect clastogenicity.

Impairment of Fertility

There was no impairment of fertility in rats given sildenafil up to 60 mg/kg/day for 36 days to females and 102 days to males, a dose producing an AUC value of more than 25 times the human male AUC.

14 CLINICAL STUDIES

In clinical studies, VIAGRA was assessed for its effect on the ability of men with erectile dysfunction (ED) to engage in sexual activity and in many cases specifically on the ability to achieve and maintain an erection sufficient for satisfactory sexual activity. VIAGRA was evaluated primarily at doses of 25 mg, 50 mg and 100 mg in 21 randomized, double-blind, placebo-controlled trials of up to 6 months in duration, using a variety of study designs (fixed dose, titration, parallel, crossover). VIAGRA was administered to more than 3,000 patients aged 19 to 87 years, with ED of various etiologies (organic, psychogenic, mixed) with a mean duration of 5 years. VIAGRA demonstrated statistically significant improvement compared to placebo in all 21 studies. The studies that established benefit demonstrated improvements in success rates for sexual intercourse compared with placebo.

Efficacy Endpoints in Controlled Clinical Studies

The effectiveness of VIAGRA was evaluated in most studies using several assessment instruments. The primary measure in the principal studies was a sexual function questionnaire (the International Index of Erectile Function - IIEF) administered during a 4-week treatment-free run-in period, at baseline, at follow-up visits, and at the end of double-blind, placebo-controlled, at-home treatment. Two of the questions from the IIEF served as primary study endpoints; categorical responses were elicited to questions about (1) the ability to achieve erections sufficient for sexual intercourse and (2) the maintenance of erections after penetration. The patient addressed both questions at the final visit for the last 4 weeks of the study. The possible categorical responses to these questions were (0) no attempted intercourse, (1) never or almost never, (2) a few times, (3) sometimes, (4) most times, and (5) almost always or always. Also collected as part of the IIEF was information about other aspects of sexual function, including information on erectile function, orgasm, desire, satisfaction with intercourse, and overall sexual satisfaction. Sexual function data were also recorded by patients in a daily diary. In addition, patients were asked a global efficacy question and an optional partner questionnaire was administered.

Efficacy Results from Controlled Clinical Studies

The effect on one of the major end points, maintenance of erections after penetration, is shown in Figure 6, for the pooled results of 5 fixed-dose, dose-response studies of greater than one month duration, showing response according to baseline function. Results with all doses have been pooled, but scores showed greater improvement at the 50 and 100 mg doses than at 25 mg. The pattern of responses was similar for the other principal question, the ability to achieve an erection sufficient for intercourse. The titration studies, in which most patients received 100 mg, showed similar results. Figure 6 shows that regardless of the baseline levels of function, subsequent function in patients treated with VIAGRA was better than that seen in patients treated with placebo. At the same time, on-treatment function was better in treated patients who were less impaired at baseline.

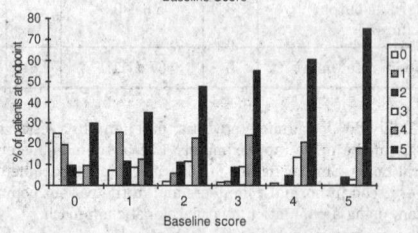

Effect of VIAGRA on Maintenance of Erection by Baseline Score

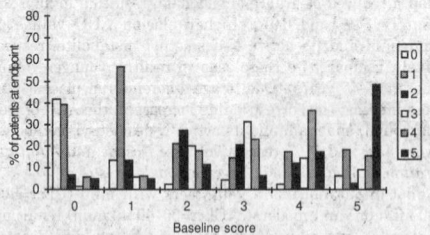

Effect of Placebo on Maintenance of Erection by Baseline Score

Figure 6. Effect of VIAGRA and Placebo on Maintenance of Erection by Baseline Score.

The frequency of patients reporting improvement of erections in response to a global question in four of the randomized, double-blind, parallel, placebo-controlled fixed dose studies (1797 patients) of 12 to 24 weeks duration is shown in Figure 7. These patients had erectile dysfunction at baseline that was characterized by median categorical scores of 2 (a few times) on principal IIEF questions. Erectile dysfunction was attributed to organic (58%; generally not characterized, but including diabetes and excluding spinal cord injury), psychogenic (17%), or mixed (24%) etiologies. Sixty-three percent, 74%, and 82% of the patients on 25 mg, 50 mg and 100 mg of VIAGRA, respectively, reported an improvement in their erections, compared to 24% on placebo. In the titration studies (n=644) (with most patients eventually receiving 100 mg), results were similar.

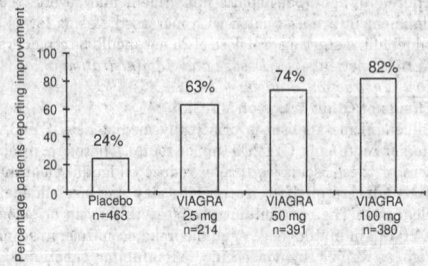

Overall treatment p<0.0001

Figure 7. Percentage of Patients Reporting an Improvement in Erections.

The patients in studies had varying degrees of ED. One-third to one-half of the subjects in these studies reported successful intercourse at least once during a 4-week, treatment-free run-in period.

In many of the studies, of both fixed dose and titration designs, daily diaries were kept by patients. In these studies, involving about 1600 patients, analyses of patient diaries showed no effect of VIAGRA on rates of attempted intercourse (about 2 per week), but there was clear treatment-related improvement in sexual function: per patient weekly success rates averaged 1.3 on 50–100 mg of VIAGRA vs 0.4 on placebo; similarly, group mean success rates (total successes divided by total attempts) were about 66% on VIAGRA vs about 20% on placebo.

During 3 to 6 months of double-blind treatment or longer-term (1 year), open-label studies, few patients withdrew from active treatment for any reason, including lack of effectiveness. At the end of the long-term study, 88% of patients reported that VIAGRA improved their erections.

Men with untreated ED had relatively low baseline scores for all aspects of sexual function measured (again using a 5-point scale) in the IIEF. VIAGRA improved these aspects of sexual function: frequency, firmness and maintenance of erections; frequency of orgasm; frequency and level of desire; frequency, satisfaction and enjoyment of intercourse; and overall relationship satisfaction.

One randomized, double-blind, flexible-dose, placebo-controlled study included only patients with erectile dysfunction attributed to complications of diabetes mellitus (n=268). As in the other titration studies, patients were started on 50 mg and allowed to adjust the dose up to 100 mg or down to 25 mg of VIAGRA; all patients, however, were receiving 50 mg or 100 mg at the end of the study. There were highly statistically significant improvements on the two principal IIEF questions (frequency of successful penetration during sexual activity and maintenance of erections after penetration) on VIAGRA compared to placebo. On a global improvement question, 57% of VIAGRA patients reported improved erections versus 10% on placebo. Diary data indicated that on VIAGRA, 48% of intercourse attempts were successful versus 12% on placebo.

One randomized, double-blind, placebo-controlled, crossover, flexible-dose (up to 100 mg) study of patients with erectile dysfunction resulting from spinal cord injury (n=178) was conducted. The changes from baseline in scoring on the two end point questions (frequency of successful penetration during sexual activity and maintenance of erections after penetration) were highly statistically significantly in favor of VIAGRA. On a global improvement question, 83% of patients reported improved erections on VIAGRA versus 12% on placebo. Diary data indicated that on VIAGRA, 59% of attempts at sexual intercourse were successful compared to 13% on placebo.

Across all trials, VIAGRA improved the erections of 43% of radical prostatectomy patients compared to 15% on placebo. Subgroup analyses of responses to a global improvement question in patients with psychogenic etiology in two fixed-dose studies (total n=179) and two titration studies (total n=149) showed 84% of VIAGRA patients reported improvement in erections compared with 26% of placebo. The changes from baseline in scoring on the two end point questions (frequency of successful penetration during sexual activity and maintenance of erections after penetration) were highly statistically significantly in favor of VIAGRA. Diary data in two of the studies (n=178) showed rates of successful intercourse per attempt of 70% for VIAGRA and 29% for placebo.

Efficacy Results in Subpopulations in Controlled Clinical Studies

A review of population subgroups demonstrated efficacy regardless of baseline severity, etiology, race and age. VIAGRA was effective in a broad range of ED patients, including those with a history of coronary artery disease, hypertension, other cardiac disease, peripheral vascular disease, diabetes mellitus, depression, coronary artery bypass graft (CABG), radical prostatectomy, transurethral resection of the prostate (TURP) and spinal cord injury, and in patients taking antidepressants/antipsychotics and antihypertensives/diuretics.

16 HOW SUPPLIED/STORAGE AND HANDLING

VIAGRA (sildenafil citrate) is supplied as blue, film-coated, rounded-diamond-shaped tablets containing sildenafil citrate equivalent to the nominally indicated amount of sildenafil and debossed on the obverse and reverse sides as follows:

[See table at bottom of next page]

Recommended Storage: Store at 25°C (77°F); excursions permitted to 15–30°C (59–86°F) [see USP Controlled Room Temperature].

17 PATIENT COUNSELING INFORMATION

See FDA-approved patient labeling (Patient Information)

Nitrates

Physicians should discuss with patients the contraindication of VIAGRA with regular and/or intermittent use of nitric oxide donors, such as organic nitrates or organic nitrites in any form [see Contraindications (4.1)].

Guanylate Cyclase (GC) Stimulators

Physicians should discuss with patients the contraindication of VIAGRA with use of guanylate cyclase stimulators such as riociguat [see Contraindications (4.3)].

Concomitant Use with Drugs Which Lower Blood Pressure

Physicians should advise patients of the potential for VIAGRA to augment the blood pressure lowering effect of alpha-blockers and anti-hypertensive medications. Concomitant administration of VIAGRA and an alpha-blocker may lead to symptomatic hypotension in some patients. Therefore, when VIAGRA is co-administered with alpha-blockers, patients should be stable on alpha-blocker therapy prior to initiating VIAGRA treatment and VIAGRA should be initiated at the lowest dose [see Warnings and Precautions (5.5)].

Cardiovascular Considerations

Physicians should discuss with patients the potential cardiac risk of sexual activity in patients with preexisting cardiovascular risk factors. Patients who experience symptoms (e.g., angina pectoris, dizziness, nausea) upon initiation of sexual activity should be advised to refrain from further activity and should discuss the episode with their physician [see Warnings and Precautions (5.1)].

Sudden Loss of Vision

Physicians should advise patients to stop use of all PDE5 inhibitors, including VIAGRA, and seek medical attention in the event of a sudden loss of vision in one or both eyes. Such an event may be a sign of non-arteritic anterior ischemic optic neuropathy (NAION), a cause of decreased vision including possible permanent loss of vision, that has been reported rarely post-marketing in temporal association with the use of all PDE5 inhibitors. It is not possible to determine whether these events are related directly to the use of PDE5 inhibitors or to other factors. Physicians should discuss with patients the increased risk of NAION in individuals who have already experienced NAION in one eye. Physicians should also discuss with patients the increased risk of NAION among the general population in patients with a "crowded" optic disc, although evidence is insufficient to support screening of prospective users of PDE5 inhibitor, including VIAGRA, for this uncommon condition [see Warnings and Precautions (5.3) and Adverse Reactions (6.2)].

Sudden Hearing Loss

Physicians should advise patients to stop taking PDE5 inhibitors, including VIAGRA, and seek prompt medical attention in the event of sudden decrease or loss of hearing. These events, which may be accompanied by tinnitus and dizziness, have been reported in temporal association to the intake of PDE5 inhibitors, including VIAGRA. It is not possible to determine whether these events are related directly to the use of PDE5 inhibitors or to other factors [see Warnings and Precautions (5.4) and Adverse Reactions (6.2)].

Priapism

Physicians should warn patients that prolonged erections greater than 4 hours and priapism (painful erections greater than 6 hours in duration) have been reported infrequently since market approval of VIAGRA. In the event of an erection that persists longer than 4 hours, the patient should seek immediate medical assistance. If priapism is not treated immediately, penile tissue damage and permanent loss of potency may result [see Warnings and Precautions (5.2)].

Avoid Use with other PDE5 Inhibitors

Physicians should inform patients not to take VIAGRA with other PDE5 inhibitors including REVATIO or other pulmonary arterial hypertension (PAH) treatments containing sildenafil. Sildenafil is also marketed as REVATIO for the treatment of PAH. The safety and efficacy of VIAGRA with other PDE5 inhibitors, including REVATIO, have not been studied [see Warnings and Precautions (5.7)].

Sexually Transmitted Disease

The use of VIAGRA offers no protection against sexually transmitted diseases. Counseling of patients about the protective measures necessary to guard against sexually transmitted diseases, including the Human Immunodeficiency Virus (HIV), may be considered [see Warnings and Precautions (5.9)].

Distributed by

Pfizer Labs

Division of Pfizer Inc, NY, NY 10017

LAB-0221-18.0

PATIENT INFORMATION

VIAGRA® (VI-AG-RAH)

(SILDENAFIL CITRATE)

TABLETS

What is the most important information I should know about VIAGRA?

VIAGRA can cause your blood pressure to drop suddenly to an unsafe level if it is taken with certain other medicines. Do not take VIAGRA if you take any other medicines called "nitrates." Nitrates are used to treat chest pain (angina). A sudden drop in blood pressure can cause you to feel dizzy, faint, or have a heart attack or stroke.

Do not take VIAGRA if you take medicines called guanylate cyclase stimulators which include:

• Riociguat (Adempas®) a medicine that treats pulmonary arterial hypertension and chronic-thromboembolic pulmonary hypertension.

Tell all your healthcare providers that you take VIAGRA. If you need emergency medical care for a heart problem, it will be important for your healthcare provider to know when you last took VIAGRA.

Stop sexual activity and get medical help right away if you get symptoms such as chest pain, dizziness, or nausea during sex.

Sexual activity can put an extra strain on your heart, especially if your heart is already weak from a heart attack or heart disease. Ask your doctor if your heart is healthy enough to handle the extra strain of having sex.

VIAGRA does not protect you or your partner from getting sexually transmitted diseases, including HIV—the virus that causes AIDS.

What is VIAGRA?

VIAGRA is a prescription medicine used to treat erectile dysfunction (ED). You will not get an erection just by taking this medicine. VIAGRA helps a man with erectile dysfunction get and keep an erection only when he is sexually excited (stimulated).

VIAGRA is not for use in women or children.

It is not known if VIAGRA is safe and effective in women or children under 18 years of age.

Who should not take VIAGRA?

Do not take VIAGRA if you:

• take medicines called nitrates (such as nitroglycerin)

• use street drugs called "poppers" such as amyl nitrate or amyl nitrite, and butyl nitrate

• take any medicines called guanylate cyclase stimulators such as riociguat (Adempas)

• are allergic to sildenafil, as contained in VIAGRA and REVATIO, or any of the ingredients in VIAGRA. See the end of this leaflet for a complete list of ingredients in VIAGRA.

What should I tell my healthcare provider before taking VIAGRA?

Before you take VIAGRA, tell your healthcare provider if you:

• have or have had heart problems such as a heart attack, irregular heartbeat, angina, chest pain, narrowing of the aortic valve or heart failure

• have had heart surgery within the last 6 months

• have pulmonary hypertension

• have had a stroke

• have low blood pressure, or high blood pressure that is not controlled

• have a deformed penis shape

• have had an erection that lasted for more than 4 hours

• have problems with your blood cells such as sickle cell anemia, multiple myeloma, or leukemia

• have retinitis pigmentosa, a rare genetic (runs in families) eye disease

• have ever had severe vision loss, including an eye problem called non-arteritic anterior ischemic optic neuropathy (NAION)

• have bleeding problems

• have or have had stomach ulcers

• have liver problems

• have kidney problems or are having kidney dialysis

• have any other medical conditions

Tell your healthcare provider about all the medicines you take[1], including prescription and over-the-counter medicines, vitamins, and herbal supplements.

VIAGRA may affect the way other medicines work, and other medicines may affect the way VIAGRA works causing side effects. Especially tell your healthcare provider if you take any of the following:

• medicines called nitrates (see "What is the most important information I should know about VIAGRA?")

• medicines called guanylate cyclase stimulators, such as riociguat (Adempas)

• medicines called alpha blockers such as Hytrin (terazosin HCl), Flomax (tamsulosin HCl), Cardura (doxazosin mesylate), Minipress (prazosin HCl), Uroxatral (alfuzosin HCl), Jalyn (dutasteride and tamsulosin HCl), or Rapaflo (silodosin). Alpha-blockers are sometimes prescribed for prostate problems or high blood pressure. In some patients, the use of VIAGRA with alpha-blockers can lead to a drop in blood pressure or to fainting.

• medicines called HIV protease inhibitors, such as ritonavir (Norvir), indinavir sulfate (Crixivan), saquinavir (Fortovase or Invirase) or atazanavir sulfate (Reyataz)

• some types of oral antifungal medicines, such as ketoconazole (Nizoral), and itraconazole (Sporanox)

• some types of antibiotics, such as clarithromycin (Biaxin), telithromycin (Ketek), or erythromycin

• other medicines that treat high blood pressure

• other medicines or treatments for ED

• VIAGRA contains sildenafil, which is the same medicine found in another drug called REVATIO. REVATIO is used to treat a rare disease called pulmonary arterial hypertension (PAH). VIAGRA should not be used with REVATIO or with other PAH treatments containing sildenafil or any other PDE5 inhibitors (such as Adcirca [tadalafil]).

Ask your healthcare provider or pharmacist for a list of these medicines, if you are not sure.

Know the medicines you take. Keep a list of them to show to your healthcare provider and pharmacist when you get a new medicine.

How should I take VIAGRA?

• Take VIAGRA exactly as your healthcare provider tells you to take it.

• Your healthcare provider will tell you how much VIAGRA to take and when to take it.

• Your healthcare provider may change your dose if needed.

• Take VIAGRA about 1 hour before sexual activity. You may take VIAGRA between 30 minutes to 4 hours before sexual activity if needed.

• VIAGRA can be taken with or without food. If you take VIAGRA after a high fat meal (such as a cheeseburger and french fries), VIAGRA may take a little longer to start working

• Do not take VIAGRA more than 1 time a day.

• If you accidentally take too much VIAGRA, call your doctor or go to the nearest hospital emergency room right away.

What are the possible side effects of VIAGRA?

VIAGRA can cause serious side effects. Rarely reported side effects include:

• **an erection that will not go away (priapism).** If you have an erection that lasts more than 4 hours, get medical help right away. If it is not treated right away, priapism can permanently damage your penis.

• **sudden vision loss in one or both eyes.** Sudden vision loss in one or both eyes can be a sign of a serious eye problem called non-arteritic anterior ischemic optic neuropathy (NAION). Stop taking VIAGRA and call your healthcare provider right away if you have sudden vision loss in one or both eyes.

• **sudden hearing decrease or hearing loss.** Some people may also have ringing in their ears (tinnitus) or dizziness. If you have these symptoms, stop taking VIAGRA and contact a doctor right away.

	25 mg	50 mg	100 mg
Obverse	VGR25	VGR50	VGR100
Reverse	PFIZER	PFIZER	PFIZER
Bottle of 30	NDC-0069-4200-30	NDC-0069-4210-30	NDC-0069-4220-30
Bottle of 100	N/A	NDC-0069-4210-66	NDC-0069-4220-66
Carton of 30 (1 tablet per Single Pack)	N/A	NDC 0069-4210-33	NDC 0069-4220-33

Continued on next page

The most common side effects of VIAGRA are:
- headache
- flushing
- upset stomach
- abnormal vision, such as changes in color vision (such as having a blue color tinge) and blurred vision
- stuffy or runny nose
- back pain
- muscle pain
- nausea
- dizziness
- rash

In addition, heart attack, stroke, irregular heartbeats and death have happened rarely in men taking VIAGRA. Most, but not all, of these men had heart problems before taking VIAGRA. It is not known if VIAGRA caused these problems. Tell your healthcare provider if you have any side effect that bothers you or does not go away.

These are not all the possible side effects of VIAGRA. For more information, ask your healthcare provider or pharmacist.

Call your doctor for medical advice about side effects. You may report side effects to FDA at 1-800-FDA-1088.

How should I store VIAGRA?
- Store VIAGRA at room temperature between 68°F to 77°F (20°C to 25°C).

Keep VIAGRA and all medicines out of the reach of children.

General information about the safe and effective use of VIAGRA.

Medicines are sometimes prescribed for purposes other than those listed in a Patient Information leaflet. Do not use VIAGRA for a condition for which it was not prescribed. Do not give VIAGRA to other people, even if they have the same symptoms that you have. It may harm them.

This Patient Information leaflet summarizes the most important information about VIAGRA. If you would like more information, talk with your healthcare provider. You can ask your healthcare provider or pharmacist for information about VIAGRA that is written for health professionals.

For more information, go to www.viagra.com, or call 1-888-4VIAGRA

What are the ingredients in VIAGRA?
Active ingredient: sildenafil citrate
Inactive ingredients: microcrystalline cellulose, anhydrous dibasic calcium phosphate, croscarmellose sodium, magnesium stearate, hypromellose, titanium dioxide, lactose, triacetin, and FD & C Blue #2 aluminum lake
This Patient Information has been approved by the U.S. Food and Drug Administration.

Distributed by
Pfizer Labs
Division of Pfizer Inc, NY, NY 10017
September 2015
This product's label may have been updated. For current full prescribing information, please visit www.pfizer.com.
Viagra (sildenafil citrate), Revatio (sildenafil), Cardura (doxazosin mesylate), and Minipress (prazosin HCl) are registered trademarks of Pfizer Inc.
LAB-0220-10.0

[1]The other brands listed are trademarks of their respective owners and are not trademarks of Pfizer Inc. The makers of these brands are not affiliated with and do not endorse Pfizer Inc or its products.

XELJANZ®   ℞
(tofacitinib)
tablets, for oral use

HIGHLIGHTS OF PRESCRIBING INFORMATION
These highlights do not include all the information needed to use XELJANZ/XELJANZ XR safely and effectively. See full prescribing information for XELJANZ.
XELJANZ ® (tofacitinib) tablets, for oral use
XELJANZ ® XR (tofacitinib) extended release tablets, for oral use
Initial U.S. Approval: 2012

WARNING: SERIOUS INFECTIONS AND MALIGNANCY
See full prescribing information for complete boxed warning.
- **Serious infections leading to hospitalization or death, including tuberculosis and bacterial, invasive**

fungal, viral, and other opportunistic infections, have occurred in patients receiving XELJANZ. (5.1)
- If a serious infection develops, interrupt XELJANZ/XELJANZ XR until the infection is controlled. (5.1)
- Prior to starting XELJANZ/XELJANZ XR, perform a test for latent tuberculosis; if it is positive, start treatment for tuberculosis prior to starting XELJANZ/XELJANZ XR. (5.1)
- Monitor all patients for active tuberculosis during treatment, even if the initial latent tuberculosis test is negative. (5.1)
- Lymphoma and other malignancies have been observed in patients treated with XELJANZ. Epstein Barr Virus-associated post-transplant lymphoproliferative disorder has been observed at an increased rate in renal transplant patients treated with XELJANZ and concomitant immunosuppressive medications. (5.2)

─────**RECENT MAJOR CHANGES**─────
Dosage and Administration (2)   2/2016
Warnings and Precautions, Serious Infections   6/2015
(5.1)
Warnings and Precautions, General (5.6)   2/2016

─────**INDICATIONS AND USAGE**─────
- XELJANZ/XELJANZ XR is an inhibitor of Janus kinases (JAKs) indicated for the treatment of adult patients with moderately to severely active rheumatoid arthritis who have had an inadequate response or intolerance to methotrexate. It may be used as monotherapy or in combination with methotrexate or other nonbiologic disease-modifying antirheumatic drugs (DMARDs). (1.1)
- Limitations of Use: Use of XELJANZ/XELJANZ XR in combination with biologic DMARDs or potent immunosuppressants such as azathioprine and cyclosporine is not recommended. (1.1)

─────**DOSAGE AND ADMINISTRATION**─────
Rheumatoid Arthritis
- Recommended dose of XELJANZ is 5 mg twice daily. (2.1)
- Recommended dose of XELJANZ XR is 11 mg once daily. (2.1)
- Recommended dose in patients with moderate and severe renal impairment and moderate hepatic impairment is XELJANZ 5 mg once daily. (2.4, 8.6, 8.7)
- Use of XELJANZ/XELJANZ XR in patients with severe hepatic impairment is not recommended. (2.4, 8.7)

─────**DOSAGE FORMS AND STRENGTHS**─────
XELJANZ Tablets: 5 mg (3)
XELJANZ XR Tablets: 11 mg (3)

─────**CONTRAINDICATIONS**─────
None (4)

─────**WARNINGS AND PRECAUTIONS**─────
- Avoid use of XELJANZ/XELJANZ XR during an active serious infection, including localized infections. (5.1)
- Gastrointestinal Perforations – Use with caution in patients that may be at increased risk. (5.3)
- Laboratory Monitoring – Recommended due to potential changes in lymphocytes, neutrophils, hemoglobin, liver enzymes and lipids. (5.4)
- Immunizations – Live vaccines: Avoid use with XELJANZ/XELJANZ XR. (5.5)

─────**ADVERSE REACTIONS**─────
The most commonly reported adverse reactions during the first 3 months in controlled clinical trials (occurring in greater than or equal to 2% of patients treated with XELJANZ monotherapy or in combination with DMARDs) were upper respiratory tract infections, headache, diarrhea and nasopharyngitis. (6.1)
To report SUSPECTED ADVERSE REACTIONS, contact Pfizer, Inc at 1-800-438-1985 or FDA at 1-800-FDA-1088 or *www.fda.gov/medwatch.*

─────**DRUG INTERACTIONS**─────
- Potent inhibitors of Cytochrome P450 3A4 (CYP3A4) (e.g., ketoconazole):
  - Recommended dose is XELJANZ 5 mg once daily. (2.3, 7.1)
- One or more concomitant medications that result in both moderate inhibition of CYP3A4 and potent inhibition of CYP2C19 (e.g., fluconazole):
  - Recommended dose is XELJANZ 5 mg once daily. (2.3, 7.2)
- Potent CYP inducers (e.g., rifampin): May result in loss of or reduced clinical response. (2.3, 7.3)

See 17 for **PATIENT COUNSELING INFORMATION** and Medication Guide.
                                                          Revised: 2/2016

FULL PRESCRIBING INFORMATION: CONTENTS*
WARNING: SERIOUS INFECTIONS AND MALIGNANCY

FULL PRESCRIBING INFORMATION

WARNING: SERIOUS INFECTIONS AND MALIGNANCY
SERIOUS INFECTIONS
Patients treated with XELJANZ/XELJANZ XR are at increased risk for developing serious infections that may lead to hospitalization or death *[see Warnings and Precautions (5.1) and Adverse Reactions (6.1)].* Most patients who developed these infections were taking concomitant immunosuppressants such as methotrexate or corticosteroids.
If a serious infection develops, interrupt XELJANZ/XELJANZ XR until the infection is controlled.
Reported infections include:
- Active tuberculosis, which may present with pulmonary or extrapulmonary disease. Patients should be tested for latent tuberculosis before XELJANZ/XELJANZ XR use and during therapy. Treatment for latent infection should be initiated prior to XELJANZ/XELJANZ XR use.
- Invasive fungal infections, including cryptococcosis and pneumocystosis. Patients with invasive fungal infections may present with disseminated, rather than localized, disease.
- Bacterial, viral, and other infections due to opportunistic pathogens.
The risks and benefits of treatment with XELJANZ/XELJANZ XR should be carefully considered prior to initiating therapy in patients with chronic or recurrent infection.

Patients should be closely monitored for the development of signs and symptoms of infection during and after treatment with XELJANZ/XELJANZ XR, including the possible development of tuberculosis in patients who tested negative for latent tuberculosis infection prior to initiating therapy *[see Warnings and Precautions (5.1)]*.

MALIGNANCIES

Lymphoma and other malignancies have been observed in patients treated with XELJANZ. Epstein Barr Virus-associated post-transplant lymphoproliferative disorder has been observed at an increased rate in renal transplant patients treated with XELJANZ and concomitant immunosuppressive medications *[see Warnings and Precautions (5.2)]*.

1 INDICATIONS AND USAGE

1.1 Rheumatoid Arthritis

• XELJANZ/XELJANZ XR (tofacitinib) is indicated for the treatment of adult patients with moderately to severely active rheumatoid arthritis who have had an inadequate response or intolerance to methotrexate. It may be used as monotherapy or in combination with methotrexate or other nonbiologic disease-modifying antirheumatic drugs (DMARDs).

• Limitations of Use: Use of XELJANZ/XELJANZ XR in combination with biologic DMARDs or with potent immunosuppressants such as azathioprine and cyclosporine is not recommended.

2 DOSAGE AND ADMINISTRATION

2.1 Dosage in Rheumatoid Arthritis

• XELJANZ/XELJANZ XR may be used as monotherapy or in combination with methotrexate or other nonbiologic disease-modifying antirheumatic drugs (DMARDs). The recommended dose of XELJANZ is 5 mg twice daily and the recommended dose of XELJANZ XR is 11 mg once daily.

• XELJANZ XR is given orally with or without food.

• Swallow XELJANZ XR tablets whole and intact. Do not crush, split, or chew.

Switching from XELJANZ Tablets to XELJANZ XR Tablets

Patients treated with XELJANZ 5 mg twice daily may be switched to XELJANZ XR 11 mg once daily the day following the last dose of XELJANZ 5 mg.

2.2 Dosage Modifications due to Serious Infections and Cytopenias

(see Tables 1, 2, and 3 below)

• It is recommended that XELJANZ/XELJANZ XR not be initiated in patients with an absolute lymphocyte count less than 500 cells/mm³, an absolute neutrophil count (ANC) less than 1000 cells/mm³ or who have hemoglobin levels less than 9 g/dL.

• Dose interruption is recommended for management of lymphopenia, neutropenia and anemia *[see Warnings and Precautions (5.4) and Adverse Reactions (6.1)]*.

• Avoid use of XELJANZ/XELJANZ XR if a patient develops a serious infection until the infection is controlled.

2.3 Dosage Modifications due to Drug Interactions

• In patients receiving:

• potent inhibitors of Cytochrome P450 3A4 (CYP3A4) (e.g., ketoconazole), or

• one or more concomitant medications that result in both moderate inhibition of CYP3A4 and potent inhibition of CYP2C19 (e.g., fluconazole), the recommended dose is XELJANZ 5 mg once daily.

• Coadministration of potent inducers of CYP3A4 (e.g., rifampin) with XELJANZ/XELJANZ XR may result in loss of or reduced clinical response to XELJANZ/XELJANZ XR.

• Coadministration of potent inducers of CYP3A4 with XELJANZ/XELJANZ XR is not recommended.

2.4 Dosage Modifications in Patients with Renal or Hepatic Impairment

• In patients with:

• moderate or severe renal insufficiency, or

• moderate hepatic impairment, the recommended dose is XELJANZ 5 mg once daily.

• Use of XELJANZ/XELJANZ XR in patients with severe hepatic impairment is not recommended.

Table 1: Dose Adjustments for Lymphopenia

Low Lymphocyte Count *[see Warnings and Precautions (5.4)]*

Lab Value (cells/mm³)	Recommendation
Lymphocyte count greater than or equal to 500	Maintain dose
Lymphocyte count less than 500 (Confirmed by repeat testing)	Discontinue XELJANZ/XELJANZ XR

Table 2: Dose Adjustments for Neutropenia

Low ANC *[see Warnings and Precautions (5.4)]*

Lab Value (cells/mm³)	Recommendation
ANC greater than 1000	Maintain dose
ANC 500–1000	For persistent decreases in this range, interrupt dosing until ANC is greater than 1000 When ANC is greater than 1000, resume XELJANZ 5 mg twice daily/XELJANZ XR 11 mg once daily
ANC less than 500 (Confirmed by repeat testing)	Discontinue XELJANZ/XELJANZ XR

Table 3: Dose Adjustments for Anemia

Low Hemoglobin Value *[see Warnings and Precautions (5.4)]*

Lab Value (g/dL)	Recommendation
Less than or equal to 2 g/dL decrease and greater than or equal to 9.0 g/dL	Maintain dose
Greater than 2 g/dL decrease or less than 8.0 g/dL (Confirmed by repeat testing)	Interrupt the administration of XELJANZ/XELJANZ XR until hemoglobin values have normalized

3 DOSAGE FORMS AND STRENGTHS

XELJANZ is provided as 5 mg tofacitinib (equivalent to 8 mg tofacitinib citrate) tablets: White, round, immediate-release film-coated tablets, debossed with "Pfizer" on one side, and "JKI 5" on the other side.

XELJANZ XR is provided as 11 mg tofacitinib (equivalent to 17.77 mg tofacitinib citrate) tablets: Pink, oval, extended release film-coated tablets with a drilled hole at one end of the tablet band and "JKI 11" printed on one side of the tablet.

4 CONTRAINDICATIONS

None

5 WARNINGS AND PRECAUTIONS

5.1 Serious Infections

Serious and sometimes fatal infections due to bacterial, mycobacterial, invasive fungal, viral, or other opportunistic pathogens have been reported in rheumatoid arthritis patients receiving XELJANZ. The most common serious infections reported with XELJANZ included pneumonia, cellulitis, herpes zoster, urinary tract infection, and diverticulitis *[see Adverse Reactions (6.1)]*. Among opportunistic infections, tuberculosis and other mycobacterial infections, cryptococcosis, esophageal candidiasis, pneumocystosis, multidermatomal herpes zoster, cytomegalovirus, and BK virus were reported with XELJANZ. Some patients have presented with disseminated rather than localized disease, and were often taking concomitant immunomodulating agents such as methotrexate or corticosteroids.

Other serious infections that were not reported in clinical studies may also occur (e.g., histoplasmosis, coccidioidomycosis, and listeriosis).

Avoid use of XELJANZ/XELJANZ XR in patients with an active, serious infection, including localized infections. The risks and benefits of treatment should be considered prior to initiating XELJANZ/XELJANZ XR in patients:

• with chronic or recurrent infection
• who have been exposed to tuberculosis
• with a history of a serious or an opportunistic infection
• who have resided or traveled in areas of endemic tuberculosis or endemic mycoses; or

• with underlying conditions that may predispose them to infection.

Patients should be closely monitored for the development of signs and symptoms of infection during and after treatment with XELJANZ/XELJANZ XR. XELJANZ/XELJANZ XR should be interrupted if a patient develops a serious infection, an opportunistic infection, or sepsis. A patient who develops a new infection during treatment with XELJANZ/XELJANZ XR should undergo prompt and complete diagnostic testing appropriate for an immunocompromised patient; appropriate antimicrobial therapy should be initiated, and the patient should be closely monitored.

Tuberculosis

Patients should be evaluated and tested for latent or active infection prior to administration of XELJANZ/XELJANZ XR.

Anti-tuberculosis therapy should also be considered prior to administration of XELJANZ/XELJANZ XR in patients with a past history of latent or active tuberculosis in whom an adequate course of treatment cannot be confirmed, and for patients with a negative test for latent tuberculosis but who have risk factors for tuberculosis infection. Consultation with a physician with expertise in the treatment of tuberculosis is recommended to aid in the decision about whether initiating anti-tuberculosis therapy is appropriate for an individual patient.

Patients should be closely monitored for the development of signs and symptoms of tuberculosis, including patients who tested negative for latent tuberculosis infection prior to initiating therapy.

Patients with latent tuberculosis should be treated with standard antimycobacterial therapy before administering XELJANZ/XELJANZ XR.

Viral Reactivation

Viral reactivation, including cases of herpes virus reactivation (e.g., herpes zoster), were observed in clinical studies with XELJANZ. The impact of XELJANZ/XELJANZ XR on chronic viral hepatitis reactivation is unknown. Patients who screened positive for hepatitis B or C were excluded from clinical trials. Screening for viral hepatitis should be performed in accordance with clinical guidelines before starting therapy with XELJANZ/XELJANZ XR. The risk of herpes zoster is increased in patients treated with XELJANZ/XELJANZ XR and appears to be higher in patients treated with XELJANZ in Japan.

5.2 Malignancy and Lymphoproliferative Disorders

Consider the risks and benefits of XELJANZ/XELJANZ XR treatment prior to initiating therapy in patients with a known malignancy other than a successfully treated non-melanoma skin cancer (NMSC) or when considering continuing XELJANZ/XELJANZ XR in patients who develop a malignancy. Malignancies were observed in clinical studies of XELJANZ *[see Adverse Reactions (6.1)]*.

In the seven controlled rheumatoid arthritis clinical studies, 11 solid cancers and one lymphoma were diagnosed in 3328 patients receiving XELJANZ with or without DMARD, compared to 0 solid cancers and 0 lymphomas in 809 patients in the placebo with or without DMARD group during the first 12 months of exposure. Lymphomas and solid cancers have also been observed in the long-term extension studies in rheumatoid arthritis patients treated with XELJANZ.

In Phase 2B, controlled dose-ranging trials in *de-novo* renal transplant patients, all of whom received induction therapy with basiliximab, high-dose corticosteroids, and mycophenolic acid products, Epstein Barr Virus-associated post-transplant lymphoproliferative disorder was observed in 5 out of 218 patients treated with XELJANZ (2.3%) compared to 0 out of 111 patients treated with cyclosporine.

Non-Melanoma Skin Cancer

Non-melanoma skin cancers (NMSCs) have been reported in patients treated with XELJANZ. Periodic skin examination is recommended for patients who are at increased risk for skin cancer.

5.3 Gastrointestinal Perforations

Events of gastrointestinal perforation have been reported in clinical studies with XELJANZ in rheumatoid arthritis patients, although the role of JAK inhibition in these events is not known.

XELJANZ/XELJANZ XR should be used with caution in patients who may be at increased risk for gastrointestinal perforation (e.g., patients with a history of diverticulitis). Pa-

Continued on next page

tients presenting with new onset abdominal symptoms should be evaluated promptly for early identification of gastrointestinal perforation *[see Adverse Reactions (6.1)]*.

5.4 Laboratory Abnormalities

Lymphocyte Abnormalities

Treatment with XELJANZ was associated with initial lymphocytosis at one month of exposure followed by a gradual decrease in mean absolute lymphocyte counts below the baseline of approximately 10% during 12 months of therapy. Lymphocyte counts less than 500 cells/mm^3 were associated with an increased incidence of treated and serious infections.

Avoid initiation of XELJANZ/XELJANZ XR treatment in patients with a low lymphocyte count (i.e., less than 500 cells/mm^3). In patients who develop a confirmed absolute lymphocyte count less than 500 cells/mm^3, treatment with XELJANZ/XELJANZ XR is not recommended.

Monitor lymphocyte counts at baseline and every 3 months thereafter. For recommended modifications based on lymphocyte counts *see Dosage and Administration (2.2)*.

Neutropenia

Treatment with XELJANZ was associated with an increased incidence of neutropenia (less than 2000 cells/mm^3) compared to placebo.

Avoid initiation of XELJANZ/XELJANZ XR treatment in patients with a low neutrophil count (i.e., ANC less than 1000 cells/mm^3). For patients who develop a persistent ANC of 500–1000 cells/mm^3, interrupt XELJANZ/XELJANZ XR dosing until ANC is greater than or equal to 1000 cells/mm^3. In patients who develop an ANC less than 500 cells/mm^3, treatment with XELJANZ/XELJANZ XR is not recommended.

Monitor neutrophil counts at baseline and after 4–8 weeks of treatment and every 3 months thereafter. For recommended modifications based on ANC results *see Dosage and Administration (2.2)*.

Anemia

Avoid initiation of XELJANZ/XELJANZ XR treatment in patients with a low hemoglobin level (i.e. less than 9 g/dL). Treatment with XELJANZ/XELJANZ XR should be interrupted in patients who develop hemoglobin levels less than 8 g/dL or whose hemoglobin level drops greater than 2 g/dL on treatment.

Monitor hemoglobin at baseline and after 4–8 weeks of treatment and every 3 months thereafter. For recommended modifications based on hemoglobin results *see Dosage and Administration (2.2)*.

Liver Enzyme Elevations

Treatment with XELJANZ was associated with an increased incidence of liver enzyme elevation compared to placebo. Most of these abnormalities occurred in studies with background DMARD (primarily methotrexate) therapy.

Routine monitoring of liver tests and prompt investigation of the causes of liver enzyme elevations is recommended to identify potential cases of drug-induced liver injury. If drug-induced liver injury is suspected, the administration of XELJANZ/XELJANZ XR should be interrupted until this diagnosis has been excluded.

Lipid Elevations

Treatment with XELJANZ was associated with increases in lipid parameters including total cholesterol, low-density lipoprotein (LDL) cholesterol, and high-density lipoprotein (HDL) cholesterol. Maximum effects were generally observed within 6 weeks. The effect of these lipid parameter elevations on cardiovascular morbidity and mortality has not been determined.

Assessment of lipid parameters should be performed approximately 4–8 weeks following initiation of XELJANZ/XELJANZ XR therapy.

Manage patients according to clinical guidelines [e.g., National Cholesterol Educational Program (NCEP)] for the management of hyperlipidemia.

5.5 Vaccinations

No data are available on the response to vaccination or on the secondary transmission of infection by live vaccines to patients receiving XELJANZ/XELJANZ XR. Avoid use of live vaccines concurrently with XELJANZ/XELJANZ XR.

Update immunizations in agreement with current immunization guidelines prior to initiating XELJANZ/XELJANZ XR therapy.

5.6 General

Specific to XELJANZ XR

As with any other non-deformable material, caution should be used when administering XELJANZ XR to patients with pre-existing severe gastrointestinal narrowing (pathologic

or iatrogenic). There have been rare reports of obstructive symptoms in patients with known strictures in association with the ingestion of other drugs utilizing a non-deformable extended release formulation.

6 ADVERSE REACTIONS

6.1 Clinical Trial Experience

Because clinical studies are conducted under widely varying conditions, adverse reaction rates observed in the clinical studies of a drug cannot be directly compared to rates in the clinical studies of another drug and may not predict the rates observed in a broader patient population in clinical practice.

The clinical studies described in the following sections were conducted using XELJANZ. Although other doses of XELJANZ have been studied, the recommended dose of XELJANZ is 5 mg twice daily.

The recommended dose for XELJANZ XR is 11 mg once daily.

The following data includes two Phase 2 and five Phase 3 double-blind, controlled, multicenter trials. In these trials, patients were randomized to doses of XELJANZ 5 mg twice daily (292 patients) and 10 mg twice daily (306 patients) monotherapy, XELJANZ 5 mg twice daily (1044 patients) and 10 mg twice daily (1043 patients) in combination with DMARDs (including methotrexate) and placebo (809 patients). All seven protocols included provisions for patients taking placebo to receive treatment with XELJANZ at Month 3 or Month 6 either by patient response (based on uncontrolled disease activity) or by design, so that adverse events cannot always be unambiguously attributed to a given treatment. Therefore some analyses that follow include patients who changed treatment by design or by patient response from placebo to XELJANZ in both the placebo and XELJANZ group of a given interval. Comparisons between placebo and XELJANZ were based on the first 3 months of exposure, and comparisons between XELJANZ 5 mg twice daily and XELJANZ 10 mg twice daily were based on the first 12 months of exposure.

The long-term safety population includes all patients who participated in a double-blind, controlled trial (including earlier development phase studies) and then participated in one of two long-term safety studies. The design of the long-term safety studies allowed for modification of XELJANZ doses according to clinical judgment. This limits the interpretation of the long-term safety data with respect to dose. The most common serious adverse reactions were serious infections *[see Warnings and Precautions (5.1)]*.

The proportion of patients who discontinued treatment due to any adverse reaction during the 0 to 3 months exposure in the double-blind, placebo-controlled trials was 4% for patients taking XELJANZ and 3% for placebo-treated patients.

Overall Infections

In the seven controlled trials, during the 0 to 3 months exposure, the overall frequency of infections was 20% and 22% in the 5 mg twice daily and 10 mg twice daily groups, respectively, and 18% in the placebo group.

The most commonly reported infections with XELJANZ were upper respiratory tract infections, nasopharyngitis, and urinary tract infections (4%, 3%, and 2% of patients, respectively).

Serious Infections

In the seven controlled trials, during the 0 to 3 months exposure, serious infections were reported in 1 patient (0.5 events per 100 patient-years) who received placebo and 11 patients (1.7 events per 100 patient-years) who received XELJANZ 5 mg or 10 mg twice daily. The rate difference between treatment groups (and the corresponding 95% confidence interval) was 1.1 (-0.4, 2.5) events per 100 patient-years for the combined 5 mg twice daily and 10 mg twice daily XELJANZ group minus placebo.

In the seven controlled trials, during the 0 to 12 months exposure, serious infections were reported in 34 patients (2.7 events per 100 patient-years) who received 5 mg twice daily of XELJANZ and 33 patients (2.7 events per 100 patient-years) who received 10 mg twice daily of XELJANZ. The rate difference between XELJANZ doses (and the corresponding 95% confidence interval) was -0.1 (-1.3, 1.2) events per 100 patient-years for 10 mg twice daily XELJANZ minus 5 mg twice daily XELJANZ.

The most common serious infections included pneumonia, cellulitis, herpes zoster, and urinary tract infection *[see Warnings and Precautions (5.1)]*.

Tuberculosis

In the seven controlled trials, during the 0 to 3 months exposure, tuberculosis was not reported in patients who received placebo, 5 mg twice daily of XELJANZ, or 10 mg twice daily of XELJANZ.

In the seven controlled trials, during the 0 to 12 months exposure, tuberculosis was reported in 0 patients who received 5 mg twice daily of XELJANZ and 6 patients (0.5 events per 100 patient-years) who received 10 mg twice daily of XELJANZ. The rate difference between XELJANZ doses (and the corresponding 95% confidence interval) was 0.5 (0.1, 0.9) events per 100 patient-years for 10 mg twice daily XELJANZ minus 5 mg twice daily XELJANZ.

Cases of disseminated tuberculosis were also reported. The median XELJANZ exposure prior to diagnosis of tuberculosis was 10 months (range from 152 to 960 days) *[see Warnings and Precautions (5.1)]*.

Opportunistic Infections (excluding tuberculosis)

In the seven controlled trials, during the 0 to 3 months exposure, opportunistic infections were not reported in patients who received placebo, 5 mg twice daily of XELJANZ, or 10 mg twice daily of XELJANZ.

In the seven controlled trials, during the 0 to 12 months exposure, opportunistic infections were reported in 4 patients (0.3 events per 100 patient-years) who received 5 mg twice daily of XELJANZ and 4 patients (0.3 events per 100 patient-years) who received 10 mg twice daily of XELJANZ. The rate difference between XELJANZ doses (and the corresponding 95% confidence interval) was 0 (-0.5, 0.5) events per 100 patient-years for 10 mg twice daily XELJANZ minus 5 mg twice daily XELJANZ.

The median XELJANZ exposure prior to diagnosis of an opportunistic infection was 8 months (range from 41 to 698 days) *[see Warnings and Precautions (5.1)]*.

Malignancy

In the seven controlled trials, during the 0 to 3 months exposure, malignancies excluding NMSC were reported in 0 patients who received placebo and 2 patients (0.3 events per 100 patient-years) who received either XELJANZ 5 mg or 10 mg twice daily. The rate difference between treatment groups (and the corresponding 95% confidence interval) was 0.3 (-0.1, 0.7) events per 100 patient-years for the combined 5 mg and 10 mg twice daily XELJANZ group minus placebo.

In the seven controlled trials, during the 0 to 12 months exposure, malignancies excluding NMSC were reported in 5 patients (0.4 events per 100 patient-years) who received 5 mg twice daily of XELJANZ and 7 patients (0.6 events per 100 patient-years) who received 10 mg twice daily of XELJANZ. The rate difference between XELJANZ doses (and the corresponding 95% confidence interval) was 0.2 (-0.4, 0.7) events per 100 patient-years for 10 mg twice daily XELJANZ minus 5 mg twice daily XELJANZ. One of these malignancies was a case of lymphoma that occurred during the 0 to 12 month period in a patient treated with XELJANZ 10 mg twice daily.

The most common types of malignancy, including malignancies observed during the long-term extension, were lung and breast cancer, followed by gastric, colorectal, renal cell, prostate cancer, lymphoma, and malignant melanoma *[see Warnings and Precautions (5.2)]*.

Laboratory Abnormalities

Lymphopenia

In the controlled clinical trials, confirmed decreases in absolute lymphocyte counts below 500 cells/mm^3 occurred in 0.04% of patients for the 5 mg twice daily and 10 mg twice daily XELJANZ groups combined during the first 3 months of exposure.

Confirmed lymphocyte counts less than 500 cells/mm^3 were associated with an increased incidence of treated and serious infections *[see Warnings and Precautions (5.4)]*.

Neutropenia

In the controlled clinical trials, confirmed decreases in ANC below 1000 cells/mm^3 occurred in 0.07% of patients for the 5 mg twice daily and 10 mg twice daily XELJANZ groups combined during the first 3 months of exposure.

There were no confirmed decreases in ANC below 500 cells/mm^3 observed in any treatment group.

There was no clear relationship between neutropenia and the occurrence of serious infections.

In the long-term safety population, the pattern and incidence of confirmed decreases in ANC remained consistent with what was seen in the controlled clinical trials *[see Warnings and Precautions (5.4)]*.

Liver Enzyme Elevations

Confirmed increases in liver enzymes greater than 3 times the upper limit of normal (3× ULN) were observed in patients treated with XELJANZ. In patients experiencing liver enzyme elevation, modification of treatment regimen, such as reduction in the dose of concomitant DMARD, interruption of XELJANZ, or reduction in XELJANZ dose, resulted in decrease or normalization of liver enzymes.

In the controlled monotherapy trials (0–3 months), no differences in the incidence of ALT or AST elevations were observed between the placebo, and XELJANZ 5 mg, and 10 mg twice daily groups.

In the controlled background DMARD trials (0–3 months), ALT elevations greater than 3× ULN were observed in 1.0%, 1.3% and 1.2% of patients receiving placebo, 5 mg, and 10 mg twice daily, respectively. In these trials, AST elevations greater than 3× ULN were observed in 0.6%, 0.5% and 0.4% of patients receiving placebo, 5 mg, and 10 mg twice daily, respectively.

One case of drug-induced liver injury was reported in a patient treated with XELJANZ 10 mg twice daily for approximately 2.5 months. The patient developed symptomatic elevations of AST and ALT greater than 3× ULN and bilirubin elevations greater than 2× ULN, which required hospitalizations and a liver biopsy.

Lipid Elevations

In the controlled clinical trials, dose-related elevations in lipid parameters (total cholesterol, LDL cholesterol, HDL cholesterol, triglycerides) were observed at one month of exposure and remained stable thereafter. Changes in lipid parameters during the first 3 months of exposure in the controlled clinical trials are summarized below:

- Mean LDL cholesterol increased by 15% in the XELJANZ 5 mg twice daily arm and 19% in the XELJANZ 10 mg twice daily arm.
- Mean HDL cholesterol increased by 10% in the XELJANZ 5 mg twice daily arm and 12% in the XELJANZ 10 mg twice daily arm.
- Mean LDL/HDL ratios were essentially unchanged in XELJANZ-treated patients.

In a controlled clinical trial, elevations in LDL cholesterol and ApoB decreased to pretreatment levels in response to statin therapy.

In the long-term safety population, elevations in lipid parameters remained consistent with what was seen in the controlled clinical trials.

Serum Creatinine Elevations

In the controlled clinical trials, dose-related elevations in serum creatinine were observed with XELJANZ treatment. The mean increase in serum creatinine was <0.1 mg/dL in the 12-month pooled safety analysis; however with increasing duration of exposure in the long-term extensions, up to 2% of patients were discontinued from XELJANZ treatment due to the protocol-specified discontinuation criterion of an increase in creatinine by more than 50% of baseline. The clinical significance of the observed serum creatinine elevations is unknown.

Other Adverse Reactions

Adverse reactions occurring in 2% or more of patients on 5 mg twice daily or 10 mg twice daily XELJANZ and at least 1% greater than that observed in patients on placebo with or without DMARD are summarized in Table 4.

Table 4: Adverse Reactions Occurring in at Least 2% or More of Patients on 5 or 10 mg Twice Daily XELJANZ With or Without DMARD (0–3 months) and at Least 1% Greater Than That Observed in Patients on Placebo

Preferred Term	XELJANZ 5 mg Twice Daily	XELJANZ 10 mg Twice Daily*	Placebo
	N = 1336 (%)	N = 1349 (%)	N = 809 (%)
Diarrhea	4.0	2.9	2.3
Nasopharyngitis	3.8	2.8	2.8
Upper respiratory tract infection	4.5	3.8	3.3
Headache	4.3	3.4	2.1
Hypertension	1.6	2.3	1.1

N reflects randomized and treated patients from the seven clinical trials

*The recommended dose of XELJANZ is 5 mg twice daily.

Other adverse reactions occurring in controlled and open-label extension studies included:

Blood and lymphatic system disorders: Anemia
Infections and infestations: Diverticulitis
Metabolism and nutrition disorders: Dehydration
Psychiatric disorders: Insomnia
Nervous system disorders: Paresthesia
Respiratory, thoracic and mediastinal disorders: Dyspnea, cough, sinus congestion
Gastrointestinal disorders: Abdominal pain, dyspepsia, vomiting, gastritis, nausea
Hepatobiliary disorders: Hepatic steatosis
Skin and subcutaneous tissue disorders: Rash, erythema, pruritus
Musculoskeletal, connective tissue and bone disorders: Musculoskeletal pain, arthralgia, tendonitis, joint swelling
Neoplasms benign, malignant and unspecified (including cysts and polyps): Non-melanoma skin cancers
General disorders and administration site conditions: Pyrexia, fatigue, peripheral edema
Clinical Experience in Methotrexate-Naïve Patients
Study VI was an active-controlled clinical trial in methotrexate-naïve patients *[see Clinical Studies (14)]*. The safety experience in these patients was consistent with Studies I–V.

7 DRUG INTERACTIONS

All information provided in this section is applicable to XELJANZ and XELJANZ XR as they contain the same active ingredient (tofacitinib).

7.1 Potent CYP3A4 Inhibitors

Tofacitinib exposure is increased when XELJANZ is coadministered with potent inhibitors of cytochrome P450 (CYP) 3A4 (e.g., ketoconazole) *[see Dosage and Administration (2.3) and Figure 3]*.

7.2 Moderate CYP3A4 and Potent CYP2C19 Inhibitors

Tofacitinib exposure is increased when XELJANZ is coadministered with medications that result in both moderate inhibition of CYP3A4 and potent inhibition of CYP2C19 (e.g., fluconazole) *[see Dosage and Administration (2.3) and Figure 3]*.

7.3 Potent CYP3A4 Inducers

Tofacitinib exposure is decreased when XELJANZ is coadministered with potent CYP3A4 inducers (e.g., rifampin) *[see Dosage and Administration (2.3) and Figure 3]*.

7.4 Immunosuppressive Drugs

There is a risk of added immunosuppression when XELJANZ/XELJANZ XR is coadministered with potent immunosuppressive drugs (e.g., azathioprine, tacrolimus, cyclosporine). Combined use of multiple-dose XELJANZ/XELJANZ XR with potent immunosuppressants has not been studied in rheumatoid arthritis. Use of XELJANZ/XELJANZ XR in combination with biologic DMARDs or potent immunosuppressants such as azathioprine and cyclosporine is not recommended.

8 USE IN SPECIFIC POPULATIONS

All information provided in this section is applicable to XELJANZ and XELJANZ XR as they contain the same active ingredient (tofacitinib).

8.1 Pregnancy

Teratogenic effects
Pregnancy Category C.
There are no adequate and well-controlled studies in pregnant women. XELJANZ/XELJANZ XR should be used during pregnancy only if the potential benefit justifies the potential risk to the fetus. Tofacitinib has been shown to be fetocidal and teratogenic in rats and rabbits when given at exposures 146 times and 13 times, respectively, the maximum recommended human dose (MRHD).

In a rat embryofetal developmental study, tofacitinib was teratogenic at exposure levels approximately 146 times the MRHD (on an AUC basis at oral doses of 100 mg/kg/day). Teratogenic effects consisted of external and soft tissue malformations of anasarca and membranous ventricular septal defects, respectively, and skeletal malformations or variations (absent cervical arch; bent femur, fibula, humerus, radius, scapula, tibia, and ulna; sternoschisis; absent rib; misshapen femur; branched rib; fused rib; fused sternebra; and hemicentric thoracic centrum). In addition, there was an increase in post-implantation loss, consisting of early and late resorptions, resulting in a reduced number of viable fetuses. Mean fetal body weight was reduced. No developmental toxicity was observed in rats at exposure levels approximately 58 times the MRHD (on an AUC basis at oral doses of 30 mg/kg/day). In the rabbit embryofetal developmental study, tofacitinib was teratogenic at exposure levels approximately 13 times the MRHD (on an AUC basis at oral doses of 30 mg/kg/day) in the absence of signs of maternal toxicity. Teratogenic effects included thoracogastroschisis, omphalocele, membranous ventricular septal defects, and cranial/skeletal malformations (microstomia, microphthalmia), mid-line and tail defects. In addition, there was an increase in post-implantation loss associated with late resorptions. No developmental toxicity was observed in rabbits at exposure levels approximately 3 times the MRHD (on an AUC basis at oral doses of 10 mg/kg/day).

Nonteratogenic effects

In a peri- and postnatal rat study, there were reductions in live litter size, postnatal survival, and pup body weights at exposure levels approximately 73 times the MRHD (on an AUC basis at oral doses of 50 mg/kg/day). There was no effect on behavioral and learning assessments, sexual maturation or the ability of the F1 generation rats to mate and produce viable F2 generation fetuses in rats at exposure levels approximately 17 times the MRHD (on an AUC basis at oral doses of 10 mg/kg/day).

Pregnancy Registry: To monitor the outcomes of pregnant women exposed to XELJANZ/XELJANZ XR, a pregnancy registry has been established. Physicians are encouraged to register patients and pregnant women are encouraged to register themselves by calling 1-877-311-8972.

8.3 Nursing Mothers

Tofacitinib was secreted in milk of lactating rats. It is not known whether tofacitinib is excreted in human milk. Because many drugs are excreted in human milk and because of the potential for serious adverse reactions in nursing infants from tofacitinib, a decision should be made whether to discontinue nursing or to discontinue the drug, taking into account the importance of the drug for the mother.

8.4 Pediatric Use

The safety and effectiveness of XELJANZ/XELJANZ XR in pediatric patients have not been established.

8.5 Geriatric Use

Of the 3315 patients who enrolled in Studies I to V, a total of 505 rheumatoid arthritis patients were 65 years of age and older, including 71 patients 75 years and older. The frequency of serious infection among XELJANZ-treated subjects 65 years of age and older was higher than among those under the age of 65. As there is a higher incidence of infections in the elderly population in general, caution should be used when treating the elderly.

8.6 Use in Diabetics

As there is a higher incidence of infection in diabetic population in general, caution should be used when treating patients with diabetes.

8.7 Hepatic Impairment

XELJANZ-treated patients with moderate hepatic impairment had greater tofacitinib levels than XELJANZ-treated patients with normal hepatic function *[see Clinical Pharmacology (12.3)]*. Higher blood levels may increase the risk of some adverse reactions, therefore, the recommended dose is XELJANZ 5 mg once daily in patients with moderate hepatic impairment *[see Dosage and Administration (2.4)]*. XELJANZ/XELJANZ XR has not been studied in patients with severe hepatic impairment; therefore, use of XELJANZ/XELJANZ XR in patients with severe hepatic impairment is not recommended. No dose adjustment is required in patients with mild hepatic impairment. The safety and efficacy of XELJANZ/XELJANZ XR have not been studied in patients with positive hepatitis B virus or hepatitis C virus serology.

8.8 Renal Impairment

XELJANZ-treated patients with moderate and severe renal impairment had greater tofacitinib blood levels than XELJANZ-treated patients with normal renal function; therefore, the recommended dose is XELJANZ 5 mg once daily in patients with moderate and severe renal impairment *[see Dosage and Administration (2.4)]*. In clinical trials, XELJANZ/XELJANZ XR was not evaluated in rheumatoid arthritis patients with baseline creatinine clearance values (estimated by the Cockroft-Gault equation) less than 40 mL/min. No dose adjustment is required in patients with mild renal impairment.

Continued on next page

Figure 1: Impact of Intrinsic Factors on Tofacitinib Pharmacokinetics

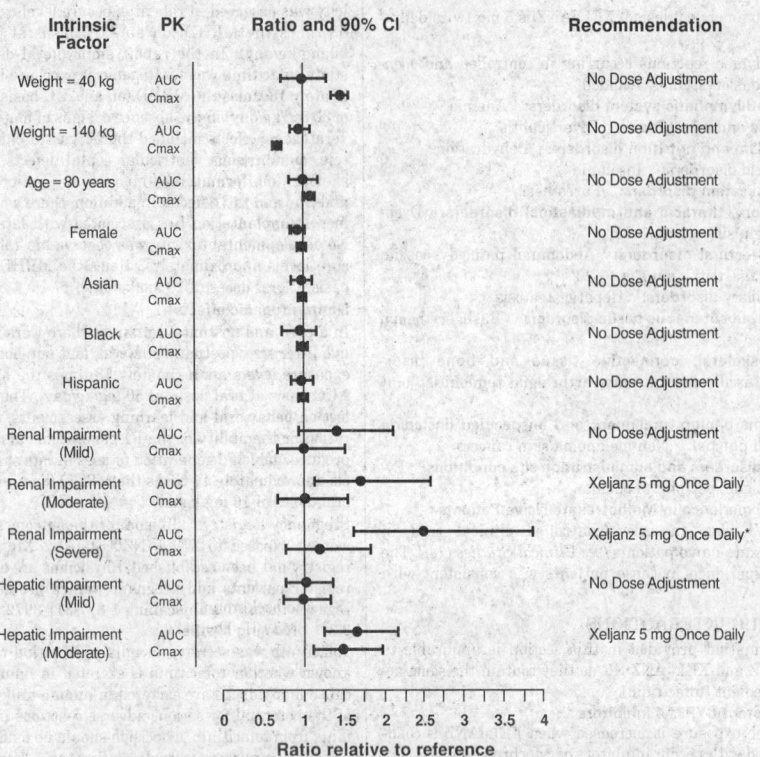

* Supplemental doses are not necessary in patients after dialysis

10   OVERDOSAGE

Signs, Symptoms, and Laboratory Findings of Acute Overdosage in Humans

There is no experience with overdose of XELJANZ/XELJANZ XR.

Treatment or Management of Overdose

Pharmacokinetic data up to and including a single dose of 100 mg in healthy volunteers indicate that more than 95% of the administered dose is expected to be eliminated within 24 hours.

There is no specific antidote for overdose with XELJANZ/ XELJANZ XR. In case of an overdose, it is recommended that the patient be monitored for signs and symptoms of adverse reactions. Patients who develop adverse reactions should receive appropriate treatment.

11   DESCRIPTION

XELJANZ/XELJANZ XR are formulated with the citrate salt of tofacitinib, a JAK inhibitor.

Tofacitinib citrate is a white to off-white powder with the following chemical name: (3R,4R)-4-methyl-3-(methyl-7H-pyrrolo   [2,3-d]pyrimidin-4-ylamino)-β-oxo-1-piperidine-propanenitrile, 2-hydroxy-1,2,3-propanetricarboxylate (1:1). The solubility of tofacitinib citrate in water is 2.9 mg/mL. Tofacitinib citrate has a molecular weight of 504.5 Daltons (or 312.4 Daltons as the tofacitinib free base) and a molecular formula of $C_{16}H_{20}N_6O \cdot C_6H_8O_7$. The chemical structure of tofacitinib citrate is:

XELJANZ is supplied for oral administration as 5 mg tofacitinib (equivalent to 8 mg tofacitinib citrate) white round, immediate-release film-coated tablet. Each tablet of XELJANZ contains the appropriate amount of tofacitinib as a citrate salt and the following inactive ingredients: microcrystalline   cellulose,   lactose   monohydrate,

croscarmellose sodium, magnesium stearate, HPMC 2910/Hypromellose 6cP, titanium dioxide, macrogol/ PEG3350, and triacetin.

XELJANZ XR is supplied for oral administration as 11 mg tofacitinib (equivalent to 17.77 mg tofacitinib citrate) pink, oval, extended release film-coated tablet with a drilled hole at one end of the tablet band. Each tablet of XELJANZ XR contains the appropriate amount of tofacitinib as a citrate salt and the following inactive ingredients: sorbitol, hydroxyethyl cellulose, copovidone, magnesium stearate, cellulose acetate, hydroxypropyl cellulose, HPMC 2910/Hypromellose, titanium dioxide, triacetin, and red iron oxide. Printing ink contains shellac glaze, ammonium hydroxide, propylene glycol, and ferrosoferric oxide/black iron oxide.

12   CLINICAL PHARMACOLOGY

12.1   Mechanism of Action

Tofacitinib is a Janus kinase (JAK) inhibitor. JAKs are intracellular enzymes which transmit signals arising from cytokine or growth factor-receptor interactions on the cellular membrane to influence cellular processes of hematopoiesis and immune cell function. Within the signaling pathway, JAKs phosphorylate and activate Signal Transducers and Activators of Transcription (STATs) which modulate intracellular activity including gene expression. Tofacitinib modulates the signaling pathway at the point of JAKs, preventing the phosphorylation and activation of STATs. JAK enzymes transmit cytokine signaling through pairing of JAKs (e.g., JAK1/JAK3, JAK1/JAK2, JAK1/TyK2, JAK2/ JAK2). Tofacitinib inhibited the *in vitro* activities of JAK1/ JAK2, JAK1/JAK3, and JAK2/JAK2 combinations with IC_{50} of 406, 56, and 1377 nM, respectively. However, the relevance of specific JAK combinations to therapeutic effectiveness is not known.

12.2   Pharmacodynamics

Treatment with XELJANZ was associated with dose-dependent reductions of circulating CD16/56+ natural killer cells, with estimated maximum reductions occurring at approximately 8–10 weeks after initiation of therapy. These changes generally resolved within 2–6 weeks after discontinuation of treatment. Treatment with XELJANZ was associated with dose-dependent increases in B cell counts. Changes in circulating T-lymphocyte counts and T-lymphocyte subsets (CD3+, CD4+ and CD8+) were small and inconsistent. The clinical significance of these changes is unknown.

Total serum IgG, IgM, and IgA levels after 6-month dosing in patients with rheumatoid arthritis were lower than placebo; however, changes were small and not dose-dependent. After treatment with XELJANZ in patients with rheumatoid arthritis, rapid decreases in serum C-reactive protein (CRP) were observed and maintained throughout dosing. Changes in CRP observed with XELJANZ treatment do not reverse fully within 2 weeks after discontinuation, indicating a longer duration of pharmacodynamic activity compared to the pharmacokinetic half-life.

12.3   Pharmacokinetics

XELJANZ

Following oral administration of XELJANZ, peak plasma concentrations are reached within 0.5–1 hour, elimination half-life is ~3 hours and a dose-proportional increase in systemic exposure was observed in the therapeutic dose range. Steady state concentrations are achieved in 24–48 hours with negligible accumulation after twice daily administration.

XELJANZ XR

Following oral administration of XELJANZ XR, peak plasma concentrations are reached at 4 hours and half-life is ~6 hours. Steady state concentrations are achieved within 48 hours with negligible accumulation after once daily administration. AUC and C_{max} of tofacitinib for XELJANZ XR 11 mg administered once daily are equivalent to those of XELJANZ 5 mg administered twice daily.

Absorption

XELJANZ

The absolute oral bioavailability of XELJANZ is 74%. Coadministration of XELJANZ with a high-fat meal resulted in no changes in AUC while C_{max} was reduced by 32%. In clinical trials, XELJANZ was administered without regard to meals.

XELJANZ XR

Coadministration of XELJANZ XR with a high-fat meal resulted in no changes in AUC while C_{max} was increased by 27% and T_{max} was extended by approximately 1 hour.

Distribution

After intravenous administration, the volume of distribution is 87 L. The protein binding of tofacitinib is ~40%. Tofacitinib binds predominantly to albumin and does not appear to bind to α1-acid glycoprotein. Tofacitinib distributes equally between red blood cells and plasma.

Metabolism and Elimination

Clearance mechanisms for tofacitinib are approximately 70% hepatic metabolism and 30% renal excretion of the parent drug. The metabolism of tofacitinib is primarily mediated by CYP3A4 with minor contribution from CYP2C19. In a human radiolabeled study, more than 65% of the total circulating radioactivity was accounted for by unchanged tofacitinib, with the remaining 35% attributed to 8 metabolites, each accounting for less than 8% of total radioactivity. The pharmacologic activity of tofacitinib is attributed to the parent molecule.

Pharmacokinetics in Rheumatoid Arthritis Patients

Population PK analysis in rheumatoid arthritis patients indicated no clinically relevant change in tofacitinib exposure, after accounting for differences in renal function (i.e., creatinine clearance) between patients, based on age, weight, gender and race (Figure 1). An approximately linear relationship between body weight and volume of distribution was observed, resulting in higher peak (C_{max}) and lower trough (C_{min}) concentrations in lighter patients. However, this difference is not considered to be clinically relevant. The between-subject variability (% coefficient of variation) in AUC of tofacitinib is estimated to be approximately 27%.

Specific Populations

The effect of renal and hepatic impairment and other intrinsic factors on the pharmacokinetics of tofacitinib is shown in Figure 1.

[See Figure 1 above]

Reference values for weight, age, gender, and race comparisons are 70 kg, 55 years, male, and White, respectively; reference groups for renal and hepatic impairment data are subjects with normal renal and hepatic function.

Drug Interactions

Potential for XELJANZ/XELJANZ XR to Influence the PK of Other Drugs

In vitro studies indicate that tofacitinib does not significantly inhibit or induce the activity of the major human drug-metabolizing CYPs (CYP1A2, CYP2B6, CYP2C8, CYP2C9, CYP2C19, CYP2D6, and CYP3A4) at concentrations exceeding 160 times the steady state C_{max} of a 5 mg twice daily dose. These *in vitro* results were confirmed by a human drug interaction study showing no changes in the PK of midazolam, a highly sensitive CYP3A4 substrate, when coadministered with XELJANZ.

In rheumatoid arthritis patients, the oral clearance of tofacitinib does not vary with time, indicating that tofacitinib does not normalize CYP enzyme activity in rheumatoid arthritis patients. Therefore, coadministration with XELJANZ/XELJANZ XR is not expected to result in clinically relevant increases in the metabolism of CYP substrates in rheumatoid arthritis patients.

In vitro data indicate that the potential for tofacitinib to inhibit transporters such as P-glycoprotein, organic anionic or cationic transporters at therapeutic concentrations is low. Dosing recommendations for coadministered drugs following administration with XELJANZ/XELJANZ XR are shown in Figure 2.

Figure 2. Impact of Tofacitinib on PK of Other Drugs

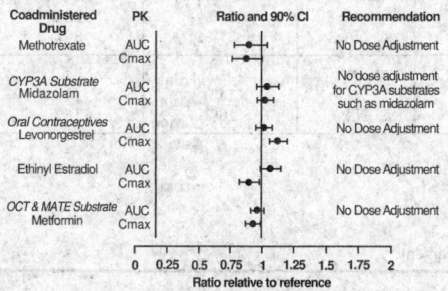

Note: Reference group is administration of concomitant medication alone; OCT = Organic Cationic Transporter; MATE = Multidrug and Toxic Compound Extrusion

Potential for Other Drugs to Influence the PK of Tofacitinib
Since tofacitinib is metabolized by CYP3A4, interaction with drugs that inhibit or induce CYP3A4 is likely. Inhibitors of CYP2C19 alone or P-glycoprotein are unlikely to substantially alter the PK of tofacitinib. Dosing recommendations for XELJANZ/XELJANZ XR for administration with CYP inhibitors or inducers are shown in Figure 3.

Figure 3. Impact of Other Drugs on PK of Tofacitinib

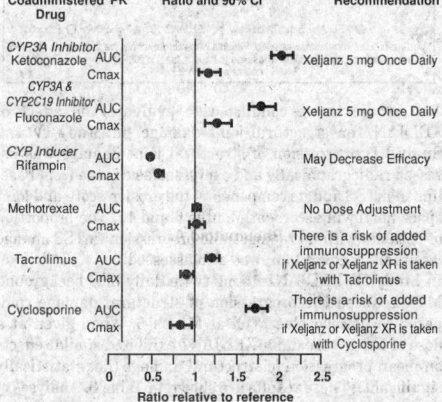

Note: Reference group is administration of tofacitinib alone

13 NONCLINICAL TOXICOLOGY

13.1 Carcinogenesis, Mutagenesis, Impairment of Fertility

In a 39-week toxicology study in monkeys, tofacitinib at exposure levels approximately 6 times the MRHD (on an AUC basis at oral doses of 5 mg/kg twice daily) produced lymphomas. No lymphomas were observed in this study at exposure levels 1 times the MRHD (on an AUC basis at oral doses of 1 mg/kg twice daily).

The carcinogenic potential of tofacitinib was assessed in 6-month rasH2 transgenic mouse carcinogenicity and 2-year rat carcinogenicity studies. Tofacitinib, at exposure levels approximately 34 times the MRHD (on an AUC basis at oral doses of 200 mg/kg/day) was not carcinogenic in mice.

In the 24-month oral carcinogenicity study in Sprague-Dawley rats, tofacitinib caused benign Leydig cell tumors, hibernomas (malignancy of brown adipose tissue), and benign thymomas at doses greater than or equal to 30 mg/kg/

day (approximately 42 times the exposure levels at the MRHD on an AUC basis). The relevance of benign Leydig cell tumors to human risk is not known.

Tofacitinib was not mutagenic in the bacterial reverse mutation assay. It was positive for clastogenicity in the *in vitro* chromosome aberration assay with human lymphocytes in the presence of metabolic enzymes, but negative in the absence of metabolic enzymes. Tofacitinib was negative in the *in vivo* rat micronucleus assay and in the *in vitro* CHO-HGPRT assay and the *in vivo* rat hepatocyte unscheduled DNA synthesis assay.

In rats, tofacitinib at exposure levels approximately 17 times the MRHD (on an AUC basis at oral doses of 10 mg/kg/day) reduced female fertility due to increased post-implantation loss. There was no impairment of female rat fertility at exposure levels of tofacitinib equal to the MRHD (on an AUC basis at oral doses of 1 mg/kg/day). Tofacitinib exposure levels at approximately 133 times the MRHD (on an AUC basis at oral doses of 100 mg/kg/day) had no effect on male fertility, sperm motility, or sperm concentration.

14 CLINICAL STUDIES

The XELJANZ clinical development program included two dose-ranging trials and five confirmatory trials. Although other doses have been studied, the recommended dose of XELJANZ is 5 mg twice daily.

Dose-Ranging Trials
Dose selection for XELJANZ was based on two pivotal dose-ranging trials.

Dose-Ranging Study 1 was a 6-month monotherapy trial in 384 patients with active rheumatoid arthritis who had an inadequate response to a DMARD. Patients who previously received adalimumab therapy were excluded. Patients were randomized to 1 of 7 monotherapy treatments: XELJANZ 1, 3, 5, 10 or 15 mg twice daily, adalimumab 40 mg subcutaneously every other week for 10 weeks followed by XELJANZ 5 mg twice daily for 3 months, or placebo.

Dose-Ranging Study 2 was a 6-month trial in which 507 patients with active rheumatoid arthritis who had an inadequate response to MTX alone received one of 6 dose regimens of XELJANZ (20 mg once daily; 1, 3, 5, 10 or 15 mg twice daily), or placebo added to background MTX.

The results of XELJANZ-treated patients achieving ACR20 responses in Studies 1 and 2 are shown in Figure 4. Although a dose-response relationship was observed in Study 1, the proportion of patients with an ACR20 response did not clearly differ between the 10 mg and 15 mg doses. In Study 2, a smaller proportion of patients achieved an ACR20 response in the placebo and XELJANZ 1 mg groups compared to patients treated with the other XELJANZ doses. However, there was no difference in the proportion of responders among patients treated with XELJANZ 3, 5, 10, 15 mg twice daily or 20 mg once daily doses.

Figure 4: Proportion of Patients with ACR20 Response at Month 3 in Dose-Ranging Studies 1 and 2

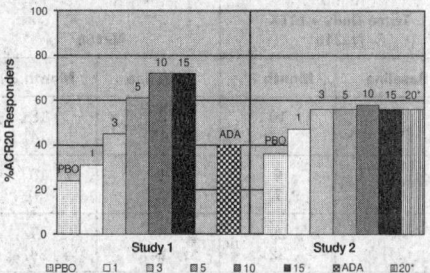

* XELJANZ twice daily dosing in mg, except for 20 mg which is once daily dosing in mg. PBO is placebo; ADA is adalimumab 40 mg subcutaneous injection every other week.

Study 1 was a dose-ranging monotherapy trial not designed to provide comparative effectiveness data and should not be interpreted as evidence of superiority to adalimumab.

Confirmatory Trials
Study I was a 6-month monotherapy trial in which 610 patients with moderate to severe active rheumatoid arthritis who had an inadequate response to a DMARD (nonbiologic or biologic) received XELJANZ 5 or 10 mg twice daily or placebo. At the Month 3 visit, all patients randomized to placebo treatment were advanced in a blinded fashion to a second predetermined treatment of XELJANZ 5 or 10 mg twice daily. The primary endpoints at Month 3 were the proportion of patients who achieved an ACR20 response, changes

in Health Assessment Questionnaire – Disability Index (HAQ-DI), and rates of Disease Activity Score DAS28-4(ESR) less than 2.6.

Study II was a 12-month trial in which 792 patients with moderate to severe active rheumatoid arthritis who had an inadequate response to a nonbiologic DMARD received XELJANZ 5 or 10 mg twice daily or placebo added to background DMARD treatment (excluding potent immunosuppressive treatments such as azathioprine or cyclosporine). At the Month 3 visit, nonresponding patients were advanced in a blinded fashion to a second predetermined treatment of XELJANZ 5 or 10 mg twice daily. At the end of Month 6, all placebo patients were advanced to their second predetermined treatment in a blinded fashion. The primary endpoints were the proportion of patients who achieved an ACR20 response at Month 6, changes in HAQ-DI at Month 3, and rates of DAS28-4(ESR) less than 2.6 at Month 6.

Study III was a 12-month trial in 717 patients with moderate to severe active rheumatoid arthritis who had an inadequate response to MTX. Patients received XELJANZ 5 or 10 mg twice daily, adalimumab 40 mg subcutaneously every other week, or placebo added to background MTX. Placebo patients were advanced as in Study II. The primary endpoints were the proportion of patients who achieved an ACR20 response at Month 6, HAQ-DI at Month 3, and DAS28-4(ESR) less than 2.6 at Month 6.

Study IV was a 2-year trial with a planned analysis at 1 year in which 797 patients with moderate to severe active rheumatoid arthritis who had an inadequate response to MTX received XELJANZ 5 or 10 mg twice daily or placebo added to background MTX. Placebo patients were advanced as in Study II. The primary endpoints were the proportion of patients who achieved an ACR20 response at Month 6, mean change from baseline in van der Heijde-modified total Sharp Score (mTSS) at Month 6, HAQ-DI at Month 3, and DAS28-4(ESR) less than 2.6 at Month 6.

Study V was a 6-month trial in which 399 patients with moderate to severe active rheumatoid arthritis who had an inadequate response to at least one approved TNF-inhibiting biologic agent received XELJANZ 5 or 10 mg twice daily or placebo added to background MTX. At the Month 3 visit, all patients randomized to placebo treatment were advanced in a blinded fashion to a second predetermined treatment of XELJANZ 5 or 10 mg twice daily. The primary endpoints at Month 3 were the proportion of patients who achieved an ACR20 response, HAQ-DI, and DAS28-4(ESR) less than 2.6.

Study VI was a 2-year monotherapy trial with a planned analysis at 1 year in which 952 MTX-naïve patients with moderate to severe active rheumatoid arthritis received XELJANZ 5 or 10 mg twice daily or MTX dose-titrated over 8 weeks to 20 mg weekly. The primary endpoints were mean change from baseline in van der Heijde-modified Total Sharp Score (mTSS) at Month 6 and the proportion of patients who achieved an ACR70 response at Month 6.

Clinical Response
The percentages of XELJANZ-treated patients achieving ACR20, ACR50, and ACR70 responses in Studies I, IV, and V are shown in Table 5. Similar results were observed with Studies III and III. In trials I–V, patients treated with either 5 or 10 mg twice daily XELJANZ had higher ACR20, ACR50, and ACR70 response rates versus placebo, with or without background DMARD treatment, at Month 3 and Month 6. Higher ACR20 response rates were observed within 2 weeks compared to placebo. In the 12-month trials, ACR response rates in XELJANZ-treated patients were consistent at 6 and 12 months.

[See table 5 at top of next page]

In Study IV, a greater proportion of patients treated with XELJANZ 5 mg or 10 mg twice daily plus MTX achieved a low level of disease activity as measured by a DAS28-4(ESR) less than 2.6 at 6 months compared to those treated with MTX alone (Table 6).

Table 6: Proportion of Patients with DAS28-4(ESR) Less Than 2.6 with Number of Residual Active Joints

Study IV

DAS28-4(ESR) Less Than 2.6	Placebo + MTX	XELJANZ 5 mg Twice Daily + MTX	XELJANZ 10 mg Twice Daily + MTX*
	160	321	316

Continued on next page

Table 5: Proportion of Patients with an ACR Response

	Percent of Patients								
	Monotherapy in Nonbiologic or Biologic DMARD Inadequate Responders*			MTX Inadequate Responders[†]			TNF Inhibitor Inadequate Responders[‡]		
	Study I			Study IV			Study V		
N[§]	PBO	XELJANZ 5 mg Twice Daily	XELJANZ 10 mg Twice Daily[¶]	PBO + MTX	XELJANZ 5 mg Twice Daily + MTX	XELJANZ 10 mg Twice Daily + MTX[¶]	PBO + MTX	XELJANZ 5 mg Twice Daily + MTX	XELJANZ 10 mg Twice Daily + MTX[¶]
	122	243	245	160	321	316	132	133	134
ACR20									
Month 3	26%	59%	65%	27%	55%	67%	24%	41%	48%
Month 6	NA[#]	69%	70%	25%	50%	62%	NA	51%	54%
ACR50									
Month 3	12%	31%	36%	8%	29%	37%	8%	26%	28%
Month 6	NA	42%	46%	9%	32%	44%	NA	37%	30%
ACR70									
Month 3	6%	15%	20%	3%	11%	17%	2%	14%	10%
Month 6	NA	22%	29%	1%	14%	23%	NA	16%	16%

*Inadequate response to at least one DMARD (biologic or nonbiologic) due to lack of efficacy or toxicity.
†Inadequate response to MTX defined as the presence of sufficient residual disease activity to meet the entry criteria.
‡Inadequate response to a least one TNF inhibitor due to lack of efficacy and/or intolerance.
§N is number of randomized and treated patients.
¶The recommended dose of XELJANZ is 5 mg twice daily.
#NA Not applicable, as data for placebo treatment is not available beyond 3 months in Studies I and V due to placebo advancement.

Proportion of responders at Month 6 (n)	1% (2)	6% (19)	13% (42)
Of responders, proportion with 0 active joints (n)	50% (1)	42% (8)	36% (15)
Of responders, proportion with 1 active joint (n)	0	5% (1)	17% (7)
Of responders, proportion with 2 active joints (n)	0	32% (6)	7% (3)

Of responders, proportion with 3 or more active joints (n)	50% (1)	21% (4)	40% (17)

*The recommended dose of XELJANZ is 5 mg twice daily.

The results of the components of the ACR response criteria for Study IV are shown in Table 7. Similar results were observed for XELJANZ in Studies I, II, III, V, and VI.
[See table 7 below]
[See figure 5 at top of next column]
The percent of ACR20 responders by visit for Study IV is shown in Figure 5. Similar responses were observed for XELJANZ in Studies I, II, III, V, and VI.
Radiographic Response

Table 7: Components of ACR Response at Month 3

	Study IV					
	XELJANZ 5 mg Twice Daily + MTX N=321		XELJANZ 10 mg* Twice Daily + MTX N=316		Placebo + MTX N=160	
Component (mean)[†]	Baseline	Month 3[†]	Baseline	Month 3[†]	Baseline	Month 3[†]
Number of tender joints (0–68)	24 (14)	13 (14)	23 (15)	10 (12)	23 (13)	18 (14)
Number of swollen joints (0–66)	14 (8)	6 (8)	14 (8)	6 (7)	14 (9)	10 (9)
Pain[‡]	58 (23)	34 (23)	58 (24)	29 (22)	55 (24)	47 (24)
Patient global assessment[‡]	58 (24)	35 (23)	57 (23)	29 (20)	54 (23)	47 (24)
Disability index (HAQ-DI)[§]	1.41 (0.68)	0.99 (0.65)	1.40 (0.66)	0.84 (0.64)	1.32 (0.67)	1.19 (0.68)
Physician global assessment[‡]	59 (16)	30 (19)	58 (17)	24 (17)	56 (18)	43 (22)
CRP (mg/L)	15.3 (19.0)	7.1 (19.1)	17.1 (26.9)	4.4 (8.6)	13.7 (14.9)	14.6 (18.7)

*The recommended dose of XELJANZ is 5 mg twice daily.
†Data shown is mean (Standard Deviation) at Month 3.
‡Visual analog scale: 0 = best, 100 = worst.
§Health Assessment Questionnaire Disability Index: 0 = best, 3 = worst; 20 questions; categories: dressing and grooming, arising, eating, walking, hygiene, reach, grip, and activities.

Figure 5: Percentage of ACR20 Responders by Visit for Study IV

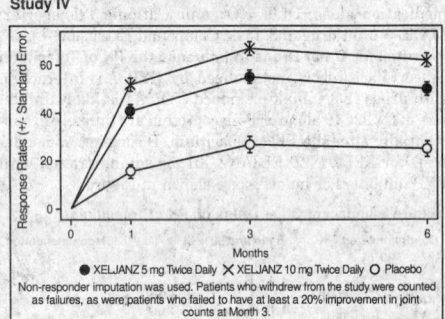

Non-responder imputation was used. Patients who withdrew from the study were counted as failures, as were patients who failed to have at least a 20% improvement in joint counts at Month 3.

- ● XELJANZ 5 mg Twice Daily ✕ XELJANZ 10 mg Twice Daily ○ Placebo

Two studies were conducted to evaluate the effect of XELJANZ on structural joint damage. In Study IV and Study VI, progression of structural joint damage was assessed radiographically and expressed as change from baseline in mTSS and its components, the erosion score and joint space narrowing score, at Months 6 and 12. The proportion of patients with no radiographic progression (mTSS change less than or equal to 0) was also assessed.

In Study IV, XELJANZ 10 mg twice daily plus background MTX reduced the progression of structural damage compared to placebo plus MTX at Month 6. When given at a dose of 5 mg twice daily, XELJANZ exhibited similar effects on mean progression of structural damage (not statistically significant). These results are shown in Table 8. Analyses of erosion and joint space narrowing scores were consistent with the overall results.

In the placebo plus MTX group, 74% of patients experienced no radiographic progression at Month 6 compared to 84% and 79% of patients treated with XELJANZ plus MTX 5 or 10 mg twice daily.

In Study VI, XELJANZ monotherapy inhibited the progression of structural damage compared to MTX at Months 6 and 12 as shown in Table 8. Analyses of erosion and joint space narrowing scores were consistent with the overall results.

In the MTX group, 55% of patients experienced no radiographic progression at Month 6 compared to 73% and 77% of patients treated with XELJANZ 5 or 10 mg twice daily.
[See table 8 at top of next page]
Physical Function Response
Improvement in physical functioning was measured by the HAQ-DI. Patients receiving XELJANZ 5 and 10 mg twice daily demonstrated greater improvement from baseline in physical functioning compared to placebo at Month 3.
The mean (95% CI) difference from placebo in HAQ-DI improvement from baseline at Month 3 in Study III was -0.22

(-0.35, -0.10) in patients receiving 5 mg XELJANZ twice daily and -0.32 (-0.44, -0.19) in patients receiving 10 mg XELJANZ twice daily. Similar results were obtained in Studies I, II, IV and V. In the 12-month trials, HAQ-DI results in XELJANZ-treated patients were consistent at 6 and 12 months.

Other Health-Related Outcomes

General health status was assessed by the Short Form health survey (SF-36). In studies I, IV, and V, patients receiving XELJANZ 5 mg twice daily or XELJANZ 10 mg twice daily demonstrated greater improvement from baseline compared to placebo in physical component summary (PCS), mental component summary (MCS) scores and in all 8 domains of the SF-36 at Month 3.

16 HOW SUPPLIED/STORAGE AND HANDLING

XELJANZ is provided as 5 mg tofacitinib (equivalent to 8 mg tofacitinib citrate) tablets: White, round, immediate-release film-coated tablets, debossed with "Pfizer" on one side, and "JKI 5" on the other side, and available in:

XELJANZ

Bottles of 28:	NDC 0069-1001-03
Bottles of 60:	NDC 0069-1001-01
Bottles of 180:	NDC 0069-1001-02

XELJANZ XR is provided as 11 mg tofacitinib (equivalent to 17.77 mg tofacitinib citrate) tablets: Pink, oval, extended release tablet with a drilled hole at one end of the tablet band and "JKI 11" printed on one side of the tablet:

XELJANZ XR

Bottles of 14:	NDC 0069-0501-14
Bottles of 30:	NDC 0069-0501-30

Storage and Handling

Store XELJANZ/XELJANZ XR at 20°C to 25°C (68°F to 77°F). [See USP Controlled Room Temperature].

XELJANZ/XELJANZ XR Do not repackage.

17 PATIENT COUNSELING INFORMATION

See FDA-approved patient labeling (Medication Guide). Advise the patient to read the FDA-approved patient labeling (Medication Guide).

Patient Counseling

Advise patients of the potential benefits and risks of XELJANZ/XELJANZ XR.

Serious Infection

Inform patients that XELJANZ/XELJANZ XR may lower the ability of their immune system to fight infections. Advise patients not to start taking XELJANZ/XELJANZ XR if they have an active infection. Instruct patients to contact their healthcare provider immediately during treatment if symptoms suggesting infection appear in order to ensure rapid evaluation and appropriate treatment [see Warnings and Precautions (5.1)].

Advise patients that the risk of herpes zoster, some cases of which can be serious, is increased in patients treated with XELJANZ [see Warnings and Precautions (5.1)].

Malignancies and Lymphoproliferative Disorders

Inform patients that XELJANZ/XELJANZ XR may increase their risk of certain cancers, and that lymphoma and other cancers have been observed in patients taking XELJANZ. Instruct patients to inform their healthcare provider if they have ever had any type of cancer [see Warnings and Precautions (5.2)].

Important Information on Laboratory Abnormalities

Inform patients that XELJANZ/XELJANZ XR may affect certain lab test results, and that blood tests are required before and during XELJANZ/XELJANZ XR treatment [see Warnings and Precautions (5.4)].

Pregnancy

Inform patients that XELJANZ/XELJANZ XR should not be used during pregnancy unless clearly necessary, and advise patients to inform their doctors right away if they become pregnant while taking XELJANZ/XELJANZ XR. Inform patients that Pfizer has a registry for pregnant women who have taken XELJANZ/XELJANZ XR during pregnancy. Advise patients to contact the registry at 1-877-311-8972 to enroll [see Use in Specific Populations (8.1)].

Residual Tablet Shell

Patients receiving XELJANZ XR may notice an inert tablet shell passing in the stool or via colostomy. Patients should be informed that the active medication has already been absorbed by the time the patient sees the inert tablet shell.

This product's label may have been updated. For current full prescribing information, please visit www.pfizer.com.

Table 8:   Radiographic Changes at Months 6 and 12

	Study IV				
	Placebo N=139 Mean (SD)[†]	XELJANZ 5 mg Twice Daily N=277 Mean (SD) [†]	XELJANZ 5 mg Twice Daily Mean Difference from Placebo[‡] (CI)	XELJANZ 10 mg Twice Daily* N=290 Mean (SD) [†]	XELJANZ 10 mg Twice Daily Mean Difference from Placebo[‡] (CI)
mTSS[§] Baseline Month 6	33 (42) 0.5 (2.0)	31 (48) 0.1 (1.7)	- -0.3 (-0.7, 0.0)	37 (54) 0.1 (2.0)	- -0.4 (-0.8, 0.0)
	Study VI				
	MTX N=166 Mean (SD)[†]	XELJANZ 5 mg Twice Daily N=346 Mean (SD) [†]	XELJANZ 5 mg Twice Daily Mean Difference from MTX[‡] (CI)	XELJANZ 10 mg Twice Daily* N=369 Mean (SD) [†]	XELJANZ 10 mg Twice Daily Mean Difference from MTX[‡] (CI)
mTSS[§] Baseline Month 6 Month 12	17 (29) 0.8 (2.7) 1.3 (3.7)	20 (40) 0.2 (2.3) 0.4 (3.0)	- -0.7 (-1.0, -0.3) -0.9 (-1.4, -0.4)	19 (39) 0.0 (1.2) 0.0 (1.5)	- -0.8 (-1.2, -0.4) -1.3 (-1.8, -0.8)

*The recommended dose of XELJANZ is 5 mg twice daily.
†SD = Standard Deviation
‡Difference between least squares means XELJANZ minus placebo or MTX (95% CI = 95% confidence interval)
§Month 6 and Month 12 data are mean change from baseline.

Distributed by
Pfizer Labs
Division of Pfizer Inc, NY, NY 10017
LAB-0445-10.0

Medication Guide
XELJANZ (ZEL' JANS')
XELJANZ XR (ZEL' JANS' EKS-AHR)
(tofacitinib)

What is the most important information I should know about XELJANZ/XELJANZ XR?
XELJANZ/XELJANZ XR may cause serious side effects including:
1. Serious infections.
XELJANZ/XELJANZ XR is a medicine that affects your immune system. XELJANZ/XELJANZ XR can lower the ability of your immune system to fight infections. Some people can have serious infections while taking XELJANZ/XELJANZ XR, including tuberculosis (TB), and infections caused by bacteria, fungi, or viruses that can spread throughout the body. Some people have died from these infections.
• Your healthcare provider should test you for TB before starting XELJANZ/XELJANZ XR.
• Your healthcare provider should monitor you closely for signs and symptoms of TB infection during treatment with XELJANZ/XELJANZ XR.
You should not start taking XELJANZ/XELJANZ XR if you have any kind of infection unless your healthcare provider tells you it is okay. You may be at a higher risk of developing shingles.
Before starting XELJANZ/XELJANZ XR, tell your healthcare provider if you:
• think you have an infection or have symptoms of an infection such as:
  ○ fever, sweating, or chills ○ muscle aches
  ○ cough ○ shortness of breath
  ○ blood in phlegm ○ weight loss
  ○ warm, red, or painful ○ diarrhea or stomach
  skin or sores on your pain
  body ○ feeling very tired
  ○ burning when you
  urinate or urinating
  more often than normal
• are being treated for an infection.
• get a lot of infections or have infections that keep coming back.
• have diabetes, HIV, or a weak immune system. People with these conditions have a higher chance for infections.
• have TB, or have been in close contact with someone with TB.
• live or have lived, or have traveled to certain parts of the country (such as the Ohio and Mississippi River valleys and the Southwest) where there is an increased chance for getting certain kinds of fungal infections (histoplasmosis, coccidioidomycosis, or blastomycosis). These infections may happen or become more severe if you use XELJANZ/XELJANZ XR. Ask your healthcare provider if you do not know if you have lived in an area where these infections are common.
• have or have had hepatitis B or C.
After starting XELJANZ/XELJANZ XR, call your healthcare provider right away if you have any symptoms of an infection. XELJANZ/XELJANZ XR can make you more likely to get infections or make worse any infection that you have.
2. Cancer and immune system problems. XELJANZ/XELJANZ XR may increase your risk of certain cancers by changing the way your immune system works.
• Lymphoma and other cancers including skin cancers can happen in patients taking XELJANZ/XELJANZ XR. Tell your healthcare provider if you have ever had any type of cancer.
• Some people who have taken XELJANZ with certain other medicines to prevent kidney transplant rejection have had a problem with certain white blood cells growing out of control (Epstein Barr Virus-associated post-transplant lymphoproliferative disorder).
3. Tears (perforation) in the stomach or intestines.
• Tell your healthcare provider if you have had diverticulitis (inflammation in parts of the large intestine) or ulcers in your stomach or intestines. Some people taking XELJANZ/XELJANZ XR can get tears in their stomach or intestines. This happens most often in people who also take nonsteroidal anti-inflammatory drugs (NSAIDs), corticosteroids, or methotrexate.
Tell your healthcare provider right away if you have fever and stomach-area pain that does not go away, and a change in your bowel habits.
4. Changes in certain laboratory test results. Your healthcare provider should do blood tests before you start receiving XELJANZ/XELJANZ XR and while you take XELJANZ/XELJANZ XR to check for the following side effects:
• **changes in lymphocyte counts.** Lymphocytes are white blood cells that help the body fight off infections.
• **low neutrophil counts.** Neutrophils are white blood cells that help the body fight off infections.
• **low red blood cell count.** This may mean that you have anemia, which may make you feel weak and tired.
Your healthcare provider should routinely check certain liver tests.
You should not receive XELJANZ/XELJANZ XR if your lymphocyte count, neutrophil count, or red blood cell count is too low or your liver tests are too high.
Your healthcare provider may stop your XELJANZ/XELJANZ XR treatment for a period of time if needed because of changes in these blood test results.
You may also have changes in other laboratory tests, such as your blood cholesterol levels. Your healthcare provider should do blood tests to check your cholesterol levels 4 to 8

Continued on next page

weeks after you start receiving XELJANZ/XELJANZ XR, and as needed after that. Normal cholesterol levels are important to good heart health.

See "What are the possible side effects of XELJANZ/XELJANZ XR?" for more information about side effects.

What is XELJANZ/XELJANZ XR?

XELJANZ/XELJANZ XR is a prescription medicine called a Janus kinase (JAK) inhibitor.

XELJANZ/XELJANZ XR is used to treat adults with moderately to severely active rheumatoid arthritis in which methotrexate did not work well.

It is not known if XELJANZ/XELJANZ XR is safe and effective in people with Hepatitis B or C.

XELJANZ/XELJANZ XR is not for people with severe liver problems.

It is not known if XELJANZ/XELJANZ XR is safe and effective in children.

What should I tell my healthcare provider before taking XELJANZ/XELJANZ XR?

XELJANZ/XELJANZ XR may not be right for you. Before taking XELJANZ/XELJANZ XR, tell your healthcare provider if you:

* have an infection. See "What is the most important information I should know about XELJANZ/XELJANZ XR?"
* have liver problems
* have kidney problems
* have any stomach area (abdominal) pain or been diagnosed with diverticulitis or ulcers in your stomach or intestines
* have had a reaction to tofacitinib or any of the ingredients in XELJANZ/XELJANZ XR
* have recently received or are scheduled to receive a vaccine. People who take XELJANZ/XELJANZ XR should not receive live vaccines. People taking XELJANZ/XELJANZ XR can receive non-live vaccines.
* have any other medical conditions.
* plan to become pregnant or are pregnant. It is not known if XELJANZ/XELJANZ XR will harm an unborn baby.
  ◦ Pregnancy Registry: Pfizer has a registry for pregnant women who take XELJANZ/XELJANZ XR. The purpose of this registry is to check the health of the pregnant mother and her baby. If you are pregnant or become pregnant while taking XELJANZ/XELJANZ XR, talk to your healthcare provider about how you can join this pregnancy registry or you may contact the registry at 1-877-311-8972 to enroll.
* plan to breastfeed or are breastfeeding. You and your healthcare provider should decide if you will take XELJANZ/XELJANZ XR or breastfeed. You should not do both.

Tell your healthcare provider about all the medicines you take, including prescription and over-the-counter medicines, vitamins, and herbal supplements. XELJANZ/XELJANZ XR and other medicines may affect each other causing side effects.

Especially tell your healthcare provider if you take:

* any other medicines to treat your rheumatoid arthritis. You should not take tocilizumab (Actemra®), etanercept (Enbrel®), adalimumab (Humira®), infliximab (Remicade®), rituximab (Rituxan®), abatacept (Orencia®), anakinra (Kineret®), certolizumab (Cimzia®), golimumab (Simponi®), azathioprine, cyclosporine, or other immunosuppressive drugs while you are taking XELJANZ or XELJANZ XR. Taking XELJANZ or XELJANZ XR with these medicines may increase your risk of infection.
* medicines that affect the way certain liver enzymes work. Ask your healthcare provider if you are not sure if your medicine is one of these.

Know the medicines you take. Keep a list of them to show your healthcare provider and pharmacist when you get a new medicine.

How should I take XELJANZ/XELJANZ XR?

* Take XELJANZ/XELJANZ XR exactly as your healthcare provider tells you to take it.
* Take XELJANZ 2 times a day with or without food.
* Take XELJANZ XR 1 time a day with or without food.
* Swallow XELJANZ XR tablets whole and intact. Do not crush, split, or chew.
* When you take XELJANZ XR, you may see something in your stool that looks like a tablet. This is the empty shell from the tablet after the medicine has been absorbed by your body.

* If you take too much XELJANZ/XELJANZ XR, call your healthcare provider or go to the nearest hospital emergency room right away.

What are possible side effects of XELJANZ/XELJANZ XR?
XELJANZ/XELJANZ XR may cause serious side effects, including:

* See "What is the most important information I should know about XELJANZ/XELJANZ XR?"
* **Hepatitis B or C activation infection** in people who carry the virus in their blood. If you are a carrier of the hepatitis B or C virus (viruses that affect the liver), the virus may become active while you use XELJANZ/XELJANZ XR. Your healthcare provider may do blood tests before you start treatment with XELJANZ and while you are using XELJANZ/XELJANZ XR. Tell your healthcare provider if you have any of the following symptoms of a possible hepatitis B or C infection:

◦ feel very tired	◦ skin or eyes look yellow
◦ little or no appetite	◦ vomiting
◦ clay-colored bowel movements	◦ fevers
◦ chills	◦ stomach discomfort
◦ muscle aches	◦ dark urine
◦ skin rash	

Common side effects of XELJANZ/XELJANZ XR include:

* upper respiratory tract infections (common cold, sinus infections)
* headache
* diarrhea
* nasal congestion, sore throat, and runny nose (nasopharyngitis)

Tell your healthcare provider if you have any side effect that bothers you or that does not go away.

These are not all the possible side effects of XELJANZ/XELJANZ XR. For more information, ask your healthcare provider or pharmacist.

Call your doctor for medical advice about side effects. You may report side effects to FDA at 1-800-FDA-1088. You may also report side effects to Pfizer at 1-800-438-1985.

How should I store XELJANZ/XELJANZ XR?

* Store XELJANZ/XELJANZ XR at room temperature between 68°F to 77°F (20°C to 25°C).
* Safely throw away medicine that is out of date or no longer needed.

Keep XELJANZ/XELJANZ XR and all medicines out of the reach of children.

General information about the safe and effective use of XELJANZ/XELJANZ XR.

Medicines are sometimes prescribed for purposes other than those listed in a Medication Guide. Do not use XELJANZ/XELJANZ XR for a condition for which it was not prescribed. Do not give XELJANZ/XELJANZ XR to other people, even if they have the same symptoms you have. It may harm them.

This Medication Guide summarizes the most important information about XELJANZ/XELJANZ XR. If you would like more information, talk to your healthcare provider. You can ask your pharmacist or healthcare provider for information about XELJANZ/XELJANZ XR that is written for health professionals.

What are the ingredients in XELJANZ?
Active ingredient: tofacitinib citrate
Inactive ingredients: microcrystalline cellulose, lactose monohydrate, croscarmellose sodium, magnesium stearate, HPMC 2910/Hypromellose 6cP, titanium dioxide, macrogol/PEG3350, and triacetin.

What are the ingredients in XELJANZ XR?
Active ingredient: tofacitinib citrate
Inactive ingredients: sorbitol, hydroxyethyl cellulose, copovidone, magnesium stearate, cellulose acetate, hydroxypropyl cellulose, HPMC 2910/Hypromellose, titanium dioxide, triacetin, and red iron oxide. Printing ink contains shellac glaze, ammonium hydroxide, propylene glycol, and ferrosoferric oxide/black iron.

Distributed by
Pfizer Labs
Division of Pfizer Inc, NY, NY 10017
LAB-0535-4.0

This Medication Guide has been approved by the U.S. Food and Drug Administration.
Revised: February 2016

Purdue Pharma L.P.
ONE STAMFORD FORUM
STAMFORD, CT 06901-3431

For Medical Inquiries:
888-726-7535
Adverse Drug Experiences:
888-726-7535
Customer Service:
800-877-5666
FAX 203-588-8850

BUTRANS®　　　　　　　　　　ⒸⅢ ℞
[*BYOO-trans*]
(buprenorphine)
Transdermal System for transdermal administration

HIGHLIGHTS OF PRESCRIBING INFORMATION
These highlights do not include all the information needed to use BUTRANS® safely and effectively. See full prescribing information for BUTRANS.
BUTRANS® (buprenorphine) Transdermal System for transdermal administration CIII
Initial U.S. Approval: 1981

> **WARNING: ADDICTION, ABUSE, and MISUSE; LIFE-THREATENING RESPIRATORY DEPRESSION; ACCIDENTAL EXPOSURE; and NEONATAL OPIOID WITHDRAWAL SYNDROME**
> *See full prescribing information for complete boxed warning.*
> * BUTRANS exposes users to risks of addiction, abuse, and misuse, which can lead to overdose and death. Assess each patient's risk before prescribing, and monitor for development of these behaviors or conditions. (5.1, 10)
> * Serious, life-threatening or fatal respiratory depression may occur. Monitor closely, especially upon initiation or following a dose increase. Instruct patients on proper administration of BUTRANS to reduce the risk. (5.2)
> * Accidental exposure to BUTRANS, especially in children, can result in fatal overdose of buprenorphine. (5.2)
> * Prolonged use of BUTRANS during pregnancy can result in neonatal opioid withdrawal syndrome, which may be life-threatening if not recognized and treated. If opioid use is required for a prolonged period in a pregnant woman, advise the patient of the risk of neonatal opioid withdrawal syndrome and ensure that appropriate treatment will be available. (5.3)

-------RECENT MAJOR CHANGES-------

Boxed Warning	04/2014
Indications and Usage (1)	04/2014
Dosage and Administration (2)	06/2014
Warnings and Precautions (5)	04/2014

-------INDICATIONS AND USAGE-------

BUTRANS is a partial opioid agonist product indicated for the management of pain severe enough to require daily, around-the-clock, long-term opioid treatment for which alternative treatment options are inadequate. (1)
Limitations of Use

* Because of the risks of addiction, abuse, and misuse with opioids, even at recommended doses, and because of the greater risks of overdose and death with extended-release opioid formulations, reserve BUTRANS for use in patients for whom alternative treatment options (e.g., non-opioid analgesics or immediate-release opioids) are ineffective, not tolerated, or would be otherwise inadequate to provide sufficient management of pain. (1)
* BUTRANS is not indicated as an as-needed (prn) analgesic. (1)

-------DOSAGE AND ADMINISTRATION-------

* BUTRANS doses of 7.5, 10, 15, and 20 mcg/hour are for opioid-experienced patients only. (2.1)
* For opioid-naïve patients, initiate with a 5 mcg/hour patch. (2.1)
* Instruct patients to wear BUTRANS for 7 days and to wait a minimum of 3 weeks before applying to the same site. (2.1)

- Do not abruptly discontinue BUTRANS in a physically dependent patient. (2.3)

————DOSAGE FORMS AND STRENGTHS————

Transdermal system: 5 mcg/hour, 7.5 mcg/hour, 10 mcg/hour, 15 mcg/hour, and 20 mcg/hour. (3)

————————CONTRAINDICATIONS————————

- Significant respiratory depression (4)
- Acute or severe bronchial asthma (4)
- Known or suspected paralytic ileus (4)
- Hypersensitivity to buprenorphine (4)

————WARNINGS AND PRECAUTIONS————

- Interactions with CNS depressants: Concomitant use may cause profound sedation, respiratory depression, and death. If coadministration is required, consider dose reduction of one or both drugs because of additive pharmacological effects. (5.4)
- Elderly, cachectic, debilitated patients, and those with chronic pulmonary disease: Monitor closely because of increased risk of respiratory depression. (5.5, 5.6)
- Avoid in patients with Long QT Syndrome, family history of Long QT Syndrome, or those taking Class IA or Class III antiarrhythmic medications. (5.7, 12.2)
- Hypotensive effects: Monitor during dose initiation and titration. (5.8)
- Patients with head injury or increased intracranial pressure: Monitor for sedation and respiratory depression and avoid use of BUTRANS in patients with impaired consciousness or coma susceptible to intracranial effects of CO_2 retention. (5.9)

————————ADVERSE REACTIONS————————

Most common adverse reactions (≥ 5%) include: nausea, headache, application site pruritus, dizziness, constipation, somnolence, vomiting, application site erythema, dry mouth, and application site rash. (6.1)

To report SUSPECTED ADVERSE REACTIONS, contact Purdue Pharma L.P. at 1-888-726-7535 or FDA at 1-800-FDA-1088 or *www.fda.gov/medwatch.*

————————DRUG INTERACTIONS————————

- Interaction with benzodiazepines: May increase buprenorphine-induced respiratory depression. Monitor patients on concurrent therapy closely. (7.1)
- CYP3A4 inhibitors/inducers: Initiating CYP3A4 inhibitors or discontinuing CYP3A4 inducers may result in an increase in buprenorphine plasma concentrations. Closely monitor patients starting CYP3A4 inhibitors or stopping CYP3A4 inducers for respiratory depression. (7.3)

————USE IN SPECIFIC POPULATIONS————

- Pregnancy: BUTRANS is not recommended for use during pregnancy. (8.1)
- Nursing Mothers: Buprenorphine has been detected in human milk. Closely monitor infants of nursing women receiving BUTRANS. (8.3)

See 17 for PATIENT COUNSELING INFORMATION and Medication Guide.

Revised: 6/2014

FULL PRESCRIBING INFORMATION: CONTENTS*
WARNING: ADDICTION, ABUSE, and MISUSE; LIFE-THREATENING RESPIRATORY DEPRESSION; ACCIDENTAL EXPOSURE; and NEONATAL OPIOID WITHDRAWAL SYNDROME

* Sections or subsections omitted from the full prescribing information are not listed.

FULL PRESCRIBING INFORMATION

> **WARNING: ADDICTION, ABUSE, and MISUSE; LIFE-THREATENING RESPIRATORY DEPRESSION; ACCIDENTAL EXPOSURE; and NEONATAL OPIOID WITHDRAWAL SYNDROME**
>
> **Addiction, Abuse, and Misuse**
> BUTRANS® exposes patients and other users to the risks of opioid addiction, abuse, and misuse, which can lead to overdose and death. Assess each patient's risk prior to prescribing BUTRANS, and monitor all patients regularly for the development of these behaviors or conditions *[see Warnings and Precautions (5.1) and Overdosage (10)]*.
> **Life-Threatening Respiratory Depression**
> Serious, life-threatening, or fatal respiratory depression may occur with use of BUTRANS. Monitor for respiratory depression, especially during initiation of BUTRANS or following a dose increase. Misuse or abuse of BUTRANS by chewing, swallowing, snorting or injecting buprenorphine extracted from the transdermal system will result in the uncontrolled delivery of buprenorphine and pose a significant risk of overdose and death *[see Warnings and Precautions (5.2)]*.
> **Accidental Exposure**
> Accidental exposure to even one dose of BUTRANS, especially by children, can result in a fatal overdose of buprenorphine *[see Warnings and Precautions (5.2)]*.
> **Neonatal Opioid Withdrawal Syndrome**
> Prolonged use of BUTRANS during pregnancy can result in neonatal opioid withdrawal syndrome, which may be life-threatening if not recognized and treated, and requires management according to protocols developed by neonatology experts. If opioid use is required for a prolonged period in a pregnant woman, advise the patient of the risk of neonatal opioid withdrawal syndrome and ensure that appropriate treatment will be available *[see Warnings and Precautions (5.3)]*.

1   INDICATIONS AND USAGE

BUTRANS is indicated for the management of pain severe enough to require daily, around-the-clock, long-term opioid treatment and for which alternative treatment options are inadequate.
Limitations of Use
- Because of the risks of addiction, abuse and misuse with opioids, even at recommended doses, and because of the greater risk of overdose and death with extended-release opioid formulations, reserve BUTRANS for use in patients for whom alternative treatment options (e.g., non-opioid analgesics or immediate-release opioids) are ineffective, not tolerated, or would be otherwise inadequate to provide sufficient management of pain.
- BUTRANS is not indicated as an as-needed (prn) analgesic

2   DOSAGE AND ADMINISTRATION
2.1   Initial Dosing
BUTRANS should be prescribed only by healthcare professionals who are knowledgeable in the use of potent opioids for the management of chronic pain.

BUTRANS doses of 7.5, 10, 15, and 20 mcg/hour are for opioid-experienced patients only.

Initiate the dosing regimen for each patient individually; take into account the patient's prior analgesic treatment experience and risk factors for addiction, abuse, and misuse *[see Warnings and Precautions (5.1)]*. Monitor patients closely for respiratory depression, especially within the first 24-72 hours of initiating therapy with BUTRANS *[see Warnings and Precautions (5.2)]*.

BUTRANS is for transdermal use (on intact skin) only. Each BUTRANS patch is intended to be worn for 7 days.

Instruct patients not to use BUTRANS if the pouch seal is broken or the patch is cut, damaged, or changed in any way and not to cut BUTRANS.

Use of BUTRANS as the First Opioid Analgesic
Initiate treatment with BUTRANS with a 5 mcg/hour patch.

Conversion from Other Opioids to BUTRANS
Discontinue all other around-the-clock opioid drugs when BUTRANS therapy is initiated.

There is a potential for buprenorphine to precipitate withdrawal in patients who are already on opioids.

Prior Total Daily Dose of Opioid Less than 30 mg of Oral Morphine Equivalents per Day:
Initiate treatment with BUTRANS 5 mcg/hour at the next dosing interval (see Table 1 below, middle column).

Prior Total Daily Dose of Opioid Between 30 mg to 80 mg of Oral Morphine Equivalents per Day:
Taper the patient's current around-the-clock opioids for up to 7 days to no more than 30 mg of morphine or equivalent per day before beginning treatment with BUTRANS. Then initiate treatment with BUTRANS 10 mcg/hour at the next dosing interval (see Table 1 below, right column). Patients may use short-acting analgesics as needed until analgesic efficacy with BUTRANS is attained.

Prior Total Daily Dose of Opioid Greater than 80 mg of Oral Morphine Equivalents per Day:
BUTRANS 20 mcg/hour may not provide adequate analgesia for patients requiring greater than 80 mg/day oral morphine equivalents. Consider the use of an alternate analgesic.

Table 1: Initial BUTRANS Dose

Previous Opioid Analgesic Daily Dose (Oral Morphine Equivalent)	<30 mg	30-80 mg
Recommended BUTRANS Starting Dose	5 mcg/ hour	10 mcg/ hour

Conversion from Methadone to BUTRANS
Close monitoring is of particular importance when converting from methadone to other opioid agonists. The ratio between methadone and other opioid agonists may vary widely as a function of previous dose exposure. Methadone has a long half-life and can accumulate in the plasma.

Continued on next page

2.2 Titration and Maintenance of Therapy

Individually titrate BUTRANS to a dose that provides adequate analgesia and minimizes adverse reactions. Continually reevaluate patients receiving BUTRANS to assess the maintenance of pain control and the relative incidence of adverse reactions, and monitor for the development of addiction, abuse, or misuse. Frequent communication is important among the prescriber, other members of healthcare team, the patient, and the caregiver/family during periods of changing analgesic requirements, including initial titration. During chronic therapy, periodically reassess the continued need for opioid analgesics.

The minimum BUTRANS titration interval is 72 hours, based on the pharmacokinetic profile and time to reach steady state levels *[see Clinical Pharmacology (12.3)]*.

The maximum BUTRANS dose is 20 mcg/hour. **Do not exceed a dose of one 20 mcg/hour BUTRANS system due to the risk of QTc interval prolongation.** In a clinical trial, BUTRANS 40 mcg/hour (given as two BUTRANS 20 mcg/hour systems) resulted in prolongation of the QTc interval *[see Warnings and Precautions (5.7) and Clinical Pharmacology (12.2)]*.

If the level of pain increases, attempt to identify the source of increased pain, while adjusting the BUTRANS dose to decrease the level of pain. Because steady-state plasma concentrations are achieved within 72 hours, BUTRANS dosage may be adjusted every 3 days. Dose adjustments may be made in 5 mcg/hour, 7.5 mcg/hour, or 10 mcg/hour increments by using no more than two patches of the 5 mcg/hour, 7.5 mcg/hour, or 10 mcg/hour system(s). The total dose from both patches should not exceed 20 mcg/hour. For the use of two patches, patients should be instructed to remove their current patch, and apply the two new patches at the same time, adjacent to one another at a different application site *[see Dosage and Administration (2.5)]*.

Patients who experience breakthrough pain may require dosage adjustment increase of BUTRANS, or may need rescue medication with an appropriate dose of an immediate-release analgesic. If the level of pain increases after dose stabilization, attempt to identify the source of increased pain before increasing the BUTRANS dose.

If unacceptable opioid-related adverse reactions are observed, the subsequent doses may be reduced. Adjust the dose to obtain an appropriate balance between the management of pain and opioid-related adverse reactions.

2.3 Cessation of Therapy

When the patient no longer requires therapy with BUTRANS, use a gradual downward titration of the dose every 7 days to prevent signs and symptoms of withdrawal in the physically dependent patient; consider introduction of an appropriate immediate-release opioid medication. Do not abruptly discontinue BUTRANS.

2.4 Patients with Hepatic Impairment

BUTRANS has not been evaluated in patients with severe hepatic impairment. As BUTRANS is only intended for 7-day application, consider use of an alternate analgesic that may permit more flexibility with the dosing in patients with severe hepatic impairment *[see Warnings and Precautions (5.10), Use in Specific Populations (8.6), and Clinical Pharmacology (12.3)]*.

2.5 Administration of BUTRANS

Instruct patients to apply immediately after removal from the individually sealed pouch. Instruct patients not to use BUTRANS if the pouch seal is broken or the patch is cut, damaged, or changed in any way. See the Instructions for Use for step-by-step instructions for applying BUTRANS.

Apply BUTRANS to the upper outer arm, upper chest, upper back or the side of the chest. These 4 sites (each present on both sides of the body) provide 8 possible application sites. Rotate BUTRANS among the 8 described skin sites. After BUTRANS removal, wait a minimum of 21 days before reapplying to the same skin site *[see Clinical Pharmacology (12.3)]*.

Apply BUTRANS to a hairless or nearly hairless skin site. If none are available, the hair at the site should be clipped, not shaven. Do not apply BUTRANS to irritated skin. If the application site must be cleaned, clean the site with water only. Do not use soaps, alcohol, oils, lotions, or abrasive devices. Allow the skin to dry before applying BUTRANS.

Incidental exposure of the BUTRANS patch to water, such as while bathing or showering is acceptable based on experience during clinical studies.

If problems with adhesion of BUTRANS occur, the edges may be taped with first aid tape. If problems with lack of adhesion continue, the patch may be covered with waterproof or semipermeable adhesive dressings suitable for 7 days of wear.

If BUTRANS falls off during the 7-day dosing interval, dispose of the transdermal system properly and place a new BUTRANS patch on at a different skin site.

When changing the system, instruct patients to remove BUTRANS and dispose of it properly *[see Dosage and Administration (2.6)]*.

If the buprenorphine-containing adhesive matrix accidentally contacts the skin, instruct patients or caregivers to wash the area with water and not to use soap, alcohol, or other solvents to remove the adhesive because they may enhance the absorption of the drug.

2.6 Disposal Instructions

Patients should refer to the Instructions for Use for proper disposal of BUTRANS. Dispose of used and unused patches by following the instructions on the Patch-Disposal Unit that is packaged with the BUTRANS patches.

Alternatively, patients can dispose of used patches by folding the adhesive side of the patch to itself, then flushing the patch down the toilet immediately upon removal. Unused patches should be removed from their pouches, the protective liners removed, the patches folded so that the adhesive side of the patch adheres to itself, and immediately flushed down the toilet.

Patients should dispose of any patches remaining from a prescription as soon as they are no longer needed.

3 DOSAGE FORMS AND STRENGTHS

BUTRANS is a rectangular or square, beige-colored system consisting of a protective liner and functional layers. BUTRANS is available in five strengths:

- BUTRANS 5 mcg/hour Transdermal System (dimensions: 45 mm by 45 mm)
- BUTRANS 7.5 mcg/hour Transdermal System (dimensions: 58 mm by 45 mm)
- BUTRANS 10 mcg/hour Transdermal System (dimensions: 45 mm by 68 mm)
- BUTRANS 15 mcg/hour Transdermal System (dimensions: 59 mm by 72 mm)
- BUTRANS 20 mcg/hour Transdermal System (dimensions: 72 mm by 72 mm)

4 CONTRAINDICATIONS

BUTRANS is contraindicated in patients with:

- Significant respiratory depression
- Acute or severe bronchial asthma in an unmonitored setting or in the absence of resuscitative equipment
- Known or suspected paralytic ileus
- Hypersensitivity (e.g., anaphylaxis) to buprenorphine *[see Warnings and Precautions (5.12) and Adverse Reactions (6)]*

5 WARNINGS AND PRECAUTIONS

5.1 Addiction, Abuse, and Misuse

BUTRANS contains buprenorphine, a Schedule III controlled substance. As an opioid, BUTRANS exposes users to the risks of addiction, abuse, and misuse. As modified-release products such as BUTRANS deliver the opioid over an extended period of time, there is a greater risk for overdose and death, due to the larger amount of buprenorphine present.

Although the risk of addiction in any individual is unknown, it can occur in patients appropriately prescribed BUTRANS and in those who obtain the drug illicitly. Addiction can occur at recommended doses and if the drug is misused or abused *[see Drug Abuse and Dependence (9)]*.

Assess each patient's risk for opioid addiction, abuse, or misuse prior to prescribing BUTRANS, and monitor all patients receiving BUTRANS for the development of these behaviors or conditions. Risks are increased in patients with a personal or family history of substance abuse (including drug or alcohol abuse or addiction) or mental illness (e.g., major depression). The potential for these risks should not, however, prevent the proper management of pain in any given patient. Patients at increased risk may be prescribed modified-release opioid formulations such as BUTRANS, but use in such patients necessitates intensive counseling about the risks and proper use of BUTRANS, along with intensive monitoring for signs of addiction, abuse, or misuse. Abuse or misuse of BUTRANS by placing it in the mouth, chewing it, swallowing it, or using it in ways other than indicated may cause choking, overdose and death *[see Overdosage (10)]*.

Opioid agonists such as BUTRANS are sought by drug abusers and people with addiction disorders and are subject to criminal diversion. Consider these risks when prescribing or dispensing BUTRANS. Strategies to reduce these risks include prescribing the drug in the smallest appropriate quantity and advising the patient on the proper disposal of unused drug *[see Patient Counseling Information (17)]*. Contact local state professional licensing board or state controlled substances authority for information on how to prevent and detect abuse or diversion of this product.

5.2 Life-Threatening Respiratory Depression

Serious, life-threatening, or fatal respiratory depression has been reported with the use of modified-release opioids, even when used as recommended. Respiratory depression, from opioid use, if not immediately recognized and treated, may lead to respiratory arrest and death. Management of respiratory depression may include close observation, supportive measures, and use of opioid antagonists, depending on the patient's clinical status *[see Overdosage (10)]*. Carbon dioxide (CO_2) retention from opioid-induced respiratory depression can exacerbate the sedating effects of opioids.

While serious, life-threatening, or fatal respiratory depression can occur at any time during the use of BUTRANS, the risk is greatest during the initiation of therapy or following a dose increase. Closely monitor patients for respiratory depression when initiating therapy with BUTRANS and following dose increases.

To reduce the risk of respiratory depression, proper dosing and titration of BUTRANS are essential *[see Dosage and Administration (2)]*. Overestimating the BUTRANS dose when converting patients from another opioid product can result in fatal overdose with the first dose.

Accidental exposure to BUTRANS, especially in children, can result in respiratory depression and death due to an overdose of buprenorphine.

5.3 Neonatal Opioid Withdrawal Syndrome

Prolonged use of BUTRANS during pregnancy can result in withdrawal signs in the neonate. Neonatal opioid withdrawal syndrome, unlike opioid withdrawal syndrome in adults, may be life-threatening if not recognized and treated, and requires management according to protocols developed by neonatology experts. If opioid use is required for a prolonged period in a pregnant woman, advise the patient of the risk of neonatal opioid withdrawal syndrome and ensure that appropriate treatment will be available.

Neonatal opioid withdrawal syndrome presents as irritability, hyperactivity and abnormal sleep pattern, high pitched cry, tremor, vomiting, diarrhea and failure to gain weight. The onset, duration, and severity of neonatal opioid withdrawal syndrome vary based on the specific opioid used, duration of use, timing and amount of last maternal use, and rate of elimination of the drug by the newborn.

5.4 Interactions with Central Nervous System Depressants

Hypotension, profound sedation, coma, respiratory depression, and death may result if BUTRANS is used concomitantly with alcohol or other (CNS) depressants (e.g., sedatives, anxiolytics, hypnotics, neuroleptics, other opioids).

When considering the use of BUTRANS in a patient taking a CNS depressant, assess the duration of use of the CNS depressant and the patient's response, including the degree of tolerance that has developed to CNS depression. Additionally, evaluate the patient's use of alcohol or illicit drugs that cause CNS depression. If the decision to begin BUTRANS therapy is made, start with BUTRANS 5 mcg/hour patch, monitor patients for signs of sedation and respiratory depression and consider using a lower dose of the concomitant CNS depressant *[see Drug Interactions (7.2)]*.

5.5 Use in Elderly, Cachectic, and Debilitated Patients

Life-threatening respiratory depression is more likely to occur in elderly, cachectic, or debilitated patients as they may have altered pharmacokinetics or altered clearance compared to younger, healthier patients. Monitor such patients closely, particularly when initiating and titrating BUTRANS and when BUTRANS is given concomitantly with other drugs that depress respiration *[see Warnings and Precautions (5.2)]*.

5.6 Use in Patients with Chronic Pulmonary Disease

Monitor patients with significant chronic obstructive pulmonary disease or cor pulmonale, and patients having a substantially decreased respiratory reserve, hypoxia, hypercapnia, or pre-existing respiratory depression for respiratory depression, particularly when initiating therapy and titrating with BUTRANS, as in these patients, even usual therapeutic doses of BUTRANS may decrease respiratory drive to the point of apnea *[see Warnings and Precautions (5.2)]*. Consider the use of alternative non-opioid analgesics in these patients if possible.

5.7 QTc Prolongation

A positive-controlled study of the effects of BUTRANS on the QTc interval in healthy subjects demonstrated no clinically meaningful effect at a BUTRANS dose of 10 mcg/hour; however, a BUTRANS dose of 40 mcg/hour (given as two BUTRANS 20 mcg/hour Transdermal Systems) was observed to prolong the QTc interval *[see Dosage and Administration (2.2) and Clinical Pharmacology (12.2)]*.

Consider these observations in clinical decisions when prescribing BUTRANS to patients with hypokalemia or clinically unstable cardiac disease, including: unstable atrial fibrillation, symptomatic bradycardia, unstable congestive heart failure, or active myocardial ischemia. Avoid the use of BUTRANS in patients with a history of Long QT Syndrome or an immediate family member with this condition, or those taking Class IA antiarrhythmic medications (e.g., quinidine, procainamide, disopyramide) or Class III antiarrhythmic medications (e.g., sotalol, amiodarone, dofetilide).

5.8 Hypotensive Effects

BUTRANS may cause severe hypotension including orthostatic hypotension and syncope in ambulatory patients. There is an increased risk in patients whose ability to maintain blood pressure has already been compromised by a reduced blood volume or concurrent administration of certain CNS depressant drugs (e.g., phenothiazines or general anesthetics) *[see Drug Interactions (7.2)]*. Monitor these patients for signs of hypotension after initiating or titrating the dose of BUTRANS.

5.9 Use in Patients with Head Injury or Increased Intracranial Pressure

Monitor patients taking BUTRANS who may be susceptible to the intracranial effects of CO_2 retention (e.g., those with evidence of increased intracranial pressure or brain tumors) for signs of sedation and respiratory depression, particularly when initiating therapy with BUTRANS. BUTRANS may reduce respiratory drive, and the resultant CO_2 retention can further increase intracranial pressure. Opioids may also obscure the clinical course in a patient with a head injury.

Avoid the use of BUTRANS in patients with impaired consciousness or coma.

5.10 Hepatotoxicity

Although not observed in BUTRANS chronic pain clinical trials, cases of cytolytic hepatitis and hepatitis with jaundice have been observed in individuals receiving sublingual buprenorphine for the treatment of opioid dependence, both in clinical trials and in post-marketing adverse event reports. The spectrum of abnormalities ranges from transient asymptomatic elevations in hepatic transaminases to case reports of hepatic failure, hepatic necrosis, hepatorenal syndrome, and hepatic encephalopathy. In many cases, the presence of pre-existing liver enzyme abnormalities, infection with hepatitis B or hepatitis C virus, concomitant usage of other potentially hepatotoxic drugs, and ongoing injection drug abuse may have played a causative or contributory role. For patients at increased risk of hepatotoxicity (e.g., patients with a history of excessive alcohol intake, intravenous drug abuse or liver disease), obtain baseline liver enzyme levels and monitor periodically and during treatment with BUTRANS.

5.11 Application Site Skin Reactions

In rare cases, severe application site skin reactions with signs of marked inflammation including "burn," "discharge," and "vesicles" have occurred. Time of onset varies, ranging from days to months following the initiation of BUTRANS treatment. Instruct patients to promptly report the development of severe application site reactions and discontinue therapy.

5.12 Anaphylactic/Allergic Reactions

Cases of acute and chronic hypersensitivity to buprenorphine have been reported both in clinical trials and in the post-marketing experience. The most common signs and symptoms include rashes, hives, and pruritus. Cases of bronchospasm, angioneurotic edema, and anaphylactic shock have been reported. A history of hypersensitivity to buprenorphine is a contraindication to the use of BUTRANS.

5.13 Application of External Heat

Advise patients and their caregivers to avoid exposing the BUTRANS application site and surrounding area to direct external heat sources, such as heating pads or electric blankets, heat or tanning lamps, saunas, hot tubs, and heated water beds while wearing the system because an increase in absorption of buprenorphine may occur *[see Clinical Pharmacology (12.3)]*. Advise patients against exposure of the BUTRANS application site and surrounding area to hot water or prolonged exposure to direct sunlight. There is a potential for temperature-dependent increases in buprenorphine released from the system resulting in possible overdose and death.

5.14 Patients with Fever

Monitor patients wearing BUTRANS systems who develop fever or increased core body temperature due to strenuous exertion for opioid side effects and adjust the BUTRANS dose if signs of respiratory or central nervous system depression occur.

5.15 Use in Patients with Gastrointestinal Conditions

BUTRANS is contraindicated in patients with paralytic ileus. Avoid the use of BUTRANS in patients with other GI obstruction.

The buprenorphine in BUTRANS may cause spasm of the sphincter of Oddi. Monitor patients with biliary tract disease, including acute pancreatitis, for worsening symptoms. Opioids may cause increases in the serum amylase.

5.16 Use in Patients with Convulsive or Seizure Disorders

The buprenorphine in BUTRANS may aggravate convulsions in patients with convulsive disorders, and may induce or aggravate seizures in some clinical settings. Monitor patients with a history of seizure disorders for worsened seizure control during BUTRANS therapy.

5.17 Driving and Operating Machinery

BUTRANS may impair the mental and physical abilities needed to perform potentially hazardous activities such as driving a car or operating machinery. Warn patients not to drive or operate dangerous machinery unless they are tolerant to the effects of BUTRANS and know how they will react to the medication.

5.18 Use in Addiction Treatment

BUTRANS has not been studied and is not approved for use in the management of addictive disorders.

6 ADVERSE REACTIONS

The following serious adverse reactions are described elsewhere in the labeling:

- Addiction, Abuse, and Misuse *[see Warnings and Precautions (5.1)]*
- Life-Threatening Respiratory Depression *[see Warnings and Precautions (5.2)]*
- QTc Prolongation *[see Warnings and Precautions (5.7)]*
- Neonatal Opioid Withdrawal Syndrome *[see Warnings and Precautions (5.3)]*
- Hypotensive Effects *[see Warnings and Precautions (5.8)]*
- Interactions with Other CNS Depressants *[see Warnings and Precautions (5.4)]*
- Application Site Skin Reactions *[see Warnings and Precautions (5.11)]*
- Anaphylactic/Allergic Reactions *[see Warnings and Precautions (5.12)]*
- Gastrointestinal Effects *[see Warnings and Precautions (5.15)]*
- Seizures *[see Warnings and Precautions (5.16)]*

6.1 Clinical Trial Experience

Because clinical trials are conducted under widely varying conditions, adverse reaction rates observed in the clinical trials of a drug cannot be directly compared to rates in the clinical trials of another drug and may not reflect the rates observed in practice.

A total of 5,415 patients were treated with BUTRANS in controlled and open-label chronic pain clinical trials. Nine hundred twenty-four subjects were treated for approximately six months and 183 subjects were treated for approximately one year. The clinical trial population consisted of patients with persistent moderate to severe pain.

The most common serious adverse drug reactions (all <0.1%) occurring during clinical trials with BUTRANS were: chest pain, abdominal pain, vomiting, dehydration, and hypertension/blood pressure increased.

The most common adverse events (≥ 2%) leading to discontinuation were: nausea, dizziness, vomiting, headache, and somnolence.

The most common adverse reactions (≥ 5%) reported by patients in clinical trials comparing BUTRANS 10 or 20 mcg/hour to placebo are shown in Table 2, and comparing BUTRANS 20 mcg/hour to BUTRANS 5 mcg/hour are shown in Table 3 below:

Table 2: Adverse Reactions Reported in ≥ 5% of Patients during the Open-Label Titration Period and Double-Blind Treatment Period: Opioid-Naïve Patients

MedDRA Preferred Term	Open-Label Titration Period BUTRANS	Double-Blind Treatment Period	
		BUTRANS	Placebo
	(N = 1024)	(N = 256)	(N = 283)
Nausea	23%	13%	10%
Dizziness	10%	4%	1%
Headache	9%	5%	5%
Application site pruritus	8%	4%	7%
Somnolence	8%	2%	2%
Vomiting	7%	4%	1%
Constipation	6%	4%	1%

Table 3: Adverse Reactions Reported in ≥ 5% of Patients during the Open-Label Titration Period and Double-Blind Treatment Period: Opioid-Experienced Patients

MedDRA Preferred Term	Open-Label Titration Period BUTRANS	Double-Blind Treatment Period	
		BUTRANS 20	BUTRANS 5
	(N = 1160)	(N = 219)	(N = 221)
Nausea	14%	11%	6%
Application site pruritus	9%	13%	5%
Headache	9%	8%	3%
Somnolence	6%	4%	2%
Dizziness	5%	4%	2%
Constipation	4%	6%	3%
Application site erythema	3%	10%	5%
Application site rash	3%	8%	6%
Application site irritation	2%	6%	2%

The following table lists adverse reactions that were reported in at least 2.0% of patients in four placebo/active-controlled titration-to-effect trials.

Table 4: Adverse Reactions Reported in Titration-to-Effect Placebo/Active-Controlled Clinical Trials with Incidence ≥ 2%

MedDRA Preferred Term	BUTRANS (N = 392)	Placebo (N = 261)
Nausea	21%	6%
Application site pruritus	15%	12%
Dizziness	15%	7%
Headache	14%	9%
Somnolence	13%	4%
Constipation	13%	5%
Vomiting	9%	1%
Application site erythema	7%	2%
Application site rash	6%	6%
Dry mouth	6%	2%
Fatigue	5%	1%
Hyperhidrosis	4%	1%
Peripheral edema	3%	1%
Pruritus	3%	0%
Stomach discomfort	2%	0%

The adverse reactions seen in controlled and open-label studies are presented below in the following manner: most common (≥ 5%), common (≥ 1% to < 5%), and less common (< 1%).

The most common adverse reactions (≥ 5%) reported by patients treated with BUTRANS in the clinical trials were nausea, headache, application site pruritus, dizziness, constipation, somnolence, vomiting, application site erythema, dry mouth, and application site rash.

The common (≥ 1% to < 5%) adverse reactions reported by patients treated with BUTRANS in the clinical trials organized by MedDRA (Medical Dictionary for Regulatory Activities) System Organ Class were:

Continued on next page

Gastrointestinal disorders: diarrhea, dyspepsia, and upper abdominal pain

General disorders and administration site conditions: fatigue, peripheral edema, application site irritation, pain, pyrexia, chest pain, and asthenia

Infections and infestations: urinary tract infection, upper respiratory tract infection, nasopharyngitis, influenza, sinusitis, and bronchitis

Injury, poisoning and procedural complications: fall

Metabolism and nutrition disorders: anorexia

Musculoskeletal and connective tissue disorders: back pain, arthralgia, pain in extremity, muscle spasms, musculoskeletal pain, joint swelling, neck pain, and myalgia

Nervous system disorders: hypoesthesia, tremor, migraine, and paresthesia

Psychiatric disorders: insomnia, anxiety, and depression

Respiratory, thoracic and mediastinal disorders: dyspnea, pharyngolaryngeal pain, and cough

Skin and subcutaneous tissue disorders: pruritus, hyperhidrosis, rash, and generalized pruritus

Vascular disorders: hypertension

Other less common adverse reactions, including those known to occur with opioid treatment, that were seen in < 1% of the patients in the BUTRANS trials include the following in alphabetical order:

Abdominal distention, abdominal pain, accidental injury, affect lability, agitation, alanine aminotransferase increased, angina pectoris, angioedema, apathy, application site dermatitis, asthma aggravated, bradycardia, chills, confusional state, contact dermatitis, coordination abnormal, dehydration, depersonalization, depressed level of consciousness, depressed mood, disorientation, disturbance in attention, diverticulitis, drug hypersensitivity, drug withdrawal syndrome, dry eye, dry skin, dysarthria, dysgeusia, dysphagia, euphoric mood, face edema, flatulence, flushing, gait disturbance, hallucination, hiccups, hot flush, hyperventilation, hypotension, hypoventilation, ileus, insomnia, libido decreased, loss of consciousness, malaise, memory impairment, mental impairment, mental status changes, miosis, muscle weakness, nervousness, nightmare, orthostatic hypotension, palpitations, psychotic disorder, respiration abnormal, respiratory depression, respiratory distress, respiratory failure, restlessness, rhinitis, sedation, sexual dysfunction, syncope, tachycardia, tinnitus, urinary hesitation, urinary incontinence, urinary retention, urticaria, vasodilatation, vertigo, vision blurred, visual disturbance, weight decreased, and wheezing.

7 DRUG INTERACTIONS

7.1 Benzodiazepines

There have been a number of reports regarding coma and death associated with the misuse and abuse of the combination of buprenorphine and benzodiazepines. In many, but not all of these cases, buprenorphine was misused by self-injection of crushed buprenorphine tablets. Preclinical studies have shown that the combination of benzodiazepines and buprenorphine altered the usual ceiling effect on buprenorphine-induced respiratory depression, making the respiratory effects of buprenorphine appear similar to those of full opioid agonists. Closely monitor patients with concurrent use of BUTRANS and benzodiazepines. Warn patients that it is extremely dangerous to self-administer benzodiazepines while taking BUTRANS, and warn patients to use benzodiazepines concurrently with BUTRANS only as directed by their physician.

7.2 CNS Depressants

The concomitant use of BUTRANS with other CNS depressants including sedatives, hypnotics, tranquilizers, general anesthetics, phenothiazines, other opioids, and alcohol can increase the risk of respiratory depression, profound sedation, coma and death. Monitor patients receiving CNS depressants and BUTRANS for signs of respiratory depression, sedation, and hypotension. When combined therapy with any of the above medications is considered, the dose of one or both agents should be reduced *[see Dosage and Administration (2.2) and Warnings and Precautions (5.4)].*

7.3 Drugs Affecting Cytochrome P450 Isoenzymes

Inhibitors of CYP3A4 and 2D6

Because the CYP3A4 isoenzyme plays a major role in the metabolism of buprenorphine, drugs that inhibit CYP3A4 activity may cause decreased clearance of buprenorphine which could lead to an increase in buprenorphine plasma concentrations and result in increased or prolonged opioid effects. These effects could be more pronounced with concomitant use of CYP2D6 and 3A4 inhibitors. If co-administration with BUTRANS is necessary, monitor patients for respiratory depression and sedation at frequent intervals and consider dose adjustments until stable drug effects are achieved *[see Clinical Pharmacology (12.3)].*

Inducers of CYP3A4

CYP450 3A4 inducers may induce the metabolism of buprenorphine and, therefore, may cause increased clearance of the drug which could lead to a decrease in buprenorphine plasma concentrations, lack of efficacy or, possibly, development of an abstinence syndrome in a patient who had developed physical dependence to buprenorphine.

After stopping the treatment of a CYP3A4 inducer, as the effects of the inducer decline, the buprenorphine plasma concentration will increase which could increase or prolong both the therapeutic and adverse effects, and may cause serious respiratory depression. If co-administration or discontinuation of a CYP3A4 inducer with BUTRANS is necessary, monitor for signs of opioid withdrawal and consider dose adjustments until stable drug effects are achieved *[see Clinical Pharmacology (12.3)].*

7.4 Muscle Relaxants

Buprenorphine may enhance the neuromuscular blocking action of skeletal muscle relaxants and produce an increased degree of respiratory depression. Monitor patients receiving muscle relaxants and BUTRANS for signs of respiratory depression that may be greater than otherwise expected.

7.5 Anticholinergics

Anticholinergics or other drugs with anticholinergic activity when used concurrently with opioid analgesics may result in increased risk of urinary retention and/or severe constipation, which may lead to paralytic ileus. Monitor patients for signs of urinary retention or reduced gastric motility when BUTRANS is used concurrently with anticholinergic drugs.

8 USE IN SPECIFIC POPULATIONS

8.1 Pregnancy

Clinical Considerations

Fetal/neonatal adverse reactions

Prolonged use of opioid analgesics during pregnancy for medical or nonmedical purposes can result in physical dependence in the neonate and neonatal opioid withdrawal syndrome shortly after birth. Observe newborns for symptoms of neonatal opioid withdrawal syndrome, such as poor feeding, diarrhea, irritability, tremor, rigidity, and seizures, and manage accordingly *[see Warnings and Precautions (5.3)].*

Teratogenic Effects - Pregnancy Category C

There are no adequate and well-controlled studies in pregnant women. BUTRANS should be used during pregnancy only if the potential benefit justifies the potential risk to the fetus.

In animal studies, buprenorphine caused an increase in the number of stillborn offspring, reduced litter size, and reduced offspring growth in rats at maternal exposure levels that were approximately 10 times that of human subjects who received one BUTRANS 20 mcg/hour, the maximum recommended human dose (MRHD).

Studies in rats and rabbits demonstrated no evidence of teratogenicity following BUTRANS or subcutaneous (SC) administration of buprenorphine during the period of major organogenesis. Rats were administered up to one BUTRANS 20 mcg/hour every 3 days (gestation days 6, 9, 12, & 15) or received daily SC buprenorphine up to 5 mg/kg (gestation days 6-17). Rabbits were administered four BUTRANS 20 mcg/hour every 3 days (gestation days 6, 9, 12, 15, 18, & 19) or received daily SC buprenorphine up to 5 mg/kg (gestation days 6-19). No teratogenicity was observed at any dose. AUC values for buprenorphine with BUTRANS application and SC injection were approximately 110 and 140 times, respectively, that of human subjects who received the MRHD of one BUTRANS 20 mcg/hour.

Non-Teratogenic Effects

In a peri- and post-natal study conducted in pregnant and lactating rats, administration of buprenorphine either as BUTRANS or SC buprenorphine was associated with toxicity to offspring. Buprenorphine was present in maternal milk. Pregnant rats were administered 1/4 of one BUTRANS 5 mcg/hour every 3 days or received daily SC buprenorphine at doses of 0.05, 0.5, or 5 mg/kg from gestation day 6 to lactation day 21 (weaning). Administration of BUTRANS or SC buprenorphine at 0.5 or 5 mg/kg caused maternal toxicity and an increase in the number of stillborns, reduced litter size, and reduced offspring growth at maternal exposure levels that were approximately 10 times that of human subjects who received the MRHD of one BUTRANS 20 mcg/hour. Maternal toxicity was also observed at the no observed adverse effect level (NOAEL) for offspring.

8.2 Labor and Delivery

Opioids cross the placenta and may produce respiratory depression in neonates. BUTRANS is not for use in women during and immediately prior to labor, when shorter acting analgesics or other analgesic techniques are more appropriate. Opioid analgesics can prolong labor through actions that temporarily reduce the strength, duration, and frequency of uterine contractions. However this effect is not consistent and may be offset by an increased rate of cervical dilatation, which tends to shorten labor.

8.3 Nursing Mothers

Buprenorphine is excreted in breast milk. The amount of buprenorphine received by the infant varies depending on the maternal plasma concentration, the amount of milk ingested by the infant, and the extent of first pass metabolism.

Withdrawal symptoms can occur in breast-feeding infants when maternal administration of buprenorphine is stopped. Because of the potential for adverse reactions in nursing infants from BUTRANS, a decision should be made whether to discontinue nursing or discontinue the drug, taking into account the importance of the drug to the mother.

8.4 Pediatric Use

The safety and efficacy of BUTRANS in patients under 18 years of age has not been established.

8.5 Geriatric Use

Of the total number of subjects in the clinical trials (5,415), BUTRANS was administered to 1,377 patients aged 65 years and older. Of those, 457 patients were 75 years of age and older. In the clinical program, the incidences of selected BUTRANS-related AEs were higher in older subjects. The incidences of application site AEs were slightly higher among subjects < 65 years of age than those ≥ 65 years of age for both BUTRANS and placebo treatment groups.

In a single-dose study of healthy elderly and healthy young subjects treated with BUTRANS 10 mcg/hour, the pharmacokinetics were similar. In a separate dose-escalation safety study, the pharmacokinetics in the healthy elderly and hypertensive elderly subjects taking thiazide diuretics were similar to those in the healthy young adults. In the elderly groups evaluated, adverse event rates were similar to or lower than rates in healthy young adult subjects, except for constipation and urinary retention, which were more common in the elderly. Although specific dose adjustments on the basis of advanced age are not required for pharmacokinetic reasons, use caution in the elderly population to ensure safe use *[see Clinical Pharmacology (12.3)].*

8.6 Hepatic Impairment

In a study utilizing intravenous buprenorphine, peak plasma levels (C_{max}) and exposure (AUC) of buprenorphine in patients with mild and moderate hepatic impairment did not increase as compared to those observed in subjects with normal hepatic function. BUTRANS has not been evaluated in patients with severe hepatic impairment. As BUTRANS is intended for 7-day dosing, consider the use of alternate analgesic therapy in patients with severe hepatic impairment *[see Dosage and Administration (2.4) and Clinical Pharmacology (12.3)].*

9 DRUG ABUSE AND DEPENDENCE

9.1 Controlled Substance

BUTRANS contains buprenorphine, a Schedule III controlled substance with an abuse potential similar to other Schedule III opioids. BUTRANS can be abused and is subject to misuse, addiction and criminal diversion *[see Warnings and Precautions (5.1)].*

9.2 Abuse

All patients treated with opioids require careful monitoring for signs of abuse and addiction, since use of opioid analgesic products carries the risk of addiction even under appropriate medical use.

Drug abuse is the intentional non-therapeutic use of an over-the-counter or prescription drug, even once, for its rewarding psychological or physiological effects. Drug abuse includes, but is not limited to the following examples: the use of a prescription or over-the-counter drug to get "high", or the use of steroids for performance enhancement and muscle build up.

Drug addiction is a cluster of behavioral, cognitive, and physiological phenomena that develop after repeated substance use and includes: a strong desire to take the drug, difficulties in controlling its use, persisting in its use despite harmful consequences, a higher priority given to drug use than to other activities and obligations, increased tolerance, and sometimes a physical withdrawal.

"Drug-seeking" behavior is very common to addicts and drug abusers. Drug-seeking tactics include emergency calls or visits near the end of office hours, refusal to undergo appropriate examination, testing or referral, repeated claims of loss of prescriptions, tampering with prescriptions and reluctance to provide prior medical records or contact information for other treating physician(s). "Doctor shopping" (visiting multiple prescribers) to obtain additional prescriptions is common among drug abusers and people suffering from untreated addiction. Preoccupation with achieving adequate pain relief can be appropriate behavior in a patient with poor pain control.

Abuse and addiction are separate and distinct from physical dependence and tolerance. Physicians should be aware that addiction may not be accompanied by concurrent tolerance and symptoms of physical dependence in all addicts. In addition, abuse of opioids can occur in the absence of true addiction.

BUTRANS, like other opioids, can be diverted for non-medical use into illicit channels of distribution. Careful record-keeping of prescribing information, including quantity, frequency, and renewal requests, as required by state law, is strongly advised.

Proper assessment of the patient, proper prescribing practices, periodic re-evaluation of therapy, and proper dispensing and storage are appropriate measures that help to reduce abuse of opioid drugs.

Risks Specific to the Abuse of BUTRANS

BUTRANS is intended for transdermal use only. Abuse of BUTRANS poses a risk of overdose and death. This risk is increased with concurrent abuse of BUTRANS with alcohol and other substances including other opioids and benzodiazepines *[see Warnings and Precautions (5.4) and Drug Interactions (7.2)]*. Intentional compromise of the transdermal delivery system will result in the uncontrolled delivery of buprenorphine and pose a significant risk to the abuser that could result in overdose and death *[see Warnings and Precautions (5.1)]*. Abuse may occur by applying the transdermal system in the absence of legitimate purpose, or by swallowing, snorting, or injecting buprenorphine extracted from the transdermal system.

9.3 Dependence

Both tolerance and physical dependence can develop during chronic opioid therapy. Tolerance is the need for increasing doses of opioids to maintain a defined effect such as analgesia (in the absence of disease progression or other external factors). Tolerance may occur to both the desired and undesired effects of drugs, and may develop at different rates for different effects.

Physical dependence results in withdrawal symptoms after abrupt discontinuation or a significant dose reduction of a drug. Withdrawal also may be precipitated through the administration of drugs with opioid antagonist activity, e.g., naloxone, nalmefene, or mixed agonist/antagonist analgesics (pentazocine, butorphanol, nalbuphine). Physical dependence may not occur to a clinically significant degree until after several days to weeks of continued opioid usage.

BUTRANS should not be abruptly discontinued *[see Dosage and Administration (2.3)]*. If BUTRANS is abruptly discontinued in a physically-dependent patient, an abstinence syndrome may occur. Some or all of the following can characterize this syndrome: restlessness, lacrimation, rhinorrhea, yawning, perspiration, chills, myalgia, and mydriasis. Other signs and symptoms also may develop, including: irritability, anxiety, backache, joint pain, weakness, abdominal cramps, insomnia, nausea, anorexia, vomiting, diarrhea, or increased blood pressure, respiratory rate, or heart rate.

Infants born to mothers physically dependent on opioids will also be physically dependent and may exhibit respiratory difficulties and withdrawal symptoms *[see Use in Specific Populations (8.1)]*.

10 OVERDOSAGE

Clinical Presentation

Acute overdosage with BUTRANS is manifested by respiratory depression, somnolence progressing to stupor or coma, skeletal muscle flaccidity, cold and clammy skin, constricted pupils, bradycardia, hypotension, partial or complete airway obstruction, atypical snoring and death. Marked mydriasis rather than miosis may be seen due to severe hypoxia in overdose situations.

Treatment of Overdose

In case of overdose, priorities are the re-establishment of a patent and protected airway and institution of assisted or controlled ventilation if needed. Employ other supportive measures (including oxygen, vasopressors) in the management of circulatory shock and pulmonary edema as indicated. Cardiac arrest or arrhythmias will require advanced life support techniques.

Naloxone may not be effective in reversing any respiratory depression produced by buprenorphine. High doses of naloxone, 10-35 mg/70 kg, may be of limited value in the management of buprenorphine overdose. The onset of naloxone effect may be delayed by 30 minutes or more. Doxapram hydrochloride (a respiratory stimulant) has also been used.

Remove BUTRANS immediately. Because the duration of reversal would be expected to be less than the duration of action of buprenorphine from BUTRANS, carefully monitor the patient until spontaneous respiration is reliably re-established. Even in the face of improvement, continued medical monitoring is required because of the possibility of extended effects as buprenorphine continues to be absorbed from the skin. After removal of BUTRANS, the mean buprenorphine concentrations decrease approximately 50% in 12 hours (range 10-24 hours) with an apparent terminal half-life of approximately 26 hours. Due to this long apparent terminal half-life, patients may require monitoring and treatment for at least 24 hours.

In an individual physically dependent on opioids, administration of an opioid receptor antagonist may precipitate an acute withdrawal. The severity of the withdrawal produced will depend on the degree of physical dependence and the dose of the antagonist administered. If a decision is made to treat serious respiratory depression in the physically dependent patient with an opioid antagonist, administration of the antagonist should be begun with care and by titration with smaller than usual doses of the antagonist.

11 DESCRIPTION

BUTRANS is a transdermal system providing systemic delivery of buprenorphine, a mu opioid partial agonist analgesic, continuously for 7 days. The chemical name of buprenorphine is 6,14-ethenomorphinan-7-methanol, 17-(cyclopropylmethyl)- α-(1,1-dimethylethyl)-4, 5-epoxy-18, 19-dihydro-3-hydroxy-6-methoxy-α-methyl-, [5α, 7α, (S)]. The structural formula is:

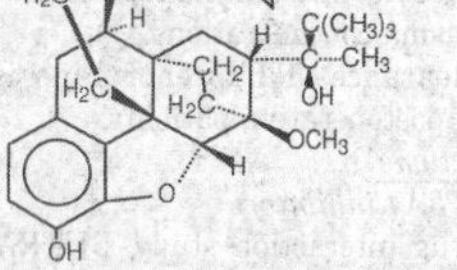

The molecular weight of buprenorphine is 467.6; the empirical formula is $C_{29}H_{41}NO_4$. Buprenorphine occurs as a white or almost white powder and is very slightly soluble in water, freely soluble in acetone, soluble in methanol and ether, and slightly soluble in cyclohexane. The pKa is 8.5 and the melting point is about 217°C.

System Components and Structure

Five different strengths of BUTRANS are available: 5, 7.5, 10, 15, and 20 mcg/hour (Table 5). The proportion of buprenorphine mixed in the adhesive matrix is the same in each of the five strengths. The amount of buprenorphine released from each system per hour is proportional to the active surface area of the system. The skin is the limiting barrier to diffusion from the system into the bloodstream.

Table 5: BUTRANS Product Specifications

Buprenorphine Delivery Rate (mcg/hour)	Active Surface Area (cm^2)	Total Buprenorphine Content (mg)
BUTRANS 5	6.25	5
BUTRANS 7.5	9.375	7.5
BUTRANS 10	12.5	10
BUTRANS 15	18.75	15
BUTRANS 20	25	20

BUTRANS is a rectangular or square, beige-colored system consisting of a protective liner and functional layers. Proceeding from the outer surface toward the surface adhering to the skin, the layers are (1) a beige-colored web backing layer; (2) an adhesive rim without buprenorphine; (3) a separating layer over the buprenorphine-containing adhesive matrix; (4) the buprenorphine-containing adhesive matrix; and (5) a peel-off release liner. Before use, the release liner covering the adhesive layer is removed and discarded.

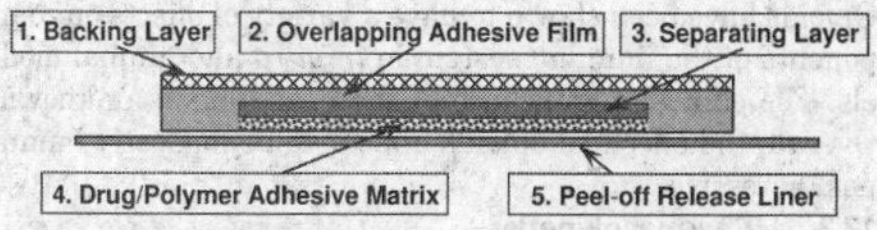

Figure 1: Cross-Section Diagram of BUTRANS (not to scale).

The active ingredient in BUTRANS is buprenorphine. The inactive ingredients in each system are: levulinic acid, oleyl oleate, povidone, and polyacrylate cross-linked with aluminum.

12 CLINICAL PHARMACOLOGY

12.1 Mechanism of Action

Buprenorphine is a partial agonist at mu opioid receptors. Buprenorphine is also an antagonist at kappa-opioid receptors, an agonist at delta-opioid receptors, and a partial agonist at ORL-1 (nociceptin) receptors. The contributions of these actions to its analgesic profile are unclear.

12.2 Pharmacodynamics

Effects on the Central Nervous System

The principal actions of therapeutic value of buprenorphine are analgesia and sedation. Specific CNS opiate receptors and endogenous compounds with morphine-like activity have been identified throughout the brain and spinal cord and are likely to play a role in the expression of analgesic effects.

Buprenorphine produces respiratory depression by direct action on brainstem respiratory centers. The mechanism of respiratory depression involves a reduction in the responsiveness of the brainstem respiratory centers to increases in carbon dioxide tension, and to electrical stimulation.

Buprenorphine causes miosis, even in total darkness, and little tolerance develops to this effect. Pinpoint pupils are a sign of opioid overdose but are not pathognomonic (e.g., pontine lesions of hemorrhagic or ischemic origins may produce similar findings). Marked mydriasis rather than miosis may be seen with worsening hypoxia in the setting of buprenorphine overdose.

Effects on the Gastrointestinal Tract and Other Smooth Muscle

Gastric, biliary, and pancreatic secretions are decreased by buprenorphine. Buprenorphine causes a reduction in motility associated with an increase in tone in the antrum of the stomach and duodenum. Digestion of food in the small intestine is delayed and propulsive contractions are decreased. Propulsive peristaltic waves in the colon are decreased, while tone is increased to the point of spasm. The end result is constipation. Buprenorphine can cause a marked increase in biliary tract pressure as a result of spasm of the sphincter of Oddi.

Effects on the Cardiovascular System

Buprenorphine may cause a reduction in blood pressure.

Effects on Cardiac Electrophysiology

The effect of BUTRANS 10 mcg/hour and 2 × BUTRANS 20 mcg/hour on QTc interval was evaluated in a double-blind (BUTRANS vs. placebo), randomized, placebo and active-controlled (moxifloxacin 400 mg, open label), parallel-group, dose-escalating, single-dose study in 132 healthy male and female subjects aged 18 to 55 years. The dose escalation sequence for BUTRANS during the titration period was: BUTRANS 5 mcg/hour for 3 days, then BUTRANS 10 mcg/hour for 3 days, then BUTRANS 20 mcg/hour for 3 days, then 2 × BUTRANS 20 mcg/hour for 4 days. The QTc evaluation was performed during the third day of BUTRANS 10 mcg/hour and the fourth day of 2 × BUTRANS 20 mcg/hour when the plasma levels of buprenorphine were at steady state for the corresponding doses *[see Warnings and Precautions (5.7)]*.

There was no clinically meaningful effect on mean QTc with a BUTRANS dose of 10 mcg/hour. A BUTRANS dose of 40 mcg/hour (given as two 20 mcg/hour BUTRANS Transdermal Systems) prolonged mean QTc by a maximum of 9.2 (90% CI: 5.2-13.3) msec across the 13 assessment time points.

Effects on the Endocrine System

Opioids inhibit the secretion of ACTH, cortisol, and lutein-

Continued on next page

izing hormone (LH) in humans. They also stimulate prolactin, growth hormone (GH) secretion, and pancreatic secretion of insulin and glucagon.

Effects on the Immune System

Opioids have been shown to have a variety of effects on components of the immune system in *in vitro* and animal models. The clinical significance of these findings is unknown. Overall, the effects of opioids appear to be modestly immunosuppressive.

12.3 Pharmacokinetics

Absorption

Each BUTRANS system provides delivery of buprenorphine for 7 days. Steady state was achieved during the first application by Day 3 (see Figure 2).

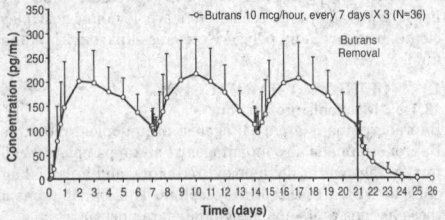

Figure 2 Mean (SD) Buprenorphine Plasma Concentrations Following Three Consecutive Applications of BUTRANS 10 mcg/hour (N = 36 Healthy Subjects)

BUTRANS 5, 10, and 20 mcg/hour provide dose-proportional total buprenorphine exposures (AUC) following 7-day applications. BUTRANS single 7-day application and steady-state pharmacokinetic parameters are summarized in Table 6. Plasma buprenorphine concentrations after titration showed no further change over the 60-day period studied.

Table 6: Pharmacokinetic Parameters of BUTRANS in Healthy Subjects, Mean (%CV)

Single 7-day Application	AUC_{inf} (pg.h/mL)	C_{max} (pg/mL)
BUTRANS 5 mcg/hour	12087 (37)	176 (67)
BUTRANS 10 mcg/hour	27035 (29)	191 (34)
BUTRANS 20 mcg/hour	54294 (36)	471 (49)

Multiple 7-day Applications	$AUC_{tau,ss}$ (pg.h/mL)	$C_{max,ss}$ (pg/mL)
BUTRANS 10 mcg/hour, steady-state	27543 (33)	224 (35)

Transdermal delivery studies showed that intact human skin is permeable to buprenorphine. In clinical pharmacology studies, the median time for BUTRANS 10 mcg/hour to deliver quantifiable buprenorphine concentrations ($\geq$ 25 pg/mL) was approximately 17 hours.

The absolute bioavailability of BUTRANS relative to IV administration, following a 7-day application, is approximately 15% for all doses (BUTRANS 5, 10, and 20 mcg/hour).

Effects of Application Site

A study in healthy subjects demonstrated that the pharmacokinetic profile of buprenorphine delivered by BUTRANS 10 mcg/hour is similar when applied to the upper outer arm, upper chest, upper back, or the side of the chest *[see Dosage and Administration (2.5)]*.

The reapplication of BUTRANS 10 mcg/hour after various rest periods to the same application site in healthy subjects showed that the minimum rest period needed to avoid variability in drug absorption is 3 weeks (21 days) *[see Dosage and Administration (2.5)]*.

Effects of Heat

In a study of healthy subjects, application of a heating pad directly on the BUTRANS 10 mcg/hour system caused a 26% - 55% increase in blood concentrations of buprenorphine. Concentrations returned to normal within 5 hours after the heat was removed. For this reason, instruct patients not to apply heating pads directly to the BUTRANS system during system wear *[see Warnings and Precautions (5.13)]*.

Fever may increase the permeability of the skin, leading to increased buprenorphine concentrations during BUTRANS treatment. As a result, febrile patients are at increased risk

for the possibility of BUTRANS-related reactions during treatment with BUTRANS. Monitor patients with febrile illness for adverse effects and consider dose adjustment *[see Warnings and Precautions (5.14)]*. In a crossover study of healthy subjects receiving endotoxin or placebo challenge during BUTRANS 10 mcg/hour wear, the AUC and C_{max} were similar despite a physiologic response of mild fever to endotoxin.

Distribution

Buprenorphine is approximately 96% bound to plasma proteins, mainly to alpha- and beta-globulin.

Studies of IV buprenorphine have shown a large volume of distribution (approximately 430 L), implying extensive distribution of buprenorphine.

CSF buprenorphine concentrations appear to be approximately 15-25% of concurrent plasma concentrations.

Metabolism

Buprenorphine metabolism in the skin following BUTRANS application is negligible.

Buprenorphine primarily undergoes *N*-dealkylation by CYP3A4 to norbuprenorphine and glucuronidation by UGT-isoenzymes (mainly UGT1A1 and 2B7) to buprenorphine 3β-*O*-glucuronide. Norbuprenorphine, the major metabolite, is also glucuronidated (mainly UGT1A3) prior to excretion. Norbuprenorphine is the only known active metabolite of buprenorphine. It has been shown to be a respiratory depressant in rats, but only at concentrations at least 50-fold greater than those observed following application to humans of BUTRANS 20 mcg/hour.

Elimination

Following IV administration, buprenorphine and its metabolites are secreted into bile and excreted in urine.

Following intramuscular administration of 2 mcg/kg dose of buprenorphine, approximately 70% of the dose was excreted in feces within 7 days. Approximately 27% was excreted in urine.

Following transdermal application, buprenorphine is eliminated via hepatic metabolism, with subsequent biliary excretion and renal excretion of soluble metabolites. After removal of BUTRANS, mean buprenorphine concentrations decrease approximately 50% within 10-24 hours, followed by decline with an apparent terminal half-life of approximately 26 hours. Since metabolism and excretion of buprenorphine occur mainly via hepatic elimination, reductions in hepatic blood flow induced by some general anesthetics (e.g., halothane) and other drugs may result in a decreased rate of hepatic elimination of the drug, leading to increased plasma concentrations.

The total clearance of buprenorphine is approximately 55 L/hour in postoperative patients.

Drug Interactions

Effect of CYP3A4 inhibitors

In a drug-drug interaction study, BUTRANS 10 mcg/hour (single dose × 7 days) was co-administered with 200 mg ketoconazole, a strong CYP3A4 inhibitor or ketoconazole placebo twice daily for 11 days and the pharmacokinetics of buprenorphine and its metabolites were evaluated. Plasma buprenorphine concentrations did not accumulate during co-medication with ketoconazole 200 mg twice daily. Based on the results from this study, metabolism during therapy with BUTRANS is not expected to be affected by co-administration of CYP3A4 inhibitors *[see Drug Interactions (7.3)]*.

Antiretroviral agents have been evaluated for CYP3A4 mediated interactions with sublingual buprenorphine. Nucleoside reverse transcriptase inhibitors (NRTIs) and nonnucleoside reverse transcriptase inhibitors (NNRTIs) do not appear to have clinically significant interactions with buprenorphine. However, certain protease inhibitors (PIs) with CYP3A4 inhibitory activity such as atazanavir and atazanavir/ritonavir resulted in elevated levels of buprenorphine and norbuprenorphine when buprenorphine and naloxone were administered sublingually. C_{max} and AUC for buprenorphine increased by up to 1.6 and 1.9 fold, and C_{max} and AUC for norbuprenorphine increased by up to 1.6 and 2.0 fold respectively, when sublingual buprenorphine was administered with these PIs. Patients in this study reported increased sedation, and symptoms of opiate excess have been found in post-marketing reports of patients receiving buprenorphine and atazanavir with and without ritonavir concomitantly. It should be noted that atazanavir is both a CYP3A4 and UGT1A1 inhibitor. As such, the drug-drug interaction potential for buprenorphine with CYP3A4 inhibitors is likely to be dependent on the route of administration as well as the specificity of enzyme inhibition *[see Drug Interactions (7.3)]*.

Effect of CYP3A4 Inducers

The interaction between buprenorphine and CYP3A4 inducers has not been studied.

Specific Populations

Geriatric Patients

Following a single application of BUTRANS 10 mcg/hour to 12 healthy young adults (mean age 32 years) and 12 healthy elderly subjects (mean age 72 years), the pharmacokinetic profile of BUTRANS was similar in healthy elderly and healthy young adult subjects, though the elderly subjects showed a trend toward higher plasma concentrations immediately after BUTRANS removal. Both groups eliminated buprenorphine at similar rates after system removal *[see Use in Specific Populations (8.5)]*.

In a study of healthy young subjects, healthy elderly subjects, and elderly subjects treated with thiazide diuretics, BUTRANS at a fixed dose-escalation schedule (BUTRANS 5 mcg/hour for 3 days, followed by BUTRANS 10 mcg/hour for 3 days and BUTRANS 20 mcg/hour for 7 days) produced similar mean plasma concentration vs. time profiles for each of the three subject groups. There were no significant differences between groups in buprenorphine C_{max} or AUC *[see Use in Specific Populations (8.5)]*.

Pediatric Patients

BUTRANS has not been studied in children and is not recommended for pediatric use.

Gender

In a pooled data analysis utilizing data from several studies that administered BUTRANS 10 mcg/hour to healthy subjects, no differences in buprenorphine C_{max} and AUC or body-weight normalized C_{max} and AUC were observed between males and females treated with BUTRANS.

Renal Impairment

No studies in patients with renal impairment have been performed with BUTRANS.

In an independent study, the effect of impaired renal function on buprenorphine pharmacokinetics after IV bolus and after continuous IV infusion administrations was evaluated. It was found that plasma buprenorphine concentrations were similar in patients with normal renal function and in patients with impaired renal function or renal failure. In a separate investigation of the effect of intermittent hemodialysis on buprenorphine plasma concentrations in chronic pain patients with end-stage renal disease who were treated with a transdermal buprenorphine product (marketed outside the US) up to 70 mcg/hour, no significant differences in buprenorphine plasma concentrations before or after hemodialysis were observed.

No notable relationship was observed between estimated creatinine clearance rates and steady-state buprenorphine concentrations among patients during BUTRANS therapy.

Hepatic Impairment

The pharmacokinetics of buprenorphine following an IV infusion of 0.3 mg of buprenorphine were compared in 8 patients with mild impairment (Child-Pugh A), 4 patients with moderate impairment (Child-Pugh B) and 12 subjects with normal hepatic function. Buprenorphine and norbuprenorphine exposure did not increase in the mild and moderate hepatic impairment patients.

BUTRANS has not been evaluated in patients with severe (Child-Pugh C) hepatic impairment *[see Dosage and Administration (2.4), Warnings and Precautions (5.10), and Use in Specific Populations (8.6)]*.

13 NONCLINICAL TOXICOLOGY

13.1 Carcinogenesis, Mutagenesis, Impairment of Fertility

Carcinogenesis

Buprenorphine administered daily by skin painting to Sprague Dawley rats for 100 weeks at dosages (20, 60, or 200 mg/kg) produced systemic exposures (based on AUC) that ranged from approximately 130 to 350 times that of human subjects administered the maximum recommended human dose (MRHD) of BUTRANS 20 mcg/hour. An increased incidence of benign testicular interstitial cell tumors, considered buprenorphine treatment-related, was observed in male rats compared with concurrent controls. The tumor incidence was also above the highest incidence in the historical control database of the testing facility. These tumors were noted at 60 mg/kg/day and higher at approximately 220 times MRHD based on AUC. The no observed effect level (NOEL) was 20 mg/kg/day (approximately 140 times the proposed MRHD based on AUC). The mechanism leading to the tumor findings and the relevance to humans is unknown.

Buprenorphine was administered by skin painting to hemizygous Tg.AC mice over a 6-month study period. At the dosages administered daily (18.75, 37.5, 150, or 600 mg/kg/day), buprenorphine was not carcinogenic or tumorigenic at systemic exposure to buprenorphine, based on AUC, of up to approximately 1000 times that of human subjects administered BUTRANS 20 mcg/hour, the MRHD.

Mutagenesis

Buprenorphine was not genotoxic in 3 *in vitro* genetic toxicology studies (bacterial mutagenicity test, mouse lymphoma assay, chromosomal aberration assay in human peripheral blood lymphocytes), and in one *in vivo* mouse micronucleus test.

Impairment of Fertility

BUTRANS (1/4 of a BUTRANS 5 mcg/hour, one BUTRANS 5 mcg/hour, or one BUTRANS 20 mcg/hour every 3 days in males for 4 weeks prior to mating for a total of 10 weeks and in females for 2 weeks prior to mating through gestation day 7) had no effect on fertility or general reproductive performance of rats at AUC-based exposure levels as high as approximately 65 times (females) and 100 times (males) that for human subjects who received BUTRANS 20 mcg/hour, the MRHD.

14   CLINICAL STUDIES

The efficacy of BUTRANS has been evaluated in four 12-week double-blind, controlled clinical trials in opioid-naïve and opioid-experienced patients with moderate to severe chronic low back pain or osteoarthritis using pain scores as the primary efficacy variable. Two of these studies, described below, demonstrated efficacy in patients with low back pain. One study in low back pain and one study in osteoarthritis did not show a statistically significant pain reduction for either BUTRANS or the respective active comparators.

12-Week Study in Opioid-Naïve Patients with Chronic Low Back Pain

A total of 1,024 patients with chronic low back pain who were suboptimally responsive to their non-opioid therapy entered an open-label, dose-titration period for up to four weeks. Patients initiated therapy with three days of treatment with BUTRANS 5 mcg/hour. After three days, if adverse events were tolerated, the dose was increased to BUTRANS 10 mcg/hour. If adverse effects were tolerated but adequate analgesia was not reached, the dose was increased to BUTRANS 20 mcg/hour for an additional 10-12 days. Patients who achieved adequate analgesia and tolerable adverse effects on BUTRANS 10 or 20 mcg/hour were then randomized to remain on their titrated dose of BUTRANS or matching placebo. Fifty-three percent of the patients who entered the open-label titration period were able to titrate to a tolerable and effective dose and were randomized into a 12-week, double-blind treatment period. Twenty-three percent of patients discontinued due to an adverse event from the open-label titration period and 14% discontinued due to lack of a therapeutic effect. The remaining 10% of patients were dropped due to various administrative reasons.

During the first seven days of double-blind treatment patients were allowed up to two tablets per day of immediate-release oxycodone 5 mg as supplemental analgesia to minimize opioid withdrawal symptoms in patients randomized to placebo. Thereafter, the supplemental analgesia was limited to either acetaminophen 500 mg or ibuprofen 200 mg at a maximum of four tablets per day. Sixty-six percent of the patients treated with BUTRANS completed the 12-week treatment compared to 70% of the patients treated with placebo. Of the 256 patients randomized to BUTRANS, 9% discontinued due to lack of efficacy and 16% due to adverse events. Of the 283 patients randomized to placebo, 13% discontinued due to lack of efficacy and 7% due to adverse events.

Of the patients who were randomized, the mean pain (SE) NRS scores were 7.2 (0.08) and 7.2 (0.07) at screening and 2.6 (0.08) and 2.6 (0.07) at pre-randomization (beginning of double-blind phase) for the BUTRANS and placebo groups, respectively.

The score for average pain over the last 24 hours at the end of the study (Week 12/Early Termination) was statistically significantly lower for patients treated with BUTRANS compared with patients treated with placebo. The proportion of patients with various degrees of improvement, from screening to study endpoint, is shown in Figure 3 below.

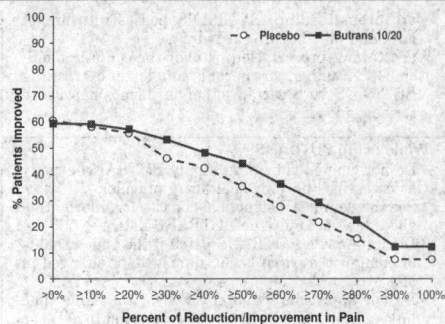

Figure 3: Percent Reduction in Pain Intensity

12-Week Study in Opioid-Experienced Patients with Chronic Low Back Pain

One thousand one hundred and sixty (1,160) patients on chronic opioid therapy (total daily dose 30-80 mg morphine equivalent) entered an open-label, dose-titration period with BUTRANS for up to 3 weeks, following taper of prior opioids. Patients initiated therapy with BUTRANS 10 mcg/hour for three days. After three days, if the patient tolerated the adverse effects, the dose was increased to BUTRANS 20 mcg/hour for up to 18 days. Patients with adequate analgesia and tolerable adverse effects on BUTRANS 20 mcg/hour were randomized to remain on BUTRANS 20 mcg/hour or were switched to a low-dose control (BUTRANS 5 mcg/hour) or an active control. Fifty-seven percent of patients who entered the open-label titration period were able to titrate to and tolerate the adverse effects of BUTRANS 20 mcg/hour and were randomized into a 12-week double-blind treatment phase. Twelve percent of patients discontinued due to an adverse event and 21% discontinued due to lack of a therapeutic effect during the open-label titration period.

During the double-blind period, patients were permitted to take ibuprofen (200 mg tablets) or acetaminophen (500 mg tablets) every 4 hours as needed for supplemental analgesia (up to 3200 mg of ibuprofen and 4 grams of acetaminophen daily). Sixty-seven percent of patients treated with BUTRANS 20 mcg/hour and 58% of patients treated with BUTRANS 5 mcg/hour completed the 12-week treatment. Of the 219 patients randomized to BUTRANS 20 mcg/hour, 11% discontinued due to lack of efficacy and 13% due to adverse events. Of the 221 patients randomized to BUTRANS 5 mcg/hour, 24% discontinued due to lack of efficacy and 6% due to adverse events.

Of the patients who were able to be randomized in the double-blind period, the mean pain (SE) NRS scores were 6.4 (0.08) and 6.5 (0.08) at screening and were 2.8 (0.08) and 2.9 (0.08) at pre-randomization (beginning of Double-Blind Period) for the BUTRANS 5 mcg/hour and BUTRANS 20 mcg/hour, respectively.

The score for average pain over the last 24 hours at Week 12 was statistically significantly lower for subjects treated with BUTRANS 20 mcg/hour compared to subjects treated with BUTRANS 5 mcg/hour. A higher proportion of BUTRANS 20 mcg/hour patients (49%) had at least a 30% reduction in pain score from screening to study endpoint when compared to BUTRANS 5 mcg/hour patients (33%). The proportion of patients with various degrees of improvement from screening to study endpoint is shown in Figure 4 below.

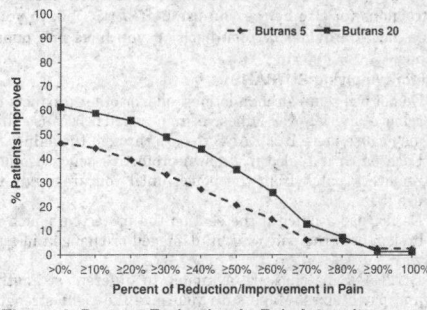

Figure 4: Percent Reduction in Pain Intensity

16   HOW SUPPLIED/STORAGE AND HANDLING

BUTRANS (buprenorphine) Transdermal System is supplied in cartons containing 4 individually-packaged systems and a pouch containing 4 Patch-Disposal Units.

BUTRANS 5 mcg/hour Transdermal System, 4-count carton
NDC 59011-750-04
BUTRANS 7.5 mcg/hour Transdermal System, 4-count carton
NDC 59011-757-04
BUTRANS 10 mcg/hour Transdermal System, 4-count carton
NDC 59011-751-04
BUTRANS 15 mcg/hour Transdermal System, 4-count carton
NDC 59011-758-04
BUTRANS 20 mcg/hour Transdermal System, 4-count carton
NDC 59011-752-04
Store at 25°C (77°F); excursions permitted between 15°C - 30°C (59°F - 86°F).

17   PATIENT COUNSELING INFORMATION

Advise the patient to read the FDA-approved patient labeling (Medication Guide and Instructions for Use).

Addiction, Abuse, and Misuse

Inform patients that the use of BUTRANS, even when taken as recommended, can result in addiction, abuse, and misuse, which could lead to overdose and death *[see Warnings and Precautions (5.1)]*. Instruct patients not to share BUTRANS with others and to take steps to protect BUTRANS from theft or misuse.

Life-Threatening Respiratory Depression

Inform patients of the risk of life-threatening respiratory depression, including information that the risk is greatest when starting BUTRANS or when the dose is increased, and that it can occur even at recommended doses *[see Warnings and Precautions (5.2)]*. Advise patients how to recognize respiratory depression and to seek medical attention if breathing difficulties develop.

Accidental Exposure

Inform patients that accidental exposure, especially in children, may result in respiratory depression or death *[see Warnings and Precautions (5.2)]*. Instruct patients to take steps to store BUTRANS securely and to dispose of unused BUTRANS by folding the patch in half and flushing it down the toilet.

Neonatal Opioid Withdrawal Syndrome

Inform female patients of reproductive potential that prolonged use of BUTRANS during pregnancy can result in neonatal opioid withdrawal syndrome, which may be life-threatening if not recognized and treated *[see Warnings and Precautions (5.3)]*.

Interaction with Alcohol and other CNS Depressants

Inform patients that potentially serious additive effects may occur if BUTRANS is used with alcohol or other CNS depressants, and not to use such drugs unless supervised by a health care provider.

Important Administration Instructions

Instruct patients how to properly use BUTRANS, including the following:
1. To carefully follow instructions for the application, removal, and disposal of BUTRANS. Each week, apply BUTRANS to a different site based on the 8 described skin sites, with a minimum of 3 weeks between applications to a previously used site.
2. To apply BUTRANS to a hairless or nearly hairless skin site. If none are available, instruct patients to clip the hair at the site and not to shave the area. Instruct patients not to apply to irritated skin. If the application site must be cleaned, use clear water only. Soaps, alcohol, oils, lotions, or abrasive devices should not be used. Allow the skin to dry before applying BUTRANS.

Hypotension

Inform patients that BUTRANS may cause orthostatic hypotension and syncope. Instruct patients how to recognize symptoms of low blood pressure and how to reduce the risk of serious consequences should hypotension occur (e.g., sit or lie down, carefully rise from a sitting or lying position).

Driving or Operating Heavy Machinery

Inform patients that BUTRANS may impair the ability to perform potentially hazardous activities such as driving a car or operating heavy machinery. Advise patients not to perform such tasks until they know how they will react to the medication.

Constipation

Advise patients of the potential for severe constipation, including management instructions and when to seek medical attention.

Continued on next page

Anaphylaxis
Inform patients that anaphylaxis has been reported with ingredients contained in BUTRANS. Advise patients how to recognize such a reaction and when to seek medical attention.

Pregnancy
Advise female patients that BUTRANS can cause fetal harm and to inform the prescriber if they are pregnant or plan to become pregnant.

Disposal
Instruct patients to refer to the Instructions for Use for proper disposal of BUTRANS. Patients can dispose of used or unused BUTRANS patches in the trash by sealing them in the Patch-Disposal Unit, following the instructions on the unit.

Alternatively, instruct patients to dispose of used patches by folding the adhesive side of the patch to itself, then flushing the patch down the toilet immediately upon removal. Unused patches should be removed from their pouches, protective liners removed, the patches folded so that the adhesive side of the patch adheres to itself, and immediately flushed down the toilet.

Instruct patients to dispose of any patches remaining from a prescription as soon as they are no longer needed.

Healthcare professionals can telephone Purdue Pharma's Medical Services Department (1-888-726-7535) for information on this product.

Distributed by: Purdue Pharma L.P., Stamford, CT 06901-3431

Manufactured by: LTS Lohmann Therapy Systems Corp., West Caldwell, NJ 07006

U.S. Patent Numbers 5681413; 5804215; 6264980; 6315854; 6344211; RE41408; RE41489; RE41571

© 2014, Purdue Pharma L.P.

Medication Guide
BUTRANS® (BYOO-trans) (buprenorphine) Transdermal System, CIII

BUTRANS is:
• A strong prescription pain medicine that contains an opioid (narcotic) that is used to manage pain severe enough to require daily, around-the-clock, long-term treatment with an opioid, when other pain treatments such as non-opioid pain medicines or immediate-release opioid medicines do not treat your pain well enough or you cannot tolerate them.
• A long-acting (extended-release) opioid pain medicine that can put you at risk for overdose and death. Even if you take your dose correctly as prescribed you are at risk for opioid addiction, abuse, and misuse that can lead to death.
• Not for use to treat pain that is not around-the-clock.

Important information about BUTRANS:
• **Get emergency help right away if you take too much BUTRANS (overdose).** When you first start taking BUTRANS, when your dose is changed, or if you take too much (overdose), serious or life-threatening breathing problems that can lead to death may occur.
• Never give anyone else your BUTRANS. They could die from taking it. Store BUTRANS away from children and in a safe place to prevent stealing or abuse. Selling or giving away BUTRANS is against the law.

Do not use BUTRANS if you have:
• severe asthma, trouble breathing, or other lung problems.
• a bowel blockage or have narrowing of the stomach or intestines.

Before applying BUTRANS, tell your healthcare provider if you have a history of:
• head injury, seizures
• liver, kidney, thyroid problems
• problems urinating
• pancreas or gallbladder problems
• heart rhythm problems (Long QT syndrome)
• abuse of street or prescription drugs, alcohol addiction, or mental health problems.

Tell your healthcare provider if you:
• have a fever
• **are pregnant or planning to become pregnant.** Prolonged use of BUTRANS during pregnancy can cause withdrawal symptoms in your newborn baby that could be life-threatening if not recognized and treated.

• **are breastfeeding.** BUTRANS passes into breast milk and may harm your baby.
• are taking prescription or over-the-counter medicines, vitamins, or herbal supplements. Taking BUTRANS with certain other medicines can cause serious side effects.

While using BUTRANS:
• Do not change your dose. Apply BUTRANS exactly as prescribed by your healthcare provider.
• See the detailed Instructions for Use for information about how to apply the BUTRANS patch.
• Do not apply a BUTRANS patch if the pouch seal is broken, or the patch is cut, damaged, or changed in any way.
• Do not apply more than 1 patch at the same time unless your healthcare provider tells you to.
• You should wear 1 BUTRANS patch continuously for 7 days.
• **Call your healthcare provider if the dose you are using does not control your pain.**
• **Do not stop using BUTRANS without talking to your healthcare provider.**
• **To properly dispose of used and unused patches, use the Patch-Disposal Unit or fold in half and flush down the toilet. See the detailed Instructions for Use.**

When using BUTRANS DO NOT:
• Take hot baths or sunbathe, use hot tubs, saunas, heating pads, electric blankets, heated waterbeds, or tanning lamps. These can cause an overdose that can lead to death.
• Drive or operate heavy machinery, until you know how BUTRANS affects you. BUTRANS can make you sleepy, dizzy, or lightheaded.
• Drink alcohol or use prescription or over-the-counter medicines containing alcohol. Using products containing alcohol during treatment with BUTRANS may cause you to overdose and die.

The possible side effects of BUTRANS are:
• constipation, nausea, sleepiness, vomiting, tiredness, headache, dizziness, itching, redness or rash where the patch is applied. Call your healthcare provider if you have any of these symptoms and they are severe.

Get emergency medical help if you have:
• trouble breathing, shortness of breath, fast heartbeat, chest pain, swelling of your face, tongue or throat, extreme drowsiness, light-headedness when changing positions, or you are feeling faint.

These are not all the possible side effects of BUTRANS. Call your doctor for medical advice about side effects. You may report side effects to FDA at 1-800-FDA-1088. **For more information go to dailymed.nlm.nih.gov**

Distributed by: Purdue Pharma L.P., Stamford, CT 06901-3431, **www.purduepharma.com or call 1-888-726-7535**

This Medication Guide has been approved by the U.S. Food and Drug Administration. Revised: April 2014

Instructions for Use
BUTRANS® (BYOO-trans) CIII
(buprenorphine)
Transdermal System

Be sure that you read, understand, and follow these Instructions for Use before you use BUTRANS. Talk to your healthcare provider or pharmacist if you have any questions.

Before Applying BUTRANS:
• Do not use soap, alcohol, lotions, oils, or other products to remove any leftover adhesive from a patch because this may cause more BUTRANS to pass through the skin.
• Each patch is sealed in its own protective pouch. Do not remove a patch from the pouch until you are ready to use it.
• Do not use a patch if the seal on the protective pouch is broken or if the patch is cut, damaged or changed in any way.
• BUTRANS patches are available in different strengths and patch sizes. Make sure you have the right strength patch that has been prescribed for you.

Where to apply BUTRANS:
• BUTRANS should be applied to the **upper outer arm, upper chest, upper back, or the side of the chest (See Figure A)**. These 4 sites (located on both sides of the body) provide 8 possible BUTRANS application sites.

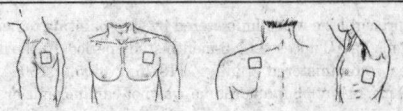
Figure A

• Do not apply more than 1 patch at the same time unless your doctor tells you to. However, if your healthcare provider tells you to do so, you may use 2 patches as prescribed, applied at the same site (**See Figure A** for application sites) right next to each other (**See Figure B** for an example of patch position when applying 2 patches). Always apply and remove the two patches together at the same time.

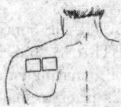
Figure B

• You should change the skin site where you apply BUTRANS each week, making sure that at least 3 weeks (21 days) pass before you re-use the same skin site.
• Apply BUTRANS to a **hairless or nearly hairless skin site**. If needed, you can clip the hair at the skin site (**See Figure C**). Do not shave the area. The skin site should not be irritated. **Use only water to clean** the application site. You should not use soaps, alcohol, oils, lotions, or abrasive devices. Allow the skin to dry before you apply the patch.

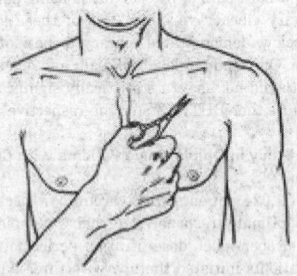
Figure C

• The skin site should be free of cuts and irritation (rashes, swelling, redness, or other skin problems).

When to apply a new patch:
• When you apply a new patch, write down the date and time that the patch is applied. Use this to remember when the patch should be removed.
• Change the patch at the same time of day, one week (exactly 7 days) after you apply it.
• After removing and disposing of the patch, write down the time it was removed and how it was disposed.

How to apply BUTRANS:
• If you are wearing a patch, remember to remove it before applying a new one.
• Each patch is sealed in its own protective pouch.
• If you are using two patches, remember to apply them at the same site right next to each other. Always apply and remove the two patches together at the same time.
• Use scissors to cut open the pouch along the dotted line (**See Figure D**) and remove the patch. Do not remove the patch from the pouch until you are ready to use it. Do not use patches that have been cut or damaged in any way.

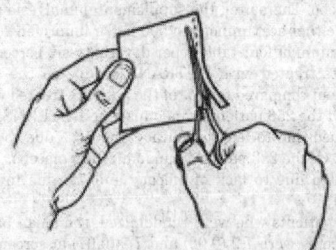
Figure D

• Hold the patch with the protective liner facing you.
• Gently bend the patch (**See Figures E and F**) along the faint line and slowly peel the larger portion of the liner, which covers the sticky surface of the patch.
[See figure E at top of next column]
[See figure F below]
• Do not touch the sticky side of the patch with your fingers.

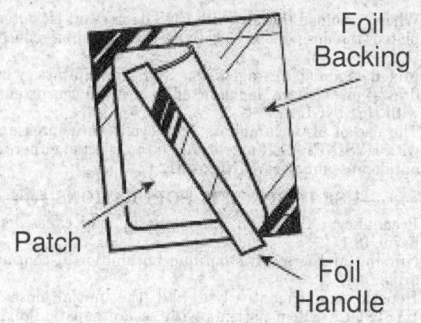

Foil Backing

Patch

Foil Handle

Figure E

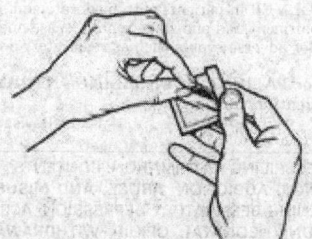

Figure F

• Using the smaller portion of the protective liner as a handle (**See Figure G**), apply the sticky side of the patch to one of the 8 body locations described above (**See "Where to apply BUTRANS"**).

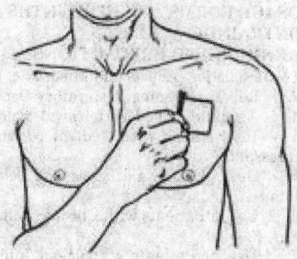

Figure G

• While still holding the sticky side down, gently fold back the smaller portion of the patch. Grasp an edge of the remaining protective liner and slowly peel it off (**See Figure H**).

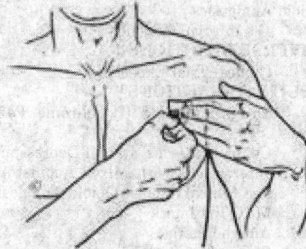

Figure H

• Press the entire patch firmly into place with the palm (**See Figure I**) of your hand over the patch, for about 15 seconds. Do not rub the patch.
• Make sure that the patch firmly sticks to the skin.
• Go over the edges with your fingers to assure good contact around the patch.
• If you are using two patches, follow the steps in this section to apply them right next to each other.
• Always wash your hands after applying or handling a patch.
• After the patch is applied, write down the date and time that the patch is applied. Use this to remember when the patch should be removed.

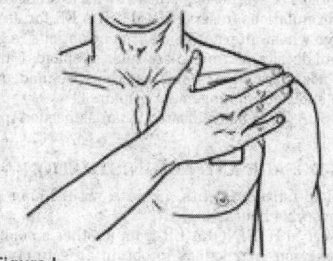

Figure I

If the patch falls off right away after applying, throw it away and put a new one on at a different skin site (**See "Disposing of BUTRANS Patch"**).
If a patch falls off, do not touch the sticky side of the patch with your fingers. A new patch should be applied to a different site. **Patches that fall off should not be re-applied.** They must be thrown away correctly.
Short-term exposure of the BUTRANS patch to water, such as when bathing or showering, is permitted.
If the edges of the BUTRANS patch start to loosen:
• Apply first aid tape only to the edges of the patch.
• If problems with the patch not sticking continue, cover the patch with special see-through adhesive dressings (for example Bioclusive or Tegaderm).
  ○ Remove the backing from the transparent adhesive dressing and place it carefully and completely over the BUTRANS patch, smoothing it over the patch and your skin.
• **Never cover a BUTRANS patch with any other bandage or tape. It should only be covered with a special see-through adhesive dressing. Talk to your healthcare provider or pharmacist about the kinds of dressing that should be used.**
If your patch falls off later, but before 1 week (7 days) of use, throw it away properly (**See "Disposing of a BUTRANS Patch"**) and apply a new patch at a different skin site. Be sure to let your healthcare provider know that this has happened. Do not replace the new patch until 1 week (7 days) after you put it on (or as directed by your healthcare provider).
Disposing of BUTRANS Patch:
BUTRANS patches should be disposed of by using the Patch-Disposal Unit. Alternatively, the patches can be flushed down the toilet.
To dispose of BUTRANS patches in household trash using the Patch-Disposal Unit:
Remove your patch and follow the directions printed on the Patch-Disposal Unit (**See Figure J**) or see complete instructions below. Use one Patch-Disposal Unit for each patch.

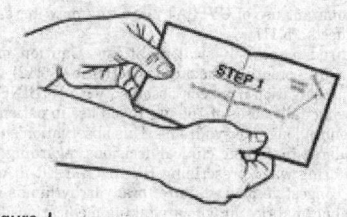

Figure J

1. Peel back the disposal unit liner to show the sticky surface (**See Figure K**).

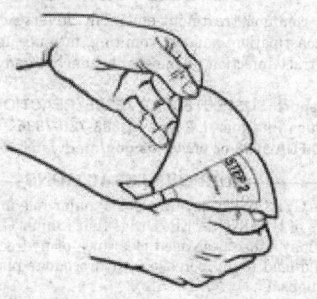

Figure K

2. Place the sticky side of the used or unused patch to the indicated area on the disposal unit (**See Figure L**).

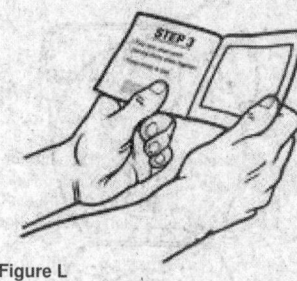

Figure L

3. Close the disposal unit by folding the sticky sides together (**See Figure M**). Press firmly and smoothly over the entire disposal unit so that the patch is sealed within.

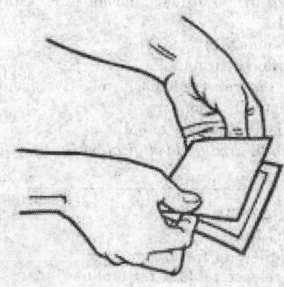

Figure M

4. The closed disposal unit, with the patch sealed inside may be thrown away in the trash (**See Figure N**).

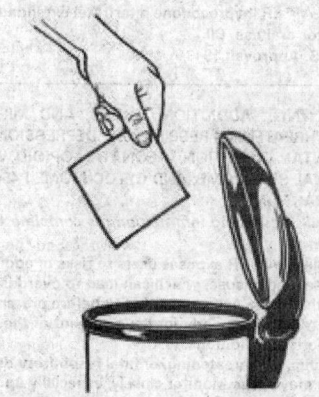

Figure N

Do not put unused patches in household trash without first sealing them in the Patch-Disposal Unit.
Always remove the leftover patches from their protective pouch and remove the protective liner. The pouch and liner can be disposed of separately in the trash and should not be sealed in the Patch-Disposal Unit.
To flush your BUTRANS patches down the toilet:
Remove your BUTRANS patch, fold the sticky sides of a used patch together and flush it down the toilet right away (**See Figure O at top of next page**).
When disposing of unused BUTRANS patches you no longer need, remove the leftover patches from their protective pouch and remove the protective liner. Fold the patches in half with the sticky sides together, and flush the patches down the toilet.
Do not flush the pouch or the protective liner down the toilet. These items can be thrown away in the trash.
If you prefer not to flush the used patch down the toilet, you must use the Patch-Disposal Unit provided to you to discard the patch.
Never put used BUTRANS patches in the trash without first sealing them in the Patch-Disposal Unit.

Continued on next page

Figure O

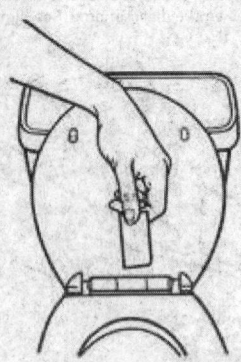

This "Instructions for Use" has been approved by the U.S. Food and Drug Administration.

Distributed by: Purdue Pharma L.P., Stamford, CT 06901-3431

Revised: June 2014

©2014, Purdue Pharma L.P.

Bioclusive is a trademark of Systagenix Wound Management (US), Inc.

Tegaderm is a trademark of 3M.

Shown in Product Identification Guide, page 509

HYSINGLA™ ER ℞ ℂⅡ

[(hye-SING-luh)]
(hydrocodone bitartrate)
extended-release tablets, for oral use

HIGHLIGHTS OF PRESCRIBING INFORMATION
These highlights do not include all the information needed to use HYSINGLA™ ER safely and effectively. See full prescribing information for HYSINGLA ER.

HYSINGLA™ ER (hydrocodone bitartrate) extended-release tablets, for oral use, CII
Initial U.S. Approval: 1943

WARNING: ADDICTION, ABUSE, AND MISUSE; LIFE-THREATENING RESPIRATORY DEPRESSION; ACCIDENTAL INGESTION; NEONATAL OPIOID WITHDRAWAL SYNDROME; AND CYTOCHROME P450 3A4 INTERACTION

See full prescribing information for complete boxed warning.

- HYSINGLA™ ER exposes users to risks of addiction, abuse, and misuse, which can lead to overdose and death. Assess each patient's risk before prescribing, and monitor regularly for development of these behaviors or conditions. (5.1)
- Serious, life-threatening, or fatal respiratory depression may occur. Monitor closely, especially upon initiation or following a dose increase. Instruct patients to swallow HYSINGLA ER whole to avoid exposure to a potentially fatal dose of hydrocodone. (5.2)
- Accidental ingestion of HYSINGLA ER, especially by children, can result in fatal overdose of hydrocodone. (5.2)
- Prolonged use of HYSINGLA ER during pregnancy can result in neonatal opioid withdrawal syndrome, which may be life-threatening if not recognized and treated. If opioid use is required for a prolonged period in a pregnant woman, advise the patient of the risk of neonatal opioid withdrawal syndrome and ensure that appropriate treatment will be available. (5.3)
- Initiation of CYP3A4 inhibitors (or discontinuation of CYP3A4 inducers) can result in a fatal overdose of hydrocodone from HYSINGLA ER. (5.11, 7.1, 12.3)

INDICATIONS AND USAGE

HYSINGLA ER is an opioid agonist indicated for the management of pain severe enough to require daily, around-the-clock, long-term opioid treatment and for which alternative treatment options are inadequate. (1)

Limitations of Use
- Because of the risks of addiction, abuse, and misuse with opioids, even at recommended doses, and because of the greater risks of overdose and death with extended-release opioid formulations, reserve HYSINGLA ER for use in patients for whom alternative treatment options (e.g., non-opioid analgesics or immediate-release opioids) are ineffective, not tolerated, or would be otherwise inadequate to provide sufficient management of pain. (1)
- HYSINGLA ER is not indicated as an as-needed (prn) analgesic. (1)

DOSAGE AND ADMINISTRATION

- For opioid-naïve patients, initiate with 20 mg tablets orally every 24 hours. (2.1)
- To convert to HYSINGLA ER from another opioid, follow the conversion instructions to obtain an estimated dose. (2.1)
- Dose titration of HYSINGLA ER may occur every 3 to 5 days (2.2)
- Tablets must be swallowed intact and are not to be crushed, dissolved, or chewed, due to the risk of overdose or death. (2.3, 5.1)
- Do not abruptly discontinue HYSINGLA ER in a physically dependent patient. (2.6)
- HYSINGLA ER tablets should be taken one tablet at a time, with enough water to ensure complete swallowing immediately after placing in the mouth (2.1, 5.9)

DOSAGE FORMS AND STRENGTHS

Extended-release Tablets: 20, 30, 40, 60, 80, 100, and 120 mg (3)

CONTRAINDICATIONS

- Significant respiratory depression (4)
- Acute or severe bronchial asthma(4)
- Known or suspected paralytic ileus and GI obstruction (4)
- Hypersensitivity to any components of HYSINGLA ER or the active ingredient, hydrocodone bitartrate (4)

WARNINGS AND PRECAUTIONS

- Misuse, abuse, and diversion: HYSINGLA ER is an opioid agonist and a Schedule II controlled substance with a high potential for abuse similar to fentanyl, methadone, morphine, oxycodone, and oxymorphone. (5.1)
- Interactions with CNS depressants: Concomitant use may cause profound sedation, respiratory depression, and death. If co-administration is required, consider dose reduction of one or both drugs. (5.4)
- Elderly, cachectic, debilitated patients, and those with chronic pulmonary disease: Monitor closely because of increased risk for life-threatening respiratory depression. (5.5, 5.6)
- Patients with head injury or increased intracranial pressure: Monitor for sedation and respiratory depression. Avoid use of HYSINGLA ER in patients with impaired consciousness or coma susceptible to intracranial effects of CO_2 retention. (5.7)
- Risk of Choking/GI Obstruction: Use with caution in patients who have difficulty swallowing or have underlying GI disorders that may predispose them to obstruction. (5.9, 5.10)
- Concomitant use of CYP3A4 inhibitors may increase opioid effects. (5.11)
- Impaired mental/physical abilities: Caution must be used with potentially hazardous activities. (5.12)
- QTc prolongation has been observed with HYSINGLA ER following daily doses of 160 mg. Avoid use in patients with congenital long QTc syndrome. This observation should be considered in making clinical decisions regarding patient monitoring when prescribing HYSINGLA ER in patients with congestive heart failure, bradyarrhythmias electrolyte abnormalities, or who are taking medications that are known to prolong the QTc interval. In patients who develop QTc prolongation, consider reducing the dose. (5.14, 12.2)

ADVERSE REACTIONS

Most common treatment-emergent adverse events (≥5%) are constipation, nausea, vomiting, fatigue, upper respiratory tract infection, dizziness, headache, and somnolence. (6.1)

To report SUSPECTED ADVERSE REACTIONS, contact Purdue Pharma L.P. at 1-888-726-7535 or FDA at 1-800-FDA-1088 or www.fda.gov/medwatch.

DRUG INTERACTIONS

- The CYP3A4 isoenzyme plays a major role in the metabolism of HYSINGLA ER. Drugs that inhibit CYP3A4 activity may cause decreased clearance of hydrocodone which could lead to an increase in hydrocodone plasma concentrations. (7.1)
- CNS depressants: Increased risk of respiratory depression, hypotension, profound sedation, coma or death.

When combined therapy with CNS depressant is contemplated, the dose of one or both agents should be reduced. (7.2)
- Mixed Agonists/Antagonists: May precipitate withdrawal or decrease analgesic effect if given concurrently with HYSINGLA ER. (7.3)
- The use of MAO inhibitors or tricyclic antidepressants with HYSINGLA ER may increase the effect of either the antidepressant or HYSINGLA ER. (7.4)

USE IN SPECIFIC POPULATIONS

- Pregnancy: Based on animal data, may cause fetal harm. (8.1)
- Nursing Mothers: Discontinue nursing or discontinue drug. (8.3)
- Hepatic impairment: Use half the initial dose of HYSINGLA ER in patients with severe hepatic impairment and monitor closely for adverse events such as respiratory depression. (8.6)
- Renal impairment: Use half the initial dose of HYSINGLA ER in patients with moderate and severe renal impairment and end-stage renal disease and monitor closely for adverse events such as respiratory depression. (8.7)

See 17 for PATIENT COUNSELING INFORMATION and Medication Guide.

Revised: 2/2015

FULL PRESCRIBING INFORMATION: CONTENTS*
WARNING: ADDICTION, ABUSE, AND MISUSE; LIFE-THREATENING RESPIRATORY DEPRESSION; ACCIDENTAL INGESTION; NEONATAL OPIOID WITHDRAWAL SYNDROME; AND CYTOCHROME P450 3A4 INTERACTION

FULL PRESCRIBING INFORMATION

WARNING: ADDICTION, ABUSE, AND MISUSE; LIFE-THREATENING RESPIRATORY DEPRESSION; ACCIDENTAL INGESTION; NEONATAL OPIOID WITHDRAWAL SYNDROME; AND CYTOCHROME P450 3A4 INTERACTION

Addiction, Abuse, and Misuse

HYSINGLA ER exposes patients and other users to the risks of opioid addiction, abuse, and misuse, which can lead to overdose and death. Assess each patient's risk prior to prescribing HYSINGLA ER, and monitor all patients regularly for the development of these behaviors or conditions [see Warnings and Precautions (5.1)].

Life-Threatening Respiratory Depression

Serious, life-threatening, or fatal respiratory depression may occur with use of HYSINGLA ER. Monitor for respiratory depression, especially during initiation of HYSINGLA ER or following a dose increase. Instruct patients to swallow HYSINGLA ER tablets whole; crushing, chewing, or dissolving HYSINGLA ER tablets can cause rapid release and absorption of a potentially fatal dose of hydrocodone [see Warnings and Precautions (5.2)].

Accidental Ingestion

Accidental ingestion of even one dose of HYSINGLA ER, especially by children, can result in a fatal overdose of hydrocodone [see Warnings and Precautions (5.2)].

Neonatal Opioid Withdrawal Syndrome

Prolonged use of HYSINGLA ER during pregnancy can result in neonatal opioid withdrawal syndrome, which may be life-threatening if not recognized and treated, and requires management according to protocols developed by neonatology experts. If opioid use is required for a prolonged period in a pregnant woman, advise the patient of the risk of neonatal opioid withdrawal syndrome and ensure that appropriate treatment will be available [see Warnings and Precautions (5.3)].

Cytochrome P450 3A4 Interaction

The concomitant use of HYSINGLA ER with all cytochrome P450 3A4 inhibitors may result in an increase in hydrocodone plasma concentrations, which could increase or prolong adverse drug effects and may cause potentially fatal respiratory depression. In addition, discontinuation of a concomitantly used cytochrome P450 3A4 inducer may result in an increase in hydrocodone plasma concentration. Monitor patients receiving HYSINGLA ER and any CYP3A4 inhibitor or inducer [see Warnings and Precautions (5.11), Drug Interactions (7.1) and Clinical Pharmacology (12.3)].

---

1 INDICATIONS AND USAGE

HYSINGLA ER is indicated for the management of pain severe enough to require daily, around-the-clock, long-term opioid treatment and for which alternative treatment options are inadequate.

Limitations of Use

• Because of the risks of addiction, abuse, and misuse with opioids, even at recommended doses, and because of the greater risks of overdose and death with extended-release opioid formulations, reserve HYSINGLA ER for use in patients for whom alternative treatment options (e.g., non-opioid analgesics or immediate-release opioids) are ineffective, not tolerated, or would be otherwise inadequate to provide sufficient management of pain.

• HYSINGLA ER is not indicated as an as-needed analgesic.

2 DOSAGE AND ADMINISTRATION

2.1 Initial Dosing

HYSINGLA ER should be prescribed only by healthcare professionals who are knowledgeable in the use of potent opioids for the management of chronic pain.

Initiate the dosing regimen for each patient individually, taking into account the patient's prior analgesic treatment experience and risk factors for addiction, abuse, and misuse [see Warnings and Precautions (5.1)]. Monitor patients closely for respiratory depression, especially within the first 24-72 hours of initiating therapy with HYSINGLA ER [see Warnings and Precautions (5.2)].

HYSINGLA ER is administered orally once daily (every 24 hours).

HYSINGLA ER tablets must be taken whole, one tablet at a time, with enough water to ensure complete swallowing immediately after placing in the mouth [see Patient Counseling Information (17)]. Crushing, chewing, or dissolving HYSINGLA ER tablets will result in uncontrolled delivery of hydrocodone and can lead to overdose or death [see Warnings and Precautions (5.1)].

Use of HYSINGLA ER as the First Opioid Analgesic

Initiate therapy with HYSINGLA ER 20 mg orally every 24 hours.

Use of HYSINGLA ER in Patients who are not Opioid Tolerant

The starting dose for patients who are not opioid tolerant is HYSINGLA ER 20 mg orally every 24 hours. Opioid tolerant patients are those receiving, for one week or longer, at least 60 mg oral morphine per day, 25 mcg transdermal fentanyl per hour, 30 mg oral oxycodone per day, 8 mg oral hydromorphone per day, 25 mg oral oxymorphone per day, or an equianalgesic dose of another opioid.

Use of higher starting doses in patients who are not opioid tolerant may cause fatal respiratory depression [see Warnings and Precautions (5.2)].

Daily doses of HYSINGLA ER greater than or equal to 80 mg are only for use in opioid tolerant patients.

Conversion from Oral Hydrocodone Formulations to HYSINGLA ER

Patients receiving other oral hydrocodone-containing formulations may be converted to HYSINGLA ER by administering the patient's total daily oral hydrocodone dose as HYSINGLA ER once daily.

Conversion from Other Oral Opioids to HYSINGLA ER

Discontinue all other around-the-clock opioid drugs when HYSINGLA ER therapy is initiated.

Although tables of oral and parenteral equivalents are readily available, there is substantial inter-patient variability in the relative potency of different opioid drugs and formulations. As such, it is preferable to underestimate a patient's 24-hour oral hydrocodone requirements and provide rescue medication (e.g., immediate-release opioid) than to overestimate the 24-hour oral hydrocodone requirements and manage an adverse reaction.

To obtain the initial HYSINGLA ER dose, first use Table 1 to convert the prior oral opioids to a total hydrocodone daily dose and then reduce the calculated daily hydrocodone dose by 25% to account for interpatient variability in relative potency of different opioids.

Consider the following when using the information found in Table 1.

• This is **not** a table of equianalgesic doses.

• The conversion factors in this table are only for the conversion **from** one of the listed oral opioid analgesics to HYSINGLA ER.

• The table **cannot** be used to convert **from** HYSINGLA ER to another opioid. Doing so will result in an overestimation of the dose of the new opioid and may result in fatal overdose

Table 1. Conversion factors to HYSINGLA ER (Not Equianalgesic Doses)

Opioid	Oral dose (mg)	Approximate oral conversion factor
Codeine	133	0.15
Hydromorphone	5	4
Methadone	13.3	1.5
Morphine	40	0.5
Oxycodone	20	1
Oxymorphone	10	2
Tramadol	200	0.1

To calculate the estimated total hydrocodone daily dose using Table 1:

• For patients on a single opioid, sum the current total daily dose of the opioid and then multiply the total daily dose by the approximate oral conversion factor to calculate the approximate oral hydrocodone daily dose.

• For patients on a regimen of more than one opioid, calculate the approximate oral hydrocodone dose for each opioid and sum the totals to obtain the approximate oral hydrocodone daily dose.

• For patients on a regimen of fixed-ratio opioid/non-opioid analgesic products, use only the opioid component of these products in the conversion.

• Reduce the calculated daily oral hydrocodone dose by 25% Always round the dose down, if necessary, to the nearest HYSINGLA ER tablet strength available and initiate therapy with that dose. If the converted HYSINGLA ER dose using Table 1 is less than 20 mg, initiate therapy with HYSINGLA ER 20 mg.

Example conversion from a single opioid to HYSINGLA ER: For example, a total daily dose of oxycodone 50 mg would be converted to hydrocodone 50 mg based on the table above, and then multiplied by 0.75 (ie, take a 25 % reduction) resulting in a dose of 37.5 mg hydrocodone. Round this down to the nearest dose strength available, HYSINGLA ER 30 mg, to initiate therapy.

Close observation and frequent titration are warranted until pain management is stable on the new opioid. Monitor patients for signs and symptoms of opioid withdrawal or for signs of over-sedation/toxicity after converting patients to HYSINGLA ER.

The dose of HYSINGLA ER can be gradually adjusted every three to five days, using increments of 10 to 20 mg, until adequate pain relief and acceptable tolerability have been achieved.

Conversion from Methadone to HYSINGLA ER

Close monitoring is of particular importance when converting from methadone to other opioid agonists. The ratio between methadone and other opioid agonists may vary widely as a function of previous dose exposure. Methadone has a long half-life and can accumulate in the plasma.

Conversion from Transdermal Fentanyl to HYSINGLA ER

Eighteen hours following the removal of the transdermal fentanyl patch, HYSINGLA ER treatment can be initiated. For each 25 mcg/hr fentanyl transdermal patch, a dose of HYSINGLA ER 20 mg every 24 hours represents a conservative initial dose. Follow the patient closely during conversion from transdermal fentanyl to HYSINGLA ER, as there is limited experience with this conversion.

Conversion from Transdermal Buprenorphine to HYSINGLA ER

All patients receiving transdermal buprenorphine (≤ 20 mcg/hr) should initiate therapy with HYSINGLA ER 20 mg every 24 hours. Follow the patient closely during conversion from transdermal buprenorphine to HYSINGLA ER, as there is limited experience with this conversion.

2.2 Titration and Maintenance of Therapy

Individually titrate HYSINGLA ER to a dose that provides adequate analgesia and minimizes adverse reactions. Continually re-evaluate patients receiving HYSINGLA ER to assess the maintenance of pain control and the relative incidence of adverse reactions as well as monitoring for the development of addiction, abuse, or misuse. Frequent communication is important among the prescriber, other members of the healthcare team, the patient, and the caregiver/family during periods of changing analgesic requirements, including initial titration. During chronic therapy, periodically reassess the continued need for the use of opioid analgesics.

Adjust the dose of HYSINGLA ER in increments of 10 mg to 20 mg every 3 to 5 days as needed to achieve adequate analgesia.

Patients who experience breakthrough pain may require a dose increase of HYSINGLA ER, or may need rescue medication with an appropriate dose of an immediate-release analgesic. If the level of pain increases after dose stabilization, attempt to identify the source of increased pain before increasing the HYSINGLA ER dose.

Continued on next page

If unacceptable opioid-related adverse reactions are observed, the next daily dose may be reduced. Adjust the dose to obtain an appropriate balance between management of pain and opioid-related adverse reactions.

2.3 Administration of HYSINGLA ER

HYSINGLA ER is administered once daily (every 24 hours). HYSINGLA ER must be taken whole, one tablet at a time, with enough water to ensure complete swallowing immediately after placing in the mouth [see Patient Counseling Information (17)].

Crushing, chewing, or dissolving HYSINGLA ER tablets will result in uncontrolled delivery of hydrocodone and can lead to overdose or death [see Warnings and Precautions (5.1)].

Multiple tablets of lower dose strengths that provide the desired total daily dose can be taken as a once daily dose.

2.4 Patients with Hepatic Impairment

Patients with severe hepatic impairment may have higher plasma concentrations than those with normal function. Initiate therapy with ½ the initial dose of HYSINGLA ER in these patients and monitor closely for respiratory depression and sedation [see Clinical Pharmacology (12.3)].

2.5 Patients with Renal Impairment

Patients with moderate to severe renal impairment and end-stage renal disease may have higher plasma concentrations than those with normal function. Initiate therapy with ½ the initial dose of HYSINGLA ER in these patients and monitor closely for respiratory depression and sedation [see Clinical Pharmacology (12.3)].

2.6 Discontinuation of HYSINGLA ER

Do not abruptly discontinue HYSINGLA ER. When the patient no longer requires opioid therapy, use a gradual downward titration of the dose to prevent signs and symptoms of withdrawal in the physically dependent patient. The dose may be reduced every 2-4 days. The next dose should be at least 50% of the prior dose. After reaching HYSINGLA ER 20 mg dose for 2-4 days, HYSINGLA ER can be discontinued.

3 DOSAGE FORMS AND STRENGTHS

- 20 mg film-coated extended-release tablets (round, green-colored, bi-convex tablets printed with "HYD 20")
- 30 mg film-coated extended-release tablets (round, yellow-colored, bi-convex tablets printed with "HYD 30")
- 40 mg film-coated extended-release tablets (round, grey-colored, bi-convex tablets printed with "HYD 40")
- 60 mg film-coated extended-release tablets (round, beige-colored, bi-convex tablets printed with "HYD 60")
- 80 mg film-coated extended-release tablets (round, pink-colored, bi-convex tablets printed with "HYD 80")
- 100 mg film-coated extended-release tablets (round, blue-colored, bi-convex tablets printed with "HYD 100")
- 120 mg film-coated extended-release tablets (round, white-colored, bi-convex tablets printed with "HYD 120")

4 CONTRAINDICATIONS

HYSINGLA ER is contraindicated in patients with:
- Significant respiratory depression
- Acute or severe bronchial asthma in an unmonitored setting or in the absence of resuscitative equipment
- Known or suspected paralytic ileus and gastrointestinal obstruction
- Hypersensitivity to any component of HYSINGLA ER or the active ingredient, hydrocodone bitartrate

5 WARNINGS AND PRECAUTIONS

5.1 Addiction, Abuse, and Misuse

HYSINGLA ER contains hydrocodone, a Schedule II controlled substance. As an opioid, HYSINGLA ER exposes users to the risks of addiction, abuse, and misuse [see Drug Abuse and Dependence (9.1)]. As extended-release products such as HYSINGLA ER deliver the opioid over an extended period of time, there is a greater risk for overdose and death due to the larger amount of hydrocodone present.

Although the risk of addiction in any individual is unknown, it can occur in patients appropriately prescribed HYSINGLA ER and in those who obtain the drug illicitly. Addiction can occur at recommended doses and if the drug is misused or abused.

Assess each patient's risk for opioid addiction, abuse, or misuse prior to prescribing HYSINGLA ER, and monitor all patients receiving HYSINGLA ER for the development of these behaviors or conditions. Risks are increased in patients with a personal or family history of substance abuse (including drug or alcohol addiction or abuse) or mental illness (e.g., major depression). The potential for these risks should not, however, prevent the prescribing of HYSINGLA ER for the proper management of pain in any given patient.

Abuse or misuse of HYSINGLA ER by crushing, chewing, snorting, or injecting the dissolved product will result in the uncontrolled delivery of the hydrocodone and can result in overdose and death [see Drug Abuse and Dependence (9.1), and Overdosage (10)].

Opioid agonists are sought by drug abusers and people with addiction disorders and are subject to criminal diversion. Consider these risks when prescribing or dispensing HYSINGLA ER. Strategies to reduce these risks include prescribing the drug in the smallest appropriate quantity and advising the patient on the proper disposal of unused drug [see Patient Counseling Information (17)]. Contact local state professional licensing board or state controlled substances authority for information on how to prevent and detect abuse or diversion of this product.

5.2 Life-Threatening Respiratory Depression

Serious, life-threatening, or fatal respiratory depression has been reported with the use of modified-release opioids, even when used as recommended. Respiratory depression from opioid use, if not immediately recognized and treated, may lead to respiratory arrest and death. Management of respiratory depression may include close observation, supportive measures, and use of opioid antagonists, depending on the patient's clinical status [see Overdosage (10.2)]. Carbon dioxide (CO_2) retention from opioid-induced respiratory depression can exacerbate the sedating effects of opioids.

While serious, life-threatening, or fatal respiratory depression can occur at any time during the use of HYSINGLA ER, the risk is greatest during the initiation of therapy or following a dose increase. Closely monitor patients for respiratory depression when initiating therapy with HYSINGLA ER and following dose increases.

To reduce the risk of respiratory depression, proper dosing and titration of HYSINGLA ER are essential [see Dosage and Administration (2.1, 2.2)]. Overestimating the HYSINGLA ER dose when converting patients from another opioid product can result in fatal overdose with the first dose.

Accidental ingestion of even one dose of HYSINGLA ER, especially by children, can result in respiratory depression and death due to an overdose of hydrocodone.

5.3 Neonatal Opioid Withdrawal Syndrome

Prolonged use of HYSINGLA ER during pregnancy can result in withdrawal signs in the neonate. Neonatal opioid withdrawal syndrome, unlike opioid withdrawal syndrome in adults, may be life-threatening if not recognized and requires management according to protocols developed by neonatology experts. If opioid use is required for a prolonged period in a pregnant woman, advise the patient of the risk of neonatal opioid withdrawal syndrome and ensure that appropriate treatment will be available.

Neonatal opioid withdrawal syndrome presents as irritability, hyperactivity and abnormal sleep pattern, high pitched cry, tremor, vomiting, diarrhea and failure to gain weight. The onset, duration, and severity of neonatal opioid withdrawal syndrome vary based on the specific opioid used, duration of use, timing and amount of last maternal use, and rate of elimination of the drug by the newborn.

5.4 Interactions with Central Nervous System Depressants

Hypotension, profound sedation, coma, respiratory depression, and death may result if HYSINGLA ER is used concomitantly with alcohol or other central nervous system (CNS) depressants (e.g., sedatives, anxiolytics, hypnotics, neuroleptics, other opioids).

When considering the use of HYSINGLA ER in a patient taking a CNS depressant, assess the duration use of the CNS depressant and the patient's response, including the degree of tolerance that has developed to CNS depression. Additionally, evaluate the patient's use of alcohol or illicit drugs that cause CNS depression. If the decision to begin HYSINGLA ER is made, start with a lower HYSINGLA ER dose than usual (i.e., 20-30% less), monitor patients for signs of sedation and respiratory depression, and consider using a lower dose of the concomitant CNS depressant [see Drug Interactions (7.2)].

5.5 Use in Elderly, Cachectic, and Debilitated Patients

Life-threatening respiratory depression is more likely to occur in elderly, cachectic, or debilitated patients as they may have altered pharmacokinetics or altered clearance compared to younger, healthier patients. Monitor such patients closely, particularly when initiating and titrating HYSINGLA ER and when HYSINGLA ER is given concomitantly with other drugs that depress respiration [see Warnings and Precautions (5.2)].

5.6 Use in Patients with Chronic Pulmonary Disease

Monitor patients with significant chronic obstructive pulmonary disease or cor pulmonale, and patients having a substantially decreased respiratory reserve, hypoxia, hypercapnia, or preexisting respiratory depression for respiratory depression, particularly when initiating therapy and titrating with HYSINGLA ER, as in these patients, even usual therapeutic doses of HYSINGLA ER may decrease respiratory drive to the point of apnea [see Warnings and Precautions (5.2)]. Consider the use of alternative non-opioid analgesics in these patients if possible.

5.7 Use in Patients with Head Injury and Increased Intracranial Pressure

In the presence of head injury, intracranial lesions or a preexisting increase in intracranial pressure, the possible respiratory depressant effects of opioid analgesics and their potential to elevate cerebrospinal fluid pressure (resulting from vasodilation following CO_2 retention) may be markedly exaggerated. Furthermore, opioid analgesics can produce effects on pupillary response and consciousness, which may obscure neurologic signs of further increases in intracranial pressure in patients with head injuries.

Monitor patients closely who may be susceptible to the intracranial effects of CO_2 retention, such as those with evidence of increased intracranial pressure or impaired consciousness. Opioids may obscure the clinical course of a patient with a head injury.

Avoid the use of HYSINGLA ER in patients with impaired consciousness or coma.

5.8 Hypotensive Effect

HYSINGLA ER may cause severe hypotension including orthostatic hypotension and syncope in ambulatory patients. There is an added risk to individuals whose ability to maintain blood pressure has been compromised by a depleted blood volume, or after concurrent administration with drugs such as phenothiazines or other agents which compromise vasomotor tone. Monitor these patients for signs of hypotension after initiating or titrating the dose of HYSINGLA ER. In patients with circulatory shock, HYSINGLA ER may cause vasodilation that can further reduce cardiac output and blood pressure. Avoid the use of HYSINGLA ER in patients with circulatory shock.

5.9 Gastrointestinal Obstruction, Dysphagia, and Choking

In the clinical studies with specific instructions to take HYSINGLA ER with adequate water to swallow the tablet, 11 out of 2476 subjects reported difficulty swallowing HYSINGLA ER. These reports included esophageal obstruction, dysphagia, and choking, one of which had required medical intervention to remove the tablet [see Adverse Reactions (6)].

Instruct patients not to pre-soak, lick, or otherwise wet HYSINGLA ER tablets prior to placing in the mouth, and to take one tablet at a time with enough water to ensure complete swallowing immediately after placing in the mouth [see Patient Counseling Information (17)].

Patients with underlying gastrointestinal disorders such as esophageal cancer or colon cancer with a small gastrointestinal lumen are at greater risk of developing these complications. Consider use of an alternative analgesic in patients who have difficulty swallowing and patients at risk for underlying gastrointestinal disorders resulting in a small gastrointestinal lumen.

5.10 Decreased Bowel Motility

HYSINGLA ER is contraindicated in patients with known or suspected gastrointestinal obstruction, including paralytic ileus. Opioids diminish propulsive peristaltic waves in the gastrointestinal tract and decrease bowel motility. Monitor for decreased bowel motility in post-operative patients receiving opioids. The administration of HYSINGLA ER may obscure the diagnosis or clinical course in patients with acute abdominal conditions. Hydrocodone may cause spasm of the sphincter of Oddi. Monitor patients with biliary tract disease, including acute pancreatitis.

5.11 Cytochrome P450 3A4 Inhibitors and Inducers

Since the CYP3A4 isoenzyme plays a major role in the metabolism of HYSINGLA ER, drugs that alter CYP3A4 activity may cause changes in clearance of hydrocodone which could lead to changes in hydrocodone plasma concentrations.

The clinical results with CYP3A4 inhibitors show an increase in hydrocodone plasma concentrations and possibly increased or prolonged opioid effects, which could be more pronounced with concomitant use of CYP3A4 inhibitors. The expected clinical result with CYP3A4 inducers is a dcrease in hydrocodone plasma concentrations, lack of efficacy or, possibly, development of an abstinence syndrome in a patient who had developed physical dependence to hydrocodone.

If co-administration is necessary, caution is advised when initiating HYSINGLA ER treatment in patients currently taking, or discontinuing, CYP3A4 inhibitors or inducers. Evaluate these patients at frequent intervals and consider dose adjustments until stable drug effects are achieved [see Drug Interactions (7.1)].

5.12 Driving and Operating Machinery

HYSINGLA ER may impair the mental and physical abilities needed to perform potentially hazardous activities such as driving a car or operating machinery. Peak blood levels of hydrocodone may occur 14 – 16 hours (range 6 – 30 hours) after initial dosing of HYSINGLA ER tablet administration. Blood levels of hydrocodone, in some patients, may be high at the end of 24 hours after repeated-dose administration. Warn patients not to drive or operate dangerous machinery unless they are tolerant to the effects of HYSINGLA ER and know how they will react to the medication [see Clinical Pharmacology (12.3)].

5.13 Interaction with Mixed Agonist/Antagonist Opioid Analgesics

Avoid the use of mixed agonist/antagonist analgesics (i.e., pentazocine, nalbuphine, and butorphanol) in patients who have received, or are receiving, a course of therapy with a full opioid agonist analgesic, including HYSINGLA ER. In these patients, mixed agonist/antagonist analgesics may reduce the analgesic effect and/or may precipitate withdrawal symptoms.

5.14 QT Interval Prolongation

QTc prolongation has been observed with HYSINGLA ER following daily doses of 160 mg [see Clinical Pharmacology (12.2)]. This observation should be considered in making clinical decisions regarding patient monitoring when prescribing HYSINGLA ER in patients with congestive heart failure, bradyarrhythmias, electrolyte abnormalities, or who are taking medications that are known to prolong the QTc interval.

HYSINGLA ER should be avoided in patients with congenital long QT syndrome. In patients who develop QTc prolongation, consider reducing the dose by 33 - 50%, or changing to an alternate analgesic.

6 ADVERSE REACTIONS

The following serious adverse reactions are described elsewhere in the labeling:
- Addiction, Abuse, and Misuse [see Warnings and Precautions (5.1)]
- Life-Threatening Respiratory Depression [see Warnings and Precautions (5.2)]
- Neonatal Opioid Withdrawal Syndrome [see Warnings and Precautions (5.3)]
- Interactions with Other CNS Depressants [see Warnings and Precautions (5.4)]
- Hypotensive Effects [see Warnings and Precautions (5.8)]
- Gastrointestinal Effects [see Warnings and Precautions (5.9, 5.10)]

6.1 Clinical Trial Experience

Because clinical trials are conducted under widely varying conditions, adverse reaction rates observed in the clinical trials of a drug cannot be directly compared to rates in the clinical trials of another drug and may not reflect the rates observed in practice.

A total of 1,827 patients were treated with HYSINGLA ER in controlled and open-label chronic pain clinical trials. Five hundred patients were treated for 6 months and 364 patients were treated for 12 months. The clinical trial population consisted of opioid-naïve and opioid-experienced patients with persistent moderate to severe chronic pain.

The common adverse reactions (≥2%) reported by patients in clinical trials comparing HYSINGLA ER (20-120 mg/day) with placebo are shown in Table 2 below:

Table 2: Adverse Reactions Reported in ≥2% of Patients during the Open-Label Titration Period and Double-Blind Treatment Period: Opioid-Naïve and Opioid-Experienced Patients

MedDRA Preferred Term	Open-label Titration Period Placebo (N=905) (%)	Double-blind Treatment Period (N=292) (%)	HYSINGLA ER (N=296) (%)
Nausea	16	5	8
Constipation	9	2	3
Vomiting	7	3	6
Dizziness	7	2	3
Headache	7	2	2
Somnolence	5	1	1
Fatigue	4	1	1
Pruritus	3	<1	0
Tinnitus	2	1	2
Insomnia	2	2	3
Decreased appetite	1	1	2
Influenza	1	1	3

The adverse reactions seen in controlled and open-label chronic pain studies are presented below in the following manner: most common (≥5%), common (≥1% to <5%), and less common (<1%).

The most common adverse reactions (≥5%) reported by patients treated with HYSINGLA ER in the chronic pain clinical trials were constipation, nausea, vomiting, fatigue, upper respiratory tract infection, dizziness, headache, somnolence.

The common (≥1% to <5%) adverse events reported by patients treated with HYSINGLA ER in the chronic pain clinical trials organized by MedDRA (Medical Dictionary for Regulatory Activities) System Organ Class were:

Ear and labyrinth disorders	tinnitus
Gastrointestinal disorders	abdominal pain, abdominal pain upper, diarrhea, dry mouth, dyspepsia, gastroesophageal reflux disease
General disorders and administration site conditions	chest pain, chills, edema peripheral, pain, pyrexia
Infections and infestations	bronchitis, gastroenteritis, gastroenteritis viral, influenza, nasopharyngitis, sinusitis, urinary tract infection
Injury, poisoning and procedural complications	fall, muscle strain
Metabolism and nutrition disorders	decreased appetite
Musculoskeletal and connective tissue disorders	arthralgia, back pain, muscle spasms, musculoskeletal pain, myalgia, pain in extremity
Nervous system disorders	lethargy, migraine, sedation
Psychiatric disorders	anxiety, depression, insomnia
Respiratory, thoracic and mediastinal disorders	cough, nasal congestion, oropharyngeal pain
Skin and subcutaneous tissue disorders	hyperhidrosis, pruritus, rash
Vascular disorders	hot flush, hypertension

Other less common adverse reactions that were seen in <1% of the patients in the HYSINGLA ER chronic pain clinical trials include the following in alphabetical order: abdominal discomfort, abdominal distention, agitation, asthenia, choking, confusional state, depressed mood, drug hypersensitivity, drug withdrawal syndrome, dysphagia, dyspnea, esophageal obstruction, flushing, hypogonadism, hypotension, hypoxia, irritability, libido decreased, malaise, mental impairment, mood altered, muscle twitching, edema, orthostatic hypotension, palpitations, presyncope, retching, syncope, thinking abnormal, thirst, tremor, and urinary retention.

7 DRUG INTERACTIONS

7.1 Drugs Affecting Cytochrome P450 Isoenzymes

Inhibitors of CYP3A4

Co-administration of HYSINGLA ER with ketoconazole, a strong CYP3A4 inhibitor, significantly increased the plasma concentrations of hydrocodone. Inhibition of CYP3A4 activity by inhibitors, such as macrolide antibiotics (e.g., erythromycin), azole-antifungal agents (e.g., ketoconazole), and protease inhibitors (e.g., ritonavir), may prolong opioid effects. Caution is advised when initiating therapy with, currently taking, or discontinuing CYP3A4 inhibitors. Evaluate these patients at frequent intervals and consider dose adjustments until stable drug effects are achieved [see Clinical Pharmacology (12.3)].

Inducers of CYP3A4

CYP3A4 inducers may induce the metabolism of hydrocodone and, therefore, may cause increased clearance of the drug which could lead to a decrease in hydrocodone plasma concentrations, lack of efficacy or, possibly, development of a withdrawal syndrome in a patient who had developed physical dependence to hydrocodone. If co-administration with HYSINGLA ER is necessary, monitor for signs of opioid withdrawal and consider dose adjustments until stable drug effects are achieved [see Clinical Pharmacology (12.3)].

7.2 Central Nervous System Depressants

The concomitant use of HYSINGLA ER with other CNS depressants including sedatives, hypnotics, tranquilizers, general anesthetics, phenothiazines, other opioids, and alcohol can increase the risk of respiratory depression, profound sedation, coma and death. Monitor patients receiving CNS depressants and HYSINGLA ER for signs of respiratory depression, sedation and hypotension.

When combined therapy with any of the above medications is considered, the dose of one or both agents should be reduced [see Warnings and Precautions (5.4)].

7.3 Interactions with Mixed Agonist/Antagonist and Partial Agonist Opioid Analgesics

Mixed agonist/antagonist analgesics (i.e., pentazocine, nalbuphine, and butorphanol) and partial agonist analgesics (buprenorphine) may reduce the analgesic effect of HYSINGLA ER or precipitate withdrawal symptoms in these patients. Avoid the use of mixed agonist/antagonist and partial agonist analgesics in patients receiving HYSINGLA ER.

7.4 MAO Inhibitors

HYSINGLA ER is not recommended for use in patients who have received MAO inhibitors within 14 days, because severe and unpredictable potentiation by MAO inhibitors has been reported with opioid analgesics. No specific interaction between hydrocodone and MAO inhibitors has been observed, but caution in the use of any opioid in patients taking this class of drugs is appropriate.

7.5 Anticholinergics

Anticholinergics or other drugs with anticholinergic activity when used concurrently with opioid analgesics may increase the risk of urinary retention or severe constipation, which may lead to paralytic ileus. Monitor patients for signs of urinary retention and constipation in addition to respiratory and central nervous system depression when HYSINGLA ER is used concurrently with anticholinergic drugs.

7.6 Strong Laxatives

Concomitant use of HYSINGLA ER with strong laxatives (e.g., lactulose), that rapidly increase gastrointestinal motility, may decrease hydrocodone absorption and result in decreased hydrocodone plasma levels. If HYSINGLA ER is used in these patients, closely monitor for the development of adverse events as well as changing analgesic requirements.

8 USE IN SPECIFIC POPULATIONS

8.1 Pregnancy

Pregnancy Category C

Risk Summary

There are no adequate and well-controlled studies of HYSINGLA ER use during pregnancy. Prolonged use of opioid analgesics during pregnancy may cause neonatal opioid withdrawal syndrome. In animal reproduction studies with hydrocodone in rats and rabbits no embryotoxicity or teratogenicity was observed. However, reduced pup survival rates, reduced fetal/pup body weights, and delayed ossification were observed at doses causing maternal toxicity. In all of the studies conducted, the exposures in animals were less than the human exposure (see Animal Data). HYSINGLA ER should be used during pregnancy only if the potential benefit justifies the potential risk to the fetus.

Clinical Considerations

Fetal/neonatal adverse reactions

Prolonged use of opioid analgesics during pregnancy for medical or nonmedical purposes can result in physical dependence in the neonate and neonatal opioid withdrawal syndrome shortly after birth. Observe newborns for symptoms of neonatal opioid withdrawal syndrome, such as poor feeding, diarrhea, irritability, tremor, rigidity, and seizures, and manage accordingly [see Warnings and Precautions (5.3)].

Data

Animal Data

No evidence of embryotoxicity or teratogenicity was ob-

Continued on next page

served after oral administration of hydrocodone throughout the period of organogenesis in rats and rabbits at doses up to 30 mg/kg/day (approximately 0.1 and 0.3-fold, respectively, the human hydrocodone dose of 120 mg/day based on AUC exposure comparisons). However, in these studies, reduced fetal body weights and delayed ossification were observed in rat at 30 mg/kg/day and reduced fetal body weights were observed in in rabbit at 30 mg/kg/day (approximately 0.1 and 0.3-fold, respectively, the human hydrocodone dose of 120 mg/day based on AUC exposure comparisons). In a pre- and post-natal development study pregnant rats were administered oral hydrocodone throughout the period of gestation and lactation. At a dose of 30 mg/kg/day decreased pup viability, pup survival indices, litter size and pup body weight were observed. This dose is approximately 0.1-fold the human hydrocodone dose of 120 mg/day based on AUC exposure comparisons.

8.2 Labor and Delivery

Opioids cross the placenta and may produce respiratory depression in neonates. HYSINGLA ER is not recommended for use in women immediately prior to and during labor, when use of shorter acting analgesics or other analgesic techniques are more appropriate. HYSINGLA ER may prolong labor through actions which temporarily reduce the strength, duration and frequency of uterine contractions. However, this effect is not consistent and may be offset by an increased rate of cervical dilatation, which tends to shorten labor.

8.3 Nursing Mothers

Hydrocodone is present in human milk. Because of the potential for serious adverse reactions in nursing infants, a decision should be made whether to discontinue nursing or to discontinue HYSINGLA ER, taking into account the importance of the drug to the mother. Infants exposed to HYSINGLA ER through breast milk should be monitored for excess sedation and respiratory depression. Withdrawal symptoms can occur in breast-fed infants when maternal administration of an opioid analgesic is stopped, or when breast-feeding is stopped.

8.4 Pediatric Use

The safety and effectiveness of HYSINGLA ER in pediatric patients have not been established.

Accidental ingestion of a single dose of HYSINGLA ER in children can result in a fatal overdose of hydrocodone *[see Warnings and Precautions (5.2)]*.

HYSINGLA ER gradually forms a viscous hydrogel (i.e., a gelatinous mass) when exposed to water or other fluids. Pediatric patients may be at increased risk of esophageal obstruction, dysphagia, and choking because of a smaller gastrointestinal lumen if they ingest HYSINGLA ER *[see Warnings and Precautions (5.9)]*.

8.5 Geriatric Use

In a controlled pharmacokinetic study, elderly subjects (greater than 65 years) compared to young adults had similar plasma concentrations of hydrocodone *[see Clinical Pharmacology (12.3)]*. Of the 1827 subjects exposed to HYSINGLA ER in the pooled chronic pain studies, 241 (13%) were age 65 and older (including those age 75 and older), while 42 (2%) were age 75 and older. In clinical trials with appropriate initiation of therapy and dose titration, no untoward or unexpected adverse reactions were seen in the elderly patients who received HYSINGLA ER.

Hydrocodone may cause confusion and over-sedation in the elderly. In addition, because of the greater frequency of decreased hepatic, renal, or cardiac function, concomitant disease and concomitant use of CNS active medications, start elderly patients on low doses of HYSINGLA ER and monitor closely for adverse events such as respiratory depression, sedation, and confusion.

8.6 Hepatic Impairment

No adjustment in starting dose with HYSINGLA ER is required in patients with mild or moderate hepatic impairment. Patients with severe hepatic impairment may have higher plasma concentrations than those with normal hepatic function. Initiate therapy with 1/2 the initial dose of HYSINGLA ER in patients with severe hepatic impairment and monitor closely for adverse events such as respiratory depression *[see Clinical Pharmacology (12.3)]*.

8.7 Renal Impairment

No dose adjustment is needed in patients with mild renal impairment. Patients with moderate or severe renal impairment or end stage renal disease have higher plasma concentrations than those with normal renal function. Initiate therapy with 1/2 the initial dose of HYSINGLA ER in these patients and monitor closely for adverse events such as respiratory depression *[see Clinical Pharmacology (12.3)]*.

9 DRUG ABUSE AND DEPENDENCE

9.1 Controlled Substance

HYSINGLA ER contains hydrocodone bitartrate, a Schedule II controlled substance with a high potential for abuse similar to fentanyl, methadone, morphine, oxycodone, and oxymorphone. HYSINGLA ER can be abused and is subject to misuse, abuse, addiction and criminal diversion. The high drug content in the extended-release formulation adds to the risk of adverse outcomes from abuse and misuse.

9.2 Abuse

All patients treated with opioids require careful monitoring for signs of abuse and addiction, because use of opioid analgesic products carries the risk of addiction even under appropriate medical use.

Drug abuse is the intentional non-therapeutic use of an over-the-counter or prescription drug, even once, for its rewarding psychological or physiological effects. Drug abuse includes, but is not limited to the following examples: the use of a prescription or over-the-counter drug to get "high," or the use of steroids for performance enhancement and muscle build up.

Drug addiction is a cluster of behavioral, cognitive, and physiological phenomena that develop after repeated substance use and include: a strong desire to take the drug, difficulties in controlling its use, persisting in its use despite harmful consequences, a higher priority given to drug use than to other activities and obligations, increased tolerance, and sometimes a physical withdrawal.

"Drug-seeking" behavior is very common to addicts and drug abusers. Drug seeking tactics include, but are not limited to, emergency calls or visits near the end of office hours, refusal to undergo appropriate examination, testing or referral, repeated claims of "loss" of prescriptions, tampering with prescriptions and reluctance to provide prior medical records or contact information for other treating physician(s). "Doctor shopping" (visiting multiple prescribers) to obtain additional prescriptions is common among drug abusers, people with untreated addiction, and criminals seeking drugs to sell. Preoccupation with achieving adequate pain relief can be appropriate behavior in a patient with poor pain control.

Abuse and addiction are separate and distinct from physical dependence and tolerance. Physicians should be aware that addiction may not be accompanied by concurrent tolerance and symptoms of physical dependence in all addicts. In addition, abuse of opioids can occur in the absence of true addiction.

HYSINGLA ER can be diverted for non-medical use into illicit channels of distribution. Careful record-keeping of prescribing information, including quantity, frequency, and renewal requests, as required by law, is strongly advised.

Proper assessment of the patient, proper prescribing practices, periodic re-evaluation of therapy, and proper dispensing and storage are appropriate measures that help to limit abuse of opioid drugs.

Abuse may occur by taking intact tablets in quantities greater than prescribed or without legitimate purpose, by crushing and chewing or snorting the crushed formulation, or by injecting a solution made from the crushed formulation. The risk is increased with concurrent use of HYSINGLA ER with alcohol or other central nervous system depressants.

Risks Specific to Abuse of HYSINGLA ER

HYSINGLA ER is for oral use only. Abuse of HYSINGLA ER poses a risk of overdose and death.. Taking cut, broken, chewed, crushed, or dissolved HYSINGLA ER increases the risk of overdose and death.

With parenteral abuse, the inactive ingredients in HYSINGLA ER can result in death, local tissue necrosis, infection, pulmonary granulomas, and increased risk of endocarditis and valvular heart injury. Parenteral drug abuse is commonly associated with transmission of infectious diseases, such as hepatitis and HIV.

Abuse Deterrence Studies

HYSINGLA ER is formulated with physicochemical properties intended to make the tablet more difficult to manipulate for misuse and abuse, and maintains some extended release characteristics even if the tablet is physically compromised. To evaluate the ability of these physicochemical properties to reduce the potential for abuse of HYSINGLA ER, a series of *in vitro*laboratory studies, pharmacokinetic studies and clinical abuse potential studies was conducted. A summary is provided at the end of this section.

In Vitro Testing

*In vitro*physical and chemical tablet manipulation studies were performed to evaluate the success of different extraction methods in defeating the extended-release formulation. Results support that HYSINGLA ER resists crushing, breaking, and dissolution using a variety of tools and solvents and retains some extended-release properties despite manipulation. When subjected to an aqueous environment, HYSINGLA ER gradually forms a viscous hydrogel (i.e., a gelatinous mass) that resists passage through a hypodermic needle.

Clinical Abuse Potential Studies

Studies in Non-dependent Opioid Abusers

Two randomized, double-blind, placebo and active-comparator studies in non-dependent opioid abusers were conducted to characterize the abuse potential of HYSINGLA ER following physical manipulation and administration via the intranasal and oral routes. For both studies, drug liking was measured on a bipolar drug liking scale of 0 to 100 where 50 represents a neutral response of neither liking nor disliking, 0 represents maximum disliking, and 100 represents maximum liking. Response to whether the subject would take the study drug again was measured on a unipolar scale of 0 to 100 where 0 represents the strongest negative response ("definitely would not take drug again") and 100 represents the strongest positive response ("definitely would take drug again").

Intranasal Abuse Potential Study

In the intranasal abuse potential study, 31 subjects were dosed and 25 subjects completed the study. Treatments studied included intranasally administered tampered HYSINGLA ER 60 mg tablets, powdered hydrocodone bitartrate 60 mg, and placebo. Incomplete dosing due to granules falling from the subjects' nostrils occurred in 82% (n = 23) of subjects receiving tampered HYSINGLA ER compared to no subjects with powdered hydrocodone or placebo. The intranasal administration of tampered HYSINGLA ER was associated with statistically significantly lower mean and median scores for drug liking and take drug again (P<0.001 for both), compared with powdered hydrocodone as summarized in Table 3.

Table 3. Summary of Maximum Scores (E_{max}) on Drug Liking and Take Drug Again VAS Following intranasal Administration of HYSINGLA ER and Hydrocodone Powder in Non-dependent Opioid Abusers

VAS Scale (100 point) *Intranasal (n=25)*	HYSINGLA ER Manipulated	Hydrocodone Powder
Drug Liking*		
Mean (SE)	65.4 (3.7)	90.4 (2.6)
Median (Range)	56 (50–100)	100 (51–100)
Take Drug Again**		
Mean (SE)	36.4 (8.2)	85.2 (5.0)
Median (Range)	14 (0-100)	100 (1-100)

*Bipolar scale (0=maximum negative response, 50=neutral response, 100=maximum positive response)

** Unipolar scale (0=maximum negative response, 100=maximum positive response)

Figure 1 demonstrates a comparison of peak drug liking scores for tampered HYSINGLA ER compared with powdered hydrocodone in subjects (n = 25) who received both treatments intranasally. The Y-axis represents the percent of subjects attaining a percent reduction in peak drug liking scores for tampered HYSINGLA ER vs. hydrocodone powder greater than or equal to the value on the X-axis.

Approximately 80% (n = 20) of subjects had some reduction in drug liking with tampered HYSINGLA ER relative to hydrocodone powder. Sixty-eight percent (n = 17) of subjects had a reduction of at least 30% in drug liking with tampered HYSINGLA ER compared with hydrocodone powder, and approximately 64% (n = 16) of subjects had a reduction of at least 50% in drug liking with tampered HYSINGLA ER compared with hydrocodone powder. Approximately 20% (n = 5) of subjects had no reduction in liking with tampered HYSINGLA ER relative to hydrocodone powder.

[See figure 1 at top of next column]

Oral Abuse Potential Study

In the oral abuse potential study, 40 subjects were dosed and 35 subjects completed the study. Treatments studied included oral administrations of chewed HYSINGLA ER 60 mg tablets, intact HYSINGLA ER 60 mg tablets, 60 mg aqueous hydrocodone bitartrate solution, and placebo.

The oral administration of chewed and intact HYSINGLA ER was associated with statistically lower

Figure 1: Percent Reduction Profiles for E$_{max}$ of Drug Liking VAS for Manipulated HYSINGLA ER vs. Hydrocodone Powder, N = 25 Following Intranasal Administration

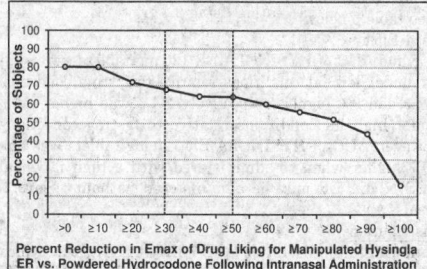

Percent Reduction in Emax of Drug Liking for Manipulated Hysingla ER vs. Powdered Hydrocodone Following Intranasal Administration

Table 4. Summary of Maximum Scores (E$_{max}$) on Drug Liking and Take Drug Again VAS Following Oral Administration of HYSINGLA ER and Hydrocodone Solution in Non-dependent Recreational Opioid Users

VAS Scale (100 point)	HYSINGLA ER		Hydrocodone Solution
Oral (n=35)	Intact	Chewed	
Drug Liking*			
Mean (SE)	63.3 (2.7)	69.0 (3.0)	94.0 (1.7)
Median (Range)	58 (50–100)	66 (50–100)	100 (51–100)
Take Drug Again**			
Mean (SE)	34.3 (6.1)	44.3 (6.9)	89.7 (3.6)
Median (Range)	24 (0-100)	55 (0-100)	100 (1-100)

*Bipolar scale (0=maximum negative response, 50=neutral response, 100=maximum positive response)
** Unipolar scale (0=maximum negative response, 100=maximum positive response)

mean and median scores on scales that measure drug liking and desire to take drug again (P<0.001), compared to hydrocodone solution as summarized in Table 4.
[See table 4 above]
Figure 2 demonstrates a comparison of peak drug liking scores for chewed HYSINGLA ER compared with hydrocodone solution in subjects who received both treatments orally. The Y-axis represents the percent of subjects attaining a percent reduction in peak drug liking scores for chewed HYSINGLA ER vs. hydrocodone solution greater than or equal to the value on the X-axis.
Approximately 80% (n = 28) of subjects had some reduction in drug liking with chewed HYSINGLA ER relative to hydrocodone solution. Approximately 69% (n = 24) of subjects had a reduction of at least 30% in drug liking with chewed HYSINGLA ER compared with hydrocodone solution, and approximately 60% (n = 21) of subjects had a reduction of at least 50% in drug liking with chewed HYSINGLA ER compared with hydrocodone solution. Approximately 20% (n = 7) of subjects had no reduction in drug liking with chewed HYSINGLA ER relative to hydrocodone solution.

Figure 2. Percent Reduction Profiles for E$_{max}$ of Drug Liking VAS for Chewed HYSINGLA ER vs. Hydrocodone Solution, N = 35 Following Oral Administration

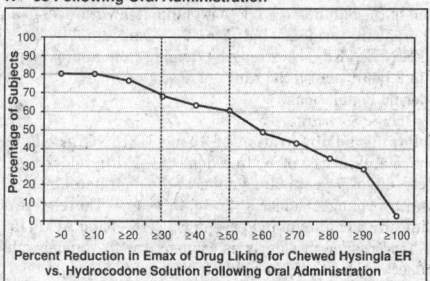

Percent Reduction in Emax of Drug Liking for Chewed Hysingla ER vs. Hydrocodone Solution Following Oral Administration

The results of a similar analysis of drug liking for intact HYSINGLA ER relative to hydrocodone solution were comparable to the results of chewed HYSINGLA ER relative to hydrocodone solution. Approximately 83% (n = 29) of subjects had some reduction in drug liking with intact HYSINGLA ER relative to hydrocodone solution. Eighty-three percent (n = 29) of subjects had a reduction of at least 30% in peak drug liking scores with intact HYSINGLA ER compared to hydrocodone solution, and approximately 74% (n = 26) of subjects had a reduction of at least 50% in peak drug liking scores with intact HYSINGLA ER compared with hydrocodone solution. Approximately 17% (n = 6) had no reduction in drug liking with intact HYSINGLA ER relative to hydrocodone solution.
Summary
The *in vitro* data demonstrate that HYSINGLA ER has physical and chemical properties that are expected to deter intranasal and intravenous abuse. The data from the clinical abuse potential studies, along with support from the *in vitro* data, also indicate that HYSINGLA ER has physicochemical properties that are expected to reduce intranasal abuse and oral abuse when chewed. However, abuse of HYSINGLA ER by the intravenous, intranasal, and oral routes is still possible.
Additional data, including epidemiological data, when available, may provide further information on the impact of HYSINGLA ER on the abuse liability of the drug. Accordingly, this section may be updated in the future as appropriate.

HYSINGLA ER contains hydrocodone, an opioid agonist and Schedule II controlled substance with an abuse liability similar to other opioid agonists, legal or illicit, including fentanyl, hydromorphone, methadone, morphine, oxycodone, and oxymorphone. HYSINGLA ER can be abused and is subject to misuse, addiction, and criminal diversion *[See Warnings and Precautions (5.1) and Drug Abuse and Dependence (9)]*.

9.3   Dependence
Both tolerance and physical dependence can develop during chronic opioid therapy. Tolerance is the need for increasing doses of opioids to maintain a defined effect such as analgesia (in the absence of disease progression or other external factors). Tolerance may occur to both the desired and undesired effects of drugs, and may develop at different rates for different effects.
Physical dependence results in withdrawal symptoms after abrupt discontinuation or a significant dose reduction of a drug. Withdrawal also may be precipitated through the administration of drugs with opioid antagonist activity, e.g., naloxone, nalmefene, or mixed agonist/antagonist analgesics (pentazocine, butorphanol, nalbuphine). Physical dependence may not occur to a clinically significant degree until after several days to weeks of continued opioid usage.
HYSINGLA ER should be discontinued by a gradual downward titration *[see Dosage and Administration (2.6)]*. If HYSINGLA ER is abruptly discontinued in a physically dependent patient, an abstinence syndrome may occur. Some or all of the following can characterize this syndrome: restlessness, lacrimation, rhinorrhea, yawning, perspiration, chills, piloerection, myalgia, mydriasis, irritability, anxiety, backache, joint pain, weakness, abdominal cramps, insomnia, nausea, anorexia, vomiting, diarrhea, increased blood pressure, respiratory rate, or heart rate.
Infants born to mothers physically dependent on opioids will also be physically dependent and may exhibit respiratory difficulties and withdrawal symptoms *[see Warnings and Precautions (5.3) and Use in Specific Populations (8.3)]*.

10   OVERDOSAGE
10.1   Symptoms
Acute overdosage with opioids is often characterized by respiratory depression, somnolence progressing to stupor or coma, skeletal muscle flaccidity, cold and clammy skin, constricted pupils, and, sometimes, pulmonary edema, bradycardia, hypotension, and death. Marked mydriasis rather than miosis may be seen due to severe hypoxia in overdose situations *[see Clinical Pharmacology (12.2)]*.
10.2   Treatment
In the treatment of HYSINGLA ER overdosage, primary attention should be given to the re-establishment of a patent airway and institution of assisted or controlled ventilation. Employ other supportive measures (including oxygen and vasopressors) in the management of circulatory shock and pulmonary edema accompanying overdose as indicated. Cardiac arrest or arrhythmias will require advanced life support techniques.
The opioid antagonist naloxone hydrochloride is a specific antidote against respiratory depression that may result from opioid overdosage. Nalmefene is an alternative opioid antagonist, which may be administered as a specific antidote to respiratory depression resulting from opioid overdose. Since the duration of action of HYSINGLA ER may exceed that of the antagonist, keep the patient under continued surveillance and administer repeated doses of the antagonist according to the antagonist labeling, as needed, to maintain adequate respiration.
Opioid antagonists should not be administered in the absence of clinically significant respiratory or circulatory de-

pression. Administer opioid antagonists cautiously to persons who are known, or suspected to be, physically dependent on HYSINGLA ER. In such cases, an abrupt or complete reversal of opioid effects may precipitate an acute abstinence syndrome. In an individual physically dependent on opioids, administration of the usual dose of the antagonist will precipitate an acute withdrawal syndrome. The severity of the withdrawal syndrome produced will depend on the degree of physical dependence and the dose of the antagonist administered. If a decision is made to treat serious respiratory depression in the physically dependent patient, administration of the antagonist should be initiated with care and by titration with smaller than usual doses of the antagonist.

11   DESCRIPTION
HYSINGLA ER (hydrocodone bitartrate) extended-release tablets are supplied in 20 mg, 30 mg, 40 mg, 60 mg, 80 mg, 100 mg and 120 mg film-coated tablets for oral administration. The tablet strengths describe the amount of hydrocodone per tablet as the bitartrate salt.
Hydrocodone bitartrate is an opioid agonist. Its chemical name is 4,5α-epoxy-3-methoxy-17-methylmorphinan-6-one tartrate (1:1) hydrate (2:5). Its structural formula is:

Empirical formula: $C_{18}H_{21}NO_3 \cdot C_4H_6O_6 \cdot 2\frac{1}{2}H_2O$; Molecular weight: 494.49.

Hydrocodone bitartrate exists as fine white crystals or a crystalline powder. It is affected by light. It is soluble in water, slightly soluble in alcohol, and insoluble in ether and chloroform.
The 20 mg, 30 mg, 40 mg, 60 mg, 80 mg, 100 mg and 120 mg tablets contain the following inactive ingredients: Butylated Hydroxytoluene (BHT, an additive in Polyethylene Oxide), Hydroxypropyl Cellulose, Macrogol/PEG 3350, Magnesium Stearate, Microcrystalline Cellulose, Polyethylene Oxide, Polysorbate 80, Polyvinyl Alcohol, Talc, Titanium Dioxide, and Black Ink.
The 20 mg tablets also contain Iron Oxide Yellow and FD&C Blue #2 Aluminum Lake/Indigo Carmine Aluminum Lake.
The 30 mg tablets also contain Iron Oxide Yellow.
The 40 mg tablets also contain Iron Oxide Yellow, Iron Oxide Red, and Iron Oxide Black.
The 60 mg tablets also contain Iron Oxide Yellow and Iron Oxide Red.
The 80 mg tablets also contain Iron Oxide Red.
The 100 mg tablets also contain FD&C Blue #2 Aluminum Lake.
Black Ink Contains: Shellac Glaze (in Ethanol), Isopropyl Alcohol, Iron Oxide Black, N-Butyl Alcohol, Propylene Glycol and Ammonium Hydroxide.

12   CLINICAL PHARMACOLOGY
12.1   Mechanism of Action
Hydrocodone is a semi-synthetic opioid agonist with relative selectivity for the mu-opioid receptor, although it can interact with other opioid receptors at higher doses. Hydrocodone acts as an agonist binding to and activating opioid receptors in the brain and spinal cord, which are coupled to G-protein complexes and modulate synaptic transmission through adenylate cyclase. The pharmacological ef-

Continued on next page

fects of hydrocodone including analgesia, euphoria, respiratory depression and physiological dependence are believed to be primarily mediated via μ opioid receptors.

12.2 Pharmacodynamics

Cardiac Electrophysiology

QTc interval prolongation was studied in a double-blind, placebo- and positive-controlled 3-treatment parallel-group, dose-escalating study of HYSINGLA ER in 196 healthy subjects. QTc interval prolongation was observed following HYSINGLA ER 160 mg per day. The maximum mean (90% upper confidence bound) difference in the QTc interval between HYSINGLA ER and placebo (after baseline-correction) at steady state was 6 (9) milliseconds, 7 (10) milliseconds, and 10 (13) milliseconds at HYSINGLA ER doses of 80 mg, 120 mg and 160mg respectively. For clinical implications of the prolonged QTc interval, see Warnings and Precautions (5.14).

Central Nervous System

The principal therapeutic action of hydrocodone is analgesia. In common with other opioids, hydrocodone causes respiratory depression, in part by a direct effect on the brainstem respiratory centers. The respiratory depression involves a reduction in the responsiveness of the brain stem respiratory centers to both increases in carbon dioxide tension and electrical stimulation. Opioids depress the cough reflex by direct effect on the cough center in the medulla. Hydrocodone causes miosis, even in total darkness. Pinpoint pupils are a sign of opioid overdose but are not pathognomonic (e.g., pontine lesions of hemorrhagic or ischemic origin may produce similar findings). Marked mydriasis rather than miosis may be seen with hypoxia in overdose situations *[see Overdosage (10.1)]*. In addition to analgesia, the widely diverse effects of hydrocodone include drowsiness, changes in mood, decreased gastrointestinal motility, nausea, vomiting, and alterations of the endocrine and autonomic nervous system *[see Clinical Pharmacology (12.2)]*.

Gastrointestinal Tract and Other Smooth Muscle

Hydrocodone causes a reduction in motility associated with an increase in smooth muscle tone in the antrum of the stomach and duodenum. Digestion of food in the small intestine is delayed and propulsive contractions are decreased. Propulsive peristaltic waves in the colon are decreased, while tone may be increased to the point of spasm resulting in constipation. Other opioid-induced effects may include a reduction in gastric, biliary and pancreatic secretions, spasm of sphincter of Oddi, and transient elevations in serum amylase.

Cardiovascular System

Hydrocodone may produce release of histamine with or without associated peripheral vasodilation. Manifestations of histamine release and/or peripheral vasodilation may include pruritus, flushing, red eyes, sweating, and/or orthostatic hypotension.

Endocrine System

Opioids may influence the hypothalamic-pituitary-adrenal or -gonadal axes. Some changes that can be seen include an increase in serum prolactin, and decreases in plasma cortisol and testosterone. Clinical signs and symptoms may be manifest from these hormonal changes.

Immune System

In vitro and animal studies indicate that opioids have a variety of effects on immune functions, depending on the context in which they are used. The clinical significance of these findings is unknown.

Concentration/Exposure—Efficacy Relationships

The minimum effective plasma concentration of hydrocodone for analgesia varies widely among patients, especially among patients who have been previously treated with agonist opioids. As a result, titrate the doses of individual patients to achieve a balance between therapeutic and adverse effects. The minimum effective analgesic concentration of hydrocodone for any individual patient may in-

crease over time due to an increase in pain, progression of disease, development of a new pain syndrome and/or potential development of analgesic tolerance.

Concentration/Exposure—Adverse Experience Relationships

There is a general relationship between increasing opioid plasma concentration and increasing frequency of adverse experiences such as nausea, vomiting, CNS effects, and respiratory depression. As with all opioids, the dose of HYSINGLA ER must be individualized *[see Dosage and Administration (2.1, 2.2)]*. The effective analgesic dose for some patients will be too high to be tolerated by other patients.

12.3 Pharmacokinetics

Absorption

HYSINGLA ER is a single-entity extended-release formulation of hydrocodone that yields a gradual increase in plasma hydrocodone concentrations with a median T_{max} of 14 – 16 hours noted for different dose strengths. Peak plasma levels may occur in the range of 6 -30 hours after single dose HYSINGLA ER administration.

Systemic exposure (AUC and C_{max}) increased linearly with doses from 20 to 120 mg. Both C_{max} and AUC increased slightly more than dose proportionally (Table 5). The mean terminal half-life ($t_{1/2}$) was similar for all HYSINGLA ER dose strengths ranging from 7 to 9 hours.

Table 5 Mean (SD) Single-Dose Pharmacokinetic Parameters of HYSINGLA ER

Dose Strength (mg)	AUCinf (ng•h/mL)	C_{max} (ng/mL)	T_{max}* (h)
20	284 (128)	14.6 (5.5)	16 (6, 24)
40	622 (252)	33.9 (11.8)	16 (6, 24)
60	1009 (294)	53.6 (15.4)	14 (10, 30)
80	1304 (375)	69.1 (17.2)	16 (10, 24)
120	1787 (679)	110 (44.1)	14 (6, 30)

* median (minimum, maximum)

As compared to an immediate-release hydrocodone combination product, HYSINGLA ER at the same daily dose results in similar bioavailability but with lower maximum concentrations at steady state. (Figure 3).

Figure 3. Mean Steady-State Plasma Hydrocodone Concentration Profile

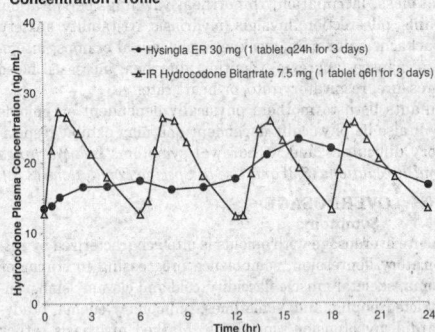

- Hysingla ER 30 mg (1 tablet q24h for 3 days)
- IR Hydrocodone Bitartrate 7.5 mg (1 tablet q6h for 3 days)

Steady-state plasma hydrocodone concentrations were confirmed on day 3 of once-daily dosing of HYSINGLA ER. The extent of accumulation of systemic exposure was 1.3 and 1.1 fold with respect to AUC and C_{max} at steady-state. The mean terminal half-life ($t_{1/2}$) at steady state was 7 hours. Median T_{max} values were 14 hours (range: 12 to 24 hours) on both Day 1 and Day 5 following once daily administration of HYSINGLA ER for five days. Daily fluctuation in

peak to trough plasma levels of hydrocodone were higher at 80 mg and 120 mg doses of HYSINGLA ER compared to 30 mg dose (Table 6).
[See table 6 below]

Food Effects

C_{max} and AUC of HYSINGLA ER 120 mg tablets were similar under low fat conditions relative to fasting conditions (17% and 9% higher, respectively). C_{max} was higher (54%) under high fat conditions relative to fasting conditions; however, AUC of HYSINGLA ER 120 mg tablets was only 20% higher when co-administered with a high fat meal. HYSINGLA ER may be administered without regard to meals.

Distribution

Following administration of HYSINGLA ER, the typical (70 kg adult) value of apparent volume of distribution (V/F) is 402 L, suggesting extensive tissue distribution. The extent of *in vivo* binding of hydrocodone to human plasma proteins was minimal with a mean % bound at 36%.

Elimination

Metabolism

Hydrocodone exhibits a complex pattern of metabolism, including N-demethylation, O-demethylation, and 6-keto reduction to the corresponding 6-α- and 6-β-hydroxy metabolites. CYP3A4 mediated N-demethylation to inactive norhydrocodone is the primary metabolic pathway of hydrocodone with a lower contribution from CYP2B6 and CYP2C19. The minor metabolite hydromorphone (<3% of the circulating parent hydrocodone) was mainly formed by CYP2D6 mediated O-demethylation with a smaller contribution by CYP2B6 and CYP2C19. Hydromorphone may contribute to the total analgesic effect of hydrocodone.

Excretion

Hydrocodone and its metabolites are cleared primarily by renal excretion. The percent of administered dose excreted unchanged as hydrocodone in urine was 6.5% in subjects with normal renal function, and 5.0%, 4.8%, and 2.3% in subjects with mild, moderate, and severe renal impairment, respectively. Renal clearance (CLr) of hydrocodone in healthy subjects was small (5.3 L/h) compared to apparent oral clearance (CL/F, 83 L/h); suggesting that non-renal clearance is the main elimination route. Ninety-nine percent of the administered dose is eliminated within 72 hours. The mean terminal half-life ($t_{1/2}$) was similar for all HYSINGLA ER dose strengths ranging from approximately 7 to 9 hours across the range of doses.

Specific Populations

Elderly (≥ 65 years)

Following administration of 40 mg HYSINGLA ER, the pharmacokinetics of hydrocodone in healthy elderly subjects (65 to 77 years) are similar to the pharmacokinetics in healthy younger subjects (20 to 45 years). There were no clinically meaningful increase in C_{max} (16%) and AUC (15%) of hydrocodone in elderly as compared with younger adult subjects *[see Use in Specific Populations (8.5)]*.

Gender

Systemic exposure of hydrocodone (C_{max} and AUC) was similar between males and females.

Hepatic Impairment

After a single dose of 20 mg HYSINGLA ER in subjects (8 each) with normal hepatic function, mild, moderate or severe hepatic impairment based on Child-Pugh classifications, mean hydrocodone C_{max} values were 16, 15, 17, and 18 ng/mL, respectively. Mean hydrocodone AUC values were 342, 310, 390, and 415 ng.hr/mL for subjects with normal hepatic function, mild, moderate or severe hepatic impairment, respectively. Geometric mean hydrocodone C_{max} values were -6%, 5%, and 5% and AUC values were -14%, 13%, and 4% in patients with mild, moderate or severe hepatic impairment, respectively, when compared with subjects with normal hepatic functions.

The mean *in vivo* plasma protein binding of hydrocodone across the groups was similar, ranging from 33% to 37% *[see Use in Specific Populations (8.6)]*.

Renal Impairment

After a single dose of 60 mg HYSINGLA ER in subjects (8 each) with normal renal function, mild, moderate, or severe renal impairment based on Cockcroft-Gault criteria and end stage renal disease (with dialysis) patients, mean hydrocodone C_{max} values were 40, 50, 51, 46, and 38 ng/mL, respectively. Mean hydrocodone AUC values were 754, 942, 1222, 1220, and 932 ng.hr/mL for subjects with normal renal function, mild, moderate or severe renal impairment and ESRD with dialysis, respectively. Hydrocodone C_{max} values were 14%, 23%, 11% and -13% and AUC values were

Table 6 Mean (SD) Steady-State Hydrocodone Pharmacokinetics Parameters

Regimen	AUC24,ss (ng•h/mL)	C_{max},ss (ng/mL)	C_{min},ss (ng/mL)	%Fluctuation*
HYSINGLA ER				
30 mg q24h	443 (128)	26.4 (7.4)	16.7 (5.2)	61 (6.4,113)
80 mg q24h	1252 (352)	82.6 (25.7)	28.2 (12)	105 (36,214)
120 mg q24h	1938 (729)	135 (50)	63.6 (29)	97.9 (32, 250)

* Mean (minimum, maximum); Percentage fluctuation in plasma concentration is derived as (C_{max},ss – C_{min}, ss)*100/ Cavg,ss.

13%, 61%, 57% and 4% higher in patients with mild, moderate or severe renal impairment or end stage renal disease with dialysis, respectively *[see Use in Specific Populations (8.7)]*.

Drug Interaction Studies

CYP3A4

Co-administration of HYSINGLA ER (20 mg single dose) and CYP3A4 inhibitor ketoconazole (200 mg BID for 6 days) increased mean hydrocodone AUC and C_{max} by 135% and 78%, respectively *[see Warnings and Precautions (5.11) and Drug Interactions (7.1)]*.

CYP2D6

The 90% confidence interval (CI) of the geometric means for hydrocodone AUC_{inf} (98 to 115%), AUC_t (98 to 115%), and C_{max} (93 to 121%) values were within the range of 80 to 125% when a single dose of HYSINGLA ER 20 mg was co-administered with CYP2D6 inhibitor paroxetine (20 mg treatment each morning for 12 days). No differences in systemic exposure of hydrocodone were observed in the presence of paroxetine.

13 NONCLINICAL TOXICOLOGY

13.1 Carcinogenesis, Mutagenesis, Impairment of Fertility

Carcinogenesis

Hydrocodone was evaluated for carcinogenic potential in rats and mice.

In a two-year bioassay in rats, doses up to 25 mg/kg in males and females were administered orally and no treatment-related neoplasms were observed (exposure is equivalent to 0.2-fold the human hydrocodone dose of 120 mg/day based on AUC exposure comparisons). In a two-year bioassay in mice, doses up to 200 mg/kg in males and 100 mg/kg in females were administered orally and no treatment-related neoplasms were observed (exposure is equivalent to 3.5-fold and 3.0-fold, respectively, the human hydrocodone dose of 120 mg/day based on AUC exposure comparisons).

Mutagenesis

Hydrocodone was genotoxic in the mouse lymphoma assay in the presence of rat S9 metabolic activation but not in the absence of rat metabolic activation. However, hydrocodone was not genotoxic in the mouse lymphoma assay with or without human S9 metabolic activation. There was no evidence of genotoxic potential with hydrocodone in an *in vitro* bacterial reverse mutation assay with Salmonella typhimurium and Escherichia coli with or without metabolic activation or in an *in vivo* mouse bone marrow micronucleus test with or without metabolic activation.

Impairment of Fertility

No effect on fertility or general reproductive performance was seen with oral administration of hydrocodone to male and female rats at doses up to 25 mg/kg/day (approximately 0.06-fold and 0.08-fold, respectively, the human hydrocodone dose of 120 mg/day based on AUC exposure comparisons).

14 CLINICAL STUDIES

The efficacy and safety of HYSINGLA ER was evaluated in a randomized double-blind, placebo-controlled, multi-center, 12-week clinical trial in both opioid-experienced and opioid-naïve patients with moderate to severe chronic low back pain.

14.1 Moderate to Severe Chronic Lower Back Pain Study

A total of 905 chronic low back pain patients (opioid naive and opioid-experienced) who were not responsive to their prior analgesic therapy entered an open-label conversion and dose-titration period for up to 45 days with HYSINGLA ER. Patients were dosed once daily with HYSINGLA ER (20 to 120 mg). Patients stopped their prior opioid analgesics and/or nonopioid analgesics prior to starting HYSINGLA ER treatment. Optional use of rescue medication (immediate-release oxycodone 5 mg) up to 2 doses (2 tablets) was permitted during the dose titration period. For inadequately controlled pain, HYSINGLA ER dose was allowed to be increased once every 3–5 days until a stabilized and tolerable dose was identified. During the dose-titration period, 65% of the patients achieved a stable HYSINGLA ER dose and entered the double-blind treatment period. The remaining subjects discontinued from the dose-titration period for the following reasons: adverse events (10%); lack of therapeutic effect (5%); confirmed or suspected diversion (3%); subject's choice (5%); lost to follow-up (2%); administrative reasons (2%); and failure to achieve protocol-defined reduction in pain score (7%).

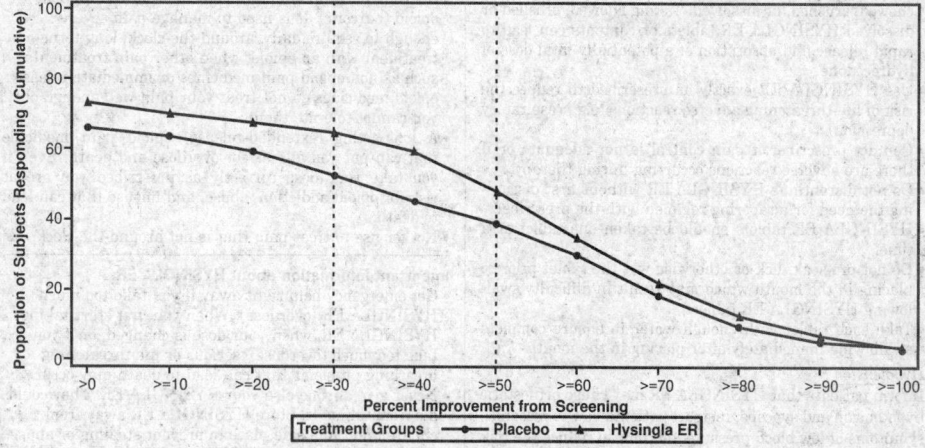

Figure 4. Percent Improvement in Pain Intensity

Following the dose titration period, 588 patients (65%) were randomized at a ratio of 1:1 into a 12-week double-blind treatment period with their fixed stabilized dose of HYSINGLA ER (or matching placebo). These patients met the study randomization criteria of adequate analgesia (pain reduction of at least 2 points to a score of 4 or less on a 0-10 numerical rating scale) and acceptable tolerability of HYSINGLA ER. Patients randomized to placebo were given a blinded taper of HYSINGLA ER according to a pre-specified tapering schedule, 3 days on each step-down dose (reduced by 25-50% from the previous dose). Patients were allowed to use rescue medication (immediate-release oxycodone 5 mg) up to 6 doses (6 tablets) per day depending on their randomized HYSINGLA ER dose. During the double-blind period, 229 treated patients (77%) completed the 12-week treatment with HYSINGLA ER and 210 patients (72%) completed on placebo. Overall, 10% of patients discontinued due to lack of therapeutic effect (5% in HYSINGLA patients and 15% in placebo patients); 5% of patients discontinued due to adverse events (6% in HYSINGLA ER treated patients and 3% in placebo patients).

HYSINGLA ER provided greater analgesia compared with placebo. There was a statistically significant difference in the weekly average pain scores at Week 12 between the two groups.

The percentage of patients (responders) in each group who demonstrated improvement in their weekly average pain scores at Week 12, as compared with screening is shown in Figure 4. The figure is cumulative, so that patients whose change from screening is, for example, 30%, are also included at every level of improvement below 30%. Patients who did not complete the study were classified as non-responders. Treatment with HYSINGLA ER resulted in a higher proportion of responders, defined as patients with at least a 30% and 50% improvement, as compared with placebo.

[See Figure 4 above]

16 HOW SUPPLIED/STORAGE AND HANDLING

HYSINGLA ER (hydrocodone bitartrate) extended-release tablets 20 mg are round, green-colored, bi-convex tablets printed with "HYD 20" and are supplied in child-resistant closure, opaque plastic bottles of 60 (NDC 59011-271-60).

HYSINGLA ER (hydrocodone bitartrate) extended-release tablets 30 mg are round, yellow-colored, bi-convex tablets printed with "HYD 30" and are supplied in child-resistant closure, opaque plastic bottles of 60 (NDC 59011-272-60).

HYSINGLA ER (hydrocodone bitartrate) extended-release tablets 40 mg are round, grey-colored, bi-convex tablets printed with "HYD 40" and are supplied in child-resistant closure, opaque plastic bottles of 60 (NDC 59011-273-60).

HYSINGLA ER (hydrocodone bitartrate) extended-release tablets 60 mg are round, beige-colored, bi-convex tablets printed with "HYD 60" and are supplied in child-resistant closure, opaque plastic bottles of 60 (NDC 59011-274-60).

HYSINGLA ER (hydrocodone bitartrate) extended-release tablets 80 mg are round, pink-colored, bi-convex tablets printed with "HYD 80" and are supplied in child-resistant closure, opaque plastic bottles of 60 (NDC 59011-275-60).

HYSINGLA ER (hydrocodone bitartrate) extended-release tablets 100 mg are round, blue-colored, bi-convex tablets

printed with "HYD 100" and are supplied in child-resistant closure, opaque plastic bottles of 60 (NDC 59011-276-60).

HYSINGLA ER (hydrocodone bitartrate) extended-release tablets 120 mg are round, white-colored, bi-convex tablets printed with "HYD 120" and are supplied in child-resistant closure, opaque plastic bottles of 60 (NDC 59011-277-60).

Store at 25°C (77°F); excursions permitted between 15°-30°C (59°-86°F).

Dispense in tight, light-resistant container, as defined by the USP.

CAUTION

DEA FORM REQUIRED

17 PATIENT COUNSELING INFORMATION

See FDA-approved patient labeling (Medication Guide)

Addiction, Abuse, and Misuse

Inform patients that the use of HYSINGLA ER, even when taken as recommended, can result in addiction, abuse, and misuse, which can lead to overdose or death *[see Warnings and Precautions (5.1)]*. Instruct patients not to share HYSINGLA ER with others and to take steps to protect HYSINGLA ER from theft or misuse.

Life-Threatening Respiratory Depression

Inform patients of the risk of life-threatening respiratory depression, including information that the risk is greatest when starting HYSINGLA ER or when the dose is increased, and that it can occur even at recommended doses *[see Warnings and Precautions (5.2)]*. Advise patients how to recognize respiratory depression and to seek medical attention if they are experiencing breathing difficulties.

Accidental Consumption

Inform patients that accidental exposure, especially in children, may result in respiratory depression or death *[see Warnings and Precautions (5.2)]*. Instruct patients to take steps to store HYSINGLA ER securely and to dispose of unused HYSINGLA ER in accordance with local state guidelines and/or regulations.

Neonatal Opioid Withdrawal Syndrome

Inform female patients of reproductive potential that chronic use of HYSINGLA ER during pregnancy can result in neonatal opioid withdrawal syndrome, which may be life-threatening if not recognized and treated *[see Warnings and Precautions (5.3)]*.

Interaction with Alcohol and other CNS Depressants

Inform patients that the concomitant use of alcohol with HYSINGLA ER can increase the risk of life-threatening respiratory depression *[see Warnings and Precautions (5.4)]*. Instruct patients not to consume alcoholic beverages, as well as prescription and over-the-counter products that contain alcohol, during treatment with HYSINGLA ER. Inform patients that potentially serious additive effects may occur if HYSINGLA ER is used with alcohol or other CNS depressants, and not to use such drugs unless supervised by a health care provider.

Important Administration Instructions

Instruct patients how to properly take HYSINGLA ER, including the following:

Continued on next page

- The tablets must be swallowed whole and must not be chewed, crushed, or dissolved. Taking chewed, crushed or dissolved HYSINGLA ER tablets or contents can lead to rapid release and absorption of a potentially fatal dose of hydrocodone.
- Use HYSINGLA ER exactly as prescribed to reduce the risk of life-threatening adverse reactions (e.g., respiratory depression).
- Contact prescriber if pain control is not adequate or if there are adverse reactions occurring during therapy.
- Do not discontinue HYSINGLA ER without first discussing the need for a tapering regimen with the prescriber.
- HYSINGLA ER tablets should be taken one tablet at a time.
- Do not pre-soak, lick or otherwise wet the tablet prior to placing in the mouth which may result in difficulty swallowing HYSINGLA ER tablets.
- Take each tablet with enough water to ensure complete swallowing immediately after placing in the mouth.

Hypotension
Inform patients that HYSINGLA ER may cause orthostatic hypotension and syncope. Instruct patients how to recognize symptoms of low blood pressure and how to reduce the risk of serious consequences should hypotension occur (e.g., sit or lie down, carefully rise from a sitting or lying position).

Driving or Operating Heavy Machinery
Inform patients that HYSINGLA ER may impair the ability to perform potentially hazardous activities such as driving a car or operating heavy machinery. Blood levels of hydrocodone, in some patients, may be high at the end of 24 hours after repeated dose administration. Advise patients not to perform such tasks until they know how they will react to the medication.

Constipation
Advise patients of the potential for severe constipation, including management instructions and when to seek medical attention. Instruct patients to monitor their analgesic response following the use of strong laxatives and to contact the prescriber if changes are noted.

QT interval prolongation
Inform patients that QT prolongation has been observed with HYSINGLA ER [see Clinical Pharmacology (12.2)]. HYSINGLA ER should be avoided in patients with congenital long QT syndrome. Instruct patients with a history of congestive heart failure or bradyarrhythmias, and patients at risk for electrolyte abnormalities or who are taking other medications known to prolong the QT interval that periodic monitoring of electrocardiograms and electrolytes may be necessary during therapy with HYSINGLA ER.

Anaphylaxis
Inform patients that anaphylaxis has been reported with ingredients contained in HYSINGLA ER. Advise patients how to recognize such a reaction and when to seek medical attention.

Pregnancy
Advise female patients that HYSINGLA ER may cause fetal harm and to inform the prescriber if they are pregnant or plan to become pregnant.

Nursing Mothers
Advise female patients that HYSINGLA ER passes into human milk. Because of the potential for serious adverse reactions in nursing infants, a decision should be made whether to discontinue nursing or to discontinue drug [see Use in Specific Populations (8.3)].

Disposal of unused HYSINGLA ER
Advise patients to dispose of any unused tablets from a prescription as soon as they are no longer needed in accordance with local state guidelines and/or regulations.
Healthcare professionals can telephone Purdue Pharma's Medical Services Department (1-888-726-7535) for information on this product.

Purdue Pharma L.P.
Stamford, CT 06901-3431
©2015, Purdue Pharma L.P.
U.S. Patent Numbers: 6,488,963; 6,733,783; 8,309,060; 8,361,499; 8,529,948; 8,551,520; 8,647,667, and 8,808,740.

Medication Guide
HYSINGLA™ ER (hye-SING-luh)
(hydrocodone bitartrate) extended-release tablets, CII

HYSINGLA ER is:

- A strong prescription pain medicine that contains an opioid (narcotic). It is used to manage pain severe enough to require daily, around-the-clock, long-term treatment with an opioid, when other pain treatments such as non-opioid pain medicines or immediate-release opioid medicines do not treat your pain well enough or you cannot tolerate them.
- A long-acting (extended-release) opioid pain medicine that can put you at risk for overdose and death. Even if you take your dose correctly as prescribed you are at risk for opioid addiction, abuse, and misuse that can lead to death.
- Not for use to treat pain that is not around-the-clock.

Important information about HYSINGLA ER:
- Get emergency help right away if you take too much HYSINGLA ER (overdose). When you first start taking HYSINGLA ER, when your dose is changed, or if you take too much (overdose), serious or life-threatening breathing problems that can lead to death may occur.
- Never give anyone else your HYSINGLA ER. They could die from taking it. Store HYSINGLA ER away from children and in a safe place to prevent stealing or abuse. Selling or giving away HYSINGLA ER is against the law.

Do not take HYSINGLA ER if you have:
- severe asthma, trouble breathing, or other lung problems.
- a bowel blockage or have narrowing of the stomach or intestines.

Before taking HYSINGLA ER, tell your healthcare provider if you have a history of:
- head injury, seizures
- liver, kidney, thyroid problems
- problems urinating
- pancreas or gallbladder problems
- heart rhythm problems (long QT syndrome)
- abuse of street or prescription drugs, alcohol addiction, or mental health problems

Tell your healthcare provider if you are:
- **pregnant or planning to become pregnant.** Prolonged use of HYSINGLA ER during pregnancy can cause withdrawal symptoms in your newborn baby that could be life-threatening if not recognized and treated.
- **breastfeeding.** HYSINGLA ER passes into breast milk and may harm your baby.
- taking prescription or over-the-counter medicines, vitamins, or herbal supplements. Taking HYSINGLA ER with certain other medicines can cause serious side effects and could lead to death.

When taking HYSINGLA ER:
- Do not change your dose. Take HYSINGLA ER exactly as prescribed by your healthcare provider.
- Take your prescribed dose every 24 hours, at the same time every day. Do not take more than your prescribed dose in 24 hours. If you miss a dose, take your next dose at your usual time the next day.
- Swallow HYSINGLA ER whole. Do not cut, break, chew, crush, dissolve, snort, or inject HYSINGLA ER because this may cause you to overdose and die.
- HYSINGLA ER should be taken 1 tablet at a time. Do not pre-soak, lick, or wet the tablet before placing it in your mouth to avoid choking on the tablet.

Call your healthcare provider if the dose you are taking does not control your pain.
- **Do not stop taking HYSINGLA ER without talking to your healthcare provider.**
- After you stop taking HYSINGLA ER, flush any unused tablets down the toilet.

While taking HYSINGLA ER, DO NOT:
- Drive or operate heavy machinery until you know how HYSINGLA ER affects you. HYSINGLA ER can make you sleepy, dizzy, or lightheaded.
- Drink alcohol or use prescription or over-the-counter medicines that contain alcohol. Using products containing alcohol during treatment with HYSINGLA ER may cause you to overdose and die.

The possible side effects of HYSINGLA ER are:
- constipation, nausea, sleepiness, vomiting, tiredness, headache, dizziness, abdominal pain. Call your healthcare provider if you have any of these symptoms and they are severe.

Get emergency medical help if you have:
- trouble breathing, shortness of breath, fast heartbeat, chest pain, swelling of your face, tongue or throat, extreme drowsiness, or you are feeling faint.

These are not all the possible side effects of HYSINGLA ER. Call your doctor for medical advice about side effects. You may report side effects to FDA at 1-800-FDA-1088.
For more information go to dailymed.nlm.nih.gov.
Manufactured by: Purdue Pharma L.P., Stamford, CT 06901-3431, **www.purduepharma.com**or call 1-888-726-7535

This Medication Guide has been approved by the U.S. Food and Drug Administration.
Issue: 11/2014
Shown in Product Identification Guide, page 509

OXYCONTIN®   Cℓ ⴽ
[(ox-e-KON-tin)]
(oxycodone hydrochloride)
extended-release tablets, for oral use, Cℓ

HIGHLIGHTS OF PRESCRIBING INFORMATION
These highlights do not include all the information needed to use OXYCONTIN® safely and effectively. See full prescribing information for OXYCONTIN.
OXYCONTIN®(oxycodone hydrochloride) extended-release tablets, for oral use, CII
Initial U.S. Approval: 1950

> **WARNING: ADDICTION, ABUSE AND MISUSE; LIFE-THREATENING RESPIRATORY DEPRESSION; ACCIDENTAL INGESTION; NEONATAL OPIOID WITHDRAWAL SYNDROME; and CYTOCHROME P450 3A4 INTERACTION**
> *See full prescribing information for complete boxed warning.*
> - **OXYCONTIN exposes users to risks of addictions, abuse and misuse, which can lead to overdose and death. Assess each patient's risk before prescribing and monitor regularly for development of these behaviors and conditions. (5.1)**
> - **Serious, life-threatening, or fatal respiratory depression may occur. Monitor closely, especially upon initiation or following a dose increase. Instruct patients to swallow OXYCONTIN tablets whole to avoid exposure to a potentially fatal dose of oxycodone. (5.2)**
> - **Accidental ingestion of OXYCONTIN, especially in children, can result in a fatal overdose of oxycodone. (5.2)**
> - **Prolonged use of OXYCONTIN during pregnancy can result in neonatal opioid withdrawal syndrome, which may be life-threatening if not recognized and treated. If opioid use is required for a prolonged period in a pregnant woman, advise the patient of the risk of neonatal opioid withdrawal syndrome and ensure that appropriate treatment will be available. (5.3)**
> - **Initiation of CYP3A4 inhibitors (or discontinuation of CYP3A4 inducers) can result in a fatal overdose of oxycodone from OXYCONTIN. (5.14, 12.3)**

————**RECENT MAJOR CHANGES**————

Indications and Usage (1)	08/2015
Dosage and Administration (2)	08/2015

————**INDICATIONS AND USAGE**————
OXYCONTIN is an opioid agonist indicated for pain severe enough to require daily, around-the-clock, long-term opioid treatment and for which alternative treatment options are inadequate in:
- Adults; and
- Opioid-tolerant pediatric patients 11 years of age and older who are already receiving and tolerate a minimum daily opioid dose of at least 20 mg oxycodone orally or its equivalent.

Limitations of Use
- Because of the risks of addiction, abuse and misuse with opioids, even at recommended doses, and because of the greater risks of overdose and death with extended-release formulations, reserve OXYCONTIN for use in patients for whom alternative treatment options (e.g. non-opioid analgesics or immediate-release opioids) are ineffective, not tolerated, or would be otherwise inadequate to provide sufficient management of pain. (1)
- OXYCONTIN is not indicated as an as-needed (prn) analgesic. (1)

5   WARNINGS AND PRECAUTIONS

5.1   Addiction, Abuse, and Misuse

OXYCONTIN contains oxycodone, a Schedule II controlled substance. As an opioid, OXYCONTIN exposes users to the risks of addiction, abuse, and misuse [see Drug Abuse and Dependence (9)]. As modified-release products such as OXYCONTIN deliver the opioid over an extended period of time, there is a greater risk for overdose and death due to the larger amount of oxycodone present [see Drug Abuse and Dependence (9)].

Although the risk of addiction in any individual is unknown, it can occur in patients appropriately prescribed OXYCONTIN. Addiction can occur at recommended doses and if the drug is misused or abused.

Assess each patient's risk for opioid addiction, abuse or misuse prior to prescribing OXYCONTIN, and monitor all patients receiving OXYCONTIN for the development of these behaviors or conditions. Risks are increased in patients with a personal or family history of substance abuse (including drug or alcohol abuse or addiction) or mental illness (e.g., major depression). The potential for these risks should not, however, prevent the proper management of pain in any given patient. Patients at increased risk may be prescribed modified-release opioid formulations such as OXYCONTIN, but use in such patients necessitates intensive counseling about the risks and proper use of OXYCONTIN along with intensive monitoring for signs of addiction, abuse, and misuse.

Abuse, or misuse of OXYCONTIN by crushing, chewing, snorting, or injecting the dissolved product will result in the uncontrolled delivery of oxycodone and can result in overdose and death [see Overdosage (10)].

Opioid agonists are sought by drug abusers and people with addiction disorders and are subject to criminal diversion. Consider these risks when prescribing or dispensing OXYCONTIN. Strategies to reduce these risks include prescribing the drug in the smallest appropriate quantity and advising the patient on the proper disposal of unused drug [see Patient Counseling Information (17)]. Contact local state professional licensing board or state controlled substances authority for information on how to prevent and detect abuse or diversion of this product.

5.2   Life-Threatening Respiratory Depression

Serious, life-threatening, or fatal respiratory depression has been reported with the use of modified-release opioids, even when used as recommended. Respiratory depression, if not immediately recognized and treated, may lead to respiratory arrest and death. Management of respiratory depression may include close observation, supportive measures, and use of opioid antagonists, depending on the patient's clinical status [see Overdosage (10)]. Carbon dioxide (CO_2) retention from opioid-induced respiratory depression can exacerbate the sedating effects of opioids.

While serious, life-threatening, or fatal respiratory depression can occur at any time during the use of OXYCONTIN, the risk is greatest during the initiation of therapy or following a dose increase. Closely monitor patients for respiratory depression when initiating therapy with OXYCONTIN and following dose increases.

To reduce the risk of respiratory depression, proper dosing and titration of OXYCONTIN are essential [see Dosage and Administration (2)]. Overestimating the OXYCONTIN dose when converting patients from another opioid product can result in a fatal overdose with the first dose.

Accidental ingestion of even one dose of OXYCONTIN, especially by children, can result in respiratory depression and death due to an overdose of oxycodone.

5.3   Neonatal Opioid Withdrawal Syndrome

Prolonged use of OXYCONTIN during pregnancy can result in withdrawal signs in the neonate. Neonatal opioid withdrawal syndrome, unlike opioid withdrawal syndrome in adults, may be life-threatening if not recognized and treated, and requires management according to protocols developed by neonatology experts. If opioid use is required for a prolonged period in a pregnant woman, advise the patient of the risk of neonatal opioid withdrawal syndrome and ensure that appropriate treatment will be available.

Neonatal opioid withdrawal syndrome presents as irritability, hyperactivity and abnormal sleep pattern, high pitched cry, tremor, vomiting, diarrhea and failure to gain weight. The onset, duration, and severity of neonatal opioid withdrawal syndrome vary based on the specific opioid used, duration of use, timing and amount of last maternal use, and rate of elimination of the drug by the newborn.

5.4   Interactions with Central Nervous System Depressants

Hypotension and profound sedation, coma, or respiratory depression may result if OXYCONTIN is used concomi-

tantly with other central nervous system (CNS) depressants (e.g., sedatives, anxiolytics, hypnotics, neuroleptics, other opioids).

When considering the use of OXYCONTIN in a patient taking a CNS depressant, assess the duration of use of the CNS depressant and the patient's response, including the degree of tolerance that has developed to CNS depression. Additionally, evaluate the patient's use of alcohol or illicit drugs that can cause CNS depression. If the decision to begin OXYCONTIN therapy is made, start with 1/3 to 1/2 the usual dose of OXYCONTIN, monitor patients for signs of sedation and respiratory depression and consider using a lower dose of the concomitant CNS depressant [see Drug Interactions (7.1) and Dosage and Administration (2.6)].

5.5   Use in Elderly, Cachectic, and Debilitated Patients

Life-threatening respiratory depression is more likely to occur in elderly, cachectic, or debilitated patients as they may have altered pharmacokinetics or altered clearance compared to younger, healthier patients. Monitor such patients closely, particularly when initiating and titrating OXYCONTIN and when OXYCONTIN is given concomitantly with other drugs that depress respiration [see Warnings and Precautions (5.2)].

5.6   Use in Patients with Chronic Pulmonary Disease

Monitor patients with significant chronic obstructive pulmonary disease or cor pulmonale, and patients having a substantially decreased respiratory reserve, hypoxia, hypercapnia, or pre-existing respiratory depression for respiratory depression, particularly when initiating therapy and titrating with OXYCONTIN, as in these patients, even usual therapeutic doses of OXYCONTIN may decrease respiratory drive to the point of apnea [see Warnings and Precautions (5.2)]. Consider the use of alternative non-opioid analgesics in these patients if possible.

5.7   Hypotensive Effects

OXYCONTIN may cause severe hypotension, including orthostatic hypotension and syncope in ambulatory patients. There is an increased risk in patients whose ability to maintain blood pressure has already been compromised by a reduced blood volume or concurrent administration of certain CNS depressant drugs (e.g., phenothiazines or general anesthetics) [see Drug Interactions (7.1)]. Monitor these patients for signs of hypotension after initiating or titrating the dose of OXYCONTIN. In patients with circulatory shock, OXYCONTIN may cause vasodilation that can further reduce cardiac output and blood pressure. Avoid the use of OXYCONTIN in patients with circulatory shock.

5.8   Use in Patients with Head Injury or Increased Intracranial Pressure

Monitor patients taking OXYCONTIN who may be susceptible to the intracranial effects of CO_2 retention (e.g., those with evidence of increased intracranial pressure or brain tumors) for signs of sedation and respiratory depression, particularly when initiating therapy with OXYCONTIN. OXYCONTIN may reduce respiratory drive, and the resultant CO_2 retention can further increase intracranial pressure. Opioids may also obscure the clinical course in a patient with a head injury.

Avoid the use of OXYCONTIN in patients with impaired consciousness or coma.

5.9   Difficulty in Swallowing and Risk for Obstruction in Patients at Risk for a Small Gastrointestinal Lumen

There have been post-marketing reports of difficulty in swallowing OXYCONTIN tablets. These reports included choking, gagging, regurgitation and tablets stuck in the throat. Instruct patients not to pre-soak, lick or otherwise wet OXYCONTIN tablets prior to placing in the mouth, and to take one tablet at a time with enough water to ensure complete swallowing immediately after placing in the mouth.

There have been rare post-marketing reports of cases of intestinal obstruction, and exacerbation of diverticulitis, some of which have required medical intervention to remove the tablet. Patients with underlying GI disorders such as esophageal cancer or colon cancer with a small gastrointestinal lumen are at greater risk of developing these complications. Consider use of an alternative analgesic in patients who have difficulty swallowing and patients at risk for underlying GI disorders resulting in a small gastrointestinal lumen.

5.10   Use in Patients with Gastrointestinal Conditions

OXYCONTIN is contraindicated in patients with GI obstruction, including paralytic ileus. The oxycodone in OXYCONTIN may cause spasm of the sphincter of Oddi. Monitor patients with biliary tract disease, including acute pancreatitis, for worsening symptoms. Opioids may cause increases in the serum amylase.

5.11   Use in Patients with Convulsive or Seizure Disorders

The oxycodone in OXYCONTIN may aggravate convulsions in patients with convulsive disorders, and may induce or aggravate seizures in some clinical settings. Monitor patients with a history of seizure disorders for worsened seizure control during OXYCONTIN therapy.

5.12   Avoidance of Withdrawal

Avoid the use of mixed agonist/antagonist (i.e., pentazocine, nalbuphine, and butorphanol) or partial agonist (buprenorphine) analgesics in patients who have received or are receiving a course of therapy with a full opioid agonist analgesic, including OXYCONTIN. In these patients, mixed agonist/antagonist and partial agonist analgesics may reduce the analgesic effect and/or may precipitate withdrawal symptoms.

When discontinuing OXYCONTIN, gradually taper the dose [see Dosage and Administration (2.9)]. Do not abruptly discontinue OXYCONTIN.

5.13   Driving and Operating Machinery

OXYCONTIN may impair the mental or physical abilities needed to perform potentially hazardous activities such as driving a car or operating machinery. Warn patients not to drive or operate dangerous machinery unless they are tolerant to the effects of OXYCONTIN and know how they will react to the medication.

5.14   Cytochrome P450 3A4 Inhibitors and Inducers

Since the CYP3A4 isoenzyme plays a major role in the metabolism of OXYCONTIN, drugs that alter CYP3A4 activity may cause changes in clearance of oxycodone which could lead to changes in oxycodone plasma concentrations.

Inhibition of CYP3A4 activity by its inhibitors, such as macrolide antibiotics (e.g., erythromycin), azole-antifungal agents (e.g., ketoconazole), and protease inhibitors (e.g., ritonavir), may increase plasma concentrations of oxycodone and prolong opioid effects.

CYP450 inducers, such as rifampin, carbamazepine, and phenytoin, may induce the metabolism of oxycodone and, therefore, may cause increased clearance of the drug which could lead to a decrease in oxycodone plasma concentrations, lack of efficacy or, possibly, development of an abstinence syndrome in a patient who had developed physical dependence to oxycodone.

If co-administration is necessary, caution is advised when initiating OXYCONTIN treatment in patients currently taking, or discontinuing, CYP3A4 inhibitors or inducers. Evaluate these patients at frequent intervals and consider dose adjustments until stable drug effects are achieved [see Drug Interactions (7.2) and Clinical Pharmacology (12.3)].

5.15   Laboratory Monitoring

Not every urine drug test for "opioids" or "opiates" detects oxycodone reliably, especially those designed for in-office use. Further, many laboratories will report urine drug concentrations below a specified "cut-off" value as "negative". Therefore, if urine testing for oxycodone is considered in the clinical management of an individual patient, ensure that the sensitivity and specificity of the assay is appropriate, and consider the limitations of the testing used when interpreting results.

6   ADVERSE REACTIONS

The following serious adverse reactions are described elsewhere in the labeling:

- Addiction, Abuse, and Misuse [see Warnings and Precautions (5.1)]
- Life-Threatening Respiratory Depression [see Warnings and Precautions (5.2)]
- Neonatal Opioid Withdrawal Syndrome [see Warnings and Precautions (5.3)]
- Interactions with Other CNS Depressants [see Warnings and Precautions (5.4)]
- Hypotensive Effects [see Warnings and Precautions (5.7)]
- Gastrointestinal Effects [see Warnings and Precautions (5.9, 5.10)]
- Seizures [see Warnings and Precautions (5.11)]

6.1   Clinical Trial Experience

Adult Clinical Trial Experience

Because clinical trials are conducted under widely varying conditions, adverse reaction rates observed in the clinical trials of a drug cannot be directly compared to rates in the clinical trials of another drug and may not reflect the rates observed in practice. The safety of OXYCONTIN was evaluated in double-blind clinical trials involving 713 patients with moderate to severe pain of various etiologies. In open-label studies of cancer pain, 187 patients received

Continued on next page

OXYCONTIN in total daily doses ranging from 20 mg to 640 mg per day. The average total daily dose was approximately 105 mg per day.

OXYCONTIN may increase the risk of serious adverse reactions such as those observed with other opioid analgesics, including respiratory depression, apnea, respiratory arrest, circulatory depression, hypotension, or shock *[see Overdosage (10)]*.

The most common adverse reactions (>5%) reported by patients in clinical trials comparing OXYCONTIN with placebo are shown in Table 2 below:

TABLE 2: Common Adverse Reactions (>5%)

Adverse Reaction	OXYCONTIN (n=227)	Placebo (n=45)
	(%)	(%)
Constipation	(23)	(7)
Nausea	(23)	(11)
Somnolence	(23)	(4)
Dizziness	(13)	(9)
Pruritus	(13)	(2)
Vomiting	(12)	(7)
Headache	(7)	(7)
Dry Mouth	(6)	(2)
Asthenia	(6)	-
Sweating	(5)	(2)

In clinical trials, the following adverse reactions were reported in patients treated with OXYCONTIN with an incidence between 1% and 5%:

Gastrointestinal disorders: abdominal pain, diarrhea, dyspepsia, gastritis

General disorders and administration site conditions: chills, fever

Metabolism and nutrition disorders: anorexia

Musculoskeletal and connective tissue disorders: twitching

Psychiatric disorders: abnormal dreams, anxiety, confusion, dysphoria, euphoria, insomnia, nervousness, thought abnormalities

Respiratory, thoracic and mediastinal disorders: dyspnea, hiccups

Skin and subcutaneous tissue disorders: rash

Vascular disorders: postural hypotension

The following adverse reactions occurred **in less than 1% of patients** involved in clinical trials:

Blood and lymphatic system disorders: lymphadenopathy

Ear and labyrinth disorders: tinnitus

Eye disorders: abnormal vision

Gastrointestinal disorders: dysphagia, eructation, flatulence, gastrointestinal disorder, increased appetite, stomatitis

General disorders and administration site conditions: withdrawal syndrome (with and without seizures), edema, peripheral edema, thirst, malaise, chest pain, facial edema

Injury, poisoning and procedural complications: accidental injury

Investigations: ST depression

Metabolism and nutrition disorders: dehydration

Nervous system disorders: syncope, migraine, abnormal gait, amnesia, hyperkinesia, hypoesthesia, hypotonia, paresthesia, speech disorder, stupor, tremor, vertigo, taste perversion

Psychiatric disorders: depression, agitation, depersonalization, emotional lability, hallucination

Renal and urinary disorders: dysuria, hematuria, polyuria, urinary retention

Reproductive system and breast disorders: impotence

Respiratory, thoracic and mediastinal disorders: cough increased, voice alteration

Skin and subcutaneous tissue disorders: dry skin, exfoliative dermatitis

Clinical Trial Experience in Pediatric Patients 11 Years and Older

The safety of OXYCONTIN has been evaluated in one clinical trial with 140 patients 11 to 16 years of age. The median duration of treatment was approximately three weeks. The most frequently reported adverse events were vomiting, nausea, headache, pyrexia, and constipation.

Table 3 includes a summary of the incidence of treatment emergent adverse events reported in ≥5% of patients.

Table 3: Incidence of Adverse Reactions Reported in ≥ 5.0% Patients 11 to 16 Years

System Organ Class Preferred Term	11 to 16 Years (N=140) n (%)
Any Adverse Event >= 5%	71 (51)
GASTROINTESTINAL DISORDERS	56 (40)
Vomiting	30 (21)
Nausea	21 (15)
Constipation	13 (9)
Diarrhea	8 (6)
GENERAL DISORDERS AND ADMINISTRATION SITE CONDITIONS	32
	(23)
Pyrexia	15 (11)
METABOLISM AND NUTRITION DISORDERS	9 (6)
Decreased appetite	7 (5)
NERVOUS SYSTEM DISORDERS	37 (26)
Headache	20 (14)
Dizziness	12 (9)
SKIN AND SUBCUTANEOUS TISSUE DISORDERS	23 (16)
Pruritus	8 (6)

The following adverse reactions occurred in a clinical trial of OXYCONTIN in patients 11 to 16 years of age with an incidence between ≥1.0% and < 5.0%. Events are listed within each System/Organ Class.

Blood and lymphatic system disorders: febrile neutropenia, neutropenia

Cardiac disorders: tachycardia

Gastrointestinal disorders: abdominal pain, gastroesophageal reflux disease

General disorders and administration site conditions: fatigue, pain, chills, asthenia

Injury, poisoning, and procedural complications: procedural pain, seroma

Investigations: oxygen saturation decreased, alanine aminotransferase increased, hemoglobin decreased, platelet count decreased, neutrophil count decreased, red blood cell count decreased, weight decreased

Metabolic and nutrition disorders: hypochloremia, hyponatraemia

Musculoskeletal and connective tissue disorders: pain in extremity, musculoskeletal pain

Nervous system disorders: somnolence, hypoesthesia, lethargy, paresthesia

Psychiatric disorders: insomnia, anxiety, depression, agitation

Renal and urinary disorders: dysuria, urinary retention

Respiratory, thoracic, and mediastinal disorders: oropharyngeal pain

Skin and subcutaneous tissue disorders: hyperhidrosis, rash

6.2 Postmarketing Experience

The following adverse reactions have been identified during post-approval use of controlled-release oxycodone: abuse, addiction, aggression, amenorrhea, cholestasis, completed suicide, death, dental caries, increased hepatic enzymes, hyperalgesia, hypogonadism, hyponatremia, ileus, intentional overdose, mood altered, muscular hypertonia, overdose, palpitations (in the context of withdrawal), seizures, suicidal attempt, suicidal ideation, syndrome of inappropriate antidiuretic hormone secretion, and urticaria.

Anaphylaxis has been reported with ingredients contained in OXYCONTIN. Advise patients how to recognize such a reaction and when to seek medical attention.

In addition to the events listed above, the following have also been reported, potentially due to the swelling and hydrogelling property of the tablet: choking, gagging, regurgitation, tablets stuck in the throat and difficulty swallowing the tablet.

7 DRUG INTERACTIONS

7.1 CNS Depressants

The concomitant use of OXYCONTIN and other CNS depressants including sedatives, hypnotics, tranquilizers, general anesthetics, phenothiazines, other opioids, and alcohol can increase the risk of respiratory depression, profound sedation, coma, or death. Monitor patients receiving CNS depressants and OXYCONTIN for signs of respiratory depression, sedation, and hypotension.

When combined therapy with any of the above medications is considered, the dose of one or both agents should be reduced *[see Dosage and Administration (2.6) and Warnings and Precautions (5.4)]*.

7.2 Drugs Affecting Cytochrome P450 Isoenzymes

Inhibitors of CYP3A4 and 2D6

Because the CYP3A4 isoenzyme plays a major role in the metabolism of oxycodone, drugs that inhibit CYP3A4 activity may cause decreased clearance of oxycodone which could lead to an increase in oxycodone plasma concentrations and result in increased or prolonged opioid effects. These effects could be more pronounced with concomitant use of CYP2D6 and 3A4 inhibitors. If co-administration with OXYCONTIN is necessary, monitor patients for respiratory depression and sedation at frequent intervals and consider dose adjustments until stable drug effects are achieved *[see Clinical Pharmacology (12.3)]*.

Inducers of CYP3A4

CYP450 3A4 inducers may induce the metabolism of oxycodone and, therefore, may cause increased clearance of the drug which could lead to a decrease in oxycodone plasma concentrations, lack of efficacy or, possibly, development of an abstinence syndrome in a patient who had developed physical dependence to oxycodone. If co-administration with OXYCONTIN is necessary, monitor for signs of opioid withdrawal and consider dose adjustments until stable drug effects are achieved.

After stopping the treatment of a CYP3A4 inducer, as the effects of the inducer decline, the oxycodone plasma concentration will increase which could increase or prolong both the therapeutic and adverse effects, and may cause serious respiratory depression *[see Clinical Pharmacology (12.3)]*.

7.3 Mixed Agonist/Antagonist and Partial Agonist Opioid Analgesics

Mixed agonist/antagonist (i.e., pentazocine, nalbuphine, and butorphanol) and partial agonist (buprenorphine) analgesics may reduce the analgesic effect of oxycodone or precipitate withdrawal symptoms. Avoid the use of mixed agonist/antagonist and partial agonist analgesics in patients receiving OXYCONTIN.

7.4 Muscle Relaxants

Oxycodone may enhance the neuromuscular blocking action of true skeletal muscle relaxants and produce an increased degree of respiratory depression. Monitor patients receiving muscle relaxants and OXYCONTIN for signs of respiratory depression that may be greater than otherwise expected.

7.5 Diuretics

Opioids can reduce the efficacy of diuretics by inducing the release of antidiuretic hormone. Opioids may also lead to acute retention of urine by causing spasm of the sphincter of the bladder, particularly in men with enlarged prostates.

7.6 Anticholinergics

Anticholinergics or other medications with anticholinergic activity when used concurrently with opioid analgesics may result in increased risk of urinary retention and/or severe constipation, which may lead to paralytic ileus. Monitor patients for signs of urinary retention or reduced gastric motility when OXYCONTIN is used concurrently with anticholinergic drugs.

8 USE IN SPECIFIC POPULATIONS

8.1 Pregnancy

Clinical Considerations

Fetal/neonatal adverse reactions

Prolonged use of opioid analgesics during pregnancy for medical or nonmedical purposes can result in physical dependence in the neonate and neonatal opioid withdrawal syndrome shortly after birth. Observe newborns for symptoms of neonatal opioid withdrawal syndrome, such as poor feeding, diarrhea, irritability, tremor, rigidity, and seizures, and manage accordingly *[see Warnings and Precautions (5.3)]*.

Teratogenic Effects - Pregnancy Category C

There are no adequate and well-controlled studies in pregnant women. OXYCONTIN should be used during pregnancy only if the potential benefit justifies the risk to the fetus.

The effect of oxycodone in human reproduction has not been adequately studied. Studies with oral doses of oxycodone hydrochloride in rats up to 8 mg/kg/day and rabbits up to 125 mg/kg/day, equivalent to 0.5 and 15 times an adult human dose of 160 mg/day, respectively on a mg/m² basis, did not reveal evidence of harm to the fetus due to oxycodone. In a pre- and postnatal toxicity study, female rats received oxycodone during gestation and lactation. There were no long-term developmental or reproductive effects in the pups *[see Nonclinical Toxicology (13.1)]*.

Non-Teratogenic Effects

Oxycodone hydrochloride was administered orally to female rats during gestation and lactation in a pre- and postnatal toxicity study. There were no drug-related effects on reproductive performance in these females or any long-term developmental or reproductive effects in pups born to these rats. Decreased body weight was found during lactation and the early post-weaning phase in pups nursed by mothers given the highest dose used (6 mg/kg/day, equivalent to approximately 0.4-times an adult human dose of 160 mg/day, on a mg/m² basis). However, body weight of these pups recovered.

8.2 Labor and Delivery

Opioids cross the placenta and may produce respiratory depression in neonates. OXYCONTIN is not recommended for use in women immediately prior to labor, when use of shorter-acting analgesics or other analgesic techniques are more appropriate. Opioid analgesics can prolong labor through actions which temporarily reduce the strength, duration and frequency of uterine contractions. However this effect is not consistent and may be offset by an increased rate of cervical dilatation, which tends to shorten labor.

8.3 Nursing Mothers

Oxycodone has been detected in breast milk. Instruct patients not to undertake nursing while receiving OXYCONTIN. Do not initiate OXYCONTIN therapy while nursing because of the possibility of sedation or respiratory depression in the infant.

Withdrawal signs can occur in breast-fed infants when maternal administration of an opioid analgesic is stopped, or when breast-feeding is stopped.

8.4 Pediatric Use

The safety and efficacy of OXYCONTIN have been established in pediatric patients ages 11 to 16 years. Use of OXYCONTIN is supported by evidence from adequate and well-controlled trials with OXYCONTIN in adults as well as an open-label study in pediatric patients ages 6 to 16 years. However, there were insufficient numbers of patients less than 11 years of age enrolled in this study to establish the safety of the product in this age group.

The safety of OXYCONTIN in pediatric patients was evaluated in 155 patients previously receiving and tolerating opioids for at least 5 consecutive days with a minimum of 20 mg per day of oxycodone or its equivalent on the two days immediately preceding dosing with OXYCONTIN. Patients were started on a total daily dose ranging between 20 mg and 100 mg depending on prior opioid dose.

The most frequent adverse events observed in pediatric patients were vomiting, nausea, headache, pyrexia, and constipation *[see Dosage and Administration (2.4), Adverse Reactions (6.1), Clinical Pharmacology (12.3) and Clinical Trials (14)]*.

8.5 Geriatric Use

In controlled pharmacokinetic studies in elderly subjects (greater than 65 years) the clearance of oxycodone was slightly reduced. Compared to young adults, the plasma concentrations of oxycodone were increased approximately 15% *[see Clinical Pharmacology (12.3)]*. Of the total number of subjects (445) in clinical studies of oxycodone hydrochloride controlled-release tablets, 148 (33.3%) were age 65 and older (including those age 75 and older) while 40 (9.0%) were age 75 and older. In clinical trials with appropriate initiation of therapy and dose titration, no untoward or unexpected adverse reactions were seen in the elderly patients who received oxycodone hydrochloride controlled-release tablets. Thus, the usual doses and dosing intervals may be appropriate for elderly patients. However, reduce the starting dose to 1/3 to 1/2 the usual dosage in debilitated, non-opioid-tolerant patients. Respiratory depression is the chief risk in elderly or debilitated patients, usually the result of large initial doses in patients who are not tolerant to opioids, or when opioids are given in conjunction with other agents that depress respiration. Titrate the dose of OXYCONTIN cautiously in these patients.

8.6 Hepatic Impairment

A study of OXYCONTIN in patients with hepatic impairment demonstrated greater plasma concentrations than those seen at equivalent doses in persons with normal hepatic function. Therefore, in the setting of hepatic impairment, start dosing patients at 1/3 to 1/2 the usual starting dose followed by careful dose titration *[see Clinical Pharmacology (12.3)]*.

8.7 Renal Impairment

In patients with renal impairment, as evidenced by decreased creatinine clearance (<60 mL/min), the concentrations of oxycodone in the plasma are approximately 50% higher than in subjects with normal renal function. Follow a conservative approach to dose initiation and adjust according to the clinical situation *[see Clinical Pharmacology (12.3)]*.

8.8 Gender Differences

In pharmacokinetic studies with OXYCONTIN, opioid-naïve females demonstrate up to 25% higher average plasma concentrations and greater frequency of typical opioid adverse events than males, even after adjustment for body weight. The clinical relevance of a difference of this magnitude is low for a drug intended for chronic usage at individualized dosages, and there was no male/female difference detected for efficacy or adverse events in clinical trials.

9 DRUG ABUSE AND DEPENDENCE

9.1 Controlled Substance

OXYCONTIN contains oxycodone, a Schedule II controlled substance with a high potential for abuse similar to other opioids including fentanyl, hydromorphone, methadone, morphine, and oxymorphone. OXYCONTIN can be abused and is subject to misuse, addiction, and criminal diversion *[see Warnings and Precautions (5.1)]*.

The high drug content in extended-release formulations adds to the risk of adverse outcomes from abuse and misuse.

9.2 Abuse

All patients treated with opioids require careful monitoring for signs of abuse and addiction, since use of opioid analgesic products carries the risk of addiction even under appropriate medical use.

Drug abuse is the intentional non-therapeutic use of an over-the-counter or prescription drug, even once, for its rewarding psychological or physiological effects. Drug abuse includes, but is not limited to, the following examples: the use of a prescription or over-the-counter drug to get "high", or the use of steroids for performance enhancement and muscle build up.

Drug addiction is a cluster of behavioral, cognitive, and physiological phenomena that develop after repeated substance use and include: a strong desire to take the drug, difficulties in controlling its use, persisting in its use despite harmful consequences, a higher priority given to drug use than to other activities and obligations, increased tolerance, and sometimes a physical withdrawal.

"Drug-seeking" behavior is very common to addicts and drug abusers. Drug-seeking tactics include emergency calls or visits near the end of office hours, refusal to undergo appropriate examination, testing or referral, repeated claims of loss of prescriptions, tampering with prescriptions and reluctance to provide prior medical records or contact information for other treating physician(s). "Doctor shopping" (visiting multiple prescribers) to obtain additional prescriptions is common among drug abusers and people suffering from untreated addiction. Preoccupation with achieving adequate pain relief can be appropriate behavior in a patient with poor pain control.

Abuse and addiction are separate and distinct from physical dependence and tolerance. Physicians should be aware that addiction may not be accompanied by concurrent tolerance and symptoms of physical dependence in all addicts. In addition, abuse of opioids can occur in the absence of true addiction.

OXYCONTIN, like other opioids, can be diverted for nonmedical use into illicit channels of distribution. Careful recordkeeping of prescribing information, including quantity, frequency, and renewal requests as required by state law, is strongly advised.

Proper assessment of the patient, proper prescribing practices, periodic reevaluation of therapy, and proper dispensing and storage are appropriate measures that help to reduce abuse of opioid drugs.

Risks Specific to Abuse of OXYCONTIN

OXYCONTIN is for oral use only. Abuse of OXYCONTIN poses a risk of overdose and death. The risk is increased with concurrent use of OXYCONTIN with alcohol and other central nervous system depressants. Taking cut, broken, chewed, crushed, or dissolved OXYCONTIN enhances drug release and increases the risk of overdose and death.

With parenteral abuse, the inactive ingredients in OXYCONTIN can be expected to result in local tissue necrosis, infection, pulmonary granulomas, and increased risk of endocarditis and valvular heart injury. Parenteral drug abuse is commonly associated with transmission of infectious diseases, such as hepatitis and HIV.

Abuse Deterrence Studies

OXYCONTIN is formulated with inactive ingredients intended to make the tablet more difficult to manipulate for misuse and abuse. For the purposes of describing the results of studies of the abuse-deterrent characteristics of OXYCONTIN resulting from a change in formulation, in this section, the original formulation of OXYCONTIN, which is no longer marketed, will be referred to as "original OxyContin" and the reformulated, currently marketed product will be referred to as "OXYCONTIN".

In Vitro Testing

In vitro physical and chemical tablet manipulation studies were performed to evaluate the success of different extraction methods in defeating the extended-release formulation. Results support that, relative to original OxyContin, there is an increase in the ability of OXYCONTIN to resist crushing, breaking, and dissolution using a variety of tools and solvents. The results of these studies also support this finding for OXYCONTIN relative to an immediate-release oxycodone. When subjected to an aqueous environment, OXYCONTIN gradually forms a viscous hydrogel (i.e., a gelatinous mass) that resists passage through a needle.

Clinical Studies

In a randomized, double-blind, placebo-controlled 5-period crossover pharmacodynamic study, 30 recreational opioid users with a history of intranasal drug abuse received intranasally administered active and placebo drug treatments. The five treatment arms were finely crushed OXYCONTIN 30 mg tablets, coarsely crushed OXYCONTIN 30 mg tablets, finely crushed original OxyContin 30 mg tablets, powdered oxycodone HCl 30 mg, and placebo. Data for finely crushed OXYCONTIN, finely crushed original OxyContin, and powdered oxycodone HCl are described below.

Drug liking was measured on a bipolar drug liking scale of 0 to 100 where 50 represents a neutral response of neither liking nor disliking, 0 represents maximum disliking and 100 represents maximum liking. Response to whether the subject would take the study drug again was also measured on a bipolar scale of 0 to 100 where 50 represents a neutral response, 0 represents the strongest negative response ("definitely would not take drug again") and 100 represents the strongest positive response ("definitely would take drug again").

Twenty-seven of the subjects completed the study. Incomplete dosing due to granules falling from the subjects' nostrils occurred in 34% (n = 10) of subjects with finely crushed OXYCONTIN, compared with 7% (n = 2) of subjects with finely crushed original OxyContin and no subjects with powdered oxycodone HCl.

The intranasal administration of finely crushed OXYCONTIN was associated with a numerically lower mean and median drug liking score and a lower mean and median score for take drug again, compared to finely crushed original OxyContin or powdered oxycodone HCl as summarized in Table 4.

Continued on next page

Table 4: Summary of Maximum Drug Liking (E_max) Data Following Intranasal Administration

VAS Scale (100 mm)*		OXYCONTIN (finely crushed)	Original OxyContin (finely crushed)	Oxycodone HCl (powdered)
Drug Liking	Mean (SE)	80.4 (3.9)	94.0 (2.7)	89.3 (3.1)
	Median (Range)	88 (36-100)	100 (51-100)	100 (50-100)
Take Drug Again	Mean (SE)	64.0 (7.1)	89.6 (3.9)	86.6 (4.4)
	Median (Range)	78 (0-100)	100 (20-100)	100 (0-100)

* Bipolar scales (0 = maximum negative response, 50 = neutral response, 100 = maximum positive response)

Figure 1 demonstrates a comparison of drug liking for finely crushed OXYCONTIN compared to powdered oxycodone HCl in subjects who received both treatments. The Y-axis represents the percent of subjects attaining a percent reduction in drug liking for OXYCONTIN vs. oxycodone HCl powder greater than or equal to the value on the X-axis. Approximately 44% (n = 12) had no reduction in liking with OXYCONTIN relative to oxycodone HCl. Approximately 56% (n = 15) of subjects had some reduction in drug liking with OXYCONTIN relative to oxycodone HCl. Thirty-three percent (n = 9) of subjects had a reduction of at least 30% in drug liking with OXYCONTIN compared to oxycodone HCl, and approximately 22% (n = 6) of subjects had a reduction of at least 50% in drug liking with OXYCONTIN compared to oxycodone HCl.

Figure 1: Percent Reduction Profiles for E_max of Drug Liking VAS for OXYCONTIN vs. oxycodone HCl, N=27 Following Intranasal Administration

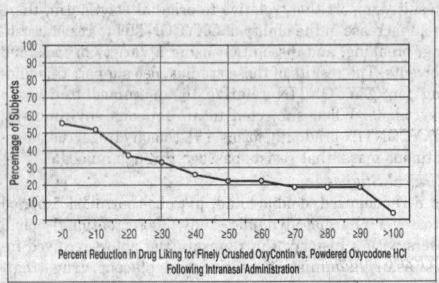

Percent Reduction in Drug Liking for Finely Crushed OxyContin vs. Powdered Oxycodone HCl Following Intranasal Administration

The results of a similar analysis of drug liking for finely crushed OXYCONTIN relative to finely crushed original OxyContin were comparable to the results of finely crushed OXYCONTIN relative to powdered oxycodone HCl. Approximately 43% (n = 12) of subjects had no reduction in liking with OXYCONTIN relative to original OxyContin. Approximately 57% (n = 16) of subjects had some reduction in drug liking, 36% (n = 10) of subjects had a reduction of at least 30% in drug liking, and approximately 29% (n = 8) of subjects had a reduction of at least 50% in drug liking with OXYCONTIN compared to original OxyContin.

Summary

The *in vitro* data demonstrate that OXYCONTIN has physicochemical properties expected to make abuse via injection difficult. The data from the clinical study, along with support from the *in vitro* data, also indicate that OXYCONTIN has physicochemical properties that are expected to reduce abuse via the intranasal route. However, abuse of OXYCONTIN by these routes, as well as by the oral route, is still possible.

Additional data, including epidemiological data, when available, may provide further information on the impact of the current formulation of OXYCONTIN on the abuse liability of the drug. Accordingly, this section may be updated in the future as appropriate.

OXYCONTIN contains oxycodone, an opioid agonist and Schedule II controlled substance with an abuse liability similar to other opioid agonists, legal or illicit, including fentanyl, hydromorphone, methadone, morphine, and oxymorphone. OXYCONTIN can be abused and is subject to misuse, addiction, and criminal diversion *[see Warnings and Precautions (5.1) and Drug Abuse and Dependence (9.1)]*.

9.3   Dependence

Both tolerance and physical dependence can develop during chronic opioid therapy. Tolerance is the need for increasing doses of opioids to maintain a defined effect such as analgesia (in the absence of disease progression or other external factors). Tolerance may occur to both the desired and undesired effects of drugs, and may develop at different rates for different effects.

Physical dependence results in withdrawal symptoms after abrupt discontinuation or a significant dose reduction of a drug. Withdrawal also may be precipitated through the administration of drugs with opioid antagonist activity, e.g., naloxone, nalmefene, mixed agonist/antagonist analgesics (pentazocine, butorphanol, nalbuphine), or partial agonists (buprenorphine). Physical dependence may not occur to a clinically significant degree until after several days to weeks of continued opioid usage.

OXYCONTIN should not be abruptly discontinued *[see Dosage and Administration (2.9)]*. If OXYCONTIN is abruptly discontinued in a physically-dependent patient, an abstinence syndrome may occur. Some or all of the following can characterize this syndrome: restlessness, lacrimation, rhinorrhea, yawning, perspiration, chills, myalgia, and mydriasis. Other signs and symptoms also may develop, including: irritability, anxiety, backache, joint pain, weakness, abdominal cramps, insomnia, nausea, anorexia, vomiting, diarrhea, or increased blood pressure, respiratory rate, or heart rate.

Infants born to mothers physically dependent on opioids will also be physically dependent and may exhibit respiratory difficulties and withdrawal signs *[see Use in Specific Populations (8.1)]*.

10   OVERDOSAGE

Clinical Presentation

Acute overdosage with OXYCONTIN can be manifested by respiratory depression, somnolence progressing to stupor or coma, skeletal muscle flaccidity, cold and clammy skin, constricted pupils, and in some cases, pulmonary edema, bradycardia, hypotension, partial or complete airway obstruction, atypical snoring and death. Marked mydriasis rather than miosis may be seen due to severe hypoxia in overdose situations.

Treatment of Overdose

In case of overdose, priorities are the reestablishment of a patent and protected airway and institution of assisted or controlled ventilation if needed. Employ other supportive measures (including oxygen, vasopressors) in the management of circulatory shock and pulmonary edema as indicated. Cardiac arrest or arrhythmias will require advanced life support techniques.

The opioid antagonists, naloxone or nalmefene, are specific antidotes to respiratory depression resulting from opioid overdose. Opioid antagonists should not be administered in the absence of clinically significant respiratory or circulatory depression secondary to oxycodone overdose. Such agents should be administered cautiously to persons who are known, or suspected to be physically dependent on OXYCONTIN. In such cases, an abrupt or complete reversal of opioid effects may precipitate an acute withdrawal syndrome.

Because the duration of reversal would be expected to be less than the duration of action of oxycodone in OXYCONTIN, carefully monitor the patient until spontaneous respiration is reliably reestablished. OXYCONTIN will continue to release oxycodone and add to the oxycodone load for 24 to 48 hours or longer following ingestion necessitating prolonged monitoring. If the response to opioid antagonists is suboptimal or not sustained, additional antagonist should be administered as directed in the product's prescribing information.

In an individual physically dependent on opioids, administration of the usual dose of the antagonist will precipitate an acute withdrawal syndrome. The severity of the withdrawal symptoms experienced will depend on the degree of physical dependence and the dose of the antagonist administered. If a decision is made to treat serious respiratory depression in the physically dependent patient, administration of the antagonist should be begun with care and by titration with smaller than usual doses of the antagonist.

11   DESCRIPTION

OXYCONTIN® (oxycodone hydrochloride) extended-release tablets is an opioid analgesic supplied in 10 mg, 15 mg, 20 mg, 30 mg, 40 mg, 60 mg, and 80 mg tablets for oral administration. The tablet strengths describe the amount of oxycodone per tablet as the hydrochloride salt. The structural formula for oxycodone hydrochloride is as follows:

$$C_{18}H_{21}NO_4 \cdot HCl \qquad MW\ 351.83$$

The chemical name is 4, 5α-epoxy-14-hydroxy-3-methoxy-17-methylmorphinan-6-one hydrochloride.

Oxycodone is a white, odorless crystalline powder derived from the opium alkaloid, thebaine. Oxycodone hydrochloride dissolves in water (1 g in 6 to 7 mL). It is slightly soluble in alcohol (octanol water partition coefficient 0.7).

The 10 mg, 15 mg, 20 mg, 30 mg, 40 mg, 60 mg and 80 mg tablets contain the following inactive ingredients: butylated hydroxytoluene (BHT), hypromellose, polyethylene glycol 400, polyethylene oxide, magnesium stearate, titanium dioxide.

The 10 mg tablets also contain hydroxypropyl cellulose.

The 15 mg tablets also contain black iron oxide, yellow iron oxide, and red iron oxide.

The 20 mg tablets also contain polysorbate 80 and red iron oxide.

The 30 mg tablets also contain polysorbate 80, red iron oxide, yellow iron oxide, and black iron oxide.

The 40 mg tablets also contain polysorbate 80 and yellow iron oxide.

The 60 mg tablets also contain polysorbate 80, red iron oxide and black iron oxide.

The 80 mg tablets also contain hydroxypropyl cellulose, yellow iron oxide and FD&C Blue #2/Indigo Carmine Aluminum Lake.

12   CLINICAL PHARMACOLOGY

Oxycodone hydrochloride is a full opioid agonist and is relatively selective for the mu receptor, although it can bind to other opioid receptors at higher doses. The principal therapeutic action of oxycodone is analgesia. Like all full opioid agonists, there is no ceiling effect to analgesia for oxycodone. Clinically, dosage is titrated to provide adequate analgesia and may be limited by adverse reactions, including respiratory and CNS depression.

12.1   Mechanism of Action

Central Nervous System

The precise mechanism of the analgesic action is unknown. However, specific CNS opioid receptors for endogenous compounds with opioid-like activity have been identified throughout the brain and spinal cord and are thought to play a role in the analgesic effects of this drug.

12.2   Pharmacodynamics

A single-dose, double-blind, placebo- and dose-controlled study was conducted using OXYCONTIN (10, 20, and 30 mg) in an analgesic pain model involving 182 patients with moderate to severe pain. OXYCONTIN doses of 20 mg and 30 mg produced statistically significant pain reduction compared to placebo.

Effects on the Central Nervous System

Oxycodone produces respiratory depression by direct action on brain stem respiratory centers. The respiratory depression involves both a reduction in the responsiveness of the brain stem respiratory centers to increases in CO_2 tension and to electrical stimulation.

Oxycodone depresses the cough reflex by direct effect on the cough center in the medulla. Antitussive effects may occur with doses lower than those usually required for analgesia. Oxycodone causes miosis, even in total darkness. Pinpoint pupils are a sign of opioid overdose but are not pathognomonic (e.g., pontine lesions of hemorrhagic or ischemic origin may produce similar findings). Marked mydriasis rather than miosis may be seen with hypoxia in the setting of oxycodone overdose *[see Overdosage (10)]*.

Effects on the Gastrointestinal Tract and Other Smooth Muscle

Oxycodone causes a reduction in motility associated with an increase in smooth muscle tone in the antrum of the stomach and duodenum. Digestion of food in the small intestine is delayed and propulsive contractions are decreased. Propulsive peristaltic waves in the colon are decreased, while tone may be increased to the point of spasm resulting in constipation. Other opioid-induced effects may include a reduction in gastric, biliary and pancreatic secretions, spasm of sphincter of Oddi, and transient elevations in serum amylase.

Effects on the Cardiovascular System
Oxycodone may produce release of histamine with or without associated peripheral vasodilation. Manifestations of histamine release and/or peripheral vasodilation may include pruritus, flushing, red eyes, sweating, and/or orthostatic hypotension.

Effects on the Endocrine System
Opioids inhibit the secretion of ACTH, cortisol, testosterone, and luteinizing hormone (LH) in humans. They also stimulate prolactin, growth hormone (GH) secretion, and pancreatic secretion of insulin and glucagon.

Effects on the Immune System
Opioids have been shown to have a variety of effects on components of the immune system in *in vitro* and animal models. The clinical significance of these findings is unknown. Overall, the effects of opioids appear to be modestly immunosuppressive.

Concentration –Efficacy Relationships
Studies in normal volunteers and patients reveal predictable relationships between oxycodone dosage and plasma oxycodone concentrations, as well as between concentration and certain expected opioid effects, such as pupillary constriction, sedation, overall subjective "drug effect", analgesia and feelings of relaxation.

The minimum effective analgesic concentration will vary widely among patients, especially among patients who have been previously treated with potent agonist opioids. As a result, patients must be treated with individualized titration of dosage to the desired effect. The minimum effective analgesic concentration of oxycodone for any individual patient may increase over time due to an increase in pain, the development of a new pain syndrome and/or the development of analgesic tolerance.

Concentration –Adverse Reaction Relationships
There is a relationship between increasing oxycodone plasma concentration and increasing frequency of dose-related opioid adverse reactions such as nausea, vomiting, CNS effects, and respiratory depression. In opioid-tolerant patients, the situation may be altered by the development of tolerance to opioid-related side effects.

The dose of OXYCONTIN must be individualized because the effective analgesic dose for some patients will be too high to be tolerated by other patients [see Dosage and Administration (2.1)].

12.3 Pharmacokinetics
The activity of OXYCONTIN is primarily due to the parent drug oxycodone. OXYCONTIN is designed to provide delivery of oxycodone over 12 hours.

Cutting, breaking, chewing, crushing or dissolving OXYCONTIN impairs the controlled-release delivery mechanism and results in the rapid release and absorption of a potentially fatal dose of oxycodone.

Oxycodone release from OXYCONTIN is pH independent. The oral bioavailability of oxycodone is 60% to 87%. The relative oral bioavailability of oxycodone from OXYCONTIN to that from immediate-release oral dosage forms is 100%. Upon repeated dosing with OXYCONTIN in healthy subjects in pharmacokinetic studies, steady-state levels were achieved within 24-36 hours. Oxycodone is extensively metabolized and eliminated primarily in the urine as both conjugated and unconjugated metabolites. The apparent elimination half-life ($t_{1/2}$) of oxycodone following the administration of OXYCONTIN was 4.5 hours compared to 3.2 hours for immediate-release oxycodone.

Absorption
About 60% to 87% of an oral dose of oxycodone reaches the central compartment in comparison to a parenteral dose. This high oral bioavailability is due to low pre-systemic and/or first-pass metabolism.

Plasma Oxycodone Concentration over Time
Dose proportionality has been established for OXYCONTIN 10 mg, 15 mg, 20 mg, 30 mg, 40 mg, 60 mg, and 80 mg tablet strengths for both peak plasma concentrations (C_{max}) and extent of absorption (AUC) *(see Table 5)*. Given the short elimination $t_{1/2}$ of oxycodone, steady-state plasma concentrations of oxycodone are achieved within 24-36 hours of initiation of dosing with OXYCONTIN. In a study comparing 10 mg of OXYCONTIN every 12 hours to 5 mg of

		TABLE 5			
		Mean [% coefficient of variation]			
Regimen	Dosage Form	AUC (ng·hr/mL)*	C_{max} (ng/mL)	T_{max} (hr)
Single Dose†	10 mg	136 [27]	11.5 [27]	5.11 [21]
	15 mg	196 [28]	16.8 [29]	4.59 [19]
	20 mg	248 [25]	22.7 [25]	4.63 [22]
	30 mg	377 [24]	34.6 [21]	4.61 [19]
	40 mg	497 [27]	47.4 [30]	4.40 [22]
	60 mg	705 [22]	64.6 [24]	4.15 [26]
	80 mg	908 [21]	87.1 [29]	4.27 [26]

*for single-dose AUC = AUC_{0-inf}
†data obtained while subjects received naltrexone, which can enhance absorption

immediate-release oxycodone every 6 hours, the two treatments were found to be equivalent for AUC and C_{max}, and similar for C_{min} (trough) concentrations.
[See table 5 above]

Food Effects
Food has no significant effect on the extent of absorption of oxycodone from OXYCONTIN.

Distribution
Following intravenous administration, the steady-state volume of distribution (Vss) for oxycodone was 2.6 L/kg. Oxycodone binding to plasma protein at 37°C and a pH of 7.4 was about 45%. Once absorbed, oxycodone is distributed to skeletal muscle, liver, intestinal tract, lungs, spleen, and brain. Oxycodone has been found in breast milk [see Use in Specific Populations (8.3)].

Metabolism
Oxycodone is extensively metabolized by multiple metabolic pathways to produce noroxycodone, oxymorphone and noroxymorphone, which are subsequently glucuronidated. Noroxycodone and noroxymorphone are the major circulating metabolites. CYP3A mediated N-demethylation to noroxycodone is the primary metabolic pathway of oxycodone with a lower contribution from CYP2D6 mediated O-demethylation to oxymorphone. Therefore, the formation of these and related metabolites can, in theory, be affected by other drugs [see Drug Interactions (7.3)].

Noroxycodone exhibits very weak anti-nociceptive potency compared to oxycodone, however, it undergoes further oxidation to produce noroxymorphone, which is active at opioid receptors. Although noroxymorphone is an active metabolite and present at relatively high concentrations in circulation, it does not appear to cross the blood-brain barrier to a significant extent. Oxymorphone is present in the plasma only at low concentrations and undergoes further metabolism to form its glucuronide and noroxymorphone. Oxymorphone has been shown to be active and possessing analgesic activity but its contribution to analgesia following oxycodone administration is thought to be clinically insignificant. Other metabolites (α- and ß-oxycodol, noroxycodol and oxymorphol) may be present at very low concentrations and demonstrate limited penetration into the brain as compared to oxycodone. The enzymes responsible for keto-reduction and glucuronidation pathways in oxycodone metabolism have not been established.

Excretion
Oxycodone and its metabolites are excreted primarily via the kidney. The amounts measured in the urine have been reported as follows: free and conjugated oxycodone 8.9%, free noroxycodone 23%, free oxymorphone less than 1%, conjugated oxymorphone 10%, free and conjugated noroxymorphone 14%, reduced free and conjugated metabolites up to 18%. The total plasma clearance was approximately 1.4 L/min in adults.

Specific Populations
Geriatric Use
The plasma concentrations of oxycodone are only nominally affected by age, being 15% greater in elderly as compared to young subjects (age 21-45).

Gender
Across individual pharmacokinetic studies, average plasma oxycodone concentrations for female subjects were up to 25% higher than for male subjects on a body weight-adjusted basis. The reason for this difference is unknown [see Use in Specific Populations (8.8)].

Renal Impairment
Data from a pharmacokinetic study involving 13 patients with mild to severe renal dysfunction (creatinine clearance

<60 mL/min) showed peak plasma oxycodone and noroxycodone concentrations 50% and 20% higher, respectively, and AUC values for oxycodone, noroxycodone, and oxymorphone 60%, 50%, and 40% higher than normal subjects, respectively. This was accompanied by an increase in sedation but not by differences in respiratory rate, pupillary constriction, or several other measures of drug effect. There was an increase in mean elimination $t_{1/2}$ for oxycodone of 1 hour.

Hepatic Impairment
Data from a study involving 24 patients with mild to moderate hepatic dysfunction show peak plasma oxycodone and noroxycodone concentrations 50% and 20% higher, respectively, than healthy subjects. AUC values are 95% and 65% higher, respectively. Oxymorphone peak plasma concentrations and AUC values are lower by 30% and 40%. These differences are accompanied by increases in some, but not other, drug effects. The mean elimination $t_{1/2}$ for oxycodone increased by 2.3 hours.

Pediatric Use
In the pediatric age group of 11 years of age and older, systemic exposure of oxycodone is expected to be similar to adults at any given dose of OXYCONTIN.

Drug-Drug Interactions
CYP3A4 Inhibitors
CYP3A4 is the major isoenzyme involved in noroxycodone formation. Co-administration of OXYCONTIN (10 mg single dose) and the CYP3A4 inhibitor ketoconazole (200 mg BID) increased oxycodone AUC and C_{max} by 170% and 100%, respectively [see Drug Interactions (7.2)].

CYP3A4 Inducers
A published study showed that the co-administration of rifampin, a drug metabolizing enzyme inducer, decreased oxycodone AUC and C_{max} values by 86% and 63%, respectively [see Drug Interactions (7.2)].

CYP2D6 Inhibitors
Oxycodone is metabolized in part to oxymorphone via CYP2D6. While this pathway may be blocked by a variety of drugs such as certain cardiovascular drugs (e.g., quinidine) and antidepressants (e.g., fluoxetine), such blockade has not been shown to be of clinical significance with OXYCONTIN [see Drug Interactions (7.2)].

13 NONCLINICAL TOXICOLOGY
13.1 Carcinogenesis, Mutagenesis, Impairment of Fertility
Carcinogenesis
No animal studies to evaluate the carcinogenic potential of oxycodone have been conducted.

Mutagenesis
Oxycodone was genotoxic in the mouse lymphoma assay at concentrations of 50 mcg/mL or greater with metabolic activation and at 400 mcg/mL or greater without metabolic activation. Clastogenicity was observed with oxycodone in the presence of metabolic activation in one chromosomal aberration assay in human lymphocytes at concentrations greater than or equal to 1250 mcg/mL at 24 but not 48 hours of exposure. In a second chromosomal aberration assay with human lymphocytes, no structural clastogenicity was observed either with or without metabolic activation; however, in the absence of metabolic activation, oxycodone increased numerical chromosomal aberrations (polyploidy). Oxycodone was not genotoxic in the following assays: Ames S. typhimurium and E. coli test with and without metabolic activation at concentrations up to 5000 µg/plate, chromosomal aberration test in human lymphocytes (in the ab-

Continued on next page

sence of metabolic activation) at concentrations up to 1500 µg/mL, and with activation after 48 hours of exposure at concentrations up to 5000 µg/mL, and in the *in vivo* bone marrow micronucleus assay in mice (at plasma levels up to 48 µg/mL).

Impairment of Fertility

In a study of reproductive performance, rats were administered a once daily gavage dose of the vehicle or oxycodone hydrochloride (0.5, 2, and 8 mg/kg/day). Male rats were dosed for 28 days before cohabitation with females, during the cohabitation and until necropsy (2-3 weeks post-cohabitation). Females were dosed for 14 days before cohabitation with males, during cohabitation and up to gestation day 6. Oxycodone hydrochloride did not affect reproductive function in male or female rats at any dose tested (≤ 8 mg/kg/day).

14 CLINICAL STUDIES

Adult clinical study

A double-blind, placebo-controlled, fixed-dose, parallel group, two-week study was conducted in 133 patients with persistent, moderate to severe pain, who were judged as having inadequate pain control with their current therapy. In this study, OXYCONTIN 20 mg, but not 10 mg, was statistically significant in pain reduction compared with placebo.

Pediatric clinical study

OXYCONTIN has been evaluated in an open-label clinical trial of 155 opioid-tolerant pediatric patients with moderate to severe chronic pain. The mean duration of therapy was 20.7 days (range 1 to 43 days). The starting total daily doses ranged from 20 mg to 100 mg based on the patient's prior opioid dose. The mean daily dose was 33.30 mg (range 20 to 140 mg/day). In an extension study, 23 of the 155 patients were treated beyond four weeks, including 13 for 28 weeks. Too few patients less than 11 years were enrolled in the clinical trial to provide meaningful safety data in this age group.

16 HOW SUPPLIED/STORAGE AND HANDLING

OXYCONTIN (oxycodone hydrochloride) extended-release tablets 10 mg are film-coated, round, white-colored, bi-convex tablets debossed with OP on one side and 10 on the other and are supplied as child-resistant closure, opaque plastic bottles of 100 (**NDC 59011-410-10**) and unit dose packaging with 10 individually numbered tablets per card; two cards per glue end carton (**NDC 59011-410-20**).

OXYCONTIN (oxycodone hydrochloride) extended-release tablets 15 mg are film-coated, round, gray-colored, bi-convex tablets debossed with OP on one side and 15 on the other and are supplied as child-resistant closure, opaque plastic bottles of 100 (**NDC 59011-415-10**) and unit dose packaging with 10 individually numbered tablets per card; two cards per glue end carton (**NDC 59011-415-20**).

OXYCONTIN (oxycodone hydrochloride) extended-release tablets 20 mg are film-coated, round, pink-colored, bi-convex tablets debossed with OP on one side and 20 on the other and are supplied as child-resistant closure, opaque plastic bottles of 100 (**NDC 59011-420-10**) and unit dose packaging with 10 individually numbered tablets per card; two cards per glue end carton (**NDC 59011-420-20**).

OXYCONTIN (oxycodone hydrochloride) extended-release tablets 30 mg are film-coated, round, brown-colored, bi-convex tablets debossed with OP on one side and 30 on the other and are supplied as child-resistant closure, opaque plastic bottles of 100 (**NDC 59011-430-10**) and unit dose packaging with 10 individually numbered tablets per card; two cards per glue end carton (**NDC 59011-430-20**).

OXYCONTIN (oxycodone hydrochloride) extended-release tablets 40 mg are film-coated, round, yellow-colored, bi-convex tablets debossed with OP on one side and 40 on the other and are supplied as child-resistant closure, opaque plastic bottles of 100 (**NDC 59011-440-10**) and unit dose packaging with 10 individually numbered tablets per card; two cards per glue end carton (**NDC 59011-440-20**).

OXYCONTIN (oxycodone hydrochloride) extended-release tablets 60 mg are film-coated, round, red-colored, bi-convex tablets debossed with OP on one side and 60 on the other and are supplied as child-resistant closure, opaque plastic bottles of 100 (**NDC 59011-460-10**) and unit dose packaging with 10 individually numbered tablets per card; two cards per glue end carton (**NDC 59011-460-20**).

OXYCONTIN (oxycodone hydrochloride) extended-release tablets 80 mg are film-coated, round, green-colored, bi-convex tablets debossed with OP on one side and 80 on the other and are supplied as child-resistant closure, opaque

plastic bottles of 100 (**NDC 59011-480-10**) and unit dose packaging with 10 individually numbered tablets per card; two cards per glue end carton (**NDC 59011-480-20**).

Store at 25°C (77°F); excursions permitted between 15°-30°C (59°-86°F).

Dispense in tight, light-resistant container.

CAUTION

DEA FORM REQUIRED

17 PATIENT COUNSELING INFORMATION

Advise the patient to read the FDA-approved patient labeling (Medication Guide).

Addiction, Abuse and Misuse

Inform patients that the use of OXYCONTIN, even when taken as recommended can result in addiction, abuse and misuse, which can lead to overdose and death *[see Warnings and Precautions (5.1)]*. Instruct patients not to share OXYCONTIN with others and to take steps to protect OXYCONTIN from theft or misuse.

Life-Threatening Respiratory Depression

Inform patients of the risk of life-threatening respiratory depression including information that the risk is greatest when starting OXYCONTIN or when the dose is increased and that it can occur even at recommended doses *[see Warnings and Precautions (5.2)]*. Advise patients how to recognize respiratory depression and to seek medical attention if breathing difficulties develop.

To guard against excessive exposure to OXYCONTIN by young children, advise caregivers to strictly adhere to recommended OXYCONTIN dosing.

Accidental Ingestion

Inform patients that accidental ingestion, especially in children, may result in respiratory depression or death *[see Warnings and Precautions (5.2)]*. Instruct patients to take steps to store OXYCONTIN securely and to dispose of unused OXYCONTIN by flushing the tablets down the toilet.

Neonatal Opioid Withdrawal Syndrome

Inform female patients of reproductive potential that prolonged use of OXYCONTIN during pregnancy can result in neonatal opioid withdrawal syndrome, which may be life-threatening if not recognized and treated *[see Warnings and Precautions (5.3)]*.

Interactions with Alcohol and other CNS Depressants

Inform patients that potentially serious additive effects may occur if OXYCONTIN is used with other CNS depressants, and not to use such drugs unless supervised by a health care provider.

Important Administration Instructions

Instruct patients how to properly take OXYCONTIN, including the following:

- OXYCONTIN is designed to work properly only if swallowed intact. Taking cut, broken, chewed, crushed, or dissolved OXYCONTIN tablets can result in a fatal overdose.
- OXYCONTIN tablets should be taken one tablet at a time.
- Do not pre-soak, lick or otherwise wet the tablet prior to placing in the mouth.
- Take each tablet with enough water to ensure complete swallowing immediately after placing in the mouth.

Hypotension

Inform patients that OXYCONTIN may cause orthostatic hypotension and syncope. Instruct patients how to recognize symptoms of low blood pressure and how to reduce the risk of serious consequences should hypotension occur (e.g., sit or lie down, carefully rise from a sitting or lying position).

Driving or Operating Heavy Machinery

Inform patients that OXYCONTIN may impair the ability to perform potentially hazardous activities such as driving a car or operating heavy machinery. Advise patients not to perform such tasks until they know how they will react to the medication.

Constipation

Advise patients of the potential for severe constipation, including management instructions and when to seek medical attention.

Anaphylaxis

Inform patients that anaphylaxis has been reported with ingredients contained in OXYCONTIN. Advise patients how to recognize such a reaction and when to seek medical attention.

Pregnancy

Advise female patients that OXYCONTIN can cause fetal harm and to inform the prescriber if they are pregnant or plan to become pregnant.

Disposal of Unused OXYCONTIN

Advise patients to flush the unused tablets down the toilet when OXYCONTIN is no longer needed.

Healthcare professionals can telephone Purdue Pharma's Medical Services Department (1-888-726-7535) for information on this product.

Purdue Pharma L.P.

Stamford, CT 06901-3431

©2015, Purdue Pharma L.P.

U.S. Patent Numbers 6,488,963; 7,129,248; 7,674,799; 7,674,800; 7,683,072; 8,114,383; 8,309,060; 8,337,888; 8,808,741; 8,821,929; 8,894,987; 8,894,988; 9,060,976 and 9,073,933.

Medication Guide

OXYCONTIN®(ox-e-KON-tin) (oxycodone hydrochloride) extended-release tablets, CII

OXYCONTIN is:

- A strong prescription pain medicine that contains an opioid (narcotic) that is used to manage pain severe enough to require daily around-the-clock, long-term treatment with an opioid, when other pain treatments such as non-opioid pain medicines or immediate-release opioid medicines do not treat your pain well enough or you cannot tolerate them.
- A long-acting (extended-release) opioid pain medicine that can put you at risk for overdose and death. Even if you take your dose correctly as prescribed you are at risk for opioid addiction, abuse, and misuse that can lead to death.
- Not for use to treat pain that is not around-the-clock.
- Not for use in children less than 11 years of age and who are not already using opioid pain medicines regularly to manage pain severe enough to require daily around-the-clock long-term treatment of pain with an opioid.

Important information about OXYCONTIN:

- Get emergency help right away if you take too much OXYCONTIN (overdose). When you first start taking OXYCONTIN, when your dose is changed, or if you take too much (overdose), serious or life-threatening breathing problems that can lead to death may occur.
- Never give anyone else your OXYCONTIN. They could die from taking it. Store OXYCONTIN away from children and in a safe place to prevent stealing or abuse. Selling or giving away OXYCONTIN is against the law.

Do not take OXYCONTIN if you have:

- severe asthma, trouble breathing, or other lung problems.
- a bowel blockage or have narrowing of the stomach or intestines.

Before taking OXYCONTIN, tell your healthcare provider if you have a history of:

- head injury, seizures
- liver, kidney, thyroid problems
- problems urinating
- pancreas or gallbladder problems
- abuse of street or prescription drugs, alcohol addiction, or mental health problems.

Tell your healthcare provider if you are:

- **pregnant or planning to become pregnant.** Prolonged use of OXYCONTIN during pregnancy can cause withdrawal symptoms in your newborn baby that could be life-threatening if not recognized and treated.
- **breastfeeding.** OXYCONTIN passes into breast milk and may harm your baby.
- taking prescription or over-the-counter medicines, vitamins, or herbal supplements. Taking OXYCONTIN with certain other medicines can cause serious side effects that could lead to death.

When taking OXYCONTIN:

- Do not change your dose. Take OXYCONTIN exactly as prescribed by your healthcare provider.
- Take your prescribed dose every 12 hours at the same time every day. Do not take more than your prescribed dose in 12 hours. If you miss a dose, take your next dose at your usual time.
- Swallow OXYCONTIN whole. Do not cut, break, chew, crush, dissolve, snort, or inject OXYCONTIN because this may cause you to overdose and die.
- OXYCONTIN should be taken 1 tablet at a time. Do not pre-soak, lick, or wet the tablet before placing in your mouth to avoid choking on the tablet.
- **Call your healthcare provider if the dose you are taking does not control your pain.**
- **Do not stop taking OXYCONTIN without talking to your healthcare provider.**

• After you stop taking OXYCONTIN, flush any unused tablets down the toilet.

While taking OXYCONTIN DO NOT:
• Drive or operate heavy machinery until you know how OXYCONTIN affects you. OXYCONTIN can make you sleepy, dizzy, or lightheaded.
• Drink alcohol, or use prescription or over-the-counter medicines that contain alcohol. Using products containing alcohol during treatment with OXYCONTIN may cause you to overdose and die.

The possible side effects of OXYCONTIN are:
• constipation, nausea, sleepiness, vomiting, tiredness, headache, dizziness, abdominal pain. Call your healthcare provider if you have any of these symptoms and they are severe.
Get emergency medical help if you have:
• trouble breathing, shortness of breath, fast heartbeat, chest pain, swelling of your face, tongue or throat, extreme drowsiness, light-headedness when changing positions, or you are feeling faint.
These are not all the possible side effects of OXYCONTIN. Call your doctor for medical advice about side effects. You may report side effects to FDA at 1-800-FDA-1088. **For more information go to dailymed.nlm.nih.gov**
Manufactured by: Purdue Pharma L.P., Stamford, CT 06901-3431, **www.purduepharma.com or call 1-888-726-7535**

This Medication Guide has been approved by the U.S. Food and Drug Administration.

Shown in Product Identification Guide, page 509

RLC Labs, Inc.
CAVE CREEK, AZ 85331

For Product Information:
(877) 797-7997
sales@rlclabs.com
For Customer Service & Ordering Information:
(877) 797-7997
(623) 879-8683 (Fax)
customerservice@rlclabs.com
www.getrealthyroid.com

NATURE-THROID®
(Thyroid USP) Tablets

R

DESCRIPTION
Nature-Throid® (Thyroid USP) Tablets, micro-coated, easy to swallow with a reduced odor, for oral use are natural preparations derived from porcine thyroid glands (T3 liothyronine is approximately four times as potent as T4 levothyroxine on a microgram for microgram basis). They provide 38 mcg levothyroxine (T4) and 9 mcg liothyronine (T3) for each 65 mg (1 Grain) of the labeled content of thyroid.
INACTIVE INGREDIENTS
Colloidal Silicon Dioxide, Dicalcium Phosphate, Lactose Monohydrate[1], Magnesium Stearate, Microcrystalline Cellulose, Croscarmellose Sodium, Stearic Acid, Opadry II 85F19316 Clear.
The structural formulas of liothyronine (T3) and levothyroxine (T4) are as follows:

[1]Present in traceable amount as part of Thyroid USP (diluent)

CLINICAL PHARMACOLOGY
The steps in the synthesis of the thyroid hormones are controlled by thyrotropin (Thyroid Stimulating Hormone, TSH) secreted by the anterior pituitary. This hormone's secretion is in turn controlled by a feedback mechanism affected by the thyroid hormones themselves and by thyrotropin releasing hormone (TRH), a tripeptide of hypothalamic origin. Endogenous thyroid hormone secretion is suppressed when exogenous thyroid hormones are administered to euthyroid individuals in excess of the normal gland's secretion.
The mechanisms by which thyroid hormones exert their physiologic action are not well understood. These hormones enhance oxygen consumption by most tissues of the body, increase the basal metabolic rate, and the metabolism of carbohydrates, lipids, and proteins. Thus, they exert a profound influence on every organ system in the body and are of particular importance in the development of the central nervous system.
The normal thyroid gland contains approximately 200 mcg of levothyroxine (T4) per gram of gland, and 15 mcg of liothyronine (T3) per gram. The ratio of these two hormones in the circulation does not represent the ratio in the thyroid gland, since about 80 percent of peripheral liothyronine (T3) comes from monodeiodination of levothyroxine (T4). Peripheral monodeiodination of levothyroxine (T4) at the 5 position (inner ring) also results in the formation of reverse liothyronine (T3), which is calorigenically inactive. Liothyronine (T3) levels are low in the fetus and newborn, in old age, in chronic caloric deprivation, hepatic cirrhosis, renal failure, surgical stress, and chronic illnesses representing what has been called the "T3 thyronine syndrome".
Pharmacokinetics
Animal studies have shown that levothyroxine (T4) is only partially absorbed from the gastrointestinal tract. The degree of absorption is dependent on the vehicle used for its administration and by the character of the intestinal contents, the intestinal flora, including plasma protein, and soluble dietary factors, all of which bind thyroid, thereby making it unavailable for diffusion. Only 41 percent is absorbed when given in a gelatin capsule, as opposed to 74 percent absorption when given with an albumin carrier.
Depending on other factors, absorption has varied from 48 to 79 percent of the administered dose. Fasting increases absorption. Malabsorption syndromes, as well as dietary factors, (children's soybean formula, concomitant use of anionic exchange resins such as cholestyramine) cause excessive fecal loss. Liothyronine (T3) is almost totally absorbed, 95 percent in 4 hours. The hormones contained in the natural preparations are absorbed in a manner similar to the synthetic hormones.
More than 99 percent of circulating hormones are bound to serum proteins, including thyroid-binding globulin (TBg), thyroid-binding pre-albumin (TBPA), and albumin (TBa), whose capacities and affinities vary for the hormones. The higher affinity of levothyroxine (T4) for both TBg and TBPA, as compared to liothyronine (T3), partially explains the higher serum levels and longer half-life of the former hormone. Both protein-bound hormones exist in reverse equilibrium with minute amounts of free hormone, the latter accounting for the metabolic activity. Deiodination of levothyroxine (T4) occurs at a number of sites, including liver, kidney, and other tissues. The conjugated hormone, in the form of glucuronide or sulfate, is found in the bile and gut where it may complete an enterohepatic circulation. Eighty-five percent of levothyroxine (T4) metabolized daily is deiodinated.

INDICATIONS AND USAGE
1. As replacement of supplemental therapy in patients with hypothyroidism of any etiology, except transient hypothyroidism during the recovery phase of subacute thyroiditis. This category includes cretinism, myxedema, and ordinary hypothyroidism in patients of any age (children, adults, the elderly), or state (including pregnancy); primary hypothyroidism resulting from functional deficiency, primary atrophy, partial or total absence of thyroid gland, or the effects of surgery, radiation, or drugs, with or without the presence of goiter; and secondary (pituitary), or tertiary (hypothalamic) hypothyroidism (See WARNINGS).
2. As pituitary TSH suppressants, in the treatment or prevention of various types of euthyroid goiters, including thyroid nodules, subacute, or chronic lymphocytic thyroiditis (Hashimoto's), multinodular goiter, and in the management of thyroid cancer.
3. As diagnostic agents in suppression tests to differentiate suspected mild hyperthyroidism or thyroid gland anatomy.

CONTRAINDICATIONS
Thyroid hormone preparations are generally contraindicated in patients with diagnosed, but as yet, uncorrected adrenal cortical insufficiency, untreated thyrotoxicosis, and apparent hypersensitivity to any of their active or extraneous constituents. There is no well documented evidence in the literature of true allergic or idiosyncratic reactions to thyroid hormone.

WARNINGS
Drugs with thyroid hormone activity, alone or together with other therapeutic agents, have been used for the treatment of obesity. In euthyroid patients, doses within the range of daily hormonal requirements are ineffective for weight reduction. Larger doses may produce serious or even life-threatening manifestations of toxicity, particularly when given in association with sympathomimetic amines such as those used for their anorectic effects.
The use of thyroid hormones in the therapy of obesity, alone or combined with other drugs, is unjustified and has been shown to be ineffective. Neither is their use justified for the treatment of male or female infertility unless this condition is accompanied by hypothyroidism.

PRECAUTIONS
General: Thyroid hormones should be used with great caution in a number of circumstances where the integrity of the cardiovascular system, particularly the coronary arteries, is suspected. These include patients with angina pectoris or the elderly, whom have a greater likelihood of occult cardiac disease. With these patients, therapy should be initiated with low doses, i.e. 16.25 - 32.5 mg. When, in such patients, a euthyroid state can only be reached at the expense of an aggravation of the cardiovascular disease, thyroid hormone dosage should be reduced.
Thyroid hormone therapy in patients with concomitant diabetes mellitus or diabetes insipidus or adrenal cortical insufficiency aggravates the intensity of their symptoms. Appropriate adjustments of the various therapeutic measures directed at these concomitant endocrine diseases are required. The therapy of myxedema coma requires simultaneous administration of glucorticoids (See DOSAGE AND ADMINISTRATION).
Hypothyroidism decreases and hyperthyroidism increases the sensitivity to oral anticoagulants. Prothrombin time should be closely monitored in thyroid treated patients on oral anticoagulants and dosage of the latter agents should be adjusted on the basis of frequent prothrombin time determinations. In infants, excessive doses of thyroid hormone preparations may produce craniosynostosis.
Information for the Patient: Patients on thyroid hormone preparations and parents of children on thyroid therapy should be informed that:
1. Replacement therapy is to be taken essentially for life, with the exception of cases of transient hypothyroidism, usually associated with thyroiditis, and in those patients receiving a therapeutic trial of the drug.
2. They should immediately report, during the course of therapy, any signs or symptoms of thyroid hormone toxicity, e.g., chest pain, increased pulse rate, palpitations, excessive sweating, heat intolerance, nervousness, or any other unusual event.
3. In case of concomitant diabetes mellitus, the daily dosage of antidiabetic medication may need readjustment as thyroid hormone replacement is achieved. If thyroid medication is stopped, a downward readjustment of the dosage of insulin or oral hypoglycemic agent may be necessary to avoid hypoglycemia. At all times, close monitoring of urinary glucose levels is mandatory in such patients.
4. In case of concomitant oral anticoagulant therapy, the prothrombin time should be measured frequently to determine if the dosage of oral anticoagulants is to be readjusted.
5. Partial loss of hair may be experienced by children in the first few months of thyroid therapy, but this is usually a transient phenomenon and later recovery is usually the rule.
Laboratory Tests: Treatment of patients with thyroid hormones requires the periodic assessment of thyroid status by means of appropriate laboratory tests, besides the full clinical evaluation. The TSH suppression test can be used to test the effectiveness of any thyroid preparation, bearing in mind the relative insensitivity of the infant pituitary to the negative feedback effect of thyroid hormones. Serum T4 levels can be used to test the effectiveness of all thyroid medi-

Continued on next page

cations except T3. When the total serum T4 is low but TSH is normal, a test specific to assess unbound (free) T4 levels is warranted. Specific measurements of T4 and T3 by competitive protein binding or radioimmunoassay are not influenced by blood levels of organic or inorganic iodine.

Drug Interactions: Oral Anticoagulants—Thyroid hormones appear to increase catabolism of vitamin K-dependent clotting factors. If oral anticoagulants are also being given, compensatory increases in clotting factor synthesis are impaired. Patients stabilized on oral anticoagulants that are found to require thyroid replacement therapy should be watched very closely when thyroid is started. If a patient is truly hypothyroid, it is likely that a reduction in anticoagulant dosage will be required. No special precautions appear to be necessary when oral anticoagulant therapy is begun in a patient already stabilized on maintenance thyroid replacement therapy.

Insulin or Oral Hypoglycemic—Initiating thyroid replacement therapy may cause increases in insulin or oral hypoglycemic requirements. The effects seen are poorly understood and depend upon a variety of factors such as dose and type of thyroid preparations and endocrine status of the patient. Patients receiving insulin or oral hypoglycemic should be closely watched during initiation of thyroid replacement therapy.

Cholestyramine or Colestipol—Cholestyramine or Colestipol binds both levothyroxine (T4) and liothyronine (T3) in the intestine, thus impairing absorption of these thyroid hormones. In vitro studies indicate that the binding is not easily removed. Therefore, four to five hours should elapse between administration of Cholestyramine or Colestipol and thyroid hormones.

Estrogen, Oral Contraceptives—Estrogens tend to increase serum thyroxine-binding globulin (TBg). In a patient with a nonfunctioning thyroid gland who is receiving thyroid replacement therapy, free levothyroxine (T4) may be decreased when estrogens are started thus increasing thyroid requirements. However, if the patient's thyroid gland has sufficient function, the decreased free levothyroxine (T4) will result in a compensatory increase in levothyroxine (T4) output by the thyroid. Therefore, patients without a functioning thyroid gland who are on thyroid replacement therapy, may need to increase their thyroid dose if estrogens or estrogen-containing oral contraceptives are given.

Drug/Laboratory Test Interactions: The following drugs or moieties are known to interfere with laboratory tests performed in patients on thyroid hormone therapy: androgens, corticosteroids, estrogens, oral contraceptives containing estrogens, iodine-containing preparations, and the numerous preparations containing salicylates.

1. Changes in TBg concentration should be taken into consideration in the interpretation of levothyroxine (T4) and liothyronine (T3) values. In such cases, the unbound (free) hormone should be measured. Pregnancy, estrogens, and estrogen-containing oral contraceptives increase TBg concentrations. TBg may also be increased during infectious hepatitis. Decreases in TBg concentrations are observed in nephrosis, acromegaly, and after androgen or corticosteroid therapy. Familial hyper or hypothyroxine-binding-globulinemias have been described. The incidence of TBg deficiency approximates 1 in 9,000. The binding of levothyroxine by TBPA is inhibited by salicylates.

2. Medicinal or dietary iodine interferes with all in vivo tests of radio-iodine uptake, producing low uptakes which may not be relative of a true decrease in hormone synthesis.

3. The persistence of clinical and laboratory evidence of hypothyroidism in spite of adequate dosage replacement indicates; either poor patient compliance, poor absorption, excessive fecal loss, or inactivity of the preparation. Intracellular resistance to thyroid hormone is quite rare.

Carcinogenesis, Mutagenesis, and Impairment of Fertility: A reportedly apparent association between prolonged thyroid therapy and breast cancer has not been confirmed and patients on thyroid for established indications should not discontinue therapy. No confirmatory long-term studies in animals have been performed to evaluate carcinogenic potential, mutagenicity, or impairment of fertility in either males or females.

Pregnancy-Category A: Thyroid hormones do not readily cross the placental barrier. The clinical experience to date does not indicate any adverse effect on fetuses when thyroid hormones are administered to pregnant women. On the basis of current knowledge, thyroid replacement therapy to hypothyroid women should not be discontinued during pregnancy.

Nursing Mothers: Minimal amounts of thyroid hormones are excreted in human milk. Thyroid is not associated with serious adverse reactions and does not have a known tumorigenic potential. However, caution should be exercised when thyroid is administered to a nursing woman.

Pediatric Use: Pregnant mothers provide little or no thyroid hormone to the fetus. The incidence of congenital hypothyroidism is relatively high (1:4,000) and the hypothyroid fetus would not derive any benefit from the small amounts of hormone crossing the placental barrier. Routine determination of serumT4 and/or TSH is strongly advised in neonates in view of the deleterious effects of thyroid deficiency on growth and development. Treatment should be initiated immediately upon diagnosis, and maintained for life, unless transient hypothyroidism is suspected; in which case, therapy may be interrupted for 2 to 8 weeks after the age of 3 years to reassess the condition. Cessation of therapy is justified in patients who have maintained a normal TSH during those 2 to 8 weeks.

Geriatric use: Clinical studies of Thyroid Tablets, USP did not include sufficient numbers of subjects aged 65 and over to determine whether they respond differently from younger subjects. Other reported clinical experience has not identified differences in responses between the elderly and younger patients. In general, dose selection for an elderly patient should be cautious, usually starting at the low end of the dosing range, reflecting the greater frequency of decreased hepatic, renal, or cardiac function, and of concomitant disease or other drug therapy.

ADVERSE REACTIONS

Adverse reactions other than those indicative of hyperthyroidism because of therapeutic overdosage, either initially or during the maintenance period, are rare (See OVERDOSAGE).

OVERDOSAGE

Signs and Symptoms: Excessive doses of thyroid result in a hypermetabolic state resembling in every respect the condition of endogenous origin. The condition may be self induced.

Treatment of Overdosage: Dosage should be reduced or therapy temporarily discontinued signs and symptoms of overdosage appear.

Treatment may be reinstituted at a lower dosage. In normal individuals, normal hypothalamic-pituitary-thyroid axis function is restored in 6 to 8 weeks after thyroid suppression.

Treatment of acute massive thyroid hormone overdosage is aimed at reducing gastrointestinal absorption of the drugs and counteracting central and peripheral effects, mainly those of increased sympathetic activity. Vomiting may be induced initially if further gastrointestinal absorption can reasonably be prevented and barring contraindications such as coma, convulsions, or loss of the gagging reflex. Treatment is symptomatic and supportive. Oxygen may be administered and ventilation maintained. Cardiac glycosides may be indicated if congestive heart failure develops. Measures to control fever, hypoglycemia, or fluid loss should be instituted if needed. Antiadrenergic agents, particularly propranolol, have been used advantageously in the treatment of increased sympathetic activity. Propranolol may be administered intravenously at a dosage of 1 to 3 mg, over a 10 minute period or orally, 80 to 160 mg/day, initially, especially when no contraindications exist for its use.

DOSAGE AND ADMINISTRATION

The dosage of thyroid hormones is determined by the indication and must in every case be individualized according to patient response and laboratory findings.

Thyroid hormones are given orally. In acute, emergency conditions, injectable levothyroxine sodium (T4) may be given intravenously when oral administration is not feasible or desirable (as in the treatment of myxedema coma, or during parenteral nutrition). Intramuscular administration is not advisable because of reported poor absorption.

Hypothyroidism: Therapy is usually instituted using low doses, with increments which depend on the cardiovascular status of the patient. The usual starting dose is 32.5 mg, with increment of 16.25 mg every 2 to 3 weeks. A lower starting dosage, 16.25 mg/day, is recommended in patients with longstanding myxedema, particularly if cardiovascular impairment is suspected, in which case extreme caution is recommended. The appearance of angina is an indication for reduction in dosage. Most patients require 65 - 130 mg/day. Failure to respond to doses of 195 mg suggests lack of com-

pliance or malabsorption. Maintenance dosages 65 - 130 mg/day usually result in normal serum T4 and T3 levels. Adequate therapy usually results in normal TSH and T4 levels after 2 or 3 weeks of therapy.

Readjustment of thyroid hormone dosage should be made within the first four weeks of therapy, after proper clinical and laboratory evaluations, including serum levels of T4, bound and free, and TSH.

Liothyronine (T3) may be used in preference to levothyroxine (T4) during radio-isotope scanning procedures, since induction of hypothyroidism in those cases is more abrupt and can be of shorter duration. It may also be preferred when impairment of peripheral conversion of levothyroxine (T4) and liothyronine (T3) is suspected.

Myxedema Coma: Myxedema coma is usually precipitated in the hypothyroid patient of longstanding by intercurrent illness or drugs such as sedatives and anesthetics and should be considered a medical emergency. Therapy should be directed at the correction of electrolyte disturbances and possible infection, besides the administration of thyroid hormones. Corticosteroids should be administered routinely. Levothyroxine (T4) and Liothyronine (T3) may be administered via a nasogastric tube, but the preferred route of administration of both hormones is intravenous. Levothyroxine sodium (T4) is given at a starting dose of 400 mcg (100 mcg/mL) given rapidly, and is usually well tolerated, even in the elderly. This initial dose is followed by daily supplements of 100 to 200 mcg given IV. Normal T4 levels are achieved in 24 hours, followed in 3 days by three-fold elevation of T3. Oral therapy with thyroid hormone would be resumed as soon as the clinical situation has been stabilized and the patient is able to take oral medication.

Thyroid Cancer: Exogenous thyroid hormone may produce regression of metastases from follicular and papillary carcinoma of the thyroid and is used as ancillary therapy of these conditions with radioactive iodine. TSH should be suppressed to low or undetectable levels. Therefore, larger amounts of thyroid hormone than those used for replacement therapy are required. Medullary carcinoma of the thyroid is usually unresponsive to this therapy.

Thyroid Suppression Therapy: Administration of thyroid hormone in doses higher than those produced physiologically by the gland results in suppression of the production of endogenous hormone. This is the basis for the thyroid suppression test and is used as an aid in the diagnosis of patients with signs of mild hyperthyroidism, in whom base line laboratory tests appear normal, or to demonstrate thyroid gland autonomy in patients with Grave's ophthalmopathy. 1 uptake is determined before and after the administration of the exogenous hormone. A fifty percent or greater suppression of uptake indicates a normal thyroid pituitary axis, and thus rules out thyroid gland autonomy.

For adults, the usual suppressive dose of levothyroxine (T4) is 1.56 mg/kg of body weight per day given for 7 to 10 days. These doses usually yield normal serum T4 and T3 levels and lack of response to TSH.

Thyroid hormones should be administered cautiously to patients in whom there is strong suspicion of thyroid gland autonomy, in view of the fact that the exogenous hormone effects will be additive to the endogenous source.

Pediatric Dosage: Pediatric dosage should follow the recommendations summarized in Table 1. In infants with congenital hypothyroidism, therapy with full doses should be instituted as soon as the diagnosis has been made.

TABLE 1. Recommended Pediatric Dosage for Congenital Hypothyroidism

Age	Dose per day	Daily dose per kg of body weight
0 - 6 months	16.25 - 32.5 mg	4.8-6.0 mg
6 - 12 months	32.5 - 48.75 mg	3.6-4.8 mg
1 - 5 years	48.75 - 65 mg	3.0-3.6 mg
6 - 12 years	65 - 97.5 mg	2.4-3.0 mg
Over 12 years	Over 97.5 mg	1.2-1.8 mg

HOW SUPPLIED

Nature-Throid® (Thyroid USP) Tablets are supplied as follows:

16.25 mg. (1/4 gr.) in bottles of 30 Count (NDC 64727-3298-4), 60 Count (NDC 64727-3298-5), 90 Count (NDC 64727-3298-6), 100 Count (NDC 64727-3298-1), 1,000 Count (NDC 64727-3298-2), 990 Count (NDC 64727-3298-3) & 1,008 Count (NDC 64727-3298-8)

32.5 mg. (1/2 gr.) in bottles of 30 Count (NDC 64727-3299-4), 60 Count (NDC 64727-3299-5), 90 Count (NDC 64727-3299-6), 100 Count (NDC 64727-3299-1), 1,000 Count (NDC 64727-3299-2), 990 Count (NDC 64727-3299-3) & 1,008 Count (NDC 64727-3299-8)

48.75 mg. (3/4 gr.) in bottles of 30 Count (NDC 64727-3302-4), 60 Count (NDC 64727-3302-5), 90 Count (NDC 64727-3302-6), 100 Count (NDC 64727-3302-1), 1,000 Count (NDC 64727-3302-2), 990 Count (NDC 64727-3302-3) & 1,008 Count (NDC 64727-3302-8)

65 mg. (1 gr.) in bottles of 30 Count (NDC 64727-3300-4), 60 Count (NDC 64727-3300-5), 90 Count (NDC 64727-3300-6), 100 Count (NDC 64727-3300-1), 1,000 Count (NDC 64727-3300-2), 990 Count (NDC 64727-3300-3) & 1,008 Count (NDC 64727-3300-8)

81.25 mg. (1 1/4 gr.) in bottles of 30 Count (NDC 64727-3303-4), 60 Count (NDC 64727-3303-5), 90 Count (NDC 64727-3303-6), 100 Count (NDC 64727-3303-1), 1,000 Count (NDC 64727-3303-2), 990 Count (NDC 64727-3303-3) & 1,008 Count (NDC 64727-3303-8)

97.5 mg. (1 1/2 gr.) in bottles of 30 Count (NDC 64727-3305-4), 60 Count (NDC 64727-3305-5), 90 Count (NDC 64727-3305-6), 100 Count (NDC 64727-3305-1), 1,000 Count (NDC 64727-3305-2), 990 Count (NDC 64727-3305-3) & 1,008 Count (NDC 64727-3305-8)

113.75 mg. (1 3/4 gr.) in bottles of 30 Count (NDC 64727-3307-4), 60 Count (NDC 64727-3307-5), 90 Count (NDC 64727-3307-6), 100 Count (NDC 64727-3307-1), 1,000 Count (NDC 64727-3307-2), 990 Count (NDC 64727-3307-3) & 1,008 Count (NDC 64727-3307-8)

130 mg. (2 gr.) in bottles of 30 Count (NDC 64727-3308-4), 60 Count (NDC 64727-3308-5), 90 Count (NDC 64727-3308-6), 100 Count (NDC 64727-3308-1), 1,000 Count (NDC 64727-3308-2), 990 Count (NDC 64727-3308-3) & 1,008 Count (NDC 64727-3308-8)

146.25 mg. (2 1/4 gr.) in bottles of 30 Count (NDC 64727-3309-4), 60 Count (NDC 64727-3309-5), 90 Count (NDC 64727-3309-6), 100 Count (NDC 64727-3309-1), 1,000 Count (NDC 64727-3309-2), 990 Count (NDC 64727-3309-3) & 1,008 Count (NDC 64727-3309-8)

162.5 mg. (2 1/2 gr.) in bottles of 30 Count (NDC 64727-3310-4), 60 Count (NDC 64727-3310-5), 90 Count (NDC 64727-3310-6), 100 Count (NDC 64727-3310-1), 1,000 Count (NDC 64727-3310-2), 990 Count (NDC 64727-3310-3) & 1,008 Count (NDC 64727-3310-8)

195 mg. (3 gr.) in bottles of 30 Count (NDC 64727-3312-4), 60 Count (NDC 64727-3312-5), 90 Count (NDC 64727-3312-6), 100 Count (NDC 64727-3312-1), 1,000 Count (NDC 64727-3312-2), 990 Count (NDC 64727-3312-3) & 1,008 Count (NDC 64727-3312-8)

260 mg. (4 gr.) in bottles of 30 Count (NDC 64727-3320-4), 60 Count (NDC 64727-3320-5), 90 Count (NDC 64727-3320-6), 100 Count (NDC 64727-3320-1), 1,000 Count (NDC 64727-3320-2), 990 Count (NDC 64727-3320-3) & 1,008 Count (NDC 64727-3320-8)

325 mg. (5 gr.) in bottles of 30 Count (NDC 64727-3340-4), 60 Count (NDC 64727-3340-5), 90 Count (NDC 64727-3340-6), 100 Count (NDC 64727-3340-1), 1,000 Count (NDC 64727-3340-2), 990 Count (NDC 64727-3340-3) & 1,008 Count (NDC 64727-3340-8)

STORAGE: Store at controlled room temperature; 15°-30°C (59°-86°F)

Dispense in tight, light-resistant containers as defined in the USP/NF

Rx Only.

Distributed by:
RLC LABS
Cave Creek, AZ 85331
Rev051309/01   SCD#700809-1
Shown in Product Identification Guide, page 510

WP THYROID®   ℞
(Thyroid USP)
Tablets

DESCRIPTION

WP Thyroid® (Thyroid USP) Tablets, for oral use, are natural preparations derived from porcine thyroid glands (T3 liothyronine is approximately four times as potent as T4 levothyroxine on a microgram for microgram basis). They provide 38 mcg levothyroxine (T4) and 9 mcg liothyronine (T3) for each 65 mg (1 Grain) of the labeled content of thyroid.

INACTIVE INGREDIENTS

Inulin, Medium Chain Triglycerides, Lactose Monohydrate[1]

The structural formulas of liothyronine (T3) and levothyroxine (T4) are as follows:

[1]Present in traceable amount as part of Thyroid USP (diluent)

CLINICAL PHARMACOLOGY

The steps in the synthesis of the thyroid hormones are controlled by thyrotropin (Thyroid Stimulating Hormone, TSH) secreted by the anterior pituitary. This hormone's secretion is in turn controlled by a feedback mechanism affected by the thyroid hormones themselves and by thyrotropin releasing hormone (TRH), a tripeptide of hypothalamic origin. Endogenous thyroid hormone secretion is suppressed when exogenous thyroid hormones are administered to euthyroid individuals in excess of the normal gland's secretion.

The mechanisms by which thyroid hormones exert their physiologic action are not well understood. These hormones enhance oxygen consumption by most tissues of the body, increase the basal metabolic rate, and the metabolism of carbohydrates, lipids, and proteins. Thus, they exert a profound influence on every organ system in the body and are of particular importance in the development of the central nervous system.

The normal thyroid gland contains approximately 200 mcg of levothyroxine (T4) per gram of gland, and 15 mcg of liothyronine (T3) per gram. The ratio of these two hormones in the circulation does not represent the ratio in the thyroid gland, since about 80 percent of peripheral liothyronine (T3) comes from monodeiodination of levothyroxine (T4). Peripheral monodeiodination of levothyroxine (T4) at the 5 position (inner ring) also results in the formation of reverse liothyronine (T3), which is calorigenically inactive. Liothyronine (T3) levels are low in the fetus and newborn, in old age, in chronic caloric deprivation, hepatic cirrhosis, renal failure, surgical stress, and chronic illnesses representing what has been called the "T3 thyronine syndrome".

Pharmacokinetics

Animal studies have shown that levothyroxine (T4) is only partially absorbed from the gastrointestinal tract. The degree of absorption is dependent on the vehicle used for its administration and by the character of the intestinal contents, the intestinal flora, including plasma protein, and soluble dietary factors, all of which bind thyroid, thereby making it unavailable for diffusion. Only 41 percent is absorbed when given in a gelatin capsule, as opposed to 74 percent absorption when given with an albumin carrier.

Depending on other factors, absorption has varied from 48 to 79 percent of the administered dose. Fasting increases absorption. Malabsorption syndromes, as well as dietary factors, (children's soybean formula, concomitant use of anionic exchange resins such as cholestyramine) cause excessive fecal loss. Liothyronine (T3) is almost totally absorbed, 95 percent in 4 hours. The hormones contained in the natural preparations are absorbed in a manner similar to the synthetic hormones.

More than 99 percent of circulating hormones are bound to serum proteins, including thyroid-binding globulin (TBg), thyroid-binding pre-albumin (TBPA), and albumin (TBa), whose capacities and affinities vary for the hormones. The higher affinity of levothyroxine (T4) for both TBg and TBPA, as compared to liothyronine (T3), partially explains the higher serum levels and longer half-life of the former hormone. Both protein-bound hormones exist in reverse equilibrium with minute amounts of free hormone, the latter accounting for the metabolic activity. Deiodination of levothyroxine (T4) occurs at a number of sites, including liver, kidney, and other tissues. The conjugated hormone, in the form of glucuronide or sulfate, is found in the bile and gut where it may complete an enterohepatic circulation. Eighty-five percent of levothyroxine (T4) metabolized daily is deiodinated.

INDICATIONS AND USAGE

1. As replacement of supplemental therapy in patients with hypothyroidism of any etiology, except transient hypothyroidism during the recovery phase of subacute thyroiditis. This category includes cretinism, myxedema, and ordinary hypothyroidism in patients of any age (children, adults, the elderly), or state (including pregnancy); primary hypothyroidism resulting from functional deficiency, primary atrophy, partial or total absence of thyroid gland, or the effects of surgery, radiation, or drugs, with or without the presence of goiter; and secondary (pituitary), or tertiary (hypothalamic) hypothyroidism (See WARNINGS).

2. As pituitary TSH suppressants, in the treatment or prevention of various types of euthyroid goiters, including thyroid nodules, subacute, or chronic lymphocytic thyroiditis (Hashimoto's), multinodular goiter, and in the management of thyroid cancer.

3. As diagnostic agents in suppression tests to differentiate suspected mild hyperthyroidism or thyroid gland anatomy.

CONTRAINDICATIONS

Thyroid hormone preparations are generally contraindicated in patients with diagnosed, but as yet, uncorrected adrenal cortical insufficiency, untreated thyrotoxicosis, and apparent hypersensitivity to any of their active or extraneous constituents. There is no well documented evidence in the literature of true allergic or idiosyncratic reactions to thyroid hormone.

WARNINGS

Drugs with thyroid hormone activity, alone or together with other therapeutic agents, have been used for the treatment of obesity. In euthyroid patients, doses within the range of daily hormonal requirements are ineffective for weight reduction. Larger doses may produce serious or even life-threatening manifestations of toxicity, particularly when given in association with sympathomimetic amines such as those used for their anorectic effects.

The use of thyroid hormones in the therapy of obesity, alone or combined with other drugs, is unjustified and has been shown to be ineffective. Neither is their use justified for the treatment of male or female infertility unless this condition is accompanied by hypothyroidism.

PRECAUTIONS

General: Thyroid hormones should be used with great caution in a number of circumstances where the integrity of the cardiovascular system, particularly the coronary arteries, is suspected. These include patients with angina pectoris or the elderly, whom have a greater likelihood of occult cardiac disease. With these patients, therapy should be initiated with low doses, i.e. 16.25 - 32.5 mg. When, in such patients, a euthyroid state can only be reached at the expense of an aggravation of the cardiovascular disease, thyroid hormone dosage should be reduced.

Thyroid hormone therapy in patients with concomitant diabetes mellitus or diabetes insipidus or adrenal cortical insufficiency aggravates the intensity of their symptoms. Appropriate adjustments of the various therapeutic measures directed at these concomitant endocrine diseases are required. The therapy of myxedema coma requires simultaneous administration of glucorticoids (See DOSAGE AND ADMINISTRATION).

Hypothyroidism decreases and hyperthyroidism increases the sensitivity to oral anticoagulants. Prothrombin time should be closely monitored in thyroid treated patients on oral anticoagulants and dosage of the latter agents should be adjusted on the basis of frequent prothrombin time determinations. In infants, excessive doses of thyroid hormone preparations may produce craniosynostosis.

Information for the Patient: Patients on thyroid hormone preparations and parents of children on thyroid therapy should be informed that:

1. Replacement therapy is to be taken essentially for life, with the exception of cases of transient hypothyroidism, usually associated with thyroiditis, and in those patients receiving a therapeutic trial of the drug.

2. They should immediately report, during the course of therapy, any signs or symptoms of thyroid hormone toxicity, e.g., chest pain, increased pulse rate, palpitations, excessive sweating, heat intolerance, nervousness, or any other unusual event.

3. In case of concomitant diabetes mellitus, the daily dosage of antidiabetic medication may need readjustment as

Continued on next page

thyroid hormone replacement is achieved. If thyroid medication is stopped, a downward readjustment of the dosage of insulin or oral hypoglycemic agent may be necessary to avoid hypoglycemia. At all times, close monitoring of urinary glucose levels is mandatory in such patients.

4. In case of concomitant oral anticoagulant therapy, the prothrombin time should be measured frequently to determine if the dosage of oral anticoagulants is to be readjusted.

5. Partial loss of hair may be experienced by children in the first few months of thyroid therapy, but this is usually a transient phenomenon and later recovery is usually the rule.

Laboratory Tests: Treatment of patients with thyroid hormones requires the periodic assessment of thyroid status by means of appropriate laboratory tests, besides the full clinical evaluation. The TSH suppression test can be used to test the effectiveness of any thyroid preparation, bearing in mind the relative insensitivity of the infant pituitary to the negative feedback effect of thyroid hormones. Serum T4 levels can be used to test the effectiveness of all thyroid medications except T3. When the total serum T4 is low but TSH is normal, a test specific to assess unbound (free) T4 levels is warranted. Specific measurements of T4 and T3 by competitive protein binding or radioimmunoassay are not influenced by blood levels of organic or inorganic iodine.

Drug Interactions: Oral Anticoagulants-Thyroid hormones appear to increase catabolism of vitamin K- dependent clotting factors. If oral anticoagulants are also being given, compensatory increases in clotting factor synthesis are impaired. Patients stabilized on oral anticoagulants that are found to require thyroid replacement therapy should be watched very closely when thyroid is started. If a patient is truly hypothyroid, it is likely that a reduction in anticoagulant dosage will be required. No special precautions appear to be necessary when oral anticoagulant therapy is begun in a patient already stabilized on maintenance thyroid replacement therapy.

Insulin or Oral Hypoglycemic-Initiating thyroid replacement therapy may cause increases in insulin or oral hypoglycemic requirements. The effects seen are poorly understood and depend upon a variety of factors such as dose and type of thyroid preparations and endocrine status of the patient. Patients receiving insulin or oral hypoglycemic should be closely watched during initiation of thyroid replacement therapy.

Cholestyramine or Colestipol- Cholestyramine or Colestipol binds both levothyroxine (T4) and liothyronine (T3) in the intestine, thus impairing absorption of these thyroid hormones. In vitro studies indicate that the binding is not easily removed. Therefore, four to five hours should elapse between administration of Cholestyramine or Colestipol and thyroid hormones.

Estrogen, Oral Contraceptives- Estrogens tend to increase serum thyroxine-binding globulin (TBg). In a patient with a nonfunctioning thyroid gland who is receiving thyroid replacement therapy, free levothyroxine (T4) may be decreased when estrogens are started thus increasing thyroid requirements. However, if the patient's thyroid gland has sufficient function, the decreased free levothyroxine (T4) will result in a compensatory increase in levothyroxine (T4) output by the thyroid. Therefore, patients without a functioning thyroid gland who are on thyroid replacement therapy, may need to increase their thyroid dose if estrogens or estrogen-containing oral contraceptives are given.

Drug/Laboratory Test Interactions: The following drugs or moieties are known to interfere with laboratory tests performed in patients on thyroid hormone therapy: androgens, corticosteroids, estrogens, oral contraceptives containing estrogens, iodine-containing preparations, and the numerous preparations containing salicylates.

1. Changes in TBg concentration should be taken into consideration in the interpretation of levothyroxine (T4) and liothyronine (T3) values. In such cases, the unbound (free) hormone should be measured. Pregnancy, estrogens, and estrogen-containing oral contraceptives increase TBg concentrations. TBg may also be increased during infectious hepatitis. Decreases in TBg concentrations are observed in nephrosis, acromegaly, and after androgen or corticosteroid therapy. Familial hyper or hypothyroxine-binding-globulinemias have been described. The incidence of TBg deficiency approximates 1 in 9,000. The binding of levothyroxine by TBPA is inhibited by salicylates.

2. Medicinal or dietary iodine interferes with all in vivo tests of radio-iodine uptake, producing low uptakes which may not be relative of a true decrease in hormone synthesis.

3. The persistence of clinical and laboratory evidence of hypothyroidism in spite of adequate dosage replacement indicates; either poor patient compliance, poor absorption, excessive fecal loss, or inactivity of the preparation. Intracellular resistance to thyroid hormone is quite rare.

Carcinogenesis, Mutagenesis, and Impairment of Fertility: A reportedly apparent association between prolonged thyroid therapy and breast cancer has not been confirmed and patients on thyroid for established indications should not discontinue therapy. No confirmatory long-term studies in animals have been performed to evaluate carcinogenic potential, mutagenicity, or impairment of fertility in either males or females.

Pregnancy-Category A: Thyroid hormones do not readily cross the placental barrier. The clinical experience to date does not indicate any adverse effect on fetuses when thyroid hormones are administered to pregnant women. On the basis of current knowledge, thyroid replacement therapy to hypothyroid women should not be discontinued during pregnancy.

Nursing Mothers: Minimal amounts of thyroid hormones are excreted in human milk. Thyroid is not associated with serious adverse reactions and does not have a known tumorigenic potential. However, caution should be exercised when thyroid is administered to a nursing woman.

Pediatric Use: Pregnant mothers provide little or no thyroid hormone to the fetus. The incidence of congenital hypothyroidism is relatively high (1:4,000) and the hypothyroid fetus would not derive any benefit from the small amounts of hormone crossing the placental barrier. Routine determination of serumT4 and/or TSH is strongly advised in neonates in view of the deleterious effects of thyroid deficiency on growth and development. Treatment should be initiated immediately upon diagnosis, and maintained for life, unless transient hypothyroidism is suspected; in which case, therapy may be interrupted for 2 to 8 weeks after the age of 3 years to reassess the condition. Cessation of therapy is justified in patients who have maintained a normal TSH during those 2 to 8 weeks.

Geriatric use: Clinical studies of Thyroid Tablets, USP did not include sufficient numbers of subjects aged 65 and over to determine whether they respond differently from younger subjects. Other reported clinical experience has not identified differences in responses between the elderly and younger patients. In general, dose selection for an elderly patient should be cautious, usually starting at the low end of the dosing range, reflecting the greater frequency of decreased hepatic, renal, or cardiac function, and of concomitant disease or other drug therapy.

ADVERSE REACTIONS

Adverse reactions other than those indicative of hyperthyroidism because of therapeutic overdosage, either initially or during the maintenance period, are rare (See OVERDOSAGE).

OVERDOSAGE

Signs and Symptoms: Excessive doses of thyroid result in a hypermetabolic state resembling in every respect the condition of endogenous origin. The condition may be self induced.

Treatment of Overdosage: Dosage should be reduced or therapy temporarily discontinued signs and symptoms of overdosage appear.

Treatment may be reinstituted at a lower dosage. In normal individuals, normal hypothalamic-pituitary-thyroid axis function is restored in 6 to 8 weeks after thyroid suppression.

Treatment of acute massive thyroid hormone overdosage is aimed at reducing gastrointestinal absorption of the drugs and counteracting central and peripheral effects, mainly those of increased sympathetic activity. Vomiting may be induced initially if further gastrointestinal absorption can reasonably be prevented and barring contraindications such as coma, convulsions, or loss of the gagging reflex. Treatment is symptomatic and supportive. Oxygen may be administered and ventilation maintained. Cardiac glycosides may be indicated if congestive heart failure develops. Measures to control fever, hypoglycemia, or fluid loss should be instituted if needed. Antiadrenergic agents, particularly propranolol, have been used advantageously in the treatment of increased sympathetic activity. Propranolol may be administered intravenously at a dosage of 1 to 3 mg, over a 10 minute period or orally, 80 to 160 mg/day, initially, especially when no contraindications exist for its use.

DOSAGE AND ADMINISTRATION

The dosage of thyroid hormones is determined by the indication and must in every case be individualized according to patient response and laboratory findings.

Thyroid hormones are given orally. In acute, emergency conditions, injectable levothyroxine sodium (T4) may be given intravenously when oral administration is not feasible or desirable (as in the treatment of myxedema coma, or during parenteral nutrition). Intramuscular administration is not advisable because of reported poor absorption.

Hypothyroidism: Therapy is usually instituted using low doses, with increments which depend on the cardiovascular status of the patient. The usual starting dose is 32.5 mg, with increment of 16.25 mg every 2 to 3 weeks. A lower starting dosage, 16.25 mg/day, is recommended in patients with longstanding myxedema, particularly if cardiovascular impairment is suspected, in which case extreme caution is recommended. The appearance of angina is an indication for reduction in dosage. Most patients require 65 - 130 mg/day. Failure to respond to doses of 195 mg suggests lack of compliance or malabsorption. Maintenance dosages 65 - 130 mg/day usually result in normal serum T4 and T3 levels. Adequate therapy usually results in normal TSH and T4 levels after 2 or 3 weeks of therapy.

Readjustment of thyroid hormone dosage should be made within the first four weeks of therapy, after proper clinical and laboratory evaluations, including serum levels of T4, bound and free, and TSH.

Liothyronine (T3) may be used in preference to levothyroxine (T4) during radio-isotope scanning procedures, since induction of hypothyroidism in those cases is more abrupt and can be of shorter duration. It may also be preferred when impairment of peripheral conversion of levothyroxine (T4) and liothyronine (T3) is suspected.

Myxedema Coma: Myxedema coma is usually precipitated in the hypothyroid patient of longstanding by intercurrent illness or drugs such as sedatives and anesthetics and should be considered a medical emergency. Therapy should be directed at the correction of electrolyte disturbances and possible infection, besides the administration of thyroid hormones. Corticosteroids should be administered routinely. Levothyroxine (T4) and Liothyronine (T3) may be administered via a nasogastric tube, but the preferred route of administration of both hormones is intravenous. Levothyroxine sodium (T4) is given at a starting dose of 400 mcg (100 mcg/mL) given rapidly, and is usually well tolerated, even in the elderly. This initial dose is followed by daily supplements of 100 to 200 mcg given IV. Normal T4 levels are achieved in 24 hours, followed in 3 days by three-fold elevation of T3. Oral therapy with thyroid hormone would be resumed as soon as the clinical situation has been stabilized and the patient is able to take oral medication.

Thyroid Cancer: Exogenous thyroid hormone may produce regression of metastases from follicular and papillary carcinoma of the thyroid and is used as ancillary therapy of these conditions with radioactive iodine. TSH should be suppressed to low or undetectable levels. Therefore, larger amounts of thyroid hormone than those used for replacement therapy are required. Medullary carcinoma of the thyroid is usually unresponsive to this therapy.

Thyroid Suppression Therapy: Administration of thyroid hormone in doses higher than those produced physiologically by the gland results in suppression of the production of endogenous hormone. This is the basis for the thyroid suppression test and is used as an aid in the diagnosis of patients with signs of mild hyperthyroidism, in whom base line laboratory tests appear normal, or to demonstrate thyroid gland autonomy in patients with Grave's ophthalmopathy. 131I uptake is determined before and after the administration of the exogenous hormone. A fifty percent or greater suppression of uptake indicates a normal thyroid pituitary axis, and thus rules out thyroid gland autonomy.

For adults, the usual suppressive dose of levothyroxine (T4) is 1.56 mg/kg of body weight per day given for 7 to 10 days. These doses usually yield normal serum T4 and T3 levels and lack of response to TSH.

Thyroid hormones should be administered cautiously to patients in whom there is strong suspicion of thyroid gland autonomy, in view of the fact that the exogenous hormone effects will be additive to the endogenous source.

Pediatric Dosage: Pediatric dosage should follow the recommendations summarized in Table 1. In infants with congenital hypothyroidism, therapy with full doses should be instituted as soon as the diagnosis has been made.

TABLE 1. Recommended Pediatric Dosage for Congenital Hypothyroidism

Age	Dose per day	Daily dose per kg of body weight
0 - 6 months	16.25 - 32.5 mg	4.8-6.0 mg
6 - 12 months	32.5 - 48.75 mg	3.6-4.8 mg
1 - 5 years	48.75 - 65 mg	3.0-3.6 mg
6 - 12 years	65 - 97.5 mg	2.4-3.0 mg
Over 12 years	Over 97.5 mg	1.2-1.8 mg

HOW SUPPLIED

WP Thyroid® (Thyroid USP) Tablets are supplied as follows:

16.25 mg. (1/4 gr.) in bottles of 30 Count (NDC 64727-5450-4), 60 Count (NDC 64727-5450-5), 90 Count (NDC 64727-5450-6), 100 Count (NDC 64727-5450-1) & 1,000 Count (NDC 64727-5450-2)

32.5 mg. (1/2 gr.) in bottles of 30 Count (NDC 64727-5550-4), 60 Count (NDC 64727-5550-5), 90 Count (NDC 64727-5550-6), 100 Count (NDC 64727-5550-1) & 1,000 Count (NDC 64727-5550-2)

48.75 mg. (3/4 gr.) in bottles of 30 Count (NDC 64727-5650-4), 60 Count (NDC 64727-5650-5), 90 Count (NDC 64727-5650-6), 100 Count (NDC 64727-5650-1) & 1,000 Count (NDC 64727-5650-2)

65 mg. (1 gr.) in bottles of 30 Count (NDC 64727-5750-4), 60 Count (NDC 64727-5750-5), 90 Count (NDC 64727-5750-6), 100 Count (NDC 64727-5750-1) & 1,000 Count (NDC 64727-5750-2)

81.25 mg. (1 1/4 gr.) in bottles of 30 Count (NDC 64727-6050-4), 60 Count (NDC 64727-6050-5), 90 Count (NDC 64727-6050-6), 100 Count (NDC 64727-6050-1) & 1,000 Count (NDC 64727-6050-2)

97.5 mg. (1 1/2 gr.) in bottles of 30 Count (NDC 64727-5850-4), 60 Count (NDC 64727-5850-5), 90 Count (NDC 64727-5850-6), 100 Count (NDC 64727-5850-1) & 1,000 Count (NDC 64727-5850-2)

113.75 mg. (1 3/4 gr.) in bottles of 30 Count (NDC 64727-6150-4), 60 Count (NDC 64727-6150-5), 90 Count (NDC 64727-6150-6), 100 Count (NDC 64727-6150-1) & 1,000 Count (NDC 64727-6150-2)

130 mg. (2 gr.) in bottles of 30 Count (NDC 64727-5950-4), 60 Count (NDC 64727-5950-5), 90 Count (NDC 64727-5950-6), 100 Count (NDC 64727-5950-1) & 1,000 Count (NDC 64727-5950-2)

146.25 mg. (2 1/4 gr.) in bottles of 30 Count (NDC 64727-6250-4), 60 Count (NDC 64727-6250-5), 90 Count (NDC 64727-6250-6), 100 Count (NDC 64727-6250-1) & 1,000 Count (NDC 64727-6250-2)

162.5 mg. (2 1/2 gr.) in bottles of 30 Count (NDC 64727-6350-4), 60 Count (NDC 64727-6350-5), 90 Count (NDC 64727-6350-6), 100 Count (NDC 64727-6350-1) & 1,000 Count (NDC 64727-6350-2)

195 mg. (3 gr.) in bottles of 30 Count (NDC 64727-6450-4), 60 Count (NDC 64727-6450-5), 90 Count (NDC 64727-6450-6), 100 Count (NDC 64727-6450-1) & 1,000 Count (NDC 64727-6450-2)

STORAGE: Store at controlled room temperature; 15°-30°C (59°-86°F)

Dispense in tight, light-resistant containers as defined in the USP/NF

Rx Only.

Distributed by:
RLC® LABS
Cave Creek, AZ 85331
Rev:063191/01
SCD#700809-3

Shown in Product Identification Guide, page 510

Supernus Pharmaceuticals, Inc.

**1550 E GUDE DR
ROCKVILLE, MD 20850**

Direct Inquiries: 1-866-398-0833

OXTELLAR XR

[(ahks-TEH-lahr eks ahr)]
(oxcarbazepine)
extended-release tablets, for oral use

℞

HIGHLIGHTS OF PRESCRIBING INFORMATION
These highlights do not include all the information needed to use OXTELLAR XR safely and effectively. See full prescribing information for OXTELLAR XR.

OXTELLAR XR® (oxcarbazepine) extended-release tablets, for oral use
Initial U.S. Approval: 2000

——————RECENT MAJOR CHANGES——————

Warnings and Precautions (5.4)   12/2015

——————INDICATIONS AND USAGE——————

Oxtellar XR® is an antiepileptic drug (AED) indicated for:
• Adults: Adjunctive therapy in the treatment of partial seizures
• Children: Adjunctive therapy in the treatment of partial seizures in children 6 to 17 years (1)

——————DOSAGE AND ADMINISTRATION——————

• Recommended daily dose is 1,200 mg to 2,400 mg once per day (2.2)
• Adults: Initiate with a dose of 600 mg once per day. Dose increases can be made at weekly intervals in 600 mg per day increments to achieve the recommended daily dose (2.2)
• Children: Target dose is based upon weight. Titrate to target dose over two to three weeks. Initiate with 8 mg/kg to 10 mg/kg once per day. Increase in weekly increments of 8 mg/kg to 10 mg/kg once daily, not to exceed 600 mg, to achieve target daily dose (2.3)
• Patients with creatinine clearance less than 30mL/minute: Start at 300 mg per day and increase slowly (2.4)
• Geriatric Patients: Start at lower dose (300 mg or 450 mg per day) and increase slowly (2.5)
• In conversion of oxcarbazepine immediate-release to Oxtellar XR®, higher doses of Oxtellar XR® may be necessary (2.8, 12.3)

——————DOSAGE FORMS AND STRENGTHS——————

Extended-release tablets: 150 mg, 300 mg and 600 mg (3)

——————CONTRAINDICATIONS——————

• Known hypersensitivity to oxcarbazepine or to any of its components (4)

——————WARNINGS AND PRECAUTIONS——————

• *Hyponatremia:* Monitor sodium as recommended. (5.1)
• *Anaphylactic Reactions and Angioedema.* Discontinue if occurs (5.2)
• *Patients with a Past History of Hypersensitivity Reaction to Carbamazepine:* Only use based upon risk benefit (5.3)
• *Serious Dermatological Reactions:* Discontinue if observed (5.4)
• *Suicidal Behavior and Ideation:* Monitor for symptoms (5.5)
• *Withdrawal of Oxtellar XR®:* Withdrawal gradually (5.6)
• *Multi-Organ Hypersensitivity:* Discontinue if suspected (5.7)
• *Hematologic Reactions:* Discontinue if suspected (5.8)

——————ADVERSE REACTIONS——————

Most commonly observed (≥5%) and more frequent than placebo adverse reactions were: dizziness, somnolence, headache, balance disorder, tremor, vomiting, diplopia, asthenia, and fatigue (6.1).

To report SUSPECTED ADVERSE REACTIONS, contact Supernus, Inc. at (1-866-398-0833) or contact FDA at 1-800-FDA-1088 or www.fda.gov/medwatch

——————DRUG INTERACTIONS——————

• *Phenytoin, Carbamazepine, and Phenobarbital:* Coadministration decreased blood levels of an active metabolite of Oxtellar XR®: Greater dose of Oxtellar XR® may be required (2.6, 7.1).
• *Oral Contraceptives:* Advise patients that Oxtellar XR® may decrease the effectiveness of hormonal contraceptives. Additional non-hormonal forms of contraception are recommended. (7.2)

——————USE IN SPECIFIC POPULATIONS——————

• *Pregnancy:* Plasma levels of active metabolite may be decreased. Monitor patients. Based on animal data, may cause fetal harm. (5.9, 8.1).
• *Severe Hepatic Impairment:* Not recommended (8.7).

See 17 for PATIENT COUNSELING INFORMATION and Medication Guide.

Revised: 12/2015

——————FULL PRESCRIBING INFORMATION: CONTENTS*——————

* Sections or subsections omitted from the full prescribing information are not listed.

FULL PRESCRIBING INFORMATION

1   INDICATIONS AND USAGE

Oxtellar XR® is indicated as adjunctive therapy of partial seizures in adults and in children 6 years to 17 years of age.

2   DOSAGE AND ADMINISTRATION

2.1   Important Administration Instructions

Administer Oxtellar XR® as a single daily dose taken on an empty stomach (at least 1 hour before or at least 2 hours after meals) [see *Clinical Pharmacology (12.3)*]. If Oxtellar XR® is taken with food, adverse reactions are more likely to occur because of increased peak levels [see *Clinical Pharmacology (12.3)*].

Swallow Oxtellar XR® tablets whole. Do not cut, crush, or chew the tablets. For ease of swallowing in pediatric patients or patients with difficulty swallowing, achieve daily dosages with multiples of appropriate lower strength tablets (e.g., 150 mg tablets).

2.2   Dosing for Adults in Adjunctive Therapy

The recommended daily dose of Oxtellar XR® is 1,200 mg to 2,400 mg per day, given once daily. The dose of 2,400 mg per day showed slightly greater efficacy than 1,200 mg per day, but was associated with an increase in adverse reactions. Initiate treatment at a dose of 600 mg per day given once daily for one week. Subsequent dose increases can be made at weekly intervals in 600 mg per day increments to achieve the recommended daily dose.

Continued on next page

2.3 Dosing for Children (6 to 17 years of age) in Adjunctive Therapy

In pediatric patients 6 years to 17 years of age, initiate treatment at a daily dose of 8 mg/kg to 10 mg/kg once daily, not to exceed 600 mg per day in the first week.

Subsequent dose increases can be made at weekly intervals in 8 mg/kg to 10 mg/kg increments once daily, not to exceed 600 mg, to achieve the target daily dose. The target maintenance dose, achieved over two to three weeks, is displayed in Table 1.

Table 1: Target Daily Dose in Pediatric Patients Aged 6 to 17 Years Old

Weight	Target Daily Dose
20 kg to 29 kg	900 mg per day
29.1 kg to 39 kg	1200 mg per day
Greater than 39 kg	1800 mg per day

2.4 Dosage Modifications in Patients with Renal Impairment

In patients with severe renal impairment (creatinine clearance less than 30 mL/minute), initiate Oxtellar XR® at one-half the usual starting dose (300 mg per day). Subsequent dose increases can be made at weekly intervals in increments of 300 mg to 450 mg per day to achieve the desired clinical response. [see *Use in Specific Populations (8.6)*].

2.5 Dosage Modifications in Geriatric Patients

In geriatric patients, consider starting at a lower dose (300 mg or 450 mg per day). Subsequent dose increases can be made at weekly intervals in increments of 300 mg to 450 mg per day to achieve the desired clinical effect [see *Use in Specific Populations (8.5)*].

2.6 Dosage Modification for Use with Concomitant Antiepileptic Drugs

Enzyme inducing antiepileptic drugs such as carbamazepine, phenobarbital, and phenytoin decrease exposure to 10-monohydroxy derivative (MHD), the active metabolite. Dosage increases may be necessary. Consider initiating dose at 900 mg once per day [see *Drug Interactions (7.1)*].

2.7 Withdrawal of AEDs

As with all antiepileptic drugs, Oxtellar XR® should be withdrawn gradually to minimize the potential of increased seizure frequency [see *Warnings and Precautions (5.6)*].

2.8 Conversion from Immediate-Release Oxcarbazepine to Oxtellar XR®

In conversion of oxcarbazepine immediate-release to Oxtellar XR®, higher doses of Oxtellar XR® may be necessary [see *Clinical Pharmacology (12.3)*].

3 DOSAGE FORMS AND STRENGTHS

Extended-release tablets:

150 mg: yellow modified-oval shaped with "150" printed on one side

300 mg: brown modified-oval shaped with "300" printed on one side

600 mg: brownish red modified-oval shaped with "600" printed on one side

4 CONTRAINDICATIONS

Oxtellar XR® is contraindicated in patients with a known hypersensitivity to oxcarbazepine or to any of its components [see *Warnings and Precautions (5.2, 5.3)*].

5 WARNINGS AND PRECAUTIONS

5.1 Hyponatremia

Clinically significant hyponatremia (sodium <125 mmol/L) may develop during Oxtellar XR® use. Serum sodium levels less than 125 mmol/L have occurred in immediate-release oxcarbazepine-treated patients generally in the first three months of treatment. However, clinically significant hyponatremia may develop more than a year after initiating therapy.

Most immediate-release oxcarbazepine-treated patients who developed hyponatremia were asymptomatic in clinical trials. However, some of these patients had their dose reduced, discontinued, or had their fluid intake restricted for hyponatremia. Serum sodium levels returned toward normal when the dosage was reduced or discontinued, or when the patient was treated conservatively (e.g., fluid restriction). Post-marketing cases of symptomatic hyponatremia have been reported during post-marketing use of immediate-release oxcarbazepine.

Among treated patients in a controlled trial of adjunctive therapy with Oxtellar XR® in 366 adults with complex par-

tial seizures, 1 patient receiving 2400 mg experienced a severe reduction in serum sodium (117 mEq/L) requiring discontinuation from treatment, while 2 other patients receiving 1200 mg experienced serum sodium concentrations low enough (125 and 126 mEq/L) to require discontinuation from treatment. The overall incidence of clinically significant hyponatremia in patients treated with Oxtellar XR® was 1.2%, although slight shifts in serum sodium concentrations from Normal to Low (<135 mEq/L) were observed for the 2400 mg (6.5%) and 1200 mg (9.8%) groups compared to placebo (1.7%). Measure serum sodium concentrations if patients develop symptoms of hyponatremia (e.g., nausea, malaise, headache, lethargy, confusion, obtunded consciousness, or increase in seizure frequency or severity). Consider measurement of serum sodium concentrations during treatment with Oxtellar XR®, particularly if the patient receives concomitant medications known to decrease serum sodium levels (for example, drugs associated with inappropriate ADH secretion).

5.2 Anaphylactic Reactions and Angioedema

Rare cases of anaphylaxis and angioedema involving the larynx, glottis, lips and eyelids have been reported in patients after taking the first or subsequent doses of immediate-release oxcarbazepine. Angioedema associated with laryngeal edema can be fatal. If a patient develops any of these reactions after treatment with Oxtellar XR®, discontinue the drug and initiate an alternative treatment. Do not rechallenge these patients with Oxtellar XR®.

5.3 Hypersensitivity Reactions in Patients with Hypersensitivity to Carbamazepine

Inform patients who have had hypersensitivity reactions to carbamazepine that approximately 25%-30% of them will experience hypersensitivity reactions with Oxtellar XR®. Question patients about any prior adverse reactions with carbamazepine. Patients with a history of hypersensitivity reactions to carbamazepine should ordinarily be treated with Oxtellar XR® only if the potential benefit justifies the potential risk. Discontinue Oxtellar XR® immediately if signs or symptoms of hypersensitivity develop [see *Warnings and Precautions (5.8)*].

5.4 Serious Dermatological Reactions

Serious dermatological reactions, including Stevens-Johnson syndrome (SJS) and toxic epidermal necrolysis (TEN), have occurred in both children and adults treated with immediate-release oxcarbazepine use. The median time of onset for reported cases was 19 days. Such serious skin reactions may be life threatening, and some patients have required hospitalization with very rare reports of fatal outcome. Recurrence of the serious skin reactions following rechallenge with immediate-release oxcarbazepine has also been reported.

The reporting rate of TEN and SJS associated with immediate-release oxcarbazepine use, which is generally accepted to be an underestimate due to underreporting, exceeds the background incidence rate estimates by a factor of 3- to 10-fold. Estimates of the background incidence rate for these serious skin reactions in the general population range between 0.5 to 6 cases per million-person years. Therefore, if a patient develops a skin reaction while taking Oxtellar XR®, consider discontinuing Oxtellar XR® use and prescribing another AED.

Association with HLA-B*1502

Patients carrying the HLA-B*1502 allele may be at increased risk for SJS/TEN with Oxtellar XR® treatment.

Human Leukocyte Antigen (HLA) allele B*1502 increases the risk for developing SJS/TEN in patients treated with carbamazepine. The chemical structures of immediate-release oxcarbazepine and Oxtellar XR® are similar to that of carbamazepine. Available clinical evidence, and data from nonclinical studies showing a direct interaction between immediate release oxcarbazepine and HLA-B*1502 protein, suggest that the HLA-B*1502 allele may also increase the risk for SJS/TEN with Oxtellar XR®.

The frequency of HLA-B*1502 allele ranges from 2 to 12% in Han Chinese populations, is about 8% in Thai populations, and above 15% in the Philippines and in some Malaysian populations. Allele frequencies up to about 2% and 6% have been reported in Korea and India, respectively. The frequency of the HLA-B*1502 allele is negligible in people from European descent, several African populations, indigenous peoples of the Americas, Hispanic populations, and in Japanese (<1%).

Testing for the presence of the HLA-B*1502 allele should be considered in patients with ancestry in genetically at-risk populations, prior to initiating treatment with Oxtellar

XR®. The use of Oxtellar XR® should be avoided in patients positive for HLA-B*1502 unless the benefits clearly outweigh the risks. Consideration should also be given to avoid the use of other drugs associated with SJS/TEN in HLA-B*1502 positive patients, when alternative therapies are otherwise equally acceptable. Screening is not generally recommended in patients from populations in which the prevalence of HLA-B*1502 is low, or in current Oxtellar XR® users, as the risk of SJS/TEN is largely confined to the first few months of therapy, regardless of HLA-B*1502 status. The use of HLA-B*1502 genotyping has important limitations and must never substitute for appropriate clinical vigilance and patient management. The role of other possible factors in the development of, and morbidity from, SJS/TEN, such as antiepileptic drug (AED) dose, compliance, concomitant medications, comorbidities, and the level of dermatologic monitoring have not been well characterized.

5.5 Suicidal Behavior and Ideation

Antiepileptic drugs (AEDs), including Oxtellar XR®, increase the risk of suicidal thoughts or behavior in patients taking these drugs for any indication. Monitor patients treated with any AED for any indication for the emergence or worsening of depression, suicidal thoughts or behavior, and/or any unusual changes in mood or behavior.

Pooled analyses of 199 placebo-controlled clinical trials (mono- and adjunctive therapy) of 11 different AEDs showed that patients randomized to one of the AEDs had approximately twice the risk (adjusted Relative Risk 1.8, 95% CI:1.2, 2.7) of suicidal thinking or behavior compared to patients randomized to placebo. In these trials, which had a median treatment duration of 12 weeks, the estimated incidence rate of suicidal behavior or ideation among 27,863 AED-treated patients was 0.43%, compared to 0.24% among 16,029 placebo-treated patients, representing an increase of approximately one case of suicidal thinking or behavior for every 530 patients treated. There were four suicides in drug-treated patients in the trials and none in placebo-treated patients, but the number is too small to allow any conclusion about drug effect on suicide.

The increased risk of suicidal thoughts or behavior with AEDs was observed as early as one week after starting drug treatment with AEDs and persisted for the duration of treatment assessed. Because most trials included in the analysis did not extend beyond 24 weeks, the risk of suicidal thoughts or behavior beyond 24 weeks could not be assessed.

The risk of suicidal thoughts or behavior was generally consistent among drugs in the data analyzed. The finding of increased risk with AEDs of varying mechanisms of action and across a range of indications suggests that the risk applies to all AEDs used for any indication. The risk did not vary substantially by age (5-100 years) in the clinical trials analyzed. Table 2 shows absolute and relative risk by indication for all evaluated AEDs.

[See table 2 at the bottom of next page]

The relative risk for suicidal thoughts or behavior was higher in clinical trials for epilepsy than in clinical trials for psychiatric or other conditions, but the absolute risk differences were similar for the epilepsy and psychiatric indications.

Anyone considering prescribing Oxtellar XR® or any other AED must balance the risk of suicidal thoughts or behavior with the risk of untreated illness. Epilepsy and many other illnesses for which AEDs are prescribed are themselves associated with morbidity and mortality and an increased risk of suicidal thoughts and behavior. Should suicidal thoughts and behavior emerge during Oxtellar XR® treatment, the prescriber needs to consider whether the emergence of these symptoms in any given patient may be related to the illness being treated.

Patients, their caregivers, and families should be informed that AEDs increase the risk of suicidal thoughts and behavior and should be advised of the need to be alert for the emergence or worsening of the signs and symptoms of depression, any unusual changes in mood or behavior, or the emergence of suicidal thoughts, behavior, or thoughts about self-harm. Behaviors of concern should be reported immediately to healthcare providers.

5.6 Withdrawal of AEDs

As with all AEDs, Oxtellar XR® should be withdrawn gradually to minimize the potential of increased seizure frequency.

5.7 Multi-Organ Hypersensitivity

Multi-organ hypersensitivity reactions have occurred in close temporal association (median time to detection 13 days: range 4-60) to the initiation of immediate-release oxcarbazepine therapy in adult and pediatric patients. Although there have been a limited number of reports, many of these cases resulted in hospitalization and some were life-threatening. Signs and symptoms of this disorder were diverse; however, patients typically, although not exclusively, presented with fever and rash associated with other organ system involvement. These included the following: hematologic and lymphatic (e.g., eosinophilia, thrombocytopenia, lymphadenopathy, leukopenia, neutropenia, splenomegaly), hepatobiliary (e.g., hepatitis, liver function test abnormalities), renal (e.g., proteinuria, nephritis, oliguria, renal failure), muscles and joints (e.g., joint swelling, myalgia, arthralgia, asthenia), nervous system (e.g., hepatic encephalopathy), respiratory (e.g., dyspnea, pulmonary edema, asthma, bronchospasm, interstitial lung disease), hepatorenal syndrome, pruritus, and angioedema. Because the disorder is variable in its expression, other organ system symptoms and signs, not noted here, may occur. If this reaction is suspected, discontinue Oxtellar XR® and initiate an alternative treatment.

5.8 Hematologic Reactions
Rare reports of pancytopenia, agranulocytosis, and leukopenia have been seen in patients treated with immediate-release oxcarbazepine during post-marketing experience. Discontinuation of Oxtellar XR® should be considered if any evidence of these hematologic reactions develops.

5.9 Risk of Seizures in the Pregnant Patient
Due to physiological changes during pregnancy, plasma concentrations of the active metabolite of oxcarbazepine, the 10-monohydroxy derivative (MHD), may gradually decrease throughout pregnancy. Monitor patients carefully during pregnancy and through the postpartum period because MHD concentrations may increase after delivery.

5.10 Laboratory Tests
Laboratory data from clinical trials suggest that immediate-release oxcarbazepine may be associated with decreases in T4, without changes in T3 or TSH.

6 ADVERSE REACTIONS
The following adverse reactions are described in other sections of the labeling:
- Hyponatremia *[see Warnings and Precautions (5.1)]*
- Anaphylactic Reactions and Angioedema *[see Warnings and Precautions (5.2)]*
- Hypersensitivity Reactions in Patients with Hypersensitivity to Carbamazepine *[see Warnings and Precautions (5.3)]*
- Serious Dermatological Reactions *[see Warnings and Precautions (5.4)]*
- Suicidal Behavior and Ideation *[see Warnings and Precautions (5.5)]*
- Withdrawal of AEDs *[see Warnings and Precautions (5.6)]*
- Multi-Organ Hypersensitivity *[see Warnings and Precautions (5.7)]*
- Hematologic Reactions *[see Warnings and Precautions (5.8)]*
- Risk of Seizures in the Pregnant Patient *[see Warnings and Precautions (5.9)]*
- Laboratory Tests *[see Warnings and Precautions (5.10)]*

6.1 Clinical Trials Experience
Because clinical trials are conducted under widely varying conditions, adverse reaction rates observed in the clinical trials of a drug cannot be directly compared to rates in the clinical trials of another drug and may not reflect the rates observed in clinical practice.
The safety data presented below are from 384 patients with partial epilepsy who received Oxtellar XR® (366 adults and 18 children) with concomitant AEDs.

Table 3: Adverse Reaction Incidence in a Controlled Clinical Study of Oxtellar XR® with Concomitant AEDs in Adults*

	Oxtellar XR® 2400 mg/day N=123 %	Oxtellar XR® 1200 mg/day N=122 %	Placebo N=121 %
Any System / Any Term	69	57	55
Nervous System Disorders			
Dizziness	41	20	15
Somnolence	14	12	9
Headache	15	8	7
Balance Disorder	7	5	5
Tremor	1	5	2
Nystagmus	3	3	1
Ataxia	1	3	1
Gastrointestinal Disorders			
Vomiting	15	6	9
Abdominal Pain Upper	0	3	1
Dyspepsia	0	3	1
Gastritis	0	3	2
Eye Disorders			
Diplopia	13	10	4
Vision Blurred	1	4	3
Visual Impairment	1	3	0
General Disorders And Administration Site Conditions			
Asthenia	7	3	1
Fatigue	3	6	1
Gait Disturbance	0	3	1
Drug Intolerance	2	0	0
Infections And Infestations			
Nasopharyngitis	0	3	0
Sinusitis	0	3	2

* Reported by ≥ 2% of Patients Treated with Oxtellar XR® and Numerically More Frequent than in the Placebo Group

In addition, safety data presented below are from a total of 2,288 patients with seizure disorders treated with immediate-release oxcarbazepine; 1,832 were adults and 456 were children.
Most Common Adverse Reactions Reported by Adult Patients Receiving Concomitant AEDs in Oxtellar XR® Clinical Studies
Table 3 lists adverse reactions that occurred in at least 2% of adult patients with epilepsy treated with Oxtellar XR® or placebo and concomitant AEDs and that were numerically more common in the patients treated with any dose of Oxtellar XR® than in patients receiving placebo.
The overall incidence of adverse reactions appeared to be dose related, particularly during the titration period. The most commonly observed (≥ 5%) adverse reactions seen in association with Oxtellar XR® and more frequent than in placebo-treated patients were: dizziness, somnolence, headache, balance disorder, tremor, vomiting, diplopia, and asthenia.
[See table 3 above]
Adverse Reactions Associated with Discontinuation of Oxtellar XR® Treatment: Approximately 23.3% of the 366 adult patients receiving Oxtellar XR® in clinical studies discontinued treatment because of an adverse reaction. The adverse reactions most commonly associated with discontinuation of Oxtellar XR® (reported by ≥2%) were: dizziness (9.8%), vomiting (5.3%), nausea (3.7%), diplopia (3.2%), and somnolence (2.4%).
Adjunctive Therapy with Oxtellar XR® in Pediatric Patients 4 to 16 Years Old Previously Treated with other AEDs
In a pharmacokinetic study in 18 children (age 4-16 years) with partial seizures treated with different doses of Oxtellar XR®, the observed adverse reactions seen in association with Oxtellar XR® were similar to those seen in adults.

Table 2: Risk by Indication for Antiepileptic Drugs in the Pooled Analysis

Indication	Placebo Patients with Events per 1,000 Patients	Drug Patients with Events per 1,000 Patients	Relative Risk: Incidence of Events in Drug Patients/Incidence in Placebo Patients	Risk Difference: Additional Drug Patients with Events per 1,000 Patients
Epilepsy	1.0	3.4	3.5	2.4
Psychiatric	5.7	8.5	1.5	2.9
Other	1.0	1.8	1.9	0.9
Total	2.4	4.3	1.8	1.9

Continued on next page

Table 4: Adverse Reaction Incidence in a Controlled Clinical Study of Immediate Release Oxcarbazepine with Concomitant AEDs in Adults*

	Immediate-Release Oxcarbazepine Dosage (mg/day)			Placebo N = 166 %
	OXC 600 N = 163 %	OXC 1200 N = 171 %	OXC 2400 N = 126 %	
Body as a Whole				
Fatigue	15	12	15	7
Asthenia	6	3	6	5
Edema Legs	2	1	2	1
Weight Increase	1	2	2	1
Feeling Abnormal	0	1	2	0
Cardiovascular System				
Hypotension	0	1	2	0
Digestive System				
Nausea	15	25	29	10
Vomiting	13	25	36	5
Pain Abdominal	10	13	11	5
Diarrhea	5	6	7	6
Dyspepsia	5	5	6	2
Constipation	2	2	6	4
Gastritis	2	1	2	1
Metabolic and Nutritional Disorders				
Hyponatremia	3	1	2	1
Musculoskeletal System				
Muscle Weakness	1	2	2	0
Sprains and Strains	0	2	2	1
Nervous System				
Headache	32	28	26	23
Dizziness	36	32	49	13
Somnolence	20	28	36	12
Ataxia	9	17	31	5
Nystagmus	7	20	26	5
Gait Abnormal	5	10	17	1
Insomnia	4	2	3	1
Tremor	3	8	16	5
Nervousness	2	4	2	1
Agitation	1	1	2	1
Coordination Abnormal	1	3	3	1
EEG Abnormal	0	0	2	0
Speech Disorder	1	1	3	0
Confusion	1	1	2	0
Cranial Injury NOS	1	0	2	1
Dysmetria	1	2	3	0
Thinking Abnormal	0	2	4	0

This table is continued on the next page

Most Common Adverse Reactions in Immediate-Release Oxcarbazepine Controlled Clinical Studies

Controlled Clinical Studies of Adjunctive Therapy with Immediate-Release Oxcarbazepine in Adults Previously Treated with other AEDs: Table 4 lists adverse reactions that occurred in at least 2% of adult patients with epilepsy treated with immediate-release oxcarbazepine or placebo with concomitant AEDs and that were numerically more common in the patients treated with any dose of immediate-release oxcarbazepine than in placebo. As immediate-release oxcarbazepine and Oxtellar XR® were not examined in the same trial, adverse event frequencies cannot be directly compared between the two formulations.

[See table 4 below and at top of next page]

Other Reactions Observed in Association with the Administration of Immediate-Release Oxcarbazepine

In the paragraphs that follow, the adverse reactions, other than those in the preceding tables or text, that occurred in a total of 565 children and 1,574 adults exposed to immediate-release oxcarbazepine and that are reasonably likely to be related to drug use are presented. Events common in the population, events reflecting chronic illness and events likely to reflect concomitant illness are omitted particularly if minor. They are listed in order of decreasing frequency. Because the reports cite reactions observed in open-label and uncontrolled trials, the role of immediate-release oxcarbazepine in their causation cannot be reliably determined.

Body as a Whole: fever, malaise, pain chest precordial, rigors, weight decrease.

Cardiovascular System: bradycardia, cardiac failure, cerebral hemorrhage, hypertension, hypotension postural, palpitation, syncope, tachycardia.

Digestive System: appetite increased, blood in stool, cholelithiasis, colitis, duodenal ulcer, dysphagia, enteritis, eructation, esophagitis, flatulence, gastric ulcer, gingival bleeding, gum hyperplasia, hematemesis, hemorrhage rectum, hemorrhoids, hiccup, mouth dry, pain biliary, pain right hypochondrium, retching, sialoadenitis, stomatitis, stomatitis ulcerative.

Hematologic and Lymphatic System: thrombocytopenia.

Laboratory Abnormality: gamma-GT increased, hyperglycemia, hypocalcemia, hypoglycemia, hypokalemia, liver enzymes elevated, serum transaminase increased.

Musculoskeletal System: hypertonia muscle.

Nervous System: aggressive reaction, amnesia, anguish, anxiety, apathy, aphasia, aura, convulsions aggravated, delirium, delusion, depressed level of consciousness, dysphonia, dystonia, emotional lability, euphoria, extrapyramidal disorder, feeling drunk, hemiplegia, hyperkinesia, hyperreflexia, hypoesthesia, hypokinesia, hyporeflexia, hypotonia, hysteria, libido decreased, libido increased, manic reaction, migraine, muscle contractions involuntary, nervousness, neuralgia, oculogyric crisis, panic disorder, paralysis, paroniria, personality disorder, psychosis, ptosis, stupor, tetany.

Respiratory System: asthma, bronchitis, coughing, dyspnea, epistaxis, laryngismus, pleurisy.

Skin and Appendages: acne, alopecia, angioedema, bruising, dermatitis contact, eczema, facial rash, flushing, folliculitis, heat rash, hot flushes, photosensitivity reaction, pruritus genital, psoriasis, purpura, rash erythematous, rash maculopapular, vitiligo, urticaria.

Special Senses: accommodation abnormal, cataract, conjunctival hemorrhage, edema eye, hemianopia, mydriasis, otitis externa, photophobia, scotoma, taste perversion, tinnitus, xerophthalmia.

Urogenital and Reproductive System: dysuria, hematuria, intermenstrual bleeding, leukorrhea, menorrhagia, micturition frequency, pain renal, pain urinary tract, polyuria, priapism, renal calculus, urinary tract infection.

Other: Systemic lupus erythematosus.

6.2   Postmarketing and Other Experience

The following adverse reactions have been observed in named patient programs or post-marketing experience with immediate-release oxcarbazepine or Oxtellar XR®. Because these reactions are reported voluntarily from a population of uncertain size, it is not always possible to reliably estimate their frequency or establish a causal relationship to drug exposure.

Body as a Whole: multi-organ hypersensitivity disorders characterized by features such as rash, fever, lymphadenopathy, abnormal liver function tests, eosinophilia and arthralgia [see *Warnings and Precautions (5.7)*]

Anaphylaxis: [see *Warnings and Precautions (5.2)*]

Digestive System: pancreatitis and/or lipase and/or amylase increase

Hematologic and Lymphatic Systems: aplastic anemia [see *Warnings and Precautions (5.8)*]

Metabolism: hypothyroidism

Skin and subcutaneous tissue disorders: erythema multiforme, Stevens-Johnson syndrome, toxic epidermal necrolysis [see *Warnings and Precautions (5.4)*], Acute Generalized Exanthematous Pustulosis (AGEP)

Musculoskeletal, connective tissue and bone disorders: There have been reports of decreased bone mineral density, osteoporosis and fractures in patients on long-term therapy with immediate-release oxcarbazepine.

7 DRUG INTERACTIONS

Oxcarbazepine and MHD induce a subgroup of the cytochrome P450 3A family (CYP3A4 and CYP3A5).

In addition, several AEDs that are cytochrome P450 inducers can decrease plasma concentrations of oxcarbazepine and MHD.

These interactions have implications when Oxtellar XR® is used with other AEDs or hormonal contraceptives.

7.1 Other Antiepileptic Drugs

Potential interactions between immediate-release oxcarbazepine and other AEDs were assessed in clinical studies. Oxtellar XR® would be expected to have the same effects on coadministered AEDs as immediate-release oxcarbazepine.

[See table 5 below]

7.2 Hormonal Contraceptives

Coadministration of immediate-release oxcarbazepine with an oral contraceptive decreased the plasma concentrations of two components of hormonal contraceptives, ethinylestradiol and levonorgestrel. Therefore, concurrent use of Oxtellar XR® with these hormonal contraceptives and other oral or implant contraceptives may render these contraceptives less effective [see *Clinical Pharmacology (12.3)*]. Additional non-hormonal forms of contraception are recommended.

8 USE IN SPECIFIC POPULATIONS

8.1 Pregnancy

Oxtellar XR® plasma concentrations may decrease during pregnancy [see *Warnings and Precautions (5.9)*]

Pregnancy Category C

There are no adequate and well-controlled clinical studies of Oxtellar XR® in pregnant women; however, Oxtellar XR® is closely related structurally to carbamazepine, which is considered to be teratogenic in humans. Given this fact, and the results of the animal studies described, it is likely that Oxtellar XR® is a human teratogen. Oxtellar XR® should be used during pregnancy only if the potential benefit justifies the potential risk to the fetus.

Increased incidences of fetal structural abnormalities and other manifestations of developmental toxicity (embryolethality, growth retardation) were observed in the offspring of animals treated with either oxcarbazepine or its active 10-hydroxy metabolite (MHD) during pregnancy at doses similar to the maximum recommended human dose.

When pregnant rats were given oxcarbazepine (30, 300, or 1000 mg/kg) orally throughout the period of organogenesis, increased incidences of fetal malformations (craniofacial, cardiovascular, and skeletal) and variations were observed at the intermediate and high doses (approximately 1.2 and 4 times, respectively, the maximum recommended human dose [MRHD] on a mg/m² basis). Increased embryofetal death and decreased fetal body weights were seen at the high dose. Doses ≥ 300 mg/kg were also maternally toxic (decreased body weight gain, clinical signs), but there is no evidence to suggest that teratogenicity was secondary to the maternal effects.

In a study in which pregnant rabbits were orally administered MHD (20, 100, or 200 mg/kg) during organogenesis, embryofetal mortality was increased at the highest dose (1.5 times the MRHD on a mg/m² basis). This dose produced only minimal maternal toxicity.

In a study in which female rats were dosed orally with oxcarbazepine (25, 50, or 150 mg/kg) during the latter part of gestation and throughout the lactation period, a persistent reduction in body weights and altered behavior (decreased activity) were observed in offspring exposed to the highest dose (0.6 times the MRHD on a mg/m² basis). Oral administration of MHD (25, 75, or 250 mg/kg) to rats during gestation and lactation resulted in a persistent reduction in offspring weights at the highest dose (equivalent to the MRHD on a mg/m² basis).

Table 4: (Cont.) Adverse Reaction Incidence in a Controlled Clinical Study of Immediate Release Oxcarbazepine with Concomitant AEDs in Adults*

	Immediate-Release Oxcarbazepine Dosage (mg/day)			Placebo N = 166 %
	OXC 600 N = 163 %	OXC 1200 N = 171 %	OXC 2400 N = 126 %	
Respiratory System				
Rhinitis	2	4	5	4
Skin and Appendages				
Acne	1	2	2	0
Special Senses				
Diplopia	14	30	40	5
Vertigo	6	12	15	2
Vision Abnormal	6	14	13	4
Accommodation Abnormal	0	0	2	0

* Events in at Least 2% of Patients Treated with 2400mg/day of Immediate-Release Oxcarbazepine and Numerically More Frequent than in the Placebo Group

Table 5: AED Drug Interactions with Oxcarbazepine

AED Coadministered (daily dose)	IR-Oxcarbazepine (daily dose)	Influence of IR-Oxcarbazepine on AED Concentration Mean Change [90% Confidence Interval]	Influence of AED on MHD Concentration (Mean Change, 90% Confidence Interval)	Recommendation
Carbamazepine (400 – 2000 mg)	900 mg	nc*	40% decrease [CI: 17% decrease, 57% decrease]	Consider initiating Oxtellar XR® at a higher dose. Monitor and titrate dose to desired clinical effect (see 2.6)
Phenobarbital (100 – 150 mg)	600 – 1800 mg	14% increase [CI: 2% increase, 24% increase]	25% decrease [CI: 12% decrease, 51% decrease]	
Phenytoin (250 – 500 mg)	600 – 1800 >1200-2400	nc*,† up to 40% increase‡ [CI: 12% increase, 60% increase]	30% decrease [CI: 3% decrease, 48% decrease]	
Valproic Acid (400 – 2800 mg)	600-1800	nc*	18% decrease [CI: 13% decrease, 40% decrease]	Monitor. Dose adjustment of Oxtellar XR® may not be needed.

* nc denotes a mean change of less than 10%
† Pediatrics
‡ Mean increase in adults at high doses of immediate-release oxcarbazepine

To provide information regarding the effects of in utero exposure to Oxtellar XR®, physicians are advised to recommend that pregnant patients taking Oxtellar XR® enroll in the NAAED Pregnancy Registry. This can be done by calling the toll free number 1-888-233-2334, and must be done by patients themselves. Information on the registry can also be found at the website http://www.aedpregnancyregistry.org/.

8.2 Labor and Delivery

The effect of Oxtellar XR® on labor and delivery in humans has not been evaluated.

8.3 Nursing Mothers

Oxcarbazepine and its active metabolite (MHD) are excreted in human milk. A milk-to-plasma concentration ratio of 0.5 was found for both. Because of the potential for serious adverse reactions to Oxtellar XR® in nursing infants, a decision should be made about whether to discontinue nursing or to discontinue the drug in nursing women, taking into account the importance of the drug to the mother.

8.4 Pediatric Use

The short term safety and effectiveness of Oxtellar XR® in pediatric patients ages 6 to 16 years with partial onset seizures is supported by:

1) An adequate and well-controlled short term safety and efficacy study of Oxtellar XR® in adults that included pharmacokinetic sampling [see *Clinical Studies (14.1)*],
2) A pharmacokinetic study of Oxtellar XR® in pediatric patients ages 4 to 16 years [see *Clinical Pharmacology (12.3)*], and
3) Safety and efficacy studies with the immediate-release formulation in adults and pediatric patients [see *Clinical Studies (14.2)* and *Adverse Reactions (6.1)*].

Oxtellar XR® is not approved for pediatric patients less than 6 years of age because the size of the tablets are inappropriate for younger children, and has not been studied in patients younger than 4 years of age.

8.5 Geriatric Use

Following administration of single (300 mg) and multiple (600 mg/day) doses of immediate-release oxcarbazepine to elderly volunteers (60-82 years of age), the maximum plasma concentrations and AUC values of MHD were 30%-60% higher than in younger volunteers (18-32 years of age). Comparisons of creatinine clearance in young and elderly volunteers indicate that the difference was due to age-

Continued on next page

related reductions in creatinine clearance. Consider starting at a lower dose and lower titration [see *Dosage and Administration (2.5)*].

8.6 Renal Impairment

There is a linear correlation between creatinine clearance and the renal clearance of MHD. [see *Clinical Pharmacology (12.3)* and *Dosage and Administration (2.4)*].

The pharmacokinetics of Oxtellar XR® has not been evaluated in patients with renal impairment. In patients with severe renal impairment (creatinine clearance <30 mL/min) given immediate release oxcarbazepine, the elimination half-life of MHD was prolonged with a corresponding two-fold increase in AUC [see *Clinical Pharmacology (12.3)*]. In these patients initiate Oxtellar XR® at a lower starting dose and increase, if necessary, at a slower than usual rate until the desired clinical response is achieved [see *Dosage and Administration (2.4)*].

In patients with end-stage renal disease on dialysis, it is recommended that immediate release oxcarbazepine be used instead of Oxtellar XR®.

8.7 Hepatic Impairment

The pharmacokinetics of oxcarbazepine and MHD has not been evaluated in severe hepatic impairment, and therefore is not recommended in these patients. [see *Clinical Pharmacology (12.3)*].

9 DRUG ABUSE AND DEPENDENCE

9.2 Abuse

The abuse potential of Oxtellar XR® has not been evaluated in human studies. Oxtellar XR® is not habit forming, and is not expected to encourage abuse.

9.3 Dependence

Intragastric injections of oxcarbazepine to four cynomolgus monkeys demonstrated no signs of physical dependence as measured by the desire to self-administer oxcarbazepine by lever pressing activity.

10 OVERDOSAGE

Human Overdose Experience

Isolated cases of overdose with immediate-release oxcarbazepine have been reported. The maximum dose taken was approximately 24,000 mg. All patients recovered with symptomatic treatment.

Treatment and Management

There is no specific antidote for Oxtellar XR® overdose. Administer symptomatic and supportive treatment as appropriate. Options include removal of the drug by gastric lavage and/or inactivation by administering activated charcoal.

11 DESCRIPTION

Oxtellar XR® is an antiepileptic drug (AED). Oxtellar XR® extended-release tablets contain oxcarbazepine for once-a-day oral administration.

Oxcarbazepine is 10,11-Dihydro-10-oxo-5H-dibenz[b,f]-azepine-5-carboxamide, and its structural formula is

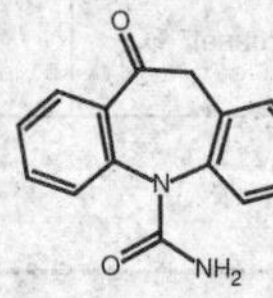

Oxcarbazepine is off-white to yellow crystalline powder. Oxcarbazepine is sparingly soluble in chloroform (30-100 g/L). In aqueous media over pH range 1 to 8, oxcarbazepine is practically insoluble and its solubility is 40 mg/L (0.04 g/L) at pH 7.0, 25°C. The molecular formula is $C_{15}H_{12}N_2O_2$ and its molecular weight is 252.27.

Oxtellar XR® tablets contain the following inactive ingredients: colloidal silicon dioxide, hypromellose, yellow iron oxide (150 mg, 300 mg tablets only), red iron oxide (300 mg, 600 mg tablets only), black iron oxide (300 mg tablet only), magnesium stearate, methacrylic acid copolymer, microcrystalline cellulose, polyethylene glycol, polyvinyl alcohol, povidone, sodium lauryl sulfate, talc, and titanium dioxide. Each tablet is printed on one side with edible black ink.

12 CLINICAL PHARMACOLOGY

12.1 Mechanism of Action

The pharmacological activity of Oxtellar XR® is primarily exerted through the 10-monohydroxy metabolite (MHD) of oxcarbazepine [see *Clinical Pharmacology (12.3)*]. The precise mechanism by which oxcarbazepine and MHD exert their antiseizure effect is unknown; however, in vitro electrophysiological studies indicate that they produce blockade of voltage-sensitive sodium channels, resulting in stabilization of hyperexcited neural membranes, inhibition of repetitive neuronal firing, and diminution of propagation of synaptic impulses. These actions are thought to be important in the prevention of seizure spread in the intact brain. In addition, increased potassium conductance and modulation of high-voltage activated calcium channels may contribute to the anticonvulsant effects of the drug. No significant interactions of oxcarbazepine or MHD with brain neurotransmitter or modulator receptor sites have been demonstrated.

12.2 Pharmacodynamics

Oxcarbazepine and its active metabolite (MHD) exhibit anticonvulsant properties in animal seizure models. They protected rodents against electrically induced tonic extension seizures and, to a lesser degree, chemically induced clonic seizures, and abolished or reduced the frequency of chronically recurring focal seizures in Rhesus monkeys with aluminum implants. No development of tolerance (i.e., attenuation of anticonvulsive activity) was observed in the maximal electroshock test when mice and rats were treated daily for five days and four weeks, respectively, with oxcarbazepine or MHD.

12.3 Pharmacokinetics

Following oral administration, oxcarbazepine is absorbed and extensively metabolized to its pharmacologically active 10-monohydroxy metabolite (MHD), which is responsible for most antiepileptic activity.

In clinical studies of Oxtellar XR®, the elimination half-life of oxcarbazepine was between 7 and 11 hours; the elimination half-life of MHD is between 9 and 11 hours.

In a mass balance study in human, only 2% of total radioactivity in plasma after administration of immediate-release oxcarbazepine was due to unchanged oxcarbazepine, with approximately 70% present as MHD, and the remainder attributable to minor metabolites.

Absorption

Oxtellar XR® administered as a once daily dose is not bioequivalent to the same total dose of the immediate release formulation given twice daily at steady state. Steady state plasma concentrations of MHD are reached within 5 days when Oxtellar XR® is given once daily. At steady state, when 1200 mg Oxtellar XR® was given once daily, MHD C_{max} occurred 7 hours post-dose. At steady state, Oxtellar XR® given once daily produced MHD exposures (AUC and C_{max}) about 19% lower and MHD minimum concentrations (C_{min}) about 16% lower than the immediate-release oxcarbazepine given twice daily when administered at the same 1200 mg total daily dose. When Oxtellar XR® was administered at an equivalent 600 mg single dose (4 × 150 mg tablets, 2 × 300 mg tablets, or 1 × 600 mg tablet), equivalent MHD exposures (AUC) were observed.

Following a single dose of Oxtellar XR® (1 × 150 mg tablets, 1 × 300 mg tablets, or 1 × 600 mg tablet), the pharmacokinetics of MHD are not linear and show greater than dose proportional increase in AUC and less than proportional increase in C_{max}: AUC increases 2.4-fold and C_{max} increases 1.9-fold with a 2-fold increase in dose.

Effect of Food: Single dose administration of 600 mg Oxtellar XR® following a high fat meal (800 – 1000 calories) produced MHD exposure (AUC) equivalent to that produced under fasting conditions. Peak MHD concentration (C_{max}) was about 60% higher and occurred 2 hours earlier under fed conditions than under fasting conditions.

The increase in C_{max}, even without a significant change in the overall exposure, should be considered by the prescriber especially during the titration phase, when some adverse reactions are most likely to occur coincidentally with peak levels.

Distribution

The apparent volume of distribution of MHD is 49 L. Approximately 40% of MHD is bound to serum proteins, predominantly to albumin. Binding is independent of the serum concentration within the therapeutically relevant range. Oxcarbazepine and MHD do not bind to alpha-1-acid glycoprotein.

Metabolism

Oxcarbazepine is rapidly reduced by cytosolic enzymes in the liver to MHD, which is primarily responsible for the pharmacological effect of Oxtellar XR®. MHD is metabolized further by conjugation with glucuronic acid. Minor amounts (4% of the dose) are oxidized to the pharmacologically inactive 10,11-dihydroxy metabolite (DHD).

Elimination

Oxcarbazepine is cleared from the body mostly in the form of metabolites which are predominantly excreted by the kidneys. More than 95% of a dose of immediate-release oxcarbazepine appears in the urine, with less than 1% as unchanged oxcarbazepine. Fecal excretion accounts for less than 4% of an administered dose. Approximately 80% of the dose is excreted in the urine either as glucuronides of MHD (49%) or as unchanged MHD (27%); the inactive DHD accounts for approximately 3% and conjugates of MHD and oxcarbazepine account for 13% of the dose.

The half-life of the parent was about two hours, while the half-life of MHD was about nine hours after the immediate release formulation. A population pharmacokinetic model for Oxtellar XR® was developed in healthy normal adults and applied to pharmacokinetic data in patients with epilepsy. For oxcarbazepine, systemic parameters were scaled allometrically, suggesting that steady state oxcarbazepine exposure will vary inversely with weight.

Special Populations

Elderly

No studies with Oxtellar XR® in elderly patients have been completed [see *Use in Specific Populations (8.5)*].

Following administration of single (300 mg) and multiple (600 mg/day) doses of immediate-release oxcarbazepine to elderly volunteers (60-82 years of age), the maximum plasma concentrations and AUC values of MHD were 30%-60% higher than in younger volunteers (18-32 years of age).

Comparisons of creatinine clearance in young and elderly volunteers indicate that the difference was due to age-related reductions in creatinine clearance.

Pediatric

Oxtellar XR® is not approved for pediatric patients less than 6 years of age because the size of the tablets are inappropriate for younger children, and has not been studied in patients younger than 4 years of age. A pharmacokinetic study of Oxtellar XR® was performed in 18 pediatric patients with epilepsy, 4 to 16 years of age, after multiple doses. The population pharmacokinetic model suggested that dosing of pediatric patients with Oxtellar XR® can be determined based on body weight. Weight-normalized doses in pediatric patients should produce MHD exposures (AUC) comparable to that in typical adults, with oxcarbazepine exposures ~40% higher in children than in adults [see *Use in Specific Populations (8.4)*].

Gender

The effects of gender have not been studied for Oxtellar XR®.

No gender-related pharmacokinetic differences have been observed in children, adults, or the elderly with immediate-release oxcarbazepine.

Race

The effects of race have not been studied for Oxtellar XR®.

Renal or Hepatic Impairment

The effects of renal or hepatic impairment have not been studied for Oxtellar XR® [see *Use in Specific Populations (8.6, 8.7)*].

Based on investigations with immediate-release oxcarbazepine, there is a linear correlation between creatinine clearance and the renal clearance of MHD. When immediate-release oxcarbazepine is administered as a single 300 mg dose in renally-impaired patients (creatinine clearance <30 mL/min), the elimination half-life of MHD is prolonged to 19 hours, with a two-fold increase in AUC. Dose adjustment is recommended in these patients [see *Dosage and Administration (2.4)* and *Use in Special Populations (8.6)*].

The pharmacokinetics and metabolism of immediate-release oxcarbazepine and MHD were evaluated in healthy volunteers and hepatically impaired subjects after a single 900 mg oral dose. Mild-to-moderate hepatic impairment did not affect the pharmacokinetics of immediate-release oxcarbazepine and MHD. The pharmacokinetics of oxcarbazepine and MHD have not been evaluated in severe hepatic impairment, and therefore it is not recommended in these patients [see *Use in Specific Populations (8.7)*].

Pregnancy

Due to physiological changes during pregnancy, MHD plasma levels may gradually decrease throughout pregnancy [see *Use in Specific Populations (8.1)*]

Drug Interaction Studies

In Vitro: Oxcarbazepine can inhibit CYP2C19 and induce CYP3A4/5 with potentially important effects on plasma concentrations of other drugs. In addition, several AEDs that are cytochrome P450 inducers can decrease plasma concentrations of oxcarbazepine and MHD.

Oxcarbazepine was evaluated in human liver microsomes to determine its capacity to inhibit the major cytochrome P450 enzymes responsible for the metabolism of other drugs. Results demonstrate that oxcarbazepine and its pharmacologically active 10-monohydroxy metabolite (MHD) have little or no capacity to function as inhibitors for most of the human cytochrome P450 enzymes evaluated (CYP1A2, CYP2A6, CYP2C9, CYP2D6, CYP2E1, CYP4A9 and CYP4A11) with the exception of CYP2C19 and CYP3A4/5. Although inhibition of CYP3A4/5 by oxcarbazepine and MHD did occur at high concentrations, it is not likely to be of clinical significance. The inhibition of CYP2C19 by oxcarbazepine and MHD, is clinically relevant.

In vitro, the UDP-glucuronyl transferase level was increased, indicating induction of this enzyme. Increases of 22% with MHD and 47% with oxcarbazepine were observed. As MHD, the predominant plasma substrate, is only a weak inducer of UDP-glucuronyl transferase, it is unlikely to have an effect on drugs that are mainly eliminated by conjugation through UDPglucuronyl transferase (e.g., valproic acid, lamotrigine).

In addition, oxcarbazepine and MHD induce a subgroup of the cytochrome P450 3A family (CYP3A4 and CYP3A5) responsible for the metabolism of dihydropyridine calcium antagonists, oral contraceptives and cyclosporine resulting in a lower plasma concentration of these drugs.

Several AEDs that are cytochrome P450 inducers can decrease plasma concentrations of oxcarbazepine and MHD. No autoinduction has been observed with immediate-release oxcarbazepine.

As binding of MHD to plasma proteins is low (40%), clinically significant interactions with other drugs through competition for protein binding sites are unlikely.

In Vivo:

Hormonal Contraceptives
Coadministration of immediate-release oxcarbazepine with an oral contraceptive has been shown to influence the plasma concentrations of two components of hormonal contraceptives, ethinylestradiol (EE) and levonorgestrel (LNG). The mean AUC values of EE were decreased by 48% [90% CI: 22-65] in one study and 52% [90% CI: 38-52] in another study. The mean AUC values of LNG were decreased by 32% [90% CI: 20-45] in one study and 52% [90% CI: 42-52] in another study. Therefore, concurrent use of oxcarbazepine with hormonal contraceptives may render these contraceptives less effective.

Calcium Channel Antagonists
After repeated coadministration of immediate-release oxcarbazepine, the AUC of felodipine was lowered by 28% [90% CI: 20-33]. Verapamil produced a decrease of 20% [90% CI: 18-27] of the plasma levels of MHD after coadministration with immediate-release oxcarbazepine.

Other Interactions
Cimetidine, erythromycin and dextropropoxyphene had no effect on the pharmacokinetics of MHD after coadministration with immediate-release oxcarbazepine. Results with warfarin show no evidence of interaction with either single or repeated doses of immediate-release oxcarbazepine.

13 NONCLINICAL TOXICOLOGY
13.1 Carcinogenesis, Mutagenesis, Impairment of Fertility
Carcinogenesis
In two-year carcinogenicity studies, oxcarbazepine was administered in the diet at doses of up to 100 mg/kg/day to mice and by gavage at doses of up to 250 mg/kg/day to rats, and the pharmacologically active 10-hydroxy metabolite (MHD) was administered orally at doses of up to 600 mg/kg/day to rats.

In mice, a dose-related increase in the incidence of hepatocellular adenomas was observed at oxcarbazepine doses ≥ 70 mg/kg/day or approximately 0.1 times the maximum recommended human dose (MRHD) on a mg/m^2 basis.

In rats, the incidence of hepatocellular carcinomas was increased in females treated with oxcarbazepine at doses ≥25 mg/kg/day (0.1 times the MRHD on a mg/m^2 basis), and incidences of hepatocellular adenomas and/or carcinomas were increased in males and females treated with MHD at doses of 600 mg/kg/day (2.4 times the MRHD on a mg/m^2 basis) and ≥ 250 mg/kg/day (equivalent to the MRHD on a mg/m^2 basis), respectively.

There was an increase in the incidence of benign testicular interstitial cell tumors in rats at 250 mg oxcarbazepine/kg/day and at ≥ 250 mg MHD/kg/day, and an increase in the incidence of granular cell tumors in the cervix and vagina in rats at 600 mg MHD/kg/day.

Mutagenesis
Oxcarbazepine increased mutation frequencies in the Ames test in vitro in the absence of metabolic activation in one of five bacterial strains. Both oxcarbazepine and MHD produced increases in chromosomal aberrations and polyploidy in the Chinese hamster ovary assay in vitro in the absence of metabolic activation. MHD was negative in the Ames test, and no mutagenic or clastogenic activity was found with either oxcarbazepine or MHD in V79 Chinese hamster cells in vitro. Oxcarbazepine and MHD were both negative for clastogenic or aneugenic effects (micronucleus formation) in an in vivo rat bone marrow assay.

Impairment of Fertility
In a fertility study in which rats were administered MHD (50, 150, or 450 mg/kg) orally prior to and during mating and early gestation, estrous cyclicity was disrupted and numbers of corpora lutea, implantations, and live embryos were reduced in females receiving the highest dose (approximately two times the MRHD on a mg/m^2 basis).

14 CLINICAL STUDIES
Oxtellar XR® has been evaluated as adjunctive therapy for partial seizures in adults. The use of Oxtellar XR® for the treatment of partial seizures in children is based on adequate and well-controlled studies of Oxtellar XR® in adults, along with clinical trials of immediate-release oxcarbazepine in children, and on pharmacokinetic evaluations of the use of Oxtellar XR® in children.

14.1 Oxtellar XR® Primary Trial
A multicenter, randomized, double-blind, placebo-controlled, three-arm, parallel-group study (Study 1) in male and female adults with refractory partial epilepsy (18 to 65 years of age, inclusive) was performed to examine the safety and efficacy of Oxtellar XR®.

Patients had at least three partial seizures per 28 days during an 8 week Baseline Period. Subjects were receiving treatment with at least one to three antiepileptic drugs and were on stable treatment for a minimum of 4 weeks. Subjects with a diagnosis other than partial epilepsy were excluded.

The study included an 8 week Baseline Period, followed by a Treatment Period, which included a 4 week Titration Phase followed by a 12 week Maintenance Phase. The primary endpoint of the study was median percentage change from baseline in seizure frequency per 28 days during the treatment period relative to the baseline period. The criterion for statistical significance was p<0.05. A total of 366 patients were enrolled at 88 sites in North America and Eastern Europe. Subjects were randomized to one of three treatment groups and took Oxtellar XR® (1200 or 2400 mg/day) or placebo.

Table 6 presents the primary efficacy results by treatment group.

[See table 6 above]

Although the 1200 mg/day-placebo contrast did not reach statistical significance, concentration-response analyses reveal that the 1200 mg/day dose is an effective dose.

14.2 Immediate-Release Oxcarbazepine Adjunctive Therapy Trials
The effectiveness of immediate-release oxcarbazepine as an adjunctive therapy for partial seizures in adults was demonstrated at doses of 600mg per day, 1200mg per day and 2400mg per day (divided twice daily) in a randomized, double-blind, placebo-controlled trial. All doses resulted in a statistically significant reduction in seizure frequency when compared to placebo (p<0.05).

The effectiveness of immediate-release oxcarbazepine in doses of 30-46 mg/kg/day, depending on baseline weight, as an adjunctive therapy for partial seizures in children 3 years to 17 years of age was studied in a randomized, double-blind, placebo-controlled trial. Oxcarbazepine in the single weight based dose group resulted in a statistically significant reduction in seizure frequency when compared to placebo (p<0.05).

16 HOW SUPPLIED/STORAGE AND HANDLING
16.1 Dosage Form Supplied
150 mg (yellow modified-oval shaped tablet printed "150" on one side with edible black ink).
Bottles of 100 tablets   NDC 17772-121-01
300 mg (brown modified-oval shaped tablet printed "300" on one side with edible black ink).
Bottles of 100 tablets   NDC 17772-122-01
600 mg (brownish red modified-oval shaped tablet printed "600" on one side with edible black ink).
Bottles of 100 tablets   NDC 17772-123-01

16.2 Storage and Handling
Store at 25°C (77°F); excursions permitted between 15°C and 30°C (59°F to 86°F) [See USP controlled room temperature]. Protect from light and moisture. Dispense in a tight, light-resistant container.

17 PATIENT COUNSELING INFORMATION
See FDA-Approved patient labeling (Medication Guide).
Inform patients and caregivers of the availability of a Medication Guide. Instruct patients and caregivers to read the Medication Guide prior to taking Oxtellar XR®.

- Advise patients to take the tablet whole with water or other liquid, and not to cut, chew or crush the tablet. Cutting, chewing or crushing Oxtellar XR® tablet could affect its performance.
- Advise patients to take Oxtellar XR® on an empty stomach. This means they should take Oxtellar XR® at least one hour before food or at least two hours after food [see *Clinical Pharmacology (12.3)*].
- Advise patients that Oxtellar XR® may reduce serum sodium concentrations especially if they are taking other medications that can lower sodium. Advise patients to report symptoms of low sodium like nausea, tiredness, lack of energy, confusion, and more frequent or more severe seizures [see *Warnings and Precautions (5.1)*].
- Anaphylactic reactions and angioedema may occur during treatment with Oxtellar XR®. Advise patients to immediately report signs and symptoms suggesting angioedema (swelling of the face, eyes, lips, tongue or difficulty in swallowing or breathing) and to stop taking the drug until they have consulted with their physician [see *Warnings and Precautions (5.2)*].
- Inform patients who have exhibited hypersensitivity reactions to carbamazepine that approximately 25%-30% of these patients may also experience hypersensitivity reactions with Oxtellar XR®. If patients experience a hyper-

Table 6: Primary Efficacy Results in Study 1: Percent Change from Baseline in Partial Seizure Frequency in the 16-week Treatment Period

	Median seizure frequency during 8-week baseline period (per 28 days)	Median seizure frequency during 16-week treatment period (per 28 days)	Median percent change in seizure frequency	Seizure frequency percent change effect size	P value vs placebo*
Placebo (N=121)	7.0	5.0	-28.7 %		
Oxtellar XR® 1200mg/day (N=122)	6.0	4.3	-38.2 %	9.5%	0.078
Oxtellar XR® 2400mg/day (N=123)	6.0	3.7	-42.9 %	14.2%	0.003

* Wilcoxon rank-sum test of the median percentage change in partial seizure frequency per 28 days during the 16-week Treatment Phase (Titration + Maintenance Periods) relative to the 8-week Baseline Phase.

Continued on next page

sensitivity reaction while taking Oxtellar XR®, advise them to consult with their physician immediately [see *Warnings and Precautions (5.3)*].
- Advise patients that serious skin reactions have been reported in association with immediate-release oxcarbazepine. If patients experience a skin reaction while taking Oxtellar XR®, advise patients to consult with their physician immediately [see *Warnings and Precautions (5.4)*].
- Instruct patients that a fever associated with other organ system involvement (rash, lymphadenopathy, etc.) occurring during treatment with Oxtellar XR® may be drug-related and advise them to consult their physician immediately [see *Warnings and Precautions (5.7)*].
- Advise patients that there have been rare reports of blood disorders reported in patients treated with immediate-release oxcarbazepine. Instruct patients to immediately consult with their physician if they experience symptoms suggestive of blood disorders during treatment with Oxtellar XR® [see *Warnings and Precautions (5.8)*].
- Warn female patients of childbearing age that the concurrent use of Oxtellar XR® with hormonal contraceptives may render this method of contraception less effective [see *Drug Interactions (7.2)*]. Additional non-hormonal forms of contraception are recommended when using Oxtellar XR®.
- Counsel patients, their caregivers, and families that AEDs, including Oxtellar XR®, may increase the risk of suicidal thoughts and behavior and that they need to be alert for the emergence or worsening of symptoms of depression, any unusual changes in mood or behavior, or the emergence of suicidal thoughts, behavior, or thoughts about self-harm. Advise them to immediately report behaviors of concern to healthcare providers.
- Advise patients to exercise caution if alcohol is taken in combination with Oxtellar XR® therapy, due to a possible additive sedative effect.
- Advise patients that Oxtellar XR® may cause dizziness and somnolence. Accordingly, advise patients not to drive or operate machinery until they have gained sufficient experience on Oxtellar XR® to gauge whether it adversely affects their ability to drive or operate machinery.
- Encourage patients to enroll in the North American Antiepileptic Drug (NAAED) Pregnancy Registry if they become pregnant. This registry is collecting information about the safety of antiepileptic drugs during pregnancy. To enroll, patients can call the toll free number 1-888-233-2334 [see *Use in Specific Populations (8.1)*].
- Advise patients that they should call their healthcare provider or poison control center (phone number 1-800-222-1222) if they take too much Oxtellar XR®.
- Discuss with your patient what they should do if they miss a dose.

Oxtellar XR® is manufactured by:
Patheon Inc.
Whitby, Ontario L1N 5Z5 CANADA
Distributed by:
Supernus Pharmaceuticals, Inc.
Rockville, MD 20850 USA
Oxtellar XR® is a trademark of Supernus Pharmaceuticals, Inc.
RA-OXT-V2
Revised: December 2015

MEDICATION GUIDE
Oxtellar XR™ (ahks-TEH-lahr eks ahr)
(oxcarbazepine)
Extended-Release Tablets

Read this Medication Guide before you start taking Oxtellar XR™ and each time you get a refill. There may be new information. This information does not take the place of talking to your healthcare provider about your medical condition or treatment.

What is the most important information I should know about Oxtellar XR™?

Do not stop taking Oxtellar XR™ without first talking to your healthcare provider.

Stopping Oxtellar XR™ suddenly can cause serious problems.

Oxtellar XR™ can cause serious side effects, including:
1. Oxtellar XR™ may cause the level of sodium in your blood to be low. Symptoms of low blood sodium include:
- nausea
- tiredness, lack of energy
- headache
- confusion
- more frequent or more severe seizures

Similar symptoms that are not related to low sodium may occur from taking Oxtellar XR™. You should tell your healthcare provider if you have any of these side effects and if they bother you or they do not go away.

Some other medicines can also cause low sodium in your blood. Be sure to tell your healthcare provider about all the other medicines that you are taking.

2. Oxtellar XR™ may also cause allergic reactions or serious problems which may affect organs and other parts of your body like the liver or blood cells. You may or may not have a rash with these types of reactions.

Call your healthcare provider right away if you have any of the following:
- swelling of your face, eyes, lips, or tongue
- trouble swallowing or breathing
- a skin rash
- hives
- fever, swollen glands, or sore throat that do not go away or come and go
- painful sores in the mouth or around your eyes
- yellowing of your skin or eyes
- unusual bruising or bleeding
- severe fatigue or weakness
- severe muscle pain
- frequent infections or infections that do not go away

Many people who are allergic to carbamazepine are also allergic to Oxtellar XR™. Tell your healthcare provider if you are allergic to carbamazepine.

3. **Like other antiepileptic drugs, Oxtellar XR™ may cause suicidal thoughts or actions in a very small number of people, about 1 in 500.**

Call your healthcare provider right away if you have any of these symptoms, especially if they are new, worse, or worry you:
- thoughts about suicide or dying
- attempts to commit suicide
- new or worse depression
- new or worse anxiety
- feeling agitated or restless
- panic attacks
- trouble sleeping (insomnia)
- new or worse irritability
- acting aggressive, being angry, or violent
- acting on dangerous impulses
- an extreme increase in activity and talking (mania)
- other unusual changes in behavior or mood

How can I watch for early symptoms of suicidal thoughts and actions?
- Pay attention to any changes, especially sudden changes, in mood, behaviors, thoughts, or feelings.
- Keep all follow-up visits with your healthcare provider as scheduled.

Call your healthcare provider between visits as needed, especially if you are worried about symptoms.

Do not stop taking Oxtellar XR™ without first talking to a healthcare provider.

Stopping Oxtellar XR™ suddenly can cause serious problems. Stopping a seizure medicine suddenly in a patient who has epilepsy may cause seizures that will not stop (status epilepticus).

Suicidal thoughts or actions may be caused by things other than medicines. If you have suicidal thoughts or actions, your healthcare provider may check for other causes.

What is Oxtellar XR™?
Oxtellar XR™ is a prescription medicine used:
- with other medicines to treat partial seizures in adults
- with other medicines to treat partial seizures in children 6 to 17 years of age.

It is not known if Oxtellar XR™ is safe and effective in children under 6 years of age.

Who should not take Oxtellar XR™?
- Do not take Oxtellar XR™ if you are allergic to oxcarbazepine or any of the other ingredients in Oxtellar XR™. See the end of this leaflet for a complete list of ingredients in Oxtellar XR™.

What should I tell my healthcare provider before taking Oxtellar XR™?
Before taking Oxtellar XR™, tell your healthcare provider about all your medical conditions, including if you:
- have or have had suicidal thoughts or actions, depression or mood problems
- have liver problems
- have kidney problems
- use birth control medicine. Oxtellar XR™ may cause your birth control medicine to be less effective. Talk to your healthcare provider about the best birth control method to use.
- are pregnant or plan to become pregnant. Oxtellar XR™ may harm your unborn baby. Tell your healthcare provider right away if you become pregnant while taking Oxtellar XR™. You and your healthcare provider will decide if you should take Oxtellar XR™ while you are pregnant.

- If you become pregnant while taking Oxtellar XR™, talk to your healthcare provider about registering with the North American Antiepileptic Drug (NAAED) Pregnancy Registry. The purpose of this registry is to collect information about the safety of antiepileptic medicine during pregnancy. You can enroll in this registry by calling 1-888-233-2334.
- are breastfeeding or plan to breastfeed. Oxtellar XR™ passes into breast milk. You and your healthcare provider should discuss whether you should take Oxtellar XR™ or breastfeed. You should not do both.

Tell your healthcare provider about all the medicines you take, including prescription and non-prescription medicines, vitamins, and herbal supplements.

Taking Oxtellar XR™ with certain other medicines may cause side effects or affect how well they work. Do not start or stop other medicines without talking to your healthcare provider.

Especially tell your healthcare provider if you take: carbamazepine, phenobarbital, phenytoin, or birth control medicine.

Ask your healthcare provider or pharmacist for a list of these medicines, if you are not sure.

Know the medicines you take. Keep a list of them and show it to your healthcare provider and pharmacist when you get a new medicine.

How should I take Oxtellar XR™?
Do not stop taking Oxtellar XR™ without talking to your healthcare provider. Stopping Oxtellar XR™ suddenly can cause serious problems, including seizures that will not stop (status epilepticus). Take Oxtellar XR™ exactly as prescribed. Your healthcare provider may change your dose. Your healthcare provider will tell you how much Oxtellar XR™ to take.

Take Oxtellar XR™ 1 time each day.

Take Oxtellar XR™ on an empty stomach. This means you should take Oxtellar XR™ at least 1 hour before or at least 2 hours after a meal. Take Oxtellar XR™ tablets whole with water or other liquid.

Do not cut, crush, or chew the tablets before swallowing.

If you take too much Oxtellar XR™ call your healthcare provider or call the poison control center at 1-800-222-1222.

Take Oxtellar XR™ at the same time each day.

Talk with your healthcare provider about what you should do if you miss a dose.

What should I avoid while taking Oxtellar XR™?
- Do not drive, operate heavy machinery, or do other dangerous activities until you know how Oxtellar XR™ affects you. Oxtellar XR™ may slow your thinking and motor skills.
- Do not drink alcohol or take other drugs that make you sleepy or dizzy while taking Oxtellar XR™ until you talk to your healthcare provider. Oxtellar XR™ taken with alcohol or drugs that cause sleepiness or dizziness may make your sleepiness or dizziness worse.

What are the possible side effects of Oxtellar XR™?
See "What is the most important information I should know about Oxtellar XR™?"

Oxtellar XR™ may cause other serious side effects including:
- your seizures can happen more often or become worse
- trouble concentrating
- problems with your speech and language
- feeling confused
- feeling sleepy and tired
- trouble walking and with coordination

Get medical help right away if you have any of the symptoms listed above or listed in "What is the most important information I should know about Oxtellar XR™?"

The most common side effects of Oxtellar XR™ include:
- dizziness
- sleepiness
- headache
- problems with walking and coordination (unsteadiness)
- shakiness
- nausea
- vomiting
- double vision
- weakness
- tiredness

These are not all the possible side effects of Oxtellar XR™. For more information, ask your healthcare provider or pharmacist.

Tell your healthcare provider if you have any side effect that bothers you or does not go away.

Call your doctor for medical advice about side effects. You may report side effects to FDA at 1-800-FDA-1088.

How should I store Oxtellar XR™?

- Store Oxtellar XR™ at room temperature 68°F to 77°F (20°C and 25°C)
- Keep Oxtellar XR™ in a tightly closed container, and keep Oxtellar XR™ out of the light.
- Keep Oxtellar XR™ tablets dry.

Keep Oxtellar XR™ and all medicines out of the reach of children.

General Information about the safe and effective use of Oxtellar XR™

Medicines are sometimes prescribed for purposes other than those listed in a Medication Guide. Do not use Oxtellar XR™ for a condition for which it was not prescribed. Do not give Oxtellar XR™ to other people, even if they have the same symptoms that you have. It may harm them.

This Medication Guide summarizes the most important information about Oxtellar XR™. If you would like more information, talk with your healthcare provider. You can ask your pharmacist or healthcare provider for the full prescribing information about Oxtellar XR™ that is written for health professionals.

For more information, go to www.supernus.com or call 1-866-398-0833.

What are the ingredients in Oxtellar XR™?

Active ingredient: oxcarbazepine

Inactive ingredients:

150 mg tablets: colloidal silicon dioxide, hypromellose, yellow iron oxide, magnesium stearate, methacrylic acid copolymer, microcrystalline cellulose, polyethylene glycol, polyvinyl alcohol, povidone, sodium lauryl sulfate, talc, and titanium dioxide.

300 mg tablets: colloidal silicon dioxide, hypromellose, yellow iron oxide, red iron oxide, black iron oxide, magnesium stearate, methacrylic acid copolymer, microcrystalline cellulose, polyethylene glycol, polyvinyl alcohol, povidone, sodium lauryl sulfate, talc, and titanium dioxide.

600 mg tablets: red iron oxide, magnesium stearate, methacrylic acid copolymer, microcrystalline cellulose, polyethylene glycol, polyvinyl alcohol, povidone, sodium lauryl sulfate, talc, and titanium dioxide.

This Medication Guide has been approved by the U.S. Food and Drug Administration.

Distributed by:
Supernus Pharmaceuticals, Inc.
© Supernus Pharmaceuticals Inc.
Issued October 2012.

Shown in Product Identification Guide, page 510

TROKENDI XR®
(topiramate)
extended-release capsules, for oral use

℞

HIGHLIGHTS OF PRESCRIBING INFORMATION
These highlights do not include all the information needed to use TROKENDI XR safely and effectively. See full prescribing information for TROKENDI XR.

TROKENDI XR (topiramate) extended-release capsules, for oral use
Initial U.S. Approval: 1996

——RECENT MAJOR CHANGES——

Indications and Usage, Monotherapy epilepsy (1.1)	8/2016
Dosage and Administration, Dosing in Monotherapy Epilepsy (2.1)	8/2016

——INDICATIONS AND USAGE——

TROKENDI XR® is indicated for:
- Monotherapy epilepsy: initial monotherapy in patients 6 years of age and older with partial onset or primary generalized tonic-clonic seizures (1.1)
- Adjunctive therapy epilepsy: adjunctive therapy in patients 6 years of age and older with partial onset, primary generalized tonic-clonic seizures, or seizures associated with Lennox-Gastaut syndrome (LGS)(1.2)

——DOSAGE AND ADMINISTRATION——

[See table above]
Swallow capsule whole and intact. Do not sprinkle on food, chew, or crush (2.9)

——DOSAGE FORMS AND STRENGTHS——

Extended-release capsules: 25 mg, 50 mg, 100 mg, and 200 mg (3)

	Initial Dose	Titration	Recommended Dose
Monotherapy: Partial Onset or Primary Generalized Tonic-Clonic Seizures			
Adults and pediatric patients 10 years and older (2.1)	50 mg orally once daily	Increase dose weekly by increments of 50 mg for first 4 weeks then 100 mg for weeks 5 to 6	400 mg once daily
Pediatric patients 6 to less than 10 (2.1)	25 mg/day nightly for the first week	Titrate over 5 to 7 weeks	Daily doses based on weight (Table 1)
Adjunctive Therapy			
Adults with partial onset seizures or LGS (2.2)	25 mg to 50 mg orally once daily	Increase dose weekly by increments of 25 mg to 50 mg to achieve an effective dose	200 mg to 400 mg once daily
Adults with primary generalized tonic-clonic seizures (2.2)	25 mg to 50 mg orally once daily	Increase dose weekly to an effective dose by increments of 25 mg to 50 mg	400 mg once daily
Pediatric patients 6 years and older with partial onset seizures, primary generalized tonic-clonic seizures, or LGS (2.2)	25 mg once at nighttime (based on a range of 1 mg/kg to 3 mg/kg once daily) for first week	Increase dosage at 1- or 2-week intervals by increments of 1 mg/kg to 3 mg/kg Dose titration should be guided by clinical outcome	5 mg/kg to 9 mg/kg once daily

——CONTRAINDICATIONS——

- With recent alcohol use ie, within 6 hours prior to and 6 hours after TROKENDI XR® use (4), (5.4)
- In patients with metabolic acidosis taking concomitant metformin (4), (5.3)

——WARNINGS AND PRECAUTIONS——

- Acute myopia and secondary angle closure glaucoma: Untreated elevated intraocular pressure can lead to permanent visual loss. Discontinue TROKENDI XR® if it occurs (5.1)
- Oligohydrosis and hyperthermia: Monitor decreased sweating and increased body temperature, especially in pediatric patients (5.2)
- Metabolic acidosis: Measure baseline and periodic measurement of serum bicarbonate. Consider dose reduction or discontinuation of TROKENDI XR® if clinically appropriate (5.3)
- Suicidal behavior and ideation: Antiepileptic drugs increase the risk of suicidal behavior or ideation (5.5)
- Cognitive/neuropsychiatric: TROKENDI XR® may cause cognitive dysfunction. Use caution when operating machinery including automobiles. Depression and mood problems may occur (5.6)
- Fetal toxicity: Topiramate use during pregnancy can cause cleft lip and/or palate and increases the risk of being small for gestational age (5.7)
- Withdrawal of AEDs: Withdrawal of TROKENDI XR® should be done gradually (5.8)
- Hyperammonemia and encephalopathy: Patients with inborn errors of metabolism or reduced mitochondrial activity may have an increased risk of hyperammonemia. Measure ammonia if encephalopathic symptoms occur (5.9)
- Kidney stones: Avoid use with other carbonic anhydrase inhibitors, other drugs causing metabolic acidosis, or in patients on a ketogenic diet (5.10)
- Hypothermia: Reported with concomitant valproic acid use (5.11)
- Visual fields defects: These have been reported independent of elevated intraocular pressure. Consider discontinuation of TROKENDI XR® (5.14)

——ADVERSE REACTIONS——

The most common (≥10% more frequent than placebo or low-dose topiramate in monotherapy and adjunctive therapy) adverse reactions in adult and pediatric patients were paresthesia, anorexia, weight decrease, speech disorders/related speech problems, fatigue, dizziness, somnolence, nervousness, psychomotor slowing, abnormal vision, difficulty with memory, difficulty with concentration/attention, and fever (6.1).

To report SUSPECTED ADVERSE REACTIONS, contact Supernus Pharmaceuticals at 1-866-398-0833- or the FDA at 1-800-FDA-1088 or www.fda.gov/medwatch.

——DRUG INTERACTIONS——

- Oral contraceptives: Decreased contraceptive efficacy and increased breakthrough bleeding, especially at doses greater than 200 mg per day (7.2)
- Phenytoin or carbamazepine: Concomitant administration with topiramate decreased plasma concentrations of topiramate (7.3)
- Lithium: Monitor lithium levels when co-administered with high-dose topiramate (7.7)

——USE IN SPECIFIC POPULATIONS——

- Renal Impairment: (creatinine clearance less than 70 mL/min/1.73m²), one-half of the adult dose is recommended (8.7)
- Patients undergoing hemodialysis: Topiramate is cleared by hemodialysis. Dosage adjustment is necessary to avoid rapid drops in topiramate plasma concentration during hemodialysis (8.8)
- Pediatric Use: Because the capsule must be swallowed whole, and may not be sprinkled on food, crushed, or chewed, TROKENDI XR® is recommended only for children ages 6 years and older (8.4)

See 17 for PATIENT COUNSELING INFORMATION and Medication Guide.

Revised: 8/2016

Continued on next page

* Sections or subsections omitted from the full prescribing information are not listed.

FULL PRESCRIBING INFORMATION

1 INDICATIONS AND USAGE
1.1 Monotherapy Epilepsy
TROKENDI XR® extended-release capsules are indicated in patients 6 years of age and older as initial monotherapy for partial onset or primary generalized tonic-clonic seizures. Safety and effectiveness in patients who were converted to monotherapy from a previous regimen of other anticonvulsant drugs have not been established in controlled trials [see *Clinical Studies (14.2)*].

1.2 Adjunctive Therapy Epilepsy
TROKENDI XR® extended-release capsules are indicated as adjunctive therapy in patients 6 years of age and older with partial onset seizures, primary generalized tonic-clonic seizures, and seizures associated with Lennox-Gastaut syndrome [see *Clinical Studies (14.3,14.4, 14.5)*].

2 DOSAGE AND ADMINISTRATION
2.1 Dosing in Monotherapy Epilepsy
Adults and Pediatric Patients 10 Years and Older with Partial Onset or Primary Generalized Tonic-Clonic Seizures
The recommended dose for topiramate monotherapy in adults and in pediatric patients 10 years of age and older is 400 mg orally once daily. Titrate TROKENDI XR® according to the following schedule:

Week 1   50 mg once daily
Week 2   100 mg once daily
Week 3   150 mg once daily
Week 4   200 mg once daily
Week 5   300 mg once daily
Week 6   400 mg once daily

Pediatric Patients Ages 6 to less than 10 Years with Partial Onset or Primary Generalized Tonic-Clonic Seizures

Dosing of topiramate as initial monotherapy in pediatric patients 6 to less than 10 years of age with partial onset or primary generalized tonic-clonic seizures was based on a pharmacometric bridging approach [see *Clinical Studies (14.1)*].
Dosing in patients 6 to less than 10 years is based on weight. During the titration period, the initial dose of TROKENDI XR® should be 25 mg/day administered nightly for the first week. Based upon tolerability, the dosage can be increased to 50 mg/day in the second week. Dosage can be increased by 25-50 mg/day each subsequent week as tolerated. Titration to the minimum maintenance dose should be attempted over 5-7 weeks of the total titration period. Based upon tolerability and clinical response, additional titration to a higher dose (up to the maximum maintenance dose) can be attempted at 25-50 mg/day weekly increments. The total daily dose should not exceed the maximum maintenance dose for each range of body weight (Table 1).

Table 1: Monotherapy Target Total Daily Maintenance Dosing for Patients 6 to less than 10 Years

Weight (kg)	Total Daily Dose (mg/day) Minimum Maintenance Dose	Total Daily Dose (mg/day) Maximum Maintenance Dose
Up to 11	150	250
12 - 22	200	300
23 - 31	200	350
32 - 38	250	350
Greater than 38	250	400

2.2 Dosing in Adjunctive Therapy Epilepsy
Adults 17 Years of Age and Over with Partial Onset Seizures, Primary Generalized Tonic-Clonic Seizures, or Lennox-Gastaut Syndrome
The recommended total daily dose of TROKENDI XR® as adjunctive therapy in adults with partial onset seizures or Lennox-Gastaut Syndrome is 200 mg to 400 mg orally once daily and with primary generalized tonic-clonic seizures is 400 mg orally once daily.
Initiate therapy at 25 mg to 50 mg once daily followed by titration to an effective dose in increments of 25 mg to 50 mg every week. Daily topiramate doses above 1600 mg have not been studied.
In the study of primary generalized tonic-clonic seizures using topiramate, the assigned dose was reached at the end of 8 weeks [see *Clinical Studies (14.4)*].
Pediatric Patients 6 to 16 Years of Age with Partial Onset Seizures, Primary Generalized Tonic-Clonic Seizures, or Lennox-Gastaut Syndrome
The recommended total daily dose of TROKENDI XR® as adjunctive therapy for pediatric patients with partial onset seizures, primary generalized tonic-clonic seizures, or seizures associated with Lennox-Gastaut syndrome is approximately 5 mg/kg to 9 mg/kg orally once daily. Begin titration at 25 mg once daily (based on a range of 1 mg/kg/day to 3 mg/kg/day) given nightly for the first week. Subsequently, increase the dosage at 1- or 2-week intervals by increments of 1 mg/kg to 3 mg/kg to achieve optimal clinical response. Dose titration should be guided by clinical outcome. If required, longer intervals between dose adjustments can be used.
In the study of primary generalized tonic-clonic seizures, the assigned dose of 6 mg/kg once daily was reached at the end of 8 weeks [see *Clinical Studies (14.4)*].

2.3 Administration with Alcohol
Alcohol use should be completely avoided within 6 hours prior to and 6 hours after TROKENDI XR® administration [see *Warnings and Precautions (5.4)*].

2.4 Dose Modifications in Patients with Renal Impairment
In patients with renal impairment (creatinine clearance less than 70 mL/min/1.73 m²), one-half of the usual adult dose is recommended. Such patients will require a longer time to reach steady-state at each dose.
Prior to dosing, obtain an estimated GFR measurement in patients at high risk for renal insufficiency (e.g., older patients, or those with diabetes mellitus, hypertension, or autoimmune disease).

2.5 Dosage Modifications in Patients Undergoing Hemodialysis
Topiramate is cleared by hemodialysis at a rate that is 4 to 6 times greater than in patients with normal renal function. Accordingly, a prolonged period of dialysis may cause topiramate concentration to fall below that required to maintain an antiseizure effect. To avoid rapid drops in topiramate plasma concentration during hemodialysis, a supplemental dose of topiramate may be required. The actual adjustment should take into account the:
• duration of dialysis period
• clearance rate of the dialysis system being used
• effective renal clearance of topiramate in the patient being dialyzed

2.6 Laboratory Testing Prior to Treatment Initiation
Measurement of baseline and periodic serum bicarbonate during TROKENDI XR® treatment is recommended [see *Warnings and Precautions (5.3)*].

2.7 Dosing Modifications in Patients Taking Phenytoin and/or Carbamazepine
The co-administration of TROKENDI XR® with phenytoin may require an adjustment of the dose of phenytoin to achieve optimal clinical outcome. Addition or withdrawal of phenytoin and/or carbamazepine during adjunctive therapy with TROKENDI XR® may require adjustment of the dose of TROKENDI XR®.

2.8 Monitoring for Therapeutic Blood Levels
It is not necessary to monitor topiramate plasma concentrations to optimize TROKENDI XR® therapy.

2.9 Administration Instructions
TROKENDI XR® can be taken without regard to meals. Swallow capsule whole and intact. Do not sprinkle on food, chew, or crush.

3 DOSAGE FORMS AND STRENGTHS
TROKENDI XR® (topiramate) extended-release capsules are available in the following strengths and colors:
25 mg: Size 2 capsules, light green opaque body/yellow opaque cap (printed "SPN" on the cap, "25" on the body)
50 mg: Size 0 capsules, light green opaque body/orange opaque cap (printed "SPN" on the cap, "50" on the body)
100 mg: Size 00 capsules, green opaque body/blue opaque cap (printed "SPN" on the cap, "100" on the body)
200 mg: Size 00 capsules, pink opaque body/blue opaque cap (printed "SPN" on the cap, "200" on the body)

4 CONTRAINDICATIONS
TROKENDI XR® is contraindicated in patients:
• With recent alcohol use (i.e., within 6 hours prior to and 6 hours after TROKENDI XR® use) [see *Warnings and Precautions (5.4)*]
• With metabolic acidosis who are taking concomitant metformin [see *Warnings and Precautions (5.3) and Drug Interactions (7.6)*]

5 WARNINGS AND PRECAUTIONS
5.1 Acute Myopia and Secondary Angle Closure Glaucoma
A syndrome consisting of acute myopia associated with secondary angle closure glaucoma has been reported in patients receiving topiramate. Symptoms include acute onset of decreased visual acuity and/or ocular pain. Ophthalmologic findings can include myopia, anterior chamber shallowing, ocular hyperemia (redness) and increased intraocular pressure. Mydriasis may or may not be present. This syndrome may be associated with supraciliary effusion resulting in anterior displacement of the lens and iris, with secondary angle closure glaucoma. Symptoms typically occur within 1 month of initiating topiramate therapy. In contrast to primary narrow angle glaucoma, which is rare under 40 years of age, secondary angle closure glaucoma associated with topiramate has been reported in pediatric patients as well as adults. The primary treatment to reverse symptoms is discontinuation of TROKENDI XR® as rapidly as possible, according to the judgment of the treating physician. Other measures, in conjunction with discontinuation of TROKENDI XR®, may be helpful.
Elevated intraocular pressure of any etiology, if left untreated, can lead to serious sequelae including permanent vision loss.

5.2 Oligohydrosis and Hyperthermia
Oligohydrosis (decreased sweating), resulting in hospitalization in some cases, has been reported in association with topiramate use. Decreased sweating and an elevation in body temperature above normal characterized these cases. Some of the cases were reported after exposure to elevated environmental temperatures.

The majority of the reports have been in pediatric patients. Patients, especially pediatric patients, treated with TROKENDI XR® should be monitored closely for evidence of decreased sweating and increased body temperature, especially in hot weather. Caution should be used when TROKENDI XR® is prescribed with other drugs that predispose patients to heat-related disorders; these drugs include, but are not limited to, other carbonic anhydrase inhibitors and drugs with anticholinergic activity.

5.3 Metabolic Acidosis

Hyperchloremic, non-anion gap, metabolic acidosis (i.e., decreased serum bicarbonate below the normal reference range in the absence of chronic respiratory alkalosis) is associated with topiramate, and can be expected with treatment with TROKENDI XR®. This metabolic acidosis is caused by renal bicarbonate loss due to the inhibitory effect of topiramate on carbonic anhydrase. Such electrolyte imbalance has been observed with the use of topiramate in placebo-controlled clinical trials and in the post-marketing period. Generally, topiramate-induced metabolic acidosis occurs early in treatment although cases can occur at any time during treatment. Bicarbonate decrements are usually mild to moderate (average decrease of 4 mEq/L at daily doses of 400 mg in adults and at approximately 6 mg/kg/day in pediatric patients); rarely, patients can experience severe decrements to values below 10 mEq/L. Conditions or therapies that predispose patients to acidosis (such as renal disease, severe respiratory disorders, status epilepticus, diarrhea, ketogenic diet or specific drugs) may be additive to the bicarbonate lowering effects of topiramate.

Manifestations of Metabolic Acidosis

Some manifestations of acute or chronic metabolic acidosis may include hyperventilation, nonspecific symptoms such as fatigue and anorexia, or more severe sequelae including cardiac arrhythmias or stupor. Chronic, untreated metabolic acidosis may increase the risk for nephrolithiasis or nephrocalcinosis, and may also result in osteomalacia (referred to as rickets in pediatric patients) and/or osteoporosis with an increased risk for fractures. Chronic metabolic acidosis in pediatric patients may also reduce growth rates. A reduction in growth rate may eventually decrease the maximal height achieved. The effect of topiramate on growth and bone-related sequelae has not been systematically investigated in long-term, placebo-controlled trials. Long-term, open-label treatment of infants/toddlers, with intractable partial epilepsy, for up to 1 year, showed reductions from baseline in Z SCORES for length, weight, and head circumference compared to age and sex-matched normative data, although these patients with epilepsy are likely to have different growth rates than normal infants. Reductions in Z SCORES for length and weight were correlated to the degree of acidosis [*see Pediatric Use (8.4)*]. Topiramate treatment that causes metabolic acidosis during pregnancy can possibly produce adverse effects on the fetus and might also cause metabolic acidosis in the neonate from possible transfer of topiramate to the fetus [*see Warnings and Precautions (5.7) and Use in Specific Populations (8.1)*].

Adults

In adults, the incidence of persistent decreases in serum bicarbonate (levels of less than 20 mEq/L at two consecutive visits or at the final visit) in controlled clinical trials for adjunctive treatment of epilepsy was 32% for 400 mg per day, and 1% for placebo. Metabolic acidosis has been observed at doses as low as 50 mg per day. The incidence of persistent decreases in serum bicarbonate in adult patients (≥16 years of age) in the epilepsy controlled clinical trial for monotherapy was 14% for 50 mg per day and 25% for 400 mg per day. The incidence of a markedly abnormally low serum bicarbonate (i.e., absolute value less than 17 mEq/L and greater than 5 mEq/L decrease from pretreatment) in the adjunctive therapy trials was 3% for 400 mg per day, and 0% for placebo, and in the monotherapy trial was 1% for 50 mg per day and 6% for 400 mg per day. Serum bicarbonate levels have not been systematically evaluated at daily doses greater than 400 mg per day.

Pediatric Patients (2 Years to 16 Years of Age)

Although TROKENDI XR® is not approved for use in patients below the age of 6, the incidence of persistent decreases in serum bicarbonate in placebo-controlled trials for adjunctive treatment of Lennox-Gastaut syndrome or refractory partial onset seizures in patients age 2 years to 16 years was 67% for topiramate (at approximately 6 mg/kg/day), and 10% for placebo. The incidence of markedly abnormally low serum bicarbonate (i.e., absolute value less than 17 mEq/L and greater than 5 mEq/L decrease from pretreatment) in these trials was 11% for topiramate and 0% for placebo. Cases of moderately severe metabolic acidosis have been reported in patients as young as 5 months old, especially at daily doses above 5 mg/kg/day.

In pediatric patients (6 years to 15 years of age), the incidence of persistent decreases in serum bicarbonate in the epilepsy controlled clinical trial for monotherapy performed with topiramate was 9% for 50 mg per day and 25% for 400 mg per day. The incidence of a markedly abnormally low serum bicarbonate (i.e., absolute value less than 17 mEq/L and greater than 5 mEq/L decrease from pretreatment) in this trial was 1% for 50 mg per day and 6% for 400 mg per day.

Pediatric Patients (Under 2 Years of Age)

Although TROKENDI XR® is not approved for use in patients less than 6 years of age, a study of topiramate as adjunctive use in patients under 2 years of age with partial onset seizures revealed that topiramate produced a metabolic acidosis that is notably greater in magnitude than that observed in controlled trials in older children and adults. The mean treatment difference (25 mg/kg/day topiramate-placebo) was -5.9 mEq/L for bicarbonate. The incidence of metabolic acidosis (defined by a serum bicarbonate less than 20 mEq/L) was 0% for placebo, 30% for 5 mg/kg/day, 50% for 15 mg/kg/day, and 45% for 25 mg/kg/day. The incidence of markedly abnormal changes (i.e., less than 17 mEq/L and greater than 5 mEq/L decrease from baseline of greater than or equal to 20 mEq/L) was 0% for placebo, 4% for 5 mg/kg/day, 5% for 15 mg/kg/day, and 5% for 25 mg/kg/day [*see Use in Specific Populations(8.4)*].

Risk Mitigation Strategies

Measurement of baseline and periodic serum bicarbonate during topiramate treatment is recommended. If metabolic acidosis develops and persists, consideration should be given to reducing the dose or discontinuing topiramate (using dose tapering). If the decision is made to continue patients on topiramate in the face of persistent acidosis, alkali treatment should be considered.

5.4 Interaction with Alcohol

In vitro data show that, in the presence of alcohol, the pattern of topiramate release from TROKENDI XR® capsules is significantly altered. As a result, plasma levels of topiramate with TROKENDI XR® may be markedly higher soon after dosing and subtherapeutic later in the day. Therefore, alcohol use should be completely avoided within 6 hours prior to and 6 hours after TROKENDI XR® administration.

5.5 Suicidal Behavior and Ideation

Antiepileptic drugs (AEDs) increase the risk of suicidal thoughts or behavior in patients taking these drugs for any indication. Patients treated with any AED, including TROKENDI XR® for any indication should be monitored for the emergence or worsening of depression, suicidal thoughts or behavior, and/or any unusual changes in mood or behavior.

Pooled analyses of 199 placebo-controlled clinical trials (mono- and adjunctive therapy) of 11 different AEDs showed that patients randomized to one of the AEDs had approximately twice the risk (adjusted Relative Risk 1.8, 95% CI:1.2, 2.7) of suicidal thinking or behavior compared to patients randomized to placebo. In these trials, which had a median treatment duration of 12 weeks, the estimated incidence rate of suicidal behavior or ideation among 27,863 AED-treated patients was 0.43%, compared to 0.24% among 16,029 placebo-treated patients, representing an increase of approximately one case of suicidal thinking or behavior for every 530 patients treated. There were four suicides in drug-treated patients in the trials and none in placebo-treated patients, but the number is too small to allow any conclusion about drug effect on suicide.

The increased risk of suicidal thoughts or behavior with AEDs was observed as early as one week after starting drug treatment with AEDs and persisted for the duration of treatment assessed. Because most trials included in the analysis did not extend beyond 24 weeks, the risk of suicidal thoughts or behavior beyond 24 weeks could not be assessed.

The risk of suicidal thoughts or behavior was generally consistent among drugs in the data analyzed. The finding of increased risk with AEDs of varying mechanisms of action and across a range of indications suggests that the risk applies to all AEDs used for any indication. The risk did not vary substantially by age (5 to 100 years) in the clinical trials analyzed.

Table 2 shows absolute and relative risk by indication for all evaluated AEDs.

[See table 2 above]

Table 2: Risk by Indication for Antiepileptic Drugs in the Pooled Analysis

Indication	Placebo Patients with Events per 1,000 Patients	Drug Patients with Events per 1,000 Patients	Relative Risk: Incidence of Events in Drug Patients/Incidence in Placebo Patients	Risk Difference: Additional Drug Patients with Events per 1,000 Patients
Epilepsy	1.0	3.4	3.5	2.4
Psychiatric	5.7	8.5	1.5	2.9
Other	1.0	1.8	1.9	0.9
Total	2.4	4.3	1.8	1.9

The relative risk for suicidal thoughts or behavior was higher in clinical trials for epilepsy than in clinical trials for psychiatric or other conditions, but the absolute risk differences were similar for the epilepsy and psychiatric indications.

Anyone considering prescribing TROKENDI XR® or any other AED must balance the risk of suicidal thoughts or behavior with the risk of untreated illness. Epilepsy and many other illnesses for which AEDs are prescribed are themselves associated with morbidity and mortality and an increased risk of suicidal thoughts and behavior. Should suicidal thoughts and behavior emerge during treatment, the prescriber needs to consider whether the emergence of these symptoms in any given patient may be related to the illness being treated.

Patients, their caregivers, and families should be informed that AEDs increase the risk of suicidal thoughts and behavior and should be advised of the need to be alert for the emergence or worsening of the signs and symptoms of depression, any unusual changes in mood or behavior or the emergence of suicidal thoughts, behavior or thoughts about self-harm. Behaviors of concern should be reported immediately to healthcare providers.

5.6 Cognitive/Neuropsychiatric Adverse Reactions

Adverse reactions most often associated with the use of topiramate, and therefore expected to be associated with the use of TROKENDI XR® were related to the central nervous system and were observed in the epilepsy population. In adults, the most frequent of these can be classified into three general categories: 1) Cognitive-related dysfunction (e.g., confusion, psychomotor slowing, difficulty with concentration/attention, difficulty with memory, speech or language problems, particularly word-finding difficulties), 2) Psychiatric/behavioral disturbances (e.g.,depression or mood problems), and 3) Somnolence or fatigue.

Adult Patients

Cognitive Related Dysfunction

The majority of cognitive-related adverse reactions were mild to moderate in severity, and they frequently occurred in isolation. Rapid titration rate and higher initial dose were associated with higher incidences of these reactions. Many of these reactions contributed to withdrawal from treatment [*see Adverse Reactions (6.1)*].

In the adjunctive epilepsy controlled trials conducted with topiramate (using rapid titration such as 100 mg per day to 200 mg per day weekly increments), the proportion of patients who experienced one or more cognitive-related adverse reactions was 42% for 200 mg per day, 41% for 400 mg per day, 52% for 600 mg per day, 56% for 800 and 1,000 mg per day, and 14% for placebo. These dose-related adverse re-

Continued on next page

actions began with a similar frequency in the titration or in the maintenance phase, although in some patients the events began during titration and persisted into the maintenance phase. Some patients who experienced one or more cognitive-related adverse reactions in the titration phase had a dose-related recurrence of these reactions in the maintenance phase.

In the monotherapy epilepsy controlled trial conducted with topiramate, the proportion of patients who experienced one or more cognitive-related adverse reactions was 19% for topiramate 50 mg per day and 26% for 400 mg per day.

Psychiatric/Behavioral Disturbances

Psychiatric/behavioral disturbances (depression or mood) were dose-related for the epilepsy population treated with topiramate.

Somnolence/Fatigue

Somnolence and fatigue were the adverse reactions most frequently reported during clinical trials of topiramate for adjunctive epilepsy. For the adjunctive epilepsy population, the incidence of somnolence did not differ substantially between 200 mg per day and 1,000 mg per day, but the incidence of fatigue was dose-related and increased at dosages above 400 mg per day. For the monotherapy epilepsy population in the 50 mg per day and 400 mg per day groups, the incidence of somnolence was dose-related (9% for the 50 mg per day group and 15% for the 400 mg per day group) and the incidence of fatigue was comparable in both treatment groups (14% each). For other uses not approved for TROKENDI XR®, somnolence and fatigue were dose-related and more common in the titration phase.

Additional nonspecific CNS events commonly observed with topiramate in the adjunctive epilepsy population include dizziness or ataxia.

Pediatric Patients

In double-blind adjunctive therapy and monotherapy epilepsy clinical studies conducted with topiramate, the incidences of cognitive/neuropsychiatric adverse reactions in pediatric patients were generally lower than observed in adults. These reactions included psychomotor slowing, difficulty with concentration/attention, speech disorders/related speech problems and language problems. The most frequently reported neuropsychiatric reactions in pediatric patients during adjunctive therapy double-blind studies were somnolence and fatigue. The most frequently reported neuropsychiatric reactions in pediatric patients in the 50 mg per day and 400 mg per day groups during the monotherapy double-blind study were headache, dizziness, anorexia, and somnolence.

No patients discontinued treatment due to any adverse reactions in the adjunctive epilepsy double-blind trials. In the monotherapy epilepsy double-blind trial conducted with immediate-release topiramate product, 1 pediatric patient (2%) in the 50 mg per day group and 7 pediatric patients (12%) in the 400 mg per day group discontinued treatment due to any adverse reactions. The most common adverse reaction associated with discontinuation of therapy was difficulty with concentration/attention; all occurred in the 400 mg per day group.

5.7   Fetal Toxicity

Topiramate can cause fetal harm when administered to a pregnant woman. Data from pregnancy registries indicate that infants exposed to topiramate *in utero* have an increased risk for cleft lip and/or cleft palate (oral clefts) and for being small for gestational age. In multiple species, oral administration of topiramate to pregnant animals at clinically relevant doses resulted in structural malformations, including craniofacial defects, and reduced body weights in offspring [*see Use in Specific Populations (8.1)*].

Consider the benefits and risks of TROKENDI XR® when administering the drug in women of childbearing potential, particularly when TROKENDI XR® is considered for a condition not usually associated with permanent injury or death [*see Use in Specific Populations (8.1)*]. TROKENDI XR® should be used during pregnancy only if the potential benefit outweighs the potential risk. If this drug is used during pregnancy, or if the patient becomes pregnant while taking this drug, the patient should be informed of the potential hazard to a fetus [*see Use in Specific Populations (8.1)*].

5.8   Withdrawal of Antiepileptic Drugs

In patients with or without a history of seizures or epilepsy, antiepileptic drugs including TROKENDI XR® should be gradually withdrawn to minimize the potential for seizures or increased seizure frequency [*see Clinical Studies (14)*]. In situations where rapid withdrawal of TROKENDI XR® is medically required, appropriate monitoring is recommended.

5.9   Hyperammonemia and Encephalopathy

Hyperammonemia/Encephalopathy Without Concomitant Valproic Acid (VPA)

Topiramate treatment has produced hyperammonemia (in some instances dose-related) in clinical investigational programs in very young pediatric patients (1 month to 24 months) who were treated with adjunctive topiramate for partial onset epilepsy (8% for placebo, 10% for 5 mg/kg/day, 0% for 15 mg/kg/day, 9% for 25 mg/kg/day). TROKENDI XR® is not approved as adjunctive treatment of partial onset seizures in pediatric patients less than 6 years old. In some patients, ammonia was markedly increased (greater than or equal to 50% above upper limit of normal). The hyperammonemia associated with topiramate treatment occurred with and without encephalopathy in placebo-controlled trials, and in an open-label, extension trial of infants with refractory epilepsy. Dose-related hyperammonemia was also observed in the extension trial in pediatric patients up to 2 years old. Clinical symptoms of hyperammonemic encephalopathy often include acute alterations in level of consciousness and/or cognitive function with lethargy or vomiting.

Hyperammonemia with and without encephalopathy has also been observed in postmarketing reports in patients who were taking topiramate without concomitant valproic acid (VPA).

Hyperammonemia/Encephalopathy With Concomitant Valproic Acid (VPA)

Concomitant administration of topiramate and valproic acid (VPA) has been associated with hyperammonemia with or without encephalopathy in patients who have tolerated either drug alone based upon postmarketing reports. Although hyperammonemia may be asymptomatic, clinical symptoms of hyperammonemic encephalopathy often include acute alterations in level of consciousness and/or cognitive function with lethargy or vomiting. In most cases, symptoms and signs abated with discontinuation of either drug. This adverse reaction is not due to a pharmacokinetic interaction.

Although TROKENDI XR® is not indicated for use in infants/toddlers (1 month to 24 months), topiramate with concomitant VPA clearly produced a dose-related increase in the incidence of hyperammonemia (above the upper limit of normal, 0% for placebo, 12% for 5 mg/kg/day, 7% for 15 mg/kg/day, 17% for 25 mg/kg/day) in an investigational program using topiramate. Markedly increased, dose-related hyperammonemia (0% for placebo and 5 mg/kg/day, 7% for 15 mg/kg/day, and 8% for 25 mg/kg/day) also occurred in these infants/toddlers. Dose-related hyperammonemia was similarly observed in a long-term, extension trial utilizing topiramate in these very young, pediatric patients [*see Use in Specific Populations (8.4)*].

Hyperammonemia with and without encephalopathy has also been observed in postmarketing reports in patients taking topiramate with valproic acid (VPA).

The hyperammonemia associated with topiramate treatment appears to be more common when used concomitantly with VPA.

Monitoring for Hyperammonemia

Patients with inborn errors of metabolism or reduced hepatic mitochondrial activity may be at an increased risk for hyperammonemia with or without encephalopathy. Although not studied, topiramate or TROKENDI XR® treatment or an interaction of concomitant topiramate-based product and valproic acid treatment may exacerbate existing defects or unmask deficiencies in susceptible persons.

In patients who develop unexplained lethargy, vomiting, or changes in mental status associated with any topiramate treatment, hyperammonemic encephalopathy should be considered and an ammonia level should be measured.

5.10   Kidney Stones

A total of 32/2086 (1.5%) of adults exposed to topiramate during its adjunctive epilepsy therapy development reported the occurrence of kidney stones, an incidence about 2 to 4 times greater than expected in a similar, untreated population. In the double-blind monotherapy epilepsy study, a total of 4/319 (1.3%) of adults exposed to topiramate reported the occurrence of kidney stones. As in the general population, the incidence of stone formation among topiramate treated patients was higher in men. Kidney stones have also been reported in pediatric patients taking topiramate for epilepsy. During long-term (up to 1 year) topiramate treatment in an open-label extension study of 284 pediatric patients 1 month to 24 months old with epilepsy, 7% developed kidney or bladder stones that were di-

agnosed clinically or by sonogram. TROKENDI XR® is not approved for pediatric patients less than 6 years old [*see Use in Specific Populations (8.4)*].

TROKENDI XR® would be expected to have the same effect as topiramate on the formation of kidney stones. An explanation for the association of topiramate and kidney stones may lay in the fact that topiramate is a carbonic anhydrase inhibitor. Carbonic anhydrase inhibitors (e.g., zonisamide, acetazolamide or dichlorphenamide) can promote stone formation by reducing urinary citrate excretion and by increasing urinary pH [*see Warnings and Precautions (5.3)*]. The concomitant use of TROKENDI XR® with any other drug producing metabolic acidosis, or potentially in patients on a ketogenic diet may create a physiological environment that increases the risk of kidney stone formation, and should therefore be avoided.

Increased fluid intake increases the urinary output, lowering the concentration of substances involved in stone formation. Hydration is recommended to reduce new stone formation.

5.11   Hypothermia with Concomitant Valproic Acid Use

Hypothermia, defined as an unintentional drop in body core temperature to less than 35°C (95°F) has been reported in association with topiramate use with concomitant valproic acid (VPA) both in the presence and in the absence of hyperammonemia. This adverse reaction in patients using concomitant topiramate and valproate can occur after starting topiramate treatment or after increasing the daily dose of topiramate [*see Drug Interactions (7.5)*]. Consideration should be given to stopping topiramate or valproate in patients who develop hypothermia, which may be manifested by a variety of clinical abnormalities including lethargy, confusion, coma, and significant alterations in other major organ systems such as the cardiovascular and respiratory systems. Clinical management and assessment should include examination of blood ammonia levels.

5.12   Paresthesia

Paresthesia (usually tingling of the extremities), an effect associated with the use of other carbonic anhydrase inhibitors, appears to be a common effect of topiramate. Paresthesia was more frequently reported in the monotherapy epilepsy trials conducted with topiramate than in the adjunctive therapy epilepsy trials conducted with the same product. In the majority of instances, paresthesia did not lead to treatment discontinuation.

5.13   Interaction with Other CNS Depressants

Topiramate is a CNS depressant. Concomitant administration of topiramate with other CNS depressant drugs can result in significant CNS depression. Patients should be watched carefully when TROKENDI XR® is co-administered with other CNS depressant drugs.

5.14   Visual Field Defects

Visual field defects (independent of elevated intraocular pressure) have been reported in clinical trials and in postmarketing experience in patients receiving topiramate. In clinical trials, most of these events were reversible after topiramate discontinuation. If visual problems occur at any time during topiramate treatment, consideration should be given to discontinuing the drug.

6   ADVERSE REACTIONS

The following serious adverse reactions are discussed in more detail in other sections of the labeling:
- Acute Myopia and Secondary Angle Closure Glaucoma [*see Warnings and Precautions (5.1)*]
- Oligohydrosis and Hyperthermia [*see Warnings and Precautions (5.2)*]
- Metabolic Acidosis [*see Warnings and Precautions (5.3)*]
- Suicidal Behavior and Ideation [*see Warnings and Precautions (5.5)*]
- Cognitive/Neuropsychiatric Adverse Reactions [*see Warnings and Precautions (5.6)*]
- Fetal Toxicity [*see Warnings and Precautions (5.7)* and *Use in Specific Populations (8.1)*]
- Withdrawal of Antiepileptic Drugs [*see Warnings and Precautions (5.8)*]
- Hyperammonemia and Encephalopathy (Without and With Concomitant Valproic Acid Use [*see Warnings and Precautions (5.9)*]
- Kidney Stones [*see Warnings and Precautions (5.10)*]
- Hypothermia with Concomitant Valproic Acid Use [*see Warnings and Precautions (5.11)*]
- Paresthesia [*see Warnings and Precautions (5.12)*]
- Visual Field Defects [*see Warnings and Precautions 5.14*]

The data described in the following sections were obtained using immediate-release topiramate tablets in studies of patients with epilepsy. TROKENDI XR® has not been studied in a randomized, placebo-controlled Phase III clinical study in the epilepsy patient population. However, it is expected that TROKENDI XR® would produce a similar adverse reaction profile as immediate-release topiramate.

6.1 Clinical Trials Experience

Because clinical trials are conducted under widely varying conditions, adverse reaction rates observed in the clinical trials of a drug cannot be directly compared to rates in the clinical trials of another drug and may not reflect the rates observed in clinical practice.

Increased Risk for Bleeding

Topiramate treatment is associated with an increased risk for bleeding. In a pooled analysis of placebocontrolled studies of approved and unapproved indications, bleeding was more frequently reported as an adverse event for topiramate than for placebo (4.5% versus 3.0% in adult patients, and 4.4% versus 2.3% in pediatric patients). In this analysis, the incidence of serious bleeding events for topiramate and placebo was 0.3% versus 0.2% for adult patients, and 0.4% versus 0% for pediatric patients.

Adverse bleeding reactions reported with topiramate ranged from mild epistaxis, ecchymosis, and increased menstrual bleeding to life-threatening hemorrhages. In patients with serious bleeding events, conditions that increased the risk for bleeding were often present, or patients were often taking drugs that cause thrombocytopenia (other antiepileptic drugs) or affect platelet function or coagulation (e.g., aspirin, nonsteroidal anti-inflammatory drugs, selective serotonin reuptake inhibitors, or warfarin or other anticoagulants).

Adverse Reactions Observed in Monotherapy Trial for Epilepsy

Adults 16 Years of Age and Older

The adverse reactions in the controlled trial (Study 1) that occurred most commonly in adults in the 400 mg per day group and at an incidence higher (≥ 5%) than in the 50 mg per day group were paresthesia, weight decrease, somnolence, anorexia, and difficulty with memory (see Table 3) [*see Clinical Studies (14.2)*].

Approximately 21% of the 159 adult patients in the 400 mg per day group who received topiramate as monotherapy in Study 1 discontinued therapy due to adverse reactions. The most common (greater than or equal to 2% more frequent than low-dose 50 mg per day topiramate) adverse reactions causing discontinuation in this trial were difficulty with memory, fatigue, asthenia, insomnia, somnolence and paresthesia.

Pediatric Patients 6 Years to Less Than 16 Years of Age

The adverse reactions in the controlled trial (Study 1) that occurred most commonly in pediatric patients in the 400 mg per day topiramate group and at an incidence higher (≥ 5%) than in the 50 mg per day group were fever, weight decrease, paresthesia, mood problems, cognitive problems, infection, and flushing (see Table 4) [*see Clinical Studies (14.2)*].

Approximately 14% of the 77 pediatric patients in the 400 mg per day group who received topiramate as monotherapy in the controlled clinical trial discontinued therapy due to adverse reactions. The most common (≥ 2% more frequent than in the 50 mg per day group) adverse reactions resulting in discontinuation in this trial were difficulty with concentration/attention, fever, flushing, and confusion.

Table 3: Incidence (%) of Adverse Reaction in the Monotherapy Epilepsy Trial in Adults[a] Where Incidence Was at Least 2% in the 400 mg/day Immediate-Release Topiramate Group and Greater Than the Rate in the 50 mg/day Immediate-Release Topiramate Group

Body System/	Immediate-release topiramate Dosage (mg/day)	
Adverse Reaction	50	400
	(N=160)	(N=159)
Body as a Whole-General Disorders		
Asthenia	4	6
Leg Pain	2	3
Chest Pain	1	2
Central & Peripheral Nervous System Disorders		
Paresthesia	21	40
Dizziness	13	14
Hypoesthesia	4	5
Ataxia	3	4
Hypertonia	0	3
Gastro-intestinal System Disorders		
Diarrhea	5	6
Constipation	1	4
Gastritis	0	3
Dry Mouth	1	3
Gastroesophageal Reflux	1	2
Liver and Biliary System Disorders		
Gamma-GT Increased	1	3
Metabolic and Nutritional Disorders		
Weight Decrease	6	16
Psychiatric Disorders		
Somnolence	9	15
Anorexia	4	14
Difficulty with Memory NOS	5	10
Insomnia	8	9
Depression	7	9
Difficulty with Concentration/Attention	7	8
Anxiety	4	6
Psychomotor Slowing	3	5
Mood Problems	2	5
Confusion	3	4
Cognitive Problem NOS	1	4
Libido Decreased	0	3
Reproductive Disorders, Female		
Vaginal Hemorrhage	0	3
Red Blood Cell Disorders		
Anemia	1	2
Resistance Mechanism Disorders		
Infection Viral	6	8
Infection	2	3
Respiratory System Disorders		
Bronchitis	3	4
Rhinitis	2	4
Dyspnea	1	2
Skin and Appendages Disorders		
Rash	1	4
Pruritus	1	4
Acne	2	3
Special Senses Other, Disorders		
Taste Perversion	3	5
Urinary System Disorders		
Cystitis	1	3
Renal Calculus	0	3
Urinary Tract Infection	1	2
Dysuria	0	2
Micturition Frequency	0	2

[a]Values represent the percentage of patients reporting a given adverse reaction. Patients may have reported more than one adverse reaction during the study and can be included in more than one adverse reaction category

Table 4: Incidence (%) of Adverse Reactions in the Monotherapy Epilepsy Trial in Pediatric Patients (Ages 6 to Less Than 16 Years)[a] Where Incidence Was at Least 2% in the 400 mg/day Immediate-Release Topiramate Group and Greater than the Rate in the 50 mg/day Immediate-Release Topiramate Group

Body System/	Immediate-release topiramate Dosage (mg/day)	
Adverse Reaction	50	400
	(N=74)	(N=77)
Body as a Whole-General Disorders		
Fever	1	12
Asthenia	0	3
Central & Peripheral Nervous System Disorders		
Paresthesia	3	12
Muscle Contractions Involuntary	0	3
Vertigo	0	3
Gastro-Intestinal System Disorders		
Diarrhea	8	9
Metabolic and Nutritional Disorders		
Weight Decrease	7	17
Platelet, Bleeding & Clotting Disorders		
Epistaxis	0	4
Psychiatric Disorders		
Difficulty with Concentration/Attention	7	10
Mood Problems	1	8
Cognitive Problems	1	6
Difficulty with Memory	1	3
Confusion	0	3
Depression	0	3
Personality Disorder (Behavior Problems)	0	3
Red Blood Cell Disorders		
Anemia	1	3

Continued on next page

Reproductive Disorders, Female[b]

Intermenstrual Bleeding	0	3

Resistance Mechanism Disorders

Infection	3	8
Infection Viral	3	6

Respiratory System Disorders

Upper Respiratory Tract Infection	16	18
Rhinitis	5	6
Bronchitis	1	5
Sinusitis	1	4

Skin and Appendages Disorders

Rash	3	4
Alopecia	1	4

Urinary System Disorders

Urinary Incontinence	1	3
Micturition Frequency	0	3

Vascular (Extracardiac) Disorders

Flushing	0	5

[a]Values represent the percentage of patients reporting a given adverse event. Patients may have reported more than one event during the study and can be included in more than one adverse event category
[b] N with Reproductive Disorders, Female-Incidence calculated relative to the number of females; Pediatric TPM 50 mg n=40; Pediatric TPM 400 mg n=33

Adverse Reactions Observed in Adjunctive Therapy Epilepsy Trials

The most commonly observed adverse reactions associated with the use of topiramate at dosages of 200 to 400 mg per day in controlled trials in adults with partial onset seizures, primary generalized tonic-clonic seizures, or Lennox-Gastaut syndrome that were seen at greater frequency in topiramate-treated patients and did not appear to be dose-related were: somnolence, ataxia, speech disorders and related speech problems, psychomotor slowing, abnormal vision, difficulty with memory, paresthesia and diplopia [*see Table 5*] [*see Clinical Studies (14.3, 14.4, and 14.5)*]. The most common dose-related adverse reactions at dosages of 200 mg to 1,000 mg per day were: fatigue, nervousness, difficulty with concentration or attention, confusion, depression, anorexia, language problems, anxiety, mood problems, and weight decrease [*see Table 7*].

Adverse reactions associated with the use of topiramate at dosages of 5 mg/kg/day to 9 mg/kg/day in controlled trials in pediatric patients with partial onset seizures, primary generalized tonic-clonic seizures, or Lennox-Gastaut syndrome that were seen at greater frequency in topiramate-treated patients were: fatigue, somnolence, anorexia, nervousness, difficulty with concentration/attention, difficulty with memory, aggressive reaction, and weight decrease [*see Table 8*].

In controlled clinical trials in adults, 11% of patients receiving topiramate 200 to 400 mg per day as adjunctive therapy discontinued due to adverse reactions. This rate appeared to increase at dosages above 400 mg per day. Adverse events associated with discontinuing therapy included somnolence, dizziness, anxiety, difficulty with concentration or attention, fatigue, and paresthesia and increased at dosages above 400 mg per day. None of the pediatric patients who received topiramate adjunctive therapy at 5 mg/kg/day to 9 mg/kg/day in controlled clinical trials discontinued due to adverse reactions.

Approximately 28% of the 1757 adults with epilepsy who received topiramate at dosages of 200 mg to 1,600 mg per day in clinical studies discontinued treatment because of adverse reactions; an individual patient could have reported more than one adverse reaction. These adverse reactions were: psychomotor slowing (4.0%), fatigue (3.2%), confusion (3.1%), somnolence (3.2%), difficulty with concentration/attention (2.9%), anorexia

(2.7%), depression (2.6%), dizziness (2.5%), weight decrease (2.5%), nervousness (2.3%), ataxia (2.1%), and paresthesia (2.0%). Approximately 11% of the 310 pediatric patients who received topiramate at dosages up to 30 mg/kg/day discontinued due to adverse reactions. Adverse reactions associated with discontinuing therapy included aggravated convulsions (2.3%), difficulty with concentration/attention (1.6%), language problems (1.3%), personality disorder (1.3%), and somnolence (1.3%).

Incidence in Epilepsy Controlled Clinical Trials – Adjunctive Therapy – Partial Onset Seizures, Primary Generalized Tonic-Clonic Seizures, and Lennox-Gastaut Syndrome
Table 5 lists adverse reactions that occurred in at least 1% of adults treated with 200 to 400 mg per day topiramate in controlled trials that were numerically more common at this dose than in the patients treated with placebo. In general, most patients who experienced adverse reactions during the first eight weeks of these trials no longer experienced them by their last visit. Table 8 lists adverse reactions that occurred in at least 1% of pediatric patients treated with 5 mg/kg to 9 mg/kg topiramate in controlled trials that were numerically more common than in patients treated with placebo.
Other Adverse Reactions Observed During Double-Blind Epilepsy Adjunctive Therapy Trials
Other adverse reactions that occurred in more than 1% of adults treated with 200 mg to 400 mg of topiramate in placebo-controlled epilepsy trials but with equal or greater frequency in the placebo group were headache, injury, anxiety, rash, pain, convulsions aggravated, coughing, fever, diarrhea, vomiting, muscle weakness, insomnia, personality disorder, dysmenorrhea, upper respiratory tract infection, and eye pain.
[See table 5 on pages 1077 to 1079]
Adverse Reactions Observed in Adjunctive Therapy Trial in Adults with Partial Onset Seizures (Study 7)
Study 7 was a randomized, double-blind, adjunctive, placebo-controlled, parallel group study with 3 treatment arms: 1) placebo; 2) topiramate 200 mg per day with a 25 mg per day starting dose, increased by 25 mg per day each week for 8 weeks until the 200 mg per day maintenance dose was reached; and 3) topiramate 200 mg per day with a 50 mg per day starting dose, increased by 50 mg per day each week for 4 weeks until the 200 mg per day maintenance dose was reached. All patients were maintained on concomitant carbamazepine with or without another concomitant antiepileptic drug.
The incidence of adverse reactions (Table 6) did not differ significantly between the 2 topiramate regimens. Because the frequencies of adverse reactions reported in this study were markedly lower than those reported in the previous epilepsy studies, they cannot be directly compared with data obtained in other studies.

Table 6: Incidence (%) of Adverse Reactions in Placebo Controlled, Adjunctive Trial in Adults with Partial Onset Seizures (Study 7)[a,b,c]

Body System/		Topiramate Dosage (mg per day)
Adverse Reaction[c]	Placebo	200
	(N=92)	(N=171)
Body as a Whole-General Disorders		
Fatigue	4	9
Chest pain	1	2
Cardiovascular Disorders, General		
Hypertension	0	2
Central & Peripheral Nervous System Disorders		
Paresthesia	2	9
Dizziness	4	7
Tremor	2	3
Hypoesthesia	0	2
Leg cramps	0	2
Language problems	0	2
Gastro-intestinal System Disorders		
Abdominal pain	3	5
Constipation	0	4
Diarrhea	1	2
Dyspepsia	0	2
Dry mouth	0	2
Hearing and Vestibular Disorders		
Tinnitus	0	2
Metabolic and Nutritional Disorders		
Weight decrease	4	8
Psychiatric Disorders		
Somnolence	9	15
Anorexia	7	9
Nervousness	2	9
Difficulty with concentration/attention	0	5
Insomnia	3	4
Difficulty with memory	1	2
Aggressive reaction	0	2
Respiratory System Disorders		
Rhinitis	0	4
Urinary System Disorders		
Cystitis	0	2
Vision Disorder		
Diplopia	0	2
Vision abnormal	0	2

[a]Patients in these adjunctive trials were receiving 1 to 2 concomitant antiepileptic drugs in addition to topiramate or placebo

[b]Values represent the percentage of patients reporting a given adverse reaction. Patients may have reported more than one adverse reaction during the study and can be included in more than one adverse reaction category

[c]Adverse reactions reported by at least 2% of patients in the topiramate 200 mg per day group and more common than in the placebo group

[See table 7 on page 1079]

Table 8: Incidence (%) of Adverse Reaction in Placebo-Controlled, Adjunctive Epilepsy Trial in Pediatric Patients (Ages 2 Years to 16 Years)[a,b,c] (Study 8)

Body System/	Placebo	Topiramate
Adverse Reaction	(N=101)	(N=98)
Body as a Whole-General Disorders		
Fatigue	5	16
Injury	13	14
Allergic reaction	1	2
Back pain	0	1
Pallor	0	1

Table 5: Incidence (%) of Adverse Reactions in Placebo-Controlled, Adjunctive Epilepsy Trials in Adults [a,b,c]

Body System/ Adverse Reaction[c]	Placebo (N=291)	Topiramate Dosage (mg per day) 200-400 (N=183)	600-1,000 (N=414)
Body as a Whole- General Disorders			
Fatigue	13	15	30
Asthenia	1	6	3
Back pain	4	5	3
Chest pain	3	4	2
Influenza-like symptoms	2	3	4
Leg pain	2	2	4
Hot flushes	1	2	1
Allergy	1	2	3
Edema	1	2	1
Body odor	0	1	0
Rigors	0	1	<1
Central & Peripheral Nervous System Disorders			
Dizziness	15	25	32
Ataxia	7	16	14
Speech disorders/Related speech problems	2	13	11
Paresthesia	4	11	19
Nystagmus	7	10	11
Tremor	6	9	9
Language problems	1	6	10
Coordination abnormal	2	4	4
Hypoesthesia	1	2	1
Gait abnormal	1	3	2
Muscle contractions involuntary	1	2	2
Stupor	0	2	1
Vertigo	1	1	2
Gastro-intestinal System Disorders			
Nausea	8	10	12
Dyspepsia	6	7	6
Abdominal pain	4	6	7
Constipation	2	4	3
Gastroenteritis	1	2	1
Dry mouth	1	2	4
Gingivitis	<1	1	1
GI disorder	<1	1	0
Hearing and Vestibular Disorders			
Hearing decreased	1	2	1
Metabolic and Nutritional Disorders			
Weight decrease	3	9	13

This table is continued on the next page

Cardiovascular Disorders, General		
Hypertension	0	1
Central & Peripheral Nervous System Disorders		
Gait abnormal	5	8
Ataxia	2	6
Hyperkinesia	4	5
Dizziness	2	4
Speech disorders/Related speech problems	2	4
Hyporeflexia	0	2
Convulsions grand mal	0	1
Fecal incontinence	0	1
Paresthesia	0	1
Gastro-Intestinal System Disorders		
Nausea	5	6
Saliva increased	4	6
Constipation	4	5
Gastroenteritis	2	3
Dysphagia	0	1
Flatulence	0	1
Gastroesophageal reflux	0	1
Glossitis	0	1
Gum hyperplasia	0	1
Heart Rate and Rhythm Disorders		
Bradycardia	0	1
Metabolic and Nutritional Disorders		
Weight decrease	1	9
Thirst	1	2
Hypoglycemia	0	1
Weight increase	0	1
Platelet, Bleeding & Clotting Disorders		
Purpura	4	8
Epistaxis	1	4
Hematoma	0	1
Prothrombin increased	0	1
Thrombocytopenia	0	1
Psychiatric Disorders		
Somnolence	16	26
Anorexia	15	24
Nervousness	7	14
Personality disorder (Behavior Problems)	9	11
Difficulty with concentration/ attention	2	10

Continued on next page

Aggressive reaction	4	9
Insomnia	7	8
Difficulty with memory	0	5
Confusion	3	4
Psychomotor slowing	2	3
Appetite increased	0	1
Neurosis	0	1
Reproductive Disorders, Female		
Leukorrhea	0	2
Resistance Mechanism Disorders		
Infection viral	3	7
Respiratory System Disorders		
Pneumonia	1	5
Respiratory disorder	0	1
Skin and Appendages Disorders		
Skin Disorder	2	3
Alopecia	1	2
Dermatitis	0	2
Hypertrichosis	1	2
Rash erythematous	0	2
Eczema	0	1
Seborrhea	0	1
Skin discoloration	0	1
Urinary System Disorders		
Urinary incontinence	2	4
Nocturia	0	1
Vision Disorders		
Eye abnormality	1	2
Vision abnormal	1	2
Diplopia	0	1
Lacrimation abnormal	0	1
Myopia	0	1
White Cell and RES Disorders		
Leukopenia	0	2

[a] Patients in these adjunctive trials were receiving 1 to 2 concomitant antiepileptic drugs in addition to topiramate or placebo
[b] Values represent the percentage of patients reporting a given adverse reaction. Patients may have reported more than one adverse reaction during the study and can be included in more than one adverse reaction category
[c] Reactions that occurred in at least 1% of topiramate-treated patients and occurred more frequently in topiramate-treated than placebo-treated patients

Laboratory Abnormalities
Topiramate decreases serum bicarbonate [*see Warnings and Precautions (5.3)*]
Topiramate treatment with or without concomitant valproic acid (VPA) can cause hyperammonemia with or without encephalopathy [*see Warnings and Precautions (5.9)*].
Immediate-release topiramate treatment was associated with changes in several clinical laboratory analytes in randomized, double-blind, placebo-controlled studies. Similar effects should be anticipated with use of TROKENDI XR®. Controlled trials of adjunctive topiramate treatment of adults for partial onset seizures showed an increased inci-

Table 5: *(Cont.)* Incidence (%) of Adverse Reactions in Placebo-Controlled, Adjunctive Epilepsy Trials in Adults [a,b,c]

Body System/	Topiramate Dosage (mg per day)		
	Placebo	200-400	600-1,000
Adverse Reaction[c]	(N=291)	(N=183)	(N=414)
Musculoskeletal System Disorders			
Myalgia	1	2	2
Skeletal pain	0	1	0
Platelet, Bleeding & Clotting Disorders			
Epistaxis	1	2	1
Psychiatric Disorders			
Somnolence	12	29	28
Nervousness	6	16	19
Psychomotor slowing	2	13	21
Difficulty with memory	3	12	14
Anorexia	4	10	12
Confusion	5	11	14
Depression	5	5	13
Difficulty with concentration/attention	2	6	14
Mood problems	2	4	9
Agitation	2	3	3
Aggressive reaction	2	3	3
Emotional liability	1	3	3
Cognitive problems	1	3	3
Libido decreased	1	2	<1
Apathy	1	1	3
Depersonalization	1	1	2
Reproductive Disorders, Female			
Breast pain	2	4	0
Amenorrhea	1	2	2
Menorrhagia	0	2	1
Menstrual disorder	1	2	1
Reproductive Disorders, Male			
Prostatic disorder	<1	2	0
Resistance Mechanism Disorders			
Infection	1	2	1
Infection viral	1	2	<1
Moniliasis	<1	1	0
Respiratory System Disorders			
Pharyngitis	2	6	3
Rhinitis	6	7	6
Sinusitis	4	5	6
Dyspnea	1	1	2

This table is continued on the next page

Table 5: *(Cont.)* Incidence (%) of Adverse Reactions in Placebo-Controlled, Adjunctive Epilepsy Trials in Adults [a,b,c]

Body System/ Adverse Reaction[c]	Topiramate Dosage (mg per day)		
	Placebo (N=291)	200-400 (N=183)	600-1,000 (N=414)
Skin and Appendages Disorders			
Skin disorder	<1	2	1
Sweating increased	<1	1	<1
Rash, erythematous	<1	1	<1
Special Senses Other, Disorders			
Taste perversion	0	2	4
Urinary System Disorders			
Hematuria	1	2	<1
Urinary tract infection	1	2	3
Micturition frequency	1	1	2
Urinary incontinence	<1	2	1
Urine abnormal	0	1	<1
Vision Disorders			
Vision abnormal	2	13	10
Diplopia	5	10	10
White Cell and RES Disorders			
Leukopenia	1	2	1

[a]Patients in these adjunctive trials were receiving 1 to 2 concomitant antiepileptic drugs in addition to topiramate or placebo

[b]Values represent the percentage of patients reporting a given reaction. Patient may have reported more than one adverse reaction during the study and can be included in more than one adverse reaction category.

[c]Adverse reactions reported by at least 1% of patients in the topiramate 200 mg to 400 mg per day group and more common than in the placebo group

Table 7: Incidence (%) of Dose-Related Adverse Reactions From Placebo-Controlled, Adjunctive Trials in Adults With Partial Onset Seizures (Studies 2 through 7)[a]

Adverse Reaction	(Topiramate) Dosage (mg per day)			
	Placebo (N=216)	200 (N=45)	400 (N=68)	600-1,000 (N=414)
Fatigue	13	11	12	30
Nervousness	7	13	18	19
Difficulty with concentration/attention	1	7	9	14
Confusion	4	9	10	14
Depression	6	9	7	13
Anorexia	4	4	6	12
Language Problems	<1	2	9	10
Anxiety	6	2	3	10
Mood Problems	2	0	6	9
Weight Decrease	3	4	9	13

[a] Dose-response studies were not conducted for other adult indications or for pediatric indications

dence of markedly decreased serum phosphorus (6% topiramate, 2% placebo), markedly increased serum alkaline phosphatase (3% topiramate, 1% placebo), and decreased serum potassium (0.4 % topiramate, 0.1 % placebo). The clinical significance of these abnormalities has not been clearly established.

Changes in several clinical laboratory results (increased creatinine, BUN, alkaline phosphatase, total protein, total eosinophil count and decreased potassium) have been observed in a clinical investigational program in very young (2 years and younger) pediatric patients who were treated with adjunctive topiramate for partial onset seizures [see *Use in Specific Populations (8.4)*].

6.2 Postmarketing Experience

The following adverse reactions have been identified during post-approval use of topiramate. Because these reactions are reported voluntarily from a population of uncertain size, it is not always possible to reliably estimate their frequency or establish a causal relationship to drug exposure. The listing is alphabetized: bullous skin reactions (including erythema multiforme, Stevens-Johnson syndrome, toxic epidermal necrolysis), hepatic failure (including fatalities), hepatitis, maculopathy, pancreatitis, and pemphigus.

7 DRUG INTERACTIONS

7.1 Alcohol

Alcohol use is contraindicated within 6 hours prior to and 6 hours after TROKENDI XR® administration [see *Contraindications (4) and Warnings and Precautions (5.4)*].

7.2 Oral Contraceptives

Exposure to ethinyl estradiol was statistically significantly decreased when topiramate (at doses above 200 mg) was given as adjunctive therapy in patients taking valproic acid. However, norethindrone exposure was not significantly affected.

In another pharmacokinetic interaction study in healthy volunteers with a concomitantly administered combination oral contraceptive product containing 1 mg norethindrone (NET) plus 35 mcg ethinyl estradiol (EE), topiramate, given in the absence of other medications at doses of 50 to 200 mg per day, was not associated with statistically significant changes in mean exposure to either component of the oral contraceptive.

The possibility of decreased contraceptive efficacy and increased breakthrough bleeding should be considered in patients taking combination oral contraceptive products with TROKENDI XR®. Patients taking estrogen-containing contraceptives should be asked to report any change in their bleeding patterns. Contraceptive efficacy can be decreased even in the absence of breakthrough bleeding [see *Clinical Pharmacology (12.3)*].

7.3 Antiepileptic Drugs

Concomitant administration of phenytoin or carbamazepine with topiramate decreased plasma concentrations of topiramate [see *Clinical Pharmacology (12.3)*].

Concomitant administration of valproic acid and topiramate has been associated with hyperammonemia with and without encephalopathy. Concomitant administration of topiramate with valproic acid has also been associated with hypothermia (with and without hyperammonemia) in patients who have tolerated either drug alone. It may be prudent to examine blood ammonia levels in patients in whom the onset of hypothermia has been reported [see *Warnings and Precautions (5.8,5.9) and Clinical Pharmacology (12.3)*].

Numerous AEDs are substrates of the CYP enzyme system. *In vitro* studies indicate that topiramate does not inhibit enzyme activity for CYP1A2, CYP2A6, CYP2B6, CYP2C9, CYP2D6, CYP2E1, and CYP3A4/5 isozymes. *In vitro* studies indicate that immediate-release topiramate is a mild inhibitor of CYP2C19 and a mild inducer of CYP3A4. The same drug interactions can be expected with the use of TROKENDI XR®.

7.4 CNS Depressants

Topiramate is a CNS depressant. Concomitant administration of topiramate with other CNS depressant drugs or alcohol can result in significant CNS depression [see *Warnings and Precautions (5.13)*].

7.5 Other Carbonic Anhydrase Inhibitors

Concomitant use of topiramate, a carbonic anhydrase inhibitor, with any other carbonic anhydrase inhibitor (e.g., zonisamide, acetazolamide or dichlorphenamide), may increase the severity of metabolic acidosis and may also increase the risk of kidney stone formation. Patient should

Continued on next page

be monitored for the appearance or worsening of metabolic acidosis when TROKENDI XR® is given concomitantly with another carbonic anhydrase inhibitor [see *Clinical Pharmacology (12.3)*].

7.6 Metformin

Topiramate treatment can frequently cause metabolic acidosis, a condition for which the use of metformin is contraindicated. The concomitant use of TROKENDI XR® and metformin is contraindicated in patients with metabolic acidosis [see *Clinical Pharmacology (12.3)*].

7.7 Lithium

In patients, there was an observed increase in systemic exposure of lithium following topiramate doses of up to 600 mg per day. Lithium levels should be monitored when co-administered with high-dose TROKENDI XR® [see *Clinical Pharmacology (12.3)*].

8 USE IN SPECIFIC POPULATIONS

8.1 Pregnancy

Pregnancy Exposure Registry

There is a pregnancy exposure registry that monitors pregnancy outcomes in women exposed to topiramate during pregnancy. Patients should be encouraged to enroll in the North American Antiepileptic Drug (NAAED) Pregnancy Registry if they become pregnant. This registry is collecting information about the safety of antiepileptic drugs during pregnancy. To enroll, patients can call the toll-free number 1-888-233-2334. Information about the North American Drug Pregnancy Registry can be found at http://www.aedpregnancyregistry.org/.

Risk Summary

Topiramate can cause fetal harm when administered to a pregnant woman. Data from pregnancy registries indicate that infants exposed to topiramate *in utero* have increased risk for cleft lip and/or cleft palate (oral clefts) and for being small for gestational age [see *Human Data*].

In multiple animal species, topiramate demonstrated developmental toxicity, including teratogenicity, in the absence of maternal toxicity at clinically relevant doses [see *Animal Data*].

In the U.S. general population, the estimated background risk of major birth defects and miscarriage in clinically recognized pregnancies is 2-4% and 15-20%, respectively.

Clinical Considerations

Fetal/Neonatal Adverse reactions

Consider the benefits and risks of topiramate when prescribing this drug to women of childbearing potential, particularly when topiramate is considered for a condition not usually associated with permanent injury or death. Because of the risk of oral clefts to the fetus, which occur in the first trimester of pregnancy before many women know they are pregnant, all women of childbearing potential should be informed of the potential risk to the fetus from exposure to topiramate. Women who are planning a pregnancy should be counseled regarding the relative risks and benefits of topiramate use during pregnancy, and alternative therapeutic options should be considered for these patients.

Labor or Delivery

Although the effect of topiramate on labor and delivery in humans has not been established, the development of topiramate-induced metabolic acidosis in the mother and/or in the fetus might affect the fetus' ability to tolerate labor [see *Use in Specific Populations (8.1)*].

Topiramate treatment can cause metabolic acidosis [see *Warnings and Precautions (5.3)*]. The effect of topiramate-induced metabolic acidosis has not been studied in pregnancy; however, metabolic acidosis in pregnancy (due to other causes) can cause decreased fetal growth, decreased fetal oxygenation, and fetal death, and may affect the fetus' ability to tolerate labor. Pregnant patients should be monitored for metabolic acidosis and treated as in the nonpregnant state [see *Warnings and Precautions (5.3)*]. Newborns of mothers treated with topiramate should be monitored for metabolic acidosis because of transfer of topiramate to the fetus and possible occurrence of transient metabolic acidosis following birth.

Data

Human Data

Data from the NAAED Pregnancy Registry indicate an increased risk of oral clefts in infants exposed to topiramate monotherapy during the first trimester of pregnancy. The prevalence of oral clefts was 1.2% compared to a prevalence of 0.39% - 0.46% in infants exposed to other AEDs, and a prevalence of 0.12% in infants of mothers without epilepsy or treatment with other AEDs. For comparison, the Centers for Disease Control and Prevention (CDC) reviewed avail-

able data on oral clefts in the United States and found a similar background rate of 0.17%. The relative risk of oral clefts in topiramate-exposed pregnancies in the NAAED Pregnancy Registry was 9.6 (95% Confidence Interval=[CI] 4.0-23.0) as compared to the risk in a background population of untreated women. The UK Epilepsy and Pregnancy Register reported a similarly increased prevalence of oral clefts of 3.2% among infants exposed to topiramate monotherapy. The observed rate of oral clefts was 16 times higher than the background rate in the UK, which is approximately 0.2%.

Data from the NAAED pregnancy registry and a population-based birth registry cohort indicate that exposure to topiramate in utero is associated with an increased risk of small for gestational age (SGA) newborns (birth weight <10th percentile). In the NAAED pregnancy registry, 18% of topiramate-exposed newborns were SGA compared to 7% of newborns exposed to a reference AED, and 5% of newborns of mothers without epilepsy and without AED exposure. In the Medical Birth Registry of Norway (MBRN), a population-based pregnancy registry, 25% of newborns in the topiramate monotherapy exposure group were SGA compared to 9 % in the comparison group who were unexposed to AEDs. The long-term consequences of the SGA findings are not known.

Animal Data

When topiramate (20, 100, and 500 mg/kg/day) was administered orally to pregnant mice during the period of organogenesis, the incidence of fetal malformations (primarily craniofacial defects) was increased at all doses. Fetal body weights and skeletal ossification were reduced at the highest dose tested in conjunction with decreased maternal body weight gain. A no-effect dose for embryofetal developmental toxicity in mice was not identified. The lowest dose tested, which was associated with teratogenic effects, is less than the maximum recommended human dose (MRHD) of 400 mg/day on a body surface area (mg/m^2) basis.

In pregnant rats administered topiramate (20, 100, and 500 mg/kg/day or 0.2, 2.5, 30, and 400 mg/kg/day) orally during the period of organogenesis, the frequency of limb malformations (ectrodactyly, micromelia, and amelia) was increased in fetuses at 400 or 500 mg/kg/day. Embryotoxicity (reduced fetal body weights, increased incidences of structural variations) was observed at doses as low as 20 mg/kg/day. Clinical signs of maternal toxicity were seen at 400 mg/kg/day and above, and maternal body weight gain was reduced at doses of 100 mg/kg/day or greater. The no-effect dose for embryofetal developmental toxicity in rats is less than the MRHD on a mg/m^2 basis.

In pregnant rabbits administered topiramate (20, 60, and 180 mg/kg/day or 10, 35, and 120 mg/kg/day) orally during organogenesis, embryofetal mortality was increased at 35 mg/kg/day and teratogenic effects (primarily rib and vertebral malformations) were observed at 120 mg/kg/day. Evidence of maternal toxicity (decreased body weight gain, clinical signs, and/or mortality) was seen at 35 mg/kg/day and above. The no-effect dose (20 mg/kg/day) for embryofetal developmental toxicity in rabbits is equivalent to the MRHD on a mg/m^2 basis.

When topiramate (0.2, 4, 20, and 100 mg/kg/day or 2, 20, and 200 mg/kg/day) was administered orally to female rats during the latter part of gestation and throughout lactation, offspring exhibited decreased viability and delayed physical development at 200 mg/kg/day and reductions in pre-and/or postweaning body weight gain at 2 mg/kg/day and above. Maternal toxicity (decreased body weight gain, clinical signs) was evident at 100 mg/kg or greater. In a rat embryofetal development study which included postnatal assessment of offspring, oral administration of topiramate (0.2, 2.5, 30, and 400 mg/kg/day) to pregnant animals during the period of organogenesis resulted in delayed physical development at 400 mg/kg/day and persistent reductions in body weight gain at 30 mg/kg/day and higher in the offspring. The no-effect dose (0.2 mg/kg/day) for pre- and postnatal developmental toxicity is less than the MRHD on a mg/m^2 basis.

8.2 Lactation

Risk Summary

Topiramate is excreted in human milk [see *Data*]. The effects of topiramate exposure in breastfed infants are unknown.

The developmental and health benefits of breastfeeding should be considered along with the mother's clinical need for TROKENDI XR® and any potential adverse effects on the breastfed infant from TROKENDI XR® or from the underlying maternal condition.

Data

Limited data from 5 women with epilepsy treated with topiramate during lactation showed drug levels in milk similar to those in maternal plasma.

8.3 Females and Males of Reproductive Potential

Contraception

Women of childbearing potential who are not planning a pregnancy should use effective contraception because of the risks to the fetus of oral clefts and of being small for gestational age [see *Drug Interactions (7.2)* and *Use in Specific Populations (8.1)*].

8.4 Pediatric Use

Seizures in Pediatric Patients 6 Years of Age and Older

The safety and effectiveness of TROKENDI XR® for treatment of partial onset seizures, primary generalized tonic-clonic seizures, or Lennox Gastaut syndromes in pediatric patients at least 6 years of age is based on controlled trials with immediate-release topiramate [see *Clinical Studies (14.2, 14.3, 14.4* and *14.5)*].

The adverse reactions in pediatric patients treated for partial onset seizure, primary generalized tonic-clonic seizures, or Lennox Gastaut syndrome are similar to those seen in adults [see *Warnings and Precautions (5)* and *Adverse Reactions (6)*].

These include, but are not limited to:

• oligohydrosis and hyperthermia [see *Warnings and Precautions (5.2)*].

• dose-related increased incidence of metabolic acidosis [see *Warnings and Precautions (5.3)*].

• dose-related increased incidence of hyperammonemia [see *Warnings and Precautions (5.9)*].

Not Recommended for Pediatric Patients Younger than 6 Years of Age

The safety and effectiveness of TROKENDI XR® for treatment of partial onset seizures, primary generalized tonic-clonic seizures, or Lennox Gastaut syndromes in pediatric patients younger than 6 years of age has not been established.

Because the capsule must be swallowed whole, and may not be sprinkled on food, crushed or chewed, TROKENDI XR® is recommended only for children age 6 or older.

The following pediatric use information for adjunctive treatment for partial onset epilepsy in infants and toddlers (1 to 24 months) is based on studies conducted with immediate-release topiramate, which failed to demonstrate efficacy.

Safety and effectiveness of immediate-release topiramate in patients below the age of 2 years have not been established for the adjunctive therapy treatment of partial onset seizures, primary generalized tonic-clonic seizures, or seizures associated with Lennox-Gastaut syndrome. In a single randomized, double-blind, placebocontrolled investigational trial, the efficacy, safety, and tolerability of immediate-release topiramate oral liquid and sprinkle formulations as an adjunct to concurrent antiepileptic drug therapy in infants 1 to 24 months of age with refractory partial onset seizures, was assessed. After 20 days of double-blind treatment, immediate-release topiramate (at fixed doses of 5 mg/kg, 15 mg/kg, and 25 mg/kg per day) did not demonstrate efficacy compared with placebo in controlling seizures.

In general, the adverse reaction profile in this population was similar to that of older pediatric patients, although results from the above controlled study, and an open-label, long-term extension study in these infants/toddlers (1 to 24 months old) suggested some adverse reactions not previously observed in older pediatric patients and adults; i.e., growth/length retardation, certain clinical laboratory abnormalities, and other adverse reactions that occurred with a greater frequency and/or greater severity than had been recognized previously from studies in older pediatric patients or adults for various indications.

These very young pediatric patients appeared to experience an increased risk for infections (any topiramate dose 12%, placebo 0%) and of respiratory disorders (any topiramate dose 40%, placebo 16%). The following adverse reactions were observed in at least 3% of patients on immediate-release topiramate and were 3% to 7% more frequent than in patients on placebo: viral infection, bronchitis, pharyngitis, rhinitis, otitis media, upper respiratory infection, cough, and bronchospasm. A generally similar profile was observed in older children [see *Adverse Reactions (6)*].

Immediate-release topiramate resulted in an increased incidence of patients with increased creatinine (any topiramate dose 5%, placebo 0%), BUN (any topiramate dose 3%, placebo 0%), and protein (any topiramate dose 34%, placebo 6%), and an increased incidence of decreased potassium (any topiramate dose 7%, placebo 0%). This increased frequency of abnormal values was not dose related. Creatinine was the only analyte showing a noteworthy increased incidence (topiramate 25 mg/kg/day 5%, placebo 0%) of a markedly abnormal increase [*see Adverse Reactions (6.1)*]. The significance of these findings is uncertain.

Immediate-release topiramate treatment also produced a dose-related increase in the percentage of patients who had a shift from normal at baseline to high/increased (above the normal reference range) in total eosinophil count at the end of treatment. The incidence of these abnormal shifts was 6% for placebo, 10% for 5 mg/kg/day, 9% for 15 mg/kg/day, 14% for 25 mg/kg/day, and 11% for any topiramate dose [*see Adverse Reactions (6.1)*]. There was a mean dose-related increase in alkaline phosphatase. The significance of these findings is uncertain.

Treatment with immediate-release topiramate for up to 1 year was associated with reductions in Z SCORES for length, weight, and head circumference [*see Warnings and Precautions (5.3) and Adverse Reactions (6)*].

In open-label, uncontrolled experience, increasing impairment of adaptive behavior was documented in behavioral testing over time in this population. There was a suggestion that this effect was dose-related. However, because of the absence of an appropriate control group, it is not known if this decrement in function was treatment related or reflects the patient's underlying disease (e.g., patients who received higher doses may have more severe underlying disease) [*see Warnings and Precautions (5.6)*].

In this open-label, uncontrolled study, the mortality was 37 deaths/1000 patient years. It is not possible to know whether this mortality rate is related to immediate-release topiramate treatment, because the background mortality rate for a similar, significantly refractory, young pediatric population (1 month to 24 months) with partial epilepsy is not known.

Other Pediatric Studies

Topiramate treatment produced a dose-related increased shift in serum creatinine from normal at baseline to an increased value at the end of 4 months treatment in adolescent patients (ages 12 years to 16 years) in a double-blind, placebo-controlled study [*see Adverse Reactions (6.1)*].

Juvenile Animal Studies

When topiramate (30, 90 and 300 mg/kg/day) was administered orally to rats during the juvenile period of development (postnatal days 12 to 50), bone growth plate thickness was reduced in males at the highest dose tested. The higher of the doses not associated with effects on bone (90 mg/kg/day) is approximately 2 times the maximum recommended pediatric dose for epilepsy (9 mg/kg/day) on a body surface area (mg/m^2) basis.

8.5 Geriatric Use

Clinical studies of immediate-release topiramate did not include sufficient numbers of subjects aged 65 and over to determine whether they respond differently than younger subjects. Dosage adjustment is necessary for elderly with creatinine clearance less than 70 mL/min/1.73 m^2. Estimate GFR should be measured prior to dosing [*see Dosage and Administration (2.4) and Clinical Pharmacology (12.3)*].

8.6 Race and Gender Effects

Evaluation of effectiveness and safety of topiramate in clinical trials has shown no race- or gender-related effects.

8.7 Renal Impairment

The clearance of topiramate was reduced by 42% in moderately renally impaired (creatinine clearance 30 to 69 mL/min/1.73m^2) and by 54% in severely renally impaired subjects (creatinine clearance less than 30 mL/min/1.73m^2) compared to normal renal function subjects (creatinine clearance greater than 70 mL/min/1.73m^2). One-half the usual starting and maintenance dose is recommended in patients with moderate or severe renal impairment [*see Dosage and Administration (2.4) and Clinical Pharmacology (12.3)*].

8.8 Patients Undergoing Hemodialysis

Topiramate is cleared by hemodialysis at a rate that is 4 to 6 times greater than a normal individual. Accordingly, a prolonged period of dialysis may cause topiramate concentration to fall below that required to maintain an anti-seizure effect. To avoid rapid drops in topiramate plasma concentration during hemodialysis, a supplemental dose of topiramate may be required. The actual adjustment should take into account the duration of dialysis period, the clearance rate of the dialysis system being used, and the effective renal clearance of topiramate in the patient being dialyzed [*see Dosage and Administration (2.5) and Clinical Pharmacology (12.3)*].

9 DRUG ABUSE AND DEPENDENCE

9.1 Controlled Substance

TROKENDI XR® (topiramate) extended-release capsule is not a controlled substance.

9.2 Abuse

The abuse and dependence potential of TROKENDI XR® has not been evaluated in human studies.

9.3 Dependence

TROKENDI XR® has not been systematically studied in animals or humans for its potential for tolerance or physical dependence.

10 OVERDOSAGE

Overdoses of topiramate have been reported. Signs and symptoms included convulsions, drowsiness, speech disturbance, blurred vision, diplopia, mentation impaired, lethargy, abnormal coordination, stupor, hypotension, abdominal pain, agitation, dizziness and depression. The clinical consequences were not severe in most cases, but deaths have been reported after polydrug overdoses involving topiramate.

Topiramate overdose has resulted in severe metabolic acidosis [*see Warnings and Precautions (5.3)*].

A patient who ingested a dose between 96 g and 110 g of topiramate was admitted to hospital with coma lasting 20 to 24 hours followed by full recovery after 3 to 4 days.

Similar signs, symptoms, and clinical consequences are expected to occur with overdosage of TROKENDI XR®. Therefore, in acute TROKENDI XR® overdose, if the ingestion is recent, the stomach should be emptied immediately by lavage or by induction of emesis. Activated charcoal has been shown to adsorb topiramate *in vitro*. Treatment should be appropriately supportive. Hemodialysis is an effective means of removing topiramate from the body.

11 DESCRIPTION

Topiramate, USP, is a sulfamate-substituted monosaccharide. TROKENDI XR® (topiramate) extended-release capsules are available as 25 mg, 50 mg, 100 mg and 200 mg capsules for oral administration.

Topiramate is a white to off-white powder. Topiramate is freely soluble in polar organic solvents such as acetonitrile and acetone; and very slightly soluble to practically insoluble in non-polar organic solvents such as hexanes. Topiramate has the molecular formula $C_{12}H_{21}NO_8S$ and a molecular weight of 339.4. Topiramate is designated chemically as 2,3:4,5-Di-*O*-isopropylidene-β-D-fructopyranose sulfamate and has the following structural formula:

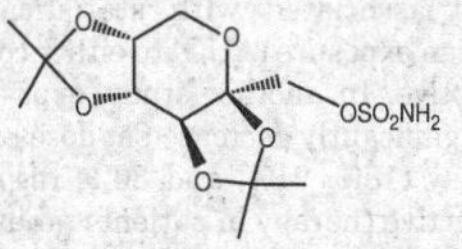

TROKENDI XR® (topiramate) is an extended-release capsule. TROKENDI XR® capsules contain the following inactive ingredients:

Sugar Spheres, NF
Hypromellose (Type 2910), USP
Mannitol, USP
Docusate Sodium, USP
Sodium Benzoate, NF
Ethylcellulose, NF
Oleic Acid, NF
Medium Chain Triglycerides, NF
Polyethylene Glycol, NF
Polyvinyl Alcohol, USP
Titanium Dioxide, USP
Talc, USP
Lecithin, NF
Xanthan Gum, NF

The capsule shells contain gelatin, USP; Titanium Dioxide, USP; and Colorants.

The colorants are:
FD&C Blue #1 (all strength capsules)
Yellow Iron Oxide, USP (25 mg and 50 mg capsules)
FD&C Red #3 (50 mg, 100 mg and 200 mg capsules)
FD&C Yellow #6 (50 mg, 100 mg and 200 mg capsules)
Riboflavin, USP (25 mg capsules)

All capsule shells are imprinted with black print that contains shellac, NF, and black iron oxide, NF.

12 CLINICAL PHARMACOLOGY

12.1 Mechanism of Action

The precise mechanisms by which topiramate exerts its anticonvulsant effects are unknown; however, preclinical studies have revealed four properties that may contribute to topiramate's efficacy for epilepsy. Electrophysiological and biochemical evidence suggests that topiramate, at pharmacologically relevant concentrations, blocks voltage-dependent sodium channels, augments the activity of the neurotransmitter gamma-aminobutyrate at some subtypes of the GABA-A receptor, antagonizes the AMPA/kainate subtype of the glutamate receptor, and inhibits the carbonic anhydrase enzyme, particularly isozymes II and IV.

12.2 Pharmacodynamics

Topiramate has anticonvulsant activity in rat and mouse maximal electroshock seizure (MES) tests. Topiramate is only weakly effective in blocking clonic seizures induced by the GABAA receptor antagonist, pentylenetetrazole. Topiramate is also effective in rodent models of epilepsy, which include tonic and absence-like seizures in the spontaneous epileptic rat (SER) and tonic and clonic seizures induced in rats by kindling of the amygdala or by global ischemia.

12.3 Pharmacokinetics

Absorption and Distribution

Linear pharmacokinetics of topiramate from TROKENDI XR® were observed following a single oral dose over the range of 50 mg to 200 mg. At 25 mg, the pharmacokinetics of TROKENDI XR® is nonlinear possibly due to the binding of topiramate to carbonic anhydrase in red blood cells.

The peak plasma concentrations (C_{max}) of topiramate occurred at approximately 24 hours following a single 200 mg oral dose of TROKENDI XR®. At steady-state, the ($AUC_{0\text{-}24}$, C_{max}, and C_{min}) of topiramate from TROKENDI XR® administered once-daily and the immediate-release tablet administered twice-daily were shown to be bioequivalent. Fluctuation of topiramate plasma concentrations at steady-state for TROKENDI XR® administered once-daily was approximately 26% and 42% in healthy subjects and in epileptic patients, respectively, compared to approximately 40% and 51%, respectively, for immediate-release topiramate [see *Clinical Pharmacology (12.6)*].

Compared to the fasted state, high-fat meal increased the C_{max} of topiramate by 37% and shortened the T_{max} to approximately 8 hours following a single dose of TROKENDI XR®, while having no effect on the AUC. Modeling of the observed single dose fed data with simulation to steady state showed that the effect on C_{max} is significantly reduced following repeat administrations. TROKENDI XR® can be taken without regard to meals.

Topiramate is 15% to 41% bound to human plasma proteins over the blood concentration range of 0.5 mcg/mL to 250 mcg/mL. The fraction bound decreased as blood concentration increased.

Carbamazepine and phenytoin do not alter the binding of immediate-release topiramate. Sodium valproate, at 500 mcg/mL (a concentration 5 to 10 times higher than considered therapeutic for valproate) decreased the protein binding of immediate-release topiramate from 23% to 13%. Immediate-release topiramate does not influence the binding of sodium valproate.

Metabolism and Excretion

Topiramate is not extensively metabolized and is primarily eliminated unchanged in the urine (approximately 70% of an administered dose). Six metabolites have been identified in humans, none of which constitutes more than 5% of an administered dose. The metabolites are formed via hydroxylation, hydrolysis, and glucuronidation. There is evidence of renal tubular reabsorption of topiramate. In rats, given probenecid to inhibit tubular reabsorption, along with topiramate, a significant increase in renal clearance of topiramate was observed. This interaction has not been evaluated in humans. Overall, oral plasma clearance (CL/F) is approximately 20 mL/min to 30 mL/min in adults following oral administration. The mean elimination half-life of topiramate was approximately 31 hours following repeat administration of TROKENDI XR®.

Specific Populations

Renal Impairment

The clearance of topiramate was reduced by 42% in moderately renally impaired (creatinine clearance 30 to 69 mL/min/1.73m^2) and by 54% in severely renally impaired subjects (creatinine clearance less than 30 mL/min/1.73m^2) compared to normal renal function subjects (creatinine clearance greater than 70 mL/min/1.73m^2). Since topiramate is presumed to undergo significant tubular reabsorption, it is uncertain whether this experience can be

Continued on next page

generalized to all situations of renal impairment. It is conceivable that some forms of renal disease could differentially affect glomerular filtration rate and tubular reabsorption resulting in a clearance of topiramate not predicted by creatinine clearance. In general, however, use of one-half the usual starting and maintenance dose is recommended in patients with creatinine clearance less than 70 mL/min/1.73 m² [*see Dosage and Administration (2.4), (2.5)*].

Hemodialysis

Topiramate is cleared by hemodialysis. Using a high-efficiency, counterflow, single pass-dialysate hemodialysis procedure, topiramate dialysis clearance was 120 mL/min with blood flow through the dialyzer at 400 mL/min. This high clearance (compared to 20 mL/min to 30 mL/min total oral clearance in healthy adults) will remove a clinically significant amount of topiramate from the patient over the hemodialysis treatment period. Therefore, a supplemental dose may be required [*see Dosage and Administration (2.5)*].

Hepatic Impairment

In hepatically impaired subjects, the clearance of topiramate may be decreased; the mechanism underlying the decrease is not well understood.

Age, Gender and Race

The pharmacokinetics of topiramate in elderly subjects (65 to 85 years of age, N=16) were evaluated in a controlled clinical study. The elderly subject population had reduced renal function (creatinine clearance [-20%]) compared to young adults. Following a single oral 100 mg dose, maximum plasma concentration for elderly and young adults was achieved at approximately 1 to 2 hours. Reflecting the primary renal elimination of topiramate, topiramate plasma and renal clearance were reduced 21% and 19%, respectively, in elderly subjects, compared to young adults. Similarly, topiramate half-life was longer (13%) in the elderly. Reduced topiramate clearance resulted in slightly higher maximum plasma concentration (23%) and AUC (25%) in elderly subjects than observed in young adults. Topiramate clearance is decreased in the elderly only to the extent that renal function is reduced.

In a study of 13 healthy elderly subjects and 18 healthy young adults who received TROKENDI XR®, 30% higher mean C_{max} and 44% higher AUC values were observed in elderly compared to young subjects. Elderly subjects exhibited shorter median T_{max} at 16 hours versus 24 hours in young subjects. The apparent elimination half-life was similar across age groups. As recommended for all patients, dosage adjustment is indicated in elderly patients with a creatinine clearance rate less than 70 mL/min/1.73 m²) [*see Dosage and Administration (2.4)*].

Clearance of topiramate in adults was not affected by gender or race.

Pediatric Pharmacokinetics

Pharmacokinetics of immediate-release topiramate were evaluated in patients ages 2 years to less than 16 years. Patients received either no or a combination of other antiepileptic drugs. A population pharmacokinetic model was developed on the basis of pharmacokinetic data from relevant topiramate clinical studies. This dataset contained data from 1217 subjects including 258 pediatric patients aged 2 years to less than 16 years (95 pediatric patients less than 10 years of age). Pediatric patients on adjunctive treatment exhibited a higher oral clearance (L/h) of topiramate com-

pared to patients on monotherapy, presumably because of increased clearance from concomitant enzyme-inducing antiepileptic drugs. In comparison, topiramate clearance per kg is greater in pediatric patients than in adults and in young pediatric patients (down to 2 years) than in older pediatric patients. Consequently, the plasma drug concentration for the same mg/kg/day dose would be lower in pediatric patients compared to adults and also in younger pediatric patients compared to older pediatric patients. Clearance was independent of dose.

As in adults, hepatic enzyme-inducing antiepileptic drugs decrease the steady state plasma concentrations of topiramate.

Drug-Drug Interaction Studies

Antiepileptic Drugs

Potential interactions between immediate-release topiramate and standard AEDs were assessed in controlled clinical pharmacokinetic studies in patients with epilepsy. The effects of these interactions on mean plasma AUCs are summarized in Table 9. Interaction of TROKENDI XR® and standard AEDs is not expected to differ from the experience with immediate-release topiramate products.

In Table 9, the second column (AED concentration) describes what happened to the concentration of the AED listed in the first column when topiramate was added. The third column (topiramate concentration) describes how the co-administration of a drug listed in the first column modified the concentration of topiramate in experimental settings when topiramate was given alone.

[See table 9 below]

In addition to the pharmacokinetic interaction described in the above table, concomitant administration of valproic acid and topiramate has been associated with hyperammonemia with and without encephalopathy and hypothermia [*see Warnings and Precautions (5.9), (5.11) and Drug Interactions (7.5)*].

CNS Depressants or Alcohol

Concomitant administration of TROKENDI XR® and other CNS depressant drugs or alcohol has not been evaluated in clinical studies [*see Contraindications (4), Warnings and Precautions (5.4), (5.13), and Drug Interactions (7.1), (7.4)*].

Oral Contraceptives

In a pharmacokinetic interaction study in healthy volunteers with a concomitantly administered combination oral contraceptive product containing 1 mg norethindrone (NET) plus 35 mcg ethinyl estradiol (EE), topiramate, given in the absence of other medications at doses of 50 to 200 mg per day, was not associated with statistically significant changes in mean exposure (AUC) to either component of the oral contraceptive. In another study, exposure to EE was statistically significantly decreased at doses of 200, 400, and 800 mg per day (18%, 21%, and 30%, respectively) when given as adjunctive therapy in patients taking valproic acid. In both studies, topiramate (50 mg per day to 800 mg per day) did not significantly affect exposure to NET. Although there was a dose-dependent decrease in EE exposure for doses between 200 to 800 mg per day, there was no significant dose-dependent change in EE exposure for doses of 50 to 200 mg per day. The clinical significance of the changes observed is not known. The possibility of decreased contraceptive efficacy and increased breakthrough bleeding should be considered in patients taking combination oral contra-

ceptive products with TROKENDI XR®. Patients taking estrogen-containing contraceptives should be asked to report any change in their bleeding patterns. Contraceptive efficacy can be decreased even in the absence of breakthrough bleeding [*see Drug Interactions (7.2)*].

Digoxin

In a single-dose study, serum digoxin AUC was decreased by 12% with concomitant topiramate administration. The clinical relevance of this observation has not been established.

Hydrochlorothiazide

A drug-drug interaction study conducted in healthy volunteers evaluated the steady-state pharmacokinetics of hydrochlorothiazide (HCTZ) (25 mg every 24 hours) and topiramate (96 mg every 12 hours) when administered alone and concomitantly. The results of this study indicate that topiramate C_{max} increased by 27% and AUC increased by 29% when HCTZ was added to topiramate. The clinical significance of this change is unknown. The addition of HCTZ to TROKENDI XR® therapy may require an adjustment of the TROKENDI XR® dose. The steady-state pharmacokinetics of HCTZ were not significantly influenced by the concomitant administration of topiramate. Clinical laboratory results indicated decreases in serum potassium after topiramate or HCTZ administration, which were greater when HCTZ and topiramate were administered in combination.

Metformin

Topiramate treatment can frequently cause metabolic acidosis, a condition for which the use of metformin is contraindicated. TROKENDI XR® is expected to exhibit the same degree of metabolic acidosis as topiramate.

A drug-drug interaction study conducted in healthy volunteers evaluated the steady-state pharmacokinetics of metformin (500 mg every 12 hr) and topiramate in plasma when metformin was given alone and when metformin and topiramate (100 mg every 12 hr) were given simultaneously. The results of this study indicated that the mean metformin C_{max} and AUC_{0-12h} increased by 17% and 25%, respectively, when topiramate was added. Topiramate did not affect metformin T_{max}. The clinical significance of the effect of topiramate on metformin pharmacokinetics is not known. Oral plasma clearance of topiramate appears to be reduced when administered with metformin. The clinical significance of the effect of metformin on topiramate or TROKENDI XR® pharmacokinetics is unclear [*see Drug Interactions (7.6)*].

Pioglitazone

A drug-drug interaction study conducted in healthy volunteers evaluated the steady-state pharmacokinetics of topiramate and pioglitazone when administered alone and concomitantly. A 15% decrease in the $AUC_{\tau,ss}$ of pioglitazone with no alteration in $C_{max,ss}$ was observed. This finding was not statistically significant. In addition, a 13% and 16% decrease in $C_{max,ss}$ and $AUC_{\tau,ss}$ respectively, of the active hydroxy-metabolite was noted as well as a 60% decrease in $C_{max,ss}$ and $AUC_{\tau,ss}$ of the active keto-metabolite. The clinical significance of these findings is not known.

When TROKENDI XR® is added to pioglitazone therapy or pioglitazone is added to TROKENDI XR® therapy, careful attention should be given to the routine monitoring of patients for adequate control of their diabetic disease state.

Glyburide

A drug-drug interaction study conducted in patients with type 2 diabetes evaluated the steady-state pharmacokinetics of glyburide (5 mg per day) alone and concomitantly with topiramate (150 mg per day). There was a 22% decrease in C_{max} and 25% reduction in AUC_{24} for glyburide during topiramate administration. Systemic exposure (AUC) of the active metabolites, 4-*trans*-hydroxy glyburide (M1) and 3-*cis*-hydroxyglyburide (M2), was also reduced by 13% and 15%, reduced C_{max} by 18% and 25%, respectively. The steady-state pharmacokinetics of topiramate were unaffected by concomitant administration of glyburide.

Lithium

In patients, the pharmacokinetics of lithium were unaffected during treatment with topiramate at doses of 200 mg per day; however, there was an observed increase in systemic exposure of lithium (27% for C_{max} and 26% for AUC) following topiramate doses up to 600 mg per day. Lithium levels should be monitored when co-administered with high-dose TROKENDI XR® [*see Drug Interactions (7.7)*].

Haloperidol

The pharmacokinetics of a single dose of haloperidol (5 mg) were not affected following multiple dosing of topiramate (100 mg every 12 hr) in 13 healthy adults (6 males, 7 females).

Table 9: Summary of AED Interactions with topiramate

AED Coadministered	AED Concentration	Topiramate Concentration
Phenytoin	NC or 25% increase*	48% decrease
Carbamazepine (CBZ)	NC	40% decrease
CBZ epoxide†	NC	NE
Valproic acid	11% decrease	14% decrease
Phenobarbital	NC	NE
Primidone	NC	NE
Lamotrigine	NC at TPM doses up to 400mg per day	13% decrease

* =Plasma concentration increased 25% in some patients, generally those on a twice a day dosing regimen of phenytoin
† =Is not administered but is an active metabolite of carbamazepine
NC=Less than 10% change in plasma concentration
AED=Antiepileptic drug
NE=Not evaluated
TPM=topiramate

Amitriptyline
There was a 12% increase in AUC and C_{max} for amitriptyline (25 mg per day) in 18 normal subjects (9 males, 9 females) receiving 200 mg per day of topiramate. Some subjects may experience a large increase in amitriptyline concentration in the presence of TROKENDI XR® and any adjustments in amitriptyline dose should be made according to the patient's clinical response and not on the basis of plasma levels.

Sumatriptan
Multiple dosing of topiramate (100 mg every 12 hrs) in 24 healthy volunteers (14 males, 10 females) did not affect the pharmacokinetics of single-dose sumatriptan either orally (100 mg) or subcutaneously (6 mg).

Risperidone
When administered concomitantly with topiramate at escalating doses of 100, 250, and 400 mg per day, there was a reduction in risperidone systemic exposure (16% and 33% for steady-state AUC at the 250 and 400 mg per day doses of topiramate). No alterations of 9-hydroxyrisperidone levels were observed. Coadministration of topiramate 400 mg per day with risperidone resulted in a 14% increase in C_{max} and a 12% increase in AUC_{12} of topiramate. There were no clinically significant changes in the systemic exposure of risperidone plus 9-hydroxyrisperidone or of topiramate; therefore, this interaction is not likely to be of clinical significance.

Propranolol
Multiple dosing of topiramate (200 mg per day) in 34 healthy volunteers (17 males, 17 females) did not affect the pharmacokinetics of propranolol following daily 160 mg doses. Propranolol doses of 160 mg per day in 39 volunteers (27 males, 12 females) had no effect on the exposure to topiramate at a dose of 200 mg per day of topiramate.

Dihydroergotamine
Multiple dosing of topiramate (200 mg per day) in 24 healthy volunteers (12 males, 12 females) did not affect the pharmacokinetics of a 1 mg subcutaneous dose of dihydroergotamine. Similarly, a 1 mg subcutaneous dose of dihydroergotamine did not affect the pharmacokinetics of a 200 mg per day dose of topiramate in the same study.

Diltiazem
Co-administration of diltiazem (240 mg Cardizem CD®) with topiramate (150 mg per day) resulted in a 10% decrease in C_{max} and 25% decrease in diltiazem AUC, 27% decrease in C_{max} and 18% decrease in des-acetyl diltiazem AUC, and no effect on N-desmethyl diltiazem. Co-administration of topiramate with diltiazem resulted in a 16% increase in C_{max} and a 19% increase in AUC_{12} of topiramate.

Venlafaxine
Multiple dosing of topiramate (150 mg per day) in healthy volunteers did not affect the pharmacokinetics of venlafaxine or O-desmethyl venlafaxine. Multiple dosing of venlafaxine (150 mg) did not affect the pharmacokinetics of topiramate.

Other Carbonic Anhydrase Inhibitors
Concomitant use of TROKENDI XR®, a carbonic anhydrase inhibitor, with any other carbonic anhydrase inhibitor (e.g., zonisamide, acetazolamide, or dichlorphenamide), may increase the severity of metabolic acidosis and may also increase the risk of kidney stone formation. Therefore, if TROKENDI XR® is given concomitantly with another carbonic anhydrase inhibitor, the patient should be monitored for the appearance or worsening of metabolic acidosis [see *Drug Interactions (7.5)*].

Drug/Laboratory Tests Interactions
There are no known interactions of TROKENDI XR® with commonly used laboratory tests.

12.6   Relative Bioavailability of TROKENDI XR® Compared to Immediate-Release Topiramate
Study in Healthy Normal Volunteers
TROKENDI XR® taken once a day provides steady state plasma levels comparable to immediate-release topiramate taken every 12 hours, when administered at the same total 200-mg daily dose. In a crossover study, 33 healthy subjects were titrated to a 200-mg dose of either TROKENDI XR® or immediate-release topiramate and were maintained at 200 mg per day for 10 days.
The 90% CI for the ratios of AUC_{0-24}, C_{max} and C_{min}, as well as partial AUC (the area under the concentration-time curve from time 0 to time p (post dose) for multiple time points were within the 80 to 125% bioequivalence limits, indicating no clinically significant difference between the two formulations. In addition, the 90% CI for the ratios of topiramate plasma concentration at each of multiple time points over 24 hours for the two formulations were within the 80 to 125% bioequivalence limits, except for the initial time points before 1.5 hour post-dose.

Study in Patients with Epilepsy
In a study in epilepsy patients treated with immediate-release topiramate alone or in combination with either enzyme-inducing or neutral AEDs who were switched to an equivalent daily dose of TROKENDI XR®, there was a 10% decrease in AUC_{0-24}, C_{max}, and C_{min} on the first day after the switch in all patients. At steady state, AUC_{0-24} and C_{max} were comparable to immediate-release topiramate in all patients. While patients treated with TROKENDI XR® alone or in combination with neutral AEDs showed comparable C_{min} at steady state, patients treated with enzyme-inducers showed a 10% decrease in C_{min}. This difference is likely not clinically significant and probably due to the small number of patients on enzyme-inducers.

13   NON-CLINICAL TOXICOLOGY
13.1   Carcinogenesis, Mutagenesis, and Impairment of Fertility
Carcinogenesis
An increase in urinary bladder tumors was observed in mice given topiramate (20, 75, and 300 mg/kg/day) in the diet for 21 months. An increase in the incidence of bladder tumors in males and females receiving 300 mg/kg was primarily due to the increased occurrence of a smooth muscle tumor considered histomorphologically unique to mice. The higher of the doses not associated with an increase in tumors (75 mg/kg/day) is equivalent to the maximum recommended human dose (MRHD) on a mg/m² basis. The relevance of this finding to human carcinogenic risk is uncertain.
No evidence of carcinogenicity was seen in rats following oral administration of topiramate for 2 years at doses up to 120 mg/kg/day (approximately 3 times the MRHD on a mg/m² basis).
Mutagenesis
Topiramate did not demonstrate genotoxic potential when tested in a battery of *in vitro* and *in vivo* assays. Topiramate was not mutagenic in the Ames test or the *in vitro* mouse lymphoma assay; it did not increase unscheduled DNA synthesis in rat hepatocytes *in vitro;* and it did not increase chromosomal aberrations in human lymphocytes *in vitro* or in rat bone marrow *in vivo*.
Impairment of Fertility
No adverse effects on male or female fertility were observed in rats administered oral doses of up to 100 mg/kg/day (2.5 times the MRHD on a mg/m² basis) prior to and during mating and early pregnancy.

14   CLINICAL STUDIES
14.1   Bridging Study to Demonstrate Pharmacokinetic Equivalence between Extended-Release and Immediate-Release Topiramate Formulations
The basis for approval of the extended-release formulation (TROKENDI XR®) included the studies described below using an immediate-release formulation and the demonstration of the pharmacokinetic equivalence of TROKENDI XR® to immediate-release topiramate through the analysis of concentrations and cumulative AUCs at multiple time points [see *Clinical Pharmacology (12.6)*].
The clinical studies described in the following sections were conducted using immediate-release topiramate.

14.2   Monotherapy Treatment in Patients with Partial Onset or Primary Generalized Tonic-Clonic Seizures
Adults and Pediatric Patients 10 Years of Age and Older
The effectiveness of topiramate as initial monotherapy in adults and children 10 years of age and older with partial onset or primary generalized tonic-clonic seizures was established in a multicenter, randomized, double-blind, dose-controlled, parallel-group trial (Study 1).
Study 1 was conducted in 487 patients diagnosed with epilepsy (6 to 83 years of age) who had 1 or 2 well-documented seizures during the 3-month retrospective baseline phase who then entered the study and received topiramate 25 mg per day for 7 days in an open-label fashion. Forty-nine percent of subjects had no prior AED treatment and 17% had a diagnosis of epilepsy for greater than 24 months. Any AED therapy used for temporary or emergency purposes was discontinued prior to randomization. In the double-blind phase, 470 patients were randomized to titrate up to 50 mg per day or 400 mg per day of topiramate. If the target dose could not be achieved, patients were maintained on the maximum tolerated dose. Fifty-eight percent of patients achieved the maximal dose of 400 mg per day for greater than 2 weeks, and patients who did not tolerate 150 mg per day were discontinued.

The primary efficacy assessment was a between-group comparison of time to first seizure during the double-blind phase. Comparison of the Kaplan-Meier survival curves of time to first seizure favored the topiramate 400 mg per day group over the topiramate 50 mg per day group (p=0.0002, log rank test; Figure 1). The treatment effects with respect to time to first seizure were consistent across various patient subgroups defined by age, sex, geographic region, baseline body weight, baseline seizure type, time since diagnosis, and baseline AED use.

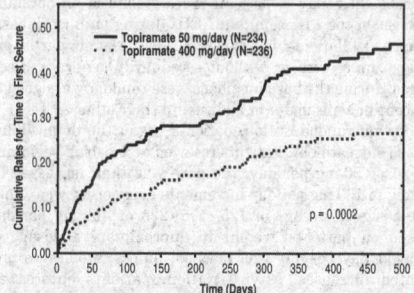

Figure 1: Kaplan-Meier Estimates of Cumulative Rates for Time to First Seizure in Study 1

Pediatric Patients 6 to Less than 10 Years of Age
The conclusion that topiramate is effective as initial monotherapy in pediatric patients 6 to less than 10 years of age with partial onset or primary generalized tonic-clonic seizures was based on a pharmacometric bridging approach using data from the controlled epilepsy trials conducted with immediate-release topiramate described in labeling. The approach consisted of first showing a similar exposure response relationship between pediatric patients down to 2 years of age and adults when immediate-release topiramate was given as adjunctive therapy [see *Use in Specific Populations (8.4)*]. Similarity of exposure-response was demonstrated in pediatric patients ages 6 to less than16 years of age and adults when topiramate was given as initial monotherapy. Specific dosing in pediatric patients 6 to less than 10 years of age was derived from simulations utilizing plasma exposure ranges observed in pediatric and adult patients treated with immediate-release topiramate initial monotherapy [see *Dosage and Administration (2.1)*].

14.3   Adjunctive Therapy in Patients with Partial Onset Seizures
Adult Patients with Partial Onset Seizures
The effectiveness of topiramate as an adjunctive treatment for adults with partial onset seizures was established in six multicenter, randomized, double-blind, placebo-controlled trials (Studies 2, 3, 4, 5, 6, and 7), two comparing several dosages of topiramate and placebo and four comparing a single dosage with placebo, in patients with a history of partial onset seizures, with or without secondarily generalized seizures.
Patients in these studies were permitted a maximum of two antiepileptic drugs (AEDs) in addition to topiramate tablets or placebo. In each study, patients were stabilized on optimum dosages of their concomitant AEDs during baseline phase lasting between 4 and 12 weeks. Patients who experienced a prespecified minimum number of partial onset seizures, with or without secondary generalization, during the baseline phase (12 seizures for 12-week baseline, 8 for 8-week baseline or 3 for 4-week baseline) were randomly assigned to placebo or a specified dose of topiramate tablets in addition to their other AEDs.
Following randomization, patients began the double-blind phase of treatment. In five of the six studies, patients received active drug beginning at 100 mg per day; the dose was then increased by 100 mg or 200 mg per day increments weekly or every other week until the assigned dose was reached, unless intolerance prevented increases. In Study 7, the 25 or 50 mg per day initial doses of topiramate were followed by respective weekly increments of 25 or 50 mg per day until the target dose of 200 mg per day was reached. After titration, patients entered a 4, 8 or 12-week stabilization period. The numbers of patients randomized to each dose, and the actual mean and median doses in the stabilization period are shown in Table 10.
[See table 10 at top of next page]

Continued on next page

Pediatric Patients Ages 2 to 16 Years with Partial Onset Seizures

The effectiveness of topiramate as an adjunctive treatment for pediatric patients ages 2 to 16 years with partial onset seizures was established in a multicenter, randomized, double-blind, placebo-controlled trial (Study 8), comparing topiramate and placebo in patients with a history of partial onset seizures, with or without secondarily generalized seizures.

Patients in Study 8 were permitted a maximum of two antiepileptic drugs (AEDs) in addition to topiramate tablets or placebo. In Study 8, patients were stabilized on optimum dosages of their concomitant AEDs during an 8-week baseline phase. Patients who experienced at least six partial onset seizures, with or without secondarily generalized seizures, during the baseline phase were randomly assigned to placebo or topiramate in addition to their other AEDs.

Following randomization, patients began the double-blind phase of treatment. Patients received active drug beginning at 25 or 50 mg per day; the dose was then increased by 25 mg to 150 mg per day increments every other week until the assigned dosage of 125, 175, 225 or 400 mg per day based on patients' weight to approximate a dosage of 6 mg/kg/day per day was reached, unless intolerance prevented increases. After titration, patients entered an 8-week stabilization period.

14.4 Adjunctive Therapy in Patients with Primary Generalized Tonic-Clonic Seizures

The effectiveness of topiramate as an adjunctive treatment for primary generalized tonic-clonic seizures in patients 2 years old and older was established in a multicenter, randomized, double-blind, placebo-controlled trial (Study 9), comparing a single dosage of topiramate and placebo.

Patients in Study 9 were permitted a maximum of two antiepileptic drugs (AEDs) in addition to topiramate or placebo. Patients were stabilized on optimum dosages of their concomitant AEDs during an 8-week baseline phase. Patients who experienced at least three primary generalized tonic-clonic seizures during the baseline phase were randomly assigned to placebo or topiramate in addition to their other AEDs.

Following randomization, patients began the double-blind phase of treatment. Patients received active drug beginning at 50 mg per day for four weeks; the dose was then increased by 50 mg to 150 mg per day increments every other week until the assigned dose of 175, 225 or 400 mg per day based on patients' body weight to approximate a dosage of 6 mg/kg/day was reached, unless intolerance prevented increases. After titration, patients entered a 12-week stabilization period.

14.5 Adjunctive Therapy in Patients with Lennox-Gastaut Syndrome

The effectiveness of topiramate as an adjunctive treatment for seizures associated with Lennox-Gastaut syndrome was established in a multicenter, randomized, double-blind, placebo-controlled trial comparing a single dosage of topiramate with placebo in patients 2 years of age and older (Study 10).

Patients in Study 10 were permitted a maximum of two antiepileptic drugs (AEDs) in addition to topiramate or placebo. Patients who were experiencing at least 60 seizures per month before study entry were stabilized on optimum dosages of their concomitant AEDs during a 4 week baseline phase. Following baseline, patients were randomly assigned to placebo or topiramate in addition to their other AEDs. Active drug was titrated beginning at 1 mg/kg/day for a week; the dose was then increased to 3 mg/kg/day for one week then to 6 mg/kg/day. After titration, patients entered an 8-week stabilization period. The primary measures of effectiveness were the percent reduction in drop attacks and a parental global rating of seizure severity.

In all adjunctive topiramate trials, the reduction in seizure rate from baseline during the entire double-blind phase was measured. The median percent reductions in seizure rates and the responder rates (fraction of patients with at least a 50% reduction) by treatment group for each study are shown below in Table 11. As described above, a global improvement in seizure severity was also assessed in the Lennox-Gastaut trial.

[See table 11 at bottom of next page]

Subset analyses of the antiepileptic efficacy of topiramate tablets in these studies showed no differences as a function of gender, race, age, baseline seizure rate, or concomitant AED.

In clinical trials for epilepsy, daily dosages were decreased in weekly intervals by 50 mg per day to 100 mg per day in

Table 10: Immediate Release Topiramate Dose Summary During the Stabilization Periods of Each of Six Double-Blind, Placebo-Controlled, Adjunctive Trials in Adults with Partial Onset Seizures[a]

Study	Stabilization Dose	Placebo[b]	200	400	600	800	1,000
2	N	42	42	40	41	--	--
2	Mean Dose	5.9	200	390	556	--	--
2	Median Dose	6.0	200	400	600	--	--
3	N	44	--	--	40	45	40
3	Mean Dose	9.7	--	--	544	739	796
3	Median Dose	10.0	--	--	600	800	1,000
4	N	23	--	19	--	--	--
4	Mean Dose	3.8	--	395	--	--	--
4	Median Dose	4.0	--	400	--	--	--
5	N	30	--	--	28	--	--
5	Mean Dose	5.7	--	--	522	--	--
5	Median Dose	6.0	--	--	600	--	--
6	N	28	--	--	--	25	--
6	Mean Dose	8.0	--	--	--	568	--
6	Median Dose	8.0	--	--	--	600	--
7	N	90	157	--	--	--	--
7	Mean Dose	8	200	--	--	--	--
7	Median Dose	8	200	--	--	--	--

a Dose-response studies were not conducted for other indications or pediatric partial-onset seizures
b Placebo dosages are given as the number of tablets. Placebo target dosages were as follows: Study 4 (4 tablets/day); Studies 2 and 5 (6 tablets/day); Studies 6 and 7 (8 tablets/day); Study 3 (10 tablets/day)

adults and over a 2- to 8-week period in children; transition was permitted to a new antiepileptic regimen when clinically indicated.

16 HOW SUPPLIED/STORAGE AND HANDLING
16.1 TROKENDI XR® Capsules

TROKENDI XR® (topiramate) extended-release capsules are available as extended-release capsules in the following strengths and colors:

Bottles

25 mg (light green opaque body/yellow opaque cap) topiramate extended-release capsules (black print "SPN" and "25") - bottles of 100 count (NDC-17772-101-01)

50 mg (light green opaque body/orange opaque cap) topiramate extended-release capsules (black print "SPN" and "50") - bottles of 100 count (NDC-17772-102-01)

100 mg (green opaque body/blue opaque cap) topiramate extended-release capsules (black print "SPN" and "100") - bottles of 100 count (NDC-17772-103-01)

200 mg (pink opaque body/blue opaque cap) topiramate extended-release capsules (black print "SPN" and "200") - bottles of 100 count (NDC-17772-104-01)

Blister package

25 mg (light green opaque body/yellow opaque cap) topiramate extended-release capsules (black print "SPN" and "25") – blister packages of 30-count (NDC-17772-101-15)

50 mg (light green opaque body/orange opaque cap) topiramate extended-release capsules (black print "SPN" and "50") – blister packages of 30-count (NDC-17772-102-15)

100 mg (green opaque body/blue opaque cap) topiramate extended-release capsules (black print "SPN" and "100") – blister packages of 30-count (NDC-17772-103-15)

200 mg (pink opaque body/blue opaque cap) topiramate extended-release capsules (black print "SPN" and "200") – blister packages of 30-count (NDC-17772-104-15)

16.2 Storage and Handling

TROKENDI XR® (topiramate) extended-release capsules should be stored in well closed containers at controlled room temperature [25°C (77°F); excursions 15°C-30°C (59°F-86°F)]. Protect from moisture and light.

17 PATIENT COUNSELING INFORMATION

Advise the patient to read the FDA-approved patient labeling (Medication Guide).

Administration Instructions

Counsel patients to swallow TROKENDI XR® capsules whole and intact. TROKENDI XR® should not be sprinkled on food, chewed or crushed [See *Dosage and Administration (2.9)*].

Consumption of Alcohol

Advise patients to completely avoid consumption of alcohol at least 6 hours prior to and 6 hours after taking TROKENDI XR®[see *Warnings and Precautions (5.4)*].

Acute Myopia and Secondary Angle Closure Glaucoma

Advise patients taking TROKENDI XR® to seek immediate medical attention if they experience blurred vision, visual disturbances or periorbital pain [see *Warnings and Precautions (5.1)*].

Oligohydrosis and Hyperthermia

Counsel patients that TROKENDI XR®, especially pediatric patients, can cause decreased sweating and increased body temperature, especially in hot weather, and they should seek medical attention if this is noticed [see *Warnings and Precautions (5.2)*].

Metabolic Acidosis

Inform patients about the potentially significant risk for metabolic acidosis that may be asymptomatic and may be associated with adverse effects on kidneys (e.g., kidney stones, nephrocalcinosis), bones (e.g., osteoporosis, osteomalacia, and/or rickets in children), and growth (e.g., growth delay/retardation) in pediatric patients, and on the fetus [see *Warnings and Precautions (5.3)*].

Suicidal Behavior and Ideation

Counsel patients, their caregivers, and families that AEDs, including TROKENDI XR®, may increase the risk of suicidal thoughts and behavior and they should be advised of the need to be alert for the emergence or worsening of the signs and symptoms of depression, any unusual changes in mood or behavior or the emergence of suicidal thoughts, behavior or thoughts about self-harm. Behaviors of concern should be reported immediately to healthcare providers [see *Warnings and Precautions (5.5)*].

Interference with Cognitive and Motor Performance

Warn patients about the potential for somnolence, dizziness, confusion, difficulty concentrating, visual effects and advise them not to drive or operate machinery until they have gained sufficient experience on TROKENDI XR® to gauge whether it adversely affects their mental performance, motor performance, and/or vision [*see Warnings and Precautions (5.6)*].

Advise patients that even when taking TROKENDI XR® or other anticonvulsants, some patients with epilepsy will continue to have unpredictable seizures. Therefore, counsel all patients taking TROKENDI XR® for epilepsy to exercise appropriate caution when engaging in any activities where loss of consciousness could result in serious danger to themselves or those around them (including swimming, driving a car, climbing in high places, etc.). Some patients with refractory epilepsy will need to avoid such activities altogether. Physicians should discuss the appropriate level of caution with their patients, before patients with epilepsy engage in such activities.

Fetal Toxicity

Counsel pregnant women and women of childbearing potential that use of topiramate during pregnancy can cause fetal harm, including an increased risk for cleft lip and/or cleft palate (oral clefts), which occur early in pregnancy before many women know they are pregnant. Also inform patients that infants exposed to topiramate monotherapy *in utero* may be small for their gestational age [*see Use in Specific Populations (8.1)*]. When appropriate, prescribers should counsel pregnant women and women of childbearing potential about alternative therapeutic options.

Advise women of childbearing potential who are not planning a pregnancy to use effective contraception while using topiramate, keeping in mind that there is a potential for decreased contraceptive efficacy when using estrogen-containing birth control with topiramate [*see Warnings and Precautions (5.7) and Drug Interactions (7.2)*].

Encourage pregnant women using topiramate to enroll in the North American Antiepileptic Drug (NAAED) Pregnancy Registry. The registry is collecting information about the safety of antiepileptic drugs during pregnancy. To enroll, patients can call the toll free number, 1-888-233-2334. Information about the North American Drug Pregnancy Registry can be found at http://www.aedpregnancyregistry.org/ [*see Use in Specific Populations (8.1)*].

Hyperammonemia and Encephalopathy

Warn patients about the possible development of hyperammonemia with or without encephalopathy. Although hyperammonemia may be asymptomatic, clinical symptoms of hyperammonemic encephalopathy often include acute alterations in level of consciousness and/or cognitive function with lethargy or vomiting. This hyperammonemia and encephalopathy can develop with topiramate treatment alone or with topiramate treatment with concomitant valproic acid (VPA). Patients should be instructed to contact their physician if they develop unexplained lethargy, vomiting, or changes in mental status [*see Warnings and Precautions (5.9)*].

Kidney Stones

Instruct patients, particularly those with predisposing factors, to maintain an adequate fluid intake in order to minimize the risk of kidney stone formation [*see Warnings and Precautions (5.10)*].

Hypothermia

Counsel patients that TROKENDI XR® can cause a reduction in body temperature, which can lead to alterations in mental status. If they note such changes, they should call their health care professional and measure their body temperature. Patients taking concomitant valproic acid should be specifically counseled on this potential adverse reaction [*see Warnings and Precautions (5.11)*].

Paresthesia

Counsel patients that they may experience tingling in the arms and legs. If this symptom occurs, they should consult with their physician [*see Warnings and Precautions (5.12)*].

Manufactured by: Catalent Pharma Solutions, Winchester, Kentucky 40391

Manufactured for: Supernus Pharmaceuticals, Inc., Rockville, Maryland 20850

RA-TRO-V4

Revised:August 2016

Table 11: Efficacy Results in Double-Blind, Placebo-Controlled, Adjunctive Epilepsy Trials

Study #	#	Target Topiramate Dosage (mg per day)						
		Placebo	200	400	600	800	1,000	≈6mg/kg/day*
Partial Onset Seizures Studies in Adults								
2	N	45	45	45	46	--	--	--
	Median % Reduction	11.6	27.2[a]	47.5[b]	44.7[c]	--	--	--
	% Responders	18	24	44[d]	46[d]	--	--	--
3	N	47	--	--	48	48	47	--
	Median % Reduction	1.7	--	--	40.8[c]	41.0[c]	36.0[c]	--
	% Responders	9	--	--	40[c]	41[c]	36[d]	--
4	N	24	--	23	--	--	--	--
	Median % Reduction	1.1	--	40.7[e]	--	--	--	--
	% Responders	8	--	35[d]	--	--	--	--
5	N	30	--	--	30	--	--	--
	Median % Reduction	-12.2	--	--	46.4[f]	--	--	--
	% Responders	10	--	--	47[c]	--	--	--
6	N	28	--	--	--	28	--	--
	Median % Reduction	-20.6	--	--	--	24.3[c]	--	--
	% Responders	0	--	--	--	43[c]	--	--
7	N	91	168	--	--	--	--	--
	Median % Reduction	20.0	44.2[c]	--	--	--	--	--
	% Responders	24	45[c]	--	--	--	--	--
Studies in Pediatric Patients								
8	N	45	--	--	--	--	--	41
	Median % Reduction	10.5	--	--	--	--	--	33.1[d]
	% Responders	20	--	--	--	--	--	39
Primary Generalized Tonic-Clonic[h]								
9	N	40	--	--	--	--	--	39
	Median % Reduction	9.0	--	--	--	--	--	56.7[d]
	% Responders	20	--	--	--	--	--	56
Lennox-Gastaut Syndrome[i]								
10	N	49	--	--	--	--	--	46
	Median % Reduction	-5.1	--	--	--	--	--	14.8[d]
	% Responders	14	--	--	--	--	--	28[g]
	Improvement in Seizure Severity[j]	28						52d

Comparisons with placebo: [a]p=0.080; [b]p ≤ 0.010; [c]p ≤ 0.001; [d]p ≤ 0.050; [e]p=0.065; [f]p ≤0.005; [g]p=0.071;
[h]Median % reduction and % responders are reported for PGTC seizures;
[i]Median % reduction and % responders are reported for drop attacks, i.e., tonic or atonic seizures
[j]Percentage of subjects who were minimally, much, or very much improved from baseline.
*For Studies 8 and 9, specified target dosages (less than 9.3 mg/kg/day) were assigned based on subject's weight to approximate a dosage of 6mg/kg per day; these dosages corresponded to mg per day dosages of 125 mg per day, 175 mg per day, 225 mg per day, and 400 mg per day

---

MEDICATION GUIDE
TROKENDI XR (tro-KEN-dee eks ahr)
(topiramate) Extended-Release Capsules

What is the most important information I should know about Trokendi XR®?

Take Trokendi XR® capsules whole. Do not sprinkle Trokendi XR® on food, or break, crush, dissolve, or chew Trokendi XR® capsules before swallowing. If you cannot swallow Trokendi XR® capsules whole, tell your healthcare provider. You may need a different medicine.

Do not drink alcohol within 6 hours prior to and 6 hours after Trokendi XR® administration.

Trokendi XR may cause eye problems. Serious eye problems include:
• any sudden decrease in vision with or without eye pain and redness.
• a blockage of fluid in the eye causing increased pressure in the eye (secondary angle closure glaucoma).
• These eye problems can lead to permanent loss of vision if not treated.
• You should call your healthcare provider right away if you have any new eye symptoms, including any new problems with your vision.

Continued on next page

Trokendi XR may cause decreased sweating and increased body temperature (fever). People, especially children, should be watched for signs of decreased sweating and fever, especially in hot temperatures. Some people may need to be hospitalized for this condition. If a high fever, a fever that does not go away, or decreased sweating develops, call your healthcare provider right away.

Trokendi XR can increase the level of acid in your blood (metabolic acidosis). If left untreated, metabolic acidosis can cause brittle or soft bones (osteoporosis, osteomalacia, osteopenia), kidney stones, can slow the rate of growth in children, and may possibly harm your baby if you are pregnant. Metabolic acidosis can happen with or without symptoms. Sometimes people with metabolic acidosis will:

- feel tired
- not feel hungry (loss of appetite)
- feel changes in heartbeat
- have trouble thinking clearly

Your healthcare provider should do a blood test to measure the level of acid in your blood before and during your treatment with Trokendi XR. If you are pregnant, you should talk to your healthcare provider about whether you have metabolic acidosis.

Like other antiepileptic drugs, Trokendi XR may cause suicidal thoughts or actions in a very small number of people, about 1 in 500.

Call a healthcare provider right away if you have any of these symptoms, especially if they are new, worse, or worry you:

- thoughts about suicide or dying
- attempts to commit suicide
- new or worse depression
- new or worse anxiety
- feeling agitated or restless
- panic attacks

- trouble sleeping (insomnia)
- new or worse irritability
- acting aggressive, being angry, or violent
- acting on dangerous impulses
- an extreme increase in activity and talking (mania)
- other unusual changes in behavior or mood

Do not stop Trokendi XR without first talking to a healthcare provider.

- Stopping Trokendi XR suddenly can cause serious problems.
- Suicidal thoughts or actions can be caused by things other than medicines. If you have suicidal thoughts or actions, your healthcare provider may check for other causes.

How can I watch for early symptoms of suicidal thoughts and actions?

- Pay attention to any changes, especially sudden changes, in mood, behaviors, thoughts, or feelings.
- Keep all follow-up visits with your healthcare provider as scheduled.
- Call your healthcare provider between visits as needed, especially if you are worried about symptoms.

Trokendi XR can harm your unborn baby.

- If you take Trokendi XR during pregnancy, your baby has a higher risk for birth defects called cleft lip and cleft palate. These defects can begin early in pregnancy, even before you know you are pregnant.
- Cleft lip and cleft palate may happen even in children born to women who are not taking any medicines and do not have other risk factors.
- Also, if you take Trokendi XR during pregnancy, your baby may be smaller than expected at birth. The long-term effects of this are not known.
- There may be other medicines to treat your condition that have a lower chance of birth defects.
- All women of childbearing age should talk to their healthcare providers about using other possible treatments instead of Trokendi XR. If the decision is made to use Trokendi XR, you should use effective birth control (contraception) unless you are planning to become pregnant. You should talk to your doctor about the best kind of birth control to use while you are taking Trokendi XR.
- Tell your healthcare provider right away if you become pregnant while taking Trokendi XR. You and your healthcare provider should decide if you will continue to take Trokendi XR while you are pregnant.
- If you take Trokendi XR during pregnancy, your baby may be smaller than expected at birth. Talk to your healthcare provider if you have questions about this risk during pregnancy.
- Metabolic acidosis may have harmful effects on your baby. Talk to your healthcare provider if Trokendi XR has caused metabolic acidosis during your pregnancy.
- Pregnancy Registry: If you become pregnant while taking Trokendi XR, talk to your healthcare provider about

registering with the North American Antiepileptic Drug Pregnancy Registry. You can enroll in this registry by calling 1-888-233-2334. The purpose of this registry is to collect information about the safety of Trokendi XR and other antiepileptic drugs during pregnancy.

What is Trokendi XR?

Trokendi XR is a prescription medicine used:

- to treat certain types of seizures (partial onset seizures and primary generalized tonic-clonic seizures) in people 6 years and older,
- with other medicines to treat certain types of seizures (partial onset seizures, primary generalized tonic-clonic seizures, and seizures associated with Lennox-Gastaut syndrome) in adults and children 6 years and older

Before taking Trokendi XR , tell your healthcare provider about all of your medical conditions, including if you:

- have or have had depression, mood problems or suicidal thoughts or behavior
- have kidney problems, kidney stones or are getting kidney dialysis
- have a history of metabolic acidosis (too much acid in the blood)
- have liver problems
- have weak, brittle or soft bones (osteomalacia, osteoporosis, osteopenia, or decreased bone density)
- have lung or breathing problems
- have eye problems, especially glaucoma
- have diarrhea
- have a growth problem
- are on a diet high in fat and low in carbohydrates, which is called a ketogenic diet
- are having surgery
- are pregnant or plan to become pregnant
- are breastfeeding. Trokendi XR passes into your breast milk. It is not known if the Trokendi XR that passes into breast milk can harm your baby. Talk to your healthcare provider about the best way to feed your baby if you take Trokendi XR.

Tell your healthcare provider about all the medicines you take, including prescription and over-the-counter medicines, vitamins, and herbal supplements. Especially, tell your healthcare provider if you take:

- Metformin (such as Glucophage)
- Valproic acid (such as DEPAKENE or DEPAKOTE)
- any medicines that impair or decrease your thinking, concentration, or muscle coordination
- birth control pills. Trokendi XR may make your birth control pills less effective. Tell your healthcare provider if your menstrual bleeding changes while you are taking birth control pills and Trokendi XR.

Ask your healthcare provider if you are not sure if your medicine is listed above.

Know the medicines you take. Keep a list of them to show your healthcare provider and pharmacist each time you get a new medicine. Do not start a new medicine without talking with your healthcare provider.

How should I take Trokendi XR?

- Take Trokendi XR exactly as prescribed.
- Your healthcare provider may change your dose. **Do not** change your dose without talking to your healthcare provider.
- Take Trokendi XR capsules whole. **Do not** sprinkle Trokendi XR on food, or break, crush, dissolve, or chew Trokendi XR capsules before swallowing.
- Trokendi XR can be taken before, during, or after a meal. Drink plenty of fluids during the day. This may help prevent kidney stones while taking Trokendi XR.
- If you take too much Trokendi XR, call your healthcare provider right away or go to the nearest emergency room.
- Talk to your health care provider on what you should do if you miss a dose.
- Do not stop taking Trokendi XR without talking to your healthcare provider.
- Stopping Trokendi XR suddenly may cause serious problems. If you have epilepsy and you stop taking Trokendi XR suddenly, you may have seizures that do not stop. Your healthcare provider will tell you how to stop taking Trokendi XR slowly.
- Your healthcare provider may do blood tests while you take Trokendi XR.

What should I avoid while taking Trokendi XR?

- Do not drink alcohol within 6 hours before or 6 hours after taking Trokendi XR capsules. Trokendi XR and alcohol can cause serious side effects such as severe sleepiness and dizziness and an increase in seizures.

- Do not drive a car or operate heavy machinery until you know how Trokendi XR affects you. Trokendi XR can slow your thinking and motor skills, and may affect vision.

What are the possible side effects of Trokendi XR?

Trokendi XR may cause serious side effects, including:

See "What is the most important information I should know about Trokendi XR?"

- **High blood ammonia levels.** High ammonia in the blood can affect your mental activities, slow your alertness, make you feel tired, or cause vomiting. This has happened when Trokendi XR is taken with a medicine called valproic acid (DEPAKENE and DEPAKOTE).
- **Kidney stones.** Drink plenty of fluids when taking Trokendi XR to decrease your chances of getting kidney stones.
- **Low body temperature.** Taking Trokendi XR when you are also taking valproic acid cause a drop in body temperature to less than 95°F, feeling tired, confusion, or coma.
- **Effects on thinking and alertness.** Trokendi XR may affect how you think, and cause confusion, problems with concentration, attention, memory, or speech. Trokendi XR may cause depression or mood problems, tiredness, and sleepiness.
- **Dizziness or loss of muscle coordination.**

Call your healthcare provider right away if you have any of the symptoms above.

The most common side effects of Trokendi XR include:

- tingling of the arms and legs (paresthesia)
- not feeling hungry
- nausea
- weight loss
- abnormal vision

- nervousness
- speech problems
- dizziness
- slow reactions
- difficulty with concentration and attention

- fever
- tiredness
- sleepiness/ drowsiness
- difficulty with memory

Tell your healthcare provider about any side effect that bothers you or that does not go away.

These are not all the possible side effects of Trokendi XR. Call your doctor for medical advice about side effects. You may report side effects to FDA at 1-800-FDA-1088.

You may also report side effects to Supernus Pharmaceuticals, Inc. at 1-866-398-0833.

How should I store Trokendi XR?

- Store Trokendi XR tablets at room temperature between 59°F to 86°F (15°C to 30°C).
- Keep Trokendi XR in a tightly closed container.
- Keep Trokendi XR dry and away from moisture and light.
- **Keep Trokendi XR and all medicines out of the reach of children.**

General information about the safe and effective use of Trokendi XR.

Medicines are sometimes prescribed for purposes other than those listed in a Medication Guide. Do not use Trokendi XR for a condition for which it was not prescribed. Do not give Trokendi XR to other people, even if they have the same symptoms that you have. It may harm them.

You can ask your pharmacist or healthcare provider for information about Trokendi XR that is written for health professionals.

What are the ingredients in Trokendi XR?

Active ingredient: topiramate

Inactive ingredients:

Sugar spheres, NF; hypromellose (Type 2910), USP; mannitol, USP; docusate sodium, USP; sodium benzoate, NF; ethylcellulose, NF; oleic acid, NF; medium chain triglycerides, NF; polyethylene glycol, NF; polyvinyl alcohol, USP; titanium dioxide, USP; talc, USP; lecithin, NF; xanthan gum, NF.

Capsule shells: Gelatin, USP; titanium dioxide, USP; colorants.

Colorants:

FD&C Blue #1 (all strength capsules)

Yellow iron oxide, USP (25 mg and 50 mg capsules)

FD&C red #3 (50 mg, 100 mg and 200 mg capsules)

FD&C yellow #6 (50 mg, 100 mg and 200 mg capsules)

Riboflavin, USP (25 mg capsules)

All capsule shells are imprinted with black print that contains shellac, NF, and black iron oxide, NF.

Manufactured by: Catalent Pharma Solutions, Winchester, KY USA 40391

Manufactured for: Supernus Pharmaceuticals, Inc. Rockville, MD USA 20850

© Supernus Pharmaceuticals

RA-TRO-MGV4

For more information, go to www.trokendixr.com or call 1-866-398-0833.

This Medication Guide has been approved by the U.S. Food and Drug Administration

Revised: AUGUST 2016

Shown in Product Identification Guide, page 510

Takeda Pharmaceuticals U.S.A., Inc.

ONE TAKEDA PARKWAY
DEERFIELD, IL 60015

Direct Inquiries to:
Sales and Ordering:
Customer Service
(877) TAKEDA7
(877) 825-3327
For Medical Information:
(877) TAKEDA7
(877) 825-3327
To Report Adverse Drug Experiences:
(877) TAKEDA7
(877) 825-3327

COLCRYS   ℞
[KOL-kris]
(colchicine, USP)
tablets, for oral use

HIGHLIGHTS OF PRESCRIBING INFORMATION
These highlights do not include all the information needed to use colchicine safely and effectively. See full prescribing information for COLCRYS.
COLCRYS (colchicine, USP) tablets, for oral use
Initial U.S. Approval: 1961

INDICATIONS AND USAGE
COLCRYS (colchicine, USP) tablets are an alkaloid indicated for:
• Prophylaxis and treatment of gout flares in adults (1.1).
• Familial Mediterranean fever (FMF) in adults and children 4 years or older (1.2).
COLCRYS is not an analgesic medication and should not be used to treat pain from other causes.

DOSAGE AND ADMINISTRATION
• **Gout Flares:**
  Prophylaxis of Gout Flares: 0.6 mg once or twice daily in adults and adolescents older than 16 years of age (2.1). Maximum dose 1.2 mg/day.
  Treatment of Gout Flares: 1.2 mg (two tablets) at the first sign of a gout flare followed by 0.6 mg (one tablet) one hour later (2.1).
• **FMF:** Adults and children older than 12 years 1.2 – 2.4 mg; children 6 to 12 years 0.9 – 1.8 mg; children 4 to 6 years 0.3 – 1.8 mg (2.2, 2.3).
  ○ Give total daily dose in one or two divided doses (2.2).
  ○ Increase or decrease the dose as indicated and as tolerated in increments of 0.3 mg/day, not to exceed the maximum recommended daily dose (2.2).
Colchicine tablets are administered orally without regard to meals.
See full prescribing information for dose adjustment regarding patients with impaired renal function (2.5), impaired hepatic function (2.6), the patient's age (2.3, 8.5) or use of coadministered drugs (2.4).

DOSAGE FORMS AND STRENGTHS
• 0.6 mg tablets (3).

CONTRAINDICATIONS
Patients with renal or hepatic impairment should not be given COLCRYS in conjunction with P-gp or strong CYP3A4 inhibitors (5.3). In these patients, life-threatening and fatal colchicine toxicity has been reported with colchicine taken in therapeutic doses (7).

WARNINGS AND PRECAUTIONS
• *Fatal overdoses* have been reported with colchicine in adults and children. Keep COLCRYS out of the reach of children (5.1, 10).

• *Blood dyscrasias:* myelosuppression, leukopenia, granulocytopenia, thrombocytopenia and aplastic anemia have been reported (5.2).
• Monitor for toxicity and if present consider temporary interruption or discontinuation of colchicine (5.2, 5.3, 5.4, 6, 10).
• *Drug interaction P-gp and/or CYP3A4 inhibitors:* Coadministration of colchicine with P-gp and/or strong CYP3A4 inhibitors has resulted in life-threatening interactions and death (5.3, 7).
• *Neuromuscular toxicity:* Myotoxicity including rhabdomyolysis may occur, especially in combination with other drugs known to cause this effect. Consider temporary interruption or discontinuation of COLCRYS (5.4, 7).

ADVERSE REACTIONS
Prophylaxis of Gout Flares: The most commonly reported adverse reaction in clinical trials for the prophylaxis of gout was diarrhea.
Treatment of Gout Flares: The most common adverse reactions reported in the clinical trial for gout were diarrhea (23%) and pharyngolaryngeal pain (3%).
FMF: Most common adverse reactions (up to 20%) are abdominal pain, diarrhea, nausea and vomiting. These effects are usually mild, transient and reversible upon lowering the dose (6).
To report SUSPECTED ADVERSE REACTIONS, contact Takeda Pharmaceuticals America, Inc. at 1-877-825-3327 or FDA at 1-800-FDA-1088 or www.fda.gov/medwatch.

DRUG INTERACTIONS
Coadministration of P-gp and/or CYP3A4 inhibitors (e.g., clarithromycin or cyclosporine) have been demonstrated to alter the concentration of colchicine. The potential for drug-drug interactions must be considered prior to and during therapy. See full prescribing information for a complete list of reported and potential interactions (2.4, 5.3, 7).

USE IN SPECIFIC POPULATIONS
• In the presence of mild to moderate renal or hepatic impairment, adjustment of dosing is not required for treatment of gout flare, prophylaxis of gout flare and FMF, but patients should be monitored closely (2.5, 8.6).
• In patients with severe renal impairment for prophylaxis of gout flares, the starting dose should be 0.3 mg/day for gout flares, no dose adjustment is required, but a treatment course should be repeated no more than once every two weeks. In FMF patients, start with 0.3 mg/day, and any increase in dose should be done with close monitoring (2.5, 8.6).
• In patients with severe hepatic impairment, a dose reduction may be needed in prophylaxis of gout flares and FMF patients; while a dose reduction may not be needed in gout flares, a treatment course should be repeated no more than once every two weeks (2.5, 2.6, 8.6, 8.7).
• For patients undergoing dialysis, the total recommended dose for prophylaxis of gout flares should be 0.3 mg given twice a week with close monitoring. For treatment of gout flares, the total recommended dose should be reduced to 0.6 mg (one tablet) × 1 dose and the treatment course should not be repeated more than once every two weeks. For FMF patients, the starting dose should be 0.3 mg/day and dosing can be increased with close monitoring (2.5, 8.6).
• Pregnancy: Use only if the potential benefit justifies the potential risk to the fetus (8.1).
• Nursing Mothers: Caution should be exercised when administered to a nursing woman (8.3).
• Geriatric Use: The recommended dose of colchicine should be based on renal function (2.5, 8.5).

See 17 for PATIENT COUNSELING INFORMATION and Medication Guide.

Revised: 12/2015

FULL PRESCRIBING INFORMATION

1   INDICATIONS AND USAGE
1.1   Gout Flares
COLCRYS (colchicine, USP) tablets are indicated for prophylaxis and the treatment of acute gout flares.
• **Prophylaxis of Gout Flares:**
  COLCRYS is indicated for prophylaxis of gout flares.
• **Treatment of Gout Flares:**
  COLCRYS tablets are indicated for treatment of acute gout flares when taken at the first sign of a flare.
1.2   Familial Mediterranean Fever (FMF)
COLCRYS (colchicine, USP) tablets are indicated in adults and children 4 years or older for treatment of familial Mediterranean fever (FMF).

2   DOSAGE AND ADMINISTRATION
The long-term use of colchicine is established for FMF and the prophylaxis of gout flares, but the safety and efficacy of repeat treatment for gout flares has not been evaluated. The dosing regimens for COLCRYS are different for each indication and must be individualized.
The recommended dosage of COLCRYS depends on the patient's age, renal function, hepatic function and use of coadministered drugs *[see Dose Modification for Coadministration of Interacting Drugs (2.4)]*.
COLCRYS tablets are administered orally without regard to meals.
COLCRYS is not an analgesic medication and should not be used to treat pain from other causes.
2.1   Gout Flares
Prophylaxis of Gout Flares
The recommended dosage of COLCRYS for prophylaxis of gout flares for adults and adolescents older than 16 years of age is 0.6 mg once or twice daily. The maximum recommended dose for prophylaxis of gout flares is 1.2 mg/day.
An increase in gout flares may occur after initiation of uric acid-lowering therapy, including pegloticase, febuxostat and allopurinol, due to changing serum uric acid levels resulting in mobilization of urate from tissue deposits. COLCRYS is recommended upon initiation of gout flare prophylaxis with uric acid-lowering therapy. Prophylactic therapy may be beneficial for at least the first six months of uric acid-lowering therapy.
Treatment of Gout Flares
The recommended dose of COLCRYS for treatment of a gout flare is 1.2 mg (two tablets) at the first sign of the flare followed by 0.6 mg (one tablet) one hour later. Higher doses have not been found to be more effective. The maximum recommended dose for treatment of gout flares is 1.8 mg over a one-hour period. COLCRYS may be administered for treatment of a gout flare during prophylaxis at doses not to exceed 1.2 mg (two tablets) at the first sign of the flare followed by 0.6 mg (one tablet) one hour later. Wait 12 hours and then resume the prophylactic dose.

Continued on next page

2.2 FMF

The recommended dosage of COLCRYS for FMF in adults is 1.2 mg to 2.4 mg daily.

COLCRYS should be increased as needed to control disease and as tolerated in increments of 0.3 mg/day to a maximum recommended daily dose. If intolerable side effects develop, the dose should be decreased in increments of 0.3 mg/day. The total daily COLCRYS dose may be administered in one to two divided doses.

2.3 Recommended Pediatric Dosage
Prophylaxis and Treatment of Gout Flares
COLCRYS is not recommended for pediatric use in prophylaxis or treatment of gout flares.

FMF
The recommended dosage of COLCRYS for FMF in pediatric patients 4 years of age and older is based on age. The following daily doses may be given as a single or divided dose twice daily:
- Children 4 to 6 years: 0.3 mg to 1.8 mg daily
- Children 6 to 12 years: 0.9 mg to 1.8 mg daily
- Adolescents older than 12 years: 1.2 mg to 2.4 mg daily

2.4 Dose Modification for Coadministration of Interacting Drugs
Concomitant Therapy
Coadministration of COLCRYS with drugs known to inhibit CYP3A4 and/or P-glycoprotein (P-gp) increases the risk of colchicine-induced toxic effects (*Table 1*). If patients are taking or have recently completed treatment with drugs listed in Table 1 within the prior 14 days, the dose adjustments are as shown in the table below [*see Drug Interactions (7)*].
[See table 1 below and at top of next page]
[See table 2 on pages 1090-1091]
Treatment of gout flares with COLCRYS is not recommended in patients receiving prophylactic dose of COLCRYS and CYP3A4 inhibitors.

2.5 Dose Modification in Renal Impairment
Colchicine dosing must be individualized according to the patient's renal function [*see Renal Impairment (8.6)*].
Cl_{cr} in mL/minute may be estimated from serum creatinine (mg/dL) determination using the following formula:

$$Cl_{cr} = \frac{[140\text{-age (years)}] \times \text{weight (kg)}}{72 \times \text{serum creatinine (mg/dL)} \times 0.85 \text{ for female patients}}$$

Gout Flares
Prophylaxis of Gout Flares
For prophylaxis of gout flares in patients with mild (estimated creatinine clearance [Cl_{cr}] 50 to 80 mL/min) to moderate (Cl_{cr} 30 to 50 mL/min) renal function impairment, adjustment of the recommended dose is not required, but patients should be monitored closely for adverse effects of colchicine. However, in patients with severe impairment, the starting dose should be 0.3 mg/day and any increase in dose should be done with close monitoring. For the prophylaxis of gout flares in patients undergoing dialysis, the starting doses should be 0.3 mg given twice a week with close monitoring [*see Clinical Pharmacology (12.3) and Renal Impairment (8.6)*].
Treatment of Gout Flares
For treatment of gout flares in patients with mild (Cl_{cr} 50 to 80 mL/min) to moderate (Cl_{cr} 30 to 50 mL/min) renal function impairment, adjustment of the recommended dose is not required, but patients should be monitored closely for adverse effects of colchicine. However, in patients with severe impairment, while the dose does not need to be adjusted for the treatment of gout flares, a treatment course should be repeated no more than once every two weeks. For patients with gout flares requiring repeated courses, consideration should be given to alternate therapy. For patients undergoing dialysis, the total recommended dose for the treatment of gout flares should be reduced to a single dose of 0.6 mg (one tablet). For these patients, the treatment course should not be repeated more than once every two weeks [*see Clinical Pharmacology (12.3) and Renal Impairment (8.6)*]. Treatment of gout flares with COLCRYS is not recommended in patients with renal impairment who are receiving COLCRYS for prophylaxis.
FMF
Caution should be taken in dosing patients with moderate and severe renal impairment and in patients undergoing dialysis. For these patients, the dosage should be reduced [*see Clinical Pharmacology (12.3)*]. Patients with mild (Cl_{cr} 50 to 80 mL/min) and moderate (Cl_{cr} 30 to 50 mL/min) renal impairment should be monitored closely for adverse effects of COLCRYS. Dose reduction may be necessary. For patients with severe renal failure (Cl_{cr} less than 30 mL/min), start with 0.3 mg/day; any increase in dose should be done with adequate monitoring of the patient for adverse effects of colchicine [*see Renal Impairment (8.6)*]. For patients undergoing dialysis, the total recommended starting dose should be 0.3 mg (half tablet) per day. Dosing can be increased with close monitoring. Any increase in dose should be done with adequate monitoring of the patient for adverse effects of colchicine [*see Clinical Pharmacology (12.3) and Renal Impairment (8.6)*].

2.6 Dose Modification in Hepatic Impairment
Gout Flares
Prophylaxis of Gout Flares
For prophylaxis of gout flares in patients with mild to moderate hepatic function impairment, adjustment of the recommended dose is not required, but patients should be monitored closely for adverse effects of colchicine. Dose reduction should be considered for the prophylaxis of gout flares in patients with severe hepatic impairment [*see Hepatic Impairment (8.7)*].
Treatment of Gout Flares
For treatment of gout flares in patients with mild to moderate hepatic function impairment, adjustment of the recommended dose is not required, but patients should be monitored closely for adverse effects of colchicine. However, for the treatment of gout flares in patients with severe impairment, while the dose does not need to be adjusted, a treatment course should be repeated no more than once every two weeks. For these patients, requiring repeated courses for the treatment of gout flares, consideration should be given to alternate therapy [*see Hepatic Impairment (8.7)*].
Treatment of gout flares with COLCRYS is not recommended in patients with hepatic impairment who are receiving COLCRYS for prophylaxis.
FMF
Patients with mild to moderate hepatic impairment should be monitored closely for adverse effects of colchicine. Dose reduction should be considered in patients with severe hepatic impairment [*see Hepatic Impairment (8.7)*].

3   DOSAGE FORMS AND STRENGTHS
0.6 mg tablets — purple capsule-shaped, film-coated with "AR 374" debossed on one side and scored on the other side.

4   CONTRAINDICATIONS
Patients with renal or hepatic impairment should not be given COLCRYS in conjunction with P-gp or strong CYP3A4 inhibitors (this includes all protease inhibitors except fosamprenavir). In these patients, life-threatening and fatal colchicine toxicity has been reported with colchicine taken in therapeutic doses.

5   WARNINGS AND PRECAUTIONS
5.1   Fatal Overdose
Fatal overdoses, both accidental and intentional, have been reported in adults and children who have ingested colchicine [*see Overdosage (10)*]. COLCRYS should be kept out of the reach of children.

Table 1. COLCRYS Dose Adjustment for Coadministration with Interacting Drugs if no Alternative Available*

Strong CYP3A4 Inhibitors†

Drug	Noted or Anticipated Outcome	Gout Flares				FMF	
		Prophylaxis of Gout Flares		Treatment of Gout Flares			
		Original Intended Dosage	Adjusted Dose	Original Intended Dosage	Adjusted Dose	Original Intended Dosage	Adjusted Dose
Atazanavir Clarithromycin Darunavir/ Ritonavir† Indinavir Itraconazole Ketoconazole Lopinavir/ Ritonavir† Nefazodone Nelfinavir Ritonavir Saquinavir Telithromycin Tipranavir/ Ritonavir†	Significant increase in colchicine plasma levels*; fatal colchicine toxicity has been reported with clarithromycin, a strong CYP3A4 inhibitor. Similarly, significant increase in colchicine plasma levels is anticipated with other strong CYP3A4 inhibitors.	0.6 mg twice a day

0.6 mg once a day | 0.3 mg once a day

0.3 mg once every other day | 1.2 mg (2 tablets) followed by 0.6 mg (1 tablet) 1 hour later. Dose to be repeated no earlier than 3 days. | 0.6 mg (1 tablet) × 1 dose, followed by 0.3 mg (1/2 tablet) 1 hour later. Dose to be repeated no earlier than 3 days. | Maximum daily dose of 1.2 – 2.4 mg | Maximum daily dose of 0.6 mg (may be given as 0.3 mg twice a day) |

Moderate CYP3A4 Inhibitors

Drug	Noted or Anticipated Outcome	Gout Flares				FMF	
		Prophylaxis of Gout Flares		Treatment of Gout Flares			
		Original Intended Dosage	Adjusted Dose	Original Intended Dosage	Adjusted Dose	Original Intended Dosage	Adjusted Dose
Amprenavir† Aprepitant Diltiazem Erythromycin Fluconazole Fosamprenavir (pro-drug of Amprenavir) Grapefruit juice Verapamil	Significant increase in colchicine plasma concentration is anticipated. Neuromuscular toxicity has been reported with diltiazem and verapamil interactions.	0.6 mg twice a day

0.6 mg once a day | 0.3 mg twice a day or 0.6 mg once a day

0.3 mg once a day | 1.2 mg (2 tablets) followed by 0.6 mg (1 tablet) 1 hour later. Dose to be repeated no earlier than 3 days. | 1.2 mg (2 tablets) × 1 dose. Dose to be repeated no earlier than 3 days. | Maximum daily dose of 1.2 – 2.4 mg. | Maximum daily dose of 1.2 mg (may be given as 0.6 mg twice a day) |

This table is continued on the next page

Table 1 *(Cont.)* COLCRYS Dose Adjustment for Coadministration with Interacting Drugs if no Alternative Available*

P-gp Inhibitors‡

Drug	Noted or Anticipated Outcome	Gout Flares				FMF	
		Prophylaxis of Gout Flares		Treatment of Gout Flares			
		Original Intended Dosage	Adjusted Dose	Original Intended Dosage	Adjusted Dose	Original Intended Dosage	Adjusted Dose
Cyclosporine Ranolazine	Significant increase in colchicine plasma levels*; fatal colchicine toxicity has been reported with cyclosporine, a P-gp inhibitor. Similarly, significant increase in colchicine plasma levels is anticipated with other P-gp inhibitors.	0.6 mg twice a day 0.6 mg once a day	0.3 mg once a day 0.3 mg once every other day	1.2 mg (2 tablets) followed by 0.6 mg (1 tablet) 1 hour later. Dose to be repeated no earlier than 3 days.	0.6 mg (1 tablet) × 1 dose. Dose to be repeated no earlier than 3 days.	Maximum daily dose of 1.2 – 2.4 mg	Maximum daily dose of 0.6 mg (may be given as 0.3 mg twice a day)

* For magnitude of effect on colchicine plasma concentrations *[see Pharmacokinetics (12.3)]*

† When used in combination with Ritonavir, see dosing recommendations for strong CYP3A4 inhibitors *[see Contraindications (4)]*

‡ Patients with renal or hepatic impairment should not be given COLCRYS in conjunction with strong CYP3A4 or P-gp inhibitors *[see Contraindications (4)]*.

5.2   Blood Dyscrasias
Myelosuppression, leukopenia, granulocytopenia, thrombocytopenia, pancytopenia and aplastic anemia have been reported with colchicine used in therapeutic doses.

5.3   Drug Interactions
Colchicine is a P-gp and CYP3A4 substrate. Life-threatening and fatal drug interactions have been reported in patients treated with colchicine given with P-gp and strong CYP3A4 inhibitors. If treatment with a P-gp or strong CYP3A4 inhibitor is required in patients with normal renal and hepatic function, the patient's dose of colchicine may need to be reduced or interrupted *[see Drug Interactions (7)]*. Use of COLCRYS in conjunction with P-gp or strong CYP3A4 inhibitors (this includes all protease inhibitors except fosamprenavir) is contraindicated in patients with renal or hepatic impairment *[see Contraindications (4)]*.

5.4   Neuromuscular Toxicity
Colchicine-induced neuromuscular toxicity and rhabdomyolysis have been reported with chronic treatment in therapeutic doses. Patients with renal dysfunction and elderly patients, even those with normal renal and hepatic function, are at increased risk. Concomitant use of atorvastatin, simvastatin, pravastatin, fluvastatin, lovastatin, gemfibrozil, fenofibrate, fenofibric acid or benzafibrate (themselves associated with myotoxicity) or cyclosporine with COLCRYS may potentiate the development of myopathy *[see Drug Interactions (7)]*. Once colchicine is stopped, the symptoms generally resolve within one week to several months.

6   ADVERSE REACTIONS
Prophylaxis of Gout Flares
The most commonly reported adverse reaction in clinical trials of colchicine for the prophylaxis of gout was diarrhea.

Treatment of Gout Flares
The most common adverse reactions reported in the clinical trial with COLCRYS for treatment of gout flares were diarrhea (23%) and pharyngolaryngeal pain (3%).
FMF

Gastrointestinal tract adverse effects are the most frequent side effects in patients initiating COLCRYS, usually presenting within 24 hours, and occurring in up to 20% of patients given therapeutic doses. Typical symptoms include cramping, nausea, diarrhea, abdominal pain and vomiting. These events should be viewed as dose-limiting if severe, as they can herald the onset of more significant toxicity.

6.1   Clinical Trials Experience in Gout
Because clinical studies are conducted under widely varying and controlled conditions, adverse reaction rates observed in clinical studies of a drug cannot be directly compared to rates in the clinical studies of another drug and may not predict the rates observed in a broader patient population in clinical practice.
In a randomized, double-blind, placebo-controlled trial in patients with a gout flare, gastrointestinal adverse reactions occurred in 26% of patients using the recommended dose (1.8 mg over one hour) of COLCRYS compared to 77% of patients taking a nonrecommended high dose (4.8 mg over six hours) of colchicine and 20% of patients taking placebo. Diarrhea was the most commonly reported drug-related gastrointestinal adverse event. As shown in Table 3, diarrhea is associated with COLCRYS treatment. Diarrhea was more likely to occur in patients taking the high-dose regimen than the low-dose regimen. Severe diarrhea occurred in 19% and vomiting occurred in 17% of patients taking the nonrecommended high-dose colchicine regimen but did not occur in the recommended low-dose COLCRYS regimen.
[See table 3 on page 1091]

6.2   Postmarketing Experience
Serious toxic manifestations associated with colchicine include myelosuppression, disseminated intravascular coagulation and injury to cells in the renal, hepatic, circulatory and central nervous systems.
These most often occur with excessive accumulation or overdosage *[see Overdosage (10)]*.
The following adverse reactions have been reported with colchicine. These have been generally reversible upon temporarily interrupting treatment or lowering the dose of colchicine.

Neurological: sensory motor neuropathy
Dermatological: alopecia, maculopapular rash, purpura, rash
Digestive: abdominal cramping, abdominal pain, diarrhea, lactose intolerance, nausea, vomiting
Hematological: leukopenia, granulocytopenia, thrombocytopenia, pancytopenia, aplastic anemia
Hepatobiliary: elevated AST, elevated ALT
Musculoskeletal: myopathy, elevated CPK, myotonia, muscle weakness, muscle pain, rhabdomyolysis
Reproductive: azoospermia, oligospermia

7   DRUG INTERACTIONS
COLCRYS (colchicine) is a substrate of the efflux transporter P-glycoprotein (P-gp). Of the cytochrome P450 enzymes tested, CYP3A4 was mainly involved in the metabolism of colchicine. If COLCRYS is administered with drugs that inhibit P-gp, most of which also inhibit CYP3A4, increased concentrations of colchicine are likely. Fatal drug interactions have been reported.
Physicians should ensure that patients are suitable candidates for treatment with COLCRYS and remain alert for signs and symptoms of toxicities related to increased colchicine exposure as a result of a drug interaction. Signs and symptoms of COLCRYS toxicity should be evaluated promptly and, if toxicity is suspected, COLCRYS should be discontinued immediately.
Table 4 provides recommendations as a result of other potentially significant drug interactions. Table 1 provides recommendations for strong and moderate CYP3A4 inhibitors and P-gp inhibitors.

Table 4. Other Potentially Significant Drug Interactions

Concomitant Drug Class or Food	Noted or Anticipated Outcome	Clinical Comment
HMG-Co A Reductase Inhibitors: atorvastatin, fluvastatin, lovastatin, pravastatin, simvastatin **Other Lipid-Lowering Drugs:** fibrates, gemfibrozil	Pharmacokinetic and/or pharmacodynamic interaction: the addition of one drug to a stable long-term regimen of the other has resulted in myopathy and rhabdomyolysis (including a fatality)	Weigh the potential benefits and risks and carefully monitor patients for any signs or symptoms of muscle pain, tenderness, or weakness, particularly during initial therapy; monitoring CPK (creatine phosphokinase) will not necessarily prevent the occurrence of severe myopathy.
Digitalis Glycosides: digoxin	P-gp substrate; rhabdomyolysis has been reported	

8   USE IN SPECIFIC POPULATIONS
8.1   Pregnancy
Pregnancy Category C
There are no adequate and well-controlled studies with colchicine in pregnant women. Colchicine crosses the human placenta. While not studied in the treatment of gout flares, data from a limited number of published studies found no evidence of an increased risk of miscarriage, stillbirth or teratogenic effects among pregnant women using colchicine to treat familial Mediterranean fever (FMF). Although animal reproductive and developmental studies were not conducted with COLCRYS, published animal reproduction and development studies indicate that colchicine causes embryofetal toxicity, teratogenicity and altered postnatal development at exposures within or above the clinical therapeutic range. COLCRYS should be used during pregnancy only if the potential benefit justifies the potential risk to the fetus.

8.2   Labor and Delivery
The effect of colchicine on labor and delivery is unknown.

8.3   Nursing Mothers
Colchicine is excreted into human milk. Limited information suggests that exclusively breastfed infants receive less than 10 percent of the maternal weight-adjusted dose. While there are no published reports of adverse effects in breastfeeding infants of mothers taking colchicine, colchicine can affect gastrointestinal cell renewal and permeability. Caution should be exercised, and breastfeeding infants should be observed for adverse effects when COLCRYS is administered to a nursing woman.

Continued on next page

8.4 Pediatric Use

The safety and efficacy of colchicine in children of all ages with FMF has been evaluated in uncontrolled studies. There does not appear to be an adverse effect on growth in children with FMF treated long-term with colchicine. Gout is rare in pediatric patients; safety and effectiveness of colchicine in pediatric patients has not been established.

8.5 Geriatric Use

Clinical studies with colchicine for prophylaxis and treatment of gout flares and for treatment of FMF did not include sufficient numbers of patients aged 65 years and older to determine whether they respond differently from younger patients. In general, dose selection for an elderly patient with gout should be cautious, reflecting the greater frequency of decreased renal function, concomitant disease or other drug therapy [see Dose Modification for Coadministration of Interacting Drugs (2.4) and Pharmacokinetics (12.3)].

8.6 Renal Impairment

Colchicine is significantly excreted in urine in healthy subjects. Clearance of colchicine is decreased in patients with impaired renal function. Total body clearance of colchicine was reduced by 75% in patients with end-stage renal disease undergoing dialysis.

Prophylaxis of Gout Flares

For prophylaxis of gout flares in patients with mild (estimated creatinine clearance Cl_{cr} 50 to 80 mL/min) to moderate (Cl_{cr} 30 to 50 mL/min) renal function impairment, adjustment of the recommended dose is not required, but patients should be monitored closely for adverse effects of colchicine. However, in patients with severe impairment, the starting dose should be 0.3 mg per day and any increase in dose should be done with close monitoring. For the prophylaxis of gout flares in patients undergoing dialysis, the starting doses should be 0.3 mg given twice a week with close monitoring [see Dose Modification in Renal Impairment (2.5)].

Treatment of Gout Flares

For treatment of gout flares in patients with mild (Cl_{cr} 50 to 80 mL/min) to moderate (Cl_{cr} 30 to 50 mL/min) renal function impairment, adjustment of the recommended dose is not required, but patients should be monitored closely for adverse effects of COLCRYS. However, in patients with severe impairment, while the dose does not need to be adjusted for the treatment of gout flares, a treatment course should be repeated no more than once every two weeks. For patients with gout flares requiring repeated courses, consideration should be given to alternate therapy. For patients undergoing dialysis, the total recommended dose for the treatment of gout flares should be reduced to a single dose of 0.6 mg (one tablet). For these patients, the treatment course should not be repeated more than once every two weeks [see Dose Modification in Renal Impairment (2.5)].

FMF

Although, pharmacokinetics of colchicine in patients with mild (Cl_{cr} 50 to 80 mL/min) and moderate (Cl_{cr} 30 to 50 mL/min) renal impairment is not known, these patients should be monitored closely for adverse effects of colchicine. Dose reduction may be necessary. In patients with severe renal failure (Cl_{cr} less than 30 mL/min) and end-stage renal disease requiring dialysis, COLCRYS may be started at the dose of 0.3 mg/day. Any increase in dose should be done with adequate monitoring of the patient for adverse effects of COLCRYS [see Pharmacokinetics (12.3) and Dose Modification in Renal Impairment (2.5)].

8.7 Hepatic Impairment

The clearance of colchicine may be significantly reduced and plasma half-life prolonged in patients with chronic hepatic impairment compared to healthy subjects [see Pharmacokinetics (12.3)].

Prophylaxis of Gout Flares

For prophylaxis of gout flares in patients with mild to moderate hepatic function impairment, adjustment of the recommended dose is not required, but patients should be monitored closely for adverse effects of colchicine. Dose reduction should be considered for the prophylaxis of gout flares in patients with severe hepatic impairment [see Dose Modification in Hepatic Impairment (2.6)].

Treatment of Gout Flares

For treatment of gout flares in patients with mild to moderate hepatic function impairment, adjustment of the recommended COLCRYS dose is not required, but patients should be monitored closely for adverse effects of COLCRYS. However, for the treatment of gout flares in patients with severe impairment, while the dose does not need to be adjusted, the treatment course should be repeated no more than once

Table 2. COLCRYS Dose Adjustment for Coadministration with Protease Inhibitors

Protease Inhibitor	Clinical Comment	w/Colchicine - Prophylaxis of Gout Flares		w/Colchicine - Treatment of Gout Flares	w/Colchicine - Treatment of FMF
Atazanavir sulfate (Reyataz)	Patients with renal or hepatic impairment should not be given colchicine with Reyataz.	**Original dose**	**Adjusted dose**	0.6 mg (1 tablet) × 1 dose, followed by 0.3 mg (1/2 tablet) 1 hour later. Dose to be repeated no earlier than 3 days.	Maximum daily dose of 0.6 mg (may be given as 0.3 mg twice a day)
		0.6 mg twice a day	0.3 mg once a day		
		0.6 mg once a day	0.3 mg once every other day		
Darunavir (Prezista)	Patients with renal or hepatic impairment should not be given colchicine with Prezista/ritonavir.	**Original dose**	**Adjusted dose**	0.6 mg (1 tablet) × 1 dose, followed by 0.3 mg (1/2 tablet) 1 hour later. Dose to be repeated no earlier than 3 days.	Maximum daily dose of 0.6 mg (may be given as 0.3 mg twice a day)
		0.6 mg twice a day	0.3 mg once a day		
		0.6 mg once a day	0.3 mg once every other day		
Fosamprenavir (Lexiva) with Ritonavir	Patients with renal or hepatic impairment should not be given colchicine with Lexiva/ritonavir.	**Original dose**	**Adjusted dose**	0.6 mg (1 tablet) × 1 dose, followed by 0.3 mg (1/2 tablet) 1 hour later. Dose to be repeated no earlier than 3 days.	Maximum daily dose of 0.6 mg (may be given as 0.3 mg twice a day)
		0.6 mg twice a day	0.3 mg once a day		
		0.6 mg once a day	0.3 mg once every other day		
Fosamprenavir (Lexiva)	Patients with renal or hepatic impairment should not be given colchicine with Lexiva/ritonavir.	**Original dose**	**Adjusted dose**	1.2 mg (2 tablets) × 1 dose. Dose to be repeated no earlier than 3 days.	Maximum daily dose of 1.2 mg (may be given as 0.6 mg twice a day)
		0.6 mg twice a day	0.3 mg twice a day or 0.6 mg once a day		
		0.6 mg once a day	0.3 mg once a day		
Indinavir (Crixivan)	Patients with renal or hepatic impairment should not be given colchicine with Crixivan.	**Original dose**	**Adjusted dose**	0.6 mg (1 tablet) × 1 dose, followed by 0.3 mg (1/2 tablet) 1 hour later. Dose to be repeated no earlier than 3 days.	Maximum daily dose of 0.6 mg (may be given as 0.3 mg twice a day)
		0.6 mg twice a day	0.3 mg once a day		
		0.6 mg once a day	0.3 mg once every other day		
Lopinavir/Ritonavir (Kaletra)	Patients with renal or hepatic impairment should not be given colchicine with Kaletra.	**Original dose**	**Adjusted dose**	0.6 mg (1 tablet) × 1 dose, followed by 0.3 mg (1/2 tablet) 1 hour later. Dose to be repeated no earlier than 3 days.	Maximum daily dose of 0.6 mg (may be given as 0.3 mg twice a day)
		0.6 mg twice a day	0.3 mg once a day		
		0.6 mg once a day	0.3 mg once every other day		
Nelfinavir mesylate (Viracept)	Patients with renal or hepatic impairment should not be given colchicine with Viracept.	**Original dose**	**Adjusted dose**	0.6 mg (1 tablet) × 1 dose, followed by 0.3 mg (1/2 tablet) 1 hour later. Dose to be repeated no earlier than 3 days.	Maximum daily dose of 0.6 mg (may be given as 0.3 mg twice a day)
		0.6 mg twice a day	0.3 mg once a day		
		0.6 mg once a day	0.3 mg once every other day		
Ritonavir (Norvir)	Patients with renal or hepatic impairment should not be given colchicine with Norvir.	**Original dose**	**Adjusted dose**	0.6 mg (1 tablet) × 1 dose, followed by 0.3 mg (1/2 tablet) 1 hour later. Dose to be repeated no earlier than 3 days.	Maximum daily dose of 0.6 mg (may be given as 0.3 mg twice a day)
		0.6 mg twice a day	0.3 mg once a day		
		0.6 mg once a day	0.3 mg once every other day		

This table is continued on the next page

[See 8 table below]
Figure 1 shows the percentage of patients achieving varying degrees of improvement in pain from baseline at 24 hours.

Figure 1

Pain Relief on Low and High Doses of COLCRYS and Placebo (Cumulative)

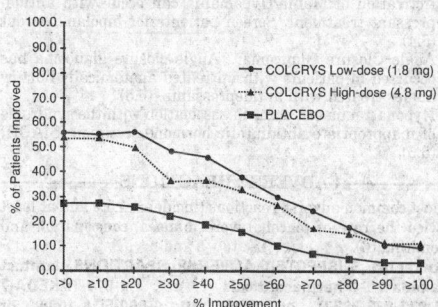

Table 8. Number (%) of Responders Based on Target Joint Pain Score at 24 Hours Post First Dose					
COLCRYS Dose Responders n (%)		Placebo n (%) (n=58)	% Differences in Proportion	
Low-Dose (n=74)	High-Dose (n=52)		Low-Dose vs Placebo (95% CI)	High-Dose vs Placebo (95% CI)
28 (38%)	17 (33%)	9 (16%)	22 (8, 37)	17 (1, 33)

The evidence for the efficacy of colchicine in patients with FMF is derived from the published literature. Three randomized, placebo-controlled studies were identified. The three placebo-controlled studies randomized a total of 48 adult patients diagnosed with FMF and reported similar efficacy endpoints as well as inclusion and exclusion criteria. One of the studies randomized 15 patients with FMF to a six-month crossover study during which five patients discontinued due to study noncompliance. The 10 patients completing the study experienced five attacks over the course of 90 days while treated with colchicine compared to 59 attacks over the course of 90 days while treated with placebo. Similarly, the second study randomized 22 patients with FMF to a four-month crossover study during which nine patients discontinued due to lack of efficacy while receiving placebo or study noncompliance. The 13 patients completing the study experienced 18 attacks over the course of 60 days while treated with colchicine compared to 68 attacks over the course of 60 days while treated with placebo. The third study was discontinued after an interim analysis of six of the 11 patients enrolled had completed the study; results could not be confirmed.

Open-label experience with colchicine in adults and children with FMF is consistent with the randomized, controlled trial experience and was utilized to support information on the safety profile of colchicine and for dosing recommendations.

16   HOW SUPPLIED/STORAGE AND HANDLING

16.1   How Supplied

COLCRYS (colchicine, USP) tablets 0.6 mg are purple, film-coated, capsule-shaped tablets debossed with "AR 374" on one side and scored on the other side.

Bottles of 30	NDC 64764-119-07
Bottles of 60	NDC 64764-119-06
Bottles of 100	NDC 64764-119-01
Bottles of 250	NDC 64764-119-03
Bottles of 500	NDC 64764-119-05
Bottles of 1000	NDC 64764-119-10

16.2   Storage

Store at 20° to 25°C (68° to 77°F) [See USP Controlled Room Temperature].
Protect from light.
DISPENSE IN TIGHT, LIGHT-RESISTANT CONTAINER.

17   PATIENT COUNSELING INFORMATION

Advise the patient to read the FDA-approved patient labeling (Medication Guide)

Dosing Instructions

Patients should be advised to take COLCRYS as prescribed, even if they are feeling better. Patients should not alter the dose or discontinue treatment without consulting with their doctor. If a dose of COLCRYS is missed:

- For treatment of a gout flare when the patient is not being dosed for prophylaxis, take the missed dose as soon as possible.
- For treatment of a gout flare during prophylaxis, take the missed dose immediately, wait 12 hours, then resume the previous dosing schedule.
- For prophylaxis without treatment for a gout flare, or FMF, take the dose as soon as possible and then return to the normal dosing schedule. However, if a dose is skipped the patient should not double the next dose.

Fatal Overdose

Instruct patient that fatal overdoses, both accidental and intentional, have been reported in adults and children who have ingested colchicine. COLCRYS should be kept out of the reach of children.

Blood Dyscrasias

Patients should be informed that bone marrow depression with agranulocytosis, aplastic anemia and thrombocytopenia may occur with COLCRYS.

Drug and Food Interactions

Patients should be advised that many drugs or other substances may interact with COLCRYS and some interactions could be fatal. Therefore, patients should report to their healthcare provider all of the current medications they are taking and check with their healthcare provider before starting any new medications, particularly antibiotics. Patients should also be advised to report the use of nonprescription medication or herbal products. Grapefruit and grapefruit juice may also interact and should not be consumed during COLCRYS treatment.

Neuromuscular Toxicity

Patients should be informed that muscle pain or weakness, tingling or numbness in fingers or toes may occur with COLCRYS alone or when it is used with certain other drugs. Patients developing any of these signs or symptoms must discontinue COLCRYS and seek medical evaluation immediately.

MEDICATION GUIDE

COLCRYS

(KOL-kris)

(colchicine) tablets

Read the Medication Guide that comes with COLCRYS before you start taking it and each time you get a refill. There may be new information. This Medication Guide does not take the place of talking to your healthcare provider about your medical condition or treatment. You and your healthcare provider should talk about COLCRYS when you start taking it and at regular checkups.

What is the most important information that I should know about COLCRYS?

COLCRYS can cause serious side effects or death if levels of COLCRYS are too high in your body.

- Taking certain medicines with COLCRYS can cause your level of COLCRYS to be too high, especially if you have kidney or liver problems.
- Tell your healthcare provider about all your medical conditions, including if you have kidney or liver problems. Your dose of COLCRYS may need to be changed.
- Tell your healthcare provider about all the medicines you take, including prescription and nonprescription medicines, vitamins and herbal supplements.
- Even medicines that you take for a short period of time, such as antibiotics, can interact with COLCRYS and cause serious side effects or death.
- Talk to your healthcare provider or pharmacist before taking any new medicine.
- Especially tell your healthcare provider if you take:

• atazanavir sulfate (Reyataz)	• clarithromycin (Biaxin)
• cyclosporine (Neoral, Gengraf, Sandimmune)	• darunavir (Prezista)
	• fosamprenavir (Lexiva)
• fosamprenavir (Lexiva) with ritonavir	• itraconazole (Sporanox)
• indinavir (Crixivan)	• lopinavir/ritonavir (Kaletra)
• ketoconazole (Nizoral)	• nelfinavir mesylate (Viracept)
• nefazodone (Serzone)	• saquinavir mesylate (Invirase)
• ritonavir (Norvir)	
• telithromycin (Ketek)	• tipranavir (Aptivus)

Ask your healthcare provider or pharmacist if you are not sure if you take any of the medicines listed above. This is not a complete list of all the medicines that can interact with COLCRYS.

- Know the medicines you take. Keep a list of them and show it to your healthcare provider and pharmacist when you get a new medicine.
- Keep COLCRYS out of the reach of children.

What is COLCRYS?

COLCRYS is a prescription medicine used to:

- prevent and treat gout flares in adults
- treat familial Mediterranean fever (FMF) in adults and children age 4 or older

COLCRYS is not a pain medicine, and it should not be taken to treat pain related to other conditions unless specifically prescribed for those conditions.

Who should not take COLCRYS?

Do not take COLCRYS if you have liver or kidney problems and you take certain other medicines. Serious side effects, including death, have been reported in these patients even when taken as directed. See "**What is the most important information that I should know about COLCRYS?**"

What should I tell my healthcare provider before starting COLCRYS?

See "**What is the most important information that I should know about COLCRYS?**"

Before you take COLCRYS, tell your healthcare provider about all your medical conditions, including if you:

- have liver or kidney problems.
- are pregnant or plan to become pregnant. It is not known if COLCRYS will harm your unborn baby. Talk to your healthcare provider if you are pregnant or plan to become pregnant.
- are breastfeeding or plan to breastfeed. COLCRYS passes into your breast milk. You and your healthcare provider should decide if you will take COLCRYS or breastfeed. If you take COLCRYS and breastfeed, you should talk to your child's healthcare provider about how to watch for side effects in your child.

Tell your healthcare provider about all the medicines you take, including ones that you may only be taking for a short time, such as antibiotics. See "**What is the most important**

Table 7. Drug Interactions: Pharmacokinetic Parameters for Coadministration of Drug in the Presence of COLCRYS (Colchicine, USP) Tablets					
Coadministered Drug	Dose of Coadministered Drug (mg)	Dose of COLCRYS (mg)	N	% Change in Coadministered Drug Concentrations from Baseline (Range: Min - Max)	
				C_{max}	AUC_{0-t}
Theophylline	300 mg (elixir) single dose	0.6 mg twice daily × 14 days	27	1.6 (-30.4 to 23.1)	1.6 (-28.5 to 27.1)
Ethinyl Estradiol (Ortho-Novum 1/35)	21-day cycle (active treatment) + 7-day placebo	0.6 mg twice daily × 14 days	27*	-6.7 (-40.3 to 44.7)	-3.0[†] (-25.3 to 24.9)
Norethindrone (Ortho-Novum 1/35)				0.94 (-37.3 to 59.4)	-1.6[†] (-32.0 to 33.7)

* Conducted in healthy adult females
[†] AUCτ

Continued on next page

information that I should know about COLCRYS?" Do not start a new medicine without talking to your healthcare provider.

Using COLCRYS with certain other medicines, such as cholesterol-lowering medications and digoxin, can affect each other, causing serious side effects. Your healthcare provider may need to change your dose of COLCRYS. Talk to your healthcare provider about whether the medications you are taking might interact with COLCRYS and what side effects to look for.

How should I take COLCRYS?

- Take COLCRYS exactly as your healthcare provider tells you to take it. **If you are not sure about your dosing**, call your healthcare provider.
- COLCRYS can be taken with or without food.
- If you take too much COLCRYS, go to the nearest hospital emergency room right away.
- Do not stop taking COLCRYS even if you start to feel better, unless your healthcare provider tells you.
- Your healthcare provider may do blood tests while you take COLCRYS.
- If you take COLCRYS daily and you miss a dose, then take it as soon as you remember. If it is almost time for your next dose, just skip the missed dose. Take the next dose at your regular time. Do not take two doses at the same time.
- If you have a gout flare while taking COLCRYS daily, report this to your healthcare provider.

What should I avoid while taking COLCRYS?

- Avoid eating grapefruit or drinking grapefruit juice while taking COLCRYS. It can increase your chances of getting serious side effects.

What are the possible side effects of COLCRYS?

COLCRYS can cause serious side effects or even cause death. See **"What is the most important information that I should know about COLCRYS?"**

Get medical help right away if you have:

- Muscle weakness or pain
- Numbness or tingling in your fingers or toes
- Unusual bleeding or bruising
- Increased infections
- Feel weak or tired
- Pale or gray color to your lips, tongue or palms of your hands
- Severe diarrhea or vomiting

Gout Flares: The most common side effect of COLCRYS in people who have gout flares is diarrhea.

FMF: The most common side effects of COLCRYS in people who have FMF are abdominal pain, diarrhea, nausea and vomiting.

Tell your healthcare provider if you have any side effect that bothers you or that does not go away.

These are not all of the possible side effects of COLCRYS. For more information, ask your healthcare provider or pharmacist.

Call your doctor for medical advice about side effects. You may report side effects to FDA at 1-800-FDA-1088.

How should I store COLCRYS?

- Store COLCRYS at room temperature between 68°F and 77°F (20°C and 25°C).
- Keep COLCRYS in a tightly closed container.
- Keep COLCRYS out of the light.

Keep COLCRYS and all medicines out of the reach of children.

General Information about COLCRYS

Medicines are sometimes prescribed for purposes other than those listed in a Medication Guide. Do not use COLCRYS for a condition for which it was not prescribed. Do not give COLCRYS to other people, even if they have the same symptoms that you have. It may harm them. This Medication Guide summarizes the most important information about COLCRYS. If you would like more information, talk with your healthcare provider. You can ask your healthcare provider or pharmacist for information about COLCRYS that is written for healthcare professionals.

For more information, go to www.COLCRYS.com or call 1-877-825-3327.

What are the ingredients in COLCRYS?

Active Ingredient: colchicine.

Inactive Ingredients: carnauba wax, FD&C blue #2, FD&C red #40, hypromellose, lactose monohydrate, magnesium stearate, microcrystalline cellulose, polydextrose, polyethylene glycol, pregelatinized starch, sodium starch glycolate, titanium dioxide and triacetin.

This Medication Guide has been approved by the U.S. Food and Drug Administration.

Distributed by:
Takeda Pharmaceuticals America, Inc.
Deerfield, IL 60015
Revised: November 2012
COLCRYS is a trademark of Takeda Pharmaceuticals U.S.A., Inc., registered with the U.S. Patent and Trademark Office and used under license by Takeda Pharmaceuticals America, Inc.
All other trademarks are the property of their respective owners.
COL243 R2

Shown in Product Identification Guide, page 510

TRINTELLIX　　　　　　　　　　　　　℞
[trin'-tel-ix]
(vortioxetine)
tablets, for oral use

HIGHLIGHTS OF PRESCRIBING INFORMATION
These highlights do not include all the information needed to use TRINTELLIX safely and effectively. See full prescribing information for TRINTELLIX.

TRINTELLIX (vortioxetine) tablets, for oral use
Initial U.S. Approval: 2013

WARNING: SUICIDAL THOUGHTS AND BEHAV-IORS
See full prescribing information for complete boxed warning.
- **Increased risk of suicidal thinking and behavior in children, adolescents, and young adults taking antidepressants (5.1).**
- **Monitor for worsening and emergence of suicidal thoughts and behaviors (5.1).**
- **TRINTELLIX has not been evaluated for use in pediatric patients (8.4).**

————RECENT MAJOR CHANGES————
Warnings and Precautions (5.5) 7/2014

————INDICATIONS AND USAGE————
TRINTELLIX is indicated for the treatment of major depressive disorder (MDD) (1, 14).

————DOSAGE AND ADMINISTRATION————
- The recommended starting dose is 10 mg administered orally once daily without regard to meals (2.1).
- The dose should then be increased to 20 mg/day, as tolerated (2.1).
- Consider 5 mg/day for patients who do not tolerate higher doses (2.1).
- TRINTELLIX can be discontinued abruptly. However, it is recommended that doses of 15 mg/day or 20 mg/day be reduced to 10 mg/day for one week prior to full discontinuation if possible (2.3).
- The maximum recommended dose is 10 mg/day in known CYP2D6 poor metabolizers (2.6).

————DOSAGE FORMS AND STRENGTHS————
TRINTELLIX is available as 5 mg, 10 mg, 15 mg, and 20 mg immediate release tablets (3).

————CONTRAINDICATIONS————
- Hypersensitivity to vortioxetine or any components of the TRINTELLIX formulation (4).
- Monoamine Oxidase Inhibitors (MAOIs): Do not use MAOIs intended to treat psychiatric disorders with TRINTELLIX or within 21 days of stopping treatment with TRINTELLIX. Do not use TRINTELLIX within 14 days of stopping an MAOI intended to treat psychiatric disorders. In addition, do not start TRINTELLIX in a patient who is being treated with linezolid or intravenous methylene blue (4).

————WARNINGS AND PRECAUTIONS————
- Serotonin Syndrome has been reported with serotonergic antidepressants (SSRIs, SNRIs, and others), including with TRINTELLIX, both when taken alone, but especially when co-administered with other serotonergic agents (including triptans, tricyclic antidepressants, fentanyl, lithium, tramadol, tryptophan, buspirone, and St. John's Wort). If such symptoms occur, discontinue TRINTELLIX and initiate supportive treatment. If concomitant use of TRINTELLIX with other serotonergic drugs is clinically warranted, patients should be made aware of a potential increased risk for serotonin syndrome, particularly during treatment initiation and dose increases (5.2).

- Treatment with serotonergic antidepressants (SSRIs, SNRIs, and others) may increase the risk of abnormal bleeding. Patients should be cautioned about the increased risk of bleeding when TRINTELLIX is coadministered with nonsteroidal anti-inflammatory drugs (NSAIDs), aspirin, or other drugs that affect coagulation (5.3).
- Activation of Mania/Hypomania can occur with antidepressant treatment. Screen patients for bipolar disorder (5.4).
- Angle Closure Glaucoma: Angle closure glaucoma has occurred in patients with untreated anatomically narrow angles treated with antidepressants. (5.5)
- Hyponatremia can occur in association with the syndrome of inappropriate antidiuretic hormone secretion (SIADH) (5.6).

————ADVERSE REACTIONS————
Most common adverse reactions (incidence ≥5% and at least twice the rate of placebo) were: nausea, constipation and vomiting (6).
To report SUSPECTED ADVERSE REACTIONS, contact Takeda Pharmaceuticals at 1-877-TAKEDA-7 (1-877-825-3327) or FDA at 1-800-FDA-1088 or www.fda.gov/medwatch.

————DRUG INTERACTIONS————
- Strong inhibitors of CYP2D6: Reduce TRINTELLIX dose by half when a strong CYP2D6 inhibitor (e.g., bupropion, fluoxetine, paroxetine, or quinidine) is coadministered (2.6 and 7.3).
- Strong CYP Inducers: Consider increasing TRINTELLIX dose when a strong CYP inducer (e.g., rifampin, carbamazepine, or phenytoin) is coadministered for more than 14 days. The maximum recommended dose should not exceed 3 times the original dose (2.7 and 7.3).

————USE IN SPECIFIC POPULATIONS————
- Pregnancy: Based on animal data, TRINTELLIX may cause fetal harm (8.1).
- Nursing Mothers: Discontinue TRINTELLIX or nursing (8.3).

See 17 for PATIENT COUNSELING INFORMATION and Medication Guide.

Revised: 5/2016

FULL PRESCRIBING INFORMATION: CONTENTS*
WARNING: SUICIDAL THOUGHTS AND BEHAVIORS

11 **DESCRIPTION**
12 **CLINICAL PHARMACOLOGY**
   12.1 Mechanism of Action
   12.2 Pharmacodynamics
   12.3 Pharmacokinetics
13 **NONCLINICAL TOXICOLOGY**
   13.1 Carcinogenesis, Mutagenesis, Impairment of Fertility
14 **CLINICAL STUDIES**
16 **HOW SUPPLIED/STORAGE AND HANDLING**
17 **PATIENT COUNSELING INFORMATION**
* Sections or subsections omitted from the full prescribing information are not listed.

FULL PRESCRIBING INFORMATION

> **WARNING: SUICIDAL THOUGHTS AND BEHAVIORS**
>
> Antidepressants increased the risk of suicidal thoughts and behavior in children, adolescents, and young adults in short-term studies. These studies did not show an increase in the risk of suicidal thoughts and behavior with antidepressant use in patients over age 24; there was a trend toward reduced risk with antidepressant use in patients aged 65 and older [see Warnings and Precautions (5.1)].
>
> In patients of all ages who are started on antidepressant therapy, monitor closely for worsening, and for emergence of suicidal thoughts and behaviors. Advise families and caregivers of the need for close observation and communication with the prescriber [see Warnings and Precautions (5.1)].
>
> TRINTELLIX has not been evaluated for use in pediatric patients [see Use in Specific Populations (8.4)].

1 INDICATIONS AND USAGE
1.1 Major Depressive Disorder
TRINTELLIX is indicated for the treatment of major depressive disorder (MDD). The efficacy of TRINTELLIX was established in six 6 to 8 week studies (including one study in the elderly) and one maintenance study in adults [see Clinical Studies (14)].

2 DOSAGE AND ADMINISTRATION
2.1 General Instruction for Use
The recommended starting dose is 10 mg administered orally once daily without regard to meals. Dosage should then be increased to 20 mg/day, as tolerated, because higher doses demonstrated better treatment effects in trials conducted in the United States. The efficacy and safety of doses above 20 mg/day have not been evaluated in controlled clinical trials. A dose decrease down to 5 mg/day may be considered for patients who do not tolerate higher doses [see Clinical Studies (14)].

2.2 Maintenance/Continuation/Extended Treatment
It is generally agreed that acute episodes of major depression should be followed by several months or longer of sustained pharmacologic therapy. A maintenance study of TRINTELLIX demonstrated that TRINTELLIX decreased the risk of recurrence of depressive episodes compared to placebo.

2.3 Discontinuing Treatment
Although TRINTELLIX can be abruptly discontinued, in placebo-controlled trials patients experienced transient adverse reactions such as headache and muscle tension following abrupt discontinuation of TRINTELLIX 15 mg/day or 20 mg/day. To avoid these adverse reactions, it is recommended that the dose be decreased to 10 mg/day for one week before full discontinuation of TRINTELLIX 15 mg/day or 20 mg/day [see Adverse Reactions (6)].

2.4 Switching a Patient To or From a Monoamine Oxidase Inhibitor (MAOI) Intended to Treat Psychiatric Disorders
At least 14 days should elapse between discontinuation of a MAOI intended to treat psychiatric disorders and initiation of therapy with TRINTELLIX to avoid the risk of Serotonin Syndrome [see Warnings and Precautions (5.2)]. Conversely, at least 21 days should be allowed after stopping TRINTELLIX before starting an MAOI intended to treat psychiatric disorders [see Contraindications (4)].

2.5 Use of TRINTELLIX with Other MAOIs such as Linezolid or Methylene Blue
Do not start TRINTELLIX in a patient who is being treated with linezolid or intravenous methylene blue because there is an increased risk of serotonin syndrome. In a patient who

requires more urgent treatment of a psychiatric condition, other interventions, including hospitalization, should be considered [see Contraindications (4)].
In some cases, a patient already receiving TRINTELLIX therapy may require urgent treatment with linezolid or intravenous methylene blue. If acceptable alternatives to linezolid or intravenous methylene blue treatment are not available and the potential benefits of linezolid or intravenous methylene blue treatment are judged to outweigh the risks of serotonin syndrome in a particular patient, TRINTELLIX should be stopped promptly, and linezolid or intravenous methylene blue can be administered. The patient should be monitored for symptoms of serotonin syndrome for 21 days or until 24 hours after the last dose of linezolid or intravenous methylene blue, whichever comes first. Therapy with TRINTELLIX may be resumed 24 hours after the last dose of linezolid or intravenous methylene blue [see Warnings and Precautions (5.2)].
The risk of administering methylene blue by non-intravenous routes (such as oral tablets or by local injection) or in intravenous doses much lower than 1 mg/kg with TRINTELLIX is unclear. The clinician should, nevertheless, be aware of the possibility of emergent symptoms of serotonin syndrome with such use [see Warnings and Precautions (5.2)].

2.6 Use of TRINTELLIX in Known CYP2D6 Poor Metabolizers or in Patients Taking Strong CYP2D6 Inhibitors
The maximum recommended dose of TRINTELLIX is 10 mg/day in known CYP2D6 poor metabolizers. Reduce the dose of TRINTELLIX by one-half when patients are receiving a CYP2D6 strong inhibitor (e.g., bupropion, fluoxetine, paroxetine, or quinidine) concomitantly. The dose should be increased to the original level when the CYP2D6 inhibitor is discontinued [see Drug Interactions (7.3)].

2.7 Use of TRINTELLIX in Patients Taking Strong CYP Inducers
Consider increasing the dose of TRINTELLIX when a strong CYP inducer (e.g., rifampin, carbamazepine, or phenytoin) is coadministered for greater than 14 days. The maximum recommended dose should not exceed three times the original dose. The dose of TRINTELLIX should be reduced to the original level within 14 days, when the inducer is discontinued [see Drug Interactions (7.3)].

3 DOSAGE FORMS AND STRENGTHS
TRINTELLIX is available as immediate-release, film-coated tablets in the following strengths:
- 5 mg: pink, almond shaped biconvex film coated tablet, debossed with "5" on one side and "TL" on the other side
- 10 mg: yellow, almond shaped biconvex film coated tablet, debossed with "10" on one side and "TL" on the other side
- 15 mg: orange, almond shaped biconvex film coated tablet, debossed with "15" on one side and "TL" on the other side
- 20 mg: red, almond shaped biconvex film coated tablet, debossed with "20" on one side and "TL" on the other side

4 CONTRAINDICATIONS
- Hypersensitivity to vortioxetine or any components of the formulation. Angioedema has been reported in patients treated with TRINTELLIX.
- The use of MAOIs intended to treat psychiatric disorders with TRINTELLIX or within 21 days of stopping treatment with TRINTELLIX is contraindicated because of an increased risk of serotonin syndrome. The use of TRINTELLIX within 14 days of stopping an MAOI intended to treat psychiatric disorders is also contraindicated [see Dosage and Administration (2.4) and Warnings and Precautions (5.2)].
Starting TRINTELLIX in a patient who is being treated with MAOIs such as linezolid or intravenous methylene blue is also contraindicated because of an increased risk of serotonin syndrome [see Dosage and Administration (2.5) and Warnings and Precautions (5.2)].

5 WARNINGS AND PRECAUTIONS
5.1 Clinical Worsening and Suicide Risk
Patients with major depressive disorder (MDD), both adult and pediatric, may experience worsening of their depression and/or the emergence of suicidal ideation and behavior (suicidality) or unusual changes in behavior, whether or not they are taking antidepressant medications, and this risk may persist until significant remission occurs. Suicide is a known risk of depression and certain other psychiatric disorders, and these disorders themselves are the strongest

predictors of suicide. There has been a long-standing concern, however, that antidepressants may have a role in inducing worsening of depression and the emergence of suicidality in certain patients during the early phases of treatment. Pooled analyses of short-term placebo-controlled studies of antidepressant drugs (selective serotonin reuptake inhibitors [SSRIs] and others) showed that these drugs increase the risk of suicidal thinking and behavior (suicidality) in children, adolescents, and young adults (ages 18 to 24) with MDD and other psychiatric disorders. Short-term studies did not show an increase in the risk of suicidality with antidepressants compared to placebo in adults beyond age 24; there was a trend toward reduction with antidepressants compared to placebo in adults aged 65 and older.
The pooled analyses of placebo-controlled studies in children and adolescents with MDD, obsessive-compulsive disorder (OCD), or other psychiatric disorders included a total of 24 short-term studies of nine antidepressant drugs in over 4,400 patients. The pooled analyses of placebo-controlled studies in adults with MDD or other psychiatric disorders included a total of 295 short-term studies (median duration of two months) of 11 antidepressant drugs in over 77,000 patients. There was considerable variation in risk of suicidality among drugs, but a tendency toward an increase in the younger patients for almost all drugs studied. There were differences in absolute risk of suicidality across the different indications, with the highest incidence in MDD. The risk differences (drug vs. placebo), however, were relatively stable within age strata and across indications. These risk differences (drug-placebo difference in the number of cases of suicidality per 1000 patients treated) are provided in *Table 1*.

Table 1. Drug-Placebo Difference in Number of Cases of Suicidality per 1000 Patients Treated

Age Range	
Increases Compared to Placebo	
<18	14 additional cases
18-24	5 additional cases
Decreases Compared to Placebo	
25-64	1 fewer case
≥65	6 fewer cases

No suicides occurred in any of the pediatric studies. There were suicides in the adult studies, but the number was not sufficient to reach any conclusion about drug effect on suicide.
It is unknown whether the suicidality risk extends to longer-term use, i.e., beyond several months. However, there is substantial evidence from placebo-controlled maintenance studies in adults with depression that the use of antidepressants can delay the recurrence of depression.
All patients being treated with antidepressants for any indication should be monitored appropriately and observed closely for clinical worsening, suicidality, and unusual changes in behavior, especially during the initial few months of a course of drug therapy, or at times of dose changes, either increases or decreases.
The following symptoms anxiety, agitation, panic attacks, insomnia, irritability, hostility, aggressiveness, impulsivity, akathisia (psychomotor restlessness), hypomania, and mania have been reported in adult and pediatric patients being treated with antidepressants for MDD as well as for other indications, both psychiatric and nonpsychiatric. Although a causal link between the emergence of such symptoms and either the worsening of depression and/or the emergence of suicidal impulses has not been established, there is concern that such symptoms may represent precursors to emerging suicidality.
Consideration should be given to changing the therapeutic regimen, including possibly discontinuing the medication, in patients whose depression is persistently worse, or who are experiencing emergent suicidality or symptoms that might be precursors to worsening depression or suicidality, especially if these symptoms are severe, abrupt in onset, or were not part of the patient's presenting symptoms.

Continued on next page

Families and caregivers of patients being treated with antidepressants for MDD or other indications, both psychiatric and nonpsychiatric, should be alerted about the need to monitor patients for the emergence of agitation, irritability, unusual changes in behavior, and the other symptoms described above, as well as the emergence of suicidality, and to report such symptoms immediately to healthcare providers. Such monitoring should include daily observation by families and caregivers.

Screening Patients for Bipolar Disorder
A major depressive episode may be the initial presentation of bipolar disorder. It is generally believed (though not established in controlled studies) that treating such an episode with an antidepressant alone may increase the likelihood of precipitation of a mixed/manic episode in patients at risk for bipolar disorder. Whether any of the symptoms described above represent such a conversion is unknown. However, prior to initiating treatment with an antidepressant, patients with depressive symptoms should be adequately screened to determine if they are at risk for bipolar disorder; such screening should include a detailed psychiatric history, including a family history of suicide, bipolar disorder, and depression. It should be noted that TRINTELLIX is not approved for use in treating bipolar depression.

5.2   Serotonin Syndrome
The development of a potentially life-threatening serotonin syndrome has been reported with serotonergic antidepressants including TRINTELLIX, when used alone but more often when used concomitantly with other serotonergic drugs (including triptans, tricyclic antidepressants, fentanyl, lithium, tramadol, tryptophan, buspirone, and St. John's Wort), and with drugs that impair metabolism of serotonin (in particular, MAOIs, both those intended to treat psychiatric disorders and also others, such as linezolid and intravenous methylene blue).

Serotonin syndrome symptoms may include mental status changes (e.g., agitation, hallucinations, delirium, and coma), autonomic instability (e.g., tachycardia, labile blood pressure, dizziness, diaphoresis, flushing, hyperthermia), neuromuscular symptoms (e.g., tremor, rigidity, myoclonus, hyperreflexia, incoordination), seizures, and/or gastrointestinal symptoms (e.g., nausea, vomiting, diarrhea). Patients should be monitored for the emergence of serotonin syndrome.

The concomitant use of TRINTELLIX with MAOIs intended to treat psychiatric disorders is contraindicated. TRINTELLIX should also not be started in a patient who is being treated with MAOIs such as linezolid or intravenous methylene blue. All reports with methylene blue that provided information on the route of administration involved intravenous administration in the dose range of 1 mg/kg to 8 mg/kg. No reports involved the administration of methylene blue by other routes (such as oral tablets or local tissue injection) or at lower doses. There may be circumstances when it is necessary to initiate treatment with a MAOI such as linezolid or intravenous methylene blue in a patient taking TRINTELLIX. TRINTELLIX should be discontinued before initiating treatment with the MAOI [see Contraindications (4) and Dosage and Administration (2.4)].

If concomitant use of TRINTELLIX with other serotonergic drugs, including triptans, tricyclic antidepressants, fentanyl, lithium, tramadol, buspirone, tryptophan, and St. John's Wort is clinically warranted, patients should be made aware of a potential increased risk for serotonin syndrome, particularly during treatment initiation and dose increases.

Treatment with TRINTELLIX and any concomitant serotonergic agents should be discontinued immediately if the above events occur and supportive symptomatic treatment should be initiated.

5.3   Abnormal Bleeding
The use of drugs that interfere with serotonin reuptake inhibition, including TRINTELLIX, may increase the risk of bleeding events. Concomitant use of aspirin, nonsteroidal anti-inflammatory drugs (NSAIDs), warfarin, and other anticoagulants may add to this risk. Case reports and epidemiological studies (case-control and cohort design) have demonstrated an association between use of drugs that interfere with serotonin reuptake and the occurrence of gastrointestinal bleeding. Bleeding events related to drugs that inhibit serotonin reuptake have ranged from ecchymosis, hematoma, epistaxis, and petechiae to life-threatening hemorrhages.

Patients should be cautioned about the increased risk of bleeding when TRINTELLIX is coadministered with NSAIDs, aspirin, or other drugs that affect coagulation or bleeding [see Drug Interactions (7.2)].

5.4   Activation of Mania/Hypomania
Symptoms of mania/hypomania were reported in <0.1% of patients treated with TRINTELLIX in pre-marketing clinical studies. Activation of mania/hypomania has been reported in a small proportion of patients with major affective disorder who were treated with other antidepressants. As with all antidepressants, use TRINTELLIX cautiously in patients with a history or family history of bipolar disorder, mania, or hypomania.

5.5   Angle Closure Glaucoma
Angle Closure Glaucoma: The pupillary dilation that occurs following use of many antidepressant drugs, including TRINTELLIX, may trigger an angle closure attack in a patient with anatomically narrow angles who does not have a patent iridectomy.

5.6   Hyponatremia
Hyponatremia has occurred as a result of treatment with serotonergic drugs. In many cases, hyponatremia appears to be the result of the syndrome of inappropriate antidiuretic hormone secretion (SIADH). One case with serum sodium lower than 110 mmol/L was reported in a subject treated with TRINTELLIX in a pre-marketing clinical study. Elderly patients may be at greater risk of developing hyponatremia with a serotonergic antidepressant. Also, patients taking diuretics or who are otherwise volume-depleted can be at greater risk. Discontinuation of TRINTELLIX in patients with symptomatic hyponatremia and appropriate medical intervention should be instituted. Signs and symptoms of hyponatremia include headache, difficulty concentrating, memory impairment, confusion, weakness, and unsteadiness, which can lead to falls. More severe and/or acute cases have included hallucination, syncope, seizure, coma, respiratory arrest, and death.

6   ADVERSE REACTIONS
The following adverse reactions are discussed in greater detail in other sections of the label.
• Hypersensitivity [see Contraindications (4)]
• Clinical Worsening and Suicide Risk [see Warnings and Precautions (5.1)]
• Serotonin Syndrome [see Warnings and Precautions (5.2)]
• Abnormal Bleeding [see Warnings and Precautions (5.3)]
• Activation of Mania/Hypomania [see Warnings and Precautions (5.4)]
• Hyponatremia [see Warnings and Precautions (5.6)]

6.1   Clinical Studies Experience
Because clinical trials are conducted under widely varying conditions, adverse reaction rates observed in the clinical trials of a drug cannot be directly compared to rates in the clinical studies of another drug and may not reflect the rates observed in clinical practice.

Patient Exposure
TRINTELLIX was evaluated for safety in 4746 patients (18 years to 88 years of age) diagnosed with MDD who participated in pre-marketing clinical studies; 2616 of those patients were exposed to TRINTELLIX in 6 to 8 week, placebo-controlled studies at doses ranging from 5 mg to 20 mg once daily and 204 patients were exposed to TRINTELLIX in a 24 week to 64 week placebo-controlled maintenance study at doses of 5 mg to 10 mg once daily. Patients from the 6 to 8 week studies continued into 12-month open-label studies. A total of 2586 patients were exposed to at least one dose of TRINTELLIX in open-label studies, 1727 were exposed to TRINTELLIX for six months and 885 were exposed for at least one year.

Adverse Reactions Reported as Reasons for Discontinuation of Treatment
In pooled 6 to 8 week placebo-controlled studies the incidence of patients who received TRINTELLIX 5 mg/day, 10 mg/day, 15 mg/day and 20 mg/day and discontinued treatment because of an adverse reaction was 5%, 6%, 8% and 8%, respectively, compared to 4% of placebo-treated patients. Nausea was the most common adverse reaction reported as a reason for discontinuation.

Common Adverse Reactions in Placebo-Controlled MDD Studies
The most commonly observed adverse reactions in MDD patients treated with TRINTELLIX in 6 to 8 week placebo-controlled studies (incidence ≥5% and at least twice the rate of placebo) were nausea, constipation and vomiting.

Table 2 shows the incidence of common adverse reactions that occurred in ≥2% of MDD patients treated with any TRINTELLIX dose and at least 2% more frequently than in placebo-treated patients in the 6 to 8 week placebo-controlled studies.
[See table 2 below]

Nausea
Nausea was the most common adverse reaction and its frequency was dose-related (Table 2). It was usually considered mild or moderate in intensity and the median duration was 2 weeks. Nausea was more common in females than males. Nausea most commonly occurred in the first week of TRINTELLIX treatment with 15 to 20% of patients experiencing nausea after 1 to 2 days of treatment. Approximately 10% of patients taking TRINTELLIX 10 mg/day to 20 mg/day had nausea at the end of the 6 to 8 week placebo-controlled studies.

Sexual Dysfunction
Difficulties in sexual desire, sexual performance and sexual satisfaction often occur as manifestations of psychiatric disorders, but they may also be consequences of pharmacologic treatment.

Table 2. Common Adverse Reactions Occurring in ≥2% of Patients Treated with any TRINTELLIX Dose and at Least 2% Greater than the Incidence in Placebo-treated Patients

System Organ Class Preferred Term	TRINTELLIX 5 mg/day	TRINTELLIX 10 mg/day	TRINTELLIX 15 mg/day	TRINTELLIX 20 mg/day	Placebo
	N=1013 %	N=699 %	N=449 %	N=455 %	N=1621 %
Gastrointestinal disorders					
Nausea	21	26	32	32	9
Diarrhea	7	7	10	7	6
Dry mouth	7	7	6	8	6
Constipation	3	5	6	6	3
Vomiting	3	5	6	6	1
Flatulence	1	3	2	1	1
Nervous system disorders					
Dizziness	6	6	8	9	6
Psychiatric disorders					
Abnormal dreams	<1	<1	2	3	1
Skin and subcutaneous tissue disorders					
Pruritus*	1	2	3	3	1

* Includes pruritus generalized

In the MDD 6 to 8 week controlled trials of TRINTELLIX, voluntarily reported adverse reactions related to sexual dysfunction were captured as individual event terms. These event terms have been aggregated and the overall incidence was as follows. In male patients the overall incidence was 3%, 4%, 4%, 5% in TRINTELLIX 5 mg/day, 10 mg/day, 15 mg/day, 20 mg/day, respectively, compared to 2% in placebo. In female patients, the overall incidence was <1%, 1%, <1%, 2% in TRINTELLIX 5 mg/day, 10 mg/day, 15 mg/day, 20 mg/day, respectively, compared to <1% in placebo.

Because voluntarily reported adverse sexual reactions are known to be underreported, in part because patients and physicians may be reluctant to discuss them, the Arizona Sexual Experiences Scale (ASEX), a validated measure designed to identify sexual side effects, was used prospectively in seven placebo-controlled trials. The ASEX scale includes five questions that pertain to the following aspects of sexual function: 1) sex drive, 2) ease of arousal, 3) ability to achieve erection (men) or lubrication (women), 4) ease of reaching orgasm, and 5) orgasm satisfaction.

The presence or absence of sexual dysfunction among patients entering clinical studies was based on their ASEX scores. For patients without sexual dysfunction at baseline (approximately 1/3 of the population across all treatment groups in each study), *Table 3* shows the incidence of patients that developed treatment-emergent sexual dysfunction when treated with TRINTELLIX or placebo in any fixed dose group. Physicians should routinely inquire about possible sexual side effects.

[See table 3 above]

Table 3. ASEX Incidence of Treatment Emergent Sexual Dysfunction*

	TRINTELLIX 5 mg/day N=65:67†	TRINTELLIX 10 mg/day N=94:86†	TRINTELLIX 15 mg/day N=57:67†	TRINTELLIX 20 mg/day N=67:59†	Placebo N=135:162†
Females	22%	23%	33%	34%	20%
Males	16%	20%	19%	29%	14%

* Incidence based on number of subjects with sexual dysfunction during the study / number of subjects without sexual dysfunction at baseline. Sexual dysfunction was defined as a subject scoring any of the following on the ASEX scale at two consecutive visits during the study: 1) total score ≥19; 2) any single item ≥5; 3) three or more items each with a score ≥4

† Sample size for each dose group is the number of patients (females:males) without sexual dysfunction at baseline

Adverse Reactions Following Abrupt Discontinuation of TRINTELLIX Treatment

Discontinuation symptoms have been prospectively evaluated in patients taking TRINTELLIX 10 mg/day, 15 mg/day, and 20 mg/day using the Discontinuation-Emergent Signs and Symptoms (DESS) scale in clinical trials. Some patients experienced discontinuation symptoms such as headache, muscle tension, mood swings, sudden outbursts of anger, dizziness, and runny nose in the first week of abrupt discontinuation of TRINTELLIX 15 mg/day and 20 mg/day.

Laboratory Tests

TRINTELLIX has not been associated with any clinically important changes in laboratory test parameters in serum chemistry (except sodium), hematology and urinalysis as measured in the 6 to 8 week placebo-controlled studies. Hyponatremia has been reported with the treatment of TRINTELLIX *[see Warnings and Precautions (5.6)]*. In the 6-month, double-blind, placebo-controlled phase of a long-term study in patients who had responded to TRINTELLIX during the initial 12-week, open-label phase, there were no clinically important changes in lab test parameters between TRINTELLIX and placebo-treated patients.

Weight

TRINTELLIX had no significant effect on body weight as measured by the mean change from baseline in the 6 to 8 week placebo-controlled studies. In the 6-month, double-blind, placebo-controlled phase of a long-term study in patients who had responded to TRINTELLIX during the initial 12-week, open-label phase, there was no significant effect on body weight between TRINTELLIX and placebo-treated patients.

Vital Signs

TRINTELLIX has not been associated with any clinically significant effects on vital signs, including systolic and diastolic blood pressure and heart rate, as measured in placebo-controlled studies.

Other Adverse Reactions Observed in Clinical Studies

The following listing does not include reactions: 1) already listed in previous tables or elsewhere in labeling, 2) for which a drug cause was remote, 3) which were so general as to be uninformative, 4) which were not considered to have significant clinical implications, or 5) which occurred at a rate equal to or less than placebo.

Ear and labyrinth disorders — vertigo
Gastrointestinal disorders — dyspepsia
Nervous system disorders — dysgeusia
Vascular disorders — flushing

7 DRUG INTERACTIONS

7.1 CNS Active Agents

Monoamine Oxidase Inhibitors

Adverse reactions, some of which are serious or fatal, can develop in patients who use MAOIs or who have recently been discontinued from an MAOI and started on a serotonergic antidepressant(s) or who have recently had SSRI or SNRI therapy discontinued prior to initiation of an MAOI *[see Dosage and Administration (2.4), Contraindications (4) and Warnings and Precautions (5.2)]*.

Serotonergic Drugs

Based on the mechanism of action of TRINTELLIX and the potential for serotonin toxicity, serotonin syndrome may occur when TRINTELLIX is coadministered with other drugs that may affect the serotonergic neurotransmitter systems (e.g., SSRIs, SNRIs, triptans, buspirone, tramadol, and tryptophan products etc.). Closely monitor symptoms of serotonin syndrome if TRINTELLIX is co-administered with other serotonergic drugs. Treatment with TRINTELLIX and any concomitant serotonergic agents should be discontinued immediately if serotonin syndrome occurs *[see Warnings and Precautions (5.2)]*.

Other CNS Active Agents

No clinically relevant effect was observed on steady state lithium exposure following coadministration with multiple daily doses of TRINTELLIX. Multiple doses of TRINTELLIX did not affect the pharmacokinetics or pharmacodynamics (composite cognitive score) of diazepam. A clinical study has shown that TRINTELLIX (single dose of 20 or 40 mg) did not increase the impairment of mental and motor skills caused by alcohol (single dose of 0.6 g/kg). Details on the potential pharmacokinetic interactions between TRINTELLIX and bupropion can be found in Section 7.3.

7.2 Drugs that Interfere with Hemostasis (e.g., NSAIDs, Aspirin, and Warfarin)

Serotonin release by platelets plays an important role in hemostasis. Epidemiological studies of case-control and cohort design have demonstrated an association between use of psychotropic drugs that interfere with serotonin reuptake and the occurrence of upper gastrointestinal bleeding. These studies have also shown that concurrent use of an NSAID or aspirin may potentiate this risk of bleeding. Altered anticoagulant effects, including increased bleeding, have been reported when SSRIs and SNRIs are coadministered with warfarin.

Following coadministration of stable doses of warfarin (1 to 10 mg/day) with multiple daily doses of TRINTELLIX, no significant effects were observed in INR, prothrombin values or total warfarin (protein bound plus free drug) pharmacokinetics for both R- and S-warfarin *[see Drug Interactions (7.4)]*. Coadministration of aspirin 150 mg/day with multiple daily doses of TRINTELLIX had no significant inhibitory effect on platelet aggregation or pharmacokinetics of aspirin and salicylic acid *[see Drug Interactions (7.4)]*. Patients receiving other drugs that interfere with hemostasis should be carefully monitored when TRINTELLIX is initiated or discontinued *[see Warnings and Precautions (5.3)]*.

7.3 Potential for Other Drugs to Affect TRINTELLIX

Reduce TRINTELLIX dose by half when a strong CYP2D6 inhibitor (e.g., bupropion, fluoxetine, paroxetine, quinidine) is coadministered. Consider increasing the TRINTELLIX dose when a strong CYP inducer (e.g., rifampicin, carbamazepine, phenytoin) is coadministered. The maximum dose is not recommended to exceed three times the original dose *[see Dosage and Administration (2.5 and 2.6)]* (Figure 1).

[See figure 1 at top of next page]

7.4 Potential for TRINTELLIX to Affect Other Drugs

No dose adjustment for the comedications is needed when TRINTELLIX is coadministered with a substrate of CYP1A2 (e.g., duloxetine), CYP2A6, CYP2B6 (e.g., bupropion), CYP2C8 (e.g., repaglinide), CYP2C9 (e.g., S-warfarin), CYP2C19 (e.g., diazepam), CYP2D6 (e.g., venlafaxine), CYP3A4/5 (e.g., budesonide), and P-gp (e.g., digoxin). In addition, no dose adjustment for lithium, aspirin, and warfarin is necessary.

Vortioxetine and its metabolites are unlikely to inhibit the following CYP enzymes and transporter based on *in vitro* data: CYP1A2, CYP2A6, CYP2B6, CYP2C8, CYP2C9, CYP2C19, CYP2D6, CYP2E1, CYP3A4/5, and P-gp. As such, no clinically relevant interactions with drugs metabolized by these CYP enzymes would be expected.

In addition, vortioxetine did not induce CYP1A2, CYP2A6, CYP2B6, CYP2C8, CYP2C9, CYP2C19, and CYP3A4/5 in an *in vitro* study in cultured human hepatocytes. Chronic administration of TRINTELLIX is unlikely to induce the metabolism of drugs metabolized by these CYP isoforms. Furthermore, in a series of clinical drug interaction studies, coadministration of TRINTELLIX with substrates for CYP2B6 (e.g., bupropion), CYP2C9 (e.g., warfarin), and CYP2C19 (e.g., diazepam), had no clinical meaningful effect on the pharmacokinetics of these substrates *(Figure 2)*.

Because vortioxetine is highly bound to plasma protein, coadministration of TRINTELLIX with another drug that is highly protein bound may increase free concentrations of the other drug. However, in a clinical study with coadministration of TRINTELLIX (10 mg/day) and warfarin (1 mg/day to 10 mg/day), a highly protein-bound drug, no significant change in INR was observed *[see Drug Interactions (7.2)]*.

[See figure 2 at top of next page]

8 USE IN SPECIFIC POPULATIONS

8.1 Pregnancy

Pregnancy Category C

Risk Summary

There are no adequate and well-controlled studies of TRINTELLIX in pregnant women. Vortioxetine caused developmental delays when administered during pregnancy to rats and rabbits at doses 15 and 10 times the maximum recommended human dose (MRHD) of 20 mg, respectively. Developmental delays were also seen after birth in rats at doses 20 times the MRHD of vortioxetine given during pregnancy and through lactation. There were no teratogenic effects in rats or rabbits at doses up to 77 and 58 times, the MRHD of vortioxetine, respectively, given during organogenesis. The incidence of malformations in human pregnancies has not been established for TRINTELLIX. All human pregnancies, regardless of drug exposure, have a background rate of 2 to 4% for major malformations, and 15 to 20% for pregnancy loss. TRINTELLIX should be used during pregnancy only if the potential benefit justifies the potential risk to the fetus.

Clinical Considerations

Neonates exposed to SSRIs or SNRIs, late in the third trimester have developed complications requiring prolonged hospitalization, respiratory support and tube feeding. Such complications can arise immediately upon delivery. Reported clinical findings have included respiratory distress, cyanosis, apnea, seizures, temperature instability, feeding difficulty, vomiting, hypoglycemia, hypotonia, hypertonia, hyperreflexia, tremor, jitteriness, irritability and constant crying. These features are consistent with either a direct toxic effect of these classes of drugs or possibly, a drug discontinuation syndrome. It should be noted that in some cases, the clinical picture is consistent with serotonin syndrome *[see Warnings and Precautions (5.2)]*. When treating a pregnant woman with TRINTELLIX during the third trimester, the physician should carefully consider the potential risks and benefits of treatment.

Neonates exposed to SSRIs in pregnancy may have an increased risk for persistent pulmonary hypertension of the newborn (PPHN). PPHN occurs in one to two per 1,000 live births in the general population and is associated with substantial neonatal morbidity and mortality. Several recent epidemiologic studies suggest a positive statistical association between SSRI use in pregnancy and PPHN. Other studies do not show a significant statistical association.

Continued on next page

A prospective longitudinal study was conducted of 201 pregnant women with a history of major depression, who were either on antidepressants or had received antidepressants less than 12 weeks prior to their last menstrual period, and were in remission. Women who discontinued antidepressant medication during pregnancy showed a significant increase in relapse of their major depression compared to those women who remained on antidepressant medication throughout pregnancy. When treating a pregnant woman with TRINTELLIX, the physician should carefully consider both the potential risks of taking a serotonergic antidepressant, along with the established benefits of treating depression with an antidepressant.

Animal Data

In pregnant rats and rabbits, no teratogenic effects were seen when vortioxetine was given during the period of organogenesis at oral doses up to 160 and 60 mg/kg/day, respectively. These doses are 77 and 58 times, in rats and rabbits, respectively, the maximum recommended human dose (MRHD) of 20 mg on a mg/m^2 basis. Developmental delay, seen as decreased fetal body weight and delayed ossification, occurred in rats and rabbits at doses equal to and greater than 30 and 10 mg/kg (15 and 10 times the MRHD, respectively) in the presence of maternal toxicity (decreased food consumption and decreased body weight gain). When vortioxetine was administered to pregnant rats at oral doses up to 120 mg/kg (58 times the MRHD) throughout pregnancy and lactation, the number of live-born pups was decreased and early postnatal pup mortality was increased at 40 and 120 mg/kg. Additionally, pup weights were decreased at birth to weaning at 120 mg/kg and development (specifically eye opening) was slightly delayed at 40 and 120 mg/kg. These effects were not seen at 10 mg/kg (5 times the MRHD).

8.3   Nursing Mothers

It is not known whether vortioxetine is present in human milk. Vortioxetine is present in the milk of lactating rats. Because many drugs are present in human milk and because of the potential for serious adverse reactions in nursing infants from TRINTELLIX, a decision should be made whether to discontinue nursing or to discontinue the drug, taking into account the importance of the drug to the mother.

8.4   Pediatric Use

Clinical studies on the use of TRINTELLIX in pediatric patients have not been conducted; therefore, the safety and effectiveness of TRINTELLIX in the pediatric population have not been established.

8.5   Geriatric Use

No dose adjustment is recommended on the basis of age *(Figure 3)*. Results from a single-dose pharmacokinetic study in elderly (>65 years old) vs. young (24 to 45 years old) subjects demonstrated that the pharmacokinetics were generally similar between the two age groups.

Of the 2616 subjects in clinical studies of TRINTELLIX, 11% (286) were 65 and over, which included subjects from a placebo-controlled study specifically in elderly patients *[see Clinical Studies (14)]*. No overall differences in safety or effectiveness were observed between these subjects and younger subjects, and other reported clinical experience has not identified differences in responses between the elderly and younger patients.

Serotonergic antidepressants have been associated with cases of clinically significant hyponatremia in elderly patients, who may be at greater risk for this adverse event *[see Warnings and Precautions (5.6)]*.

8.6   Use in Other Patient Populations

No dose adjustment of TRINTELLIX on the basis of race, gender, ethnicity, or renal function (from mild renal impairment to end-stage renal disease) is necessary. In addition, the same dose can be administered in patients with mild to moderate hepatic impairment *(Figure 3)*. TRINTELLIX has not been studied in patients with severe hepatic impairment. Therefore, TRINTELLIX is not recommended in patients with severe hepatic impairment.

[See figure 3 at bottom of next page]

9   DRUG ABUSE AND DEPENDENCE

TRINTELLIX is not a controlled substance.

10   OVERDOSAGE

10.1   Human Experience

There is limited clinical trial experience regarding human overdosage with TRINTELLIX. In pre-marketing clinical studies, cases of overdose were limited to patients who ac-

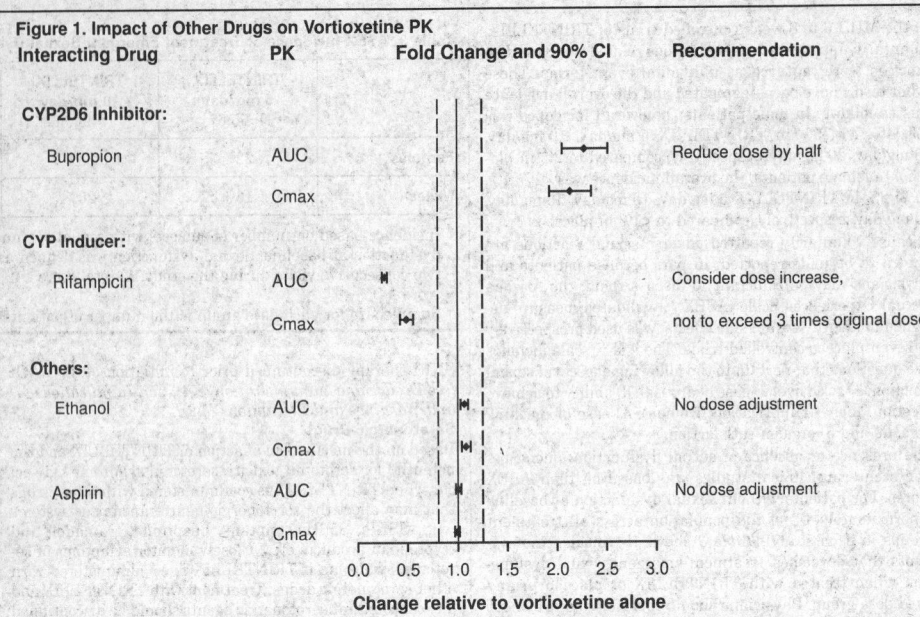

Figure 1. Impact of Other Drugs on Vortioxetine PK

Interacting Drug	PK	Fold Change and 90% CI	Recommendation
CYP2D6 Inhibitor:			
Bupropion	AUC		Reduce dose by half
	Cmax		
CYP Inducer:			
Rifampicin	AUC		Consider dose increase,
	Cmax		not to exceed 3 times original dose
Others:			
Ethanol	AUC		No dose adjustment
	Cmax		
Aspirin	AUC		No dose adjustment
	Cmax		

Change relative to vortioxetine alone

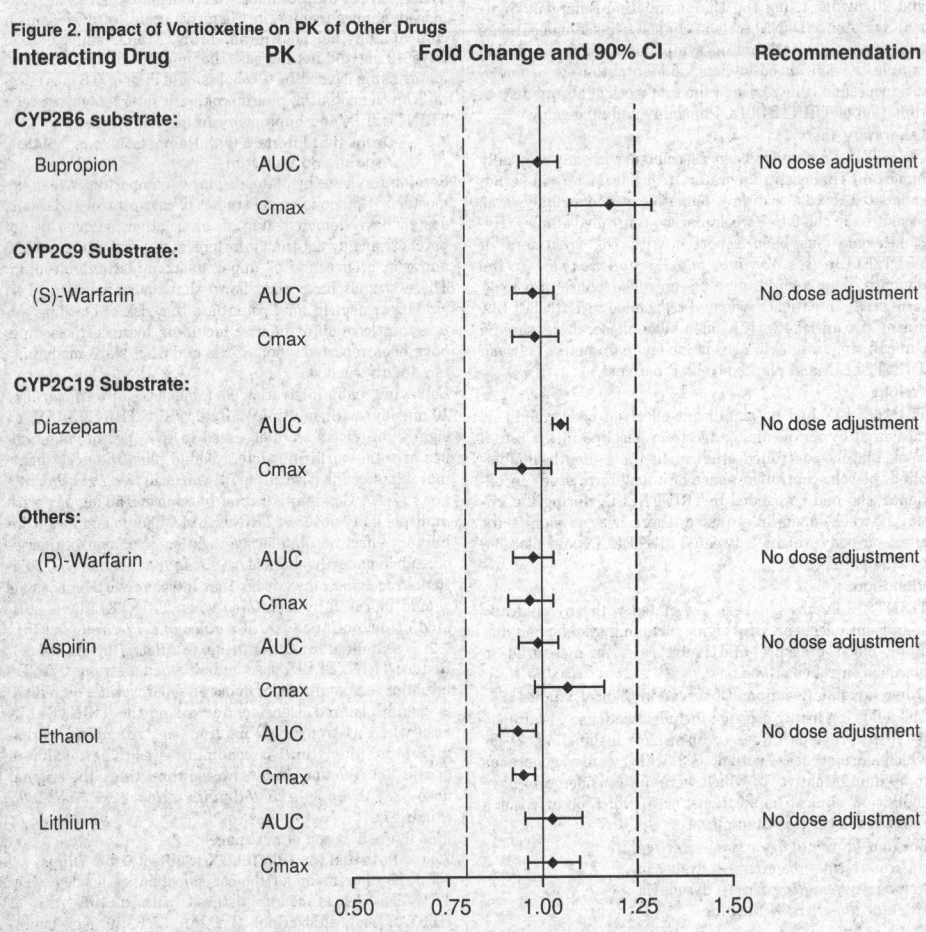

Figure 2. Impact of Vortioxetine on PK of Other Drugs

Interacting Drug	PK	Fold Change and 90% CI	Recommendation
CYP2B6 substrate:			
Bupropion	AUC		No dose adjustment
	Cmax		
CYP2C9 Substrate:			
(S)-Warfarin	AUC		No dose adjustment
	Cmax		
CYP2C19 Substrate:			
Diazepam	AUC		No dose adjustment
	Cmax		
Others:			
(R)-Warfarin	AUC		No dose adjustment
	Cmax		
Aspirin	AUC		No dose adjustment
	Cmax		
Ethanol	AUC		No dose adjustment
	Cmax		
Lithium	AUC		No dose adjustment
	Cmax		

Change relative to interacting drug alone

cidentally or intentionally consumed up to a maximum dose of 40 mg of TRINTELLIX. The maximum single dose tested was 75 mg in men. Ingestion of TRINTELLIX in the dose range of 40 to 75 mg was associated with increased rates of nausea, dizziness, diarrhea, abdominal discomfort, generalized pruritus, somnolence, and flushing.

10.2 Management of Overdose
No specific antidotes for TRINTELLIX are known. In managing over dosage, consider the possibility of multiple drug involvement. In case of overdose, call Poison Control Center at 1-800-222-1222 for latest recommendations.

11 DESCRIPTION
TRINTELLIX is an immediate-release tablet for oral administration that contains the beta (β) polymorph of vortioxetine hydrobromide (HBr), an antidepressant. Vortioxetine HBr is known chemically as 1-[2-(2,4-Dimethyl-phenylsulfanyl)-phenyl]-piperazine, hydrobromide. The empirical formula is $C_{18} H_{22} N_2 S$, HBr with a molecular weight of 379.36 g/mol. The structural formula is: [See structural formula at top of next column]
Vortioxetine HBr is a white to very slightly beige powder that is slightly soluble in water.
Each TRINTELLIX tablet contains 6.355 mg, 12.71 mg, 19.065 mg, or 25.42 mg of vortioxetine HBr equivalent to 5 mg, 10 mg, 15 mg, or 20 mg of vortioxetine, respectively.

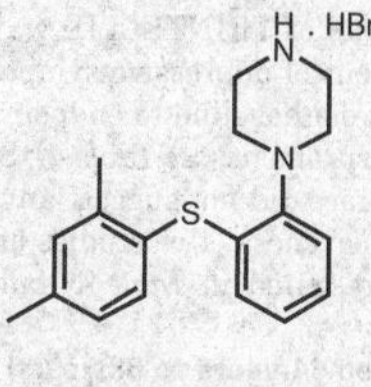

The inactive ingredients in TRINTELLIX tablets include mannitol, microcrystalline cellulose, hydroxypropyl cellulose, sodium starch glycolate, magnesium stearate and film coating which consists of hypromellose, titanium dioxide, polyethylene glycol 400, iron oxide red (5 mg, 15 mg, and 20 mg) and iron oxide yellow (10 mg and 15 mg).

12 CLINICAL PHARMACOLOGY
12.1 Mechanism of Action
The mechanism of the antidepressant effect of vortioxetine is not fully understood, but is thought to be related to its enhancement of serotonergic activity in the CNS through inhibition of the reuptake of serotonin (5-HT). It also has several other activities including 5-HT3 receptor antagonism and 5-HT1A receptor agonism. The contribution of these activities to vortioxetine's antidepressant effect has not been established.

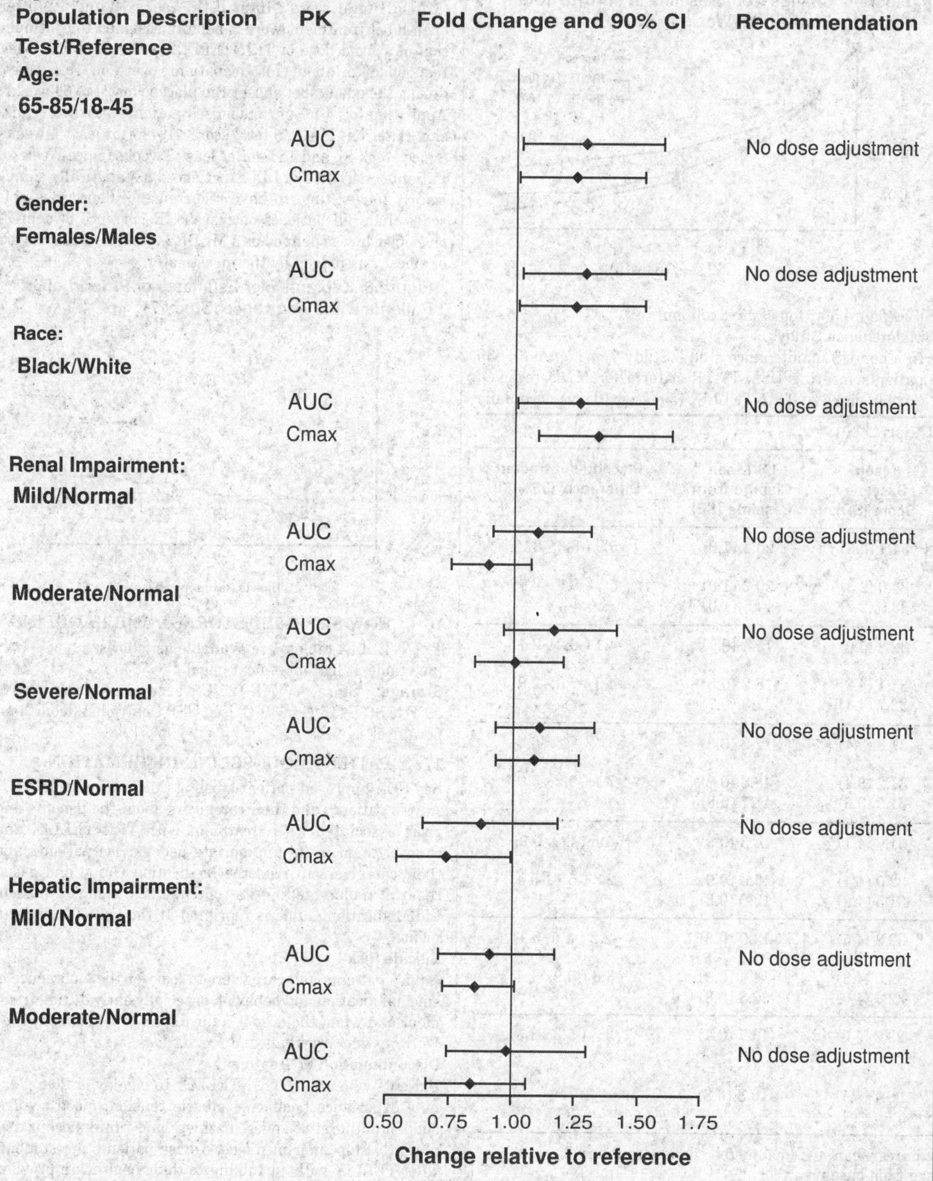

12.2 Pharmacodynamics
Vortioxetine binds with high affinity to the human serotonin transporter (Ki=1.6 nM), but not to the norepinephrine (Ki=113 nM) or dopamine (Ki>1000 nM) transporters. Vortioxetine potently and selectively inhibits reuptake of serotonin (IC50=5.4 nM). Vortioxetine binds to 5-HT3 (Ki=3.7 nM), 5-HT1A (Ki=15 nM), 5-HT7 (Ki=19 nM), 5-HT1D (Ki=54 nM), and 5-HT1B (Ki=33 nM), receptors and is a 5-HT3, 5-HT1D, and 5-HT7 receptor antagonist, 5-HT1B receptor partial agonist, and 5-HT1A receptor agonist.

In humans, the mean 5-HT transporter occupancy, based on the results from 2 clinical PET studies using 5-HTT ligands ([11C]-MADAM or [11C]-DASB), was approximately 50% at 5 mg/day, 65% at 10 mg/day and approximately 80% at 20 mg/day in the regions of interest.

Effect on Cardiac Repolarization
The effect of vortioxetine 10 mg and 40 mg administered once daily on QTc interval was evaluated in a randomized, double-blind, placebo-, and active-controlled (moxifloxacin 400 mg), four-treatment-arm parallel study in 340 male subjects. In the study the upper bound of the one-sided 95% confidence interval for the QTc was below 10 ms, the threshold for regulatory concern. The oral dose of 40 mg is sufficient to assess the effect of metabolic inhibition.

Effect on Driving Performance
In a clinical study in healthy subjects, TRINTELLIX did not impair driving performance, or have adverse psychomotor or cognitive effects following single and multiple doses of 10 mg/day. Because any psychoactive drug may impair judgment, thinking, or motor skills, however, patients should be cautioned about operating hazardous machinery, including automobiles, until they are reasonably certain that TRINTELLIX therapy does not affect their ability to engage in such activities.

12.3 Pharmacokinetics
Vortioxetine pharmacological activity is due to the parent drug. The pharmacokinetics of vortioxetine (2.5 mg to 60 mg) are linear and dose-proportional when vortioxetine is administered once daily. The mean terminal half-life is approximately 66 hours, and steady-state plasma concentrations are typically achieved within two weeks of dosing.

Absorption
The maximal plasma vortioxetine concentration (C_{max}) after dosing is reached within 7 to 11 hours postdose (T_{max}). Steady-state mean C_{max} values were 9, 18, and 33 ng/mL following doses of 5, 10, and 20 mg/day. Absolute bioavailability is 75%. No effect of food on the pharmacokinetics was observed.

Distribution
The apparent volume of distribution of vortioxetine is approximately 2600 L, indicating extensive extravascular distribution. The plasma protein binding of vortioxetine in humans is 98%, independent of plasma concentrations. No apparent difference in the plasma protein binding between healthy subjects and subjects with hepatic (mild, moderate) or renal (mild, moderate, severe, ESRD) impairment is observed.

Metabolism and Elimination
Vortioxetine is extensively metabolized primarily through oxidation via cytochrome P450 isozymes CYP2D6, CYP3A4/5, CYP2C19, CYP2C9, CYP2A6, CYP2C8 and CYP2B6 and subsequent glucuronic acid conjugation. CYP2D6 is the primary enzyme catalyzing the metabolism of vortioxetine to its major, pharmacologically inactive, carboxylic acid metabolite, and poor metabolizers of CYP2D6 have approximately twice the vortioxetine plasma concentration of extensive metabolizers.

Following a single oral dose of [14C]-labeled vortioxetine, approximately 59% and 26% of the administered radioactivity was recovered in the urine and feces, respectively as metabolites. Negligible amounts of unchanged vortioxetine were excreted in the urine up to 48 hours. The presence of hepatic (mild or moderate) or renal impairment (mild, moderate, severe and ESRD) did not affect the apparent clearance of vortioxetine.

13 NONCLINICAL TOXICOLOGY
13.1 Carcinogenesis, Mutagenesis, Impairment of Fertility
Carcinogenesis
Carcinogenicity studies were conducted in which CD-1 mice and Wistar rats were given oral doses of vortioxetine up to 50 and 100 mg/kg/day for male and female mice, respec-

Figure 3. Impact of Intrinsic Factors on Vortioxetine PK

Population Description Test/Reference	PK	Fold Change and 90% CI	Recommendation
Age: 65-85/18-45			
	AUC		No dose adjustment
	Cmax		
Gender: Females/Males			
	AUC		No dose adjustment
	Cmax		
Race: Black/White			
	AUC		No dose adjustment
	Cmax		
Renal Impairment: Mild/Normal			
	AUC		No dose adjustment
	Cmax		
Moderate/Normal			
	AUC		No dose adjustment
	Cmax		
Severe/Normal			
	AUC		No dose adjustment
	Cmax		
ESRD/Normal			
	AUC		No dose adjustment
	Cmax		
Hepatic Impairment: Mild/Normal			
	AUC		No dose adjustment
	Cmax		
Moderate/Normal			
	AUC		No dose adjustment
	Cmax		

Change relative to reference (0.50 0.75 1.00 1.25 1.50 1.75)

Continued on next page

tively, and 40 and 80 mg/kg/day for male and female rats, respectively, for 2 years. The doses in the two species were approximately 12, 24, 20, and 39 times the maximum recommended human dose (MRHD) of 20 mg on a mg/m² basis.

In rats, the incidence of benign polypoid adenomas of the rectum was statistically significantly increased in females at doses 39 times the MRHD, but not at 15 times the MRHD. These were considered related to inflammation and hyperplasia and possibly caused by an interaction with a vehicle component of the formulation used for the study. The finding did not occur in male rats at 20 times the MRHD.

In mice, vortioxetine was not carcinogenic in males or females at doses up to 12 and 24 times, respectively, the MRHD.

Mutagenicity

Vortioxetine was not genotoxic in the *in vitro* bacterial reverse mutation assay (Ames test), an *in vitro* chromosome aberration assay in cultured human lymphocytes, and an *in vivo* rat bone marrow micronucleus assay.

Impairment of Fertility

Treatment of rats with vortioxetine at doses up to 120 mg/kg/day had no effect on male or female fertility, which is 58 times the maximum recommended human dose (MRHD) of 20 mg on a mg/m² basis.

14   CLINICAL STUDIES

The efficacy of TRINTELLIX in treatment for MDD was established in six 6 to 8 week randomized, double-blind, placebo-controlled, fixed-dose studies (including one study in the elderly) and one maintenance study in adult inpatients and outpatients who met the Diagnostic and Statistical Manual of Mental Disorders (DSM-IV-TR) criteria for MDD.

Adults (aged 18 years to 75 years)

The efficacy of TRINTELLIX in patients aged 18 years to 75 years was demonstrated in five 6 to 8 week, placebo-controlled studies (Studies 1 to 5 in *Table 4*). In these studies, patients were randomized to TRINTELLIX 5 mg, 10 mg, 15 mg or 20 mg or placebo once daily. For patients who were randomized to TRINTELLIX 15 mg/day or 20 mg/day, the final doses were titrated up from 10 mg/day after the first week.

The primary efficacy measures were the Hamilton Depression Scale (HAMD-24) total score in Study 2 and the Montgomery-Asberg Depression Rating Scale (MADRS) total score in all other studies. In each of these studies, at

least one dose group of TRINTELLIX was superior to placebo in improvement of depressive symptoms as measured by mean change from baseline to endpoint visit on the primary efficacy measurement (*see Table 4*). Subgroup analysis by age, gender or race did not suggest any clear evidence of differential responsiveness. Two studies of the 5 mg dose in the U.S. (not represented in *Table 4*) failed to show effectiveness.

Elderly Study (aged 64 years to 88 years)

The efficacy of TRINTELLIX for the treatment of MDD was also demonstrated in a randomized, double-blind, placebo-controlled, fixed-dose study of TRINTELLIX in elderly patients (aged 64 years to 88 years) with MDD (Study 6 in *Table 4*). Patients meeting the diagnostic criteria for recurrent MDD with at least one previous major depressive episode before the age of 60 years and without comorbid cognitive impairment (Mini Mental State Examination score <24) received TRINTELLIX 5 mg or placebo.

[See table 4 below]

Time Course of Treatment Response

In the 6 to 8 week placebo-controlled studies, an effect of TRINTELLIX based on the primary efficacy measure was generally observed starting at Week 2 and increased in subsequent weeks with the full antidepressant effect of TRINTELLIX generally not seen until Study Week 4 or later. *Figure 4* depicts time course of response in U.S. based on the primary efficacy measure (MADRS) in Study 5.

Figure 4. Change from Baseline in MADRS Total Score by Study Visit (Week) in Study 5

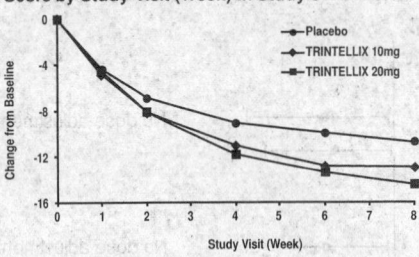

[See figure 5 at top of next column]

Maintenance Study

In a non-US maintenance study (Study 7 *in Figure 6*), 639 patients meeting DSM-IV-TR criteria for MDD received flexible doses of TRINTELLIX (5 mg or 10 mg) once daily

Figure 5. Difference from Placebo in Mean Change from Baseline in MADRS Total Score at Week 6 or Week 8

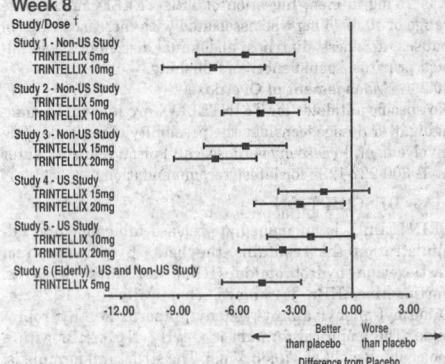

†Results (point estimate and unadjusted 95% confidence interval) are from mixed model for repeated measures (MMRM) analysis. In Studies 1 and 6, the primary analysis was not based on MMRM and in Studies 2 and 6 the primary efficacy measure was not based on MADRS.

during an initial 12 week open-label treatment phase; the dose of TRINTELLIX was fixed during Weeks 8 to 12. Three hundred ninety six (396) patients who were in remission (MADRS total score ≤10 at both Weeks 10 and 12) after open-label treatment were randomly assigned to continuation of a fixed dose of TRINTELLIX at the final dose they responded to (about 75% of patients were on 10 mg/day) during the open-label phase or to placebo for 24 to 64 weeks. Approximately 61% of randomized patients satisfied remission criterion (MADRS total score ≤10) for at least 4 weeks (since Week 8), and 15% for at least 8 weeks (since Week 4). Patients on TRINTELLIX experienced a statistically significantly longer time to have recurrence of depressive episodes than did patients on placebo. Recurrence of depressive episode was defined as a MADRS total score ≥22 or lack of efficacy as judged by the investigator.

Figure 6. Kaplan-Meier Estimates of Proportion of Patients with Recurrence (Study 7)

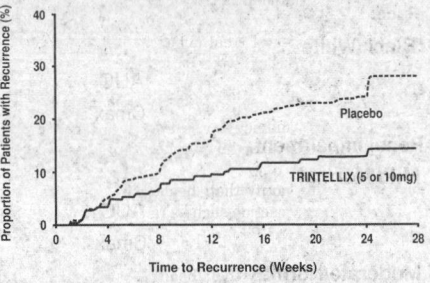

16   HOW SUPPLIED/STORAGE AND HANDLING

TRINTELLIX tablets are available as follows:
[See table at bottom of next page]
Storage: Store at 77°F (25°C); excursions permitted to 59°F to 86°F (15°C to 30°C) [see USP Controlled Room Temperature].

17   PATIENT COUNSELING INFORMATION

See FDA-approved patient labeling (Medication Guide) Advise patients and their caregivers about the benefits and risks associated with treatment with TRINTELLIX and counsel them in its appropriate use. Advise patients and their caregivers to read the Medication Guide and assist them in understanding its contents. The complete text of the Medication Guide is reprinted at the end of this document.

Suicide Risk

Advise patients and caregivers to look for the emergence of suicidal ideation and behavior, especially during treatment and when the dose is adjusted up or down [see Boxed Warning and Warnings and Precautions (5.1)].

Discontinuation of Treatment

Patients who are on TRINTELLIX 15 mg/day or 20 mg/day may experience headache, muscle tension, mood swings, sudden outburst of anger, dizziness and runny nose if they abruptly stop their medicine. Advise patients not stopping TRINTELLIX without talking to their healthcare provider [see Adverse Reactions (6)].

Table 4. Primary Efficacy Results of 6 Week to 8 Week Clinical Trials

Study No. [Primary Measure]	Treatment Group	Number of Patients	Mean Baseline Score (SD)	LS Mean Change from Baseline (SE)	Placebo-subtracted Difference*(95% CI)
Study 1 [MADRS] Non-US Study	TRINTELLIX (5 mg/day)†	108	34.1 (2.6)	-20.4 (1.0)	-5.9 (-8.6, -3.2)
	TRINTELLIX (10 mg/day)†	100	34.0 (2.8)	-20.2 (1.0)	-5.7 (-8.5, -2.9)
	Placebo	105	33.9 (2.7)	-14.5 (1.0)	--
Study 2 [HAMD-24] Non-US Study	TRINTELLIX (5 mg/day)	139	32.2 (5.0)	-15.4 (0.7)	-4.1 (-6.2, -2.1)
	TRINTELLIX (10 mg/day)†	139	33.1 (4.8)	-16.2 (0.8)	-4.9 (-7.0, -2.9)
	Placebo	139	32.7 (4.4)	-11.3 (0.7)	--
Study 3 [MADRS] Non-US Study	TRINTELLIX (15 mg/day)†	149	31.8 (3.4)	-17.2 (0.8)	-5.5 (-7.7, -3.4)
	TRINTELLIX (20 mg/day)†	151	31.2 (3.4)	-18.8 (0.8)	-7.1 (-9.2, -5.0)
	Placebo	158	31.5 (3.6)	-11.7 (0.8)	--
Study 4 [MADRS] US Study	TRINTELLIX (15 mg/day)	145	31.9 (4.1)	-14.3 (0.9)	-1.5 (-3.9, 0.9)
	TRINTELLIX (20 mg/day)†	147	32.0 (4.4)	-15.6 (0.9)	-2.8 (-5.1, -0.4)
	Placebo	153	31.5 (4.2)	-12.8 (0.8)	--
Study 5 [MADRS] US Study	TRINTELLIX (10 mg/day)	154	32.2 (4.5)	-13.0 (0.8)	-2.2 (-4.5, 0.1)
	TRINTELLIX (20 mg/day)†	148	32.5 (4.3)	-14.4 (0.9)	-3.6 (-5.9, -1.4)
	Placebo	155	32.0 (4.0)	-10.8 (0.8)	--
Study 6 (elderly) [HAMD-24] US and Non-US	TRINTELLIX (5 mg/day)†	155	29.2 (5.0)	-13.7 (0.7)	-3.3 (-5.3, -1.3)
	Placebo	145	29.4 (5.1)	-10.3 (0.8)	--

SD: standard deviation; SE: standard error; LS Mean: least-squares mean; CI: unadjusted confidence interval.
* Difference (drug minus placebo) in least-squares mean change from baseline.
† Doses that are statistically significantly superior to placebo after adjusting for multiplicity.

Concomitant Medication

Advise patients to inform their physicians if they are taking, or plan to take, any prescription or over-the-counter medications because of a potential for interactions. Instruct patients not to take TRINTELLIX with an MAOI or within 14 days of stopping an MAOI and to allow 21 days after stopping TRINTELLIX before starting an MAOI *[see Dosage and Administration (2.4), Contraindications (4), Warnings and Precautions (5.2), and Drug Interactions (7.1)].*

Serotonin Syndrome

Caution patients about the risk of serotonin syndrome, particularly with the concomitant use of TRINTELLIX and triptans, tricyclic antidepressants, fentanyl, Lithium, tramadol, tryptophan supplements, and St. John's Wort supplements *[see Warnings and Precautions (5.2) and Drug Interactions (7.1, 7.2)].*

Abnormal Bleeding

Caution patients about the increased risk of abnormal bleeding when TRINTELLIX is given with NSAIDs, aspirin, warfarin, or other drugs that affect coagulation *[see Warnings and Precautions (5.3)].*

Activation of Mania/Hypomania

Advise patients and their caregivers to look for signs of activation of mania/hypomania *[see Warnings and Precautions (5.4)].*

Angle Closure Glaucoma

Patients should be advised that taking TRINTELLIX can cause mild pupillary dilation, which in susceptible individuals, can lead to an episode of angle closure glaucoma. Pre-existing glaucoma is almost always open-angle glaucoma because angle closure glaucoma, when diagnosed, can be treated definitively with iridectomy. Open-angle glaucoma is not a risk factor for angle closure glaucoma. Patients may wish to be examined to determine whether they are susceptible to angle closure, and have a prophylactic procedure (e.g., iridectomy), if they are susceptible *[see Warnings and Precautions (5.5)].*

Hyponatremia

Advise patients that if they are treated with diuretics, or are otherwise volume depleted, or are elderly, they may be at greater risk of developing hyponatremia while taking TRINTELLIX *[see Warnings and Precautions (5.6)].*

Nausea

Advise patients that nausea is the most common adverse reaction, and is dose related. Nausea commonly occurs within the first week of treatment, then decreases in frequency but can persist in some patients.

Alcohol

A clinical study has shown that TRINTELLIX (single dose of 20 or 40 mg/day) did not increase the impairment of mental and motor skills caused by alcohol.

Allergic Reactions

Advise patients to notify their healthcare provider if they develop an allergic reaction such as rash, hives, swelling, or difficulty breathing.

Pregnancy

Advise patients to notify their healthcare provider if they become pregnant or intend to become pregnant during therapy with TRINTELLIX *[see Use in Specific Populations (8.1)].*

Nursing Mothers

Advise patients to notify their healthcare provider if they are breast-feeding an infant and would like to continue or start TRINTELLIX *[see Use in Specific Populations (8.3)].*

Distributed and marketed by:
Takeda Pharmaceuticals America, Inc.
Deerfield, IL 60015

Marketed by:
Lundbeck
Deerfield, IL 60015
TRINTELLIX is a trademark of H. Lundbeck A/S registered with the U.S. Patent and Trademark Office and used under license by Takeda Pharmaceuticals America, Inc.
©2013-2016 Takeda Pharmaceuticals America, Inc.
LUN205 R7 May 2016

MEDICATION GUIDE
TRINTELLIX [trin'-tel-ix]
(vortioxetine) Tablets

Read this Medication Guide before you start taking TRINTELLIX and each time you get a refill. There may be new information. This information does not take the place of talking to your healthcare provider about your medical condition or your treatment.

What is the most important information I should know about TRINTELLIX?

TRINTELLIX and other antidepressant medicines may cause serious side effects.

1. **Antidepressant medicines may increase suicidal thoughts or actions in some children, teenagers, or young adults within the first few months of treatment.**
2. **Depression or other serious mental illnesses are the most important causes of suicidal thoughts or actions. Some people may have a particularly high risk of having suicidal thoughts or actions.** These include people who have (or have a family history of) bipolar illness (also called manic-depressive illness) or suicidal thoughts or actions.
3. **How can I watch for and try to prevent suicidal thoughts and actions?**
- Pay close attention to any changes, especially sudden changes in mood, behavior, thoughts, or feelings. This is very important when an antidepressant medicine is started or when the dose is changed.
- Call your healthcare provider right away to report new or sudden changes in mood, behavior, thoughts, or feelings.
- Keep all follow-up visits with your healthcare provider as scheduled. Call your healthcare provider between visits as needed, especially if you have concerns about symptoms.

Call your healthcare provider right away if you have any of the following symptoms, especially if they are new, worse, or worry you:

- attempts to commit suicide
- acting on dangerous impulses
- acting aggressive, being angry or violent
- thoughts about suicide or dying
- new or worse depression
- new or worse anxiety
- feeling agitated, restless, angry or irritable
- trouble sleeping
- an extreme increase in activity or talking (mania)
- other unusual changes in behavior or mood
- panic attacks
- new or worse irritability

What is TRINTELLIX?

TRINTELLIX is a prescription medicine used to treat a certain type of depression called Major Depressive Disorder (MDD).

It is important to talk with your healthcare provider about the risks of treating depression and also the risk of not treating it. You should discuss all treatment choices with your healthcare provider.

- Talk to your healthcare provider if you do not think that your condition is getting better with TRINTELLIX treatment.

Who should not take TRINTELLIX?

Do not take TRINTELLIX if you:

- are allergic to vortioxetine, or any of the ingredients in TRINTELLIX. See the end of this Medication Guide for a complete list of ingredients in TRINTELLIX.
- take a Monoamine Oxidase Inhibitor (MAOI). Ask your healthcare provider or pharmacist if you are not sure if you take an MAOI, including the antibiotic linezolid.
- Do not take an MAOI within 21 days of stopping TRINTELLIX.
- Do not start TRINTELLIX if you stopped taking an MAOI in the last 14 days.

What should I tell my healthcare provider before taking TRINTELLIX?

Tell your healthcare provider if you:

- have liver problems
- have or had seizures or convulsions
- have mania or bipolar disorder (manic depression)
- have low salt (sodium) levels in your blood
- have or had bleeding problems
- drink alcohol
- have any other medical conditions
- are pregnant or plan to become pregnant. It is not known if TRINTELLIX will harm your unborn baby.
- are breastfeeding or plan to breastfeed. It is not known if TRINTELLIX passes into breast milk. Talk to your healthcare provider about the best way to feed your baby if you take TRINTELLIX.

Tell your healthcare provider about all the medicines that you take, including prescription and over-the-counter medicines, vitamins, and herbal supplements. TRINTELLIX and some medicines may interact with each other, may not work as well, or may cause serious side effects when taken together.

Especially tell your healthcare provider if you take:

- medicines used to treat migraine headache (e.g. triptans)
- medicines used to treat mood, anxiety, psychotic or thought disorders, including tricyclics, lithium, selective serotonin reuptake inhibitors (SSRIs), serotonin norepinephrine reuptake inhibitors (SNRIs), buspirone, or antipsychotics
- MAOIs (including linezolid, an antibiotic)
- Tramadol or fentanyl
- over-the-counter supplements such as tryptophan or St. John's Wort
- nonsteroidal anti-inflammatory drugs (NSAIDs)
- aspirin
- warfarin (Coumadin, Jantoven)
- diuretics
- rifampicin
- carbamazepine
- phenytoin
- quinidine

Ask your healthcare provider if you are not sure if you are taking any of these medicines.

Before you take TRINTELLIX with any of these medicines, talk to your healthcare provider about serotonin syndrome. See "What are the possible side effects of TRINTELLIX?"

Know the medicines you take. Keep a list of them to show your healthcare provider or pharmacist when you get new medicine.

How should I take TRINTELLIX?

- Take TRINTELLIX exactly as your healthcare provider tells you to take it.
- Take TRINTELLIX at about the same time each day.
- Your healthcare provider may need to change the dose of TRINTELLIX until it is the right dose for you.
- Do not start or stop taking TRINTELLIX without talking to your healthcare provider first. Suddenly stopping TRINTELLIX when you take higher doses may cause you to have side effects, including:
- headache
- stiff muscles
- mood swings
- sudden outburst of anger
- dizziness or feeling lightheaded
- runny nose
- TRINTELLIX may be taken with or without food.
- If you take too much TRINTELLIX, call the Poison Control Center at 1-800-222-1222 or go to the nearest hospital emergency room right away.

What should I avoid while taking TRINTELLIX?

- Do not drive, operate heavy machinery, or do other dangerous activities until you know how TRINTELLIX affects you.
- Avoid drinking alcohol while taking TRINTELLIX.

What are the possible side effects of TRINTELLIX?

Features	Strengths			
	5 mg	10 mg	15 mg	20 mg
Color	pink	yellow	orange	red
Debossment	"5" on one side of tablet "TL" on other side of tablet	"10" on one side of tablet "TL" on other side of tablet	"15" on one side of tablet "TL" on other side of tablet	"20" on one side of tablet "TL" on other side of tablet
Presentations and NDC Codes				
Bottles of 30	64764-720-30	64764-730-30	64764-740-30	64764-750-30
Bottles of 90	64764-720-90	64764-730-90	64764-740-90	64764-750-90
Bottles of 500	64764-720-77	64764-730-77	64764-740-77	64764-750-77

Continued on next page

TRINTELLIX may cause serious side effects, including:

- See "What is the most important information I should know about TRINTELLIX?"
- **serotonin syndrome.** A potentially life-threatening problem called serotonin syndrome can happen when medicines such as TRINTELLIX are taken with certain other medicines. Symptoms of serotonin syndrome may include:
  - agitation, hallucinations, coma or other changes in mental status
  - problems controlling your movements or muscle twitching
  - fast heartbeat
  - high or low blood pressure
  - sweating or fever
  - nausea or vomiting
  - diarrhea
  - muscle stiffness or tightness
- **abnormal bleeding or bruising.** TRINTELLIX may increase your risk of bleeding or bruising, especially if you take the blood thinner warfarin (Coumadin®, Jantoven®), a non-steroidal anti-inflammatory drug (NSAID), or aspirin.
- **hypomania** (manic episodes). Symptoms of manic episodes include:
  - greatly increased energy
  - severe problems sleeping
  - racing thoughts
  - reckless behavior
  - unusually grand ideas
  - excessive happiness or irritability
  - talking more or faster than usual
- **visual problems**
  - eye pain
  - changes in vision
  - swelling or redness in or around the eye

Only some people are at risk for these problems. You may want to undergo an eye examination to see if you are at risk and receive preventative treatment if you are.

- **low levels of salt (sodium) in your blood.** Symptoms of this may include: headache, difficulty concentrating, memory changes, confusion, weakness and unsteadiness on your feet. Symptoms of severe or sudden cases of low salt levels in your blood may include: hallucinations (seeing or hearing things that are not real), fainting, seizures and coma. If not treated, severe low sodium levels can cause death.

Common side effects in people who take TRINTELLIX include:
- nausea
- constipation
- vomiting

Tell your healthcare provider if you have any side effect that bothers you or that does not go away. These are not all the possible side effects of TRINTELLIX. For more information, ask your healthcare provider or pharmacist.

Call your doctor for medical advice about side effects. You may report side effects to FDA at 1-800-FDA-1088.

How should I store TRINTELLIX?

Store TRINTELLIX at room temperature between 59°F to 86°F (15°C to 30°C).

Keep TRINTELLIX and all medicines out of the reach of children.

General information about the safe and effective use of TRINTELLIX.

Medicines are sometimes prescribed for purposes other than those listed in a Medication Guide. Do not use TRINTELLIX for a condition for which it was not prescribed. Do not give TRINTELLIX to other people, even if they have the same condition. It may harm them.

This Medication Guide summarizes the most important information about TRINTELLIX. If you would like more information, talk with your healthcare provider. You may ask your healthcare provider or pharmacist for information about TRINTELLIX that is written for healthcare professionals.

For more information, go to www.TRINTELLIX.com or call 1-877-TAKEDA-7 (1-877-825-3327).

What are the ingredients in TRINTELLIX?

Active ingredient: vortioxetine hydrobromide

Inactive ingredients: mannitol, microcrystalline cellulose, hydroxypropyl cellulose, sodium starch glycolate, magnesium stearate and film coating consisting of hypromellose, titanium dioxide, polyethylene glycol 400, iron oxide red (5 mg, 15 mg, and 20 mg) and iron oxide yellow (10 mg and 15 mg)

This Medication Guide has been approved by the U.S. Food and Drug Administration.

Distributed and Marketed by:

Takeda Pharmaceuticals America, Inc.
Deerfield, IL 60015
Marketed by:
Lundbeck
Deerfield, IL 60015
TRINTELLIX is a trademark of H. Lundbeck A/S registered with the U.S. Patent and Trademark Office and used under license by Takeda Pharmaceuticals America, Inc.
All other trademarks are the property of their respective owners.
©2013-2016 Takeda Pharmaceuticals America, Inc.
LUN205 R7 May 2016
Shown in Product Identification Guide, page 510

ULORIC   ℞
[*U–'lor–ik*]
(febuxostat)
tablet for oral use

HIGHLIGHTS OF PRESCRIBING INFORMATION
These HIGHLIGHTS do not include all the information needed to use ULORIC safely and effectively. See full prescribing information for ULORIC.
ULORIC (febuxostat) tablet for oral use
Initial U.S. Approval: 2009

———RECENT MAJOR CHANGES———
Warnings and Precautions
Hepatic Effects (5.3)   11/2012

———INDICATIONS AND USAGE———
ULORIC is a xanthine oxidase (XO) inhibitor indicated for the chronic management of hyperuricemia in patients with gout. (1)
ULORIC is not recommended for the treatment of asymptomatic hyperuricemia. (1)

———DOSAGE AND ADMINISTRATION———
- ULORIC is recommended at 40 mg or 80 mg once daily. The recommended starting dose of ULORIC is 40 mg once daily. For patients who do not achieve a serum uric acid (sUA) less than 6 mg/dL after 2 weeks with 40 mg, ULORIC 80 mg is recommended. (2.1)
- ULORIC can be administered without regard to food or antacid use. (2.1)
- No dose adjustment is necessary when administering ULORIC to patients with mild to moderate renal or hepatic impairment. (2.2)

———DOSAGE FORMS AND STRENGTHS———
Tablet: 40 mg, 80 mg. (3)

———CONTRAINDICATIONS———
ULORIC is contraindicated in patients being treated with azathioprine or mercaptopurine. (4)

———WARNINGS AND PRECAUTIONS———
- Gout Flare: An increase in gout flares is frequently observed during initiation of anti-hyperuricemic agents, including ULORIC. If a gout flare occurs during treatment, ULORIC need not be discontinued. Prophylactic therapy (i.e., non-steroidal anti-inflammatory drug [NSAID] or colchicine upon initiation of treatment) may be beneficial for up to six months. (2.4, 5.1)
- Cardiovascular Events: A higher rate of cardiovascular thromboembolic events was observed in patients treated with ULORIC than allopurinol in clinical trials. Monitor for signs and symptoms of MI and stroke. (5.2)
- Hepatic Effects: Postmarketing reports of hepatic failure, sometimes fatal. Causality cannot be excluded. If liver injury is detected, promptly interrupt ULORIC and assess patient for probable cause, then treat cause if possible, to resolution or stabilization. Do not restart ULORIC if liver injury is confirmed and no alternate etiology can be found. (5.3)

———ADVERSE REACTIONS———
Adverse reactions occurring in at least 1% of ULORIC-treated patients, and at least 0.5% greater than placebo, are liver function abnormalities, nausea, arthralgia, and rash. (6.1)

To report SUSPECTED ADVERSE REACTIONS, contact Takeda Pharmaceuticals at 1-877-TAKEDA-7 (1-877-825-3327) or FDA at 1-800-FDA-1088 or www.fda.gov/medwatch.

———DRUG INTERACTIONS———
Concomitant administration of ULORIC with XO substrate drugs, azathioprine or mercaptopurine could increase plasma concentrations of these drugs resulting in severe toxicity. (7)

———USE IN SPECIFIC POPULATIONS———
- There is insufficient data in patients with severe renal impairment. No studies have been conducted in patients with severe hepatic impairment. Caution should be exercised in these patients. (8.6, 8.7)
- No studies have been conducted in patients with secondary hyperuricemia (including patients being treated for Lesch-Nyhan syndrome or malignant disease, or in organ transplant recipients); therefore, ULORIC is not recommended for use in these patients. (8.8)

See 17 for PATIENT COUNSELING INFORMATION and FDA-approved patient labeling.

     Revised: 11/2013

FULL PRESCRIBING INFORMATION

1   INDICATIONS AND USAGE
ULORIC is a xanthine oxidase (XO) inhibitor indicated for the chronic management of hyperuricemia in patients with gout.
ULORIC is not recommended for the treatment of asymptomatic hyperuricemia.

2   DOSAGE AND ADMINISTRATION
2.1   Recommended Dose
For treatment of hyperuricemia in patients with gout, ULORIC is recommended at 40 mg or 80 mg once daily.
The recommended starting dose of ULORIC is 40 mg once daily. For patients who do not achieve a serum uric acid (sUA) less than 6 mg/dL after two weeks with 40 mg, ULORIC 80 mg is recommended.
ULORIC can be taken without regard to food or antacid use *[see Clinical Pharmacology (12.3)]*.
2.2   Special Populations
No dose adjustment is necessary when administering ULORIC in patients with mild to moderate renal impair-

ment *[see Use in Specific Populations (8.6) and Clinical Pharmacology (12.3)]*. The recommended starting dose of ULORIC is 40 mg once daily. For patients who do not achieve a sUA less than 6 mg/dL after two weeks with 40 mg, ULORIC 80 mg is recommended.

No dose adjustment is necessary in patients with mild to moderate hepatic impairment *[see Use in Specific Populations (8.7) and Clinical Pharmacology (12.3)]*.

2.3 Uric Acid Level

Testing for the target serum uric acid level of less than 6 mg/dL may be performed as early as two weeks after initiating ULORIC therapy.

2.4 Gout Flares

Gout flares may occur after initiation of ULORIC due to changing serum uric acid levels resulting in mobilization of urate from tissue deposits. Flare prophylaxis with a nonsteroidal anti-inflammatory drug (NSAID) or colchicine is recommended upon initiation of ULORIC. Prophylactic therapy may be beneficial for up to six months *[see Clinical Studies (14.1)]*.

If a gout flare occurs during ULORIC treatment, ULORIC need not be discontinued. The gout flare should be managed concurrently, as appropriate for the individual patient *[see Warnings and Precautions (5.1)]*.

3 DOSAGE FORMS AND STRENGTHS

- 40 mg tablets, light green to green, round, debossed with "TAP" and "40"
- 80 mg tablets, light green to green, teardrop shaped, debossed with "TAP" and "80"

4 CONTRAINDICATIONS

ULORIC is contraindicated in patients being treated with azathioprine or mercaptopurine *[see Drug Interactions (7)]*.

5 WARNINGS AND PRECAUTIONS

5.1 Gout Flare

After initiation of ULORIC, an increase in gout flares is frequently observed. This increase is due to reduction in serum uric acid levels, resulting in mobilization of urate from tissue deposits.

In order to prevent gout flares when ULORIC is initiated, concurrent prophylactic treatment with an NSAID or colchicine is recommended *[see Dosage and Administration (2.4)]*.

5.2 Cardiovascular Events

In the randomized controlled studies, there was a higher rate of cardiovascular thromboembolic events (cardiovascular deaths, non-fatal myocardial infarctions, and non-fatal strokes) in patients treated with ULORIC (0.74 per 100 P-Y [95% Confidence Interval (CI) 0.36-1.37]) than allopurinol (0.60 per 100 P-Y [95% CI 0.16-1.53]) *[see Adverse Reactions (6.1)]*. A causal relationship with ULORIC has not been established. Monitor for signs and symptoms of myocardial infarction (MI) and stroke.

5.3 Hepatic Effects

There have been postmarketing reports of fatal and nonfatal hepatic failure in patients taking ULORIC, although the reports contain insufficient information necessary to establish the probable cause. During randomized controlled studies, transaminase elevations greater than three times the upper limit of normal (ULN) were observed (AST: 2%, 2%, and ALT: 3%, 2% in ULORIC and allopurinol-treated patients, respectively). No dose-effect relationship for these transaminase elevations was noted *[see Clinical Pharmacology (12.3)]*.

Obtain a liver test panel (serum alanine aminotransferase [ALT], aspartate aminotransferase [AST], alkaline phosphatase, and total bilirubin) as a baseline before initiating ULORIC.

Measure liver tests promptly in patients who report symptoms that may indicate liver injury, including fatigue, anorexia, right upper abdominal discomfort, dark urine or jaundice. In this clinical context, if the patient is found to have abnormal liver tests (ALT greater than three times the upper limit of the reference range), ULORIC treatment should be interrupted and investigation done to establish the probable cause. ULORIC should not be restarted in these patients without another explanation for the liver test abnormalities.

Patients who have serum ALT greater than three times the reference range with serum total bilirubin greater than two times the reference range without alternative etiologies are at risk for severe drug-induced liver injury and should not be restarted on ULORIC. For patients with lesser elevations of serum ALT or bilirubin and with an alternate probable cause, treatment with ULORIC can be used with caution.

Table 1: Adverse Reactions Occurring in ≥1% of ULORIC-Treated Patients and at Least 0.5% Greater than Seen in Patients Receiving Placebo in Controlled Studies

Adverse Reactions	Placebo (N=134)	ULORIC 40 mg daily (N=757)	ULORIC 80 mg daily (N=1279)	allopurinol* (N=1277)
Liver Function Abnormalities	0.7%	6.6%	4.6%	4.2%
Nausea	0.7%	1.1%	1.3%	0.8%
Arthralgia	0%	1.1%	0.7%	0.7%
Rash	0.7%	0.5%	1.6%	1.6%

* Of the subjects who received allopurinol, 10 received 100 mg, 145 received 200 mg, and 1122 received 300 mg, based on level of renal impairment.

6 ADVERSE REACTIONS

6.1 Clinical Trials Experience

Because clinical trials are conducted under widely varying conditions, adverse reaction rates observed in the clinical trials of a drug cannot be directly compared to rates in the clinical trials of another drug and may not reflect the rates observed in practice.

A total of 2757 subjects with hyperuricemia and gout were treated with ULORIC 40 mg or 80 mg daily in clinical studies. For ULORIC 40 mg, 559 patients were treated for ≥6 months. For ULORIC 80 mg, 1377 subjects were treated for ≥6 months, 674 patients were treated for ≥1 year and 515 patients were treated for ≥2 years.

Most Common Adverse Reactions

In three randomized, controlled clinical studies (Studies 1, 2 and 3), which were six to 12 months in duration, the following adverse reactions were reported by the treating physician as related to study drug. Table 1 summarizes adverse reactions reported at a rate of at least 1% in ULORIC treatment groups and at least 0.5% greater than placebo.

[See table 1 above]

The most common adverse reaction leading to discontinuation from therapy was liver function abnormalities in 1.8% of ULORIC 40 mg, 1.2% of ULORIC 80 mg, and in 0.9% of allopurinol-treated subjects.

In addition to the adverse reactions presented in Table 1, dizziness was reported in more than 1% of ULORIC-treated subjects although not at a rate more than 0.5% greater than placebo.

Less Common Adverse Reactions

In Phase 2 and 3 clinical studies the following adverse reactions occurred in less than 1% of subjects and in more than one subject treated with doses ranging from 40 mg to 240 mg of ULORIC. This list also includes adverse reactions (less than 1% of subjects) associated with organ systems from Warnings and Precautions.

Blood and Lymphatic System Disorders: anemia, idiopathic thrombocytopenic purpura, leukocytosis/leukopenia, neutropenia, pancytopenia, splenomegaly, thrombocytopenia.

Cardiac Disorders: angina pectoris, atrial fibrillation/flutter, cardiac murmur, ECG abnormal, palpitations, sinus bradycardia, tachycardia.

Ear and Labyrinth Disorders: deafness, tinnitus, vertigo.

Eye Disorders: vision blurred.

Gastrointestinal Disorders: abdominal distention, abdominal pain, constipation, dry mouth, dyspepsia, flatulence, frequent stools, gastritis, gastroesophageal reflux disease, gastrointestinal discomfort, gingival pain, haematemesis, hyperchlorhydria, hematochezia, mouth ulceration, pancreatitis, peptic ulcer, vomiting.

General Disorders and Administration Site Conditions: asthenia, chest pain/discomfort, edema, fatigue, feeling abnormal, gait disturbance, influenza-like symptoms, mass, pain, thirst.

Hepatobiliary Disorders: cholelithiasis/cholecystitis, hepatic steatosis, hepatitis, hepatomegaly.

Immune System Disorder: hypersensitivity.

Infections and Infestations: herpes zoster.

Procedural Complications: contusion.

Metabolism and Nutrition Disorders: anorexia, appetite decreased/increased, dehydration, diabetes mellitus, hypercholesterolemia, hyperglycemia, hyperlipidemia, hypertriglyceridemia, hypokalemia, weight decreased/increased.

Musculoskeletal and Connective Tissue Disorders: arthritis, joint stiffness, joint swelling, muscle spasms/twitching/tightness/weakness, musculoskeletal pain/stiffness, myalgia.

Nervous System Disorders: altered taste, balance disorder, cerebrovascular accident, Guillain-Barré syndrome, headache, hemiparesis, hypoesthesia, hyposmia, lacunar infarction, lethargy, mental impairment, migraine, paresthesia, somnolence, transient ischemic attack, tremor.

Psychiatric Disorders: agitation, anxiety, depression, insomnia, irritability, libido decreased, nervousness, panic attack, personality change.

Renal and Urinary Disorders: hematuria, nephrolithiasis, pollakiuria, proteinuria, renal failure, renal insufficiency, urgency, incontinence.

Reproductive System and Breast Changes: breast pain, erectile dysfunction, gynecomastia.

Respiratory, Thoracic and Mediastinal Disorders: bronchitis, cough, dyspnea, epistaxis, nasal dryness, paranasal sinus hypersecretion, pharyngeal edema, respiratory tract congestion, sneezing, throat irritation, upper respiratory tract infection.

Skin and Subcutaneous Tissue Disorders: alopecia, angioedema, dermatitis, dermographism, ecchymosis, eczema, hair color changes, hair growth abnormal, hyperhidrosis, peeling skin, petechiae, photosensitivity, pruritus, purpura, skin discoloration/altered pigmentation, skin lesion, skin odor abnormal, urticaria.

Vascular Disorders: flushing, hot flush, hypertension, hypotension.

Laboratory Parameters: activated partial thromboplastin time prolonged, creatine increased, bicarbonate decreased, sodium increased, EEG abnormal, glucose increased, cholesterol increased, triglycerides increased, amylase increased, potassium increased, TSH increased, platelet count decreased, hematocrit decreased, hemoglobin decreased, MCV increased, RBC decreased, creatinine increased, blood urea increased, BUN/creatinine ratio increased, creatine phosphokinase (CPK) increased, alkaline phosphatase increased, LDH increased, PSA increased, urine output increased/decreased, lymphocyte count decreased, neutrophil count decreased, WBC increased/decreased, coagulation test abnormal, low density lipoprotein (LDL) increased, prothrombin time prolonged, urinary casts, urine positive for white blood cells and protein.

Cardiovascular Safety

Cardiovascular events and deaths were adjudicated to one of the pre-defined endpoints from the Anti-Platelet Trialists' Collaborations (APTC) (cardiovascular death, non-fatal myocardial infarction, and non-fatal stroke) in the randomized controlled and long-term extension studies. In the Phase 3 randomized controlled studies, the incidences of adjudicated APTC events per 100 patient-years of exposure were: Placebo 0 (95% CI 0.00-6.16), ULORIC 40 mg 0 (95% CI 0.00-1.08), ULORIC 80 mg 1.09 (95% CI 0.44-2.24), and allopurinol 0.60 (95% CI 0.16-1.53).

In the long-term extension studies, the incidences of adjudicated APTC events were: ULORIC 80 mg 0.97 (95% CI 0.57-1.56), and allopurinol 0.58 (95% CI 0.02-3.24).

Overall, a higher rate of APTC events was observed in ULORIC than in allopurinol-treated patients. A causal relationship with ULORIC has not been established. Monitor for signs and symptoms of MI and stroke.

Continued on next page

6.2 Postmarketing Experience

Adverse reactions have been identified during postapproval use of ULORIC. Because these reactions are reported voluntarily from a population of uncertain size, it is not always possible to reliably estimate their frequency or establish a causal relationship.

Hepatobiliary Disorders: hepatic failure (some fatal), jaundice, serious cases of abnormal liver function test results, liver disorder.

Immune System Disorders: anaphylaxis, anaphylactic reaction.

Musculoskeletal and Connective Tissue Disorders: rhabdomyolysis.

Psychiatric Disorders: psychotic behavior including aggressive thoughts.

Renal and Urinary Disorders: tubulointerstitial nephritis.

Skin and Subcutaneous Tissue Disorders: generalized rash, Stevens Johnson Syndrome, hypersensitivity skin reactions.

7 DRUG INTERACTIONS

7.1 Xanthine Oxidase Substrate Drugs

ULORIC is an XO inhibitor. Based on a drug interaction study in healthy subjects, febuxostat altered the metabolism of theophylline (a substrate of XO) in humans *[see Clinical Pharmacology (12.3)]*. Therefore, use with caution when coadministering ULORIC with theophylline.

Drug interaction studies of ULORIC with other drugs that are metabolized by XO (e.g., mercaptopurine and azathioprine) have not been conducted. Inhibition of XO by ULORIC may cause increased plasma concentrations of these drugs leading to toxicity *[see Clinical Pharmacology (12.3)]*. ULORIC is contraindicated in patients being treated with azathioprine or mercaptopurine *[see Contraindications (4)]*.

7.2 Cytotoxic Chemotherapy Drugs

Drug interaction studies of ULORIC with cytotoxic chemotherapy have not been conducted. No data are available regarding the safety of ULORIC during cytotoxic chemotherapy.

7.3 *In Vivo* Drug Interaction Studies

Based on drug interaction studies in healthy subjects, ULORIC does not have clinically significant interactions with colchicine, naproxen, indomethacin, hydrochlorothiazide, warfarin or desipramine *[see Clinical Pharmacology (12.3)]*. Therefore, ULORIC may be used concomitantly with these medications.

8 USE IN SPECIFIC POPULATIONS

8.1 Pregnancy

Pregnancy Category C: There are no adequate and well-controlled studies in pregnant women. ULORIC should be used during pregnancy only if the potential benefit justifies the potential risk to the fetus.

Febuxostat was not teratogenic in rats and rabbits at oral doses up to 48 mg/kg (40 and 51 times the human plasma exposure at 80 mg/day for equal body surface area, respectively) during organogenesis. However, increased neonatal mortality and a reduction in the neonatal body weight gain were observed when pregnant rats were treated with oral doses up to 48 mg/kg (40 times the human plasma exposure at 80 mg/day) during organogenesis and through lactation period.

8.3 Nursing Mothers

Febuxostat is excreted in the milk of rats. It is not known whether this drug is excreted in human milk. Because many drugs are excreted in human milk, caution should be exercised when ULORIC is administered to a nursing woman.

8.4 Pediatric Use

Safety and effectiveness in pediatric patients under 18 years of age have not been established.

8.5 Geriatric Use

No dose adjustment is necessary in elderly patients. Of the total number of subjects in clinical studies of ULORIC, 16% were 65 and over, while 4% were 75 and over. Comparing subjects in different age groups, no clinically significant differences in safety or effectiveness were observed but greater sensitivity of some older individuals cannot be ruled out. The C_{max} and AUC_{24} of febuxostat following multiple oral doses of ULORIC in geriatric subjects (≥65 years) were similar to those in younger subjects (18 to 40 years) *[see Clinical Pharmacology (12.3)]*.

8.6 Renal Impairment

No dose adjustment is necessary in patients with mild or moderate renal impairment (Cl_{cr} 30 to 89 mL/min). The recommended starting dose of ULORIC is 40 mg once daily. For patients who do not achieve a sUA less than 6 mg/dL after two weeks with 40 mg, ULORIC 80 mg is recommended.

There are insufficient data in patients with severe renal impairment (Cl_{cr} less than 30 mL/min); therefore, caution should be exercised in these patients *[see Clinical Pharmacology (12.3)]*.

8.7 Hepatic Impairment

No dose adjustment is necessary in patients with mild or moderate hepatic impairment (Child-Pugh Class A or B). No studies have been conducted in patients with severe hepatic impairment (Child-Pugh Class C); therefore, caution should be exercised in these patients *[see Clinical Pharmacology (12.3)]*.

8.8 Secondary Hyperuricemia

No studies have been conducted in patients with secondary hyperuricemia (including organ transplant recipients); ULORIC is not recommended for use in patients whom the rate of urate formation is greatly increased (e.g., malignant disease and its treatment, Lesch-Nyhan syndrome). The concentration of xanthine in urine could, in rare cases, rise sufficiently to allow deposition in the urinary tract.

10 OVERDOSAGE

ULORIC was studied in healthy subjects in doses up to 300 mg daily for seven days without evidence of dose-limiting toxicities. No overdose of ULORIC was reported in clinical studies. Patients should be managed by symptomatic and supportive care should there be an overdose.

11 DESCRIPTION

ULORIC (febuxostat) is a xanthine oxidase inhibitor. The active ingredient in ULORIC is 2-[3-cyano-4-(2-methylpropoxy) phenyl]-4-methylthiazole-5-carboxylic acid, with a molecular weight of 316.38. The empirical formula is $C_{16}H_{16}N_2O_3S$.

The chemical structure is:

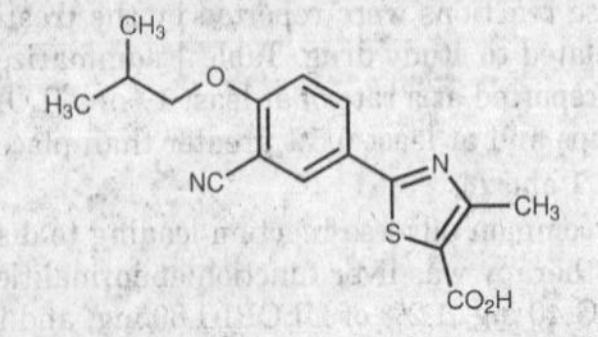

Febuxostat is a non-hygroscopic, white crystalline powder that is freely soluble in dimethylformamide; soluble in dimethylsulfoxide; sparingly soluble in ethanol; slightly soluble in methanol and acetonitrile; and practically insoluble in water. The melting range is 205°C to 208°C.

ULORIC tablets for oral use contain the active ingredient, febuxostat, and are available in two dosage strengths, 40 mg and 80 mg. Inactive ingredients include lactose monohydrate, microcrystalline cellulose, hydroxypropyl cellulose, sodium croscarmellose, silicon dioxide and magnesium stearate. ULORIC tablets are coated with Opadry II, green.

12 CLINICAL PHARMACOLOGY

12.1 Mechanism of Action

ULORIC, a xanthine oxidase inhibitor, achieves its therapeutic effect by decreasing serum uric acid. ULORIC is not expected to inhibit other enzymes involved in purine and pyrimidine synthesis and metabolism at therapeutic concentrations.

12.2 Pharmacodynamics

Effect on Uric Acid and Xanthine Concentrations: In healthy subjects, ULORIC resulted in a dose dependent decrease in 24-hour mean serum uric acid concentrations and an increase in 24-hour mean serum xanthine concentrations. In addition, there was a decrease in the total daily urinary uric acid excretion. Also, there was an increase in total daily urinary xanthine excretion. Percent reduction in 24-hour mean serum uric acid concentrations was between 40% and 55% at the exposure levels of 40 mg and 80 mg daily doses.

Effect on Cardiac Repolarization: The effect of ULORIC on cardiac repolarization as assessed by the QTc interval was evaluated in normal healthy subjects and in patients with gout. ULORIC in doses up to 300 mg daily, at steady-state, did not demonstrate an effect on the QTc interval.

12.3 Pharmacokinetics

In healthy subjects, maximum plasma concentrations (C_{max}) and AUC of febuxostat increased in a dose proportional manner following single and multiple doses of 10 mg to 120 mg. There is no accumulation when therapeutic doses are administered every 24 hours. Febuxostat has an apparent mean terminal elimination half-life ($t_{1/2}$) of approximately 5 to 8 hours. Febuxostat pharmacokinetic parameters for patients with hyperuricemia and gout estimated by population pharmacokinetic analyses were similar to those estimated in healthy subjects.

Absorption: The absorption of radiolabeled febuxostat following oral dose administration was estimated to be at least 49% (based on total radioactivity recovered in urine). Maximum plasma concentrations of febuxostat occurred between 1 and 1.5 hours post-dose. After multiple oral 40 mg and 80 mg once daily doses, C_{max} is approximately 1.6 ± 0.6 mcg/mL (N=30), and 2.6 ± 1.7 mcg/mL (N=227), respectively. Absolute bioavailability of the febuxostat tablet has not been studied.

Following multiple 80 mg once daily doses with a high fat meal, there was a 49% decrease in C_{max} and an 18% decrease in AUC, respectively. However, no clinically significant change in the percent decrease in serum uric acid concentration was observed (58% fed vs. 51% fasting). Thus, ULORIC may be taken without regard to food.

Concomitant ingestion of an antacid containing magnesium hydroxide and aluminum hydroxide with an 80 mg single dose of ULORIC has been shown to delay absorption of febuxostat (approximately one hour) and to cause a 31% decrease in C_{max} and a 15% decrease in AUC_{∞}. As AUC rather than C_{max} was related to drug effect, change observed in AUC was not considered clinically significant. Therefore, ULORIC may be taken without regard to antacid use.

Distribution: The mean apparent steady state volume of distribution (V_{ss}/F) of febuxostat was approximately 50 L (CV ~40%). The plasma protein binding of febuxostat is approximately 99.2% (primarily to albumin), and is constant over the concentration range achieved with 40 mg and 80 mg doses.

Metabolism: Febuxostat is extensively metabolized by both conjugation via uridine diphosphate glucuronosyltransferase (UGT) enzymes including UGT1A1, UGT1A3, UGT1A9, and UGT2B7 and oxidation via cytochrome P450 (CYP) enzymes including CYP1A2, 2C8 and 2C9 and non-P450 enzymes. The relative contribution of each enzyme isoform in the metabolism of febuxostat is not clear. The oxidation of the isobutyl side chain leads to the formation of four pharmacologically active hydroxy metabolites, all of which occur in plasma of humans at a much lower extent than febuxostat.

In urine and feces, acyl glucuronide metabolites of febuxostat (~35% of the dose), and oxidative metabolites, 67M-1 (~10% of the dose), 67M-2 (~11% of the dose), and 67M-4, a secondary metabolite from 67M-1 (~14% of the dose), appeared to be the major metabolites of febuxostat *in vivo*.

Elimination: Febuxostat is eliminated by both hepatic and renal pathways. Following an 80 mg oral dose of ^{14}C-labeled febuxostat, approximately 49% of the dose was recovered in the urine as unchanged febuxostat (3%), the acyl glucuronide of the drug (30%), its known oxidative metabolites and their conjugates (13%), and other unknown metabolites (3%). In addition to the urinary excretion, approximately 45% of the dose was recovered in the feces as the unchanged febuxostat (12%), the acyl glucuronide of the drug (1%), its known oxidative metabolites and their conjugates (25%), and other unknown metabolites (7%).

The apparent mean terminal elimination half-life ($t_{1/2}$) of febuxostat was approximately 5 to 8 hours.

Special Populations

Pediatric Use: The pharmacokinetics of ULORIC in patients under the age of 18 years have not been studied.

Geriatric Use: The C_{max} and AUC of febuxostat and its metabolites following multiple oral doses of ULORIC in geriatric subjects (≥65 years) were similar to those in younger subjects (18 to 40 years). In addition, the percent decrease in serum uric acid concentration was similar between elderly and younger subjects. No dose adjustment is necessary in geriatric patients *[see Use in Specific Populations (8.5)]*.

Renal Impairment: Following multiple 80 mg doses of ULORIC in healthy subjects with mild (Cl_{cr} 50 to 80 mL/min), moderate (Cl_{cr} 30 to 49 mL/min) or severe renal impairment (Cl_{cr} 10 to 29 mL/min), the C_{max} of febuxostat did not change relative to subjects with normal renal function (Cl_{cr} greater than 80 mL/min). AUC and half-life of febuxostat increased in subjects with renal impairment in comparison to subjects with normal renal function, but values were similar among three renal impairment groups. Mean febuxostat AUC values were up to 1.8 times higher in subjects with renal impairment compared to those with normal renal function. Mean C_{max} and AUC values for three active metabolites increased up to 2- and 4-fold, respectively. However, the percent decrease in serum uric acid concentration for subjects with renal impairment was comparable to those with normal renal function (58% in normal renal function group and 55% in the severe renal function group).

No dose adjustment is necessary in patients with mild to moderate renal impairment *[see Dosage and Administration (2) and Use in Specific Populations (8.6)]*. The recommended starting dose of ULORIC is 40 mg once daily. For patients who do not achieve a sUA less than 6 mg/dL after two weeks with 40 mg, ULORIC 80 mg is recommended. There is insufficient data in patients with severe renal impairment; caution should be exercised in those patients *[see Use in Specific Populations (8.6)]*.

ULORIC has not been studied in end stage renal impairment patients who are on dialysis.

Hepatic Impairment: Following multiple 80 mg doses of ULORIC in patients with mild (Child-Pugh Class A) or moderate (Child-Pugh Class B) hepatic impairment, an average of 20% to 30% increase was observed for both C_{max} and AUC_{24} (total and unbound) in hepatic impairment groups compared to subjects with normal hepatic function. In addition, the percent decrease in serum uric acid concentration was comparable between different hepatic groups (62% in healthy group, 49% in mild hepatic impairment group, and 48% in moderate hepatic impairment group). No dose adjustment is necessary in patients with mild or moderate hepatic impairment. No studies have been conducted in subjects with severe hepatic impairment (Child-Pugh Class C); caution should be exercised in those patients *[see Use in Specific Populations (8.7)]*.

Gender: Following multiple oral doses of ULORIC, the C_{max} and AUC_{24} of febuxostat were 30% and 14% higher in females than in males, respectively. However, weight-corrected C_{max} and AUC were similar between the genders. In addition, the percent decrease in serum uric acid concentrations was similar between genders. No dose adjustment is necessary based on gender.

Race: No specific pharmacokinetic study was conducted to investigate the effects of race.

Drug-Drug Interactions
Effect of ULORIC on Other Drugs
Xanthine Oxidase Substrate Drugs-Azathioprine, Mercaptopurine, and Theophylline: Febuxostat is an XO inhibitor. A drug-drug interaction study evaluating the effect of ULORIC upon the pharmacokinetics of theophylline (an XO substrate) in healthy subjects showed that coadministration of febuxostat with theophylline resulted in an approximately 400-fold increase in the amount of 1-methylxanthine, one of the major metabolites of theophylline, excreted in the urine. Since the long-term safety of exposure to 1-methylxanthine in humans is unknown, use with caution when coadministering febuxostat with theophylline.

Drug interaction studies of ULORIC with other drugs that are metabolized by XO (e.g., mercaptopurine and azathioprine) have not been conducted. Inhibition of XO by ULORIC may cause increased plasma concentrations of these drugs leading to toxicity. ULORIC is contraindicated in patients being treated with azathioprine or mercaptopurine *[see Contraindications (4) and Drug Interactions (7)]*.

Azathioprine and mercaptopurine undergo metabolism via three major metabolic pathways, one of which is mediated by XO. Although ULORIC drug interaction studies with azathioprine and mercaptopurine have not been conducted, concomitant administration of allopurinol [a xanthine oxidase inhibitor] with azathioprine or mercaptopurine has been reported to substantially increase plasma concentrations of these drugs. Because ULORIC is a xanthine oxidase inhibitor, it could inhibit the XO-mediated metabolism of azathioprine and mercaptopurine leading to increased plasma concentrations of azathioprine or mercaptopurine that could result in severe toxicity.

P450 Substrate Drugs: In vitro studies have shown that febuxostat does not inhibit P450 enzymes CYP1A2, 2C9, 2C19, 2D6, or 3A4 and it also does not induce CYP1A2, 2B6, 2C9, 2C19, or 3A4 at clinically relevant concentrations. As such, pharmacokinetic interactions between ULORIC and drugs metabolized by these CYP enzymes are unlikely.

Effect of Other Drugs on ULORIC

Febuxostat is metabolized by conjugation and oxidation via multiple metabolizing enzymes. The relative contribution of each enzyme isoform is not clear. Drug interactions between ULORIC and a drug that inhibits or induces one particular enzyme isoform is in general not expected.

In Vivo Drug Interaction Studies
Theophylline: No dose adjustment is necessary for theophylline when coadministered with ULORIC. Administration of ULORIC (80 mg once daily) with theophylline resulted in an increase of 6% in C_{max} and 6.5% in AUC of theophylline. These changes were not considered statistically significant. However, the study also showed an approximately 400-fold increase in the amount of 1-methylxanthine (one of the major theophylline metabolites) excreted in urine as a result of XO inhibition by ULORIC. The safety of long-term exposure to 1-methylxanthine has not been evaluated. This should be taken into consideration when deciding to coadminister ULORIC and theophylline.

Colchicine: No dose adjustment is necessary for either ULORIC or colchicine when the two drugs are coadministered. Administration of ULORIC (40 mg once daily) with colchicine (0.6 mg twice daily) resulted in an increase of 12% in C_{max} and 7% in AUC_{24} of febuxostat. In addition, administration of colchicine (0.6 mg twice daily) with ULORIC (120 mg daily) resulted in a less than 11% change in C_{max} or AUC of colchicine for both AM and PM doses. These changes were not considered clinically significant.

Naproxen: No dose adjustment is necessary for ULORIC or naproxen when the two drugs are coadministered. Administration of ULORIC (80 mg once daily) with naproxen (500 mg twice daily) resulted in a 28% increase in C_{max} and a 40% increase in AUC of febuxostat. The increases were not considered clinically significant. In addition, there were no significant changes in the C_{max} or AUC of naproxen (less than 2%).

Indomethacin: No dose adjustment is necessary for either ULORIC or indomethacin when these two drugs are coadministered. Administration of ULORIC (80 mg once daily) with indomethacin (50 mg twice daily) did not result in any significant changes in C_{max} or AUC of febuxostat or indomethacin (less than 7%).

Hydrochlorothiazide: No dose adjustment is necessary for ULORIC when coadministered with hydrochlorothiazide. Administration of ULORIC (80 mg) with hydrochlorothiazide (50 mg) did not result in any clinically significant changes in C_{max} or AUC of febuxostat (less than 4%), and serum uric acid concentrations were not substantially affected.

Warfarin: No dose adjustment is necessary for warfarin when coadministered with ULORIC. Administration of ULORIC (80 mg once daily) with warfarin had no effect on the pharmacokinetics of warfarin in healthy subjects. INR and Factor VII activity were also not affected by the coadministration of ULORIC.

Desipramine: Coadministration of drugs that are CYP2D6 substrates (such as desipramine) with ULORIC are not expected to require dose adjustment. Febuxostat was shown to be a weak inhibitor of CYP2D6 *in vitro* and *in vivo*. Administration of ULORIC (120 mg once daily) with desipramine (25 mg) resulted in an increase in C_{max} (16%) and AUC (22%) of desipramine, which was associated with a 17% decrease in the 2-hydroxydesipramine to desipramine metabolic ratio (based on AUC).

13 NONCLINICAL TOXICOLOGY
13.1 Carcinogenesis, Mutagenesis, Impairment of Fertility
Carcinogenesis: Two-year carcinogenicity studies were conducted in F344 rats and B6C3F1 mice. Increased transitional cell papilloma and carcinoma of urinary bladder was observed at 24 mg/kg (25 times the human plasma exposure at maximum recommended human dose of 80 mg/day) and 18.75 mg/kg (12.5 times the human plasma exposure at 80 mg/day) in male rats and female mice, respectively. The urinary bladder neoplasms were secondary to calculus formation in the kidney and urinary bladder.

Mutagenesis: Febuxostat showed a positive mutagenic response in a chromosomal aberration assay in a Chinese hamster lung fibroblast cell line with and without metabolic activation *in vitro*. Febuxostat was negative in the *in vitro* Ames assay and chromosomal aberration test in human peripheral lymphocytes, and L5178Y mouse lymphoma cell line, and *in vivo* tests in mouse micronucleus, rat unscheduled DNA synthesis and rat bone marrow cells.

Impairment of Fertility: Febuxostat at oral doses up to 48 mg/kg/day (approximately 35 times the human plasma exposure at 80 mg/day) had no effect on fertility and reproductive performance of male and female rats.

13.2 Animal Toxicology
A 12-month toxicity study in beagle dogs showed deposition of xanthine crystals and calculi in kidneys at 15 mg/kg (approximately four times the human plasma exposure at 80 mg/day). A similar effect of calculus formation was noted in rats in a six-month study due to deposition of xanthine crystals at 48 mg/kg (approximately 35 times the human plasma exposure at 80 mg/day).

14 CLINICAL STUDIES
A serum uric acid level of less than 6 mg/dL is the goal of anti-hyperuricemic therapy and has been established as appropriate for the treatment of gout.

14.1 Management of Hyperuricemia in Gout
The efficacy of ULORIC was demonstrated in three randomized, double-blind, controlled trials in patients with hyperuricemia and gout. Hyperuricemia was defined as a baseline serum uric acid level ≥8 mg/dL.

Study 1 randomized patients to: ULORIC 40 mg daily, ULORIC 80 mg daily, or allopurinol (300 mg daily for patients with estimated creatinine clearance (Cl_{cr}) ≥60 mL/min or 200 mg daily for patients with estimated Cl_{cr} ≥30 mL/min and ≤59 mL/min). The duration of Study 1 was six months.

Study 2 randomized patients to: placebo, ULORIC 80 mg daily, ULORIC 120 mg daily, ULORIC 240 mg daily or allopurinol (300 mg daily for patients with a baseline serum creatinine ≤1.5 mg/dL or 100 mg daily for patients with a baseline serum creatinine greater than 1.5 mg/dL and ≤2 mg/dL). The duration of Study 2 was six months.

Study 3, a 1-year study, randomized patients to: ULORIC 80 mg daily, ULORIC 120 mg daily, or allopurinol 300 mg daily. Subjects who completed Study 2 and Study 3 were eligible to enroll in a phase 3 long-term extension study in which subjects received treatment with ULORIC for over three years.

In all three studies, subjects received naproxen 250 mg twice daily or colchicine 0.6 mg once or twice daily for gout flare prophylaxis. In Study 1 the duration of prophylaxis was six months; in Study 2 and Study 3 the duration of prophylaxis was eight weeks.

The efficacy of ULORIC was also evaluated in a four week dose ranging study which randomized patients to: placebo, ULORIC 40 mg daily, ULORIC 80 mg daily, or ULORIC 120 mg daily. Subjects who completed this study were eligible to enroll in a long-term extension study in which subjects received treatment with ULORIC for up to five years.

Patients in these studies were representative of the patient population for which ULORIC use is intended. Table 2 summarizes the demographics and baseline characteristics for the subjects enrolled in the studies.

Table 2: Patient Demographics and Baseline Characteristics in Study 1, Study 2 and Study 3

Male		95%
Race:	Caucasian	80%
	African American	10%
Ethnicity: Hispanic or Latino		7%
Alcohol User		67%
Mild to Moderate Renal Insufficiency (percent with estimated Cl_{cr} less than 90 mL/min)		59%
History of Hypertension		49%
History of Hyperlipidemia		38%
BMI ≥30 kg/m²		63%
Mean BMI		33 kg/m²
Baseline sUA ≥10 mg/dL		36%
Mean baseline sUA		9.7 mg/dL
Experienced a gout flare in previous year		85%

Serum Uric Acid Level less than 6 mg/dL at Final Visit: ULORIC 80 mg was superior to allopurinol in lowering se-

Continued on next page

Table 3: Proportion of Patients with Serum Uric Acid Levels less than 6 mg/dL at Final Visit

Study*	ULORIC 40 mg daily	ULORIC 80 mg daily	allopurinol	Placebo	Difference in Proportion (95% CI)	
					ULORIC 40 mg vs allopurinol	ULORIC 80 mg vs allopurinol
Study 1 (6 months) (N=2268)	45%	67%	42%		3% (-2%, 8%)	25% (20%, 30%)
Study 2 (6 months) (N=643)		72%	39%	1%		33% (26%, 42%)
Study 3 (12 months) (N=491)		74%	36%			38% (30%, 46%)

* Randomization was balanced between treatment groups, except in Study 2 in which twice as many patients were randomized to each of the active treatment groups compared to placebo.

rum uric acid to less than 6 mg/dL at the final visit. ULORIC 40 mg daily, although not superior to allopurinol, was effective in lowering serum uric acid to less than 6 mg/dL at the final visit *(Table 3)*.
[See table 3 above]

In 76% of ULORIC 80 mg patients, reduction in serum uric acid levels to less than 6 mg/dL was noted by the Week 2 visit. Average serum uric acid levels were maintained at 6 mg/dL or below throughout treatment in 83% of these patients.

In all treatment groups, fewer subjects with higher baseline serum urate levels (≥10 mg/dL) and/or tophi achieved the goal of lowering serum uric acid to less than 6 mg/dL at the final visit; however, a higher proportion achieved a serum uric acid less than 6 mg/dL with ULORIC 80 mg than with ULORIC 40 mg or allopurinol.

Study 1 evaluated efficacy in patients with mild to moderate renal impairment (i.e., baseline estimated Cl_{cr} less than 90 mL/min). The results in this sub-group of patients are shown in Table 4.
[See table 4 below]

16   HOW SUPPLIED/STORAGE AND HANDLING

ULORIC 40 mg tablets are light green to green in color, round, debossed with "TAP" on one side and "40" on the other side and supplied as:

NDC Number	Size
64764-918-11	Hospital Unit Dose Pack of 100 Tablets
64764-918-30	Bottle of 30 Tablets
64764-918-90	Bottle of 90 Tablets
64764-918-18	Bottle of 500 Tablets

ULORIC 80 mg tablets are light green to green in color, teardrop shaped, debossed with "TAP" on one side and "80" on the other side and supplied as:

NDC Number	Size
64764-677-11	Hospital Unit Dose Pack of 100 Tablets
64764-677-30	Bottle of 30 Tablets

| 64764-677-13 | Bottle of 100 Tablets |
| 64764-677-19 | Bottle of 1000 Tablets |

Protect from light. Store at 25°C (77°F); excursions permitted to 15° to 30°C (59° to 86°F) [See USP Controlled Room Temperature].

17   PATIENT COUNSELING INFORMATION

See FDA-Approved Patient Labeling (Patient Information)

17.1   General Information

Patients should be advised of the potential benefits and risks of ULORIC. Patients should be informed about the potential for gout flares, elevated liver enzymes and adverse cardiovascular events after initiation of ULORIC therapy.

Concomitant prophylaxis with an NSAID or colchicine for gout flares should be considered.

Patients should be instructed to inform their healthcare professional if they develop a rash, chest pain, shortness of breath or neurologic symptoms suggesting a stroke. Patients should be instructed to inform their healthcare professional of any other medications they are currently taking with ULORIC, including over-the-counter medications.

Patient Information

ULORIC (Ū-'lor–ik)
(febuxostat) tablets

Read the Patient Information that comes with ULORIC before you start taking it and each time you get a refill. There may be new information. This information does not take the place of talking with your healthcare provider about your medical condition or your treatment.

What is ULORIC?

ULORIC is a prescription medicine called a xanthine oxidase (XO) inhibitor, used to lower blood uric acid levels in adults with gout.

It is not known if ULORIC is safe and effective in children under 18 years of age.

Who should not take ULORIC?

Do not take ULORIC if you:

• take azathioprine (Azasan, Imuran)
• take mercaptopurine (Purinethol)

It is not known if ULORIC is safe and effective in children under 18 years of age.

What should I tell my healthcare provider before taking ULORIC?

Before taking ULORIC tell your healthcare provider about all of your medical conditions, including if you:

• have liver or kidney problems
• have a history of heart disease or stroke
• are pregnant or plan to become pregnant. It is not known if ULORIC will harm your unborn baby. Talk with your healthcare provider if you are pregnant or plan to become pregnant.
• are breastfeeding or plan to breastfeed. It is not known if ULORIC passes into your breast milk. You and your healthcare provider should decide if you should take ULORIC while breastfeeding.

Tell your healthcare provider about all the medicines you take, including prescription and non-prescription medicines, vitamins, and herbal supplements. ULORIC may affect the way other medicines work, and other medicines may affect how ULORIC works.

Know the medicines you take. Keep a list of them and show it to your healthcare provider and pharmacist when you get a new medicine.

How should I take ULORIC?

• Take ULORIC exactly as your healthcare provider tells you to take it.
• ULORIC can be taken with or without food.
• ULORIC can be taken with antacids.
• Your gout may flare up when you start taking ULORIC, do not stop taking your ULORIC even if you have a flare. Your healthcare provider may give you other medicines to help prevent your gout flares.
• Your healthcare provider may do certain tests while you take ULORIC.

What are the possible side effects of ULORIC?

Heart problems. A small number of heart attacks, strokes and heart-related deaths were seen in clinical studies. It is not certain that ULORIC caused these events.

The most common side effects of ULORIC include:

• liver problems
• nausea
• gout flares
• joint pain
• rash

Tell your healthcare provider if you develop a rash, have any side effect that bothers you, or that does not go away. These are not all of the possible side effects of ULORIC. For more information, ask your healthcare provider or pharmacist.

Call your doctor for medical advice about side effects. You may report side effects to the FDA at 1-800-FDA-1088.

How should I store ULORIC?

Store ULORIC between 59°F and 86°F (15°C to 30°C).
Keep ULORIC out of the light.
Keep ULORIC and all medicines out of the reach of children.

General information about the safe and effective use of ULORIC.

Medicines are sometimes prescribed for purposes other than those listed in a patient information leaflet. Do not use ULORIC for a condition for which it was not prescribed. Do not give ULORIC to other people, even if they have the same symptoms that you have. It may harm them.

This patient information leaflet summarizes the most important information about ULORIC. If you would like more information about ULORIC talk with your healthcare provider. You can ask your healthcare provider or pharmacist for information about ULORIC that is written for health professionals. For more information go to www.uloric.com, or call 1-877-825-3327.

What are the ingredients in ULORIC?

Active Ingredient: febuxostat

Inactive ingredients include: lactose monohydrate, microcrystalline cellulose, hydroxypropyl cellulose, sodium croscarmellose, silicon dioxide, magnesium stearate, and Opadry II, green

Distributed by:
Takeda Pharmaceuticals America, Inc.
Deerfield, IL 60015
Revised: March 2013
ULORIC is a registered trademark of Teijin Limited registered in the U.S. Patent and Trademark Office and used under license by Takeda Pharmaceuticals America, Inc.
All other trademarks are the property of their respective owners.
©2009-2013 Takeda Pharmaceuticals America, Inc.
ULR015 R4

Shown in Product Identification Guide, page 510

Table 4: Proportion of Patients with Serum Uric Acid Levels less than 6 mg/dL in Patients with Mild or Moderate Renal Impairment at Final Visit

ULORIC 40 mg daily (N=479)	ULORIC 80 mg daily (N=503)	allopurinol* 300 mg daily (N=501)	Difference in Proportion (95% CI)	
			ULORIC 40 mg vs allopurinol	ULORIC 80 mg vs allopurinol
50%	72%	42%	7% (1%, 14%)	29% (23%, 35%)

* Allopurinol patients (n=145) with estimated Clcr ≥30 mL/min and Clcr ≤59 mL/min were dosed at 200 mg daily.

Vanda Pharmaceuticals, Inc.
2200 PENNSYLVANIA AVE NW SUITE 300E
WASHINGTON, DC 20037

Tel: 202-734-3400
Fax: 202-296-1450

FANAPT®   ℞
(iloperidone)
tablets

HIGHLIGHTS OF PRESCRIBING INFORMATION
These highlights do not include all the information needed to use FANAPT safely and effectively. See full prescribing information for FANAPT.
FANAPT® (iloperidone) tablets, for oral use
Initial U.S. Approval: 2009

> **WARNING: INCREASED MORTALITY IN ELDERLY PATIENTS WITH DEMENTIA-RELATED PSYCHOSIS**
> *See full prescribing information for complete boxed warning.*
> Elderly patients with dementia-related psychosis treated with antipsychotic drugs are at an increased risk of death. FANAPT is not approved for use in patients with dementia-related psychosis. (5.1)

RECENT MAJOR CHANGES

Boxed Warning	5/2016
Indications and Usage (1)	5/2016
Dose and Administration (2.3)	5/2016
Contraindications (4)	1/2016
Warnings and Precautions (5.1 , 5.2)	5/2016

INDICATIONS AND USAGE

FANAPT is an atypical antipsychotic indicated for the treatment of schizophrenia in adults. (1, 14) In choosing among treatments, prescribers should consider the ability of FANAPT to prolong the QT interval and the use of other drugs first. Prescribers should also consider the need to titrate FANAPT slowly to avoid orthostatic hypotension, which may lead to delayed effectiveness compared to some other drugs that do not require similar titration. (2, 5, 14)

DOSAGE AND ADMINISTRATION

The recommended target dosage of FANAPT tablets is 12 to 24 mg/day administered twice daily. This target dosage range is achieved by daily dosage adjustments, alerting patients to symptoms of orthostatic hypotension, starting at a dose of 1 mg twice daily, then moving to 2 mg, 4 mg, 6 mg, 8 mg, 10 mg, and 12 mg twice daily on Days 2, 3, 4, 5, 6, and 7 respectively, to reach the 12 mg/day to 24 mg/day dose range. FANAPT can be administered without regard to meals. (2.1)

DOSAGE FORMS AND STRENGTHS

1 mg, 2 mg, 4 mg, 6 mg, 8 mg, 10 mg and 12 mg tablets. (3)

CONTRAINDICATIONS

Known hypersensitivity to FANAPT or to any components in the formulation. (4 , 6.2)

WARNINGS AND PRECAUTIONS

• Cerebrovascular Adverse Reactions in Elderly Patients with Dementia- Related Psychosis: Increased incidence of cerebrovascular adverse reactions (e.g., stroke, transient ischemic attack). (5.2)
• QT prolongation: Prolongs QT interval and may be associated with arrhythmia and sudden death—consider using other antipsychotics first.
Avoid use of FANAPT in combination with other drugs that are known to prolong QTc; use caution and consider dose modification when prescribing FANAPT with other drugs that inhibit FANAPT metabolism. Monitor serum potassium and magnesium in patients at risk for electrolyte disturbances. (1, 5.3, 7.1, 7.3, 12.3)
• Neuroleptic Malignant Syndrome: Manage with immediate discontinuation of drug and close monitoring. (5.4)
• Tardive dyskinesia: Discontinue if clinically appropriate. (5.5)
• Metabolic Changes: Monitor for hyperglycemia/diabetes mellitus, dyslipidemia and weight gain. (5.6)

• Seizures: Use cautiously in patients with a history of seizures or with conditions that lower seizure threshold. (5.7)
• Orthostatic hypotension: Dizziness, tachycardia, and syncope can occur with standing. (5.8)
• Leukopenia, Neutropenia, and Agranulocytosis have been reported with antipsychotics. Patients with a pre-existing low white blood cell count (WBC) or a history of leukopenia/neutropenia should have their complete blood count (CBC) monitored frequently during the first few months of therapy and should discontinue FANAPT at the first sign of a decline in WBC in the absence of other causative factors. (5.9)
• Suicide: Close supervision of high risk patients. (5.13)
• Priapism: Cases have been reported in association with FANAPT treatment. (5.14)
• Potential for cognitive and motor impairment: Use caution when operating machinery. (5.15)

ADVERSE REACTIONS

Commonly observed adverse reactions (incidence ≥5% and 2-fold greater than placebo) were: dizziness, dry mouth, fatigue, nasal congestion, orthostatic hypotension, somnolence, tachycardia, and weight increased. (6.1)
To report SUSPECTED ADVERSE REACTIONS, contact Vanda Pharmaceuticals Inc. at 1-844-GO-VANDA (1-844-468-2632) or FDA at 1-800-FDA-1088 or www.fda.gov/medwatch.

DRUG INTERACTIONS

• The dose of FANAPT should be reduced in patients co-administered a strong CYP2D6 or CYP3A4 inhibitor. (2.2, 7.1)

USE IN SPECIFIC POPULATIONS

• Pregnancy: May cause extrapyramidal and/or withdrawal symptoms in neonates with third trimester exposure. (8.1)
• Lactation: Advise not to breast feed. (8.2)
• Pediatric Use: Safety and effectiveness not established in children and adolescents. (8.3)
• Hepatic Impairment: FANAPT is not recommended for patients with severe hepatic impairment. (2.2 , 8.6)
• The dose of FANAPT should be reduced in patients who are poor metabolizers of CYP2D6. (2.2, 12.3)

See 17 for PATIENT COUNSELING INFORMATION.

Revised: 5/2016

FULL PRESCRIBING INFORMATION

> **WARNING: INCREASED MORTALITY IN ELDERLY PATIENTS WITH DEMENTIA-RELATED PSYCHOSIS**
> Elderly patients with dementia-related psychosis treated with antipsychotic drugs are at an increased risk of death. FANAPT is not approved for the treatment of patients with dementia-related psychosis *[see Warnings and Precautions (5.1)]*.

---

1   INDICATIONS AND USAGE

FANAPT® is indicated for the treatment of schizophrenia in adults.
When deciding among the alternative treatments available for this condition, the prescriber should consider the finding that FANAPT is associated with prolongation of the QTc interval *[see Warnings and Precautions (5.3)]*. Prolongation of the QTc interval is associated in some other drugs with the ability to cause torsade de pointes-type arrhythmia, a potentially fatal polymorphic ventricular tachycardia which can result in sudden death. In many cases this would lead to the conclusion that other drugs should be tried first. Whether FANAPT will cause torsade de pointes or increase the rate of sudden death is not yet known.
Patients must be titrated to an effective dose of FANAPT. Thus, control of symptoms may be delayed during the first 1 to 2 weeks of treatment compared to some other antipsychotic drugs that do not require a similar titration. Prescribers should be mindful of this delay when selecting an antipsychotic drug for the treatment of schizophrenia *[see Dosage and Administration (2.1) and Clinical Studies (14)]*.

2   DOSAGE AND ADMINISTRATION

2.1   Usual Dose
FANAPT must be titrated slowly from a low starting dose to avoid orthostatic hypotension due to its alpha-adrenergic blocking properties. The recommended starting dose for FANAPT tablets is 1 mg orally twice daily. Dose increases to reach the target range of 6-12 mg twice daily (12_24 mg/day) may be made with daily dosage adjustments not to exceed 2 mg twice daily (4 mg/day). The maximum recommended dose is 12 mg twice daily (24 mg/day). FANAPT doses above 24 mg/day have not been systematically evaluated in the clinical trials. Efficacy was demonstrated with FANAPT in a dose range of 6 to 12 mg twice daily. Prescribers should be mindful of the fact that patients need to be titrated to an effective dose of FANAPT. Thus, control of symptoms may be delayed during the first 1 to 2 weeks of treatment compared to some other antipsychotic drugs that do not require similar titration. Prescribers should also be aware that some adverse effects associated with FANAPT use are dose related *[see Adverse Reactions (6.1)]*.
FANAPT can be administered without regard to meals.

2.2   Dosage in Special Populations
Dosage adjustment for patients taking FANAPT concomitantly with potential CYP2D6 inhibitors: FANAPT dose

Continued on next page

should be reduced by one-half when administered concomitantly with strong CYP2D6 inhibitors such as fluoxetine or paroxetine. When the CYP2D6 inhibitor is withdrawn from the combination therapy, FANAPT dose should then be increased to where it was before [see Drug Interactions (7)].

Dosage adjustment for patients taking FANAPT concomitantly with potential CYP3A4 inhibitors: FANAPT dose should be reduced by one-half when administered concomitantly with strong CYP3A4 inhibitors such as ketoconazole or clarithromycin. When the CYP3A4 inhibitor is withdrawn from the combination therapy, FANAPT dose should be increased to where it was before [see Drug Interactions (7)].

Dosage adjustment for patients taking FANAPT who are poor metabolizers of CYP2D6: FANAPT dose should be reduced by one-half for poor metabolizers of CYP2D6 [see Clinical Pharmacology (12.3)].

Hepatic Impairment: No dose adjustment to FANAPT is needed in patients with mild hepatic impairment. Patients with moderate hepatic impairment may require dose reduction, if clinically indicated. FANAPT is not recommended for patients with severe hepatic impairment [see Use in Specific Populations (8.7)].

2.3   Maintenance Treatment

In a longer-term study, FANAPT was effective in delaying time to relapse in patients with schizophrenia who were stabilized on FANAPT up to 24 mg/day [see Clinical Studies (14)]. Patients should be periodically reassessed to determine the need for maintenance treatment.

2.4   Reinitiation of Treatment in Patients Previously Discontinued

Although there are no data to specifically address reinitiation of treatment, it is recommended that the initiation titration schedule be followed whenever patients have had an interval off FANAPT of more than 3 days.

3   DOSAGE FORMS AND STRENGTHS

FANAPT tablets are available in the following strengths: 1 mg, 2 mg, 4 mg, 6 mg, 8 mg, 10 mg, and 12 mg. The tablets are white, round, flat, beveled-edged and identified with

a logo "⬡" debossed on one side and tablet strength "1", "2", "4", "6", "8", "10", or "12" debossed on the other side.

4   CONTRAINDICATIONS

FANAPT is contraindicated in individuals with a known hypersensitivity reaction to the product. Anaphylaxis, angioedema, and other hypersensitivity reactions have been reported [see Adverse Reactions (6.2)].

5   WARNINGS AND PRECAUTIONS

5.1   Increased Mortality in Elderly Patients with Dementia-Related Psychosis

Antipsychotic drugs increase the all-cause risk of death in elderly patients with dementia-related psychosis. Analyses of 17 dementia-related psychosis placebo-controlled trials (modal duration of 10 weeks and largely in patients taking atypical antipsychotic drugs) revealed a risk of death in the drug-treated patients of between 1.6 to 1.7 times that in placebo-treated patients. Over the course of a typical 10-week controlled trial, the rate of death in drug-treated patients was about 4.5%, compared to a rate of about 2.6% in placebo-treated patients.

Although the causes of death were varied, most of the deaths appeared to be either cardiovascular (e.g., heart failure, sudden death) or infectious (e.g., pneumonia) in nature. FANAPT is not approved for the treatment of patients with dementia-related psychosis [see Boxed Warning, Warnings and Precautions (5.2)].

5.2   Cerebrovascular Adverse Reactions, Including Stroke, in Elderly Patients with Dementia-Related Psychosis

In placebo-controlled trials in elderly subjects with dementia, patients randomized to risperidone, aripiprazole, and olanzapine had a higher incidence of stroke and transient ischemic attack, including fatal stroke. FANAPT is not approved for the treatment of patients with dementia-related psychosis [see Boxed Warning, Warnings and Precautions (5.1)].

5.3   QT Prolongation

In an open-label QTc study in patients with schizophrenia or schizoaffective disorder (n=160), FANAPT was associated with QTc prolongation of 9 msec at an iloperidone dose of 12 mg twice daily. The effect of FANAPT on the QT interval was augmented by the presence of CYP450 2D6 or 3A4 metabolic inhibition (paroxetine 20 mg once daily and ketoconazole 200 mg twice daily, respectively). Under conditions of metabolic inhibition for both 2D6 and 3A4, FANAPT 12 mg twice daily was associated with a mean QTcF increase from baseline of about 19 msec.

No cases of torsade de pointes or other severe cardiac arrhythmias were observed during the pre-marketing clinical program.

The use of FANAPT should be avoided in combination with other drugs that are known to prolong QTc including Class 1A (e.g., quinidine, procainamide) or Class III (e.g., amiodarone, sotalol) antiarrhythmic medications, antipsychotic medications (e.g., chlorpromazine, thioridazine), antibiotics (e.g., gatifloxacin, moxifloxacin), or any other class of medications known to prolong the QTc interval (e.g., pentamidine, levomethadyl acetate, methadone). FANAPT should also be avoided in patients with congenital long QT syndrome and in patients with a history of cardiac arrhythmias.

Certain circumstances may increase the risk of torsade de pointes and/or sudden death in association with the use of drugs that prolong the QTc interval, including (1) bradycardia; (2) hypokalemia or hypomagnesemia; (3) concomitant use of other drugs that prolong the QTc interval; and (4) presence of congenital prolongation of the QT interval; (5) recent acute myocardial infarction; and/or (6) uncompensated heart failure.

Caution is warranted when prescribing FANAPT with drugs that inhibit FANAPT metabolism [see Drug Interactions (7.1)], and in patients with reduced activity of CYP2D6 [see Clinical Pharmacology (12.3)].

It is recommended that patients being considered for FANAPT treatment who are at risk for significant electrolyte disturbances have baseline serum potassium and magnesium measurements with periodic monitoring. Hypokalemia (and/or hypomagnesemia) may increase the risk of QT prolongation and arrhythmia. FANAPT should be avoided in patients with histories of significant cardiovascular illness, e.g., QT prolongation, recent acute myocardial infarction, uncompensated heart failure, or cardiac arrhythmia. FANAPT should be discontinued in patients who are found to have persistent QTc measurements >500 msec.

If patients taking FANAPT experience symptoms that could indicate the occurrence of cardiac arrhythmias, e.g., dizziness, palpitations, or syncope, the prescriber should initiate further evaluation, including cardiac monitoring.

5.4   Neuroleptic Malignant Syndrome (NMS)

A potentially fatal symptom complex sometimes referred to as Neuroleptic Malignant Syndrome (NMS) has been reported in association with administration of antipsychotic drugs, including FANAPT. Clinical manifestations include hyperpyrexia, muscle rigidity, altered mental status (including catatonic signs) and evidence of autonomic instability (irregular pulse or blood pressure, tachycardia, diaphoresis, and cardiac dysrhythmia). Additional signs may include elevated creatine phosphokinase, myoglobinuria (rhabdomyolysis), and acute renal failure.

The diagnostic evaluation of patients with this syndrome is complicated. In arriving at a diagnosis, it is important to identify cases in which the clinical presentation includes both serious medical illness (e.g., pneumonia, systemic infection, etc.) and untreated or inadequately treated extrapyramidal signs and symptoms (EPS). Other important considerations in the differential diagnosis include central anticholinergic toxicity, heat stroke, drug fever, and primary central nervous system (CNS) pathology.

The management of this syndrome should include: (1) immediate discontinuation of the antipsychotic drugs and other drugs not essential to concurrent therapy, (2) intensive symptomatic treatment and medical monitoring, and (3) treatment of any concomitant serious medical problems for which specific treatments are available. There is no general agreement about specific pharmacological treatment regimens for NMS.

If a patient requires antipsychotic drug treatment after recovery from NMS, the potential reintroduction of drug therapy should be carefully considered. The patient should be carefully monitored, since recurrences of NMS have been reported.

5.5   Tardive Dyskinesia

Tardive dyskinesia is a syndrome consisting of potentially irreversible, involuntary, dyskinetic movements, which may develop in patients treated with antipsychotic drugs. Although the prevalence of the syndrome appears to be highest among the elderly, especially elderly women, it is impossible to rely on prevalence estimates to predict, at the inception of antipsychotic treatment, which patients are likely to develop the syndrome. Whether antipsychotic drug products differ in their potential to cause tardive dyskinesia is unknown.

The risk of developing tardive dyskinesia and the likelihood that it will become irreversible are believed to increase as the duration of treatment and the total cumulative dose of antipsychotic administered increases. However, the syndrome can develop, although much less commonly, after relatively brief treatment periods at low doses.

There is no known treatment for established cases of tardive dyskinesia, although the syndrome may remit, partially or completely, if antipsychotic treatment is withdrawn. Antipsychotic treatment itself, however, may suppress (or partially suppress) the signs and symptoms of the syndrome and thereby may possibly mask the underlying process. The effect that symptomatic suppression has upon the long-term course of the syndrome is unknown.

Given these considerations, FANAPT should be prescribed in a manner that is most likely to minimize the occurrence of tardive dyskinesia. Chronic antipsychotic treatment should generally be reserved for patients who suffer from a chronic illness that (1) is known to respond to antipsychotic drugs, and (2) for whom alternative, equally effective, but potentially less harmful treatments are not available or appropriate. In patients who do require chronic treatment, the smallest dose and the shortest duration of treatment producing a satisfactory clinical response should be sought. The need for continued treatment should be reassessed periodically.

If signs and symptoms of tardive dyskinesia appear in a patient on FANAPT, drug discontinuation should be considered. However, some patients may require treatment with FANAPT despite the presence of the syndrome.

5.6   Metabolic Changes

Atypical antipsychotic drugs have been associated with metabolic changes that may increase cardiovascular/cerebrovascular risk. These metabolic changes include hyperglycemia, dyslipidemia, and body weight gain. While all atypical antipsychotic drugs have been shown to produce some metabolic changes, each drug in the class has its own specific risk profile.

Hyperglycemia and Diabetes Mellitus

Hyperglycemia, in some cases extreme and associated with ketoacidosis or hyperosmolar coma or death, has been reported in patients treated with atypical antipsychotics including FANAPT. Assessment of the relationship between atypical antipsychotic use and glucose abnormalities is complicated by the possibility of an increased background risk of diabetes mellitus in patients with schizophrenia and the increasing incidence of diabetes mellitus in the general population. Given these confounders, the relationship between atypical antipsychotic use and hyperglycemia-related adverse events is not completely understood. However, epidemiological studies suggest an increased risk of hyperglycemia-related adverse events in patients treated with the atypical antipsychotics included in these studies. Patients with an established diagnosis of diabetes mellitus who are started on atypical antipsychotics should be monitored regularly for worsening of glucose control. Patients with risk factors for diabetes mellitus (e.g., obesity, family history of diabetes) who are starting treatment with atypical antipsychotics should undergo fasting blood glucose testing at the beginning of treatment and periodically during treatment. Any patient treated with atypical antipsychotics should be monitored for symptoms of hyperglycemia including polydipsia, polyuria, polyphagia, and weakness. Patients who develop symptoms of hyperglycemia during treatment with atypical antipsychotics should undergo fasting blood glucose testing. In some cases, hyperglycemia has resolved when the atypical antipsychotic was discontinued; however, some patients required continuation of antidiabetic treatment despite discontinuation of the suspect drug. Data from a 4- week, fixed-dose study in adult subjects with schizophrenia, in which fasting blood samples were drawn, are presented in Table 1.

Table 1: Change in Fasting Glucose

	Placebo	FANAPT 24 mg/day
	Mean Change from Baseline(mg/dL)	
	n=114	n=228
Serum Glucose Change from Baseline	-0.5	6.6
	Proportion of Patients with Shifts	
Serum Glucose Normal to High (<100 mg/dL to ≥126 mg/dL)	2.5 % (2/80)	10.7 % (18/169)

Pooled analyses of glucose data from clinical studies including longer term trials are shown in Table 2.

Table 2: Change in Glucose

	Mean Change from Baseline (mg/dL)		
	3-6 months	6-12 months	>12 months
FANAPT 10-16 mg/day	1.8 (N=773)	5.4 (N=723)	5.4 (N=425)
FANAPT 20-24 mg/day	-3.6 (N=34)	-9.0 (N=31)	-18.0 (N=20)

Dyslipidemia

Undesirable alterations in lipids have been observed in patients treated with atypical antipsychotics.

Data from a placebo-controlled, 4-week, fixed-dose study, in which fasting blood samples were drawn, in adult subjects with schizophrenia are presented in Table 3 .

Table 3: Change in Fasting Lipids

	Placebo	FANAPT 24 mg/day
	Mean Change from Baseline (mg/dL)	
Cholesterol	n= 114	n=228
Change from baseline	-2.17	8.18
LDL	n=109	n=217
Change from baseline	-1.41	9.03
HDL	n= 114	n=228
Change from baseline	-3.35	0.55
Triglycerides	n= 114	n=228
Change from baseline	16.47	-0.83
	Proportion of Patients with Shifts	
Cholesterol Normal to High (<200 mg/dL to ≥240 mg/dL)	1.4% (1/72)	3.6% (5/141)
LDL Normal to High (<100 mg/dL to ≥160 mg/dL)	2.4% (1/42)	1.1% (1/90)
HDL Normal to Low (≥40 mg/dL to <40 mg/dL)	23.8% (19/80)	12.1% (20/166)
Triglycerides Normal to High (<150 mg/dL to ≥200 mg/dL)	8.3% (6/72)	10.1% (15/148)

Pooled analyses of cholesterol and triglyceride data from clinical studies including longer term trials are shown in Table 4 and Table 5 .

Table 4: Change in Cholesterol

	Mean Change from Baseline (mg/dL)		
	3-6 months	6-12 months	>12 months
FANAPT 10-16 mg/day	-3.9 (N=783)	-3.9 (N=726)	-7.7 (N=428)
FANAPT 20-24 mg/day	-19.4 (N=34)	-23.2 (N=31)	-19.4 (N=20)

Table 5: Change in Triglycerides

	Mean Change from Baseline (mg/dL)		
	3-6 months	6-12 months	>12 months
FANAPT 10-16 mg/day	-8.9 (N=783)	-8.9 (N=726)	-17.7 (N=428)
FANAPT 20-24 mg/day	-26.6 (N=34)	-35.4 (N=31)	-17.7 (N=20)

Weight Gain

Weight gain has been observed with atypical antipsychotic use. Clinical monitoring of weight is recommended.

Across all short- and long-term studies, the overall mean change from baseline at endpoint was 2.1 kg.

Changes in body weight (kg) and the proportion of subjects with ≥7% gain in body weight from 4 placebo-controlled, 4- or 6-week, fixed- or flexible-dose studies in adult subjects are presented in Table 6.

Table 6: Change in Body Weight

	Placebo n=576	FANAPT 10-16 mg/day n=481	FANAPT 20-24 mg/day n=391
Weight (kg) Change from Baseline	-0.1	2.0	2.7
Weight Gain ≥7% increase from Baseline	4%	12%	18%

5.7   Seizures

In short-term placebo-controlled trials (4- to 6-weeks), seizures occurred in 0.1% (1/1344) of patients treated with FANAPT compared to 0.3% (2/587) on placebo. As with other antipsychotics, FANAPT should be used cautiously in patients with a history of seizures or with conditions that potentially lower the seizure threshold. Conditions that lower the seizure threshold may be more prevalent in a population of 65 years or older.

5.8   Orthostatic Hypotension and Syncope

FANAPT can induce orthostatic hypotension associated with dizziness, tachycardia, and syncope. This reflects its alpha1-adrenergic antagonist properties. In double-blind placebo-controlled short-term studies, where the dose was increased slowly, as recommended above, syncope was reported in 0.4% (5/1344) of patients treated with FANAPT, compared with 0.2% (1/587) on placebo. Orthostatic hypotension was reported in 5% of patients given 20-24 mg/day, 3% of patients given 10-16 mg/day, and 1% of patients given placebo. More rapid titration would be expected to increase the rate of orthostatic hypotension and syncope.

FANAPT should be used with caution in patients with known cardiovascular disease (e.g., heart failure, history of myocardial infarction, ischemia, or conduction abnormalities), cerebrovascular disease, or conditions that predispose the patient to hypotension (dehydration, hypovolemia, and treatment with antihypertensive medications). Monitoring of orthostatic vital signs should be considered in patients who are vulnerable to hypotension.

5.9   Leukopenia, Neutropenia and Agranulocytosis

In clinical trial and postmarketing experience, events of leukopenia/neutropenia have been reported temporally related to antipsychotic agents. Agranulocytosis (including fatal cases) has also been reported.

Possible risk factors for leukopenia/neutropenia include preexisting low white blood cell count (WBC) and history of drug induced leukopenia/neutropenia. Patients with a pre-existing low WBC or a history of drug induced leukopenia/neutropenia should have their complete blood count (CBC) monitored frequently during the first few months of therapy and should discontinue FANAPT at the first sign of a decline in WBC in the absence of other causative factors. Patients with neutropenia should be carefully monitored for fever or other symptoms or signs of infection and treated promptly if such symptoms or signs occur. Patients with severe neutropenia (absolute neutrophil count <1000/mm³) should discontinue FANAPT and have their WBC followed until recovery.

5.10   Hyperprolactinemia

As with other drugs that antagonize dopamine D2 receptors, FANAPT elevates prolactin levels.

Hyperprolactinemia may suppress hypothalamic GnRH, resulting in reduced pituitary gonadotropin secretion. This, in turn, may inhibit reproductive function by impairing gonadalsteroidogenesis in both female and male patients. Galactorrhea, amenorrhea, gynecomastia, and impotence have been reported with prolactin-elevating compounds. Long-standing hyperprolactinemia when associated with hypogonadism may lead to decreased bone density in both female and male patients.

Tissue culture experiments indicate that approximately one-third of human breast cancers are prolactin-dependent in vitro, a factor of potential importance if the prescription of these drugs is contemplated in a patient with previously detected breast cancer. Mammary gland proliferative changes and increases in serum prolactin were seen in mice and rats treated with FANAPT [see Nonclinical Toxicology (13)]. Neither clinical studies nor epidemiologic studies conducted to date have shown an association between chronic administration of this class of drugs and tumorigenesis in humans; the available evidence is considered too limited to be conclusive at this time.

In a short-term placebo-controlled trial (4-weeks), the mean change from baseline to endpoint in plasma prolactin levels for the FANAPT 24 mg/day-treated group was an increase of 2.6 ng/mL compared to a decrease of 6.3 ng/mL in the placebo-group. In this trial, elevated plasma prolactin levels were observed in 26% of adults treated with FANAPT compared to 12% in the placebo group. In the short-term trials, FANAPT was associated with modest levels of prolactin elevation compared to greater prolactin elevations observed with some other antipsychotic agents. In pooled analysis from clinical studies including longer term trials, in 3210 adults treated with iloperidone, gynecomastia was reported in 2 male subjects (0.1%) compared to 0% in placebo-treated patients, and galactorrhea was reported in 8 female subjects (0.2%) compared to 3 female subjects (0.5%) in placebo-treated patients.

5.11   Body Temperature Regulation

Disruption of the body's ability to reduce core body temperature has been attributed to antipsychotic agents. Appropriate care is advised when prescribing FANAPT for patients who will be experiencing conditions which may contribute to an elevation in core body temperature, e.g., exercising strenuously, exposure to extreme heat, receiving concomitant medication with anticholinergic activity, or being subject to dehydration.

5.12   Dysphagia

Esophageal dysmotility and aspiration have been associated with antipsychotic drug use. Aspiration pneumonia is a common cause of morbidity and mortality in elderly patients. FANAPT and other antipsychotic drugs should be used cautiously in patients at risk for aspiration pneumonia [see Boxed Warning].

5.13   Suicide

The possibility of a suicide attempt is inherent in psychotic illness, and close supervision of high-risk patients should accompany drug therapy. Prescriptions for FANAPT should be written for the smallest quantity of tablets consistent with good patient management in order to reduce the risk of overdose.

5.14   Priapism

Three cases of priapism were reported in the pre-marketing FANAPT program. Drugs with alpha-adrenergic blocking effects have been reported to induce priapism. FANAPT shares this pharmacologic activity. Severe priapism may require surgical intervention.

5.15   Potential for Cognitive and Motor Impairment

FANAPT, like other antipsychotics, has the potential to impair judgment, thinking or motor skills. In short-term, placebo-controlled trials, somnolence (including sedation) was reported in 11.9% (104/874) of adult patients treated with FANAPT at doses of 10 mg/day or greater versus 5.3% (31/587) treated with placebo. Patients should be cautioned about operating hazardous machinery, including automobiles, until they are reasonably certain that therapy with FANAPT does not affect them adversely.

6   ADVERSE REACTIONS

6.1   Clinical Studies Experience

Because clinical trials are conducted under widely varying conditions, adverse reaction rates observed in the clinical trial of a drug cannot be directly compared to rates in the clinical trials of another drug and may not reflect the rates observed in clinical practice. The information below is de-

Continued on next page

rived from a clinical trial database for FANAPT consisting of 3229 patients exposed to FANAPT at doses of 10 mg/day or greater, for the treatment of schizophrenia. Of these, 999 received FANAPT for at least 6 months, with 657 exposed to FANAPT for at least 12 months. All of these patients who received FANAPT were participating in multiple-dose clinical trials. The conditions and duration of treatment with FANAPT varied greatly and included (in overlapping categories), open-label and double-blind phases of studies, inpatients and outpatients, fixed-dose and flexible-dose studies, and short-term and longer-term exposure.

The information presented in these sections was derived from pooled data from 4 placebo-controlled, 4- or 6-week, fixed- or flexible-dose studies in patients who received FANAPT at daily doses within a range of 10 to 24 mg (n=874).

Adverse Reactions Occurring at an Incidence of 2% or More among FANAPT-Treated Patients and More Frequent than Placebo

Table 7 enumerates the pooled incidences of adverse reactions that were spontaneously reported in four placebo-controlled, 4- or 6-week, fixed- or flexible-dose studies, listing those reactions that occurred in 2% or more of patients treated with FANAPT in any of the dose groups, and for which the incidence in FANAPT-treated patients in any dose group was greater than the incidence in patients treated with placebo.

Table 7: Percentage of Adverse Reactions in Short-Term, Fixed- or Flexible-Dose, Placebo-Controlled Trials in Adult Patients*

Body System or Organ Class Dictionary-derived Term	Placebo % (N=587)	FANAPT 10-16 mg/day % (N=483)	FANAPT 20-24 mg/day % (N=391)
Body as a Whole			
Arthralgia	2	3	3
Fatigue	3	4	6
Musculoskeletal Stiffness	1	1	3
Weight Increased	1	1	9
Cardiac Disorders			
Tachycardia	1	3	12
Eye Disorders			
Vision Blurred	2	3	1
Gastrointestinal Disorders			
Nausea	8	7	10
Dry Mouth	1	8	10
Diarrhea	4	5	7
Abdominal Discomfort	1	1	3
Infections			
Nasopharyngitis	3	4	3
Upper Respiratory Tract Infection	1	2	3
Nervous System Disorders			
Dizziness	7	10	20
Somnolence	5	9	15
Extrapyramidal Disorder	4	5	4
Tremor	2	3	3
Lethargy	1	3	1
Reproductive System			
Ejaculation Failure	<1	2	2
Respiratory			
Nasal Congestion	2	5	8
Dyspnea	<1	2	2
Skin			
Rash	2	3	2
Vascular Disorders			
Orthostatic Hypotension	1	3	5
Hypotension	<1	<1	3

*Table includes adverse reactions that were reported in 2% or more of patients in any of the FANAPT dose groups and which occurred at greater incidence than in the placebo group. Figures rounded to the nearest integer.

Dose-Related Adverse Reactions in Clinical Trials

Based on the pooled data from 4 placebo-controlled, 4- or 6-week, fixed- or flexible-dose studies, adverse reactions that occurred with a greater than 2% incidence in the patients treated with FANAPT, and for which the incidence in patients treated with FANAPT 20-24 mg/day were twice than the incidence in patients treated with FANAPT 10-16 mg/day were: abdominal discomfort, dizziness, hypotension, musculoskeletal stiffness, tachycardia, and weight increased.

Common and Drug-Related Adverse Reactions in Clinical Trials

Based on the pooled data from 4 placebo-controlled, 4- or 6-week, fixed- or flexible-dose studies, the following adverse reactions occurred in ≥5% incidence in the patients treated with FANAPT and at least twice the placebo rate for at least 1 dose: dizziness, dry mouth, fatigue, nasal congestion, somnolence, tachycardia, orthostatic hypotension, and weight increased. Dizziness, tachycardia, and weight increased were at least twice as common on 20-24 mg/day as on 10-16 mg/day.

Extrapyramidal Symptoms (EPS) in Clinical Trials

Pooled data from the 4 placebo-controlled, 4- or 6-week, fixed- or flexible-dose studies provided information regarding EPS. Adverse event data collected from those trials showed the following rates of EPS-related adverse events as shown in Table 8 .

Table 8: Percentage of EPS Compared to Placebo

Adverse Event Term	Placebo (%) (N=587)	FANAPT 10-16 mg/day (%) (N=483)	FANAPT 20-24 mg/day (%) (N=391)
All EPS events	11.6	13.5	15.1
Akathisia	2.7	1.7	2.3
Bradykinesia	0	0.6	0.5
Dyskinesia	1.5	1.7	1.0
Dystonia	0.7	1.0	0.8
Parkinsonism	0	0.2	0.3
Tremor	1.9	2.5	3.1

Adverse Reactions Associated with Discontinuation of Treatment in Clinical Trials

Based on the pooled data from 4 placebo-controlled, 4- or 6-week, fixed- or flexible-dose studies, there was no difference in the incidence of discontinuation due to adverse events between FANAPT-treated (5%) and placebo-treated (5%) patients. The types of adverse events that led to discontinuation were similar for the FANAPT- and placebo-treated patients.

Demographic Differences in Adverse Reactions in Clinical Trials

An examination of population subgroups in the 4 placebo-controlled, 4- or 6-week, fixed- or flexible-dose studies did not reveal any evidence of differences in safety on the basis of age, gender or race.

Laboratory Test Abnormalities in Clinical Trials

There were no differences between FANAPT and placebo in the incidence of discontinuation due to changes in hematology, urinalysis, or serum chemistry.

In short-term placebo-controlled trials (4- to 6-weeks), there were 1.0% (13/1342) iloperidone-treated patients with hematocrit at least one time below the extended normal range during post-randomization treatment, compared to 0.3% (2/585) on placebo. The extended normal range for lowered hematocrit was defined in each of these trials as the value 15% below the normal range for the centralized laboratory that was used in the trial.

Other Reactions During the Pre-marketing Evaluation of FANAPT

The following is a list of MedDRA terms that reflect adverse reactions in patients treated with FANAPT at multiple doses ≥ 4 mg/day during any phase of a trial with the database of 3210 FANAPT-treated patients. All reported reactions are included except those already listed in Table 7, or other parts of the *Adverse Reactions (6)*, those considered in the *Warnings and Precautions (5)*, those reaction terms which were so general as to be uninformative, reactions reported in fewer than 3 patients and which were neither se-

rious nor life-threatening, reactions that are otherwise common as background reactions, and reactions considered unlikely to be drug related.

Reactions are further categorized by MedDRA system organ class and listed in order of decreasing frequency according to the following definitions: frequent adverse events are those occurring in at least 1/100 patients (only those not listed in Table 7 appear in this listing); infrequent adverse reactions are those occurring in 1/100 to 1/1000 patients; rare events are those occurring in fewer than 1/1000 patients.

Blood and Lymphatic Disorders: Infrequent – anemia, iron deficiency anemia; *Rare* – leukopenia

Cardiac Disorders: Frequent – palpitations; *Rare* – arrhythmia, atrioventricular block first degree, cardiac failure (including congestive and acute)

Ear and Labyrinth Disorders: Infrequent – vertigo, tinnitus

Endocrine Disorders: Infrequent – hypothyroidism

Eye Disorders: Frequent - conjunctivitis (including allergic); *Infrequent* – dry eye, blepharitis, eyelid edema, eye swelling, lenticular opacities, cataract, hyperemia (including conjunctival)

Gastrointestinal Disorders: Infrequent – gastritis, salivary hypersecretion, fecal incontinence, mouth ulceration; *Rare* - aphthous stomatitis, duodenal ulcer, hiatus hernia, hyperchlorhydria, lip ulceration, reflux esophagitis, stomatitis

General Disorders and Administrative Site Conditions: Infrequent – edema (general, pitting, due to cardiac disease), difficulty in walking, thirst; *Rare* - hyperthermia

Hepatobiliary Disorders: Infrequent – cholelithiasis

Investigations: Frequent: weight decreased; *Infrequent* – hemoglobin decreased, neutrophil count increased, hematocrit decreased

Metabolism and Nutrition Disorders: Infrequent – increased appetite, dehydration, hypokalemia, fluid retention

Musculoskeletal and Connective Tissue Disorders: Frequent – myalgia, muscle spasms; *Rare* – torticollis

Nervous System Disorders: Infrequent – paresthesia, psychomotor hyperactivity, restlessness, amnesia, nystagmus; *Rare* – restless legs syndrome

Psychiatric Disorders: Frequent – restlessness, aggression, delusion; *Infrequent* – hostility, libido decreased, paranoia, anorgasmia, confusional state, mania, catatonia, mood swings, panic attack, obsessive-compulsive disorder, bulimia nervosa, delirium, polydipsia psychogenic, impulse-control disorder, major depression

Renal and Urinary Disorders: Frequent – urinary incontinence; *Infrequent* – dysuria, pollakiuria, enuresis, nephrolithiasis; *Rare* – urinary retention, renal failure acute

Reproductive System and Breast Disorders: Frequent – erectile dysfunction; *Infrequent* – testicular pain, amenorrhea, breast pain; *Rare* – menstruation irregular, gynecomastia, menorrhagia, metrorrhagia, postmenopausal hemorrhage, prostatitis.

Respiratory, Thoracic and Mediastinal Disorders: Infrequent – epistaxis, asthma, rhinorrhea, sinus congestion, nasal dryness; *Rare* – dry throat, sleep apnea syndrome, dyspnea exertional

6.2 Postmarketing Experience

The following adverse reactions have been identified during post-approval use of FANAPT: retrograde ejaculation and hypersensitivity reactions (including anaphylaxis; angioedema; throat tightness; oropharyngeal swelling; swelling of the face, lips, mouth, and tongue; urticaria; rash; and pruritus). Because these reactions were reported voluntarily from a population of uncertain size, it is not possible to reliably estimate their frequency or establish a causal relationship to drug exposure.

7   DRUG INTERACTIONS

Given the primary CNS effects of FANAPT, caution should be used when it is taken in combination with other centrally acting drugs and alcohol. Due to its - alpha1-adrenergic receptor antagonism, FANAPT has the potential to enhance the effect of certain antihypertensive agents.

7.1   Potential for Other Drugs to Affect FANAPT

Iloperidone is not a substrate for CYP1A1, CYP1A2, CYP2A6, CYP2B6, CYP2C8, CYP2C9, CYP2C19, or CYP2E1 enzymes. This suggests that an interaction of iloperidone with inhibitors or inducers of these enzymes, or other factors, like smoking, is unlikely.

Both CYP3A4 and CYP2D6 are responsible for iloperidone metabolism. Inhibitors of CYP3A4 (e.g., ketoconazole) or

CYP2D6 (e.g., fluoxetine, paroxetine) can inhibit iloperidone elimination and cause increased blood levels.

Ketoconazole: Co-administration of ketoconazole (200 mg twice daily for 4 days), a potent inhibitor of CYP3A4, with a 3 mg single dose of iloperidone to 19 healthy volunteers, ages 18-45 years, increased the area under the curve (AUC) of iloperidone and its metabolites P88 and P95 by 57%, 55% and 35%, respectively. Iloperidone doses should be reduced by about one-half when administered with ketoconazole or other strong inhibitors of CYP3A4 (e.g., itraconazole). Weaker inhibitors (e.g., erythromycin, grapefruit juice) have not been studied. When the CYP3A4 inhibitor is withdrawn from the combination therapy, the iloperidone dose should be returned to the previous level.

Fluoxetine: Coadministration of fluoxetine (20 mg twice daily for 21 days), a potent inhibitor of CYP2D6, with a single 3 mg dose of iloperidone to 23 healthy volunteers, ages 29-44 years, who were classified as CYP2D6 extensive metabolizers, increased the AUC of iloperidone and its metabolite P88, by about 2- to 3-fold, and decreased the AUC of its metabolite P95 by one-half. Iloperidone doses should be reduced by one-half when administered with fluoxetine. When fluoxetine is withdrawn from the combination therapy, the iloperidone dose should be returned to the previous level. Other strong inhibitors of CYP2D6 would be expected to have similar effects and would need appropriate dose reductions. When the CYP2D6 inhibitor is withdrawn from the combination therapy, iloperidone dose could then be increased to the previous level.

Paroxetine: Coadministration of paroxetine (20 mg/day for 5-8 days), a potent inhibitor of CYP2D6, with multiple doses of iloperidone (8 or 12 mg twice daily) to patients with schizophrenia ages 18-65 years resulted in increased mean steady-state peak concentrations of iloperidone and its metabolite P88, by about 1.6 fold, and decreased mean steady-state peak concentrations of its metabolite P95 by one-half. Iloperidone doses should be reduced by one-half when administered with paroxetine. When paroxetine is withdrawn from the combination therapy, the iloperidone dose should be returned to the previous level. Other strong inhibitors of CYP2D6 would be expected to have similar effects and would need appropriate dose reductions. When the CYP2D6 inhibitor is withdrawn from the combination therapy, iloperidone dose could then be increased to previous levels.

Paroxetine and Ketoconazole: Coadministration of paroxetine (20 mg once daily for 10 days), a CYP2D6 inhibitor, and ketoconazole (200 mg twice daily) with multiple doses of iloperidone (8 or 12 mg twice daily) to patients with schizophrenia ages 18-65 years resulted in a 1.4 fold increase in steady-state concentrations of iloperidone and its metabolite P88 and a 1.4 fold decrease in the P95 in the presence of paroxetine. So giving iloperidone with inhibitors of both of its metabolic pathways did not add to the effect of either inhibitor given alone. Iloperidone doses should therefore be reduced by about one-half if administered concomitantly with both a CYP2D6 and CYP3A4 inhibitor.

7.2 Potential for FANAPT to Affect Other Drugs

In vitro studies in human liver microsomes showed that iloperidone does not substantially inhibit the metabolism of drugs metabolized by the following cytochrome P450 isozymes: CYP1A1, CYP1A2, CYP2A6, CYP2B6, CYP2C8, CYP2C9, or CYP2E1. Furthermore, *in vitro* studies in human liver microsomes showed that iloperidone does not have enzyme inducing properties, specifically for the following cytochrome P450 isozymes: CYP1A2, CYP2C8, CYP2C9, CYP2C19, CYP3A4 and CYP3A5.

Dextromethorphan: A study in healthy volunteers showed that changes in the pharmacokinetics of dextromethorphan (80 mg dose) when a 3 mg dose of iloperidone was co-administered resulted in a 17% increase in total exposure and a 26% increase in the maximum plasma concentrations C_{max} of dextromethorphan. Thus, an interaction between iloperidone and other CYP2D6 substrates is unlikely.

Fluoxetine: A single 3 mg dose of iloperidone had no effect on the pharmacokinetics of fluoxetine (20 mg twice daily).

Midazolam (a sensitive CYP 3A4 substrate): A study in patients with schizophrenia showed a less than 50% increase in midazolam total exposure at iloperidone steady state (14 days of oral dosing at up to 10 mg iloperidone twice daily) and no effect on midazolam C_{max}. Thus, an interaction between iloperidone and other CYP3A4 substrates is unlikely.

7.3 Drugs that Prolong the QT Interval

FANAPT should not be used with any other drugs that prolong the QT interval *[see Warnings and Precautions (5.3)]*.

8 USE IN SPECIFIC POPULATIONS

8.1 Pregnancy

Pregnancy Exposure Registry

There is a pregnancy exposure registry that monitors pregnancy outcomes in women exposed to FANAPT during pregnancy. For more information contact the National Pregnancy Registry for Atypical Antipsychotics at 1-866-961-2388 or visit http://womensmentalhealth.org/clinical-and-research-programs/pregnancyregistry/.

Risk Summary

Neonates whose mothers are exposed to antipsychotic drugs, including FANAPT, during the third trimester of pregnancy are at risk for extrapyramidal and/or withdrawal symptoms following delivery *[see Clinical Considerations]*. The limited available data with FANAPT in pregnant women are not sufficient to inform a drug-associated risk for major birth defects and miscarriage. Iloperidone was not teratogenic when administered orally to pregnant rats during organogenesis at doses up to 26 times the maximum recommended human dose of 24 mg/day on mg/m2 basis. However, it prolonged the duration of pregnancy and parturition, increased still births, early intrauterine deaths, increased incidence of developmental delays, and decreased post-partum pup survival. Iloperidone was not teratogenic when administered orally to pregnant rabbits during organogenesis at doses up to 20-times the MRHD on mg/m2 basis. However, it increased early intrauterine deaths and decreased fetal viability at term at the highest dose which was also a maternally toxic dose *[see Data]*.

The background risk of major birth defects and miscarriage for the indicated population is unknown. In the U.S. general population, the estimated background risk of major birth defects and miscarriage in clinically recognized pregnancies is 2-4% and 15-20%, respectively.

Clinical Considerations

Fetal/Neonatal Adverse Reactions

Extrapyramidal and/or withdrawal symptoms, including agitation, hypertonia, hypotonia, tremor, somnolence, respiratory distress and feeding disorder have been reported in neonates whose mothers were exposed to antipsychotic drugs during the third trimester of pregnancy. These symptoms have varied in severity. Some neonates recovered within hours or days without specific treatment; others required prolonged hospitalization. Monitor neonates for extrapyramidal and/or withdrawal symptoms and manage symptoms appropriately.

Data

Animal Data

In an embryo-fetal development study, pregnant rats were given 4, 16, or 64 mg/kg/day (1.6, 6.5, and 26 times the maximum recommended human dose (MRHD) of 24 mg/day on a mg/m^2 basis) of iloperidone orally during the period of organogenesis. The highest dose caused increased early intrauterine deaths, decreased fetal weight and length, decreased fetal skeletal ossification, and an increased incidence of minor fetal skeletal anomalies and variations; this dose also caused decreased maternal food consumption and weight gain.

In an embryo-fetal development study, pregnant rabbits were given 4, 10, or 25 mg/kg/day (3, 8, and 20 times the MRHD on a mg/m^2 basis) of iloperidone during the period of organogenesis. The highest dose caused increased early intrauterine deaths and decreased fetal viability at term; this dose also caused maternal toxicity.

In additional studies in which rats were given iloperidone at doses similar to the above beginning from either pre-conception or from day 17 of gestation and continuing through weaning, adverse reproductive effects included prolonged pregnancy and parturition, increased stillbirth rates, increased incidence of fetal visceral variations, decreased fetal and pup weights, and decreased post-partum pup survival. There were no drug effects on the neurobehavioral or reproductive development of the surviving pups. No-effect doses ranged from 4 to 12 mg/kg except for the increase in stillbirth rates which occurred at the lowest dose tested of 4 mg/kg, which is 1.6 times the MRHD on a mg/m^2 basis. Maternal toxicity was seen at the higher doses in these studies.

The iloperidone metabolite P95, which is a major circulating metabolite of iloperidone in humans but is not present in significant amounts in rats, was given to pregnant rats during the period of organogenesis at oral doses of 20, 80, or 200 mg/kg/day. No teratogenic effects were seen. Delayed skeletal ossification occurred at all doses. No significant ma-

ternal toxicity was produced. Plasma levels of P95 (AUC) at the highest dose tested were 2 times those in humans receiving the MRHD of iloperidone.

8.2 Lactation

Risk Summary

There is no information regarding the presence of iloperidone or its metabolites in human milk, the effects of iloperidone on a breastfed child, nor the effects of iloperidone on human milk production. Iloperidone is present in rat milk *[see Data]*. Because of the potential for serious adverse reactions in breastfed infants, advise a woman not to breastfeed during treatment with FANAPT.

Data

The transfer of radioactivity into the milk of lactating rats was investigated following a single dose of [14C] iloperidone at 5 mg/kg. The concentration of radioactivity in milk at 4 hours post-dose was near 10-fold greater than that in plasma at the same time. However, by 24 hours after dosing, concentrations of radioactivity in milk had fallen to values slightly lower than plasma. The metabolic profile in milk was qualitatively similar to that in plasma.

8.4 Pediatric Use

Safety and effectiveness in pediatric and adolescent patients have not been established.

8.5 Geriatric Use

Clinical Studies of FANAPT in the treatment of schizophrenia did not include sufficient numbers of patients aged 65 years and over to determine whether or not they respond differently than younger adult patients. Of the 3210 patients treated with FANAPT in premarketing trials, 25 (0.5%) were ≥65 years old and there were no patients ≥75 years old.

Elderly patients with dementia-related psychosis treated with FANAPT are at an increased risk of death compared to placebo. FANAPT is not approved for the treatment of patients with dementia-related psychosis *[see Boxed Warning and Warnings and Precautions (5.1, 5.2)]*.

8.6 Renal Impairment

Because FANAPT is highly metabolized, with less than 1% of the drug excreted unchanged, renal impairment alone is unlikely to have a significant impact on the pharmacokinetics of FANAPT. Renal impairment (creatinine clearance <30 mL/min) had minimal effect on C_{max} of iloperidone (given in a single dose of 3 mg) and its metabolites P88 and P95 in any of the 3 analytes measured. $AUC_{0-\infty}$ was increased by 24%, decreased by 6%, and increased by 52% for iloperidone, P88 and P95, respectively, in subjects with renal impairment.

8.7 Hepatic Impairment

No dose adjustment to FANAPT is needed in patients with mild hepatic impairment. Patients with moderate hepatic impairment may require dose reduction. FANAPT is not recommended for patients with severe hepatic impairment *[see Dosage and Administration (2.2)]*.

In adult subjects with mild hepatic impairment no relevant difference in pharmacokinetics of iloperidone, P88 or P95 (total or unbound) was observed compared to healthy adult controls. In subjects with moderate hepatic impairment a higher (2-fold) and more variable free exposure to the active metabolites P88 was observed compared to healthy controls, whereas exposure to iloperidone and P95 was generally similar (less than 50% change compared to control). Since a study in severe liver impaired subjects has not been conducted, FANAPT is not recommended for patients with severe hepatic impairment.

8.8 Smoking Status

Based on *in vitro* studies utilizing human liver enzymes, FANAPT is not a substrate for CYP1A2; smoking should therefore not have an effect on the pharmacokinetics of FANAPT.

9 DRUG ABUSE AND DEPENDENCE

9.1 Controlled Substance

FANAPT is not a controlled substance.

9.2 Abuse

FANAPT has not been systematically studied in animals or humans for its potential for abuse, tolerance, or physical dependence. While the clinical trials did not reveal any tendency for drug-seeking behavior, these observations were not systematic and it is not possible to predict on the basis of this experience the extent to which a CNS active drug, FANAPT, will be misused, diverted, and/or abused once marketed. Consequently, patients should be evaluated carefully for a history of drug abuse, and such patients should

Continued on next page

be observed closely for signs of FANAPT misuse or abuse (e.g. development of tolerance, increases in dose, drug-seeking behavior).

10 OVERDOSAGE

10.1 Human Experience

In pre-marketing trials involving over 3210 patients, accidental or intentional overdose of FANAPT was documented in 8 patients ranging from 48 mg to 576 mg taken at once and 292 mg taken over a 3-day period. No fatalities were reported from these cases. The largest confirmed single ingestion of FANAPT was 576 mg; no adverse physical effects were noted for this patient. The next largest confirmed ingestion of FANAPT was 438 mg over a 4-day period; extrapyramidal symptoms and a QTc interval of 507 msec were reported for this patient with no cardiac sequelae. This patient resumed FANAPT treatment for an additional 11 months. In general, reported signs and symptoms were those resulting from an exaggeration of the known pharmacological effects (e.g., drowsiness and sedation, tachycardia and hypotension) of FANAPT.

10.2 Management of Overdose

There is no specific antidote for FANAPT. Therefore appropriate supportive measures should be instituted. In case of acute overdose, the physician should establish and maintain an airway and ensure adequate oxygenation and ventilation. Gastric lavage (after intubation, if patient is unconscious) and administration of activated charcoal together with a laxative should be considered. The possibility of obtundation, seizures or dystonic reaction of the head and neck following overdose may create a risk of aspiration with induced emesis. Cardiovascular monitoring should commence immediately and should include continuous ECG monitoring to detect possible arrhythmias. If antiarrhythmic therapy is administered, disopyramide, procainamide and quinidine should not be used, as they have the potential for QT-prolonging effects that might be additive to those of FANAPT. Similarly, it is reasonable to expect that the alpha-blocking properties of bretylium might be additive to those of FANAPT, resulting in problematic hypotension. Hypotension and circulatory collapse should be treated with appropriate measures such as intravenous fluids or sympathomimetic agents (epinephrine and dopamine should not be used, since beta stimulation may worsen hypotension in the setting of FANAPT-induced alpha blockade). In cases of severe extrapyramidal symptoms, anticholinergic medication should be administered. Close medical supervision should continue until the patient recovers.

11 DESCRIPTION

FANAPT is an atypical antipsychotic belonging to the chemical class of piperidinyl-benzisoxazole derivatives. Its chemical name is 4'-[3-[4-(6-Fluoro-1,2-benzisoxazol-3-yl)piperidino]propoxy]-3'-methoxyacetophenone. Its molecular formula is $C_{24}H_{27}FN_2O_4$ and its molecular weight is 426.48. The structural formula is:

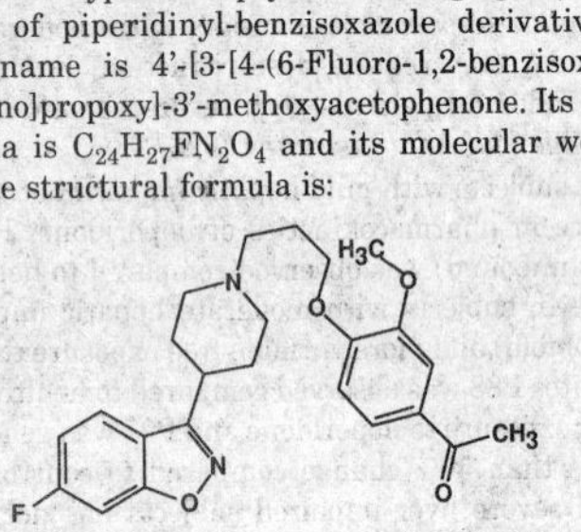

Iloperidone is a white to off-white finely crystalline powder. It is practically insoluble in water, very slightly soluble in 0.1 N HCl and freely soluble in chloroform, ethanol, methanol, and acetonitrile.

FANAPT tablets are intended for oral administration only. Each round, uncoated tablet contains 1 mg, 2 mg, 4 mg, 6 mg, 8 mg, 10 mg, or 12 mg of iloperidone. Inactive ingredients are: lactose monohydrate, microcrystalline cellulose, hydroxypropylmethylcellulose, crospovidone, magnesium stearate, colloidal silicon dioxide, and purified water (removed during processing). The tablets are white, round, flat, beveled-edged and identified with a logo " " debossed on one side and tablet strength "1", "2", "4", "6", "8", "10", or "12" debossed on the other side.

12 CLINICAL PHARMACOLOGY

12.1 Mechanism of Action

The mechanism of action of iloperidone in schizophrenia is unknown. However the efficacy of iloperidone could be mediated through a combination of dopamine type 2 (D_2) and serotonin type 2 ($5\text{-}HT_2$) antagonism.

Iloperidone forms an active metabolite, P88, that has an in vitro receptor binding profile similar to the parent drug.

12.2 Pharmacodynamics

Iloperidone acts as an antagonist with high (nM) affinity binding to serotonin $5\text{-}HT_{2A}$ dopamine D_2 and D_3 receptors, and norepinephrine $NE\alpha1$ receptors (K_i values of 5.6, 6.3, 7.1, and 0.36 nM, respectively). Iloperidone has moderate affinity for dopamine D_4, and serotonin $5\text{-}HT_6$ and $5\text{-}HT_7$ receptors (K_i values of 25, 43, and 22, nM respectively), and low affinity for the serotonin $5\text{-}HT_{1A}$, dopamine D_1, and histamine H_1 receptors (K_i values of 168, 216 and 437 nM, respectively). Iloperidone has no appreciable affinity (K_i>1000 nM) for cholinergic muscarinic receptors. The affinity of iloperidone metabolite P88 is generally equal to or less than that of the parent compound, while the metabolite P95 only shows affinity for $5\text{-}HT_{2A}$ (K_i value of 3.91) and the $NE_{\alpha1A}$, $NE_{\alpha1B}$, $NE_{\alpha1D}$, and $NE_{\alpha2C}$ receptors (K_i values of 4.7, 2.7, 8.8 and 4.7 nM respectively).

12.3 Pharmacokinetics

The observed mean elimination half-lives for iloperidone, P88 and P95 in CYP2D6 extensive metabolizers (EM) are 18, 26, and 23 hours, respectively, and in poor metabolizers (PM) are 33, 37 and 31 hours, respectively. Steady-state concentrations are attained within 3 -4 days of dosing. Iloperidone accumulation is predictable from single-dose pharmacokinetics. The pharmacokinetics of iloperidone is more than dose proportional. Elimination of iloperidone is mainly through hepatic metabolism involving 2 P450 isozymes, CYP2D6 and CYP3A4.

Absorption: Iloperidone is well absorbed after administration of the tablet with peak plasma concentrations occurring within 2 to 4 hours; while the relative bioavailability of the tablet formulation compared to oral solution is 96%. Administration of iloperidone with a standard high-fat meal did not significantly affect the C_{max} or AUC of iloperidone, P88, or P95, but delayed T_{max} by 1 hour for iloperidone, 2 hours for P88 and 6 hours for P95. FANAPT can be administered without regard to meals.

Distribution: Iloperidone has an apparent clearance (clearance / bioavailability) of 47 to 102 L/h, with an apparent volume of distribution of 1340-2800 L. At therapeutic concentrations, the unbound fraction of iloperidone in plasma is ~3% and of each metabolite (P88 and P95) it is ~8%.

Metabolism and Elimination: Iloperidone is metabolized primarily by 3 biotransformation pathways: carbonyl reduction, hydroxylation (mediated by CYP2D6) and *O*-demethylation (mediated by CYP3A4). There are 2 predominant iloperidone metabolites, P95 and P88. The iloperidone metabolite P95 represents 47.9% of the AUC of iloperidone and its metabolites in plasma at steady-state for extensive metabolizers (EM) and 25% for poor metabolizers (PM). The active metabolite P88 accounts for 19.5% and 34.0% of total plasma exposure in EM and PM, respectively. Approximately 7% - 10% of Caucasians and 3% - 8% of black/African Americans lack the capacity to metabolize CYP2D6 substrates and are classified as poor metabolizers (PM), whereas the rest are intermediate, extensive or ultrarapid metabolizers. Coadministration of FANAPT with known strong inhibitors of CYP2D6 like fluoxetine results in a 2.3- fold increase in iloperidone plasma exposure, and therefore one-half of the FANAPT dose should be administered.

Similarly, PMs of CYP2D6 have higher exposure to iloperidone compared with EMs and PMs should have their dose reduced by one-half. Laboratory tests are available to identify CYP2D6 PMs.

The bulk of the radioactive materials were recovered in the urine (mean 58.2% and 45.1% in EM and PM, respectively), with feces accounting for 19.9% (EM) to 22.1% (PM) of the dosed radioactivity.

Transporter Interaction: Iloperidone and P88 are not substrates of P-gp and iloperidone is a weak P-gp inhibitor.

13 NONCLINICAL TOXICOLOGY

13.1 Carcinogenesis, Mutagenesis, Impairment of Fertility

Carcinogenesis: Lifetime carcinogenicity studies were conducted in CD-1 mice and Sprague Dawley rats. Iloperidone was administered orally at doses of 2.5, 5.0 and 10 mg/kg/day to CD-1 mice and 4, 8, and 16 mg/kg/day to Sprague Dawley rats (0.5, 1.0 and 2.0 times and 1.6, 3.2 and 6.5 times, respectively, the MRHD of 24 mg/day on a mg/m² basis). There was an increased incidence of malignant mammary gland tumors in female mice treated with the lowest dose (2.5 mg/kg/day) only. There were no treatment-related increases in neoplasia in rats.

The carcinogenic potential of the iloperidone metabolite P95, which is a major circulating metabolite of iloperidone in humans but is not present at significant amounts in mice or rats, was assessed in a lifetime carcinogenicity study in Wistar rats at oral doses of 25, 75 and 200 mg/kg/day in males and 50, 150, and 250 (reduced from 400) mg/kg/day in females.

Drug-related neoplastic changes occurred in males, in the pituitary gland (pars distalis adenoma) at all doses and in the pancreas (islet cell adenoma) at the high dose. Plasma levels of P95 (AUC) in males at the tested doses (25, 75, and 200 mg/kg/day) were approximately 0.4, 3, and 23 times, respectively, the human exposure to P95 at the MRHD of iloperidone.

Mutagenesis: Iloperidone was negative in the Ames test and in the *in vivo* mouse bone marrow and rat liver micronucleus tests. Iloperidone induced chromosomal aberrations in Chinese Hamster Ovary (CHO) cells *in vitro* at concentrations which also caused some cytotoxicity.

The iloperidone metabolite P95 was negative in the Ames test, the V79 chromosome aberration test, and an *in vivo* mouse bone marrow micronucleus test.

Impairment of Fertility: Iloperidone decreased fertility at 12 and 36 mg/kg in a study in which both male and female rats were treated. The no-effect dose was 4 mg/kg, which is 1.6 times the MRHD of 24 mg/day on a mg/m² basis.

14 CLINICAL STUDIES

The efficacy of FANAPT in the treatment of schizophrenia was supported by 2 placebo- and active-controlled short-term (4- and 6-week) trials and one long-term placebo-controlled randomized withdrawal trial. All trials enrolled patients who met the DSM-III/IV criteria for schizophrenia.

Three instruments were used for assessing psychiatric signs and symptoms in these studies. The Positive and Negative Syndrome Scale (PANSS) and Brief Psychiatric Rating Scale (BPRS) are both multi-item inventories of general psychopathology usually used to evaluate the effects of drug treatment in schizophrenia. The Clinical Global Impression (CGI) assessment reflects the impression of a skilled observer, fully familiar with the manifestations of schizophrenia, about the overall clinical state of the patient.

A 6-week, placebo-controlled trial (n=706) involved 2 flexible dose ranges of FANAPT (12-16 mg/day or 20- 24 mg/day) compared to placebo and an active control (risperidone). For the 12-16 mg/day group, the titration schedule of FANAPT was 1 mg twice daily on Days 1 and 2, 2 mg twice daily on Days 3 and 4, 4 mg twice daily on Days 5 and 6, and 6 mg twice daily on Day 7. For the 20-24 mg/day group, the titration schedule of FANAPT was 1 mg twice daily on Day 1, 2 mg twice daily on Day 2, 4 mg twice daily on Day 3, 6 mg twice daily on Days 4 and 5, 8 mg twice daily on Day 6, and 10 mg twice daily on Day 7. The primary endpoint was change from baseline on the BPRS total score at the end of treatment (Day 42). Both the 12-16 mg/day and the 20-24 mg/day dose ranges of FANAPT were superior to placebo on the BPRS total score. The active control antipsychotic drug appeared to be superior to FANAPT in this trial within the first 2 weeks, a finding that may in part be explained by the more rapid titration that was possible for that drug. In patients in this study who remained on treatment for at least 2 weeks, iloperidone appeared to have had comparable efficacy to the active control.

A 4-week, placebo-controlled trial (n=604) involved one fixed dose of FANAPT (24 mg/day) compared to placebo and an active control (ziprasidone). The titration schedule for this study was similar to that for the 6-week study. This study involved titration of FANAPT starting at 1 mg twice daily on Day 1 and increasing to 2, 4, 6, 8, 10 and 12 mg twice daily on Days 2, 3, 4, 5, 6, and 7. The primary endpoint was change from baseline on the PANSS total score at the end of treatment (Day 28). The 24 mg/day FANAPT dose was superior to placebo in the PANSS total score. FANAPT appeared to have similar efficacy to the active control drug which also needed a slow titration to the target dose.

In a longer-term trial, clinically stable adult outpatients (n=303) meeting DSM-IV criteria for schizophrenia who remained stable following 12 weeks of open-label treatment with flexible doses of FANAPT (8 mg/day – 24 mg/day administered as twice daily doses) were randomized to placebo or to continue on their current FANAPT dose (8 mg/day – 24 mg/day administered as twice daily doses) for observation for possible relapse during the double-blind relapse prevention phase. Stabilization during the open-label phase was defined as being on an established dose of FANAPT that was unchanged due to efficacy in the 4 weeks prior to randomization, having CGI-Severity score of ≤4 and PANSS total score ≤70, a score of ≤4 on each of the following individual PANSS items (P1-delusions, P2-conceptual disorganization, P3-hallucinatory behavior, P6-suspiciousness/persecution, P7-hostility, or G8-uncooperativeness), and no hospitalization or increase in level of care to treat exacerbations. Relapse or impending relapse during the double-blind relapse prevention phase was defined as any of the following: hospitalization due to worsening of schizophrenia, increase (worsening) of the PANSS total score ≥30%, CGI-Improvement score ≥6, patient had suicidal, homicidal, or aggressive behavior, or need for any other antipsychotic medication.

Figure 1: Kaplan Meier Estimation of Percent Relapse/Impending Relapse for iloperidone (Ilo) and placebo (Pbo)

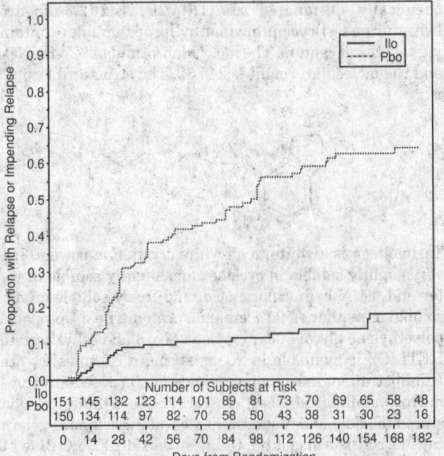

Package Configuration	Tablet Strength (mg)	NDC Code
Bottles of 60	1 mg	43068-101-02
Bottles of 60	2 mg	43068-102-02
Bottles of 60	4 mg	43068-104-02
Bottles of 60	6 mg	43068-106-02
Bottles of 60	8 mg	43068-108-02
Bottles of 60	10 mg	43068-110-02
Bottles of 60	12 mg	43068-112-02
Titration Pack	2×1 mg, 2×2 mg, 2×4 mg, 2×6 mg (Total of 8 tablets)	43068-113-04

Based on the interim analysis, an independent data monitoring committee decided the study should be discontinued early due to evidence of efficacy. Based on results from the interim analysis, which were confirmed by the final analysis dataset, patients treated with FANAPT experienced a statistically significant longer time to relapse or impending relapse than patients who received placebo. Figure 1 displays the estimated cumulative proportion of patients with relapse or impending relapse based on the final data set.

16 HOW SUPPLIED/STORAGE AND HANDLING

FANAPT tablets are white, round and identified with a logo " ⬡ " debossed on one side and tablet strength "1", "2", "4", "6", "8", "10", or "12" debossed on the other side. Tablets are supplied in the following strengths and package configurations:
[See table above]

Storage
Store FANAPT tablets at controlled room temperature, 25°C (77°F); excursions permitted to 15°to 30 °C (59° to 86°F) [See USP Controlled Room Temperature]. Protect FANAPT tablets from exposure to light and moisture.

17 PATIENT COUNSELING INFORMATION

Physicians are advised to discuss the following issues with patients for whom they prescribe FANAPT:

QT Interval Prolongation
Patients should be advised to consult their physician immediately if they feel faint, lose consciousness or have heart palpitations. Patients should be counseled not to take FANAPT with other drugs that cause QT interval prolongation [see Warnings and Precautions (5.3)]. Patients should be told to inform physicians that they are taking FANAPT before any new drug is taken.

Neuroleptic Malignant Syndrome
Patients and caregivers should be counseled that a potentially fatal symptom complex sometimes referred to as NMS has been reported in association with administration of antipsychotic drugs, including FANAPT. Signs and symptoms of NMS include hyperpyrexia, muscle rigidity, altered mental status, and evidence of autonomic instability (irregular pulse or blood pressure, tachycardia, diaphoresis, and cardiac dysrhythmia) [see Warnings and Precautions (5.4)].

Metabolic Changes

Patients should be aware of the symptoms of hyperglycemia (high blood sugar) and diabetes mellitus. Patients who are diagnosed with diabetes, those with risk factors for diabetes, or those who develop these symptoms during treatment should have their blood glucose monitored at the beginning of and periodically during treatment. Patients should be counseled that weight gain has occurred during treatment with FANAPT. Clinical monitoring of weight is recommended. [see Warnings and Precautions (5.6)].

Orthostatic Hypotension
Patients should be advised of the risk of orthostatic hypotension, particularly at the time of initiating treatment, reinitiating treatment, or increasing the dose [see Warnings and Precautions (5.8)].

Interference with Cognitive and Motor Performance
Because FANAPT may have the potential to impair judgment, thinking, or motor skills, patients should be cautioned about operating hazardous machinery, including automobiles, until they are reasonably certain that FANAPT therapy does not affect them adversely [see Warnings and Precautions (5.15)].

Pregnancy
Advise patients that third trimester use of Fanapt may cause extrapyramidal and/or withdrawal symptoms in a neonate. Advise patients to notify their healthcare provider with known or suspected pregnancy [see Use in Specific Populations (8.1)].

Pregnancy Registry
Advise patients that there is a pregnancy exposure registry that monitors pregnancy outcomes in women exposed to FANAPT during pregnancy [see Use in Specific Populations (8.1)].

Lactation
Advise women not to breastfeed during treatment with FANAPT [see Use in Specific Populations (8.2)].

Concomitant Medication
Patients should be advised to inform their physicians if they are taking, or plan to take, any prescription or over-the-counter drugs, since there is a potential for interactions [see Drug Interactions (7)].

Alcohol
Patients should be advised to avoid alcohol while taking FANAPT.

Heat Exposure and Dehydration
Patients should be advised regarding appropriate care in avoiding overheating and dehydration.

Distributed by:
Vanda Pharmaceuticals Inc.
Washington, D.C. 20037 USA
Vanda and Fanapt® are registered trademarks of Vanda Pharmaceuticals Inc. in the United States and other countries.
May 2016

Shown in Product Identification Guide, page 511

HETLIOZ®
(tasimelteon)
capsules, for oral use   ℞

HIGHLIGHTS OF PRESCRIBING INFORMATION
These highlights do not include all the information needed to use HETLIOZ safely and effectively. See full prescribing information for HETLIOZ.
HETLIOZ® (tasimelteon) capsules, for oral use
Initial U.S. Approval: 2014

INDICATIONS AND USAGE
HETLIOZ is a melatonin receptor agonist indicated for the treatment of Non-24-Hour Sleep-Wake Disorder (Non-24) (1)

DOSAGE AND ADMINISTRATION
• 20 mg prior to bedtime, at same time every night (2)
• Take without food (2)

DOSAGE FORMS AND STRENGTHS
Capsules: 20 mg (3)

CONTRAINDICATIONS
None (4)

WARNINGS AND PRECAUTIONS
May cause somnolence: After taking HETLIOZ, patients should limit their activity to preparing for going to bed, because HETLIOZ can impair the performance of activities requiring complete mental alertness (5.1)

ADVERSE REACTIONS
The most common adverse reactions (incidence >5% and at least twice as high on HETLIOZ than on placebo) were headache, increased alanine aminotransferase, nightmares or unusual dreams, and upper respiratory or urinary tract infection (6.1)
To report SUSPECTED ADVERSE REACTIONS, contact Vanda Pharmaceuticals Inc. at 1-844-438-5469 or www.hetlioz.com or FDA at 1-800-FDA-1088 or *www.fda.gov/medwatch*.

DRUG INTERACTIONS
• Strong CYP1A2 inhibitors (e.g., fluvoxamine): Avoid use of HETLIOZ in combination with strong CYP1A2 inhibitors because of increased exposure (7.1, 12.3)
• Strong CYP3A4 inducers (e.g., rifampin): Avoid use of HETLIOZ in combination with rifampin or other CYP3A4 inducers, because of decreased exposure (7.2, 12.3)

USE IN SPECIFIC POPULATIONS
• Pregnancy: Based on animal data, may cause fetal harm (8.1)
• Hepatic impairment: HETLIOZ has not been studied in patients with severe hepatic impairment and is not recommended in these patients (8.6)
See 17 for PATIENT COUNSELING INFORMATION.

Revised: 12/2014

FULL PRESCRIBING INFORMATION: CONTENTS*

Continued on next page

FULL PRESCRIBING INFORMATION

1.   INDICATIONS AND USAGE

HETLIOZ is indicated for the treatment of Non-24-Hour Sleep-Wake Disorder (Non-24).

2.   DOSAGE AND ADMINISTRATION

The recommended dosage of HETLIOZ is 20 mg per day taken before bedtime, at the same time every night. Because of individual differences in circadian rhythms, drug effect may not occur for weeks or months.
HETLIOZ should be taken without food [see Clinical Pharmacology (12.3)].

3.   DOSAGE FORMS AND STRENGTHS

Capsules: 20 mg size 1 dark blue opaque, hard gelatin capsules printed with "VANDA 20 mg" in white.

4.   CONTRAINDICATIONS

None.

5.   WARNINGS AND PRECAUTIONS

5.1   Somnolence
After taking HETLIOZ, patients should limit their activity to preparing for going to bed. HETLIOZ can potentially impair the performance of activities requiring complete mental alertness.

6.   ADVERSE REACTIONS

6.1   Clinical Trials Experience
Because clinical trials are conducted under widely varying conditions, adverse reaction rates observed in the clinical trials of a drug cannot be directly compared to rates in the clinical trials of another drug and may not reflect the rates observed in clinical practice.
A total of 1346 subjects were treated with at least one dose of HETLIOZ, of which 139 were treated for > 26 weeks and 93 were treated for > 1 year.
A 26-week, parallel-arm placebo-controlled study (Study 1) evaluated HETLIOZ (n=42) compared to placebo (n=42) in patients with Non-24. A randomized-withdrawal, placebo-controlled study of 8 weeks duration (Study 2) also evaluated HETLIOZ (n=10), compared to placebo (n=10), in patients with Non-24.
In placebo-controlled studies, 6% of patients exposed to HETLIOZ discontinued treatment due to an adverse event, compared with 4% of patients who received placebo.
Table 1 shows the incidence of adverse reactions from Study 1.

Table 1: Adverse Reactions in Study 1

	HETLIOZ N=42	Placebo N=42
Headache	17 %	7 %
Alanine aminotransferase increased	10 %	5 %
Nightmare/abnormal dreams	10 %	0 %
Upper respiratory tract infection	7 %	0 %
Urinary tract infection	7 %	2 %

*Adverse reactions with an incidence > 5% and at least twice as high on HETLIOZ than on placebo are displayed.

7.   DRUG INTERACTIONS

7.1   Strong CYP1A2 Inhibitors (e.g., fluvoxamine)
Avoid use of HETLIOZ in combination with fluvoxamine or other strong CYP1A2 inhibitors because of a potentially large increase in tasimelteon exposure and greater risk of adverse reactions [see Clinical Pharmacology (12.3)].

7.2   Strong CYP3A4 Inducers (e.g., rifampin)
Avoid use of HETLIOZ in combination with rifampin or other CYP3A4 inducers because of a potentially large decrease in tasimelteon exposure with reduced efficacy [see Clinical Pharmacology (12.3)].

8.   USE IN SPECIFIC POPULATIONS

8.1   Pregnancy
Pregnancy Category C
There are no adequate and well-controlled studies of HETLIOZ in pregnant women. In animal studies, administration of tasimelteon during pregnancy resulted in developmental toxicity (embryofetal mortality, neurobehavioral impairment, and decreased growth and development in offspring) at doses greater than those used clinically. HETLIOZ should be used during pregnancy only if the potential benefit justifies the potential risks.
In pregnant rats administered tasimelteon at oral doses of 5, 50, or 500 mg/kg/day during the period of organogenesis, there were no effects on embryofetal development. The highest dose tested is approximately 240 times the recommended human dose (RHD) of 20 mg/day, on a mg/m^2 basis. In pregnant rabbits administered tasimelteon at oral doses of 5, 30, or 200 mg/kg/day during the period of organogenesis, embryolethality and embryofetal toxicity (reduced fetal body weight and delayed ossification) were observed at the highest dose tested. The highest dose not associated with adverse effects (30 mg/kg/day) is approximately 30 times the RHD on a mg/m^2 basis.
Oral administration of tasimelteon (50, 150, or 450 mg/kg/day) to rats throughout organogenesis and lactation resulted in persistent reductions in body weight, delayed sexual maturation and physical development, and neurobehavioral impairment in offspring at the highest dose tested. Reduced body weight in offspring was also observed at the mid-dose. The no effect dose (50 mg/kg/day) is approximately 25 times the RHD on a mg/m^2 basis.

8.3   Nursing Mothers
It is not known whether this drug is excreted in human milk. Because many drugs are excreted in human milk, caution should be exercised when HETLIOZ is administered to a nursing woman.

8.4   Pediatric Use
Safety and effectiveness in pediatric patients have not been established.

8.5   Geriatric Use
The risk of adverse reactions may be greater in elderly (>65 years) patients than younger patients because exposure to tasimelteon is increased by approximately 2-fold compared with younger patients.

8.6   Hepatic Impairment
Dose adjustment is not necessary in patients with mild or moderate hepatic impairment. HETLIOZ has not been studied in patients with severe hepatic impairment (Child-Pugh Class C). Therefore, HETLIOZ is not recommended for use in patients with severe hepatic impairment [see Clinical Pharmacology (12.3)].

8.7   Smokers
Smoking causes induction of CYP1A2 levels. The exposure of tasimelteon in smokers was lower than in non-smokers and therefore the efficacy of HETLIOZ may be reduced in smokers [see Clinical pharmacology (12.3)].

9.   DRUG ABUSE AND DEPENDENCE

9.1   Controlled Substance
Tasimelteon is not a controlled substance under the Controlled Substances Act.

9.2   Abuse
Tasimelteon did not produce any abuse-related signals in animal behavioral studies. Rats did not self-administer tasimelteon, suggesting that the drug does not have rewarding properties. There were also no signs or symptoms indicative of abuse potential in clinical studies with HETLIOZ.

9.3   Dependence
Discontinuation of HETLIOZ in humans following chronic administration did not produce withdrawal signs. HETLIOZ does not appear to produce physical dependence.

10.   OVERDOSAGE

There is limited premarketing clinical experience with the effects of an overdosage of HETLIOZ.

As with the management of any overdose, general symptomatic and supportive measures should be used, along with immediate gastric lavage where appropriate. Intravenous fluids should be administered as needed. Respiration, pulse, blood pressure, and other appropriate vital signs should be monitored, and general supportive measures employed.
While hemodialysis was effective at clearing HETLIOZ and the majority of its major metabolites in patients with renal impairment, it is not known if hemodialysis will effectively reduce exposure in the case of overdose.
As with the management of any overdose, the possibility of multiple drug ingestion should be considered. Contact a poison control center for current information on the management of overdose.

11.   DESCRIPTION

HETLIOZ (tasimelteon) is a melatonin receptor agonist, chemically designated as (1R, 2R)-N-[2-(2,3-dihydrobenzofuran-4-yl)cyclopropylmethyl]propanamide, containing two chiral centers. The molecular formula is $C_{15}H_{19}NO_2$, and the molecular weight is 245.32. The structural formula is:

Tasimelteon is a white to off-white crystalline powder. It is very slightly soluble in cyclohexane, slightly soluble in water and 0.1 N hydrochloric acid, and freely soluble or very soluble in methanol, 95% ethanol, acetonitrile, isopropanol, polyethylene glycol 300, propylene glycol and ethyl acetate. HETLIOZ is available in 20 mg strength capsules for oral administration. Inactive ingredients are: lactose anhydrous, microcrystalline cellulose, croscarmellose sodium, colloidal silicon dioxide, and magnesium stearate. Each hard gelatin capsule consists of gelatin, titanium dioxide, FD&C Blue #1, FD&C Red #3, and FD&C Yellow #6.

12.   CLINICAL PHARMACOLOGY

12.1   Mechanism of Action
The precise mechanism by which tasimelteon exerts its therapeutic effect in patients with Non-24 is not known. Tasimelteon is an agonist at melatonin MT$_1$ and MT$_2$ receptors. These receptors are thought to be involved in the control of circadian rhythms.

12.2   Pharmacodynamics
HETLIOZ is an agonist at MT$_1$ and MT$_2$ receptors. HETLIOZ exhibits a greater affinity for the MT$_2$ as compared to the MT$_1$ receptor. The most abundant metabolites of HETLIOZ have less than one-tenth of the binding affinity of the parent molecule for both the MT$_1$ and MT$_2$ receptors.

12.3   Pharmacokinetics
The pharmacokinetics of HETLIOZ is linear over doses ranging from 3 to 300 mg (0.15 to 15 times the recommended daily dosage). The pharmacokinetics of HETLIOZ and its metabolites did not change with repeated daily dosing.

Absorption
The absolute oral bioavailability is 38.3%. The peak concentration (T$_{max}$) of tasimelteon occurred approximately 0.5 to 3 hours after fasted oral administration.
When administered with a high-fat meal, the C$_{max}$ of tasimelteon was 44% lower than when given in a fasted state, and the median T$_{max}$ was delayed by approximately 1.75 hours. Therefore, HETLIOZ should be taken without food.

Distribution
The apparent oral volume of distribution of tasimelteon at steady state in young healthy subjects is approximately 59 - 126 L. At therapeutic concentrations, tasimelteon is about 90% bound to proteins.

Metabolism
Tasimelteon is extensively metabolized. Metabolism of tasimelteon consists primarily of oxidation at multiple sites and oxidative dealkylation resulting in opening of the dihydrofuran ring followed by further oxidation to give a carboxylic acid. CYP1A2 and CYP3A4 are the major isozymes involved in the metabolism of tasimelteon.
Phenolic glucuronidation is the major phase II metabolic route.
Major metabolites had 13-fold or less activity at melatonin receptors compared to tasimelteon.

Elimination

Following oral administration of radiolabeled tasimelteon, 80% of total radioactivity was excreted in urine and approximately 4% in feces, resulting in a mean recovery of 84%. Less than 1% of the dose was excreted in urine as the parent compound.

The observed mean elimination half-life for tasimelteon is 1.3 ± 0.4 hours. The mean terminal elimination half-life ± standard deviation of the main metabolites ranges from 1.3 ± 0.5 to 3.7 ± 2.2.

Repeated once daily dosing with HETLIOZ does not result in changes in pharmacokinetic parameters or significant accumulation of tasimelteon.

Studies in Specific Populations

Elderly

In elderly subjects, tasimelteon exposure increased by approximately two-fold compared with non-elderly adults.

Gender

The mean overall exposure of tasimelteon was approximately 20-30% greater in female than in male subjects.

Race

The effect of race on exposure of HETLIOZ was not evaluated.

Hepatic Impairment

The pharmacokinetic profile of a 20 mg dose of HETLIOZ was compared among eight subjects with mild hepatic impairment (Child-Pugh Score ≥5 and ≤6 points), eight subjects with moderate hepatic impairment (Child-Pugh Score ≥7 and ≤9 points), and 13 healthy matched controls. Tasimelteon exposure was increased less than two-fold in subjects with moderate hepatic impairment. Therefore, no dose adjustment is needed in patients with mild or moderate hepatic impairment. HETLIOZ has not been studied in patients with severe hepatic impairment (Child-Pugh Class C) and is not recommended in these patients.

Renal Impairment

The pharmacokinetic profile of a 20 mg dose of HETLIOZ was compared among eight subjects with severe renal impairment (estimated glomerular filtration rate [eGFR] ≤ 29 mL/min/$1.73m^2$), eight subjects with end-stage renal disease (ESRD) (GFR < 15 mL/min/$1.73m^2$) requiring hemodialysis, and sixteen healthy matched controls. There was no apparent relationship between tasimelteon CL/F and renal function, as measured by either estimated creatinine clearance or eGFR. Subjects with severe renal impairment had a 30% lower clearance, and clearance in subjects with ESRD was comparable to that of healthy subjects. No dose adjustment is necessary for patients with renal impairment.

Smokers (smoking is a moderate CYP1A2 inducer)

Tasimelteon exposure decreased by approximately 40% in smokers, compared to non- smokers *[see Use in Specific Populations (8.7)]*.

Drug Interaction Studies

No potential drug interactions were identified in *in vitro* studies with CYP inducers or inhibitors of CYP1A1, CYP1A2, CYP2B6, CYP2C9/2C19, CYP2E1, CYP2D6 and transporters including P-glycoprotein, OATP1B1, OATP1B3, OCT2, OAT1 and OAT3.

Effect of Other Drugs on HETLIOZ

Drugs that inhibit CYP1A2 and CYP3A4 are expected to alter the metabolism of tasimelteon.

Fluvoxamine (strong CYP1A2 inhibitor): the AUC_{0-inf} and C_{max} of tasimelteon increased by 7-fold and 2-fold, respectively, when co-administered with fluvoxamine 50 mg (after 6 days of fluvoxamine 50 mg per day) *[see Drug Interactions (7.1)]*.

Ketoconazole (strong CYP3A4 inhibitor): tasimelteon exposure increased by approximately 50% when co-administered with ketoconazole 400 mg (after 5 days of ketoconazole 400 mg per day) *[see Drug Interactions (7.2)]*.

Rifampin (strong CYP3A4 and moderate CYP2C19 inducer): the exposure of tasimelteon decreased by approximately 90% when co-administered with rifampin 600 mg (after 11 days of rifampin 600 mg per day). Efficacy may be reduced when HETLIOZ is used in combination with strong CYP3A4 inducers, such as rifampin *[see Drug Interactions (7.2)]*.

Effect of HETLIOZ on Other Drugs

Midazolam (CYP3A4 substrate): Administration of HETLIOZ 20 mg once a day for 14 days did not produce any significant changes in the T_{max}, C_{max}, or AUC of midazolam or 1-OH midazolam. This indicates there is no induction of CYP3A4 by tasimelteon at this dose.

Rosiglitazone (CYP2C8 substrate): Administration of HETLIOZ 20 mg once a day for 16 days did not produce any clinically significant changes in the T_{max}, C_{max}, or AUC of rosiglitazone after oral administration of 4 mg. This indicates that there is no induction of CYP2C8 by tasimelteon at this dose.

Effect of Alcohol on HETLIOZ

In a study of 28 healthy volunteers, a single dose of ethanol (0.6 g/kg for women and 0.7 g/kg for men) was co-administered with a 20 mg dose of HETLIOZ. There was a trend for an additive effect of HETLIOZ and ethanol on some psychomotor tests.

13. NONCLINICAL TOXICOLOGY

13.1 Carcinogenesis, Mutagenesis, Impairment of Fertility

Carcinogenesis

Tasimelteon was administered orally for up to two years to mice (30, 100, and 300 mg/kg/day) and rats (20, 100, and 250 mg/kg/day). No evidence of carcinogenic potential was observed in mice; the highest dose tested is approximately 75 times the recommended human dose (RHD) of 20 mg/day, on a mg/m^2 basis. In rats, the incidence of liver tumors was increased in males (adenoma and carcinoma) and females (adenoma) at 100 and 250 mg/kg/day; the incidence of tumors of the uterus (endometrial adenocarcinoma) and uterus and cervix (squamous cell carcinoma) were increased at 250 mg/kg/day. There was no increase in tumors at the lowest dose tested in rats, which is approximately 10 times the RHD on a mg/m^2 basis.

Mutagenesis

Tasimelteon was negative in an *in vitro* bacterial reverse mutation (Ames) assay, an *in vitro* cytogenetics assay in primary human lymphocytes, and an *in vivo* micronucleus assay in rats.

Impairment of Fertility

When male and female rats were given tasimelteon at oral doses of 5, 50, or 500 mg/kg/day prior to and throughout mating and continuing in females to gestation day 7, estrus cycle disruption and decreased fertility were observed at all but the lowest dose tested. The no-effect dose for effects on female reproduction (5 mg/kg/day) is approximately 2 times the RHD on a mg/m^2 basis.

14. CLINICAL STUDIES

The effectiveness of HETLIOZ in the treatment of Non-24-Hour Sleep-Wake Disorder (Non-24) was established in two randomized double-masked, placebo-controlled, multicenter, parallel-group studies (Studies 1 and 2) in totally blind patients with Non-24.

In study 1, 84 patients with Non-24 (median age 54 years) were randomized to receive HETLIOZ 20 mg or placebo, one hour prior to bedtime, at the same time every night for up to 6 months.

Study 2 was a randomized withdrawal trial in 20 patients with Non-24 (median age 55 years) that was designed to evaluate the maintenance of efficacy of HETLIOZ after 12-weeks. Patients were treated for approximately 12 weeks with HETLIOZ 20 mg one hour prior to bedtime, at the same time every night. Patients in whom the calculated time of peak melatonin level (melatonin acrophase) occurred at approximately the same time of day (in contrast to the expected daily delay) during the run-in phase were randomized to receive placebo or continue treatment with HETLIOZ 20 mg for 8 weeks.

Study 1 and Study 2 evaluated the duration and timing of nighttime sleep and daytime naps via patient-recorded diaries. During Study 1, patient diaries were recorded for an average of 88 days during screening, and 133 days during randomization. During Study 2, patient diaries were recorded for an average of 57 days during the run-in phase, and 59 days during the randomized-withdrawal phase.

Because symptoms of nighttime sleep disruption and daytime sleepiness are cyclical in patients with Non-24, with severity varying according to the state of alignment of the individual patient's circadian rhythm with the 24-hour day (least severe when fully aligned, most severe when 12 hours out of alignment), efficacy endpoints for nighttime total sleep time and daytime nap duration were based on the 25% of nights with the least nighttime sleep, and the 25% of days with the most daytime nap time. In Study 1, patients in the HETLIOZ group had, at baseline, an average 195 minutes of nighttime sleep and 137 minutes of daytime nap time on the 25% of most symptomatic nights and days, respectively. Treatment with HETLIOZ resulted in a significant improvement, compared with placebo, for both of these endpoints in Study 1 and Study 2 (see Table 2).

Table 2: Effects of HETLIOZ 20 MG on Nighttime Sleep Time and Daytime Nap Time in Study 1 and Study 2

Change from Baseline	Study 1		Study 2	
	HETLIOZ 20 MG N=42	Placebo N=42	HETLIOZ 20 MG N=10	Placebo N=10
Nighttime sleep time on 25% most symptomatic nights (minutes)	50	22	-7	-74
Daytime nap time on 25% most symptomatic days (minutes)	-49	-22	-9	50

A responder analysis of patients with both ≥ 45 minutes increase in nighttime sleep and ≥ 45 minutes decrease in daytime nap time was conducted in Study 1: 29% (n=12) of patients treated with HETLIOZ, compared with 12% (n=5) of patients treated with placebo met the responder criteria. The efficacy of HETLIOZ in treating Non-24 may be reduced in subjects with concomitant administration of beta adrenergic receptor antagonists.

16. HOW SUPPLIED/STORAGE AND HANDLING

HETLIOZ 20 mg capsules are available as size 1, dark blue opaque, hard gelatin capsules printed with "VANDA 20 mg" in white, containing 20 mg of tasimelteon per capsule.

• NDC 43068-220-01   Bottles of 30

Storage

Store HETLIOZ 20 mg capsules at controlled room temperature, 25°C (77°F); excursions permitted to 15°C to 30°C (59°F to 86°F) [See USP Controlled Room Temperature]. Protect HETLIOZ 20 mg capsules from exposure to light and moisture.

17. PATIENT COUNSELING INFORMATION

Advise patients

• To take HETLIOZ before bedtime at the same time every night.

• To skip the dose that night if they cannot take HETLIOZ at approximately the same time on a given night.

• To limit their activities to preparing for going to bed after taking HETLIOZ because HETLIOZ can potentially impair the performance of activities requiring complete mental alertness.

• That because of individual differences in circadian rhythms, daily use for several weeks or months may be necessary before benefit from HETLIOZ is observed.

• To swallow the capsule whole.

Distributed by:

Vanda Pharmaceuticals Inc.

Washington, D.C. 20037 USA

www.hetlioz.com

Vanda and HETLIOZ are registered trademarks of Vanda Pharmaceuticals Inc. in the United States and other countries.

Shown in Product Identification Guide, page 511

To purchase the new *Clinical Lipid Management* drug reference, and other PDR® clinical references handbooks, visit PDRbooks.com.

SECTION 8

DIETARY SUPPLEMENTS

This section presents information on natural remedies and nutritional supplements marketed under the Dietary Supplement Health and Education Act (DSHEA) of 1994. The information on each product described has been provided by the manufacturer and contains the latest information available when the *PDR*® went to press. Listings are arranged alphabetically by manufacturer.

The function of PDR is solely the compilation, organization, and distribution of this information on natural remedies and nutritional supplements. PDR does not assume, and expressly disclaims, any obligation to obtain and include any information on natural remedies and nutritional supplements other than that provided to it by the manufacturers. It should be understood that by making this material available, PDR is not advocating the use of any product described herein, nor is PDR responsible for misuse of a product due to typographical error. Additional information on any natural remedy and/or nutritional supplement product may be obtained from the manufacturer.

Products found in this section include herbal preparations, vitamins, minerals, and other substances intended to supplement the diet. The descriptions of these products are designed to provide the information necessary for informed use. Dietary supplements marketed inder the DSHEA do not receive formal evaluation or approval from the FDA. The fillowing disclaimer applies to all product information listed in this section, as mandated by the federal government: *These statements have not been evaluated by the Food and Drug Administration. This product is not intended to diagnose, treat, cure, or prevent any disease.*

4Life Research USA, LLC

9850 SOUTH 300 WEST
SANDY, UT 84070

Direct Inquiries to:
(801) 562-3600
productsupport@4life.com
www.4life.com

4LIFE TRANSFER FACTOR® TRI-FACTOR® FORMULA DS

PRODUCT DESCRIPTION

4Life Transfer Factor Tri-Factor Formula combines proprietary transfer factors and NanoFactor® molecules extracted from bovine colostrum and chicken egg yolk sources. These molecules contain antigen information which educates, enhances, and helps maintain immune system balance.

TECHNICAL DESCRIPTION

Transfer factors are molecules that communicate antigenic immunological information intercellularly and from a donor to a recipient. They support immune function through cell mediated immunity. Transfer factors, which carry antigen specific information to which all tested immune cells respond, are produced by mononuclear cells and serve to support and improve immune mediated pathways. Mammalian transfer factors, including those of humans are small molecules between 3,500 and 10,000 daltons. (1; 2) Transfer factors are polypeptides that consist of 40 to 44 amino acids (3) and have a conserved region and a variable region. From a molecular biological standpoint, these two properties are analogous to antibodies; however transfer factor's functions of cell mediated immunity (CMI) and non-specific immunological activity differ almost completely from the functions of antibodies. The molecules that have a molecular weight of less than 3,500 daltons modulate immune response but they do not transfer delayed-type hypersensitivity (DTH). (1)

4Life's transfer factors are sourced from the ultra-filtration of colostrum and from egg yolks. (4; 5) The molecules obtained from the spray dried ultra-filtrate of bovine colostrum are of two classes; the transfer factors present in the ultra-filtrate of ≤10,000 daltons and the nanofraction molecules that are present in the nano-filtrate of ≤3,500 daltons.

Transfer factors were first discovered in 1949 by H. Sherwood Lawrence when he demonstrated that CMI could be transferred from one individual to another by way of low molecular weight extracts of white blood cells. Transfer factors could transfer DTH of a specific form from a skin test positive individual to a skin test negative individual who subsequent to the transfer would skin test positive for that antigen. (6) In a subsequent study in 1955 he demonstrated that DTH could be passed serially, first from a skin test positive individual to a test negative individual, who became test positive, then 6 months later from the second individual to another test negative individual who became test positive. (7) At the time antibodies were the focus of immune research and little was known of the importance of DTH and of the involvement of T-cells in immune response. Transfer factors promote wellness via cell mediated immunity. These compounds are components of colostrum, an infant's first meal. They bridge the generational gap by passing cell mediated immunity from mother to infant.

BIOLOGICAL AND PHYSIOLOGICAL ACTION

Transfer factors' preparations contain more than 200 different moieties of polypeptide molecules with a molecular weight of <10,000 daltons; each moiety potentially having a great number of epitotic variations. These antigen specific factors are synthesized in monocytes and stored in the cytoplasm or on the cell membrane. A significant body of evidence indicates that the primary biological function of transfer factors is to recruit and specifically sensitize previously uncommitted lymphocytes. These sensitized T-lymphocytes initiate the events of cell-mediated immunity, thereby, promoting immunity not only at the site of antigen challenge but also throughout the body. (8) The effect of transfer factors on antigen mediated immunity, via B-cells, is not completely understood; however, a clinical test has reported an increase in particular antibodies, such as IgA and IgG, during transfer factor administration.

Clinical studies have demonstrated that transfer factors' unique ability to express DTH and promote cell-mediated immunity can be transferred from a sensitized donor to a non-immune recipient. (1; 9) This antigen specific effect is well documented and is likely produced through activation of the CD3-antigen site of T-cells, increased macrophage activation, and interleukin production—which can also enhance natural killer cell function. (1; 10)

Although the exact mechanism of action is unknown, research has shown that transfer factors will bind to antigens. However, the antigen specificity that is "transferred" to recipients is mediated by T-lymphocytes. (3) Current structure function models propose that transfer factors have a variable region and a conserved amino acid region, which determines the antigenic specificity for an estimated 8^{18} epitopes (1) and serves as a binding target for immune cell receptors respectively. (2; 11) These highly conserved regions presumably allow transfer factors to be administered across a species barrier without any loss of potency. In fact, research has demonstrated that bovine transfer factors are structurally analogous to human-derived transfer factors with equivalent physiological activity. This is further supported by several studies, which used transfer factors extracted from bovine lymph nodes and colostrum to confer cell-mediated immunity to specific antigens in animals and human recipients. (12; 13)

Although most clinical trials with transfer factors have used parental administration; oral administration has also demonstrated successful transfer of DTH and cell mediated immunity I recipients. (14) Dose response studies, which compare in various routes of administration, have been performed in both human and animals. Results of these experiments refute any arguments that the acidic or enzymatic environment of gastrointestinal tract effects oral administration of transfer factors. (14)

CLINICAL AND EXPERIMENTAL STUDIES

Natural Killer Cell Activity

Peripheral blood mononuclear cells were isolated and pooled from several healthy donors. Sixty thousand cells were added to each well of 96-well microtiter plate. Various immune modulating ingredients, including 4Life Transfer Factor Tri-Factor Formula, were added to select wells on the plate and 48 hour incubation started. At the end of the incubation period 30 thousand K562 cells were added to each well. MTT assay techniques were used to determine the cytotoxic index. The various 4Life Transfer Factor products resulted in cytotoxic indices of 80-98%. By comparison, mononuclear cells incubated with IL-2 for the same 48 hour period produced a cytotoxic index of 88%.

CD4 T Helper Cell Research

Multiple studies were performed using the FDA-approved diagnostic CD4 T Helper cell assay kit and/or a T Cell Memory (CD8) assay kit under development by the same company. Similar to the NK cell research described above these *in vitro* studies were performed on 96-well microtiter plates measuring ATP production via a luciferase-based luminescence reaction.

The CD4 assay utilizes PHA-stimulated cells isolated from whole blood via the use of Dynabeads™. An 18 hour incubation of these isolated, stimulated CD4 cells with the 4Life Transfer Factor products has resulted in a modulation of immune cell activity as exhibited by a decrease in ATP production without a negative impact on cell viability. It is hypothesized that this reduction on ATP production is a result of a redirection in immune cell focus, essentially diminishing the distraction induced by the addition of PHA to the microtiter wells.

Salivary Secretory IgA-Preliminary Investigation

Twenty-four subjects naïve to transfer factor supplementation were enrolled in a small-scale, preliminary test. Twenty-one were included in the final analysis. Salivary samples were collected from each subject weekly at roughly the same time of day and day of the week. Saliva was collected over a 5 minute period via passive drool while subjects chewed on a piece of Parafilm™. The samples were put on ice and then frozen at -70°C until assay. The commercial Salimetrics™ salivary IgA assay kit was used for analysis. Subjects were given 4Life Transfer Factor Tri-Factor Formula at 2 capsules per day for two weeks and then transitioned to 4Life Transfer Factor RioVida Tri-Factor Formula at 60ml per day for an additional 2 weeks. At the end of the 4 week supplementation period the group showed an average 73% increase in salivary secretory IgA (SIgA) production over their baseline value. Furthermore, none of the 21 subjects showed SIgA production rate less than their baseline value at the end of the test.

Wellness Research

A study conducted with 30 college students found that either 1x 15 days or 2x 15 days (with 2 weeks break in between) of transfer factor administered according to label dose helped them maintain their health. In both groups, transfer factor administration improved the number of CD8+ T cells and NK cells to healthier levels. Particularly, those that took the product for 2x 15 days showed prolonged health maintenance and improvement of immune cells markers than those who took it for 15 days. Specifically, the maintenance of good health and improvement of immune cells markers remained for up to 3 months after stopping transfer factor administration in those that took the product for 2x 15 days in comparison to 1 month in those that took the product for 1x 15 days. (15)

Safety

In a study of acute toxicity rats were assessed for fourteen days following a single gavage of 4Life Transfer Factor. Five female SD rats were each gavaged with a dose of 2,000mg/kg. No treatment-related mortalities occurred and there were no clinical signs of toxicity. No significant difference in body weight occurred. No gross lesions were found at necropsy in any of the animals. Thus, acute toxicity is considered to be greater than 2,000mg/kg (human equivalent dose of approximately 320 mg/kg). (16)

Another similar single-dose oral toxicity study was conducted in mice. Six female Wistar mice each received 2,000mg/kg via oral gavage and monitored for fourteen days. No observable toxicity occurred as assessed by mortality, body weight gain, histopathology of brain, liver, kidneys and lungs, and clinical signs of aggression, lethargy, breathing difficulties, diarrhea, mobility and shivering. Thus, the no-observed adverse effect level was considered to be greater than 2,000mg/kg in mice, which is equivalent to approximately 9.7g/kg in humans. (17) The use of transfer factors is contraindicated in person receiving immunosuppressive therapy, though actual interactions have not been documented. The use of transfer factors during pregnancy and nursing has not been evaluated.

How Supplied

4Life Transfer Factor® can be found in the following products:

4Life Transfer Factor® Tri-Factor® Formula
4Life® Transfer Factor Plus® Tri-Factor® Formula
4Life Transfer Factor® RioVida® Tri-Factor® Formula
4Life Transfer Factor Renuvo®
4Life Transfer Factor® Chewable Tri-Factor® Formula
4Life Transfer Factor® Classic
4Life Transfer Factor® Immune Spray
4Life Transfer Factor® KBU®
4Life Transfer Factor® Belle Vie®
4Life Transfer Factor® Cardio
4Life Transfer Factor® GluCoach®
4Life Transfer Factor® MalePro®
4Life Transfer Factor® ReCall®
4Life Transfer Factor Reflexion™
4Life Transfer Factor Vista®
RiteStart® Men
RiteStart® Women
RiteStart® Kids & Teens
PRO-TF®

REFERENCES

1. **Fundenberg, H. and G. Pizza.** 1994, *Progress in Drug Research*, Vol. 42, pp. 309-400.
2. **Lawrence, H.S. and W. Borkowsjy.** (1-3), 1996, Biotherapy, Vol. 9, pp. 1-5.
3. **Kirkpatrick, C.H.** 4, 2000, Mol Med, Vol. 6, pp. 332-41.
4. **Hennen, W. and D. Lisonbee.** s.l. : U.P. Office, Editor., 2002, 4Life Research, LC:USA.
5. **Wilson, G. and G. Paddock.** s.l. : U.P. Office, Editor., 1989, Amtron, Inc: USA.
6. **Lawrence, H.S.** 4, 1949, Proc Soc Exp Biol Med, Vol. 71, pp. 516-22.
7. **Lawrence, H.S.** 2, 1955, J Clin Invest, Vol. 34, pp. 219-30.
8. **Levin, A.S., L.E. Spitler, and H.H. Fundenberg.** 1973, Annu Rev Med, Vol. 24, pp. 175-208.
9. **Fudenberg, H. and H. Fudenberg.** 1989, Ann Rev Pharmacol Toxicol, Vol. 29, pp. 475-516.
10. **See, D., S. Mason, and R. Roshan.** 2, 2002, Immunol Invest, Vol. 31, pp. 137-53.

11. **Dwyer, John M.** 1-3, 1996, Biotherapy, Vol. 9, pp. 7-11.
12. **Wilson, G.B., R.T. Newell, and N.M. Burdash.** 1, 1979, Cell Immunol, Vol. 47, pp. 1-18.
13. **Radosevich, J.K., G.H. Scott, and G.B. Olson.** 4, 1985, Am J Vet Res, Vol. 46, pp. 875-8.
14. **Kirkpatrick, C.H.** 1-3, 1996, Biotherapy, Vol. 9, pp. 13-6.
15. **Klimov, V. and E. Oganova.** *in Euromedica Hannover 2004.* Hannover, Germany : s.n., 2004. pp. 15-16.
16. **Kabirov, K.K.** 2009, unpublished: University of Illinois at Chicago.
17. **Burbano, Z. and G. Sarmiento.** 2013. Facultad de Ciencias Quimicas, Universidad de Guayaquil, Ecuador.
These statements have not been evaluated by the Food and Drug Administration. This product is not intended to diagnose, treat, cure of prevent any disease.

Shown in Product Identification Guide, page 505

Alto Pharmaceuticals, Inc.

P.O. BOX 271150
TAMPA, FL 33688-1150
3172 LAKE ELLEN DRIVE
TAMPA, FL 33618
www.altopharm.com

Direct Inquiries to:
John J. Cullaro
Customer Service
JOHNC@ALTOPHARM.COM
(813) 968-0522
Fax (813) 968-0527

ZINC-220®   DS
DIETARY SUPPLEMENT
(Zinc Sulfate 220 mg. USP)

UNIT DOSE
100 CAPSULES

Supplement Facts
Serving Size 1 Capsule

Amount Per Serving		% Daily Value*
Zinc	50mg	333%

(From Zinc Sulfate Heptahydrate 220mg)

INGREDIENTS: Each blue and pink capsule contains 50 mg. of elemental zinc. Zinc-220 capsules are gluten free and do not contain dextrose or glucose. Inactive ingredients: rice flour, magnesium stearate, D&C red #22, D&C red #28, FD&C blue #1, titanium dioxide and gelatin (capsule shell).

ACTION AND USES: Zinc-220® Capsules are indicated as a dietary supplement. Normal growth and tissue repair are directly dependent upon an adequate supply of zinc in the diet. Zinc functions as an integral part of a number of enzymes important to protein and carbohydrate metabolism. Zinc-220® Capsules are recommended for deficiencies or the prevention of deficiencies of zinc.

WARNINGS: Zinc-220® if administered in stat dosages of 2 grams (9 capsules) will cause an emetic effect. As with any supplement, if you are pregnant, nursing or taking medication, consult your physician before use.

PRECAUTION: It is recommended that Zinc-220® Capsules be taken with meals to avoid gastric distress.

ADULTS: Take one capsule daily with meals or as directed by a physician.

ALTO®
Pharmaceuticals, Inc.
Tampa, Florida 33688
For Customer Service: 1-813-968-0522
Dist. U.S.A   REV 3/11
Shown in Product Identification Guide, page 507

Andorra Life LLC
18635 GALE AVENUE
CITY OF INDUSTRY, CA 91748

Direct Inquiries to:
(Tel) 1-855-558-8088
(Email): info@andorralife.com

ADVANCED BLOOD SUGAR CONTROL   DS

Benefits:
• Helps Maintain Healthy Blood Sugar Levels
• Supports Healthy Blood Vessels
• Supports Sensory/Nerve Function
Why high blood sugar level is bad for you?
Balanced blood sugar is critical for our bodies to function; it is important for healthy blood vessels, optimal circulation and nerve functions. Persistently elevated blood sugar level leads to Diabetes. Diabetes damages the body and can lead to the multiple health problems.
A normal sugar level is currently considered to be less than 100 mg/dL when fasting and less than 140 mg/dL two hours after eating. But in most healthy people, sugar levels are even lower. During the day, our blood glucose levels tend to be at their lowest just before meals. For most people without diabetes, blood sugar levels before meals hover around 70 to 80 mg/dL. In some, 60 is normal; in others, 90. Again, anything less than 100 mg/dL while fasting is considered normal by today's standards.
High blood sugar (Hyperglycemia) is caused by many factors:
• **Type I Diabetes:** The body does not produce insulin.
• **Type II Diabetes:** The body does not produce enough insulin for proper function. (most common)
• **Gestational Diabetes:** This type affects about 9.2% of females during pregnancy.
People with Diabetes are in special need to lower their blood sugar levels. People who have irregular life styles are also in need to regulate their blood sugar levels. Stress, lack of exercise and eating more than planned, all trigger high blood glucose.
Why choose Andorra Life?
Andorra's Advanced Blood Sugar Control uses the finest ingredients which are specially formulated to keep your blood sugar level in line.
Premium Pine Bark:
Advanced scientific research has revealed that pine bark has potent blood sugar benefits, including lowering fasting and post-meal glucose levels as well as promoting insulin sensitivity. Pine bark can significantly lowered fasting and post meal blood glucose levels compared to baseline. Furthermore, insulin levels remained unchanged at all doses, indicating Pine bark facilitated blood sugar uptake by previously insulin resistant cells. In another study Pine bark was shown to significantly lower fasting blood glucose.
Alpha Lipoic Acid (ALA):
Studies have shown that ALA significantly improves insulin stimulated glucose uptake in patients with type II diabetes. Not only does it help lower blood sugar levels by reducing the secretion of insulin, it also increases insulin sensitivity at the cell level and thus, even LESS insulin is required.
Cinnamon Powder:
Cinnamon powders may help improve glucose and lipids levels in patients with type 2 diabetes, according to a study published in Diabetics Care.
The study authors concluded that consuming up to 6 grams of cinnamon per day "reduces serum glucose, triglyceride, LDL cholesterol, and total cholesterol in people with type 2 diabetes." and that "the inclusion of cinnamon in the diet of people with type 2 diabetes will reduce risk factors associated with diabetes and cardiovascular diseases."
In addition, cinnamon extract can reduce fasting blood sugar levels in patients, researchers reported in the European Journal of Clinical Investigation.
Berberine:
A plant alkaloid and naturally occurring compound found in the roots, rhizomes, and stem bark of various plants, berberine works by targeting a key regulator of metabolism, the AMP-activated protein kinase (AMPK) enzyme. AMPK regulates glucose uptake and the synthesis of glucose transporters— which move glucose out of your blood and into your cells, where it is converted to energy. Berberine may also increase the number and activity of the insulin recep-

tors, promoting insulin sensitivity. On top of that, AMPK facilitates the burning of fatty acids in your cells, which is why it is a powerful tool for helping keep blood lipid levels in check.
Chromium:
This essential trace element is required for normal fat and carbohydrate metabolism and healthy glucose tolerance. Chromium may help promote insulin sensitivity by increasing the number of insulin binding sites on cells, which allow for better transport of glucose into cells for energy.
Vitamin B6:
Pyridoxamine is a specialized form of vitamin B6 easily converted in the body to pyridoxal 5-phosphate (PLP), the active form of the vitamin. Pyridoxamine may help prevent diabetic complications by blocking formation of advanced glycation end products (AGEs) and advanced lipoxidation end products (ALEs) underlying loss of structure and function accompanying aging. AGEs are implicated in diabetes-related conditions including kidney disease (nephropathy), visual loss (retinopathy), and neuropathy. It has been described as "the most potent natural substance for inhibiting AGE formation."
Vitamin B12:
Vitamin B12 supports the digestive system in keeping glucose levels stable. Vitamin B12 is bound to protein in food. The activity of hydrochloric acid and gastric protease in the stomach releases vitamin B12 from its protein. Once it is released, vitamin B12 begins to work quickly. B12 deficiency can cause permanent nerve damage. Neuropathy is a common problem for people with diabetes, who experience pain, tingling, and numbness in their arms, hands, legs, and feet, resulting in sores.

Supplement Facts Serving Size: 1 capsule	Per Serving
Servings Per Container: 30	
Vitamin B$_6$	10 mg
Vitamin B$_{12}$	100 mcg
Chromium	200 mcg
Cinnamon Bark	200 mg
Alpha Lipoic Acid	50 mg
Pine Bark Extract	50 mg
Berberine	200 mg

Free of: milk or milk by-products, egg or egg by-products, fish or fish by-products, shellfish and by-products, tree nuts, peanut or peanut by-products, wheat or wheat by-products, soybeans and soy byproducts.
Suggested Use: take one (1) capsule daily as a dietary supplement or as recommended by your healthcare professional.
• **KEEP OUT OF REACH OF CHILDREN.**
• Consult your doctor before use if you are pregnant, nursing or taking medication.
• Keep tightly closed at a cool dry place.
• Store at Room temperature.
• For your protection, do not use if imprinted safety seal under cap is broken or missing.
Manufactured in a FDA Licensed cGMP facility.

REFERENCES
1. Alam Khan, MS, PHD, Mahpara Safdar, MS, Mohammad Muzaffar Ali Khan, MS, PHD, Khan Nawaz Khattak, MS and Richard A. Anderson, PHD. *"Cinnamon Improves Glucose and Lipids of People With Type 2 Diabetes". Diabetes Care.* December 2003 vol. 26 no. 12 3215-3218. Accessed October 14th 2013.
2. Cameron NE, Gibson TM, Nangle MR, Cotter MA. Inhibitors of advanced glycation end product formation and neurovascular dysfunction in experimental diabetes. Ann NY Acad Sci. 2005 Jun;1043:784-92.
3. Giusti C, Gargiulo P. Advances in biochemical mechanisms of diabetic retinopathy. Eur Rev Med Pharmacol Sci. 2007 May;11(3):155-63.
4. Head KA. Peripheral neuropathy: pathogenic mechanisms and alternative therapies. Altern Med Rev. 2006 Dec;11(4):294-329.

Continued on next page

5. Karachalias N, Babaei-Jadidi R, Ahmed N, Thornalley PJ. Accumulation of fructosyl-lysine and advanced glycation end products in the kidney, retina and peripheral nerve of streptozotocin-induced diabetic rats. Biochem Soc Trans. 2003 Dec;31(Pt 6):1423-5.

6. Ahmed N, Thornalley PJ. Advanced glycation endproducts: what is their relevance to diabetic complications? Diabetes Obes Metab. 2007 May;9(3):233-45.

7. Vasdev S, Gill V, Singal P. Role of advanced glycation end products in hypertension and atherosclerosis: therapeutic implications. Cell Biochem Biophys. 2007;49(1):48-63.

8. Theodoratou E, Farrington SM, Tenesa A, et al. Dietary vitamin B6 intake and the risk of colorectal cancer. Cancer Epidemiol Biomarkers Prev. 2008 Jan;17(1):171-82.

9. Nawale RB, Mourya VK, Bhise SB. Non-enzymatic glycation of proteins: a cause for complications in diabetes. Indian J Biochem Biophys. 2006 Dec;43(6):337-44.

10. Perricone N. Ageless Face, Ageless Mind. New York, New York: Ballantine Books; 2007.

11. Chetyrkin SV, Mathis ME, Ham AJ, et al. Propagation of protein glycation damage involves modification of tryptophan residues via reactive oxygen species: inhibition by pyridoxamine. Free Radic Biol Med. 2008 Apr 1;44(7):1276-85.

12. Ahmed N, Thornalley PJ. Advanced glycation endproducts: what is their relevance to diabetic complications? Diabetes Obes Metab. 2007 May;9(3):233-45.

13. Voziyan PA, Metz TO, Baynes JW, Hudson BG. A post-Amadori inhibitor pyridoxamine also inhibits chemical modification of proteins by scavenging carbonyl intermediates of carbohydrate and lipid degradation. J Biol Chem. 2002 Feb 1;277(5):3397-403.

14. Chetyrkin SV, Zhang W, Hudson BG, Serianni AS, Voziyan PA. Pyridoxamine protects proteins from functional damage by 3-deoxyglucosone: mechanism of action of pyridoxamine. Biochemistry. 2008 Jan 22;47(3):997-1006.

15. Jain SK, Lim G. Pyridoxine and pyridoxamine inhibits superoxide radicals and prevents lipid peroxidation, protein glycosylation, and (Na+ + K+)-ATPase activity reduction in high glucose-treated human erythrocytes. Free Radic Biol Med. 2001 Feb 1;30(3):232-7.

16. Metz TO, Alderson NL, Thorpe SR, Baynes JW. Pyridoxamine, an inhibitor of advanced glycation and lipoxidation reactions: a novel therapy for treatment of diabetic complications. Arch Biochem Biophys. 2003 Nov 1;419(1):41-9.

17. Onorato JM, Jenkins AJ, Thorpe SR, Baynes JW. Pyridoxamine, an inhibitor of advanced glycation reactions, also inhibits advanced lipoxidation reactions. Mechanism of action of pyridoxamine. J Biol Chem. 2000 Jul 14;275(28):21177-84.

18. Higuchi O, Nakagawa K, Tsuzuki T, et al. Aminophospholipid glycation and its inhibitor screening system: a new role of pyridoxal 5'-phosphate as the inhibitor. J Lipid Res. 2006 May;47(5):964-74.

19. Takatori A, Ishii Y, Itagaki S, Kyuwa S, Yoshikawa Y. Amelioration of the beta-cell dysfunction in diabetic APA hamsters by antioxidants and AGE inhibitor treatments. Diabetes Metab Res Rev. 2004 May;20(3):211-8.

20. Alderson NL, Chachich ME, Youssef NN, et al. The AGE inhibitor pyridoxamine inhibits lipemia and development of renal and vascular disease in Zucker obese rats. Kidney Int. 2003 Jun;63(6):2123-33.

21. Araghi-Niknam M, Hosseini S, Larson D, Rohdewald P, Watson RR. Pine bark extract reduces platelet aggregation. *Integr Med*. 2000;2:73-77.

22. Summary of data for chemical selection: oligomeric proanthocyanidins from grape seeds and pine bark. National Toxicology Program Web site. Accessed at http://ntp.niehs.nih.gov/ntp/htdocs/Chem_Background/ExSumPdf/GrapeSeeds_PineBark.pdf on June 6, 2008.

23. Devaraj S, Vega-López S, Kaul N, et al. Supplementation with a pine bark extract rich in polyphenols increase plasma antioxidant capacity and alters the plasma lipoprotein profile. Lipids. 2002;37:931-934.

Shown in Product Identification Guide, page 507

ADVANCED LUNG CLEANSE   DS

Benefits:
• Supports Healthy Respiration
• Supports Healthy Bronchial Sinus Function
• Maintain Healthy Lung Function
Why our lungs need protection?
The lungs are different from most of the other organs in our bodies because their delicate tissues are directly connected to the outside environment. Anything we breathe in can af-

fect the lungs. Germs, tobacco smoke and other harmful substances can cause damage to the airways and threaten the lungs ability to work properly.

Our bodies have the natural defense systems designed to protect the lungs. This works very well most of the time to keep out dirt and fight off germs. But there are some important things we have to do to reduce the risk of lung disease. Cigarette smoking, Secondhand smoke, outdoor air pollution, chemicals in the home and workplace, and radon can all cause or worsen lung disease. Regular check-ups are an important part of disease prevention, even when you are feeling well. This is especially true for lung disease, which sometimes goes undetected until it is serious.

Without any extra effort, our lungs are in a near-constant state of inhaling and exhaling. Like all active areas of our bodies, the lungs require a fair share of vitamins to help them create new cells, repair DNA and fight damage from oxidation. In addition to a healthy diet, consuming the best vitamins for lungs can help promote lung health.

Why choose Andorra Life?

Andorra's Lung Cleanse is scientifically formulated and tested to shield your lung from air pollutants, smoking damages, detoxifies, and promotes the healthy lung blood circulation.

N-Acetyl Cysteine (NAC):

NAC is a compound that is converted by the body into the naturally occurring amino acid cysteine. NAC has been shown to lower blood levels of homocysteine, an effect that is potentially beneficial for heart disease prevention.

NAC also can break up trapped mucus and enhance its clearance from the bronchial passages, thereby improving the flow of air in and out of the lungs in people with COPD. In addition, NAC is the precursor of glutathione, one of the major antioxidants in lung tissue. Although the mucus-clearing effect of NAC occurs mainly when the compound is administered by inhalation, oral NAC has repeatedly been shown to prevent flare-ups in people with chronic bronchitis.

Supplementing with N-Acetylcysteine (NAC) can reduce the need for hospitalization among people suffering from chronic obstructive pulmonary disease (COPD), according to a study in the *European Respiratory Journal* (2003;21:795-8).

In the study, 1,219 people who had been hospitalized for COPD were observed for an average of nine months after they were discharged from the hospital. Those who were prescribed NAC were approximately one-third less likely to be readmitted to the hospital, compared with those who were not given NAC. The risk of hospitalization decreased with increasing doses of NAC. Excluding those who were prescribed less than 400 mg per day, treatment with NAC was associated with an 85% reduction in the rate of readmission.

A large number of studies have used 600 mg per day of NAC for prevention of chronic bronchitis. Although a few of participants in some studies experienced side effects, including nausea, vomiting, abdominal pain, indigestion, dyspepsia, dry mouth, headache, dizziness, or abnormal taste, most people tolerated the treatment well. Long-term use of NAC has the potential to increase the requirement for zinc and copper. Some doctors, therefore, advise people who are taking NAC also to take a multivitaminmineral preparation that provides approximately 15 mg of zinc and 2 mg of copper per day.

Vitamin A:

Vitamin A is the name of a group of fat-soluble retinoids, including retinol, retinal, retinoic acid, and retinyl esters. Vitamin A is involved in immune function, vision, reproduction, and cellular communication . Vitamin A is critical for vision as an essential component of rhodopsin, a protein that absorbs light in the retinal receptors, and because it supports the normal differentiation and functioning of the conjunctival membranes and cornea. Vitamin A also supports cell growth and differentiation, playing a critical role in the normal formation and maintenance of the heart, lungs, kidneys, and other organs.

One of the most important functions of vitamin A is to repair and re-build all the internal mucosal membranes, from the top orifice to the bottom one. Thus Vitamin A is recommended for sinus problems, leaky gut syndrome and even interstitial cystitis. Vitamin A is helpful for anything that has to do with internal mucous membranes.

In these days of constantly increasing air pollution, and the spread of airborne bacteria and viruses, it is important to realize that the lining of the sinuses and lungs are the first

line of defense. Thus vitamin A is essential for protection against colds, influenza and infections of the kidneys, bladder, lungs and mucous membranes.

Vitamin B-6 and Vitamin B-12:

Vitamin B6 is also called pyridoxine. Vitamin B6 has been studied for the treatment of many conditions, including anemia (low amounts of healthy red blood cells). A new study has shown that to have higher blood levels of vitamin B6 and the amino acid methionine both appear to reduce lung cancer risk in smokers and nonsmokers alike.

Vitamin B12 is a B vitamin. It can be found in foods such as meat, fish, and dairy products. Vitamin B12 is used for treating and preventing vitamin B12 deficiency that could cause pernicious anemia. Vitamin B12 is also used for asthma, allergies and skin infections.

Vitamin C:

Vitamin C was identified in the early 1900s in the search for a deficient substance responsible for scurvy, which was a serious disease of sailors in the Age of Sail. Starting in the 1930s, some German and US physicians proposed that vitamin C would be beneficial in the treatment of pneumonia. Although the burden of pneumonia has decreased dramatically in developed countries during the past century, lung infections are still a leading cause of mortality and morbidity globally. Many infections, including pneumonia, lead to reduced vitamin C levels in plasma, leukocytes and urine. Because of these changes in metabolism, vitamin C might have a therapeutic effect on pneumonia patients. Thus there is a biological rationale to examine the effect of vitamin C on infections in humans.

The researchers agreed that a diet rich in the foods that provide vitamin C is likely to be beneficial for lung health. By reducing the amount of decline in lung function over time, consuming ample amounts of these foods could lower the risk of COPD - a COPD can be due to chronic bronchitis, emphysema, or both. Risk factors for COPD include history of smoking or passive smoke exposure, allergy and asthma, exposure to environmental pollution, recurrent respiratory illness, or a family history of chronic bronchitis or emphysema.

Vitamin D:

Many people associate vitamin D strictly with the health of their bones. However, vitamin D is also important for immune health, hormone production and lung health. According to research published in the May 2011 "American Journal of Respiratory and Critical Care Medicine," vitamin D deficiency can lead to poor lung function.

Coenzyme Q10, Ginger Extract and Tumeric Extract:

Coenzyme Q10 (CoQ10) is a substance similar to a vitamin. It is found in every cell of the body. The body makes CoQ10, and the cells use it to produce energy that the body needs for cell growth and maintenance. It also functions as an antioxidant, which protects the body from damage caused by harmful molecules known as free radicals.

Ginger is an herb. The rhizome (underground stem) is used as a spice and also as a medicine to improve conditions on many diseases. Ginger is used here for its anti inflammation effect on upper respiratory tract infections, cough, and bronchitis.

Turmeric is a plant. It has a warm, bitter taste and is frequently used to flavor or color curry powders, mustards, butters, and cheeses. But the root of turmeric is also used widely to make medicine. Turmeric is used for arthritis, heartburn (dyspepsia), stomach pain, bronchitis, colds, lung infections, fibromyalgia, leprosy, and fever. Turmeric has also been recognized for its anti inflammatory effect.

Hawthorn Berry Extract and Elecampane Root:

Hawthorn is used for Cadiovascular health and a powerfully antioxidant. Hawthorn can help improve the amount of blood pumped out of the heart during contractions, widen the blood vessels, and increase the transmission of nerve signals. It can relax the tiniest lung blood vessels hence increased blood flow farther from the heart, due to a component in hawthorn called proanthocyanidin.

Elecampane, also known as horse heal and marchalan, is a plant common in Great Britain, central and southern Europe, and Asia. Elecampane, has been long valued as an effective respiratory support herb, even being listed in the U.S. Pharmacopeia. Traditional Chinese and Indian Ayurvedic medicine use elecampane for bronchitis and asthma, as did ancient Greeks and Romans. In the 1800's, lozenges, candy, and cough drops were all produced from elecampane root.

Elecampane has actions, which are expectorant, antitussive, sedative, anti-fungal, relaxing, warming, and antimicrobial. Elecampane can soothe bronchial tube linings and act as an expectorant for lung cleansing. For this reason, elecampane is beneficial in supporting any respiratory condition which produces copious mucus discharge.

Supplement Facts Serving Size: 2 Capsules Servings Per Container: 30	Per Serving
Vitamin A	5000 IU
Vitamin C	250 mg
Vitamin D	400 IU
Vitamin B-6 (Pyridoxine)	10 mg
Vitamin B-12	100 mcg
Calcium	94 mg
Coenzyme Q10	10 mg
Ginger Extract	50 mg
Hawthorn Berry Extract	25 mg
N-Acetyl Cysteine	200 mg
Tumeric Extract (Curcumin)	10 mg
Elecampane Root Extract	100 mg

Free of: milk or milk by-products, egg or egg by-products, fish or fish by-products, shellfish and by-products, tree nuts, peanut or peanut by-products, wheat or wheat by-products, soybeans and soy by-products.

Suggested Use: take two (2) capsules daily as a dietary supplement or as recommended by your healthcare professional.

● **KEEP OUT OF REACH OF CHILDREN.**
● Consult your doctor before use if you are pregnant, nursing or taking medication.
● Keep tightly closed at a cool dry place.
● Store at Room temperature.
● For your protection, do not use if imprinted safety seal under cap is broken or missing.

Manufactured in a FDA Licensed cGMP facility.

REFERENCES

1. Tokarski S, Rutkowski M, Godala M, Mejer A, Kowalski J. [The impact of ascorbic acid on the concentrations of antioxidative vitamins in the plasma of patients with non-small cell lung cancer undergoing first-line chemotherapy]. Pol Merkur Lekarski. 2013 Sep;35(207):136-40. Polish.

2. Cheng TY, Lacroix AZ, Beresford SA, Goodman GE, Thornquist MD, Zheng Y, Chlebowski RT, Ho GY, Neuhouser ML. Vitamin D intake and lung cancer risk in the Women's Health Initiative. Am J Clin Nutr. 2013 Oct;98(4):1002-11. doi: 10.3945/ajcn.112.055905. Epub 2013 Aug 21.

3. Arrieta Ó, Hernández-Pedro N, Fernández-González-Aragón MC, Saavedra-Pérez D, Campos- Parra AD, Ríos-Trejo MÁ, Cerón-Lizárraga T, Martínez-Barrera L, Pineda B, Ordóñez G, Ortiz-Plata A, Granados-Soto V, Sotelo J. Retinoic acid reduces chemotherapy-induced neuropathy in an animal model and patients with lung cancer. Neurology. 2011 Sep 6;77(10):987-95. doi: 10.1212/WNL.0b013e31822e045c. Epub 2011 Aug 24.

4. Neuhouser ML, Barnett MJ, Kristal AR, Ambrosone CB, King IB, Thornquist M, Goodman GG. Dietary supplement use and prostate cancer risk in the Carotene and Retinol Efficacy Trial. Cancer Epidemiol Biomarkers Prev. 2009 Aug;18(8):2202-6. doi: 10.1158/1055-9965.EPI-09-0013.

5. Ito Y, Wakai K, Suzuki K, Ozasa K, Watanabe Y, Seki N, Ando M, Nishino Y, Kondo T, Ohno Y, Tamakoshi A; JACC Study Group. Lung cancer mortality and serum levels of carotenoids, retinol, tocopherols, and folic acid in men and women: a case-control study nested in the JACC Study. J Epidemiol. 2005 Jun;15 Suppl 2:S140-9.

6. Galluzzi L, Vitale I, Senovilla L, Olaussen KA, Pinna G, Eisenberg T, Goubar A, Martins I, Michels J, Kratassiouk G, Carmona-Gutierrez D, Scoazec M, Vacchelli E, Schlemmer F, Kepp O, Shen S, Tailler M, Niso-Santano M, Morselli E, Criollo A, Adjemian S, Jemaà M, Chaba K, Pailleret C, Michaud M, Pietrocola F, Tajeddine N, de La Motte Rouge T, Araujo N, Morozova N, Robert T, Ripoche H, Commo F,

Besse B, Validire P, Fouret P, Robin A, Dorvault N, Girard P, Gouy S, Pautier P, Jägemann N, Nickel AC, Marsili S, Paccard C, Servant N, Hupé P, Behrens C, Behnam-Motlagh P, Kohno K, Cremer I, Damotte D, Alifano M, Midttun O, Ueland PM, Lazar V, Dessen P, Zischka H, Chatelut E, Castedo M, Madeo F, Barillot E, Thomale J, Wistuba II, Sautès-Fridman C, Zitvogel L, Soria JC, Harel-Bellan A, Kroemer G. Prognostic impact of vitamin B6 metabolism in lung cancer. Cell Rep. 2012 Aug 30;2(2):257-69. doi: 10.1016/j.celrep.2012.06.017. Epub 2012 Jul 26.

7. Mooney LA, Madsen AM, Tang D, Orjuela MA, Tsai WY, Garduno ER, Perera FP. Antioxidant vitamin supplementation reduces benzo(a)pyrene-DNA adducts and potentialcancer risk in female smokers. Cancer Epidemiol Biomarkers Prev. 2005 Jan;14(1):237-42.

8. Yang TY, Chang GC, Hsu SL, Huang YR, Chiu LY, Sheu GT. Effect of folic acid and vitamin B12 on pemetrexed antifolate chemotherapy in nutrientlung cancer cells. Biomed Res Int. 2013;2013:389046. doi: 10.1155/2013/389046. Epub 2013 Jul 31.

9. Takata Y, Cai Q, Beeghly-Fadiel A, Li H, Shrubsole MJ, Ji BT, Yang G, Chow WH, Gao YT, Zheng W, Shu XO. Dietary B vitamin and methionine intakes and lung cancer risk among female never smokers in China. Cancer Causes Control. 2012 Dec;23(12):1965-75. doi: 10.1007/s10552-012-0074-z. Epub 2012 Oct 12.

10. Cobanoglu U, Demir H, Cebi A, Sayir F, Alp HH, Akan Z, Gur T, Bakan E. Lipid peroxidation, DNA damage and coenzyme Q10 in lung cancer patients--markers for risk assessment? Asian Pac J Cancer Prev. 2011;12(6):1399-403.

11. Miyamae T, Seki M, Naga T, Uchino S, Asazuma H, Yoshida T, Iizuka Y, Kikuchi M, Imagawa T, Natsumeda Y, Yokota S, Yamamoto Y. Increased oxidative stress and coenzyme Q10 deficiency in juvenile fibromyalgia: amelioration of hypercholesterolemia and fatigue by ubiquinol-10 supplementation. Redox Rep. 2013;18(1):12-9. doi: 10.1179/1351000212Y.0000000036.

12. Cooney RV, Dai Q, Gao YT, Chow WH, Franke AA, Shu XO, Li H, Ji B, Cai Q, Chai W, Zheng W. Low plasma coenzyme Q(10) levels and breast cancer risk in Chinese women. Cancer Epidemiol Biomarkers Prev. 2011 Jun;20(6):1124-30. doi: 10.1158/1055-9965.EPI-10-1261. Epub 2011 Apr 5.

13. Ryan JL, Heckler CE, Roscoe JA, Dakhil SR, Kirshner J, Flynn PJ, Hickok JT, Morrow GR. Ginger (Zingiber officinale) reduces acute chemotherapy-induced nausea: a URCC CCOP study of 576 patients. Support Care Cancer. 2012 Jul;20(7):1479-89. doi: 10.1007/s00520-011-1236-3. Epub 2011 Aug 5.

14. Walker AF, Marakis G, Morris AP, Robinson PA. Promising hypotensive effect of hawthorn extract: a randomized double-blind pilot study of mild, essential hypertension. Phytother Res. 2002 Feb;16(1):48-54.

15. De Backer J, Vos W, Van Holsbeke C, Vinchurkar S, Claes R, Parizel PM, De Backer W. Effect of high-dose N-acetylcysteine on airway geometry, inflammation, and oxidative stress in COPD patients. Int J Chron Obstruct Pulmon Dis. 2013;8:569-79. doi: 10.2147/COPD.S49307. Epub 2013 Nov 22.

16. Tse HN, Raiteri L, Wong KY, Yee KS, Ng LY, Wai KY, Loo CK, Chan MH. High-dose N-acetylcysteine in stable COPD: the 1-year, double-blind, randomized, placebo-controlled HIACE study. Chest. 2013 Jul;144(1):106-18. doi: 10.1378/chest.12-2357.

17. Stav D, Raz M. Effect of N-acetylcysteine on air trapping in COPD: a randomized placebocontrolled study. Chest. 2009 Aug;136(2):381-6. doi: 10.1378/chest.09-0421. Epub 2009 May 15.

18. Moradi M, Mojtahedzadeh M, Mandegari A, Soltan-Sharifi MS, Najafi A, Khajavi MR, Hajibabayee M, Ghahremani MH. The role of glutathione-S-transferase polymorphisms on clinical outcome of ALI/ARDS patient treated with N-acetylcysteine. Respir Med. 2009 Mar;103(3):434-41. doi: 10.1016/j.rmed.2008.09.013. Epub 2008 Nov 7.

19. Panahi Y, Sahebkar A, Parvin S, Saadat A. A randomized controlled trial on the anti-inflammatory effects of curcumin in patients with chronic sulphur mustard-induced cutaneous complications. Ann Clin Biochem. 2012 Nov;49(Pt 6):580-8. doi: 10.1258/acb.2012.012040. Epub 2012 Oct 4.

20. Pinsornsak P, Niempoog S. The efficacy of Curcuma Longa L. extract as an adjuvant therapy in primary knee osteoarthritis: a randomized control trial. J Med Assoc Thai. 2012 Jan;95 Suppl 1:S51-8.

21. Satoskar RR, Shah SJ, Shenoy SG. Evaluation of anti-inflammatory property of curcumin (diferuloyl methane) in patients with postoperative inflammation. Int J Clin Pharmacol Ther Toxicol. 1986 Dec;24(12):651-4.

22. Lim SS, Kim JR, Lim HA, Jang CH, Kim YK, Konishi T, Kim EJ, Park JH, Kim JS. Induction of detoxifying enzyme by sesquiterpenes present in Inula helenium. J Med Food. 2007 Sep;10(3):503-10. Erratum in: J Med Food. 2007 Dec;10(4):739. Lim, Soon Sung.

23. Supplementing with N-Acetylcysteine (NAC) can reduce the need for hospitalization among people suffering from chronic obstructive pulmonary disease (COPD), *European Respiratory Journal* (2003;21:795-8).

Shown in Product Identification Guide, page 507

CHOLESTERIGHT   DS

Benefits:
● Reduces the Risk of Coronary Heart Disease
● Supports Healthy Cholesterol, LDL & Triglyceride Levels
● Natural Formula

What is Cholesterol?
Cholesterol is an important substance made by the liver. It is necessary for the production of hormones, bile that is necessary for digestion, and maintains cell membranes within the body.

Cholesterol moves around in the body is special molecules called lipoproteins. The low density lipoproteins (LDL) bring cholesterol from the liver to the rest of the body. The high density lipoproteins (HDL) carry excess cholesterol back to the liver. Both are critical for a normal functioning body.

However, it is important to regulate lipoprotein levels and rations to maintain a healthy cardiovascular system. Ideally you should maintain LDL cholesterol under 130 and HDL cholesterol at 60 or above. While your genetics plays a big role in determining your cholesterol levels, a diet high in certain fats (mainly saturated and trans fats) is a significant factor as well.

Changing your diet and getting enough exercise is the first step toward maintaining healthy cholesterol levels, but for those who need extra support, nature has several solutions with scientific research showing their benefits.

Why choose Andorra Life?
Andorra Life's Cholesteright fights cholesterol powerfully. The ingredients in Cholesteright are tested to be effective in helping you reach and maintain healthy cholesterol levels - without medication.

A daily serving of Two Cholesteright includes:

800mg of Phytosterols Concentrate:
Phytosterols Concentrate is a source of plant sterols including beta sitosterol, campesterol and stigmasterol, it helps absorb excess cholesterol from the diet so it can be excreted. 800mg is the effective dosage that can help our bodies to fight off the bad Cholesterol and to reduce risk of coronary heart disease.

Policosanol:
Helps to lower LDL cholesterol ("bad" cholesterol) and increase HDL cholesterol ("good" or "healthy" cholesterol) and to help prevent atherosclerosis (thickening of the arteries).

Vitamin C
Is superb at fighting free radicals—one of the main contributors to LDL cholesterol oxidation. It also helps to reduce lipid peroxidation, including that of cholesterol and unsaturated fatty acids, such as EPA and DHA, which make up cell membranes. Vitamin C helps maintain healthy blood vessels, another important factor for total cholesterol health.

Tocotrienols Complex:
In nature, there are eight types of Vitamin E, 4 types of tocopherols and 4 types of tocotrienols. They differ in cellular uptake and bioavailability. Tocotrienols are mainly transported in triglyceride-rich particles such as very low density lipoproteins (VLDLs) and chylomicrons. Tocopherols are mainly transported in low-density lipoproteins (LDLs).

Most importantly, tocotrienols have unique and additional health properties with a much more potent antioxidant effect than the more "common" forms of tocopherols. It is also believed that tocotrienols may help reduce serum cholesterol and reverse arterial blockage in Carotid Stenosis patients. These unique additional health benefits are not associated with the use of alpha-tocopherol by itself.

Continued on next page

Supplement Facts Serving Size: 2 capsules Servings Per Container: 30	Per Serving
Vitamin C	50 mg
Vitamin E (Tocotrienols Complex)	10 mg
Phytosterols	800 mg
Policosanol	10 mg

Free of: milk or milk by-products, egg or egg by-products, fish or fish by-products, shellfish and by-products, tree nuts, peanut or peanut by-products, wheat or wheat by-products, soybeans and soy by-products.

Suggested Use: take two (2) capsules daily as a dietary supplement or as recommended by your healthcare professional.

- **KEEP OUT OF REACH OF CHILDREN.**
- Consult your doctor before use if you are pregnant, nursing or taking medication.
- Keep tightly closed at a cool dry place.
- Store at Room temperature.
- For your protection, do not use if imprinted safety seal under cap is broken or missing.

Manufactured in a FDA Licensed cGMP facility.

REFERENCES

1. Desvarieux M, Demmer RT, Jacobs DR, Papapanou PN, Sacco RL, Rundek T. Changes in clinical and microbiological periodontal profiles relate to progression of carotid intima-media thickness: the oral infections and vascular disease epidemiology study. J Am Heart Assoc. 2013 Oct 28
2. Mathunjwa M, Semple S, Preez Cd. The effect of 10-week tae-bo intervention programme on physical fitness and health related risk factors in overweight/obese females. Br J Sports Med. 2013 Nov
3. Burg VK, Grimm HS, Rothhaar TL, Grösgen S, Hundsdörfer B, Haupenthal VJ, Zimmer VC, Mett J, Weingärtner O, Laufs U, Broersen LM, Tanila H, Vanmierlo T, Lütjohann D, Hartmann T, Grimm MO. Plant sterols the better cholesterol in Alzheimer's disease? A mechanistical study. J Neurosci. 2013 Oct 9
4. Nunes D, Eskinazi B, Camboim Rockett F, Delgado VB, Schweigert Perry ID. Nutritional status, food intake and cardiovascular disease risk in individuals with schizophrenia in southern Brazil: A case-control study. Rev Psiquiatr Salud Ment. 2013 Sep 17.
5. Barbosa SP, Lins LC, Fonseca FA, Matos LN, Aguirre AC, Bianco HT, Amaral JB, França CN, Santana JM, Izar MC. Effects of ezetimibe on markers of synthesis and absorption of cholesterol in high-risk patients with elevated C-reactive protein. Life Sci. 2013 May 2
6. Grattan BJ Jr. Plant sterols as anticancer nutrients: evidence for their role in breast cancer. Nutrients. 2013 Jan 31;5(2):359-87.
7. Tang M, Wu SZ, Gong X. Effects of policosanol combined with simvastatin on serum lipids and sex hormones in male patients with hyperlipidemia. Zhonghua Xin Xue Guan Bing Za Zhi. 2013 Jun;41(6):488-92.
8. Zanardi M, Quirico E, Benvenuti C, Pezzana A. Use of a lipid-lowering food supplement in patients on hormone therapy following breast cancer. Minerva Ginecol. 2012 Oct;64(5):431-5.
9. Becker DJ, Gordon RY, Morris PB, et al. Simvastatin vs therapeutic lifestyle changes and supplements: randomized primary prevention trial. Mayo Clin Proc. 2008 Jul;83(7):758-64.
10. Li JJ, Lu ZL, Kou WR, et al. Beneficial Impact of Xuezhikang on Cardiovascular Events and Mortality in Elderly Hypertensive Patients With Previous Myocardial Infarction From the China Coronary Secondary Prevention Study (CCSPS). J Clin Pharmacol. 2009;49:947-56.
11. Lu Z, Kou W, Du B, et al. Effect of Xuezhikang, an extract from red yeast Chinese rice, on coronary events in a Chinese population with previous myocardial infarction. Am J Cardiol. 2008;101:1689-93.
12. Keithley JK, Swanson B, Sha BE, Zeller JM, Kessler HA, Smith KY. A pilot study of the safety and efficacy of cholestin in treating HIV-related dyslipidemia. Nutrition. 2002;18:201-4.
13. Liu J, Zhang J, Shi Y, et al. Chinese red yeast rice (Monascus purpureus) for primary hyperlipidemia: a meta-analysis of randomized controlled trials. Chin Med. 2006;1:4.
14. Becker DJ, Gordon RY, et al. Red yeast rice for dyslipidemia in statin-intolerant patients. Annals Int Med. 2009 Jun;150(16):830-9.
15. Zhao SP, Liu L, Cheng YC, Li YL. Effect of xuezhikang, a cholestin extract, on reflecting postprandial triglyceridemia after a high-fat meal in patients with coronary heart disease. Atherosclerosis. 2003;168:375-80.
16. Binaghi P, Cellina G, Lo Cicero G, Bruschi F, Porcaro E, Penotti M. Evaluation of the cholesterol-lowering effectiveness of pantethine in women in perimenopausal age. Minerva Med. 1990;81:475-9.
17. Bertolini S, Donati C, Elicio N, et al. Lipoprotein changes induced by pantethine in hyperlipoproteinemic patients: adults and children. Int J Clin Pharmacol Ther Toxicol. 1986;24:630-7.
18. Gensini GF, Prisco D, Rogasi PG, Matucci M, Neri Serneri GG. Changes in fatty acid composition of the single platelet phospholipids induced by pantethine treatment. Int J Clin Pharmacol Res. 1985;5:309-18.
19. Lau VW, Journoud M, Jones PJ. Plant sterols are efficacious in lowering plasma LDL and non-HDL cholesterol in hypercholesterolemic type 2 diabetic and nondiabetic persons. Am J Clin Nutr. 2005 Jun;81(6):1351-8.
20. Law MR. Plant sterol and stanol margarines and health. West J Med. 2000 Jul;173(1):43-7.
21. Bouic PJ. The role of phytosterols and phytosterolins in immune modulation: a review of the past 10 years. Curr Opin Clin Nutr Metab Care. 2001 Nov;4(6):471-5.
22. Bouic PJ, Clark A, Lamprecht J, et al. The effects of [f0992d73]itosterol (BSS) and—sitosterol glucoside (BSSG) mixture on selected immune parameters of marathon runners: inhibition of post marathon immune suppression and inflammation. Int J Sports Med. 1999;20:258-62.
23. Castaño G, Fernández L, Mas R, et al. Effects of addition of policosanol to omega-3 fatty acid therapy on the lipid profile of patients with type II hypercholesterolaemia. Drugs R D. 2005;6(4):207-19.
24. Kassis AN, Marinangeli CP, Jain D, Ebine N, Jones PJ. Lack of effect of sugar cane policosanol on plasma cholesterol in Golden Syrian hamsters. Atherosclerosis. 2007;194:153-8.
25. Gamez R, Maz, R, Arruzazabala ML, Mendoza S, Castano G. Effects of concurrent therapy with policosanol and omega-3 fatty acids on lipid profile and platelet aggregation in rabbits. Drugs R D. 2005;6(1):11-9.
26. Hanai J, Cao P, Tanksale P, et al. The muscle-specific ubiquitin ligase atrogin-1/MAFbx mediates statin-induced muscle toxicity. J Clin Invest. 2007 Dec;117(12):3940-51.
27. King DS, Wilburn AJ, Wofford MR, Harrell TK, Lindley BJ, Jones DW. Cognitive impairment associated with atorvastatin and simvastatin. Pharmacotherapy. 2003;23:1663-7.
28. Fraunfelder FW, Richards AB. Diplopia, blepharoptosis, and ophthalmoplegia and 3-hydroxy-3-methyl-glutaryl-CoA reductase inhibitor use. Ophthalmology. 2008;115:2282-5.
29. Gaist D, Garca Rodrguez LA, Huerta C, Hallas J, Sindrup SH. Are users of lipid-lowering drugs at increased risk of peripheral neuropathy? Eur J Clin Pharmacol. 2001;56:931-3.
30. de Langen JJ, van Puijenbroek EP. HMG-CoA-reductase inhibitors and neuropathy: reports to the Netherlands Pharmacovigilance Centre. Neth J Med. 2006;64:334-8.
31. Chong PH, Boskovich A, Stevkovic N, Bartt RE. Statin-associated peripheral neuropathy: review of the literature. Pharmacotherapy. 2004;24:1194-203.
32. Yang HT, Lin SH, Huang SY, Chou HJ. Acute administration of red yeast rice (Monascus purpureus) depletes tissue coenzyme Q(10) levels in ICR mice. Br J Nutr. 2005;93:131-5.
33. Prasad GV, Wong T, Meliton G, et al. Rhabdomyolysis due to red yeast rice (Monascus purpureus) in a renal transplant recipient. Transplantation. 2002;74:1200-1.
34. Yang HT, Lin SH, Huang SY, et al. Acute administration of red yeast rice (Monascus purpureus) depletes tissue coenzyme Q(10) levels in ICR mice. Br J Nutr. 2005;93:131-5.

Shown in Product Identification Guide, page 507

CIRCULATION PLUS — DS

Benefits:

- Supports Healthy Blood Pressure and Circulation
- Supports Healthy Blood Vessel Function
- Supports Healthy Blood Flow

Circulation Plus addresses three top cardiovascular factors all at the same time: blood pressure, cholesterol, and circulation in just two capsules per day.

Andorra's Circulation Plus helps to:

- Support normal circulation, blood flow, and blood viscosity (thickness)
- Support your body's production of plasmin, which reduces fibrin
- Maintain normal blood pressure levels
- Support optimal LDL to HDL cholesterol ratio
- Support healthy HDL cholesterol levels
- Maintain the health of artery walls
- Provide powerful antioxidant protection to your entire body

Andorra life's Circulation Plus contains the following ingredients:

Nattokinase:

Nattokinase is a natural enzyme. It is one of the best nutrients to keep your blood flow in check. Healthy blood flow means maintaining proper blood thickness or viscosity. Fibrin is one of the most important components of blood viscosity. It acts like a net to stop bleeding and is a normal and necessary part of the healing process when you cut your fingers. Plasmin is an enzyme that helps dissolve and break down fibrin to keep your blood flowing normally. Its production, however, slows as you age. Nattokinase resembles plasmin closely enough so that it actually breaks down fibrin. Plus, it stimulates your body's natural ability to produce plasmin on its own, to help support normal circulation, blood flow and blood viscosity.

L-Arginine:

L-arginine is an amino acid functioning as a building block of proteins. Our body produces L-arginine and it plays a significant role in multiple areas of our physiology and metabolism. L-Arginine significantly affects the cardiovascular system by maintaining the blood vessel vitality by maintaining the natural, healthy functions of the vascular endothelium (vessel lining).

L-Arginine also promotes blood vessel relaxation and flexibility from the nitric oxide created by the vascular endothelium. Without enough L-arginine, the endothelial cells may not create enough nitric oxide to promote optimal blood flow and cardiovascular health. When the immune system does not have enough L-arginine, it could desensitize important white cell components called neutrophils, which is vital in a healthy immune system response.

L-Arginine deficiencies are likely caused by:

- Might not consume and digest enough protein
- Could require more L-arginine in the body due to inherited genetics
- Prone to lower levels of antioxidants and excessive free radicals

Making sure we are getting enough protein in our system and eating the right natural foods to increase antioxidant nutrients can help with the L-Arginine deficiencies.

Vitamin C:

Vitamin C is the most popular single vitamin. Besides taking it to treat colds, it helps to improve conditions of numerous other ailments. As with the other antioxidants, vitamin C helps to prevent heart disease by preventing free radicals from damaging artery walls, which could lead to plaque formation. Vitamin C also keeps cholesterol in the bloodstream from oxidizing, another early step in the progression towards heart disease and stroke. Vitamin C may help people who have marginal vitamin C status to obtain favorable blood cholesterol levels. High blood pressure may also improve in the presence of vitamin C.

Vitamin E:

In nature, there are 8 types of Vitamin E, 4 types of tocopherols and 4 types of tocotrienols. They differ in cellular uptake and bioavailability. Tocotrienols are mainly transported in triglyceride-rich particles such as very low density lipoproteins (VLDLs) and chylomicrons. Tocopherols are mainly transported in low-density lipoproteins (LDLs). Alpha tocopherol is a strong antioxidant that may help reduce serum cholesterol and reverse arterial blockage in Carotid Stenosis patients.

Vitamin K

Vitamin K is a group of structurally similar, fat-soluble vitamins that the human body needs for complete synthesis of certain proteins required for blood coagulation, and also of certain proteins that the body uses to manipulate binding of calcium in bone and other tissues. The vitamin K related modification of the proteins allows them to bind calcium ions, which they cannot do otherwise. Without vitamin K, blood coagulation is seriously impaired, and uncontrolled bleeding occurs. Low levels of vitamin K also weaken bones and promote calcification of arteries and other soft tissues.

Vitamin K is actually a group of compounds. The most important of these compounds appears to be vitamin K1 and vitamin K2. Vitamin K1 is obtained from leafy greens and some other vegetables. Vitamin K2 is a group of compounds largely obtained from meats, cheeses and eggs, synthesized by bacteria.

Ginko Biloba:

Ginkgo biloba has been used medicinally for thousands of years. Today, it is one of the top-selling herbs in the United States. Ginkgo is used for the treatment of numerous conditions, many of which are under scientific investigation. Available evidence supports ginkgo for managing dementia, anxiety, schizophrenia, and cerebral insufficiency (insufficient blood flow to brain).

Although ginkgo is generally well tolerated, it should be used cautiously in people with clotting disorders or taking blood thinners, or prior to some surgical or dental procedures, due to reports of bleeding.

Garlic Extract:

Garlic is an herb. It is best known as a flavoring for food. But over the years, garlic has been used as a medicine to prevent or treat a wide range of diseases and conditions. The fresh clove or supplements made from the clove are used for medicine.

Garlic is used for many conditions related to the heart and blood system. These conditions include high blood pressure, high cholesterol, coronary heart disease, heart attack, and "hardening of the arteries" (atherosclerosis). Some of these uses are supported by science. Garlic actually may be effective in slowing the development of atherosclerosis and seems to be able to modestly reduce blood pressure.

Supplement Facts	
Serving Size: 2 capsules Servings Per Container: 30	Per Serving
Vitamin C (as ascorbic acid)	100mg
Vitamin E (as dl-alpha tocopheryl acetate)	200IU
Vitamin K1 (as phytonadione)	50mcg
Ginko Bilboa Extract	40mg
Garlic Extract	150mg
L-Arginine (as HCl)	400mg
Nattokinase (from soy)	50mg

Other Ingredients:

Gelatin, corn starch, silicon dioxide, magnesium stearate, soybean oil, sucrose, sorbic acid, calcium carbonate, sodium benzoate, ascorbyl palmitate and mixed tocopherols.

Contains Soy

Free of: milk or milk by-products, egg or egg by-products, fish or fish by-products, shellfish and byproducts, tree nuts, peanut or peanut by-products, wheat or wheat by-products.

Suggested Use: take two (2) capsules daily as a dietary supplement or as recommended by your healthcare professional.

- **KEEP OUT OF REACH OF CHILDREN.**
- Consult your doctor before use if you are pregnant, nursing or taking medication.
- Keep tightly closed at a cool dry place.
- Store at Room temperature.
- For your protection, do not use if imprinted safety seal under cap is broken or missing

Manufactured in a FDA Licensed cGMP facility.

REFERENCES

1. Godala M, Materek-Kuśmierkiewicz I, Moczulski D, Rutkowski M, Szatko F, Gaszyńska E, Kowalski J. [Estimation of plasma vitamin A, C and E levels in patients with metabolic syndrome]. Pol Merkur Lekarski. 2014 May; 36(215):320-3. Polish.

2. Otero-Losada M, Vila S, Azzato F, Milei J. Antioxidants supplementation in elderly cardiovascular patients. Oxid Med Cell Longev. 2013;2013:408260. doi: 10.1155/2013/408260. Epub 2013 Dec 29.

3. Moreau KL, Stauffer BL, Kohrt WM, Seals DR. Essential role of estrogen for improvements in vascular endothelial function with endurance exercise in postmenopausal women. J Clin Endocrinol Metab. 2013 Nov;98(11):4507-15. doi: 10.1210/jc.2013-2183. Epub 2013 Oct 3.

4. Laubscher B, Bänziger O, Schubiger G; Swiss Paediatric Surveillance Unit (SPSU). Prevention of vitamin K deficiency bleeding with three oral mixed micellar phylloquinone doses: results of a 6-year (2005-2011) surveillance in Switzerland. Eur J Pediatr. 2013 Mar;172(3):357-60. doi: 10.1007/s00431-012-1895-1. Epub 2012 Nov 29.

5. Cornelissen M, von Kries R, Loughnan P, Schubiger G. Prevention of vitamin K deficiency bleeding: efficacy of different multiple oral dose schedules of vitamin K. Eur J Pediatr. 1997 Feb;156(2):126-30.

6. Holden RM, Booth SL, Tuttle A, James PD, Morton AR, Hopman WM, Nolan RL, Garland JS. Sequence variation in vitamin K epoxide reductase gene is associated with survival and progressive coronary calcification in chronic kidney disease. Arterioscler Thromb Vasc Biol. 2014 Jul;34(7):1591-6. doi: 10.1161/ATVBAHA.114.303211. Epub 2014 May 22

7. Arsenault BJ, Boekholdt SM, Mora S, DeMicco DA, Bao W, Tardif JC, Amarenco P, Pedersen T, Barter P, Waters DD. Impact of high-dose atorvastatin therapy and clinical risk factors on incident aortic valve stenosis in patients with cardiovascular disease (from TNT, IDEAL, and SPARCL). Am J Cardiol. 2014 Apr 15;113(8):1378-82. doi: 10.1016/j.amjcard.2014.01.414. Epub 2014 Feb 1.

8. Ng BH, Karuthan C, Yuen KH. Gopalan Y, Shuaib IL, Magosso E, Ansari MA, Abu Bakar MR, Wong JW, Khan NA, Liong WC, Sundram K. Clinical investigation of the protective effects of palm vitamin E tocotrienols on brain white matter. Stroke. 2014 May;45(5):1422-8. doi: 10.1161/STROKEAHA.113.004449. Epub 2014 Apr 3.

9. Hsia CH, Shen MC, Lin JS, Wen YK, Hwang KL, Cham TM, Yang NC. Nattokinase decreases plasma levels of fibrinogen, factor VII, and factor VIII in human subjects. Nutr Res. 2009 Mar;29(3):190- 6. doi: 10.1016/j.nutres.2009.01.009.

10. Kim JY, Gum SN, Paik JK, Lim HH, Kim KC, Ogasawara K, Inoue K, Park S, Jang Y, Lee JH. Effects of nattokinase on blood pressure: a randomized, controlled trial. Hypertens Res. 2008 Aug;31(8):1583-8. doi: 10.1291/hypres.31.1583.

11. Cesarone MR, Belcaro G, Nicolaides AN, Ricci A, Geroulakos G, Ippolito E, Brandolini R, Vinciguerra G, Dugall M, Griffin M, Ruffini I, Acerbi G, Corsi M, Riordan NH, Stuard S, Bavera P, Di Renzo A, Kenyon J, Errichi BM. Prevention of venous thrombosis in long-haul flights with Flite Tabs: the LONFLIT-FLITE randomized, controlled trial. Angiology. 2003 Sep-Oct;54(5):531-9.

12. Balderas-Munoz K, Castillo-Martínez L, Orea-Tejeda A, Infante-Vázquez O, Utrera-Lagunas M, Martínez-Memije R, Keirns-Davis C, Becerra-Luna B, Sánchez-Vidal G. Improvement of ventricular function in systolic heart failure patients with oral L-citrulline supplementation. Cardiol J. 2012;19(6):612-7.

13. Ashraf R, Khan RA, Ashraf I, Qureshi AA. Effects of Allium sativum (garlic) on systolic and diastolic blood pressure in patients with essential hypertension. Pak J Pharm Sci. 2013 Sep;26(5):859-63.

14. Ashraf R, Khan RA, Ashraf I, Qureshi AA. Effects of Allium sativum (garlic) on systolic and diastolic blood pressure in patients with essential hypertension. Pak J Pharm Sci. 2013 Sep;26(5):859-63.

15. Ried K, Frank OR, Stocks NP. Aged garlic extract reduces blood pressure in hypertensives: a doseresponse trial. Eur J Clin Nutr. 2013 Jan;67(1):64-70. doi: 10.1038/ejcn.2012.178. Epub 2012 Nov 21.

16. Ried K, Frank OR, Stocks NP. Aged garlic extract lowers blood pressure in patients with treated but uncontrolled hypertension: a randomised controlled trial. Maturitas. 2010 Oct;67(2):144-50. doi: 10.1016/j.maturitas.2010. 06.001. Epub 2010 Jul 1.

17. Sobenin IA, Andrianova IV, Fomchenkov IV, Gorchakova TV, Orekhov AN. Time-released garlic powder tablets lower systolic and diastolic blood pressure in men with mild and moderate arterial hypertension. Hypertens Res. 2009 Jun;32(6):433-7. doi: 10.1038/hr.2009.36. Epub 2009 Apr 24.

18. Zhang SJ, Xue ZY. Effect of Western medicine therapy assisted by Ginkgo biloba tablet on vascular cognitive impairment of non dementia. Asian Pac J Trop Med. 2012 Aug;5(8):661-4. doi: 10.1016/S1995-7645(12)60135-7.

Shown in Product Identification Guide, page 507

GOUT SUPPORT   DS

Benefits:
- Tart Cherry to Promote Healthy Uric Acid Levels
- Support Healthy Kidney Function
- Clinically Proven Bospure Boswellia

Key Ingredients:

Tart Cherry Extract:

Tart cherries contain powerful antioxidants called anthocyanins. Anthocyanins give cherries their distinctive red color. Tart cherries are actually one of the richest sources of anthocyanins 1 and 2, which help block pro-inflammatory COX-1 and COX-2.

Cherries have traditionally been used to promote normal levels of uric acid and alleviate the pain associated with this condition.

Bromelain:

Bromelain is an enzyme found in pineapple juice and in the pineapple stem. Bromelain is used for reducing inflammation. Bromelain causes the uric acid crystals to decompose thus relieving you from the pain associated with gout. If taken regularly, bromelain may also prevent repeated gout attacks.

Quercetin Anhydrate:

Quercetin is a flavonoid that reduces high uric acid levels that causes the inflammation and pain during a gout attack. Bromelain assists in increasing your body's absorption and utilization of quercetin, working very well together.

Quercetin is anti-inflammatory, anti-viral, and antioxidant, so there are many quercetin benefits for your health.

Alfalfa Herb Powder:

Alfalfa works by helping to neutralize and reduce high uric acid levels in your body, but it also has natural anti-inflammatory and antioxidant properties, making it a good choice to consume alfalfa for the gout sufferer. What alfalfa does very well is increase uric acid levels in your urine which can help reduce the excess amount of uric acid available to crystallize and give you a gout attack.

BosPure® (Boswellia Serrata):

Boswellia serrata is a tree of family Burseraceae which grows in the dry mountainous regions of India, Northern Africa and Middle East. Boswellia Serrata or frankincense has been used for centuries. This powerful herb is known for providing pain relief from joint inflammation, arthritis and gout.

It is mostly known to help people who suffer from arthritis like osteoarthritis or gout. Boswellia serrata is a natural pain killer since it has active ingredients like boswellic acids (acetyl-11-keto-β-boswellic acid) that are super powerful anti-inflammatories that actually prevent inflammatory white cells from getting into the damaged tissue. They also increase blood supply to the inflamed joints helping repair any damage caused by the inflammation or gout attack and help stimulate the growth of cartilage.

Suggested Use: Take two (2) capsules daily as dietary supplement or as recommended by your healthcare professional.

Supplement Facts	Amount Per Serving	% of Daily Value*
Serving Size: 2 capsules Servings Per Container: 60		
Tart Cherry Extract	500mg	*
Bromelain (2000 GDU/gm)	300mg	*
Quercetin Anhydrate	50mg	*
Alfalfa Herb Powder (Aerial Parts) (Medicago Sativa)	300mg	*
BosPure (Boswellia Serrata) (Gum Resin)	150mg	*

*Daily Value not established.

Other Ingredients: gelatin, maltodextrin, silicon dioxide and magnesium stearate.

Free of: Milk or milk by-products, egg or egg by-products, fish or fish by-products, shellfish or shellfish by-products, tree nuts, wheat or wheat by-products, peanuts or peanuts by-products and soybeans or soy by-products.

Continued on next page

**This statement has not been evaluated by the Food and Drug Administration. This product is not intended to diagnose, treat, cure, or prevent any disease.

- **KEEP OUT OF REACH OF CHILDREN**.
- Consult your doctor before use if you are pregnant, nursing or taking medication.
- Keep tightly closed at a cool dry place.
- Store at Room temperature.
- For your protection, do not use if imprinted safety seal under cap is broken or missing.

Manufactured in a FDA Licensed cGMP facility.

Distributed by: Andorra Life LLC, City of Industry, CA 91748 USA

REFERENCES:

1. Schumacher HR, Pullman-Mooar S, Gupta SR, Dinnella JE, Kim R, McHugh MP; Randomized double-blind crossover study of the efficacy of a tart cherry juice blend in treatment of osteoarthritis (OA) of the knee.; Osteoarthritis Cartilage. 2013 Aug;21(8):1035-41. doi: 10.1016/j.joca.2013.05.009. Epub 2013 May 31.; PMID: 23727631

2. Howatson G, McHugh MP, Hill JA, Brouner J, Jewell AP, van Someren KA, Shave RE, Howatson SA.; Influence of tart cherry juice on indices of recovery following marathon running.; Scand J Med Sci Sports. 2010 Dec;20(6):843-52. doi: 10.1111/j.1600-0838.2009.01005.x.; PMID: 19883392

3. Conrozier T, Mathieu P, Bonjean M, Marc JF, Renevier JL, Balblanc JC.; A complex of three natural anti-inflammatory agents provides relief of osteoarthritis pain.; Altern Ther Health Med. 2014 Winter;20 Suppl 1:32-7.; PMID: 24473984

4. Szczurko O, Cooley K, Mills EJ, Zhou Q, Perri D, Seely D.; Naturopathic treatment of rotator cuff tendinitis among Canadian postal workers: a randomized controlled trial. Arthritis Rheum. 2009 Aug 15;61(8):1037-45. doi: 10.1002/art.24675.; PMID: 19644905

5. Tsui T, Boon H, Boecker A, Kachan N, Krahn M.; Understanding the role of scientific evidence in consumer evaluation of natural health products for osteoarthritis an application of the means end chain approach.; BMC Complement Altern Med. 2012 Oct 30;12:198. doi: 10.1186/1472-6882-12-198.; PMID: 23107559

6. Walker AF, Bundy R, Hicks SM, Middleton RW.; Bromelain reduces mild acute knee pain and improves wellbeing in a dose-dependent fashion in an open study of otherwise healthy adults. Phytomedicine. 2002 Dec;9(8):681-6.; PMID: 12587686

7. Shi Y, Williamson G.; Quercetin lowers plasma uric acid in pre-hyperuricaemic males: a randomised, double-blinded, placebo-controlled, cross-over trial.; Br J Nutr. 2016 Mar 14;115(5):800-6. doi: 10.1017/S0007114515005310. Epub 2016 Jan 20.; PMID: 26785820

8. Cao H, Pauff JM, Hille R.; X-ray crystal structure of a xanthine oxidase complex with the flavonoid inhibitor quercetin.; J Nat Prod. 2014 Jul 25;77(7):1693-9. doi: 10.1021/np500320g. Epub 2014 Jul 1.; PMID: 25060641

9. Choi KC, Hwang JM, Bang SJ, Kim BT, Kim DH, Chae M, Lee SA, Choi GJ, Kim da H, Lee JC.; Chloroform extract of alfalfa (Medicago sativa) inhibits lipopolysaccharide-induced inflammationby downregulating ERK/NF-κB signaling and cytokine production.; J Med Food. 2013 May;16(5):410-20. doi: 10.1089/jmf.2012.2679. Epub 2013 Apr 30.; PMID: 23631491

10. Umar S, Umar K, Sarwar AH, Khan A, Ahmad N, Ahmad S, Katiyar CK, Husain SA, Khan HA; Boswellia serrata extract attenuates inflammatory mediators and oxidative stress in collagen induced arthritis.; Phytomedicine. 2014 May 15;21(6):847-56. doi: 10.1016/j.phymed.2014.02.001. Epub 2014 Mar 22.

11. Ammon HP, Modulation of the immune system by Boswellia serrata extracts and boswellic acids.; Phytomedicine. 2010 Sep;17(11):862-7. doi: 10.1016/j.phymed.2010.03.003. Epub 2010 Aug 8.

12. Etzel R, Special extract of BOSWELLIA serrata (H 15) in the treatment of rheumatoid arthritis.; Phytomedicine. 1996 May;3(1):91-4. doi: 10.1016/S0944-7113(96)80019-5.

Shown in Product Identification Guide, page 507

OPC SUPREME   DS

Benefits:
- Mega Antioxidant Blends of Supreme Ingredients
- Supports Energy and Overall Health
- Anti-stress, Anti-aging

Why we need antioxidants?

Antioxidants are natural compounds found in some foods that help neutralize free radicals in our bodies.

Free radicals are substances that occur naturally in our bodies that attack the fats, protein and the DNA in our cells, ultimately causing different types of diseases by accelerating the aging process. Therefore, antioxidants play an important role in our overall health.

Why choose Andorra Life?

Andorra's OPC Supreme contains 4 types natural's most powerful antioxidants extract.

Grapeseed extract:

Grapeseed extract is an excellent source of specific polyphenol antioxidants called OPCs, which have been clinically proven to fight free radicals and provide many healthy-aging benefits. Grapeseed extract supports production and stability of collagen and elastin, the two proteins which are very important to connective tissue health. Grapeseed extract also supports cardiovascular health and a healthy immune system.

All parts of red grapes contain some proanthocyanidins, including the juice, skins and seeds, and the highest source of small molecule and highly bioactive oligomeric proanthocyanidins (OPCs) are found in red grape seeds. Misleading marketers market their white grape products and lower quality red grape products as red grape seed extracts. For the purpose of dietary supplements, only red grape seed extracts have the overwhelming science behind them.

Vitamin C:

Vitamin C is an essential nutrient for humans and certain other animal species. Vitamin C is a cofactor in at least eight enzymatic reactions, including several collagen synthesis reactions. Ascorbate (a form of Vitamin C) may also act as an antioxidant against oxidative stress, it is required for a range of essential metabolic reactions in all animals and plants. It is made internally by almost all organisms but not humans. Humans absorb Vitamin C from the diet. A major deficiency of vitamin c can cause the most severe symptoms of scurvy.

Andorra Life's Nature C is the new form of Vitamin C, clinically proven superior to standard vitamin c supplements. It contains vitamin C-lipid metabolites for enhanced delivery, absorption and utilization throughout your body. Nature C also improves blood plasma and tissue retention of vitamin C.

Green Tea Extract:

A green tea extract is an herbal derivative from green tea leaves. Containing antioxidant ingredients - mainly green tea catechins (GTC) - green tea and its derivatives are sought-after amongst people who pursue good health. The Indian and Chinese have used the green tea for hundreds of years for a wide variety of health related functions. These cultures have used green tea to treat headaches, aching body parts to improve life expectancy and more.

Pine Bark Extract:

Pine bark extract is made from the bark of the maritime pine tree, which contains naturally occurring OPCs. Pine bark extract is used for its antioxidant properties and multiple anti-aging benefits, such as improving the hearts condition, providing joint support, skin care, eye and vision support, and to ameliorate the condition of chronic venous insufficiency (blood circulation).

Andorra's OPC Supreme brings you:
- Highest quality ingredients: All Natural, Non GMO
- Maximum Strength and science based grapeseed extract formulation for optimal health
- Made in the USA in an FDA inspected and registered facility to meet the stringent standards of US Pharmacopeia (USP) for quality, purity and potency.

Supplement Facts Serving Size: 2 capsules Servings Per Container: 60	Per Serving
Vitamin C	500 mg
Grape Seed Extract	250 mg
Green Tea Extract	50 mg
Pine Bark Extract	20 mg

Free of: milk or milk by-products, egg or egg by-products, fish or fish by-products, shellfish and by-products, tree nuts, peanut or peanut by-products, wheat or wheat by-products, soybeans and soy by-products.

Suggested Use: take two (2) capsules daily as a dietary supplement or as recommended by your healthcare professional.

- **KEEP OUT OF REACH OF CHILDREN**.
- Consult your doctor before use if you are pregnant, nursing or taking medication.
- Keep tightly closed at a cool dry place.
- Store at Room temperature.
- For your protection, do not use if imprinted safety seal under cap is broken or missing.

Manufactured in a FDA Licensed cGMP facility.

REFERENCES

1. Araghi-Niknam M, Hosseini S, Larson D, Rohdewald P, Watson RR. Pine bark extract reduces platelet aggregation. Integr Med. 2000;2:73-77.

2. Summary of data for chemical selection: oligomeric proanthocyanidins from grape seeds and pine bark. National Toxicology Program Web site. Accessed at http://ntp-.niehs.nih.gov/ntp/htdocs/Chem_Background/ExSumPdf/GrapeSeeds_PineBark.pdf on June 6, 2008.

3. Devaraj S, Vega-López S, Kaul N, et al. Supplementation with a pine bark extract rich in polyphenols increase plasma antioxidant capacity and alters the plasma lipoprotein profile. Lipids. 2002;37:931-934.

4. Downs AM, Sansom JE. Colophony allergy: a review. Contact Dermatitis.1999;41:305-310.

5. Fetrow CW, Avila JR. Professional's Handbook of Complementary & Alternative Medicines. Springhouse, PA: Springhouse Corp; 1999.

6. Pine Bark. PDRhealth Web site. Accessed at www.pdrhealth.com/drugs/altmed/altmedmono.aspx?contentFileName=ame0425.xml&contentName=Pine+Bark+ on June 6, 2008.

7. Kushi LH, Doyle C, McCullough M, et al; American Cancer Society 2010 Nutrition and Physical Activity Guidelines Advisory Committee. American Cancer Society guidelines on Nutrition and Physical Activity for cancer prevention: reducing the risk of cancer with healthy food choices and physical activity. CA Cancer J Clin. 2012;62:30-67.

8. McEvoy CT, Schilling D, Clay N, Jackson K, Go MD, Spitale P, Bunten C, Leiva M, Gonzales D, Hollister-Smith J, Durand M, Frei B, Buist AS, Peters D, Morris CD, Spindel ER. Vitamin C supplementation for pregnant smoking women and pulmonary function in their newborn infants: a randomized clinical trial. JAMA. 2014 May;311(20):2074-82. doi: 10.1001/jama.2014.5217.

9. Jubiz W, Ramirez M. Effect of vitamin C on the absorption of levothyroxine in patients with hypothyroidism and gastritis. J Clin Endocrinol Metab. 2014 Jun;99(6):E1031-4. doi: 10.1210/jc.2013-4360. Epub 2014 Mar 6.

10. Mazloom Z, Ekramzadeh M, Hejazi N. Pak. Efficacy of supplementary vitamins C and E on anxiety, depression and stress in type 2 diabetic patients: a randomized, single-blind, placebo-controlled trial. J Biol Sci. 2013 Nov 15;16(22):1597-600.

11. Hong YH, Jung EY, Shin KS, Yu KW, Chang UJ, Suh HJ. Tannase-converted green tea catechins and their anti-wrinkle activity in humans. J Cosmet Dermatol. 2013 Jun;12(2):137-43. doi: 10.1111/jocd.12038.

12. Basu A, Betts NM, Mulugeta A, Tong C, Newman E, Lyons TJ. Green tea supplementation increases glutathione and plasma antioxidant capacity in adults with the metabolic syndrome. Nutr Res. 2013 Mar;33(3):180-7. doi: 10.1016/j.nutres.2013.01.010. Epub 2013 Jan 30.

13. Bogdanski P, Suliburska J, Szulinska M, Stepien M, Pupek-Musialik D, Jablecka A. Green tea extract reduces blood pressure, inflammatory biomarkers, and oxidative stress and improves parameters associated with insulin resistance in obese, hypertensive patients. Nutr Res. 2012 Jun;32(6):421-7. doi: 10.1016/j.nutres.2012.05.007. Epub 2012 Jun 20.

14. Razavi SM, Gholamin S, Eskandari A, Mohsenian N, Ghorbanihaghjo A, Delazar A, Rashtchizadeh N, Keshtkar-Jahromi M, Argani H. Red grape seed extract improves lipid profiles and decreases oxidized low-density lipoprotein in patients with mild hyperlipidemia. J Med Food. 2013 Mar;16(3):255-8. doi: 10.1089/jmf.2012.2408. Epub 2013 Feb 25.

15. De Groote D, Van Belleghem K, Devière J, Van Brussel W, Mukaneza A, Amininejad L. Effect of the intake of resveratrol, resveratrol phosphate, and catechin-rich grape seed extract on markers of oxidative stress and gene expression in adult obese subjects. Ann Nutr Metab. 2012;61(1):15-24. doi: 10.1159/000338634. Epub 2012 Jul 5.
16. Sano A, Tokutake S, Seo A. Proanthocyanidin-rich grape seed extract reduces leg swelling in healthy women during prolonged sitting. J Sci Food Agric. 2013 Feb;93(3):457-62. doi: 10.1002/jsfa.5773. Epub 2012 Jul 2.
17. Kar P, Laight D, Rooprai HK, Shaw KM, Cummings M. Effects of grape seed extract in Type 2 diabetic subjects at high cardiovascular risk: a double blind randomized placebo controlled trial examining metabolic markers, vascular tone, inflammation, oxidative stress and insulin sensitivity. Diabet Med. 2009 May;26(5):526-31. doi: 10.1111/j.1464-5491.2009.02727.x.
18. Yubero N, Sanz-Buenhombre M, Guadarrama A, Villanueva S, Carrión JM, Larrarte E, Moro C. LDL cholesterol-lowering effects of grape extract used as a dietary supplement on healthy volunteers. Int J Food Sci Nutr. 2013 Jun;64(4):400-6. doi: 10.3109/09637486.2012.753040. Epub 2012 Dec 19.

Shown in Product Identification Guide, page 507

Ariix
563 WEST 500 SOUTH, SUITE 300
BOUNTIFUL, UT 84010

Direct Inquiries to:
Telephone: 1-801-813-3000 Toll Free: 855-GO-ARIIX (855-462-7449)
Fax: 801.813.3001

OPTIMALS   DS
OPTIMAL-V™
OPTIMAL-M™

Overall Support For Your Body And Life

Nutrifii Optimals contain a comprehensive array of vitamins, minerals and antioxidants, including nutrients and other beneficial ingredients which university studies have shown to be critical in maintaining healthy cellular function, support heart, eye, skin and lung function, as well as promoting improved bone, muscle and nerve health.[1]

[1]These statements have not been evaluated by the Food and Drug Administration. These products are not intended to diagnose, treat, cure, or prevent any disease.

FOR YOUR VISION

Studies have shown the effectiveness of vitamins and minerals such as beta carotene, vitamin C, E, zinc and lutein in supporting the maintenance of healthy vision.[1]

FOR YOUR HEART AND LUNGS

Both B and E vitamins, plus an arsenal of antioxidants in our special blends, work together to complement your diet in supporting a healthy cardiovascular system. Also antioxidants vitamin C and vitamin E, combined with carotenoids, have been shown to help support healthy pulmonary and respiratory function.[1]

FOR YOUR BONES AND JOINTS

Getting enough calcium in your diet is crucial for bone health. While bones increase in size and mass during your childhood and adolescence, as you age, your bones naturally become more fragile. Nutrifii Optimals support bone and joint health with a signature blend of calcium, vitamin C, manganese, magnesium, vitamin D, vitamin K, and silicon.[1]

FOR YOUR LIFE

The benefits of ensuring that essential vitamins are in your diet can make a very long list. As a few examples, vitamin C plays a vital role in protecting cells and tissues from damaging oxidation. Studies have also shown that it plays an important role in retaining sound cardiovascular function. Vitamin E is a family of essential nutrients that act as powerful antioxidants. Vitamin B is also known for improving mental function, especially in the elderly.[1]

Optimal-V
Supplement Facts
Serving Size: 3 Capsules Twice Daily
Servings Per Container: 56

	Amount Per Serving	%DV
Vitamin A (as beta-carotene)	7500 IU	150%
Vitamin C (as calcium ascorbate, magnesium ascorbate, zinc ascorbate, potassium ascorbate, acerola cherry)	650 mg	1083%
Vitamin D3 (as cholecalciferol)	1000 IU	250%
Vitamin E (as D alpha tocopheryl succinate, mixed tocopherols 50 mg)	150 IU	500%
Vitamin K (as phylloquinone)	45 mcg	57%
Thiamin (as thiamin HCl)	14 mg	900%
Riboflavin	14 mg	794%
Niacin (50% as niacinamide)	20 mg	100%
Vitamin B6 (as pyridoxine HCl)	16 mg	750%
Folate (folic acid)	500 mcg	125%
Vitamin B12 (as methylcobalamin)	200 mcg	3333%
Biotin	150 mcg	50%
Pantothenic Acid (as D calcium pantothenate)	45 mg	450%
Calcium (as calcium ascorbate)	75 mg	8%
Molybdenum (as molybdenum citrate complex)	25 mcg	33%
Inositol	75 mg	*
Grape Seed Extract (95% anthocyanins)	50 mg	*
Bromelain	25 mg	*
Vegetable Blend	10 mg	*

(broccoli leaf and flower, carrot, tomato, beet root, spinach leaf, cucumber, brussels sprout, cabbage leaf, celery leaf, kale leaf, asparagus shoot, green bell pepper, cauliflower, parsley, wheat grass)

*Daily Value (DV) Not Established.

Other Ingredients: Gelatin, rice bran, mica, sodium copper chlorophyllin.

Optimal-M
Supplement Facts
Serving Size: 2 Capsules Twice Daily
Servings Per Container: 56

	Amount Per Serving	%DV
Calcium (as calcium citrate)	75 mg	8%
Iodine (as potassium iodide)	150 mcg	100%
Magnesium (as magnesium amino acid chelate)	100 mg	25%
Zinc (as zinc citrate)	10 mg	67%
Selenium (as selenomethionine, selenium methionate)	100 mcg	142%
Copper (as copper gluconate)	1 mg	50%
Manganese (as manganese gluconate)	2.5 mg	125%
Chromium (as chromium niacinate)	200 mcg	167%
Citrus bioflavonoids	100 mg	*
N-Acetyl Cysteine	50 mg	*
Rutin	30 mg	*
Resveratrol	15 mg	*
Green Tea Leaf Extract (90% polyphenols / 50% EGCG)	20 mg	*
Quercetin	6 mg	*
Hesperidin	6 mg	*
Pomegranate Fruit Extract (40% ellagic acid)	5 mg	*
Choline (as choline bitartrate)	50 mg	*
Alpha Lipoic Acid	50 mg	*
Inland Sea Trace Minerals	1500 mcg	*
Boron (as boron citrate)	1.5 mg	*
Superplant Blend	98 mg	*

(broccoli leaf and flower, carrot, tomato, beet root, spinach leaf, cucumber, brussels sprout, cabbage leaf, celery leaf, kale leaf, asparagus shoot, green bell pepper, cauliflower, parsley, wheat grass, rosemary leaf extract, olive leaf extract, cinnamon bark extract, lutein, lycopene)

*Daily Value (DV) Not Established.

Other Ingredients: Gelatin, rice bran, mica.
Shown in Product Identification Guide, page 507

VINÁLI   DS

Vináli is a comprehensive antioxidant blend of bioflavonoids, vitamin C, and grape seed extract, which studies show are critical for cardiovascular and immune system support, with superior anti-aging and anti-inflammatory properties.

Recommended Use

Take 1 capsule, twice daily, preferably with meals.

Supplement Facts
Serving Size: 1 Capsule
Servings Per Container: 56

	Amount Per Capsule	%DV
Vitamin C (as calcium, magnesium, zinc, potassium ascorbate, acerola cherry, ascorbyl palmitate)	300 mg	500%
Calcium (as calcium ascorbate)	36 mg	4%
Grape Seed Extract	100 mg	*
Citrus Bioflavonoids	10 mg	*

* Daily Value (DV) Not Established.

Other Ingredients: Gelatin, Rice Bran, Natural Color

For Your Heart

Both vitamin C[1] and the anti-oxidative properties of bioflavonoids[2] have been shown to reduce the risk factors associated with cardiovascular disease. In fact, populations that consume higher amounts of bioflavonoids have decreased

Continued on next page

rates of cardiovascular mortality and comorbidity.[2] Grape seed extract also helps protect blood vessels from damage, which can lead to high blood pressure.[4]

For Your Immunity

Time and again both vitamin C[1] and grape seed extract[3] have been shown to improve immunity[3] and are even credited with protection against immune system deficiencies[1].

For Anti-Aging

Research reveals that grape seed extract provides exceptional skin protection from damaging UV radiation.[4] Furthermore, one of the compounds in grape seed extract is proven to promote the skin's elasticity and increase the appearance of youthfulness.[5] The bioflavonoids in Vináli also improve connective tissue structure, helping to diminish wrinkles and enhance the skin's appearance.[6]

For Healing

Many people suffer from swelling, known as edema, following trauma. Studies show that people regularly taking superior grape seed extract, like that found in Vináli, experienced significantly reduced edema to promote quicker healing following surgery or injury.[7]

[1] Katherleen M. Zleman *The Benefits of Vitamin C.* http://www.webmd.com/diet/the-benefits-of-vitamin-c
[2] Denise Slayback & Ronald Ross. Journal of American Medical Association.*Bioflavonoids and cardiovascular health: tea, red wine, cocoa, and Pycnogenol.* http://enaonline.org/files/artikel/75/Bioflavonoids.pdf
[3] Dr. David Jockers. (2013). *Health benefits of grape seed extract.* http://www.naturalnews.com/042417_grape_seed _extract_health_benefits_antioxid ants.html#
[4] University of Maryland Medical Center. (2013). http://umm.edu/health/medical/altmed/herb/grape-seed
[5] Preventative Health Guide. *Grape seed extract and the prevention of chronic dengerative disease.* http:// www.preventive-health-guide.com/grape-seedextract. html
[6] Daniel Gastelu *All About Bioflavonoids.* http://www.supplementfacts.com/BioflavonoidBook.htm
[7] National Center for Complementary and Integrative Health. (2012). https://nccih.nih.gov/health/grapeseed/ataglance.htm

Shown in Product Identification Guide, page 507

Essentia Water, LLC
**22833 BOTHELL EVERETT HIGHWAY
SUITE 220
BOTHELL, WA 98021**

For general inquiries
425.402.9555 or toll free 877.293.2239

Essentia® Water   OTC
Ionized Alkaline Water

PRODUCT CLASS
Water (Ionized Alkaline Water)

INGREDIENTS
Purified water, sodium bicarbonate, dipotassium phosphate, magnesium sulfate and calcium chloride (electrolyte sources added for taste).

DEA CLASS
N/A

INDICATIONS
For hydration of healthy adults.

PEDIATRIC DOSAGE
Pediatrics:
>1 yr.: Consume 32-64 fl. oz./day for rehydration. Take as frequently as desired.

HOW SUPPLIED
20oz, 700ml with Sports cap, 1.0L (33.8oz.) and 1.5L (50.7oz) PET bottles.

WARNINGS/PRECAUTIONS
Notify and use only under medical supervision if experiencing vomiting, fever, and/or diarrhea.

PREGNANCY
Safe for pregnancy/nursing. Category A.

MECHANISM OF ACTION
Hydration. Essentia, an ionized high-pH bottled water, performed an independent randomized, double-blind, parallel arm study on the systolic blood viscosity (SBV) and other hydration biomarkers in healthy subjects. Essentia® demonstrated significantly better rehydration overall when compared with the leading brand of bottled water.

ASSESSMENT
Assess hydration status.

MONITORING
Monitor for dehydration, vomiting, fever, and persistence of diarrhea.

PATIENT COUNSELING
Advise to notify physician if diarrhea continues beyond 24 hrs or if vomiting or fever occurs.

ADMINISTRATION/STORAGE
Administration: Oral route. See label for directions for use.
Storage: Store unopened product in a cool place. Do not reuse plastic bottle. Avoid excessive heat. After opening, replace cap, and refrigerate to chill if desired.
Shown in Product Identification Guide, page 508

Immunotec Inc.
**300 JOSEPH CARRIER
VAUDREUIL-DORION, QC
CANADA J7V 5V5**

For Direct Inquiries Contact:
450-424-9992 Ext 4453

IMMUNOCAL®   DS
Nutraceutical
Glutathione precursor (Bonded cysteine™ supplement)
Powder Sachets

DESCRIPTION and CLINICAL PHARMACOLOGY
IMMUNOCAL® is a specially formulated undenatured whey protein isolate. It holds several patents in the USA and worldwide and is listed by the FDA in the category of GRAS (generally recognized as safe). It assists the body in maintaining optimal concentrations of glutathione (GSH) by supplying the precursors required for intracellular glutathione synthesis. It is clinically proven to raise glutathione values.

Glutathione is a tripeptide made intracellularly from its constituent amino acids L-glutamate, L-cysteine and glycine. The sulfhydryl (thiol) group (SH) of cysteine is responsible for the biological activity of glutathione. Provision of this amino acid is the rate-limiting factor in glutathione synthesis by the cells since bioavailable cysteine is relatively rare in foodstuffs.

Immunocal® is a bovine whey protein isolate specially prepared so as to provide a rich source of bioavailable cysteine. Immunocal® can thus be viewed as a cysteine delivery system.

The disulphide bond in cystine is pepsin and trypsin resistant but may be split by heat, low pH or mechanical stress releasing free cysteine. When subject to heat or shearing forces (inherent in most extraction processes), the fragile disulfide bonds within the peptides are broken and the bioavailablility of cysteine is greatly diminished.

Glutathione is a tightly regulated intracellular constituent and is limited in its production by negative feedback inhibition of its own synthesis through the enzyme gamma-glutamylcysteine synthetase, thus greatly minimizing any possibility of overdosage.

Glutathione has multiple functions:
1. It is the major endogenous antioxidant produced by the cells, participating directly in the neutralization of free radicals and reactive oxygen compounds, as well as maintaining exogenous antioxidants such as vitamins C and E in their reduced (active) forms.
2. Through direct conjugation, it detoxifies many xenobiotics (foreign compounds) and carcinogens, both organic and inorganic.
3. It is essential for the immune system to exert its full potential, e.g. (1) modulating antigen presentation to lymphocytes, thereby influencing cytokine production and type of response (cellular or humoral) that develops, (2) enhancing proliferation of lymphocytes thereby increasing magnitude of response, (3) enhancing killing activity of cytotoxic T cells and NK cells, and (4) regulating apoptosis, thereby maintaining control of the immune response.
4. It plays a fundamental role in numerous metabolic and biochemical reactions such as DNA synthesis and repair, protein synthesis, prostaglandin synthesis, amino acid transport and enzyme activation. Thus, most systems in the body can be affected by the state of the glutathione system, especially the immune system, the nervous system, the gastrointestinal system and the lungs.

INDICATIONS AND USAGE
IMMUNOCAL® is a natural food supplement and as such is limited from stating medical claims per se. Statements have not been evaluated by the FDA. As such, this product is thus not intended to diagnose, cure, prevent or treat any disease. Glutathione augmentation is a strategy developed to address states of glutathione deficiency, high oxidative stress, immune deficiency, and xenobiotic overload in which glutathione plays a part in the detoxification of the xenobiotic in question. Glutathione deficiency states include, but are not limited to: HIV/AIDS, infectious hepatitis, certain types of cancers, cataracts, Alzheimer's Disease, Parkinsons, chronic obstructive pulmonary disease, asthma, radiation, poisoning by acetaminophen and related agents, malnutritive states, arduous physical stress, aging, and has been associated with sub-optimal immune response. Many clinical pathologies are associated with oxidative stress and are elaborated upon in numerous medical references.

Low glutathione is also strongly implicated in wasting and negative nitrogen balance, notably as seen in cancer, AIDS, sepsis, trauma, burns and even athletic overtraining. Cysteine supplementation can oppose this process and in AIDS, for example, result in improved survival rates.

CONTRAINDICATIONS
IMMUNOCAL® is contraindicated in individuals who develop or have known hypersensitivity to specific milk proteins.

PRECAUTIONS
Each sachet of IMMUNOCAL® contains nine grams of protein. Patients on a protein-restricted diet need to take this into account when calculating their daily protein load. Although a bovine milk derivative, IMMUNOCAL® contains less than 1% lactose and therefore is generally well tolerated by lactose-intolerant individuals.

WARNINGS
Patients undergoing immunosuppressive therapy should discuss the use of this product with their health professional. Individuals with the autosomal-recessive metabolic disorder cystinuria, are at higher risk of developing cysteine nephrolithiasis (1–2% of renal calculi).

ADVERSE REACTIONS
Gastrointestinal bloating and cramps if not sufficiently rehydrated. Transient urticarial-like rash in rare individuals undergoing severe detoxification reaction. Rash abates when product intake stopped or reduced.

OVERDOSAGE
Overdosing on IMMUNOCAL® has not been reported.

DOSAGE AND ADMINISTRATION
For mild to moderate health challenges, 20 grams per day is recommended. Clinical trials in patients with AIDS, COPD, cancer and chronic fatigue syndrome have used 30–40 grams per day without ill effect. IMMUNOCAL® is best administered on an empty stomach or with a light meal. Concomitant intake of another high protein load may adversely affect absorption.

RECONSTITUTION
IMMUNOCAL® is a dehydrated powdered protein isolate. It must be appropriately rehydrated before use. Ideally consumed after mixing. If it is premixed for later consumption, it should be refrigerated and consumed shortly after mixing. DO NOT heat or use a hot liquid to rehydrate the product. DO NOT use a high-speed blender for reconstitution. These methods will decrease the activity of the product.

Proper mixing is imperative. Consult instructions included in packaging.

HOW SUPPLIED

10 grams of bovine milk protein isolate powder per sachet. 30 sachets per box.

STORAGE

Store in a cool dry environment. Refrigeration is not necessary.

REFERENCES

1. Baruchel S, Viau G, Olivier R. et al. Nutraceutical modulation of glutathione with a humanized native milk serum protein isolate, Immunocal®: application in AIDS and cancer. *In*: Oxidative Stress in Cancer, AIDS and Neurodegenerative Diseases. Ed.; Montagnier L, Olivier R, Pasquier C. Marcel Dekker Inc. New York, 447–461, 1998
2. Bounous G, Kongshavn P. Influence of protein type in nutritionally adequate diets on the development of immunity. *In* Absorption and Utilization of Amino Acids Vol.II. Ed. M. Friedman. CRC Press, Inc., Fla. 2:219–32, 1989
3. Bounous G, Gold P. The biological activity of undenatured whey proteins: role of glutathione. Clin Invest Med 14:296–309, 1991
4. Bounous G, Baruchel S, Falutz J. Gold P. Whey proteins as a food supplement in HIV-seropositive individuals. Clin Invest Med. 16:3; 204–209, 1992
5. Bounous G. Whey protein concentrate (WPC) and glutathione modulation in cancer treatment. Anticancer Res. 20:4785–4792, 2000
6. Bounous G. Immunoenhancing properties of undenatured milk serum protein isolate in HIV patients. Int. Dairy Fed; Whey: 293–305, 1998
7. Bray,T, Taylor C. Enhancement of tissue glutathione for antioxidant and immune functions in malnutrition. Biochem. Pharmacol. 47:2113–2123, 1994.
8. Droge W, Holm E. Role of cysteine and glutathione in HIV infection and other diseases associated with muscle wasting and immunological dysfunction. FASEB J: 11(13):1077–1089, 1997
9. Herzenberg LA, De Rosa SC, Dubs JG et al. Glutathione deficiency is associated with impaired survival in HIV disease. Proc Natl Acad Sci 94:1967–72, 1997
10. Kennedy R, Konok G, Bounous G et al.. The use of a whey protein concentrate in the treatment of patients with metastatic carcinoma: A phase 1-II clinical study. Anticancer Res. 15:2643–50, 1995
11. Lands LC, Grey VL, Smountas AA. Effect of supplementation with a cysteine donor on muscular performance. J. Appl. Physiol. 87:1381–1385, 1999
12. Locigno R, Castronovo V. Reduced glutathione System: Role in cancer development, prevention and treatment. International Journal of Oncology 19:221–236, 2001
13. Lomaestro B, Malone M. Glutathione in health and disease: pharmacotherapeutic issues. Ann Pharmacother 29: 1263–73, 1995
14. Lothian B, Grey V, Kimoff RJ, Lands. Treatment of obstructive airway disease with a cysteine donor protein supplement: a case report. Chest 117:914–916, 2000
15. Meister A. Glutathione. Ann Rev Biochem 52:711–60, 1983
16. Peterson JD, Herzenberg LA, Vasquez KK, Waltenbaugh C. Glutathione levels in antigen-presenting cells modulate Th1 versus Th2 response patterns. Proc. Natl. Acad. Sci. 95:3071–3076, 1998
17. Tozer RG, Tai P, Falconer W, Ducruet T, Karabadjian A, Bounous G, Molson J, Dröge W. Cysteine-rich protein reverses weight loss in lung cancer patients receiving chemotherapy or radiotherapy. Antioxidants & redox signalling. 10: 395–402, 2008.
18. Watanabe A, Higachi K, Yasumura S. et al. Nutritional modulation of glutathione level and cellular immunity in chronic hepatitis B and C. Hepatology. 24:597A, 1996
19. Witschi A, Reddy S, Stofer B, Lauterberg B. The systemic availability of oral glutathione. Eur. J. Clin. Pharmacol. 43:667–669, 1992.
20. Grey V, Mohammed SR, Smountas AA, Bahlool R, Lands LC. Improved glutathione status in young adult patients with cystic fibrosis supplemented with whey protein. J Cyst Fibros. 2(4):195-8, Dec 2003.
21. Baumann JM, Rundell KW, Evans TM, Levine AM. Effects of cysteine donor supplementation on exercise-induced bronchoconstriction. Med Sci Sports Exerc. 37(9):1468-73, Sep 2005.
22. Chitapanarux T, Tienboon P, Pojchamarnwiputh S, Leelarungrayub D. Open-labeled pilot study of cysteine-rich whey protein isolate supplementation for nonalcoholic steatohepatitis patients. J Gastroenterol Hepatol. 24(6):1045-50, Jun 2009.
23. Karelis AD, Messier V, Suppère C, Briand P, Rabasa-Lhoret R. Effect of cysteine-rich whey protein (immunocal®) supplementation in combination with resistance training on muscle strength and lean body mass in non-frail elderly subjects: a randomized, double-blind controlled study. J Nutr Health Aging. 19(5):531-6, May 2015.

Manufactured by Immunotec Inc.
Tel: 450-424-9992 Ext. 4453
www.immunocal.com

LifePharm

**32 RANCHO CIRCLE
LAKE FOREST, CA 92630
UNITED STATES OF AMERICA**

Phone:
949.216.9600 • 800.400.1287
Fax: 949.216.9601
Email: CustomerService@LifePharmGlobal.com

LAMININE®   DS

LifePharm

RECOMMENDED USE

Laminine® is a dietary supplement intended for anti-aging. Laminine® capsules are to be administered orally. Recommended usage for adults is 1 to 4 capsules daily.
Do not take if you have a known allergy to eggs or fish.
If you are pregnant or nursing do NOT consume this product.

PRODUCT DESCRIPTION

Ingredients & Supplement Facts

Serving size: 1 capsule
Serving per container: 30

	Amount Per Serving	% Daily Value
OPT9 Proprietary Blend	620 mg	*

(Fertilized Avian Egg Extract, Marine Protein, Phyto Protein)

* Daily Value (%DV) Not Established

The proprietary formula in Laminine® is called OPT9™. This formula is composed of three (3) ingredients: Fertilized Avian Egg Extract (FAEE), Phyto Proteins, and Marine Proteins.

Other Ingredients
Laminine® contains the following inactive carriers: Vegetable Capsule, Silicon Dioxide, and Magnesium Stearate.

PRODUCT DESCRIPTION

Laminine contains fertilized avian egg extract, along with a blend of marine and phyto proteins added to make it unique with all essential amino acids.

TECHNICAL DESCRIPTION

The health benefits of the hen egg have been known for centuries. Investigation of the mechanism of the development of an egg after fertilization revealed certain health benefits. In earlier studies, whilst monitoring weight gain of the egg during their development, scientists (1) found very little gain in the first 9-10 days (7.5%), and then a sharp increase (1190% by day 23), suggesting rapid development of a body. The potency of the nutrients available to the fertilized avian egg at this stage has always been assumed to be high, but it was only recently that the chemical structure of the original egg solids for these critical stages, termed blastodermal to protoembryoinic stages was obtained. During the blastodermal to protoembryonic stages of embryogenesis, oligopeptides with molecular weights from 0.5 to 1.0 kD were identified. Oligopeptides are compounds, which have 2 to 20 amino acids joined by a peptide bond. These short chains of amino acids are able to cross the digestive barrier without breaking down or changing the ratios and proportions (2). Peptides are far more potent than other neurotransmitters, requiring only small amounts to produce a profound effect. Additionally, the uptake of the Fibroblast Growth Factor (FGF) (present in the protoembryonic fluid) by the developing avian egg sharply increases between days 11 & 12. These peptides and the FGF have been isolated through a proprietary process precisely at the right stage of development, using a proprietary drying technique to bring the health benefits to humans. The extract is termed Fertilized Avian Egg Extract (FAEE).

In 1929, John R. Davidson, a Canadian Doctor, discovered an extract derived from fertilized avian eggs when they were at a critical stage of development. He used this extract to restore health in his patients. Dr. Davidson spent well over a decade developing and researching his theory. However, when Dr. Davidson passed away in 1943, his research on fertilized avian eggs was not passed on and was soon forgotten. Nearly 50 years later, the pursuit of fertilized avian egg extract was revived by Norway's foremost expert on egg research: Dr. Bjoedne Eskeland. He took Dr. Davidson's original research a step further and hypothesized that fertilized avian eggs contained a special combination of amino acids, peptides and protein fractions that could help provide an incredible array of health benefits when consumed by humans. This included vitamins, minerals and proteins, as well as important defense elements, growth factors, hormones and other biologically active components.

MECHANISM OF ACTION

The bioactive peptides in Laminine stimulate the dormant stem cells to utilize the phyto amino acids and marine protein to repair damaged aged cells.

Drying the protoembryonic fluid before the peptides are "used up" to build organs and bones, allows us to provide this building, repairing, maintenance mechanism of perfectly balanced amino acids, peptides and growth factors to humans.

Nature has devised an extremely versatile mechanism to provide nutrition with miraculous precision to the embryo of living creatures. The precise blend of oligopeptides may be seen as building blocks, without a bridge, or a director. The role of such a director is fulfilled by a growth factor known as the Fibroblast Growth Factor, or FGF, also a bioactive peptide. FGF is prolific in protoembryonic liquid as well as the human placenta. On the 11th day of the incubation cycle of a chicken egg, the chicken tissue shows a steep increase in these bioactive peptides, with the appropriate peptides to form the solid organs and bones (3). A detailed day-by-day study was performed in 1988 (5; 7). Discovered only in the seventies, FGF and bioactive peptides are critical in the development of embryos, including humans.

Bioactive peptides are responsible for building the linings in the blood vessels, creating the infrastructure for the nutrients to flow to critical areas of the brain and organs. Research credits bioactive peptides with the potential to directly affect many neuro disorders because of clear results of the ability of bioactive peptides to affect the growth of neurites (4). Neurites are signal senders (Axons) and signal receivers (dendrites) attached to the brain neurons.

Research (6) has also shown clearly that new cell cultures show a dramatic increase in peptide and amino acid uptake in the presence of FGF. This result gives credence to the hypothesis that embryonic growth is influenced by a very precise mechanism, which combines unique combinations of amino acids, peptides and FGF.

BENEFITS

The beneficial impacts of Laminine® are: positive effects on memory, skin, libido, energy, joints, muscles, stress, sleep and emotional stability.

CLINICAL AND EXPERIMENTAL STUDIES

Wound Healing Activity

In a 1997 study, immediately following surgery, (animal) subjects were randomized to receive either an amino acid diet or a peptide diet for 10 days and the strength of the wound was measured. Wound bursting pressure was found to be significantly higher in subjects receiving the peptide diets than in those just receiving amino acid diets. The authors suggest that dietary peptides may stimulate the production of growth factors such as growth hormone, insulin, or insulin growth factor (IGF-1). They also postulate that it is possible that the amino acid entry into the cell via peptide transporters is more efficient for stimulation of protein synthesis than entry in the form of just amino acids. Other possible mechanisms suggested by the authors for the increased wound healing with peptide versus non peptide diets include stimulation of collagen synthesis, increased

Continued on next page

blood flow to the wound, free radical scavenging, and generation of cytokine profiles which better support wound healing.

Cortisol Study

This study was designed to ascertain the effect of the nutritional supplement, Laminine on cortisol levels in the body. During the experiment, 28 subjects, 16 women and 12 men, between the ages of 36 and 83 took part in the study. Salivary cortisol level content of each participant was measured prior to him/her taking part in the study. This figure is known as "pre-Laminine usage level." The salivary cortisol level was also measured every fifth day three times throughout the study when each participant's intake amount was changed. Overall, study participants' cortisol levels were reduced by an average of 23.7 percent, where 16 started on a higher intake of Laminine—four capsules, twice a day—and 12 started on one capsule twice per day. Participants that initially started on a higher intake of Laminine saw their cortisol level reduced significantly over the first four days as compared to subjects that began the study with a lower usage amount. However, at the end of the study, there was a small, although insignificant, difference in favor of the high initial intake. The total cortisol reduction by the end of the study was 27.3 percent in women and 19.2 percent in men.

While the results of this study are encouraging, additional tests with a larger sample size are needed to validate the findings.

CLINICAL EXPERIENCE

The Effects of Laminine on Normal Blood Sugar Levels

ABSTRACT

A pilot study was undertaken to observe a possible trend of the effects of Laminine, a dietary supplement, on normalizing blood sugar levels in subjects beginning to experience unhealthy blood sugar levels. Subjects' Hgb A1c (hemoglobin marker for blood sugar levels) were assessed at the beginning of the study and after 12 weeks taking two supplements daily. Eleven individuals participated in the study. Three subjects took a placebo, four subjects with slightly higher than normal Hgb A1c levels took two Laminine daily. Four subjects who were on blood sugar lowering medications that had been previously prescribed for them took two Laminine daily.

Although sample sizes were small, statistical evaluation using matched pairs T test showed that the group experiencing slightly higher than normal blood sugar levels were significantly downregulated with supplementation ($p < 0.05$). The unit change in down-regulation of blood sugar was also statistically significant ($p < 0.05$). No significant change was observed in the group that was also taking blood sugar medication with supplements. The results indicated that Laminine supplementation may have supported the normalization of blood sugar levels in individuals who are experiencing higher than normal blood sugar levels. A study is warranted to observe this effect in a larger population. No untoward side effects were observed in either group supplementing with Laminine for 12 weeks.

INTRODUCTION

Although metabolic syndrome was primarily a condition of middle-aged populations, it is becoming a condition of children, adolescents and young adults all over the world.[9] Its criteria are overweight, sedentary lifestyle, and "modern diets" of too much food and poor lifestyle habits. Obesity, which is part of the metabolic syndrome, is the fastest growing health-related problem worldwide. The urgent need for preventive measures aimed at reducing the significantly increased health risk is underscored.[10] The metabolic syndrome is an entity, made up of a cluster of cardiovascular risk factors, which increase the risk of future coronary heart disease, type II diabetes, and stroke.[10] The prevalence varies between countries but runs about 20 percent in most westernized cultures (i.e. 24 percent in the middle-aged population in Europe).[11] Lifestyle has been closely associated with the development of metabolic syndrome, with diet and physical activity identified as two of the most important modifiable lifestyle factors, in this regard.[11]

The physician provides the primary counsel to help turn these conditions around by discouraging high fat diets, overweight and a sedentary lifestyle. Physicians welcome any additional tools they can use besides traditional pharmaceuticals to counteract high cholesterol, high blood pressure, unhealthy blood sugar levels and overweight. Besides encouraging low calorie diets and adequate exercise, certain dietary supplements may support maintaining healthier blood glucose levels. Laminine contains two categories of supplemental ingredients. A substantial amount of egg from a nine-day fertilized egg is high in levels of particular growth stimulants and rare antioxidants. This egg product is not heat processed or heat dried so as to not alter structural changes in the proteins and hormone substances (i.e. fibroblast growth factors). Receptor sites on fibroblast growth factor may stimulate receptor sites on somatic cells or stem cells, encouraging cell responses. Additional marine and plant proteins (also Spirulina) round out the amino acid profile.

METHODS

All participants signed a voluntary consent form and were informed of the dietary supplement's ingredients and safety. The Hgb A1c test was chosen to measure the effects of Laminine on normal blood sugar levels as opposed to other blood sugar tests because of its accuracy. Hgb A1c measures the percentage of hemoglobin (a protein in red blood cells that carries oxygen throughout the body) coated in sugar (glycated hemoglobin) over the previous 60-90 days. Therefore, it is not affected by shortterm glycemic fluctuations (heavy meal, medications, etc.) that may impact the accuracy of other tests. The study lasted 12 weeks (84 days) in order to measure changes in Hgb A1c levels properly. Normal/healthy Hgb A1c levels are 5.6 percent and below, Hgb A1c levels between 5.7 to 6.4 percent may indicate an increased risk for unhealthy blood sugar levels and Hgb A1c levels of 6.5 percent or above may indicate unhealthy blood sugar levels.

Standards for Hgb A1c Levels

	HGB A1C LEVELS
NORMAL/HEALTHY	5.6% or below
INCREASED RISK OF UNHEALTHY BLOOD SUGAR LEVELS	5.7% to 6.4%
UNHEALTHY BLOOD SUGAR LEVELS	6.5% or above

As the difference between healthy blood sugar levels and an increased risk for unhealthy levels can be as minute as 0.1 percent, even a slight drop in Hgb A1c levels proves beneficial for maintaining normal blood sugar.

The dietary supplement, Laminine is a proprietary blend of Fertilized Avian Egg Extract, phyto proteins and marine proteins. Together, this combination provides the body with all 22 amino acids, including both the essential and nonessential required for protein synthesis.

Group A took one placebo in the morning and one in the evening.

Group B took one Laminine capsule in the morning and one in the evening.

Participants in Group C took one Laminine capsule in the morning and one in the evening in addition to their blood sugar medication. All of the participants in Group C were taking their blood sugar medication prior to participating in the study. Participants in this group were on as few as one and as many as three different medications during the course of the study. These medications included insulin and oral medications.

Group A and the two groups receiving Laminine were tested initially at week 0 before administration of placebo or dietary supplement and then at week 12.

Neither diet nor exercise was monitored during the study period.

PARTICIPANT RESULTS

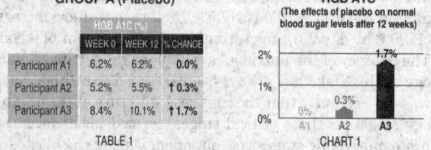

Participants with Unhealthy Blood Sugar Taking no Medication Received Two Placebo Tablets Daily (n=3)

GROUP A (Placebo)

	HGB A1C (%)		
	WEEK 0	WEEK 12	% CHANGE
Participant A1	6.2%	6.2%	0.0%
Participant A2	5.2%	5.5%	↑0.3%
Participant A3	8.4%	10.1%	↑1.7%

TABLE 1

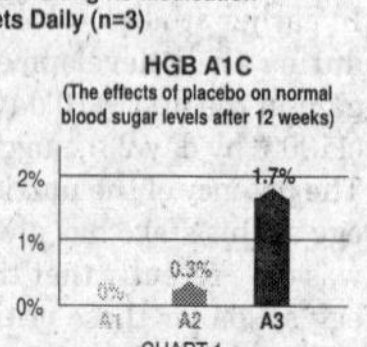

CHART 1

Of the three random participants in Group A, one experienced no change in Hgb A1c levels while the other two saw their levels rise over the 12-week period.

EVALUATION

The four subjects in Group B (at risk for unhealthy blood sugar levels) consuming two Laminine daily were evaluated using two sample matched pairs T test with a significant result (p=0.0273). Using one sample test, only on the differences, there was an average change of 0.475, which was also significant (p=0.0382).

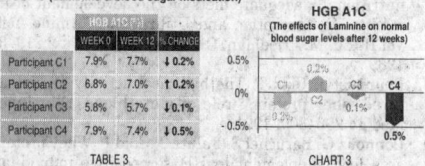

Participants with Unhealthy Blood Sugar Taking no Medication Received Two Laminine Capsules Daily (n=4)

GROUP B (Laminine)

	HGB A1C (%)		
	WEEK 0	WEEK 12	% CHANGE
Participant B1	6.3%	5.8%	↓0.5%
Participant B2	6.4%	5.8%	↓0.6%
Participant B3	6.1%	5.8%	↓0.3%
Participant B4	6.2%	6.0%	↓0.2%

TABLE 2

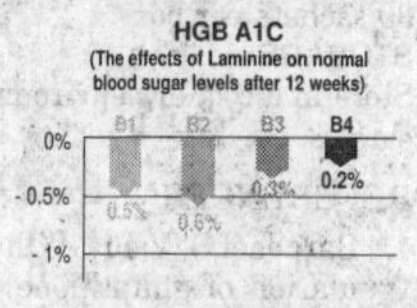

CHART 2

Each of the four participants in Group B (Laminine) experienced a down-regulation in Hgb A1c levels after 12 weeks, with the greatest normalization exhibited in participant B2.

Participants with Unhealthy Blood Sugar Taking Previously Prescribed Medication Received Two Laminine Capsules Daily (n=4)

GROUP C (Laminine & blood sugar medication)

	HGB A1C (%)		
	WEEK 0	WEEK 12	% CHANGE
Participant C1	7.9%	7.7%	↓0.2%
Participant C2	6.8%	7.0%	↑0.2%
Participant C3	5.8%	5.7%	↓0.1%
Participant C4	7.9%	7.4%	↓0.5%

TABLE 3

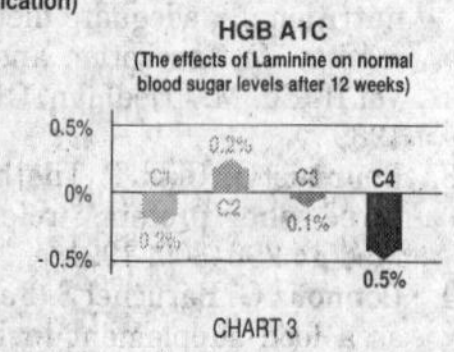

CHART 3

In Group C (Laminine + blood sugar medication), three of the four participants showed normalizing Hgb A1c levels.

STATISTICAL RESULTS

Participants with Unhealthy Blood Sugar Taking no Medication Received two Laminine capsules daily showed statistical significance in blood sugar down-regulation (n=4)

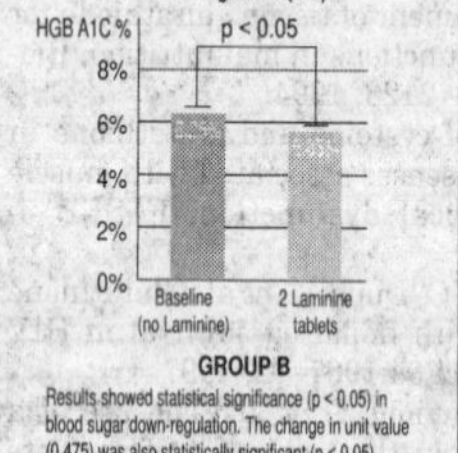

GROUP B

Results showed statistical significance ($p < 0.05$) in blood sugar down-regulation. The change in unit value (0.475) was also statistically significant ($p < 0.05$).

Participants with Unhealthy Blood Sugar Taking Previously Prescribed Medication Received two Laminine capsules daily showed no statistical significance in blood sugar down-regulation (n=4)

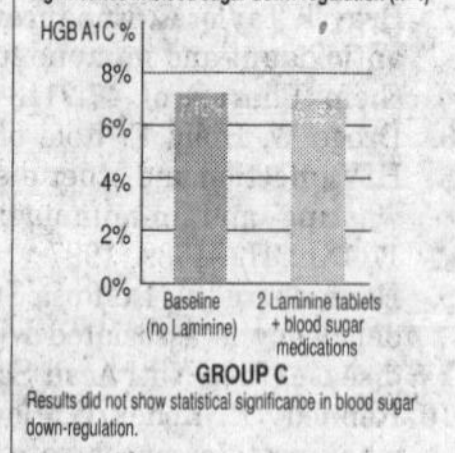

GROUP C

Results did not show statistical significance in blood sugar down-regulation.

The group of subjects who were experiencing blood sugar levels controlled by medication (Group C) consuming two Laminine daily were also evaluated using two sample matched pairs T test with no significant results.

Both statistical evaluations assumed the data was normally distributed. Subject groups were extremely small, but each subject had measurements taken before and after 12 weeks of supplementation, therefore these differences could be evaluated.

CONCLUSION

Metabolic syndrome often shows increasing levels of glucose intolerance. Measures to support persons who are overweight, have sedentary lifestyles and are showing higher than normal glucose levels but are not classified as diabetic, could possibly benefit from taking Laminine. Although the sample size was small, this preliminary investigation did show significant difference between glucose levels before and after 12 weeks of supplementation with Laminine. The difference in the Hgb A1c marker measurements before and after supplementation (a change of 0.475 units) was also statistically significant in Group B, adding additional credence of the noted effect. This preliminary evaluation shows the possibility that this supplement may have a beneficial effect towards helping maintain normal blood glucose in subjects at risk for developing high blood glucose and warrants further study with a larger population.

The statistical evaluation of Group C individuals, taking medicines for normalizing high blood glucose levels, illustrated safety of the supplement as it did not interfere with medication or alter significantly the measurements as a group. Only one subject showed a higher rather than lower effect while on the supplement. Noticeably, one participant in Group C had been taking insulin with Laminine at the start of the study, and per this participant's personal physician's recommendation had tapered off insulin and maintained stable blood sugar levels by the conclusion of the 12 weeks.

All participants in Group B experienced a normalized down-regulation in Hgb A1c levels and three out of the four participants experienced a positive change in their levels in Group C.

It is known that nine-day fertilized avian egg extract that is not denatured with heat processing could retain fibroblast growth factor (FGF) activity. Because growth factors react with receptor sites on somatic cells or stem cells, this activity could support glucose absorption. Laminine also contains fish and vegetable protein, which may have an effect on glucose tolerance when added to the diet continuously. Continuing studies are warranted on clinical effectiveness and also on mechanism of action of Laminine.

J.B. Spalding, Ph. D. retired statistics professor from University of North Texas, Denton, Texas performed the statistical analysis.

Cholesterol Profiles Study

The study was designed to test the effects of the nutritional supplement, Laminine, independently and in combination with Laminine OMEGA+++, on cholesterol, low density lipoproteins (LDL), high density lipoproteins (HDL), triglycerides and blood pressure. There were 15 individuals in the study, broken into three groups of five. This was a double-blind placebo-controlled study that took place over a total period of 12 weeks.

The study took place during two phases. The first lasted eight weeks and included Groups A, B, and C. Cholesterol serum profiles and blood pressure were taken from participants in each group at the start of week one and at the conclusion of week eight. During this phase of the study, participants took a total of four supplements a day—two in the morning and two in the evening. The second phase of the study only included participants from Group A and lasted an additional four weeks, after which time cholesterol serum profiles were measured again. During phase II, participants in Group A consumed eight supplements a day—four in the morning and four in the evening.

During the first phase of the study, results showed that the average cholesterol down-regulation in Group B was about 9.8 percent, compared to 11.5 percent in Group C. Meanwhile, cholesterol levels in Group A actually rose by 1.0 percent over the first eight weeks but normalized by 11 percent between weeks nine and 12. Results for LDL and triglycerides generally followed a similar pattern.

Phase I	CHOLESTEROL*	LDL*	TRIGLYCERIDES*
GROUP A (Placebo/Placebo)	↑1.04%	↓ 9.7%	↑140.3%
GROUP B (Laminine OMEGA+++/Placebo)	↓ 9.8%	↓ 19.6%	↓ 32.2%
GROUP C (Laminine/Laminine OMEGA+++)	↓ 11.5%	↓ 20.9%	↓ 16.7%

* Measured in mg/dl
Percentages reflect average change after eight weeks

Phase II	CHOLESTEROL	LDL*	TRIGLYCERIDES*
GROUP A (Laminine/Laminine OMEGA+++)	↓ 11%	↓ 2.6%	↓ 58.2%

* Measured in mg/dl
Percentages reflect average change after four weeks

Subjects in Group A were also given a subjective survey at the conclusion of Phase II, when they were asked to rate improvement in their joints, memory, skin, sexual drive, muscle tone and strength, stress levels, sleep and emotional wellbeing. Of the five subjects in Group A, only four chose to be a part of the survey. After Phase II, the average improvement in all categories was about 5.75 on a scale of 0-10, with zero representing no change and 10 representing a significant improvement. These are subjective results but nonetheless notable.

	AVERAGE IMPROVEMENT AT WEEK 12
JOINTS	5.8
MEMORY	6
SKIN	5.8
SEXUAL DRIVE	5.8
MUSCLE TONE AND STRENGTH	5.5
STRESS	5
SLEEP	6.2
EMOTIONAL WELL-BEING	6.2

Cholesterol Profiles Study Discussion

Triglyceride levels in Group A normalized by 267 mg/dl or 58.2 percent during Phase II, the most substantial change throughout the duration of the study. However, participants

in Group C experienced the best and most consistent overall results. HDL levels were within normal limits both at the beginning and end of the study for all participants.

Although participants in Group A took double the Laminine and Laminine OMEGA+++ during Phase II, results were not drastic enough to recommend doubling the suggested usage for Laminine OMEGA+++ for all individuals. The down-regulation in LDL was not significant in Group A during Phase II as compared to Group C during Phase I. Nevertheless, for individuals that do have high triglyceride concerns, doubling the intake of Laminine and Laminine OMEGA+++ can yield a normalization in a short period of time.

These data suggest that Laminine OMEGA+++ helps to down-regulate cholesterol, LDL, triglyceride and blood pressure levels (Group B), but when taken with Laminine, the benefits are more significant as a whole (Group C after Phase I and Group A after Phase II).

A study of this size has an estimated margin of error of approximately 30 percent. Therefore, while the results of this study are encouraging, additional tests with a larger sample size are needed to validate the findings.

SAFETY

People with egg allergies should consult a physician before taking Laminine®. Pregnant women should consult with a physician before taking Laminine®.

THE EFFECTS OF IMMUNE+++ AND LAMININE ON NORMAL WHITE BLOOD CELL COUNT LEVELS

INTRODUCTION

The study was designed to test the effects of LifePharm IMMUNE+++, independently and in combination with Laminine on total white blood cell (lymphocyte) count, which includes natural killer cells, B cells and T cells. This was a placebo-controlled study that took place over a 12-week period.

Ten individuals participated in the study, divided into three groups: A, B and C. Group A was on placebo, Group B took only IMMUNE+++ and Group C took IMMUNE+++ in concert with Laminine.

A rise in white blood cell count can be considered indicative of a positive effect of the nutritional supplements. Overall, white blood cell count down-regulated in the placebo group but marked notable increases in Group B and Group C.

METHODS

White blood cell count vacillates daily, even hourly, and can be affected by a number of factors, notably illness caused by bacterial and viral infections. Therefore, all participants in this sample were evaluated during the initial blood draw at week zero and at the conclusion of week 12 and deemed to be healthy and not

NORMAL RANGE (µl)	
TOTAL WHITE CELLS	850 - 3,900
NATURAL KILLER CELLS	70 - 760
B CELLS	110 - 660
T CELLS	840 - 3,060

DETAILS

IMMUNE+++ is a proprietary combination of:
- Opti-Shield Blend: a polysaccharide complex, reishi, maitake and turkey tail mushrooms
- Life-C blend: Pure vitamin C with citrus bioflavonoids and lip id metabolites
- Herb and Botanical Blend: Camu camu, acerola, ashwagandha, sea buckthorn and pomegranate

IMMUNE+++ comes in tablet form with an enteric coating. Laminine is a proprietary blend of Fertilized Avian Egg Extract, phyto proteins and fish proteins. Together, this combination provides the body with the full chain of 22 amino acids essential for cellular health. Laminine is a powder in capsule form.

Group A took one placebo in the morning and one in the evening. This portion of the study was double blind.

Group B took one IMMUNE+++ tablet in the morning and one in the evening. This portion of the study was double blind.

Group C took one Laminine capsule and one IMMUNE+++ tablet in the morning and one of each in the evening. This portion of the study was not double blind. Both the partici-

pants and the administering physician knew that individuals in this group were taking both Laminine and IMMUNE+++.

Subjects in the study ranged in age from 18 to 85 years.

PARTICIPANT RESULTS

TOTAL WHITE BLOOD CELL COUNT

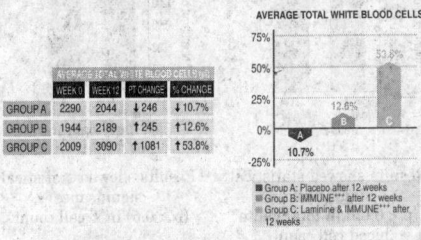

AVERAGE TOTAL WHITE BLOOD CELLS (µl)				
	WEEK 0	WEEK 12	PT CHANGE	% CHANGE
GROUP A	2290	2044	↓ 246	↓ 10.7%
GROUP B	1944	2189	↑ 245	↑ 12.6%
GROUP C	2009	3090	↑ 1081	↑ 53.8%

Overall, Group B (supplemented with only IMMUNE+++ for 12 weeks) noticed a 12.6 percent improvement in total while blood cell count, but Group C (supplemented with Laminine and IMMUNE+++ for 12 weeks) experienced the most significant positive change of 53.8 percent.

B CELL COUNT

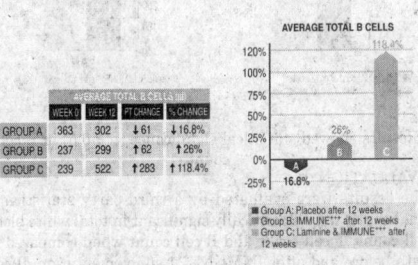

AVERAGE TOTAL B CELLS (µl)				
	WEEK 0	WEEK 12	PT CHANGE	% CHANGE
GROUP A	363	302	↓ 61	↓ 16.8%
GROUP B	237	299	↑ 62	↑ 26%
GROUP C	239	522	↑ 283	↑ 118.4%

The average number of B cells in Group A (supplemented with placebo for 12 weeks) down-regulated by 16.8 percent, compared to more significant, positive changes in Group B (IMMUNE+++ for 12 weeks) and Group C (Laminine and IMMUNE+++ for 12 weeks).

T CELL COUNT

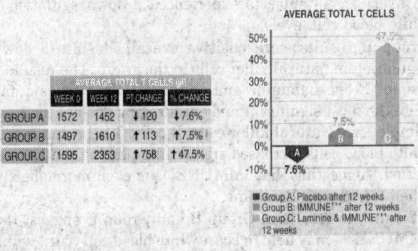

AVERAGE TOTAL T CELLS (µl)				
	WEEK 0	WEEK 12	PT CHANGE	% CHANGE
GROUP A	1572	1452	↓ 120	↓ 7.6%
GROUP B	1497	1610	↑ 113	↑ 7.5%
GROUP C	1595	2353	↑ 758	↑ 47.5%

T cell count in Groups A (Placebo), B (IMMUNE+++) and C (Laminine and IMMUNE+++) followed a similar trend with participants in Group C experiencing the most notable changes.

NATURAL KILLER CELL COUNT

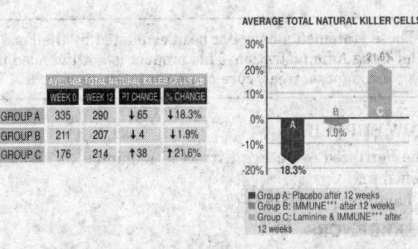

AVERAGE TOTAL NATURAL KILLER CELLS (µl)				
	WEEK 0	WEEK 12	PT CHANGE	% CHANGE
GROUP A	335	290	↓ 65	↓ 18.3%
GROUP B	211	207	↓ 4	↓ 1.9%
GROUP C	176	214	↑ 38	↑ 21.6%

The total number of natural killer cells fell an average of 1.9 percent within the normal range for Group B and 21.6 percent for Group C.

Continued on next page

STATISTICAL RESULTS

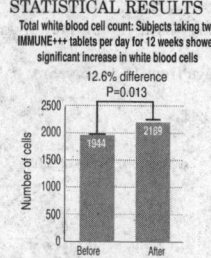

Total white blood cell count: Subjects taking two IMMUNE+++ tablets per day for 12 weeks showed significant increase in white blood cells

12.6% difference
P=0.013

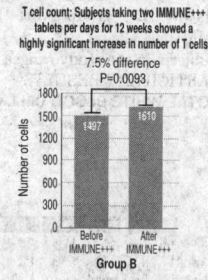

T cell count: Subjects taking two IMMUNE+++ tablets per days for 12 weeks showed a highly significant increase in number of T cells

7.5% difference
P=0.0093

Results showed statistical significance (p < 0.05) in total white blood cell count.

Subjects taking two IMMUNE+++ tablets and two Laminine capsules per day for 12 weeks compared to Placebo

124% difference
P=0.0139

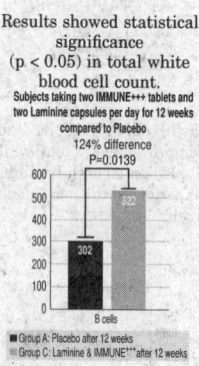

Results showed statistical significance (p < 0.5) in T cell count.

Subjects taking both IMMUNE+++ with Laminine showed greater results than only taking IMMUNE+++

61.25% difference
P=0.0059

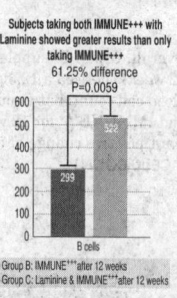

■ Group A: Placebo after 12 weeks
■ Group C: Laminine & IMMUNE+++ after 12 weeks

Results showed statistical significance (p < 0.5) in B cell count.

EVALUATION

The results were evaluated by a third-party statistician. The results were statistically significant in total white blood cell count, T cell count and B cell count when compared to data before and after IMMUNE+++ supplementation. B cell count was shown to be statistically significant when comparing Group A to Group C and Group B to Group C.

Both statistical evaluations assumed the data was normally distributed. Subject groups were small, but each subject had measurements taken before and after 12 weeks of supplementation; therefore, these differences could be evaluated.

CONCLUSION

Expectedly, individual results in Group A were mixed, but on average, all subjects experienced a downregulation in white blood cell levels.

Group B results were positive overall, despite a down-regulation in natural killer cells in the group. The results in Group C (one Laminine and one IMMUNE+++twice a day) were the most significant and encouraging despite the small sample size. Natural killer cells, B cells, T cells and overall white blood cells increased significantly during the 12-week period, suggesting that IMMUNE+++ is even more effective when taken with Laminine.

Overall, the results in Group B and Group C suggest that IMMUNE+++ may help to boost white blood cell count within the normal range. When combined with Laminine, IMMUNE+++ boosts the count within the normal range and is even more effective at supporting healthy immune function in individuals at a variety of ages and genders.

J.B. Spalding, Ph. D. retired statistics professor from University of North Texas, Denton, Texas performed the statistical analysis.

These statements have not been evaluated by the Food and Drug Administration. This product is not intended to diagnose, treat, cure or prevent any disease.

HOW SUPPLIED

The Fertilized Avian Egg Extract in Laminine® is also contained in:

Laminine® OMEGA+++

REFERENCES

1. Roberts, Pamela R, et al. Nutrition Vol. 14, No. 3, 1998
2. Arvanitakis, Constantine. Am. Jour. of Physiology, Vol. 231, No. 1, July 1976.
3. Joseph-Silverstein, Jacquelyn, et al (June 1989) Basic Fibroblast Growth Factor in the Chick Embryo: Immunolocalization to Striated Muscle Cells and Their Precursors. The Journal of Cell Biology, 108: 2459-2466.
4. Hatten, M. E., et al (1988) In Vitro Neurite Extension by Granule Neurons is Dependent upon Astroglial-Derived Fibroblast Growth Factor. Developmental Biology, 125:280-289.
5. Seed, Jennifer, et al (1988) Fibroblast Growth Factor Levels in the Whole Embryo and Limb Bud during Chick Development. Developmental Biology, 128:50-57.
6. Gospodarowicz, D, et al (1986) Molecular and Biological Characterization of Fibroblast Growth Factor, an Angiogenic Factor Which Also Controls the Proliferation and Differentiation of Mesoderm and Neuroectoderm Derived Cells. Cell Differentiation, 19: 1-17.
7. Seed, Jennifer, et al (1988) Fibroblast Growth Factor Levels in the Whole Embryo and Limb Bud during Chick Development. Developmental Biology, 128:50-57.
8. Jin, Kunlin, et al (Dec 2005) FGF-2 Promotes Neurogenesis and Neuroprotection and Prolongs Survival in a Transgenic Mouse Model of Huntington's disease, Vol. 102.
9. Ekelund U, Anderssen SA, Froberg K, Sardinha LB, Andersen LB, Brage S, et al. (2007) Independent associations of physical activity and cardiorespiratory fitness with metabolic risk factors in children: the European youth heart study. Diabetologia 50: 1832–1840.
10. Healy GN, Matthews CE, Dunstan DW, Winkler EA, Owen N (2011) Sedentary time and cardio-metabolic biomarkers in US adults: NHANES 2003–06. Eur Heart J 32: 590–597.
11. Elin Ekblom-Bak, Annika Rosengren, Mattias Hallsten, Göran Bergström, and Mats Börjesson. Cardiorespiratory Fitness, Sedentary Behaviour and Physical Activity Are Independently Associated with the Metabolic Syndrome, Results from the SCAPIS Pilot Study. PLoS One. 2015; 10(6): e0131586.

Shown in Product Identification Guide, page 509

NSE Products, Inc. (Pharmanex)

75 WEST CENTER STREET
PROVO, UT 84601

For Information and Product Support:
Phone: 1-800-487-1000
Website: www.nuskin.com

ageLOC R²   DS

Description

ageLOC® R² is delivered as alternating Day and Night formulas to help balance two interconnected aspects of youthfulness. ageLOC R² Day resets youthful gene expression related to cellular energy production while ageLOC R² Night resets youthful gene expression related to cellular purification. Together, ageLOC R² targets aging at its source to promote physical vigor, mental acuity, and sexual health, as well as to support the body's ability to neutralize and remove cellular waste and metabolic byproducts.*

Benefits

ageLOC R² Day and Night were developed to address cellular energy production (primarily mitochondrial functions) and cellular purification mechanisms. The cellular mechanisms of energy production and cellular purification are mutually supporting. ageLOC R² Day and Night work synergistically by targeting both mechanisms of cellular energy production and mechanisms of cellular purification.*

Ingredients

Each ageLOC R² Day capsule provides 378 mg of a proprietary blend of Cordyceps Cs-4 Mushroom Mycelia (*Cordyceps sinensis* [Berk.] Sacc.), Pomegranate (*Punica granatum*) Fruit Extract, and Pharmanex Asian Ginseng Rb1 (*Panax ginseng*) Root Extract. Each ageLOC R² Night capsule provides 225 mg of a proprietary blend of Grape (*Vitis vinifera L.*) Seed Extract, Red Orange (*Citrus sinensis*) Fruit Extract, and Broccoli (*Brassica oleracea italica*) Seed Extract.

Recommended Use

Take six (6) ageLOC R² Day capsules in the morning, and take two (2) ageLOC R² Night capsules in the evening. May be taken with or without meals.

Warnings

Keep this product out of reach of children. Consult a physician prior to use if pregnant or lactating, or taking a prescription medication. Discontinue use of this product 2 weeks prior to and after surgery. Discontinue use and consult a physician if any adverse reactions occur. May contain soy and/or peanuts.

How Supplied

One box of ageLOC R² delivers 180 capsules of ageLOC R² Day, and 60 capsules of ageLOC R² Night, providing a 30 day supply of each.

*These statements have not been evaluated by the Food and Drug Administration. This product is not intended to diagnose, treat, cure or prevent any disease.

---

ageLOC® TR90™   DS

Description

The ageLOC TR90 program is a weight management system which consists of three dietary supplements, protein shake formulations, a simple eating plan, and physical activity recommendations. The ageLOC TR90 product regimen includes a powder mix-in beverage supplement known as ageLOC TR90 JumpStart, two encapsulated dietary supplements known as ageLOC TR90 Fit and ageLOC TR90 Control, and ageLOC TR90 TrimShakes formulated to meet specific protein requirements. ageLOC TR90 JumpStart is used during the first 15 days of the program. The eating plan provides optimal portions of protein, fruits, vegetables, and complex carbohydrates based on hand sizes so intake is proportional to an individual's body size. The central design of the eating plan is to create a caloric deficit without creating a protein deficit, with the intent to minimize diet-induced lean muscle loss, and increase healthy metabolism. Emerging weight management research indicates that most westernized diets consume adequate daily protein but only with the largest meal of the day (typically dinner). Key points of the TR90 eating plan include: 1) equal distribution of protein intake among each of three daily meals (approximately 30 grams of protein per meal), 2) limiting intake of excess carbohydrates including grains, pastas, and breads, 3) consuming small healthy snacks two to three times each day, 4) consuming large portion sizes of fruits and vegetables to remain in line with recommended intakes of 5-9 servings of fruits and vegetables per day. Exercise recommendations strive for regular physical activity from aerobic and resistance training.

Benefits

ageLOC TR90 is a program designed to create a healthy body transformation. The ageLOC TR90 program helps support the maintenance of lean muscle, increase healthy metabolism, and improve mood and mindset while reducing cravings. The TR90 dietary supplements were formulated using typical dietary supplement methodologies as well as gene expression research. ageLOC TR90 supplements, including ageLOC TR90 JumpStart, Control and Fit, provide ingredients designed to support appetite control, healthy metabolism, and lean muscle to optimize weight management.* The ageLOC TR90 TrimShakes provide high-quality protein and help reduce calories and control appetite.* The ageLOC TR90 eating plan and exercise programs are complementary to the benefits of the supplements and are essential to the program.

Ingredients

Each ageLOC TR90 JumpStart packet provides 2000 mg of Prickly Pear (Opuntia ficus-indica) fruit powder, 177 mg of Satiereal® Saffron (Crocus sativus L.) stigma extract, 150 mg of Pomegranate (Punica granatum) fruit extract, and 125 mg of Red Orange (Citrus sinensis) fruit extract. Each ageLOC TR90 Fit capsule provides 83.3 mg of Red Orange (Citrus sinensis) fruit extract, 83.3 mg of Brown Seaweed (Undaria pinnatifida) Extract, 50 mg of Green Tea (Camellia sinensis) leaf extract, 33.3 mg of Citrus Bioflavonoids (from citrus fruits), 25 mg of Quercetin (from Onion (Allium cepa alliaceae) bulb extract), and 16.7 mg of Cayenne (Capsicum annum L.) fruit powder. Each ageLOC TR90 Control capsule provides 187.5 mg of Cocoa (Theobroma Cacao) bean powder, 75 mg of Tart Cherry (Prunus cerasus) fruit powder, 62.5 mg of Pomegranate (Punica granatum) fruit extract, and 107.5 mg of Green Tea (Camellia sinensis) leaf extract with added L-Theanine. Each TR90 TrimShake serving provides 15 grams of Protein, 0 grams of Total fat, and 10-11 grams of Total Carbohydrate including 3 grams of dietary fiber and 6 grams of sugar.

Recommended Use

Exact dosage varies from market to market. Please consult local labels for instructions.

ageLOC TR90 Fit and TR90 Control usage instructions:

ageLOC TR90 Fit and ageLOC TR90 Control should be taken 15 to 20 minutes prior to meals, per label instructions. 90 count bottles recommend taking one (1) capsule 15 to 20 minutes before meals three times per day, while 120 count bottles recommend taking two (2) capsules 15 to 20 minutes before meals twice per day.

ageLOC TR90 JumpStart usage instructions:

Mix packet with 2-8 ounces (60-240 mL) of water or other beverage. Drink each morning for the first 15 days of the ageLOC TR90 program.

ageLOC TR90 TrimShakes:

ageLOC TR90 TrimShakes can be taken one or two times per day. Each serving provides one portion of six daily portions of protein.

Warnings

Keep out of reach of children. Pregnant or lactating women and people with known medical conditions should consult a physician prior to use. Discontinue use and consult a physician if any adverse reactions occur. If you have any questions or concerns or any medical conditions you should consult your physician prior to starting any diet or change in exercise program.

*These statements have not been evaluated by the Food and Drug Administration. This product is not intended to diagnose, treat, cure or prevent any disease.

---

ageLOC® YOUTH   DS

Description

ageLOC® Youth is a formula to provide enhanced nutritional benefits based on proprietary gene expression insights into healthy aging, and promote the years an individual can enjoy life being physically active, energetic, and healthy.* It works by modulating the body's Aging Defense Mechanisms (ADMs) which result in broad spectrum, systemic youth preservation benefits.*

ADMs are mechanisms which function to maintain resistance to internal and external stressors known to accelerate aging (aging aggressors). These mechanisms are active in all tissues, but require healthy gene expression to function youthfully. ADMs are classified into six categories, including mechanisms which support: antioxidant defense/protection, detoxification and stress response, DNA protection/repair and apoptosis, regulation of inflammation, tissue renewal, and regulation of metabolism. ADMs make up a network of mechanisms which work synergistically to defend against the effects of aging aggressors, resulting in systemic youth preservation benefits, for broad spectrum health.

A unique formulation approach reviews independent scientific research, and screens a library of ingredients for compounds that positively influence gene expression related to ADMs. Although individual ageLOC Youth ingredients are found in the diets of some distinct populations, it is the combination of ingredients that is not likely to be achieved solely through dietary intake of any one population.

Benefits

ageLOC Youth modulates Aging Defense Mechanisms (ADMs) resulting in systemic youth preservation benefits, including:*

Cellular Health
• Reinforces the body's protection and repair mechanisms at the cellular level
• Helps balance healthy cellular response. Disruption of cellular response can spark a cascade of other aging effects
• Positively modulates systemic cytokine responses
• Supports cellular DNA damage protection/repair
• Provides cellular antioxidant protection

Brain Health
• Supports healthy brain structure and function
• Promotes cognition and memory
• Promotes sense of wellbeing and healthy mood

Heart Health
• Sustains overall cardiovascular health
• Promotes blood vessel integrity/elasticity, essential for healthy blood circulation
• Supports normal blood glucose control
• Supports healthy blood pressure regulation

Metabolic Health
• Supports healthy lipid metabolism
• Supports normal glucose metabolism

Skin Health
• Promotes optimal skin barrier function and protection
• Maintains optimal skin health

Bone Health
• Boosts bone health and supports bone structure and integrity

Joint Health
• Supports healthy joints and promotes healthy joint fluidity

Eye Health
• Provides ingredients important for healthy eye composition and protection
• Promotes eye health and supports healthy vision

Physical Performance
• Enables optimal physical performance

Immune Health
• Promotes healthy immune function and response
• Supports a healthy immune system

Ingredients

Each ageLOC Youth capsule provides 250 IU of vitamin D3, 10 mcg of vitamin K2, 50 mg of citrus bioflavonoids including hesperidin and naringin, 33.33 mg of purple corn, 25 mg of alpha lipoic acid, 18.75 mg of quercetin, 12.5 mg of d-limonene, 9.375 mg of rosemary extract including carnosic acid, 7.5 mg of resveratrol, 7.5 mg of coenzyme Q10, 1.25 mg of lycopene, 1 mg of lutein, 0.25 mg of astaxanthin, and 527.5 mg of ultra-pure fish oil concentrate with 150 mg of EPA and 100 mg of DHA.

Recommended Use

Take two capsules twice daily with morning and evening meals.

Warnings

Keep out of reach of children. Consult a physician prior to use if pregnant or lactating, or using prescription medication. Contains fish derived ingredients (anchovies, sardines, mackerel). Discontinue use of this product 2 weeks prior to and after surgery. Discontinue use and consult a physician if any adverse reactions occur.

How Supplied

30 day supply, 120 count bottle.

*These statements have not been evaluated by the Food and Drug Administration. This product is not intended to diagnose, treat, cure or prevent any disease.

---

g3   DS

Description

g3 is a proprietary, nutrient-rich juice from the prized Gâc superfruit of Southern Asia, blended with three additional superfruits— Chinese lycium, Siberian pineapple, and Cili fruit. g3 has a unique red-orange color which signifies its carotenoid content (predominantly lycopene and beta-carotene in unique lipocarotene delivery form). It has a refreshing taste, and is suitable for the whole family. Unlike typical fruit juices, it is a unique blend of fruits selected for their extraordinary antioxidant and nutritional content, and backed by scientific data. Each of the four superfruits are impressive in their own right, yet Gâc is one of the most unique and beneficial of these superfruits.

• Gâc (*Momordica cochinchinnensis*) is a large red fruit and is prized by natives of Southern Asia. Modern research shows Gâc naturally contains concentrated amounts of a unique, highly bioavailable form of carotenoids in a matrix of fatty acids (termed *lipocarotenes*). Owing to the use and harvesting practices of Gâc, the indigenous people of Southern Asia have dubbed Gâc as *the fruit from heaven*.
• Siberian Pineapple (*Hippophae rhamnoides*) or Sea Buckthorn is a small shrub with pea-size orange or yellow berries, and has a 2000-year history of traditional use in Siberia, Tibet, China, and Europe.
• Chinese lycium (*Lycium barbarum L.*), also known as wolfberry, is a perennial shrub with small red fruits that has over 2000 years of traditional Chinese medicine history.
• Cili fruit (*Rosa roxburghii*) is the fruit of a deciduous shrub, also known as Chestnut Rose; the fruit is yellow-orange with a spiny exterior.

In addition to scientific substantiation of the antioxidant and nutritional content of the four superfruits, the formulators of g3 (Pharmanex) have used a scientific method which leverages light physics— to confirm the unique absorptive characteristics of Gâc fruit lipocarotenes within g3 juice. The BioPhotonic Scanner non-invasively measures carotenoid levels in living tissue, providing an immediate indication of a person's overall antioxidant status. By placing the palm of one's hand in front of the scanner's safe, low energy blue light, one can obtain a reading of their carotenoid antioxidant levels; this reading known as the skin carotenoid score (SCS). The technology of the BioPhotonic Scanner is based on an optical method known as Resonant Raman Spectroscopy, which has been used for decades in research laboratories, but recently adapted for measurements in living tissues. To determine the bioavailability of lipocarotenes in g3, a clinical study was conducted comparing skin carotenoid scores over 2 months of g3 consumption. g3 was found to increase SCS by approximately 9000 points after 8 weeks of consuming 6 oz. daily. Contact Nu Skin for more information regarding research that validates g3.

Benefits
• Helps support cellular rejuvenation*
• Helps slow the common effects of aging through DNA protection*
• Improves Skin Carotenoid Score (SCS) as verified by the Pharmanex BioPhotonic Scanner*
• Fortifies antioxidant defense against cellular free radical damage*
• Supports healthy skin and eyes*
• Supports healthy immune function*
• Supports prostate health*

Ingredients

Water, Proprietary Juice Blend (Gâc, Siberian Pineapple, Chinese Lycium, Cili), Grape Concentrate, Pear Concentrate, Apple Concentrate, Acerola, Natural Flavor, Citric Acid, Ascorbic Acid, Sodium Benzoate, Xanthan Gum, Pectin.

Recommended Use

g3 bottle: Shake well to ensure proper mixture of lipocarotenes. Drink 1-3 oz. (30-90 mL) with morning and evening meal. For optimal results, take with ageLOC Youth. Refrigerate up to 14 days after opening. Prior to opening– store in a cool, dark place.

g3 pouch: Shake before using. Drink the entire contents of the pouch anytime, anyplace. For optimal results, take with ageLOC Youth. Prior to opening– store in a cool, dark place.

*These statement shave not been evaluated by the Food and Drug Administration. This product is not intended to diagnose treat, cure or prevent any disease.

LIFEPAK® ANTI-AGING FORMULA   DS

Description

LifePak® is a comprehensive nutritional wellness program, delivering the optimum types and amounts of vitamins, minerals, trace elements, antioxidants, and phytonutrients for general health and well-being. LifePak addresses all common nutrient deficiencies, and provides key anti-aging nutrients that promote cellular protection. Additionally, it supports cardiovascular health, bone nutrition, nutrient metabolism, and normal immune function.*

Benefits

Addresses common nutrient deficiencies: LifePak was formulated in consideration of typical dietary intakes, and when consumed with a typical diet ensures meeting the RDAs for all vitamins and minerals.

Provides ingredients that promote cellular protection: LifePak, with its broad spectrum of vitamins and phytonutrients, is optimally formulated to provide comprehensive protection of cellular and mitochondrial DNA as well as the body's lipids and proteins.

Supports cardiovascular health: LifePak addresses many aspects of cardiovascular health by offering the recommended amounts of key cardiovascular nutrients, including vitamin E, vitamin C, carotenoids, flavonoids, B vitamins, magnesium, and calcium.

Supports bone nutrition: LifePak addresses bone health with a comprehensive array of bone nutrients, including nutritionally significant amounts of calcium, magnesium, and vitamin D.

Continued on next page

Supports nutrient metabolism: LifePak provides nutritionally meaningful amounts of vitamins and minerals that promote normal glucose metabolism and insulin function, including chromium, zinc, and antioxidants.

Supports normal immune function: LifePak provides nutritionally significant amounts of vitamins A, C, E, and B₆, zinc and selenium. Since the immune system depends on adequate nutritional status of these nutrients, it is expected that LifePak effectively promotes healthy immune function in multiple ways. Deficiency of single nutrients results in altered immune responses, which can be observed even when the deficiency state is relatively mild.

Protects cells with a powerful antioxidant network: LifePak contains more than 40 antioxidants for cell health, including both water- and fat-soluble antioxidants. As part of this antioxidant support, LifePak provides a balanced carotenoid combination in amounts similar to those provided by diets high in fruits and vegetables.

Pharmanex BioPhotonic Scanner:
The BioPhotonic Scanner program may be used in conjunction with LifePak usage. Nu Skin has licensed a scientifically validated method to non-invasively measure the levels of carotenoids present in the skin. These fat-soluble carotenoids have been shown in third party literature to be a reliable indicator of overall antioxidant status. The BioPhotonic Scanner can be used to track overall antioxidant status over time as well as track the effect of LifePak on an individual's skin carotenoid status.

Ingredients
LifePak provides an optimal blend of vitamins, minerals, trace elements, antioxidants, and phytonutrients.
Each LifePak packet contains 1 vitamin capsule, two mineral capsules, and 1 phytonutrient capsule, together providing 1250 IU Vitamin A, 6250 IU Beta Carotene, 200 mg Vitamin C, 200 IU Vitamin D, 75 IU Vitamin E, 20 mcg Vitamin K, 3.75 mg Thiamin, 4.25 mg Riboflavin, 17.5 mg Niacin, 5 mg Vitamin B6, 300 mcg Folate, 15 mcg Vitamin B12, 75 mcg Biotin, 15 mg Pantothenic acid, 250 mg Calcium, 50 mcg Iodine, 125 mg Magnesium, 7.5 mg Zinc, 70 mcg Selenium, 0.5 mg Copper, 1 mg Manganese, 100 mcg Chromium, 37.5 mcg Molybdenum, 45 mg Catechins (from green tea), 25 mg Quercetin, 12.5 mg Grape Seed Extract, 12.5 mg Citrus Bioflavonoids, 2.5 mg Reseveratrol, 37.5 mg Gamma Tocopherol, 16 mg Beta- and Delta-Tocopherols, 15 mg Alpha-Lipoic Acid, 5 mg Inositol, 2.5 mg Lycopene, 1 mg Alpha Carotene, 1 mg Lutein, 1.5 mg Boron, and 10 mcg Vanadium.

Recommended Use
Take 1 packet bid with water and food.

Warnings
Keep this product out of reach of children. Consult a physician prior to use if pregnant or lactating, or taking a prescription medication. Discontinue use of this product 2 weeks prior to and after surgery. Discontinue use and consult a physician if any adverse reactions occur.

How Supplied
60 individual packets, 30 day supply. Additional LifePak® products include: LifePak® Nano, LifePak Prime, LifePak Women, LifePak Prenatal, LifePak Teen, and Jungamals.

Research using Pharmanex LifePak
LifePak has been used in over 13 published studies. Contact Nu Skin for a list of references of studies which have used Pharmanex LifePak.

*These statements have not been evaluated by the Food and Drug Administration. This product is not intended to diagnose, treat, cure or prevent any disease.

REISHIMAX GLp®   DS

Description
ReishiMax GLp® is a proprietary, standardized extract of reishi (*Ganoderma lucidum*) mushroom. This standardized product also incorporates cracked spores, a novel technology that releases reishi's active ingredient, providing unique immune activity.*
ReishiMax is produced through solid wood log cultivation. This method is preferred to sawdust and liquid cultivation because it yields both polysaccharides and triterpenes from the fruiting body and is less prone to contamination and quality control issues than other methods.

Reishi spores are minute reproductive cells that are released by the mushroom at maturity. The spores are protected by an extremely hard shell, which prevents the polysaccharides and triterpenes contained in the spore from being absorbed. Pharmanex uses technology which mechanically 'cracks' the spores, making the active ingredients bioavailable.

Benefits
ReishiMax has been demonstrated to support healthy immune system function by stimulating cell-mediated immunity. According to the results of animal and *in vitro* studies, ReishiMax has been demonstrated to stimulate the formation of antibodies, stimulate the proliferation of immune cells, and modulate the functions of T cells. ReishiMax is intended for adults who wish to maintain a healthy immune system.*
In addition to animal and *in vitro* studies conducted with ReishiMax, third party clinical studies have established the ability of reishi mushroom to support immune function in humans.*

Ingredients
Each capsule contains 495 mg of standardized reishi mushroom extract and 5 mg of reishi cracked spores and is standardized to 6% triterpenes and 13.5% polysaccharides.

Warnings
Keep out of reach of children. If you are pregnant or nursing, or taking a prescription medication, including immunosuppressive therapies, consult a physician before using this product. Discontinue use of this product 2 weeks prior to and after surgery. Discontinue use and consult a physician if any adverse reactions occur.

Recommended Use
Take 1-2 capsules bid with water and food.

How Supplied
15-30 day supply, 60 count bottle.

Research using Pharmanex ReishiMax Glp
ReishiMax has been used as the source of reishi mushroom in over 29 published studies. Contact Nu Skin for a list of references of studies which have used Pharmanex ReishiMax Glp.

*These statements have not been evaluated by the Food and Drug Administration. This product is not intended to diagnose, treat, cure or prevent any disease.

TEGREEN 97   DS

Description
Tegreen® is a standardized, decaffeinated polyphenol extract of fresh green tea leaves, with proven free radical scavenging and antioxidant properties.*

Benefits
Studies have demonstrated that the polyphenols in green tea, particularly the catechin component, offer potent antioxidant activity through the scavenging of free radicals. More specifically, numerous experiments and studies indicate that green tea polyphenols, especially EGCg, may help block the formation of some potentially toxic compounds such as nitrosamines, suppress the activation of free radicals, detoxify or trap free radicals, inhibit spontaneous and photo-enhanced lipid peroxidation, and increase the activity of natural antioxidants and detoxifying enzymes (e.g., glutathione peroxidase and catalase).*
Antioxidant supplementation may also offer some protective benefits to the skin from free radical damage and the effects of ultraviolet rays. Among the polyphenols that are antioxidants in green tea, EGCg and ECG show the strongest effect in reducing collagenase activity—an enzyme that breaks down collagen.*
Additional third party research shows that green tea supplementation may help improve lipid and glucose metabolism, maintain normal insulin sensitivity, and support a healthy metabolic rate.*

Ingredients
Each capsule contains 250 mg of extract of green tea leaves (*Camellia sinensis*) standardized to a minimum 97% pure polyphenols including 162 mg catechins, of which 95 mg is EGCg.

Recommended Use
Take 1-2 capsules bid with water and food. Maximum recommended dose of 4 capsules daily (1,000 mg). Do not exceed 1,200 mg green tea extract in combination with other green tea-containing supplements.

Warnings
Keep out of reach of children. Consult a physician prior to use if pregnant or lactating, taking anticoagulants, or taking any other prescription medications. Discontinue use of this product 2 weeks prior to and after surgery. Discontinue use and consult a physician if any adverse reactions occur.

How Supplied
30-day supply, 30 and 120 count bottles.

Research using Pharmanex Tegreen 97
Tegreen 97 has been used as the source of green tea in over 13 published studies. Contact Nu Skin for a list of references of studies which have used Pharmanex Tegreen 97.

* These statements have not been evaluated by the Food and Drug Administration. This product is not intended to diagnose, treat, cure or prevent any disease.

PERQUE Integrative Health
44621 GUILFORD DRIVE, SUITE 150
ASHBURN, VA 20147

Telephone:
1-(800)-525-7372

PERQUE LIFE GUARD™   DS
Tabsules

40 Essential Nutrients Protects Heart, Body, and Brain
Full Disclosure Label
(no hidden or inactive ingredients)
Directions: As a dietary supplement, take two (2) tabsules with meals or as directed by your health professional.
Best if taken with meals. Alternative daily doses as follows:

Low stress, healthy	1-2 tabsules/day
Moderate stress, unwell	3-4 tabsules/day
High stress, training	5-6 tabsules/day

SUPPLEMENT FACTS
Serving size: 2 Tabsules
Servings per container: 90

Energized Nutrients	Amount per serving	% Daily Value
Vitamins:		
Vitamin A (beta-carotene)	5,000 IU	100
Vitamin B-1 (thiamine HCl)	100 mg.	6,666
Vitamin B-2 (riboflavin 40 mg: riboflavin 5'-phosphate, 10 mg)	50 mg.	2,941
Vitamin B-3 (niacin)	25 mg.	125
Vitamin B-3 (niacinamide)	75 mg.	375
Vitamin B-5 (calcium d-pantothenate)	100 mg.	1,000
Vitamin B-6 (pyridoxine HCl, 160 mg. pyridoxol 5'-phosphate, 40 mg	200 mg.	10,000
Vitamin B-12 (hydroxocobalamin)	200 mcg	3,333
Folinate (as calcium folinate)	200 mcg	100
(6S)-5-Methyltetrahydrofolate (as Quatrefolic™)	200 mcg	
PABA (para-aminobenzoic acid)	30 mg.	*
Biotin (pure crystalline)	500 mcg	166
Vitamin C (100% l-ascorbate, fully reduced, corn free)	150 mg.	250
Vitamin D-3 (cholecalciferol)	400 IU	100
Vitamins E (from mixed natural tocopherols)	200 IU	667
Vitamin K-1 (phylloquinone)	500 mcg	625
Elemental Minerals:		
Potassium (as citrate)	99 mg.	3
Calcium (as ascorbate, pantothenate, citrate, fumarate, malate and succinate)	50 mg.	5
Magnesium (as C16 and C18 alkyls†)	100 mg.	25
Zinc (as picolinate)	25 mg.	167
Boron (as ascorbate)	2 mg	*
Chromium (as picolinate 50%, ascorbate 50%)	200 mcg	167

Manganese (as ascorbate)	15 mg.	750
Molybdenum (as ascorbate)	100 mcg	133
Selenium (as l-selenomethionine)	50 mcg	71
Vanadium (as ascorbate)	100 mcg	*

Active Cofactors:

Quercetin dihydrate (water-soluble bioflavonoid)	100 mg.	*
L-aspartic acid (magnesium aspartate)	50 mg.	*
Trimethylglycine (betaine HCl)	50 mg.	*
Tocotrienols:		
Triacontanol (polycosonol)	774 mcg	*
Hexacosanol (polycosonol)	33 mcg	*
Tetracosanol (polycosonol)	193 mcg	*
Octacosanol (polycosonol)	500 mcg	*
Citrate	59 mg.	*
Fumarate	59 mg.	*
Malate	59 mg.	*
Succinate	59 mg.	*
Vegetable fiber (organic croscarmellose)	170 mg.	*
Natural Vanilla	120 mg.	*

†from whole, untreated palm fruit and leaf

*Daily value not established by FDA

OTHER INGREDIENTS: None
KEEP OUT OF REACH OF CHILDREN. Must be stored with cap on tightly in a cool, dry place . Do not use product if the tamper-resist shrink band around the cap or the inner seal beneath the cap appears to have been tampered with or is missing.
WARNING: Pregnant and nursing mothers need to check with their health professional before taking supplements.
How Supplied: 180 Count
Patents Pending
Researched, uniquely formulated,
& exclusively distributed by:
PERQUE Integrative Health, USA
These statements have not been evaluated by the Food and Drug Administration. This product is not intended to diagnose, treat, cure, or prevent any disease.

PERQUE POTENT C GUARD™   DS
Buffered Ascorbate Powder

Enhances Cell Energy and Helps Reduce Oxidative Stress
Full Disclosure Label
(no hidden or inactive ingredients)
Directions: Take one (1) rounded half-teaspoon mixed with two (2) to four (4) ounces of liquid or as directed by your health professional. Use only **dry** transfer spoons to remove powder from bottle. Keep tightly capped and moisture free. Please take a few deep, relaxing breaths while the natural effervescence subsides (~1 min.). May be kept on the counter, in refrigerator or freezer to maintain dryness.

SUPPLEMENT FACTS
Serving Size: 1 Rounded Half-Teaspoon
Servings per container: 287

Energized Nutrients	Amount per serving	% Daily Value
Vitamin C (as 100% l-ascorbates, fully reduced and buffered)	1,584 mg.	2,640
Potassium (as ascorbate)	99 mg.	3
Calcium (as ascorbate)	40 mg.	5
Magnesium (as ascorbate)	16 mg.	4
Zinc (as ascorbate)	600 mcg	4

Other Ingredients: None
3/13
KEEP OUT OF REACH OF CHILDREN. Must be stored with cap on tightly in a cool, dry place. Do not use product if the tamper-resist shrink band around the cap or the inner seal beneath the cap appears to have been tampered with or is missing.
WARNING: Pregnant and nursing mothers need to check with their health professional before taking supplements.
How Supplied: 16 oz./454 grams net weight
Patents Pending
Researched, uniquely formulated,
& exclusively distributed by:
PERQUE Integrative Health, USA

These statements have not been evaluated by the Food and Drug Administration. This product is not intended to diagnose, treat, cure, or prevent any disease.

PERQUE REPAIR GUARD™   DS
Tabsules

Eases Oxidative Stress, Pain, and Inflammation
Full Disclosure Label
(no hidden or inactive ingredients)
Directions:
Mild condition: 1 tabsule daily
Moderate condition: 2-4 tabsules daily
Severe condition: 4-12 tabsules daily

SUPPLEMENT FACTS
Serving size:1 Tabsule
Servings per container: 180

Energized Nutrients	Amount per serving	% Daily Value
Quercetin dihydrate (water-soluble bioflavonoid)	1,000 mg.	*
Pomegranate juice powder (high ORAC)	60 mg.	*
OPC (soluble LMW ActiVin®1294™)	10 mg.	*
Magnesium (as c16 and C18 alkyls from whole, untreated palm fruit and leaf)	35 mg.	*
Vegetable fiber (organic croscarmellose)	10 mg.	*
Chlorophyll	100 mcg	*
Turmeric	4 mcg	*

* Daily value not established by FDA

Other Ingredients: None
3/13
KEEP OUT OF REACH OF CHILDREN. Must be stored with cap on tightly in a cool, dry place. Do not use product if the tamper-resist shrink band around the cap or the inner seal beneath the cap appears to have been tampered with or is missing.
WARNING: Pregnant and nursing mothers need to check with their health professional before taking supplements.
How Supplied: 180 Count
U.S. Pat. No. 6,620,798
Researched, uniquely formulated,
& exclusively distributed by:
PERQUE Integrative Health, USA
These statements have not been evaluated by the Food and Drug Administration. This product is not intended to diagnose, treat, cure, or prevent any disease.

PERQUE VESSEL HEALTH GUARD™   DS

90 LOZENGES
Promotes Healthy Homocysteine Levels
Full disclosure label (no hidden or inactive ingredients)
Directions: As a dietary supplement, take one (1) to six (6) lozenges daily or as directed by your health professional.

SUPPLEMENT FACTS
Serving size:1 Lozenge
Servings per container: 90

Energized Nutrients	Amount per serving	% Daily Value
B-12 (hydroxocobalamin)	2 mg.	33,330
Folinate (as calcium folinate)	2.5 mg.	625
Magnesium ascorbate	50 mg.	13
B-6 (pyridoxine)	10 mg.	500
Mannitol	198 mg.	*
Magnesium (as C16 and C18 alkyls†)	3 mg.	1
100% Whole cherry fruit extract	10 mg.	*
Sucanat® (organic, whole cane juice)	5 mg	*
Xylitol	20 mg.	*

† from whole, untreated palm fruit and leaf
* Daily value not established by FDA

KEEP OUT OF REACH OF CHILDREN. Must be stored with cap on tightly in a cool, dry place. Do not use product if the tamper-resist shrink band around the cap or the inner seal beneath the cap appears to have been tampered with or is missing. **WARNING:** Pregnant and nursing mothers need to check with their health professional before taking supplements.
Unique PERQUE Features
Pure, hypoallergenic components • Organic base •Biochemically formulated • Includes cofactors that are usable in generating high-energy compounds •Vitamins, minerals, synergistic cofactors • **DOES NOT CONTAIN:** citrus, MSG, wheat, gluten, corn, starch, sugar, soy, yeast, zein, sulfate, phosphates (other than coenzymes), preservatives, casein or other milk derivatives • No GMOs
Dietary Supplement
90 Lozenges
Patents Pending
Researched, uniquely formulated, & exclusively distributed by:
PERQUE LLC
Ashburn, VA 20147
These statements have not been evaluated by the Food and Drug Administration. This product is not intended to diagnose, treat, cure, or prevent any disease.

PERQUE WHEY GUARD REPAIR

100 Percent Native Whey Protein
Contains Quercetin Dihydrate and OPC
Directions for Use:
Replace 1 meal per day (or as directed by your healthcare practitioner) with 1 serving of PERQUE Whey Guard REPAIR. Add 2 scoops (40g) of powder to 6-8 oz. of cold water and shake or blend. May also be mixed with milk, juice or fruit smoothie of your choice.

Nutrition Facts
Serving Size: 2 scoops (40g)
Servings Per Container: 14

Amount Per Serving

Calories 150		Calories from Fat 13
	Amt	% Daily Value*
Total Fat	14 g	2%
Saturated Fat	0.5 g	3%
Trans Fats	0 g	0%
Cholesterol	42.5 mg	14%
Sodium	85.8 mg	4%
Potassium	179.4 mg	5%
Total Carbohydrates	18.7 g	6%
Dietary Fiber	10.3 g	41%
Sugars	8 g	
Protein	15.4 g	
Quercetin dihydrate (water soluble bioflavonoid)	500 mg	
OPC (ActiVin®)	500 mg	

* Percent Daily Values are based on a 2,000 calorie diet. Calories per gram: Fat – 9 Carbohydrate – 4 Protein – 4

Native Whey Protein Concentrate by Cross Flow, fibers (dahlian, guar gum, xanthan gum), sugars (organic evaporated cane juice, maple flakes), natural vanilla extract, quercetin dihydrate, OPC (ActiVin®), milk buds, potassium chloride, natural cream extract (butyrate rich butter fat), cinnamon, nutmeg, monk fruit concentrate, Equisetum arvense (natural silica), MCT (from raw coconut and palm)

Continued on next page

Actual Amino Acid Profile*

in mg per serving (40g)

Branch chain amino acid; BCAA

Isoleucine (enhanced alertness; BCAA)	2567
Leucine (enhanced alertness; BCAA)	4278
Valine (enhanced alertness; BCAA)	3935

Communication, detox, energy and neurochemicals

Alanine (energy source)	1344
Aspartate (nerve energy source)	2394
Arginine (nitric oxide [NO] source)	295
Cysteine/Cystine (detox sulfur source)	1170
Glutamine/Glutamate (energy source)	9036
Glycine (detox & soothing neurotransmitter)	539
Methionine (detox sulfur source)	1240
Phenylalanine (noradrenaline source)	1113
Serine (phosphoserine source)	1317
Threonine (phosphothreonine source)	1912
Tyrosine (adrenaline source)	1234

Specialized functions

Histidine (stomach digestive source)	518
Lysine (collagen cross link source)	1938
Proline (structure source)	4223

*Analysis by H. Stone (BUMC) April 2010. Data on file.

PERQUE Whey Guard REPAIR contains NO:

Corn	Phthalates	Melamine
Soy	GMOs	Toxic Metals
Eggs	BSE	Pesticide Residues
Gluten	BPA	Solvent Residues

KEEP OUT OF REACH OF CHILDREN.

Must be stored with cap on tightly in a cool, dry place
Do not use product if the tamper-resistant shrink band around the cap or the inner seal beneath the cap appears to have been tampered with or is missing.
14 servings
NET WT.
20 oz. 573g
Vanilla flavored

These statements have not been evaluated by the Food and Drug Administration. This product is not intended to diagnose, treat, cure or prevent any disease.

PureTrim

1201 SOUTH ALMA SCHOOL ROAD #8550
MESA, AZ 85210

Direct Inquiries to:
800-69AWARE (9273)
http://www.puretrim.net

BOOST TEA   DS

DESCRIPTION
PureTrim Boost Tea will help boost your metabolism and reduce your appetite and food cravings.
Boost Tea comes in an amazing passionfruit or strawberry lemonade flavor, with 31 organic greens, fruits, vegetables, and seeds designed to help you lose weight by fighting food cravings and supporting your metabolism.
INGREDIENTS
Organic acacia, Raspberry extract, Cinnamon bark, Brown seaweed, Mango seed extract, Potato tuber extract, Organic blue green algae (Spirulina), Organic chlorella, Organic beet, Organic cranberry, Organic red raspberry, Organic strawberry, Organic carrot, Organic blueberry, Organic pomegranate, Organic acai (Euterpe oleracea), Organic blackberry, Organic black raspberry, Organic cherry, Organic acerola extract, Organic apple, Organic apple pectin, Organic banana, Organic flax seed, Organic mango, Organic papaya, Organic peach, Organic pear, Organic pineapple, Organic tomato, Organic watermelon, Organic alfalfa sprouts, Organic barley grass, Organic broccoli, Organic green tea leaf (Decaffeinated), Organic kale, Organic wheat grass, Resveratrol, Bacillus coagulans, Protease, Amylase, Lipase, Acid Protease, Cellulase, Glucoamylase.

DIRECTIONS
Take twice daily. Add one scoop to 8 ounces of cold water with ice, and drink twice a day between meals. Have a third glass of PureTrim Boost Tea later in the evening if needed.
WARNINGS
Do not use if you are pregnant or nursing. Must be 18 years or older to use. Keep out of reach of children.
HOW SUPPLIED
7.4 oz per jar (30 servings)
Shown in Product Identification Guide, page 509

EXPERIENCE   DS

Description:
Promotes Regularity and Cleanses the Colon.*
Ingredients:
A Mediterranean Proprietary Blend of Senna (leaf), Psyllium (Blonde) Seed Husk, Fennel (Seed), Kelp (entire plant), Cornsilk (stigmas), Polygonatum (many flower Solomon's seal) (rhizome), Black Seed (Nigella sativa), Rhubarb (root).
Directions:
Take 1 capsule with a full glass of water before bedtime. Increase your serving size by one capsule every other day until you achieve your desired results.
Warnings:
Do not use if pregnant or nursing. Keep out of reach of children.
If you are under 18, consult your physician before use.
How Supplied:
90 Capsules per bottle.
Shown in Product Identification Guide, page 509

LIQUID DAILY COMPLETE   DS

Description
Mediterranean Liquid Supplement. 243 Vitamins, Minerals & Special Nutrients which Provide Energy, Reduce Stress & Support Healthy Joints*. Contains 100% RDA of key Vitamins and Minerals, and other Nutrients.

Ingredients
A Food-based Blend of Organic Mediterranean Super Seed Blend, Organic Fruit & Vegetable Whole Juice Complex, 100% RDA Of Essential Vitamins & Minerals, With Vitamins D3 & K1, Antioxidants With Resveratrol & Acai Berry, Whole Superfood Green Complex, Proprietary Ocean Blend With Pure Phytoplankton, Ionic Plant Minerals, 34 Mediterranean Herbal Ingredients, Essential Fatty Acid Complex, Vegetarian Wellness Formula

Directions
Take 1 ounce (2 tbsp) only once per day, during or immediately after a meal. Less than 4 calories per ounce, less than 1 gram of sugar.

Warnings
Do not use if Pregnant. Keep out of reach of children.

How Supplied
30 ounces per bottle.
Shown in Product Identification Guide, page 509

LIVERMASTER   DS

Cleanses and supports a healthy liver, thyroid, and pancreas.

Mediterranean Ingredients
Proprietary Mediterranean Liver/Thyroid/Pancreas Blend
Milk thistle seed extract, Blessed thistle, Milk thistle seed, Chlorophyll, Eucommia leaf extract, Cordyceps extract, N-acetyl-L-tyrosine, Red beet root extract, Artichoke leaf extract, Enzyme concentrate (a proprietary blend of cellulases, hemicellulase, invertase, alpha-galactosidase, amylase, protease and lipase), Bacillus coagulans (Lactospore® probiotic, 100 million CFU), Black pepper extract, Organic blend [Organic Acai fruit (Euterpe oleracea), Organic Alfalfa grass (leaf), Organic Amla fruit, Organic Burdock root, Organic Carrot root, Organic Chlorella (cracked cell wall), Organic Ginger root extract, Organic Lycium (goji) fruit, Organic Kale (aerial parts), Organic Kelp (Ascophyllum nodosum), Organic Moringa leaf, Organic Nopal (clade), Organic Oat grass, Organic Pomegranate fruit, Organic Purple corn, Organic Spirulina (whole algae)], Organic Rosemary leaf extract, Pycnogenol® French Maritime pine tree bark extract.

Directions
1 capsule with water right after your morning meal then take 1 capsule with water right after your evening meal. Take Liver Master for 90 days. You can do up to two 90 day cleanses a year.

Warnings
Do not use if Pregnant. Keep out of reach of children.

How Supplied
60 capsules per box
Shown in Product Identification Guide, page 509

PURETRIM JOINT TEA   DS

DESCRIPTION
PureTrim Joint Tea supports healthy joint function, improves flexibility & mobility. You can get results in just 72 hours!
Joint Tea comes in an amazing tropical fruit flavor, blended with 19 organic greens and 14 organic sprouts to support healthy joint and muscle function.

INGREDIENTS
Organic Acacia, Organic Kale, Organic Collard Greens, Organic Turnip Greens, Organic cabbage, Organic Swiss Chard, Spinach, Organic Mustard Greens, Organic Rapini (Broccoli Rabe), Organic Red and Green Leaf and Romaine Lettuce, Quinoa, Organic Chia, Organic Banana, Organic Inulin, Organic Tomato, Organic Flax Seed, Organic Spirulina, Organic Amaranth Sprout, Organic Quinoa Sprout, Organic Millet Sprout, Curcuma longa (Turmeric extra) Organic Buckwheat Sprout, Organic Garbanzo Bean Sprout, Organic Lentil Sprout, Organic Adzuki Sprout, Organic Flax Sprout, Organic Sunflower Sprout, Organic Pumpkin Sprout, Organic Chia Sprout, Organic Sesame Sprout, Organic Alfalfa Grass, Organic Sweet Potato, Organic Beet, Organic Stevia, Organic Strawberry, Organic Blueberry, Organic Cherry, Organic Apple, Organic Pineapple, Avocado, Organic Elderberry, Organic Carrot, Organic Broccoli, Organic Spinach, Hyaluronic acid, Organic Broccoli Sprout, Organic Daikon Radish Sprout, Organic Chlorella, Organic Barley Grass, Organic Wheat Grass, Seaweed, Organic Green Tea (decaffeinated)
Other ingredients: citric acid, magnesium citrate, natural berry flavor, silica, monk fruit extract and rebaudioside-A (stevia).

DIRECTIONS
For the first 7 days: Add one scoop to 8 ounces of cold water with ice, and drink once in the morning, once in the evening.
After 7 days: Drink once a day.
Be consistent daily, and for the best results, also use Daily Complete®, Experience®, and SynergyDefense®.

WARNINGS
Do not use if you are pregnant or nursing. Must be 18 years or older to use. Keep out of reach of children.

HOW SUPPLIED
5.4 oz per jar (30 servings)
Shown in Product Identification Guide, page 509

PURETRIM MEDITERRANEAN WELLNESS SHAKES   DS

Description
Natural, Vegetarian Weight Loss Shake, High Protein, Low Carbs, Less than 1 gram of Sugar. No Soy, No Whey, No Dairy, and No Aspartame. Less than 200 calories per shake.

Ingredients
21 Gram Protein Blend: NON-GMO Vegetable Pea, Organic Brown Rice, Organic Lentil, and Organic Flaxseed. Blend of Antioxidants, Prebiotics, 500mg of Plant Calcium, 8000mg of Essential Fatty Acids & 1100mg of Super Raw Greens Blend.

Directions
Mix contents of shake in 10-12 oz. of chilled water.
Have 2 shakes a day (one for breakfast & one for your evening meal.) Drink 2 glasses of water after you drink your shake for best results. Once weight loss is achieved, reduce to 1 shake a day for maintenance.

Warnings

Do not use if you are pregnant or nursing. Must be 18 years or older to use. Do not use as a replacement for more than two meals per day.

How Supplied

10 Packets (Net Weight 500g)

Shown in Product Identification Guide, page 509

Synergy WorldWide

**1955 WEST GROVE PARKWAY, SUITE 100
PLEASANT GROVE UT 84062**

(801) 769-7800

PROARGI-9⁺   DS
**L-arginine Complexer
Dietary Supplement**

ProArgi-9⁺ is the highest quality l-arginine supplement in the world. This proprietary formulation combines the powerful cardiovascular benefits of l-arginine with a variety of superior heart health ingredients to give your cardiovascular system optimum support.

ProArgi-9⁺ was formulated in collaboration with leading scientists and cardiovascular specialists who have conducted extensive research on the proper application of l-arginine in promoting heart health. With ProArgi-9⁺, you're giving your heart the supplementation it needs for a long, healthy life.*

*These statements have not been evaluated by the Food and Drug Administration. This product is not intended to diagnose, treat, cure or prevent any disease.

Supplement Facts
Serving Size: 10.5 g (approx. 1 level scoop)
Servings per container: 30

Amount Per Serving		% Daily Value
Calories 15		
Total Carbohydrate	5 g	2%*
Vitamin C (Ascorbic Acid)	60 mg	100%
Vitamin D3 (Cholecalciferol)	2,500 IU	625%
Vitamin K (Menaquinone)	20 mcg	25%
Vitamin B6 (Pyridoxine HCl)	2 mg	100%
Folate (Folic Acid)	200 mcg	50%
Vitamin B12 (Cyanocobalamin)	6 mcg	100%
Proprietary Blend	6.5 g	**

L-arginine, xylitol, pomegranate fruit concentrate (*Punica granatum*), L-citrulline, d-ribose, grape skin extract (*Vitis vinifera*), red wine extract

*Percent daily values are based on a 2,000 calorie diet.
**Daily value not established.

Other Ingredients: Citric Acid, Malic Acid, Natural Citrus Sweetener, Silicon Dioxide, Natural Citrus and Huckleberry Flavors, Stevia leaf extract (*Stevia rebaudiana*).

DIRECTIONS: Mix 1 serving (1 scoop providing 5 g pure, free form L-arginine) with 4-8 oz. water (depending on individual taste). Stir to dissolve. If water is very cold, mixture will take about one minute to dissolve. One serving (1 scoop) may be taken twice per day.

Store in a cool, dry place. Slight color changes may occur over time due to the natural fruit flavor. There is no change in the efficacy or potency of the product.

Shake Well Before Dispensing

Consult your physician prior to use if you have a preexisting medical condition including: myocardial infarction (heart attack), cardiovascular disease or diabetes, or take medications for any reasons including erectile dysfunction. Not recommended for use in children or pregnant or lactating women.

Manufactured Exclusively for Synergy Worldwide®
Pleasant Grove, UT 84062 • (801) 769-7700
www.synergyworldwide.com
Item Code: Isu74154 ©2012 Made in U.S.A. REV1112
Shown in Product Identification Guide, page 510

Unicity International, Inc.
**THE MAKE LIFE BETTER COMPANY
1201 NORTH 800 EAST
OREM, UT 84097**

Direct Inquiries to:
(801) 226-2600
www.unicity.com
science@unicity.com
Products of Unicity International, Inc. are distributed through independent distributors.

BIO-C™   DS
[*bīo sē*]

DESCRIPTION
Bio-C™ is a vitamin C nutritional supplement.

Bio-C™ is a yellow, water-soluble, crystalline powder pressed into a tablet. Each Bio-C™ tablet consists of a proprietary blend of ascorbyl palmitate, calcium ascorbate, ascorbic acid, magnesium ascorbate, and 37.5 mg of citrus bioflavonoids. In addition to the active ingredients, each tablet contains cellulose, stearic acid, silicon dioxide, croscarmellose sodium, and magnesium stearate.

BENEFITS AND RESEARCH
Vitamin C (ascorbic acid) is a water-soluble vitamin that is used in the body to form cartilage, collagen, muscles, and blood vessels. Vitamin C is a potent antioxidant that can protect small molecules such as proteins, carbohydrates, nucleic acids, and lipids from damage caused by free radicals that are generated through the course of normal metabolism or through exposure to external toxins and pollutants (e.g. ultraviolet radiation from the sun or smoking). Vitamin C can also regenerate other antioxidants like vitamin E. Additionally, vitamin C is required for the synthesis of carnitine, a molecule involved in the transport of fats across the mitochondrial membrane, as well as the synthesis of norepinephrine, a neurotransmitter.[1]

USAGE
Take one tablet morning and night with a meal.

SAFETY AND WARNINGS
Bio-C™ is well tolerated. Some gastrointestinal discomfort may be experienced as with any dietary supplement.

HOW SUPPLIED
Available in tablets.

REFERENCES
Carr, AC and Frei B. (1999), American Journal of Clinical Nutrition 96: 1086-1107.
Jacob, RA and Sotoudeh G. (2002), Nutrition in Clinical Care 5: 66-74.
Deruelle F, Baron B. (2008), Journal of Alternative and Complementary Medicine 14:1291-1298.
Levine M, Rumsey SC, Daruwala R, Park JB, Wang Y. (1999), The Journal of the American Medical Association 281: 1415-1423.

---

[1] THESE STATEMENTS HAVE NOT BEEN EVALUATED BY THE FOOD AND DRUG ADMINISTRATION. THIS PRODUCT IS NOT INTENDED TO DIAGNOSE, TREAT, CURE, OR PREVENT ANY DISEASE.

BIOS LIFE® C PLUS (BIOS LIFE® C)   DS
Advanced Fiber and Nutrient Drink

DESCRIPTION
Bios Life® C Plus is a fiber-based, vitamin rich dietary supplement. Bios Life® C Plus contains a blend of soluble and insoluble fibers, phytosterols, policosanol, an extract of *Chrysanthemum morifolium*, vitamins, and minerals that when combined with a healthy diet and exercise may lower total serum cholesterol and triglyceride levels.

Bios Life® C Plus is light orange in color. It is a hygroscopic crystalline powder that is generally soluble in water. Each serving of Bios Life® C Plus contains 3 g of fiber, 1 g of phytosterols, 6 mg of policosanol, and 12.5 mg of an extract of *Chrysamthemum morifolium*. In addition to these active ingredients, each serving of Bios Life® C Plus contains maltodextrin, citric acid, orange juice powder, sucralose, and orange flavor.

BENEFITS AND RESEARCH
It's estimated that Americans consume 10-12 g of total fiber per day, less than half the amount of the recommended daily intake. Epidemiological and clinical studies have correlated high daily fiber intake with an improvement in overall health.

Bios Life® C Plus is a dietary supplement designed to increased daily fiber intake. Each serving of Bios Life® C Plus contains three grams of dietary fiber. When taken three times daily, Bios Life® C Plus contributes nearly half of the recommended daily value of fiber. Fiber supplementation has been shown to decrease preprandial and postprandial glucose levels and lower LDL cholesterol and apolipoprotein B levels.

In addition to fiber supplementation, Bios Life® C Plus contains a patented blend of phytosterols, policosanol, *Chrysanthemum morifolium*, vitamins, and minerals. This blend of ingredients optimizes cholesterol levels through a combination of four mechanisms. First, the soluble fiber matrix prevents cholesterol reabsorption in the gastrointestinal tract through bile-acid sequestration. Second, the phytosterols reduce dietary absorption of cholesterol. Third, policosanol inhibits hepatic synthesis of cholesterol mediated through HMG-CoA reductase. Fourth, *Chrysanthemum morifolium* provides phytonutrients that enhance conversion of cholesterol to 7-α-hydryoxycholesterol. The four mechanisms provide a synergistic approach to optimizing cholesterol levels.

SUGGESTED USAGE
Dissolve the contents of one packet or one scoop into 8 to 10 fl. oz. of liquid (water or juice) and stir vigorously. Drink immediately. Use 15-20 minutes prior to meals up to three times daily.

SAFETY AND WARNINGS
Bios Life® C Plus is well tolerated. There may be mild gastrointestinal discomfort, such as increased flatulence or loose stools, during the first month of initial use due to the increased uptake of dietary fiber. This GI disturbance usually disappears within the first thirty days. If the GI discomfort persists, reduce the number of servings of Bios Life® C Plus. If the GI discomfort further persists, stop taking the product and consult your physician. Taking this product without adequate liquid can result in complications.

HOW SUPPLIED
Bios Life® C Plus is packaged in single-serving foil packets or in bulk canisters.

REFERENCES
Sprecher, DL and Pearce GL (2002), Metabolism 51: 1166–70.
Verdegem, PJE; Freed, S and Joffe D (2005), American Diabetes Assocation 65th Scientific Sessions, San Diego, CA.
Duenas, V; Duenas, J; Burke, E and Verdegem, PJE (2006), 7th International Conference on Arteriosclerosis, Thrombosis, and Vascular Biology, American Heart Association, Denver, CO.
Verdegem, PJE (2007), Current Topics in Nutraceutical Research 5: 1-6
US Patent 6,933,291.

* THESE STATEMENTS HAVE NOT BEEN EVALUATED BY THE FOOD AND DRUG ADMINISTRATION. THIS PRODUCT IS NOT INTENDED TO DIAGNOSE, TREAT, CURE, OR PREVENT ANY DISEASE.

Shown in Product Identification Guide, page 510

BIOS LIFE® E (UNICITY MATCHA)   DS

Supports a Healthy Metabolism

Description
Bios Life® E (Unicity Matcha) is a nutritional supplement used to supply necessary vitamins, minerals, and electrolytes, as well as provide energy, amino acids, and antioxi-

Continued on next page

dants on a daily basis. Bios life® E is a flavored powdered drink mix, delivered in a single-serve packet for convenience and ease of use.

Benefits and Research

Bios Life® E (Unicity Matcha) is a refreshing ingredient blend that may boost energy and concentration, lower stress levels, and increase the metabolism. The principle ingredient in Bios Life® E is a high-quality Matcha, a uniquely-grown green tea from Japan, which delivers a powerful dose of antioxidants in each serving.

Research shows Matcha delivers as much as 137 times more antioxidants than other green or black teas available on the market. Matcha contains especially high amounts of green tea antioxidants called catechins, a class of polyphenols, which may produce thermogenic effects by increasing the body's metabolism. Catechins and other green tea polyphenols may also protect against cell damage.

Matcha is derived from *Camellia sinesis*, one of the few plants that naturally produce high levels of L-theanine and caffeine which may supply an increase in energy as well as enhance cognitive ability. Matcha is a unique tea leaf because it is shade-grown, forcing the plant to grow at a much slower rate. This greatly increases the catechins and amino acids available in an equivalent serving of Matcha green tea compared to standard tea. Additionally, because Matcha tea leaves are powdered and consumed whole and not just steeped, a cup of Matcha tea contains a larger variety and quantity of nutrients. This includes soluble and insoluble components such as chlorophyll, protein, and dietary fiber. The catechins in Matcha have strong antioxidant properties and measured benefits in humans. These antioxidants work to speed up the metabolism, provide more energy over a longer period of time, and even decrease muscle fatigue. Research shows the amino acid L-theanine, found in Matcha, has a calming effect on the human brain without causing drowsiness. This relaxation, paired with the stimulant effects of caffeine and theophylline, creates a heightened mental state that improves concentration.

Suggested Use

The contents of the packet can be mixed with 8-12 fl. oz. of water, shaken or stirred vigorously, and consumed. It can be served with ice if desired. Use one packet daily.

Safety and Warnings

Bios Life® E (Unicity Matcha) is generally well tolerated. As with any dietary supplement, some gastrointestinal discomfort may be experienced. Bios Life® E contains moderate amounts of caffeine; as such, caffeine-sensitive individuals should maintain caution when using this product.

How Supplied

Bios Life® E is packaged in single-serve foil packets.

References

Weiss DJ, et al. Determination of catechins in matcha green tea by micellar electrokinetic chromatography. J Chromatogr A. 2003;1011(1-2):173-80.

Dulloo A. et al. Efficacy of a green tea extract rich in catechins polyphenols and caffeine in increasing 24-h energy expenditure and fat oxidation in humans. American Journal of Clinical Nutrition. 1999; 70(6): 1040-1045.

Gomez-Ramirez M, et al. The effects of L-theanine on alpha-band oscillatory brain activity during a visuo-spatial attention task. Brain Topogr 2009;22(1):44-51.

Cabrera C, et al. Beneficial Effects of Green Tea—A Review. J Am Coll Nutr 2006;25(2):79-99.

[1]THESE STATEMENTS HAVE NOT BEEN EVALUATED BY THE FOOD AND DRUG ADMINISTRATION. THIS PRODUCT IS NOT INTENDED TO DIAGNOSE, TREAT, CURE OR PREVENT ANY DISEASE.

BIOS LIFE PROBIONIC®   OTC

Description

ProBionic® contains four strands of live, healthy bacteria that enter the digestive system and help balance bacterial populations in the intestinal tract. This supplement is for individuals with symptoms of poor digestive health such as constipation, diarrhea, bloating, and inflammation.

ProBionic® is a water-soluble, light-pink crystalline powder. The proprietary encapsulation used for ProBionic® allows the healthy bacteria to be delivered to the small intestines alive, ensuring the bacteria can confer health benefits for the user. Each packet of ProBionic® contains a 100 mg Pro-

biotic Blend of *Lactobacillus acidophilus LA 02, Lactobacillus rhamnosus LR 04, Bifidobacterium breve BR 03,* and *Bifidobacterium lactis BS 01,* with a total of 5 billion cells. In addition to these live bacteria, each 2 g packet also contains xylitol, natural berry flavor, citric acid, and silica.

Benefits and Research

Your body needs good bacteria to help with detoxification, food digestion, waste removal, production of vitamins, and protection from harmful organisms. When the intestinal bacteria is imbalanced and unhealthy bacteria dominate, the body is less able to fight off infection resulting in inflammation. The individual strains used in ProBionic® are helpful for maintaining overall gut health.

The proprietary encapsulation used in ProBionic® allows healthy strains of bacteria to be delivered to the digestive system alive and undisturbed. This also ensures the bacteria will remain alive throughout their shelf life.

Suggested Use

The contents of the packet can be taken dry, or they can be mixed with 8-10 fl. oz. of liquid (water or juice) and consumed. Use one packet daily

Safety and Warnings

ProBionic® is generally well tolerated. As with any dietary supplement, some gastrointestinal discomfort may be experienced.

How Supplied

ProBionic® is packaged in single-serve foil packets.

References

Saggioro A. Probiotics in the treatment of Irritable Bowel Syndrome. Journal of Clinical Gastroenterology, 2004; 38(8): S104-106.

Del Piano M, Carmagnola S, Andorno S, Pagliarulo M, Tari R, Mogna L, Strozzi GP, Sforza F, Capurso L. Evaluation of the intestinal colonization by microencapsulated probiotic bacteria in comparison to the same uncoated strains. Under pubblication in supplement of the Journal of Clinical Gastroenterology.

Del Piano M, Carmagnola S, Anderloni A, Andorno S, Ballare M, Balzarini M, Montino F, Orsello M, Pagliarulo M, Stratori M, Tari R, Sforza F, Capurso L. The use of probiotics in healthy volunteers with evacuation disorders and hard stools. A double blind, randomized, placebo-controlled study. Under pubblication in a supplement of the Journal of Clinical Gastroenterology.

Pregliasco F, Anselmi G, Fonte L, Giussani F, Schieppati S, Soletti L. A New Chance of Preventing Winter Diseases by the Administration of Symbiotic Formulations. Journal of Clinical Gastroenterology, 2008; 42(2): 224-233.

* THESE STATEMENTS HAVE NOT BEEN EVALUATED BY THE FOOD AND DRUG ADMINISTRATION. THIS PRODUCT IS NOT INTENDED TO DIAGNOSE, TREAT, CURE, OR PREVENT ANY DISEASE.

BIOS LIFE® VISION ESSENTIALS™   DS
[bī-ōs līf vizh-uhn ē-sen-shuhls]

Clinically proven to support healthy eyes and vision.*

DESCRIPTION

Bios Life® Vision Essentials™ is a nutritional supplement for maintaining healthy eyes. Bios Life® Vision Essentials™contains the following active ingredients: vitamin C, vitamin E, zinc, natural beta carotene, lutein, zeaxanthin, and anthocyanidins from wild bilberry, wild blueberry, strawberry, cranberry, grape seed extract, elderberry, and raspberries.

Bios Life® Vision Essentials™ is a purple crystalline powder that is water-soluble. In addition to the active ingredients, each capsule contains silicon dioxide, microcrystalline cellulose, and is packaged in vegetarian capsules.

BENEFITS AND RESEARCH

Antioxidants from the carotenoid chemical family, such as beta carotene, lutein, and zeaxanthin, play an important role in eye health. Clinical studies have demonstrated that lutein and zeaxanthin are concentrated to the retina and lens of the eye. Supplementation with high levels of lutein can restore the lutein concentration in the retina. Further supplementation of vitamins C, E, and A (in the form of beta-carotene) along with zinc and copper aid with the healthy function of the eyes. Additional support for the eyes comes from a proprietary berry blend included in Bios Life®

Vision Essentials™. This proprietary berry blend contains anthocyanidins, antioxidant compounds that support the vasculature within the eye.

USAGE

Take two capsules per day with a meal.

SAFETY AND WARNINGS

Bios Life® Vision Essentials™ is well tolerated. As with any dietary supplement, some gastrointestinal discomfort may be experienced.

HOW SUPPLIED

Available in capsules.

REFERENCES

Krishnadev N, Meleth AD, Chew EY (2010) "Nutritional supplements for age-related macular degeneration." Current Opinion in Opthamology 21:184-189.

Ma L, Lin XM, Zou ZY, Xu XR, Li Y, Xu R. (2009) "A 12-week lutein supplementation improves visual function in Chinese people with long-term computer display light exposure." British Journal of Nutrition 102: 186-190.

Yagi, A, Fujimoto, K, Michihiro, K, Goh, B, Tsi, D, Nagai, H, (2009) "The effect of lutein supplementation on visual fatigue: A psychophysiological analysis". Applied Ergonomics 40:1047-1054.

Age Related Eye Disease Study Group, (2001) "A randomized, placebo-controlled, clinical trial of high-dose supplementation with vitamins C and E, beta carotene, and zinc for age-related macular degeneration and vision loss: AREDS report no. 8". Archives of Ophthalmology. 10: 1417-36.

* THESE STATEMENTS HAVE NOT BEEN EVALUATED BY THE FOOD AND DRUG ADMINISTRATION. THIS PRODUCT IS NOT INTENDED TO DIAGNOSE, TREAT CURE, OR PREVENT ANY DISEASE.

CARDIO-BASICS™   DS
Essential Cardiovascular Nutrients*

DESCRIPTION

Cardio-Basics™ is a nutritional supplement that combines multivitamins, minerals, and antioxidants to support the cardiovascular system.

Cardio-Basics™ is a light orange, water-soluble powder pressed into tablets. Each tablet of Cardio-Basics™ contains the following vitamins, minerals, amino acids, and antioxidants: beta-carotene (vitamin A), thiamine (vitamin B1), riboflavin (vitamin B2), niacin (vitamin B3), calcium d-pantothenate (vitamin B5), pyridoxine hydrochloride (vitamin B6), folate (vitamin B9), cyanocobalamin (vitamin B12), ascorbic acid and ascorbyl palmitate (vitamin C), cholecalciferol (vitamin D), d-alpha-tocopherol (vitamin E), biotin, calcium, chromium, copper, magnesium, manganese, molybdenum, phosphorus, potassium, selenium, sodium, zinc, L-arginine, L-carnitine, L-cysteine, L-lysine, L-proline, inositol, coenzyme Q10, and maritime pine extract. In addition to those active ingredients, each tablet also contains cellulose, croscarmellose sodium, stearic acid, silicon dioxide, and magnesium stearate.

BENEFITS AND RESEARCH

Cardio-Basics™ provides the vitamins, minerals, and antioxidants needed for a healthy heart. In clinical studies, participants using Cardio-Basics™ and Bio-C™ saw a significant reduction in arterial wall thickness and removal of calcification deposits when compared to the placebo group. Cardio-Basics™ provides the body with the necessary vitamins and minerals needed to support a healthy vascular system.*

SUGGESTED USE

Take two tablets daily with food.

SAFETY AND WARNINGS

Cardio-Basics™ is well tolerated. Contains chromium and niacin. Do not use if pregnant, nursing, diabetic, or when taking other niacin-containing supplements.

HOW SUPPLIED

Available in tablets

REFERENCES

Niedzwiekcki A, Rath, M. (1996) Journal of Applied Nutrition, 48: 67-78.

Jeejeebhoy F, Keith M, Freeman M, Barr A, McCall M, Kurian R, Mazer D, Errett L, (2002), American Heart Journal 143: 1092-1100.

Verdgem PJE, Lonky S, Curley S. (2005) 7th Conference on Arteriosclerosis, Thrombosis and Vascular Biology.
Lloyd-Jones D, Adams R, Carnethon M, DeSimone G, Ferguson TB, Flegal K, Ford E, Furie K, Go A, Greenlund K, Haase N, Hailpern S, Ho M, Howard V, Kissela B, Kittner S, Lackland D, Lisabeth L, Marelli A, McDermott M, Meigs J, Mozaffarian D, Nichol G, O'Donnell C, Roger V, Rosamond W, Sacco R, Sorlie P, Stafford R, Steinberger J, Hong Y; (2009) Circulation, 119: 480-486.

* THESE STATEMENTS HAVE NOT BEEN EVALUATED BY THE FOOD AND DRUG ADMINISTRATION. THIS PRODUCT IS NOT INTENDED TO DIAGNOSE, TREAT, CURE, OR PREVENT ANY DISEASE.

CARDIO-ESSENTIALS™   DS
Caring for your heart*

DESCRIPTION
Cardio-Essentials™ is a dietary supplement for the heart. Cardio-Essentials™ contains Coenzyme Q-10, L-carnitine, L-taurine, and Hawthorn berry.
Cardio-Essentials™ is a light tan, water-soluble powder. Each serving of Cardio-Essentials™ contains 100 mg of Coenzyme Q-10 and 3.5 g of a blend of L-carnitine, L-taurine, and Hawthorn berry. In addition to these active ingredients, each capsule also contains silicon dioxide, stearic acid, and calcium silicate.

BENEFITS AND RESEARCH
The ventricles of the heart requires specific nutrients to maintain overall health. These important nutrients are included in Cardio-Essentials™: Coenzyme Q10, L-carnitine, and L-taurine. In a clinical study, the combination of L-carnitine, L-taurine, and Coenzyme Q10 was shown to reduce the size of the left ventricle, which is important to maintain heart health. These ingredients are known to be important in providing adequate energy for heart muscle. Cardio-Essentials™ provides adequate amounts of these ingredients, i.e. 100 mg of CoQ10. Hawthorn extract is traditionally used in supporting the heart function.

SUGGESTED USE
Take three capsules twice daily with food.

SAFETY AND WARNINGS
Cardio-Essentials™ is well tolerated. As with any dietary supplement, some gastrointestinal discomfort may be experienced.

HOW SUPPLIED
Available in capsules.

REFERENCES
Lee, JH. et al. (2011) Congestive Heart Failure 4 199-203.
* THESE STATEMENTS HAVE NOT BEEN EVALUATED BY THE FOOD AND DRUG ADMINISTRATION. THIS PRODUCT IS NOT INTENDED TO DIAGNOSE, TREAT, CURE, OR PREVENT ANY DISEASE.

CM PLEX® AND CM CREAM   DS
[CM plĕks]
Supports Joint Health and Mobility*

DESCRIPTION
CM Plex® and CM Cream are a softgel and topical cream, respectively, that contain a proprietary blend of cetylated fatty acids, soy, and fish oil.
CM Plex® is an opaque oil that is insoluble in water. One softgel capsule of CM Plex® contains 350 mg of cetylated fatty acids, 160 mg of soy oil, and 25 mg of salmon oil. In addition to these active ingredients, each softgel capsule contains glycerin and St. John's Bread.
CM Cream is an off-white cream that is insoluble in water. One gram of CM Cream contains 7.7 mg of cetylated fatty acids and olive oil. In addition to these active ingredients, CM Cream also contains glyceryl stearate, glycerin, lecithin, tocopheryl acetate, benzyl alcohol, phenoxyethanol, carbomer, PEG-100 stearate, sodium hydroxide, methylparaben, propylparaben, butylparaben, ethylparaben, isobutylparaben, and citrus aurantium bergamia (Bergamot) fruit oil.

BENEFITS AND RESEARCH
Cetyl myristoleate and related fatty acids have been proven to improve joint health through their anti-inflammatory ef-

fects. A clinical study indicated that subjects exhibited improvements in knee flexion compared to placebo. A second study indicated the cream is effective for improving knee range of motion, ability to climb stairs, rise from a chair and walk, balance, strength, and endurance.*

SUGGESTED USE
Softgels: Take one to two softgels three times daily with meals.
Cream: Apply generously onto clean skin and gently massage until the cream disappears. Repeat 3 to 4 times daily as necessary. For maximum results, use both products concurrently.

SAFETY AND WARNINGS
CM Plex® Softgels and CM Cream are well tolerated. As with any dietary supplement, some gastrointestinal discomfort may be experienced with CM Plex® Softgels.

HOW SUPPLIED
CM Plex® is available in softgels and as a topical cream.

REFERENCES
Hesslink, R et al (2002), Journal of Rheumatology 29, 1708-1712.
Kraemer, WJ et al (2004), Journal of Rheumatology 31, 767-774.
* THESE STATEMENTS HAVE NOT BEEN EVALUATED BY THE FOOD AND DRUG ADMINISTRATION. THIS PRODUCT IS NOT INTENDED TO DIAGNOSE, TREAT, CURE, OR PREVENT ANY DISEASE.

Shown in Product Identification Guide, page 510

CORE HEALTH   DS
Supports Overall Health*

DESCRIPTION
Core Health is a patent-pending multivitamin designed to maintain overall health and wellness. This product consists of three tablets, namely a Day tablet, a Night tablet, and a Genome tablet. Core Health is the flagship product of Unicity International's Genomeceutical™ line of products. The Day tablet is a dark yellow color. The active ingredients in the Day tablet are as follows: vitamin A, beta-carotene, vitamin C, vitamin E, vitamin B1, riboflavin, niacinamide, vitamin B6, folic acid, vitamin B12, biotin, vitamin B5, iron, zinc, CoQ10, phosphatidyl serine, green tea extract (standardized to 38% EGCG), quercetin, turmeric extract (standardized to 20% total curcuminoids), and sugar cane extract (standardized to 60% octacosanol). Other ingredients in the Day tablet are as follows: Silicified microcrystalline cellulose, acacia gum, sodium carboxymethyl starch, potato starch, stearic acid, coating (dextrin, dextrose, soy lecithin, sodium carboxymethylcellulose, sodium citrate), silicon dioxide, and magnesium stearate.
The Night tablet is a light greenish color. The active ingredients in the Night tablet are as follows: vitamin D3, calcium, magnesium, L-theanine, and lavender. Other ingredients in the Night tablet are as follows: Acacia gum, potato starch, stearic acid, coating (dextrin, dextrose, soy lecithin, sodium carboxymethylcellulose, sodium citrate), silicon dioxide, and magnesium stearate.
The Genome tablet is a dark brown color. The active ingredients in the Genome tablet are as follows: vitamin K, iodine, copper, manganese, potassium, hesperidin, grape seed extract (standardized to 95% polyphenols), broccoli powder (standardized to 0.5% sulphoraphane), cranberry juice extract (standardized to 10% proanthocyanidins), apple extract (standardized to 70% polyphenols), citrus bioflavonoids (standardized to 50% flavanoids), and a proprietary Unicity Phyto Blend containing green coffee extract, broccoli sprout concentrate, green tea extract, onion extract, apple extract, quercetin, camu camu concentrate, acerola concentrate, tomato concentrate, broccoli concentrate, acai concentrate, basil concentrate, cinnamon concentrate, garlic concentrate, oregano concentrate, turmeric extract, elderberry concentrate, carrot concentrate, mangosteen concentrate, black currant extract, soybean extract, corn extract, blueberry extract, chokeberry concentrate, blackberry concentrate, raspberry concentrate, sweet cherry concentrate, spinach concentrate, kale concentrate, bilberry extract, and brussels sprout concentrate, maltodextrin, corn starch, silicon dioxide, lecithin. Other ingredients in the Genome tablet are as follows: Silicified microcrystalline cellulose, acacia gum, sodium carboxymethyl starch, stearic acid, potato

starch, coating (dextrin, dextrose, soy lecithin, sodium carboxymethylcellulose, sodium citrate), and magnesium stearate.

BENEFITS AND RESEARCH
Core Health contains efficacious amounts of vitamins and minerals known to act as cofactors in enzymatic reactions and help to maintain the thousands of chemical reactions the body performs every second. Secondary metabolites in standardized amounts from forty different botanical sources are also included. Certain plant secondary metabolites have been implicated in maintaining healthy gene expression through interaction with microRNA.*
Phosphatidylserine included in the Day tablet has been shown in the scientific literature to maintain healthy memory function. Clinical studies have shown that Octacosanol can improve stamina and exercise capability in athletes. CoQ10 helps to maintain good cellular energy in the body by interaction with the mitochondria.*
The Night tablet contains vitamin D3—which has been shown to help maintain healthy calcium absorption in the body. L-Theanine in the Night tablet helps in reduction and healthy maintenance of the stress response. The relaxation and sleep promoting effects of lavender flower are well known in the scientific literature.*

*THESE STATEMENTS HAVE NOT BEEN EVALUATED BY THE FOOD AND DRUG ADMINISTRATION. THIS PRODUCT IS NOT INTENDED TO DIAGNOSE, TREAT, CURE, OR PREVENT ANY DISEASE.

USAGE
Take 1 Day (D) packet (6 tablets—3 Day and 3 Genome) in the morning and 1 Night (N) packet (6 tablets—3 Night and 3 Genome) in the evening daily with water. Do not exceed recommended dosage.

SAFETY AND WARNINGS
Core Health is generally well tolerated. As with any dietary supplement, some gastrointestinal discomfort may be experienced.

HOW SUPPLIED
Available as tablets in single-serve foil packets.

REFERENCES
Palmer JD, Soule BP, Simone BA, Zaorsky NG, Jin J, Simone NL: MicroRNA Expression Altered by Diet: Can Food be Medicinal? Aging Res Rev 2014, 17: 16-24.
Kato-Kataoka K, Sakai M, Ebina R, Nonaka C, Asano T, Miyamori T: Soybean-Derived Phosphatidylserine Improves Memory Function of the Elderly Japanese Subjects with Memory Complaints. J Clin Biochem Nutr 2010, 47: 246-255.
Taylor TC, Rapport L, Lockwood GB: Octacosanol in Human Health. Nutrition 2003, 19: 192-195. Christakos S, Dhawan P, Porta A, Mady LJ, Seth T: Vitamin D and Intestinal Calcium Absorption. Mol Cell Endocrinol 2011, 347: 25-29.
Kimura K, Ozeki M, Juneja LR, Ohara H: L-Theanine Reduces Psychological and Physiological Stress Responses. Biol Psychol 2007, 74: 39-45.
Hirokawa K, Nishimoto T: Effects of Lavender Aroma on Sleep Quality in Healthy Japanese Students. Percept Mot Skills 2012, 114: 111-122.

ENZYGEN® PLUS   DS
Support a Healthy Digestive System*

Description
In digestion, enzymes liberate and break down nutrients from food that become the building blocks for cell growth and regeneration. Proper enzyme levels are crucial to a healthy body. In order to provide a balanced blend of specific enzymes and help break down foods in digestion, Enzygen® Plus contains a wide variety of unique enzymes that aid in digestion. The enzymes found in Enzygen® Plus help break down various types of fats, carbohydrates, and proteins to help convert food into useful nutrients for the body. Additionally, Enzygen® Plus helps to promote proper digestion and helps the stomach maintain proper acidity.
The five basic categories of enzymes include lipase for breaking down oils and fats, cellulase to break down fibers, amylase for breaking down starches, lactase for dairy products, and protease to break down proteins.

Continued on next page

There are many different enzymes in Unicity's proprietary blend of enzymes found in Enzygen® Plus. These include different forms of amylase, protease, lipase, catalase, lactase, cellulase, hemicellulase, invertase, peptidase, bromelain, papain, superoxide dismutase, beta-glucanase, and phytase.

Benefits and Research

Our bodies need proper levels of active enzymes in order to conduct a variety of tasks, including digestion. While enzymes occur naturally in our bodies and in plants, they can be destroyed by pesticides, pollution, processes used to cook or irradiate foods, and chemical additives. Enzygen® Plus supplements your enzyme supply to help your body break down fats, carbohydrates, and proteins, convert foods to useful nutrients, and complete proper digestion.

Enzymes are natural substances created in plant, animal and human cells, and they play a vital role in digestion. There are more than 2,700 identified enzymes in the human body, and each affects a unique chemical reaction. The body relies on properly functioning enzymes to assist with breathing, digestion, growth, blood coagulation, sensory perception, reproduction, and other functions.

Enzygen® Plus contains a wide variety of enzymes and other ingredients that may aid digestion by breaking down food in the digestive system, stimulating the release of essential nutrients from food.

Suggested Use

Take one capsule three times daily with food.

Safety and Warnings

Enzygen® Plus is generally well tolerated. As with any dietary supplement, some gastrointestinal discomfort may be experienced.

How Supplied

Available in capsules.

References

Roxas M. The Role of Enzyme Supplementation in Digestive Disorders. Alternative Medicine Review. 2008; 13(4): 307-314.

Shastri D, Kumar M, Kumar A. Modulation of lead toxicity by Spirulina fusiformis.Phytother Res 1999;13:258-60.

The Review of Natural Products by Facts and Comparisons. St. Louis, MO: Wolters Kluwer Co., 1999.

Peirce A. The American Pharmaceutical Association Practical Guide to Natural Medicines. New York, NY: William Morrow and Co., 1999.

*THESE STATEMENTS HAVE NOT BEEN EVALUATED BY THE FOOD AND DRUG ADMINISTRATION. THIS PRODUCT IS NOT INTENDED TO DIAGNOSE, TREAT, CURE, OR PREVENT ANY DISEASE.

IMMUNIZEN®   DS
[ĭm mōō nĭ zĕn]
Support a Healthy Immune System*

DESCRIPTION

Immunizen® is a dietary supplement for strengthening and fortifying the immune system.

Immunizen® is a modestly water-soluble, white crystalline powder. Immunizen® consists of a proprietary ingredient blend of colostrum, arabinogalactan, 1,3, 1,6 yeast beta-glucans, and lactoferrin. In addition to the active ingredients, each 835 mg capsule of Immunizen® contains natural gelatin, stearic acid, and silicon dioxide.

BENEFITS AND RESEARCH

Immunizen® combines the positive immune modulating effects of colostrum, arabinogalactans, yeast beta-glucans, and lactoferrin to boost your body's natural defenses to foreign antigens. Colostrum is composed of immunoglobulins that bolster the body's immune system by providing immunity against various pathogens.

Beta-glucans are generally derived from the cell walls of the yeast species *Saccharomyces cerevisiae*. Beta-glucans are potent immuno-modulating agents that prime both the innate and adaptive immune systems.

USAGE

As a dietary supplement, take two capsules daily with water one to two hours before a meal.

SAFETY AND WARNINGS

Immunizen® is well tolerated. As with any dietary supplement, some gastrointestinal discomfort may be experienced.

HOW SUPPLIED

Available in capsules.

REFERENCES

Lilius EM, Marnila P. (2001), Current Opinion in Infectious Diseases 14:295-300.

Hammarström L, Weiner CK. (2008), Advances in Experimental Medicine and Biology 606: 321-343.

Chan GC, Chan WK, Sze DM. (2009), The Journal of Hematology and Oncology, 2: 25-

* THESE STATEMENTS HAVE NOT BEEN EVALUATED BY THE FOOD AND DRUG ADMINISTRATION. THIS PRODUCT IS NOT INTENDED TO DIAGNOSE, TREAT, CURE, OR PREVENT ANY DISEASE.

JOINT MOBILITY™   DS
Promotes Healthy Joints*

Description

Joint Mobility is a nutritional supplement for overall joint health.

Joint Mobility contains Undenatured Type II Collagen, Turmeric Extract (95% Curcumin), Boswellia Extract and Vitamin D3 as active ingredients, and also includes microcrystalline cellulose and silicon dioxide. This supplement is for individuals with joint pain and discomfort caused from normal wear and tear.

Joint Mobility is a powder filled capsule that takes on the yellow color of Turmeric. Compared to more traditional joint supplements, Joint Mobility is a small dose at just 881 mg per day. These smaller capsules are ideal for individuals who have trouble taking large capsules or pills.

Benefits and Research

Many people suffer daily from joint pain and discomfort caused from years of overuse or from being overweight or obese. Joint pain and a loss of mobility can dramatically affect quality of life, making simple everyday activity difficult and painful. The ingredients contained in Joint Mobility work in several different ways to help maintain overall joint health. Curcumin and Boswellia extract have been shown to downregulate the genes involved in chronic inflammation. Vitamin D3 has been shown to help increase collagen production which is needed to maintain overall joint health. Joint Mobility works in several different ways for a multifaceted approach to joint health. The ingredients contained have been shown to inhibit proinflammatory pathways, and also help to prevent the breakdown of joint collagen allowing the body to repair and heal itself.[1]

Usage

Take two capsules daily.

Safety and Warnings

Joint Mobility is generally well tolerated. As with any dietary supplement, some gastrointestinal discomfort may be experienced.

How Supplied

Available in capsules.

References

Crowley DC, Lau FC, Sharma P, *et al.*: Safety and efficacy of undenatured type II collagen in the treatment of osteoarthritis of the knee: a clinical trial. Int J Med Sci 2009; **6**:312-321.

Chandran B, Goel A.: A randomized, pilot study to assess the efficacy and safety of curcumin in patients with active rheumatoid arthritis. Phytother. Res. 2012 Nov; 26(11): 1719-25. Doi: 10.1002/ptr.4639.Epub 2012 Mar 9.

Dobak J1, Grzybowski J, et al.: 1,25-Dihydroxyvitamin D3 increases collagen production in dermal fibroblasts. J Dermatol Sci. 1994 Aug;8(1):18-24.

Kimmatkar N, Thawani V, et al.: Efficacy and tolerability of Boswellia serrate extract in treatment of osteoarthritis of knee—a randomized double bling placebo controlled trial. Phytomedicine 2003 Jan; 10(1):3-7.

Reuter S, Gupta S, et al.: Epigenetic changes induced by curcumin and other natural compounds. Genes Nutr (2011) 6:93–108.

Takada Y, Ichikawa H, et al.: Acetyl-11-Keto-β-Boswellic Acid Potentiates Apoptosis, Inhibits Invasion, and Abolishes Osteoclastogenesis by Suppressing NF-κB and NF-κB-Regulated Gene Expression. J Immunol 2006; 176:3127-3140.

---

*THESE STATEMENTS HAVE NOT BEEN EVALUATED BY THE FOOD AND DRUG ADMINISTRATION. THIS PRODUCT IS NOT INTENDED TO DIAGNOSE, TREAT, CURE, OR PREVENT ANY DISEASE.

Shown in Product Identification Guide, page 510

OMEGALIFE-3™   DS
[ōmĕgā-līf 3]
Omega-3 Fatty Acid Supplementation

DESCRIPTION

OmegaLife-3™ is a blend of omega-3 fatty acids designed to help maintain healthy cardiovascular and cerebral function. OmegaLife-3™ is an amber-colored, semi-viscous, fat-soluble liquid. Each serving of OmegaLife-3™ contains the following active ingredients: 800 mg eicosapentaenoic acid (EPA), 400 mg docosahexaenoic acid (DHA), and vitamin E. In addition, it also contains the inactive ingredients gelatin, glycerin, purified water, and orange oil. OmegaLife-3™ has been molecularly distilled to ensure exceptionally pure oil and includes orange oil to prevent a fishy aftertaste.

BENEFITS AND RESEARCH

Clinical research suggests fish oil can help support proper brain and visual function. In 2002 the FDA approved supplementation of DHA in infant formula. DHA is potentially important in fetal and infant neural development, in that DHA and arachidonic acid have been shown to be incorporated into brain and retinal cell membranes—particularly during the third trimester of pregnancy and early infant life.

DHA is the predominant structural fatty acid in the central nervous system and in the retina of the eyes.

EPA supports the synthesis of important compounds in the body. EPA is the precursor of thromboxane and leukotriene, compounds involved in supporting healthy circulation. They also promote healthy blood vessels.

Evidence is accumulating that increasing intakes of EPA and DHA can decrease the risk thrombosis, decrease triglyceride levels, and decrease inflammation.[1]

The U.S. Food and Drug Administration (FDA) has stated, "Supportive but not conclusive research shows that consumption of EPA and DHA omega-3 fatty acids may reduce the risk of coronary heart disease."

USAGE

Take two softgels twice daily with a meal.

SAFETY AND WARNINGS

OmegaLife-3™ is well tolerated. As with any dietary supplement, some gastrointestinal discomfort may be experienced. Common side effects include a "fishy" taste upon eructation.

HOW SUPPLIED

Available in softgels.

REFERENCES

Barter P, Ginsberg HN. Effectiveness of combined statin plus omega-3 fatty acid therapy for mixed dyslipidemia. Am J Cardiol. 2008 Oct 15:102(8):1040-5

Lee JH, Harris WS, et al. Omega-3 fatty acids for cardioprotection. Mayo Clin Proc. 2008 Mar;83(3):324-32.

SanGiovanni JP, Chew EY, Sperduto RD, et al. The relationship of dietary omega-3 long-chain polyunsaturated fatty acid intake with incident age-related macular degeneration: AREDS report no. 23. Arch Ophthalmol. 2008 Sep;126(9):1274-9.

SanGiovanni JP, Parra-Cabrera S, Colditz GA, Berkey CS, Dwyer JT. Meta-analysis of dietary essential fatty acids and long-chain polyunsaturated fatty acids as they relate to visual resolution acuity in healthy preterm infants. Pediatrics 2000;105:1292-8.

Kris-Etherton PM, Harris WS, Appel LJ. Omega-3 fatty acids and cardiovascular disease: new recommendations from the American Heart Association. Arterioscler Thromb Vasc Biol. 2003;23(2):151-152.

---

[1] THESE STATEMENTS HAVE NOT BEEN EVALUATED BY THE FOOD AND DRUG ADMINISTRATION. THIS PRODUCT IS NOT INTENDED TO DIAGNOSE, TREAT, CURE, OR PREVENT ANY DISEASE.

UBIQUINOL-CoQ10   DS
(Also known as CoQ10 Advanced Formula)

Description

As we age, levels of CoQ10 in the body decrease, causing the degeneration of cells. This may contribute to age-related conditions. Ubiquinol CoQ10 provides essential nutrients that may benefit the heart; it also contains antioxidants that may combat free-radical damage as well as help to naturally sustain healthy levels of CoQ10 in people as they age. Ubiquinol CoQ10 is a high-potency formula of Ubiquinol along with sunflower oil, yellow beeswax, and sunflower lecithin to increase solubility and bioavailability. CoenzymeQ10 (CoQ10) is found naturally in the body and plays an essential role in the production of energy in all cells.

Benefits and Research

Ubiquinol (CoQ10) is found naturally in the body and plays an essential role in the production of energy in all cells. The body requires a sufficient amount of CoQ10 in order to function optimally. This product may help enhance the effectiveness of the immune system. Some research has shown that a CoQ10 deficiency may contribute to possible side effects in persons taking statin medications. CoQ10 may support heart health and may assist the body in energy production in cells. CoQ10 is also an antioxidant that may protect cells from free radicals.

Suggested Use

Take one softgel daily. Do not take while on blood thinning medication without consulting a doctor.

Safety and Warnings

Ubiquinol CoQ10 is generally well tolerated. As with any dietary supplement, some gastrointestinal discomfort may be experienced.

How Supplied

Available in softgels.

References

Resenfeldt, Franklin, Francis Miller, Phillip Nagley, Anthony Hadj, Silvana Marasco, Deahne Quick, Freya Sheeran, Michelle Wowk, Salvatore Pepe. 2004. Response of the Senescent Heart to Stress: Clinical Therapeutic Strategies and Quest for Mitochondrial Predictors of Biological Age. *Annals of the New York Academy of Sciences* 1019

[1]THESE STATEMENTS HAVE NOT BEEN EVALUATED BY THE FOOD AND DRUG ADMINISTRATION. THIS PRODUCT IS NOT INTENDED TO DIAGNOSE, TREAT, CURE OR PREVENT ANY DISEASE.

UNICITY BALANCE™   DS
(Also known as Bios Life® Slim or Bios Life® S)
Formula for Healthy Cholesterol Support

DESCRIPTION

Unicity Balance™ (also known as Bios Life® Slim or Bios Life® S) is a fiber-based, vitamin-rich nutritional supplement. Unicity Balance™ contains a blend of soluble and insoluble fibers, Unicity® 7× technology, phytosterols, policosanol, an extract of *Chrysanthemum morifolium*, vitamins, and minerals that when combined with a healthy diet and exercise may lower total serum cholesterol, and help achieve and maintain a healthy body weight.

Unicity Balance™ is light orange in color. It is a hygroscopic crystalline powder that is generally soluble in water. Each serving of Unicity Balance™ contains 4 g of fiber, 1 g of phytosterols, 750 mg of Unicity 7×, 6 mg of policosanol, and 12.5 mg of an extract of *Chrysanthemum morifolium*. In addition to these active ingredients, each serving of Unicity Balance™ contains maltodextrin, citric acid, orange juice powder, sweeteners, and orange flavor.

BENEFITS AND RESEARCH

It's estimated that Americans consume 10-12 g of total fiber per day, less than half the amount of the recommended daily intake. Epidemiological and clinical studies have correlated high daily fiber intake with an improvement in overall health.

Unicity Balance™ is a nutritional supplement designed to increase fiber intake. Each serving of Unicity Balance™ contains four grams of fiber. When taken three times daily, Unicity Balance™ contributes half of the recommended daily value of fiber. Fiber supplementation has been shown to decrease preprandial and postprandial glucose levels, lower LDL cholesterol and apolipoprotein B levels, increase satiety, and facilitate weight loss.

In addition to fiber supplementation, Unicity Balance™ contains a patented blend of phytosterols, policosanol, *Chrysanthemum morifolium*, vitamins, and minerals. Unicity Balance™ facilitates weight loss through five distinct mechanisms. First, the soluble fiber matrix promotes an increase in satiety. Second, Unicity Balance™ improves cholesterol levels. Reduction in LDL content removes a potent inhibitor of lipolysis. Third, Unicity Balance™ improves blood glucose levels. Appropriate serum glucose levels help maintain many metabolic processes in the body. Reducing insulin levels permits fatty acid oxidation to occur. Fourth, Unicity Balance™ restores appropriate leptin signaling. Lastly, Unicity Balance™ reduces triglyceride levels allowing for leptin to cross the blood-brain barrier and affect its mechanism of action.

SUGGESTED USAGE

Dissolve the contents of one packet or one scoop into 8 to 10 fl. oz. of liquid (water or juice) and stir vigorously. Drink immediately. Use 15-20 minutes before meals up to three times daily.

SAFETY AND WARNINGS

Unicity Balance™ is well tolerated. There may be mild gastrointestinal discomfort, such as increased flatulence or loose stools, during the first month of initial use due to the increased uptake of dietary fiber. This GI disturbance usually disappears within the first thirty days. If the GI discomfort persists, reduce the number of servings of Unicity Balance™. If the GI discomfort further persists, stop taking the product and consult your physician. Taking this product without adequate liquid can result in complications.

HOW SUPPLIED

Unicity Balance™ is packaged in single-serving foil packets or in bulk canisters.

REFERENCES

Sprecher, DL and Pearce GL (2002), Metabolism 51: 1166-70.
Verdegem, PJE; Freed, S and Joffe D (2005), American Diabetess Assocation 65th Scientific Sessions, San Diego, CA.
Slavin, JL, (2005) Nutrition 21: 411-418.
Delzenne NM, Cani PD, (2005) Current Opinion Clincal Nutrition & Metabolic Care 8: 636-640
Duenas, V; Duenas, J; Burke, E and Verdegem, PJE (2006), 7th International Conference on Arteriosclerosis, Thrombosis, and Vascular Biology, American Heart Association, Denver, CO.
Verdegem, PJE (2007), Current Topics in Nutraceutical Research 5: 1-6
US Patent 6,933,291.

* THESE STATEMENTS HAVE NOT BEEN EVALUATED BY THE FOOD AND DRUG ADMINISTRATION. THIS PRODUCT IS NOT INTENDED TO DIAGNOSE, TREAT, CURE, OR PREVENT ANY DISEASE.

Shown in Product Identification Guide, page 510

Unilever Thai Trading Limited
161 RAMA 9 ROAD
HUAI KHWANG, HUAI KHWANG,
BANGKOK 10310 THAILAND

Direct Inquiries to:
www.unilevernetwork.com
unilevernetwork.th@unilever.com

---

aviance Perfec Radiance   DS

DESCRIPTION

aviance Perfec Radiance (aviance Pycno Plus in some countries), is a dietary supplement formulated from a proprietary combination of 7 nutritive ingredients. It contains the main ingredient Pycnogenol® (French maritime pine bark extract), Pomegranate extract, Borage seeds oil, Alpha lipoic acid (ALA), Zinc amino acid chelate, Vitamin C and Vitamin E, which help prevent oxidative damage in blood vessel & skin tissue.

BENEFITS AND RESEARCH

Pycnogenol® is the patented extract selected from pine barks grown in an unpolluted environment in the southwest of France, Gascony region. It contains various antioxidants, mainly Proanthocyanidins, and has been proven for preventing oxidative damage. Its safety is guaranteed with a GRAS (Generally Recognized As Safe) from USA. A 6 weeks study of 150 mg treatment in 45 subjects demonstrated that Pycnogenol® increases Oxygen Radical Absorbance Capacity in blood. Pycnogenol® significantly contributes to the improvement of heart health risk factors due to its antioxidant properties and other actions e.g. normalizing blood pressure, improving blood lipids, lowering blood sugar, controlling inflammation and decreasing platelet aggregation. An ever increasing number of clinical study demonstrates the efficacy of Pycnogenol® in keeping cardiovascular health problems at bay. In addition to its antioxidant activity in blood, Pycnogenol® also involves in blood circulation, oxygen and nutrients supply within the skin, and supports following activities;
- Production of glutathione, a natural antioxidant that regulates skin pigmentation
- Formation of collagen and elastin in the skin
- Skin recovery from UV damages.

Pomegranate Extract supports & maintains optimal cardiovascular health by Punicalagins, compounds primarily responsible for the fruit's antioxidant capacity and benefit for heart health. The sum effects of its phenolic compounds, including flavonoids, anthocyanins, and phenolic glycosides, offers pronounced effects on cardiovascular health e.g. increase endothelial nitric oxide, decrease oxidation of LDL cholesterol and maintain healthy HDL cholesterol level. Pomegranate extract can also enhance the production of collagen and increase the skin resistance to UVA and UVB radiations. Consequently, it prevents collagen damages, preserves collagen, and prevents aging signs.

Borage Seed Oil contains gamma-linolenic acid (GLA) which helps reducing risk of inflammation and maintain blood pressure. Many studies showed that it also helps boost immunity, lower serum cholesterol, phospholipids and triglyceride levels, lower blood pressure and prevent blood platelets aggregation. GLA can also improve skin structure, softness, suppleness, hydration, and reduce irritation.

ALA (Alpha lipoic Acid) is a natural compound found to mitigate oxidative stress in heart tissue, and has been used to prevent vascular disease, hypertension, and inflammation, as well as supplement diabetes treatment. A study showed that ALA may possess a lipid-lowering effect by significantly lower total cholesterol and low density lipoprotein (LDL) levels in blood.

ALA is beneficial for skin as it helps preserve vitamin C and E in the body, and prevents glutathione in the body from being damaged.

Zinc Amino Acid Chelate. Zinc plays important roles in maintaining structures and functions of endothelial cells, as well as strengthening and healing the vessels. Zinc is an essential mineral involved for the production of skin, hair, nails, and various tissues, as well as wound healing process.

Vitamin C is a water-soluble antioxidant which supports skin collagen formation and promotes blood cell and vessel strength.

Vitamin E is a lipid-soluble antioxidant that protects cells, tissues, and skin lipids from free radicals. There is evidence of synergistic effects for vitamin E and ALA to prevent excessive production of oxidant radicals in certain pathological processes. Regular consumption of both vitamin E and vitamin C helps increase skin resistance to sunlight.

USAGE

1 capsule daily after meal.

SAFETY AND WARNINGS

The product is well tolerated. Some gastrointestinal discomfort may be experienced as with any dietary supplement. All individual nutrient levels in Perfec Radiance are documented to be safe.

HOW SUPPLIED

Available in 30 packets of 2 capsules in carton box.

REFERENCES

1. Belcaro G et al. Venous ulcers: microcirculatory improvement and faster healing with local use of Pycnogenol®. *Angiology* 56:699-705, 2005.

Continued on next page

2. Belcaro G, Cesarone MR, Rohdewald P, Ricci A, Ippolito E, Dugall M, Griffin M, Ruffini I, Acerbi G, Vinciguerra MG, Bavera P, DiRenzo A, Errichi BM, Cerritelli F.Prevention of venous thrombosis and thrombophlebitis in long-haul flights with Pycnogenol®, *Clin Appl Thromb Hemost* 10: 373-377, 2004.
3. Blazsó G et al. Pycnogenol® accelerates wound healing and reduces scar formation. *Phytother Res* 18:579-581, 2004.
4. Brosche, T ; Platt, D., Effect of borage oil consumption on fatty acid metabolism, transepidermal water loss and skin parameters in elderly people, *Archives of Gerontology and Geriatrics*, 2000, Vol.30(2), pp.139-150
5. Cesarone MR, Belcaro G, Stuard S, Schönlau F, DiRenzo A, Grossi MG, Dugall M, Cornelli U, Cacchio M, Gizzi G, Pellegrini L.Kidney Flow and Function in Hypertension: Protective Effects of Pycnogenol® in Hypertensive Participants – A Controlled Study. *J Cardiovasc Pharmacol Ther* 15: 41-46, 2010.
6. De Spirt, S. ; Stahl, W. ; Tronnier, H. ; Sies, H. ; Bejot, M. ; Maurette, J. ; Heinrich, U., Intervention with flaxseed and borage oil supplements modulates skin condition in women, *British Journal of Nutrition,* 2008, Vol.101(3), pp.440-445
7. Devaraj S et al. Supplementation with a pine bark extract rich in polyphenols increases plasma antioxidant capacity and alters the plasma lipoprotein profile. *Lipids* 37: 931-934, 2002.
8. Enseleit, F ; Sudano, I ; Périat, D ; Winnik, S ; Wolfrum, M ; Flammer, A J ; Fröhlich, GM ; Kaiser, P; Hirt, A ; Haile, SR ; Krasniqi, N ; Matter, CM ; Uhlenhut, K; Högger, P ; Neidhart, M ; Lüscher, TF ; Ruschitzka, F ; Noll, G, Effects of Pycnogenol on endothelial function in patients with stable coronary artery disease: a double-blind, randomized, placebo-controlled, crossover study, *European Heart Journal*, 2012, Vol. 33(13), pp.1589-1597
9. Ephraim P. L, Robert A. N, *Punica granatum* (pomegranate) and its potential for prevention and treatment of inflammation and cancer, *Journal of Ethnopharmacology*, Volume 109, Issue 2, 19 January 2007, Pages 177–206
10. Fan , Y.Y. ; Chapkin , R.S., Importance of dietary gamma-linolenic acid in human health and nutrition, *Journal of nutrition*, 1998, Vol.128(9), pp.1411-1414
11. Fitzpatrick et al. Endothelium-dependent vascular effects of Pycnogenol®, *J Cardiovas Pharmacol* 32: 509-515, 1998.
12. Gilani , A.H. ; Bashir , S. ; Khan , A.U., Pharmacological basis for the use of Borago officinalis in gastrointestinal, respiratory and cardiovascular disorders, *Journal of Ethnopharmacology*, 2007, Vol.114, pp.393-399
13. Grimm T et al. Inhibition of NF-kB activation and MMP-9 secretion by plasma of human volunteers after ingestion of maritime pine bark extract (Pycnogenol®). *J Inflamm* 3: 1-15, 2006.
14. Hosseini S, Lee J, Sepulveda RT, Fagan T, Rohdewald P, Watson RR.A Randomized, double blind, placebo controlled, prospective, 16 week crossover study to determine the role of Pycnogenol® inmodifying blood pressure in mildly hypertensive patients. *Nutr Res* 21: 67-76, 2001.
15. Ismail, T.; Sestili, P.; Akhtar, S., Pomegranate peel and fruit extracts: A review of potential anti-inflammatory and antiinfective effects , *Journal of Ethnopharmacology*, 28 September 2012, Vol.143(2), pp.397-405.
16. Jameel, N.; Shekhar, M. A. ; Vishwanath, B. S., α-lipoic acid: An inhibitor of secretory phospholipase A 2 with antiinflammatory activity, *Life Sciences*, 2006, Vol.80(2), pp.146-153.
17. Liu X, Wei J, Tan F, Zhou S, Wurthwein G, Rohdewald P. Pycnogenol®, French maritime pine bark extract, improves endothelial function of hypertensive patients. *Life Sciences* 74: 855-862, 2004.
18. Maret, W.; Sandstead, H.H., Zinc requirements and the risks and benefits of zinc supplementation. *Journal of Trace Elements in Medicine and Biology*, 2006, Vol.20(1), pp.3-18.
19. Meydani, M., Vitamin E, *The Lancet*, 1995, Vol.345(8943), pp.170-175.
20. Nishioka K, Hidaka T, Takemoto H, Nakamura S, Umemura T, Jitsuiki D, Soga J, Goto C, Chayama K, Yoshizumi M, Higashi Y.Pycnogenol®, French maritime pinebarkextract,augmentsendothelium-dependentvasodilation in humans. *Hypertens Res* 30: 775-780, 2007.
21. Pumori S Telang, Vitamin C in dermatology, *Indian Dermatol Online J.* 2013 Apr-Jun; 4(2): 143–146.
22. Rohdewald P. A review of the French maritime pine bark extract (Pycnogenol®), a herbal medication with a diverse pharmacology. *Int J Clin Pharmacol Ther* 40(4): 158-168, 2002.
23. Saliou C et al. Solar ultraviolet-induced erythema in human skin and nuclear factor-kappa-B-dependent gene expression in keratinocytes are modulated by a French maritime pine bark extract. *Free Rad Biol Med* 30: 154-160, 2001.
24. Shay, KP ; Moreau, RF. ; Smith, E J. ; Smith, A R. ; Hagen, TM, Alpha-lipoic acid as a dietary supplement: Molecular mechanisms and therapeutic potential, *BBA - General Subjects*, 2009, Vol.1790(10), pp.1149-1160.
25. Stuard S, Belcaro G, Cesarone MR, Ricci A, Dugall M, Cornelli U, Gizzi G, Pellegrini L, Rohdewald PJ.,Kidney function in metabolic syndrome may be improved with Pycnogenol®. *Panminerva Med* 52(Suppl. 1): 27-32, 2010.
26. Wollin , S D. ; Jones , P J.H., α-Lipoic Acid and Cardiovascular Disease, *Journal of nutrition*, 2003, Vol.133(11), pp.3327-3330.
27. Yasumuro M et al. Inhibition of melanogenesis by pine (*Pinus pinaster*) bark extract containing procyanidins. *Manuscript in preparation* 2006.
28. Zibadi S, Qianli Y, Rohdewald P, Larson DF, Watson RR., Impact of Pycnogenol® on left ventricular remodeling induced by LNAME administration. *Cardiovasc Toxicol* 7:10-18. 2007.

Shown in Product Identification Guide, page 510

---

beyonde Algae Calcium-D — DS

Chicory Fiber,
Calcium plus vitamin D Dietary supplement

DESCRIPTION

beyonde algae calcium D is one of the breakthrough innovations of nutritional supplement as an instant drink powder format with "CALCIUM PRO-ABSORPTION" technology – a nutrient cocktail which improves gastrointestinal balance and enhances calcium absorption to help restore bone calcium deficiency. The product mainly contains calcium from red algae, selective mixed inulin & fructo-oligofructose from chicory fiber and vitamin D3.

In addition, it also contains permitted food conditioners & additives; dextrose, malic acid, gum arabic, orange powder, erythritol, sodium citrate, betacarotene, glycine, sucralose.

BENEFITS AND RESEARCH

Calcium from diets can increase blood calcium and prevent bone loss. It helps maintain bone calcium, protect bone density and strengthen bone mass. In addition, calcium is also essential for muscles and nerves. Lack of calcium can cause muscles malfunction and lead to cramping.

Calcium from red algae, *Lithothamnion calcareum*, growing naturally under the sea of Iceland, provides bioactive calcium, magnesium and 72 other minerals. It is derived from the calcified structure of red algae, which absorbs trace minerals from the surrounding seawater. Calcium from red algae has a unique structure similar to plant cells, and possesses larger surface area than conventional calcium from limestones. This mineral-rich product is neutral taste, free of chalky texture, and absorbable by the human body.

Minerals and other nutrients are also essential for calcium absorption, and building strong bones and muscles. Vitamin D is the most important nutrient to help promoting calcium absorption in intestine. A combination of vitamin D and calcium can increase calcium absorptivity by 3-4 times compared to single calcium supplementation. The study in a sample group of 389 patients, aged 70-75 years, receiving calcium 500 mg + Vit D 700 IU every night before bedtime for three years was found that the group with supplementation has lower rate of bone fractures than those who did not take (Bess Dawson, 1997). Another study in a sample group of 120 women, aged 45-55 years, had been taking calcium 500 mg + Vit. D 200 IU every day for three years was found to have the higher bone mineral than those who did not consume (Nicola Di Daniele, 2004).

Inulin & fructo-oligofructose are prebiotics beneficially for health. They are selectively fermented by bifidobacteria and lactobacilli which are beneficial microorganisms in the colon. Their fermentation generates end products such as lactic acid and short chain fatty acids, which allow the colonic condition to increase calcium absorption.

A study of 8 weeks supplementation with 8 grams of selective mixed inulin & fructo-oligofructose from chicory fiber (Abrams, 2007) showed that it can enhance the calcium absorption occurred principally in the colon. In addition, calcium absorption can still be traced over 24 hour period after oral supplementation of the mixed inulin & fructooligofructose.

In postmenopausal women, the high risk group for bone mineral loss & osteoporosis, there is a study on 6 weeks supplementation of selective mixed inulin & fructo-oligofructose from chicory fiber on intestinal absorption of calcium and bone turnover markers (Holloway, 2007). It demonstrated that the absorption of calcium is significantly increased (123%) after 5g per day treatment with the selective mixed inulin & fructo-oligofructose from chicory fiber.

USAGE

Mix 1 sachet with 120-150 ml of water and drink instantly. It is recommended to take 1-2 sachets a day.

SAFETY AND WARNINGS

For children, the recommended intake level for less than 15kg body weight is 1 sachet a day. It may possibly induce laxation in the 4-10 year old children consuming calcium drink due to the aggregate exposure to erythritol from different sources of food.

HOW SUPPLIED

Available in 15 sachets in a pouch.

REFERENCES

1) Abrams , Steven A ; Griffin , Ian J ; Hawthorne , Keli M ; Liang , Lily ; Gunn , Sheila K ; Darlington , Gretchen ; Ellis , Kenneth J, Combination of Prebiotic Short- and Long-chain Inulin-type Fructans Enhances Calcium Absorption and Bone Mineralization in Young Adolescents, *American journal of clinical nutrition*, 2005, Vol.82(2), pp.471-476
2) Abrams , Steven A. ; Hawthorne , Keli M. ; Aliu , Oluseyi ; Hicks , Penni D. ; Chen , Zhensheng ; Griffin , Ian J.Inulin-Type Fructan Enhances Calcium Absorption Primarily via an Effect on Colonic Absorption in Humans, *Journal of nutrition*, 2007, Vol.137(10), pp.2208-2212.
3) Aquamin Nutrition test certificate.
4) Bess Dawson-Hughes, M.D., Susans. Harris D.Sc. Elizabeth A. Krall, Ph.D. and Gerard E. Dallal, Ph.D., Effect of Calcium and Vitamin D Supplement on Bone Density in Men and Women 65 Years of Age or Older (1997).
5) Bronner, Felix ; Pansu, Danielle, Nutritional Aspects of Calcium Absorption, *Journal of Nutrition*, 2000, Vol.130(1), pp.9-12.
6) C Coudray ; J Bellanger ; C Castiglia-Delavaud ; C Rémésy ; M Vermorel ; Y Rayssignuier, Effect of soluble or partly soluble dietary fibers supplementation on absorption and balance of calcium, magnesium, iron and zinc in healthy young men, *European Journal of Clinical Nutrition*, 1997, Vol.51(6), p.375.
7) Connie M , Robert P; Calcium in Human Health,2006, (chapter9 Food Sources Supplement and bioavailability)
8) Daniele, Nicola Di ; Carbonelli, Maria Grazia ; Candeloro, Nicola ; Iacopino, Leonardo ; De Lorenzo, Antonino ; Andreoli, Angela, Effect of supplementation of calcium and Vitamin D on bone mineral density and bone mineral content in peri- and post-menopause women: A double-blind, randomized, controlled trial, *Pharmacological Research*, 2004, Vol.50(6), pp.637-641.
9) Fleet, James C. ; Schoch, Ryan D., Molecular mechanisms for regulation of intestinal calcium absorption by vitamin D and other factors, *Critical Reviews in Clinical Laboratory Sciences*, 2010, Vol.47(4), p.181-195.
10) Griffin, I. J ; Davila, P. M ; Abrams, S. A, Non-digestible oligosaccharides and calcium absorption in girls with adequate calcium intakes, *British Journal of Nutrition*, 2002, Vol.87(S2), pp.S187-S191.
11) Griffin, Ian J ; Hicks, Penni M.D ; Heaney, Robert P ; Abrams, Steven A, Enriched chicory inulin increases calcium absorption mainly in girls with lower calcium absorption, *Nutrition Research*, 2003, Vol.23(7), pp.901-909.
12) Heaney, Robert ; Recker, Robert ; Weaver, Connie, Absorbability of calcium sources: The limited role of solubility, Calcified Tissue International, 1990, Vol.46(5), pp.300-304.
13) Heuvel , E.G.H.M. Van Den ; Muys , T. ; Dokkum , W. Van. ; Schaafsma , G., Oligofructose stimulates calcium absorption in adolescents, *American Journal of Clinical Nutrition*, 1999, Vol.69(3), pp.544-548.
14) Holloway, Leah ; Moynihan, Sharon ; Abrams, Steven A ; Kent, Kyla ; Hsu, Andrew R ; Friedlander, Anne L, Effects of oligofructoseenriched inulin on intestinal absorption of calcium and magnesium and bone turnover markers in postmenopausal women, *British Journal of Nutrition*, 2007, Vol.97(2), pp.365-372.
15) http://www.kidneyatlas.org/book1/adk1_05.pdf(search on April 1,2006).
16) Keiko Sakuma, Molecular Mechanism of the Effect of Fructo-oligosaccharides on Calcium Absorption, *Bioscience and Microflora*, 2002, Vol.21(1), pp.13-20.

17) Lacour, B ; Tardivel, S ; Drüeke, T, Stimulation by citric acid of calcium and phosphorus bioavailability in rats fed a calcium-rich diet. *Mineral and electrolyte metabolism*, 1997, Vol.23(2), pp.79-87.

18) Meiron, Oren E ; Bar-david, Elad ; Aflalo, Eliahu D ; Shechter, Assaf ; Stepensky, David ; Berman, Amir ; Sagi, Amir, Solubility and bioavailability of stabilized amorphous calcium carbonate, *Journal of Bone and Mineral Research*, 2011,Vol.26(2), pp.364-372.

19) Nicola Di Daniele, Maria Grazia Carbonelli, Nicola Candeloro, Leonardo Iacopino, Antonino De Lorenzo, Angela Andreoli. Effect of supplementation of calcium and Vitamin D on bone mineral density and bone mineral content in peri- and post-menopause women A double-blind, randomized, controlled trial, *Pharmacological Research 50* , 2004, 637–641.

20) Souza, Maria Cristina Corrêa de ; Lajolo, Franco Maria ; Martini, Ligia de Araujo ; Correa, Nelton Bespalez ; Dan, Milana Cara ; Menezes, Elizabete Wenzel de, Effect of oligofructose-enriched inulin on bone metabolism in girls with low calcium intakes, 2010, Vol.53(1), p.193-201.

21) Vavrusova, Martina ; Skibsted, Leif H., Calcium nutrition. Bioavailability and fortification LWT - *Food Science and Technology*, 2014, Vol.59(2), pp.1198-1204.

22) Yotsanan Weerapol ; Kamonrak Cheewatanakornkool ; Pornsak Sriamornsak, Impact of Gastric pH and Dietary Fiber on Calcium Availability of Various Calcium Salts, *Silpakorn University Science and Technology Journal*, 2010, Vol.4(1), pp.15-23.

Shown in Product Identification Guide, page 510

---

beyonde Life Sential   DS
Multivitamins Plus Minerals / S-O-D Plus Coenzyme Q10 / Chlorella Plus Shiitake

DESCRIPTION
beyonde Life Sential is a revolutionary dietary supplement which contains Vitamins, Minerals, Amino Acids and *Phytomolecules* for helping restore strength, defend against stress and fatigue and protect immunity at the cellular level.
The product contains 3 tablets which are;

1) **Multivitamins and Minerals plus Amino Acids** (Vitamin A, Vitamin C, Vitamin E, Vitamin B1, Vitamin B2, Vitamin B3, Vitamin B5, Vitamin B6, Vitamin B12, Folic acid, Magnesium, Chromium, Iron, Selenium, Copper, Manganese, Zinc, Iodine, Calcium, L-Leucine, L-Isoleucine, L-Valine, L-Arginine, L-Methionine).

2) **SOD plus Coenzyme Q10** (Superoxide Dismutase from French Melon Juice Extract, Coenzyme Q10, Sodium Copper Chlorophyllin)

3) **Chlorella Plus Shiitake** (Nucleotides complex from *Chlorella vulgaris* & Bioactive Beta -glucan from Shiitake mycelium)

In addition to those active ingredients, beyonde Life Sential also contains microcrystalline cellulose, calcium carbonate, croscarmellose sodium, colloidal silicon dioxide, pregelatinized starch, caramel powdered color, magnesium stearate, hydroxypropyl methylcellulose, hydroxypropyl cellulose-L, talcum and polyethylene glycol.

BENEFITS AND RESEARCH
Multivitamins and Minerals play many important roles in human body such as; delivering nutrients to cells and organs for cellular metabolism & energy production, regulating neurological processes and supporting eye sight, heart, skin, immunity, blood cell, muscles and bone functions.

Leucine, Iso-leucine, Valine, Arginine and Methionine are amino acids which help improve complication in chronic fatigue. A research found that the plasma levels of Leucine, Iso-leucine, Valine, Arginine and Methionine are decreased in chronic fatigue subjects. Supplementation of these amino acids is possibly positive effect. Fatigues has been found to affect the neurotransmitter level, in particular 5-Hydroxytryptamine (5-HT), decrease metabolism in brain, sleep quality, mood and emotion. **Branched-chain amino acids (L-Leucine, L-Isoleucine, L-Valine)** can elevate 5-HT balance which then relieve fatigue and stress, and enhance cell functions and physical endurance. **L-Arginine** serves as a precursor for the synthesis of growth hormone, supports vascular and heart functions, regulates nitric oxide level and blood flow, and promotes energy expenditure function of mitochondria. **L-Methionine** is a major amino acid for brain functions, as being previously been used for treatment of depression.

Superoxide Dismutase or SOD enzyme is one of the most crucial antioxidants found in cells. It helps prolong cell lifespan, reduce body & brain stress, increase attention span and memory. A clinical study in 61 healthy subjects, 30 to 65 years old, with a certain level of stress and fatigue but without any depressive symptoms, demonstrated the significant reduction of stress induced by a one-month supplementation with 140 IU of SOD from French melon juice extract. According to the study, French melon SOD enzyme supplementation can be also very beneficial for the complete fatigue condition, by reducing both physical and cognitive fatigue. beyonde Life Sential contains 140 IU of SOD from French melon juice extract per serving.

Co-enzyme Q 10 (CoQ10) helps prolong life and enhances energy production in cells of important organs such as heart, brain, liver, kidney, and muscle. CoQ10 level in human starts to decrease after the age of 20. Supplementation of CoQ10 can slow down cell aging and reduce risks of chronic diseases that might occur in aging people. **Chlorophyll** has been found to protect cells from damages by free radicals, radiations, and toxins. **Sodium copper chlorophyllin** is better absorbed than chlorophyll existed in fruits and vegetables.

Nucleotides complex from *Chlorella vulgaris* is the concentrated nutrient specially extracted from the nucleus of *Chlorella vulgaris* algae. It is full of amino acids, vitamins, and minerals, especially "Nucleotide complex". Nucleotide complex improves natural immunity and protects DNA in the cells from various toxins that lead to tumors and cancers. A study in healthy subjects showed that the extract from *Chlorella vulgaris* can significantly increase the production of cytokines in a human cell line.

Bioactive Beta-glucan from Shiitake mycelium cultivated with a special technique to obtain bioactive beta-glucan with special 3D helix structure, so called Lentinan. This bioactive beta-glucan possesses the biological efficiency in stimulating the production of Lymphocytes, Macrophages, NK-cells, Interferon and were found to suppress cancer recurrence, prolong the lifespan of Cancer & HIV patients. A double-blind, cross-over, placebo-controlled trial in 42 subjects revealed that Beta-glucan from Shiitake mycelium can increase the number of B-cells which help produce antibody to fight off infections.

USAGE
Take 1 sachet containing 3 tablets after meal with a glass of water.

SAFETY AND WARNINGS
While there are no acute toxicity concerns, continuous exposure to some components of this product at the levels provided by the maximum recommended dose should be done with the knowledge of the consumer's health care provider. Do not exceed 4 sachets per day. Not recommended for children and pregnant women. The product contains Mushroom and Soy.

HOW SUPPLIED
Available in 30 packets of 3 tablets in carton box

REFERENCES
1) da Luz, C.R.; Nicastro, H.; Zanchi, N.E.; Chaves, D.F.S.; Lancha Jr, A.H. Potential therapeutic effects of branched-chain amino acids supplementation on resistance exercise-based muscle damage in humans. Journal of the International Society of Sports Nutrition, 14 December 2011, Vol.8.

2) Ewart HS, Bloch O, Girouard GS, Kralovec J, Barrow CJ, Ben-Yehudah G, Suárez ER, Rapoport MJ, Stimulation of cytokine production in human peripheral blood mononuclear cells by an aqueous Chlorella extract., Planta Medica [2007, 73(8):762-768].

3) French, Glyn N. "Exercise-induced muscle damage is reduced in resistance-trained males by branched chain amino acids: a randomized, double-blind, placebo controlled study." Journal of the International Society of Sports Nutrition 9.1 (2012): 20-20.

4) Gad, M.Z., Anti-aging effects of L-arginine, Journal of Advanced Research, July 2010, Vol.1(3), pp.169-177.

5) Garlick, P.J., Toxicity of methionine in humans, Journal of Nutrition, June 2006, Vol.136(6), pp.1722S-1725S.

6) Giroux, I.; Kurowska, E.M.; Carroll, K.K. Role of dietary lysine, methionine, and arginine in the regulation of hypercholesterolemia in rabbits. Journal of Nutritional Biochemistry, March 1999, Vol.10(3), pp.166-171.

7) Humberto J. Morrisa, Olimpia Carrillob, Angel Almaralesc, Rosa C. Bermúdeza, Yamila Lebequea, Roberto Fontainea, Gabriel Llauradóa, Yaixa Beltrána, Immunostimulant activity of an enzymatic protein hydrolysate from green microalga Chlorella vulgaris on undernourished mice, Enzyme and Microbial Technology, Volume 40, Issue 3, 5 February 2007, Pages 456–460.

8) Hyo-Jin An, Hong-Kun Rim, Jong-Hyun Lee, Jin-Woo Hong, Na-Hyung Kim, Noh-Yil Myung, Phil-Dong Moon, In-Young Choi, Ho-Jeong Na, Hyun-Ja Jeong, Hyeung-Suk Park, Jae-Gab Han, Jae-Young Um, Hyung-Min Kim, Effect of *Chlorella vulgaris* on Immune-enhancement and Cytokine Production in vivo and in vitro, Food Science and Biotechnology 2008; 17(5): 953-958.

9) Isoda N1, Eguchi Y, Nukaya H, Hosho K, Suga Y, Suga T, Nakazawa S, Sugano K., Clinical efficacy of superfine dispersed lentinan (beta-1,3-glucan) in patients with hepatocellular carcinoma., Hepatogastroenterology. 2009 Mar-Apr;56(90):437-41.

10) JM. Gaullier, J. Sleboda, E. Snorre Ø, E. Ulvestad, M. Nurminiemi, C. Moe, T. Albrektsen, O.Gudmundsen., Six weeks supplementation with a beta-glucan exported from shiitake mycelium, induce immune response in healthy, elderly humans.- A cross-over, placebo-controlled study. (Unpublished).

11) Konishi F, Tanaka K, Himeno K, Taniguchi K, Nomoto K.,Antitumor effect induced by a hot water extract of *Chlorella vulgaris* (CE): resistance to Meth-A tumor growth mediated by CE-induced polymorphonuclear leukocytes., Cancer Immunol Immunother. 1985;19(2):73-8.

12) Konishi F1, Mitsuyama M, Okuda M, Tanaka K, Hasegawa T, Nomoto K., Protective effect of an acidic glycoprotein obtained from culture of *Chlorella vulgaris* against myelosuppression by 5-fluorouracil. Cancer Immunol Immunother. 1996 Jun;42(5):268-74.

13) Konishi F1, Tanaka K, Kumamoto S, Hasegawa T, Okuda M, Yano I, Yoshikai Y, Nomoto K., Enhanced resistance against Escherichia coli infection by subcutaneous administration of the hot-water extract of *Chlorella vulgaris* in cyclophosphamide-treated mice. Cancer Immunol Immunother. 1990;32(1):1-7.

14) Lanfer-Marquez, U.M.; Barros, R.M.C.; Sinnecker, P. Antioxidant activity of chlorophylls and their derivatives ,Food Research International, October 2005, Vol. 38 (8-9), pp.885-891.

15) Milesi, M.-A.; Lacan, D.; Brosse, H .; Desor, D.; Notin, C., Effect of an oral supplementation with a proprietary melon juice concentrate (Extramel ®) on stress and fatigue in healthy people: A pilot, double-blind, placebo-controlled clinical trial, Nutrition Journal, 2009, Vol.8(1).

16) Mischoulon, D.; Fava, M., Role of S-adenosyl-L-methionine in the treatment of depression: A review of the evidence, American Journal of Clinical Nutrition, 1 November 2002, Vol.76(5), pp.1158S-1161S

17) Rodney L. Levine, Jackob Moskovitz and Earl R. Stadtman, Oxidation of Methionine in Proteins: Roles in Antioxidant Defense and Cellular Regulation, IUBMB LIFE Volume 50, Issue 4-5, October 2000, Pages: 301–307,

18) Sia GM, Candlish JK., Effects of shiitake (*Lentinus edodes*) extract on human neutrophils and the U937 monocytic cell line., Phytother Res. 1999 Mar;13(2):133-7.

19) Takashi Hasegawa, a, Yuki Kimurab, Kenji Hiromatsub, Noritada Kobayashib, Akira Yamadac, Masahiko Makinod, Masao Okudaa, Toshihiko Sanoa, Kikuo Nomotoe, Yasunobu Yoshikaib, Effect of hot water extract of *Chlorella vulgaris* on cytokine expression patterns in mice with murine acquired immunodeficiency syndrome after infection with Listeria monocytogenes, Immunopharmacology, Volume 35, Issue 3, January 1997, Pages 273–282.

20) Tanaka K1, Yamada A, Noda K, Hasegawa T, Okuda M, Shoyama Y, Nomoto K., A novel glycoprotein obtained from *Chlorella vulgaris* strain CK22 shows antimetastatic immunopotentiation., Cancer Immunol Immunother. 1998 Feb;45(6):313-20.

21) Yasmin Anum Mohd Yusof, I Suhana Md. Saad, II Suzana Makpol, I Nor Aripin Shamaan,III and Wan Zurinah Wan NgahI, Hot water extract of *Chlorella vulgaris* induced DNA damage and apoptosis, Clinics (Sao Paulo). Dec 2010; 65(12): 1371–1377.

22) Yoshiharu Shimomura, Yuko Yamamoto, Gustavo Bajotto, Juichi Sato, Taro Murakami, Noriko Shimomura, Hisamine Kobayashi, and Kazunori Mawatari, Nutraceutical Effects of Branched-Chain Amino Acids on Skeletal Muscle, The Journal of Nutrition. Page:529S-532S.

Shown in Product Identification Guide, page 510

---

beyonde Maqui Plus⁺   DS
Multi Fruits & Berries Concentrate Drink

DESCRIPTION
beyonde Maqui Plus⁺ is the concentrate antioxidant drink from the proprietary natural combination of Multi Fruits &

Continued on next page

Berries Concentrate which contains 12 fruits including Maqui Berry, Artichoke, Goji Berry, Acai, Acerola Cherry, Raspberry, Red Grape & Grape Seed Extract, Chokeberry, Cranberry, Apple, Strawberry and Cherry.

Regular consumption of Maqui Plus⁺, a combination of multi-fruits and berries concentrate, provides high levels of natural antioxidants which help reduce free radicals in the body, prevent oxidative stress, reduce risks of age-related diseases, and promote overall well-being.

In addition, it also contains fructose, pectin and sodium benzoate. The product is aseptic bottled in amber glass container in order to preserve its antioxidant capacity.

BENEFITS AND RESEARCH

Maqui berry is an exotic deep purple berry found in Chile, known as Chilean wineberry. It is reported that Maqui berry has exceptionally high antioxidant capacity. The major antioxidants in Maqui berry are anthocyanins, the group of deep-purple phytonutrients found in blue and purple color fruits. Anthocyanins have antioxidative property which can fight against free radicals, thus delay the aging of cells due to exposure of free radicals. Research indicates that anthocyanins can reduce risks of aging diseases such as heart disease, cancer, Alzheimer's disease, Parkinson's disease and reduce diabetes complications. It also helps improve blood circulation in the eye peripheral capillary and slows down degeneration of eye and vision. Many *in vitro & in vivo* studies also showed that high anthocyanins content enables Maqui berry to promote insulin functions and regulate blood sugar levels.

Artichoke is widely cultivated in Mediterranean, Europe, Australia and North America. It is a medicinal plant with high antioxidants, minerals and fibers. The important antioxidant in Artichoke is Cynarin which has been proven beneficial for health, in particular, improving liver functions. It enhances antioxidant capacity of the liver, hence aiding in its detoxification functions.

Gojiberry is a small orange-red berry which is well known in traditional Chinese herbal medicine. It is rich in vitamins and antioxidants e.g. Betacarotene, Lycopene, *L.barbarum* Polysaccharides. Gojiberry is widely used as functional food with broad health benefits such as aiding detoxification process in the liver, promoting the liver regeneration, antitumor and inhibit cancer cell growth (e.g. colon cancer, prostate cancer and liver cancer).

A study in 20 adults who smoke or drink alcohol regularly showed that Maqui Plus+ supplementation significantly increased glutathione (GSH), the activities of glutathione peroxidase (GSH-Px), glutathione reductase (GSH-Rd), superoxide dismutase (SOD) and decreased thiobarbituric acid reactive substances (TBARS) compared with the placebo. Additionally, hepatic and renal functions were not adversely altered in Maqui Plus+ ingested subjects. It is suggested that Maqui Plus+ effectively promotes the endogenous antioxidant activity, and can be consumed as a functional supplement for people who are in danger of suffering oxidative-related chronic diseases.

USAGE

Take 1 shot (25 ml) twice daily, morning & evening. Consumption can be increased to 2 shots (50 ml) twice daily as required.

SAFETY AND WARNINGS

Allergies to fruits (e.g., berries) and other plant components of this product could occur, but would be rare. Ingestion of large amounts of concentrate could occur which may result in gastrointestinal distress such as vomiting, cramping and diarrhea. This could be a concern for an accidental ingestion of large amounts of concentrate, especially by a child.

HOW SUPPLIED

50 ml & 750 ml bottle

REFERENCES

1. Güldal Mehmetçik, Gül Özdemirler, Necla Koçak-Toker, Ugur Çevikbas, Müjdat Uysal, Effect of pretreatment with artichoke extract on carbon tetrachloride-induced liver injury and oxidative stress, Experimental and *Toxicologic Pathology*, Volume 60, Issue 6, 18 September 2008, Pages 475-480.
2. Bo-Han Wu, Wen-Chao Wang, Hsin-Yu Kuo, Effect of Multi-berries Drink on Endogenous Antioxidant Activity in Subjects Who Are Regular Smokers or Drinkers, *Journal of Food and Nutrition Research*, Vol. 4, No. 5, 2016, pp 289-295. doi: 10.12691/jfnr-4-5-4 | A Clinical Study
3. BoKang Cui, YanFeng Chen, Su Liu, Jun Wang, ShuHong Li, QiBo Wang, ShengPing Li, MinShan Chen,

XiaoJun Lin, Antitumour activity of *Lycium chinensis* polysaccharides in liver cancer rats, International *Journal of Biological Macromolecules*, Volume 51, Issue 3, October 2012, Pages 314-318.
4. Carolina Fredes, Gloria Montenegro, Juan Pablo Zoffoli, Miguel Gómez, and Paz Rober, Chilean Journal of Agricultural Research 72(4) October-December 2012 Scientific Note's Polyphenol Content and Anti-oxidant Activity of Maqui (*Aristotelia chilensis* (Molina) Stuntz) During Fruit Development and Maturation in Central Chile, *Chilean Journal of Agricultural Research* 72(4) October-December 2012, pages 582-589.
5. Escribano-Bailón MT, Alcalde-Eon C, Muñoz O, Rivas-Gonzalo JC, Santos-Buelga C., Anthocyanins in berries of Maqui (*Aristotelia chilensis* (Mol.) Stuntz).,*Phytochem Anal.* 2006 Jan-Feb;17(1):8-14.
6. K. Kraft, Artichoke leaf extract — Recent findings reflecting effects on lipid metabolism, liver and gastrointestinal tracts, *Phytomedicine*, Volume 4, Issue 4, December 1997, Pages 369-378.
7. Leonel E. Rojo, David Ribnicky, Sithes Logendra, Alex Poulev, Patricio Rojas-Silva, Peter Kuhn, Ruth Dorn, Mary H. Grace, Mary Ann Lila, Ilya Raskin, In vitro and in vivo anti-diabetic effects of anthocyanins from Maqui Berry (*Aristotelia chilensis*), *Food Chemistry*, Volume 131, Issue 2, 15 March 2012, Pages 387-396.
8. Mingliang Jin, Qingsheng Huang, Ke Zhao, Peng Shang, Biological activities and potential health benefit effects of polysaccharides isolated from *Lycium barbarum* L., *International Journal of Biological Macromolecules*, Volume 54, March 2013, Pages 16-23.
9. Miranda-Rottmann S, Aspillaga AA, Pérez DD, Vasquez L, Martinez AL, Leighton F, Juice and phenolic fractions of the berry *Aristotelia chilensis* inhibit LDL oxidation in vitro and protect human endothelial cells against oxidative stress., *J Agric Food Chem.* 2002 Dec 18;50(26):7542-7.
10. Nello Ceccarelli, Maurizio Curadi, Piero Picciarelli, Luca Martelloni, Cristiana Sbrana, Manuela Giovannetti, Globe artichoke as a functional food, *Mediterranean Journal of Nutrition and Metabolism*, December 2010, Volume 3, Issue 3, Pages 197-201.
11. Qiong Luo, Yizhong Cai, Jun Yan, Mei Sun, Harold Corke, Hypoglycemic and hypolipidemic effects and antioxidant activity of fruit extracts from *Lycium barbarum*, Life Sciences, Volume 76, Issue 2, 26 November 2004, Pages 137-149
12. Tanaka J, Kadekaru T, Ogawa K, Hitoe S, Shimoda H, Hara H., Maqui berry (*Aristotelia chilensis*) and the constituent delphinidin glycoside inhibit photoreceptor cell death induced by visible light., *Food Chem.* 2013 Aug 15;139(1-4):129-37.
13. Vincenzo Lattanzio, Paul A. Kroon, Vito Linsalata, Angela Cardinali, Globe artichoke: A functional food and source of nutraceutical ingredients, *Journal of Functional Foods*, Volume 1, Issue 2, April 2009, Pages 131-144.

Shown in Product Identification Guide, page 510

USANA Health Sciences, Inc.
3838 WEST PARKWAY BOULEVARD
SALT LAKE CITY, UT 84120-6336

Direct Inquiries to:
Ph: (801) 954 7860
Fax: (801) 954 7658

ACTIVE CALCIUM™ CHEWABLE   OTC

COMPOSITION

Each Active Calcium™ Chewable contains the following:

Active Ingredients		Purpose
Calcium Carbonate	356 mg	Antacid
Magnesium Oxide	100 mg	Antacid

OTHER INGREDIENTS

Honey powder, calcium citrate, fructose, soy lecithin, magnesium citrate, xylitol, vegetable fatty acid, citric acid, guar gum, malic acid, rice protein hydrolysate, natural citrus flavor, calcium silicate, natural vanilla flavor, cholecalciferol (100 IU).

ADVANTAGES

This over-the-counter antacid utilizes calcium carbonate and magnesium oxide to neutralize stomach acid and provide supplemental calcium. In addition to calcium and magnesium, each tablet also vitamin D; each of which are required for bone development, bone remodeling and skeletal health. This product is certified Kosher by OK Kosher. This over-the-counter product meets USP guidelines for potency (as applicable), uniformity and disintegration, and is manufactured according to pharmaceutical cGMP standards.

DIRECTIONS:

Chew 2-4 tablets as symptoms occur, or as directed by a doctor.

WARNINGS

Ask a doctor or pharmacist before use if you are taking a prescription drug. Antacids may interact with certain prescription drugs. When using this product, do not take more than 6 tablets in a 24-hour period. Do not use the maximum dosage for more than 2 weeks. Consult your physician if you are pregnant, nursing, have kidney disease, or have a medical condition.

SUPPLIED

Round wafer with no imprinting or distinguishing marks, pale, cream-colored with faint yellow mottling. Some color variation is normal. In a bottle of 112 tablets.

ACTIVE CALCIUM™   DS

COMPOSITION

Each Active Calcium contains the following minerals:

Vitamin D3 (as Cholecalciferol)	100 IU
Vitamin K (as Phylloquinone)	15 mcg
Calcium (as Calcium Citrate and Carbonate)	200 mg
Magnesium (as Magnesium Citrate, Amino Acid Chelate and Oxide)	100 mg
Boron (as Boron Citrate)	0.33 mg

ADVANTAGES

Each tablet contains a balanced blend of calcium, magnesium, vitamin D, vitamin K, boron and silicon; six nutrients required for bone development, bone remodeling and skeletal health. This non-prescription product meets USP guidelines for potency (as applicable), uniformity and disintegration, and is manufactured according to pharmaceutical cGMP standards.

RECOMMENDED USE

Take 4 tablets by mouth daily, preferably with meals.

SUPPLIED

Capsule-shaped tablet, white to off white color, with clear film coating, and with USANA imprint. In bottle of 112 tablets.

COQUINONE® 30   DS
[*cō'-kwi-nōn*]

COMPOSITION

Each CoQuinone 30 capsule contains the following:

Coenzyme Q₁₀	30 mg
Alpha Lipoic Acid	12.5 mg

ADVANTAGES

CoQuinone 30 contains a hydrosoluble form of Coenzyme Q₁₀ (CoQ₁₀) that is 2.5 times more bioavailable than material supplied in dry tablet/capsule formulas. The higher blood levels of CoQ₁₀ supplied enhance mitochondrial production of ATP. CoQ₁₀ is a rate-limiting factor in the electron transport chain involved in mitochondrial production of ATP. It is also involved in neutralizing free radicals generated during ATP production. As such, CoQ₁₀ helps the body maintain healthy skeletal and cardiac muscle. Alpha lipoic acid is included in the formula as a lipid-soluble antioxidant to recycle CoQ₁₀ from the prooxidant form to the antioxidant form. This non-prescription product meets USP guidelines for potency (where applicable), uniformity and disintegration, and is manufactured according to cGMP standards.

RECOMMENDED USE

Take 1 or 2 capsules by mouth daily.

SUPPLIED

Oval shaped, soft gelatin capsule, annatto-colored, opaque. Capsules contain an orange colored liquid. In bottle of 56 soft-gel capsules.

CORE MINERALS DS

COMPOSITION

Each Core Minerals contains the following:

Vitamin C (as Magnesium Ascorbate and Calcium Ascorbate)	150 mg
Calcium (as Calcium Citrate and Magnesium Ascorbate)	56.25 mg
Iodine (as Potassium Iodide)	125 µg
Magnesium (as Magnesium Citrate and Magnesium Ascorbate)	56.25 mg
Zinc (as Zinc Citrate)	5 mg
Selenium (as L-Selenomethionine and Sodium Selenite)	50 µg
Copper (as Copper Gluconate)	.5 mg
Manganese (as Manganese Gluconate)	.5 mg
Chromium (as Chromium Polynicotinate)	75 µg
Molybdenum (as Molybdenum Citrate)	12.5 µg
Boron (as Boron Citrate)	750 µg
Silicon (as Calcium Silicate)	1 mg
Vanadium (as Vanadium Citrate)	10 µg
Ultra Trace Minerals	750 µg
N-Acetyl L-Cysteine	80 mg

ADVANTAGES

Each tablet contains a complete and balanced blend of essential minerals in bioavailable forms. The Core Minerals is designed to be taken with USANA's Vita-Antioxidant to provide a full complement of essential nutrients required for health. This product is certified kosher by OK Kosher. This nonprescription product meets USP guidelines for potency (as applicable), uniformity and disintegration, and is manufactured according to pharmaceutical cGMP standards.

RECOMMENDED USE

Take two (2) tablets twice daily, preferably with food.

SUPPLIED

Shaped as a medium caplet; is film-coated with USANA imprinted. Off white with light blue hue; some color variation is normal. In a bottle of 112 tablets.

PRENATAL CORE MINERALS DS

COMPOSITION

Each Prenatal Core Minerals contains the following:

Vitamin C (as Magnesium Ascorbate and Calcium Ascorbate)	150 mg
Calcium (as Calcium Citrate and Calcium Ascorbate)	56.25 mg
Iron (as Ferrous Fumarate)	7 mg
Iodine (as Potassium Iodide)	60 µg
Magnesium (as Magnesium Citrate and Magnesium Ascorbate)	56.25 mg
Zinc (as Zinc Citrate)	5 mg
Copper (as Copper Gluconate)	.50 mg
Selenium (as L-Selenomethionine and Sodium Selenite)	50 µg
Manganese (as Manganese Gluconate)	.50 mg
Chromium (as Chromium Polynicotinate)	75 µg
Molybdenum (as Molybdenum Citrate)	12.5 µg
Silicon (as Calcium Silicate)	1 mg
Vanadium (as Vanadium Citrate)	10 µg
Ultra Trace Minerals	750 µg
L-Cysteine HCL	40 mg

ADVANTAGES

USANA Prenatal Core Minerals is a multi-mineral product supplement designed to improve the nutritional status of women during pregnancy. It contains iron and calcium to help assure that adequate doses of these minerals are consumed during pregnancy.

RECOMMENDED USE

Take two (2) tablets twice daily, preferably with food.

SUPPLIED

Shaped as a medium, film-coated tablet with USANA imprinted. Off white with light blue hue; some color variation is normal. In a bottle of 112 tablets.

PRENATAL VITA-ANTIOXIDANT DS

COMPOSITION

Each Prenatal Vita-Antioxidant contains the following:

Vitamin A (as Beta Carotene and Mixed Carotenoids)	2500 IU
Vitamin C (as Poly C® Blend: Potassium, Calcium, Magnesium, and Zinc Ascorbates)	100 mg
Vitamin D3 (as Cholecalciferol)	250 IU
Vitamin E (as D-Alpha Tocopheryl Succinate)	50 IU
Niacin (as Niacinamide and Niacin)	10 mg
Vitamin B6 (as Pyridoxine HCl)	8 mg
Folate (as Folic Acid)	150 µg
Vitamin B12 (as Cyanocobalamin)	50 µg
Biotin	75 µg
Pantothenic Acid (as D-Calcium Pantothenate)	22.5 mg
Vitamin K (as K1 [Phytonadione] and K2 [Mk-7 Menaquinone])	30 µg
Vitamin B1 (as Thiamin HCl)	7.5 mg
Vitamin B2 (as Riboflavin)	7.5 mg
Mixed Tocopherols (D-Gamma, D-Delta, D-Beta Tocopherol)	20 mg
Incelligence™ Complex	
Alpha Lipoic Acid	25 mg
Meriva® Bioavailable Curcumin Complex [Curcuma Longa L., Root]	18mg
Green Tea Extract [Camellia Sinensis Hunt., Leaves]	17.5 mg
Quercitin Dihydrate	15 mg
Rutin	10 mg
Hesperidin [Citrus Spp.L., Fruit]	10 mg
Resveratrol	10 mg
Olivol ® [Olive Fruit Extract, Olea Europaea L., Fruit]	7.5 mg
Inositol	32 mg
Choline Bitartrate	62.5 mg
Coenzyme Q10	3 mg
Lutein (Tagetes Erecta L., Flower)	150 µg
Lycopene	250 µg

ADVANTAGES

USANA Prenatal Vita-Antioxidant is a multi-vitamin supplement designed to improve the nutritional status of women during pregnancy. It contains folic acid to help assure adequate doses of this vitamin during the early stages of pregnancy.

RECOMMENDED USE

Take two (2) tablets twice daily, preferably with food.

SUPPLIED

Shaped as a medium, film-coated tablet with USANA imprinted. Mottled orange-brown; some color variation is normal. In a bottle of 112 tablets.

PROCOSA® DS

COMPOSITION

Each Procosa® contains the following:

Vitamin C (As Calcium Ascorbate)	75 mg
Manganese (As Manganese Gluconate)	1.67 mg
Magnesium (As Magnesium Sulphate)	14.5 mg
Potassium (As Potassium Sulphate)	31.4 mg
Incelligence™ Joint-Support Complex	
Glucosamine HCL(Vegetarian)	500 mg
Meriva® Bioavailable Curcumin Complex	82.5 mg

ADVANTAGES

USANA's Procosa is comprehensive joint health formula with a blend of glucosamine, manganese, vitamin C, and silicon — building blocks for healthy cartilage. The combination of glucosamine with Meriva® bioavailable curcumin complex, manganese, vitamin C, and silicon represents a more comprehensive approach to joint health. Over the long term, these ingredients help retain healthy cartilage. Meriva, the new curcumin phytosome used in Procosa, dramatically increases human absorption of curcumin, delivering the same effectiveness at a much lower dose.

RECOMMENDED USE

Take three (3) tablets daily, preferably with meals.

SUPPLIED

Modified rectangle, orange-colored tablet, scored on one side. In bottle of 84 tablets.

PROFLAVANOL® C 100 DS

[prō-flā' vi-nol]

COMPOSITION

Each Proflavanol C 100 tablet contains the following:

POLY C® VITAMIN BLEND (As Calcium, Potassium, Magnesium, Zinc Ascorbates)	300 mg
Grape Seed Extract (*Vitis Vinifera L.*, Seeds)	100 mg

ADVANTAGES

A potent antioxidant formula combining the proanthocyanidins (bioflavonoids) from standardized grape seed extract with vitamin C in the form of ascorbate salts and ascorbyl palmitate. Proflavanol C 100 is designed to be taken as a stand-alone antioxidant, or preferably in combination with USANA's CellSentials to provide additional antioxidant protection. This non-prescription product meets USP guidelines for potency (where applicable), uniformity and disintegration, and is manufactured according to pharmaceutical cGMP standards.

RECOMMENDED USE

Adults, take two (2) to four (4) tablets daily, preferably with meals.

SUPPLIED

Oblong, bilayer tablet, with clear film coating, with USANA imprint, with bisect. In bottles of 56 tablets.

USANA® HEALTHPAK™ DS

COMPOSITION

Each USANA® HealthPak™ contains the following:

Vitamin A (as Retinyl Acetate, as Beta Carotene and Mixed Carotenoids)	6000 IU
Vitamin C (as Calcium, Potassium, Magnesium and Zinc Ascorbates)	500 mg
Vitamin D3 (as Cholecalciferol)	1250 IU
Vitamin E (as D-Alpha Tocopheryl Succinate)	100 IU
Vitamin K (as K1 [Phylloquinone] and K2 [Mk-7 Menaquinone])	270 µg
Thiamin (Vitamin B1)	15 mg
Riboflavin (Vitamin B2)	15 mg
Niacin (as Niacinamide and Niacin)	20 mg
Vitamin B6 (as Pyridoxine Hcl)	16 mg
Folate (as Folic Acid)	300 µg
Vitamin B12 (as Cyanocobalimin)	100 µg
Biotin	150 µg
Pantothinic Acid (as D-Calcium Pantothenate)	45 mg
Calcium (as Calcium Citrate, Carbonate, and Ascorbate)	238 mg
Iodine (as Potassium Iodide)	10 mg
Magnesium (as Magnesium Citrate, Carbonate, and Ascorbate)	238 mg
Zinc (as Zinc Citrate)	10 Mg
Selenium (as L-Selenomethionine and Selenium Sodium Selenite)	100 µg
Copper (as Copper Gluconate)	1 mg
Manganese (as Manganese Gluconate)	1 mg
Chromium (as Chromium Polynicotinate)	150 µg
Molybdenum (as Molybdenujm Citrate)	25 µg
Mixed Natural Tocopherols (D Gamma, D-Delta, D-Beta Tocopherol)	40 mg
Inositol	64 mg
Choline Bitartrate	125 mg
N-Acetyl L-Cysteine	80 mg
Coenzyme Q10	6 mg
Lutein (Tagetes Erecta L., Flower)	300 µg
Lycopene	500 µg
Silicon (as Calcium Silicate)	4.25 mg
Boron (as Boron Citrate)	1.83 mg
Vanadium (as Vanadium Citrate)	20 µg
Ultra Trace Minerals	1500 µg

Continued on next page

Incelligence™ Complex

Alpha Lipoic Acid	125 mg
Quercetin Dihydrate	90 mg
Pterocarpus Marsupium Extract	50 mg
(Containing Pterostilbene [Pterocarpus Marsupium, Wood])	
Meriva® Bioavailable Circumin Complex (Curcuma Longa L., Root)	36 mg
Green Tea Extract – Decaffeinated (Camellia Sinensis Hunt, Leaves)	35 mg
Olivol® (Olive Fruit Extract [Olea Europea L., Fruit])	25 mg
Resveratrol	20 mg
Rutin	20 mg
Hesperidin (Citrus Spp. L., Fruit)	20 mg

ADVANTAGES

This product contains a selection of USANA's products, which includes USANA's core multivitamin/mineral products (Core Minerals and Vita-Antioxidant). It includes MagneCal D, a bone health supplement that contains Magnesium, Calcium, and Vitamin D. It contains the CellSentials Booster, an antioxidant complex. This non-prescription product meets USP guidelines for potency (as applicable), uniformity and disintegration, and is manufactured according to pharmaceutical cGMP standards.

RECOMMENDED USE

Take one (1) packet in the morning and one (1) packet in the evening, preferably with meals.

SUPPLIED

Two (2) Vita Antioxidant tablets
Shaped as medium, film coated tablets with USANA imprinted. Mottled orange brown; some color variation is normal. In a bottle of 112 tablets.
Two (2) Core Minerals tablets
Shaped as medium, film-coated tablets with USANA imprinted. Off white with light blue hue; some color variation is normal. In a bottle of 112 tablets.
One (1) MagneCal D tablet
Shaped as modified, film coated tablet with USANA imprinted. White to off-white; some color variation is normal. In a bottle of 112 tablets.
One (1) CellSentials Booster tablet
Shaped as a small, film coated tablet with no imprinting or distinguishing marks. Brown to dark brown; some color variation is normal.

VISIONEX®   DS

COMPOSITION

Each Visionex® contains the following:

Vitamin C (as Calcium, Potassium, Magnesium, And Zinc Ascorbates)	250 mg
Zinc (as Zinc Citrate)	5 mg
Lutein (Tagetes Erecta L. Flower)	5 mg
Zeaxanthin (Tagetes Erecta L, Petals)	1000 µg
Bilberry Extract (Vaccinum Myrtillus L., Fruit)	25 mg

ADVANTAGES

This product contains a blend of antioxidants specifically designed to protect the tissues of the eye from photo-oxidation. This product is certified kosher by OK Kosher. This non-prescription product meets USP guidelines for potency (as applicable), uniformity and disintegration, and is manufactured according to pharmaceutical cGMP standards.

RECOMMENDED USE

Adults take two (2) tablets daily, preferably with a meal.

SUPPLIED

Medium caplet, clear film coated tablet with bisecting line. Purplish; some color variation is normal. In a bottle of 56 tablets.

VITA-ANTIOXIDANT   DS

COMPOSITION

Each Vita-Antioxidant contains the following:

Vitamin A (as 25% Retinyl Acetate, and 75 % [4500 IU] as Beta Carotene and Mixed Carotenoids)	3000 IU
Vitamin C (as Poly C® Blend: Potassium, Calcium, Magnesium, and Zinc Ascorbates)	100 mg
Vitamin D3 (as Cholecalciferol)	500 IU
Vitamin E (as D-Alpha Tocipheryl Succinate)	500 IU
Vitamin K (as K1 [Phytonadione] And K2 [Mk-7 Menaquinone])	135 µg

Vitamin B1 (as Thiamin HCl)	7.5 mg
Vitamin B2 (as Riboflavin)	7.5 mg
Niacin (as Niacinamide and Niacin)	10 mg
Vitamin B6 (as Pyridoxine HCl)	8 mg
Folate (as Folic Acid)	150 µg
Vitamin B12 (as Cyanocobalim)	50 µg
Biotin	75 µg
Pantothenic Acid (as D-Calcium Pantothenate)	22.5 mg
Mixed Tocopherols (D-Gamma, D-Delta, D-Beta Tocopherol)	20 mg

InCelligence™ Complex

Alpha Lipoic Acid	25 mg
Meriva® Bioavailable Curcumin Complex [Curcuma Longa L., Root]	18 mg
Green Tea Extract [Camellia Sinesis Hunt., Leaves]	17.5 mg
Quercitin Dihydrate	15 mg
Rutin	10 mg
Hesperidin [Citrus Spp.L., Fruit]	10 mg
Resveratrol	10 mg
Olivol® [Olive Fruit Extract, Olea Europaea L., Fruit]	15 mg
Inositol	32 mg
Choline Bitartrate	62.5 mg
Coenzyme Q10	3 mg
Lutein (Tagetes Erecta L., Flower)	150 µg
Lycopene	250 µg

ADVANTAGES

Each tablet contains a complete and balanced blend of essential vitamins. In addition to the traditionally recognized essential vitamins, this product contains a blend of dietary antioxidants, other beneficial ingredients, and USANA's InCelligence Complex. These ingredients include mixed carotenoids and tocopherols, USANA's patented Olivol® olive extract, Meriva® bioavailable curcumin, resveratrol, and other ingredients. This product is certified kosher by OK Kosher. This non-prescription product meets USP guidelines for potency (as applicable), uniformity and disintegration, and is manufactured according to pharmaceutical cGMP standards.

RECOMMENDED USE

Adults take two (2) tablets twice daily, preferably with food.

SUPPLIED

Medium caplet, film-coated tablet with USANA imprinted. Mottled orange-brown. Some color variation is normal. In a bottle of 112 tablets.

SECTION 9

DRUG SUMMARIES

This all-new section provides quick reference to concise information for the latest updated and newly approved FDA-regulated drugs. Each alphabetically ordered drug summary provides easy access to key details from current FDA-approved labeling, including: brand and generic names; pharmacological class; boxed warning; indications/dosage (organized by adult and pediatric patients in a streamlined, two-column format); dosing considerations; administration information; specifics on safe storage and handling; how supplied details; contraindications; relevant warnings and precautions; key adverse reactions;

drug interactions; pregnancy and lactation details; mechanism of action; pharmacokinetics; and information on assessment, monitoring, and counseling.

Abbreviations used within these drug summaries are defined in the *Abbreviations, Acronyms, and Symbols* table on page S-1449.

For additional detailed information, please refer to full FDA-approved labeling. Visit PDR.net® for further drug listings.

ABELCET — amphotericin B lipid complex   Rx
Class: Polyene antifungal

ADULT DOSAGE	PEDIATRIC DOSAGE
Fungal Infections	**Fungal Infections**
Invasive fungal infections in patients who are refractory to or intolerant of conventional amphotericin B therapy	Invasive fungal infections in patients who are refractory to or intolerant of conventional amphotericin B therapy
5mg/kg/day given as a single IV infusion at a rate of 2.5mg/kg/hr	5mg/kg/day given as a single IV infusion at a rate of 2.5mg/kg/hr

ADMINISTRATION
IV route

Do not dilute w/ saline sol or mix w/ other drugs or electrolytes
Flush existing IV lines w/ D5 inj before infusion of therapy or use a separate infusion line
Do not use an in-line filter
Shake the infusion bag q2h if the infusion time exceeds 2 hrs

Preparation
1. Withdraw appropriate dose into 1 or more sterile syringes using an 18-gauge needle
2. Remove needle and replace w/ supplied 5-micron filter needle to empty contents of syringe into an IV bag containing D5 inj
3. Final infusion concentration should be 1mg/mL (2mg/mL for pediatric patients and patients w/ cardiovascular disease)
4. Shake the bag until contents are thoroughly mixed; discard unused material

STORAGE
2-8°C (36-46°F). Protect from light. Do not freeze. Diluted Ready-For-Use Admixture: Stable for up to 48 hrs at 2-8°C (36-46°F) and an additional 6 hrs at room temperature. Do not freeze. Discard any unused material.

HOW SUPPLIED
Inj: 5mg/mL

CONTRAINDICATIONS
Hypersensitivity to amphotericin B or any other component in the formulation.

WARNINGS/PRECAUTIONS
Anaphylaxis reported; d/c immediately infusion and avoid further infusions if severe respiratory distress occurs. Should be administered by medically trained personnel during the initial dosing of therapy. Acute reactions, including fever and chills, may occur 1-2 hrs after starting IV infusion. Infusion has been associated with hypotension, bronchospasm, arrhythmias, and shock (rare). Dose-dependent renal toxicity reported.

ADVERSE REACTIONS
Chills, fever, increased SrCr, multiple organ failure, N/V, hypotension, respiratory failure, dyspnea, sepsis, diarrhea, headache, cardiac arrest, HTN, hypokalemia, kidney failure.

DRUG INTERACTIONS
Caution with antineoplastic agents; may enhance the potential for renal toxicity, bronchospasm, and hypotension. Corticosteroids and corticotropin may potentiate hypokalemia; monitor serum electrolytes and cardiac function if used concomitantly. Concurrent initiation with cyclosporine A within several days of bone marrow ablation may be associated with increased nephrotoxicity. May induce hypokalemia and potentiate digitalis toxicity with digitalis glycosides; closely monitor serum K^+ levels. May increase flucytosine toxicity; use with caution. Antagonism with imidazole derivatives (eg, miconazole, ketoconazole, clotrimazole) reported. Acute pulmonary toxicity reported with leukocyte transfusions; avoid concurrent use. May enhance the potential for drug-induced renal toxicity with nephrotoxic agents (eg, aminoglycosides, pentamidine); use with caution and monitor renal function intensively. Amphotericin B-induced hypokalemia may enhance curariform effect of skeletal muscle relaxants (eg, tubocurarine) due to hypokalemia; closely monitor serum K^+ levels. Monitor renal and hematologic function with zidovudine.

PREGNANCY AND LACTATION
Category B, not for use in nursing.

MECHANISM OF ACTION
Polyene antifungal; acts by binding to sterols in the cell membrane of susceptible fungi, with a resultant change in membrane permeability.

PHARMACOKINETICS
Absorption: C_{max}=1.7mcg/mL; AUC_{0-24}=14mcg•hr/mL. **Distribution:** V_d=131L/kg. **Elimination:** Urine (0.9%); $T_{1/2}$=173.4 hrs.

PATIENT CONSIDERATIONS
Assessment: Assess for previous hypersensitivity to the drug, pregnancy/nursing status, and possible drug interactions.

Monitoring: Monitor for signs and symptoms of anaphylaxis, severe respiratory distress, acute reactions, and other adverse reactions. Monitor for overall clinical condition. Frequently monitor SrCr. Regularly monitor LFTs, serum electrolytes (particularly Mg^{2+} and K^+), and CBCs.

Counseling: Inform about the risks and benefits of therapy. Advise to seek medical attention if pregnant or nursing, and if any adverse reactions occur.

ABILIFY — aripiprazole   Rx
Class: Atypical antipsychotic

> Elderly patients w/ dementia-related psychosis treated w/ antipsychotic drugs are at an increased risk of death. Not approved for treatment of patients w/ dementia-related psychosis. Antidepressants increased the risk of suicidal thoughts and behavior in children, adolescents, and young adults in short-term studies. Monitor closely for worsening, and for emergence of suicidal thoughts and behaviors in patients who are started on antidepressant therapy.

OTHER BRAND NAMES
Abilify Discmelt

ADULT DOSAGE	PEDIATRIC DOSAGE
Schizophrenia	**Schizophrenia**
Initial/Target: 10mg or 15mg qd	**13-17 Years:**
Titrate: Should not increase dose before 2 weeks	**Initial:** 2mg/day
Range: 10-30mg/day	**Titrate:** May increase to 5mg/day after 2 days and to the target dose of 10mg/day after 2 additional days. Administer subsequent dose increases in 5mg increments
Bipolar I Disorder	**Max:** 30mg/day
Manic and Mixed Episodes: Monotherapy:	**Bipolar I Disorder**
Initial/Target: 15mg qd	**Monotherapy or Adjunct to Lithium/ Valproate for Manic and Mixed Episodes:**
Titrate: May increase to 30mg/day based on clinical response	**10-17 Years:**
Max: 30mg/day	**Initial:** 2mg/day
Adjunct to Lithium or Valproate:	**Titrate:** May increase to 5mg/day after 2 days and to the target dose of 10mg/day after 2 additional days. Administer subsequent dose increases, if needed, in 5mg increments
Initial: 10-15mg qd	**Autistic Disorder**
Target: 15mg/day	**Irritability Associated w/ Autistic Disorder:**
Titrate: May increase to 30mg/day based on clinical response	**6-17 Years:**
Max: 30mg/day	**Initial:** 2mg/day
Major Depressive Disorder	**Titrate:** Increase to 5mg/day, w/ subsequent increases to 10 or 15mg/day, if needed. Dose adjustments of up to 5mg/day should occur gradually at intervals of ≥1 week
Adjunct to Antidepressants:	**Range:** 5-15mg/day
Initial: 2-5mg/day	**Tourette's Disorder**
Titrate: Dose adjustments of up to 5mg/day should occur gradually at intervals of ≥1 week	**6-18 Years:**
Range: 2-15mg/day	**Range:** 5-20mg/day
Agitation	**<50kg:**
Agitation Associated w/ Schizophrenia or Bipolar Mania: Inj:	**Initial:** 2mg/day w/ a target dose of 5mg/day after 2 days
9.75mg IM	**Titrate:** Increase to 10mg/day in patients who do not achieve optimal control of tics. Dose adjustments should occur gradually at intervals of ≥1 week
Range: 5.25-15mg	**≥50kg:**
A lower dose of 5.25mg may be considered when clinical factors warrant. If agitation warranting a 2nd dose persists following the initial dose, cumulative doses of up to a total of 30mg/day may be given	**Initial:** 2mg/day for 2 days
Max: 30mg/day or more frequently than q2h	**Titrate:** Increase to 5mg/day for 5 days w/ a target dose of 10mg/day on Day 8; increase up to 20mg/day for patients who do not achieve optimal control of tics. Dose adjustments should occur gradually in increments of 5mg/day at intervals of ≥1 week
If ongoing treatment is clinically indicated, replace w/ oral aripiprazole in a range of 10-30mg/day as soon as possible	

DOSING CONSIDERATIONS
Concomitant Medications
Strong CYP2D6 or CYP3A4 Inhibitors:
Administer 1/2 of usual dose

Strong CYP2D6 and CYP3A4 Inhibitors:
Administer 1/4 of the usual dose

Strong CYP3A4 Inducers:
Double usual dose over 1-2 weeks; when coadministered inducer is withdrawn, reduce aripiprazole dose to original level over 1-2 weeks

Combination of Strong, Moderate, and Weak Inhibitors of CYP3A4 and CYP2D6:
Reduce to 1/4 of usual dose initially, then adjust to achieve a favorable clinical response

Other Important Considerations
Known CYP2D6 Poor Metabolizers:
Administer 1/2 of usual dose

Known CYP2D6 Poor Metabolizers Taking Concomitant Strong CYP3A4 Inhibitors:
Administer 1/4 of usual dose

ADMINISTRATION
Oral/IM route

PO
Administer w/o regard to meals.
Oral sol can be substituted for tabs on a mg-per-mg basis up to 25mg dose level. Patients receiving 30mg tabs should receive 25mg of the sol.

Inj
Inject slowly, deep into the muscle mass.

STORAGE
25°C (77°F); excursions permitted to 15-30°C (59-86°F). **Sol:** May be used for up to 6 months after opening. **Inj:** Protect from light.

HOW SUPPLIED
Inj: 7.5mg/mL [1.3mL]; **Sol:** 1mg/mL [150mL]; **Tab:** 2mg, 5mg, 10mg, 15mg, 20mg, 30mg; **Tab, Disintegrating:** (Discmelt) 10mg, 15mg

CONTRAINDICATIONS
History of a hypersensitivity reaction to aripiprazole.

WARNINGS/PRECAUTIONS
Neuroleptic malignant syndrome (NMS) reported; d/c immediately, institute symptomatic treatment, and monitor. May cause tardive dyskinesia (TD), especially in the elderly; d/c if this occurs. Hyperglycemia, in some cases extreme and associated w/ ketoacidosis or hyperosmolar coma or death, reported. Dyslipidemia and weight gain reported. May cause orthostatic hypotension; caution w/ known cardiovascular disease (history of MI or ischemic heart disease, heart failure, or conduction abnormalities), cerebrovascular disease, or conditions that would predispose patients to hypotension (dehydration, hypovolemia). Leukopenia, neutropenia, and agranulocytosis reported; consider discontinuation at 1st sign of a clinically significant decline in WBC counts in the absence of other causative factors. D/C therapy and follow WBC counts until recovery in patients w/ severe neutropenia (ANC <1000/mm^3). Caution w/ history of seizures or w/ conditions that lower seizure threshold. May impair physical/mental abilities. May disrupt body's ability to reduce core body temperature; caution when exposed to conditions that may contribute to an elevation in core body temperature (eg, exercising strenuously, exposure to extreme heat, receiving concomitant medication w/ anticholinergic activity, or being subject to dehydration). May cause esophageal dysmotility and aspiration; caution in patients at risk for aspiration pneumonia.

ADVERSE REACTIONS
Adults: N/V, constipation, headache, dizziness, akathisia, anxiety, insomnia, restlessness.
Pediatrics: Somnolence, headache, N/V, extrapyramidal disorder, fatigue, increased appetite, insomnia, nasopharyngitis, weight increased.

DRUG INTERACTIONS
See Dosing Considerations. Strong CYP3A4 inhibitors (eg, itraconazole, clarithromycin) or strong CYP2D6 inhibitors (eg, quinidine, fluoxetine, paroxetine) may increase exposure. Strong CYP3A4 inducers (eg, carbamazepine, rifampin) may decrease exposure. May potentiate the effect of certain antihypertensive agents; monitor BP and adjust dose accordingly. Greater sedation and orthostatic hypotension observed w/ lorazepam; monitor sedation and BP and adjust dose accordingly in patients on concomitant therapy w/ benzodiazepines.

PREGNANCY AND LACTATION
Pregnancy: Category C.
Lactation: Found in breast milk; not for use in nursing.

MECHANISM OF ACTION
Partial D$_2$/5HT$_{1A}$ agonist/5HT$_{2A}$ antagonist; mechanism not established. Efficacy may be mediated through a combination of partial agonist activity at D$_2$ and 5-HT$_{1A}$ receptors and antagonist activity at 5-HT$_{2A}$ receptors.

PHARMACOKINETICS
Absorption: Well-absorbed (tab/sol). Absolute bioavailability (87%, tab), (100%, IM); T$_{max}$=3-5 hrs (tab), 1-3 hrs (IM, median). **Distribution:** V$_d$=404L (IV); plasma protein binding (>99%, albumin); found in breast milk. **Metabolism:** Hepatic via dehydrogenation, hydroxylation (CYP2D6 and CYP3A4), and N-dealkylation (CYP3A4). Dehydro-aripiprazole (active metabolite). **Elimination:** (PO) Urine (approx 25%, <1% unchanged), feces (approx 55%, approx 18% unchanged); T$_{1/2}$=75 hrs, 94 hrs (metabolite), 146 hrs (CYP2D6 poor metabolizers).

PATIENT CONSIDERATIONS
Assessment: Assess for dementia-related psychosis, drug hypersensitivity, any other conditions where treatment is cautioned, pregnancy/nursing status, and possible drug interactions. Obtain baseline FPG in patients w/ diabetes mellitus (DM) or at risk for DM. Obtain baseline CBC if at risk for leukopenia/neutropenia.

Monitoring: Monitor for clinical worsening of depression, suicidality, unusual changes in behavior, NMS, TD, hyperglycemia, dyslipidemia, orthostatic hypotension, seizures/convulsions, esophageal dysmotility, aspiration, weight gain, and other adverse reactions. Monitor CBC frequently during the 1st few months of therapy in patients w/ a history of a clinically significant low WBC count/ANC or drug-induced leukopenia/neutropenia. Monitor for fever or other signs/symptoms of infection in patients w/ neutropenia. Monitor for worsening of glucose control in patients w/ DM and FPG in patients at risk for DM periodically during therapy. Periodically reassess patient to determine the continued need for maintenance treatment.

Counseling: Inform about the risks and benefits of treatment. Instruct patients, families, and caregivers to be alert for the emergence of anxiety, agitation, panic attacks, insomnia, irritability, hostility, aggressiveness, impulsivity, akathisia, hypomania, mania, other unusual changes in behavior, worsening of depression, and suicidal ideation; advise to contact physician if these symptoms occur. Instruct to use caution when operating hazardous machinery. Counsel to avoid overheating and dehydration. Advise to notify physician if patient is taking or plans to take any prescription or OTC drugs. Instruct to not breastfeed during therapy. (Discmelt) Inform phenylketonurics that product contains phenylalanine. Instruct to not open blister until ready to administer. Instruct not push the tab through the foil because this could damage the tab. Advise that immediately upon opening the blister, using dry hands, remove the tab and place the entire tab on the tongue. Inform that tab disintegration occurs rapidly in saliva. Instruct that drug is to be taken w/o liquid, but that if needed, can be taken w/ liquid. Advise not to split the tab. (Sol) Inform that sol contains sucrose and fructose.

ABILIFY MAINTENA — *aripiprazole*   Rx
Class: Atypical antipsychotic

> Elderly patients w/ dementia-related psychosis treated w/ antipsychotic drugs are at an increased risk of death. Not approved for the treatment of patients w/ dementia-related psychosis.

ADULT DOSAGE
Schizophrenia

Initial/Maint: 400mg monthly (no sooner than 26 days after the previous inj); establish tolerability w/ oral aripiprazole prior to initiating treatment in aripiprazole-naive patients

After the 1st inj, administer oral aripiprazole (10-20mg) for 14 consecutive days, or if already stable on another oral antipsychotic (and known to tolerate aripiprazole), continue treatment w/ the antipsychotic for 14 consecutive days

Missed Dose

2nd or 3rd Doses are Missed:
>4 Weeks and <5 Weeks Since Last Inj: Administer inj as soon as possible
>5 Weeks Since Last Inj: Restart concomitant oral aripiprazole for 14 days w/ next administered inj

4th or Subsequent Doses are Missed:
>4 Weeks and <6 Weeks Since Last Inj: Administer inj as soon as possible
>6 Weeks Since Last Inj: Restart concomitant oral aripiprazole for 14 days w/ next administered inj

PEDIATRIC DOSAGE
Pediatric use may not have been established

DOSING CONSIDERATIONS
Concomitant Medications
Concomitant Use for >14 Days:

Patients Taking 300mg:
Strong CYP2D6 or CYP3A4 Inhibitors: 200mg
CYP2D6 and CYP3A4 Inhibitors: 160mg
CYP3A4 Inducers: Avoid use

Patients Taking 400mg:
Strong CYP2D6 or CYP3A4 Inhibitors: 300mg
CYP2D6 and CYP3A4 Inhibitors: 200mg
CYP3A4 Inducers: Avoid use

Adverse Reactions
If adverse reactions occur w/ the 400mg dose, consider reducing dose to 300mg once monthly

Other Important Considerations
CYP2D6 Poor Metabolizers: 300mg
CYP2D6 Poor Metabolizers Taking Concomitant CYP3A4 Inhibitors: 200mg

ADMINISTRATION
IM route

For deep IM deltoid or gluteal inj by healthcare professionals only; do not administer by any other route.
Use 23-gauge, 1-inch needle for deltoid administration in non-obese patients; use 22-gauge, 1.5-inch needle for gluteal administration in non-obese patients or deltoid administration in obese patients; use 21-gauge, 2-inch needle for gluteal administration in obese patients.
Inject immediately following reconstitution.
Inject slowly; do not massage inj site.
Rotate inj sites between the 2 deltoid or gluteal muscles.
To obtain 200mg and 160mg dosage adjustments, use 300mg or 400mg strength vials.

Preparation
Prefilled Dual Chamber Syringe:
1. Reconstitute at room temperature.
2. Push plunger rod slightly to engage threads, then rotate plunger rod until the rod stops rotating to release diluent. Middle stopper will be at the indicator line after plunger rod is at a complete stop.
3. Vertically shake syringe vigorously for 20 sec until drug is uniformly milky white; reconstituted sus is a uniform, homogenous sus that is opaque and milky white.
4. Attach appropriate needle; hold syringe upright and advance plunger rod slowly to expel air until sus fills needle base.

Vial:
1. Reconstitute at room temperature.
2. Reconstitute 400mg vial w/ 1.9mL sterile water for inj (SWFI) and 300mg vial w/ 1.5mL SWFI.
3. Shake vigorously for 30 sec until sus appears uniform; reconstituted sus is a uniform, homogenous sus that is opaque and milky white.
4. If not injected immediately after reconstitution, keep vial at room temperature and shake vigorously for at least 60 sec to re-suspend prior to inj.
5. Inject 2mL for 400mg dose (400mg vial only), 1.5mL for 300mg dose, 1mL for 200mg dose, and 0.8mg for 160mg dose.

Refer to PI for further preparation and administration instructions.

STORAGE
Prefilled Dual Chamber Syringe: <30°C (86°F). Do not freeze. Protect from light.
Vial: 25°C (77°F); excursions permitted to 15-30°C (59-86°F).

HOW SUPPLIED
Inj, Extended-Release: 300mg, 400mg [vial, prefilled dual chamber syringe]

CONTRAINDICATIONS
Known hypersensitivity to aripiprazole.

WARNINGS/PRECAUTIONS
Do not substitute w/ other aripiprazole formulation. Neuroleptic malignant syndrome (NMS) may occur; d/c immediately and institute symptomatic treatment and medical monitoring. May cause tardive dyskinesia (TD), especially in the elderly; consider discontinuation if this occurs. Hyperglycemia, in some cases extreme and associated w/ ketoacidosis or hyperosmolar coma or death, reported w/ atypical antipsychotics. Dyslipidemia and weight gain reported w/ atypical antipsychotics. May cause orthostatic hypotension. Leukopenia, neutropenia, and agranulocytosis reported; consider discontinuation at 1st sign of clinically significant decline in WBC counts w/o causative factors in patients w/ history of clinically significant low WBC count/ANC or drug-induced leukopenia/neutropenia. D/C therapy and follow WBC counts until recovery in patients w/ severe neutropenia (ANC <1000/mm³). Caution w/ history of seizures or w/ conditions that lower seizure threshold. May impair mental/physical abilities. May disrupt body's ability to reduce core body temperature. May cause esophageal dysmotility and aspiration; caution in patients at risk for aspiration pneumonia.

ADVERSE REACTIONS
Increased weight, akathisia, injection-site pain, sedation.

DRUG INTERACTIONS
See Dosing Considerations. Concomitant oral aripiprazole w/ strong CYP3A4/CYP2D6 inhibitors increased concentration of aripiprazole. Concomitant oral aripiprazole and carbamazepine decreased concentration of aripiprazole. May enhance effect of certain antihypertensives; monitor BP and adjust dose accordingly. Greater sedation and orthostatic hypotension observed w/ oral aripiprazole and lorazepam; monitor sedation and BP and adjust dose accordingly w/ benzodiazepines.

PREGNANCY AND LACTATION
Pregnancy: There is a pregnancy exposure registry that monitors pregnancy outcomes in women exposed to aripiprazole during pregnancy. Neonates exposed to antipsychotic drugs during the 3rd trimester of pregnancy are at risk for extrapyramidal and/or withdrawal symptoms; monitor and manage symptoms appropriately.
Lactation: Found in breast milk; however, there are insufficient data to assess the amount in milk, the effects on the breastfed infant, or the effects on milk production. Caution in nursing.

MECHANISM OF ACTION
Atypical antipsychotic; mechanism not established. Efficacy may be mediated through a combination of partial agonist activity at D_2 and $5\text{-}HT_{1A}$ receptors and antagonist activity at $5\text{-}HT_{2A}$ receptors.

PHARMACOKINETICS
Absorption: Slow and prolonged. T_{max} (median)=5-7 days (gluteal), 4 days (deltoid). **Distribution:** Found in breast milk. **Metabolism:** Hepatic via CYP2D6 and CYP3A4; dehydro-aripiprazole (major metabolite). **Elimination:** $T_{1/2}$=29.9 days (300mg, gluteal), 46.5 days (400mg, gluteal).

PATIENT CONSIDERATIONS
Assessment: Assess for history of dementia-related psychosis, diabetes mellitus (DM), drug hypersensitivity, any other conditions where treatment is cautioned, pregnancy/nursing status, and possible drug interactions. Obtain baseline FPG in patients at risk for DM. Obtain baseline CBC if at risk for leukopenia/neutropenia.
Monitoring: Monitor for NMS, TD, hyperglycemia, orthostatic hypotension, seizures, weight gain, dyslipidemia, esophageal dysmotility, aspiration, and other adverse reactions. Monitor CBC frequently during the 1st few months of therapy in patients w/ a history of a clinically significant low WBC count/ANC or drug-induced leukopenia/neutropenia. Monitor for fever or other symptoms/signs of infection in patients w/ neutropenia. Monitor for worsening of glucose control in patients w/ DM and FPG in patients at risk for DM. Periodically reassess need for continued treatment.
Counseling: Inform of the risks/benefits of therapy. Inform about NMS; advise to contact healthcare provider or report to emergency room if signs/symptoms develop. Instruct to notify healthcare provider if any movements that cannot be controlled in the face, tongue, or other body part develop. Inform about risk of metabolic changes, symptoms of hyperglycemia/DM, and the need for specific monitoring. Inform about risk of orthostatic hypotension and syncope especially early in treatment and at times of treatment reinitiation or dosage increases. Advise patients w/ preexisting low WBC count or history of drug-induced leukopenia/neutropenia to have their CBC monitored. Advise to use caution when operating hazardous machinery. Instruct to avoid overheating and dehydration. Instruct to notify healthcare provider of any changes to prescription or OTC drugs.

ABRAXANE — paclitaxel protein-bound   Rx

Class: Antimicrotubule agent

> Do not administer to patients who have baseline neutrophil counts of <1500 cells/mm³. Perform frequent peripheral blood cell counts to monitor occurrence of bone marrow suppression, primarily neutropenia. Do not substitute for or w/ other paclitaxel formulations.

ADULT DOSAGE
Non-Small Cell Lung Cancer

Locally Advanced or Metastatic:
100mg/m² IV infusion over 30 min on Days 1, 8, and 15 of each 21-day cycle. Give carboplatin on Day 1 of each 21-day cycle immediately after paclitaxel.

Do not administer on Day 1 of a cycle until ANC is at least 1500 cells/mm³ and platelet count is at least 100,000 cells/mm³

Metastatic Pancreatic Adenocarcinoma

125mg/m² IV infusion over 30-40 min on Days 1, 8, and 15 of each 28-day cycle
Give gemcitabine immediately after paclitaxel on Days 1, 8, and 15 of each 28-day cycle

Metastatic Breast Cancer

After failure of combination chemotherapy or relapse w/in 6 months of adjuvant chemotherapy
260mg/m² IV over 30 min every 3 weeks

PEDIATRIC DOSAGE
Pediatric use may not have been established

DOSING CONSIDERATIONS
Hepatic Impairment
Metastatic Breast Cancer:
Moderate (AST <10X ULN and Bilirubin >1.5 to ≤3X ULN):
Initial: 200mg/m² for the 1st course of therapy
Titrate: May increase up to 260mg/m² in subsequent courses if reduced dose tolerated for 2 cycles
Severe (AST <10X ULN and Bilirubin >3 to ≤5X ULN):
Initial: 200mg/m² for the 1st course of therapy
Titrate: May increase up to 260mg/m² in subsequent courses if reduced dose tolerated for 2 cycles
AST >10X ULN or Bilirubin >5X ULN: Not recommended

Non-Small Cell Lung Cancer:
Moderate (AST <10X ULN and Bilirubin >1.5 to ≤3X ULN):
Initial: 80mg/m² for the 1st course of therapy
Titrate: May increase up to 100mg/m² in subsequent courses if reduced dose tolerated for 2 cycles
Severe (AST <10X ULN and Bilirubin >3 to ≤5X ULN):
Initial: 80mg/m² for the 1st course of therapy
Titrate: May increase up to 100mg/m² in subsequent courses if reduced dose tolerated for 2 cycles
AST >10X ULN or Bilirubin >5X ULN: Not recommended

Adverse Reactions
Metastatic Breast Cancer:
Severe Neutropenia (Neutrophil <500 cells/mm³ for ≥1 Week) or Severe Sensory Neuropathy: Reduce to 220mg/m²
Recurrence of Severe Neutropenia or Severe Sensory Neuropathy: Reduce to 180mg/m²
Grade 3 Sensory Neuropathy: Hold treatment until resolution to Grade 1 or 2, followed by a dose reduction for all subsequent courses

Non-Small Cell Lung Cancer:
Severe Neutropenia or Thrombocytopenia: Withhold treatment until ANC at least 1500 cells/mm³ and platelet count at least 100,000 cells/mm³ on Day 1 or to ANC of at least 500 cells/mm³ and platelet count of at least 50,000 cells/mm³ on Days 8 or 15 of the cycle; upon resumption of dosing, permanently reduce as outlined below
Grade 3-4 Peripheral Neuropathy: Withhold; resume at reduced dose w/ improvement to Grade 1 or complete resolution

Neutropenic Fever (ANC <500/mm³ w/ Fever >38°C) or Delay of Next Cycle by >7 Days for ANC <1500/mm³ or ANC <500/mm³ for >7 Days:
1st Occurrence: Reduce to 75mg/m² weekly
2nd Occurrence: Reduce to 50mg/m² weekly
3rd Occurrence: D/C treatment

Platelet Count <50,000/mm³:
1st Occurrence: Reduce to 75mg/m² weekly
2nd Occurrence: D/C treatment

Severe Sensory Neuropathy (Grade 3 or 4):
1st Occurrence: Reduce to 75mg/m² weekly
2nd Occurrence: Reduce to 50mg/m² weekly
3rd Occurrence: D/C treatment

Pancreatic Adenocarcinoma:
Dose Level Reductions:
1st Dose Reduction: 100mg/m²

2nd Dose Reduction: 75mg/m²
Additional Dose Reduction Required: D/C
Febrile Neutropenia (Grade 3 or 4): Withhold until fever resolves and ANC ≥1500; resume at next lower dose level
Peripheral Neuropathy (Grade 3 or 4): Withhold until improvement to ≤Grade 1; resume at next lower dose level
Cutaneous Toxicity (Grade 2 or 3): Reduce to next lower dose level; d/c treatment if toxicity persists
GI Toxicity (Grade 3 Mucositis or Diarrhea): Withhold until improvement to ≤Grade 1; resume at next lower level
Neutropenia and/or Thrombocytopenia at the Start of a Cycle or w/in a Cycle: Refer to PI

ADMINISTRATION
IV route

If paclitaxel (lyophilized cake or reconstituted sus) contacts the skin, wash the skin immediately and thoroughly w/ soap and water; if contact occurs w/ mucous membranes, flush the membranes thoroughly w/ water.
Limit the infusion to 30 min to reduce infusion-related reactions.

Preparation
Reconstitute each vial by slowly injecting 20mL of 0.9% NaCl inj onto the inside wall of the vial over a minimum of 1 min.
Allow vial to sit for a minimum of 5 min after inj into vial; gently swirl and/or invert the vial slowly for at least 2 min.
If foaming/clumping occurs, stand sol for at least 15 min until foam subsides.
Reconstituted sus should be milky and homogenous. Inj the appropriate amount of reconstituted sus into an empty, sterile IV bag.
Discard reconstituted sus if proteinaceous strands are observed.

Stability
Reconstituted paclitaxel in the vial should be used immediately, but may be refrigerated at 2-8°C (36-46°F) for a max of 24 hrs if necessary.
If not used immediately, each vial of reconstituted sus should be replaced in the original carton to protect it from bright light.
The sus for infusion when prepared in an infusion bag should be used immediately but may be refrigerated at 2-8°C (36-46°F) and protected from light for a max of 24 hrs. Total combined refrigerated storage time of sus and in the infusion bag is 24 hrs; this may be followed by storage in the infusion bag at ambient temperature (approx 25°C [77°F]) and lighting conditions for a maximum of 4 hrs.
Discard any unused portion.

STORAGE
20-25°C (68-77°F). Retain in original packaging to protect from bright light.

HOW SUPPLIED
Inj: 100mg

CONTRAINDICATIONS
Patients w/ baseline neutrophil counts of <1500 cells/mm³. Severe hypersensitivity reaction to this product should not be rechallenged w/ the drug.

WARNINGS/PRECAUTIONS
Bone marrow suppression (primarily neutropenia) is dose-dependent and a dose-limiting toxicity. Withhold therapy if ANC <500 cells/mm³ and platelets are <50,000 cells/mm³ and delay initiation of the next cycle if ANC is <1500 cells/mm³ or platelets are <100,000 cells/mm³ on Day 1 of the cycle in patients w/ pancreatic adenocarcinoma. Sensory neuropathy is dose- and schedule-dependent. Sepsis reported; initiate treatment w/ broad-spectrum antibiotics if patient becomes febrile (regardless of ANC). Pneumonitis reported; interrupt treatment and gemcitabine during evaluation of suspected pneumonitis. After ruling out infectious etiology and upon making a diagnosis of pneumonitis, permanently d/c combination therapy. Severe and sometimes fatal hypersensitivity reactions, including anaphylactic reactions, reported. Caution w/ hepatic impairment; not recommended in patients who have total bilirubin >5X ULN or AST >10X ULN and in patients w/ metastatic adenocarcinoma of the pancreas who have moderate to severe hepatic impairment (total bilirubin >1.5X ULN and AST ≤10X ULN). Contains human albumin; may carry a remote risk for transmission of viral diseases. May cause fetal harm. Men should be advised not to father a child while receiving treatment.

ADVERSE REACTIONS
Alopecia, neutropenia, thrombocytopenia, sensory/peripheral neuropathy, abnormal ECG, fatigue/asthenia, myalgia/arthralgia, AST elevation, alkaline phosphatase elevation, anemia, nausea, infections, diarrhea.

DRUG INTERACTIONS
Caution w/ medicines known to inhibit (eg, ketoconazole and other imidazole antifungals, erythromycin, fluoxetine, gemfibrozil, ritonavir) or induce (eg, rifampicin, carbamazepine, phenytoin, efavirenz, nevirapine) either CYP2C8 or CYP3A4.

PREGNANCY AND LACTATION
Category D, not for use in nursing.

MECHANISM OF ACTION
Antimicrotubule agent; promotes assembly of microtubules from tubulin dimers and stabilizes microtubules by preventing depolymerization. This stability results in inhibition of the normal dynamic reorganization of the microtubule network that is essential for vital interphase and mitotic cellular functions.

PHARMACOKINETICS
Distribution: V_d=1741L; plasma protein binding (94%). **Metabolism:** Liver via CYP2C8 to 6α-hydroxypaclitaxel (major metabolite), and CYP3A4.
Elimination: Urine (4% unchanged, <1% metabolites), feces (20%); $T_{1/2}$=13-27 hrs.

PATIENT CONSIDERATIONS
Assessment: Assess for previous hypersensitivity reactions to drug, hepatic impairment, pregnancy/nursing status, and possible drug interactions. Obtain baseline CBC, including neutrophil counts, and LFTs.

Monitoring: Monitor for bone marrow suppression, sensory neuropathy, sepsis, pneumonitis, hypersensitivity reactions, and other adverse reactions. Frequently monitor CBC (including neutrophil counts); perform prior to dosing on Day 1 (for metastatic breast cancer) and Days 1, 8, and 15 (for non-Small cell lung cancer and pancreatic cancer).

Counseling: Inform that drug may cause fetal harm; advise women of childbearing potential to avoid becoming pregnant. Advise men not to father a child while on therapy. Inform of the risk of low blood cell counts and severe and life-threatening infections; instruct to contact physician immediately for fever or evidence of infection. Advise to contact physician for persistent vomiting, diarrhea, or signs of dehydration. Inform that sensory neuropathy occurs frequently and instruct to report to physician any numbness, tingling, pain, or weakness involving the extremities. Inform that alopecia, fatigue/asthenia, and myalgia/arthralgia occur frequently w/ therapy. Instruct to contact physician for signs of an allergic reaction and for sudden onset of dry, persistent cough or SOB.

ABSORICA — isotretinoin   Rx
Class: Retinoid

> Not for use by females who are or may become pregnant. Severe birth defects, including death, have been documented. Increased risk of spontaneous abortion and premature births reported. D/C immediately if pregnancy occurs during treatment and refer to an obstetrician-gynecologist experienced in reproductive toxicity for further evaluation and counseling. Available only through a restricted program under a Risk Evaluation and Mitigation Strategy called iPLEDGE. Prescribers, patients, pharmacies, and distributors must enroll and be registered in the program.

ADULT DOSAGE
Severe Recalcitrant Nodular Acne

Unresponsive to Conventional Therapy, Including Systemic Antibiotics:
0.5-1mg/kg/day given in 2 divided doses for 15-20 weeks
Titrate: May adjust dose according to response of disease and/or appearance of clinical side effects

Very Severe Disease w/ Scarring or Primarily Manifested on Trunk:
May adjust dose up to 2mg/kg/day, as tolerated

May d/c if total nodule count has been reduced by >70% prior to completing 15-20 weeks of treatment

After a period of ≥2 months off therapy, and if warranted by persistent or recurring severe nodular acne, a 2nd course of therapy may be initiated; the optimal interval before retreatment has not been defined for patients who have not completed skeletal growth

PEDIATRIC DOSAGE
Severe Recalcitrant Nodular Acne

Unresponsive to Conventional Therapy, Including Systemic Antibiotics:
≥12 Years:
0.5-1mg/kg/day given in 2 divided doses for 15-20 weeks
Titrate: May adjust dose according to response of disease and/or appearance of clinical side effects

May d/c if total nodule count has been reduced by >70% prior to completing 15-20 weeks of treatment

After a period of ≥2 months off therapy, and if warranted by persistent or recurring severe nodular acne, a 2nd course of therapy may be initiated; the optimal interval before retreatment has not been defined for patients who have not completed skeletal growth

ADMINISTRATION
Oral route
Take w/o regard to meals.
Swallow caps w/ a full glass of liquid.

STORAGE
20-25°C (68-77°F); excursions permitted to 15-30°C (59-86°F). Protect from light.

HOW SUPPLIED
Cap: 10mg, 20mg, 25mg, 30mg, 35mg, 40mg

CONTRAINDICATIONS
Pregnancy, hypersensitivity to this product (or Vitamin A) or to any of its components.

WARNINGS/PRECAUTIONS
Avoid long-term use. 25mg capsule contains tartrazine, which may cause allergic-type reactions (including bronchial asthma) in certain susceptible persons. Do not donate blood during therapy and for 1 month following discontinuation of therapy. Micro-dosed progesterone preparations are an inadequate method of contraception during therapy. May cause depression, psychosis, suicidal ideation/attempts, suicide, and aggressive and/or violent behaviors; d/c if symptoms occur. Associated w/ pseudotumor cerebri (benign intracranial HTN). Erythema multiforme and severe skin reactions (eg, Stevens-Johnson syndrome, toxic epidermal necrolysis) reported; closely monitor for severe skin reactions and consider discontinuation of therapy if warranted. Acute pancreatitis reported; d/c if hypertriglyceridemia cannot be controlled at an acceptable level or if symptoms of pancreatitis occur. Hypersensitivity reactions reported; d/c therapy and institute appropriate management if a severe allergic reaction occurs. Increased TG levels, increased cholesterol levels, decreased HDL levels, impaired hearing, hepatotoxicity, inflammatory bowel disease, premature epiphyseal closure, skeletal hyperostosis, dry eye, decreased night vision, corneal opacities, and impaired glucose control reported. D/C if symptoms of pseudotumor cerebri and papilledema are present, significant decrease in WBC count, tinnitus or hearing impairment, visual impairment, abdominal pain, rectal bleeding, severe diarrhea, or if liver enzyme levels do not normalize or if hepatitis is suspected. May have a negative effect on bone mineral density; caution w/ history of

childhood osteoporosis conditions, osteomalacia, other bone metabolism disorders, or anorexia nervosa. Anaphylactic reactions and other allergic reactions reported; d/c and institute appropriate management if a severe allergic reaction occurs. Increased CPK levels and rhabdomyolysis reported. Osteoporosis, osteopenia, bone fractures, and/or delayed fracture healing reported; increased risk in patients participating in sports w/ repetitive impact.

ADVERSE REACTIONS
Cheilitis, hypertriglyceridemia, fatigue, irritability, pain, allergic reactions, vascular thrombotic disease, stroke, decreased appetite, weight fluctuation, chapped lips, N/V, nasopharyngitis, anemia, colitis.

DRUG INTERACTIONS
Avoid use w/ tetracyclines or vitamin supplements containing vitamin A. Caution w/ drugs that cause drug-induced osteoporosis/osteomalacia and/or affect vitamin D metabolism (eg, systemic corticosteroids, any anticonvulsant).

PREGNANCY AND LACTATION
Pregnancy: Category X; refer to PI for further information on pregnancy precautions that must be taken in females of reproductive potential.
Lactation: Not for use in nursing.

MECHANISM OF ACTION
Retinoid; not established. Suspected to inhibit sebaceous gland function and keratinization.

PHARMACOKINETICS
Absorption: AUC=6095ng•hr/mL (fed), 4055ng•hr/mL (fasted); C_{max}= 395ng/mL (fed), 314ng/mL (fasted); T_{max}=6.4 hrs (fed), 2.9 hrs (fasted). **Distribution:** Plasma protein binding (>99.9%). **Metabolism:** Liver via CYP2C8, 2C9, 3A4, and 2B6; 4-oxo-isotretinoin, retinoic acid, and 4-oxo-retinoic acid (active metabolites). **Elimination:** Feces and urine (total of 65%-83%); $T_{1/2}$=22 hrs (fed), 24 hrs (fasted), 18 hrs (fed, isotretinoin), 38 hrs (fed, 4-oxo-isotretinoin).

PATIENT CONSIDERATIONS
Assessment: Assess that females have had 2 negative urine or serum pregnancy tests separated by at least 19 days, and are on 2 forms of effective contraception. Assess for hypersensitivity to the drug or vitamin A, history of psychiatric disorder, depression, risk of hyperlipidemia, pregnancy/nursing status, and possible drug interactions. Obtain blood lipids and LFTs.

Monitoring: Monitor for signs/symptoms of psychiatric disorders, pseudotumor cerebri, lipid abnormalities, acute pancreatitis, hearing/visual impairment, inflammatory bowel disease (regional ileitis), hepatotoxicity, premature epiphyseal closure, hyperostosis, musculoskeletal symptoms/abnormalities, hypersensitivity reactions, and other adverse reactions. Monitor lipid levels and LFTs (weekly or biweekly), glucose levels, and CPK levels until response is established. Monitor that females remain on 2 forms of contraception during and for 1 month following discontinuation of therapy.

Counseling: Instruct to read the iPLEDGE and sign the Patient Information/Informed Consent form. Inform male patients and female patients not of childbearing potential about the risks and benefits of the drug. Inform females of childbearing potential that 2 forms of contraception are required starting 1 month prior to initiation, during treatment, and for 1 month following discontinuation. Inform that monthly pregnancy tests are required before new prescription is issued. Instruct patients to d/c therapy if signs/symptoms of pseudotumor cerebri (eg, papilledema, headache, N/V) occur. Counsel not to share drug w/ anyone and not to donate blood during therapy and 1 month following discontinuation. Inform that transient exacerbation (flare) of acne may occur. Instruct to notify physician if depression, mood disturbances, psychosis, or aggression occurs. Instruct to avoid wax epilation and skin resurfacing procedures during and for at least 6 months thereafter. Instruct to avoid prolonged UV rays or sunlight exposure. Inform that dry eye, corneal opacities, and decreased night vision may be experienced, and decreased tolerance to contact lenses during and after therapy may occur. Inform that musculoskeletal symptoms, transient chest pain, back pain in pediatric patients, arthralgias, neutropenia, agranulocytosis, anaphylactic/allergic/severe skin reactions, and inflammatory bowel disease may occur. Inform adolescent patients who participate in sports w/ repetitive impact that medication may increase their risk of spondylolisthesis or hip growth plate injuries.

ABSTRAL — fentanyl

Class: Opioid analgesic

CII

> Fatal respiratory depression may occur. Contraindicated in the management of acute or postoperative pain (eg, headache/migraine) and in opioid-nontolerant patients. Keep out of reach of children. Concomitant use with CYP3A4 inhibitors may increase plasma levels, and may cause fatal respiratory depression. Do not convert patients on a mcg-per-mcg basis from any other fentanyl products to Abstral or substitute for any fentanyl products; may result in fatal overdose. Contains fentanyl with abuse liability similar to other opioid analgesics. Available only through a restricted program called Transmucosal Immediate Release Fentanyl (TIRF) Risk Evaluation Mitigation Strategy (REMS) Access program due to risk of misuse, abuse, addiction, and overdose. Outpatients, healthcare professionals who prescribe to outpatients, pharmacies, and distributors must enroll in this program.

ADULT DOSAGE
Pain

Management of breakthrough pain in cancer patients already receiving and are tolerant to opioid therapy for their underlying persistent cancer pain

PEDIATRIC DOSAGE
Pediatric use may not have been established

Initial: 100mcg
Adequate Analgesia Obtained w/ in 30 Min of Initial Dose: Continue to treat subsequent episodes of breakthrough pain with this dose
Adequate Analgesia Not Obtained After Initial Dose: Use 2nd dose (30 min after initial dose)
Titrate:
Continue dose escalation in a stepwise manner over consecutive breakthrough episodes until adequate analgesia with tolerable side effects is achieved.
Increase dose by 100mcg multiples up to 400mcg prn.
If adequate analgesia is not obtained w/ 400mcg dose, titrate to 600mcg.
If adequate analgesia is not obtained w/ a 600mcg dose, titrate to 800mcg.
During titration, patients may use multiples of 100mcg tabs and/or 200mcg tabs for any single dose.
May repeat the same dose if adequate analgesia is not obtained 30 min after use.
May use rescue medication if adequate analgesia not achieved.
Do not use more than 4 tabs at one time.

Maint:
Once an appropriate dose for pain management has been established, use only one tab of the appropriate strength per dose

Do not use more than 2 doses to treat an episode of breakthrough pain and wait at least 2 hrs before treating another episode

Conversions
Conversion from Actiq to Abstral:
200mcg: 100mcg
400mcg: 200mcg
600mcg: 200mcg
800mcg: 200mcg
1200mcg: 200mcg
1600mcg: 400mcg

DOSING CONSIDERATIONS
Discontinuation
Patients Who No Longer Require Opioid Therapy: Consider discontinuing w/ a gradual downward titration of other opioids
Patients Who No Longer Require Treatment for Breakthrough Pain: D/C immediately

ADMINISTRATION
SL route
Allow tabs to completely dissolve in the SL cavity; do not chew, suck, or swallow. Do not eat or drink until tab is completely dissolved.
In patients who have dry mouth, water may be used to moisten buccal mucosa before taking dose.

STORAGE
20-25°C (68-77°F); excursions permitted between 15-30°C (59-86°F). Protect from moisture.

HOW SUPPLIED
Tab, SL: 100mcg, 200mcg, 300mcg, 400mcg, 600mcg, 800mcg

CONTRAINDICATIONS
Opioid-nontolerant patients, management of acute or postoperative pain (eg, headache/migraine, dental pain, or use in emergency room), known intolerance or hypersensitivity to any of its components or the drug fentanyl.

WARNINGS/PRECAUTIONS
May cause anaphylaxis and hypersensitivity reactions. Increased risk of respiratory depression in patients with underlying respiratory disorders and in elderly/debilitated. May impair mental/physical abilities. Caution with chronic obstructive pulmonary disease or preexisting medical conditions predisposing to hypoventilation; may further decrease respiratory drive to the point of respiratory failure. Extreme caution in patients who may be susceptible to intracranial effects of CO_2 retention (eg, with evidence of increased intracranial pressure or impaired consciousness). May obscure clinical course of head injuries. Caution with bradyarrhythmias. Caution with hepatic/renal impairment.

ADVERSE REACTIONS
Respiratory depression, nausea, somnolence, dizziness, headache, constipation, stomatitis, dry mouth, dysgeusia, fatigue, dyspnea, hyperhidrosis, bradycardia, asthenia, anxiety.

DRUG INTERACTIONS

See Boxed Warning. May produce increased depressant effects with other CNS depressants (eg, other opioids, sedatives or hypnotics, general anesthetics, phenothiazines, tranquilizers, skeletal muscle relaxants, sedating antihistamines, and alcoholic beverages); adjust dose if warranted. CYP3A4 inducers (eg, barbiturates, carbamazepine, efavirenz, glucocorticoids, modafinil, nevirapine, oxcarbazepine, phenobarbital, phenytoin, pioglitazone, rifabutin, rifampin, St. John's wort, troglitazone) may decrease levels and efficacy. Not recommended with MAOIs or within 14 days of discontinuation of MAOIs. Respiratory depression is more likely to occur when given with other drugs that depress respiration.

PREGNANCY AND LACTATION

Category C, not for use in nursing.

MECHANISM OF ACTION

Opioid analgesic; μ-opioid receptor agonist. Exact mechanism not established. Specific CNS opioid receptors for endogenous compounds with opioid-like activity have been identified throughout the brain and spinal cord and play a role in analgesic effects.

PHARMACOKINETICS

Absorption: Bioavailability (54%). Administration of variable doses resulted in different pharmacokinetic parameters. **Distribution:** V_d=4L/kg; plasma protein binding (80-85%); crosses placenta; found in breast milk. **Metabolism:** Liver and intestinal mucosa via CYP3A4; norfentanyl (metabolite). **Elimination:** Urine (<7% unchanged), feces (1% unchanged); $T_{1/2}$=5.02 hrs (100mcg), 6.67 hrs (200mcg), 13.5 hrs (400mcg), 10.1 hrs (800mcg).

PATIENT CONSIDERATIONS

Assessment: Assess for degree of opioid tolerance, previous opioid dose, level of pain intensity, type of pain, patient's general condition and medical status, and for any other conditions where treatment is contraindicated or cautioned. Assess for hypersensitivity to the drug, renal/hepatic function, pregnancy/nursing status, and possible drug interactions.

Monitoring: Monitor for signs/symptoms of respiratory depression, bradycardia, impairment of mental/physical abilities, drug abuse/addiction, hypersensitivity reactions, and other adverse reactions.

Counseling: Inform outpatients to enroll in the TIRF REMS Access program. Counsel that therapy may be fatal in children, in individuals for whom it is not prescribed, and who are not opioid tolerant. Counsel on proper administration and disposal. Advise to take drug as prescribed and avoid sharing it with anyone else. Instruct not to take medication for acute or postoperative pain, pain from injuries, headache, migraine, or any other short-term pain. Instruct to notify physician if breakthrough pain is not alleviated or worsens after taking the drug. Inform that drug may impair mental/physical abilities; caution against performing activities that require high level of attention (eg, driving/using heavy machinery). Advise not to combine with alcohol, sleep aids, or tranquilizers except if ordered by the physician. Instruct to notify physician if pregnant or planning to become pregnant.

ACANYA — benzoyl peroxide/clindamycin phosphate　　Rx

Class: Antibacterial/keratolytic

ADULT DOSAGE	PEDIATRIC DOSAGE
Acne Vulgaris	**Acne Vulgaris**
Apply a pea-sized amount to face qd	**≥12 Years:**
	Apply a pea-sized amount to face qd

ADMINISTRATION

Topical route

STORAGE

Prior to Dispensing: 2-8°C (36-46°F). After Dispensing: Room temperature up to 25°C (77°F). Do not freeze.

HOW SUPPLIED

Gel: (Clindamycin-Benzoyl Peroxide) 1.2%-2.5% [50g]

CONTRAINDICATIONS

Previous hypersensitivity to clindamycin, benzoyl peroxide, any components of the formulation, or lincomycin. History of regional enteritis, ulcerative colitis, or antibiotic-associated colitis.

WARNINGS/PRECAUTIONS

Not for oral, ophthalmic, or intravaginal use. Diarrhea, bloody diarrhea, and colitis (including pseudomembranous colitis) reported; d/c if significant diarrhea occurs. Minimize sun exposure including use of tanning beds or sun lamps, following application.

ADVERSE REACTIONS

Erythema, scaling, itching, burning, stinging.

DRUG INTERACTIONS

Caution with topical acne therapy; possible cumulative irritancy effect may occur, especially with the use of peeling, desquamating, or abrasive agents. Caution with other neuromuscular blocking agents. Antiperistaltic agents (eg, opiates, diphenoxylate with atropine) may prolong and/or worsen severe colitis. Avoid with topical or oral erythromycin-containing products.

PREGNANCY AND LACTATION

Category C, not for use in nursing.

MECHANISM OF ACTION

Clindamycin: Lincosamide antibacterial; binds to the 50S ribosomal subunits of susceptible bacteria and prevents elongation of peptide chains by interfering with peptidyl transfer, thereby suppressing bacterial protein synthesis. Benzoyl Peroxide: Not established; an oxidizing agent with bactericidal and keratolytic effects.

PHARMACOKINETICS

Absorption: Clindamycin: (Day 1) C_{max}=0.78ng/mL; AUC_{0-t}=5.29 hr•ng/mL. (Day 30) C_{max}=1.22ng/mL, AUC_{0-t}=8.42 hr•ng/mL. **Distribution:** Clindamycin: (PO/Parenteral) Found in breast milk. **Metabolism:** Benzoyl peroxide: Converted to benzoic acid.

PATIENT CONSIDERATIONS

Assessment: Assess for history of hypersensitivity to drug/lincomycin, regional enteritis, ulcerative colitis, antibiotic-associated colitis, pregnancy/nursing status, and possible drug interactions.

Monitoring: Monitor for local skin reactions, diarrhea, bloody diarrhea, colitis, and other adverse reactions.

Counseling: Instruct to d/c use and contact physician immediately if allergic reactions (eg, severe swelling, SOB) develop. Inform that medication may cause irritation (eg, erythema, scaling, itching, burning), especially when used with other topical acne therapies. Instruct to limit excessive/prolonged exposure to sunlight by wearing a hat or other clothing and using sunscreen. Inform that medication may bleach hair or colored fabric.

ACCUNEB — albuterol sulfate　　Rx

Class: Short-acting beta₂ agonist (SABA)

PEDIATRIC DOSAGE
Bronchospasm
2-12 Years w/ Asthma:
Initial: 0.63mg or 1.25mg tid-qid prn
6-12 Years w/ More Severe Asthma (Baseline FEV_1 <60% Predicted), Weight >40kg, or 11-12 Years: May achieve better initial response w/ 1.25mg dose

---

ADMINISTRATION

Inh route

Administer using a jet nebulizer connected to an air compressor w/ adequate air flow, equipped w/ a mouthpiece or suitable face mask
Use the entire contents of one unit-dose vial (3mL of 1.25mg or 0.63mg inh sol)
Adjust nebulizer flow rate to deliver over 5 to 15 min

STORAGE

2-25°C (36-77°F). Protect from light and excessive heat. Store in protective foil pouch at all times. Once removed, use within 1 week. Discard if sol not colorless.

HOW SUPPLIED

Sol, Inhalation: 0.63mg/3mL, 1.25mg/3mL

CONTRAINDICATIONS

History of hypersensitivity to any of its components.

WARNINGS/PRECAUTIONS

Can produce paradoxical bronchospasm; d/c if this occurs. Consider adding anti-inflammatory agents (eg, corticosteroids) to adequately control asthma. Reevaluate patient and treatment regimen if deterioration of asthma observed. Can produce clinically significant cardiovascular (CV) effect (eg, ECG changes); caution with CV disorders (eg, coronary insufficiency, cardiac arrhythmias, HTN). Immediate hypersensitivity reactions reported. Aggravation of preexisting diabetes mellitus (DM) and ketoacidosis reported with large doses of IV albuterol. May cause hypokalemia. Has not been studied with acute attacks of bronchospasm.

ADVERSE REACTIONS

Asthma exacerbation, otitis media, allergic reaction, gastroenteritis, cold symptoms.

DRUG INTERACTIONS

Avoid other short-acting sympathomimetic aerosol bronchodilators and epinephrine. Extreme caution with MAOIs or TCAs, or within 2 weeks of discontinuation of such agents; action of albuterol may be potentiated. May decrease serum levels of digoxin; monitor levels. May worsen ECG changes and/or hypokalemia caused by non-K sparing diuretics (eg, loop/thiazide); caution is advised. Pulmonary effect blocked by β-blockers; caution with cardioselective β-blockers.

PREGNANCY AND LACTATION

Category C, not for use in nursing.

MECHANISM OF ACTION

β₂-adrenergic agonist; stimulates intracellular adenyl cyclase, which catalyzes conversion of ATP to cAMP to produce relaxation of bronchial smooth muscle.

PHARMACOKINETICS

Absorption: Bioavailability (<20%); (Inh) C_{max}=2.1ng/mL, T_{max}=0.5 hrs. **Elimination:** Urine; (PO) $T_{1/2}$=5-6 hrs.

PATIENT CONSIDERATIONS

Assessment: Assess for previous hypersensitivity to the drug, CV disorders, HTN, DM, pregnancy/nursing status, and possible drug interactions.

Monitoring: Monitor for signs/symptoms of CV effects (measured by pulse rate and BP), worsening of symptoms, paradoxical bronchospasm, deterioration of asthma, hypokalemia, and hypersensitivity reactions.

Counseling: Instruct not to use more frequently than recommended. Advise not to increase dose or frequency without consulting physician. Counsel to seek medical attention if symptoms worsen, if therapy becomes less effective, or if there is need to use the drug more frequently than usual. Inform of the common effects (eg, palpitations, chest pain, rapid HR, tremor, nervousness). Advise not to use if the contents of vial change color or become cloudy. Inform that drug compatibility, clinical efficacy, and safety, when mixed with other drugs in nebulizer, have not been established.

ACCUPRIL — quinapril hydrochloride   Rx

Class: ACE inhibitor

> D/C if pregnancy is detected. Drugs that act directly on the renin-angiotensin system (RAS) can cause injury/death to the developing fetus.

ADULT DOSAGE	PEDIATRIC DOSAGE
Hypertension	Pediatric use may not have been established
Monotherapy:	
Initial: 10mg or 20mg qd	
Titrate: May adjust dosage at intervals of at least 2 weeks	
Most patients have required doses of 20, 40, or 80mg/day, given as a single dose or in 2 equally divided doses	
Concomitant Diuretics:	
May add a diuretic if BP is uncontrolled w/ monotherapy In patients currently treated w/ a diuretic, d/c diuretic, if possible, 2-3 days before beginning treatment w/ quinapril, to reduce likelihood of hypotension; may then resume diuretic if BP is not controlled w/ monotherapy	
Initial: 5mg qd if diuretic therapy cannot be discontinued	
Heart Failure	
Adjunctive therapy when added to conventional therapy, including diuretics and/or digitalis	
Initial: 5mg bid	
Titrate: Adjust weekly	
Usual: 20-40mg/day given in 2 equally divided doses	

DOSING CONSIDERATIONS
Renal Impairment
HTN:
CrCl >60mL/min:
Max Initial: 10mg/day
CrCl 30-60mL/min:
Max Initial: 5mg/day
CrCl 10-30mL/min:
Max Initial: 2.5mg/day
Heart Failure (HF) and Renal Impairment or Hyponatremia:
CrCl >30mL/min:
Initial: 5mg/day
CrCl 10-30mL/min:
Initial: 2.5mg/day
Titrate: May increase dose at weekly intervals
Elderly
≥65 Years:
HTN:
Initial: 10mg qd
ADMINISTRATION
Oral route
STORAGE
15-30°C (59-86°F). Protect from light.
HOW SUPPLIED
Tab: 5mg*, 10mg, 20mg, 40mg *scored
CONTRAINDICATIONS
Hypersensitivity to quinapril HCl, history of ACE inhibitor-associated angioedema. Coadministration w/ aliskiren in patients w/ diabetes.
WARNINGS/PRECAUTIONS
Less effect on BP and higher incidence of angioedema in blacks than nonblacks. Head/neck angioedema reported; d/c and administer appropriate therapy if laryngeal stridor or angioedema of the face, tongue, or glottis occurs. Intestinal angioedema reported; monitor for abdominal pain. Patients w/ history of angioedema unrelated to ACE inhibitor therapy may be at increased risk of angioedema during therapy. Anaphylactoid reactions reported during desensitization w/ hymenoptera venom, dialysis w/ high-flux membranes, and LDL apheresis w/ dextran sulfate absorption. Associated w/ syndrome that starts w/ cholestatic jaundice and progresses to fulminant hepatic necrosis and,

sometimes, death (rare); d/c if jaundice or marked hepatic enzyme elevations occur. Excessive hypotension sometimes associated w/ oliguria, azotemia, and (rarely) acute renal failure and/or death may occur. Risk factors for excessive hypotension include HF, hyponatremia, high-dose diuretic therapy, recent intensive diuresis, dialysis, or severe volume and/or salt depletion; eliminate or reduce the diuretic dose or cautiously increase salt intake (except w/ HF) prior to therapy and monitor closely. If symptomatic hypotension develops, reduce dose or d/c therapy or concomitant diuretic. May cause agranulocytosis and bone marrow depression; consider periodic monitoring of WBC counts in patients w/ collagen vascular disease and/or renal disease. May cause renal function changes. May be associated w/ oliguria and/or progressive azotemia and rarely acute renal failure and/or death in patients w/ severe HF whose renal function may depend on the activity of the renin-angiotensin-aldosterone system. May increase BUN and SrCr levels in hypertensive patients w/ unilateral/bilateral renal artery stenosis; monitor renal function during the 1st few weeks of therapy. Minor/transient increases in BUN/SrCr reported in patients w/ no apparent renal vascular disease, when therapy was given concomitantly w/ a diuretic; dose reduction and/or discontinuation of any diuretic and/or quinapril may be required. Hyperkalemia reported; risk factors include renal insufficiency and diabetes mellitus (DM). Persistent nonproductive cough reported. Hypotension may occur w/ surgery or during anesthesia. Caution in elderly.

ADVERSE REACTIONS
Headache, dizziness, cough.

DRUG INTERACTIONS
See Contraindications. Excessive reduction of BP may occur after initiation of treatment in patients on diuretics, especially those on recently instituted diuretic therapy; d/c the diuretic or cautiously increase salt intake prior to initiation of treatment. If not possible to d/c the diuretic, reduce starting dose of quinapril. Coadministration w/ other drugs that raise serum K+ levels may result in hyperkalemia; monitor serum K+ in such patients. Reduces tetracycline absorption (possibly due to Mg2+ content in quinapril) during simultaneous administration; consider this interaction w/ concomitant tetracycline or other drugs that interact w/ Mg2+. May increase serum lithium levels and symptoms of lithium toxicity; use caution and monitor serum lithium levels. If a diuretic is also used, may increase the risk of lithium toxicity. Nitritoid reactions reported rarely w/ injectable gold (eg, sodium aurothiomalate). NSAIDs, including selective COX-2 inhibitors, may result in deterioration of renal function, including possible acute renal failure in patients who are elderly, volume-depleted, or w/ compromised renal function; monitor renal function periodically during coadministration. NSAIDs may attenuate the antihypertensive effect. Coadministration w/ mTOR inhibitors (eg, temsirolimus) may increase risk for angioedema. Dual blockade of the RAS is associated w/ increased risks of hypotension, hyperkalemia, and changes in renal function (including acute renal failure); avoid combined use of RAS inhibitors. Closely monitor BP, renal function, and electrolytes w/ other agents that also affect the RAS. Avoid concomitant use of aliskiren in patients w/ renal impairment (GFR <60mL/min). Hypotension risk and increased BUN and SrCr w/ diuretics.

PREGNANCY AND LACTATION
Pregnancy: Category D.
Lactation: Caution in nursing.

MECHANISM OF ACTION
ACE inhibitor; decreases plasma angiotensin II, which leads to decreased aldosterone secretion.

PHARMACOKINETICS
Absorption: T_{max}=1 hr, 2 hrs (quinaprilat). **Distribution:** Plasma protein binding (97%); crosses placenta; found in breast milk. **Metabolism:** Deesterification to quinaprilat (major active metabolite). **Elimination:** (IV) Renal (≤96% quinaprilat); $T_{1/2}$=2 hrs (quinaprilat).

PATIENT CONSIDERATIONS
Assessment: Assess for history of angioedema, hypersensitivity to drug, volume/salt depletion, collagen vascular disease, DM, renal artery stenosis, ischemic heart disease, cerebrovascular disease, renal function, pregnancy/nursing status, and possible drug interactions.

Monitoring: Monitor for signs/symptoms of hypotension, anaphylactoid or hypersensitivity reactions, head/neck/intestinal angioedema, agranulocytosis, neutropenia, bone marrow depression, cholestatic jaundice, fulminant hepatic necrosis, and hyperkalemia. Monitor BP and renal function. Monitor WBC count periodically in patients w/ collagen vascular disease and/or renal disease.

Counseling: Inform about the consequences of exposure to therapy during pregnancy; discuss treatment options w/ women planning to become pregnant. Instruct to report pregnancies to physician as soon as possible. Instruct to d/c therapy and immediately report signs/symptoms of angioedema. Caution about lightheadedness, especially during the 1st few days of therapy and advise to report to physician. Instruct to d/c and consult physician if syncope occurs. Caution that inadequate fluid intake or excessive perspiration, diarrhea, or vomiting may lead to an excessive fall in BP, w/ the same consequences of lightheadedness and syncope. Instruct to inform physician about therapy if planning to undergo surgery/anesthesia. Instruct not to use K+ supplements or salt substitutes containing K+ w/o consulting physician. Advise to report any symptoms of infection.

ACCURETIC — hydrochlorothiazide/quinapril hydrochloride   Rx

Class: ACE inhibitor/thiazide diuretic

> D/C if pregnancy is detected. Drugs that act directly on the renin-angiotensin system (RAS) can cause injury/death to the developing fetus.

ADULT DOSAGE

Hypertension

BP Uncontrolled w/ Quinapril Monotherapy:
10mg/12.5mg or 20mg/12.5mg qd. Further increases of either or both components depends on clinical response; may increase HCTZ after 2-3 weeks

BP Controlled w/ HCTZ 25mg/day w/ Significant K+ Loss:
10mg/12.5mg or 20mg/12.5mg qd

Replacement Therapy:
Patients adequately treated w/ 20mg quinapril and 25mg HCTZ w/o significant electrolyte disturbances may switch to 20mg/25mg qd

Not for initial therapy; begin combination therapy only after a patient fails to achieve desired effect w/ monotherapy

PEDIATRIC DOSAGE

Pediatric use may not have been established

DOSING CONSIDERATIONS

Renal Impairment
CrCl ≤30mL/min: Not recommended; loop diuretics preferred

Elderly
Start at lower end of dosing range

ADMINISTRATION
Oral route

STORAGE
20-25°C (68-77°F).

HOW SUPPLIED
Tab: (Quinapril/HCTZ) 10mg/12.5mg*, 20mg/12.5mg*, 20mg/25mg *scored

CONTRAINDICATIONS
Anuria, hypersensitivity to other sulfonamide-derived drugs, hypersensitivity to quinapril or hydrochlorothiazide, history of ACE inhibitor-associated angioedema. Coadministration w/ aliskiren in patients w/ diabetes.

WARNINGS/PRECAUTIONS
Not for initial therapy of HTN. May cause symptomatic hypotension; reduce dose or d/c if symptomatic hypotension occurs. Correct volume/salt depletion prior to therapy. Monitor patients at risk of excessive hypotension closely for the first 2 weeks of treatment and whenever dose of quinapril or diuretic is increased. Caution w/ ischemic heart or cerebrovascular disease in whom an excessive fall in BP could result in MI or cerebrovascular accident. Caution w/ impaired hepatic function or progressive liver disease; may precipitate hepatic coma. **Quinapril:** Higher incidence of angioedema and less effect on BP in blacks than nonblacks. Head/neck angioedema reported; d/c immediately and administer appropriate therapy if laryngeal stridor or angioedema of the face/tongue/glottis occurs. Intestinal angioedema reported; monitor for abdominal pain. Patients w/ history of angioedema unrelated to ACE inhibitor therapy may be at increased risk of angioedema during therapy. Anaphylactoid reactions reported during desensitization w/ hymenoptera venom, dialysis w/ high-flux membranes, and LDL apheresis w/ dextran sulfate absorption. Associated w/ syndrome that starts w/ cholestatic jaundice and progresses to fulminant hepatic necrosis, and sometimes death (rare); d/c if jaundice or marked hepatic enzyme elevation occurs. May cause changes in renal function. May be associated w/ oliguria and/or progressive azotemia and rarely w/ acute renal failure and/or death in patients w/ severe CHF whose renal function may depend on the activity of the renin-angiotensin-aldosterone system. May increase BUN and SrCr in patients w/ unilateral renal artery stenosis; monitor renal function during 1st few weeks of therapy. May increase BUN/SrCr in patients w/o preexisting renal vascular disease; may require dose reduction. May cause agranulocytosis and bone marrow depression; consider periodic monitoring of WBC counts in patients w/ collagen vascular disease and/or renal disease. Hyperkalemia reported; risk factors include renal insufficiency and diabetes mellitus. Persistent nonproductive cough reported. Hypotension may occur w/ surgery or during anesthesia. **HCTZ:** Antihypertensive effects may be enhanced in postsympathectomy patients. May precipitate azotemia w/ renal disease. May exacerbate/activate systemic lupus erythematosus (SLE). May cause idiosyncratic reaction, resulting in acute transient myopia and acute angle-closure glaucoma; d/c as rapidly as possible. May cause hyponatremia, hypokalemia, hyperkalemia, and hypomagnesemia. May alter glucose tolerance and raise serum levels of cholesterol, TG, and Ca2+. May raise serum uric acid level and may cause/exacerbate hyperuricemia and precipitate gout in susceptible patients. May decrease protein-bound iodine levels w/o signs of thyroid disturbance. Interrupt treatment for a few days prior to carrying out parathyroid function tests.

ADVERSE REACTIONS
Headache, dizziness, cough, fatigue.

DRUG INTERACTIONS
See Contraindications. Coadministration w/ other drugs that raise serum K+ levels may result in hyperkalemia; monitor serum K+ in such patients. May increase lithium levels and risk of toxicity; use caution and monitor lithium levels. Avoid w/ aliskiren in patients w/ renal impairment (GFR <60mL/min). Coadministration w/ mTOR inhibitors (eg, temsirolimus) may increase risk for angioedema. **Quinapril:** Dual blockade of the RAS is associated w/ increased risk of hypotension, hyperkalemia, and changes in renal function (including acute renal failure); in general, avoid combined use of RAS inhibitors. Closely monitor BP, renal function, and electrolytes w/ concomitant agents that also affect the RAS. Reduces tetracycline absorption (possibly due to Mg2+ content in quinapril); consider this interaction if coadministering w/ tetracycline or other drugs that interact w/ Mg2+. Nitritoid reactions reported rarely w/ injectable gold (eg, sodium aurothiomalate). NSAIDs, including selective COX-2 inhibitors, may result in deterioration of renal function, including possible acute renal failure, in patients who are elderly, volume depleted, or w/ compromised renal function. NSAIDs may attenuate the antihypertensive effects. **HCTZ:** Thiazide-induced electrolyte disturbances (eg, hypokalemia, hypomagnesemia) increase the risk of digoxin toxicity, which may lead to fatal arrhythmic events. May potentiate orthostatic hypotension w/ alcohol, barbiturates, and narcotics. Dose adjustment of the antidiabetic drug (oral agents and insulin) may be required. Cholestyramine and colestipol resins impair absorption. Corticosteroids and ACTH may intensify electrolyte depletion, particularly hypokalemia. May decrease response to pressor amines (eg, norepinephrine). May increase responsiveness to nondepolarizing skeletal muscle relaxants (eg, tubocurarine). NSAIDs may reduce diuretic, natriuretic, and antihypertensive effects of thiazide diuretics. May potentiate action of other antihypertensives, especially ganglionic or peripheral adrenergic-blocking drugs.

PREGNANCY AND LACTATION
Pregnancy: Category D.
Lactation: Not for use in nursing.

MECHANISM OF ACTION
Quinapril: ACE inhibitor; decreases plasma angiotensin II, which leads to decreased aldosterone secretion. **HCTZ:** Thiazide diuretic; has not been established. Affects renal tubular mechanism of electrolyte reabsorption, directly increasing excretion of Na+ and Cl-, and indirectly reducing plasma volume.

PHARMACOKINETICS
Absorption: Quinapril: T_{max}=1 hr, 2 hrs (quinaprilat). **Distribution:** Crosses placenta; found in breast milk. Quinapril: Plasma protein binding (97%). HCTZ: V_d=3.6-7.8L/kg; plasma protein binding (67.9%). **Metabolism:** Quinapril: Deesterification. Quinaprilat (major active metabolite). **Elimination:** Quinapril: (IV) Renal (≤96% quinaprilat); $T_{1/2}$=2 hrs (quinaprilat). HCTZ: Kidney (≥61% unchanged); $T_{1/2}$=4-15 hrs.

PATIENT CONSIDERATIONS

Assessment: Assess for hypersensitivity to drug or sulfonamides, anuria, history of angioedema, volume/salt depletion, heart failure, SLE, any other conditions where treatment is contraindicated or cautioned, pregnancy/nursing status, and possible drug interactions. Assess renal/hepatic function and electrolyte levels.

Monitoring: Monitor for angioedema, agranulocytosis, hyperkalemia, anaphylactoid reactions, hypotension, jaundice, hypersensitivity/idiosyncratic reactions, SLE, gout, myopia, and angle-closure glaucoma. Periodically monitor WBC counts in patients w/ collagen vascular disease and/or renal disease. Monitor serum electrolytes, BP, LFTs, BUN, SrCr, uric acid levels, and cholesterol/TG levels. Monitor Ca2+ levels in patients w/ hypercalcemia.

Counseling: Inform females of childbearing age of the consequences of exposure during pregnancy and of the treatment options for women planning to become pregnant. Instruct to report pregnancy to the physician as soon as possible. Instruct to d/c therapy and immediately report signs/symptoms of angioedema. Caution about lightheadedness, especially during the 1st days of therapy and advise to report to physician. Instruct to d/c and consult physician if syncope occurs. Caution that inadequate fluid intake or excessive perspiration, diarrhea, or vomiting may lead to an excessive fall in BP, resulting in lightheadedness or syncope. Instruct to inform physician about therapy if planning to undergo surgery/anesthesia. Instruct to avoid K+ supplements or salt substitutes containing K+ w/o consulting physician. Instruct to report any symptoms of infection.

ACEON — perindopril erbumine   Rx

Class: ACE inhibitor

> D/C if pregnancy is detected. Drugs that act directly on the renin-angiotensin system (RAS) can cause injury/death to the developing fetus.

ADULT DOSAGE

Hypertension

Initial: 4mg qd
Titrate: May titrate prn to max of 16mg/day
Maint: 4-8mg/day given in 1 or 2 divided doses

Stable Coronary Artery Disease

Initial: 4mg qd for 2 weeks
Maint: Increase as tolerated to 8mg qd

PEDIATRIC DOSAGE

Pediatric use may not have been established

DOSING CONSIDERATIONS
Concomitant Medications
Concomitant Diuretics:
Consider reducing diuretic dose prior to start of treatment

Renal Impairment
CrCl <30mL/min: Not recommended

CrCl ≥30mL/min:
Initial: 2mg/day
Max: 8mg/day
Elderly
HTN:
Initial: 4mg/day given in 1 or 2 divided doses
Monitor BP and titrate carefully w/ doses >8mg

>70 Years:
Stable CAD:
Initial: 2mg qd in the 1st week, followed by 4mg qd in the 2nd week
Maint: 8mg qd if tolerated

ADMINISTRATION
Oral route
STORAGE
20-25°C (68-77°F). Protect from moisture.
HOW SUPPLIED
Tab: 2mg*, 4mg*, 8mg* *scored
CONTRAINDICATIONS
Known hypersensitivity (eg, angioedema) to this product or to any other ACE inhibitor. Hereditary or idiopathic angioedema. Coadministration w/ aliskiren in patients w/ diabetes.
WARNINGS/PRECAUTIONS
Higher incidence of angioedema in blacks than nonblacks. Angioedema of the face, extremities, lips, tongue, glottis, or larynx reported; d/c and administer appropriate therapy. Intestinal angioedema reported; monitor for abdominal pain. Symptomatic hypotension may occur and is most likely in patients w/ volume/salt depletion. Closely monitor patients at risk for excessive hypotension, especially during the first 2 weeks of treatment and whenever dose is increased. May cause agranulocytosis and bone marrow depression, most frequently in renal impairment patients, especially w/ collagen vascular disease (eg, systemic lupus erythematosus [SLE] or scleroderma). May cause changes in renal function. Oliguria, progressive azotemia, and (rarely) acute renal failure and death may occur in patients w/ severe CHF. May increase BUN and SrCr in patients w/ renal artery stenosis. May cause hyperkalemia; risk factors include renal insufficiency and diabetes mellitus (DM). Persistent nonproductive cough reported. Rarely, associated w/ syndrome that starts w/ cholestatic jaundice and progresses to fulminant necrosis and sometimes death; d/c if jaundice or marked elevations of hepatic enzymes develop. Hypotension may occur w/ major surgery or during anesthesia.
ADVERSE REACTIONS
Cough, headache, asthenia, dizziness, hypotension.
DRUG INTERACTIONS
See Contraindications and Dosing Considerations. Dual blockade of the RAS is associated w/ increased risks of hypotension, hyperkalemia, and changes in renal function (including acute renal failure); avoid combined use of RAS inhibitors, or closely monitor BP, renal function, and electrolytes w/ concomitant agents that affect the RAS. Avoid w/ aliskiren in patients w/ renal impairment (GFR <60mL/min). Hypotension risk, increased BUN and SrCr, and reduced perindoprilat bioavailability w/ diuretics. Increased risk of hyperkalemia w/ K^+-sparing diuretics, drugs that increase serum K^+ (eg, indomethacin, heparin, cyclosporine), K^+ supplements and/or K^+-containing salt substitutes. May increase lithium levels and risk of toxicity; monitor lithium levels. Nitritoid reactions reported w/ injectable gold (sodium aurothiomalate). Caution w/ digoxin. Coadministration w/ NSAIDs, including selective COX-2 inhibitors, may attenuate antihypertensive effect of ACE inhibitors and may further deteriorate renal function.
PREGNANCY AND LACTATION
Category D, caution in nursing.
MECHANISM OF ACTION
ACE inhibitor; inhibits ACE activity, resulting in decreased plasma angiotensin II, leading to decreased vasoconstriction, increased plasma renin activity, and decreased aldosterone secretion.
PHARMACOKINETICS
Absorption: Absolute bioavailability (75%, 25% perindoprilat); T_{max}=1 hr, 3-7 hrs (perindoprilat). **Distribution:** Plasma protein binding (approx 60%, 10-20% perindoprilat); crosses placenta. **Metabolism:** Hepatic (extensive); hydrolysis, glucuronidation, cyclization via dehydration; perindoprilat (active metabolite). **Elimination:** Urine (4-12%, unchanged); $T_{1/2}$=approx 0.8-1 hr, 3-10 hrs (perindoprilat).

PATIENT CONSIDERATIONS
Assessment: Assess for hereditary or idiopathic angioedema, volume and/or salt depletion, CHF, renal artery stenosis, ischemic heart disease, cerebrovascular disease, hepatic/renal impairment, DM, collagen vascular disease (eg, SLE), previous hypersensitivity to the drug, pregnancy/nursing status, and possible drug interactions.

Monitoring: Monitor for signs/symptoms of anaphylactoid reactions, head/neck/intestinal angioedema, hypotension, agranulocytosis, bone marrow depression, cholestatic jaundice, fulminant hepatic necrosis, hepatic failure, hyperkalemia, persistent nonproductive cough, hypersensitivity reactions, and neutropenia. Monitor hepatic/renal function, BP, and K^+ levels.

Counseling: Inform of pregnancy risks and discuss treatment options w/ women planning to become pregnant; advise to report pregnancy to physician as soon as possible. Instruct to d/c and immediately report to physician if any signs/symptoms of angioedema develop. Counsel to report any signs of infection (eg, sore throat, fever).

ACETAMINOPHEN AND CODEINE
TABLETS — acetaminophen/codeine phosphate   CIII
Class: Opioid analgesic

> Associated with cases of acute liver failure, at times resulting in liver transplant and death. Most cases of liver injury are associated with acetaminophen (APAP) use at doses >4000mg/day, and often involve >1 APAP-containing product. Respiratory depression and death reported in children who received codeine following tonsillectomy and/or adenoidectomy and had evidence of being ultra-rapid metabolizers of codeine due to a CYP2D6 polymorphism.

OTHER BRAND NAMES
Tylenol with Codeine

ADULT DOSAGE
Mild to Moderately Severe Pain
Usual Range (Single Dose): 15mg-60mg codeine; 300mg-1000mg acetaminophen (APAP); may repeat doses up to q4h
Max: 360mg/24 hrs codeine; 4000mg/24 hrs APAP

PEDIATRIC DOSAGE
Pediatric use may not have been established

ADMINISTRATION
Oral route
STORAGE
20-25°C (68-77°F).
HOW SUPPLIED
Tab: (APAP/Codeine) 300mg/15mg; (Tylenol with Codeine) 300mg/30mg, 300mg/60mg
CONTRAINDICATIONS
Postoperative pain management in children who have undergone tonsillectomy and/or adenoidectomy. Previously exhibited hypersensitivity to codeine or acetaminophen.
WARNINGS/PRECAUTIONS
Increased risk of acute liver failure in patients with underlying liver disease. May cause serious skin reactions (eg, acute generalized exanthematous pustulosis, Stevens-Johnson syndrome, toxic epidermal necrolysis), which can be fatal; d/c at the 1st appearance of skin rash or any other sign of hypersensitivity. Deaths reported in nursing infants exposed to high levels of morphine because their mothers were ultra-rapid metabolizers of codeine. Ultra-rapid metabolizers, due to specific CYP2D6 genotype (gene duplications denoted as *1/*1xN or *1/*2xN), may have life-threatening or fatal respiratory depression or experience signs of overdose (eg, extreme sleepiness, confusion, shallow breathing). Choose lowest effective dose for the shortest period of time. Hypersensitivity and anaphylaxis reported; d/c if signs/symptoms occur. Respiratory-depressant effects and capacity for elevating CSF pressure may be markedly enhanced in the presence of head injury or other intracranial lesions. May obscure diagnosis or clinical course of head injuries and acute abdominal conditions. Habit-forming and potentially abusable; extended use is not recommended. Caution with severe renal/hepatic impairment, head injuries, elevated intracranial pressure, acute abdominal conditions, hypothyroidism, urethral stricture, Addison's disease, prostatic hypertrophy, and in the elderly or debilitated. May increase serum amylase levels. Lab test interactions may occur. Avoid during labor if delivery of a premature infant is anticipated. (Tylenol with Codeine) Contains sodium metabisulfite; may cause allergic-type reactions in certain susceptible people.
ADVERSE REACTIONS
Acute liver failure, drowsiness, lightheadedness, dizziness, sedation, SOB, N/V.
DRUG INTERACTIONS
Increased risk of acute liver failure with alcohol ingestion. May enhance effects of other narcotic analgesics, alcohol, general anesthetics, tranquilizers (eg, chlordiazepoxide), sedative-hypnotics, or other CNS depressants; may increase CNS depression.
PREGNANCY AND LACTATION
Category C, not for use in nursing.
MECHANISM OF ACTION
Codeine: Narcotic analgesic; centrally acting analgesic. APAP: Nonopiate, nonsalicylate analgesic; peripherally acting analgesic.
PHARMACOKINETICS
Absorption: Rapid. **Distribution:** Found in breast milk. Codeine: Crosses placenta. **Metabolism:** Codeine: CYP2D6; morphine (active metabolite). APAP: Liver (conjugation). **Elimination:** Codeine: Urine (90%), feces; $T_{1/2}$=2.9 hrs. APAP: Urine (85%); $T_{1/2}$=1.25-3 hrs.

PATIENT CONSIDERATIONS
Assessment: Assess for hypersensitivity to drug, hepatic/renal impairment, head injury, intracranial lesions, acute abdominal conditions, any other conditions where treatment is contraindicated or cautioned, pregnancy/nursing status, and possible drug interactions.

Monitoring: Monitor for signs/symptoms of hepatotoxicity, respiratory depression, skin reactions, hypersensitivity, anaphylaxis, elevation in CSF pressure, drug abuse, tolerance, dependence, and other adverse reactions. Monitor effects of therapy with serial LFTs and/or renal function tests in patients with severe hepatic/renal disease. Closely monitor newborn infants for signs of respiratory depression if the mother received the drug during labor.

Counseling: Instruct to d/c therapy and contact physician immediately if signs of allergy develop. Instruct to look for APAP on package labels and not to use >1 APAP-containing product. Instruct to seek medical attention immediately upon ingestion of >4000mg/day APAP, even if patient is feeling well. Advise that drug may impair mental/physical abilities. Instruct to avoid performing potentially hazardous tasks (eg, driving, operating machinery), drinking alcohol, or taking other CNS depressants while on therapy. Inform that drug may be habit-forming; instruct to take ud.

ACIPHEX — rabeprazole sodium   Rx

Class: Proton pump inhibitor (PPI)

ADULT DOSAGE

Helicobacter pylori Eradication

Treatment of *H. pylori* infection and duodenal ulcer disease (active or history w/in past 5 yrs) for *H. pylori* eradication to reduce the risk of duodenal ulcer recurrence

20mg tab + clarithromycin 500mg + amoxicillin 1000mg, all bid w/ am and pm meals for 7 days

Pathological Hypersecretory Conditions

Treatment of pathological hypersecretory conditions, including Zollinger-Ellison syndrome

Initial: 60mg qd or in divided doses
Titrate: Adjust to individual needs and continue for as long as clinically indicated

Doses up to 100mg qd and 60mg bid have been administered. Some patients w/ Zollinger-Ellison syndrome have been treated continuously for up to 1 yr

Gastroesophageal Reflux Disease

Healing of Erosive or Ulcerative GERD:
20mg tab qd for 4-8 weeks; consider an additional 8 weeks if not healed after 8 weeks of treatment

Maint of Healing of Erosive or Ulcerative GERD:
20mg tab qd; controlled studies do not extend beyond 12 months

Symptomatic GERD:
Treatment of daytime and nighttime heartburn and other symptoms associated w/ GERD

20mg tab qd for up to 4 weeks; consider an additional course of treatment if symptoms do not resolve completely after 4 weeks

Duodenal Ulcers

Healing and Symptomatic Relief of Duodenal Ulcers:
20mg tab qd after am meal for up to 4 weeks; some patients may need additional therapy to achieve healing

PEDIATRIC DOSAGE

Gastroesophageal Reflux Disease

Symptomatic:
≥12 Years:
20mg qd for up to 8 weeks

DOSING CONSIDERATIONS
Hepatic Impairment
Severe (Child-Pugh Class C): Avoid use; monitor for adverse reactions if treatment is necessary

ADMINISTRATION
Oral route
Swallow tabs whole; do not chew, crush, or split.
Take after a meal for the treatment of duodenal ulcers.
Take w/ food for *H. pylori* eradication.
May be taken w/ or w/o food for all other indications.

STORAGE
25°C (77°F); excursions permitted to 15-30°C (59-86°F). Protect from moisture.

HOW SUPPLIED
Tab, Delayed-Release: 20mg

CONTRAINDICATIONS
Known hypersensitivity to rabeprazole, substituted benzimidazoles, or to any component of the formulation. Concomitant use w/ rilpivirine-containing products. When used w/ clarithromycin and amoxicillin, refer to the prescribing information for each product.

WARNINGS/PRECAUTIONS
Symptomatic response to therapy does not preclude the presence of gastric malignancy. Acute interstitial nephritis reported; d/c if this develops. Cyanocobalamin (vitamin B12) deficiency may occur w/ daily long-term treatment (eg, >3 yrs). May increase risk of *Clostridium difficile*-associated diarrhea (CDAD), especially in hospitalized patients. May increase risk of osteoporosis-related fractures of the hip, wrist, or spine, especially w/ high-dose and long-term therapy (≥1 yr). Use lowest dose and shortest duration appropriate to the condition being treated. Hypomagnesemia reported in patients treated for ≥3 months; may require Mg^{2+} replacement and discontinuation of therapy. Consider monitoring Mg^{2+} levels prior to and periodically during therapy for patients expected to be on prolonged treatment or if taking medications such as digoxin or drugs that may cause hypomagnesemia (eg, diuretics).

ADVERSE REACTIONS
Adults: Pain, pharyngitis, flatulence, infection, constipation.
Adolescents: Headache, diarrhea, N/V, abdominal pain.

DRUG INTERACTIONS
See Contraindications. May decrease exposure of some antiretroviral drugs (eg, rilpivirine, atazanavir, nelfinavir) and may reduce antiviral effect and promote the development of drug resistance; refer to atazanavir prescribing information for dosing information. Avoid use w/ nelfinavir and refer to the prescribing information for nelfinavir and other antiretrovirals. May increase exposure of other antiretroviral drugs (eg, saquinavir) and may increase toxicity; monitor for potential saquinavir toxicities and refer to the prescribing information for saquinavir. Increased INR and PT reported w/ warfarin; monitor INR and PT. Refer to warfarin prescribing information; dose adjustment of warfarin may be needed. May elevate and prolong levels of methotrexate (MTX) and/or its metabolite hydroxymethotrexate, possibly leading to MTX toxicities; consider temporary withdrawal of rabeprazole in some patients receiving high-dose MTX. May increase digoxin exposure. Monitor digoxin concentrations; dose adjustment of digoxin may be needed. Refer to digoxin prescribing information. May reduce absorption of drugs dependent on gastric pH for absorption (eg, iron salts, erlotinib, dasatinib, nilotinib, mycophenolate mofetil, ketoconazole, itraconazole); refer to the prescribing information for concomitantly used drugs. Coadministration in patients receiving mycophenolate mofetil has been reported to reduce the exposure to the active metabolite, mycophenolic acid; use w/ caution in transplant patients. Concomitant administration of clarithromycin w/ other drugs can lead to serious adverse reactions (eg, potentially fatal arrhythmias); refer to the prescribing information of clarithromycin and amoxicillin if used concomitantly w/ rabeprazole.

PREGNANCY AND LACTATION
Pregnancy: There are no available human data on use in pregnant women to inform the drug-associated risk.
Lactation: Studies have not been conducted to assess the presence of rabeprazole in human milk, the effects on the breastfed infant, or the effects on milk production; caution in nursing.

MECHANISM OF ACTION
PPI; substituted benzimidazole that suppresses gastric acid secretion by inhibiting the gastric H^+/K^+-ATPase at the secretory surface of the gastric parietal cell. Blocks the final step of gastric acid secretion.

PHARMACOKINETICS
Absorption: T_{max}=2-5 hrs; absolute bioavailability (52%). **Distribution:** Plasma protein binding (96.3%). **Metabolism:** Liver (extensive) via CYP3A, CYP2C19; thioether and sulphone (primary metabolites). **Elimination:** Urine (90%, metabolites), feces; $T_{1/2}$=1-2 hrs.

PATIENT CONSIDERATIONS

Assessment: Assess for hypersensitivity to the drug, hepatic impairment, risk for osteoporosis-related fractures, pregnancy/nursing status, and possible drug interactions. Obtain baseline Mg^{2+} levels.

Monitoring: Monitor for signs/symptoms of acute interstitial nephritis, cyanocobalamin deficiency, CDAD, bone fractures, hypersensitivity reactions, and other adverse reactions. Monitor Mg^{2+} levels periodically. Monitor INR and PT when given w/ warfarin.

Counseling: Instruct to take ud. Advise to contact physician if any adverse reaction develops, if taking any other concomitant drug (eg, warfarin, high-dose MTX), or if pregnant or nursing.

ACIPHEX SPRINKLE — rabeprazole sodium   Rx

Class: Proton pump inhibitor (PPI)

PEDIATRIC DOSAGE
Gastroesophageal Reflux Disease
1-11 Years:
<15kg: 5mg qd for up to 12 weeks w/ the option to increase to 10mg qd if inadequate response
≥15kg: 10mg qd for up to 12 weeks

DOSING CONSIDERATIONS
Hepatic Impairment
Severe (Child-Pugh Class C): Avoid use; monitor for adverse reactions if treatment is necessary

ADMINISTRATION
Oral route
Take dose 30 min ac.
Open cap and sprinkle entire contents on a small amount of soft food (eg, applesauce, fruit- or vegetable-based baby food, yogurt) or empty contents into a small amount of liquid (eg, infant formula, apple juice, pediatric electrolyte sol); do not swallow the cap whole or chew/crush the granules.
Take entire dose w/in 15 min of preparation; do not store mixture for future use. Food or liquid should be at or below room temperature.

STORAGE
25°C (77°F); excursions permitted to 15-30°C (59-86°F). Protect from moisture.

HOW SUPPLIED
Cap, Delayed-Release: 5mg, 10mg

CONTRAINDICATIONS
Known hypersensitivity to rabeprazole, substituted benzimidazoles, or to any component of the formulation. Concomitant use w/ rilpivirine-containing products.

WARNINGS/PRECAUTIONS
Symptomatic response to therapy does not preclude the presence of gastric malignancy. Acute interstitial nephritis reported; d/c if this develops. Cyanocobalamin (vitamin B12) deficiency may occur w/ daily long-term treatment (eg, >3 yrs). May increase risk of *Clostridium difficile*-associated diarrhea (CDAD), especially in hospitalized patients. May increase risk of osteoporosis-related fractures of the hip, wrist, or spine, especially w/ high-dose and long-term therapy (≥1 yr). Use lowest dose and shortest duration appropriate to the condition being treated. Hypomagnesemia reported in adult patients treated for ≥3 months; may require Mg²⁺ replacement and discontinuation of therapy. Consider monitoring Mg²⁺ levels prior to and periodically during therapy for patients expected to be on prolonged treatment or if taking medications such as digoxin or drugs that may cause hypomagnesemia (eg, diuretics).

ADVERSE REACTIONS
N/V, abdominal pain, diarrhea, headache.

DRUG INTERACTIONS
See Contraindications. May decrease exposure of some antiretroviral drugs (eg, rilpivirine, atazanavir, nelfinavir) and may reduce antiviral effect and promote the development of drug resistance; refer to atazanavir prescribing information for dosing information. Avoid use w/ nelfinavir and refer to the prescribing information for nelfinavir and other antiretrovirals. May increase exposure of other antiretroviral drugs (eg, saquinavir) and may increase toxicity; refer to the prescribing information for saquinavir and monitor for potential saquinavir toxicities. Increased INR and PT reported w/ warfarin; monitor INR and PT. Dose adjustment of warfarin may be needed; refer to warfarin prescribing information. May elevate and prolong levels of methotrexate (MTX) and/or its metabolite hydroxymethotrexate, possibly leading to MTX toxicities; consider temporary withdrawal of rabeprazole in some patients receiving high-dose MTX. May increase digoxin exposure. Monitor digoxin concentrations; may need to adjust dose. Refer to digoxin prescribing information. May reduce absorption of drugs dependent on gastric pH for absorption (eg, iron salts, erlotinib, dasatinib, nilotinib, mycophenolate mofetil, ketoconazole, itraconazole); refer to the prescribing information for concomitantly used drugs. Coadministration in patients receiving mycophenolate mofetil has been reported to reduce the exposure to the active metabolite, mycophenolic acid; use w/ caution in transplant patients.

PREGNANCY AND LACTATION
Pregnancy: There are no available human data on use in pregnant women to inform the drug-associated risk.
Lactation: Studies have not been conducted to assess the presence of rabeprazole in human milk, the effects on the breastfed infant, or the effects on milk production; caution in nursing.

MECHANISM OF ACTION
PPI; substituted benzimidazole that suppresses gastric acid secretion by inhibiting the gastric H⁺/K⁺-ATPase at the secretory surface of the gastric parietal cell. Blocks the final step of gastric acid secretion.

PHARMACOKINETICS
Absorption: T_{max}=2.5 hrs (median). **Distribution:** Plasma protein binding (96.3%). **Metabolism:** Liver (extensive) via CYP3A, CYP2C19; thioether and sulphone (primary metabolites). **Elimination:** Urine (90%, metabolites), feces; $T_{1/2}$=1-2 hrs.

PATIENT CONSIDERATIONS
Assessment: Assess for hypersensitivity to the drug, hepatic impairment, risk for osteoporosis-related fractures, pregnancy/nursing status, and possible drug interactions. Obtain baseline Mg²⁺ levels.

Monitoring: Monitor for signs/symptoms of acute interstitial nephritis, cyanocobalamin deficiency, CDAD, bone fractures, hypersensitivity reactions, and other adverse reactions. Monitor Mg²⁺ levels periodically. Monitor INR and PT when given w/ warfarin.

Counseling: Instruct to take ud. Advise to contact physician if any adverse reaction develops, if taking any other concomitant drug (eg, warfarin, high-dose MTX), or if pregnant or nursing.

ACTEMRA — tocilizumab   Rx

Class: Monoclonal antibody/interleukin-6 (IL-6) receptor antagonist

> Increased risk for developing serious infections (eg, active tuberculosis (TB), invasive fungal infections, bacterial/viral infections due to opportunistic pathogens) that may lead to hospitalization or death. Most patients who developed these infections were taking concomitant immunosuppressants (eg, methotrexate [MTX], corticosteroids). If serious infection develops, interrupt treatment until infection is controlled. Test for latent TB prior to and during therapy; initiate latent TB treatment prior to therapy. Consider risks and benefits prior to initiating therapy in patients w/ chronic or recurrent infection. Monitor for development of signs/symptoms of infection during and after treatment.

ADULT DOSAGE
Rheumatoid Arthritis
Moderately to Severely Active:
IV:
4mg/kg every 4 weeks; may increase to 8mg/kg every 4 weeks based on clinical response
Max: 800mg/infusion
SQ:
<100kg: 162mg every other week, followed by an increase to every week based on response
≥100kg: 162mg every week

Transition from IV to SQ:
Administer 1st SQ dose instead of the next scheduled IV dose

May be used alone or in combination w/ methotrexate or other nonbiologic disease-modifying antirheumatic drugs

PEDIATRIC DOSAGE
Juvenile Idiopathic Arthritis
≥2 Years:
IV:
Active Polyarticular Juvenile Idiopathic Arthritis:
<30kg: 10mg/kg every 4 weeks
≥30kg: 8mg/kg every 4 weeks

Active Systemic Juvenile Idiopathic Arthritis:
<30kg: 12mg/kg every 2 weeks
≥30 kg: 8mg/kg every 2 weeks

May be used alone or in combination w/ methotrexate
Do not change dose based on a single visit body weight measurement

---

DOSING CONSIDERATIONS
Adverse Reactions
Rheumatoid Arthritis:
Liver Enzyme Abnormalities:
>1-3X ULN: Modify dose of concomitant disease-modifying antirheumatic drugs if appropriate. For persistent increases in this range, reduce dose to 4mg/kg or hold until ALT or AST have normalized if receiving IV. If receiving SQ, reduce inj frequency to every other week and hold dosing until ALT/AST have normalized and resume at every other week and increase frequency
>3-5X ULN: Hold until <3X ULN and follow recommendations above for >1-3X ULN. If persistent increases in this range, d/c therapy
>5X ULN: D/C

Low ANC:
ANC <500/mm³: D/C
ANC 500-1000/mm³: Hold dosing until ANC >1000/mm³. If receiving IV, resume at 4mg/kg and increase to 8mg/kg; if receiving SQ, resume at every other week and increase to every week

Low Platelet Counts:
<50,000/mm³: D/C
50,000-100,000/mm³: Hold until >100,000/mm³. If receiving IV, resume at 4mg/kg and increase to 8mg/kg. If receiving SQ, resume at every other week and increase to every week

Polyarticular/Systemic Juvenile Idiopathic Arthritis:
Dose reduction recommended for liver enzyme abnormalities, low neutrophil counts, and low platelet counts at levels similar to patients w/ rheumatoid arthritis
If appropriate, modify dose or stop methotrexate and/or other medications and hold therapy until clinical situation has been evaluated
Decision to d/c for a lab abnormality should be based on medical assessment of patient

ADMINISTRATION
IV/SQ route

Do not initiate therapy in patients w/ an ANC <2000/mm³, platelet count <100,000/mm³, or who have ALT or AST >1.5X ULN.
Do not administer as IV bolus/push.

IV
Preparation:
Polyarticular and Systemic Juvenile Idiopathic Arthritis:
<30kg: Use a 50mL infusion bag/bottle of 0.9% NaCl
≥30kg: Use a 100mL infusion bag/bottle of 0.9% NaCl
Rheumatoid Arthritis:
≥30kg: Use a 100mL infusion bag/bottle of 0.9% NaCl

Dilution:
Withdraw a volume of 0.9% NaCl inj, equal to volume of tocilizumab inj required for patient's dose from infusion bag/bottle.
Withdraw amount of tocilizumab for IV infusion from vial(s) and add slowly into NaCl infusion bag/bottle; gently invert bag to avoid foaming to mix sol.

Administration:
Administer infusion over 60 min, and must be administered w/ an infusion set.
Do not infuse concomitantly in same IV line w/ other drugs.
Fully diluted sol are compatible w/ polypropylene, polyethylene and polyvinyl chloride infusion bags and polypropylene, polyethylene, and glass infusion bottles.

SQ
Inject full amount in syringe (0.9mL), which provides 162mg of tocilizumab. Rotate inj sites w/ each inj and never inj into moles, scars, or areas where the skin is tender, bruised, red, hard, or not intact.

STORAGE
2-8°C (36-46°F). Do not freeze. Protect from light; store in original package until time of use. Keep syringes dry. Diluted Sol for Infusion: 2-8°C (36-46°F) or room temperature for up to 24 hrs. Protect from light. Discard unused portion.

HOW SUPPLIED
Inj: 20mg/mL [4mL, 10mL, 20mL vials]; 162mg/0.9mL [prefilled syringe]

CONTRAINDICATIONS
Known hypersensitivity to tocilizumab.

WARNINGS/PRECAUTIONS
Avoid w/ active infection, including localized infections. Caution in patients who have been exposed to TB, w/ history of serious/opportunistic infection, who resided or traveled in areas of endemic TB/mycoses, or w/ underlying conditions that may predispose them to infection. Viral reactivation and herpes zoster exacerbation observed. GI perforation reported; caution in patients at risk for GI perforation. Neutropenia, thrombocytopenia, elevation of liver enzymes, and increase in lipid parameters reported; do not initiate treatment if ANC <2000/mm^3, platelets <100,000/mm^3, or ALT/AST >1.5X ULN. D/C treatment w/ ANC <500/mm^3, platelets <50,000/mm^3, or ALT/AST >5X ULN. May increase risk of malignancies. Hypersensitivity reactions, including anaphylaxis and death, reported; d/c immediately and permanently if anaphylaxis or other hypersensitivity reaction occurs. Should only be infused IV by a healthcare professional w/ appropriate medical support to manage anaphylaxis. MS and chronic inflammatory demyelinating polyneuropathy reported rarely in RA studies; caution w/ preexisting or recent onset demyelinating disorders. Not recommended in patients w/ active hepatic disease or hepatic impairment. Caution in elderly.

ADVERSE REACTIONS
URTIs, nasopharyngitis, headache, HTN, increased ALT/AST, dizziness, bronchitis, infusion reaction, neutropenia, diarrhea, inj-site reaction, total cholesterol elevation, increased LDL.

DRUG INTERACTIONS
See Boxed Warning. Avoid w/ live vaccines. May increase metabolism of CYP450 substrates (eg, 1A2, 2B6, 2C9, 2C19, 2D6, 3A4). Upon initiation or discontinuation of tocilizumab, monitor therapeutic effect (eg, warfarin) or drug concentrations (eg, cyclosporine, theophylline) and adjust dose prn. Caution w/ CYP3A4 substrates where decrease in effectiveness is undesirable (eg, oral contraceptives, lovastatin, atorvastatin). Avoid w/ biological DMARDs (eg, TNF antagonists, interleukin [IL]-1R antagonists, anti-CD20 monoclonal antibodies, selective costimulation modulators) due to increased immunosuppression and risk of infection. Increased frequency and magnitude of transaminase elevations w/ hepatotoxic drugs (eg, MTX). Decreased exposure of simvastatin and omeprazole.

PREGNANCY AND LACTATION
Category C, not for use in nursing.

MECHANISM OF ACTION
IL-6 receptor antagonist monoclonal antibody; binds specifically to both soluble and membrane-bound IL-6 receptors (sIL-6R and mIL-6R) and inhibits IL-6-mediated signaling through these receptors.

PHARMACOKINETICS
Absorption: Administration of variable doses resulted in different pharmacokinetic parameters. **Distribution:** V$_d$=6.4L (RA), 4.08L (PJIA), 2.54L (SJIA). **Elimination:** (RA) T$_{1/2}$=Up to 11 days (4mg/kg IV); up to 13 days (8mg/kg IV, 162mg every week); 5 days (162mg every other week SQ). (SJIA) T$_{1/2}$=Up to 23 days. (PJIA) T$_{1/2}$=Up to 16 days.

PATIENT CONSIDERATIONS
Assessment: Assess for infections (eg, bacteria, fungi, viruses), including latent TB. Assess for demyelinating disorders, risk of GI perforation, active hepatic disease or impairment, hypersensitivity to drug, pregnancy/nursing status, and possible drug interactions. Obtain baseline lipid levels and platelet, liver transaminases, and neutrophil counts.

Monitoring: Monitor for signs/symptoms of TB and other infections. Monitor for hypersensitivity reactions, GI perforation, malignancies, and demyelinating disorders. Monitor neutrophil counts, platelet counts, and LFTs, after 4-8 weeks after initiation and every 3 months thereafter in RA patients, or at the time of 2nd infusion and every 4-8 weeks thereafter in PJIA patients, or every 2-4 weeks thereafter in SJIA patients. Monitor lipid levels 4-8 weeks after initiation then at approx 24-week intervals.

Counseling: Advise of the potential risks/benefits of therapy. Inform that therapy may lower resistance to infections and may cause serious GI side effects; instruct to contact physician if symptoms of infection or severe, persistent abdominal pain appear. Advise to inform physician of travel history, especially to places that are endemic for TB/mycoses. Inform that some patients have developed serious allergic reactions, including anaphylaxis. Advise to seek immediate medical attention if any symptoms of serious allergic reactions develop. Inform of inj techniques and procedures. Advise not to reuse needles/syringes and instruct on proper disposal procedures.

ACTICLATE — doxycycline hyclate   Rx
Class: Tetracyclines

OTHER BRAND NAMES
Acticlate CAP

ADULT DOSAGE
General Dosing
Usual: 100mg q12h on 1st day
Maint: 100mg qd or 50mg q12h

More Severe Infections (eg, Chronic UTIs): 100mg q12h

Streptococcal Infections: Continue therapy for 10 days

Chlamydia trachomatis Infections
Uncomplicated Urethral/Endocervical/Rectal Infections: 100mg bid for 7 days

Gonococcal Infections
Uncomplicated Gonococcal Infections (Except Anorectal Infections in Men): 100mg bid for 7 days or as an alternate single visit dose of 300mg stat followed in 1 hr by a second 300mg dose

Nongonococcal Urethritis
Caused by *C. trachomatis* and *Ureaplasma urealyticum*: 100mg bid for 7 days

Syphilis
Patients Allergic to Penicillin (PCN):
Early Syphilis: 100mg bid for 2 weeks
>1-Year Duration: 100mg bid for 4 weeks

Acute Epididymo-Orchitis
Caused by *Neisseria gonorrhoeae/C. trachomatis*: 100mg bid for at least 10 days

Malaria
Prophylaxis:
100mg qd, beginning 1 or 2 days before travel to the malarious area, continuing daily during travel and for 4 weeks after departure from malarious area

Inhalational Anthrax (Postexposure)
100mg bid for 60 days

Other Indications
- Rocky Mountain spotted fever
- Typhus fever and the typhus group
- Q fever
- Rickettsialpox
- Tick fevers
- Lymphogranuloma venereum
- Granuloma inguinale
- Chancroid
- Respiratory tract infections
- Psittacosis (ornithosis)
- Relapsing fever
- Plague
- Tularemia
- Cholera
- *Campylobacter fetus* infections
- Brucellosis (in conjunction w/ streptomycin)
- Bartonellosis
- UTIs
- Trachoma
- Inclusion conjunctivitis
- Infections caused by susceptible strains of *Escherichia coli*, *Enterobacter aerogenes*, *Shigella* species, and *Acinetobacter* species
- When PCN is contraindicated, treatment of the following infections caused by susceptible microorganisms: yaws, listeriosis, Vincent's infection, actinomycosis, and infections caused by *Clostridium* species
- Adjunct to amebicides in acute intestinal amebiasis
- Adjunctive therapy in severe acne

PEDIATRIC DOSAGE
General Dosing
W/ Severe or Life-Threatening Infections (eg, Anthrax, Rocky Mountain Spotted Fever):
<45kg:
2.2mg/kg q12h
≥45kg:
Use adult dose

W/ Less Severe Disease:
>8 Years and <45kg:
4.4mg/kg divided into 2 doses on the 1st day of treatment
Maint: 2.2mg/kg (given as a single daily dose or divided into bid doses)
>45kg:
Use adult dose

Malaria
≥8 Years:
Prophylaxis:
2mg/kg qd, beginning 1 or 2 days before travel to the malarious area, continuing daily during travel and for 4 weeks after departure from malarious area

≥45kg:
Use adult dose

Inhalational Anthrax (Postexposure)
<45kg:
2.2mg/kg bid for 60 days
≥45kg:
Use adult dose

ACTICLATE — doxycycline hyclate   Rx

ADMINISTRATION
Oral route

Administer w/ adequate amounts of fluid to wash down drug and reduce the risk of esophageal irritation/ulceration.
May be given w/ food or milk if gastric irritation occurs.

Cap
Swallow whole; do not break, open, crush, dissolve or chew the cap.

Tab
150mg tab can be broken into 2/3 or 1/3 to provide a 100mg and 50mg strength, respectively.

STORAGE
20-25°C (68-77°F); excursions permitted to 15-30°C (59-86°F). Protect from light and moisture.

HOW SUPPLIED
Tab: 75mg, 150mg*; **Cap:** (Acticlate CAP) 75mg *scored

CONTRAINDICATIONS
Hypersensitivity to any of the tetracyclines.

WARNINGS/PRECAUTIONS
May cause permanent discoloration of the teeth (yellow-gray-brown) if used during tooth development (last 1/2 of pregnancy, infancy, and childhood to 8 yrs of age); enamel hypoplasia also reported. Use in pediatric patients ≤8 years only when the potential benefits outweigh the risks in severe or life-threatening conditions (eg, anthrax, Rocky Mountain spotted fever), particularly when there are no alternative therapies. *Clostridium difficile*-associated diarrhea (CDAD) reported; may need to d/c if CDAD is suspected or confirmed. Photosensitivity, manifested by an exaggerated sunburn reaction, reported; d/c at the 1st evidence of skin erythema. May result in overgrowth of non-susceptible organisms, including fungi; d/c use and institute appropriate therapy if such infections occur. May result in bacterial resistance if used in the absence of proven or suspected bacterial infection or a prophylactic indication. Associated w/ intracranial HTN (pseudotumor cerebri); increased risk in women of childbearing age who are overweight or have a history of intracranial HTN. If visual disturbance occurs, prompt ophthalmologic evaluation is warranted. Intracranial pressure can remain elevated for weeks after drug cessation; monitor patients until they stabilize. May decrease fibula growth rate in prematures. May cause fetal harm. May cause an increase in BUN. When used for malaria prophylaxis, patient may still transmit the infection to mosquitoes outside endemic areas. False elevations of urinary catecholamines may occur due to interference w/ the fluorescence test.

ADVERSE REACTIONS
Anorexia, N/V, diarrhea, glossitis, hepatotoxicity, maculopapular and erythematous rashes, Stevens-Johnson syndrome, toxic epidermal necrolysis, urticaria, angioneurotic edema, anaphylaxis, hemolytic anemia, thrombocytopenia, neutropenia.

DRUG INTERACTIONS
Avoid concomitant use w/ isotretinoin; may also cause pseudotumor cerebri. May depress plasma prothrombin activity; may require downward adjustment of anticoagulant dose. May interfere w/ bactericidal action of PCN; avoid concurrent use. Impaired absorption w/ bismuth subsalicylate, antacids containing aluminum, Ca^{2+}, or Mg^{2+}, and iron-containing preparations. May render oral contraceptives less effective. Decreased $T_{1/2}$ w/ barbiturates, carbamazepine, and phenytoin. Fatal renal toxicity reported w/ methoxyflurane.

PREGNANCY AND LACTATION
Pregnancy: Category D.
Lactation: Tetracyclines are excreted in human milk; not for use in nursing.

MECHANISM OF ACTION
Tetracycline; has bacteriostatic activity. Inhibits bacterial protein synthesis by binding to the 30S ribosomal subunit.

PHARMACOKINETICS
Absorption: Virtually complete. (300mg single dose) C_{max}=3mcg/mL (tab), 2.8mcg/mL (cap); T_{max}=3 hrs (tab/cap). **Distribution:** Found in breast milk. **Elimination:** Urine (40%/72 hrs in CrCl 75mL/min, 1-5%/72 hrs in CrCl <10mL/min), feces; $T_{1/2}$=18-22 hrs.

PATIENT CONSIDERATIONS

Assessment: Assess for hypersensitivity to drug or any tetracyclines, risk for intracranial HTN, pregnancy/nursing status, and possible drug interactions. Perform culture and susceptibility testing.

Monitoring: Monitor for CDAD, photosensitivity, skin erythema, intracranial HTN, visual disturbance, and other adverse reactions. In long-term therapy, perform periodic lab evaluation of organ systems, including hematopoietic, renal, and hepatic studies.

Counseling: Apprise of the potential hazard to fetus if used during pregnancy. Inform that therapy does not guarantee protection against malaria; advise to use measures that help avoid contact w/ mosquitoes. Advise to avoid excessive sunlight or artificial UV light and to d/c therapy if phototoxicity occurs; instruct to consider use of sunscreen or sunblock. Inform that absorption of drug is reduced when taken w/ bismuth subsalicylate, antacids containing aluminum, Ca^{2+}, or Mg^{2+}, iron-containing preparations, and w/ foods, especially those that contain Ca^{2+}. Inform that drug may increase the incidence of vaginal candidiasis. Inform that diarrhea may be experienced and instruct to immediately contact physician if watery and bloody stools (w/ or w/o stomach cramps and fever) occur, even as late as ≥2 months after the last dose. Inform that therapy should only be used to treat bacterial, not viral, infections. Instruct to take exactly ud even if the patient feels better early in the course of therapy. Inform that skipping doses or not completing the full course of therapy may decrease effectiveness of treatment and increase bacterial resistance.

ACTIQ — fentanyl citrate   CII
Class: Opioid analgesic

> Fatal respiratory depression may occur. Contraindicated in the management of acute or postoperative pain (eg, headache/migraine) and in opioid-nontolerant patients. Death reported upon accidental ingestion in children; keep out of reach of children. Concomitant use with CYP3A4 inhibitors may increase plasma levels, and may cause fatal respiratory depression. Do not convert patients on a mcg-per-mcg basis from any other fentanyl products to Actiq. Do not substitute for any other fentanyl products; may result in fatal overdose. Contains fentanyl with abuse liability similar to other opioid analgesics. Available only through a restricted program called Transmucosal Immediate Release Fentanyl (TIRF) Risk Evaluation Mitigation Strategy (REMS) Access program due to risk of misuse, abuse, addiction, and overdose. Outpatients, healthcare professionals who prescribe to outpatients, pharmacies, and distributors must enroll in the program.

ADULT DOSAGE
Cancer Pain

Breakthrough pain in patients already receiving and tolerant to around-the-clock opioid therapy

Initial: 200mcg; dispense no more than 6 units initially
Titrate:
If signs of excessive opioid effects appear before unit is consumed, remove dosage unit, dispose properly, and decrease subsequent doses
If breakthrough pain is not relieved 15 min after completion of previous dose, give only 1 additional dose of the same strength
Maint: Once titrated to an effective dose, use only 1 unit of the appropriate strength per breakthrough pain episode; limit to ≤4 units/day
Max: 2 doses/breakthrough pain episode; wait ≥4 hrs before treating another breakthrough pain episode

Increase dose only when a single administration of current dose fails to adequately treat breakthrough pain episode for several consecutive episodes

If >4 breakthrough pain episodes/day are experienced, reevaluate maint dose (around-the-clock) used for persistent pain

PEDIATRIC DOSAGE
Cancer Pain

Breakthrough pain in patients already receiving and tolerant to around-the-clock opioid therapy

≥16 Years:
Initial: 200mcg; dispense no more than 6 units initially
Titrate:
If signs of excessive opioid effects appear before unit is consumed, remove dosage unit, dispose properly, and decrease subsequent doses
If breakthrough pain is not relieved 15 min after completion of previous dose, give only 1 additional dose of the same strength
Maint: Once titrated to an effective dose, use only 1 unit of the appropriate strength per breakthrough pain episode; limit to ≤4 units/day
Max: 2 doses/breakthrough pain episode; wait ≥4 hrs before treating another breakthrough pain episode

Increase dose only when a single administration of current dose fails to adequately treat breakthrough pain episode for several consecutive episodes

If >4 breakthrough pain episodes/day are experienced, reevaluate maint dose (around-the-clock) used for persistent pain

DOSING CONSIDERATIONS
Discontinuation
Gradually titrate dose downward

ADMINISTRATION
Oral route

Place unit in mouth between cheek and lower gum, occasionally moving the drug matrix from one side to the other using the handle
Do not suck or chew
Consume unit over a 15-min period

STORAGE
20-25°C (68-77°F); excursions permitted between 15-30°C (59-86°F). Protect from freezing and moisture.

HOW SUPPLIED
Loz: 200mcg, 400mcg, 600mcg, 800mcg, 1200mcg, 1600mcg

CONTRAINDICATIONS
Opioid-nontolerant patients, management of acute or postoperative pain including headache/migraine and dental pain, known intolerance or hypersensitivity to any of its components or the drug fentanyl.

WARNINGS/PRECAUTIONS
Increased risk of respiratory depression in patients with underlying respiratory disorders and in elderly/debilitated. May impair mental/physical abilities. Caution with chronic obstructive pulmonary disease or preexisting medical conditions predisposing to respiratory depression; may further decrease respiratory drive to the point of respiratory failure. Extreme caution in patients who may be susceptible to the intracranial effects of CO_2 retention (eg, with evidence of increased intracranial pressure or impaired consciousness). May obscure clinical course of head injuries. Caution with bradyarrhythmias. Anaphylaxis and hypersensitivity reported. Avoid use during labor and delivery. Caution with renal/hepatic impairment.

ADVERSE REACTIONS
Respiratory depression, circulatory depression, hypotension, shock, N/V, headache, constipation, dizziness, dyspnea, anxiety, somnolence, asthenia, confusion, depression.

DRUG INTERACTIONS
See Boxed Warning. Respiratory depression is more likely to occur when given with other drugs that depress respiration. Increased depressant effects with other CNS depressants (eg, other opioids, sedatives, hypnotics, general anesthetics, phenothiazines, tranquilizers, skeletal muscle relaxants, sedating antihistamines,

alcoholic beverages); adjust dose if warranted. Avoid with grapefruit and grapefruit juice. CYP3A4 inducers may decrease levels. Not recommended with MAOIs or within 14 days of discontinuation of MAOIs.

PREGNANCY AND LACTATION
Category C, not for use in nursing.

MECHANISM OF ACTION
Opioid analgesic; has not been established. Known to be µ-opioid receptor agonist; specific CNS opioid receptors for endogenous compounds with opioid-like activity have been identified throughout the brain and spinal cord and play a role in analgesic effects.

PHARMACOKINETICS
Absorption: Rapidly absorbed from buccal mucosa; more prolonged absorption of swallowed fentanyl from GI tract. Absolute bioavailability (50%). Administration of variable doses resulted in different pharmacokinetic parameters. **Distribution:** V_d=4L/kg; plasma protein binding (80-85%); crosses the placenta; found in breast milk. **Metabolism:** Liver and intestinal mucosa via CYP3A4; norfentanyl (metabolite). **Elimination:** Urine (<7%, unchanged), feces (1%, unchanged); $T_{1/2}$=7 hrs.

PATIENT CONSIDERATIONS

Assessment: Assess for degree of opioid tolerance, previous opioid dose, level of pain intensity, type of pain, patient's general condition and medical status, and any other conditions where treatment is contraindicated or cautioned. Assess for hypersensitivity to the drug, renal/hepatic function, pregnancy/nursing status, and possible drug interactions.

Monitoring: Monitor for signs/symptoms of respiratory depression, impairment of mental/physical abilities, bradycardia, anaphylaxis/hypersensitivity, abuse/addiction, and other adverse reactions.

Counseling: Advise to enroll in TIRF REMS Access program. Instruct to keep drug out of reach of children. Advise to take drug as prescribed and avoid sharing it with anyone else. Instruct to notify physician if breakthrough pain is not alleviated or worsens after taking the drug. Inform that drug may impair mental/physical abilities; caution against performing activities that require high level of attention (eg, driving/using heavy machinery). Advise not to combine with alcohol, sleep aids, or tranquilizers, except if ordered by the physician. Instruct to notify physician if pregnant or planning to become pregnant. Inform that frequent consumption may increase risk of dental decay; advise to consult dentist to ensure appropriate oral hygiene. Inform diabetics that drug contains approximately 2g sugar/U. Inform of proper storage, administration, and disposal.

ACTIVELLA — estradiol/norethindrone acetate   Rx
Class: Estrogen/progestogen combination

> Should not be used for the prevention of cardiovascular (CV) disease or dementia. Increased risk of MI, stroke, invasive breast cancer, pulmonary embolism (PE), and deep vein thrombosis (DVT) in postmenopausal women (50-79 yrs of age) reported. Increased risk of developing probable dementia in postmenopausal women ≥65 yrs of age reported. Increased risk of endometrial cancer in women with a uterus who use unopposed estrogens. Perform adequate diagnostic measures, including endometrial sampling, to rule out malignancy in postmenopausal women with undiagnosed persistent or recurrent abnormal genital bleeding. Should be prescribed at the lowest effective dose and for the shortest duration consistent with treatment goals and risks.

ADULT DOSAGE	PEDIATRIC DOSAGE
Menopausal Vasomotor Symptoms	Pediatric use may not have been established
Moderate to Severe:	
Usual: 1 tab (1mg/0.5mg or 0.5mg/0.1mg) once daily	
Menopausal Vulvar/Vaginal Atrophy	
Moderate to Severe:	
Usual: 1 tab (1mg/0.5mg) once daily	
Postmenopausal Osteoporosis	
Prevention:	
Usual: 1 tab (1mg/0.5mg or 0.5mg/0.1mg) once daily	

ADMINISTRATION
Oral route

STORAGE
20-25°C (68-77°F); excursions permitted to 15-30°C (59-86°F). Protect from light.

HOW SUPPLIED
Tab: (Estradiol/Norethindrone) 1mg/0.5mg, 0.5mg/0.1mg

CONTRAINDICATIONS
Undiagnosed abnormal genital bleeding, known/suspected/history of breast cancer, known/suspected estrogen-dependent neoplasia, active/history of DVT/PE, active/history of arterial thromboembolic disease (eg, stroke, MI), known anaphylactic reaction or angioedema or hypersensitivity to this medication, liver impairment or disease, known protein C/protein S/antithrombin deficiency or other known thrombophilic disorders, known/suspected pregnancy.

WARNINGS/PRECAUTIONS
D/C immediately if stroke, DVT, PE, or MI occurs or is suspected. Caution with risk factors for arterial vascular disease and/or venous thromboembolism. If feasible, d/c at least 4-6 weeks before surgery of the type associated with an increased risk of thromboembolism, or during periods of prolonged immobilization. May increase risk of ovarian cancer and gallbladder disease. May lead to severe hypercalcemia in patients with breast cancer and bone metastases; d/c and

take appropriate measures if hypercalcemia occurs. Retinal vascular thrombosis reported; d/c therapy pending exam if sudden partial/complete loss of vision, or sudden onset of proptosis, diplopia, or migraine occurs. D/C permanently if exam reveals papilledema or retinal vascular lesions. May elevate BP and thyroid-binding globulin levels. May elevate plasma TG levels leading to pancreatitis in women with preexisting hypertriglyceridemia; consider discontinuation if pancreatitis occurs. Caution with history of cholestatic jaundice associated with past estrogen use or with pregnancy; d/c in case of recurrence. May cause fluid retention; caution with conditions that might be influenced by this factor (eg, cardiac/renal impairment). Caution with hypoparathyroidism as estrogen-induced hypocalcemia may occur. May exacerbate endometriosis, asthma, diabetes mellitus, epilepsy, migraine, porphyria, systemic lupus erythematosus, and hepatic hemangiomas; use with caution. May exacerbate symptoms of angioedema in women with hereditary angioedema. May affect certain endocrine and blood components in lab tests.

ADVERSE REACTIONS
Back pain, headache, nasopharyngitis, sinusitis, insomnia, upper respiratory tract infection, breast pain, postmenopausal bleeding, vaginal hemorrhage, endometrial thickening, uterine fibroid, pain in extremities, nausea, diarrhea, viral infection.

DRUG INTERACTIONS
CYP3A4 inducers (eg, St. John's wort preparations, phenobarbital, carbamazepine) may decrease levels, which may decrease therapeutic effects and/or change uterine bleeding profile. CYP3A4 inhibitors (eg, erythromycin, ketoconazole, ritonavir) may increase levels, which may result in side effects. Patients concomitantly receiving thyroid hormone replacement therapy and estrogens may require increased doses of their thyroid replacement therapy; monitor thyroid function.

PREGNANCY AND LACTATION
Contraindicated in pregnancy, not for use in nursing.

MECHANISM OF ACTION
Estradiol: Estrogen; binds to nuclear receptors in estrogen-responsive tissues. Reduces elevated levels of gonadotropins, luteinizing hormone and follicle-stimulating hormone, in postmenopausal women. Norethindrone: Progestin; enhances cellular differentiation and opposes actions of estrogens by decreasing estrogen receptor levels, increasing local metabolism of estrogens to less active metabolites, or inducing gene products that blunt cellular responses to estrogen.

PHARMACOKINETICS
Absorption: Administration of various doses resulted in different parameters. **Distribution:** Found in breast milk. Estradiol: Sex hormone-binding globulin (SHBG) (37%); albumin (61%). Norethindrone: SHBG (36%); albumin (61%). **Metabolism:** Estradiol: Liver to estrone (metabolite); estriol (major urinary metabolite); enterohepatic recirculation via sulfate and glucuronide conjugation; biliary secretion of conjugates into the intestine; hydrolysis in the intestine followed by reabsorption. Norethindrone: isomers of 5α-dihydro-norethindrone, tetrahydro-norethindrone (metabolites). **Elimination:** Estradiol: Urine (unchanged and metabolites); $T_{1/2}$=12-14 hrs. Norethindrone: $T_{1/2}$=8-11 hrs.

PATIENT CONSIDERATIONS

Assessment: Assess for undiagnosed abnormal genital bleeding, presence/history of breast cancer, estrogen-dependent neoplasia, active/history of DVT/PE/arterial thromboembolic disease, liver impairment/disease, thrombophilic disorders, drug hypersensitivity, pregnancy/nursing status, any other conditions where treatment is contraindicated or cautioned, and for possible drug interactions.

Monitoring: Monitor for signs/symptoms of CV disease, malignant neoplasms, dementia, gallbladder disease, hypercalcemia, visual abnormalities, BP and plasma TG level elevations, pancreatitis, cholestatic jaundice, fluid retention, exacerbation of endometriosis and other conditions, and other adverse reactions. Perform annual breast exam; schedule mammography based on age, risk factors, and prior mammogram results. Perform adequate diagnostic measures (eg, endometrial sampling) to rule out malignancies in cases of undiagnosed, persistent, or recurring abnormal genital bleeding. Regularly monitor thyroid function if on thyroid hormone replacement therapy.

Counseling: Inform of the importance of reporting vaginal bleeding to physician as soon as possible. Advise of possible serious adverse reactions of therapy (eg, CV disorders, malignant neoplasms, probable dementia) and of possible less serious, but common adverse reactions (eg, headache, breast pain and tenderness, N/V). Instruct to have yearly breast examinations by a healthcare provider and to perform monthly breast self-examinations.

ACTONEL — risedronate sodium   Rx
Class: Bisphosphonate

ADULT DOSAGE	PEDIATRIC DOSAGE
Osteoporosis	Pediatric use may not have been established
Treatment/Prevention of Postmenopausal Osteoporosis:	
Usual: 5mg qd, or 35mg once a week, or 75mg taken on 2 consecutive days for a total of 2 tabs/month, or 150mg once a month	
Osteoporosis in Men:	
Usual: 35mg once a week	
Treatment/Prevention of Glucocorticoid-Induced Osteoporosis:	
Usual: 5mg qd	

Paget's Disease

Treatment in Men/Women:

Usual: 30mg qd for 2 months

May consider retreatment (following post-treatment observation of at least 2 months) if relapse occurs, or if treatment fails to normalize serum alkaline phosphatase; dose and duration of therapy are the same as for initial treatment

Missed Dose

35mg Once a Week is Missed:
Take 1 tab on the am after remembering and return to taking 1 tab once a week as originally scheduled on chosen day; do not take 2 tabs on same day

One or Both 75mg Tabs (Taken on 2 Consecutive Days/Month) are Missed:
If Next Month's Scheduled Doses are >7 Days Away:
If both tabs are missed, take one 75mg tab in the am after the day it is remembered, then take the other tab on the next consecutive am. If only one 75mg tab is missed, take the missed tab in the am after the day it is remembered. Return to taking 75mg on 2 consecutive days/month as originally scheduled. Do not take more than two 75mg tabs w/in 7 days
If Next Month's Scheduled Doses are w/in 7 Days:
Wait until the next month's scheduled doses and then continue taking 75mg on 2 consecutive days/month as originally scheduled

150mg Once a Month is Missed:
If Next Month's Scheduled Dose is >7 Days Away:
Take missed tab in the am after the day it is remembered, then return to taking 150mg once a month as originally scheduled; do not take more than one 150mg tab w/in 7 days
If Next Month's Scheduled Doses are w/in 7 Days:
Wait until the next month's scheduled dose and then continue taking 150mg once a month as originally scheduled

- -

DOSING CONSIDERATIONS
Renal Impairment
Severe (CrCl <30mL/min): Not recommended

ADMINISTRATION
Oral route

Take at least 30 min before the 1st food or drink of the day other than water, and before taking any oral medication or supplementation
Swallow tabs whole w/ a full glass of plain water (6-8 oz); avoid lying down for 30 min after taking medication
Do not chew or suck tab
Avoid water w/ supplements (including mineral water)
Take Ca^{2+} supplements, antacids, Mg^{2+}-based supplements/laxatives, and iron preparations at a different time of the day

STORAGE
20-25°C (68-77°F).

HOW SUPPLIED
Tab: 5mg, 30mg, 35mg, 75mg, 150mg

CONTRAINDICATIONS
Esophageal abnormalities that delay esophageal emptying (eg, stricture or achalasia), inability to stand or sit upright for at least 30 min, hypocalcemia, known hypersensitivity to risedronate sodium or any of its excipients.

WARNINGS/PRECAUTIONS
Consider discontinuation after 3-5 yrs of use in patients at low risk for fracture; periodically reevaluate risk for fracture in patients who d/c therapy. Contains same active ingredient as Atelvia; do not treat w/ Actonel if on concomitant therapy w/ Atelvia. May cause local irritation of the upper GI mucosa; caution w/ active upper GI problems (eg, Barrett's esophagus, dysphagia, esophageal diseases, gastritis, duodenitis, ulcers). Esophageal reactions (eg, esophagitis, esophageal ulcers/erosions) reported; d/c if dysphagia, odynophagia, retrosternal pain, or new/worsening heartburn develops. Use therapy under appropriate supervision in patients who cannot comply w/ dosing instructions due to mental disability. Gastric and duodenal ulcers reported. Hypocalcemia reported; treat hypocalcemia and other disturbances of bone and mineral metabolism before starting therapy, and ensure adequate Ca^{2+} and vitamin D intake. Osteonecrosis of the jaw (ONJ) reported; risk may increase w/ duration of exposure to drug. For patients requiring invasive dental procedures, discontinuation of treatment may reduce risk for ONJ. Consider discontinuation if ONJ develops. Severe and occasionally incapacitating bone, joint, and/or muscle pain reported; consider discontinuation if severe symptoms develop. Atypical, low-energy, or low-trauma fractures of the femoral shaft reported; evaluate any patient w/ a history of bisphosphonate exposure who presents w/ thigh/groin pain to rule out an incomplete femur fracture, and consider interruption of therapy. Ascertain sex steroid hormonal status and consider appropriate replacement before initiating therapy for the treatment and prevention of glucocorticoid-induced osteoporosis. May interfere w/ the use of bone-imaging agents.

ADVERSE REACTIONS
Back pain, arthralgia, abdominal pain, dyspepsia, acute phase reaction, allergic reaction, arthritis, diarrhea, headache, infection, UTI, bronchitis, HTN, nausea, rash.

DRUG INTERACTIONS
Coadministration w/ Ca^{2+} supplements, antacids, or oral medications containing divalent cations will interfere w/ absorption.

PREGNANCY AND LACTATION
Category C, not for use in nursing.

MECHANISM OF ACTION
Bisphosphonate; has an affinity for hydroxyapatite crystals in bone and acts as an antiresorptive agent. Inhibits osteoclasts.

PHARMACOKINETICS
Absorption: Absolute bioavailability (0.63%) (30mg); T$_{max}$=approx 1 hr. **Distribution:** V$_d$=13.8L/kg; plasma protein binding (24%). **Elimination:** Urine (approx 1/2 of the absorbed dose), feces (unchanged [unabsorbed drug]); T$_{1/2}$=561 hrs (osteopenic postmenopausal women).

PATIENT CONSIDERATIONS

Assessment: Assess for esophageal abnormalities, ability to stand or sit upright for at least 30 min, active upper GI problems, mental disability, hypocalcemia, disturbances of bone and mineral metabolism, risk for ONJ, renal impairment, drug hypersensitivity, any other conditions where treatment is contraindicated or cautioned, pregnancy/nursing status, and possible drug interactions. For glucocorticoid-induced osteoporosis treatment/prevention, assess sex steroid hormonal status.

Monitoring: Monitor for signs/symptoms of ONJ, atypical femoral fracture, esophageal reactions, hypocalcemia, musculoskeletal pain, and other adverse events. Periodically reevaluate the need for continued therapy.

Counseling: Instruct to pay particular attention to dosing instructions and counsel about missed dose instructions. Advise to take at least 30 min before 1st food or drink of the day other than water. Instruct to take while in an upright position w/ a full glass of plain water (6-8 oz) and to avoid lying down for 30 min after taking the drug. Advise to consult physician before continuing treatment if symptoms of esophageal disease develop. Instruct to take supplemental Ca^{2+} and vitamin D if dietary intake is inadequate; instruct to take Ca^{2+} supplements or Ca^{2+}-, aluminum-, and Mg^{2+}-containing medications at a different time of the day. Counsel to consider weight-bearing exercise along w/ the modification of certain behavioral factors (eg, excessive cigarette smoking and/or alcohol consumption) if these factors exist. Instruct to inform physician about medication history. Advise to consult physician any time they have a medical problem they think may be from treatment.

ACTOPLUS MET XR — metformin hydrochloride/pioglitazone **Rx**

Class: Biguanide/thiazolidinedione (glitazone)

> Thiazolidinediones, including pioglitazone, cause or exacerbate CHF in some patients. After initiation and dose increases, monitor carefully for signs and symptoms of heart failure (HF); manage accordingly and consider discontinuation or dose reduction if HF develops. Not recommended w/ symptomatic HF. Contraindicated w/ established NYHA Class III or IV HF. Cases of metformin-associated lactic acidosis resulting in death, hypothermia, hypotension, and resistant bradyarrhythmias reported; risk factors include renal impairment, concomitant use of certain drugs (eg, cationic drugs such as topiramate), age ≥65 years, having a radiological study w/ contrast, surgery, and other procedures, hypoxic states (eg, acute CHF), excessive alcohol intake, and hepatic impairment. D/C therapy immediately and institute general supportive measures in a hospital setting if metformin-associated lactic acidosis is suspected. Prompt hemodialysis is recommended.

OTHER BRAND NAMES
Actoplus Met

ADULT DOSAGE	PEDIATRIC DOSAGE
Type 2 Diabetes Mellitus When treatment w/ both pioglitazone and metformin is appropriate **Initial:** **Actoplus Met:** 15mg/500mg bid or 15mg/850mg qd **Actoplus Met XR:** 15mg/1000mg or 30mg/1000mg qd **NYHA Class I or II CHF:** **Actoplus Met:** 15mg/500mg or 15mg/850mg qd **Actoplus Met XR:** 15mg/1000mg or 30mg/1000mg qd **Inadequately Controlled on Metformin Monotherapy:** **Actoplus Met:** 15mg/500mg bid or 15mg/850mg qd or bid, depending on metformin dose already being taken	Pediatric use may not have been established

Actoplus Met XR: 15mg/1000mg bid or 30mg/1000mg qd, depending on metformin dose already being taken

Inadequately Controlled on Pioglitazone Monotherapy:
Actoplus Met: 15mg/500mg bid or 15mg/850mg bid
Actoplus Met XR: 15mg/1000mg bid or 30mg/1000mg qd

Switching from Combination Therapy of Pioglitazone Plus Metformin as Separate Tabs:
Actoplus Met/Actoplus Met XR: Take at doses that are as close as possible to the dose of pioglitazone and metformin already being taken

Titrate:
Gradually adjust, as needed, after assessing adequacy of response and tolerability

Max:
Actoplus Met: (45mg/2550mg)/day
Actoplus Met XR: (45mg/2000mg)/day
Metformin doses >2000mg may be better tolerated given tid

DOSING CONSIDERATIONS
Concomitant Medications
Strong CYP2C8 Inhibitors (eg, Gemfibrozil):
Max:
Actoplus Met: (15mg/850mg)/day
Actoplus Met XR: (15mg/1000mg)/day
Renal Impairment
eGFR 30-45mL/min/1.73m²: Initiation of therapy is not recommended
eGFR <30mL/min/1.73m²: Contraindicated

If eGFR Falls <45mL/min/1.73m² During Therapy: Assess benefit/risk of continuing therapy
If eGFR Falls <30mL/min/1.73m² During Therapy: D/C

Hepatic Impairment
Not recommended
Other Important Considerations
Iodinated Contrast Imaging Procedures:
D/C therapy at the time of, or prior to, an iodinated contrast imaging procedure in patients w/ an eGFR 30-60mL/min/1.73m²; in patients w/ a history of liver disease, alcoholism, or HF; or in patients who will be administered intra-arterial iodinated contrast. Reevaluate eGFR 48 hrs after the imaging procedure and restart therapy if renal function is stable

ADMINISTRATION
Oral route
Take w/ meals to reduce GI side effects associated w/ metformin.

Actoplus Met XR
Swallow whole; do not chew, cut, or crush.

STORAGE
25°C (77°F); excursions permitted to 15-30°C (59-86°F). Keep container tightly closed, and protect from moisture and humidity.

HOW SUPPLIED
(Pioglitazone/Metformin) **Tab, ER:** (Actoplus Met XR) 15mg/1000mg, 30mg/1000mg; **Tab:** (Actoplus Met) 15mg/500mg, 15mg/850mg

CONTRAINDICATIONS
NYHA Class III or IV HF; severe renal impairment (eGFR <30mL/min/1.73m²); metabolic acidosis, including diabetic ketoacidosis; known hypersensitivity to pioglitazone, metformin, or any other component of this medication.

WARNINGS/PRECAUTIONS
See Dosing Considerations. Not for the treatment of type 1 diabetes mellitus (DM) or diabetic ketoacidosis. Hypoglycemia may occur when caloric intake is deficient or when strenuous exercise is not compensated by caloric supplementation; elderly, debilitated, or malnourished patients and those w/ adrenal or pituitary insufficiency or alcohol intoxication are particularly susceptible to hypoglycemic effects. Hypoglycemia may be difficult to recognize in the elderly. Not for use in patients w/ active bladder cancer; consider benefits versus risks in patients w/ a prior history of bladder cancer. **Metformin:** Temporarily d/c while patient has restricted food and fluid intake. D/C if a condition associated w/ hypoxemia occurs (eg, cardiovascular collapse, acute MI, sepsis). May decrease vitamin B12 levels; monitor hematologic parameters annually. **Pioglitazone:** Dose-related edema reported; caution in patients w/ edema or at risk for CHF. Fatal and nonfatal hepatic failure reported; caution w/ abnormal liver tests. Measure LFTs promptly in patients who report symptoms that may indicate liver injury. Interrupt treatment if ALT >3X ULN; do not restart in patients w/o another explanation for the liver test abnormalities. Patients w/ ALT >3X the reference range w/ serum total bilirubin >2X the reference range w/o alternative etiologies are at risk for severe drug-induced liver injury and should not be restarted on therapy. May use w/ caution in patients w/ lesser elevations of ALT or bilirubin and w/ an alternate probable cause. Increased incidence of bone fracture reported in females. Macular

edema reported; promptly refer to an ophthalmologist if visual symptoms occur. May result in ovulation in some premenopausal anovulatory women, which may increase risk for pregnancy; adequate contraception is recommended.

ADVERSE REACTIONS
Diarrhea, headache, edema, URTI, weight gain.

DRUG INTERACTIONS
See Boxed Warning and Dosing Considerations. Risk for hypoglycemia w/ insulin or other antidiabetic medications (particularly insulin secretagogues such as sulfonylureas); may require a reduction in the dose of the concomitant antidiabetic medication. May be difficult to recognize hypoglycemia w/ β-adrenergic blocking drugs. **Pioglitazone:** Increased exposure and T₁/₂ w/ strong CYP2C8 inhibitors (eg, gemfibrozil). CYP2C8 inducers (eg, rifampin) may decrease exposure; if a CYP2C8 inducer is started or stopped during treatment, changes in diabetes treatment may be needed, based on clinical response. May cause dose-related fluid retention when used w/ other antidiabetic medications, most commonly w/ insulin. **Metformin:** Topiramate and other carbonic anhydrase inhibitors (eg, zonisamide, acetazolamide, dichlorphenamide) may increase the risk of lactic acidosis; consider more frequent monitoring of these patients. Drugs that are eliminated by renal tubular secretion, drugs that impair renal function, drugs that result in significant hemodynamic change, drugs that interfere w/ acid-base balance, or drugs that increase metformin accumulation may increase the risk of metformin-associated lactic acidosis; consider more frequent monitoring of these patients. Avoid excessive alcohol intake. Thiazides and other diuretics, corticosteroids, phenothiazines, thyroid products, estrogens, oral contraceptives, phenytoin, nicotinic acid, sympathomimetics, calcium channel blockers, and isoniazid may produce hyperglycemia and lead to loss of glycemic control; observe closely for loss of blood glucose control when such drugs are administered and observe closely for hypoglycemia when such drugs are withdrawn.

PREGNANCY AND LACTATION
Pregnancy: Category C.
Lactation: Not for use in nursing.

MECHANISM OF ACTION
Pioglitazone: Thiazolidinedione; insulin-sensitizing agent that acts primarily by enhancing peripheral glucose utilization. Decreases insulin resistance in the periphery and in the liver, resulting in increased insulin-dependent glucose disposal and decreased hepatic glucose output. **Metformin:** Biguanide; decreases endogenous hepatic glucose production, decreases intestinal absorption of glucose, and improves insulin sensitivity by increasing peripheral glucose uptake and utilization.

PHARMACOKINETICS
Absorption: Pioglitazone: T_{max}=w/in 2 hrs, 3-4 hrs (w/ food). Metformin: Absolute bioavailability (50-60%) (fasted). **Distribution:** Pioglitazone: V_d=0.63L/kg; plasma protein binding (>99%). Metformin: V_d=654L (immediate-release). **Metabolism:** Pioglitazone: Hydroxylation and oxidation (extensive), CYP2C8, CYP3A4; M-III [keto derivative] and M-IV [hydroxyl derivative] (major active metabolites). **Elimination:** Pioglitazone: Urine (15-30%), bile and feces; $T_{1/2}$=3-7 hrs, 16-24 hrs (metabolites). Metformin: Urine (90%); $T_{1/2}$=6.2 hrs (plasma), 17.6 hrs (blood).

PATIENT CONSIDERATIONS

Assessment: Assess for acute/chronic metabolic acidosis (including diabetic ketoacidosis), type of DM, risk factors for lactic acidosis, renal/hepatic impairment, previous hypersensitivity to the drug, HF or risk factors for HF, active/history of bladder cancer, predisposition to developing subnormal vitamin B12 levels, any other conditions where treatment is contraindicated or cautioned, pregnancy/nursing status, and possible drug interactions. Assess if patient is planning to undergo any surgical procedure. Obtain baseline LFTs, FPG, HbA1c, eGFR, and hematologic parameters.

Monitoring: Monitor for signs/symptoms of lactic acidosis, CHF, edema, hepatic effects, fractures, visual symptoms, and other adverse reactions. Monitor eGFR at least annually; monitor more frequently in patients at risk of developing renal impairment. Monitor FPG, HbA1c, and hepatic function periodically. Monitor hematologic parameters annually. Perform routine serum vitamin B12 measurements at 2- to 3-yr intervals in patients predisposed to developing subnormal vitamin B12 levels. Perform regular eye exams.

Counseling: Advise on the importance of adherence to dietary instructions and regular testing of blood glucose, HbA1c, renal function, and hematologic parameters. Advise to seek medical advice promptly during periods of stress, as medication requirements may change. Instruct to promptly report any signs/symptoms of bladder cancer or HF. Advise of the risks of lactic acidosis, its symptoms, and conditions that predispose to its development; instruct to d/c therapy immediately and contact physician if unexplained hyperventilation, myalgia, malaise, unusual somnolence, or other nonspecific symptoms occur. Counsel against excessive alcohol intake while on therapy. Instruct to d/c use and seek medical advice promptly if signs/symptoms of hepatotoxicity occur. Counsel premenopausal women to use adequate contraception during treatment. Inform that hypoglycemia can occur; explain the risks, symptoms, and appropriate management. Instruct to take drug as prescribed and explain that any change in dosing should only be done if directed by physician. **Actoplus Met XR:** Inform that the inactive ingredients may occasionally be eliminated in the feces as a soft mass that may resemble the original tab.

ACTOS — pioglitazone   Rx

Class: Thiazolidinedione (glitazone)

> Thiazolidinediones cause or exacerbate congestive heart failure (CHF) in some patients. After initiation and dose increases, monitor carefully for signs and symptoms of heart failure (HF) and manage accordingly; consider discontinuation or dose reduction. Not recommended in patients with symptomatic HF. Contraindicated with established NYHA Class III or IV HF.

ADULT DOSAGE

Type 2 Diabetes Mellitus

W/O CHF:
Initial: 15mg or 30mg qd
Titrate: In increments of 15mg
Max: 45mg qd

W/ CHF (NYHA Class I or II):
Initial: 15mg qd
Titrate: In increments of 15mg
Max: 45mg qd

PEDIATRIC DOSAGE
Pediatric use may not have been established

DOSING CONSIDERATIONS
Concomitant Medications
Insulin Secretagogue:
Reduce dose of insulin secretagogue if hypoglycemia occurs

Insulin:
Decrease insulin dose by 10-25% if hypoglycemia occurs

Gemfibrozil/Other Strong CYP2C8 Inhibitors:
Max: 15mg qd

ADMINISTRATION
Oral route

Take w/o regard to meals

STORAGE
25°C (77°F); excursions permitted to 15-30°C (59-86°F). Protect from light, moisture, and humidity.

HOW SUPPLIED
Tab: 15mg, 30mg, 45mg

CONTRAINDICATIONS
Established NYHA Class III or IV HF, known hypersensitivity to pioglitazone or any other component of this medication.

WARNINGS/PRECAUTIONS
Not for use in treatment of type 1 DM or diabetic ketoacidosis. Fatal and nonfatal hepatic failure reported. May use with caution in patients with lesser ALT elevations or bilirubin and with an alternate probable cause. Obtain LFTs prior to initiation; caution with liver disease/abnormal LFTs. D/C if ALT >3X ULN; do not restart if cause of abnormal LFTs not established or if ALT remains >3X ULN with total bilirubin >2X ULN without alternative etiologies. Not for use in patients with active bladder cancer; consider benefits versus risks in patients with a prior history of bladder cancer. New onset or worsening of edema reported; caution in patients with edema and in patients at risk for CHF. Increased incidence of bone fractures reported in females. Macular edema reported; refer to an ophthalmologist if visual symptoms develop. Ovulation in premenopausal anovulatory patients may occur; use adequate contraception.

ADVERSE REACTIONS
CHF, URTI, hypoglycemia, edema, headache, cardiac failure, pain in extremity, sinusitis, back pain, myalgia, pharyngitis, chest pain.

DRUG INTERACTIONS
Increased exposure and $T_{1/2}$ with CYP2C8 inhibitors (eg, gemfibrozil). Decreased exposure with CYP2C8 inducers (eg, rifampin). Risk of fluid retention and hypoglycemia with insulin and other antidiabetic medications (eg, insulin secretagogues such as sulfonylureas).

PREGNANCY AND LACTATION
Category C, not for use in nursing.

MECHANISM OF ACTION
Thiazolidinedione; decreases insulin resistance in the periphery and liver, resulting in increased insulin-dependent glucose disposal and decreased hepatic glucose output.

PHARMACOKINETICS
Absorption: T_{max}=Within 2 hrs, 3-4 hrs (with food). **Distribution:** V_d=0.63L/kg; plasma protein binding (>99%). **Metabolism:** Hydroxylation and oxidation (extensive), CYP2C8, CYP3A4; M-III [keto derivative] and M-IV [hydroxyl derivative] (active metabolites). **Elimination:** Urine (15-30%), bile and feces; $T_{1/2}$=3-7 hrs (pioglitazone), 16-24 hrs (metabolites).

PATIENT CONSIDERATIONS

Assessment: Assess for previous hypersensitivity, HF, edema, risk factors for developing HF, liver disease, bone health, active/history of bladder cancer, pregnancy/nursing status, and possible drug interactions. Obtain baseline LFTs.

Monitoring: Monitor for signs and symptoms of HF, edema, weight gain, hematological changes (eg, decreases in Hgb, Hct), liver injury, macular edema, bone fractures, ovulation in premenopausal anovulatory women, and other adverse reactions. Perform periodic measurements of FPG and HbA1c. Periodically monitor LFTs in patients with liver disease. Perform periodic eye exams.

Counseling: Advise to adhere to dietary instructions and have blood glucose and glycosylated Hgb levels tested regularly. Instruct to seek medical advice promptly during periods of stress and report rapid increase in weight or edema, SOB, or other symptoms of HF to physician. Instruct to d/c and consult physician if unexplained N/V, abdominal pain, anorexia, fatigue, or dark urine occurs. Advise to report any signs of macroscopic hematuria or other symptoms such as dysuria or urinary urgency. Advise to take qd with or without meals. If dose is missed, advise to not double the dose the following day. Inform about the risk of hypoglycemia when using with insulin or other antidiabetic medications. Inform that therapy may result in ovulation in some premenopausal anovulatory women; recommend adequate contraception for all premenopausal women.

ACULAR LS — ketorolac tromethamine   Rx

Class: NSAID

ADULT DOSAGE
Corneal Refractive Surgery
Reduction of Ocular Pain and Burning/Stinging:
1 drop qid in the operated eye prn for up to 4 days following surgery

PEDIATRIC DOSAGE
Corneal Refractive Surgery
Reduction of Ocular Pain and Burning/Stinging:
≥3 Years:
1 drop qid in the operated eye prn for up to 4 days following surgery

DOSING CONSIDERATIONS
Concomitant Medications
Safely administered w/ other topical ophthalmic medications (eg, alpha-agonists, antibiotics, beta-blockers, carbonic anhydrase inhibitors, cycloplegics, mydriatics); administer drops at least 5 min apart.

ADMINISTRATION
Ocular route

STORAGE
15-25°C (59-77°F). Protect from light.

HOW SUPPLIED
Sol: 0.4% [5mL]

CONTRAINDICATIONS
Previously demonstrated hypersensitivity to any of the ingredients in the formulation.

WARNINGS/PRECAUTIONS
Potential cross-sensitivity to acetylsalicylic acid, phenylacetic acid derivatives, and other NSAIDs; caution w/ previous sensitivities to these drugs. May increase bleeding of ocular tissues (including hyphemas) in conjunction w/ ocular surgery; caution w/ known bleeding tendencies. May slow/delay healing or result in keratitis. Continued use may result in epithelial breakdown, corneal thinning, erosion, ulceration, or perforation; d/c if corneal epithelium breakdown occurs and closely monitor for corneal health. Caution w/ complicated ocular surgeries, corneal denervation, corneal epithelial defects, diabetes mellitus (DM), ocular surface diseases (eg, dry eye syndrome), rheumatoid arthritis (RA), or repeat ocular surgeries w/in a short period of time. Use for >1 day prior to surgery or beyond 14 days postsurgery may increase risk for occurrence and severity of corneal adverse events. Do not administer while wearing contact lenses.

ADVERSE REACTIONS
Conjunctival hyperemia, corneal infiltrates, headache, ocular edema/pain.

DRUG INTERACTIONS
Concomitant use of topical NSAIDs and topical steroids may increase potential for healing problems. Caution w/ other medications that may prolong bleeding time.

PREGNANCY AND LACTATION
Pregnancy: No evidence of teratogenicity has been observed in animal studies.
Lactation: Not known if topical ketorolac is present in human milk; caution in nursing.

MECHANISM OF ACTION
NSAID; inhibits prostaglandin biosynthesis.

PATIENT CONSIDERATIONS

Assessment: Assess for drug hypersensitivity, cross-sensitivity reactions, bleeding tendencies, corneal denervation, corneal epithelial defects, DM, ocular surface diseases, RA, and possible drug interactions.

Monitoring: Monitor for bleeding of ocular tissues, healing problems, keratitis, corneal epithelial breakdown, and corneal thinning/erosion/ulceration/perforation.

Counseling: Inform of the possibility that slow or delayed healing may occur. Instruct to avoid allowing tip of bottle to contact eye or surrounding structures. Instruct to use one bottle for each eye following bilateral ocular surgery. Advise not to use while wearing contact lenses. Advise to immediately seek physician's advice concerning continued use if intercurrent ocular conditions (eg, trauma, infection) occur or if having ocular surgery. Advise to administer topical medications at least 5 min apart.

ACUVAIL — ketorolac tromethamine   Rx

Class: NSAID

ADULT DOSAGE
Ocular Pain and Inflammation
Instill 1 drop to the affected eye bid beginning 1 day prior to cataract surgery, continued on the day of surgery, and through the first 2 weeks of the postoperative period

PEDIATRIC DOSAGE
Pediatric use may not have been established

DOSING CONSIDERATIONS
Concomitant Medications
With Other Topical Ophthalmic Medications:
Administer drops ≥5 min apart
ADMINISTRATION
Ocular route
STORAGE
15-30°C (59-86°F). Protect from light.
HOW SUPPLIED
Sol: 0.45% [0.4mL]
CONTRAINDICATIONS
Prior hypersensitivity to any of the ingredients in the formulation.
WARNINGS/PRECAUTIONS
May slow or delay healing. Potential for cross-sensitivity to acetylsalicylic acid (ASA), phenylacetic acid derivatives, and other NSAIDs; caution with previous sensitivities to these drugs. Bronchospasm or exacerbation of asthma reported in patients with known hypersensitivity to ASA/NSAIDs or past history of asthma. Potential for increased bleeding time due to interference with thrombocyte aggregation. May cause increased bleeding of ocular tissues (including hyphemas) in conjunction with ocular surgery; caution with known bleeding tendencies. May result in keratitis. Continued use may result in sight-threatening epithelial breakdown or corneal thinning/erosion/ulceration/perforation; d/c use and monitor for corneal health if corneal epithelial breakdown occurs. Increased risk for corneal adverse events which may become sight-threatening in patients with complicated ocular surgeries, corneal denervation, corneal epithelial defects, diabetes mellitus (DM), ocular surface diseases (eg, dry eye syndrome), rheumatoid arthritis (RA), or repeat ocular surgeries within a short period; caution in these patients. Use of therapy >1 day prior to surgery or beyond 14 days postsurgery may increase risk for occurrence and severity of corneal adverse events. Do not administer while wearing contact lenses. Avoid use during late pregnancy.
ADVERSE REACTIONS
Increased intraocular pressure, conjunctival hyperemia and/or hemorrhage, corneal edema, ocular pain, headache, tearing, vision blurred.
DRUG INTERACTIONS
Caution with medications that may prolong bleeding time. Increased potential for healing problems with topical steroids.
PREGNANCY AND LACTATION
Category C, caution in nursing.
MECHANISM OF ACTION
NSAID; inhibits prostaglandin biosynthesis.
PATIENT CONSIDERATIONS
Assessment: Assess for previous hypersensitivity to the drug or to ASA, phenylacetic acid derivatives, and other NSAIDs, history of asthma, bleeding tendencies, complicated ocular surgeries, corneal denervation, corneal epithelial defects, DM, ocular surface diseases, RA, repeated ocular surgeries within a short period, contact lens use, pregnancy/nursing status, and possible drug interactions.
Monitoring: Monitor for hypersensitivity reactions, healing problems, increased bleeding of ocular tissues in conjunction with ocular surgery, keratitis, corneal epithelial breakdown, and other adverse reactions.
Counseling: Inform of the possibility that slow or delayed healing may occur. Advise to use 1 vial for each eye immediately after opening and discard the remaining contents after use. Instruct to avoid allowing the tip of the vial to contact the eye or surrounding structures. Advise not to administer while wearing contact lenses, and to seek physician's advice if an intercurrent ocular condition (eg, trauma or infection) develops or in the case of ocular surgery. Advise to administer at least 5 min apart if >1 ophthalmic medication is being used.

ACZONE 5% — dapsone   Rx

Class: Sulfone

ADULT DOSAGE	**PEDIATRIC DOSAGE**
Acne Vulgaris	**Acne Vulgaris**
Apply a pea-sized amount of gel in a thin layer to the affected areas bid	**≥12 Years:** Apply a pea-sized amount of gel in a thin layer to the affected areas bid
If no improvement seen after 12 weeks, reassess treatment	If no improvement seen after 12 weeks, reassess treatment

ADMINISTRATION
Topical route
Not for oral, ophthalmic, or intravaginal use.
Apply the gel after skin is gently washed and patted dry; rub in gently and completely.
Wash hands after application.
STORAGE
20-25°C (68-77°F); excursions permitted to 15-30°C (59-86°F). Protect from freezing.
HOW SUPPLIED
Gel: 5% [30g, 60g, 90g]
WARNINGS/PRECAUTIONS
Cases of methemoglobinemia reported; avoid use in patients w/ congenital or idiopathic methemoglobinemia. D/C and seek immediate medical attention in

the event of cyanosis. Laboratory changes suggestive of hemolysis reported in some patients w/ G6PD deficiency using dapsone gel. Dose-related hemolysis and hemolytic anemia, peripheral neuropathy (motor loss, muscle weakness) and skin reactions (toxic epidermal necrolysis, erythema multiforme, morbilliform/scarlatiniform reactions, bullous/exfoliative dermatitis, erythema nodosum, urticaria) reported w/ oral dapsone; d/c if signs/symptoms suggestive of hemolytic anemia occur.
ADVERSE REACTIONS
Oiliness/peeling, dryness, erythema.
DRUG INTERACTIONS
Avoid w/ patients taking oral dapsone or antimalarial medications due to potential for hemolytic reactions. Trimethoprim/sulfamethoxazole may increase levels. Trimethoprim/sulfamethoxazole may increase likelihood of hemolysis in patients w/ G6PD deficiency. Topical benzoyl peroxide reported to cause a temporary local yellow or orange discoloration of the skin and facial hair. Folic acid antagonists (eg, pyrimethamine) may increase hematologic reactions w/ oral dapsone treatment. Coadministration of oral dapsone w/ certain medications (eg, rifampin, anticonvulsants, St. John's wort) may increase dapsone hydroxylamine formation, a metabolite of dapsone associated w/ hemolysis. Concomitant use w/ drugs that induce methemoglobinemia (eg, sulfonamides, acetaminophen, phenytoin) may increase risk for developing methemoglobinemia.
PREGNANCY AND LACTATION
Pregnancy: Category C.
Lactation: Not for use in nursing.
MECHANISM OF ACTION
Sulfone; not established.
PHARMACOKINETICS
Absorption: AUC_{0-24}=415ng•h/mL. Distribution: Found in breast milk.
PATIENT CONSIDERATIONS
Assessment: Assess for congenital or idiopathic methemoglobinemia, G6PD deficiency, previous allergic reactions to the drug, pregnancy/nursing status, and for possible drug interactions.
Monitoring: Monitor for signs/symptoms of methemoglobinemia, hemolytic anemia, skin reactions, and other adverse reactions. Monitor for response to treatment; reevaluate if no improvement is seen after 12 weeks of therapy.
Counseling: Advise to seek immediate medical attention for cyanosis. Instruct to use externally and ud. Inform that drug is not for oral, ophthalmic or intravaginal use. Instruct to notify physician if any signs of adverse reactions occur.

ADALAT CC — nifedipine   Rx

Class: Calcium channel blocker (CCB) (dihydropyridine)

OTHER BRAND NAMES
Nifediac CC, Afeditab CR

ADULT DOSAGE	**PEDIATRIC DOSAGE**
Hypertension	Pediatric use may not have been established
Initial: 30mg qd	
Titrate: Increase dose over a 7- to 14-day period based on therapeutic efficacy and safety	
Maint: 30-60mg qd	
Max: 90mg qd	

DOSING CONSIDERATIONS
Elderly
Start at low end of dosing range
Discontinuation
Decrease dose gradually w/ close physician supervision
ADMINISTRATION
Oral route
Take PO on empty stomach
Swallow tab whole; do not chew, crush, or divide
STORAGE
Adalat CC/Afeditab CR: <30°C (86°F). Nifediac CC: 25°C (77°F); excursions permitted to 15-30°C (59-86°F). Protect from light and moisture.
HOW SUPPLIED
Tab, Extended-Release: (Adalat CC) 30mg, 60mg, 90mg, (Afeditab CR) 30mg, 60mg, (Nifediac CC) 30mg, 60mg, 90mg
CONTRAINDICATIONS
Known hypersensitivity to nifedipine or any component of the tablet. (Adalat CC) Cardiogenic shock and concomitant use with strong P450 inducers (eg, rifampin).
WARNINGS/PRECAUTIONS
May cause hypotension; monitor BP initially or with titration. May increase frequency, duration, and/or severity of angina or acute myocardial infarction (MI) upon starting or at time of dose increase, particularly with severe obstructive coronary artery disease (CAD). May develop congestive heart failure (CHF), especially with tight aortic stenosis or β-blockers. Peripheral edema may occur; rule out peripheral edema caused by left ventricular dysfunction if HTN is complicated by CHF. Transient elevations of enzymes (eg, alkaline phosphatase, CPK, LDH, SGOT, SGPT), cholestasis with/without jaundice, and allergic hepatitis reported rarely. May decrease platelet aggregation and increase bleeding time. Lab test interactions may occur. Reversible elevations in BUN

and SrCr reported rarely in patients with chronic renal insufficiency. Caution with renal/hepatic impairment and in elderly. Adalat CC: Reduced clearance in cirrhosis; initiate lowest dose possible. Contains lactose; avoid with hereditary galactose intolerance problems, Lapp lactase deficiency, and glucose-galactose malabsorption. Nifediac CC: Contains tartrazine, which may cause allergic-type reactions in certain susceptible persons (eg, patients with aspirin hypersensitivity).

ADVERSE REACTIONS
Peripheral edema, headache, flushing, heat sensation, dizziness, fatigue, asthenia, nausea, constipation.

DRUG INTERACTIONS
See Contraindications. β-blockers may increase risk of CHF, severe hypotension, or angina exacerbation; avoid abrupt β-blocker withdrawal. Severe hypotension and/or increased fluid volume may occur with β-blockers and fentanyl or other narcotic analgesics. May increase plasma levels of digoxin; monitor digoxin levels when initiating, adjusting, and discontinuing therapy. May increase PT with coumarin anticoagulants. Monitor with other medications known to lower BP. Enhanced hypotensive effect with benazepril and timolol. Avoid with grapefruit juice; stop grapefruit juice intake at least 3 days prior to therapy. Increased exposure with CYP3A inhibitors (eg, ketoconazole, itraconazole, fluconazole, erythromycin, clarithromycin, nefazodone, fluoxetine, diltiazem, verapamil, cimetidine, quinupristin/dalfopristin, amprenavir, atazanavir, delavirdine, fosamprenavir, indinavir, nelfinavir, ritonavir, saquinavir), valproic acid, and doxazosin; monitor BP and consider dose reduction. Increased levels with quinidine; monitor HR and adjust dose if necessary. Monitor blood glucose levels and consider dose adjustment with acarbose. May increase plasma levels of metformin. May increase exposure of tacrolimus; monitor blood levels and consider dose reduction. May decrease doxazosin levels; monitor BP and reduce dose. May inhibit metabolism of CYP3A substrates. Afeditab CR/Nifediac CC: Decreased exposure with CYP3A4 inducers (eg, rifampin, rifapentine, phenytoin, phenobarbitone, carbamazepine, St. John's wort); monitor BP and consider dose adjustment. Adalat CC: May increase the BP-lowering effects of diuretics, PDE-5 inhibitors, and α-methyldopa. Magnesium sulfate IV in pregnant women may cause excessive fall in BP. Increased plasma concentrations with cisapride.

PREGNANCY AND LACTATION
Category C, not for use in nursing.

MECHANISM OF ACTION
Calcium channel blocker (dihydropyridine); inhibits the transmembrane influx of Ca^{2+} ions into vascular smooth muscle and cardiac muscle. Involves peripheral arterial vasodilation and reduction in peripheral vascular resistance, resulting in reduced arterial BP.

PHARMACOKINETICS
Absorption: Complete; T_{max}=2.5-5 hrs; (90mg) C_{max}=115ng/mL. **Distribution:** Plasma protein binding (92-98%); found in breast milk. **Metabolism:** Liver via CYP3A4. **Elimination:** Urine (60-80%, metabolite; <0.1%, unchanged); feces (metabolite); $T_{1/2}$=7 hrs.

PATIENT CONSIDERATIONS
Assessment: Assess for previous hypersensitivity to the drug, CHF, severe obstructive CAD, aortic stenosis, hepatic/renal impairment, pregnancy/nursing status, and possible drug interactions. (Adalat CC) Assess for cirrhosis, hereditary galactose intolerance problems, Lapp lactase deficiency, and glucose-galactose malabsorption. (Nifediac CC) Assess for susceptibility for tartrazine hypersensitivity (eg, aspirin hypersensitivity).

Monitoring: Monitor for excessive hypotension, increased frequency, duration and/or severity of angina and/or acute MI (especially during initiation and dose titration), CHF, peripheral edema, cholestasis with/without jaundice, and allergic hepatitis. Monitor BP, LFTs, BUN, SrCr, and increased bleeding time.

Counseling: Inform about potential benefits/risks of therapy. Instruct to notify physician if pregnant/nursing or if any adverse reactions occur. (Afeditab CR) Advise patients that empty matrix "ghost" tab may pass via colostomy or in the stool and this should not be a concern.

ADASUVE — loxapine   Rx

Class: Typical antipsychotic

> May cause bronchospasm with potential to lead to respiratory distress and respiratory arrest; monitor for signs/symptoms of bronchospasm. Administer only in an enrolled healthcare facility that has immediate access on-site to equipment and personnel trained to manage acute bronchospasm, including advanced airway management (intubation and mechanical ventilation). Prior to administering, screen for current diagnosis, history, or symptoms of asthma, COPD and other lung diseases, and examine (including chest auscultation) for respiratory signs. Available only through a restricted program under a Risk Evaluation and Mitigation Strategy (REMS) because of the risk of bronchospasm. Elderly patients with dementia-related psychosis treated with atypical antipsychotic drugs are at an increased risk for death. Not approved for the treatment of patients with dementia-related psychosis.

ADULT DOSAGE
Agitation

Acute Treatment of Agitation Associated w/ Schizophrenia or Bipolar I Disorder:
Usual: 10mg, by oral inh, using a single use inhaler; administer only a single dose w/in a 24-hr period

PEDIATRIC DOSAGE
Pediatric use may not have been established

ADMINISTRATION
Oral inh route

Administration Instructions
1. When ready to use, tear open foil pouch and remove inhaler from the package; when inhaler is removed from pouch, the indicator light is on
2. Firmly pull the plastic tab from the rear of the inhaler; check that the green light turns on. Use inhaler w/in 15 min after removing the tab to prevent automatic deactivation. Green light will turn off, indicating that the inhaler is not usable. Discard after 1 use
3. Hold inhaler away from mouth and breathe out fully to empty the lungs
4. Put mouthpiece of the inhaler between lips, close lips, and inhale through the mouthpiece w/ a steady deep breath; check that the green light turns off indicating that the dose has been delivered
5. Remove mouthpiece from mouth and hold the breath for as long as possible, up to 10 sec
6. If the green light remains on after inhalation, the dose has not been delivered; repeat steps 3, 4, and 5 up to 2 additional times. If the green light still does not turn off, discard inhaler and use a new one

STORAGE
15-30°C (59-86°F).

HOW SUPPLIED
Powder, Inhalation: 10mg

CONTRAINDICATIONS
Current diagnosis or history of asthma, COPD, or other lung disease associated w/ bronchospasm, acute respiratory symptoms/signs (eg, wheezing), history of bronchospasm following loxapine treatment or known hypersensitivity to loxapine or amoxapine. Current use of medications to treat airways disease (eg, asthma, COPD).

WARNINGS/PRECAUTIONS
May cause sedation, which can mask symptoms of bronchospasm. May cause neuroleptic malignant syndrome (NMS); d/c and treat immediately if this occurs. May cause hypotension, orthostatic hypotension, and syncope; caution with known cardiovascular (CVD) or cerebrovascular disease, or conditions that would predispose to hypotension (eg, dehydration, hypovolemia). Do not use epinephrine in presence of severe hypotension requiring vasopressor therapy; preferred drugs may be norepinephrine or phenylephrine. May lower seizure threshold; seizures reported with oral loxapine. May impair mental/physical abilities. Has anticholinergic activity; potential to cause anticholinergic adverse reactions, including exacerbation of glaucoma or urinary retention.

ADVERSE REACTIONS
Bronchospasm, dysgeusia, sedation, throat irritation.

DRUG INTERACTIONS
See Contraindications. Caution with antihypertensives or other drugs that affect BP or reduce HR. CNS depressants (eg, alcohol, opioid analgesics, benzodiazepines) may increase risk of respiratory depression, hypotension, profound sedation, and syncope; consider reducing dose of CNS depressants. Concomitant use with other anticholinergic drugs (eg, antiparkinson drugs) may increase risk of anticholinergic adverse reactions, including exacerbation of glaucoma and urinary retention.

PREGNANCY AND LACTATION
Category C, not for use in nursing.

MECHANISM OF ACTION
Dibenzapine derivative; typical antipsychotic agent; not established. Efficacy could be mediated through a combination of antagonism of central dopamine D_2 and serotonin 5-HT_{2A} receptors.

PHARMACOKINETICS
Absorption: Rapid. AUC_{0-2h}=66.7ng•hr/mL, AUC_{inf}=188ng•hr/mL; C_{max}=257ng/mL; T_{max}=1.13 min. **Distribution:** Plasma protein binding (96.6%). **Metabolism:** Liver (extensive); hydroxylation via CYP1A2, CYP3A4 and CYP2D6, N-oxidation via flavanoid monoamine oxidases, and demethylation; 8-OH-loxapine, loxapine N-oxide, 7-OH-loxapine, amoxapine (metabolites). **Elimination:** Urine (conjugates), feces (unconjugated). $T_{1/2}$=7.61 hrs.

PATIENT CONSIDERATIONS
Assessment: Assess for dementia-related psychosis, history of bronchospasm following loxapine treatment, CVD, cerebrovascular disease, or conditions that would predispose to hypotension, seizure disorder, hypersensitivity to the drug, pregnancy/nursing status, and possible drug interactions. Screen for current diagnosis, history, or symptoms of asthma, COPD, or other lung diseases, and acute respiratory signs/symptoms or signs. Examine for respiratory abnormalities (eg, wheezing).

Monitoring: Monitor for sedation, NMS, hypotension, orthostatic hypotension, syncope, seizures, cognitive/motor impairment, anticholinergic reactions, and other adverse reactions. Monitor for signs/symptoms of bronchospasm at least every 15 min for a minimum of 1 hr following administration.

Counseling: Advise of the risk of bronchospasm; instruct to inform physician if breathing problems develop. Caution patient against performing activities requiring mental alertness (eg, operating machinery/motor vehicle), until reasonably certain that drug does not adversely affect him or her. Inform about the potential for sedation, especially when used concurrently with other CNS antidepressants. Counsel that NMS may occur. Advise of the risk of hypotension or orthostatic hypotension and the potential risk of anticholinergic reactions. Inform about the potential risks if taken while pregnant or breastfeeding.

ADCETRIS — brentuximab vedotin Rx

Class: CD30-directed antibody-drug conjugate

> JC virus infection resulting in progressive multifocal leukoencephalopathy (PML) and death may occur.

ADULT DOSAGE

Hodgkin Lymphoma

Treatment of patients w/ classical Hodgkin lymphoma after failure of autologous hematopoietic stem cell transplant (auto-HSCT) or after failure of ≥2 prior multi-agent chemotherapy regimens in patients who are not auto-HSCT candidates

Initial: 1.8mg/kg IV (up to 180mg) over 30 min every 3 weeks until disease progression or unacceptable toxicity

Hodgkin Lymphoma Post-auto-HSCT Consolidation

Treatment of patients w/ classical Hodgkin lymphoma at high risk of relapse or progression as post-auto-HSCT consolidation

Initial: 1.8mg/kg IV (up to 180mg) over 30 min every 3 weeks

Initiate treatment w/in 4-6 weeks post-auto-HSCT or upon recovery from auto-HSCT; continue treatment until a max of 16 cycles, disease progression, or unacceptable toxicity

Systemic Anaplastic Large Cell Lymphoma

Use after failure of ≥1 prior multi-agent chemotherapy regimen

Initial: 1.8mg/kg IV (up to 180mg) over 30 min every 3 weeks until disease progression or unacceptable toxicity

PEDIATRIC DOSAGE

Pediatric use may not have been established

DOSING CONSIDERATIONS

Renal Impairment
Severe (CrCl <30mL/min): Avoid use

Hepatic Impairment
Mild (Child-Pugh A):
Initial: 1.2mg/kg up to 120mg
Moderate (Child-Pugh B)/Severe (Child-Pugh C): Avoid use

Adverse Reactions
Peripheral Neuropathy:
New or Worsening Grade 2 or 3: Hold dosing until neuropathy improves to Grade 1 or baseline, then restart at 1.2mg/kg
Grade 4: D/C therapy

Neutropenia:
Grade 3 or 4: Hold dose until resolution to baseline or Grade 2 or lower; consider granulocyte colony-stimulating factor (G-CSF) prophylaxis for subsequent cycles if Grade 3 or 4 neutropenia was experienced in the previous cycle
Recurrent Grade 4 Neutropenia Despite G-CSF Prophylaxis: Consider discontinuation or reduce dose to 1.2mg/kg

ADMINISTRATION

IV route
For IV infusion only.
Do not mix w/, or administer as an infusion w/, other medicinal products.
If sol is not diluted/used immediately, store at 2-8°C (36-46°F) and use w/in 24 hrs of reconstitution. Do not freeze.

Reconstitution
1. Reconstitute each 50mg vial w/ 10.5mL sterile water for inj to yield 5mg/mL.
2. Direct the stream toward vial wall and not directly at the cake or powder.
3. Swirl the vial gently to aid dissolution; do not shake.
4. Dilute immediately into an infusion bag following reconstitution.

Dilution
1. Withdraw required calculated reconstituted amount of sol from the vial and immediately add it to an infusion bag containing a minimum volume of 100mL of 0.9% NaCl, D5 or lactated Ringer's inj to a final concentration of 0.4mg/mL to 1.8mg/mL.
2. Invert the bag gently to mix sol.
3. Infuse sol immediately following dilution.

STORAGE
2-8°C (36-46°F). Protect from light.

HOW SUPPLIED
Inj: 50mg

CONTRAINDICATIONS
Concomitant bleomycin due to pulmonary toxicity.

WARNINGS/PRECAUTIONS

See Dosing Considerations. Peripheral neuropathy (sensory and motor) reported. Infusion-related reactions, including anaphylaxis, reported; d/c immediately and permanently and institute appropriate therapy if anaphylaxis occurs. Interrupt treatment if an infusion-related reaction occurs and institute appropriate medical management; patients who have experienced a prior infusion-related reaction should be premedicated for subsequent infusions. Prolonged (≥1 week) severe neutropenia, Grade 3 or 4 thrombocytopenia, anemia, or febrile neutropenia reported; monitor CBCs prior to each dose and consider more frequent monitoring for patients w/ Grade 3 or 4 neutropenia. Serious infections and opportunistic infections (eg, pneumonia, bacteremia, sepsis, septic shock) reported; closely monitor during treatment for the emergence of possible bacterial, fungal, or viral infections. Increased risk of tumor lysis syndrome in patients w/ rapidly proliferating tumor and high tumor burden; monitor closely and take appropriate measures. Increased risk of ≥Grade 3 adverse reactions and deaths in patients w/ severe renal impairment and w/ moderate or severe hepatic impairment. Serious hepatotoxicity, including fatal outcomes, may occur after the 1st dose or after rechallenge; preexisting liver disease, elevated baseline LFTs, and concomitant medications may increase risk. Patients experiencing new/worsening/recurrent hepatotoxicity may require a delay, change in dose, or discontinuation of therapy. Hold dosing for any suspected case of PML and d/c if diagnosis is confirmed. Events of noninfectious pulmonary toxicity (eg, pneumonitis, interstitial lung disease, acute respiratory distress syndrome) reported; in the event of new/worsening pulmonary symptoms, hold dosing during evaluation and until symptomatic improvement. Stevens-Johnson syndrome (SJS) and toxic epidermal necrolysis (TEN) reported; d/c and administer appropriate therapy if SJS or TEN occurs. Fatal and serious GI complications (eg, perforation, hemorrhage, intestinal obstruction) reported; in the event of new/worsening GI symptoms, perform a prompt diagnostic evaluation and treat appropriately. May cause fetal harm.

ADVERSE REACTIONS

Classical Hodgkin Lymphoma: Neutropenia, peripheral sensory neuropathy, fatigue, URTI, N/V, diarrhea, anemia, pyrexia, thrombocytopenia, rash, abdominal pain, cough.
Classical Hodgkin Lymphoma Post-auto-HSCT Consolidation: Neutropenia, peripheral sensory neuropathy, thrombocytopenia, anemia, URTI, fatigue, peripheral motor neuropathy, nausea, cough, diarrhea.
Systemic Anaplastic Large Cell Lymphoma: Neutropenia, anemia, peripheral sensory neuropathy, fatigue, nausea, pyrexia, rash, diarrhea, pain.

DRUG INTERACTIONS

See Contraindications. Concomitant ketoconazole (potent CYP3A4 inhibitor) or P-gp inhibitors may increase exposure to monomethyl auristatin E (MMAE); monitor closely for adverse reactions when given concomitantly w/ strong CYP3A4 or P-gp inhibitors. Coadministration w/ rifampin (potent CYP3A4 inducer) may decrease exposure to MMAE.

PREGNANCY AND LACTATION

Pregnancy: Can cause fetal harm based on the findings from animal studies and the drug's mechanism of action.
Lactation: Not for use in nursing.
Reproductive Potential: Verify pregnancy status of females of reproductive potential prior to initiating therapy. Females of reproductive potential should avoid pregnancy during treatment and for at least 6 months after the final dose of therapy; females should immediately report pregnancy. May damage spermatozoa and testicular tissue, resulting in possible genetic abnormalities. Males w/ female sexual partners of reproductive potential should use effective contraception during treatment and for at least 6 months after the final dose of therapy. Male fertility may be compromised by treatment.

MECHANISM OF ACTION

CD30-directed antibody-drug conjugate (ADC); binds to CD30-expressing cells, followed by internalization of ADC-CD30 complex, and release of MMAE via proteolytic cleavage. Binding of MMAE to tubulin disrupts the microtubule network w/in the cell, inducing cell cycle arrest and apoptotic death of the cell.

PHARMACOKINETICS

Absorption: (MMAE) T_{max}=1-3 days. **Distribution:** (MMAE) Plasma protein binding (68-82%); (ADC) V_d=6-10L. **Metabolism:** (MMAE) Oxidation via CYP3A4/5. **Elimination:** (MMAE) Urine, feces (24%); $T_{1/2}$=4-6 days (ADC).

PATIENT CONSIDERATIONS

Assessment: Assess for history of infusion-related reactions, renal/hepatic impairment, pregnancy/nursing status, and for possible drug interactions. Assess for rapidly proliferating tumors and high tumor burden. Obtain baseline CBC, liver enzymes, and bilirubin.

Monitoring: Monitor for peripheral neuropathy, anaphylaxis, infusion reactions, tumor lysis syndrome, SJS, TEN, fever, opportunistic infections, PML, pulmonary toxicity, GI complications, and other adverse reactions. Monitor CBCs prior to each dose and perform more frequent monitoring w/ Grade 3 or 4 neutropenia. Monitor liver enzymes and bilirubin.

Counseling: Inform that therapy may cause peripheral neuropathy; advise to report to physician any numbness/tingling of hands or feet, or any muscle weakness. Advise to contact physician if a fever of ≥38.05°C (100.5°F) or other evidence of potential infection develops; if signs/symptoms of infusion reactions w/in 24 hrs of infusion are experienced; or if severe abdominal pain, chills, fever, N/V, or diarrhea develop. Advise to report symptoms that may indicate liver injury/hepatotoxicity, or pulmonary toxicity. Instruct to immediately report changes in mood/usual behavior; confusion, thinking problems, or loss of memory; changes in vision, speech, or walking; or decreased strength or weakness on 1 side of the body. Inform that therapy can cause fetal harm. Advise women to avoid pregnancy during treatment and for at least 6 months after the final dose; advise males w/ female sexual partners of reproductive potential to use effective contraception during treatment and for at least 6 months after the final dose. Instruct to report pregnancy immediately; advise to avoid breastfeeding while receiving therapy.

ADCIRCA — tadalafil   Rx

Class: Phosphodiesterase-5 (PDE-5) inhibitor

ADULT DOSAGE	PEDIATRIC DOSAGE
Pulmonary Arterial Hypertension	Pediatric use may not have been established
Treatment of pulmonary arterial HTN (WHO Group 1) to improve exercise ability	
40mg (two 20mg tabs) qd	

DOSING CONSIDERATIONS
Concomitant Medications
Patients on Ritonavir (RTV) for at Least 1 Week:
Initial: 20mg qd
Titrate: Increase to 40mg qd based on individual tolerability

Adding RTV:
Avoid use of tadalafil during the initiation of RTV
Stop tadalafil at least 24 hrs prior to starting RTV
After at least 1 week following RTV initiation, resume tadalafil at 20mg qd
Increase to 40mg qd based on individual tolerability

Renal Impairment
Mild (CrCl 51-80mL/min) or Moderate (CrCl 31-50mL/min):
Initial: 20mg qd
Titrate: Increase to 40mg qd based on individual tolerability
Severe (CrCl <30mL/min and on Hemodialysis): Avoid use

Hepatic Impairment
Mild or Moderate Hepatic Cirrhosis (Child-Pugh Class A or B):
Initial: Consider 20mg qd
Severe Hepatic Cirrhosis (Child-Pugh Class C): Avoid use

ADMINISTRATION
Oral route

Take w/ or w/o food
Dividing the dose (40mg) over the course of the day is not recommended

STORAGE
25°C (77°F); excursions permitted to 15-30°C (59-86°F).

HOW SUPPLIED
Tab: 20mg

CONTRAINDICATIONS
Patients using any form of organic nitrate, either regularly or intermittently, or guanylate cyclase (GC) stimulator (eg, riociguat), known serious hypersensitivity to tadalafil (Adcirca or Cialis).

WARNINGS/PRECAUTIONS
Patients who experience anginal chest pain after taking tadalafil should seek immediate medical attention. May cause a transient decrease in BP; caution w/ underlying cardiovascular disease (CVD). Patients w/ severely impaired autonomic control of BP or w/ left ventricular outflow obstruction may be particularly sensitive to vasodilatory effects. May significantly worsen cardiovascular status of patients w/ pulmonary veno-occlusive disease (PVOD); not recommended w/ veno-occlusive disease. Consider PVOD if signs of pulmonary edema occur. Nonarteritic anterior ischemic optic neuropathy (NAION) reported; seek immediate medical attention if sudden loss of vision in 1 or both eyes occurs. Not recommended in patients w/ hereditary degenerative retinal disorders (eg, retinitis pigmentosa). Seek immediate medical attention in the event of sudden decrease or loss of hearing. Prolonged erections >4 hrs and priapism reported rarely; caution w/ conditions that might predispose to priapism (eg, sickle cell anemia, multiple myeloma, leukemia) or in patients w/ anatomical penile deformation (eg, angulation, cavernosal fibrosis, Peyronie's disease). Caution w/ bleeding disorders or significant active peptic ulceration.

ADVERSE REACTIONS
Headache, myalgia, nasopharyngitis, flushing, respiratory tract infection, pain in extremity, nausea, back pain, dyspepsia, nasal congestion.

DRUG INTERACTIONS
See Contraindications and Dosing Considerations. If nitrate administration is deemed medically necessary in a life-threatening situation, at least 48 hrs should elapse after the last dose of tadalafil before nitrate administration is considered; administer nitrates only under close medical supervision w/ appropriate hemodynamic monitoring. Additive hypotensive effects w/ α-adrenergic blockers, antihypertensives (eg, amlodipine, ARBs, bendroflumethiazide, enalapril, metoprolol), and alcohol. Avoid w/ potent CYP3A inhibitors (eg, ketoconazole, itraconazole) or chronic therapy of potent CYP3A inducers (eg, rifampin). Do not give w/ Cialis or other PDE-5 inhibitors.

PREGNANCY AND LACTATION
Category B, caution in nursing.

MECHANISM OF ACTION
PDE-5 inhibitor; increases the concentrations of cGMP, resulting in relaxation of pulmonary vascular smooth muscle cells and vasodilation of the pulmonary vascular bed.

PHARMACOKINETICS
Absorption: T_{max}=4 hrs (median). **Distribution:** V_d=77L; plasma protein binding (94%). **Metabolism:** Liver via CYP3A to a catechol metabolite, which undergoes extensive methylation and glucuronidation; methylcatechol glucuronide (major circulating metabolite). **Elimination:** Feces (61%), urine (36%); $T_{1/2}$=35 hrs.

PATIENT CONSIDERATIONS
Assessment: Assess for CVD, PVOD, renal/hepatic impairment, history of NAION, hereditary degenerative retinal disorders, conditions that might predispose to priapism, anatomical deformation of the penis, bleeding disorders, active peptic ulceration, hypersensitivity to drug, pregnancy/nursing status, and possible drug interactions.

Monitoring: Monitor for signs/symptoms of anginal chest pain, pulmonary edema, NAION, hearing loss, prolonged erections >4 hrs, priapism, and other adverse reactions. Monitor BP.

Counseling: Inform of contraindication of treatment w/ any use of organic nitrates or GC stimulators. Instruct not to take Cialis or other PDE-5 inhibitors. Advise to seek immediate medical attention if sudden loss of vision in 1 or both eyes, sudden decrease/loss of hearing, or erection lasting >4 hrs occurs. Counsel about appropriate action to take if anginal chest pain requiring nitroglycerin occurs following intake of therapy.

ADDERALL — amphetamine aspartate monohydrate/amphetamine sulfate/dextroamphetamine saccharate/dextroamphetamine sulfate   CII

Class: CNS stimulant

> High potential for abuse; prolonged use may lead to drug dependence and must be avoided. Misuse of amphetamine may cause sudden death and serious cardiovascular (CV) adverse events.

ADULT DOSAGE	PEDIATRIC DOSAGE
Narcolepsy	**Narcolepsy**
Initial: 10mg/day	**Usual:** 5-60mg/day in divided doses
Titrate: May increase in increments of 10mg at weekly intervals until optimal response is obtained	**6-12 Years:**
Usual: 5-60mg/day in divided doses	**Initial:** 5mg/day
	Titrate: May increase in increments of 5mg at weekly intervals until optimal response is obtained
Give 1st dose on awakening; additional doses (1 or 2) at intervals of 4-6 hrs	**≥12 Years:**
Attention-Deficit Hyperactivity Disorder	**Initial:** 10mg/day
Refer to pediatric dosing	**Titrate:** May increase in increments of 10mg at weekly intervals until optimal response is obtained
	Give 1st dose on awakening; additional doses (1 or 2) at intervals of 4-6 hrs
	Attention-Deficit Hyperactivity Disorder
	3-5 Years:
	Initial: 2.5mg/day
	Titrate: May increase in increments of 2.5mg at weekly intervals until optimal response is obtained
	≥6 Years:
	Initial: 5mg qd or bid
	Titrate: May increase in increments of 5mg at weekly intervals until optimal response is obtained. Only in rare cases will it be necessary to exceed a total of 40mg/day
	Give 1st dose on awakening; additional doses (1 or 2) at intervals of 4-6 hrs
	Interrupt occasionally to determine the need for continued therapy

DOSING CONSIDERATIONS
Adverse Reactions
Narcolepsy Patients:
Reduce dose if bothersome adverse reactions appear (eg, insomnia or anorexia)

ADMINISTRATION
Oral route

Give 1st dose on awakening; avoid late pm doses due to potential for insomnia.

STORAGE
20-25°C (68-77°F).

HOW SUPPLIED
Tab: 5mg*, 7.5mg*, 10mg*, 12.5mg*, 15mg*, 20mg*, 30mg* *scored

CONTRAINDICATIONS
Advanced arteriosclerosis, symptomatic CV disease, moderate to severe HTN, hyperthyroidism, known hypersensitivity or idiosyncrasy to the sympathomimetic amines, glaucoma, agitated states, history of drug abuse, during or w/in 14 days of MAOI use.

WARNINGS/PRECAUTIONS

Sudden death reported in children and adolescents w/ structural cardiac abnormalities or other serious heart problems. Sudden death, stroke, and MI reported in adults. Avoid use in patients w/ serious structural cardiac abnormalities, cardiomyopathy, serious heart rhythm abnormalities, coronary artery disease, or other serious cardiac problems. May cause modest increase in average BP and HR. Perform prompt cardiac evaluation when symptoms suggestive of cardiac disease develop. May exacerbate symptoms of behavior disturbance and thought disorder in patients w/ preexisting psychotic disorder. Caution in patients w/ comorbid bipolar disorder; may induce mixed/manic episodes. May cause treatment-emergent psychotic/manic symptoms in children and adolescents w/o prior history of psychotic illness or mania; consider discontinuation if such symptoms occur. Aggressive behavior or hostility reported in children and adolescents w/ ADHD. May cause long-term suppression of growth in children; may need to interrupt treatment if patients are not growing or gaining weight as expected. May lower convulsive threshold; d/c if seizures develop. Associated w/ peripheral vasculopathy, including Raynaud's phenomenon. Difficulties w/ accommodation and blurring of vision reported. May exacerbate motor and phonic tics and Tourette's syndrome. May cause a significant elevation in plasma corticosteroid levels or interfere w/ urinary steroid determinations.

ADVERSE REACTIONS

Palpitations, tachycardia, BP elevation, psychotic episodes, tremor, blurred vision, mydriasis, dry mouth, unpleasant taste, anorexia, urticaria, rash, libido changes, alopecia, rhabdomyolysis.

DRUG INTERACTIONS

See Contraindications. GI alkalinizing agents (eg, sodium bicarbonate, antacids) and urinary alkalinizing agents (eg, acetazolamide, some thiazides) may increase blood levels and potentiate effects; avoid w/ GI alkalinizing agents. GI acidifying agents (eg, guanethidine, reserpine, glutamic acid HCl) and urinary acidifying agents (eg, ammonium chloride, sodium acid phosphate) may lower blood levels and efficacy. May inhibit adrenergic blockers. May enhance activity of TCAs or sympathomimetic agents; caution w/ other sympathomimetic drugs. Increased d-amphetamine levels in the brain w/ desipramine or protriptyline and possibly other tricyclics. May counteract sedative effect of antihistamines. May antagonize the hypotensive effects of antihypertensives. Chlorpromazine and haloperidol may inhibit the central stimulant effects. Lithium carbonate may inhibit the anorectic and stimulatory effects. May delay intestinal absorption of ethosuximide, phenobarbital, and phenytoin; may produce a synergistic anticonvulsant action if coadministered w/ phenobarbital or phenytoin. May potentiate analgesic effect of meperidine. May enhance the adrenergic effect of norepinephrine. Use in cases of propoxyphene overdose may potentiate CNS stimulation and cause fatal convulsions. Monitor for changes in clinical effect when coadministered w/ proton pump inhibitors. May inhibit the hypotensive effect of veratrum alkaloids.

PREGNANCY AND LACTATION

Pregnancy: Category C. Infants born to mothers dependent on amphetamines have an increased risk of premature delivery and low birth weight; also, these infants may experience symptoms of withdrawal as demonstrated by dysphoria, including agitation, and significant lassitude. **Lactation:** Found in breast milk; not for use in nursing.

MECHANISM OF ACTION

Sympathomimetic amine w/ CNS stimulant activity; has not been established. Thought to block the reuptake of norepinephrine and dopamine into the presynaptic neuron and increase the release of these monoamines into the extraneuronal space.

PHARMACOKINETICS

Absorption: T_{max}=3 hrs (fasted). **Distribution:** Found in breast milk. **Metabolism:** CYP2D6 (oxidation); 4-hydroxy-amphetamine and norephedrine (active metabolites). **Elimination:** Urine (30-40%, unchanged; 50%, α-hydroxy-amphetamine derivatives). $T_{1/2}$=9.77-11 hrs (d-amphetamine), 11.5-13.8 hrs (l-amphetamine).

PATIENT CONSIDERATIONS

Assessment: Assess for advanced arteriosclerosis, symptomatic CV disease, moderate to severe HTN, hyperthyroidism, hypersensitivity or idiosyncrasy to sympathomimetic amines, glaucoma, agitation, history of drug abuse, psychiatric history, history of seizure, tics or Tourette's syndrome, pregnancy/nursing status, and possible drug interactions. Prior to treatment, adequately screen patients to determine risk for bipolar disorder.

Monitoring: Monitor for CV abnormalities, exacerbations of behavior disturbances and thought disorder, psychotic or manic symptoms, aggressive behavior, hostility, seizures, visual disturbances, exacerbation of motor and phonic tics and Tourette's syndrome, and other adverse reactions. Monitor BP and HR. Monitor growth and weight in children. Periodically reevaluate long-term usefulness of therapy. Observe carefully for signs and symptoms of peripheral vasculopathy; further clinical evaluation (eg, rheumatology referral) may be appropriate for certain patients.

Counseling: Inform about benefits and risks of treatment, appropriate use, and about the potential for abuse/dependence. Instruct to use caution when engaging in potentially hazardous activities (eg, operating machinery or vehicles). Inform about the risk of peripheral vasculopathy, including Raynaud's phenomenon; instruct to report to physician any new numbness, pain, skin color change, or sensitivity to temperature in fingers or toes, and to call physician immediately if any signs of unexplained wounds appear on fingers or toes while on therapy.

ADDERALL XR — amphetamine aspartate monohydrate/amphetamine sulfate/dextroamphetamine saccharate/dextroamphetamine sulfate

CII

Class: CNS stimulant

> High potential for abuse; prolonged use may lead to drug dependence. Misuse may cause sudden death and serious cardiovascular (CV) adverse reactions.

ADULT DOSAGE	PEDIATRIC DOSAGE
Attention-Deficit Hyperactivity Disorder	**Attention-Deficit Hyperactivity Disorder**
Amphetamine-Naïve/Switching from Another Medication: 20mg qam	**Amphetamine-Naïve/Switching from Another Medication:**
Switching from Amphetamine Immediate-Release: Give the same total daily dose, qd	**6-12 Years:** **Initial:** 10mg qam or 5mg qam when lower initial dose is appropriate
Titrate at weekly intervals as indicated	**Titrate:** Adjust daily dosage in increments of 5mg or 10mg at weekly intervals **Max:** 30mg/day
	13-17 Years: **Initial:** 10mg qam **Titrate:** May increase to 20mg/day after 1 week if symptoms are not controlled
	Switching from Amphetamine Immediate-Release: **≥6 Years:** Give the same total daily dose, qd Titrate at weekly intervals as indicated

ADMINISTRATION

Oral route

Give upon awakening; avoid pm doses due to potential for insomnia
Take w/ or w/o food
Take caps whole or sprinkle entire contents on applesauce. Consume sprinkled applesauce immediately w/o chewing the sprinkled beads
Do not divide the dose of a single cap or take anything <1 cap/day

STORAGE

25°C (77°F); excursions permitted to 15-30°C (59-86°F).

HOW SUPPLIED

Cap, Extended-Release: 5mg, 10mg, 15mg, 20mg, 25mg, 30mg

CONTRAINDICATIONS

Advanced arteriosclerosis, symptomatic CV disease, moderate to severe HTN, hyperthyroidism, known hypersensitivity or idiosyncrasy to the sympathomimetic amines (eg, anaphylaxis, angioedema, serious skin rashes), glaucoma, agitated states, history of drug abuse, during or w/in 14 days following MAOI use.

WARNINGS/PRECAUTIONS

Sudden death, stroke, and MI reported in adults. Sudden death reported in children and adolescents w/ structural cardiac abnormalities or other serious heart problems. Avoid use in patients w/ known serious structural cardiac and heart rhythm abnormalities, cardiomyopathy, coronary artery disease, or other serious cardiac problems. May cause modest increase in BP and HR. May exacerbate symptoms of behavior disturbance and thought disorder in patients w/ preexisting psychotic disorder. Caution in patients w/ comorbid bipolar disorder; may cause induction of mixed/manic episode. May cause treatment-emergent psychotic/manic symptoms in children and adolescents w/o a prior history of psychotic illness or mania; consider discontinuation if such symptoms occur. Aggressive behavior or hostility reported; monitor for appearance or worsening. May cause long-term suppression of growth in children; may need to d/c if patients are not growing or gaining weight as expected. May lower convulsive threshold; d/c if seizures develop. Associated w/ peripheral vasculopathy, including Raynaud's phenomenon. Difficulties w/ accommodation and blurring of vision reported. Exacerbation of motor and phonic tics and Tourette's syndrome reported. May significantly elevate plasma corticosteroid levels or interfere w/ urinary steroid determinations. Where possible, interrupt occasionally to determine the need for continued therapy.

ADVERSE REACTIONS

Dry mouth, loss of appetite, insomnia, headache, abdominal pain, weight loss, agitation, anxiety, N/V, dizziness, tachycardia, nervousness, asthenia, diarrhea, UTI.

DRUG INTERACTIONS

See Contraindications. Avoid w/ GI alkalinizing agents (eg, sodium bicarbonate, antacids). Urinary alkalinizing agents (eg, acetazolamide, some thiazides) may increase blood levels and potentiate effects. GI acidifying agents (eg, guanethidine, reserpine, ascorbic acid) and urinary acidifying agents (eg, ammonium chloride, sodium acid phosphate, methenamine salts) may lower blood levels and efficacy. May reduce CV effects of adrenergic blockers. May counteract sedative effects of antihistamines. May antagonize effects of antihypertensives. May inhibit hypotensive effect of veratrum alkaloids. May delay intestinal absorption of phenobarbital, phenytoin, and ethosuximide. May enhance activity of TCAs or sympathomimetic agents. Increased d-amphetamine levels in the brain w/ desipramine or protriptyline and possibly other tricyclics. May potentiate analgesic effect of meperidine. May enhance the adrenergic effect of norepinephrine. Chlorpromazine and haloperidol may inhibit central stimulant effects. Lithium carbonate may inhibit anorectic and stimulatory effects. Norepinephrine may enhance the adrenergic effect. Use in cases of propoxyphene overdose may potentiate CNS stimulation and cause fatal convulsions. Monitor for changes in clinical effect when coadministered w/ proton pump inhibitors.

PREGNANCY AND LACTATION
Category C, not for use in nursing.

MECHANISM OF ACTION
Sympathomimetic amine; has not been established. Thought to block the reuptake of norepinephrine and dopamine into the presynaptic neuron and increase the release of these monoamines into the extraneuronal space.

PHARMACOKINETICS
Absorption: T_{max}=7 hrs. **Distribution:** Found in breast milk. **Metabolism:** CYP2D6 (oxidation); 4-hydroxy-amphetamine and norephedrine (active metabolites). **Elimination:** Urine (normal pH) (30-40%, unchanged; 50%, α-hydroxy-amphetamine derivatives). (20mg single dose) d-amphetamine: $T_{1/2}$=10 hrs (adults), 11 hrs (13-17 yrs of age), 9 hrs (6-12 yrs of age). l-amphetamine: $T_{1/2}$=13 hrs (adults), 13-14 hrs (13-17 yrs of age), 11 hrs (6-12 yrs of age).

PATIENT CONSIDERATIONS
Assessment: Assess for advanced arteriosclerosis, symptomatic CV disease, moderate to severe HTN, hyperthyroidism, hypersensitivity or idiosyncrasy to sympathomimetic amines, glaucoma, agitation, history of drug abuse, psychiatric history, history of seizure, tics or Tourette's syndrome, hepatic/renal dysfunction, pregnancy/nursing status, and possible drug interactions.

Monitoring: Monitor for CV abnormalities, exacerbations of behavior disturbances and thought disorder, psychotic or manic symptoms, aggressive behavior, hostility, seizures, visual disturbances, exacerbation of motor and phonic tics and Tourette's syndrome, and other adverse reactions. Monitor BP and HR. Monitor height and weight in children. Observe carefully for signs and symptoms of peripheral vasculopathy; further clinical evaluation (eg, rheumatology referral) may be appropriate for certain patients.

Counseling: Inform about benefits and risks of treatment, appropriate use, and about the potential for abuse/dependence. Advise about serious CV risks. Inform that treatment-emergent psychotic or manic symptoms may occur. Instruct to report signs/symptoms of peripheral vasculopathy, including Raynaud's phenomenon. Advise parents or guardians of pediatric patients to monitor growth and weight during treatment. Advise to notify physician if pregnant or planning to become pregnant. Advise to avoid breastfeeding. Advise to use caution when engaging in potentially hazardous activities (eg, operating machinery or vehicles).

ADDYI — flibanserin   Rx
Class: Mixed 5-HT$_{1A}$ agonist/5-HT$_{2A}$ antagonist

> **Alcohol increases the risk of severe hypotension and syncope; alcohol use is contraindicated. Before prescribing, assess the likelihood of abstaining from alcohol, taking into account current/past drinking behavior, and other pertinent social and medical history. Available only through a restricted program under a Risk Evaluation and Mitigation Strategy (REMS) called the Addyi REMS Program. Contraindicated w/ concomitant moderate or strong CYP3A4 inhibitors and in patients w/ hepatic impairment due to increases in flibanserin concentrations and potential for severe hypotension and syncope.**

ADULT DOSAGE
Hypoactive Sexual Desire Disorder

Treatment of premenopausal women w/ acquired, generalized hypoactive sexual desire disorder (HSDD); as characterized by low sexual desire that causes marked distress or interpersonal difficulty and is not caused by a coexisting medical or psychiatric condition, problems w/ in the relationship, or the effects of a medication or other drug substance

100mg qhs; d/c after 8 weeks if no improvement in symptoms

Missed Dose

If dose is missed at hs; take next dose at hs on the next day; do not double the next dose

PEDIATRIC DOSAGE
Pediatric use may not have been established

DOSING CONSIDERATIONS
Concomitant Medications
If initiating flibanserin following moderate/strong CYP3A4 inhibitor use, start 2 weeks after last dose of the CYP3A4 inhibitor

If initiating a moderate or strong CYP3A4 inhibitor following flibanserin use, start moderate or strong CYP3A4 inhibitor 2 days after the last dose of flibanserin

ADMINISTRATION
Oral route

STORAGE
25°C (77°F); excursions permitted to 15-30°C (59-86°F).

HOW SUPPLIED
Tab: 100mg

CONTRAINDICATIONS
Concomitant use w/ alcohol, moderate or strong CYP3A4 inhibitors, and in patients w/ hepatic impairment.

WARNINGS/PRECAUTIONS
Not indicated to enhance sexual performance. May cause CNS depression (eg, somnolence, sedation), hypotension, and syncope; increased risk if taken during waking hrs. May impair mental/physical abilities; wait ≥6 hrs after taking therapy before driving or engaging in activities requiring full alertness. Consider the benefits of use and the risks of hypotension and syncope in patients w/ preexisting conditions that predispose them to hypotension. Immediately lie supine if experiencing presyncope and promptly seek medical help if the symptoms do not resolve or if experiencing syncope. CYP2C19 poor metabolizers had increased flibanserin exposures; increase monitoring for adverse reactions.

ADVERSE REACTIONS
Dizziness, somnolence, nausea, fatigue, insomnia, dry mouth.

DRUG INTERACTIONS
See Boxed Warning/Dosing Considerations. If benefit of initiating a moderate/strong CYP3A4 inhibitor (eg, ketoconazole, clarithromycin, ciprofloxacin) w/in 2 days of stopping flibanserin outweighs risk, monitor patient for signs of hypotension and syncope. Concomitant use of multiple weak CYP3A4 inhibitors (eg, cimetidine, fluoxetine, ginkgo) may increase flibanserin concentrations and the risk of adverse reactions. CNS depressants (eg, diphenhydramine, opioids, hypnotics) may increase the risk of CNS depression. Strong CYP2C19 inhibitors (eg, proton pump inhibitors, SSRIs, benzodiazepines) may increase flibanserin exposure which may increase the risk of hypotension, syncope, and CNS depression. CYP3A4 inducers (eg, carbamazepine, phenobarbital, rifampin) decrease flibanserin exposure; concomitant use is not recommended. May increase concentrations of digoxin or other P-gp substrates (eg, sirolimus); increase monitoring of concentrations of drugs transported by P-gp that have a narrow therapeutic index.

PREGNANCY AND LACTATION
Pregnancy: There are no studies in pregnant women to inform whether there is a drug-associated risk in humans.
Lactation: It is unknown whether flibanserin is present in human milk; not for use in nursing.

MECHANISM OF ACTION
5-HT$_{1A}$ agonist/5-HT$_{2A, 2B, 2C}$ antagonist/Dopamine D$_4$ antagonist; mechanism of action is unknown.

PHARMACOKINETICS
Absorption: Absolute bioavailability (33%); C_{max}=419ng/mL; AUC_{0-inf}=1543ng•hr/mL; T_{max}=0.75 hrs (median). **Distribution:** Plasma protein binding (98%). **Metabolism:** CYP3A4 (major), CYP2C19. **Elimination:** (50mg oral sol) Feces (51%), urine (44%); $T_{1/2}$=11 hrs.

PATIENT CONSIDERATIONS
Assessment: Assess for coexisting medical or psychiatric conditions, problems w/ in the relationship, or effects of a medication or other drug substance that may be contributing to HSDD. Assess for alcohol use and likelihood of the patient abstaining from alcohol, taking into account the patient's current and past drinking behavior, and other pertinent social and medical history. Assess if patient is a poor CYP2C19 metabolizer. Assess for preexisting conditions that predispose to hypotension, hepatic impairment, pregnancy/nursing status, and for possible drug interactions.

Monitoring: Monitor for CNS depression, hypotension, syncope, and other adverse reactions. Perform increased monitoring for adverse reactions in patients who are CYP2C19 poor metabolizers. If on concomitant therapy w/ digoxin or another P-gp substrate that has a narrow therapeutic index, perform increased monitoring of the P-gp substrate concentration.

Counseling: Advise to take at hs and not any other time of the day. Inform that drug may cause severe hypotension and syncope, particularly w/ alcohol or w/ moderate and strong CYP3A4 inhibitors; inform that concomitant use is contraindicated. Notify about the importance of abstaining from alcohol and to consult w/ physician before starting a new prescription, nonprescription medication, or using other products that contain CYP3A4 inhibitors (eg, grapefruit juice, St. John's wort). Advise patients who experience presyncope or lightheadedness to lie down and to call for help if symptoms persist. Inform patients that they can only obtain the drug from certified pharmacies participating in the Addyi REMS Program. Inform that drug may cause CNS depression and that risk is increased if taken during waking hrs; advise to avoid engaging in activities requiring full alertness until ≥6 hrs after taking the drug and until the patient knows how it affects her. Advise not to breastfeed.

ADEMPAS — riociguat   Rx
Class: Soluble guanylate cyclase (sGC) stimulator

> **Do not administer to a pregnant female; may cause fetal harm. Exclude pregnancy before the start of treatment, monthly during treatment, and 1 month after stopping treatment. Prevent pregnancy during and for 1 month after stopping treatment; use acceptable methods of contraception. For all female patients, available only through a restricted program called the Adempas Risk Evaluation and Mitigation Strategy (REMS) Program.**

ADULT DOSAGE
Chronic-Thromboembolic Pulmonary Hypertension

Treatment of persistent/recurrent chronic thromboembolic pulmonary hypertension (CTEPH) WHO Group 4 after surgical treatment, or inoperable CTEPH, to improve exercise capacity and WHO functional class

PEDIATRIC DOSAGE
Pediatric use may not have been established

Initial: 1mg tid; consider 0.5mg tid for patients who may not tolerate the hypotensive effect

Titrate: Increase by 0.5mg tid if systolic BP remains >95mmHg and patient has no signs/symptoms of hypotension

Dose increases should be no sooner than 2 weeks apart

Max: 2.5mg tid; if patient has symptoms of hypotension, decrease the dose by 0.5mg tid

Dose Interruption:
Retitrate if treatment is interrupted for ≥3 days

Pulmonary Arterial Hypertension

Treatment of pulmonary arterial HTN, (WHO Group 1), to improve exercise capacity, WHO functional class, and to delay clinical worsening

Initial: 1mg tid; consider 0.5mg tid for patients who may not tolerate the hypotensive effect

Titrate: Increase by 0.5mg tid if systolic BP remains >95mmHg and patient has no signs/symptoms of hypotension

Dose increases should be no sooner than 2 weeks apart

Max: 2.5mg tid; if patient has symptoms of hypotension, decrease the dose by 0.5mg tid

Dose Interruption:
Retitrate if treatment is interrupted for ≥3 days

DOSING CONSIDERATIONS
Concomitant Medications
Strong CYP and P-gp/Breast Cancer Resistance Protein (P-gp/BCRP) Inhibitors (eg, Azole Antimycotics, HIV Protease Inhibitors):
Initial: 0.5mg tid

Other Important Considerations
Patients Who Smoke:
Consider titrating to dosages >2.5mg tid, if tolerated
May require a dose decrease in patients who stop smoking

ADMINISTRATION
Oral route

Take PO w/ or w/o food

STORAGE
25°C (77°F); excursions permitted from 15-30°C (59-86°F).

HOW SUPPLIED
Tab: 0.5mg, 1mg, 1.5mg, 2mg, 2.5mg

CONTRAINDICATIONS
Pregnancy. Coadministration with nitrates or nitric oxide (NO) donors (eg, amyl nitrite) in any form, specific PDE-5 inhibitors (eg, sildenafil, tadalafil, vardenafil), or nonspecific PDE inhibitors (eg, dipyridamole, theophylline).

WARNINGS/PRECAUTIONS
Reduces BP; consider the potential for symptomatic hypotension or ischemia in patients with hypovolemia, severe left ventricular outflow obstruction, resting hypotension, or autonomic dysfunction. Serious bleeding/hemoptysis/hemorrhagic events reported. May significantly worsen the cardiovascular status of patients with pulmonary veno-occlusive disease (PVOD); administration to such patients is not recommended. If signs of pulmonary edema occur, consider possibility of associated PVOD and, if confirmed, d/c treatment. Caution in elderly.

ADVERSE REACTIONS
Headache, dyspepsia, gastritis, dizziness, N/V, diarrhea, hypotension, anemia, gastroesophageal reflux disease, constipation.

DRUG INTERACTIONS
See Contraindications and Dosing Considerations. Consider the potential for symptomatic hypotension or ischemia with concomitant antihypertensives. Smoking may reduce concentrations. Strong CYP inhibitors and P-gp/BCRP inhibitors increase exposure and may result in hypotension. Strong CYP3A inducers (eg, rifampin, phenytoin, carbamazepine) may significantly reduce exposure. Antacids (eg, aluminum hydroxide, magnesium hydroxide) decrease absorption and should not be taken within 1 hr of taking riociguat.

PREGNANCY AND LACTATION
Category X, not for use in nursing.

MECHANISM OF ACTION
sGC stimulator; sensitizes sGC to endogenous NO by stabilizing the NO-sGC binding. Also, directly stimulates sGC via a different binding site, independently of NO. Stimulates the NO-sGC-cGMP pathway and leads to increased generation of cGMP with subsequent vasodilation.

PHARMACOKINETICS
Absorption: Absolute bioavailability (94%); T_{max}=1.5 hrs. **Distribution:** V_d=30L; plasma protein binding (95%). **Metabolism:** CYP1A1, CYP3A, CYP2C8, CYP2J2; M1 (major active metabolite) (catalyzed by CYP1A1). **Elimination:** Urine (40%); feces (53%); $T_{1/2}$=12 hrs.

PATIENT CONSIDERATIONS
Assessment: Assess for hypovolemia, severe left ventricular outflow obstruction, resting hypotension, autonomic dysfunction, PVOD, pregnancy/nursing status, and possible drug interactions.

Monitoring: Monitor for signs/symptoms of hypotension, bleeding, pulmonary edema, and other adverse reactions. Obtain pregnancy tests monthly during treatment and 1 month after discontinuation of treatment.

Counseling: Counsel on the risk of fetal harm when used during pregnancy; instruct females of reproductive potential to use effective contraception during therapy and for 1 month after stopping treatment. Instruct to contact physician immediately if pregnancy is suspected. Inform female patients that they must enroll in the Adempas REMS Program. Advise about the potential risks/signs of hemoptysis and to report any potential signs of hemoptysis to physician. Instruct to report all current and new medications, and smoking history to physician. Advise that antacids should not be taken within 1 hr of taking the drug. Inform that drug can cause dizziness, which can affect the ability to drive and use machines.

ADLYXIN — lixisenatide   Rx

Class: Glucagon-like peptide-1 (GLP-1) receptor agonist

ADULT DOSAGE	PEDIATRIC DOSAGE
Type 2 Diabetes Mellitus	Pediatric use may not have been established
Initial: 10mcg qd for 14 days	
Maint: Increase to 20mcg qd starting on Day 15	
Missed Dose	
If a dose is missed, administer w/in 1 hr prior to the next meal	

DOSING CONSIDERATIONS
Renal Impairment
Mild (eGFR: 60 to 89mL/min/1.73m²): No dosage adjustment required; closely monitor for lixisenatide-related adverse reactions and for changes in renal function
Moderate (eGFR: 30 to <60mL/min/1.73 m²): No dosing adjustment is recommended; closely monitor for lixisenatide-related adverse GI reactions
Severe (eGFR 15 to <30mL/min/1.73 m²): Limited clinical experience; closely monitor for GI adverse reactions and for changes in renal function
ESRD (eGFR <15 mL/min/1.73 m²): Use not recommended

Other Important Considerations
Gastroparesis: Do not initiate in patients w/ severe gastroparesis

ADMINISTRATION
SQ route

- Administer in the abdomen, thigh, or upper arm.
- Rotate inj site w/ each dose; do not use the same site.
- Administer w/in 1 hr before the first meal of the day, preferably the same meal each day.
- Protect pen from light.
- Discard pen 14 days after its first use.

STORAGE
Prior to First Use: 2-8°C (36-46°F) Do not freeze. Protect from light. **After First Use:** <30°C (86°F). Replace pen cap after each use to protect from light. Discard pen 14 days after first use.

HOW SUPPLIED
Inj: 50mcg/mL [3mL], 100mcg/mL [3mL]

CONTRAINDICATIONS
Known hypersensitivity to lixisenatide or to any component of this product.

WARNINGS/PRECAUTIONS
Consider other antidiabetic therapies in patients w/ a history of pancreatitis. Not a substitute for insulin; not indicated for use in type 1 diabetes mellitus or for treatment of diabetic ketoacidosis. Not recommended in patients w/ gastroparesis. Anaphylaxis and other serious hypersensitivity reactions (eg, angioedema) reported. Closely monitor patients w/ a history of anaphylaxis or angioedema w/ another GLP-1 receptor agonist for allergic reactions; d/c therapy and promptly seek medical attention if a hypersensitivity reaction occurs. Acute pancreatitis, including fatal and nonfatal hemorrhagic or necrotizing pancreatitis, reported; d/c if suspected and initiate appropriate management. Do not restart if pancreatitis is confirmed. Pen-sharing poses a risk for transmission of blood-borne pathogens; never share pens between patients, even if the needle is changed. Acute kidney injury and worsening of chronic renal failure, sometimes requiring hemodialysis, reported. Monitor renal function when initiating or escalating doses in patients w/ renal impairment and in patients reporting severe GI reactions. May develop antibodies; consider alternative antidiabetic therapy if there is worsening glycemic control or failure to achieve targeted glycemic control.

ADVERSE REACTIONS
N/V, headache, diarrhea, dizziness, hypoglycemia.

DRUG INTERACTIONS

Concurrent use w/ short-acting insulin is not recommended. Increased risk of hypoglycemia w/ concomitant use of basal insulin or a sulfonylurea; dose reduction of the sulfonylurea or basal insulin may be necessary. Lixisenatide delays gastric emptying, which may reduce the rate of absorption of orally administered medications; caution when coadministering oral medications that have a narrow therapeutic ratio or that require careful clinical monitoring. If such medications are to be administered w/ food, they should be taken w/ a meal or snack when lixisenatide is not administered. Administer oral medications that are particularly dependent on threshold concentrations for efficacy (eg, antibiotics), or medications for which a delay in effect is undesirable (eg, acetaminophen), at least 1 hr before lixisenatide. Oral contraceptives should be taken at least 1 hr before lixisenatide administration or at least 11 hrs after the lixisenatide dose.

PREGNANCY AND LACTATION

Pregnancy: Based on animal reproduction studies, there may be risks to the fetus from exposure to lixisenatide during pregnancy; should only be used during pregnancy if the potential benefit justifies the potential risk to the fetus.
Lactation: There is no information regarding the presence of lixisenatide in human milk, the effects on the breastfed infant, or the effects on milk production. Caution in nursing.

MECHANISM OF ACTION

GLP-1 receptor agonist; increases glucose-dependent insulin release, decreases glucagon secretion, and slows gastric emptying.

PHARMACOKINETICS

Absorption: T_{max}=1-3.5 hrs (median). **Distribution:** V_d=100L. **Elimination:** $T_{1/2}$= approx 3 hrs.

PATIENT CONSIDERATIONS

Assessment: Assess for known hypersensitivity to lixisenatide or to any component of this product, history of anaphylaxis or angioedema w/ another GLP-1 receptor agonist, history of pancreatitis, gastroparesis, renal impairment, pregnancy/nursing status, and for possible drug interactions. Assess renal function in patients w/ renal impairment. Obtain baseline blood glucose levels.

Monitoring: Monitor for anaphylaxis and other serious hypersensitivity reactions, pancreatitis, acute kidney injury, worsening of chronic renal failure, development of antibodies to lixisenatide, and other adverse reactions. Monitor renal function when escalating doses of therapy in patients w/ renal impairment and in patients reporting severe GI reactions. Monitor blood glucose levels.

Counseling: Inform about risks/benefits of therapy. Advise on how to administer therapy. Instruct to d/c therapy and to seek prompt medical advice if symptoms of a hypersensitivity reaction occur. Inform that persistent severe abdominal pain that may radiate to the back and which may or may not be accompanied by vomiting is the hallmark symptom of acute pancreatitis; instruct to promptly d/c therapy and contact physician if persistent severe abdominal pain occurs. Advise never to share lixisenatide pen w/ another person, even if the needle is changed, because doing so carries a risk for transmission of blood-borne pathogens. Inform that the risk of hypoglycemia is increased when therapy is used in combination w/ a sulfonylurea or basal insulin. Advise of the risk of dehydration due to GI adverse reactions and instruct to take precautions to avoid fluid depletion. Inform of risk for worsening renal function, which in some cases may require dialysis. Advise to inform physician if patient is pregnant, intends to become pregnant, or is nursing.

ADOXA — doxycycline   Rx

Class: Tetracyclines

ADULT DOSAGE

General Dosing

Initial: 100mg q12h or 50mg q6h on 1st day
Maint: 100mg qd or 50mg q12h

More Severe Infections (eg, Chronic UTIs): 100mg q12h

Streptococcal Infections: Continue therapy for 10 days

Gonococcal Infections

Uncomplicated Infections (Except Anorectal Infections in Men): 100mg bid for 7 days

Alternate Dosing:
Single visit dose of 300mg stat followed in 1 hr by a second 300mg dose

Acute Epididymo-Orchitis

Caused by *Neisseria gonorrhoeae*/ *Chlamydia trachomatis*:
100mg bid for at least 10 days

Syphilis

Patients Allergic to Penicillin: Primary and Secondary:
300mg/day in divided doses for at least 10 days

PEDIATRIC DOSAGE

General Dosing

>8 Years:

≤100 lbs:
2mg/lb divided into 2 doses on 1st day, followed by 1mg/lb qd or as 2 divided doses, on subsequent days
More Severe Infections: Up to 2mg/lb

>100 lbs:
Initial: 100mg q12h or 50mg q6h on 1st day
Maint: 100mg qd or 50mg q12h
More Severe Infections (eg, Chronic UTIs): 100mg q12h

Streptococcal Infections:
Continue therapy for 10 days

Inhalational Anthrax (Postexposure)

<100 lbs:
1mg/lb bid for 60 days
≥100 lbs:
100mg bid for 60 days

Other Indications

The following infections caused by susceptible microorganisms: Rocky Mountain spotted fever, typhus fever and the typhus group, Q fever,

Chlamydia trachomatis Infections

Uncomplicated Urethral/ Endocervical/Rectal Infections Caused by *Chlamydia trachomatis*:
100mg bid for at least 7 days

Nongonococcal Urethritis

Caused by *Chlamydia trachomatis* and *Ureaplasma urealyticum*:
100mg bid for at least 7 days

Inhalational Anthrax (Postexposure)

100mg bid for 60 days

Other Indications

The following infections caused by susceptible microorganisms: Rocky Mountain spotted fever, typhus fever and the typhus group, Q fever, rickettsialpox, tick fevers, respiratory tract infections, lymphogranuloma venereum, psittacosis (ornithosis), trachoma, inclusion conjunctivitis, relapsing fever, chancroid, plague, tularemia, cholera, *Campylobacter fetus* infections, brucellosis, bartonellosis, granuloma inguinale, UTIs, skin and skin structure infections, and anthrax

Infections caused by *Escherichia coli*, *Enterobacter aerogenes*, *Shigella* species, or *Acinetobacter* species

When penicillin is contraindicated, treatment of the following infections caused by susceptible microorganisms: yaws, listeriosis, Vincent's infection, actinomycosis, and infections caused by *Clostridium* species

Adjunct to amebicides in acute intestinal amebiasis

Adjunctive therapy in severe acne

rickettsialpox, tick fevers, respiratory tract infections, lymphogranuloma venereum, psittacosis (ornithosis), trachoma, inclusion conjunctivitis, relapsing fever, chancroid, plague, tularemia, cholera, *Campylobacter fetus* infections, brucellosis, bartonellosis, granuloma inguinale, UTIs, skin and skin structure infections, and anthrax

Infections caused by *Escherichia coli*, *Enterobacter aerogenes*, *Shigella* species, or *Acinetobacter* species

When penicillin is contraindicated, treatment of the following infections caused by susceptible microorganisms: uncomplicated gonorrhea, syphilis, yaws, listeriosis, Vincent's infection, actinomycosis, and infections caused by *Clostridium* species

Adjunct to amebicides in acute intestinal amebiasis

Adjunctive therapy in severe acne

ADMINISTRATION

Oral route

Administer w/ adequate amounts of fluid
May be given w/ food if gastric irritation occurs

STORAGE

20-25°C (68-77°F).

HOW SUPPLIED

Cap: 150mg

CONTRAINDICATIONS

Hypersensitivity to any of the tetracyclines.

WARNINGS/PRECAUTIONS

May cause permanent discoloration of the teeth (yellow-gray-brown) if used during tooth development (last 1/2 of pregnancy, infancy, and childhood to 8 yrs of age); do not use in this age group, except for anthrax. Enamel hypoplasia reported. *Clostridium difficile*-associated diarrhea (CDAD) reported; may need to d/c if CDAD is suspected or confirmed. May decrease fibula growth rate in prematures. May cause an increase in BUN. Photosensitivity manifested by an exaggerated sunburn reaction reported; d/c at the 1st evidence of skin erythema. May result in bacterial resistance if used in the absence of proven or suspected bacterial infection, or a prophylactic indication; take appropriate measures if superinfection develops. Bulging fontanels in infants and benign intracranial HTN in adults reported. False elevations of urinary catecholamine levels may occur due to interference w/ the fluorescence test.

ADVERSE REACTIONS

Anorexia, N/V, diarrhea, hepatotoxicity, maculopapular/erythematous rash, Stevens-Johnson syndrome, toxic epidermal necrolysis, urticaria, anaphylaxis, pericarditis, hemolytic anemia, thrombocytopenia, neutropenia, eosinophilia.

DRUG INTERACTIONS

Depresses plasma prothrombin activity; may require downward adjustment of anticoagulant dose. May interfere w/ bactericidal action of PCN; avoid concurrent use. Impaired absorption w/ antacids containing aluminum, Ca^{2+}, or Mg^{2+}, and iron-containing preparations. Decreased $T_{1/2}$ w/ barbiturates, carbamazepine, and phenytoin. Fatal renal toxicity reported w/ methoxyflurane. May render oral contraceptives less effective.

PREGNANCY AND LACTATION

Category D, not for use in nursing.

MECHANISM OF ACTION

Tetracycline; primarily bacteriostatic and thought to exert antimicrobial effect by inhibition of protein synthesis.

PHARMACOKINETICS

Absorption: Readily absorbed; virtually complete. (200mg) C_{max}=3.61mcg/mL; T_{max}=2.6 hrs. **Distribution:** Plasma protein binding in varying degrees; found in breast milk. **Elimination:** Urine (40%/72 hrs in CrCl 75mL/min, 1-5%/72 hrs in CrCl <10mL/min), feces; $T_{1/2}$=18-22 hrs.

PATIENT CONSIDERATIONS

Assessment: Assess for hypersensitivity to drug or any tetracyclines, pregnancy/nursing status, and possible drug interactions. Perform culture and susceptibility tests. In venereal disease when coexistent syphilis is suspected, perform a dark-field examination and blood serology.

Monitoring: Monitor for signs/symptoms of CDAD, photosensitivity, skin erythema, superinfection, bulging fontanels in infants, intracranial HTN in adults, and other adverse reactions. In long-term therapy, perform periodic lab evaluations of organ systems, including hematopoietic, renal, and hepatic studies. In venereal disease when coexistent syphilis is suspected, repeat blood serology monthly for at least 4 months.

Counseling: Apprise of the potential hazard to fetus if used during pregnancy; instruct to notify physician if pregnant. Advise to avoid excessive sunlight or artificial UV light and to d/c therapy if phototoxicity (eg, skin eruptions) occurs; advise to consider use of sunscreen or sunblock. Inform that absorption of drug is reduced when taken w/ bismuth subsalicylate and w/ foods, especially those that contain Ca^{2+}. Inform that drug may increase the incidence of vaginal candidiasis. Inform that diarrhea may be experienced and instruct to immediately contact physician if watery and bloody stools (w/ or w/o stomach cramps and fever) occur, even as late as ≥2 months after the last dose. Counsel that therapy should only be used to treat bacterial, not viral, infections. Instruct to take exactly ud even if the patient feels better early in the course of therapy. Inform that skipping doses or not completing the full course of therapy may decrease effectiveness of treatment and increase bacterial resistance.

ADRENACLICK — *epinephrine*   Rx

Class: Sympathomimetic catecholamine

ADULT DOSAGE	PEDIATRIC DOSAGE
Emergency Treatment of Type I Allergic Reactions	**Emergency Treatment of Type I Allergic Reactions**
Includes anaphylaxis to stinging and biting insects, allergen immunotherapy, foods, drugs, diagnostic testing substances, and other allergens, as well as idiopathic anaphylaxis or exercise-induced anaphylaxis	Includes anaphylaxis to stinging and biting insects, allergen immunotherapy, foods, drugs, diagnostic testing substances, and other allergens, as well as idiopathic anaphylaxis or exercise-induced anaphylaxis
15-30kg: 0.15mg IM/SQ	**15-30kg:** 0.15mg IM/SQ
≥30kg: 0.3mg IM/SQ	**≥30kg:** 0.3mg IM/SQ
Severe Persistent Anaphylaxis: Repeat inj may be necessary	**Severe Persistent Anaphylaxis:** Repeat inj may be necessary

---

ADMINISTRATION
IM/SQ route

Inject into the anterolateral aspect of the thigh, through clothing if necessary. Caregivers of young children who may be uncooperative and kick or move during an inj should hold the leg firmly in place and limit movement prior to and during administration.

Consider using other forms of injectable epinephrine if doses <0.15mg are deemed necessary.

STORAGE
20-25°C (68-77°F); excursions permitted to 15-30°C (59-86°F). Store in the carrying-case provided. Protect from light. Do not refrigerate.

HOW SUPPLIED
Inj: 0.15mg/0.15mL, 0.3mg/0.3mL

WARNINGS/PRECAUTIONS
Intended for immediate administration in patients who are determined to be at increased risk for anaphylaxis, including those w/ a history of anaphylactic reactions. Intended for immediate administration as emergency supportive therapy only and is not a substitute for immediate medical care. More than 2 sequential doses should only be administered under direct medical supervision. Do not inject IV. Large doses or accidental IV inj may result in cerebral hemorrhage due to sharp rise in BP; rapidly acting vasodilators can counteract the marked pressor effects of epinephrine. Do not inject into buttock; may not provide effective treatment of anaphylaxis. Do not inject into digits, hands, or feet; may result in loss of blood flow to the affected area. Lacerations, bent needles, and embedded needles reported in children who were uncooperative, kicking, or moving during administration; hold child's leg firmly in place and limit movement prior to and during inj. Rare cases of serious skin and soft tissue infections, including necrotizing fasciitis and myonecrosis caused by Clostridia, reported; do not inject into the buttock to decrease the risk of *Clostridium* infection. Contains sodium bisulfite; should not deter administration of the drug for treatment of serious allergic or other emergency situations, even in certain susceptible persons. Caution in elderly, pregnant women, and patients w/ heart disease, hyperthyroidism, or diabetes mellitus (DM). May temporarily worsen symptoms of Parkinson's disease.

ADVERSE REACTIONS
Anxiety, apprehensiveness, restlessness, tremor, weakness, dizziness, sweating, palpitations, pallor, N/V, headache, respiratory difficulties.

DRUG INTERACTIONS
May precipitate/aggravate angina pectoris as well as produce ventricular arrhythmias w/ drugs that may sensitize the heart to arrhythmias; use w/ caution. Monitor for cardiac arrhythmias w/ antiarrhythmics, cardiac glycosides, and diuretics. Effects of epinephrine may be potentiated by TCAs, MAOIs, levothyroxine sodium, and certain antihistamines (eg, chlorpheniramine, tripelennamine, diphenhydramine). Cardiostimulating and bronchodilating effects are antagonized by β-adrenergic blockers (eg, propranolol). Vasoconstricting and hypertensive effects are antagonized by α-adrenergic blockers (eg, phentolamine). Ergot alkaloids may reverse pressor effects.

PREGNANCY AND LACTATION
Pregnancy: Category C.
Lactation: It is not known whether epinephrine is excreted in human milk; caution in nursing.

MECHANISM OF ACTION
Sympathomimetic catecholamine; acts on α-adrenergic receptors and lessens the vasodilation and increased vascular permeability that occurs during anaphylaxis. Acts on β-adrenergic receptors, causing bronchial smooth muscle relaxation. Also may alleviate GI and genitourinary symptoms associated w/ anaphylaxis due to relaxer effects on smooth muscle of the stomach, intestine, uterus, and urinary bladder.

PATIENT CONSIDERATIONS

Assessment: Assess for risk of anaphylaxis, heart disease, hyperthyroidism, DM, Parkinson's disease, pregnancy/nursing status, and for possible drug interactions.

Monitoring: Monitor for allergic-type reactions, angina pectoris, ventricular arrhythmias, cerebral hemorrhage, serious skin and soft tissue infections, and other adverse reactions. Monitor HR and BP.

Counseling: Review patient instructions and operation of drug w/ patient and caregiver. Advise that therapy may produce signs/symptoms that include increased HR, sensation of more forceful heartbeat, palpitations, sweating, N/V, difficulty breathing, pallor, dizziness, weakness or shakiness, headache, apprehension, nervousness, or anxiety; advise that these signs and symptoms usually subside rapidly, especially w/ rest, quiet, and recumbency. Inform that patients may develop more severe or persistent effects if they have HTN or hyperthyroidism. Inform that patient may experience angina if they have coronary artery disease. Advise that patients may develop increased blood glucose levels following administration if they have DM. Advise that a temporary worsening of symptoms may be noticed if patient has Parkinson's disease. Instruct to seek immediate medical care in case of accidental inj or if signs/symptoms of an infection develop at the inj site.

ADVAIR DISKUS — *fluticasone propionate/salmeterol*   Rx

Class: Corticosteroid/long-acting beta₂ agonist (LABA)

> Long-acting β₂-adrenergic agonists (LABAs), such as salmeterol, increase the risk of asthma-related death. LABAs may increase the risk of asthma-related hospitalization in pediatric and adolescent patients. Use only for patients not adequately controlled on a long-term asthma control medication (eg, inhaled corticosteroid) or whose disease severity clearly warrants initiation of treatment w/ both an inhaled corticosteroid and a LABA. Once asthma control is achieved and maintained, assess the patient at regular intervals and step down therapy (eg, d/c Advair Diskus) if possible w/o loss of asthma control and maintain the patient on a long-term asthma control medication. Do not use if asthma is adequately controlled on low- or medium-dose inhaled corticosteroids.

ADULT DOSAGE	PEDIATRIC DOSAGE
Asthma	**Asthma**
1 inh bid, approx 12 hrs apart	**4-11 Years:**
Titrate: May replace current strength w/ a higher strength if response to initial dose after 2 weeks is inadequate	1 inh of 100/50 bid, approx 12 hrs apart
Max: 500/50 bid	**≥12 Years:**
Chronic Obstructive Pulmonary Disease	1 inh bid, approx 12 hrs apart
Maint Treatment of Airflow Obstruction:	**Titrate:** May replace current strength w/ a higher strength if response to initial dose after 2 weeks is inadequate
1 inh of 250/50 bid, approx 12 hrs apart	**Max:** 500/50 bid
An inhaled, short-acting β₂-agonist (SABA) should be taken for immediate relief if SOB occurs in the period between doses	

DOSING CONSIDERATIONS
Hepatic Impairment
Closely monitor patient

ADMINISTRATION
Oral inh route

After inh, rinse mouth w/ water w/o swallowing.

STORAGE
20-25°C (68-77°F); excursions permitted from 15-30°C (59-86°F). Store in a dry place away from direct heat or sunlight. Store inside the unopened moisture-protective foil pouch and only remove from the pouch immediately before initial use. Discard 1 month after opening the foil pouch or when the counter reads "0," whichever comes 1st.

HOW SUPPLIED
Powder, Inh: (Fluticasone Propionate/Salmeterol) (100/50) (100mcg/50mcg)/blister, (250/50) (250mcg/50mcg)/blister, (500/50) (500mcg/50mcg)/blister [14, 60 blisters]

CONTRAINDICATIONS
Primary treatment of status asthmaticus or other acute episodes of asthma or COPD where intensive measures are required. Severe hypersensitivity to milk proteins.

WARNINGS/PRECAUTIONS
Not indicated for acute bronchospasm relief. Do not initiate during rapidly deteriorating or potentially life-threatening episodes of asthma or COPD; serious acute respiratory events reported. D/C regular use of oral/inhaled SABAs when beginning treatment. May produce paradoxical bronchospasm; treat immediately w/ an inhaled, short acting bronchodilator; d/c Advair Diskus, and institute alternative therapy. Upper airway symptoms reported. Immediate hypersensitivity reactions (eg, anaphylaxis) may occur. **Fluticasone:** *Candida albicans* infections of mouth and pharynx reported; treat and if needed, interrupt therapy. Lower respiratory tract infections (eg, pneumonia) reported in patients w/ COPD. Increased susceptibility to infections. May lead to serious/fatal course of chickenpox or measles; avoid exposure and, if exposed, consider prophylaxis/treatment. Use w/ caution, if at all, in patients w/ active/quiescent tuberculosis (TB), systemic fungal, bacterial, viral, or parasitic infections, or ocular herpes simplex. Deaths due to adrenal insufficiency reported during and after transfer from systemic to inhaled corticosteroids. Resume oral corticosteroids (in large doses) immediately during periods of stress or a severe asthma attack in patients previously withdrawn from systemic corticosteroids. Patients requiring oral corticosteroids should be weaned slowly from systemic corticosteroid use after transferring to therapy. Transfer from systemic to inhaled corticosteroids may unmask allergic conditions previously suppressed by systemic therapy (eg, rhinitis, conjunctivitis, eczema). Systemic corticosteroid effects (eg, hypercorticism and adrenal suppression) may occur in patients sensitive to these effects; if such effects occur, reduce therapy slowly and consider other treatments for management of asthma symptoms. Decreases in bone mineral density (BMD) reported w/ long-term use. Monitor patients w/ major risk factors for decreased bone mineral content (eg, prolonged immobilization, tobacco use, advanced age, poor nutrition, chronic use of drugs that can reduce bone mass) and treat w/ established standards of care. Assess BMD in COPD patients prior to initiating therapy and periodically thereafter; if significant reductions are seen and therapy is still considered medically important, consider using medicine to treat or prevent osteoporosis. May reduce growth velocity in pediatric patients; routinely monitor growth. Glaucoma, increased IOP, and cataracts reported w/ long-term use. Systemic eosinophilic conditions and vasculitis consistent w/ Churg-Strauss syndrome may occur. **Salmeterol:** Clinically significant cardiovascular (CV) effects and fatalities reported w/ excessive use. CNS effects associated w/ excessive β-adrenergic stimulation. Caution w/ CV disorders, convulsive disorders, thyrotoxicosis, and in patients unusually responsive to sympathomimetic amines. Doses of IV albuterol reported to aggravate preexisting diabetes mellitus (DM) and ketoacidosis. May produce significant hypokalemia and hyperglycemia.

ADVERSE REACTIONS
Asthma: URTI, pharyngitis, upper respiratory inflammation, dysphonia, oral candidiasis, bronchitis, cough, headaches, N/V.
COPD: Pneumonia, oral candidiasis, throat irritation, dysphonia, viral respiratory infections, headaches, musculoskeletal pain.

DRUG INTERACTIONS
Do not use w/ other medicines containing LABAs. Not recommended w/ strong CYP3A4 inhibitors (eg, ritonavir, clarithromycin, ketoconazole); increased systemic corticosteroid and increased CV adverse effects may occur. **Salmeterol:** Extreme caution w/ TCAs or MAOIs, or w/in 2 weeks of discontinuation of such agents; action on the vascular system may be potentiated. β-blockers may block pulmonary effects and produce severe bronchospasm; if such therapy is needed, consider cardioselective β-blockers and use w/ caution. Caution w/ non-K+-sparing diuretics (eg, loop, thiazide); may acutely worsen ECG changes and/or hypokalemia that may result from non-K+-sparing diuretics.

PREGNANCY AND LACTATION
Pregnancy: Category C.
Lactation: Caution in nursing.

MECHANISM OF ACTION
Fluticasone: Corticosteroid; effects in COPD treatment not established. Shown to have a wide range of actions on multiple cell types (eg, mast cells, eosinophils, neutrophils, macrophages, lymphocytes) and mediators (eg, histamine, eicosanoids, leukotrienes, cytokines) involved in inflammation. **Salmeterol:** Selective LABA; attributable to stimulation of intracellular adenyl cyclase, the enzyme that catalyzes the conversion of ATP to cAMP. Increased cAMP levels cause relaxation of bronchial smooth muscle and inhibition of release of mediators of immediate hypersensitivity from cells, especially from mast cells.

PHARMACOKINETICS
Absorption: Administration of multiple doses in healthy, asthmatic, and COPD patients resulted in different pharmacokinetic parameters. **Distribution:** Fluticasone: V_d=4.2L/kg (IV); plasma protein binding (99%). Salmeterol: Plasma protein binding (96%). **Metabolism:** Fluticasone: Liver via CYP3A4; 17β-carboxylic acid derivative (metabolite). Salmeterol: Liver (extensive) by hydroxylation; α-hydroxysalmeterol (aliphatic oxidation) via CYP3A4. **Elimination:** Fluticasone: Urine (<5%, metabolites), feces (unchanged and metabolites); $T_{1/2}$=5.6 hrs. Salmeterol: Urine (25%), feces (60%); $T_{1/2}$=5.5 hrs.

PATIENT CONSIDERATIONS
Assessment: Assess for hypersensitivity to drug or to milk proteins; COPD/asthma status; active/quiescent TB; systemic infections; ocular herpes simplex; CV disorders; risk factors for decreased bone mineral content; convulsive disorders; thyrotoxicosis; DM; ketoacidosis; history of increased IOP, glaucoma, and/or cataracts; hepatic impairment; pregnancy/nursing status; and possible drug interactions. Assess BMD in patients w/ COPD.

Monitoring: Monitor for deteriorating disease, localized oropharyngeal *C. albicans* infections, pneumonia, infections, systemic corticosteroid effects (eg, hypercorticism, adrenal suppression), paradoxical bronchospasm, upper airway symptoms, immediate hypersensitivity reactions, CV and CNS effects, glaucoma, cataracts, increased IOP, eosinophilic conditions, changes in blood glucose and/or serum K+, and other adverse reactions. Periodically monitor BMD in patients w/ COPD and in patients w/ major risk factors for decreased bone mineral content. Monitor growth of pediatric patients routinely. Closely monitor patients w/ hepatic disease.

Counseling: Counsel about the risks and benefits of therapy. Inform that drug is not meant to relieve acute asthma symptoms or exacerbations of COPD; advise to treat acute symptoms w/ an inhaled SABA (eg, albuterol). Instruct to seek medical attention immediately if experiencing a decrease in effectiveness of inhaled SABAs, a need for more inhalations than usual of inhaled SABAs, or a significant decrease in lung function. Advise not to d/c therapy w/o physician guidance and not to use other LABA. Instruct to contact physician if oropharyngeal candidiasis or symptoms of pneumonia develop. Instruct to rinse mouth w/ water w/o swallowing after inhalation of therapy. Advise to avoid exposure to chickenpox or measles, and, if exposed, to consult physician w/o delay. Inform about risk of immunosuppression, hypercorticism, adrenal suppression, reduction in BMD, reduced growth velocity in pediatric patients, ocular effects, and about adverse effects associated w/ β-agonists (eg, palpitations, chest pain, rapid HR, tremor, nervousness). Instruct to d/c therapy if immediate hypersensitivity reactions occur. Inform that the inhaler is not reusable and advise not to take the inhaler apart.

ADVAIR HFA — fluticasone propionate/salmeterol   Rx
Class: Corticosteroid/long-acting beta₂ agonist (LABA)

> LABAs, such as salmeterol, increase the risk of asthma-related death. LABAs may increase the risk of asthma-related hospitalization in pediatric and adolescent patients. Use only for patients not adequately controlled on a long-term asthma control medication (eg, inhaled corticosteroid) or whose disease severity clearly warrants initiation of treatment w/ both an inhaled corticosteroid and a LABA. Once asthma control is achieved and maintained, assess the patient at regular intervals and step down therapy (eg, d/c Advair HFA) if possible w/o loss of asthma control and maintain the patient on a long-term asthma control medication. Do not use if asthma is adequately controlled on low- or medium-dose inhaled corticosteroids.

ADULT DOSAGE	PEDIATRIC DOSAGE
Asthma	**Asthma**
2 inh bid, approx 12 hrs apart	**≥12 Years:**
Titrate: Replace w/ higher strength if response is inadequate after 2 weeks	2 inh bid, approx 12 hrs apart
Max: 2 inh of 230/21 bid	**Titrate:** Replace w/ higher strength if response is inadequate after 2 weeks
	Max: 2 inh of 230/21 bid

DOSING CONSIDERATIONS
Renal Impairment
Formal pharmacokinetic studies have not been conducted

Hepatic Impairment
Formal pharmacokinetic studies have not been conducted; closely monitor patients w/ hepatic disease

Elderly
Start at lower end of dosing range

ADMINISTRATION
Oral inh route
Rinse mouth w/ water (w/o swallowing) after inh.
Shake well for 5 sec before each spray.

Priming Instructions
Prime before using for the 1st time by releasing 4 sprays into the air away from the face; if the inhaler has not been used for >4 weeks or has been dropped, prime the inhaler by releasing 2 sprays into the air away from the face

STORAGE
20-25°C (68-77°F); excursions permitted from 15-30°C (59-86°F). Store w/ the mouthpiece down. Do not puncture, use/store near heat or open flame, or throw into fire/incinerator. Exposure to temperatures >49°C (120°F) may cause bursting. Discard when the counter reads "000."

HOW SUPPLIED
MDI: (Fluticasone/Salmeterol) (45/21) (45mcg/21mcg)/inh, (115/21) (115mcg/21mcg)/inh, (230/21) (230mcg/21mcg)/inh [60, 120 inh]

CONTRAINDICATIONS
Primary treatment of status asthmaticus or other acute episodes of asthma where intensive measures are required. Hypersensitivity to any of the ingredients.

WARNINGS/PRECAUTIONS
Not indicated for acute bronchospasm relief. Do not initiate during rapidly deteriorating or potentially life-threatening episodes of asthma. D/C regular use of oral/inhaled short-acting β₂-agonists (SABAs) when beginning treatment. May produce paradoxical bronchospasm; treat immediately, d/c Advair HFA, and institute alternative therapy. Upper airway symptoms reported. Immediate hypersensitivity reactions (eg, anaphylaxis) may occur. **Fluticasone:** *Candida*

albicans infections of the mouth and pharynx reported; treat and, if needed, interrupt therapy. Lower respiratory tract infections (eg, pneumonia) reported in patients w/ COPD. Increased susceptibility to infections. May lead to serious/fatal course of chickenpox or measles; avoid exposure and, if exposed, consider prophylaxis/treatment. Use w/ caution, if at all, in patients w/ active/quiescent tuberculosis (TB); systemic fungal, bacterial, viral, or parasitic infections; or ocular herpes simplex. Deaths due to adrenal insufficiency reported during and after transfer from systemic to inhaled corticosteroids. Resume oral corticosteroids (in large doses) immediately during periods of stress or a severe asthma attack in patients previously withdrawn from systemic corticosteroids. Patients requiring oral corticosteroids should be weaned slowly from systemic corticosteroid use after transferring to therapy. Transfer from systemic to inhaled corticosteroids may unmask allergic conditions previously suppressed by systemic therapy (eg, rhinitis, conjunctivitis, eczema). Systemic corticosteroid effects (eg, hypercorticism and adrenal suppression) may occur in patients sensitive to these effects; if such effects occur, reduce therapy slowly and consider other treatments for management of asthma symptoms. Decreases in bone mineral density (BMD) reported w/ long-term use. May reduce growth velocity in pediatric patients. Glaucoma, increased IOP, and cataracts reported w/ long-term use. Systemic eosinophilic conditions and vasculitis consistent w/ Churg-Strauss syndrome may occur. **Salmeterol:** Clinically significant cardiovascular (CV) effects and fatalities reported w/ excessive use. CNS effects associated w/ excessive β-adrenergic stimulation. Caution w/ convulsive disorders, thyrotoxicosis, and in patients unusually responsive to sympathomimetic amines. Large doses of IV albuterol reported to aggravate preexisting diabetes mellitus (DM) and ketoacidosis. May produce significant hypokalemia and hyperglycemia.

ADVERSE REACTIONS
URTI, upper respiratory inflammation, headache, throat irritation, musculoskeletal pain, N/V, dizziness, viral GI infection, hoarseness/dysphonia, muscle pain, GI signs/symptoms.

DRUG INTERACTIONS
Do not use w/ other medicines containing LABAs. Not recommended w/ strong CYP3A4 inhibitors (eg, ritonavir, clarithromycin, ketoconazole); increased systemic corticosteroid and increased CV adverse effects may occur. **Salmeterol:** Extreme caution w/ TCAs or MAOIs, or w/in 2 weeks of discontinuation of such agents; action on the vascular system may be potentiated. β-blockers may block pulmonary effects and produce severe bronchospasm; if such therapy is needed, consider cardioselective β-blockers and use w/ caution. Caution w/ non-K⁺-sparing diuretics (eg, loop, thiazide); may acutely worsen ECG changes and/or hypokalemia that may result from non-K⁺-sparing diuretics.

PREGNANCY AND LACTATION
Pregnancy: Category C.
Lactation: Caution in nursing.

MECHANISM OF ACTION
Fluticasone: Corticosteroid; shown to have a wide range of actions on multiple cell types (eg, mast cells, eosinophils, neutrophils, macrophages, lymphocytes) and mediators (eg, histamine, eicosanoids, leukotrienes, cytokines) involved in inflammation. **Salmeterol:** Selective LABA; attributable to stimulation of intracellular adenyl cyclase, the enzyme that catalyzes the conversion of ATP to cAMP. Increased cAMP levels cause relaxation of bronchial smooth muscle and inhibition of release of mediators of immediate hypersensitivity from cells, especially from mast cells.

PHARMACOKINETICS
Absorption: Administration of multiple doses in healthy and asthmatic patients resulted in different pharmacokinetic parameters. **Distribution:** Fluticasone: V_d=4.2L/kg (IV); plasma protein binding (99%). Salmeterol: Plasma protein binding (96%). **Metabolism:** Fluticasone: Liver via CYP3A4; 17β-carboxylic acid derivative (metabolite). Salmeterol: Liver (extensive) by hydroxylation; α-hydroxysalmeterol (aliphatic oxidation) via CYP3A4. **Elimination:** Fluticasone: Urine (<5%, metabolites), feces (unchanged and metabolites); $T_{1/2}$=5.6 hrs. Salmeterol: Urine (25%), feces (60%); $T_{1/2}$=5.5 hrs.

PATIENT CONSIDERATIONS
Assessment: Assess for hypersensitivity to drug; asthma status; active/quiescent TB; systemic infections; ocular herpes simplex; CV disorders; risk factors for decreased bone mineral content; convulsive disorders; thyrotoxicosis; DM; ketoacidosis; history of increased IOP, glaucoma, and/or cataracts; hepatic impairment; pregnancy/nursing status; and possible drug interactions.

Monitoring: Monitor for deteriorating disease, localized oropharyngeal *C. albicans* infections, pneumonia, infections, systemic corticosteroid effects (eg, hypercorticism, adrenal suppression), paradoxical bronchospasm, upper airway symptoms, immediate hypersensitivity reactions, CV and CNS effects, decreases in BMD, glaucoma, cataracts, increased IOP, eosinophilic conditions, changes in blood glucose and/or serum K⁺, and other adverse reactions. Monitor growth of pediatric patients routinely. Closely monitor patients w/ hepatic disease.

Counseling: Counsel about the risks and benefits of therapy. Inform that drug is not meant to relieve acute asthma symptoms; advise to treat acute symptoms w/ an inhaled SABA (eg, albuterol). Instruct to seek medical attention immediately if experiencing a decrease in effectiveness of inhaled SABAs, a need for more inhalations than usual of inhaled SABAs, or a significant decrease in lung function. Advise not to d/c therapy w/o physician guidance and not to use other LABA. Instruct to contact physician if oropharyngeal candidiasis or symptoms of pneumonia develop. Instruct to rinse mouth w/ water w/o swallowing after inhalation of therapy. Advise to avoid exposure to chickenpox or measles, and, if exposed, to consult physician w/o delay. Inform about risk

of immunosuppression, hypercorticism, adrenal suppression, reduction in BMD, reduced growth velocity in pediatric patients, ocular effects, and about adverse effects associated w/ β-agonists (eg; palpitations, chest pain, rapid HR, tremor, nervousness). Instruct to d/c therapy if immediate hypersensitivity reactions occur.

ADVICOR — lovastatin/niacin Rx
Class: HMG-CoA reductase inhibitor (statin)/nicotinic acid

ADULT DOSAGE	PEDIATRIC DOSAGE
Primary Hypercholesterolemia/Mixed Dyslipidemia	Pediatric use may not have been established
Not Currently on Niacin ER:	
Initial: 500mg-20mg qhs	
Titrate: Increase by no more than 500mg qd (based on niacin ER component) every 4 weeks	
Max: 2000mg-40mg qhs	
Stable on Niacin ER:	
May be directly switched to niacin-equivalent dose of Advicor	
Should not be substituted for other modified-release (sustained-release or time-release) niacin preparations or other IR (crystalline) niacin preparations	
If therapy is discontinued for an extended period (>7 days), reinstitution should begin with lowest dose	
Advicor tab strengths are not interchangeable	
Women may respond at lower niacin doses than men	

DOSING CONSIDERATIONS
Concomitant Medications
Danazol, Diltiazem, or Verapamil:
Lovastatin Content:
Initial: 10mg/day
Max: 20mg/day

Amiodarone:
Lovastatin Content:
Max: 40mg/day

Gemfibrozil:
Avoid lovastatin use w/ gemfibrozil

Renal Impairment
Severe (CrCl <30mL/min):
Carefully consider lovastatin dose increases >20mg/day; give cautiously if deemed necessary

ADMINISTRATION
Oral route

Take at hs w/ a low-fat snack
Take tab whole; do not break, crush, or chew
Avoid administration on an empty stomach and slowly increase niacin dose to reduce flushing, pruritus, and GI distress
May take ASA (up to 325mg) 30 min prior to treatment to reduce flushing

STORAGE
20-25°C (68-77°F).

HOW SUPPLIED
Tab: (Niacin ER-Lovastatin) 500mg-20mg, 750mg-20mg, 1000mg-20mg, 1000mg-40mg

CONTRAINDICATIONS
Known hypersensitivity to Advicor or any component of this medication. Active liver disease or unexplained persistent elevations in serum transaminases, active peptic ulcer disease (PUD), arterial bleeding, pregnancy, women of childbearing age who may become pregnant, and nursing mothers. Concomitant administration with strong CYP3A4 inhibitors (eg, itraconazole, ketoconazole, posaconazole, HIV protease inhibitors, boceprevir, telaprevir, erythromycin, clarithromycin, telithromycin, nefazodone).

WARNINGS/PRECAUTIONS
Do not substitute for equivalent doses of immediate-release (IR) (crystalline) niacin or other modified-release (sustained-release or time-release) niacin preparations other than Niaspan. Severe hepatic toxicity, including fulminant hepatic necrosis, reported when substituting sustained-release niacin for IR niacin at equivalent doses. If switching from IR niacin, initiate with low doses (500mg qhs) and titrate to desired therapeutic response. Caution with renal impairment, or with substantial alcohol consumption and/or history of liver disease. Associated with abnormal LFTs; obtain LFTs prior to initiation and repeat as clinically indicated. Fatal and nonfatal hepatic failure (rare) reported; promptly interrupt therapy if serious liver injury with clinical symptoms and/or hyperbilirubinemia or jaundice occurs and do not restart if no alternate etiology found. Myopathy and/or rhabdomyolysis reported when lovastatin is used with lipid-altering doses (≥1g/day) of niacin; d/c if markedly elevated CPK levels occur or myopathy is diagnosed/suspected, and temporarily withhold in any patient experiencing acute

or serious condition predisposing to development of renal failure secondary to rhabdomyolysis. Immune-mediated necrotizing myopathy (IMNM) reported. Closely observe patients with history of jaundice, hepatobiliary disease, or peptic ulcer. Increases in HbA1c and FPG levels reported; closely monitor diabetic/ potentially diabetic patients, and adjust diet and/or hypoglycemic therapy if necessary. May increase PT and reduce platelet counts; carefully evaluate patients undergoing surgery. Associated with dose-related reductions in phosphorus (P) levels; periodically monitor P levels in patients at risk for hypophosphatemia. Caution with unstable angina or in the acute phase of MI, particularly when such patients are also receiving vasoactive drugs (eg, nitrates, calcium channel blockers, adrenergic blocking agents). Elevated uric acid levels reported; caution in patients predisposed to gout. Evaluate patients who develop endocrine dysfunction. Lab test interactions may occur.

ADVERSE REACTIONS
Flushing, infection, headache, pain, N/V, pruritus, flu syndrome, diarrhea, back pain, asthenia, rash, hyperglycemia, abdominal pain, myalgia, dyspepsia.

DRUG INTERACTIONS
See Contraindications and Dosage. Lovastatin: Due to the risk of myopathy, avoid with gemfibrozil, cyclosporine, and large quantities of grapefruit juice (>1 quart/day); caution with fibrates, colchicine, danazol, diltiazem, verapamil, and amiodarone. Voriconazole may increase concentrations and may increase risk of myopathy/rhabdomyolysis; consider dose adjustment of lovastatin. Ranolazine may increase risk of myopathy/rhabdomyolysis; consider dose adjustment of lovastatin. Caution with drugs (eg, spironolactone, cimetidine) that may decrease the levels or activity of endogenous steroid hormones. Determine PT before initiation and frequently during therapy with coumarin anticoagulants. Niacin ER: Avoid ingestion of alcohol, hot drinks, or spicy foods around the time of administration; may increase flushing and pruritus. May potentiate the effects of ganglionic blocking agents and vasoactive drugs, resulting in postural hypotension. ASA may decrease the metabolic clearance. Separate dosing from bile acid-binding resins (eg, colestipol, cholestyramine) by at least 4-6 hrs. Vitamins or other nutritional supplements containing large doses of niacin or related compounds (eg, nicotinamide) may potentiate adverse effects.

PREGNANCY AND LACTATION
Category X, not for use in nursing.

MECHANISM OF ACTION
Niacin ER: Nicotinic acid; has not been established. May partially inhibit release of free fatty acids from adipose tissue, and increase lipoprotein lipase activity (which may increase the rate of chylomicron TG removal from plasma). Decreases the rate of hepatic synthesis of VLDL and LDL. Lovastatin: HMG-CoA reductase inhibitor; may involve both reduction of VLDL concentration and induction of LDL receptor, leading to reduced production and/or increased catabolism of LDL.

PHARMACOKINETICS
Absorption: Niacin ER: C_{max}=18mcg/mL, T_{max}=5 hrs. Lovastatin: Incomplete. C_{max}=11ng/mL, T_{max}=2 hrs. **Distribution:** Niacin ER: Plasma protein binding (<20%); found in breast milk. Lovastatin: Plasma protein binding (>95%). **Metabolism:** Niacin ER: Liver (rapid and extensive 1st-pass); nicotinuric acid (via conjugation), nicotinamide adenine dinucleotide (metabolites). Lovastatin: Liver (extensive 1st-pass) via CYP3A4; β-hydroxyacid and 6'-hydroxy derivative (major active metabolites). **Elimination:** Niacin ER: Urine (≥60%); $T_{1/2}$=20-48 min. Lovastatin: (Mevacor) Urine (10%), feces (83%); $T_{1/2}$=4.5 hrs.

PATIENT CONSIDERATIONS
Assessment: Assess for history of/active liver disease or PUD, unexplained persistent hepatic transaminase elevations, arterial bleeding, history of jaundice or hepatobiliary disease, renal impairment, diabetes, risk for hypophosphatemia, any other conditions where treatment is contraindicated or cautioned, drug hypersensitivity, pregnancy/nursing status, and possible drug interactions. Assess lipid profile and LFTs.

Monitoring: Monitor for signs/symptoms of myopathy (including IMNM), rhabdomyolysis, liver/renal/endocrine dysfunction, decreases in platelet counts, increases in PT and uric acid levels, and other adverse reactions. Monitor LFTs, blood glucose, and CPK levels. Perform lipid determinations at intervals of ≥4 weeks. Periodically monitor P levels in patients at risk for hypophosphatemia. Check PT with coumarin anticoagulants.

Counseling: Instruct to report promptly any unexplained muscle pain, tenderness, or weakness, particularly if accompanied by malaise or fever or if muscle signs and symptoms persist after discontinuation. Instruct to report promptly any symptoms that may indicate liver injury (eg, fatigue, anorexia, right upper abdominal discomfort, dark urine, jaundice). Advise to carefully follow the prescribed dosing regimen. Inform that flushing may occur, but usually subsides after several weeks of consistent use of therapy. Instruct that if awakened by flushing, especially if taking antihypertensives, to rise slowly to minimize the potential for dizziness and/or syncope. Instruct to avoid ingestion of alcohol, hot beverages, or spicy foods around the time of administration to minimize flushing. Counsel to avoid administration with grapefruit juice. Instruct to contact physician prior to restarting therapy if therapy is discontinued for an extended length of time. Advise to notify physician if taking vitamins or other nutritional supplements containing niacin or related compounds, and if symptoms of dizziness occur. Instruct diabetic patients to notify physician of changes in blood glucose. Instruct to immediately d/c use and notify physician as soon as pregnancy is recognized.

ADZENYS XR-ODT — amphetamine   CII
Class: CNS stimulant

> High potential for abuse and dependence; assess risk of abuse prior to prescribing and monitor for signs of abuse and dependence while on therapy.

ADULT DOSAGE
Attention-Deficit Hyperactivity Disorder

12.5mg qam

Conversions

Adderall XR:
May be switched to Adzenys XR-ODT at the equivalent dose taken qd

Equivalent Doses:
Adzenys XR-ODT 3.1mg = Adderall XR 5mg
Adzenys XR-ODT 6.3mg = Adderall XR 10mg
Adzenys XR-ODT 9.4mg = Adderall XR 15mg
Adzenys XR-ODT 12.5mg = Adderall XR 20mg
Adzenys XR-ODT 15.7mg = Adderall XR 25mg
Adzenys XR-ODT 18.8mg = Adderall XR 30mg

Other Amphetamine Products:
D/C other treatment, and titrate w/ Adzenys XR-ODT using usual titration schedule
Do not substitute for other amphetamine products on mg-per-mg basis

PEDIATRIC DOSAGE
Attention-Deficit Hyperactivity Disorder

≥6 Years:
Initial: 6.3mg qam
Titrate: Increase in increments of 3.1mg or 6.3mg at weekly intervals
Max: 18.8mg/day (6-12 years) and 12.5mg/day (13-17 years)

Conversions

Adderall XR:
May be switched to Adzenys XR-ODT at the equivalent dose taken qd

Equivalent Doses:
Adzenys XR-ODT 3.1mg = Adderall XR 5mg
Adzenys XR-ODT 6.3mg = Adderall XR 10mg
Adzenys XR-ODT 9.4mg = Adderall XR 15mg
Adzenys XR-ODT 12.5mg = Adderall XR 20mg
Adzenys XR-ODT 15.7mg = Adderall XR 25mg
Adzenys XR-ODT 18.8mg = Adderall XR 30mg

Other Amphetamine Products:
D/C other treatment, and titrate w/ Adzenys XR-ODT using usual titration schedule
Do not substitute for other amphetamine products on mg-per-mg basis

---

DOSING CONSIDERATIONS
Concomitant Medications
- Agents that alter urinary pH may impact urinary excretion and alter blood levels
- Acidifying agents (eg, ascorbic acid) decrease blood levels, while alkalinizing agents (eg, sodium bicarbonate) increase blood levels; adjust Adzenys XR-ODT dose accordingly

ADMINISTRATION
Oral route

- Take w/ or w/o food.
- Keep in blister pack until ready for use.
- Use dry hands to open blister.
- Tab should not be pushed through foil; peel back of blister.
- Place whole tab on tongue and allow to disintegrate w/o chewing/crushing.

STORAGE
20-25°C (68-77°F); excursions permitted to 15-30°C (59-86°F).

HOW SUPPLIED
Tab, Disintegrating: 3.1mg, 6.3mg, 9.4mg, 12.5mg, 15.7mg, 18.8mg

CONTRAINDICATIONS
Hypersensitivity to amphetamine, or other components of the product. Treatment w/ MAOIs, and also w/in 14 days following discontinuation of treatment w/ an MAOI.

WARNINGS/PRECAUTIONS
Sudden death, stroke, and MI reported in adults. Sudden death reported in pediatric patients w/ structural cardiac abnormalities or other serious heart problems. Avoid w/ known structural cardiac abnormalities, cardiomyopathy, serious heart arrhythmia, coronary artery disease, or other serious heart problems. Further evaluate patients who develop exertional chest pain, unexplained syncope, or arrhythmias during treatment. May cause increase in BP/HR; monitor for tachycardia and HTN. May exacerbate symptoms of behavior disturbance and thought disorder in patients w/ preexisting psychotic disorder. May induce a mixed or manic episode in patients w/ bipolar disorder; prior to initiation, screen for risk factors for developing a manic episode. May cause psychotic/manic symptoms w/o a prior history of psychotic illness or mania; consider discontinuation if such symptoms occur. Associated w/ weight loss and slowing of growth rate in pediatric patients; closely monitor growth (weight/height). Associated w/ peripheral vasculopathy, including Raynaud's phenomenon; carefully observe for digital changes. May cause significant elevation in plasma corticosteroid levels; may interfere w/ urinary steroid determinations.

ADVERSE REACTIONS
6-12 Years: Loss of appetite, insomnia, abdominal pain, emotional lability, N/V, nervousness, fever.
13-17 Years: Loss of appetite, insomnia, abdominal pain, weight loss.
Adults: Dry mouth, loss of appetite, insomnia, headache, weight loss, nausea, anxiety, agitation, dizziness, tachycardia, diarrhea, asthenia, UTI.

DRUG INTERACTIONS

See Dosing Considerations and Contraindications. Alkalinizing agents (eg, sodium bicarbonate, acetazolamide, some thiazides) may increase blood levels and potentiate effects; avoid coadministration. Acidifying agents (guanethidine, reserpine, glutamic acid HCl, ascorbic acid) may lower blood levels and efficacy; increase dose based on response. May enhance activity of TCAs (eg, desipramine, protriptyline) or sympathomimetic agents causing striking and sustained increases in the concentration of d-amphetamine in the brain; may potentiate cardiovascular (CV) effects; monitor frequently and adjust or use alternative therapy based on clinical response. Proton pump inhibitors (eg, omeprazole) may increase T_{max} of amphetamine; monitor for changes in clinical effect and adjust therapy based on clinical response.

PREGNANCY AND LACTATION

Pregnancy: Category C.
Lactation: Not for use in nursing.

MECHANISM OF ACTION

CNS stimulant; has not been established. Thought to block the reuptake of norepinephrine and dopamine into the presynaptic neuron and increase the release of these monoamines into the extraneuronal space.

PHARMACOKINETICS

Absorption: C_{max}=44.9ng/mL, T_{max}=5 hrs (median) (d-amphetamine); C_{max}=14.5ng/mL, T_{max}=5.25 hrs (median) (l-amphetamine). **Distribution:** Found in breast milk. **Metabolism:** CYP2D6 (oxidation); 4-hydroxy-amphetamine and norephedrine (active metabolites). **Elimination:** Urine (30-40%, unchanged; approx 50%, α-hydroxy-amphetamine derivatives). $T_{1/2}$=11 hrs (adults), 9-10 hrs (6-12 years) (d-amphetamine:); 14 hrs (adults), 10-11 hrs (6-12 years) (l-amphetamine).

PATIENT CONSIDERATIONS

Assessment: Assess for drug hypersensitivity, cardiac problems/disease, psychotic disorders, bipolar disorder, pregnancy/nursing status, and for possible drug interactions. Obtain baseline height/weight in pediatric patients. Screen patients for risk factors for developing a manic episode and the risk of abuse before starting therapy.

Monitoring: Monitor for stroke, MI, HTN, tachycardia, exacerbations of behavior disturbances and thought disorders, psychotic or manic symptoms, digital changes, and other adverse reactions. Monitor height/weight in pediatric patients. Monitor for signs of abuse and dependence. Periodically reevaluate the need for use.

Counseling: Instruct to take ud. Inform that product is a federally controlled substance that can be abused or lead to dependence; advise to store in a safe place, preferably locked. Instruct to dispose of remaining, unused, or expired tabs by a medicine take-back program if available. Advise of serious CV risk; instruct to contact a healthcare provider immediately if CV symptoms (eg, exertional chest pain, unexplained syncope) develop. Instruct that elevations in BP/HR may occur. Advise that treatment may cause psychotic symptoms or mania and may cause slowing of growth and weight loss. Instruct about the risk of peripheral vasculopathy, including Raynaud's phenomenon, and associated signs/symptoms; instruct to report any new numbness, pain, skin color change, or sensitivity to temperature in fingers/toes. Instruct to call physician immediately w/ any signs of unexplained wounds appearing on fingers/toes while on therapy. Advise to notify healthcare provider if pregnant or intending to become pregnant during treatment; advise of potential fetal effects. Instruct not to breastfeed. Advise to avoid alcohol.

AFINITOR — everolimus   Rx

Class: Kinase inhibitor

OTHER BRAND NAMES

Afinitor Disperz

ADULT DOSAGE

Breast Cancer

Treatment of postmenopausal women w/ advanced hormone receptor (HR)-positive, HER2-negative breast cancer in combination w/ exemestane, after failure of treatment w/ letrozole or anastrozole

Tab:
10mg qd; continue until disease progression or unacceptable toxicity occurs

Advanced Neuroendocrine Tumors

Treatment of progressive neuroendocrine tumors of pancreatic origin w/ unresectable, locally advanced or metastatic disease; also indicated for progressive, well-differentiated, non-functional neuroendocrine tumors of GI or lung origin w/ unresectable, locally advanced or metastatic disease

Tab:
10mg qd; continue until disease progression or unacceptable toxicity occurs

PEDIATRIC DOSAGE

Subependymal Giant Cell Astrocytoma with Tuberous Sclerosis Complex

Requiring Therapeutic Intervention but Cannot Be Curatively Resected: Tab/Tab for Oral Sus:
≥1 Year:
Initial: 4.5mg/m² qd
Adjust dose at 2-week intervals prn to achieve/maintain trough concentrations of 5-15ng/mL

Continue until disease progression or unacceptable toxicity occurs

Therapeutic Drug Monitoring:
Assess trough levels 2 weeks after initiation, a change in dose, a change in coadministration of CYP3A4/P-gp inducers/inhibitors, a change in hepatic function, or a change in dosage form.
Once a stable dose is attained, monitor trough levels every 3-6 months in patients w/ changing BSA or every 6-12 months in patients w/ stable BSA.

Advanced Renal Cell Carcinoma

After Failure of Treatment w/ Sunitinib or Sorafenib:
Tab:
10mg qd; continue until disease progression or unacceptable toxicity occurs

Renal Angiomyolipoma with Tuberous Sclerosis Complex

In Patients Not Requiring Immediate Surgery:
Tab:
10mg qd; continue until disease progression or unacceptable toxicity occurs

Subependymal Giant Cell Astrocytoma with Tuberous Sclerosis Complex

Requiring Therapeutic Intervention but Cannot Be Curatively Resected: Tab/Tab for Oral Sus:
Initial: 4.5mg/m² qd
Adjust dose at 2-week intervals prn to achieve/maintain trough concentrations of 5-15ng/mL

Continue until disease progression or unacceptable toxicity occurs

Therapeutic Drug Monitoring:
Assess trough levels 2 weeks after initiation, a change in dose, a change in coadministration of CYP3A4/P-gp inducers/inhibitors, a change in hepatic function, or a change in dosage form.
Once a stable dose is attained, monitor trough levels every 3-6 months in patients w/ changing BSA or every 6-12 months in patients w/ stable BSA.
Titrate (Based on Trough Levels):
<5ng/mL: Increase daily dose by 2.5mg (tab) or 2mg (tab for oral sus)
>15ng/mL: Reduce daily dose by 2.5mg (tab) or 2mg (tab for oral sus)

If dose reduction is required for patients receiving the lowest available strength, administer qod

Titrate (Based on Trough Levels):
<5ng/mL: Increase daily dose by 2.5mg (tab) or 2mg (tab for oral sus)
>15ng/mL: Reduce daily dose by 2.5mg (tab) or 2mg (tab for oral sus)

If dose reduction is required for patients receiving the lowest available strength, administer qod

---

DOSING CONSIDERATIONS

Concomitant Medications

Advanced HR-Positive, HER2-Negative Breast Cancer, Advanced Neuroendocrine Tumors (NET), Advanced Renal Cell Carcinoma (RCC), Renal Angiomyolipoma w/ Tuberous Sclerosis Complex (TSC):

Strong CYP3A4/P-gp Inhibitors: Avoid use
Moderate CYP3A4/P-gp Inhibitors (If Coadministration Is Necessary):
- Reduce to 2.5mg qd; may increase to 5mg if tolerated
- 2-3 days after discontinuation of the moderate inhibitor, return to dose used prior to initiating the inhibitor

Avoid grapefruit, grapefruit juice, and other foods known to inhibit CYP450 and P-gp activity during treatment

Strong CYP3A4/P-gp Inducers: Avoid use
If Coadministration Is Required:
- Consider doubling daily dose by increments of ≤5mg
- 3-5 days after discontinuation of the strong inducer, return to dose used prior to initiating the inducer

Avoid St. John's wort during treatment

Subependymal Giant Cell Astrocytoma (SEGA) w/ TSC:

Strong CYP3A4/P-gp Inhibitors: Avoid use
Moderate CYP3A4/P-gp Inhibitors (If Coadministration Is Necessary):
Initial: 2.5mg/m² qd (reduce dose by approx 50%); administer qod if receiving the lowest available strength
- 2-3 days after discontinuation of the moderate inhibitor, return to dose used prior to initiating the inhibitor

Avoid ingestion of foods or nutritional supplements (eg, grapefruit, grapefruit juice) known to inhibit CYP450 or P-gp activity

Strong CYP3A4/P-gp Inducers: Avoid use
If Necessary: Double the dose and assess tolerability
Initial: 9mg/m² qd
Return to dose used prior to initiating the inducer if the strong inducer is discontinued

Avoid ingestion of foods or nutritional supplements (eg, St. John's wort) known to induce CYP450 activity

Hepatic Impairment
Advanced HR-Positive, HER2-Negative Breast Cancer, Advanced NET, Advanced RCC, Renal Angiomyolipoma w/ TSC:
Mild (Child-Pugh Class A): 7.5mg qd; reduce to 5mg qd if not tolerated
Moderate (Child-Pugh Class B): 5mg qd; reduce to 2.5mg qd if not tolerated
Severe (Child-Pugh Class C): 2.5mg qd if benefit outweighs the risk
SEGA w/ TSC:
Severe (Child-Pugh Class C):
Initial: $2.5mg/m^2$ qd (reduce starting dose by approx 50%)

Adverse Reactions
Advanced HR-Positive, HER2-Negative Breast Cancer, Advanced NET, Advanced RCC, Renal Angiomyolipoma w/ TSC:
If dose reduction is required, administer approx 50% lower than the previously administered daily dose
Noninfectious Pneumonitis:
Grade 1 (Asymptomatic, Radiographic Findings Only):
- Initiate appropriate monitoring
Grade 2 (Symptomatic, Not Interfering w/ Activities of Daily Living [ADL]):
- Consider interrupting therapy, rule out infection, and consider treatment w/ corticosteroids until symptoms improve to Grade ≤1
- Reinitiate at a lower dose
- D/C if failure to recover w/in 4 weeks
Grade 3 (Symptomatic, Interfering w/ ADL; O₂ Indicated):
- Interrupt therapy until symptoms resolve to Grade ≤1, rule out infection, and consider treatment w/ corticosteroids
- Consider reinitiating at a lower dose
- Consider discontinuation if toxicity recurs at Grade 3
Grade 4 (Life-Threatening, Ventilator Support Indicated):
- D/C, rule out infection, and consider treatment w/ corticosteroids
Stomatitis:
Grade 1 (Minimal Symptoms, Normal Diet):
- Manage w/ nonalcoholic or salt water (0.9%) mouthwash several times a day
Grade 2 (Symptomatic but Can Eat and Swallow Modified Diet):
- Temporarily interrupt dose until recovery to Grade ≤1; reinitiate at the same dose
- If stomatitis recurs at Grade 2, interrupt dose until recovery to Grade ≤1; reinitiate at a lower dose
- Manage w/ topical analgesic mouth treatments (eg, benzocaine, butyl aminobenzoate, tetracaine, menthol, phenol) ± topical corticosteroids (eg, triamcinolone oral paste); avoid agents w/ alcohol, hydrogen peroxide, iodine, and thyme derivatives
Grade 3 (Symptomatic and Unable to Aliment or Hydrate Orally):
- Temporarily interrupt dose until recovery to Grade ≤1
- Reinitiate at a lower dose
- Manage w/ topical analgesic mouth treatments (eg, benzocaine, butyl aminobenzoate, tetracaine, menthol, phenol) ± topical corticosteroids (eg, triamcinolone oral paste); avoid agents w/ alcohol, hydrogen peroxide, iodine, and thyme derivatives
Grade 4 (Symptoms Associated w/ Life-Threatening Consequences):
- D/C and treat appropriately
Other Nonhematologic Toxicities (Excluding Metabolic Events):
Grade 1:
- If toxicity is tolerable, no dose adjustment required; initiate appropriate medical therapy and monitor
Grade 2:
- If toxicity is tolerable, no dose adjustment required; initiate appropriate medical therapy and monitor
- If toxicity becomes intolerable, temporarily interrupt dose until recovery to Grade ≤1; reinitiate at same dose
- If toxicity recurs at Grade 2, interrupt until recovery to Grade ≤1; reinitiate at lower dose
Grade 3:
- Temporarily interrupt dose until recovery to Grade ≤1
- Initiate appropriate therapy and monitor
- Consider reinitiating at a lower dose
- If toxicity recurs at Grade 3, consider discontinuation
Grade 4:
- D/C and treat appropriately
Metabolic Events (eg, Hyperglycemia, Dyslipidemia):
Grade 1:
- Initiate appropriate medical therapy and monitor
Grade 2:
- Manage w/ appropriate medical therapy and monitor
Grade 3:
- Temporarily interrupt dose
- Reinitiate at a lower dose
- Manage w/ appropriate therapy and monitor
Grade 4:
- D/C and treat appropriately
SEGA w/ TSC:
- Temporarily interrupt or permanently d/c for severe or intolerable adverse reactions
- If dose reduction is required when reinitiating therapy, reduce dose by 50%
- If dose reduction is required for patients receiving the lowest available strength, administer qod

ADMINISTRATION
Oral route

Take qd at the same time every day.
Take consistently either w/ or w/o food.

Do not combine the 2 dosage forms to achieve the desired total dose.
Do not break or crush.
Tab
Swallow whole w/ a glass of water.
Tab for Oral Sus
Wear gloves to avoid possible contact w/ drug when preparing sus for another person.
Administer as sus only.
Administer sus immediately after preparation and discard if not given w/in 60 min after preparation.
Prepare sus in water only.
Preparation Using an Oral Syringe:
1. Place prescribed dose into a 10mL syringe; do not exceed a total of 10mg/syringe and if higher doses are required, prepare an additional syringe.
2. Draw approx 5mL of water and 4mL of air into syringe.
3. Place the filled syringe into a container (tip up) for 3 min, until the tabs are in sus.
4. Gently invert the syringe 5X immediately prior to administration.
5. After administration of the prepared sus, draw approx 5mL of water and 4mL of air into the same syringe, and swirl the contents to suspend remaining particles; administer entire contents of the syringe.
Preparation Using a Small Drinking Glass:
1. Place prescribed dose into a small drinking glass (max size 100mL) containing approx 25mL of water; do not exceed a total of 10mg/glass and if higher doses are required, prepare an additional glass.
2. Allow 3 min for sus to occur.
3. Stir contents gently w/ a spoon, immediately prior to drinking.
4. After administration of the prepared sus, add 25mL of water and stir w/ the same spoon to resuspend remaining particles; administer entire contents of glass.

STORAGE
25°C (77°F); excursions permitted between 15-30°C (59-86°F). Protect from light and moisture.

HOW SUPPLIED
Tab for Oral Sus: (Afinitor Disperz) 2mg, 3mg, 5mg; **Tab:** (Afinitor) 2.5mg, 5mg, 7.5mg, 10mg

CONTRAINDICATIONS
Hypersensitivity to the active substance, to other rapamycin derivatives, or to any of the excipients of this product.

WARNINGS/PRECAUTIONS
See Dosing Considerations. Not indicated for the treatment of functional carcinoid tumors in NET. Noninfectious pneumonitis reported; some cases reported w/ pulmonary HTN as a secondary event. Immunosuppressive properties may predispose patients to infections, including infections w/ opportunistic pathogens. Localized and systemic infections, including reactivation of hepatitis B, reported. Complete treatment of preexisting invasive fungal infections prior to therapy. Institute appropriate treatment if diagnosis of an infection is made and consider interruption or discontinuation of therapy. If a diagnosis of invasive systemic fungal infection is made, d/c therapy. *Pneumocystis jiroveci* pneumonia (PJP) reported; consider prophylaxis of PJP when concomitant use of corticosteroids or other immunosuppressive agents are required. Mouth ulcers, stomatitis, and oral mucositis reported. Cases of renal failure (including acute renal failure), some w/ fatal outcome, observed. May delay wound healing and increase the occurrence of wound-related complications (eg, wound dehiscence, wound infection, incisional hernia); use caution in the perisurgical period. Elevated SrCr, proteinuria, hyperglycemia, hyperlipidemia, hypertriglyceridemia, and decreased Hgb, lymphocytes, neutrophils, and platelets reported. Exposure is increased in patients w/ hepatic impairment. Avoid close contact w/ those who have received live vaccines during treatment. In pediatric patients w/ SEGA who do not require immediate treatment, complete the recommended childhood series of live virus vaccinations prior to therapy; an accelerated vaccination schedule may be appropriate. Can cause fetal harm; advise females of reproductive potential to avoid becoming pregnant and to use effective contraception during and for 8 weeks after ending treatment. Caution in elderly.

ADVERSE REACTIONS
Advanced HR-Positive, HER2-Negative Breast Cancer/Advanced NET/Advanced RCC: Stomatitis, infections, rash, fatigue, diarrhea, edema, abdominal pain, nausea, fever, asthenia, cough, headache, decreased appetite.
Renal Angiomyolipoma w/ TSC: Stomatitis.
SEGA w/ TSC: Stomatitis, respiratory tract infection.

DRUG INTERACTIONS
See Dosing Considerations. ACE inhibitors may increase risk for angioedema. Avoid use of live vaccines while on therapy. More frequent monitoring is recommended when coadministered w/ other drugs that may induce hyperglycemia. Significant increases in everolimus exposure reported when coadministered w/ ketoconazole (a strong CYP3A4 inhibitor and a P-gp inhibitor), erythromycin (a moderate CYP3A4 inhibitor and a P-gp inhibitor), and verapamil (a moderate CYP3A4 inhibitor and a P-gp inhibitor). Decreased everolimus levels reported when coadministered w/ rifampin (a strong inducer of CYP3A4 and an inducer of P-gp). St. John's wort may decrease everolimus exposure unpredictably. May increase levels of midazolam, octreotide, and exemestane.

PREGNANCY AND LACTATION
Pregnancy: May cause fetal harm.
Lactation: Do not breastfeed during treatment and for 2 weeks after the last dose.
Reproductive Potential: Females of reproductive potential should use effective contraception during and for 8 weeks after ending treatment. Menstrual irregularities, secondary amenorrhea, and increases in luteinizing hormone and follicle-stimulating hormone reported. Female fertility may be compromised. May impair male fertility.

MECHANISM OF ACTION

Kinase inhibitor; inhibitor of mammalian target of rapamycin (mTOR), a serine-threonine kinase, downstream of the PI3K/AKT pathway. Binds to an intracellular protein, FKBP-12, resulting in an inhibitory complex formation w/ mTOR complex 1, inhibiting mTOR kinase activity. Inhibition of mTOR has been shown to reduce cell proliferation, angiogenesis, and glucose uptake. Also, inhibits the expression of hypoxia-inducible factor and reduces the expression of vascular endothelial growth factor.

PHARMACOKINETICS

Absorption: T_{max}=1-2 hrs. **Distribution:** Plasma protein binding (74%). **Metabolism:** CYP3A4 and P-gp. **Elimination:** (3mg single dose) Urine (5%), feces (80%); $T_{1/2}$=30 hrs.

PATIENT CONSIDERATIONS

Assessment: Assess for hypersensitivity, preexisting fungal infections, pregnancy/nursing status, and possible drug interactions. Assess hepatic function and renal function, including measurement of BUN, urinary protein, or SrCr. Obtain FPG, lipid profile, and CBC prior to start of therapy. Assess vaccination history in pediatric patients w/ SEGA.

Monitoring: Monitor for signs/symptoms of hypersensitivity reactions, noninfectious pneumonitis, infections, mouth ulcers, stomatitis, oral mucositis, and other adverse reactions. Monitor FPG, lipid profile, CBC count, and renal function, including measurement of BUN, urinary protein, or SrCr, periodically. Routine therapeutic drug monitoring is recommended in SEGA w/ TSC.

Counseling: Inform that noninfectious pneumonitis or infections may develop; advise to report new or worsening respiratory symptoms or any signs or symptoms of infection. Inform patients that they are more susceptible to angioedema if concomitantly taking ACE inhibitors; advise to be aware of any signs/symptoms of angioedema and to seek prompt medical attention. Inform of the possibility of developing mouth ulcers, stomatitis, and oral mucositis; instruct to use topical treatments and mouthwashes (w/o alcohol, peroxide, iodine, or thyme) in such cases. Inform of the possibility of developing kidney failure and the need to monitor kidney function. Inform of the possibility of impaired wound healing or dehiscence during therapy. Inform of the need to monitor blood chemistry and hematology prior to therapy and periodically thereafter. Advise to notify healthcare provider of all concomitant medications, including OTC medications and dietary supplements. Advise to avoid the use of live vaccines and close contact w/ those who have received live vaccines. Advise of risk of fetal harm. Advise female patients of reproductive potential to use effective contraception during treatment and for 8 weeks after the last dose. Advise not to breastfeed during treatment and for 2 weeks after the last dose. Advise males and females of reproductive potential of the potential risk for impaired fertility. Instruct to follow the dosing instructions ud; inform that missed doses may be taken up to 6 hrs after scheduled time but that if >6 hrs have elapsed, dose should be skipped and resumed at next scheduled time. Advise to read and carefully follow the FDA-approved "Instructions for Use."

AFLURIA — influenza vaccine   Rx

Class: Vaccine

ADULT DOSAGE	PEDIATRIC DOSAGE
Influenza	**Influenza**
Active Immunization Against Influenza Virus Subtypes A and Type B: 1 dose of 0.5mL	**Active Immunization Against Influenza Virus Subtypes A and Type B:** **5-8 Years:** 1 or 2 doses (at least 1 month apart) of 0.5mL, depending on vaccination history **≥9 Years:** 1 dose of 0.5mL

ADMINISTRATION

IM route

May be administered by needle and syringe (≥5 yrs) or by PharmaJet Stratis Needle-Free Injection System (18-64 yrs).
The preferred site for IM inj is the deltoid muscle of the upper arm.
If given at the same time as another injectable vaccine(s), administer in separate syringes and use a separate arm.
Do not mix w/ any other vaccine in the same syringe or vial.

Single-Dose Prefilled Syringe
Shake syringe thoroughly and administer immediately.

Multidose Vial
Shake vial thoroughly before withdrawing each dose, and administer immediately. Draw up the exact dose using a separate sterile needle and syringe for each individual patient; small syringes (0.5mL or 1mL) are recommended to minimize any product loss.
Refer to PI for further administration instructions.

STORAGE

2-8°C (36-46°F). Do not freeze; discard if it has been frozen. Protect from light. Discard vial w/in 28 days once stopper has been pierced.

HOW SUPPLIED

Inj: 0.5mL [prefilled syringe], 5mL [multidose vial]

CONTRAINDICATIONS

Known severe allergic reactions (eg, anaphylaxis) to any component of the vaccine including egg protein, or to a previous dose of any influenza vaccine.

WARNINGS/PRECAUTIONS

Increased rates of fever and febrile seizures reported in children predominantly <5 yrs of age; febrile events were also reported in children 5-8 yrs of age. Caution if Guillain-Barre syndrome (GBS) has occurred w/in 6 weeks of previous influenza vaccination. Appropriate medical treatment and supervision must be available to manage possible anaphylactic reactions. Immune response may be diminished if vaccine is administered to immunocompromised persons, including those receiving immunosuppressive therapy. May not protect all individuals.

ADVERSE REACTIONS

Needle and Syringe:
5-17 Years: Inj-site reactions (pain, redness, swelling), headache, myalgia, irritability, malaise, fever.
18-64 Years: Inj-site reactions (tenderness, pain, swelling, redness, itching), muscle aches, headache, malaise.

PharmaJet Stratis Needle-Free Inj System:
18-64 Years: Inj-site reactions (tenderness, swelling, pain, redness, itching, bruising), myalgia, malaise, headache.
≥65 Years: Inj-site reactions (tenderness, pain).

DRUG INTERACTIONS

Immune response may be diminished if administered in patients receiving immunosuppressive therapy.

PREGNANCY AND LACTATION

Pregnancy: Category B. An exposure and surveillance study that monitors pregnancy outcomes in women exposed to Afluria during pregnancy has been established.
Lactation: Caution in nursing.

MECHANISM OF ACTION

Vaccine; elicits the formation of antibodies that may protect against influenza virus subtypes A and type B.

PATIENT CONSIDERATIONS

Assessment: Review vaccination history. Assess for known severe allergic reactions to any component of the vaccine (eg, egg protein) or to a previous influenza vaccine, development of GBS following a prior dose of influenza vaccine, immunosuppression, pregnancy/nursing status, and possible drug interactions.

Monitoring: Monitor for signs/symptoms of fever, febrile seizures, GBS, allergic reactions, and other adverse reactions.

Counseling: Inform of the potential benefits and risks of immunization. Inform that vaccine cannot cause influenza but stimulates the immune system to produce antibodies that protect against influenza and that the full effect of the vaccine is achieved approximately 3 weeks after vaccination. Instruct to report any severe or unusual adverse reactions to physician. Encourage women who receive vaccine while pregnant to participate in the exposure and surveillance study. Instruct that annual revaccination is recommended.

AFREZZA — insulin human   Rx

Class: Insulin (rapid-acting)

> Acute bronchospasm reported in patients w/ asthma and COPD. Contraindicated w/ chronic lung disease (eg, asthma, COPD). Perform a detailed medical history, physical examination, and spirometry before initiating therapy.

ADULT DOSAGE	PEDIATRIC DOSAGE
Diabetes Mellitus	Pediatric use may not have been established
Initial Mealtime Dose:	
Insulin Naive: 4 U at each meal	
Using SQ Mealtime (Prandial) Insulin: Determine appropriate dose for each meal by converting from the injected dose (see Conversions)	
Using SQ Premixed Insulin: Estimate mealtime injected dose by dividing 1/2 of total daily premixed insulin dose equally among the 3 meals of the day then. Convert each estimated injected mealtime dose to Afrezza dose (see Conversions). Administer 1/2 of total daily injected premixed dose as an injected basal insulin dose	
In patients requiring high doses, if blood glucose control is not achieved w/ increased doses, consider use of SQ mealtime insulin	
Conversions	
Injected Mealtime Insulin Dose to Afrezza Dose Conversion:	
Up to 4 U SQ: 4 U	
5-8 U SQ: 8 U	
9-12 U SQ: 12 U	
13-16 U SQ: 16 U	
17-20 U SQ: 20 U	
21-24 U SQ: 24 U	

DOSING CONSIDERATIONS
Renal Impairment
Dose adjustment may be necessary
Hepatic Impairment
Dose adjustment may be necessary

ADMINISTRATION
Oral inh route

Administer using a single inh per cartridge
Administer at the beginning of the meal

Doses >12 U
Inhalations from multiple cartridges are necessary; administer using a combination of 4 U, 8 U, and 12 U cartridges to achieve required total mealtime dose

Keep inhaler level w/ the white mouthpiece on top and purple base on the bottom after a cartridge has been inserted into the inhaler; loss of drug effect can occur if the inhaler is turned upside down, held w/ the mouthpiece pointing down, or shaken (or dropped) after the cartridge has been inserted but before the dose has been administered. If any of the above occur, the cartridge should be replaced before use

STORAGE
Not in Use: 2-8°C (36-46°F). Sealed (Unopened) Foil Package: May be stored until the expiration date. Sealed (Unopened) Blister Cards + Strips: May be stored for 1 month. If a foil package, blister card, or strip is not refrigerated, use w/in 10 days. In Use: 25°C (77°F); excursions permitted to 15-30°C (59-86°F). Sealed (Unopened) Blister Cards + Strips: Use w/in 10 days. Opened Strips: Use w/in 3 days. Do not put a blister card or strip back into the refrigerator after being stored at room temperature. Inhaler: 2-25°C (36-77°F); excursions permitted. May refrigerate, but should be at room temperature before use. May be used for up to 15 days from date of first use; discard and replace w/ a new inhaler after 15 days of use. Handling: Before use, cartridges should be at room temperature for 10 min.

HOW SUPPLIED
Powder, Inh: 4 U, 8 U, 12 U

CONTRAINDICATIONS
During episodes of hypoglycemia, chronic lung disease (eg, asthma, COPD), hypersensitivity to regular human insulin or any of the excipients to this medication.

WARNINGS/PRECAUTIONS
Not a substitute for long-acting insulin; use in combination w/ long-acting insulin w/ type 1 diabetes mellitus. Not recommended for the treatment of diabetic ketoacidosis (DKA) or in patients who smoke or who have recently stopped smoking. Increase the frequency of glucose monitoring and consider alternative route of delivery of insulin in patients at risk for DKA. Changes in strength, manufacturer, type, or method of administration may affect glycemic control and predispose to hypo/hyperglycemia; these changes should be made under close medical supervision and w/ increased frequency of blood glucose monitoring. Hypoglycemia may occur; increased risk w/ renal/hepatic impairment. May cause a decline in lung function over time as measured by FEV_1; consider discontinuing therapy w/ decline of ≥20% in FEV_1. Consider more frequent monitoring of pulmonary function w/ pulmonary symptoms; d/c if symptoms persist. Consider benefits and potential risk in patients w/ active, prior history of, or at risk for lung cancer. Severe, life-threatening, generalized allergy, including anaphylaxis, may occur; if hypersensitivity reactions occur, d/c therapy, treat, and monitor until symptoms/signs resolve. May cause hypokalemia; monitor K^+ levels in patients at risk for hypokalemia. Patients w/ renal/hepatic impairment may require more frequent blood glucose monitoring.

ADVERSE REACTIONS
Cough, throat pain/irritation, headache, hypoglycemia.

DRUG INTERACTIONS
Concomitant oral antidiabetic treatment may need to be adjusted. Thiazolidinediones (TZDs) may cause fluid retention and lead to or exacerbate heart failure (HF); observe for signs and symptoms of HF and consider dose reduction or discontinuation of TZDs. Risk of hypoglycemia may be increased w/ antidiabetic agents, ACE inhibitors, ARBs, disopyramide, fibrates, fluoxetine, MAOIs, pentoxifylline, pramlintide, propoxyphene, salicylates, somatostatin analogues (eg, octreotide), and sulfonamide antibiotics. Glucose lowering effect may be decreased w/ atypical antipsychotics (eg, olanzapine, clozapine), corticosteroids, danazol, diuretics, estrogens, glucagon, isoniazid, niacin, oral contraceptives, phenothiazines, progestogens, protease inhibitors, somatropin, sympathomimetic agents (eg, albuterol, epinephrine, terbutaline), and thyroid hormones. Glucose lowering effect may be increased or decreased when coadministered w/ alcohol, β-blockers, clonidine, and lithium salts. Pentamidine may cause hypoglycemia, sometimes followed by hyperglycemia. Signs/symptoms of hypoglycemia may be blunted w/ β-blockers, clonidine, guanethidine, and reserpine. Dose adjustment and increased frequency of glucose monitoring may be required when administered w/ drugs that increase/decrease glucose lowering effect or increase hypoglycemia risk.

PREGNANCY AND LACTATION
Category C, not for use in nursing.

MECHANISM OF ACTION
Insulin, human (rDNA origin); lowers blood glucose levels by stimulating peripheral glucose uptake by skeletal muscle and fat, and by inhibiting hepatic glucose production. Inhibits lipolysis in adipocytes, inhibits proteolysis, and enhances protein synthesis.

PHARMACOKINETICS
Absorption: T_{max}=12-15 min (8 U). **Distribution:** Highly likely to be excreted in breast milk. **Elimination:** (Median) $T_{1/2}$=28-39 min (4 U, 32 U).

PATIENT CONSIDERATIONS
Assessment: Assess for drug hypersensitivity, risk of hypoglycemia, chronic lung disease, lung cancer, renal/hepatic impairment, pregnancy/nursing status, and possible drug interactions. Obtain baseline blood glucose. Assess pulmonary function at baseline. Perform medical history, physical examination, and spirometry.

Monitoring: Monitor for signs/symptoms of hypoglycemia, hypokalemia, allergic reactions, decline in lung function, and other adverse reactions. Monitor for acute bronchospasm in patients w/ asthma or COPD. Monitor pulmonary function after 6 months of therapy and annually thereafter. Increase frequency of glucose monitoring in patients at increased risk for hypoglycemia or who have reduced symptomatic awareness of hypoglycemia.

Counseling: Inform of the potential risks and benefits and of alternative modes of therapy. Inform about the importance of adherence to dietary instructions, regular physical activity, periodic blood glucose monitoring and HbA1c testing, recognition and management of hypo/hyperglycemia, and assessment for diabetes complications. Instruct to promptly seek medical advice during periods of stress (eg, fever, trauma, infection, surgery) as medication requirements may change. Instruct to use only w/ inhaler. Instruct to inform physician of any history of lung disease, if any unusual symptom develops, or if any known symptom persists or worsens. Inform that the most common adverse reactions associated w/ therapy are hypoglycemia, cough, and throat pain/irritation. Advise women w/ diabetes to inform physician if pregnant or planning to become pregnant. Advise to immediately report to physician if any respiratory difficulty occurs after inhalation. Instruct on self-management procedures and on handling of special situations. Inform that ability to concentrate and react may be impaired as a result of hypoglycemia; advise to use caution when driving or operating machinery. Inform that therapy may cause a decline in lung function. Instruct to promptly report any signs or symptoms potentially related to lung cancer. Instruct to monitor blood glucose during illness, infection, and other risk situations for DKA; advise to contact physician if blood glucose control worsens. Educate on the symptoms of hypersensitivity reactions.

AGGRENOX — aspirin/dipyridamole   **Rx**
Class: Antiplatelet agent

ADULT DOSAGE	PEDIATRIC DOSAGE
Stroke To reduce risk of stroke in patients who have had transient ischemia of the brain or completed ischemic stroke due to thrombosis 1 cap bid (1 in am and 1 in pm)	Pediatric use may not have been established

DOSING CONSIDERATIONS
Adverse Reactions
Intolerable Headaches During Initial Treatment:
Switch to 1 cap at hs and low-dose aspirin (ASA) in am
Return to usual regimen as soon as possible, usually w/in 1 week

ADMINISTRATION
Oral route

Take PO w/ or w/o food.
Swallow whole; do not chew or crush.

STORAGE
25°C (77°F); excursions permitted to 15-30°C (59-86°F). Protect from excessive moisture.

HOW SUPPLIED
Cap: (ASA/Dipyridamole Extended-Release) 25mg/200mg

CONTRAINDICATIONS
NSAID allergy; syndrome of asthma, rhinitis, and nasal polyps; children or teenagers w/ viral infections; known hypersensitivity to any of the product components.

WARNINGS/PRECAUTIONS
May increase risk of bleeding. Intracranial hemorrhage reported. Risk of GI side effects (eg, stomach pain, heartburn, N/V, gross GI bleeding, dyspepsia); monitor for signs of ulceration and bleeding. May cause fetal harm; avoid in 3rd trimester of pregnancy. Not interchangeable w/ individual components of ASA and dipyridamole tabs. **ASA:** Avoid w/ history of active peptic ulcer disease (PUD) or w/ severe hepatic or severe renal (GFR <10mL/min) dysfunction. Bleeding risks reported w/ chronic, heavy alcohol use (≥3 alcoholic drinks/day). May not provide adequate treatment for cardiac indications for stroke/transient ischemic attack patients for whom ASA is indicated to prevent recurrent MI or angina pectoris. **Dipyridamole:** Elevations of hepatic enzymes and hepatic failure reported. Has a vasodilatory effect; may precipitate/aggravate chest pain in patients w/ underlying coronary artery disease (CAD). May exacerbate preexisting hypotension.

ADVERSE REACTIONS
Headache, dyspepsia, abdominal pain, N/V, diarrhea, fatigue, arthralgia, pain, back pain, GI bleeding, hemorrhage.

DRUG INTERACTIONS
Increased risk of bleeding w/ other drugs that increase the risk of bleeding (eg, anticoagulants, antiplatelet agents, heparin, fibrinolytics, NSAIDs). **Dipyridamole:** May increase plasma levels and cardiovascular (CV) effects of adenosine. May counteract effect of cholinesterase inhibitors, potentially aggravating myasthenia gravis. **ASA:** May decrease effects of ACE inhibitors and β-blockers.

Concurrent use w/ acetazolamide may lead to high serum concentrations of acetazolamide (and toxicity). May displace warfarin from protein binding sites, leading to prolongation of both PT and bleeding time. May decrease total concentration of phenytoin. May increase serum valproic acid levels. May decrease effects of diuretics in renal or CV disease. May inhibit renal clearance of methotrexate, leading to bone marrow toxicity (especially in elderly/renally impaired). Decreased renal function w/ NSAIDs. May increase effectiveness of oral hypoglycemics. May antagonize uricosuric agents (probenecid and sulfinpyrazone).

PREGNANCY AND LACTATION
Pregnancy: Category D.
Lactation: Both dipyridamole and ASA are excreted in human milk; caution in nursing.

MECHANISM OF ACTION
Dipyridamole: Platelet aggregation inhibitor. Inhibits uptake of adenosine into platelets, endothelial cells, and erythrocytes. **ASA:** Platelet aggregation inhibitor. Irreversibly inhibits platelet cyclooxygenase and thus inhibits the generation of thromboxane A_2, a powerful inducer of platelet aggregation and vasoconstriction.

PHARMACOKINETICS
Absorption: Dipyridamole: C_{max}=1.98mcg/mL; T_{max}=2 hrs. ASA: C_{max}=319ng/mL; T_{max}=0.63 hrs. **Distribution:** Found in breast milk. Dipyridamole: V_d=92L; plasma protein binding (99%). ASA: V_d=10L; plasma protein binding (concentration-dependent). **Metabolism:** Dipyridamole: Liver (conjugation); monoglucuronide (primary metabolite). ASA: Plasma (hydrolysis) into salicylic acid (metabolite) then liver (conjugation). **Elimination:** Dipyridamole: Feces, urine; $T_{1/2}$=13.6 hrs. ASA: Urine (10% salicylic acid, 75% salicyluric acid); $T_{1/2}$=0.33 hrs, 1.71 hrs (salicylic acid).

PATIENT CONSIDERATIONS

Assessment: Assess for NSAID allergy, syndrome of asthma, rhinitis and nasal polyps, renal/hepatic dysfunction, history of active PUD, alcohol use, CAD, hypotension, hypersensitivity, pregnancy/nursing status, and possible drug interactions.

Monitoring: Monitor for signs/symptoms of allergic reactions, GI effects, elevated hepatic enzymes, hepatic failure, and bleeding.

Counseling: Inform of risk and signs/symptoms of bleeding (eg, occult bleeding). Instruct to notify physician of all medications and supplements being taken, especially drugs that may increase risk of bleeding. Counsel patients who consume ≥3 alcoholic drinks daily about the bleeding risks. Inform that transient headache may occur; instruct to notify physician if an intolerable headache develops. Inform about signs and symptoms of GI side effects and what steps to take if they occur. Advise that if a dose is missed, to take next dose on regular schedule and not to take a double dose. Inform of potential hazard to fetus if used during pregnancy; instruct to notify physician if patient is pregnant or becomes pregnant.

AKYNZEO — netupitant/palonosetron   Rx

Class: Substance P/neurokinin-1 (NK1) receptor antagonist and 5-HT₃ receptor antagonist

ADULT DOSAGE	PEDIATRIC DOSAGE
Chemotherapy-Induced Nausea/Vomiting	Pediatric use may not have been established
Highly Emetogenic Chemotherapy (Including Cisplatin Based):	
Day 1: 1 cap approx 1 hr prior to the start of chemotherapy w/ dexamethasone 12mg PO 30 min prior to chemotherapy	
Days 2-4: Dexamethasone 8mg PO qd	
Anthracyclines and Cyclophosphamide Based/Non-Highly Emetogenic Chemotherapy:	
Day 1: 1 cap approx 1 hr prior to the start of chemotherapy w/ dexamethasone 12mg PO 30 min prior to chemotherapy	
Days 2-4: Administration of dexamethasone is not necessary	

ADMINISTRATION
Oral route
Take w/ or w/o food

STORAGE
20-25°C (68-77°F); excursions permitted from 15-30°C (59-86°F).

HOW SUPPLIED
Cap: (Netupitant-Palonosetron) 300mg-0.5mg

WARNINGS/PRECAUTIONS
Hypersensitivity reactions, including anaphylaxis, reported. Serotonin syndrome reported; d/c and initiate supportive treatment if symptoms occur. Avoid with severe hepatic/renal impairment and end-stage renal disease. Caution in elderly.

ADVERSE REACTIONS
Dyspepsia, fatigue, constipation, erythema, headache, asthenia.

DRUG INTERACTIONS
Serotonin syndrome reported with concomitant use of other serotonergic drugs (eg, SSRIs, SNRIs, MAOIs); d/c and initiate supportive treatment if symptoms

occur. May increase levels of CYP3A4 substrates; use with caution. Increased exposure of dexamethasone. Increased exposure to midazolam; consider the potential effects of increased levels of midazolam or other benzodiazepines metabolized via CYP3A4 (alprazolam, triazolam). May increase exposure of chemotherapy agents metabolized by CYP3A4 (eg, docetaxel, imatinib, vinblastine); use with caution and monitor for chemotherapeutic-related adverse reactions. Strong CYP3A4 inducers may decrease efficacy; avoid with chronic strong CYP3A4 inducers (eg, rifampin). Strong CYP3A4 inhibitors (eg, ketoconazole) may increase exposure.

PREGNANCY AND LACTATION
Category C, not for use in nursing.

MECHANISM OF ACTION
Netupitant: Substance P/neurokinin 1 receptor antagonist; Palonosetron: 5-HT₃ receptor antagonist.

PHARMACOKINETICS
Absorption: T_{max} (median)=5 hrs. Netupitant: C_{max}=434ng/mL; AUC=14,401ng•hr/mL. Palonosetron: Well absorbed. Absolute bioavailability (97%); C_{max}=1.53ng/mL; AUC=56.7ng•hr/mL. **Distribution:** Netupitant: V_d=1982L; plasma protein binding (>99.5%). Palonosetron: V_d=8.3L/kg; plasma protein binding (62%). **Metabolism:** Netupitant: Extensive via CYP3A4 (primary), CYP2C9 and CYP2D6 (lesser extent); desmethyl derivative, N-oxide derivative, and OH-methyl derivative (major metabolites). Palonosetron: Via CYP2D6, CYP3A4 and CYP1A2 (lesser extent); N-oxide-palonosetron and 6-S-hydroxy-palonosetron (primary metabolites). **Elimination:** Netupitant: Urine and feces (50% [120 hrs]). Urine (3.95%, <1% unchanged [336 hrs]; 4.7% [30 days post-dose]), feces (70.7% [336 hrs]; 86.5% [30 days post-dose]); $T_{1/2}$=80 hrs. Palonosetron: (Single 0.75mg dose) Urine (85-93%, 40% unchanged), feces (5-8%); $T_{1/2}$=48 hrs.

PATIENT CONSIDERATIONS

Assessment: Assess for hypersensitivity to drug, renal/hepatic impairment, pregnancy/nursing status, and possible drug interactions.

Monitoring: Monitor for hypersensitivity reactions, serotonin syndrome, and other adverse reactions.

Counseling: Instruct to seek immediate medical attention if any signs/symptoms of a hypersensitivity reaction or serotonin syndrome (eg, changes in mental status, autonomic instability, neuromuscular symptoms, with or without GI symptoms) occur.

ALDACTAZIDE — hydrochlorothiazide/spironolactone   Rx

Class: Aldosterone blocker/thiazide diuretic

> Tumorigenic in chronic toxicity animal studies; avoid unnecessary use. Not for initial therapy of edema or HTN. Edema or HTN requires therapy titration, and treatment must be reevaluated as conditions in each patient warrant.

ADULT DOSAGE	PEDIATRIC DOSAGE
Edema	Pediatric use may not have been established
For patients w/ congestive heart failure, cirrhosis of the liver accompanied by edema and/or ascites, nephrotic syndrome	
Maint: 100mg of each component daily, as a single dose or in divided doses	
Range: 25-200mg/day of each component depending on response to initial titration	
Hypertension	
Usual: 50-100mg of each component daily, as single dose or in divided doses	
Other Indications	
Edema during pregnancy due to pathologic causes	

ADMINISTRATION
Oral route

STORAGE
<25°C (77°F).

HOW SUPPLIED
Tab: (Spironolactone/HCTZ) 25mg/25mg, 50mg/50mg* *scored

CONTRAINDICATIONS
Anuria, acute renal insufficiency, significant impairment of renal excretory function, hypercalcemia, hyperkalemia, Addison's disease, allergy to thiazide diuretics or sulfonamide-derived drug hypersensitivity, acute or severe hepatic failure.

WARNINGS/PRECAUTIONS
Administration with conditions known to cause hyperkalemia may lead to severe hyperkalemia. Caution with hepatic dysfunction; alterations of fluid and electrolyte balance may precipitate hepatic coma. Somnolence and dizziness reported; may impair mental/physical abilities. HCTZ: Caution with severe renal disease; may precipitate azotemia. Sensitivity reactions with or without a history of allergy or bronchial asthma may occur. May exacerbate or activate systemic

lupus erythematosus (SLE). Idiosyncratic reaction, resulting in acute transient myopia and acute angle-closure glaucoma may occur; d/c treatment as rapidly as possible and consider medical/surgical treatment if intraocular pressure remains uncontrolled. Hypokalemia, hyponatremia, and hypercalcemia may occur. May alter glucose tolerance and increase cholesterol and TG levels. May increase uric acid levels and cause or exacerbate hyperuricemia and precipitate gout in susceptible patients. Spironolactone: May cause hyperkalemia; increased risk in patients with renal insufficiency and diabetes mellitus (DM). Gynecomastia may occur. (Rare) Breast enlargement may persist when therapy is discontinued.

ADVERSE REACTIONS
Gastric bleeding, ulceration, gynecomastia, leukopenia, fever, urticaria, mental confusion, ataxia, renal dysfunction, electrolyte disturbances, weakness, irregular menses, toxic epidermal necrolysis, vertigo, muscle spasm.

DRUG INTERACTIONS
Avoid with K+ supplements, K+-sparing diuretics, or a diet rich in K+; hyperkalemia may occur. Extreme caution with NSAIDs (eg, indomethacin), ACE inhibitors, angiotensin II receptor antagonists, aldosterone blockers, heparin, low molecular weight heparin, other drugs known to cause hyperkalemia, and salt substitutes containing K+; severe hyperkalemia may occur. Alcohol, barbiturates, or narcotics may potentiate orthostatic hypotension. Dose adjustment of antidiabetic drugs (eg, oral agents, insulin) may be required. Intensified electrolyte depletion, particularly hypokalemia, may occur with corticosteroids and adrenocorticotropic hormone. Reduced vascular responsiveness to norepinephrine. Caution with regional or general anesthesia. Increased responsiveness to nondepolarizing skeletal muscle relaxants (eg, tubocurarine). Increased risk of lithium toxicity; avoid with lithium. NSAIDs may reduce the effects of therapy. HCTZ: May add to or potentiate the action of other antihypertensive drugs. Electrolyte disturbances (eg, hypokalemia, hypomagnesemia) may increase risk of digoxin toxicity. Spironolactone: May increase levels of digoxin; monitor digoxin levels and adjust dose accordingly. Hyperkalemic metabolic acidosis reported with cholestyramine.

PREGNANCY AND LACTATION
Category C, not for use in nursing.

MECHANISM OF ACTION
Spironolactone: Aldosterone antagonist; acts primarily by competitive binding of receptors at the aldosterone-dependent Na^+-K^+ exchange site in the distal convoluted renal tubule. HCTZ: Thiazide diuretic and antihypertensive; promotes the excretion of Na^+ and water by inhibiting reabsorption in the cortical diluting segment of the distal renal tubule.

PHARMACOKINETICS
Absorption: Spironolactone; C_{max}=80ng/mL, 181ng/mL (canrenone); T_{max}=2.6 hrs, 4.3 hrs (canrenone); AUC_{0-24}=1.30ng•hr/mL, 1.41ng•hr/mL (canrenone). HCTZ: Rapid; T_{max}=1-2 hrs. **Distribution:** Spironolactone: Plasma protein binding (>90%). Canrenone: Found in breast milk. **Metabolism:** Spironolactone: Rapid and extensive; canrenone (active metabolite). **Elimination:** Spironolactone: Urine (major), bile (minor); $T_{1/2}$=1.4 hrs, 16.5 hrs (canrenone). HCTZ: Urine; $T_{1/2}$=4-5 hrs.

PATIENT CONSIDERATIONS
Assessment: Assess for anuria, acute renal insufficiency, hypercalcemia, renal/hepatic impairment, risk factors for acute angle-closure glaucoma (eg, history of sulfonamide/penicillin allergy), hyperkalemia, SLE, DM, history of allergy or bronchial asthma, any other conditions where treatment is contraindicated or cautioned, pregnancy/nursing status, and possible drug interactions.

Monitoring: Monitor for signs/symptoms of serum electrolyte abnormalities, hyperkalemia, gynecomastia, exacerbation or activation of SLE, hyperuricemia or precipitation of gout, hypersensitivity reactions, idiosyncratic reactions, and other adverse reactions. Monitor serum electrolytes, TG, cholesterol, and Ca^{2+} levels, and renal/hepatic function.

Counseling: Instruct to avoid K+ supplements and foods containing high levels of K+, including salt substitutes. Inform of pregnancy risks. Advise to seek medical attention if signs/symptoms of serum electrolyte abnormalities, hypersensitivity reactions, or other adverse events occur.

ALDACTONE — spironolactone   Rx
Class: Aldosterone blocker

> Tumorigenic in chronic toxicity animal studies; avoid unnecessary use.

ADULT DOSAGE
Primary Hyperaldosteronism

As a Diagnostic Agent:
Long Test: 400mg/day for 3-4 weeks
Short Test: 400mg/day for 4 days
Short-Term Preoperative Treatment:
100-400mg/day
Unsuitable for Surgery/Long-Term Maint:
Lowest effective dose individualized for patient

Edema

Due to CHF, Hepatic Cirrhosis, or Nephrotic Syndrome:
Initial: 100mg/day given in either single or divided doses for at least 5 days

PEDIATRIC DOSAGE
Pediatric use may not have been established

Range: 25-200mg/day
May adjust to optimal therapeutic or maintenance level in single or divided daily doses.
May add 2nd diuretic that acts more proximally in the renal tubule if no adequate diuretic response after 5 days.
Do not change spironolactone dose when other diuretic therapy is added.

Hypertension
Initial: 50-100mg/day given in single or divided doses for at least 2 weeks. Adjust dose according to response.

Hypokalemia
Diuretic-Induced:
25-100mg/day

Severe Heart Failure
In Conjunction w/ Standard Therapy (Serum K+ ≤5.0mEq/L, SrCr ≤2.5mg/dL):
Initial: 25mg qd
Titrate: If tolerated, may increase to 50mg qd as clinically indicated; may reduce to 25mg qod if not tolerated

---

ADMINISTRATION
Oral route
STORAGE
<25°C (77°F).
HOW SUPPLIED
Tab: 25mg, 50mg*, 100mg* *scored
CONTRAINDICATIONS
Anuria, acute renal insufficiency, significant impairment of renal excretory function, hyperkalemia, Addison's disease. Concomitant use of eplerenone.
WARNINGS/PRECAUTIONS
Administration in patients with conditions known to cause hyperkalemia may lead to severe hyperkalemia. Hyperkalemia may be fatal; monitor and manage serum K+ in patients with severe HF. If hyperkalemia is suspected, obtain an ECG, monitor serum K+, and d/c or interrupt treatment for serum K+ >5mEq/L or SrCr >4mg/dL. Monitor for fluid/electrolyte balance (eg, hypomagnesemia, hyponatremia, hypochloremic alkalosis, hyperkalemia). Caution with hepatic impairment; may precipitate hepatic coma. Reversible hyperchloremic metabolic acidosis reported in patients with decompensated hepatic cirrhosis. Dilutional hyponatremia may occur in edematous patients in hot weather. May cause transient BUN elevation, especially with preexisting renal impairment. Mild acidosis and dose-related gynecomastia may occur. Somnolence and dizziness reported; may impair mental/physical abilities.
ADVERSE REACTIONS
Gastric bleeding, ulceration, inability to achieve or maintain erection, leukopenia, fever, urticaria, hyperkalemia, mental confusion, ataxia, renal dysfunction, irregular menses, postmenopausal bleeding, N/V, diarrhea, breast pain.
DRUG INTERACTIONS
See Contraindications. Concomitant administration of K+ supplements, other K+-sparing diuretics, ACE inhibitors, angiotensin II antagonists, aldosterone blockers, NSAIDs (eg, indomethacin), heparin and low molecular weight heparin, other drugs known to cause hyperkalemia, diet rich in K+, or salt substitutes containing K+, may lead to severe hyperkalemia; avoid with other K+-sparing diuretics. Avoid using oral K+ supplements in patients with serum K+ >3.5mEq/L. Alcohol, barbiturates, or narcotics may potentiate orthostatic hypotension. Corticosteroids and adrenocorticotropic hormone may intensify electrolyte depletion, particularly hypokalemia. Reduced vascular responsiveness to norepinephrine, a pressor amine; caution with regional/general anesthesia. May increase responsiveness to nondepolarizing skeletal muscle relaxants (eg, tubocurarine). May increase digoxin levels and subsequent digitalis toxicity; may need to reduce maintenance and digitalization doses and carefully monitor. Avoid with lithium; may reduce clearance of lithium and cause lithium toxicity. NSAIDs may reduce the effects of therapy. Dilutional hyponatremia may be caused or aggravated with other diuretics. Hyperkalemic metabolic acidosis reported with cholestyramine.
PREGNANCY AND LACTATION
Category C, not for use in nursing.
MECHANISM OF ACTION
Aldosterone antagonist; competitively binds to receptors at aldosterone-dependent Na^+-K^+ exchange site in distal convoluted renal tubule, causing increased Na^+ and water excretion, and K+ retention.
PHARMACOKINETICS
Absorption: (Healthy) C_{max}=80ng/mL, 181ng/mL (canrenone); T_{max}=2.6 hrs, 4.3 hrs (canrenone). **Distribution:** Plasma protein binding (>90%); found in breast milk (canrenone). **Metabolism:** Rapid and extensive; canrenone (active metabolite). **Elimination:** Urine (major), bile (minor); $T_{1/2}$=1.4 hrs, 16.5 hrs (canrenone).
PATIENT CONSIDERATIONS
Assessment: Assess for renal/hepatic impairment, hyperkalemia, Addison's disease or other conditions associated with hyperkalemia, anuria, any other

conditions where treatment is contraindicated or cautioned, pregnancy/nursing status, and for possible drug interactions.

Monitoring: Monitor for signs/symptoms of fluid/electrolyte imbalance, dilutional hyponatremia, BUN elevation, hyperchloremic metabolic acidosis, somnolence, dizziness, gynecomastia, and other adverse reactions. Monitor serum electrolytes periodically at appropriate intervals particularly in the elderly and with significant renal/hepatic impairment. Monitor serum K⁺ and SrCr one week after initiation or dose increase, monthly for the first 3 months, then quarterly for a yr, and then every 6 months with severe HF.

Counseling: Instruct to avoid K⁺ supplements and foods containing high levels of K⁺, including salt substitutes. Inform that somnolence and dizziness may occur; advise to use caution when driving or operating machinery, until response to initial treatment has been determined.

ALDARA — imiquimod   Rx

Class: Immune response modifier

ADULT DOSAGE

Actinic Keratosis

Clinically Typical, Nonhyperkeratotic, Nonhypertrophic Actinic Keratoses on Face or Scalp:

Apply 2X/week (eg, Monday, Thursday) before hs for a full 16 weeks to defined treatment area (contiguous area 25cm² [eg, 5cm x 5cm]) on face (forehead or 1 cheek) or on scalp (but not both concurrently)
Max: 36 pkts for 16 weeks

Superficial Basal Cell Carcinomas

Biopsy-confirmed, primary carcinoma, w/ a max tumor diameter of 2cm, located on trunk (excluding anogenital skin), neck, or extremities (excluding hands and feet)

Tumor Diameter:
0.5-<1cm: 4mm cre droplet (10mg)
1-<1.5cm: 5mm cre droplet (25mg)
1.5-2cm: 7mm cre droplet (40mg)
Max: 36 pkts for 6 weeks

Apply before hs 5X/week for a full 6 weeks
Use only when surgical methods are medically less appropriate and follow-up can be assured

External Genital and Perianal Warts

Apply a thin layer 3X/week before hs until warts are totally cleared
Max: 16 weeks

PEDIATRIC DOSAGE

External Genital and Perianal Warts

≥12 Years:
Apply a thin layer before hs and rub in until no longer visible 3X/week until warts are totally cleared
Max: 16 weeks

ADMINISTRATION

Topical route

Prior to application, wash treatment area w/ mild soap and water and allow to dry thoroughly for at least 10 min
Wash hands before and after application
Use 1 pkt/application
Rub in until no longer visible
Wash off w/ mild soap and water
Do not occlude treatment area

Actinic Keratosis

Wash off after 8 hrs

Superficial Basal Cell Carcinoma

Apply a sufficient amount to cover treatment area including 1cm of skin surrounding tumor
Wash off after 8 hrs

External Genital and Perianal Warts/Condyloma Acuminata

Wash off after 6-10 hrs

STORAGE

4-25°C (39-77°F). Do not freeze. Discard unused and partially used pkts; do not reuse partially used pkts.

HOW SUPPLIED

Cre: 5% [250mg, 12ˢ]

WARNINGS/PRECAUTIONS

Caution in patients with preexisting autoimmune conditions. Not recommended for treatment of BCC subtypes other than sBCC. Not for oral, ophthalmic, or intravaginal use. Not recommended until completely healed from any previous drug/surgical treatment or sunburn. Avoid contact with eyes, lips, and nostrils. Local skin reactions are common; a rest period of several days may be taken if required by patient's discomfort or severity of local skin reaction. Do not extend treatment beyond 16 weeks due to missed doses or rest periods. Non-occlusive dressings (eg, cotton gauze, cotton underwear) may be used in the management of skin reactions. Early clinical clearance cannot be adequately assessed until resolution of local skin reactions (eg, 12 weeks post-treatment). Consider biopsy

or other alternative interventions if there is evidence of persistent tumor. Carefully reevaluate treatment and reconsider management with lesions that do not respond to treatment. Avoid or minimize exposure to sunlight (including sunlamps); sunburn susceptibility may be heightened. Caution in patients with considerable sun exposure (eg, due to occupation) and in those with inherent sensitivity to sunlight. Intense local inflammatory reactions (eg, skin weeping or erosion, severe vulvar swelling that can lead to urinary retention) may occur and may be accompanied or preceded by flu-like signs/symptoms. May exacerbate inflammatory skin conditions, including chronic graft versus host disease. Interruption of dosing should be considered if systemic/local inflammatory reactions occur.

ADVERSE REACTIONS

Application-site reaction, local skin reactions, URTI, sinusitis, headache, squamous cell carcinoma, diarrhea, back pain, rhinitis, lymphadenopathy, influenza-like symptoms.

PREGNANCY AND LACTATION

Category C, caution in nursing.

MECHANISM OF ACTION

Immune response modifier; has not been established. In actinic keratosis, suspected to increase biomarker levels (CD3, CD4, CD8, CD11c, CD68). In sBCC, suspected to increase infiltration of lymphocytes, dendritic cells, and macrophages into the tumor lesion. In external genital warts, suspected to induce mRNA encoding cytokines, including interferon-α at the treatment site.

PHARMACOKINETICS

Absorption: C_{max}=0.1ng/mL (12.5mg face), 0.2ng/mL (25mg scalp), 3.5ng/mL (75mg hands/arms), 0.4ng/mL (4.6mg average dose). **Elimination:** Urine (4.6mg average dose) (0.11% [males], 2.41% [females]); (75mg dose) (0.08% [males], 0.15% [females]).

PATIENT CONSIDERATIONS

Assessment: Assess for preexisting autoimmune conditions, immunosuppression, previous drug/surgical treatment, sunburn, inherent sensitivity to sunlight, and pregnancy/nursing status. For treatment of sBCC, perform biopsy to confirm diagnosis.

Monitoring: Monitor for local inflammatory reactions (eg, weeping or erosion, vulvar swelling), application-site reactions, systemic reactions (eg, flu-like symptoms), and other adverse reactions. For sBCC, monitor treatment site regularly; assess at 12 weeks post-treatment for clinical clearance.

Counseling: Instruct on proper application technique and to use ud. Instruct to avoid contact with eyes, lips, and nostrils. Instruct not to bandage or occlude treatment area. Inform that local skin reactions may occur; instruct to contact physician promptly if experiencing any sign/symptom at application site that restricts/prohibits daily activities or makes continued application difficult. For patients being treated for actinic keratosis and sBCC, encourage using sunscreen and minimizing or avoiding exposure to natural or artificial sunlight (tanning beds, UVA/B treatment) while on therapy. Inform that subclinical lesions may appear in treatment area and may subsequently resolve. For patients being treated for external genital warts, instruct to avoid sexual (genital, anal, oral) contact while cream is on the skin. Advise female patients to avoid vaginal application and caution when applying cream at the vaginal opening. Instruct uncircumcised males treating warts under the foreskin to retract foreskin and clean area daily. Inform that new warts may develop during therapy, as drug is not a cure. Inform that drug may also weaken condoms and vaginal diaphragms and that concurrent use is not recommended.

ALECENSA — alectinib   Rx

Class: Kinase inhibitor

ADULT DOSAGE

Metastatic Non-Small Cell Lung Cancer

W/ anaplastic lymphoma kinase (ALK)-positive, metastatic non-small cell lung cancer (NSCLC) who have progressed on or are intolerant to crizotinib

600mg bid until disease progression or unacceptable toxicity

Missed Dose

If a dose is missed or vomiting occurs after taking a dose, take the next dose at the scheduled time

PEDIATRIC DOSAGE

Pediatric use may not have been established

DOSING CONSIDERATIONS

Adverse Reactions

Dose Reduction Schedule:
Starting Dose: 600mg bid
1st Dose Reduction: 450mg bid
2nd Dose Reduction: 300mg bid
D/C if patients are unable to tolerate the 300mg twice daily dose

ALT or AST >5X ULN w/ Total Bilirubin ≤2X ULN: Temporarily withhold until recovery to baseline or to ≤3X ULN, then resume at reduced dose as per dose reduction schedule

ALT or AST >3X ULN w/ Total Bilirubin >2X ULN in the Absence of Cholestasis or Hemolysis: Permanently d/c

Total Bilirubin Elevation of >3X ULN: Temporarily withhold until recovery to baseline or to ≤1.5X ULN, then resume at reduced dose as per dose reduction schedule

Any Grade Treatment-Related Interstitial Lung Disease (ILD)/Pneumonitis: Permanently d/c

Symptomatic Bradycardia: Withhold until recovery to asymptomatic bradycardia or to a HR ≥60 bpm
- If contributing concomitant medication is identified and discontinued, or its dose is adjusted, resume alectinib at previous dose upon recovery to asymptomatic bradycardia or to a HR ≥60 bpm
- If no contributing concomitant medication is identified, or if contributing concomitant medications are not discontinued or dose modified, resume alectinib at reduced dose as per dose reduction schedule upon recovery to asymptomatic bradycardia or to HR ≥60 bpm

Bradycardia (Life-Threatening Consequences, Urgent Intervention Indicated): Permanently d/c alectinib if no contributing concomitant medication is identified
- If contributing concomitant medication is identified and discontinued, or its dose is adjusted, resume alectinib at reduced dose upon recovery to asymptomatic bradycardia or to a HR ≥60 bpm w/ frequent monitoring as clinically indicated; permanently d/c in case of recurrence

Creatine Phosphokinase (CPK) Elevation>5X ULN: Temporarily withhold until recovery to baseline or to ≤2.5X ULN, then resume at same dose

CPK Elevation >10X ULN or 2nd Occurrence of CPK Elevation of >5X ULN: Temporarily withhold until recovery to baseline or ≤2.5X ULN, then resume at reduced dose as per dose reduction schedule

ADMINISTRATION
Oral route

Take w/ food.
Do not open or dissolve the contents of the capsule.

STORAGE
≤30°C (86°F); protect from light and moisture.

HOW SUPPLIED
Cap: 150mg

WARNINGS/PRECAUTIONS
See Dosing Considerations. Elevations of AST >5X ULN, ALT >5X ULN, and bilirubin >3X ULN reported; monitor LFTs including ALT, AST, and total bilirubin q2 weeks during the first 2 months of treatment, then periodically, w/ more frequent testing if transaminase/ bilirubin elevations occur. Severe ILD reported; promptly investigate for ILD/pneumonitis in any patient who presents w/ worsening of respiratory symptoms (eg, dyspnea, cough, fever). Immediately withhold treatment in patients diagnosed w/ ILD/pneumonitis and permanently d/c if no other potential causes of ILD/pneumonitis have been identified. Symptomatic bradycardia may occur; monitor HR and BP regularly. Myalgia or musculoskeletal pain and elevations of CPK levels reported. Assess CPK levels every 2 weeks during 1st month of treatment and in patients reporting unexplained muscle pain, tenderness, or weakness. May cause fetal harm.

ADVERSE REACTIONS
Fatigue, constipation, edema, myalgia, cough, rash, N/V, headache, diarrhea, dyspnea, back pain, increased weight, vision disorder.

PREGNANCY AND LACTATION
Pregnancy: Can cause fetal harm.
Lactation: Do not breastfeed during treatment and for 1 week after the final dose.
Reproductive Risk Potential:
Females: Use effective contraception during treatment and for 1 week after the final dose.
Males: Males w/ female partners of reproductive potential should use effective contraception during treatment and for 3 months following the final dose.

MECHANISM OF ACTION
Tyrosine kinase inhibitor; targets ALK and RET. Inhibits ALK phosphorylation and ALK-mediated activation of the downstream signaling proteins STAT3 and AKT, and decreases tumor cell viability in multiple cell lines harboring ALK fusions, amplifications, or activating mutations.

PHARMACOKINETICS
Absorption: Absolute bioavailability (37%), T_{max}=4 hrs, AUC: 7430ng•h/mL; 2810ng•h/mL (M4). **Distribution:** V_d=4016L, 10,093L (M4); plasma protein binding (>99%, parent drug and M4). **Metabolism:** Via CYP3A4 to M4 (major active metabolite). **Elimination:** Urine (<0.5%), Feces (98%; 84% unchanged, 6% M4). $T_{1/2}$=33 hrs, 31 hrs (M4).

PATIENT CONSIDERATIONS
Assessment: Assess for hepatic impairment, pregnancy/nursing status, and possible drug interactions.

Monitoring: Monitor LFTs including ALT, AST, and total bilirubin every 2 weeks during the first 2 months of treatment, then periodically w/ more frequent testing in patients who develop transaminase and bilirubin elevations. Monitor for worsening of respiratory symptoms indicative of ILD/pneumonitis (eg, dyspnea, cough, fever) and monitor for unexplained muscle pain, tenderness, or weakness. Assess CPK levels every 2 weeks for the 1st month of treatment and as clinically indicated in patients reporting symptoms. Monitor HR and BP regularly.

Counseling: Advise about the signs/symptoms of bilirubin and hepatic transaminase elevations. Inform about the risks of severe ILD/pneumonitis. Instruct to report new or worsening respiratory symptoms, symptoms of bradycardia (eg, dizziness, lightheadedness, syncope), and to report about the use of any heart or BP medications. Advise of signs/symptoms of myalgia and instruct

to report new or worsening symptoms of muscle pain or weakness. Advise to avoid prolonged sun exposure while taking this medication and for at least 7 days after discontinuation. Advise to use a broad spectrum UVA/UVB sunscreen and lip balm (SPF ≥50) to help protect against potential sunburn. Inform that therapy may cause fetal harm; advise females of reproductive potential to use effective contraception during treatment and for at least 1 week after the last dose. Advise male patients w/ female partners of reproductive potential to use effective contraception during treatment and for 3 months after the last dose. Advise women not to breastfeed during treatment and for 1 week after the last dose. Instruct to take alectinib twice a day w/ food, and to swallow whole. Advise that if a dose is missed or if the patient vomits after taking a dose, not to take an extra dose, but to take the next dose at the regular time.

ALENDRONATE — alendronate sodium   Rx

Class: Bisphosphonate

OTHER BRAND NAMES
Fosamax

ADULT DOSAGE	PEDIATRIC DOSAGE
Osteoporosis	Pediatric use may not have been established
In Postmenopausal Women:	
Treatment:	
70mg tab/sol once weekly or 10mg tab qd	
Prevention:	
35mg tab once weekly or 5mg tab qd	
Treatment to Increase Bone Mass in Men w/ Osteoporosis:	
70mg tab/sol once weekly or 10mg tab qd	
Treatment of Glucocorticoid-Induced Osteoporosis:	
In men and women receiving glucocorticoids in a daily dosage equivalent to 7.5mg or greater of prednisone and who have low bone mineral density	
5mg tab qd; 10mg tab qd for postmenopausal women not on estrogen	
Paget's Disease	
Treatment of Paget's Disease of Bone in Men and Women:	
40mg tab qd for 6 months	
Retreatment: Following a 6-month post-treatment evaluation period, may consider retreatment if relapse occurs (based on increases in serum alkaline phosphatase). May also consider retreatment if treatment fails to normalize serum alkaline phosphatase	
Missed Dose	
If once-weekly dose is missed, administer 1 dose on am after patient remembers; do not administer 2 doses on same day but return to 1 dose once a week, as originally scheduled on chosen day	

DOSING CONSIDERATIONS
Renal Impairment
CrCl <35mL/min: Not recommended

ADMINISTRATION
Oral route

Take upon arising for the day.
Swallow tabs w/ full glass of water (6-8 oz); do not chew or suck on the tab.
Oral sol should be followed by at least 2 oz of water.
Take at least 1/2 hr before the 1st food, beverage, or medication of the day w/ plain water only.
Do not lie down for at least 30 min and until after 1st food of the day.

STORAGE
Oral Sol: 25°C (77°F); excursions permitted to 15-30°C (59-86°F). Do not freeze.
Tab: 20-25°C (68-77°F); (Fosamax) 15-30°C (59-86°F).

HOW SUPPLIED
Oral Sol: 70mg [75mL]; **Tab:** 5mg, 10mg, 35mg, 40mg; (Fosamax) 70mg

CONTRAINDICATIONS
Esophageal abnormalities that delay esophageal emptying (eg, stricture, achalasia), inability to stand or sit upright for at least 30 min, hypocalcemia, hypersensitivity to any component of the medication. **Oral Sol:** Patients at increased risk of aspiration.

WARNINGS/PRECAUTIONS
May cause local irritation of the upper GI mucosa; caution w/ active upper GI problems (eg, Barrett's esophagus, dysphagia, other esophageal diseases, gastritis, duodenitis, ulcers). Esophageal reactions (eg, esophagitis, esophageal ulcers/

erosions) reported; d/c and seek medical attention if dysphagia, odynophagia, retrosternal pain, or new/worsening heartburn develops. Use therapy under appropriate supervision in patients who cannot comply w/ dosing instructions due to mental disability. Gastric and duodenal ulcers reported. Treat hypocalcemia and other disorders affecting mineral metabolism (eg, vitamin D deficiency) prior to therapy. Asymptomatic decreases in serum Ca^{2+} and phosphate may occur; ensure adequate Ca^{2+} and vitamin D intake especially in patients w/ Paget's disease of bone and in patients taking glucocorticoids. Severe and occasionally incapacitating bone, joint, and/or muscle pain reported; d/c if severe symptoms develop. Osteonecrosis of the jaw (ONJ) reported; risk may increase w/ duration of exposure to drug. If invasive dental procedures are required, discontinuation of treatment may reduce risk for ONJ. Consider discontinuation if ONJ develops. Atypical, low-energy, or low-trauma fractures of the femoral shaft reported; evaluate any patient w/ a history of bisphosphonate exposure who presents w/ thigh/groin pain to rule out incomplete femur fracture, and consider interruption of therapy. **Tab:** Consider discontinuation after 3-5 yrs of use in patients at low risk for fracture; periodically reevaluate risk for fracture in patients who d/c therapy. Ascertain gonadal hormonal status and consider appropriate replacement before initiating therapy for glucocorticoid-induced osteoporosis.

ADVERSE REACTIONS
Nausea, abdominal pain, musculoskeletal pain, dyspepsia, constipation, diarrhea.

DRUG INTERACTIONS
Ca^{2+} supplements, antacids, or oral medications containing multivalent cations will interfere w/ absorption; wait at least 1/2 hr after taking alendronate before taking any other oral medications. Increased incidence of upper GI adverse events in patients receiving concomitant therapy w/ daily doses of alendronate >10mg and aspirin-containing products. NSAID use is associated w/ GI irritation; use w/ caution.

PREGNANCY AND LACTATION
Pregnancy: Category C. There are no data on fetal risk in humans; however, there is a theoretical risk of fetal harm, predominantly skeletal, if a woman becomes pregnant after completing a course of bisphosphonate therapy.
Lactation: It is not known whether alendronate is excreted in human milk. Caution in nursing.

MECHANISM OF ACTION
Bisphosphonate; binds to hydroxyapatite found in bone, and specifically inhibits osteoclast-mediated bone resorption.

PHARMACOKINETICS
Absorption: Absolute bioavailability (0.64% in women), (0.59% in men).
Distribution: V_d= at least 28L; plasma protein binding (78%). **Elimination:** (IV) Urine (50%); $T_{1/2}$ >10 yrs.

PATIENT CONSIDERATIONS
Assessment: Assess for esophageal abnormalities, ability to stand or sit upright for at least 30 min, hypocalcemia, risk for ONJ, active upper GI problems, mental disability, renal impairment, drug hypersensitivity, any other conditions where treatment is contraindicated or cautioned, pregnancy/nursing status, and possible drug interactions. **Tab:** For glucocorticoid-induced osteoporosis treatment, assess gonadal hormonal status and obtain bone mineral density.

Monitoring: Monitor for signs/symptoms of ONJ, atypical fractures, esophageal reactions, musculoskeletal pain, hypocalcemia, and other adverse reactions. Monitor serum Ca^{2+} levels. Periodically reevaluate the need for continued therapy. **Tab:** Monitor bone mineral density after 6-12 months of combined alendronate and glucocorticoid treatment. For Paget's disease treatment, monitor serum alkaline phosphatase periodically.

Counseling: Inform about benefits/risks of therapy. Instruct to follow all dosing instructions and inform that failure to follow them may increase risk of esophageal problems. Instruct to take upon arising for the day and at least 1/2 hr before the 1st food, beverage, or medication of the day w/ plain water only; advise to swallow tab w/ 6-8 oz of water and to follow oral sol by at least 2 oz of water. Advise to avoid lying down for at least 30 min after taking the drug and until after 1st food of the day. Instruct to take supplemental Ca^{2+} and vitamin D if daily dietary intake is inadequate. Advise to consider weight-bearing exercise along w/ the modification of certain behavioral factors (eg, cigarette smoking, excessive alcohol use), if these factors exist. Advise to d/c and consult physician if symptoms of esophageal disease develop. Instruct that if a once-weekly dose is missed, to take 1 dose the am after patient remembers and to return to taking the dose as originally scheduled on patient's chosen day; instruct not to take 2 doses on the same day.

ALIMTA — pemetrexed disodium   **Rx**
Class: Antifolate

ADULT DOSAGE
Nonsquamous Non-Small Cell Lung Cancer

Initial treatment of locally advanced or metastatic nonsquamous non-small cell lung cancer (NSCLC) in combination w/ cisplatin. Maint treatment of patients w/ locally advanced or metastatic nonsquamous NSCLC whose disease has not progressed after 4 cycles of platinum-based first-line chemotherapy. Single-agent for the treatment of patients w/ locally advanced or metastatic nonsquamous NSCLC after prior chemotherapy

PEDIATRIC DOSAGE
Pediatric use may not have been established

Combination w/ Cisplatin:
$500mg/m^2$ IV infused over 10 min on Day 1 of each 21-day cycle.
Give cisplatin $75mg/m^2$ infused over 2 hrs beginning 30 min after the end of administration

Single Agent:
$500mg/m^2$ IV infused over 10 min on Day 1 of each 21-day cycle

Malignant Pleural Mesothelioma

Patients whose disease is unresectable or who are otherwise not candidates for curative surgery in combination w/ cisplatin

Combination w/ Cisplatin:
$500mg/m^2$ IV infused over 10 min on Day 1 of each 21-day cycle.
Give cisplatin $75mg/m^2$ infused over 2 hrs beginning 30 min after the end of administration

Premedication

Initiate folic acid (400-1000mcg) PO qd beginning 7 days before the 1st dose; continue during the full course of therapy and for 21 days after the last dose of therapy.
Administer vitamin B12 1mg IM 1 week prior to the 1st dose and every 3 cycles thereafter.
Subsequent vitamin B12 inj may be given the same day as treatment.
Give dexamethasone 4mg PO bid the day before, the day of, and the day after administration of therapy.

DOSING CONSIDERATIONS
Adverse Reactions
As a Single Agent or in Combination:
Hematologic Toxicities:
Nadir ANC <500/mm³ and Nadir Platelets ≥50,000/mm³: 75% of previous dose (pemetrexed and cisplatin)
Nadir Platelets <50,000/mm³ w/o Bleeding Regardless of Nadir ANC: 75% of previous dose (pemetrexed and cisplatin)
Nadir Platelets <50,000/mm³ w/ Bleeding Regardless of Nadir ANC: 50% of previous dose (pemetrexed and cisplatin)

Nonhematologic Toxicities:
≥Grade 3 (Excluding Neurotoxicity): Withhold treatment until resolution to ≤pre-therapy value
Any Grade 3 or 4 Toxicities Except Mucositis: 75% of previous dose (pemetrexed and cisplatin)
Any Diarrhea Requiring Hospitalization (Irrespective of Grade) or Grade 3 or 4 Diarrhea: 75% of previous dose (pemetrexed and cisplatin)
Grade 3 or 4 Mucositis: 50% of previous pemetrexed dose, 100% of previous cisplatin dose

Neurotoxicity:
CTC Grade 1: 100% of previous pemetrexed and cisplatin dose
CTC Grade 2: 100% of previous pemetrexed dose, 50% of previous cisplatin dose

Discontinuation
For Any of the Following:
1. Experiences any hematologic or nonhematologic Grade 3 or 4 toxicity after 2 dose reductions
2. Grade 3 or 4 neurotoxicity is observed

ADMINISTRATION
IV route

Preparation
1. Calculate dose and determine the number of vials needed.
2. Reconstitute each 100mg vial w/ 4.2mL of 0.9% NaCl (preservative free). Reconstitute each 500mg vial w/ 20mL of 0.9% NaCl (preservative free).
3. Gently swirl each vial until the powder is completely dissolved. The resulting sol is clear and ranges in color from colorless to yellow or green-yellow w/o adversely affecting product quality.
4. An appropriate quantity of the reconstituted sol must be further diluted into a sol of 0.9% NaCl (preservative free), so that the total volume of sol is 100mL.
5. Administered as an IV infusion over 10 min.

Compatibility and Stability
Compatible w/ standard polyvinyl chloride administration sets and IV sol bags. Stable for up to 24 hrs following initial reconstitution, when refrigerated.

Handling Precautions
If sol contacts the skin, wash the skin immediately and thoroughly w/ soap and water.
If sol contacts the mucous membranes, flush thoroughly w/ water.

STORAGE
Unreconstituted: 25°C (77°F); excursions permitted to 15-30°C (59-86°F).
Reconstituted and Infusion Sol: Stable at 2-8°C (36-46°F) for up to 24 hrs.

HOW SUPPLIED
Inj: 100mg, 500mg

CONTRAINDICATIONS
History of severe hypersensitivity reaction to pemetrexed.

WARNINGS/PRECAUTIONS
Not indicated for the treatment of patients with squamous cell NSCLC. Premedicate with folic acid and vitamin B12 to reduce hematologic/GI toxicity, and with dexamethasone. Do not substitute oral vitamin B12 for IM vitamin B12. Bone marrow suppression may occur; myelosuppression is usually the dose-limiting toxicity. Caution with renal/hepatic impairment and in elderly. Avoid in patients with CrCl <45mL/min. D/C if hematologic or nonhematologic Grade 3 or 4 toxicity after two dose reductions or immediately if Grade 3 or 4 neurotoxicity is observed. Do not start a cycle of treatment unless CrCl is ≥45mL/min, ANC is ≥1500 cells/mm³, and platelet count is ≥100,000 cells/mm³; obtain CBC and renal function tests at the beginning of each cycle and prn. May cause fetal harm; use effective contraception to prevent pregnancy.

ADVERSE REACTIONS
Anemia, anorexia, fatigue, leukopenia, N/V, stomatitis, neutropenia, rash/desquamation, thrombocytopenia, constipation, pharyngitis, diarrhea.

DRUG INTERACTIONS
Reduced clearance with ibuprofen. In patients with mild to moderate renal insufficiency (CrCl 45-79mL/min), caution with NSAIDs; avoid NSAIDs with short $T_{1/2}$ (eg, diclofenac, indomethacin) for 2 days before, the day of, and 2 days following therapy. Interrupt dosing of NSAIDs with longer $T_{1/2}$ (eg, meloxicam, nabumetone) for at least 5 days before, the day of, and 2 days following therapy. If concomitant NSAID administration is necessary, monitor for toxicity. Delayed clearance with nephrotoxic or tubularly secreted drugs (eg, probenecid).

PREGNANCY AND LACTATION
Category D, not for use in nursing.

MECHANISM OF ACTION
Antifolate; disrupts folate-dependent metabolic processes essential for cell replication. Inhibits thymidylate synthase, dihydrofolate reductase, and glycinamide ribonucleotide formyltransferase.

PHARMACOKINETICS
Distribution: V_d=16.1L; plasma protein binding (81%). **Elimination:** Urine (70-90% unchanged); $T_{1/2}$=3.5 hrs (normal renal function).

PATIENT CONSIDERATIONS
Assessment: Assess for drug hypersensitivity, renal/hepatic impairment, pregnancy/nursing status, and possible drug interactions. Obtain CBC and renal function tests at the beginning of each cycle.

Monitoring: Monitor for signs and symptoms of hematologic/nonhematologic toxicities, bone marrow suppression (eg, neutropenia, thrombocytopenia, anemia), GI toxicity, neurotoxicity, and other adverse events. Monitor CBC with platelet counts and for nadir and recovery. Perform renal and hepatic function tests periodically.

Counseling: Inform about benefits and risks of therapy. Instruct on the need for folic acid and vitamin B12 supplementation to reduce treatment-related hematological and GI toxicity, and of the need for corticosteroids to reduce treatment-related dermatologic toxicity. Inform about risks of low blood cell counts and instruct to contact physician immediately if signs of infection (eg, fever, bleeding or symptoms of anemia) occur. Instruct to contact physician if persistent vomiting, diarrhea, or signs of dehydration appear. Instruct to inform physician of all concomitant prescription or OTC medications (eg, NSAIDs). Inform female patients of the potential hazard to fetus; advise to avoid pregnancy and to use effective contraceptive measures to prevent pregnancy during treatment.

ALINIA — nitazoxanide   Rx

Class: Antiprotozoal agent

ADULT DOSAGE	**PEDIATRIC DOSAGE**
Diarrhea	**Diarrhea**
Caused by *Giardia lamblia* or *Cryptosporidium parvum*: 500mg (1 tab or 25mL of sus) q12h for 3 days	**Caused by *Giardia lamblia* or *Cryptosporidium parvum*:** **1-3 Years:** 100mg (5mL of sus) q12h for 3 days **4-11 Years:** 200mg (10mL of sus) q12h for 3 days **≥12 Years:** 500mg (1 tab or 25mL of sus) q12h for 3 days

---

ADMINISTRATION
Oral route
Take w/ food.
Sus
- Measure 48mL of water for preparation of the 100 mg/5 mL suspension.
- Tap bottle until all powder flows freely.
- Add approx 1/2 of the 48mL of water required for reconstitution and shake vigorously to suspend powder.
- Add remainder of water and again shake vigorously.
- Keep container tightly closed, and shake sus well before each administration.
- Reconstituted sus may be stored for 7 days at room temperature, after which any unused portion must be discarded.

Tab
Do not use in pediatric patients ≤11 years.

STORAGE
25°C (77°F); excursions permitted to 15-30°C (59-86°F). **Reconstituted Sus:** May be stored for 7 days at room temperature; discard any unused portion.

HOW SUPPLIED
Sus: 100mg/5mL [60mL]; **Tab:** 500mg

CONTRAINDICATIONS
Prior hypersensitivity to nitazoxanide or any other ingredient in the formulations.

WARNINGS/PRECAUTIONS
Not shown to be effective for the treatment of diarrhea caused by *Cryptosporidium parvum* in HIV-infected or immunodeficient patients. Caution in elderly.

ADVERSE REACTIONS
Abdominal pain, headache, chromaturia, nausea.

DRUG INTERACTIONS
Caution w/ other highly plasma protein-bound drugs w/ narrow therapeutic indices (eg, warfarin), as competition for binding sites may occur.

PREGNANCY AND LACTATION
Pregnancy: There are no data w/ nitazoxanide in pregnant women to inform a drug-associated risk.
Lactation: No information regarding the presence of nitazoxanide in human milk, the effects on the breastfed infant, or the effects on milk production is available; caution in nursing.

MECHANISM OF ACTION
Antiprotozoal agent; believed to be due to interference w/ the pyruvate:ferredoxin oxidoreductase enzyme-dependent electron transfer reaction which is essential to anaerobic energy metabolism.

PHARMACOKINETICS
Absorption: (Tizoxanide) 12-17 Years: C_{max}=9.1μg/mL, T_{max}=4 hrs, AUC=39.5μg•hr/mL; ≥18 Years: C_{max}=10.6 μg/mL, T_{max}=3 hrs, AUC=41.9μg•hr/mL. (Tizoxanide Glucuronide) 12-17 Years: C_{max}=7.3 μg/mL, T_{max}=4 hrs, AUC=46.5μg•hr/mL; ≥18 Years: C_{max}=10.5μg/mL, T_{max}=4.5 hrs, AUC=63μg•hr/mL. **Distribution:** Plasma protein binding (>99.9%, tizoxanide). **Metabolism:** Tizoxanide and tizoxanide glucuronide (active metabolites).

PATIENT CONSIDERATIONS
Assessment: Assess for hypersensitivity to drug, pregnancy/nursing status, and possible drug interactions.

Monitoring: Monitor for adverse reactions.

Counseling: Instruct to take w/ food and to avoid concurrent warfarin use.

ALLERNAZE — triamcinolone acetonide   Rx

Class: Corticosteroid

ADULT DOSAGE	**PEDIATRIC DOSAGE**
Seasonal/Perennial Allergic Rhinitis	**Seasonal/Perennial Allergic Rhinitis**
Initial: 2 sprays/nostril qd; if a faster onset of relief is desired, may consider 4 sprays/nostril qd or 2 sprays/nostril bid	**≥12 Years:** **Initial:** 2 sprays/nostril qd; if a faster onset of relief is desired, may consider 4 sprays/nostril qd or 2 sprays/nostril bid
Max: 4 sprays/nostril qd or 2 sprays/nostril bid	**Max:** 4 sprays/nostril qd or 2 sprays/nostril bid
Titrate to lowest effective dose after control of symptoms	Titrate to lowest effective dose after control of symptoms
D/C and consider alternative diagnosis/therapies if relief of symptoms is not achieved after 14-21 days	D/C and consider alternative diagnosis/therapies if relief of symptoms is not achieved after 14-21 days

---

DOSING CONSIDERATIONS
Elderly
Start at lower end of dosing range

ADMINISTRATION
Intranasal route

Priming
Prime pump before initial use or if not used for >14 days by releasing 3 sprays or until a fine mist is observed

STORAGE
20-25°C (68-77°F). Protect from freezing. Use within 2 months after opening of the protective foil pouch or before expiration date, whichever comes 1st. Discard after 120 sprays following initial priming.

HOW SUPPLIED
Spray: 50mcg/spray [15mL]

CONTRAINDICATIONS
Hypersensitivity to any of the ingredients in the product.

WARNINGS/PRECAUTIONS
Risk of adrenal insufficiency and withdrawal symptoms when replacing systemic corticosteroids with topical corticosteroids. May increase susceptibility to infections. Avoid exposure to chickenpox and measles. May reduce growth velocity in pediatrics. Development of localized infections of the nose and pharynx

with Candida albicans may occur; may require appropriate local treatment and d/c of therapy. Caution with active or quiescent tuberculosis (TB), untreated fungal, bacterial, or systemic viral infections, or ocular herpes simplex. Caution with recent nasal septal ulcers, nasal surgery, or nasal trauma. Nasal septal perforations reported in rare instances. D/C slowly if hypercorticism and adrenal suppression occur. Caution in elderly.

ADVERSE REACTIONS
Headache, back pain, pharyngitis, asthma, dyspepsia, nausea, taste perversion, conjunctivitis, myalgia.

PREGNANCY AND LACTATION
Category C, caution in nursing.

MECHANISM OF ACTION
Corticosteroid; not established. Shown to have a wide range of effects on multiple cell types (eg, mast cells, eosinophils, neutrophils, macrophages, lymphocytes) and mediators (eg, histamines, eicosanoids, leukotrienes, cytokines) involved in inflammation.

PHARMACOKINETICS
Absorption: (400mcg single dose) C_{max}=1.12ng/mL; T_{max}=0.5 hrs (median). **Distribution:** V_d=99.5L. **Elimination:** (400mcg single dose) $T_{1/2}$=2.26 hrs.

PATIENT CONSIDERATIONS
Assessment: Assess for drug hypersensitivity, patients who have not been exposed to infections (eg, measles or chickenpox), active or quiescent TB, untreated fungal/bacterial/systemic viral infections, ocular herpes simplex, recent nasal surgery/trauma/septal ulcers, and pregnancy/nursing status.

Monitoring: Monitor for acute adrenal insufficiency and withdrawal symptoms when replacing systemic corticosteroid with topical corticosteroid. Monitor for hypercorticism, chickenpox, measles, nasal or pharyngeal *Candida* infections, hypoadrenalism (in infants born to a mother who received corticosteroids during pregnancy), and other adverse effects. Routinely monitor growth of pediatrics.

Counseling: Instruct to avoid exposure to chickenpox or measles and to consult physician if exposed. Instruct to use as directed, at regular intervals, and not to exceed the prescribed dosage. Advise to contact physician if symptoms do not improve after 3 weeks, if condition worsens, or if recurrent episodes of epistaxis or nasal septum discomfort occur. Inform that transient nasal irritation and/or burning or stinging may occur upon instillation. Instruct to avoid spraying directly into the eyes or onto the nasal septum.

ALOMIDE — lodoxamide tromethamine   Rx

Class: Mast cell stabilizer

ADULT DOSAGE	PEDIATRIC DOSAGE
Ocular Conditions	**Ocular Conditions**
Vernal Keratoconjunctivitis, Vernal Conjunctivitis, and Vernal Keratitis: 1-2 drops in each affected eye qid for up to 3 months	**Vernal Keratoconjunctivitis, Vernal Conjunctivitis, and Vernal Keratitis:** >2 Years: 1-2 drops in each affected eye qid for up to 3 months

---

ADMINISTRATION
Ocular route

STORAGE
15-27°C (59-80°F).

HOW SUPPLIED
Sol: 0.1% [10mL]

CONTRAINDICATIONS
Hypersensitivity to any component of this product.

WARNINGS/PRECAUTIONS
Do not wear soft contacts during treatment. Transient burning and stinging upon instillation. Do not touch container tip to any surface to avoid contamination.

ADVERSE REACTIONS
Ocular pruritus, blurred vision, dry eye, tearing, discharge, hyperemia, crystalline deposits, foreign body sensation.

PREGNANCY AND LACTATION
Category B, caution in nursing.

MECHANISM OF ACTION
Mast cell stabilizer; not established; suspected to inhibit the Type I immediate hypersensitivity reaction, decrease cutaneous vascular permeability associated with reagin or IgE and antigen-mediated reactions, and prevent calcium influx into mast cells upon stimulation.

PHARMACOKINETICS
Elimination: Urine; $T_{1/2}$=8.5 hrs.

PATIENT CONSIDERATIONS
Assessment: Assess for drug hypersensitivity.

Monitoring: Monitor for transient burning, stinging or discomfort, itching, blurred vision, dry eye, tearing/discharge, hyperemia, crystalline deposits, and foreign body sensation.

Counseling: Instruct not to wear soft contact lenses during treatment and not to touch dropper tip to any surface to prevent contamination. Advise to notify physician of adverse reactions.

ALOPRIM — allopurinol sodium   Rx

Class: Xanthine oxidase inhibitor

ADULT DOSAGE	PEDIATRIC DOSAGE
Chemotherapy-Induced Hyperuricemia	**Chemotherapy-Induced Hyperuricemia**
Management of patients w/ leukemia, lymphoma, and solid tumor malignancies who are receiving cancer therapy that causes elevations of serum and urinary uric acid levels and who cannot tolerate oral therapy	Management of patients w/ leukemia, lymphoma, and solid tumor malignancies who are receiving cancer therapy that causes elevations of serum and urinary uric acid levels and who cannot tolerate oral therapy
Usual: 200-400mg/m²/day, as a single infusion or in equally divided infusions at 6-, 8-, or 12-hr intervals **Max:** 600mg/day	**Initial:** 200mg/m²/day, as a single infusion or in equally divided infusions at 6-, 8-, or 12-hr intervals
Whenever possible, initiate therapy 24-48 hrs before the start of chemotherapy known to cause tumor cell lysis (including adrenocortical steroids)	Whenever possible, initiate therapy 24-48 hrs before the start of chemotherapy known to cause tumor cell lysis (including adrenocortical steroids)

DOSING CONSIDERATIONS
Renal Impairment
CrCl 10-20mL/min: 200mg/day
CrCl 3-10mL/min: 100mg/day
CrCl <3mL/min: 100mg/day at extended intervals
Elderly
Start at lower end of dosing range

ADMINISTRATION
IV route

Hydration
Fluid intake sufficient to yield a daily urinary output of ≥2L in adults and the maint of a neutral or, preferably, slightly alkaline urine are desirable

Preparation of Sol
1. Dissolve the contents of each 30mL vial w/ 25mL of sterile water for inj; reconstitution yields a concentrated sol w/ a pH of 11.1-11.8
2. Dilute the sol to the desired concentration w/ 0.9% NaCl inj or D5 for inj; refer to PI for drugs that are physically incompatible in sol w/ allopurinol
3. A final concentration of ≤6mg/mL is recommended

Administration
Begin administration w/in 10 hrs after reconstitution
The rate of infusion depends on the volume of infusate
Do not mix w/ or administer through the same IV port w/ agents that are incompatible in sol w/ allopurinol

STORAGE
20-25°C (68-77°F). Do not refrigerate reconstituted/diluted sol.

HOW SUPPLIED
Inj: 500mg

CONTRAINDICATIONS
Re-initiation in patients who developed a severe reaction to allopurinol.

WARNINGS/PRECAUTIONS
D/C at 1st appearance of skin rash or other signs of an allergic reaction. Hepatotoxicity and elevated serum alkaline phosphatase/transaminase reported with PO allopurinol. Bone marrow suppression reported. Evaluate liver function if anorexia, weight loss, or pruritus develops. Periodically monitor LFTs during early stages of therapy in patients with preexisting liver disease. May impair mental/physical abilities. Maintain sufficient fluid intake to yield a daily urinary output in adults of at least 2L and maintain neutral or slightly alkaline urine. Caution with renal impairment or concurrent illnesses affecting renal function (eg, HTN, diabetes mellitus); periodically monitor renal function. Caution in elderly.

ADVERSE REACTIONS
Rash, eosinophilia, local inj-site reaction, diarrhea, nausea, decreased renal function, generalized seizure.

DRUG INTERACTIONS
Inhibits oxidation of mercaptopurine and azathioprine; reduce mercaptopurine or azathioprine dose to 1/3-1/4 of usual dose when given with 300-600mg of allopurinol. May prolong $T_{1/2}$ of dicumarol; monitor PT with concomitant use. Inhibition of xanthine oxidase by oxypurinol may be decreased and urinary excretion of uric acid may be increased with concomitant uricosuric agents. May increase toxicity and occurrence of hypersensitivity reactions with concomitant thiazide diuretics in patients with decreased renal function; monitor renal function. May increase frequency of skin rash when used with ampicillin or amoxicillin. Bone marrow suppression may be enhanced with cyclophosphamide and other cytotoxic agents among patients with neoplastic disease, except leukemia. May increase risk of hypoglycemia in the presence of renal insufficiency with concomitant chlorpropamide. May increase cyclosporine levels; monitor cyclosporine levels and consider possible adjustment of cyclosporine dose.

PREGNANCY AND LACTATION
Category C, caution in nursing.

MECHANISM OF ACTION

Xanthine oxidase inhibitor; reduces production of uric acid by inhibiting the biochemical reactions immediately preceding its formation.

PHARMACOKINETICS

Absorption: Allopurinol: C_{max}=1.58mcg/mL (100mg), 5.12mcg/mL (300mg); T_{max}=0.5 hr; AUC=1.99 hr•mcg/mL (100mg), 7.1 hr•mcg/mL (300mg). Oxypurinol: C_{max}=2.2mcg/mL (100mg), 6.18mcg/mL (300mg); T_{max}=3.89 hrs (100mg), 4.16 hrs (300mg); AUC=80 hr•mcg/mL (100mg), 231 hr•mcg/mL (300mg). **Distribution:** Found in breast milk. Allopurinol: V_d=0.84L/kg (100mg), 0.87L/kg (300mg). **Metabolism:** Oxidation; oxypurinol (active metabolite). **Elimination:** Urine (12% unchanged, 76% oxypurinol). Allopurinol: $T_{1/2}$=1 hr (100mg); 1.21 hrs (300mg). Oxypurinol: $T_{1/2}$=24.1 hrs (100mg), 23.5 hrs (300mg).

PATIENT CONSIDERATIONS

Assessment: Assess for renal/hepatic disease, concurrent illnesses affecting renal function, previous severe reaction to the drug, pregnancy/nursing status, and possible drug interactions. Obtain serum uric acid level to provide correct dosage and schedule.

Monitoring: Monitor for signs/symptoms of hypersensitivity/allergic reactions, drowsiness, bone marrow suppression, and other adverse reactions. Monitor fluid intake, LFTs, renal function (BUN, SrCr, CrCl), and serum uric acid level.

Counseling: Inform of risks and benefits of therapy. Counsel that drug may impair mental/physical abilities. Advise to take sufficient fluid to yield urinary output of at least 2L/day in adults and inform of the need to maintain a neutral or, preferably, slightly alkaline urine. Instruct to report any adverse events to physician.

ALOXI — palonosetron hydrochloride Rx

Class: 5-HT$_3$ receptor antagonist

ADULT DOSAGE	PEDIATRIC DOSAGE
Chemotherapy-Induced Nausea/ Vomiting	**Chemotherapy-Induced Nausea/ Vomiting**
Moderately Emetogenic Chemotherapy: Prevention of acute and delayed N/V associated w/ initial and repeat courses	**Prevention of Acute N/V Associated w/ Initial and Repeat Courses of Emetogenic Cancer Chemotherapy, Including Highly Emetogenic Cancer Chemotherapy:**
0.25mg IV as a single dose over 30 sec; begin approx 30 min before the start of chemotherapy	**1 Month to <17 Years:** 20mcg/kg IV as a single dose over 15 min; begin approx 30 min before the start of chemotherapy
Highly Emetogenic Chemotherapy: Prevention of acute N/V associated w/ initial and repeat courses	**Max Dose:** 1.5mg
0.25mg IV as a single dose over 30 sec; begin approx 30 min before the start of chemotherapy	
Postoperative Nausea/Vomiting	
Prevention for up to 24 hrs Following Surgery: 0.075mg IV as single dose over 10 sec immediately before induction of anesthesia	

ADMINISTRATION

IV route

Do not mix w/ other drugs.
Flush infusion line w/ normal saline before and after administration.

STORAGE

20-25°C (68-77°F); excursions permitted to 15-30°C (59-86°F). Protect from light and freezing.

HOW SUPPLIED

Inj: 0.075mg/1.5mL, 0.25mg/5mL

CONTRAINDICATIONS

Known hypersensitivity to the drug or any of its components.

WARNINGS/PRECAUTIONS

Hypersensitivity reactions, including anaphylaxis, reported w/ or w/o known hypersensitivity to other 5-HT$_3$ receptor antagonists. Serotonin syndrome reported; d/c treatment and initiate supportive treatment if symptoms occur. Routine prophylaxis is not recommended in patients in whom there is little expectation that nausea and/or vomiting will occur postoperatively. Therapy is recommended in patients where N/V must be avoided during the postoperative period, even where the incidence of postoperative nausea and/or vomiting is low.

ADVERSE REACTIONS

Chemotherapy-Induced N/V: Headache, constipation.
Postoperative N/V: QT prolongation, bradycardia, headache.

DRUG INTERACTIONS

Serotonin syndrome reported w/ concomitant use of serotonergic drugs (eg, SSRIs, SNRIs, MAOIs, mirtazapine, fentanyl); d/c if symptoms of serotonin syndrome occur.

PREGNANCY AND LACTATION

Pregnancy: Category B.
Lactation: Not for use in nursing.

MECHANISM OF ACTION

5-HT$_3$ receptor antagonist; antiemetic and antinauseant agent.

PHARMACOKINETICS

Absorption: (3mcg/kg single dose) C_{max}=5630ng/L, AUC=35.8mcg•hr/L. **Distribution:** V_d=8.3L/kg; plasma protein binding (62%). **Metabolism:** Via CYP2D6 and to a lesser extent, CYP3A4, CYP1A2; N-oxide-palonosetron and 6-S-hydroxy-palonosetron (primary metabolites). **Elimination:** (10mcg/kg single dose) Urine (80%, 40% unchanged); $T_{1/2}$=40 hrs.

PATIENT CONSIDERATIONS

Assessment: Assess for hypersensitivity to drug, risk/possibility of postoperative N/V, emetogenicity of cancer chemotherapy, pregnancy/nursing status, and possible drug interactions.

Monitoring: Monitor for hypersensitivity reactions, emergence of serotonin syndrome, and other adverse reactions.

Counseling: Inform of the benefits/risks of therapy. Advise to report to physician all medical conditions, including any pain, redness, or swelling in and around infusion site. Advise of the possibility of serotonin syndrome, especially w/ concomitant use of other serotonergic agents; instruct to seek immediate medical attention if changes in mental status, autonomic instability, or neuromuscular symptoms w/ or w/o GI symptoms occur.

ALPHAGAN P — brimonidine tartrate Rx

Class: Selective alpha$_2$ agonist

ADULT DOSAGE	PEDIATRIC DOSAGE
Elevated Intraocular Pressure	**Elevated Intraocular Pressure**
Reduction of Elevated IOP in Patients w/ Open-Angle Glaucoma or Ocular HTN: Instill 1 drop in affected eye(s) tid (8 hrs apart)	**Reduction of Elevated IOP in Patients w/ Open-Angle Glaucoma or Ocular HTN:** **≥2 Years:** Instill 1 drop in affected eye(s) tid (8 hrs apart)

ADMINISTRATION

Ocular route

Space by at least 5 min if using >1 topical ophthalmic drug

STORAGE

15-25°C (59-77°F).

HOW SUPPLIED

Sol: 0.1%, 0.15% [5mL, 10mL, 15mL]

CONTRAINDICATIONS

Neonates and infants <2 yrs of age, hypersensitivity reaction to any component of this medication.

WARNINGS/PRECAUTIONS

May potentiate syndromes associated with vascular insufficiency. Caution with severe cardiovascular disease (CVD), depression, cerebral or coronary insufficiency, Raynaud's phenomenon, orthostatic hypotension, or thromboangiitis obliterans. Bacterial keratitis reported with multidose containers.

ADVERSE REACTIONS

Allergic conjunctivitis, conjunctival hyperemia, eye pruritus, burning sensation, conjunctival folliculosis, HTN, oral dryness, ocular allergic reaction, visual disturbance, somnolence, decreased alertness.

DRUG INTERACTIONS

May potentiate effect with CNS depressants (alcohol, barbiturates, opiates, sedatives, anesthetics). Caution with antihypertensives, cardiac glycosides, and TCAs. May increase systemic side effects (eg, hypotension) with MAOIs; caution is advised.

PREGNANCY AND LACTATION

Category B, not for use in nursing.

MECHANISM OF ACTION

Selective α_2 agonist; reduces aqueous humor production and increases uveoscleral outflow.

PHARMACOKINETICS

Absorption: T_{max}=0.5-2.5 hrs. **Metabolism:** Liver (extensive). **Elimination:** (Oral) Urine (74% unchanged and metabolites); $T_{1/2}$=2 hrs.

PATIENT CONSIDERATIONS

Assessment: Assess for hypersensitivity, severe CVD, depression, cerebral or coronary insufficiency, Raynaud's phenomenon, orthostatic hypotension, thromboangiitis obliterans, pregnancy/nursing, and possible drug interactions.

Monitoring: Monitor vascular insufficiency, bacterial keratitis, and other adverse reactions.

Counseling: Advise to avoid touching tip of applicator to eye or surrounding areas. Instruct patient to notify physician if they have ocular surgery or develop an intercurrent ocular condition (eg, trauma or infection). Inform patients that fatigue and/or drowsiness may occur; may impair physical or mental abilities. Instruct to space by at least 5 min if using >1 topical ophthalmic drug.

ALPRAZOLAM — alprazolam   CIV

Class: Benzodiazepine

OTHER BRAND NAMES
Niravam (Discontinued)

ADULT DOSAGE

Generalized Anxiety Disorder
Initial: 0.25-0.5mg tid
Titrate: May increase at intervals of 3-4 days
Max: 4mg/day in divided doses
Periodically reassess need for continued treatment

Panic Disorder
W/ or w/o Agoraphobia:
Initial: 0.5mg tid
Titrate: May increase in increments of no more than 1mg/day at intervals of 3-4 days; slower titration to dose levels >4mg/day may be advisable. Advance dose until acceptable therapeutic response is achieved, intolerance occurs, or max recommended dose is attained
Maint: For patients receiving >4mg/day, periodically reassess treatment and consider dose reduction
Range: 1-10mg/day

PEDIATRIC DOSAGE
Pediatric use may not have been established

DOSING CONSIDERATIONS
Hepatic Impairment
Advanced Liver Disease:
Initial: 0.25mg bid-tid; if adverse reactions occur, may lower initial dose
Titrate: May gradually increase if needed/tolerated

Elderly
Elderly or Patients w/ Debilitating Disease:
Initial: 0.25mg bid-tid; if adverse reactions occur, may lower initial dose
Titrate: May gradually increase if needed/tolerated

Discontinuation
Generalized Anxiety Disorder:
Gradually reduce when discontinuing therapy/decreasing daily dosage. Decrease by no more than 0.5mg every 3 days; some patients may require an even slower dosage reduction
Panic Disorder:
Avoid abrupt discontinuation and gradually reduce dose when discontinuing therapy/decreasing daily dosage
Decrease by no more than 0.5mg every 3 days; some patients may require an even slower dosage reduction
If significant withdrawal symptoms develop, reinstitute previous stable dosing schedule; after stabilization, consider less rapid discontinuation schedule
Some patients may prove resistant to all discontinuation regimens

ADMINISTRATION
Oral route
Just prior to administration, remove tab from blister w/ dry hands
Immediately place tab on top of tongue where it will disintegrate and will be swallowed w/ saliva

STORAGE
20-25°C (68-77°F); excursions permitted between 15-30°C (59-86°F). Protect from moisture.

HOW SUPPLIED
Tab, Disintegrating: 0.25mg*, 0.5mg*, 1mg*, 2mg* *scored

CONTRAINDICATIONS
Acute narrow-angle glaucoma, coadministration w/ potent CYP3A4 inhibitors (eg, ketoconazole, itraconazole).

WARNINGS/PRECAUTIONS
Caution w/ administration and size of prescription in severely depressed patients or those in whom there is reason to expect concealed suicidal ideation or plan. Seizures, including status epilepticus, reported w/ dose reduction or abrupt discontinuation. Use may lead to physical and psychological dependence; prescribe for short periods and periodically reassess the need for continued treatment. Increased risk of dependence w/ doses >4mg/day, treatment for >12 weeks, and in panic disorder patients. May cause fetal harm. Avoid use during 1st trimester of pregnancy; may increase risk of congenital abnormalities. May impair mental/physical abilities. Hypomania and mania reported in patients w/ depression. Early morning anxiety and emergence of anxiety symptoms between doses reported; give same total daily dose divided as more frequent administrations. Withdrawal reactions may occur when dosage reduction occurs; reduce dose or d/c therapy gradually. Has a weak uricosuric effect. Decreased systemic elimination rate w/ alcoholic liver disease and obesity. Deaths reported in patients w/ severe pulmonary disease shortly after the initiation of therapy. Caution w/ impaired renal/hepatic/pulmonary function, elderly, and debilitated. Diseases that cause dry mouth or raise stomach pH might slow tab disintegration or dissolution, resulting in slowed or decreased absorption.

ADVERSE REACTIONS
Sedation, impaired coordination, dysarthria, decreased/increased libido, fatigue/tiredness, dry mouth, irritability, memory impairment, increased/decreased appetite, cognitive disorder, weight gain/loss, constipation, lightheadedness.

DRUG INTERACTIONS
See Contraindications. Not recommended w/ azole-type antifungals. Caution w/ alcohol, other CNS depressants, diltiazem, INH, macrolide antibiotics (eg, erythromycin, clarithromycin), grapefruit juice, sertraline, paroxetine, ergotamine, cyclosporine, amiodarone, nicardipine, nifedipine, and other CYP3A inhibitors. Additive CNS depressant effects w/ psychotropics, anticonvulsants, antihistaminics, alcohol, and other drugs that produce CNS depression. Concomitant use w/ drugs that cause dry mouth or raise stomach pH might slow disintegration or dissolution of alprazolam, resulting in slowed or decreased absorption. May increase plasma levels of imipramine and desipramine. Nefazodone, fluvoxamine, and cimetidine may increase levels; consider dose reduction of alprazolam. Fluoxetine and oral contraceptives may increase levels; use w/ caution. CYP3A inducers (eg, carbamazepine) and propoxyphene may decrease levels.

PREGNANCY AND LACTATION
Category D, not for use in nursing.

MECHANISM OF ACTION
Benzodiazepine; not established. Binds to GABA receptors in the brain and enhances GABA-mediated synaptic inhibition; such actions may be responsible for the efficacy in anxiety disorder and panic disorder.

PHARMACOKINETICS
Absorption: Readily absorbed; C_{max}=8-37ng/mL (0.5-3mg); T_{max}=1.5-2 hrs.
Distribution: Plasma protein binding (80%); crosses placenta; found in breast milk. **Metabolism:** Extensive. Liver via CYP3A4; 4-hydroxyalprazolam and α-hydroxyalprazolam (major metabolites). **Elimination:** Urine; $T_{1/2}$=12.5 hrs.

PATIENT CONSIDERATIONS
Assessment: Assess for drug hypersensitivity, acute narrow-angle glaucoma, depression, suicidal ideation, renal/hepatic/pulmonary impairment, debilitation, obesity, diseases that cause dry mouth or raise stomach pH, history of alcohol/substance abuse, history of seizures/epilepsy, pregnancy/nursing status, and possible drug interactions.

Monitoring: Monitor for dependence, rebound/withdrawal symptoms (eg, seizures), early morning anxiety and emergence of anxiety symptoms between doses, CNS depression, hypomania/mania, suicidality, and other adverse reactions. Periodically reassess usefulness of therapy.

Counseling: Instruct on how to administer tab. Advise to inform physician about any alcohol consumption, medicines taken, and pregnancy/nursing status. Instruct to avoid alcohol during treatment. Advise not to drive or operate dangerous machinery until familiar with the effects of therapy. Advise not to increase/decrease dose or abruptly d/c therapy w/o consulting physician; instruct to follow gradual dosage tapering schedule. Inform of risks associated w/ doses >4mg/day.

ALSUMA — sumatriptan   Rx

Class: 5-HT$_{1B/1D}$ agonist (triptans)

ADULT DOSAGE

Migraine
W/ or w/o Aura:
Max Single Dose: 6mg SQ
Max Dose/24 Hrs: 2 doses separated by at least 1 hr; only consider 2nd dose if there was some response to the 1st inj

Cluster Headache
Acute Treatment:
Max Single Dose: 6mg SQ
Max Dose/24 Hrs: 2 doses separated by at least 1 hr; only consider 2nd dose if there was some response to the 1st inj

PEDIATRIC DOSAGE
Pediatric use may not have been established

DOSING CONSIDERATIONS
Elderly
Start at lower end of dosing range

ADMINISTRATION
SQ route

STORAGE
25°C (77°F); excursions permitted to 15-30°C (59-86°F). Protect from light. Do not refrigerate.

HOW SUPPLIED
Inj: 6mg/0.5mL

CONTRAINDICATIONS
Ischemic coronary artery disease (CAD) (eg, angina pectoris, history of myocardial infarction [MI], or documented silent ischemia), coronary artery vasospasm (eg, Prinzmetal's angina), Wolff-Parkinson-White syndrome or arrhythmias associated with other cardiac accessory conduction pathway disorders, history of stroke or transient ischemic attack (TIA), hemiplegic/basilar migraine or history thereof, peripheral vascular disease, ischemic bowel disease, uncontrolled HTN, hypersensitivity to sumatriptan, and severe hepatic impairment.

Recent use (within 24 hrs) of ergotamine-containing or ergot-type medication (eg, dihydroergotamine, methysergide) or another 5-HT$_1$ agonist. Concurrent administration or recent use (within 2 weeks) of an MAO-A inhibitor.

WARNINGS/PRECAUTIONS
Reconsider the diagnosis of migraine before treating any subsequent attacks if patient has no response to the 1st dose of therapy. Serious cardiac adverse reactions (eg, acute MI) reported. May cause coronary artery vasospasm and sensations of tightness, pain, pressure, and heaviness in the precordium, throat, neck, and jaw, usually noncardiac in origin. Perform cardiovascular (CV) evaluation in triptan-naive patients with multiple CV risk factors prior to therapy; if (-), consider administering 1st dose under medical supervision and perform an ECG immediately following administration. Consider periodic CV evaluation in intermittent long-term users with risk factors for CAD. Life-threatening cardiac rhythm disturbances (eg, ventricular tachycardia, ventricular fibrillation leading to death) reported; d/c if these occur. Cerebral/subarachnoid hemorrhage and stroke reported; d/c therapy if a cerebrovascular event occurs. Exclude other potentially serious neurological conditions before therapy in patients not previously diagnosed as migraineurs, and in migraineurs who present with atypical symptoms. May cause noncoronary vasospastic reactions (eg, peripheral vascular ischemia, GI vascular ischemia/infarction, splenic infarction, Raynaud's syndrome); rule out a vasospastic reaction before giving additional doses. Transient/permanent blindness and significant partial vision loss reported. Overuse of acute migraine drugs may lead to exacerbation of headache; detoxification may be necessary. Serotonin syndrome may occur; d/c if suspected. Significant elevation in BP, including hypertensive crisis with acute impairment of organ systems, reported. Anaphylactic/anaphylactoid/hypersensitivity reactions and seizures reported.

ADVERSE REACTIONS
Inj-site reactions, tingling, warm/burning/pressure sensation, dizziness, feeling of heaviness/tightness, flushing, numbness, chest discomfort/tightness, throat discomfort, weakness, neck pain.

DRUG INTERACTIONS
See Contraindications. Serotonin syndrome reported with SSRIs, SNRIs, TCAs, or MAOIs.

PREGNANCY AND LACTATION
Category C, caution in nursing.

MECHANISM OF ACTION
Selective 5-HT$_{1B/1D}$ agonist; thought to be due to the agonist effects at the 5-HT$_{1B/1D}$ receptors on intracranial blood vessels and sensory nerves of the trigeminal system, which result in cranial vessel constriction and inhibition of proinflammatory neuropeptide release.

PHARMACOKINETICS
Absorption: Bioavailability (97%); (Deltoid) C_{max}=74ng/mL, T_{max}=12 min. (Thigh) C_{max}=61ng/mL (manual inj), 52ng/mL (auto-injector). **Distribution:** V_d=50L; plasma protein binding (14-21%), found in breast milk. **Metabolism:** Via MAO-A; indole acetic acid (IAA) (major metabolite). **Elimination:** Urine (22% unchanged, 38% IAA); $T_{1/2}$=115 min.

PATIENT CONSIDERATIONS
Assessment: Confirm diagnosis of migraine or cluster headache and exclude other potentially serious neurologic conditions prior to therapy. Assess for CV disease, HTN, hemiplegic/basilar migraine, hypersensitivity to drug, and any other conditions where treatment is cautioned or contraindicated. Assess hepatic function, pregnancy/nursing status, and for possible drug interactions.

Monitoring: Monitor for signs/symptoms of cardiac events, cerebrovascular events, noncoronary vasospastic reactions, serotonin syndrome, hypersensitivity reactions, HTN, ophthalmic changes, and other adverse reactions. Perform periodic CV evaluation in intermittent long-term users with risk factors for CAD.

Counseling: Inform that therapy may cause serious CV side effects and anaphylactic/anaphylactoid reactions. Instruct to seek medical attention if signs/symptoms of chest pain, SOB, weakness, or slurring of speech occur. Caution about the risk of serotonin syndrome. Inform that use of acute migraine drugs for ≥10 days/month may lead to an exacerbation of headache; encourage to record headache frequency and drug use (eg, by keeping a headache diary). Inform that drug should not be used during pregnancy; instruct to notify physician if breastfeeding/planning to breastfeed. Inform that drug may cause somnolence and dizziness; instruct to evaluate ability to perform complex tasks during migraine attacks and after administration of drug. Instruct on proper use of product, to avoid IM or intravascular delivery, and to use inj sites with adequate skin and SQ thickness (eg, lateral thigh, upper arms) to accommodate the length of the needle.

ALTACE — ramipril   Rx
Class: ACE inhibitor

> D/C when pregnancy is detected. Drugs that act directly on the renin-angiotensin system (RAS) can cause injury/death to the developing fetus.

ADULT DOSAGE
Hypertension

Not Receiving a Diuretic:
Initial: 2.5mg qd
Maint: 2.5-20mg/day as single dose or in 2 equally divided doses

May add a diuretic if BP is not controlled

PEDIATRIC DOSAGE
Pediatric use may not have been established

Risk Reduction of Myocardial Infarction, Stroke, Cardiovascular Death

High Risk Patients ≥55 Years:
Initial: 2.5mg qd for 1 week
Titrate: Increase to 5mg qd for next 3 weeks, then increase as tolerated
Maint: 10mg qd
May be given as a divided dose if patient is hypertensive or recently post-MI

Congestive Heart Failure Post-Myocardial Infarction

Stable patients w/ signs of CHF w/in 1st few days after sustaining acute MI

Initial: 2.5mg bid; may switch to 1.25mg bid if patient becomes hypotensive at this dose
Titrate: After 1 week at initial dose, increase dose, if tolerated, to target dose of 5mg bid, w/ dose increases being about 3 weeks apart

After initial dose, observe for at least 2 hrs and until BP has stabilized for at least an additional hr
Reduce dose of any concomitant diuretic, if possible, to decrease incidence of hypotension

---

DOSING CONSIDERATIONS
Renal Impairment
CrCl ≤40mL/min:
HTN:
Initial: 1.25mg qd
Max: 5mg/day

Heart Failure Post MI:
Initial: 1.25mg qd
Titrate: May increase to 1.25mg bid
Max: 2.5mg bid

Other Important Considerations
Renal Artery Stenosis/Volume Depletion (eg, Past and Current Diuretic Use):
Initial: 1.25mg qd

ADMINISTRATION
Oral route

Swallow caps whole.
May also open cap and sprinkle content on a small amount (about 4 oz) of applesauce or mix in 4 oz (120mL) of water or apple juice; consume mixture in its entirety.
May pre-prepare mixture and store for up to 24 hrs at room temperature or up to 48 hrs under refrigeration.

STORAGE
15-30°C (59-86°F).

HOW SUPPLIED
Cap: 1.25mg, 2.5mg, 5mg, 10mg

CONTRAINDICATIONS
Hypersensitivity to this product or any other ACE inhibitor (eg, history of ACE inhibitor-associated angioedema), coadministration w/ aliskiren in patients w/ diabetes.

WARNINGS/PRECAUTIONS
Increased risk of angioedema in patients w/ history of angioedema unrelated to ACE inhibitor therapy. Head/neck angioedema reported; d/c and institute appropriate therapy if laryngeal stridor or angioedema of the face, tongue, or glottis occurs. Higher rate of angioedema in blacks than nonblacks. Intestinal angioedema reported; monitor for abdominal pain. Anaphylactoid reactions reported during desensitization w/ hymenoptera venom, dialysis w/ high-flux membranes, and LDL apheresis w/ dextran sulfate absorption. Rarely, associated w/ a syndrome that starts w/ cholestatic jaundice and progresses to fulminant hepatic necrosis and sometimes death; d/c if jaundice or marked hepatic enzyme elevations develop. May cause changes in renal function. May be associated w/ oliguria or progressive azotemia and rarely w/ acute renal failure or death, in patients w/ severe CHF whose renal function may depend on the activity of the RAS. Increases in BUN and SrCr may occur in hypertensive patients w/ unilateral or bilateral renal artery stenosis; monitor renal function during the 1st few weeks of therapy. Increases in BUN and SrCr reported in some hypertensive patients w/ no apparent preexisting renal vascular disease; dose reduction of ramipril and/or discontinuation of the diuretic may be required. Agranulocytosis, pancytopenia, bone marrow depression, and mild reductions in RBC count and Hgb content, blood cell or platelet counts may occur; consider monitoring WBCs in patients w/ collagen vascular disease (eg, systemic lupus erythematosus, scleroderma), especially w/ renal impairment. Symptomatic hypotension may occur and is most likely to occur in patients w/ volume and/or salt depletion; correct depletion prior to therapy. May cause excessive hypotension, which may be associated w/ oliguria or azotemia and rarely, w/ acute renal failure and death, in patients with CHF, w/ or w/o associated renal insufficiency; follow patients closely for the first 2 weeks of treatment and whenever the dose of therapy or diuretic is increased. Hypotension may occur w/ surgery or during anesthesia. Hyperkalemia reported;

monitor serum K^+ in patients w/ risk factors (eg, renal insufficiency, diabetes mellitus). Persistent nonproductive cough reported.

ADVERSE REACTIONS
Hypotension, cough increased, dizziness, headache, asthenia, fatigue.

DRUG INTERACTIONS
See Contraindications. Dual blockade of the RAS is associated w/ increased risks of hypotension, hyperkalemia, and changes in renal function (including acute renal failure); avoid combined use of RAS inhibitors, or closely monitor BP, renal function, and electrolytes w/ other agents that also affect the RAS. Not recommended w/ telmisartan; increased risk of renal dysfunction. Avoid w/ aliskiren in patients w/ renal impairment (GFR <60mL/min). Initiation of therapy in patients on diuretics (especially those in whom diuretic therapy was recently instituted) may result in excessive reduction of BP. Decrease or d/c diuretic or increase the salt intake prior to initiation of therapy; if this is not possible, reduce the starting dose of ramipril. Increased risk of hyperkalemia w/ K^+-sparing diuretics, K^+ supplements, and/or K^+-containing salt substitutes; monitor serum K^+. Increased lithium levels and symptoms of lithium toxicity reported; frequently monitor serum lithium levels. Diuretics may further increase risk of lithium toxicity. Nitritoid reactions reported rarely w/ injectable gold (sodium aurothiomalate). NSAIDs, including selective COX-2 inhibitors, may result in deterioration of renal function, including possible acute renal failure in elderly, volume depleted or patients w/ compromised renal function. Antihypertensive effect may be attenuated by NSAIDs. Coadministration w/ mTOR inhibitors (eg, temsirolimus) may increase risk for angioedema. Increased BUN and SrCr w/ diuretics.

PREGNANCY AND LACTATION
Pregnancy: Category D.
Lactation: Not for use in nursing.

MECHANISM OF ACTION
ACE inhibitor; decreases plasma angiotensin II, which leads to decreased vasopressor activity and aldosterone secretion.

PHARMACOKINETICS
Absorption: Absolute bioavailability (28%, 44% ramiprilat); T_{max}=1 hr, 2-4 hrs (ramiprilat). **Distribution:** Plasma protein binding (73%, 56% ramiprilat); crosses placenta. **Metabolism:** Cleavage of ester group (primarily in the liver); ramiprilat (active metabolite). **Elimination:** Urine (60%, <2% unchanged), feces (40%); $T_{1/2}$>50 hrs (ramiprilat), 13-17 hrs (multiple daily doses, ramiprilat).

PATIENT CONSIDERATIONS
Assessment: Assess for history of angioedema, CHF, renal artery stenosis, collagen vascular disease, volume/salt depletion, risk factors for hyperkalemia, renal/hepatic impairment, hypersensitivity to drug, pregnancy/nursing status, and possible drug interactions.

Monitoring: Monitor for signs/symptoms of angioedema, anaphylactoid reactions, hyperkalemia, cough, jaundice, and other adverse reactions. Consider monitoring WBCs in patients w/ collagen vascular disease, especially w/ renal impairment. Monitor BP and renal/hepatic function.

Counseling: Instruct to d/c therapy and to immediately report any signs/symptoms of angioedema. Advise to promptly report any indication of infection. Instruct to report lightheadedness, especially during 1st days of therapy; advise to d/c and consult w/ a physician if syncope occurs. Inform that inadequate fluid intake or excessive perspiration, diarrhea, or vomiting may lead to an excessive fall in BP, w/ the same consequences of lightheadedness and possible syncope. Inform females of childbearing age about the consequences of exposure during pregnancy and discuss treatment options in women planning to become pregnant; instruct to report pregnancy to physician as soon as possible. Advise not to use salt substitutes containing K^+ w/o consulting physician.

ALTOPREV — lovastatin
Rx

Class: HMG-CoA reductase inhibitor (statin)

ADULT DOSAGE	PEDIATRIC DOSAGE
Hyperlipidemia/Mixed Dyslipidemia	Pediatric use may not have been established
Usual: 20-60mg/day given qhs	
Prevention of Coronary Heart Disease	
Dose based on current clinical practice	

DOSING CONSIDERATIONS
Concomitant Medications
Danazol, Diltiazem, Dronedarone, or Verapamil:
Max: 20mg/day
Amiodarone:
Max: 40mg/day
Renal Impairment
Severe (CrCl <30mL/min): Consider dosage increases >20mg/day only if the expected benefit exceeds the increased risk of myopathy/rhabdomyolysis
Elderly
Initial: 20mg qhs

ADMINISTRATION
Oral route

STORAGE
20-25°C (68-77°F); excursions permitted to 15-30°C (59-86°F). Avoid excessive heat and humidity.

HOW SUPPLIED
Tab, Extended-Release: 20mg, 40mg, 60mg

CONTRAINDICATIONS
Concomitant strong CYP3A inhibitors and erythromycin, hypersensitivity to any component of this product. Active liver disease (eg, unexplained persistent elevations of hepatic transaminase levels), women who are or may become pregnant, nursing mothers.

WARNINGS/PRECAUTIONS
Myopathy (including immune-mediated necrotizing myopathy) and rhabdomyolysis with acute renal failure secondary to myoglobinuria reported; d/c if markedly elevated creatine kinase levels occur or myopathy is diagnosed/suspected and temporarily withhold in any patient experiencing an acute or serious condition predisposing to development of renal failure secondary to rhabdomyolysis. Increases in serum transaminases reported. Fatal and nonfatal hepatic failure rarely reported; promptly interrupt therapy if serious liver injury with clinical symptoms and/or hyperbilirubinemia or jaundice occurs and do not restart if no alternate etiology found. Caution in patients who consume substantial quantities of alcohol and/or have history of chronic liver disease. Increases in HbA1c and FPG levels reported. Evaluate patients who develop endocrine dysfunction. Caution in elderly.

ADVERSE REACTIONS
Infection, pain, headache, asthenia, myalgia, back pain, flu syndrome, arthralgia, sinusitis, diarrhea.

DRUG INTERACTIONS
See Dosing Considerations and Contraindications. Ranolazine may increase risk of myopathy/rhabdomyolysis; consider dose adjustment of lovastatin. Due to the risk of myopathy, avoid with gemfibrozil, cyclosporine, and grapefruit juice, and caution with other fibrates, lipid-lowering doses (≥1g/day) of niacin, colchicine, danazol, diltiazem, dronedarone, verapamil, or amiodarone. Determine PT before initiation and frequently enough during early therapy with anticoagulants; bleeding and/or increased PT reported with coumarin anticoagulants. Caution with drugs that may decrease the levels or activity of endogenous steroid hormones (eg, spironolactone, cimetidine).

PREGNANCY AND LACTATION
Category X, not for use in nursing.

MECHANISM OF ACTION
HMG-CoA reductase inhibitor; a strong inhibitor of HMG-CoA reductase, the enzyme that catalyzes the conversion of HMG-CoA to mevalonate, which is an early step in the biosynthetic pathway for cholesterol.

PHARMACOKINETICS
Absorption: Lovastatin: C_{max}=5.5ng/mL; T_{max}=14.2 hrs; AUC=77ng•hr/mL. Lovastatin Acid: C_{max}=5.8ng/mL; T_{max}=11.8 hrs; AUC=87ng•hr/mL. **Distribution:** Plasma protein binding (>95%). **Metabolism:** Liver (extensive 1st-pass); CYP3A4, hydrolysis; β-hydroxyacid and 6'-hydroxy derivative (major active metabolites). **Elimination:** Bile.

PATIENT CONSIDERATIONS
Assessment: Assess for drug hypersensitivity, active/history of liver disease, alcohol consumption, renal impairment, pregnancy/nursing status, and possible drug interactions. Obtain baseline LFTs, lipid profile, and check PT with coumarin anticoagulants.

Monitoring: Monitor for signs/symptoms of myopathy, rhabdomyolysis, endocrine/renal dysfunction, and other adverse effects. Monitor LFTs. Monitor PT with coumarin anticoagulants.

Counseling: Instruct to promptly report any unexplained muscle pain, tenderness, or weakness, particularly if accompanied by malaise or fever or if muscle signs/symptoms persist after discontinuation. Inform about substances that should be avoided during therapy, and advise to discuss all medications, both prescription and OTC, with physician. Inform that liver enzyme tests should be performed before the initiation of therapy and if signs/symptoms of liver injury occur; advise to promptly report any symptoms that may indicate liver injury. Advise women of childbearing age to use an effective method of birth control, to stop taking the drug if they become pregnant, and not to breastfeed while on therapy.

ALVESCO — ciclesonide
Rx

Class: Non-halogenated glucocorticoid

ADULT DOSAGE	PEDIATRIC DOSAGE
Asthma	**Asthma**
Previous Therapy:	**≥12 Years:**
	Previous Therapy:
Bronchodilators Alone:	
Initial: 80mcg bid	**Bronchodilators Alone:**
Max: 160mcg bid	**Initial:** 80mcg bid
	Max: 160mcg bid
Inhaled Corticosteroids:	
Initial: 80mcg bid	**Inhaled Corticosteroids:**
Max: 320mcg bid	**Initial:** 80mcg bid
	Max: 320mcg bid
Oral Corticosteroids:	
Initial/Max: 320mcg bid	**Oral Corticosteroids:**
Titrate: Reduce to lowest effective dose once asthma stability is achieved. May increase to higher dose if response to initial dose is inadequate after 4 weeks	**Initial/Max:** 320mcg bid
	Titrate: Reduce to lowest effective dose once asthma stability is achieved. May increase to higher dose if response to initial dose is inadequate after 4 weeks

DOSING CONSIDERATIONS
Elderly
Start at lower end of dosing range

ADMINISTRATION
Oral inh route

Refer to PI for further administration instructions

Priming
Prime inhaler before using for the 1st time or when inhaler has not been used for >10 days by actuating 3 times

STORAGE
25°C (77°F); excursions permitted to 15-30°C (59-86°F). Do not puncture or use/store near heat or open flame. Exposure to temperatures >49°C (120°F) may cause bursting. Discard when dose indicator display window shows zero.

HOW SUPPLIED
MDI: 80mcg/actuation, 160mcg/actuation [60 actuations]

CONTRAINDICATIONS
Primary treatment of status asthmaticus or other acute episodes of asthma where intensive measures are required, known hypersensitivity to ciclesonide or any of the ingredients of this medication.

WARNINGS/PRECAUTIONS
Localized *Candida albicans* infections of mouth and pharynx reported; treat appropriately while remaining on treatment, or interrupt treatment if needed. Not indicated for rapid relief of bronchospasm or other acute episodes of asthma. Increased susceptibility to infections (eg, chickenpox, measles); may lead to serious/fatal course. Avoid exposure to chickenpox and measles; if exposed, consider prophylaxis/treatment. Caution w/ active/quiescent tuberculosis (TB), untreated systemic fungal, bacterial, viral, or parasitic infections, or ocular herpes simplex. Deaths due to adrenal insufficiency reported w/ transfer from systemic to inhaled corticosteroids; if oral corticosteroid is required, wean slowly from systemic corticosteroid use after transferring to therapy. Resume oral corticosteroids immediately during periods of stress or a severe asthma attack if previously withdrawn from systemic corticosteroids. Transferring from systemic to inhalation therapy may unmask allergic conditions previously suppressed (eg, rhinitis, conjunctivitis, eczema, arthritis, eosinophilic conditions). Systemic corticosteroid withdrawal effects may occur during withdrawal from oral steroids. Reduce dose slowly if hypercorticism and adrenal suppression occur. Decreases in bone mineral density (BMD) reported w/ long-term use; caution w/ major risk factors for decreased bone mineral content. May reduce growth velocity in pediatric patients; monitor growth of pediatric patients routinely (eg, via stadiometry). Glaucoma, increased intraocular pressure (IOP), and cataracts reported. Bronchospasm may occur; d/c use, treat immediately, and institute alternative treatment. Caution in elderly.

ADVERSE REACTIONS
Headache, nasopharyngitis, sinusitis, pharyngolaryngeal pain, upper respiratory infection, arthralgia, nasal congestion, pain in extremity, back pain.

DRUG INTERACTIONS
Oral ketoconazole may increase the exposure of the active metabolite des-ciclesonide.

PREGNANCY AND LACTATION
Category C, caution in nursing.

MECHANISM OF ACTION
Nonhalogenated glucocorticoid; not established. Has anti-inflammatory activity w/ affinity for glucocorticoid receptors. Shown to inhibit multiple cell types (eg, mast cells, eosinophils, basophils, lymphocytes, macrophages, neutrophils) and mediators (eg, histamine, eicosanoids, leukotrienes, cytokines) involved in the asthmatic response.

PHARMACOKINETICS
Absorption: Ciclesonide: Absolute bioavailability (22%). Des-ciclesonide: $AUC=2.18ng \cdot hr/mL$; $C_{max}=0.369ng/mL$; $T_{max}=1.04$ hrs. **Distribution:** Plasma protein binding (≥99%). Ciclesonide: (IV) $V_d=2.9L/kg$. Des-ciclesonide: (IV) $V_d=12.1L/kg$. **Metabolism:** Hydrolyzed to des-ciclesonide (active metabolite); further metabolism in liver via CYP3A4 (major) and CYP2D6 (minor). **Elimination:** Ciclesonide: (IV) Feces (66%); $T_{1/2}=0.71$ hrs. Des-ciclesonide: (IV) Urine (≤20%); $T_{1/2}=6-7$ hrs.

PATIENT CONSIDERATIONS
Assessment: Assess for status asthmaticus or other acute episodes of asthma, active/quiescent TB, untreated systemic infections, ocular herpes simplex, risk factors for decreased bone mineral content, previous hypersensitivity, pregnancy/nursing status, and possible drug interactions. Assess for history of increased IOP, glaucoma, and/or cataracts.

Monitoring: Monitor for infections, TB, chickenpox, measles, hypercorticism, adrenal suppression, decreased BMD, glaucoma, increased IOP, cataracts, bronchospasm, and other adverse events. Monitor growth routinely (eg, via stadiometry) in pediatric patients.

Counseling: Advise that localized infections w/ *C. albicans* may occur in the mouth and pharynx; advise to rinse mouth after use and to notify physician if oropharyngeal candidiasis develops. Inform that drug is not a bronchodilator and is not for use as rescue medication for acute asthma exacerbations; instruct to contact physician immediately if deterioration of asthma occurs. Advise to avoid exposure to chickenpox or measles, and, if exposed, to consult physician immediately. Counsel on risks of immunosuppression, hypercorticism, adrenal suppression, and decreased BMD. Inform of risk of reduced growth velocity in pediatric patients. Advise to use medication at regular intervals, not to increase the prescribed dosage, not to stop use abruptly, and to contact physician if symptoms do not improve, condition worsens, or if use is discontinued. Inform to use only w/ the actuator supplied w/ the product.

AMANTADINE — amantadine hydrochloride   Rx
Class: Dopamine receptor agonist

ADULT DOSAGE	PEDIATRIC DOSAGE
Influenza A	**Influenza A**
Prophylaxis/Treatment: 200mg qd	**Prophylaxis/Treatment:**
May split into 100mg bid if CNS effects develop	**1-9 Years:** 4.4-8.8mg/kg/day **Max:** 150mg/day
Initiate treatment within 24-48 hrs after onset of signs/symptoms	**9-12 Years:** 100mg bid
Continue treatment for 24-48 hrs after signs/symptoms disappear	Initiate treatment within 24-48 hrs after onset of signs/symptoms
Parkinsonism	Continue treatment for 24-48 hrs after signs/symptoms disappear
Usual: 100mg bid	
Serious Associated Illness/ Concomitant High-Dose Antiparkinson Agent:	
Initial: 100mg qd	
Titrate: May increase to 100mg bid after one to several weeks	
Max: 400mg/day in divided doses	
Drug-Induced Extrapyramidal Reactions	
Usual: 100mg bid	
Max: 300mg/day in divided doses	

DOSING CONSIDERATIONS
Concomitant Medications
Combination with Levodopa: Hold dose constant at 100mg qd or bid while gradually increasing daily dose of levodopa

Renal Impairment
CrCl 30-50mL/min: 200mg on Day 1, then 100mg qd
CrCl 15-29mL/min: 200mg on Day 1, then 100mg qod
CrCl <15mL/min or Hemodialysis: 200mg every 7 days

Elderly
≥65 Years: 100mg/day

Other Important Considerations
Intolerant to 200mg/day: 100mg/day

ADMINISTRATION
Oral route

Continue for ≥10 days following known exposure
Administer for 2-4 weeks after inactivated influenza A virus vaccine has been given if used chemoprophylactically with vaccine until protective antibody responses develop

STORAGE
20-25°C (68-77°F). (Cap) Protect from moisture.

HOW SUPPLIED
Cap: 100mg; **Sol:** 50mg/5mL; **Tab:** 100mg

CONTRAINDICATIONS
Known hypersensitivity to amantadine hydrochloride or to any of the other ingredients in this medication.

WARNINGS/PRECAUTIONS
May need dose reduction with congestive heart failure (CHF), peripheral edema, orthostatic hypotension, or renal impairment. Deaths reported from overdose. Neuroleptic malignant syndrome (NMS) reported in association with dose reduction or withdrawal. Impulse control/compulsive behaviors reported; consider dose reduction or d/c if such behaviors develop. Suicide attempts reported. May exacerbate mental problems in patients with history of psychiatric disorder or substance abuse. May increase seizure activity. May impair mental/physical abilities. May cause mydriasis; avoid with untreated angle-closure glaucoma. Do not d/c abruptly in Parkinson's disease patients. Caution with liver disease, history of recurrent eczematoid rash, and uncontrolled psychosis or severe psychoneurosis. Monitor for melanomas frequently and regularly. Not shown to prevent complications secondary to influenza-like symptoms or concurrent bacterial infections.

ADVERSE REACTIONS
Nausea, dizziness, insomnia, depression, anxiety, hallucinations, confusion, anorexia, dry mouth, constipation, ataxia, livedo reticularis, peripheral edema, orthostatic hypotension, headache.

DRUG INTERACTIONS
Avoid live attenuated influenza vaccines within 2 weeks before or 48 hrs after therapy. Caution with neuroleptics and drugs having CNS effects. Triamterene/HCTZ may increase concentration. Quinine or quinidine may reduce renal clearance. Urine acidifying drugs may increase elimination. Anticholinergic agents may potentiate the anticholinergic-like side effects. May worsen tremor in elderly Parkinson's patients with thioridazine.

PREGNANCY AND LACTATION
Category C, not for use in nursing.

MECHANISM OF ACTION
Dopamine receptor agonist; not established. Antiviral: Appears to prevent release of infectious viral nucleic acid into host cell by interfering with function of transmembrane domain of viral M2 protein. Also prevents virus assembly during

replication. Parkinson's disease: May have direct/indirect effect on dopamine neurons and is a weak, noncompetitive N-methyl D-aspartate receptor antagonist.

PHARMACOKINETICS
Absorption: Well-absorbed. (Cap) C_{max}=0.22mcg/mL, T_{max}=3.3 hrs. (Sol) C_{max}=0.24mcg/mL (single dose), 0.47mcg/mL (multiple dose). (Tab) C_{max}=0.51mcg/mL, T_{max}=2-4 hrs. **Distribution:** V_d=3-8L/kg (IV); plasma protein binding (67%); found in breast milk. **Metabolism:** N-acetylation; acetylamantadine (metabolite). **Elimination:** Urine (unchanged); $T_{1/2}$=16 hrs.

PATIENT CONSIDERATIONS
Assessment: Assess for CHF, peripheral edema, orthostatic hypotension, history of psychiatric disorders, substance abuse, epilepsy or other "seizures," and recurrent eczematoid rash, untreated angle-closure glaucoma, renal/hepatic impairment, hypersensitivity to the drug, pregnancy/nursing status, and possible drug interactions.

Monitoring: Monitor for signs/symptoms of suicide attempt, increased seizures, CNS and anticholinergic effects, NMS, impulse control/compulsive behaviors, melanoma, and renal/hepatic dysfunction.

Counseling: Advise that blurry vision and/or impaired mental acuity may occur. Instruct to avoid excessive alcohol use, getting up suddenly from sitting or lying position, and taking more than prescribed. Instruct to notify physician if mood/mental changes, swelling of extremities, difficulty urinating, SOB, and intense urges occur, no improvement in a few days or drug appears less effective after a few weeks, or if suspicious that overdose has been taken. Advise to consult physician before discontinuing medication. Instruct Parkinson's disease patients to gradually increase physical activity as symptoms improve.

AMBIEN – zolpidem tartrate   CIV
Class: GABA$_A$ agonist

ADULT DOSAGE	**PEDIATRIC DOSAGE**
Insomnia	Pediatric use may not have been established
Difficulties w/ Sleep Initiation:	
Initial:	
Women: 5mg qhs	
Men: 5mg or 10mg qhs	
Titrate: May increase to 10mg if the 5mg dose is not effective	
Max: 10mg qhs	

DOSING CONSIDERATIONS
Concomitant Medications
CNS Depressants: May need to adjust dose of zolpidem
Hepatic Impairment
5mg qhs
Elderly
Elderly/Debilitated: 5mg qhs

ADMINISTRATION
Oral route
Take immediately before hs w/ at least 7-8 hrs remaining before the planned time of awakening
Do not administer w/ or immediately after a meal

STORAGE
20-25°C (68-77°F).

HOW SUPPLIED
Tab: 5mg, 10mg

CONTRAINDICATIONS
Known hypersensitivity to zolpidem.

WARNINGS/PRECAUTIONS
Increased risk of next-day psychomotor impairment if taken with less than a full night of sleep remaining (7-8 hrs). May impair mental/physical abilities. Initiate only after careful evaluation; failure of insomnia to remit after 7-10 days of treatment may indicate presence of a primary psychiatric and/or medical illness. Angioedema and anaphylaxis reported; do not rechallenge if such reactions develop. Abnormal thinking, behavior changes, and visual and auditory hallucinations reported. Complex behaviors (eg, sleep-driving) while not fully awake reported; consider discontinuation if a sleep-driving episode occurs. Amnesia, anxiety, and other neuropsychiatric symptoms may occur. Worsening of depression and suicidal thoughts and actions (including completed suicides) reported primarily in depressed patients; prescribe the lowest feasible number of tabs at a time. Caution with compromised respiratory function; prior to prescribing, consider the risk of respiratory depression in patients with respiratory impairment (eg, sleep apnea, myasthenia gravis). Withdrawal signs and symptoms reported following rapid dose decrease or abrupt discontinuation; monitor for tolerance, abuse, and dependence. May cause drowsiness and a decreased level of consciousness, which may lead to falls and consequently to severe injuries (eg, hip fractures, intracranial hemorrhage).

ADVERSE REACTIONS
Drowsiness, dizziness, headache, diarrhea, drugged feeling, lethargy, dry mouth, back pain, pharyngitis, sinusitis, allergy.

DRUG INTERACTIONS
See Dosing Considerations. Increased risk of CNS depression and complex behaviors with other CNS depressants (eg, benzodiazepines, opioids, TCAs, alcohol). Use with other sedative-hypnotics (eg, other zolpidem products) at

hs or the middle of the night is not recommended. Increased risk of next-day psychomotor impairment with other CNS depressants or drugs that increase zolpidem levels. May decrease peak levels of imipramine. Additive effect of decreased alertness with imipramine or chlorpromazine. Additive adverse effect on psychomotor performance with chlorpromazine or alcohol. Sertraline and CYP3A inhibitors may increase exposure. Fluoxetine may increase $T_{1/2}$. Rifampin (a CYP3A4 inducer) may reduce exposure, pharmacodynamic effects, and efficacy. Ketoconazole (a potent CYP3A4 inhibitor) may increase pharmacodynamic effects; consider lower dose of zolpidem.

PREGNANCY AND LACTATION
Category C, caution in nursing.

MECHANISM OF ACTION
Imidazopyridine, nonbenzodiazepine hypnotic; interacts with a gamma-aminobutyric acid-BZ receptor complex. Binds the BZ$_1$ receptor preferentially with a high affinity ratio of the α_1/α_5 subunits.

PHARMACOKINETICS
Absorption: Rapid. C_{max}=59ng/mL (5mg), 121ng/mL (10mg); T_{max}=1.6 hrs (5mg, 10mg). **Distribution:** Plasma protein binding (92.5%); found in breast milk. **Elimination:** Renal; $T_{1/2}$=2.6 hrs (5mg), 2.5 hrs (10mg).

PATIENT CONSIDERATIONS
Assessment: Assess for physical and/or psychiatric disorder, depression, compromised respiratory function, sleep apnea, myasthenia gravis, hepatic impairment, history of drug/alcohol addiction or abuse, hypersensitivity to the drug, pregnancy/nursing status, and possible drug interactions.

Monitoring: Monitor for angioedema, anaphylaxis, emergence of any new behavioral signs/symptoms of concern, respiratory depression, withdrawal signs/symptoms, tolerance, abuse, dependence, drowsiness, decreased level of consciousness, and other adverse reactions.

Counseling: Inform about the benefits and risks of treatment. Instruct to take only as prescribed; advise to wait at least 8 hrs after dosing before driving or engaging in other activities requiring full mental alertness. Instruct to contact physician immediately if any adverse reactions (eg, severe anaphylactic/anaphylactoid reactions, sleep-driving, other complex behaviors, suicidal thoughts) develop. Advise not to use the drug if patient drank alcohol that pm or before bed. Instruct not to increase the dose and to inform physician if it is believed that the drug does not work.

AMBIEN CR – zolpidem tartrate   CIV
Class: GABA$_A$ agonist

ADULT DOSAGE	**PEDIATRIC DOSAGE**
Insomnia	Pediatric use may not have been established
Difficulties w/ Sleep Onset and/or Sleep Maintenance:	
Initial:	
Women: 6.25mg qhs	
Men: 6.25mg or 12.5mg qhs	
Titrate: May increase to 12.5mg if the 6.25mg dose is not effective	
Max: 12.5mg qhs	

DOSING CONSIDERATIONS
Concomitant Medications
CNS Depressants: May need to adjust dose of zolpidem
Hepatic Impairment
6.25mg qhs
Elderly
Elderly/Debilitated: 6.25mg qhs

ADMINISTRATION
Oral route
Swallow whole; do not divide, crush, or chew
Take immediately before hs w/ at least 7-8 hrs remaining before the planned time of awakening
Do not administer w/ or immediately after a meal

STORAGE
15-25°C (59-77°F); limited excursions permissible up to 30°C (86°F).

HOW SUPPLIED
Tab, Extended-Release: 6.25mg, 12.5mg

CONTRAINDICATIONS
Known hypersensitivity to zolpidem.

WARNINGS/PRECAUTIONS
May impair daytime function; monitor for excess depressant effects. May impair mental/physical abilities. Increased risk of next-day psychomotor impairment if taken with less than a full night of sleep remaining (7-8 hrs). Initiate only after careful evaluation; failure of insomnia to remit after 7-10 days of treatment may indicate presence of a primary psychiatric and/or medical illness. Angioedema and anaphylaxis reported; do not rechallenge if such reactions develop. Abnormal thinking, behavior changes, and visual and auditory hallucinations reported. Complex behaviors (eg, sleep-driving) while not fully awake reported; consider discontinuation if a sleep-driving episode occurs. Amnesia, anxiety, and other neuropsychiatric symptoms may occur. Worsening of depression and suicidal thoughts and actions (including completed suicides) reported primarily in depressed patients; prescribe the lowest feasible number of tabs at a time. Caution

with compromised respiratory function; prior to prescribing, consider the risk of respiratory depression in patients with respiratory impairment (eg, sleep apnea, myasthenia gravis). Withdrawal signs and symptoms reported following rapid dose decrease or abrupt discontinuation; monitor for tolerance, abuse, and dependence. May cause drowsiness and a decreased level of consciousness, which may lead to falls and consequently to severe injuries (eg, hip fractures, intracranial hemorrhage).

ADVERSE REACTIONS
Headache, somnolence, dizziness, anxiety, nausea, influenza, hallucinations, back pain, myalgia, fatigue, disorientation, memory disorder, visual disturbance, nasopharyngitis.

DRUG INTERACTIONS
See Dosing Considerations. Additive effects with other CNS depressants (eg, benzodiazepines, opioids, TCAs, alcohol), including daytime use. Use with other sedative-hypnotics (eg, other zolpidem products) at hs or the middle of the night is not recommended. Increased risk of next-day psychomotor impairment with other CNS depressants or drugs that increase zolpidem levels. Increased risk of complex behaviors with alcohol and other CNS depressants. May decrease peak levels of imipramine. Additive effect of decreased alertness with imipramine or chlorpromazine. Additive adverse effect on psychomotor performance with chlorpromazine or alcohol. Sertraline and CYP3A inhibitors may increase exposure. Fluoxetine may increase $T_{1/2}$. Rifampin (a CYP3A4 inducer) may reduce exposure, pharmacodynamic effects, and efficacy. Ketoconazole (a potent CYP3A4 inhibitor) may increase pharmacodynamic effects; consider lower dose of zolpidem.

PREGNANCY AND LACTATION
Category C, caution in nursing.

MECHANISM OF ACTION
Imidazopyridine, nonbenzodiazepine hypnotic; interacts with a gamma-aminobutyric acid-BZ receptor complex. Binds the BZ_1 receptor preferentially with a high affinity ratio of the α_1/α_5 subunits.

PHARMACOKINETICS
Absorption: Biphasic. C_{max}=134ng/mL; T_{max}=1.5 hrs (median); AUC=740ng•hr/mL. **Distribution:** Plasma protein binding (92.5%); found in breast milk. **Elimination:** Renal; $T_{1/2}$=2.8 hrs.

PATIENT CONSIDERATIONS
Assessment: Assess for physical and/or psychiatric disorder, depression, compromised respiratory function, sleep apnea, myasthenia gravis, hepatic impairment, history of drug/alcohol addiction or abuse, hypersensitivity to the drug, pregnancy/nursing status, and possible drug interactions.

Monitoring: Monitor for angioedema, anaphylaxis, emergence of any new behavioral signs/symptoms of concern, respiratory depression, withdrawal signs/symptoms, tolerance, abuse, dependence, drowsiness, decreased level of consciousness, and other adverse reactions. Monitor for excess depressant effects.

Counseling: Inform about the benefits and risks of treatment. Instruct to take only as prescribed. Caution against driving and other activities requiring complete mental alertness the day after use. Instruct to contact physician immediately if any adverse reactions (eg, severe anaphylactic/anaphylactoid reactions, sleep-driving, other complex behaviors, suicidal thoughts) develop. Advise not to use the drug if patient drank alcohol that pm or before bed. Instruct not to increase the dose and to inform physician if it is believed that the drug does not work.

AmBisome — amphotericin B liposome   Rx
Class: Polyene antifungal

ADULT DOSAGE	PEDIATRIC DOSAGE
Fungal Infections	**Fungal Infections**
Empirical therapy for presumed fungal infection in febrile, neutropenic patients	Empirical therapy for presumed fungal infection in febrile, neutropenic patients
Initial: 3mg/kg/day IV	**≥1 Month of Age:** **Initial:** 3mg/kg/day IV
Systemic Infections	**Systemic Infections**
Aspergillus species, *Candida* species, and/or *Cryptococcus* species infections refractory to amphotericin B deoxycholate, or in patients where renal impairment or unacceptable toxicity precludes the use of amphotericin B deoxycholate	*Aspergillus* species, *Candida* species, and/or *Cryptococcus* species infections refractory to amphotericin B deoxycholate, or in patients where renal impairment or unacceptable toxicity precludes the use of amphotericin B deoxycholate
Initial: 3-5mg/kg/day IV	**≥1 Month of Age:** **Initial:** 3-5mg/kg/day IV
Cryptococcal Meningitis	**Cryptococcal Meningitis**
HIV-Infected Patients: **Initial:** 6mg/kg/day IV	**HIV-Infected Patients:** **Initial:** 6mg/kg/day IV
Visceral Leishmaniasis	**Visceral Leishmaniasis**
Immunocompetent Patients: 3mg/kg/day IV on Days 1-5, 14, 21; may repeat course if parasitic clearance is not achieved w/ recommended dose	**≥1 Month of Age:** **Immunocompetent Patients:** 3mg/kg/day IV on Days 1-5, 14, 21; may repeat course if parasitic clearance is not achieved w/ recommended dose
Immunocompromised Patients: 4mg/kg/day IV on Days 1-5, 10, 17, 24, 31, 38	**Immunocompromised Patients:** 4mg/kg/day IV on Days 1-5, 10, 17, 24, 31, 38

ADMINISTRATION
IV route

Infuse over 120 min; may reduce to 60 min if well tolerated or increase duration if experiencing discomfort.
An in-line membrane filter may be used provided the mean pore diameter of the filter is not <1.0 micron.
Flush existing IV line w/ D5W prior to infusion; if not feasible, administer through a separate line.

Preparation
Reconstitute w/ 12mL of sterile water for inj and shake vial vigorously for 30 sec. Do not reconstitute w/ saline or add saline to reconstituted sol or mix w/ other drugs.
Calculate appropriate volume of reconstituted sol to be further diluted and withdraw amount into syringe.
Attach provided 5-micron filter to syringe and inject contents through filter into appropriate amount of D5 inj diluent for a final concentration of 1-2mg/mL (lower concentrations [0.2-0.5mg/mL] may be appropriate for infants and small children). Use only 1 filter per vial and discard partially used vials.

STORAGE
Unopened Vials: ≤25°C (77°F). Reconstituted Concentrate: 2-8°C (36-46°F) for up to 24 hrs. Do not freeze. Diluted Product: Inj should commence within 6 hrs of dilution with D5W.

HOW SUPPLIED
Inj: 50mg

CONTRAINDICATIONS
Known hypersensitivity to amphotericin B deoxycholate or any other constituents of the product.

WARNINGS/PRECAUTIONS
Anaphylaxis reported; d/c immediately and do not give further infusions if severe anaphylactic reaction occurs. Should be administered by medically trained personnel; monitor closely during the initial dosing period. Significantly less toxic than amphotericin B deoxycholate. False elevations of serum phosphate seen with PHOSm assays.

ADVERSE REACTIONS
Hypokalemia, chills/rigors, SrCr elevation, anemia, N/V, diarrhea, hypomagnesemia, rash, dyspnea, bilirubinemia, BUN increased, headache, abdominal pain.

DRUG INTERACTIONS
Antineoplastic agents may enhance potential for renal toxicity, bronchospasm, and hypotension. Corticosteroids and adrenocorticotropic hormone may potentiate hypokalemia; closely monitor serum electrolytes and cardiac function. May induce hypokalemia and potentiate digitalis toxicity with digitalis glycosides; closely monitor serum K^+ levels. May increase flucytosine toxicity. Imidazoles (eg, ketoconazole, miconazole, clotrimazole, fluconazole) may induce fungal resistance; use with caution, especially in immunocompromised patients. Acute pulmonary toxicity reported with simultaneous leukocyte transfusions. Nephrotoxic drugs may enhance drug-induced renal toxicity; intensive monitoring of renal function is recommended. Amphotericin B-induced hypokalemia may enhance curariform effect of skeletal muscle relaxants (eg, tubocurarine); closely monitor serum K^+ levels.

PREGNANCY AND LACTATION
Category B, not for use in nursing.

MECHANISM OF ACTION
Polyene antifungal; acts by binding to the sterol component, ergosterol, of the cell membrane in susceptible fungi, leading to alterations in cell permeability and cell death. Also binds to the cholesterol component of the mammalian cell, leading to cytotoxicity. Has been shown to penetrate the cell wall of both extracellular and intracellular forms of susceptible fungi.

PHARMACOKINETICS
Absorption: IV administration of variable doses resulted in different pharmacokinetic parameters. **Elimination:** $T_{1/2}$=7-10 hrs (24-hr dosing interval), 100-153 hrs (49 days after dosing).

PATIENT CONSIDERATIONS
Assessment: Assess for hypersensitivity, health status, pregnancy/nursing status, and possible drug interactions.

Monitoring: Monitor for severe anaphylactic and other adverse reactions. Monitor renal, hepatic and hematopoietic function, and serum electrolytes (particularly Mg^{2+} and K^+).

Counseling: Inform of risks and benefits of therapy. Advise to seek medical attention if any adverse reactions occur.

Amerge — naratriptan hydrochloride   Rx
Class: 5-HT$_{1B/1D}$ agonist (triptans)

ADULT DOSAGE	PEDIATRIC DOSAGE
Migraine	Pediatric use may not have been established
W/ or w/o Aura:	
1mg or 2.5mg; may repeat once after 4 hrs if migraine returns or if patient has only partial response	
Max: 5mg/24 hrs	
Safety of treating an average of >4 migraine attacks in a 30-day period has not been established	

DOSING CONSIDERATIONS
Renal Impairment
Mild-Moderate:
Initial: 1mg
Max: 2.5mg/24 hrs
Hepatic Impairment
Mild or Moderate (Child-Pugh Grade A or B):
Initial: 1mg
Max: 2.5mg/24 hrs
Elderly
Start at lower end of dosing range

ADMINISTRATION
Oral route

STORAGE
20-25°C (68-77°F).

HOW SUPPLIED
Tab: 1mg, 2.5mg

CONTRAINDICATIONS
Ischemic coronary artery disease (CAD) (angina pectoris, history of MI, documented silent ischemia), or coronary artery vasospasm, including Prinzmetal's angina; Wolff-Parkinson-White syndrome or arrhythmias associated w/ other cardiac accessory conduction pathway disorders; history of stroke or transient ischemic attack or history of hemiplegic or basilar migraine; peripheral vascular disease; ischemic bowel disease; uncontrolled HTN; recent use (eg, w/ in 24 hrs) of another 5-HT$_1$ agonist, ergotamine-containing medication, ergot-type medication (eg, dihydroergotamine, methysergide); severe renal/hepatic impairment; hypersensitivity to naratriptan HCl.

WARNINGS/PRECAUTIONS
Rare reports of serious cardiac adverse reactions, including acute MI, occurring w/in a few hrs following administration. May cause coronary artery vasospasm (Prinzmetal's angina). Perform cardiovascular (CV) evaluation in triptan-naive patients w/ multiple CV risk factors; if CV evaluation is negative, consider administering 1st dose in a medically supervised setting, performing an ECG immediately following administration, and consider periodic CV evaluation w/ long-term intermittent use. Life-threatening disturbances of cardiac rhythm, including ventricular tachycardia and ventricular fibrillation leading to death, reported; d/c if these disturbances occur. Sensations of tightness, pain, and pressure in the chest, throat, neck, and jaw may occur after treatment and are usually noncardiac in origin; perform a cardiac evaluation if these patients are at high cardiac risk. Cerebral hemorrhage, subarachnoid hemorrhage, and stroke reported; d/c if a cerebrovascular event occurs. Exclude other potentially serious neurological conditions before treating headaches in patients not previously diagnosed as migraineurs and in migraineurs who present w/ symptoms atypical for migraine. May cause noncoronary vasospastic reactions (eg, peripheral vascular ischemia, GI vascular ischemia and infarction, splenic infarction, Raynaud's syndrome); rule out a vasospastic reaction in patients who experience signs/symptoms before administering additional doses. Transient and permanent blindness and significant partial vision loss reported. Overuse of acute migraine drugs may lead to exacerbation of headache; detoxification, including withdrawal of overused drugs, and treatment of withdrawal symptoms may be necessary. Serotonin syndrome may occur; d/c if suspected. Significant BP elevation, including hypertensive crisis w/ acute impairment of organ systems reported. Anaphylaxis/anaphylactoid/hypersensitivity reactions, including angioedema reported.

ADVERSE REACTIONS
Paresthesias, nausea, dizziness, drowsiness, malaise/fatigue, throat and neck symptoms.

DRUG INTERACTIONS
See Contraindications. Serotonin syndrome reported during coadministration of triptans and SSRIs, SNRIs, TCAs, and MAOIs.

PREGNANCY AND LACTATION
Pregnancy: Category C.
Lactation: Not for use in nursing.

MECHANISM OF ACTION
Selective 5-HT$_{1B/1D}$ receptor agonist; binds w/ high affinity to human cloned 5-HT$_{1B/1D}$ receptors. Therapeutic activity is thought to be due to the agonist effects at the 5-HT$_{1B/1D}$ receptors on intracranial blood vessels (including the arteriovenous anastomoses) and sensory nerves of the trigeminal system, which result in cranial vessel constriction and inhibition of pro-inflammatory neuropeptide release.

PHARMACOKINETICS
Absorption: Well-absorbed; oral bioavailability (70%); T$_{max}$=2-3 hrs (2.5mg), 3-4 hrs (during a migraine attack). **Distribution:** V$_d$=170L, plasma protein binding (28-31%). **Metabolism:** Via CYP450 isoenzymes. **Elimination:** Urine (50% unchanged, 30% as metabolites); T$_{1/2}$=6 hrs.

PATIENT CONSIDERATIONS
Assessment: Confirm diagnosis of migraine before therapy. Assess for CAD, uncontrolled HTN, history of hemiplegic/basilar migraine, ECG changes, renal/hepatic impairment, or any conditions where treatment is cautioned or contraindicated. Assess for pregnancy/nursing status and for possible drug interactions. Exclude other potentially serious neurological conditions before therapy. Perform a CV evaluation in triptan-naive patients who have multiple CV risk factors (eg, increased age, diabetes, HTN, smoking, obesity, strong family history of CAD).

Monitoring: Monitor for serious cardiac adverse reactions, arrhythmias, cerebrovascular events, noncoronary vasospastic reactions, exacerbation of headache, serotonin syndrome, increase in BP, anaphylactic/anaphylactoid reactions, and other adverse reactions. Perform ECG immediately after administration of 1st dose in patients w/ multiple CV risk factors. Consider periodic cardiac evaluation in patients who have multiple CV risk factors and are long-term intermittent users.

Counseling: Inform that drug may cause serious CV effects; instruct to be alert for signs/symptoms of chest pain, SOB, irregular heartbeat, significant rise in BP, weakness, and slurring of speech, and ask for medical advice if any indicative sign/symptoms are observed. Inform that anaphylactic/anaphylactoid reactions may occur. Inform that use of drug w/in 24 hrs of another triptan or an ergot-type medication is contraindicated. Caution about the risk of serotonin syndrome, particularly during combined use w/ SSRIs, SNRIs, TCAs, and MAOIs. Inform that use of acute migraine drugs for ≥10 days/month may lead to an exacerbation of headache, and encourage to record headache frequency and drug use (eg, by keeping a headache diary). Inform that drug should not be used during pregnancy unless the potential benefit justifies the potential risk to the fetus. Advise to notify physician if breastfeeding or planning to breastfeed. Inform that treatment may cause somnolence and dizziness; instruct to evaluate the ability to perform complex tasks after drug administration.

AMIKACIN — amikacin sulfate   Rx
Class: Aminoglycoside

> Potential ototoxicity/nephrotoxicity associated w/ therapy; safety for treatment periods >14 days has not been established. Increased risk of nephrotoxicity in patients w/ impaired renal function and in those who receive high doses or prolonged therapy. Neurotoxicity can occur in patients w/ preexisting renal damage and in patients w/ normal renal function treated at higher doses and/or periods longer than those recommended. Increased risk of ototoxicity w/ renal damage. Increased risk of hearing loss w/ degree of exposure to either high peak or high trough serum concentrations. Total/partial irreversible bilateral deafness may occur after therapy has been discontinued. D/C therapy or adjust the dose upon evidence of ototoxicity or nephrotoxicity. Neuromuscular blockade and respiratory paralysis reported following parenteral inj, topical instillation, and following oral use of therapy; consider possibility of these phenomena if therapy is administered by any route, especially in patients taking anesthetics, neuromuscular blocking agents (eg, tubocurarine, succinylcholine, decamethonium), or massive transfusions of citrate-anticoagulated blood. If blockage occurs, Ca^{2+} salts may reverse these phenomena, but mechanical respiratory assistance may be necessary. Closely monitor renal and 8th nerve function. Monitor serum concentrations of amikacin to assure adequate levels and to avoid potentially toxic levels and prolonged peak concentrations >35mcg/mL. Examine urine for decreased specific gravity, increased protein excretion, and presence of cells/casts. Obtain serial audiograms in patients old enough to be tested. Avoid concurrent and/or sequential systemic, oral, or topical use of other neurotoxic/nephrotoxic products (eg, bacitracin, cisplatin, amphotericin B). Advanced age and dehydration may increase risk of toxicity. Avoid concurrent use w/ potent diuretics (eg, furosemide, ethacrynic acid).

OTHER BRAND NAMES
Amikin (Discontinued)

ADULT DOSAGE
General Dosing
15mg/kg/day IM/IV divided into 2 or 3 equal doses given at equally divided intervals
Max: 15mg/kg/day
Max for Heavier Weight Patients: 1.5g/day

Avoid peak levels >35mcg/mL and trough levels >10mcg/mL

Urinary Tract Infections
Uncomplicated:
250mg IM/IV bid

Avoid peak levels >35mcg/mL and trough levels >10mcg/mL

Treatment Duration
Usual: 7-10 days; d/c therapy if definite clinical response does not occur w/in 3-5 days

Reevaluate if considering therapy beyond 10 days in difficult and complicated infections

Other Indications
Treatment of the Following Infections Caused by Susceptible Microorganisms:
Serious infections due to gram-negative bacteria
Bacterial septicemia (including neonatal sepsis)
Serious respiratory tract infections
Serious bone and joint infections
Serious CNS infections (including meningitis)
Serious skin and soft tissue infections
Serious intra-abdominal infections (including peritonitis)

PEDIATRIC DOSAGE
General Dosing
Newborns:
LD: 10mg/kg IM/IV
Maint: 7.5mg/kg IM/IV q12h
Older Infants and Children:
15mg/kg/day IM/IV divided into 2 or 3 equal doses given at equally divided intervals
Max: 15mg/kg/day
Max for Heavier Weight Patients: 1.5g/day

Avoid peak levels >35mcg/mL and trough levels >10mcg/mL

Treatment Duration
Usual: 7-10 days; d/c therapy if definite clinical response does not occur w/in 3-5 days

Reevaluate if considering therapy beyond 10 days in difficult and complicated infections

Burns and postoperative infections
(including post-vascular surgery)
Serious complicated and recurrent
UTIs
Staphylococcal infections

Infections caused by gentamicin- and/
or tobramycin-resistant strains of
gram-negative organisms, particularly
Proteus rettgeri, *Providencia
stuartii*, *Serratia marcescens*, and
Pseudomonas aeruginosa

Certain severe infections in
combination w/ a penicillin-type drug

DOSING CONSIDERATIONS
Renal Impairment
Reduce dose or prolong intervals
Normal Dosage at Prolonged Intervals:
If CrCl is unavailable and patient's condition is stable, may calculate dosage interval in hrs by multiplying patient's SrCr by 9 (eg, if SrCr concentration is 2mg/100mL, recommended single dose (7.5mg/kg) should be administered q18h)
Reduced Dosage at Fixed Intervals:
Initial LD: 7.5mg/kg
Maint Dose q12h: (Observed CrCl [mL/min]/Normal CrCl [mL/min]) x Calculated LD (mg)
Alternatively, may determine reduced q12h dose (if steady state SrCr known) by dividing normal recommended dose by SrCr

ADMINISTRATION
IM/IV route
IV
Add contents of a 500mg vial to 100 or 200mL of sterile diluent (eg, 0.9% NaCl inj, D5 inj).
Administer over a period of 30-60 min; infuse over 1-2 hrs in infants.
Do not physically premix w/ other drugs; administer separately.
Stability:
Stable for 24 hrs at room temperature (at concentrations of 0.25 and 5mg/mL) in D5 inj, D5 and 0.2% or 0.45% NaCl inj, 0.9% NaCl inj, lactated Ringer's inj, Normosol M in D5 inj (or Plasma-Lyte 56 inj in D5W), and Normosol R in D5 inj (or Plasma-Lyte inj 148 in D5W).
At same concentrations, sol frozen and aged for 30 days at -15°C, thawed, and stored at 25°C had utility times of 24 hrs.
At same concentrations, sol aged for 60 days at 4°C and then stored at 25°C had utility times of 24 hrs.

STORAGE
20-25°C (68-77°F).

HOW SUPPLIED
Inj: 250mg/mL [2mL, 4mL]

CONTRAINDICATIONS
History of hypersensitivity to amikacin, history of hypersensitivity or serious toxic reactions to aminoglycosides.

WARNINGS/PRECAUTIONS
May cause fetal harm. Not for uncomplicated initial episodes of UTI unless the causative organisms are not susceptible to antibiotics having less potential toxicity. Contains sodium metabisulfite; allergic-type reactions may occur more frequently in asthmatics. *Clostridium difficile*-associated diarrhea (CDAD) reported; may need to d/c if CDAD is suspected or confirmed. May result in overgrowth of nonsusceptible organisms; institute appropriate therapy if this occurs. Use in the absence of a proven or strongly suspected bacterial infection or prophylactic indication is unlikely to provide benefit and increases the risk of the development of drug-resistant bacteria. Irreversible deafness, renal failure, and death due to neuromuscular blockade reported following irrigation of surgical fields w/ an aminoglycoside preparation. If signs of renal irritation appear (eg, casts, white/red cells, albumin), increase hydration; if azotemia increases or if progressive decrease in urinary output occurs, d/c treatment. May aggravate muscle weakness; caution w/ muscular disorders (eg, myasthenia gravis, parkinsonism). Cross-allergenicity among aminoglycosides demonstrated. Caution in elderly and in premature and neonatal infants. Specimens of body fluids collected for assay should be properly handled.

ADVERSE REACTIONS
Ototoxicity, neurotoxicity, nephrotoxicity.

DRUG INTERACTIONS
See Boxed Warning. Increased nephrotoxicity w/ parenteral administration of aminoglycosides, antibiotics, and cephalosporins. Concomitant cephalosporins may falsely elevate creatinine determinations. Significant mutual inactivation may occur w/ β-lactam antibiotics.

PREGNANCY AND LACTATION
Pregnancy: Category D.
Lactation: Not for use in nursing.

MECHANISM OF ACTION
Aminoglycoside; binds to prokaryotic ribosome, inhibiting protein synthesis in susceptible bacteria.

PHARMACOKINETICS
Absorption: (IM) Rapid. T_{max}=1 hr. Administration of different doses resulted in different parameters. (IV) C_{max}=38mcg/mL. **Distribution:** V_d=24L; plasma protein binding (0-11%); crosses placenta. **Elimination:** Urine (91.9-98.2% unchanged, IM), (84-94% IV); $T_{1/2}$=>2 hrs.

PATIENT CONSIDERATIONS
Assessment: Obtain pretreatment body weight for calculation of correct dosage. Assess and document bacterial infection using culture and susceptibility techniques. Assess for history of hypersensitivity to drug, other aminoglycosides, or to sulfites. Assess for muscular disorders, pregnancy/nursing status, and possible drug interactions. Assess renal function.

Monitoring: Monitor for signs/symptoms of nephrotoxicity, neurotoxicity, ototoxicity, hypersensitivity reactions, neuromuscular blockade, respiratory paralysis, and other adverse reactions. Periodically monitor hydration status, BUN, SrCr, CrCl, 8th nerve function, and peak and trough concentrations. Perform urinalysis.

Counseling: Inform about potential risks/benefits of therapy. Inform that drug only treats bacterial, not viral, infections. Instruct to take exactly ud even if patient feels better early in the course of therapy. Inform that skipping doses or not completing the full course of therapy may decrease effectiveness and increase the likelihood of bacterial resistance. Inform that diarrhea may occur and to contact physician as soon as possible if watery/bloody stools (w/ or w/o stomach cramps, fever) develop even as late as ≥2 months after the last dose.

AMITIZA — lubiprostone   **Rx**
Class: Chloride channel activator

ADULT DOSAGE	PEDIATRIC DOSAGE
Chronic Idiopathic Constipation 24mcg bid **Opioid-Induced Constipation** **Chronic Non-Cancer Pain:** 24mcg bid **Irritable Bowel Syndrome with Constipation** **Women:** 8mcg bid	Pediatric use may not have been established

---

DOSING CONSIDERATIONS
Hepatic Impairment
Chronic Idiopathic Constipation/Opioid-Induced Constipation (OIC):
Moderate (Child-Pugh Class B):
Initial: 16mcg bid
Severe (Child-Pugh Class C):
Initial: 8mcg bid
Titrate: If dose is tolerated but adequate response not obtained, may escalate to full dose w/ appropriate monitoring
Irritable Bowel Syndrome w/ Constipation:
Severe (Child-Pugh Class C):
Initial: 8mcg qd
Titrate: If dose is tolerated but adequate response not obtained, may escalate to full dose w/ appropriate monitoring

ADMINISTRATION
Oral route
Take w/ food and water.
Swallow caps whole; do not break or chew.

STORAGE
25°C (77°F); excursions permitted to 15-30°C (59-86°F). Protect from light and extreme temperatures.

HOW SUPPLIED
Cap: 8mcg, 24mcg

CONTRAINDICATIONS
Known or suspected mechanical GI obstruction.

WARNINGS/PRECAUTIONS
Effectiveness not established in treatment of OIC in patients taking diphenylheptane opioids (eg, methadone). May cause nausea; give with food to reduce symptoms of nausea. Diarrhea may occur; avoid in patients with severe diarrhea and d/c therapy if severe diarrhea occurs. Dyspnea reported; resolves within a few hrs after dose but may recur with subsequent doses. Thoroughly evaluate patients with symptoms suggestive of mechanical GI obstruction prior to initiation of therapy.

ADVERSE REACTIONS
N/V, diarrhea, headache, abdominal pain/distention, flatulence, loose stools, dizziness, edema, dyspnea, abdominal discomfort.

DRUG INTERACTIONS
Diphenylheptane opioids (eg, methadone) may cause dose-dependent decrease in efficacy.

PREGNANCY AND LACTATION
Category C, caution in nursing.

MECHANISM OF ACTION
Chloride channel activator; enhances chloride-rich intestinal fluid secretion, increasing motility in the intestine, thereby facilitating the passage of stool.

PHARMACOKINETICS
Absorption: (24mcg single dose) (M3) C_{max}=41.5pg/mL, T_{max}=1.1 hrs, AUC_{0-t}=57.1pg•hr/mL. **Distribution:** Plasma protein binding (94%).

Metabolism: Rapid and extensive; reduction and oxidation by carbonyl reductase; M3 (active metabolite). **Elimination:** Urine (60%), feces (30%); (M3) $T_{1/2}$=0.9-1.4 hrs.

PATIENT CONSIDERATIONS

Assessment: Assess for known or suspected mechanical GI obstruction, severe diarrhea, pregnancy/nursing status, and possible drug interactions.

Monitoring: Monitor for nausea, dyspnea, severe diarrhea, and other adverse reactions. Periodically assess the need for continued therapy.

Counseling: Instruct to notify physician if experiencing severe nausea, diarrhea, or dyspnea during treatment. Inform that dyspnea may occur within an hr after 1st dose and resolves within 3 hrs, but may recur with repeat dosing. Advise lactating women to monitor their breastfed infants for diarrhea while on therapy.

AMITRIPTYLINE — amitriptyline hydrochloride   Rx

Class: Tricyclic antidepressant (TCA)

> Antidepressants increased the risk of suicidal thinking and behavior (suicidality) in children, adolescents, and young adults in short-term studies of major depressive disorder and other psychiatric disorders. Monitor and observe closely for clinical worsening, suicidality, or unusual changes in behavior in patients who are started on antidepressant therapy. Not approved for use in pediatric patients.

OTHER BRAND NAMES

Elavil (Discontinued)

ADULT DOSAGE	PEDIATRIC DOSAGE
Depression	**Depression**
Outpatients:	**≥12 Years:**
Initial (Divided Dose): 75mg/day in divided doses	10mg tid w/ 20mg at hs
Titrate: May increase to 150mg/day; increases are made preferably in the late afternoon and/or hs doses	
Initial (Single Dose): 50-100mg at hs	
Titrate: May increase by 25mg or 50mg in the hs dose, to a total of 150mg/day	
Hospitalized Patients:	
Initial: 100mg/day	
Titrate: May increase gradually to 200mg/day; some patients may need as much as 300mg/day	
Maint: 50-100mg/day (40mg/day is sufficient in some patients); total daily dose may be given in a single dose, preferably at hs. Continue ≥3 months	

DOSING CONSIDERATIONS

Elderly
10mg tid w/ 20mg at hs

ADMINISTRATION

Oral route

STORAGE

20-25°C (68-77°F). Protect from light.

HOW SUPPLIED

Tab: 10mg, 25mg, 50mg, 75mg, 100mg, 150mg

CONTRAINDICATIONS

Prior hypersensitivity to the product, use of an MAOI concomitantly, treatment w/in 14 days of discontinuing an MAOI, coadministration w/ cisapride, during the acute recovery phase following MI.

WARNINGS/PRECAUTIONS

Not approved for the treatment of bipolar depression. May precipitate a mixed/manic episode in patients at risk for bipolar disorder; screen for risk for bipolar disorder prior to initiating treatment. Caution w/ history of seizures, history of urinary retention, angle-closure glaucoma, or increased IOP. Caution w/ cardiovascular disorders (CVD); high doses reported to produce arrhythmias, sinus tachycardia, and prolongation of the conduction time. Caution w/ hyperthyroidism, liver dysfunction, and in elderly. Pupillary dilation that occurs following therapy may trigger an angle-closure attack in a patient w/ anatomically narrow angles who does not have a patent iridectomy. Dose may be reduced or a major tranquilizer (eg, perphenazine) may be administered concurrently if schizophrenic patients develop increased symptoms of psychosis (patients w/ paranoid symptomatology may have an exaggeration of such symptoms), or if depressed patients, particularly those w/ known manic-depressive illness, experience a shift to mania or hypomania. Hazards may be increased w/ electroshock therapy. D/C several days before elective surgery. May alter blood glucose levels.

ADVERSE REACTIONS

Arrhythmias, tachycardia, seizures, extrapyramidal symptoms, anxiety, insomnia, dizziness, headache, constipation, dry mouth, skin rash, N/V, diarrhea, increased/decreased libido, weight gain/loss.

DRUG INTERACTIONS

See Contraindications. May block antihypertensive action of guanethidine or similarly acting compounds. Caution in patients receiving thyroid medication. May enhance the response to alcohol and the effects of barbiturates and other CNS depressants. Delirium reported w/ disulfiram. Topiramate may increase levels; adjust amitriptyline dose according to patient's clinical response and not based on plasma levels. Drugs that inhibit CYP2D6 (eg, quinidine, cimetidine, many CYP2D6 substrates [other antidepressants, phenothiazines, propafenone, flecainide]) may increase plasma concentrations; may require lower doses for either TCA or the other drug, and monitoring of TCA plasma levels. Caution w/ SSRI coadministration and when switching between TCAs and SSRIs (eg, fluoxetine, sertraline, paroxetine); sufficient time must elapse before starting therapy when switching from fluoxetine (at least 5 weeks may be necessary). Close supervision and careful dose adjustment is required when given w/ anticholinergic agents or sympathomimetic drugs, including epinephrine combined w/ local anesthetics. Hyperpyrexia reported w/ anticholinergics or neuroleptics, particularly during hot weather. Paralytic ileus may occur w/ anticholinergic-type drugs. Caution w/ large doses of ethchlorvynol; transient delirium reported.

PREGNANCY AND LACTATION

Pregnancy: Category C. Although a causal relationship has not been established, there have been a few reports of adverse events, including CNS effects, limb deformities, or developmental delay, in infants whose mothers had taken amitriptyline during pregnancy.

Lactation: Excreted into breast milk. Not for use in nursing.

MECHANISM OF ACTION

TCA; has not been established. Inhibits the membrane pump mechanism responsible for uptake of norepinephrine and serotonin in adrenergic and serotonergic neurons.

PHARMACOKINETICS

Absorption: Rapid. **Distribution:** Found in breast milk; crosses the placenta.
Metabolism: N-demethylation and bridge hydroxylation. **Elimination:** Urine.

PATIENT CONSIDERATIONS

Assessment: Assess for acute recovery phase following MI, hypersensitivity to drug, risk for bipolar disorder, history of seizures or urinary retention, susceptibility to angle-closure glaucoma, increased IOP, CVD, hyperthyroidism, liver dysfunction, schizophrenia, paranoid symptomatology, manic-depressive illness, pregnancy/nursing status, and possible drug interactions.

Monitoring: Monitor for signs/symptoms of clinical worsening, suicidality, unusual changes in behavior, angle-closure glaucoma, increased psychosis symptoms, exaggeration of paranoid symptoms, hypomanic/manic episodes, changes in blood glucose levels, and other adverse reactions.

Counseling: Inform about benefits, risks, and appropriate use of therapy. Advise that drug may impair mental/physical abilities required for the performance of hazardous tasks (eg, operating machinery, driving). Caution about the risk of angle-closure glaucoma. Advise patients, families, and caregivers to monitor for unusual changes in behavior, worsening of depression, and suicidal ideation on a day-to-day basis, and to report such symptoms to physician.

AMNESTEEM — isotretinoin   Rx

Class: Retinoid

> Not for use by females who are or may become pregnant. Severe birth defects, including death, have been documented. Increased risk of spontaneous abortion and premature births reported. D/C immediately if pregnancy occurs during treatment and refer to an obstetrician-gynecologist experienced in reproductive toxicity for evaluation and counseling. Approved only under special restricted distribution program called iPLEDGE. Prescribers and pharmacies must be registered and activated w/ the program. Patients must be registered and meet all the requirements of iPLEDGE.

OTHER BRAND NAMES

Sotret, Claravis

ADULT DOSAGE	PEDIATRIC DOSAGE
Severe Recalcitrant Nodular Acne	**Severe Recalcitrant Nodular Acne**
Unresponsive to Conventional Therapy, Including Systemic Antibiotics:	**≥12 Years:**
0.5-1mg/kg/day given in 2 divided doses for 15-20 weeks	**Unresponsive to Conventional Therapy, Including Systemic Antibiotics:**
Titrate: Adjust dose according to response of the disease and/or the appearance of clinical side effects	0.5-1mg/kg/day given in 2 divided doses for 15-20 weeks
Very Severe Disease w/ Scarring or Primarily Manifested on Trunk:	**Titrate:** Adjust dose according to response of the disease and/or the appearance of clinical side effects
May adjust dose up to 2mg/kg/day, as tolerated	May d/c if total nodule count has been reduced by >70% prior to completing 15-20 weeks
May d/c if total nodule count has been reduced by >70% prior to completing 15-20 weeks	After a period of ≥2 months off therapy, and if warranted by persistent or recurring severe nodular acne, a 2nd course of therapy may be initiated; the optimal interval before retreatment has not been defined for patients who have not completed skeletal growth
After a period of ≥2 months off therapy, and if warranted by persistent or recurring severe nodular acne, a 2nd course of therapy may be initiated; the optimal interval before retreatment has not been defined for patients who have not completed skeletal growth	

ADMINISTRATION
Oral route
Take w/ a meal.
Swallow caps w/ a full glass of liquid.

STORAGE
20-25°C (68-77°F). Protect from light.

HOW SUPPLIED
Cap: 10mg, 20mg, 40mg, (Claravis, Sotret) 10mg, 20mg, 30mg, 40mg

CONTRAINDICATIONS
Pregnancy, hypersensitivity to this medication or to any of its components. (Sotret) Paraben sensitivity.

WARNINGS/PRECAUTIONS
Avoid long-term use. Do not donate blood during therapy and for 1 month following discontinuation of therapy. May cause depression, psychosis, suicidal ideation/attempts, suicide, and aggressive and/or violent behaviors. Associated w/ pseudotumor cerebri (benign intracranial HTN). Erythema multiforme and severe skin reactions (eg, Stevens-Johnson syndrome, toxic epidermal necrolysis) reported; closely monitor for severe skin reactions and consider discontinuation of therapy. Acute pancreatitis reported; d/c if hypertriglyceridemia cannot be controlled at an acceptable level or if symptoms of pancreatitis occur. Increased TG levels, increased cholesterol levels, decreased HDL levels, impaired hearing, inflammatory bowel disease, hepatotoxicity, premature epiphyseal closure, skeletal hyperostosis, corneal opacities, decreased night vision, and impaired glucose control reported. D/C if symptoms of pseudotumor cerebri and papilledema are present, significant decrease in WBC count, tinnitus or hearing impairment, visual impairment, abdominal pain, rectal bleeding, severe diarrhea, or if liver enzyme levels do not normalize or if hepatitis is suspected. Spontaneous osteoporosis, osteopenia, bone fractures, and delayed fracture healing reported; caution w/ genetic predisposition for age related osteoporosis, history of childhood osteoporosis conditions, osteomalacia, other bone metabolism disorders, anorexia nervosa, and in patients participating in sports w/ repetitive impact. Anaphylactic reactions and other allergic reactions reported; d/c and institute appropriate management if a severe allergic reaction occurs. Micro-dosed progesterone preparations may be an inadequate method of contraception during therapy.

ADVERSE REACTIONS
Cheilitis, hypertriglyceridemia, allergic reactions, inflammatory bowel disease, skeletal hyperostosis, pseudotumor cerebri, suicidal ideation/attempt, abnormal menses, bronchospasms, hearing impairment, corneal opacities, tachycardia, drowsiness, respiratory infection.

DRUG INTERACTIONS
Avoid use w/ tetracyclines or vitamin supplements containing vitamin A. Caution w/ drugs that cause drug-induced osteoporosis/osteomalacia and/or affect vitamin D metabolism (eg, systemic corticosteroids, any anticonvulsant).

PREGNANCY AND LACTATION
Pregnancy: Category X; refer to PI for further information on pregnancy precautions that must be taken in females of reproductive potential.
Lactation: Not for use in nursing.

MECHANISM OF ACTION
Retinoid; mechanism not established. Inhibits sebaceous gland function and keratinization.

PHARMACOKINETICS
Absorption: (Adult, fed) AUC=10,004ng•hr/mL, C_{max}=862ng/mL, T_{max}=5.3 hrs. (12-15 years of age, multiple doses) C_{max}=731.98ng/mL, AUC_{0-12}=5082ng•hr/mL, T_{max}=4 hrs. **Distribution:** Plasma protein binding (>99.9%). **Metabolism:** Liver via CYP2C8, 2C9, 3A4, and 2B6; 4-*oxo*-isotretinoin, retinoic acid, and 4-*oxo*-retinoic acid (active metabolites). **Elimination:** Feces and urine (65%-83%); (Adult, fed) $T_{1/2}$=21 hrs (isotretinoin), 24 hrs (4-*oxo*-isotretinoin). (12-15 years of age, multiple doses) $T_{1/2}$=15.7 hrs (isotretinoin), 23.1 hrs (4-*oxo*-isotretinoin).

PATIENT CONSIDERATIONS
Assessment: Assess that females have had 2 (-) urine or serum pregnancy tests separated by at least 19 days, and are on 2 forms of effective contraception. Assess for hypersensitivity to the drug or any other component in the cap, history of psychiatric disorder, depression, risk of hyperlipidemia, nursing status, and possible drug interactions. Obtain blood lipids and LFTs.

Monitoring: Monitor for signs/symptoms of psychiatric disorders, pseudotumor cerebri, lipid abnormalities, serious skin reactions, acute pancreatitis, hearing impairment, hepatotoxicity, inflammatory bowel disease, decreased bone mineral density, hyperostosis, premature epiphyseal closure, visual difficulties, and other adverse reactions. Monitor lipid levels and LFTs (weekly or biweekly) until response to drug is established. Monitor glucose levels and creatine phosphokinase levels. Monitor that females remain on 2 forms of contraception 1 month before, during, and for 1 month following discontinuation of therapy.

Counseling: Instruct to read the Medication Guide/iPLEDGE educational materials and sign the Patient Information/Informed Consent form. Instruct females who can get pregnant to also sign a 2nd Patient Information/Informed Consent About Birth Defects form. Inform females of reproductive potential that 2 forms of effective contraception are required starting 1 month prior to initiation, during treatment, and for 1 month following discontinuation. Inform that monthly pregnancy tests are required before new prescription is issued. Advise to notify physician if depression, mood disturbances, psychosis, or aggression occurs. Counsel not to share drug w/ anyone and not to donate blood during therapy and for 1 month following discontinuation. Instruct to take w/ a meal and swallow cap w/ a full glass of liquid. Inform that transient exacerbation (flare) of acne may occur. Instruct to avoid wax epilation and skin resurfacing procedures during and for at least 6 months following therapy. Instruct to avoid prolonged exposure to UV rays or sunlight. Inform that decreased tolerance to contact lenses during and after therapy may occur. Inform that musculoskeletal symptoms, transient pain in chest, back pain, arthralgias, neutropenia, agranulocytosis, severe skin reactions, and anaphylactic reactions and other allergic reactions may occur. Advise to use caution when driving or operating any vehicle at night.

AMOXICILLIN — amoxicillin   Rx
Class: Semisynthetic ampicillin derivative

OTHER BRAND NAMES
Amoxil (Discontinued), Trimox (Discontinued)

ADULT DOSAGE

Helicobacter pylori Eradication
W/ (Active or 1-Year History) Duodenal Ulcer Disease:
Dual Therapy: 1g + 30mg lansoprazole, each q8h for 14 days
Triple Therapy: 1g + 30mg lansoprazole + 500mg clarithromycin, all q12h for 14 days

Ear/Nose/Throat Infection
Mild/Moderate: 500mg q12h or 250mg q8h
Severe: 875mg q12h or 500mg q8h

Genitourinary Tract Infections
Mild/Moderate: 500mg q12h or 250mg q8h
Severe: 875mg q12h or 500mg q8h

Skin and Skin Structure Infections
Mild/Moderate: 500mg q12h or 250mg q8h
Severe: 875mg q12h or 500mg q8h

Lower Respiratory Tract Infections
Mild/Moderate or Severe: 875mg q12h or 500mg q8h

Treatment Duration
Continue for a minimum of 48-72 hrs beyond the time the patient becomes asymptomatic or evidence of bacterial eradication has been obtained

***Streptococcus pyogenes* Infections:** Treat for at least 10 days

PEDIATRIC DOSAGE

Lower Respiratory Tract Infections
≤12 Weeks of Age:
Max: 30mg/kg/day divided q12h
>3 Months of Age:
<40kg: 45mg/kg/day divided q12h or 40mg/kg/day divided q8h
≥40kg: 875mg q12h or 500mg q8h

Ear/Nose/Throat Infection
≤12 Weeks of Age:
Max: 30mg/kg/day divided q12h
>3 Months of Age:
<40kg:
Mild/Moderate: 25mg/kg/day divided q12h or 20mg/kg/day divided q8h
Severe: 45mg/kg/day divided q12h or 40mg/kg/day divided q8h
≥40kg:
Mild/Moderate: 500mg q12h or 250mg q8h
Severe: 875mg q12h or 500mg q8h

Genitourinary Tract Infections
≤12 Weeks of Age:
Max: 30mg/kg/day divided q12h
>3 Months of Age:
<40kg:
Mild/Moderate: 25mg/kg/day divided q12h or 20mg/kg/day divided q8h
Severe: 45mg/kg/day divided q12h or 40mg/kg/day divided q8h
≥40kg:
Mild/Moderate: 500mg q12h or 250mg q8h
Severe: 875mg q12h or 500mg q8h

Skin and Skin Structure Infections
≤12 Weeks of Age:
Max: 30mg/kg/day divided q12h
>3 Months of Age:
<40kg:
Mild/Moderate: 25mg/kg/day divided q12h or 20mg/kg/day divided q8h
Severe: 45mg/kg/day divided q12h or 40mg/kg/day divided q8h
≥40kg:
Mild/Moderate: 500mg q12h or 250mg q8h
Severe: 875mg q12h or 500mg q8h

Treatment Duration
Continue for a minimum of 48-72 hrs beyond the time that patient becomes asymptomatic or evidence of bacterial eradication has been obtained

***S. pyogenes* Infections:** Treat for at least 10 days

DOSING CONSIDERATIONS
Renal Impairment
Adults:
GFR <30mL/min: Should not receive an 875mg dose
GFR 10-30mL/min: 250mg or 500mg q12h, depending on severity of infection
GFR <10mL/min: 250mg or 500mg q24h, depending on severity of infection
Hemodialysis: 250mg or 500mg q24h, depending on severity of infection; give an additional dose during and at end of dialysis

Other Important Considerations
Bacteria that are intermediate in their susceptibility to amoxicillin should follow the recommendations for severe infections

ADMINISTRATION
Oral route

Oral Sus
Can be added to formula, milk, fruit juice, water, ginger ale, or cold drinks; take immediately.
Shake well before use.
Discard any unused portion of the reconstituted sus after 14 days; refrigeration is preferable, but not required.

Reconstitution:
125mg/5mL: Reconstitute 80mL, 100mL, or 150mL bottle size w/ 62mL, 77mL, or 113mL of water, respectively.
200mg/5mL: Reconstitute 50mL, 75mL, or 100mL bottle size w/ 39mL, 57mL, or 75mL of water, respectively.
250mg/5mL: Reconstitute 80mL, 100mL, or 150mL bottle size w/ 47mL, 60mL, or 90mL of water, respectively.
400mg/5mL: Reconstitute 50mL, 75mL, or 100mL bottle size w/ 35mL, 51mL, or 67mL of water, respectively.
Add approximately 1/3 of the total amount of water to wet powder, then shake vigorously.
Add the remainder of the water and shake vigorously.
Place directly on tongue for swallowing.

STORAGE
20-25°C (68-77°F).

HOW SUPPLIED
Cap: 250mg, 500mg; **Oral Sus:** 125mg/5mL [80mL, 100mL, 150mL], 200mg/5mL [50mL, 75mL, 100mL], 250mg/5mL [80mL, 100mL, 150mL], 400mg/5mL [50mL, 75mL, 100mL]; **Tab:** 500mg, 875mg*; **Tab, Chewable:** 125mg, 250mg *scored

CONTRAINDICATIONS
Serious hypersensitivity reaction to amoxicillin or to other β-lactam antibiotics.

WARNINGS/PRECAUTIONS
Serious and occasionally fatal hypersensitivity (anaphylactic) reactions reported; increased risk w/ a history of penicillin (PCN) hypersensitivity and/or history of sensitivity to multiple allergens. D/C and institute appropriate therapy if an allergic reaction occurs. *Clostridium difficile*-associated diarrhea (CDAD) reported; may need to d/c if CDAD is suspected or confirmed. Avoid use w/ mononucleosis; erythematous skin rash may develop in these patients. May result in bacterial resistance if used in the absence of a proven/suspected bacterial indication. Lab test interactions may occur. Caution in elderly; monitor renal function.

ADVERSE REACTIONS
N/V, diarrhea, rash.

DRUG INTERACTIONS
Decreased renal tubular secretion and increased/prolonged levels w/ probenecid. May reduce efficacy of combined oral estrogen/progesterone contraceptives. Chloramphenicol, macrolides, sulfonamides, and tetracyclines may interfere w/ bactericidal effects of PCN. PT prolongation (increased INR) reported w/ oral anticoagulants; dose adjustments of oral anticoagulants may be necessary. Increased incidence of rashes w/ allopurinol.

PREGNANCY AND LACTATION
Pregnancy: Category B.
Lactation: PCNs have been shown to be excreted in human milk; may lead to sensitization of infants. Caution in nursing.

MECHANISM OF ACTION
Ampicillin analogue; has bactericidal action against susceptible bacteria during the stage of active multiplication; acts through inhibition of biosynthesis of cell wall.

PHARMACOKINETICS
Absorption: Rapid. Cap: T_{max}=1-2 hrs; C_{max}=3.5-5mcg/mL (250mg), C_{max}=5.5-7.5mcg/mL (500mg). Tab: (875mg) C_{max}=13.8mcg/mL, AUC=35.4mcg•hr/mL. Sus: T_{max}=1-2 hrs (125mg/5mL, 250mg/5mL); C_{max}=1.5-3mcg/mL (125mg/5mL), C_{max}=3.5-5mcg/mL (250mg/5mL); (400mg/5mL) T_{max}=1 hr, C_{max}=5.92mcg/mL, AUC=17.1mcg•hr/mL. Tab, Chewable: (400mg) T_{max}=1 hr, C_{max}=5.18mcg/mL, AUC=17.9mcg•hr/mL. **Distribution:** Plasma protein binding (20%); found in breast milk. **Elimination:** Urine (60%, unchanged); $T_{1/2}$=61.3 min.

PATIENT CONSIDERATIONS
Assessment: Assess for history of allergic reaction to PCNs, cephalosporins, or other allergens, mononucleosis, renal function, pregnancy/nursing status, and possible drug interactions. Obtain culture and susceptibility information.

Monitoring: Monitor for serious anaphylactic reactions, erythematous skin rash, development of drug-resistant bacteria, and CDAD. Monitor renal function. Monitor PT and INR if coadministered w/ an oral anticoagulant.

Counseling: Inform that drug treats only bacterial, not viral, infections. Instruct to take exactly ud; inform that skipping doses or not completing the full course of therapy may decrease effectiveness and increase resistance. Instruct to notify physician as soon as possible if watery and bloody stools (w/ or w/o stomach cramps and fever) develop, even as late as ≥2 months after having last dose. Advise patients that drug may cause allergic reactions.

AMOXICILLIN/CLAVULANATE 600/42.9 –
amoxicillin/clavulanate potassium   **Rx**

Class: Aminopenicillin/beta lactamase inhibitor

OTHER BRAND NAMES
Augmentin ES- 600 (Discontinued)

> **PEDIATRIC DOSAGE**
> **Acute Otitis Media**
>
> Recurrent or persistent acute otitis media due to *Streptococcus pneumoniae*, *Haemophilus influenzae*, or *Moraxella catarrhalis*, characterized by antibiotic exposure for acute otitis media w/in the preceding 3 months, and if ≤2 yrs of age or attend daycare
>
> **≥3 Months of Age:**
> **<40kg:**
> 90mg/kg/day divided q12h for 10 days; dose based on amoxicillin component (600mg/5mL)

ADMINISTRATION
Oral route
Take at the start of a meal
Shake well before use
Do not substitute (600mg/42.9mg)/5mL w/ (200mg/28.5mg)/5mL or (400mg/57mg)/5mL sus; not interchangeable

Preparation
Add approx 2/3 of the total amount of water for reconstitution and shake, then add remainder of the water and shake again
Reconstitute 75mL, 125mL, and 200mL bottle sizes w/ 68mL, 108mL, and 170mL of water, respectively

STORAGE
20-25°C (68-77°F). Refrigerate reconstituted sus; discard after 10 days.

HOW SUPPLIED
Sus: (Amoxicillin/Clavulanate) (600mg/42.9mg)/5mL [75mL, 125mL, 200mL]

CONTRAINDICATIONS
History of serious hypersensitivity reactions (eg, anaphylaxis or Stevens-Johnson syndrome) to amoxicillin, clavulanate or to other beta-lactam antibacterial drugs (eg, penicillins and cephalosporins), history of amoxicillin/clavulanate-associated cholestatic jaundice/hepatic dysfunction.

WARNINGS/PRECAUTIONS
Serious, occasionally fatal, hypersensitivity reactions reported; increased risk w/ history of penicillin (PCN) hypersensitivity and/or a history of sensitivity to multiple allergens. D/C if allergic reaction occurs and institute appropriate therapy. Caution w/ hepatic dysfunction. *Clostridium difficile* associated diarrhea (CDAD) reported; may need to d/c if CDAD is suspected or confirmed. Avoid w/ mononucleosis. May result in bacterial resistance w/ use in the absence of a proven/suspected bacterial infection; d/c and/or institute appropriate therapy if superinfection develops. Each 5mL of 600mg/42.9mg sus contains 1.4mg of phenylalanine. Lab test interactions may occur.

ADVERSE REACTIONS
Contact dermatitis (diaper rash), URTI, diarrhea, vomiting, cough, fever.

DRUG INTERACTIONS
Probenecid may increase/prolong levels; coadministration not recommended. Abnormal prolongation of PT (increased INR) reported w/ anticoagulants; may require oral anticoagulant dose adjustment. Allopurinol may increase incidence of rashes. May reduce efficacy of oral contraceptives.

PREGNANCY AND LACTATION
Category B, caution in nursing.

MECHANISM OF ACTION
Amoxicillin: Aminopenicillin; binds to PCN-binding proteins w/in the bacterial cell wall and inhibits its synthesis. Clavulanate: β-lactamase inhibitor; possesses ability to inactivate a wide range of β-lactamase enzymes commonly found in microorganisms resistant to PCN and cephalosporins.

PHARMACOKINETICS
Absorption: Amoxicillin: C_{max}=15.7mcg/mL, T_{max}=2 hrs; AUC=59.8mcg•hr/mL. Clavulanate: C_{max}=1.7mcg/mL, T_{max}=1.1 hrs; AUC=4mcg•hr/mL. **Distribution:** Plasma protein binding: Amoxicillin (approx 18%), clavulanate (approx 25%). Amoxicillin: Found in breast milk. **Elimination:** Amoxicillin: Urine (approx 50-70% unchanged); $T_{1/2}$=1.4 hrs. Clavulanate: Urine (approx 25-40% unchanged); $T_{1/2}$=1.1 hrs.

PATIENT CONSIDERATIONS
Assessment: Assess for history of serious hypersensitivity reactions to other β-lactam antibacterial drugs (eg, PCNs, cephalosporins) or other allergens, history of amoxicillin/clavulanate-associated cholestatic jaundice/hepatic dysfunction, mononucleosis, phenylketonuria, pregnancy/nursing status, and possible drug interactions.

Monitoring: Monitor hepatic function at regular intervals. Monitor for anaphylactic reactions, development of superinfection, skin rash, CDAD, and other adverse reactions.

Counseling: Instruct to take q12h w/ a meal or snack to reduce possibility of GI upset. Advise to consult physician if severe diarrhea or watery and bloody stools occur (even as late as ≥2 months after having taken the last dose). Counsel that therapy should only be used to treat bacterial infections. Instruct to take ud; inform that skipping doses or not completing the full course of therapy may decrease effectiveness of the drug and increase bacterial resistance. Instruct to use a dosing spoon or medicine dropper when dosing, and to rinse them after each use. Instruct to discard any unused medicine. Counsel patients w/ phenylketonuria that therapy contains 1.4mg of phenylalanine.

AMPHOTEC — amphotericin B cholesteryl sulfate complex   Rx
Class: Polyene antifungal

ADULT DOSAGE	PEDIATRIC DOSAGE
Aspergillosis	**Aspergillosis**
Invasive aspergillosis in patients where renal impairment or unacceptable toxicity precludes the use of amphotericin B deoxycholate in effective doses, and in patients w/ invasive aspergillosis where prior amphotericin B deoxycholate therapy has failed	Invasive aspergillosis in patients where renal impairment or unacceptable toxicity precludes the use of amphotericin B deoxycholate in effective doses, and in patients w/ invasive aspergillosis where prior amphotericin B deoxycholate therapy has failed
3-4mg/kg as required, qd, at infusion rate of 1mg/kg/hr	3-4mg/kg as required, qd, at infusion rate of 1mg/kg/hr
Test Dose: Infuse small amount (eg, 10mL of the final preparation containing between 1.6-8.3mg) over 15-30 min immediately preceding the first dose; carefully observe for next 30 min	**Test Dose:** Infuse small amount (eg, 10mL of the final preparation containing between 1.6-8.3mg) over 15-30 min immediately preceding the first dose; carefully observe for next 30 min

ADMINISTRATION
IV route

May shorten infusion time to a minimum of 2 hrs if no evidence of intolerance or infusion-related reactions

If acute reactions or intolerance to infusion volume occurs, may extend infusion time

Do not reconstitute w/ saline or dextrose sol, or admix reconstituted liquid w/ saline or electrolytes

Avoid addition of sol containing a bacteriostatic agent (eg, benzyl alcohol)

Do not mix infusion admixture w/ other drugs; if administered through existing IV line, flush w/ D5 for inj prior to and following infusion of therapy

Do not filter or use an in-line filter

Preparation
Reconstitute w/ 10mL or 20mL of sterile water for inj in 50mg or 100mg vial, respectively, using a sterile syringe and a 20-gauge needle

Further dilute reconstituted liquid to final concentration of 0.6mg/mL (range 0.16-0.83mg/mL) by adding appropriate reconstituted volume to D5 for inj infusion bag

STORAGE
Unopened Vials: 15-30°C (59-86°F). Retain in carton until time of use. Reconstituted: 2-8°C (36-46°F). Use within 24 hrs. Do not freeze. Further Diluted with D5W for Inj: 2-8°C (36-46°F). Use within 24 hrs.

HOW SUPPLIED
Inj: 50mg [20mL], 100mg [50mL]

CONTRAINDICATIONS
Documented hypersensitivity to any component of Amphotec, unless benefit outweighs risk.

WARNINGS/PRECAUTIONS
Anaphylaxis reported; administer epinephrine, oxygen, IV steroids, and airway management as indicated. D/C if severe respiratory distress occurs; do not give further infusions. Acute infusion-related reactions may occur 1-3 hrs after starting IV infusion; manage by pretreatment with antihistamines and corticosteroids and/or by reducing the rate of infusion and by prompt administration of antihistamines and corticosteroids. Avoid rapid IV infusion. Monitor renal and hepatic function, serum electrolytes, CBC, and PT as medically indicated.

ADVERSE REACTIONS
Chills, fever, tachycardia, N/V, increased creatinine, hypotension, HTN, headache, thrombocytopenia, hypokalemia, hypomagnesemia, hypoxia, abnormal LFTs, dyspnea.

DRUG INTERACTIONS
Caution with antineoplastic agents; may enhance potential for renal toxicity, bronchospasm, hypotension. Corticosteroids and corticotropin may potentiate hypokalemia; monitor serum electrolytes and cardiac function. Cyclosporine and tacrolimus may cause renal toxicity. Concurrent use with digitalis glycosides may induce hypokalemia and may potentiate digitalis toxicity of digitalis glycosides; closely monitor serum K⁺ levels. May increase flucytosine toxicity; use with caution. Antagonism with imidazole derivatives (eg, miconazole, ketoconazole) reported. Nephrotoxic agents (eg, aminoglycosides, pentamidine) may enhance the potential for drug-induced renal toxicity; use with caution and intensively monitor renal function. Amphotericin B-induced hypokalemia may enhance curariform effect of skeletal muscle relaxants (eg, tubocurarine) due to hypokalemia; closely monitor serum K⁺ levels.

PREGNANCY AND LACTATION
Category B, not for use in nursing.

MECHANISM OF ACTION
Polyene antifungal; binds to sterols (primarily ergosterol) in cell membranes of sensitive fungi, with subsequent leakage of intracellular contents and cell death due to changes in membrane permeability. Also binds to cholesterol in mammalian cell membranes, which may account for human toxicity.

PHARMACOKINETICS
Absorption: (3mg/kg/day) AUC=29mcg/mL•hr; C_{max}=2.6mcg/mL. (4mg/kg/day) AUC=36mcg/mL•hr; C_{max}=2.9mcg/mL. **Distribution:** V_d=3.8L/kg (3mg/kg/day), 4.1L/kg (4mg/kg/day). **Elimination:** $T_{1/2}$=27.5 hrs (3mg/kg/day), 28.2 hrs (4mg/kg/day).

PATIENT CONSIDERATIONS
Assessment: Assess for previous hypersensitivity to the drug, pregnancy/nursing status, and for possible drug interactions. Assess renal function.

Monitoring: Monitor for anaphylaxis, respiratory distress, and acute infusion-related reactions. Monitor renal and hepatic function, serum electrolytes, CBC, and PT. Monitor patients for 30 min after administering the test dose.

Counseling: Inform of risks and benefits of therapy. Advise to seek medical attention if any adverse reactions occur.

AMPHOTERICIN B — amphotericin B   Rx
Class: Polyene antifungal

> Used primarily for treatment of progressive and potentially life-threatening fungal infections; do not use to treat noninvasive forms of fungal disease (eg, oral thrush, vaginal and esophageal candidiasis) in patients with normal neutrophil counts. Do not give in doses >1.5mg/kg. Exercise caution to prevent inadvertent overdosage; may result in potentially fatal cardiac or cardiopulmonary arrest. Verify product name and dosage preadministration, especially if dose exceeds 1.5mg/kg.

ADULT DOSAGE	PEDIATRIC DOSAGE
Fungal Infections	Pediatric use may not have been established
Potentially life-threatening fungal infections: aspergillosis, cryptococcosis (torulosis), North American blastomycosis, systemic candidiasis, coccidioidomycosis, histoplasmosis, zygomycosis including mucormycosis due to susceptible species of the genera *Absidia*, *Mucor*, and *Rhizopus*, and infections due to related susceptible species of *Conidiobolus* and *Basidiobolus*, and sporotrichosis; may be useful for treatment of American mucocutaneous leishmaniasis, but not the drug of choice as primary therapy	
Test Dose: 1mg in 20mL of D5W over 20-30 min	
Initial Treatment Dose: Good Cardio-Renal Function and Well-Tolerated Test Dose: 0.25mg/kg/day	
Severe and Rapidly Progressive Infection: 0.3mg/kg/day	
Impaired Cardio-Renal Function or Severe Reaction to Test Dose: Initiate w/ smaller daily dose (eg, 5-10mg)	
Titrate: May increase by 5-10mg/day to final dose of 0.5-0.7mg/kg/day, depending on cardio-renal status	
Total Daily Dose: May range up to 1mg/kg/day or up to 1.5mg/kg/day when given on alternate days	
Max: 1.5mg/kg/day	
Sporotrichosis: Total dose up to 2.5g for up to 9 months	
Aspergillosis: Total dose up to 3.6g for up to 11 months	
Rhinocerebral Phycomycosis: Cumulative dose of at least 3g is recommended; if there is evidence of deep tissue invasion, may use total dose of 3-4g	

ADMINISTRATION
IV route

Administer by slow IV infusion over a period of approx 2-6 hrs (depending on dose). Recommended concentration for IV infusion is 0.1mg/mL (1mg/10mL).

Preparation of Sol
1. Rapidly express 10mL sterile water for inj (w/o a bacteriostatic agent) directly into the lyophilized cake, using a needle (minimum diameter of 20 gauge) and a syringe
2. Shake the vial immediately until sol is clear
3. Infusion sol is obtained by further dilution (1:50) w/ D5 inj (pH >4.2)

Do not reconstitute w/ saline sol or use any diluent other than the ones recommended.
May use an in-line membrane filter for IV infusion; however, the mean pore diameter of the filter should not be <1.0 micron.

STORAGE
Prior to Reconstitution: 2-8°C (36-46°F). Protect against exposure to light. Concentrate (5mg/mL after reconstitution with 10mL Sterile Water for Inj USP): May be stored in the dark, at room temperature for 24 hrs, or refrigerate for 1 week with minimal loss of potency and clarity. Sol for IV Infusion (≤0.1mg/mL): Use promptly after preparation and protect from light during administration.

HOW SUPPLIED
Inj: 50mg

CONTRAINDICATIONS
Hypersensitivity to amphotericin B or any other component in the formulation, unless condition requiring treatment is life-threatening and amenable only to amphotericin B therapy.

WARNINGS/PRECAUTIONS
Balance possible life-saving benefit against untoward and dangerous side effects. Administer IV under close clinical observation by medically trained personnel. Acute reactions, including fever, shaking chills, hypotension, anorexia, N/V, headache, tachypnea may occur 1-3 hrs after starting IV infusion. Avoid rapid IV infusion; may cause hypotension, hypokalemia, arrhythmias, and shock. Caution with reduced renal function; frequently monitor renal function. Hydration and Na+ repletion prior to administration may reduce the risk of developing nephrotoxicity. Supplemental alkali medication may decrease renal tubular acidosis complications. Leukoencephalopathy reported; total body irradiation may be a predisposition.

ADVERSE REACTIONS
Fever, malaise, weight loss, hypotension, tachypnea, anorexia, N/V, diarrhea, dyspepsia, cramping epigastric pain, normochromic normocytic anemia, inj-site pain, generalized pain, headache, decreased renal function.

DRUG INTERACTIONS
Antineoplastic agents (eg, nitrogen mustard) may enhance potential for renal toxicity, bronchospasm, hypotension; use with great caution. Corticosteroids and corticotropin may potentiate drug-induced hypokalemia; avoid use unless necessary to control side effects of the drug; if used concomitantly, closely monitor serum electrolytes and cardiac function. Drug-induced hypokalemia may potentiate digitalis toxicity with digitalis glycosides; closely monitor serum K+ levels and cardiac function, and promptly correct any deficit. May increase flucytosine toxicity. Imidazoles (eg, ketoconazole, miconazole, clotrimazole) may induce fungal resistance; use with caution, especially in immunocompromised patients. Nephrotoxic agents (eg, aminoglycosides, cyclosporine, pentamidine) may enhance the potential for drug-induced renal toxicity; use with great caution and intensively monitor renal function. Drug-induced hypokalemia may enhance curariform effect of skeletal muscle relaxants (eg, tubocurarine); monitor serum K+ levels and correct deficiencies. Acute pulmonary reactions/toxicity reported with leukocyte transfusions; separate infusions as far as possible and monitor pulmonary function.

PREGNANCY AND LACTATION
Category B, not for use in nursing.

MECHANISM OF ACTION
Polyene antifungal; fungistatic or fungicidal depending on concentration. Binds to sterols in the cell membrane of susceptible fungi with a resultant change in membrane permeability allowing leakage of intracellular components.

PHARMACOKINETICS
Absorption: C_{max}=0.5-2mcg/mL. **Distribution:** Plasma protein binding (>90%). **Elimination:** Urine (40%, 2-5% unchanged); $T_{1/2}$=15 days.

PATIENT CONSIDERATIONS
Assessment: Assess for type of fungal disease, previous hypersensitivity to the drug, reduced renal function, pregnancy/nursing status, and possible drug interactions.

Monitoring: Monitor clinical status, and for overdosage, acute reactions, nephrotoxicity, and other adverse reactions. Monitor temperature, pulse, respiration, and BP every 30 min for 2-4 hrs after test dose. Frequently monitor renal function. Regularly monitor LFTs, serum electrolytes (particularly Mg^{2+} and K+), blood counts, and Hgb concentrations.

Counseling: Inform of risks and benefits of therapy. Advise to seek medical attention if any adverse reactions occur.

AMPICILLIN INJECTION — ampicillin   Rx
Class: Semisynthetic penicillin (PCN) derivative

ADULT DOSAGE

Respiratory Tract/Soft Tissue Infections
<40kg:
25-50mg/kg/day in equally divided doses q6-8h
≥40kg:
250-500mg q6h

Gastrointestinal Infections
<40kg:
50mg/kg/day given in equally divided doses q6-8h
≥40kg:
500mg q6h

Use higher doses for stubborn or severe infections; stubborn infections may require therapy for several weeks

Genitourinary Tract Infections
Including *Neisseria gonorrhoeae* Infections in Females:
<40kg:
50mg/kg/day given in equally divided doses q6-8h
≥40kg:
500mg q6h

Use higher doses for stubborn or severe infections; stubborn infections may require therapy for several weeks

Urethral Infections
Urethritis in Males Caused by *N. gonorrhoeae*:
2 doses of 500mg at an interval of 8-12 hrs; may be repeated if necessary or extended if required

Prolonged and intensive therapy recommended for gonorrheal urethritis (eg, prostatitis, epididymitis)

Bacterial Meningitis
150-200mg/kg/day in equally divided doses q3-4h; may initiate w/ IV drip and continued w/ IM inj

Septicemia
150-200mg/kg/day; start w/ IV administration for at least 3 days and continue w/ IM route q3-4h

Treatment Duration
Continue for a minimum of 48-72 hrs beyond the time the patient becomes asymptomatic or evidence of bacterial eradication has been obtained

Group A β-Hemolytic Streptococci Infections:
Treatment recommended for a minimum of 10 days

PEDIATRIC DOSAGE

Bacterial Meningitis
150-200mg/kg/day in equally divided doses q3-4h; may initiate w/ IV drip and continued w/ IM inj

Septicemia
150-200mg/kg/day; start w/ IV administration for at least 3 days and continue w/ IM route q3-4h

Respiratory Tract/Soft Tissue Infections
<40kg:
25-50mg/kg/day in equally divided doses q6-8h
≥40kg:
250-500mg q6h

Gastrointestinal Infections
<40kg:
50mg/kg/day given in equally divided doses q6-8h
≥40kg:
500mg q6h

Use higher doses for stubborn or severe infections; stubborn infections may require therapy for several weeks

Genitourinary Tract Infections
Including *N. gonorrhoeae* Infections in Females:
<40kg:
50mg/kg/day given in equally divided doses q6-8h
≥40kg:
500mg q6h

Use higher doses for stubborn or severe infections; stubborn infections may require therapy for several weeks

Treatment Duration
Continue for a minimum of 48-72 hrs beyond the time the patient becomes asymptomatic or evidence of bacterial eradication has been obtained

Group A β-Hemolytic Streptococci Infections:
Treatment recommended for a minimum of 10 days

ADMINISTRATION
IM/IV routes

Administer w/in 1 hr after preparation.

IM
125mg/mL: Reconstitute 125mg vial w/ 1.2mL of sterile water for inj (SWFI) or bacteriostatic water for inj.
250mg/mL: Reconstitute 250mg, 500mg, 1g, or 2g vials w/ 1mL, 1.8mL, 3.5mL, or 6.8mL, respectively, w/ SWFI or bacteriostatic water for inj.

IV
Direct IV Use:
Dissolve 125mg, 250mg, or 500mg vial w/ 5mL of SWFI or bacteriostatic water for inj and administer slowly over 3-5 min.
Dissolve 1g or 2g vial w/ 7.4mL or 14.8mL of SWFI or bacteriostatic water for inj, respectively, and administer slowly over at least 10-15 min to avoid convulsive seizures.
IV Drip:
Reconstitute as directed above prior to diluting w/ compatible IV sol.

IV Diluents
SWFI, bacteriostatic water for inj, 0.9% NaCl inj, D5 inj, D5 and 0.45% NaCl inj, lactated Ringer's inj.

Refer to PI for additional administration and storage instructions.

STORAGE
20-25°C (68-77°F). Protect the constituted sol from freezing.

HOW SUPPLIED
Inj: 125mg, 250mg, 500mg, 1g, 2g. Also available as a Pharmacy Bulk Package. Refer to individual package insert for more information.

CONTRAINDICATIONS
History of a previous hypersensitivity reaction to any of the penicillins (PCNs).

WARNINGS/PRECAUTIONS
Reserve the parenteral form of this drug for moderately severe and severe infections and for patients unable to take the oral forms; a change to oral ampicillin may be made as soon as appropriate. Serious and occasionally fatal hypersensitivity (anaphylactoid) reactions w/ PCN therapy reported. Prior to therapy, assess for previous hypersensitivity reactions to PCNs, cephalosporins, and other allergens. D/C and institute appropriate therapy if an allergic reaction occurs. *Clostridium difficile*-associated diarrhea (CDAD) reported; d/c therapy if CDAD is suspected/confirmed. Avoid in infectious mononucleosis; skin rash reported. Use in the absence of a proven or strongly suspected bacterial infection or a prophylactic indication is unlikely to provide benefit and increases the risk of development of drug-resistant bacteria; d/c and substitute appropriate treatment if superinfection occurs. Lab test interactions may occur. More rapid administration may result in convulsive seizures.

ADVERSE REACTIONS
Skin rashes, urticaria, glossitis, N/V, diarrhea, black hairy tongue, stomatitis, enterocolitis, anemia, thrombocytopenia, eosinophilia, leukopenia, agranulocytosis.

DRUG INTERACTIONS
Increased incidence of skin rash w/ allopurinol.

PREGNANCY AND LACTATION
Pregnancy: Category B.
Lactation: Caution in nursing.

MECHANISM OF ACTION
PCN derivative; bactericidal against PCN-susceptible gram-positive organisms and many common gram-negative pathogens.

PHARMACOKINETICS
Distribution: Plasma protein binding (20%), found in breast milk. Penetrates to CSF and brain only when meninges are inflamed. **Elimination:** Urine (unchanged).

PATIENT CONSIDERATIONS

Assessment: Assess for hypersensitivity to PCNs/cephalosporins or other allergens, infectious mononucleosis, pregnancy/nursing status, and possible drug interactions. Conduct culture and susceptibility testing prior to therapy. In gonorrhea w/ a suspected primary lesion of syphilis, perform a dark-field exam before therapy.

Monitoring: Monitor for signs/symptoms of hypersensitivity reactions, CDAD, superinfection, skin rashes, and other adverse reactions. Perform periodic monitoring of organ system function, including renal, hepatic, and hematopoietic function w/ prolonged therapy. Where concomitant syphilis is suspected, perform serological tests monthly for at least 4 months.

Counseling: Inform that drug treats bacterial, not viral, infections. Instruct to take exactly ud; skipping dose or not completing full course of therapy may decrease effectiveness and increase the likelihood of bacterial resistance. Instruct to contact physician as soon as possible if watery and bloody stools (w/ or w/o stomach cramps, fever) develop even as late as 2 or more months after having taken the last dose of therapy.

AMPICILLIN ORAL — ampicillin trihydrate   Rx

Class: Semisynthetic penicillin (PCN) derivative

ADULT DOSAGE

Genitourinary Tract Infections
Usual: 500mg qid in equally spaced doses; severe or chronic infections may require larger doses

Prolonged intensive therapy is needed for complications (eg, prostatitis, epididymitis)

Gonorrhea
Usual: 3.5g single dose w/ 1g probenecid; use no less than the recommended dosage

Gastrointestinal Infections
Usual: 500mg qid in equally spaced doses; severe or chronic infections may require larger doses

Respiratory Tract Infections
Usual: 250mg qid in equally spaced doses; severe or chronic infections may require larger doses

Treatment Duration
Except for single dose regimen of gonorrhea, continue therapy for a minimum of 48-72 hrs after patient becomes asymptomatic or evidence of bacterial eradication has been obtained; stubborn infections may require treatment for several weeks

PEDIATRIC DOSAGE

Genitourinary Tract Infections
≤20kg:
100mg/kg/day total, qid in equally divided and spaced doses
>20kg:
500mg qid in equally spaced doses
Severe or chronic infections may require larger doses
Prolonged intensive therapy is needed for complications (eg, prostatitis, epididymitis)

Gastrointestinal Infections
≤20kg:
100mg/kg/day total, qid in equally divided and spaced doses
>20kg:
500mg qid in equally spaced doses
Severe or chronic infections may require larger doses

Gonorrhea
>20kg:
3.5g single dose w/ 1g probenecid; use no less than the recommended dosage

Respiratory Tract Infections
≤20kg:
Usual: 50mg/kg/day total, in equally divided and spaced doses tid-qid

Hemolytic Strains of Streptococci:
Treat for a minimum of 10 days

Other Indications
Meningitis

Max: Do not exceed adult doses
>20kg:
250mg qid in equally spaced doses
Severe or chronic infections may require larger doses

Treatment Duration
Except for single dose regimen of gonorrhea, continue therapy for a minimum of 48-72 hrs after patient becomes asymptomatic or evidence of bacterial eradication has been obtained; stubborn infections may require treatment for several weeks

Hemolytic Strains of Streptococci:
Treat for a minimum of 10 days

ADMINISTRATION
Oral route
Take at least 30 min ac or 2 hrs pc w/ a full glass of water.

Sus Preparation
125mg/5mL: Reconstitute 100mL and 200mL package sizes w/ 86mL and 170mL of water respectively.
250mg/5mL: Reconstitute 100mL and 200mL package sizes w/ 70mL and 139mL of water respectively.
Add water in 2 portions; shake well after each addition.

STORAGE
Cap/Dry Powder: 20-25°C (68-77°F). **Sus:** Store reconstituted sus in the refrigerator; discard unused portion after 14 days.

HOW SUPPLIED
Cap: 250mg, 500mg; **Sus:** 125mg/5mL, 250mg/5mL [100mL, 200mL]

CONTRAINDICATIONS
History of a previous hypersensitivity reaction to any of the penicillins, infections caused by penicillinase-producing organisms.

WARNINGS/PRECAUTIONS
Serious and fatal hypersensitivity reactions reported w/ PCN therapy; increased risk w/ history of sensitivity to multiple allergens. Anaphylactoid reactions require immediate treatment w/ appropriate management. Possible cross-sensitivity w/ cephalosporins. Pseudomembranous colitis reported; initiate therapeutic measures if diagnosed and consider discontinuation of treatment. May result in bacterial resistance w/ prolonged use or use in the absence of a proven or suspected bacterial infection or a prophylactic indication; take appropriate measures if superinfection develops. Give additional parenteral PCN in patients w/ gonorrhea who also have syphilis. Treatment does not preclude the need for surgical procedures, particularly in staphylococcal infections. Lab test interactions may occur.

ADVERSE REACTIONS
Glossitis, stomatitis, N/V, diarrhea, skin rash, pruritus, urticaria, erythema multiforme, agranulocytosis, anemia, eosinophilia, leukopenia, thrombocytopenia, thrombocytopenic purpura.

DRUG INTERACTIONS
Increased risk of rash w/ allopurinol. Bacteriostatic antibiotics (eg, chloramphenicol, erythromycins, sulfonamides, tetracyclines) may interfere w/ bactericidal activity. May increase breakthrough bleeding w/ oral contraceptives and decrease oral contraceptive effectiveness. Probenecid may increase levels and toxicity.

PREGNANCY AND LACTATION
Pregnancy: Category B.
Lactation: Not for use in nursing.

MECHANISM OF ACTION
PCN derivative; has bactericidal action during the stage of active multiplication by inhibiting cell wall biosynthesis, leading to the death of the bacteria.

PHARMACOKINETICS
Absorption: Well-absorbed; C_{max}=3mcg/mL (500mg Cap); C_{max}=2.3mcg/mL (250mg Sus). **Distribution:** Plasma protein binding (20%); found in breast milk. **Elimination:** Urine (unchanged).

PATIENT CONSIDERATIONS

Assessment: Assess for previous hypersensitivity reactions to PCNs, cephalosporins, or other allergens; history of allergy; pregnancy/nursing status; syphilis; and possible drug interactions. Perform appropriate culture and susceptibility tests.

Monitoring: Monitor for hypersensitivity reactions, pseudomembranous colitis, and overgrowth of nonsusceptible organisms. Evaluate renal/hepatic/hematopoietic systems periodically w/ prolonged therapy. Upon completion, obtain cultures to determine organism eradication. Monitor for masked syphilis; perform follow-up serologic test for each month for 4 months for syphilis in patients w/o suspected lesions of syphilis.

Counseling: Instruct to notify physician of history of hypersensitivity to PCNs, cephalosporins, or other allergens. Advise diabetics to consult w/ physician prior to changing diet or dosage of diabetic medication. Instruct to take exactly ud; explain that skipping doses or not completing full course decreases effectiveness and increases bacterial resistance. Instruct to d/c and notify physician if side effects occur. Inform that therapy only treats bacterial, and not viral, infections.

AMPYRA — dalfampridine   Rx

Class: Potassium channel blocker

ADULT DOSAGE	PEDIATRIC DOSAGE
Multiple Sclerosis	Pediatric use may not have been established
To Improve Walking:	
Max: 10mg bid (approx 12 hrs apart)	

ADMINISTRATION

Oral route

Take w/ or w/o food
Take tab whole; do not divide, crush, chew, or dissolve

STORAGE

25°C (77°F); excursions permitted to 15-30°C (59-86°F).

HOW SUPPLIED

Tab, Extended-Release: 10mg

CONTRAINDICATIONS

History of seizure, moderate or severe renal impairment (CrCl ≤50mL/min), history of hypersensitivity to this medication or 4-aminopyridine.

WARNINGS/PRECAUTIONS

May cause seizures; d/c and do not restart in patients who experience a seizure while on therapy. Caution with mild renal impairment (CrCl 51-80mL/min). Avoid with other forms of 4-aminopyridine; d/c use of any product containing 4-aminopyridine prior to initiating therapy. May cause anaphylaxis and severe allergic reactions; d/c if signs and symptoms occur. Urinary tract infections (UTIs) reported; evaluate and treat patients as clinically indicated.

ADVERSE REACTIONS

UTI, insomnia, dizziness, headache, nausea, asthenia, back pain, balance disorder, MS relapse, paresthesia, nasopharyngitis, constipation.

PREGNANCY AND LACTATION

Category C, not for use in nursing.

MECHANISM OF ACTION

Broad-spectrum K^+ channel blocker; has not been established. Has been shown to increase conduction of action potentials in demyelinated axons through inhibition of K^+ channels.

PHARMACOKINETICS

Absorption: Rapid and complete. C_{max}=17.3-21.6ng/mL (fasted), T_{max}=3-4 hrs (fasted). **Distribution:** Plasma protein binding (1-3%); V_d=2.6L/kg. **Metabolism:** Hydroxylation; CYP2E1 (major). **Elimination:** Urine (95.9%, 90.3% parent drug), feces (0.5%); $T_{1/2}$=5.2-6.5 hrs.

PATIENT CONSIDERATIONS

Assessment: Assess for hypersensitivity to the drug or 4-aminopyridine, history of seizures, and pregnancy/nursing status. Obtain baseline CrCl.

Monitoring: Monitor for seizures, anaphylaxis, severe allergic reactions, UTIs, and other adverse reactions. Monitor CrCl at least annually.

Counseling: Inform that therapy may cause seizures and to d/c treatment if seizure is experienced. Instruct to take exactly ud and not take a double dose if a dose is missed. Instruct not to take more than 2 tabs in a 24-hr period and to make sure that there is an approximate 12-hr interval between doses. Inform of the signs/symptoms of anaphylaxis; instruct to d/c therapy and seek medical care if anaphylaxis develops.

AMRIX — cyclobenzaprine hydrochloride   Rx

Class: Skeletal muscle relaxant (centrally acting)

ADULT DOSAGE	PEDIATRIC DOSAGE
Muscle Spasms	Pediatric use may not have been established
Relief of Muscle Spasm Associated w/ Acute, Painful Musculoskeletal Conditions:	
15mg qd; may require up to 30mg/day	
Use for periods longer than 2 or 3 weeks is not recommended	

DOSING CONSIDERATIONS

Hepatic Impairment
Mild, Moderate, or Severe: Not recommended

Elderly
Not recommended

ADMINISTRATION

Oral route

Take at approx the same time each day.
Swallow caps intact. Alternatively, the contents of the cap may be sprinkled over applesauce and then swallowed; appropriate only for patients able to reliably swallow the applesauce w/o chewing.
- Sprinkle contents of the cap onto a tbsp of applesauce and consume immediately w/o chewing.
- Rinse mouth to ensure all of the contents have been swallowed.
- Discard any unused portion of the cap after the contents have been sprinkled on applesauce.

STORAGE

25°C (77°F); excursions permitted to 15-30°C (59-86°F).

HOW SUPPLIED

Cap, Extended-Release: 15mg, 30mg

CONTRAINDICATIONS

Hypersensitivity to any component of this product, concomitant use of MAOIs or w/in 14 days after their discontinuation, arrhythmias, heart block or conduction disturbances, CHF, hyperthyroidism, during the acute recovery phase of MI.

WARNINGS/PRECAUTIONS

Not effective in the treatment of spasticity associated w/ cerebral or spinal cord disease or in children w/ cerebral palsy. May produce arrhythmias, sinus tachycardia, and conduction time prolongation leading to MI and stroke. Serious CNS reactions may occur; consider discontinuation if clinically significant CNS symptoms develop. Caution w/ history of urinary retention, angle-closure glaucoma, and increased IOP.

ADVERSE REACTIONS

Dry mouth, dizziness, fatigue, constipation, nausea, dyspepsia, somnolence.

DRUG INTERACTIONS

See Contraindications. Serotonin syndrome reported when used w/ SSRIs, SNRIs, TCAs, tramadol, bupropion, meperidine, verapamil, or MAOIs; d/c therapy and any concomitant serotonergic agents immediately if this occurs. Observe carefully, particularly during treatment initiation or dose increases, if concomitant use w/ other serotonergic drugs is warranted. May enhance effects of alcohol, barbiturates, and other CNS depressants. Caution w/ anticholinergic medication. May block the antihypertensive action of guanethidine and similarly acting compounds. May enhance seizure risk w/ tramadol.

PREGNANCY AND LACTATION

Pregnancy: Category B.
Lactation: It is not known whether this drug is excreted in human milk; caution in nursing.

MECHANISM OF ACTION

Skeletal muscle relaxant (central-acting); relieves skeletal muscle spasm of local origin w/o interfering w/ muscle function. Reduces tonic somatic motor activity, influencing both gamma and α motor systems.

PHARMACOKINETICS

Absorption: T_{max}=7-8 hrs. **Metabolism:** Extensive; N-demethylation via CYP3A4, 1A2, and, to a lesser extent, 2D6. **Elimination:** Kidney (glucuronides); $T_{1/2}$=32 hrs.

PATIENT CONSIDERATIONS

Assessment: Assess for arrhythmias; heart block or conduction disturbances; CHF; hyperthyroidism; acute recovery phase of MI; history of urinary retention, angle-closure glaucoma, or increased IOP; hepatic impairment; drug hypersensitivity; pregnancy/nursing status; and possible drug interactions.

Monitoring: Monitor for arrhythmias, sinus tachycardia, conduction time prolongation, CNS symptoms, and other adverse reactions.

Counseling: Instruct to take ud and at approx the same time each day. Advise to d/c use and notify physician immediately if experiencing symptoms of an allergic reaction (eg, difficulty breathing, hives, swelling of face/tongue, itching), arrhythmias, or tachycardia. Caution about the risk of serotonin syndrome; instruct to seek medical care immediately if signs/symptoms occur. Inform that drug may enhance impairment effects of alcohol and other CNS depressants. Caution about operating an automobile or other hazardous machinery until accustomed to effects of medication.

AMTURNIDE — aliskiren/amlodipine/hydrochlorothiazide   Rx

Class: Calcium channel blocker (CCB) (dihydropyridine)/renin inhibitor/thiazide diuretic

> D/C when pregnancy is detected. Drugs that act directly on the renin-angiotensin system can cause injury/death to the developing fetus.

ADULT DOSAGE	PEDIATRIC DOSAGE
Hypertension	Pediatric use may not have been established
Dose qd; may increase dose after 2 weeks of therapy	
Max: 300mg/10mg/25mg	
Add-On/Switch Therapy:	
Use if not adequately controlled w/ any 2 of the following: aliskiren, dihydropyridine calcium channel blockers, and thiazide diuretics. W/ dose-limiting adverse reactions to any component on dual therapy, switch to triple therapy at a lower dose of that component.	
Replacement Therapy:	
Switch from separate tabs to Amturnide containing the same component doses	

DOSING CONSIDERATIONS

Renal Impairment
Consider lower doses; safety and effectiveness in patients w/ severe renal impairment (CrCl <30mL/min) have not been established

Hepatic Impairment
Consider lower doses

Elderly
Consider starting w/ the lowest available dose of amlodipine; the lowest strength of Amturnide contains 5mg of amlodipine

ADMINISTRATION
Oral route

Establish a routine pattern for taking the drug, either w/ or w/o a meal; high-fat meals decrease absorption of aliskiren substantially.

STORAGE
25°C (77°F); excursions permitted to 15-30°C (59-86°F). Protect from heat and moisture.

HOW SUPPLIED
Tab: (Aliskiren/Amlodipine/Hydrochlorothiazide [HCTZ]) 150mg/5mg/12.5mg, 300mg/5mg/12.5mg, 300mg/5mg/25mg, 300mg/10mg/12.5mg, 300mg/10mg/25mg

CONTRAINDICATIONS
Anuria, known hypersensitivity to sulfonamide-derived drugs (eg, hydrochlorothiazide) or to any of the components. Concomitant use w/ ARBs or ACE inhibitors in patients w/ diabetes.

WARNINGS/PRECAUTIONS
Not indicated for initial therapy of HTN. Symptomatic hypotension may occur in patients w/ marked volume depletion or w/ salt depletion; correct volume/ salt depletion prior to administration, or start treatment under close medical supervision. May cause changes in renal function, including acute renal failure; caution in patients whose renal function may depend in part on the activity of the renin-angiotensin-aldosterone system (RAAS) (eg, renal artery stenosis, severe heart failure [HF], post-MI, volume depletion). Consider withholding or discontinuing therapy if clinically significant decrease in renal function develops. May cause serum electrolyte abnormalities (eg, hyper/hypokalemia, hyponatremia, hypomagnesemia); correct hypokalemia and any coexisting hypomagnesemia prior to initiation. D/C if hypokalemia is accompanied by clinical signs (eg, muscular weakness, paresis, ECG alterations). **Aliskiren:** Hypersensitivity reactions and head/neck angioedema reported; d/c therapy immediately and do not readminister if anaphylactic reactions or angioedema develops. **Amlodipine:** May cause symptomatic hypotension, particularly in patients w/ severe aortic stenosis. May develop worsening of angina and acute MI after starting or increasing the dose, particularly w/ severe obstructive coronary artery disease (CAD). **HCTZ:** May cause hypersensitivity reactions and exacerbation of systemic lupus erythematosus (SLE). Minor alterations of fluid and electrolyte balance may precipitate hepatic coma in patients w/ hepatic impairment or progressive liver disease. May cause idiosyncratic reaction, resulting in transient myopia and acute angle-closure glaucoma; d/c as rapidly as possible. May alter glucose tolerance, increase serum cholesterol/TG levels, and increase serum Ca^{2+}. May cause or exacerbate hyperuricemia and precipitate gout in susceptible patients.

ADVERSE REACTIONS
Peripheral edema, dizziness, headache.

DRUG INTERACTIONS
See Contraindications. **Aliskiren:** Cyclosporine or itraconazole may increase levels; avoid concomitant use w/ such drugs. NSAIDs, including selective COX-2 inhibitors, may deteriorate renal function and attenuate antihypertensive effect. Dual blockade of the RAAS is associated w/ increased risk of hypotension, hyperkalemia, and changes in renal function (including acute renal failure); in general, avoid combined use w/ ACE inhibitors or ARBs, particularly in patients w/ CrCl <60mL/min. Oral coadministration w/ furosemide reduced exposure to furosemide; monitor diuretic effects when coadministered. Risk of developing hyperkalemia w/ NSAIDs, K$^+$ supplements, or K$^+$-sparing diuretics. **Amlodipine:** May increase simvastatin exposure; limit simvastatin dose to 20mg/ day. Increased systemic exposure w/ CYP3A inhibitors (moderate and strong) warranting dose reduction; monitor for symptoms of hypotension and edema w/ CYP3A4 inhibitors to determine the need for dose adjustment. Monitor BP when coadministered w/ CYP3A4 inducers. **HCTZ:** Dosage adjustment of antidiabetic drugs (insulin or oral agents) may be required. Space dosing ≥4 hrs before or 4-6 hrs after the administration of ion-exchange resins (eg, cholestyramine, colestipol). May increase risk of lithium toxicity; monitor serum lithium levels.

PREGNANCY AND LACTATION
Pregnancy: Category D.
Lactation: Thiazides are excreted in breast milk; not for use in nursing.

MECHANISM OF ACTION
Aliskiren: Direct renin inhibitor; decreases plasma renin activity and inhibits conversion of angiotensinogen to angiotensin I. **Amlodipine:** Dihydropyridine calcium channel blocker; inhibits the transmembrane influx of Ca^{2+} ions into vascular smooth muscle and cardiac muscle, causing a reduction in peripheral vascular resistance and BP. **HCTZ:** Thiazide diuretic; has not been established. Affects renal tubular mechanisms of electrolyte reabsorption, directly increasing excretion of Na$^+$ and Cl$^-$ in approx equivalent amounts.

PHARMACOKINETICS
Absorption: Aliskiren: Poor; T_{max}=1-2 hrs; bioavailability (2.5%). Amlodipine: Absolute bioavailability (64-90%); T_{max}=6-12 hrs. HCTZ: Absolute bioavailability (70%); T_{max}=1-4 hrs. **Distribution:** Amlodipine: Plasma protein binding (approx 93%); V_d=21L/kg. HCTZ: Albumin binding (40-70%). Crosses the placenta; found in breast milk. **Metabolism:** Aliskiren: via CYP3A4. Amlodipine: Hepatic; extensive. **Elimination:** Aliskiren: Urine (25% parent drug). Amlodipine: Urine (10% parent compound, 60% metabolites), $T_{1/2}$=30-50 hrs. HCTZ: Urine (70% unchanged), $T_{1/2}$=10 hrs.

PATIENT CONSIDERATIONS
Assessment: Assess for diabetes, sulfonamide-derived drug hypersensitivity, hepatic/renal impairment, anuria, CAD, renal artery stenosis, HF, post-MI status, history of penicillin allergy, volume/salt depletion, SLE, severe aortic stenosis, bronchial asthma, pregnancy/nursing status, and possible drug interactions. Correct electrolyte imbalances prior to initiation of therapy.

Monitoring: Monitor for hypersensitivity/anaphylactic reactions, head/neck angioedema, airway obstruction, worsening of angina and MI, exacerbation of SLE, idiosyncratic reaction, transient myopia, acute angle-closure glaucoma, and other adverse reactions. Monitor BP, hepatic/renal function, serum uric acid, serum electrolytes, and glucose/cholesterol/TG levels.

Counseling: Advise female patients of childbearing age about consequences of exposure during pregnancy and discuss the treatment options w/ women planning to become pregnant. Advise to report pregnancy to physician as soon as possible. Caution that lightheadedness may occur, especially during the 1st days of therapy; instruct to contact physician if lightheadedness occurs. Advise to d/c treatment and to consult physician if syncope occurs. Caution that inadequate fluid intake, excessive perspiration, diarrhea, or vomiting can lead to excessive fall in BP. Advise to d/c and immediately report any signs/symptoms of severe allergic reaction or angioedema. Inform that angioedema, including laryngeal edema, may occur anytime during treatment. Instruct not to use K$^+$ supplements or salt substitutes containing K$^+$ w/o consulting physician.

ANAGRELIDE — anagrelide   **Rx**
Class: Platelet-reducing agent

OTHER BRAND NAMES
Agrylin

ADULT DOSAGE	PEDIATRIC DOSAGE
Thrombocythemia	**Thrombocythemia**
Treatment of thrombocythemia secondary to myeloproliferative neoplasms, to reduce the elevated platelet count and risk of thrombosis and to ameliorate associated symptoms including thrombo-hemorrhagic events	Treatment of thrombocythemia secondary to myeloproliferative neoplasms, to reduce the elevated platelet count and risk of thrombosis and to ameliorate associated symptoms including thrombo-hemorrhagic events
Initial: 0.5mg qid or 1mg bid for at least 1 week	**Initial:** 0.5mg qd for at least 1 week
Titrate: Adjust to reduce and maintain platelet count to <600,000/µL, and ideally between 150,000-400,000/µL; dose increment should not exceed 0.5mg/day in any 1 week	**Titrate:** Adjust to reduce and maintain platelet count to <600,000/µL, and ideally between 150,000-400,000/µL; dose increment should not exceed 0.5mg/day in any 1 week
Max: 10mg/day or 2.5mg/dose	**Max:** 10mg/day or 2.5mg/dose
Most patients will experience an adequate response at a dose of 1.5-3mg/day	Most patients will experience an adequate response at a dose of 1.5-3mg/day

- -

DOSING CONSIDERATIONS
Hepatic Impairment
Moderate (Child-Pugh Score 7-9):
Initial: 0.5mg/day
Titrate: May increase dose in patients who have tolerated initial dose for 1 week; increase by not more than 0.5mg/day in any 1 week
Severe: Avoid use

ADMINISTRATION
Oral route

STORAGE
20-25°C (68-77°F). (Agrylin) 25°C (77°F); excursions permitted to 15-30°C (59-86°F).

HOW SUPPLIED
Cap: 1mg; (Agrylin) 0.5mg

WARNINGS/PRECAUTIONS
Torsades de pointes and ventricular tachycardia reported. Increases QTc interval and HR; do not use in patients w/ known risk factors for QT interval prolongation (eg, congenital long QT syndrome, history of acquired QTc prolongation, hypokalemia). Hepatic impairment increases exposure and could increase the risk of QTc prolongation; monitor patients w/ hepatic impairment for QTc prolongation and other cardiovascular (CV) adverse reactions. Consider periodic monitoring w/ ECGs in patients w/ heart failure (HF), bradyarrhythmias, or electrolyte abnormalities. May cause vasodilation, tachycardia, palpitations, and CHF; use only when benefits outweigh the risks in patients w/ cardiac disease. Interstitial lung diseases (eg, allergic alveolitis, eosinophilic pneumonia, interstitial pneumonitis) reported; if suspected, d/c therapy and evaluate.

ADVERSE REACTIONS
Headache, palpitations, diarrhea, asthenia, edema, N/V, abdominal pain, dizziness, pain, dyspnea, flatulence, fever, peripheral edema, rash.

DRUG INTERACTIONS
Do not use w/ medications that may prolong QTc interval (eg, chloroquine, clarithromycin, haloperidol). Concomitant use w/ aspirin (ASA) increased major hemorrhagic events; assess potential risks and benefits for concomitant use, and monitor patients for bleeding, particularly those receiving concomitant therapy w/ other drugs known to cause bleeding (eg, anticoagulants, PDE3 inhibitors, NSAIDs, antiplatelet agents, SSRIs). Avoid use w/ drug products w/ similar properties such

as inotropes and other PDE3 inhibitors (eg, cilostazol, milrinone). CYP1A2 inhibitors (eg, fluvoxamine, ciprofloxacin) may increase exposure; monitor for CV events and titrate doses accordingly when CYP1A2 inhibitors are coadministered. CYP1A2 inducers (eg, omeprazole) may decrease exposure; may need to titrate dose of therapy in patients taking concomitant CYP1A2 inducers. May alter exposure of CYP1A2 substrates (eg, theophylline, fluvoxamine, ondansetron).

PREGNANCY AND LACTATION
Pregnancy: Category C.
Lactation: Not for use in nursing.

MECHANISM OF ACTION
Platelet-reducing agent; has not been established. Suppresses expression of transcription factors including GATA-1 and FOG-1 required for megakaryocytopoiesis, ultimately leading to reduced platelet production.

PHARMACOKINETICS
Absorption: T_{max}=1 hr. **Metabolism:** Via CYP1A2; 3-hydroxy anagrelide (active metabolite). **Elimination:** Urine (<1%, unchanged; 3%, 3-hydroxy anagrelide); $T_{1/2}$=1.5 hrs, 2.5 hrs (3-hydroxy anagrelide).

PATIENT CONSIDERATIONS
Assessment: Assess for risk factors for QT interval prolongation, pregnancy/nursing status, and possible drug interactions. Assess hepatic/renal function and electrolytes. Perform CV exam, including ECG.

Monitoring: Monitor for CV effects, interstitial lung diseases, and other adverse reactions. Consider periodic monitoring w/ ECGs in patients w/ HF, bradyarrhythmias, or electrolyte abnormalities. Monitor for bleeding w/ ASA or other drugs known to cause bleeding. Monitor hepatic/renal function and electrolytes. Monitor CBCs; monitor platelet counts every 2 days during the 1st week of treatment and at least weekly thereafter until the maintenance dosage is reached, then monthly or as necessary.

Counseling: Inform patients that their dose will be adjusted on a weekly basis until they are on a dose that lowers their platelets to an appropriate level; advise to contact physician if tolerability issues develop. Instruct to contact physician immediately if chest pain, palpitations, or irregular heartbeat occurs. Inform of the risk of bleeding w/ concomitant ASA or other medications that affect blood clotting; advise to contact physician immediately if patient experiences signs/symptoms of bleeding or unexplained bruising/bruise more easily than usual.

ANAVIP — crotalidae immune F(ab')2 (equine)   Rx
Class: Venom specific immunoglobulin F(ab')$_2$ fragment

ADULT DOSAGE	PEDIATRIC DOSAGE
North American Rattlesnake Envenomation	**North American Rattlesnake Envenomation**
Administer as soon as possible after rattlesnake bite	Administer as soon as possible after rattlesnake bite
Initial: 10 vials IV over 60 min	**Initial:** 10 vials IV over 60 min
For the first 10 min infuse at 25-50mL/hr, carefully monitoring for any allergic reaction. If no reaction occurs, may increase infusion rate to the full 250mL/hr rate until completion.	For the first 10 min infuse at 25-50mL/hr, carefully monitoring for any allergic reactions. If no reaction occurs, may increase infusion rate to the full 250mL/hr rate until completion.
Monitor for at least 60 min following completion of infusion for any allergic reaction and to determine that local signs of envenomation are not progressing (leading edge of local injury not progressing), systemic symptoms are resolved, and coagulation parameters have normalized or are trending toward normal	Monitor for at least 60 min following completion of infusion for any allergic reaction and to determine that local signs of envenomation are not progressing (leading edge of local injury not progressing), systemic symptoms are resolved, and coagulation parameters have normalized or are trending toward normal
Additional Dosing to Achieve Initial Control:	**Additional Dosing to Achieve Initial Control:**
Administer additional 10-vial doses if needed to arrest the progressive symptoms, and repeat every hr Repeat above steps for initial dose as many times prn until local signs of envenomation are not progressing, systemic symptoms are resolved, and coagulation parameters have normalized or are trending toward normal.	Administer additional 10-vial doses if needed to arrest the progressive symptoms, and repeat every hr Repeat above steps for initial dose as many times prn until local signs of envenomation are not progressing, systemic symptoms are resolved, and coagulation parameters have normalized or are trending toward normal.
Once initial control has been achieved, observe patient to determine any need for further dosing, as described below	Once initial control has been achieved, observe patient to determine any need for further dosing, as described below
Observation and Late Dosing:	**Observation and Late Dosing:**
Monitor patients in a healthcare setting at least 18 hrs following initial control of signs/symptoms Reemerging symptoms including coagulopathies may be suppressed w/ additional 4-vial doses prn	Monitor patients in a healthcare setting at least 18 hrs following initial control of signs/symptoms Reemerging symptoms including coagulopathies may be suppressed w/ additional 4-vial doses prn

DOSING CONSIDERATIONS
Adverse Reactions
D/C infusion if any allergic reaction occurs during the first 10 min of the initial infusion, or at any time while infusing at the full 250mL/hr infusion rate; reassess the risk to benefit before continuing therapy

ADMINISTRATION
IV route
Reconstitution
Reconstitute contents of each vial w/ 10mL of sterile normal saline; reconstitution time should be <1 min when using continuous gentle swirling
Combine contents of reconstituted vials promptly and further dilute to a total volume of 250mL w/ sterile normal saline
Fluid volumes may need to be adjusted for very small children or infants

STORAGE
≤25°C (77°F); brief excursions permitted up to 40°C (104°F). Do not freeze.

HOW SUPPLIED
Inj: 120mg/vial

WARNINGS/PRECAUTIONS
May cause allergic reactions; patients w/ known allergies to horse protein are particularly at risk for an anaphylactic reaction. Monitor patients w/ follow-up visits for signs/symptoms of delayed allergic reactions or serum sickness and treat appropriately if necessary. Made from equine plasma; may carry a risk of transmitting infectious agents (eg, viruses). Contains trace amounts of cresol; localized reactions and generalized myalgias reported w/ use of cresol as an injectable excipient.

ADVERSE REACTIONS
Pruritus, rash, blister, erythema, N/V, arthralgia, myalgia, pain in extremity, peripheral edema, chills, pyrexia, headache.

PREGNANCY AND LACTATION
Category C, caution in nursing.

MECHANISM OF ACTION
Venom-specific immunoglobulin F(ab')$_2$ fragment; binds and neutralizes venom toxins, facilitating redistribution away from target tissues and elimination from the body.

PHARMACOKINETICS
Absorption: AUC=4144µg•hr/mL. **Distribution:** V_d=3.3L. **Elimination:** $T_{1/2}$=133 hrs.

PATIENT CONSIDERATIONS
Assessment: Assess for known allergies to horse protein, and pregnancy/nursing status. Perform lab analyses, including CBC, platelet count, PT, PTT, serum fibrinogen level, and routine serum chemistries.

Monitoring: Monitor for hypersensitivity/allergic reactions, delayed allergic reactions or serum sickness, infection, localized reactions, generalized myalgias, and other adverse reactions. Monitor patients in a healthcare setting at least 18 hrs following initial control of signs/symptoms. Repeat lab analyses, including CBC, platelet count, PT, PTT, serum fibrinogen level, and routine serum chemistries at regular intervals to gauge response to therapy and anticipate additional dosing.

Counseling: Advise to contact physician immediately if unusual bruising or bleeding (eg, nosebleeds, excessive bleeding after brushing teeth, appearance of blood in stools/urine) or any signs/symptoms of delayed allergic reactions or serum sickness (eg, rash, fever, myalgias, urticaria) after hospital discharge occur.

ANCOBON — flucytosine   Rx
Class: 5-fluorocytosine antifungal

> Extreme caution in patients with renal impairment. Monitor hematologic, renal, and hepatic status closely.

ADULT DOSAGE	PEDIATRIC DOSAGE
General Dosing	Pediatric use may not have been established
Serious infections caused by susceptible strains of *Candida* (eg, septicemia, endocarditis, urinary system infections) and/or *Cryptococcus* (eg, meningitis, pulmonary infections)	
Usual: 50-150mg/kg/day in divided doses at 6-hr intervals in combination w/ amphotericin B	

DOSING CONSIDERATIONS
Renal Impairment
Initial: Give at a lower level

ADMINISTRATION
Oral route
Give a few caps at a time over a 15-min period to reduce or avoid N/V

STORAGE
25°C (77°F); excursions permitted to 15-30°C (59-86°F).

HOW SUPPLIED
Cap: 250mg, 500mg

CONTRAINDICATIONS
Known hypersensitivity to flucytosine.

WARNINGS/PRECAUTIONS
Extreme caution with bone marrow depression. Patients with hematologic disease, patients being treated with radiation or drugs that depress bone marrow, or patients who have a history of treatment with such drugs or radiation may be more prone to bone marrow depression. Bone marrow toxicity can be irreversible and may lead to death in immunosuppressed patients.

ADVERSE REACTIONS
Myocardial toxicity, chest pain, dyspnea, rash, pruritus, urticaria, nausea, jaundice, renal failure, azotemia, crystalluria, anemia, leukopenia, ataxia, confusion.

DRUG INTERACTIONS
Cytosine arabinoside reported to inactivate antifungal activity by competitive inhibition. Drugs that impair glomerular filtration may prolong the biological $T_{1/2}$.

PREGNANCY AND LACTATION
Category C, not for use in nursing.

MECHANISM OF ACTION
5-fluorocytosine antifungal; exerts antifungal activity through the subsequent conversion into several active metabolites, which inhibit protein synthesis by being falsely incorporated into fungal RNA or interfere with biosynthesis of fungal DNA through inhibition of enzyme thymidylate synthetase.

PHARMACOKINETICS
Absorption: Rapid and complete. Absolute bioavailability (78-89%); (2g, Healthy) C_{max}=30-40mcg/mL, T_{max}=2 hrs. **Distribution:** Plasma protein binding (2.9-4%). **Metabolism:** Deamination (by gut bacteria) to 5-fluorouracil; α-fluoro-β-ureido-propionic acid (metabolite). **Elimination:** Urine (>90% unchanged, 1% metabolite), feces; $T_{1/2}$=2.4-4.8 hrs (healthy), 85 hrs (nephrectomized/anuric).

PATIENT CONSIDERATIONS
Assessment: Assess for hypersensitivity to the drug, renal impairment, bone marrow depression, immunosuppressed patients, pregnancy/nursing status, and possible drug interactions. Determine serum electrolytes and hematologic status prior to treatment.

Monitoring: Monitor for adverse reactions. Monitor renal function and blood concentrations. Monitor hematologic status (leukocyte and thrombocyte count) and hepatic function frequently.

Counseling: Inform of the risks and benefits of therapy. Advise to take a few caps at a time over a 15-min period to reduce or avoid N/V.

ANDRODERM — testosterone   CIII
Class: Androgen

ADULT DOSAGE	PEDIATRIC DOSAGE
Testosterone Replacement Therapy	Pediatric use may not have been established
Congenital/Acquired Primary Hypogonadism or Hypogonadotropic Hypogonadism in Males:	
Initial: One 4mg/day system applied nightly for 24 hrs	
Titrate: Measure early am serum testosterone concentrations, approx 2 weeks after starting therapy	
If outside the range of 400-930ng/dL, increase daily dose to 6mg (one 4mg/day and one 2mg/day system) or decrease daily dose to 2mg (one 2mg/day system), maintaining nightly application	
Patients currently maintained on 2.5mg/day, 5mg/day, and 7.5mg/day systems may be switched to 2mg/day, 4mg/day, or 6mg/day (2mg/day and 4mg/day) systems respectively, at the next scheduled dose	
Measure early am serum testosterone concentration approx 2 weeks after switching to ensure proper dosing	

ADMINISTRATION
Transdermal route

Apply adhesive side of the system to a clean, dry area of the skin on the back, abdomen, upper arms, or thighs
Avoid swimming, showering, or washing the administration site for a minimum of 3 hrs after application
Rotate application site w/ an interval of 7 days between applications to the same site
Refer to PI for further application instructions

STORAGE
20-25° (68-77°F). Do not store outside the pouch provided. Drug reservoir may be burst by excessive pressure or heat.

HOW SUPPLIED
Patch: 2mg/day [60ˢ], 4mg/day [30ˢ]

CONTRAINDICATIONS
Men w/ breast carcinoma or known/suspected prostate carcinoma; women who are or may become pregnant, or who are breastfeeding.

WARNINGS/PRECAUTIONS
Monitor patients w/ BPH for worsening of signs/symptoms of BPH. May increase risk for prostate cancer. Increases in Hct/RBC mass may increase risk for thromboembolic events; d/c therapy if Hct becomes elevated; may restart therapy when Hct decreases to acceptable level. Venous thromboembolic events (eg, deep vein thrombosis, pulmonary embolism) reported; d/c treatment and initiate appropriate workup and management if suspected. Increased risk of major adverse cardiovascular events (MACE) (eg, non-fatal stroke, non-fatal, MI reported. Suppression of spermatogenesis may occur at large doses. Edema w/ or w/o CHF may be a complication in patients w/ preexisting cardiac/renal/hepatic disease. Gynecomastia may develop and persist. May potentiate sleep apnea. Changes in serum lipid profile may require dose adjustment or discontinuation of therapy. Caution in cancer patients at risk of hypercalcemia (and associated hypercalciuria); monitor serum Ca^{2+} concentrations regularly. May decrease concentrations of thyroxine-binding globulins, resulting in decreased total T4 serum concentrations and increased resin uptake of T3 and T4. Skin burns reported at application site in patients wearing an aluminized transdermal system during a magnetic resonance imaging scan (MRI); remove the system before patient undergoes an MRI.

ADVERSE REACTIONS
Application-site reactions (eg, pruritus, blistering, erythema, vesicles, burning, induration), back pain, prostate abnormalities, headache, contact dermatitis, depression.

DRUG INTERACTIONS
Changes in insulin sensitivity or glycemic control may occur; may decrease blood glucose and therefore, decrease insulin requirements in diabetic patients. Changes in anticoagulant activity may occur; monitor INR and PT more frequently in patients taking anticoagulants, especially at initiation and termination of androgen therapy. Concurrent use w/ adrenocorticotropic hormone or corticosteroids may increase fluid retention; caution in patients w/ cardiac/renal/hepatic disease. Pretreatment w/ triamcinolone oint formulation reported to significantly reduce testosterone absorption.

PREGNANCY AND LACTATION
Category X, not for use in nursing.

MECHANISM OF ACTION
Androgen; responsible for normal growth and development of male sex organs and for maintenance of secondary sex characteristics.

PHARMACOKINETICS
Absorption: T_{max}=8 hrs (median). **Distribution:** Sex hormone-binding globulin binding (40%), albumin and plasma protein binding (58%). **Metabolism:** Estradiol and dihydrotestosterone (major active metabolites). **Elimination:** (IM) Urine (90% glucuronic and sulfuric acid conjugates), feces (6% unconjugated); $T_{1/2}$=10-100 min, $T_{1/2}$=70 min (upon removal).

PATIENT CONSIDERATIONS
Assessment: Assess for breast/prostate cancer, BPH, cardiac/renal/hepatic disease, risk factors for sleep apnea, cancer patients at risk for hypercalcemia, upcoming MRI exam, any other conditions where treatment is contraindicated or cautioned, and possible drug interactions. Obtain baseline Hct, and lipid levels. Confirm diagnosis of hypogonadism by measuring testosterone levels in am on at least 2 separate days prior to initiating therapy.

Monitoring: Monitor for signs/symptoms of edema w/ or w/o CHF, MACE, venous thromboembolic events, gynecomastia, sleep apnea, worsening of BPH and other adverse reactions. Monitor Hct, prostate-specific antigen, serum lipid profile, liver function, and serum testosterone levels periodically. In cancer patients at risk for hypercalcemia, regularly monitor serum Ca^{2+} levels. Reevaluate for prostate cancer 3-6 months after initiation of therapy, and then in accordance w/ prostate cancer screening practices. Reevaluate Hct 3-6 months after start of therapy, then annually. Monitor PT/INR more frequently w/ concomitant anticoagulants.

Counseling: Inform that men w/ known or suspected prostate/breast cancer should not use androgen therapy. Inform about potential adverse reactions. Instruct to apply ud. Advise not to apply to the scrotum, over a bony prominence, or any part of the body that could be subject to prolonged pressure during sleep or sitting. Advise that patch does not need to be removed during sexual intercourse, nor while taking a shower or bath. Inform that strenuous exercise or excessive perspiration may loosen a patch or cause it to fall off; if patch falls off, advise not to tape to skin. Advise to avoid swimming or showering until 3 hrs following application. Instruct to use OTC topical hydrocortisone cream after system removal in order to ameliorate mild skin irritation. Advise to remove the patch before undergoing MRI. Instruct not to cut the patches.

ANDROGEL — testosterone   CIII
Class: Androgen

> Virilization reported in children secondarily exposed to testosterone gel. Children should avoid contact w/ unwashed or unclothed application sites in men using testosterone gel. Advise to strictly adhere to recommended instructions for use.

ADULT DOSAGE	PEDIATRIC DOSAGE
Testosterone Replacement Therapy	Pediatric use may not have been established
Congenital/Acquired Primary Hypogonadism or Hypogonadotropic Hypogonadism in Males:	
1%:	
Initial: Apply 50mg (4 pump actuations, two 25mg pkts, or one 50mg pkt) qd in am (preferably at the same time every day)	

Titrate: May increase to 75mg qd and then to 100mg qd if serum testosterone is below normal range
May decrease daily dose if serum testosterone exceeds normal range
D/C therapy if serum testosterone consistently exceeds the normal range at a daily dose of 50mg
Refer to PI for specific dosing guidelines using the multidose pump

1.62%:
Initial: Apply 40.5mg (2 pump actuations or a single 40.5mg pkt) qd in am
Titrate: May adjust dose between a minimum of 20.25mg (1 pump actuation or a single 20.25mg pkt) and a max of 81mg (4 pump actuations or two 40.5mg pkts)
Titrate based on the predose am serum testosterone concentration from a single blood draw at approx 14 days and 28 days after starting treatment or following dose adjustment
Titration Based on Predose AM Serum Testosterone:
Serum Testosterone >750ng/dL:
Decrease daily dose by 20.25mg (1 pump actuation or a single 20.25mg pkt)
Serum Testosterone 350-750ng/dL:
Continue current dose
Serum Testosterone <350ng/dL:
Increase daily dose by 20.25mg (1 pump actuation or a single 20.25mg pkt)

ADMINISTRATION
Topical route

Apply to clean, dry, healthy, intact skin
Refer to PI for additional administration and priming instructions

1%
Apply to right and left upper arms/shoulders and/or right and left abdomen; do not apply to any other parts of the body (eg, genitals, chest)
Avoid swimming or showering for at least 5 hrs after application

1.62%
Apply to upper arms and shoulders; do not apply to any other parts of the body (eg, abdomen, genitals)
Avoid swimming, showering, or washing the administration site for a minimum of 2 hrs after application

STORAGE
(1%) 25°C (77°F); excursions permitted to 15-30°C (59-86°F). (1.62%) 20-25°C (68-77°F); excursions permitted to 15-30°C (59-86°F).

HOW SUPPLIED
Gel: 1% [2.5g pkt, 5g pkt (30ˢ); 75g pump (60 pumps)], 1.62% [1.25g pkt, 2.5g pkt (30ˢ); 88g pump (60 pumps)]

CONTRAINDICATIONS
Breast carcinoma or known/suspected prostate carcinoma in men; women who are or may become pregnant, or are breastfeeding.

WARNINGS/PRECAUTIONS
Topical testosterone products may have different doses, strengths, or application instructions that may result in different systemic exposure. Application site and dose are not interchangeable w/ other topical testosterone products. Patients w/ BPH treated w/ androgens, may be at increased risk for worsening of signs/ symptoms of BPH. May increase risk for prostate cancer. Increases in Hct, reflective of increases in RBC mass, may require lowering or discontinuation of therapy; increase in RBC mass may increase risk for thromboembolic events. Venous thromboembolic events reported; d/c and initiate appropriate workup and management if a venous thromboembolic event is suspected. Suppression of spermatogenesis may occur w/ large doses. Edema w/ or w/o CHF may be a serious complication in patients w/ preexisting cardiac, renal, or hepatic disease. Gynecomastia may develop and persist. May potentiate sleep apnea. Changes in serum lipid profile may require dose adjustment or discontinuation of therapy. Caution in cancer patients at risk of hypercalcemia and associated hypercalciuria. May decrease levels of thyroxin-binding globulins, resulting in decreased total T4 serum concentrations and increased resin uptake of T3 and T4. Flammable; avoid fire, flame, or smoking until the gel has dried.

ADVERSE REACTIONS
(1.62%) Prostate specific antigen (PSA) increase. (1%) Acne, application-site reactions, prostatic/urinary/testicular disorders, abnormal lab tests, headache, emotional lability, gynecomastia, HTN, nervousness, asthenia, decreased libido.

DRUG INTERACTIONS
Changes in insulin sensitivity or glycemic control may occur; may decrease blood glucose and, therefore, may decrease insulin requirements in diabetic patients. Changes in anticoagulant activity may occur; frequently monitor INR and PT in patients taking anticoagulants, especially at initiation and termination of androgen therapy. Adrenocorticotropic hormone or corticosteroids may increase fluid retention; caution in patients w/ cardiac, renal, or hepatic disease.

PREGNANCY AND LACTATION
Category X, not for use in nursing.

MECHANISM OF ACTION
Androgen; responsible for normal growth and development of male sex organs and for maintenance of secondary sex characteristics.

PHARMACOKINETICS
Distribution: Sex hormone-binding globulin binding (40%), albumin and other plasma protein binding (58%), unbound (2%). **Metabolism:** Estradiol and dihydrotestosterone (major active metabolites). **Elimination:** $T_{1/2}$=10-100 min; (IM) Urine (90% glucuronic and sulfuric acid conjugates), feces (6% unconjugated).

PATIENT CONSIDERATIONS
Assessment: Assess for BPH, breast/prostate cancer, cardiac/renal/hepatic disease, risk factors for sleep apnea, cancer patients at risk for hypercalcemia, any conditions where treatment is contraindicated or cautioned, and possible drug interactions. Obtain baseline Hct and serum testosterone levels.

Monitoring: Monitor for prostate cancer, edema w/ or w/o CHF, venous thromboembolic events, gynecomastia, sleep apnea, worsening of signs/ symptoms of BPH, and other adverse reactions. Perform periodic monitoring of Hgb, PSA, serum lipid profile, LFTs, and serum testosterone concentrations. In cancer patients at risk for hypercalcemia, regularly monitor serum Ca^{2+} levels. Reevaluate Hct 3-6 months after start of therapy, then annually. Frequently monitor PT/INR w/ anticoagulants. Assess serum testosterone concentrations periodically.

Counseling: Inform that men w/ known or suspected prostate/breast cancer should not use androgen therapy. Advise to report signs and symptoms of secondary exposure in children and women to the physician. Instruct women and children to avoid contact w/ unwashed or unclothed application sites of men. Instruct to apply ud and to wash hands w/ soap and water after application, cover application site w/ clothing after gel dries, and wash application site w/ soap and water prior to direct skin-to-skin contact w/ others. Counsel about possible adverse reactions. Advise to read Medication Guide before therapy and reread each time prescription is renewed. Inform that drug is flammable; instruct to avoid fire, flame, or smoking until the gel has dried. Advise not to share the medication w/ anyone. Inform patients about importance of adhering to all the recommended monitoring and instruct to report changes in their state of health and to wait 5 hrs (1%) or 2 hrs (1.62%) before swimming or bathing.

ANDROID — methyltestosterone   CIII

Class: Androgen

ADULT DOSAGE	PEDIATRIC DOSAGE
Testosterone Replacement Therapy	**Testosterone Replacement Therapy**
Congenital/Acquired Primary Hypogonadism or Hypogonadotropic Hypogonadism in Males: 10-50mg/day; adjust according to response and appearance of adverse reactions	**Congenital/Acquired Primary Hypogonadism or Hypogonadotropic Hypogonadism in Males:** 10-50mg/day; adjust according to response and appearance of adverse reactions
Consider chronological and skeletal age in determining the initial dose and in adjusting the dose	Consider chronological and skeletal age in determining the initial dose and in adjusting the dose
Metastatic Breast Cancer Used secondarily in women w/ advancing inoperable metastatic (skeletal) mammary cancer who are 1-5 yrs postmenopausal. Also used in premenopausal women w/ breast cancer who have benefitted from oophorectomy and are considered to have a hormone-responsive tumor	**Delayed Puberty in Males** Doses used are generally in the lower range of that given during testosterone replacement therapy, and for a limited duration (eg, 4-6 months)
50-200mg/day; adjust according to response and appearance of adverse reactions	Consider chronological and skeletal age in determining the initial dose and in adjusting the dose

---

ADMINISTRATION
Oral route

STORAGE
25°C (77°F); excursions permitted to 15-30°C (59-86°F).

HOW SUPPLIED
Cap: 10mg

CONTRAINDICATIONS
Males w/ carcinomas of the breast or w/ known/suspected carcinomas of the prostate. Females who are or may become pregnant.

WARNINGS/PRECAUTIONS
May cause hypercalcemia in patients w/ breast cancer; d/c if this occurs. Peliosis hepatis and hepatic neoplasms, including hepatocellular carcinoma, reported w/ prolonged use of high doses. D/C if cholestatic hepatitis w/ jaundice, or if abnormal LFTs occur. May increase risk of prostatic hypertrophy and prostatic carcinoma in elderly. Venous thromboembolic events (VTEs) reported; evaluate patients who report symptoms of pain, edema, warmth, and erythema in the

lower extremity for deep vein thrombosis and those who present w/ acute SOB for pulmonary embolism. D/C treatment and initiate appropriate workup and management if a VTE is suspected. May increase risk of major adverse cardiovascular (CV) events (eg, nonfatal MI, nonfatal stroke, CV death). Edema w/ or w/o CHF may be a serious complication in patients w/ preexisting cardiac, renal, or hepatic disease; may require diuretic therapy in addition to discontinuation of therapy. Gynecomastia may develop and persist in patients being treated for hypogonadism. Caution in healthy males w/ delayed puberty; monitor bone maturation by assessing bone age of wrist and hand every 6 months. May accelerate bone maturation w/o producing compensatory gain in linear growth in children; compromised adult stature may result. Should not be used for enhancement of athletic performance. Monitor for signs of virilization in females; d/c therapy at evidence of mild virilism to prevent irreversible virilization. May decrease levels of thyroxine-binding globulin.

ADVERSE REACTIONS
Females: Amenorrhea, menstrual irregularities, inhibition of gonadotropin secretion, virilization.
Males: Gynecomastia, excessive frequency and duration of penile erections, oligospermia (if at high doses), hirsutism, male pattern baldness, acne, increased/decreased libido, headache, anxiety, depression, generalized paresthesia.

DRUG INTERACTIONS
May decrease oral anticoagulant requirement; close monitoring is required especially when androgens are started or stopped. May increase oxyphenbutazone levels. May decrease blood glucose and insulin requirements in diabetics.

PREGNANCY AND LACTATION
Pregnancy: Category X.
Lactation: Not for use in nursing.

MECHANISM OF ACTION
Androgen; responsible for normal growth and development of male sex organs and for maintenance of secondary sex characteristics.

PHARMACOKINETICS
Distribution: (Testosterone) Plasma protein binding (98% bound to a specific testosterone-estradiol binding globulin). **Metabolism:** Liver. **Elimination:** (Testosterone) Urine (90% [glucuronic and sulfuric acid conjugates]); feces (6% [unconjugated]); $T_{1/2}$=10-100 min.

PATIENT CONSIDERATIONS
Assessment: Assess for breast/prostate carcinoma in males, cardiac/renal/hepatic disease, pregnancy/nursing status, any other conditions where treatment is contraindicated/cautioned, and possible drug interactions.

Monitoring: Monitor for signs/symptoms of hypercalcemia, edema w/ or w/o CHF, prostatic hypertrophy/carcinoma in elderly, virilization in females, VTEs, and other adverse reactions. Monitor LFTs periodically. Frequently monitor urine and serum Ca^{2+} in women w/ disseminated breast carcinoma. Perform periodic (every 6 months) x-ray exam of bone age of prepubertal males. Periodically check Hgb and Hct for polycythemia in patients receiving high androgen doses.

Counseling: Instruct to report to physician any of the following side effects: too frequent or persistent erections of the penis (adult/adolescent males); hoarseness, acne, changes in menstrual period, more hair on the face (females); and N/V, changes in skin color, or ankle swelling (all patients). Inform that any male adolescent patient receiving androgens for delayed puberty should have bone development checked every 6 months.

ANECTINE — succinylcholine chloride   Rx
Class: Skeletal muscle relaxant (depolarizing)

> Rare reports of acute rhabdomyolysis w/ hyperkalemia followed by ventricular dysrhythmias, cardiac arrest, and death in healthy pediatric patients w/ undiagnosed skeletal muscle myopathy; most frequently Duchenne's muscular dystrophy. Often presented w/ peaked T-waves and sudden cardiac arrest w/in min after administration to healthy-appearing pediatric patients (most frequently ≤8 yrs of age) and adolescents. Treatment of hyperkalemia should be instituted; administer IV Ca^{2+}, bicarbonate, and glucose w/ insulin, w/ hyperventilation. Appropriate treatment should be instituted when signs of malignant hyperthermia are present. Reserve use in pediatric patients for emergency intubation where securing airway is necessary (eg, laryngospasm, difficult airway, full stomach, or for IM use when suitable vein is inaccessible).

OTHER BRAND NAMES
Quelicin

ADULT DOSAGE
Adjunct to General Anesthesia
Facilitates tracheal intubation and provides skeletal muscle relaxation during surgery or mechanical ventilation

IV:
Short Surgical Procedure:
Average Dose: 0.6mg/kg
Optimum Dose: 0.3-1.1mg/kg

Very large doses may result in more prolonged blockade; a 5-10mg test dose may be used to determine the sensitivity of the patient and the individual recovery time

PEDIATRIC DOSAGE
Adjunct to General Anesthesia
Facilitates tracheal intubation and provides skeletal muscle relaxation during surgery or mechanical ventilation

IV:
Emergency Tracheal Intubation/ Immediate Securing of Airway:
Infants and Small Children: 2mg/kg
Older Children and Adolescents: 1mg/kg

IM:
May be given when a suitable vein is inaccessible

Long Surgical Procedure:
The dose administered depends upon the duration of the surgical procedure and the need for muscle relaxation

Average Rate: 2.5-4.3mg/min

Sol containing 1-2mg/mL have commonly been used for continuous infusion; 1mg/mL preferable due to ease of control of the rate of administration and, hence, of relaxation and may be administered at a rate of 0.5-10mg/min (0.5-10mL/min) to obtain the required amount of relaxation

Intermittent IV inj may also be used for long procedures; 0.3-1.1mg/kg may be given initially, followed, at appropriate intervals, by 0.04-0.07mg/kg

IM:
May be given when a suitable vein is inaccessible
Up to 3-4mg/kg may be given, but no more than 150mg total dose should be administered IM

Up to 3-4mg/kg may be given, but no more than 150mg total dose should be administered IM

ADMINISTRATION
IV/IM route
Compatibility and Admixtures
Do not mix w/ alkaline sol having a pH >8.5 (eg, barbiturate sol)
Stable for 24 hrs after dilution to a final concentration of 1-2mg/mL in D5 inj or 0.9% NaCl inj
Admixtures should be prepared for single patient use only; discard unused portion of diluted sol

STORAGE
2-8°C (36-46°F). Stable for up to 14 days at room temperature.

HOW SUPPLIED
Inj: 20mg/mL; (Quelicin) 20mg/mL, 100mg/mL

CONTRAINDICATIONS
Personal or familial history of malignant hyperthermia, skeletal muscle myopathies, known hypersensitivity to succinylcholine chloride, acute phase of injury following major burns, multiple trauma, extensive skeletal muscle denervation, upper motor neuron injury.

WARNINGS/PRECAUTIONS
Should only be used by those skilled in the management of artificial respiration and only when facilities are instantly available. To avoid distress, do not administer before unconsciousness has been induced except in emergency situations. Life-threatening and fatal anaphylactic reactions reported; caution w/ previous anaphylactic reactions to other neuromuscular blocking agents. Caution when used in patients known or suspected homozygous for the atypical plasma cholinesterase gene. Caution in patients suffering from electrolyte abnormalities and those who may have massive digitalis toxicity; may induce cardiac arrhythmias or cardiac arrest. Caution w/ chronic abdominal infection, subarachnoid hemorrhage, conditions causing degeneration of central and peripheral nervous system, fractures, muscle spasms, reduced plasma cholinesterase activity, or acute phase of injury. D/C if skin mottling, rising temperature, and coagulopathies occur. Higher incidence of bradycardia progressing to asystole w/ 2nd dose; pretreatment w/ anticholinergic agents (eg, atropine) may reduce bradyarrhythmias. May increase intraocular, intracranial, or intragastric pressure. Avoid w/ narrow-angle glaucoma or penetrating eye injury unless potential benefit outweighs potential risk. W/ prolonged therapy, Phase I block will progress to Phase II block associated w/ prolonged respiratory paralysis and weakness. Hypokalemia or hypocalcemia may prolong neuromuscular blockade. (Quelicin) Caution in elderly.

ADVERSE REACTIONS
Respiratory depression, apnea, cardiac arrest, malignant hyperthermia, arrhythmia, bradycardia, tachycardia, HTN, hypotension, hyperkalemia, increased IOP, muscle fasciculation, jaw rigidity, postoperative muscle pains.

DRUG INTERACTIONS
Enhanced effects w/ promazine, oxytocin, certain non-penicillin antibiotics, quinidine, β-blockers, procainamide, lidocaine, trimethaphan, lithium carbonate, Mg^{2+} salts, quinine, aprotinin, chloroquine, diethylether, isoflurane, desflurane, metoclopramide, terbutaline, and drugs that reduce plasma cholinesterase activity (eg, chronically administered oral contraceptives, glucocorticoids, certain MAOIs) or inhibit plasma cholinesterase (eg, organophosphate insecticides, echothiophate, certain antineoplastic drugs). Increased risk of malignant hyperthermia w/ volatile anesthetics. Consider synergistic or antagonistic effect w/ other neuromuscular blocking agents.

PREGNANCY AND LACTATION
Category C, caution in nursing.

MECHANISM OF ACTION
Depolarizing skeletal muscle relaxant; combines w/ cholinergic receptors of motor end plate to produce depolarization, and subsequent neuromuscular transmission inhibition.

PHARMACOKINETICS

Distribution: Crosses the placenta. **Metabolism:** Rapid; via plasma cholinesterases through hydrolysis to succinylmonocholine and to succinic acid and choline. **Elimination:** Urine (10% unchanged).

PATIENT CONSIDERATIONS

Assessment: Assess for drug hypersensitivity, familial or personal history of malignant hyperthermia, skeletal muscle myopathy, extensive denervation of skeletal muscle or upper motor neuron injury, acute phase of injury following major burns, multiple trauma, electrolyte abnormalities, patients known to be or suspected of being homozygous/heterozygous for the atypical plasma cholinesterases gene, Duchenne's muscular dystrophy, digitalis toxicity, chronic abdominal infection, subarachnoid hemorrhage, degeneration of central and peripheral nervous system, narrow-angle glaucoma or penetrating eye injury, fracture or muscle spasm, hypokalemia/hypocalcemia, concomitant use of drugs or conditions that may reduce plasma cholinesterase activity, previous anaphylactic reactions to other neuromuscular blocking agents, pregnancy/nursing status, and possible drug interactions.

Monitoring: Monitor for signs/symptoms of malignant hyperthermia, acute rhabdomyolysis, hyperkalemia, ventricular dysrhythmias, bradycardia, cardiac arrest, prolonged respiratory muscle paralysis or weakness, increased intragastric pressure, IOP, increased intracranial pressure, anaphylactic reactions, and other adverse reactions. Monitor ECG changes, neuromuscular function, temperature, expired CO_2.

Counseling: Inform that therapy is to be administered only by those skilled in management of artificial respiration and only when facilities are immediately available to provide artificial intubation and adequate ventilation for patients.

ANGELIQ — drospirenone/estradiol Rx

Class: Estrogen/progestogen combination

> Estrogens increase the risk of endometrial cancer. Perform adequate diagnostic measures, including endometrial sampling, to rule out malignancy in postmenopausal women w/ undiagnosed persistent or recurring abnormal genital bleeding. Should not be used for the prevention of cardiovascular disease (CVD) or dementia. Increased risk of MI, stroke, invasive breast cancer, pulmonary embolism (PE), and deep vein thrombosis (DVT) in postmenopausal women (50-79 yrs of age) reported. Increased risk of developing probable dementia in postmenopausal women ≥65 yrs of age reported. Should be prescribed at the lowest effective dose and for the shortest duration consistent w/ treatment goals and risks.

ADULT DOSAGE	PEDIATRIC DOSAGE
Menopausal Vasomotor Symptoms	Pediatric use may not have been established
Moderate to Severe:	
1 tab (0.25mg/0.5mg or 0.5mg/1mg) qd	
Menopausal Vulvar/Vaginal Atrophy	
Moderate to Severe:	
1 tab (0.5mg/1mg) qd	
Missed Dose	
If a tab is forgotten, it should be taken as soon as possible	
If >24 hrs have elapsed, the missed tab should not be taken	
If several tabs are forgotten, bleeding may occur	

ADMINISTRATION

Oral route
Swallow whole w/ some liquid, irrespective of food intake
Take at the same time qd

STORAGE

25°C (77°F); excursions permitted to 15-30°C (59-86°F).

HOW SUPPLIED

Tab: (Drospirenone [DRSP]/Estradiol [E2]) 0.25mg/0.5mg, 0.5mg/1mg

CONTRAINDICATIONS

Undiagnosed abnormal genital bleeding, known/suspected/history of breast cancer, known/suspected estrogen-dependent neoplasia, active or history of DVT/PE/arterial thromboembolic disease (eg, stroke, MI), renal impairment, liver impairment/disease, adrenal insufficiency, protein C, protein S, antithrombin deficiency, or other known thrombophilic disorders; known/suspected pregnancy. Known anaphylactic reaction, angioedema, or hypersensitivity to Angeliq or any of its ingredients.

WARNINGS/PRECAUTIONS

D/C immediately if PE, DVT, stroke, or MI occurs or is suspected. Caution in patients w/ risk factors for arterial vascular disease (eg, HTN, diabetes mellitus [DM], tobacco use, hypercholesterolemia, obesity) and/or venous thromboembolism (VTE) (eg, personal/family history of VTE, obesity, systemic lupus erythematosus [SLE]). May increase risk of ovarian cancer. May cause fluid retention; caution w/ cardiac/renal dysfunction. May affect certain endocrine and blood components in lab tests. DRSP: Potential for hyperkalemia development in high-risk patients; contraindicated w/ conditions that predispose to hyperkalemia. May increase possibility of hyponatremia in high-risk patients. E2: If feasible, d/c therapy at least 4-6 weeks before surgery of the type associated w/ increased risk of thromboembolism, or during periods of prolonged immobilization. Increased risk of gallbladder disease reported. May lead to severe hypercalcemia in patients w/ breast cancer and bone metastases; d/c and take appropriate measures if hypercalcemia occurs. Retinal vascular thrombosis reported; d/c therapy pending examination if sudden partial or complete loss of vision, sudden onset of proptosis, diplopia, or migraine occurs. D/C permanently if examination reveals papilledema or retinal vascular lesions. May elevate BP, thyroid-binding globulin levels, and plasma TG levels (w/ preexisting hypertriglyceridemia); d/c if pancreatitis occurs. Caution w/ history of cholestatic jaundice associated w/ past estrogen use or w/ pregnancy; d/c in case of recurrence. Caution w/ hypoparathyroidism; hypocalcemia may occur. May induce or exacerbate symptoms of angioedema in women w/ hereditary angioedema. May exacerbate endometriosis, asthma, DM, epilepsy, migraine, porphyria, SLE, otosclerosis, chorea minor, and hepatic hemangiomas; use w/ caution.

ADVERSE REACTIONS

GI and abdominal pain, female genital tract bleeding, headache, breast pain, vulvovaginal fungal infections, nausea.

DRUG INTERACTIONS

CYP3A4 inducers (eg, St. John's wort, phenobarbital, carbamazepine, rifampin) may decrease levels, which may decrease therapeutic effects and/or change uterine bleeding profile. Moderate or strong CYP3A4 inhibitors (eg, erythromycin, clarithromycin, verapamil, grapefruit juice) may increase levels. Significant changes (increase/decrease) in levels reported w/ HIV/hepatitis C virus protease inhibitors or non-nucleoside reverse transcriptase inhibitors. DRSP: Potential for an increase in serum K^+ concentration w/ other drugs that may increase serum K^+ concentration (eg, ACE inhibitors, heparin, aldosterone antagonists, NSAIDs); consider monitoring serum K^+ concentration during 1st month of therapy in high-risk patients who take a strong CYP3A4 inhibitor long-term and concomitantly. E2: Acute alcohol ingestion may elevate circulating E2 concentrations. May need to increase dose of thyroid hormone in patients dependent on thyroid hormone replacement therapy due to increased thyroid-binding globulin.

PREGNANCY AND LACTATION

Contraindicated in pregnancy, not for use in nursing.

MECHANISM OF ACTION

Estrogen/progestogen combination. E2: Binds to nuclear receptors in estrogen-responsive tissues. Modulates pituitary secretion of gonadotropins, luteinizing hormone and follicle-stimulating hormone, through a (-) feedback mechanism. DRSP: Synthetic progestin and spironolactone analogue w/ antimineralocorticoid activity. Possesses antiandrogenic activity. Counters estrogenic effects by decreasing number of nuclear estradiol receptors and suppressing epithelial DNA synthesis in endometrial tissue.

PHARMACOKINETICS

Absorption: DRSP: Absolute bioavailability (76-85%). Administration of variable doses resulted in different pharmacokinetic parameters. **Distribution:** Found in breast milk. DRSP: V_d=4.2L/kg; serum protein binding (97%). E2: Sex hormone-binding globulin (37%); albumin binding (61%). **Metabolism:** DRSP: Reduction, subsequent sulfation, oxidation catalyzed by CYP3A4. E2: Gut and liver, conjugation w/ sulfate and glucuronide, hydroxylation. **Elimination:** DRSP: Urine, feces; $T_{1/2}$=36-42 hrs. E2: Urine.

PATIENT CONSIDERATIONS

Assessment: Assess for undiagnosed abnormal genital bleeding, presence/history of breast cancer, estrogen-dependent neoplasia, arterial thromboembolic disease, pregnancy/nursing status, other conditions where treatment is cautioned/contraindicated, and possible drug interactions.

Monitoring: Monitor for signs/symptoms of CVD, malignant neoplasms, dementia, gallbladder disease, visual abnormalities, BP and plasma TG elevations, pancreatitis, cholestatic jaundice, hypothyroidism, fluid retention, hyperkalemia, hyponatremia, and exacerbation of endometriosis and other conditions. Perform annual breast examination; schedule mammography based on patient's age, risk factors, and prior mammogram results. Monitor K^+ levels and thyroid function if patient is receiving thyroid replacement therapy. Perform adequate diagnostic measures (eg, endometrial sampling) in patients w/ undiagnosed persistent or recurrent genital bleeding. Perform periodic evaluation to determine treatment need.

Counseling: Inform postmenopausal women of the importance of reporting abnormal vaginal bleeding as soon as possible. Advise of possible adverse reactions. Instruct to have yearly breast exams by a healthcare provider and to perform monthly breast self-examinations.

ANGIOMAX — bivalirudin Rx

Class: Direct thrombin inhibitor (DTI)

ADULT DOSAGE	PEDIATRIC DOSAGE
Percutaneous Transluminal Coronary Angioplasty/Percutaneous Coronary Intervention	Pediatric use may not have been established
Anticoagulant in patients w/ unstable angina undergoing percutaneous transluminal coronary angioplasty (PTCA). Anticoagulant in patients undergoing percutaneous coronary intervention (PCI) w/ provisional use of glycoprotein IIb/IIIa inhibitor (GPI). Indicated for patients w/, or at risk of, heparin-induced thrombocytopenia (HIT) or heparin-induced thrombocytopenia and thrombosis syndrome (HITTS) undergoing PCI	
Give w/ aspirin (300-325mg/day)	

Patients w/o HIT/HITTS:
0.75mg/kg IV bolus, then 1.75mg/kg/hr infusion for the duration of the PCI/PTCA procedure

An activated clotting time should be performed 5 min after the bolus dose and an additional bolus of 0.3mg/kg should be given if needed

Consider GPI administration in the event that any conditions listed in the REPLACE-2 clinical trial description is present; refer to PI

Patients w/ HIT/HITTS Undergoing PCI:
0.75mg/kg IV bolus, then 1.75mg/kg/hr infusion for the duration of the procedure

Ongoing Treatment Post-Procedure:
May continue infusion following PCI/PTCA for up to 4 hrs post-procedure

In patients w/ ST segment elevation myocardial infarction (STEMI), consider continuation of the infusion at a rate of 1.75mg/kg/hr following PCI/PTCA for up to 4 hrs post-procedure to mitigate the risk of stent thrombosis

After 4 hrs, an additional infusion may be initiated at a rate of 0.2mg/kg/hr (low-rate infusion), for up to 20 hrs, if needed

DOSING CONSIDERATIONS
Renal Impairment
Reduction in bolus dose not needed
Severe (CrCl <30mL/min): Consider reducing infusion to 1mg/kg/hr
Hemodialysis: 0.25mg/kg/hr infusion
ADMINISTRATION
IV route
Reconstitution and Dilution
1. To each 250mg vial, add 5mL of sterile water for inj.
2. Gently swirl until all material is dissolved.
3. Withdraw and discard 5mL from a 50mL infusion bag containing D5W or 0.9% NaCl for inj.
4. Add the contents of the reconstituted vial to the infusion bag containing D5W or 0.9% NaCl for inj to yield a final concentration of 5mg/mL.

If the low-rate infusion is used after the initial infusion, a lower concentration bag should be prepared; refer to PI for further details.
Incompatibilities
Alteplase, amiodarone HCl, amphotericin B, chlorpromazine HCl, diazepam, prochlorperazine edisylate, reteplase, streptokinase, and vancomycin HCl. Dobutamine compatibility varies w/ concentration; see PI.
STORAGE
20-25°C (68-77°F); excursions permitted to 15-30°C (59-86°F). **Reconstituted:** 2-8°C (36-46°F) for up to 24 hrs, Diluted concentration of between 0.5mg/mL and 5mg/mL is stable at room temperature for up to 24 hrs. Do not freeze.
HOW SUPPLIED
Inj: 250mg
CONTRAINDICATIONS
Active major bleeding, hypersensitivity (eg, anaphylaxis) to bivalirudin or its components.
WARNINGS/PRECAUTIONS
Hemorrhage may occur at any site; caution w/ disease states associated w/ increased risk of bleeding. D/C w/ unexplained fall in BP or Hct. Increased incidence of acute stent thrombosis (AST) in STEMI patients undergoing primary PCI; patients should remain for at least 24 hrs in a facility capable of managing ischemic complications and should be carefully monitored following primary PCI for signs/symptoms consistent w/ myocardial ischemia. Associated w/ increased risk of thrombus formation, including fatal outcomes in gamma brachytherapy; maintain meticulous catheter technique, w/ frequent aspiration and flushing, paying special attention to minimize conditions of stasis w/in the catheter/vessels. May need to reduce infusion dose and monitor anticoagulant status in patients w/ renal impairment. Affects INR; INR measurements may not be useful for determining the appropriate dose of warfarin.
ADVERSE REACTIONS
Bleeding, headache, fever.
DRUG INTERACTIONS
Increased risk of major bleeding events w/ heparin, warfarin, thrombolytics, or GPIs.
PREGNANCY AND LACTATION
Pregnancy: Category B.
Lactation: It is not known whether bivalirudin is excreted in human milk; caution in nursing.
MECHANISM OF ACTION
Direct thrombin inhibitor; inhibits thrombin by specifically binding both to the catalytic site and to the anion-binding exosite of circulating and clot-bound thrombin.

PHARMACOKINETICS
Metabolism: Proteolytic cleavage. **Elimination:** Renal. $T_{1/2}$=25 min (plasma).
PATIENT CONSIDERATIONS
Assessment: Assess for drug hypersensitivity, active major bleeding, renal impairment, disease states associated w/ increased risk of bleeding, pregnancy/nursing status, and for possible drug interactions.
Monitoring: Monitor for signs/symptoms of hemorrhage, AST in patients w/ STEMI undergoing PCI, thrombus formation in gamma brachytherapy, and other adverse reactions. For patients w/ renal impairment, monitor anticoagulant status.
Counseling: Advise to watch for any signs of bleeding/bruising and to report to physician if these occur. Advise to inform physician about the use of any other medications (eg, warfarin and heparin), including OTC medicines or herbal products, prior to therapy.

ANORO ELLIPTA — umeclidinium/vilanterol   Rx
Class: Anticholinergic/long-acting beta₂ agonist (LABA)

> Long-acting β_2-adrenergic agonists (LABAs) (eg, vilanterol) increase the risk of asthma-related death. Not indicated for the treatment of asthma.

ADULT DOSAGE	PEDIATRIC DOSAGE
Chronic Obstructive Pulmonary Disease **Long-Term Maint Treatment of Airflow Obstruction:** 1 inh qd; do not use >1 time q24h	Pediatric use may not have been established

ADMINISTRATION
Oral inh route
Take at the same time every day.
STORAGE
20-25°C (68-77°F); excursions permitted from 15-30°C (59-86°F). Store in a dry place away from direct heat or sunlight. Store inside the unopened moisture-protective foil tray and only remove from the tray immediately before initial use. Discard 6 weeks after opening the foil tray or when the counter reads "0" (after all blisters have been used), whichever comes 1st.
HOW SUPPLIED
Powder, Inh: (Umeclidinium/Vilanterol) (62.5mcg/25mcg)/blister [7, 30 blisters]
CONTRAINDICATIONS
Severe hypersensitivity to milk proteins or hypersensitivity to umeclidinium, vilanterol, or any of the excipients.
WARNINGS/PRECAUTIONS
Not indicated for acute bronchospasm relief. Should not be initiated in patients during rapidly deteriorating or potentially life-threatening episodes of COPD. D/C regular use of oral/inhaled short-acting β_2-agonist when beginning treatment. May produce paradoxical bronchospasm; treat immediately w/ an inhaled, short-acting bronchodilator; immediately d/c Anoro Ellipta and institute alternative therapy. Hypersensitivity reactions (eg, anaphylaxis, angioedema, rash) may occur; d/c if such reactions occur. Caution w/ narrow-angle glaucoma and urinary retention. **Vilanterol:** Do not use more often or at higher doses than recommended; clinically significant cardiovascular (CV) effects and fatalities reported w/ excessive use. CV effects may occur; may need to d/c if such effects occur. Caution w/ CV disorders, convulsive disorders, thyrotoxicosis, diabetes mellitus (DM), ketoacidosis, and in patients unusually responsive to sympathomimetic amines. May produce significant hypokalemia and transient hyperglycemia.
ADVERSE REACTIONS
Pharyngitis, diarrhea, pain in extremity, sinusitis, lower respiratory tract infection, constipation, muscle spasms, neck pain, chest pain.
DRUG INTERACTIONS
Umeclidinium: Avoid w/ other anticholinergics; may increase anticholinergic adverse effects. **Vilanterol:** Do not use w/ other medicines containing LABAs. Caution w/ long-term ketoconazole and other strong CYP3A4 inhibitors (eg, ritonavir, clarithromycin, conivaptan); increased vilanterol exposure and increased CV adverse effects may occur. Extreme caution w/ MAOIs, TCAs, or drugs known to prolong the QTc interval or w/in 2 weeks of discontinuation of such agents; effect on CV system may be potentiated. β-blockers may block pulmonary effects and produce severe bronchospasm in patients w/ COPD; avoid treatment w/ β-blockers. If such therapy is needed, consider cardioselective β-blockers and administer w/ caution. Caution w/ non-K⁺-sparing diuretics (eg, loop or thiazide diuretics).
PREGNANCY AND LACTATION
Pregnancy: Category C.
Lactation: Not for use in nursing.
MECHANISM OF ACTION
Umeclidinium: Anticholinergic (long-acting); exhibits effects through inhibition of M3 receptor at the smooth muscle, leading to bronchodilation. **Vilanterol:** LABA; attributable to stimulation of intracellular adenyl cyclase, the enzyme that catalyzes the conversion of ATP to cAMP. Increased cAMP levels cause relaxation of bronchial smooth muscle and inhibition of release of mediators of immediate hypersensitivity from cells, especially from mast cells.
PHARMACOKINETICS
Absorption: Umeclidinium: T_{max}=5-15 min. Vilanterol: T_{max}=5-15 min. **Distribution:** Umeclidinium: V_d=86L (IV); plasma protein binding (89%). Vilanterol: V_d=165L (IV); plasma protein binding (94%). **Metabolism:** Umeclidinium: Via CYP2D6, substrate

for P-gp; oxidative (hydroxylation, O-dealkylation) followed by conjugation (eg, glucuronidation). Vilanterol: Via CYP3A4, substrate for P-gp. **Elimination:** Umeclidinium (PO, IV): Feces (92%, 58%), urine (<1%, 22%); $T_{1/2}$=11 hrs. Vilanterol (PO): Urine (70%), feces (30%); $T_{1/2}$=11 hrs.

PATIENT CONSIDERATIONS
Assessment: Assess for hypersensitivity to milk proteins; hypersensitivity to umeclidinium, vilanterol, or any of the excipients; COPD status; CV/convulsive disorders; thyrotoxicosis; DM; ketoacidosis; narrow-angle glaucoma; urinary retention; prostatic hyperplasia; bladder-neck obstruction; pregnancy/nursing status; and possible drug interactions. Evaluate use in patients unusually responsive to sympathomimetic amines.

Monitoring: Monitor for deteriorating disease, paradoxical bronchospasm, hypersensitivity reactions, CV effects, worsening of narrow-angle glaucoma, worsening of urinary retention, hypokalemia, hyperglycemia, and other adverse reactions.

Counseling: Inform that drug is not for treatment of asthma or to relieve acute symptoms of COPD. Advise that acute symptoms should be treated w/ an inhaled short-acting β_2-agonist (eg, albuterol). Instruct to seek medical attention immediately if experiencing decreasing effectiveness of inhaled, short-acting β_2-agonists, a need for more inhalations than usual of inhaled, short-acting β_2-agonists, or if a significant decrease in lung function develops. Advise not to d/c therapy w/o physician guidance and not to use an additional LABA. Instruct to d/c therapy and contact physician if paradoxical bronchospasm occurs. Inform about adverse effects (eg, palpitations, chest pain, rapid HR, tremor, nervousness) and other risks (eg, worsening of narrow-angle glaucoma, worsening of urinary retention) associated w/ therapy; instruct to consult physician immediately if any signs/symptoms develop. Advise to contact physician if pregnancy occurs while on therapy. Inform that the inhaler is not reusable and advise not to take the inhaler apart.

ANTARA — fenofibrate   Rx
Class: Fibric acid derivative

ADULT DOSAGE	PEDIATRIC DOSAGE
Primary Hypercholesterolemia/Mixed Dyslipidemia	Pediatric use may not have been established
Initial/Max: 90mg/day	
Titrate: May consider dose reduction if lipid levels fall significantly below the targeted range	
D/C if no adequate response after 2 months of therapy w/ max dose	
Severe Hypertriglyceridemia	
Initial: 30-90mg/day	
Titrate: Adjust dose if necessary following repeat lipid determinations at 4- to 8-week intervals; may consider dose reduction if lipid levels fall significantly below the targeted range	
Max: 90mg/day	
D/C if no adequate response after 2 months of therapy w/ max dose	

DOSING CONSIDERATIONS
Renal Impairment
Mild to Moderate:
Initial: 30mg/day
Titrate: Increase only after evaluation of effects on renal function and lipid levels

ADMINISTRATION
Oral route

May be taken w/o regard to meals
Swallow cap whole; do not open, crush, dissolve, or chew

STORAGE
25°C (77°F); excursions permitted to 15-30°C (59-86°F).

HOW SUPPLIED
Cap: 30mg, 90mg

CONTRAINDICATIONS
Severe renal impairment (including dialysis), active liver disease (including primary biliary cirrhosis and unexplained persistent liver function abnormalities), preexisting gallbladder disease, nursing mothers, known hypersensitivity to fenofibric acid or fenofibrate.

WARNINGS/PRECAUTIONS
Not shown to reduce coronary heart disease morbidity and mortality in patients with type 2 diabetes mellitus (DM). Increased risk of myopathy and rhabdomyolysis; risk increased with diabetes, renal failure, hypothyroidism, and in elderly. D/C therapy if markedly elevated CPK levels occur or myopathy/myositis is suspected or diagnosed. Increases in serum transaminases, hepatocellular, chronic active and cholestatic hepatitis, and cirrhosis (extremely rare) reported; perform baseline and regular monitoring of LFTs, and d/c therapy if enzyme levels persist >3X the normal limit. Elevations in SrCr reported; monitor renal function in patients with renal impairment or at risk for renal insufficiency. May cause cholelithiasis; d/c if gallstones are found. Acute hypersensitivity reactions and pancreatitis reported. Mild to moderate decreases in Hgb, Hct, and WBCs, thrombocytopenia, and

agranulocytosis reported; periodically monitor RBC and WBC counts during the first 12 months of therapy. May cause venothromboembolic disease (eg, pulmonary embolism [PE], deep vein thrombosis [DVT]). Severe decreases in HDL levels reported; check HDL levels within the 1st few months after initiation of therapy. If a severely depressed HDL level is detected, withdraw therapy, monitor HDL level until it has returned to baseline, and do not reinitiate therapy. Estrogen therapy, thiazide diuretics, and β-blockers may be associated with massive rises in plasma TG levels; discontinuation of the specific etiologic agent may obviate the need for specific drug therapy of hypertriglyceridemia.

ADVERSE REACTIONS
Abdominal pain, back pain, headache, abnormal LFTs, respiratory disorder, increased AST/ALT/CPK.

DRUG INTERACTIONS
May potentiate coumarin anticoagulant effects; use with caution, reduce anticoagulant dose, and monitor PT/INR frequently. Increased risk of rhabdomyolysis with HMG-CoA reductase inhibitors (statins); avoid combination unless benefits outweigh risks. Bile acid-binding resins may bind other drugs given concurrently; take at least 1 hr before or 4-6 hrs after the bile acid-binding resin. Immunosuppressants (eg, cyclosporine, tacrolimus) may produce nephrotoxicity; consider benefits and risks of use with immunosuppressants and other potentially nephrotoxic agents, and use lowest effective dose. Cases of myopathy, including rhabdomyolysis, reported when coadministered with colchicine; caution when prescribing with colchicine.

PREGNANCY AND LACTATION
Category C, not for use in nursing.

MECHANISM OF ACTION
Fibric acid derivative; activates peroxisome proliferator activated receptor α. Increases lipolysis and elimination of TG-rich particles from plasma by activating lipoprotein lipase and reducing production of apoprotein C-III (lipoprotein lipase activity inhibitor). Also, induces an increase in the synthesis of apoproteins A-I, A-II, and HDL.

PHARMACOKINETICS
Absorption: Well-absorbed. T_{max}=2-6 hrs (90mg dose). **Distribution:** Plasma protein binding (99%). **Metabolism:** Rapid via ester hydrolysis to fenofibric acid (active metabolite); conjugation with glucuronic acid. **Elimination:** Urine (60%, primarily fenofibric acid and glucuronate conjugate), feces (25%); $T_{1/2}$=23 hrs.

PATIENT CONSIDERATIONS
Assessment: Assess for hypersensitivity to the drug, renal impairment, active liver disease, preexisting gallbladder disease, other medical conditions (eg, DM, hypothyroidism), pregnancy/nursing status, and for possible drug interactions. Obtain baseline LFTs.

Monitoring: Monitor for cholelithiasis, pancreatitis, hypersensitivity reactions, PE, and DVT. Monitor renal function, LFTs, CBC, and lipid levels. Monitor for signs/symptoms of myositis, myopathy, or rhabdomyolysis; measure CPK levels in patients reporting such symptoms. Monitor PT/INR frequently with coumarin anticoagulants.

Counseling: Advise of potential risks and benefits of therapy and medications to avoid during treatment. Instruct to continue to follow appropriate lipid-modifying diet during therapy and to take drug ud. Instruct to inform physician of all medications, supplements, and herbal preparations being taken; any changes in medical condition; development of muscle pain, tenderness, or weakness; onset of abdominal pain; or any other new symptoms. Advise to return to the physician's office for routine monitoring.

ANTHRASIL — anthrax immune globulin intravenous (human)   Rx
Class: Immune globulin

> Maltose in immune globulin products may give falsely high blood glucose levels w/ some point-of-care blood glucose testing systems (eg, those based on the GDH-PQQ or glucose-dye-oxidoreductase methods) resulting in inappropriate administration of insulin and life-threatening hypoglycemia. To avoid interference by maltose, perform blood glucose measurement in patients w/ a glucose-specific method (monitor and test strips). Thrombosis may occur, and may occur in the absence of known risk factors (eg, advanced age, prolonged immobilization, hypercoagulable conditions, history of venous or arterial thrombosis, use of estrogens). Administer at the minimum infusion rate practicable in patients at risk of thrombosis. Ensure adequate hydration in patients before administration. Monitor for signs/symptoms of thrombosis and assess blood viscosity in patients at risk of hyperviscosity.

ADULT DOSAGE	PEDIATRIC DOSAGE
Inhalational Anthrax	**Inhalational Anthrax**
Treatment of inhalational anthrax in combination w/ appropriate antibacterial drugs	Treatment of inhalational anthrax in combination w/ appropriate antibacterial drugs
≥17 Years:	**<1 Year to ≤16 Years:**
7 vials (420 U)	1-7 vials (60-420 U) based on patient weight
Select initial dose based on clinical severity; severe cases may warrant use of 14 vials (840 U)	Select initial dose based on clinical severity; severe cases may warrant use of 2-14 vials (based on weight) in pediatric patients weighing >5kg
Initial Infusion Rate (First 30 min): 0.5mL/min	**Initial Infusion Rate (First 30 min):** 0.01mL/kg/min (do not exceed adult rate)
Incremental Infusion Rate if Tolerated (Every 30 min): 1mL/min	**Incremental Infusion Rate if Tolerated (Every 30 min):** 0.02mL/kg/min
Max Infusion Rate: 2mL/min	

Max Infusion Rate:
0.04mL/kg/min (do not exceed adult rate)

Number of Vials per Dose:
<10kg: 1
10 to <18kg: 2
18 to <25kg: 3
25 to <35kg: 4
35 to <50kg: 5
50 to <60kg: 6
≥60kg: 7
Dose may be doubled for severe cases in patients >5kg

ADMINISTRATION
IV route
Slow the rate of infusion or temporarily stop the infusion if adverse reactions occur (eg, flushing, headache, nausea, changes in pulse rate or BP).

Preparation
1. Bring vials to room temperature. Thaw frozen vials rapidly for immediate use by placing at room temperature for 1 hr followed by a water bath at 37°C (98.6°F) until thawed; alternatively, thaw vials by placing the required number of vials in a refrigerator at 2-8°C (36-46°F) until the vials are thawed (approx 14 hrs). Do not thaw in a microwave oven and do not refreeze vials.
2. Bring thawed vials to room temperature by letting sit on a bench for a few min prior to infusion.
3. Gently swirl upright vials by hand to ensure uniformity; do not shake vial during preparation.
4. Withdraw contents of vial into a syringe, aseptically transfer into an appropriately sized IV bag, and label w/ the volume to be infused. No further dilution is required.
5. Administer in an IV line w/ constant infusion pump. Use of an in-line filter is optional.
6. Discard any unused portion.

STORAGE
Store frozen at or below -15°C (5°F) until required for use; do not refreeze, reuse, or save for future use.

HOW SUPPLIED
Inj: Minimum potency of ≥60 U/vial

CONTRAINDICATIONS
History of anaphylactic or severe systemic reaction to this product or other human immune globulins, IgA-deficient patients w/ antibodies against IgA and a history of IgA hypersensitivity.

WARNINGS/PRECAUTIONS
Hypersensitivity reactions may occur; d/c immediately and administer appropriate emergency care if a severe hypersensitivity reaction occurs. Administer in a setting where appropriate equipment, medication (including epinephrine) and personnel trained in the management of hypersensitivity, anaphylaxis, and shock are available. Consider baseline assessment of blood viscosity in patients at risk for hyperviscosity (eg, those w/ cryoglobulins, fasting chylomicronemia/markedly high TGs, monoclonal gammopathies). Acute renal dysfunction, acute renal failure, osmotic nephropathy, acute tubular necrosis, proximal tubular nephropathy, and death may occur. Caution in patients w/ any degree of pre-existing renal insufficiency and in patients at risk of developing renal insufficiency (eg, those w/ diabetes mellitus, >65 years of age, volume depletion, paraproteinemia, sepsis, receiving known nephrotoxic drugs); administer at the minimum rate of infusion practicable. Ensure that patients are not volume depleted before infusion. Consider discontinuation if renal function deteriorates. Adverse reactions (eg, chills, fever, headache, N/V) may be related to the rate of infusion; closely monitor and carefully observe patients and their vital signs for any symptoms throughout the infusion period and immediately following an infusion. Hemolytic anemia and hemolysis may develop; consider appropriate laboratory testing in higher risk patients (including measurement of Hgb or Hct) prior to infusion and w/in approx 36-96 hrs and again approx 7-10 days post infusion. Perform additional confirmatory laboratory testing if signs/symptoms of hemolysis or a significant drop in Hgb or Hct have been observed after infusion. Aseptic meningitis syndrome (AMS) may occur. Transfusion-related acute lung injury (TRALI) may occur; perform tests for the presence of anti-HLA and anti-neutrophil antibodies in the product if TRALI is suspected. Antibodies present in Anthrasil may interfere w/ some serological tests; after administration, a transitory increase of passively transferred antibodies in the patient's blood may result in positive results in serological tests (eg, Coombs' test). Urinalysis after administration may result in elevated glucose levels; repeat testing to determine if further action is warranted since this is a known transient effect. May carry a risk of transmitting blood-borne infectious agents (eg, viruses, the variant Creutzfeldt-Jakob disease agent, and theoretically, the Creutzfeldt-Jakob disease agent).

ADVERSE REACTIONS
Headache, infusion-site pain, nausea, infusion-site swelling, back pain.

DRUG INTERACTIONS
May impair efficacy of live attenuated vaccines (eg, measles, rubella, mumps, and varicella); defer vaccination w/ live virus vaccines until approx 3 months after administration of Anthrasil. Revaccinate those who received Anthrasil shortly after live virus vaccination 3 months after the administration of Anthrasil.

PREGNANCY AND LACTATION
Pregnancy: There are no human data to establish the presence or absence of an associated risk w/ Anthrasil.

Lactation: There are no data to assess the presence or absence of Anthrasil in human milk, the effects on the breastfed child, or the effects on milk production/ excretion.

MECHANISM OF ACTION
Immune globulin; passive immunizing agent that neutralizes anthrax toxin by binding to protective antigen (PA) to prevent PA mediated cellular entry of anthrax edema factor and lethal factor.

PHARMACOKINETICS
Absorption: (210 U) AUC_{0-t}=1031.8 mU•d/mL; C_{max}=83mU/mL; T_{max}=0.116 days; (420 U) AUC_{0-t}=2176.7mU•d/mL; C_{max}=156.4mU/mL; T_{max}=0.120 days.
Distribution: (210 U) V_d=5714.8mL; (420 U) V_d=6837.2mL. **Elimination:** (210 U) $T_{1/2}$=24.3 days; (420 U) $T_{1/2}$=28.3 days. Refer to PI for further information.

PATIENT CONSIDERATIONS
Assessment: Assess for history of hypersensitivity to this therapy or other human immune globulin preparations, IgA-deficiency, risk factors for thrombosis, renal insufficiency or risk of developing renal insufficiency, volume depletion, pregnancy/nursing status, and for possible drug interactions. Consider baseline assessment of blood viscosity in patients at risk for hyperviscosity. Assess for risk of hemolysis; consider appropriate laboratory testing in higher risk patients. Ensure adequate hydration before administration.

Monitoring: Monitor for thrombosis, acute renal dysfunction/failure, hemolysis, AMS, TRALI, transmission of infectious agents, and for other adverse reactions. Monitor for signs/symptoms of an acute allergic reactions (eg, urticaria, pruritus, erythema) during and following the infusion. Monitor renal function at appropriate intervals. Monitor urine output in patients judged to be at increased risk of developing acute renal failure. Monitor vital signs throughout the infusion period and immediately following an infusion. In patients at higher risk of hemolysis, consider appropriate laboratory testing w/in approx 36-96 hrs and again approx 7-10 days post infusion. Conduct a detailed neurological examination in patients exhibiting signs/symptoms of AMS to rule out other causes of meningitis. If TRALI is suspected, perform tests for the presence of anti-HLA and anti-neutrophil antibodies in the product.

Counseling: Inform of the risks and benefits of therapy. Advise of the potential for hypersensitivity reactions, especially in individuals w/ previous reactions to human immune globulin and in individuals deficient in IgA; instruct to seek immediate medical attention if experiencing signs/symptoms of hypersensitivity. Advise that maltose is contained in the product and can interfere w/ some types of blood glucose monitoring systems; advise to use only testing systems that are glucose-specific. Inform that therapy may cause thrombosis, hemolysis, AMS, TRALI, acute respiratory distress syndrome, and acute renal dysfunction or failure. Advise that the product may impair the effectiveness of certain live virus vaccines. Inform that product is prepared from human plasma and that products made from human plasma may contain infectious agents (eg, viruses).

ANTIVERT — meclizine hydrochloride   Rx

Class: Antihistamine

ADULT DOSAGE	PEDIATRIC DOSAGE
Motion Sickness	**Motion Sickness**
25-50mg 1 hr prior to embarkation Thereafter, may repeat dose q24h for the duration of the journey	**≥12 Years:** 25-50mg 1 hr prior to embarkation Thereafter, may repeat dose q24h for the duration of the journey
Vertigo	**Vertigo**
25-100mg/day in divided doses, depending upon clinical response	**≥12 Years:** 25-100mg/day in divided doses, depending upon clinical response

---

ADMINISTRATION
Oral route

STORAGE
<30°C (86°F).

HOW SUPPLIED
Tab: 12.5mg, 25mg, 50mg

CONTRAINDICATIONS
Previous hypersensitivity.

WARNINGS/PRECAUTIONS
Caution with asthma, glaucoma, enlargement of the prostate gland, hepatic/renal impairment, and in elderly. Drowsiness may occur. May impair physical/mental abilities.

ADVERSE REACTIONS
Anaphylactoid reaction, drowsiness, dry mouth, headache, fatigue, vomiting.

DRUG INTERACTIONS
Avoid alcohol use. Increased CNS depression with other CNS depressants (eg, alcohol, tranquilizers, sedatives). Possible interaction with CYP2D6 inhibitors.

PREGNANCY AND LACTATION
Category B, caution in nursing.

MECHANISM OF ACTION
Antihistamine; has marked effect in blocking the vasodepressor response to histamine, but only a slight blocking action against acetylcholine.

PHARMACOKINETICS
Absorption: T_{max}=3 hrs. **Metabolism:** Via CYP2D6. **Elimination:** $T_{1/2}$=5-6 hrs.

PATIENT CONSIDERATIONS

Assessment: Assess for previous hypersensitivity to the drug, asthma, glaucoma, prostate gland enlargement, renal/hepatic impairment, pregnancy/nursing status, and possible drug interactions.

Monitoring: Monitor for drowsiness and other adverse reactions.

Counseling: Inform that drowsiness may occur; instruct to use caution when driving a vehicle or operating machinery. Advise to avoid alcohol use. Advise to notify physician if pregnant/nursing.

ANUSOL-HC SUPPOSITORY — hydrocortisone acetate   Rx

Class: Corticosteroid

OTHER BRAND NAMES
Anucort HC

ADULT DOSAGE
Colorectal Disorders

For use in inflamed hemorrhoids, post-irradiation (factitial) proctitis, as an adjunct in the treatment of chronic ulcerative colitis, cryptitis, other inflammatory conditions of the anorectum, and pruritus ani

Usual: 1 sup rectally bid (am and pm) for 2 weeks, in nonspecific proctitis. In more severe cases, 1 sup rectally tid or 2 sup rectally bid. In factitial proctitis, recommended therapy is 6-8 weeks or less, according to response

PEDIATRIC DOSAGE
Pediatric use may not have been established

ADMINISTRATION
Rectal route

STORAGE
Store at 20-25°C (68-77°F). Store away from heat. Protect from freezing.

HOW SUPPLIED
Sup: (Anusol-HC) 25mg [12^s 24^s]

CONTRAINDICATIONS
History of hypersensitivity to any of the components.

WARNINGS/PRECAUTIONS
D/C if irritation develops. D/C if infection develops that does not respond to appropriate therapy. May stain fabric. Only use after adequate proctologic exam.

ADVERSE REACTIONS
Burning, itching, irritation, dryness, folliculitis, hypopigmentation, allergic contact dermatitis, secondary infection.

PREGNANCY AND LACTATION
Category C, not for use in nursing.

MECHANISM OF ACTION
Corticosteroid; suspected to produce anti-inflammatory, anti-pruritic, and vasoconstrictive action.

PHARMACOKINETICS
Absorption: Rectum (26%).

PATIENT CONSIDERATIONS
Assessment: Proctologic examination should be done. Assess for drug hypersensitivity and presence of infection.

Monitoring: Monitor possible local adverse reactions including burning, itching, irritation, dryness, folliculitis, hypopigmentation, allergic contact dermatitis, and secondary infection.

Counseling: Advise that staining of fabric may occur with use of sup; precautionary measures recommended. If irritation develops, d/c therapy and institute appropriate therapy. Report adverse effects.

ANZEMET — dolasetron mesylate   Rx

Class: 5-HT$_3$ receptor antagonist

ADULT DOSAGE
Postoperative Nausea/Vomiting

Inj:
Prevention/Treatment of Postoperative Nausea and Vomiting (PONV):
12.5mg IV as a single dose approx 15 min before cessation of anesthesia (prevention) or as soon as N/V presents (treatment)

Chemotherapy-Induced Nausea/ Vomiting

Tab:
Prevention of N/V Associated w/ Moderately Emetogenic Cancer Chemotherapy, Including Initial and Repeat Courses:
100mg w/in 1 hr before chemotherapy

PEDIATRIC DOSAGE
Postoperative Nausea/Vomiting

Inj:
2-16 Years:
Prevention/Treatment of PONV:

IV Administration:
0.35mg/kg IV as a single dose approx 15 min before cessation of anesthesia or as soon as N/V presents
Max Dose: 12.5mg

Oral Administration of the IV Product:
May mix inj sol into apple or apple-grape juice for oral dosing
Usual: 1.2mg/kg up to a max 100mg dose given w/in 2 hrs before surgery

Chemotherapy-Induced Nausea/ Vomiting

Tab:
2-16 Years:
Prevention of N/V Associated w/ Moderately Emetogenic Cancer Chemotherapy, Including Initial and Repeat Courses:
1.8mg/kg w/in 1 hr before chemotherapy
Max: 100mg

DOSING CONSIDERATIONS
Elderly
Inj:
Start at lower end of dosing range

ADMINISTRATION
IV/oral route

Tab
Pediatric Patients:
In children for whom the 100mg tab is not appropriate based on weight or ability to swallow tabs, dolasetron inj sol may be mixed into apple or apple-grape juice for oral dosing.
The diluted product may be kept up to 2 hrs at room temperature before use; however, dolasetron inj sol when administered IV is contraindicated in adult and pediatric patients for the prevention of N/V associated w/ initial/repeat courses of emetogenic cancer chemotherapy.

Inj
Administration:
May be safely infused IV as rapidly as 30 sec or diluted in a compatible IV sol to 50mL and infused over a period of up to 15 min.
Do not mix w/ other drugs.
Flush infusion line before and after administration.

Stability:
After dilution, inj is stable under normal lighting conditions at room temperature for 24 hrs or under refrigeration for 48 hrs w/ the following compatible IV fluids:
0.9% NaCl inj
D5 inj
D5 and 0.45% NaCl inj
D5 and lactated Ringer's inj
Lactated Ringer's inj
10% mannitol inj

Oral Administration of the IV Product:
Diluted product may be kept up to 2 hrs at room temperature before use.

STORAGE
Inj: 20-25°C (68-77°F); excursions permitted to 15-30°C (59-86°F). Protect from light. **Tab:** 20-25°C (68-77°F). Protect from light.

HOW SUPPLIED
Inj: 20mg/mL [0.625mL, 5mL, 25mL]; **Tab:** 50mg, 100mg

CONTRAINDICATIONS
Known hypersensitivity to the drug. **Inj:** Prevention of N/V associated w/ initial and repeat courses of emetogenic cancer chemotherapy in adults and pediatric patients due to dose-dependent QT prolongation.

WARNINGS/PRECAUTIONS
QT interval prolongation (in a dose-dependent fashion) and torsades de pointes reported; avoid in patients w/ congenital long QT syndrome, hypokalemia, or hypomagnesemia. Correct hypokalemia and hypomagnesemia prior to administration and monitor these electrolytes after administration. Monitor ECG in patients w/ CHF, bradycardia, or renal impairment, and in elderly. Shown to cause dose-dependent prolongation of the PR and QRS interval and reports of 2nd- or 3rd-degree atrioventricular block, cardiac arrest, and serious ventricular arrhythmias including fatalities. Caution in patients w/ underlying structural heart disease and preexisting conduction system abnormalities, sick sinus syndrome, A-fib w/ slow ventricular response, or myocardial ischemia, and in elderly; monitor ECG in these patients. Avoid in patients w/ or at risk for complete heart block, unless implanted pacemaker is present. Serotonin syndrome reported; d/c and initiate supportive treatment if symptoms occur. **Inj:** Routine prophylaxis is not recommended in patients in whom there is little expectation that nausea and/or vomiting will occur postoperatively. Therapy is recommended in patients where N/V must be avoided postoperatively, even where the incidence of postoperative nausea and/or vomiting is low. When prophylaxis has failed, a repeat dose should not be initiated as rescue therapy.

ADVERSE REACTIONS
Inj: Headache, dizziness.
Tab: Headache, fatigue, diarrhea, bradycardia, dizziness, pain, tachycardia, dyspepsia.

DRUG INTERACTIONS
Caution w/ drugs that prolong the PR interval (eg, verapamil) and QRS interval (eg, flecainide, quinidine), diuretics w/ potential for inducing electrolyte abnormalities, antiarrhythmics or other drugs which lead to QT prolongation, cumulative high-dose anthracycline therapy, and drugs that cause hypokalemia or hypomagnesemia. May cause serotonin syndrome w/ other serotonergic drugs (eg, SSRIs, SNRIs, MAOIs, mirtazapine, fentanyl); d/c if symptoms of serotonin syndrome occur. **Inj:** Atenolol may decrease clearance of hydrodolasetron. **Oral Dolasetron:** Cimetidine may increase exposure and levels of hydrodolasetron. Rifampin may decrease exposure and levels of hydrodolasetron.

PREGNANCY AND LACTATION
Pregnancy: Category B.
Lactation: It is not known whether dolasetron mesylate is excreted in human milk. Caution in nursing.

MECHANISM OF ACTION
5-HT₃ receptor antagonist; antiemetic and antinauseant agent.

PHARMACOKINETICS
Absorption: Various age groups resulted in different parameters. (IV) T_{max}=0.6 hr (hydrodolasetron). (Tab) Well-absorbed. Absolute bioavailability (75%); T_{max}=1 hr (hydrodolasetron). **Distribution:** V_d=5.8L/kg (hydrodolasetron); plasma protein binding (69-77% hydrodolasetron). **Metabolism:** Complete. Reduction via carbonyl reductase to hydrodolasetron (active, major metabolite); CYP2D6 (hydroxylation of hydrodolasetron); CYP3A and flavin monooxygenase (N-oxidation of hydrodolasetron). **Elimination:** (IV) Urine (53%, unchanged hydrodolasetron), feces; $T_{1/2}$= <10 min, 7.3 hrs (hydrodolasetron). (Tab) Urine (61%, unchanged hydrodolasetron), feces; $T_{1/2}$=8.1 hrs (hydrodolasetron). Refer to PI for hydrodolasetron pharmacokinetic values in special and targeted patient populations.

PATIENT CONSIDERATIONS
Assessment: Assess for presence or possibility of cardiac conduction interval prolongation, renal impairment, pregnancy/nursing status, possible drug interactions, and other conditions where treatment is cautioned or contraindicated. Correct hypokalemia and hypomagnesemia prior to administration.

Monitoring: Monitor for QT/PR/QRS interval prolongation, torsades de pointes, serotonin syndrome, and other adverse reactions. Monitor ECG in patients w/ CHF, bradycardia or renal impairment; at risk for cardiac conduction interval prolongation; or who are elderly. Monitor serum electrolytes (K⁺, Mg²⁺).

Counseling: Inform about potential benefits/risks of therapy. Inform that drug may cause serious cardiac arrhythmias; instruct patients to contact physician immediately if they perceive a change in their HR, feel lightheaded, or have a syncopal episode. Inform that chances of developing severe cardiac arrhythmias are higher in patients w/ a personal/family history of abnormal heart rhythms; personal history of sick sinus syndrome; atrial fibrillation w/ slow ventricular response or myocardial ischemia; taking medications that may prolong PR interval, QRS interval, or that may cause electrolyte abnormalities; w/ hypokalemia or hypomagnesemia; or who are elderly. Advise of the possibility of serotonin syndrome w/ concomitant use w/ another serotonergic agent such as medications to treat depression and migraines; instruct to seek immediate medical attention if changes in mental status, autonomic instability, and neuromuscular symptoms w/ or w/o GI symptoms occur.

APIDRA — insulin glulisine (rDNA origin)   Rx
Class: Insulin (rapid-acting)

OTHER BRAND NAMES
Apidra Solostar

ADULT DOSAGE
Diabetes Mellitus
Total Daily Insulin Requirement:
Usual: 0.5-1 U/kg/day; give SQ w/in 15 min ac or w/in 20 min after starting a meal
IV:
Use at concentrations of 0.05-1 U/mL in infusion systems using polyvinyl chloride bags

PEDIATRIC DOSAGE
Type 1 Diabetes Mellitus
≥4 Years:
Total Daily Insulin Requirement:
Usual: 0.5-1 U/kg/day; give SQ w/in 15 min ac or w/in 20 min after starting a meal

DOSING CONSIDERATIONS
Renal Impairment
May require dose reduction
Hepatic Impairment
May require dose reduction

ADMINISTRATION
SQ/IV route
SQ
Inject SQ in the abdominal wall, thigh, or upper arm; rotate inj sites w/in the same region.
Use w/ an intermediate or long-acting insulin.
Do not mix w/ insulin preparations other than NPH insulin; if mixed w/ NPH insulin, draw Apidra into syringe 1st, and inject mixture immediately after mixing.

Continuous SQ Insulin Infusion by External Pump
Read the pump label to make sure the pump has been evaluated w/ Apidra.
Administer by continuous SQ infusion in the abdominal wall by an external insulin pump; rotate infusion sites w/in the same region.
Must have an alternative insulin delivery system in case of pump system failure.
Do not mix w/ other insulins.

IV
Do not mix w/ other insulins
Stable only in 0.9% NaCl

STORAGE
Unopened: 2-8°C (36-46°F). Do not freeze; discard if frozen. Protect from light.
Must be used within 28 days if not stored in a refrigerator. Open (In-Use): <25°C (77°F). Discard after 28 days. Protect from direct heat and light. Do not refrigerate opened (in-use) SoloStar. Discard infusion sets and insulin in reservoir after 48 hrs of use or after exposure to temperatures >37°C (98.6°F). Prepared Infusion Bags: Room temperature for 48 hrs.

HOW SUPPLIED
Inj: 100 U/mL [3mL, SoloStar; 10mL, vial]

CONTRAINDICATIONS
During episodes of hypoglycemia, known hypersensitivity to Apidra or its excipients.

WARNINGS/PRECAUTIONS
Insulin pens must never be shared between patients; poses a risk for transmission of blood-borne pathogens. Any change in insulin regimen should be made cautiously and only under medical supervision. Changes in insulin strength, manufacturer, type, or method of administration may result in the need for a change in dosage or adjustment in concomitant oral antidiabetic treatment. Insulin requirements may be altered during stress, major illness, or w/ changes in exercise, meal patterns, or coadministered drugs. Hypoglycemia may occur and may impair ability to concentrate and react; caution in patients w/ hypoglycemia unawareness and in those predisposed to hypoglycemia. Severe, life-threatening, generalized allergy, including anaphylaxis, may occur. Hypokalemia may occur; caution in patients who may be at risk. May be administered IV under medical supervision w/ close monitoring of glucose and K⁺ levels to avoid potentially fatal hypoglycemia and hypokalemia. Malfunction of insulin pump or infusion set, handling errors, or insulin degradation can rapidly lead to hyperglycemia, ketosis, and diabetic ketoacidosis; prompt identification/correction of the cause is necessary and interim SQ inj may be required. Train patients using CSII pump therapy how to administer by inj and have alternate insulin therapy available. Caution in elderly.

ADVERSE REACTIONS
Allergic reactions, infusion-site reactions, hypoglycemia, influenza, nasopharyngitis, URTI, arthralgia, HTN, headache, peripheral edema.

DRUG INTERACTIONS
Dose adjustment and close monitoring may be necessary w/ drugs that may increase blood-glucose-lowering effect and susceptibility to hypoglycemia (eg, oral antidiabetic products, pramlintide, ACE inhibitors), drugs that may reduce blood-glucose-lowering effect (eg, corticosteroids, danazol, niacin), or drugs that may either increase or decrease blood-glucose-lowering effect (eg, β-blockers, clonidine, lithium salts, alcohol). Pentamidine may cause hypoglycemia, sometimes followed by hyperglycemia. Hypoglycemic signs may be reduced or absent w/ antiadrenergic drugs (eg, β-blockers, clonidine, guanethidine, reserpine). Caution w/ K⁺-lowering drugs and drugs sensitive to serum K⁺ levels. Concomitant use w/ thiazolidinediones (TZDs) may cause dose-related fluid retention and heart failure (HF); observe for signs/symptoms of HF and consider dose reduction or discontinuation of TZDs if HF occurs.

PREGNANCY AND LACTATION
Category C, caution in nursing.

MECHANISM OF ACTION
Insulin glulisine (rDNA origin); regulates glucose metabolism. Lowers blood glucose by stimulating peripheral glucose uptake by skeletal muscle and fat, and by inhibiting hepatic glucose production. Also inhibits lipolysis and proteolysis, and enhances protein synthesis.

PHARMACOKINETICS
Absorption: (SQ) Absolute bioavailability (70%); (0.15 U/kg, 0.2 U/kg) C_{max}= 83 microU/mL, 84 microU/mL (median); T_{max}=60 min (median), 100 min (median). **Distribution:** (IV) V_d=13L. **Elimination:** (SQ, IV) $T_{1/2}$=42 min, 13 min.

PATIENT CONSIDERATIONS
Assessment: Assess for predisposition to hypoglycemia, risk of hypokalemia, hypersensitivity to drug or to any of its excipients, renal/hepatic impairment, pregnancy/nursing status, and possible drug interactions. Obtain baseline blood glucose and HbA1c levels.

Monitoring: Monitor for signs/symptoms of hypoglycemia, hypokalemia, allergic reactions, and other adverse reactions. Monitor blood glucose, HbA1c levels, and renal/hepatic function. Frequent glucose monitoring may be required w/ renal/hepatic impairment. Monitor glucose and K⁺ levels frequently during IV administration.

Counseling: Advise never to share insulin pen w/ another person, even if needle is changed. Counsel on self-management procedures including glucose monitoring, proper inj technique, and management of hypo/hyperglycemia. Instruct on handling of special situations (eg, intercurrent conditions, inadequate or skipped dose, inadvertent administration of increased dose, inadequate food intake, skipped meals). Advise to inform physician if pregnant or contemplating pregnancy. Instruct to always check the label before each inj to avoid medication errors. Instruct on how to use an external infusion pump.

APLENZIN — bupropion hydrobromide   Rx
Class: Aminoketone

Antidepressants increased the risk of suicidal thoughts and behavior in children, adolescents, and young adults in short-term trials. Monitor closely for worsening, and for emergence of suicidal thoughts and behaviors. Serious neuropsychiatric reactions reported in patients taking bupropion for smoking cessation; not approved for smoking cessation. Observe all patients for neuropsychiatric reactions.

ADULT DOSAGE

Major Depressive Disorder

Initial: 174mg qam
Titrate: May increase to target dose of 348mg qam after 4 days

Periodically reassess need for maint treatment and the appropriate dose for such treatment

Seasonal Affective Disorder

Prevention of seasonal major depressive episodes in patients w/ seasonal affective disorder

Initial: 174mg qam
Titrate: May increase to target dose of 348mg qam after 7 days

Initiate treatment in the autumn, prior to the onset of depressive symptoms, and continue through the winter season. Taper and d/c therapy in early spring

Individualize timing of initiation and treatment duration

Conversions

Equivalent Daily Doses of Aplenzin and Bupropion HCl:
522mg Aplenzin: 450mg bupropion HCl
348mg Aplenzin: 300mg bupropion HCl
174mg Aplenzin: 150mg bupropion HCl

Dosing Considerations with MAOIs

Switching to/from an MAOI Antidepressant:
Allow at least 14 days between discontinuation of an MAOI and initiation of treatment and allow at least 14 days between discontinuation of treatment and initiation of an MAOI

W/ Reversible MAOIs (eg, Linezolid, IV Methylene Blue):
Do not start Aplenzin in a patient being treated w/ a reversible MAOI. In patients already receiving Aplenzin, if acceptable alternatives are not available and benefits outweigh risks, d/c Aplenzin promptly and administer linezolid or IV methylene blue; monitor for 2 weeks or until 24 hrs after the last dose of linezolid or IV methylene blue, whichever comes 1st. May resume Aplenzin therapy 24 hrs after the last dose of linezolid or IV methylene blue

---

DOSING CONSIDERATIONS

Renal Impairment
GFR <90mL/min:
Consider reducing dose and/or frequency

Hepatic Impairment
Mild (Child-Pugh Score 5-6):
Consider reducing dose and/or frequency

Moderate to Severe (Child-Pugh Score 7-15):
Max: 174mg qod

Discontinuation
Patients Treated w/ 348mg/day:
Decrease dose to 174mg qd prior to discontinuation

ADMINISTRATION
Oral route

Swallow whole; do not crush, divide, or chew.
Administer in the am.
May be taken w/ or w/o regard to meals.

STORAGE
25°C (77°F); excursions permitted to 15-30°C (59-86°F).

HOW SUPPLIED
Tab, Extended-Release: 174mg, 348mg, 522mg

CONTRAINDICATIONS
Seizure disorder or current/prior diagnosis of bulimia or anorexia nervosa. Patients undergoing abrupt discontinuation of alcohol, benzodiazepines, barbiturates, and antiepileptic drugs. Known hypersensitivity to bupropion or other ingredients of the medication. Use of MAOIs (intended to treat psychiatric disorders) either concomitantly or w/in 14 days of discontinuing treatment. Treatment w/in 14 days of discontinuing treatment w/ an MAOI. Starting treatment in patients being treated w/ reversible MAOIs (eg, linezolid, IV methylene blue).

PEDIATRIC DOSAGE
Pediatric use may not have been established

WARNINGS/PRECAUTIONS
Dose-related risk of seizures; do not exceed 522mg qd, and gradually increase dose. D/C and do not restart treatment if seizure occurs. Contraindicated in patients w/ conditions that increase the risk of seizure (eg, severe head injury, arteriovenous malformation, CNS tumor or CNS infection, severe stroke). May result in elevated BP and HTN. May precipitate a manic, mixed, or hypomanic manic episode; not approved for treatment of bipolar depression. Neuropsychiatric signs and symptoms (eg, delusions, hallucinations, psychosis, concentration disturbance) reported; d/c if these reactions occur. Pupillary dilation that occurs following use may trigger an angle-closure attack in a patient w/ anatomically narrow angles who does not have a patent iridectomy. D/C treatment if an allergic or anaphylactoid/anaphylactic reaction occurs. Arthralgia, myalgia, fever w/ rash, and other symptoms of serum sickness suggestive of delayed hypersensitivity reported. Caution in elderly. False (+) urine immunoassay screening tests for amphetamines reported.

ADVERSE REACTIONS
Dry mouth, nausea, insomnia, dizziness, pharyngitis, abdominal pain, agitation, anxiety, tremor, palpitation, sweating, tinnitus, myalgia, anorexia, urinary frequency.

DRUG INTERACTIONS
See Contraindications. CYP2B6 inhibitors (eg, ticlopidine, clopidogrel) may increase bupropion exposure but decrease hydroxybupropion exposure; dose adjustment of bupropion may be necessary. CYP2B6 inducers (eg, ritonavir, lopinavir, efavirenz) may decrease bupropion and hydroxybupropion exposure; may need to increase bupropion dose. Other CYP inducers (eg, carbamazepine, phenobarbital, phenytoin) may decrease bupropion exposure; may need to increase bupropion dose. May increase exposure of CYP2D6 substrates (eg, venlafaxine, haloperidol, metoprolol, propafenone); may need to decrease the dose of CYP2D6 substrates, particularly for drugs w/ a narrow therapeutic index. May reduce efficacy of drugs that require metabolic activation by CYP2D6 to be effective (eg, tamoxifen); may require increased doses of the drug when used concomitantly w/ bupropion. Use extreme caution w/ other drugs that lower the seizure threshold (eg, other bupropion products, antipsychotics, antidepressants, theophylline, systemic corticosteroids); use low initial doses of bupropion and increase the dose gradually. Increased risk of seizure w/ use of illicit drugs (eg, cocaine); abuse/misuse of prescription drugs (eg, CNS stimulants); oral hypoglycemic drugs or insulin; use of anorectic drugs; or excessive use of benzodiazepines, sedative/hypnotics, or opiates. CNS toxicity reported when coadministered w/ levodopa or amantadine; use w/ caution. Adverse neuropsychiatric events or reduced alcohol tolerance reported during treatment; minimize or avoid alcohol consumption. Altered PT and/or INR, associated w/ hemorrhagic or thrombotic complication, reported w/ warfarin.

PREGNANCY AND LACTATION
Pregnancy: Category C.
Lactation: Bupropion and its metabolites are present in human milk; caution in nursing.

MECHANISM OF ACTION
Aminoketone antidepressant; mechanism not established. Relatively weak inhibitor of the neuronal uptake of norepinephrine and dopamine. Presumed that action is mediated by noradrenergic and/or dopaminergic mechanisms.

PHARMACOKINETICS
Absorption: C_{max}=134.3ng/mL; AUC=1409ng•hr/mL; T_{max}=5 hrs (median), 6 hrs (hydroxybupropion). **Distribution:** Plasma protein binding (84%); found in breast milk. **Metabolism:** Extensive. Hydroxylation (CYP2B6) and reduction of carbonyl group; hydroxybupropion, threohydrobupropion, and erythrohydrobupropion (active metabolites). **Elimination:** Urine (87%), feces (10%), (0.5% unchanged); $T_{1/2}$=21.3 hrs, 24.3 hrs (hydroxybupropion), 31.1 hrs (erythrohydrobupropion), 50.8 hrs (threohydrobupropion).

PATIENT CONSIDERATIONS
Assessment: Assess for seizure disorders or conditions that may increase risk of seizure, bipolar disorder or risk factors for bipolar disorder, susceptibility to angle-closure glaucoma, hypersensitivity to bupropion or other ingredients of the medication, hepatic/renal impairment, any other conditions where treatment is contraindicated or cautioned, pregnancy/nursing status, and possible drug interactions. Obtain baseline BP.

Monitoring: Monitor for clinical worsening, suicidality, or unusual changes in behavior, seizures, activation of mania or hypomania, neuropsychiatric signs/symptoms, angle-closure glaucoma, anaphylactoid/anaphylactic reactions, delayed hypersensitivity reactions, and other adverse reactions. Monitor hepatic/renal function and BP.

Counseling: Inform about benefits/risks of therapy. Advise patients and caregivers of need for close observation for clinical worsening, suicidality, or unusual changes in behavior. Inform that product contains same active ingredient found in Zyban. Educate on the symptoms of hypersensitivity and advise to d/c if a severe allergic reaction occurs. Instruct to d/c and not restart if a seizure occurs while on therapy. Inform that excessive use or abrupt discontinuation of alcohol, benzodiazepines, antiepileptic drugs, or sedative/hypnotics may increase seizure risk; advise to minimize or avoid alcohol use. Caution about risk of angle-closure glaucoma. Inform that therapy may impair mental/physical abilities; advise to refrain from operating hazardous machinery/driving until effects of therapy are known. Instruct to notify physician if taking/planning to take any prescription or OTC medications. Advise to contact physician if pregnancy occurs or is intended during therapy.

APOKYN — apomorphine hydrochloride   Rx

Class: Dopamine receptor agonist

ADULT DOSAGE

Parkinson's Disease

Acute, intermittent treatment of hypomobility, "off" episodes ("end-of-dose wearing off" and unpredictable "on/off" episodes) in patients w/ advanced Parkinson's disease

Initial Test Dose:
0.2mL (2mg); begin dosing when patients are in an "off" state
Check both supine and standing BP and pulse predose and at 20, 40, and 60 min postdose (and after 60 min, if there is significant hypotension at 60 min)
If significant orthostatic hypotension develops in response to test dose, do not consider patients candidates for treatment

If Initial Test Dose Tolerated:
Initial: 0.2mL (2mg) prn to treat recurring "off" episodes
Titrate: Increase in increments of 0.1mL (1mg) every few days, if needed, on an outpatient basis

Subsequent Dosing:
Determine that patient needs and tolerates a higher test dose (0.3mL [3mg] or 0.4mL [4mg]), under close medical supervision; outpatient dosing trial may follow using a dose 0.1mL (1mg) lower than the tolerated test dose

If Patient Tolerates 0.2mL (2mg) Test Dose but Responds Inadequately:
May administer 0.4mL (4mg) at the next observed "off" period (at least 2 hrs after initial test dose)

If Patient Tolerates and Responds to 0.4mL (4mg) Test Dose:
Initial Maint: 0.3mL (3mg) prn to treat recurring "off" episodes
Titrate: May increase in 0.1mL (1mg) increments every few days, if needed, on an outpatient basis

If Patient Does Not Tolerate 0.4mL (4mg) Test Dose:
May administer 0.3mL (3mg) during a separate "off" period (at least 2 hrs after the previous dose)

If Patient Tolerates 0.3mL (3mg) Test Dose:
Initial Maint: 0.2mL (2mg) prn to treat existing "off" episodes
Titrate: May increase to 0.3mL (3mg) after a few days, if needed and if the 0.2mL (2mg) dose is tolerated; do not increase to 0.4mL (4mg) on an outpatient basis in such patients

Max: 0.6mL (6mg)/dose

Re-treatment and Interruption in Therapy:
If a single dose of therapy is ineffective for a particular "off" period, do not give a 2nd dose for that "off" episode
Do not administer a repeat dose sooner than 2 hrs after last dose
If therapy is interrupted for >1 week, restart on 0.2mL (2mg) dose and gradually titrate to effect and tolerability

Premedication

Initiate therapy w/ a concomitant antiemetic; oral trimethobenzamide (300mg tid) should be started 3 days prior to initial dose and continued at least during the first 2 months of therapy

PEDIATRIC DOSAGE

Pediatric use may not have been established

DOSING CONSIDERATIONS

Renal Impairment
Mild/Moderate: Reduce test dose and starting dose to 0.1mL (1mg)

Hepatic Impairment
Mild/Moderate: Closely monitor

ADMINISTRATION

SQ route
Administer only by a multiple-dose pen w/ supplied cartridges
Initial dose and dose titrations should be performed by a healthcare provider
Rotate inj site

STORAGE

25°C (77°F); excursions permitted to 15-30°C (59-86°F).

HOW SUPPLIED

Inj: 10mg/mL [3mL]

CONTRAINDICATIONS

Concomitant use w/ 5HT3 antagonists, including antiemetics (eg, ondansetron, granisetron, dolasetron, palonosetron) and alosetron; hypersensitivity to apomorphine and its excipients, including sulfite (eg, sodium metabisulfite).

WARNINGS/PRECAUTIONS

Serious adverse reactions (eg, thrombus formation, pulmonary embolism) following IV use reported; not for IV administration. N/V, syncope, orthostatic hypotension, and falling reported. Falling asleep during activities of daily living may occur; d/c if daytime sleepiness or episodes of falling asleep develop. May impair mental/physical abilities. Hallucinations/psychotic-like behavior reported; avoid w/ major psychotic disorder. May cause or worsen dyskinesias. May cause intense urges to gamble, increased sexual urges, intense urges to spend money uncontrollably, and other intense urges and the inability to control these urges while on therapy; consider dose reduction or discontinuation of therapy. Coronary events (eg, angina, MI, cardiac arrest, sudden death) reported; caution w/ known cardiovascular (CV)/cerebrovascular disease. May prolong the QT interval and increase potential for proarrhythmic effects; caution w/ hypokalemia, hypomagnesemia, bradycardia, or genetic predisposition (eg, congenital prolongation of the QT interval). Monitor for withdrawal-emergent hyperpyrexia and confusion, fibrotic complications (eg, retroperitoneal fibrosis, pulmonary infiltrates, pleural effusion/thickening, cardiac valvulopathy), and melanoma. May cause priapism. Potential for abuse.

ADVERSE REACTIONS

Yawning, dyskinesia, N/V, somnolence, dizziness, rhinorrhea, hallucinations, edema, chest pain, inj-site reaction, fall, arthralgia, insomnia, headache, depression.

DRUG INTERACTIONS

See Contraindications. Antihypertensives and vasodilators may increase risk of hypotension, MI, serious pneumonia, serious falls, and bone and joint injuries. Dopamine antagonists, such as neuroleptics (eg, phenothiazines, butyrophenones, thioxanthenes) or metoclopramide, may diminish effectiveness. Caution w/ drugs that prolong QT/QTc interval. May increase drowsiness w/ sedating medications. Avoid w/ alcohol.

PREGNANCY AND LACTATION

Category C, not for use in nursing.

MECHANISM OF ACTION

Non-ergoline dopamine agonist; not established, suspected to stimulate postsynaptic dopamine D_2-type receptors w/in the caudate-putamen in the brain.

PHARMACOKINETICS

Absorption: Rapid; T_{max}=10-60 min. **Distribution:** V_d=218L. **Metabolism:** Sulfation, N-demethylation, glucuronidation, and oxidation. **Elimination:** $T_{1/2}$=40 min.

PATIENT CONSIDERATIONS

Assessment: Assess for hypersensitivity to the drug, sulfite sensitivity, asthma, risk for QT prolongation, history of psychotic disorders, CV/cerebrovascular disease, dyskinesia, hepatic/renal impairment, pregnancy/nursing status, and possible drug interactions. Obtain baseline BP (supine and standing position).

Monitoring: Monitor for N/V, syncope, QT/QTc interval prolongation and other proarrhythmic effects, hypotension, hallucinations/psychotic-like behavior, coronary/cerebral ischemia, dyskinesia (or exacerbation), impulse control/compulsive behaviors, hepatic/renal impairment, withdrawal-emergent hyperpyrexia and confusion, fibrotic complications, priapism, and other adverse reactions. Perform periodic skin exams to monitor for melanomas. Monitor BP closely.

Counseling: Instruct to use only as prescribed. Instruct to rotate the inj site and observe proper aseptic technique. Inform of the potential risks and benefits of therapy. Inform that hypersensitivity/allergic reaction may occur; advise patients to avoid taking the drug again if a reaction occurs. Advise not to drive a car or engage in any other potentially dangerous activities while on treatment. Advise to limit alcohol intake. Alert patients that they may have increased risk for falling when using the drug. Inform of the potential for hallucinations, psychotic-like behavior, hypotension, sedating effects including somnolence and the possibility of falling asleep, coronary events, dyskinesias, and other adverse events. Instruct to rise slowly after sitting or lying down after taking the drug. Advise to inform physician if new or increased gambling urges, increased sexual urges, or other intense urges develop while on treatment. Instruct to notify physician if pregnancy occurs, or if intending to become pregnant and/or breastfeed.

APRISO — mesalamine   Rx

Class: 5-aminosalicylic acid derivative

ADULT DOSAGE	PEDIATRIC DOSAGE
Ulcerative Colitis	Pediatric use may not have been established
Maint of Remission:	
1.5g (4 caps) qam	

ADMINISTRATION
Oral route

May be taken w/o regard to meals.

STORAGE
20-25°C (68-77°F); excursions permitted between 15-30°C (59-86°F).

HOW SUPPLIED
Cap, Extended-Release: 0.375g

CONTRAINDICATIONS
Hypersensitivity to salicylates, aminosalicylates, or any of the components of this medication.

WARNINGS/PRECAUTIONS
Renal impairment, including minimal change nephropathy, acute and chronic interstitial nephritis, and, rarely, renal failure, reported; caution w/ renal dysfunction or history of renal disease. Evaluate renal function prior to initiation of therapy and periodically thereafter. May cause acute intolerance syndrome (eg, acute abdominal pain, cramping, bloody diarrhea) that may be difficult to distinguish from a flare of inflammatory bowel disease; d/c if suspected. Hepatic failure reported in patients w/ preexisting liver disease; caution w/ liver disease. Caution w/ sulfasalazine hypersensitivity and in elderly.

ADVERSE REACTIONS
Headache, diarrhea, upper abdominal pain, nausea, nasopharyngitis, influenza/influenza-like illness, sinusitis.

DRUG INTERACTIONS
Avoid w/ antacids.

PREGNANCY AND LACTATION
Pregnancy: Category B.
Lactation: Caution in nursing.

MECHANISM OF ACTION
5-aminosalicylic acid; has not been established. Suspected to diminish inflammation by blocking production of arachidonic acid metabolites.

PHARMACOKINETICS
Absorption: (Single dose) T_{max}=4 hrs, C_{max}=2.1mcg/mL, AUC_{0-24}=11mcg·h/mL, AUC_{0-inf}=14mcg·h/mL. Refer to PI for parameters using multiple doses and of major metabolite. **Distribution:** Plasma protein binding (43%); crosses placenta; found in breast milk. **Metabolism:** Liver and intestinal mucosa; N-acetyl-5-aminosalicylic acid (major metabolite). **Elimination:** Urine (2% unchanged; 30% N-acetyl-5-aminosalicylic acid); $T_{1/2}$=9-10 hrs.

PATIENT CONSIDERATIONS
Assessment: Assess for previous hypersensitivity to sulfasalazine or salicylates, history of or known renal/hepatic dysfunction, phenylketonuria, pregnancy/nursing status, and possible drug interactions. Evaluate renal function prior to initiation of therapy.

Monitoring: Monitor for renal impairment, hepatic failure, acute intolerance syndrome, and hypersensitivity reactions. Perform periodic monitoring of renal function and blood cell counts (in elderly).

Counseling: Inform patients w/ phenylketonuria or their caregivers that each cap contains aspartame. Instruct not to take w/ antacids. Instruct to contact a healthcare provider if symptoms of ulcerative colitis worsen.

APTENSIO XR — methylphenidate hydrochloride   CII

Class: CNS stimulant

> **High potential for abuse and dependence. Assess the risk of abuse prior to prescribing, and monitor for signs of abuse and dependence while on therapy.**

ADULT DOSAGE	PEDIATRIC DOSAGE
Attention-Deficit Hyperactivity Disorder	**Attention-Deficit Hyperactivity Disorder**
Initial: 10mg qam	**≥6 Years:**
Titrate: May titrate weekly in increments of 10mg	**Initial:** 10mg qam
Max: 60mg/day	**Titrate:** May titrate weekly in increments of 10mg
D/C if no improvement observed after appropriate dosage adjustment over 1 month	**Max:** 60mg/day
	D/C if no improvement observed after appropriate dosage adjustment over 1 month

DOSING CONSIDERATIONS
Elderly
Start at lower end of dosing range

Adverse Reactions
Reduce dose or, if necessary, d/c if paradoxical aggravation of symptoms or other adverse events occur

ADMINISTRATION
Oral route

Take w/ or w/o food; establish a routine pattern w/ regard to meals.
Caps may be swallowed whole or opened and the entire contents sprinkled onto applesauce.
Consume sprinkled applesauce immediately w/o chewing the sprinkled beads.
Do not divide the dose of a single cap or take anything <1 cap/day.

STORAGE
20-25°C (68-77°F). Protect from moisture.

HOW SUPPLIED
Cap, Extended-Release: 10mg, 15mg, 20mg, 30mg, 40mg, 50mg, 60mg

CONTRAINDICATIONS
Hypersensitivity to methylphenidate or other components of the product, concomitant use w/ an MAOI or w/in 14 days following discontinuation of an MAOI.

WARNINGS/PRECAUTIONS
Sudden death, stroke, and MI reported in adults w/ CNS stimulants. Sudden death reported in pediatric patients w/ structural cardiac abnormalities and other serious heart problems taking CNS stimulants. Avoid w/ known structural cardiac abnormalities, cardiomyopathy, serious heart arrhythmia, coronary artery disease, or other serious heart problems. May increase BP and HR. May exacerbate symptoms of behavior disturbance and thought disorder in patients w/ a preexisting psychotic disorder. May induce a manic or mixed episode in patients w/ bipolar disorder. May cause psychotic or manic symptoms in patients w/o a prior history of psychotic illness or mania; consider discontinuation. Priapism reported; seek immediate medical attention. Associated w/ peripheral vasculopathy, including Raynaud's phenomenon; monitor for digital changes. May cause weight loss and long-term suppression of growth in pediatric patients; may need to interrupt treatment in patients not growing or gaining height or weight as expected.

ADVERSE REACTIONS
Abdominal pain, pyrexia, headache, decreased appetite, insomnia, N/V.

DRUG INTERACTIONS
See Contraindications. Avoid alcohol; may result in more rapid release of the dose of methylphenidate.

PREGNANCY AND LACTATION
Pregnancy: Can cause vasoconstriction and thereby decrease placental perfusion. Premature delivery and low birth weight infants reported in amphetamine-dependent mothers.
Lactation: Found in breast milk; caution in nursing. Monitor breastfeeding infants for adverse reactions.

MECHANISM OF ACTION
Sympathomimetic amine; CNS stimulant. Thought to block the reuptake of norepinephrine and dopamine into the presynaptic neuron and increase the release of these monoamines into the extraneuronal space.

PHARMACOKINETICS
Absorption: (80mg) C_{max}=23.47ng/mL (cap), 21.78ng/mL (sprinkle); T_{max}=2 hrs (median); AUC=258.1ng·hr/mL (cap), 258ng·hr/mL (sprinkle). **Distribution:** Found in breast milk. **Metabolism:** Deesterification to α-phenyl-piperidine acetic acid [PPAA] (metabolite). **Elimination:** Urine (90%, approx 80% PPAA); (80mg) $T_{1/2}$=5.09 hrs (cap), 5.43 hrs (sprinkle).

PATIENT CONSIDERATIONS
Assessment: Assess for drug hypersensitivity, cardiac problems/disease, psychotic disorders, bipolar disorder, pregnancy/nursing status, and for possible drug interactions. Obtain baseline height/weight in children. Screen patients for risk factors for developing a manic episode and the risk of abuse before starting therapy.

Monitoring: Monitor for stroke, MI, HTN, tachycardia, exacerbations of behavior disturbances and thought disorders, psychotic or manic symptoms, digital changes, priapism, and other adverse reactions. Monitor growth in children. Monitor for signs of abuse and dependence. Periodically reevaluate the need for use.

Counseling: Inform about risks, benefits, and appropriate use of treatment. Counsel that drug has potential for abuse or dependence. Instruct to keep medication in a safe place to prevent abuse. Advise of the potential for serious cardiovascular risks, including sudden death, MI, stroke, and HTN. Instruct to contact physician immediately if symptoms, such as exertional chest pain, unexplained syncope, or other symptoms suggestive of cardiac disease develop. Advise that the drug can elevate BP and pulse rate, can cause psychotic or manic symptoms even in patients w/o a prior history of psychotic symptoms or mania, and in pediatric patients can cause slowing of growth and weight loss. Advise of the possibility of priapism. Instruct to seek immediate medical attention in the event of priapism. Inform about the risk of peripheral vasculopathy, including Raynaud's phenomenon. Instruct to report to the physician any new numbness, pain, skin color change, sensitivity to temperature in fingers or toes, and any signs of unexplained wounds appearing on fingers or toes. Advise to avoid alcohol while taking therapy.

APTIOM — eslicarbazepine acetate   Rx

Class: Dibenzazepine

ADULT DOSAGE
Partial Onset Seizures

Monotherapy or Adjunctive Therapy:
Initial: 400mg qd; may initiate at 800mg qd if need for additional seizure reduction outweighs increased risk of adverse reactions during initiation
Titrate: Increase in weekly increments of 400-600mg, based on response/tolerability
Maint: 800-1600mg qd

For patients on monotherapy, consider the 800mg qd maint dose in patients who are unable to tolerate a 1200mg daily dose
For patients on adjunctive therapy, consider the 1600mg daily dose in patients who did not achieve a satisfactory response w/ a 1200mg daily dose

PEDIATRIC DOSAGE
Pediatric use may not have been established

DOSING CONSIDERATIONS
Concomitant Medications
Carbamazepine: Dose of eslicarbazepine or carbamazepine may need to be adjusted
Other Enzyme-Inducing Antiepileptic Drugs: May need higher doses of eslicarbazepine
Oxcarbazepine: Do not administer eslicarbazepine as an adjunctive therapy w/ oxcarbazepine
Renal Impairment
Moderate and Severe (CrCl <50mL/min): Reduce the initial, titration, and maint doses by 50%; titration and maint doses may be adjusted according to clinical response
Hepatic Impairment
Severe: Not recommended
Discontinuation
Reduce dose gradually and avoid abrupt discontinuation

ADMINISTRATION
Oral route
Administer as whole or crushed tabs.
Take w/ or w/o food.

STORAGE
20-25°C (68-77°F); excursions permitted to 15-30°C (59-86°F).

HOW SUPPLIED
Tab: 200mg*, 400mg, 600mg*, 800mg* *scored

CONTRAINDICATIONS
Hypersensitivity to eslicarbazepine acetate or oxcarbazepine.

WARNINGS/PRECAUTIONS
Increased risk of suicidal thoughts or behavior; monitor for emergence/worsening of depression, suicidal thoughts or behavior, and/or any unusual changes in mood or behavior. Serious dermatological reactions (eg, Stevens-Johnson syndrome) reported; d/c use if dermatologic reaction develops, unless the reaction is not drug related. Drug reaction w/ eosinophilia and systemic symptoms (DRESS), also known as multiorgan hypersensitivity, reported; evaluate immediately if signs/symptoms of hypersensitivity (eg, fever, lymphadenopathy) are present and d/c if alternative etiology cannot be established. Anaphylaxis and angioedema reported; d/c if any of these reactions develop. Avoid in patients w/ prior dermatological reaction, DRESS reaction, or anaphylactic-type reaction w/ either the drug or oxcarbazepine. Consider measuring serum Na+ and Cl- levels during maintenance treatment; clinically significant hyponatremia w/ concurrent hypochloremia may develop, requiring dose reduction/discontinuation. Associated w/ dose-related increases in adverse reactions related to dizziness and disturbance in gait and coordination, somnolence and fatigue, cognitive dysfunction, and visual changes. May impair mental/physical abilities. Withdraw gradually due to risk of increased seizure frequency and status epilepticus. Hepatic effects reported; d/c in patients w/ jaundice or other evidence of significant liver injury. Dose-dependent decreases in serum T3 and T4 (free and total) observed. Caution in elderly.

ADVERSE REACTIONS
Dizziness, somnolence, N/V, headache, diplopia, fatigue, vertigo, ataxia, blurred vision, tremor.

DRUG INTERACTIONS
See Dosing Considerations. Greater incidence of dizziness reported w/ the concomitant use of carbamazepine. Several antiepileptic drugs (eg, carbamazepine, phenobarbital, phenytoin, primidone) can induce enzymes that metabolize eslicarbazepine and can cause decreased plasma concentrations. May increase levels of CYP2C19 substrates (eg, phenytoin, clobazam, omeprazole). Monitor plasma phenytoin concentration; in epilepsy, dose adjustment may be needed based on clinical response and serum levels of phenytoin. May decrease levels of CYP3A4 substrates (eg, simvastatin). Adjust dose of simvastatin or rosuvastatin if a clinically significant change in lipids is noted. May decrease levels of oral contraceptives (eg, ethinyl estradiol, levonorgestrel); use additional or alternative nonhormonal birth control. Monitor to maintain INR in patients on warfarin.

PREGNANCY AND LACTATION
Pregnancy: Category C. Physicians are advised to recommend that pregnant patients enroll in the North American Antiepileptic Drug Pregnancy Registry.
Lactation: Not for use in nursing.
Reproductive Potential: Females of reproductive potential should use additional or alternative nonhormonal birth control.

MECHANISM OF ACTION
Dibenzazepine; has not been established. Thought to involve inhibition of voltage-gated Na+ channels.

PHARMACOKINETICS
Absorption: T_{max}=1-4 hrs (post-dose). **Distribution:** Found in breast milk. V_d=61L; plasma protein binding (<40%). **Metabolism:** Rapid and extensive by hydrolytic 1st pass metabolism to eslicarbazepine (major active metabolite); (R)-licarbazepine and oxcarbazepine (minor active metabolites). **Elimination:** Urine (90% metabolites; 2/3 unchanged, 1/3 glucuronide conjugate, and 10% minor metabolites); $T_{1/2}$=13-20 hrs.

PATIENT CONSIDERATIONS
Assessment: Assess for history of hypersensitivity to the drug or oxcarbazepine, renal/hepatic impairment, pregnancy/nursing status, and possible drug interactions.

Monitoring: Monitor for suicidal thoughts or behavior, any unusual changes in mood or behavior, dermatologic reactions, multiorgan hypersensitivity reaction, hyponatremia, anaphylaxis, angioedema, dizziness, disturbance in gait and coordination, somnolence, fatigue, cognitive dysfunction, visual changes; and other adverse reactions. Monitor Na+ and Cl- levels. Monitor to maintain INR in patients on warfarin.

Counseling: Inform of the availability of a Medication Guide and instruct to read the Medication Guide prior to treatment. Instruct to take ud. Advise of the need to be alert for the emergence/worsening of symptoms of depression, any unusual changes in mood/behavior, or the emergence of suicidal thoughts, behavior, or thoughts about self-harm; instruct to immediately report behaviors of concern to physician. Educate about signs/symptoms of a skin reaction; instruct to consult physician immediately if a skin reaction occurs. Inform that a fever associated w/ signs of other organ system involvement may be drug-related; instruct to contact physician immediately if such signs/symptoms occur. Instruct to d/c and contact physician immediately if signs/symptoms suggesting angioedema develop. Advise to report symptoms of low Na+ to physician. Inform that drug may cause dizziness, gait disturbance, somnolence/fatigue, cognitive dysfunction, and visual changes; advise not to drive or operate machinery until effects have been determined. Instruct not to d/c use w/o consulting physician. Recommend female patients of childbearing age to use additional or alternative nonhormonal forms of contraception during treatment and after treatment has been discontinued for at least 1 menstrual cycle or until otherwise instructed by physician. Encourage to enroll in the North American Antiepileptic Drug Pregnancy Registry if patient becomes pregnant.

APTIVUS — tipranavir   Rx

Class: Protease inhibitor

> Both fatal and nonfatal intracranial hemorrhage (ICH) reported. Clinical hepatitis and hepatic decompensation, including some fatalities, reported. Extra vigilance is warranted in patients w/ chronic hepatitis B or hepatitis C coinfection due to an increased risk of hepatotoxicity.

ADULT DOSAGE
HIV-1 Infection

Coadministered w/ ritonavir (RTV) in treatment-experienced patients infected w/ HIV-1 strains resistant to >1 protease inhibitor

Cap:
Usual: 500mg (two 250mg caps) + 200mg RTV bid

Sol:
Usual: 500mg (5mL) + 200mg RTV bid

PEDIATRIC DOSAGE
HIV-1 Infection

Coadministered w/ ritonavir (RTV) in treatment-experienced patients infected w/ HIV-1 strains resistant to >1 protease inhibitor

2-18 Years:
Usual: 14mg/kg + 6mg/kg RTV (or 375mg/m² + 150mg/m² RTV) bid
Max: 500mg + 200mg RTV bid

DOSING CONSIDERATIONS
Adverse Reactions
Pediatrics:
Development of Intolerance/Toxicity: Decrease dose to 12mg/kg + 5mg/kg ritonavir (RTV) (or 290mg/m² + 115mg/m² RTV) bid

ADMINISTRATION
Oral route
Coadministered w/ Ritonavir (RTV) Caps/Sol
May be taken w/ or w/o meals
Coadministered w/ RTV Tabs
Must only be taken w/ meals

STORAGE
Must be used w/in 60 days after 1st opening the bottle. (Cap) Prior to Opening the Bottle: 2-8°C (36-46°F). After Opening the Bottle: 25°C (77°F); excursions permitted to 15-30°C (59-86°F). (Sol) 25°C (77°F); excursions permitted to 15-30°C (59-86°F). Do not refrigerate or freeze.

HOW SUPPLIED
Cap: 250mg; **Sol:** 100mg/mL [95mL]

CONTRAINDICATIONS
Moderate or severe (Child-Pugh Class B or C) hepatic impairment. Coadministration w/ drugs that are highly dependent on CYP3A for clearance or are potent CYP3A inducers (eg, amiodarone, bepridil, flecainide, propafenone, quinidine, rifampin, dihydroergotamine, ergonovine, ergotamine, methylergonovine, cisapride, St. John's wort, lovastatin, simvastatin, pimozide, oral midazolam, triazolam, alfuzosin, and sildenafil [for treatment of pulmonary arterial HTN]). Refer to the individual monograph for RTV.

WARNINGS/PRECAUTIONS
Not recommended for treatment-naive patients. Caution w/ elevated transaminases, hepatitis B or C coinfection, mild hepatic impairment (Child-Pugh Class A), supplemental high doses of vitamin E, known sulfonamide allergy, patients at risk of increased bleeding from trauma, surgery, or other medical conditions, and in elderly. D/C if signs and symptoms of clinical hepatitis develop. D/C if asymptomatic elevations in AST or ALT >10X the ULN or if asymptomatic elevations in AST or ALT between 5-10X the ULN and increases in total bilirubin >2.5X the ULN occur. Rash (eg, urticarial, maculopapular, possible photosensitivity) accompanied by joint pain/stiffness, throat tightness, or generalized pruritus reported; d/c and initiate appropriate treatment if severe skin rash develops. New onset diabetes mellitus (DM), exacerbation of preexisting DM, hyperglycemia, and diabetic ketoacidosis reported. Increased total cholesterol and TG levels reported. Immune reconstitution syndrome reported; autoimmune disorders (eg, Graves' disease, polymyositis, and Guillain-Barre syndrome) have also been reported in the setting of immune reconstitution. Redistribution/accumulation of body fat may occur. Increased bleeding in patients w/ hemophilia type A and B reported; additional factor VIII may be given. (Sol) Avoid supplemental vitamin E greater than a standard multivitamin as oral sol contains 116 IU/mL of vitamin E, which is higher than the Reference Daily Intake (adults 30 IU, pediatrics approx 10 IU). Refer to individual monograph for RTV.

ADVERSE REACTIONS
ICH, clinical hepatitis, hepatic decompensation, diarrhea, N/V, abdominal pain, pyrexia, fatigue, headache, cough, rash, anemia, weight decreased, hypertriglyceridemia, bleeding.

DRUG INTERACTIONS
See Contraindications. Not recommended w/ other protease inhibitors, boceprevir, telaprevir, salmeterol, and fluticasone. Concomitant colchicine is contraindicated in renally/hepatically impaired patients. Avoid w/ atorvastatin and etravirine. Caution w/ medications known to increase the risk of bleeding (eg, antiplatelets, anticoagulants, or high doses of vitamin E). May increase levels of rilpivirine, SSRIs (eg, fluoxetine, paroxetine, sertraline), atorvastatin, rosuvastatin, trazodone, desipramine, colchicine, bosentan, itraconazole, ketoconazole, clarithromycin, rifabutin, quetiapine, parenteral midazolam, normeperidine, and PDE-5 inhibitors. May decrease levels of etravirine, abacavir, atazanavir, didanosine, zidovudine, amprenavir, lopinavir, saquinavir, raltegravir, valproic acid, methadone, meperidine, and omeprazole. Increased levels w/ fluconazole, enfuvirtide, clarithromycin, and atazanavir. Decreased levels w/ buprenorphine/naloxone, carbamazepine, phenobarbital, and phenytoin. May alter levels of voriconazole, calcium channel blockers, and immunosuppressants. May decrease levels of ethinyl estradiol by 50%; use alternative methods of nonhormonal contraception. Monitor glucose w/ hypoglycemic agents. Monitor INR w/ warfarin. (Cap) May produce disulfiram-like reactions w/ disulfiram or other drugs that produce the reaction (eg, metronidazole). See Prescribing Information for detailed information.

PREGNANCY AND LACTATION
Category C, not for use in nursing.

MECHANISM OF ACTION
Protease inhibitor; inhibits virus-specific processing of viral Gag and Gag-Pol polyproteins in HIV-1 infected cells, thus preventing formation of mature virions.

PHARMACOKINETICS
Absorption: Tipranavir/RTV: (Female) C_{max}=94.8μM, T_{max}=2.9 hrs, AUC_{0-12h}=851μM•hr; (Male) C_{max}=77.6μM, T_{max}=3 hrs, AUC_{0-12h}=710μM•hr. Refer to Prescribing Information for pediatric parameters by age. **Distribution:** Plasma protein binding (>99.9%). **Metabolism:** Liver via CYP3A4. **Elimination:** Tipranavir/RTV: Feces (82.3% [median], 79.9% unchanged), urine (4.4%, 0.5% unchanged); $T_{1/2}$=5.5 hrs (females), 6 hrs (males).

PATIENT CONSIDERATIONS
Assessment: Assess for hepatitis B or C infection, hepatic impairment, increased bleeding risk, hemophilia, sulfonamide allergy, DM, pregnancy/nursing status, and possible drug interactions. Assess LFTs and lipid levels. Assess the ability to swallow caps in pediatric patients.

Monitoring: Monitor for signs and symptoms of clinical hepatitis, hepatic decompensation, ICH, rash, DM, hyperglycemia, diabetic ketoacidosis, bleeding, immune reconstitution syndrome, autoimmune disorders, fat redistribution, and other adverse reactions. Monitor for LFTs and lipid levels periodically during treatment. Monitor INR w/ warfarin.

Counseling: Inform of the risks and benefits of therapy. Advise to seek medical attention for symptoms of hepatitis (eg, fatigue, malaise, anorexia, nausea), any unusual/unexplained bleeding, and rash. Advise to report use of all medications, including prescription or nonprescription medications (eg, St. John's wort). Instruct to avoid vitamin E supplements greater than a standard multivitamin when taking oral sol. Instruct to report any history of sulfonamide allergy. Instruct to use additional or alternative contraceptive measures for patients taking estrogen-based hormonal contraceptives. Inform that redistribution/accumulation of body fat may occur. Instruct to take medication ud. Inform that therapy is not a cure for HIV-1 infection and that illness associated w/ HIV-1 infection may continue, including opportunistic infection; advise to remain under the care of a physician during therapy. Advise to avoid doing things that can spread HIV-1 infection to others.

ARANESP — darbepoetin alfa   Rx
Class: Erythropoiesis-stimulating agent (ESA)

> Increased risk of death, MI, stroke, venous thromboembolism, thrombosis of vascular access, and tumor progression or recurrence. Use the lowest dose sufficient to reduce/avoid the need for RBC transfusions. **Chronic Kidney Disease (CKD):** Greater risks for death, serious adverse cardiovascular (CV) reactions, and stroke when administered ESAs to target Hgb level of >11g/dL. **Cancer:** Shortened overall survival and/or increased risk of tumor progression or recurrence in patients w/ breast, non-small cell lung, head and neck, lymphoid, and cervical cancers. Must enroll in and comply w/ the ESA APPRISE Oncology Program to prescribe and/or dispense drug to patients. Use only for anemia from myelosuppressive chemotherapy. Not indicated for patients receiving myelosuppressive chemotherapy when anticipated outcome is cure. D/C following completion of chemotherapy course.

ADULT DOSAGE
Anemia Due to Chronic Kidney Disease
On Dialysis:
Initiate when Hgb is <10g/dL
Initial: 0.45mcg/kg IV/SQ weekly or 0.75mcg/kg IV/SQ once every 2 weeks; IV route is recommended for hemodialysis patients
Titrate: Adjust dose based on Hgb levels. If Hgb approaches or exceeds 11g/dL, reduce or interrupt dose

Not on Dialysis:
Initiate when Hgb is <10g/dL, the rate of Hgb decline indicates likelihood of a RBC transfusion, and when reducing the risk of alloimmunization and/or other RBC transfusion-related risks is a goal
Initial: 0.45mcg/kg IV/SQ once every 4 weeks
Titrate: Adjust dose based on Hgb levels. If Hgb exceeds 10g/dL, reduce or interrupt dose and use lowest dose sufficient to reduce RBC transfusion

All Patients:
Titrate:
Do not increase dose more frequently than once every 4 weeks; dose decreases may occur more frequently
Rapid Increase in Hgb (>1g/dL in Any 2-Week Period): Reduce by ≥25% prn to reduce rapid responses
Hgb Has Not Increased by >1g/dL After 4 Weeks of Therapy: Increase by 25%
No Adequate Response Over a 12-Week Escalation Period: Further dose increase is unlikely to improve response and may increase risks. Use lowest dose to maintain Hgb level sufficient to reduce the need of RBC transfusion; d/c if responsiveness does not improve

Anemia Due to Chemotherapy
Anemia in Patients w/ Nonmyeloid Malignancies:
Initiate when Hgb is <10g/dL and if there is a minimum of 2 additional months of chemotherapy
Initial: 2.25mcg/kg SQ weekly or 500mcg SQ every 3 weeks until completion of chemotherapy course
Titrate:
Hgb Increases >1g/dL in Any 2-Week Period/Hgb Reaches a Level Needed to Avoid RBC Transfusion: Reduce dose by 40%
Hgb Exceeds Level Needed to Avoid RBC Transfusion: Withhold until Hgb approaches a level where RBC transfusions may be required; reinitiate at a dose 40% below previous dose
Hgb Increases by <1g/dL and Remains <10g/dL After 6 Weeks of Therapy: Increase dose to 4.5mcg/kg/week (weekly schedule) or no dose adjustment (3-week schedule)

PEDIATRIC DOSAGE
Anemia Due to Chronic Kidney Disease
Initiate when Hgb is <10g/dL
Initial: 0.45mcg/kg IV/SQ weekly; patients not receiving dialysis may be initiated at a dose of 0.75mcg/kg once every 2 weeks
Titrate:
Adjust dose based on Hgb levels. If Hgb approaches or exceeds 12g/dL, reduce or interrupt dose.
Do not increase dose more frequently than once every 4 weeks; dose decreases may occur more frequently.
Rapid Increase in Hgb (>1g/dL in Any 2-Week Period): Reduce by ≥25% prn to reduce rapid responses
Hgb Has Not Increased by >1g/dL After 4 Weeks of Therapy: Increase by 25%
No Adequate Response Over a 12-Week Escalation Period: Further dose increase is unlikely to improve response and may increase risks. Use lowest dose to maintain Hgb level sufficient to reduce the need of RBC transfusion; d/c if responsiveness does not improve

Conversions
On Dialysis:
Conversion from Epoetin Alfa:
Administer less frequently than epoetin alfa; administer once weekly or every 2 weeks in patients who were receiving epoetin alfa 2-3X weekly or once weekly, respectively

Estimate the starting weekly dose based on weekly epoetin alfa dose at the time of substitution
Epoetin Alfa Dose (U/Week):
1500-2499: 6.25mcg/week
2500-4999: 10mcg/week
5000-10,999: 20mcg/week
11,000-17,999: 40mcg/week
18,000-33,999: 60mcg/week
34,000-89,999: 100mcg/week
≥90,000: 200mcg/week

Maintain the route of administration

Not on Dialysis:
The dose conversion above does not accurately estimate the once monthly dose of darbepoetin alfa

No Response in Hgb Levels/Still Require RBC Transfusions After 8 Weeks of Therapy/Following Completion of Chemotherapy Course: D/C therapy

Conversions

On Dialysis:

Conversion from Epoetin Alfa: Administer less frequently than epoetin alfa; administer once weekly or every 2 weeks in patients who were receiving epoetin alfa 2-3X weekly or once weekly, respectively

Estimate the starting weekly dose based on weekly epoetin alfa dose at the time of substitution

Epoetin Alfa Dose (U/Week):
<1500: 6.25mcg/week
1500-2499: 6.25mcg/week
2500-4999: 12.5mcg/week
5000-10,999: 25mcg/week
11,000-17,999: 40mcg/week
18,000-33,999: 60mcg/week
34,000-89,999: 100mcg/week
≥90,000: 200mcg/week

Maintain the route of administration

Not on Dialysis:
The dose conversion above does not accurately estimate the once monthly dose of darbepoetin alfa

ADMINISTRATION

IV/SQ route

Do not shake.
Do not use if it has been frozen or shaken.
Do not dilute and do not administer in conjunction w/ other drug sol.
Discard any unused portion in vials or prefilled syringes; do not re-enter vial.

Self-Administration of Prefilled Syringe

If patient or caregiver is unable to demonstrate successful measuring of dose and administration of product, consider whether patient is an appropriate candidate for self-administration or whether patient would benefit from a different darbepoetin alfa presentation.

STORAGE

2-8°C (36-46°F). Do not freeze. Protect from light.

HOW SUPPLIED

Inj: 25mcg/mL, 40mcg/mL, 60mcg/mL, 100mcg/mL, 150mcg/0.75mL, 200mcg/mL, 300mcg/mL [single-dose vial]; 10mcg/0.4mL, 25mcg/0.42mL, 40mcg/0.4mL, 60mcg/0.3mL, 100mcg/0.5mL, 150mcg/0.3mL, 200mcg/0.4mL, 300mcg/0.6mL, 500mcg/mL [single-dose prefilled syringe]

CONTRAINDICATIONS

Uncontrolled HTN, pure red cell aplasia (PRCA) that begins after treatment w/ darbepoetin alfa or other erythropoietin protein drugs, serious allergic reactions to darbepoetin alfa.

WARNINGS/PRECAUTIONS

Not indicated for use in patients w/ cancer receiving hormonal agents, biologic products, or radiotherapy, unless also receiving concomitant myelosuppressive chemotherapy, nor indicated as a substitute for RBC transfusions in patients requiring immediate correction of anemia. Evaluate transferrin saturation and serum ferritin prior to and during treatment; administer supplemental iron when serum ferritin is <100mcg/L or serum transferrin saturation is <20%. Correct/exclude other causes of anemia (eg, vitamin deficiency, metabolic/chronic inflammatory conditions, bleeding) before initiating therapy. Caution in patients w/ coexistent CV disease and stroke. Not approved for reduction of RBC transfusions in patients scheduled for surgical procedures. Hypertensive encephalopathy reported in patients w/ CKD. Appropriately control HTN prior to initiation of and during treatment; reduce/withhold therapy if BP becomes difficult to control. Increased risk of seizures. Cases of PRCA and severe anemia, w/ or w/o other cytopenias that arise following development of neutralizing antibodies to erythropoietin, reported. Withhold and evaluate for neutralizing antibodies to erythropoietin if severe anemia and low reticulocyte count develop; d/c permanently if PRCA develops, and do not switch to other ESAs. Serious allergic reactions may occur; immediately and permanently d/c treatment and administer appropriate therapy if a serious allergic/anaphylactic reaction occurs. Patients may require adjustments in dialysis prescriptions after initiation of therapy, or may require increased anticoagulation w/ heparin to prevent clotting of extracorporeal circuit during hemodialysis. Needle cover of the prefilled syringe contains dry natural rubber (a derivative of latex), which may cause allergic reactions.

ADVERSE REACTIONS

Patients w/ CKD: (Adults) HTN, dyspnea, peripheral edema, cough, procedural hypotension. (Pediatrics) HTN, inj-site pain, rash, convulsions.
Patients w/ Cancer Receiving Chemotherapy: Abdominal pain, edema, thrombovascular events.

PREGNANCY AND LACTATION

Pregnancy: Category C.
Lactation: It is not known if darbepoetin alfa is present in human milk; caution in nursing.

MECHANISM OF ACTION

Erythropoiesis-stimulating protein; stimulates erythropoiesis by the same mechanism as endogenous erythropoietin.

PHARMACOKINETICS

Absorption: Adults w/ CKD: (SQ) Slow. Bioavailability (37%) (on dialysis); T_{max}=48 hrs. Pediatric Patients w/ CKD: (SQ) Bioavailability (54%). Adults w/ Cancer: (SQ, 6.75mcg/kg) T_{max}=71 hrs. **Elimination:** Adults w/ CKD: (IV) $T_{1/2}$=21 hrs (on dialysis). (SQ) $T_{1/2}$=46 hrs (on dialysis), 70 hrs (not on dialysis). Adults w/ Cancer: (SQ, 6.75mcg/kg) $T_{1/2}$=74 hrs.

PATIENT CONSIDERATIONS

Assessment: Assess for uncontrolled HTN, previous hypersensitivity to the drug, latex allergy, causes of anemia, pregnancy/nursing status, and other conditions where treatment is cautioned/contraindicated. Obtain baseline Hgb levels, transferrin saturation, and serum ferritin.

Monitoring: Monitor for signs/symptoms of an allergic reaction; CV/thromboembolic events, stroke, PRCA, severe anemia, progression/recurrence of tumor, HTN, and other adverse reactions. Monitor BP, transferrin saturation, and serum ferritin. Monitor closely for premonitory neurologic symptoms during the 1st several months following initiation of treatment. Following initiation of therapy and after each dose adjustment, monitor Hgb weekly until Hgb is stable and sufficient to minimize need for RBC transfusion, and then monitor Hgb less frequently (at least monthly in CKD patients), provided Hgb levels remain stable.

Counseling: Inform of the risks/benefits of therapy, including the increased risks of mortality, serious CV reactions, thromboembolic reactions, stroke, and tumor progression. Advise of the need to have regular lab tests for Hgb. Inform cancer patients that they must sign the patient-healthcare provider acknowledgment form prior to the start of each treatment course. Instruct to undergo regular BP monitoring, adhere to prescribed antihypertensive regimen, and follow recommended dietary restrictions. Advise to contact healthcare provider for new-onset neurologic symptoms or change in seizure frequency. Instruct patients who self-administer regarding proper disposal; dangers of reusing needles, syringes, or unused portions of single-dose vials; and the importance of informing healthcare provider if difficulty occurs when measuring or administering partial doses from the prefilled syringe.

ARAVA — leflunomide   Rx

Class: Pyrimidine synthesis inhibitor

Contraindicated for use in pregnant women due to the potential for fetal harm; exclude pregnancy before start of treatment in females of reproductive potential. Advise females of reproductive potential to use effective contraception during treatment and during an accelerated drug elimination procedure after treatment. If patient becomes pregnant, d/c therapy and use an accelerated drug elimination procedure. Severe liver injury, including fatal liver failure, reported; contraindicated in patients w/ severe hepatic impairment. Concomitant use w/ other potentially hepatotoxic drugs may increase risk of liver injury. Not for use in patients w/ preexisting acute or chronic liver disease, or those w/ serum ALT >2X ULN before initiating treatment. Monitor ALT levels at least monthly for 6 months after starting therapy, and thereafter every 6-8 weeks. If leflunomide-induced liver injury is suspected, d/c treatment, start an accelerated drug elimination procedure, and monitor liver tests weekly until normalized.

ADULT DOSAGE	PEDIATRIC DOSAGE
Rheumatoid Arthritis	Pediatric use may not have been established
Recommended Dose: 20mg qd	
Max: 20mg qd	
Consider dose reduction to 10mg qd if unable to tolerate 20mg qd	
May initiate treatment w/ or w/o LD, depending on risk of drug-associated hepatotoxicity and drug-associated myelosuppression	
Low Risk for Hepatotoxicity and Myelosuppression:	
LD: 100mg qd for 3 days	
Maint: 20mg qd	
High Risk for Hepatotoxicity (eg, Concomitant Methotrexate [MTX]) or Myelosuppression (eg, Concomitant Immunosuppressants):	
20mg qd w/o LD	

DOSING CONSIDERATIONS

Hepatic Impairment
Not recommended

Discontinuation

Procedure for Accelerated Elimination of Leflunomide and its Active Metabolite:
- Use of an accelerated drug elimination procedure will rapidly reduce plasma levels of leflunomide and its active metabolite, teriflunomide; w/o use of an accelerated drug elimination procedure, it may take up to 2 yrs to reach plasma teriflunomide levels of <0.02mg/L
- Consider an accelerated elimination procedure at any time after discontinuation of leflunomide, and in particular, when a patient has experienced a severe adverse reaction (eg, hepatotoxicity, serious infection, bone marrow suppression, Stevens-Johnson syndrome [SJS], toxic epidermal necrolysis [TEN], peripheral neuropathy, interstitial lung disease [ILD]), suspected hypersensitivity, or has become pregnant; all women of childbearing potential should undergo an accelerated elimination procedure after stopping treatment

Elimination Can Be Accelerated by the Following Procedures:
1. Administer cholestyramine 8g PO tid for 11 days, or alternatively, administer 50g of activated charcoal powder (made into a sus) PO q12h for 11 days
2. Verify plasma teriflunomide levels of <0.02mg/L by 2 separate tests at least 14 days apart; if plasma teriflunomide levels are higher than 0.02mg/L, repeat cholestyramine and/or activated charcoal treatment

The duration of accelerated drug elimination treatment may be modified based on the clinical status and tolerability of the elimination procedure; may repeat procedure as needed, based on teriflunomide levels and clinical status

ADMINISTRATION
Oral route

STORAGE
25°C (77°F); excursions permitted to 15-30°C (59-86°F). Protect from light.

HOW SUPPLIED
Tab: 10mg, 20mg, 100mg

CONTRAINDICATIONS
Pregnant women, severe hepatic impairment, known hypersensitivity to leflunomide or any of the other components in this medication, patients being treated w/ teriflunomide.

WARNINGS/PRECAUTIONS
See Dosing Considerations. Interrupt therapy if ALT elevation >3X ULN occurs; if likely leflunomide-induced, perform the accelerated drug elimination procedure and monitor liver tests weekly until normalized. If leflunomide-induced liver injury is unlikely, may consider resumption of therapy. Use of the accelerated drug elimination procedure may result in return of disease activity if patient had been responding to treatment. Not recommended w/ severe immunodeficiency, bone marrow dysplasia, or severe, uncontrolled infections; consider interrupting therapy and initiating the accelerated drug elimination procedure if a serious infection occurs. May cause immunosuppression and increased susceptibility to infections, including opportunistic infections, especially *Pneumocystis jiroveci* pneumonia, tuberculosis (TB), and aspergillosis. Screen all patients for active and inactive (latent) TB infection prior to initiating therapy; treat patients testing positive in TB screening prior to therapy and monitor carefully during treatment w/ leflunomide for possible reactivation of the infection. Pancytopenia, agranulocytosis, and thrombocytopenia reported; monitor platelets, WBC count, and Hgb or Hct at baseline and monthly for 6 months following initiation of therapy and every 6-8 weeks thereafter. D/C therapy if evidence of bone marrow suppression occurs. Monitor for hematologic toxicity if switching to another antirheumatic agent w/ a known potential for hematologic suppression. Rare cases of SJS and TEN, and drug reaction w/ eosinophilia and systemic symptoms (DRESS) reported; d/c therapy if any of these occur. May increase risk of malignancy, particularly lymphoproliferative disorders. Peripheral neuropathy reported; age >60 yrs and diabetes may increase risk for peripheral neuropathy. Consider discontinuing if peripheral neuropathy develops. ILD and worsening of preexisting ILD reported. New onset or worsening of pulmonary symptoms (eg, cough, dyspnea), w/ or w/o associated fever, may be a reason for discontinuation of therapy and for further investigation as appropriate. BP elevation reported. Caution w/ renal impairment.

ADVERSE REACTIONS
Diarrhea, abnormal liver enzymes, alopecia, headache, N/V, rash, HTN, asthenia, back pain, GI/abdominal pain, allergic reaction, bronchitis, dizziness, mouth ulcer, pruritus.

DRUG INTERACTIONS
See Boxed Warning and Contraindications. Concomitant use w/ rifampin increased levels of teriflunomide; caution if receiving both leflunomide and rifampin. May increase exposure of drugs metabolized by CYP2C8 (eg, paclitaxel, pioglitazone, repaglinide); monitor and adjust the dose of the concomitant drug as required. Closely monitor INR w/ warfarin; teriflunomide may decrease peak INR. Teriflunomide may increase exposures of ethinyl estradiol and levonorgestrel. May reduce exposure of drugs metabolized by CYP1A2 (eg, alosetron, duloxetine, theophylline); monitor and adjust the dose of the concomitant drug as required. May increase exposure of OAT3 substrates (eg, cefaclor, cimetidine, ciprofloxacin); monitor and adjust the dose of the concomitant drug as required. For a patient taking leflunomide, the dose of rosuvastatin should not exceed 10mg qd. For other substrates of breast cancer resistance protein (eg, mitoxantrone) and drugs in the OATP family (eg, MTX, rifampin), especially HMG-Co reductase inhibitors (eg, atorvastatin, nateglinide, pravastatin), consider reducing the dose of these drugs and monitor closely for signs/symptoms of increased exposures to the drugs while taking leflunomide. Vaccination w/ live vaccines is not recommended; consider long $T_{1/2}$ of the active metabolite when contemplating administration of live vaccine after stopping therapy. May increase risk of peripheral neuropathy w/ neurotoxic medications. If given concomitantly w/ MTX, follow the American College of Rheumatology guidelines for monitoring MTX liver toxicity w/ ALT, AST, and serum albumin testing.

PREGNANCY AND LACTATION
Pregnancy: Contraindicated for use in pregnant women. If used during pregnancy, or if patient becomes pregnant while on treatment, d/c use, apprise of the potential hazard to a fetus, and perform the accelerated drug elimination procedure to achieve teriflunomide concentrations of <0.02mg/L; this may decrease the risk to the fetus. There is a pregnancy exposure registry that monitors pregnancy outcomes in women exposed to leflunomide during pregnancy; healthcare providers and patients are encouraged to report pregnancies.
Lactation: Not for use in nursing.
Reproductive Potential: Females of reproductive potential should use effective contraception during treatment and while undergoing a drug elimination procedure until verification that the plasma teriflunomide concentration is <0.02mg/L.

MECHANISM OF ACTION
Pyrimidine synthesis inhibitor; isoxazole immunomodulatory agent that inhibits dihydroorotate dehydrogenase and has antiproliferative activity. Has demonstrated an anti-inflammatory effect.

PHARMACOKINETICS
Absorption: T_{max}=6-12 hrs (teriflunomide). **Distribution:** (Teriflunomide) Plasma protein binding (>99%); V_d=11L (IV). **Metabolism:** Via CYP1A2, 2C19 and 3A4; teriflunomide (active metabolite). **Elimination:** (Teriflunomide) Urine (22.6%), feces (60.1%); (median) $T_{1/2}$=18-19 days.

PATIENT CONSIDERATIONS
Assessment: Assess for hypersensitivity to drug or any of the other components of the drug, severe immunodeficiency, bone marrow dysplasia, severe uncontrolled infections, hepatic/renal impairment, any other conditions where treatment is contraindicated or cautioned, pregnancy/nursing status, and possible drug interactions. Evaluate for active TB and screen for latent TB infection. Obtain baseline BP, platelet counts, WBC count, Hgb or Hct, and ALT levels. Perform pregnancy testing for females of reproductive potential to exclude pregnancy before the start of treatment.

Monitoring: Monitor for signs/symptoms of hepatotoxicity, immunosuppression, infections (including opportunistic infections), pancytopenia, agranulocytosis, thrombocytopenia, SJS, TEN, DRESS, peripheral neuropathy, ILD, malignancy, and other adverse reactions. Monitor BP periodically. Monitor platelets, WBC count, and Hgb or Hct monthly for 6 months following initiation of therapy and every 6-8 weeks thereafter; chronic monitoring should be monthly if used w/ concomitant MTX and/or other potential immunosuppressive agents. Monitor ALT levels monthly for 6 months after starting treatment and every 6-8 weeks thereafter. Monitor carefully after dose reduction and after stopping therapy. Monitor for hematologic toxicity when switching to another antirheumatic agent w/ known potential for hematologic suppression.

Counseling: Advise females of reproductive potential of the potential for fetal harm if drug is taken during pregnancy. Instruct to notify physician immediately if a pregnancy occurs/is suspected and to use effective contraception during treatment and until plasma concentration of the active metabolite is verified to be <0.02mg/L. Advise nursing women to d/c breastfeeding during treatment. Inform of the possibility of rare, serious skin reactions; instruct to promptly report development of any skin rash or mucous membrane lesions. Advise of the potential hepatotoxic effects and of the need for monitoring liver enzymes; instruct to notify physician if symptoms such as unusual tiredness, abdominal pain, or jaundice develop. Advise that lowering of blood counts may develop; instruct to have frequent hematologic monitoring, particularly in patients who are receiving other concurrent immunosuppressive therapy or who have had a history of significant hematologic abnormality. Instruct to notify physician if symptoms of pancytopenia develop. Inform about the early warning signs of ILD and instruct to contact physician promptly if these symptoms appear/worsen during therapy.

ARCAPTA — indacaterol   Rx
Class: Long-acting beta₂ agonist (LABA)

> Long-acting β_2-adrenergic agonists (LABAs) may increase the risk of asthma-related death. Not indicated for treatment of asthma.

ADULT DOSAGE	PEDIATRIC DOSAGE
Chronic Obstructive Pulmonary Disease **Long-Term Maint Treatment of Airflow Obstruction:** 1 inh (75mcg) qd	Pediatric use may not have been established

ADMINISTRATION
Oral inh route
Use only w/ Neohaler device
Do not swallow caps
Administer at the same time every day
Remove cap from blister immediately before use

STORAGE
25°C (77°F); excursions permitted to 15-30°C (59-86°F). Protect from light and moisture.

HOW SUPPLIED
Cap, Inh: 75mcg

CONTRAINDICATIONS
Asthma without use of a long-term asthma control medication. Not indicated for treatment of asthma. History of hypersensitivity to indacaterol or to any of the ingredients.

WARNINGS/PRECAUTIONS
Not for acutely deteriorating COPD, or relief of acute symptoms (eg, as rescue therapy for treatment of acute episodes of bronchospasm). Cardiovascular (CV) effects and fatalities reported with excessive use; do not use excessively or with other LABA. D/C if paradoxical bronchospasm or CV effects occur. ECG changes reported. Caution with CV disorders (eg, coronary insufficiency, cardiac arrhythmias, HTN), convulsive disorders, thyrotoxicosis, and in patients unusually responsive to sympathomimetic amines. Hypokalemia, hyperglycemia, and immediate hypersensitivity reactions may occur. D/C immediately and institute alternative therapy if signs suggesting allergic reactions occur.

ADVERSE REACTIONS
Cough, nasopharyngitis, headache, COPD exacerbation, pneumonia, angina pectoris, A-fib.

DRUG INTERACTIONS
Adrenergic drugs may potentiate effects; use with caution. Xanthine derivatives, steroids, or diuretics may potentiate any hypokalemic effect. ECG changes or hypokalemia that may result from non-K⁺-sparing diuretics (eg, loop/thiazide diuretics) can be acutely worsened; use with caution. MAOIs, TCAs, and drugs known to prolong QTc interval may potentiate effect on CV system; use with extreme caution. Drugs that are known to prolong the QTc interval may increase risk of ventricular arrhythmias. β-blockers may block effects and produce severe bronchospasm in COPD patients; if needed, consider cardioselective β-blocker with caution. May result in overdose if used in conjunction with other medications containing LABAs. Increased plasma levels with ketoconazole, verapamil, erythromycin, and ritonavir.

PREGNANCY AND LACTATION
Category C, caution in nursing.

MECHANISM OF ACTION
LABA; stimulates intracellular adenyl cyclase, the enzyme that catalyzes the conversion of ATP to cAMP. Increases cAMP levels, causing relaxation of bronchial smooth muscles.

PHARMACOKINETICS
Absorption: Absolute bioavailability (43-45%); T_{max}=15 min. **Distribution:** (IV) V_d=2361-2557L; plasma protein binding (95.1-96.2%). **Metabolism:** Hydroxylation, glucuronidation, N-dealkylation; CYP3A4, UGT1A1; hydroxylated indacaterol (most prominent metabolite). **Elimination:** Urine (<2% unchanged), feces (54% unchanged, 23% metabolites); $T_{1/2}$=45.5-126 hrs.

PATIENT CONSIDERATIONS
Assessment: Assess for previous hypersensitivity to the drug, acute COPD deteriorations, asthma and use of control medication, CV disorders, convulsive disorders, thyrotoxicosis, diabetes mellitus, pregnancy/nursing status, and possible drug interactions. Assess use in patients unusually responsive to sympathomimetic amines. Obtain baseline serum K⁺ and blood glucose levels.

Monitoring: Monitor lung function periodically. Monitor for signs of worsening asthma, CV effects, paradoxical bronchospasm, and immediate hypersensitivity reactions. Monitor pulse rate, BP, ECG changes, and serum K⁺ and glucose levels.

Counseling: Inform of the risks and benefits of therapy. Instruct on proper administration of caps using the inhaler device and not to swallow caps. Caution that inhaler cannot be used more than once a day. Advise to d/c the regular use of short acting β₂-agonist (SABA) and use them only for the symptomatic relief of acute symptoms. Instruct to notify physician immediately if worsening of symptoms, decreasing effectiveness of inhaled SABA, need for more inhalations than usual of inhaled SABA, and significant decrease in lung function occur. Instruct not to stop therapy without physician's guidance. Inform patients not to use other inhaled medications containing LABAs. Inform about associated adverse effects, such as palpitations, chest pain, rapid HR, tremor, or nervousness.

ARGATROBAN — argatroban   **Rx**
Class: Direct thrombin inhibitor (DTI)

ADULT DOSAGE

Heparin-Induced Thrombocytopenia
Prophylaxis or treatment of thrombosis in patients w/ heparin-induced thrombocytopenia (HIT)

Initial: 2mcg/kg/min as a continuous infusion
Titrate: Adjust dose as necessary to obtain a steady-state aPTT in the target range
Max: 10mcg/kg/min

Before administration, d/c heparin and obtain a baseline aPTT

Percutaneous Coronary Intervention
In patients w/ or at risk for HIT undergoing percutaneous coronary intervention (PCI)

Initial: Initiate an infusion at 25mcg/kg/min and administer a bolus of 350mcg/kg via a large bore IV line over 3-5 min

Check activated clotting time (ACT) 5-10 min after bolus dose is completed; PCI procedure may proceed if ACT is >300 sec

Titrate:
ACT <300 Sec: Administer additional 150mcg/kg IV bolus and increase infusion dose to 30mcg/kg/min; check ACT 5-10 min later
ACT >450 Sec: Decrease infusion rate to 15mcg/kg/min; check ACT 5-10 min later

PEDIATRIC DOSAGE

Heparin-Induced Thrombocytopenia (HIT)/HIT and Thrombosis Syndrome

Patients Requiring an Alternative to Heparin:
Initial: 0.75mcg/kg/min continuous infusion; check aPTT 2 hrs after initiation
Titrate: May adjust in increments of 0.1-0.25mcg/kg/min

Dose recommendations are based upon a goal of aPTT prolongation of 1.5-3X the baseline value and avoidance of an aPTT >100 sec

Conversions

Initiating Oral Anticoagulant Therapy:
Initiate therapy using the expected daily dose of warfarin; do not use a LD of warfarin

Overlap argatroban and warfarin therapy to avoid prothrombotic effects and to ensure continuous anticoagulation when initiating warfarin

Coadministration w/ Warfarin: Argatroban Inj at Doses up to 2mcg/kg/min:
Measure INR daily during coadministration; d/c argatroban when INR is >4 on combined therapy

After argatroban is discontinued, repeat INR measurement in 4-6

Continue titrating the dose until a therapeutic ACT (300-450 sec) has been achieved; continue the same infusion rate for the duration of the PCI procedure

In case of dissection, impending abrupt closure, thrombus formation during the procedure, or inability to achieve or maintain an ACT >300 sec, additional bolus doses of 150mcg/kg may be administered and the infusion dose increased to 40mcg/kg/min; check ACT after each additional bolus or change in the rate of infusion

Continued Anticoagulation After PCI:
If a patient requires anticoagulation after the procedure, argatroban inj may be continued at a rate of 2mcg/kg/min and adjusted as needed to maintain the aPTT in the desired range

Conversions

Initiating Oral Anticoagulant Therapy:
Initiate therapy using the expected daily dose of warfarin; do not use a LD of warfarin

Overlap argatroban and warfarin therapy to avoid prothrombotic effects and to ensure continuous anticoagulation when initiating warfarin

Coadministration w/ Warfarin: Argatroban Inj at Doses up to 2mcg/kg/min:
Measure INR daily during coadministration; d/c argatroban when INR is >4 on combined therapy

After argatroban is discontinued, repeat INR measurement in 4-6 hrs; if repeat INR is below desired therapeutic range, resume infusion of argatroban and repeat the procedure daily until the desired therapeutic range on warfarin alone is reached

Argatroban Inj at Doses >2mcg/kg/min:
Temporarily reduce argatroban dose to 2mcg/kg/min; repeat INR 4-6 hrs after dose reduction and follow the process for administering argatroban at doses up to 2mcg/kg/min

---

hrs; if repeat INR is below desired therapeutic range, resume infusion of argatroban and repeat the procedure daily until the desired therapeutic range on warfarin alone is reached

Argatroban Inj at Doses >2mcg/kg/min:
Temporarily reduce argatroban dose to 2mcg/kg/min; repeat INR 4-6 hrs after dose reduction and follow the process for administering argatroban at doses up to 2mcg/kg/min

---

DOSING CONSIDERATIONS
Hepatic Impairment
Adults:
Moderate or Severe Impairment:
HIT:
Initial: 0.5mcg/kg/min; adjust dose as clinically indicated

Patients w/ or at Risk for HIT Undergoing PCI:
Titrate: Carefully titrate until desired level of anticoagulation is achieved

Clinically Significant Hepatic Disease or AST/ALT ≥3X ULN:
PCI Patients: Avoid use

Pediatrics:
HIT/HIT and Thrombosis Syndrome:
Initial: 0.2mcg/kg/min continuous infusion; check aPTT 2 hrs after initiation
Titrate: May adjust in increments of ≤0.05mcg/kg/min

ADMINISTRATION
IV route

250mg/2.5mL (100mg/mL) Vial
Preparation for IV Administration:
- Dilute in 0.9% NaCl inj, D5 inj, or lactated Ringer's inj to a final concentration of 1mg/mL. The contents of each 2.5mL vial should be diluted 100-fold by mixing w/ 250mL of diluent; use 250mg (2.5mL) per 250mL of diluent or 500mg (5mL) per 500mL of diluent.
- Mix the constituted sol by repeated inversion of the diluent bag for 1 min; upon preparation, the sol may show slight but brief haziness due to the formation of microprecipitates that rapidly dissolve upon mixing.
- Use of diluent at room temperature is recommended; colder temperatures can slow down the rate of dissolution of precipitates.
- The pH of the IV sol prepared as recommended is 3.2-7.5.
- Sol is physically and chemically stable for up to 96 hrs when protected from light and stored at 20-25°C (68-77°F), or 5°C ± 3°C (41°F ± 5°F). Do not expose prepared sol to direct sunlight.

STORAGE
(50mg/50mL, 125mg/125mL) 20-25°C (68-77°F). Do not freeze. Protect from light. (50mg/50mL) Do not refrigerate. (100mg/mL) **Undiluted Vial:** 25°C (77°F); excursions permitted to 15-30°C (59-86°F). Do not freeze. Protect from light. **Diluted Sol:** 20-25°C (68-77°F) in ambient indoor light for 24 hrs; or stable for up to 96 hrs when protected from light at 20-25°C (68-77°F) or at 5°C (41°F). Do not expose to direct sunlight.

HOW SUPPLIED
Inj: 100mg/mL [2.5mL]; 1mg/mL [50mL]; (NaCl) 1mg/mL [125mL]

CONTRAINDICATIONS
Major bleeding, history of hypersensitivity to argatroban.

WARNINGS/PRECAUTIONS
Hemorrhage may occur at any site in the body; use extreme caution in disease states and other circumstances in which there is an increased danger of hemorrhage (eg, severe HTN, immediately following lumbar puncture, spinal anesthesia, major surgery [especially involving the brain, spinal cord, or eye], hematologic conditions associated w/ increased bleeding tendencies [eg, congenital or acquired bleeding disorders], GI lesions). Caution w/ hepatic impairment; full reversal of anticoagulant effects may require >4 hrs upon cessation of infusion. Avoid use in PCI patients w/ significant hepatic disease or AST/ALT ≥3X ULN.

ADVERSE REACTIONS
HIT Patients: Bleeding, dyspnea, hypotension, fever, diarrhea, sepsis, cardiac arrest, N/V, ventricular tachycardia, pain, UTI, infection, pneumonia, A-fib.
PCI Patients: Bleeding, chest pain, hypotension, back pain, N/V, headache, bradycardia, abdominal pain, fever, MI.

DRUG INTERACTIONS
If therapy is to be initiated after cessation of heparin, allow sufficient time for heparin's effect on the aPTT to decrease prior to initiation of argatroban therapy. Prolonged PT and INR w/ warfarin. Antiplatelet agents, thrombolytics, and other anticoagulants may increase risk of bleeding.

PREGNANCY AND LACTATION
Pregnancy: Category B.
Lactation: Not for use in nursing.

MECHANISM OF ACTION
DTI. Inhibits thrombin-catalyzed or thrombin-induced reactions, including fibrin formation; activation of coagulation factors V, VIII, and XIII; activation of protein C; and platelet aggregation. Capable of inhibiting both free and clot-associated thrombin.

PHARMACOKINETICS
Distribution: V_d=174mL/kg; plasma protein binding (54%). **Metabolism:** Liver via hydroxylation and aromatization; CYP3A4/5; M1 (primary metabolite). **Elimination:** Feces (65%, ≥14% unchanged), urine (22%, 16% unchanged); $T_{1/2}$=39-51 min.

PATIENT CONSIDERATIONS

Assessment: Assess for hypersensitivity to drug, hepatic impairment, major bleeding, any disease state or other circumstance that increases the risk of hemorrhage, pregnancy/nursing status, and possible drug interactions. Obtain baseline aPTT and ACT.

Monitoring: Monitor for signs/symptoms of hemorrhagic events and other adverse reactions. In patients w/ HIT, monitor aPTT 2 hrs after initiation of therapy and after any dose changes. In patients undergoing a PCI, monitor ACT 5-10 min after bolus dosing, after changes in infusion rate, at the end of the PCI procedure, and every 20-30 min during a prolonged procedure. Monitor PT/INR when coadministered w/ warfarin.

Counseling: Inform of the risks of therapy as well as the plan for regular monitoring during therapy. Instruct to tell physician if using any other products known to affect bleeding, if any medical history exists that may increase the risk for bleeding, if experiencing any bleeding signs/symptoms, or if any signs/symptoms of an allergic reaction develop.

ARICEPT — donepezil hydrochloride   Rx

Class: Acetylcholinesterase (AChE) inhibitor

ADULT DOSAGE	**PEDIATRIC DOSAGE**
Alzheimer's Disease	Pediatric use may not have been established
Treatment of Dementia of the Alzheimer's Type:	
Mild to Moderate:	
Initial: 5mg qhs	
Max: 10mg/day	
Moderate to Severe:	
Initial: 5mg qhs	
Max: 23mg/day	
Do not administer 10mg/day dose until patients have been on 5mg/day for 4-6 weeks	
Do not administer 23mg/day dose until patients have been on 10mg/day for at least 3 months	

ADMINISTRATION
Oral route
Take qhs.
Take w/ or w/o food.
23mg Tab
Do not split, crush, or chew.
ODT
Allow to dissolve on the tongue and follow w/ water.

STORAGE
15-30°C (59-86°F).

HOW SUPPLIED
Tab: 5mg, 10mg, 23mg; **Tab, Disintegrating:** (ODT) 5mg, 10mg

CONTRAINDICATIONS
Known hypersensitivity to donepezil HCl or to piperidine derivatives.

WARNINGS/PRECAUTIONS
May exaggerate succinylcholine-type muscle relaxation during anesthesia. May have vagotonic effects on sinoatrial (SA) and atrioventricular (AV) nodes, manifesting as bradycardia or heart block. Syncopal episodes reported. May produce N/V and diarrhea; observe closely at initiation of treatment and after dose increases. May increase gastric acid secretion; monitor closely for symptoms of active or occult GI bleeding, especially in patients at increased risk for developing ulcers (eg, concurrent NSAID use). Weight loss reported. May cause bladder outflow obstruction and generalized convulsions. Caution w/ history of asthma or obstructive pulmonary disease.

ADVERSE REACTIONS
Diarrhea, anorexia, N/V, ecchymosis, insomnia, muscle cramps, fatigue, headache, dizziness, weight loss, abnormal dreams, infection, HTN, back pain.

DRUG INTERACTIONS
May interfere w/ activity of anticholinergic medications. Synergistic effect when given concurrently w/ succinylcholine, similar neuromuscular blocking agents, or cholinergic agonists (eg, bethanechol).

PREGNANCY AND LACTATION
Category C, caution in nursing.

MECHANISM OF ACTION
Acetylcholinesterase inhibitor; postulated to exert its therapeutic effect by enhancing cholinergic function, by increasing acetylcholine concentrations through reversible inhibition of its hydrolysis by acetylcholinesterase.

PHARMACOKINETICS
Absorption: T_{max}=3 hrs (10mg), 8 hrs (23mg). **Distribution:** V_d=12-16L/kg; plasma protein binding (96%). **Metabolism:** Hepatic (extensive) via CYP2D6, CYP3A4, and glucuronidation to 4 major metabolites (2 of which are active). **Elimination:** Urine (57%, 17% unchanged), feces (15%); $T_{1/2}$=70 hrs.

PATIENT CONSIDERATIONS

Assessment: Assess for hypersensitivity to the drug or to piperidine derivatives, underlying cardiac conduction abnormalities, risks for developing ulcers, history of asthma or obstructive pulmonary disease, pregnancy/nursing status, and possible drug interactions.

Monitoring: Monitor for vagotonic effects on SA and AV nodes, syncopal episodes, diarrhea, N/V, active/occult GI bleeding, weight loss, bladder outflow obstruction, generalized convulsions, and other possible adverse reactions.

Counseling: Instruct to take as prescribed. Advise that N/V, diarrhea, insomnia, muscle cramps, fatigue, and decreased appetite may occur.

ARIMIDEX — anastrozole   Rx

Class: Nonsteroidal aromatase inhibitor

ADULT DOSAGE	**PEDIATRIC DOSAGE**
Breast Cancer	Pediatric use may not have been established
In postmenopausal women for adjuvant treatment of hormone receptor-positive early breast cancer; 1st-line treatment of hormone receptor-positive or hormone receptor unknown locally advanced or metastatic breast cancer; and treatment of advanced breast cancer w/ disease progression following tamoxifen therapy	
Advanced Breast Cancer: 1mg qd; continue until tumor progression	
Adjuvant Treatment of Early Breast Cancer: 1mg qd; administered for 5 years in a clinical trial	

ADMINISTRATION
Oral route
Take w/ or w/o food

STORAGE
20-25°C (68-77°F).

HOW SUPPLIED
Tab: 1mg

CONTRAINDICATIONS
Women who are or may become pregnant, premenopausal women, hypersensitivity reaction to the drug or to any of the excipients.

WARNINGS/PRECAUTIONS
Increased incidence of ischemic cardiovascular (CV) events in women with preexisting ischemic heart disease reported. Decreases in bone mineral density (BMD) may occur. Elevated serum cholesterol reported.

ADVERSE REACTIONS
Hot flashes, asthenia, arthritis, pain, pharyngitis, HTN, depression, N/V, rash, osteoporosis, fractures, headache, bone pain, peripheral edema.

DRUG INTERACTIONS
Tamoxifen may decrease levels; avoid concomitant use. Avoid with estrogen-containing therapies.

PREGNANCY AND LACTATION
Category X, not for use in nursing.

MECHANISM OF ACTION
Nonsteroidal aromatase inhibitor; lowers serum estradiol concentrations and has no detectable effect on formation of adrenal corticosteroids or aldosterone.

PHARMACOKINETICS
Absorption: (Fasted state) Rapid. T_{max}=2 hrs. **Distribution:** Plasma protein binding (40%). **Metabolism:** Liver via N-dealkylation, hydroxylation, and glucuronidation; triazole (major metabolite). **Elimination:** Urine and feces (85%); $T_{1/2}$=50 hrs.

PATIENT CONSIDERATIONS
Assessment: Assess for hypersensitivity to drug, preexisting ischemic cardiac disease, premenopausal status, pregnancy/nursing status, and possible drug interactions.

Monitoring: Monitor for hypersensitivity reactions and other adverse reactions. Monitor BMD and serum cholesterol levels.

Counseling: Inform that drug may cause fetal harm and is not for use in premenopausal women; instruct to d/c therapy if patient becomes pregnant and to immediately contact physician. Instruct to seek medical attention immediately if serious allergic reactions occur. Inform patients with preexisting ischemic heart disease that an increased incidence of CV events has been observed; advise to seek medical attention immediately if new or worsening chest pain or SOB occurs. Inform that drug may lower estrogen level, which may lead to a loss of the mineral content of bones, possibly decreasing the bone strength, leading to an increased risk of fractures. Inform that an increased level of cholesterol might be seen while receiving therapy. Instruct to notify physician if tickling, tingling, or numbness is experienced. Advise not to take drug with tamoxifen.

ARISTADA — aripiprazole lauroxil
Rx

Class: Atypical antipsychotic

> Elderly patients w/ dementia-related psychosis treated w/ antipsychotic drugs are at an increased risk of death. Not approved for the treatment of patients w/ dementia-related psychosis.

ADULT DOSAGE
Schizophrenia

Establish tolerability w/ oral aripiprazole prior to initiating treatment in patients who have never taken aripiprazole; it may take up to 2 weeks to fully assess tolerability

Dosing Frequency and Site of Inj:
441mg: Administer monthly in the deltoid or gluteal muscle
662mg: Administer monthly in the gluteal muscle
882mg: Administer monthly or every 6 weeks in the gluteal muscle

Dose Based on Oral Aripiprazole Total Daily Dose:
10mg/day PO: 441mg/month inj
15mg/day PO: 662mg/month inj
≥20mg/day PO: 882mg/month inj

In conjunction w/ the 1st Aristada inj, administer treatment w/ oral aripiprazole for 21 consecutive days

In the event of early dosing, an inj should not be given earlier than 14 days after the previous inj

Missed Dose

Concomitant Oral Aripiprazole Supplementation Following Missed Doses:
441mg Monthly:
≤6 Weeks Since Last Inj: No oral aripiprazole required; administer next inj as soon as possible
>6 and ≤7 Weeks Since Last Inj: Supplement next inj dose w/ 7 days oral aripiprazole

PEDIATRIC DOSAGE
Pediatric use may not have been established

>7 Weeks Since Last Inj: Supplement next inj dose w/ 21 days oral aripiprazole

662mg & 882mg Monthly or 882mg Every 6 Weeks:
≤8 Weeks Since Last Inj: No oral aripiprazole required; administer next inj as soon as possible
>8 and ≤12 Weeks Since Last Inj: Supplement next inj dose w/ 7 days oral aripiprazole
>12 Weeks Since Last Inj: Supplement next inj dose w/ 21 days oral aripiprazole

Supplement w/ the same dose of oral aripiprazole as when the patient began therapy

DOSING CONSIDERATIONS
Concomitant Medications
CYP450 Modulators (Added for <2 Weeks):
No dosage changes recommended.

CYP450 Modulators (Added for >2 Weeks):
Strong CYP3A4 Inhibitor:
Reduce Aristada dose to the next lower strength. No adjustment is necessary in patients taking 441mg, if tolerated.
Poor Metabolizers of CYP2D6: Reduce dose to 441mg from 662mg or 882mg; no dosage adjustment is necessary in patients taking 441mg, if tolerated.
Strong CYP2D6 Inhibitor:
Reduce Aristada dose to the next lower strength. No adjustment is necessary in patients taking 441mg, if tolerated.
Poor Metabolizers of CYP2D6: No dose adjustment required.
Both Strong CYP3A4 Inhibitor and Strong CYP2D6 Inhibitor:
Avoid use for patients at 662mg or 882mg dose. No dosage adjustment is necessary in patients taking 441mg, if tolerated.
CYP3A4 Inducers:
No dose adjustment for 662mg and 882mg dose. Increase the 441mg dose to 662mg.

For the 882mg dose administered every 6 weeks, the next lower strength should be 441mg administered every 4 weeks.

ADMINISTRATION
IM route

Inj Site and Associated Needle Length:
441mg Dose:
Deltoid: 21 gauge, 1 inch or 20 gauge, 1.5 inch
Gluteal: 20 gauge, 1.5 inch or 20 gauge, 2 inch
662mg Dose:
Gluteal: 20 gauge, 1.5 inch or 20 gauge, 2 inch
882mg Dose:
Gluteal: 20 gauge, 1.5 inch or 20 gauge, 2 inch

STORAGE
20-25°C (68-77°F); excursions permitted between 15-30°C (59-86°F).

HOW SUPPLIED
Inj, Extended-Release: 441mg/1.6mL, 662mg/2.4mL, 882mg/3.2mL

CONTRAINDICATIONS
Known hypersensitivity reaction to aripiprazole.

WARNINGS/PRECAUTIONS
Neuroleptic malignant syndrome (NMS) may occur; d/c immediately and institute intensive symptomatic treatment and medical monitoring. If patient appears to require antipsychotic treatment after recovery from NMS, reintroduction of therapy should be closely monitored, since recurrences of NMS have been reported. May cause tardive dyskinesia (TD), especially in the elderly; consider discontinuation if signs/symptoms appear. Associated w/ metabolic changes (eg, hyperglycemia/diabetes mellitus [DM], dyslipidemia, weight gain). May experience intense urges, particularly for gambling, and the inability to control these urges while on this medication. Other compulsive urges, reported less frequently include: sexual urges, shopping, eating or binge eating, and other impulsive or compulsive behaviors; consider dose reduction or discontinuation if such urges develop. May cause orthostatic hypotension, w/ greatest risk at therapy initiation and during dose escalation; consider using a lower starting dose and monitor orthostatic vital signs in patients at increased risk of adverse reactions related to orthostatic hypotension or at increased risk of developing complications from hypotension. Leukopenia, neutropenia, and agranulocytosis reported; frequently monitor CBC during the first few months of therapy in patients w/ a history of a clinically significant low WBC count/ANC or drug-induced leukopenia/neutropenia, and consider discontinuation at the 1st sign of a clinically significant decline in WBC counts w/o other causative factors. D/C therapy in patients w/ severe neutropenia (ANC <1000/mm³) and follow their WBC count until recovery. Caution w/ history of seizures or w/ conditions that lower seizure threshold. May impair mental/physical abilities and disrupt body temperature regulation. May cause esophageal dysmotility and aspiration; caution in patients at risk for aspiration pneumonia.

ADVERSE REACTIONS
Akathisia.

DRUG INTERACTIONS

See Dosing Considerations. Use of oral aripiprazole w/ strong CYP3A4 inhibitors (eg, itraconazole, clarithromycin) or strong CYP2D6 inhibitors (eg, quinidine, fluoxetine, paroxetine) increased exposure of aripiprazole. Use of oral aripiprazole w/ carbamazepine, a strong CYP3A4 inducer, decreased exposure of aripiprazole. May enhance effect of certain antihypertensives; monitor BP and adjust dose accordingly. Intensity of sedation and orthostatic hypotension observed was greater w/ the combination of oral aripiprazole and lorazepam; monitor sedation and BP and adjust dose accordingly w/ concomitant benzodiazepines.

PREGNANCY AND LACTATION

Pregnancy: A pregnancy registry that monitors pregnancy outcomes in women exposed to Aristada during pregnancy is available. Neonates exposed to antipsychotic drugs during the 3rd trimester are at risk for extrapyramidal and/or withdrawal symptoms following delivery; monitor and manage symptoms appropriately.
Lactation: Found in breast milk; however, there are insufficient data to assess the amount in milk, the effects on the breastfed infant, or the effects on milk production. Caution in nursing.

MECHANISM OF ACTION

Atypical antipsychotic; prodrug of aripiprazole. Mechanism of aripiprazole is unknown; efficacy could be mediated through a combination of partial agonist activity at D_2 and $5\text{-}HT_{1A}$ receptors and antagonist activity at $5\text{-}HT_{2A}$ receptors.

PHARMACOKINETICS

Distribution: V_d=268L; serum protein binding (>99%, primarily to albumin); found in breast milk. **Metabolism:** Prodrug via enzyme-mediated hydrolysis to N-hydroxymethyl aripiprazole; water-mediated hydrolysis to aripiprazole. Hepatic metabolism of aripiprazole via CYP3A4 and CYP2D6. **Elimination:** $T_{1/2}$=29.2-34.9 days (after monthly inj).

PATIENT CONSIDERATIONS

Assessment: Assess for dementia-related psychosis, DM, dehydration, hypovolemia, cardiovascular disease, cerebrovascular disease, seizures, risk for aspiration pneumonia, drug hypersensitivity, any other conditions where treatment is cautioned, pregnancy/nursing status, and possible drug interactions. Obtain baseline FPG in patients at risk for DM. Obtain baseline CBC in patients w/ a history of a clinically significant low WBC counts/ANC or drug-induced leukopenia/neutropenia.

Monitoring: Monitor for NMS, TD, hyperglycemia/DM, dyslipidemia, weight gain, orthostatic hypotension, leukopenia, neutropenia, agranulocytosis, seizures, disruption of body temperature regulation, esophageal dysmotility, aspiration, and other adverse reactions. Monitor for worsening of glucose control in patients w/ DM and FPG in patients at risk for DM. Monitor CBC frequently during the 1st few months of therapy in patients w/ a history of a clinically significant low WBC counts/ANC or drug-induced leukopenia/neutropenia. Monitor for fever or other symptoms/signs of infection in patients w/ clinically significant neutropenia. Periodically reassess need for continued treatment.

Counseling: Advise patients and caregivers of the possibility of experiencing intense urges to spend money or gamble, increased sexual urges, binge eating and/or other intense urges and the inability to control these urges while taking aripiprazole. Educate about NMS; advise to contact a healthcare provider or report to the emergency room if signs/symptoms develop. Instruct to notify healthcare provider if any movements that cannot be controlled in the face, tongue, or other body part develop. Educate about the risk of metabolic changes, how to recognize symptoms of hyperglycemia/DM, and the need for specific monitoring. Educate about the risk of orthostatic hypotension, particularly at the time of initiating treatment, reinitiating treatment, or increasing the dose. Advise patients w/ preexisting low WBC count or a history of drug-induced leukopenia/neutropenia to have their CBC monitored during treatment. Instruct to use caution when operating hazardous machinery. Instruct to avoid overheating and dehydration. Instruct to notify healthcare provider of any changes to prescription or OTC drugs. Advise that therapy may cause extrapyramidal and/or withdrawal symptoms in a neonate and to notify healthcare provider w/ a known or suspected pregnancy.

ARIXTRA — fondaparinux sodium Rx

Class: Selective factor Xa inhibitor

> Epidural or spinal hematomas may occur in patients who are anticoagulated with low molecular weight heparins (LMWHs), heparinoids, or fondaparinux sodium and who are receiving neuraxial anesthesia or undergoing spinal puncture; long-term or permanent paralysis may result. Increased risk of developing epidural or spinal hematomas in patients using indwelling epidural catheters, concomitant use of other drugs that affect hemostasis (eg, NSAIDs, platelet inhibitors, other anticoagulants), history of traumatic or repeated epidural or spinal puncture, history of spinal deformity or spinal surgery, or unknown optimal timing between the administration of therapy and neuraxial procedures. Monitor frequently for signs/symptoms of neurologic impairment; if neurologic compromise noted, urgent treatment is necessary. Consider benefit and risks before neuraxial intervention in patients anticoagulated or to be anticoagulated for thromboprophylaxis.

ADULT DOSAGE

Deep Vein Thrombosis/Pulmonary Embolism

DVT Prophylaxis Following Hip Fracture Surgery, Hip Replacement Surgery, Knee Replacement Surgery, or Abdominal Surgery (in Patients at Risk for Thromboembolic Complications):
≥50kg: 2.5mg SQ qd after hemostasis has been established; administer initial

PEDIATRIC DOSAGE

Pediatric use may not have been established

---

dose no earlier than 6-8 hrs after surgery
Usual Duration: 5-9 days (administered up to 11 days following hip replacement or knee replacement surgery and administered up to 10 days following abdominal surgery in clinical trials); extended prophylaxis course of up to 24 additional days recommended for patients undergoing hip fracture surgery (total of 32 days administered in clinical trials)

DVT/PE Treatment:
Treatment of acute DVT w/ warfarin sodium, and treatment of acute PE w/ warfarin sodium when initial therapy is administered in the hospital
<50kg: 5mg SQ qd
50-100kg: 7.5mg SQ qd
>100kg: 10mg SQ qd
Initiate concomitant treatment w/ warfarin sodium as soon as possible, usually w/in 72 hrs
Continue fondaparinux for at least 5 days and until therapeutic oral anticoagulant effect is established (INR 2-3)
Usual Duration: 5-9 days (administered up to 26 days in clinical trials)

DOSING CONSIDERATIONS
Renal Impairment
CrCl 30-50mL/min: Use caution

ADMINISTRATION
SQ route

Do not mix w/ other medications or sol
Do not expel air bubble from syringe before the inj
Administer in fatty tissue, alternating inj sites
Refer to PI for further instructions for use

STORAGE
25°C (77°F); excursions permitted to 15-30°C (59-86°F).

HOW SUPPLIED
Inj: 2.5mg/0.5mL, 5mg/0.4mL, 7.5mg/0.6mL, 10mg/0.8mL

CONTRAINDICATIONS
Severe renal impairment (CrCl <30mL/min), active major bleeding, bacterial endocarditis, thrombocytopenia associated w/ a (+) in vitro test for antiplatelet antibody in the presence of fondaparinux sodium, body weight <50kg (venous thromboembolism prophylaxis only), history of serious hypersensitivity reaction (eg, angioedema, anaphylactoid/anaphylactic reactions) to fondaparinux.

WARNINGS/PRECAUTIONS
Extreme caution in conditions with increased risk of hemorrhage (eg, congenital or acquired bleeding disorders, active ulcerative and angiodysplastic GI disease, hemorrhagic stroke, uncontrolled arterial HTN, diabetic retinopathy, or shortly after brain, spinal, or ophthalmological surgery). Elevated activated PTT temporally associated with bleeding events reported. Administration of initial dose earlier than 6 hrs after surgery increases risk of major bleeding. Increased risk of bleeding in patients with impaired renal function; d/c therapy immediately if severe renal impairment develops. Caution with CrCl 30-50mL/min. Increased risk of bleeding in patients who weigh <50kg; caution in treatment of PE and DVT. Thrombocytopenia reported. D/C if platelet count falls <100,000/mm³. D/C if unexpected changes in coagulation parameters or major bleeding occur during therapy. Needle guard of the prefilled syringe contains dry natural latex rubber that may cause allergic reactions in latex-sensitive individuals. Caution with moderate hepatic impairment (Child-Pugh Category B) and in elderly.

ADVERSE REACTIONS
Bleeding complications, thrombocytopenia, local irritation (eg, inj-site bleeding, rash, pruritus), anemia, insomnia, increased wound drainage, hypokalemia, dizziness, purpura, hypotension, confusion.

DRUG INTERACTIONS
See Boxed Warning. Agents that may enhance the risk of hemorrhage should be discontinued prior to initiation of therapy unless these agents are essential; if coadministration is necessary, monitor closely for hemorrhage.

PREGNANCY AND LACTATION
Category B, caution in nursing.

MECHANISM OF ACTION
Selective factor Xa inhibitor; selectively binds to antithrombin III (ATIII) and potentiates the innate neutralization of FXa by ATIII, thereby interrupting the blood coagulation cascade and inhibiting thrombin formation and thrombus development.

PHARMACOKINETICS
Absorption: Rapid, complete. Absolute bioavailability (100%). (2.5mg qd) C_{max}=0.39-0.50mg/L, T_{max}=3 hrs. (5mg, 7.5mg, 10mg qd) C_{max}=1.2-1.26mg/L. **Distribution:** V_d=7-11L; plasma protein binding (≥94%, bound to ATIII). **Elimination:** Urine (≤77%, unchanged); $T_{1/2}$=17-21 hrs.

PATIENT CONSIDERATIONS

Assessment: Assess for history of serious hypersensitivity reaction to the drug, conditions that increase the risk of hemorrhage, or any other conditions where treatment is cautioned or contraindicated, renal/hepatic impairment, latex sensitivity, pregnancy/nursing status, and for possible drug interactions.

Monitoring: Monitor for signs/symptoms of bleeding, thrombocytopenia, and other adverse reactions. In patients undergoing neuraxial anesthesia or spinal puncture, monitor for epidural or spinal hematomas and neurologic impairment. Perform periodic CBC (including platelet count), stool occult blood tests, and SrCr level tests.

Counseling: Advise patients who have had neuraxial anesthesia or spinal puncture to watch for signs and symptoms of spinal/epidural hematoma, especially if concomitantly taking NSAIDs, platelet inhibitors, or other anticoagulants; instruct to contact physician immediately if symptoms occur. Advise that the use of aspirin and other NSAIDs may enhance the risk of hemorrhage. Instruct on proper administration technique. Counsel on signs/symptoms of possible bleeding. Inform patients that it may take longer than usual to stop bleeding and that they may bruise and/or bleed more easily while on therapy. Instruct to report any unusual bleeding, bruising, or signs of thrombocytopenia to the physician. Instruct to notify physician or dentist of all prescription and nonprescription medications currently being taken.

ARMOUR THYROID — thyroid   Rx

Class: Thyroid replacement hormone

> Do not use for the treatment of obesity or weight loss; doses within range of daily hormonal requirements are ineffective for weight reduction in euthyroid patients. Serious or life-threatening manifestations of toxicity may occur when given in larger doses, particularly when given in association with sympathomimetic amines.

ADULT DOSAGE	PEDIATRIC DOSAGE
Hypothyroidism	**Hypothyroidism**
Replacement/supplemental therapy in hypothyroidism of any etiology, except transient hypothyroidism during the recovery phase of subacute thyroiditis	**Congenital:** **0-6 Months of Age:** 4.8-6mg/kg/day **6-12 Months of Age:** 3.6-4.8mg/kg/day **1-5 Years:** 3-3.6mg/kg/day **6-12 Years:** 2.4-3mg/kg/day **>12 Years:** 1.2-1.8mg/kg/day
Initial: 30mg/day; 15mg/day in patients w/ long-standing myxedema	
Titrate: Increase by 15mg every 2-3 weeks	
Readjust dose w/in the first 4 weeks	
Maint: 60-120mg/day	
Myxedema Coma: Resume oral therapy when clinical situation has been stabilized after IV administration and patient is able to take oral medications	
Pituitary TSH Suppressant	
Used to treat/prevent various types of euthyroid goiters (eg, thyroid nodules, subacute or chronic lymphocytic thyroiditis [Hashimoto's], multinodular goiter) and to manage thyroid cancer	
Thyroid Suppression Therapy: 1.56mcg/kg/day T4 for 7-10 days	
Thyroid Cancer: Give larger doses than those used for replacement therapy	

ADMINISTRATION
Oral route

STORAGE
15-30°C (59-86°F). Protect from light and moisture.

HOW SUPPLIED
Tab: 15mg, 30mg, 60mg, 90mg, 120mg, 180mg*, 240mg, 300mg* *scored

CONTRAINDICATIONS
Uncorrected adrenal cortical insufficiency, untreated thyrotoxicosis, apparent hypersensitivity to any of the active or extraneous constituents of this medication.

WARNINGS/PRECAUTIONS
Use is unjustified for the treatment of male or female infertility unless accompanied by hypothyroidism. Caution with cardiovascular (CV) disorders (eg, angina pectoris) and elderly with risk of occult cardiac disease; initiate at low doses (eg, 15-30mg/day) and reduce dose if euthyroid state can only be reached at the expense of aggravation of CV disease. May aggravate diabetes mellitus (DM), diabetes insipidus (DI), and adrenal cortical insufficiency. Treatment of myxedema coma requires simultaneous administration of glucocorticoids. Excessive doses in infants may cause craniosynostosis. Caution with strong suspicion of thyroid gland autonomy. Androgens, corticosteroids, estrogens, iodine-containing preparations, and salicylates may interfere with lab tests.

DRUG INTERACTIONS
See Boxed Warning. Closely monitor PT in patients on oral anticoagulants; dose reduction of anticoagulant may be required. May increase insulin or oral hypoglycemic requirements. Impaired absorption with cholestyramine and colestipol; space dosing by 4-5 hrs. Estrogens may increase thyroxine-binding globulin and may decrease free T4; increase in thyroid dose may be needed.

PREGNANCY AND LACTATION
Category A, caution in nursing.

MECHANISM OF ACTION
Thyroid hormone; not established. Enhances oxygen consumption by most body tissues, increases basal metabolic rate and metabolism of carbohydrates, lipids, and proteins.

PHARMACOKINETICS
Absorption: (T3) Almost total; (T4) partial. **Distribution:** Plasma protein binding (>99%), found in breast milk. **Metabolism:** (T4) Deiodination in liver, kidneys, other tissues.

PATIENT CONSIDERATIONS

Assessment: Assess for adrenal cortical insufficiency, thyrotoxicosis, previous hypersensitivity to the drug, CV disorders (eg, coronary artery disease, angina pectoris), DM, DI, myxedema coma, nursing status, and possible drug interactions.

Monitoring: Monitor response to treatment, urinary glucose levels in patients with DM, PT in patients receiving anticoagulants, and aggravation of diabetes or CV disease. Monitor thyroid function periodically.

Counseling: Inform that replacement therapy is to be taken essentially for life, except in transient hypothyroidism. Instruct to immediately report any signs/symptoms of thyroid hormone toxicity. Inform about the importance of frequent/close monitoring of PT and urinary glucose and the need for dose adjustment of antidiabetic and/or oral anticoagulant medication. Inform that partial hair loss may be seen in children in 1st few months of therapy. Inform that drug is not for treatment of obesity or weight loss.

ARNUITY ELLIPTA — fluticasone furoate   Rx

Class: Corticosteroid

ADULT DOSAGE	PEDIATRIC DOSAGE
Asthma	**Asthma**
Prophylactic Maint Treatment: **Initial:**	**Prophylactic Maint Treatment:** **≥12 Years:** **Initial:**
Not on an Inhaled Corticosteroid: 100mcg qd	**Not on an Inhaled Corticosteroid:** 100mcg qd
All Other Patients: Dose based on previous asthma drug therapy and disease severity	**All Other Patients:** Dose based on previous asthma drug therapy and disease severity
Titrate: May replace w/ 200mcg in patients who do not respond to 100mcg after 2 weeks of therapy	**Titrate:** May replace w/ 200mcg in patients who do not respond to 100mcg after 2 weeks of therapy
Max: 200mcg/day	**Max:** 200mcg/day

DOSING CONSIDERATIONS
Elderly
Start at lower end of dosing range

ADMINISTRATION
Oral inh route

Administer as 1 inh qd, at the same time every day; do not use >1X q24h
Rinse mouth w/ water w/o swallowing after each dose

STORAGE
20-25°C (68-77°F); excursions permitted from 15-30°C (59-86°F). Store in a dry place away from direct heat or sunlight. Store inside the unopened moisture-protective foil tray and only remove from the tray immediately before initial use. Discard 6 weeks after opening the foil tray or when the counter reads "0" (after all blisters have been used), whichever comes 1st.

HOW SUPPLIED
Powder, Inh: 100mcg/blister, 200mcg/blister [14, 30 inh]

CONTRAINDICATIONS
Primary treatment of status asthmaticus or other acute episodes of asthma where intensive measures are required, known severe hypersensitivity to milk proteins or demonstrated hypersensitivity to fluticasone furoate or any of the excipients.

WARNINGS/PRECAUTIONS
Not indicated for acute bronchospasm relief. *Candida albicans* infections of mouth and pharynx reported; treat and, if needed, interrupt therapy. Increased susceptibility to infections. May lead to serious/fatal course of chickenpox or measles; avoid exposure and if exposed, consider prophylaxis/treatment. Use w/ caution, if at all, in patients w/ active/quiescent tuberculosis (TB); untreated systemic fungal, bacterial, viral, or parasitic infections; or ocular herpes simplex. Deaths due to adrenal insufficiency reported during and after transfer from systemic to inhaled corticosteroids; wean slowly from systemic corticosteroid use after transferring to therapy. Resume oral corticosteroids during periods of stress or a severe asthma attack in patients previously withdrawn from systemic corticosteroids. Transfer from systemic corticosteroids to therapy may unmask allergic conditions previously suppressed by systemic therapy (eg, rhinitis, conjunctivitis, eczema). Monitor for systemic corticosteroid effects; reduce dose slowly if hypercorticism and adrenal suppression occur. Bronchospasm may occur w/ an immediate increase in wheezing after dosing; treat immediately w/ an inhaled, short acting bronchodilator; d/c Arnuity Ellipta immediately, and institute alternative therapy. Hypersensitivity reactions may occur; d/c if such reactions occur. Decreases in bone mineral density (BMD) reported w/ long-term use; caution w/ major risk factors for decreased bone mineral content,

including chronic use of drugs that can reduce bone mass (eg, anticonvulsants, oral corticosteroids). May reduce growth velocity in children and adolescents. Glaucoma, increased IOP, and cataracts reported w/ long-term use. Caution w/ moderate or severe hepatic impairment.

ADVERSE REACTIONS

Nasopharyngitis, bronchitis, URTI, headache, pharyngitis, sinusitis, toothache, viral gastroenteritis, oral candidiasis, oropharyngeal candidiasis/pain, influenza, back pain, dysphonia, rhinitis, throat irritation.

DRUG INTERACTIONS

Ketoconazole increases exposure. Caution w/ long-term ketoconazole and other known strong CYP3A4 inhibitors (eg, ritonavir, clarithromycin, itraconazole); increased systemic corticosteroid adverse effects may occur.

PREGNANCY AND LACTATION

Category C, caution in nursing.

MECHANISM OF ACTION

Corticosteroid; has not been established. Shown to have a wide range of actions on multiple cell types (eg, mast cells, eosinophils, neutrophils, macrophages, lymphocytes) and mediators (eg, histamine, eicosanoids, leukotrienes, cytokines) involved in inflammation.

PHARMACOKINETICS

Absorption: Absolute bioavailability (13.9%); T_{max}=0.5-1 hr. **Distribution:** V_d=661L (IV); plasma protein binding (99.6%). **Metabolism:** Liver via CYP3A4. **Elimination:** Feces (101% [PO], 90% [IV]), urine (1% [PO], 2% [IV]); $T_{1/2}$=24 hrs.

PATIENT CONSIDERATIONS

Assessment: Assess for status asthmaticus; acute episodes of asthma; hypersensitivity to drug or to milk proteins; active/quiescent TB; untreated systemic infections; ocular herpes simplex; risk factors for decreased bone mineral content; history of increased IOP, glaucoma, and/or cataracts; hepatic impairment; pregnancy/nursing status; and possible drug interactions.

Monitoring: Monitor for localized oropharyngeal infections w/ *C. albicans*, infections, systemic corticosteroid effects (eg, hypercorticism, adrenal suppression), paradoxical bronchospasm, hypersensitivity reactions, decreases in BMD, glaucoma, cataracts, increased IOP, and other adverse reactions. Monitor growth of children and adolescents routinely (eg, via stadiometry). Closely monitor patients w/ moderate to severe hepatic disease.

Counseling: Inform that drug is not meant to relieve acute asthma symptoms; advise to treat acute symptoms w/ an inhaled short-acting β_2-agonist (SABA). Instruct to seek medical attention immediately if experiencing worsening of symptoms, a significant decrease in lung function, or a need for more inhalations than usual of inhaled SABAs. Advise to use at regular intervals, not to increase the dose or frequency of therapy, and not to d/c or reduce therapy w/o physician guidance. Instruct to contact physician if oropharyngeal candidiasis develops, or if symptoms do not improve after 2 weeks. Advise to rinse mouth w/ water w/o swallowing after inhalation. Advise to avoid exposure to chickenpox or measles, and, if exposed, to consult physician w/o delay. Inform about risk of immunosuppression, hypercorticism, adrenal suppression, reduction in BMD, reduced growth velocity in pediatric patients, ocular effects, and hypersensitivity reactions, including anaphylaxis; instruct to d/c if hypersensitivity reactions occur. Inform that the inhaler is not reusable and advise not to take the inhaler apart.

AROMASIN — exemestane   Rx

Class: Aromatase inactivator

ADULT DOSAGE	PEDIATRIC DOSAGE
Estrogen-Receptor Positive Early Breast Cancer	Pediatric use may not have been established
Adjuvant treatment of postmenopausal women who have received 2-3 years of tamoxifen and are switched to exemestane for completion of a total of 5 consecutive years of adjuvant hormonal therapy	
Usual: 25mg qd	
Advanced Breast Cancer	
In postmenopausal women whose disease has progressed following tamoxifen therapy	
Usual: 25mg qd	

DOSING CONSIDERATIONS
Concomitant Medications
Strong CYP3A4 Inducers: 50mg qd

ADMINISTRATION
Oral route

Take after a meal

STORAGE
25°C (77°F); excursions permitted to 15-30°C (59-86°F).

HOW SUPPLIED
Tab: 25mg

CONTRAINDICATIONS
Known hypersensitivity to the drug or to any of the excipients.

WARNINGS/PRECAUTIONS

Reductions in bone mineral density (BMD) over time reported. During adjuvant treatment, assess BMD in women w/ osteoporosis or at risk of osteoporosis at the commencement of treatment. Monitor patients for BMD loss and treat as appropriate. Perform routine assessment of 25-hydroxy vitamin D levels prior to treatment; give vitamin D supplementation in women w/ vitamin D deficiency. Lymphocytopenia (common toxicity criteria [CTC] Grade 3 or 4) reported w/ advanced breast cancer; most had a preexisting lower grade lymphopenia. Elevations of serum levels of AST, ALT, alkaline phosphatase, and gamma-glutamyl transferase >5X ULN (eg, ≥CTC Grade 3) have been rarely reported w/ advanced breast cancer, but appear mostly attributable to the underlying presence of liver and/or bone metastases. Elevations in bilirubin, alkaline phosphatase, and creatinine reported w/ early breast cancer. Not indicated for the treatment of breast cancer in premenopausal women. May cause fetal harm when administered to a pregnant woman; females of reproductive potential should use effective contraception during treatment and for 1 month after the last dose.

ADVERSE REACTIONS

Adjuvant Treatment of Early Breast Cancer: Hot flushes, fatigue, arthralgia, headache, insomnia.
Treatment of Advanced Breast Cancer: Hot flushes, nausea, fatigue, increased sweating, increased appetite.

DRUG INTERACTIONS

See Dosing Considerations. Avoid coadministration w/ estrogen-containing agents. CYP3A4 inducers (eg, rifampicin, phenytoin, carbamazepine, phenobarbital, St. John's wort) may significantly decrease exposure; dose modification is recommended w/ a strong CYP3A4 inducer.

PREGNANCY AND LACTATION

Pregnancy: Based on findings in animal studies and its mechanism of action, exemestane can cause fetal harm when administered to a pregnant woman.
Lactation: Women should not breastfeed during treatment and for 1 month after the final dose.
Reproductive Potential: Pregnancy testing is recommended for females of reproductive potential w/in 7 days prior to initiating exemestane. Females of reproductive potential should use effective contraception during treatment and for 1 month after the final dose. Male and female fertility may be impaired by treatment.

MECHANISM OF ACTION

Irreversible, steroidal aromatase inactivator; acts as false substrate for aromatase enzyme and is processed to an intermediate that binds irreversibly to the active site of the enzyme, causing its inactivation. Significantly lowers circulating estrogen concentrations in postmenopausal women.

PHARMACOKINETICS

Absorption: Rapid. T_{max}=1.2 hrs; AUC=75.4ng•hr/mL. **Distribution:** Plasma protein binding (90%). **Metabolism:** Extensive. Oxidation and reduction; CYP3A4, aldoketoreductases. **Elimination:** Urine (42%, <1% unchanged), feces (42%); $T_{1/2}$=24 hrs.

PATIENT CONSIDERATIONS

Assessment: Assess for hypersensitivity, preexisting lower grade lymphopenia, liver and/or bone metastases, osteoporosis/risk of osteoporosis, pregnancy/nursing status, and for possible drug interactions. Perform routine assessment of 25-hydroxy vitamin D levels prior to treatment. Assess BMD in women w/ osteoporosis/at risk of osteoporosis.

Monitoring: Monitor for hematological abnormalities, BMD loss, osteoporosis, and other adverse reactions. Monitor LFTs, creatinine, alkaline phosphatase, and bilirubin levels.

Counseling: Advise that drug lowers the estrogen level in the body, which may lead to reduction in BMD over time, and that the lower the BMD, the greater the risk of osteoporosis and fracture. Inform not to take concomitant estrogen-containing agents while on therapy. Advise that drug is not for use for the treatment of breast cancer in premenopausal women. Advise pregnant women and females of reproductive potential that exposure during pregnancy or w/in 1 month prior to conception can result in fetal harm. Instruct to inform physician of a known or suspected pregnancy. Advise females of reproductive potential to use effective contraception during treatment and for 1 month after the last dose. Instruct women not to breastfeed during treatment and for 1 month after the last dose.

ARRANON — nelarabine   Rx

Class: Deoxyguanosine analogue

> Severe neurologic adverse reactions reported, including altered mental states (eg, severe somnolence), CNS effects (eg, convulsions), and peripheral neuropathy, ranging from numbness and paresthesias to motor weakness and paralysis. Adverse reactions associated with demyelination and ascending peripheral neuropathies similar in appearance to Guillain-Barre syndrome also reported. Close monitoring for neurologic adverse reactions is strongly recommended. D/C if neurologic adverse reactions of NCI Common Toxicity Criteria ≥Grade 2 occur.

ADULT DOSAGE	PEDIATRIC DOSAGE
T-Cell Acute Lymphoblastic Leukemia	**T-Cell Acute Lymphoblastic Leukemia**
In patients whose disease has not responded to or has relapsed following treatment w/ ≥2 chemotherapy regimens	In patients whose disease has not responded to or has relapsed following treatment w/ ≥2 chemotherapy regimens

1500mg/m² IV over 2 hrs on Days 1, 3, and 5, repeated every 21 days

T-Cell Lymphoblastic Lymphoma

In patients whose disease has not responded to or has relapsed following treatment w/ ≥2 chemotherapy regimens

1500mg/m² IV over 2 hrs on Days 1, 3, and 5, repeated every 21 days

650mg/m²/day IV over 1 hr for 5 consecutive days, repeated every 21 days

T-Cell Lymphoblastic Lymphoma

In patients whose disease has not responded to or has relapsed following treatment w/ ≥2 chemotherapy regimens

650mg/m²/day IV over 1 hr for 5 consecutive days, repeated every 21 days

---

DOSING CONSIDERATIONS

Adverse Reactions

Neurologic Reactions ≥Grade 2: D/C treatment
Dosage may be delayed for other toxicity including hematologic toxicity

ADMINISTRATION

IV route

Preparation

Do not dilute nelarabine prior to administration
Transfer the appropriate dose of nelarabine into polyvinylchloride infusion bags or glass containers for administration

STORAGE

25°C (77°F); excursions permitted to 15-30°C (59-86°F). Stable in polyvinylchloride infusion bags or glass containers for up to 8 hrs at up to 30°C.

HOW SUPPLIED

Inj: 5mg/mL [50mL]

WARNINGS/PRECAUTIONS

Leukopenia, thrombocytopenia, anemia, and neutropenia, including febrile neutropenia, reported; regularly monitor CBC including platelets. May cause fetal harm. IV hydration should be given for the management of hyperuricemia in patients at risk for tumor lysis syndrome; may also consider giving allopurinol in patients at risk for hyperuricemia. Closely monitor for toxicities in patients with moderate or severe renal impairment (CrCl ≤50mL/min) or severe hepatic impairment (total bilirubin >3X ULN). Caution in elderly.

ADVERSE REACTIONS

Altered mental status, CNS effects, peripheral neuropathy, anemia, thrombocytopenia, neutropenia, leukopenia, N/V, diarrhea, constipation, fatigue, pyrexia, cough, headache.

DRUG INTERACTIONS

Use with adenosine deaminase inhibitors (eg, pentostatin) is not recommended. Patients treated previously or concurrently with intrathecal chemotherapy or previously with craniospinal irradiation may be at increased risk for neurologic adverse events. Avoid administration of live vaccines to immunocompromised patients.

PREGNANCY AND LACTATION

Category D, not for use in nursing.

MECHANISM OF ACTION

Deoxyguanosine analogue; nucleoside metabolic inhibitor; demethylated by adenosine deaminase to ara-G, mono-phosphorylated by deoxyguanosine kinase and deoxycytidine kinase, and subsequently converted to the active 5'-triphosphate, ara-GTP. Accumulation of ara-GTP in leukemic blasts allows for incorporation into DNA, leading to inhibition of DNA synthesis and cell death.

PHARMACOKINETICS

Absorption: C_{max}=5µg/mL, 31.4µg/mL (ara-G); AUC=4.4µg•hr/mL, 162µg•hr/mL (ara-G). **Distribution:** Plasma protein binding (<25%). (Adults) V_{ss}=197L/m², 50L/m² (ara-G); (Pediatrics) V_{ss}=213L/m², 33L/m² (ara-G). **Metabolism:** O-demethylation via adenosine deaminase; ara-G (metabolite). **Elimination:** Urine (6.6%, 27% ara-G); (Adults) $T_{1/2}$=18 min, 3.2 hrs (ara-G), (Pediatrics) $T_{1/2}$=13 min, 2 hrs (ara-G).

PATIENT CONSIDERATIONS

Assessment: Assess for renal/hepatic impairment, risk of tumor lysis syndrome or hyperuricemia, pregnancy/nursing status, and possible drug interactions.

Monitoring: Monitor for signs/symptoms of neurotoxicity (eg, somnolence, confusion, convulsions, ataxia, peripheral neuropathy, hypoesthesia), hyperuricemia, leukopenia, thrombocytopenia, anemia, neutropenia, and other adverse reactions. Perform regular monitoring of CBC, including platelets.

Counseling: Inform that therapy may cause somnolence and therefore caution should be taken when operating hazardous machinery or driving. Instruct to contact physician if new or worsening symptoms of peripheral neuropathy develop (eg; tingling or numbness in fingers, hands, toes or feet; difficulty with fine motor coordination tasks; unsteadiness while walking, weakness arising from a low chair/climbing stairs, increased tripping). Instruct to contact physician if seizures, fever, or signs of infection develop. Advise to use effective contraceptive measures to prevent pregnancy and to avoid breastfeeding during treatment.

ARTHROTEC — diclofenac sodium/misoprostol   Rx

Class: NSAID/prostaglandin E₁ analogue

> **Misoprostol:** Administration of misoprostol to women who are pregnant can cause abortion, premature birth, or birth defects. Uterine rupture reported when used to induce labor or to induce abortion beyond the 8th week of pregnancy. Arthrotec should not be taken by pregnant women. Patient must be advised of the abortifacient property and warned not to give drug to others. Should not be used in women of childbearing potential unless patient requires NSAID therapy and is at high risk for developing gastric or duodenal ulcers or complications from NSAID-associated gastric or duodenal ulcers. In such patients, may prescribe if patient has had a (-) serum pregnancy test w/in 2 weeks prior to beginning therapy; is capable of complying w/ effective contraceptive measures; has received both oral and written warnings of the hazards of misoprostol, the risk of possible contraception failure, and the danger to other women of childbearing potential should the drug be taken by mistake; and will begin therapy only on the 2nd or 3rd day of the next normal menstrual period. **Diclofenac:** NSAIDs cause an increased risk of serious cardiovascular (CV) thrombotic events, including MI and stroke, which can be fatal. This risk may occur early in treatment and may increase w/ duration of use. Contraindicated in the setting of CABG surgery. NSAIDs cause an increased risk of serious GI adverse events (eg, bleeding, ulceration, stomach/intestinal perforation), which can be fatal and can occur at any time during use and w/o warning symptoms; elderly patients and patients w/ a prior history of peptic ulcer disease and/or GI bleeding are at a greater risk.

ADULT DOSAGE

Osteoarthritis

Treatment of signs/symptoms of osteoarthritis in patients at high risk of developing NSAID-induced gastric and duodenal ulcers and their complications

50mg/200mcg tab tid; for patients who experience intolerance, may use 50mg/200mcg tab bid or 75mg/200mcg tab bid

Max:
Diclofenac: 150mg/day
Misoprostol: 200mcg/dose or 800mcg/day

Rheumatoid Arthritis

Treatment of the signs/symptoms of rheumatoid arthritis in patients at high risk of developing NSAID-induced gastric and duodenal ulcers and their complications

50mg/200mcg tab tid or qid; for patients who experience intolerance, may use 50mg/200mcg tab bid or 75mg/200mcg tab bid

Max:
Diclofenac: 225mg/day
Misoprostol: 200mcg/dose or 800mcg/day

PEDIATRIC DOSAGE

Pediatric use may not have been established

DOSING CONSIDERATIONS

Concomitant Medications

CYP2C9 Inhibitors: When concomitant use is necessary, diclofenac total daily dose should not exceed the lowest recommended dose of 50mg/200mcg bid

Elderly

If the anticipated benefit outweighs the potential risks, start at lower end of dosing range; monitor for adverse effects

Other Important Considerations

Fixed combination product; not recommended for patients who would not receive the appropriate dose of both ingredients

ADMINISTRATION

Oral route

STORAGE

≤25°C (77°F), in a dry area.

HOW SUPPLIED

Tab: (Diclofenac/Misoprostol) 50mg/200mcg, 75mg/200mcg

CONTRAINDICATIONS

Known hypersensitivity (eg, anaphylactic reactions, serious skin reactions) to diclofenac sodium/misoprostol, other prostaglandins, or any components of the drug product; history of asthma, urticaria, or other allergic-type reactions after taking aspirin (ASA) or other NSAIDs; in the setting of CABG surgery; pregnancy; active GI bleeding.

WARNINGS/PRECAUTIONS

Use lowest effective dose for the shortest duration possible. Associated w/ anaphylactic reactions. **Diclofenac:** Increased CV thrombotic risk w/ higher doses reported. Avoid in patients w/ a recent MI unless benefits outweigh the risks of recurrent CV thrombotic events; if used, monitor for signs of cardiac ischemia. Increased risk for GI bleeding w/ longer duration of NSAID therapy, older age, poor general health status, and advanced liver disease and/or coagulopathy; avoid use in patients at higher risk unless benefits are expected to outweigh the increased risk of bleeding. Consider alternate therapies other than NSAIDs for patients at higher risk and patients w/ active GI bleeding. Promptly initiate evaluation and treatment if a serious GI adverse event is suspected; d/c until a serious GI adverse event is ruled out. Hepatotoxicity reported; d/c immediately and perform a clinical evaluation if clinical signs/

symptoms consistent w/ liver disease develop, if systemic manifestations occur, or if abnormal liver tests persist/worsen. May cause new onset HTN or worsen preexisting HTN. Fluid retention and edema reported. Avoid use in patients w/ severe heart failure (HF) unless benefits outweigh risks; monitor for signs of worsening HF if used. Renal papillary necrosis and other renal injury reported w/ long-term use. Renal toxicity also reported in patients in whom renal prostaglandins have a compensatory role in the maintenance of renal perfusion; increased risk w/ renal/hepatic dysfunction, dehydration, hypovolemia, and HF, and in the elderly. Correct volume status in dehydrated or hypovolemic patients prior to initiating therapy. Avoid use in patients w/ advanced renal disease unless the benefits are expected to outweigh the risk; monitor for signs of worsening renal function if used. Hyperkalemia reported. Monitor for changes in the signs/symptoms of asthma in patients w/ preexisting asthma (w/o known ASA sensitivity). May cause serious skin reactions (eg, exfoliative dermatitis, Stevens-Johnson syndrome, toxic epidermal necrolysis); d/c at 1st appearance of skin rash/hypersensitivity. Anemia reported. May increase the risk of bleeding events; coagulation disorders may increase this risk. May mask inflammation and fever.

ADVERSE REACTIONS
Abdominal pain, diarrhea, dyspepsia, nausea, flatulence.

DRUG INTERACTIONS
See Dosing Considerations. Concomitant use w/ Mg^{2+}-containing antacids is not recommended. Caution w/ concomitant drugs known to be potentially hepatotoxic (eg, antibiotics, antiepileptics). **Diclofenac:** Drugs that interfere w/ serotonin reuptake may potentiate the risk of bleeding. Synergistic effect on bleeding w/ anticoagulants (eg, warfarin); monitor for signs of bleeding w/ concomitant anticoagulants, antiplatelet agents (eg, ASA), SSRIs, and SNRIs. May increase risk of GI bleeding w/ use of oral corticosteroids, anticoagulants, and SSRIs; smoking; and alcohol use. ASA may increase risk of bleeding and serious GI events; concomitant use w/ analgesic doses of ASA is not recommended. Monitor patients more closely for GI bleeding w/ concomitant use of low-dose ASA for cardiac prophylaxis. May diminish antihypertensive effect of ACE inhibitors, ARBs, and β-blockers (eg, propranolol); monitor BP. Coadministration w/ ACE inhibitors or ARBs may result in deterioration of renal function (including possible acute renal failure) in patients who are elderly or volume-depleted (including those on diuretic therapy), or who have renal impairment; monitor for worsening renal function when these drugs are administered concomitantly and adequately hydrate patients. May reduce the natriuretic effect of loop diuretics (eg, furosemide) and thiazide diuretics; observe for signs of worsening renal function, in addition to assuring diuretic efficacy including antihypertensive effects. May increase digoxin serum concentrations and prolong the $T_{1/2}$ of digoxin; monitor digoxin levels. May elevate plasma lithium levels and reduce renal lithium clearance; monitor for signs of lithium toxicity. May increase the risk for methotrexate (MTX) toxicity; monitor for MTX toxicity. May increase cyclosporine's nephrotoxicity; monitor for signs of worsening renal function. Concomitant use w/ other NSAIDs or salicylates (eg, diflunisal, salsalate) increases the risk of GI toxicity; not recommended w/ other NSAIDs or salicylates. Concomitant use w/ pemetrexed may increase the risk of pemetrexed-associated myelosuppression, renal, and GI toxicity; refer to PI for further information. Antacids may delay absorption. Concomitant use w/ corticosteroids may increase the risk of GI ulceration or bleeding; monitor for signs of bleeding. Coadministration w/ CYP2C9 inhibitors (eg, voriconazole) may enhance the exposure and toxicity of diclofenac. Coadministration w/ CYP2C9 inducers (eg, rifampin) may lead to compromised efficacy of diclofenac. A dosage adjustment may be warranted when administered w/ CYP2C9 inducers; administer the separate products of misoprostol and diclofenac if a higher dose of diclofenac is deemed necessary. **Misoprostol:** Antacids may reduce bioavailability. Mg^{2+}-containing antacids exacerbate misoprostol-associated diarrhea.

PREGNANCY AND LACTATION
Pregnancy: Contraindicated in pregnant women.
Lactation: No lactation studies have been conducted w/ Arthrotec; however, limited published literature reports that diclofenac and the active metabolite of misoprostol are present in breast milk. Caution in nursing.
Reproductive Potential: Verify pregnancy status for females of reproductive potential w/in 2 weeks prior to initiating therapy. Advise females of reproductive potential to use effective contraception during treatment. Based on the mechanism of action, the use of prostaglandin-mediated NSAIDs may delay or prevent rupture of ovarian follicles, which has been associated w/ reversible infertility in some women. Small studies in women treated w/ NSAIDs have also shown a reversible delay in ovulation. Consider withdrawal of Arthrotec in women who have difficulties conceiving or who are undergoing investigation of infertility.

MECHANISM OF ACTION
Diclofenac: NSAID; mechanism not completely understood but involves inhibition of COX-1 and COX-2. Has analgesic, anti-inflammatory, and antipyretic properties. Mode of action may be due to a decrease of prostaglandins in peripheral tissues.
Misoprostol: Synthetic prostaglandin E_1 analogue w/ gastric antisecretory and mucosal protective properties. Inhibits basal and nocturnal gastric acid secretion and acid secretion in response to stimuli (eg, meals, histamine, pentagastrin, coffee).

PHARMACOKINETICS
Absorption: Diclofenac: Complete. Misoprostol: Extensive, rapid. Administration of variable doses resulted in different parameters; refer to PI. **Distribution:** Found in breast milk. Diclofenac: V_d=0.55L/kg; plasma protein binding (>99%). Misoprostol: Plasma protein binding (<90%, misoprostol acid). **Metabolism:** Diclofenac: 4'-hydroxy diclofenac (major metabolite) via CYP2C9; glucuronidation or sulfation, and acylglucuronidation (via UGT2B7) and oxidation (via CYP2C8). Misoprostol: Rapid; misoprostol acid (active metabolite). **Elimination:** Diclofenac: Urine (65%, 5-10% conjugates of unchanged drug, 20-30% conjugates of the principal metabolite), bile (35%, <5% conjugates of unchanged drug, 10-20%

conjugates of the principal metabolite); $T_{1/2}$=2 hrs. Misoprostol: Urine (70%); $T_{1/2}$=30 min.

PATIENT CONSIDERATIONS

Assessment: Assess for known hypersensitivity to diclofenac sodium/misoprostol, other prostaglandins, or any components of the drug product; history of asthma, urticaria, or other allergic-type reactions after taking ASA or other NSAIDs; active GI bleeding; CV disease (CVD) or risk factors for CVD; HTN; history of peptic ulcer disease; coagulation disorders; renal/hepatic impairment; pregnancy/nursing status; or any other conditions where treatment is contraindicated or cautioned. Assess volume status. Assess for possible drug interactions. Obtain baseline BP, CBC, and chemistry profile.

Monitoring: Monitor for signs/symptoms of CV thrombotic events; cardiac ischemia in patients w/ a recent MI; GI bleeding/ulceration and perforation; hepatotoxicity; new or worsening HTN; HF; edema; renal papillary necrosis and other renal injury; hyperkalemia; anaphylactic reactions; serious skin reactions; anemia; and other adverse reactions. Monitor BP during initiation of therapy and throughout the course of therapy. Monitor for signs of bleeding in patients on concomitant therapy w/ anticoagulants, antiplatelet agents, SSRIs, or SNRIs. Monitor renal function in patients w/ renal/hepatic impairment, HF, dehydration, or hypovolemia. Monitor CBC and chemistry profiles periodically during long-term treatment.

Counseling: Advise females that use of therapy during pregnancy can result in maternal and fetal harm (eg, abortion, premature birth, birth defects, uterine rupture); instruct not to give to other females of reproductive potential. Instruct females of reproductive potential of the potential to use effective contraception during treatment. Advise females to inform physician of a known/suspected pregnancy. Advise females of reproductive potential that therapy may be associated w/ reversible infertility. Inform of potential for CV thrombotic events, GI adverse events, and worsening CHF/edema, and advise of symptoms; instruct to report any symptoms to healthcare provider immediately. Inform of the potential for hepatotoxicity, and advise of signs/symptoms; if signs/symptoms occur, instruct to d/c and seek immediate medical therapy. Instruct to seek immediate emergency help if signs of an anaphylactic reaction occur. Advise to d/c immediately if rash develops and to contact healthcare provider as soon as possible. Instruct patient not to use other NSAIDs or salicylates concomitantly; notify of the presence of NSAIDs in OTC medications for colds, fever, or insomnia. Advise patient not to use low-dose ASA concomitantly w/o talking to healthcare provider.

ARZERRA — ofatumumab   Rx
Class: Monoclonal antibody/CD20 blocker

> Hepatitis B virus (HBV) reactivation may occur, in some cases resulting in fulminant hepatitis, hepatic failure, and death. Progressive multifocal leukoencephalopathy (PML) resulting in death may occur.

ADULT DOSAGE	PEDIATRIC DOSAGE
Chronic Lymphocytic Leukemia	Pediatric use may not have been established
Previously Untreated:	
In combination w/ chlorambucil, for the treatment of patients for whom fludarabine-based therapy is considered inappropriate	
Day 1: 300mg	
Day 8: 1000mg (Cycle 1)	
Subsequent Doses: 1000mg on Day 1 of subsequent 28-day cycles for a minimum of 3 cycles until best response or a max of 12 cycles	
Extended Treatment:	
For patients who are in complete or partial response after at least 2 lines of therapy for recurrent/progressive chronic lymphocytic leukemia (CLL)	
Day 1: 300mg	
Day 8: 1000mg	
Subsequent Doses: 1000mg 7 weeks later and every 8 weeks thereafter for up to a max of 2 yrs	
Infusion Rates for Previously Untreated CLL and Extended Treatment in CLL:	
Initial 300mg Dose: Initiate at a rate of 3.6mg/hr (12mL/hr)	
Subsequent Infusions of 1000mg: Initiate at a rate of 25mg/hr (25mL/hr); initiate at a rate of 12mg/hr if a Grade ≥3 infusion-related adverse event occurred during the previous infusion	
The rate of infusion may be increased every 30 mins in the absence of an infusion-related adverse event; refer to PI for further infusion rate information	

Refractory to Fludarabine and Alemtuzumab:
300mg initially on Day 1, followed 1 week later by 2000mg/week for 7 doses (Infusions 2 through 8), followed 4 weeks later by 2000mg every 4 weeks for 4 doses (Infusions 9-12)

Infusion Rates for Refractory CLL:
Infusion 1 (300mg Dose): Initiate at a rate of 3.6mg/hr (12mL/hr)
Infusion 2 (2000mg Dose): Initiate at a rate of 24mg/hr (12mL/hr)
Infusions 3-12 (2000mg Doses): Initiate at a rate of 50mg/hr (25mL/hr)
The rate of infusion may be increased every 30 mins in the absence of an infusion-related adverse event; refer to PI for further infusion rate information

Premedication
Administer 30 min to 2 hrs prior to each infusion

Previously Untreated CLL/Extended Treatment in CLL:
Infusion 1 and 2:
IV corticosteroid (prednisolone or equivalent) 50mg + oral acetaminophen 1000mg + oral/ IV antihistamine (diphenhydramine 50mg, cetirizine 10mg, or equivalent)
Infusion 3-13 (Previously Untreated CLL)/Infusion 3-14 (Extended Treatment in CLL):
IV corticosteroid (prednisolone or equivalent) 0-50mg (may be reduced/omitted for subsequent infusions if a Grade ≥3 infusion-related adverse event did not occur w/ the preceding infusion[s]) + oral acetaminophen 1000mg + oral/ IV antihistamine (diphenhydramine 50mg, cetirizine 10mg, or equivalent)

Refractory CLL:
Infusion 1, 2, 9:
IV corticosteroid (prednisolone or equivalent) 100mg + oral acetaminophen 1000mg + oral/ IV antihistamine (diphenhydramine 50mg, cetirizine 10mg, or equivalent)
Infusion 3-8:
IV corticosteroid (prednisolone or equivalent) 0-100mg (may be reduced/omitted for subsequent infusions if a Grade ≥3 infusion-related adverse event did not occur w/ the preceding infusion[s]) + oral acetaminophen 1000mg + oral/ IV antihistamine (diphenhydramine 50mg, cetirizine 10mg, or equivalent)
Infusion 10-12:
IV corticosteroid (prednisolone or equivalent) 50-100mg (prednisolone may be reduced to 50-100mg [or equivalent] if a Grade ≥3 infusion-related adverse event did not occur w/ Infusion 9) + oral acetaminophen 1000mg + oral/IV antihistamine (diphenhydramine 50mg, cetirizine 10mg, or equivalent)

DOSING CONSIDERATIONS
Adverse Reactions
Infusion Reactions:
Interrupt infusion for reactions of any severity.
If infusion reaction resolves/remains ≤Grade 2, resume infusion according to initial grade of reaction:
Grade 1 or 2: Infuse at 1/2 of the previous infusion rate.
Grade 3 or 4: Infuse at a rate of 12mL/hr.
After resuming infusion, increase infusion rate as specified in the PI, based on patient tolerance.
Consider permanent discontinuation if severity of infusion reaction does not resolve to ≤Grade 2 despite adequate clinical intervention; permanently d/c therapy if anaphylactic reaction develops.

ADMINISTRATION
IV route
Do not administer as IV push or bolus, or as SQ inj.
Do not shake.

Preparation of Sol
300mg Dose:
1. Withdraw and discard 15mL from a 1000mL bag of 0.9% NaCl inj.
2. Withdraw 5mL from each of 3 single-use 100mg vials and add to the bag.
3. Mix diluted sol by gentle inversion.
1000mg Dose:
1. Withdraw and discard 50mL from a 1000mL bag of 0.9% NaCl inj.
2. Withdraw 50mL from 1 single-use 1000mg vial and add to the bag.
3. Mix diluted sol by gentle inversion.
2000mg Dose:
1. Withdraw and discard 100mL from a 1000mL bag of 0.9% NaCl inj.
2. Withdraw 50mL from each of 2 single-use 1000mg vials and add to the bag.
3. Mix diluted sol by gentle inversion.
Store diluted sol at 2-8°C (36-46°F).
No incompatibilities between therapy and polyvinylchloride or polyolefin bags and administration sets have been observed.

Administration Instructions
Do not mix w/, or administer as an infusion w/, other medicinal products.
Administer using an infusion pump and an administration set.
Flush the IV line w/ 0.9% NaCl inj before and after each dose.
Start infusion w/in 12 hrs of preparation.
Discard prepared sol after 24 hrs.

STORAGE
2-8°C (36-46°F). Do not freeze. Protect from light.

HOW SUPPLIED
Inj: 20mg/mL [5mL, 50mL]

WARNINGS/PRECAUTIONS
Administer in an environment where facilities to adequately monitor and treat infusion reactions are available. May cause serious, including fatal, infusion reactions; interrupt for infusion reactions of any severity and institute medical management for severe reactions. Permanently d/c if an anaphylactic reaction occurs. Screen for HBV infection before initiating treatment. Monitor patients w/ evidence of current or prior HBV infection for clinical and laboratory signs of hepatitis or HBV reactivation during and for several months following treatment. Immediately d/c therapy and any concomitant chemotherapy, and institute appropriate treatment if HBV reactivation develops. Fatal infection due to hepatitis B in patients who have not been previously infected reported. Consider PML in any patient w/ new onset of or changes in preexisting neurological signs/symptoms; if PML is suspected, d/c therapy and initiate evaluation for PML. Tumor lysis syndrome (TLS), including the need for hospitalization, reported; increased risk w/ high tumor burden and/or high circulating lymphocyte counts (>25 x 10^9/L). Consider tumor lysis prophylaxis w/ antihyperuricemics and hydration beginning 12-24 hrs prior to infusion. Severe cytopenias, including neutropenia, thrombocytopenia, and anemia, may occur.

ADVERSE REACTIONS
Previously Untreated CLL: Infusion reactions, neutropenia.
Extended Treatment in CLL: Infusion reactions, neutropenia, URTIs.
Refractory CLL: Neutropenia, pneumonia, pyrexia, cough, diarrhea, anemia, fatigue, dyspnea, rash, nausea, bronchitis, URTIs.

DRUG INTERACTIONS
Pancytopenia, agranulocytosis, and fatal neutropenic sepsis reported w/ chlorambucil. Do not administer live viral vaccines to recently treated patients.

PREGNANCY AND LACTATION
Pregnancy: There are no data on the use of therapy in pregnant women to inform a drug-associated risk. May cause fetal B-cell depletion; avoid administering live vaccines to neonates and infants exposed to ofatumumab in utero until B-cell recovery occurs.
Lactation: There is no information regarding the presence of ofatumumab in human milk, the effects on the breastfed infant, or the effects on milk production. Human IgG is known to be present in human milk. Published data suggest that antibodies in breast milk do not enter the neonatal and infant circulations in substantial amounts. Caution in nursing.

MECHANISM OF ACTION
CD20-directed cytolytic monoclonal antibody; binds specifically to both the small and large extracellular loops of CD20 molecule. The Fab domain of ofatumumab binds to the CD20 molecule and the Fc domain mediates immune effector functions to result in B-cell lysis in vitro. Possible mechanisms of cell lysis include complement-dependent cytotoxicity and antibody-dependent, cell-mediated cytotoxicity.

PHARMACOKINETICS
Distribution: V_d=5.8L. **Elimination:** $T_{1/2}$=17.1 days.

PATIENT CONSIDERATIONS
Assessment: Assess for current/prior HBV infection, risk for TLS, pregnancy/ nursing status, and possible drug interactions.

Monitoring: Monitor for signs/symptoms of HBV reactivation, hepatitis, PML, infusion reactions, TLS, and other adverse reactions. Monitor CBC at regular intervals during and after conclusion of therapy, and at increased frequency in patients who develop Grade 3 or 4 cytopenias.

Counseling: Instruct to inform physician of signs/symptoms of infusion reactions; symptoms of hepatitis (eg, worsening fatigue, yellow discoloration of skin/eyes); new neurological symptoms (eg, confusion, dizziness, loss of balance); bleeding, easy bruising, petechiae, pallor, worsening weakness, or fatigue; or signs of infections. Advise to notify physician if pregnant/nursing. Advise of the need for monitoring and possible need for treatment if patient has a history of hepatitis B infection, for periodic monitoring of blood counts, and for avoiding vaccination w/ live viral vaccines.

ASACOL HD — mesalamine   Rx

Class: 5-aminosalicylic acid derivative

ADULT DOSAGE	**PEDIATRIC DOSAGE**
Ulcerative Colitis	Pediatric use may not have been established
Moderately Active:	
1600mg (two 800mg tabs) tid for 6 weeks	

ADMINISTRATION
Oral route

Take on an empty stomach, at least 1 hr before and 2 hrs after a meal.
Swallow tab whole; do not cut, break, or chew.
Do not substitute one Asacol HD 800 tab for two mesalamine delayed-release 400mg oral products.
Intact, partially intact, and/or tab shells have been reported in the stool.
Protect tabs from moisture; close the container tightly and leave desiccant pouches in the bottle along w/ the tabs.

STORAGE
20-25°C (68-77°F); excursions permitted from 15-30°C (59-86°F). Protect from moisture.

HOW SUPPLIED
Tab, Delayed-Release: 800mg

CONTRAINDICATIONS
Known or suspected hypersensitivity to salicylates or aminosalicylates or to any of the ingredients of this medication.

WARNINGS/PRECAUTIONS
Renal impairment, including minimal change nephropathy, acute and chronic interstitial nephritis, and, rarely, renal failure, reported; evaluate renal function prior to therapy and periodically thereafter. Has been associated w/ an acute intolerance syndrome that may be difficult to distinguish from an exacerbation of ulcerative colitis. Exacerbation of symptoms of colitis reported; symptoms usually abate when therapy is discontinued. Hypersensitivity reactions reported in patients taking sulfasalazine; patients may have a similar reaction to Asacol HD tabs or to other compounds that contain or are converted to mesalamine. Mesalamine-induced hypersensitivity reactions may present as internal organ involvement; evaluate patients immediately if signs/symptoms of a hypersensitivity reaction are present, and d/c if an alternative etiology cannot be established. Hepatic failure reported in patients w/ preexisting liver disease; caution w/ liver impairment. Caution in elderly.

ADVERSE REACTIONS
Headache, nausea, nasopharyngitis, abdominal pain, diarrhea, dyspepsia.

DRUG INTERACTIONS
Known nephrotoxic agents, including NSAIDs, may increase the risk of nephrotoxicity; monitor for changes in renal function and mesalamine-related adverse reactions. Azathioprine or 6-mercaptopurine may increase the risk for blood disorders; if concomitant use cannot be avoided, monitor blood tests, including complete blood cell counts and platelet counts.

PREGNANCY AND LACTATION
Pregnancy: Limited published data on mesalamine use in pregnant women are insufficient to inform a drug-associated risk.
Lactation: Mesalamine is present in human milk in undetectable to small amounts. There are limited reports of diarrhea in breastfed infants. Caution in nursing. Monitor breastfed infants for diarrhea.

MECHANISM OF ACTION
5-aminosalicylic acid derivative; has not been established. Suspected to diminish inflammation by blocking cyclooxygenase and inhibiting prostaglandin production in the colon.

PHARMACOKINETICS
Absorption: T_{max}=approx 24 hrs (median), C_{max}=208ng/mL; AUC_{8-48h}=2296ng•hr/mL; AUC_{0-tldc}=2533ng•hr/mL. **Distribution:** Found in breast milk. **Metabolism:** Gut mucosal wall and liver via acetylation; N-acetyl-5-aminosalicylic acid (metabolite). **Elimination:** Urine (absorbed mesalamine as N-acetyl-5-aminosalicylic acid); feces (unabsorbed mesalamine).

PATIENT CONSIDERATIONS
Assessment: Assess for hypersensitivity to sulfasalazine, salicylates, or aminosalicylates; hepatic impairment; pregnancy/nursing status; and possible drug interactions. Evaluate renal function prior to initiation of therapy.

Monitoring: Monitor for acute intolerance syndrome, exacerbation of symptoms of colitis, hepatic failure, hypersensitivity reactions, and other adverse reactions. Perform periodic monitoring of renal function. Monitor blood cell counts in elderly patients.

Counseling: Inform that if switching from a previous oral mesalamine therapy to Asacol HD, to d/c previous oral mesalamine therapy and follow the dosing instructions for Asacol HD. Inform to take on an empty stomach, at least 1 hr before and 2 hrs after a meal. Instruct to swallow tabs whole, and not to break, cut, or chew tabs. Inform that intact, partially intact, and/or tab shells have been reported in the stool; instruct to contact physician if this occurs repeatedly. Instruct to protect tabs from moisture, and to close the container tightly and to leave desiccant pouches in the bottle along w/ the tabs. Inform that therapy may decrease renal function, and to complete all blood tests ordered by physician. Instruct to report if experiencing new or worsening symptoms of cramping, abdominal pain, bloody diarrhea, and sometimes fever, headache, and rash. Inform of the signs/symptoms of hypersensitivity reactions, and advise to seek

---

immediate medical care if signs/symptoms occur. Inform patients w/ known liver disease of the signs/symptoms of worsening liver function, and advise to report to physician if experiencing such signs/symptoms. Inform elderly patients and those taking azathioprine or 6-mercaptopurine of the risk for blood disorders and the need for periodic monitoring of complete blood cell counts and platelet counts while on therapy.

ASMANEX — mometasone furoate   Rx

Class: Corticosteroid

ADULT DOSAGE	**PEDIATRIC DOSAGE**
Asthma	**Asthma**
Maint Treatment of Asthma as Prophylactic Therapy:	**Maint Treatment of Asthma as Prophylactic Therapy:**
Previous Therapy:	**4-11 Years:**
Bronchodilators Alone or Inhaled Corticosteroids:	**Initial/Max:** 110mcg qpm
Initial: 220mcg qpm	**≥12 Years:**
Titrate: Higher doses may provide additional control if inadequate response after 2 weeks of therapy; adjust to lowest effective dose once asthma stability is achieved	**Previous Therapy:**
	Bronchodilators Alone or Inhaled Corticosteroids:
Max: 440mcg qpm or 220mcg bid	**Initial:** 220mcg qpm
Oral Corticosteroids:	**Titrate:** Higher doses may provide additional control if inadequate response after 2 weeks of therapy; adjust to lowest effective dose once asthma stability is achieved
Initial: 440mcg bid	
Titrate: Higher doses may provide additional control if inadequate response after 2 weeks of therapy; adjust to lowest effective dose once asthma stability is achieved	**Max:** 440mcg qpm or 220mcg bid
	Oral Corticosteroids:
Max: 880mcg/day	**Initial:** 440mcg bid
	Titrate: Higher doses may provide additional control if inadequate response after 2 weeks of therapy; adjust to lowest effective dose once asthma stability is achieved
	Max: 880mcg/day

ADMINISTRATION
Orally inhaled powder

When administered qd, Asmanex should be taken only in the pm
Inhale rapidly and deeply
Rinse mouth after inh

STORAGE
25°C (77°F); excursions permitted to 15-30°C (59-86°F). Store in dry place.
Discard inhaler 45 days after opening foil pouch or when dose counter reads "00," whichever comes 1st.

HOW SUPPLIED
Powder, Inhalation: 110mcg/actuation; 220mcg/actuation

CONTRAINDICATIONS
Primary treatment of status asthmaticus or other acute episodes of asthma where intensive measures are required, known hypersensitivity to milk proteins or any ingredients of this medication.

WARNINGS/PRECAUTIONS
Not for the relief of acute bronchospasm. Localized *Candida albicans* infections of the mouth and pharynx reported; treat accordingly or interrupt therapy if needed. D/C if hypersensitivity reactions occur. Contains small amount of lactose that contains milk proteins; anaphylactic reactions with milk protein allergy reported. May increase susceptibility to infections; caution with active or quiescent tuberculosis (TB) infection, untreated systemic fungal, bacterial, viral, or parasitic infections, or ocular herpes simplex. Avoid exposure to chickenpox and measles. Deaths due to adrenal insufficiency have occurred with transfer from systemic to inhaled corticosteroids; wean slowly from systemic corticosteroid therapy. Resume oral corticosteroids immediately during periods of stress or severe asthma attack. Transferring from systemic corticosteroid may unmask allergic conditions (eg, rhinitis, conjunctivitis, eczema, arthritis, eosinophilic conditions). Monitor for systemic corticosteroid effects, such as hypercorticism and adrenal suppression; reduce dose slowly when the effects occur. Prolonged use may result in decrease of bone mineral density (BMD); caution in patients at risk (eg, prolonged immobilization, family history of osteoporosis, chronic use of drugs that reduce bone mass [eg, anticonvulsants, corticosteroids]). May cause reduction in growth velocity in pediatric patients; monitor growth routinely. Glaucoma, increased IOP, and cataracts reported. Bronchospasm may occur with an increase in wheezing after dosing; d/c treatment and institute alternative therapy.

ADVERSE REACTIONS
Headache, allergic rhinitis, pharyngitis, URTI, sinusitis, oral candidiasis, dysmenorrhea, musculoskeletal pain, back pain, dyspepsia, myalgia, abdominal pain, nausea.

DRUG INTERACTIONS
Ketoconazole may increase plasma levels.

PREGNANCY AND LACTATION
Category C, caution in nursing.

MECHANISM OF ACTION
Corticosteroid; not established. Shown to have inhibitory effects on multiple cell types (eg, mast cells, eosinophils, neutrophils, macrophages, and lymphocytes)

and mediators (eg, histamine, eicosanoids, leukotrienes, and cytokines) involved in inflammatory and asthmatic response.

PHARMACOKINETICS
Absorption: Absolute bioavailability (<1%); C_{max}=94-114pcg/mL; T_{max}=1-2.5 hrs. **Distribution:** (IV) V_d=152L; plasma protein binding (98-99%). **Metabolism:** Liver via CYP3A4. **Elimination:** Feces (74%), urine (8%); (IV) $T_{1/2}$=5 hrs.

PATIENT CONSIDERATIONS

Assessment: Assess for status asthmaticus, acute asthma episodes, known hypersensitivity to milk proteins or to any drug component, risk factors for decreased BMD, history of increased IOP/glaucoma/cataracts, active or quiescent pulmonary TB, ocular herpes simplex, untreated systemic infections, chickenpox, measles, pregnancy/nursing status, and possible drug interactions.

Monitoring: Monitor for localized infections of mouth and pharynx with *C. albicans*, decreased BMD, asthma instability, growth in pediatrics routinely, development of glaucoma, increased IOP, cataracts, change in vision, hypercorticism, signs and symptoms of adrenal insufficiency, paradoxical bronchospasm, hypersensitivity reactions, and immunosuppression. Monitor for lung function, β-agonist use, and asthma symptoms during withdrawal of oral corticosteroids

Counseling: Advise that localized infection with *C. albicans* may occur in mouth and pharynx; instruct to rinse mouth after inhalation. Inform that therapy should not be used to treat status asthmaticus or to relieve acute asthma symptoms. Counsel to d/c if hypersensitivity reactions occur. Advise to avoid exposure to chickenpox or measles and to seek medical attention if exposed. Inform of potential worsening of existing TB, other infections, or ocular herpes simplex. Inform that drug may cause systemic corticosteroid effects of hypercorticism and adrenal suppression, may reduce BMD, and may cause reduction in growth rate (pediatrics). Advise to take ud, to use medication at regular intervals, and to contact physician if symptoms do not improve or if condition worsens. Instruct on proper administration procedures and on when to discard inhaler.

Asmanex HFA — mometasone furoate   Rx

Class: Corticosteroid

ADULT DOSAGE	PEDIATRIC DOSAGE
Asthma	**Asthma**
Maint Treatment:	**Maint Treatment:**
	≥12 Years:
Previously Taking Inhaled Medium-Dose Corticosteroids:	**Previously Taking Inhaled Medium-Dose Corticosteroids:**
Recommended: 2 inh of 100mcg bid (am and pm)	**Recommended:** 2 inh of 100mcg bid (am and pm)
Max: 400mcg bid	**Max:** 400mcg bid
Previously Taking Inhaled High-Dose Corticosteroids:	**Previously Taking Inhaled High-Dose Corticosteroids:**
Recommended: 2 inh of 200mcg bid (am and pm)	**Recommended:** 2 inh of 200mcg bid (am and pm)
Max: 400mcg bid	**Max:** 400mcg bid
Previously Taking Oral Corticosteroids:	**Previously Taking Oral Corticosteroids:**
Recommended: 2 inh of 200mcg bid (am and pm)	**Recommended:** 2 inh of 200mcg bid (am and pm)
Max: 400mcg bid	**Max:** 400mcg bid
Reduce oral prednisone slowly, beginning after at least 1 week of Asmanex HFA therapy	Reduce oral prednisone slowly, beginning after at least 1 week of Asmanex HFA therapy
If inadequate response after 2 weeks of therapy, higher strength may provide additional asthma control	If inadequate response after 2 weeks of therapy, higher strength may provide additional asthma control

ADMINISTRATION
Oral inh route
Rinse mouth after each dose w/ water w/o swallowing.
Shake well prior to each inh.

Priming
Prime the inhaler before using for the 1st time by releasing 4 test sprays into the air, shaking well before each spray.
If the inhaler has not been used for >5 days, prime inhaler again.

STORAGE
20-25°C (68-77°F); excursions permitted to 15-30°C (59-86°F). Do not puncture, use/store near heat or open flame, or throw into fire/incinerator. Exposure to temperatures >49°C (120°F) may cause bursting. Discard when the labeled number of actuations has been used (the dose counter reads "0").

HOW SUPPLIED
MDI: 100mcg/inh, 200mcg/inh [120 inh]

CONTRAINDICATIONS
Primary treatment of status asthmaticus or other acute episodes of asthma where intensive measures are required, known hypersensitivity to mometasone furoate or any of the ingredients in this product.

WARNINGS/PRECAUTIONS
Not indicated for the relief of acute symptoms. *Candida albicans* infections of mouth and pharynx reported; treat and/or interrupt therapy if needed. Increased susceptibility to infections. May lead to serious/fatal course of chickenpox or

measles; avoid exposure, and if exposed, consider prophylaxis/treatment. Caution w/ active/quiescent tuberculosis (TB), untreated systemic fungal/bacterial/viral/parasitic infections, or ocular herpes simplex. Deaths due to adrenal insufficiency reported during and after transfer from systemic to inhaled corticosteroids; wean slowly from oral or other systemic corticosteroid use after transferring to therapy. Resume oral corticosteroids during periods of stress or a severe asthma attack in patients previously withdrawn from systemic corticosteroids. Transfer from systemic to inhaled corticosteroids may unmask conditions previously suppressed by systemic therapy (eg, rhinitis, conjunctivitis, eczema). Observe for systemic corticosteroid withdrawal effects. Hypercorticism and adrenal suppression may appear; reduce dose slowly. May produce inhalation induced bronchospasm w/ an immediate increase in wheezing after dosing that may be life-threatening; treat immediately w/ an inhaled, short-acting bronchodilator and d/c therapy and institute alternative therapy. Hypersensitivity reactions may occur; d/c if such reactions occur. Decreases in bone mineral density (BMD) reported w/ long-term use; caution w/ major risk factors for decreased bone mineral content, including chronic use of drugs that can reduce bone mass (eg, anticonvulsants, corticosteroids). May cause reduction in growth velocity in pediatric patients. Glaucoma, increased IOP, and cataracts reported w/ long-term use. Drug concentrations appear to increase w/ severity of hepatic impairment.

ADVERSE REACTIONS
Nasopharyngitis, headache, influenza, sinusitis, bronchitis.

DRUG INTERACTIONS
Ketoconazole may increase levels. Inhibition of metabolism and increased exposure w/ CYP3A4 inhibitors; caution w/ long-term ketoconazole and other known strong CYP3A4 inhibitors (eg, ritonavir, clarithromycin, itraconazole).

PREGNANCY AND LACTATION
Pregnancy: In women w/ poorly/moderately controlled asthma, there is an increased risk of several perinatal adverse outcomes such as preeclampsia in the mother and prematurity, low birth weight, and small for gestational age in the neonate. Pregnant women w/ asthma should be closely monitored and medication adjusted as necessary to maintain optimal asthma control.
Lactation: There are no available data on the presence of the drug in human milk, the effects on the breastfed child, or the effects on milk production. Caution in nursing.

MECHANISM OF ACTION
Corticosteroid; has not been established. Shown to have a wide range of inhibitory effects on multiple cell types (eg, mast cells, eosinophils, neutrophils, macrophages, lymphocytes) and mediators (eg, histamine, eicosanoids, leukotrienes, cytokines) involved in inflammation and in the asthmatic response.

PHARMACOKINETICS
Absorption: (Healthy) Systemic bioavailability (<1%). (Asthma Patients) T_{max}= 1-2 hrs (median). **Distribution:** (IV 400mcg) V_d=152L; plasma protein binding (98-99%). **Metabolism:** Liver via CYP3A4. **Elimination:** (1000mcg) Urine (8%), feces (74%); (IV) $T_{1/2}$=5 hrs.

PATIENT CONSIDERATIONS
Assessment: Assess for hypersensitivity to drug, status asthmaticus, acute asthma symptoms, active/quiescent TB of the respiratory tract, ocular herpes simplex, untreated systemic infections, risk factors for decreased bone mineral content, history of increased IOP, glaucoma, cataracts, hepatic impairment, pregnancy/nursing status, and possible drug interactions.

Monitoring: Monitor for signs of infection, systemic corticosteroid effects (eg, hypercorticism, adrenal suppression), hypersensitivity reactions, decreased BMD, glaucoma, increased IOP, cataracts, paradoxical bronchospasm, and other adverse reactions. Monitor growth in pediatric patients routinely. Monitor patients w/ hepatic impairment for signs of increased drug exposure.

Counseling: Inform about the risks and benefits of therapy. Inform that product is not a bronchodilator and is not to be used to treat status asthmaticus or to relieve acute asthma symptoms; advise to treat acute symptoms w/ an inhaled short-acting β₂-agonist (SABA). Instruct to seek medical attention immediately if experiencing a significant decrease in lung function, a need for more inhalations than usual of inhaled SABAs, or if symptoms worsen. Advise not to increase the dose or frequency of therapy. Advise not to d/c or reduce therapy w/o physician guidance. Advise to contact physician if oropharyngeal candidiasis develops. Instruct to avoid exposure to chickenpox or measles and to consult physician w/o delay if exposed. Inform about risks of immunosuppression, hypercorticism, adrenal suppression, reduction in BMD, reduced growth velocity in pediatric patients, glaucoma, and cataracts. Instruct to d/c therapy if a hypersensitivity reaction occurs. Advise to use at regular intervals; instruct to contact physician if symptoms do not improve after 2 weeks of therapy or if condition worsens.

Astelin — azelastine hydrochloride   Rx

Class: H₁ antagonist

ADULT DOSAGE	PEDIATRIC DOSAGE
Vasomotor Rhinitis	**Vasomotor Rhinitis**
Usual: 2 sprays/nostril bid	**≥12 Years:**
	Usual: 2 sprays/nostril bid
Seasonal Allergic Rhinitis	**Seasonal Allergic Rhinitis**
Usual: 1-2 sprays/nostril bid	**5-11 Years:**
	Usual: 1 spray/nostril bid
	≥12 Years:
	Usual: 1-2 sprays/nostril bid

DOSING CONSIDERATIONS
Elderly
Start at lower end of dosing range

ADMINISTRATION
Intranasal route

Priming
Prime before initial use by releasing 4 sprays or until a fine mist appears. When not used for ≥3 days, reprime w/ 2 sprays or until a fine mist appears.

STORAGE
20-25°C (68-77°F). Store upright. Protect from freezing.

HOW SUPPLIED
Spray: 137mcg/spray [30mL]

WARNINGS/PRECAUTIONS
Occurrence of somnolence reported. May impair physical/mental abilities. Caution in elderly.

ADVERSE REACTIONS
Bitter taste, headache, somnolence, dysesthesia, rhinitis, cough, conjunctivitis, asthma, epistaxis, sinusitis, nasal burning, pharyngitis, paroxysmal sneezing.

DRUG INTERACTIONS
Avoid alcohol or other CNS depressants; additional reductions in alertness and CNS performance impairment may occur.

PREGNANCY AND LACTATION
Category C, caution in nursing.

MECHANISM OF ACTION
Antihistamine; exhibits histamine H_1-receptor antagonist activity in isolated tissues.

PHARMACOKINETICS
Absorption: T_{max}=2-3 hrs; bioavailability (40%). **Distribution:** V_d=14.5L/kg (PO/IV); plasma protein binding (88%, 97% metabolite). **Metabolism:** Oxidation via CYP450; desmethylazelastine (major active metabolite). **Elimination:** (PO) Feces (75%, <10% unchanged); $T_{1/2}$=22 hrs (PO/IV).

PATIENT CONSIDERATIONS
Assessment: Assess for pregnancy/nursing status and possible drug interactions.
Monitoring: Monitor for somnolence and other adverse reactions.
Counseling: Instruct to use only as prescribed. Caution patients against engaging in hazardous occupations requiring complete mental alertness and motor coordination (eg, driving a car or operating machinery). Instruct to avoid concurrent use with alcohol or other CNS depressants because additional reductions in alertness or CNS performance impairment may occur. Inform that therapy may lead to adverse reactions (eg, bitter taste, headache, somnolence). Instruct to consult physician if pregnant/nursing or planning to become pregnant. Instruct to keep out of reach of children and to seek medical help or call a poison control center immediately if a child accidentally ingests the medication.

ASTEPRO — azelastine hydrochloride   Rx
Class: H_1 antagonist

ADULT DOSAGE	PEDIATRIC DOSAGE
Seasonal/Perennial Allergic Rhinitis	**Seasonal/Perennial Allergic Rhinitis**
Seasonal Allergic Rhinitis:	**Seasonal Allergic Rhinitis:**
0.1%, 0.15%:	**2-5 Years:**
Usual: 1 or 2 sprays/nostril bid or 2 sprays (0.15%)/nostril qd	0.1%:
	Usual: 1 spray/nostril bid
Perennial Allergic Rhinitis:	**6-11 Years:**
0.15%:	0.1%, 0.15%:
Usual: 2 sprays/nostril bid	**Usual:** 1 spray/nostril bid
	≥12 Years:
	0.1%, 0.15%:
	Usual: 1 or 2 sprays/nostril bid or 2 sprays (0.15%)/nostril qd
	Perennial Allergic Rhinitis:
	6 Months-5 Years:
	0.1%:
	Usual: 1 spray/nostril bid
	6-11 Years:
	0.1%, 0.15%:
	Usual: 1 spray/nostril bid
	≥12 Years:
	0.15%:
	Usual: 2 sprays/nostril bid

DOSING CONSIDERATIONS
Elderly
Start at lower end of dosing range

ADMINISTRATION
Intranasal route

Avoid spraying into eyes.
Discard after 200 sprays have been used.

Priming
Prime before initial use by releasing 6 sprays or until a fine mist appears.
When not used for ≥3 days, reprime w/ 2 sprays or until a fine mist appears.

STORAGE
20-25°C (68-77°F). Protect from freezing.

HOW SUPPLIED
Spray: 0.1%, 0.15% [30mL]

WARNINGS/PRECAUTIONS
Somnolence reported. May impair mental/physical abilities. Caution in elderly.

ADVERSE REACTIONS
Bitter taste, nasal discomfort, headache, sinusitis, epistaxis, dysgeusia, URI, sneezing, cough, rhinalgia, vomiting, otitis media, contact dermatitis, oropharyngeal pain.

DRUG INTERACTIONS
Avoid w/ alcohol or other CNS depressants; additional reductions in alertness and additional impairment of CNS performance may occur. Cimetidine increased levels of orally administered azelastine.

PREGNANCY AND LACTATION
Category C, caution in nursing.

MECHANISM OF ACTION
H_1-receptor antagonist; phthalazinone derivative.

PHARMACOKINETICS
Absorption: Bioavailability (40%). C_{max}=409pg/mL; T_{max}=4 hrs (median); AUC=9312pg•hr/mL. Desmethylazelastine: C_{max}=38pg/mL; T_{max}=24 hrs (median); AUC=3824pg•hr/mL. **Distribution:** V_d=14.5L/kg (IV/PO); plasma protein binding (88%). Desmethylazelastine: Plasma protein binding (97%). **Metabolism:** Oxidation via CYP450; desmethylazelastine (major active metabolite). **Elimination:** $T_{1/2}$=25 hrs; (PO) feces (75%, <10% unchanged). Desmethylazelastine: $T_{1/2}$=57 hrs.

PATIENT CONSIDERATIONS
Assessment: Assess pregnancy/nursing status and for possible drug interactions.
Monitoring: Monitor for somnolence and other adverse reactions.
Counseling: Caution against engaging in hazardous occupations requiring complete mental alertness and motor coordination (eg, driving, operating machinery). Advise to avoid alcohol or other CNS depressants. Inform that treatment may lead to adverse reactions, the most common of which include pyrexia, dysgeusia, nasal discomfort, epistaxis, headache, sneezing, fatigue, somnolence, URI, cough, rhinalgia, vomiting, otitis media, contact dermatitis, and oropharyngeal pain. Advise to avoid spraying into eyes.

ATACAND — candesartan cilexetil   Rx
Class: Angiotensin II receptor blocker (ARB)

> D/C when pregnancy is detected. Drugs that act directly on the renin-angiotensin system (RAS) can cause injury/death to the developing fetus.

ADULT DOSAGE	PEDIATRIC DOSAGE
Hypertension	**Hypertension**
Initial: 16mg qd as monotherapy in patients who are not volume depleted	**1 to <6 Years:**
Dose Range: 8-32mg/day given qd or bid	**Initial:** 0.20mg/kg (Sus)
	Dose Range: 0.05-0.4mg/kg/day
May add diuretic if BP not controlled and may be administered w/ other antihypertensive agents	**6 to <17 Years:**
	<50kg:
Heart Failure	**Initial:** 4-8mg
Heart Failure (HF) (NYHA Class II-IV) w/ Left Ventricular Systolic Dysfunction (Ejection Fraction ≤40%):	**Dose Range:** 2-16mg/day
Initial: 4mg qd	**>50kg:**
Titrate: Double the dose at 2-week intervals, as tolerated, to the target dose of 32mg qd	**Initial:** 8-16mg
	Dose Range: 4-32mg/day
	May be administered qd or divided into 2 equal doses

DOSING CONSIDERATIONS
Renal Impairment
Pediatric Patients:
GFR <30mL/min/1.73m²: Do not use; has not been studied in this population

Hepatic Impairment
Adults:
Moderate:
Initial: 8mg
Dosing recommendations cannot be provided for severe hepatic insufficiency

Other Important Considerations
Intravascular Volume Depletion in Pediatric Patients:
Consider initiating at a lower dose

ADMINISTRATION
Oral route

Take w/ or w/o food.
For children who cannot swallow tabs, oral sus may be substituted.

Oral Sus
Shake well before each use.
Store at room temperature (<30°C [86°F]); use w/in 30 days after opening.

Preparation of Oral Sus:
The number of tabs and volume of vehicle specified below will yield 160mL of a 1mg/mL sus.
1. Prepare the vehicle by adding equal volumes of Ora-Plus (80mL) and Ora-Sweet SF (80mL) or, alternatively, use Ora-Blend SF (160mL).
2. Add a small amount of vehicle to five 32mg tabs and grind into a smooth paste using a mortar and pestle.
3. Add the paste to a preparation vessel of suitable size.
4. Rinse the mortar and pestle clean using the vehicle and add this to the vessel. Repeat, if necessary.
5. Prepare the final volume by adding the remaining vehicle.
6. Mix thoroughly and dispense into suitably sized amber PET bottles.
7. Label w/ an expiration date of 100 days.

STORAGE
25°C (77°F); excursions permitted to 15-30°C (59-86°F).

HOW SUPPLIED
Tab: 4mg*, 8mg*, 16mg*, 32mg* *scored

CONTRAINDICATIONS
Hypersensitivity to candesartan, coadministration w/ aliskiren in patients w/ diabetes.

WARNINGS/PRECAUTIONS
Symptomatic hypotension may occur; most likely in patients who have been volume- and/or salt-depleted (eg, prolonged diuretic therapy, dietary salt restriction, dialysis, diarrhea, vomiting); correct volume and/or salt depletion prior to therapy and temporary dose reduction of candesartan, diuretic, or both may be required. Hypotension may occur during major surgery and anesthesia. Renal function changes including acute renal failure may occur. Oliguria, progressive azotemia, or acute renal failure may occur in patients whose renal function is dependent on the RAS (eg, renal artery stenosis, chronic kidney disease, severe HF, volume depletion); consider withholding or discontinuing therapy if clinically significant decrease in renal function develops. May cause hyperkalemia.

ADVERSE REACTIONS
HTN: URTI, dizziness, back pain.
HF: Hypotension, abnormal renal function, hyperkalemia.

DRUG INTERACTIONS
See Contraindications. Dual blockade of the RAS w/ ARBs, ACE inhibitors, or aliskiren, is associated w/ increased risk of hypotension, hyperkalemia, and changes in renal function (eg, acute renal failure); closely monitor BP, renal function, and electrolytes w/ concomitant agents that also affect the RAS. Avoid concomitant aliskiren in patients w/ renal impairment (GFR <60mL/min). NSAIDs, (eg, selective COX-2 inhibitors), may deteriorate renal function in patients who are elderly, volume-depleted, or w/ compromised renal function; monitor renal function periodically. NSAIDs may attenuate antihypertensive effect of candesartan. Increased lithium levels and toxicity reported; monitor serum lithium levels. May result in hyperkalemia w/ K^+-sparing diuretics, K^+ supplements, K^+-containing salt substitutes, or other drugs that raise serum K^+ levels.

PREGNANCY AND LACTATION
Pregnancy: Category D. Use of drugs that act on the RAS during the 2nd and 3rd trimesters of pregnancy reduces fetal renal function and increases fetal and neonatal morbidity and death.
Lactation: Not for use in nursing.

MECHANISM OF ACTION
Angiotensin II receptor antagonist; blocks vasoconstrictor and aldosterone-secreting effects of angiotensin II by selectively blocking the binding of angiotensin II to the AT_1 receptor in many tissues.

PHARMACOKINETICS
Absorption: Rapid and complete. Absolute bioavailability (15%); T_{max}=3-4 hrs.
Distribution: V_d=0.13L/kg; plasma protein binding (>99%). **Metabolism:** Ester hydrolysis, liver via O-deethylation (minor). **Elimination:** Feces (67%), urine (33%, 26% unchanged); $T_{1/2}$=9 hrs.

PATIENT CONSIDERATIONS
Assessment: Assess for hypersensitivity to drug, volume/salt depletion, diabetes, HF, hepatic/renal impairment, pregnancy/nursing status, and possible drug interactions.

Monitoring: Monitor for signs/symptoms of hypotension, renal function changes, and other adverse reactions. Monitor serum K^+ periodically and BP during dose escalation and periodically thereafter.

Counseling: Inform of risks/benefits of therapy. Inform of pregnancy risks; instruct to notify physician as soon as possible if pregnant.

ATACAND HCT — candesartan cilexetil/hydrochlorothiazide   Rx
Class: Angiotensin II receptor blocker (ARB)/thiazide diuretic

> D/C when pregnancy is detected. Drugs that act directly on the renin-angiotensin system (RAS) can cause injury/death to developing fetus.

ADULT DOSAGE	PEDIATRIC DOSAGE
Hypertension	Pediatric use may not have been established
16-32mg candesartan/12.5-25mg hydrochlorothiazide (HCTZ) qd	
Replacement Therapy: May be substituted for its titrated components	

Dose Titration by Clinical Effect:
BP Not Controlled on 25mg HCTZ
QD: Can expect an incremental effect from Atacand HCT 16mg/12.5mg

BP Controlled on 25mg HCTZ but Experiencing Decreases in Serum K^+:
Can expect the same or incremental BP effects from Atacand HCT 16mg/12.5mg and serum K^+ may improve

BP Not Controlled on 32mg Atacand:
Can expect incremental BP effects from Atacand HCT 32mg/12.5mg and then 32mg/25mg

May be administered w/ other antihypertensive agents

DOSING CONSIDERATIONS
Renal Impairment
CrCl <30mL/min: Dosing recommendations cannot be provided

Hepatic Impairment
Moderate to Severe: Not recommended for initiation

ADMINISTRATION
Oral route
Take w/ or w/o food.

STORAGE
25°C (77°F); excursions permitted to 15-30°C (59-86°F).

HOW SUPPLIED
Tab: (Candesartan/HCTZ) 16mg/12.5mg*, 32mg/12.5mg*, 32mg/25mg* *scored

CONTRAINDICATIONS
Hypersensitivity to candesartan, HCTZ, or other sulfonamide-derived drugs; coadministration w/ aliskiren in patients w/ diabetes, anuria.

WARNINGS/PRECAUTIONS
See Dosing Considerations. Not for initial therapy. Symptomatic hypotension may occur in patients who have been volume- and/or salt-depleted (eg, prolonged diuretic therapy, dietary salt restriction, dialysis, diarrhea, vomiting); may require temporary dose reduction. Correct volume and/or salt depletion prior to therapy. May cause excessive hypotension leading to oliguria, azotemia, and (rarely) w/ acute renal failure and death in patients w/ heart failure (HF); monitor closely for the first 2 weeks of therapy and whenever dose is increased. Oliguria, progressive azotemia, or acute renal failure may occur in patients whose renal function is dependent on the RAS (eg, severe HF, renal artery stenosis, chronic kidney disease, volume depletion); consider withholding or discontinuing therapy if clinically significant decrease in renal function develops. **HCTZ:** May cause hypokalemia and hyponatremia. May cause idiosyncratic reaction, resulting in acute transient myopia and acute angle-closure glaucoma; d/c as rapidly as possible. May cause hypersensitivity reactions (w/ or w/o history of allergy or bronchial asthma), alter glucose tolerance, raise serum levels of cholesterol/TG/uric acid, cause/exacerbate hyperuricemia and precipitate gout, and exacerbate/activate systemic lupus erythematosus (SLE). May decrease urinary Ca^{2+} excretion and cause elevation of serum Ca^{2+}; avoid w/ hypercalcemia.

ADVERSE REACTIONS
URTI, back pain.

DRUG INTERACTIONS
See Contraindications. NSAIDs, including selective COX-2 inhibitors, may deteriorate renal function and attenuate the antihypertensive effect; monitor renal function periodically. Increased lithium levels and lithium toxicity reported; monitor serum lithium levels. **Candesartan:** Dual blockade of the RAS is associated w/ increased risk of hypotension, hyperkalemia, and changes in renal function (including acute renal failure); closely monitor BP, renal function, and electrolytes w/ concomitant agents that also affect the RAS. Coadministration w/ K^+-sparing diuretics, K^+ supplements, K^+-containing salt substitutes, or other drugs that raise serum K^+ levels may result in hyperkalemia; monitor serum K^+. Avoid w/ aliskiren in patients w/ renal impairment (GFR <60mL/min). **HCTZ:** Alcohol, barbiturates, or narcotics may potentiate orthostatic hypotension. Dose adjustment of antidiabetic drugs (oral agents and insulin) may be required. Hyperglycemic effect of diazoxide may be enhanced. Single doses of either cholestyramine or colestipol resins may impair absorption; administer therapy at least 4 hrs before or 4-6 hrs after administration of resins. May increase responsiveness to nondepolarizing skeletal muscle relaxants (eg, tubocurarine). Thiazide-induced hypokalemia or hypomagnesemia may predispose to digoxin toxicity. May decrease arterial responsiveness to noradrenaline, but not enough to preclude effectiveness of the pressor agent for therapeutic use. Hypokalemia may develop during concomitant use of steroids or ACTH. May reduce the renal excretion of cytotoxic medicinal products (eg, cyclophosphamide, methotrexate) and potentiate their myelosuppressive effects. Concomitant treatment w/ cyclosporine may increase the risk of hyperuricemia and gout-type complications.

PREGNANCY AND LACTATION
Pregnancy: Category D. Use of drugs that act on the RAS during the 2nd and 3rd trimesters reduces fetal renal function and increases fetal and neonatal morbidity and death.
Lactation: Found in breast milk; not for use in nursing.

MECHANISM OF ACTION
Candesartan: ARB; blocks vasoconstrictor and aldosterone-secreting effects of angiotensin II by selectively blocking the binding of angiotensin II to AT_1 receptor

in many tissues. **HCTZ:** Thiazide diuretic; has not been established. Affects renal tubular mechanisms of electrolyte reabsorption, directly increasing excretion of Na^+ and Cl^- and indirectly reducing plasma volume.

PHARMACOKINETICS

Absorption: Candesartan: Rapid and complete. Absolute bioavailability (15%); T_{max}=3-4 hrs. **Distribution:** Candesartan: Plasma protein binding (>99%); V_d=0.13L/kg. HCTZ: Crosses placenta; found in breast milk. **Metabolism:** Candesartan: Ester hydrolysis, liver via O-deethylation (minor). **Elimination:** Candesartan: Feces (67%), urine (33%, 26% unchanged); $T_{1/2}$=9 hrs. HCTZ: Urine (61% unchanged); $T_{1/2}$=5.6-14.8 hrs.

PATIENT CONSIDERATIONS

Assessment: Assess for hypersensitivity to the drugs and their components, anuria, sulfonamide-derived drug hypersensitivity, history of penicillin allergy, volume/salt depletion, SLE, diabetes, HF, hepatic/renal impairment, renal artery stenosis, pregnancy/nursing status, and possible drug interactions.

Monitoring: Monitor for signs/symptoms of fluid/electrolyte imbalance, exacerbation or activation of SLE, hypotension, hypersensitivity reactions, idiosyncratic reaction, renal function changes, and other adverse reactions. Monitor BP and serum electrolytes periodically.

Counseling: Inform females of childbearing potential of the consequences of exposure during pregnancy and of the treatment options for women planning to become pregnant; instruct to notify physician as soon as possible if pregnant. Inform that lightheadedness may occur, especially during the 1st days of therapy; instruct to d/c therapy if syncope occurs and seek consult. Caution that inadequate fluid intake, excessive perspiration, diarrhea, or vomiting may lead to an excessive fall in BP, w/ the same consequences of lightheadedness and possible syncope. Instruct not to use K^+ supplements, salt substitutes containing K^+, or other drugs that may increase serum K^+ levels w/o consulting physician.

ATELVIA — risedronate sodium   Rx

Class: Bisphosphonate

ADULT DOSAGE	PEDIATRIC DOSAGE
Postmenopausal Osteoporosis	Pediatric use may not have been established
Usual: 1 tab once a week	
Missed Dose	
If the once-weekly dose is missed, administer 1 tab on the am after patient remembers and return to 1 tab once a week, as originally scheduled on chosen day; do not administer 2 tabs on the same day	

DOSING CONSIDERATIONS

Renal Impairment

Severe (CrCl <30mL/min): Not recommended

ADMINISTRATION

Oral route

Take in the am immediately following breakfast
Swallow tabs whole in upright position w/ at least 4 oz of plain water. Avoid lying down for 30 min after taking medication
Do not chew, cut, or crush tabs
Take Ca^{2+} supplements, antacids, Mg^{2+}-based supplements or laxatives, and iron preparations at a different time of the day

STORAGE

20-25°C (68-77°F).

HOW SUPPLIED

Tab, Delayed-Release: 35mg

CONTRAINDICATIONS

Esophageal abnormalities that delay esophageal emptying (eg, stricture, achalasia), inability to stand or sit upright for at least 30 min, hypocalcemia, known hypersensitivity to any components of the product.

WARNINGS/PRECAUTIONS

Consider discontinuation after 3-5 yrs of use in patients at low risk for fracture; periodically reevaluate risk for fracture in patients who d/c therapy. Contains same active ingredient as Actonel; do not treat w/ Atelvia if on concomitant therapy w/ Actonel. May cause local irritation of the upper GI mucosa; caution w/ active upper GI problems (eg, Barrett's esophagus, dysphagia, other esophageal diseases, gastritis, duodenitis, ulcers). Esophageal reactions (eg, esophagitis, esophageal ulcers/erosions) reported; d/c if dysphagia, odynophagia, retrosternal pain, or new/worsening heartburn develops. Use therapy under appropriate supervision in patients who cannot comply w/ dosing instructions due to mental disability. Gastric and duodenal ulcers reported. Hypocalcemia reported; treat hypocalcemia and other disturbances of bone and mineral metabolism before therapy, and ensure adequate Ca^{2+} and vitamin D intake. Osteonecrosis of the jaw (ONJ) reported; risk may increase w/ duration of exposure to drug. If invasive dental procedures are required, discontinuation of treatment may reduce risk for ONJ. Consider discontinuation if ONJ develops. Severe and occasionally incapacitating bone, joint, and/or muscle pain reported; consider discontinuing use if severe symptoms develop. Atypical, low-energy, or low-trauma fractures of the femoral shaft reported; evaluate any patient w/ a history of bisphosphonate exposure who presents w/ thigh/groin pain to rule out incomplete femur fracture, and consider interruption of therapy. May interfere w/ the use of bone-imaging agents.

ADVERSE REACTIONS

Diarrhea, influenza, arthralgia, back pain, abdominal pain, constipation, N/V, dyspepsia, bronchitis, URTI, pain in extremity.

DRUG INTERACTIONS

Ca^{2+} supplements, antacids, Mg^{2+}-based supplements or laxatives, and iron preparations interfere w/ absorption; take such medications at a different time of the day. Drugs that raise stomach pH (eg, proton pump inhibitors [PPIs], H_2 blockers) may cause faster drug release from the enteric coating. Increased bioavailability w/ esomeprazole. Not recommended w/ H_2 blockers or PPIs. Upper GI adverse reactions reported w/ NSAIDs.

PREGNANCY AND LACTATION

Category C, not for use in nursing.

MECHANISM OF ACTION

Bisphosphonate; has an affinity for hydroxyapatite crystals in bone and acts as an antiresorptive agent. Inhibits osteoclasts.

PHARMACOKINETICS

Absorption: Absolute bioavailability (0.63%) (30mg immediate-release); T_{max}=3 hrs. **Distribution:** V_d=13.8L/kg; plasma protein binding (24%). **Elimination:** Urine (1/2 of the absorbed dose), feces (unchanged [unabsorbed drug]); $T_{1/2}$=561 hrs (osteopenic postmenopausal women).

PATIENT CONSIDERATIONS

Assessment: Assess for esophageal abnormalities, ability to stand or sit upright for at least 30 min, active upper GI problems, mental disability, hypocalcemia, disturbances of bone and mineral metabolism, risk for ONJ, renal impairment, drug hypersensitivity, any other conditions where treatment is contraindicated or cautioned, pregnancy/nursing status, and possible drug interactions.

Monitoring: Monitor for signs/symptoms of esophageal reactions, hypocalcemia, ONJ, musculoskeletal pain, atypical femoral fractures, and other adverse events. Periodically reevaluate the need for continued therapy.

Counseling: Instruct to pay particular attention to the dosing instructions. Advise to take in the am w/ at least 4 oz of plain water immediately following breakfast. Advise to avoid lying down for 30 min after taking the drug. Advise to consult physician before continuing treatment if symptoms of esophageal disease develop. Instruct to take supplemental Ca^{2+} and vitamin D if dietary intake is inadequate. Advise to consult physician any time they have a medical problem they think may be from treatment.

ATIVAN INJECTION — lorazepam   CIV

Class: Benzodiazepine

ADULT DOSAGE	PEDIATRIC DOSAGE
Status Epilepticus	Pediatric use may not have been established
Usual: 4mg IV (given slowly at 2mg/min); may repeat 1 dose after 10-15 min if seizures recur or fail to cease	
Preanesthetic	
To produce sedation, anxiety relief, and to decrease ability to recall events related to the day of surgery	
Usual:	
IM:	
0.05mg/kg given at least 2 hrs prior to anticipated operative procedure	
IV:	
2mg or 0.044mg/kg IV (whichever is smaller) 15-20 min prior to anticipated operative procedure. Larger doses as high as 0.05mg/kg up to a total of 4mg may be administered in patients in whom a greater likelihood of lack of recall for perioperative events would be beneficial.	
Max (IM/IV): 4mg	

DOSING CONSIDERATIONS

Concomitant Medications

Probenecid or Valproate: Reduce lorazepam dose by 50%

Oral Contraceptives: May be necessary to increase lorazepam dose

Elderly

Start at the low end of the dosing range

ADMINISTRATION

IM/IV route

Can be used w/ atropine sulfate, narcotic analgesics, other parenterally used analgesics, commonly used anesthetics, and muscle relaxants.

IM

Inject undiluted deep in muscle mass.

IV

Must be diluted immediately prior to use w/ an equal volume of compatible sol (sterile water for inj, NaCl inj, D5 inj).
Mix thoroughly by gently inverting container repeatedly until a homogenous solution results; do not shake vigorously.

When properly diluted, the drug may be injected directly into a vein or into the tubing of an existing IV infusion.
Rate of inj should not exceed 2mg/min.

STORAGE
Refrigerate; protect from light.

HOW SUPPLIED
Inj: 2mg/mL, 4mg/mL [1mL, 10mL]

CONTRAINDICATIONS
Known sensitivity to benzodiazepines or its vehicle (polyethylene glycol, propylene glycol, and benzyl alcohol), acute narrow-angle glaucoma, sleep apnea syndrome, severe respiratory insufficiency. Not for intra-arterial inj.

WARNINGS/PRECAUTIONS
Airway obstruction and respiratory depression may occur; ensure airway patency and monitor respiration. May produce heavy sedation; equipment necessary to maintain a patent airway and support respiration/ventilation should be available. May impair mental/physical abilities. Avoid in patients w/ hepatic and/or renal failure; caution in patients w/ hepatic and/or renal disease. May cause fetal damage during pregnancy. When used for peroral endoscopic procedures, adequate topical/regional anesthesia is recommended to minimize reflex activity. Extreme caution when administering inj to elderly, very ill, or to patients w/ limited pulmonary reserve; hypoventilation and/or hypoxic cardiac arrest may occur. Possibility of excessive sleepiness/drowsiness may interfere w/ patient cooperation in determining levels of anesthesia when used as the premedicant prior to regional/local anesthesia. Paradoxical reaction may occur; caution w/ further use of the drug in these patients. Propylene glycol toxicity (eg, lactic acidosis, hyperosmolality, hypotension) and polyethylene glycol toxicity (eg, acute tubular necrosis) reported at higher than recommended doses. Repeated doses over a prolonged period may result in physical and psychological dependence and withdrawal symptoms following abrupt discontinuation.

ADVERSE REACTIONS
Status Epilepticus: Hypotension, somnolence, respiratory failure.
Preanesthetic: CNS depression, skin rash, N/V. (IM) Inj-site pain, burning sensation, redness in inj-site.

DRUG INTERACTIONS
See Dosing Considerations. Additive CNS depression w/ other CNS depressants (eg, ethyl alcohol, phenothiazines, barbiturates, MAOIs, antidepressants). Increased sedation, hallucinations, and irrational behavior w/ scopolamine. Significant respiratory depression, stupor, and/or hypotension reported w/ concomitant use w/ clozapine. Marked sedation, excessive salivation, ataxia, and death (rarely) reported w/ concomitant use w/ clozapine. Apnea, coma, bradycardia, arrhythmia, heart arrest, and death reported w/ concomitant use w/ haloperidol. Increased clearance w/ oral contraceptives. Valproate decreases total clearance and increases plasma levels. Oral contraceptives increases total clearance. Probenecid prolongs $T_{1/2}$ and decreases total clearance. Prolonged and profound effect w/ concomitant sedatives, tranquilizers, narcotic analgesics.

PREGNANCY AND LACTATION
Pregnancy: Category D. May cause fetal damage.
Lactation: Lorazepam has been detected in human breast milk; not for use in nursing.

MECHANISM OF ACTION
Benzodiazepine; antianxiety, sedative, and anticonvulsant effects. Interacts w/ GABA-benzodiazepine receptor complex in the human brain. Exhibits relatively high and specific affinity for its recognition site but does not displace GABA. Attachment to the specific binding site enhances the affinity of GABA for its receptor site on the same receptor complex.

PHARMACOKINETICS
Absorption: Complete, rapid; (IM) C_{max}=48ng/mL, T_{max}=w/in 3 hrs. **Distribution:** V_d=1.3L/kg, plasma protein binding (91%), crosses blood brain barrier and placenta. **Metabolism:** Liver. **Elimination:** (2mg oral dose) Urine (88%), feces (7%), (0.3% unchanged); $T_{1/2}$=14 hrs.

PATIENT CONSIDERATIONS

Assessment: Perform a comprehensive review of benefits/risks in status epilepticus. Assess for hypersensitivity to benzodiazepine or its vehicle, acute-angle glaucoma, preexisting respiratory impairment, hepatic/renal impairment, pregnancy/nursing status, and possible drug interactions.

Monitoring: Monitor for respiratory depression; heavy sedation; drowsiness; excessive sleepiness; hypoglycemia, hyponatremia, or other metabolic/toxic derangement in status epilepticus; seizures; and paradoxical reactions. Monitor for signs of toxicity to the vehicle's components (eg, lactic acidosis, hyperosmolarity, hypotension, acute tubular necrosis). Monitor vital signs and maintain an unobstructed airway.

Counseling: Inform of risks/benefits of therapy. Advise that driving a motor vehicle, operating machinery, or engaging in hazardous or other activities requiring attention and coordination should be delayed for 24-48 hrs following the inj or until effects of drug have subsided. Instruct to not get out of bed unassisted w/in 8 hrs of therapy. Advise to avoid alcoholic beverages for at least 24-48 hrs after receiving drug. Inform elderly patients that the drug may make them very sleepy for a period longer than 6-8 hrs following surgery. Advise about potential for physical/psychological dependence and withdrawal symptoms.

ATRIDOX — doxycycline hyclate   **Rx**
Class: Tetracyclines

ADULT DOSAGE	PEDIATRIC DOSAGE
Chronic Periodontitis	Pediatric use may not have been established
• For a gain in clinical attachment, reduction in probing depth, and reduction in bleeding on probing	
• Dose varies depending on the size, shape, and number of pockets being treated	

ADMINISTRATION
Subgingival route
Does not require local anesthesia for placement
Each syringe system is intended for use in only one patient; refer to PI for preparation instructions

Administration
1. Bend the cannula to resemble a periodontal probe and explore the periodontal pocket in a manner similar to periodontal probing
2. Keeping the cannula tip near the base of the pocket, express the product into the pocket until the formulation reaches the top of the gingival margin
3. Withdraw the cannula tip from the pocket
4. In order to separate the tip from the formulation, turn the tip of the cannula towards the tooth, press the tip against the tooth surface, and pinch the string of formulation from the tip of the cannula
5. If desired, using an appropriate dental instrument, pack Atridox into the pocket. Dipping the edge of the instrument in water before packing will help keep Atridox from sticking to the instrument, and will help speed coagulation of Atridox. A few drops of water dripped onto the surface of Atridox once in the pocket will also aid in coagulation
6. If necessary, add more Atridox as described above and pack it into the pocket until the pocket is full
7. Cover the pockets containing Atridox w/ either Coe-Pak periodontal dressing or a cyanoacrylate dental adhesive
8. Application may be repeated 4 months after initial treatment

STORAGE
2-30°C (36-86°F). Do not use if packaging has been previously opened/damaged. Coupled syringes can be stored at room temperature for a maximum of 3 days.

HOW SUPPLIED
Syringe Delivery System, Controlled Release: 10% (50mg)

CONTRAINDICATIONS
Hypersensitivity to doxycycline or any other drug in the tetracycline class.

WARNINGS/PRECAUTIONS
May cause permanent discoloration of the teeth during tooth development. Unless other drugs are not likely to be effective or are contraindicated, do not use in infants, children <8 yrs, or pregnant women. Enamel hypoplasia reported. Photosensitivity manifested by sunburn reaction has been observed; avoid exposure to direct sunlight or ultraviolet light. May result in overgrowth of nonsusceptible microorganisms including fungi. Caution with a history of predisposition to oral candidiasis. Not clinically tested for use in the regeneration of alveolar bone, either in preparation for/in conjunction with the placement of dental implants or in the treatment of failing implants, in pregnant women, immunocompromised patients. Not clinically evaluated with conditions involving extremely severe periodontal defects with very little remaining periodontium.

ADVERSE REACTIONS
Headache, gum discomfort (pain/soreness), toothache, periodontal (abscess, exudate, infection, drainage, extreme mobility, suppuration), thermal tooth sensitivity, sore mouth, premenstrual tension syndrome, muscle aches, common cold, respiratory flu, stuffy head, post nasal drip, congestion, sore throat.

DRUG INTERACTIONS
May decrease effectiveness of birth control pills.

PREGNANCY AND LACTATION
Category D, not for use in nursing.

MECHANISM OF ACTION
Tetracycline derivative; bacteriostatic, inhibiting bacterial protein synthesis due to disruption of transfer RNA and messenger RNA at ribosomal sites.

PHARMACOKINETICS
Absorption: T_{max}=2 hrs.

PATIENT CONSIDERATIONS

Assessment: Assess for hypersensitivity to tetracyclines, pregnancy/nursing status, and history of predisposition to oral candidiasis. Assess use in infants and children <8 yrs.

Monitoring: Monitor for hypersensitivity reactions, photosensitivity, and enamel hypoplasia.

Counseling: Advise to avoid mechanical oral hygiene procedures (eg, tooth brushing, flossing) on any treated areas for 7 days. Advise to avoid excessive sunlight/artificial ultraviolet light while on therapy. Inform that therapy may decrease the effectiveness of birth control pills.

ATRIPLA — efavirenz/emtricitabine/tenofovir disoproxil fumarate   Rx

Class: Non-nucleoside reverse transcriptase inhibitor (NNRTI)/nucleoside reverse transcriptase inhibitor (NRTI) combination

> Lactic acidosis and severe hepatomegaly w/ steatosis, including fatal cases, reported w/ the use of nucleoside analogues. Not approved for the treatment of chronic hepatitis B virus (HBV) infection and safety and efficacy have not been established in patients coinfected w/ HBV and HIV. Severe acute exacerbations of hepatitis B reported in patients coinfected w/ HBV upon discontinuation of emtricitabine or tenofovir disoproxil fumarate (TDF); closely monitor hepatic function for at least several months after stopping therapy. If appropriate, initiation of antihepatitis B therapy may be warranted.

ADULT DOSAGE	PEDIATRIC DOSAGE
HIV-1 Infection	**HIV-1 Infection**
Alone/Combination w/ Other Antiretrovirals:	**Alone/Combination w/ Other Antiretrovirals:**
1 tab qd	**≥12 Years and ≥40kg:**
	1 tab qd

DOSING CONSIDERATIONS
Concomitant Medications
Rifampin:
≥50kg: Additional 200mg/day of efavirenz is recommended

Renal Impairment
Moderate or Severe (CrCl <50mL/min): Not recommended for use

Hepatic Impairment
Moderate or Severe: Not recommended for use

ADMINISTRATION
Oral route

Take on an empty stomach.
Bedtime dosing may improve tolerability of nervous system symptoms.

STORAGE
25°C (77°F); excursions permitted to 15-30°C (59-86°F).

HOW SUPPLIED
Tab: (Efavirenz/Emtricitabine/TDF) 600mg/200mg/300mg

CONTRAINDICATIONS
Hypersensitivity to efavirenz. Coadministration w/ voriconazole.

WARNINGS/PRECAUTIONS
Hepatic failure reported; monitor liver enzymes w/ underlying hepatic diseases. In patients w/ persistent elevations of serum transaminases >5X ULN, weigh benefit of continued therapy against risks of significant liver toxicity. Immune reconstitution syndrome and autoimmune disorders (eg, Graves' disease, polymyositis, Guillain-Barre syndrome) in the setting of immune reconstitution reported. Redistribution/accumulation of body fat has been observed. Caution in elderly. **Efavirenz:** Serious psychiatric adverse events and CNS symptoms reported; if serious psychiatric adverse events occur, evaluate to assess if they are related to therapy and determine risks and benefits of continued therapy. May impair mental/physical abilities. May cause fetal harm if administered during 1st trimester of pregnancy; avoid pregnancy during use. Use adequate contraceptive measures for 12 weeks after discontinuation. Skin rash reported; d/c if severe rash associated w/ blistering, desquamation, mucosal involvement, or fever develops. Consider alternative therapy in patients who have had a life-threatening cutaneous reaction (eg, Stevens-Johnson syndrome). Consider appropriate antihistamine prophylaxis in pediatric patients before initiating therapy. Convulsions reported; caution w/ history of seizures. **TDF:** Obesity and prolonged nucleoside exposure may be risk factors for lactic acidosis and severe hepatomegaly w/ steatosis. Caution w/ known risk factors for liver disease. D/C if lactic acidosis or pronounced hepatotoxicity occurs. Renal impairment, including acute renal failure and Fanconi syndrome, reported. Decreased bone mineral density (BMD), increased biochemical markers of bone metabolism, and osteomalacia reported; consider assessment of BMD in patients w/ a history of pathologic bone fracture or other risk factors for osteoporosis or bone loss. Arthralgias and muscle pain/weakness reported in cases of proximal renal tubulopathy. Consider hypophosphatemia and osteomalacia secondary to proximal renal tubulopathy in patients at risk of renal dysfunction who present w/ persistent or worsening bone or muscle symptoms.

ADVERSE REACTIONS
Diarrhea, nausea, fatigue, headache, dizziness, depression, insomnia, abnormal dreams, rash.

DRUG INTERACTIONS
See Contraindications. Avoid w/ adefovir dipivoxil, drugs which contain the same active components as Atripla, atazanavir, drugs containing same component or lamivudine, other NNRTIs, boceprevir, posaconazole, or nephrotoxic agents (eg, high-dose or multiple NSAIDs). Potential additive CNS effects w/ alcohol or psychoactive drugs. May increase levels of didanosine and ritonavir (RTV). May decrease levels of amprenavir, indinavir, lopinavir, saquinavir, maraviroc, raltegravir, simeprevir, carbamazepine, anticonvulsants, bupropion, sertraline, itraconazole, ketoconazole, clarithromycin, rifabutin, diltiazem or other calcium channel blockers, atorvastatin, pravastatin, simvastatin, norelgestromin, levonorgestrel, etonogestrel, immunosuppressants, and methadone. May decrease levels of artemether, dihydroartemisinin, and/or lumefantrine resulting in a decrease antimalarial efficacy of artemether/lumefantrine; use w/ caution. **Efavirenz:** RTV may increase levels. Avoid w/ simeprevir. Carbamazepine, anticonvulsants, rifabutin, and rifampin may decrease levels. CYP3A substrates, inhibitors, or inducers may alter levels. May alter plasma levels of warfarin or drugs metabolized by CYP3A or CYP2B6. **TDF/Emtricitabine:** Coadministration of drugs that reduce renal function or compete for active tubular secretion (eg, acyclovir, adefovir dipivoxil, cidofovir, ganciclovir, valacyclovir, valganciclovir, valganciclovir, aminoglycosides [eg, gentamicin], and high-dose or multiple NSAIDs) may increase levels of emtricitabine, TDF, and/or other renally eliminated drugs. Monitor closely for didanosine-associated adverse reactions w/ TDF. Atazanavir, darunavir w/ RTV, and lopinavir/RTV may increase TDF levels. An increase in absorption may be observed when TDF is coadministered w/ an inhibitor of P-gp or breast cancer resistance protein. Refer to PI for further information on drug interactions.

PREGNANCY AND LACTATION
Pregnancy: Category D. Physicians are encouraged to register patients who become pregnant in the Antiretroviral Pregnancy Registry.
Lactation: Excreted in human milk; not for use in nursing.

MECHANISM OF ACTION
Efavirenz: NNRTI; noncompetitive inhibition of HIV-1 reverse transcriptase (RT). **Emtricitabine:** Nucleoside analogue of cytidine; inhibits activity of HIV-1 RT by competing w/ natural substrate deoxycytidine 5'-triphosphate and incorporating into nascent viral DNA, resulting in chain termination. **TDF:** Acyclic nucleoside phosphonate diester analogue of adenosine monophosphate; inhibits activity of HIV-1 RT by competing w/ the natural substrate deoxyadenosine 5'-triphosphate and, after incorporation into the DNA, by DNA chain termination.

PHARMACOKINETICS
Absorption: Efavirenz: C_{max}=12.9µM, T_{max}=3-5 hrs, AUC=184µM•hr. Emtricitabine: Rapid; absolute bioavailability (93%), C_{max}=1.8mcg/mL, T_{max}=1-2 hrs, AUC=10mcg•hr/mL. TDF: Bioavailability (25%, fasted), C_{max}=296ng/mL, T_{max}=1 hr, AUC=2287ng•hr/mL. **Distribution:** Efavirenz: Plasma protein binding (99.5-99.75%); found in breast milk. Emtricitabine: Plasma protein binding (<4%); found in breast milk. TDF: Plasma protein binding (<0.7%); found in breast milk. **Metabolism:** Efavirenz: Via CYP3A and CYP2B6. Emtricitabine: 3'-sulfoxide diastereomers and glucuronic acid conjugate (metabolites). **Elimination:** Efavirenz: Urine (14-34% mostly metabolites), feces (16-61% mostly unchanged); $T_{1/2}$=52-76 hrs (single dose), 40-55 hrs (multiple doses). Emtricitabine: Urine (86%, 13% metabolites); $T_{1/2}$=10 hrs (single dose). TDF: (IV) Urine (70-80% unchanged); $T_{1/2}$=17 hrs (single dose).

PATIENT CONSIDERATIONS

Assessment: Assess for obesity, prolonged nucleoside exposure, liver dysfunction or risk factors for liver disease, renal dysfunction, HBV infection, psychiatric history, history of injection drug use/seizures/cutaneous reaction, drug hypersensitivity, pregnancy/nursing status, and possible drug interactions. Assess BMD in patients w/ a history of pathological bone fracture or w/ other risk factors for osteoporosis or bone loss. Assess estimated CrCl, serum P, urine glucose and urine protein in patients at risk for renal dysfunction.

Monitoring: Monitor for signs/symptoms of lactic acidosis, severe hepatomegaly w/ steatosis, psychiatric/nervous system symptoms, new onset/worsening renal impairment, decreased BMD, increased biochemical markers for bone metabolism, osteomalacia, convulsions, immune reconstitution syndrome (eg, opportunistic infections), fat redistribution/accumulation, skin rash, and other adverse reactions. Monitor for acute exacerbations of hepatitis B in patients w/ coinfection upon discontinuation of therapy. Monitor LFTs. Monitor estimated CrCl, serum P, urine glucose, and urine protein periodically in patients at risk for renal dysfunction.

Counseling: Inform that therapy is not a cure for HIV-1 infection and illnesses associated w/ HIV-1 infection may still be experienced. Advise to practice safe sex, use latex or polyurethane condoms, not to share personal items (eg, toothbrush, razor blades), needles, or other inj equipment, and not to breastfeed. Inform that lactic acidosis, severe hepatomegaly w/ steatosis, and renal impairment have occurred. Instruct to avoid potentially hazardous tasks such as driving or operating machinery if CNS symptoms occur. Instruct to contact physician if severe psychiatric adverse experiences or a rash occur. Advise that fat redistribution/accumulation and decreases in BMD may occur. Advise to avoid pregnancy while on therapy and to use adequate contraceptive measures for 12 weeks after discontinuation; instruct that barrier contraception must always be used in combination w/ other methods of contraception. Advise to avoid potentially hazardous tasks if experiencing CNS/psychiatric symptoms or taking alcohol or psychoactive drugs. Advise that severe acute exacerbation of hepatitis B may occur if coinfected. Advise to report use of any prescription, nonprescription medication, vitamins, and herbal supplements.

ATROPINE INJECTION — atropine sulfate   Rx

Class: Anticholinergic

ADULT DOSAGE	PEDIATRIC DOSAGE
General Dosing	**General Dosing**
Temporary blockade of severe or life-threatening muscarinic effects	Dosing in pediatric populations has not been well studied
Antisialagogue or Other Antivagal Effects:	**Initial:** 0.01-0.03mg/kg
0.5-1mg; repeat in 1-2 hrs	
Antidote for Organophosphorus or Muscarinic Mushroom Poisoning:	
2-3mg; repeat in 20-30 min	
Bradyasystolic Cardiac Arrest:	
1mg; repeat in 3-5 min	
Max: 3mg	
Titrate based on HR, PR interval, BP, and symptoms	

DOSING CONSIDERATIONS
Elderly
Start at lower end of dosing range

ADMINISTRATION
IV (preferred)/IM/SQ/Endotracheal route

Endotracheal Administration
Dilute 1-2mg in no more than 10mL of sterile water or normal saline.

STORAGE
20-25°C (68-77°F); excursions permitted between 15-30°C (59-86°F).

HOW SUPPLIED
Inj: 0.05mg/mL [5mL], 0.1mg/mL [5mL, 10mL]

WARNINGS/PRECAUTIONS
Restrict total dose to 2-3mg (maximum 0.03-0.04mg/kg) when recurrent use is essential in patients w/ coronary artery disease. May precipitate acute glaucoma, convert partial organic pyloric stenosis into complete obstruction, lead to complete urinary retention in patients w/ prostatic hypertrophy, or cause inspissation of bronchial secretions and formation of viscid plugs in patients w/ chronic lung disease.

ADVERSE REACTIONS
Dry mouth, blurred vision, photophobia, tachycardia.

DRUG INTERACTIONS
May decrease the absorption rate of mexiletine.

PREGNANCY AND LACTATION
Pregnancy: Category C.
Lactation: Trace amounts found in breast milk; clinical impact not known.

MECHANISM OF ACTION
Anticholinergic; inhibits muscarinic actions of acetylcholine on structures innervated by postganglionic cholinergic nerves, and on smooth muscles, which respond to endogenous acetylcholine but are not so innervated. Major action is by competitive or surmountable antagonism.

PHARMACOKINETICS
Distribution: Plasma protein binding (44%); found in breast milk; crosses placenta. Metabolism: Liver via enzymatic hydrolysis; noratropine, atropin-n-oxide, tropine, and tropic acid (major metabolites). Elimination: Urine (13-50% unchanged).

PATIENT CONSIDERATIONS
Assessment: Assess for glaucoma, pyloric stenosis, prostatic hypertrophy, chronic lung disease, pregnancy/nursing status, and possible drug interactions.

Monitoring: Monitor for acute glaucoma, conversion of partial organic pyloric stenosis into complete obstruction, complete urinary retention, inspissation of bronchial secretions, formation of viscid plugs, and other possible adverse effects.

Counseling: Inform about the risks and benefits of the treatment.

ATROVENT HFA — ipratropium bromide Rx

Class: Anticholinergic

ADULT DOSAGE	PEDIATRIC DOSAGE
Chronic Obstructive Pulmonary Disease	Pediatric use may not have been established
Maint Treatment of Bronchospasm:	
Initial: 2 inh qid; may take additional inh as required	
Max: 12 inh/24 hrs	

ADMINISTRATION
Oral inh route

Priming
Prime inhaler before using for the 1st time or if inhaler has not been used for >3 days by releasing 2 test sprays into the air, away from the face

STORAGE
25°C (77°F); excursions permitted to 15-30°C (59-86°F). Do not puncture, use/store near heat or open flame, or throw into fire/incinerator. Exposure to temperatures >49°C (120°F) may cause bursting. Discard when indicator displays "0."

HOW SUPPLIED
MDI: 17mcg/inh [200 inhalations]

CONTRAINDICATIONS
Hypersensitivity to ipratropium bromide or other components in this medication, hypersensitivity to atropine or any of its derivatives.

WARNINGS/PRECAUTIONS
Not for initial treatment of acute episodes of bronchospasm. Hypersensitivity reactions and/or paradoxical bronchospasm may occur; d/c therapy and consider alternative treatment if these occur. May increase IOP, which may result in precipitation/worsening of narrow-angle glaucoma; caution with narrow-angle glaucoma. Avoid spraying in eyes. May cause urinary retention; caution with prostatic hyperplasia or bladder neck obstruction.

ADVERSE REACTIONS
Bronchitis, COPD exacerbation, sinusitis, UTI, influenza-like symptoms, dyspnea, back pain, dyspepsia, headache, dizziness, nausea, dry mouth.

DRUG INTERACTIONS
Avoid with other anticholinergic-containing drugs; may lead to an increase in anticholinergic adverse effects.

PREGNANCY AND LACTATION
Category B, caution in nursing.

MECHANISM OF ACTION
Anticholinergic bronchodilator; appears to inhibit vagally-mediated reflexes by antagonizing the action of acetylcholine. Prevents the increases in intracellular concentration of Ca^{2+} that is caused by interaction of acetylcholine with the muscarinic receptors on bronchial smooth muscle.

PHARMACOKINETICS
Absorption: Not readily absorbed. C_{max}=59pg/mL (4 inh, single dose), 82pg/mL (4 inh, qid). Distribution: Plasma protein binding (0-9%). Metabolism: Partial; ester hydrolysis. Elimination: Urine (1/2 of the IV dose, unchanged); $T_{1/2}$=2 hrs.

PATIENT CONSIDERATIONS
Assessment: Assess for hypersensitivity to drug or to atropine or any of its derivatives, narrow-angle glaucoma, prostatic hyperplasia, bladder neck obstruction, pregnancy/nursing status, and possible drug interactions.

Monitoring: Monitor for hypersensitivity reactions, paradoxical bronchospasm, increased IOP, urinary retention, and other adverse reactions.

Counseling: Inform that drug is not for initial treatment of acute episodes of bronchospasm where rescue therapy is required for rapid response. Instruct to d/c use if paradoxical bronchospasm occurs. Instruct to avoid spraying the aerosol into the eyes; advise to consult physician immediately if ocular effects develop. Inform that dizziness, accommodation disorder, mydriasis, and blurred vision may occur; caution about engaging in activities requiring balance and visual acuity (eg, driving, operating appliances/machinery). Advise to consult physician if experiencing difficulty with urination. Instruct to use consistently as prescribed throughout the course of therapy. Counsel not to increase the dose or frequency without consulting physician, and to seek immediate medical attention if treatment becomes less effective for symptomatic relief, symptoms become worse, and/or there is a need to use the product more frequently than usual. Advise on the use of medication in relation to other inhaled drugs.

AUBAGIO — teriflunomide Rx

Class: Pyrimidine synthesis inhibitor

Severe liver injury, including fatal liver failure, reported in patients treated w/ leflunomide; similar risk would be expected because recommended doses of teriflunomide and leflunomide result in a similar range of plasma concentrations of teriflunomide. Concomitant use w/ other potentially hepatotoxic drugs may increase risk of severe liver injury. Obtain transaminase and bilirubin levels w/in 6 months before initiation of therapy. Monitor ALT levels at least monthly for 6 months after starting therapy. D/C therapy and start an accelerated elimination procedure w/ cholestyramine or charcoal if drug-induced liver injury is suspected. Contraindicated in patients w/ severe hepatic impairment. Increased risk of developing elevated serum transaminases in patients w/ preexisting liver disease. May cause major birth defects if used during pregnancy. Pregnancy must be excluded before initiation; contraindicated in pregnant women or women of childbearing potential who are not using reliable contraception. Avoid pregnancy during treatment or before completion of an accelerated elimination procedure after treatment.

ADULT DOSAGE	PEDIATRIC DOSAGE
Multiple Sclerosis	Pediatric use may not have been established
Relapsing Forms:	
Usual: 7mg or 14mg qd	

ADMINISTRATION
Oral route

May take w/ or w/o food.

STORAGE
20-25°C (68-77°F); excursions permitted between 15-30°C (59-86°F).

HOW SUPPLIED
Tab: 7mg, 14mg

CONTRAINDICATIONS
Severe hepatic impairment, women who are pregnant or of childbearing potential not using reliable contraception, concomitant use of leflunomide, history of hypersensitivity reaction to teriflunomide, leflunomide, or to any of its inactive ingredients.

WARNINGS/PRECAUTIONS
Not for use w/ preexisting acute or chronic liver disease, or those w/ serum ALT >2X ULN before initiating therapy. Consider discontinuing therapy if serum transaminase >3X ULN. Consider resumption of therapy if liver injury is not drug induced. Consider additional monitoring if given w/ other potentially hepatotoxic drugs. Eliminated slowly from the plasma. An accelerated elimination procedure can be used at any time after discontinuation of therapy; refer to PI. Decrease in WBC count and platelet count reported; obtain CBC w/in 6 months before initiation of treatment, and base further monitoring on signs and symptoms of bone marrow suppression. Avoid starting treatment until active acute or chronic infections are resolved. Consider suspending treatment and using an accelerated elimination procedure if serious infection develops. Not recommended w/ severe immunodeficiency, bone marrow disease, or severe, uncontrolled infections. May cause immunosuppression and increased susceptibility to infections. Screen patients for latent tuberculosis (TB) infection; if positive treat by standard medical practice prior to initiating therapy w/ teriflunomide. May increase risk of malignancy. May cause anaphylaxis and severe allergic reactions (eg, Stevens-Johnson syndrome, toxic epidermal necrolysis, drug reaction w/ eosinophilia and systemic symptoms); d/c treatment and begin accelerated elimination process immediately if reactions are clearly drug related. Do not re-expose after such reactions. Peripheral neuropathy reported; increased risk w/ >60 yrs of

age, concomitant neurotoxic medications, and diabetes. Consider discontinuing and performing an accelerated elimination procedure if peripheral neuropathy symptoms develop. HTN was reported. Interstitial lung disease (ILD) (eg, acute interstitial pneumonitis) and worsening of preexisting ILD reported. New onset or worsening of pulmonary symptoms, w/ or w/o associated fever, may be a reason for discontinuation; consider initiation of an accelerated elimination procedure. Monitor for hematologic toxicity if switching to another agent w/ a known potential for hematologic suppression.

ADVERSE REACTIONS
Headache, diarrhea, nausea, alopecia, increase in ALT.

DRUG INTERACTIONS
See Boxed Warning and Contraindications. May increase exposure of drugs metabolized by CYP2C8 (eg, paclitaxel, pioglitazone, rosiglitazone. May decrease exposure of drugs metabolized by CYP1A2 (eg, alosetron, duloxetine, theophylline). May increase exposure of OAT3 substrates (eg, cefaclor, cimetidine, ciprofloxacin). Monitor and adjust the dose of OAT3 substrates and drugs metabolized by CYP2C8/CYP1A2 as required. Vaccination w/ live vaccines is not recommended. Coadministration w/ warfarin requires close monitoring of the INR; may decrease peak INR. May increase the systemic exposures of ethinyl estradiol and levonorgestrel; consider the type or dose of contraceptives to be used. Inhibits activity of breast cancer resistance protein (BCRP) and OATP1B1/1B3; do not exceed rosuvastatin dose of 10mg qd if used concomitantly. Consider reducing the dose of other BCRP substrates (eg, mitoxantrone) and drugs in the OATP family (eg, methotrexate, rifampin), especially HMG-CoA reductase inhibitors (eg, atorvastatin, nateglinide, pravastatin); monitor closely for signs and symptoms of increased exposures.

PREGNANCY AND LACTATION
Pregnancy: Category X. Detected in human semen; men should use reliable contraception. Men wishing to father a child should d/c treatment and undergo an accelerated elimination procedure.
Lactation: Not for use in nursing.

MECHANISM OF ACTION
Pyrimidine synthesis inhibitor; immunomodulatory agent w/ anti-inflammatory properties that inhibits dihydroorotate dehydrogenase. Exact mechanism is unknown but may involve a reduction in the number of activated lymphocytes in CNS.

PHARMACOKINETICS
Absorption: T_{max}=1-4 hrs (median). **Distribution:** V_d=11L (IV); plasma protein binding (>99%). **Metabolism:** Hydrolysis (primary), oxidation (minor), N-acetylation, sulfate conjugation. **Elimination:** Urine (22.6%), feces (37.5%).

PATIENT CONSIDERATIONS
Assessment: Assess for previous hypersensitivity, severe immunodeficiency, bone marrow disease, severe uncontrolled infections, ILD, hepatic impairment, diabetes, any other conditions where treatment is cautioned or contraindicated, pregnancy/nursing status, and for possible drug interactions. Obtain transaminase levels, bilirubin levels, and CBC w/in 6 months before initiation of therapy. Obtain BP. Screen for latent TB infection w/ a tuberculin skin test or blood test for mycobacterium TB infection.

Monitoring: Monitor for signs/symptoms of hypersensitivity and skin reactions, immunosuppression and infections, bone marrow suppression, severe liver injury, peripheral neuropathy, skin reactions, ILD, new onset or worsening of pulmonary symptoms, malignancy, and other adverse reactions. Monitor ALT levels at least monthly for 6 months after starting therapy. Monitor BP periodically thereafter.

Counseling: Instruct to contact physician if unexplained N/V, abdominal pain, fatigue, anorexia, jaundice, dark urine, or symptoms of infection develop. Advise women of childbearing potential and men and their female partners to use effective contraception during treatment and until completion of an accelerated elimination procedure. Instruct to immediately report pregnancy if suspected or confirmed. Advise that therapy may stay in the blood for up to 2 yrs after the last dose and that an accelerated elimination procedure may be used if needed. Instruct to avoid some vaccines during treatment and for at least 6 months after discontinuation. Advise to contact physician if symptoms of peripheral neuropathy develop. Inform that treatment may increase BP. Advise to either d/c breastfeeding or d/c therapy. Advise to d/c and seek immediate medical attention if signs/symptoms of a hypersensitivity reaction occur.

AUGMENTIN — amoxicillin/clavulanate potassium   Rx
Class: Aminopenicillin/beta lactamase inhibitor

ADULT DOSAGE
General Dosing

Usual: One 500mg tab q12h or one 250mg tab q8h
Severe Infections: One 875mg tab q12h or one 500mg tab q8h

Lower Respiratory Tract Infections

Usual: One 875mg tab q12h or one 500mg tab q8h

Other Indications

- Skin and skin structure infections
- UTIs
- Acute bacterial otitis media
- Sinusitis

PEDIATRIC DOSAGE
General Dosing

<12 Weeks of Age:
Usual: 30mg/kg/day divided q12h (125mg/5mL sus)

≥12 Weeks of Age:
Less Severe Infections:
25mg/kg/day q12h (200mg/5mL or 400mg/5mL sus; 200mg or 400mg chewable tab) or 20mg/kg/day q8h (125mg/5mL or 250mg/5mL sus; 125mg or 250mg chewable tab)
Severe Infections:
45mg/kg/day q12h (200mg/5mL or 400mg/5mL sus; 200mg or 400mg chewable tab) or 40mg/kg/day q8h (125mg/5mL or 250mg/5mL sus; 125mg or 250mg chewable tab)
≥40kg:
Use adult dose

Otitis Media

≥12 Weeks of Age:
45mg/kg/day q12h (200mg/5mL or 400mg/5mL sus; 200mg or 400mg chewable tab) or 40mg/kg/day q8h (125mg/5mL or 250mg/5mL sus; 125mg or 250mg chewable tab) for 10 days

Sinusitis

≥12 Weeks of Age:
45mg/kg/day q12h (200mg/5mL or 400mg/5mL sus; 200mg or 400mg chewable tab) or 40mg/kg/day q8h (125mg/5mL or 250mg/5mL sus; 125mg or 250mg chewable tab)

Lower Respiratory Tract Infections

≥12 Weeks of Age:
45mg/kg/day q12h (200mg/5mL or 400mg/5mL sus; 200mg or 400mg chewable tab) or 40mg/kg/day q8h (125mg/5mL or 250mg/5mL sus; 125mg or 250mg chewable tab)

DOSING CONSIDERATIONS
Renal Impairment
GFR <30mL/min: Do not give the 875mg dose
GFR 10-30mL/min: 500mg or 250mg q12h
GFR <10mL/min: 500mg or 250mg q24h
Hemodialysis: 500mg or 250mg q24h; give additional dose during and at the end of dialysis

ADMINISTRATION
Oral route

Doses are based on amoxicillin component
Take w/ or w/o food
Take at start of a meal to reduce GI intolerance

Sus
Shake well before use
Reconstituted sus must be stored under refrigeration and discarded after 10 days
Refer to PI for mixing directions

Adults:
May use 125mg/5mL or 250mg/5mL sus in place of 500mg tab
May use 200mg/5mL or 400mg/5mL sus in place of 875mg tab

STORAGE
≤25°C (77°F).

HOW SUPPLIED
(Amoxicillin-Clavulanic Acid) Sus: 125mg-31.25mg/5mL, 250mg-62.5mg/5mL [75mL, 100mL, 150mL], 200mg-28.5mg/5mL, 400mg-57mg/5mL [50mL, 75mL, 100mL]; **Tab:** 250mg-125mg, 500mg-125mg, 875mg-125mg*; **Tab, Chewable:** 125mg-31.25mg, 200mg-28.5mg, 250mg-62.5mg, 400mg-57mg *scored

CONTRAINDICATIONS
History of amoxicillin/clavulanate-associated cholestatic jaundice/hepatic dysfunction.

WARNINGS/PRECAUTIONS
Serious and occasionally fatal hypersensitivity (anaphylactic) reactions reported; d/c if an allergic reaction occurs and institute appropriate therapy. Hepatic dysfunction, including hepatitis and cholestatic jaundice, may occur. *Clostridium difficile*-associated diarrhea (CDAD) reported; d/c if CDAD is suspected or confirmed. Avoid with mononucleosis. May result in bacterial resistance with prolonged use in the absence of a proven/suspected bacterial infection; take appropriate measures if superinfection develops. The 200mg and 400mg chewable tabs and 200mg/5mL and 400mg/5mL sus contain phenylalanine; avoid with phenylketonurics. The 250mg tab and 250mg chewable tab are not interchangeable due to unequal clavulanic acid amounts; do not use 250mg tab in pediatric patients until child weighs at least 40kg. Do not substitute two 250mg tabs for one 500mg tab. May decrease estrogen levels in pregnant women. Lab test interactions may occur. Caution in elderly.

ADVERSE REACTIONS
Diarrhea/loose stools, nausea, skin rashes, urticaria

DRUG INTERACTIONS
Probenecid may increase/prolong levels of amoxicillin; coadministration not recommended. Abnormal prolongation of PT (increased INR) reported with oral anticoagulants; may require oral anticoagulant dose adjustment. Allopurinol may increase incidence of rashes. May reduce efficacy of combined oral estrogen/progesterone contraceptives.

PREGNANCY AND LACTATION
Category B, caution in nursing.

MECHANISM OF ACTION
Amoxicillin: Aminopenicillin; semisynthetic antibiotic with broad spectrum of bactericidal activity against gram-positive and gram-negative organisms.

Clavulanate: β-lactamase inhibitor; possesses ability to inactivate a wide range of β-lactamase enzymes commonly found in microorganisms resistant to penicillin (PCN) and cephalosporins.

PHARMACOKINETICS
Absorption: Refer to PI for absorption parameters. **Distribution:** Plasma protein binding: Amoxicillin (18%); clavulanic acid (25%). Amoxicillin: Found in breast milk. **Elimination:** Amoxicillin: Urine (50-70% unchanged); $T_{1/2}$=1.3 hrs. Clavulanic Acid: Urine (25-40% unchanged); $T_{1/2}$=1 hr.

PATIENT CONSIDERATIONS
Assessment: Assess for history of serious hypersensitivity reactions to other β-lactam antibacterial drugs (eg, PCN, cephalosporins) or other allergens, history of amoxicillin/clavulanate-associated cholestatic jaundice/hepatic dysfunction, hepatic/renal impairment, mononucleosis, phenylketonuria, pregnancy/nursing status, and possible drug interactions.

Monitoring: Monitor for anaphylactic reactions, superinfection, skin rash, CDAD, and other adverse reactions. Periodically monitor renal (especially in elderly) and hepatic function. Monitor PT/INR with oral anticoagulants.

Counseling: Instruct to take each dose with a meal or snack to reduce possibility of GI upset. Counsel that drug only treats bacterial, not viral (eg, common cold), infections. Instruct to take ud; inform that skipping doses or not completing the full course of therapy may decrease effectiveness of the drug and increase resistance of bacteria. Advise to consult physician if severe diarrhea or watery/bloody stools occur (even as late as ≥2 months after treatment). Instruct to use a dosing spoon or medicine dropper when dosing a child with sus, and rinse measuring device after each use. Instruct to discard any unused medicine.

AUGMENTIN XR — amoxicillin/clavulanate potassium   Rx
Class: Aminopenicillin/beta lactamase inhibitor

ADULT DOSAGE	PEDIATRIC DOSAGE
Acute Bacterial Sinusitis	**Acute Bacterial Sinusitis**
2 tabs q12h for 10 days	**≥40kg (Able to Swallow Tab):**
Community-Acquired Pneumonia	2 tabs q12h for 10 days
2 tabs q12h for 7-10 days	**Community-Acquired Pneumonia**
	≥40kg (Able to Swallow Tab):
	2 tabs q12h for 7-10 days

DOSING CONSIDERATIONS
Hepatic Impairment
Caution and monitor hepatic function at regular intervals

ADMINISTRATION
Oral route
Take at the start of a meal; not recommended w/ a high-fat meal.

STORAGE
≤25°C (77°F).

HOW SUPPLIED
Tab, Extended-Release: (Amoxicillin/Clavulanic Acid) 1000mg/62.5mg* *scored

CONTRAINDICATIONS
History of serious hypersensitivity reactions (eg, anaphylaxis or Stevens-Johnson syndrome) to amoxicillin, clavulanate, or to other beta-lactam antibacterial drugs (eg, penicillins and cephalosporins). Severe renal impairment (CrCl <30mL/min), hemodialysis, history of amoxicillin/clavulanate-associated cholestatic jaundice/hepatic dysfunction.

WARNINGS/PRECAUTIONS
Serious, occasionally fatal, hypersensitivity reactions reported with PCN therapy; d/c if allergic reaction occurs and institute appropriate therapy. *Clostridium difficile*-associated diarrhea (CDAD) reported; d/c if CDAD is suspected or confirmed. Caution with hepatic dysfunction. Avoid with mononucleosis. May result in bacterial resistance with prolonged use or use in the absence of a proven/suspected bacterial infection or a prophylactic indication; take appropriate measures if superinfection develops. May decrease estrogen levels in pregnant women. Lab test interactions may occur.

ADVERSE REACTIONS
Diarrhea, vaginal mycosis.

DRUG INTERACTIONS
Probenecid may increase/prolong levels; coadministration not recommended. Abnormal prolongation of PT (increased INR) reported with oral anticoagulants; may require anticoagulant dose adjustment. Allopurinol may increase incidence of rashes. May reduce efficacy of oral contraceptives.

PREGNANCY AND LACTATION
Category B, caution in nursing.

MECHANISM OF ACTION
Amoxicillin: Aminopenicillin; semisynthetic antibiotic that binds to penicillin-binding proteins within the bacterial cell wall and inhibits its synthesis.
Clavulanate: β-lactamase inhibitor; possesses ability to inactivate a wide range of β-lactamase enzymes commonly found in microorganisms resistant to PCN and cephalosporins.

PHARMACOKINETICS
Absorption: Well-absorbed. Refer to PI for absorption parameters in adults and pediatric patients. **Distribution:** Plasma protein binding: Amoxicillin (18%), clavulanate (25%). Amoxicillin: Found in breast milk. **Elimination:** Amoxicillin: Urine (60-80% unchanged); $T_{1/2}$=1.3 hrs. Clavulanate: Urine (30-50% unchanged); $T_{1/2}$=1 hr.

PATIENT CONSIDERATIONS
Assessment: Assess for history of serious hypersensitivity reactions to other β-lactam antibacterial drugs (eg, PCN, cephalosporins) or other allergens, history of amoxicillin/clavulanate-associated cholestatic jaundice/hepatic dysfunction, hepatic/renal impairment, mononucleosis, pregnancy/nursing status, and possible drug interactions.

Monitoring: Monitor for anaphylactic reactions, hepatic toxicity, superinfection, skin rash, diarrhea, CDAD, and other adverse reactions. Monitor PT/INR with oral anticoagulants. Monitor renal function in elderly. Monitor renal, hepatic, and hematopoietic functions with prolonged use.

Counseling: Instruct to take q12h with a meal or snack to reduce possibility of GI upset. Advise to consult physician if severe diarrhea or watery/bloody stools occur (even as late as ≥2 months after treatment). Instruct to take ud; skipping doses or not completing the full course of therapy may decrease effectiveness of the drug and increase resistance of bacteria. Instruct to discard any unused medicine.

AUVI-Q — epinephrine   Rx
Class: Sympathomimetic catecholamine

ADULT DOSAGE	PEDIATRIC DOSAGE
Allergic Reactions	**Allergic Reactions**
Emergency treatment of allergic reactions (Type I) including anaphylaxis to allergens, as well as idiopathic anaphylaxis or exercise-induced anaphylaxis	Emergency treatment of allergic reactions (Type I) including anaphylaxis to allergens, as well as idiopathic anaphylaxis or exercise-induced anaphylaxis
15-30kg: 0.15mg **≥30kg:** 0.3mg	**15-30kg:** 0.15mg **≥30kg:** 0.3mg
Repeat inj may be necessary in patients w/ severe persistent anaphylaxis; >2 sequential doses should only be administered under direct medical supervision	Repeat inj may be necessary in patients w/ severe persistent anaphylaxis; >2 sequential doses should only be administered under direct medical supervision

ADMINISTRATION
IM/SQ route
- Inject into the anterolateral aspect of the thigh, through clothing if necessary.
- Hold uncooperative child's leg firmly in place and limit movement prior to and during an inj.

STORAGE
20-25°C (68-77°F); excursions permitted to 15-30°C (59-86°F). Protect from light; store in the outer case provided. Do not refrigerate. Replace auto-injector if sol is discolored or cloudy, or contains particles.

HOW SUPPLIED
Inj: 0.15mg/0.15mL, 0.3mg/0.3mL

WARNINGS/PRECAUTIONS
Intended for immediate administration in patients who are determined to be at increased risk for anaphylaxis, including those w/ a history of anaphylactic reactions. Intended for immediate self-administration as emergency supportive therapy only and is not a substitute for immediate medical care. More than two sequential doses should only be administered under direct medical supervision. Do not inject IV. Large doses or accidental IV inj use may result in cerebral hemorrhage due to sharp rise in BP; rapidly acting vasodilators can counteract the marked pressor effect of epinephrine. Do not inject into buttock; may not provide effective treatment of anaphylaxis. Inj into buttock associated w/ Clostridial infections (gas gangrene). Do not inject into digits, hands, or feet as this may result in loss of blood flow to the affected area. Rare cases of serious skin and soft tissue infections (eg, necrotizing fasciitis, myonecrosis) caused by Clostridia (gas gangrene), reported at inj site. Contains sodium bisulfite; may cause allergic-type reactions, including anaphylactic symptoms or life-threatening or less severe asthmatic episodes in certain susceptible persons. Caution w/ heart disease (eg, cardiac arrhythmias, coronary artery or organic heart disease, or HTN), hyperthyroidism, diabetes, the elderly, and pregnant women. May temporarily worsen symptoms of Parkinson's disease.

ADVERSE REACTIONS
Anxiety, apprehensiveness, restlessness, tremor, weakness, dizziness, sweating, palpitations, pallor, N/V, headache, respiratory difficulties.

DRUG INTERACTIONS
May precipitate/aggravate angina pectoris as well as produce ventricular arrhythmias w/ drugs that may sensitize the heart to arrhythmias; use w/ caution. Monitor for cardiac arrhythmias w/ anti-arrhythmics, cardiac glycosides, and diuretics. Effects may be potentiated by TCAs, MAOIs, levothyroxine sodium, and certain antihistamines (notably, chlorpheniramine, tripelennamine, diphenhydramine). Cardiostimulating and bronchodilating effects antagonized by β-adrenergic blockers (eg, propranolol). Vasoconstricting and hypertensive effects antagonized by α-adrenergic blockers (eg, phentolamine). Ergot alkaloids may reverse pressor effects.

PREGNANCY AND LACTATION
Pregnancy: Category C.
Lactation: Caution in nursing.

MECHANISM OF ACTION

Sympathomimetic catecholamine; acts on α-adrenergic receptors and lessens the vasodilation and increased vascular permeability that occurs during anaphylaxis. Acts on β-adrenergic receptors, causes bronchial smooth muscle relaxation, and helps alleviate bronchospasm, wheezing, and dyspnea that may occur during anaphylaxis. Also alleviates pruritus, urticaria, and angioedema and may relieve GI and genitourinary symptoms associated w/ anaphylaxis because of its relaxer effects on the smooth muscle of the stomach, intestine, uterus, and urinary bladder.

PATIENT CONSIDERATIONS

Assessment: Assess for risk of anaphylaxis, heart disease, HTN, diabetes mellitus (DM), hyperthyroidism, Parkinson's disease, pregnancy/nursing status, and for possible drug interactions.

Monitoring: Monitor for allergic-type reactions, angina pectoris, ventricular arrhythmias, cerebral hemorrhage, and for other adverse reactions. Monitor HR and BP.

Counseling: Instruct on proper use and storage. Advise that therapy may produce signs and symptoms that include increased HR, sensation of more forceful heartbeat, palpitations, sweating, N/V, difficulty breathing, pallor, dizziness, weakness or shakiness, headache, apprehension, nervousness, or anxiety; advise that these signs and symptoms usually subside rapidly, especially w/ rest, quiet, and recumbency. Inform that patients may develop more severe or persistent effects if they have HTN or hyperthyroidism. Inform that patients may experience angina if they have coronary artery disease. Advise that patients may develop increased blood glucose levels following administration if they have DM. Advise that a temporary worsening of symptoms may occur if patient has Parkinson's disease. Instruct to seek immediate medical care in case of accidental inj. Advise to seek medical care if signs/symptoms of infection develop at inj site. Instruct caregivers of young, uncooperative children to hold leg firmly in place and limit movement prior to and during an inj.

AVALIDE — hydrochlorothiazide/irbesartan Rx

Class: Angiotensin II receptor blocker (ARB)/thiazide diuretic

> D/C when pregnancy is detected. Drugs that act directly on the renin-angiotensin system (RAS) can cause injury/death to the developing fetus.

ADULT DOSAGE	PEDIATRIC DOSAGE
Hypertension	Pediatric use may not have been established
May use w/ other antihypertensive agents	
Add-On Therapy:	
Use if not controlled on monotherapy w/ irbesartan or HCTZ	
Recommended doses in order of increasing mean effect are 150mg/12.5mg, 300mg/12.5mg, 300mg/25mg	
Replacement Therapy:	
May be substituted for titrated components	
Initial Therapy:	
Usual: 150mg/12.5mg qd	
Titrate: May increase after 1-2 weeks of therapy	
Max: 300mg/25mg qd	

DOSING CONSIDERATIONS
Renal Impairment
Severe (CrCl ≤30mL/min): Not recommended
ADMINISTRATION
Oral route

Take w/ or w/o food.
STORAGE
25°C (77°F); excursions permitted to 15-30°C (59-86°F).
HOW SUPPLIED
Tab: (Irbesartan/HCTZ) 150mg/12.5mg, 300mg/12.5mg
CONTRAINDICATIONS
Hypersensitivity to any component of this product, anuria, hypersensitivity to sulfonamide-derived drugs, coadministration w/ aliskiren in patients w/ diabetes.
WARNINGS/PRECAUTIONS
Not for initial therapy w/ intravascular volume depletion. Symptomatic hypotension may occur in intravascular volume- or Na+-depleted patients (eg, patients treated vigorously w/ diuretics or on dialysis); correct volume depletion prior to therapy. Hypokalemia and hyperkalemia reported. **Irbesartan:** Oliguria and/or progressive azotemia and (rarely) acute renal failure and/or death may occur in patients whose renal function may depend on the renin-angiotensin-aldosterone system activity (eg, severe congestive heart failure [CHF]). May increase BUN or SrCr levels in patients w/ renal artery stenosis. **HCTZ:** May cause hypersensitivity reactions in patients w/ or w/o a history of allergy or bronchial asthma, but are more likely in patients w/ such a history. May cause exacerbation or activation of systemic lupus erythematosus (SLE). May cause hyponatremia, hypomagnesemia, hyperuricemia, or precipitation of frank gout. May alter

glucose tolerance and increase cholesterol and TG. Antihypertensive effects may be enhanced in the post-sympathectomy patient. May increase serum Ca²⁺; d/c before testing for parathyroid function. Caution w/ hepatic impairment or progressive liver disease; may precipitate hepatic coma. May precipitate azotemia in patients w/ renal disease. May cause idiosyncratic reaction, resulting in transient myopia and acute angle-closure glaucoma; d/c as rapidly as possible.

ADVERSE REACTIONS

Dizziness, fatigue, musculoskeletal pain, influenza, edema, N/V.

DRUG INTERACTIONS

See Contraindications. Coadministration w/ K⁺-sparing diuretics, K⁺ supplements, K⁺-containing salt substitutes, or other drugs that raise serum K⁺ levels may result in hyperkalemia. Increases in lithium concentrations and lithium toxicity reported; monitor lithium levels. **Irbesartan:** NSAIDs, including selective COX-2 inhibitors, may result in deterioration of renal function (including possible acute renal failure) in the elderly, volume-depleted (eg, those on diuretic therapy), or w/ compromised renal function; monitor renal function periodically. Dual blockade of the RAS w/ ARBs, ACE inhibitors, or aliskiren is associated w/ increased risks of hypotension, hyperkalemia, and changes in renal function (including acute renal failure); avoid combined use of RAS inhibitors. Closely monitor BP, renal function, and electrolytes w/ concomitant agents that also affect the RAS. Avoid w/ aliskiren in patients w/ renal impairment (GFR <60mL/min). **HCTZ:** NSAIDs, including COX-2 inhibitors may reduce the diuretic, natriuretic, and antihypertensive effects. Dosage adjustment of antidiabetic drugs (oral agents and insulin) may be required. Anionic exchange resins (eg, cholestyramine, colestipol) may impair absorption; take at least 4 hrs before or 4-6 hrs after these medications. Risk of symptomatic hyponatremia w/ carbamazepine; monitor electrolytes.

PREGNANCY AND LACTATION

Pregnancy: Category D. Use of drugs that act on the RAS during the 2nd and 3rd trimesters of pregnancy reduces fetal renal function and increases fetal and neonatal morbidity and death.

Lactation: Thiazides appear in human milk; not for use in nursing.

MECHANISM OF ACTION

Irbesartan: Angiotensin II receptor antagonist; blocks the vasoconstrictor and aldosterone-secreting effects of angiotensin II by selectively binding to the AT₁ angiotensin II receptor. **HCTZ:** Thiazide diuretic; not established. Affects renal tubular mechanisms of electrolyte reabsorption, directly increasing Na⁺ and Cl⁻ excretion in approximately equivalent amounts, and indirectly reducing plasma volume.

PHARMACOKINETICS

Absorption: Irbesartan: Rapid and complete. Absolute bioavailability (60-80%); T_{max}=1.5-2 hrs. **Distribution:** Irbesartan: V_d=53-93L; plasma protein binding (90%). HCTZ: Crosses placenta; found in breast milk. **Metabolism:** Irbesartan: Oxidation by CYP2C9 and glucuronide conjugation. **Elimination:** Irbesartan: Urine (20%), feces; $T_{1/2}$=11-15 hrs. HCTZ: Kidney (at least 61%, unchanged); $T_{1/2}$=5.6-14.8 hrs.

PATIENT CONSIDERATIONS

Assessment: Assess for hypersensitivity to drug and its components, anuria, sulfonamide-derived drug hypersensitivity, diabetes, volume/salt depletion, SLE, CHF, renal/hepatic impairment, renal artery stenosis, postsympathectomy status, pregnancy/nursing status, and possible drug interactions.

Monitoring: Monitor for hypersensitivity/idiosyncratic reactions, exacerbation/activation of SLE, hyperuricemia, precipitation of gout, myopia, angle-closure glaucoma, and other adverse reactions. Monitor BP, serum electrolytes, cholesterol and TG levels, and renal/hepatic function.

Counseling: Inform females of childbearing age about the consequences of exposure during pregnancy. Discuss treatment options w/ women planning to become pregnant. Instruct to report pregnancies to physician as soon as possible. Inform that lightheadedness may occur, especially during 1st days of use; instruct to d/c use and contact physician if fainting occurs. Inform that dehydration, which may occur w/ excessive sweating, diarrhea, vomiting, and not drinking enough liquids, may lower BP too much and lead to lightheadedness and possible fainting. Advise patients not to use K⁺ supplements or salt substitutes containing K⁺ w/o consulting the physician. Instruct to d/c therapy and seek immediate medical attention if symptoms of acute myopia or secondary angle-closure glaucoma occur.

AVANDAMET — metformin hydrochloride/rosiglitazone maleate Rx

Class: Biguanide/thiazolidinedione (glitazone)

> Thiazolidinediones, including rosiglitazone, cause or exacerbate CHF in some patients. After initiation and dose increases, observe for signs and symptoms of heart failure (HF); manage accordingly and consider discontinuation or dose reduction if signs/symptoms develop. Not recommended in patients with symptomatic HF. Contraindicated with established NYHA Class III or IV HF. Lactic acidosis may occur due to metformin accumulation; risk increases with conditions such as sepsis, dehydration, excess alcohol intake, hepatic/renal impairment, and acute CHF. If acidosis is suspected, d/c therapy and hospitalize patient immediately.

ADULT DOSAGE	PEDIATRIC DOSAGE
Type 2 Diabetes Mellitus	Pediatric use may not have been established
Initial: 2mg/500mg qd or bid; may consider a starting dose of 2mg/500mg bid w/ HbA1c >11% or FPG >270mg/dL	
Titrate: May increase in increments of (2mg/500mg)/day given in divided	

doses if inadequately controlled after 4 weeks

Max: (8mg/2000mg)/day

Start the rosiglitazone component at the lowest recommended dose

Inadequately Controlled on Rosiglitazone or Metformin Monotherapy:
Initial:
On Metformin 1000mg/day:
2mg/500mg bid
On Metformin 2000mg/day:
2mg/1000mg bid
On Rosiglitazone 4mg/day:
2mg/500mg bid
On Rosiglitazone 8mg/day:
4mg/500mg bid
Individualize therapy if on metformin 1000-2000mg/day

Titrate:
If additional glycemic control is needed, may increase daily dose by increments of 4mg rosiglitazone and/or 500mg metformin
After an increase in metformin dose, if inadequately controlled, titrate after 1-2 weeks
After an increase in rosiglitazone dose, if inadequately controlled, titrate after 8-12 weeks

Max: (8mg/2000mg)/day taken in divided doses bid

DOSING CONSIDERATIONS
Hepatic Impairment
Active Liver Disease/Increased Serum Transaminase Levels (ALT >2.5X ULN): Do not initiate therapy

Elderly
Elderly/Debilitated/Malnourished: Dose conservatively; do not titrate to max dose

ADMINISTRATION
Oral route
Take in divided doses w/ meals

STORAGE
25°C (77°F); excursions permitted to 15-30°C (59-86°F).

HOW SUPPLIED
Tab: (Rosiglitazone/Metformin) 2mg/500mg, 4mg/500mg, 2mg/1000mg, 4mg/1000mg

CONTRAINDICATIONS
NYHA Class III or IV HF, renal disease or dysfunction (eg, SrCr ≥1.5mg/dL [males], ≥1.4mg/dL [females], abnormal CrCl), acute/chronic metabolic acidosis including diabetic ketoacidosis w/ or w/o coma, use in patients undergoing radiologic studies involving intravascular administration of iodinated contrast materials, history of a hypersensitivity reaction to rosiglitazone or any of the product's ingredients.

WARNINGS/PRECAUTIONS
Assess renal function before initiation of therapy and at least annually thereafter; d/c with evidence of renal impairment. Promptly withhold in the presence of any condition associated with hypoxemia, dehydration, or sepsis. Temporarily d/c at the time of or prior to radiologic studies involving the use of intravascular iodinated contrast materials, withhold for 48 hrs subsequent to the procedure, and reinstitute only if renal function is normal. Temporarily suspend for any surgical procedure (except minor procedures not associated with restricted food and fluid intake); restart when oral intake is resumed and renal function is normal. Evaluate patients previously well-controlled on therapy who develop laboratory abnormalities or clinical illness for evidence of ketoacidosis or lactic acidosis; d/c if acidosis occurs. Increased risk of cardiovascular events in patients with CHF NYHA Class I and II. Treatment initiation is not recommended for patients experiencing an acute coronary event; consider discontinuation during this acute phase. Increased risk for myocardial infarction (MI) reported. Caution in patients with edema or at risk for HF. Edema and dose-related weight gain reported. Macular edema reported; promptly refer to an ophthalmologist if visual symptoms develop. Increased incidence of bone fracture, particularly in females. Dose-related decreases in Hgb and Hct reported. May decrease serum vitamin B12 levels. Temporary loss of glycemic control may occur when exposed to stress (eg, fever, trauma, infection, surgery); may be necessary to withhold therapy and temporarily administer insulin. Caution in patients susceptible to hypoglycemic effects, such as elderly, debilitated/malnourished patients, and those with adrenal/pituitary insufficiency, or alcohol intoxication. May result in ovulation in some premenopausal anovulatory women, which may increase risk for pregnancy; adequate contraception is recommended. Review benefits of continued therapy if unexpected menstrual dysfunction occurs. Do not initiate in patients ≥80 yrs of age unless renal function is not reduced. Not recommended for use in pregnancy. Avoid with active liver disease or if ALT levels >2.5X ULN. Caution in patients with mild LFT elevations (ALT levels ≤2.5X ULN). If ALT levels increase to >3X ULN during therapy, recheck LFTs as soon as possible; d/c if ALT levels remain >3X ULN. Check LFTs if symptoms suggesting hepatic dysfunction develop; d/c if jaundice is observed.

ADVERSE REACTIONS
CHF, lactic acidosis, N/V, upper respiratory tract infection, headache, diarrhea, arthralgia, dyspepsia, dizziness, edema, nasopharyngitis, abdominal pain, loose stools, constipation, anemia.

DRUG INTERACTIONS
Caution with drugs that may affect renal function or result in significant hemodynamic change or may interfere with the disposition of metformin, such as cationic drugs eliminated by renal tubular secretion (eg, cimetidine, amiloride, digoxin, morphine, procainamide); monitor and adjust dose of Avandamet and/or the interfering drug. Alcohol potentiates the effects of metformin on lactate metabolism; avoid excessive alcohol intake. Increased risk of CHF with insulin; coadministration is not recommended. Hypoglycemia may occur with other hypoglycemic agents (eg, sulfonylureas, insulin) or ethanol; may need to reduce dose of the concomitant agent. May be difficult to recognize hypoglycemia with β-adrenergic blocking drugs. CYP2C8 inhibitors (eg, gemfibrozil) may increase exposure and CYP2C8 inducers (eg, rifampin) may decrease exposure; if an inhibitor or an inducer of CYP2C8 is started or stopped during treatment, changes in diabetes treatment may be needed based upon clinical response. Observe for loss of glycemic control with drugs that produce hyperglycemia.

PREGNANCY AND LACTATION
Category C, not for use in nursing.

MECHANISM OF ACTION
Rosiglitazone: Thiazolidinedione; insulin-sensitizing agent that acts primarily by enhancing peripheral glucose utilization. Metformin: Biguanide; decreases endogenous hepatic glucose production, decreases intestinal absorption of glucose, and increases peripheral glucose uptake and utilization.

PHARMACOKINETICS
Absorption: Rosiglitazone: Absolute bioavailability (99%). (4mg) AUC_{0-inf}=1442ng•hr/mL; C_{max}=242ng/mL; T_{max}=0.95 hr (median). Metformin: (500mg) Absolute bioavailability (50-60%) (fasted); AUC_{0-inf}=7116ng•hr/mL; C_{max}=1106ng/mL; T_{max}=2.97 hrs (median). **Distribution:** Rosiglitazone: V_d=17.6L; plasma protein binding (99.8%); crosses the placenta. Metformin: (850mg) V_d=654L. **Metabolism:** Rosiglitazone: Extensive by N-demethylation and hydroxylation, followed by conjugation with sulfate and glucuronic acid; CYP2C8 (major), 2C9 (minor). **Elimination:** Rosiglitazone: Urine (64%), feces (23%); $T_{1/2}$=3-4 hrs. Metformin: Urine (90%); $T_{1/2}$=6.2 hrs (plasma), 17.6 hrs (blood).

PATIENT CONSIDERATIONS
Assessment: Assess for HF or risk of HF, metabolic acidosis, diabetic ketoacidosis, risk factors for lactic acidosis, previous hypersensitivity to the drug, presence of an acute coronary event, cardiac status, edema, bone health, inadequate vitamin B12 or Ca^{2+} intake/absorption, any other conditions where treatment is cautioned, pregnancy/nursing status, and possible drug interactions. Assess if patient is planning to undergo any surgical procedure, radiologic studies involving the use of intravascular iodinated contrast materials, or is under any form of stress. Assess baseline renal function, LFTs, FPG, and HbA1c levels, and hematologic parameters.

Monitoring: Monitor for signs/symptoms of HF, lactic acidosis, hypoxic states, MI, edema, weight gain, visual symptoms, fractures, menstrual dysfunction, and other adverse reactions. Monitor for changes in clinical status. Monitor renal function, especially in elderly, at least annually. Monitor hematologic parameters annually. Perform routine serum vitamin B12 measurements at 2- to 3-yr intervals in patients predisposed to developing subnormal vitamin B12 levels. Periodically monitor LFTs, FPG, and HbA1c levels.

Counseling: Inform of the risks and benefits of therapy. Inform of the risk of lactic acidosis; instruct to d/c therapy immediately and notify physician if unexplained hyperventilation, myalgia, malaise, unusual somnolence, or other nonspecific symptoms occur. Counsel against excessive alcohol intake. Advise on the importance of adherence to dietary instructions and regular testing of blood glucose, HbA1c, renal/hepatic function, and hematologic parameters. Instruct to immediately report any signs/symptoms of hepatotoxicity or HF to physician. Counsel premenopausal women to use adequate contraception during treatment.

AVANDARYL — glimepiride/rosiglitazone maleate   **Rx**
Class: Sulfonylurea/thiazolidinedione (glitazone)

> Thiazolidinediones, including rosiglitazone, cause or exacerbate CHF in some patients. After initiation and dose increases, observe for signs and symptoms of heart failure (HF); manage accordingly and consider discontinuation or dose reduction if signs/symptoms develop. Not recommended in patients w/ symptomatic HF. Contraindicated w/ established NYHA Class III or IV HF.

ADULT DOSAGE
Type 2 Diabetes Mellitus
Initial: 4mg/1mg qd w/ 1st meal of the day; may consider 4mg/2mg for patients already treated w/ a sulfonylurea or rosiglitazone
Max: (8mg/4mg)/day

Start the rosiglitazone component at the lowest recommended dose; if hypoglycemia occurs, may consider dose reduction of glimepiride component

PEDIATRIC DOSAGE
Pediatric use may not have been established

Switching from Combination Therapy of Rosiglitazone Plus Glimepiride as Separate Tablets:
Initial: Start at the dose of rosiglitazone and glimepiride already being taken

Conversions

Switching to Avandaryl in Patients Currently Treated w/ Rosiglitazone:
If not adequately controlled after 1-2 weeks, may increase glimepiride component of Avandaryl in no >2mg increments; afterwards, may titrate Avandaryl if not adequately controlled after 1-2 weeks

Switching to Avandaryl in Patients Currently Treated w/ Sulfonylurea:
If not adequately controlled after 8-12 weeks, may titrate rosiglitazone component of Avandaryl; afterwards, may titrate Avandaryl if not adequately controlled after 2-3 months

---

DOSING CONSIDERATIONS
Concomitant Medications
Colesevelam: Administer therapy at least 4 hrs prior to colesevelam

ADMINISTRATION
Oral route

Take w/ the 1st meal of the day

STORAGE
25°C (77°F); excursions permitted to 15-30°C (59-86°F).

HOW SUPPLIED
Tab: (Rosiglitazone/Glimepiride) 4mg/1mg, 4mg/2mg, 4mg/4mg, 8mg/2mg, 8mg/4mg

CONTRAINDICATIONS
NYHA Class III or IV HF. History of a hypersensitivity reaction to rosiglitazone or glimepiride or any of the product's ingredients.

WARNINGS/PRECAUTIONS
Not for use in patients w/ type 1 DM or for the treatment of diabetic ketoacidosis. Treatment initiation is not recommended in patients experiencing an acute coronary event; consider discontinuation during this acute phase. May cause severe hypoglycemia; caution in patients susceptible to hypoglycemic action, such as elderly, debilitated, or malnourished patients, and those w/ adrenal, pituitary, renal, or hepatic insufficiency. Temporary loss of glycemic control may occur when exposed to stress (eg, fever, trauma, infection, surgery); may be necessary to withhold therapy and temporarily administer insulin. Should not be used during pregnancy. Rosiglitazone: Increased risk of CHF w/ insulin; coadministration is not recommended. Caution in patients w/ edema or at risk for HF. Edema and dose-related weight gain reported. Elevation of LFTs may occur; hepatic impairment and hepatitis reported. Do not initiate in patients w/ increased baseline LFTs (ALT levels >2.5X ULN). Caution in patients w/ mild LFT elevations (ALT levels ≤2.5X ULN). If ALT levels increase to >3X ULN during therapy, recheck LFTs as soon as possible; d/c if ALT levels remain >3X ULN. Check LFTs if symptoms suggesting hepatic dysfunction develop; d/c if jaundice is observed. Increased risk of cardiovascular (CV) events in patients w/ CHF NYHA Class I and II. Increased risk for MI reported. Macular edema reported; promptly refer to an ophthalmologist if visual symptoms develop. Increased incidence of bone fracture, particularly in females. Dose-related decreases in Hgb and Hct reported. May result in ovulation in some premenopausal anovulatory women, which may increase risk for pregnancy; adequate contraception is recommended. Review benefits of continued therapy if unexpected menstrual dysfunction occurs. Glimepiride: May be associated w/ increased CV mortality. Hypersensitivity reactions (eg, anaphylaxis, angioedema, Stevens-Johnson syndrome) reported; if suspected, promptly d/c therapy, assess for other potential causes for the reaction, and institute alternative treatment. May cause hemolytic anemia; caution w/ G6PD deficiency and consider the use of a non-sulfonylurea alternative.

ADVERSE REACTIONS
CHF, headache, hypoglycemia, nasopharyngitis, HTN, edema.

DRUG INTERACTIONS
See Dosing Considerations. May require dose adjustment and close monitoring for hypoglycemia or worsening glycemic control w/ drugs that may increase glucose-lowering effect (eg, ACE inhibitors, fibrates, somatostatin analogues, highly protein-bound drugs), drugs that may reduce glucose-lowering effect (eg, protease inhibitors, corticosteroids, oral contraceptives), or drugs that may either increase or decrease glucose-lowering effect (eg, β-blockers, clonidine, reserpine). Signs of hypoglycemia may be reduced or absent w/ sympatholytic drugs (eg, β-blockers, clonidine, guanethidine, reserpine). Glimepiride: Alcohol may also potentiate or weaken glucose-lowering action. Colesevelam may reduce levels. Potential interaction leading to severe hypoglycemia reported w/ oral miconazole. Potential interaction may occur w/ other drugs metabolized by CYP2C9 (eg, phenytoin, ibuprofen, mefenamic acid), and w/ CYP2C9 inhibitors (eg, fluconazole) or inducers (eg, rifampin). Rosiglitazone: CYP2C8 inhibitors (eg, gemfibrozil) may increase AUC and CYP2C8 inducers (eg, rifampin) may decrease AUC; if an inhibitor or an inducer of CYP2C8 is started or stopped during

treatment, changes in diabetes treatment may be needed based upon clinical response. Refer to PI for additional drug interactions.

PREGNANCY AND LACTATION
Category C, not for use in nursing.

MECHANISM OF ACTION
Rosiglitazone: Thiazolidinedione; improves glycemic control by improving insulin sensitivity. Glimepiride: Sulfonylurea; lowers blood glucose by stimulating insulin release from pancreatic β cells.

PHARMACOKINETICS
Absorption: Glimepiride: Complete. T_{max}=2-3 hrs; (4mg) C_{max}=151ng/mL; $AUC_{(0-inf, 0-t)}$=1052ng•hr/mL, 944ng•hr/mL. Rosiglitazone: Absolute bioavailability (99%); T_{max}=1 hr; (4mg) C_{max}=257ng/mL; $AUC_{(0-inf, 0-t)}$=1259ng•hr/mL, 1231ng•hr/mL. **Distribution:** Glimepiride: V_d=8.8L (IV); plasma protein binding (>99.5%). Rosiglitazone: V_d=17.6L; plasma protein binding (99.8%); crosses the placenta. **Metabolism:** Glimepiride: Complete by oxidation; cyclohexyl hydroxy methyl derivative (M1) (via CYP2C9) and carboxyl derivative (M2) (major metabolites). Rosiglitazone: Extensive by N-demethylation and hydroxylation, followed by conjugation w/ sulfate and glucuronic acid; CYP2C8 (major), 2C9 (minor). **Elimination:** Glimepiride: Urine (60%, 80-90% major metabolites), feces (40%, 70% major metabolites); (4mg) $T_{1/2}$=7.63 hrs. Rosiglitazone: Urine (64%), feces (23%); $T_{1/2}$=3-4 hrs.

PATIENT CONSIDERATIONS
Assessment: Assess for HF or risk of HF, presence of acute coronary event, cardiac status, susceptibility to hypoglycemia, edema, bone health, G6PD deficiency, previous hypersensitivity to the drug or sulfonamide derivatives, pregnancy/nursing status, and possible drug interactions. Assess if patient is under any form of stress. Obtain baseline renal function, LFTs, FPG, and HbA1c levels.

Monitoring: Monitor for signs/symptoms of HF, MI, hypoglycemia, edema, weight gain, visual symptoms, fractures, hypersensitivity reactions, hematologic effects, menstrual dysfunction, and other adverse reactions. Periodically monitor LFTs, FPG, and HbA1c levels.

Counseling: Inform of the risks and benefits of therapy. Advise on the importance of adherence to dietary instructions and regular testing of blood glucose, HbA1c, and liver function. Inform about the risk of hypoglycemia, its symptoms and treatment, and conditions that predispose to its development. Instruct to immediately report to physician any symptoms of HF or hepatic dysfunction. Counsel premenopausal women to use adequate contraception during treatment.

AVANDIA — rosiglitazone maleate   Rx
Class: Thiazolidinedione (glitazone)

> Thiazolidinediones, including rosiglitazone, cause or exacerbate congestive heart failure (CHF) in some patients. After initiation and dose increases, observe for signs and symptoms of heart failure (HF); manage accordingly and consider discontinuation or dose reduction if signs/symptoms develop. Not recommended in patients with symptomatic HF. Contraindicated with established NYHA Class III or IV HF.

ADULT DOSAGE
Type 2 Diabetes Mellitus
Initial: 4mg as qd dose or in 2 divided doses
Titrate: May increase to 8mg/day if response is inadequate after 8-12 weeks
Max: 8mg/day

PEDIATRIC DOSAGE
Pediatric use may not have been established

DOSING CONSIDERATIONS
Concomitant Medications
Other Hypoglycemic Agents: May need to reduce dose of the concomitant agent
Hepatic Impairment
Do not initiate therapy in patients w/ clinical evidence of active liver disease or increased serum transaminase levels (ALT >2.5X ULN at start of therapy)

ADMINISTRATION
Oral route

Take w/ or w/o food

STORAGE
25°C (77°F); excursions permitted to 15-30°C (59-86°F).

HOW SUPPLIED
Tab: 2mg, 4mg, 8mg

CONTRAINDICATIONS
NYHA Class III or IV HF, history of a hypersensitivity reaction to rosiglitazone or any of the product's ingredients.

WARNINGS/PRECAUTIONS
Not for use in patients with type 1 DM or for the treatment of diabetic ketoacidosis. Increased risk of cardiovascular events in patients with CHF NYHA Class I and II. Treatment initiation is not recommended for patients experiencing an acute coronary event; consider discontinuation during this acute phase. Increased risk for myocardial infarction (MI) reported. Caution in patients with edema or at risk for HF. Edema and dose-related weight gain reported. Do not initiate in patients with active liver disease or increased baseline LFTs (ALT levels >2.5X ULN). Caution in patients with mild LFT elevations (ALT levels ≤2.5X ULN). If ALT levels increase to >3X ULN during therapy, recheck LFTs as soon as possible; d/c if ALT levels remain >3X ULN. Check LFTs if symptoms suggesting

hepatic dysfunction develop; d/c if jaundice is observed. Macular edema reported; promptly refer to an ophthalmologist if visual symptoms develop. Increased incidence of bone fracture, particularly in females. Dose-related decreases in Hgb and Hct reported. May result in ovulation in some premenopausal anovulatory women, which may increase risk for pregnancy; adequate contraception is recommended. Review benefits of continued therapy if unexpected menstrual dysfunction occurs.

ADVERSE REACTIONS
CHF, upper respiratory tract infection, headache, back pain, hyperglycemia, fatigue, sinusitis, edema.

DRUG INTERACTIONS
See Dosing Considerations. Risk for hypoglycemia when given with other hypoglycemic agents; a reduction in the dose of concomitant agent may be necessary. CYP2C8 inhibitors (eg, gemfibrozil) may increase exposure and CYP2C8 inducers (eg, rifampin) may decrease exposure; if an inhibitor or an inducer of CYP2C8 is started or stopped during treatment, changes in diabetes treatment may be needed based upon clinical response. Increased risk of CHF with insulin; coadministration is not recommended.

PREGNANCY AND LACTATION
Category C, not for use in nursing.

MECHANISM OF ACTION
Thiazolidinedione; improves glycemic control by improving insulin sensitivity.

PHARMACOKINETICS
Absorption: Administration of variable doses resulted in different parameters. Absolute bioavailability (99%); T_{max}=1 hr. **Distribution:** V_d=17.6L; plasma protein binding (99.8%); crosses the placenta. **Metabolism:** Extensive by N-demethylation and hydroxylation, followed by conjugation with sulfate and glucuronic acid; CYP2C8 (major), 2C9 (minor). **Elimination:** Urine (64%), feces (23%). $T_{1/2}$=3-4 hrs.

PATIENT CONSIDERATIONS
Assessment: Assess for HF or risk factors for HF, presence of an acute coronary event, cardiac status, edema, drug hypersensitivity, pregnancy/nursing status, and possible drug interactions. Obtain baseline LFTs, FPG and HbA1c levels, and bone health.

Monitoring: Monitor for signs/symptoms of HF, MI, edema, weight gain, macular edema, fractures, hematologic effects, menstrual dysfunction, and other adverse reactions. Periodically monitor LFTs, FPG, and HbA1c levels.

Counseling: Inform of the risks and benefits of therapy. Advise on the importance of adherence to dietary instructions and regular testing of blood glucose, HbA1c, and liver function. Instruct to immediately report to physician any symptoms of HF or hepatic dysfunction. Inform about the risk of hypoglycemia, its symptoms and treatment, and conditions that predispose to its development when using in combination with other hypoglycemic agents. Counsel premenopausal women to use adequate contraception during treatment.

AVAPRO — irbesartan　　　　　　　　　　　Rx
Class: Angiotensin II receptor blocker (ARB)

> D/C when pregnancy is detected. Drugs that act directly on the renin-angiotensin system (RAS) can cause injury/death to the developing fetus.

ADULT DOSAGE
Hypertension
Initial: 150mg qd
Titrate: May increase to 300mg qd
Max: 300mg qd

Diabetic Nephropathy
Type 2 Diabetes and HTN w/ Elevated SrCr/Proteinuria (>300mg/day):
Recommended Dose: 300mg qd

PEDIATRIC DOSAGE
Pediatric use may not have been established

DOSING CONSIDERATIONS
Other Important Considerations
Intravascular Volume- or Salt-Depleted Patients:
Initial: 75mg qd

ADMINISTRATION
Oral route
May be administered w/ other antihypertensive agents.
May take w/ or w/o food.

STORAGE
25°C (77°F); excursions permitted to 15-30°C (59-86°F).

HOW SUPPLIED
Tab: 75mg, 150mg, 300mg

CONTRAINDICATIONS
Hypersensitivity to any component of this product, coadministration w/ aliskiren in patients w/ diabetes.

WARNINGS/PRECAUTIONS
Symptomatic hypotension may occur in patients w/ an activated RAS (eg, volume- or salt-depleted patients receiving high doses of diuretic); correct volume or salt depletion prior to therapy or use a lower starting dose. Changes in renal function may occur. Patients whose renal function may depend in part on the activity of the RAS may be at particular risk of developing acute renal failure or

death; monitor renal function periodically in these patients. Consider withholding or discontinuing therapy in patients who develop a clinically significant decrease in renal function on irbesartan.

ADVERSE REACTIONS
Hyperkalemia, dizziness, orthostatic dizziness, orthostatic hypotension.

DRUG INTERACTIONS
See Contraindications. Coadministration w/ other drugs that raise serum K+ levels may result in hyperkalemia; monitor serum K+ levels. Increases in serum lithium concentrations and lithium toxicity reported; monitor lithium levels. In patients who are elderly, volume-depleted (including those on diuretic therapy), or w/ compromised renal function, coadministration w/ NSAIDs, including selective COX-2 inhibitors, may result in deterioration in renal function, including possible acute renal failure; monitor renal function periodically. Dual blockade of the RAS is associated w/ increased risk of hypotension, hyperkalemia, and changes in renal function (including acute renal failure); avoid combined use of RAS inhibitors. Closely monitor BP, renal function, and electrolytes w/ concomitant agents that affect the RAS. Avoid w/ aliskiren in patients w/ renal impairment (GFR <60mL/min).

PREGNANCY AND LACTATION
Pregnancy: Category D.
Lactation: Not for use in nursing.

MECHANISM OF ACTION
Angiotensin II receptor antagonist; blocks the vasoconstrictor and aldosterone-secreting effects of angiotensin II by selectively binding to the AT₁ angiotensin II receptor.

PHARMACOKINETICS
Absorption: Rapid and complete. Absolute bioavailability (60-80%); T_{max}=1.5-2 hrs. **Distribution:** V_d=53-93L; plasma protein binding (90%). **Metabolism:** Oxidation by CYP2C9 and glucuronide conjugation. **Elimination:** Urine (20%), feces; $T_{1/2}$=11-15 hrs.

PATIENT CONSIDERATIONS
Assessment: Assess for hypersensitivity, volume/salt depletion, renal impairment, CHF, renal artery stenosis, diabetes, pregnancy/nursing status, and possible drug interactions.

Monitoring: Monitor for signs/symptoms of hypotension, changes in renal function, and other adverse reactions. Monitor BP and renal function periodically.

Counseling: Inform of pregnancy risks and discuss treatment options w/ women planning to become pregnant; instruct to report pregnancy to physician as soon as possible. Instruct not to use K+ supplements or salt substitutes containing K+ w/o consulting physician.

AVAR — sodium sulfacetamide/sulfur　　　　　Rx
Class: Sulfonamide/sulfur combination

OTHER BRAND NAMES
Avar-e LS, Avar-e, Avar LS

ADULT DOSAGE
Acne Vulgaris/Acne Rosacea

Cre:
Apply a thin layer to the affected area qd-tid or ud

Sol:
Wash affected areas qd-bid or ud

Foam:
Treat affected area qd-tid or ud

Seborrheic Dermatitis

Cre:
Apply a thin layer to the affected area qd-tid or ud

Sol:
Wash affected areas qd-bid or ud

Foam:
Treat affected area qd-tid or ud

PEDIATRIC DOSAGE
Acne Vulgaris/Acne Rosacea

≥12 Years:
Cre:
Apply a thin layer to the affected area qd-tid or ud

Sol:
Wash affected areas qd-bid or ud

Foam:
Treat affected area qd-tid or ud

Seborrheic Dermatitis

≥12 Years:
Cre:
Apply a thin layer to the affected area qd-tid or ud

Sol:
Wash affected areas qd-bid or ud

Foam:
Treat affected area qd-tid or ud

ADMINISTRATION
Topical route

Cre
Wash hands and cleanse affected area.
Massage cre completely and uniformly into skin.

Sol
Wet skin and liberally apply to areas to be cleansed.
Massage gently into skin for 10-20 sec working into a full lather, then rinse thoroughly and pat dry.
Rinse off sooner or use less frequently if drying occurs.

Foam
Shake well before use.
Clean affected skin thoroughly and pat dry before each application.
Dispense product into palm of hand, holding can upright.
Massage into the affected area and wait for 10 min.
Rinse thoroughly w/ water and pat dry.

STORAGE

Protect from freezing and excessive heat. (Sol) 25°C (77°F); excursions permitted to 15-30°C (59-86°F). (Cre, Foam) 20-25°C (68-77°F); excursions permitted between 15-30°C (59-86°F). Brief exposures up to 40°C (104°F) may be tolerated provided the mean kinetic temperature does not exceed 25°C (77°F); minimize such exposure. (Foam) Contents under pressure. Do not puncture or incinerate.

HOW SUPPLIED

(Sodium Sulfacetamide/Sulfur) **Sol:** 10%/5% [227g]; (LS) 10%/2% [227g]; **Cre:** (E) 10%/5% [45g tube, 57g bottle]; (E LS) 10%/2% [45g tube, 57g bottle]; **Foam:** 9.5%/5% [100g]; (LS) 10%/2% [100g]

CONTRAINDICATIONS

Kidney disease, known hypersensitivity to sulfonamides, sulfur, or any other component of this preparation.

WARNINGS/PRECAUTIONS

Carefully supervise and use caution in patients who may be prone to hypersensitivity to topical sulfonamides; systemic toxic reactions (eg, agranulocytosis, acute hemolytic anemia, purpura hemorrhagica, drug fever, jaundice, contact dermatitis) indicate sulfonamide hypersensitivity. Caution if areas of denuded or abraded skin are involved. Stevens-Johnson syndrome (SJS) and drug induced systemic lupus erythematosus (SLE) reported. Carefully observe for possible local irritation or sensitization during long-term therapy. D/C and institute appropriate therapy if irritation develops. May cause reddening and scaling of the epidermis. (Foam) Nonsusceptible organisms, including fungi, may proliferate w/ the use of this preparation. D/C use if product produces signs of hypersensitivity or other untoward reaction. Systemic absorption is greater following application to larger, infected, abraded, denuded, or severely burned areas; under these circumstances, any of the adverse effects produced by the systemic administration of these agents could potentially occur, and appropriate observations and lab determinations should be performed.

ADVERSE REACTIONS

Local irritation.

DRUG INTERACTIONS

(Foam) Incompatible w/ silver preparations.

PREGNANCY AND LACTATION

Category C, caution in nursing.

MECHANISM OF ACTION

Sodium Sulfacetamide: Sulfonamide; acts as competitive antagonist to para-aminobenzoic acid, an essential component for bacterial growth. Sulfur: Keratolytic; not established. Reported to inhibit the growth of *Propionibacterium acnes* and the formation of free fatty acids.

PHARMACOKINETICS

Absorption: Sodium sulfacetamide: (Oral) Readily absorbed from GI tract. **Distribution:** Found in breast milk (orally administered sulfonamides). **Elimination:** Sodium sulfacetamide: Urine; $T_{1/2}$=7-12.8 hrs.

PATIENT CONSIDERATIONS

Assessment: Assess for hypersensitivity to sulfonamides or sulfur, kidney disease, and pregnancy/nursing status. Assess if affected areas involve denuded or abraded skin.

Monitoring: Monitor for hypersensitivity reactions, local irritation or sensitization, reddening and scaling of epidermis, SJS, drug-induced SLE, and other possible adverse reactions. Following application to large, infected, abraded, denuded or severely burned areas, perform appropriate observations and lab determinations.

Counseling: Advise to avoid contact w/ eyes, lips, and mucous membranes. Inform that reddening and scaling of epidermis may occur. Instruct to notify physician if any sensitivity/systemic toxic reaction (eg, agranulocytosis, acute hemolytic anemia, purpura hemorrhagica, drug fever, jaundice, contact dermatitis) occurs. Advise to use particular caution when applying to affected skin areas that are denuded or abraded. Advise to notify physician if irritation occurs. Advise to d/c if the condition worsens or if rash develops in the area being treated or elsewhere. Advise to promptly d/c and notify physician if any arthritis, fever or sores in the mouth develop.

AVASTIN — bevacizumab
Rx

Class: Vascular endothelial growth factor (VEGF) inhibitor

> GI perforation reported; d/c w/ GI perforation. Increased incidence of wound-healing and surgical complications; d/c at least 28 days prior to elective surgery. Do not initiate for at least 28 days after surgery and until surgical wound is fully healed. D/C in patients w/ wound dehiscence. Severe or fatal hemorrhage, including hemoptysis, GI bleeding, CNS hemorrhage, epistaxis, and vaginal bleeding, may occur; do not administer to patients w/ serious hemorrhage or recent hemoptysis.

ADULT DOSAGE

Metastatic Colorectal Cancer

1st- or 2nd-line treatment in combination w/ IV 5-fluorouracil-based chemotherapy; 2nd-line treatment in combination w/ fluoropyrimidine-irinotecan- or fluoropyrimidine-oxaliplatin-based chemotherapy, in patients who have progressed on a 1st-line bevacizumab-containing regimen

In Combination w/ Bolus-IFL:

5mg/kg every 2 weeks

PEDIATRIC DOSAGE

Pediatric use may not have been established

In Combination w/ FOLFOX4:

10mg/kg every 2 weeks

In Combination w/ Fluoropyrimidine-Irinotecan- or Fluoropyrimidine-Oxaliplatin-Based Chemotherapy:

5mg/kg every 2 weeks or 7.5mg/kg every 3 weeks

Nonsquamous Non-Small Cell Lung Cancer

1st-line treatment of unresectable, locally advanced, recurrent, or metastatic nonsquamous non-small cell lung cancer in combination w/ carboplatin and paclitaxel

15mg/kg every 3 weeks

Glioblastoma

W/ progressive disease following prior therapy as a single agent

10mg/kg every 2 weeks

Metastatic Renal Cell Carcinoma

10mg/kg every 2 weeks w/ Interferon Alfa

Cervical Cancer

Treatment of persistent, recurrent, or metastatic carcinoma of the cervix in combination w/ paclitaxel and cisplatin or paclitaxel and topotecan

15mg/kg every 3 weeks

Ovarian, Fallopian Tube, or Peritoneal Cancer

Treatment of patients w/ platinum-resistant recurrent epithelial ovarian, fallopian tube, or primary peritoneal cancer who received no more than 2 prior chemotherapy regimens in combination w/ paclitaxel, pegylated liposomal doxorubicin, or topotecan

10mg/kg every 2 weeks w/ 1 of the following IV chemotherapy regimens: paclitaxel, pegylated liposomal doxorubicin, or topotecan (weekly); or 15mg/kg every 3 weeks in combination w/ topotecan (every 3 weeks)

- -

DOSING CONSIDERATIONS

Discontinuation

D/C For:

1. GI perforations, fistula formation in the GI tract or involving an internal organ, intra-abdominal abscess
2. Wound dehiscence and wound healing complications requiring medical intervention
3. Serious hemorrhage (requiring medical intervention)
4. Severe arterial thromboembolic events
5. Life-threatening (Grade 4) venous thromboembolic events, including pulmonary embolism
6. Hypertensive crisis or hypertensive encephalopathy
7. Posterior reversible encephalopathy syndrome
8. Nephrotic syndrome

Temporarily Suspend For:

1. At least 4 weeks prior to elective surgery
2. Severe HTN not controlled w/ medical management
3. Moderate to severe proteinuria
4. Severe infusion reactions

ADMINISTRATION

IV route

Do not administer as an IV push/bolus; administer only as an IV infusion.
Do not initiate until ≥28 days following major surgery and after surgical incision has fully healed.
Give 1st infusion over 90 min.
Give 2nd infusion over 60 min if 1st infusion is tolerated.
Give all subsequent infusions over 30 min if infusion over 60 min is tolerated.

Preparation

Withdraw necessary amount and dilute in a total volume of 100mL of 0.9% NaCl inj.
Discard any unused portion left in a vial, as the product contains no preservatives. Do not administer or mix w/ dextrose sol.

STORAGE

2-8°C (36-46°F). Protect from light. Do not freeze or shake. **Diluted Sol:** May be stored at 2-8°C (36-46°F) for up to 8 hrs. Store in original carton until time of use.

HOW SUPPLIED

Inj: 100mg/4mL, 400mg/16mL

WARNINGS/PRECAUTIONS

Not indicated for adjuvant treatment of colon cancer. Avoid use in patients w/ ovarian cancer w/ evidence of recto-sigmoid involvement by pelvic examination or bowel involvement on CT scan or clinical symptoms of bowel obstruction. GI fistula reported. Serious and sometimes fatal non-GI fistula formation involving tracheoesophageal (TE), bronchopleural, biliary, vaginal, renal, and bladder sites may occur; d/c permanently in patients w/ TE fistula or any Grade 4 fistula. Necrotizing fasciitis, usually secondary to wound-healing complications, GI perforation, or fistula formation, reported; d/c therapy if necrotizing fasciitis develops. Arterial thromboembolic events (ATEs) (eg, cerebral infarction, transient ischemic attacks, MI, angina) reported; increased risk w/ history of arterial thromboembolism, diabetes, or age >65 yrs. May increase risk of venous thromboembolic events (VTEs) in patients treated for persistent, recurrent, or metastatic cervical cancer. Increased incidence of severe HTN. Posterior reversible encephalopathy syndrome (PRES) reported. Increased incidence and severity of proteinuria; suspend therapy for ≥2g proteinuria/24 hrs and resume when proteinuria is <2g/24 hrs. Nephrotic syndrome may occur. Infusion reactions reported. May cause fetal harm. Increases the risk of ovarian failure.

ADVERSE REACTIONS

Epistaxis, headache, HTN, rhinitis, proteinuria, taste alteration, dry skin, rectal hemorrhage, lacrimation disorder, back pain, exfoliative dermatitis.

DRUG INTERACTIONS

May decrease paclitaxel exposure w/ paclitaxel/carboplatin.

PREGNANCY AND LACTATION

Pregnancy: May cause fetal harm; animal models link angiogenesis, VEGF and VEGF Receptor 2 to critical aspects of female reproduction, embryofetal development, and postnatal development. Advise pregnant women of the potential risk to a fetus. **Lactation:** No data are available regarding the presence of bevacizumab in human milk; not for use in nursing. **Reproductive Potential:** Females of reproductive potential should use effective contraception during treatment and for 6 months following the last dose of therapy. Increases the risk of ovarian failure and may impair fertility.

MECHANISM OF ACTION

VEGF inhibitor; binds VEGF and prevents the interaction of VEGF to its receptors (Flt-1, KDR) on the surface of endothelial cells. The interaction of VEGF w/ its receptors leads to endothelial cell proliferation and new blood vessel formation.

PHARMACOKINETICS

Elimination: $T_{1/2}$=20 days.

PATIENT CONSIDERATIONS

Assessment: Assess for recent hemoptysis, serious hemorrhage, HTN, proteinuria, history of ATEs, diabetes, pregnancy/nursing status, and possible drug interactions. Assess for prior surgical history and for any scheduled elective surgeries. Assess for evidence of recto-sigmoid involvement in patients w/ ovarian cancer.

Monitoring: Monitor for GI perforation, fistula formation, wound-healing complications, hemorrhage, ATEs, VTEs, hypertensive crisis, hypertensive encephalopathy, PRES, nephrotic syndrome, severe infusion reactions, and other adverse reactions. Monitor BP every 2-3 weeks, treat w/ appropriate anti-hypertensive therapy, and monitor BP regularly; continue to monitor BP at regular intervals w/ drug-induced or -exacerbated HTN after drug discontinuation. Monitor for proteinuria by dipstick urine analysis for the development or worsening of proteinuria w/ serial urinalyses.

Counseling: Advise to undergo routine BP monitoring and to contact physician if BP is elevated. Instruct to immediately seek medical attention for unusual bleeding, high fever, rigors, sudden onset of worsening neurological function, persistent/severe abdominal pain, severe constipation, or vomiting. Inform of the increased risk of wound-healing complications, ovarian failure, and ATE. Advise females of reproductive potential to use effective contraception during treatment and for 6 months after therapy, and to inform physician of a known/suspected pregnancy. Advise nursing women that breastfeeding is not recommended during treatment.

AVEED — testosterone undecanoate   CIII

Class: Androgen

> Serious pulmonary oil microembolism (POME) reactions, involving urge to cough, dyspnea, throat tightening, chest pain, dizziness, and syncope; and episodes of anaphylaxis, including life-threatening reactions, reported to occur during or immediately after administration. Following each inj, observe patients in healthcare setting for 30 min. Available only through a restricted program under a Risk Evaluation and Mitigation Strategy (REMS) called the Aveed REMS Program.

ADULT DOSAGE

Testosterone Replacement Therapy

Congenital/Acquired Primary Hypogonadism or Hypogonadotropic Hypogonadism in Males:
Usual: 3mL (750mg) IM, followed by 3mL (750mg) after 4 weeks, then 3mL (750mg) every 10 weeks thereafter

PEDIATRIC DOSAGE

Pediatric use may not have been established

ADMINISTRATION

IM route

Inject deeply into the gluteal muscle (gluteus medius); avoid intravascular inj. Between consecutive inj, alternate the inj site between left and right buttock. Following each inj, observe patients for 30 min in order to provide appropriate medical treatment in the event of serious POME reactions or anaphylaxis.

Preparation and Administration Instructions

1. Remove only the gray plastic cap while leaving the aluminum metal ring and clamp seal in place
2. Withdraw 3mL (750mg) of sol from the vial
3. Replace the syringe needle used to draw up the sol from the vial w/ a new IM needle to inj
4. Discard any unused portion of the vial
5. Enter the muscle and maintain the syringe at a 90° angle w/ the needle in its deeply imbedded position
6. Aspirate for several sec to ensure that no blood appears
7. If no blood is aspirated, reinforce the current needle position to avoid any movement of the needle and slowly (over 60-90 sec) depress the plunger carefully and at a constant rate, until all the medication has been delivered

STORAGE

25°C (77°F); excursions permitted to 15-30°C (59-86°F).

HOW SUPPLIED

Inj: 750mg/3mL

CONTRAINDICATIONS

Men w/ breast carcinoma or known/suspected prostate carcinoma; women who are or may become pregnant, or who are breastfeeding; men w/ known hypersensitivity to this product or any of its ingredients (eg, testosterone undecanoate, refined castor oil, benzyl benzoate).

WARNINGS/PRECAUTIONS

Patients w/ BPH and geriatric patients are at an increased risk of worsening of signs and symptoms of BPH. May increase risk for prostate cancer. Increases in Hct/RBC mass, may require discontinuation; may increase the risk of thromboembolic events. If Hct becomes elevated, d/c therapy until Hct decreases to an acceptable level. Venous thromboembolic events (VTEs), including deep vein thrombosis and pulmonary embolism, reported; d/c treatment and initiate appropriate workup and management if a VTE is suspected. Increased risk of major adverse cardiovascular events (MACE) reported. Not indicated for use in women. Suppression of spermatogenesis may occur w/ large doses. Monitor for signs/symptoms of hepatic dysfunction; if these occur, promptly d/c therapy while the cause is evaluated. May promote retention of Na⁺ and water. Edema w/ or w/o CHF in patients w/ preexisting cardiac/renal/hepatic disease may occur; in addition to discontinuation of therapy, diuretic therapy may be required. Gynecomastia may develop and persist. May potentiate sleep apnea. Changes in serum lipid profile may require dose adjustment of lipid lowering drugs or discontinuation of testosterone therapy. Caution in cancer patients at risk of hypercalcemia (and associated hypercalciuria); regularly monitor serum Ca^{2+} concentrations. May decrease concentrations of thyroxine-binding globulin (TBG), resulting in decreased total T4 serum concentrations and increased resin uptake of T3 and T4.

ADVERSE REACTIONS

POME, anaphylaxis, acne, inj-site pain, prostate specific antigen increased.

DRUG INTERACTIONS

Changes in insulin sensitivity or glycemic control may occur; may decrease blood glucose, which may necessitate a decrease in the dose of antidiabetic medication in diabetic patients. Changes in anticoagulant activity may occur; frequently monitor INR and PT in patients taking warfarin, especially at the initiation and termination of androgen therapy. Concurrent use w/ corticosteroids may result in increased fluid retention; caution in patients w/ cardiac/renal/hepatic disease.

PREGNANCY AND LACTATION

Category X, not for use in nursing.

MECHANISM OF ACTION

Androgen; responsible for the normal growth and development of male sex organs and for maintenance of secondary sex characteristics.

PHARMACOKINETICS

Absorption: T_{max}=7 days (median); C_{max}=90.9ng/dL. **Distribution:** Plasma protein binding (40%, sex hormone-binding globulin). **Metabolism:** Via ester cleavage of the undecanoate group; estradiol and dihydrotestosterone (major active metabolites). **Elimination:** Urine (90%, glucuronic and sulfuric acid-conjugates or metabolites), feces (6%, unconjugated); $T_{1/2}$=10-100 min.

PATIENT CONSIDERATIONS

Assessment: Assess for breast/prostate cancer, BPH, cardiac/renal/hepatic disease, obesity, chronic lung diseases, any other conditions where treatment is contraindicated or cautioned, and possible drug interactions. Check Hct prior to therapy. Confirm diagnosis of hypogonadism by measuring testosterone levels in am on at least 2 separate days prior to initiation.

Monitoring: Monitor for worsening signs/symptoms of BPH, prostate cancer, VTE, MACE, hepatic dysfunction, Na⁺/water retention, gynecomastia, sleep apnea, and other adverse reactions. Monitor serum lipid profile and TBG. Regularly monitor serum Ca^{2+} concentrations in cancer patients at risk of hypercalcemia. Reevaluate Hct 3-6 months after starting therapy, then annually. Frequently monitor INR and PT in patients taking warfarin, especially at the initiation and termination of androgen therapy.

Counseling: Advise of the risks of serious POME and anaphylaxis; instruct to remain at the healthcare setting for 30 min after each inj. Inform that treatment may lead to adverse reactions (eg, changes in urinary habits, breathing disturbances, too frequent or persistent erections of the penis, N/V, changes in skin color, ankle swelling). Instruct to adhere to all recommended monitoring and report any changes in state of health (eg, changes in urinary habits, breathing, sleep, mood). Inform of the possible risk of MACE when deciding whether to use or continue to use drug.

AVELOX — moxifloxacin hydrochloride   Rx
Class: Fluoroquinolone

> Fluoroquinolones have been associated w/ disabling and potentially irreversible serious adverse reactions that have occurred together, including tendinitis and tendon rupture, peripheral neuropathy, CNS effects; d/c immediately and avoid fluoroquinolone use in patients who experience any of these serious adverse reactions. May exacerbate muscle weakness in patients w/ myasthenia gravis; avoid w/ known history of myasthenia gravis. Because fluoroquinolones have been associated w/ serious adverse reactions, reserve moxifloxacin for use in patients who have no alternative treatment options for the following indications: acute bacterial sinusitis and acute bacterial exacerbation of chronic bronchitis.

ADULT DOSAGE

Skin and Skin Structure Infections
Uncomplicated: 400mg PO/IV q24h for 7 days

Complicated: 400mg PO/IV q24h for 7-21 days

Intra-Abdominal Infections
Complicated: 400mg PO/IV q24h for 5-14 days

Acute Bacterial Sinusitis
400mg PO/IV q24h for 10 days

Reserve moxifloxacin for treatment in patients who have no alternative treatment options

Acute Bacterial Exacerbation of Chronic Bronchitis
400mg PO/IV q24h for 5 days

Reserve moxifloxacin for treatment in patients who have no alternative treatment options

Community-Acquired Pneumonia
400mg PO/IV q24h for 7-14 days

Plague
Treatment of Plague (Including Pneumonic and Septicemic Plague) and Prophylaxis of Plague:
400mg PO/IV q24h for 10-14 days

Drug administration should begin as soon as possible after suspected or confirmed exposure to *Yersinia pestis*

Conversions
IV to Oral Dosing:
No dose adjustment is necessary; patients started w/ moxifloxacin inj may be switched to moxifloxacin tabs when clinically indicated

PEDIATRIC DOSAGE
Pediatric use may not have been established

ADMINISTRATION
Oral/IV route

Tab
W/ Multivalent Cations:
Administer at least 4 hrs before or 8 hrs after products containing Mg^{2+}, aluminum, iron, or zinc, including antacids, sucralfate, multivitamins, and didanosine buffered tabs for oral sus or the pediatric powder for oral sol.

W/ Food:
Take w/ or w/o food.
Drink fluids liberally.

IV
Administer by IV infusion only; infuse IV over 60 min by direct infusion or through a Y-type IV infusion set.
Avoid rapid or bolus IV infusion.

Drug and Diluent Compatibilities:
Limited data on compatibility w/ other IV substances; additives or other medications should not be added to inj or infused simultaneously through same IV line.
If the same IV line or a Y-type line is used for sequential infusion of other drugs, or if the "piggyback" method of administration is used, flush the line before and after infusion of moxifloxacin w/ an infusion sol compatible w/ the inj as well as w/ other drug(s) administered via this common line.

Compatible IV Sol:
0.9% NaCl inj
1M NaCl inj
D5 inj
Sterile water for inj
D10 for inj
Lactated Ringer's for inj
Refer to PI for preparation for administration of inj.

STORAGE
25°C (77°F); excursions permitted to 15-30°C (59-86°F). **Tab:** Avoid high humidity. **Inj:** Do not refrigerate.

HOW SUPPLIED
Inj: 400mg/250mL; **Tab:** 400mg

CONTRAINDICATIONS
History of hypersensitivity to moxifloxacin or any member of the quinolone class.

WARNINGS/PRECAUTIONS
Tendinitis or tendon rupture can occur w/in hours or days of starting therapy or as long as several months after completion of therapy and may occur bilaterally; increased risk in patients >60 yrs and in patients w/ kidney, heart, or lung transplants. Avoid in patients who have a history of tendon disorders or who have experienced tendinitis or tendon rupture. Cases of sensory or sensorimotor axonal polyneuropathy, resulting in paresthesias, hypoesthesias, dysesthesias, and weakness reported; symptoms may occur soon after initiation of therapy and may be irreversible in some patients. Avoid in patients who have previously experienced peripheral neuropathy. Use moxifloxacin when benefits exceed the risks in patients w/ known or suspected CNS disorders (eg, severe cerebral arteriosclerosis, epilepsy) or in the presence of other risk factors that may predispose to seizures or lower the seizure threshold. May prolong QT interval; avoid w/ known QT interval prolongation, ventricular arrhythmias including torsades de pointes, ongoing proarrhythmic conditions (eg, clinically significant bradycardia, acute myocardial ischemia), or uncorrected hypokalemia or hypomagnesemia. Elderly using IV formulation may be more susceptible to drug-associated QT prolongation. In patients w/ mild, moderate, or severe liver cirrhosis, metabolic disturbances associated w/ hepatic insufficiency may lead to QT prolongation; monitor ECG in patients w/ liver cirrhosis. Magnitude of QT prolongation may increase w/ increasing drug concentrations or increasing infusion rates of the IV formulation; do not exceed recommended dose or infusion rate. Serious anaphylactic reactions and other serious and sometimes fatal adverse reactions reported; d/c immediately and institute supportive measures at the 1st appearance of a skin rash, jaundice, or any other sign of hypersensitivity. *Clostridium difficile*-associated diarrhea (CDAD) reported; may need to d/c if CDAD is suspected or confirmed. Blood glucose disturbances (eg, hypo/hyperglycemia) reported, predominantly in elderly diabetic patients receiving concomitant treatment w/ an oral hypoglycemic agent (eg, sulfonylurea) or w/ insulin; d/c therapy and immediately initiate appropriate therapy if hypoglycemic reaction occurs. May cause moderate to severe photosensitivity/phototoxicity reactions; d/c if phototoxicity occurs. Avoid excessive exposure to sun/UV light. May result in bacterial resistance if used in the absence of a proven/strongly suspected bacterial infection or a prophylactic indication.

ADVERSE REACTIONS
Nausea, diarrhea, headache, dizziness.

DRUG INTERACTIONS
See Administration. Oral administration of moxifloxacin w/ antacids containing Mg^{2+} or aluminum, sucralfate, metal cations (eg, iron), multivitamins containing iron or zinc, or formulations containing divalent and trivalent cations such as didanosine buffered tabs for oral sus or the pediatric powder for oral sol, may substantially interfere w/ absorption of moxifloxacin and lower systemic concentrations. May enhance anticoagulant effects of warfarin or its derivatives. Disturbances of blood glucose in diabetic patients receiving a concomitant antidiabetic agent reported. NSAIDs may increase risk of CNS stimulation and convulsions. Avoid w/ Class IA (eg, quinidine, procainamide) or Class III (eg, amiodarone, sotalol) antiarrhythmics, or other drugs that prolong the QT interval (eg, cisapride, erythromycin, antipsychotics, TCAs). Increased risk of developing fluoroquinolone-associated tendinitis and tendon rupture in patients taking corticosteroid drugs.

PREGNANCY AND LACTATION
Pregnancy: Category C.
Lactation: May be excreted in human milk; not for use in nursing.

MECHANISM OF ACTION
Fluoroquinolone; bactericidal action results from inhibiting topoisomerase II (DNA gyrase) and topoisomerase IV, which are required for bacterial DNA replication, transcription, repair, and recombination.

PHARMACOKINETICS
Absorption: (PO) Well-absorbed; absolute bioavailability (approx 90%). Administration of variable doses in different patient populations resulted in different pharmacokinetic parameters. **Distribution:** V_d=1.7-2.7L/kg; plasma protein binding (approx 30-50%). May be found in breast milk. **Metabolism:** Glucuronide and sulfate conjugation. **Elimination:** approx 45% unchanged; urine (20%), feces (25%). Single dose: $T_{1/2}$=11.5-15.6 hrs (PO), 8.2-15.4 hrs (IV). Refer to PI for additional pharmacokinetic parameters.

PATIENT CONSIDERATIONS
Assessment: Assess for risk factors for developing tendinitis and tendon rupture; history of myasthenia gravis, tendon disorders, or peripheral neuropathy; drug hypersensitivity; known QT interval prolongation; ventricular arrhythmias including torsades de pointes; uncorrected hypokalemia or hypomagnesemia; ongoing proarrhythmic conditions; liver cirrhosis; CNS disorders or risk factors that may predispose to seizures or lower seizure threshold; diabetes; pregnancy/nursing status; and possible drug interactions. Obtain baseline culture and susceptibility tests.

Monitoring: Monitor for tendinitis, tendon rupture, peripheral neuropathy, CNS effects, exacerbation of myasthenia gravis, QT prolongation, hypersensitivity reactions, CDAD, photosensitivity/phototoxicity reactions, and other adverse reactions. Monitor ECG in patients w/ liver cirrhosis. Carefully monitor blood glucose in diabetic patients. Monitor PT and INR if administered w/ warfarin or its derivatives.

Counseling: Inform about benefits/risks of therapy. Advise to d/c if an adverse reaction is experienced and to call physician for advice on completing the full course of treatment w/ another antibacterial drug. Inform about the risks of tendinitis and tendon rupture, peripheral neuropathies, CNS effects, exacerbation of myasthenia gravis, QT interval prolongation. Instruct to d/c and contact physician if pain, swelling, or inflammation of a tendon, or weakness or inability to use joints is experienced; advise to rest and refrain from exercise. Instruct to d/c immediately and contact physician if symptoms of peripheral neuropathy (eg, pain, burning, tingling, numbness and/or weakness) develop. Advise to inform physician if patient has history of convulsions or myasthenia gravis. Inform patients that they should know how they react to therapy before operating an automobile or machinery or engaging in other activities requiring mental alertness/coordination. Instruct to notify physician if persistent headache w/ or w/o blurred vision occurs. Advise to notify physician if symptoms of muscle weakness, including respiratory difficulties, are experienced. Instruct to d/c at the 1st sign of a skin rash, hives, or other skin reactions, a rapid heartbeat, difficulty in swallowing or breathing, any swelling suggesting angioedema, or other symptoms of an allergic reaction. Instruct to notify physician if experiencing any signs or symptoms of liver injury. Inform that diarrhea is a common problem; instruct to notify physician if experiencing watery and bloody stools (w/ or w/o stomach cramps/fever) even as late as ≥2 months after having taken the last dose of treatment. Instruct to inform physician of any personal or family history of QT prolongation or proarrhythmic conditions. Advise to minimize or avoid exposure to natural or artificial light (eg, tanning beds or UVA/B treatment); instruct to contact physician if a sunburn-like reaction or skin eruption occurs. Instruct diabetic patients being treated w/ insulin or an oral hypoglycemic agent to d/c therapy and notify physician if hypoglycemia occurs. Inform that drug treats only bacterial, not viral, infections. Instruct to take exactly ud; inform that skipping doses or not completing full course may decrease effectiveness and increase bacterial resistance. Instruct to take at least 4 hrs before or 8 hrs after multivitamins (containing iron or zinc), antacids (containing Mg^{2+} or aluminum), sucralfate, or didanosine buffered tabs for oral sus or the pediatric powder for oral sol.

AVIANE — ethinyl estradiol/levonorgestrel   Rx

Class: Estrogen/progestogen combination

> Cigarette smoking increases the risk of serious cardiovascular side effects. This risk increases with age (>35 yrs of age) and with extent of smoking (≥15 cigarettes/day). Women who use oral contraceptives should be strongly advised not to smoke.

OTHER BRAND NAMES
Orsythia

ADULT DOSAGE
Contraception
1 tab qd for 28 days at the same time each day, then repeat

Start on 1st Sunday after onset of menses or on Day 1 of menses

Conversions
Switching from 21-Day Regimen Tabs:
Wait 7 days after last tab before starting therapy

Switching from 28-Day Regimen Tabs:
Start on the day after the last tab is taken; do not wait any days between packs

Switching from a Progestin-Only Pill:
May switch any day from progestin-only pill and begin therapy the next day; use a nonhormonal backup method for the first 7 days

Switching from an Implant/Inj:
Start on the day of implant removal or the day the next inj would be due; use a nonhormonal backup method for the first 7 days

PEDIATRIC DOSAGE
Contraception
Not indicated for use premenarche; refer to adult dosing

DOSING CONSIDERATIONS
Other Important Considerations
Use After Pregnancy/Abortion/Miscarriage:
Initiate no earlier than 28 days postpartum in the nonlactating mother or after a 2nd trimester abortion; use a nonhormonal backup method for the first 7 days
May initiate immediately after a 1st trimester abortion/miscarriage; backup contraception is not needed

ADMINISTRATION
Oral route
Take exactly ud and at intervals not exceeding 24 hrs
If therapy is started later than Day 1 of 1st menstrual cycle or postpartum, use a nonhormonal backup method of birth control during the first 7 days of therapy

STORAGE
20-25°C (68-77°F).

HOW SUPPLIED
Tab: (Ethinyl Estradiol [EE]-Levonorgestrel) 0.02mg-0.1mg

CONTRAINDICATIONS
Thrombophlebitis or history of deep vein thrombophlebitis, presence or history of thromboembolic disorders, presence or history of cerebrovascular or coronary artery disease, valvular heart disease with thrombogenic complications, thrombogenic rhythm disorders, hereditary or acquired thrombophilias, major surgery with prolonged immobilization, uncontrolled HTN, diabetes mellitus (DM) with vascular involvement, headaches with focal neurological symptoms, presence or history of breast cancer, carcinoma of the endometrium or other known or suspected estrogen-dependent neoplasia, undiagnosed abnormal genital bleeding, cholestatic jaundice of pregnancy or jaundice with prior pill use, hepatic adenomas/carcinomas or active liver disease, known/suspected pregnancy, hypersensitivity to any of the components of this product.

WARNINGS/PRECAUTIONS
Increased risk of MI, vascular disease, thromboembolism, stroke, hepatic neoplasia, and gallbladder disease. Increased risk of morbidity and mortality with certain inherited/acquired thrombophilias, HTN, hyperlipidemia, obesity, DM, and surgery or trauma with increased risk of thrombosis. If feasible, d/c at least 4 weeks prior to and for 2 weeks after elective surgery of a type associated with an increase in risk of thromboembolism, and during and following prolonged immobilization. Start use no earlier than four weeks after delivery in women who elect not to breastfeed or after a midtrimester pregnancy termination. May increase risk of breast cancer and cancer of the reproductive organs. Contact lens wearers who develop visual changes or changes in lens tolerance should be assessed by an ophthalmologist. Retinal thrombosis reported; d/c if unexplained partial/complete loss of vision; onset of proptosis or diplopia; papilledema; or retinal vascular lesions develop. Should not be used to induce withdrawal bleeding as a test for pregnancy, nor to treat threatened or habitual abortion during pregnancy. Rule out pregnancy if 2 consecutive periods are missed. May cause glucose intolerance; monitor prediabetic and diabetic patients. May elevate serum TG and LDL levels and may render the control of hyperlipidemias more difficult. Caution with history of depression; d/c if depression recurs to a serious degree. May cause increased BP and fluid retention; d/c if a significant BP elevation occurs. Onset/exacerbation of migraine, or recurrent, persistent, severe headache may develop; d/c if this occurs. Breakthrough bleeding and spotting reported; rule out malignancy or pregnancy. Post-pill amenorrhea or oligomenorrhea may occur. Ectopic and intrauterine pregnancy may occur in contraceptive failures. D/C if jaundice develops. Diarrhea and/or vomiting may reduce hormone absorption, resulting in decreased serum concentrations. May affect certain endocrine function tests, LFTs, and blood components.

ADVERSE REACTIONS
N/V, dizziness, spotting, amenorrhea, change in menstrual flow, mood changes, vaginal candidiasis, edema, weight changes, melasma, breast changes, changes in cervical erosion and secretion, allergic rash, change in appetite.

DRUG INTERACTIONS
May reduce contraceptive effectiveness, resulting in unintended pregnancy or breakthrough bleeding when used concomitantly with antibiotics, anticonvulsants, and other drugs that increase the metabolism of contraceptive steroids (eg, rifampin, barbiturates, dexamethasone); consider a backup nonhormonal method of birth control. Several cases of contraceptive failure and breakthrough bleeding reported with concomitant administration of antibiotics (eg, ampicillin and other penicillins, tetracyclines). Anti-HIV protease inhibitors may increase or decrease plasma levels. Herbal products containing St. John's wort (*Hypericum perforatum*) may induce hepatic enzymes (cytochrome P450) and P-gp transporter; may reduce effectiveness of contraceptive steroids and may also result in breakthrough bleeding. Atorvastatin may increase EE exposure. Ascorbic acid and acetaminophen (APAP) may increase bioavailability of EE. CYP3A4 inhibitors (eg, indinavir, ketoconazole, troleandomycin) may increase plasma hormone levels. Troleandomycin may increase risk of intrahepatic cholestasis. Increased plasma levels of cyclosporine, prednisolone and other corticosteroids, and theophylline have been reported. Decreased plasma concentrations of APAP and increased clearance of temazepam, salicylic acid, morphine, and clofibric acid reported.

PREGNANCY AND LACTATION
Category X, not for use in nursing.

MECHANISM OF ACTION
Estrogen/progestogen combination; acts by suppressing gonadotropins, primarily inhibiting ovulation, and causing other alterations, including changes in the cervical mucus (increases difficulty of sperm entry into the uterus) and the endometrium (reduces likelihood of implantation).

PHARMACOKINETICS
Absorption: Levonorgestrel: Rapid and complete. Bioavailability (100%); C_{max}=2.8ng/mL (single dose), 6ng/mL (multiple doses); T_{max}=1.6 hrs (single dose), 1.5 hrs (multiple doses). EE: Rapid. Bioavailability (38-48%); C_{max}=62pg/mL (single dose), 77pg/mL (multiple doses); T_{max}=1.5 hrs (single dose), 1.3 hrs (multiple doses). **Distribution:** Found in breast milk. Levonorgestrel: Primarily bound to sex hormone-binding globulin. EE: Plasma protein binding (97%). **Metabolism:** Levonorgestrel: Reduction, hydroxylation, and conjugation. EE: Hepatic, via CYP3A4 (hydroxylation), methylation, and glucuronidation. **Elimination:** Levonorgestrel: Urine (40-68%), feces (16-48%); $T_{1/2}$=36 hrs. EE: $T_{1/2}$=18 hrs.

PATIENT CONSIDERATIONS
Assessment: Assess for hypersensitivity to drug, thrombophlebitis or thromboembolic disorders, HTN, hyperlipidemia, diabetes, breast cancer,

endometrial cancer or other estrogen-dependent neoplasia, undiagnosed abnormal genital bleeding, cholestatic jaundice of pregnancy or jaundice with prior pill use, pregnancy/nursing status, and for any other conditions where treatment is contraindicated/cautioned. Assess for possible drug interactions.

Monitoring: Monitor for MI, thromboembolism, stroke, hepatic neoplasia, and other adverse effects. Monitor BP with history of HTN, serum glucose levels in diabetic or prediabetic patients, lipid levels with hyperlipidemia, and for signs of worsening depression with previous history. Monitor liver function. Refer contact lens wearer to an ophthalmologist if visual changes or changes in lens tolerance develop. Monitor women with a strong family history of breast cancer or who have breast nodules. Perform periodic personal and family medical history and complete physical examination.

Counseling: Inform that the drug does not protect against transmission of HIV and other sexually transmitted diseases. Counsel about potential adverse effects. Advise to avoid smoking. Instruct to take exactly ud and at intervals not exceeding 24 hrs. Advise about risks of pregnancy if dose is missed; counsel to have a back up nonhormonal birth control method (eg, condoms, spermicide) at all times. Instruct that if one dose is missed, take as soon as possible and take next pill at regular scheduled time. Inform that spotting, light bleeding, or nausea may occur during the first 1-3 packs of pills; advise not to d/c medication and if symptoms persist, to notify physician. Instruct to d/c if pregnancy is confirmed/suspected.

AVINZA — morphine sulfate

CII

Class: Opioid analgesic

> Exposes users to risks of addiction, abuse, and misuse, leading to overdose and death; assess each patient's risk prior to prescribing, and monitor regularly for development of these behaviors/conditions. Serious, life-threatening, or fatal respiratory depression may occur; monitor during initiation or following a dose increase. Crushing, chewing, or dissolving can cause rapid release and absorption of a potentially fatal dose; instruct to swallow caps whole or sprinkle contents on applesauce. Accidental ingestion, especially by children, can result in fatal overdose. Prolonged use during pregnancy can result in neonatal opioid withdrawal syndrome; advise pregnant women of the risk and ensure availability of appropriate treatment. Avoid alcohol consumption or medications containing alcohol; may result in increased plasma levels and potentially fatal overdose of morphine.

ADULT DOSAGE

Severe Pain (Daily, Around-the-Clock Management)

1st Opioid Analgesic:
Initial: 30mg q24h
Titrate: Adjust dose in increments of ≥30mg every 3-4 days

Opioid Intolerant:
Initial: 30mg q24h

Titration/Maint:
Individually titrate to a dose that provides adequate analgesia and minimizes adverse reactions; dose adjustments may be dose every 3-4 days
Max Daily Dose: 1600mg/day

Breakthrough Pain:
May require a dose increase or may need rescue medication w/ an appropriate dose of an immediate-release analgesic

Conversions

From Other Opioids:
Initial: 30mg q24h; d/c all other around-the-clock opioids

From Other Oral Morphine Formulations:
Administer total daily oral morphine dose once daily; do not give more frequently than q24h

From Parenteral Morphine:
Between 2-6mg of oral morphine may be required to provide analgesia equivalent to 1mg of parenteral morphine

From Other Non-Morphine Opioids (Parenteral or Oral):
Initial: 1/2 the estimated daily morphine requirement

PEDIATRIC DOSAGE

Pediatric use may not have been established

DOSING CONSIDERATIONS

Discontinuation
Do not abruptly d/c; use a gradual downward titration of dose every 2-4 days to prevent signs/symptoms of withdrawal

ADMINISTRATION
Oral route

Take caps whole; do not crush, chew, or dissolve the pellets in the caps

Alternative Administration
Sprinkle over applesauce and consume immediately w/o chewing
Rinse mouth to ensure all pellets have been swallowed
Discard any unused portion of caps after contents have been sprinkled on applesauce
Do not administer through a NG or gastric tubes

STORAGE
25°C (77°F); excursions permitted to 15-30°C (59-86°F). Protect from light and moisture.

HOW SUPPLIED
Cap, Extended-Release: 30mg, 45mg, 60mg, 75mg, 90mg, 120mg

CONTRAINDICATIONS
Significant respiratory depression, acute or severe bronchial asthma in an unmonitored setting or in the absence of resuscitative equipment, known/suspected paralytic ileus, hypersensitivity (eg, anaphylaxis) to morphine.

WARNINGS/PRECAUTIONS
Reserve use in patients for whom alternative treatment options are ineffective, not tolerated, or would be otherwise inadequate to provide sufficient management of pain. Should be prescribed only by healthcare professionals knowledgeable in the use of potent opioids for management of chronic pain. 90mg and 120mg caps are for use in opioid-tolerant patients only. Doses >1600mg/day contain a quantity of fumaric acid that may cause serious renal toxicity. Life-threatening respiratory depression is more likely to occur in elderly, cachectic, or debilitated patients. Consider alternative nonopioid analgesics in patients with significant chronic obstructive pulmonary disease (COPD) or cor pulmonale, and in patients having a substantially decreased respiratory reserve, hypoxia, hypercapnia, or preexisting respiratory depression. May cause severe hypotension, including orthostatic hypotension and syncope; increased risk in patients whose ability to maintain BP has already been compromised by a reduced blood volume or concurrent administration of certain CNS depressants. Avoid with circulatory shock, impaired consciousness, coma, or GI obstruction. Monitor patients who may be susceptible to intracranial effects of carbon dioxide retention (eg, those with evidence of increased intracranial pressure, brain tumors) for signs of sedation and respiratory depression, particularly when initiating therapy. May obscure clinical course in patients with head injury. May cause spasm of sphincter of Oddi and increases in serum amylase; monitor patients with biliary tract disease, including acute pancreatitis, for worsening symptoms. May aggravate convulsions and induce/aggravate seizures. May impair mental/physical abilities. Not recommended for use during and immediately prior to labor.

ADVERSE REACTIONS
Respiratory depression, constipation, N/V, somnolence, headache, peripheral edema, diarrhea, abdominal pain, infection, urinary tract infection, flu syndrome, back pain, rash, insomnia, depression, dyspnea.

DRUG INTERACTIONS
See Boxed Warning. Concomitant use with other CNS depressants (eg, sedatives, anxiolytics, neuroleptics) may increase risk of respiratory depression, profound sedation, hypotension, coma and death; if coadministration is required, consider dose reduction of one or both agents. Monitor use in elderly, cachectic, and debilitated patients when coadministered with other drugs that depress respiration. Mixed agonist/antagonists (eg, pentazocine, nalbuphine, butorphanol) and partial agonist (buprenorphine) analgesics may reduce analgesic effect or precipitate withdrawal symptoms; avoid coadministration. May enhance neuromuscular blocking action of skeletal muscle relaxants and produce an increased degree of respiratory depression. MAOIs may potentiate effects of morphine; avoid use with MAOIs or within 14 days of stopping such treatment. Cimetidine may potentiate morphine-induced respiratory depression. Confusion and severe respiratory depression in a patient undergoing hemodialysis reported with concurrent cimetidine. May reduce efficacy of diuretics and lead to acute urinary retention. Anticholinergics or other medications with anticholinergic activity may increase risk of urinary retention and/or severe constipation and lead to paralytic ileus. Absorption/exposure may be increased with p-glycoprotein inhibitors (eg, quinidine).

PREGNANCY AND LACTATION
Category C, not for use in nursing.

MECHANISM OF ACTION
Opioid analgesic; acts as a full agonist, binds with and activates opioid receptors at sites in the periaqueductal and periventricular grey matter, the ventromedial medulla and the spinal cord to produce analgesia.

PHARMACOKINETICS
Absorption: C_{max}=18.65ng/mL; AUC=273.25ng/mL•hr. **Distribution:** V_d=1-6L/kg, plasma protein binding (20-35%); crosses the placenta; found in breast milk. **Metabolism:** Liver via glucuronidation and sulfation; (metabolites) morphine-3-glucuronide (M3G, about 50%), morphine-6-glucuronide (M6G, about 5-15%), morphine-3-etheral sulfate. **Elimination:** Urine (M3G/M6G, 10% unchanged), bile, feces (7-10%); $T_{1/2}$=approximately 24 hrs.

PATIENT CONSIDERATIONS

Assessment: Assess for abuse/addiction risk, pain intensity, prior opioid therapy, opioid tolerance, respiratory depression, drug hypersensitivity, pregnancy/nursing status, possible drug interactions, or any other condition where treatment is contraindicated or cautioned.

Monitoring: Monitor for respiratory depression (especially within first 24-72 hrs of initiation), hypotension, seizures/convulsions, and other adverse reactions. Monitor BP and serum amylase levels. Routinely monitor for signs of misuse, abuse, and addiction. Periodically reassess the continued need for therapy.

Counseling: Inform that use of drug can result in addiction, abuse, and misuse; instruct not to share with others and to take steps to protect from theft or misuse. Inform about risk of respiratory depression and advise to seek medical attention if breathing difficulties develop. Advise to store securely and dispose unused caps by flushing down the toilet. Inform female patients of reproductive potential that prolonged use during pregnancy may result in neonatal opioid withdrawal syndrome and instruct to inform physician if pregnant or planning to become pregnant. Inform that potentially serious additive effects may occur when used with alcohol or other CNS depressants, and not to use such drugs unless supervised by physician. Instruct about proper administration instructions. Inform that drug may cause orthostatic hypotension, syncope, and impair the ability to perform potentially hazardous activities; advise to not perform such tasks until patients know how they will react to medication. Advise of potential for severe constipation, including management instructions. Advise how to recognize anaphylaxis and when to seek medical attention.

AVODART — dutasteride   Rx

Class: Type I and II 5 alpha-reductase inhibitor (5-ARI) (2nd generation)

ADULT DOSAGE	**PEDIATRIC DOSAGE**
Benign Prostatic Hyperplasia	Pediatric use may not have been
Monotherapy:	established
1 cap (0.5mg) qd	
W/ Tamsulosin:	
1 cap (0.5mg) qd and tamsulosin	
0.4mg qd	

ADMINISTRATION
Oral route
Swallow whole; do not chew or open.
Take w/ or w/o food.

STORAGE
25°C (77°F); excursions permitted to 15-30°C (59-86°F).

HOW SUPPLIED
Cap: 0.5mg

CONTRAINDICATIONS
Pregnancy; women of childbearing potential; pediatric patients; previously demonstrated, clinically significant hypersensitivity (eg, serious skin reactions, angioedema) to dutasteride or other 5 alpha-reductase inhibitors.

WARNINGS/PRECAUTIONS
Not approved for the prevention of prostate cancer. May decrease serum prostate specific antigen (PSA) concentration during therapy or in the presence of prostate cancer; establish a new baseline PSA at least 3 months after starting treatment and monitor PSA periodically thereafter. Any confirmed increase from the lowest PSA value while on treatment may signal presence of prostate cancer. May increase risk of high-grade prostate cancer. Prior to initiating treatment, consider other urological conditions that may cause similar symptoms; BPH and prostate cancer may coexist. Risk to male fetus; caps should not be handled by pregnant women or women who could become pregnant. Avoid donating blood until at least 6 months after last dose. Reduced total sperm count, semen volume, and sperm motility reported.

ADVERSE REACTIONS
Impotence, decreased libido, breast disorders, ejaculation disorders.

DRUG INTERACTIONS
Caution w/ potent, chronic CYP3A4 inhibitors (eg, ritonavir).

PREGNANCY AND LACTATION
Category X, not for use in nursing.

MECHANISM OF ACTION
Selective type I and II 5α-reductase inhibitor (2nd generation); inhibits conversion of testosterone to dihydrotestosterone, the androgen primarily responsible for initial development and subsequent enlargement of the prostate gland.

PHARMACOKINETICS
Absorption: Absolute bioavailability (60%); T_{max}=2-3 hrs. **Distribution:** V_d=300-500L; plasma protein binding (99% albumin, 96.6% α-1 acid glycoprotein). **Metabolism:** Liver (extensive) via CYP3A4, 3A5; 4'-hydroxydutasteride, 1,2-dihydrodutasteride, 6-hydroxydutasteride (major metabolites). **Elimination:** Feces (5% unchanged, 40% metabolites), urine (<1% unchanged); $T_{1/2}$=5 weeks.

PATIENT CONSIDERATIONS
Assessment: Assess for urological conditions that may cause similar symptoms, previous hypersensitivity to the drug, and for possible drug interactions.
Monitoring: Monitor for signs/symptoms of prostate cancer and other urological diseases. Obtain new PSA baseline at least 3 months after starting treatment and monitor PSA periodically thereafter.
Counseling: Inform of the importance of periodic PSA monitoring. Advise that therapy may increase risk of high-grade prostate cancer. Counsel that drug should not be handled by women who are pregnant or who could become pregnant, due to potential fetal risks; advise to wash area immediately w/ soap and water if contact is made. Instruct not to donate blood until at least 6 months after last dose.

AVYCAZ — avibactam/ceftazidime   Rx

Class: Beta-lactamase inhibitor/cephalosporin

ADULT DOSAGE	**PEDIATRIC DOSAGE**
Intra-Abdominal Infections	Pediatric use may not have been
Complicated Infections:	established
2.5g (2g/0.5g) IV q8h for 5-14 days in	
combination w/ metronidazole	
Urinary Tract Infections	
Complicated Infections, Including	
Pyelonephritis:	
2.5g (2g/0.5g) IV q8h for 7-14 days	

DOSING CONSIDERATIONS
Renal Impairment
CrCl 31-50mL/min: 1.25g (1g/0.25g) IV q8h
CrCl 16-30mL/min: 0.94g (0.75g/0.19g) IV q12h
CrCl 6-15mL/min: 0.94g (0.75g/0.19g) IV q24h
CrCl ≤5mL/min: 0.94g (0.75g/0.19g) IV q48h
Administer after hemodialysis on hemodialysis days
For patients w/ changing renal function, monitor CrCl at least daily and adjust the dose accordingly

ADMINISTRATION
IV route
Administer by IV infusion over 2 hrs.

Preparation of Sol for Administration
1. Constitute powder in the vial w/ 10mL of 1 of the following sol: sterile water for inj (SWFI); 0.9% NaCl inj; D5 inj; all combinations of dextrose inj and NaCl inj, containing up to 2.5% dextrose, and 0.45% NaCl; or lactated Ringer's inj.
2. Mix gently; constituted sol will have an approx ceftazidime level of 0.167g/mL and an approx avibactam level of 0.042g/mL. The constituted sol is not for direct injection; must be diluted before IV infusion.
3. Prepare the required dose for IV infusion by withdrawing the appropriate volume from the constituted vial; refer to PI for volume to withdraw.
4. Before infusion, dilute the withdrawn volume of the constituted sol further w/ the same diluent used for constitution of the powder (except SWFI), to achieve total volume between 50mL (0.04g/mL ceftazidime and 0.01g/mL avibactam) to 250mL (0.008g/mL ceftazidime and 0.002g/mL avibactam) in an infusion bag. If SWFI was used for constitution, use any of the other appropriate constitution diluents for dilution.
5. Mix gently and ensure contents are dissolved completely.

Drug Compatibility
The sol for administration at the range of diluted concentrations of ceftazidime 0.008g/mL and avibactam 0.002g/mL to ceftazidime 0.04g/mL and avibactam 0.01g/mL is compatible w/ the more commonly used IV infusion fluids in infusion bags such as:
1. 0.9% NaCl inj
2. D5 inj
3. All combinations of dextrose inj and NaCl inj, containing up to 2.5% dextrose, and 0.45% NaCl
4. Lactated Ringer's inj
5. Baxter Mini-Bag Plus containing 0.9% NaCl inj or D5 inj

Stability
Upon constitution w/ appropriate diluent, the constituted sol may be held for no longer than 30 min prior to transfer and dilution in a suitable infusion bag. Following dilution of the constituted sol w/ the appropriate diluents, sol in the infusion bags are stable for 12 hrs when stored at room temperature; may also be refrigerated at 2-8°C (36-46°F) for up to 24 hrs; and then should be used w/in 12 hrs of subsequent storage at room temperature.

STORAGE
25°C (77°F); excursions permitted between 15-30°C (59-86°F). Protect from light.

HOW SUPPLIED
Inj: (Ceftazidime/Avibactam) 2g/0.5g

CONTRAINDICATIONS
Known serious hypersensitivity to the components of Avycaz (ceftazidime and avibactam), avibactam-containing products, or other members of the cephalosporin class.

WARNINGS/PRECAUTIONS
In the treatment of complicated UTIs, reserve for use in patients who have limited or no alternative treatment options. Decreased clinical response in patients w/ baseline CrCl 30 to ≤50mL/min. Serious and occasionally fatal hypersensitivity (anaphylactic) reactions and serious skin reactions reported; d/c if an allergic reaction occurs. Cross-sensitivity among β-lactam antibacterials reported; caution in penicillin (PCN) or other β-lactam allergic patients. *Clostridium difficile*-associated diarrhea (CDAD) reported; may need to d/c if CDAD is suspected or confirmed. Seizures, nonconvulsive status epilepticus, encephalopathy, coma, asterixis, neuromuscular excitability, and myoclonia reported, particularly in the setting of renal impairment; adjust dosing based on CrCl. Use in the absence of a proven or strongly suspected bacterial infection is unlikely to provide benefit and increases the risk of development of drug-resistant bacteria. Caution in elderly. Lab test interactions may occur.

ADVERSE REACTIONS
Complicated Intra-Abdominal Infections: Diarrhea, N/V.
Complicated UTIs: Constipation, anxiety.

DRUG INTERACTIONS
Not recommended w/ probenecid.

PREGNANCY AND LACTATION

Pregnancy: There are no adequate and well-controlled studies of Avycaz, ceftazidime, or avibactam in pregnant women.

Lactation: Ceftazidime is excreted in human milk in low concentrations. It is not known whether avibactam is excreted into human milk, although avibactam was shown to be excreted in the milk of rats. Caution in nursing.

MECHANISM OF ACTION

Ceftazidime: Cephalosporin; binds to essential PCN-binding proteins. **Avibactam:** β-lactamase inhibitor; inactivates some β-lactamases and protects ceftazidime form degradation by certain β-lactamases.

PHARMACOKINETICS

Absorption: Administration of variable doses resulted in different parameters. **Distribution:** Ceftazidime: Plasma protein binding (<10%); V_d=17L; found in breast milk. Avibactam: Plasma protein binding (5.7-8.2%); V_d=22.2L. **Elimination:** Single Dose: $T_{1/2}$=3.27 hrs (ceftazidime), 2.22 hrs (avibactam). Multiple Doses: $T_{1/2}$=2.76 hrs (ceftazidime), 2.71 hrs (avibactam). Ceftazidime: Urine (Approx 80-90%, unchanged). Avibactam: Urine (97%), feces (0.20%).

PATIENT CONSIDERATIONS

Assessment: Assess for hypersensitivity to drug, cephalosporins, PCNs, carbapenems, or other β-lactam antibiotics; renal impairment; pregnancy/nursing status; and possible drug interactions. Perform culture and susceptibility testing.

Monitoring: Monitor for signs/symptoms of hypersensitivity reactions, CDAD, seizures, nonconvulsive status epilepticus, encephalopathy, coma, asterixis, neuromuscular excitability, myoclonia, and other adverse reactions. Monitor CrCl at least daily w/ changing renal function.

Counseling: Advise that allergic reactions, including serious allergic reactions, may occur and require immediate treatment. Advise that diarrhea is a common problem caused by antibacterial drugs; instruct to contact physician if severe watery or bloody diarrhea develops. Inform that neurological adverse reactions may occur; instruct to inform physician immediately if any neurological signs and symptoms develop. Inform that therapy should only be used to treat bacterial, not viral, infections. Advise to take exactly ud; inform that skipping doses or not completing full course of therapy may decrease effectiveness of therapy and increase bacterial resistance.

AXERT — almotriptan malate

Class: 5-HT$_{1B/1D}$ agonist (triptans)

Rx

ADULT DOSAGE

Migraine

Acute Treatment w/ or w/o Aura:
Initial: 6.25-12.5mg at onset of headache; may repeat after 2 hrs
Max: 25mg/day

PEDIATRIC DOSAGE

Migraine

Acute Treatment w/ or w/o Aura:
12-17 Years:
Initial: 6.25-12.5mg at onset of headache; may repeat after 2 hrs
Max: 25mg/day

DOSING CONSIDERATIONS

Renal Impairment
Severe:
Initial: 6.25mg
Max: 12.5mg/day

Hepatic Impairment
Initial: 6.25mg
Max: 12.5mg/day

Elderly
Use caution; start at lower end of dosing range

ADMINISTRATION
Oral route

STORAGE
25°C (77°F); excursions permitted to 15-30°C (59-86°F).

HOW SUPPLIED
Tab: 6.25mg, 12.5mg

CONTRAINDICATIONS
Ischemic heart disease (angina pectoris, history of MI, documented silent ischemia), symptoms or findings consistent w/ ischemic heart disease, coronary artery vasospasm, including Prinzmetal's variant angina, or other significant underlying cardiovascular disease (CVD); cerebrovascular syndromes (eg, stroke of any type, transient ischemic attacks); peripheral vascular disease (eg, ischemic bowel disease); uncontrolled HTN; hemiplegic or basilar migraine; hypersensitivity to almotriptan or any of its ingredients. Use w/in 24 hrs of other 5-HT$_1$ agonists (eg, triptans) or ergotamine-containing or ergot-derived medications (eg, dihydroergotamine, ergotamine tartrate, methysergide).

WARNINGS/PRECAUTIONS
Use only where a clear diagnosis of migraine has been established. If no response after the 1st migraine attack, reconsider diagnosis before treating subsequent attacks. Not intended for prophylactic therapy of migraine or for use in the management of hemiplegic/basilar migraine. Serious adverse cardiac events, including acute MI, reported. May cause coronary artery vasospasm. Perform cardiovascular (CV) evaluation prior to therapy. In patients with CV risk factors, consider administering 1st dose in a medically-supervised setting and perform ECG immediately after. Consider periodic CV evaluation in intermittent long-term users who have CV risk factors. Sensations of tightness, pain, pressure, and heaviness in the precordium, throat, neck, and jaw reported. Evaluate if cardiac origin is suspected. May cause cerebral/subarachnoid hemorrhage, stroke, and other cerebrovascular events. May cause vasospastic reactions other than coronary

artery vasospasm (eg, peripheral and GI vascular ischemia with abdominal pain and bloody diarrhea). Transient/permanent blindness and significant partial vision loss reported rarely. Serotonin syndrome may occur. Overuse of acute migraine drugs may lead to exacerbation of headache; detoxification, including withdrawal of the overused drugs, and treatment of withdrawal symptoms may be necessary. Significant elevations in systemic BP reported (rare). Caution with known hypersensitivity to sulfonamides. Caution with renal or hepatic impairment. May bind to melanin in the eye. Caution in elderly.

ADVERSE REACTIONS
N/V, dizziness, somnolence, headache, paresthesia, dry mouth.

DRUG INTERACTIONS
See Contraindications. Life-threatening serotonin syndrome reported with SSRIs (eg, fluoxetine, paroxetine, sertraline, fluvoxamine, citalopram, escitalopram) or SNRIs (eg, venlafaxine, duloxetine). Increased exposure with potent CYP3A4 inhibitors (eg, oral ketoconazole); the recommended starting dose of almotriptan is 6.25mg and max daily dose is 12.5mg/24 hrs. Avoid concomitant use with potent CYP3A4 inhibitors in patients with renal/hepatic impairment.

PREGNANCY AND LACTATION
Category C, caution in nursing.

MECHANISM OF ACTION
Selective 5-HT$_{1B/1D}$ receptor agonist; thought to be due to agonist effects at 5-HT$_{1B/1D}$ receptors on extracerebral, intracranial blood vessels, and on nerve terminals in the trigeminal system, which results in cranial vessel constriction, inhibition of neuropeptide release, and reduced transmission in trigeminal pain pathways.

PHARMACOKINETICS
Absorption: Absolute bioavailability (70%); T_{max}=1-3 hrs. **Distribution:** V_d=180-200L; plasma protein binding (35%). **Metabolism:** Oxidative deamination via MAO-A and oxidation via CYP450 (major pathway), flavin monooxygenase (minor pathway). **Elimination:** Urine (75%, 40% unchanged), feces (13%, unchanged and metabolites); $T_{1/2}$=3-4 hrs.

PATIENT CONSIDERATIONS

Assessment: Confirm diagnosis of migraine and exclude other potentially serious neurologic conditions prior to therapy. Assess for CVD, HTN, hemiplegic/basilar migraine, hypersensitivity to the drug or to sulfonamides, and any other conditions where treatment is cautioned or contraindicated. Assess renal/hepatic function, pregnancy/nursing status, and possible drug interactions.

Monitoring: Monitor for signs/symptoms of cardiac/cerebrovascular events, peripheral/GI vascular ischemia, serotonin syndrome, hypersensitivity reactions, HTN, and other adverse reactions. Perform periodic CV evaluation in intermittent long-term users with risk factors for coronary artery disease.

Counseling: Advise to talk with physician or pharmacist before taking any new medicines. Instruct to inform physician if rash, itching, or breathing difficulties develop. Inform that therapy may cause serious CV side effects; instruct to seek medical attention if signs/symptoms of chest pain, SOB, weakness, or slurring of speech occur. Caution about the risk of serotonin syndrome, particularly during combined use with SSRIs or SNRIs. Inform that use of acute migraine drugs for ≥10 days/month may lead to an exacerbation of headache; encourage to record headache frequency and drug use. Advise to notify physician if pregnant or intend to become pregnant or if breastfeeding/planning to breastfeed. Inform that drug may cause dizziness, somnolence, visual disturbances, and other CNS symptoms; advise not to drive, operate complex machinery, or engage in other hazardous activities until patients gain sufficient experience with medication to gauge whether it affects their mental/visual performance adversely.

AXIRON — testosterone

Class: Androgen

CIII

> Virilization reported in children secondarily exposed to topical testosterone. Children should avoid contact w/ unwashed or unclothed application sites in men using topical testosterone. Advise patients to strictly adhere to recommended instructions for use.

ADULT DOSAGE

Testosterone Replacement Therapy

Congenital/Acquired Primary Hypogonadism or Hypogonadotropic Hypogonadism in Males:
Initial: Apply 60mg (2 pump actuations) qam
Titrate: May adjust dose based on serum testosterone concentration from a single blood draw 2-8 hrs after application, and at least 14 days after starting treatment or following dose adjustment
If Serum Testosterone Concentration <300ng/dL: May increase from 60mg to 90mg or from 90mg to 120mg
If Serum Testosterone Concentration >1050ng/dL: Decrease from 60mg to 30mg

D/C if serum testosterone concentration is consistently >1050ng/dL at lowest daily dose of 30mg

PEDIATRIC DOSAGE
Pediatric use may not have been established

ADMINISTRATION
Topical route

Apply to clean, dry, intact skin of axilla, preferably at the same time each am
Do not apply to other parts of the body, including the scrotum, penis, abdomen, shoulders, or upper arms
Prime pump in upright position, depress actuator 3X prior to 1st use

Application
30mg Dose: Apply once to 1 axilla only
60mg Dose: Apply once to the left axilla and then once to the right axilla
90mg Dose: Apply once to the left and once to the right axilla, wait for the product to dry, and then apply once again to the left or right axilla
120mg: Apply once to the left and once to the right axilla, wait for the product to dry, and then apply once again to the left and right axilla

STORAGE
25°C (77°F); excursions permitted to 15-30°C (59-86°F). Discard used bottles and applicators in household trash in a manner that prevents accidental exposure of children or pets.

HOW SUPPLIED
Sol: 30mg/actuation [110mL]

CONTRAINDICATIONS
Breast carcinoma or known/suspected prostate carcinoma in men; women who are or may become pregnant, or are breastfeeding.

WARNINGS/PRECAUTIONS
Application site and dose are not interchangeable w/ other topical testosterone products. Monitor patients w/ BPH for worsening of signs and symptoms of BPH. May increase risk for prostate cancer. Risk of virilization in women due to secondary exposure. Increases in Hct/RBC mass may occur; if Hct elevates, lower dose or d/c therapy until Hct decreases to acceptable level. Increases in RBC mass may increase risk of thromboembolic events. Venous thromboembolic events (eg, deep vein thrombosis, pulmonary embolism) reported; d/c treatment and initiate appropriate workup and management if suspected. Increased risk of major adverse cardiovascular events (MACE) reported. Suppression of spermatogenesis may occur w/ large doses. Hepatic adverse effects reported w/ prolonged use of high doses of orally active 17-α-alkyl androgens and long-term therapy w/ IM testosterone enanthate. May promote retention of Na⁺ and water. Edema w/ or w/o CHF may be a serious complication w/ preexisting cardiac/renal/hepatic disease. Gynecomastia may develop and persist. May potentiate sleep apnea, especially w/ risk factors such as obesity or chronic lung disease. Changes in serum lipid profile may require dose adjustment or discontinuation. Caution in cancer patients at risk of hypercalcemia and associated hypercalciuria. May decrease concentrations of thyroxine-binding globulins, resulting in decreased total T4 serum concentrations and increased resin uptake of T3 and T4. Flammable; avoid fire, flame, or smoking until applied dose has dried.

ADVERSE REACTIONS
Application-site irritation, application-site erythema, headache, Hct increase, diarrhea, vomiting, increases in prostate specific antigen.

DRUG INTERACTIONS
Changes in insulin sensitivity or glycemic control may occur; may decrease blood glucose and insulin requirements in diabetic patients. Changes in anticoagulant activity may occur; frequently monitor INR and PT in patients taking anticoagulants, especially at initiation and termination of androgen therapy. ACTH or corticosteroids may increase fluid retention; caution in patients w/ cardiac, renal, or hepatic disease.

PREGNANCY AND LACTATION
Category X, not for use in nursing.

MECHANISM OF ACTION
Androgen; responsible for normal growth and development of male sex organs and for maintenance of secondary sex characteristics.

PHARMACOKINETICS
Absorption: Systemic. **Distribution:** Plasma protein binding (40% sex hormone-binding globulin). **Metabolism:** Estradiol and dihydrotestosterone (major active metabolites). **Elimination:** (IM) Urine (90% glucuronic/sulfuric acid conjugates and metabolites), feces (6% unconjugated); $T_{1/2}$=10-100 min.

PATIENT CONSIDERATIONS
Assessment: Assess for prostate cancer, breast carcinoma, BPH, cardiac/renal/hepatic disease, risk factors for sleep apnea, and any other conditions where treatment is contraindicated or cautioned, and possible drug interactions. Obtain baseline Hct, lipid, and serum testosterone levels. Confirm diagnosis of hypogonadism by measuring testosterone levels in am on at least 2 separate days prior to initiation.

Monitoring: Monitor for worsening of BPH, edema, gynecomastia, sleep apnea, venous thromboembolic events, MACE, and other adverse reactions. Perform periodic monitoring of serum lipid profile and serum testosterone levels. In cancer patients at risk for hypercalcemia, regularly monitor serum Ca²⁺ levels. Reevaluate Hct 3-6 months after start of therapy, then annually. Reevaluate for prostate cancer 3-6 months after initiation of treatment, and then in accordance w/ screening practices.

Counseling: Inform that men w/ known or suspected prostate/breast cancer should not use androgen therapy. Advise to report signs/symptoms of secondary exposure in children and in women. Inform that children and women should avoid contact w/ unwashed or unclothed application sites of men using topical testosterone. Instruct to apply only to axilla and not to any other part of the body, to wash hands immediately after application, and to cover application site w/ clothing after waiting 3 min for the sol to dry. Instruct to wash application site w/ soap and water prior to any situation in which direct skin-to-skin contact is anticipated, and to immediately wash area of contact if unwashed/unclothed skin comes in direct contact w/ skin of another person. Inform of the potential adverse reactions. Instruct to prime the pump by depressing 3X prior to 1st use; advise that no priming is needed w/ subsequent uses of the pump. Instruct patient to allow the sol to dry after the 1st application before the 2nd. Instruct to apply to clean, dry skin at approx the same time each day. Inform that antiperspirant or deodorant may be used before applying the medication. Counsel to avoid swimming or washing application site until 2 hrs following application. Advise to avoid splashing in the eyes; instruct to flush thoroughly w/ water in case of contact and to seek medical advice if irritation persists.

AZACTAM — aztreonam   Rx

Class: Monobactam

ADULT DOSAGE
Urinary Tract Infections
500mg or 1g q8h or q12h
Max: 8g/day

Systemic Infections
Lower respiratory tract infections (eg, pneumonia, bronchitis), septicemia, skin and skin-structure infections (eg, postoperative wounds, ulcers, burns), intra-abdominal infections (eg, peritonitis), and gynecologic infections (eg, endometritis, pelvic cellulitis) caused by susceptible gram-negative microorganisms; adjunctive therapy to surgery in the management of infections caused by susceptible organisms (eg, abscesses, hollow viscus perforation infections, cutaneous infections, infections of serous surfaces); and concurrent initial therapy w/ other antimicrobial agents before causative organism(s) is known in seriously ill patients who are also at risk of having gram-positive aerobic/anaerobic infection

Moderately Severe: 1g or 2g q8h or q12h
Max: 8g/day

Severe or Life-Threatening: 2g q6h or q8h
Max: 8g/day

IV route is recommended for single doses >1g or w/ bacterial septicemia, localized parenchymal abscess, peritonitis, or other severe systemic or life-threatening infections

Pseudomonas aeruginosa Infections
2g q6h or q8h, at least upon initiation of therapy
Max: 8g/day

Treatment Duration
Continue treatment for at least 48 hrs after the patient becomes asymptomatic or evidence of bacterial eradication has been obtained; persistent infections may require treatment for several weeks

PEDIATRIC DOSAGE
General Dosing
9 Months-16 Years:
IV:

Mild to Moderate Infections: 30mg/kg q8h
Max: 120mg/kg/day

Moderate to Severe Infections: 30mg/kg q6h or q8h
Max: 120mg/kg/day

Patients w/ cystic fibrosis may require higher doses

Treatment Duration
Continue treatment for at least 48 hrs after the patient becomes asymptomatic or evidence of bacterial eradication has been obtained; persistent infections may require treatment for several weeks

---

DOSING CONSIDERATIONS
Renal Impairment
CrCl 10-30mL/min:
Initial LD: 1g or 2g
Maint: 50% of dose
CrCl <10mL/min (eg, Hemodialysis):
Initial: 500mg, 1g, or 2g
Maint: 25% of initial dose given at fixed intervals of 6, 8, or 12 hrs; for serious/life-threatening infections, in addition to the maint doses, give 1/8 of the initial dose after each hemodialysis session

ADMINISTRATION
IM/IV route

Aztreonam sol (at concentrations >2% w/v) prepared w/ sterile water for inj (SWFI) or NaCl inj must be used w/in 48 hrs (stored at room temperature) or w/in 7 days (refrigerated); all other prepared sol must be used promptly after preparation

IM
Reconstitute 15mL vial w/ at least 3mL of appropriate diluent
Appropriate diluents are SWFI, Sterile Bacteriostatic Water for inj, 0.9% NaCl inj, or Bacteriostatic NaCl inj
Inject deep into a large muscle mass (eg, gluteus maximus)

IV

Reconstitute 15mL vial w/ 6-10mL of SWFI for a bolus inj; if contents of 15mL vial are to be transferred to an appropriate infusion sol, each gram of aztreonam should be initially constituted w/ at least 3mL of SWFI
Refer to PI for appropriate diluents for further dilution
Inject bolus slowly over 3-5 min
Infuse aztreonam infusion over 20-60 min
If administering multiple drug sol, do not deliver simultaneously; flush delivery tube before and after delivery w/ any appropriate infusion sol compatible w/ both drug sol

Galaxy

Intermittent IV infusion only
Thaw frozen container; do not force thawing by immersion in water baths or by microwave irradiation
Do not add supplementary medication
Do not freeze thawed antibiotics
Do not use plastic containers in series connects
Aztreonam infusion should be completed w/in 20-60 min; discard any unused portion
Refer to PI for compatible infusion sol
Refer to PI for further preparation/administration instructions and compatibility information

STORAGE

Vial: Room temperature. Avoid excessive heat. Galaxy Container: ≤-20°C (-4°F). Thawed Sol: Stable for 14 days at 2-8°C (36-46°F) or 48 hrs at 25°C (77°F). Do not refreeze. Refer to PI for diluted/reconstituted sol storage information.

HOW SUPPLIED

Inj: 1g, 2g; 1g/50mL, 2g/50mL [Galaxy]

CONTRAINDICATIONS

Known hypersensitivity to aztreonam or any other component in the formulation.

WARNINGS/PRECAUTIONS

Hypersensitivity reactions may occur; d/c and institute appropriate supportive treatment. Caution w/ history of hypersensitivity to β-lactams (eg, penicillins, cephalosporins, carbapenems). *Clostridium difficile*-associated diarrhea (CDAD) reported; d/c if CDAD is suspected or confirmed. Toxic epidermal necrolysis (TEN) reported (rare) in patients undergoing bone marrow transplant w/ multiple risk factors (eg, sepsis, radiation therapy, concomitant drugs associated w/ TEN). May result in bacterial resistance w/ prolonged use in the absence of proven or suspected bacterial infection, or a prophylactic indication; take appropriate measures if superinfection develops. Caution w/ renal/hepatic impairment and in elderly.

ADVERSE REACTIONS

ALT/AST elevation, rash, eosinophilia, neutropenia, pain at inj site, increased SrCr, thrombocytosis.

DRUG INTERACTIONS

Avoid w/ β-lactamase inducing antibiotics (eg, cefoxitin, imipenem). Potential nephrotoxicity and ototoxicity w/ aminoglycosides; monitor renal function.

PREGNANCY AND LACTATION

Category B, not for use in nursing.

MECHANISM OF ACTION

Monobactam; inhibits bacterial cell-wall synthesis. Has activity in the presence of some β-lactamases, both penicillinases and cephalosporinases, of gram-negative and gram-positive bacteria.

PHARMACOKINETICS

Absorption: Administration of variable doses resulted in different pharmacokinetic parameters. **Distribution:** Plasma protein binding (56%); V_d=12.6L; crosses placenta; found in breast milk. **Metabolism:** Ring hydrolysis. **Elimination:** Urine (60-70% unchanged and metabolites), (IV)feces (12% unchanged and metabolites); $T_{1/2}$=1.7 hrs.

PATIENT CONSIDERATIONS

Assessment: Assess for drug hypersensitivity (eg, β-lactams), hypersensitivity to any allergens, hepatic/renal impairment, pregnancy/nursing status, and for possible drug interactions. Assess use in patients undergoing bone marrow transplant w/ multiple risk factors. Confirm diagnosis of causative organisms.

Monitoring: Monitor for signs/symptoms of hypersensitivity reactions, CDAD, superinfection, TEN in patients undergoing bone marrow transplant, and hepatic/renal function.

Counseling: Inform that therapy should only be used to treat bacterial and not viral infections (eg, common cold). Advise to take exactly ud; inform that skipping doses or not completing full course may decrease effectiveness and increase resistance. Inform that diarrhea is a common problem caused by therapy and will usually end upon discontinuation of therapy. Inform that diarrhea may occur, even as late as ≥2 months after last dose of therapy; instruct to notify physician as soon as possible if watery/bloody stools (w/ or w/o stomach cramps and fever) occur.

AZASITE — azithromycin

Class: Macrolide

Rx

ADULT DOSAGE
Bacterial Conjunctivitis

Instill 1 drop in affected eye(s) bid, 8-12 hrs apart for the first 2 days, then 1 drop qd for the next 5 days

PEDIATRIC DOSAGE
Bacterial Conjunctivitis
≥1 Year:

Instill 1 drop in affected eye(s) bid, 8-12 hrs apart for the first 2 days, then 1 drop qd for the next 5 days

ADMINISTRATION

Ocular route

STORAGE

Unopened Bottle: 2-8°C (36-46°F). Opened Bottle: 2-25°C (36-77°F) for up to 14 days. Discard after 14 days.

HOW SUPPLIED

Sol: 1% [2.5mL]

CONTRAINDICATIONS

Hypersensitivity to any component of this product.

WARNINGS/PRECAUTIONS

Not for inj. Do not administer systemically, inject subconjunctivally, or introduce directly into the anterior chamber of the eye. Serious allergic reactions, including angioedema, anaphylaxis, and dermatologic reactions (eg, Stevens-Johnson syndrome, toxic epidermal necrolysis), rarely reported when administered systemically. May result in bacterial resistance with prolonged use; take appropriate measures if superinfection develops. Avoid wearing contact lenses if signs or symptoms of bacterial conjunctivitis exist.

ADVERSE REACTIONS

Eye irritation, blurred vision, burning/stinging upon instillation, contact dermatitis, corneal erosion, dry eye, eye pain, ocular discharge, dysgeusia, facial swelling, hives, nasal congestion, periocular swelling, rash.

PREGNANCY AND LACTATION

Category B, caution in nursing.

MECHANISM OF ACTION

Macrolide; binds to the 50S ribosomal subunit of susceptible microorganisms and interferes with microbial protein synthesis.

PATIENT CONSIDERATIONS

Assessment: Assess for hypersensitivity, proper diagnosis of causative organisms, use of contact lenses, and pregnancy/nursing status.

Monitoring: Monitor for hypersensitivity reactions, superinfection, eye irritation, and other adverse reactions.

Counseling: Advise to avoid contaminating the applicator tip by allowing it to touch the eye, fingers, or other sources. Instruct to d/c and contact physician if any signs of allergic reaction occur. Instruct to use exactly ud; skipping doses or not completing full course may decrease effectiveness of treatment and increase bacterial resistance. Advise not to wear contact lenses if patient has signs/symptoms of bacterial conjunctivitis. Advise to wash hands thoroughly before instillation. Counsel on proper administration; shake bottle once before each use.

AZILECT — rasagiline mesylate

Class: Monoamine oxidase inhibitor (MAOI) (type B)

Rx

ADULT DOSAGE
Parkinson's Disease

Monotherapy or Adjunctive Therapy in Patients Not Taking Levodopa:
Initial: 1mg qd

Patients Taking Levodopa w/ or w/o Other Parkinson's Disease Drugs:
Initial: 0.5mg qd
Titrate: May increase to 1mg qd if a sufficient clinical response is not achieved. May consider dose reduction of concomitant levodopa based upon individual response

PEDIATRIC DOSAGE

Pediatric use may not have been established

DOSING CONSIDERATIONS
Concomitant Medications
Ciprofloxacin or Other CYP1A2 Inhibitors:
Max: 0.5mg qd

Hepatic Impairment
Mild:
Max: 0.5mg qd

ADMINISTRATION

Oral route

May be administered w/ or w/o food

STORAGE

25°C (77°F); excursions permitted to 15-30°C (59-86°F).

HOW SUPPLIED

Tab: 0.5mg, 1mg

CONTRAINDICATIONS

Concomitant use with any other MAOI, meperidine, tramadol, methadone, or propoxyphene; at least 14 days should elapse between discontinuation of rasagiline and initiation of treatment with these medications. Concomitant use with St. John's wort, cyclobenzaprine, or dextromethorphan.

WARNINGS/PRECAUTIONS

Avoid with moderate/severe hepatic impairment. Exacerbation of HTN may occur; medication adjustment may be necessary if BP elevation is sustained. Falling asleep during activities of daily living and somnolence reported; d/c therapy if significant daytime sleepiness or episodes of falling asleep during activities that require active participation (eg, driving a motor vehicle, conversations, eating) develop. May potentiate dopaminergic side effects and cause/exacerbate dyskinesia when used as an adjunct to levodopa; reducing levodopa dose may mitigate effect. Hypotension (eg, orthostatic hypotension) and hallucinations reported. New/worsening mental status and behavioral changes, which may be severe, including psychotic-like behavior, may occur; consider dose reduction or discontinuation if these symptoms develop. Do not use in patients with a major psychotic disorder. Increased sexual urges, binge eating, intense urges to gamble or spend money, and/or other intense urges, and the inability to control these urges may occur; consider dose reduction or discontinuation if such urges develop. A symptom complex resembling neuroleptic malignant syndrome reported with rapid dose reduction, withdrawal of, or changes in drugs that increase central dopaminergic tone. Patients with PD have a higher risk of developing melanoma.

ADVERSE REACTIONS
Headache, arthralgia, dyspepsia, depression, fall, flu syndrome, conjunctivitis, fever, gastroenteritis, rhinitis, dyskinesia, weight loss, N/V, dizziness, abdominal pain.

DRUG INTERACTIONS
See Contraindications and Dosage. Not recommended with antidepressants; serotonin syndrome reported. At least 14 days should elapse between discontinuation of therapy and initiation of an SSRI, SNRI, TCA, tetracyclic, or triazolopyridine antidepressant. At least 5 weeks (longer with chronic/high-dose fluoxetine) should elapse between discontinuation of fluoxetine and initiation of rasagiline due to the long $T_{1/2}$ of fluoxetine and its active metabolite. Ciprofloxacin and other CYP1A2 inhibitors may increase levels. Hypertensive crisis/reactions reported with sympathomimetics or tyramine-rich foods; caution with sympathomimetics (eg, nasal/oral/ophthalmic decongestants, cold remedies), and avoid foods containing a very large amount of tyramine (eg, aged cheese). Dopamine antagonists (eg, antipsychotics, metoclopramide) may diminish effectiveness.

PREGNANCY AND LACTATION
Category C, caution in nursing.

MECHANISM OF ACTION
MAOI (Type B); has not been established. Inhibits MAO type B, which causes an increase in extracellular dopamine levels in the striatum, subsequently increasing dopaminergic activity.

PHARMACOKINETICS
Absorption: Rapid. Absolute bioavailability (36%); T_{max}=1 hr. **Distribution:** V_d=87L; plasma protein binding (88-94%). **Metabolism:** Liver; N-dealkylation and/or hydroxylation via CYP1A2 (major); 1-aminoindan, 3-hydroxy-N-propargyl-1 aminoindan and 3-hydroxy-1-aminoindan (metabolites). **Elimination:** Urine (62% over 7 days, <1% unchanged), feces (7% over 7 days); $T_{1/2}$=3 hrs.

PATIENT CONSIDERATIONS
Assessment: Assess for hepatic impairment, HTN, dyskinesia, major psychotic disorder, pregnancy/nursing status, and possible drug interactions.

Monitoring: Monitor for HTN, drowsiness/sleepiness, dyskinesia, hypotension, hallucinations, new/worsening mental status and behavioral changes, psychotic-like behavior, intense urges, and other adverse reactions. Monitor for melanomas frequently and on a regular basis.

Counseling: Inform of the risk of using higher than recommended daily doses; provide a brief description of the tyramine-associated hypertensive reaction. Advise to avoid foods containing a very large amount of tyramine while on therapy. Instruct to inform physician if taking or planning to take any prescription or OTC drugs. Instruct not to drive a car or engage in other potentially dangerous activities until patient has gained sufficient experience with therapy and other dopaminergic medications; advise to exercise caution when taking alcohol. Inform that orthostatic hypotension may develop; caution against standing up rapidly after sitting or lying down for prolonged periods and at the initiation of treatment. Instruct to contact physician if discontinuation of therapy is desired, or if BP elevation, hallucinations, new/increased gambling urges, increased sexual urges, or other intense urges develop. Instruct to take drug as prescribed. Advise to undergo periodic skin examinations.

AZOPT — brinzolamide   Rx
Class: Carbonic anhydrase inhibitor

ADULT DOSAGE	PEDIATRIC DOSAGE
Elevated Intraocular Pressure	Pediatric use may not have been established
Ocular HTN/Open-Angle Glaucoma: 1 drop in the affected eye(s) tid	
May be used concomitantly w/ other topical ophthalmic drugs to lower IOP	

- -

DOSING CONSIDERATIONS
Concomitant Medications
Space dosing by at least 10 min if using >1 topical ophthalmic drug

ADMINISTRATION
Ocular route

Shake well before use.

STORAGE
4-30°C (39-86°F).

HOW SUPPLIED
Ophthalmic Sus: 1% [10mL, 15mL]

CONTRAINDICATIONS
Hypersensitivity to any component of this product.

WARNINGS/PRECAUTIONS
Systemically absorbed. Fatalities occurred (rarely) due to severe reactions to sulfonamides including Stevens-Johnson syndrome, toxic epidermal necrolysis, fulminant hepatic necrosis, agranulocytosis, aplastic anemia, and other blood dyscrasias. Sensitization may recur when a sulfonamide is readministered irrespective of route. D/C if signs of serious reactions or hypersensitivity occur. Caution w/ low endothelial cell counts; increased potential for corneal edema. Not recommended w/ severe renal impairment (CrCl <30mL/min). Contains benzalkonium chloride, which may be absorbed by soft contact lenses; contact lenses should be removed during instillation, but may be reinserted 15 min after instillation.

ADVERSE REACTIONS
Blurred vision, bitter/sour/unusual taste.

DRUG INTERACTIONS
Potential additive systemic effects w/ oral carbonic anhydrase inhibitors; coadministration is not recommended. Acid-base alterations reported w/ high-dose salicylate therapy in patients treated w/ oral carbonic anhydrase inhibitors.

PREGNANCY AND LACTATION
Pregnancy: Category C.
Lactation: Not for use in nursing.

MECHANISM OF ACTION
Carbonic anhydrase II inhibitor; inhibits aqueous humor formation and reduces elevated IOP.

PHARMACOKINETICS
Absorption: Systemic. **Distribution:** Plasma protein binding (60%). **Metabolism:** N-desethyl brinzolamide (metabolite). **Elimination:** Urine (unchanged, metabolites); $T_{1/2}$=111 days (whole blood).

PATIENT CONSIDERATIONS
Assessment: Assess for hypersensitivity to drug or to sulfonamides, low endothelial cell counts, renal impairment, contact lens use, pregnancy/nursing status, and possible drug interactions.

Monitoring: Monitor for sulfonamide/hypersensitivity reactions, and other adverse reactions.

Counseling: Advise to d/c use and consult physician if serious or unusual ocular or systemic reactions or signs of hypersensitivity occur. Inform that vision may be temporarily blurred following administration; instruct to use caution in operating machinery or driving a motor vehicle. Instruct to avoid allowing the container tip to contact the eye or surrounding structures or other surfaces. Instruct to consult physician about the continued use of the present multidose container if undergoing ocular surgery or if an intercurrent ocular condition (eg, trauma, infection) develops. Instruct that if using >1 topical ophthalmic drug, to administer the drugs at least 10 min apart. Advise that contact lenses should be removed during instillation, but may be reinserted 15 min after instillation.

AZOR — amlodipine/olmesartan medoxomil   Rx
Class: Angiotensin II receptor blocker (ARB)/calcium channel blocker (CCB) (dihydropyridine)

> D/C when pregnancy is detected. Drugs that act directly on the renin-angiotensin system (RAS) can cause death/injury to the developing fetus.

ADULT DOSAGE	PEDIATRIC DOSAGE
Hypertension	Pediatric use may not have been established
Initial Therapy:	
Initial: 5mg/20mg qd	
Titrate: May increase dose after 1-2 weeks	
Max: 10mg/40mg qd	
Replacement Therapy: May be substituted for individually titrated components. When substituting for individual components, the dose of 1 or both of the components may be increased if BP control has not been satisfactory.	
Add-On Therapy: May be used to provide additional BP lowering for patients not adequately controlled w/ amlodipine (or another dihydropyridine CCB) alone or w/ olmesartan (or another ARB) alone.	
May be administered w/ other antihypertensive agents	

- -

DOSING CONSIDERATIONS
Hepatic Impairment
Initial therapy is not recommended

Elderly
≥75 Years: Initial therapy is not recommended

ADMINISTRATION
Oral route

Take w/ or w/o food.

STORAGE
25°C (77°F); excursions permitted to 15-30°C (59-86°F).

HOW SUPPLIED
Tab: (Amlodipine/Olmesartan) 5mg/20mg, 5mg/40mg, 10mg/20mg, 10mg/40mg

CONTRAINDICATIONS
Coadministration w/ aliskiren in patients w/ diabetes.

WARNINGS/PRECAUTIONS
May decrease Hct and Hgb levels. **Amlodipine:** Acute hypotension rarely reported; caution w/ severe aortic stenosis. May develop increased frequency, duration, or severity of angina or acute MI w/ dosage initiation or increase, particularly in patients w/ severe obstructive coronary artery disease (CAD). May cause hepatic enzyme elevations. Caution w/ severe hepatic impairment and in elderly. **Olmesartan:** Symptomatic hypotension may occur after initiation of treatment; patients w/ an activated RAS, such as volume- and/or salt-depleted patients (eg, those being treated w/ high doses of diuretics) may be particularly vulnerable. May cause changes in renal function. Associated w/ oliguria or progressive azotemia and (rarely) w/ acute renal failure and/or death in patients whose renal function may depend upon the activity of the renin-angiotensin-aldosterone system (eg, patients w/ severe CHF). May increase SrCr or BUN in patients w/ renal artery stenosis. Sprue-like enteropathy w/ symptoms of severe, chronic diarrhea w/ substantial weight loss reported; exclude other etiologies if these symptoms develop, and consider discontinuation in cases where no other etiology is identified. May cause hyperkalemia; monitor serum electrolytes periodically.

ADVERSE REACTIONS
Edema, headache, palpitation, dizziness, flushing.

DRUG INTERACTIONS
See Contraindications. **Amlodipine:** May increase simvastatin exposure; limit simvastatin dose to 20mg/day. **Olmesartan:** NSAIDs, including selective COX-2 inhibitors, may result in deterioration of renal function, including possible acute renal failure in patients who are elderly, volume-depleted (including those on diuretic therapy), or w/ compromised renal function; monitor renal function periodically. Antihypertensive effect may be attenuated by NSAIDs including selective COX-2 inhibitors. Dual blockade of the RAS is associated w/ increased risks of hypotension, hyperkalemia, and changes in renal function (including acute renal failure); in general, avoid combined use of RAS inhibitors, or closely monitor BP, renal function, and electrolytes w/ other agents that affect the RAS. Avoid w/ aliskiren in patients w/ renal impairment (GFR <60mL/min). Colesevelam reduces exposure and levels; consider administering olmesartan at least 4 hrs before colesevelam dose. Increases in serum lithium levels and lithium toxicity reported; monitor lithium levels.

PREGNANCY AND LACTATION
Pregnancy: Category D. Use of drugs that act on the RAS during the 2nd and 3rd trimesters of pregnancy reduces fetal renal function and increases fetal and neonatal morbidity and death. Resulting oligohydramnios can be associated w/ fetal lung hypoplasia and skeletal deformations. When pregnancy is detected, d/c therapy as soon as possible.
Lactation: Not for use in nursing.

MECHANISM OF ACTION
Amlodipine: Dihydropyridine CCB; inhibits transmembrane influx of Ca^{2+} ions into vascular smooth muscle and cardiac muscle. Peripheral arterial vasodilator that acts directly on vascular smooth muscle to cause a reduction in peripheral vascular resistance and reduction in BP. **Olmesartan:** ARB; blocks the vasoconstrictor effects of angiotensin II by selectively blocking the binding of angiotensin II to the AT_1 receptor in vascular smooth muscle.

PHARMACOKINETICS
Absorption: Amlodipine: Absolute bioavailability (64-90%); T_{max}=6-12 hrs. Olmesartan: Absolute bioavailability (26%); T_{max}=1-2 hrs. **Distribution:** Amlodipine: Plasma protein binding (93%). Olmesartan: V_d=17L; plasma protein binding (99%). **Metabolism:** Amlodipine: Liver (extensive). Olmesartan: Rapid and complete by ester hydrolysis to olmesartan. **Elimination:** Amlodipine: Urine (10% parent compound, 60% metabolites); $T_{1/2}$=30-50 hrs. Olmesartan: Urine (35-50%), feces; $T_{1/2}$=13 hrs.

PATIENT CONSIDERATIONS

Assessment: Assess for severe aortic stenosis, severe obstructive CAD, renal artery stenosis, volume/salt depletion, diabetes, renal/hepatic impairment, pregnancy/nursing status, and possible drug interactions.

Monitoring: Monitor for signs/symptoms of hypotension, sprue-like enteropathy, and other adverse reactions. Monitor for symptoms of angina or MI, particularly in patients w/ severe obstructive CAD, after dosage initiation or increase. Monitor for decrease in Hct/Hgb and for increase in SrCr, BUN, and K^+ levels. Monitor hepatic enzymes and serum electrolytes.

Counseling: Inform about the consequences of exposure during pregnancy and of the treatment options in women if planning to become pregnant; instruct to report pregnancy to the physician as soon as possible.

AZULFIDINE — sulfasalazine

Class: 5-aminosalicylic acid derivative/sulfapyridine

Rx

ADULT DOSAGE	PEDIATRIC DOSAGE
Ulcerative Colitis	**Ulcerative Colitis**
Treatment of mild to moderate ulcerative colitis (UC), adjunctive therapy in severe UC, and to prolong remission period between acute attacks of UC	Treatment of mild to moderate ulcerative colitis (UC), adjunctive therapy in severe UC, and to prolong remission period between acute attacks of UC

Initial: 3-4g/day in evenly divided doses w/ intervals not >8 hrs; may initiate w/ a lower dose (eg, 1-2g/day) to reduce GI intolerance
Maint: 2g/day

When endoscopic examination confirms satisfactory improvement, reduce dose to a maint level; if diarrhea recurs, increase dose to previously effective level

Desensitization Regimen:
Initial: 50-250mg/day
Titrate: Double dose every 4-7 days until desired therapeutic level is achieved; d/c if sensitivity symptoms recur

≥6 Years:
Initial: 40-60mg/kg/24 hrs divided into 3-6 doses
Maint: 30mg/kg/24 hrs divided into 4 doses

When endoscopic examination confirms satisfactory improvement, reduce dose to a maint level; if diarrhea recurs, increase dose to previously effective level

Desensitization Regimen:
Initial: 50-250mg/day
Titrate: Double dose every 4-7 days until desired therapeutic level is achieved; d/c if sensitivity symptoms recur

---

DOSING CONSIDERATIONS
Other Important Considerations
Gastric Intolerance:
If symptoms of gastric intolerance (eg, anorexia, N/V) occur after 1st few doses, may be alleviated by halving daily dose and subsequently increasing gradually over several days; if gastric intolerance continues, stop drug for 5-7 days, then reintroduce at a lower daily dose

ADMINISTRATION
Oral route
Take in evenly divided doses, preferably pc.

STORAGE
25°C (77°F); excursions permitted to 15-30°C (59-86°F).

HOW SUPPLIED
Tab: 500mg* *scored

CONTRAINDICATIONS
Intestinal or urinary obstruction; porphyria; hypersensitivity to sulfasalazine, its metabolites, sulfonamides, or salicylates.

WARNINGS/PRECAUTIONS
Caution with hepatic/renal damage, blood dyscrasias, severe allergy, bronchial asthma, history of recurring/chronic infections, or with underlying conditions or concomitant drugs that may predispose patients to infections. Deaths reported from hypersensitivity reactions, agranulocytosis, aplastic anemia, other blood dyscrasias, renal and liver damage, irreversible neuromuscular and CNS changes, and fibrosing alveolitis. Perform CBC, including differential WBC count, and LFTs before starting therapy, every 2nd week for the first 3 months, monthly for the next 3 months, then every 3 months thereafter, and as clinically indicated; d/c while awaiting the results of blood tests. Monitor urinalysis and renal function periodically. Oligospermia and infertility reported in males. Serious infections (eg, fatal sepsis, pneumonia) reported. D/C if serious infection or toxic/hypersensitivity reactions develop. Closely monitor for signs and symptoms of infection during and after treatment; if a new infection develops, perform a prompt and complete diagnostic workup for infection and myelosuppression. Serious skin reactions, some fatal (eg, exfoliative dermatitis, Stevens-Johnson syndrome, toxic epidermal necrolysis), reported; d/c at 1st appearance of skin rash, mucosal lesions, or any other sign of hypersensitivity. Severe, life-threatening, systemic hypersensitivity reactions (eg, drug rash with eosinophilia and systemic symptoms) reported; evaluate immediately if signs/symptoms develop, and d/c if an alternative etiology cannot be established. Maintain adequate fluid intake to prevent crystalluria and stone formation. Closely monitor patients with G6PD deficiency for signs of hemolytic anemia. Do not attempt desensitization in patients who have a history of agranulocytosis, or who have experienced an anaphylactoid reaction with previous sulfasalazine (SSZ) therapy. Serum sulfapyridine (SP) levels >50mcg/mL appear to be associated with increased incidence of adverse reactions. Lab test interactions may occur.

ADVERSE REACTIONS
Anorexia, headache, N/V, gastric distress, reversible oligospermia.

DRUG INTERACTIONS
May reduce absorption of folic acid and digoxin.

PREGNANCY AND LACTATION
Category B, caution in nursing.

MECHANISM OF ACTION
5-aminosalicylic acid (5-ASA) derivative/SP; not established. May be related to anti-inflammatory and/or immunomodulatory properties, to its affinity for connective tissue, and/or to the relatively high concentration it reaches in serous fluids, the liver, and intestinal walls.

PHARMACOKINETICS
Absorption: SSZ: Absolute bioavailability (<15%); C_{max}=6mcg/mL; T_{max}=6 hrs. SP: Well absorbed from colon. Bioavailability (60%); T_{max}=10 hrs. 5-ASA: Much less well absorbed from GI tract. Bioavailability (10-30%); T_{max}=10 hrs. **Distribution:** Crosses placenta; found in breast milk. SSZ: V_d=7.5L (IV); plasma protein binding (>99.3%). SP: Plasma protein binding (70%, 90% [acetylsulfapyridine]). **Metabolism:** SSZ: Intestinal bacteria and liver to SP (active) and 5-ASA (metabolites). SP: Acetylation to acetylsulfapyridine (principal metabolite). 5-ASA: Liver and intestine to N-acetyl-5-ASA. **Elimination:** Urine, feces. SSZ: $T_{1/2}$=7.6 hrs (IV). SP: $T_{1/2}$=10.4 hrs (fast acetylators), 14.8 hrs (slow acetylators).

PATIENT CONSIDERATIONS
Assessment: Assess for intestinal or urinary obstruction, porphyria, renal dysfunction, severe allergy, bronchial asthma, G6PD deficiency, pregnancy/nursing status, possible drug interactions, history of hypersensitivity to the drug,

its metabolites, sulfonamides, or salicylates, history of recurring/chronic infections, and underlying conditions which may predispose patients to infections. Obtain CBC, including differential WBC count, and LFTs.

Monitoring: Monitor for GI intolerance, hypersensitivity/skin reactions, neuromuscular and CNS changes, fibrosing alveolitis, infection, signs of hemolytic anemia (in patients with G6PD deficiency), and other adverse reactions. Monitor CBC, including differential WBC count, and LFTs every 2nd week for the first 3 months, monthly for the next 3 months, then every 3 months thereafter, and as clinically indicated. Monitor urinalysis and renal function periodically, and serum SP levels. Monitor for diarrhea and/or bloody stools in infants fed milk from mothers taking SSZ. Monitor newborns for kernicterus.

Counseling: Inform of possible adverse reactions and need for careful medical supervision. Instruct to seek medical advice if sore throat, fever, pallor, purpura, or jaundice occurs. Inform that UC rarely remits completely and that risk of relapse can be reduced by continued administration at a maintenance dosage. Advise that orange-yellow discoloration of urine or skin may occur.

AZULFIDINE EN-TABS — sulfasalazine   Rx

Class: 5-aminosalicylic acid derivative/sulfapyridine

ADULT DOSAGE

Ulcerative Colitis

Treatment of mild to moderate ulcerative colitis (UC), adjunctive therapy in severe UC, and to prolong remission period between acute attacks of UC

Initial: 3-4g/day in evenly divided doses w/ intervals not >8 hrs; may initiate w/ a lower dose (eg, 1-2g/day) to reduce GI intolerance
Maint: 2g/day

When endoscopic exam confirms satisfactory improvement, reduce dose to a maint level; if diarrhea recurs, increase dose to previously effective levels

Indicated particularly in patients w/ UC who cannot take uncoated sulfasalazine tabs because of GI intolerance, and in whom there is evidence that this intolerance is not primarily the result of high blood levels of sulfapyridine and its metabolites

Desensitization Regimen:
Initial: 50-250mg/day
Titrate: Double dose every 4-7 days until desired therapeutic level is achieved; d/c if sensitivity recurs

Rheumatoid Arthritis

Treatment of Patients Who Have Responded Inadequately to Salicylates or Other NSAIDs:
Initial: 0.5-1g/day
Usual: 2g/day in 2 evenly divided doses; may consider increasing to 3g/day if clinical response after 12 weeks is inadequate

Suggested Dosing Schedule:
Week 1: 1 tab qpm
Week 2: 1 tab qam and 1 tab qpm
Week 3: 1 tab qam and 2 tabs qpm
Week 4: 2 tabs qam and 2 tabs qpm

Desensitization Regimen:
Initial: 50-250mg/day
Titrate: Double dose every 4-7 days until desired therapeutic level is achieved; d/c if sensitivity recurs

Concurrent treatment w/ analgesics and/or NSAIDs is recommended at least until effect is apparent

PEDIATRIC DOSAGE

Ulcerative Colitis

Treatment of mild to moderate ulcerative colitis (UC), adjunctive therapy in severe UC, and to prolong remission period between acute attacks of UC

≥6 Years:
Initial: 40-60mg/kg/24 hrs divided into 3-6 doses
Maint: 30mg/kg/24 hrs divided into 4 doses

When endoscopic exam confirms satisfactory improvement, reduce dose to a maint level; if diarrhea recurs, increase dose to previously effective levels

Indicated particularly in patients w/ UC who cannot take uncoated sulfasalazine tabs because of GI intolerance, and in whom there is evidence that this intolerance is not primarily the result of high blood levels of sulfapyridine and its metabolites

Desensitization Regimen:
Initial: 50-250mg/day
Titrate: Double dose every 4-7 days until desired therapeutic level is achieved; d/c if sensitivity recurs

Juvenile Rheumatoid Arthritis

Treatment of Patients w/ Polyarticular-Course Juvenile Rheumatoid Arthritis Who Have Responded Inadequately to Salicylates or Other NSAIDs:
≥6 Years:
Usual: 30-50mg/kg/day in 2 evenly divided doses; begin w/ 1/4-1/3 of planned maint dose and increase weekly until reaching maint dose at 1 month
Max: 2g/day

Desensitization Regimen:
Initial: 50-250mg/day
Titrate: Double dose every 4-7 days until desired therapeutic level is achieved; d/c if sensitivity recurs

Concurrent treatment w/ analgesics and/or NSAIDs is recommended at least until effect is apparent

---

DOSING CONSIDERATIONS
Other Important Considerations
Gastric Intolerance:
If symptoms of gastric intolerance (eg, anorexia, N/V) occur after 1st few doses, may be alleviated by halving daily dose and subsequently increasing gradually over several days; if gastric intolerance continues, stop drug for 5-7 days, then reintroduce at a lower daily dose

ADMINISTRATION
Oral route

Take in evenly divided doses, preferably pc.
Swallow tabs whole.
Careful monitoring is recommended for doses >2g/day.

STORAGE
25°C (77°F); excursions permitted to 15-30°C (59-86°F).

HOW SUPPLIED
Tab, Delayed-Release: 500mg

CONTRAINDICATIONS
Hypersensitivity to sulfasalazine, its metabolites, sulfonamides, or salicylates; intestinal or urinary obstruction; porphyria.

WARNINGS/PRECAUTIONS
Caution with hepatic/renal damage, blood dyscrasias, severe allergy, bronchial asthma, history of recurring/chronic infections, or with underlying conditions or concomitant drugs that may predispose patients to infections. Deaths reported from hypersensitivity reactions, agranulocytosis, aplastic anemia, other blood dyscrasias, renal and liver damage, irreversible neuromuscular and CNS changes, and fibrosing alveolitis. Perform CBC, including differential WBC count, and LFTs before starting therapy, every 2nd week for the first 3 months, monthly for the next 3 months, then every 3 months thereafter, and as clinically indicated; d/c while awaiting the results of blood tests. Monitor urinalysis and renal function periodically. Oligospermia and infertility reported in males. Serious infections (eg, fatal sepsis, pneumonia) reported. D/C if serious infection or toxic/hypersensitivity reactions develop. Closely monitor for signs and symptoms of infection during and after treatment; if a new infection develops, perform a prompt/complete diagnostic workup for infection and myelosuppression. Serious skin reactions, some fatal (eg, exfoliative dermatitis, Stevens-Johnson syndrome, toxic epidermal necrolysis), reported; d/c at 1st appearance of skin rash, mucosal lesions, or any other sign of hypersensitivity. Severe, life-threatening, systemic hypersensitivity reactions (eg, drug rash with eosinophilia and systemic symptoms) reported; evaluate immediately if signs/symptoms develop, and d/c if an alternative etiology cannot be established. Maintain adequate fluid intake to prevent crystalluria and stone formation. Closely monitor patients with G6PD deficiency for signs of hemolytic anemia. Do not attempt desensitization in patients who have a history of agranulocytosis, or have experienced an anaphylactoid reaction with previous sulfasalazine (SSZ) therapy. Serum sulfapyridine (SP) levels >50mcg/mL appear to be associated with increased incidence of adverse reactions. D/C immediately if tabs pass without disintegrating. Lab test interactions may occur.

ADVERSE REACTIONS
Anorexia, headache, N/V, gastric distress, reversible oligospermia, dyspepsia, rash, abdominal pain, fever, dizziness, stomatitis, pruritus, abnormal LFTs, leukopenia.

DRUG INTERACTIONS
May reduce absorption of folic acid and digoxin. Increased incidence of GI adverse events (especially nausea) with methotrexate.

PREGNANCY AND LACTATION
Category B, caution in nursing.

MECHANISM OF ACTION
5-aminosalicylic acid (5-ASA) derivative/SP; not established. May be related to the anti-inflammatory and/or immunomodulatory properties, to its affinity for connective tissue, and/or to the relatively high concentration it reaches in serous fluids, liver, and intestinal walls.

PHARMACOKINETICS
Absorption: SSZ: Absolute bioavailability (<15%); C_{max}=6mcg/mL; T_{max}=6 hrs. SP: Well absorbed from colon. Bioavailability (60%); T_{max}=10 hrs. 5-ASA: Much less well absorbed from GI tract. Bioavailability (10-30%); T_{max}=10 hrs.
Distribution: Crosses placenta; found in breast milk. SSZ: V_d=7.5L (IV); plasma protein binding (>99.3%). SP: Plasma protein binding (70%, 90% [acetylsulfapyridine]). **Metabolism:** SSZ: Intestinal bacteria and liver to SP (active) and 5-ASA (metabolites). SP: Acetylation to acetylsulfapyridine (principal metabolite). 5-ASA: Liver and intestine to N-acetyl-5-ASA.
Elimination: Urine, feces. SSZ: $T_{1/2}$=7.6 hrs (IV). SP: $T_{1/2}$=10.4 hrs (fast acetylators), 14.8 hrs (slow acetylators).

PATIENT CONSIDERATIONS

Assessment: Assess for intestinal or urinary obstruction, porphyria, renal dysfunction, severe allergy, bronchial asthma, G6PD deficiency, pregnancy/nursing status, possible drug interactions, history of hypersensitivity to the drug, its metabolites, sulfonamides, or salicylates, history of recurring/chronic infections, and underlying conditions which may predispose patients to infections. Obtain CBC, including differential WBC count, and LFTs.

Monitoring: Monitor for GI intolerance, hypersensitivity/skin reactions, neuromuscular and CNS changes, fibrosing alveolitis, infection, signs of hemolytic anemia (in patients with G6PD deficiency), and other adverse reactions. Monitor CBC, including differential WBC count, and LFTs every 2nd week for the first 3 months, monthly for the next 3 months, then every 3 months thereafter, and as clinically indicated. Monitor urinalysis and renal function periodically, and serum SP levels. Monitor for tabs passing without disintegrating. Monitor for diarrhea and/or bloody stools in infants fed milk from mothers taking SSZ. Monitor newborns for kernicterus.

Counseling: Inform of possible adverse effects and need for careful medical supervision. Instruct to seek medical advice if sore throat, fever, pallor, purpura, or jaundice occurs. Advise that orange-yellow discoloration of urine or skin may occur. Inform that UC rarely remits completely and that risk of relapse can be substantially reduced by continued administration at a maintenance dosage. Inform that RA rarely remits; instruct to follow up with physician to determine the need for continued administration.

BACLOFEN — baclofen   Rx
Class: GABA analogue

ADULT DOSAGE
Spasticity
Alleviation of signs and symptoms of spasticity resulting from multiple sclerosis. May be effective in spinal cord injuries and other spinal cord diseases

Initial: 5mg tid for 3 days
Titrate: May increase by 5mg tid every 3 days
Usual: 40-80mg/day
Max: 80mg/day (20mg qid)

PEDIATRIC DOSAGE
Spasticity
Alleviation of signs and symptoms of spasticity resulting from multiple sclerosis. May be effective in spinal cord injuries and other spinal cord diseases

≥12 Years:
Initial: 5mg tid for 3 days
Titrate: May increase by 5mg tid every 3 days
Usual: 40-80mg/day
Max: 80mg/day (20mg qid)

DOSING CONSIDERATIONS
Renal Impairment
Dose reduction may be necessary

ADMINISTRATION
Oral route

STORAGE
20-25°C (68-77°F); excursions permitted to 15-30°C (59-86°F).

HOW SUPPLIED
Tab: 10mg*, 20mg* *scored

CONTRAINDICATIONS
Hypersensitivity to baclofen.

WARNINGS/PRECAUTIONS
Not recommended w/ stroke, cerebral palsy, and Parkinson's disease. Hallucinations and seizures reported w/ abrupt withdrawal; reduce dose slowly when therapy is discontinued except for serious adverse reactions. Caution w/ impaired renal function. Should be used during pregnancy only if the benefit clearly justifies the potential risk to fetus. May impair physical/mental abilities. Caution where spasticity is utilized to sustain upright posture and balance in locomotion or to obtain increased function. Deterioration in seizure control and EEG reported; monitor clinical state and EEG at regular intervals in patients w/ epilepsy. Ovarian cysts reported in patients treated for up to 1 yr; in most cases these cysts disappeared spontaneously while patients continued therapy.

ADVERSE REACTIONS
Drowsiness, dizziness, weakness, fatigue, confusion, headache, insomnia, hypotension, nausea, constipation, urinary frequency.

DRUG INTERACTIONS
Additive CNS effects w/ alcohol and other CNS depressants.

PREGNANCY AND LACTATION
Safety not known in pregnancy, not for use in nursing.

MECHANISM OF ACTION
GABA analogue; not established. Capable of inhibiting both monosynaptic and polysynaptic reflexes at the spinal level, possibly by hyperpolarization of afferent terminals, although actions at supraspinal sites may also occur and contribute to its clinical effect.

PHARMACOKINETICS
Absorption: Rapid and extensive. **Elimination:** Kidney (unchanged).

PATIENT CONSIDERATIONS
Assessment: Assess for drug hypersensitivity, stroke, cerebral palsy, Parkinson's disease, epilepsy, renal impairment, pregnancy/nursing status, and possible drug interactions.

Monitoring: Monitor for hallucinations, seizures, ovarian cysts, and other adverse reactions. Monitor clinical state and EEG at regular intervals in patients w/ epilepsy.

Counseling: Instruct to take ud. Instruct to notify physician of any adverse effects. Caution against performing hazardous tasks (eg, operating machinery/driving). Instruct to notify physician if pregnant/nursing.

BACTROBAN NASAL — mupirocin calcium   Rx
Class: Bacterial protein synthesis inhibitor

ADULT DOSAGE
Methicillin-Resistant *Staphylococcus aureus*
Eradication of nasal colonization w/ methicillin-resistant *Staphylococcus aureus* as part of a comprehensive infection control program to reduce risk of infection among patients at high risk

Apply approx 1/2 tube into each nostril bid (am and pm) for 5 days

PEDIATRIC DOSAGE
Methicillin-Resistant *Staphylococcus aureus*
Eradication of nasal colonization w/ methicillin-resistant *Staphylococcus aureus* as part of a comprehensive infection control program to reduce risk of infection among patients at high risk

≥12 Years:
Apply approx 1/2 tube into each nostril bid (am and pm) for 5 days

DOSING CONSIDERATIONS
Concomitant Medications
Do not apply concurrently w/ any other intranasal products

ADMINISTRATION
Intranasal route

Spread oint by pressing together and releasing the sides of the nose repetitively for approx 1 min
Do not reuse

STORAGE
20-25°C (68-77°F); excursions permitted to 15-30°C (59-86°F). Do not refrigerate.

HOW SUPPLIED
Oint: 2% [1g]

CONTRAINDICATIONS
Known hypersensitivity to mupirocin or any of the excipients of this product.

WARNINGS/PRECAUTIONS
Systemic allergic reactions (eg, anaphylaxis, urticaria, angioedema, generalized rash) reported. Avoid contact w/ eyes; rinse well w/ water in case of accidental contact. D/C if sensitization or severe local irritation occurs. *Clostridium difficile*-associated diarrhea (CDAD) reported; may need to d/c if CDAD is suspected or confirmed. Prolonged use may result in overgrowth of nonsusceptible microorganisms, including fungi.

ADVERSE REACTIONS
Headache, rhinitis, respiratory disorder (eg, upper respiratory tract congestion), pharyngitis, taste perversion.

PREGNANCY AND LACTATION
Category B, caution in nursing.

MECHANISM OF ACTION
Bacterial protein synthesis inhibitor; inhibits bacterial protein synthesis by reversibly and specifically binding to bacterial isoleucyl transfer-RNA synthetase.

PHARMACOKINETICS
Distribution: Plasma protein binding (>97%). **Metabolism:** (IV/Oral) Rapid. **Elimination:** Urine. (IV) $T_{1/2}$=20-40 min.

PATIENT CONSIDERATIONS
Assessment: Assess for drug hypersensitivity and possible drug interactions.

Monitoring: Monitor for sensitization, severe local irritation, CDAD, and other adverse reactions.

Counseling: Instruct to avoid contact w/ eyes; advise to rinse thoroughly w/ water if oint gets in or near the eyes. Advise to take ud and d/c use and contact physician if sensitization or severe local irritation occurs. Advise to take the full course of treatment and not to stop early because the amount of bacteria in the nose may not be reduced.

BACTROBAN TOPICAL — mupirocin   Rx
Class: Bacterial protein synthesis inhibitor

ADULT DOSAGE
Secondarily Infected Traumatic Skin Lesions
Lesions up to 10cm in length or 100cm² in area due to *Staphylococcus aureus* and *Streptococcus pyogenes*

Cre:
Apply a small amount to the affected area tid for 10 days; reevaluate if no clinical response observed w/in 3-5 days

Impetigo
Due to *S. aureus* and *S. pyogenes*

Oint:
Apply a small amount to the affected area tid for up to 10 days; reevaluate if no clinical response observed w/in 3-5 days

PEDIATRIC DOSAGE
Secondarily Infected Traumatic Skin Lesions
Lesions up to 10cm in length or 100cm² in area due to *S. aureus* and *S. pyogenes*

3 Months-16 Years:
Cre:
Apply a small amount to the affected area tid for 10 days; reevaluate if no clinical response observed w/in 3-5 days

Impetigo
Due to *S. aureus* and *S. pyogenes*

2 Months-16 Years:
Oint:
Apply a small amount to the affected area tid for up to 10 days; reevaluate if no clinical response observed w/in 3-5 days

DOSING CONSIDERATIONS
Concomitant Medications
Do not apply concurrently w/ any other lotions, creams, or ointments

ADMINISTRATION
Topical route

Apply w/ a cotton swab or gauze pad.
Cover treated area w/ gauze dressing if desired.

STORAGE
Cre: ≤25°C (77°F). Do not freeze. **Oint:** 20-25°C (68-77°F).

HOW SUPPLIED
Cre: 2% [15g, 30g]; **Oint:** 2% [22g]

CONTRAINDICATIONS
Known hypersensitivity to mupirocin or any of the excipients of cre/oint.

WARNINGS/PRECAUTIONS

Systemic allergic reactions reported. Avoid contact w/ eyes; rinse well w/ water in case of accidental contact. D/C and institute appropriate alternative therapy if sensitization or severe local irritation occurs. *Clostridium difficile*-associated diarrhea (CDAD) reported; may need to d/c if CDAD is suspected/confirmed. Prolonged use may result in overgrowth of nonsusceptible microorganisms, including fungi. Not for use on mucosal surfaces. **Oint:** Polyethylene glycol can be absorbed from open wounds and damaged skin and is excreted by the kidneys; avoid use in conditions where absorption of large quantities of polyethylene glycol is possible, especially if there is evidence of moderate or severe renal impairment. Avoid use w/ IV cannulae or at central IV sites; may promote fungal infections and antimicrobial resistance.

ADVERSE REACTIONS

Cre: Headache, burning at application site, nausea, rash.
Oint: Burning, stinging, pain, itching.

PREGNANCY AND LACTATION

Pregnancy: Category B.
Lactation: It is not known whether this drug is excreted in human milk. Caution in nursing.

MECHANISM OF ACTION

RNA synthetase inhibitor antibacterial; inhibits bacterial protein synthesis by reversibly and specifically binding to bacterial isoleucyl-transfer RNA synthetase.

PHARMACOKINETICS

Absorption: (Cre) Minimal systemic absorption. **Distribution:** Plasma protein binding (>97%). **Metabolism:** (IV/Oral) Rapid. **Elimination:** Urine. (IV) $T_{1/2}$=20-40 min.

PATIENT CONSIDERATIONS

Assessment: Assess for hypersensitivity to the drug and pregnancy/nursing status.

Monitoring: Monitor for systemic allergic reactions, sensitization, severe local irritation, CDAD, and other adverse reactions.

Counseling: Instruct to use only ud. Inform that medication is for external use only. Instruct to avoid contact w/ eyes; advise to rinse thoroughly w/ water if product gets in the eyes. Advise not to use in the nose. Instruct to wash hands before and after applying the product. Inform that treated area can be covered w/ a gauze dressing if desired. Advise to d/c medication and contact physician if irritation, severe itching, or rash occurs. Instruct to report to physician or go to the nearest emergency room if severe allergic reactions (eg, swelling of the lips/face/tongue, wheezing) occur. Advise to notify physician if no improvement is seen in 3-5 days.

BANZEL — rufinamide   Rx

Class: Triazole derivative

ADULT DOSAGE	PEDIATRIC DOSAGE
Seizures	**Seizures**
Associated w/ Lennox-Gastaut Syndrome:	**Associated w/ Lennox-Gastaut Syndrome:**
≥17 Years:	**1-<17 Years:**
Initial: 400-800mg/day given in 2 equally divided doses	**Initial:** 10mg/kg/day given in 2 equally divided doses
Titrate: Increase by 400-800mg qod until max dose is reached	**Titrate:** Increase by 10mg/kg increments qod until max dose is reached
Max: 3200mg/day	**Max:** 45mg/kg/day, not to exceed 3200mg/day

---

DOSING CONSIDERATIONS
Concomitant Medications
Valproate:
Initial: <400mg/day (adults) or <10mg/kg/day (pediatric patients)

Renal Impairment
Hemodialysis may reduce exposure; consider dose adjustment during the dialysis process

Hepatic Impairment
Severe (Child-Pugh Score 10-15): Not recommended

Elderly
Start at lower end of dosing range

ADMINISTRATION
Oral route

Take w/ food.

Tab
May be administered whole, as 1/2 tabs, or crushed.

Oral Sus
Shake well before every administration.
Use the provided adapter and calibrated oral dosing syringe to administer the oral sus; firmly insert the adapter into the neck of the bottle before use and leave in place for the duration of the usage of the bottle.
Insert the dosing syringe into the adapter and withdraw the dose from the inverted bottle.
Replace the cap after each use; the cap fits properly when the adapter is in place.

STORAGE

25°C (77°F); excursions permitted to 15-30°C (59-86°F). (Tab) Protect from moisture. (Sus) Store in an upright position. Use w/in 90 days of 1st opening the bottle.

HOW SUPPLIED

Oral Sus: 40mg/mL [460mL]; **Tab:** 200mg*, 400mg* *scored

CONTRAINDICATIONS

Familial short QT syndrome.

WARNINGS/PRECAUTIONS

May increase risk of suicidal thoughts or behavior. CNS-related adverse effects (eg, somnolence, fatigue, dizziness, ataxia, gait disturbance) reported; may impair mental/physical abilities. QT interval shortening and leukopenia reported. Drug reaction w/ eosinophilia and systemic symptoms (DRESS), also known as multiorgan hypersensitivity, reported; evaluate immediately, d/c treatment, and initiate alternative treatment if DRESS is suspected. Withdraw gradually to minimize risk of precipitating seizures, seizure exacerbation, or status epilepticus. If abrupt discontinuation is necessary, transition to another antiepileptic drug should be made under close medical supervision. Caution w/ mild (Child-Pugh score 5-6) to moderate (Child-Pugh score 7-9) hepatic impairment.

ADVERSE REACTIONS

Somnolence, N/V, headache, fatigue, dizziness, influenza, nasopharyngitis, decreased appetite, rash, ataxia, diplopia, tremor, nystagmus, blurred vision.

DRUG INTERACTIONS

See Dosing Considerations. Potent CYP450 inducers (eg, carbamazepine, phenytoin, primidone, phenobarbital) may increase clearance and decrease levels. Valproate may increase levels. May increase phenytoin or phenobarbital levels. May decrease levels of lamotrigine or carbamazepine. Concurrent use w/ hormonal contraceptives may render this method of contraception less effective; additional forms of nonhormonal contraception are recommended during coadministration. Caution w/ other drugs that shorten QT interval.

PREGNANCY AND LACTATION

Category C, not for use in nursing.

MECHANISM OF ACTION

Triazole derivative; not established. Suspected to modulate activity of Na+ channels and, in particular, prolongation of the inactive state of the channel. Slows Na+ channel recovery from inactivation after prolonged prepulse in cultured cortical neurons, and limits sustained repetitive firing of Na+-dependent action potentials.

PHARMACOKINETICS

Absorption: Well-absorbed; T_{max}=4-6 hrs. **Distribution:** V_d=50L (3200mg/day); plasma protein binding (34%; 27% bound to albumin); likely found in breast milk. **Metabolism:** Extensive; via carboxylesterase mediated hydrolysis. **Elimination:** Urine (85%; 2% unchanged and ≥66% as the acid metabolite CGP 47292); $T_{1/2}$=6-10 hrs.

PATIENT CONSIDERATIONS

Assessment: Assess for familial short QT syndrome, depression, hepatic/renal impairment, pregnancy/nursing status, and possible drug interactions.

Monitoring: Monitor for CNS reactions, QT interval shortening, DRESS, leukopenia, emergence or worsening of depression, suicidal thoughts/behavior, unusual changes in mood/behavior, and other adverse reactions. Upon withdrawal of therapy, monitor for precipitation/exacerbation of seizures and status epilepticus.

Counseling: Inform patients, caregivers, and families of the increased risk of suicidal thoughts/behavior; advise to be alert for emergence or worsening of signs/symptoms of depression, any unusual changes in mood/behavior, or emergence of suicidal thoughts, behavior, or thoughts about self-harm. Instruct to immediately report behaviors of concern to physician. Inform of the potential for somnolence or dizziness; advise not to drive or operate machinery until the effects of drug are known. Advise to notify physician if rash associated w/ fever develops. Inform females of childbearing age that concurrent use w/ hormonal contraceptives may render this method of contraception less effective and recommend using additional nonhormonal forms of contraception during therapy. Inform that alcohol may cause additive CNS effects. Advise to notify physician if pregnant or intending to become pregnant; encourage enrollment in the North American Antiepileptic Drug Pregnancy Registry if pregnancy occurs. Advise to notify physician if breastfeeding or intending to breastfeed.

BARACLUDE — entecavir   Rx

Class: Nucleoside reverse transcriptase inhibitor (NRTI)

> Severe acute exacerbations of hepatitis B reported upon discontinuation of therapy; monitor liver function for at least several months after discontinuation. If appropriate, may initiate antihepatitis B therapy. Potential for development of resistance to HIV nucleoside reverse transcriptase inhibitors if entecavir is used to treat chronic hepatitis B virus (HBV) infection in patients with untreated HIV infection. Not recommended for HIV/HBV coinfected patients not receiving highly active antiretroviral therapy (HAART). Lactic acidosis and severe hepatomegaly with steatosis, including fatal cases, have been reported with the use of nucleoside analogue inhibitors.

ADULT DOSAGE	PEDIATRIC DOSAGE
Chronic Hepatitis B	**Chronic Hepatitis B**
In patients w/ evidence of active viral replication and either evidence of persistent elevations in serum aminotransferases (ALT/AST) or histologically active disease	In patients w/ evidence of active viral replication and either evidence of persistent elevations in serum aminotransferases (ALT/AST) or histologically active disease

Compensated Liver Disease:
Nucleoside-Inhibitor Treatment-Naive:
0.5mg qd

History of Hepatitis B Viremia While Receiving Lamivudine or Known Lamivudine- or Telbivudine-Resistant Substitutions:
1mg qd

Decompensated Liver Disease:
1mg qd

≥2 Years:
Treatment-Naive:
10-11kg: 3mL qd
>11-14kg: 4mL qd
>14-17kg: 5mL qd
>17-20kg: 6mL qd
>20-23kg: 7mL qd
>23-26kg: 8mL qd
>26-30kg: 9mL qd
>30kg: 10mL or 0.5mg tab qd

Lamivudine-Experienced:
10-11kg: 6mL qd
>11-14kg: 8mL qd
>14-17kg: 10mL qd
>17-20kg: 12mL qd
>20-23kg: 14mL qd
>23-26kg: 16mL qd
>26-30kg: 18mL qd
>30kg: 20mL or 1mg tab qd

Compensated Liver Disease:
Nucleoside-Inhibitor Treatment-Naive:
≥16 Years:
0.5mg qd

History of Hepatitis B Viremia While Receiving Lamivudine or Known Lamivudine- or Telbivudine-Resistant Substitutions:
≥16 Years:
1mg qd

- - - - - - - - - -

DOSING CONSIDERATIONS
Renal Impairment
CrCl 30-<50mL/min:
Usual: 0.25mg qd or 0.5mg q48h
Lamivudine-Refractory or Decompensated Liver Disease: 0.5mg qd or 1mg q48h

CrCl 10-<30mL/min:
Usual: 0.15mg qd or 0.5mg q72h
Lamivudine-Refractory or Decompensated Liver Disease: 0.3mg qd or 1mg q72h

CrCl <10mL/min or CAPD:
Usual: 0.05mg qd or 0.5mg every 7 days
Lamivudine-Refractory or Decompensated Liver Disease: 0.1mg qd or 1mg every 7 days

Hemodialysis:
Usual: 0.05mg qd or 0.5mg every 7 days (after session if administered on hemodialysis day)
Lamivudine-Refractory or Decompensated Liver Disease: 0.1mg qd or 1mg every 7 days (after session if administered on hemodialysis day)

ADMINISTRATION
Oral route
Take on an empty stomach (at least 2 hrs pc and 2 hrs before the next meal)

STORAGE
25°C (77°F); excursions permitted between 15-30°C (59-86°F). Protect from light.

HOW SUPPLIED
Sol: 0.05mg/mL [210mL]; **Tab:** 0.5mg, 1mg

WARNINGS/PRECAUTIONS
Dosage adjustment is recommended in renal dysfunction (CrCl <50mL/min), including patients on hemodialysis or continuous ambulatory peritoneal dialysis. May require HIV antibody testing prior to treatment. Caution with known risk factors for liver disease. D/C if lactic acidosis or pronounced hepatotoxicity occurs. Caution in elderly.

ADVERSE REACTIONS
Hepatitis B exacerbation, lactic acidosis, hepatomegaly, headache, fatigue, dizziness, nausea, ALT/lipase/total bilirubin elevation, hyperglycemia, glycosuria, hematuria.

DRUG INTERACTIONS
May increase levels of either entecavir or concomitant drugs that reduce renal function or compete for active tubular secretion; closely monitor for adverse events.

PREGNANCY AND LACTATION
Category C, not for use in nursing.

MECHANISM OF ACTION
Guanosine nucleoside analogue; inhibits base priming, reverse transcription of negative strand from pregenomic mRNA, and synthesis of positive strand of HBV DNA.

PHARMACOKINETICS
Absorption: C_{max}=4.2ng/mL (0.5mg), 8.2ng/mL (1mg); T_{max}=0.5-1.5 hrs.
Distribution: Serum protein binding (13%). **Metabolism:** Glucuronidation and sulfate conjugation. **Elimination:** Urine (62-73% unchanged); $T_{1/2}$=128-149 hrs.

PATIENT CONSIDERATIONS
Assessment: Assess for hepatic/renal impairment, pregnancy/nursing status, and possible drug interactions. Perform HIV antibody testing before initiating therapy.

Monitoring: Monitor for signs/symptoms of lactic acidosis, hepatotoxicity, renal/hepatic impairment, and other adverse reactions.

Counseling: Advise to remain under care of physician during therapy and report any new symptoms or concurrent medications. Advise that treatment has not been shown to reduce risk of transmission of HBV to others through sexual contact or blood contamination. Advise to take the missed dose as soon as remembered unless it is almost time for the next dose and not to take 2 doses at the same time. Inform that treatment may lower the amount of HBV in the body and improve the condition of the liver, but will not cure HBV. Counsel that it is not known whether treatment will reduce risk of liver cancer or cirrhosis. Inform that deterioration of liver disease may occur in some cases if treatment is discontinued, and instruct to discuss any change in regimen with physician. Inform that drug may increase the chance of HIV resistance to HIV medication if HIV-infected patient is not receiving effective HIV treatment.

BASAGLAR — insulin glargine   Rx
Class: Insulin (long-acting)

ADULT DOSAGE
Type 1 Diabetes Mellitus
Initial: Approx 1/3 of total daily insulin requirement; must be used w/ short-acting insulin

Use short- or rapid-acting, premeal insulin to satisfy remainder of the daily insulin requirements

Type 2 Diabetes Mellitus
Initial: 0.2 U/kg or up to 10 U qd

May need to adjust amount and timing of short- or rapid-acting insulins and dosages of any anti-diabetic drugs

Conversions
From Another Insulin Glargine (100 U/mL):
Basaglar dose should be the same as other insulin glargine product, 100 U/mL, and time of day for administration should be determined by the physician

From Once-Daily Insulin Glargine (300 U/mL):
Initial Basaglar dose is 80% of the insulin glargine product that is being discontinued

From Intermediate- or Long-Acting Insulin (Other Than an Insulin Glargine Product 100 U/mL):
Change in basal insulin dose may be required and amount and timing of the shorter-acting insulins and doses of any antidiabetic drugs may need to be adjusted

From BID NPH Insulin:
Initial Basaglar dose is 80% of total NPH dose that is being discontinued

PEDIATRIC DOSAGE
Type 1 Diabetes Mellitus
≥6 Years:
Initial: Approx 1/3 of total daily insulin requirement; must be used w/ short-acting insulin

Use short- or rapid-acting, premeal insulin to satisfy remainder of the daily insulin requirements

Conversions
From Another Insulin Glargine (100 U/mL):
Basaglar dose should be the same as the other insulin glargine product, 100 U/mL, and time of day for administration should be determined by the physician

From Once-Daily Insulin Glargine (300 U/mL):
Initial Basaglar dose is 80% of the insulin glargine product that is being discontinued

From Intermediate- or Long-Acting Insulin (Other Than an Insulin Glargine Product 100 U/mL):
Change in basal insulin dose may be required and amount and timing of the shorter-acting insulins and doses of any antidiabetic drugs may need to be adjusted

From BID NPH Insulin:
Initial Basaglar dose is 80% of total NPH dose that is being discontinued

- - - - - - - - - -

DOSING CONSIDERATIONS
Renal Impairment
Frequent glucose monitoring and dose adjustments may be necessary

Hepatic Impairment
More frequent glucose monitoring and dose adjustments may be necessary

Elderly
Dose conservatively

Other Important Considerations
Dosage adjustments may be needed w/ changes in physical activity, changes in meal patterns (eg, macronutrient content, timing of food intake), changes in hepatic/renal function, or during acute illness

ADMINISTRATION
SQ route

Inject 1-80 U/inj.
Inject SQ qd at any time of day but at the same time every day.
Administer into the abdominal area, thigh, or deltoid, and rotate inj sites w/in the same region from one inj to the next.
Do not dilute or mix w/ any other insulin or sol.
Do not administer IV or via an insulin pump.

STORAGE
Do not freeze; discard if frozen. Protect from direct heat and light. **Not in Use: Unopened:** ≤30°C (86°F) for 28 days or 2-8°C (36-46°F) until expiration date. **In Use: Opened:** ≤30°C (86°F) for 28 days. Do not refrigerate.

HOW SUPPLIED
Inj: 100 U/mL [3mL]

CONTRAINDICATIONS
During episodes of hypoglycemia. Hypersensitivity to insulin glargine or one of its excipients.

WARNINGS/PRECAUTIONS
Not recommended for the treatment of diabetic ketoacidosis. KwikPens must never be shared between patients, even if the needle is changed; may carry a risk for transmission of blood-borne pathogens. Changes in insulin strength, manufacturer, type, or method of administration may affect glycemic control and predispose

to hypo/hyperglycemia. Hypoglycemia may occur and may impair concentration ability and reaction time. Symptomatic awareness of hypoglycemia may be less pronounced in patients w/ longstanding diabetes, w/ diabetic nerve disease, using medications that block the sympathetic nervous system (eg, β-blockers), or who experience recurrent hypoglycemia. The long-acting effect of insulin glargine may delay recovery from hypoglycemia. Accidental mix-ups among insulin products reported. Severe, life-threatening, generalized allergy, including anaphylaxis, may occur. If hypersensitivity reactions occur, d/c therapy; treat per standard of care and monitor until signs/symptoms resolve. May cause hypokalemia; monitor K⁺ levels in patients at risk for hypokalemia (eg, patients using K⁺-lowering medications or medications sensitive to serum K⁺ concentrations) if indicated.

ADVERSE REACTIONS
Hypoglycemia, allergic reactions, inj-site reaction, lipodystrophy, pruritus, rash, edema, weight gain.

DRUG INTERACTIONS
Dose adjustment and increased frequency of glucose monitoring may be required w/ drugs that may increase the risk of hypoglycemia (eg, antidiabetic agents, ACE inhibitors, ARBs, disopyramide, fibrates, fluoxetine, MAOIs, pentoxifylline, pramlintide, propoxyphene, salicylates, somatostatin analogues [eg, octreotide], sulfonamide antibiotics), drugs that may decrease blood glucose-lowering effect (eg, atypical antipsychotics [eg, olanzapine, clozapine], corticosteroids, danazol, diuretics, estrogens, glucagon, isoniazid, niacin, oral contraceptives, phenothiazines, progestogens [eg, in oral contraceptives], protease inhibitors, somatropin, sympathomimetic agents [eg, albuterol, epinephrine, terbutaline], thyroid hormones), or drugs that may increase/decrease blood glucose-lowering effect (eg, alcohol, β-blockers, clonidine, lithium salts, pentamidine). Signs/symptoms of hypoglycemia may be blunted w/ β-blockers, clonidine, guanethidine, or reserpine. Observe for signs/symptoms of heart failure (HF) if treated concomitantly w/ a peroxisome proliferator-activated receptor (PPAR)-gamma agonist (eg, thiazolidinedione); consider discontinuation or dose reduction of the PPAR-gamma agonist if HF develops.

PREGNANCY AND LACTATION
Pregnancy: Category C.
Lactation: It is not known if insulin glargine is excreted in human milk; caution in nursing. Use is compatible w/ breastfeeding, but women may require adjustments of insulin doses.

MECHANISM OF ACTION
Insulin glargine; regulates glucose metabolism. Lowers blood glucose by stimulating peripheral glucose uptake and by inhibiting hepatic glucose production. Inhibits lipolysis and proteolysis, and enhances protein synthesis.

PHARMACOKINETICS
Absorption: C_{max}=103 pmol/L; T_{max} (median)=12 hrs; AUC=1720 pmol•hr/L.
Metabolism: M1 (21ᴬ-Gly-insulin) and M2 (21ᴬ-Gly-des-30ᴮ-Thr-insulin) (active metabolites).

PATIENT CONSIDERATIONS
Assessment: Assess for hypoglycemia, diabetic ketoacidosis, predisposition to hypo/hyperglycemia, risk factors for hypokalemia, hypersensitivity, renal/hepatic impairment, pregnancy/nursing status, and possible drug interactions. Obtain baseline blood glucose and HbA1c levels.

Monitoring: Monitor for signs/symptoms of hypoglycemia, hypersensitivity/allergic reactions, and other adverse reactions. Monitor for changes in physical activity, changes in meal patterns, changes in renal/hepatic function, or acute illness. Monitor blood glucose and HbA1c levels; increase frequency of blood glucose monitoring in patients at higher risk for hypoglycemia and in those w/ reduced symptomatic awareness of hypoglycemia. Monitor K⁺ levels in patients at risk for hypokalemia if indicated.

Counseling: Inform of the risks/benefits of therapy. Advise to never share a KwikPen w/ another person, even if needle is changed. Inform of the symptoms of hypoglycemia, including impairment of the ability to concentrate and react; advise to use caution when driving/operating machinery. Advise that changes in insulin regimen can predispose to hyper- or hypoglycemia. Instruct to always check the label before each inj to avoid medication errors. Instruct on self-management procedures, including glucose monitoring, proper inj technique, management of hypo/hyperglycemia, and on handling of special situations (eg, intercurrent conditions, inadequate or skipped dose, inadvertent administration of increased insulin dose, inadequate food intake, skipped meals). Advise to inform physician if pregnant or contemplating pregnancy.

BECONASE AQ — beclomethasone dipropionate monohydrate   Rx
Class: Corticosteroid

ADULT DOSAGE
Rhinitis

Relief of Symptoms of Seasonal or Perennial Allergic and Nonallergic (Vasomotor) Rhinitis:
1-2 sprays per nostril bid
Max: 2 sprays per nostril bid

Should not be continued beyond 3 weeks in the absence of significant symptomatic improvement

Other Indications
Prevention of nasal polyps recurrence following surgical removal

PEDIATRIC DOSAGE
Rhinitis

Relief of Symptoms of Seasonal or Perennial Allergic and Nonallergic (Vasomotor) Rhinitis:

6-12 Years:
Initial: 1 spray per nostril bid
Titrate: May increase to 2 sprays per nostril. Once adequate control is achieved, decrease to 1 spray per nostril bid
Max: 2 sprays per nostril bid

>12 Years:
1-2 sprays per nostril bid
Max: 2 sprays per nostril bid

Should not be continued beyond 3 weeks in the absence of significant symptomatic improvement

Other Indications
Prevention of nasal polyps recurrence following surgical removal

---

DOSING CONSIDERATIONS
Elderly
Start at lower end of dosing range

ADMINISTRATION
Intranasal route

STORAGE
15-30°C (59-86°F).

HOW SUPPLIED
Spray: 42mcg/spray [25g]

CONTRAINDICATIONS
Hypersensitivity to any ingredients of this preparation.

WARNINGS/PRECAUTIONS
May use a nasal vasoconstrictor during the first 2 to 3 days of therapy in the presence of excessive nasal mucous secretion or edema of the nasal mucosa. Risk of adrenal insufficiency and withdrawal symptoms when replacing systemic corticosteroids with topical corticosteroids. Caution with active or quiescent tuberculous (TB), ocular herpes simplex, or untreated bacterial, fungal and systemic viral or parasitic infections. Avoid with recent nasal trauma/surgery or septum ulcers. Risk for more severe/fatal course of infections (eg, chickenpox, measles) and for *Candida* infections of nose and pharynx. Potential for reduced growth velocity in pediatrics. Rare cases of nasal septum perforation, wheezing, cataracts, glaucoma, increased intraocular pressure reported. Hypersensitivity reactions may occur. D/C if nasopharyngeal irritation persists. Caution in elderly.

ADVERSE REACTIONS
Nasopharyngeal irritation, sneezing, headache, nausea, lightheadedness, irritated/dry nose and throat, unpleasant taste/smell.

DRUG INTERACTIONS
Concomitant systemic corticosteroids increase risk of hypercorticism and/or HPA axis suppression.

PREGNANCY AND LACTATION
Category C, caution in nursing.

MECHANISM OF ACTION
Corticosteroid; mechanism not established; anti-inflammatory and vasoconstrictor effects.

PHARMACOKINETICS
Absorption: Absolute bioavailability (44%) (for the active metabolite B-17-MP). C_{max}<50pg/mL. **Distribution:** V_d=20L (parent drug); V_d=424L (B-17-MP). Plasma protein binding (87%). **Metabolism:** B-17-MP (active metabolite) via esterase enzymes. **Elimination:** Urine (12% metabolites), feces (60% metabolites). $T_{1/2}$=0.5 hrs (parent drug), 2.7 hrs (B-17-MP).

PATIENT CONSIDERATIONS
Assessment: Assess for associated asthma with history of long-term therapy with systemic steroids, active or quiescent TB of upper respiratory tract, untreated local or systemic fungal or bacterial infections, systemic viral or parasitic infections, ocular herpes simplex, nasal polyps or recent nasal septal ulcers, nasal surgery/trauma, and possible drug interactions.

Monitoring: Monitor for reduced growth velocity (in pediatrics), nasal septum perforation, localized infection, *Candida* infection, exacerbation of infections, nasopharyngeal irritation, signs of adrenal insufficiency, and symptoms of hypercorticism.

Counseling: Instruct to take as directed at regular intervals and to avoid exposure to chickenpox or measles. Consult physician immediately if exposed to infection or symptoms do not improve, if the condition worsens, or if sneezing or nasal irritation occurs. Advise to avoid spraying in the eyes.

BELBUCA — buprenorphine   CIII
Class: Partial opioid agonist

> Exposes patients and other users to risks of opioid addiction, abuse, and misuse, which can lead to overdose and death; assess each patient's risk prior to prescribing, and monitor regularly for development of these behaviors/conditions. Serious, life-threatening, or fatal respiratory depression may occur; monitor for respiratory depression, especially during initiation or following a dose increase. Misuse or abuse by chewing, swallowing, snorting, or injecting buprenorphine extracted from the buccal film will result in uncontrolled delivery of buprenorphine and pose a significant risk of overdose and death. Accidental exposure, especially in children, can result in a fatal overdose. Prolonged use during pregnancy can result in neonatal opioid withdrawal syndrome; advise of the risk and ensure availability of appropriate treatment if opioid use is required for a prolonged period in a pregnant woman.

ADULT DOSAGE

Severe Pain (Daily, Around-the-Clock Management)

Management of pain severe enough to require daily, around-the-clock, long-term opioid treatment and for which alternative treatment options are inadequate

Initial:

Opioid-Naïve Patients: 75mcg qd or, if tolerated, q12h for at least 4 days, then increase to 150mcg q12h
Conversion from Other Opioids: See conversions section below

Titrate:

Increase in increments of 150mcg q12h, no more frequently than every 4 days, to a dose that provides adequate analgesia and minimizes adverse reactions

Doses up to 450mcg q12h were studied in opioid-naïve patients

Max:

900mcg q12h

Consider an alternate analgesic if pain is not adequately managed on 900mcg

Conversions

From Other Opioids:
To reduce the risk of opioid withdrawal, taper to no more than 30mg oral morphine sulfate equivalents (MSE) daily before beginning Belbuca. Following analgesic taper, base the starting dose on patient's daily opioid dose prior to taper; may require additional short-acting analgesics during the taper period and during titration

Initial Belbuca Dose Based on Prior Daily Opioid Analgesic Dose Before Taper:
<30mg Oral MSE: 75mcg qd or q12h
30-89mg Oral MSE: 150mcg q12h
90-160mg Oral MSE: 300mcg q12h
>160mg Oral MSE: Consider alternate analgesic

Doses of 600mcg, 750mcg, and 900mcg are only for use following titration from lower doses of Belbuca

From Methadone:
The ratio between methadone and other opioid agonists may vary widely as a function of previous dose exposure. Methadone has a long $T_{1/2}$ and can accumulate in the plasma; monitor closely during conversion

---

DOSING CONSIDERATIONS
Hepatic Impairment
Mild to Moderate (Child-Pugh Class A and B): Dose reduction not needed
Severe (Child-Pugh Class C): Reduce initial and titration dose by 1/2 that of patients w/ normal liver function (from 150mcg to 75mcg)

Discontinuation
Use gradual downward titration; do not abruptly d/c

Other Important Considerations
Oral Mucositis: Reduce initial dose and titration incremental dose by 1/2 compared to patients w/o mucositis

ADMINISTRATION
Buccal route

Apply to the buccal mucosa q12h.
Avoid applying to areas of the mouth w/ any open sores or lesions.
Use the tongue to wet the inside of the cheek or rinse mouth w/ water to wet the area for placement.
Apply immediately after removal from the individually sealed package.
Place the yellow side of the film against the inside of the cheek.
Hold the entire film in place w/ clean, dry fingers for 5 sec and then leave in place on the inside of the cheek until fully dissolved.
Film will completely dissolve after application, usually w/in 30 min. Do not manipulate film w/ tongue or finger(s).
Avoid eating food and drinking liquids until the film has dissolved.
Dispose of unused film as soon as it is no longer needed; refer to PI for disposal instructions.

STORAGE
25°C (77°F); excursions permitted to 15-30°C (59-86°F).

PEDIATRIC DOSAGE
Pediatric use may not have been established

HOW SUPPLIED
Film, Buccal: 75mcg, 150mcg, 300mcg, 450mcg, 600mcg, 750mcg, 900mcg [60s]

CONTRAINDICATIONS
Significant respiratory depression, acute or severe bronchial asthma in an unmonitored setting or in the absence of resuscitative equipment, known/suspected GI obstruction (eg, paralytic ileus), hypersensitivity (eg, anaphylaxis) to buprenorphine.

WARNINGS/PRECAUTIONS
Reserve use in patients for whom alternative treatment options are ineffective, not tolerated, or would be otherwise inadequate to provide sufficient management of pain. Should be prescribed only by healthcare professionals who are knowledgeable in the use of potent opioids for the management of chronic pain. Life-threatening respiratory depression is more likely to occur in elderly, cachectic, or debilitated patients; monitor closely (particularly when initiating/titrating therapy and w/ concomitant drugs that depress respiration). Increased risk of decreased respiratory drive, including apnea, even at recommended doses in patients w/ significant COPD or cor pulmonale, and those w/ substantially decreased respiratory reserve, hypoxia, hypercapnia, or preexisting respiratory depression; monitor closely (especially when initiating/titrating therapy) or, alternatively, consider other nonopioid analgesics. QTc prolongation reported; caution in patients w/ hypokalemia, hypomagnesemia, or clinically unstable cardiac disease, and periodically monitor ECG in these patients. Avoid use in patients w/ history of or immediate family w/ long QT syndrome. May cause severe hypotension, including orthostatic hypotension and syncope in ambulatory patients. Increased risk for severe hypotension in patients whose ability to maintain BP has already been compromised by a reduced blood volume or concurrent administration of certain CNS depressants; monitor for hypotension during initiation and titration. Avoid in patients w/ circulatory shock. Monitor patients who may be susceptible to intracranial effects of carbon dioxide retention (eg, those w/ evidence of increased intracranial pressure or brain tumors) for signs of sedation and respiratory depression, particularly when initiating therapy. May obscure clinical course in patients w/ a head injury. Avoid w/ impaired consciousness or coma. Cases of cytolytic hepatitis and hepatitis w/ jaundice reported in patients receiving SL buprenorphine for opioid dependence treatment. Obtain baseline liver enzyme levels in patients at increased risk of hepatotoxicity (eg, history of excessive alcohol intake, IV drug abuse, or liver disease), and monitor periodically during treatment. Monitor for signs/symptoms of toxicity or overdose in patients w/ moderate or severe hepatic impairment. Cases of acute and chronic hypersensitivity, bronchospasm, angioneurotic edema, and anaphylactic shock reported. May cause spasm of the sphincter of Oddi. May increase serum amylase; monitor patients w/ biliary tract disease, including acute pancreatitis, for worsening symptoms. May increase seizure frequency in patients w/ seizure disorders and may increase the risk of seizures occurring in other clinical settings associated w/ seizures. Cancer patients w/ oral mucositis may absorb buprenorphine more rapidly than intended; monitor for signs/symptoms of toxicity/overdose. May impair mental/physical abilities. Caution in elderly.

ADVERSE REACTIONS
N/V, constipation, headache, dizziness, somnolence, fatigue, diarrhea, dry mouth, URTI.

DRUG INTERACTIONS
Hypotension, profound sedation, coma, or respiratory depression may occur if used concomitantly w/ alcohol or other CNS depressants (eg, sedatives, anxiolytics, hypnotics); monitor and consider dose reduction of one or both drugs. Closely monitor elderly, cachectic, and debilitated patients when therapy is coadministered w/ other drugs that depress respiration. Avoid w/ Class IA antiarrhythmics (eg, quinidine, procainamide, disopyramide) or Class III antiarrhythmics (eg, sotalol, amiodarone, dofetilide), or other medications that prolong the QT interval. Closely monitor w/ concomitant benzodiazepines; coma and death associated w/ the misuse/abuse of the combination reported. CYP3A4 inhibitors may increase levels, resulting in increased/prolonged opioid effects, particularly when an inhibitor is added after a stable dose of therapy is achieved. If concomitant use of a CYP3A4 inhibitor is necessary, consider dose reduction of Belbuca and monitor for respiratory depression/sedation at frequent intervals; if a CYP3A4 inhibitor is discontinued, consider increasing Belbuca dose and monitor for signs of opioid withdrawal. CYP3A4 inducers may decrease levels, potentially resulting in decreased efficacy or onset of a withdrawal syndrome. If concomitant use of a CYP3A4 inducer is necessary, consider increasing Belbuca dose and monitor for signs of opioid withdrawal; if a CYP3A4 inducer is discontinued, consider Belbuca dose reduction and monitor for signs of respiratory depression. Avoid w/ mixed agonist/antagonist and partial agonist opioid analgesics (eg, butorphanol, nalbuphine, pentazocine); may reduce analgesic effect and/or precipitate withdrawal symptoms. May enhance neuromuscular blocking action of skeletal muscle relaxants and produce an increased degree of respiratory depression; monitor and decrease dose of therapy and/or the muscle relaxant as necessary. May reduce efficacy of diuretics; monitor for signs of diminished diuresis and/or effects on BP and increase diuretic dose prn. Concomitant use w/ anticholinergics may increase risk of urinary retention and/or severe constipation, which may lead to paralytic ileus; monitor for signs of urinary retention or reduced gastric motility. Monitor dose of patients on chronic treatment if non-nucleoside reverse transcriptase inhibitors are added to treatment regimen. Certain protease inhibitors w/ CYP3A4 inhibitory activity (atazanavir and atazanavir/ritonavir [RTV]) resulted in elevated levels of buprenorphine and norbuprenorphine; monitor patients taking atazanavir w/ and w/o RTV, and dose reduction of Belbuca may be warranted.

PREGNANCY AND LACTATION
Pregnancy: There are no adequate and well-controlled studies in pregnant women. Prolonged use of opioid analgesics during pregnancy can result in physical dependence in the neonate and neonatal opioid withdrawal syndrome shortly after birth; observe newborns for symptoms of neonatal opioid withdrawal

syndrome and manage accordingly. Not recommended for use in women immediately prior to labor, when shorter-acting analgesics or other analgesic techniques are more appropriate.

Lactation: Present in low levels in human milk and infant urine; breastfeeding is not recommended during treatment. Monitor infants exposed to therapy through breast milk for excess sedation/respiratory depression. Withdrawal symptoms can occur in breastfed infants when maternal administration of buprenorphine is stopped or when breastfeeding is stopped.

MECHANISM OF ACTION
Opioid analgesic; partial agonist at the mu-opioid receptor and an antagonist at the kappa-opioid receptor.

PHARMACOKINETICS
Absorption: Absolute bioavailability (46-65%). 75mcg Single Dose: C_{max}=0.17ng/mL; T_{max} (median)=3 hrs; AUC_{0-inf}=0.63 hr•ng/mL. 300mcg Single Dose: C_{max}=0.47ng/mL; T_{max} (median)=2.5 hrs; AUC_{0-inf}=2.3 hr•ng/mL. 1200mcg Single Dose: C_{max}=1.43ng/mL; T_{max} (median)=3 hrs; AUC_{0-inf}=10.5 hr•ng/mL. **Distribution:** Plasma protein binding (96%, primarily to α and β globulin). Crosses placenta; found in breast milk. **Metabolism:** Extensive in the liver. Undergoes both N-dealkylation (primarily via CYP3A4) to norbuprenorphine (major metabolite) and glucuronidation. **Elimination:** Urine (30%; unchanged and metabolites), feces (69%; unchanged and metabolites). $T_{1/2}$=27.6 hrs.

PATIENT CONSIDERATIONS
Assessment: Assess for hypersensitivity to therapy, risk of addiction/abuse/misuse, respiratory depression, mucositis, GI obstruction, circulatory shock, chronic pulmonary disease, long QT syndrome, impaired consciousness or coma, biliary tract disease, seizure disorders, hepatic impairment, other conditions where treatment is contraindicated or cautioned, pregnancy/nursing status, and possible drug interactions. Obtain baseline liver enzyme levels in patients at increased risk of hepatotoxicity.

Monitoring: Monitor for respiratory depression (especially w/in the first 24-72 hrs of initiating therapy and following dose increases), misuse/abuse, QTc prolongation, severe hypotension, hepatotoxicity, hypersensitivity, bronchospasm, angioneurotic edema, anaphylactic shock, spasm of the sphincter of Oddi, serum amylase increases, worsened seizure control in patients w/ history of seizure disorders, and other adverse reactions. Monitor cancer patients w/ oral mucositis for signs/symptoms of toxicity/overdose. Periodically monitor ECG in patients w/ hypokalemia, hypomagnesemia, or clinically unstable cardiac disease. Periodically monitor liver enzyme levels in patients at increased risk of hepatotoxicity. Periodically reassess the continued need for therapy.

Counseling: Advise about risks/benefits of therapy. Inform that use of therapy, even when taken as recommended, can result in addiction, abuse, and misuse; instruct not to share w/ others and to take steps to protect from theft or misuse. Inform of the risk of life-threatening respiratory depression; advise how to recognize respiratory depression and instruct to seek medical attention if breathing difficulties develop. Inform that accidental exposure, especially in children, may result in respiratory depression or death; instruct to store securely and to dispose of unused product by opening unused packages and flushing the film down the toilet. Inform about interaction w/ alcohol, other CNS depressants, and benzodiazepines. Inform that therapy may cause orthostatic hypotension and syncope; instruct how to recognize symptoms of low BP and how to reduce risk of serious consequences should hypotension occur (eg, sit or lie down, carefully rise from a sitting or lying position). Advise of the risk for severe constipation and anaphylaxis. Inform that therapy may impair ability to perform potentially hazardous activities (eg, driving a car or operating heavy machinery); advise not to perform such tasks until effects of medication are known. Inform of risk of neonatal opioid withdrawal syndrome, and inform that therapy may cause fetal harm; instruct to inform healthcare provider of a known or suspected pregnancy. Inform that breastfeeding is not recommended during treatment. Inform about important administration and disposal instructions.

BELEODAQ — belinostat   Rx
Class: Histone deacetylase (HDAC) inhibitor

▲ADULT DOSAGE
Peripheral T-Cell Lymphoma

Relapsed or Refractory:
1000mg/m² IV infusion over 30 min qd on Days 1-5 of a 21-day cycle

May repeat cycles every 21 days until disease progression or unacceptable toxicity

Dosing Based on Genotype Consideration

Patients Homozygous for the UGT1A1*28 Allele:
Reduce starting dose to 750mg/m²

▲PEDIATRIC DOSAGE
Pediatric use may not have been established

DOSING CONSIDERATIONS
Adverse Reactions
Hematologic Toxicities:
Nadir ANC <0.5 x 10⁹/L (Any Platelet Count): Decrease dose by 25% (750mg/m²)
Platelet Count <25 x 10⁹/L (Any Nadir ANC): Decrease dose by 25% (750mg/m²)
Recurrent Nadir ANC <0.5 x 10⁹/L and/or Recurrent Platelet Count <25 x 10⁹/L
After 2 Dosage Reductions: D/C therapy

Nonhematologic Toxicities:
Any CTCAE Grade 3 or 4 Adverse Reaction: Decrease dose by 25% (750mg/m²); for N/V, and diarrhea, only dose modify if the duration is >7 days w/ supportive management
Recurrence of CTCAE Grade 3 or 4 Adverse Reaction After 2 Dosage Reductions: D/C therapy

ADMINISTRATION
IV route

Reconstitution and Infusion Instructions
1. Add 9mL of sterile water for inj into the vial w/ a suitable syringe to achieve a concentration of 50mg/mL
2. Swirl the contents of the vial until there are no visible particles in the resulting sol
3. Withdraw the volume needed for the required dosage (based on the 50mg/mL concentration and the patient's BSA) and transfer to an infusion bag containing 250mL of 0.9% NaCl inj
4. Connect the infusion bag containing drug sol to an infusion set w/ a 0.22μm in-line filter for administration
5. Infuse over 30 min; may extend to 45 min if infusion-site pain or other symptoms potentially attributable to the infusion occur

STORAGE
20-25°C (68-77°F); excursions permitted between 15-30°C (59-86°F). Retain in original package until use. Reconstituted Sol: 15-25°C (59-77°F) for up to 12 hrs. Infusion Bag with Drug Sol: 15-25°C (59-77°F) for up to 36 hrs including infusion time.

HOW SUPPLIED
Inj: 500mg

WARNINGS/PRECAUTIONS
May cause thrombocytopenia, leukopenia (neutropenia and lymphopenia), and/or anemia. Serious and sometimes fatal infections, including pneumonia and sepsis, reported; do not administer to patients with an active infection. Patients with a history of extensive or intensive chemotherapy may be at higher risk of life-threatening infections. May cause fatal hepatotoxicity and LFT abnormalities. Tumor lysis syndrome (TLS) reported; caution with advanced stage disease and/or high tumor burden. N/V and diarrhea reported and may require the use of antiemetic and antidiarrheal medications. May cause fetal harm.

ADVERSE REACTIONS
N/V, fatigue, pyrexia, anemia, constipation, diarrhea, dyspnea, rash, peripheral edema, cough, thrombocytopenia, pruritus, chills, increased blood lactate dehydrogenase, decreased appetite.

DRUG INTERACTIONS
Avoid with strong UGT1A1 inhibitors.

PREGNANCY AND LACTATION
Category D, not for use in nursing.

MECHANISM OF ACTION
Histone deacetylase inhibitor; causes the accumulation of acetylated histones and other proteins, inducing cell cycle arrest and/or apoptosis of some transformed cells. Shows preferential cytotoxicity towards tumor cells compared to normal cells.

PHARMACOKINETICS
Distribution: Plasma protein binding (92.9-95.8%). **Metabolism:** Liver by UGT1A1 (primary); belinostat amide and belinostat acid (by CYP2A6, CYP2C9, and CYP3A4), methyl belinostat, 3-(anilinosulfonyl)-benzenecarboxylic acid, and belinostat glucuronide (major metabolites). **Elimination:** Urine (<2%, unchanged); $T_{1/2}$=1.1 hrs.

PATIENT CONSIDERATIONS
Assessment: Assess for active infection, history of extensive or intensive chemotherapy, advanced stage disease and/or high tumor burden, reduced UGT1A1 activity, pregnancy/nursing status, and possible drug interactions. Obtain baseline CBCs. Perform serum chemistry tests, including renal and hepatic functions, prior to the start of the 1st dose of each cycle.

Monitoring: Monitor for signs/symptoms of hematologic/hepatic/GI toxicity, infections, TLS, and other adverse reactions. Monitor CBCs weekly.

Counseling: Instruct to report symptoms of N/V, diarrhea, thrombocytopenia, leukopenia, anemia, and infection. Inform of the potential risk to the fetus and for women to avoid pregnancy while receiving therapy. Advise to understand the importance of monitoring LFT abnormalities and to immediately report potential symptoms of liver injury.

BELSOMRA — suvorexant   CIV
Class: Orexin receptor antagonist

ADULT DOSAGE
Insomnia

Treatment of insomnia characterized by difficulties w/ sleep onset and/or sleep maintenance

10mg, taken no more than once per night and w/in 30 min of going to bed, w/ at least 7 hrs remaining before planned time of awakening
Titrate: May increase dose if 10mg is well tolerated but not effective
Max: 20mg qd

PEDIATRIC DOSAGE
Pediatric use may not have been established

DOSING CONSIDERATIONS
Concomitant Medications
Other CNS Depressants:
Dose adjustment of suvorexant and/or the other drug(s) may be necessary

Moderate CYP3A Inhibitors:
Recommended Dose: 5mg
Max: 10mg

Strong CYP3A Inhibitors:
Not recommended

Hepatic Impairment
Severe: Not recommended

ADMINISTRATION
Oral route

May be taken w/ or w/o food; however, for faster sleep onset, do not administer w/ or soon after a meal.

STORAGE
20-25°C (68-77°F); excursions permitted to 15-30°C (59-86°F). Protect from light and moisture.

HOW SUPPLIED
Tab: 5mg, 10mg, 15mg, 20mg

CONTRAINDICATIONS
Narcolepsy.

WARNINGS/PRECAUTIONS
Exposure is increased in obese patients and in women. Particularly in obese women, the increased risk of exposure-related adverse effects should be considered before increasing the dose. May impair mental/physical abilities. Risk of next-day impairment, including impaired driving, is increased if taken w/ less than a full night of sleep remaining or if a higher than recommended dose is taken. Initiate only after careful evaluation of patient; failure of insomnia to remit after 7-10 days of treatment may indicate presence of a primary psychiatric and/or medical illness. Variety of cognitive and behavioral changes (eg, amnesia, anxiety, hallucinations) reported. Complex behaviors (eg, sleep-driving) may occur; strongly consider discontinuation for patients who report any complex sleep behavior. Worsening of depression and suicidal thoughts and actions (including completed suicides) reported in primarily depressed patients treated w/ sedative-hypnotics; immediately evaluate patients w/ suicidal ideation or any new behavioral sign/symptom. Increase in suicidal ideation was observed to be dose-dependent in patients taking suvorexant. Consider effects on respiratory function when prescribing to patients w/ compromised respiratory function. Sleep paralysis and hypnagogic/hypnopompic hallucinations, including vivid and disturbing perceptions by the patient, may occur. Symptoms similar to mild cataplexy may occur, w/ risk increasing w/ the dose. Has an abuse potential; carefully monitor patients w/ a history of abuse or addiction to alcohol or other drugs.

ADVERSE REACTIONS
Somnolence, headache, dizziness.

DRUG INTERACTIONS
See Dosing Considerations. Coadministration w/ other CNS depressants (eg, benzodiazepines, opioids, TCAs, alcohol) increases the risk of CNS depression, abnormal thinking, and behavioral changes. Avoid w/ alcohol. The risk of next-day impairment is increased if coadministered w/ other CNS depressants or other drugs that increase suvorexant levels. Not recommended w/ other drugs used to treat insomnia. Strong CYP3A inducers (eg, rifampin, carbamazepine, phenytoin) may substantially decrease exposure and reduce efficacy. Concomitant administration w/ digoxin slightly increased digoxin levels; monitor digoxin levels during coadministration.

PREGNANCY AND LACTATION
Pregnancy: Category C.
Lactation: Caution in nursing.

MECHANISM OF ACTION
Selective orexin receptor antagonist; blocks the binding of wake-promoting neuropeptides orexin A and orexin B to receptors OX1R and OX2R, thereby suppressing wake drive.

PHARMACOKINETICS
Absorption: Absolute bioavailability (82%); T_{max}=2 hrs (median). **Distribution:** V_d=49L; plasma protein binding (>99%, albumin and α1-acid glycoprotein). **Metabolism:** Liver via CYP3A (primary) and CYP2C19 (minor); hydroxy-suvorexant (inactive metabolite). **Elimination:** Feces (approx 66%), urine (23%); $T_{1/2}$=12 hrs.

PATIENT CONSIDERATIONS
Assessment: Assess for narcolepsy, physical and/or psychiatric disorders, depression, suicidal ideation, compromised respiratory function, severe hepatic impairment, history of abuse/addiction to alcohol or other drugs, pregnancy/nursing status, and possible drug interactions.

Monitoring: Monitor for somnolence, CNS depressant effects, next-day impairment, cognitive and behavioral changes, complex behaviors, worsening of depression/suicidal ideation, sleep paralysis, hypnagogic/hypnopompic hallucinations, cataplexy-like symptoms, abuse, and other adverse reactions.

Counseling: Caution against driving or engaging in other activities requiring full alertness w/in 8 hrs of taking suvorexant. Instruct to contact physician if sleep-driving or other complex behaviors occur. Advise to report any worsening of depression or suicidal thoughts immediately. Advise not to take suvorexant if patient drank alcohol that evening or before bed. Advise to take only when preparing for or getting into bed and only if patient can stay in bed for a full night before being active again. Advise to report all prescription and nonprescription medicines to the physician.

BELVIQ — lorcaserin hydrochloride **CIV**
Class: Serotonin 2C receptor agonist

ADULT DOSAGE
Weight Loss
Adjunct to reduced-calorie diet and increased physical activity for chronic weight management in patients w/ initial BMI ≥30kg/m², or ≥27kg/m² in the presence of ≥1 weight-related comorbid condition

Usual: 10mg bid

Evaluate response to therapy by Week 12; d/c therapy if patient has not lost at least 5% of baseline weight

PEDIATRIC DOSAGE
Pediatric use may not have been established

ADMINISTRATION
Oral route

Take w/ or w/o food

STORAGE
25°C (77°F); excursions permitted to 15-30°C (59-86°F).

HOW SUPPLIED
Tab: 10mg

CONTRAINDICATIONS
Pregnancy.

WARNINGS/PRECAUTIONS
Potentially life-threatening serotonin syndrome or neuroleptic malignant syndrome (NMS)-like reactions reported; monitor for emergence of serotonin syndrome or NMS-like signs/symptoms. Regurgitant cardiac valvular disease reported; evaluate and consider discontinuation of therapy if signs/symptoms of valvular heart disease develop. Caution with chronic heart failure (CHF). May impair mental/physical abilities. Monitor for emergence or worsening of depression, suicidal thoughts or behavior, and/or any unusual changes in mood or behavior; d/c in patients who experience suicidal thoughts or behaviors. Hypoglycemia reported; measure blood glucose levels prior to and during therapy in patients with type 2 diabetes. Caution in men who have conditions that might predispose them to priapism, or in men with anatomical deformation of the penis. Caution with bradycardia or history of heart block >1st degree, moderate renal impairment, and severe hepatic impairment. Not recommended with severe renal impairment or ESRD. Decrease in WBCs and RBCs reported; consider monitoring CBC periodically during therapy. May elevate prolactin levels. May increase risk for pulmonary HTN.

ADVERSE REACTIONS
Nasopharyngitis, headache, constipation, diarrhea, hypoglycemia, cough, dizziness, fatigue, back pain, N/V, dry mouth, URTI, peripheral edema, UTI, muscle spasms.

DRUG INTERACTIONS
Use extreme caution, particularly during initiation and dose increases, with drugs that may affect the serotonergic neurotransmitter system (eg, triptans, drugs that impair metabolism of serotonin including MAOIs [eg, linezolid], SSRIs, SNRIs, dextromethorphan, TCAs, bupropion, lithium, tramadol, tryptophan, St. John's wort, antipsychotics, other dopamine antagonists); d/c lorcaserin and any concomitant serotonergic or antidopaminergic agents immediately if serotonin syndrome occurs. Consider decreasing dose of non-glucose dependent antidiabetic medications in order to mitigate risk of hypoglycemia. Caution with CYP2D6 substrates. Avoid with serotonergic and dopaminergic drugs that are potent $5-HT_{2B}$ receptor agonists and are known to increase the risk for cardiac valvulopathy (eg, cabergoline). Caution with medications indicated for erectile dysfunction (eg, PDE-5 inhibitors).

PREGNANCY AND LACTATION
Category X, not for use in nursing.

MECHANISM OF ACTION
Serotonin 2C receptor agonist; not established. Believed to decrease food consumption and promote satiety by selectively activating $5-HT_{2C}$ receptors on anorexigenic pro-opiomelanocortin neurons located in the hypothalamus.

PHARMACOKINETICS
Absorption: T_{max}=1.5-2 hrs. **Distribution:** Plasma protein binding (70%). **Metabolism:** Liver (extensive); lorcaserin sulfamate (M1) (major circulating metabolite), N-carbamoyl glucuronide lorcaserin (major metabolite in urine). **Elimination:** Urine (92.3%), feces (2.2%); $T_{1/2}$=11 hrs.

PATIENT CONSIDERATIONS
Assessment: Assess for CHF, bradycardia or history of heart block >1st degree, renal/hepatic impairment, pregnancy/nursing status, and possible drug interactions. Assess for conditions in men that might predispose them to priapism and assess for anatomical deformities of the penis. Assess baseline body weight and CBC. Assess baseline blood glucose levels in patients with type 2 diabetes.

Monitoring: Monitor for signs/symptoms of serotonin syndrome or NMS-like reactions, valvular heart disease, emergence or worsening of depression, suicidal thoughts or behavior, any unusual changes in mood or behavior, and other adverse reactions. Monitor CBC periodically during therapy. Monitor blood glucose levels in patients with type 2 diabetes. Evaluate response to treatment by Week 12 of therapy.

Counseling: Inform about the risk and benefits of the drug. Inform that therapy is indicated for chronic weight management only in conjunction with a reduced-calorie diet and increased physical activity. Instruct to d/c therapy if patient has not achieved 5% weight loss by 12 weeks of therapy. Inform of the possibility of serotonin or NMS-like reactions. Instruct to use caution when operating hazardous machinery, including automobiles, until aware of the effects of the medication. Instruct not to increase the dose. Instruct to notify physician if signs/symptoms of valvular heart disease, emergence or worsening of depression, suicidal thoughts or behavior, or if any unusual changes in mood or behavior develop. Instruct men who have an erection lasting >4 hrs to immediately d/c and seek emergency medical attention. Advise to avoid pregnancy/breastfeeding while on therapy and to inform physician if planning to get pregnant/breastfeed. Instruct to inform physician about all medications, nutritional supplements, and vitamins that patient is taking while on therapy.

BENAZEPRIL — benazepril hydrochloride　　Rx

Class: ACE inhibitor

> D/C when pregnancy is detected. Drugs that act directly on the renin-angiotensin system (RAS) can cause injury/death to the developing fetus.

OTHER BRAND NAMES
Lotensin

ADULT DOSAGE
Hypertension

Initial: 10mg qd; 5mg qd in patients on a diuretic
Maint: 20-40mg/day as single dose or in 2 equally divided doses. A dose of 80mg gives an increased response, but experience w/ this dose is limited
May add a low dose of diuretic if BP is not controlled

PEDIATRIC DOSAGE
Hypertension

≥6 Years:
Initial: 0.2mg/kg qd
Max: 0.6mg/kg qd (or 40mg/day)

DOSING CONSIDERATIONS
Renal Impairment
Adults:
GFR <30mL/min/1.73m² (SrCr >3mg/dL):
Initial: 5mg qd
Titrate: May increase until BP is controlled
Max: 40mg/day
Pediatric Patients:
GFR <30mL/min/1.73m²: Not recommended

ADMINISTRATION
Oral route
Preparation of Sus (for 150mL of a 2mg/mL Sus):
1. Add 75mL of Ora-Plus oral suspending vehicle to an amber polyethylene terephthalate (PET) bottle containing 15 benazepril 20mg tabs, and shake for at least 2 min.
2. Allow the sus to stand for a minimum of 1 hr.
3. After the standing time, shake the sus for a minimum of 1 additional min.
4. Add 75mL of Ora-Sweet oral syrup vehicle to the bottle and shake the sus to disperse the ingredients.
5. Store the sus at 2-8°C (36-46°F) for up to 30 days in the PET bottle.
6. Shake before each use.

STORAGE
20-25°C (68-77°F); excursions permitted to 15-30°C (59-86°F). Protect from moisture. **Lotensin:** ≤30°C (86°F). Protect from moisture.

HOW SUPPLIED
Tab: 5mg; (Lotensin) 10mg, 20mg, 40mg

CONTRAINDICATIONS
Hypersensitivity to benazepril or to any other ACE inhibitors, history of angioedema w/ or w/o previous ACE inhibitor treatment, coadministration w/ aliskiren in patients w/ diabetes.

WARNINGS/PRECAUTIONS
Head/neck angioedema reported; d/c and institute appropriate therapy immediately. Patients w/ a history of angioedema unrelated to ACE inhibitor therapy may be at increased risk of angioedema during therapy. Higher rate of angioedema in blacks than nonblacks. Intestinal angioedema reported. Anaphylactoid reactions reported during desensitization w/ hymenoptera venom, dialysis w/ high-flux membranes, and LDL apheresis w/ dextran sulfate absorption. May cause changes in renal function, including acute renal failure, especially in patients whose renal function may depend on the activity of the RAS; consider withholding or discontinuing therapy if a clinically significant decrease in renal function develops. May cause symptomatic hypotension, sometimes complicated by oliguria, progressive azotemia, acute renal failure, or death; closely monitor patients at risk of excessive hypotension for the first 2 weeks of treatment and whenever the dose of benazepril and/or diuretic is increased; correct by volume expansion if hypotension occurs. Avoid in patients who are hemodynamically unstable after acute MI. Hypotension may occur w/ major surgery or during anesthesia. May cause hyperkalemia; periodically monitor serum K⁺ during therapy. Associated w/ a syndrome that starts w/ cholestatic jaundice and progresses to fulminant hepatic necrosis and (sometimes) death; d/c therapy if jaundice or marked hepatic enzymes elevations develop. Less antihypertensive effect in blacks than in nonblacks as monotherapy. Caution in elderly.

ADVERSE REACTIONS
Headache, dizziness.

DRUG INTERACTIONS
See Contraindications. Initiation of therapy in patients on diuretics (especially those in whom diuretic therapy was recently instituted) may result in excessive reduction of BP; d/c or decrease the dose of diuretic prior to initiation of treatment w/ benazepril to minimize the possibility of hypotensive effects. K⁺-sparing diuretics (eg, spironolactone, amiloride, triamterene) may increase risk of hyperkalemia; frequently monitor serum K⁺ if concomitant use of such agents is indicated. Attenuates K⁺ loss caused by thiazide-type diuretics. Increased risk of hyperkalemia w/ K⁺-containing salt substitutes or K⁺ supplements. Concomitant administration w/ antidiabetic medicines (insulins, oral hypoglycemic agents) may increase risk of hypoglycemia. Coadministration of NSAIDs, including selective COX-2 inhibitors, in patients who are elderly, volume-depleted, or w/ compromised renal function, may result in deterioration of renal function, including possible acute renal failure; monitor renal function periodically in patients receiving concomitant therapy w/ NSAIDs. Antihypertensive effect may be attenuated by NSAIDs. Dual blockade of the RAS is associated w/ increased risks of hypotension, hyperkalemia, and changes in renal function (including acute renal failure); in general, avoid combined use of RAS inhibitors, or closely monitor BP, renal function, and electrolytes w/ concomitant agents that affect the RAS. Avoid w/ aliskiren in patients w/ renal impairment (GFR <60mL/min). Coadministration w/ mammalian target of rapamycin (mTOR) inhibitor (eg, temsirolimus, sirolimus, everolimus) therapy may increase risk for angioedema; monitor for signs of angioedema. Lithium toxicity reported; monitor serum lithium levels during concurrent use. Nitritoid reactions reported w/ injectable gold.

PREGNANCY AND LACTATION
Pregnancy: Category D.
Lactation: Safety not known in nursing.

MECHANISM OF ACTION
ACE inhibitor; decreases plasma angiotensin II, leading to decreased vasopressor activity and aldosterone secretion.

PHARMACOKINETICS
Absorption: T_{max}=0.5-1 hr, 1-2 hrs (benazeprilat). **Distribution:** Plasma protein binding (96.7%, 95.3% benazeprilat); crosses placenta; found in breast milk. **Metabolism:** Liver, cleavage of ester group; benazeprilat (active metabolite). Both benazepril and benazeprilat undergo glucuronidation. **Elimination:** Urine (20% benazeprilat, 8% benazeprilat glucuronide, 4% benazepril glucuronide, and as trace amounts of benazepril), bile (11-12%, benazeprilat); $T_{1/2}$=10-11 hrs (benazeprilat).
Refer to PI for PK parameters in pediatric patients.

PATIENT CONSIDERATIONS
Assessment: Assess for history of angioedema w/ or w/o previous ACE inhibitor treatment, hypersensitivity to drug, risk factors for hyperkalemia, risk of excessive hypotension, renal impairment, pregnancy/nursing status, and possible drug interactions.

Monitoring: Monitor for angioedema, anaphylactoid reactions, hyperkalemia, and other adverse reactions. Monitor BP, LFTs, serum K⁺, and renal function.

Counseling: Inform female patients of childbearing age about the consequences of exposure to benazepril during pregnancy and discuss treatment options w/ women planning to become pregnant; instruct to report pregnancies to physician as soon as possible. Advise to d/c therapy and to immediately report to physician signs/symptoms of angioedema. Instruct to report to physician lightheadedness, especially during the 1st few days of therapy; if syncope occurs, advise to d/c therapy until physician is consulted. Inform that excessive perspiration, dehydration, and other causes of volume depletion (eg, vomiting, diarrhea) may lead to an excessive fall in BP. Instruct not to use K⁺ supplements or salt substitutes containing K⁺ w/o consulting physician. Advise diabetic patients treated w/ oral antidiabetic agents or insulin to closely monitor for hypoglycemia, especially during the 1st month of combined use.

BENDEKA — bendamustine hydrochloride　　Rx

Class: Alkylating agent

ADULT DOSAGE
Chronic Lymphocytic Leukemia

100mg/m² IV over 10 min on Days 1 and 2 of a 28-day cycle, up to 6 cycles

B-Cell Non-Hodgkin Lymphoma

Indolent B-cell non-Hodgkin lymphoma that has progressed during or w/in 6 months of treatment w/ rituximab or a rituximab-containing regimen

120mg/m² IV over 10 min on Days 1 and 2 of a 21-day cycle, up to 8 cycles

PEDIATRIC DOSAGE
Pediatric use may not have been established

DOSING CONSIDERATIONS
Renal Impairment
CrCl <40mL/min: Not recommended for use
Hepatic Impairment
Moderate (AST or ALT 2.5-10X ULN and Total Bilirubin 1.5-3X ULN): Not recommended for use
Severe (Total Bilirubin >3X ULN): Not recommended for use

Adverse Reactions

Treatment Delay:

Grade 4 Hematologic Toxicity: Delay administration

Clinically Significant ≥Grade 2 Nonhematologic Toxicity: Delay administration

May reinitiate once nonhematologic toxicity has recovered to ≤Grade 1 and/or blood counts have improved (ANC ≥1 x 10^9/L, platelets ≥75 x 10^9/L); dose reduction may be warranted

Chronic Lymphocytic Leukemia (CLL):

Hematologic Toxicity:

≥Grade 3: Reduce to 50mg/m² on Days 1 and 2 of each cycle; if ≥Grade 3 toxicity recurs, reduce to 25mg/m² on Days 1 and 2 of each cycle

Nonhematologic Toxicity:

≥Grade 3: Reduce to 50mg/m² on Days 1 and 2 of each cycle

May consider dose re-escalation in subsequent cycles

B-Cell Non-Hodgkin Lymphoma:

Hematologic Toxicity:

Grade 4: Reduce to 90mg/m² on Days 1 and 2 of each cycle; if Grade 4 toxicity recurs, reduce dose to 60mg/m² on Days 1 and 2 of each cycle

Nonhematologic Toxicity:

≥Grade 3: Reduce to 90mg/m² on Days 1 and 2 of each cycle; if ≥Grade 3 toxicity recurs, reduce to 60mg/m² on Days 1 and 2 of each cycle

ADMINISTRATION

IV route

Cytotoxic drug; follow applicable special handling and disposal procedures.

Preparation

Allow vial to reach room temperature (15-30°C or 59-86°F) prior to use. Contents may partially freeze when refrigerated; if particulate matter is observed after achieving room temperature, do not use.

Aseptically withdraw the volume needed for the required dose from the 25mg/mL sol and immediately transfer the sol to a 50mL infusion bag of 0.9% NaCl inj, or 2.5% dextrose/0.45% NaCl inj, or D5 inj.

After transferring, thoroughly mix the contents of the infusion bag; the resulting final concentration should be w/in 1.85-5.6mg/mL.

Admixture Stability

Contains no antimicrobial preservative; prepare admixture as close as possible to the time of administration.

If diluted w/ 0.9% NaCl or 2.5% dextrose/0.45% NaCl inj, the final admixture is stable for 24 hrs when stored at 2-8°C (36-46°F) or for 6 hrs when stored at 15-30°C (59-86°F) and room light; administration must be completed w/in this period of time.

If diluted w/ D5 inj, the final admixture is stable for 24 hrs when stored at 2-8°C (36-46°F) or for 3 hrs when stored at 15-30°C (59-86°F) and room light; administration must be completed w/in this period of time.

Stability of Partially Used Vials

Stable for up to 28 days when stored in original carton at 2-8°C (36-46°F); each vial is not recommended for >6 dose withdrawals.

Refer to PI for further administration instructions.

STORAGE

2-8°C (36-46°F). Protect from light.

HOW SUPPLIED

Inj: 100mg/4mL

CONTRAINDICATIONS

Known hypersensitivity (eg, anaphylactic and anaphylactoid reactions) to bendamustine, polyethylene glycol 400, propylene glycol, or monothioglycerol.

WARNINGS/PRECAUTIONS

Severe myelosuppression reported; may require dose delays and/or subsequent dose reductions if recovery to the recommended values has not occurred by the 1st day of the next scheduled cycle. Frequently monitor CBC, including leukocytes, platelets, Hgb, and neutrophils. Infection (eg, pneumonia, sepsis, septic shock, hepatitis) and death reported. Increased risk for reactivation of infections (eg, hepatitis B, cytomegalovirus, mycobacterium tuberculosis, herpes zoster); perform appropriate measures for infection and infection reactivation prior to administration. Infusion reactions and severe anaphylactic/anaphylactoid reactions reported; monitor clinically and d/c for severe reactions. Consider measures to prevent severe reactions (eg, antihistamines, antipyretics, corticosteroids) in subsequent cycles in patients who have experienced Grade 1 or 2 infusion reactions. Consider discontinuation for Grade 3 infusion reactions as clinically appropriate; d/c for Grade 4 infusion reactions. Patients who experience ≥Grade 3 allergic-type reactions were not typically rechallenged. Tumor lysis syndrome reported; preventive measures include vigorous hydration and close monitoring of blood chemistry, particularly K⁺ and uric acid levels. Skin reactions (eg, rash, toxic skin reactions, bullous exanthema) reported; monitor closely and withhold or d/c if skin reactions are severe or progressive. Premalignant and malignant diseases (eg, myelodysplastic syndrome, myeloproliferative disorders, acute myeloid leukemia, bronchial carcinoma) reported. Extravasations reported; assure good venous access prior to starting infusion and monitor for infusion-site redness, swelling, pain, infection, and necrosis during and after administration. May cause fetal harm. Caution w/ mild/moderate renal impairment and w/ mild hepatic impairment.

ADVERSE REACTIONS

CLL: Pyrexia, N/V.

Non-Hodgkin Lymphoma: N/V, fatigue, diarrhea, pyrexia.

DRUG INTERACTIONS

CYP1A2 inhibitors (eg, fluvoxamine, ciprofloxacin) may increase plasma concentrations of bendamustine and may decrease plasma concentrations of active metabolites. CYP1A2 inducers (eg, omeprazole, smoking) may decrease plasma concentrations of bendamustine and may increase plasma concentrations of active

metabolites. Use caution or consider alternative treatments if treatment w/ CYP1A2 inhibitors/inducers is needed. May increase risk of severe skin toxicity w/ allopurinol.

PREGNANCY AND LACTATION

Pregnancy: Category D. Avoid becoming pregnant during treatment and for 3 months after therapy has stopped; men should use reliable contraception for the same time period.

Lactation: Not for use in nursing.

MECHANISM OF ACTION

Alkylating agent; has not been established. Bifunctional mechlorethamine derivative containing a purine-like benzimidazole ring; forms electrophilic alkyl groups that form covalent bonds w/ electron-rich nucleophilic moieties, resulting in interstrand DNA crosslinks. Bifunctional covalent linkage can lead to cell death via several pathways. Active against both quiescent and dividing cells.

PHARMACOKINETICS

Absorption: C_{max}=35μg/mL. **Distribution:** Plasma protein binding (94-96%); V_d=20-25L. **Metabolism:** Extensive via hydrolytic (primary), oxidative, and conjugative pathways; gamma-hydroxy-bendamustine (M3), N-desmethyl-bendamustine (M4) (active minor metabolites) via CYP1A2. **Elimination:** Urine (50%, 3.3% unchanged, <1% as M3 and M4), feces (25%); $T_{1/2}$=40 min, 3 hrs (M3), 30 min (M4).

PATIENT CONSIDERATIONS

Assessment: Assess for renal/hepatic impairment, hypersensitivity to bendamustine and components of the product, pregnancy/nursing status, and possible drug interactions. Obtain baseline CBC and ANC should be ≥1 x 10^9/L and platelet count should be ≥75 x 10^9/L.

Monitoring: Monitor for signs/symptoms of myelosuppression, infections, anaphylaxis/infusion reactions, tumor lysis syndrome, skin reactions, premalignant/malignant diseases, extravasation, lab abnormalities, and other adverse reactions. Monitor CBCs and blood chemistry, particularly K⁺ and uric acid levels.

Counseling: Inform of the possibility of mild/serious allergic reactions and instruct to immediately report such symptoms. Inform that therapy may cause a decrease in WBC counts, platelets, and RBC counts, and of the need for frequent monitoring of blood counts; instruct to report SOB, significant fatigue, bleeding, fever, or other signs of infection. Advise that therapy may cause tiredness; instruct to avoid driving or operating dangerous tools or machinery if tiredness occurs. Inform that therapy may cause N/V, diarrhea, and mild rash or itching; instruct to report any adverse reactions immediately to physician. Advise women to avoid becoming pregnant and to use reliable contraception throughout treatment and for 3 months after discontinuation of therapy; instruct to immediately report pregnancy and to avoid nursing while on therapy. Advise men to use reliable contraception throughout treatment and for 3 months after discontinuation of therapy.

BENICAR — olmesartan medoxomil   Rx

Class: Angiotensin II receptor blocker (ARB)

> D/C when pregnancy is detected. Drugs that act directly on the renin-angiotensin system (RAS) can cause injury/death to the developing fetus.

ADULT DOSAGE	PEDIATRIC DOSAGE
Hypertension	**Hypertension**
Initial: 20mg qd when used as monotherapy in patients who are not volume-contracted	**6-16 Years:**
	20 to <35kg:
Titrate: May increase to 40mg qd after 2 weeks if needed.	**Initial:** 10mg qd
Doses >40mg do not appear to have greater effect.	**Titrate:** May increase to 20mg qd after 2 weeks if needed
	Max: 20mg qd
May add a diuretic if BP is not controlled.	**≥35kg:**
May be administered w/ other antihypertensive agents.	**Initial:** 20mg qd
	Titrate: May increase to 40mg qd after 2 weeks if needed
	Max: 40mg qd

- -

DOSING CONSIDERATIONS

Other Important Considerations

Intravascular Volume-Depleted Patients (eg, Treated w/ Diuretics):

Consider a lower initial dose and monitor closely

ADMINISTRATION

Oral route

May be administered w/ or w/o food.

For children who cannot swallow tabs, the same dose can be given using an extemporaneous sus.

Preparation of Sus (for 200mL of a 2mg/mL Sus):

1. Add 50mL of purified water to an amber polyethylene terephthalate bottle containing twenty Benicar 20mg tabs and allow to stand for a minimum of 5 min.
2. Shake the container for at least 1 min and allow the sus to stand for at least 1 min.
3. Repeat 1 min shaking and 1 min standing for 4 additional times.
4. Add 100mL of Ora-Sweet and 50mL of Ora-Plus to the sus and shake well for at least 1 min.
5. The sus should be refrigerated at 2-8°C (36-46°F) and can be stored for up to 4 weeks.
6. Shake the sus well before each use and return promptly to the refrigerator.

STORAGE

20-25°C (68-77°F).

HOW SUPPLIED

Tab: 5mg, 20mg, 40mg

CONTRAINDICATIONS

Coadministration w/ aliskiren in patients w/ diabetes.

WARNINGS/PRECAUTIONS

Children <1 year must not receive olmesartan for HTN; drugs that act directly on the renin-angiotensin aldosterone system (RAAS) can have effects on the development of immature kidneys. Symptomatic hypotension may occur after treatment initiation in patients w/ an activated RAAS, such as volume- and/or salt-depleted patients (eg, those being treated w/ high doses of diuretics). Changes in renal function may occur. Associated w/ oliguria and/or progressive azotemia and rarely w/ acute renal failure and/or death in patients whose renal function may depend on the activity of the RAAS (eg, patients w/ severe CHF). May increase SrCr or BUN levels in patients w/ renal artery stenosis. Sprue-like enteropathy w/ symptoms of severe, chronic diarrhea w/ substantial weight loss reported; exclude other etiologies if these symptoms develop, and consider discontinuation in cases where no other etiology is identified. May cause hyperkalemia; monitor serum electrolytes periodically.

ADVERSE REACTIONS

Dizziness.

DRUG INTERACTIONS

See Contraindications. NSAIDs, including selective COX-2 inhibitors, may result in deterioration of renal function, including possible acute renal failure in patients who are elderly, volume-depleted (including those on diuretic therapy), or w/ compromised renal function; monitor renal function periodically. Antihypertensive effect may be attenuated by NSAIDs including selective COX-2 inhibitors. Dual blockade of the RAS is associated w/ increased risks of hypotension, hyperkalemia, and changes in renal function (including acute renal failure); in general, avoid combined use of RAS inhibitors, or closely monitor BP, renal function, and electrolytes w/ other agents that also affect the RAS. Avoid w/ aliskiren in patients w/ renal impairment (GFR <60mL/min). Colesevelam reduces exposure and levels; consider administering olmesartan at least 4 hrs before colesevelam dose. Increases in serum lithium levels and lithium toxicity reported; monitor lithium levels.

PREGNANCY AND LACTATION

Pregnancy: Category D. Use of drugs that act on the RAS during the 2nd and 3rd trimesters of pregnancy reduces fetal renal function and increases fetal and neonatal morbidity and death. Resulting oligohydramnios can be associated w/ fetal lung hypoplasia and skeletal deformations. When pregnancy is detected, d/c therapy as soon as possible. **Lactation:** Not for use in nursing.

MECHANISM OF ACTION

ARB; blocks the vasoconstrictor effects of angiotensin II by selectively blocking the binding of angiotensin II to the AT_1 receptor in vascular smooth muscle.

PHARMACOKINETICS

Absorption: Absolute bioavailability (26%); T_{max}=1-2 hrs. **Distribution:** V_d=17L; plasma protein binding (99%). **Metabolism:** Rapid and complete by ester hydrolysis to olmesartan during absorption from the GI tract. **Elimination:** Urine (35-50%), feces; $T_{1/2}$=13 hrs.

PATIENT CONSIDERATIONS

Assessment: Assess for diabetes, CHF, renal artery stenosis, volume/salt depletion, renal impairment, pregnancy/nursing status, and possible drug interactions.

Monitoring: Monitor for signs/symptoms of hypotension, renal dysfunction, sprue-like enteropathy, and other adverse reactions. Periodically monitor electrolytes.

Counseling: Inform females of childbearing potential about the consequences of exposure to drug during pregnancy and of the treatment options for women planning to become pregnant. Instruct to report pregnancy to the physician as soon as possible.

BENICAR HCT — hydrochlorothiazide/olmesartan medoxomil   Rx

Class: Angiotensin II receptor blocker (ARB)/thiazide diuretic

> When pregnancy is detected, d/c as soon as possible. Drugs that act directly on the renin-angiotensin system (RAS) can cause injury/death to the developing fetus.

ADULT DOSAGE

Hypertension

May be used alone or in combination w/ other antihypertensive drugs

Uncontrolled BP on Olmesartan Monotherapy:
Initial: 40mg/12.5mg qd
Titrate: Dose may be titrated up to 40mg/25mg if necessary

Uncontrolled BP on HCTZ Monotherapy or Patients Experiencing Dose-Limiting Adverse Reactions w/ HCTZ:
Initial: 20mg/12.5mg qd
Titrate: Dose may be titrated up to 40mg/25mg if necessary

Patients titrated to the individual components may instead receive the corresponding dose of Benicar HCT

PEDIATRIC DOSAGE

Pediatric use may not have been established

DOSING CONSIDERATIONS

Elderly
Start at lower end of dosing range

ADMINISTRATION

Oral route

STORAGE

20-25°C (68-77°F).

HOW SUPPLIED

Tab: (Olmesartan/HCTZ) 20mg/12.5mg, 40mg/12.5mg, 40mg/25mg

CONTRAINDICATIONS

Hypersensitivity to any component of this product, anuria, coadministration w/ aliskiren in patients w/ diabetes.

WARNINGS/PRECAUTIONS

Not indicated for initial therapy. Symptomatic hypotension may occur after treatment initiation in patients w/ an activated RAS (eg, volume- or salt-depleted patients [eg, those being treated w/ high doses of diuretics]); may continue therapy w/o difficulty when electrolyte and fluid imbalances have been corrected. May cause changes in renal function, including acute renal failure; periodically monitor renal function in patients whose renal function may depend in part on the activity of the RAS (eg, patients w/ renal artery stenosis, chronic kidney disease, severe congestive heart failure, volume depletion). Consider withholding or discontinuing therapy in patients who develop a clinically significant decrease in renal function. **HCTZ:** Hypersensitivity reactions may occur in patients w/ or w/o a history of allergy or bronchial asthma, but are more likely in patients w/ such a history. May cause hypokalemia, hyponatremia, and hypomagnesemia. May alter glucose tolerance and raise serum levels of cholesterol and triglycerides. Hyperuricemia may occur or frank gout may be precipitated. Decreases urinary Ca^{2+} excretion and may cause serum Ca^{2+} elevations; monitor Ca^{2+} levels. May cause an idiosyncratic reaction, resulting in acute transient myopia and acute angle-closure glaucoma; d/c as rapidly as possible. Risk factors for developing acute angle-closure glaucoma may include a history of sulfonamide or penicillin allergy. May cause exacerbation or activation of systemic lupus erythematosus (SLE). May precipitate hepatic coma in patients w/ hepatic impairment or progressive liver disease. **Olmesartan:** May cause hyperkalemia. Sprue-like enteropathy w/ symptoms of severe, chronic diarrhea w/ substantial weight loss reported; exclude other etiologies if these symptoms develop during treatment, and consider discontinuation in cases where no other etiology is identified.

ADVERSE REACTIONS

Dizziness, URTI, hyperuricemia, nausea.

DRUG INTERACTIONS

See Contraindications. Coadministration w/ other drugs that raise serum K^+ levels may result in hyperkalemia. Increases in serum lithium concentrations and lithium toxicity reported; monitor lithium levels during concomitant use. Avoid w/ aliskiren in patients w/ renal impairment (GFR <60mL/min). **Olmesartan:** NSAIDs, including selective COX-2 inhibitors, may result in deterioration of renal function (eg, possible acute renal failure) in patients who are elderly, volume-depleted (eg, those on diuretic therapy), or w/ compromised renal function; monitor renal function periodically. NSAIDs may attenuate antihypertensive effect of olmesartan. Dual blockade of the RAS w/ ARBs, ACE inhibitors, or aliskiren, is associated w/ increased risks of hypotension, hyperkalemia, and changes in renal function (including acute renal failure); avoid combined use of RAS inhibitors, and closely monitor BP, renal function, and electrolytes w/ concomitant agents that also affect the RAS. Colesevelam reduces levels of olmesartan; consider administering olmesartan at least 4 hrs before the colesevelam dose. **HCTZ:** NSAID may reduce the diuretic, natriuretic, and antihypertensive effects of thiazide diuretics; closely monitor BP. Dose adjustment of antidiabetic drugs (eg, oral agents and insulin) may be required. Staggering the HCTZ dose and ion exchange resins (eg, cholestyramine, colestipol) such that HCTZ is administered at least 4 hrs before or 4-6 hrs after the administration of resins would potentially minimize the interaction. Corticosteroids and adrenocorticotropic hormone may intensify electrolyte depletion, particularly hypokalemia.

PREGNANCY AND LACTATION

Pregnancy: Category D. Use of drugs that act on the RAS during the 2nd and 3rd trimesters of pregnancy reduces fetal renal function and increases fetal and neonatal morbidity and death. **Lactation:** Thiazides appear in human milk. Not for use in nursing.

MECHANISM OF ACTION

Olmesartan: Angiotensin II receptor antagonist; blocks the vasoconstrictor effects of angiotensin II by selectively blocking the binding of angiotensin II to the AT_1 receptor in vascular smooth muscle. **HCTZ:** Thiazide diuretic; has not been established. Affects renal tubular mechanisms of electrolyte reabsorption, directly increasing excretion of Na^+ and Cl^- in approximately equivalent amounts, and indirectly reducing plasma volume.

PHARMACOKINETICS

Absorption: Olmesartan: Absolute bioavailability (26%); T_{max}=1-2 hrs. HCTZ: Absolute bioavailability (70%); T_{max}=2-5 hrs. **Distribution:** Olmesartan: V_d=17L; plasma protein binding (99%). HCTZ: plasma protein binding (40-70%); crosses placenta; found in breast milk. **Metabolism:** Olmesartan: Completely bioactivated by ester hydrolysis to olmesartan during absorption from the GI tract. **Elimination:** Olmesartan: Urine (35-50%), feces; $T_{1/2}$=13 hrs. HCTZ: Urine (70% unchanged); $T_{1/2}$=10 hrs.

PATIENT CONSIDERATIONS

Assessment: Assess for hypersensitivity to any components of the product, anuria, history of allergy or bronchial asthma, history of sulfonamide or penicillin allergy, volume/salt depletion, patients whose renal function may depend on the activity of the RAS, SLE, hepatic/renal impairment, pregnancy/nursing status, and possible drug interactions.

Monitoring: Monitor for symptomatic hypotension, changes in renal function, hypersensitivity reactions, electrolyte and metabolic imbalances, acute myopia and secondary angle-closure glaucoma, SLE, sprue-like enteropathy, and other adverse reactions. Periodically monitor serum electrolytes. Monitor serum K$^+$ in patients receiving other drugs that raise K$^+$ levels, and monitor Ca^{2+} levels.

Counseling: Inform females of childbearing potential of the consequences of exposure to treatment during pregnancy and of the treatment options for women planning to become pregnant. Instruct to report pregnancy to the physician as soon as possible. Inform that lightheadedness may occur, especially during the 1st days of therapy; instruct to report this symptom to physician. Advise that dehydration from inadequate fluid intake, excessive perspiration, vomiting, or diarrhea may lead to an excessive fall in BP. Instruct to contact physician if syncope occurs. Advise not to use K$^+$ supplements or salt substitutes containing K$^+$ w/o consulting physician. Instruct to d/c therapy and seek immediate medical attention if symptoms of acute myopia or secondary angle-closure glaucoma are experienced.

BENLYSTA — belimumab   Rx

Class: Monoclonal antibody/BLyS blocker

ADULT DOSAGE	PEDIATRIC DOSAGE
Systemic Lupus Erythematosus	Pediatric use may not have been established
Treatment of Patients w/ Active, Autoantibody-Positive, Systemic Lupus Erythematosus Receiving Standard Therapy:	
10mg/kg at 2-week intervals for the first 3 doses, and at 4-week intervals thereafter	
Infuse IV over a period of 1 hr	
Premedication	
Consider administering premedication for prophylaxis against infusion reactions and hypersensitivity reactions	

DOSING CONSIDERATIONS

Adverse Reactions
May slow or interrupt the infusion rate if patient develops an infusion reaction. D/C infusion immediately if patient experiences a serious hypersensitivity reaction

ADMINISTRATION
IV route

Administer by IV infusion only; do not administer as an IV push or bolus.
Must be reconstituted and diluted prior to administration.
Do not infuse concomitantly in the same IV line w/ other agents.

Reconstitution Instructions
1. Remove vial from the refrigerator and allow to stand for 10-15 min to reach room temperature.
2. Reconstitute the 120mg vial w/ 1.5mL sterile water for inj (SWFI) and the 400mg vial w/ 4.8mL SWFI; reconstituted sol will contain a concentration of 80mg/mL belimumab.
3. Direct the stream of sterile water toward the side of the vial to minimize foaming.
4. Gently swirl the vial for 60 sec.
5. Allow the vial to sit at room temperature during reconstitution, gently swirling the vial for 60 sec every 5 min until the powder is dissolved; do not shake.
6. Reconstitution is typically complete w/in 10-15 min after the sterile water has been added, but it may take up to 30 min. Protect the reconstituted sol from sunlight.
7. If a mechanical reconstitution device (swirler) is used to reconstitute belimumab, it should not exceed 500 rpm and the vial swirled for no longer than 30 min.
8. Once reconstitution is complete, the sol should be opalescent and colorless to pale yellow, and w/o particles; small air bubbles, however, are expected and acceptable.

Dilution Instructions
9. Dilute the reconstituted product to 250mL in 0.9% NaCl inj (normal saline) for IV infusion. From a 250mL infusion bag or bottle of normal saline, withdraw and discard a volume equal to the volume of the reconstituted sol required for the patient's dose, then add the required volume of the reconstituted sol into the infusion bag or bottle.
10. Gently invert the bag or bottle to mix the sol; any unused sol in the vials must be discarded.
11. If reconstituted sol is not used immediately, it should be stored protected from direct sunlight at 2-8°C (36-46°F); sol diluted in normal saline may be stored at 2-8°C (36-46°F) or room temperature. The total time from reconstitution of belimumab to completion of infusion should not exceed 8 hrs.
12. No incompatibilities between belimumab and polyvinylchloride or polyolefin bags have been observed.

STORAGE
2-8°C (36-46°F). Do not freeze. Protect from light and store vials in original carton until use. Avoid exposure to heat.

HOW SUPPLIED
Inj: 120mg [5mL], 400mg [20mL]

CONTRAINDICATIONS
History of anaphylaxis w/ belimumab.

WARNINGS/PRECAUTIONS
Deaths reported; etiologies included infection, cardiovascular disease, and suicide. Serious and sometimes fatal infections reported; caution w/ chronic infections and consider interrupting therapy if a new infection develops while undergoing treatment. Patients receiving any therapy for chronic infection should not begin therapy. JC virus-associated progressive multifocal leukoencephalopathy (PML) resulting in neurological deficits, including fatal cases, reported. Consider diagnosis of PML in any patient presenting w/ new-onset or deteriorating neurological signs/symptoms. Consider stopping therapy in patients w/ confirmed PML. Malignancies (including non-melanoma skin cancers), infusion reactions, psychiatric events (eg, depression) reported. Hypersensitivity reactions, including anaphylaxis and death, reported; d/c immediately if serious hypersensitivity reactions occur. Monitor patients during and for an appropriate period of time after administration. Caution in elderly and in black/African-American patients. Not recommended w/ severe active lupus nephritis or severe active CNS lupus.

ADVERSE REACTIONS
Serious infections, nausea, diarrhea, pyrexia, nasopharyngitis, bronchitis, insomnia, pain in extremity, depression, migraine, pharyngitis, cystitis, leukopenia, viral gastroenteritis.

DRUG INTERACTIONS
Not recommended w/ other biologics or IV cyclophosphamide. Live vaccines should not be given for 30 days before or concurrently w/ therapy; may interfere w/ the response to immunizations.

PREGNANCY AND LACTATION
Pregnancy: Category C. Women of childbearing potential should use adequate contraception during treatment and for ≥4 months after the final treatment. A pregnancy registry has been established; physicians are encouraged to register patients and pregnant women are encouraged to enroll themselves.
Lactation: Not for use in nursing.

MECHANISM OF ACTION
Monoclonal antibody/BLyS blocker; blocks binding of soluble human BLyS, a B-cell survival factor, to its receptors on B cells. Inhibits survival of B cells, including autoreactive B cells, and reduces the differentiation of B cells into immunoglobulin-producing plasma cells.

PHARMACOKINETICS
Absorption: AUC=3083mcg•day/mL; C$_{max}$=313mcg/mL. Distribution: V$_d$=5.29L; crosses placenta. Elimination: T$_{1/2}$=19.4 days.

PATIENT CONSIDERATIONS

Assessment: Assess for chronic infection, history of depression or other serious psychiatric disorders, previous anaphylaxis w/ the drug, history of multiple drug allergies or significant hypersensitivity, pregnancy/nursing status, and possible drug interactions.

Monitoring: Monitor for infusion and hypersensitivity reactions, infections, PML, malignancy, psychiatric events, and other adverse reactions.

Counseling: Inform about risks/benefits of therapy. Advise that drug may decrease ability to fight infections; instruct to notify physician if signs/symptoms of an infection develop. Advise to contact physician if new or worsening neurological symptoms (eg, memory loss, confusion, dizziness/loss of balance, difficulty talking/walking, vision problems) are experienced. Educate on the signs/symptoms of hypersensitivity and infusion reactions; instruct to immediately report symptoms of an allergic reaction during or after the administration of therapy. Instruct to contact physician if new or worsening depression, suicidal thoughts, or other mood changes develop. Inform patients that they should not receive live vaccines while on therapy. Instruct to notify physician if pregnant/planning on becoming pregnant or breastfeeding; encourage pregnant patients to enroll in the pregnancy registry.

BENZACLIN — benzoyl peroxide/clindamycin   Rx

Class: Antibacterial/keratolytic

ADULT DOSAGE	PEDIATRIC DOSAGE
Acne Vulgaris	**Acne Vulgaris**
Apply bid (am and pm) or ud to affected areas	**≥12 Years:**
	Apply bid (am and pm) or ud to affected areas

ADMINISTRATION
Topical route

Prior to application, wash skin gently, then rinse w/ warm water and pat dry. Reconstitute before dispensing; refer to PI for reconstitution instructions.

STORAGE
Room temperature up to 25°C (77°F). Do not freeze. Discard product 3 months following reconstitution.

HOW SUPPLIED
Gel: (Clindamycin/Benzoyl Peroxide) 1%/5% [25g, jar; 35g, 50g, pump]

CONTRAINDICATIONS
Hypersensitivity to any of its components or to lincomycin, history of regional enteritis, ulcerative colitis (UC), or antibiotic-associated colitis.

WARNINGS/PRECAUTIONS
Severe colitis, which may result in death, reported following oral and parenteral clindamycin administration. Diarrhea, bloody diarrhea, and colitis (including pseudomembranous colitis) reported; d/c if significant diarrhea occurs. Not for ophthalmic use. May cause overgrowth of nonsusceptible organisms, including fungi; d/c use and take appropriate measures if this occurs. Avoid contact with eyes and mucous membranes.

ADVERSE REACTIONS
Dry skin, application-site reaction.

DRUG INTERACTIONS
Antiperistaltic agents (eg, opiates, diphenoxylate with atropine) may prolong and/or worsen colitis. Caution with concomitant topical acne therapy (eg, peeling, desquamating, or abrasive agents) because of possible cumulative irritancy effect. Do not use with erythromycin-containing products.

PREGNANCY AND LACTATION
Category C, not for use in nursing.

MECHANISM OF ACTION
Antibacterial/keratolytic; individual components act against *Propionibacterium acnes*, an organism associated with acne vulgaris.

PHARMACOKINETICS
Absorption: Clindamycin: Systemic bioavailability (<1%). Benzoyl peroxide: Skin. **Distribution:** Clindamycin: (PO/Parenteral) Found in breast milk. **Metabolism:** Benzoyl peroxide: Converted to benzoic acid.

PATIENT CONSIDERATIONS
Assessment: Assess for hypersensitivity to drug or to lincomycin, history of regional enteritis, UC, or antibiotic-associated colitis, pregnancy/nursing status, and possible drug interactions.

Monitoring: Monitor for signs/symptoms of diarrhea, colitis, overgrowth of nonsusceptible organisms, and other adverse reactions. For colitis, perform stool culture and assay for *Clostridium difficile* toxin. Consider large bowel endoscopy in cases of severe diarrhea.

Counseling: Instruct to use externally ud and to avoid contact with eyes, and inside the nose, mouth, and all mucous membranes. Advise not to use for any disorder other than for which it was prescribed and not to use any other topical acne preparation unless otherwise directed by physician. Counsel to minimize or avoid exposure to natural or artificial sunlight (tanning beds or UVA/B treatment) while using medication; instruct to wear a wide-brimmed hat or other protective clothing, and use a sunscreen with SPF ≥15 to minimize exposure to sunlight. Instruct to report any signs of local adverse reactions to physician. Inform that drug may bleach hair or colored fabric.

BENZAMYCIN — benzoyl peroxide/erythromycin   Rx
Class: Antibacterial/keratolytic

ADULT DOSAGE	PEDIATRIC DOSAGE
Acne Vulgaris	**Acne Vulgaris**
Apply bid (am and pm) or ud	**≥12 Years:** Apply bid (am and pm) or ud

ADMINISTRATION
Topical route
Wash and dry skin prior to administration.
Requires thorough mixing immediately prior to each use.

STORAGE
Prior to reconstitution: 15°-30°C (59°-86°F). After reconstitution: 2°-8°C (36°-46°F). Do not freeze. Keep tightly closed. Discard after 3 months.

HOW SUPPLIED
Gel: (Benzoyl Peroxide-Erythromycin) 5%-3% [46.6g]

CONTRAINDICATIONS
Hypersensitivity to any of its components.

WARNINGS/PRECAUTIONS
D/C if severe irritation or overgrowth of nonsusceptible organisms (eg, fungi) occurs. Avoid eyes, mouth, and mucous membranes. Pseudomembranous colitis reported with nearly all antibacterial agents, including erythromycin.

ADVERSE REACTIONS
Dryness, urticaria.

DRUG INTERACTIONS
Additive irritation with peeling, desquamating, or abrasive agents. Lincomycin, chloramphenicol, and clindamycin antagonizes protein inhibition of erythromycin *in vitro*.

PREGNANCY AND LACTATION
Category C, caution in nursing.

MECHANISM OF ACTION
Antibacterial/keratolytic agent. Erythromycin: Antibacterial agent; exact mechanism of acne lesion reduction has not been established; inhibits protein synthesis by reversibly binding to 50S ribosomal subunits, thereby inhibiting translocation of aminoacyl transfer-RNA and inhibiting polypeptide synthesis. Benzoyl peroxide: Believed to act by releasing active oxygen.

PHARMACOKINETICS
Absorption: Benzoyl peroxide shown to be absorbed by skin, where it is converted to benzoic acid. **Distribution:** Orally and parenterally administered erythromycin found in breast milk.

PATIENT CONSIDERATIONS
Assessment: Assess proper diagnosis of acne vulgaris. Assess use in patients who are using other concomitant topical acne therapies. Assess use in pregnant/nursing patients.

Monitoring: Monitor for occurrence of cumulative irritancy effect when using other concomitant topical acne agents. Monitor for development of severe skin irritation and for overgrowth of nonsusceptible organisms that is associated with antibiotic usage.

Counseling: Counsel to report to physician signs of local adverse reactions (eg, skin irritation, photosensitivity reaction). Advise not to use any other topical acne preparation unless directed by physician. Advise that contact with hair or fabrics may bleach them.

BENZEFOAM — benzoyl peroxide   Rx
Class: Antibacterial/keratolytic

ADULT DOSAGE	PEDIATRIC DOSAGE
Acne Vulgaris	**Acne Vulgaris**
Mild to Moderate: Dispense into palm of hand and rub into affected area qd or ud until completely absorbed; may adjust frequency of use to obtain desired clinical response	**Mild to Moderate:** **≥12 Years:** Dispense into palm of hand and rub into affected area qd or ud until completely absorbed; may adjust frequency of use to obtain desired clinical response
Facial Acne: Use a dollop the size of a marble	**Facial Acne:** Use a dollop the size of a marble
Back/Chest Acne: Use a dollop the size of a whole walnut	**Back/Chest Acne:** Use a dollop the size of a whole walnut

---

ADMINISTRATION
Topical route

Gently cleanse affected area prior to application
Prime container before initial use
Shake vigorously before each use and gently tap bottom of can onto palm of other hand or a solid surface at least 3 times
Wipe off any excess foam from actuator after use
Wash hands with soap and water after application

Priming
1. Shake vigorously, then gently tap bottom of can onto palm of other hand or a solid surface at least 3 times
2. Remove cap and hold can upright over sink
3. Avoid contact with hair, fabrics, or carpeting as benzoyl peroxide will cause bleaching/discoloration
4. Firmly depress the actuator for 1 to 3 seconds until tab breaks and foam begins to dispense
5. If foam does not dispense within 3 seconds, repeat entire process and depress the actuator again until foam begins to dispense

STORAGE
15-25°C (59-77°F). Avoid exposure to temperatures >49°C (120°F). Protect from freezing. Store upright. Contents under pressure; do not puncture or incinerate container.

HOW SUPPLIED
Foam: 5.3% [60g]

CONTRAINDICATIONS
Hypersensitivity to benzoyl peroxide or to any of the other ingredients in the product.

WARNINGS/PRECAUTIONS
For external use only. Not for ophthalmic use. Avoid contact with eyes, eyelids, lips, and mucous membranes; rinse with water if accidental contact occurs. Avoid unnecessary sun exposure; apply sunscreen. D/C use if hypersensitivity or severe irritation develops.

ADVERSE REACTIONS
Allergic contact dermatitis, dryness.

PREGNANCY AND LACTATION
Category C, caution in nursing.

MECHANISM OF ACTION
Antibacterial/keratolytic; not established. Demonstrated antibacterial activity against *Propionibacterium acnes*.

PHARMACOKINETICS
Metabolism: Benzoic acid (metabolite). **Elimination:** Urine (as benzoate).

PATIENT CONSIDERATIONS
Assessment: Assess for previous hypersensitivity to the drug and pregnancy/nursing status.

Monitoring: Monitor for hypersensitivity reactions, allergic contact dermatitis, dryness, and irritation. Monitor clinical response.

Counseling: Instruct to use only ud and not to use to treat any condition other than that for which it was prescribed. Instruct to avoid contact with eyes, eyelids, lips, and mucous membranes; counsel to rinse with water if accidental contact occurs. Advise to d/c and consult physician if excessive redness or irritation develops. Advise to avoid contact with hair, fabrics, or carpeting; bleaching or discoloration may occur. Instruct to avoid unnecessary sun exposure and to use sunscreen.

BenzEFoam Ultra — benzoyl peroxide

Rx

Class: Antibacterial/keratolytic

ADULT DOSAGE	PEDIATRIC DOSAGE
Acne Vulgaris	**Acne Vulgaris**
Mild to Moderate:	**Mild to Moderate:**
Initial: Apply qd	**≥12 Years:**
Titrate: Gradually increase to bid-tid prn; if bothersome dryness or peeling occurs, reduce frequency to qd or qod	**Initial:** Apply qd
	Titrate: Gradually increase to bid-tid prn; if bothersome dryness or peeling occurs, reduce frequency to qd or qod

ADMINISTRATION

Topical route

Priming

1. Gently push up on actuator w/ thumb until tab breaks
2. Shake vigorously (until product moves inside can), then firmly strike bottom of can onto palm/solid surface at least 3X
3. Direct initial spray to a non-skin surface
4. Press down on actuator for 1-3 sec until foam begins to dispense
5. If foam does not dispense w/in 3 sec, prime can again

Do not spray directly on the skin as the initial spray until primed
Before each use, shake can vigorously and firmly strike bottom of can onto palm/hard surface at least 3X
Holding can upright, dispense into palm of hand and cover entire affected area w/ thin layer
Rub in until completely absorbed, then rinse off after 2 min
Wash hands w/ soap and water after application

STORAGE

15-25°C (59-77°F). Avoid exposure to temperatures >49°C (120°F). Protect from freezing. Store upright. Contents under pressure; do not puncture or incinerate container.

HOW SUPPLIED

Foam: 9.8% [100g]

CONTRAINDICATIONS

Hypersensitivity to benzoyl peroxide or to any of the other ingredients in the product.

WARNINGS/PRECAUTIONS

For external use only. Not for ophthalmic use. Skin irritation (redness, burning, itching, peeling, swelling) and dryness are more likely to occur if foam is left on skin longer than directed. Use less frequently if irritation occurs. Do not use w/ very sensitive skin or if sensitive to benzoyl peroxide. D/C if irritation becomes severe or if hypersensitivity occurs. Avoid unnecessary sun exposure; apply sunscreen. Avoid contact w/ eyes, lips, and mouth. Avoid contact w/ hair and dyed fabrics; bleaching may occur.

ADVERSE REACTIONS

Allergic contact dermatitis, dryness.

DRUG INTERACTIONS

Skin irritation and dryness are more likely to occur if another topical acne medication is used at the same time; use 1 topical acne medication at a time if irritation occurs.

PREGNANCY AND LACTATION

Category C, caution in nursing.

MECHANISM OF ACTION

Antibacterial/keratolytic; not established. Demonstrated antibacterial activity against *Propionibacterium acnes*.

PHARMACOKINETICS

Metabolism: Benzoic acid (metabolite). **Elimination:** Urine (as benzoate).

PATIENT CONSIDERATIONS

Assessment: Assess for previous hypersensitivity to the drug, pregnancy/nursing status, and use of another topical acne medication.

Monitoring: Monitor for hypersensitivity reactions, allergic contact dermatitis, skin dryness, and irritation. Monitor for clinical response.

Counseling: Instruct to use only ud and not to use to treat any condition other than that for which it was prescribed. Instruct to avoid contact w/ eyes, eyelids, lips, and mucous membranes; counsel to rinse w/ water if accidental contact occurs. Advise to d/c and consult physician if excessive redness or irritation develops. Advise to avoid contact w/ hair, fabrics, or carpeting; bleaching or discoloration may occur. Instruct to avoid unnecessary sun exposure and to use sunscreen if going outside. Inform that use w/ another topical acne medication at the same time may increase likelihood of skin irritation and dryness; counsel to use 1 topical acne medication at a time if irritation occurs.

Benzonatate — benzonatate

Rx

Class: Non-narcotic antitussive

OTHER BRAND NAMES

Tessalon

ADULT DOSAGE	PEDIATRIC DOSAGE
Cough	**Cough**
Usual: 100mg, 150mg, or 200mg tid prn	**>10 Years:**
Max: 600mg/day in 3 divided doses	**Usual:** 100mg, 150mg, or 200mg tid prn
	Max: 600mg/day in 3 divided doses

ADMINISTRATION

Oral route
Swallow whole; do not break, chew, dissolve, cut, or crush.

STORAGE

Protect from light. (150mg, 200mg Cap) 20-25°C (68-77°F). **Tessalon:** 25°C (77°F); excursions permitted to 15-30°C (59-86°F).

HOW SUPPLIED

Cap: 150mg, 200mg; (Tessalon) 100mg

CONTRAINDICATIONS

Hypersensitivity to benzonatate or related compounds.

WARNINGS/PRECAUTIONS

Severe hypersensitivity reactions (eg, bronchospasm, laryngospasm, cardiovascular collapse) reported, possibly related to local anesthesia from sucking or chewing the cap instead of swallowing. Accidental ingestion resulting in death reported in children <10 yrs of age. May cause adverse CNS effects; caution w/ prior sensitivity to related agents, such as para-aminobenzoic acid (PABA) based anesthetics (eg, procaine, tetracaine).

ADVERSE REACTIONS

Hypersensitivity reactions, sedation, headache, dizziness, mental confusion, visual hallucinations, constipation, nausea, GI upset, pruritus, skin eruptions, nasal congestion, numbness of the chest, sensation of burning in the eyes, vague "chilly" sensation.

DRUG INTERACTIONS

Bizarre behavior (eg, mental confusion, visual hallucinations) reported when taken in combination w/ other prescribed drugs. May cause adverse CNS effects w/ concomitant medications.

PREGNANCY AND LACTATION

Pregnancy: Category C.
Lactation: Caution in nursing.

MECHANISM OF ACTION

Non-narcotic antitussive; acts peripherally by anesthetizing the stretch receptors located in the respiratory passages, lungs, and pleura by dampening their activity, thereby reducing cough reflex at its source.

PATIENT CONSIDERATIONS

Assessment: Assess for hypersensitivity to the drug or previous sensitivity to related compounds such as PABA based anesthetics, pregnancy/nursing status, and possible drug interactions.

Monitoring: Monitor for hypersensitivity reactions, CNS adverse effects, and other adverse reactions.

Counseling: Inform to take ud. Inform that release of benzonatate from the cap in the mouth can produce a temporary local anesthesia of the oral mucosa and choking may occur. Instruct to refrain from oral ingestion of food or liquids if numbness or tingling of the tongue, mouth, throat, or face occurs until numbness resolves. Advise to seek medical attention if symptoms worsen/persist. Inform that overdosage resulting in death may occur in adults; instruct not to exceed a single dose of 200mg and a total daily dosage of 600mg.

Benztropine — benztropine mesylate

Rx

Class: Anticholinergic

OTHER BRAND NAMES

Cogentin

ADULT DOSAGE	PEDIATRIC DOSAGE
Parkinsonism	**Parkinsonism**
Adjunct in the Therapy of All Forms of Parkinsonism:	**Adjunct in the Therapy of All Forms of Parkinsonism:**
Initiate w/ a low dose	**>3 Years:**
Titrate: May increase in increments of 0.5mg, to a max of 6mg, or until optimal results obtained, at 5- to 6-day intervals	Initiate w/ a low dose
	Titrate: May increase in increments of 0.5mg, to a max of 6mg, or until optimal results obtained, at 5- to 6-day intervals
Idiopathic Parkinsonism:	**Idiopathic Parkinsonism:**
Initial: 0.5-1mg qhs; 4-6mg/day may be required in other patients	**Initial:** 0.5-1mg qhs; 4-6mg/day may be required in other patients
Postencephalitic Parkinsonism:	**Postencephalitic Parkinsonism:**
Initial: 2mg/day given in 1 or more doses; 0.5mg qhs and increase as necessary in highly sensitive patients	**Initial:** 2mg/day given in 1 or more doses; 0.5mg qhs and increase as necessary in highly sensitive patients
Postencephalitic and Idiopathic Parkinsonism:	**Postencephalitic and Idiopathic Parkinsonism:**
Usual: 1-2mg/day	**Usual:** 1-2mg/day
Range: 0.5-6mg/day	**Range:** 0.5-6mg/day
Inj:	**Inj:**
Emergency Situations:	**Emergency Situations:**
1-2mL	1-2mL
Dose can be repeated if the parkinsonian effect begins to return	Dose can be repeated if the parkinsonian effect begins to return
Do not terminate other antiparkinsonian agents abruptly when therapy is started; gradually reduce or d/c other agents	Do not terminate other antiparkinsonian agents abruptly when therapy is started; gradually reduce or d/c other agents

Drug-Induced Extrapyramidal Reactions

Control of extrapyramidal disorders (except tardive dyskinesia) due to neuroleptic drugs (eg, phenothiazines)

Usual: 1-4mg qd or bid
1-2mg bid or tid for extrapyramidal disorders that develop soon after initiation of neuroleptic drugs

Tab:
D/C to determine continued need after 1 or 2 weeks
May reinstitute therapy if disorders recur

Acute Dystonic Reactions:
1-2mL IM/IV relieves the condition quickly
After the inj, 1-2mg tab bid usually prevents recurrence

Drug-Induced Extrapyramidal Reactions

Control of extrapyramidal disorders (except tardive dyskinesia) due to neuroleptic drugs (eg, phenothiazines)

>3 Years:
Usual: 1-4mg qd or bid
1-2mg bid or tid for extrapyramidal disorders that develop soon after initiation of neuroleptic drugs

Tab:
D/C to determine continued need after 1 or 2 weeks
May reinstitute therapy if disorders recur

Acute Dystonic Reactions:
1-2mL IM/IV relieves the condition quickly
After the inj, 1-2mg tab bid usually prevents recurrence

DOSING CONSIDERATIONS
Concomitant Medications
Concomitant Carbidopa-Levodopa or Levodopa: May require periodic dose adjustment

Elderly
Start at lower end of dosing range, and increase dose prn w/ monitoring for the emergence of adverse events

ADMINISTRATION
IV/IM/Oral route

STORAGE
Inj: 20-25°C (68-77°F). **Tab:** 15-30°C (59-86°F).

HOW SUPPLIED
Inj: (Cogentin) 1mg/mL [2mL, ampul]; **Tab:** 0.5mg*, 1mg*, 2mg* *scored

CONTRAINDICATIONS
Hypersensitivity to benztropine mesylate tablets or to any component of the tablets, pediatric patients <3 yrs of age.

WARNINGS/PRECAUTIONS
May impair mental/physical abilities. Caution with use during hot weather, especially when given with other atropine-like drugs to the chronically ill, alcoholics, those who have CNS disease, or those who do manual labor in a hot environment; severe anhidrosis and hyperthermia may occur; consider dose reduction. Continued supervision is advisable. Closely monitor patients with a tendency to tachycardia and those with prostatic hypertrophy. Dysuria may occur. Urinary retention reported. May cause weakness and inability to move particular muscle groups, especially in large doses; may require dose adjustment. Mental confusion and excitement may occur with large doses, or in susceptible patients. Visual hallucinations reported occasionally. In the treatment of extrapyramidal disorders due to neuroleptic drugs, may intensify mental symptoms in patients with mental disorders and precipitate toxic psychosis; monitor patients with mental disorders, especially at start of therapy or if dose is increased. Not recommended for use in patients with TD; may aggravate TD symptoms. Glaucoma may develop; avoid with angle-closure glaucoma. Certain drug-induced extrapyramidal disorders that develop slowly may not respond to therapy. Caution in pediatric patients >3 yrs of age.

ADVERSE REACTIONS
Tachycardia, paralytic ileus, constipation, N/V, dry mouth, toxic psychosis, blurred vision, dilated pupils, urinary retention, dysuria, allergic reaction, heat stroke, hyperthermia, fever.

DRUG INTERACTIONS
May cause GI complaints, fever, or heat intolerance with phenothiazines, haloperidol, or other drugs with anticholinergic/antidopaminergic activity. Paralytic ileus, hyperthermia, and heat stroke reported with phenothiazines and/ or TCAs.

PREGNANCY AND LACTATION
Safety not known in pregnancy/nursing.

MECHANISM OF ACTION
Anticholinergic agent; therapeutically significant in the management of parkinsonism. Also possesses antihistaminic activity.

PATIENT CONSIDERATIONS
Assessment: Assess for drug hypersensitivity, exposure to hot weather, tachycardia, prostatic hypertrophy, mental disorders, TD, angle-closure glaucoma, chronic illness, alcohol consumption, CNS disease, pregnancy/nursing status, and for possible drug interactions.

Monitoring: Monitor for anhidrosis, hyperthermia, tachycardia, dysuria, urinary retention, weakness, inability to move muscles, mental confusion and excitement, toxic psychosis, visual hallucinations, glaucoma, and other adverse reactions. Monitor patients with mental disorders at start of therapy or if dose is increased.

Counseling: Inform of the risks/benefits of therapy. Advise to use with caution during hot weather. Inform that drug may impair mental/physical abilities; caution against performing hazardous tasks (eg, operating machinery/driving). Advise to report GI complaints, fever, or heat intolerance promptly.

BEPREVE — bepotastine besilate　　　　**Rx**
Class: H₁ antagonist

ADULT DOSAGE **Allergic Conjunctivitis**	**PEDIATRIC DOSAGE** **Allergic Conjunctivitis**
Itching: 1 drop into the affected eye(s) bid	**Itching:** **≥2 Years:** 1 drop into the affected eye(s) bid

ADMINISTRATION
Ocular route

STORAGE
15-25°C (59-77°F). Keep bottle tightly closed when not in use.

HOW SUPPLIED
Sol: 1.5% [5mL, 10mL]

CONTRAINDICATIONS
History of hypersensitivity reactions to bepotastine or any of the other ingredients in this product.

WARNINGS/PRECAUTIONS
For topical ophthalmic use only. Avoid touching the eyelids or surrounding areas with dropper tip of the bottle. Not for the treatment of contact lens-related irritation. Contains benzalkonium chloride, which may be absorbed by soft contact lenses; remove contact lenses prior to instillation and may reinsert 10 min after administration.

ADVERSE REACTIONS
Mild taste, eye irritation, headache, nasopharyngitis.

PREGNANCY AND LACTATION
Category C, caution in nursing.

MECHANISM OF ACTION
H₁-antagonist; antagonizes H₁ receptor and inhibits release of histamine from mast cells.

PHARMACOKINETICS
Absorption: T_{max}=1-2 hrs; C_{max}=7.3ng/mL. **Distribution:** Plasma protein binding (55%). **Metabolism:** Liver via CYP450 (minimal). **Excretion:** Urine (75-90%, unchanged).

PATIENT CONSIDERATIONS
Assessment: Assess for previous hypersensitivity to the drug, contact lens use, and pregnancy/nursing status.

Monitoring: Monitor for hypersensitivity and other adverse reactions.

Counseling: Counsel that therapy is not for the treatment of lens-related irritation and advise not to instill while wearing contact lenses; inform that they may reinsert contact lenses 10 min after instillation. Advise not to touch the dropper tip to any surface, as this may contaminate the contents. Inform that sol is for topical ophthalmic use only.

BESIVANCE — besifloxacin　　　　**Rx**
Class: Fluoroquinolone

ADULT DOSAGE **Bacterial Conjunctivitis**	**PEDIATRIC DOSAGE** **Bacterial Conjunctivitis**
1 drop in affected eye(s) tid, 4-12 hrs apart for 7 days	**≥1 Year:** 1 drop in affected eye(s) tid, 4-12 hrs apart for 7 days

ADMINISTRATION
Ocular route
Invert closed bottle and shake once before use

STORAGE
15-25°C (59-77°F). Protect from light.

HOW SUPPLIED
Sus: 0.6% [5mL]

WARNINGS/PRECAUTIONS
For topical ophthalmic use only; should not be injected subconjunctivally, nor should it be introduced directly into the anterior chamber of the eye. May result in overgrowth of nonsusceptible organisms (eg, fungi) with prolonged use; d/c and institute alternative therapy if superinfection occurs. Avoid wearing contact lenses if signs or symptoms of bacterial conjunctivitis occur and avoid wearing contact lenses during the course of therapy.

ADVERSE REACTIONS
Conjunctival redness.

PREGNANCY AND LACTATION
Category C, caution in nursing.

MECHANISM OF ACTION
Fluoroquinolone antibacterial; inhibits both bacterial DNA gyrase and topoisomerase IV. DNA gyrase is an essential enzyme required for replication, transcription, and repair of bacterial DNA. Topoisomerase IV is an essential enzyme required for partitioning of the chromosomal DNA during bacterial cell division.

PHARMACOKINETICS
Absorption: C_{max}=0.37ng/mL (Day 1), 0.43ng/mL (Day 6). **Elimination:** $T_{1/2}$=7 hrs.

PATIENT CONSIDERATIONS

Assessment: Assess for previous hypersensitivity to the drug, use of contact lenses, and pregnancy/nursing status. Assess for proper diagnosis of causative organisms.

Monitoring: Monitor for superinfection; examine with magnification (eg, slit-lamp biomicroscopy) and fluorescein staining, where appropriate. Monitor for hypersensitivity reactions and other adverse reactions.

Counseling: Advise to avoid contaminating applicator tip with material from the eye, fingers, or other source. Advise to d/c use immediately and contact physician at first sign of a rash or allergic reaction. Instruct to use medication exactly ud. Inform that skipping doses or not completing the full course of therapy may decrease effectiveness and increase bacterial resistance. Advise to avoid wearing contact lenses if having signs or symptoms of bacterial conjunctivitis and avoid wearing during the course of therapy. Advise to thoroughly wash hands before use. Instruct to invert closed bottle and shake once before each use. Instruct to remove cap with bottle still in inverted position. Instruct to tilt head back, and with bottle inverted, gently squeeze bottle to instill 1 drop into the affected eye(s).

BETAGAN — levobunolol hydrochloride

Rx

Class: Nonselective beta blocker

ADULT DOSAGE
Elevated Intraocular Pressure
Chronic Open-Angle Glaucoma/Ocular HTN:
0.25%:
1-2 drops bid
0.5%:
1-2 drops qd; may increase to bid for more severe or uncontrolled glaucoma

Dosages >1 drop of 0.5% bid are not generally more effective; if IOP is not at a satisfactory level on this regimen, may institute concomitant therapy

PEDIATRIC DOSAGE
Pediatric use may not have been established

DOSING CONSIDERATIONS
Concomitant Medications
Should not typically use ≥2 topical ophthalmic β-adrenergic blocking agents simultaneously

ADMINISTRATION
Ocular route

STORAGE
15-25°C (59-77°F). Protect from light.

HOW SUPPLIED
Ophthalmic Sol: 0.25% [10mL], 0.5% [5mL, 10mL, 15mL]

CONTRAINDICATIONS
Bronchial asthma, history of bronchial asthma, severe COPD, sinus bradycardia, 2nd- and 3rd-degree atrioventricular (AV) block, overt cardiac failure, cardiogenic shock; hypersensitivity to any component of the product.

WARNINGS/PRECAUTIONS
May be absorbed systemically. Severe respiratory reactions and cardiac reactions, including death due to bronchospasm in patients w/ asthma, and rarely death in association w/ cardiac failure, reported. May precipitate more severe failure in individuals w/ diminished myocardial contractility. In patients w/o a history of cardiac failure, continued depression of the myocardium w/ β-blocking agents over a period of time can, in some cases, lead to cardiac failure; d/c at the 1st sign/symptom of cardiac failure. Avoid w/ COPD (eg, chronic bronchitis, emphysema) of mild or moderate severity, bronchospastic disease, or a history of bronchospastic disease; use w/ caution if administration is necessary in such patients. Impairs the ability of the heart to respond to β-adrenergically mediated reflex stimuli and may augment the risk of general anesthesia in surgical procedures; consider gradual withdrawal of therapy in patients undergoing elective surgery. May mask signs/symptoms of acute hypoglycemia; caution in patients subject to spontaneous hypoglycemia and in diabetic patients (especially those w/ labile diabetes) receiving insulin or hypoglycemic agents. May mask certain clinical signs of hyperthyroidism (eg, tachycardia); carefully manage patients suspected of developing thyrotoxicosis to avoid abrupt withdrawal that may precipitate a thyroid storm. Contains sodium metabisulfite; may cause allergic-type reactions in certain susceptible people. Caution in patients w/ diminished pulmonary function or w/ known hypersensitivity to other β-adrenoceptor blocking agents. Caution w/ cerebrovascular insufficiency; consider alternative therapy if signs/symptoms suggesting reduced cerebral blood flow develop. Should not be used alone in the treatment of angle-closure glaucoma. May potentiate muscle weakness consistent w/ certain myasthenic symptoms (eg, diplopia, ptosis, generalized weakness). While taking β-blockers, patients w/ a history of severe anaphylactic reactions to a variety of allergens may be more reactive to repeated challenge; may be unresponsive to the usual doses of epinephrine.

ADVERSE REACTIONS
Ocular burning, ocular stinging, decreased HR, decreased BP.

DRUG INTERACTIONS
See Dosing Considerations. Caution w/ oral β-blockers; potential for additive effects on systemic beta-blockade or on IOP. Mydriasis may occur w/ concomitant epinephrine. Closely observe patients receiving catecholamine-depleting drugs (eg, reserpine) because of possible additive effects and the production of hypotension and/or marked bradycardia. Monitor for possible AV conduction disturbances, left ventricular failure, and hypotension w/ oral or IV calcium antagonists; avoid simultaneous use in patients w/ impaired cardiac function. Concomitant use w/ digitalis or calcium antagonists may have additive effects in prolonging AV conduction time. May have additive hypotensive effects w/ phenothiazine-related compounds.

PREGNANCY AND LACTATION
Pregnancy: There are no adequate and well-controlled studies in pregnant women; should be used during pregnancy only if the potential benefit justifies the potential risk to the fetus.
Lactation: Caution in nursing.

MECHANISM OF ACTION
Noncardioselective β-adrenoceptor blocking agent; equipotent at both β_1 and β_2 receptors. Lowers elevated as well as normal IOP, whether or not accompanied by glaucoma. Primary mechanism of the ocular hypotensive action in reducing IOP is most likely a decrease in aqueous humor production.

PATIENT CONSIDERATIONS
Assessment: Assess for presence or history of bronchial asthma, COPD (eg, bronchitis, emphysema), or any other conditions where treatment is contraindicated or cautioned. Assess pregnancy/nursing status and for possible drug interactions.

Monitoring: Monitor for signs/symptoms of cardiac failure, masking of signs/symptoms of hypoglycemia or hyperthyroidism, reduced cerebral blood flow, muscle weakness, and other adverse reactions.

Counseling: Counsel to notify physician immediately if any signs of anaphylactic reaction, cardiac, or respiratory symptoms develop while on medication. Counsel patients w/ diabetes mellitus that medication may mask symptoms of hypoglycemia.

BETAPACE — sotalol hydrochloride

Rx

Class: Beta blocker (group II/III antiarrhythmic)

> To minimize risk of arrhythmia, for a minimum of 3 days, place patients initiated or reinitiated on therapy in a facility that can provide cardiac resuscitation and continuous ECG monitoring. Calculate CrCl prior to dosing. Not approved for A-fib or A-flutter; do not substitute for Betapace AF.

OTHER BRAND NAMES
Sorine

ADULT DOSAGE
Ventricular Arrhythmias
Documented Ventricular Arrhythmias (eg, Sustained Ventricular Tachycardia):
Initial: 80mg bid
Titrate: May increase after appropriate evaluation to 240 or 320mg/day (120-160mg bid); adjust dose gradually, allowing 3 days between dosing increments
Total Daily Dose: 160-320mg/day in 2 or 3 divided doses

Refractory Ventricular Arrhythmia:
480-640mg/day when benefit outweighs risk

Transferring to Betapace/Sorine:
Withdraw previous antiarrhythmic therapy for a minimum of 2-3 plasma half-lives before initiating therapy After discontinuation of amiodarone, do not initiate therapy until QT interval is normalized

PEDIATRIC DOSAGE
Ventricular Arrhythmias
Documented Ventricular Arrhythmias (eg, Sustained Ventricular Tachycardia):
<2 Years:
Refer to PI for dosing chart
≥2 Years:
Initial: 30mg/m² tid (90mg/m² total daily dose)
Titrate: Allow at least 36 hrs between dose increments; guide titration by response, HR, and QTc
Max: 60mg/m²

Reduce dose or d/c if QTc >550 msec

Transferring to Betapace/Sorine:
Withdraw previous antiarrhythmic therapy for a minimum of 2-3 plasma half-lives before initiating therapy After discontinuation of amiodarone, do not initiate therapy until QT interval is normalized

---

DOSING CONSIDERATIONS
Renal Impairment
Adults:
CrCl >60mL/min: Dose q12h
CrCl 30-59mL/min: Dose q24h
CrCl 10-29mL/min: Dose q36-48h
CrCl <10mL/min: Dose should be individualized
Pediatrics:
Lower doses or increase intervals between doses

ADMINISTRATION
Oral route

Preparation of Extemporaneous Oral Sol
1. Measure 120mL of simple syrup containing 0.1% sodium benzoate.
2. Transfer the syrup to a 6-oz amber plastic (polyethylene terephthalate) prescription bottle.
3. Add 5 sotalol 120mg tabs to the bottle. These tabs are added intact; it is not necessary to crush the tabs.
4. Shake the bottle to wet the entire surface of the tabs. If the tabs have been crushed, shake the bottle until the endpoint is achieved.

5. Allow the tabs to hydrate for at least 2 hrs. After at least 2 hrs have elapsed, shake the bottle intermittently over the course of at least another 2 hrs until the tabs are completely disintegrated.

6. The procedure results in a sol containing 5mg/mL of sotalol HCl.

STORAGE
Betapace: 25°C (77°F); excursions permitted to 15-30°C (59-86°F). **Sorine:** 15-30°C (59-86°F). **Sus:** Stable for 3 months at 15-30°C (59-86°F) and ambient humidity.

HOW SUPPLIED
Tab: (Betapace) 80mg*, 120mg*, 160mg*; (Sorine) 80mg*, 120mg*, 160mg*, 240mg* *scored

CONTRAINDICATIONS
Bronchial asthma, sinus bradycardia, 2nd- and 3rd-degree atrioventricular (AV) block (unless a functioning pacemaker is present), congenital or acquired long QT syndrome, cardiogenic shock, uncontrolled CHF, previous evidence of hypersensitivity to sotalol.

WARNINGS/PRECAUTIONS
May provoke new or worsen ventricular arrhythmias (eg, sustained ventricular tachycardia or ventricular fibrillation). Torsades de pointes, QT interval prolongation, and new or worsened CHF reported. Anticipate proarrhythmic events upon initiation and every upward dose adjustment. Caution in patients w/ QTc >500 msec on-therapy and consider reducing dose or discontinuing therapy when QTc >550 msec. Avoid w/ uncorrected hypokalemia or hypomagnesemia. Give special attention to electrolyte and acid-base balance in patients w/ severe/prolonged diarrhea or w/ concomitant diuretic drugs. May cause further depression of myocardial contractility and precipitate more severe failure; caution w/ CHF controlled by digitalis and/or diuretics. Caution w/ left ventricular dysfunction, sick sinus syndrome associated w/ symptomatic arrhythmias, and renal impairment (especially w/ hemodialysis). Caution during the first 2 weeks post-MI; careful dose titration is especially important (eg, in patients w/ markedly impaired ventricular function). Exacerbation of angina pectoris, arrhythmias, and MI reported after abrupt discontinuation; reduce dose gradually over 1-2 weeks. May unmask latent coronary insufficiency in patients w/ arrhythmias. Avoid in patients w/ bronchospastic diseases; use lowest effective dose. Impaired ability of the heart to respond to reflex adrenergic stimuli may augment the risks of general anesthesia and surgical procedures; chronically administered therapy should not be routinely withdrawn prior to major surgery. Patients w/ a history of anaphylactic reaction to various allergens may have a more severe reaction on repeated challenge and may be unresponsive to usual doses of epinephrine. Caution in patients w/ diabetes (especially labile diabetes) or w/ a history of episodes of spontaneous hypoglycemia; may mask premonitory signs of acute hypoglycemia (eg, tachycardia). May mask certain clinical signs (eg, tachycardia) of hyperthyroidism.

ADVERSE REACTIONS
Torsades de pointes, dyspnea, fatigue, dizziness, bradycardia, chest pain, palpitation, asthenia, abnormal ECG, hypotension, headache, light-headedness, edema, N/V, pulmonary problems.

DRUG INTERACTIONS
Avoid w/ Class Ia (eg, disopyramide, quinidine, procainamide) and Class III (eg, amiodarone) antiarrhythmics. Additive Class II effects w/ other β-blockers. Proarrhythmic events were more common when concomitantly used w/ digoxin. May increase risk of bradycardia w/ digitalis glycosides. Possible additive effects on AV conduction or ventricular function and BP w/ calcium-blocking agents. May produce excessive reduction of resting sympathetic nervous tone w/ catecholamine-depleting drugs (eg, reserpine, guanethidine). Hyperglycemia may occur; may require dose adjustment of insulin or antidiabetic agents. β2-agonists (eg, salbutamol, terbutaline, isoprenaline) may need dose increase. May potentiate rebound HTN w/ clonidine withdrawal. Avoid administration w/in 2 hrs of antacids containing aluminum oxide and magnesium hydroxide; may reduce levels. Caution w/ drugs that prolong QT interval (eg, Class I and III antiarrhythmics, phenothiazines, TCAs, astemizole, bepridil, certain oral macrolides, certain quinolone antibiotics).

PREGNANCY AND LACTATION
Pregnancy: Category B.
Lactation: Not for use in nursing.

MECHANISM OF ACTION
β-blocker (group II/III antiarrhythmic); has both β-adrenoreceptor blocking and cardiac action potential duration prolongation properties.

PHARMACOKINETICS
Absorption: Bioavailability (90-100%); T_{max}=2.5-4 hrs. **Distribution:** Crosses placenta; found in breast milk. **Elimination:** Urine (unchanged); $T_{1/2}$=12 hrs.

PATIENT CONSIDERATIONS
Assessment: Assess for hypersensitivity to drug, bronchial asthma, sinus bradycardia, sick sinus syndrome, 2nd- and 3rd-degree AV block, pacemaker, long QT syndromes, cardiogenic shock, left ventricular dysfunction or uncontrolled CHF, recent MI, ischemic heart disease, hypokalemia or hypomagnesemia, bronchospastic disease, diabetes, episodes of hypoglycemia, upcoming major surgery, hyperthyroidism, renal impairment, any other conditions where treatment is contraindicated or cautioned, pregnancy/nursing status, and possible drug interactions.

Monitoring: Monitor for ECG changes, tachycardia, arrhythmias, depressed myocardial contractility, severe CHF, anaphylaxis, hypoglycemia, electrolyte imbalance, hyperthyroidism, and other adverse reactions.

Counseling: Inform of the benefits/risks of therapy. Advise not to d/c therapy w/o consulting physician. Instruct to report any adverse reactions to physician.

BETAXOLOL — betaxolol hydrochloride   **Rx**
Class: Selective beta₁ blocker

ADULT DOSAGE
Hypertension
Initial: 10mg qd
Titrate: May increase to 20mg qd after 7-14 days if desired response is not achieved

Doses >20mg has not shown a statistically significant additional antihypertensive effect; however the 40-mg dose has been studied and is well tolerated

If monotherapy does not produce the desired response, consider addition of a diuretic or other antihypertensive

Cessation of Therapy:
If withdrawal of therapy is planned, it should be achieved gradually over a period of 2 weeks

PEDIATRIC DOSAGE
Pediatric use may not have been established

DOSING CONSIDERATIONS
Renal Impairment
Severe Impairment/Dialysis:
Initial: 5mg qd
Titrate: May increase by 5mg/day increments every 2 weeks
Max: 20mg/day

Elderly
Initial: Consider reducing to 5mg qd

ADMINISTRATION
Oral route

STORAGE
20-25°C (68-77°F).

HOW SUPPLIED
Tab: 10mg*, 20mg *scored

CONTRAINDICATIONS
Known hypersensitivity to the drug, sinus bradycardia, >1st-degree heart block, cardiogenic shock, overt cardiac failure.

WARNINGS/PRECAUTIONS
Caution in congestive heart failure controlled by digitalis and diuretics. May cause cardiac failure; consider discontinuation at the 1st sign/symptom of cardiac failure. Exacerbation of angina pectoris and, in some cases, MI reported upon abrupt discontinuation in patients w/ coronary artery disease (CAD); avoid abrupt withdrawal and carefully observe and reinstitute therapy, at least temporarily, if withdrawal symptoms occur during planned discontinuation of therapy. Should generally not be given to patients w/ bronchospastic disease; cautiously use lowest possible dose (5-10mg qd) in patients who do not respond to or cannot tolerate alternative treatment and have a bronchodilator available. If dosage must be increased, consider divided dosage to avoid higher peak blood levels associated w/ qd dosing. Chronically administered therapy should not be routinely withdrawn prior to major surgery; however, may augment risks of general anesthesia and surgical procedures; titrate betaxolol dose to maintain effective HR control while avoiding frank hypotension and bradycardia. Caution in diabetic patients; may mask tachycardia occurring w/ hypoglycemia. May mask certain clinical signs of hyperthyroidism (eg, tachycardia) and abrupt withdrawal may precipitate thyroid storm. Do not give to patients w/ untreated pheochromocytoma. May cause reduction of intraocular pressure (IOP) and interfere w/ glaucoma-screening test; withdrawal of therapy may lead to return of increased IOP. Aggravation in psoriasis reported. Caution w/ renal/hepatic impairment. May produce bradycardia more frequently in elderly. Severe allergic reactions including anaphylaxis reported in patients exposed to a variety of allergens either by repeated challenge or accidental contact, and in those exposed to diagnostic or therapeutic agents while receiving β-blockers; such patients may be unresponsive to usual doses of epinephrine used to treat allergic reactions.

ADVERSE REACTIONS
Bradycardia, headache, dizziness, dyspepsia, arthralgia.

DRUG INTERACTIONS
Observe for potential additive effects either on IOP or on the known systemic effects when used concomitantly w/ β-blocking ophthalmic solutions. Possible additive effect w/ catecholamine-depleting drugs (eg, reserpine); monitor closely. If discontinuing betaxolol and clonidine concurrently, d/c betaxolol slowly over several days before gradual clonidine withdrawal. Avoid oral calcium antagonists in patients w/ impaired cardiac function; hypotension is more likely to occur w/ dihydropyridine derivatives (eg, nifedipine), while left ventricular failure and atrioventricular conduction disturbances, including complete heart block, are more likely to occur w/ either verapamil or diltiazem. May increase risk of bradycardia w/ digitalis glycosides. Additive negative chronotropic properties w/ amiodarone. Coadministration w/ disopyramide has been associated w/ severe bradycardia, asystole, and heart failure. Caution w/ anesthetic agents that depress myocardium (eg, ether, cyclopropane, trichloroethylene). May be refractory to epinephrine in the treatment of anaphylactic shock.

PREGNANCY AND LACTATION
Pregnancy: Category C. β-blockers reduce placental perfusion and adverse effects (especially hypoglycemia and bradycardia) may occur in fetus. β-blocker action persists in the neonate for several days after birth to a treated mother.
Lactation: Excreted in human milk. Caution in nursing.

MECHANISM OF ACTION
Selective β1-blocker; has not been established. Possible mechanisms proposed include: competitive antagonism of catecholamines at peripheral adrenergic-neuronal sites, leading to a decreased cardiac output; a central effect leading to reduced sympathetic outflow to periphery; and suppression of renin activity.

PHARMACOKINETICS
Absorption: Complete. Absolute bioavailability (89%) (10mg) C_{max}=21.6ng/mL, T_{max}=3 hrs. **Distribution:** Plasma protein binding (50%); found in breast milk. **Metabolism:** Liver. **Elimination:** Urine (>80%, 15% unchanged); $T_{1/2}$=14-22 hrs.

PATIENT CONSIDERATIONS
Assessment: Assess for hypersensitivity to the drug, sinus bradycardia, >1st-degree heart block, cardiogenic shock, overt cardiac failure, bronchospastic disease, untreated pheochromocytoma, psoriasis, CAD, thyrotoxicosis/hyperthyroidism, diabetes, hepatic/renal impairment, pregnancy/nursing status, any other conditions where treatment is contraindicated or cautioned, and possible drug interactions.

Monitoring: Monitor for signs/symptoms of cardiac failure, tachycardia occurring w/ hypoglycemia, decreased IOP, exacerbation of angina pectoris upon withdrawal, MI, and other adverse reactions. Monitor closely patients known or suspected of being thyrotoxic from whom therapy is to be withdrawn. Monitor patients w/ hepatic insufficiency.

Counseling: Instruct not to interrupt or d/c therapy w/o physician's advice, especially if there is evidence of coronary artery insufficiency. Advise to consult physician at the 1st sign or symptom of cardiac failure. Advise patients that they should know how they react to therapy before operating automobiles and machinery or engaging in other tasks requiring alertness. Advise to contact physician if any difficulty in breathing occurs, and before surgery of any type. Instruct to inform physicians, ophthalmologists, or dentists that patient is taking betaxolol. Warn patients w/ diabetes that therapy may mask tachycardia occurring w/ hypoglycemia.

BETHKIS — tobramycin
Class: Aminoglycoside
Rx

ADULT DOSAGE	**PEDIATRIC DOSAGE**
Pseudomonas aeruginosa **Infections**	_Pseudomonas aeruginosa_ **Infections**
In Cystic Fibrosis Patients:	**In Cystic Fibrosis Patients:**
300mg bid by oral inh (as close to 12 hrs apart as possible; not <6 hrs apart) in repeated cycles of 28 days on drug, followed by 28 days off drug	**≥6 Years:**
	300mg bid by oral inh (as close to 12 hrs apart as possible; not <6 hrs apart) in repeated cycles of 28 days on drug, followed by 28 days off drug

ADMINISTRATION
Oral inh route

Administer by using a hand-held Pari LC Plus reusable nebulizer w/ a Pari Vios air compressor over approx 15 min and until sputtering from the output of the nebulizer has occurred for at least 1 min
Do not mix w/ other medicines in the nebulizer
Administer other inhaled medicines (eg, bronchodilators) before administration of therapy
Refer to PI for further preparation and administration instructions

STORAGE
2-8°C (36-46°F). Upon removal from the refrigerator, or if refrigeration is unavailable, may be stored at room temperature (up to 25°C [77°F]) for up to 28 days. Do not expose to intense light.

HOW SUPPLIED
Sol, Inhalation: 300mg/4mL

CONTRAINDICATIONS
Known hypersensitivity to any aminoglycoside.

WARNINGS/PRECAUTIONS
Ototoxicity (eg, tinnitus) may occur; caution with auditory or vestibular dysfunction. Nephrotoxicity may occur; caution with renal dysfunction. If nephrotoxicity occurs, d/c therapy until serum concentrations fall <2mcg/mL. If an increase in SrCr develops, closely monitor renal function. May aggravate muscle weakness; caution with muscular disorders (eg, myasthenia gravis, Parkinson's disease). Bronchospasm and wheezing reported. Consider an audiogram for patients with any evidence of or at increased risk for auditory dysfunction. May cause fetal harm.

ADVERSE REACTIONS
Decreased forced expiratory volume, rales, increased RBC sedimentation rate, dysphonia, wheezing, epistaxis, pharyngolaryngeal pain, bronchitis.

DRUG INTERACTIONS
Avoid concurrent and/or sequential use with other drugs with neurotoxic or ototoxic potential. Some diuretics may enhance toxicity by altering concentrations in serum and tissue; do not administer with ethacrynic acid, furosemide, urea, or mannitol.

PREGNANCY AND LACTATION
Category D, not for use in nursing.

MECHANISM OF ACTION
Aminoglycoside; acts primarily by disrupting protein synthesis in the bacterial cell, which eventually leads to death of the cell.

PHARMACOKINETICS
Distribution: Crosses placenta. **Elimination:** Expectorated sputum (unabsorbed); $T_{1/2}$=4.4 hrs.

PATIENT CONSIDERATIONS
Assessment: Assess for auditory, vestibular, or renal dysfunction, muscular disorders, drug hypersensitivity, pregnancy/nursing status, and possible drug interactions. Consider a baseline audiogram for patients at increased risk for auditory dysfunction.

Monitoring: Monitor for ototoxicity, nephrotoxicity, muscle weakness, bronchospasm, wheezing, and other adverse reactions. Consider an audiogram for patients who show any evidence of auditory dysfunction.

Counseling: Instruct to take drug ud, and to complete a full 28-day course of therapy even if feeling better. Inform of the adverse reactions associated with therapy, such as ototoxicity, bronchospasm, nephrotoxicity, and neuromuscular disorders. Inform of the need to monitor hearing, serum concentrations, and renal function during treatment. Advise to inform physician if pregnant/nursing or planning to become pregnant. Counsel on proper storage of the drug.

BEXSERO — meningococcal group B vaccine
Class: Vaccine
Rx

ADULT DOSAGE	**PEDIATRIC DOSAGE**
Meningococcal Vaccine	**Meningococcal Vaccine**
Active Immunization to Prevent Invasive Disease Caused by _Neisseria meningitidis_ Serogroup B:	**Active Immunization to Prevent Invasive Disease Caused by _Neisseria meningitidis_ Serogroup B:**
<25 Years:	**>10 Years:**
2 doses (0.5mL/dose) at least 1 month apart	2 doses (0.5mL/dose) at least 1 month apart
Sufficient data not available on the safety and effectiveness of using interchangeably w/ other meningococcal group B vaccines to complete vaccination series	Sufficient data not available on the safety and effectiveness of using interchangeably w/ other meningococcal group B vaccines to complete vaccination series

ADMINISTRATION
IM route

Shake syringe immediately before use; do not use if vaccine cannot be resuspended
Administer into the deltoid muscle of upper arm

STORAGE
2-8°C (36-46°F). Do not freeze; discard if the vaccine has been frozen. Protect from light.

HOW SUPPLIED
Inj: 0.5mL

CONTRAINDICATIONS
Hypersensitivity, including severe allergic reaction, to any component of the vaccine, or after a previous dose of Bexsero.

WARNINGS/PRECAUTIONS
Appropriate observation and medical treatment should always be readily available in case of an anaphylactic event. Syncope may occur; procedures should be in place to avoid injury from falling. Tip caps of prefilled syringes contain natural rubber latex; may cause allergic reactions in latex sensitive individuals. May not protect all vaccine recipients. May not provide protection against all meningococcal serogroup B strains. Individuals w/ altered immunocompetence may have reduced immune responses to therapy.

ADVERSE REACTIONS
Inj-site pain, myalgia, erythema, fatigue, headache, induration, nausea, arthralgia.

PREGNANCY AND LACTATION
Category B, caution in nursing.

MECHANISM OF ACTION
Vaccine; protection against invasive meningococcal disease is conferred mainly by complement-mediated antibody-dependent killing of _N. meningitidis_.

PATIENT CONSIDERATIONS
Assessment: Assess for hypersensitivity, vaccination history, latex sensitivity, altered immunocompetence, and pregnancy/nursing status.

Monitoring: Monitor for allergic/anaphylactic reactions, syncope, and other adverse reactions. Monitor immune response to vaccine.

Counseling: Inform patients and parents/guardians about the importance of completing the immunization series. Instruct to report any adverse reactions to physician. Inform women who receive therapy while pregnant that they will need to be registered in the vaccine's pregnancy registry.

BEYAZ — drospirenone/ethinyl estradiol/levomefolate calcium   Rx

Class: Estrogen/progestogen combination

> Cigarette smoking increases the risk of serious cardiovascular (CV) events from combination oral contraceptive (COC) use. Risk increases w/ age (>35 yrs) and w/ the number of cigarettes smoked. Should not be used by women who are >35 yrs of age and smoke.

ADULT DOSAGE

Contraception

1 tab qd at the same time each day for 28 days, then repeat

Start either on 1st day of menses or on 1st Sunday after onset of menses

Premenstrual Dysphoric Disorder

In Women Who Desire Oral Contraception:

1 tab qd at the same time each day for 28 days, then repeat

Start either on 1st day of menses or on 1st Sunday after onset of menses

Acne Vulgaris

Moderate Acne in Women Who Desire Oral Contraception:

1 tab qd at the same time each day for 28 days, then repeat

Start either on 1st day of menses or on 1st Sunday after onset of menses

Other Indications

May be used to raise folate levels for the purpose of reducing the risk of neural tube defect in a pregnancy conceived while taking the product or shortly after discontinuation

Conversions

Switching from a Different Birth Control Pill:

Start on the same day that a new pack of the previous oral contraceptive would have been started

Switching from a Method Other than a Birth Control Pill:

Transdermal Patch/Vaginal Ring/Inj: Start when the next application/inj would have been due

Intrauterine Contraceptive/Implant: Start on day of removal

PEDIATRIC DOSAGE

Contraception

Not indicated for use premenarche; refer to adult dosing

Premenstrual Dysphoric Disorder

Not indicated for use premenarche; refer to adult dosing

Acne Vulgaris

Moderate Acne in Postpubertal Women ≥14 Years Who Desire Oral Contraception:

1 tab qd at the same time each day for 28 days, then repeat

Start either on 1st day of menses or on 1st Sunday after onset of menses

---

DOSING CONSIDERATIONS

Adverse Reactions

GI Disturbances: If vomiting occurs w/in 3-4 hrs after taking tab, may regard as missed tab

Other Important Considerations

Postpartum Women Who Elect Not to Breastfeed/After 2nd Trimester Abortion: Start therapy no earlier than 4 weeks postpartum; if patient initiates therapy postpartum and has not yet had a period, use an additional method of contraception until patient has taken 7 consecutive days of therapy

ADMINISTRATION

Oral route

Take tabs in the order directed on the package, at the same time each day, preferably after pm meal or hs

Take w/o regard to meals

If 1st taken later than the 1st day of menstrual cycle, use a nonhormonal contraceptive as backup during the first 7 days

STORAGE

25°C (77°F); excursions permitted to 15-30°C (59-86°F).

HOW SUPPLIED

Tab: (Drospirenone [DRSP]/Ethinyl Estradiol [EE]/Levomefolate calcium) 3mg/0.02mg/0.451mg; **Tab:** (Levomefolate calcium) 0.451mg

CONTRAINDICATIONS

Renal impairment, adrenal insufficiency, high risk of arterial/venous thrombotic disease (eg, smoking if >35 yrs of age, history/presence of deep vein thrombosis/pulmonary embolism, cerebrovascular disease, coronary artery disease, thrombogenic valvular or thrombogenic rhythm diseases of the heart [eg, subacute bacterial endocarditis w/ valvular disease, A-fib], inherited/acquired hypercoagulopathies, uncontrolled HTN, diabetes mellitus [DM] w/ vascular disease, headaches w/ focal neurological symptoms or migraine w/ or w/o aura if >35 yrs of age), undiagnosed abnormal uterine bleeding, history/presence of breast or other estrogen-/progestin-sensitive cancer, benign/malignant liver tumors, liver disease, pregnancy.

WARNINGS/PRECAUTIONS

May increase risk of venous thromboembolism (VTE) and arterial thromboses (eg, stroke, MI); d/c if unexplained loss of vision, proptosis, diplopia, papilledema, or retinal vascular lesions occur; evaluate for retinal vein thrombosis immediately. If feasible, d/c at least 4 weeks before and through 2 weeks after major surgery or other surgeries known to have an elevated risk of thromboembolism. Potential for hyperkalemia in high-risk patients; contraindicated in patients predisposed to hyperkalemia. May increase risk of cervical cancer or intraepithelial neoplasia, and gallbladder disease. D/C if jaundice develops. May increase risk of hepatic adenomas and hepatocellular carcinoma. Cholestasis may occur w/ history of pregnancy-related cholestasis; women w/ a history of COC-related cholestasis may have the condition recur w/ subsequent COC use. Increased BP reported; d/c if BP rises significantly. May decrease glucose tolerance; monitor prediabetic and diabetic women. Consider alternative contraception for women w/ uncontrolled dyslipidemia. May increase risk of pancreatitis in women w/ hypertriglyceridemia or family history thereof. Evaluate the cause and d/c if indicated; if new headaches that are recurrent, persistent, or severe develop; increase in frequency/severity of migraines may be a reason for immediate discontinuation of therapy. Unscheduled bleeding and spotting may occur; rule out pregnancy or malignancy. Post-pill amenorrhea or oligomenorrhea may occur. Caution w/ history of depression; d/c if depression recurs to a serious degree. May change results of some lab tests (eg, coagulation factors, binding proteins). Folate may mask vitamin B12 deficiency. May induce/exacerbate angioedema in patients w/ hereditary angioedema. Chloasma may occur, especially w/ history of chloasma gravidarum; avoid sun or UV radiation exposure in women w/ a tendency to chloasma. Absorption may not be complete and additional contraceptive measures should be taken in case of severe vomiting or diarrhea; if vomiting occurs w/in 3-4 hrs after tab taking, regard this as a missed tab.

ADVERSE REACTIONS

Menstrual irregularities, N/V, headache/migraine, breast pain/tenderness, fatigue.

DRUG INTERACTIONS

Consider monitoring serum K^+ levels in high-risk patients who take a strong CYP3A4 inhibitor long-term and concomitantly. Potential for an increase in serum K^+ levels w/ use of other drugs that may increase serum K^+ levels (eg, ACE inhibitors, heparin, aldosterone antagonists, NSAIDs); monitor serum K^+ levels during 1st treatment cycle in women receiving daily, long-term treatment for chronic conditions/diseases. May reduce effectiveness or increase breakthrough bleeding when used w/ drugs or herbal products that induce certain enzymes, including CYP3A4 (eg, phenytoin, barbiturates, carbamazepine); use an alternative or backup method of contraception when using enzyme inducers and continue backup contraception for 28 days after discontinuation of the enzyme inducer. Atorvastatin may increase EE exposure; ascorbic acid and acetaminophen may increase EE levels. Moderate or strong CYP3A4 inhibitors (eg, itraconazole, verapamil, clarithromycin, diltiazem) may increase plasma levels of estrogen or progestin or both. Significant changes (increase/decrease) in plasma estrogen and progestin levels w/ HIV/hepatitis C virus protease inhibitors or non-nucleoside reverse transcriptase inhibitors. Pregnancy reported w/ antibiotics. May decrease levels of lamotrigine and reduce seizure control; may need to adjust dose of lamotrigine. May increase levels of CYP3A4 substrates (eg, midazolam), CYP2C19 substrates (eg, omeprazole, voriconazole), and CYP1A2 substrates (eg, theophylline, tizanidine). Increases thyroid-binding globulin levels; may need to increase dose of thyroid hormone in women on thyroid hormone replacement therapy. May decrease pharmacological effect of antifolate drugs (eg, antiepileptics [phenytoin], methotrexate, pyrimethamine). Reduced folate levels reported via inhibition of dihydrofolate reductase enzyme (eg, methotrexate, sulfasalazine), reduced folate absorption (eg, cholestyramine), or unknown mechanism (eg, antiepileptics [carbamazepine, phenytoin, primidone]).

PREGNANCY AND LACTATION

Contraindicated in pregnancy, not for use in nursing.

MECHANISM OF ACTION

Estrogen/progestogen oral contraceptive; acts by primarily suppressing ovulation. Also causes cervical mucus changes that inhibit sperm penetration and endometrial changes that reduce the likelihood of implantation. (Levomefolate calcium) Folate supplementation.

PHARMACOKINETICS

Absorption: DRSP: Absolute bioavailability (76%); (Cycle 1/Day 21) C_{max}=70.3ng/mL; T_{max}=1.5 hrs; AUC=763ng•h/mL. EE: Absolute bioavailability (40%); (Cycle 1/Day 21) C_{max}=45.1pg/mL; T_{max}=1.5 hrs; AUC=220pg•h/mL. Levomefolate: T_{max}=0.5-1.5 hrs. Refer to PI for additional parameters. **Distribution:** Found in breast milk; DRSP: V_d=4L/kg; serum protein binding (97%). EE: V_d=4-5L/kg; serum albumin binding (98.5%). **Metabolism:** DRSP: Reduction, subsequent sulfation, oxidation catalyzed by CYP3A4. EE: Gut and liver (1st-pass), conjugation w/ glucuronide or sulfate, hydroxylation (via CYP3A4). **Elimination:** DRSP: Urine, feces; $T_{1/2}$=30 hrs. EE: Urine, feces; $T_{1/2}$=24 hrs. Levomefolate (L-5-methyl-THF): Urine, feces; $T_{1/2}$=4-5 hrs.

PATIENT CONSIDERATIONS

Assessment: Assess for renal impairment, abnormal uterine bleeding, adrenal insufficiency, predisposition to hyperkalemia, pregnancy/nursing status, other conditions where treatment is cautioned or contraindicated, and for possible drug interactions.

Monitoring: Monitor for bleeding irregularities, thromboembolic disorders and other vascular problems, cervical cancer or intraepithelial neoplasia, retinal vein thrombosis or any other ophthalmic changes, jaundice, acute/chronic disturbances in liver function, new/worsening headaches or migraines, serious depression, cholestasis w/ history of pregnancy-related cholestasis, pancreatitis, and other adverse reactions. Monitor K^+ levels, thyroid function if receiving thyroid replacement therapy, glucose levels in diabetic and prediabetic women, and lipids levels w/ dyslipidemia. Check BP annually.

Counseling: Inform of risks/benefits of therapy. Explain that cigarette smoking increases the risk of serious CV events. Inform of the risk of VTE. Inform that drug does not protect against HIV infection and other STDs. Instruct to take ud and at the same time every day. Instruct on what to do if pills are missed or vomiting occurs w/in 3-4 hrs after taking tab. Advise to inform physician of preexisting medical conditions and of all concomitant medications and herbal supplements currently being taken. Instruct to d/c if pregnancy occurs during treatment. Instruct to use a backup or alternative method of contraception when enzyme inducers are used concomitantly. Inform that therapy may reduce breast milk production. Inform that amenorrhea may occur and pregnancy should be ruled out if amenorrhea occurs in ≥2 consecutive cycles. Counsel women who start therapy postpartum and have not yet had a period to use additional method of contraception until a pink tab has been taken for 7 consecutive days. Advise to report if taking folate supplements and to maintain folate supplementation upon discontinuation due to pregnancy.

Biaxin — clarithromycin   Rx

Class: Macrolide

OTHER BRAND NAMES
Biaxin XL

ADULT DOSAGE

Mycobacterial Infections

Treatment and Prophylaxis of Disseminated Infection Due to *Mycobacterium avium* Complex (MAC) in Patients w/ Advanced HIV Infection:

Tab/Sus:
Recommended Dose: 500mg q12h; continue therapy if clinical response is observed. D/C when the patient is considered at low risk of disseminated infection.

Pharyngitis/Tonsillitis
Due to *Streptococcus pyogenes*:
Tab/Sus:
250mg q12h for 10 days

Acute Maxillary Sinusitis
Due to *Haemophilus influenzae*, *Moraxella catarrhalis*, or *Streptococcus pneumoniae*:
Tab/Sus:
500mg q12h for 14 days
XL Tab:
1000mg q24h for 14 days

Community-Acquired Pneumonia
Tab/Sus:
H. influenzae:
250mg q12h for 7 days
S. pneumoniae, *Chlamydophila pneumoniae*, or *Mycoplasma pneumoniae*: 250mg q12h for 7-14 days
XL Tab:
H. influenzae, *Haemophilus parainfluenzae*, *M. catarrhalis*, *S. pneumoniae*, *C. pneumoniae*, or *M. pneumoniae*:
1000mg q24h for 7 days

Skin and Skin Structure Infections
Uncomplicated Infections Due to *Staphylococcus aureus* or *S. pyogenes*:
Tab/Sus:
250mg q12h for 7-14 days

Helicobacter pylori Eradication
Tab:
Triple Therapy:
500mg + 1g amoxicillin + 20mg omeprazole, all q12h for 10 days; give additional 20mg omeprazole qd for 18 days for ulcer healing/symptom relief if an ulcer was present at the time of initiation
or
500mg + 1g amoxicillin + 30mg lansoprazole, all q12h for 10 or 14 days
Dual Therapy:
500mg q8h + 40mg omeprazole qam for 14 days; give additional 20mg omeprazole qd for 14 days for ulcer healing/symptom relief

Acute Bacterial Exacerbation of Chronic Bronchitis
Tab/Sus:
M. catarrhalis or *S. pneumoniae*:
250mg q12h for 7-14 days

PEDIATRIC DOSAGE

General Dosing

Pharyngitis/tonsillitis due to *S. pyogenes*; community-acquired pneumonia due to *M. pneumoniae*, *S. pneumoniae*, or *C. pneumoniae*; acute maxillary sinusitis or acute otitis media due to *H. influenzae*, *M. catarrhalis*, or *S. pneumoniae*; or uncomplicated skin and skin structure infections due to *S. aureus* or *S. pyogenes*

Tab/Sus:
≥6 Months of Age:
Recommended Dose: 15mg/kg/day divided q12h for 10 days
Max: Up to adult dose

Mycobacterial Infections

Treatment and Prophylaxis of Disseminated Infection Due to MAC in Patients w/ Advanced HIV Infection:

Tab/Sus:
≥20 Months of Age:
Recommended Dose: 7.5mg/kg q12h, up to 500mg q12h; continue therapy if clinical response is observed. D/C when the patient is considered at low risk of disseminated infection.

H. influenzae:
500mg q12h for 7-14 days
H. parainfluenzae:
500mg q12h for 7 days
XL Tab:
H. influenzae, *H. parainfluenzae*, *M. catarrhalis*, or *S. pneumoniae*:
1000mg q24h for 7 days

- -

DOSING CONSIDERATIONS
Concomitant Medications
Atazanavir: Decrease clarithromycin dose by 50%

Renal Impairment
Severe (CrCl <30mL/min): Reduce dose by 50%

Concomitant Atazanavir or Ritonavir:
CrCl 30-60mL/min: Reduce dose by 50%
CrCl <30mL/min: Reduce dose by 75%

ADMINISTRATION
Oral route

Tab/Sus
- Take w/ or w/o food; may be taken w/ milk.

Sus
- Shake well before each use.
- Reconstitute 50mL bottle sizes w/ 27mL of water and 100mL bottle sizes w/ 55mL of water.
- Add half the volume of water to the bottle and shake vigorously. Add the remainder of water to the bottle and shake.
- Keep tightly closed.
- Do not refrigerate. After mixing, store at 15-30°C (59-86°F) and use w/in 14 days.

XL Tab
- Take w/ food.
- Swallow whole; do not chew, crush, or break.

STORAGE
250mg Tab: 15-30°C (59-86°F). Protect from light. **500mg Tab:** 20-25°C (68-77°F). **Sus:** <25°C (77°F). Do not refrigerate reconstituted granules. **XL Tab:** 20-25°C (68-77°F); excursions permitted between 15-30°C (59-86°F).

HOW SUPPLIED
Sus: 125mg/5mL, 250mg/5mL [50mL, 100mL]; **Tab:** 250mg, 500mg; **Tab, Extended-Release (XL):** 500mg

CONTRAINDICATIONS
Known hypersensitivity to clarithromycin, erythromycin, or any of the macrolide antibiotics. History of cholestatic jaundice/hepatic dysfunction associated w/ prior use of clarithromycin. Concomitant use w/ cisapride, pimozide, ergotamine, or dihydroergotamine, and w/ HMG-CoA reductase inhibitors that are extensively metabolized by CYP3A4 (lovastatin or simvastatin). Concomitant use w/ colchicine in patients w/ renal/hepatic impairment.

WARNINGS/PRECAUTIONS
D/C therapy immediately and institute appropriate treatment if severe acute hypersensitivity reactions (eg, anaphylaxis, Stevens-Johnson syndrome, toxic epidermal necrolysis, drug rash w/ eosinophilia and systemic symptoms, Henoch-Schonlein purpura) occur. QT interval prolongation, arrhythmia (infrequent), and torsades de pointes reported; avoid w/ known prolongation of the QT interval, ventricular cardiac arrhythmia (including torsades de pointes), ongoing proarrhythmic conditions (eg, uncorrected hypokalemia, hypomagnesemia) and clinically significant bradycardia. Hepatic dysfunction, including increased liver enzymes, and hepatocellular and/or cholestatic hepatitis, w/ or w/o jaundice, reported; d/c immediately if signs/symptoms of hepatitis occur. *Clostridium difficile*-associated diarrhea (CDAD) reported; may need to d/c if CDAD is suspected or confirmed. Avoid in pregnancy, except in clinical circumstances where no alternative therapy is appropriate. Exacerbation of symptoms of myasthenia gravis and new onset of symptoms of myasthenic syndrome reported. May result in bacterial resistance w/ prolonged use in the absence of a proven/suspected bacterial infection or a prophylactic indication. Caution in elderly.

ADVERSE REACTIONS
Abdominal pain, diarrhea, N/V, dysgeusia.

DRUG INTERACTIONS
See Contraindications and Dosing Considerations. Avoid Class IA (quinidine, procainamide) or Class III (dofetilide, amiodarone, sotalol) antiarrhythmic agents, and w/ drugs known to prolong the QT interval. Torsades de pointes reported w/ quinidine or disopyramide; monitor serum levels and monitor ECG for QT prolongation. May increase digoxin and carbamazepine levels. Serious adverse reactions have been reported w/ CYP3A4 substrates (eg, colchicine toxicity w/ colchicine; rhabdomyolysis w/ simvastatin, lovastatin, and atorvastatin; hypoglycemia w/ disopyramide; hypotension and acute kidney injury w/ calcium channel blockers metabolized by CYP3A4). CYP3A inducers (eg, efavirenz, nevirapine, rifampicin, rifapentine) may decrease levels; consider alternative antibacterial treatment. Caution w/ colchicine in patients w/ normal renal and hepatic function; reduce the dose of colchicine. Suspend therapy w/ lovastatin or simvastatin if treatment w/ clarithromycin cannot be avoided. Caution w/ atorvastatin and pravastatin; do not exceed 20mg/day of atorvastatin and 40mg/day of pravastatin if concomitant use cannot be avoided. Significant hypoglycemia may occur w/ oral hypoglycemic agents (eg, nateglinide, pioglitazone, repaglinide, rosiglitazone) and/or insulin. May increase quetiapine exposure and possible quetiapine related toxicities; refer to quetiapine prescribing information for recommendations on dose reduction. Risk of serious hemorrhage and significant elevations in PT/INR w/ warfarin; monitor PT/INR frequently when oral anticoagulants are administered concurrently. Increased

sedation and prolongation of sedation reported w/ triazolobenzodiazepines (eg, triazolam, midazolam). Dose adjustments may be necessary when coadministered w/ midazolam. Caution and appropriate dose adjustments should be considered when triazolam or alprazolam is coadministered. Erythromycin reported to decrease the clearance of triazolam and midazolam and may consequently increase the pharmacologic effect of these benzodiazepines. Concomitant use w/ itraconazole may increase itraconazole and clarithromycin levels; monitor for increased or prolonged adverse reactions. Caution w/ tolterodine in patients deficient in CYP2D6 activity; dose of tolterodine 1mg bid is recommended. Caution w/ atazanavir; consider alternative antibacterial therapy for indications other than MAC infections. Caution w/ saquinavir in patients w/ decreased renal function. Caution w/ ritonavir in patients w/ decreased renal function; consider alternative antibacterial therapy for indications other than *M. avium* infections. Doses of clarithromycin greater than 1000mg/day should not be coadministered w/ protease inhibitors. Caution w/ etravirine; may have reduced activity against MAC and alternatives should be considered for the treatment of MAC. May increase maraviroc exposure; refer to Selzentry prescribing information for dose recommendation. Concomitant use w/ boceprevir may affect both boceprevir and clarithromycin levels. Hypotension, bradyarrhythmias, and lactic acidosis reported w/ verapamil; caution w/ use. Hypotension and peripheral edema reported w/ nifedipine; caution w/ use. Interactions may occur w/ cyclosporine and tacrolimus. Not recommended w/ sildenafil, tadalafil, or vardenafil; consider a dose reduction for these phosphodiesterase inhibitors. Concomitant use w/ omeprazole may affect both omeprazole and clarithromycin levels. May increase theophylline levels; consider monitoring theophylline concentrations for patients receiving high doses of theophylline or w/ baseline concentrations in the upper therapeutic range. Concomitant use w/ rifabutin may increase rifabutin levels, decrease clarithromycin levels, and increase the risk of uveitis; consider alternative antibacterial therapy. Caution w/ alfentanil, methylprednisolone, cilostazol, bromocriptine, vinblastine, phenobarbital, St. John's wort, hexobarbital, phenytoin, and valproate. **Tab:** May decrease levels of zidovudine; separate zidovudine administration by at least 2 hrs. Refer to Biaxin prescribing information for further details on drug interactions.

PREGNANCY AND LACTATION
Pregnancy: Category C.
Lactation: Excreted in breast milk; caution in nursing.

MECHANISM OF ACTION
Semisynthetic macrolide antibiotic; exerts antibacterial action by binding to the 50S ribosomal subunit of susceptible bacteria, resulting in inhibition of protein synthesis.

PHARMACOKINETICS
Absorption: Rapid; (250mg tab) absolute bioavailability (50%). Administration of variable doses resulted in different parameters. **Distribution:** Found in breast milk. **Metabolism:** 14-OH clarithromycin (primary metabolite). **Elimination:** Urine (20-40% unchanged, 10-15% metabolite). $T_{1/2}$=3-4 hrs (250mg tab, XL tab), 5-7 hrs (500mg tab); $T_{1/2}$ (metabolite)=5-6 hrs (250mg tab), 7-9 hrs (500mg tab), 5-7 hrs (XL tab).

PATIENT CONSIDERATIONS
Assessment: Assess for hypersensitivity to clarithromycin, erythromycin, or any of the macrolide antibacterial drugs; history of cholestatic jaundice/hepatic dysfunction associated w/ prior use of clarithromycin; hepatic/renal impairment; QT interval prolongation; ongoing proarrhythmic conditions; clinically significant bradycardia; ventricular cardiac arrhythmia; torsades de pointes; myasthenia gravis; pregnancy/nursing status; and possible drug interactions.

Monitoring: Monitor for development of severe acute hypersensitivity reactions, QT prolongation, hepatotoxicity, CDAD, drug-resistant bacteria, exacerbation of myasthenia gravis, new onset of symptoms of myasthenic syndrome, and other adverse reactions. Monitor LFTs and renal function. Frequently monitor INR/PT w/ oral anticoagulants.

Counseling: Inform about potential benefits/risks of therapy. Counsel that therapy should only be used to treat bacterial, not viral, infections. Instruct to take exactly ud; inform that skipping doses or not completing full course may decrease effectiveness and increase antibiotic resistance. Instruct to notify physician if watery/bloody diarrhea (w/ or w/o stomach cramps and fever) develops, even as late as ≥2 months after treatment. Advise about the potential for dizziness, vertigo, confusion, and disorientation w/ therapy; instruct to consider these adverse reactions before driving or using machines. Instruct to notify physician if pregnant/nursing and of all medications currently being taken.

BINOSTO — alendronate sodium   Rx
Class: Bisphosphonate

ADULT DOSAGE
Osteoporosis
Treatment in Postmenopausal Women:
One 70mg effervescent tab once weekly

Treatment to Increase Bone Mass in Men w/ Osteoporosis:
One 70mg effervescent tab once weekly

Missed Dose
If once-weekly dose is missed, administer 1 dose on am after patient remembers; do not take 2 doses on same day, but return to taking 1 dose once a week, as originally scheduled on chosen day

PEDIATRIC DOSAGE
Pediatric use may not have been established

DOSING CONSIDERATIONS
Renal Impairment
CrCl <35mL/min: Not recommended

ADMINISTRATION
Oral route

Take upon arising for the day and at least 30 min before the 1st food, beverage, or medication of the day
Dissolve the effervescent tab in 4 oz room temperature plain water only (not mineral water or flavored water)
Wait at least 5 min after the effervescence stops and then stir the sol for approx 10 sec and ingest
Do not lie down for at least 30 min and until after 1st food of the day

STORAGE
20-25°C (68-77°F); excursions permitted to 15-30°C (59-86°F). Protect from moisture.

HOW SUPPLIED
Tab, Effervescent: 70mg

CONTRAINDICATIONS
Esophageal abnormalities that delay esophageal emptying (eg, stricture, achalasia), inability to stand or sit upright for at least 30 min, hypocalcemia, patients at increased risk of aspiration, hypersensitivity to any component of this product.

WARNINGS/PRECAUTIONS
Consider discontinuation after 3-5 yrs of use in patients at low risk for fracture; periodically reevaluate risk for fracture in patients who d/c therapy. May cause local irritation of the upper GI mucosa; caution w/ active upper GI problems (eg, Barrett's esophagus, dysphagia, gastritis). Esophageal reactions (eg, esophagitis, esophageal ulcers/erosions) reported; d/c if dysphagia, odynophagia, retrosternal pain, or new/worsening heartburn develops. Use therapy under appropriate supervision in patients who cannot comply w/ dosing instructions due to mental disability. Gastric and duodenal ulcers reported. Treat hypocalcemia and other disorders affecting mineral metabolism (eg, vitamin D deficiency) prior to therapy. Asymptomatic decreases in serum Ca^{2+} and phosphate may occur; ensure adequate Ca^{2+} and vitamin D intake. Severe and occasionally incapacitating bone, joint, and/or muscle pain reported; d/c if severe symptoms develop. Osteonecrosis of the jaw (ONJ) reported; risk may increase w/ duration of exposure to drug. If invasive dental procedures are required, discontinuation of treatment may reduce risk for ONJ. Consider discontinuation if ONJ develops. Atypical, low-energy, or low-trauma fractures of the femoral shaft reported; evaluate any patient w/ a history of bisphosphonate exposure who presents w/ thigh/groin pain to rule out incomplete femur fracture, and consider interruption of therapy. Contains 650mg of Na^+; caution in patients who have Na^+-intake restrictions.

ADVERSE REACTIONS
Nausea, abdominal pain, musculoskeletal pain, acid regurgitation, dyspepsia, constipation, diarrhea.

DRUG INTERACTIONS
Ca^{2+} supplements, antacids, or oral medications containing multivalent cations will interfere w/ absorption; wait at least 1/2 hr after taking alendronate before taking any other oral medications. Increased incidence of upper GI adverse events in patients receiving concomitant therapy w/ daily doses of alendronate >10mg and aspirin-containing products. NSAID use is associated w/ GI irritation; use w/ caution. Slightly decreased bioavailability w/ levothyroxine.

PREGNANCY AND LACTATION
Category C, caution in nursing.

MECHANISM OF ACTION
Bisphosphonate; binds to hydroxyapatite found in bone and specifically inhibits the osteoclast-mediated bone resorption.

PHARMACOKINETICS
Absorption: Absolute bioavailability (0.64% in women), (0.59% in men).
Distribution: V_d=at least 28L (exclusive of bone); plasma protein binding (78%).
Elimination: (IV) Urine (50%); $T_{1/2}$>10 yrs.

PATIENT CONSIDERATIONS
Assessment: Assess for esophageal abnormalities, ability to stand or sit upright for at least 30 min, hypocalcemia, risk for aspiration or ONJ, active upper GI problems, mental disability, Na^+-intake restriction, renal impairment, drug hypersensitivity, any other conditions where treatment is contraindicated or cautioned, pregnancy/nursing status, and possible drug interactions.

Monitoring: Monitor for signs/symptoms of ONJ, atypical fractures, esophageal reactions, musculoskeletal pain, hypocalcemia, and other adverse events. Monitor serum Ca^{2+} levels. Periodically reevaluate the need for continued therapy.

Counseling: Inform about benefits/risks of therapy. Instruct to follow all dosing instructions and inform that failure to follow them may increase risk of esophageal problems. Instruct to take supplemental Ca^{2+} and vitamin D if daily dietary intake is inadequate. Counsel to consider weight-bearing exercise along w/ modification of certain behavioral factors (eg, cigarette smoking, excessive alcohol use), if these factors exist. Instruct to take upon arising for the day and at least 30 min before the 1st food, beverage, or medication of the day. Advise to avoid lying down for at least 30 min after taking the drug and until after 1st food of the day. Instruct not to attempt to swallow, chew, or suck on the tab because of a potential for oropharyngeal ulceration. Advise to d/c and consult physician if symptoms of esophageal disease develop. Instruct that if the once-weekly dose is missed, to take 1 dose on the am after patient remembers and to return to taking the dose, as originally scheduled on their chosen day; instruct not to take 2 doses on the same day. Inform patients on Na^+-restricted diet that each tab contains 650mg Na^+, equivalent to 1650mg NaCl.

BIVIGAM — immune globulin intravenous (human)

Rx

Class: Immune globulin

> Thrombosis may occur. Renal dysfunction, acute renal failure, osmotic nephrosis, and death reported w/ immune globulin intravenous (IGIV) products, particularly those containing sucrose; this product does not contain sucrose. For patients at risk of thrombosis (eg, advanced age, prolonged immobilization, hypercoagulable conditions, history of venous/arterial thrombosis, use of estrogens, indwelling central vascular catheters, hyperviscosity, cardiovascular risk factors), renal dysfunction, or renal failure (eg, preexisting renal insufficiency, diabetes mellitus, age >65 yrs, volume depletion, sepsis, paraproteinemia, or receiving known nephrotoxic drugs), administer at the minimum dose and infusion rate practicable. Ensure adequate hydration before administration. Monitor for signs/symptoms of thrombosis and assess blood viscosity if at risk for hyperviscosity.

ADULT DOSAGE

Primary Humoral Immunodeficiency

Replacement Therapy:
Recommended Dose: 300-800mg/kg every 3-4 weeks
Titrate: May adjust to achieve desired trough levels and clinical response
Initial Infusion Rate:
0.5mg/kg/min (0.005mL/kg/min) for the first 10 min
Maint Infusion Rate:
Increase every 20 min (if tolerated) by 0.8mg/kg/min up to 6mg/kg/min

PEDIATRIC DOSAGE

Pediatric use may not have been established

DOSING CONSIDERATIONS

Elderly

Do not exceed recommended doses; administer at minimum infusion rate practicable

Adverse Reactions

Slow or stop the infusion if adverse reactions occur; may resume at a lower rate if symptoms subside

ADMINISTRATION

IV route

Allow refrigerated product to come to room temperature before use and maintain at room temperature during administration.
Do not freeze or heat; do not use any sol that has been frozen or heated.
Do not shake.
Do not mix w/ other IGIV products or other IV medications.
If large doses are to be administered, several vials may be pooled using aseptic technique into sterile infusion bags and infused.
Do not dilute.

STORAGE

2-8°C (36-46°F). Do not freeze or heat; do not use any sol that has been frozen or heated.

HOW SUPPLIED

Inj: 10% [50mL, 100mL]

CONTRAINDICATIONS

History of an anaphylactic or severe systemic reaction to the administration of human immune globulin, IgA-deficient patients w/ antibodies to IgA and a history of hypersensitivity.

WARNINGS/PRECAUTIONS

Contains trace amounts of IgA; severe hypersensitivity reactions may occur. D/C infusion immediately and institute appropriate treatment if hypersensitivity develops. Consider discontinuation if renal function deteriorates. Hyperproteinemia, increased serum viscosity, and hyponatremia may occur. Distinguish true hyponatremia from pseudohyponatremia that is associated w/ or related to hyperproteinemia w/ concomitant decreased calculated serum osmolality or elevated osmolar gap; treatment aimed at decreasing serum free water in patients w/ pseudohyponatremia may lead to volume depletion, a further increase in serum viscosity, and a possible predisposition to thrombotic events. Aseptic meningitis syndrome (AMS) may occur; may occur more frequently w/ high doses (eg, 2g/kg) and/or rapid infusion; rule out other causes of meningitis. Delayed hemolytic anemia may develop and acute hemolysis reported. Noncardiogenic pulmonary edema may occur; if transfusion-related acute lung injury (TRALI) is suspected, perform tests for presence of antineutrophil antibodies in both the product and patient's serum. May carry a risk of transmitting infectious agents (eg, viruses, Creutzfeldt-Jakob disease agent). May interfere w/ some serological tests.

ADVERSE REACTIONS

Headache, fatigue, infusion-site reaction, nausea, sinusitis, BP increased, diarrhea, dizziness, lethargy.

DRUG INTERACTIONS

See Boxed Warning. Passive transfer of antibodies may transiently interfere w/ the immune response to live virus vaccines (eg, measles, mumps, rubella, varicella).

PREGNANCY AND LACTATION

Pregnancy: Category C.
Lactation: Caution in nursing.

MECHANISM OF ACTION

Immune globulin; not established. Replacement therapy in patients w/ primary humoral immunodeficiency. The broad spectrum of neutralizing IgG antibodies against bacterial and viral pathogens and their toxins helps to avoid recurrent serious opportunistic infections.

PHARMACOKINETICS

Absorption: C_{max}=2137mg/dL; T_{max}=3.5 hrs; AUC=33,592 day•mg/dL. **Distribution:** V_d=0.626dL/kg. **Elimination:** $T_{1/2}$=30 days.

PATIENT CONSIDERATIONS

Assessment: Assess for history of anaphylactic or severe systemic reactions to human immune globulin, IgA deficiency, risk of thrombosis/renal dysfunction/renal failure, pregnancy/nursing status, and possible drug interactions. Assess renal function. Consider baseline assessment of blood viscosity in patients at risk for hyperviscosity, including those w/ cryoglobulins, fasting chylomicronemia/markedly high TGs, or monoclonal gammopathies.

Monitoring: Monitor for thrombosis, hypersensitivity reactions, hyperproteinemia, increased serum viscosity, hyponatremia, hemolytic anemia, pulmonary adverse reactions, infection, and other adverse reactions. Monitor renal function and urine output periodically. Perform neurological exam, including CSF studies, if AMS is suspected. Perform confirmatory lab testing if signs/symptoms of hemolysis are present after an infusion. Perform tests for the presence of antineutrophil antibodies in both product and patient's serum if TRALI is suspected. Monitor vital signs throughout the infusion.

Counseling: Instruct to immediately report signs/symptoms of acute renal dysfunction/failure, thrombosis, AMS, hemolysis, TRALI, and infection. Inform that drug is made from human plasma and may contain infectious agents that can cause disease. Inform that product can interfere w/ immune response to live viral vaccines; instruct to notify physician of this potential interaction when receiving vaccinations.

BLINCYTO — blinatumomab

Rx

Class: CD19-directed CD3 T-cell engager

> Cytokine release syndrome (CRS), which may be life-threatening or fatal, reported; interrupt or d/c therapy as recommended. Neurological toxicities, which may be severe, life-threatening, or fatal, reported; interrupt or d/c therapy as recommended.

ADULT DOSAGE

Acute Lymphoblastic Leukemia

Philadelphia Chromosome-Negative: Relapsed or Refractory B-Cell Precursor:
>45kg:
Cycle 1: 9mcg/day on Days 1-7, and 28mcg/day on Days 8-28
Subsequent Cycles: 28mcg/day on Days 1-28

Single cycle of treatment consists of 4 weeks of continuous IV infusion followed by a 2-week treatment-free interval
Treatment course consists of up to 2 cycles for induction followed by 3 additional cycles for consolidation treatment (up to a total of 5 cycles)

PEDIATRIC DOSAGE

Acute Lymphoblastic Leukemia

Philadelphia Chromosome-Negative: Relapsed or Refractory B-Cell Precursor:

Limited experience in pediatric patients

Evaluated in a dose-escalation study of 41 pediatric patients with relapsed or refractory B-precursor acute lymphoblastic leukemia (median age was 6 yrs [range: 2-17 yrs]). Administered at doses of 5-30mcg/m²/day. Recommended phase 2 regimen was 5mcg/m²/day on Days 1-7 and 15mcg/m²/day on Days 8-28 for cycle 1, and 15mcg/m²/day on Days 1-28 for subsequent cycles

Steady-state concentrations were comparable in adult and pediatric patients at the equivalent dose levels based on BSA-based regimens

DOSING CONSIDERATIONS

Adverse Reactions

If interruption after an adverse event is no longer than 7 days, continue same cycle to a total of 28 days of infusion inclusive of days before and after the interruption in that cycle. If an interruption due to an adverse event is >7 days, start a new cycle

Cytokine Release Syndrome:

Grade 3: Withhold until resolved, then restart at 9mcg/day. Escalate to 28mcg/day after 7 days if the toxicity does not recur
Grade 4: D/C permanently

Neurological Toxicity:

Seizure: D/C permanently if >1 seizure occurs
Grade 3: Withhold until no more than Grade 1 (mild) for at least 3 days, then restart at 9mcg/day. Escalate to 28mcg/day after 7 days if the toxicity does not recur. If the toxicity occurred at 9mcg/day, or if the toxicity takes >7 days to resolve, d/c permanently
Grade 4: D/C permanently

Other Clinically Relevant Adverse Reactions:

Grade 3: Withhold until no more than Grade 1 (mild), then restart at 9mcg/day. Escalate to 28mcg/day after 7 days if the toxicity does not recur. If the toxicity takes >14 days to resolve, d/c permanently
Grade 4: Consider discontinuing permanently

ADMINISTRATION

IV route

Premedicate with dexamethasone 20mg IV 1 hr prior to the 1st dose of each cycle, prior to a step dose (eg, Cycle 1 day 8), or when restarting an infusion after an interruption of ≥4 hrs.
Administer as a continuous IV infusion at a constant flow rate using an infusion pump that is programmable, lockable, non-elastomeric, and has an alarm.

Infusion bags should be infused over 24 hrs or 48 hrs.
Infuse the total 240mL sol according to the instructions on the pharmacy label on the bag at 1 of the following constant infusion rates:
Infusion rate of 10mL/hr for a duration of 24 hrs, or 5mL/hr for a duration of 48 hrs.
Refer to PI for further administration, reconstitution, and preparation instructions.

STORAGE
2-8°C (36-46°F). Protect from light until time of use. Do not freeze. May store lyophilized vial and IV sol stabilizer for a max of 8 hrs at room temperature. **Reconstituted Vial:** 23-27°C (73-81°F) for 4 hrs, or 2-8°C (36-46°F) for 24 hrs. Protect from light. **Prepared IV Bag Containing Sol for Infusion:** 23-27°C (73-81°F) for 48 hrs (storage time includes infusion time; if not administered within the time frames and temperatures indicated, discard and do not refrigerate again), or 2-8°C (36-46°F) for 8 days. Ship in packaging that has been validated to maintain temperature of the contents at 2-8°C (36-46°F). Do not freeze.

HOW SUPPLIED
Inj: 35mcg

CONTRAINDICATIONS
Known hypersensitivity to blinatumomab or to any component of the product formulation.

WARNINGS/PRECAUTIONS
Hospitalization is recommended for the first 9 days of the 1st cycle and the first 2 days of the 2nd cycle. For all subsequent cycle starts and reinitiation (eg, if treatment is interrupted for ≥4 hrs), supervision by a healthcare professional or hospitalization is recommended. Infusion reactions may occur and may be clinically indistinguishable from manifestations of CRS. Disseminated intravascular coagulation (DIC), capillary leak syndrome (CLS), and hemophagocytic lymphohistiocytosis/macrophage activation syndrome (HLH/MAS) reported in the setting of CRS. Serious infections (eg, sepsis, pneumonia, bacteremia, opportunistic infections, catheter-site infections) reported; administer prophylactic antibiotics and employ surveillance testing during treatment as appropriate. Tumor lysis syndrome (TLS) reported; use appropriate prophylactic measures, including pretreatment nontoxic cytoreduction and on-treatment hydration; may require either temporary interruption or discontinuation of therapy. Neutropenia and febrile neutropenia, including life-threatening cases, reported; interrupt therapy if prolonged neutropenia occurs. Risk for loss of consciousness. Associated with transient elevations in liver enzymes; interrupt therapy if the transaminases rise to >5X ULN or if bilirubin rises to >3X ULN. Cranial magnetic resonance imaging changes showing leukoencephalopathy observed, especially in patients with prior treatment with cranial irradiation and antileukemic chemotherapy (including systemic high-dose methotrexate or intrathecal cytarabine); clinical significance of this is unknown. Preparation and administration errors reported; follow instructions strictly to minimize medication errors. Potential for immunogenicity. Caution in elderly.

ADVERSE REACTIONS
CRS, neurological toxicities, pyrexia, headache, peripheral edema, febrile neutropenia, nausea, hypokalemia, constipation, anemia, diarrhea, fatigue, bacterial infections, tremor, cough.

DRUG INTERACTIONS
May suppress CYP450 enzymes; highest risk during the first 9 days of the 1st cycle and the first 2 days of the 2nd cycle in patients receiving concomitant CYP450 substrates, particularly those with a narrow therapeutic index; monitor for toxicity (eg, warfarin) or drug concentrations (eg, cyclosporine) and adjust dose of concomitant drug PRN.

PREGNANCY AND LACTATION
Category C, not for use in nursing.

MECHANISM OF ACTION
Bispecific CD19-directed CD3 T-cell engager; binds to CD19 expressed on the surface of cells of B-lineage origin and CD3 expressed on the surface of T-cells. Activates endogenous T-cells by connecting CD3 in the T-cell receptor complex with CD19 on benign and malignant B cells. Mediates formation of a synapse between the T-cell and the tumor cell, up-regulation of cell adhesion molecules, production of cytolytic proteins, release of inflammatory cytokines, and proliferation of T-cells, resulting in redirected lysis of CD19+ cells.

PHARMACOKINETICS
Distribution: V_d=4.52L. **Elimination:** $T_{1/2}$=2.11 hrs.

PATIENT CONSIDERATIONS
Assessment: Assess for known hypersensitivity to drug or to any component of the formulation, prior treatment with cranial irradiation and antileukemic chemotherapy, pregnancy/nursing status, and possible drug interactions. Obtain baseline WBC count, absolute neutrophil count (ANC), ALT, AST, gamma-glutamyl transferase (GGT), and total bilirubin.

Monitoring: Monitor for signs/symptoms of CRS, DIC, CLS, HLH/MAS, neurological toxicities, infections, TLS, loss of consciousness, and other adverse reactions. Monitor for neutropenia/febrile neutropenia; monitor lab parameters (eg, WBC count, ANC) during infusion. Monitor ALT, AST, GGT, and total blood bilirubin during therapy.

Counseling: Advise to contact physician for any signs/symptoms of CRS or infusion reactions, neurological toxicities, or infections (eg, pneumonia). Advise to refrain from driving and engaging in hazardous occupations/activities (eg, operating heavy/potentially dangerous machinery) while on therapy and inform that neurological events may be experienced. Inform that it is very important to keep area around the IV catheter clean to reduce the risk of infection. Advise to not adjust setting on the infusion pump; inform that any changes to pump function may result in dosing errors. Instruct to contact physician or nurse immediately if there is a problem with the infusion pump or the pump alarms.

BONIVA — ibandronate   Rx
Class: Bisphosphonate

ADULT DOSAGE
Osteoporosis

Inj:
Treatment in Postmenopausal Women:
3mg IV over 15-30 sec every 3 months

Tab:
Treatment and Prevention in Postmenopausal Women:
150mg once monthly on the same date each month

Missed Dose

Inj:
If dose is missed, administer as soon as it can be rescheduled
Thereafter, schedule every 3 months from date of last inj

Tab:
If next scheduled ibandronate day is >7 days away, take one 150mg tab in am following date that it is remembered
If next scheduled ibandronate day is 1-7 days away, wait until subsequent month's scheduled ibandronate day to take tab
For both scenarios, return to original schedule by taking one 150mg tab every month on previous chosen day for subsequent doses

---

DOSING CONSIDERATIONS
Renal Impairment
Severe (CrCl <30mL/min): Not recommended

ADMINISTRATION
IV/Oral route

Inj
Do not mix w/ Ca^{2+}-containing sol or other IV administered drugs.
Do not use prefilled syringes w/ particulate matter or discoloration.
Administer only w/ the enclosed needle.
Do not administer more frequently than once every 3 months.

Tab
Take at least 60 min before the 1st food or drink of the day other than water or before taking any oral medication or supplementation.
Swallow tabs whole; do not chew or suck.
Swallow tabs w/ full glass of plain water (6-8 oz) while standing or sitting in upright position; avoid lying down for 60 min after taking medication.
Do not eat, drink anything except plain water, or take other medications for at least 60 min after taking ibandronate.

STORAGE
25°C (77°F); excursions permitted to 15-30°C (59-86°F).

HOW SUPPLIED
Inj: 3mg/3mL [prefilled syringe]; **Tab:** 150mg

CONTRAINDICATIONS
Hypocalcemia. **Tab:** Esophageal abnormalities that delay esophageal emptying (eg, stricture or achalasia), inability to stand or sit upright for at least 60 min, known hypersensitivity to ibandronate sodium or to any of its excipients.

WARNINGS/PRECAUTIONS
Consider discontinuation after 3-5 yrs of use in patients at low-risk for fracture; periodically reevaluate risk for fracture in patients who d/c therapy. Hypocalcemia reported; treat hypocalcemia and other disturbances of bone and mineral metabolism before therapy. Osteonecrosis of the jaw (ONJ) reported; risk may increase w/ duration of exposure to drug or w/ concomitant administration of drugs associated w/ ONJ. Consider a dental examination w/ appropriate preventive dentistry prior to treatment in patients w/ a history of concomitant risk factors (eg, cancer, chemotherapy, angiogenesis inhibitors, radiotherapy, corticosteroids, poor oral hygiene) and if possible, avoid invasive dental procedures while on treatment. For patients requiring invasive dental procedures, discontinuation of treatment may reduce risk for ONJ. Consider discontinuation if ONJ develops. Severe and occasionally incapacitating bone, joint, and/or muscle pain reported; d/c if severe symptoms develop. Atypical, low-energy, or low-trauma fractures of the femoral shaft reported; evaluate any patient w/ a history of bisphosphonate exposure who presents w/ thigh/groin pain to rule out an incomplete femur fracture, and consider interruption of therapy. (Inj) Caution not to administer intra-arterially or paravenously as this could lead to tissue damage. Anaphylaxis reported; d/c and initiate appropriate treatment if anaphylactic or other severe hypersensitivity/allergic reactions occur. **Tab:** May cause local irritation of the upper GI mucosa; caution w/ active upper GI problems (eg, Barrett's esophagus, dysphagia, esophageal diseases, gastritis, duodenitis, ulcers). Esophageal reactions (eg, esophagitis, esophageal ulcers/erosions) reported; d/c if dysphagia, odynophagia, retrosternal pain, or new/worsening heartburn develops. Use therapy under appropriate supervision in patients who cannot comply w/ dosing instructions due to mental disability. Gastric and duodenal ulcers reported.

PEDIATRIC DOSAGE
Pediatric use may not have been established

ADVERSE REACTIONS

Influenza, nasopharyngitis, abdominal pain, dyspepsia, constipation, arthralgia, back pain, pain in extremity, headache, diarrhea, UTI, myalgia.

DRUG INTERACTIONS

May interfere w/ the use of bone-imaging agents. **Tab:** Products containing Ca^{2+} and other multivalent cations (eg, aluminum, Mg^{2+}, iron) may interfere w/ absorption; do not take these products w/in 60 min of dosing. Caution w/ aspirin or NSAIDs due to GI irritation.

PREGNANCY AND LACTATION

Category C, caution in nursing.

MECHANISM OF ACTION

Bisphosphonate; has an affinity for hydroxyapatite, which is part of the mineral matrix of bone. Inhibits osteoclast activity and reduces bone resorption and turnover. In postmenopausal women, it reduces the elevated rate of bone turnover, leading to, on average, net gain in bone mass.

PHARMACOKINETICS

Absorption: (Tab) Bioavailability (0.6%); T_{max}=0.5-2 hrs. **Distribution:** V_d=at least 90L. (Inj) Plasma protein binding (86%). (Tab) Plasma protein binding (90.9-99.5% [2-10ng/mL concentration]; 85.7% [0.5-10ng/mL concentration]). **Elimination:** Kidney (50-60%, unchanged). (Inj) $T_{1/2}$=4.6-15.3 hrs (2mg), 5-25.5 hrs (4mg). (Tab) Feces (unchanged); $T_{1/2}$=37-157 hrs.

PATIENT CONSIDERATIONS

Assessment: Assess for hypocalcemia, disturbances of bone and mineral metabolism, risk for ONJ, renal impairment, drug hypersensitivity, any other conditions where treatment is contraindicated or cautioned, pregnancy/nursing status, and possible drug interactions. **Inj:** Obtain SrCr before each dose. Perform routine oral exam, and consider appropriate preventive dentistry in patients w/ history of concomitant risk factors for ONJ. **Tab:** Assess for esophageal abnormalities, ability to stand or sit upright for at least 60 min, active upper GI problems, and mental disability.

Monitoring: Monitor for signs/symptoms of ONJ, musculoskeletal pain, hypocalcemia, atypical femoral fracture, and other adverse reactions. Monitor renal function and periodically reevaluate the need for continued therapy. **Tab:** Monitor for esophageal reactions. **Inj:** Monitor for severe hypersensitivity/allergic reactions.

Counseling: Inform about benefits/risks of therapy. Instruct to take supplemental Ca^{2+} and vitamin D if dietary intake is inadequate. **Tab:** Instruct to carefully follow dosing instructions and on what to do if doses are missed. Advise to d/c and seek medical attention if symptoms of esophageal irritation develop. Instruct on appropriate administration of drug.

BOOSTRIX — tetanus toxoid, reduced diphtheria toxoid and acellular pertussis vaccine, adsorbed

Rx

Class: Toxoid/vaccine combination

ADULT DOSAGE	PEDIATRIC DOSAGE
Active Booster Immunization Against Tetanus, Diphtheria, and Pertussis	**Active Booster Immunization Against Tetanus, Diphtheria, and Pertussis**
0.5mL IM single dose	**≥10 Years:**
	0.5mL IM single dose
Wound Management:	
May be given as a tetanus prophylaxis if no previous dose of any tetanus toxoid, reduced diphtheria toxoid, and acellular pertussis vaccine, adsorbed (Tdap) has been administered	**Wound Management:**
	May be given as a tetanus prophylaxis if no previous dose of any tetanus toxoid, reduced diphtheria toxoid, and acellular pertussis vaccine, adsorbed (Tdap) has been administered

ADMINISTRATION

IM route

5 yrs should elapse between the last dose of the recommended series of diphtheria and tetanus toxoids and acellular pertussis vaccine adsorbed (DTaP) and/or tetanus and diphtheria toxoids adsorbed for adult use (Td) vaccine and administration of Boostrix.

Shake vigorously to obtain a homogeneous, turbid, white sus before administration; do not use if resuspension does not occur w/ vigorous shaking. Inject into the deltoid muscle of the upper arm.
Do not administer IV, intradermally, or SQ.
Do not mix w/ any other vaccine in the same syringe or vial.

STORAGE

2-8°C (36-46°F). Do not freeze; discard if has been frozen.

HOW SUPPLIED

Inj: 0.5mL [vial, prefilled syringe]

CONTRAINDICATIONS

A severe allergic reaction (eg, anaphylaxis) after a previous dose of any tetanus toxoid-, diphtheria toxoid-, or pertussis antigen-containing vaccine or any component of this vaccine. Encephalopathy (eg, coma, decreased level of consciousness, prolonged seizures) w/in 7 days of administration of a previous dose of a pertussis antigen-containing vaccine that is not attributable to another identifiable cause.

WARNINGS/PRECAUTIONS

Tip caps of prefilled syringes contain natural rubber latex; may cause allergic reactions. May cause brachial neuritis and Guillain-Barre syndrome. Risk of

Guillain-Barre syndrome may increase if Guillain-Barre syndrome occurred w/ in 6 weeks of receipt of a prior tetanus toxoid-containing vaccine. Syncope may occur and can be accompanied by transient neurological signs (eg, visual disturbance, paresthesia, tonic-clonic limb movements). Defer vaccination in patients w/ progressive/unstable neurologic conditions (eg, cerebrovascular events, acute encephalopathic conditions). Avoid if patient experienced an Arthus-type hypersensitivity reaction following a prior dose of tetanus toxoid-containing vaccine unless at least 10 yrs have elapsed since last dose of tetanus toxoid-containing vaccine. Expected immune response may not be obtained in immunosuppressed persons. Review immunization history for possible vaccine sensitivity and previous vaccination-related adverse reactions; epinephrine and other appropriate agents should be immediately available for control of allergic reactions.

ADVERSE REACTIONS

Adolescents (10-18 Years): Inj-site reactions (eg, pain, redness, swelling), increase in arm circumference of injected arm, headache, fatigue, GI symptoms.
Adults (19-64 Years): Inj-site reactions (eg, pain, redness, swelling), headache, fatigue, GI symptoms.
Elderly (≥65 Years): Pain at inj site.

DRUG INTERACTIONS

Lower postvaccination geometric mean antibody concentrations (GMCs) to pertactin observed following concomitant administration w/ meningococcal conjugate vaccine as compared to Boostrix administered 1st. Lower GMCs for antibodies to the pertussis antigens filamentous hemagglutinin and pertactin observed when concomitantly administered w/ influenza virus vaccine as compared w/ Boostrix alone. Immunosuppressive therapies, including irradiation, antimetabolites, alkylating agents, cytotoxic drugs, and corticosteroids (used in greater than physiologic doses), may reduce the immune response to vaccine.

PREGNANCY AND LACTATION

Pregnancy: Category B. A pregnancy registry is available.
Lactation: Caution in nursing.

MECHANISM OF ACTION

Vaccine/toxoid combination; develops neutralizing antibodies to tetanus, diphtheria, and pertussis.

PATIENT CONSIDERATIONS

Assessment: Assess for history of encephalopathy, latex hypersensitivity, development of Guillain-Barre syndrome following a prior vaccine containing tetanus toxoid, progressive/unstable neurologic conditions, immunosuppression, pregnancy/nursing status, and for possible drug interactions. Review immunization history for possible vaccine sensitivity and previous vaccination-related adverse reactions.

Monitoring: Monitor for signs and symptoms of Guillain-Barre syndrome, brachial neuritis, allergic reactions, syncope, neurological signs, and other adverse reactions. Monitor immune response.

Counseling: Inform about benefits/risks of immunization. Advise about the potential for adverse reactions. Instruct to notify physician if any adverse reactions occur, if pregnant, or if planning to become pregnant. Encourage pregnant women receiving the vaccine to contact the pregnancy registry.

BOSULIF — bosutinib

Rx

Class: Kinase inhibitor

ADULT DOSAGE	PEDIATRIC DOSAGE
Chronic Myelogenous Leukemia	Pediatric use may not have been established
Chronic, accelerated, or blast phase Philadelphia chromosome-positive chronic myelogenous leukemia w/ resistance or intolerance to prior therapy	
500mg qd until disease progression or patient intolerance	
Titrate: Consider escalation to 600mg qd in patients who do not reach complete hematological response by Week 8 or a complete cytogenetic response by Week 12, who did not have Grade 3 or higher adverse reactions, and who are currently taking 500mg qd	

DOSING CONSIDERATIONS

Concomitant Medications
CYP3A Strong or Moderate Inducers/Inhibitors: Avoid use
Renal Impairment
CrCl 30-50mL/min:
Initial: 400mg qd

CrCl <30mL/min:
Initial: 300mg qd

Declining Renal Function/Not Tolerating 500mg: Follow recommendations for toxicity

Hepatic Impairment
Mild (Child-Pugh A), Moderate (Child-Pugh B), or Severe (Child-Pugh C): 200mg qd

Adverse Reactions

Elevated Liver Transaminases:
≥3X ULN w/ Bilirubin elevations >2X ULN and Alkaline Phosphatase <2X ULN: D/C therapy
>5X ULN: Withhold therapy until recovery to ≤2.5X ULN and resume at 400mg qd thereafter; if recovery takes longer than 4 weeks, d/c therapy

Diarrhea:
Grade 3-4: Withhold therapy until recovery to Grade ≤1; may resume at 400mg qd

Other Significant, Moderate/Severe Nonhematologic Toxicity:
Withhold until toxicity has resolved, then consider 400mg qd; if clinically appropriate, consider re-escalating to 500mg qd

Myelosuppression:
ANC <1000 x 10^6/L or Platelets <50,000 x 10^6/L:
Withhold therapy until ANC ≥1000 x 10^6/L and platelets ≥50,000 x 10^6/L; resume therapy at the same dose if recovery occurs w/in 2 weeks
If blood counts remain low for >2 weeks, upon recovery, reduce dose by 100mg and resume treatment
If cytopenia recurs, reduce dose by an additional 100mg upon recovery and resume treatment

Doses less than 300 mg/day have not been evaluated

ADMINISTRATION
Oral route

Take w/ food.

Do not crush or cut tab; do not touch or handle crushed or broken tabs.

STORAGE
20-25°C (68-77°F); excursions permitted to 15-30°C (59-86°F).

HOW SUPPLIED
Tab: 100mg, 500mg

CONTRAINDICATIONS
Hypersensitivity to bosutinib.

WARNINGS/PRECAUTIONS
Diarrhea, N/V, and abdominal pain reported; monitor and manage patients using standards of care. Thrombocytopenia, anemia, and neutropenia reported; withhold, reduce dose, or d/c therapy as necessary. Hepatic toxicity reported. Fluid retention reported and may manifest as pericardial effusion, pleural effusion, pulmonary edema, and/or peripheral edema; monitor and manage patients using standards of care. Consider dose adjustment w/ baseline and treatment emergent renal impairment. May cause fetal harm.

ADVERSE REACTIONS
Diarrhea, N/V, thrombocytopenia, abdominal pain, rash, anemia, pyrexia, fatigue, neutropenia, edema, asthenia, respiratory tract infection, decreased appetite, headache, dyspnea.

DRUG INTERACTIONS
See Dosing Considerations. Lansoprazole may decrease levels; consider using short-acting antacids or H_2-blockers instead of proton pump inhibitors, but separate dosing by >2 hrs. May increase concentrations of drugs that are P-gp substrates (eg, digoxin).

PREGNANCY AND LACTATION
Category D, not for use in nursing.

MECHANISM OF ACTION
Tyrosine kinase inhibitor; inhibits the Bcr-Abl kinase that promotes CML. Also inhibits Src-family kinases, including Src, Lyn, and Hck.

PHARMACOKINETICS
Absorption: (500mg, Multiple-dose) C_{max}=200ng/mL; AUC=3650ng•hr/mL. (500mg, Single-dose) T_{max}=4-6 hrs (median). **Distribution:** Plasma protein binding (94%, in vitro; 96%, ex vivo [healthy]); (500mg, Single-dose) V_d=6080L. **Metabolism:** Via CYP3A4; oxydechlorinated bosutinib and N-desmethylated bosutinib (major circulating metabolites). **Elimination:** (Healthy) Feces (91.3%), urine (3%); (500mg, Single-dose) $T_{1/2}$=22.5 hrs.

PATIENT CONSIDERATIONS

Assessment: Assess for hypersensitivity to drug, hepatic/renal impairment, pregnancy/nursing status, and possible drug interactions.

Monitoring: Monitor for signs/symptoms of GI toxicity, fluid retention, and other adverse reactions. Perform CBC weekly for the 1st month and then monthly thereafter, or as clinically indicated. Perform monthly LFTs for the first 3 months and as clinically indicated; monitor more frequently in patients w/ transaminase elevations. Monitor renal function during therapy w/ particular attention to patients w/ preexisting renal impairment or risk factors for renal dysfunction.

Counseling: Instruct to take medication exactly as prescribed and not to change the dose or d/c unless directed by physician. Instruct that if a dose is missed beyond 12 hrs, to skip the dose and take the usual prescribed dose on the following day. Advise to seek medical attention promptly if symptoms of GI problems or fluid retention develop, developing renal problems or if symptoms of other adverse reactions (eg, respiratory tract infections, rash, fatigue) are significant. Instruct to immediately report fever, any suggestion of infection, signs/symptoms of bleeding or easy bruising, or jaundice. Inform that drug may cause fetal harm; counsel females of reproductive potential to use effective contraceptive measures to prevent pregnancy during and for at least 30 days after completing treatment. Instruct to contact physician immediately if pregnancy occurs during treatment. Advise not to breastfeed or provide breast milk to infants while on therapy; if a patient wishes to restart breastfeeding after treatment, advise to discuss the appropriate timing w/ physician. Inform that drug and certain other medicines, including OTC drugs and herbal supplements (eg, St. John's wort), can interact w/ each other and may alter the effects of treatment.

Botox — onabotulinumtoxinA
Class: Acetylcholine release inhibitor   **Rx**

> Effects may spread from the area of inj to produce symptoms consistent w/ botulinum toxin effects (eg, asthenia, generalized muscle weakness, diplopia, ptosis, dysphagia, dysphonia, dysarthria, urinary incontinence, breathing difficulties). Symptoms have been reported hrs to weeks after inj. Swallowing and breathing difficulties can be life threatening and there have been reports of death. Risk of symptoms is probably greatest in children treated for spasticity but can also occur in adults treated for spasticity and other conditions, particularly in patients who have an underlying condition that would predispose them to these symptoms. In unapproved uses and approved indications, cases of spread of effect have been reported at doses comparable to those used to treat cervical dystonia and spasticity and at lower doses.

ADULT DOSAGE

Bladder Dysfunction

Overactive Bladder (OAB):
W/ symptoms of urge urinary incontinence, urgency, and frequency, in patients who have an inadequate response to or are intolerant of an anticholinergic medication

100 U; recommended dilution is 100 U/10mL w/ preservative-free 0.9% NaCl inj
Max: 100 U

Detrusor Overactivity:
Treatment of urinary incontinence due to detrusor overactivity associated w/ a neurologic condition in patients who have an inadequate response to or are intolerant of an anticholinergic medication

200 U per treatment; do not exceed

Consider for reinjection when the clinical effect of the previous inj has diminished, but no sooner than 12 weeks from the prior bladder inj

Refer to PI for further dosing and administration instructions

Migraine
Prophylaxis of headaches in patients w/ chronic migraine (≥15 days per month w/ headache lasting ≥4 hrs/day)

155 U IM using a sterile 30-gauge, 0.5-inch needle as 0.1mL (5 U) inj per each site; recommended dilution is 200 U/4mL or 100 U/2mL, w/ a final concentration of 5 U/0.1mL

Inj should be divided across 7 specific head/neck muscle areas as follows:
Frontalis: 20 U divided in 4 sites
Corrugator: 10 U divided in 2 sites
Procerus: 5 U in 1 site
Occipitalis: 30 U divided in 6 sites
Temporalis: 40 U divided in 8 sites
Trapezius: 30 U divided in 6 sites
Cervical Paraspinal: 20 U divided in 4 sites

Recommended re-treatment schedule is every 12 weeks

Refer to PI for further dosing and administration instructions

Spasticity
Recommended Dilution: 200 U/4mL or 100 U/2mL w/ preservative-free 0.9% NaCl inj

Tailor dosing based on individual size, number, and location of muscles involved, severity of spasticity, presence of local muscle weakness, patient's previous response, or adverse event history w/ therapy. Repeat treatment may be administered when the effect of a previous inj has diminished, but generally no sooner than 12 weeks after the previous inj

Upper Limb:
To decrease the severity of increased muscle tone in elbow flexors (biceps), wrist flexors (flexor carpi radialis and flexor carpi ulnaris), finger flexors (flexor digitorum profundus and flexor digitorum sublimis), and thumb flexors (adductor pollicis and flexor pollicis longus)

PEDIATRIC DOSAGE

Blepharospasm and Strabismus
Associated w/ dystonia, including benign essential blepharospasm or VII nerve disorders

≥12 Years:
Blepharospasm:
Initial: 1.25-2.5 U (0.05-0.1mL at each site)
Dose may be increased up to 2-fold if response from initial treatment does not last longer than 2 months; little benefit obtainable from injecting >5 U/site
Max: 200 U in a 30-day period

Recommended Dilution:
For 1.25 U: 100 U/8mL
For 2.5 U: 100 U/4mL

Strabismus:
Inject between 0.05-0.15mL/muscle

Initial Doses in Units:
Use the lower listed doses for treatment of small deviations. Use the larger doses only for large deviations
Vertical Muscles and Horizontal Strabismus <20 Prism Diopters: 1.25-2.5 U in any 1 muscle
Horizontal Strabismus of 20-50 Prism Diopters: 2.5-5 U in any 1 muscle
Persistent VI Nerve Palsy of ≥1 Month Duration: 1.25-2.5 U in the medial rectus muscle

Subsequent Doses for Residual/ Recurrent Strabismus:
1. Reexamine patients 7-14 days after each inj to assess the effect of that dose
2. Patients experiencing adequate paralysis of the target muscle that require subsequent inj should receive a dose comparable to the initial dose
3. Subsequent doses for patients experiencing incomplete paralysis of the target muscle may be increased up to 2-fold compared to the previously administered dose
4. Do not administer subsequent inj until effects of the previous dose have dissipated as evidenced by substantial function in the injected and adjacent muscles

Max: 25 U single inj for any 1 muscle

Refer to PI for further dosing and administration instructions

Dosing by Muscle for Upper Limb:
Biceps Brachii: 100-200 U divided in 4 sites
Flexor Carpi Radialis: 12.5-50 U in 1 site
Flexor Carpi Ulnaris: 12.5-50 U in 1 site
Flexor Digitorum Profundus: 30-50 U in 1 site
Flexor Digitorum Sublimis: 30-50 U in 1 site
Adductor Pollicis: 20 U in 1 site
Flexor Pollicis Longus: 20 U in 1 site
Max: 50 U/site

Lower Limb:
To decrease the severity of increased muscle tone in ankle and toe flexors (gastrocnemius, soleus, tibialis posterior, flexor hallucis longus, and flexor digitorum longus)

Dosing by Muscle for Lower Limb:
Gastrocnemius Medial Head: 75 U divided in 3 sites
Gastrocnemius Lateral Head: 75 U divided in 3 sites
Soleus: 75 U divided in 3 sites
Tibialis Posterior: 75 U divided in 3 sites
Flexor Hallucis Longus: 50 U divided in 2 sites
Flexor Digitorum Longus: 50 U divided in 2 sites

Refer to PI for further dosing and administration instructions

Cervical Dystonia

To reduce the severity of abnormal head position and neck pain associated w/ cervical dystonia

≥16 Years:
Tailor dose based on patient's head and neck position, localization of pain, muscle hypertrophy, patient response, and adverse event history
Initial: Start at a lower dose for a patient w/o prior use of Botox
Recommended Dilution: 200 U/2mL, 200 U/4mL, 100 U/1mL, or 100 U/2mL w/ preservative-free 0.9% NaCl inj, depending on volume and number of inj sites desired to achieve treatment objectives; refer to PI for dilution instructions for Botox vials
Max: 50 U/site

Refer to PI for further dosing and administration instructions

Hyperhidrosis

Severe Primary Axillary Hyperhidrosis Inadequately Managed w/ Topical Agents:
50 U/axilla; recommended dilution is 100 U/4mL w/ 0.9% preservative-free sterile saline

Administer repeat inj when the clinical effect of previous inj diminishes

Refer to PI for further dosing and administration instructions

Blepharospasm and Strabismus

Associated w/ dystonia, including benign essential blepharospasm or VII nerve disorders

Blepharospasm:
Initial: 1.25-2.5 U (0.05-0.1mL at each site)
Dose may be increased up to 2-fold if response from initial treatment does not last longer than 2 months; little benefit obtainable from injecting >5 U/site
Max: 200 U in a 30-day period

Recommended Dilution:
For 1.25 U: 100 U/8mL
For 2.5 U: 100 U/4mL

Strabismus:
Inject between 0.05-0.15mL/muscle

Initial Doses in Units:
Use the lower listed doses for treatment of small deviations. Use the larger doses only for large deviations
Vertical Muscles and Horizontal Strabismus <20 Prism Diopters:
1.25-2.5 U in any 1 muscle
Horizontal Strabismus of 20-50 Prism Diopters: 2.5-5 U in any 1 muscle
Persistent VI Nerve Palsy of ≥1 Month Duration: 1.25-2.5 U in the medial rectus muscle

Subsequent Doses for Residual/Recurrent Strabismus:
1. Reexamine patients 7-14 days after each inj to assess the effect of that dose
2. Patients experiencing adequate paralysis of the target muscle that require subsequent inj should receive a dose comparable to the initial dose
3. Subsequent doses for patients experiencing incomplete paralysis of the target muscle may be increased up to 2-fold compared to the previously administered dose
4. Do not administer subsequent inj until effects of the previous dose have dissipated as evidenced by substantial function in the injected and adjacent muscles

Max: 25 U single inj for any 1 muscle
Refer to PI for further dosing and administration instructions

----

DOSING CONSIDERATIONS
Elderly
Start at lower end of dosing range

Other Important Considerations
In treating adult patients for ≥1 indication, the max cumulative dose should not exceed 400 U in a 3-month interval

ADMINISTRATION
Intradermal/IM/Intradetrusor route
Refer to PI for further administration instructions.

Preparation/Dilution
1. Prior to inj, reconstitute each vial w/ only sterile, preservative-free 0.9% NaCl inj.
2. Draw up the proper amount of diluent in the appropriate size syringe; refer to PI for dilution instructions for Botox vials.
3. Slowly inject the diluent into the vial.
4. Discard the vial if a vacuum does not pull the diluent into the vial.
5. Gently mix w/ the saline by rotating the vial.
6. Draw into an appropriately sized sterile syringe an amount of the reconstituted toxin slightly greater than the intended dose.
7. Expel air bubbles in the syringe barrel.
8. Attach the syringe to an appropriate inj needle; confirm patency of the needle.
9. A new, sterile needle and syringe should be used to enter the vial on each occasion for removal.
10. Reconstituted Botox should be stored at 2-8°C (36-46°F) and should be administered w/in 24 hrs.

Overactive Bladder
Administration Instructions:
1. Fill (prime) inj needle w/ approx 1mL of reconstituted Botox prior to the start of inj (depending on the needle length) to remove any air.
2. Insert the needle approx 2mm into the detrusor, and space 20 inj of 0.5mL each (total volume of 10mL) approx 1cm apart.
3. For the final inj, inject approx 1mL of sterile normal saline so that the remaining Botox in the needle is delivered to the bladder.
4. After the inj are given, patients should demonstrate their ability to void prior to leaving the clinic; observe patient for at least 30 min post-inj and until a spontaneous void has occurred.

Detrusor Overactivity
200 U Vial of Botox:
1. Reconstitute a 200 U vial w/ 6mL of preservative-free 0.9% NaCl inj and mix vial gently.
2. Draw 2mL from the vial into each of three 10mL syringes.
3. Complete reconstitution by adding 8mL of preservative-free 0.9% NaCl inj into each of 10mL syringes, and mix gently; this will result in three 10mL syringes each containing 10mL (approx 67 U in each), for a total of 200 U of reconstituted Botox.
4. Use immediately after reconstitution in the syringe; dispose of any unused saline.

100 U Vial of Botox:
1. Reconstitute two 100 U vials, each w/ 6mL of preservative-free 0.9% NaCl inj and mix vials gently.
2. Draw 4mL from each vial into each of two 10mL syringes; draw the remaining 2mL from each vial into a third 10mL syringe for a total of 4mL in each syringe.

3. Complete reconstitution by adding 6mL of preservative-free 0.9% NaCl inj into each of the 10mL syringes, and mix gently; this will result in three 10mL syringes each containing 10mL (approx 67 U in each), for a total of 200 U of reconstituted Botox.
4. Use immediately after reconstitution in the syringe; dispose of any unused saline.

Administration Instructions:
1. Fill (prime) inj needle w/ approx 1mL of reconstituted Botox prior to the start of inj (depending on the needle length) to remove any air.
2. Insert the needle approx 2mm into the detrusor, and space 30 inj of 1mL each (total volume of 30mL) approx 1cm apart.
3. For the final inj, inject approx 1mL of sterile normal saline so that the remaining Botox in the needle is delivered to the bladder.
4. After the inj are given, the saline used for bladder wall visualization should be drained; observe patient for at least 30 min post-inj.

Migraine
A 1-inch needle may be needed in the neck region for patients w/ thick neck muscles.
W/ the exception of the procerus muscle, which should be injected at 1 site (midline), all muscles should be injected bilaterally w/ half the number of inj sites administered to the left, and half to the right side of the head and neck.

Spasticity
An appropriately sized needle (eg, 25-30 gauge) may be used for superficial muscles, and a longer 22-gauge needle may be used for deeper musculature; localization of the involved muscles w/ techniques such as needle electromyographic guidance or nerve stimulation is recommended.

Cervical Dystonia
Use a sterile needle (eg, 25-30 gauge) of an appropriate length; localization of the involved muscles w/ electromyographic guidance may be useful.

Primary Axillary Hyperhidrosis
Define the hyperhidrotic area to be injected using standard staining techniques (eg, Minor's Iodine-Starch Test); refer to PI for instructions.
Using a 30-gauge needle, inject 50 U (2mL) intradermally in 0.1-0.2mL aliquots to each axilla evenly distributed in multiple sites (10-15) approx 1-2cm apart.
Each inj site has a ring of effect of up to approx 2cm in diameter; evenly space inj sites to minimize the area of no effect.
Inject each dose to a depth of approx 2mm and at a 45° angle to the skin surface, w/ the bevel side up to minimize leakage and to ensure the inj remain intradermal; if inj sites are marked in ink, do not inject Botox directly through the ink mark to avoid a permanent tattoo effect.

Blepharospasm
Use a sterile, 27- to 30-gauge needle w/o electromyographic guidance to inject into the medial and lateral pre-tarsal orbicularis oculi of upper lid and into the lateral pre-tarsal orbicularis oculi of the lower lid.
Avoiding inj near levator palpebrae superioris may reduce complication of ptosis. Avoiding medial lower lid inj, and thereby reducing diffusion into inferior oblique, may reduce the complication of diplopia.
Ecchymosis occurs easily in soft eyelid tissues; prevent by applying pressure at inj site immediately after inj.

Strabismus
Inject into extraocular muscles utilizing electrical activity recorded from tip of inj needle as a guide to placement w/in the target muscle; inj w/o surgical exposure or electromyographic guidance should not be attempted.
To prepare the eye for inj, it is recommended that several drops of a local anesthetic and an ocular decongestant be given several min prior to inj.

STORAGE
Unopened Vials: 2-8°C (36-46°F) for up to 36 months. Administer w/in 24 hrs of reconstitution; during this time period, store reconstituted sol at 2-8°C (36-46°F).

HOW SUPPLIED
Inj: 100 U, 200 U

CONTRAINDICATIONS
Infection at the proposed inj site(s). Intradetrusor inj is contraindicated in patients w/ OAB or detrusor overactivity associated w/ a neurologic condition who have a UTI, in patients w/ urinary retention, and in patients w/ post-void residual (PVR) urine volume >200mL who are not routinely performing clean intermittent self-catheterization (CIC). Hypersensitivity to any botulinum toxin preparation or to any of the components in the medication.

WARNINGS/PRECAUTIONS
Not interchangeable w/ other botulinum toxin products; cannot be compared to nor converted into U of any other botulinum toxin products. Serious adverse reactions reported w/ unapproved uses. Serious and/or immediate hypersensitivity reactions reported; d/c and institute appropriate medical therapy immediately. Patients w/ neuromuscular disorders may be at increased risk of clinically significant effects; monitor patients w/ peripheral motor neuropathic diseases, amyotrophic lateral sclerosis, or neuromuscular junction disorders. May cause swallowing or breathing difficulties; increased risk of dysphagia in patients w/ smaller neck muscle mass and in those who require bilateral inj into the sternocleidomastoid muscle for treatment of cervical dystonia. Inj into levator scapulae may increase risk of URI and dysphagia. Closely monitor patients w/ compromised respiratory status being treated for spasticity. Reduced blinking from inj of orbicularis muscle may lead to corneal exposure, persistent epithelial defect, and corneal ulceration, especially in patients w/ VII nerve disorders; employ vigorous treatment for any epithelial defect. Retrobulbar hemorrhages sufficient to compromise retinal circulation reported in patients being treated for strabismus; appropriate instruments to decompress the orbit should be accessible. Bronchitis was reported more frequently in patients being treated for upper limb spasticity and URTIs were reported more frequently in patients being treated for upper/lower limb spasticity. Autonomic dysreflexia associated w/ intradetrusor inj may occur in patients treated for detrusor overactivity associated w/ a neurological condition. Increases the incidence of UTI in patients w/ OAB. In patients who are not catheterizing, assess PVR urine volume w/in 2 weeks post-treatment and periodically as medically appropriate up to 12 weeks, particularly in patients w/ multiple sclerosis (MS) or diabetes mellitus (DM). Depending on patient symptoms, institute catheterization if PVR urine volume exceeds 200mL and continue until PVR falls to <200mL. Contains albumin; carries an extremely remote risk for transmission of viral diseases and Creutzfeldt-Jakob disease.

ADVERSE REACTIONS
OAB: UTI, dysuria, urinary retention, bacteriuria, residual urine volume.
Detrusor Overactivity Associated w/ a Neurologic Condition: UTI, urinary retention, hematuria, constipation, muscular weakness, dysuria, gait disturbance.
Chronic Migraine: Neck pain, headache, migraine, eyelid ptosis, musculoskeletal stiffness, muscular weakness, myalgia, inj-site pain, bronchitis, musculoskeletal pain.
Upper Limb Spasticity: Nausea, fatigue, bronchitis, pain in extremity, muscular weakness.
Lower Limb Spasticity: Arthralgia, back pain.
Cervical Dystonia: Dysphagia, URI, neck pain, headache.
Primary Axillary Hyperhidrosis: Inj-site pain/hemorrhage, non-axillary sweating, infection, pharyngitis, flu syndrome, headache, fever, neck/back pain, pruritus, anxiety.

DRUG INTERACTIONS
Potentiation of toxin effect may occur w/ aminoglycosides or other agents interfering w/ neuromuscular transmission (eg, curare-like compounds). Use of anticholinergic drugs after administration may potentiate systemic anticholinergic effects. Excessive neuromuscular weakness may be exacerbated by administration of another botulinum toxin prior to the resolution of the effects of a previously administered botulinum toxin. Use of a muscle relaxant before/ after administration may exaggerate excessive weakness.

PREGNANCY AND LACTATION
Pregnancy: Category C.
Lactation: Caution in nursing.

MECHANISM OF ACTION
Purified neurotoxin complex; blocks neuromuscular transmission by binding to acceptor sites on motor or sympathetic nerve terminals, entering the nerve terminals, and inhibiting release of acetylcholine.

PATIENT CONSIDERATIONS
Assessment: Assess for infection at proposed inj site(s), muscle weakness/ hypertrophy, neuromuscular disorders, compromised swallowing or respiratory function, increased risk for dysphagia, VII nerve disorders, MS, DM, potential causes of secondary hyperhidrosis (eg, hyperthyroidism), hypersensitivity, pregnancy/nursing status, and possible drug interactions. In patients undergoing intradetrusor inj, assess for UTI, urinary retention, and if PVR urine volume is >200mL and not routinely performing CIC.

Monitoring: Monitor for spread of toxin effects, hypersensitivity reactions, weakening of neck muscles, swallowing/speech/respiratory disorders, UTI, and other adverse reactions. Monitor patients w/ peripheral motor neuropathic diseases, amyotrophic lateral sclerosis, neuromuscular junction disorders, or compromised respiratory status. In patients w/ strabismus, monitor for retrobulbar hemorrhages. Monitor for bronchitis and URTIs in patients w/ spasticity. Monitor PVR urine volume (in patients who are not catheterizing) w/in 2 weeks post-treatment and periodically as medically appropriate up to 12 weeks, particularly in patients w/ MS or DM.

Counseling: Advise to inform physician if unusual symptoms (eg, swallowing, speaking, breathing difficulty) develop, or if any existing symptom worsens. Instruct to avoid driving or engaging in other potentially hazardous activities if loss of strength, muscle weakness, blurred vision, or drooping eyelids occur. Advise to contact physician if experiencing difficulties in voiding or burning sensation upon voiding after bladder inj for urinary incontinence.

Botox Cosmetic — onabotulinumtoxinA   Rx
Class: Acetylcholine release inhibitor

> Distant spread of toxin effects (eg, asthenia, generalized muscle weakness, diplopia, ptosis, dysphagia, dysphonia, dysarthria, urinary incontinence, breathing difficulties) reported hrs to weeks after inj. Swallowing and breathing difficulties can be life threatening; reports of death. Risk of symptoms greatest in children treated for spasticity; may also occur in adults treated for spasticity and other conditions, particularly in patients who have an underlying condition that would predispose them to these symptoms. In unapproved uses, including spasticity in children, and in approved indications, cases of spread of effect have been reported at doses comparable to those used to treat cervical dystonia and upper limb spasticity and at lower doses.

ADULT DOSAGE
Correction of Moderate to Severe Facial Wrinkles and Folds

Glabellar Lines:
For temporary improvement in appearance of moderate to severe glabellar lines associated w/ corrugator and/or procerus muscle activity

Inject 4 U/0.1mL IM into each of 5 sites; 2 in each corrugator muscle and 1 in the procerus muscle, for a total dose of 20 U

PEDIATRIC DOSAGE
Pediatric use may not have been established

Lateral Canthal Lines:

For temporary improvement in appearance of moderate to severe lateral canthal lines associated w/ orbicularis oculi activity

Inject 4 U/0.1mL into 3 sites/side (6 total inj points) in lateral orbicularis oculi muscle for a total of 24 U/0.6mL (12 U/side)

Max Cumulative Dose When Treating for ≥1 Indication: 360 U in a 3-month interval

For simultaneous treatment w/ glabellar lines, the dose is 24 U for lateral canthal lines and 20 U for glabellar lines, w/ a total dose of 44 U

ADMINISTRATION
IM route

Dilution
2.5mL diluent added to 100 U vial results in 4 U/0.1mL.
1.25mL diluent added to 50 U vial results in 4 U/0.1mL.

Preparation
1. Prior to IM inj, reconstitute each vial w/ sterile, preservative-free 0.9% NaCl inj.
2. Draw up proper amount of diluent to obtain a reconstituted sol at a concentration of 4 U/0.1mL and a total treatment dose of 20 U in 0.5mL for glabellar lines and 24 U in 0.6mL for lateral canthal lines.
3. Slowly inject diluent into vial; discard vial if vacuum does not pull diluent into vial.
4. Gently mix by rotating vial.

Administration
Administer w/in 24 hrs after reconstitution; store at 2-8°C (36-46°F) during this time period.
Use a 30- to 33-gauge needle.

Glabellar Lines:
Avoid inj near the levator palpebrae superioris, particularly in patients w/ larger brow depressor complexes.
Lateral corrugator inj should be placed at least 1cm above the bony supraorbital ridge.
Do not inject toxin closer than 1cm above the central eyebrow.

Lateral Canthal Lines:
Inj should be given w/ needle bevel tip up and oriented away from the eye.
The 1st inj should be approximately 1.5-2.0cm temporal to the lateral canthus and just temporal to the orbital rim.
Refer to PI for diagrams depicting proper administration.

STORAGE
2-8°C (36-46°F).

HOW SUPPLIED
Inj: 50 U, 100 U

CONTRAINDICATIONS
Infection at proposed inj site(s), known hypersensitivity to any botulinum toxin preparation or to any of the components in the formulation.

WARNINGS/PRECAUTIONS
Not interchangeable w/ other botulinum toxin products; cannot be compared nor converted into U of any other botulinum toxin products. Serious/fatal adverse reactions (eg, excessive weakness, dysphagia, aspiration pneumonia) reported in patients who received inj for unapproved uses. Serious and/or immediate hypersensitivity reactions reported; d/c further injections and institute appropriate medical therapy immediately. Caution w/ preexisting cardiovascular (CV) disease; adverse events involving CV system (eg, arrhythmia, MI) reported. Increased risk of clinically significant effects (eg, severe dysphagia, respiratory compromise) in patients w/ neuromuscular disorders; monitor patients w/ peripheral motor neuropathic diseases, amyotrophic lateral sclerosis, or neuromuscular junction disorders. May result in swallowing or breathing difficulties; increased risk of dysphagia in patients w/ smaller neck muscle mass and those who require bilateral inj into the sternocleidomastoid muscle for treatment of cervical dystonia. Caution w/ inflammation at the proposed inj site(s), ptosis, or when excessive weakness or atrophy is present in the targeted muscle(s). Reduced blinking from inj of orbicularis muscle may lead to corneal exposure, persistent epithelial defect, and corneal ulceration, especially in patients w/ VII nerve disorders; vigorously treat any epithelial defect. Inducing paralysis in one or more extraocular muscles may produce spatial disorientation, double vision, or past pointing; covering affected eye may alleviate symptoms. Contains albumin; carries an extremely remote risk for transmission of viral diseases and Creutzfeldt-Jakob disease.

ADVERSE REACTIONS
Eyelid ptosis.

DRUG INTERACTIONS
Potentiation of toxic effects may occur w/ aminoglycosides or other agents interfering w/ neuromuscular transmission (eg, curare-like compounds); use w/ caution. Use of anticholinergic drugs after administration may potentiate systemic anticholinergic effects. Excessive neuromuscular weakness may be exacerbated by administration of another botulinum toxin prior to the resolution of the effects of a previously administered botulinum toxin. Excessive weakness may be exaggerated by administration of muscle relaxant before or after administration of onabotulinumtoxinA.

PREGNANCY AND LACTATION
Pregnancy: Category C.
Lactation: Caution in nursing.

MECHANISM OF ACTION
Purified neurotoxin complex; blocks neuromuscular transmission by binding to acceptor sites on motor nerve terminals, entering the nerve terminals, and inhibiting the release of acetylcholine. Produces partial chemical denervation of the muscle resulting in a localized reduction in muscle activity if injected IM at therapeutic doses.

PATIENT CONSIDERATIONS
Assessment: Assess for hypersensitivity to any botulinum toxin preparation or any components of the product, infection/inflammation at proposed inj site(s), ptosis, weakness/atrophy in targeted muscle(s), CV disease, neuromuscular disorders, preexisting swallowing/breathing difficulties, smaller neck muscle mass, patients w/ required bilateral inj into the sternocleidomastoid muscle, VII nerve disorders, pregnancy/nursing status, and possible drug interactions.

Monitoring: Monitor for spread of toxin effects, swallowing/speech/respiratory difficulties, hypersensitivity reactions, CV system adverse events, dysphagia, infections, epithelial defects, and other adverse reactions. Monitor patients w/ peripheral motor neuropathic diseases, amyotrophic lateral sclerosis, neuromuscular junction disorders, or compromised respiratory status.

Counseling: Advise to seek immediate medical attention if any unusual symptoms (eg, swallowing/speaking/breathing difficulty) develop, or if any existing symptom worsens. Instruct to avoid driving a car or engaging in other potentially hazardous activities if loss of strength, muscle weakness, blurred vision, or drooping eyelids occur.

BRAVELLE — urofollitropin   Rx
Class: Follicle-stimulating hormone (FSH)

ADULT DOSAGE	PEDIATRIC DOSAGE
Ovulation Induction	Pediatric use may not have been established

ADULT DOSAGE

Ovulation Induction

In Women Who Have Previously Received Pituitary Suppression:
1st Cycle of Treatment:
Initial: 150 IU per day for 5 days

Subsequent Cycles:
Initial/Titrate: Based on history of the ovarian response to therapy
Do not make adjustments more frequently than once every 2 days
Do not exceed >75-150 IU per adjustment
Max: 450 IU per day
Max Duration: Do not exceed 12 days of treatment

When pre-ovulatory conditions are reached, administer human chorionic gonadotropin (hCG) to induce final oocyte maturation and ovulation
Withhold hCG in cases where the ovarian monitoring on the last day of treatment suggests an increased risk of ovarian hyperstimulation syndrome (OHSS)
Encourage woman and her partner to have intercourse daily, beginning on the day prior to the administration of hCG and until ovulation becomes apparent
Discourage intercourse when the risk of OHSS is increased

Assisted Reproductive Technology

Development of multiple follicles as part of an assisted reproductive technology cycle in ovulatory women who previously received pituitary suppression

Initial: 225 IU/day starting on cycle day 2 or 3 and continued until sufficient follicular development; should not exceed 12 days
May be administered together w/ menotropins for inj; total initial dose for combined therapy should not exceed 225 IU (150 IU of urofollitropin and 75 IU of menotropins or 75 IU of urofollitropin and 150 IU of menotropins)
Titrate: Adjust dose after 5 days based on ovarian response
Do not make additional dose adjustments more frequently than every 2 days or by more than 75-150 IU/ per adjustment

PEDIATRIC DOSAGE
Pediatric use may not have been established

Max: 450 IU (w/ or w/o menotropins)

Continue treatment until adequate follicular development is evident, then administer human chorionic gonadotropin (hCG)
Withhold hCG if, on the last day of therapy, ovarian monitoring suggests an increased risk of ovarian hyperstimulation syndrome

ADMINISTRATION
SQ/IM route

Administer SQ in the abdomen

STORAGE
3-25°C (37-77°F). Protect from light. Use immediately after reconstitution.

HOW SUPPLIED
Inj: 75 IU

CONTRAINDICATIONS
Hypersensitivity to urofollitropins, high follicle stimulating hormone (FSH) levels indicating primary ovarian failure, presence of uncontrolled non-gonadal endocrinopathies (eg, thyroid, adrenal, pituitary disorders), sex hormone dependent tumors of the reproductive tract and accessory organ, tumors of pituitary gland or hypothalamus, abnormal uterine bleeding of undetermined origin, ovarian cysts or enlargement of undetermined origin not due to polycystic ovary syndrome, pregnancy.

WARNINGS/PRECAUTIONS
Should only be used by physicians who are experienced in infertility treatment. May cause OHSS with or without pulmonary/vascular complications and multiple births. Hypersensitivity/anaphylactic reactions reported. Abnormal ovarian enlargement may occur; use lowest effective dose. Prohibit intercourse in women with significant ovarian enlargement; hemoperitoneum resulting from rupture of ovarian cysts may occur. Transient LFT abnormalities suggestive of hepatic dysfunction reported in association with OHSS. Withhold hCG if ovaries are abnormally enlarged on the last day of therapy; monitor patients for at least 2 weeks after hCG administration. D/C therapy and consider whether patient needs to be hospitalized if severe OHSS occurs. Serious pulmonary conditions (eg, atelectasis, acute respiratory distress syndrome), thromboembolic events, ovarian torsion, and multi-fetal gestation/births reported. Risk of congenital malformations or ectopic pregnancy may be increased in women undergoing ART. May increase risk of spontaneous abortions and ovarian neoplasms.

ADVERSE REACTIONS
OHSS, headache, nausea, vaginal hemorrhage, ovarian disorder, pelvic pain/cramps, respiratory disorder, hot flashes, abdominal pain/cramps/fullness/enlargement, inj-site reaction, pain.

PREGNANCY AND LACTATION
Category X, not for use in nursing.

MECHANISM OF ACTION
FSH; produces ovarian follicular growth in women who do not have primary ovarian failure.

PHARMACOKINETICS
Absorption: Multiple Dose (150 IU for 7 days): C_{max} =14.8 mIU/mL (SQ), 11.5 mIU/mL (IM); T_{max}=9.6 hrs (SQ), 11.3 hrs (IM); AUC=234.7 mIU•hr/mL (SQ), 192.1 mIU•hr/mL (IM). **Elimination:** Multiple Dose (150 IU for 7 days): $T_{1/2}$=20.6 hrs (SQ), 15.2 hrs (IM).

PATIENT CONSIDERATIONS
Assessment: Assess for previous hypersensitivity to the drug, primary ovarian failure, uncontrolled non-gonadal endocrinopathies, tumors of pituitary gland or hypothalamus, pregnancy/nursing status, and any other conditions where treatment is contraindicated or cautioned. Perform a complete gynecologic/endocrinologic evaluation, and diagnose the cause of infertility.

Monitoring: Monitor for hypersensitivity/anaphylactic reactions, OHSS, ovarian enlargement, ovarian torsion, pulmonary conditions, thromboembolic events, and other adverse reactions. Monitor for signs of ovulation and ovarian response. Monitor serum estradiol levels and perform vaginal ultrasound.

Counseling: Instruct on the correct usage and dosing of therapy; caution not to change dosage or the schedule of administration unless instructed to do so by physician. Prior to therapy, inform about the time commitment and monitoring procedures necessary for treatment. Instruct to contact physician if dose is missed and not to double next dose. Inform of the risks of OHSS, OHSS-associated symptoms, ovarian torsion, and multi-fetal gestation/birth with the use of the drug.

BREO ELLIPTA — fluticasone furoate/vilanterol   Rx

Class: Corticosteroid/long-acting beta₂ agonist (LABA)

Long-acting β₂-adrenergic agonists (LABAs) increase the risk of asthma-related death. LABAs may increase the risk of asthma-related hospitalization in pediatric and adolescent patients. Use only for patients not adequately controlled on a long-term asthma control medication (eg, inhaled corticosteroid [ICS]) or whose disease severity clearly warrants initiation of treatment w/ both an ICS and a LABA. Once asthma control is achieved and maintained, assess the patient at regular intervals and step down therapy (eg, d/c Breo Ellipta) if possible w/o loss of asthma control and maintain the patient on a long-term asthma control medication. Do not use if asthma is adequately controlled on low- or medium-dose ICS.

ADULT DOSAGE
Chronic Obstructive Pulmonary Disease
Long-term maint treatment of airflow obstruction; also indicated to reduce COPD exacerbations in patients w/ history of exacerbations

1 inh of 100mcg/25mcg qd
Max: 1 inh of 100mcg/25mcg qd

If shortness of breath occurs in the period between doses, an inhaled, short-acting β₂-agonist (eg, albuterol) should be taken for immediate relief

Asthma
Initial: 1 inh of 100mcg/25mcg or 200mcg/25mcg qd
Previous Low- to Mid-Dose Corticosteroid-Containing Treatment: Consider 1 inh of 100mcg/25mcg qd
Previous Mid- to High-Dose Corticosteroid-Containing Treatment: Consider 1 inh of 200mcg/25mcg qd
Titrate: Increase dose to 200mcg/25mcg for patients who do not respond adequately to the 100mcg/25mcg dose
Max: 1 inh of 200mcg/25mcg qd

If asthma symptoms arise in the period between doses, an inhaled, short-acting β₂-agonist (eg, albuterol) should be taken for immediate relief

---

ADMINISTRATION
Oral inh route

After inh, patient should rinse mouth w/ water w/o swallowing.
Take at the same time every day; do not use >1 inh q24h.

STORAGE
20-25°C (68-77°F); excursions permitted from 15-30°C (59-86°F). Store in a dry place away from direct heat or sunlight. Store inside the unopened moisture-protective foil tray and only remove from the tray immediately before initial use. Discard 6 weeks after opening the foil tray or when the counter reads "0" (after all blisters have been used), whichever comes 1st.

HOW SUPPLIED
Powder, Inh: (Fluticasone/Vilanterol) (100mcg/25mcg)/blister, (200mcg/25mcg)/blister [14, 30 inh]

CONTRAINDICATIONS
Primary treatment of status asthmaticus or other acute episodes of COPD or asthma where intensive measures are required. Severe hypersensitivity to milk proteins or demonstrated hypersensitivity to fluticasone furoate, vilanterol, or any of the excipients.

WARNINGS/PRECAUTIONS
Not indicated for acute bronchospasm relief. Do not initiate during rapidly deteriorating or potentially life-threatening episodes of COPD or asthma. D/C regular use of oral/inhaled short-acting β₂-agonists when beginning treatment; use them only for symptomatic relief of acute respiratory symptoms. Increased incidence of pneumonia reported in COPD patients receiving 100mcg/25mcg. May produce paradoxical bronchospasm; treat immediately, d/c Breo Ellipta, and institute alternative therapy. Hypersensitivity reactions may occur; d/c if such reactions occur. **Fluticasone:** *Candida albicans* infections of mouth and pharynx reported; treat and, if needed, interrupt therapy. Increased susceptibility to infections. Chickenpox or measles may have a more serious/fatal course; avoid exposure and, if exposed, consider prophylaxis/treatment. Use w/ caution, if at all, in patients w/ active/quiescent tuberculosis (TB); systemic fungal, bacterial, viral, or parasitic infections; or ocular herpes simplex. Deaths due to adrenal insufficiency reported in asthma patients during and after transfer from a systemic corticosteroid to an ICS. Patients who have been withdrawn from systemic corticosteroids should resume oral corticosteroids immediately during periods of stress, a severe COPD exacerbation, or a severe asthma attack. Patients requiring oral corticosteroids should be weaned slowly from systemic corticosteroid use after transferring to therapy. Systemic corticosteroid effects (eg, hypercorticism and adrenal suppression) may occur in patients sensitive to these effects; if such effects occur, reduce therapy slowly and consider other treatments for management of COPD or asthma symptoms. Decreases in bone mineral density (BMD) reported w/ long-term use. Assess BMD in COPD patients prior to initiating therapy and periodically thereafter; if significant reductions are seen and therapy is still considered medically important, consider using medicine to treat or prevent osteoporosis. Glaucoma, increased IOP, and cataracts reported w/ long-term use. Caution w/ moderate/severe hepatic impairment. May cause reduction in growth velocity in children and adolescents. **Vilanterol:** Clinically significant cardiovascular (CV) effects may occur (eg, increases in pulse rate, BP, cardiac arrhythmias); if such effects occur, therapy may need to be discontinued. Caution w/ CV disorders, convulsive disorders, and thyrotoxicosis, and in patients unusually responsive to sympathomimetic amines. Doses of IV albuterol reported to aggravate preexisting diabetes mellitus (DM) and ketoacidosis. May produce significant hypokalemia or transient hyperglycemia.

PEDIATRIC DOSAGE
Pediatric use may not have been established

ADVERSE REACTIONS

Nasopharyngitis, URTI, oral candidiasis, headache, sinusitis, cough, oropharyngeal pain, dysphonia, influenza, bronchitis.

DRUG INTERACTIONS

Do not use w/ another medicine containing a LABA; clinically significant CV effects and fatalities reported w/ excessive use of inhaled sympathomimetic drugs. Caution w/ long-term ketoconazole and other strong CYP3A4 inhibitors (eg, ritonavir, clarithromycin, conivaptan); increased systemic corticosteroid and increased CV adverse effects may occur. **Vilanterol:** Extreme caution w/ MAOIs, TCAs, or drugs known to prolong the QTc interval or w/in 2 weeks of discontinuation of such agents; effect on CV system may be potentiated by these agents. β-blockers block pulmonary effects and may produce severe bronchospasm in COPD or asthma patients; if such therapy is needed, consider cardioselective β-blockers and use w/ caution. Caution is advised when coadministered w/ non-K+-sparing diuretics; may acutely worsen ECG changes and/or hypokalemia that may result from non-K+-sparing diuretics.

PREGNANCY AND LACTATION

Pregnancy: Category C; there are no adequate and well-controlled trials w/ Breo Ellipta in pregnant women.
Lactation: It is not known whether fluticasone furoate or vilanterol are excreted in human breast milk. However, other corticosteroids and β2 agonists have been detected in human milk; caution in nursing.

MECHANISM OF ACTION

Fluticasone: Corticosteroid; precise mechanism unknown. Shown to have a wide range of actions on multiple cell types (eg, mast cells, eosinophils, neutrophils, macrophages, lymphocytes) and mediators (eg, histamine, eicosanoids, leukotrienes, cytokines) involved in inflammation. **Vilanterol:** LABA; attributable to stimulation of intracellular adenyl cyclase, the enzyme that catalyzes the conversion of ATP to cAMP. Increased cAMP levels cause relaxation of bronchial smooth muscle and inhibition of release of mediators of immediate hypersensitivity from cells, especially from mast cells.

PHARMACOKINETICS

Absorption: Fluticasone: Absolute bioavailability (15.2%); T_{max}=0.5-1 hr. Vilanterol: Absolute bioavailability (27.3%); T_{max}=10 min. **Distribution:** Fluticasone: V_d=661L (IV); plasma protein binding (99.6%). Vilanterol: V_d=165L (IV); plasma protein binding (93.9%). **Metabolism:** Via CYP3A4. **Elimination:** Fluticasone: Feces (101% [PO], 90% [IV]), urine (1% [PO], 2% [IV]); $T_{1/2}$=24 hrs. Vilanterol: (PO) Urine (70%), feces (30%); $T_{1/2}$=21.3 hrs (w/ COPD), 16 hrs (w/ asthma).

PATIENT CONSIDERATIONS

Assessment: Assess for hypersensitivity to drug or to milk proteins; COPD/asthma status; active/quiescent TB; systemic infections; ocular herpes simplex; CV disorders; risk factors for decreased bone mineral content; convulsive disorders; thyrotoxicosis; DM; ketoacidosis; history of increased IOP, glaucoma, and/or cataracts; hepatic impairment; pregnancy/nursing status; and possible drug interactions. Assess BMD.

Monitoring: Monitor for deteriorating disease, localized oropharyngeal *C. albicans* infections, pneumonia, infections, systemic corticosteroid effects, paradoxical bronchospasm, hypersensitivity reactions, CV effects, glaucoma, cataracts, increased IOP, hypokalemia, hyperglycemia, and other adverse reactions. Periodically monitor BMD.

Counseling: Advise patients w/ asthma that LABAs increase the risk of asthma-related death and may increase the risk of asthma-related hospitalization in pediatric and adolescent patients. Inform that drug is not meant to relieve acute symptoms of COPD or asthma and extra doses should not be used for that purpose; advise to treat acute symptoms w/ an inhaled, short-acting β2-agonist (eg, albuterol). Instruct to seek medical attention immediately if patient experiences decreasing effectiveness of inhaled, short-acting β2-agonist; a need for more inhalations than usual of inhaled, short-acting β2-agonist; or a significant decrease in lung function. Advise not to d/c therapy w/o physician guidance and not to use additional LABAs. Instruct to contact physician if oropharyngeal candidiasis or symptoms of pneumonia develop. Advise to rinse mouth w/ water w/o swallowing after inhalation. Advise to avoid exposure to chickenpox or measles, and, if exposed, to consult physician w/o delay. Inform about risk of immunosuppression, hypercorticism, adrenal suppression, reduction in BMD, ocular effects, and adverse effects (eg, palpitations, chest pain, rapid HR, tremor, nervousness). Instruct to taper slowly from systemic corticosteroids if transferring to Breo Ellipta. Advise that hypersensitivity reactions may occur; instruct to d/c therapy if any occur. Inform that the inhaler is not reusable and advise not to take the inhaler apart.

BREVIBLOC — esmolol hydrochloride

Rx

Class: Selective beta₁ blocker

ADULT DOSAGE

Supraventricular Tachycardia/Noncompensatory Sinus Tachycardia

Short-term use for rapid control of ventricular rate in patients w/ A-fib or A-flutter in perioperative, postoperative, or other emergent circumstances, and for noncompensatory sinus tachycardia

Administer by continuous IV infusion w/ or w/o LD

PEDIATRIC DOSAGE

Pediatric use may not have been established

Additional LD and/or titration of maint infusion (step-wise dosing) may be necessary based on desired ventricular response

Step 1: Optional LD (500mcg/kg over 1 min), then 50mcg/kg/min for 4 min
Step 2: Optional LD if necessary, then 100mcg/kg/min for 4 min
Step 3: Optional LD if necessary, then 150mcg/kg/min for 4 min
Step 4: If necessary, increase dose to 200mcg/kg/min
Maint: 50-200mcg/kg/min; may continue maint infusions for up to 48 hrs
Max: 200mcg/kg/min

Intraoperative/Postoperative Tachycardia and/or Hypertension

Short-term treatment of tachycardia and HTN that occur during induction and tracheal intubation, during surgery, on emergence from anesthesia, and in the postoperative period

Immediate Control:
1mg/kg bolus over 30 sec followed by 150mcg/kg/min infusion, if necessary
Titrate: Adjust infusion rate as required to maintain desired HR and BP

Gradual Control:
500mcg/kg bolus over 1 min followed by maint infusion of 50mcg/kg/min for 4 min
Continue dosing as for supraventricular tachycardia, depending on response

Maint Infusion:
Tachycardia:
Max: 200mcg/kg/min
HTN:
May require higher maint infusion dosages (250-300mcg/kg/min)
Max: 300mcg/kg/min

Conversions

Transition to Alternative Drugs:
Reduce infusion rate by 50%, 30 min following 1st dose of alternative drug. After administration of 2nd dose of alternative drug, monitor response and if satisfactory control is maintained for 1st hr, d/c infusion

---

DOSING CONSIDERATIONS

Elderly
Start at lower end of dosing range

ADMINISTRATION
IV route

Premixed Bag
Medication port is used solely for withdrawing initial bolus from the bag
Do not add any additional medications to the bag

Ready-to-Use Vial
May be used to administer LD by hand-held syringe while maint infusion is being prepared

Compatible IV Fluids
D5 inj
D5 in Lactated Ringer's inj
D5 in Ringer's inj
D5 and NaCl 0.45% inj
D5 and NaCl 0.9% inj
Lactated Ringer's inj
Potassium Chloride (40mEq/L) in D5 inj
NaCl 0.45% inj
NaCl 0.9% inj

Refer to PI for additional administration and preparation instructions

STORAGE
25°C (77°F); excursions permitted to 15-30°C (59-86°F). Protect from freezing. Avoid excessive heat. **Ready to Use Bag:** Use w/in 24 hrs once drug has been withdrawn; discard any unused portion. Do not use plastic containers in series connections. Do not remove unit from overwrap until time of use.

HOW SUPPLIED
Inj: 10mg/mL [10mL, vial; 250mL, premixed inj bag], 20mg/mL [100mL, double strength premixed inj bag]

CONTRAINDICATIONS

Severe sinus bradycardia, heart block >1st degree, sick sinus syndrome, decompensated heart failure (HF), cardiogenic shock, pulmonary HTN, IV administration of cardiodepressant calcium channel antagonists (eg, verapamil) and esmolol in close proximity (eg, while cardiac effects from the other are still present), hypersensitivity reactions, including anaphylaxis, to esmolol or any of the inactive ingredients of the product (cross-sensitivity between beta blockers is possible).

WARNINGS/PRECAUTIONS

Not for prevention of intraoperative/postoperative tachycardia and/or HTN. Dose-related hypotension, loss of consciousness, cardiac arrest, and death may occur; reduce dose or d/c in case of an unacceptable drop in BP. Bradycardia, including sinus pause, heart block, and severe bradycardia, may occur; patients w/ 1st-degree AV block, sinus node dysfunction, or conduction disorders may be at increased risk. Reduce dose or d/c if severe bradycardia develops. May cause cardiac failure and cardiogenic shock; d/c at 1st sign/symptom of impending cardiac failure and start supportive therapy. Monitor vital signs closely and titrate slowly in the treatment of patients whose BP is primarily driven by vasoconstriction associated w/ hypothermia. Should generally not be given to patients w/ reactive airways disease; titrate to lowest possible effective dose and d/c immediately in the event of bronchospasm. Caution in patients w/ hypoglycemia and in diabetics; may mask tachycardia occurring w/ hypoglycemia. Infusion-site reactions may develop; use an alternative infusion site and avoid extravasation if a local infusion-site reaction develops. Avoid infusions into small veins or through a butterfly-catheter. May exacerbate anginal attacks in patients w/ Prinzmetal's angina; do not use nonselective β-blockers. If used in the setting of pheochromocytoma, give in combination w/ an α-blocker, and only after α-blocker has been initiated; may cause a paradoxical increase in BP if administered alone. Can attenuate reflex tachycardia and increase risk of hypotension in hypovolemic patients. May aggravate peripheral circulatory disorders (eg, Raynaud's disease or syndrome, peripheral occlusive vascular disease). Severe exacerbations of angina, MI, and ventricular arrhythmias reported upon abrupt discontinuation in patients w/ CAD; observe for signs of myocardial ischemia when discontinued. Hyperkalemia reported; increased risk in patients w/ renal impairment. May cause hyperkalemic renal tubular acidosis. May mask clinical signs of hyperthyroidism (eg, tachycardia). May precipitate thyroid storm w/ abrupt withdrawal. Patients at risk of anaphylactic reactions may be more reactive to allergen exposure (accidental, diagnostic, or therapeutic). Caution in elderly.

ADVERSE REACTIONS

Hypotension, dizziness, somnolence, nausea, infusion-site reactions.

DRUG INTERACTIONS

See Contraindications. May exaggerate effects on BP, contractility, and impulse propagation w/ other drugs that can lower BP, reduce myocardial contractility, or interfere w/ sinus node function or electrical impulse propagation in the myocardium. Concomitant use w/ digoxin may increase the risk of bradycardia and may increase digoxin levels. May prolong effects of succinylcholine-induced neuromuscular blockade. May moderately prolong effects and recovery index of mivacurium. Increased risk of clonidine-, guanfacine-, moxonidine-withdrawal rebound HTN; d/c β-blocker gradually 1st if antihypertensive therapy needs to be interrupted or discontinued. In patients w/ depressed myocardial function, use w/ cardiodepressant calcium channel antagonists (eg, verapamil) can lead to fatal cardiac arrests. Sympathomimetic drugs having β-adrenergic agonist activity will counteract effects. Do not use to control tachycardia in patients receiving drugs that are vasoconstrictive and have positive inotropic effects (eg, dopamine, epinephrine, norepinephrine) because of risk of reducing cardiac contractility in presence of high systemic vascular resistance. May be unresponsive to usual doses of epinephrine used to treat anaphylactic/anaphylactoid reactions. May enhance the effect of antidiabetic agents.

PREGNANCY AND LACTATION

Category C, not for use in nursing.

MECHANISM OF ACTION

Selective β₁-blocker; inhibits β₁-receptors located chiefly in cardiac muscle, and at higher doses begins to inhibit β₂-receptors located chiefly in the bronchial and vascular musculature.

PHARMACOKINETICS

Distribution: Plasma protein binding (55%). **Metabolism:** Rapid through hydrolysis of the ester linkage in cytosol of RBCs to methanol and free acid. **Elimination:** Urine (73-88% acid metabolite, <2% unchanged); $T_{1/2}$=9 min (esmolol HCl), 3.7 hrs (acid metabolite).

PATIENT CONSIDERATIONS

Assessment: Assess for severe sinus bradycardia, heart block >1st degree, sick sinus syndrome, decompensated HF, cardiogenic shock, pulmonary HTN, hypersensitivity, or any other conditions where treatment is contraindicated or cautioned. Assess pregnancy/nursing status and for possible drug interactions. Obtain baseline BP, HR and rhythm, and serum electrolytes.

Monitoring: Monitor for hypotension, bradycardia, signs/symptoms of impending cardiac failure, bronchospasm, infusion-site reactions, and other adverse reactions. Monitor for signs of thyrotoxicosis when withdrawing therapy in patients w/ hyperthyroidism. Monitor BP, HR and rhythm, and serum electrolytes.

Counseling: Inform about benefits/risks of therapy. Instruct to report any adverse reactions to physician.

BRIDION — sugammadex

Class: Antidote

Rx

ADULT DOSAGE

Reversal of Neuromuscular Blockade

Reversal of Blockade Induced by Rocuronium Bromide and Vecuronium Bromide in Adults Undergoing Surgery:

Base doses/timing of administration on twitch responses and extent of spontaneous recovery that has occurred

Satisfactory recovery should be determined through assessment of skeletal muscle tone and respiratory measurements in addition to the response to peripheral nerve stimulation

Rocuronium + Vecuronium:

4mg/kg if spontaneous recovery of twitch response has reached 1-2 post-tetanic counts and there are no twitch responses to train-of-four (TOF) stimulation following rocuronium- or vecuronium-induced neuromuscular blockade

2mg/kg if spontaneous recovery has reached the reappearance of the second twitch in response to TOF stimulation following rocuronium- or vecuronium-induced neuromuscular blockade

Rocuronium Only:

16mg/kg if there is a clinical need to reverse neuromuscular blockade soon (approx 3 min) after administration of a single dose of 1.2mg/kg of rocuronium

Re-Administration of Neuromuscular Blocking Agents for Intubation Following Reversal

Re-Administration After Reversal w/ ≤4mg/kg of Sugammadex:

1.2mg/kg Rocuronium: Wait ≥5 min

0.6mg/kg Rocuronium or 0.1mg/kg Vecuronium: Wait ≥4 hrs. Wait 24 hrs w/ mild or moderate renal impairment. If shorter wait time is required, give a 1.2mg/kg rocuronium dose

When rocuronium 1.2mg/kg is administered w/in 30 min after reversal, onset of neuromuscular blockade may be delayed ≤4 min and duration may be shortened ≤15 min

For re-administration of rocuronium or administration of vecuronium after reversal of rocuronium w/ 16mg/kg sugammadex, wait 24 hrs

Use a nonsteroidal neuromuscular blocking agent if neuromuscular blockade is required before recommended waiting time has elapsed

---

DOSING CONSIDERATIONS

Renal Impairment

Severe/Dialysis: Not recommended

ADMINISTRATION

IV route

Administer as single bolus inj; may be given over 10 sec, into an existing IV line. Ensure infusion line is adequately flushed (eg, w/ 0.9% NaCl) between administration of sugammadex and other drugs.

Compatibility

May inject into IV line of a running infusion w/ the following IV sol (do not mix w/ other products):
0.9% NaCl
D5
0.45% NaCl and 2.5% dextrose
D5 in 0.9% NaCl
isolyte P w/ D5
Ringer's lactate sol
Ringer's sol
Physically incompatible w/ verapamil, ondansetron, and ranitidine.

PEDIATRIC DOSAGE

Pediatric use may not have been established

STORAGE
25°C (77°F); excursions permitted to 15-30°C (59-86°F). Protect from light. When not protected from light, use w/in 5 days.

HOW SUPPLIED
Inj: 200mg/2mL, 500mg/5mL

CONTRAINDICATIONS
Hypersensitivity to sugammadex or any of its components.

WARNINGS/PRECAUTIONS
Serious hypersensitivity reactions, including anaphylaxis, reported. Marked bradycardia reported, some resulting in cardiac arrest; closely monitor for hemodynamic changes during and after reversal of neuromuscular blockade. Ventilatory support is mandatory until adequate spontaneous respiration is restored and the ability to maintain a patent airway is assured; should neuromuscular blockade persist after administration or recur following extubation, provide adequate ventilation. Delayed or minimal response to sugammadex reported in a small number of patients. Use of lower than recommended dose is not recommended; may lead to an increased risk of recurrence of neuromuscular blockade after initial reversal. Doses ≤16mg/kg reported to be associated w/ increases in aPTT and PT/INR; carefully monitor coagulation parameters in patients w/ known coagulopathies, being treated w/ therapeutic anticoagulation, receiving thromboprophylaxis drugs other than heparin and low molecular weight heparin (LMWH), or receiving thromboprophylaxis drugs and who then receive a dose of 16mg/kg sugammadex. Signs of light anesthesia noted occasionally when neuromuscular blockade was reversed intentionally in the middle of anesthesia. Do not use to reverse blockade induced by nonsteroidal neuromuscular blocking agents (eg, succinylcholine/benzylisoquinolinium compounds) and steroidal neuromuscular blocking agents other than rocuronium or vecuronium.

ADVERSE REACTIONS
N/V, pain, hypotension, headache.

DRUG INTERACTIONS
Certain drugs may become less effective due to a lowering of (free) plasma concentrations; consider re-administration of other drug, administration of a therapeutically equivalent drug, and/or non-pharmacological interventions. Administration of a bolus dose of sugammadex is equivalent to missing dose(s) of oral contraceptives containing an estrogen or progestogen; if an oral contraceptive is taken on same day that sugammadex is administered or non-oral hormonal contraception is being used, use additional, non-hormonal contraceptive method or back-up method of contraception for the next 7 days. May interfere w/ serum progesterone assay. Certain drugs may displace rocuronium or vecuronium from sugammadex; d/c drug causing displacement and provide adequate ventilation if required. Recovery of TOF ratio to 0.9 could be delayed in patients who have received toremifene on the same day of surgery. Drugs that potentiate neuromuscular blockade used postoperatively may cause recurrence of neuromuscular blockade; may require mechanical ventilation.

PREGNANCY AND LACTATION
Pregnancy: There are no data on use in pregnant women to inform any drug-associated risks.
Lactation: No data are available regarding the presence of sugammadex in human milk, the effects of sugammadex on the breastfed infant, or the effects of sugammadex on milk production; caution in nursing.
Reproductive Potential: Efficacy of hormonal contraceptives may be reduced for ≤7 days; see Drug Interactions.

MECHANISM OF ACTION
Modified gamma cyclodextrin; forms a complex w/ the neuromuscular blocking agents rocuronium and vecuronium, and reduces amount of neuromuscular blocking agent available to bind to nicotinic cholinergic receptors in the neuromuscular junction, resulting in reversal of neuromuscular blockade.

PHARMACOKINETICS
Distribution: V_d=11-14L. **Elimination:** Urine (96%, ≥95% unchanged); $T_{1/2}$=2 hrs.

PATIENT CONSIDERATIONS
Assessment: Assess for drug hypersensitivity, renal impairment, known coagulopathies, pregnancy/nursing status, hormonal contraception use, and for other possible drug interactions.

Monitoring: Monitor twitch responses and the extent of spontaneous recovery that has occurred. Monitor patient to assure adequate ventilation and maintenance of a patent airway from the time of administration of sugammadex until complete recovery of neuromuscular function. Monitor for hemodynamic changes during and after neuromuscular blockade. Monitor for hypersensitivity reactions and for other adverse reactions. Monitor coagulation parameters in patients w/ known coagulopathies, being treated w/ therapeutic anticoagulation, receiving thromboprophylaxis drugs other than heparin and LMWH, or receiving thromboprophylaxis drugs and who then receive a dose of 16mg/kg sugammadex.

Counseling: Advise females of reproductive potential using hormonal contraceptives that concomitant use may reduce contraceptive effect. Instruct females to use an additional, non-hormonal method of contraception for the next 7 days following administration of sugammadex.

BRILINTA — ticagrelor
Class: Antiplatelet agent

Rx

May cause significant, sometimes fatal, bleeding. Do not use in patients w/ active pathological bleeding or a history of intracranial hemorrhage. Do not start therapy in patients undergoing urgent CABG. If possible, manage bleeding w/o discontinuing therapy; stopping therapy increases the risk of subsequent cardiovascular (CV) events. Maintenance doses of aspirin (ASA) >100mg reduce the effectiveness of ticagrelor and should be avoided.

ADULT DOSAGE
Acute Coronary Syndrome
To reduce the rate of CV death, MI, and stroke in patients w/ acute coronary syndrome or a history of MI; also reduces the rate of stent thrombosis in patients who have been stented for treatment of acute coronary syndrome

LD: 180mg
Maint: 90mg bid during 1st year; 60mg bid after 1 year
Use w/ daily maint dose of ASA of 75-100mg

Missed Dose
If a dose is missed, take 1 tab (next dose) at its scheduled time

----

DOSING CONSIDERATIONS
Hepatic Impairment
Severe: Avoid use

ADMINISTRATION
Oral route
Take w/ or w/o food.
If unable to swallow tab(s) whole, tab can be crushed, mixed w/ water, and drunk; the mixture can also be administered via a NG tube (≥CH8).
Do not administer w/ another oral P2Y12 platelet inhibitor.

STORAGE
25°C (77°F); excursions permitted to 15-30°C (59-86°F).

HOW SUPPLIED
Tab: 60mg, 90mg

CONTRAINDICATIONS
History of intracranial hemorrhage, active pathological bleeding (eg, peptic ulcer, intracranial hemorrhage), hypersensitivity (eg, angioedema) to ticagrelor or any component of the product.

WARNINGS/PRECAUTIONS
Dyspnea reported. If new, prolonged, or worsened dyspnea is determined to be related to therapy, no specific treatment is required; continue therapy w/o interruption. In the case of intolerable dyspnea requiring discontinuation of therapy, consider another antiplatelet agent. Discontinuation of therapy increases risk of MI, stroke, and death; if therapy must be temporarily discontinued, restart it as soon as possible. When possible, interrupt therapy for 5 days prior to surgery that has major risk of bleeding; resume as soon as hemostasis is achieved.

ADVERSE REACTIONS
Bleeding, dyspnea, dizziness, nausea, diarrhea.

DRUG INTERACTIONS
See Boxed Warning. Strong CYP3A inhibitors substantially increase ticagrelor exposure and may increase adverse events; avoid w/ strong CYP3A inhibitors (eg, atazanavir, clarithromycin, ketoconazole). Strong CYP3A inducers substantially reduce ticagrelor exposure and may decrease efficacy; avoid w/ strong CYP3A inducers (eg, rifampin, phenytoin, carbamazepine). May increase concentrations of simvastatin and lovastatin (CYP3A4 substrates); avoid simvastatin and lovastatin doses >40mg. Inhibits P-gp transporter; monitor digoxin levels w/ initiation of or any change in ticagrelor therapy.

PREGNANCY AND LACTATION
Pregnancy: Category C.
Lactation: Not for use in nursing.

MECHANISM OF ACTION
Platelet activation and aggregation inhibitor; reversibly interacts w/ the platelet P2Y12 adenosine diphosphate receptor to prevent signal transduction and platelet activation.

PHARMACOKINETICS
Absorption: Absolute bioavailability (36%); T_{max} (median)=1.5 hrs, 2.5 hrs (AR-C124910XX). **Distribution:** V_d=88L; plasma protein binding (>99%). **Metabolism:** Liver via CYP3A4; AR-C124910XX (major active metabolite). **Elimination:** Urine (26%, <1% unchanged, <1% AR-C124910XX), feces (58%); $T_{1/2}$=approx 7 hrs, 9 hrs (AR-C124910XX).

PATIENT CONSIDERATIONS
Assessment: Assess for history of intracranial hemorrhage, active pathological bleeding, risk factors for bleeding, severe hepatic impairment, hypersensitivity to drug, pregnancy/nursing status, and possible drug interactions.

Monitoring: Monitor for bleeding, dyspnea, and other adverse reactions.

Counseling: Advise that daily doses of ASA should not exceed 100mg and to avoid taking any other medications that contain ASA. Advise that patients may experience bleeding and bruising more easily and will take longer than usual to stop bleeding; instruct to report any unanticipated, prolonged, or excessive bleeding, or blood in the stool or urine. Advise to contact physician if unexpected shortness of breath occurs. Advise to inform physicians and dentists of ticagrelor therapy before any surgery or dental procedure.

PEDIATRIC DOSAGE
Pediatric use may not have been established

BRISDELLE — paroxetine   Rx

Class: Selective serotonin reuptake inhibitor (SSRI)

> Antidepressants increase the risk of suicidal thoughts and behavior in pediatrics and young adults when used to treat major depressive disorder and other psychiatric disorders. Monitor closely for worsening and for emergence of suicidal thoughts and behaviors.

ADULT DOSAGE
Menopausal Vasomotor Symptoms
Moderate to Severe:
7.5mg qhs

Dosing Considerations with MAOIs
Use Before or After an MAOI:
Wait at least 14 days after discontinuation of an MAOI before initiating therapy, and allow at least 14 days after stopping therapy before starting an MAOI

PEDIATRIC DOSAGE
Pediatric use may not have been established

ADMINISTRATION
Oral route
Take w/ or w/o food.

STORAGE
20-25°C (68-77°F); excursions permitted to 15-30°C (59-86°F). Protect from light and humidity.

HOW SUPPLIED
Cap: 7.5mg

CONTRAINDICATIONS
Concomitant use of an MAOI or w/in 14 days of stopping treatment, starting treatment in a patient being treated w/ linezolid or IV methylene blue. Concomitant use w/ thioridazine or pimozide, pregnancy, history of hypersensitivity to paroxetine or any of the other ingredients in this product.

WARNINGS/PRECAUTIONS
Not indicated for treatment of any psychiatric condition. Serotonin syndrome reported; d/c immediately and initiate supportive symptomatic treatment. May increase risk of bleeding events. Hyponatremia may occur; caution in elderly and volume-depleted patients. Bone fracture risk reported. May increase the likelihood of precipitation of a mixed/manic episode in patients at risk for bipolar disorder. Caution in patients with a history of seizures or with conditions that potentially lower the seizure threshold. Akathisia may develop; d/c if this occurs. Pupillary dilation that occurs following use may trigger an angle closure attack in a patient with anatomically narrow angles who does not have a patent iridectomy. May impair physical/mental abilities.

ADVERSE REACTIONS
Headache, fatigue/malaise/lethargy, N/V.

DRUG INTERACTIONS
See Contraindications. Increased risk of serotonin syndrome with other serotonergic drugs (eg, triptans, TCAs, fentanyl) and with drugs that impair metabolism of serotonin; d/c therapy and any concomitant serotonergic agents immediately if serotonin syndrome occurs and initiate supportive symptomatic treatment. Not recommended with tryptophan or other paroxetine products. May decrease effectiveness of tamoxifen; consider avoiding concomitant use. Increased risk of bleeding with aspirin, NSAIDs, warfarin, and other anticoagulants reported. Carefully monitor patients receiving warfarin therapy when paroxetine is initiated or discontinued. Increased risk of hyponatremia with diuretics. May increase levels of risperidone, atomoxetine, or theophylline; dosage of coadministered drug may need to be decreased. May increase levels and elimination T$_{1/2}$ of TCAs (eg, desipramine); may need to monitor levels and reduce dose of TCAs. May decrease digoxin levels; monitor digoxin levels and digoxin dosage may need to be increased. Caution with other drugs metabolized by CYP2D6 (eg, fluoxetine, risperidone, propafenone) and with CYP2D6 inhibitors (eg, quinidine). Increased levels with highly protein-bound drugs (eg, warfarin); monitor INR. Increased levels with cimetidine. Decreased exposure with phenobarbital or phenytoin. Decreased plasma levels with fosamprenavir/ritonavir.

PREGNANCY AND LACTATION
Category X, not for use in nursing.

MECHANISM OF ACTION
SSRI; mechanism for the treatment of VMS is unknown.

PHARMACOKINETICS
Absorption: Complete; C$_{max}$=13.10ng/mL; T$_{max}$=6 hrs (median); AUC$_{0\text{-last}}$=237hr•ng/mL. **Distribution:** Plasma protein binding (93-95%); found in breast milk. **Metabolism:** Extensive; oxidation and methylation via CYP2D6. **Elimination:** (30mg of oral sol) Urine (64%, 2% unchanged, 62% metabolites); feces (36%, mostly metabolites, <1% unchanged).

PATIENT CONSIDERATIONS
Assessment: Assess for hypersensitivity to drug, history of seizures or conditions that potentially lower the seizure threshold, risk of bipolar disorder, volume depletion, susceptibility to angle-closure glaucoma, pregnancy/nursing status, and possible drug interactions.

Monitoring: Monitor for signs/symptoms of worsening and emergence of suicidal thoughts and behaviors, serotonin syndrome, abnormal bleeding, hyponatremia, bone fractures, mania/hypomania, seizures, akathisia, angle-closure glaucoma, and other adverse reactions.

Counseling: Advise patients, families, and caregivers to look for the emergence of suicidality, especially early during treatment, and to observe for signs of activation of mania/hypomania. Caution about the risk of serotonin syndrome and hypernatremia. Inform of the possibility for an increased risk of fracture. Advise to notify physician if patient becomes pregnant during therapy. Caution about the risk of angle closure glaucoma. Caution about operating hazardous machinery, including motor vehicles, until reasonably certain that therapy does not affect ability to engage in such activities. Advise to inform physician if taking or planning to take any prescription or OTC drugs, including herbal supplements.

BRIVIACT — brivaracetam   CV

Class: Pyrrolidine derivative

ADULT DOSAGE
Partial Onset Seizures
Adjunctive Therapy in Patients w/ Epilepsy:
≥16 Years:
Initial: 50mg bid
Titrate: May adjust down to 25mg bid or up to 100mg bid based on tolerability and therapeutic response

Inj may be used when oral administration is temporarily not feasible; administer at same dosage and frequency as tab and oral sol

Clinical study experience w/ inj is limited to 4 consecutive days of treatment

PEDIATRIC DOSAGE
Pediatric use may not have been established

DOSING CONSIDERATIONS
Concomitant Medications
Increase the dosage in patients on concomitant rifampin by up to 100%

Hepatic Impairment
Initial: 25mg bid
Max: 75mg bid

Elderly
Start at low end of dosing range

Discontinuation
Avoid abrupt withdrawal

ADMINISTRATION
Oral/IV route
May initiate w/ either IV or tab/oral sol.
Take w/ or w/o food.

Tab
Swallow whole w/ liquid; do not crush or chew.

Oral Sol
Use calibrated measuring device.
No dilution is necessary.
May be administered using a NG or gastrostomy tube.
Discard any unused sol remaining after 5 months of first opening the bottle.

Inj
Administer IV over 2-15 min.
Diluted sol should not be stored for >4 hrs at room temperature and may be stored in PVC bags.
Discard any unused portion of inj vial contents.
Administer w/o dilution or may be mixed w/ diluents listed below:
- 0.9% NaCl
- Lactated Ringer's inj
- 5% dextrose inj

STORAGE
25°C (77°F); excursions permitted between 15-30°C (59-86°F). Do not freeze inj or oral sol.

HOW SUPPLIED
Inj: 50mg/5mL; **Oral Sol:** 10mg/mL; **Tab:** 10mg, 25mg, 50mg, 75mg, 100mg

CONTRAINDICATIONS
Hypersensitivity to brivaracetam or any of the inactive ingredients in the product.

WARNINGS/PRECAUTIONS
Increased risk of suicidal thoughts/behavior. May cause somnolence, fatigue, dizziness, and disturbance in coordination; may impair mental/physical abilities. Psychiatric adverse reactions reported. May cause hypersensitivity reactions; d/c if a reaction occurs. Withdraw gradually to minimize potential of increased seizure frequency and status epilepticus.

ADVERSE REACTIONS
Somnolence/sedation, dizziness, fatigue, N/V.

DRUG INTERACTIONS
See Dosing Considerations. Rifampin decreases plasma concentrations due to CYP2C19 induction. Carbamazepine may increase exposure to carbamazepine-epoxide; consider carbamazepine dose reduction if tolerability issues arise. Increases plasma concentrations of phenytoin; monitor phenytoin levels or d/c ongoing phenytoin therapy.

PREGNANCY AND LACTATION
Pregnancy: Category C. Physicians are advised to recommend that pregnant patients enroll in the North American Antiepileptic Drug (NAAED) Pregnancy Registry.
Lactation: Not for use in nursing.

MECHANISM OF ACTION
Anticonvulsant; not established. Displays a high and selective affinity for synaptic vesicle protein 2A (SV2A) in the brain.

PHARMACOKINETICS
Absorption: Rapid and almost complete; T_{max}=1 hr (median) (Tab, w/o food).
Distribution: Plasma protein binding (≤20%); V_d=0.5L/kg. **Metabolism:** Primarily by hydrolysis (via hepatic/extra hepatic amidase) of amide moiety to form a carboxylic acid metabolite; secondarily by hydroxylation (via CYP2C19) on the propyl side chain to form a hydroxy metabolite. **Elimination:** Urine (>95%, <10% unchanged); feces (<1%); $T_{1/2}$=9 hrs.

PATIENT CONSIDERATIONS
Assessment: Assess for hypersensitivity to the drug, hepatic impairment, suicidal thoughts/behavior, pregnancy/nursing status, and for possible drug interactions.
Monitoring: Monitor for emergence or worsening of depression, suicidal thoughts/behavior, and/or any unusual changes in mood or behavior; somnolence/fatigue; coordination difficulties; hypersensitivity reactions; and other adverse reactions.
Counseling: Counsel patients, their caregivers, and/or families that drug may increase risk of suicidal thoughts/behavior; instruct to immediately report emergence or worsening of symptoms of depression, any unusual changes in mood/behavior, or suicidal thoughts, behavior, or thoughts about self-harm to physician. Advise patients that treatment causes somnolence, fatigue, dizziness, and gait disturbance; advise not to drive or operate machinery until they have gained sufficient experience on therapy. Advise that medication may cause changes in behavior (eg, aggression, agitation, anger, anxiety, irritability) and psychotic symptoms; instruct to report these symptoms immediately. Advise that symptoms of hypersensitivity may occur and to seek immediate medical care if symptoms occur. Advise not to d/c use w/o consulting healthcare provider. Advise to notify physician if pregnancy occurs or is intended while on therapy; encourage to enroll in the North American Antiepileptic Drug Pregnancy Registry if pregnant.

BROMDAY — bromfenac
Rx

Class: NSAID

ADULT DOSAGE	PEDIATRIC DOSAGE
Ocular Pain and Inflammation	Pediatric use may not have been established
Instill 1 drop qd in affected eye(s), starting 1 day prior to cataract surgery, continued on day of surgery, and through first 14 days of postoperative period	

DOSING CONSIDERATIONS
Concomitant Medications
Space dosing ≥5 min apart with other topical ophthalmic medications

ADMINISTRATION
Ocular route

STORAGE
15-25°C (59-77°F).

HOW SUPPLIED
Sol: 0.09% [1.7mL]

WARNINGS/PRECAUTIONS
Contains sodium sulfite; may cause allergic-type reactions (eg, anaphylactic symptoms, asthmatic episodes). Sulfite sensitivity is seen more frequently in asthmatics. May slow or delay healing. Potential cross-sensitivity to acetylsalicylic acid, phenylacetic acid derivatives, and other NSAIDs. Caution when treating individuals who previously exhibited sensitivity to these drugs. May increase bleeding of ocular tissues (eg, hyphemas) in conjunction with ocular surgery. Caution in patients with known bleeding tendencies. May result in keratitis. Continued use may lead to sight-threatening epithelial breakdown, corneal thinning, corneal erosion, corneal ulceration, or corneal perforation; d/c if corneal epithelium breakdown occurs. Caution in patients with complicated ocular surgeries, corneal denervation, corneal epithelial defects, diabetes mellitus (DM), ocular surface diseases (eg, dry eye syndrome), rheumatoid arthritis (RA), or repeat ocular surgeries within a short period of time. Increased risk for occurrence and severity of corneal adverse events if used >24 hrs prior to surgery or use beyond 14 days postsurgery. Avoid use with contact lenses. Avoid use during late pregnancy because of the known effects on the fetal cardiovascular system (closure of ductus arteriosus).

ADVERSE REACTIONS
Abnormal sensation in eye, conjunctival hyperemia, eye irritation (burning/stinging), eye pain, eye pruritus, eye redness, headache, iritis.

DRUG INTERACTIONS
Concomitant use of topical NSAIDs and topical steroids may increase potential for healing problems. Caution with other medications that may prolong bleeding time.

PREGNANCY AND LACTATION
Category C, caution in nursing.

MECHANISM OF ACTION
NSAID; thought to block prostaglandin synthesis by inhibiting cyclooxygenase 1 and 2.

PATIENT CONSIDERATIONS
Assessment: Assess for hypersensitivity (eg, sodium sulfite) or cross-sensitivity (eg, aspirin) reactions, history of complicated or repeated ocular surgeries, corneal denervation, corneal epithelial defects, DM, ocular surface diseases (eg, dry eye syndrome), RA, bleeding tendencies, pregnancy/nursing status, and possible drug interactions.
Monitoring: Monitor for anaphylactic symptoms, severe asthma attacks, wound-healing problems, keratitis, corneal epithelial breakdown, corneal thinning/erosion/ulceration/perforation, increased bleeding time, and bleeding of ocular tissues (hyphemas) in conjunction with ocular surgery.
Counseling: Advise not to wear contact lenses during therapy. Advise of the possibility of slow or delayed healing that may occur while using this product. Advise not to touch the dropper tip to any surface, as this may contaminate the contents. If >1 topical ophthalmic medication is used, instruct to administer 5 min apart.

BROMFED DM — brompheniramine maleate/ dextromethorphan hydrobromide/pseudoephedrine hydrochloride
Rx

Class: Antihistamine/antitussive/decongestant

ADULT DOSAGE	PEDIATRIC DOSAGE
Antihistamine/Cough Suppressant/ Nasal Decongestant	**Antihistamine/Cough Suppressant/ Nasal Decongestant**
Relief of coughs and upper respiratory symptoms, including nasal congestion, associated w/ allergy or the common cold	Relief of coughs and upper respiratory symptoms, including nasal congestion, associated w/ allergy or the common cold
10mL (2 tsp) q4h **Max:** 6 doses/24 hrs	**6 Months to <2 Years:** Dosage to be established by physician
	2 to <6 Years: 2.5mL (1/2 tsp) q4h **Max:** 6 doses/24 hrs
	6 to <12 Years: 5mL (1 tsp) q4h **Max:** 6 doses/24 hrs
	≥12 Years: 10mL (2 tsp) q4h **Max:** 6 doses/24 hrs

DOSING CONSIDERATIONS
Elderly
Start at the low end of the dosing range

ADMINISTRATION
Oral route

STORAGE
20-25°C (68-77°F). Keep tightly closed.

HOW SUPPLIED
Syrup: (Brompheniramine Maleate/Pseudoephedrine HCl/Dextromethorphan HBr) (2mg/30mg/10mg)/5mL [118mL, 473mL]

CONTRAINDICATIONS
Hypersensitivity to any of the ingredients, newborn, premature infants, nursing mothers, severe HTN, severe coronary artery disease (CAD), lower respiratory tract conditions (including asthma), coadministration w/ MAOIs.

WARNINGS/PRECAUTIONS
Overdosage may cause hallucinations, convulsions, and death, especially in infants and small children. May diminish mental alertness. May produce excitation in the young child. Caution w/ diabetes, HTN, heart or thyroid disease, history of bronchial asthma, narrow-angle glaucoma, or GI or urinary bladder neck obstruction. Caution in the elderly.

ADVERSE REACTIONS
Sedation, dryness of mouth, nose and throat, thickening of bronchial secretions, dizziness.

DRUG INTERACTIONS
See Contraindications. Additive effects w/ alcohol and other CNS depressants (eg, hypnotics, sedatives, tranquilizers, antianxiety agents). May reduce effects of antihypertensive drugs.

PREGNANCY AND LACTATION
Pregnancy: Category C.
Lactation: Contraindicated in nursing mothers.

MECHANISM OF ACTION
Brompheniramine: Antihistamine (H_1-receptor-blocking agent); appears to compete w/ histamine for receptor sites on effector cells. Antagonizes the allergic response (vasodilation, increased vascular permeability, increased mucus secretion) of nasal tissue. **Pseudoephedrine:** Nasal decongestant; acts on sympathetic nerve endings and also on smooth muscle. Effect is mediated by the action on α-sympathetic receptors, producing vasoconstriction of the dilated nasal arterioles. **Dextromethorphan:** Antitussive; acts centrally to elevate the threshold for coughing.

PHARMACOKINETICS
Absorption: Brompheniramine: Well absorbed from GI tract. T_{max}=5 hrs.
Metabolism: Brompheniramine: Liver. **Elimination:** Brompheniramine: Urine.

PATIENT CONSIDERATIONS
Assessment: Assess for HTN, CAD, lower respiratory tract conditions, diabetes, heart/thyroid disease, history of bronchial asthma, narrow-angle glaucoma, GI or

urinary bladder neck obstruction, drug hypersensitivity, pregnancy/nursing status, and possible drug interactions.

Monitoring: Monitor for excitation in the young child, diminished mental alertness, and other adverse reactions.

Counseling: Warn about engaging in activities requiring mental alertness (eg, driving a car, operating dangerous machinery). Advise to notify physician if taking any other medications, and if pregnant/breastfeeding.

BromSite — bromfenac   Rx

Class: NSAID

ADULT DOSAGE	**PEDIATRIC DOSAGE**
Ocular Pain and Inflammation	Pediatric use may not have been established
1 drop bid to the affected eye 1 day prior to cataract surgery, the day of surgery, and through 14 days postsurgery	

DOSING CONSIDERATIONS

Concomitant Medications
Administer at least 5 min after instillation of other topical medications

ADMINISTRATION
Ocular route

STORAGE
15-25°C (59-77°F). Discard after treatment completion.

HOW SUPPLIED
Sol: 0.075%

WARNINGS/PRECAUTIONS
May slow or delay healing. Potential for cross-sensitivity to acetylsalicylic acid (ASA), phenylacetic acid derivatives, and other NSAIDs; caution w/ previous sensitivities to these drugs. May cause increased bleeding of ocular tissues (eg, hyphemas) in conjunction w/ ocular surgery; caution w/ known bleeding tendencies. May result in keratitis. Continued use in some susceptible patients may result in epithelial breakdown or corneal thinning/erosion/ulceration/perforation; immediately d/c and monitor for corneal health if corneal epithelial breakdown occurs. Caution in patients w/ complicated ocular surgeries, corneal denervation, corneal epithelial defects, diabetes mellitus (DM), ocular surface diseases (eg, dry eye syndrome), rheumatoid arthritis (RA), or repeat ocular surgeries w/in a short period. Use >24 hrs prior to surgery or use beyond 14 days postsurgery may increase risk for occurrence and severity of corneal adverse events. Do not administer while wearing contact lenses.

ADVERSE REACTIONS
Anterior chamber inflammation, headache, vitreous floaters, iritis, eye pain, ocular HTN.

DRUG INTERACTIONS
Increased potential for healing problems w/ topical steroids. Caution w/ medications that may prolong bleeding time.

PREGNANCY AND LACTATION
Pregnancy: Avoid during late pregnancy due to the known effects on the fetal cardiovascular system.
Lactation: Systemic exposure to bromfenac is low; caution in nursing.

MECHANISM OF ACTION
NSAID; thought to block prostaglandin synthesis by inhibiting cyclooxygenase 1 and 2.

PATIENT CONSIDERATIONS
Assessment: Assess for hypersensitivity or cross-sensitivity (eg, ASA, phenylacetic acid derivatives, other NSAIDs) reactions, bleeding tendencies, history of complicated or repeated ocular surgeries, corneal denervation, corneal epithelial defects, DM, ocular surface diseases (eg, dry eye syndrome), RA, pregnancy/nursing status, and possible drug interactions.

Monitoring: Monitor for slow or delayed healing, increased bleeding of ocular tissues, keratitis, corneal epithelial breakdown, corneal thinning/erosion/ulceration/perforation, and other adverse reactions.

Counseling: Inform of the possibility that slow or delayed healing may occur. Advise to administer at least 5 min after instillation of other topical medications if >1 topical ophthalmic medication is being used. Instruct not to wear contact lenses during administration. Advise to replace bottle cap after use and not to touch dropper tip to any surface. Instruct to thoroughly wash hands prior to administering therapy.

Brovana — arformoterol tartrate   Rx

Class: Long-acting beta₂ agonist (LABA)

> Long-acting β₂-adrenergic agonists (LABAs) increase the risk of asthma-related death. Contraindicated in asthma without use of a long-term asthma control medication.

ADULT DOSAGE	**PEDIATRIC DOSAGE**
Chronic Obstructive Pulmonary Disease	Pediatric use may not have been established
Long-Term Maint Treatment of Bronchoconstriction:	
15mcg bid (am and pm) by nebulization	
Max: 30mcg/day (15mcg bid)	

ADMINISTRATION
Oral inh route
Administer via a standard jet nebulizer connected to an air compressor
Refer to PI for further administration instructions

STORAGE
2-8°C (36-46°F). Store in the protective foil pouch. Protect from light and excessive heat. After opening the pouch, unused vials should be returned to, and stored in, the pouch. Use opened vial immediately; discard if sol is not colorless. Unopened foil pouches can also be stored at 20-25°C (68-77°F) for up to 6 weeks.

HOW SUPPLIED
Sol, Inhalation: 15mcg base/2mL [30ˢ, 60ˢ]

CONTRAINDICATIONS
History of hypersensitivity to arformoterol, racemic formoterol, or to any other components of this product, asthma w/o use of a long-term asthma control medication.

WARNINGS/PRECAUTIONS
Not indicated to treat asthma, acute deteriorations of COPD, or acute episodes of bronchospasm (eg, as rescue therapy). D/C regular use of inhaled short-acting β₂-agonist (SABA) when beginning treatment; use only for symptomatic relief of acute respiratory symptoms. Do not use more often or at higher doses than recommended; fatalities reported with excessive use. May produce paradoxical bronchospasm; d/c therapy immediately and institute alternative therapy. Cardiovascular (CV) effects may occur; d/c if such effects occur. Caution with CV disorders, convulsive disorders, thyrotoxicosis, diabetes mellitus (DM), ketoacidosis, hepatic impairment, and in patients unusually responsive to sympathomimetic amines. May produce significant hypokalemia or transient hyperglycemia. Immediate hypersensitivity reactions may occur.

ADVERSE REACTIONS
Pain, chest/back pain, diarrhea, sinusitis, leg cramps, dyspnea, rash, flu syndrome, peripheral edema.

DRUG INTERACTIONS
Do not use with other medications containing LABAs. Adrenergic drugs may potentiate sympathetic effects; use with caution. Methylxanthine (aminophylline, theophylline), steroids, or diuretics may potentiate hypokalemic effect. Increased HR and systolic BP with theophylline. ECG changes and/or hypokalemia that may result from non-K⁺-sparing diuretics (eg, loop or thiazide diuretics) may be acutely worsened; use with caution. Extreme caution with MAOIs, TCAs, or drugs known to prolong the QTc interval; effect on CV system may be potentiated by these agents. Drugs known to prolong the QTc interval have an increased risk of ventricular arrhythmias. β-blockers and arformoterol may inhibit the effect of each other when administered concurrently. β-blockers may block therapeutic effects and produce severe bronchospasm in COPD patients; if such therapy is needed, consider cardioselective β-blockers and use with caution.

PREGNANCY AND LACTATION
Category C, caution in nursing.

MECHANISM OF ACTION
LABA; stimulates intracellular adenyl cyclase, the enzyme that catalyzes the conversion of adenosine triphosphate to cAMP. Increased cAMP levels cause relaxation of bronchial smooth muscle and inhibition of release of mediators of immediate hypersensitivity from cells, especially from mast cells.

PHARMACOKINETICS
Absorption: C_{max}=4.3pg/mL; T_{max}=30 min (median); AUC_{0-12h}=34.5pg•hr/mL.
Distribution: Plasma protein binding (52-65%). **Metabolism:** Glucuronidation (primary) via uridine diphosphoglucuronosyltransferase isozymes, and O-demethylation (secondary) via CYP2D6 and CYP2C19 (secondary). **Elimination:** (Within 48 hrs) Urine (63%), feces (11%); $T_{1/2}$=26 hrs.

PATIENT CONSIDERATIONS
Assessment: Assess for asthma and use of control medication, acutely deteriorating COPD, CV disorders, convulsive disorders, thyrotoxicosis, DM, ketoacidosis, hepatic impairment, history of hypersensitivity to drug, pregnancy/nursing status, and possible drug interactions. Assess use in patients unusually responsive to sympathomimetic amines.

Monitoring: Monitor for deteriorating disease, paradoxical bronchospasm, CV effects, hypokalemia, hyperglycemia, immediate hypersensitivity reactions, and other adverse reactions.

Counseling: Inform that drug is not for treatment of asthma. Advise not to use to relieve acute respiratory symptoms; inform that acute symptoms should be treated with an inhaled SABA. Instruct to seek medical attention if symptoms worsen despite recommended doses, if treatment becomes less effective, or if experiencing a need for more inhalations of a SABA than usual. Advise not to stop therapy unless directed by physician, not to inhale >1 dose at any 1 time, and not to exceed recommended daily dosage. Instruct to d/c the regular use of inhaled SABAs (eg, levalbuterol) when beginning treatment. Counsel not to use with other inhaled medications containing a LABA, and not to stop or change the dose of other concomitant COPD therapy without medical advice, even if symptoms improve after initiating treatment. Inform of the common adverse reactions with therapy. Instruct on how to properly use the medication. Advise to contact physician if pregnancy occurs, or if nursing.

BUMETANIDE — bumetanide   Rx

Class: Loop diuretic

> May lead to profound diuresis with water and electrolyte depletion if given in excessive amounts; careful medical supervision required and dose and dosage schedule must be adjusted to individual patient's needs.

OTHER BRAND NAMES
Bumex (Discontinued)

ADULT DOSAGE

Edema

Associated w/ CHF, Hepatic/Renal Disease (Nephrotic Syndrome):

Tab:
Usual: 0.5-2mg/day as single dose; may give a 2nd or 3rd dose at 4- to 5-hr intervals if response is not adequate
Maint: Give on alternate days or for 3-4 days w/ rest periods of 1-2 days in between
Max: 10mg/day

Inj:
Initial: 0.5-1mg IV/IM (give IV over 1-2 min); may give a 2nd or 3rd dose at 2- to 3-hr intervals if response is insufficient
Max: 10mg/day
Initiate oral treatment as soon as possible

PEDIATRIC DOSAGE
Pediatric use may not have been established

DOSING CONSIDERATIONS

Hepatic Impairment
Tab: Give minimum dose, and if necessary, increase dose very carefully

Elderly
Tab/Inj: Start at lower end of dosing range

ADMINISTRATION
Oral/IV/IM route

Compatibility
5% dextrose sol; 0.9% NaCl; lactated Ringer's inj

STORAGE
20-25°C (68-77°F). Protect from light. **Inj:** Excursions permitted to 15-30°C (59-86°F).

HOW SUPPLIED
Inj: 0.25mg/mL [4mL, 10mL]; **Tab:** 0.5mg*, 1mg*, 2mg* *scored

CONTRAINDICATIONS
Anuria, hepatic coma, severe electrolyte depletion, hypersensitivity to this product.

WARNINGS/PRECAUTIONS
Excessive doses may cause dehydration, blood volume reduction, and circulatory collapse with possible vascular thrombosis and embolism, particularly in elderly. Hypokalemia may occur; caution with hepatic cirrhosis and ascites, states of aldosterone excess with normal renal function, K+-losing nephropathy, certain diarrheal states, other states where hypokalemia represents added risks, or in patients receiving digitalis and diuretics for CHF. Sudden alterations of electrolyte balance may precipitate hepatic encephalopathy and coma in patients with hepatic cirrhosis and ascites; initiate therapy in hospital. Ototoxicity, thrombocytopenia, hypocalcemia, hypomagnesemia, and hyperuricemia may occur. May affect glucose metabolism; monitor glucose levels in patients with diabetes or suspected latent diabetes. Monitor for blood dyscrasias, hepatic damage, or idiosyncratic reactions. Caution with sulfonamide allergy. Reversible elevations of BUN and creatinine may occur; d/c if marked increase in BUN or creatinine occurs, or if oliguria develops in patients with progressive renal disease. Tab may be substituted at approximately a 1:40 ratio of bumetanide tabs to furosemide in patients allergic to furosemide.

ADVERSE REACTIONS
Muscle cramps, dizziness, hypotension, headache, nausea, encephalopathy, hyperuricemia, hypochloremia, hypokalemia, hyponatremia, hyperglycemia, azotemia, increased SrCr.

DRUG INTERACTIONS
Avoid with drugs known to have a nephrotoxic potential. Not recommended for use with indomethacin. High risk of lithium toxicity; avoid coadministration. Pretreatment with probenecid reduces effects; do not administer concurrently. May potentiate the effect of various antihypertensives; reduction in the dose of these drugs may be necessary. **Inj:** Avoid with aminoglycosides (except in life-threatening situations).

PREGNANCY AND LACTATION
Category C, not for use in nursing.

MECHANISM OF ACTION
Loop diuretic; inhibits Na+ reabsorption in the ascending limb of the loop of Henle.

PHARMACOKINETICS
Absorption: T_{max}=15-30 min (IV), 1-2 hrs (PO). **Distribution:** Plasma protein binding (94-96%). **Metabolism:** Oxidation. **Elimination:** (PO) Urine (81%, 45% unchanged), bile (2%); $T_{1/2}$=1-1.5 hrs.

PATIENT CONSIDERATIONS
Assessment: Assess for progressive renal disease, severe electrolyte depletion, anuria, diabetes or suspected latent diabetes, sulfonamide allergy, liver disease (hepatic coma), any other conditions where treatment is contraindicated or cautioned, pregnancy/nursing status, and possible drug interactions.

Monitoring: Monitor for ototoxicity, blood dyscrasias, liver damage or idiosyncratic reactions, hypersensitivity reactions, hyperuricemia, oliguria, thrombocytopenia, and other adverse reactions. Periodically monitor serum K+, serum electrolytes, blood glucose, and renal function.

Counseling: Inform of the risks/benefits of therapy. Advise to seek medical attention if adverse reactions occur.

BUNAVAIL — buprenorphine/naloxone   CIII

Class: Partial opioid agonist/opioid antagonist

ADULT DOSAGE

Opioid Dependence

Maint Treatment:
Use as part of a complete treatment plan to include counseling and psychosocial support
Target Dose: (8.4mg/1.4mg)/day as a single dose
Titrate: Adjust dose in increments/decrements of 2.1mg/0.3mg to maintain treatment and suppress opioid withdrawal signs/symptoms
Range: (2.1mg/0.3mg)/day to (12.6mg/2.1mg)/day

Apply film to the buccal mucosa as a single daily dose in patients who have been initially inducted using buprenorphine SL tabs

Conversions

Switching Between Suboxone SL Tab/Film:
4mg/1mg Suboxone: 2.1mg/0.3mg Bunavail
8mg/2mg Suboxone: 4.2mg/0.7mg Bunavail
12mg/3mg Suboxone: 6.3mg/1mg Bunavail

PEDIATRIC DOSAGE
Pediatric use may not have been established

DOSING CONSIDERATIONS

Hepatic Impairment
Moderate: Therapy may not be appropriate
Severe: Avoid use

Elderly
Start at the lower end of the dosing range

Discontinuation
Taper to avoid withdrawal signs/symptoms

ADMINISTRATION
Buccal route

Do not eat or drink until film(s) dissolves; do not chew or swallow film
Do not cut or tear the film; use the entire film
Avoid manipulating film(s) w/ tongue or finger(s)

Application
Use the tongue to wet the inside of the cheek or rinse the mouth w/ water to moisten the area immediately before placing the film
Hold the film w/ clean, dry fingers w/ the text (BN2, BN4, or BN6) facing up, then place the side w/ the text (BN2, BN4, or BN6) against the inside of the cheek; press and hold in place for 5 sec
If multiple films need to be administered, immediately apply the next film; no more than 2 films should be applied to the inside of 1 cheek at a time
If 2 films are required for 1 dose, place each film on separate cheeks

STORAGE
20-25°C (68-77°F); excursions permitted to 15-30°C (59-86°F). Protect from freezing and moisture.

HOW SUPPLIED
Film, Buccal: (Buprenorphine/Naloxone) 2.1mg/0.3mg, 4.2mg/0.7mg, 6.3mg/1mg

CONTRAINDICATIONS
Hypersensitivity to buprenorphine or naloxone.

WARNINGS/PRECAUTIONS
Not appropriate for the treatment of neonatal abstinence syndrome in neonates and as an analgesic. Hypersensitivity reactions, bronchospasm, angioneurotic edema, and anaphylactic shock reported. May precipitate opioid withdrawal signs and symptoms if administered before the agonist effects of the opioid have subsided. May impair mental/physical abilities. May produce orthostatic hypotension in ambulatory patients. Caution with debilitated patients, and in those with myxedema, hypothyroidism, adrenal cortical insufficiency (eg, Addison's disease), CNS depression or coma, toxic psychoses, prostatic hypertrophy or urethral stricture, acute alcoholism, delirium tremens, kyphoscoliosis, and in elderly. Not recommended with severe hepatic impairment and may not be appropriate with moderate hepatic impairment. Buprenorphine: Potential for abuse. Significant respiratory depression

reported; caution with compromised respiratory function. To manage overdose, higher than normal doses and repeated administration of naloxone may be necessary. Accidental pediatric exposure can cause severe, possibly fatal, respiratory depression. Chronic use produces physical dependence. Cytolytic hepatitis and hepatitis with jaundice reported; obtain LFTs prior to initiation and periodically thereafter. Evaluate cause if a hepatic event is suspected; careful discontinuation may be needed. Caution with preexisting liver enzyme abnormalities, hepatitis B or C infection, use with other potentially hepatotoxic drugs, and ongoing injecting drug use. Neonatal withdrawal reported when used during pregnancy. May elevate CSF pressure; caution with head injury, intracranial lesions, and other circumstances when cerebrospinal pressure may be increased. May produce miosis and changes in consciousness level that may interfere with patient evaluation. May increase intracholedochal pressure; caution with biliary tract dysfunction. May obscure diagnosis or clinical course of patients with acute abdominal conditions.

ADVERSE REACTIONS
Headache, withdrawal syndrome, pain, N/V, insomnia, sweating, constipation, abdominal pain, vasodilation, chills, asthenia, infection, rhinitis, back pain, diarrhea.

DRUG INTERACTIONS
May cause respiratory depression, coma, and death with benzodiazepines or other CNS depressants (eg, alcohol); caution when used concurrently. May cause increased CNS depression with opioid analgesics, general anesthetics, benzodiazepines, phenothiazines, other tranquilizers, sedative/hypnotics, or other CNS depressants (eg, alcohol); consider dose reduction of 1 or both agents. Concomitant use with CYP3A4 inhibitors (eg, azole antifungals, macrolides, HIV protease inhibitors) should be monitored and may require dose reduction of 1 or both agents. Monitor for signs and symptoms of opioid withdrawal with CYP3A4 inducers (eg, efavirenz, phenobarbital, carbamazepine). Monitor dose if non-nucleoside reverse transcriptase inhibitors are added to treatment regimen. Atazanavir and atazanavir/ritonavir may increase levels; monitor and consider dose reduction of buprenorphine.

PREGNANCY AND LACTATION
Category C, caution in nursing.

MECHANISM OF ACTION
Buprenorphine: Partial agonist at the μ-opioid receptor and antagonist at the kappa-opioid receptor. Naloxone: Potent antagonist at μ-opioid receptors.

PHARMACOKINETICS
Distribution: Plasma protein binding (96%, buprenorphine; 45%, naloxone); found in breast milk (buprenorphine). **Metabolism:** Buprenorphine: N-dealkylation (by CYP3A4) and glucuronidation; norbuprenorphine (major metabolite). Naloxone: Glucuronidation, N-dealkylation, and reduction. **Elimination:** Buprenorphine: Urine (30%), feces (69%); $T_{1/2}$=16.4-27.5 hrs. Naloxone: $T_{1/2}$=1.9-2.4 hrs.

PATIENT CONSIDERATIONS
Assessment: Assess for history of hypersensitivity reactions, debilitation, myxedema, hypothyroidism, acute alcoholism, adrenal cortical insufficiency (eg, Addison's disease), CNS depression or coma, toxic psychoses, prostatic hypertrophy, urethral stricture, delirium tremens, kyphoscoliosis, biliary tract dysfunction, hepatic impairment, compromised respiratory function, hepatitis B or C infection, head injury, intracranial lesions and other circumstances in which cerebrospinal pressure may be increased, acute abdominal conditions, pregnancy/nursing status, and possible drug interactions. Obtain baseline LFTs.

Monitoring: Monitor for hypersensitivity reactions, signs/symptoms of opioid withdrawal, impaired mental/physical ability, orthostatic hypotension, respiratory depression, drug abuse/dependence, cytolytic hepatitis, hepatitis with jaundice, elevation of CSF, miosis, changes in consciousness levels, and other adverse reactions. Monitor LFTs periodically.

Counseling: Warn patient on danger of self-administration of benzodiazepines and other CNS depressants, including alcohol, while on therapy. Advise that films contain an opioid that can be a target for abuse; instruct to keep films in safe place protected from theft and children. Instruct to seek medical attention immediately if a child is exposed to the drug. Caution that the drug may impair mental/physical abilities and cause orthostatic hypotension. Advise to take film qd and not to change dose without consulting physician. Inform that treatment can cause dependence and withdrawal syndrome may occur upon discontinuation. Advise patients seeking to d/c treatment with buprenorphine, to work closely with physician on a tapering schedule, and apprise of the potential to relapse to illicit drug use associated with discontinuation of treatment. Advise to inform physician of all medications prescribed or currently being used. Advise women regarding possible effects during pregnancy and not to breastfeed. Advise to instruct family members that, in event of emergency, the treating physician or staff should be informed that patient is physically dependent on an opioid. Advise to dispose of unused drugs as soon as they are no longer needed by flushing down the toilet.

BUPRENEX — buprenorphine hydrochloride   CIII
Class: Partial opioid agonist

ADULT DOSAGE Moderate to Severe Pain	PEDIATRIC DOSAGE Moderate to Severe Pain
Usual: 0.3mg IM/IV q6h prn; repeat once (up to 0.3mg) if needed, 30-60 min after initial dose May use single doses up to 0.6mg IM if not in a high-risk category	**2-12 Years:** 2-6mcg/kg IM/IV q4-6h **≥13 Years:** **Usual:** 0.3mg IM/IV q6h prn; repeat once (up to 0.3mg) if needed, 30-60 min after initial dose May use single doses up to 0.6mg IM if not in a high-risk category

DOSING CONSIDERATIONS
Concomitant Medications
Reduce dose by approximately 50% in patients taking other CNS depressants

Other Important Considerations
High-Risk Patients (eg, Elderly, Debilitated, Presence of Respiratory Disease):
Reduce dose by approximately 50%

ADMINISTRATION
IM/IV route
Administer deep IM or slow IV route (over at least 2 min).

STORAGE
20-25°C (68-77°F); excursions permitted between 15-30°C (59-86°F). Protect from prolonged exposure to light.

HOW SUPPLIED
Inj: 0.3mg/mL

CONTRAINDICATIONS
Hypersensitivity to the product.

WARNINGS/PRECAUTIONS
Clinically significant respiratory depression may occur; caution with compromised respiratory function. Naloxone may not be effective in reversing respiratory depression. May increase CSF pressure; caution with head injury, intracranial lesions, and other circumstances where cerebrospinal pressure may be increased. Can produce miosis and changes in level of consciousness. May impair mental or physical abilities; caution in ambulatory patients. May result in withdrawal effects in physically dependent patients. Caution in elderly, debilitated, and pediatric patients. Caution with hepatic/renal/pulmonary impairment, myxedema or hypothyroidism, adrenal cortical insufficiency, CNS depression or coma, toxic psychoses, prostatic hypertrophy or urethral stricture, acute alcoholism, delirium tremens, kyphoscoliosis, or biliary tract dysfunction.

ADVERSE REACTIONS
Sedation, N/V, dizziness, sweating, hypotension, headache, miosis, hypoventilation.

DRUG INTERACTIONS
Caution with MAOIs and CNS and respiratory depressants. Increased CNS depression with other narcotic analgesics, general anesthetics, antihistamines, benzodiazepines, phenothiazines, other tranquilizers, sedative-hypnotics, or other CNS depressants (eg, alcohol); reduce dose of one or both agents. Respiratory and cardiovascular collapse reported with diazepam. Suspected interaction with phenprocoumon resulting in purpura. Decreased clearance with CYP3A4 inhibitors (eg, macrolides, azole antifungals, protease inhibitors). Increased clearance with CYP3A4 inducers (eg, rifampin, carbamazepine, phenytoin).

PREGNANCY AND LACTATION
Category C, not for use in nursing.

MECHANISM OF ACTION
Partial opioid agonist/opioid antagonist; high affinity binding to μ-opiate receptors in CNS. Also possesses narcotic antagonist activity.

PHARMACOKINETICS
Distribution: Found in breast milk. **Metabolism:** Liver. **Elimination:** (IV) $T_{1/2}$=1.2-7.2 hrs.

PATIENT CONSIDERATIONS
Assessment: Assess for compromised respiratory function (eg, chronic obstructive pulmonary disease, hypoxia), head injury, intracranial lesions, hepatic/renal function, any condition where treatment is cautioned, pregnancy/nursing status, and possible drug interactions.

Monitoring: Monitor for signs/symptoms of respiratory depression, CNS depression, elevation of CSF pressure, increased intracholedochal pressure, drug abuse/dependence, and withdrawal effects.

Counseling: Counsel that effects (eg, drowsiness) may be potentiated by other centrally acting agents (eg, alcohol); advise not to drive/operate machinery under these circumstances. Advise that medication may lead to dependence. Counsel to not exceed prescribed dosage. Advise to notify physician of all medications currently being taken.

BUPRENORPHINE AND NALOXONE SUBLINGUAL TABLETS (2 MG/0.5 MG, 8 MG/2 MG) — buprenorphine/naloxone   CIII
Class: Partial opioid agonist/opioid antagonist

OTHER BRAND NAMES
Suboxone Sublingual Tablets (Discontinued)

ADULT DOSAGE Opioid Dependence	PEDIATRIC DOSAGE
Use as part of a complete treatment plan to include counseling and psychosocial support Administer SL as a single daily dose; use in patients initially inducted using buprenorphine SL tab **Maint:** **Target Dose:** (16mg/4mg)/day as single dose	Pediatric use may not have been established

Titrate: Adjust dose progressively in increments/decrements of 2mg/0.5mg or 4mg/1mg to maintain treatment and suppress opioid withdrawal signs/symptoms
Range: (4mg/1mg)/day to (24mg/6mg)/day depending on the patient

Conversions
Switching Between SL Film and SL Tab:
Start on the same dose as the previously administered product; dose adjustments may be necessary
From SL Tabs to SL Film: Monitor for over-medication
From SL Film to SL Tabs: Monitor for withdrawal or other indications of underdosing

----

DOSING CONSIDERATIONS
Hepatic Impairment
Moderate: Use may not be appropriate
Severe: Avoid use
Elderly
Start at lower end of dosing range
Discontinuation
Decision to d/c therapy should be made as part of a comprehensive treatment plan; both gradual and abrupt discontinuation of buprenorphine has been used, but data are insufficient to determine best method of dose taper at the end of treatment

ADMINISTRATION
SL route

Place tab under tongue until dissolved; for doses requiring use of >2 tabs, place all the tabs at once or alternatively (if unable to fit in >2 tabs comfortably), place 2 tabs at a time under the tongue.

STORAGE
20-25°C (68-77°F); excursions permitted to 15-30°C (59-86°F).

HOW SUPPLIED
Tab, SL: (Buprenorphine/Naloxone) 2mg/0.5mg, 8mg/2mg

CONTRAINDICATIONS
Hypersensitivity to buprenorphine or naloxone.

WARNINGS/PRECAUTIONS
Not appropriate as an analgesic. Hypersensitivity reactions, bronchospasm, angioneurotic edema, and anaphylactic shock reported. May precipitate opioid withdrawal signs and symptoms if administered before the agonist effects of the opioid have subsided. May be used w/ caution for maintenance treatment in patients w/ moderate hepatic impairment who have initiated treatment on a buprenorphine product w/o naloxone. May impair mental/physical abilities. May produce orthostatic hypotension in ambulatory patients. Caution w/ debilitated patients, myxedema, hypothyroidism, adrenal cortical insufficiency (eg, Addison's disease), CNS depression or coma, toxic psychoses, prostatic hypertrophy or urethral stricture, acute alcoholism, delirium tremens, kyphoscoliosis, and in elderly. **Buprenorphine:** Potential for abuse. Significant respiratory depression reported; caution w/ compromised respiratory function. To manage overdose, higher than normal doses and repeated administration of naloxone may be necessary. Accidental pediatric exposure can cause severe, possibly fatal, respiratory depression. Chronic use produces physical dependence. Cytolytic hepatitis and hepatitis w/ jaundice reported; obtain LFTs prior to initiation and periodically thereafter. If a hepatic event is suspected, biological and etiological evaluation is recommended; careful discontinuation may be needed depending on the case. Caution w/ preexisting liver enzyme abnormalities, hepatitis B or C infection, use w/ other potentially hepatotoxic drugs, and ongoing injecting drug use. Neonatal withdrawal reported when used during pregnancy. May elevate CSF pressure; caution w/ head injury, intracranial lesions, and other circumstances when cerebrospinal pressure may be increased. May produce miosis and changes in consciousness level that may interfere w/ patient evaluation. May increase intracholedochal pressure; caution w/ biliary tract dysfunction. May obscure diagnosis or clinical course of patients w/ acute abdominal conditions.

ADVERSE REACTIONS
Headache, withdrawal syndrome, pain, N/V, insomnia, sweating, constipation, abdominal pain, vasodilation, chills, asthenia, infection, rhinitis, back pain, diarrhea.

DRUG INTERACTIONS
May cause respiratory depression, coma, and death w/ benzodiazepines or other CNS depressants (eg, alcohol); caution when used concurrently. May cause increased CNS depression w/ opioid analgesics, general anesthetics, benzodiazepines, phenothiazines, other tranquilizers, sedative/hypnotics, or other CNS depressants (eg, alcohol); consider dose reduction of 1 or both agents. Concomitant use w/ CYP3A4 inhibitors (eg, azole antifungals, macrolides, HIV protease inhibitors) should be monitored and may require dose reduction of 1 or both agents. Monitor for signs and symptoms of opioid withdrawal w/ CYP3A4 inducers (eg, efavirenz, phenobarbital, carbamazepine, phenytoin, rifampicin). Monitor dose if non-nucleoside reverse transcriptase inhibitors are added to treatment regimen. Atazanavir and atazanavir/ritonavir may increase levels; monitor and consider dose reduction of buprenorphine.

PREGNANCY AND LACTATION
Pregnancy: Category C.
Lactation: Not for use in nursing.

MECHANISM OF ACTION
Buprenorphine: Partial agonist at the μ-opioid receptor and antagonist at the kappa-opioid receptor. **Naloxone:** Potent antagonist at μ-opioid receptors.

PHARMACOKINETICS
Absorption: Administration of variable doses resulted in different parameters.
Distribution: Plasma protein binding (96%, buprenorphine; 45%, naloxone); found in breast milk (buprenorphine). **Metabolism:** Buprenorphine: N-dealkylation (by CYP3A4) and glucuronidation; norbuprenorphine (major metabolite). Naloxone: Glucuronidation, N-dealkylation, and reduction; naloxone-3-glucuronide (metabolite). **Elimination:** Buprenorphine: Urine (30%), feces (69%); $T_{1/2}$=24-42 hrs. Naloxone: $T_{1/2}$=2-12 hrs.

PATIENT CONSIDERATIONS
Assessment: Assess for history of hypersensitivity reactions, debilitation, myxedema, hypothyroidism, acute alcoholism, adrenal cortical insufficiency (eg, Addison's disease), CNS depression or coma, toxic psychoses, prostatic hypertrophy, urethral stricture, delirium tremens, kyphoscoliosis, biliary tract dysfunction, hepatic impairment, compromised respiratory function, hepatitis B or C infection, head injury, intracranial lesions and other circumstances in which cerebrospinal pressure may be increased, acute abdominal conditions, pregnancy/nursing status, and possible drug interactions. Obtain baseline LFTs.

Monitoring: Monitor for hypersensitivity reactions, signs/symptoms of opioid withdrawal, impaired mental/physical ability, orthostatic hypotension, respiratory depression, drug abuse/dependence, cytolytic hepatitis, hepatitis w/ jaundice, elevation of CSF, miosis, changes in consciousness levels, and other adverse reactions. Monitor LFTs periodically. Monitor for over-medication as well as withdrawal or other indications of underdosing when switching between SL film and SL tab.

Counseling: Warn patient on danger of self-administration of benzodiazepines and other CNS depressants, including alcohol, while on therapy. Advise that tabs contain an opioid that can be a target for abuse; instruct to keep tabs in safe place protected from theft and children. Instruct to seek medical attention immediately if a child is exposed to the drug. Caution that the drug may impair mental/physical abilities and cause orthostatic hypotension. Advise to take tab qd and not to change dose w/o consulting physician. Inform that treatment can cause dependence and that withdrawal syndrome may occur upon discontinuation. Advise patients seeking to d/c treatment w/ buprenorphine for opioid dependence to work closely w/ physician on a tapering schedule, and apprise of the potential to relapse to illicit drug use associated w/ discontinuation of treatment. Advise to inform physician of all medications prescribed or currently being used. Advise women regarding possible effects during pregnancy and not to breastfeed. Advise to instruct family members that, in event of emergency, the treating physician or staff should be informed that patient is physically dependent on an opioid. Advise to dispose of unused drugs as soon as they are no longer needed by flushing the tabs down the toilet.

BUPROBAN — bupropion hydrochloride   **Rx**
Class: Aminoketone

> Serious neuropsychiatric reactions reported in patients taking bupropion for smoking cessation. Weigh risks against benefits of use. Antidepressants increased the risk of suicidal thoughts and behavior in children, adolescents, and young adults in short-term trials. Monitor closely for worsening and emergence of suicidal thoughts and behaviors. Advise families and caregivers of the need for close observation and communication with the prescriber.

ADULT DOSAGE	PEDIATRIC DOSAGE
Smoking Cessation Aid Initiate treatment while patient is still smoking Patients should set a "target quit date" w/in the first 2 weeks of treatment **Initial:** 150mg qd for first 3 days **Titrate:** Increase to 300mg/day, given as 150mg bid w/ an interval of at least 8 hrs between each dose **Max:** 300mg/day Continue treatment for 7-12 weeks; if patient has not quit smoking after 7-12 weeks, d/c and reassess treatment plan May consider continuing therapy in patients who successfully quit smoking after 12 weeks of treatment but do not feel ready to d/c treatment; base longer treatment on individual patient benefits/risks **Dosing Considerations with MAOIs** **Use w/ Reversible MAOIs (eg, Linezolid, IV Methylene Blue):** Do not start bupropion in patients being treated w/ reversible MAOIs If acceptable alternatives are not available, d/c bupropion and	Pediatric use may not have been established

administer linezolid or IV methylene blue; monitor for 2 weeks or until 24 hrs after the last dose of linezolid or IV methylene blue, whichever comes 1st May resume bupropion 24 hrs after the last dose of linezolid or IV methylene blue

DOSING CONSIDERATIONS
Renal Impairment
GFR <90mL/min: Consider reducing dose and/or frequency

Hepatic Impairment
Mild (Child-Pugh Score 5-6): Consider reducing dose and/or frequency
Moderate-Severe (Child-Pugh Score 7-15): Max: 150mg qod

ADMINISTRATION
Oral route

Swallow tab whole; do not crush, divide, or chew
Take w/ or w/o food
Avoid hs dosing to minimize insomnia
May be used w/ a nicotine transdermal system

STORAGE
20-25°C (68-77°F). Protect from light and moisture.

HOW SUPPLIED
Tab, Extended-Release: 150mg

CONTRAINDICATIONS
Seizure disorder, current/prior diagnosis of bulimia or anorexia nervosa. Undergoing abrupt discontinuation of alcohol, benzodiazepines, barbiturates, or antiepileptic drugs. Use of MAOIs (intended to treat psychiatric disorders) either concomitantly or w/in 14 days of discontinuing treatment. Treatment w/ in 14 days of discontinuing treatment w/ an MAOI. Starting treatment in patients being treated w/ reversible MAOIs (eg, linezolid, IV methylene blue). Known hypersensitivity to bupropion or other ingredients of this medication.

WARNINGS/PRECAUTIONS
Dose-related risk of seizures; do not exceed 300mg/day, and titrate gradually. D/C and do not restart if seizure occurs. May result in elevated BP and HTN. May precipitate a manic, mixed, or hypomanic episode; risk appears to be increased in patients with bipolar disorder or who have risk factors for bipolar disorder. Not approved for use in treating bipolar depression. D/C if an allergic or anaphylactoid/anaphylactic reaction occurs. Arthralgia, myalgia, fever with rash, and other serum sickness-like symptoms suggestive of delayed hypersensitivity reported. False (+) urine immunoassay screening tests for amphetamines reported. Caution with renal/hepatic impairment and in the elderly.

ADVERSE REACTIONS
Neuropsychiatric reactions, insomnia, rhinitis, dry mouth, dizziness, nausea, disturbed concentration, nervousness, constipation, anxiety, dream abnormality, rash, diarrhea, myalgia, anorexia.

DRUG INTERACTIONS
See Contraindications. CYP2B6 inhibitors (eg, ticlopidine, clopidogrel) may increase bupropion exposure but decrease hydroxybupropion exposure; may need to adjust bupropion dose. CYP2B6 inducers (eg, ritonavir, lopinavir, efavirenz) may decrease exposure; may need to increase bupropion dose but not to exceed max dose. Carbamazepine, phenytoin, and phenobarbital may induce metabolism and decrease exposure; may be necessary to increase dose of bupropion, but max recommended dose should not be exceeded if used concomitantly with a CYP inducer. May increase exposure of CYP2D6 substrates (eg, venlafaxine, haloperidol, metoprolol); may need to decrease dose of CYP2D6 substrate, particularly for drugs with a narrow therapeutic index. May reduce efficacy of drugs that require metabolic activation by CYP2D6 to be effective (eg, tamoxifen); may require increased doses of the drug. Extreme caution with other drugs that lower seizure threshold (eg, antipsychotics, theophylline, systemic corticosteroids); use low initial doses and increase the dose gradually. Increased risk of seizure with illicit drugs (eg, cocaine), abuse or misuse of prescription drugs (eg, CNS stimulants), oral hypoglycemic drugs, insulin, anorectic drugs, excessive use of alcohol, benzodiazepines, sedative/hypnotics, and opiates. CNS toxicity reported when coadministered with levodopa or amantadine; use with caution. Minimize or avoid alcohol. Increased risk of HTN with MAOIs or other drugs that increase dopaminergic or noradrenergic activity. Monitor for HTN with nicotine replacement therapy. Altered PT and/or INR, infrequently associated with hemorrhagic or thrombotic complication, reported with warfarin. Physiological changes resulting from smoking cessation, with or without bupropion, may alter the pharmacokinetics or pharmacodynamics of certain drugs (eg, theophylline, warfarin, insulin) for which dosage adjustment may be necessary.

PREGNANCY AND LACTATION
Category C, caution in nursing.

MECHANISM OF ACTION
Aminoketone; has not been established. Presumed that action is related to noradrenergic and/or dopaminergic mechanisms. Weak inhibitor of the neuronal reuptake of norepinephrine and dopamine.

PHARMACOKINETICS
Absorption: T_{max}=3 hrs. **Distribution:** Plasma protein binding (84%); found in breast milk. **Metabolism:** Liver (extensive); hydroxylation, hydroxybupropion (active metabolite) (CYP2B6). Reduction of carbonyl group, threohydrobupropion, and erythrohydrobupropion (active metabolites). **Elimination:** Urine (87%) and feces (10%), (0.5% unchanged); $T_{1/2}$=21 hrs (bupropion), 20 hrs (hydroxybupropion), 33 hrs (erythrohydrobupropion), 37 hrs (threohydrobupropion).

PATIENT CONSIDERATIONS
Assessment: Assess for bipolar disorder, hepatic/renal dysfunction, seizure disorder or conditions that may increase the risk of seizure, hypersensitivity to the drug, any other conditions where treatment is contraindicated or cautioned, pregnancy/nursing status, and possible drug interactions. Assess BP.

Monitoring: Monitor for seizures, suicidality, activation of mania or hypomania, neuropsychiatric reactions, anaphylactoid/anaphylactic reactions, delayed hypersensitivity, and other adverse reactions. Monitor hepatic/renal function and BP.

Counseling: Inform about benefits/risks of therapy. Inform that quitting smoking may be associated with nicotine withdrawal symptoms or exacerbation of preexisting psychiatric illness. Advise to notify physician immediately if agitation, hostility, depressed mood, changes in thinking or behavior, or suicidal ideation/behavior occurs. Educate on the symptoms of hypersensitivity and to d/c if a severe allergic reaction occurs. Instruct to d/c and not restart if a seizure occurs while on therapy. Inform that excessive use or abrupt discontinuation of alcohol or sedatives may alter the seizure threshold; advise to minimize or avoid alcohol use. Inform that therapy may impair mental/physical abilities; advise to use caution while operating hazardous machinery/driving. Counsel to notify physician if taking/planning to take any prescription or OTC medications. Advise to notify physician if pregnant, intending to become pregnant, or if nursing. If taking >150mg/day, instruct to take in 2 doses at least 8 hrs apart, to minimize the risk of seizures. Instruct on what to do if a dose is missed. Inform that tab may have an odor.

BUSPIRONE — buspirone hydrochloride   Rx

Class: Atypical anxiolytic

OTHER BRAND NAMES
Buspar (Discontinued)

ADULT DOSAGE	PEDIATRIC DOSAGE
Anxiety Disorders	Pediatric use may not have been established
Management of Disorders or Short-Term Relief of Symptoms:	
Initial: 7.5mg bid	
Titrate: May increase by 5mg/day at intervals of 2-3 days, prn	
Usual: 20-30mg/day in divided doses	
Max: 60mg/day	
Periodically reassess usefulness of drug if used for extended periods	

DOSING CONSIDERATIONS
Renal Impairment
Severe: Not recommended

Hepatic Impairment
Severe: Not recommended

ADMINISTRATION
Oral route

Take in a consistent manner w/ regard to the timing of dosing; either always w/ or always w/o food.

STORAGE
(5mg, 10mg, 15mg, 30mg) 20-25°C (68-77°F). (7.5mg) 25°C (77°F); excursions permitted between 15-30°C (59-86°F).

HOW SUPPLIED
Tab: 5mg*, 7.5mg*, 10mg*, 15mg*, 30mg* *scored

CONTRAINDICATIONS
Hypersensitivity to buspirone HCl.

WARNINGS/PRECAUTIONS
May impair mental/physical abilities. Does not exhibit cross-tolerance with benzodiazepines and other common sedatives/hypnotics; before starting therapy, withdraw gradually from prior treatment, especially in patients using a CNS depressant chronically. May cause acute and chronic changes in dopamine-mediated neurological function; syndrome of restlessness, appearing shortly after initiation, reported. May interfere with urinary metanephrine/catecholamine assay; d/c therapy for at least 48 hrs prior to undergoing urine collection for catecholamines. Not recommended with severe hepatic/renal impairment.

ADVERSE REACTIONS
Dizziness, nausea, headache, nervousness, lightheadedness, excitement, drowsiness, fatigue, insomnia, dry mouth.

DRUG INTERACTIONS
See Dosage. Elevated BP reported with MAOI; avoid concomitant use. Avoid with alcohol. Dizziness, headache, nausea, and increased nordiazepam reported with diazepam. May increase serum concentrations of haloperidol. ALT elevations reported with trazodone. Caution with CNS-active drugs. CYP3A4 inhibitors (eg, diltiazem, ketoconazole, ritonavir) may increase concentrations; may require dose adjustment. CYP3A4 inducers (eg, dexamethasone, phenytoin, rifampin), including potent inducers, may decrease concentrations; may require dose adjustment of buspirone. Avoid with large amounts of grapefruit juice. Nefazodone may decrease concentrations of metabolite 1-pyrimidinylpiperazine (1-PP). May increase levels of nefazodone. Cimetidine may increase C_{max} and T_{max}. Prolonged PT reported with warfarin. May displace less firmly bound drugs like digoxin.

PREGNANCY AND LACTATION
Category B, not for use in nursing.

MECHANISM OF ACTION

Atypical anxiolytic; has not been established. Has a high affinity to 5-HT$_{1A}$ receptors and moderate affinity for brain D$_2$-dopamine receptors; may have indirect effects on other neurotransmitter systems.

PHARMACOKINETICS

Absorption: Rapid. (20mg, single dose) C$_{max}$=1-6ng/mL; T$_{max}$=40-90 min.
Distribution: Plasma protein binding (86%). **Metabolism:** Liver (extensive 1st-pass), primarily by oxidation via CYP3A4, and by hydroxylation; 1-PP (active metabolite). **Elimination:** Urine (29-63%), feces (18-38%); (10-40mg, single dose) T$_{1/2}$=2-3 hrs.

PATIENT CONSIDERATIONS

Assessment: Assess for hypersensitivity to drug, hepatic/renal impairment, pregnancy/nursing status, and possible drug interactions.

Monitoring: Monitor for CNS effects, syndrome of restlessness, and other adverse reactions. Periodically reassess usefulness of drug if used for extended periods.

Counseling: Instruct to inform physician about any medications, prescription or nonprescription, alcohol, or drugs patient is taking or planning to take, and if patient is pregnant/breastfeeding, becomes pregnant, or is planning to become pregnant. Advise not to drive a car or operate potentially dangerous machinery until effects have been determined. Instruct to avoid drinking large amounts of grapefruit juice.

BUSULFEX — busulfan   Rx

Class: Alkylating agent

> Causes severe and prolonged myelosuppression at the recommended dosage. Hematopoietic progenitor cell transplantation is required to prevent potentially fatal complications of the prolonged myelosuppression.

ADULT DOSAGE	PEDIATRIC DOSAGE
Chronic Myeloid Leukemia	Pediatric use may not have been established
In Combination w/ Cyclophosphamide as a Conditioning Regimen Prior to Allogeneic Hematopoietic Progenitor Cell Transplantation:	
Initial:	
>12kg: 0.8mg/kg (ideal body weight [IBW] or actual body weight [whichever is lower]) q6h IV for 4 days for a total of 16 doses (Days -7, -6, -5, and -4)	
Obese/Severely Obese: Dose based on adjusted IBW; refer to PI for calculation	
Give 60mg/kg of cyclophosphamide IV as a 1-hr infusion on each of the 2 days beginning no sooner than 6 hrs following the 16th dose of treatment (Days -3 and -2)	
Premedication	
Administer anticonvulsants (eg, benzodiazepines, phenytoin, valproic acid, or levetiracetam) 12 hrs prior to treatment to 24 hrs after the last dose of treatment.	
Administer antiemetics prior to 1st dose of treatment and continue on a fixed schedule throughout treatment.	

ADMINISTRATION

IV route

Use an administration set w/ minimal residual hold-up volume (2-5mL) for product administration.
Use gloves when preparing; if sol contacts the skin/mucosa, wash thoroughly w/ water.
Dilute w/ 0.9% NaCl or D5W; final concentration should be approx 0.5mg/mL.
Do not put into an IV bag or large-volume syringe that does not contain NaCl or D5W.
Always add busulfan to the diluent, not the diluent to the busulfan; mix thoroughly by inverting several times.
Use infusion pumps to administer diluted sol.
Set flow rate of the pump to deliver the entire prescribed dose over 2 hrs; rapid infusion not tested/not recommended.
Prior to and following each infusion, flush indwelling catheter line w/ approx 5mL of NaCl or D5W.
Do not infuse concomitantly w/ another IV sol of unknown compatibility.

STORAGE

Unopened: 2-8°C (36-46°F). **Diluted in 0.9% NaCl or D5W:** 25°C (77°F) for up to 8 hrs; complete the infusion w/in that time. **Diluted in 0.9% NaCl:** 2-8°C (36-46°F) for up to 12 hrs; complete the infusion w/in that time.

HOW SUPPLIED

Inj: 6mg/mL [10mL]

CONTRAINDICATIONS

History of hypersensitivity to any of its components.

WARNINGS/PRECAUTIONS

Use antibiotic therapy and platelet and RBC support when medically indicated. Seizures reported; caution in patients w/ history of a seizure disorder or head trauma. May be associated w/ increased risk of developing hepatic veno-occlusive disease; increased risk in patients who have received prior radiation therapy, ≥3 cycles of chemotherapy, or a prior progenitor cell transplant. Can cause fetal harm. Cardiac tamponade reported in pediatric patients w/ thalassemia; monitor for signs/symptoms and promptly evaluate/treat if suspected. Bronchopulmonary dysplasia w/ pulmonary fibrosis may occur following chronic therapy. May cause cellular dysplasia in many organs.

ADVERSE REACTIONS

N/V, stomatitis (mucositis), anorexia, insomnia, diarrhea, fever, hypomagnesemia, anxiety, abdominal pain, headache, hyperglycemia, hypokalemia, rash, asthenia, chills.

DRUG INTERACTIONS

Itraconazole decreases clearance. Phenytoin increases clearance. Use of acetaminophen prior to (<72 hrs) or concurrent w/ therapy may result in reduced busulfan clearance. Caution w/ other potentially epileptogenic drugs.

PREGNANCY AND LACTATION

Pregnancy: Can cause fetal harm based on animal data.
Lactation: It is not known if busulfan is present in human milk; d/c breastfeeding during treatment.
Reproductive Potential: Females of reproductive potential and males w/ female partners of reproductive potential should use effective contraception during and after treatment. Ovarian suppression and amenorrhea reported in premenopausal women. Sterility, azoospermia, and testicular atrophy reported in males.

MECHANISM OF ACTION

Alkylating agent; hydrolyzes to release the methanesulfonate groups, producing reactive carbonium ions that can alkylate DNA.

PHARMACOKINETICS

Absorption: C$_{max}$=1222ng/mL; AUC=1167μM•min. **Distribution:** Plasma protein binding (32.4%). **Metabolism:** Conjugation w/ glutathione; conjugate undergoes extensive oxidative metabolism in liver. **Elimination:** Urine (30%).

PATIENT CONSIDERATIONS

Assessment: Assess for history of hypersensitivity to any of the components, history of seizure disorder or head trauma, risk of developing hepatic veno-occlusive disease, pregnancy/nursing status, and possible drug interactions.

Monitoring: Monitor for seizures, hepatic veno-occlusive disease, cardiac tamponade, bronchopulmonary/cellular dysplasia, and other adverse reactions. Monitor CBCs, including WBC differentials, and quantitative platelet counts daily during treatment and until engraftment is demonstrated. Monitor serum transaminases, alkaline phosphatase, and bilirubin daily through bone marrow transplant Day +28 to detect hepatotoxicity.

Counseling: Inform of the possibility of developing low blood cell counts and the need for hematopoietic progenitor cell infusion; instruct to immediately report to physician if fever develops. Inform of the risks associated w/ therapy (eg, veno-occlusive liver disease) as well as the plan for regular blood monitoring during therapy. Advise females of reproductive potential of the potential risk to a fetus and to inform physician w/ a known or suspected pregnancy. Advise females and males of reproductive potential to use effective contraception during and after treatment. Instruct to d/c breastfeeding during treatment. Advise females and males of reproductive potential that drug may cause temporary or permanent infertility.

BUTORPHANOL INJECTION — butorphanol tartrate   Rx

Class: Partial opioid agonist

OTHER BRAND NAMES

Stadol (Discontinued)

ADULT DOSAGE	PEDIATRIC DOSAGE
Pain	Pediatric use may not have been established
IV:	
Usual: 1mg q3-4h prn	
Range: 0.5-2mg q3-4h	
IM:	
Usual: 2mg q3-4h prn	
Range: 1-4mg q3-4h	
Max: 4mg/dose	
Preoperative/Preanesthetic Medication	
Usual: 2mg IM 60-90 min before surgery	
Anesthesia	
Supplement to Balanced Anesthesia:	
Usual: 2mg IV shortly before induction and/or 0.5-1mg IV in increments during anesthesia; increment may be higher, up to 0.06mg/kg (4mg/70kg), depending on previous sedative, analgesic, and hypnotic drugs administered	

Labor Pain
Initial: 1-2mg IV/IM in patients at full term in early labor; may repeat after 4 hrs
Use alternative analgesia for pain associated w/ delivery or if delivery is expected to occur w/in 4 hrs

DOSING CONSIDERATIONS
Renal Impairment
Initial: 1/2 the recommended adult dose (0.5mg IV and 1mg IM)
Repeat doses will generally be ≥6 hrs apart
Hepatic Impairment
Initial: 1/2 the recommended adult dose (0.5mg IV and 1mg IM)
Repeat doses should be ≥6 hrs apart
Elderly
Initial: 1/2 the recommended adult dose (0.5mg IV and 1mg IM)
Repeat doses will generally be ≥6 hrs apart

ADMINISTRATION
IM/IV route
Ordinary care should be taken to avoid aerosol generation while preparing for syringe use
Rinse w/ cool water following skin contact

STORAGE
20-25°C (68-77°F). Protect from light.

HOW SUPPLIED
Inj: 1mg/mL [1mL], 2mg/mL [1mL]

CONTRAINDICATIONS
Hypersensitivity to butorphanol tartrate or the preservative benzethonium chloride (multiple dose vial).

WARNINGS/PRECAUTIONS
Not recommended for use in narcotic-dependent patients; may precipitate withdrawal symptoms (eg, anxiety, agitation, mood changes). Caution in patients who have recently received repeated doses of narcotic analgesic medication. Episodes of abuse reported. Prolonged, continuous use of therapy may result in physical dependence or tolerance; abrupt discontinuation may result in withdrawal symptoms. May obscure the interpretation of the clinical course of patients with head injuries; use with caution. May produce respiratory depression, especially in patients with CNS diseases or respiratory impairment. May increase the work of the heart, especially the pulmonary circuit; caution in patients with acute myocardial infarction, ventricular dysfunction, or coronary insufficiency. Severe HTN reported rarely; d/c if this occurs. May impair mental/physical abilities. Caution with hepatic/renal disease, history of drug abuse, in labor, and in elderly.

ADVERSE REACTIONS
Somnolence, dizziness, N/V.

DRUG INTERACTIONS
Increased CNS depressant effects with drugs that affect the CNS (eg, alcohol, barbiturates, tranquilizers, antihistamines); use the smallest effective dose when used concurrently with such drugs and reduce dosing frequency as much as possible when administered concomitantly with drugs that potentiate the action of opioids. Do not consume alcohol during therapy. Potential for interaction with medications that affect hepatic metabolism of drugs (eg, erythromycin, theophylline); smaller initial dose and longer intervals between doses may be needed. May produce respiratory depression with other CNS active agents.

PREGNANCY AND LACTATION
Category C, safety not known in nursing.

MECHANISM OF ACTION
Opioid agonist-antagonist analgesic; has low intrinsic activity at receptors of μ-opioid type (morphine-like). Also an agonist at kappa-opioid receptors.

PHARMACOKINETICS
Absorption: (IM) Rapid. T_{max}=20-40 min. (IV) AUC=7.24ng•hr/mL (young), 8.71ng•hr/mL (elderly). **Distribution:** V_d=305-901L; plasma protein binding (80%); crosses placenta; found in breast milk. **Metabolism:** Liver (extensive); hydroxybutorphanol (major metabolite). **Elimination:** Urine (70-80%; 5%, unchanged; 49% as hydroxybutorphanol, feces (15%); $T_{1/2}$=4.56 hrs (IV, young), 5.61 hrs (IV, elderly), 18 hrs (hydroxybutorphanol).

PATIENT CONSIDERATIONS
Assessment: Assess for hypersensitivity to the drug, narcotic dependence, head injury, CNS diseases, respiratory/hepatic/renal impairment, or any other conditions where treatment is contraindicated or cautioned, pregnancy/nursing status, and possible drug interactions.

Monitoring: Monitor for signs/symptoms of abuse/dependence/tolerance, respiratory depression, HTN, withdrawal symptoms, and other adverse reactions.

Counseling: Inform that therapy may impair mental/physical abilities required for the performance of potentially dangerous tasks; instruct not to drive or operate dangerous machinery for at least 1 hr and until effects of drug are no longer present. Advise not to consume alcohol while on therapy. Inform that therapy has potential for abuse and should be handled accordingly.

BUTRANS — buprenorphine   CIII
Class: Partial opioid agonist

> Exposes users to risks of addiction, abuse, and misuse, which can lead to overdose and death; assess each patient's risk prior to prescribing, and monitor regularly for development of these behaviors/conditions. Serious, life-threatening, or fatal respiratory depression may occur; monitor during initiation or following a dose increase. Chewing, swallowing, snorting, or injecting buprenorphine extracted from the transdermal system will result in uncontrolled delivery and pose risk of overdose and death. Accidental exposure, especially in children, can result in a fatal overdose. Prolonged use during pregnancy can result in neonatal opioid withdrawal syndrome; advise pregnant women of the risk and ensure availability of appropriate treatment.

ADULT DOSAGE
Severe Pain (Daily, Around-the-Clock Management)
Long-Term Opioid Treatment for Which Alternative Treatment Options are Inadequate:
First Opioid Analgesic:
Initial: 5mcg/hr
Titrate: Individualize dose
Minimum Titration Interval: 72 hrs; may adjust dose every 3 days
Max: 20mcg/hr

Dose adjustments may be made in 5mcg/hr, 7.5mcg/hr, or 10mcg/hr increments by using no more than 2 patches of the 5mcg/hr, 7.5mcg/hr, or 10mcg/hr systems

Conversions
From Other Opioids to Buprenorphine Transdermal System: D/C all other around-the-clock opioid drugs when therapy is initiated

Prior Total Daily Dose of Opioid <30mg of Oral Morphine Equivalents/Day:
Initiate treatment w/ 5mcg/hr at the next dosing interval

Prior Total Daily Dose of Opioid Between 30mg to 80mg of Oral Morphine Equivalents/Day:
Taper the patient's current around-the-clock opioids for up to 7 days to no more than 30mg of morphine or equivalent/day before beginning treatment
Then initiate treatment w/ 10mcg/hr at the next dosing interval
Patients may use short-acting analgesics prn until efficacy is attained

Prior Total Daily Dose of Opioid >80mg of Oral Morphine Equivalents/Day:
20mcg/hr may not provide adequate analgesia for patients requiring >80mg/day oral morphine equivalents
Consider the use of an alternate analgesic

PEDIATRIC DOSAGE
Pediatric use may not have been established

DOSING CONSIDERATIONS
Hepatic Impairment
Severe: Consider use of an alternate analgesic that may permit more flexibility w/ dosing
Discontinuation
Use gradual downward titration every 7 days
Consider introduction of an appropriate immediate-release opioid medication
ADMINISTRATION
Transdermal route
Each patch is intended to be worn for 7 days.
Do not cut patch.
Apply immediately after removal from individually sealed pouch.
Apply to intact skin on upper outer arm, upper chest, upper back, or side of chest; rotate application site w/ a minimum of 21 days before reapplying to the same skin site.
For use of 2 patches, remove current patch and apply the 2 new patches at the same time, adjacent to one another at a different application site.
Refer to PI for further administration and disposal instructions.
STORAGE
25°C (77°F); excursions permitted between 15-30°C (59-86°F).
HOW SUPPLIED
Patch: 5mcg/hr, 7.5mcg/hr, 10mcg/hr, 15mcg/hr, 20mcg/hr

CONTRAINDICATIONS

Significant respiratory depression, acute or severe bronchial asthma in an unmonitored setting or in the absence of resuscitative equipment, known or suspected paralytic ileus. Hypersensitivity (eg, anaphylaxis) to buprenorphine.

WARNINGS/PRECAUTIONS

Reserve use in patients for whom alternative treatment options are ineffective, not tolerated, or would be otherwise inadequate to provide sufficient management of pain. Should only be prescribed by healthcare professionals who are knowledgeable in the use of potent opioids for management of chronic pain. Doses of 7.5, 10, 15, and 20mcg/hr are for opioid-experienced patients only. Life-threatening respiratory depression is more likely to occur in elderly, cachectic, or debilitated patients. Consider alternative nonopioid analgesics in patients with significant chronic obstructive pulmonary disease or cor pulmonale, and in patients who have a substantially decreased respiratory reserve, hypoxia, hypercapnia, or preexisting respiratory depression. QTc interval prolongation observed at dose of 40mcg/hr; caution with hypokalemia or clinically unstable cardiac disease. Avoid use with history/immediate family history of long QT syndrome. May cause severe hypotension, orthostatic hypotension, and syncope; increased risk in patients whose ability to maintain BP has already been compromised by a reduced blood volume or concurrent administration of certain CNS depressants. Monitor patients who may be susceptible to intracranial effects of carbon dioxide retention for signs of sedation and respiratory depression when initiating therapy. Therapy may obscure clinical course in patients with head injury. Avoid with impaired consciousness or coma. Obtain baseline liver enzyme levels and monitor periodically during treatment in patients at increased risk of hepatotoxicity (eg, history of excessive alcohol intake, IV drug abuse). Application-site skin reactions with signs of marked inflammation reported; d/c if severe application-site reactions develop. Cases of acute and chronic hypersensitivity, bronchospasm, angioneurotic edema, and anaphylactic shock reported. Potential for temperature-dependent increases in drug release, resulting in possible overdose and death; avoid exposure of application site and surrounding area to direct external heat sources. If fever or increased core body temperature due to strenuous exertion develops, monitor for side effects and adjust dose if signs of respiratory/CNS depression occur. Avoid with GI obstruction. May cause spasm of sphincter of Oddi and increase in serum amylase; monitor patients with biliary tract disease. May aggravate convulsions and induce/aggravate seizures. May impair mental/physical abilities. Not approved for management of addictive disorders. Not for use during and immediately prior to labor. Caution in elderly.

ADVERSE REACTIONS

Respiratory depression, N/V, dizziness, headache, application-site pruritus/irritation/erythema/rash, constipation, somnolence, dry mouth, fatigue, hyperhidrosis, peripheral edema.

DRUG INTERACTIONS

Respiratory depression, hypotension, profound sedation, or coma may occur with alcohol and other CNS depressants (eg, sedatives, anxiolytics, neuroleptics); if coadministration is required, consider dose reduction of one or both agents. Monitor use in elderly, cachectic, and debilitated patients when coadministered with other drugs that depress respiration. Monitor closely with benzodiazepines. CYP3A4 inhibitors may increase levels and prolong opioid effects; these effects could be more pronounced with concomitant use of CYP2D6 and 3A4 inhibitors; if coadministration is necessary, monitor for respiratory depression and sedation at frequent intervals and consider dose adjustments. CYP3A4 inducers may decrease levels and cause lack of efficacy or development of abstinence syndrome; if coadministration or discontinuation of a CYP3A4 inducer is necessary, monitor for signs of opioid withdrawal and consider dose adjustments. May enhance neuromuscular blocking action of skeletal muscle relaxants and increase respiratory depression. Avoid with Class IA antiarrhythmics (eg, quinidine, procainamide, disopyramide) or Class III antiarrhythmics (eg, sotalol, amiodarone, dofetilide). Anticholinergics or other drugs with anticholinergic activity may increase risk of urinary retention and/or severe constipation and lead to paralytic ileus.

PREGNANCY AND LACTATION

Category C, not for use in nursing.

MECHANISM OF ACTION

Opioid analgesic; partial agonist at μ-opioid and ORL-1 (nociceptin) receptors, antagonist at kappa-opioid receptors, and agonist at delta-opioid receptors. Contributions of these actions to its analgesic profile are unclear.

PHARMACOKINETICS

Absorption: Absolute bioavailability (15%). Administration of variable doses resulted in different parameters. **Distribution:** Plasma protein binding (96%); found in breast milk; crosses placenta. (IV) V_d=430L. **Metabolism:** Liver; N-dealkylation via CYP3A4 to norbuprenorphine and glucuronidation by UGT-isoenzymes (mainly UGT1A1 and 2B7) to buprenorphine 3β-O-glucuronide; norbuprenorphine (active, major metabolite). **Elimination:** (2mcg/kg IM) Urine (27%), feces (70%). $T_{1/2}$=26 hrs.

PATIENT CONSIDERATIONS

Assessment: Assess for abuse/addiction risk, pain intensity, prior opioid therapy, opioid tolerance, respiratory depression, drug hypersensitivity, pregnancy/nursing status, possible drug interactions, or any other conditions where treatment is contraindicated or cautioned. Obtain baseline liver enzyme levels in patients at increased risk of hepatotoxicity.

Monitoring: Monitor for respiratory depression (especially within first 24-72 hrs of initiation), hypotension, application-site skin reactions, seizures/convulsions, and other adverse reactions. Monitor BP and serum amylase levels. Regularly monitor for signs of misuse, abuse, and addiction. Periodically reassess the continued need for therapy. Monitor liver enzyme levels periodically in patients at increased risk of hepatotoxicity.

Counseling: Inform that use of drug can result in addiction, abuse, and misuse; instruct not to share with others and to take steps to protect from theft or misuse. Inform patients about risk of respiratory depression. Advise to store securely and dispose unused patch by folding the patch in 1/2 and flushing down the toilet. Inform women of reproductive potential that prolonged use during pregnancy may result in neonatal opioid withdrawal syndrome and instruct to inform physician if pregnant or planning to become pregnant. Inform that potentially serious additive effects may occur when used with alcohol or CNS depressants, and not to use such drugs unless supervised by healthcare provider. Instruct about proper application, removal, and disposal instructions. Inform that drug may cause orthostatic hypotension, syncope, impair the ability to perform potentially hazardous activities; advise to not perform such tasks until patients know how they will react to medication. Advise of potential for severe constipation, including management instructions. Advise how to recognize anaphylaxis and when to seek medical attention.

BYDUREON — exenatide　　　　Rx

Class: Glucagon-like peptide-1 (GLP-1) receptor agonist

> Causes an increased incidence in thyroid C-cell tumors at clinically relevant exposures in animal studies. It is unknown whether drug causes thyroid C-cell tumors (eg, medullary thyroid carcinoma [MTC]) in humans. Contraindicated in patients w/ a personal/family history of MTC and w/ multiple endocrine neoplasia syndrome type 2 (MEN 2). Counsel patients on the potential risk for MTC w/ exenatide use and inform them of symptoms of thyroid tumors (eg, mass in the neck, dysphagia, dyspnea, persistent hoarseness). Routine monitoring of serum calcitonin or using thyroid ultrasound is of uncertain value for detection of MTC in patients treated w/ exenatide.

ADULT DOSAGE	PEDIATRIC DOSAGE
Type 2 Diabetes Mellitus 2mg/dose SQ once every 7 days, at any time of day **Changing Weekly Dosing Schedule:** May change the day of weekly administration if necessary as long as the last dose was given ≥3 days before **Conversions** **Changing from Byetta to Bydureon:** Prior treatment w/ Byetta is not required when initiating Bydureon therapy D/C Byetta if the decision is made to start Bydureon in a patient already taking Byetta Patients changing from Byetta to Bydureon may experience transient (approx 2 weeks) elevations in blood glucose concentrations **Missed Dose** If a dose is missed, administer it as soon as noticed, provided the next regularly scheduled dose is due at least 3 days later. Thereafter, may resume usual dosing schedule of once every 7 days (weekly) If a dose is missed and the next regularly scheduled dose is due 1 or 2 days later, do not administer the missed dose and instead resume therapy w/ the next regularly scheduled dose	Pediatric use may not have been established

---

DOSING CONSIDERATIONS

Renal Impairment

Moderate (CrCl 30-50mL/min): Use w/ caution
Severe (CrCl <30mL/min) or ESRD: Not recommended
Patients w/ Renal Transplantation: Use w/ caution

Elderly

Caution when initiating treatment

ADMINISTRATION

SQ route

Administer at any time of day, w/ or w/o meals.
Inject in the abdomen, thigh, or upper arm region; use a different inj site each week when injecting in the same region.
Do not administer IV or IM.
Intended for patient self-administration.
Administer immediately after powder is suspended in diluent.
Refer to PI for further administration instructions.

STORAGE

2-8°C (36-46°F).May store at room temperature not exceeding 25°C (77°F) for ≤4 weeks, if needed. Do not freeze; do not use if product has been frozen. Protect from light.

HOW SUPPLIED

Inj, Extended-Release: 2mg [vial, pen]

CONTRAINDICATIONS
MEN 2, personal/family history of MTC, prior serious hypersensitivity reaction to exenatide or to any of its components.

WARNINGS/PRECAUTIONS
Not recommended as 1st-line therapy for patients who have inadequate glycemic control on diet and exercise. Not a substitute for insulin; do not use in type 1 DM or for treatment of diabetic ketoacidosis. Not studied and cannot be recommended w/ insulin. Acute pancreatitis, including fatal and nonfatal hemorrhagic or necrotizing pancreatitis, reported; d/c promptly if suspected, and do not restart therapy if confirmed. Consider other antidiabetic therapies in patients w/ history of pancreatitis. Patients w/ elevated calcitonin levels and those w/ thyroid nodules noted on physical examination or neck imaging should be further evaluated. Altered renal function, including increased SrCr, renal impairment, worsened chronic renal failure, and acute renal failure reported. Not recommended w/ severe GI disease. May develop antibodies; consider alternative antidiabetic therapy if there is worsening glycemic control or failure to achieve targeted glycemic control. Serious hypersensitivity reactions reported; d/c if a hypersensitivity reaction occurs. Serious inj-site reactions (eg, abscess, cellulitis, necrosis), w/ or w/o subcutaneous nodules reported; isolated cases required surgical intervention.

ADVERSE REACTIONS
Constipation, diarrhea, dyspepsia, headache, N/V, inj-site nodule, fatigue, decreased appetite, inj-site pruritus, viral gastroenteritis, GERD, inj-site erythema, inj-site hematoma.

DRUG INTERACTIONS
Increased risk of hypoglycemia w/ insulin secretagogues (eg, sulfonylureas) or insulin; may require a lower dose of the secretagogue or insulin. May reduce the rate of absorption of orally administered drugs; caution w/ oral medications. May increase INR w/ warfarin, sometimes associated w/ bleeding; monitor INR more frequently after initiation of exenatide. Should not be used w/ other drugs containing the same active ingredient (eg, Byetta).

PREGNANCY AND LACTATION
Pregnancy: Category C. A Pregnancy Registry has been implemented; physicians are encouraged to register patients.
Lactation: Not for use in nursing.

MECHANISM OF ACTION
GLP-1 receptor agonist; enhances glucose-dependent insulin secretion by the pancreatic β-cell, suppresses inappropriately elevated glucagon secretion, and slows gastric emptying.

PHARMACOKINETICS
Absorption: Gradual release over 6-7 weeks. **Distribution:** V_d=28.3L. **Elimination:** Kidney.

PATIENT CONSIDERATIONS
Assessment: Assess for previous hypersensitivity reactions, MEN 2, personal/family history of MTC, history of pancreatitis, type of DM, diabetic ketoacidosis, renal impairment, severe GI disease, pregnancy/nursing status, and possible drug interactions. Assess glucose and HbA1c levels.

Monitoring: Monitor for signs/symptoms of thyroid tumor, pancreatitis, elevated serum calcitonin levels, hypoglycemia, GI events, immunogenicity, hypersensitivity reactions, inj-site reactions, and other adverse reactions. Monitor renal function, blood glucose levels, and HbA1c levels. Monitor INR more frequently after initiation of therapy in patients receiving warfarin.

Counseling: Counsel on potential risks/benefits of therapy and alternative modes of therapy. Inform of importance of adhering to dietary instructions, regular physical activity, periodic blood glucose monitoring and HbA1c testing, recognition/management of hypo/hyperglycemia, and assessment for diabetes complications. Advise to report symptoms of thyroid tumors (eg, lump in the neck, hoarseness, dysphagia, dyspnea) to physician. Inform of potential risk for pancreatitis, worsening of renal function, and serious hypersensitivity reactions. Instruct to d/c therapy promptly and contact physician if persistent severe abdominal pain and/or symptoms of a hypersensitivity reaction occur. Inform that serious inj-site reactions w/ or w/o subcutaneous nodules may occur; advise to seek medical advice if symptomatic nodules occur, or for any signs/symptoms of abscess, cellulitis, or necrosis. Instruct to never share a prefilled syringe/pen w/ another person, even if the needle is changed. Inform that therapy may result in nausea, particularly upon initiation of therapy. Advise that if a dose is missed, administer as soon as noticed, provided that the next regularly scheduled dose is due at least 3 days later. Instruct to then resume the usual dosing schedule thereafter. Inform that if a dose is missed and the next regularly scheduled dose is due in 1 or 2 days, to not administer the missed dose and instead resume w/ the next regularly scheduled dose. Advise to inform physician if pregnant/intending to become pregnant. Inform about the importance of proper storage, inj technique, and dosing.

BYETTA — exenatide   Rx
Class: Glucagon-like peptide-1 (GLP-1) receptor agonist

ADULT DOSAGE
Type 2 Diabetes Mellitus

Initial: 5mcg SQ bid, at any time w/in 60 min before am and pm meals (or before the 2 main meals of the day, approx 6 hrs or more apart).
Titrate: May increase to 10mcg bid after 1 month based on response

PEDIATRIC DOSAGE
Pediatric use may not have been established

DOSING CONSIDERATIONS
Renal Impairment
Moderate (CrCl 30-50mL/min): Caution when initiating or escalating doses from 5mcg to 10mcg
Severe (CrCl <30mL/min) or ESRD: Not recommended
Renal Transplantation: Use w/ caution

ADMINISTRATION
SQ route

Inject into thigh, abdomen, or upper arm.
Do not mix w/ insulin.
Do not transfer from the pen to a syringe or a vial.

STORAGE
Prior to 1st Use: 2-8°C (36-46°F). After 1st Use: <25°C (77°F). Do not freeze. Do not use if it has been frozen. Protect from light. Discard pen 30 days after 1st use.

HOW SUPPLIED
Inj: 5mcg/dose, 10mcg/dose [60 doses]

CONTRAINDICATIONS
Prior serious hypersensitivity reaction to exenatide or to any of its components.

WARNINGS/PRECAUTIONS
Not a substitute for insulin; do not use in type 1 DM or for the treatment of diabetic ketoacidosis. Not studied and cannot be recommended w/ prandial insulin. Evaluate dose of insulin if used in combination; consider dose reduction in patients at risk of hypoglycemia. Do not share pens between patients, even if needle is changed; risk of transmission of blood-borne pathogens. Acute pancreatitis, including fatal and nonfatal hemorrhagic or necrotizing pancreatitis, reported; observe for signs/symptoms of pancreatitis after initiation of therapy and dose increases, d/c promptly if suspected, and do not restart therapy if confirmed. Consider other antidiabetic therapies in patients w/ history of pancreatitis. Altered renal function, including increased SrCr, renal impairment, worsened chronic renal failure, and acute renal failure, reported. Not recommended w/ severe GI disease. May develop antibodies; consider alternative antidiabetic therapy if there is worsening glycemic control or failure to achieve targeted glycemic control. Serious hypersensitivity reactions (eg, anaphylaxis, angioedema) reported; d/c if a hypersensitivity reaction occurs.

ADVERSE REACTIONS
Hypoglycemia, N/V, immunogenicity, dyspepsia, diarrhea, feeling jittery, dizziness, headache, constipation, asthenia, GERD, hyperhidrosis, abdominal distension, decreased appetite.

DRUG INTERACTIONS
Increased risk of hypoglycemia w/ a sulfonylurea or other glucose-independent insulin secretagogues (eg, meglitinides); may require a lower dose of the sulfonylurea. May reduce the extent and rate of absorption of orally administered drugs; caution w/ oral medications w/ narrow therapeutic index or that require rapid GI absorption. Oral medications that are dependent on threshold concentrations for efficacy (eg, contraceptives, antibiotics) should be taken at least 1 hr before inj. May increase INR w/ warfarin, sometimes associated w/ bleeding; monitor PT more frequently after initiation or alteration of therapy.

PREGNANCY AND LACTATION
Category C, not for use in nursing.

MECHANISM OF ACTION
Glucagon-like peptide-1 receptor agonist; enhances glucose-dependent insulin secretion by the pancreatic β-cell, suppresses inappropriately elevated glucagon secretion, and slows gastric emptying.

PHARMACOKINETICS
Absorption: C_{max}=211pg/mL (10mcg), AUC=1036pg•hr/mL (10mcg), T_{max}=2.1 hrs (median). **Distribution:** V_d=28.3L. **Elimination:** $T_{1/2}$=2.4 hrs.

PATIENT CONSIDERATIONS
Assessment: Assess for history of hypersensitivity to drug or any product components, type of DM, diabetic ketoacidosis, history of pancreatitis, renal impairment, severe GI disease, pregnancy/nursing status, and possible drug interactions.

Monitoring: Monitor for signs/symptoms of hypoglycemia, pancreatitis, GI events, immunogenicity, hypersensitivity reactions, and other adverse reactions. Monitor renal function, blood glucose levels, and HbA1c levels. Monitor PT more frequently after initiation or alteration of therapy in patients receiving warfarin.

Counseling: Counsel on the potential risks/benefits of therapy and alternative modes of therapy. Inform of importance of proper storage of drug, inj technique, timing of dosage and concomitant oral drugs, adherence to meal planning, regular physical activity, periodic blood glucose monitoring and HbA1c testing, recognition/management of hypo/hyperglycemia, and assessment for diabetes complications. Advise to never share inj pen w/ another person, even if needle is changed. Inform that pen needles are purchased separately and advise on proper needle selection and disposal. Inform that if a dose is missed, treatment regimen should be resumed as prescribed w/ the next scheduled dose. Instruct to inform physician if pregnant or intending to become pregnant. Advise that treatment may result in reduction in appetite, food intake, and/or body weight, and that there is no need to modify the dosing regimen due to such effects. Inform that nausea, particularly upon initiation of therapy, may occur. Instruct to contact a physician if signs/symptoms of acute pancreatitis (eg, severe abdominal pain), renal dysfunction, or hypersensitivity reactions develop.

BYSTOLIC — nebivolol   Rx

Class: Selective beta₁ blocker

ADULT DOSAGE	**PEDIATRIC DOSAGE**
Hypertension	Pediatric use may not have been established
Initial: 5mg qd	
Titrate: May increase at 2-week intervals	
Max: 40mg	

DOSING CONSIDERATIONS

Renal Impairment
Severe (CrCl <30mL/min):
Initial: 2.5mg qd; titrate up slowly if needed

Hepatic Impairment
Moderate:
Initial: 2.5mg qd; titrate up slowly if needed

ADMINISTRATION
Oral route
Take w/ or w/o food.

STORAGE
20-25°C (68-77°F).

HOW SUPPLIED
Tab: 2.5mg, 5mg, 10mg, 20mg

CONTRAINDICATIONS
Severe bradycardia, heart block >1st degree, cardiogenic shock, decompensated cardiac failure, sick sinus syndrome (unless permanent pacemaker in place), severe hepatic impairment (Child-Pugh >B), hypersensitivity to any component of this product.

WARNINGS/PRECAUTIONS
Severe exacerbation of angina, myocardial infarction, and ventricular arrhythmias reported in patients with coronary artery disease (CAD) following abrupt discontinuation; taper over 1-2 weeks when possible. Restart therapy promptly, at least temporarily, if angina worsens or acute coronary insufficiency develops. Caution patients without overt CAD against interruption or abrupt discontinuation of therapy. Avoid with bronchospastic disease. Treatment should generally be continued throughout perioperative period. If therapy is to be continued perioperatively, monitor closely when anesthetic agents that depress myocardial function (eg, ether, cyclopropane, trichloroethylene) are used. If therapy is withdrawn prior to major surgery, impaired ability of the heart to respond to reflex adrenergic stimuli may augment the risks of general anesthesia and surgical procedures; difficulty in restarting and maintaining heartbeat reported. May mask manifestations of hypoglycemia/hyperthyroidism, particularly tachycardia; abrupt withdrawal may be followed by exacerbation of the symptoms of hyperthyroidism or may precipitate a thyroid storm. May precipitate/aggravate symptoms of arterial insufficiency with peripheral vascular disease (PVD). Patients with history of severe anaphylactic reactions to variety of allergens may be more reactive to repeated accidental/diagnostic/therapeutic challenge; may be unresponsive to usual doses of epinephrine. Initiate an α-blocker prior to use of any β-blocker in patients with known/suspected pheochromocytoma.

ADVERSE REACTIONS
Headache, fatigue, dizziness, diarrhea, nausea.

DRUG INTERACTIONS
Avoid with other β-blockers. D/C for several days before the gradual tapering of clonidine. Caution with CYP2D6 inhibitors (eg, quinidine, propafenone, paroxetine, fluoxetine); may need to reduce dose of nebivolol. May produce excessive reduction of sympathetic activity with catecholamine-depleting drugs (eg, reserpine, guanethidine). May increase risk of bradycardia with digitalis glycosides. May exacerbate effects of myocardial depressants/inhibitors of atrioventricular conduction (eg, antiarrhythmics, certain Ca²⁺ antagonists). May potentiate hypoglycemic effect of insulin and oral hypoglycemics. Significant negative inotropic and chronotropic effects may occur with verapamil and diltiazem type; monitor ECG and BP.

PREGNANCY AND LACTATION
Category C, not for use in nursing.

MECHANISM OF ACTION
Selective β₁-blocker; has not been established. Possible factors include decreased HR and myocardial contractility, diminution of tonic sympathetic outflow to the periphery from cerebral vasomotor centers, suppression of renin activity, vasodilation, and decreased peripheral vascular resistance.

PHARMACOKINETICS
Absorption: T_{max}=1.5-4 hrs. **Distribution:** Plasma protein binding (98%, albumin). **Metabolism:** Glucuronidation, N-dealkylation, and oxidation via CYP2D6. **Elimination:** Urine (38%, extensive metabolizers [EM]), (67%, poor metabolizers [PM]); feces (44%, EM), (13%, PM); $T_{1/2}$=12 hrs (EM), 19 hrs (PM).

PATIENT CONSIDERATIONS
Assessment: Assess for CAD, bronchospastic disease, diabetes mellitus, hypoglycemia, hyperthyroidism, PVD, pheochromocytoma, hepatic/renal impairment, pregnancy/nursing status, any other conditions where treatment is contraindicated or cautioned, and possible drug interactions.

Monitoring: Monitor for precipitation/aggravation of arterial insufficiency, hypersensitivity, and other adverse reactions. Monitor ECG, BP, and serum glucose levels.

Counseling: Inform of the risks and benefits of therapy. Advise to take drug regularly and continuously, ud. Instruct to take only the next scheduled dose, without doubling it, if a dose is missed, and not to interrupt or d/c without consulting physician. Advise to consult physician if any difficulty in breathing occurs, or signs/symptoms of worsening congestive heart failure develop. Caution about operating automobiles, using machinery, or engaging in tasks requiring alertness. Caution patients subject to spontaneous hypoglycemia, or diabetic patients receiving insulin or oral hypoglycemics, that the drug may mask some of the manifestations of hypoglycemia, particularly tachycardia.

BYVALSON — nebivolol/valsartan   Rx

Class: Angiotensin II receptor blocker (ARB)/beta adrenergic receptor blocker

> D/C when pregnancy is detected. Drugs that act directly on the renin-angiotensin system (RAS) can cause injury/death to the developing fetus.

ADULT DOSAGE	**PEDIATRIC DOSAGE**
Hypertension	Pediatric use may not have been established
Initial Therapy/Inadequately Controlled on Valsartan 80mg or Nebivolol ≤10mg:	
1 tab qd	
May substitute for its components in patients already receiving 5mg nebivolol and 80mg valsartan	

DOSING CONSIDERATIONS

Renal Impairment
Mild/Moderate: No dosage adjustment is required
Severe: Not recommended as initial treatment

Hepatic Impairment
Mild: No initial dosage adjustment is required
Moderate: Not recommended as initial treatment
Severe: Not recommended

STORAGE
20-25°C (68-77°F).

HOW SUPPLIED
Tab: (Nebivolol/Valsartan) 5mg/80mg

CONTRAINDICATIONS
Severe bradycardia, heart block >1st degree, cardiogenic shock, decompensated cardiac failure, sick sinus syndrome (unless permanent pacemaker in place), severe hepatic impairment (Child-Pugh >B), hypersensitivity to any component of this product, coadministration w/ aliskiren in patients w/ diabetes.

WARNINGS/PRECAUTIONS
Nebivolol: Severe exacerbation of angina, MI, and ventricular arrhythmias reported in patients w/ coronary artery disease (CAD) following abrupt discontinuation; taper nebivolol using monotherapy over 1-2 weeks when possible. If angina worsens, restart nebivolol promptly, at least temporarily. Worsening heart failure (HF) or fluid retention may occur during nebivolol therapy because of its β-blocking effects; consider diuretic therapy and treat HF appropriately. Avoid w/ bronchospastic disease. Chronically administered therapy should not be withdrawn prior to major surgery, however impaired ability of the heart to respond to reflex adrenergic stimuli may augment the risks of general anesthesia and surgical procedures; monitor closely when anesthetic agents that depress myocardial function (eg, ether, cyclopropane, trichloroethylene) are used. May mask manifestations of hypoglycemia/hyperthyroidism, particularly tachycardia. Abrupt withdrawal may be followed by exacerbation of the symptoms of hyperthyroidism or may precipitate a thyroid storm. May precipitate/aggravate symptoms of arterial insufficiency w/ peripheral vascular disease (PVD). Patients w/ history of severe anaphylactic reactions to variety of allergens may be more reactive to repeated accidental/diagnostic/therapeutic challenge; may be unresponsive to usual doses of epinephrine. Initiate an α-blocker prior to use of any β-blocker in patients w/ known/suspected pheochromocytoma. **Valsartan:** Symptomatic hypotension may occur in patients w/ an activated RAS (eg, volume- and/or salt-depleted patients receiving high doses of diuretics); correct this condition prior to therapy, or start treatment under close medical supervision. Renal function changes may occur; caution in patients whose renal function depend in part on the activity of the RAS (eg, renal artery stenosis, chronic kidney disease, severe CHF, volume depletion). Consider withholding or discontinuing therapy if clinically significant decrease in renal function develops. Increased K⁺ reported; discontinuation of therapy may be required.

ADVERSE REACTIONS
Hypotension, hyperkalemia

DRUG INTERACTIONS
Nebivolol: Avoid concomitant use w/ CYP2D6 inhibitors (eg, quinidine, propafenone, paroxetine, fluoxetine, paroxetine). Do not use w/ other β-blockers; closely monitor patients receiving catecholamine-depleting drugs (eg, reserpine, guanethidine. D/C for several days before the gradual tapering of clonidine. May increase risk of bradycardia w/ digitalis glycosides. May exacerbate effects of myocardial depressants/inhibitors of atrioventricular conduction (eg, certain Ca²⁺ antagonists [eg, phenylalkylamine (verapamil) and benzothiazepine (diltiazem) classes], antiarrhythmic agents [eg, disopyramide]); monitor for effects on HR and cardiac conduction. **Valsartan:** Hyperkalemia may occur w/ concomitant use w/ other agents that block the RAS, K⁺-sparing diuretics (eg, spironolactone, triamterene, amiloride), K⁺ supplements, salt substitutes containing K⁺, or

other agents that may increase K+ levels (eg, heparin); monitor serum K+ levels. Coadministration of NSAIDs, including selective COX-2 inhibitors, in patients who are elderly, volume-depleted (eg, on diuretic therapy), or w/ compromised renal function may result in deterioration of renal function, including possible acute renal failure; monitor renal function periodically. Concomitant use w/ NSAIDs including selective COX-2 inhibitors may attenuate the antihypertensive effect. Use of ARB w/ ACE inhibitors or w/ aliskiren is associated w/ increased risks of hypotension, hyperkalemia, and changes in renal function (eg, acute renal failure); closely monitor BP, renal function, and electrolytes in patients on valsartan and ACE inhibitors or aliskiren. Avoid concomitant use w/ aliskiren in patients w/ renal impairment (GFR <60mL/min). Increased lithium levels and lithium toxicity reported; monitor serum lithium levels during concomitant use.

PREGNANCY AND LACTATION

Pregnancy: May cause fetal harm; use of drugs that act on the RAS during second and third trimesters of pregnancy reduces fetal renal function and increases fetal and neonatal morbidity and death. Closely observe infants w/ histories of in utero exposure to Byvalson for hypotension, oliguria, and hyperkalemia. If oliguria or hypotension occur in such neonates, support BP and renal perfusion. Exchange transfusions or dialysis may be required as a means of reversing hypotension and substituting for disordered renal function.
Lactation: There is no information regarding the presence of Byvalson or its individual components in human milk, the effects on the breastfed infant, or the effects on milk production; not for use in nursing.

MECHANISM OF ACTION

Nebivolol: Selective β1-blocker; has not been established. Possible factors include decreased HR, decreased myocardial contractility, decreased sympathetic activity, suppression of renin activity, vasodilation, and decreased peripheral vascular resistance. **Valsartan:** ARB; blocks vasoconstrictor and aldosterone-secreting effects of angiotensin II by selectively blocking the binding of angiotensin II to the AT1 receptor in many tissues (eg, vascular smooth muscle, adrenal gland).

PHARMACOKINETICS

Absorption: Nebivolol: T_{max}=1-6 hrs. Valsartan: T_{max}=2-4 hrs. **Distribution:** Nebivolol: Plasma protein binding (98%, albumin). Valsartan: Plasma protein binding (95%, albumin). (IV) V_d=17L. **Metabolism:** Nebivolol: Glucuronidation, N-dealkylation, and oxidation via CYP2D6. Valsartan: Via CYP2C9; valeryl 4-hydroxy valsartan (primary metabolite). **Elimination:** Nebivolol: Urine (38%, extensive metabolizers [EM]), (67%, poor metabolizers [PM]); feces (44%, EM), (13%, PM); $T_{1/2}$=12 hrs (EM), 19 hrs (PM). Valsartan: (Sol) Feces (83%), urine (13%). (IV) $T_{1/2}$=6 hrs.

PATIENT CONSIDERATIONS

Assessment: Assess for hypersensitivity to the drug and its components, hepatic/renal impairment, volume/salt depletion, renal artery stenosis, HF, CAD, bronchospastic disease, diabetes, hypoglycemia, hyperthyroidism, PVD, pheochromocytoma, pregnancy/nursing status, other conditions where treatment is contraindicated or cautioned, and possible drug interactions.

Monitoring: Monitor for signs/symptoms of hypotension, precipitation/ aggravation of arterial insufficiency, hypersensitivity, and other adverse reactions. Monitor electrolytes, ECG, BP, serum glucose levels, and renal function.

Counseling: Counsel about the risk/benefits of therapy and possible adverse effects. Advise pregnant women and females of reproductive potential of the potential risk to a fetus. Advise females of reproductive potential to notify their physician w/ known or suspected pregnancy. Advise women not to breastfeed during therapy. Advise that lightheadedness can occur, especially during the first days of therapy, and that it should be reported to their physician. Advise to d/c therapy if syncope occurs, until a physician is consulted. Inform that inadequate fluid intake, excessive perspiration, diarrhea, or vomiting can lead to excessive fall in BP. Advise patents not to use salt substitutes containing K+ w/o consulting their physician.

CABOMETYX ← cabozantinib   Rx

Class: Kinase inhibitor

ADULT DOSAGE

Advanced Renal Cell Carcinoma

Use in patients who have received prior anti-angiogenic therapy

60mg qd until patient no longer experiences clinical benefit or experiences unacceptable toxicity

Missed Dose

Do not take a missed dose w/in 12 hrs of next dose

PEDIATRIC DOSAGE

Pediatric use may not have been established

DOSING CONSIDERATIONS

Concomitant Medications
Strong CYP3A4 Inhibitor:
Reduce daily Cabometyx dose by 20mg; resume dose that was used prior to initiating CYP3A4 inhibitor 2-3 days after discontinuation of the strong inhibitor
Do not ingest foods (eg, grapefruit, grapefruit juice) or nutritional supplements that are known to inhibit CYP450 during treatment

Strong CYP3A4 Inducer:
Increase daily Cabometyx dose by 20mg as tolerated; resume dose that was used prior to initiating CYP3A4 inducer 2-3 days after discontinuation of the strong inducer
Max: 80mg

Renal Impairment
Mild or Moderate: No dosage adjustment is required
Severe: There is no experience in patients w/ severe renal impairment

Hepatic Impairment
Mild/Moderate (Child-Pugh Score A or B): Initial: 40mg qd
Severe: Not recommended for use

Adverse Reactions
Withhold for NCI CTCAE Grade 4 adverse reactions, and for Grade 3 or intolerable Grade 2 adverse reactions that cannot be managed w/ a dose reduction or supportive care

Upon resolution/improvement (eg, return to baseline or resolution to Grade 1), reduce dose as follows:
- If previously receiving 60mg qd, resume at 40mg qd
- If previously receiving 40mg qd, resume at 20mg qd
- If previously receiving 20mg qd, resume at 20mg if tolerated, otherwise, d/c

Discontinuation
Permanently d/c for any of the following:
- Development of unmanageable fistula or GI perforation
- Severe hemorrhage
- Arterial thromboembolic event (eg, MI, cerebral infarction)
- Hypertensive crisis or severe hypertension despite optimal medical management
- Nephrotic syndrome
- Reversible posterior leukoencephalopathy syndrome (RPLS)

Other Important Modifications
Stop treatment at least 28 days prior to scheduled surgery, including dental surgery

ADMINISTRATION
Oral route

- Do not substitute Cabometyx tabs w/ cabozantinib caps.
- Do not administer w/ food; do not eat for at least 2 hrs before and at least 1 hr after taking tab.
- Swallow tab whole; do not crush.

STORAGE
20-25°C (68-77°F); excursions permitted from 15-30°C (59-86°F).

HOW SUPPLIED
Tab: 20mg, 40mg, 60mg

WARNINGS/PRECAUTIONS
See Dosing Considerations. Severe hemorrhage reported; do not administer to patients that have or are at risk for severe hemorrhage. GI perforations/fistulas reported; monitor for symptoms and d/c use in patients who experience a fistula which cannot be appropriately managed or a GI perforation. Increased incidence of thrombotic events; d/c if acute MI or any other arterial thromboembolic complication develops. Increased incidence of treatment-emergent HTN; monitor BP prior to initiation and regularly during treatment. Withhold for HTN that is not adequately controlled w/ medical management; when controlled, resume at reduced dose. Diarrhea reported; withhold in patients who develop intolerable Grade 2 diarrhea or Grade 3-4 diarrhea that cannot be managed w/ standard antidiarrheal treatments until improvement to Grade 1; resume at a reduced dose. Palmar-plantar erythrodysesthesia syndrome (PPES) reported; withhold in patients who develop intolerable Grade 2 PPES or Grade 3 PPES until improvement to Grade 1; resume at a reduced dose. RPLS reported; perform an evaluation for RPLS if presenting w/ seizures, headache, visual disturbances, confusion, or altered mental function. May cause fetal harm.

ADVERSE REACTIONS
Diarrhea, fatigue, N/V, decreased appetite, PPES, HTN, decreased weight, constipation.

DRUG INTERACTIONS
See Dosing Considerations. Strong CYP3A4 inhibitors (eg, boceprevir, clarithromycin, saquinavir) may increase exposure and may increase the risk of exposure-related toxicity. Strong CYP3A4 inducers (eg, rifampin, phenytoin, carbamazepine) may decrease exposure and this may lead to reduced efficacy.

PREGNANCY AND LACTATION
Pregnancy: May cause fetal harm.
Lactation: Not for use in nursing.
Females and Males of Reproductive Potential: Females of reproductive potential should use effective contraception during treatment and for 4 months after final dose. May impair fertility in females and males.

MECHANISM OF ACTION
Kinase inhibitor; inhibits the tyrosine kinase activity of MET, VEGFR-1, -2, and -3, AXL, RET, ROS1, TYRO3, MER, KIT, TRKB, FLT-3, and TIE-2. These receptor tyrosine kinases are involved in both normal cellular function and pathologic processes (eg, oncogenesis, metastasis, tumor angiogenesis, drug resistance, maintenance of tumor microenvironment).

PHARMACOKINETICS
Absorption: T_{max}=2-3 hrs (median). **Distribution:** V_d=319L; plasma protein binding (≥99.7%). **Metabolism:** Via CYP3A4. **Elimination:** Urine (27%), feces (54%, 43% unchanged); $T_{1/2}$=99 hrs.

PATIENT CONSIDERATIONS

Assessment: Assess for risk for severe hemorrhage, hepatic impairment, pregnancy/nursing status, and possible drug interactions. Assess BP.

Monitoring: Monitor for severe hemorrhage, fistulas, GI perforations, thrombotic events, diarrhea, PPES, RPLS, and other adverse reactions. Monitor BP.

Counseling: Instruct on proper use. Instruct to contact healthcare provider to seek immediate medical attention for signs or symptoms of unusual severe bleeding/hemorrhage. Instruct to contact healthcare provider at the first signs of poorly formed or loose stool or an increased frequency of bowel movements; for progressive or intolerable rash; before any planned surgeries, including dental surgery; and if significant weight loss occurs. Advise to inform healthcare provider of all prescription or nonprescription medication or herbal products that the patient is taking. Advise females of reproductive potential of the potential risk to a fetus and instruct to contact healthcare provider if pregnancy occurs or is suspected during treatment. Advise patients of reproductive potential to use effective contraception during treatment and for at least 4 months after the final dose. Advise not to breastfeed during treatment and for 4 months following the last dose.

CADUET — amlodipine besylate/atorvastatin calcium   Rx

Class: Calcium channel blocker (CCB)/HMG-CoA reductase inhibitor (statin)

ADULT DOSAGE

Hypertension

Treatment alone or in combination w/ other antihypertensive agents

Amlodipine:
Initial: 5mg qd
Max: 10mg qd

Adjust dose according to BP goals. In general, wait 7-14 days between titration steps; titration may proceed more rapidly if clinically warranted

Angina

Chronic stable angina or confirmed or suspected vasospastic (Prinzmetal's/variant) angina, alone or in combination w/ other antianginals

Amlodipine:
5-10mg qd

Coronary Artery Disease

Reduces the risk of hospitalization due to angina and reduces risk of coronary revascularization procedures in patients w/ recently documented coronary artery disease (CAD) by angiography and w/o heart failure or an ejection fraction <40%

Amlodipine:
5-10mg qd

Hyperlipidemia/Mixed Dyslipidemia

Adjunct to diet for treatment of primary hypercholesterolemia (heterozygous familial and nonfamilial) and mixed dyslipidemia (Types IIa and IIb); adjunct to diet for treatment of patients w/ elevated serum TG levels (Type IV); primary dysbetalipoproteinemia (Type III) inadequately responding to diet; adjunct to other lipid-lowering treatments or if treatments are unavailable, for treatment of homozygous familial hypercholesterolemia

Atorvastatin:
Hyperlipidemia (Heterozygous Familial and Nonfamilial) and Mixed Dyslipidemia (Fredrickson Types IIa and IIb):
Initial: 10 or 20mg qd; patients who require ≥45% reduction in LDL-C may be started at 40mg qd
Titrate: Analyze lipid levels w/in 2-4 weeks and adjust dose accordingly
Range: 10-80mg qd

Homozygous Familial Hypercholesterolemia:
Range: 10-80mg qd
Atorvastatin should be used as an adjunct to other lipid-lowering treatments (eg, LDL apheresis)

Risk Reduction of Myocardial Infarction, Stroke, Cardiovascular Death

Reduces the risk of MI, stroke, revascularization procedures, and angina in adults w/o clinically evident coronary heart disease (CHD), but w/ multiple risk factors for CHD; reduces the risk of MI and stroke in patients w/ type 2 diabetes, and w/o clinically evident CHD, but w/ multiple risk factors for CHD; reduces the risk of nonfatal MI, fatal and nonfatal stroke, revascularization procedures, hospitalization for CHF, and angina in patients w/ clinically evident CHD

PEDIATRIC DOSAGE

Hypertension

Treatment alone or in combination w/ other antihypertensive agents

Amlodipine:
6-17 Years:
Usual: 2.5-5mg qd
Max: 5mg qd

Heterozygous Familial Hypercholesterolemia

As an adjunct to diet if after an adequate trial of diet therapy LDL remains ≥190mg/dL or LDL remains ≥160mg/dL and there is a positive family history of premature cardiovascular disease (CVD) or 2 or more other CVD risk factors are present in the pediatric patient

Atorvastatin:
Heterozygous Familial Hypercholesterolemia:
10-17 Years (Postmenarchal):
Initial: 10mg/day
Max: 20mg/day
Dose adjustments should be made at intervals of ≥4 weeks

DOSING CONSIDERATIONS

Concomitant Medications

Antihypertensives: Start w/ 2.5mg qd amlodipine
Cyclosporine or HIV Protease Inhibitors (Tipranavir Plus Ritonavir [RTV]) or Telaprevir: Avoid therapy w/ atorvastatin
Lopinavir Plus RTV: Use lowest necessary dose of atorvastatin
Clarithromycin, Itraconazole, Fosamprenavir, or Combination of Saquinavir/Darunavir/Fosamprenavir Plus RTV: Limit therapy w/ atorvastatin to 20mg and ensure lowest dose needed is employed
Nelfinavir or Boceprevir: Limit therapy w/ atorvastatin to 40mg and ensure lowest dose needed is employed

Hepatic Impairment
Hepatic Insufficiency:
Initial: 2.5mg qd amlodipine

Elderly
Initial: 2.5mg qd amlodipine

Other Important Considerations
Small Adults or Fragile Patients:
Initial: 2.5mg qd amlodipine

ADMINISTRATION

Oral route

Take w/ or w/o food.

STORAGE

25°C (77°F); excursions permitted to 15-30°C (59-86°F).

HOW SUPPLIED

Tab: (Amlodipine/Atorvastatin) 2.5mg/10mg, 2.5mg/20mg, 2.5mg/40mg, 5mg/10mg, 5mg/20mg, 5mg/40mg, 5mg/80mg, 10mg/10mg, 10mg/20mg, 10mg/40mg, 10mg/80mg

CONTRAINDICATIONS

Active liver disease, which may include unexplained persistent elevations in hepatic transaminases, women who are pregnant or may become pregnant, and nursing mothers.

WARNINGS/PRECAUTIONS

Amlodipine: Worsening angina and acute MI may develop after starting or increasing the dose, particularly w/ severe obstructive CAD. Symptomatic hypotension may occur, particularly in patients w/ severe aortic stenosis. **Atorvastatin:** Rare cases of rhabdomyolysis w/ acute renal failure secondary to myoglobinuria reported. Increased risk of rhabdomyolysis in patients w/ history of renal impairment; closely monitor for skeletal muscle effects. Myopathy (including immune-mediated necrotizing myopathy [IMNM]) reported; predisposing factor includes advanced age (≥65 yrs of age). D/C if markedly elevated creatine phosphokinase (CPK) levels occur or if myopathy is diagnosed or suspected. Withhold or d/c if an acute, serious condition suggestive of a myopathy occurs or if there is a risk factor predisposing to development of renal failure secondary to rhabdomyolysis. Persistent increases in serum transaminases reported; perform LFTs prior to initiation and repeat as clinically indicated. Fatal and nonfatal hepatic failure (rare) reported; promptly interrupt therapy if serious liver injury w/ clinical symptoms and/or hyperbilirubinemia or jaundice occurs and do not restart if no alternate etiology found. Increases in HbA1c and FPG levels reported. May blunt adrenal and/or gonadal steroid production. Increased risk of hemorrhagic stroke in patients w/ recent stroke or transient ischemic attack (TIA).

ADVERSE REACTIONS

Amlodipine: Dizziness, edema.
Atorvastatin: Nasopharyngitis, arthralgia, diarrhea, pain in extremity, UTI.

DRUG INTERACTIONS

See Dosing Considerations. **Amlodipine:** CYP3A inhibitors (moderate and strong) may increase systemic exposure to amlodipine and may require dose reduction; monitor for symptoms of hypotension and edema to determine the need for dose adjustment. Closely monitor BP if coadministered w/ CYP3A inducers. Monitor for hypotension when coadministered w/ sildenafil. May increase systemic exposure of cyclosporine or tacrolimus; monitor trough blood levels of cyclosporine and tacrolimus frequently and adjust dose when appropriate. **Atorvastatin:** Avoid w/ gemfibrozil and drugs that decrease levels or activity of endogenous steroid hormones (eg, ketoconazole, spironolactone, cimetidine). Increased risk of myopathy w/ fibric acid derivatives, erythromycin, strong CYP3A4 inhibitors, clarithromycin, combinations of HIV protease inhibitors, and azole antifungals; consider lower initial and maintenance doses of atorvastatin. Increased risk of myopathy w/ cyclosporine and telaprevir. Risk of skeletal muscle effects may be enhanced when used w/ niacin; consider a reduction in atorvastatin dose. Strong CYP3A4 inhibitors (eg, clarithromycin, several combinations of HIV protease inhibitors, telaprevir, itraconazole, boceprevir) and grapefruit juice may increase levels. CYP3A4 inducers (eg, efavirenz, rifampin) may decrease levels; simultaneous coadministration w/ rifampin is recommended. May increase digoxin levels; monitor appropriately. May increase exposure of norethindrone and ethinyl estradiol. Myopathy, including rhabdomyolysis, reported w/ colchicine; use w/ caution. OATP1B1 inhibitors (eg, cyclosporine) may increase bioavailability.

PREGNANCY AND LACTATION

Pregnancy: Category X.
Lactation: Not for use in nursing.

MECHANISM OF ACTION
Amlodipine: Calcium channel blocker (dihydropyridine); inhibits transmembrane influx of Ca^{2+} ions into vascular smooth muscle and cardiac muscle. Acts directly on vascular smooth muscle to cause a reduction in peripheral vascular resistance and reduction in BP. **Atorvastatin:** HMG-CoA reductase inhibitor; inhibits conversion of HMG-CoA to mevalonate (precursor of sterols, including cholesterol).

PHARMACOKINETICS
Absorption: Amlodipine: Absolute bioavailability (64-90%); T_{max}=6-12 hrs. Atorvastatin: Rapid; absolute bioavailability (14%); T_{max}=1-2 hrs. **Distribution:** Amlodipine: Plasma protein binding (93%). Atorvastatin: V_d=381L; plasma protein binding ($\geq$98%). **Metabolism:** Amlodipine: Hepatic (extensive). Atorvastatin: CYP3A4 (extensive); ortho- and parahydroxylated derivatives (active metabolites). **Elimination:** Amlodipine: Urine (10% parent compound; 60% metabolites); $T_{1/2}$=30-50 hrs. Atorvastatin: Bile (major), urine (<2%); $T_{1/2}$=14 hrs (parent drug), 20-30 hrs (active metabolites).

PATIENT CONSIDERATIONS
Assessment: Assess for active liver disease, unexplained and persistent elevations in serum transaminase levels, history of renal impairment, risk factors for developing renal failure secondary to rhabdomyolysis, recent stroke or TIA, CAD, aortic stenosis, hypersensitivity to the drug, pregnancy/nursing status, and possible drug interactions. Obtain baseline lipid profile (total-C, LDL, HDL, TG), liver function (eg, AST, ALT) parameters, and BP.

Monitoring: Monitor for signs/symptoms of rhabdomyolysis, myopathy (eg, IMNM), worsening angina, MI, and other adverse reactions. Monitor lipid profile, and CPK levels. Monitor LFTs as clinically indicated, and for increases in HbA1c and FPG levels. Monitor BP.

Counseling: Advise to adhere to medication, along w/ the National Cholesterol Education Program-recommended diet, a regular exercise program, and periodic fasting lipid panel testing. Inform of the substances that should not be taken concomitantly w/ the drug. Advise patients to inform other healthcare professionals that they are taking the drug. Inform of the risk of myopathy; instruct to report promptly any unexplained muscle pain, tenderness, or weakness, particularly if accompanied by malaise or fever, or if muscle signs and symptoms persist after discontinuation. Instruct to report promptly any symptoms that may indicate liver injury. Instruct women of childbearing potential to use effective contraceptive methods to prevent pregnancy and to d/c therapy and contact physician if pregnancy occurs. Instruct not to use the drug if breastfeeding.

CALAN — verapamil hydrochloride   Rx

Class: Calcium channel blocker (CCB) (nondihydropyridine)

ADULT DOSAGE
Hypertension
Initial (Monotherapy): 80mg tid (240mg/day)
Range: 360-480mg/day; no evidence that dosages >360mg/day provided added effect
Titrate: Based upward titration on therapeutic efficacy, assessed at the end of the dosing interval

Angina
Angina at rest including vasospastic (Prinzmetal's variant) angina and unstable (crescendo, pre-infarction) angina/chronic stable angina (classic effort-associated angina)
Usual: 80-120mg tid
Titrate: Base upward titration on therapeutic efficacy and safety evaluated approx 8 hrs after dosing; may increase daily (eg, patients w/ unstable angina) or at weekly intervals until optimum response is obtained

Arrhythmias
In association w/ digitalis, for the control of ventricular rate at rest and during stress in patients w/ chronic A-flutter/A-fib
Range: 240-320mg/day in divided doses tid or qid

Paroxysmal Supraventricular Tachycardia
Prophylaxis (Non-Digitalized):
Range: 240-480mg/day in divided doses tid or qid
Max effects for any given dosage will be apparent during the first 48 hrs of therapy

PEDIATRIC DOSAGE
Pediatric use may not have been established

DOSING CONSIDERATIONS
Hepatic Impairment
Severe Dysfunction: Give 30% of normal dose

Other Important Considerations
Patients Who May Respond to Lower Doses (eg, Elderly, People of Small Stature):
HTN: Consider beginning titration at 40mg tid
Angina: 40mg tid may be warranted

ADMINISTRATION
Oral route

STORAGE
15-25°C (59-77°F). Protect from light.

HOW SUPPLIED
Tab: 40mg, 80mg*, 120mg* *scored

CONTRAINDICATIONS
Severe left ventricular dysfunction, hypotension (systolic pressure <90mmHg) or cardiogenic shock, sick sinus syndrome or 2nd- or 3rd-degree atrioventricular (AV) block (except with functioning ventricular artificial pacemaker), A-fib/flutter and an accessory bypass tract (eg, Wolff-Parkinson-White, Lown-Ganong-Levine syndromes), hypersensitivity to verapamil HCl.

WARNINGS/PRECAUTIONS
Has negative inotropic effect; avoid with severe left ventricular dysfunction (eg, ejection fraction <30%) or moderate to severe symptoms of cardiac failure. Patients with milder ventricular dysfunction should, if possible, be controlled with optimum doses of digitalis and/or diuretics before treatment. May cause congestive heart failure (CHF), pulmonary edema, hypotension, asymptomatic 1st-degree AV block, transient bradycardia, and PR interval prolongation. Marked 1st-degree AV block or progressive development to 2nd- or 3rd-degree AV block requires dose reduction, or in rare instances, discontinuation and institution of appropriate therapy. Hepatocellular injury as well as elevated transaminases with or without concomitant elevations in alkaline phosphatase and bilirubin reported; monitor LFTs periodically. Sinus bradycardia, 2nd-degree AV block, pulmonary edema, severe hypotension, and sinus arrest reported in patients with hypertrophic cardiomyopathy. Caution with renal/hepatic impairment; monitor for abnormal PR interval prolongation or other signs of overdosage. 30% of normal dose should be given to patients with severe hepatic dysfunction. May decrease neuromuscular transmission in patients with Duchenne muscular dystrophy and may cause worsening of myasthenia gravis; may be necessary to decrease dose when administered to patients with attenuated neuromuscular transmission. Caution in elderly.

ADVERSE REACTIONS
Constipation, dizziness.

DRUG INTERACTIONS
CYP3A4 inhibitors (eg, erythromycin, ritonavir) and grapefruit juice may increase levels. CYP3A4 inducers (eg, rifampin) may decrease levels. May cause myopathy/rhabdomyolysis with HMG-CoA reductase inhibitors that are CYP3A4 substrates and may increase levels of such drugs; limit dose of simvastatin to 10mg/day and lovastatin to 40mg/day, and lower starting/maintenance doses of other CYP3A4 substrates (eg, atorvastatin) may be required. Increased bleeding times with aspirin. Additive negative effects on HR, AV conduction, and/or cardiac contractility with β-blockers; monitor closely and avoid with any degree of ventricular dysfunction. Combined therapy with propranolol should usually be avoided in patients with AV conduction abnormalities and those with depressed left ventricular function. May produce asymptomatic bradycardia with a wandering atrial pacemaker with timolol eye drops. Decreased metoprolol and propranolol clearance and variable effect with atenolol reported. Chronic treatment may increase digoxin levels, which may result in digitalis toxicity; reduce maintenance and digitalization doses and monitor carefully to avoid over-/under-digitalization. May reduce total body/extra renal clearance of digitoxin. Additive effects with other oral antihypertensives (eg, vasodilators, ACE inhibitors, diuretics); monitor appropriately. Coadmination with agents that attenuate α-adrenergic function (eg, prazosin) may excessively reduce BP. Avoid disopyramide within 48 hrs before or 24 hrs after administration. Coadministration with flecainide may result in additive negative inotropic effect and AV conduction prolongation. May counteract effects of quinidine on AV conduction and increase levels of quinidine; avoid concomitant use in patients with hypertrophic cardiomyopathy. Reduced or unchanged clearance with cimetidine. Increased sensitivity to effects of lithium (neurotoxicity) when used concomitantly; monitor carefully. May increase carbamazepine, theophylline, cyclosporine, and alcohol levels. Increased clearance with phenobarbital. Rifampin may reduce oral bioavailability. Titrate both verapamil and inhalation anesthetics carefully, in order to avoid excessive cardiovascular depression. May potentiate neuromuscular blockers (eg, curare-like and depolarizing); verapamil or both agents may need dose reduction. Hypotension and bradyarrhythmias reported with telithromycin. Sinus bradycardia resulting in hospitalization and pacemaker insertion reported with clonidine; monitor HR.

PREGNANCY AND LACTATION
Category C, not for use in nursing.

MECHANISM OF ACTION
Calcium channel blocker (nondihydropyridine); modulates the influx of ionic Ca^{2+} across the cell membrane of the arterial smooth muscle, as well as in conductile and contractile myocardial cells.

PHARMACOKINETICS
Absorption: Bioavailability (20-35%); T_{max}=1-2 hrs. **Distribution:** Plasma protein binding (90%); crosses the placenta, found in breast milk. **Metabolism:** Liver (extensive); norverapamil (metabolite). **Elimination:** Urine (70% metabolites, 3-4% unchanged), feces ($\geq$16%); $T_{1/2}$=4.5-12 hrs (repetitive dosing).

PATIENT CONSIDERATIONS
Assessment: Assess for known hypersensitivity to the drug, cardiac failure, severe left ventricular dysfunction, hypertrophic cardiomyopathy, hepatic/renal

impairment, attenuated neuromuscular transmission (eg, Duchenne muscular dystrophy), any conditions where treatment is contraindicated or cautioned, pregnancy/nursing status, and possible drug interactions.

Monitoring: Monitor for CHF, hypotension, AV block, abnormal prolongation of the PR interval, transient bradycardia, and other adverse reactions. Monitor LFTs periodically.

Counseling: Inform of the risks/benefits of therapy. Advise to seek medical attention if any adverse reactions occur.

CALAN SR — verapamil hydrochloride   Rx

Class: Calcium channel blocker (CCB) (nondihydropyridine)

ADULT DOSAGE	PEDIATRIC DOSAGE
Hypertension	Pediatric use may not have been established
Initial: 180mg qam	
Titrate: If response is inadequate, increase to 240mg qam, then 180mg bid (am and pm) or 240mg qam plus 120mg qpm, then 240mg q12h. Upward titration should be based on therapeutic efficacy and safety evaluated weekly and approx 24 hrs after the previous dose	
Switching from IR Calan to Calan SR: Total daily dose in mg may remain the same	

DOSING CONSIDERATIONS
Hepatic Impairment
Severe Dysfunction: Give 30% of normal dose

Other Important Considerations
Increased Response to Verapamil (eg, Elderly, Small Stature):
Initial: 120mg qam may be warranted

ADMINISTRATION
Oral route
Take w/ food.

STORAGE
15-25°C (59-77°F). Protect from light and moisture.

HOW SUPPLIED
Tab, Extended-Release: 120mg, 180mg*, 240mg* *scored

CONTRAINDICATIONS
Severe left ventricular dysfunction, hypotension (systolic pressure <90mmHg) or cardiogenic shock, sick sinus syndrome or 2nd- or 3rd-degree AV block (except with functioning artificial ventricular pacemaker), A-flutter/A-fib and an accessory bypass tract (eg, Wolff-Parkinson-White, Lown-Ganong-Levine syndromes), hypersensitivity to verapamil HCl.

WARNINGS/PRECAUTIONS
Has negative inotropic effect; avoid with severe left ventricular dysfunction (eg, ejection fraction <30%) or moderate to severe symptoms of cardiac failure. Patients with milder ventricular dysfunction should, if possible, be controlled with optimum doses of digitalis and/or diuretics before treatment. May cause hypotension, CHF, pulmonary edema, asymptomatic 1st-degree AV block, transient bradycardia, and PR-interval prolongation. Marked 1st-degree AV block or progressive development to 2nd- or 3rd-degree AV block requires dose reduction, or in rare instances, discontinuation and institution of appropriate therapy. Sinus bradycardia, pulmonary edema, severe hypotension, 2nd-degree AV block, and sinus arrest reported in patients with hypertrophic cardiomyopathy. Hepatocellular injury as well as elevated transaminases with or without concomitant elevations in alkaline phosphatase and bilirubin reported; monitor LFTs periodically. Caution with renal/hepatic impairment; monitor for abnormal PR interval prolongation or other signs of overdosage. 30% of normal dose should be given to patients with severe hepatic dysfunction. May decrease neuromuscular transmission in patients with Duchenne muscular dystrophy; may be necessary to decrease dose when administered to patients with attenuated neuromuscular transmission. Caution in elderly.

ADVERSE REACTIONS
Constipation, dizziness.

DRUG INTERACTIONS
May cause myopathy/rhabdomyolysis with HMG-CoA reductase inhibitors that are CYP3A4 substrates and may increase levels of such drugs; limit dose of simvastatin to 10mg/day or lovastatin to 40mg/day, and consider lower starting/maintenance doses of other CYP3A4 substrates (eg, atorvastatin). Additive negative effects on HR, AV conduction, and/or cardiac contractility with β-blockers; monitor closely and avoid with any degree of ventricular dysfunction. May produce asymptomatic bradycardia with a wandering atrial pacemaker with timolol eye drops. Decreased metoprolol and propranolol clearance and variable effect with atenolol reported. Additive effects with other oral antihypertensives (eg, vasodilators, ACE inhibitors, diuretics); monitor appropriately. Coadministration with agents that attenuate α-adrenergic function (eg, prazosin) may excessively reduce BP. May increase carbamazepine, theophylline, and cyclosporine levels. Chronic treatment may increase digoxin levels, which may result in digitalis toxicity; reduce maintenance and digitalization doses and monitor carefully to avoid over-/under-digitalization. May reduce total body/extrarenal clearance of digitoxin. Avoid disopyramide within 48 hrs before or 24 hrs after administration. Coadministration with flecainide may result in additive negative inotropic effect and AV conduction prolongation. May

counteract effects of quinidine on AV conduction and increase levels of quinidine; avoid concomitant use in patients with hypertrophic cardiomyopathy. May increase ethanol concentrations that may prolong the intoxicating effects of alcohol. Increased sensitivity to effects of lithium (neurotoxicity) when used concomitantly; monitor carefully. Increased clearance with phenobarbital. Rifampin may reduce oral bioavailability. May potentiate neuromuscular blockers (eg, curare-like and depolarizing); verapamil or both agents may need dose reduction. Titrate both verapamil and inhalation anesthetics carefully to avoid excessive cardiovascular depression. Hypotension and bradyarrhythmias reported with telithromycin. Sinus bradycardia resulting in hospitalization and pacemaker insertion reported with clonidine; monitor HR. Reduced or unchanged clearance with cimetidine.

PREGNANCY AND LACTATION
Category C, not for use in nursing.

MECHANISM OF ACTION
Calcium channel blocker (nondihydropyridine); modulates influx of ionic Ca^{2+} across the cell membrane of the arterial smooth muscle, as well as in conductile and contractile myocardial cells.

PHARMACOKINETICS
Absorption: (Fed) (240mg) T_{max}=7.71 hrs, C_{max}=79ng/mL, $AUC_{(0-24\ hr)}$=841ng•hr/mL. (Fasted) T_{max}=5.21 hrs, C_{max}=164ng/mL, $AUC_{(0-24\ hr)}$=1478ng•hr/mL. **Distribution:** Plasma protein binding (90%); crosses placenta; found in breast milk. **Metabolism:** Liver (extensive); norverapamil (metabolite). **Elimination:** Urine (70% metabolites, 3-4% unchanged); feces (≥16%).

PATIENT CONSIDERATIONS
Assessment: Assess for known hypersensitivity to drug, severe left ventricular dysfunction, attenuated neuromuscular transmission (eg, Duchenne muscular dystrophy), cardiac failure, hypertrophic cardiomyopathy, hepatic/renal impairment, and for any other conditions where treatment is contraindicated or cautioned. Assess pregnancy/nursing status and for possible drug interactions.

Monitoring: Monitor for abnormal prolongation of PR-interval, hypotension, CHF, pulmonary edema, AV block, transient bradycardia, and other adverse reactions. Monitor LFTs periodically.

Counseling: Inform of the risks/benefits of therapy. Advise to seek medical attention if any adverse reactions occur.

CALCIPOTRIENE OINTMENT — calcipotriene   Rx

Class: Vitamin D3 derivative

OTHER BRAND NAMES
Dovonex Ointment (Discontinued)

ADULT DOSAGE	PEDIATRIC DOSAGE
Plaque Psoriasis	Pediatric use may not have been established
Usual: Apply a thin layer qd-bid and rub in gently and completely	

ADMINISTRATION
Topical route
Wash hands thoroughly after use

STORAGE
15-25°C (59-77°F). Do not freeze.

HOW SUPPLIED
Oint: 0.005% [60g, 120g]

CONTRAINDICATIONS
History of hypersensitivity to any of the components of the preparation, hypercalcemia, evidence of vitamin D toxicity. Do not use on the face.

WARNINGS/PRECAUTIONS
For external use only; not for ophthalmic, oral, or intravaginal use. May cause irritation of lesions and surrounding uninvolved skin; d/c if irritation develops. Transient, rapidly reversible elevation of serum Ca^{2+} reported; d/c until normal Ca^{2+} levels are restored.

ADVERSE REACTIONS
Burning, itching, skin irritation, erythema, dry skin, peeling, rash, dermatitis, worsening of psoriasis.

PREGNANCY AND LACTATION
Category C, caution in nursing.

MECHANISM OF ACTION
Vitamin D3 derivative; synthetic analog of vitamin D3.

PHARMACOKINETICS
Metabolism: Liver (rapid). **Elimination:** Bile.

PATIENT CONSIDERATIONS
Assessment: Assess for history of hypersensitivity to any of the components of the preparation, hypercalcemia, evidence of vitamin D toxicity, and pregnancy/nursing status.

Monitoring: Monitor for irritation, serum Ca^{2+} elevation, and other adverse reactions.

Counseling: Instruct to use externally ud, to avoid contact with face or eyes, and to wash hands after application. Counsel that the medication should not be used for any disorder other than for which it was prescribed. Instruct to report any signs of local adverse reactions to the physician. Counsel patients that apply medication to exposed portions of the body to avoid excessive exposure to either natural or artificial sunlight (eg, tanning booths, sun lamps).

CALCIPOTRIENE TOPICAL SOLUTION — calcipotriene   Rx

Class: Vitamin D3 derivative

OTHER BRAND NAMES
Dovonex Scalp Solution

ADULT DOSAGE	PEDIATRIC DOSAGE
Psoriasis	Pediatric use may not have been established
Chronic, Moderately Severe Psoriasis of Scalp:	
Apply only to lesions bid and rub in gently and completely	
Safety and efficacy demonstrated in patients treated for 8 weeks	

ADMINISTRATION
Topical route

Comb the hair to remove scaly debris and suitably part hair to expose lesions prior to application
Avoid application to uninvolved scalp margins; prevent spreading of sol onto the forehead
Wash hands thoroughly after use

STORAGE
20-25°C (68-77°F); excursions permitted to 15-30°C (59-86°F). Avoid sunlight. Do not freeze.

HOW SUPPLIED
Sol: 0.005% [60mL]

CONTRAINDICATIONS
Acute psoriatic eruptions, history of hypersensitivity to any of the components of the preparation, hypercalcemia, evidence of vitamin D toxicity.

WARNINGS/PRECAUTIONS
Avoid contact w/ the eyes or mucous membranes. D/C if sensitivity reaction occurs or if excessive irritation develops on uninvolved skin areas; may cause transient irritation of both lesions and surrounding uninvolved skin. Flammable; keep away from open flame. Reversible elevation of serum Ca^{2+} may occur; d/c treatment until normal Ca^{2+} levels are restored.

ADVERSE REACTIONS
Transient burning/stinging/tingling, rash, dry skin, irritation, worsening of psoriasis.

PREGNANCY AND LACTATION
Category C, caution in nursing.

MECHANISM OF ACTION
Vitamin D3 derivative; has not been established. Suggested to be roughly equipotent to the natural vitamin in its effects on proliferation and differentiation of a variety of cell types.

PHARMACOKINETICS
Metabolism: Liver. **Elimination:** Bile.

PATIENT CONSIDERATIONS

Assessment: Assess for history of hypersensitivity to any of the components of the preparation, acute psoriatic eruptions, hypercalcemia, evidence of vitamin D toxicity, and pregnancy/nursing status.

Monitoring: Monitor for sensitivity reactions, irritation of lesions or surrounding uninvolved skin areas, serum Ca^{2+} elevation, and other adverse reactions.

Counseling: Advise to use drug only ud by the physician. Inform that medication is for external use only; instruct to avoid contact w/ face or eyes. Advise to wash hands after application. Inform that medication should not be used for any disorder other than for which it was prescribed. Instruct to report any signs of adverse reactions to the physician. Instruct patients who apply medication to exposed portions of the body, to avoid excessive exposure to either natural or artificial sunlight (eg, tanning booths, sun lamps).

CALDOLOR — ibuprofen   Rx

Class: NSAID

> NSAIDs cause an increased risk of serious cardiovascular (CV) thrombotic events (eg, MI, stroke) which can be fatal; risk may occur early in treatment and may increase w/ duration of use. Contraindicated in the setting of CABG surgery. NSAIDs cause an increased risk of serious GI adverse events (eg, bleeding, ulceration, perforation of the stomach/intestines) which can be fatal; these events may occur at any time during use and w/o warning symptoms. Elderly patients and patients w/ a prior history of peptic ulcer disease and/or GI bleeding are at greater risk for serious GI events.

ADULT DOSAGE	PEDIATRIC DOSAGE
Mild to Moderate Pain	**Mild to Moderate Pain**
400-800mg IV q6h prn	**6 Months to <12 Years:**
Max: 3200mg/day	10mg/kg IV q4-6h prn
Moderate to Severe Pain	**Max Single Dose:** 400mg
Adjunct to Opioid Analgesics:	**Max Daily Dose:** 40mg/kg or 2400mg, whichever is less
400-800mg IV q6h prn	**12-17 Years:**
Max: 3200mg/day	400mg IV q4-6h prn
Fever	**Max Daily Dose:** 2400mg
400mg IV, followed by 400mg q4-6h or 100-200mg q4h prn	
Max: 3200mg/day	

Moderate to Severe Pain
Adjunct to Opioid Analgesics:
6 Months to <12 Years:
10mg/kg IV q4-6h prn
Max Single Dose: 400mg
Max Daily Dose: 40mg/kg or
2400mg, whichever is less

12-17 Years:
400mg IV q4-6h prn
Max Daily Dose: 2400mg

Fever
6 Months to <12 Years:
10mg/kg IV q4-6h prn
Max Single Dose: 400mg
Max Daily Dose: 40mg/kg or
2400mg, whichever is less

12-17 Years:
400mg IV q4-6h prn
Max Daily Dose: 2400mg

DOSING CONSIDERATIONS
Elderly
Use caution; start at low end of dosing range

ADMINISTRATION
IV route

- Hydrate well prior to administration to reduce risk of renal adverse reactions.
- Infusion time must be ≥30 min in adults and ≥10 min in pediatric patients.

Dilution
Must be diluted to a final concentration of ≤4mg/mL.
100mg Dose: Dilute 1mL of Caldolor in at least 100mL of diluent.
200mg Dose: Dilute 2mL of Caldolor in at least 100mL of diluent.
400mg Dose: Dilute 4mL of Caldolor in at least 100mL of diluent.
800mg Dose: Dilute 8mL of Caldolor in at least 200mL of diluent.
Diluted sol are stable for up to 24 hrs at ambient temperature (approx 20-25°C [68-77°F]) and room lighting.

Appropriate Diluents:
0.9% NaCl
D5W
Lactated Ringer's sol

STORAGE
20-25°C (68-77°F); excursions permitted between 15-30°C (59-86°F).

HOW SUPPLIED
Inj: 100mg/mL [8mL]

CONTRAINDICATIONS
History of asthma, urticaria, or other allergic-type reactions to aspirin (ASA) or other NSAIDs. In the setting of CABG surgery. Known hypersensitivity (eg, anaphylactic reactions and serious skin reactions) to ibuprofen or any components of this product.

WARNINGS/PRECAUTIONS
Use the lowest effective dosage for the shortest duration. Avoid use in patients w/ a recent MI unless the benefits are expected to outweigh the risk of recurrent CV thrombotic events; monitor for signs of cardiac ischemia if used in patients w/ a recent MI. Increased risk for GI bleeding w/ longer duration of therapy, older age, poor general health status, and advanced liver disease and/or coagulopathy. Avoid use in patients at higher risk for GI bleeding unless benefits are expected to outweigh the risks. If a serious GI adverse event is suspected, promptly initiate evaluation and treatment, and d/c ibuprofen until a serious GI adverse event is ruled out. Hepatotoxicity reported; d/c if signs/symptoms of liver disease develop or if systemic manifestations occur. May lead to onset of new HTN or worsening of preexisting HTN. In patients w/ heart failure (HF), may increase risk of MI, hospitalization for HF, and death. Fluid retention and edema reported. Avoid w/ severe HF unless benefits are expected to outweigh the risks; monitor for worsening HF if used in patients w/ severe HF. Renal papillary necrosis and other renal injury reported after long-term use. Renal toxicity also seen in patients in whom renal prostaglandins have a compensatory role in the maintenance of renal perfusion. Avoid use in patients w/ advanced renal disease unless the benefits are expected to outweigh the risks; monitor for worsening renal function if used in patients w/ advanced renal disease. Correct volume status prior to initiating. Hyperkalemia and anaphylactic reactions reported. Monitor patients w/ preexisting asthma (w/o ASA sensitivity). May cause serious skin adverse reactions; d/c at 1st appearance of skin rash or any other sign of hypersensitivity. Anemia may occur. May increase risk of bleeding events. Infusion of ibuprofen w/o dilution may cause hemolysis. May mask signs of inflammation and fever. Caution in elderly. Blurred or diminished vision, scotomata, and changes in color vision reported; d/c use and conduct ophthalmologic examinations (eg, central visual fields, color vision testing). Aseptic meningitis w/ fever and coma observed w/ oral ibuprofen; give consideration to whether or not signs/symptoms are related to therapy.

ADVERSE REACTIONS
Adults: N/V, flatulence, headache, hemorrhage, dizziness, anemia.
Pediatrics: Infusion-site pain, N/V, anemia, headache.

DRUG INTERACTIONS
Synergistic effect on bleeding w/ anticoagulants (eg, warfarin). Drugs that interfere w/ serotonin reuptake may potentiate the risk of bleeding. May increase risk of GI bleeding w/ use of oral corticosteroids, anticoagulants, or SSRIs;

smoking; and alcohol use. Monitor patients on anticoagulants (eg, warfarin), antiplatelet agents, SSRIs, or SNRIs for signs of bleeding. ASA may increase risk of bleeding and serious GI events; concomitant use w/ analgesic doses of ASA is not recommended. May diminish antihypertensive effect of ACE inhibitors, ARBs, or β-blockers (eg, propranolol); monitor BP. Coadministration w/ ACE inhibitors or ARBs may result in deterioration of renal function in patients who are elderly or volume-depleted (including those on diuretic therapy), or who have renal impairment; monitor for worsening renal function. Adequately hydrate and assess renal function at the beginning of the concomitant treatment and periodically thereafter. May decrease natriuretic effects of loop diuretics (eg, furosemide) and thiazide diuretics; monitor for signs of worsening renal function, in addition to assuring diuretic efficacy including antihypertensive effects. May increase digoxin levels and prolong the $T_{1/2}$ of digoxin; monitor serum digoxin levels. May increase lithium levels and reduce renal lithium clearance; monitor for signs of lithium toxicity. May increase risk of methotrexate toxicity; monitor for methotrexate toxicity. May increase cyclosporine's nephrotoxicity; monitor for worsening renal function. Avoid use w/ other NSAIDs or salicylates (eg, diflunisal, salsalate); increased risk of GI toxicity, w/ little or no increase in efficacy. Concomitant use w/ pemetrexed may increase the risk of pemetrexed-associated myelosuppression, renal, and GI toxicity; refer to pemetrexed prescribing information for further information.

PREGNANCY AND LACTATION
Pregnancy: Use during the 3rd trimester of pregnancy increases the risk of premature closure of the fetal ductus arteriosus; avoid use in pregnant women starting at 30 weeks of gestation (3rd trimester).
Lactation: Present in human milk at relative infant doses of 0.06-0.6% of the maternal weight-adjusted daily dose. There are no reports of adverse effects on the breastfed infant and no effects on milk production; caution in nursing.
Reproductive Potential: May delay or prevent rupture of ovarian follicles, which has been associated w/ reversible infertility in some women; consider withdrawal of therapy in women who have difficulties conceiving or who are undergoing investigation of infertility.

MECHANISM OF ACTION
NSAID; has not been established. Possesses analgesic, anti-inflammatory, and antipyretic properties. Mechanism of action involves inhibition of COX-1 and COX-2. Because ibuprofen is an inhibitor of prostaglandin synthesis, its mode of action may be due to a decrease of prostaglandins in peripheral tissues.

PHARMACOKINETICS
Absorption: AUC=109.3mcg•hr/mL (400mg), 192.8mcg•hr/mL (800mg); C_{max}=39.2mcg/mL (400mg), 72.6mcg/mL (800mg). **Distribution:** Plasma protein binding (>99%); found in breast milk. **Elimination:** $T_{1/2}$=2.22 hrs (400mg), 2.44 hrs (800mg). Refer to PI for pediatric parameters.

PATIENT CONSIDERATIONS
Assessment: Assess for history of asthma, urticaria, or other allergic-type reactions w/ previous use of ASA or other NSAIDs; asthma; CV disease (CVD) or risk factors for CVD; HTN; history of peptic ulcer disease or GI bleeding; coagulation disorders; renal/hepatic impairment; pregnancy/nursing status; or any other conditions where treatment is contraindicated or cautioned. Assess volume status. Assess for possible drug interactions. Obtain baseline BP, CBC, and chemistry profile.

Monitoring: Monitor for signs/symptoms of CV thrombotic events; cardiac ischemia in patients w/ a recent MI; GI bleeding/ulceration and perforation; hepatotoxicity; new or worsening HTN; HF; edema; renal papillary necrosis and other renal injury; hyperkalemia; anaphylactic reactions; serious skin reactions; anemia; and other adverse reactions. Monitor BP during initiation of therapy and throughout the course of therapy. Monitor for signs of bleeding in patients on concomitant therapy w/ anticoagulants, antiplatelet agents, SSRIs, or SNRIs. Monitor renal function in patients w/ renal/hepatic impairment, HF, dehydration, or hypovolemia. Monitor CBC and chemistry profiles periodically during long-term treatment.

Counseling: Inform of potential for CV thrombotic events, GI adverse events, and worsening CHF/edema, and advise of symptoms; if symptoms occur, instruct to report symptoms to healthcare provider. Inform of the potential for hepatotoxicity, and advise of signs/symptoms; if signs/symptoms occur, instruct to d/c and seek immediate medical therapy. Instruct to seek immediate emergency help if signs of an anaphylactic reaction occur. Advise to d/c immediately if rash develops and to contact healthcare provider as soon as possible. Inform pregnant women to avoid use starting at 30 weeks of gestation. Inform patient to not use other NSAIDs or salicylates concomitantly; notify of the presence of NSAIDs in OTC medications for colds, fever, or insomnia. Inform patient to not use low-dose ASA concomitantly w/o talking to healthcare provider. Advise females of reproductive potential who desire pregnancy that treatment may be associated w/ a reversible delay in ovulation.

CANASA — mesalamine   Rx
Class: 5-aminosalicylic acid derivative

ADULT DOSAGE	PEDIATRIC DOSAGE
Ulcerative Proctitis	Pediatric use may not have been established
Mild to Moderately Active:	
1 sup rectally qhs for 3-6 weeks depending on symptoms and sigmoidoscopic findings. Retain sup for at least 1-3 hrs	

DOSING CONSIDERATIONS
Elderly
Start at lower end of dosing range
ADMINISTRATION
Rectal route
STORAGE
<25°C (77°F). May be refrigerated. Keep away from direct heat, light, or humidity.
HOW SUPPLIED
Sup: 1000mg
CONTRAINDICATIONS
Hypersensitivity to mesalamine (5-aminosalicylic acid) or to the sup vehicle (saturated vegetable fatty acid esters), or to salicylates (including ASA).
WARNINGS/PRECAUTIONS
Renal impairment, including minimal change nephropathy, acute and chronic interstitial nephritis, and renal failure (rare), reported; evaluate renal function prior to initiation and periodically during therapy. Caution w/ known renal dysfunction or history of renal disease. Associated w/ acute intolerance syndrome (eg, cramping, acute abdominal pain and bloody diarrhea, fever, headache, rash); observe closely for worsening of these symptoms, and promptly d/c therapy if acute intolerance syndrome is suspected. Patients w/ sulfasalazine hypersensitivity may have similar reaction to therapy. Drug-induced cardiac hypersensitivity reactions (myocarditis, pericarditis) reported. Hepatic failure in patients w/ preexisting liver disease reported; caution w/ liver disease. Possible interference w/ measurements, by liquid chromatography, of urinary normetanephrine in patients exposed to sulfasalazine or its metabolite, mesalamine/mesalazine.
ADVERSE REACTIONS
Dizziness, headache, flatulence, abdominal pain, diarrhea, nausea.
DRUG INTERACTIONS
Concurrent use w/ nephrotoxic agents (eg, NSAIDs) may increase risk of renal reactions. Concurrent use w/ azathioprine or 6-mercaptopurine may increase risk for blood disorders.
PREGNANCY AND LACTATION
Category B, caution in nursing.
MECHANISM OF ACTION
5-aminosalicylic acid (5-ASA) derivative; not established. Suspected to act topically rather than systemically.
PHARMACOKINETICS
Absorption: Variable. (500mg q8h) C_{max}=361ng/mL. **Distribution:** Found in breast milk. **Metabolism:** Extensive, mainly to N-acetyl-5-ASA (metabolite). **Elimination:** (500mg q8h) Urine (≤11% unchanged, 3-35% N-acetyl-5-ASA); $T_{1/2}$=7 hrs.
PATIENT CONSIDERATIONS
Assessment: Assess for hypersensitivity to drug, sup vehicle, salicylates, or sulfasalazine. Assess renal/hepatic function, pregnancy/nursing status, and possible drug interactions.

Monitoring: Monitor for acute intolerance syndrome, hypersensitivity reactions (eg, myocarditis, pericarditis), hepatic failure, and other adverse reactions. Monitor renal function periodically. Monitor blood cell counts in elderly.

Counseling: Instruct to notify physician of all medications being taken and if patient is allergic to sulfasalazine, salicylates, or mesalamine; experiences cramping, abdominal pain, bloody diarrhea, fever, headache, or rash; has a history of myocarditis/pericarditis or stomach blockage; has kidney/liver disease; or is pregnant, intends to become pregnant, or is breastfeeding. Inform that sup will cause staining of direct contact surfaces (eg, fabrics, flooring, painted surfaces, marble, granite, vinyl, enamel).

CANCIDAS — caspofungin acetate   Rx
Class: Echinocandin

ADULT DOSAGE	PEDIATRIC DOSAGE
Aspergillosis	**Fungal Infections**
Invasive Aspergillosis, Refractory/Intolerant of Other Therapies:	**Empirical Therapy for Presumed Fungal Infections in Febrile, Neutropenic Patients:**
LD: 70mg on Day 1	**3 Months-17 Years:**
Maint: 50mg qd thereafter	**LD:** 70mg/m² on Day 1
Duration of treatment should be based upon severity of underlying disease, recovery from immunosuppression, and clinical response	**Maint:** 50mg/m² qd thereafter; may increase to 70mg/m² qd if 50mg/m² dose is well tolerated but provides inadequate clinical response
	Max: 70mg/day (regardless of calculated dose)
Fungal Infections	
Empirical Therapy for Presumed Fungal Infections in Febrile, Neutropenic Patients:	Continue until resolution of neutropenia for empiric therapy; treat for a minimum of 14 days after the last positive culture and continue for at least 7 days after neutropenia and clinical symptoms are resolved
LD: 70mg on Day 1	
Maint: 50mg qd thereafter; may increase to 70mg/day if 50mg dose is well tolerated but provides inadequate clinical response	
	***Candida* Infections**
Continue until resolution of neutropenia for empiric therapy; treat for a minimum of 14 days after the last positive culture and continue for at least 7 days after neutropenia and clinical symptoms are resolved	**Candidemia, Intra-Abdominal Abscesses, Peritonitis, and Pleural Space Infections:**
	3 Months-17 Years:
	LD: 70mg/m² on Day 1
	Maint: 50mg/m² qd thereafter; may

Candida Infections
Candidemia, Intra-Abdominal Abscesses, Peritonitis, and Pleural Space Infections:
LD: 70mg on Day 1
Maint: 50mg qd thereafter

Continue for at least 14 days after the last positive culture; may warrant a longer course of therapy pending resolution of neutropenia in patients who remain persistently neutropenic

Esophageal Candidiasis
50mg qd for 7-14 days after symptom resolution

Consider suppressive oral therapy in patients w/ HIV infections due to risk of relapse

increase to 70mg/m² qd if 50mg/m² dose is well tolerated but provides inadequate clinical response
Max: 70mg/day (regardless of calculated dose)

Continue for at least 14 days after the last positive culture; may warrant a longer course of therapy pending resolution of neutropenia in patients who remain persistently neutropenic

Esophageal Candidiasis
3 Months-17 Years:
LD: 70mg/m² on Day 1
Maint: 50mg/m² qd thereafter; may increase to 70mg/m² qd if 50mg/m² dose is well tolerated but provides inadequate clinical response
Max: 70mg/day (regardless of calculated dose)

Treat for 7-14 days after symptom resolution

Consider suppressive oral therapy in patients w/ HIV infections due to risk of relapse

Aspergillosis
Invasive Aspergillosis, Refractory/Intolerant of Other Therapies:
3 Months-17 Years:
LD: 70mg/m² on Day 1
Maint: 50mg/m² qd thereafter; may increase to 70mg/m² qd if 50mg/m² dose is well tolerated but provides inadequate clinical response
Max: 70mg/day (regardless of calculated dose)

Duration of treatment should be based upon severity of underlying disease, recovery from immunosuppression, and clinical response

DOSING CONSIDERATIONS
Concomitant Medications
Adults:
Concomitant Rifampin: 70mg qd
Concomitant CYP Inducers (eg, Nevirapine, Efavirenz, Carbamazepine, Dexamethasone, Phenytoin): Consider 70mg qd
Pediatrics:
Concomitant Rifampin: 70mg/m² qd (not to exceed 70mg)
Concomitant Inducers of CYP Enzymes (eg, Efavirenz, Nevirapine, Phenytoin, Dexamethasone, Carbamazepine): Consider 70mg/m² qd (not to exceed 70mg)

Hepatic Impairment
Adults:
Moderate Impairment (Child-Pugh Score 7-9):
Maint: 35mg qd; still administer 70mg LD on Day 1 if recommended
Severe Impairment (Child-Pugh Score >9): No clinical experience in adult patients

ADMINISTRATION
IV route

Not for IV bolus administration.
Give by slow IV infusion over approx 1 hr.
Do not mix or coinfuse w/ other medications or use diluents containing dextrose (α-D-glucose).

Preparation
Reconstitution:
1. Equilibrate product vials to room temperature.
2. Reconstitute 50mg or 70mg vials w/ 10.8mL of 0.9% NaCl inj, sterile water for inj, bacteriostatic water for inj w/ methylparaben and propylparaben, or bacteriostatic water for inj w/ 0.9% benzyl alcohol.
3. Mix gently until a clear sol is obtained.
4. Reconstituted sol may be stored for up to 1 hr at ≤25°C (≤77°F) prior to preparation of the infusion sol in the IV bag or bottle.
5. Vials are for single use only; discard unused portion.
Dilution of Reconstituted Sol in IV Bag for Infusion:
1. Transfer the appropriate volume of the reconstituted sol to an IV bag/bottle containing 250mL of 0.9%, 0.45%, or 0.225% NaCl inj or lactated Ringer's inj.
2. Alternatively, reconstituted volume may be added to a reduced volume of 0.9%, 0.45%, or 0.225% NaCl inj or lactated Ringer's inj, not to exceed a final concentration of 0.5mg/mL.
3. The diluted infusion sol in the IV bag/bottle must be used w/in 24 hrs if stored at ≤25°C (≤77°F) or w/in 48 hrs if refrigerated at 2-8°C (36-46°F).

Special Considerations for Pediatrics ≥3 Months of Age:
Reconstitute as above using the 70mg or 50mg vial, then remove volume of drug equal to calculated LD/maint dose based on a concentration of 7mg/mL or 5mg/mL.
For doses <50mg, use 50mg vials; for doses >50mg, use 70mg vials.

STORAGE
2-8°C (36-46°F).
HOW SUPPLIED
Inj: 50mg, 70mg
CONTRAINDICATIONS
Known hypersensitivity (eg, anaphylaxis) to any component of this product.
WARNINGS/PRECAUTIONS
Anaphylaxis reported; d/c and administer appropriate treatment if this occurs. Possible histamine-mediated adverse reactions (eg, rash, facial swelling, angioedema) reported and may require discontinuation and/or administration of appropriate treatment. Abnormal LFTs reported; monitor patients who develop abnormal LFTs for evidence of worsening hepatic function and evaluate risk/benefit of continuing therapy. Isolated cases of significant hepatic dysfunction, hepatitis, and hepatic failure reported w/ multiple concomitant medications in patients w/ serious underlying conditions.
ADVERSE REACTIONS
Pyrexia, chills, hypokalemia, hypotension, diarrhea, increased blood alkaline phosphatase, increased ALT/AST, N/V, abdominal pain, peripheral edema, headache, rash, increased blood bilirubin, pneumonia, cough.
DRUG INTERACTIONS
See Dosing Considerations. Increased exposure and transient increases in ALT and AST reported w/ concomitant cyclosporine. Limit concomitant use w/ cyclosporine to patients for whom potential benefit outweighs the potential risk. Monitor tacrolimus trough blood concentrations and adjust tacrolimus dosage appropriately. Rifampin reduces plasma levels. Inducers of CYP enzymes (eg, efavirenz, nevirapine, phenytoin, rifampin, dexamethasone, carbamazepine) may decrease levels.
PREGNANCY AND LACTATION
Pregnancy: Category C.
Lactation: It is not known whether caspofungin is present in human milk; caution in nursing.
MECHANISM OF ACTION
Echinocandin; inhibits the synthesis of β (1,3)-D-glucan, an essential component of the cell wall of susceptible *Aspergillus* and *Candida* species.
PHARMACOKINETICS
Absorption: Administration to different age groups resulted in different parameters. **Distribution:** Plasma protein binding (97%). **Metabolism:** Hydrolysis and N-acetylation. **Elimination:** Urine (41%, 1.4% unchanged), feces (35%); $T_{1/2}$=9-11 hrs (β-phase), 40-50 hrs (gamma-phase).

PATIENT CONSIDERATIONS
Assessment: Assess for drug hypersensitivity, hepatic function, pregnancy/nursing status, and possible drug interactions.
Monitoring: Monitor for anaphylaxis, histamine-mediated adverse reactions, resolution of neutropenia, and other adverse reactions. Monitor LFTs.
Counseling: Inform that anaphylactic reactions have been reported; instruct to report signs/symptoms of hypersensitivity to physician. Inform that there have been isolated reports of serious hepatic effects.

CAPRELSA — vandetanib　　　Rx
Class: Kinase inhibitor

> May prolong the QT interval. Torsades de pointes and sudden death reported. Avoid w/ hypocalcemia, hypokalemia, hypomagnesemia, or long QT syndrome; correct hypocalcemia, hypokalemia, and/or hypomagnesemia prior to therapy. Monitor electrolytes periodically. Avoid drugs known to prolong QT interval. Only prescribers and pharmacies certified w/ the restricted distribution program are able to prescribe and dispense this therapy.

ADULT DOSAGE
Medullary Thyroid Cancer

Symptomatic or progressive cancer in patients w/ unresectable locally advanced or metastatic disease

300mg qd until disease progression or unacceptable toxicity occurs

Missed Dose

Do not take a missed dose w/in 12 hrs of the next dose

PEDIATRIC DOSAGE
Pediatric use may not have been established

DOSING CONSIDERATIONS
Renal Impairment
Moderate (CrCl ≥30 to <50mL/min) and Severe (CrCl <30mL/min):
Initial: 200mg qd

Hepatic Impairment
Moderate and Severe: Not recommended for use

Adverse Reactions
Corrected QT Interval, Fridericia (QTcF) >500 ms:
Interrupt therapy, then resume at a reduced dose when the QTcF returns to <450 ms

CTCAE Grade ≥3 Toxicities:
Interrupt therapy, then resume at 200mg (two 100mg tabs) when toxicity resolves or improves to CTCAE Grade 1

For recurrent toxicities, reduce the dose to 100mg after resolution or improvement to CTCAE Grade 1 severity, if continued treatment is warranted

ADMINISTRATION
Oral route

Take w/ or w/o food.
Do not crush tabs.
May disperse in 2 oz of water by stirring for approx 10 min (will not completely dissolve); do not use other liquids for dispersion. Swallow immediately and mix any remaining residue w/ additional 4 oz of water and swallow. The dispersion can also be administered through nasogastric or gastrostomy tubes.

STORAGE
25°C (77°F); excursions permitted to 15-30°C (59-86°F).

HOW SUPPLIED
Tab: 100mg, 300mg

CONTRAINDICATIONS
Congenital long QT syndrome.

WARNINGS/PRECAUTIONS
See Dosing Considerations. Caution in patients w/ indolent, asymptomatic, or slowly progressing disease. Do not start therapy w/ QTcF interval >450 ms. Avoid w/ history of torsades de pointes, bradyarrhythmias, or uncompensated heart failure (HF). Severe and sometimes fatal skin reactions (eg, Stevens-Johnson syndrome, toxic epidermal necrosis) reported; permanently d/c and refer the patient for urgent medical evaluation. Photosensitivity reactions may occur during treatment and up to 4 months after discontinuation. Interstitial lung disease (ILD) or pneumonitis reported; interrupt treatment for acute/worsening pulmonary symptoms and d/c if ILD is confirmed. Ischemic cerebrovascular events and serious hemorrhagic events reported; d/c if severe. Avoid w/ recent history of hemoptysis of ≥1/2 tsp of red blood. HF reported; monitor for signs/symptoms of HF and consider discontinuation in patients w/ HF. Diarrhea of ≥Grade 3 reported; interrupt therapy for severe diarrhea and resume at a reduced dose upon improvement. HTN, including hypertensive crisis, may occur; monitor for HTN. Reduce dose or interrupt therapy if HTN occurs; do not resume therapy if BP cannot be controlled. Reversible posterior leukoencephalopathy syndrome (RPLS) reported; d/c in patients w/ RPLS. Increased exposure w/ impaired renal function. May cause fetal harm.

ADVERSE REACTIONS
Diarrhea/colitis, rash, acneiform dermatitis, HTN, nausea, headache, URTIs, decreased appetite, abdominal pain.

DRUG INTERACTIONS
See Boxed Warning. Rifampicin, a strong CYP3A4 inducer, decreases levels. Avoid use w/ strong CYP3A4 inducers, St. John's wort, antiarrhythmic drugs (eg, amiodarone, disopyramide, procainamide), and other drugs that may prolong QT interval (eg, chloroquine, clarithromycin, dolasetron). Increased plasma levels of metformin that is transported by organic cation transporter type 2 (OCT2); use caution and closely monitor for toxicities when administering w/ drugs that are transported by OCT2. Increases digoxin levels; use w/ caution and closely monitor for toxicities. May require dose increase of thyroid replacement therapy; if signs or symptoms of hypothyroidism occur, examine thyroid hormone levels and adjust thyroid replacement therapy accordingly.

PREGNANCY AND LACTATION
Pregnancy: Category D.
Lactation: Not for use in nursing.
Reproductive Potential: Females of reproductive potential should avoid pregnancy. Use effective contraception during treatment and up to 4 months after the last dose.

MECHANISM OF ACTION
Multikinase inhibitor; inhibits the tyrosine kinase activity of the epidermal growth factor receptor and vascular endothelial growth factor receptor families, RET, BRK, TIE2, and members of the EPH receptor and Src kinase families, which are involved in both normal cellular function and pathologic processes such as oncogenesis, metastasis, tumor angiogenesis, and maintenance of the tumor microenvironment.

PHARMACOKINETICS
Absorption: Slow; T_{max}=6 hrs (median). **Distribution:** V_d=7450L; plasma protein binding (90% in vitro). **Metabolism:** Via CYP3A4; vandetanib N-oxide and N-desmethyl vandetanib (metabolites). **Elimination:** Urine (25%), feces (44%); $T_{1/2}$=19 days (median).

PATIENT CONSIDERATIONS
Assessment: Assess for congenital long QT syndrome, history of torsades de pointes or hemoptysis, bradyarrhythmias, uncompensated HF, renal/hepatic impairment, pregnancy/nursing status, and possible drug interactions. Obtain baseline ECG, serum K^+, Ca^{2+}, Mg^{2+}, and TSH levels.

Monitoring: Monitor for QT interval prolongation, torsades de pointes, skin/photosensitivity reactions, ILD, ischemic cerebrovascular events, hemorrhage, HF, diarrhea, hypothyroidism, HTN, RPLS, and other adverse reactions. Monitor ECG, serum K^+, Ca^{2+}, Mg^{2+}, and TSH levels at 2-4 weeks and 8-12 weeks after initial therapy, every 3 months thereafter, and following any dose reduction for QT prolongation, or any dose interruptions >2 weeks. Monitor renal function.

Counseling: Advise to take ud. Instruct to contact physician in the event of syncope, pre-syncopal symptoms, and cardiac palpitations. Inform patients that the physician will monitor electrolytes and ECGs during treatment. Advise to contact physician in the event of skin reactions or rash, sudden onset or worsening of breathlessness, persistent cough or fever, diarrhea, seizures, headaches, visual disturbances, confusion, or difficulty thinking. Advise patients of reproductive potential to use effective contraception during therapy and for

at least 4 months after the last dose and to immediately contact physician if pregnancy is suspected or confirmed. Advise to d/c nursing while on therapy. Instruct to use appropriate sun protection due to the increased susceptibility to sunburn while on therapy and for at least 4 months after drug discontinuation.

CAPTOPRIL — captopril   Rx
Class: ACE inhibitor

> **D/C when pregnancy is detected. Drugs that act directly on the renin-angiotensin system (RAS) can cause injury and death to the developing fetus.**

ADULT DOSAGE

Hypertension
D/C previous antihypertensive drug regimen for 1 week before starting captopril therapy, if possible

Initial: 25mg bid or tid
Titrate: May increase to 50mg bid or tid if satisfactory BP reduction is not achieved after 1 or 2 weeks. Add a modest dose of a thiazide diuretic (eg, hydrochlorothiazide, 25mg/day) if BP is not controlled after 1-2 weeks at 50mg tid and patient is not already receiving a diuretic; diuretic dose may be increased at 1- to 2-week intervals until its highest usual antihypertensive dose is reached. If further BP reduction is required, may increase captopril dose to 100mg bid or tid and then, if necessary, to 150mg bid or tid (while continuing the diuretic)
Usual Range: 25-150mg bid or tid
Max: 450mg/day

Severe HTN (eg, Accelerated or Malignant HTN):
When temporary discontinuation of current antihypertensive therapy is not practical or desirable, or when prompt titration to more normotensive blood pressure levels is indicated, continue the diuretic but d/c other current antihypertensive medication and promptly initiate captopril at 25mg bid or tid

Congestive Heart Failure
Initial: 25mg tid; 6.25mg or 12.5mg tid in patients w/ normal/low BP, who have been vigorously treated w/ diuretics and who may be hyponatremic and/or hypovolemic
Titrate: After a dose of 50mg tid is reached, delay further increases in dosage, where possible, for at least 2 weeks to determine if a satisfactory response occurs. Most patients studied have had a satisfactory clinical improvement at 50mg or 100mg tid
Max: 450mg/day

Captopril should generally be used in conjunction w/ a diuretic and digitalis

Left Ventricular Dysfunction Post-Myocardial Infarction
May initiate therapy as early as 3 days following MI

Initial: 6.25mg single dose, then 12.5mg tid
Titrate: Increase to 25mg tid during the next several days, then to 50mg tid over next several weeks
Maint: 50mg tid

May be used in patients treated w/ other post-MI therapies (eg, thrombolytics, aspirin, beta blockers)

Diabetic Neuropathy
25mg tid

Other antihypertensives (eg, diuretics, beta blockers, centrally acting agents, or vasodilators) may be used in conjunction w/ captopril if additional therapy is required

PEDIATRIC DOSAGE
Pediatric use may not have been established

DOSING CONSIDERATIONS
Renal Impairment
Patients may respond to smaller or less frequent doses
Significant Impairment:
Reduce initial daily dosage, and utilize smaller increments for titration, which should be quite slow (1- to 2-week intervals)
After desired effect is achieved, slowly back-titrate dose to determine the minimal effective dose
When concomitant diuretic therapy is required, administer a loop diuretic (eg, furosemide) rather than a thiazide diuretic
ADMINISTRATION
Oral route
Take 1 hr ac.
STORAGE
20-25°C (68-77°F). Protect from moisture.
HOW SUPPLIED
Tab: 12.5mg*, 25mg*, 50mg*, 100mg* *scored
CONTRAINDICATIONS
Hypersensitivity to this product or any other ACE inhibitor (ACE inhibitor-associated angioedema). Coadministration w/ aliskiren in patients w/ diabetes.
WARNINGS/PRECAUTIONS
Head/neck angioedema reported; promptly institute appropriate therapy if this occurs. Intestinal angioedema reported; monitor for abdominal pain. Higher rate of angioedema in black patients than in nonblack patients. Anaphylactoid reactions reported during desensitization w/ hymenoptera venom, dialysis w/ high-flux membranes, and LDL apheresis w/ dextran sulfate absorption. Consider using a different type of dialysis membrane or a different class of medication in patients undergoing hemodialysis w/ high-flux dialysis membranes. Neutropenia/agranulocytosis reported; risk of neutropenia is dependent on the clinical status of the patient. In patients w/ collagen vascular disease or who are exposed to other drugs known to affect the white cells or immune response, particularly w/ impaired renal function, use captopril only after an assessment of benefit and risk, and then w/ caution. Perform WBC counts if infection is suspected. Withdraw therapy and closely follow patient's course if neutropenia (neutrophil count <1000/mm^3) is confirmed. Total urinary proteins >1g/day reported. Excessive hypotension may occur in patients w/ salt/volume depletion, heart failure (HF), or those undergoing renal dialysis; initiate therapy under very close medical supervision in these patients. Rarely, associated w/ a syndrome that starts w/ cholestatic jaundice and progresses to fulminant hepatic necrosis and sometimes death; d/c if jaundice or marked elevations of hepatic enzymes develop. May increase BUN/SrCr after reduction of BP or upon long-term HF treatment. Hyperkalemia and persistent nonproductive cough reported. Patients w/ aortic stenosis may be at particular risk of decreased coronary perfusion. Hypotension may occur w/ major surgery or during anesthesia. Lab test interactions may occur.
ADVERSE REACTIONS
Anemia, thrombocytopenia, pancytopenia, rash, diminution/loss of taste perception.
DRUG INTERACTIONS
Coadministration w/ mTOR (mammalian target of rapamycin) inhibitors (eg, temsirolimus, sirolimus, everolimus) may increase risk for angioedema. Dual blockade of the RAS is associated w/ increased risks of hypotension, hyperkalemia, and changes in renal function (including acute renal failure); avoid combined use of RAS inhibitors. Closely monitor BP, renal function, and electrolytes w/ concomitant agents that also block the RAS. Do not coadminister w/ aliskiren in patients w/ diabetes or renal impairment (GFR <60mL/min). Coadministration w/ NSAIDs, including selective COX-2 inhibitors, may cause deterioration of renal function, including possible acute renal failure, in patients who are elderly, volume-depleted, or w/ compromised renal function. NSAIDs may also attenuate antihypertensive effect. Precipitous BP reduction may occur w/ diuretics, usually w/in the 1st hr after the initial dose of captopril. Nitroglycerin, other nitrates, or drugs having vasodilator activity should, if possible, be discontinued before starting captopril; administer such agents cautiously, and perhaps at lower dosage if resumed during captopril therapy. Antihypertensive agents that cause renin release may augment effect of captopril (eg, diuretics [eg, thiazides] may activate renin-angiotensin-aldosterone system [RAAS]). Caution w/ agents affecting sympathetic activity (eg, ganglionic-blocking agents, adrenergic neuron-blocking agents); β-adrenergic blocking drugs may add further antihypertensive effect. Increased risk of hyperkalemia w/ K$^+$-sparing diuretics (eg, spironolactone, triamterene, amiloride), K$^+$ supplements, K$^+$-containing salt substitutes, or other drugs associated w/ increases in serum K$^+$; use w/ caution. Increased serum lithium levels and symptoms of lithium toxicity reported; coadminister w/ caution and frequently monitor serum lithium levels. Nitritoid reactions reported w/ injectable gold.
PREGNANCY AND LACTATION
Pregnancy: Category D.
Lactation: Not for use in nursing.
MECHANISM OF ACTION
ACE inhibitor; mechanism not established. Effects in HTN and HF appear to result primarily from suppression of the RAAS.
PHARMACOKINETICS
Absorption: Rapid. T_{max}=1 hr. **Distribution:** Plasma protein binding (approx 25-30%); found in breast milk. **Elimination:** Urine (>95%; 40-50% unchanged); $T_{1/2}$<3 hrs, <2 hrs (unchanged).
PATIENT CONSIDERATIONS
Assessment: Assess for hypersensitivity to drug, history of ACE inhibitor-associated angioedema, diabetes, collagen vascular disease, volume/salt

depletion, HF, renal artery stenosis, risk factors for hyperkalemia, renal function, aortic stenosis, pregnancy/nursing status, and possible drug interactions. In patients w/ renal impairment, evaluate WBC and differential counts.
Monitoring: Monitor for angioedema, anaphylactoid reactions, neutropenia/agranulocytosis, hyperkalemia, and other adverse reactions. Monitor BP, LFTs, and renal function. In patients w/ renal impairment, evaluate WBC and differential counts at approx 2-week intervals for about 3 months, then periodically.
Counseling: Instruct to d/c therapy and to immediately report to physician any signs/symptoms of angioedema. Advise to report promptly any indication of infection (eg, sore throat, fever) or of progressive edema. Inform that excessive perspiration, dehydration, and other causes of volume depletion (eg, vomiting, diarrhea) may lead to excessive fall in BP; advise to consult w/ physician. Instruct not to use K$^+$-sparing diuretics, K$^+$ supplements, or K$^+$-containing salt substitutes w/o consulting physician. Warn against interruption or discontinuation of medication unless instructed by physician. Caution HF patients against rapid increases in physical activity. Inform female patients of childbearing age about the consequences of exposure to captopril during pregnancy and discuss treatment options w/ those planning to become pregnant; instruct to report pregnancies to physician as soon as possible.

CAPTOPRIL/HCTZ — captopril/hydrochlorothiazide   Rx
Class: ACE inhibitor/thiazide diuretic

> ACE inhibitors can cause injury and death to the developing fetus during 2nd and 3rd trimesters. D/C when pregnancy is detected.

OTHER BRAND NAMES
Capozide (Discontinued)

ADULT DOSAGE	PEDIATRIC DOSAGE
Hypertension	Pediatric use may not have been established
May be substituted for previously titrated individual components	
Initial: 25mg-15mg qd	
Titrate: Adjust dosage at 6-week intervals, unless situation demands more rapid adjustment	
Additional captopril or HCTZ may be added as individual components or by using 50mg-15mg, 25mg-25mg or 50mg-25mg, or divided doses may be used	
Max: 150mg captopril and 50mg HCTZ per day	

DOSING CONSIDERATIONS
Renal Impairment
May respond to smaller or less frequent doses
After the desired effect has been achieved, increase dose intervals or reduce total daily dose until the minimal effective dose is achieved
ADMINISTRATION
Oral route
Take 1 hr ac
STORAGE
20-25°C (68-77°F). Protect from moisture.
HOW SUPPLIED
Tab: (Captopril-HCTZ) 25mg-15mg*, 25mg-25mg*, 50mg-15mg*, 50mg-25mg* *scored
CONTRAINDICATIONS
Captopril: Hypersensitivity to captopril or history of ACE inhibitor-associated angioedema. **HCTZ:** Anuria, hypersensitivity to HCTZ or sulfonamide-derived drugs.
WARNINGS/PRECAUTIONS
May be used as initial therapy. Higher rate of angioedema in blacks than nonblacks. Not recommended with severe renal dysfunction. Lab test interactions may occur. Captopril: Head/neck angioedema reported; institute appropriate therapy promptly. Intestinal angioedema reported; monitor for abdominal pain. Anaphylactoid reactions reported during desensitization with hymenoptera venom, dialysis with high-flux membranes, and LDL apheresis with dextran sulfate absorption; consider using a different type of dialysis membrane or a different class of medication in patients undergoing hemodialysis with high-flux dialysis membranes. Neutropenia/agranulocytosis reported. In patients with renal impairment, evaluate WBC and differential counts prior to starting therapy and at approximately 2-week intervals for about 3 months, then periodically. In patients with collagen vascular disease or those exposed to other drugs known to affect the white cells or immune response, particularly impaired renal function, use therapy only after an assessment of benefit and risk, and then with caution. Perform WBC count if infection is suspected. Withdraw therapy and closely follow patient's course if neutropenia (neutrophil count <1000/mm^3) is confirmed. Total urinary proteins >1g/day reported. Excessive hypotension may occur, most likely in patients with salt/volume depletion, heart failure (HF), or undergoing renal dialysis. Rarely, associated with syndrome that starts with cholestatic jaundice and progresses to fulminant hepatic necrosis and sometimes death; d/c if jaundice or marked elevations of hepatic enzymes develop. May increase BUN/SrCr levels in patients with severe renal artery stenosis. Hyperkalemia and persistent nonproductive cough reported. Hypotension may occur with major

surgery or during anesthesia. HCTZ: May precipitate azotemia in patients with renal disease. Caution with hepatic impairment or progressive liver disease; may precipitate hepatic coma. Sensitivity reactions may occur in patients with or without a history of allergy or bronchial asthma. May cause exacerbation or activation of systemic lupus erythematosus (SLE), hyperuricemia or precipitation of frank gout, manifestations of latent diabetes mellitus (DM), hypercalcemia, hypophosphatemia, and hypomagnesemia. Observe for signs of fluid/electrolyte imbalance. Hypokalemia may sensitize or exaggerate the response of the heart to toxic effects of digitalis. Enhanced antihypertensive effect in postsympathectomy patients. D/C or withhold if progressive renal impairment becomes evident. May decrease serum protein-bound iodine levels without signs of thyroid disturbance. D/C before testing for parathyroid function.

ADVERSE REACTIONS
Anemia, thrombocytopenia, pancytopenia, rash, diminution/loss of taste perception.

DRUG INTERACTIONS
NSAIDs (eg, indomethacin, aspirin) may reduce antihypertensive effects. May increase risk of lithium toxicity; avoid concomitant use or use with caution and frequent monitoring of serum lithium levels. Captopril: Precipitous BP reduction may occur with diuretics. Nitroglycerin, other nitrates, or drugs having vasodilator activity should, if possible, be discontinued before starting captopril; if resumed during captopril therapy, administer such agents cautiously, and perhaps at lower dosage. Antihypertensive agents that cause renin release may augment effect (eg, diuretics [eg, thiazides] may activate renin-angiotensin-aldosterone system [RAAS]). Caution with agents affecting sympathetic activity (eg, ganglionic-blocking agents, adrenergic neuron-blocking agents). Increased risk of hyperkalemia with K^+-sparing diuretics (eg, spironolactone, triamterene, amiloride), K^+ supplements, K^+-containing salt substitutes, or other drugs associated with increases in serum K^+; use with caution. HCTZ: Potentiation of orthostatic hypotension may occur with alcohol, barbiturates, or narcotics. Amphotericin B, corticosteroids, or corticotropin (adrenocorticotropic hormone) may intensify electrolyte imbalance, particularly hypokalemia; monitor K^+ levels, and use K^+ replacements if necessary. May increase blood glucose and uric acid levels; may decrease effects of oral anticoagulants; dosage adjustment of the anticoagulant may be necessary. Dosage adjustments of antigout medications or antidiabetic agents (oral agents and insulin) may be necessary. May potentiate effects of other antihypertensive medications (eg, ganglionic or peripheral adrenergic-blocking agents); dosage adjustments may be necessary. Monitor serum Ca^{2+} levels and adjust Ca^{2+} dosage accordingly if Ca^{2+} must be prescribed. Anionic exchange resins (eg, cholestyramine, colestipol) may impair absorption. Enhanced hyperglycemic, hyperuricemic, and antihypertensive effects with diazoxide; monitor blood glucose and serum uric acid levels. Enhanced hypotensive effects with MAOIs; dosage adjustments of one or both agents may be necessary. May potentiate effects of nondepolarizing muscle relaxants, preanesthetics and anesthetics used in surgery (eg, tubocurarine chloride, gallamine triethiodide); may require dosage adjustments, and monitor and correct any fluid and electrolyte imbalances prior to surgery if feasible. May decrease effectiveness of methenamine. May decrease response to pressor amines (eg, norepinephrine); use caution in patients taking both medications who undergo surgery, and administer preanesthetic and anesthetic agents in reduced dosage, and if possible, d/c HCTZ therapy 1 week prior to surgery. Increased dosage of probenecid or sulfinpyrazone may be necessary.

PREGNANCY AND LACTATION
Category C (1st trimester) and D (2nd and 3rd trimesters), not for use in nursing.

MECHANISM OF ACTION
Captopril: ACE inhibitor; not established. Effects appear to result primarily from suppression of the RAAS. Decreases plasma angiotensin II, which leads to decreased aldosterone secretion. HCTZ: Thiazide diuretic; not established. Affects renal tubular mechanism of electrolyte reabsorption. Increases excretion of Na^+ and Cl^- in approximately equivalent amounts.

PHARMACOKINETICS
Absorption: Captopril: Rapid; T_{max}=1 hr. **Distribution:** Found in breast milk. Captopril: Plasma protein binding (25-30%). **Elimination:** Captopril: Urine (>95%; 40-50% unchanged); $T_{1/2}$<3 hrs, <2 hrs (unchanged). HCTZ: Kidney; $T_{1/2}$=2.5 hrs (fasted).

PATIENT CONSIDERATIONS
Assessment: Assess for history of ACE inhibitor-associated angioedema, anuria, hypersensitivity to drug or sulfonamide-derived drugs, history of allergy or bronchial asthma, collagen vascular disease, volume/salt depletion, HF, renal artery stenosis, risk factors for hyperkalemia, SLE, hepatic/renal function, postsympathectomy status, pregnancy/nursing status, and possible drug interactions. In patients with renal impairment, evaluate WBC and differential counts.

Monitoring: Monitor for signs/symptoms of fluid/electrolyte imbalance, angioedema, anaphylactoid reactions, neutropenia/agranulocytosis, sensitivity reactions, exacerbation/activation of SLE, hyperuricemia or precipitation of frank gout, latent DM, and other adverse reactions. Monitor BP, serum electrolytes, and renal/hepatic function. In patients with renal impairment, evaluate WBC and differential counts during therapy at approximately 2-week intervals for about 3 months, then periodically.

Counseling: Instruct to d/c therapy and to immediately report to physician any signs/symptoms of angioedema. Advise to report promptly any indication of infection or of progressive edema. Inform that excessive perspiration, dehydration, and other causes of volume depletion may lead to excessive fall in BP; advise to consult with physician. Instruct not to use K^+-sparing diuretics, K^+ supplements, or K^+-containing salt substitutes without consulting physician. Warn against interruption or discontinuation of medication unless instructed by physician.

Caution HF patients against rapid increases in physical activity. Inform female patients of childbearing age about the consequences of 2nd- and 3rd-trimester exposure to therapy and instruct to report pregnancies to physician as soon as possible.

CARAFATE — sucralfate   Rx
Class: Duodenal ulcer adherent complex

ADULT DOSAGE	PEDIATRIC DOSAGE
Active Duodenal Ulcer	Pediatric use may not have been established
1g qid on an empty stomach; continue for 4-8 weeks unless healing has been demonstrated by x-ray or endoscopic exam	
Antacids may be prescribed prn for relief of pain but should not be taken w/in 1/2 hr before or after administration	
Tab:	
Maint: 1g bid	

DOSING CONSIDERATIONS
Elderly
Start at the lower end of dosing range

ADMINISTRATION
Oral route
Sus
Shake well before use.

STORAGE
(Sus) 20-25°C (68-77°F). Avoid freezing. (Tab) 15-30°C (59-86°F).

HOW SUPPLIED
Sus: 1g/10mL [14 fl oz]; **Tab:** 1g* *scored

CONTRAINDICATIONS
Hypersensitivity reactions to the active substance or to any of the excipients.

WARNINGS/PRECAUTIONS
DU is a chronic, recurrent disease; a successful course of treatment should not be expected to alter post healing frequency or severity of duodenal ulceration. May impair excretion of absorbed aluminum with chronic renal failure or those receiving dialysis; aluminum accumulation and toxicity (aluminum osteodystrophy, osteomalacia, encephalopathy) reported with renal impairment. Caution with chronic renal failure and in elderly. (Sus) Episodes of hyperglycemia reported in diabetic patients; may need to adjust dose of antidiabetic treatment during therapy. (Tab) Aspiration with accompanying respiratory complications reported; caution with known conditions that may impair swallowing (eg, recent or prolonged intubation, tracheostomy, prior history of aspiration, dysphagia), or any other conditions that may alter gag and cough reflexes, or diminish oropharyngeal coordination or motility.

ADVERSE REACTIONS
Constipation, diarrhea, N/V, pruritus, rash, dizziness, insomnia, back pain, headache, dry mouth, flatulence, gastric discomfort, indigestion, sleepiness, vertigo.

DRUG INTERACTIONS
Simultaneous administration may reduce the extent of absorption of single doses of cimetidine, digoxin, fluoroquinolone antibiotics, ketoconazole, l-thyroxine, phenytoin, quinidine, ranitidine, tetracycline, and theophylline; administer separately when alterations in bioavailability are felt to be critical and monitor patients appropriately. Subtherapeutic PT with concomitant warfarin reported. Concomitant use with other products that contain aluminum (eg, aluminum-containing antacids) may increase the total body burden of aluminum.

PREGNANCY AND LACTATION
Category B, caution in nursing.

MECHANISM OF ACTION
DU-adherent complex; not established. Forms an ulcer-adherent complex that covers the ulcer site and protects it against further attack by acid, pepsin, and bile salts.

PHARMACOKINETICS
Absorption: GI (minimal). **Elimination:** Urine.

PATIENT CONSIDERATIONS
Assessment: Assess for hypersensitivity to the drug or to any of the excipients, chronic renal failure or if patient is receiving dialysis, pregnancy/nursing status, and possible drug interactions. (Sus) Assess for diabetes mellitus. (Tab) Assess for known conditions that may impair swallowing or any other conditions that may alter gag and cough reflexes, or diminish oropharyngeal coordination or motility.

Monitoring: Monitor for aluminum accumulation and toxicity in patients with renal impairment and other adverse reactions. Monitor renal function. (Sus) Monitor for episodes of hyperglycemia. (Tab) Monitor for aspiration with accompanying respiratory complications.

Counseling: Inform about the risks/benefits of treatment. Instruct to take exactly ud. Advise to contact physician if any side effects develop. Counsel about the possible drug interactions. Advise to notify physician if pregnant/nursing or planning to become pregnant.

CARBAMAZEPINE — carbamazepine　　　Rx

Class: Carboxamide

> Serious and sometimes fatal dermatologic reactions, including toxic epidermal necrolysis (TEN) and Stevens-Johnson syndrome (SJS) reported; increased risk w/ presence of HLA-B*1502 allele. Screen patients w/ ancestry in genetically at-risk populations for the presence of HLA-B*1502 prior to initiation of therapy. Avoid in patients testing positive for the allele unless benefits clearly outweigh risks. Aplastic anemia and agranulocytosis reported; obtain complete pretreatment hematological testing as a baseline and monitor closely if a patient exhibits low/decreased WBC or platelet counts during treatment. Consider discontinuation if evidence of significant bone marrow depression develops.

OTHER BRAND NAMES
Tegretol, Tegretol-XR, Epitol

ADULT DOSAGE

Trigeminal Neuralgia
Initial (Day 1): 100mg bid (tab/tab, extended-release [ER]) or 1/2 tsp qid (200mg/day) (sus)
Titrate: May increase by up to 200mg/day using increments of 100mg q12h (tab/tab, ER) or 50mg (1/2 tsp) qid (sus) prn
Maint: 400-800mg/day. Attempt to reduce dose to minimum effective level or even to d/c therapy at least once every 3 months
Max: 1200mg/day

Beneficial results have also been reported in glossopharyngeal neuralgia

Epilepsy
Partial Seizures w/ Complex Symptomatology (Psychomotor, Temporal Lobe), Generalized Tonic-Clonic Seizures (Grand Mal), and Mixed Seizure Patterns of These, or Other Partial or Generalized Seizures:
Initial: 200mg bid (tab/tab, ER) or 1 tsp qid (400mg/day) (sus)
Titrate: Increase at weekly intervals by adding up to 200mg/day bid (tab, ER) or tid or qid (all other formulations)
Maint: 800-1200mg/day
Max: 1200mg/day; doses up to 1600mg/day have been used in rare instances

Combination Therapy:
When added to existing anticonvulsant therapy, add gradually while other anticonvulsants are maintained or gradually decreased (except phenytoin, which may have to be increased)

Conversions
From Oral Carbamazepine Tabs to Carbamazepine Sus:
Patients should be converted by administering the same number of mg/day in smaller, more frequent doses (eg, bid tabs to tid sus)

From Carbamazepine Conventional Tabs to Carbamazepine ER Tabs:
The same total daily mg dose of carbamazepine ER tabs should be administered

PEDIATRIC DOSAGE

Epilepsy
Partial Seizures w/ Complex Symptomatology (Psychomotor, Temporal Lobe), Generalized Tonic-Clonic Seizures (Grand Mal), and Mixed Seizure Patterns of These, or Other Partial or Generalized Seizures:

<6 Years:
Initial: 10-20mg/kg/day bid or tid (tab) or qid (sus)
Titrate: Increase weekly to tid or qid (tab/sus)
Maint: Optimal clinical response is achieved at daily doses <35mg/kg; no recommendation regarding safety at doses >35mg/kg/24 hrs

6-12 Years:
Initial: 100mg bid (tab/tab, ER) or 1/2 tsp qid (200mg/day) (sus)
Titrate: Increase at weekly intervals by adding up to 100mg/day bid (tab, ER) or tid or qid (all other formulations)
Maint: 400-800mg/day
Max: 1000mg/day

>12 Years:
Initial: 200mg bid (tab/tab, ER) or 1 tsp qid (400mg/day) (sus)
Titrate: Increase at weekly intervals by adding up to 200mg/day bid (tab, ER) or tid or qid (all other formulations)
Maint: 800-1200mg/day
Max:
12-15 Years: 1000mg/day
>15 Years: 1200mg/day

Combination Therapy:
When added to existing anticonvulsant therapy, add gradually while other anticonvulsants are maintained or gradually decreased (except phenytoin, which may have to be increased)

Conversions
From Oral Carbamazepine Tabs to Carbamazepine Sus:
Patients should be converted by administering the same number of mg/day in smaller, more frequent doses (eg, bid tabs to tid sus)

From Carbamazepine Conventional Tabs to Carbamazepine ER Tabs:
The same total daily mg dose of carbamazepine ER tabs should be administered

ADMINISTRATION
Oral route

Take w/ meals.
Sus will produce higher peak levels than the same dose given as the tab; start patients given sus on lower doses and increase slowly to avoid unwanted side effects.

Sus
Do not administer simultaneously w/ other liquid medications or diluents.
Shake well before using.

Tab, ER
Swallow whole; do not chew or crush.

STORAGE
Tab, Chewable: 20-25°C (68-77°F). Protect from light/moisture. (Tegretol) **Tab, Chewable:** ≤30°C (86°F). Protect from light/moisture. **Sus:** ≤30°C (86°F). **Tab:** ≤30°C (86°F). Protect from moisture. **Tab, ER:** 25°C (77°F); excursions permitted to 15-30°C (59-86°F). Protect from moisture. (Epitol) **Tab:** 20-25°C (68-77°F). Protect from moisture.

HOW SUPPLIED
Tab, Chewable: 200mg*, (Tegretol) 100mg*; **Sus:** (Tegretol) 100mg/5mL [450mL]; **Tab:** (Tegretol, Epitol) 200mg*; **Tab, ER:** (Tegretol-XR) 100mg, 200mg, 400mg *scored

CONTRAINDICATIONS
History of previous bone marrow depression; hypersensitivity to the drug, or sensitivity to any of the tricyclic compounds (eg, amitriptyline, desipramine, imipramine, protriptyline, nortriptyline); coadministration w/ nefazodone; concomitant use w/ an MAOI or w/in 14 days after discontinuing an MAOI.

WARNINGS/PRECAUTIONS
D/C at 1st sign of rash; do not resume treatment and consider alternative therapy if signs/symptoms suggest SJS/TEN. Consider risks and benefits of therapy in patients known to be positive for HLA-A*3101. Patients w/ a history of adverse hematologic reaction to any drug may be particularly at risk of bone marrow depression. Drug reaction w/ eosinophilia and systemic symptoms (DRESS), also known as multiorgan hypersensitivity, reported; evaluate immediately if signs/symptoms (eg, fever, lymphadenopathy) are present and d/c if an alternative etiology cannot be established. Caution in patients w/ history of hypersensitivity reactions to anticonvulsants (eg, phenytoin, primidone, phenobarbital). Increased risk of suicidal thoughts or behavior reported. Has mild anticholinergic activity that may be associated w/ increased IOP; closely observe patients w/ increased IOP during therapy. Consider the possibility of activation of latent psychosis and, in elderly patients, of confusion or agitation. Avoid in patients w/ history of hepatic porphyria (eg, acute intermittent porphyria, variegate porphyria, porphyria cutanea tarda); acute attacks reported. Withdraw gradually to minimize potential of increased seizure frequency. Hyponatremia may occur and in many cases, appears to be caused by the syndrome of inappropriate antidiuretic hormone secretion; consider discontinuing therapy in patients w/ symptomatic hyponatremia. May cause fetal harm and symptoms representing neonatal withdrawal syndrome. Caution in patients w/ a mixed seizure disorder that includes atypical absence seizures; therapy associated w/ increased frequency of generalized convulsions in these patients. Caution in patients w/ history of cardiac conduction disturbance, cardiac/hepatic/renal damage, adverse hematologic or hypersensitivity reaction to other drugs, and interrupted courses of therapy w/ carbamazepine. Atrioventricular heart block (eg, 2nd- and 3rd-degree block) and hepatic effects (ranging from slight elevations in liver enzymes to rare cases of hepatic failure) reported. D/C if new or worsening clinical/lab evidence of liver dysfunction/hepatic damage, or active liver disease develops. Interference w/ some pregnancy tests, decreased values of thyroid function tests, renal dysfunction, and eye changes reported. Higher prevalence of teratogenic effects w/ the use of anticonvulsants in combination therapy; if therapy is to be continued, monotherapy may be preferable for pregnant women. **Sus/Tab, Chewable 200mg:** Contains sorbitol; avoid w/ rare hereditary problems of fructose intolerance. **Tab, ER:** Coating is not absorbed and is excreted in the feces; may be noticeable in the stool.

ADVERSE REACTIONS
Dizziness, drowsiness, unsteadiness, N/V.

DRUG INTERACTIONS
See Contraindications. Close monitoring of carbamazepine levels is indicated and dosage adjustment may be required when given w/ drugs that increase/decrease levels. CYP3A4 inhibitors (eg, azole antifungals, erythromycin, protease inhibitors) may increase levels. Coadministration of inhibitors of human microsomal epoxide hydrolase may result in increased carbamazepine-10,11 epoxide levels; adjust dose and/or monitor levels of carbamazepine when used w/ loxapine, quetiapine, or valproic acid. CYP3A4 inducers (eg, cisplatin, doxorubicin, rifampin) may decrease levels. May decrease levels of CYP1A2, 2B6, 2C9/19, and 3A4 substrates; monitoring of concentrations or dosage adjustment of the concomitant agents may be necessary. When added to aripiprazole therapy, double aripiprazole dose and if carbamazepine is later withdrawn, reduce aripiprazole dose. When used w/ tacrolimus, monitoring of tacrolimus levels and appropriate dosage adjustments are recommended. Avoid w/ temsirolimus; consider dose adjustment of temsirolimus if coadministration is a must. Avoid w/ lapatinib; gradually titrate up dose of lapatinib if carbamazepine is started in a patient already taking lapatinib and reduce lapatinib dose when carbamazepine is discontinued. Monitor concentrations of valproate when carbamazepine is introduced or withdrawn in patients using valproic acid. May cause, or would be expected to cause, decreased levels of the following drugs, for which monitoring of concentrations or dosage adjustment may be necessary: acetaminophen, albendazole, alprazolam, aprepitant, buprenorphine, bupropion, citalopram, clonazepam, clozapine, corticosteroids (eg, prednisolone, dexamethasone), cyclosporine, dicumarol, dihydropyridine calcium channel blockers (eg, felodipine), doxycycline, ethosuximide, everolimus, haloperidol, imatinib, itraconazole, lamotrigine, levothyroxine, methadone, methsuximide, mianserin, midazolam, olanzapine, oxcarbazepine, paliperidone, phensuximide, phenytoin, praziquantel, protease inhibitors, risperidone, sertraline, sirolimus, tadalafil, theophylline, tiagabine, topiramate, tramadol, trazodone, TCAs (eg, imipramine, amitriptyline, nortriptyline), valproate, warfarin, ziprasidone, zonisamide. May increase cyclophosphamide toxicity. May increase risk of neurotoxic side effects w/ lithium. Increased isoniazid-induced hepatotoxicity reported w/ isoniazid. Alterations of thyroid function reported w/ other anticonvulsant medications. May decrease levels of hormonal contraceptive products (eg, oral and levonorgestrel subdermal implant contraceptives) that may render contraceptives less effective; consider alternative or back-up method of contraception. Resistance to the neuromuscular blocking action of the nondepolarizing neuromuscular blocking agents (eg, pancuronium, vecuronium, rocuronium) reported w/ chronic carbamazepine administration; monitor closely for more rapid recovery from neuromuscular blockade than expected, and infusion rate requirements may be higher. Increased risk of developing hyponatremia w/ diuretics. **Sus:** Occurrence of stool precipitate reported w/ liquid chlorpromazine or thioridazine.

PREGNANCY AND LACTATION
Pregnancy: Category D. Physicians are advised to recommend that pregnant patients enroll in the North American Antiepileptic Drug (NAAED) Pregnancy Registry.
Lactation: Not for use in nursing.

MECHANISM OF ACTION
Carboxamide; has not been established. Appears to act by reducing polysynaptic responses and blocking the post-tetanic potentiation. Depresses thalamic potential and bulbar and polysynaptic reflexes.

PHARMACOKINETICS
Absorption: T_{max}=1.5 hrs (sus), 4-5 hrs (tab), 3-12 hrs (tab, ER). **Distribution:** Plasma protein binding (76%); crosses the placenta; found in breast milk.
Metabolism: Liver via CYP3A4; carbamazepine-10,11-epoxide (active metabolite).
Elimination: Urine (72%; 3% unchanged), feces (28%); $T_{1/2}$=25-65 hrs (initial), 12-17 hrs (repeated doses).

PATIENT CONSIDERATIONS
Assessment: Assess for hypersensitivity to the drug, known sensitivity to any of the tricyclic compounds, mixed seizure disorder, history of cardiac conduction disturbance, renal/hepatic impairment, any other conditions where treatment is contraindicated or cautioned, pregnancy/nursing status, and possible drug interactions. Perform detailed history and physical exam prior to treatment. Screen for HLA-B*1502 and HLA-A*3101 allele in suspected populations. Obtain baseline CBCs w/ platelets and reticulocytes and serum iron, LFTs, complete urinalysis, BUN determinations, and eye examination (including slit-lamp exam, funduscopy, and tonometry).

Monitoring: Monitor for signs/symptoms of dermatologic reactions, DRESS, bone marrow depression, aplastic anemia, agranulocytosis, increase in seizure frequency, emergence or worsening of depression, suicidal thoughts/behavior, unusual changes in mood/behavior, latent psychosis, confusion or agitation in elderly patients, hepatic effects, and other adverse reactions. Periodically monitor WBC and platelet counts, LFTs, serum drug levels, complete urinalysis, BUN determinations, and eye examinations.

Counseling: Inform of the early toxic signs and symptoms of a potential hematologic problem, as well as dermatologic, hypersensitivity, or hepatic reactions; advise to report to physician even if the signs and symptoms are mild or when occurring after extended use. Instruct to immediately contact physician if a skin reaction occurs. Inform about the increased risk of suicidal thoughts and behavior; advise to report behaviors of concern immediately and to be alert for the emergence/worsening of symptoms of depression, any unusual changes in mood or behavior, the emergence of suicidal thoughts, or behavior/thoughts about self-harm. Advise to report the use of any other prescription or nonprescription medications or herbal products. Instruct to exercise caution when taken w/ alcohol due to a possible additive sedative effect. Inform that drowsiness or dizziness may occur; caution against hazardous tasks. Encourage patients to enroll in the NAAED Pregnancy Registry.

CARBATROL — carbamazepine   Rx
Class: Carboxamide

> Serious and fatal dermatologic reactions, including toxic epidermal necrolysis (TEN) and Stevens-Johnson syndrome (SJS) reported; increased risk with presence of HLA-B*1502 allele. Screen patients with ancestry in genetically at risk populations for the presence of HLA-B*1502 prior to initiation of therapy. Avoid in patients testing positive for the allele unless the benefits clearly outweigh the risks. Aplastic anemia and agranulocytosis reported. Obtain complete pretreatment hematological testing as a baseline. Consider discontinuation if evidence of bone marrow depression develops.

ADULT DOSAGE
Epilepsy
Partial Seizures w/ Complex Symptomatology (Psychomotor, Temporal Lobe), Generalized Tonic-Clonic Seizures (Grand Mal), and Mixed Seizure Patterns of These, or Other Partial or Generalized Seizures:
Initial: 200mg bid
Titrate: Increase at weekly intervals by adding up to 200mg/day until optimal response is obtained
Maint: 800-1200mg/day
Max: 1200mg/day; doses up to 1600mg/day have been used

Combination Therapy:
When added to existing anticonvulsant therapy, add gradually while other anticonvulsants are maintained or gradually decreased (except phenytoin, which may have to be increased)

Trigeminal Neuralgia
Initial (Day 1): One 200mg cap
Titrate: May increase by up to 200mg/day q12h prn
Maint: 400-800mg/day. Attempt to reduce dose to minimum effective level or even to d/c therapy at least once every 3 months

PEDIATRIC DOSAGE
Epilepsy
Partial Seizures w/ Complex Symptomatology (Psychomotor, Temporal Lobe), Generalized Tonic-Clonic Seizures (Grand Mal), and Mixed Seizure Patterns of These, or Other Partial or Generalized Seizures:
>12 Years:
Initial: 200mg bid
Titrate: Increase at weekly intervals by adding up to 200mg/day until optimal response is obtained
Maint: 800-1200mg/day
Max:
12-15 Years: 1000mg/day
>15 Years: 1200mg/day

Combination Therapy:
When added to existing anticonvulsant therapy, add gradually while other anticonvulsants are maintained or gradually decreased (except phenytoin, which may have to be increased)

Conversions
From Immediate-Release (IR) Carbamazepine:
<12 Years:
If receiving ≥400mg/day of IR carbamazepine, may be converted to same total daily dose of extended-

Max: 1200mg/day
Beneficial results have also been reported in glossopharyngeal neuralgia

Conversions
From Immediate-Release Carbamazepine:
Administer the same total daily mg dose. Closely monitor for seizure control following conversion; may need to adjust total daily dose, depending on response

---

release carbamazepine, using bid regimen. Optimal response usually achieved at doses <35mg/kg/day
>12 Years:
Administer the same total daily mg dose
Closely monitor for seizure control following conversion; may need to adjust total daily dose, depending on response

---

ADMINISTRATION
Oral route
Take w/ or w/o food
Caps may be swallowed whole or opened and all the beads sprinkled on a tsp of soft food (eg, applesauce); make sure all food/medicine mixture is swallowed
Do not crush/chew caps or the sprinkled beads

STORAGE
25°C (77°F); excursions permitted to 15-30°C (59-86°F). Protect from light and moisture.

HOW SUPPLIED
Cap, Extended-Release: 100mg, 200mg, 300mg

CONTRAINDICATIONS
History of previous bone marrow depression, hypersensitivity to the drug or known sensitivity to TCAs (eg, amitriptyline, desipramine, imipramine, protriptyline, nortriptyline), coadministration w/ nefazodone or delavirdine. Concomitant use of an MAOI or w/in 14 days after discontinuing an MAOI.

WARNINGS/PRECAUTIONS
D/C at first sign of rash; do not resume treatment and consider alternative therapy if signs/symptoms suggest SJS/TEN. Consider risks and benefits of therapy in patients known to be positive for HLA-A*3101. Drug reaction with eosinophilia and systemic symptoms (DRESS), also known as multiorgan hypersensitivity, may occur; evaluate immediately if signs/symptoms (eg, fever, lymphadenopathy) are present and d/c if alternative etiology cannot be established. Caution in patients with history of hypersensitivity reactions to anticonvulsants (eg, phenytoin, primidone, phenobarbital). Abrupt discontinuation of antiepileptic drugs may increase seizure frequency, including status epilepticus; reduce dose gradually. Increased risk of suicidal thoughts or behavior reported; monitor for the emergence/worsening of depression, suicidal thoughts/behavior, or any changes in mood or behavior. May cause fetal harm and symptoms representing neonatal withdrawal syndrome. Has mild anticholinergic activity; closely observe patients with increased intraocular pressure (IOP). Consider the possibility of activation of latent psychosis and, in the elderly, of confusion or agitation. Avoid in patients with history of hepatic porphyria (eg, acute intermittent porphyria, variegate porphyria, porphyria cutanea tarda); acute attacks reported. Caution in patients with history of cardiac/hepatic/renal damage, adverse hematologic reactions to drugs, interrupted courses of therapy with carbamazepine, and mixed seizure disorder. Hyponatremia may occur; consider discontinuation in patients with symptomatic hyponatremia. Hepatic failure reported. Caution with history of liver disease; d/c immediately in cases of aggravated liver dysfunction or active liver disease. Interference with some pregnancy tests, decreased values of thyroid function tests, renal dysfunction, eye changes, increased total cholesterol, LDL, and HDL reported.

ADVERSE REACTIONS
Dizziness, drowsiness, unsteadiness, N/V, aplastic anemia, agranulocytosis, SJS, TEN.

DRUG INTERACTIONS
See Contraindications. CYP3A4 and/or epoxide hydrolase inhibitors (eg, azole antifungals, cimetidine, erythromycin, protease inhibitors) may increase plasma levels. CYP3A4 inducers (eg, cisplatin, doxorubicin, rifampin) may decrease plasma levels. May decrease plasma levels of CYP1A2 and CYP3A4 substrates (eg, acetaminophen, alprazolam, trazodone, warfarin). May decrease plasma levels of hormonal contraceptive products (eg, oral and levonorgestrel subdermal implant contraceptives) that may render contraceptives less effective. May reduce warfarin's anticoagulant effect. May increase plasma levels of clomipramine HCl and primidone. May increase or decrease plasma level of phenytoin. Increased risk of neurotoxic side effects with lithium. Antimalarial drugs (eg, chloroquine, mefloquine) may antagonize activity. Caution with other centrally acting drugs and alcohol.

PREGNANCY AND LACTATION
Category D, not for use in nursing.

MECHANISM OF ACTION
Carboxamide; has not been established. Appears to act by reducing polysynaptic responses and blocking the post-tetanic potentiation. Depresses thalamic potential and bulbar and polysynaptic reflexes.

PHARMACOKINETICS
Absorption: (Single 200mg dose) C_{max}=1.9μg/mL, 0.11μg/mL carbamazepine-10,11-epoxide (CBZ-E); T_{max}=19 hrs, 36 hrs (CBZ-E). (Multiple 800mg dose) C_{max}=11μg/mL, 2.2μg/mL (CBZ-E); T_{max}=5.9 hrs, 14 hrs (CBZ-E). **Distribution:** Plasma protein binding (76%), (50% CBZ-E); crosses the placenta; found in breast milk. **Metabolism:** Liver via CYP3A4; CBZ-E (active metabolite). **Elimination:** Urine (72%, 3% unchanged), feces (28%); $T_{1/2}$=35-40 hrs (single dose), 12-17 hrs (multiple doses), 34 hrs (CBZ-E).

PATIENT CONSIDERATIONS

Assessment: Assess for conditions where treatment is contraindicated or cautioned, pregnancy/nursing status, and possible drug interactions. Perform detailed history and physical exam prior to treatment. Screen for HLA-B*1502 and HLA-A*3101 allele in suspected populations. Obtain baseline CBC with platelet and reticulocyte counts, serum iron, LFTs, complete urinalysis, BUN determinations, lipid profile, and eye examinations (eg, including slit-lamp exam, funduscopy, and tonometry).

Monitoring: Monitor for signs/symptoms of dermatologic reactions, hypersensitivity reactions, aplastic anemia, agranulocytosis, bone marrow depression, worsening of seizure frequency, multiorgan hypersensitivity reactions, emergence or worsening of depression, suicidal thoughts/behavior, unusual changes in mood or behavior, hyponatremia, hepatic failure, liver dysfunction aggravation or active liver disease, DRESS, and other adverse reactions. Periodically monitor WBC count, platelet count, LFTs, complete urinalysis, BUN determinations, lipid profile, serum drug levels, and eye examinations. Monitor patients with increased IOP.

Counseling: Instruct to read Medication Guide prior to therapy. Inform of the early toxic signs and symptoms of potential hematologic, dermatologic, hypersensitivity, or hepatic reactions; advise to report to physician even if the signs and symptoms are mild or when occurring after extended use. Counsel about the increased risk of suicidal thoughts and behavior; advise to report behaviors of concern immediately and to be alert for the emergence/worsening of depression, unusual changes in mood or behavior, the emergence of suicidal thoughts, or for behavior/thoughts about self-harm. Caution against hazardous tasks. Advise to exercise caution if consuming alcohol. Advise to report the use of any other prescription or nonprescription medication or herbal products. Instruct to notify physician if pregnant or intending to become pregnant. Encourage patients to enroll in the North American Antiepileptic Drug (NAAED) Pregnancy Registry.

CARDENE IV — nicardipine hydrochloride   Rx

Class: Calcium channel blocker (CCB) (dihydropyridine)

ADULT DOSAGE	PEDIATRIC DOSAGE
Hypertension	Pediatric use may not have been established
Short-term treatment when oral therapy is not feasible or not desirable	

Patients Not Receiving Oral Nicardipine:
Initial: 5mg/hr IV infusion
Titrate: May increase by 2.5mg/hr every 5 min (for rapid titration) to 15 min (for gradual titration) if desired BP reduction is not achieved
Max: 15mg/hr
Decrease infusion rate to 3mg/hr after BP goal is achieved w/ rapid titration

IV Dosage as a Substitute for Oral Nicardipine Therapy:
20mg PO q8h=0.5mg/hr IV infusion
30mg PO q8h=1.2mg/hr IV infusion
40mg PO q8h=2.2mg/hr IV infusion

Transition to Oral Antihypertensives:
Transfer to Oral Nicardipine: Give 1st dose 1 hr prior to discontinuation of infusion
Transfer to Oral Antihypertensive Other Than Nicardipine: Initiate therapy upon discontinuation of IV nicardipine

DOSING CONSIDERATIONS
Renal Impairment
Titrate slowly

Hepatic Impairment
Impaired Function/Reduced Hepatic Blood Flow: Consider lower dosages and titrate slowly

Elderly
Use low initial doses

Other Important Considerations
Heart Failure: Titrate slowly

D/C infusion if there is concern of impending hypotension/tachycardia; may restart infusion at low doses (3-5mg/hr) when BP has stabilized and adjust to maintain desired BP

ADMINISTRATION
IV route

Administer by a central line or through a large peripheral vein; change infusion site q12h if administered via peripheral vein

Premixed Sol
No further dilution is required
Do not combine w/ any product in the same IV line or premixed container; do not add supplementary medication to the bag
Do not use plastic containers in series connections

Ampules
Administer by slow continuous infusion at a concentration of 0.1mg/mL
Dilute each ampule (25mg) w/ 240mL of compatible IV fluid (yielding 250mL of sol at a concentration of 0.1mg/mL); diluted sol is stable for 24 hrs at room temperature

IV Compatibilities:
Compatible and stable in glass or polyvinyl chloride containers for 24 hrs at controlled room temperature w/:
D5 inj
D5 and NaCl 0.45% inj
D5 and NaCl 0.9% inj
D5 w/ 40mEq K+
NaCl 0.45% inj
NaCl 0.9% inj

IV Incompatibilities:
Sodium bicarbonate (5%) inj
Lactated Ringer's inj

STORAGE
20-25°C (68-77°F). Avoid excessive heat. Protect from light. Premixed Sol: Protect from freezing.

HOW SUPPLIED
Inj: 2.5mg/mL [10mL, ampule]; 0.1mg/mL, 0.2mg/mL [200mL, premixed sol]

CONTRAINDICATIONS
Advanced aortic stenosis.

WARNINGS/PRECAUTIONS
May occasionally produce symptomatic hypotension or tachycardia. Avoid systemic hypotension when administering drug to patients who have sustained an acute cerebral infarction or hemorrhage. May induce or exacerbate angina in coronary artery disease (CAD) patients. Caution w/ heart failure (HF) or significant left ventricular dysfunction. To reduce possibility of venous thrombosis, phlebitis, local irritation, swelling, extravasation, and occurrence of vascular impairment, administer through large peripheral or central veins; change IV site q12h to minimize risk of peripheral venous irritation.

ADVERSE REACTIONS
Headache, hypotension, tachycardia, N/V.

DRUG INTERACTIONS
Titrate slowly when used in combination w/ β-blockers in patients w/ HF or significant left ventricular dysfunction due to possible negative inotropic effects. Increased nicardipine levels when oral nicardipine is given w/ cimetidine; frequently monitor response in patients receiving both drugs. Elevated cyclosporine levels reported w/ oral nicardipine; closely monitor cyclosporine levels and reduce cyclosporine dose accordingly.

PREGNANCY AND LACTATION
Category C, caution in nursing.

MECHANISM OF ACTION
Calcium channel blocker (dihydropyridine); inhibits transmembrane influx of Ca^{2+} ions into cardiac muscle and smooth muscle w/o changing serum Ca^{2+} concentrations.

PHARMACOKINETICS
Distribution: V_d=8.3L/kg; plasma protein binding (>95%); minimally excreted in breast milk. **Metabolism:** Liver (rapid and extensive). **Elimination:** Urine (49%), feces (43%); $T_{1/2}$=14.4 hrs.

PATIENT CONSIDERATIONS
Assessment: Assess for advanced aortic stenosis, HF, left ventricular dysfunction, acute cerebral infarction or hemorrhage, hepatic/renal impairment, pregnancy/nursing status, and possible drug interactions.

Monitoring: Monitor for symptomatic hypotension, tachycardia, induction or exacerbation of angina, and other adverse reactions. Monitor BP and HR during administration. Closely monitor responses w/ impaired liver function or reduced hepatic blood flow.

Counseling: Advise to seek medical attention if adverse reactions occur.

CARDIZEM CD — diltiazem hydrochloride   Rx

Class: Calcium channel blocker (CCB) (nondihydropyridine)

OTHER BRAND NAMES
Cartia XT

ADULT DOSAGE	PEDIATRIC DOSAGE
Hypertension	Pediatric use may not have been established
Initial (Monotherapy): 180-240mg qd	
Titrate: Max antihypertensive effect usually observed by 14 days of chronic therapy; schedule dose adjustments accordingly	
Usual Range: 240-360mg qd	
Max: 480mg qd	
Angina	
Chronic Stable Angina and Angina Due to Coronary Artery Spasm:	
Initial: 120mg or 180mg qd	
Titrate: Adjust to each patient's needs; may be carried out over a 7- to 14-day period when necessary	
Max: 480mg qd	

DOSING CONSIDERATIONS
Concomitant Medications
SL Nitroglycerin: May take as required to abort acute anginal attacks during therapy
Prophylactic Nitrate Therapy: May be coadministered w/ short- and long-acting nitrates
Other Antihypertensives: Diltiazem or the concomitant antihypertensives may need to be adjusted when adding 1 to the other

Elderly
Start at lower end of dosing range

ADMINISTRATION
Oral route

STORAGE
Avoid excessive humidity. **Cardizem CD:** 25°C (77°F); excursions permitted to 15-30°C (59-86°F). **Cartia XT:** 20-25°C (68-77°F).

HOW SUPPLIED
Cap, Extended-Release: (Cartia XT) 120mg, 180mg, 240mg, 300mg, (Cardizem CD) 360mg

CONTRAINDICATIONS
Sick sinus syndrome and 2nd- or 3rd-degree atrioventricular block (AV) block (except w/ functioning ventricular pacemaker), hypotension (<90mmHg systolic), demonstrated hypersensitivity to the drug, acute MI and pulmonary congestion documented by x-ray on admission.

WARNINGS/PRECAUTIONS
May cause abnormally slow HR(s) (particularly in patients w/ sick sinus syndrome) or 2nd- or 3rd-degree AV block. Periods of asystole (2-5 sec) reported in a patient w/ Prinzmetal's angina. Worsening of CHF reported in patients w/ preexisting impairment of ventricular function. Symptomatic hypotension may occur. Mild transaminase elevation w/ or w/o concomitant alkaline phosphatase and bilirubin elevation reported. Significant enzyme elevations and other phenomena consistent w/ acute hepatic injury reported in rare instances. Dermatologic events (eg, erythema multiforme, exfoliative dermatitis) may occur; d/c if a dermatologic reaction persists.

ADVERSE REACTIONS
Headache, dizziness, bradycardia, 1st-degree AV block, edema, asthenia.

DRUG INTERACTIONS
See Dosing Considerations. May increase levels of propranolol, carbamazepine, buspirone, and lovastatin. Increased levels w/ cimetidine; carefully monitor for a change in pharmacological effect when initiating and discontinuing therapy w/ cimetidine. Monitor digoxin and cyclosporine levels. Depression of cardiac contractility, conductivity, automaticity, and vascular dilation potentiated w/ anesthetics. Additive cardiac conduction effects w/ digitalis or β-blockers. Potential additive effects w/ agents known to affect cardiac contractility and/or conduction; caution and slow titration is warranted. May have significant impact on efficacy and side effect profile w/ CYP3A4 substrates, inducers, and inhibitors. Avoid w/ CYP3A4 inducers (eg, rifampin). Patients taking other drugs that are CYP3A4 substrates, especially patients w/ renal and/or hepatic impairment, may require dosage adjustment when starting or stopping concomitantly administered diltiazem. Sinus bradycardia resulting in hospitalization and pacemaker insertion reported w/ clonidine; monitor HR. Increased exposure of simvastatin; limit daily doses of simvastatin to 10mg and diltiazem to 240mg. Risk of myopathy and rhabdomyolysis w/ statins metabolized by CYP3A4 may be increased; when possible, use a non-CYP3A4 metabolized statin or consider dose adjustments for both diltiazem and the statin. May increase elimination of half-lives and levels of midazolam, triazolam, and quinidine. **Cardizem CD:** Concomitant use w/ alcohol may lead to more rapid absorption and an increase in the systemic exposure of diltiazem, and associated dose-related adverse reactions; avoid consumption of alcohol.

PREGNANCY AND LACTATION
Pregnancy: There are no well-controlled studies in pregnant women; only use in pregnant women if the potential benefit justifies the potential risk.
Lactation: Diltiazem is excreted in human milk; not for use in nursing.

MECHANISM OF ACTION
Calcium channel blocker; inhibits cellular influx of Ca^{2+} ions during membrane depolarization of cardiac and vascular smooth muscle. **HTN:** Relaxes vascular smooth muscle, resulting in decreased peripheral vascular resistance. **Angina:** Produces increases in exercise tolerance by its ability to reduce myocardial oxygen demand; accomplished via reduction in HR and systemic BP at submaximal and maximal workloads.

PHARMACOKINETICS
Absorption: Well-absorbed. Absolute bioavailability (40%); T_{max}=10-14 hrs. **Distribution:** Plasma protein binding (70-80%); found in breast milk. **Metabolism:** Liver (extensive). **Elimination:** Urine (2-4%, unchanged), bile. $T_{1/2}$=5-8 hrs.

PATIENT CONSIDERATIONS
Assessment: Assess for previous hypersensitivity to the drug, sick sinus syndrome, 2nd- or 3rd-degree AV block, presence of a functioning ventricular pacemaker, hypotension, acute MI and pulmonary congestion, ventricular dysfunction, hepatic/renal impairment, pregnancy/nursing status, and possible drug interactions.

Monitoring: Monitor for bradycardia, AV block, symptomatic hypotension, dermatological events, and other adverse reactions. Perform regular monitoring of liver and renal function.

Counseling: Advise to report any adverse reactions to physician and to notify physician if pregnant or nursing.

CARDIZEM LA — diltiazem hydrochloride   Rx
Class: Calcium channel blocker (CCB) (nondihydropyridine)

ADULT DOSAGE	PEDIATRIC DOSAGE
Hypertension	Pediatric use may not have been established
Initial: 180-240mg qd; some patients may respond to lower doses	
Titrate: Adjust according to BP	
Max: 540mg/day	
Angina	
Improve exercise tolerance in patients w/ chronic stable angina	
Initial: 180mg qd	
Titrate: Increase dose at intervals of 7-14-days if adequate response is not obtained	
Max: 360mg	
Conversions	
Switching from Diltiazem Alone or in Combination w/ Other Medications: May switch to Cardizem LA qd at the nearest equivalent total daily dose. Higher doses may be needed in some patients based on clinical response	

DOSING CONSIDERATIONS
Elderly
Start at lower end of dosing range

ADMINISTRATION
Oral route

Take at approx the same time each day
Swallow tab whole; do not chew or crush

STORAGE
25°C (77°F); excursions permitted to 15-30°C (59-86°F). Avoid excessive humidity and temperatures >30°C (86°F).

HOW SUPPLIED
Tab, Extended-Release: 120mg, 180mg, 240mg, 300mg, 360mg, 420mg

CONTRAINDICATIONS
Sick sinus syndrome and 2nd- or 3rd-degree atrioventricular (AV) block (except w/ functioning ventricular pacemaker), hypotension (<90mmHg systolic), demonstrated hypersensitivity to the drug, acute MI and pulmonary congestion.

WARNINGS/PRECAUTIONS
May cause abnormally slow HR(s) or 2nd- or 3rd-degree AV block. Patients w/ sick sinus syndrome are at increased risk of bradycardia. Periods of asystole (2-5 sec) reported in a patient w/ Prinzmetal's angina. Worsening of heart failure (HF) reported in patients w/ ventricular impairment. Significant elevations in liver enzymes (eg, alkaline phosphatase, lactate dehydrogenase, AST, ALT) and signs of acute hepatic injury reported; mild elevations of transaminases w/ and w/o concomitant elevation in alkaline phosphatase and bilirubin also observed. Stevens-Johnson syndrome (SJS), toxic epidermal necrolysis (TEN), erythema multiforme, and/or exfoliative dermatitis reported.

ADVERSE REACTIONS
Edema lower limb, dizziness, fatigue, bradycardia, 1st degree AV block.

DRUG INTERACTIONS
Use w/ other agents known to affect cardiac conduction or contractility may increase risk of bradycardia, AV block, and HF. β-blockers or digitalis may result in additive effects on cardiac conduction. Increased exposure of simvastatin; limit daily dose of simvastatin to 10mg and diltiazem to 240mg if coadministration is required. Avoid w/ rifampin.

PREGNANCY AND LACTATION
Pregnancy: Category C.
Lactation: Not for use in nursing.

MECHANISM OF ACTION
Calcium channel blocker; inhibits cellular influx of Ca^{2+} ions during membrane depolarization of cardiac and vascular smooth muscle. HTN: Relaxes vascular smooth muscle, resulting in decreased peripheral vascular resistance. Angina: Produces increases in exercise tolerance by its ability to reduce myocardial oxygen demand; accomplished via reduction in HR and systemic BP at submaximal and maximal workloads.

PHARMACOKINETICS
Absorption: Well-absorbed from GI tract. Absolute bioavailability (40%); T_{max}=11-18 hrs. **Distribution:** Plasma protein binding (70-80%); found in breast milk. **Metabolism:** Liver (extensive). **Elimination:** Urine (2-4%, unchanged); $T_{1/2}$=6-9 hrs (single/multiple dose), 2-5 hrs (IV).

PATIENT CONSIDERATIONS
Assessment: Assess for previous hypersensitivity to the drug, sick sinus syndrome, 2nd- or 3rd-degree AV block, presence of a functioning ventricular pacemaker, hypotension, acute MI and pulmonary congestion, ventricular impairment, pregnancy/nursing status, and possible drug interactions. Obtain baseline hepatic function.

Monitoring: Monitor for elevation of liver enzymes, signs of acute hepatic injury, SJS, TEN, erythema multiforme, exfoliative dermatitis, and other adverse reactions. Monitor effects on HR and cardiac conduction. Monitor for worsening of HF in patients w/ ventricular impairment.

Counseling: Advise to consult prescribing physician before taking/stopping any other medications (eg, OTC products, nutritional supplements [eg, St. John's wort]). Advise to contact physician immediately if possible adverse reactions (eg, bradycardia, arrhythmias, symptoms indicative of hypotension or HF, hepatic/skin reactions) develop. Advise to consult physician if pregnant/planning to become pregnant.

CARDURA — doxazosin mesylate   Rx

Class: Alpha₁ blocker (quinazoline)

ADULT DOSAGE

Hypertension
Initial: 1mg qd
Titrate: May double daily dose up to 16mg qd, prn, to achieve desired reduction in BP

If discontinued for several days, restart using the initial dosing regimen

Benign Prostatic Hyperplasia
Initial: 1mg qd (am or pm)
Titrate: May increase to 2mg and thereafter to 4mg, and 8mg qd in 1- to 2-week intervals, depending on urodynamics and BPH symptomatology
Max: 8mg qd

If discontinued for several days, restart using the initial dosing regimen

PEDIATRIC DOSAGE
Pediatric use may not have been established

DOSING CONSIDERATIONS
Hepatic Impairment
Child Pugh Class A and B: Monitor BP and for symptoms of hypotension
Child Pugh Class C: Not recommended

Elderly
Start at lower end of dosing range

ADMINISTRATION
Oral route

Monitor BP for at least 6 hrs after administering the initial dose and w/ each dose increase.

STORAGE
25°C (77°F); excursions permitted to 15-30°C (59-86°F).

HOW SUPPLIED
Tab: 1mg*, 2mg*, 4mg*, 8mg* *scored

CONTRAINDICATIONS
Hypersensitivity to doxazosin, other quinazolines (eg, prazosin, terazosin), or any components of this product.

WARNINGS/PRECAUTIONS
Postural hypotension w/ or w/o symptoms (eg, dizziness) and syncope may develop. Intraoperative floppy iris syndrome (IFIS) has been observed during cataract surgery in some patients on, or previously treated w/, α₁-blockers. Rule out carcinoma of the prostate prior to therapy. Associated w/ priapism; may lead to permanent impotence if not promptly treated.

ADVERSE REACTIONS
Fatigue, malaise, hypotension, dizziness.

DRUG INTERACTIONS
Strong CYP3A inhibitors may increase doxazosin exposure; monitor BP and for symptoms of hypotension when used concomitantly w/ strong CYP3A inhibitors. May result in additive BP-lowering effects and symptomatic hypotension w/ PDE-5 inhibitors; monitor BP and for symptoms of hypotension.

PREGNANCY AND LACTATION
Pregnancy: The limited available data w/ doxazosin in pregnant women are not sufficient to inform a drug-associated risk for major birth defects and miscarriage; untreated HTN during pregnancy can result in increased maternal risks.
Lactation: Data is insufficient to confirm the presence of doxazosin in human milk.

MECHANISM OF ACTION
α₁-blocker. **BPH:** Decreases urethral resistance and may relieve the obstruction and BPH symptoms and improve urine flow. **HTN:** Decreases systemic vascular resistance.

PHARMACOKINETICS
Absorption: Bioavailability (65%); T_{max}=2-3 hrs. **Distribution:** Plasma protein binding (98%). **Metabolism:** Liver (extensive); O-demethylation or hydroxylation. **Elimination:** Feces (63%, 4.8% unchanged), urine (9%, trace amounts unchanged); $T_{1/2}$=22 hrs.

PATIENT CONSIDERATIONS
Assessment: Assess for hypersensitivity to doxazosin, other quinazolines (eg, prazosin, terazosin), or any components of this product; hepatic impairment; prostate cancer; pregnancy/nursing status; and possible drug interactions. Assess BP.

Monitoring: Monitor for signs/symptoms of postural hypotension, syncope, IFIS during cataract surgery, priapism, and other adverse reactions. Monitor BP for at least 6 hrs after administering the initial dose and w/ each dose increase.

Counseling: Inform of the possibility of syncopal and orthostatic symptoms, especially at the initiation of therapy; urge to avoid driving or hazardous tasks for 24 hrs after the 1st dose, dose increase, and interruption of therapy when treatment is resumed. Instruct to report to physician if symptoms of postural hypotension develop. Advise of possibility of priapism and to seek immediate medical attention if this occurs. Counsel to inform surgeon of drug use prior to cataract surgery.

CARDURA XL — doxazosin mesylate   Rx

Class: Alpha₁ blocker (quinazoline)

ADULT DOSAGE

Benign Prostatic Hyperplasia
Initial: 4mg qd w/ breakfast
Titrate: May increase to 8mg after 3-4 weeks based on symptomatic response and tolerability
Max: 8mg

If discontinued for several days, restart using 4mg qd dose

Conversions
Switching from Cardura Immediate-Release to Cardura XL:
Initial: 4mg qd; final pm dose of Cardura should not be taken prior to starting therapy w/ Cardura XL

PEDIATRIC DOSAGE
Pediatric use may not have been established

DOSING CONSIDERATIONS
Concomitant Medications
PDE-5 Inhibitors: Initiate PDE-5 inhibitor therapy at the lowest dose

Hepatic Impairment
Severe: Not recommended
Mild or Moderate: Use caution

ADMINISTRATION
Oral route

Swallow tab whole; do not chew, divide, cut, or crush

STORAGE
25°C (77°F); excursions permitted to 15-30°C (59-86°F).

HOW SUPPLIED
Tab, Extended-Release: 4mg, 8mg

CONTRAINDICATIONS
Known hypersensitivity to doxazosin, other quinazolines (eg, prazosin, terazosin), or any inert ingredients.

WARNINGS/PRECAUTIONS
Postural hypotension w/ or w/o symptoms (eg, dizziness) and syncope may develop; caution w/ symptomatic hypotension or patients who have had a hypotensive response to other medications. Intraoperative floppy iris syndrome has been observed during cataract surgery in some patients on, or previously treated w/, α₁-blockers. Caution w/ preexisting severe GI narrowing (pathologic or iatrogenic). Prostate cancer causes many of the same symptoms associated w/ BPH; rule out prostate cancer prior to therapy. D/C if symptoms of worsening of or new onset of angina pectoris develop. Priapism reported (rarely); may lead to permanent impotence if not promptly treated.

ADVERSE REACTIONS
Dizziness, asthenia, headache, respiratory tract infection, abdominal pain, hypotension, somnolence, vertigo, dyspepsia, myalgia, UTI, postural hypotension, nausea, dyspnea.

DRUG INTERACTIONS
Caution w/ strong CYP3A4 inhibitors (eg, atazanavir, clarithromycin, itraconazole). Additive BP-lowering effects and symptomatic hypotension w/ PDE-5 inhibitors.

PREGNANCY AND LACTATION
Pregnancy: Category C, not indicated for use in women.
Lactation: Not for use in nursing.

MECHANISM OF ACTION
α₁-blocker; antagonizes α₁-agonist-induced contractions in the prostate, decreasing urethral resistance, which may relieve BPH symptoms and improve urine flow.

PHARMACOKINETICS
Absorption: (4mg) C_{max}=10.1ng/mL, AUC=183ng•hr/mL, T_{max}=8 hrs. (8mg) C_{max}=25.8ng/mL, AUC=472ng•hr/mL, T_{max}=9 hrs. **Distribution:** Plasma protein binding (98%). **Metabolism:** Liver (extensive) via CYP3A4 (major) and CYP2D6, CYP2C19 (minor). **Elimination:** $T_{1/2}$=15-19 hrs.

PATIENT CONSIDERATIONS
Assessment: Assess for hepatic impairment, symptomatic hypotension, history of hypotensive response to other medications, severe GI narrowing (chronic constipation), coronary insufficiency, and possible drug interactions. Rule out prostate cancer.

Monitoring: Monitor for signs/symptoms of postural hypotension, new onset or worsening of angina pectoris, and priapism.

Counseling: Instruct to take exactly ud. Advise that symptoms related to postural hypotension (eg, dizziness, syncope) may occur; caution about driving, operating machinery, or performing hazardous tasks, until drug's effect has been determined. Inform about the possibility of priapism. Explain that there is no need for concern if something that looks like a tab is occasionally noticed in the stool. Instruct to inform ophthalmologist of drug use prior to cataract surgery.

CASODEX — bicalutamide　　　　　　　　　Rx

Class: Antiandrogen

ADULT DOSAGE

D_2 Metastatic Prostate Carcinoma

Combination w/ Luteinizing Hormone-Releasing Hormone (LHRH) Analogue:
50mg qd (am or pm) at the same time as LHRH analogue

Missed Dose
If a dose is missed, take the next dose at the scheduled time; do not take the missed dose and do not double the next dose

PEDIATRIC DOSAGE
Pediatric use may not have been established

ADMINISTRATION
Oral route
Take w/ or w/o food
Take at the same time each day

STORAGE
20-25°C (68-77°F).

HOW SUPPLIED
Tab: 50mg

CONTRAINDICATIONS
Hypersensitivity reaction to the drug or any of the tab's components, women, pregnancy.

WARNINGS/PRECAUTIONS
Death or hospitalization due to severe liver injury (hepatic failure) reported. Hepatitis or marked increases in liver enzymes leading to discontinuation reported. Measure serum ALT immediately if signs/symptoms of liver dysfunction occur; d/c immediately w/ close follow-up of liver function if jaundice occurs or ALT rises >2X ULN. Reduction in glucose tolerance reported. Regularly assess serum prostate-specific antigen (PSA) to monitor response; evaluate for clinical progression if PSA levels rise during therapy. For patients w/ objective disease progression w/ an elevated PSA, consider a treatment period free of antiandrogen while continuing the LHRH analogue. Caution w/ moderate-severe hepatic impairment.

ADVERSE REACTIONS
Pain, hot flashes, asthenia, infection, back pain, constipation, nausea, diarrhea, anemia, peripheral edema, dizziness, dyspnea, rash, nocturia, hematuria.

DRUG INTERACTIONS
Can displace coumarin anticoagulants from binding sites; closely monitor PT and consider anticoagulant dose adjustment. Caution w/ CYP3A4 substrates. May increase levels of midazolam.

PREGNANCY AND LACTATION
Pregnancy: Category X.
Lactation: Not for use in nursing.

MECHANISM OF ACTION
Nonsteroidal antiandrogen; inhibits the action of androgens by binding to cytosol androgen receptors in target tissue.

PHARMACOKINETICS
Absorption: Well-absorbed; C_{max}=0.768µg/mL; T_{max}=31.3 hrs. **Distribution:** Plasma protein binding (96%). **Metabolism:** Liver via oxidation and glucuronidation. **Elimination:** Urine, feces; $T_{1/2}$=5.8 days.

PATIENT CONSIDERATIONS
Assessment: Assess for drug hypersensitivity, diabetes, hepatic impairment, and possible drug interactions. Measure serum transaminase levels.

Monitoring: Measure serum transaminase levels at regular intervals for the first 4 months of treatment, then periodically thereafter. Measure serum ALT for signs/ symptoms of liver dysfunction. Monitor LFTs in hepatically impaired patients on long-term therapy. Regularly monitor serum PSA levels. Monitor blood glucose levels.

Counseling: Advise not to interrupt or d/c medication w/o consulting physician. Inform that somnolence may occur; advise to use caution when driving or operating machinery. Advise to monitor blood glucose levels while on therapy. Inform that photosensitivity has been reported during treatment; advise to avoid direct exposure to excessive sunlight or UV-light exposure and to consider using sunscreen.

CATAFLAM — diclofenac potassium　　　　　　Rx

Class: NSAID

> NSAIDs cause an increased risk of serious cardiovascular (CV) thrombotic events (eg, MI, stroke), which can be fatal; risk may occur early in treatment and may increase w/ duration of use. Contraindicated in the setting of CABG surgery. NSAIDs cause an increased risk of serious GI adverse events (eg, bleeding, ulceration, stomach/intestinal perforation), which can be fatal and may occur at any time during use w/o warning symptoms; elderly patients and patients w/ a prior history of peptic ulcer disease and/or GI bleeding are at greater risk.

ADULT DOSAGE

Osteoarthritis
100-150mg/day in divided doses (50mg bid or tid)

Rheumatoid Arthritis
150-200mg/day in divided doses (50mg tid or qid)

Mild to Moderate Pain
50mg tid; may give initial dose of 100mg followed by 50mg doses in some patients

Primary Dysmenorrhea
50mg tid; may give initial dose of 100mg followed by 50mg doses in some patients

PEDIATRIC DOSAGE
Pediatric use may not have been established

DOSING CONSIDERATIONS
Elderly
If the anticipated benefit outweighs the potential risks, start at lower end of dosing range; monitor for adverse effects

ADMINISTRATION
Oral route
Different formulations of diclofenac are not necessarily bioequivalent even if the mg strength is the same.

STORAGE
20-25°C (68-77°F); excursions permitted between 15-30°C (59-86°F).

HOW SUPPLIED
Tab: 50mg

CONTRAINDICATIONS
Known hypersensitivity (eg, anaphylactic reactions, serious skin reactions) to diclofenac or any other component of the drug product, history of asthma, urticaria, or allergic-type reactions after taking aspirin (ASA) or other NSAIDs. In the setting of CABG surgery.

WARNINGS/PRECAUTIONS
Use the lowest effective dose for the shortest duration possible. Increased CV thrombotic risk w/ higher doses reported. Avoid in patients w/ a recent MI unless benefits outweigh the risks of recurrent CV thrombotic events; if used, monitor for signs of cardiac ischemia. Increased risk for GI bleeding w/ longer duration of therapy, older age, poor general health status, and advanced liver disease and/ or coagulopathy; avoid use in patients at higher risk unless benefits are expected to outweigh the increased risk. Consider alternate therapies other than NSAIDs for patients at higher risk and patients w/ active GI bleeding. Promptly initiate evaluation and treatment if a serious GI adverse event is suspected; d/c until a serious GI adverse event is ruled out. Hepatotoxicity reported; d/c immediately and perform a clinical evaluation if clinical signs/symptoms consistent w/ liver disease develop, if systemic manifestations occur, or if abnormal liver tests persist or worsen. May cause new onset HTN or worsen preexisting HTN. Fluid retention and edema reported. Avoid use in patients w/ severe heart failure (HF) unless benefits outweigh risks; monitor for signs of worsening HF if used. Renal papillary necrosis and other renal injury reported w/ long-term use. Renal toxicity also reported in patients in whom renal prostaglandins have a compensatory role in the maintenance of renal perfusion; increased risk w/ renal/hepatic dysfunction, dehydration, hypovolemia, or HF, and in the elderly. Correct volume status in dehydrated or hypovolemic patients prior to initiating therapy. Avoid use in patients w/ advanced renal disease unless the benefits are expected to outweigh the risk; monitor for signs of worsening renal function if used in patients w/ advanced renal disease. Hyperkalemia reported. Associated w/ anaphylactic reactions in patients w/ and w/o known hypersensitivity to diclofenac and in patients w/ ASA-sensitive asthma. Monitor for changes in the signs/symptoms of asthma in patients w/ preexisting asthma (w/o known ASA sensitivity). May cause serious skin reactions (eg, exfoliative dermatitis, Stevens-Johnson syndrome, toxic epidermal necrolysis); d/c at 1st appearance of skin rash/hypersensitivity. May cause premature closure of the fetal ductus arteriosus. Anemia reported. May increase the risk of bleeding events; coagulation disorders may increase this risk. Monitor for signs of bleeding. Do not substitute for corticosteroids or use to treat corticosteroid insufficiency. May mask inflammation and fever.

ADVERSE REACTIONS
Abdominal pain, constipation, diarrhea, dyspepsia, flatulence, heartburn, N/V, GI ulcers (gastric/duodenal), anemia, dizziness, edema, headaches, pruritus, rashes, tinnitus.

DRUG INTERACTIONS
Synergistic effect on bleeding w/ anticoagulants (eg, warfarin); monitor for signs of bleeding w/ concomitant anticoagulants, antiplatelet agents (eg, ASA), SSRIs, and SNRIs. Drugs that interfere w/ serotonin reuptake may potentiate the risk of bleeding. May increase risk of GI bleeding w/ use of oral corticosteroids, anticoagulants, and SSRIs; smoking; and alcohol use. ASA may increase risk of bleeding and serious GI events; concomitant use w/ analgesic doses of ASA is not recommended. Not a substitute for ASA for CV prophylaxis; monitor patients more closely for GI bleeding w/ concomitant use of low-dose ASA for cardiac prophylaxis. May diminish antihypertensive effect of ACE inhibitors, ARBs, and β-blockers (eg, propranolol); monitor BP. Coadministration w/ ACE inhibitors or ARBs may result in deterioration of renal function (including possible acute renal failure) in patients who are elderly or volume-depleted (including those on diuretic therapy), or who have renal impairment; monitor for worsening renal function and adequately hydrate patient when these drugs are administered

concomitantly. May reduce the natriuretic effect of loop diuretics (eg, furosemide) and thiazide diuretics; observe for signs of worsening renal function, in addition to assuring diuretic efficacy including antihypertensive effects. May increase digoxin serum concentrations and prolong the $T_{1/2}$ of digoxin; monitor digoxin levels. May elevate plasma lithium levels and reduce renal lithium clearance; monitor for signs of lithium toxicity. May increase the risk for methotrexate (MTX) toxicity; monitor for MTX toxicity. May increase cyclosporine's nephrotoxicity; monitor for signs of worsening renal function. Concomitant use w/ other NSAIDs or salicylates (eg, diflunisal, salsalate) increases the risk of GI toxicity; not recommended w/ other NSAIDs or salicylates. Concomitant use w/ pemetrexed may increase the risk of pemetrexed-associated myelosuppression, renal, and GI toxicity; refer to prescribing information for further information. CYP2C9 inhibitors (eg, voriconazole) may enhance exposure and toxicity. CYP2C9 inducers (eg, rifampin) may lead to compromised efficacy. Dose adjustment may be warranted if administered w/ CYP2C9 inhibitors or inducers. Caution w/ concomitant drugs known to be potentially hepatotoxic (eg, acetaminophen, antibiotics, anti-epileptics).

PREGNANCY AND LACTATION
Pregnancy: Use during the 3rd trimester of pregnancy increases the risk of premature closure of the fetal ductus arteriosus. Avoid use starting at 30 weeks of gestation (3rd trimester).
Lactation: May be present in human milk; caution in nursing.

MECHANISM OF ACTION
NSAID; mechanism is not completely understood but involves inhibition of COX-1 and COX-2. Has analgesic, anti-inflammatory, and antipyretic properties.

PHARMACOKINETICS
Absorption: Absolute bioavailability (55%), T_{max}=1 hr. **Distribution:** V_d=1.3L/kg; serum protein binding (>99%). **Metabolism:** 4'-hydroxy-diclofenac (major metabolite) via CYP2C9. Both diclofenac and its oxidative metabolites undergo glucuronidation or sulfation. **Elimination:** Urine (65%), bile (35%); $T_{1/2}$=2 hrs.

PATIENT CONSIDERATIONS
Assessment: Assess for history of hypersensitivity; history of asthma, urticaria, or other allergic-type reactions w/ ASA or other NSAIDs; asthma; CV disease (CVD) or risk factors for CVD; HTN; history of peptic ulcer disease or GI bleeding; coagulation disorders; renal/hepatic impairment; pregnancy/nursing status; or any other conditions where treatment is contraindicated or cautioned. Assess volume status. Assess for possible drug interactions. Obtain baseline LFTs, BP, CBC, and chemistry profile.

Monitoring: Monitor for signs/symptoms of CV thrombotic events; cardiac ischemia in patients w/ a recent MI; GI bleeding/ulceration and perforation; hepatotoxicity; new or worsening HTN; HF; edema; renal papillary necrosis and other renal injury; hyperkalemia; anaphylactic reactions; serious skin reactions; anemia; and other adverse reactions. Monitor BP during initiation of therapy and throughout the course of therapy. Monitor for signs of bleeding in patients on concomitant therapy w/ anticoagulants, antiplatelet agents, SSRIs, or SNRIs. Monitor renal function in patients w/ renal/hepatic impairment, HF, dehydration, or hypovolemia. Monitor LFTs, CBC, and chemistry profiles periodically during long-term treatment.

Counseling: Inform of potential for CV thrombotic events, GI adverse events, and worsening HF/edema, and advise of symptoms; instruct to report any symptoms to healthcare provider immediately. Inform of the potential for hepatotoxicity, and advise of signs/symptoms; if signs/symptoms occur, instruct to d/c and seek immediate medical therapy. Instruct to seek immediate emergency help if signs of an anaphylactic reaction occur. Advise to d/c immediately if rash develops and to contact healthcare provider as soon as possible. Advise females of reproductive potential who desire pregnancy that therapy may be associated w/ a reversible delay in ovulation. Advise pregnant women to avoid use starting at 30 weeks of gestation. Advise patient not to use other NSAIDs or salicylates concomitantly; notify of the presence of NSAIDs in OTC medications for colds, fever, or insomnia. Advise patient not to use low-dose ASA concomitantly w/o talking to healthcare provider.

CATAPRES — clonidine   Rx
Class: Alpha-adrenergic agonist

OTHER BRAND NAMES
Catapres-TTS

ADULT DOSAGE
Hypertension
Tab:
Initial: 0.1mg bid (am and hs)
Maint: May increase by 0.1mg/day at weekly intervals prn until desired response is achieved
Range: 0.2-0.6mg/day in divided doses
Max: 2.4mg/day

Patch:
Initial: Apply 1 patch every 7 days; start w/ TTS-1
Titrate: If inadequate reduction in BP after 1-2 weeks, increase dosage by adding another TTS-1 or changing to a larger system

PEDIATRIC DOSAGE
Pediatric use may not have been established

No usual additional efficacy w/ dose increase above 2 TTS-3

When substituting for PO clonidine or other antihypertensives, gradually reduce prior drug dose; effect of patch may not commence until 2-3 days after initial application

---

DOSING CONSIDERATIONS
Renal Impairment
Patch/Tab:
May benefit from lower initial dose
Elderly
Tab:
May benefit from lower initial dose

ADMINISTRATION
Oral/Transdermal route

Patch
Apply to hairless area of intact skin of upper outer arm or chest once every 7 days
Apply each new patch on different skin site from previous location
If the system loosens during 7-day wearing, the adhesive cover should be applied directly over the system to ensure good adhesion

STORAGE
(Patch) Below 30°C (86°F). (Tab) 25°C (77°F); excursions permitted to 15-30°C (59-86°F).

HOW SUPPLIED
Patch, Extended-Release (TTS): (TTS-1) 0.1mg, (TTS-2) 0.2mg, (TTS-3) 0.3mg; **Tab:** 0.1mg, 0.2mg, 0.3mg

CONTRAINDICATIONS
Known hypersensitivity to clonidine or to any other components of the medication.

WARNINGS/PRECAUTIONS
Sudden cessation of treatment may cause nervousness, agitation, headache, confusion, and tremor accompanied or followed by a rapid rise in BP and elevated catecholamine concentrations; if discontinuing therapy, reduce dose gradually over 2 to 4 days to avoid withdrawal symptoms. Rare instances of hypertensive encephalopathy, cerebrovascular accidents (CVAs), and death reported after withdrawal. Continuation of clonidine transdermal system or substitution to PO may cause generalized skin rash and elicit an allergic reaction if with localized contact sensitization or allergic reaction to clonidine transdermal system. Monitor BP during surgery; additional measures to control BP should be available. No therapeutic effect can be expected in HTN caused by pheochromocytoma. May worsen sinus node dysfunction and atrioventricular (AV) block, especially with other sympatholytic drugs; patients with conduction abnormalities and/or taking other sympatholytic drugs may develop severe bradycardia. (Tab) Continue administration to within 4 hrs of surgery and resume as soon as possible thereafter. (Patch) Loss of BP control reported (rare). Do not remove during surgery. Remove before defibrillation or cardioversion due to potential for altered electrical conductivity, and before undergoing an MRI due to the occurrence of skin burns.

ADVERSE REACTIONS
Dry mouth, drowsiness, dizziness, constipation, sedation.

DRUG INTERACTIONS
May potentiate CNS depressive effects of alcohol, barbiturates, or other sedating drugs. Hypotensive effect may be reduced by TCAs; may need to increase clonidine dose. Neuroleptics may induce or exacerbate orthostatic regulation disturbances (eg, orthostatic hypotension, dizziness, fatigue). Monitor HR with agents that affect sinus node function or AV nodal conduction (eg, digitalis, calcium channel blockers, β-blockers). D/C concurrent β-blockers several days before the gradual withdrawal of clonidine. Reports of sinus bradycardia and pacemaker insertion with diltiazem or verapamil. High IV doses of clonidine may increase the arrhythmogenic potential (QT prolongation, ventricular fibrillation) of high IV doses of haloperidol as observed in patients in a state of alcoholic delirium.

PREGNANCY AND LACTATION
Pregnancy: Category C.
Lactation: Caution in nursing.

MECHANISM OF ACTION
Centrally acting α-agonist; stimulates α-adrenoreceptors in brain stem, reducing sympathetic outflow from CNS and decreasing peripheral resistance, renal vascular resistance, HR, and BP.

PHARMACOKINETICS
Absorption: (Patch) Absolute bioavailability (60%); (Tab) absolute bioavailability (70-80%); T_{max}=1-3 hrs. **Distribution:** Crosses placenta; found in breast milk. **Metabolism:** Liver. **Elimination:** Urine (40-60%, unchanged); (Patch) $T_{1/2}$=20 hrs.

PATIENT CONSIDERATIONS
Assessment: Assess for pheochromocytoma, renal impairment, allergic reactions/contact sensitization, pregnancy/nursing status, and for possible drug interactions.

Monitoring: Monitor BP and renal function periodically. Monitor for withdrawal signs/symptoms (eg, hypertensive encephalopathy, CVA), presence of generalized skin rash, and allergic reactions.

Counseling: Caution patients against interrupting therapy without physician's advice and engaging in hazardous activities (eg, driving, operating appliances/machinery). Inform that sedative effect may be increased by concomitant use of alcohol, barbiturates, or other sedating drugs. Caution patients who wear contact lenses that drug may cause dryness of eyes. (Patch) Instruct to consult physician promptly about possible need to remove or replace patch if skin reactions develop. Inform that if patch begins to loosen, place adhesive cover directly over the patch to ensure adhesion for 7 days total. Advise to keep used and unused patch out of reach of children; instruct to fold in half with adhesive sides together and discard.

CAYSTON — aztreonam   Rx

Class: Monobactam

ADULT DOSAGE

Cystic Fibrosis

To Improve Respiratory Symptoms in Patients w/ *Pseudomonas aeruginosa*:
75mg tid via nebulizer for a 28-day course (followed by 28 days off therapy); take doses at least 4 hrs apart

PEDIATRIC DOSAGE

Cystic Fibrosis

To Improve Respiratory Symptoms in Patients w/ *Pseudomonas aeruginosa*:
≥7 Years:
75mg tid via nebulizer for a 28-day course (followed by 28 days off therapy); take doses at least 4 hrs apart

---

ADMINISTRATION
Inh route

Do not mix w/ any other drugs
Use bronchodilator before administration

Reconstitution
Administer immediately after reconstitution; do not reconstitute until ready to administer a dose
To open the glass vial, carefully remove the metal ring by lifting or pulling the tab and remove the gray rubber stopper
Twist the tip off the diluent ampule and squeeze the liquid into the glass vial
Replace the rubber stopper, then gently swirl the vial until contents have completely dissolved

Administration
Administer only using an Altera nebulizer system
Pour reconstituted sol into the handset of the nebulizer system
Turn the unit on and place the mouthpiece of the handset in the mouth and breathe normally only through the mouth
Administration typically takes between 2-3 min

Refer to PI for further instructions on how to test and clean the nebulizer

STORAGE
2-8°C (36-46°F). Once removed from refrigerator, store at room temperature up to 25°C (77°F) for up to 28 days. Protect from light.

HOW SUPPLIED
Sol, Inhalation: 75mg/vial

CONTRAINDICATIONS
Known allergy to aztreonam.

WARNINGS/PRECAUTIONS
Severe allergic reactions reported; d/c and initiate treatment as appropriate if allergic reaction occurs. Caution with history of β-lactam allergy (eg, penicillins [PCNs], cephalosporins, carbapenems); cross-reactivity may occur. Treatment is associated with bronchospasm. Decrease in forced expiratory volume in 1 sec (FEV$_1$) after treatment course reported; assess baseline FEV and other pulmonary symptoms prior to therapy. May result in bacterial resistance with use in the absence of known *P. aeruginosa* infection.

ADVERSE REACTIONS
Cough, nasal congestion, wheezing, pharyngolaryngeal pain, pyrexia, chest discomfort, abdominal pain, vomiting, bronchospasm.

PREGNANCY AND LACTATION
Category B, safe in nursing.

MECHANISM OF ACTION
Monobactam; binds to PCN-binding proteins of susceptible bacteria, which leads to inhibition of bacterial cell-wall synthesis and death of the cell.

PHARMACOKINETICS
Absorption: C$_{max}$=0.55mcg/mL, 0.67mcg/mL, 0.65mcg/mL (Days 0, 14, and 28, respectively). **Distribution:** Serum protein binding (56%); (IV) found in breast milk, crosses the placenta. **Metabolism:** Hydrolysis. **Elimination:** Urine (10%, unchanged), (IV) feces (12%); T$_{1/2}$=2.1 hrs.

PATIENT CONSIDERATIONS
Assessment: Assess for previous hypersensitivity to the drug, history of β-lactam allergy, presence of pulmonary symptoms, and pregnancy/nursing status. Obtain baseline FEV$_1$.

Monitoring: Monitor for signs/symptoms of allergic reactions, bronchospasm, and other adverse reactions. Monitor for pulmonary exacerbations.

Counseling: Counsel that therapy should only be used to treat bacterial, not viral, infections. Instruct to take exactly ud; inform that skipping doses or not completing full course of therapy may decrease effectiveness and increase resistance. Advise that therapy is for inhalation use and only using an Altera nebulizer system. Inform that if a dose is missed, all 3 daily doses should be taken as long as doses are at least 4 hrs apart. Advise to contact physician if allergic reaction or new/worsening symptoms develop. Advise to use a bronchodilator prior to administration. Instruct patients taking several medications to administer drugs in the following order: bronchodilator, mucolytics, and lastly, aztreonam.

CEFACLOR — cefaclor   Rx

Class: Cephalosporin (2nd generation)

OTHER BRAND NAMES
Ceclor (Discontinued)

ADULT DOSAGE

General Dosing

Usual: 250mg q8h

More Severe Infections (eg, Pneumonia)/Infections Caused by Less Susceptible Organisms: May double the dose

β-Hemolytic Streptococcal Infections: Administer for at least 10 days

Other Indications

Treatment of the Following Infections Caused by Susceptible Organisms:
Otitis media
Lower respiratory tract infections, including pneumonia
Pharyngitis
Tonsillitis
UTIs, including pyelonephritis and cystitis
Skin and skin structure infections

PEDIATRIC DOSAGE

General Dosing

≥1 Month of Age:
Usual: 20mg/kg/day in divided doses q8h

More Serious Infections/Infections Caused by Less Susceptible Organisms:
Usual: 40mg/kg/day in divided doses q8h
Max: 1g/day

β-Hemolytic Streptococcal Infections:
Administer for at least 10 days

Total daily dosage may be divided and administered q12h for pharyngitis

Otitis Media

≥1 Month of Age:
Usual: 40mg/kg/day in divided doses q8h
Max: 1g/day

Alternatively, total daily dosage may be divided and administered q12h

---

ADMINISTRATION
Oral route

Sus
Shake well before using.

Directions for Mixing:
Add appropriate water volume in 2 portions to dry mixture in bottle; shake well after each addition.
Refer to PI for the appropriate water volume to add.

STORAGE
20-25°C (68-77°F). **Oral Sus:** Store in refrigerator after mixing. Discard unused portion after 14 days.

HOW SUPPLIED
Cap: 250mg, 500mg; **Oral Sus:** 125mg/5mL [75mL, 150mL], 187mg/5mL [50mL, 100mL], 250mg/5mL [75mL, 150mL], 375mg/5mL [50mL, 100mL]

CONTRAINDICATIONS
Known allergy to the cephalosporin group of antibiotics.

WARNINGS/PRECAUTIONS
Caution in penicillin (PCN)-sensitive patients; cross-hypersensitivity among β-lactam antibiotics reported. D/C if an allergic reaction occurs. *Clostridium difficile*-associated diarrhea (CDAD) reported; may need to d/c if CDAD is suspected or confirmed. May result in bacterial resistance w/ prolonged use or if used in the absence of proven/ suspected bacterial infection or a prophylactic indication; take appropriate measures if superinfection develops. Lab test interactions may occur. Caution w/ markedly impaired renal function, history of GI disease (particularly colitis), and in elderly.

ADVERSE REACTIONS
GI symptoms, hypersensitivity reactions, eosinophilia, genital pruritus, moniliasis, vaginitis, serum-sickness-like reactions.

DRUG INTERACTIONS
Probenecid inhibits renal excretion. Increased anticoagulant effect reported when cefaclor and oral anticoagulants were administered concomitantly.

PREGNANCY AND LACTATION
Pregnancy: Category B.
Lactation: Caution in nursing.

MECHANISM OF ACTION
Cephalosporin (2nd generation); bactericidal action results from inhibition of cell-wall synthesis.

PHARMACOKINETICS
Absorption: Fasting: Well-absorbed; C$_{max}$=7mcg/mL (250mg), 13mcg/mL (500mg), 23mcg/mL (1g); T$_{max}$=30-60 min. **Distribution:** Found in breast milk. **Elimination:** Urine (60-85% unchanged); T$_{1/2}$=0.6-0.9 hrs (normal subjects), 2.3-2.8 hrs (anuria/complete absence of renal function).

PATIENT CONSIDERATIONS
Assessment: Assess for hypersensitivity to cephalosporins/PCNs/other drugs, history of GI disease (particularly colitis), renal impairment, pregnancy/ nursing status, and possible drug interactions. Perform appropriate culture and susceptibility tests to determine susceptible causative organisms.

Monitoring: Monitor for hypersensitivity reactions, CDAD, development of superinfection, and other adverse reactions.

Counseling: Inform that drug only treats bacterial, not viral, infections. Instruct to take exactly ud and inform that skipping doses or not completing full course of therapy may decrease effectiveness and increase the likelihood of bacterial resistance. Inform that diarrhea may occur and will usually end when therapy is discontinued. Instruct to contact physician as soon as possible if watery/bloody stools (w/ or w/o stomach cramps and fever) develop, even as late as ≥2 months after having taken the last dose.

CEFACLOR ER — cefaclor   Rx

Class: Cephalosporin (2nd generation)

OTHER BRAND NAMES
Ceclor CD (Discontinued)

ADULT DOSAGE

Acute Bacterial Exacerbation of Chronic Bronchitis

Due to *Haemophilus influenzae* (non-β-lactamase-producing strains only), *Moraxella catarrhalis* (including β-lactamase-producing strains), or *Streptococcus pneumoniae*

≥16 Years:
Mild to Moderate: 500mg q12h for 7 days

Bronchitis

Secondary bacterial infection of acute bronchitis due to *H. influenzae* (non-β-lactamase producing strains only), *M. catarrhalis* (including β-lactamase-producing strains), or *S. pneumoniae*

≥16 Years:
Mild to Moderate: 500mg q12h for 7 days

Pharyngitis/Tonsillitis

Due to *Streptococcus pyogenes*:
≥16 Years:
Mild to Moderate: 375mg q12h for 10 days

Skin and Skin Structure Infections

Uncomplicated Infections Due to *Staphylococcus aureus* (Methicillin-Susceptible):
≥16 Years:
Mild to Moderate: 375mg q12h for 7-10 days

PEDIATRIC DOSAGE
Pediatric use may not have been established

ADMINISTRATION
Oral route
Take w/ meals (at least w/in 1 hr of eating).
Do not crush, cut, or chew tab.

STORAGE
20-25°C (68-77°F).

HOW SUPPLIED
Tab, Extended-Release: 500mg

CONTRAINDICATIONS
Known hypersensitivity to cefaclor and other cephalosporins.

WARNINGS/PRECAUTIONS
Caution in penicillin (PCN)-sensitive patients; cross-sensitivity among β-lactam antibiotics reported. D/C if an allergic reaction occurs. *Clostridium difficile*-associated diarrhea (CDAD) reported; may need to d/c if CDAD is suspected or confirmed. May result in bacterial resistance if used in the absence of proven/suspected bacterial infection or a prophylactic indication; take appropriate measures if superinfection develops. Lab test interactions may occur.

ADVERSE REACTIONS
Headache, rhinitis, diarrhea, nausea.

DRUG INTERACTIONS
Extent of absorption is diminished if magnesium or aluminum hydroxide-containing antacids are taken w/in 1 hr of administration. Probenecid inhibits renal excretion. Concomitant use w/ warfarin may increase PT.

PREGNANCY AND LACTATION
Pregnancy: Category B.
Lactation: Caution in nursing.

MECHANISM OF ACTION
Cephalosporin (2nd generation); bactericidal action results from inhibition of cell-wall synthesis.

PHARMACOKINETICS
Absorption: Fed: (375mg) C_{max}=3.7mcg/mL; T_{max}=2.7 hrs. (500mg) C_{max}=8.2mcg/mL; T_{max}=2.5 hrs. Fasting: (500mg) C_{max}=5.4mcg/mL; T_{max}=1.5 hrs. Refer to PI for additional pharmacokinetic parameters. **Distribution:** Found in breast milk. **Elimination:** $T_{1/2}$=1 hr.

PATIENT CONSIDERATIONS
Assessment: Assess for hypersensitivity to cephalosporins/PCNs/other drugs, pregnancy/nursing status, and possible drug interactions. Perform appropriate culture and susceptibility tests to determine susceptible causative organisms.

Monitoring: Monitor for allergic reactions, CDAD, development of superinfection, and other adverse reactions.

Counseling: Inform that drug only treats bacterial, not viral, infections. Instruct to take exactly ud and inform that skipping doses or not completing full course of therapy may decrease effectiveness and increase the likelihood of bacterial resistance. Inform that diarrhea may occur and will usually end when therapy is discontinued. Instruct to contact physician as soon as possible if watery/bloody stools (w/ or w/o stomach cramps and fever) develop, even as late as ≥2 months after having taken the last dose.

CEFADROXIL — cefadroxil   Rx

Class: Cephalosporin (1st generation)

OTHER BRAND NAMES
Duricef (Discontinued)

ADULT DOSAGE

Urinary Tract Infections
Uncomplicated Lower UTIs (eg, Cystitis):
Usual: 1 or 2g/day given qd or bid
Other UTIs:
Usual: 2g/day given bid

Skin and Skin Structure Infections
Usual: 1g/day given qd or bid

Tonsillitis and/or Pharyngitis
Caused by Group A β-Hemolytic Streptococci:
1g/day given qd or bid for 10 days

PEDIATRIC DOSAGE

Urinary Tract Infections
Usual: 30mg/kg/day in divided doses q12h

Skin and Skin Structure Infections
Impetigo:
Usual: 30mg/kg/day given qd or in equally divided doses q12h
Other SSSIs:
Usual: 30mg/kg/day in divided doses q12h

Tonsillitis and/or Pharyngitis
Usual: 30mg/kg/day given qd or in equally divided doses q12h

Streptococcal Infections
β-Hemolytic Infections:
Administer for at least 10 days

DOSING CONSIDERATIONS
Renal Impairment
Adults:
Initial: 1g
Maint:
CrCl 25-50mL/min: 500mg q12h
CrCl 10-25mL/min: 500mg q24h
CrCl 0-10mL/min: 500mg q36h

ADMINISTRATION
Oral route
Take w/o regard to meals

Sus
Suspend 50mL bottle size in a total of 34mL water, 75mL bottle size in a total of 51mL water, 100mL bottle size in a total of 67mL water; add water in two portions and shake well after each addition
Shake well before using
Refer to PI for daily dosage of oral sus

STORAGE
(Cap/Tab) 20-25°C (68-77°F). (Sus) Before Reconstitution: 25°C (77°F); excursions permitted to 15-30°C (59-86°F). After Reconstitution: Store in refrigerator; discard unused portion after 14 days.

HOW SUPPLIED
Cap: 500mg; **Sus:** 250mg/5mL [50mL, 100mL], 500mg/5mL [50mL, 75mL, 100mL]; **Tab:** 1000mg* *scored

CONTRAINDICATIONS
Known allergy to cephalosporins.

WARNINGS/PRECAUTIONS
Caution in penicillin (PCN)-sensitive patients; cross-sensitivity among β-lactam antibiotics may occur. D/C if an allergic reaction occurs. *Clostridium difficile*-associated diarrhea (CDAD) reported; may need to d/c if CDAD is suspected or confirmed. Caution w/ renal impairment (CrCl <50mL/min); monitor prior to and during therapy. May result in bacterial resistance if used in the absence of proven or suspected bacterial infection, or a prophylactic indication. May result in overgrowth of nonsusceptible organisms w/ prolonged use; take appropriate measures if superinfection develops. Caution w/ history of GI disease, particularly colitis. Lab test interactions may occur. D/C if seizures associated w/ drug therapy occur. Caution in elderly.

ADVERSE REACTIONS
Diarrhea, allergies, hepatic dysfunction, genital moniliasis, vaginitis, moderate transient neutropenia, fever, toxic epidermal necrolysis, abdominal pain, superinfection, renal dysfunction, toxic nephropathy, aplastic anemia, hemolytic anemia, hemorrhage.

PREGNANCY AND LACTATION
Pregnancy: Category B.
Lactation: Caution in nursing.

MECHANISM OF ACTION
Cephalosporin (1st generation); bactericidal activity results from its inhibition of cell-wall synthesis.

PHARMACOKINETICS
Absorption: Rapid. C_{max}=16mcg/mL (500mg), 28mcg/mL (1000mg). **Elimination:** Urine (>90% unchanged).

PATIENT CONSIDERATIONS
Assessment: Assess for allergy to other cephalosporins, PCN, or to other drugs, renal impairment, history of GI disease, and pregnancy/nursing status. Initiate culture and susceptibility tests prior to therapy.

Monitoring: Monitor for signs/symptoms of an allergic reaction, CDAD, seizure, and superinfection. Carefully observe patients w/ known or suspected renal impairment.

Counseling: Inform that therapy only treats bacterial, not viral, infections. Instruct to take exactly ud; inform that skipping doses or not completing full course of therapy may decrease effectiveness and increase risk of bacterial resistance. Inform that diarrhea is a common problem that usually ends upon discontinuation. Instruct to notify physician as soon as possible if watery and bloody stools (w/ or w/o stomach cramps/fever) occur, even as late as ≥2 months after last dose.

CEFAZOLIN — cefazolin sodium   Rx

Class: Cephalosporin (1st generation)

ADULT DOSAGE

General Dosing

Mild Infections Caused by Gram-Positive Cocci:
250-500mg IV/IM q8h

Moderate to Severe Infections:
500mg-1g IV/IM q6-8h

Severe/Life-Threatening Infections (eg, Endocarditis, Septicemia):
1-1.5g IV/IM q6h; doses up to 12g/day have been used in rare instances

Urinary Tract Infections

Acute/Uncomplicated:
1g IV/IM q12h

Pneumonia

Pneumococcal Pneumonia:
500mg IV/IM q12h

Prophylaxis of Postoperative Infections

Preoperative:
1g IV/IM, 0.5-1 hr prior to the start of surgery

Lengthy Procedures (eg, ≥2 hrs):
500mg-1g IV/IM during surgery

Postoperative:
500mg-1g IV/IM q6-8h for 24 hrs

D/C w/in 24 hrs after the surgical procedure; continue for 3-5 days after the completion of surgery where occurrence of infection may be particularly devastating (eg, open-heart surgery, prosthetic arthroplasty)

Other Indications

Treatment of the Following Infections Caused by Susceptible Microorganisms:
Respiratory tract
Skin and skin structure
Biliary tract
Bone and joint
Genital infections

PEDIATRIC DOSAGE

General Dosing

>1 Month of Age:

Mild to Moderately Severe Infections:
25-50mg/kg/day (approx 10-20mg/lb) IV/IM, divided tid or qid in equal doses

Severe Infections:
May increase to 100mg/kg/day IV/IM

DOSING CONSIDERATIONS

Renal Impairment

Apply reduced dosage recommendations after initial LD is given

Adults:
CrCl 35-54mL/min or SrCr 1.6-3mg%: Full dose q8h or longer
CrCl 11-34mL/min or SrCr 3.1-4.5mg%: 1/2 usual dose q12h
CrCl ≤10mL/min or SrCr ≥4.6mg%: 1/2 usual dose q18-24h

Pediatrics:
CrCl 41-70mL/min: 60% of usual dose given in equally divided doses q12h
CrCl 21-40mL/min: 25% of usual dose given in equally divided doses q12h
CrCl ≤5-20mL/min: 10% of usual dose given in equally divided doses q24h

ADMINISTRATION

IV/IM route

Shake well.

Preparation

For IM inj, IV direct (bolus) inj, or IV infusion, reconstitute 500mg or 1g vial size w/ 2mL or 2.5mL of sterile water for inj (SWFI) respectively, for a concentration of 225mg/mL (500g vial) or 330mg/mL (1g vial).

Stable for 24 hrs at room temperature or for 10 days if stored under refrigeration (5°C [41°F]) when reconstituted or diluted according to instructions.

IM

Shake well until dissolved.
Inject into a large muscle mass.

IV

Direct (Bolus) Inj:
Further dilute reconstituted sol w/ 5mL SWFI.
Inject sol slowly over 3-5 min directly or through tubing in patients receiving parenteral fluids.

Intermittent/Continuous Infusion:
Dilute reconstituted sol in 50-100mL of a compatible IV sol.

Compatible IV Sol

NaCl inj, D5 or D10 inj, D5 in lactated Ringer's inj, D5 and 0.9% NaCl inj, D5 and 0.45% NaCl inj, D5 and 0.2% NaCl inj, lactated Ringer's inj, invert sugar 5% or 10% in SWFI, Ringer's inj, or 5% sodium bicarbonate inj.

STORAGE

Before Reconstitution: 20-25°C (68-77°F). Protect from light.

HOW SUPPLIED

Inj: 500mg, 1g

CONTRAINDICATIONS

Known allergy to cephalosporins.

WARNINGS/PRECAUTIONS

Caution w/ penicillin (PCN)-sensitive patients; cross-hypersensitivity among β-lactam antibiotics may occur. D/C if an allergic reaction occurs and initiate appropriate treatment. *Clostridium difficile*-associated diarrhea (CDAD) reported; d/c if CDAD suspected or confirmed. Institute appropriate fluid and electrolyte management, protein supplementation, and antibacterial drug treatment of *C. difficile* as clinically indicated. Use in the absence of a proven or strongly suspected bacterial infection or prophylactic indication is unlikely to provide benefit and increases the risk of the development of drug-resistant bacteria. May result in overgrowth of nonsusceptible microorganisms w/ prolonged use; take appropriate measures if superinfection develops. Seizures may occur if inappropriately high doses are administered to patients w/ impaired renal function. Caution w/ renal impairment, history of GI disease, and in elderly. Lab test interactions may occur. Not recommended for premature infants and neonates.

ADVERSE REACTIONS

Diarrhea, oral candidiasis, stomach cramps, anorexia, anaphylaxis, eosinophilia, itching, skin rash, leukopenia, thrombocytopenia, hepatitis, increased BUN and creatinine levels, genital/anal pruritus.

DRUG INTERACTIONS

Probenecid may decrease renal tubular secretion, increasing levels of cephalosporins. May be associated w/ fall in prothrombin activity; monitor PT in patients previously stabilized on anticoagulant therapy and administer exogenous vitamin K as indicated.

PREGNANCY AND LACTATION

Pregnancy: Category B.
Lactation: Present in very low concentrations in milk of nursing mothers; caution in nursing.

MECHANISM OF ACTION

Cephalosporin (1st generation); bactericidal agent that acts by inhibition of bacterial cell wall synthesis.

PHARMACOKINETICS

Absorption: (IV) C_{max}=185mcg/mL. **Distribution:** Crosses placenta; found in breast milk. **Elimination:** Urine (unchanged); $T_{1/2}$=2 hrs (IM), 1.8 hrs (IV).

PATIENT CONSIDERATIONS

Assessment: Assess for hypersensitivity to cephalosporin class of antibacterial drugs/PCN/other β-lactams, renal impairment, history of GI disease, pregnancy/nursing status, and possible drug interactions. Perform appropriate culture and susceptibility tests to determine susceptible causative organisms.

Monitoring: Monitor for hypersensitivity reactions, CDAD, development of superinfection, drug resistance, and other adverse reactions. Monitor renal function in elderly. Monitor for seizures in patients w/ renal dysfunction.

Counseling: Instruct to notify physician of any previous allergic reactions to the drug, cephalosporins, PCNs, or other similar antibacterials. Advise that diarrhea is a common problem that usually ends when therapy is discontinued; however, if watery and bloody stools (w/ or w/o stomach cramps and fever) occur, even as late as 2 or more months after last dose, instruct to contact physician as soon as possible. Inform that therapy only treats bacterial, not viral, infections. Instruct to take exactly ud even if the patient feels better early in the course of therapy. Inform that skipping doses or not completing the full course of therapy may decrease effectiveness and increase risk of bacterial resistance.

CEFDINIR — cefdinir   Rx

Class: Cephalosporin (3rd generation)

OTHER BRAND NAMES

Omnicef (Discontinued)

ADULT DOSAGE

Community-Acquired Pneumonia

Cap:
300mg q12h for 10 days

Acute Bacterial Exacerbation of Chronic Bronchitis

Cap:
300mg q12h for 5-10 days or 600mg q24h for 10 days

Acute Maxillary Sinusitis

Cap:
300mg q12h or 600mg q24h for 10 days

PEDIATRIC DOSAGE

Skin and Skin Structure Infections

Uncomplicated:

Sus:
6 Months-12 Years:
7mg/kg q12h for 10 days
≥43kg: 600mg/day
Max: 600mg/day

Cap:
≥13 Years:
300mg q12h for 10 days

Acute Otitis Media

Sus:
6 Months-12 Years:
7mg/kg q12h for 5-10 days or 14mg/kg q24h for 10 days

Pharyngitis/Tonsillitis

Cap:
300mg q12h for 5-10 days or 600mg q24h for 10 days

Skin and Skin Structure Infections

Uncomplicated:
Cap:
300mg q12h for 10 days

≥43kg: 600mg/day
Max: 600mg/day

Community-Acquired Pneumonia

Cap:
≥13 Years:
300mg q12h for 10 days

Acute Bacterial Exacerbation of Chronic Bronchitis

Cap:
≥13 Years:
300mg q12h for 5-10 days or 600mg q24h for 10 days

Acute Maxillary Sinusitis

Sus:
6 Months-12 Years:
7mg/kg q12h or 14mg/kg q24h for 10 days
≥43kg: 600mg/day
Max: 600mg/day

Cap:
≥13 Years:
300mg q12h or 600mg q24h for 10 days

Pharyngitis/Tonsillitis

Sus:
6 Months-12 Years:
7mg/kg q12h for 5-10 days or 14mg/kg q24h for 10 days
≥43kg: 600mg/day
Max: 600mg/day

Cap:
≥13 Years:
300mg q12h for 5-10 days or 600mg q24h for 10 days

DOSING CONSIDERATIONS

Renal Impairment

Adults:
CrCl <30mL/min: 300mg qd
Hemodialysis:
Initial: 300mg or 7mg/kg qod; give 300mg or 7mg/kg at the end of each hemodialysis session
Subsequent Doses: 300mg or 7mg/kg qod

Pediatrics:
CrCl <30mL/min/1.73m^2: 7mg/kg (up to 300mg) qd
Hemodialysis:
Initial: 300mg or 7mg/kg qod; give 300mg or 7mg/kg at the end of each hemodialysis session
Subsequent Doses: 300mg or 7mg/kg qod

ADMINISTRATION

Oral route

May take w/o regard to food.

Oral Sus

Shake well before use.
Reconstitute w/ 37mL of water (for final volume of 60mL) or 62mL of water (for final volume of 100mL); add water in 2 portions, shake well after each aliquot. After mixing, store at room temperature (20-25°C [68-77°F]).
May use for 10 days and discard any unused portion.

STORAGE

Cap/Unsuspended Powder: 20-25°C (68-77°F). **Reconstituted Oral Sus:** Can be stored at controlled room temperature for 10 days.

HOW SUPPLIED

Cap: 300mg; **Oral Sus:** 125mg/5mL, 250mg/5mL [60mL, 100mL]

CONTRAINDICATIONS

Known allergy to cephalosporins.

WARNINGS/PRECAUTIONS

Caution in penicillin (PCN)-sensitive patients; cross-hypersensitivity among β-lactam antibiotics may occur. D/C use if an allergic reaction occurs. Serious acute hypersensitivity reactions may require the use of SQ epinephrine and other emergency measures. *Clostridium difficile*-associated diarrhea (CDAD) reported; may need to d/c if CDAD is suspected/confirmed. May result in bacterial resistance w/ prolonged use in the absence of a proven or suspected bacterial infection, or a prophylactic indication; take appropriate measures if superinfection develops. Caution in patients w/ a history of colitis. Reduce dose in patients w/ transient or persistent renal insufficiency (CrCl <30mL/min). Lab test interactions may occur.

ADVERSE REACTIONS

Cap: Diarrhea, vaginal moniliasis, nausea.
Oral Sus: Diarrhea, rash.

DRUG INTERACTIONS

Iron-fortified foods (except iron-fortified infant formula), iron supplements, and aluminum- or Mg^{2+}-containing antacids reduce absorption; take dose at least 2 hrs before or after these medications. Inhibited renal excretion w/ probenecid. Reddish stools reported w/ iron-containing products.

PREGNANCY AND LACTATION

Pregnancy: Category B.
Lactation: Following administration of single 600mg doses, cefdinir was not detected in human breast milk.

MECHANISM OF ACTION

Cephalosporin (3rd generation); bactericidal activity results from its inhibition of cell-wall synthesis.

PHARMACOKINETICS

Absorption: Cap: (300mg) C_{max}=1.60mcg/mL, T_{max}=2.9 hrs, AUC=7.05mcg•hr/mL. (600mg) C_{max}=2.87mcg/mL, T_{max}=3 hrs, AUC=11.1mcg•hr/mL. Sus: Absolute bioavailability (25%); (7mg/kg) C_{max}=2.30mcg/mL, T_{max}=2.2 hrs, AUC=8.31mcg•hr/mL. (14mg/kg) C_{max}=3.86mcg/mL, T_{max}=1.8 hrs, AUC=13.4mcg•hr/mL. **Distribution:** V_d=0.35L/kg (adults), 0.67L/kg (pediatrics); plasma protein binding (60-70%). **Elimination:** (300mg) Urine (18.4% unchanged); (600mg) Urine (11.6% unchanged); $T_{1/2}$=1.7 hrs.

PATIENT CONSIDERATIONS

Assessment: Assess for allergy to other cephalosporins, PCN, or to other drugs, history of colitis, renal impairment, and for possible drug interactions. Assess for diabetes if planning to use sus formulation.

Monitoring: Monitor for signs/symptoms of hypersensitivity reactions, CDAD, and development of superinfection.

Counseling: Inform that therapy only treats bacterial, not viral, infections. Instruct to take ud; skipping doses or not completing full course may decrease drug effectiveness and increase risk of bacterial resistance. Instruct to take dose at least 2 hrs before or after antacid or iron supplements. Inform diabetic patients and caregivers that oral sus contains 2.86g of sucrose/tsp. Instruct to contact physician as soon as possible if watery and bloody stools (w/ or w/o stomach cramps and fever) develop even as late as ≥2 months after having taken the last dose.

CEFOTETAN — cefotetan disodium   Rx

Class: Cephalosporin (2nd generation)

ADULT DOSAGE	PEDIATRIC DOSAGE
General Dosing	Pediatric use may not have been established
Usual: 1g or 2g IM/IV	
Other Sites: 1g or 2g q12h IV/IM	
Severe Infections: 2g IV q12h	
Life-Threatening Infections: 3g IV q12h	
Max: 6g/day	
Urinary Tract Infections	
500mg IV/IM q12h or 1g or 2g IV/IM q12h or q24h	
Skin and Skin Structure Infections	
Mild to Moderate: 2g IV q24h or 1g IV/IM q12h; for *Klebsiella pneumoniae*, give 1g or 2g IV/IM q12h	
Severe: 2g IV q12h	
Prophylaxis of Postoperative Infections	
1g or 2g IV once, 30-60 min prior to surgery	
Cesarean Section: Administer as soon as umbilical cord is clamped	
Other Indications	
Lower respiratory tract, gynecologic, intra-abdominal, and bone and joint infections caused by susceptible strains of microorganisms	
May be used concomitantly w/ an aminoglycoside in cases of sepsis or other serious infections in which causative organism has not been identified	

DOSING CONSIDERATIONS

Renal Impairment

CrCl >30mL/min: Usual dose q12h
CrCl 10-30mL/min: Usual dose q24h or 1/2 the dose given q12h
CrCl <10mL/min: Usual dose q48h or 1/4 of usual dose q12h
Intermittent Hemodialysis: 1/4 of usual dose q24h on days between dialysis and 1/2 of usual dose on the day of dialysis

ADMINISTRATION

IM/IV route

IM

Inject well w/in the body of a relatively large muscle (eg, gluteus maximus)
Aspiration is necessary to avoid inadvertent inj into a blood vessel
Reconstitute w/ sterile water for inj (SWFI), bacteriostatic water for inj, 0.9% NaCl, 0.5% lidocaine HCl, or 1% lidocaine HCl
Add 2mL of diluent to the 1g vial size or add 3mL of diluent to the 2g vial size

IV

May inject over a period of 3-5 min; may give for a longer period using an infusion system

Reconstitute w/ SWFI

Add 10mL of diluent to the 1g vial size or add 10-20mL of diluent to the 2g vial size

Compatibility and Stability

Thaw frozen samples at room temperature before use

Do not admix sol w/ sol containing aminoglycosides; must administer separately, not as a mixed inj

Do not add supplementary medication

Maintains satisfactory potency for 24 hrs at room temperature 25°C (77°F), 96 hrs under refrigeration 5°C (41°F), and for at least 1 week in the frozen state -20°C (-4°F)

STORAGE

≤22°C (72°F). Protect from light.

HOW SUPPLIED

Inj: 1g, 2g

CONTRAINDICATIONS

Known allergy to the cephalosporin group of antibiotics, history of cephalosporin-associated hemolytic anemia.

WARNINGS/PRECAUTIONS

Cross-hypersensitivity among β-lactam antibiotics reported; caution in penicillin (PCN)-sensitive patients. D/C if an allergic reaction occurs. Immune-mediated hemolytic anemia reported; if anemia develops anytime w/in 2-3 weeks subsequent to administration, consider the diagnosis of cephalosporin-associated anemia and d/c therapy until certain etiology is determined. *Clostridium difficile*-associated diarrhea (CDAD) reported; may need to d/c if CDAD is suspected or confirmed. May cause a fall in prothrombin activity and subsequent bleeding; increased risk w/ renal/hepatobiliary impairment, poor nutritional state, cancer, and in the elderly. May result in bacterial resistance w/ prolonged use or use in the absence of proven or suspected bacterial infection, or a prophylactic indication; take appropriate measures if superinfection develops. Caution w/ history of GI disease, particularly colitis. Lab test interactions may occur. Caution in elderly.

ADVERSE REACTIONS

Diarrhea, nausea, hematologic abnormalities, hepatic enzyme elevations, hypersensitivity reactions, local effects (eg, phlebitis at inj site, discomfort).

DRUG INTERACTIONS

Aminoglycosides may potentiate nephrotoxicity; monitor renal function.

PREGNANCY AND LACTATION

Category B, caution in nursing.

MECHANISM OF ACTION

Cephalosporin (2nd generation); bactericidal action results from inhibition of cell wall synthesis.

PHARMACOKINETICS

Distribution: V_d=10.3L (1g IV bolus dose); plasma protein binding (88%); found in breast milk. **Elimination:** Urine (51-81% unchanged); $T_{1/2}$=3-4.6 hrs.

PATIENT CONSIDERATIONS

Assessment: Assess for hypersensitivity to cephalosporins, PCNs, or other drugs, history of cephalosporin-associated hemolytic anemia, renal/hepatobiliary impairment, nutritional status, cancer, history of GI disease, pregnancy/nursing status, and possible drug interactions. Perform culture and susceptibility testing.

Monitoring: Monitor for signs/symptoms of allergic reactions, hemolytic anemia, CDAD, bleeding, superinfection, and other adverse reactions. Monitor renal function, PT and hematological parameters.

Counseling: Inform that diarrhea is a common problem caused by therapy, which usually ends when therapy is discontinued. Instruct to immediately contact physician if watery and bloody stools (w/ or w/o stomach cramps and fever) occur, even as late as ≥2 months after the last dose. Inform that therapy should only be used to treat bacterial, not viral (eg, common cold) infections. Instruct to take exactly ud even if the patient feels better early in the course of therapy. Inform that skipping doses or not completing the full course of therapy may decrease effectiveness and increase bacterial resistance. Counsel that disulfiram-like reaction, characterized by flushing, sweating, headache, and tachycardia, may occur when alcohol is ingested w/in 72 hrs after administration of the drug; caution about ingestion of alcoholic beverages.

CEFOXITIN — cefoxitin sodium   Rx

Class: Cephalosporin (2nd generation)

ADULT DOSAGE

General Dosing

Lower respiratory tract/urinary tract/intra-abdominal/gynecological/skin and skin structure/bone and joint infections and septicemia caused by susceptible strains of microorganisms

Usual:
1-2g IV q6-8h

Uncomplicated Infections (eg, Pneumonia, UTI, Cutaneous):
1g IV q6-8h

PEDIATRIC DOSAGE

General Dosing

≥3 Months of Age:
80-160mg/kg/day divided into 4-6 equal doses; use higher doses for more severe/serious infections

Max: 12g/day

Group A β-Hemolytic Streptococcal Infections:
Administer for at least 10 days

Moderately Severe/Severe Infections:
1g IV q4h or 2g IV q6-8h

Gas Gangrene/Other Infections Requiring Higher Dose:
2g IV q4h or 3g IV q6h

Group A β-Hemolytic Streptococcal Infections:
Administer for at least 10 days

Prophylaxis of Postoperative Infections

For Uncontaminated GI Surgery, Abdominal/Vaginal Hysterectomy:
2g IV prior to surgery (0.5-1 hr before initial incision), then 2g IV q6h after 1st dose for ≤24 hrs

Cesarean Section:
Single dose of 2g IV as soon as umbilical cord is clamped, or 2g IV as soon as umbilical cord is clamped, followed by 2g IV at 4 and 8 hrs after initial dose

Prophylaxis of Postoperative Infections

≥3 Months of Age:

For Uncontaminated GI Surgery, Abdominal/Vaginal Hysterectomy:
30-40mg/kg IV prior to surgery (0.5-1 hr before initial incision) and q6h after 1st dose for ≤24 hrs

---

DOSING CONSIDERATIONS

Renal Impairment

Adults:
LD: 1-2g IV
Maint:
CrCl 30-50mL/min: 1-2g IV q8-12h
CrCl 10-29mL/min: 1-2g IV q12-24h
CrCl 5-9mL/min: 0.5-1g IV q12-24h
CrCl <5mL/min: 0.5-1g q24-48h

Hemodialysis:
LD: 1-2g IV after each hemodialysis
Maint: See renal impairment maintenance dose above

Pediatrics:
Modify dosage and frequency of dosage consistent w/ recommendations for adults

ADMINISTRATION

IV route

Preparation

1g vial should be constituted w/ at least 10mL of diluent, and 2g vial w/ 10mL or 20mL of diluent

May use sterile water for inj (SWFI), bacteriostatic water for inj, 0.9% NaCl inj, or D5 inj for initial dilution

Further dilute in 50-1000mL of compatible diluents

IV

Intermittent IV:

May inject 1g or 2g sol in 10mL of SWFI over 3-5 min

May give over a longer period of time through the tubing system if receiving other IV sol

D/C administration of any other sol at the same site

Higher Doses by Continuous Infusion:

May add to an IV bottle containing D5 inj, 0.9% NaCl inj, or D5 and 0.9% NaCl inj; butterfly or scalp vein-type needles are preferred

Do not add to aminoglycoside sol; administer separately

Compatibility

0.9% NaCl

D5 or D10 inj

D5 and 0.9% NaCl inj

D5 inj w/ 0.2% or 0.45% saline sol

Lactated Ringer's inj

D5 in lactated Ringer's inj

5% sodium bicarbonate inj

M/6 sodium lactate sol

Mannitol 5% and 10%

STORAGE

Dry State: 2-25°C (36-77°F). Avoid >50°C (122°F). Reconstituted Sol: Maintains satisfactory potency at room temperature for 6 hrs or for 1 week under refrigeration (<5°C [41°F]). Further Diluted Sol: Room temperature for additional 18 hrs or additional 48 hrs under refrigeration.

HOW SUPPLIED

Inj: 1g, 2g

CONTRAINDICATIONS

Hypersensitivity to cefoxitin and the cephalosporin group of antibiotics.

WARNINGS/PRECAUTIONS

Caution with previous hypersensitivity to cephalosporins, penicillins (PCNs), or other drugs. D/C if allergic reaction occurs. *Clostridium difficile*-associated diarrhea (CDAD) reported; d/c if CDAD suspected or confirmed. May result in overgrowth of nonsusceptible organisms with prolonged use or use in the absence of a proven or strongly suspected bacterial infection or prophylactic indication; take appropriate measures if superinfection develops. Appropriate anti-chlamydial coverage should be added when used in the treatment of pelvic inflammatory disease and *Chlamydia trachomatis* is the suspected pathogen. Lab test interactions may occur. Caution with impaired renal function, history of GI disease (particularly colitis), and in elderly.

ADVERSE REACTIONS
Local reactions, rash, pruritus, fever, dyspnea, hypotension, diarrhea, pseudomembranous colitis, exacerbation of myasthenia gravis, eosinophilia, leukopenia, thrombocytopenia, bone marrow depression, elevated LFTs, SrCr elevation.

DRUG INTERACTIONS
Increased nephrotoxicity with aminoglycoside antibiotics.

PREGNANCY AND LACTATION
Category B, caution in nursing.

MECHANISM OF ACTION
Cephalosporin (2nd generation); bactericidal, inhibits cell-wall synthesis.

PHARMACOKINETICS
Distribution: Found in breast milk. **Elimination:** Urine (85% unchanged); $T_{1/2}$=41-59 min.

PATIENT CONSIDERATIONS

Assessment: Assess for previous hypersensitivity reactions to cephalosporins, PCNs, or other drugs, renal impairment, GI disease (eg, colitis), pregnancy/ nursing status, and possible drug interactions. Perform appropriate culture and susceptibility studies to determine susceptible causative organisms.

Monitoring: Monitor for signs/symptoms of an allergic reaction, CDAD, development of superinfection or drug resistance, and other adverse reactions. Periodically monitor renal/hepatic/hematopoietic functions, especially with prolonged therapy.

Counseling: Inform that drug only treats bacterial, not viral, infections. Instruct to take exactly ud; skipping doses or not completing full course of therapy may decrease effectiveness and increase the likelihood of bacterial resistance. Inform that diarrhea may occur and will usually end if therapy is discontinued. Instruct to contact physician as soon as possible if watery/bloody stools (with/ without stomach cramps, fever) develop even as late as 2 or more months after discontinuation.

CEFPODOXIME — cefpodoxime proxetil   Rx

Class: Cephalosporin (3rd generation)

OTHER BRAND NAMES
Vantin (Discontinued)

ADULT DOSAGE

Tonsillitis and/or Pharyngitis
100mg q12h for 5-10 days

Community-Acquired Pneumonia
200mg q12h for 14 days

Acute Bacterial Exacerbation of Chronic Bronchitis
Tab:
200mg q12h for 10 days

Gonorrhea
Uncomplicated Gonorrhea (Men and Women):
Single 200mg dose

Rectal Infections
Gonococcal Infections (Women):
Single 200mg dose

Skin and Skin Structure Infections
400mg q12h for 7-14 days

Acute Maxillary Sinusitis
200mg q12h for 10 days

Urinary Tract Infections
Uncomplicated:
100mg q12h for 7 days

PEDIATRIC DOSAGE

Acute Otitis Media
2 Months-12 Years:
Sus:
5mg/kg q12h for 5 days
Max: 200mg/dose

Tonsillitis and/or Pharyngitis
2 Months-12 Years:
Sus:
5mg/kg/dose q12h for 5-10 days
Max: 100mg/dose
≥12 Years:
100mg q12h for 5-10 days

Acute Maxillary Sinusitis
2 Months-12 Years:
Sus:
5mg/kg q12h for 10 days
Max:
200mg/dose
≥12 Years:
200mg q12h for 10 days

Community-Acquired Pneumonia
≥12 Years:
200mg q12h for 14 days

Gonorrhea
Uncomplicated (Men and Women):
≥12 Years:
Single 200mg dose

Rectal Infections
Gonococcal Infections (Women):
≥12 Years:
Single 200mg dose

Skin and Skin Structure Infections
≥12 Years:
400mg q12h for 7-14 days

Urinary Tract Infections
Uncomplicated:
≥12 Years:
100mg q12h for 7 days

Acute Bacterial Exacerbation of Chronic Bronchitis
≥12 Years:
200mg q12h for 10 days

DOSING CONSIDERATIONS
Renal Impairment
Severe (CrCl <30mL/min): Increase dosing interval to q24h
Hemodialysis: Dose 3X/week after hemodialysis

ADMINISTRATION
Oral route

Tab
Take w/ food

Sus
May be given w/o regard to food
Shake well before using

Preparation of Sus
50mL of 50mg/5mL: Suspend in 32mL of distilled water
100mL of 50mg/5mL: Suspend in 63mL of distilled water
50mL of 100mg/5mL: Suspend in 32mL of distilled water
100mL of 100mg/5mL: Suspend in 63mL of distilled water
Add water in approx 2 equal portions, shaking vigorously after each aliquot

STORAGE
20-25°C (68-77°F). (Sus) After Constitution: 2-8°C (36-46°F). Discard unused portion after 14 days.

HOW SUPPLIED
Sus: 50mg/5mL, 100mg/5mL [50mL, 100mL]; **Tab:** 100mg, 200mg

CONTRAINDICATIONS
Known allergy to cefpodoxime or to the cephalosporin group of antibiotics.

WARNINGS/PRECAUTIONS
Cross hypersensitivity among β-lactam antibiotics reported; caution in patients with penicillin (PCN) sensitivity. D/C if an allergic reaction occurs. Serious acute hypersensitivity reactions may require treatment with epinephrine and other emergency measures. *Clostridium difficile*-associated diarrhea (CDAD) reported; d/c if CDAD is suspected or confirmed. Pseudomembranous colitis reported. May result in bacterial resistance with prolonged use or in the absence of proven or suspected bacterial infection, or a prophylactic indication; take appropriate measures if superinfection develops. Lab test interactions may occur.

ADVERSE REACTIONS
Diarrhea, nausea.

DRUG INTERACTIONS
High doses of antacids (sodium bicarbonate and aluminum hydroxide) or H_2 blockers reduce C_{max} and the extent of absorption. Oral anticholinergics (eg, propantheline) delay C_{max}. Probenecid inhibits renal excretion; monitor renal function with nephrotoxic agents. Caution with potent diuretics.

PREGNANCY AND LACTATION
Category B, not for use in nursing.

MECHANISM OF ACTION
Cephalosporin (3rd generation); bactericidal agent that acts by inhibition of bacterial cell-wall synthesis.

PHARMACOKINETICS
Absorption: (Tab) C_{max}=1.4mcg/mL (100mg), 2.3mcg/mL (200mg), 3.9mcg/mL (400mg); T_{max}=2-3 hrs. (Sus) C_{max}=1.5mcg/mL (100mg). **Distribution:** Plasma protein binding (21-29%); found in breast milk. **Metabolism:** Via deesterification; cefpodoxime (active metabolite). **Elimination:** Urine (29-33% unchanged). (Tab) $T_{1/2}$=2.09-2.84 hrs.

PATIENT CONSIDERATIONS

Assessment: Assess for history of hypersensitivity to cephalosporins, PCNs, or other drugs, renal impairment, pregnancy/nursing status, and possible drug interactions. Perform culture and susceptibility testing.

Monitoring: Monitor for signs/symptoms of hypersensitivity reactions, CDAD, pseudomembranous colitis, development of superinfection, and other adverse reactions.

Counseling: Inform that therapy should only be used to treat bacterial, not viral (eg, common cold), infections. Instruct to take exactly ud even if the patient feels better early in the course of therapy. Inform that skipping doses or not completing the full course of therapy may decrease effectiveness of immediate treatment and increase bacterial resistance. Inform that diarrhea is a common problem caused by therapy, which usually ends when therapy is discontinued. Instruct to immediately contact physician if watery and bloody stools (with or without stomach cramps and fever) occur, even as late as ≥2 months after the last dose. (Sus) Inform that drug contains phenylalanine.

CEFPROZIL — cefprozil   Rx

Class: Cephalosporin (2nd generation)

ADULT DOSAGE

Pharyngitis/Tonsillitis
500mg q24h for 10 days; administer for >10 days for *Streptococcus pyogenes* infections

Acute Bacterial Sinusitis
250mg or 500mg q12h for 10 days; use the higher dose for moderate to severe infections

PEDIATRIC DOSAGE

Acute Otitis Media
6 Months-12 Years:
15mg/kg q12h for 10 days
Do not exceed recommended adult doses

Acute Bacterial Sinusitis
6 Months-12 Years:
7.5mg/kg or 15mg/kg q12h for 10 days

Lower Respiratory Tract Infections

Secondary Bacterial Infection of Acute Bronchitis/Acute Bacterial Exacerbation of Chronic Bronchitis:
500mg q12h for 10 days

Skin and Skin Structure Infections

Uncomplicated:
250mg or 500mg q12h or 500mg q24h for 10 days

≥13 Years:
250mg or 500mg q12h for 10 days; use the higher dose for moderate to severe infections
Do not exceed recommended adult doses

Pharyngitis/Tonsillitis

2-12 Years:
7.5mg/kg q12h for 10 days
≥13 Years:
500mg q24h for 10 days

Administer for >10 days for *Streptococcus pyogenes* infections
Do not exceed recommended adult doses

Skin and Skin Structure Infections

Uncomplicated:
2-12 Years:
20mg/kg q24h for 10 days
≥13 Years:
250mg or 500mg q12h or 500mg q24h for 10 days

Lower Respiratory Tract Infections

Acute Bacterial Exacerbation of Chronic Bronchitis/Secondary Bacterial Infection of Acute Bronchitis:
≥13 Years:
500mg q12h for 10 days

DOSING CONSIDERATIONS
Renal Impairment
CrCl 0-29mL/min: Give 50% of standard dose

ADMINISTRATION
Oral route

Shake sus well before use
Administer after completion of hemodialysis

Reconstitution
Final Concentration of 125mg/5mL:
Add 36mL, 54mL, or 72mL of water to the 50mL, 75mL, or 100mL bottle size respectively
Final Concentration of 250mg/5mL:
Add 36mL, 54mL, or 72mL of water to the 50mL, 75mL, or 100mL bottle size respectively

STORAGE
Tab/Dry Powder: 20-25°C (68-77°F). Reconstituted Sus: Refrigerate after mixing and discard unused portion after 14 days.

HOW SUPPLIED
Sus: 125mg/5mL, 250mg/5mL [50mL, 75mL, 100mL]; **Tab:** 250mg, 500mg

CONTRAINDICATIONS
Known allergy to cephalosporins.

WARNINGS/PRECAUTIONS
Caution with previous hypersensitivity to cephalosporins, penicillins (PCNs), or other drugs; cross-sensitivity may occur with history of PCN allergy. D/C if allergic reaction occurs. *Clostridium difficile*-associated diarrhea (CDAD) reported. May result in bacterial resistance with prolonged use or use in the absence of a proven/suspected bacterial infection or a prophylactic indication; take appropriate measures if superinfection develops. Caution with GI disease, particularly colitis. Caution with renal impairment and elderly. Lab test interactions may occur.

ADVERSE REACTIONS
Diarrhea, N/V, ALT/AST elevation, eosinophilia, genital pruritus, vaginitis, superinfection, diaper rash, dizziness, abdominal pain.

DRUG INTERACTIONS
Nephrotoxicity with aminoglycosides reported. Probenecid may increase plasma levels. Caution with potent diuretics.

PREGNANCY AND LACTATION
Pregnancy: Category B.
Lactation: Caution in nursing.

MECHANISM OF ACTION
Cephalosporin (2nd generation); bactericidal activity results from its inhibition of cell-wall synthesis.

PHARMACOKINETICS
Absorption: C_{max}=6.1mcg/mL (250mg), 10.5mcg/mL (500mg), 18.3mcg/mL (1g); T_{max}=1.5 hrs (adults), 1-2 hrs (peds). Plasma concentration (peds) at 7.5, 15, and 30mg/kg doses similar to those observed within same time frame in normal adults at 250, 500, and 1000mg doses, respectively. **Distribution:** V_d=0.23L/kg; plasma protein binding (36%); found in breast milk. **Elimination:** Urine (60%); $T_{1/2}$=1.3 hrs (adults), 1.5 hrs (peds).

PATIENT CONSIDERATIONS
Assessment: Assess for previous hypersensitivity reactions to PCNs/cephalosporins or other drugs, renal/hepatic function, GI disease, pregnancy/

nursing status, and possible drug interactions. Perform appropriate culture and susceptibility studies to determine susceptible causative organisms.

Monitoring: Periodically monitor renal/hepatic/hematopoietic functions. Monitor for CDAD (may range from mild diarrhea to fatal colitis), development of superinfections or drug resistance, allergic reactions, and other adverse reactions.

Counseling: Inform that the oral sus contains phenylalanine. Inform that drug only treats bacterial, not viral, infections. Instruct to take ud and that skipping doses or not completing full course may decrease effectiveness and increase resistance. Inform about potential benefits/risks. Notify physician if watery/bloody stools (with/without stomach cramps/fever) occur even ≥2 months after therapy. Notify if pregnant/nursing.

CEFTIN — cefuroxime axetil   Rx

Class: Cephalosporin (2nd generation)

ADULT DOSAGE

Pharyngitis/Tonsillitis
Mild to Moderate:
250mg tab q12h for 10 days

Acute Maxillary Sinusitis
Mild to Moderate:
250mg tab q12h for 10 days

Bronchitis
Mild to Moderate:
Acute Bacterial Exacerbations of Chronic Bronchitis: 250mg tab or 500mg tab q12h for 10 days
Secondary Bacterial Infections of Acute Bronchitis: 250mg tab or 500mg tab q12h for 5-10 days

Skin and Skin Structure Infections
Uncomplicated:
250mg tab or 500mg tab q12h for 10 days

Urinary Tract Infections
Uncomplicated:
250mg tab q12h for 7-10 days

Gonorrhea
Uncomplicated (Urethral, Endocervical, Rectal [in Females]):
1g tab as a single dose

Lyme Disease
Early Lyme Disease (Erythema Migrans):
500mg tab q12h for 20 days

PEDIATRIC DOSAGE

Skin and Skin Structure Infections
≥13 Years:
Uncomplicated: 250mg tab or 500mg tab q12h for 10 days

Urinary Tract Infections
≥13 Years:
Uncomplicated: 250mg tab q12h for 7-10 days

Gonorrhea
≥13 Years:
Uncomplicated (Urethral, Endocervical, Rectal [in Females]): 1g tab as a single dose

Lyme Disease
Early Lyme Disease (Erythema Migrans):
≥13 Years:
500mg tab q12h for 20 days

Pharyngitis/Tonsillitis
Mild to Moderate:
3 Months-12 Years: 20mg/kg/day sus divided bid for 10 days
Max: 500mg/day sus
≥13 Years: 250mg tab q12h for 10 days

Acute Otitis Media
3 Months-12 Years:
30mg/kg/day sus divided bid for 10 days
Max: 1g/day sus
Patients Who Can Swallow Tabs Whole: 250mg tab q12h for 10 days

Acute Maxillary Sinusitis
Mild to Moderate:
3 Months-12 Years: 30mg/kg/day sus divided bid for 10 days
Max: 1g/day sus
≥13 Years or Pediatric Patients <13 Years Who Can Swallow Tabs Whole: 250mg tab q12h for 10 days

Impetigo
3 Months-12 Years:
30mg/kg/day sus divided bid for 10 days
Max: 1g/day sus

Bronchitis
≥13 Years:
Mild to Moderate:
Acute Bacterial Exacerbations of Chronic Bronchitis: 250mg tab or 500mg tab q12h for 10 days
Secondary Bacterial Infections of Acute Bronchitis: 250mg tab or 500mg tab q12h for 5-10 days

---

DOSING CONSIDERATIONS
Renal Impairment
CrCl 10 to <30mL/min: Standard individual dose given q24h
CrCl <10mL/min (w/o Hemodialysis): Standard individual dose given q48h
Hemodialysis: Give a single additional standard dose at the end of each dialysis

ADMINISTRATION
Oral route

Tabs and sus are not bioequivalent and are not substitutable on a mg-per-mg basis
Pediatric patients ≥13 years who cannot swallow tabs whole should receive sus because the tab has a strong, persistent bitter taste when crushed

Sus

Take w/ food

Reconstitute 125mg/5mL w/ 37mL of water (for a volume of 100mL after reconstitution)

Reconstitute 250mg/5mL w/ 19mL of water (for a volume of 50mL after reconstitution) or 35mL of water (for a volume of 100mL after reconstitution)

Shake well before each use

Store reconstituted sus refrigerated between 2-8°C (36-46°F); discard reconstituted sus after 10 days

Tab

Take w/ or w/o food

Swallow whole w/o crushing

STORAGE

Tab: 15-30°C (59-86°F). Dry Powder: 2-30°C (36-86°F). Reconstituted Sus: Immediately store refrigerated between 2-8°C (36-46°F); discard after 10 days.

HOW SUPPLIED

Sus: 125mg/5mL [100mL], 250mg/5mL [50mL, 100mL]; **Tab:** 250mg, 500mg

CONTRAINDICATIONS

Known hypersensitivity (eg, anaphylaxis) to cefuroxime axetil or to other β-lactam antibacterial drugs (eg, penicillins and cephalosporins).

WARNINGS/PRECAUTIONS

Serious and occasionally fatal hypersensitivity (anaphylactic) reactions reported; d/c and institute appropriate therapy if an allergic reaction occurs. *Clostridium difficile*-associated diarrhea (CDAD) reported; may need to d/c if CDAD is suspected or confirmed. May result in bacterial resistance if used in the absence of proven or strongly suspected bacterial infection, or a prophylactic indication; consider possibility of superinfections w/ fungal or bacterial pathogens during therapy. Lab test interactions may occur. Caution in elderly. (Sus) Contains phenylalanine.

ADVERSE REACTIONS

Diarrhea, N/V, dislike of taste, diaper rash, Jarisch-Herxheimer reaction, vaginitis.

DRUG INTERACTIONS

May affect the gut flora, leading to lower estrogen reabsorption and reduced efficacy of combined oral estrogen/progesterone contraceptives. Drugs that reduce gastric acidity may result in a lower bioavailability; administer at least 1 hr before or 2 hrs after administration of short-acting antacids. Avoid H₂ antagonists and proton pump inhibitors. Probenecid increases plasma levels; coadministration is not recommended.

PREGNANCY AND LACTATION

Category B, caution in nursing.

MECHANISM OF ACTION

Cephalosporin (2nd generation); bactericidal agent that acts by inhibition of bacterial cell-wall synthesis.

PHARMACOKINETICS

Absorption: Absolute bioavailability (37% before food, 52% after food). **Distribution:** Plasma protein binding (50%); found in breast milk. **Metabolism:** Rapid hydrolysis via nonspecific esterases in the intestinal mucosa and blood. **Elimination:** Urine (50% unchanged).

Administration of variable doses resulted in different pharmacokinetic parameters.

PATIENT CONSIDERATIONS

Assessment: Assess for known hypersensitivity to therapy, other β-lactam antibacterial drugs (eg, penicillins, cephalosporins), or other allergens, renal impairment, pregnancy/nursing status, and possible drug interactions. For patients planning on using sus formulation, assess for phenylketonuria.

Monitoring: Monitor for anaphylactic reactions, CDAD, development of superinfection, and other adverse reactions.

Counseling: Advise of potential benefits/risks of therapy. Inform that drug only treats bacterial, not viral, infections. Instruct to take exactly ud; inform that skipping doses or not completing full course of therapy may decrease effectiveness and increase the likelihood of bacterial resistance. Inform that diarrhea may occur and will usually end when therapy is discontinued. Instruct to contact physician as soon as possible if watery and bloody stools (w/ or w/o stomach cramps and fever) develop even as late as ≥2 months after having taken the last dose. Inform that therapy may cause allergic reactions in some individuals. Inform that sus contains phenylalanine (a component of aspartame). Counsel patients to consider alternate supplementary (non-hormonal) contraceptive measures during treatment.

CEFTRIAXONE — ceftriaxone   Rx

Class: Cephalosporin (3rd generation)

OTHER BRAND NAMES

Rocephin

ADULT DOSAGE

General Dosing

Usual: 1-2g IV/IM qd or in equally divided doses bid depending on the type and severity of infection

Max: 4g/day

Usual Duration of Therapy: 4-14 days; complicated infections may require longer therapy

Continue for ≥2 days after signs and symptoms of infection have disappeared

PEDIATRIC DOSAGE

Skin and Skin Structure Infections

50-75mg/kg IV/IM qd or in equally divided doses bid

Max: 2g/day

Acute Otitis Media

Single dose of 50mg/kg IM

Max: 1g

Serious Infections

50-75mg/kg IV/IM in divided doses q12h

Streptococcus pyogenes Infections:

Continue therapy for ≥10 days

Appropriate coverage should be added for *Chlamydia trachomatis* infections

Gonococcal Infections

Uncomplicated:

250mg IM single dose

Prophylaxis of Postoperative Infections

Single dose of 1g IV, 0.5-2 hrs before surgery

Other Indications

Treatment of the Following Infections Caused by Susceptible Organisms:

Lower respiratory tract infections

Acute bacterial otitis media

Skin and skin structure infections

UTIs

Pelvic inflammatory disease

Bacterial septicemia

Bone and joint infections

Intra-abdominal infections

Meningitis

Max: 2g/day

Meningitis

100mg/kg IV/IM initially, then 100mg/kg IV/IM qd or in equally divided doses q12h for 7-14 days

Max: 4g/day

DOSING CONSIDERATIONS

Hepatic Impairment

Hepatic Dysfunction w/ Significant Renal Disease Max Dose: 2g/day

ADMINISTRATION

IV/IM route

Do not use diluents containing Ca²⁺ (eg, Ringer's sol or Hartmann's sol) to reconstitute or to further dilute a reconstituted vial for IV administration.

Do not simultaneously administer w/ Ca²⁺-containing IV sol; may administer sequentially of one another if the infusion lines are thoroughly flushed between infusions w/ a compatible fluid in patients other than neonates.

IM

Reconstitute 250mg, 500mg, 1g, or 2g vial w/ 0.9mL, 1.8mL, 3.6mL, or 7.2mL (respectively) of compatible diluent for a concentration of approx 250mg/mL.

Reconstitute 500mg, 1g, or 2g vial w/ 1mL, 2.1mL, or 4.2mL (respectively) of compatible diluent for a concentration of approx 350mg/mL.

Inject well w/in the body of a relatively large muscle; avoid unintentional inj into a blood vessel.

Compatible IM Diluents:

Sterile water for inj

0.9% NaCl sol

D5 sol

Bacteriostatic water + 0.9% benzyl alcohol

1% lidocaine sol (w/o epinephrine)

IV

Infuse over a 30-min period and administer over 60 min in neonates.

Concentrations of 10-40mg/mL are recommended; lower concentrations may be used if desired.

Reconstitute 250mg, 500mg, 1g, or 2g vial w/ 2.4mL, 4.8mL, 9.6mL, or 19.2mL (respectively) of compatible IV diluent for a concentration of approx 100mg/mL.

Withdraw entire contents of vial and dilute to desired concentration w/ appropriate IV diluent.

Compatibility:

Compatible w/ metronidazole HCl; do not exceed 5-7.5mg/mL of metronidazole HCl w/ 10mg/mL ceftriaxone as an admixture.

Physically incompatible w/ vancomycin, amsacrine, aminoglycosides, and fluconazole; when administered concomitantly by intermittent IV infusion, give sequentially, w/ thorough flushing of the IV lines between administrations.

Avoid physically mixing w/ or piggybacking into sol containing other antimicrobial drugs or into diluent sol.

Compatible IV Sol:

Sterile water

0.9% NaCl

D5 sol

D10 sol

D5 + 0.9% or 0.45% NaCl sol (incompatible when refrigerated)

Sodium lactate

10% invert sugar

5% sodium bicarbonate

Freamine III

Normosol-M in D5

Ionosol-B in D5

5% mannitol

10% mannitol

Refer to PI for further administration and stability instructions.

STORAGE

20-25°C (68-77°F). Protect from light. **Rocephin:** (Powder) ≤25°C (77°F).

HOW SUPPLIED

Inj: 250mg, 2g; (Rocephin) 500mg, 1g

CONTRAINDICATIONS

Known hypersensitivity to ceftriaxone, any of its excipients or to any other cephalosporin. Premature neonates up to a postmenstrual age of 41 weeks (gestational age + chronological age); hyperbilirubinemic neonates; neonates (≤28 days) that require (or are expected to require) treatment w/ Ca^{2+}-containing IV sol, including continuous Ca^{2+}-containing infusions; IV administration of ceftriaxone sol containing lidocaine.

WARNINGS/PRECAUTIONS

Anaphylactic reactions reported; caution in penicillin (PCN)- and other β-lactam agent-sensitive patients. *Clostridium difficile*-associated diarrhea (CDAD) reported; may need to d/c therapy if CDAD is suspected/confirmed. Severe cases of hemolytic anemia reported; consider if the diagnosis is associated w/ therapy and d/c until cause is determined. May result in overgrowth of nonsusceptible organisms w/ prolonged use or use in the absence of a proven or strongly suspected bacterial infection or prophylactic indication; take appropriate measures if superinfection develops. Alterations in PT may occur rarely; monitor w/ impaired vitamin K synthesis or low vitamin K stores during treatment (eg, chronic hepatitis disease, malnutrition). Gallbladder sonographic abnormalities reported; d/c if signs and symptoms of gallbladder disease develop. Pancreatitis reported. Ceftriaxone-calcium precipitates in the urinary tract reported; may develop symptoms of urolithiasis, ureteral obstruction, and post-renal acute renal failure. Ensure adequate hydration; d/c if signs and symptoms suggestive of urolithiasis, oliguria, or renal failure, and/or sonographic abnormalities occur. Lab test interactions may occur.

ADVERSE REACTIONS

Inj-site reactions (eg, warmth, tightness, induration), eosinophilia, thrombocytosis, AST/ALT elevation.

DRUG INTERACTIONS

See Contraindications and Administration. Vitamin K antagonist may increase risk of bleeding; monitor coagulation parameters and adjust dose of the anticoagulant accordingly.

PREGNANCY AND LACTATION

Pregnancy: Category B.
Lactation: Caution in nursing.

MECHANISM OF ACTION

Cephalosporin (3rd generation); bactericidal agent that acts by inhibition of bacterial cell-wall synthesis.

PHARMACOKINETICS

Absorption: (IM) Complete; T_{max}=2-3 hrs. (Pediatrics) Bacterial meningitis: C_{max}=216mcg/mL (50mg/kg IV), 275mcg/mL (75mg/kg IV). Middle Ear Fluid: C_{max}=35mcg/mL; T_{max}=24 hrs. **Distribution:** Found in breast milk, crosses placenta; plasma protein binding (95% at <25mcg/mL), (85% at 300mcg/mL); (Adults, healthy) V_d=5.78-13.5L. (Pediatrics) Bacterial Meningitis: V_d=338mL/kg (50mg/kg IV), 373mL/kg (75mg/kg IV). **Elimination:** Urine (33-67%, unchanged), feces, bile. (Adults, healthy) $T_{1/2}$=5.8-8.7 hrs. (Pediatrics) Bacterial Meningitis: $T_{1/2}$=4.6 hrs (50mg/kg IV), 4.3 hrs (75mg/kg IV). Middle Ear Fluid: $T_{1/2}$=25 hrs.

PATIENT CONSIDERATIONS

Assessment: Assess for hyperbilirubinemic neonates, hypersensitivity to cephalosporins/PCNs/other β-lactam agents, presence of both hepatic dysfunction and significant renal disease, impaired vitamin K synthesis or low vitamin K stores, pregnancy/nursing status, and possible drug interactions. Obtain appropriate specimens for isolation of the causative organism and for determination of susceptibility to the drug.

Monitoring: Monitor for signs/symptoms of hypersensitivity reactions, CDAD, hemolytic anemia, overgrowth of nonsusceptible organisms (eg, superinfection), gallbladder disease, pancreatitis, and other adverse reactions. Monitor PT levels in patients w/ impaired vitamin K synthesis or low vitamin K stores. Monitor for urolithiasis, oliguria, renal failure, or sonographic abnormalities. Monitor coagulation parameters.

Counseling: Inform that therapy only treats bacterial, not viral, infections. Instruct to take exactly ud even if feeling better early in the course of therapy; inform that skipping doses or not completing full course may decrease drug effectiveness and increase the likelihood of bacterial resistance. Instruct to contact physician as soon as possible if watery and bloody stools (w/ or w/o stomach cramps, fever) develop even as late as 2 or more months after having taken the last dose of therapy.

CELEBREX — celecoxib   Rx

Class: COX-2 inhibitor

ADULT DOSAGE

Osteoarthritis
200mg qd or 100mg bid

Rheumatoid Arthritis
100-200mg bid

Ankylosing Spondylitis
200mg qd or 100mg bid
Titrate: May increase to 400mg/day if no effect is observed after 6 weeks;

PEDIATRIC DOSAGE

Juvenile Rheumatoid Arthritis
≥2 Years:
10-25kg:
50mg bid
>25kg:
100mg bid

consider alternative treatment if no effect is observed after 6 weeks on 400mg/day

Acute Pain
Initial: 400mg initially, then 200mg if needed on 1st day
Maint: 200mg bid prn on subsequent days

Primary Dysmenorrhea
Initial: 400mg initially, then 200mg if needed on 1st day
Maint: 200mg bid prn on subsequent days

DOSING CONSIDERATIONS

Renal Impairment
Severe: Not recommended

Hepatic Impairment
Moderate (Child-Pugh Class B): Reduce daily dose by 50%
Severe: Not recommended

Elderly
If the anticipated benefit outweighs the potential risks, start at lower end of dosing range; monitor for adverse effects

Other Important Considerations
Poor Metabolizers of CYP2C9 Substrates:
Adults:
Initial: Consider 1/2 the lowest recommended dose
Juvenile Rheumatoid Arthritis (JRA) Patients:
Consider using alternative treatments.

ADMINISTRATION

Oral route

May be given w/o regard to timing of meals.
For patients w/ difficulty swallowing caps, contents may be added to applesauce; entire cap contents should be emptied onto a level tsp of cool or room temperature applesauce and ingested immediately w/ water.

STORAGE

20-25°C (68-77°F); excursions permitted to 15-30°C (59-86°F). Sprinkled contents on applesauce are stable for up to 6 hrs at 2-8°C (35-45°F).

HOW SUPPLIED

Cap: 50mg, 100mg, 200mg, 400mg

CONTRAINDICATIONS

Known hypersensitivity to celecoxib or any components of the drug product; history of asthma, urticaria, or allergic-type reactions w/ aspirin (ASA) or other NSAIDs; in the setting of CABG surgery; allergic-type reactions to sulfonamides.

WARNINGS/PRECAUTIONS

Use lowest effective dose for the shortest duration possible. Avoid in patients w/ a recent MI unless benefits outweigh the risks; if used, monitor for signs of cardiac ischemia. Increased risk for GI bleeding w/ longer duration of therapy, older age, poor general health status, and advanced liver disease and/or coagulopathy; avoid use in patients at higher risk unless benefits are expected to outweigh the increased risk, and consider alternate therapies. Promptly initiate evaluation and treatment if a serious GI adverse event is suspected; d/c until a serious GI adverse event is ruled out. Hepatotoxicity reported; d/c immediately and perform a clinical evaluation if clinical signs/symptoms consistent w/ liver disease develop, or if systemic manifestations occur. May cause new onset HTN or worsen preexisting HTN. Fluid retention and edema reported. Avoid use in patients w/ severe heart failure (HF) unless benefits outweigh risks; monitor for signs of worsening HF if used. Renal papillary necrosis and other renal injury reported w/ long-term use. Renal toxicity also reported in patients in whom renal prostaglandins have a compensatory role in the maintenance of renal perfusion; increased risk w/ renal/hepatic dysfunction, dehydration, hypovolemia, HF, and in the elderly. Correct volume status in dehydrated or hypovolemic patients prior to initiating therapy. Avoid use in patients w/ advanced renal disease unless the benefits are expected to outweigh the risk; monitor for signs of worsening renal function if used in patients w/ advanced renal disease. Hyperkalemia reported. Associated w/ anaphylactic reactions. Monitor for changes in the signs/symptoms of asthma in patients w/ preexisting asthma (w/o known ASA sensitivity). May cause serious skin reactions (eg, exfoliative dermatitis, Stevens-Johnson syndrome, toxic epidermal necrolysis); d/c at 1st appearance of skin rash/hypersensitivity. Anemia reported. May increase the risk of bleeding events; coagulation disorders may increase this risk. May mask inflammation and fever. Risk of disseminated intravascular coagulation in pediatric patients w/ systemic onset JRA; monitor for signs and symptoms of abnormal clotting or bleeding.

ADVERSE REACTIONS

Abdominal pain, diarrhea, dyspepsia, flatulence, peripheral edema, dizziness, pharyngitis, rhinitis, sinusitis, URTI, rash.

DRUG INTERACTIONS

Synergistic effect on bleeding w/ anticoagulants (eg, warfarin); monitor for signs of bleeding w/ concomitant anticoagulants, antiplatelet agents (eg, ASA), SSRIs, and SNRIs. Drugs that interfere w/ serotonin reuptake may potentiate the risk of bleeding. May increase risk of GI bleeding w/ use of anticoagulants, SSRIs, smoking, and alcohol use. ASA may increase risk of bleeding and serious GI events; concomitant use w/ analgesic doses of ASA is not recommended. Not a substitute for ASA for CV prophylaxis. May diminish antihypertensive effect of ACE inhibitors, ARBs, and β-blockers (eg, propranolol); monitor BP.

Coadministration w/ ACE inhibitors or ARBs may result in deterioration of renal function (including possible acute renal failure) in patients who are elderly, volume-depleted (including those on diuretic therapy), or have renal impairment; monitor for worsening renal function and adequately hydrate patient when these drugs are administered concomitantly. May reduce the natriuretic effect of loop diuretics (eg, furosemide) and thiazide diuretics; observe for signs of worsening renal function, in addition to assuring diuretic efficacy including antihypertensive effects. May increase digoxin serum concentrations and prolong the $T_{1/2}$ of digoxin; monitor digoxin levels. May elevate plasma lithium levels and reduce renal lithium clearance; monitor for signs of lithium toxicity. May increase the risk for methotrexate (MTX) toxicity; monitor for MTX toxicity. May increase cyclosporine's nephrotoxicity; monitor for signs of worsening renal function. Concomitant use w/ other NSAIDs or salicylates (eg, diflunisal, salsalate) increases the risk of GI toxicity; not recommended w/ other NSAIDs or salicylates. Concomitant use w/ pemetrexed may increase the risk of pemetrexed-associated myelosuppression, renal, and GI toxicity; refer to prescribing information for further information. CYP2C9 inhibitors (eg, fluconazole) may enhance the exposure and toxicity of celecoxib and CYP2C9 inducers (eg, rifampin) may lead to compromised efficacy of celecoxib; a dosage adjustment may be warranted. Corticosteroids may increase the risk of GI ulceration or bleeding; monitor for signs of bleeding.

PREGNANCY AND LACTATION
Pregnancy: Category C (<30 weeks of gestation) and D (≥30 weeks of gestation). Use during the 3rd trimester of pregnancy increases the risk of premature closure of the fetal ductus arteriosus; avoid use in pregnant women starting at 30 weeks of gestation.
Lactation: Found in breast milk; caution in nursing.
Reproductive Potential: May delay or prevent rupture of ovarian follicles, which has been associated w/ reversible infertility in some women. Small studies in women treated w/ NSAIDs have also shown a reversible delay in ovulation. Consider withdrawal of therapy in women who have difficulties conceiving or who are undergoing investigation of infertility.

MECHANISM OF ACTION
NSAID (COX-2 inhibitor); inhibits prostaglandin synthesis, primarily via inhibition of COX-2. Has anti-inflammatory, analgesic, and antipyretic activities.

PHARMACOKINETICS
Absorption: C_{max}=705ng/mL, T_{max}=2.8 hrs (fasted, 200mg). **Distribution:** V_d=429L (fasted, 200mg); plasma protein binding (97%); found in breast milk. **Metabolism:** CYP2C9. **Elimination:** Feces (57%), urine (27%), urine and feces (<3% unchanged); $T_{1/2}$=11.2 hrs (fasted, 200mg).

PATIENT CONSIDERATIONS
Assessment: Assess for history of allergic-type reactions to sulfonamides, history of asthma, urticaria, other allergic-type reactions w/ ASA or other NSAIDs; asthma; CV disease (CVD) or risk factors for CVD; HTN; history of peptic ulcer disease or GI bleeding; coagulation disorders; renal/hepatic impairment; pregnancy/nursing status; or any other conditions where treatment is contraindicated or cautioned. Assess volume status. Assess for possible drug interactions. Obtain baseline BP, CBC, and chemistry profile.

Monitoring: Monitor for signs/symptoms of CV thrombotic events; cardiac ischemia in patients w/ a recent MI; GI bleeding/ulceration and perforation; hepatotoxicity; new or worsening HTN; HF; edema; renal papillary necrosis and other renal injury; hyperkalemia; anaphylactic reactions; serious skin reactions; anemia; and other adverse reactions. Monitor for development of abnormal clotting or bleeding in patients w/ systemic onset JRA. Monitor BP during initiation of therapy and throughout the course of therapy. Monitor for signs of bleeding in patients on concomitant therapy w/ anticoagulants, antiplatelet agents, SSRIs, or SNRIs. Monitor renal function in patients w/ renal/hepatic impairment, HF, dehydration, or hypovolemia. Monitor CBC and chemistry profiles periodically during long-term treatment.

Counseling: Inform of potential for CV thrombotic events, GI adverse events, and worsening CHF/edema, and advise of symptoms; instruct to report symptoms to healthcare provider if any occur. Inform of the potential for hepatotoxicity, and advise of signs/symptoms; if signs/symptoms occur, instruct to call healthcare provider. Instruct to seek immediate emergency help if signs of an anaphylactic reaction occur. Advise to d/c immediately if rash develops and to contact healthcare provider as soon as possible. Advise females of reproductive potential who desire pregnancy that therapy may be associated w/ a reversible delay in ovulation. Instruct pregnant women to avoid use starting at 30 weeks of gestation. Instruct patient not to use other NSAIDs or salicylates concomitantly; notify of the presence of NSAIDs in OTC medications for colds, fever, or insomnia. Inform patient to not use low-dose ASA concomitantly w/o talking to healthcare provider.

CELLCEPT — mycophenolate mofetil   Rx
Class: Inosine monophosphate dehydrogenase (IMPDH) inhibitor

Use during pregnancy is associated w/ increased risks of 1st trimester pregnancy loss and congenital malformations; counsel females of reproductive potential regarding pregnancy prevention and planning. Immunosuppression may lead to increased susceptibility to infection and possible development of lymphoma. Should only be prescribed by physicians experienced in immunosuppressive therapy and management of organ transplant patients. Manage patients in facilities equipped and staffed w/ adequate lab and supportive medical resources.

ADULT DOSAGE
Renal Transplant
Prophylaxis of organ rejection in patients receiving allogeneic renal transplants; use concomitantly w/ cyclosporine and corticosteroids

1g PO/IV bid

Cardiac Transplant
Prophylaxis of organ rejection in patients receiving allogeneic cardiac transplants; use concomitantly w/ cyclosporine and corticosteroids

1.5g PO/IV bid

Hepatic Transplant
Prophylaxis of organ rejection in patients receiving allogeneic hepatic transplants; use concomitantly w/ cyclosporine and corticosteroids

1.5g PO bid or 1g IV bid

PEDIATRIC DOSAGE
Renal Transplant
Prophylaxis of organ rejection in patients receiving allogeneic renal transplants; use concomitantly w/ cyclosporine and corticosteroids

3 Months-18 Years:
Sus:
$600mg/m^2$ bid
Max Daily Dose: 2g/10mL
Cap:
BSA $1.25-1.5m^2$: 750mg bid
Cap/Tab:
BSA $>1.5m^2$: 1g bid

DOSING CONSIDERATIONS
Renal Impairment
Renal Transplant:
Severe Chronic Renal Impairment (GFR <25mL/min) Outside the Immediate Post-Transplant Period: Avoid doses >1g bid

No dose adjustments needed in renal transplant patients experiencing delayed graft function postoperatively

Adverse Reactions
Neutropenia (ANC $<1.3 \times 10^3/\mu L$): Interrupt or reduce dose

ADMINISTRATION
Oral/IV route

Exercise caution in handling; refer to PI.

Oral
Give initial dose as soon as possible after transplant.
Administer on an empty stomach; may administer w/ food if necessary in stable renal transplant patients.
Do not crush tab; do not open or crush cap.
Sus may be given via NG tube (minimum size of 8 French).

IV
Administer w/in 24 hrs following transplant.
Administer by slow IV infusion over no less than 2 hrs by either peripheral or central vein.
May administer for up to 14 days; switch to oral therapy as soon as patient can tolerate oral medication.
Start administration w/in 4 hrs from reconstitution and dilution.
Do not mix or administer concurrently via same infusion catheter w/ other IV drugs or infusion admixtures.

Preparation
Sus:
1. Measure 94mL of water in a graduated cylinder.
2. Add approx 1/2 the total amount of water to bottle and shake closed bottle well for about 1 min.
3. Add remainder of water and shake closed bottle well for about 1 min.
4. Remove child-resistant cap and push bottle adapter into neck of bottle; close bottle w/ child-resistant cap tightly.

IV Reconstitution:
2 vials are needed to prepare a 1g dose; 3 vials are needed for a 1.5g dose. Reconstitute contents of each vial by injecting 14mL of D5 inj; gently shake vials to dissolve.

IV Dilution:
For a 1g dose, further dilute contents of the 2 reconstituted vials into 140mL of D5 inj.
For a 1.5g dose, further dilute contents of the 3 reconstituted vials into 210mL of D5 inj.
Final concentration of both sol is 6mg/mL.

STORAGE
25°C (77°F); excursions permitted to 15-30°C (59-86°F). Constituted Sus: Stable up to 60 days; may also be refrigerated at 2-8°C (36-46°F). Do not freeze.

HOW SUPPLIED
Cap: 250mg; Inj: 500mg/20mL; Sus: 200mg/mL; Tab: 500mg

CONTRAINDICATIONS
Hypersensitivity to mycophenolate mofetil, mycophenolic acid, or any component of the medication. Inj: Allergy to Polysorbate 80.

WARNINGS/PRECAUTIONS
Do not administer IV sol by rapid or bolus inj. May increase risk of developing malignancies, particularly of the skin; limit exposure to sunlight and UV light in patients w/ increased risk for skin cancer. Polyomavirus-associated nephropathy (PVAN), JC virus-associated progressive multifocal leukoencephalopathy (PML), cytomegalovirus infections, and reactivation of hepatitis B virus (HBV) or hepatitis C virus (HCV) reported; consider dose reduction if new or reactivated viral infection develops. PVAN, especially due to BK virus infection, may lead to deteriorating renal function and renal graft loss. Consider PML in differential diagnosis in patients reporting neurological symptoms and consider consultation w/ a neurologist. Severe neutropenia reported; interrupt or reduce dose if

neutropenia develops. Cases of pure red cell aplasia (PRCA) reported when used w/ other immunosuppressive agents. Acceptable birth control must be used during therapy and for 6 weeks after discontinuation. GI bleeding, ulceration, and perforation reported; caution w/ active serious digestive system disease. Avoid doses >1g bid in renal transplant patients w/ severe chronic renal impairment (GFR <25mL/min); caution w/ delayed renal graft function post-transplant. More reports of opportunistic/herpes virus infections in cardiac transplant patients in comparison w/ azathioprine. Avoid w/ rare hereditary deficiency of hypoxanthine-guanine phosphoribosyl-transferase (HGPRT) (eg, Lesch-Nyhan and Kelley-Seegmiller syndromes). Oral sus contains 0.56mg phenylalanine/mL; caution w/ phenylketonurics. Caution in elderly.

ADVERSE REACTIONS
Infection, diarrhea, leukopenia, sepsis, N/V, HTN, peripheral edema, abdominal pain, fever, headache, constipation, hyperglycemia, anemia, insomnia.

DRUG INTERACTIONS
Avoid w/ azathioprine, drugs that interfere w/ enterohepatic recirculation (eg, cholestyramine), and norfloxacin-metronidazole combination. Vaccinations may be less effective; avoid live, attenuated vaccines. Decreased exposure w/ rifampin; concomitant use not recommended unless benefit outweighs risk. Increased levels of both drugs w/ drugs that compete w/ renal tubular secretion (eg, acyclovir/valacyclovir, ganciclovir/valganciclovir, probenecid). Oral ciprofloxacin and amoxicillin plus clavulanic acid may decrease levels. Mean mycophenolic acid (MPA) exposure may be 30-50% greater when mycophenolate mofetil is administered w/o cyclosporine compared to when coadministered w/ cyclosporine. Expect changes in exposure when switching from cyclosporine A to an immunosuppressant that does not interfere w/ the enterohepatic cycle (eg, tacrolimus, belatacept). Telmisartan decreases levels. May decrease levels and effectiveness of hormonal contraceptives; use w/ caution and must use additional barrier contraceptive methods. Drugs that alter GI flora may reduce levels available for absorption. Decreased levels w/ proton pump inhibitors (eg, lansoprazole, pantoprazole), Mg^{2+}- and aluminum-containing antacids, and Ca^{2+} free phosphate binders (eg, sevelamer). Do not administer simultaneously w/ antacids containing aluminum and magnesium hydroxides. Do not administer Ca^{2+} free phosphate binders simultaneously; may give 2 hrs after intake. Combination immunosuppressant therapy should be used w/ caution.

PREGNANCY AND LACTATION
Pregnancy: Category D.
Lactation: Not for use in nursing.

MECHANISM OF ACTION
Inosine monophosphate dehydrogenase inhibitor; inhibits the de novo pathway of guanosine nucleotide synthesis w/o incorporation into deoxyribonucleic acid.

PHARMACOKINETICS
Absorption: Rapid and complete; (oral) absolute bioavailability (94%). Refer to PI for parameters in different populations. **Distribution:** V_d=3.6L/kg (IV), 4L/kg (oral); plasma albumin binding (97% MPA, 82% phenolic glucuronide of MPA [MPAG]). **Metabolism:** Complete hydrolysis to MPA (active metabolite). MPA is metabolized by glucuronyl transferase to MPAG, which is converted to MPA via enterohepatic recirculation. **Elimination:** (Oral) Urine (93%; <1% MPA, 87% MPAG), feces (6%); MPA: $T_{1/2}$=17.9 hrs (oral), 16.6 hrs (IV).

PATIENT CONSIDERATIONS
Assessment: Assess for hypersensitivity to the drug or its components, hepatic/renal impairment, delayed renal graft function post-transplant, phenylketonuria, hereditary deficiency of HGPRT (eg, Lesch-Nyhan and Kelley-Seegmiller syndromes), active digestive disease, vaccination history, nursing status, and possible drug interactions. Assess pregnancy status using serum or urine test of at least 25 mIU/mL sensitivity, immediately before starting therapy.

Monitoring: Monitor for signs/symptoms of lymphomas, skin cancer, and other malignancies, infections, HCV/HBV reactivation, neutropenia, PRCA, GI bleeding/perforation/ulceration, and other adverse reactions. Monitor CBC weekly during the 1st month, twice monthly for the 2nd and 3rd months of therapy, and then monthly through the 1st yr. Monitor pregnancy status by obtaining pregnancy test 8-10 days after initiation of therapy and repeatedly during follow-up visits.

Counseling: Inform that use during pregnancy is associated w/ an increased risk of 1st trimester pregnancy loss and congenital malformations; discuss pregnancy testing, prevention (including acceptable contraception methods), and planning. Discuss appropriate alternative immunosuppressants w/ less potential for embryofetal toxicity if patient is considering pregnancy. Advise of complete dosage instructions and inform about increased risk of lymphoproliferative disease and certain other malignancies. Inform of the need for repeated appropriate lab tests during therapy. Instruct patients to report immediately any evidence of infection, unexpected bruising, bleeding, or any other manifestation of bone marrow depression. Advise not to breastfeed during therapy. Encourage to enroll in the pregnancy registry if patient becomes pregnant while on medication.

CEPHALEXIN — cephalexin   Rx
Class: Cephalosporin (1st generation)

OTHER BRAND NAMES
Keflex

ADULT DOSAGE
General Dosing

Usual: 250mg q6h; may administer a dose of 500mg q12h. Treat for 7-14 days

PEDIATRIC DOSAGE
General Dosing

>1 Year:
Recommended Dose: 25-50mg/kg/day in equally divided doses for 7-14 days

More Severe Infections:
May need larger doses, up to 4g/day in 2-4 equally divided doses

Other Indications
- Respiratory tract infections
- Otitis media
- Skin and skin structure infections
- Bone infections
- Genitourinary tract infections, including acute prostatitis

Severe Infections:
May administer 50-100mg/kg/day in equally divided doses

β-Hemolytic Streptococcal Infections:
Administer for at least 10 days

≥15 Years:
Usual: 250mg q6h; may administer a dose of 500mg q12h. Treat for 7-14 days

More Severe Infections:
May need larger doses, up to 4g/day in 2-4 equally divided doses

Otitis Media
>1 Year:
75-100mg/kg/day given in equally divided doses

DOSING CONSIDERATIONS
Renal Impairment
Adults and Pediatric Patients ≥15 Years:
CrCl 30-59mL/min: No dose adjustment; max dose should not exceed 1g/day
CrCl 15-29mL/min: 250mg q8h or q12h
CrCl 5-14mL/min Not Yet on Dialysis: 250mg q24h
CrCl 1-4mL/min Not Yet on Dialysis: 250mg q48h or q60h
Hemodialysis: Insufficient information to make dose adjustment recommendation

ADMINISTRATION
Oral route

Take w/o regard to meals.

Oral Sus
Shake well before using.
After mixing, store in refrigerator; may be kept for 14 days w/o significant loss of potency.

Directions for Mixing:
125mg/5mL: Add to the bottle a total of 71mL (for 100mL when mixed) or 140mL (for 200mL when mixed) of water in 2 portions. Shake well after each addition.
250mg/5mL: Add to the bottle a total of 71mL (for 100mL when mixed) or 140mL (for 200mL when mixed) of water in 2 portions. Shake well after each addition.

STORAGE
20-25°C (68-77°F). **Keflex:** 25°C (77°F); excursions permitted to 15-30°C (59-86°F).

HOW SUPPLIED
Oral Sus: 125mg/5mL [100mL, 200mL], 250mg/5mL [100mL, 200mL]; **Tab:** 250mg*, 500mg*; **Cap:** (Keflex) 250mg, 500mg, 750mg *scored

CONTRAINDICATIONS
Known hypersensitivity to cephalexin or other cephalosporins.

WARNINGS/PRECAUTIONS
Allergic reactions reported. Prior to therapy, inquire about hypersensitivity reactions to cephalexin, cephalosporins, penicillins (PCNs), or other drugs; cross-hypersensitivity among β-lactam antibacterials may occur in patients w/ history of PCN allergy. D/C therapy and institute appropriate treatment if an allergic reaction occurs. *Clostridium difficile*-associated diarrhea (CDAD) reported; may need to d/c if CDAD is suspected or confirmed. Positive direct Coombs' tests and acute intravascular hemolysis induced by cephalexin therapy reported; if anemia develops during or after therapy, perform a diagnostic work-up for drug-induced hemolytic anemia, d/c cephalexin, and institute appropriate therapy. May trigger seizures (particularly w/ renal impairment when dose is not reduced); d/c if seizures occur. May be associated w/ prolonged PT; patients w/ renal/hepatic impairment, poor nutritional state, or who are receiving a protracted course of antibacterial therapy and anticoagulant therapy may be at risk. May result in bacterial resistance w/ prolonged use or if used in the absence of a proven/suspected bacterial infection or a prophylactic indication; take appropriate measures if superinfection develops. Lab test interactions may occur. Caution in elderly.

ADVERSE REACTIONS
Diarrhea, N/V, dyspepsia, gastritis, abdominal pain.

DRUG INTERACTIONS
Increased metformin levels and decreased renal clearance of metformin; monitor patient carefully and adjust dose of metformin. Probenecid inhibits renal excretion; coadministration w/ probenecid is not recommended.

PREGNANCY AND LACTATION
Pregnancy: Category B.
Lactation: Cephalexin is excreted in human milk; caution in nursing.

MECHANISM OF ACTION
Cephalosporin (1st generation); bactericidal agent that acts by the inhibition of bacterial cell-wall synthesis.

PHARMACOKINETICS
Absorption: C_{max}=9mcg/mL (250mg), 18mcg/mL (500mg), 32mcg/mL (1g); T_{max}=1 hr. **Distribution:** Plasma protein binding (approx 10-15%). Found in breast milk. **Elimination:** Urine (>90% unchanged).

PATIENT CONSIDERATIONS
Assessment: Assess for previous hypersensitivity to cephalexin, cephalosporins, PCNs, or other drugs. Assess renal/hepatic function, pregnancy/nursing status, and possible drug interactions. Obtain baseline culture and susceptibility tests.

Monitoring: Monitor for signs/symptoms of hypersensitivity reactions, CDAD, superinfection, and other adverse reactions. Monitor PT and renal function when indicated. Perform culture and susceptibility tests.

Counseling: Advise that allergic reactions, including serious allergic reactions, may occur and that serious reactions require immediate treatment. Inform that drug only treats bacterial, not viral, infections. Instruct to take exactly ud; inform that skipping doses or not completing full course of therapy may decrease effectiveness and increase likelihood of bacterial resistance. Advise that diarrhea is a common problem caused by therapy and usually resolves when the drug is discontinued; instruct to contact physician if severe watery or bloody diarrhea (w/ or w/o stomach cramps and fever) develops even as late as ≥2 months after taking last dose.

CERDELGA — eliglustat   Rx

Class: Glucosylceramide synthase inhibitor

ADULT DOSAGE	PEDIATRIC DOSAGE
Type 1 Gaucher Disease Long-term treatment of patients who are CYP2D6 extensive metabolizers (EMs), intermediate metabolizers (IMs), or poor metabolizers (PMs) as detected by an FDA-cleared test **Usual:** **CYP2D6 EMs/IMs:** 84mg bid **CYP2D6 PMs:** 84mg qd	Pediatric use may not have been established

---

DOSING CONSIDERATIONS
Concomitant Medications
Strong/Moderate CYP2D6 Inhibitors:
CYP2D6 EMs/IMs: Reduce dose to 84mg qd
Strong/Moderate CYP3A Inhibitors:
Grapefruit/Grapefruit Juice: Avoid
CYP2D6 EMs: Reduce dose to 84mg qd
Renal Impairment
Moderate to Severe Impairment/ESRD: Use not recommended
Hepatic Impairment
All Stages/Cirrhosis: Use not recommended
Other Important Considerations
Administer therapy 24 hrs after the last dose of the previous enzyme replacement therapy (eg, imiglucerase, velaglucerase alfa, taliglucerase alfa)

ADMINISTRATION
Oral route
Swallow caps whole, preferably w/ water; do not crush, dissolve, or open
May be taken w/ or w/o food

STORAGE
20-25°C (68-77°F); excursions permitted between 15-30°C (59-86°F).

HOW SUPPLIED
Cap: 84mg

CONTRAINDICATIONS
EMs or IMs taking a strong or moderate CYP2D6 inhibitor concomitantly with a strong or moderate CYP3A inhibitor. IMs or PMs taking a strong CYP3A inhibitor.

WARNINGS/PRECAUTIONS
May cause increases in ECG intervals (PR, QTc, and QRS) at substantially elevated eliglustat plasma concentrations; not recommended in patients with preexisting cardiac disease (congestive heart failure, recent acute myocardial infarction, bradycardia, heart block, ventricular arrhythmia) or long QT syndrome. Not recommended with moderate to severe renal impairment, end-stage renal disease, and in all stages of hepatic impairment or cirrhosis. Patients who are CYP2D6 ultra-rapid metabolizers may not achieve adequate concentrations of eliglustat to achieve a therapeutic effect.

ADVERSE REACTIONS
Fatigue, headache, nausea, diarrhea, back pain, pain in extremities, upper abdominal pain, flatulence, oropharyngeal pain, dizziness, asthenia, cough, dyspepsia, gastroesophageal reflux disease, constipation.

DRUG INTERACTIONS
See Dosing Considerations and Contraindications. Avoid consumption of grapefruit or grapefruit juice. For patients currently treated with imiglucerase, velaglucerase alfa, or taliglucerase alfa, eliglustat may be administered 24 hrs after the last dose of the previous enzyme replacement therapy (ERT). Not recommended with class IA (eg, quinidine, procainamide) and class III (eg, amiodarone, sotalol) antiarrhythmic medications. CYP2D6 and CYP3A inhibitors may significantly increase exposure and result in prolongation of the PR, QTc, and/or QRS cardiac interval which could result in cardiac arrhythmias; not recommended with moderate CYP3A inhibitors (eg, fluconazole) in IMs and PMs, or weak CYP3A inhibitors (eg, ranitidine) in PMs. Strong CYP3A inducers (eg, rifampin, carbamazepine, St. John's wort) significantly decrease exposure; coadministration is not recommended in EMs, IMs, and PMs. May increase concentrations of P-glycoprotein (eg, digoxin, phenytoin, colchicine, dabigatran etexilate) or CYP2D6 (eg, metoprolol, nortriptyline, perphenazine) substrates; monitor therapeutic drug concentrations, as indicated, or consider reducing the dosage of the concomitant drug and titrate to clinical effect. Measure serum digoxin concentrations before initiating eliglustat, reduce digoxin dose by 30%, and continue monitoring.

PREGNANCY AND LACTATION
Category C, not for use in nursing.

MECHANISM OF ACTION
Glucosylceramide synthase inhibitor; acts as a substrate reduction therapy for GD1.

PHARMACOKINETICS
Absorption: Administration to patients with different CYP2D6 metabolizer statuses resulted in different parameters. **Distribution:** Plasma protein binding (76-83%); (IV) V_d=835L (EMs). **Metabolism:** Extensive via CYP2D6 (major) and CYP3A4 (minor); sequential oxidation of the octanoyl moiety followed by oxidation of the 2,3-dihydro-1,4-benzodioxane moiety, or a combination of the two pathways. **Elimination:** (PO) Urine (41.8%), feces (51.4%). $T_{1/2}$=6.5 hrs (EMs), 8.9 hrs (PMs).

PATIENT CONSIDERATIONS
Assessment: Assess for preexisting cardiac disease, long QT syndrome, renal/hepatic impairment, CYP2D6 metabolizer status, pregnancy/nursing status, and possible drug interactions.
Monitoring: Monitor for ECG changes and other adverse reactions.
Counseling: Advise to discuss all the medications being taken, including any herbal supplements or vitamins, with physician. Advise to inform physician if new symptoms (eg, palpitations, fainting, dizziness) develop. Instruct to avoid consumption of grapefruit or its juice. Inform patients currently treated with imiglucerase, velaglucerase alfa, or taliglucerase alfa, that drug may be administered 24 hrs after the last dose of the previous ERT.

CERVARIX — human papillomavirus bivalent
(types 16, 18) vaccine, recombinant   Rx

Class: Vaccine

ADULT DOSAGE	PEDIATRIC DOSAGE
Prevention of Cervical Cancer Prevention of cervical cancer, cervical intraepithelial neoplasia (CIN) Grade 2 or worse and adenocarcinoma in situ, and CIN Grade 1, caused by oncogenic human papillomavirus (HPV) types 16 and 18 **≤25 Years:** 3 IM doses (0.5mL each) at 0, 1, and 6 months	**Prevention of Cervical Cancer** Prevention of cervical cancer, CIN Grade 2 or worse and adenocarcinoma in situ, and CIN Grade 1, caused by oncogenic HPV types 16 and 18 **≥9 Years:** 3 IM doses (0.5mL each) at 0, 1, and 6 months

---

ADMINISTRATION
IM route
Inject preferably in the deltoid region of the upper arm.
Do not mix w/ any other vaccine in the same syringe or vial.
Shake well before withdrawal and use.

STORAGE
2-8°C (36-46°F). Do not freeze; discard if frozen.

HOW SUPPLIED
Inj: 0.5mL

CONTRAINDICATIONS
Severe allergic reactions (eg, anaphylaxis) to any component of this vaccine.

WARNINGS/PRECAUTIONS
Does not provide protection against disease due to all HPV types or from vaccine and non-vaccine HPV types to which a woman has previously been exposed through sexual activity. May not result in protection in all vaccine recipients. Females should continue to adhere to recommended cervical cancer screening procedures. Syncope sometimes associated w/ falling w/ injury, tonic-clonic movements, and other seizure-like activity reported; observe for 15 min after administration. Tip cap of prefilled syringe contains natural rubber latex; may cause allergic reactions. Review immunization history for possible vaccine hypersensitivity and previous vaccination-related adverse reactions; appropriate treatment and supervision must be available for possible anaphylactic reactions. Immunocompromised individuals may have diminished immune response.

ADVERSE REACTIONS
Inj-site reactions (eg, pain, redness, swelling), fatigue, headache, myalgia, GI symptoms, arthralgia.

DRUG INTERACTIONS
Immunosuppressive therapies, including irradiation, antimetabolites, alkylating agents, cytotoxic drugs, and corticosteroids (used in greater than physiologic doses), may reduce immune response to vaccine.

PREGNANCY AND LACTATION
Pregnancy: Category B.
Lactation: Excretion of vaccine-induced antibodies in human milk has not been studied for Cervarix. Caution in nursing.

MECHANISM OF ACTION
Vaccine; may be mediated by the development of IgG-neutralizing antibodies directed against HPV-L1 capsid proteins generated as a result of vaccination.

PATIENT CONSIDERATIONS
Assessment: Assess for latex hypersensitivity, immunosuppression, pregnancy/nursing status, and possible drug interactions. Review immunization history for possible vaccine hypersensitivity and for previous vaccination-related adverse reactions.
Monitoring: Monitor for syncope, tonic-clonic movements, seizure-like activity, anaphylactic reactions, and other adverse reactions.

Counseling: Inform that vaccine does not substitute for routine cervical cancer screening; advise women who receive the vaccine to continue to undergo cervical screening per standard of care. Counsel that vaccine does not protect against disease from HPV types to which a woman has previously been exposed through sexual activity. Inform that since syncope has been reported following vaccination in young females, observation for 15 min after administration is recommended.

CESAMET — nabilone   CII

Class: Cannabinoid

ADULT DOSAGE

Chemotherapy-Induced Nausea/Vomiting

In patients who have failed to respond adequately to conventional antiemetics

Usual: 1 or 2mg bid
Give initial dose 1-3 hrs before chemotherapeutic agent; use lower starting dose and increase as necessary to minimize side effects. May be useful to give a dose of 1 or 2mg the night before
Max: 6mg/day in divided doses tid

May be administered bid or tid during the entire course of each cycle of chemotherapy and, if needed, for 48 hrs after the last dose of each cycle of chemotherapy

PEDIATRIC DOSAGE
Pediatric use may not have been established

DOSING CONSIDERATIONS
Elderly
Start at lower end of dosing range

ADMINISTRATION
Oral route

STORAGE
25°C (77°F); excursions permitted to 15-30°C (59-86°F).

HOW SUPPLIED
Cap: 1mg

CONTRAINDICATIONS
History of hypersensitivity to any cannabinoid.

WARNINGS/PRECAUTIONS
Not for use on prn basis or as 1st antiemetic product prescribed. High potential for abuse. Adverse psychiatric reactions can persist for 48-72 hrs following discontinuation of treatment. May cause dizziness, drowsiness, euphoria, disorientation, depression, hallucinations, psychosis, tachycardia, and orthostatic hypotension. May alter mental states; keep patients under adult supervision, especially during initial use and dose adjustments. May impair mental/physical abilities. May elevate HR and cause postural hypotension. Caution w/ HTN, heart disease, current or previous psychiatric disorders (eg, manic depressive illness, depression, schizophrenia) and history of substance abuse. Caution in pregnant/nursing patients and pediatrics.

ADVERSE REACTIONS
Drowsiness, vertigo, dizziness, dry mouth, euphoria, ataxia, headache, concentration difficulties, dysphoria, visual disturbance, asthenia, anorexia, depression, hypotension.

DRUG INTERACTIONS
Avoid w/ alcohol, sedatives, hypnotics, or other psychoactive drugs. Additive HTN, tachycardia, and possible cardiotoxicity w/ sympathomimetics (eg, amphetamines, cocaine). Additive or super-additive tachycardia and drowsiness w/ anticholinergics (eg, atropine, scopolamine, antihistamines). Additive tachycardia, HTN, and drowsiness w/ TCAs (eg, amitriptyline, amoxapine, desipramine). Additive drowsiness and CNS depression w/ CNS depressants (eg, barbiturates, benzodiazepines, ethanol). May result in hypomanic reaction w/ disulfiram and fluoxetine and increase theophylline metabolism in patients who smoked marijuana. May decrease clearance of antipyrine and barbiturates. Cross-tolerance and mutual potentiation w/ opioids. Enhanced tetrahydrocannabinol effects w/ naltrexone. Increase in the positive subjective mood effects of smoked marijuana w/ alcohol. Impaired psychomotor function w/ diazepam. May displace highly protein-bound drugs; monitor for dose requirement changes.

PREGNANCY AND LACTATION
Category C, not for use in nursing.

MECHANISM OF ACTION
Cannabinoid; interacts w/ the cannabinoid receptor system, CB (1) receptor.

PHARMACOKINETICS
Absorption: Complete, C_{max}=approx 2ng/mL, T_{max}=2 hrs. **Distribution:** V_d=12.5L/kg. **Metabolism:** Liver (extensive) via reduction and oxidation; CYP450. **Elimination:** (IV) Feces (60%), urine (24%); $T_{1/2}$=2 hrs (identified metabolites), 35 hrs (unidentified metabolites).

PATIENT CONSIDERATIONS
Assessment: Assess for history of hypersensitivity to the drug, heart disease, HTN, previous/current psychiatric disorders, history of substance abuse (eg, alcohol abuse/dependence, marijuana use), pregnancy/nursing status, and possible drug interactions.

Monitoring: Monitor for adverse psychiatric reactions or unmasking of symptoms of psychiatric disorders, signs/symptoms of CNS effects, postural hypotension. Monitor BP and HR. Monitor for signs of excessive use, abuse, and misuse. Monitor for signs/symptoms of hypersensitivity and other adverse reactions.

Counseling: Inform about additive CNS depression effect if taken concomitantly w/ alcohol or other CNS depressants; advise to avoid this combination. Advise not to engage in hazardous activity (eg, operating machinery/driving). Inform of possible mood changes and other adverse behavioral effects that may occur during therapy. Instruct to remain under supervision of responsible adult during treatment.

CHANTIX — varenicline   Rx

Class: Nicotinic acetylcholine receptor agonist

> Serious neuropsychiatric events including, but not limited to, depression, suicidal ideation, suicide attempt, and completed suicide reported. Some reported cases might have been complicated by nicotine withdrawal symptoms in patients who stopped smoking. Monitor for neuropsychiatric symptoms, including changes in behavior, hostility, agitation, depressed mood, and suicide-related events. Worsening of preexisting psychiatric illness and completed suicide reported in some patients attempting to quit smoking while on therapy. Advise patients and caregivers that the patient should stop taking therapy and contact a healthcare provider immediately if agitation, hostility, depressed mood, changes in behavior or thinking, suicidal ideation, or suicidal behavior occurs. Weigh risks against benefits of use.

ADULT DOSAGE
Smoking Cessation Aid

Set quit date and start 1 week before quit date. Alternatively, may begin therapy and then quit smoking between Days 8 and 35 of treatment

Days 1-3: 0.5mg qd
Days 4-7: 0.5mg bid
Day 8-End of Treatment: 1mg bid
Treat for 12 weeks

If patient has successfully stopped smoking at end of 12 weeks, additional course of 12-week treatment is recommended to further increase the likelihood of long-term abstinence

If patient is sure that he or she is not able or willing to quit abruptly, consider a gradual approach to quitting smoking w/ varenicline. Begin varenicline dosing and reduce smoking by 50% from baseline w/in the first 4 weeks, by an additional 50% in the next 4 weeks, and continue reducing w/ the goal of reaching complete abstinence by 12 weeks. Continue varenicline for an additional 12 weeks, for a total of 24 weeks of treatment. Encourage to attempt quitting sooner if patient feels ready

If patient is motivated to quit and not successful in stopping smoking during prior therapy for reasons other than intolerability due to adverse events, or if relapse occurs after treatment, should make another attempt once factors contributing to failed attempt are identified and addressed

PEDIATRIC DOSAGE
Pediatric use may not have been established

DOSING CONSIDERATIONS
Renal Impairment
Severe (CrCl <30mL/min):
Initial: 0.5mg qd
Titrate: May titrate prn to a max dose of 0.5mg bid
ESRD w/ Hemodialysis:
Max: 0.5mg qd if tolerated

Adverse Reactions
Consider a temporary/permanent dose reduction in patients who cannot tolerate adverse effects

ADMINISTRATION
Oral route

Take pc and w/ a full glass of water.
Provide patients w/ appropriate educational materials and counseling to support the quit attempt.

STORAGE
25°C (77°F); excursions permitted to 15-30°C (59-86°F).

HOW SUPPLIED
Tab: 0.5mg, 1mg

CONTRAINDICATIONS
Known history of serious hypersensitivity reactions or skin reactions to varenicline.

WARNINGS/PRECAUTIONS
Seizures reported; consider discontinuing therapy if this occurs. Caution w/ history of seizures or other factors that can lower the seizure threshold. Somnolence,

dizziness, loss of consciousness, and difficulty concentrating reported; may impair physical/mental abilities. Cardiovascular (CV) events reported in patients w/ stable CV disease. Cases of somnambulism reported; consider discontinuing therapy if this occurs. Hypersensitivity reactions, including angioedema, reported; d/c if symptoms develop. Serious skin reactions (eg, Stevens-Johnson syndrome, erythema multiforme) reported; d/c at the first appearance of a skin rash w/ mucosal lesions or any other signs of hypersensitivity. Nausea reported; consider dose reduction for patients w/ intolerable nausea. Caution in elderly.

ADVERSE REACTIONS
N/V, abnormal dreams, constipation, flatulence.

DRUG INTERACTIONS
May increase intoxicating effects of alcohol. Nicotine replacement therapy (transdermal nicotine) may increase incidence of N/V, headache, dizziness, dyspepsia, and fatigue. Physiological changes resulting from smoking cessation may alter pharmacokinetics or pharmacodynamics of certain drugs (eg, theophylline, warfarin, insulin) for which dosage adjustment may be necessary.

PREGNANCY AND LACTATION
Pregnancy: Available human data on the use of varenicline in pregnant women are not sufficient to inform a drug-associated risk.
Lactation: There are no data on the presence of varenicline in human milk, the effects on the breastfed infant, or the effects on milk production. Caution in nursing; monitor infants for seizures and excessive vomiting.

MECHANISM OF ACTION
Nicotinic acetylcholine receptor agonist; binds w/ high affinity and selectivity at α4β2 neuronal nicotinic acetylcholine receptors. The binding produces agonist activity while simultaneously preventing nicotine binding to these receptors.

PHARMACOKINETICS
Absorption: T_{max}=3-4 hrs. **Distribution:** Plasma protein binding (≤20%). **Metabolism:** Minimal. **Elimination:** Urine (92% unchanged); $T_{1/2}$=24 hrs.

PATIENT CONSIDERATIONS
Assessment: Assess for preexisting psychiatric illness, history of seizures or other factors that can lower the seizure threshold, CV disease, history of hypersensitivity to the drug, renal impairment, pregnancy/nursing status, and for possible drug interactions.

Monitoring: Monitor for neuropsychiatric symptoms or worsening of preexisting psychiatric illness, seizures, somnolence, dizziness, loss of consciousness, difficulty concentrating, CV events, somnambulism, skin reactions, hypersensitivity reactions, nausea, and other adverse reactions. Monitor renal function.

Counseling: Inform about risks and benefits of treatment. Instruct to set a date to quit smoking and initiate treatment 1 week before quit date. Alternatively, inform that patient can begin therapy and then set a date to quit smoking between Days 8 and 35 of treatment. Encourage to continue to attempt to quit even w/ early lapses after quit day. Advise patients who are sure that they are not able or willing to quit abruptly that a gradual approach to quitting w/ therapy may be considered. Encourage patients who are motivated to quit and who did not succeed in stopping smoking during prior therapy for reasons other than intolerability due to adverse events, or who relapsed after treatment, to make another attempt w/ therapy once factors contributing to the failed attempt have been identified and addressed. Provide educational materials and necessary counseling to support attempt at quitting smoking. Instruct to notify physician if persistent nausea or insomnia develops. Advise to d/c and notify physician if agitation, hostility, depressed mood, changes in behavior/thinking, or somnambulism occurs. Advise to notify physician prior to treatment of any history of psychiatric illness. Inform that quitting smoking may be associated w/ nicotine withdrawal symptoms or exacerbation of preexisting psychiatric illness. Advise to inform physician of any history of seizures or other factors that can lower seizure threshold; instruct patient to d/c treatment and contact physician immediately if seizure is experienced. Instruct patient to reduce amount of alcohol they consume while on therapy until they know whether therapy affects their tolerance for alcohol. Advise to use caution when driving or operating machinery until patients know how quitting smoking and/or therapy may affect them. Advise to notify physician if symptoms of new or worsening CV events develop and to seek immediate medical attention if signs/symptoms of a MI or stroke are experienced. Instruct to d/c and seek immediate medical care if angioedema or a skin reaction occurs. Inform that vivid, unusual, or strange dreams may occur. If patient is pregnant, planning to become pregnant, or breastfeeding, advise about the risks of smoking, the potential risks of therapy, and the benefits of smoking cessation.

CHENODAL — chenodiol
Rx

Class: Bile acid

ADULT DOSAGE
Gallbladder Stones

Use in patients w/ radiolucent stones in well-opacifying gallbladders, in whom selective surgery would be undertaken except for the presence of increased surgical risk due to systemic disease or age

Initial: 250mg bid for the first 2 weeks
Titrate: Increase by 250mg/day each week thereafter until recommended or max tolerated dose is reached
Range: 13-16mg/kg/day in 2 divided doses (am and pm)

PEDIATRIC DOSAGE
Pediatric use may not have been established

Weight/Dosage Guide:
45-58kg: 3 tabs/day
59-75kg: 4 tabs/day
76-90kg: 5 tabs/day
91-107kg: 6 tabs/day
108-125kg: 7 tabs/day
D/C if no response by 18 months

DOSING CONSIDERATIONS
Adverse Reactions
Diarrhea: If diarrhea occurs during dosage buildup or later in treatment, may be controlled by temporary dosage adjustment until symptoms abate, after which, previous dose is usually tolerated

If Cholesterol Rises Above Acceptable Age-Adjusted Limit: May be advisable to d/c therapy

If Aminotransferase Elevations Over 3X ULN Occur: May require immediate discontinuation of therapy

ADMINISTRATION
Oral route

STORAGE
20-25°C (68-77°F).

HOW SUPPLIED
Tab: 250mg

CONTRAINDICATIONS
Presence of known hepatocyte dysfunction or bile ductal abnormalities (eg, intrahepatic cholestasis, primary biliary cirrhosis, sclerosing cholangitis); a nonvisualizing gallbladder after two consecutive single doses of dye; radiopaque stones; or gallstone complications or compelling reasons for gallbladder surgery including unremitting acute cholecystitis, cholangitis, biliary obstruction, gallstone pancreatitis, or biliary GI fistula. Women who are or may become pregnant.

WARNINGS/PRECAUTIONS
Has the potential to cause hepatotoxicity or may increase rate of need for cholecystectomy. Treatment should be reserved for carefully selected patients and must be accompanied by systemic monitoring for liver function alterations. Will not dissolve calcified or radiolucent bile pigment stones. May cause serious hepatic disease and fetal harm. May contribute to colon cancer in susceptible individuals. Use in patient w/o preexisting liver disease; monitor serum aminotransferase levels to detect drug-induced liver toxicity. Caution in patients w/ history of jaundice. Stone recurrence may occur; maintenance of reduced weight recommended. Safety of use beyond 24 months not established.

ADVERSE REACTIONS
Aminotransferase elevations (mainly SGPT), intrahepatic cholestasis, diarrhea, gastrointestinal side effects, increase in serum total cholesterol and LDL, decrease in WBC count.

DRUG INTERACTIONS
Bile acid sequestering agents (eg, cholestyramine, colestipol) and aluminum-based antacids may reduce absorption. Estrogen, oral contraceptives, and clofibrate (and perhaps other lipid-lowering drugs) may counteract the effectiveness of chenodiol. May cause unexpected prolongation of PT and hemorrhages w/ coumarin and its derivatives; may need to readjust coumarin dosage and may need to d/c chenodiol.

PREGNANCY AND LACTATION
Pregnancy: Category X.
Lactation: Caution in nursing.

MECHANISM OF ACTION
Bile acid; suppresses hepatic synthesis of both cholesterol and cholic acid, gradually replacing the latter and its metabolite, deoxycholic acid, in an expanded bile acid pool that contributes to biliary cholesterol desaturation and gradual dissolution of radiolucent cholesterol gallstone.

PHARMACOKINETICS
Absorption: Well absorbed. **Metabolism:** Liver, converted in the colon by bacterial action to lithocholic acid (metabolite). **Elimination:** (Lithocholate) Feces (80%).

PATIENT CONSIDERATIONS
Assessment: Assess for hepatocyte dysfunction or bile ductal abnormalities or any other diseases or conditions where treatment is contraindicated or cautioned. Assess for pregnancy/nursing status and possible drug interactions. Obtain LFTs (AST/ALT), serum cholesterol, and TG levels.

Monitoring: Monitor for patient's weight, increased risk for cholecystectomy, and for signs and symptoms of hepatotoxicity, colon cancer, or other adverse reactions. Monitor liver function alterations. Monitor serum aminotransferase levels monthly for the first 3 months, and every 3 months thereafter. Monitor serum cholesterol at 6-month intervals. Monitor response and/or recurrence w/ cholecystograms or ultrasonograms at 6- to 9-month intervals.

Counseling: Inform of the importance of periodic visits for LFTs and oral cholecystograms (or ultrasonograms) for monitoring stone dissolution. Inform about the symptoms of gallstone complications and advise to notify physician immediately if symptoms occur. Instruct on ways to facilitate faithful compliance w/ the dosage regimen throughout the usual long term of therapy, and on temporary dose reduction if episodes of diarrhea occur. Advise to maintain reduced weight to forestall stone recurrence.

CHLORDIAZEPOXIDE/AMITRIPTYLINE —
amitriptyline hydrochloride/chlordiazepoxide   **CIV**

Class: Benzodiazepine/tricyclic antidepressant (TCA)

> Antidepressants increased the risk of suicidal thinking and behavior (suicidality) in children, adolescents, and young adults in short-term studies of major depressive disorder and other psychiatric disorders. Monitor and observe closely for clinical worsening, suicidality, or unusual changes in behavior. Not approved for use in pediatric patients.

ADULT DOSAGE
Depression/Anxiety

Moderate-Severe Depression Associated w/ Moderate-Severe Anxiety:

Initial: 3 or 4 tabs/day in divided doses

10mg/25mg Tab:
May increase to 6 tabs/day as required; some patients respond to smaller doses and may be maintained on 2 tabs/day

Reduce dose to the smallest amount needed to maintain remission, when a satisfactory response is obtained

PEDIATRIC DOSAGE
Pediatric use may not have been established

DOSING CONSIDERATIONS
Elderly
Start at lower end of dosing range

ADMINISTRATION
Oral route
The larger portion of the total daily dose may be taken hs.

STORAGE
20-25°C (68-77°F).

HOW SUPPLIED
Tab: (Chlordiazepoxide/Amitriptyline) 5mg/12.5mg, 10mg/25mg

CONTRAINDICATIONS
Hypersensitivity to benzodiazepines or TCAs; during or w/in 14 days of MAOI use; acute recovery phase following MI.

WARNINGS/PRECAUTIONS
Not approved for the treatment of bipolar depression. May precipitate mixed/manic episodes in patients at risk for bipolar disorder. Pupillary dilation that occurs following therapy may trigger an angle-closure attack in a patient w/ anatomically narrow angles who does not have a patent iridectomy. Caution w/ history of urinary retention or angle-closure glaucoma; may precipitate an attack w/ glaucoma. Caution w/ cardiovascular disorders; arrhythmias, sinus tachycardia, and prolongation of conduction time reported, particularly w/ high doses. MI and stroke reported. May impair mental/physical abilities. Caution w/ history of seizures, hyperthyroidism, renal/hepatic impairment, and in elderly. D/C several days prior to elective surgery. Increased risk of congenital malformation during the 1st trimester of pregnancy reported w/ use of minor tranquilizers (chlordiazepoxide); use during this period should almost always be avoided. Withdrawal symptoms of the barbiturate type have occurred after discontinuation.

ADVERSE REACTIONS
Drowsiness, dry mouth, constipation, blurred vision, dizziness, bloating, anorexia, fatigue, weakness, restlessness, lethargy.

DRUG INTERACTIONS
See Contraindications. May block the antihypertensive action of guanethidine or similarly acting agents. Drugs that inhibit CYP2D6 (eg, quinidine, cimetidine, CYP2D6 substrates [other antidepressants, phenothiazines, propafenone, and flecainide]) may increase plasma concentration; may require lower doses of either TCA or the other drug and monitoring of TCA levels. Caution w/ SSRI coadministration and when switching between TCAs and SSRIs (eg, fluoxetine, sertraline, paroxetine); sufficient time must elapse before starting therapy when switching from fluoxetine (at least 5 weeks may be necessary). Caution w/ thyroid medications. Sedative effects may be additive w/ psychotropic drugs. May delay elimination and increase levels w/ cimetidine. Caution w/ alcohol and CNS depressants; additive effects may produce a harmful level of sedation and CNS depression. May cause severe constipation w/ anticholinergics. Topiramate may cause large increases in amitriptyline concentrations; adjustments in amitriptyline dose should be made according to clinical response and not on the basis of plasma levels.

PREGNANCY AND LACTATION
Safety not known in pregnancy, not for use in nursing.

MECHANISM OF ACTION
Chlordiazepoxide: Benzodiazepine; acts in limbic system producing taming action. **Amitriptyline:** Dibenzocycloheptadiene derivative; has not been established. Appears to interfere w/ the reuptake of norepinephrine into adrenergic nerve endings, leading to prolongation of sympathetic activity of biogenic amines.

PATIENT CONSIDERATIONS
Assessment: Assess for acute recovery phase following MI, hypersensitivity to drug, risk of bipolar depression, cardiovascular disorders, history of seizures, hypothyroidism, susceptibility to angle-closure glaucoma, renal/hepatic impairment, pregnancy/nursing status, and possible drug interactions.

Monitoring: Monitor for signs/symptoms of clinical worsening, suicidality, unusual changes in behavior, mixed/manic episodes, MI, stroke, arrhythmias, sinus tachycardia, prolongation of conduction time, angle-closure glaucoma, and other adverse reactions. Monitor renal/hepatic function. Monitor blood counts and LFTs periodically w/ long-term therapy.

Counseling: Inform patients, families, and caregivers about benefits/risks of therapy and counsel on its appropriate use. Advise families and caregivers to be alert for unusual changes in behavior, worsening of depression, and suicidal ideation; instruct to report symptoms to physician. Inform that the drug may produce psychological/physical dependence and advise not to change dose or abruptly d/c therapy w/o consulting physician. Inform that drug may impair physical/mental ability. Instruct to notify physician if pregnant or planning to become pregnant. Caution about the risk of angle-closure glaucoma.

CHLOROTHIAZIDE — chlorothiazide   **Rx**

Class: Thiazide diuretic

OTHER BRAND NAMES
Diuril, Sodium Diuril

ADULT DOSAGE
Edema

IV/PO:
Usual: 0.5-1g qd-bid; may be given qod or 3-5 days/week
When medication can be taken PO, substitute PO for IV using same dosage

Hypertension

PO:
Initial: 0.5-1g/day given qd or in divided doses
Titrate: Adjust dose based on BP response
Max: 2g/day in divided doses

PEDIATRIC DOSAGE
Diuresis

PO:
Usual: 10-20mg/kg/day given qd-bid
Max:
<6 Months of Age: Up to 30mg/kg/day given bid
Infants Up to 2 Years: 375mg/day
2-12 Years: 1g/day

Hypertension

PO:
Usual: 10-20mg/kg/day given qd-bid
Max:
<6 Months of Age: Up to 30mg/kg/day given bid
Infants Up to 2 Years: 375mg/day
2-12 Years: 1g/day

DOSING CONSIDERATIONS
Elderly
Start at lower end of dosing range

ADMINISTRATION
Oral, IV route

IV
Extravasation must be rigidly avoided

Directions for Reconstitution
1) Add 18mL of sterile water to the vial to form an isotonic sol for IV inj. Never add <18mL
2) When reconstituted w/ 18mL of sterile water, the final concentration of IV Sodium Diuril is 28mg/mL. The reconstituted sol is clear and essentially free from visible particles
3) The sol is compatible w/ dextrose or NaCl sol for IV infusion
4) Avoid simultaneous administration of sol of chlorothiazide w/ whole blood or its derivatives

STORAGE
(PO) 15-30°C (59-86°F); (Sus) protect from freezing. (IV) 20-25°C (68-77°F).

HOW SUPPLIED
Inj: (Sodium Diuril) 0.5g; **Sus:** (Diuril) 250mg/5mL [237mL]; **Tab:** 250mg*, 500mg*
*scored

CONTRAINDICATIONS
Anuria, hypersensitivity to this product or to other sulfonamide-derived drugs.

WARNINGS/PRECAUTIONS
Caution in severe renal disease; may precipitate azotemia. Caution in impaired hepatic function or progressive liver disease; may precipitate hepatic coma. Sensitivity reactions may occur. May exacerbate or activate systemic lupus erythematosus (SLE). Observe for evidence of electrolyte/fluid imbalance. Hypokalemia may develop; may cause arrhythmias and may also sensitize or exaggerate the response of the heart to toxic effects of digitalis (eg, increased ventricular irritability). Hyponatremia, hypochloremic alkalosis, hyperuricemia or precipitation of acute gout, hyperglycemia, hypomagnesemia, and hypercalcemia may occur. May enhance antihypertensive effects in postsympathectomy patients. May cause increases in cholesterol and TG levels. If progressive renal impairment becomes evident, consider withholding or d/c therapy. D/C prior to parathyroid test. IV use not recommended in infants or children.

ADVERSE REACTIONS
Weakness, hypotension, pancreatitis, jaundice, diarrhea, vomiting, rash, photosensitivity, electrolyte imbalance, impotence.

DRUG INTERACTIONS
May potentiate orthostatic hypotension with alcohol, barbiturates, narcotics. Dosage adjustment of antidiabetic drugs (eg, insulin, oral agents) may be required. Antihypertensives may produce an additive effect or potentiation. May reduce GI absorption with cholestyramine and colestipol. Corticosteroid, adrenocorticotropic hormone may intensify electrolyte depletion, particularly hypokalemia. Possible decreased response to pressor amines (eg, norepinephrine). May increase responsiveness to nondepolarizing skeletal muscle relaxants (eg,

tubocurarine). Avoid use with lithium; may produce lithium toxicity. NSAIDs may decrease diuretic, natriuretic, and antihypertensive effects of thiazides.

PREGNANCY AND LACTATION
Category C, not for use in nursing.

MECHANISM OF ACTION
Thiazide diuretic; has not been established. Affects the distal renal tubular mechanism of electrolyte reabsorption.

PHARMACOKINETICS
Distribution: Crosses the placenta; found in breast milk. **Elimination:** (PO) Urine (10-15%, unchanged); (IV) Urine (96%, unchanged). $T_{1/2}$=45-120 min.

PATIENT CONSIDERATIONS
Assessment: Assess for anuria, sulfonamide hypersensitivity, diabetes mellitus, SLE, history of allergy or bronchial asthma, hepatic/renal impairment, pregnancy/nursing status, and possible drug interactions.

Monitoring: Monitor for signs/symptoms of electrolyte imbalance (eg, hyponatremia, hypochloremic alkalosis, hypokalemia, hypomagnesemia), exacerbation or activation of SLE, hypotension, hyperglycemia, hypercalcemia, hyperuricemia or precipitation of gout, hypersensitivity reactions, renal/hepatic dysfunction, and for increases in cholesterol and TG levels. In patients with renal disease, monitor for signs/symptoms of azotemia. Perform periodic monitoring of renal function and serum electrolytes.

Counseling: Advise to seek medical attention if hypotension, electrolyte imbalance (eg, dry mouth, thirst, weakness), or hypersensitivity reactions occur.

Chlorpromazine — chlorpromazine hydrochloride   Rx
Class: Typical antipsychotic

> Elderly patients with dementia-related psychosis treated with antipsychotic drugs are at increased risk of death; most deaths appeared to be cardiovascular (eg, heart failure, sudden death) or infectious (eg, pneumonia) in nature. Not approved for the treatment of patients with dementia-related psychosis.

ADULT DOSAGE
Psychotic Disorders
Hospitalized Patients:

Acute Schizophrenic or Manic States:
Initial treatment should be w/ chlorpromazine inj until patient is controlled
IM:
Initial: 25mg; give additional 25-50mg inj in 1 hr, if necessary
Titrate: Increase gradually over several days up to 400mg q4-6h until controlled, then switch to PO

PO:
Generally, 500mg/day is sufficient; gradual increases to 2000mg/day or more may be necessary
Less Acutely Disturbed:
Initial: 25mg tid
Titrate: Increase gradually to effective dose
Usual: 400mg/day

More Severe Cases:
Initial: 25mg tid
Titrate: After 1-2 days, may increase by 20-50mg at semi-weekly intervals until calm and cooperative

Outpatients:
Usual: 10mg tid-qid or 25mg bid-tid

Prompt Control of Severe Symptoms:
Initial treatment should be w/ IM chlorpromazine; subsequent doses should be oral, 25-50 mg tid
IM:
Usual: 25mg; repeat in 1 hr, if necessary

Nausea/Vomiting
PO:
Usual: 10-25mg q4-6h prn; increase, if necessary

IM:
Usual: 25mg; give 25-50mg q3-4h prn if no hypotension occurs until vomiting stops, then switch to PO

Preoperative Medication
For Relief of Restlessness and Apprehension Before Surgery:
Presurgical Apprehension:
PO:
Usual: 25-50mg, given 2-3 hrs before operation

PEDIATRIC DOSAGE
Behavioral Problems
6 Months-12 Years:
Outpatient:
Select route of administration according to severity of condition
PO:
1/4mg/lb q4-6h prn
IM:
1/4mg/lb q6-8h prn

Inpatient:
PO/IM:
Initial: Start low and may increase gradually to 50-100mg/day; ≥200mg/day in older children

Max:
PO:
500mg/day
IM:
Up to 5 Years (or 50 lbs): ≤40mg/day
5-12 Years (or 50-100 lbs): ≤75mg/day except in unmanageable cases

Nausea/Vomiting
6 Months-12 Years:
Adjust dosage/frequency according to severity of symptoms and patient response
PO:
1/4mg/lb q4-6h
IM:
1/4mg/lb q6-8h, prn
Max:
IM:
6 Months-5 Years (or 50 lbs):
≤40mg/day
5-12 Years (or 50-100 lbs): ≤75mg/day except in severe cases

Preoperative Medication
For Relief of Restlessness and Apprehension Before Surgery:
6 Months-12 Years:
Presurgical Apprehension:
PO:
Usual: 1/4mg/lb, given 2-3 hrs before operation
IM:
Usual: 1/4mg/lb, given 1-2 hrs before operation

IM:
Usual: 12.5-25mg, given 1-2 hrs before operation
During Surgery:
IM:
Usual: 12.5mg; repeat in 1/2 hr, if necessary, if no hypotension occurs
IV:
Usual: 2mg per fractional inj, at 2-min intervals
Max: 25mg
Dilute to 1mg/mL (eg, 1mL [25mg] mixed w/ 24mL of saline)

Intractable Hiccups
Initial: 25-50mg PO tid-qid; if symptoms persist for 2-3 days, give 25-50mg IM; if symptoms still persist, give 25-50mg in 500-1000mL of saline as slow IV infusion w/ patient flat in bed

Porphyria
Acute Intermittent Porphyria:
PO:
Usual: 25-50mg tid-qid; maint therapy may be necessary in some patients
IM:
Usual: 25mg tid-qid until patient can take PO therapy

Tetanus
Adjunct Treatment:
IM:
Usual: 25-50mg tid-qid, usually in conjunction w/ barbiturates; determine total doses and frequency by patient's response
IV:
Usual: 25-50mg; dilute to at least 1mg/mL and administer at a rate of 1mg/min

During Surgery:
IM:
Usual: 1/8mg/lb; repeat in 1/2 hr, if necessary, if no hypotension occurs
IV:
Usual: 1mg per fractional inj, at 2-min intervals and not exceeding recommended IM dosage.
Dilute to 1mg/mL (eg, 1mL [25mg] mixed w/ 24mL of saline)

Tetanus
Adjunct Treatment:
6 Months-12 Years:
IM/IV:
1/4mg/lb q6-8h
When given IV, dilute to at least 1mg/mL and administer at a rate of 1mg/2 min
Max:
≤50 lbs: ≤40mg/day
50-100 lbs: ≤75mg/day except in severe cases

DOSING CONSIDERATIONS
Elderly
Elderly/Debilitated:
Start at lower end of dosing range; increase gradually and monitor closely

ADMINISTRATION
Oral/IM/IV route

Inj
Inject slowly, deep into upper outer quadrant of buttock
Reserve parenteral administration for bedfast patients or for acute ambulatory cases, and keep patient lying down for at least 1/2 hr after inj
If irritation is a problem, dilute inj w/ saline or 2% procaine; do not mix w/ other agents in syringe
Avoid injecting undiluted inj into vein
Avoid getting sol on hands or clothing, because of possibility of contact dermatitis

STORAGE
(Inj) 20-25°C (68-77°F); excursions permitted to 15-30°C (59-86°F). Protect from light and freezing. (Tab) 20-25°C (68-77°F). Protect from moisture.

HOW SUPPLIED
Inj: 25mg/mL [1mL, 2mL]; **Tab:** 10mg, 25mg, 50mg, 100mg, 200mg

CONTRAINDICATIONS
Known hypersensitivity to phenothiazines. Comatose states or the presence of large amounts of CNS depressants (eg, alcohol, barbiturates, narcotics).

WARNINGS/PRECAUTIONS
Extrapyramidal symptoms may be confused with CNS signs of undiagnosed primary disease responsible for vomiting; avoid in children/adolescents with signs of Reye's syndrome. Risk of tardive dyskinesia (TD), especially in elderly; consider d/c if signs/symptoms appear. Neuroleptic malignant syndrome (NMS) reported; d/c therapy and carefully monitor for recurrences if therapy is reintroduced. May impair mental/physical abilities. Neonates exposed during 3rd trimester of pregnancy are at risk for extrapyramidal and/or withdrawal symptoms. Leukopenia, neutropenia, and agranulocytosis reported. Monitor for fever or infection with neutropenia; d/c in patients with severe neutropenia (absolute neutrophil count <1000/mm³). Caution with chronic respiratory disorders, acute respiratory infections (especially in children), glaucoma, cardiovascular, hepatic, or renal disease. May suppress cough reflex; aspiration of vomitus possible. Caution if exposed to extreme heat. May elevate prolactin levels. May produce α-adrenergic blockade. May mask signs and symptoms of overdosage of other drugs and obscure diagnosis and treatment of other conditions (eg, intestinal obstruction, brain tumor, Reye's syndrome). Avoid abrupt withdrawal of high-dose therapy. Evaluate patients with a history of long-term therapy on whether the maint dose could be lowered or d/c therapy to lessen likelihood of adverse reactions related to cumulative drug effect. May produce false-(+) phenylketonuria test results. (Inj) Contains sulfites.

ADVERSE REACTIONS

Drowsiness, jaundice, agranulocytosis, hypotensive effects, ECG changes, dystonia, motor restlessness, pseudo-parkinsonism, TD, anticholinergic effects, NMS, ocular changes, skin pigmentation, allergic reactions.

DRUG INTERACTIONS

See Contraindications. Monitor for neurological toxicity with lithium; d/c if signs occur. Prolongs and intensifies action of CNS depressants (eg, anesthetics, barbiturates, narcotics); administer about 1/4 to 1/2 the usual dose of such agents when used concomitantly. Caution with organophosphorus insecticides, atropine or related drugs. Avoid use of alcohol due to possible additive effects and hypotension. May counteract the antihypertensive effect of guanethidine and related compounds. Diminished effect of oral anticoagulants reported. May lower convulsive threshold; anticonvulsant dose adjustment may be needed. May interfere with phenytoin metabolism and precipitate phenytoin toxicity. Increased plasma levels of both agents with propranolol. Thiazide diuretics may potentiate orthostatic hypotension. Do not use with metrizamide; d/c at least 48 hrs before myelography and should not be resumed for at least 24 hrs after; do not administer for control of N/V prior to or after procedure with metrizamide. May obscure vomiting as a sign of toxicity of chemotherapeutic drugs. Certain pressor agents, such as epinephrine, may cause paradoxical further lowering of BP; do not use to control hypotension.

PREGNANCY AND LACTATION

Safety not known in pregnancy, not for use in nursing.

MECHANISM OF ACTION

Phenothiazine; not established. Suspected to act at all levels of CNS, primarily at subcortical levels as well as on multiple organ systems.

PHARMACOKINETICS

Distribution: Found in breast milk.

PATIENT CONSIDERATIONS

Assessment: Assess for Reye's syndrome in children and adolescents prior to initiation, mental status, renal/hepatic/cardiovascular function, glaucoma, respiratory disorders, bone marrow depression, use of large amounts of CNS depressants, heat exposure, hypersensitivity to drug, pregnancy/nursing status, and possible drug interactions.

Monitoring: Monitor for hypersensitivity reactions, TD, NMS, hypotension, leukopenia/neutropenia/agranulocytosis, fever, infection, and other adverse reactions. Monitor CBC frequently during the 1st few months of therapy.

Counseling: Counsel on risks/benefits of therapy. Instruct to immediately report signs of infection and to avoid exposure to extreme heat. Inform that drug may impair mental/physical abilities, especially during first few days of therapy; caution with activities requiring alertness (eg, operating vehicles or machinery). Advise to avoid alcohol and abrupt withdrawal of therapy.

CHOLBAM — cholic acid   Rx

Class: Bile acid

ADULT DOSAGE

Bile Acid Synthesis Disorders

Treatment of bile acid synthesis disorders due to single enzyme defects

Usual: 10-15mg/kg qd, or in 2 divided dose

Peroxisomal Disorders

Adjunctive treatment of peroxisomal disorders including Zellweger spectrum disorders in patients who exhibit manifestations of liver disease, steatorrhea, or complications from decreased fat soluble vitamin absorption

Usual: 10-15mg/kg qd, or in 2 divided doses

PEDIATRIC DOSAGE

Bile Acid Synthesis Disorders

Treatment of bile acid synthesis disorders due to single enzyme defects

≥3 Weeks of Age:
Usual: 10-15mg/kg qd, or in 2 divided doses

Peroxisomal Disorders

Adjunctive treatment of peroxisomal disorders including Zellweger spectrum disorders in patients who exhibit manifestations of liver disease, steatorrhea, or complications from decreased fat soluble vitamin absorption

≥3 Weeks of Age:
Usual: 10-15mg/kg qd, or in 2 divided doses

DOSING CONSIDERATIONS

Discontinuation

D/C if liver function does not improve w/in 3 months of the start of treatment or complete biliary obstruction develops

D/C at any time if there are persistent clinical or lab indicators of worsening liver function or cholestasis. Concurrent elevations of serum gamma glutamyltransferase and serum ALT may indicate overdose. Continue to monitor lab parameters of liver function and consider restarting dose when the parameters return to baseline

Other Important Considerations
Familial Hypertriglyceridemia:
Patients w/ newly diagnosed, or a family history of, familial hypertriglyceridemia may have a poor absorption of therapy from the intestine and require a 10% increase in the recommended dosage
Usual: 11-17mg/kg qd, or in 2 divided doses

Monitor clinical response including steatorrhea, and lab values including transaminases, bilirubin, and PT/INR to determine the adequacy of the dosage regimen

Administer the lowest dose of therapy that effectively maintains liver function

ADMINISTRATION

Oral route

Take w/ food

Take at least 1 hr before or 4-6 hrs (or at as great an interval as possible) after a bile acid binding resin or aluminum-based antacid

Do not crush or chew the caps

Refer to PI for number of caps needed to achieve dosage of 10mg/kg/day and 15mg/kg/day

Patients Unable to Swallow Caps

Caps can be opened and the contents mixed w/ either infant formula or expressed breast milk (for younger children), or soft food such as mashed potatoes or apple puree (for older children and adults) in order to mask any unpleasant taste:
1. Hold the cap over the prepared liquid/food, gently twist open, and allow the contents to fall into the liquid/food
2. Mix the entire cap contents w/ 1 or 2 tbsp (15-30mL) of infant formula, expressed breast milk, or soft food
3. Stir for 30 sec
4. Cap contents will remain as fine granules in the milk or food, and will not dissolve
5. Administer the mixture immediately

STORAGE

20-25°C (68-77°F); excursions permitted between 15-30°C (59-86°F).

HOW SUPPLIED

Cap: 50mg, 250mg

WARNINGS/PRECAUTIONS

Should be initiated and monitored by an experienced hepatologist or pediatric gastroenterologist. Monitor liver function and d/c in patients who develop worsening of liver function while on treatment.

ADVERSE REACTIONS

Diarrhea, reflux esophagitis, malaise, jaundice, skin lesion, nausea, abdominal pain, intestinal polyp, UTI, peripheral neuropathy.

DRUG INTERACTIONS

Concomitant medications that inhibit canalicular membrane bile acid transporters such as bile salt efflux pump (eg, cyclosporine) may exacerbate accumulation of conjugated bile salts in the liver and result in clinical symptoms; avoid concomitant use, and if concomitant use is necessary, monitor serum transaminases and bilirubin. Bile acid binding resins (eg, cholestyramine, colestipol, colesevelam) adsorb and reduce bile acid absorption and may reduce efficacy of cholic acid; take cholic acid at least 1 hr before or 4-6 hrs (or at as great an interval as possible) after a bile acid binding resin. Aluminum-based antacids may reduce the bioavailability of cholic acid; take cholic acid at least 1 hr before or 4-6 hrs (or at as great an interval as possible) after an aluminum-based antacid.

PREGNANCY AND LACTATION

Pregnancy: There is a pregnancy surveillance program that monitors pregnancy outcomes in women exposed to cholic acid during pregnancy (COCOA Registry [Cholbam: Child and mother's health]); women who become pregnant during treatment are encouraged to enroll. Limited published case reports discuss pregnancies in women taking cholic acid for 3β-hydroxysteroid dehydrogenase deficiency resulting in healthy infants; these reports may not adequately inform the presence or absence of drug-associated risk w/ the use of cholic acid during pregnancy.
Lactation: Endogenous cholic acid is present in human milk. Caution in nursing.

MECHANISM OF ACTION

Bile acid; has not been established. It is known that cholic acid and its conjugates are endogenous ligands of the nuclear receptor, farnesoid X receptor (FXR). FXR regulates enzymes and transporters that are involved in bile acid synthesis and in the enterohepatic circulation to maintain bile acid homeostasis under normal physiologic conditions.

PHARMACOKINETICS

Absorption: Passive diffusion along the length of the GI tract. **Metabolism:** Liver; conjugated w/ glycine or taurine by bile acid-CoA synthetase and bile acid-CoA: amino acid N-acetyltransferase. Conjugated cholic acid is secreted into bile, reabsorbed in the ileum, and enters another cycle of enterohepatic circulation. **Elimination:** Feces.

PATIENT CONSIDERATIONS

Assessment: Assess for newly diagnosed or a family history of familial hypertriglyceridemia, hepatic impairment, pregnancy/nursing status, and possible drug interactions. Assess serum or urinary bile acid levels using mass spectrometry.

Monitoring: Monitor for worsening liver function or cholestasis, complete biliary obstruction, and other adverse reactions. Monitor serum AST/ALT/gamma-glutamyl transpeptidase, alkaline phosphatase, bilirubin, and INR every month for the first 3 months, every 3 months for the next 9 months, every 6 months during the subsequent 3 yrs, and annually thereafter. Monitor liver function more frequently during periods of rapid growth, concomitant disease, and pregnancy. Monitor clinical response to therapy.

Counseling: Advise the need to undergo lab testing periodically while on treatment to assess liver function. Advise that therapy may worsen liver impairment; instruct to immediately report to physician any symptoms associated w/ liver impairment (eg, skin or the whites of eyes turn yellow, urine turns dark or brown [tea colored], pain on the right side of stomach, bleeding or bruising occurs more easily than normal, increased lethargy). Instruct to take exactly ud. Advise that there is a pregnancy surveillance program that monitors pregnancy outcomes in women exposed to cholic acid during pregnancy.

CIALIS — tadalafil

Rx

Class: Phosphodiesterase-5 (PDE-5) inhibitor

ADULT DOSAGE

Erectile Dysfunction

PRN Use:
Initial: 10mg prior to sexual activity
Titrate: May increase to 20mg or decrease to 5mg, based on individual efficacy and tolerability
Max Dosing Frequency: Once daily

Once-Daily Use:
Initial: 2.5mg qd
Titrate: May increase to 5mg qd based on individual efficacy and tolerability

Benign Prostatic Hyperplasia

W/ or w/o Erectile Dysfunction (ED): 5mg qd

Initiated w/ Finasteride: 5mg qd for ≤26 weeks

PEDIATRIC DOSAGE

Pediatric use may not have been established

DOSING CONSIDERATIONS

Concomitant Medications

α-Blockers:
ED:
Initial: Use lowest recommended dose; should be stable on α-blocker therapy prior to initiating treatment
BPH:
Not recommended

Potent CYP3A4 Inhibitors (eg, Ketoconazole, Ritonavir):
PRN Use:
Max: 10mg/72 hrs
Once-Daily Use:
Max: 2.5mg

Renal Impairment

PRN Use:
CrCl 30-50mL/min:
Initial: 5mg qd
Max: 10mg/48 hrs
CrCl <30mL/min or Hemodialysis:
Max: 5mg/72 hrs
Once-Daily Use:
ED:
CrCl <30mL/min or Hemodialysis:
Not recommended
BPH or ED/BPH:
CrCl 30-50mL/min:
Initial: 2.5mg
Titrate: May increase to 5mg based on individual response
CrCl <30mL/min or Hemodialysis:
Not recommended

Hepatic Impairment

PRN Use:
Mild or Moderate (Child-Pugh Class A or B):
Max: 10mg qd
Severe (Child-Pugh Class C):
Not recommended
Once-Daily Use:
Mild or Moderate (Child-Pugh Class A or B): Use caution
Severe (Child-Pugh Class C): Not recommended

ADMINISTRATION

Oral route
May be taken w/o regard to food.
Do not split tabs; entire dose should be taken.

Once-Daily Use
Take at approx the same time every day.

STORAGE

25°C (77°F); excursions permitted to 15-30°C (59-86°F).

HOW SUPPLIED

Tab: 2.5mg, 5mg, 10mg, 20mg

CONTRAINDICATIONS

Any form of organic nitrate, either regularly and/or intermittently used. Known serious hypersensitivity to tadalafil. Concomitant guanylate cyclase (GC) stimulators (eg, riociguat).

WARNINGS/PRECAUTIONS

Consider cardiovascular (CV) status of patients due to cardiac risk associated w/ sexual activity; avoid in men for whom sexual activity is inadvisable due to underlying CV status. Caution in patients w/ left ventricular outflow obstruction (eg, aortic stenosis, idiopathic hypertrophic subaortic stenosis) and w/ severely impaired autonomic control of BP. Avoid w/ MI (w/in last 90 days), unstable angina or angina occurring during sexual intercourse, NYHA Class 2 or greater HF (in the last 6 months), uncontrolled arrhythmias, hypotension (<90/50mmHg), uncontrolled HTN, and stroke (w/in the last 6 months). Mild systemic vasodilatory properties may result in transient decreases in BP. Prolonged erections (>4 hrs) and priapism (painful erections >6 hrs in duration) reported; caution in patients who have conditions predisposing to priapism (eg, sickle cell anemia, multiple myeloma, leukemia), or w/ anatomical deformation of the penis (eg, angulation, cavernosal fibrosis, Peyronie's disease). Nonarteritic anterior ischemic optic neuropathy (NAION) reported; d/c if sudden loss of vision is experienced in one or both eyes. Caution in patients w/ underlying NAION risk factors, individuals who have experienced NAION, and individuals w/ "crowded" optic disc. Sudden decrease or loss of hearing reported, which may be accompanied by tinnitus and dizziness; d/c if this occurs. Avoid qd use in patients w/ CrCl <30mL/min or on hemodialysis. Avoid use w/ severe hepatic impairment (Child-Pugh Class C) and hereditary degenerative retinal disorders, including retinitis pigmentosa. Caution w/ mild to moderate hepatic impairment (Child-Pugh Class A/B), bleeding disorders, or significant active peptic ulceration. Consider other urological conditions that may cause similar symptoms prior to initiating treatment for BPH; prostate cancer and BPH may coexist.

ADVERSE REACTIONS

Headache, dyspepsia, back pain, myalgia, nasal congestion, flushing, limb pain, nasopharyngitis, URTI, gastroenteritis, cough, GERD, HTN.

DRUG INTERACTIONS

See Contraindications and Dosing Considerations. Avoid concomitant use w/ other PDE-5 inhibitors, including Adcirca. In patients who have taken tadalafil, where nitrate administration is deemed medically necessary in a life-threatening situation, at least 48 hrs should elapse after the last dose of tadalafil before nitrate administration is considered; in such circumstances, administer nitrates only under close medical supervision w/ appropriate hemodynamic monitoring. Potential additive BP-lowering effects w/ α-blockers and selected antihypertensives (amlodipine, ARBs, bendrofluazide, enalapril, metoprolol). Concomitant use not recommended w/ α-blockers for the treatment of BPH. BP-lowering effects of each individual compound may be increased w/ alcohol. Antacids (eg, magnesium hydroxide/aluminum hydroxide) may reduce the apparent rate of absorption. CYP3A4 inhibitors (eg, ketoconazole, erythromycin, itraconazole, grapefruit juice), ritonavir, and other HIV protease inhibitors may increase exposure. CYP3A4 inducers (eg, rifampin, carbamazepine, phenytoin, phenobarbital) may decrease exposure. A small increase in HR reported w/ theophylline.

PREGNANCY AND LACTATION

Not for use in women.
Pregnancy: Category B.

MECHANISM OF ACTION

PDE-5 inhibitor; increases amount of cGMP that causes smooth muscle relaxation and increased blood flow into the corpus cavernosum.

PHARMACOKINETICS

Absorption: T_{max}=2 hrs (median). **Distribution:** V_d=63L; plasma protein binding (94%). **Metabolism:** Liver, via CYP3A4 to a catechol metabolite, which undergoes extensive methylation and glucuronidation; methylcatechol glucuronide (major metabolite). **Elimination:** Urine (36%), feces (61%); $T_{1/2}$=17.5 hrs.

PATIENT CONSIDERATIONS

Assessment: Assess for previous hypersensitivity to drug, CV disease, hereditary degenerative retinal disorders, bleeding disorders, significant active peptic ulceration, anatomical deformation of the penis or presence of conditions that would predispose to priapism, underlying NAION risk factors, "crowded" optic disc, potential underlying causes of ED, other urological conditions, renal/hepatic impairment, pregnancy/nursing status, and possible drug interactions.

Monitoring: Monitor for hypersensitivity reactions, BP decrease, decrease/loss of hearing or vision, prolonged erection, priapism, and other adverse reactions.

Counseling: Instruct to seek emergency medical attention if erection persists >4 hrs. Advise of potential BP-lowering effect of α-blockers, antihypertensive medications, and alcohol. Inform of the potential cardiac risk of sexual activity in patients w/ preexisting CV disease; instruct patients who experience symptoms upon initiation of sexual activity to refrain from further sexual activity and seek immediate medical attention. Counsel about the protective measures necessary to guard against STDs (including HIV) that should be considered. Inform about contraindication w/ regular and/or intermittent use of organic nitrates and potential interactions w/ medications. Instruct to d/c and seek medical attention if sudden decrease or loss of vision or hearing occurs. Inform of the increased risk of NAION in individuals who have already experienced NAION in 1 eye and in patients w/ a "crowded" optic disc. Counsel to take 1 tab at least 30 min before anticipated sexual activity for prn use in men w/ ED, and at approx the same time every day w/o regard to timing of sexual activity for qd use in men w/ ED, BPH, or ED/BPH.

CILOXAN — ciprofloxacin hydrochloride

Rx

Class: Fluoroquinolone

ADULT DOSAGE

Bacterial Conjunctivitis

Sol:
1-2 drops into the conjunctival sac q2h while awake for 2 days, then 1-2 drops q4h while awake for the next 5 days

PEDIATRIC DOSAGE

Bacterial Conjunctivitis

Sol:
≥1 Year:
1-2 drops into the conjunctival sac q2h while awake for 2 days, then 1-2 drops q4h while awake for the next 5 days

Oint:
Apply 1/2-inch ribbon into the conjunctival sac tid on the first 2 days, then 1/2-inch ribbon bid for the next 5 days

Corneal Ulcers

Sol:
Day 1: 2 drops into the affected eye every 15 min for the first 6 hrs, then 2 drops every 30 min for the remainder of the day
Day 2: 2 drops every hr
Days 3-14: 2 drops q4h

May continue treatment after 14 days if reepithelialization has not occurred

Oint:
≥2 Years:
Apply 1/2-inch ribbon tid into the conjunctival sac on the first 2 days, then bid for the next 5 days

Corneal Ulcers

Sol:
≥1 Year:
Day 1: 2 drops into the affected eye every 15 min for the first 6 hrs, then 2 drops every 30 min for the remainder of the day
Day 2: 2 drops every hr
Days 3-14: 2 drops q4h

May continue treatment after 14 days if reepithelialization has not occurred

ADMINISTRATION
Ocular route

STORAGE
2-25°C (36-77°F). (Sol) Protect from light.

HOW SUPPLIED
Oint: 0.3% [3.5g]; **Sol:** 0.3% [2.5mL, 5mL, 10mL]

CONTRAINDICATIONS
History of hypersensitivity to ciprofloxacin, to other quinolones, or any other component of the medication.

WARNINGS/PRECAUTIONS
For topical ophthalmic use only; do not inject into eye. Serious and occasionally fatal hypersensitivity (anaphylactic) reactions reported in patients receiving systemic therapy; immediate emergency treatment with epinephrine and other resuscitation measures may be required as clinically indicated. Prolonged use may result in overgrowth of nonsusceptible organisms, including fungi; initiate appropriate therapy if superinfection occurs. D/C at 1st appearance of skin rash or other signs of hypersensitivity reaction. Remove contact lenses before use; avoid wearing contact lenses when signs/symptoms of bacterial conjunctivitis are present. (Oint) May retard corneal healing and cause visual blurring. (Sol) May form a white crystalline precipitate in the superficial portion of the corneal defect.

ADVERSE REACTIONS
Local discomfort, keratopathy, allergic reactions, corneal staining, foreign body sensation. (Oint) Blurred vision, irritation, lid margin hyperemia. (Sol) Local burning, white crystalline precipitate formation, lid margin crusting, conjunctival hyperemia, crystals/scales, itching, bad taste.

DRUG INTERACTIONS
Systemic quinolone therapy may increase theophylline levels, interfere with caffeine metabolism, enhance effects of warfarin and its derivatives, and elevate SrCr with cyclosporine.

PREGNANCY AND LACTATION
Category C, caution in nursing.

MECHANISM OF ACTION
Fluoroquinolone; bactericidal, interferes with the enzyme DNA gyrase, which is needed for synthesis of bacterial DNA.

PHARMACOKINETICS
Absorption: (Sol) C_{max}=<5ng/mL.

PATIENT CONSIDERATIONS
Assessment: Assess for previous hypersensitivity to the drug and other quinolones, use of contact lenses, pregnancy/nursing status, and possible drug interactions.

Monitoring: Monitor for signs/symptoms of hypersensitivity/anaphylactic reactions, and other adverse reactions. Monitor for superinfection; examine with magnification (eg, slit-lamp biomicroscopy) and fluorescein staining, where appropriate.

Counseling: Instruct to use as prescribed. Instruct not to touch dropper tip to any surface because it may contaminate sol. Advise to contact physician if hypersensitivity reaction occurs (eg, rash). Instruct to remove contact lenses before use and not to wear contact lenses if signs/symptoms of bacterial conjunctivitis are present.

CIMETIDINE — cimetidine   Rx

Class: H₂ blocker

OTHER BRAND NAMES
Tagamet (Discontinued)

ADULT DOSAGE
Duodenal Ulcers

Short-Term Treatment of Active Ulcer:
800mg qhs (preferred) or 300mg qid (w/ meals and qhs) or 400mg bid (qam and qhs) for 4-6 weeks

PEDIATRIC DOSAGE
Duodenal Ulcers

≥16 Years:
Short-Term Treatment of Active Ulcer:
800mg qhs (preferred) or 300mg qid (w/ meals and qhs) or 400mg bid (qam and qhs) for 4-6 weeks

Maint Therapy After Healing of Active Ulcer:
400mg qhs

Concomitant antacids should be given prn for relief of pain; however, simultaneous administration not recommended

Gastric Ulcers
Short-Term Treatment of Active, Benign Ulcer:
800mg qhs (preferred) or 300mg qid (w/ meals and qhs) for 6 weeks

Gastroesophageal Reflux Disease
Erosive Esophagitis Diagnosed by Endoscopy:
800mg bid or 400mg qid for 12 weeks
Max: 12 weeks

Pathological Hypersecretory Conditions
Treatment of Pathological Hypersecretory Conditions (eg, Zollinger-Ellison Syndrome, Systemic Mastocytosis, Multiple Endocrine Adenomas):
Usual: 300mg qid (w/ meals and qhs)
Max: 2400mg/day
Continue as long as clinically indicated

Maint Therapy After Healing of Active Ulcer:
400mg qhs

Concomitant antacids should be given prn for relief of pain; however, simultaneous administration not recommended

Gastric Ulcers
Short-Term Treatment of Active, Benign Ulcer:
≥16 Years:
800mg qhs or 300mg qid (w/ meals and qhs) for 6 weeks

Gastroesophageal Reflux Disease
Erosive Esophagitis Diagnosed by Endoscopy:
≥16 Years:
800mg bid or 400mg qid for 12 weeks
Max: 12 weeks

Pathological Hypersecretory Conditions
Treatment of Pathological Hypersecretory Conditions (eg, Zollinger-Ellison Syndrome, Systemic Mastocytosis, Multiple Endocrine Adenomas):
≥16 Years:
Usual: 300mg qid (w/ meals and qhs)
Max: 2400mg/day
Continue as long as clinically indicated

DOSING CONSIDERATIONS
Renal Impairment
Severe: 300mg q12h; may increase to q8h or further w/ caution if required
Hemodialysis: Adjust so that timing of scheduled dose coincides w/ end of hemodialysis

ADMINISTRATION
Oral route

STORAGE
20-25°C (68-77°F). (Tab) Protect from light.

HOW SUPPLIED
Sol: 300mg/5mL [237mL]; **Tab:** 200mg, 300mg, 400mg*, 800mg* *scored

CONTRAINDICATIONS
Known hypersensitivity to the product.

WARNINGS/PRECAUTIONS
Symptomatic response does not preclude the presence of gastric malignancy. Reversible confusional states observed on occasion, predominantly in severely ill patients; contributing factors include advancing age (≥50 yrs) and preexisting liver and/or renal disease. Increased possibility of a hyperinfection of strongyloidiasis in immunocompromised patients. Cardiac arrhythmias and hypotension reported (rare) following rapid administration of inj by IV bolus.

ADVERSE REACTIONS
Headache, reversible confusional states, reversible impotence, increased serum transaminase, gynecomastia.

DRUG INTERACTIONS
Increases blood levels of warfarin-type anticoagulants, phenytoin, propranolol, nifedipine, chlordiazepoxide, diazepam, certain TCAs, lidocaine, theophylline, and metronidazole. Closely monitor PT and adjust dose of warfarin anticoagulants. Adverse effects reported with phenytoin, lidocaine, and theophylline. May affect absorption of certain drugs due to alteration of pH (eg, ketoconazole); give at least 2 hrs before cimetidine. Antacids may interfere with absorption; simultaneous administration of oral cimetidine with antacids is not recommended.

PREGNANCY AND LACTATION
Category B, not for use in nursing.

MECHANISM OF ACTION
H₂-blocker; competitively inhibits the action of histamine at the histamine H₂ receptors of the parietal cells. Also inhibits gastric acid secretion.

PHARMACOKINETICS
Absorption: Rapid. T_{max}=45-90 min. **Distribution:** Found in breast milk.
Metabolism: Extensive; sulfoxide (major metabolite). **Elimination:** Urine (48% unchanged); $T_{1/2}$=2 hrs.

PATIENT CONSIDERATIONS
Assessment: Assess for hypersensitivity to drug, immunosuppression, renal/hepatic impairment, pregnancy/nursing status, and possible drug interactions.

Monitoring: Monitor for hypersensitivity reactions and other adverse reactions.

Counseling: Inform that antacids may be given PRN for pain relief; however, concomitant use of antacids is not recommended. Instruct to contact physician if hypersensitivity or other adverse reactions develop.

CIMZIA — certolizumab pegol   Rx

Class: Tumor necrosis factor (TNF) blocker

Increased risk for developing serious infections (eg, active tuberculosis [TB], latent TB reactivation, invasive fungal infections, bacterial/viral and other opportunistic infections) leading to hospitalization or death, mostly w/ concomitant use w/ immunosuppressants (eg, methotrexate or corticosteroids). D/C if serious infection or sepsis develops. Active TB/reactivation of latent TB may present w/ disseminated or extrapulmonary disease; test for latent TB before and during therapy and initiate treatment for latent TB prior to therapy. Invasive fungal infections reported; consider empiric antifungal therapy in patients at risk who develop severe systemic illness. Consider risks and benefits prior to therapy in patients w/ chronic or recurrent infection. Monitor patients for development of infection during and after treatment, including development of TB in patients who tested (-) for latent TB infection prior to therapy. Lymphoma and other malignancies, some fatal, reported in children and adolescents. Not indicated for pediatric patients.

ADULT DOSAGE

Crohn's Disease

Moderately to Severely Active Disease w/ Inadequate Response to Conventional Therapy:
Initial: 400mg (given as 2 SQ inj of 200mg) initially, and at Weeks 2 and 4
Maint: 400mg every 4 weeks

Rheumatoid Arthritis

Moderately to Severely Active:
Recommended: 400mg (given as 2 SQ inj of 200mg) initially and at Weeks 2 and 4, followed by 200mg every other week
Maint: Consider 400mg every 4 weeks

Psoriatic Arthritis

Active:
Recommended: 400mg (given as 2 SQ inj of 200mg) initially and at Weeks 2 and 4, followed by 200mg every other week
Maint: Consider 400mg every 4 weeks

Ankylosing Spondylitis

Active:
Recommended: 400mg (given as 2 SQ inj of 200mg) initially and at Weeks 2 and 4, followed by 200mg every 2 weeks or 400mg every 4 weeks

PEDIATRIC DOSAGE

Pediatric use may not have been established

DOSING CONSIDERATIONS
Concomitant Medications
Not recommended in combination w/ biological disease-modifying anti-rheumatic drugs (DMARDs) or other TNF blocker therapy

ADMINISTRATION
SQ route

Rotate inj sites; avoid areas where the skin is tender, bruised, red, or hard. Once reconstituted, can store in the vials for up to 24 hrs between 2-8°C (36-46°F) prior to inj; do not freeze.

Lyophilized Powder for Inj
Preparation:
1. Bring to room temperature for 30 min before reconstituting; do not warm the vial in any other way.
2. Reconstitute vial(s) w/ 1mL of sterile water for inj (SWFI) using 20-gauge needle provided; direct SWFI at the vial wall rather than directly on the product.
3. Gently swirl each vial for 1 min w/o shaking, assuring that all of the powder comes in contact w/ SWFI.
4. Continue swirling every 5 min as long as non-dissolved particles are observed; full reconstitution may take as long as 30 min.
5. Final reconstituted sol contains 200mg/mL.

Administration:
1. Prior to injecting, reconstituted sol should be at room temperature (but not for >2 hrs prior to administration).
2. Withdraw reconstituted sol into a separate syringe for each vial using a new 20-gauge needle for each vial so that each syringe contains 1mL of sol (200mg of certolizumab pegol).
3. Replace 20-gauge needle(s) on syringes w/ a 23-gauge(s) for administration.
4. Inject full contents of syringe(s) SQ by pinching the skin of the thigh or abdomen; when a 400mg dose is needed (given as 2 SQ inj of 200mg), inj should occur at separate sites in the thigh or abdomen.

Prefilled Syringe
After proper training in SQ inj technique, a patient may self-inject w/ a prefilled syringe if appropriate.
Patients using prefilled syringes should be instructed to inject full amount in syringe (1mL), according to the directions provided in Instructions for Use booklet.

STORAGE
2-8°C (36-46°F). Do not freeze. Protect sol from light.

HOW SUPPLIED
Inj: 200mg/mL [prefilled syringe, vial]

WARNINGS/PRECAUTIONS
May be used as monotherapy or concomitantly w/ non-biological DMARDs. Do not initiate w/ an active infection. Increased risk of infection in elderly patients and in patients w/ comorbid conditions; consider the risks prior to therapy for those who have been exposed to TB, w/ a history of an opportunistic infection, who have resided or traveled in areas of endemic TB or mycoses, or w/ any underlying conditions predisposing to infection. Postmarketing cases of aggressive and fatal hepatosplenic T-cell lymphoma (HSTCL) reported; the majority of cases occurred in adolescent and young adult males w/ Crohn's disease or ulcerative colitis. Acute and chronic leukemia, melanoma, and Merkel cell carcinoma reported. Perform periodic skin examination, particularly in patients w/ risk factors for skin cancer. New onset and worsening of CHF reported; caution in patients w/ heart failure (HF) and monitor carefully. Hypersensitivity reactions reported (rare); d/c and institute appropriate therapy if such reactions occur. Hepatitis B virus (HBV) reactivation reported; if reactivation occurs, d/c and initiate antiviral therapy w/ appropriate supportive treatment. Monitor patients closely and exercise caution when considering resumption of therapy. Associated w/ rare cases of new onset or exacerbation of clinical symptoms and/or radiographic evidence of CNS and peripheral demyelinating disease; caution w/ preexisting or recent-onset central or peripheral nervous system demyelinating disorders. Rare cases of neurological disorders (eg, seizure disorder, optic neuritis, peripheral neuropathy) reported. Hematological reactions (eg, leukopenia, pancytopenia, thrombocytopenia) reported; caution in patients w/ ongoing, or a history of, significant hematologic abnormalities, and consider discontinuation in patients w/ confirmed significant hematologic abnormalities. May result in the formation of autoantibodies and rarely, in the development of a lupus-like syndrome; d/c if lupus-like syndrome develops. Lab test interactions may occur.

ADVERSE REACTIONS
URTIs, rash, UTIs.

DRUG INTERACTIONS
See Boxed Warning and Dosing Considerations. Avoid concurrent use w/ live (eg, attenuated) vaccines. Not recommended w/ anakinra, abatacept, rituximab, or natalizumab; may increase risk of serious infections. Carefully consider the potential risk of HSTCL w/ the combination of azathioprine or 6-mercaptopurine.

PREGNANCY AND LACTATION
Pregnancy: Category B; may be eliminated at a slower rate in exposed infants than in adult patients. There is a pregnancy exposure registry that monitors pregnancy outcomes in women exposed to the drug during pregnancy.
Lactation: Not for use in nursing.

MECHANISM OF ACTION
TNF-blocker; binds to and selectively neutralizes TNF-α, which has a central role in inflammatory processes.

PHARMACOKINETICS
Absorption: C_{max}=approx 43-49mcg/mL; T_{max}=54-171 hrs; bioavailability (approx 80%). **Distribution:** V_d=6-8L. **Elimination:** $T_{1/2}$=approx 14 days.

PATIENT CONSIDERATIONS
Assessment: Assess for active/chronic/recurrent infection (eg, TB, HBV), TB exposure, history of an opportunistic infection, recent travel to areas of endemic TB or endemic mycoses, underlying conditions that may predispose to infection, HF, presence or history of significant hematologic abnormalities, neurologic disorders, risk factors for skin cancer, pregnancy/nursing status, and possible drug interactions. Perform test for latent TB infection.

Monitoring: Monitor for sepsis, TB (active, reactivation, or latent), invasive fungal infections, bacterial/viral/other infections, lymphoma/other malignancies, new onset/worsening of CHF, active HBV infection, hematological events, hypersensitivity reactions, CNS demyelinating disorders, lupus-like syndrome, and other adverse reactions. Perform periodic skin examination, particularly in patients w/ risk factors for skin cancer and test for latent TB infection.

Counseling: Advise of potential risks and benefits of therapy. Inform that therapy may lower the ability of the immune system to fight infections; instruct to immediately contact physician if any signs/symptoms of an infection develop, including TB and HBV reactivation. Inform about the risks of lymphoma and other malignancies while on therapy. Advise to seek immediate medical attention if any symptoms of severe allergic reactions occur. Advise to report to physician signs of new or worsening medical conditions (eg, heart disease, neurological diseases, autoimmune disorders) and symptoms of cytopenia (eg, bruising, bleeding, persistent fever). Instruct about proper administration techniques.

CINQAIR — reslizumab   Rx

Class: Monoclonal antibody/interleukin-5 (IL-5) receptor antagonist

---

Anaphylaxis has been observed as early as the second dose; observe for an appropriate period of time after administration by a healthcare professional prepared to manage anaphylaxis. D/C immediately if signs/symptoms of anaphylaxis occur.

ADULT DOSAGE
Asthma
Add-on maint treatment of severe asthma in patients w/ an eosinophilic phenotype
3mg/kg IV once q4 weeks

PEDIATRIC DOSAGE
Pediatric use may not have been established

DOSING CONSIDERATIONS
Adverse Reactions
Severe Systemic Reaction: D/C infusion immediately

ADMINISTRATION
IV route

Preparation
1. Remove from refrigerator; do not shake.
2. Withdraw proper volume of from the vial(s), based on the recommended weight-based dosage; discard any unused portion.
3. Dispense syringe contents slowly into infusion bag containing 50mL of 0.9% NaCl inj to minimize foaming (compatible w/ PVC or polyolefin infusion bags). Gently invert bag to mix sol; do not shake. Do not mix/dilute w/ other drugs.
4. Administer immediately after preparation. If not used immediately, store diluted sol at 2-8°C (36-46°F) or at ≤25°C (77°F), protected from light, for ≤16 hrs. Time between preparation and administration should not exceed 16 hrs.

Administration
1. If refrigerated, allow diluted sol to reach room temperature.
2. Use an infusion set w/ an inline, low protein binding filter (pore size of 0.2 micron). Compatible w/ polyethersulfone, polyvinylidene fluoride, nylon, and cellulose acetate inline infusion filters.
3. Infuse diluted sol over a 20-50 min period. Infusion time may vary depending on the total volume to be infused as based upon patient weight. Do not administer as IV push or bolus.
4. Do not infuse concomitantly in same IV line w/ other agents.
5. Observe patient during infusion and for an appropriate period of time following infusion.
6. Upon completion of the infusion, flush the IV set w/ 0.9% NaCl inj.

STORAGE
2-8°C (36-46°F). Do not freeze. Do not shake. Protect from light.

HOW SUPPLIED
Inj: 100mg/10mL

CONTRAINDICATIONS
Known hypersensitivity to reslizumab or any of its excipients.

WARNINGS/PRECAUTIONS
Not indicated for treatment of other eosinophilic conditions or relief of acute bronchospasm or status asthmaticus. Do not use to treat acute asthma symptoms/exacerbations/bronchospasm or status asthmaticus. Malignancies observed. Do not d/c systemic or inhaled corticosteroids abruptly upon initiation of therapy; reductions in corticosteroid dose, if appropriate, should be gradual and performed under the direct supervision of a physician. Reduction in corticosteroid dose may be associated w/ systemic withdrawal symptoms and/or unmask conditions previously suppressed by systemic corticosteroid therapy. It is unknown if treatment will influence immune response against parasitic infections; treat preexisting helminth infections before initiating reslizumab. If patients become infected while receiving reslizumab and does not respond to anti-helminth treatment, d/c reslizumab treatment until infection resolves.

ADVERSE REACTIONS
Oropharyngeal pain.

PREGNANCY AND LACTATION
Pregnancy: Insufficient data to inform on drug-associated risk. Monoclonal antibodies are transported across the placenta in a linear fashion as pregnancy progresses; potential effects on a fetus are likely to be greater during the 2nd/3rd trimester of pregnancy.
Lactation: It is not known whether reslizumab is present in human milk, and the effects on the breastfed infant and on milk production are not known.

MECHANISM OF ACTION
IL-5 antagonist monoclonal antibody; mechanism not definitively established. Reduces the production and survival of eosinophils by inhibiting IL-5 signaling.

PHARMACOKINETICS
Distribution: V_d=5L. **Metabolism:** Degraded by enzymatic proteolysis. **Elimination:** $T_{1/2}$=24 days.

PATIENT CONSIDERATIONS
Assessment: Assess for other eosinophilic conditions, acute bronchospasm or status asthmaticus, preexisting helminth infections, hypersensitivity to drug or excipients in the formulation, and pregnancy/nursing status.

Monitoring: Monitor for hypersensitivity reactions, acute asthma symptoms or acute exacerbations, and other adverse reactions.

Counseling: Inform that hypersensitivity reactions, including anaphylaxis, have occurred. Educate on the signs and symptoms of hypersensitivity reactions and anaphylaxis; instruct to contact a healthcare professional immediately if experiencing symptoms of an allergic reaction after receiving infusion. Inform that therapy is not used to treat acute asthma symptoms or acute exacerbations. Instruct to seek medical advice if asthma remains uncontrolled or worsens after initiation of treatment. Counsel about the risk of malignancies. Inform not to d/c systemic or inhaled corticosteroids except under the direct supervision of a physician. Inform that reduction in corticosteroid dose may be associated w/ withdrawal symptoms and/or may unmask conditions previously suppressed by systemic corticosteroid therapy.

CIPRO XR — ciprofloxacin   Rx
Class: Fluoroquinolone

> Fluoroquinolones have been associated w/ disabling and potentially irreversible serious adverse reactions that have occurred together, including tendinitis and tendon rupture, peripheral neuropathy, and CNS effects; d/c immediately and avoid use in patients who experience any of these serious adverse reactions. May exacerbate muscle weakness in patients w/ myasthenia gravis; avoid in patients w/ known history of myasthenia gravis. Due to the association w/ serious adverse reactions, reserve use in patients who have no alternative treatment options for uncomplicated UTIs.

ADULT DOSAGE	PEDIATRIC DOSAGE
Urinary Tract Infections	Pediatric use may not have been established
Uncomplicated (Acute Cystitis): 500mg q24h for 3 days	
Reserve for patients w/ no alternative treatment options	
Complicated UTI/Acute Uncomplicated Pyelonephritis: 1000mg q24h for 7-14 days	
Cipro XR tabs and ciprofloxacin immediate-release (IR) tabs are not interchangeable. May switch from Cipro IV to Cipro XR at discretion of physician.	

DOSING CONSIDERATIONS
Renal Impairment
Hemodialysis/Peritoneal Dialysis: Give after procedure is completed
Max: 500mg q24h
Continuous Ambulatory Peritoneal Dialysis:
Max: 500mg q24h

Complicated UTI/Acute Uncomplicated Pyelonephritis:
CrCl ≤30mL/min: Reduce dose from 1000mg to 500mg qd

ADMINISTRATION
Oral route

Swallow tab whole; do not split, crush, or chew.
Take w/ or w/o food.
Avoid w/ dairy products or w/ Ca^{2+}-fortified products; space Ca^{2+} intake (>800mg) by 2 hrs. May take w/ a meal that contains these products.
Administer ≥2 hrs before or 6 hrs after antacids containing Mg^{2+} or aluminum, polymeric phosphate binders, sucralfate, didanosine chewable/buffered tabs or pediatric powder, other highly buffered drugs, metal cations such as iron, and multivitamin preparations w/ zinc.

STORAGE
25°C (77°F); excursions permitted to 15-30°C (59-86°F).

HOW SUPPLIED
Tab, Extended-Release: 500mg, 1000mg

CONTRAINDICATIONS
History of hypersensitivity to ciprofloxacin, any member of the quinolone class of antibacterials, or any of the product components. Concomitant administration w/ tizanidine.

WARNINGS/PRECAUTIONS
Tendinitis or tendon rupture can occur w/in hours or days of starting therapy or as long as several months after completion of therapy and may occur bilaterally; increased risk in patients >60 yrs and in patients w/ kidney, heart, or lung transplants. Avoid in patients who have a history of tendon disorders or who have experienced tendinitis or tendon rupture. Cases of sensory or sensorimotor axonal polyneuropathy resulting in paresthesias, hypoesthesias, dysesthesias, and weakness reported; symptoms may occur soon after initiation of therapy and may be irreversible in some patients. Avoid in patients who have previously experienced peripheral neuropathy. May trigger seizures or lower the seizure threshold; caution in epileptic patients, w/ known/suspected CNS disorders that may predispose to seizures or lower the seizure threshold, or in the presence of other risk factors that may predispose to seizures or lower the seizure threshold. Status epilepticus reported. D/C if seizures occur. Hypersensitivity (anaphylactic) reactions and other serious and sometimes fatal adverse reactions reported; d/c immediately at 1st appearance of skin rash, jaundice, or any other sign of hypersensitivity. Severe hepatotoxicity, including hepatic necrosis, life-threatening hepatic failure, and fatal events, reported; d/c immediately if signs and symptoms of hepatitis occur. Temporary increase in transaminases, alkaline phosphatase, or cholestatic jaundice possible. Clostridium difficile-associated diarrhea (CDAD) reported; may need to d/c if CDAD is suspected or confirmed. May prolong QT interval; avoid w/ known QT interval prolongation and w/ risk factors for QT prolongation/torsades de pointes (eg, congenital long QT syndrome, uncorrected hypokalemia/hypomagnesemia, cardiac disease). Musculoskeletal disorders seen in pediatric patients. May cause photosensitivity/phototoxicity reactions; d/c if phototoxicity occurs. Avoid excessive exposure to sun/UV light. May result in bacterial resistance if used in the absence of a proven or strongly suspected bacterial infection or a prophylactic indication. Has not been shown to be effective in the treatment of syphilis; antimicrobial agents used in high dose for short periods to treat gonorrhea may mask or delay symptoms of incubating syphilis. Crystalluria reported; maintain hydration and avoid alkalinity of urine. Caution in elderly.

ADVERSE REACTIONS
N/V, headache, dizziness, diarrhea, vaginal moniliasis.

DRUG INTERACTIONS

See Administration and Contraindications. May increase levels of CYP1A2 substrates (eg, theophylline, methylxanthines, olanzapine), duloxetine, or sildenafil. Increased theophylline levels may increase the risk of developing CNS or other adverse reactions; if coadministration cannot be avoided, monitor theophylline levels and adjust dose. Avoid w/ Class IA (eg, quinidine, procainamide) and Class III (eg, amiodarone, sotalol) antiarrhythmics, TCAs, macrolides, and antipsychotics; may further prolong the QT interval. May potentiate glucose-lowering effect of oral antidiabetic agents; monitor blood glucose. May alter serum levels of phenytoin; monitor phenytoin therapy, including phenytoin levels during and shortly after coadministration. Transient SrCr elevations w/ cyclosporine; monitor renal function. May increase effects of anticoagulants; monitor PT and INR frequently during and shortly after coadministration w/ an oral anticoagulant. May increase levels and risk of toxic reactions of methotrexate; carefully monitor w/ concomitant use. Monitor for clozapine- or ropinirole-related adverse reactions and adjust dose of clozapine or ropinirole during and shortly after coadministration. High-dose quinolones in combination w/ NSAIDs (not acetyl salicylic acid) may provoke convulsions. Monitor for sildenafil toxicity. Avoid use w/ duloxetine; monitor for duloxetine toxicity if coadministration is unavoidable. May inhibit the formation of paraxanthine after caffeine administration (or pentoxifylline-containing products); monitor for xanthine toxicity and adjust dose as necessary. Antacids, sucralfate, multivitamins, and other multivalent cation-containing products (eg, Mg^{2+}/aluminum antacids, polymeric phosphate binders, products containing Ca^{2+}, iron, or zinc and dairy products) may decrease absorption, resulting in lower serum and urine levels lower than desired. Probenecid may increase levels. Increased risk of fluoroquinolone-associated tendinitis and tendon rupture w/ corticosteroids. Caution w/ drugs that may lower seizure threshold.

PREGNANCY AND LACTATION

Pregnancy: Category C.
Lactation: Found in breast milk; not for use in nursing.

MECHANISM OF ACTION

Fluoroquinolone; inhibits the enzymes topoisomerase II (DNA gyrase) and topoisomerase IV (both Type II topoisomerases), which are required for bacterial DNA replication, transcription, repair, and recombination.

PHARMACOKINETICS

Absorption: (500mg) C_{max}=1.59mg/L; T_{max}=1.5 hrs; AUC_{0-24h}=7.97mg•hr/L. (1000mg) C_{max}=3.11mg/L; T_{max}=2 hrs; AUC_{0-24h}=16.83mg•hr/L. **Distribution:** V_d=2.1-2.7L/kg (IV); plasma protein binding (20-40%); found in breast milk. **Metabolism:** Oxociprofloxacin (M_3), sulfociprofloxacin (M_2) (primary metabolites). **Elimination:** Urine (35%, unchanged), (IR) feces (20-35%); $T_{1/2}$=6.6 hrs (500mg), 6.31 hrs (1000mg).

PATIENT CONSIDERATIONS

Assessment: Assess for risk factors for developing tendinitis and tendon rupture; history of myasthenia gravis, tendon disorders, or peripheral neuropathy; drug hypersensitivity; CNS disorders or other risk factors that may predispose to seizures or lower seizure threshold; QT interval prolongation; renal/hepatic impairment; pregnancy/nursing status; and possible drug interactions. Obtain baseline culture and susceptibility tests. Perform serologic test for syphilis in patients w/ gonorrhea.

Monitoring: Monitor for tendinitis or tendon rupture, peripheral neuropathy, CNS effects, exacerbation of myasthenia gravis, hypersensitivity reactions, hepatotoxicity, CDAD, QT prolongation, photosensitivity/phototoxicity reactions, crystalluria, and other adverse reactions. Monitor PT and INR if coadministered w/ an oral anticoagulant (eg, warfarin). Perform periodic culture and susceptibility testing. Perform follow-up serologic test for syphilis 3 months after treatment in patients w/ gonorrhea.

Counseling: Inform about benefits/risks of therapy. Advise to d/c if an adverse reaction is experienced and to contact physician. Inform about the risk of disabling and potentially irreversible serious adverse reactions that may occur together, including tendinitis and tendon rupture, peripheral neuropathies, and CNS effects. Inform about the risk of exacerbation of myasthenia gravis, hypersensitivity reactions, hepatotoxicity, diarrhea, QT interval prolongation, and photosensitivity/phototoxicity. Instruct to d/c and contact physician if pain, swelling, or inflammation of a tendon or weakness or inability to use joints is experienced; advise to rest and refrain from exercise. Instruct to d/c immediately and contact physician if symptoms of peripheral neuropathy (eg, pain, burning, tingling, numbness, and/or weakness) develop. Advise to inform physician if patient has history of convulsions or myasthenia gravis. Inform patients that they should know how they react to therapy before operating an automobile or machinery or engaging in other activities requiring mental alertness/coordination. Instruct to notify physician if persistent headache w/ or w/o blurred vision occurs. Advise to notify physician if symptoms of muscle weakness, including respiratory difficulties, are experienced. Instruct to d/c at the 1st sign of a skin rash, hives, or other skin reactions; a rapid heartbeat; difficulty in swallowing or breathing; any swelling suggesting angioedema; or other symptoms of an allergic reaction. Advise to notify physician if experiencing any signs or symptoms of liver injury. Inform that diarrhea is a common problem; instruct to notify physician if experiencing watery and bloody stools (w/ or w/o stomach cramps/fever) even as late as ≥2 months after having taken the last dose of treatment. Instruct to inform physician of any personal or family history of QT prolongation or proarrhythmic conditions and if symptoms of QT prolongation are experienced. Counsel caregiver to inform physician if child has joint-related problems prior to, during, or after therapy. Inform of drug interactions (eg, tizanidine, theophylline, caffeine). Advise to minimize or avoid exposure to natural or artificial light (eg, tanning beds or UVA/B treatment); instruct to contact physician if a sunburn-like reaction or skin eruption occurs. Inform that drug treats only bacterial, not viral infections. Instruct to take exactly ud; inform that skipping doses or not completing full course may decrease effectiveness and increase bacterial resistance. Advise to drink fluids liberally. Advise on administration w/ antacids, sucralfate, multivitamins, multivalent cation-containing products, dairy products, and Ca^{2+}-fortified products. Instruct patients being treated w/ oral antidiabetic agents to notify physician if hypoglycemia occurs.

CIPRODEX — ciprofloxacin/dexamethasone   Rx

Class: Antibacterial/corticosteroid combination

ADULT DOSAGE	PEDIATRIC DOSAGE
Acute Otitis Externa	**Acute Otitis Media**
4 drops into the affected ear bid for 7 days	**≥6 Months of Age w/ Tympanostomy Tubes:**
	4 drops into the affected ear bid for 7 days
	Acute Otitis Externa
	≥6 Months of Age:
	4 drops into the affected ear bid for 7 days

ADMINISTRATION

Otic route
Shake well immediately before use.

Instructions

1. Warm sus by holding bottle in hand for 1 or 2 min to avoid dizziness, which may result from instillation of cold sus.
2. Lie w/ affected ear upward, and then instill drops.
3. For treatment of otitis media in patients w/ tympanostomy tubes, the tragus should be pumped 5X by pushing inward to facilitate penetration of the drops into the middle ear.
4. Maintain position for 60 sec and repeat, if necessary, for the opposite ear.

STORAGE

20-25°C (68-77°F); excursions permitted to 15-30°C (59-86°F). Avoid freezing. Protect from light.

HOW SUPPLIED

Otic Sus: (Ciprofloxacin/Dexamethasone) 0.3%/0.1% [7.5mL]

CONTRAINDICATIONS

History of hypersensitivity to ciprofloxacin, other quinolones, or any components in this medication. Viral infections of the external canal (eg, herpes simplex infections) and fungal otic infections.

WARNINGS/PRECAUTIONS

For otic use only; not for ophthalmic use, or for injection. D/C at 1st appearance of skin rash or any other sign of hypersensitivity. Serious and occasionally fatal hypersensitivity (anaphylactic) reactions reported in patients receiving systemic quinolones. Prolonged use may result in overgrowth of nonsusceptible bacteria and fungi; perform culture testing if infection is not improved after 1 week and d/c and institute alternative therapy if such infections occur. If otorrhea persists after full course of therapy, or if ≥2 episodes of otorrhea occur w/in 6 months, evaluate further to exclude an underlying condition (eg, cholesteatoma, foreign body, tumor).

ADVERSE REACTIONS

Ear discomfort/pain/precipitate/pruritus/debris/congestion, irritability, taste perversion, superimposed ear infection, erythema.

PREGNANCY AND LACTATION

Pregnancy: Category C.
Lactation: Not for use in nursing.

MECHANISM OF ACTION

Ciprofloxacin: Fluoroquinolone antibacterial; bactericidal action results from interference w/ the enzyme, DNA gyrase, which is needed for the synthesis of bacterial DNA. **Dexamethasone:** Corticosteroid; has been shown to suppress inflammation by inhibiting multiple inflammatory cytokines, resulting in decreased edema, fibrin deposition, capillary leakage, and migration of inflammatory cells.

PHARMACOKINETICS

Absorption: Ciprofloxacin: C_{max}=1.39ng/mL; T_{max}=15 min-2 hrs. Dexamethasone: C_{max}=1.14ng/mL; T_{max}=15 min-2 hrs.

PATIENT CONSIDERATIONS

Assessment: Assess for history of drug hypersensitivity, viral infection of the external canal (eg, herpes simplex infections), fungal otic infections, and pregnancy/nursing status.

Monitoring: Monitor for hypersensitivity reactions, skin rash, overgrowth of nonsusceptible bacteria and fungi, continued/recurrent otorrhea, and other adverse reactions. Perform culture testing if infection is not improved after 1 week of treatment.

Counseling: Inform that drug is for otic use only. Advise to avoid contaminating the tip w/ material from the ear, fingers, or other sources. Instruct to d/c immediately and consult physician if rash or allergic reaction occurs. Advise to warm bottle in hand for 1-2 min prior to use and to shake well immediately before using. Instruct to take ud, even if symptoms improve. Instruct to protect product from light and to discard unused portion after therapy is completed.

CIPROFLOXACIN INJECTION — ciprofloxacin   Rx
Class: Fluoroquinolone

> Fluoroquinolones have been associated w/ disabling and potentially irreversible serious adverse reactions that have occurred together, including tendinitis and tendon rupture, peripheral neuropathy, and CNS effects; d/c immediately and avoid fluoroquinolone use in patients who experience any of these serious adverse reactions. May exacerbate muscle weakness in patients w/ myasthenia gravis; avoid w/ known history of myasthenia gravis. Because fluoroquinolones have been associated w/ serious adverse reactions, reserve ciprofloxacin for use in patients who have no alternative treatment options for the following indications: acute exacerbation of chronic bronchitis, and acute bacterial sinusitis.

OTHER BRAND NAMES
Cipro IV

ADULT DOSAGE
Intra-Abdominal Infections
Complicated:
400mg q12h for 7-14 days, concomitantly w/ metronidazole
Sinusitis
Acute:
400mg q12h for 10 days
Chronic Bacterial Prostatitis
400mg q12h for 28 days
Febrile Neutropenia
Empirical Therapy:
400mg q8h + piperacillin 50mg/kg q4h for 7-14 days
Inhalational Anthrax (Postexposure)
400mg q12h for 60 days
Drug administration should begin as soon as possible after suspected or confirmed exposure
Urinary Tract Infections
200-400mg q8-12h for 7-14 days
Lower Respiratory Tract Infections
400mg q8-12h for 7-14 days
Also used to treat acute exacerbations of chronic bronchitis
Pneumonia
Nosocomial:
400mg q8h for 10-14 days
Skin and Skin Structure Infections
400mg q8-12h for 7-14 days
Bone/Joint Infections
400mg q8-12h for 4-8 weeks
Plague
400mg q8-12h for 14 days
Drug administration should begin as soon as possible after suspected or confirmed exposure
Conversions
IV to PO:
200mg IV q12h: 250mg tab q12h
400mg IV q12h: 500mg tab q12h
400mg IV q8h: 750mg tab q12h

PEDIATRIC DOSAGE
Urinary Tract Infections
Complicated UTI/Pyelonephritis:
1-17 Years:
6-10mg/kg q8h for 10-21 days
Max: 400mg/dose; even in patients >51kg
Inhalational Anthrax (Postexposure)
10mg/kg q12h for 60 days
Max: 400mg/dose
Drug administration should begin as soon as possible after suspected or confirmed exposure
Plague
10mg/kg q8-12h for 10-21 days
Max: 400mg/dose
Drug administration should begin as soon as possible after suspected or confirmed exposure

DOSING CONSIDERATIONS
Renal Impairment
Adults:
CrCl 5-29mL/min: 200-400mg q18-24h

ADMINISTRATION
IV route
- Infuse IV over 60 min; slow infusion of a dilute sol into larger vein will minimize discomfort and reduce risk of venous irritation.
- Maintain adequate hydration.

Cipro IV
Flexible Containers: Do not need to be diluted.

Ciprofloxacin Inj
- Dilute w/ a suitable IV sol to a final concentration of 1-2mg/mL.
- Infuse resulting sol over a period of 60 min by direct infusion or through a Y-type IV infusion set which may already be in place.
- If Y-type method is used, temporarily d/c administration of any other sol during the infusion.
- If concomitant use w/ another drug is necessary, give separately.

Compatibility and Stability:
Stable for up to 14 days refrigerated or room temperature storage when diluted w/ the following IV sol to concentrations of 0.5-2mg/mL:
- 0.9% NaCl inj
- D5 inj
- Sterile water for inj
- D10 for inj
- D5 and 0.225% NaCl for inj
- D5 and 0.45% NaCl for inj
- Lactated Ringer's for inj

STORAGE
20-25°C (68-77°F). Protect from light and freezing. Avoid excessive heat. **Cipro IV:** 5-25°C (41-77°F). Protect from light and freezing. Avoid excessive heat.

HOW SUPPLIED
Inj: 10mg/mL [20mL, 40mL]; (Cipro IV) 2mg/mL [200mL]

CONTRAINDICATIONS
History of hypersensitivity to ciprofloxacin, other quinolones, or any of the product components; concomitant administration w/ tizanidine.

WARNINGS/PRECAUTIONS
Not a drug of 1st choice in the treatment of presumed or confirmed pneumonia secondary to *Streptococcus pneumoniae*. Tendinitis or tendon rupture can occur w/in hours or days of starting therapy or as long as several months after completion of therapy and may occur bilaterally; increased risk in patients >60 yrs and in patients w/ kidney, heart, or lung transplants. Avoid in patients who have a history of tendon disorders or who have experienced tendinitis or tendon rupture. Cases of sensory or sensorimotor axonal polyneuropathy, resulting in paresthesias, hypoesthesias, dysesthesias, and weakness, reported; symptoms may occur soon after initiation of therapy and may be irreversible in some patients. Avoid in patients who have previously experienced peripheral neuropathy. May trigger seizures or lower the seizure threshold; caution in epileptic patients, w/ known/suspected CNS disorders that may predispose to seizures or lower the seizure threshold, or in the presence of other risk factors that may predispose to seizures or lower the seizure threshold. Status epilepticus reported. D/C if seizures occur. Serious anaphylactic reactions and other serious and sometimes fatal adverse reactions reported; d/c immediately and institute supportive measures at the 1st appearance of a skin rash, jaundice, or any other sign of hypersensitivity. Severe hepatotoxicity, including hepatic necrosis, life-threatening hepatic failure, and fatal events, reported; d/c immediately if signs and symptoms of hepatitis occur. May temporarily increase transaminases, alkaline phosphatase, or cholestatic jaundice, especially w/ previous liver damage. *Clostridium difficile*-associated diarrhea (CDAD) reported; may need to d/c if CDAD is suspected or confirmed. Prolongation of the QT interval and cases of torsades de pointes reported; avoid w/ known QT interval prolongation and risk factors for QT prolongation/torsades de pointes (eg, congenital long QT syndrome, uncorrected electrolyte imbalance, cardiac disease). Not a drug of 1st choice in pediatric patients due to reported increased incidence of adverse events, including events related to joints and/or surrounding tissues. Crystalluria reported; maintain hydration and avoid alkalinity of urine. May cause photosensitivity/phototoxicity reactions; d/c if phototoxicity occurs. Avoid excessive exposure to sun/UV light. May result in bacterial resistance if used in the absence of a proven or strongly suspected bacterial infection or a prophylactic indication. Caution in elderly.

ADVERSE REACTIONS
N/V, diarrhea, abnormal LFTs, CNS disturbances, local IV site reactions, eosinophilia, headache, restlessness, rash.

DRUG INTERACTIONS
See Contraindications. Increased risk of developing fluoroquinolone-associated tendinitis and tendon rupture in patients taking corticosteroid drugs. May increase levels of CYP1A2 substrates (eg, theophylline, methylxanthines, olanzapine). Avoid w/ theophylline; increased theophylline levels may increase the risk of developing CNS or other adverse reactions; if coadministration cannot be avoided, monitor theophylline levels and adjust dose. Avoid w/ Class IA (eg, quinidine, procainamide) and Class III (eg, amiodarone, sotalol) antiarrhythmics, TCAs, macrolides, antipsychotics, or other drugs that prolong the QT interval. Hypoglycemia reported w/ oral antidiabetic agents, mainly sulfonylureas (eg, glyburide, glimepiride); monitor blood glucose. May alter serum levels of phenytoin; monitor phenytoin therapy, including phenytoin levels during and shortly after coadministration. Transient SrCr elevations w/ cyclosporine; monitor renal function. May increase effects of oral anticoagulants; monitor PT and INR frequently during and shortly after coadministration. May increase levels and toxic reactions of methotrexate (MTX); carefully monitor w/ MTX therapy. Monitor for clozapine- or ropinirole-related adverse reactions and adjust dose of clozapine or ropinirole during and shortly after coadministration. High-dose quinolones in combination w/ NSAIDs (not acetyl salicylic acid) may provoke convulsions. Use w/ caution w/ sildenafil; monitor for sildenafil toxicity. Avoid use w/ duloxetine; if unavoidable, monitor for duloxetine toxicity. May inhibit the formation of paraxanthine after caffeine administration (or pentoxifylline-containing products) and may increase levels and prolong serum $T_{1/2}$ of caffeine/xanthine derivatives; monitor for xanthine toxicity and adjust dose as necessary. Probenecid may increase levels and potentiate ciprofloxacin toxicity; use w/ caution. Caution w/ drugs that may lower the seizure threshold.

PREGNANCY AND LACTATION
Pregnancy: Category C.
Lactation: Not for use in nursing.

MECHANISM OF ACTION
Fluoroquinolone; inhibits the enzymes topoisomerase II (DNA gyrase) and topoisomerase IV (both Type II topoisomerases) that are required for bacterial DNA replication, transcription, repair, and recombination.

PHARMACOKINETICS
Absorption: Absolute bioavailability (Oral) (70-80%). Administration of various doses resulted in different pharmacokinetic parameters. **Distribution:** Found in breast milk. **Elimination:** Bile (<1%, unchanged), urine (50-70%, unchanged), feces (15%); $T_{1/2}$=5-6 hrs.

PATIENT CONSIDERATIONS

Assessment: Assess for risk factors for developing tendinitis and tendon rupture; history of myasthenia gravis, tendon disorders, or peripheral neuropathy; drug hypersensitivity; CNS disorders or other risk factors that may predispose to seizures or lower seizure threshold; QT interval prolongation; renal/hepatic/hematopoietic function; pregnancy/nursing status; and possible drug interactions. Obtain baseline culture and susceptibility tests.

Monitoring: Monitor for tendinitis or tendon rupture, peripheral neuropathy, CNS effects, exacerbation of myasthenia gravis, hypersensitivity reactions, hepatotoxicity, CDAD, QT prolongation, photosensitivity/phototoxicity reactions, crystalluria, and other adverse reactions. Monitor PT and INR if coadministered w/ an oral anticoagulant (eg, warfarin). Perform periodic culture and susceptibility testing. Periodically monitor organ system function (eg, renal/hepatic/hematopoietic function), particularly during prolonged therapy.

Counseling: Inform about benefits/risks of therapy. Advise to d/c if an adverse reaction is experienced and to contact physician. Inform about the risk of disabling and potentially irreversible serious adverse reactions that may occur together, including tendinitis and tendon rupture, peripheral neuropathies, and CNS effects. Inform about the risk of exacerbation of myasthenia gravis, hypersensitivity reactions, hepatotoxicity, diarrhea, QT interval prolongation, and photosensitivity/phototoxicity. Instruct to d/c and contact physician if pain, swelling, or inflammation of a tendon, or weakness or inability to use joints is experienced; advise to rest and refrain from exercise. Instruct to d/c immediately and contact physician if symptoms of peripheral neuropathy (eg, pain, burning, tingling, numbness, and/or weakness) develop. Advise to inform physician if patient has history of convulsions or myasthenia gravis. Inform patients that they should know how they react to therapy before operating an automobile or machinery or engaging in other activities requiring mental alertness/coordination. Instruct to notify physician if persistent headache w/ or w/o blurred vision occurs. Advise to notify physician if symptoms of muscle weakness, including respiratory difficulties, are experienced. Instruct to d/c at the 1st sign of a skin rash, hives, or other skin reactions; a rapid heartbeat; difficulty in swallowing or breathing; any swelling suggesting angioedema; or other symptoms of an allergic reaction. Advise to notify physician if experiencing any signs or symptoms of liver injury. Inform that diarrhea is a common problem; instruct to notify physician if experiencing watery and bloody stools (w/ or w/o stomach cramps/fever) even as late as ≥2 months after having taken the last dose of treatment. Instruct to inform physician of any personal or family history of QT prolongation or proarrhythmic conditions and if symptoms of QT prolongation are experienced. Counsel caregiver to inform physician if child has joint-related problems prior to, during, or after therapy. Inform of drug interactions (eg, tizanidine, theophylline, caffeine). Advise to minimize or avoid exposure to natural or artificial light (eg, tanning beds or UVA/B treatment); instruct to contact physician if a sunburn-like reaction or skin eruption occurs. Inform that drug treats only bacterial, not viral, infections. Instruct to take exactly ud; inform that skipping doses or not completing full course may decrease effectiveness and increase bacterial resistance. Advise to drink fluids liberally. Instruct patients being treated w/ oral antidiabetic agents to notify physician if hypoglycemia occurs. Inform that efficacy studies of ciprofloxacin could not be conducted in humans w/ plague and anthrax for feasibility reasons and that approval for these conditions was based on an efficacy study conducted in animals.

CIPROFLOXACIN ORAL — ciprofloxacin   **Rx**

Class: Fluoroquinolone

> Fluoroquinolones have been associated w/ disabling and potentially irreversible serious adverse reactions that have occurred together, including tendinitis and tendon rupture, peripheral neuropathy, and CNS effects; d/c immediately and avoid use in patients who experience any of these serious adverse reactions. May exacerbate muscle weakness in patients w/ myasthenia gravis; avoid in patients w/ known history of myasthenia gravis. Because fluoroquinolones have been associated w/ serious adverse reactions, reserve ciprofloxacin for use in patients who have no alternative treatment options for the following indications: acute exacerbation of chronic bronchitis, acute uncomplicated cystitis, and acute sinusitis.

OTHER BRAND NAMES
Cipro

ADULT DOSAGE

Urinary Tract Infections
250-500mg q12h for 7-14 days

Uncomplicated Cystitis

Acute Infection in Female Patients:
250mg q12h for 3 days

Reserve ciprofloxacin for treatment in patients who have no alternative treatment options

Chronic Bacterial Prostatitis
500mg q12h for 28 days

Lower Respiratory Tract Infections
500-750mg q12h for 7-14 days

Indicated for treatment of acute exacerbations of chronic bronchitis; reserve ciprofloxacin for treatment in patients who have no alternative treatment options

PEDIATRIC DOSAGE

Urinary Tract Infections

Complicated UTIs or Pyelonephritis:
1-17 Years:
10-20mg/kg q12h for 10-21 days
Max: 750mg/dose; not to be exceeded even if >51kg

Inhalational Anthrax (Postexposure)
15mg/kg q12h for 60 days
Max: 500mg/dose

Plague

Treatment of Plague (Including Pneumonic and Septicemic Plague) and Prophylaxis of Plague:
15mg/kg q8-12h for 10-21 days
Max: 500mg/dose

Acute Bacterial Sinusitis
500mg q12h for 10 days
Reserve ciprofloxacin for treatment in patients who have no alternative treatment options

Skin and Skin Structure Infections
500-750mg q12h for 7-14 days

Bone/Joint Infections
500-750mg q12h for 4-8 weeks

Intra-Abdominal Infections

Complicated:
500mg q12h for 7-14 days, in combination w/ metronidazole

Diarrhea

Infectious:
500mg q12h for 5-7 days

Typhoid Fever
500mg q12h for 10 days

Gonococcal Infections

Uncomplicated Urethral and Cervical:
250mg single dose

Inhalational Anthrax (Postexposure)
500mg q12h for 60 days

Plague

Treatment of Plague (Including Pneumonic and Septicemic Plague) and Prophylaxis of Plague:
500-750mg q12h for 14 days

Conversions

Switching from Ciprofloxacin IV to Oral Therapy:
200mg IV q12h: 250mg tab q12h
400mg IV q12h: 500mg tab q12h
400mg IV q8h: 750mg tab q12h

DOSING CONSIDERATIONS

Renal Impairment

Adults:
CrCl 30-50mL/min: 250-500mg q12h
CrCl 5-29mL/min: 250-500mg q18h
Hemodialysis/Peritoneal Dialysis: 250-500mg q24h (after dialysis)
Severe Impairment w/ Severe Infections: A unit dose of 750mg may be administered at the intervals noted above

Pediatric Patients:
No information is available on dosing adjustments necessary for patients w/ moderate to severe renal insufficiency (CrCl <50mL/min/1.73m^2)

ADMINISTRATION
Oral route

Take w/ or w/o food.
Assure adequate hydration.

W/ Multivalent Cations
Administer ≥2 hrs before or 6 hrs after Mg^{2+}/aluminum antacids; polymeric phosphate binders or sucralfate; Videx (didanosine) chewable/buffered tabs or pediatric powder for oral sol; other highly buffered drugs; or other products containing Ca^{2+}, iron, or zinc.

W/ Dairy Products
Avoid concomitant administration w/ dairy products or Ca^{2+}-fortified juices alone; may take w/ a meal that contains these products.

Reconstitution of the Cipro Microcapsules for Oral Sus
1. Pour the microcapsules (small bottle) completely into the larger bottle of diluent; do not add water to the sus.
2. Close the larger bottle completely and shake vigorously for about 15 sec.
3. May store reconstituted product below 30°C (86°F) for 14 days; protect from freezing.
4. No additions should be made to the mixed final sus; should not be administered through feeding or NG tubes due to its physical characteristics.

Refer to PI for appropriate dosing volumes of the reconstituted oral sus.

STORAGE
Tab: 20-25°C (68-77°F). (Cipro) Excursions permitted to 15-30°C (59-86°F). **Microcapsules and Diluent:** <25°C (77°F); excursions permitted from 15-30°C (59-86°F). Protect from freezing. **Reconstituted Sus:** 25°C (77°F); excursions permitted from 15-30°C (59-86°F). Store reconstituted product for 14 days. Protect from freezing.

HOW SUPPLIED
Oral Sus: (Cipro) 250mg/5mL, 500mg/5mL [100mL]; **Tab:** 100mg, 750mg; (Cipro) 250mg, 500mg

CONTRAINDICATIONS
History of hypersensitivity to ciprofloxacin, any member of the quinolone class of antibacterials, or any of the product components. Concomitant administration w/ tizanidine.

WARNINGS/PRECAUTIONS

Not a drug of 1st choice in the treatment of presumed or confirmed pneumonia secondary to *Streptococcus pneumoniae*. Not a drug of 1st choice in the pediatric population due to an increased incidence of adverse events, including reactions related to joints and/or surrounding tissues. Tendinitis or tendon rupture can occur w/in hours or days of starting therapy or as long as several months after completion of therapy and may occur bilaterally; increased risk in patients >60 yrs and in patients w/ kidney, heart, or lung transplants. Avoid in patients who have a history of tendon disorders or who have experienced tendinitis or tendon rupture. Cases of sensory or sensorimotor axonal polyneuropathy resulting in paresthesias, hypoesthesias, dysesthesias, and weakness reported; symptoms may occur soon after initiation of therapy and may be irreversible in some patients. Avoid in patients who have previously experienced peripheral neuropathy. Known to trigger seizures or lower the seizure threshold and cases of status epilepticus reported; d/c if seizures occur. Caution in epileptic patients and patients w/ known or suspected CNS disorders that may predispose to seizures or lower the seizure threshold (eg, severe cerebral arteriosclerosis, previous history of convulsion, reduced cerebral blood flow, altered brain structure, stroke), or in the presence of other risk factors that may predispose to seizures or lower the seizure threshold (eg, certain drug therapy, renal dysfunction). Serious anaphylactic reactions and other serious and sometimes fatal adverse reactions reported; d/c immediately and institute supportive measures at the 1st appearance of a skin rash, jaundice, or any other sign of hypersensitivity. Severe hepatotoxicity, including hepatic necrosis, life-threatening hepatic failure, and fatal events, reported; d/c immediately if signs and symptoms of hepatitis occur. *Clostridium difficile*-associated diarrhea (CDAD) reported; may need to d/c if CDAD is suspected or confirmed. Associated w/ QT interval prolongation and cases of arrhythmia; cases of torsades de pointes reported. Avoid w/ known QT interval prolongation and risk factors for QT prolongation/torsades de pointes (eg, congenital long QT syndrome, uncorrected electrolyte imbalance, cardiac disease). Elderly patients may also be more susceptible to drug-associated effects on the QT interval. May cause moderate to severe photosensitivity/phototoxicity reactions; d/c if phototoxicity occurs. Avoid excessive exposure to sun/UV light. May result in bacterial resistance if used in the absence of a proven or strongly suspected bacterial infection or a prophylactic indication. Has not been shown to be effective in the treatment of syphilis; antimicrobial agents used in high dose for short periods to treat gonorrhea may mask or delay symptoms of incubating syphilis. Crystalluria reported; maintain hydration and avoid alkalinity of urine. Caution in elderly.

ADVERSE REACTIONS

N/V, diarrhea, abnormal LFTs, rash.

DRUG INTERACTIONS

See Boxed Warning, and Contraindications. Avoid concomitant administration w/ dairy products (eg, milk, yogurt), or Ca^{2+}-fortified juices alone; absorption may be reduced. May increase levels of CYP1A2 substrates (eg, theophylline, methylxanthines, olanzapine), duloxetine, or sildenafil. Use w/ caution and monitor for sildenafil toxicity. Avoid use w/ duloxetine; if unavoidable, monitor for duloxetine toxicity. Concurrent administration w/ theophylline may increase the risk of developing CNS or other adverse reactions; if coadministration cannot be avoided, monitor theophylline levels and adjust dose. Avoid w/ Class IA (eg, quinidine, procainamide) and Class III (eg, amiodarone, sotalol) antiarrhythmics, TCAs, macrolides, antipsychotics, and any other drug known to prolong the QT interval; may further prolong the QT interval. Hypoglycemia reported w/ oral antidiabetic agents, mainly sulfonylureas (eg, glyburide, glimepiride); monitor blood glucose. May alter serum levels of phenytoin; monitor phenytoin therapy, including phenytoin levels during and shortly after coadministration. Transient SrCr elevations w/ cyclosporine; monitor renal function. May increase effects of oral anticoagulants; monitor PT and INR frequently during and shortly after coadministration. May increase levels and toxic reactions of methotrexate; carefully monitor w/ concomitant use. Monitor for clozapine- or ropinirole-related adverse reactions and adjust dose of clozapine or ropinirole during and shortly after coadministration w/ ciprofloxacin. High-dose quinolones in combination w/ NSAIDs (not acetyl salicylic acid) may provoke convulsions. May inhibit the formation of paraxanthine after caffeine administration (or pentoxifylline-containing products); monitor for xanthine toxicity and adjust dose as necessary. Antacids, sucralfate, multivitamins, and other multivalent cation-containing products (eg, Mg^{2+}/aluminum antacids; polymeric phosphate binders; Videx [didanosine] chewable/buffered tab or pediatric powder; products containing Ca^{2+}, iron, or zinc; dairy products) may decrease absorption, resulting in lower serum and urine levels than desired; administer ≥2 hrs before or 6 hrs after multivalent cation-containing products administration. Probenecid may increase levels; use w/ caution. Caution w/ drugs that may lower seizure threshold. Increased risk of developing fluoroquinolone-associated tendinitis and tendon rupture in patients taking corticosteroid drugs.

PREGNANCY AND LACTATION

Pregnancy: Category C.
Lactation: Found in breast milk; not for use in nursing.

MECHANISM OF ACTION

Fluoroquinolone; inhibits the enzymes topoisomerase II (DNA gyrase) and topoisomerase IV (both Type II topoisomerases), which are required for bacterial DNA replication, transcription, repair, and recombination.

PHARMACOKINETICS

Absorption: T_{max}=1-2 hrs. (Tab) Absolute bioavailability (approx 70%). Administration of various doses resulted in different pharmacokinetic parameters. **Distribution:** Plasma protein binding (20-40%); found in breast milk. **Elimination:** Urine (approx 40-50%, unchanged), feces (approx 20-35%), bile; $T_{1/2}$=4 hrs.

PATIENT CONSIDERATIONS

Assessment: Assess for risk factors for developing tendinitis and tendon rupture; history of myasthenia gravis, tendon disorders, or peripheral neuropathy; drug hypersensitivity; QT interval prolongation; CNS disorders or risk factors that may predispose to seizures or lower seizure threshold; renal/hepatic impairment; pregnancy/nursing status; and possible drug interactions. Obtain baseline culture and susceptibility tests. Perform serologic test for syphilis in patients w/ gonorrhea.

Monitoring: Monitor for tendinitis, tendon rupture, peripheral neuropathy, CNS effects, exacerbation of myasthenia gravis, hypersensitivity reactions, hepatotoxicity, CDAD, QT prolongation, arrhythmias, musculoskeletal disorders (pediatric patients), crystalluria, photosensitivity/phototoxicity reactions, and other adverse reactions. Monitor hydration status, blood glucose levels, and renal function. Monitor PT and INR if coadministered w/ an oral anticoagulant. Perform follow-up serologic test for syphilis after 3 months in patients w/ gonorrhea.

Counseling: Inform about benefits/risks of therapy. Advise to d/c if an adverse reaction is experienced and to contact physician. Inform about the risks of tendinitis and tendon rupture, peripheral neuropathies, CNS effects, exacerbation of myasthenia gravis, and QT interval prolongation. Instruct to d/c and contact physician if pain, swelling, or inflammation of a tendon, or weakness or inability to use joints is experienced; advise to rest and refrain from exercise. Instruct to d/c immediately and contact physician if symptoms of peripheral neuropathy (eg, pain, burning, tingling, numbness and/or weakness) develop. Advise to inform physician if patient has history of convulsions or myasthenia gravis. Inform patients that they should know how they react to therapy before operating an automobile or machinery or engaging in other activities requiring mental alertness/coordination. Instruct to notify physician if persistent headache w/ or w/o blurred vision occurs. Advise to notify physician if symptoms of muscle weakness, including respiratory difficulties are experienced. Instruct to d/c at the 1st sign of a skin rash, hives, or other skin reactions; a rapid heartbeat; difficulty in swallowing or breathing; any swelling suggesting angioedema; or other symptoms of an allergic reaction. Inform to notify physician if experiencing any signs or symptoms of liver injury. Inform that diarrhea is a common problem; instruct to notify physician if experiencing watery and bloody stools (w/ or w/o stomach cramps/fever) even as late as ≥2 months after having taken the last dose of treatment. Instruct to inform physician of any personal or family history of QT prolongation or proarrhythmic conditions. Counsel caregiver to inform physician if child has joint-related problems prior to, during, or after therapy. Advise to seek medical help immediately if experiencing seizures, palpitations, or breathing difficulty. Advise to minimize or avoid exposure to natural or artificial light (eg, tanning beds or UVA/B treatment); instruct to contact physician if a sunburn-like reaction or skin eruption occurs. Instruct diabetic patients being treated w/ oral hypoglycemic agents to notify physician if hypoglycemia occurs. Inform that drug treats only bacterial, not viral, infections. Instruct to take exactly ud; inform that skipping doses or not completing full course may decrease effectiveness and increase bacterial resistance. Inform that antacids (containing Mg^{2+} or aluminum), sucralfate, metal cations (eg, iron), multivitamin preparations w/ zinc, or didanosine should be taken at least 2 hrs before or 6 hrs after ciprofloxacin administration. Advise to drink fluids liberally. Instruct to avoid concomitant use w/ dairy products or Ca^{2+}-fortified juices alone, but explain that drug may be taken w/ a meal that contains these products. Inform that efficacy studies of ciprofloxacin could not be conducted in humans w/ plague and anthrax for feasibility reasons and that approval for these conditions was therefore based on efficacy studies conducted in animals.

CITALOPRAM — citalopram   **Rx**

Class: Selective serotonin reuptake inhibitor (SSRI)

> Antidepressants increased the risk of suicidal thinking and behavior (suicidality) in children, adolescents, and young adults in short-term studies of major depressive disorder and other psychiatric disorders. Monitor and observe closely for clinical worsening, suicidality, or unusual changes in behavior. Not approved for use in pediatric patients.

OTHER BRAND NAMES

Celexa

ADULT DOSAGE	PEDIATRIC DOSAGE
Depression	Pediatric use may not have been established
Initial Treatment:	
Initial: 20mg qd	
Titrate: Increase dose to 40mg/day at an interval of no less than 1 week	
Max: 40mg/day	
Maint Treatment:	
Consider decreasing dose to 20mg/day if adverse reactions are bothersome	
Periodically reevaluate long-term usefulness of drug if used for extended periods	
Dosing Considerations with MAOIs	
Switching to/from an MAOI for Psychiatric Disorders:	
Allow at least 14 days between discontinuation of an MAOI and initiation of treatment, and allow at least 14 days between discontinuation of treatment and initiation of an MAOI	

W/ Other MAOIs (eg, Linezolid, IV Methylene Blue):
Do not start citalopram in patient being treated w/ linezolid or IV methylene blue.
In patients already receiving citalopram, if acceptable alternatives are not available and benefits outweigh risks, d/c citalopram and administer linezolid or IV methylene blue; monitor for serotonin syndrome for 2 weeks or until 24 hrs after the last dose of linezolid or IV methylene blue, whichever comes 1st. May resume citalopram therapy 24 hrs after the last dose of linezolid or IV methylene blue.

DOSING CONSIDERATIONS
Concomitant Medications
Cimetidine or Another CYP2C19 Inhibitor:
Max: 20mg/day

Hepatic Impairment
Max: 20mg/day

Elderly
>60 Years:
Max: 20mg/day

Discontinuation
Gradually reduce dose to d/c; if intolerable symptoms occur following a decrease in dose or upon discontinuation of treatment, may consider resuming previously prescribed dose or continue decreasing dose at a more gradual rate

Other Important Considerations
CYP2C19 Poor Metabolizers:
Max: 20mg/day

ADMINISTRATION
Oral route
Administer qd, in am or pm, w/ or w/o food.

STORAGE
(Tab) 25°C (77°F); excursions permitted to 15-30°C (59-86°F). (Sol) 20-25°C (68-77°F); excursions permitted to 15-30°C (59-86°F).

HOW SUPPLIED
Sol: 10mg/5mL [240mL]; **Tab:** (Celexa) 10mg, 20mg*, 40mg* *scored

CONTRAINDICATIONS
Use of an MAOI for psychiatric disorders either concomitantly or w/in 14 days of stopping treatment. Treatment w/in 14 days of stopping an MAOI for psychiatric disorders. Starting treatment in a patient being treated w/ MAOIs (eg, linezolid, IV methylene blue). Concomitant use w/ pimozide. Hypersensitivity to citalopram or any of the inactive ingredients in the medication.

WARNINGS/PRECAUTIONS
Not approved for the treatment of bipolar depression. May cause dose-dependent QTc prolongation. Avoid in patients w/ congenital long QT syndrome, bradycardia, hypokalemia or hypomagnesemia, recent acute MI (AMI), or uncompensated HF; monitor ECG if therapy is needed. Correct hypokalemia and/or hypomagnesemia prior to initiation of therapy and monitor periodically. D/C therapy w/ persistent QTc measurements >500 msec. May precipitate mixed/manic episode in patients at risk for bipolar disorder; screen for risk for bipolar disorder prior to initiating treatment. Serotonin syndrome reported; d/c immediately and initiate supportive symptomatic treatment. Pupillary dilation that occurs following use may trigger an angle-closure attack in a patient w/ anatomically narrow angles who does not have a patent iridectomy. Adverse events reported upon discontinuation; gradually reduce dose. May increase risk of bleeding events. Hyponatremia may occur; caution in elderly and volume-depleted patients. Consider discontinuation in patients w/ symptomatic hyponatremia and institute appropriate medical intervention. Activation of mania/hypomania reported; caution w/ history of mania. Seizures reported; caution w/ history of seizure disorder. Caution w/ hepatic impairment, severe renal impairment, and in pregnancy (3rd trimester). May impair mental/physical abilities.

ADVERSE REACTIONS
N/V, dyspepsia, diarrhea, dry mouth, somnolence, insomnia, increased sweating, ejaculation disorder, fatigue, URTI, rhinitis, anxiety, anorexia, tremor, agitation.

DRUG INTERACTIONS
See Contraindications and Dosage. Avoid w/ alcohol and drugs that prolong the QTc interval (eg, Class 1A [eg, quinidine, procainamide] or Class III [eg, amiodarone, sotalol] antiarrhythmic medications, antipsychotic medications [eg, chlorpromazine, thioridazine], antibiotics [eg, gatifloxacin, moxifloxacin], pentamidine, levomethadyl acetate, methadone). Caution w/ other centrally acting drugs or TCAs (eg, imipramine). Risk of QT prolongation w/ CYP2C19 inhibitors (eg, cimetidine). May cause serotonin syndrome w/ other serotonergic drugs (eg, triptans, TCAs, fentanyl) and w/ drugs that impair metabolism of serotonin; d/c immediately if this occurs. Risk of bleeding may be increased w/ aspirin, NSAIDs, warfarin, and other drugs that affect coagulation. May increase PT w/ warfarin. Monitor lithium levels and adjust its dose appropriately. Rare reports of weakness, hyperreflexia, and incoordination w/ sumatriptan. Possible increased clearance w/ carbamazepine. May decrease

levels of ketoconazole. May increase levels of metoprolol. Increased risk of hyponatremia w/ diuretics.

PREGNANCY AND LACTATION
Pregnancy: Category C.
Lactation: Not for use in nursing.

MECHANISM OF ACTION
SSRI; presumed to be linked to potentiation of serotonergic activity in the CNS resulting from its inhibition of CNS neuronal reuptake of serotonin.

PHARMACOKINETICS
Absorption: Absolute bioavailability (80%). (40mg single-dose tab) T_{max}=4 hrs.
Distribution: Plasma protein binding (80%); V_d=12L/kg; found in breast milk.
Metabolism: Hepatic; N-demethylation via CYP3A4, 2C19; demethylcitalopram (DCT), didemethylcitalopram, citalopram-N-oxide, deaminated propionic acid derivative (metabolites) **Elimination:** (IV) Urine (10% unchanged, 5% DCT); $T_{1/2}$=35 hrs.

PATIENT CONSIDERATIONS
Assessment: Assess for drug hypersensitivity, risk for bipolar disorder, history of mania, history of seizures, susceptibility to angle-closure glaucoma, volume depletion, congenital long QT syndrome, hypokalemia, hypomagnesemia, bradycardia, recent AMI, uncompensated HF, hepatic/renal impairment, pregnancy/nursing status, and possible drug interactions. Obtain baseline serum K^+ and Mg^{2+} measurements for patients being considered for therapy who are at risk for significant electrolyte disturbances.

Monitoring: Monitor for signs/symptoms of clinical worsening, suicidality, unusual changes in behavior, serotonin syndrome, bleeding events, hyponatremia, seizures, angle-closure glaucoma, activation of mania/hypomania, discontinuation symptoms, and other adverse reactions. Monitor electrolytes in patients w/ diseases or conditions that cause hypokalemia or hypomagnesemia. Monitor ECG in patients w/ cardiac conditions/disorders and in patients on concomitant QTc interval prolonging agents. Periodically reevaluate long-term usefulness.

Counseling: Inform about risks, benefits, and appropriate use of therapy. Caution about operating hazardous machinery, including automobiles, until reasonably certain that therapy does not affect ability to engage in such activities. Inform about serotonin syndrome and bleeding risks. Caution about risk of angle-closure glaucoma. Instruct to avoid alcohol. Advise to notify physician if taking or planning to take any prescription or OTC drugs. Instruct to notify physician if pregnant, intending to become pregnant, or breastfeeding. Encourage to be alert to unusual changes in behavior, worsening of depression, and suicidal ideation, especially early during treatment and when dose is adjusted up/down; instruct to report such symptoms, especially if severe, abrupt in onset, or not part of presenting symptoms.

CitraNatal 90 DHA — calcium citrate/cupric oxide/docosahexaenoic acid (DHA)/docusate sodium/eicosapentaenoic acid (EPA)/ferrous gluconate/iron carbonyl/potassium iodide/vitamin B1 (thiamine)/vitamin B2 (riboflavin)/vitamin B3 (niacinamide)/vitamin B6 (pyridoxine)/vitamin B9 (folic acid)/vitamin C (ascorbic acid)/vitamin D3 (cholecalciferol)/vitamin E (dl-alpha tocopheryl acetate)/zinc oxide   **Rx**

Class: Prenatal vitamin

> Accidental overdose of iron-containing products is a leading cause of fatal poisoning in children <6 yrs of age. Keep out of reach of children. In case of accidental overdose, call a doctor or poison control center immediately.

OTHER BRAND NAMES
CitraNatal Assure, CitraNatal DHA

ADULT DOSAGE	PEDIATRIC DOSAGE
Dietary/Nutritional Supplement	Pediatric use may not have been established
For use prior to conception, throughout pregnancy, and during postnatal period (lactating and nonlactating mothers)	
1 tab and 1 cap qd or ud	

ADMINISTRATION
Oral route

STORAGE
20-25°C (68-77°F). Contact with moisture can discolor or erode tab. (DHA) 20-25°C (68-77°F); excursions permitted between 15-30°C (59-86°F). Brief exposure to temperatures up to 40°C (104°F) may be tolerated provided the mean kinetic temperature does not exceed 25°C (77°F); however, such exposure should be minimized.

HOW SUPPLIED
(90 DHA) Cap: Docosahexaenoic acid (DHA) 300mg-Eicosapentaenoic acid (EPA) ≤0.75mg; **Tab:** Ascorbic acid 120mg-Calcium 159mg-Iron 90mg-Cholecalciferol 400 IU-Vitamin E 30 IU-Thiamin 3mg-Riboflavin 3.4mg-Niacinamide 20mg-Pyridoxine 20mg-Folic acid 1mg-Potassium iodide 150mcg-Zinc 25mg-Cupric oxide 2mg-Docusate 50mg*. **(Assure) Cap:** DHA 300mg-EPA ≤0.75mg; **Tab:** Ascorbic acid 120mg-Calcium 124mg-Iron 35mg-Cholecalciferol

400 IU-Vitamin E 30 IU-Thiamin 3mg-Riboflavin 3.4mg-Niacinamide 20mg-Pyridoxine 25mg-Folic acid 1mg-Potassium iodide 150mcg-Zinc 25mg-Cupric oxide 2mg-Docusate 50mg. **(DHA) Cap:** DHA 250mg-EPA ≤0.625mg; **Tab:** Ascorbic acid 120mg-Calcium 124mg-Iron 27mg-Cholecalciferol 400 IU-Vitamin E 30 IU-Thiamin 3mg-Riboflavin 3.4mg-Niacinamide 20mg-Pyridoxine 20mg-Folic acid 1mg-Potassium iodide 150mcg-Zinc 25mg-Cupric oxide 2mg-Docusate 50mg* *scored

CONTRAINDICATIONS
Known hypersensitivity to any of the ingredients in this product.

WARNINGS/PRECAUTIONS
Ingestion of >3g/day of omega-3 fatty acids has been shown to have potential antithrombotic effects, including an increased bleeding time and INR; avoid in patients with an inherited or acquired bleeding diathesis. Folic acid alone is improper therapy in the treatment of pernicious anemia and other megaloblastic anemias where vitamin B12 is deficient. Folic acid in doses >0.1mg/day may obscure pernicious anemia; hematologic remission may occur while neurological manifestations progress.

ADVERSE REACTIONS
Allergic sensitization.

DRUG INTERACTIONS
Avoid administration of omega-3 fatty acids in patients on anticoagulants.

MECHANISM OF ACTION
Prenatal and postnatal vitamin/minerals.

PATIENT CONSIDERATIONS
Assessment: Assess for inherited or acquired bleeding diathesis, pernicious anemia and other megaloblastic anemias, hypersensitivity to drug, and possible drug interactions.

Monitoring: Monitor for antithrombotic effects, allergic sensitization, and masking of pernicious anemia.

Counseling: Instruct to take ud. Advise to immediately call a doctor or poison control center in case of accidental overdose.

CITRANATAL HARMONY — calcium citrate/docosahexaenoic acid (DHA)/docusate sodium/ferrous fumarate/iron carbonyl/vitamin B6 (pyridoxine hydrochloride)/vitamin B9 (folic acid)/vitamin D3 (cholecalciferol)/vitamin E (dl-alpha tocopheryl acetate) **Rx**

Class: Prenatal vitamin

> Accidental overdose of iron-containing products is a leading cause of fatal poisoning in children <6 yrs of age. Keep out of reach of children. In case of accidental overdose, call a doctor or poison control center immediately.

ADULT DOSAGE	PEDIATRIC DOSAGE
Dietary/Nutritional Supplement	Pediatric use may not have been established
For use prior to conception, throughout pregnancy, and during postnatal period (lactating and nonlactating mothers)	
1 cap qd or ud	

ADMINISTRATION
Oral route

STORAGE
Controlled room temperature. Contact with moisture can discolor or erode the cap.

HOW SUPPLIED
Cap: Calcium 104mg-Iron 27mg-Cholecalciferol 400 IU-Vitamin E 30 IU-Pyridoxine 25mg-Folic acid 1mg-Docusate 50mg-Docosahexaenoic acid (DHA) 260mg

CONTRAINDICATIONS
Known hypersensitivity to any of the ingredients in this product.

WARNINGS/PRECAUTIONS
Ingestion of >3g/day of omega-3 fatty acids has been shown to have potential antithrombotic effects, including an increased bleeding time and INR; avoid in patients with an inherited or acquired bleeding diathesis. Folic acid alone is improper therapy in the treatment of pernicious anemia and other megaloblastic anemias where vitamin B12 is deficient. Folic acid in doses >0.1mg/day may obscure pernicious anemia; hematologic remission may occur while neurological manifestations progress. Exercise caution to ensure that the prescribed DHA dosage does not exceed 1000mg/day.

ADVERSE REACTIONS
Allergic sensitization.

DRUG INTERACTIONS
Avoid administration of omega-3 fatty acids in patients on anticoagulants.

MECHANISM OF ACTION
Prenatal and postnatal vitamins/minerals.

PATIENT CONSIDERATIONS
Assessment: Assess for inherited or acquired bleeding diathesis, pernicious anemia and other megaloblastic anemias, hypersensitivity to drug, and possible drug interactions.

MONITORING / COUNSELING (right column top)
Monitoring: Monitor for antithrombotic effects, allergic sensitization, and masking of pernicious anemia.

Counseling: Instruct to take ud. Advise to immediately call a doctor or poison control center in case of accidental overdose.

CLARINEX-D — desloratadine/pseudoephedrine sulfate **Rx**

Class: H₁ antagonist/sympathomimetic amine

ADULT DOSAGE	PEDIATRIC DOSAGE
Seasonal Allergic Rhinitis	**Seasonal Allergic Rhinitis**
Relief of Nasal and Non-Nasal Symptoms, Including Nasal Congestion:	**Relief of Nasal and Non-Nasal Symptoms, Including Nasal Congestion:**
12 Hour:	**≥12 Years:**
Usual/Max: 1 tab bid, approx 12 hrs apart	**12 Hour:**
24 Hour:	**Usual/Max:** 1 tab bid, approx 12 hrs apart
Usual/Max: 1 tab qd	**24 Hour:**
	Usual/Max: 1 tab qd

ADMINISTRATION
Oral route
Take w/ or w/o a meal
Swallow tab whole; do not break, chew, or crush

STORAGE
25°C (77°F); excursions permitted to 15-30°C (59-86°F). Heat sensitive; avoid exposure at or >30°C (86°F). Protect from excessive moisture and light.

HOW SUPPLIED
Tab, Extended-Release: (Desloratadine/Pseudoephedrine) (12 Hour) 2.5mg/120mg, (24 Hour) 5mg/240mg

CONTRAINDICATIONS
Narrow-angle glaucoma, urinary retention, MAOI therapy or within 14 days of stopping an MAOI, severe HTN, or severe coronary artery disease (CAD). Hypersensitivity to any of its ingredients, or to loratadine.

WARNINGS/PRECAUTIONS
Can produce cardiovascular (CV) and CNS effects (eg, insomnia, dizziness, weakness, tremor, arrhythmias). CNS stimulation with convulsions or CV collapse with hypotension reported. Caution with CV disorders, diabetes, hyperthyroidism, prostatic hypertrophy, or increased intraocular pressure (IOP). Hypersensitivity reactions (eg, rash, pruritus, urticaria, edema, dyspnea, anaphylaxis) reported; d/c and consider alternative treatment if this occurs. Avoid in patients with hepatic/renal impairment. Caution in elderly patients.

ADVERSE REACTIONS
Dry mouth, headache, insomnia, fatigue, pharyngitis, somnolence, dizziness.

DRUG INTERACTIONS
See Contraindications. May reduce the antihypertensive effects of β-adrenergic blocking agents, methyldopa, and reserpine; use caution with these agents. Increased ectopic pacemaker activity may occur with concomitant digitalis; use caution with these agents.

PREGNANCY AND LACTATION
Category C, not for use in nursing.

MECHANISM OF ACTION
Desloratadine: H₁-receptor antagonist; inhibits histamine release from human mast cells in vitro. Pseudoephedrine: Sympathomimetic amine; exerts a decongestant action on nasal mucosa.

PHARMACOKINETICS
Absorption: Desloratadine: (24 Hour) C_{max}=1.79ng/mL, T_{max}=6-7 hrs, AUC=61.1ng•hr/mL. (12 Hour) C_{max}=1.09ng/mL, T_{max}=4-5 hrs, AUC=31.6ng•hr/mL. Pseudoephedrine: (24 Hour) C_{max}=328ng/mL, T_{max}=8-9 hrs, AUC=6438ng•hr/mL. (12 Hour) C_{max}=263ng/mL, T_{max}=6-7 hrs, AUC=4588ng•hr/mL. **Distribution:** Desloratadine: Plasma protein binding (82-87%, 85-89% active metabolite); found in breast milk. Pseudoephedrine: Found in breast milk. **Metabolism:** Desloratadine: Extensive; 3-hydroxydesloratadine (active metabolite). Pseudoephedrine: Liver (incomplete), by N-demethylation. **Elimination:** Desloratadine: Urine and feces (87%); $T_{1/2}$=24 hrs (24 Hour), 27 hrs (12 Hour). Pseudoephedrine: Urine (55-96% unchanged); $T_{1/2}$=3-6 hrs (urinary pH=5), 9-16 hrs (urinary pH=8).

PATIENT CONSIDERATIONS
Assessment: Assess for drug hypersensitivity, increased IOP, prostatic hypertrophy, CV disorders, diabetes, hyperthyroidism, narrow-angle glaucoma, urinary retention, HTN, CAD, hepatic/renal impairment, pregnancy/nursing status, and possible drug interactions.

Monitoring: Monitor for CV/CNS effects, hypersensitivity reactions, and other adverse reactions. Monitor for urinary retention and narrow-angle glaucoma in patients with prostatic hypertrophy or increased IOP.

Counseling: Inform that CV or CNS effects may occur. Advise not to increase the dose or dosing frequency. Advise not to use with other antihistamines and/or decongestants. Advise not to use with an MAOI or within 14 days of stopping an MAOI. Advise patients with severe HTN or severe CAD, narrow-angle glaucoma, or urinary retention not to use this drug.

CLEOCIN — clindamycin

Rx

Class: Lincomycin derivative

Clostridium difficile-associated diarrhea (CDAD) reported and may range in severity from mild diarrhea to fatal colitis. Due to the association w/ severe colitis, which may be fatal, reserve use for serious infections where less toxic agents are inappropriate. Not for use w/ nonbacterial infections such as most URTIs. CDAD must be considered in all patients w/ diarrhea following antibiotic use. Careful medical history is necessary since CDAD has been reported to occur over 2 months after the administration of antibacterial agents. If CDAD is suspected or confirmed, ongoing antibiotic use not directed against *C. difficile* may need to be discontinued. Appropriate fluid and electrolyte management, protein supplementation, antibiotic treatment of *C. difficile*, and surgical evaluation should be instituted as clinically indicated.

OTHER BRAND NAMES
Cleocin Pediatric

ADULT DOSAGE
Serious Infections
Respiratory tract/skin and skin structure/intra-abdominal/ gynecological infections and septicemia; (Inj) bone and joint infections and adjunctive therapy in the surgical treatment of chronic bone and joint infections

Cap:
150-300mg PO q6h
More Severe: 300-450mg PO q6h

Inj:
Aerobic Gram-Positive Cocci and More Susceptible Anaerobes:
600-1200mg/day IV/IM given in 2, 3, or 4 equal doses
More Severe (Particularly Due to *Bacteroides fragilis*, *Peptococcus* species, or *Clostridium* species other than *Clostridium perfringens*):
1200-2700mg/day IV/IM given in 2, 3, or 4 equal doses
More Serious/Life-Threatening:
May have to increase dose; as much as 4800mg/day IV have been given

Single IM inj >600mg are not recommended

Alternative Administration:
Administer 1st dose as a single rapid infusion, followed by continuous IV infusion as follows:
To Maintain Serum Clindamycin Levels >4mcg/mL:
Rapid Infusion Rate: 10mg/min for 30 min
Maint Infusion Rate: 0.75mg/min

To Maintain Serum Clindamycin Levels >5mcg/mL:
Rapid Infusion Rate: 15mg/min for 30 min
Maint Infusion Rate: 1mg/min

To Maintain Serum Clindamycin Levels >6mcg/mL:
Rapid Infusion Rate: 20mg/min for 30 min
Maint Infusion Rate: 1.25mg/min

β-Hemolytic Streptococcal Infections:
Continue treatment for at least 10 days

ADMINISTRATION
Oral/IM/IV route

Cap
Take w/ full glass of water to avoid esophageal irritation.

Oral Sol
Reconstitute 100mL bottles w/ 75mL of water.
Do not refrigerate the reconstituted sol; stable at room temperature for 2 weeks.
Reconstitution Instructions:
1. Add a large portion of water and shake vigorously.
2. Add the remainder of the water and shake until sol is uniform.

Inj
IM administration should be used undiluted.
IV administration should be diluted.

Dilution for IV Use and IV Infusion Rates:
Concentration of clindamycin in diluent should not exceed 18mg/mL.
Infusion rates should not exceed 30mg/min.
300mg Dose: Dilute w/ 50mL; infuse over 10 min
600mg Dose: Dilute w/ 50mL; infuse over 20 min

PEDIATRIC DOSAGE
Serious Infections
Cap:
8-16mg/kg/day (4-8mg/lb/day) PO divided into 3 or 4 equal doses
More Severe: 16-20mg/kg/day (8-10mg/lb/day) PO divided into 3 or 4 equal doses

Oral Sol:
8-12mg/kg/day (4-6mg/lb/day) PO divided into 3 or 4 equal doses
Severe: 13-16mg/kg/day (6.5-8mg/lb/day) PO divided into 3 or 4 equal doses
More Severe: 17-25mg/kg/day (8.5-12.5mg/lb/day) PO divided into 3 or 4 equal doses
≤10kg:
Minimum Dose: 1/2 tsp (37.5mg) tid

Inj:
Neonates (<1 Month):
15-20mg/kg/day given in 3-4 equal doses; lower dosage may be adequate for small prematures

1 Month-16 Years:
20-40mg/kg/day IV/IM given in 3 or 4 equal doses; use higher dose for more severe infections
Alternative Dosing:
350mg/m^2/day for serious infections; 450mg/m^2/day for more severe infections

β-Hemolytic Streptococcal Infections:
Continue treatment for at least 10 days

900mg Dose: Dilute w/ 50-100mL; infuse over 30 min
1200mg Dose: Dilute w/ 100mL; infuse over 40 min
Administration of >1200mg in a single 1-hr infusion is not recommended.
Physical Incompatibilities:
- Ampicillin sodium
- Phenytoin sodium
- Barbiturates
- Aminophylline
- Calcium gluconate
- Magnesium sulfate

Do not add supplementary medication to Galaxy container.
Refer to PI for stability information of diluted sol and further directions for use.

STORAGE
20-25°C (68-77°F). **Inj:** (Galaxy Container) 25°C (77°F); avoid temperatures >30°C (86°F).

HOW SUPPLIED
Cap: (HCl) 75mg, 150mg, 300mg; **Inj:** (Phosphate) 150mg/mL [2mL, 4mL, 6mL vial]; 150mg/mL [2mL, 4mL, 6mL ADD-Vantage vial]; 300mg/50mL, 600mg/50mL, 900mg/50mL [Galaxy plastic container]; (Pediatric) **Oral Sol:** (Palmitate HCl) 75mg/5mL [100mL]

CONTRAINDICATIONS
History of hypersensitivity to preparations containing clindamycin or lincomycin.

WARNINGS/PRECAUTIONS
D/C use if significant diarrhea occurs during therapy. Reserve use for penicillin (PCN)-allergic patients or other patients for whom a PCN is inappropriate. Severe hypersensitivity reactions, including severe skin reactions (eg, toxic epidermal necrolysis, drug reaction w/ eosinophilia and systemic symptoms [DRESS], and Stevens-Johnson syndrome), reported; permanently d/c treatment in case of such an event. May increase bacterial resistance if used in the absence of a proven/strongly suspected bacterial infection or a prophylactic indication; take appropriate measures if superinfection develops. Not for treatment of meningitis. Caution w/ severe liver disease, history of GI disease (eg, colitis), and in atopic or elderly patients. Indicated surgical procedures should be performed in conjunction w/ antibiotic therapy. **Cap (75mg, 150mg):** Contains tartrazine, which may cause allergic-type reactions (eg, bronchial asthma); caution w/ aspirin hypersensitivity. **Inj:** Do not inject IV undiluted as bolus; infuse over at least 10-60 min. Contains benzyl alcohol; benzyl alcohol preservative has been associated w/ serious adverse events, including "gasping syndrome" and death in pediatric patients. Premature infants and low birth weight infants may be more likely to develop benzyl alcohol toxicity.

ADVERSE REACTIONS
Abdominal pain, pseudomembranous colitis, N/V, maculopapular skin rash, pruritus, vaginitis, jaundice, abnormal LFTs, transient neutropenia, eosinophilia, DRESS, azotemia, oliguria, polyarthritis.

DRUG INTERACTIONS
May enhance the action of neuromuscular blockers; use w/ caution. Antagonism reported between clindamycin and erythromycin; avoid concurrent use.

PREGNANCY AND LACTATION
Pregnancy: Category B. (Inj) Contains benzyl alcohol that can cross the placenta.
Lactation: Not for use in nursing. Reported to appear in breast milk.

MECHANISM OF ACTION
Lincomycin-derivative antibiotic; inhibits bacterial protein synthesis by binding to the 23S RNA of the 50S subunit of the ribosome.

PHARMACOKINETICS
Absorption: Cap (150mg): Rapid; virtually complete (90%). C_{max}=2.5mcg/mL, T_{max}=45 min. Inj: T_{max}=3 hrs (Adults, IM), 1 hr (Pediatric Patients, IM). Inj/Oral Sol: Administration of variable doses resulted in different parameters. **Distribution:** Wide; distributed in body fluids, tissues, and bones; found in breast milk. **Elimination:** Cap: Urine (10%), feces (3.6%); $T_{1/2}$=2.4 hrs. Inj: $T_{1/2}$=3 hrs (Adults), 2.5 hrs (Pediatric Patients). Oral Sol: $T_{1/2}$=2 hrs.

PATIENT CONSIDERATIONS
Assessment: Assess for history of hypersensitivity to drug or lincomycin, aspirin hypersensitivity, history of GI disease, presence of meningitis, atopy, and possible drug interactions. Assess hepatic function and pregnancy/nursing status. Obtain baseline culture and susceptibility tests.

Monitoring: Monitor for CDAD, superinfection, allergic reactions, severe skin reactions, and other adverse reactions. Monitor for changes in bowel frequency in older patients w/ severe illness. If available, consider culture and susceptibility information when modifying antibacterial therapy. If on prolonged therapy, perform periodic LFTs, renal function tests, and blood counts. Perform periodic liver enzyme determinations in patients w/ severe liver disease.

Counseling: Inform about potential benefits/risks of therapy. Inform that therapy only treats bacterial, not viral, infections. Instruct to take exactly ud and inform that skipping doses or not completing full course may decrease effectiveness and increase likelihood of bacterial resistance. Instruct to contact physician if an allergic reaction develops. Inform that diarrhea is a common problem; instruct to contact physician if watery and bloody stools (w/ or w/o stomach cramps and fever) occur, even as late as ≥2 months after last dose of therapy. Advise to notify physician if pregnant/nursing.

CLEOCIN VAGINAL — clindamycin phosphate   Rx
Class: Lincomycin derivative

ADULT DOSAGE	PEDIATRIC DOSAGE
Bacterial Vaginosis	**Bacterial Vaginosis**
Cre:	**Postmenarchal:**
Nonpregnant and Pregnant Women During 2nd and 3rd Trimesters:	1 sup intravaginally qhs for 3 consecutive days
1 applicatorful (5g) intravaginally qhs for 3 or 7 consecutive days in nonpregnant patients and for 7 consecutive days in pregnant patients	
Sup:	
Nonpregnant:	
1 sup intravaginally qhs for 3 consecutive days	

ADMINISTRATION
Intravaginal route

Instructions for Use
Cre:
1. Remove cap from cre tube; screw a plastic applicator on the threaded end of the tube.
2. Rolling tube from the bottom, squeeze gently and force the medication into the applicator; applicator is filled when the plunger reaches its predetermined stopping point.
3. Unscrew the applicator from the tube and replace the cap.
4. Firmly grasp the applicator barrel and insert into vagina as far as possible w/o causing discomfort while lying on your back.
5. Slowly push the plunger until it stops.
6. Carefully withdraw applicator from vagina, and discard applicator.

Sup:
W/ Applicator:
1. Remove the ovule from its packaging.
2. Pull back the plunger about an inch and place the ovule in the wider end of the applicator barrel.
3. Gently insert the end of the applicator into the vagina as far as it will go comfortably while lying on back w/ knees bent, or while standing w/ feet apart and knees bent.
4. While holding the barrel of the applicator in place, push the plunger in until it stops to release the ovule.
5. Remove the applicator from the vagina and lie down as soon as possible to minimize leakage.
6. Clean the applicator after each use; pull the 2 pieces apart and wash them w/ soap and warm water then rinse well and dry.

W/O Applicator:
1. Hold the ovule w/ thumb and a finger and insert it into the vagina.
2. Gently push the ovule into the vagina as far as it will comfortably go.
3. Lie down as soon as possible to minimize leakage.

STORAGE
Cre: 20-25°C (68-77°F). Protect from freezing. **Sup:** 25°C (77°F); excursions permitted to 15-30°C (59-86°F). Avoid heat >30°C (86°F). Avoid high humidity.

HOW SUPPLIED
Cre: 2% [40g]; **Sup:** (Ovules) 100mg [3ˢ]

CONTRAINDICATIONS
History of hypersensitivity to clindamycin, lincomycin, or any components of the medication. History of regional enteritis, ulcerative colitis, or a history of antibiotic-associated colitis.

WARNINGS/PRECAUTIONS
Diarrhea, bloody diarrhea, and colitis (including pseudomembranous colitis) reported w/ oral, parenteral, and topical formulations; consider this diagnosis in patients who present w/ diarrhea subsequent to clindamycin administration. May cause overgrowth of nonsusceptible organisms in the vagina. Use only during the 1st trimester of pregnancy if clearly needed. **Cre:** Burning and irritation of the eye may occur w/ accidental contact.

ADVERSE REACTIONS
Cre: Vulvovaginal disorder, vulvovaginitis, vaginal moniliasis.
Sup: Vulvovaginal disorder.

DRUG INTERACTIONS
Systemic clindamycin may enhance the action of neuromuscular blocking agents; use w/ caution.

PREGNANCY AND LACTATION
Pregnancy: Category B.
Lactation: Not for use in nursing.

MECHANISM OF ACTION
Lincomycin derivative; inhibits bacterial protein synthesis at the level of the bacterial ribosome. Binds preferentially to the 50S ribosomal subunit and affects the process of peptide chain initiation.

PHARMACOKINETICS
Absorption: (Cre) C_{max}=13ng/mL (Day 1), 16ng/mL (Day 7); T_{max}=14 hrs. (Sup) AUC=3.2mcg•hr/mL, C_{max}=0.27mcg/mL (Day 3), T_{max}=5 hrs. **Distribution:** (Oral/Parenteral) Found in breast milk. **Elimination:** (Cre) $T_{1/2}$=1.5-2.6 hrs. (Sup) $T_{1/2}$=11 hrs.

PATIENT CONSIDERATIONS
Assessment: Assess for clinical diagnosis of bacterial vaginosis, history of hypersensitivity to the drug or lincomycin, history of regional enteritis, ulcerative colitis, history of antibiotic-associated colitis, pregnancy/nursing status, and for possible drug interactions.

Monitoring: Monitor for signs/symptoms of diarrhea, colitis, overgrowth of nonsusceptible organisms, burning/irritation of the eye, and other adverse reactions.

Counseling: Instruct not to engage in vaginal intercourse, or use other vaginal products (eg, tampons, douches) during therapy. Inform that product contains mineral oil/oleaginous base that may weaken latex or rubber products (eg, condoms, vaginal contraceptive diaphragms); instruct not to use such products w/in 72 hrs following treatment. **Cre:** Instruct to rinse the eye w/ copious amounts of cool tap water if accidental contact w/ the eye occurs.

CLEVIPREX — clevidipine   Rx
Class: Calcium channel blocker (CCB) (dihydropyridine)

ADULT DOSAGE	PEDIATRIC DOSAGE
Hypertension	Pediatric use may not have been established
Oral Therapy Not Feasible/Desirable:	
Initial: 1-2mg/hr	
Titrate: May double the dose at 90-sec intervals initially; as BP approaches goal, increase in doses should be less than doubling and the time between dose adjustments should be lengthened to every 5-10 min	
Maint: 4-6mg/hr	
Max: 1000mL or 21mg/hr per 24 hrs	

DOSING CONSIDERATIONS
Elderly
Start at the lower end of dosing range

Discontinuation
Transition to PO Therapy:
D/C or titrate downward until PO therapy is established
Consider the lag time of onset of the PO agent's effect when PO antihypertensive is instituted
Continue BP monitoring until desired effect is reached

ADMINISTRATION
IV route

Compatible IV Sol
- Water for inj
- 0.9% NaCl inj
- Dextrose 5% inj
- Dextrose 5% in NaCl inj
- Dextrose 5% in Ringer's lactate inj
- Lactated Ringer's inj
- 10% amino acid

Administration Instructions
Use within 12 hrs once the stopper is punctured; discard any unused portion.
Invert vial gently several times before use.
Administer using an infusion device allowing calibrated infusion rates.
Commercially available standard plastic cannulae may be used to administer infusion.
Administer via central or peripheral line.
Should not be diluted.

STORAGE
2-8°C (36-46°F). Do not freeze. Leave vials in cartons until use; may be transferred to 25°C (77°F) for a period not to exceed 2 months. Do not return to refrigerated storage after beginning room temperature storage. Discard any unused portion within 12 hrs of stopper puncture.

HOW SUPPLIED
Inj: 0.5mg/mL [50mL, 100mL, 250mL]

CONTRAINDICATIONS
Allergies to soybeans, eggs, soy or egg products, severe aortic stenosis, defective lipid metabolism (eg, pathologic hyperlipemia, lipoid nephrosis, or acute pancreatitis if it is accompanied by hyperlipidemia).

WARNINGS/PRECAUTIONS
Systemic hypotension and reflex tachycardia may occur; decrease dose if either occurs. Lipid intake restrictions may be necessary with significant disorders of lipid metabolism; a reduction in the quantity of concurrently administered lipids may be necessary to compensate for the amount of lipid infused as part of the drug's formulation. May produce negative inotropic effects and exacerbation of heart failure (HF). Does not reduce HR and does not protect against the effects of abrupt β-blocker withdrawal. Monitor for the possibility of rebound HTN for at least 8 hrs after discontinuation of infusion in patients who receive prolonged infusions and are not transitioned to other antihypertensive therapies. Caution in elderly.

ADVERSE REACTIONS
Atrial fibrillation, acute renal failure, headache, N/V.

PREGNANCY AND LACTATION
Category C, safety not known in nursing.

MECHANISM OF ACTION
Calcium channel blocker (dihydropyridine); mediates the influx of Ca^{2+} during depolarization in arterial smooth muscle and reduces mean arterial BP by decreasing systemic vascular resistance; does not reduce cardiac filling pressure (preload).

PHARMACOKINETICS
Distribution: V_d=0.17L/kg; plasma protein binding (>99.5%). **Metabolism:** Hydrolysis of the ester linkage, glucuronidation or oxidation; carboxylic acid metabolite and formaldehyde (primary metabolites). **Elimination:** Urine (63-74%), feces (7-22%); $T_{1/2}$=15 min.

PATIENT CONSIDERATIONS
Assessment: Assess for allergies to soybeans, eggs or soy/egg products, defective lipid metabolism, β-blocker usage, and pregnancy/nursing status. Obtain baseline parameters for BP, HR, and lipid profile.

Monitoring: Monitor for hypotension, reflex tachycardia, rebound HTN, HF exacerbation, and other adverse reactions. Monitor BP and HR during infusion, and until vital signs are stable.

Counseling: Advise patients with underlying HTN that they require continued follow up for their medical condition, and, if applicable, to continue taking oral antihypertensive medication(s) ud. Instruct to report any signs of new hypertensive emergency (eg, neurological symptoms, visual changes, evidence of congestive HF) to a healthcare provider immediately.

CLIMARA PRO — estradiol/levonorgestrel　　　　Rx
Class: Estrogen/progestogen combination

> **Estrogen Plus Progestin Therapy:** Should not be used for the prevention of cardiovascular disease (CVD) or dementia. Increased risk of deep vein thrombosis (DVT), pulmonary embolism (PE), stroke, and MI in postmenopausal women (50-79 yrs of age) reported. Increased risk of developing probable dementia in postmenopausal women ≥65 yrs of age reported. Increased risk of invasive breast cancer reported. Estrogens w/ or w/o progestins should be prescribed at the lowest effective dose and for the shortest duration consistent w/ treatment goals and risks. **Estrogen-Alone Therapy:** Increased risk of endometrial cancer in women w/ a uterus who uses unopposed estrogens. Adding a progestin to estrogen therapy has been shown to reduce the risk of endometrial hyperplasia. Perform adequate diagnostic measures, including directed or random endometrial sampling when indicated, to rule out malignancy in postmenopausal women w/ undiagnosed persistent or recurring abnormal genital bleeding. Should not be used for the prevention of CVD or dementia. Increased risks of stroke and DVT in postmenopausal women (50-79 yrs of age) reported. Increased risk of developing probable dementia in postmenopausal women ≥65 yrs of age reported.

ADULT DOSAGE

Menopausal Vasomotor Symptoms

1 patch applied to the skin once weekly

May start therapy at any time in women not currently using continuous estrogen-alone therapy or estrogen plus progestin therapy

Women currently using continuous estrogen-alone therapy or estrogen plus progestin therapy should complete current cycle of therapy before initiating estradiol-levonorgestrel therapy

Attempts to d/c therapy should be made at 3- to 6-month intervals

Postmenopausal Osteoporosis

1 patch applied to the skin once weekly

May start therapy at any time in women not currently using continuous estrogen-alone therapy or estrogen plus progestin therapy

Women currently using continuous estrogen-alone therapy or estrogen plus progestin therapy should complete current cycle of therapy before initiating estradiol-levonorgestrel therapy

PEDIATRIC DOSAGE
Pediatric use may not have been established

ADMINISTRATION
Transdermal route

Site Selection
Adhesive side of patch should be placed on a smooth (fold free), clean, dry area of the skin on the lower abdomen or upper quadrant of the buttock.
Application area should not be oily, damaged, or irritated.
Avoid the waistline and do not apply on or near the breasts.
Rotate application sites w/ an interval of at least 1 week between application to the same site.

Application
Apply immediately upon removal from the protective pouch.
Press patch firmly in place w/ fingers for at least 10 sec.

If the patch falls off, apply the same patch to another area of the lower abdomen. If the patch cannot be reapplied, a new patch may be applied w/ the original treatment schedule.
Do not expose treatment area to sun for prolonged periods.

Removal
Removal should be done carefully and slowly to avoid irritation.
If adhesive remains on skin after removal, allow area to dry for 15 min.
Gently rub area w/ and oil-based cre or lot to remove residue.
Fold each used patch in 1/2 so it sticks to itself before disposing.

STORAGE
20-25°C (68-77°F); excursions permitted to 15-30°C (59-86°F). Do not store unpouched.

HOW SUPPLIED
Patch: (Estradiol/Levonorgestrel) (0.045mg/0.015mg)/day [4^s]

CONTRAINDICATIONS
Undiagnosed abnormal genital bleeding, known/suspected/history of breast cancer, known/suspected estrogen-dependent neoplasia, active/history of DVT/PE, active/history of arterial thromboembolic disease (eg, stroke, MI), known anaphylactic reaction or angioedema w/ this medication, known liver impairment or disease, known protein C/protein S/antithrombin deficiency or other known thrombophilic disorders, known/suspected pregnancy.

WARNINGS/PRECAUTIONS
D/C immediately if PE, DVT, stroke, or MI occurs or is suspected. If feasible, d/c at least 4-6 weeks before surgery of the type associated w/ an increased risk of thromboembolism, or during periods of prolonged immobilization. May increase risk of ovarian cancer. May cause fluid retention. May affect certain endocrine and blood components in lab tests. **Estrogen:** May increase risk of gallbladder disease requiring surgery. May lead to severe hypercalcemia in patients w/ breast cancer and bone metastases; d/c and take appropriate measures if hypercalcemia occurs. Retinal vascular thrombosis reported; d/c therapy pending exam if sudden partial/complete loss of vision, or sudden onset of proptosis, diplopia, or migraine occurs. D/C estrogens permanently if exam reveals papilledema or retinal vascular lesions. May elevate BP and thyroid-binding globulin levels. May elevate plasma TGs leading to pancreatitis in patients w/ preexisting hypertriglyceridemia; consider discontinuation if pancreatitis occurs. Caution w/ history of cholestatic jaundice associated w/ past estrogen use or w/ pregnancy; d/c in case of recurrence. Caution w/ hypoparathyroidism; hypocalcemia may occur. Cases of malignant transformation of residual endometrial implants reported in women treated post-hysterectomy w/ estrogen-alone therapy; consider addition of progestin to estrogen-alone therapy for women w/ residual endometriosis post-hysterectomy. May exacerbate symptoms of angioedema in women w/ hereditary angioedema. May exacerbate asthma, diabetes mellitus, epilepsy, migraine, porphyria, systemic lupus erythematosus, and hepatic hemangiomas. Conventional transdermal doses used in patients w/ normal renal function may be excessive for women w/ ESRD receiving maintenance hemodialysis.

ADVERSE REACTIONS
Application-site reaction, vaginal bleeding, breast pain, URTI, back pain, pain, headache, depression, arthralgia, flu syndrome, abdominal pain, flatulence, edema, bronchitis, sinusitis.

DRUG INTERACTIONS
Estradiol: CYP3A4 inducers (eg, St. John's wort preparations, carbamazepine, rifampin) may decrease levels, which may decrease therapeutic effects and/or change uterine bleeding profile. CYP3A4 inhibitors (eg, erythromycin, ketoconazole, ritonavir) may increase levels, which may result in side effects. Patients concomitantly receiving thyroid hormone replacement therapy and estrogens may require increased doses of their thyroid replacement therapy; monitor thyroid function. **Levonorgestrel:** Inducers or inhibitors of CYP3A, CYP2E, and CYP2C may either, respectively, decrease the therapeutic effects or result in side effects.

PREGNANCY AND LACTATION
Contraindicated in pregnancy, not for use in nursing.

MECHANISM OF ACTION
Estradiol: Estrogen; binds to nuclear receptors in estrogen-responsive tissues. Circulating estrogens modulate pituitary secretion of gonadotropins, luteinizing hormone and follicle-stimulating hormone, through (-) feedback mechanism. Reduces elevated levels of these hormones seen in postmenopausal women. **Levonorgestrel:** Progestogen; inhibits gonadotropin production resulting in retardation of follicular growth and inhibition of ovulation. Counteracts the proliferative effects of estrogens on the endometrium.

PHARMACOKINETICS
Absorption: Transdermal administration following single and multiple application resulted in different parameters. **Distribution:** Found in breast milk. Estradiol: Largely bound to sex hormone-binding globulin (SHBG) and albumin. Levonorgestrel: Bound to SHBG and albumin. **Metabolism:** Estradiol: Liver to estrone (metabolite), estriol (major urinary metabolite); sulfate and glucuronide conjugation (liver); biliary secretion of conjugates into the intestine, hydrolysis (intestine), reabsorption; CYP3A4 (partial metabolism). Levonorgestrel: Reduction, hydroxylation, conjugation. **Elimination:** Estradiol: Urine; $T_{1/2}$=3 hrs. Levonorgestrel: Urine; $T_{1/2}$=28 hrs.

PATIENT CONSIDERATIONS
Assessment: Assess for undiagnosed abnormal genital bleeding, presence/history of breast cancer, estrogen-dependent neoplasia, active/history of DVT/PE/arterial thromboembolic disease, liver impairment/disease, history of cholestatic jaundice associated w/ past estrogen use or w/ pregnancy, drug hypersensitivity, pregnancy/nursing status, any other conditions where treatment may be contraindicated or cautioned, and possible drug interactions.

Monitoring: Monitor for signs/symptoms of CVD, malignant neoplasms, dementia, gallbladder disease, hypercalcemia, visual abnormalities, BP and plasma TG elevations, pancreatitis, cholestatic jaundice, hypothyroidism, fluid retention, and other adverse reactions. Perform annual breast exam; schedule mammography based on age, risk factors, and prior mammogram results. Perform adequate diagnostic measures (eg, endometrial sampling) in patients w/ undiagnosed persistent or recurring genital bleeding. Periodically reevaluate to determine if treatment is still necessary. Regularly monitor thyroid function if on thyroid hormone replacement therapy.

Counseling: Inform of the importance of reporting abnormal vaginal bleeding to physician as soon as possible. Inform of possible serious reactions of therapy including CV disorders, malignant neoplasms, and probable dementia. Inform of the possible less serious but common adverse reactions (eg, headache, breast pain and tenderness, N/V).

CLINDAGEL — clindamycin phosphate   Rx

Class: Lincomycin derivative

ADULT DOSAGE	PEDIATRIC DOSAGE
Acne Vulgaris	**Acne Vulgaris**
Apply thin film qd; cover entire affected area lightly	**≥12 Years:** Apply thin film qd; cover entire affected area lightly

ADMINISTRATION
Topical route

STORAGE
Controlled room temperature, 20-25°C (68-77°F); excursions permitted to 15-30°C (59-86°F). Keep container tightly closed, out of direct sunlight.

HOW SUPPLIED
Gel: 1% [40mL, 75mL]

CONTRAINDICATIONS
Hypersensitivity to clindamycin or lincomycin. History of regional enteritis, ulcerative colitis, or antibiotic-associated colitis.

WARNINGS/PRECAUTIONS
D/C if significant diarrhea occurs. Caution in atopic individuals.

ADVERSE REACTIONS
Peeling, pruritus, pseudomembranous colitis (rare).

DRUG INTERACTIONS
May potentiate neuromuscular blockers.

PREGNANCY AND LACTATION
Category B, not for use in nursing.

MECHANISM OF ACTION
Lincomycin derivative; inhibits bacteria protein synthesis at ribosomal level by binding to the 50S ribosomal subunit and affecting the process of peptide chain initiation.

PHARMACOKINETICS
Absorption: C_{max}=≤5.5ng/mL. **Distribution:** Orally and parenterally administered clindamycin appears in breast milk. **Elimination:** Urine (<0.4% of total dose).

PATIENT CONSIDERATIONS

Assessment: Assess for hypersensitivity to lincomycin, history of regional or ulcerative colitis, antibiotic-associated colitis, nursing status. Assess use in atopic individuals and for possible drug interactions.

Monitoring: Monitor for signs/symptoms of colitis (pseudomembranous colitis), diarrhea, and bloody diarrhea. In patients with diarrhea, consider stool culture for *Clostridium difficile* and stool assay for *C. difficile* toxin. In patients with significant diarrhea, consider large bowel endoscopy.

Counseling: Instruct to notify physician of significant diarrhea during therapy or up to several weeks following end of therapy.

CLOBETASOL — clobetasol propionate   Rx

Class: Corticosteroid

ADULT DOSAGE	PEDIATRIC DOSAGE
Inflammatory and Pruritic Manifestations of Corticosteroid-Responsive Dermatoses	**Inflammatory and Pruritic Manifestations of Corticosteroid-Responsive Dermatoses**
Cre/Gel/Oint: Apply a thin layer to affected skin areas bid and rub in gently and completely	**≥12 Years:** **Cre/Gel/Oint:** Apply a thin layer to affected skin areas bid and rub in gently and completely
Max: 50g/week; limit treatment to 2 consecutive weeks	**Max:** 50g/week; limit treatment to 2 consecutive weeks
D/C therapy when control is achieved; reassess diagnosis if no improvement is seen w/in 2 weeks	D/C therapy when control is achieved; reassess diagnosis if no improvement is seen w/in 2 weeks
Moderate to Severe Dermatoses of the Scalp: **Sol:** Apply to affected scalp areas bid (am and pm)	**Moderate to Severe Dermatoses of the Scalp:** **Sol:** Apply to affected scalp areas bid (am and pm)
Max: 50mL/week; limit treatment to 2 consecutive weeks	**Max:** 50mL/week; limit treatment to 2 consecutive weeks

ADMINISTRATION
Topical route
Avoid use w/ occlusive dressings

STORAGE
(Cre/Gel/Oint) 15-30°C (59-86°F). Do not refrigerate. (Sol) 20-25°C (68-77°F); excursions permitted to 15-30°C (59-86°F). Do not refrigerate or use near an open flame.

HOW SUPPLIED
Cre/Oint: 0.05% [15g, 30g, 45g, 60g]; **Gel:** 0.05% [15g, 30g, 60g]; **Sol:** 0.05% [50mL]

CONTRAINDICATIONS
History of hypersensitivity to any of the components of the preparations. (Sol) Primary infections of the scalp.

WARNINGS/PRECAUTIONS
Systemic absorption may produce reversible hypothalamic-pituitary-adrenal (HPA) axis suppression, manifestations of Cushing's syndrome, hyperglycemia, and glucosuria. Application of more potent corticosteroids, use over large surface areas, prolonged use, and the addition of occlusive dressings may augment systemic absorption. Evaluate periodically for evidence of HPA axis suppression when large dose is applied to large surface area or under occlusive dressings; if noted, withdraw treatment, reduce frequency of application, or substitute w/ a less potent steroid. Infrequently, signs/symptoms of steroid withdrawal may occur, requiring supplemental systemic corticosteroids. Pediatric patients may be more susceptible to systemic toxicity. D/C and institute appropriate therapy if irritation develops. Use appropriate antifungal or antibacterial agent if concomitant skin infections are present or develop; if favorable response does not occur promptly, d/c until infection is controlled. Not for use in rosacea and perioral dermatitis. Caution in elderly. (Cre/Gel/Oint) Allergic contact dermatitis may occur; confirm by patch testing. Do not use on the face, groin, or axillae. (Sol) Certain areas of the body (eg, face, groin, axillae) are more prone to atrophic changes than other areas of the body following therapy; monitor frequently if these areas are to be treated. Should not be used for acne treatment or as sole therapy in widespread plaque psoriasis. May cause eye irritation if sol contacts the eye; flush eye w/ a large volume of water immediately.

ADVERSE REACTIONS
Burning/stinging sensation, irritation, itching, folliculitis. (Sol) Scalp pustules, tingling.

PREGNANCY AND LACTATION
Category C, caution in nursing.

MECHANISM OF ACTION
Corticosteroid; possesses anti-inflammatory, antipruritic, and vasoconstrictive actions. Anti-inflammatory mechanism not established. Thought to act by induction of phospholipase A_2 inhibitory proteins, collectively called lipocortins, which control the biosynthesis of potent mediators of inflammation (eg, prostaglandins, leukotrienes) by inhibiting the release of arachidonic acid.

PHARMACOKINETICS
Absorption: Percutaneous; extent of absorption is determined by many factors (eg, vehicle, integrity of epidermal barrier, use of occlusive dressings). **Distribution:** Bound to plasma proteins in varying degrees; found in breast milk (systemic administration). **Metabolism:** Liver. **Elimination:** Kidneys, bile.

PATIENT CONSIDERATIONS

Assessment: Assess for hypersensitivity to the drug, conditions that augment systemic absorption, concomitant skin infections, rosacea, perioral dermatitis, and pregnancy/nursing status. (Sol) Assess for primary infections of the scalp, acne, and widespread plaque psoriasis.

Monitoring: Monitor for signs/symptoms of HPA axis suppression, Cushing's syndrome, hyperglycemia, glucosuria, skin irritation, and other adverse reactions. Perform periodic monitoring of HPA axis suppression by using urinary free cortisol and adrenocorticotropic hormone stimulation tests.

Counseling: Instruct to use externally and ud, to avoid contact w/ eyes, and not to use for any disorder other than that for which it was prescribed. Counsel not to bandage, cover, or wrap treated skin area, unless directed by physician. Advise to report any signs of local adverse reactions to physician. (Cre/Gel/Oint) Instruct to inform physician of clobetasol use if contemplating surgery.

CLOLAR — clofarabine   Rx

Class: Antimetabolite

PEDIATRIC DOSAGE
Acute Lymphoblastic Leukemia
Treatment of relapsed or refractory acute lymphoblastic leukemia after at least 2 prior regimens
1-21 Years: 52mg/m² IV infusion over 2 hrs daily for 5 consecutive days
Repeat treatment cycles following recovery or return to baseline organ function, approx every 2-6 weeks
Consider prophylactic antiemetic medications and steroids

DOSING CONSIDERATIONS

Concomitant Medications

Drugs w/ Known Renal Toxicity: Minimize exposure to these during the 5 days of clofarabine administration

Drugs Known to Induce Hepatic Toxicity: Consider avoiding concomitant use

Renal Impairment

CrCl 30-60mL/min: Reduce dose by 50%

Adverse Reactions

Hypotension: D/C therapy if hypotension develops during the 5 days of administration

Hematologic Toxicity:
Administer subsequent cycles no sooner than 14 days from the starting day of the previous cycle and provided the patient's ANC is ≥0.75 x 10^9/L

Grade 4 Neutropenia (ANC <0.5 x 10^9/L) Lasting ≥4 Weeks: Reduce dose by 25% for the next cycle

Non-Hematologic Toxicity:

Clinically Significant Infection: Withhold until infection is controlled, then restart at full dose

Grade 3 Non-Infectious Toxicity (Excluding Transient Elevations in Serum Transaminases and/or Serum Bilirubin and/or N/V Controlled by Antiemetic Therapy): Withhold, then reinstitute at a 25% dose reduction when resolution or return to baseline

Grade 4 Non-Infectious Toxicity: D/C administration

Early Signs/Symptoms of Systemic Inflammatory Response Syndrome/Capillary Leak: D/C administration and provide appropriate supportive measures

≥Grade 3 Increase in Creatinine/Bilirubin: D/C administration, then reinstitute w/ a 25% dose reduction when patient is stable and organ function has returned to baseline. If hyperuricemia is anticipated (tumor lysis), initiate measures to control uric acid

ADMINISTRATION

IV route

Do not administer any other medications through the same IV line.

Provide supportive care (eg, IV fluids, antihyperuricemic treatment, alkalinization of urine) throughout the 5 days of clofarabine administration to reduce the effects of tumor lysis and other adverse events.

Preparation

1. Filter clofarabine through sterile 0.2 micron syringe filter.
2. Dilute w/ D5 inj or 0.9% NaCl inj prior to IV infusion to a final concentration between 0.15mg/mL and 0.4mg/mL.
3. Use w/in 24 hrs of preparation.

STORAGE

Undiluted: 25°C (77°F); excursions permitted to 15-30°C (59-86°F). **Diluted:** Room temperature; must be used w/in 24 hrs of preparation.

HOW SUPPLIED

Inj: 20mg/20mL

WARNINGS/PRECAUTIONS

Causes myelosuppression, which may be severe and prolonged. Serious and fatal hemorrhage, including cerebral, GI, and pulmonary hemorrhage, reported; majority of cases were associated w/ thrombocytopenia. Increases the risk of infection (eg, severe and fatal sepsis, opportunistic infections); monitor for signs/symptoms of infection, d/c therapy, and treat promptly. May result in tumor lysis syndrome; monitor and initiate preventive measures including adequate IV fluids and measures to control uric acid. May cause a cytokine release syndrome (eg, tachypnea, tachycardia, hypotension, pulmonary edema) that may progress to systemic inflammatory response syndrome (SIRS) w/ capillary leak syndrome and organ impairment, which may be fatal; d/c immediately and provide appropriate supportive measures. Consider prophylactic steroids to mitigate SIRS or capillary leak syndrome; consider use of diuretics and/or albumin. Patients who have previously received hematopoietic stem cell transplant may be at higher risk for veno-occlusive disease (VOD) of the liver following administration of therapy in combination w/ etoposide and cyclophosphamide; monitor and d/c therapy if suspected. Severe and fatal hepatotoxicity, including hepatitis and hepatic failure, reported; monitor hepatic function and for signs/symptoms of hepatitis and hepatic failure, and d/c therapy for ≥Grade 3 liver enzyme elevations and/or bilirubin elevations. Elevated creatinine, acute renal failure, and hematuria reported; monitor patients for renal toxicity and interrupt or d/c therapy as necessary. Fatal and serious cases of enterocolitis (eg, neutropenic colitis, cecitis, *Clostridium difficile* colitis) reported; monitor for signs/symptoms and treat promptly. Serious and fatal cases of Stevens-Johnson syndrome (SJS) and toxic epidermal necrolysis (TEN) reported; d/c for exfoliative or bullous rash, or if SJS or TEN is suspected. May cause fetal harm. Monitor cardiac function during administration and monitor patients taking medications known to affect BP. Moderately emetogenic; consider prophylactic antiemetic medications.

ADVERSE REACTIONS

N/V, diarrhea, febrile neutropenia, headache, rash, pruritus, pyrexia, fatigue, palmar-plantar erythrodysesthesia syndrome, anxiety, flushing, mucosal inflammation.

DRUG INTERACTIONS

Minimize exposure to drugs w/ known renal toxicity during the 5 days of therapy; risk of renal toxicity may be increased. Consider avoiding concomitant use of medications known to induce hepatic toxicity.

PREGNANCY AND LACTATION

Pregnancy: Category D. May cause fetal harm. Women of childbearing potential should avoid becoming pregnant while receiving treatment; all patients should use effective contraceptive measures to prevent pregnancy.

Lactation: Not for use in nursing.

MECHANISM OF ACTION

Antimetabolite; purine nucleoside metabolic inhibitor. Inhibits DNA synthesis by decreasing cellular deoxynucleotide triphosphate pools through an inhibitory action on ribonucleotide reductase, and by terminating DNA chain elongation and inhibiting repair through incorporation into DNA chain by competitive inhibition of DNA polymerases. Also disrupts the integrity of mitochondrial membrane, leading to release of the pro-apoptotic mitochondrial proteins, cytochrome C and apoptosis-inducing factor, leading to programmed cell death.

PHARMACOKINETICS

Distribution: V_d=172L/m^2; plasma protein binding (47%). **Metabolism:** 5'-triphosphate clofarabine (active metabolite). **Elimination:** Urine (49-60%, unchanged); $T_{1/2}$=5.2 hrs.

PATIENT CONSIDERATIONS

Assessment: Assess for renal impairment, pregnancy/nursing status, and possible drug interactions.

Monitoring: Monitor for signs and symptoms of infection, myelosuppression, hemorrhage, tumor lysis syndrome, cytokine release syndrome, SIRS, capillary leak syndrome, VOD, hepatotoxicity, enterocolitis, SJS, TEN, exfoliative or bullous rash, and other adverse reactions. Monitor CBCs, platelets and coagulation parameters, cardiac function, and renal/hepatic function.

Counseling: Advise to return for regular blood counts and to report any symptoms associated w/ hematological toxicity to physician. Inform to report to physician immediately if signs or symptoms of infection occur. Advise of the signs/symptoms of SIRS. Instruct to avoid medications, including OTC and herbal medications, that may be hepatotoxic or nephrotoxic, during the 5 days of treatment. Advise patients of the possibility of developing liver function abnormalities and to immediately report signs/symptoms of jaundice. Advise male and female patients w/ reproductive potential to use effective contraceptive measures to prevent pregnancy. Instruct female patients to avoid breastfeeding during treatment. Advise patients that N/V, diarrhea, or skin rash may be experienced, and to seek medical attention if these symptoms are significant.

CLOMID — clomiphene citrate   Rx

Class: Ovulatory stimulant

OTHER BRAND NAMES

Serophene

ADULT DOSAGE

Ovulatory Dysfunction

Initial: 50mg qd for 5 days
If progestin-induced bleeding is planned, or if spontaneous uterine bleeding occurs prior to therapy, start on 5th day of cycle; may start at any time if w/o recent uterine bleeding

Titrate: Increase to 100mg qd for 5 days only in patients who do not ovulate in response to cyclic 50mg after the 1st course of therapy; may start as early as 30 days after 1st course

Max: 100mg/day for 5 days
Long-term cyclic therapy beyond a total of 6 cycles is not recommended

If ovulation does not occur after 3 courses of therapy or if 3 ovulatory responses occur but pregnancy is not achieved, further treatment is not recommended

If menses does not occur after an ovulatory response, reevaluate patient

PEDIATRIC DOSAGE

Pediatric use may not have been established

DOSING CONSIDERATIONS

Other Important Considerations

Polycystic Ovary Syndrome (PCOS)/Unusual Pituitary Gonadotropin Sensitivity: Use lowest recommended dose and shortest treatment duration for the 1st course of therapy

ADMINISTRATION

Oral route

STORAGE

15-30°C (59-86°F). Protect from heat, light, and excessive humidity.

HOW SUPPLIED

Tab: 50mg* *scored

CONTRAINDICATIONS

Known hypersensitivity or allergy to clomiphene or to any of its components, pregnancy, liver disease or history of liver dysfunction, abnormal uterine bleeding of undetermined origin, ovarian cysts or enlargement not due to PCOS, uncontrolled thyroid or adrenal dysfunction or in the presence of an organic intracranial lesion (eg, pituitary tumor).

WARNINGS/PRECAUTIONS

Workup and treatment should be supervised by physician experienced in management of gynecologic or endocrine disorders. Visual symptoms (eg, blurring, spots, flashes), some occurring after discontinuation of therapy, reported; d/c treatment and perform complete ophthalmological evaluation promptly if visual symptoms develop. Visual disturbances may be irreversible, especially w/ increased dosage or duration of therapy. Ovarian hyperstimulation syndrome (OHSS), which may progress rapidly (w/in 24 hrs to several days) reported; monitor for abdominal pain/distention, N/V, diarrhea, weight gain, and for other warning signs. If conception results, rapid progression to severe form of the syndrome may occur. Use lowest effective dose consistent w/ expected clinical results to minimize the hazard of abnormal ovarian enlargement. If ovarian enlargement occurs, do not give additional therapy until the ovaries have returned to pretreatment size, and reduce the dosage or duration of the next course. Ovarian enlargement and cyst formation usually regresses spontaneously w/in a few days or weeks after discontinuing treatment; manage cystic enlargement conservatively unless surgical indication for laparotomy exists. Perform a thorough evaluation to rule out ovarian neoplasia if ovarian cysts do not regress spontaneously. Prolonged use may increase risk of borderline/invasive ovarian tumor. Perform pelvic exam prior to initiating therapy and before each subsequent course. Carefully evaluate to exclude pregnancy, ovarian enlargement, or ovarian cyst formation between each treatment cycle. Caution w/ uterine fibroids; potential for further enlargement.

ADVERSE REACTIONS
Ovarian enlargement, vasomotor flushes, abdominal-pelvic discomfort/distention/bloating.

PREGNANCY AND LACTATION
Category X, caution in nursing.

MECHANISM OF ACTION
Ovulatory stimulant; may compete w/ estrogen for estrogen-receptor-binding sites and may delay replenishment of intracellular estrogen receptors. Increases release of pituitary gonadotropins, thereby initiating steroidogenesis and folliculogenesis, resulting in ovarian follicle growth and increased circulating estradiol levels.

PHARMACOKINETICS
Absorption: Readily absorbed. **Elimination:** Feces (42%), urine (8%).

PATIENT CONSIDERATIONS
Assessment: Assess for hypersensitivity to drug, ovarian cysts/enlargement, abnormal vaginal/uterine bleeding, presence of organic intracranial lesion, primary pituitary/ovarian failure, endometriosis/endometrial carcinoma, liver disease or history of liver dysfunction, impediments to pregnancy (eg, thyroid/adrenal disorders, hyperprolactinemia, male factor infertility), uterine fibroids, preexisting or family history of hyperlipidemia, and pregnancy/nursing status. Perform pelvic exam prior to treatment. Assess estrogen levels.

Monitoring: Monitor for signs/symptoms of visual symptoms (eg, blurring, spots, flashes), OHSS, ovarian neoplasia, and other adverse reactions. Monitor plasma TG levels periodically in patients w/ preexisting or family history of hyperlipidemia. Exclude pregnancy, ovarian enlargement, or ovarian cyst formation between each treatment cycle. Perform pelvic exam before each subsequent course.

Counseling: Advise that blurring or other visual symptoms may occur during or shortly after therapy and inform that in some instances, visual disturbances may be prolonged, and possibly irreversible, especially w/ increased dosage or duration of therapy. Advise that visual symptoms may render such activities as driving a car or operating machinery more hazardous than usual, particularly under conditions of variable lighting. Instruct to inform physician whenever any unusual visual symptoms occur and to d/c therapy. Advise that ovarian enlargement may occur during or shortly after therapy; instruct to inform physician if any abdominal/pelvic pain, weight gain, discomfort, or distention occurs after taking therapy. Inform that preexisting or family history of hyperlipidemia and use of higher than recommended dose and/or longer duration of treatment may increase risk of hypertriglyceridemia. Inform of the increased chance of multiple pregnancy (eg, bilateral tubal pregnancy, coexisting tubal and intrauterine pregnancy), and the potential complications/hazards of multiple pregnancy.

Clonazepam — clonazepam   CIV

Class: Benzodiazepine

OTHER BRAND NAMES
Klonopin

ADULT DOSAGE

Seizures

Treatment of Lennox-Gastaut syndrome (petit mal variant), akinetic, and myoclonic seizures. May be useful in patients w/ absence seizures (petit mal) who have failed to respond to succinimides

Initial: Not to exceed 1.5mg/day divided into 3 doses
Titrate: May increase in increments of 0.5-1mg every 3 days until seizures are controlled or until side effects preclude any further increase
Maint: Individualize dose
Max: 20mg/day

Panic Disorder

Initial: 0.25mg bid
Titrate: May increase to target dose of 1mg/day after 3 days; for some, may increase in increments of

PEDIATRIC DOSAGE

Seizures

Treatment of Lennox-Gastaut syndrome (petit mal variant), akinetic, and myoclonic seizures. May be useful in patients w/ absence seizures (petit mal) who have failed to respond to succinimides

≤10 Years or ≤30kg:
Initial: 0.01-0.03mg/kg/day up to 0.05mg/kg/day given in 2 or 3 divided doses
Titrate: May increase by no more than 0.25-0.5mg every 3 days until daily maintenance dose is reached, unless seizures are controlled or until side effects preclude further increase
Maint: 0.1-0.2mg/kg/day divided into 3 doses. Whenever possible, divide daily dose into 3 equal doses; give the largest dose qhs if doses are not equally divided

0.125-0.25mg bid every 3 days until panic disorder is controlled or until side effects make further increases undesired
Max: 4mg/day

ADMINISTRATION
Oral route

To reduce somnolence, may give 1 dose at hs.

Tab, Disintegrating
Peel back foil on blister; do not push tab through foil.
Using dry hands, remove tab and place it in mouth.

Tab
Swallow whole w/ water.

STORAGE
(Tab, Disintegrating) 20-25°C (68-77°F). (Tab) 25°C (77°F); excursions permitted to 15-30°C (59-86°F).

HOW SUPPLIED
Tab, Disintegrating: 0.125mg, 0.25mg, 0.5mg, 1mg, 2mg; (Klonopin) **Tab:** 0.5mg*, 1mg, 2mg *scored

CONTRAINDICATIONS
History of sensitivity to benzodiazepines, significant liver disease, acute narrow angle glaucoma.

WARNINGS/PRECAUTIONS
May be used w/ treated open angle glaucoma. May impair mental/physical abilities. May increase risk of suicidal thoughts/behavior. Caution w/ use in pregnancy and women of childbearing potential; may increase risk of congenital malformations. Avoid use during the 1st trimester of pregnancy. May increase incidence or precipitate the onset of generalized tonic-clonic seizures in patients in whom several different types of seizure disorders coexist; addition of appropriate anticonvulsants or increase in their dosages may be required. Withdrawal symptoms reported after discontinuation. Abrupt withdrawal of therapy may precipitate status epilepticus; gradual withdrawal is essential, and simultaneous substitution of another anticonvulsant may be indicated while therapy is being gradually withdrawn. May produce an increase in salivation; caution w/ compromised respiratory function. Caution w/ renal impairment, addiction-prone individuals, and in elderly. May have porphyrogenic effect; caution w/ porphyria. (Tab, Disintegrating) Contains phenylalanine.

ADVERSE REACTIONS
CNS depression, ataxia, drowsiness, abnormal coordination, depression, somnolence, behavior problems, dizziness, URTI, memory disturbance, dysmenorrhea, fatigue, influenza, nervousness, sinusitis.

DRUG INTERACTIONS
CYP450 inducers (eg, phenytoin, carbamazepine, phenobarbital) and propantheline may decrease levels. Caution w/ CYP3A inhibitors (eg, oral antifungals). Alcohol, narcotics, barbiturates, nonbarbiturate hypnotics, antianxiety agents, phenothiazines, thioxanthene and butyrophenone antipsychotics, MAOIs, TCAs, other anticonvulsant drugs, and other CNS depressant drugs may potentiate CNS-depressant effects. May produce absence status w/ valproic acid.

PREGNANCY AND LACTATION
Pregnancy: Category D.
Lactation: Not for use in nursing.

MECHANISM OF ACTION
Benzodiazepine; has not been established. Suspected to be related to its ability to enhance activity of gamma-aminobutyric acid, the major inhibitory neurotransmitter in the CNS.

PHARMACOKINETICS
Absorption: Rapid and complete. Absolute bioavailability (90%); T_{max}=1-4 hrs.
Distribution: Plasma protein binding (85%). **Metabolism:** Liver via CYP450 (including CYP3A), acetylation, hydroxylation, and glucuronidation. **Elimination:** Urine (<2% unchanged); $T_{1/2}$=30-40 hrs.

PATIENT CONSIDERATIONS
Assessment: Assess for drug/benzodiazepine hypersensitivity, significant liver disease, acute narrow angle glaucoma, mental depression, history of drug or alcohol addiction, renal/hepatic impairment, chronic respiratory diseases, pregnancy/nursing status, and possible drug interactions.

Monitoring: Monitor for CNS depression, emergence or worsening of depression, suicidal thoughts/behavior, unusual changes in mood or behavior, worsening of seizures, withdrawal symptoms upon discontinuation, and other adverse reactions. Periodically monitor blood counts and LFTs during long-term therapy.

Counseling: Instruct to take only as prescribed. Inform that therapy may produce psychological and physical dependence; instruct to consult physician before either increasing the dose or abruptly discontinuing the drug. Caution about operating hazardous machinery, including automobiles. Counsel that drug may increase risk of suicidal thoughts and behavior; advise of the need to be alert for the emergence/worsening of symptoms of depression, any unusual changes in mood or behavior, or the emergence of suicidal thoughts, behavior, or thoughts of self-harm, and instruct to immediately report behaviors of concern to physician. Advise to notify physician if pregnancy occurs or is intended during therapy; encourage enrollment in the North American Antiepileptic Drug Pregnancy Registry. Advise not to breastfeed while on therapy. Advise to inform physician if taking, or planning to take, any prescription or OTC drugs and to avoid alcohol while on therapy. (Tab, Disintegrating) Inform that drug contains phenylalanine.

CLOZAPINE — clozapine   Rx

Class: Atypical antipsychotic

> Severe neutropenia, defined as an ANC <500/μL, reported; may lead to serious infection and death. Prior to initiating treatment, a baseline ANC must be ≥1500/μL for the general population, and ≥1000/μL for patients w/ documented benign ethnic neutropenia (BEN). Regularly monitor ANC during treatment. Available only through a restricted program under a Risk Evaluation Mitigation Strategy (REMS) called the Clozapine REMS program. Orthostatic hypotension, bradycardia, syncope, and cardiac arrest reported; risk is highest during the initial titration period, particularly w/ rapid dose escalation. Caution w/ cardiovascular (CV)/cerebrovascular disease or conditions predisposing to hypotension (eg, dehydration, use of antihypertensives). Seizures reported and risk is dose related; caution w/ history of seizures or other predisposing risk factors for seizure (eg, CNS pathology, medications that lower seizure threshold, alcohol abuse). Fatal myocarditis and cardiomyopathy reported; d/c and obtain cardiac evaluation upon suspicion of these reactions. Do not rechallenge patients w/ clozapine-related myocarditis or cardiomyopathy. Elderly patients w/ dementia-related psychosis treated w/ antipsychotic drugs are at an increased risk of death. Not approved for the treatment of dementia-related psychosis.

OTHER BRAND NAMES
Clozaril

ADULT DOSAGE

Schizophrenia
Treatment of severely ill patients w/ schizophrenia who fail to respond adequately to standard antipsychotic treatment. Reduction in risk of recurrent suicidal behavior in patients w/ schizophrenia or schizoaffective disorder who are judged to be at chronic risk for reexperiencing suicidal behavior

Initial: 12.5mg qd or bid
Titrate: May increase total daily dose in increments of 25-50mg/day, if well tolerated
Target Dose: 300-450mg/day (in divided doses) by the end of 2 weeks. Subsequently, may increase dose once weekly or twice weekly, in increments of up to 100mg
Max: 900mg/day

Patients responding to treatment should generally continue maint treatment on their effective dose beyond the acute episode

Reinitiation of Treatment:
When restarting in patients who have discontinued clozapine (≥2 days since last dose), reinitiate w/ 12.5mg qd or bid; if well tolerated, may increase to previous therapeutic dose more quickly than recommended for initial treatment

PEDIATRIC DOSAGE
Pediatric use may not have been established

DOSING CONSIDERATIONS
Concomitant Medications
Strong CYP1A2 Inhibitors:
During coadministration, use 1/3 of clozapine dose; when discontinuing comedication, increase clozapine dose based on clinical response

Moderate or Weak CYP1A2 Inhibitors:
During coadministration, monitor for adverse reactions and consider reducing clozapine dose if necessary; when discontinuing comedication, monitor for lack of effectiveness and consider increasing clozapine dose if necessary

CYP2D6 or CYP3A4 Inhibitors:
During coadministration, monitor for adverse reactions and consider reducing clozapine dose if necessary; when discontinuing comedication, monitor for lack of effectiveness and consider increasing clozapine dose if necessary

Strong CYP3A4 Inducers:
Concomitant use is not recommended; however, if the inducer is necessary, may need to increase clozapine dose and monitor for decreased effectiveness. When discontinuing comedication, reduce clozapine dose based on clinical response

Moderate or Weak CYP1A2 or CYP3A4 Inducers:
During coadministration, monitor for decreased effectiveness and consider increasing clozapine dose if necessary; when discontinuing comedication, monitor for adverse reactions and consider reducing clozapine dose if necessary

Renal Impairment
May need to reduce dose w/ significant renal impairment

Hepatic Impairment
May need to reduce dose w/ significant hepatic impairment

Discontinuation
Method of treatment discontinuation will vary depending on patient's last ANC:
1. If abrupt treatment discontinuation is necessary due to moderate-severe neutropenia, refer to PI for appropriate ANC monitoring based on the level of neutropenia
2. If termination of therapy is planned and there is no evidence of moderate-severe neutropenia, reduce dose gradually over 1-2 weeks

3. For abrupt discontinuation for a reason unrelated to neutropenia, continue existing ANC monitoring for general population patients until ANC is ≥1500/μL and for BEN patients until ANC is ≥1000/μL or above baseline
4. During the 2 weeks after discontinuation, additional ANC monitoring is required for any patient reporting onset of fever (temperature of ≥38.5°C [≥101.3°F])

Other Important Considerations
CYP2D6 Poor Metabolizers:
May need to reduce dose

ADMINISTRATION
Oral route

Administer in divided doses.
May be taken w/ or w/o food.

STORAGE
20-25°C (68-77°F). **Clozaril:** Should not exceed 30°C (86°F).

HOW SUPPLIED
Tab: 50mg*, 200mg*; (Clozaril) 25mg*, 100mg* *scored

CONTRAINDICATIONS
History of serious hypersensitivity to clozapine (eg, photosensitivity, vasculitis, erythema multiforme, or Stevens-Johnson syndrome) or any other component of the medication.

WARNINGS/PRECAUTIONS
Interrupt therapy as a precautionary measure in any patient who develops fever, defined as a temperature of ≥38.5°C (101.3°F), and obtain an ANC level; fever is often the 1st sign of neutropenic infection. In general, do not rechallenge patients who develop severe neutropenia w/ clozapine; for some patients, the risk of serious psychiatric illness from discontinuing treatment may be greater than the risk of rechallenge. Eosinophilia may occur and may be associated w/ myocarditis, pancreatitis, hepatitis, colitis, and nephritis. Evaluate promptly for signs/symptoms of systemic reactions if eosinophilia develops and d/c immediately if clozapine-related systemic disease is suspected. QT prolongation, torsades de pointes, and other life-threatening ventricular arrhythmias, cardiac arrest, and sudden death reported. D/C if QTc interval exceeds 500 msec or symptoms consistent w/ torsades de pointes or other arrhythmias develop. Caution in patients at risk for significant electrolyte disturbance, particularly hypokalemia; correct electrolyte abnormalities before initiating treatment. Associated w/ metabolic changes (eg, hyperglycemia sometimes associated w/ ketoacidosis or hyperosmolar coma, dyslipidemia, weight gain) that may increase CV and cerebrovascular risk. Neuroleptic malignant syndrome (NMS) reported; d/c therapy immediately and institute symptomatic treatment. Transient fever may occur and may necessitate discontinuing treatment; carefully evaluate patients to rule out severe neutropenia or infection, and consider the possibility of NMS. Pulmonary embolism (PE), deep vein thrombosis (DVT), and tardive dyskinesia (TD) reported; consider discontinuation if TD occurs. Has potent anticholinergic effects; may result in CNS and peripheral anticholinergic toxicity. Caution w/ narrow-angle glaucoma, prostatic hypertrophy, or other conditions in which anticholinergic effects can lead to significant adverse reactions. May result in GI adverse reactions (eg, constipation, intestinal obstruction, fecal impaction, paralytic ileus). May impair mental/physical abilities. Consider dose reduction if sedation, or impairment of cognitive/motor performance occurs. Caution in patients w/ risk factors for cerebrovascular adverse reactions. If abrupt discontinuation is necessary, monitor carefully for the recurrence of psychotic symptoms and adverse reactions related to cholinergic rebound (eg, profuse sweating, headache, N/V, diarrhea). Caution in elderly. Refer to PI for treatment recommendations based on ANC monitoring for the general patient population and for patients w/ BEN.

ADVERSE REACTIONS
CNS reactions (eg, sedation, dizziness/vertigo, headache, tremor), CV reactions (eg, tachycardia, hypotension, syncope), autonomic nervous system reactions (eg, hypersalivation, sweating, dry mouth, visual disturbances), GI reactions (eg, constipation, nausea), fever.

DRUG INTERACTIONS
See Boxed Warning and Dosing Considerations. Caution w/ drugs that are inducers or inhibitors of CYP1A2, CYP3A4, and CYP2D6. CYP1A2 inhibitors (eg, fluvoxamine, ciprofloxacin, oral contraceptives), CYP2D6 or CYP3A4 inhibitors (eg, cimetidine, escitalopram, erythromycin) may increase levels, potentially resulting in adverse reactions. CYP1A2 inducers (eg, tobacco) or CYP3A4 inducers (eg, carbamazepine, phenytoin, St. John's wort) may decrease levels, resulting in decreased effectiveness. Caution w/ medications that prolong the QT interval (eg, ziprasidone, erythromycin, quinidine) or inhibit the metabolism of clozapine. Use caution when coadministering w/ other drugs metabolized by CYP2D6 (eg, phenothiazines, carbamazepine, propafenone) and may be necessary to use lower doses of such drugs; concomitant use may increase levels these CYP2D6 substrates. Caution w/ anticholinergic medications. NMS reported w/ CNS-active medications, including lithium. If used concurrently w/ an agent known to cause neutropenia (eg, some chemotherapeutic agents), consider monitoring more closely than the treatment guidelines.

PREGNANCY AND LACTATION
Pregnancy: Category B.
Lactation: Clozapine is present in human milk. Not for use in nursing.

MECHANISM OF ACTION
Atypical antipsychotic; tricyclic dibenzodiazepine derivative. Has not been established. Efficacy proposed to be mediated through antagonism of the dopamine type 2 and the serotonin type 2A receptors. Also acts as an antagonist at adrenergic, cholinergic, histaminergic, and other dopaminergic and serotonergic receptors.

PHARMACOKINETICS

Absorption: (100mg bid) C_{max}=319ng/mL; T_{max}=2.5 hrs. **Distribution:** Plasma protein binding (97%); found in breast milk. **Metabolism:** CYP1A2, CYP2D6, CYP3A4; demethylation, hydroxylation, N-oxidation. Norclozapine (limited metabolite). **Elimination:** Urine (50%), feces (30%); $T_{1/2}$=8 hrs (75mg single dose), 12 hrs (100mg bid).

PATIENT CONSIDERATIONS

Assessment: Assess for hypersensitivity to drug, history of seizures or other predisposing factors for seizure, risk factors for QT prolongation and serious CV reactions, narrow-angle glaucoma, prostatic hypertrophy, renal/hepatic impairment, any other conditions where treatment is cautioned, pregnancy/nursing status, and possible drug interactions. Obtain baseline ANC, lipid evaluations, ECG, and serum chemistry panel (K^+ and Mg^{2+}). Obtain baseline FPG in patients w/ diabetes mellitus (DM) or at risk for DM.

Monitoring: Monitor for signs/symptoms of severe neutropenia, orthostatic hypotension, bradycardia, syncope, cardiac arrest, seizures, myocarditis, cardiomyopathy, cognitive/motor impairment, eosinophilia, NMS, recurrence of psychosis and cholinergic rebound after abrupt discontinuation, metabolic changes (hyperglycemia, DM, dyslipidemia, weight gain), QT interval prolongation, fever, PE, DVT, TD, cerebrovascular adverse reactions, and other adverse reactions. Monitor serum electrolyte levels, glucose control in patients w/ DM and periodic FPG levels if at risk for hyperglycemia. Monitor ANC regularly to continue treatment; refer to PI for monitoring frequency.

Counseling: Inform about benefits/risks of therapy. Advise about risk of developing severe neutropenia and infection. Instruct to immediately report any sign/symptom of infection occurring at any time during therapy. Inform that drug is available only through a restricted program called the Clozapine REMS Program designed to ensure the required blood monitoring; advise of the importance of having blood tested ud. Inform about risks of orthostatic hypotension and syncope, especially during the period of initial dose titration; instruct to strictly follow the instructions of the physician for dosage and administration. Advise to consult physician immediately if patients feel faint, lose consciousness, or have signs/symptoms suggestive of bradycardia or arrhythmia. Inform about significant risk of seizure during therapy; caution about driving and any other potentially hazardous activity while taking treatment. Instruct to inform physician if taking clozapine before any new drug. Educate about the risk of metabolic changes and the need for specific monitoring. If dose was missed for >2 days, instruct not to restart medication at same dose but to contact physician for dosing instructions. Advise to notify physician if taking/planning to take any prescription or OTC drugs. Instruct to notify physician if pregnant/intending to become pregnant during therapy. Advise not to breastfeed if taking the drug.

COAGADEX — coagulation factor X (human)   Rx

Class: Coagulation factor X (human)

ADULT DOSAGE
Hereditary Factor X Deficiency

Indicated for hereditary factor X deficiency for on-demand treatment and control of bleeding episodes, and for perioperative management of bleeding in patients w/ mild hereditary factor X deficiency

Dose and duration of the treatment depend on the severity of the Factor X deficiency, location and extent of the bleeding, and on the patient's clinical condition

Base dose and frequency on the individual clinical response; do not administer >60 IU/kg daily

Each vial of therapy is labeled w/ the actual Factor X potency/content in IU

Estimate the expected in vivo peak increase in Factor X level expressed as IU/dL (or % of normal) using the following formula:
Estimated Increment of Factor X (IU/dL or % of normal) = [Total Dose (IU)/Body Weight (kg)] x 2

Dose to achieve a desired in vivo peak increase in Factor X level may be calculated using the following formula:
Dose (IU) = Body Weight (kg) x Desired Factor X Rise (IU/dL) x 0.5

Desired Factor X rise is the difference between the patient's plasma Factor X level and the desired level. The dosing formula is based on the observed recovery of 2 IU/dL per IU/kg

PEDIATRIC DOSAGE
Hereditary Factor X Deficiency

Indicated for hereditary factor X deficiency for on-demand treatment and control of bleeding episodes, and for perioperative management of bleeding in patients w/ mild hereditary factor X deficiency

≥12 Years:

Dose and duration of the treatment depend on the severity of the Factor X deficiency, location and extent of the bleeding, and on the patient's clinical condition

Base dose and frequency on the individual clinical response; do not administer >60 IU/kg daily

Each vial of therapy is labeled w/ the actual Factor X potency/content in IU

Estimate the expected in vivo peak increase in Factor X level expressed as IU/dL (or % of normal) using the following formula:
Estimated Increment of Factor X (IU/dL or % of normal) = [Total Dose (IU)/Body Weight (kg)] x 2

Dose to achieve a desired in vivo peak increase in Factor X level may be calculated using the following formula:
Dose (IU) = Body Weight (kg) x Desired Factor X Rise (IU/dL) x 0.5

Desired Factor X rise is the difference between the patient's plasma Factor X level and the desired level. The dosing formula is based on the observed recovery of 2 IU/dL per IU/kg

On-Demand Treatment and Control of Bleeding Episodes:
Infuse 25 IU/kg when the first sign of bleeding occurs; repeat at intervals of 24 hrs until bleed stops

Perioperative Management of Bleeding:
To ensure that hemostatic levels are obtained and maintained, measure post-infusion plasma Factor X levels before and after surgery

Presurgery: Calculate the dose to raise plasma Factor X levels to 70-90 IU/dL using the following formula: Required dose (IU) = Body Weight (kg) x Desired Factor X Rise (IU/dL) x 0.5

Postsurgery: Repeat dose as necessary to maintain plasma Factor X levels at a minimum of 50 IU/dL until the patient is no longer at risk of bleeding due to surgery

On-Demand Treatment and Control of Bleeding Episodes:
Infuse 25 IU/kg when the first sign of bleeding occurs; repeat at intervals of 24 hrs until bleed stops

Perioperative Management of Bleeding:
To ensure that hemostatic levels are obtained and maintained, measure post-infusion plasma Factor X levels before and after surgery

Presurgery: Calculate the dose to raise plasma Factor X levels to 70-90 IU/dL using the following formula: Required dose (IU) = Body Weight (kg) x Desired Factor X Rise (IU/dL) x 0.5

Postsurgery: Repeat dose as necessary to maintain plasma Factor X levels at a minimum of 50 IU/dL until the patient is no longer at risk of bleeding due to surgery

---

ADMINISTRATION
IV route

Administer by IV infusion at a rate of 10mL/min, but no more than 20mL/min. Refer to PI for preparation and reconstitution instructions.

STORAGE
Store in a refrigerator or at room temperature (2-30°C [36-86°F]). Do not freeze. Protect from light. Use reconstituted sol w/in 1 hr of reconstitution.

HOW SUPPLIED
Inj: 250 IU, 500 IU

CONTRAINDICATIONS
Life-threatening hypersensitivity reactions to Coagadex or any of the components.

WARNINGS/PRECAUTIONS
Allergic-type hypersensitivity reactions, including anaphylaxis, are possible; d/c immediately and administer appropriate emergency treatment if hypersensitivity symptoms occur. Contains traces of human proteins other than Factor X. Formation of neutralizing antibodies (inhibitors) to Factor X may occur; perform an assay that measures Factor X inhibitor concentration if expected Factor X activity levels are not attained, or if bleeding is not controlled w/ an expected dose. May carry a risk of transmitting infectious agents (eg, viruses, the variant Creutzfeldt-Jakob disease agent and, theoretically, the Creutzfeldt-Jakob disease agent).

ADVERSE REACTIONS
Infusion-site erythema, infusion-site pain, fatigue, back pain.

DRUG INTERACTIONS
Caution in patients who are receiving other plasma products that may contain Factor X (eg, fresh frozen plasma, prothrombin complex concentrates). Likely to be counteracted by direct and indirect Factor Xa inhibitors.

PREGNANCY AND LACTATION
Pregnancy: It is not known whether therapy can cause fetal harm; give only if clearly needed.
Lactation: There is no information regarding the presence of drug in human milk; caution in nursing.

MECHANISM OF ACTION
Plasma-derived human blood coagulation factor; temporarily replaces the missing Factor X needed for effective hemostasis.

PHARMACOKINETICS
Absorption: C_{max}=0.504 IU/mL; AUC_{0-144h}=17.1 IU•hr/mL. **Distribution:** V_d=56.3 mL/kg. **Elimination:** $T_{1/2}$=30.3 hrs.

PATIENT CONSIDERATIONS

Assessment: Assess for life threatening hypersensitivity reactions to any constituent of the product, location and extent of bleeding, patient's clinical condition, pregnancy/nursing status, and for possible drug interactions.

Monitoring: Monitor for signs/symptoms of hypersensitivity reactions, transmission of infectious agents, and other adverse reactions. Monitor plasma Factor X activity by performing a validated test (eg, one-stage clotting assay), to confirm that adequate Factor X levels have been achieved and maintained. Monitor for the development of Factor X inhibitors. Perform a Nijmegen-Bethesda inhibitor assay if expected Factor X plasma levels are not attained or if bleeding is not controlled w/ the expected dose of therapy.

Counseling: Instruct to immediately report to healthcare professional the early signs/symptoms of a hypersensitivity reaction (eg, burning, stinging, erythema, chills, cough, dizziness, fever, generalized urticaria, headache, hives, hypotension, lethargy, N/V, tightness of the chest). Inform that the development of inhibitors to Factor X is a possible complication of treatment; advise to contact healthcare provider for further treatment and/or assessment if a lack of clinical response to therapy is experienced. Inform that therapy is made from human plasma and may contain infectious agents that can cause diseases; instruct to report any symptoms that concern the patient.

COARTEM — artemether/lumefantrine Rx

Class: Artemisinin-based combination therapy

ADULT DOSAGE	PEDIATRIC DOSAGE
Malaria	**Malaria**
Acute, Uncomplicated Infection:	**Acute, Uncomplicated Infection:**
>16 Years:	**5-<15kg:**
<35kg:	1 tab as an initial dose, 1 tab again
Refer to pediatric dosage	after 8 hrs, and then 1 tab bid (am and
	pm) for the following 2 days (total
≥35kg:	course of 6 tabs)
4 tabs as a single initial dose, 4 tabs	
again after 8 hrs, and then 4 tabs bid	**15-<25kg:**
(am and pm) for the following 2 days	2 tabs as an initial dose, 2 tabs again
(total course of 24 tabs)	after 8 hrs, and then 2 tabs bid (am
	and pm) for the following 2 days
	(total course of 12 tabs)
	25-<35kg:
	3 tabs as an initial dose, 3 tabs again
	after 8 hrs, and then 3 tabs bid (am
	and pm) for the following 2 days
	(total course of 18 tabs)
	≥35kg:
	4 tabs as a single initial dose, 4 tabs
	again after 8 hrs, and then 4 tabs bid
	(am and pm) for the following 2 days
	(total course of 24 tabs)

ADMINISTRATION

Oral route

Take w/ food; resume normal eating as soon as food can be tolerated
If vomiting occurs w/in 1-2 hrs of administration, give a repeat dose; if the repeat dose is vomited, give an alternative antimalarial for treatment

Patients Unable to Swallow Tabs

1. Crush tabs and mix w/ small amount of water (1-2 tsp) in a clean container for immediate administration
2. Container can be rinsed w/ more water and contents swallowed by the patient
3. Crushed tab preparation should be followed whenever possible by food/drink (eg, milk, formula, pudding, broth, porridge)

STORAGE

25°C (77°F); excursions permitted to 15-30°C (59-86°F).

HOW SUPPLIED

Tab: (Artemether/Lumefantrine) 20mg/120mg* *scored

CONTRAINDICATIONS

Known hypersensitivity to artemether, lumefantrine, or to any of the excipients of this medication, coadministration w/ strong CYP3A4 inducers (eg, rifampin, carbamazepine, phenytoin, St. John's wort).

WARNINGS/PRECAUTIONS

Not approved for prevention of malaria or for patients w/ severe or complicated *Plasmodium falciparum* malaria. May prolong the QT interval; avoid w/ congenital QT interval prolongation (eg, long QT syndrome) or any other clinical condition known to prolong the QT interval (eg, history of symptomatic cardiac arrhythmias, clinically relevant bradycardia, severe cardiac disease), family history of congenital QT interval prolongation or sudden death, or known disturbances of electrolyte balance (eg, hypokalemia, hypomagnesemia). Closely monitor patients who remain averse to food during treatment as risk of recrudescence may be greater; if recrudescent *P. falciparum* infection develops after treatment, treat patient w/ a different antimalarial drug. Caution w/ severe hepatic/renal impairment.

ADVERSE REACTIONS

Headache, dizziness, anorexia, asthenia, pyrexia, chills, fatigue, arthralgia, myalgia, N/V, abdominal pain, sleep disorder, palpitations, cough.

DRUG INTERACTIONS

See Contraindications. Avoid w/ other medications that prolong the QT interval (eg, Class IA [quinidine, procainamide, disopyramide] or Class III [amiodarone, sotalol] antiarrhythmic agents, antipsychotics [pimozide, ziprasidone], antidepressants, certain antibiotics [macrolide/fluoroquinolone antibiotics, imidazole/triazole antifungal agents]); monitor ECG if concomitant use w/ a drug that prolongs the QT interval, including antimalarials such as quinine, is medically required. Avoid w/ medications metabolized by CYP2D6 that also have cardiac effects (eg, flecainide, imipramine, amitriptyline, clomipramine). Do not administer with halofantrine w/in 1 month of each other. Do not give w/ antimalarials, unless there is no other treatment option. Mefloquine administered immediately prior to therapy may lead to decreased exposure to lumefantrine. May decrease concentrations and efficacy of CYP3A4 substrates. CYP3A4 inhibitors (eg, grapefruit juice, ketoconazole) may increase concentrations and potentiate QT prolongation. CYP3A4 inducers may decrease concentrations and antimalarial efficacy. Caution w/ drugs that have a mixed effect on CYP3A4, especially antiretroviral drugs (eg, HIV protease inhibitors and non-nucleoside reverse transcriptase inhibitors), and those that have an effect on the QT interval. May reduce effectiveness of hormonal contraceptives; use an additional nonhormonal method of birth control. May increase concentrations of CYP2D6 substrates and increase risk of adverse effects.

PREGNANCY AND LACTATION

Category C, caution in nursing.

MECHANISM OF ACTION

Artemether: Artemisinin derivative; antimalarial activity attributed to endoperoxide moiety. Lumefantrine: Antimalarial agent; not established. Suspected to inhibit the formation of β-hematin by forming a complex w/ hemin. Both artemether and lumefantrine inhibit nucleic acid and protein synthesis.

PHARMACOKINETICS

Absorption: Administration of variable doses resulted in different parameters. **Distribution:** Artemether: Plasma protein binding (95.4%, 47-76% dihydroartemisinin [DHA]). Lumefantrine: Plasma protein binding (99.7%). **Metabolism:** Artemether: Liver via CYP3A4/5 (major), CYP2B6, CYP2C9, CYP2C19 (minor); DHA (active metabolite). Lumefantrine: Liver via CYP3A4; desbutyl-lumefantrine (metabolite). **Elimination:** Artemether and DHA: $T_{1/2}$=2 hrs. Lumefantrine: $T_{1/2}$=3-6 days.

PATIENT CONSIDERATIONS

Assessment: Assess for hypersensitivity to the drug, congenital QT interval prolongation or any other clinical condition known to prolong the QT interval, family history of congenital QT interval prolongation or sudden death, known disturbances of electrolyte balance, severe hepatic/renal impairment, pregnancy/nursing status, and possible drug interactions.

Monitoring: Monitor for QT interval prolongation, recrudescent *P. falciparum* infection, and other adverse reactions.

Counseling: Instruct to inform physician of any personal/family history of QT prolongation or proarrhythmic conditions, if taking any other medications, and if symptoms of QT interval prolongation occur. Advise patients using hormonal contraceptives to use an additional nonhormonal method of birth control. Instruct to d/c therapy at the 1st sign of a skin rash, hives or other skin reactions, a rapid heartbeat, difficulty in swallowing or breathing, any swelling suggesting angioedema, or other symptoms of an allergic reaction.

COLAZAL — balsalazide disodium Rx

Class: 5-aminosalicylic acid derivative

ADULT DOSAGE	PEDIATRIC DOSAGE
Ulcerative Colitis	**Ulcerative Colitis**
Mild to Moderately Active:	**Mild to Moderately Active:**
3 caps tid (6.75g/day) for up to	**5-17 Years:**
8 weeks; some patients required	1 cap tid (2.25g/day) or 3 caps tid
treatment for up to 12 weeks	(6.75g/day) for up to 8 weeks

ADMINISTRATION

Oral route

May also be administered by carefully opening cap and sprinkling contents on applesauce.
Entire drug/applesauce mixture should be swallowed immediately; may chew contents if necessary.
Do not store mixture for future use.

STORAGE

20-25°C (68-77°F); excursions permitted to 15-30°C (59-86°F).

HOW SUPPLIED

Cap: 750mg

CONTRAINDICATIONS

Hypersensitivity to salicylates or to any of the components of this medication or to balsalazide metabolites.

WARNINGS/PRECAUTIONS

May exacerbate symptoms of colitis. May prolong gastric retention w/ pyloric stenosis. Caution w/ renal dysfunction or history of renal disease.

ADVERSE REACTIONS

Headache, abdominal pain, diarrhea, N/V, respiratory infection, arthralgia.

PREGNANCY AND LACTATION

Pregnancy: Category B.
Lactation: Caution in nursing.

MECHANISM OF ACTION

Not established; a prodrug enzymatically cleaved in colon to produce mesalamine (5-ASA), an anti-inflammatory drug that acts locally to block production of arachidonic acid metabolites in the colon.

PHARMACOKINETICS

Absorption: Different dosing conditions (fasted, fed, sprinkled) resulted in variable parameters. **Distribution:** Plasma protein binding (≥99%). **Metabolism:** Key metabolites: 5-ASA and N-acetyl-5-ASA. **Elimination:** Urine, feces.

PATIENT CONSIDERATIONS

Assessment: Assess for pyloric stenosis and history of renal/hepatic disease.
Monitoring: Monitor renal function, and for signs/symptoms of prolonged gastric retention w/ pyloric stenosis, worsening of colitis symptoms, and hypersensitivity.
Counseling: Advise that teeth and/or tongue may get stained when using sprinkle form w/ food. Instruct to contact physician if experiencing a worsening of ulcerative colitis symptoms, if diagnosed w/ pyloric stenosis, or if diagnosed w/ renal dysfunction. Instruct not to take drug if patient has hypersensitivity to salicylates (eg, aspirin).

COLCRYS — colchicine

Rx

Class: Miscellaneous gout agent

ADULT DOSAGE

Gout Flares

Prophylaxis:
>16 Years:
Usual: 0.6mg qd or bid
Max: 1.2mg/day

Treatment:
Usual: 1.2mg at the 1st sign of flare followed by 0.6mg 1 hr later
Max: 1.8mg over a 1-hr period
May administer for treatment of gout flare during prophylaxis at doses not to exceed 1.2mg at the 1st sign of the flare followed by 0.6mg 1 hr later; wait 12 hrs, then resume prophylactic dose

Familial Mediterranean Fever

Usual Range: 1.2-2.4mg/day in 1-2 divided doses
Titrate: Increase or decrease dose in 0.3mg increments based on disease control or intolerable side effects

PEDIATRIC DOSAGE

Familial Mediterranean Fever

4-6 Years: 0.3-1.8mg/day
6-12 Years: 0.9-1.8mg/day
>12 Years: 1.2-2.4mg/day

May be given qd or bid

DOSING CONSIDERATIONS

Concomitant Medications

Strong CYP3A4 Inhibitors:

Gout Flare Prophylaxis:
Original Dose 0.6mg BID: Adjust to 0.3mg qd
Original Dose 0.6mg QD: Adjust to 0.3mg qod

Gout Flare Treatment:
0.6mg for 1 dose, followed by 0.3mg 1 hr later; repeat dose no earlier than 3 days

Familial Mediterranean Fever:
Max: 0.6mg/day (may be given as 0.3mg bid)

Moderate CYP3A4 Inhibitors:

Gout Flare Prophylaxis:
Original Dose 0.6mg BID: Adjust to 0.3mg bid or 0.6mg qd
Original Dose 0.6mg QD: Adjust to 0.3mg qd

Gout Flare Treatment:
1.2mg for 1 dose; repeat dose no earlier than 3 days

Familial Mediterranean Fever:
Max: 1.2mg/day (may be given as 0.6mg bid)

P-gp Inhibitors:

Gout Flare Prophylaxis:
Original Dose 0.6mg BID: Adjust to 0.3mg qd
Original Dose 0.6mg QD: Adjust to 0.3mg qod

Gout Flare Treatment:
0.6mg for 1 dose; repeat dose no earlier than 3 days

Familial Mediterranean Fever:
Max: 0.6mg/day (may be given as 0.3mg bid)

Renal Impairment

Gout Flare Prophylaxis:
Severe Impairment:
Initial: 0.3mg/day
Titrate: Increase dose w/ close monitoring
Dialysis:
Initial: 0.3mg twice a week w/ close monitoring

Gout Flare Treatment:
Severe Impairment: Repeat treatment course no more than once every 2 weeks; consider alternate therapy if repeat treatment courses are required
Dialysis: Reduce to 0.6mg single dose; do not repeat treatment course more than once every 2 weeks

Familial Mediterranean Fever:
Mild (CrCl 50-80mL/min) to Moderate (CrCl 30-50mL/min): Consider reducing dose
Severe (CrCl <30mL/min)/Dialysis:
Initial: 0.3mg/day
Titrate: Increase dose w/ close monitoring

Hepatic Impairment

Gout Flare Prophylaxis:
Severe Impairment: Consider reducing dose

Gout Flare Treatment:
Severe Impairment: Repeat treatment course no more than once every 2 weeks; consider alternate therapy if repeat treatment courses are required

Familial Mediterranean Fever:
Severe Impairment: Consider reducing dose

ADMINISTRATION

Oral route

Take w/o regard to meals.

STORAGE

20-25°C (68-77°F). Protect from light.

HOW SUPPLIED

Tab: 0.6mg* *scored

CONTRAINDICATIONS

Concomitant use w/ P-gp or strong CYP3A4 inhibitors (includes all protease inhibitors, except fosamprenavir) in patients w/ renal/hepatic impairment.

WARNINGS/PRECAUTIONS

Not an analgesic medication and should not be used to treat pain from other causes. Fatal overdoses (accidental/intentional), myelosuppression, leukopenia, granulocytopenia, thrombocytopenia, pancytopenia, and aplastic anemia reported. Drug-induced neuromuscular toxicity and rhabdomyolysis reported w/ chronic use; increased risk in elderly and in patients w/ renal dysfunction. Treatment of gout flare w/ Colcrys is not recommended in patients w/ renal/hepatic impairment who are receiving Colcrys for prophylaxis. Caution w/ renal/hepatic impairment and in elderly.

ADVERSE REACTIONS

Diarrhea, pharyngolaryngeal pain, cramping, abdominal pain, N/V, fatigue.

DRUG INTERACTIONS

See Dosing Considerations and Contraindications. Significant increase in plasma levels reported w/ strong CYP3A4 inhibitors (eg, atazanavir, clarithromycin, itraconazole), moderate CYP3A4 inhibitors (eg, amprenavir, aprepitant, diltiazem, erythromycin), and P-gp inhibitors (eg, cyclosporine, ranolazine); see PI for dose adjustments. Fatal toxicity reported w/ clarithromycin and cyclosporine. Neuromuscular toxicity reported w/ diltiazem and verapamil. May potentiate the development of myopathy and rhabdomyolysis when used w/ HMG-CoA reductase inhibitors (eg, atorvastatin, simvastatin), gemfibrozil, and fibrates. May potentiate the development of myopathy when used w/ cyclosporine. Rhabdomyolysis reported w/ digoxin.

PREGNANCY AND LACTATION

Pregnancy: Category C.
Lactation: Caution in nursing.

MECHANISM OF ACTION

Alkaloid; not established. May interfere w/ the intracellular assembly of the inflammasome complex present in neutrophils and monocytes that mediates activation of interleukin-1β in patients w/ familial Mediterranean fever. Disrupts cytoskeletal functions through inhibition of β-tubulin polymerization into microtubules, consequently preventing the activation, degranulation, and migration of neutrophils thought to mediate some gout symptoms.

PHARMACOKINETICS

Absorption: Administration of variable doses resulted in different pharmacokinetic parameters. Absolute bioavailability (45%). **Distribution:** V_d=5-8L/kg; plasma protein binding (39%). Crosses placenta; found in breast milk. **Metabolism:** CYP3A4; demethylation; 2-O-demethylcolchicine and 3-O-demethylcolchicine (primary metabolites); 10-O-demethylcolchicine (minor metabolite). **Elimination:** Urine (40-65%, unchanged); $T_{1/2}$=26.6-31.2 hrs.

PATIENT CONSIDERATIONS

Assessment: Assess for renal/hepatic impairment, pregnancy/nursing status, and possible drug interactions.

Monitoring: Monitor for myelosuppression, leukopenia, granulocytopenia, thrombocytopenia, pancytopenia, aplastic anemia, neuromuscular toxicity, rhabdomyolysis, and other adverse reactions.

Counseling: Instruct to take medication ud. If a dose is missed for treatment of gout flare, instruct to take missed dose as soon as possible. If a dose is missed for treatment of gout flare during prophylaxis, instruct to take missed dose immediately, wait 12 hrs, and then resume previous schedule. If a dose is missed for prophylaxis w/o treatment of gout flares or familial Mediterranean fever, instruct to take next dose as soon as possible, then return to normal dosing schedule, and not to double the next dose. Inform that fatal overdoses were reported. Instruct to avoid grapefruit/grapefruit juice consumption during treatment. Inform that bone marrow depression w/ agranulocytosis, aplastic anemia, and thrombocytopenia may occur. Advise to notify physician of all medications currently being taken and to notify physician before starting any new medications, particularly antibiotics. Advise to d/c therapy and notify physician if experiencing muscle pain/weakness and/or tingling/numbness of fingers/toes.

COLESTID — colestipol hydrochloride

Rx

Class: Bile acid sequestrant

ADULT DOSAGE

Primary Hypercholesterolemia

Tab:
Initial: 2g qd-bid
Titrate: Increase by 2g qd or bid at 1- or 2-month intervals
Usual: 2-16g/day qd or in divided doses

Granules:
Initial: 1 pkt or 1 scoopful qd-bid
Titrate: May increase at an increment of 1 dose/day (1 pkt or 1 level tsp of granules) at 1- or 2-month intervals
Usual: 1-6 pkts or scoopfuls qd or in divided doses

Significant Rise in TG Levels:
Consider dose reduction, drug discontinuation, or combined/alternate therapy

PEDIATRIC DOSAGE

Pediatric use may not have been established

ADMINISTRATION
Oral route
Tab
Take 1 tab at a time and promptly swallow tabs whole using plenty of water or other appropriate liquid
Do not cut, crush, or chew
Granules
Always mix granules with water or other fluids before ingesting
Refer to PI for mixing and administration guide (with beverages/cereals/soups/fruits)

STORAGE
20-25°C (68-77°F).

HOW SUPPLIED
Granules: 5g/pkt [30ˢ 90ˢ], 5g/scoopful [300g, 500g]; **Tab:** 1g

CONTRAINDICATIONS
Hypersensitivity to any of the components.

WARNINGS/PRECAUTIONS
Exclude secondary causes of hypercholesterolemia. May interfere with normal fat absorption. Chronic use may be associated with an increase bleeding tendency due to hypoprothrombinemia from vitamin K deficiency. May cause hypothyroidism. May produce or severely worsen preexisting constipation. Avoid constipation with symptomatic coronary artery disease. Constipation associated with colestipol may aggravate hemorrhoids. May produce hyperchloremic acidosis with prolonged use. (Granules) Flavored form contains phenylalanine. Avoid taking in dry form; always mix granules with water or other fluids before ingesting.

ADVERSE REACTIONS
Constipation, abdominal discomfort, indigestion/heartburn, musculoskeletal pain, headache, AST/ALT/alkaline phosphatase elevation, chest pain, rash, anorexia, fatigue, tachycardia, SOB.

DRUG INTERACTIONS
May interfere the absorption of folic acid, fat-soluble vitamins (eg, A, D, K), oral phosphate supplements, and hydrocortisone. May delay or reduce absorption of concomitant oral medication; take other drugs at least 1 hr before or 4 hrs after colestipol. Reduces absorption of chlorothiazide, tetracycline, furosemide, penicillin G, HCTZ, and gemfibrozil. Caution with digitalis preparations, propranolol. Reduce mycophenolic acid exposure and potentially reduce efficacy of mycophenolate mofetil.

PREGNANCY AND LACTATION
Pregnancy: Safety is not known in pregnancy.
Lactation: Caution in nursing.

MECHANISM OF ACTION
Bile acid sequestrant; binds bile acids in the intestine forming a complex that is excreted in the feces, leading to increased fecal loss of bile acids and increased oxidation of cholesterol to bile acids, a decrease in β lipoprotein or LDL/serum cholesterol levels.

PHARMACOKINETICS
Elimination: Feces.

PATIENT CONSIDERATIONS
Assessment: Assess for hypersensitivity to the drug, secondary causes of hypercholesterolemia (eg, hypothyroidism, poorly controlled diabetes mellitus, nephrotic syndrome, dysproteinemias, obstructive liver disease, alcoholism), preexisting constipation, pregnancy/nursing status, and possible drug interactions. Determine baseline lipid profile.

Monitoring: Monitor for signs/symptoms of vitamin K deficiency (eg, tendency for bleeding), constipation, hypothyroidism, hyperchloremic acidosis, and other adverse reactions. Monitor serum cholesterol, lipoprotein, and TG levels.

Counseling: Inform about benefits/risks of therapy. Instruct to take ud. Advise to take other medications at least 1 hr before or 4 hrs after taking colestipol. Instruct to report any adverse reactions to physician.

COMBIGAN — brimonidine tartrate/timolol maleate   Rx

Class: Alpha₂ agonist/beta blocker

ADULT DOSAGE	PEDIATRIC DOSAGE
Elevated Intraocular Pressure	**Elevated Intraocular Pressure**
Reduction of elevated IOP in patients w/ glaucoma or ocular HTN requiring adjunctive or replacement therapy due to inadequately controlled IOP	Reduction of elevated IOP in patients w/ glaucoma or ocular HTN requiring adjunctive or replacement therapy due to inadequately controlled IOP
Instill 1 drop in affected eye(s) bid q12h	**≥2 Years:** Instill 1 drop in affected eye(s) bid q12h

DOSING CONSIDERATIONS
Concomitant Medications
Space by at least 5 min if using >1 topical ophthalmic product

ADMINISTRATION
Ocular route

STORAGE
15-25°C (59-77°F). Protect from light.

HOW SUPPLIED
Ophthalmic Sol: (Brimonidine/Timolol) 0.2%/0.5% [5mL, 10mL, 15mL]

CONTRAINDICATIONS
Reactive airway disease including bronchial asthma, history of bronchial asthma, severe COPD. Sinus bradycardia, 2nd- or 3rd-degree atrioventricular (AV) block, overt cardiac failure, cardiogenic shock. Neonates and infants (<2 yrs of age). History of hypersensitivity reaction to any component of the medication.

WARNINGS/PRECAUTIONS
May potentiate syndromes associated w/ vascular insufficiency; caution w/ depression, cerebral or coronary insufficiency, Raynaud's phenomenon, orthostatic hypotension, or thromboangiitis obliterans. Bacterial keratitis reported w/ use of multiple-dose containers of topical ophthalmic products. **Timolol:** May be absorbed systemically. Severe respiratory reactions and cardiac reactions including death due to bronchospasm in patients w/ asthma, and rarely death in association w/ cardiac failure, reported following systemic or ophthalmic administration of timolol. Ophthalmic β-blockers may impair compensatory tachycardia and increase risk of hypotension. May precipitate more severe failure in patients w/ diminished myocardial contractility. Continued depression of the myocardium w/ β-blocking agents over a period of time may lead to cardiac failure in patients w/o a history of cardiac failure; d/c at the 1st sign/symptom of cardiac failure. Avoid in patients w/ mild to moderate COPD (eg, chronic bronchitis, emphysema), bronchospastic disease, or a history of bronchospastic disease. May increase reactivity to allergens. May potentiate muscle weakness consistent w/ certain myasthenic symptoms (eg, diplopia, ptosis, generalized weakness). Increased muscle weakness in some patients w/ myasthenia gravis or myasthenic symptoms reported rarely w/ timolol. May mask signs/symptoms of acute hypoglycemia; caution in patients subject to spontaneous hypoglycemia and in diabetic patients (especially those w/ labile diabetes) receiving insulin or hypoglycemic agents. May mask certain clinical signs of hyperthyroidism (eg, tachycardia); carefully manage patients suspected of developing thyrotoxicosis to avoid abrupt withdrawal that may precipitate a thyroid storm. May impair the ability of the heart to respond to β-adrenergically mediated reflex stimuli during surgery; gradual withdrawal of β-blocking agents is recommended in patients undergoing elective surgery. **Brimonidine:** Ocular hypersensitivity reactions reported.

ADVERSE REACTIONS
Allergic conjunctivitis, conjunctival folliculosis, conjunctival hyperemia, eye pruritus, ocular burning/stinging.

DRUG INTERACTIONS
May reduce BP; caution w/ antihypertensives and/or cardiac glycosides. Monitor for potentially additive effects, both systemic and on IOP w/ concomitant oral or IV β-blockers; concomitant use of 2 topical β-blocking agents is not recommended. Possibility of additive or potentiating effect w/ CNS depressants (eg, alcohol, barbiturates, opiates, sedatives, anesthetics). May affect the metabolism and uptake of circulating amines w/ TCAs and/or MAOIs; caution w/ TCAs and MAOIs. **Timolol:** Possible AV conduction disturbances, left ventricular failure, and hypotension may occur w/ oral or IV calcium antagonists; use w/ caution and avoid coadministration in patients w/ impaired cardiac function. Closely observe patients receiving catecholamine-depleting drugs (eg, reserpine) because of possible additive effects and the production of hypotension and/or marked bradycardia. Concomitant use of β-blockers w/ digitalis or calcium antagonists may have additive effects in prolonging AV conduction time. Potentiated systemic β-blockade (eg, decreased HR, depression) reported w/ concomitant CYP2D6 inhibitors (eg, quinidine, SSRIs).

PREGNANCY AND LACTATION
Pregnancy: There are no adequate and well-controlled studies in pregnant women. Brimonidine crossed placenta and entered into the fetal circulation to a limited extent, in animal studies. Use Combigan during pregnancy only if the potential benefit justifies the potential risk. **Lactation:** Not for use in nursing. Timolol has been detected in human milk.

MECHANISM OF ACTION
Decreases elevated IOP. **Brimonidine:** Selective α-2 adrenergic receptor agonist. **Timolol:** Nonselective β-blocker.

PHARMACOKINETICS
Absorption: Brimonidine: C_{max}=30pg/mL; T_{max}=1-4 hrs; AUC=128pg•hr/mL. Timolol: C_{max}=400pg/mL; T_{max}=1-3 hrs; AUC=2919pg•hr/mL. **Distribution:** Timolol: Plasma protein binding (60%); found in breast milk. Brimonidine: Crosses placenta. **Metabolism:** Brimonidine: Liver (extensive). Timolol: Liver (partial). **Elimination:** Brimonidine: $T_{1/2}$=3 hrs. Timolol: $T_{1/2}$=7 hrs.

PATIENT CONSIDERATIONS
Assessment: Assess for reactive airway disease, sinus bradycardia, AV block, cardiac failure, or any other conditions where treatment is contraindicated or cautioned. Assess pregnancy/nursing status, and for possible drug interactions.

Monitoring: Monitor for respiratory or cardiac reactions, potentiation of syndromes associated w/ vascular insufficiency, muscle weakness, increased reactivity to allergens, masking of signs/symptoms of hypoglycemia or hyperthyroidism, ocular hypersensitivity reactions, bacterial keratitis, and other adverse reactions.

Counseling: Inform that ocular infections may occur if handled improperly or if the tip of dispensing container contacts the eye or surrounding structures. Advise that serious damage to the eye and subsequent loss of vision may result from using contaminated sol or by inadvertent contact w/ dropper tip. Instruct to always replace cap after using. Advise not to use if sol changes color or becomes cloudy. Advise to immediately consult physician concerning continued use of multidose container if undergoing ocular surgery or if an intercurrent ocular condition (eg, trauma, infection) develops. Instruct to space dosing by at least 5 min apart if >1 topical ophthalmic drug is being used. Inform that drug contains benzalkonium chloride, which may be absorbed by soft contact lenses; instruct to remove contact lenses prior to administration and explain that lenses may be reinserted 15 min following administration. Inform that drug may cause fatigue and/or drowsiness in some patients; advise to use caution in engaging in hazardous activities because of the potential for a decrease in mental alertness.

COMBIPATCH — estradiol/norethindrone acetate   Rx

Class: Estrogen/progestogen combination

> Should not be used for prevention of cardiovascular (CV) disease or dementia. Increased risk of MI, stroke, pulmonary embolism (PE), and deep vein thrombosis (DVT) in postmenopausal women (50-79 yrs of age) reported. Increased risk of developing probable dementia in postmenopausal women ≥65 yrs of age reported. Increased risk of invasive breast cancer reported. Increased risk of endometrial cancer in women w/ a uterus who use unopposed estrogens. Perform adequate diagnostic measures to rule out malignancy in postmenopausal women w/ undiagnosed persistent or recurrent abnormal vaginal bleeding. Should be prescribed at the lowest effective dose and for the shortest duration consistent w/ treatment goals and risks.

ADULT DOSAGE
Menopausal Vasomotor Symptoms

Moderate to Severe:
Initiation of Therapy:
Start at lowest dose. Women not currently using continuous estrogen or combination estrogen + progestin therapy may start therapy w/ CombiPatch at any time. However, women currently using continuous estrogen or combination estrogen + progestin therapy should complete current cycle of therapy prior to initiating CombiPatch therapy

Women often experience withdrawal bleeding at the completion of the cycle. The first day of this bleeding would be an appropriate time to begin CombiPatch therapy

Continuous Combined Regimen:
Wear a (0.05mg/0.14mg)/day patch for continuous uninterrupted treatment twice weekly on the lower abdomen; replace every 3-4 days (twice weekly) during a 28-day cycle

Use 0.05mg/0.25mg if a greater progestin dose is desired

Continuous Sequential Regimen:
CombiPatch can be applied as a sequential regimen in combination w/ an estradiol-only patch

Days 1-14: Wear a 0.05mg/day estradiol patch (Vivelle-Dot); replace every 3-4 days (twice weekly)
Days 15-28: Wear CombiPatch (0.05mg/0.14mg)/day patch continuously on the lower abdomen; replace every 3-4 days (twice weekly)

Use 0.05mg/0.25mg if a greater progestin dose is desired

Use the lowest effective dose for the shortest duration; reevaluate at 3- to 6-month intervals

Menopausal Vulvar/Vaginal Atrophy

Moderate to Severe:
Initiation of Therapy:
Start at lowest dose. Women not currently using continuous estrogen or combination estrogen + progestin therapy may start therapy w/ CombiPatch at any time. However, women currently using continuous estrogen or combination estrogen + progestin therapy should complete current cycle of therapy prior to initiating CombiPatch therapy

Women often experience withdrawal bleeding at the completion of the cycle. The first day of this bleeding would be an appropriate time to begin CombiPatch therapy

Continuous Combined Regimen:
Wear a (0.05mg/0.14mg)/day patch for continuous uninterrupted treatment twice weekly on the lower abdomen; replace every 3-4 days (twice weekly) during a 28-day cycle

PEDIATRIC DOSAGE
Pediatric use may not have been established

Use 0.05mg/0.25mg if a greater progestin dose is desired

Continuous Sequential Regimen:
CombiPatch can be applied as a sequential regimen in combination w/ an estradiol-only patch

Days 1-14: Wear a 0.05mg/day estradiol patch (Vivelle-Dot); replace every 3-4 days (twice weekly)
Days 15-28: Wear CombiPatch (0.05mg/0.14mg)/day patch continuously on the lower abdomen; replace every 3-4 days (twice weekly)

Use 0.05mg/0.25mg if a greater progestin dose is desired

Use the lowest effective dose for the shortest duration; reevaluate at 3- to 6-month intervals

Hypoestrogenism

Due to Hypogonadism, Castration, or Primary Ovarian Failure:
Initiation of Therapy:
Start at lowest dose. Women not currently using continuous estrogen or combination estrogen + progestin therapy may start therapy w/ CombiPatch at any time. However, women currently using continuous estrogen or combination estrogen + progestin therapy should complete current cycle of therapy prior to initiating CombiPatch therapy

Women often experience withdrawal bleeding at the completion of the cycle. The first day of this bleeding would be an appropriate time to begin CombiPatch therapy

Continuous Combined Regimen:
Wear a (0.05mg/0.14mg)/day patch for continuous uninterrupted treatment twice weekly on the lower abdomen; replace every 3-4 days (twice weekly) during a 28-day cycle

Use 0.05mg/0.25mg if a greater progestin dose is desired

Continuous Sequential Regimen:
CombiPatch can be applied as a sequential regimen in combination w/ an estradiol-only patch

Days 1-14: Wear a 0.05mg/day estradiol patch (Vivelle-Dot); replace every 3-4 days (twice weekly)
Days 15-28: Wear CombiPatch (0.05mg/0.14mg)/day patch continuously on the lower abdomen; replace every 3-4 days (twice weekly)

Use 0.05mg/0.25mg if a greater progestin dose is desired

Use the lowest effective dose for the shortest duration; reevaluate at 3- to 6-month intervals

---

ADMINISTRATION
Transdermal route

Site Selection
Place on a smooth (fold-free), clean, dry area of the skin on the lower abdomen. Do not apply to or near the breasts. Area selected should not be oily, damaged, or irritated. Avoid application to the waistline, as tight clothing may rub the system off or modify drug delivery. Rotate site of application, w/ an interval of at least 1 week allowed between applications to the same site.

Application
1. After opening the pouch, remove 1 side of the protective liner, taking care not to touch the adhesive part of the patch w/ the fingers.
2. Immediately apply the patch to a smooth (fold-free) area of skin on the lower abdomen.
3. Remove the 2nd side of the protective liner and press the patch firmly in place for at least 10 sec, making sure there is good contact, especially around the edges.

If a patch falls off, reapply the same patch to another area of the lower abdomen. If necessary, a new patch may be applied, in which case the original treatment schedule should be continued. Only 1 system should be worn at any 1 time during the 3- to 4-day dosing interval.

Once in place, the patch should not be exposed to the sun for prolonged periods of time.

Removal
Remove the patch carefully and slowly to avoid skin irritation. Should any adhesive remain on the skin after removal of the patch, allow the area to dry for 15 min, then gently rub the area w/ an oil-based cream or lotion to remove adhesive residue.

STORAGE
Prior to Dispensing: 2-8°C (36-46°F). **After Dispensing:** 20-25°C (66-77°F) for up to 6 months. Store the systems in the sealed foil pouch. Do not store in areas where extreme temperatures may occur.

HOW SUPPLIED
Patch: (Estradiol/Norethindrone Acetate) (0.05mg/0.14mg)/day, (0.05mg/0.25mg)/day [8^s]

CONTRAINDICATIONS
Undiagnosed abnormal genital bleeding, known/suspected/history of breast cancer, known/suspected estrogen-dependent neoplasia, active/history of DVT/PE, active/history of arterial thromboembolic disease (eg, stroke, MI), known anaphylactic reaction/angioedema/hypersensitivity to CombiPatch, known liver impairment/disease, known protein C/protein S/antithrombin deficiency or other known thrombophilic disorders, known/suspected pregnancy.

WARNINGS/PRECAUTIONS
In some cases, hysterectomized women w/ a history of endometriosis may need a progestin. D/C immediately if stroke, DVT, PE, or MI occurs or is suspected. Manage risk factors for arterial vascular disease and/or venous thromboembolism appropriately. If feasible, d/c at least 4-6 weeks before surgery of the type associated w/ an increased risk of thromboembolism, or during periods of prolonged immobilization. May increase risk of ovarian cancer and gallbladder disease. May lead to severe hypercalcemia in patients w/ breast cancer and bone metastases; d/c and take appropriate measures if hypercalcemia occurs. Retinal vascular thrombosis reported in women; d/c therapy pending exam if sudden partial/complete loss of vision or sudden onset of proptosis, diplopia, or migraine occurs. D/C permanently if exam reveals papilledema or retinal vascular lesions. Angioedema involving eye/eyelid, face, larynx, pharynx, tongue, and extremity w/ or w/o urticaria requiring medical intervention reported. Women who develop angioedema anytime during the course of treatment should not receive treatment again. May exacerbate symptoms of angioedema in women w/ hereditary angioedema. Cases of anaphylactic/anaphylactoid reactions, which developed anytime during the course of treatment and required emergency medical management reported; involvement of skin (hives, pruritus, swollen lips-tongue-face) and either respiratory tract (respiratory compromise) or GI tract (abdominal pain, vomiting) has been noted. May elevate BP and thyroid-binding globulin levels. May elevate plasma TGs in women w/ preexisting hypertriglyceridemia, leading to pancreatitis; consider discontinuation if pancreatitis occurs. Caution w/ history of cholestatic jaundice associated w/ past estrogen use or w/ pregnancy; d/c in case of recurrence. May cause fluid retention. Caution w/ hypoparathyroidism as estrogen-induced hypocalcemia may occur. May exacerbate endometriosis, asthma, diabetes mellitus, epilepsy, migraine, porphyria, systemic lupus erythematosus, and hepatic hemangiomas. May affect certain endocrine and blood components in lab tests.

ADVERSE REACTIONS
Abdominal pain, back pain, asthenia, flu syndrome, headache, application-site reaction, diarrhea, nausea, nervousness, pharyngitis, respiratory disorder, breast pain, dysmenorrhea, menstrual disorder, vaginitis.

DRUG INTERACTIONS
CYP3A4 inducers (eg, St. John's wort preparations, phenobarbital, phenylbutazone, rifabutin) may decrease levels and may decrease therapeutic effects and/or change uterine bleeding profile. CYP3A4 inhibitors (eg, erythromycin, clarithromycin, ketoconazole, nelfinavir) may increase levels, which may result in side effects. Women concomitantly receiving thyroid hormone replacement therapy and estrogens may require increased doses of their thyroid replacement therapy; monitor thyroid function.

PREGNANCY AND LACTATION
Pregnancy: Contraindicated in pregnancy.
Lactation: Not for use in nursing.

MECHANISM OF ACTION
Estrogen/progestogen combination; estrogen binds to nuclear receptors in estrogen-responsive tissues. Reduces elevated levels of luteinizing hormone and follicle-stimulating hormone in postmenopausal women.

PHARMACOKINETICS
Absorption: Transdermal administration of variable doses resulted in different parameters. **Distribution:** Found in breast milk. Estradiol: Largely bound to sex hormone-binding globulin (SHBG) and albumin. Norethindrone: Approx 90% bound to SHBG and albumin. **Metabolism:** Estradiol: Liver to estrone (metabolite), estriol (major urinary metabolite). Also undergoes enterohepatic recirculation via sulfate and glucuronide conjugation in the liver, biliary secretion of conjugates into the intestine, and hydrolysis in the intestine followed by reabsorption. Norethindrone: Liver. **Elimination:** Estradiol: Urine; $T_{1/2}$=2-3 hrs. Norethindrone: $T_{1/2}$=6-8 hrs.

PATIENT CONSIDERATIONS
Assessment: Assess for undiagnosed abnormal genital bleeding, presence/history of breast cancer, estrogen-dependent neoplasia, active/history of DVT/PE/arterial thromboembolic disease, liver impairment/disease, thrombophilic disorders, drug hypersensitivity, pregnancy/nursing status, any other conditions where treatment is contraindicated or cautioned, and possible drug interactions.

Monitoring: Monitor for signs/symptoms of CV disease, malignant neoplasms, dementia, gallbladder disease, hypercalcemia, visual abnormalities, BP and plasma TG elevations, pancreatitis, cholestatic jaundice, fluid retention, exacerbation of

endometriosis and other conditions, angioedema, anaphylactic/anaphylactoid reactions, and other adverse reactions. Perform annual breast exam; schedule mammography based on age, risk factors, and prior mammogram results. Periodically reevaluate (every 3-6 months) to determine need for continued therapy. Perform adequate diagnostic measures (eg, endometrial sampling) to rule out malignancies in postmenopausal women w/ undiagnosed, persistent, or recurring abnormal genital bleeding. Regularly monitor thyroid function if on thyroid hormone replacement therapy.

Counseling: Inform of the importance of reporting abnormal vaginal bleeding to physician as soon as possible. Inform of possible serious adverse reactions of therapy (eg, CV disorders, malignant neoplasms, probable dementia) and of possible less serious, but common adverse reactions (eg, headache, breast pain and tenderness, nausea). Instruct to have yearly breast exams by a healthcare provider and to perform monthly breast self-exams. Advise that monthly withdrawal bleeding often occurs w/ the continuous sequential regimen.

COMBIVENT RESPIMAT — albuterol/ipratropium bromide   **Rx**
Class: Anticholinergic/short-acting beta$_2$ agonist (SABA)

ADULT DOSAGE	PEDIATRIC DOSAGE
Chronic Obstructive Pulmonary Disease **Bronchospasm Requiring a 2nd Bronchodilator:** **Recommended:** 1 inh qid. May take additional inh as required **Max:** 6 inh/24 hrs	Pediatric use may not have been established

ADMINISTRATION
Oral inh route
Priming
- Prior to 1st use, insert cartridge into the inhaler and prime the unit; actuate the inhaler toward the ground until an aerosol cloud is visible and then repeat the process 3 more times.
- If not used for >3 days, actuate the inhaler once.
- If not used for >21 days, actuate the inhaler until an aerosol cloud is visible and then repeat the process 3 more times.

STORAGE
25°C (77°F); excursions permitted to 15-30°C (59-86°F). Avoid freezing.

HOW SUPPLIED
Spray, Inhalation: (Ipratropium/Albuterol) (20mcg/100mcg)/actuation [120 actuations]

CONTRAINDICATIONS
Hypersensitivity to any of the ingredients in the medication or to atropine or any of its derivatives.

WARNINGS/PRECAUTIONS
May produce paradoxical bronchospasm; d/c and institute alternative therapy if this occurs. Hypersensitivity reactions may occur; d/c and consider alternative treatment if such a reaction occurs. **Albuterol:** May produce significant cardiovascular (CV) effects (eg, ECG changes); may need to d/c if symptoms occur. Caution w/ CV disorders (eg, coronary insufficiency, cardiac arrhythmias, HTN). Fatalities reported w/ excessive use of inhaled sympathomimetic drugs in patients w/ asthma. Caution w/ convulsive disorders, hyperthyroidism, and diabetes mellitus (DM), and in patients who are unusually responsive to sympathomimetic amines. May produce significant but usually transient hypokalemia. **Ipratropium:** May increase IOP and result in precipitation/worsening of narrow-angle glaucoma. May cause urinary retention; caution w/ prostatic hyperplasia or bladder-neck obstruction.

ADVERSE REACTIONS
Nasopharyngitis, cough, headache, bronchitis, URI, dyspnea.

DRUG INTERACTIONS
Potential for an additive interaction w/ other anticholinergic-containing drugs; avoid coadministration. Increased risk of adverse CV effects w/ other sympathomimetic agents; use w/ caution. β-blockers and albuterol inhibit the effect of each other; use β-blockers w/ caution in patients w/ hyperreactive airways. ECG changes and/or hypokalemia that may result from non-K$^+$-sparing diuretics (eg, loop or thiazide diuretics) may be acutely worsened; use w/ caution and consider monitoring K$^+$ levels. Administration w/ MAOIs or TCAs or w/in 2 weeks of discontinuation of such agents may potentiate the action of albuterol on CV system; use w/ extreme caution and consider alternative therapy.

PREGNANCY AND LACTATION
Pregnancy: Category C.
Lactation: Not for use in nursing.

MECHANISM OF ACTION
Ipratropium: Anticholinergic bronchodilator; appears to inhibit vagally mediated reflexes by antagonizing the action of acetylcholine. Prevents the increases in intracellular concentration of Ca^{2+}, which is caused by interaction of acetylcholine w/ the muscarinic receptors on bronchial smooth muscle. **Albuterol:** Selective β$_2$-adrenergic bronchodilator; activates β$_2$-receptors on airway smooth muscle, resulting in activation of protein kinase, which inhibits phosphorylation of myosin and lowers intracellular ionic Ca^{2+} concentrations, resulting in relaxation.

PHARMACOKINETICS
Absorption: Ipratropium: Not readily absorbed. C$_{max}$=33.5pg/mL. **Distribution:** Ipratropium: Plasma protein binding (0-9%). **Metabolism:** Ipratropium: Partial;

ester hydrolysis. Albuterol: Conjugation; albuterol 4'-O-sulfate (metabolite).
Elimination: Ipratropium: $T_{1/2}$=2 hrs.

PATIENT CONSIDERATIONS

Assessment: Assess for hypersensitivity to drug or to atropine or any of its derivatives, CV disorders, narrow-angle glaucoma, prostatic hyperplasia, bladder-neck obstruction, convulsive disorders, hyperthyroidism, DM, pregnancy/nursing status, and possible drug interactions. Assess if unusually responsive to sympathomimetic amines.

Monitoring: Monitor for signs/symptoms of hypersensitivity reactions, paradoxical bronchospasm, CV effects (measured by pulse rate and BP), hypokalemia, unexpected development of severe acute asthmatic crisis, hypoxia, and other adverse reactions.

Counseling: Instruct to use caution to avoid spraying the product into eyes. Instruct to consult physician if ocular symptoms or difficulty w/ urination develops. Instruct to exercise caution when engaging in activities requiring balance and visual acuity (eg, driving a car, operating appliances/machinery). Instruct not to increase dose or frequency w/o consulting physician. Instruct to seek immediate medical attention if therapy lessens in effectiveness, symptoms worsen, and/or product is needed more frequently than usual. Counsel to take other inhaled drugs only ud by physician. Counsel to d/c if paradoxical bronchospasm occurs. Inform of possible adverse effects (eg, palpitations, chest pain, rapid HR, tremor, nervousness). Instruct to contact physician if pregnant/nursing.

COMETRIQ — cabozantinib   Rx

Class: Kinase inhibitor

> GI perforations and fistulas reported; d/c if perforation or fistula develops. Severe, sometimes fatal, hemorrhage (eg, hemoptysis, GI hemorrhage) reported; monitor for signs and symptoms of bleeding. Do not administer w/ severe hemorrhage.

ADULT DOSAGE	PEDIATRIC DOSAGE
Medullary Thyroid Cancer	Pediatric use may not have been established
Progressive, Metastatic: 140mg (one 80mg and three 20mg caps) qd until disease progression or unacceptable toxicity occurs	

DOSING CONSIDERATIONS
Concomitant Medications
Strong CYP3A4 Inhibitors:
Reduce the daily dose by 40mg (eg, from 140mg to 100mg qd).
Resume the dose that was used prior to initiating the CYP3A4 inhibitor 2-3 days after discontinuation of the strong inhibitor.

Strong CYP3A4 Inducers:
Increase the daily dose by 40mg (eg, from 140mg to 180mg qd) as tolerated.
Resume the dose that was used prior to initiating the CYP3A4 inducer 2-3 days after discontinuation of the strong inducer.
Max: 180mg/day

Hepatic Impairment
Mild to Moderate:
Initial: 80mg
Severe: Not recommended

Adverse Reactions
Withhold for Any of the Following:
- NCI CTCAE Grade 4 hematologic adverse reactions
- Grade ≥3 nonhematologic adverse reactions
- Intolerable Grade 2 adverse reactions

Upon Improvement (eg, Return to Baseline or Resolution to Grade 1), Reduce as Follows:
- If previously receiving 140mg qd, resume at 100mg qd (one 80mg and one 20mg cap)
- If previously receiving 100mg qd, resume at 60mg qd (three 20mg caps)
- If previously receiving 60mg qd, resume at 60mg if tolerated, otherwise d/c

Permanently D/C for Any of the Following:
- Development of visceral perforation or fistula formation
- Severe hemorrhage
- Serious arterial thromboembolic event (eg, MI, cerebral infarction)
- Nephrotic syndrome
- Malignant HTN, hypertensive crisis, persistent uncontrolled HTN despite optimal medical management
- Osteonecrosis of the jaw (ONJ)
- Reversible posterior leukoencephalopathy syndrome (RPLS)

Other Important Considerations
Do not ingest foods (eg, grapefruit, grapefruit juice) or nutritional supplements that are known to inhibit CYP450 while on therapy

ADMINISTRATION
Oral route

Do not substitute Cometriq caps w/ cabozantinib tabs.
Do not take w/ food; do not eat for at least 2 hrs before and at least 1 hr after taking the dose.
Take w/ a full glass (at least 8 fl oz) of water.
Do not take a missed dose w/in 12 hrs of the next dose.
Swallow caps whole; do not open or crush the caps.

STORAGE
20-25°C (68-77°F); excursions are permitted from 15-30°C (59-86°F).

HOW SUPPLIED
Cap: 20mg, 80mg

WARNINGS/PRECAUTIONS
See Dosing Considerations. Avoid w/ recent history of hemorrhage or hemoptysis. Increased incidence of thrombotic events reported; d/c if an acute MI, cerebral infarction, or any other clinically significant arterial thromboembolic complication occurs. Wound complications reported; d/c at least 28 days prior to scheduled surgery; may resume therapy after surgery if wound healing is adequate. Withhold therapy in patients w/ dehiscence or wound healing complications requiring medical intervention. Increased incidence of HTN reported; withhold w/ uncontrolled HTN then resume at reduced dose when controlled. ONJ reported; d/c if ONJ occurs and withhold at least 28 days prior to invasive dental procedures. Palmar-plantar erythrodysesthesia syndrome (PPES) reported; withhold w/ intolerable Grade 2 PPES or Grade 3 PPES until improvement to Grade 1; resume at reduced dose. Proteinuria reported. RPLS reported; evaluate for RPLS in patients presenting w/ seizures, headache, visual disturbances, confusion, or altered mental function. May cause fetal harm; use effective contraception during and up to 4 months after completion of therapy.

ADVERSE REACTIONS
Diarrhea, stomatitis, PPES, decreased weight, decreased appetite, nausea, fatigue, oral pain, hair color changes, dysgeusia, HTN, abdominal pain, constipation, increased AST, increased ALT.

DRUG INTERACTIONS
See Dosing Considerations. Strong CYP3A4 inhibitors (eg, ketoconazole, itraconazole, clarithromycin) may increase exposure; avoid coadministration or reduce dose of cabozantinib if concomitant use cannot be avoided. Strong CYP3A4 inducers (eg, dexamethasone, phenytoin, carbamazepine) may decrease exposure; avoid chronic coadministration or increase dose of cabozantinib if concomitant use cannot be avoided. Avoid w/ foods (eg, grapefruits, grapefruit juice) or nutritional supplements known to inhibit CYP450 activity. MRP2 inhibitors (eg, abacavir, cidofovir, furosemide) may increase exposure; monitor for increased toxicity w/ concomitant MRP2 inhibitors.

PREGNANCY AND LACTATION
Pregnancy: May cause fetal harm.
Lactation: Not for use in nursing during treatment and for 4 months after the final dose.
Reproductive Potential: Females of reproductive potential should use effective contraception during treatment and for 4 months after the final dose. May impair fertility in females and males of reproductive potential.

MECHANISM OF ACTION
Kinase inhibitor; inhibits the tyrosine kinase activity of RET, MET, VEGFR-1, -2, and -3, KIT, TRKB, FLT-3, AXL, ROS1, TYRO3, MER, and TIE-2, involved in both normal cellular function and pathologic processes such as oncogenesis, metastasis, tumor angiogenesis, drug resistance, and maintenance of the tumor microenvironment.

PHARMACOKINETICS
Absorption: T_{max}=2-5 hrs. **Distribution:** V_d=349L; plasma protein binding (≥99.7%). **Metabolism:** Via CYP3A4. **Elimination:** Urine (27%), feces (54%; 43% unchanged); $T_{1/2}$=55 hrs.

PATIENT CONSIDERATIONS
Assessment: Assess for history of hemorrhage/hemoptysis, scheduled/recent surgery or invasive dental procedure, wounds, HTN, hepatic impairment, pregnancy/nursing status, and possible drug interactions. Obtain baseline BP and perform an oral examination.

Monitoring: Monitor for signs and symptoms of GI perforations and fistulas, hemorrhage, thrombotic events, dehiscence, wound healing complications, ONJ, PPES, nephrotic syndrome, RPLS (eg, seizures, headache, visual disturbances), and other adverse reactions. Monitor BP and urine protein regularly, and perform oral examinations periodically.

Counseling: Advise to notify physician if severe diarrhea, progressive or intolerable rash, mouth sores, oral pain, changes in taste, N/V, weight loss, or other adverse reactions occur. Instruct to contact physician prior to any planned surgeries, including dental procedures. Advise females of reproductive potential of the potential risk to fetus and instruct to contact physician if pregnancy occurs or is suspected during treatment. Instruct to use effective contraception during therapy and for at least 4 months after the last dose. Advise women not to breastfeed during treatment and for 4 months following the last dose. Instruct not to consume grapefruits or grapefruit juice while taking treatment.

COMPLERA — emtricitabine/rilpivirine/tenofovir disoproxil fumarate   Rx

Class: Non-nucleoside reverse transcriptase inhibitor (NNRTI)/nucleoside reverse transcriptase inhibitor (NRTI) combination

> Lactic acidosis and severe hepatomegaly w/ steatosis, including fatal cases, reported w/ the use of nucleoside analogues in combination w/ other antiretrovirals. Not approved for the treatment of chronic hepatitis B virus (HBV) infection. Severe acute exacerbations of hepatitis B reported in patients coinfected w/ HBV upon discontinuation of therapy; closely monitor hepatic function for at least several months. If appropriate, initiation of antihepatitis B therapy may be warranted.

ADULT DOSAGE
HIV-1 Infection

As a complete regimen for the treatment of HIV-1 infection in patients w/ no antiretroviral treatment history and w/ HIV-1 RNA ≤100,000 copies/mL at the start of therapy, and in certain virologically-suppressed (HIV-1 RNA <50 copies/mL) patients on a stable antiretroviral regimen at start of therapy

Recommended Dose: 1 tab qd

PEDIATRIC DOSAGE
HIV-1 Infection

As a complete regimen for the treatment of HIV-1 infection in patients w/ no antiretroviral treatment history and w/ HIV-1 RNA ≤100,000 copies/mL at the start of therapy, and in certain virologically-suppressed (HIV-1 RNA <50 copies/mL) patients on a stable antiretroviral regimen at start of therapy

≥12 Years:
≥35kg:
Recommended Dose: 1 tab qd

DOSING CONSIDERATIONS
Concomitant Medications
W/ Rifabutin: Additional 25mg tab of rilpivirine qd recommended to be taken concomitantly w/ Complera

Renal Impairment
Moderate or Severe (CrCl <50mL/min): Not recommended for use

ADMINISTRATION
Oral route

Take w/ food.

STORAGE
25°C (77°F); excursions permitted to 15-30°C (59-86°F).

HOW SUPPLIED
Tab: (Emtricitabine/Rilpivirine/Tenofovir Disoproxil Fumarate [TDF]) 200mg/25mg/300mg

CONTRAINDICATIONS
Coadministration w/ CYP3A inducers or agents that increase gastric pH causing decreased plasma concentrations, which may result in loss of virologic response and possible resistance (eg, carbamazepine, oxcarbazepine, phenobarbital, phenytoin, rifampin, rifapentine, proton pump inhibitors [eg, dexlansoprazole, esomeprazole, lansoprazole, omeprazole, pantoprazole, rabeprazole], systemic dexamethasone [more than a single dose], St. John's wort).

WARNINGS/PRECAUTIONS
When considering replacing the current regimen in virologically-suppressed patients, patients should have no history of virologic failure, have been stably suppressed for at least 6 months prior to switching therapy, currently be on the 1st or 2nd antiretroviral regimen prior to switching therapy, and have no current/past history of resistance to any of the 3 drug components. Additional monitoring of HIV-1 RNA and regimen tolerability is recommended after replacing therapy to assess for potential virologic failure or rebound. Immune reconstitution syndrome, autoimmune disorders (eg, Graves' disease, polymyositis, Guillain-Barre syndrome) in the setting of immune reconstitution, and redistribution/accumulation of body fat reported. Caution in elderly. **Rilpivirine:** Severe skin and hypersensitivity reactions reported, including cases of drug reaction w/ eosinophilia and systemic symptoms; d/c immediately and initiate appropriate therapy if signs/symptoms develop. Depressive disorders reported; immediate medical evaluation is recommended if severe depressive symptoms occur. Hepatic adverse events reported; increased risk for worsening/development of liver-associated test elevations in patients w/ underlying hepatitis B or C, or marked liver-associated test elevations prior to treatment. Consider liver-associated test monitoring for patients w/o preexisting hepatic dysfunction or other risk factors. **TDF:** Caution w/ known risk factors for liver disease. D/C if lactic acidosis or pronounced hepatotoxicity occurs. Renal impairment (eg, acute renal failure, Fanconi syndrome) reported. Decreased bone mineral density (BMD), increased biochemical markers of bone metabolism, and osteomalacia reported. Consider assessment of BMD in patients w/ history of pathologic bone fracture or other risk factors for osteoporosis or bone loss. Arthralgias and muscle pain/weakness reported in cases of proximal renal tubulopathy. Consider hypophosphatemia and osteomalacia secondary to proximal renal tubulopathy in patients at risk of renal dysfunction who present w/ persistent or worsening bone or muscle symptoms.

ADVERSE REACTIONS
Rilpivirine w/ Emtricitabine/TDF: Nausea, headache, dizziness, depressive disorders, insomnia, abnormal dreams, rash.
Emtricitabine/TDF: Diarrhea, nausea, fatigue, headache, dizziness, depression, insomnia, abnormal dreams, rash.

DRUG INTERACTIONS
See Dosing Considerations and Contraindications. Avoid w/ concurrent or recent use of nephrotoxic agents (eg, high-dose or multiple NSAIDs). Avoid administration w/ other antiretrovirals, adefovir dipivoxil, or drugs containing any of the same active components or lamivudine. Avoid w/ rilpivirine unless needed for dose adjustment (eg, w/ rifabutin). **Rilpivirine:** Caution w/ drugs that may reduce exposure or drugs w/ a known risk of torsades de pointes. Decreased levels, loss of virologic response, and possible resistance w/ CYP3A inducers or drugs increasing gastric pH (eg, antacids, H_2-receptor antagonists [H_2-RAs]). Administer antacids at least 2 hrs before or at least 4 hrs after dosing, and H_2-RAs at least 12 hrs before or at least 4 hrs after dosing. Decreased levels w/ rifabutin. CYP3A inhibitors, azole antifungals, clarithromycin, erythromycin, or telithromycin may increase levels. May decrease levels of ketoconazole and methadone. **Emtricitabine and TDF:** Drugs that reduce renal function or compete for active tubular secretion (eg, acyclovir, aminoglycosides [eg, gentamicin], high-dose or multiple NSAIDs) may increase levels of emtricitabine, TDF, and/or other renally eliminated drugs. **TDF:** Cases of acute renal failure after initiation of high-dose or multiple NSAIDs reported in HIV-infected patients w/ risk factors for renal dysfunction who appeared stable on TDF; consider alternatives to NSAIDs, if needed. Increased levels w/ ledipasvir/sofosbuvir; monitor for adverse reactions.

PREGNANCY AND LACTATION
Pregnancy: Category B. An Antiretroviral Pregnancy Registry has been established to monitor fetal outcomes of pregnant women.
Lactation: Emtricitabine and TDF are found in breast milk. Not for use in nursing.

MECHANISM OF ACTION
Emtricitabine: Nucleoside analogue of cytidine; inhibits activity of HIV-1 reverse transcriptase (RT) by competing w/ natural substrate deoxycytidine 5'-triphosphate and being incorporated into nascent viral DNA, resulting in chain termination. **Rilpivirine:** Non-nucleoside reverse transcriptase inhibitor; inhibits HIV-1 replication by noncompetitive inhibition of HIV-1 RT. **TDF:** Acyclic nucleoside phosphonate diester analogue of adenosine monophosphate; inhibits activity of HIV-1 RT by competing w/ the natural substrate deoxyadenosine 5'-triphosphate and, after incorporation into DNA, by DNA chain termination.

PHARMACOKINETICS
Absorption: Emtricitabine: Absolute bioavailability (93%), C_{max}=1.8mcg/mL, T_{max}=1-2 hrs, AUC=10mcg•hr/mL. Rilpivirine: T_{max}=4-5 hrs, AUC=2235ng•hr/mL. TDF: Bioavailability (25%, fasted), C_{max}=0.30mcg/mL, T_{max}=1 hr, AUC=2.29mcg•hr/mL. **Distribution:** Emtricitabine: Plasma protein binding (<4%); found in breast milk. Rilpivirine: Plasma protein binding (99.7%). TDF: Plasma protein binding (<0.7%); found in breast milk. **Metabolism:** Emtricitabine: 3'-sulfoxide diastereomers, glucuronic acid conjugate (metabolites). Rilpivirine: Oxidative metabolism by CYP3A system. **Elimination:** Emtricitabine: Feces (14%), urine (86%, 13% metabolites); $T_{1/2}$=10 hrs. Rilpivirine: Feces (85%, 25% unchanged), urine (6.1%, <1% unchanged); $T_{1/2}$=50 hrs. TDF: (IV) Urine (70-80% unchanged); $T_{1/2}$=17 hrs.

PATIENT CONSIDERATIONS
Assessment: Assess for history of virologic failure, current/past history of resistance to any of the drug components, obesity, prolonged nucleoside exposure, liver dysfunction or risk factors for liver disease, renal impairment, HBV infection, pregnancy/nursing status, and possible drug interactions. Assess BMD in patients w/ a history of pathological bone fracture or w/ other risk factors for osteoporosis/bone loss. Assess estimated CrCl, serum phosphorus (P), urine glucose, and urine protein in patients at risk for renal dysfunction.

Monitoring: Monitor for signs/symptoms of lactic acidosis, severe skin and hypersensitivity reactions, severe hepatomegaly w/ steatosis, depressive symptoms, hepatotoxicity, decreased BMD, increased biochemical markers for bone metabolism, osteomalacia, fat redistribution/accumulation, immune reconstitution syndrome (eg, opportunistic infections), autoimmune disorders, renal impairment, and other adverse reactions. Monitor patients coinfected w/ HBV and HIV-1 w/ clinical and lab follow-up for acute exacerbations of hepatitis B for at least several months upon discontinuation of therapy. Monitor estimated CrCl, serum P, urine glucose, and urine protein periodically in patients at risk for renal dysfunction. Additional monitoring of HIV-1 RNA and regimen tolerability is recommended after replacing therapy to assess for potential virologic failure or rebound.

Counseling: Inform that therapy is not a cure for HIV infection; advise that continuous therapy is necessary to control HIV infection and decrease HIV-related illnesses. Advise to practice safer sex and use latex or polyurethane condoms. Inform that there is a pregnancy exposure registry to monitor outcomes in women exposed to therapy during pregnancy. Instruct to never reuse or share needles. Advise not to breastfeed. Advise to take on a regular dosing schedule w/ food and avoid missing doses. Inform that a protein drink is not a substitute for food. Advise on missed dose instructions. Instruct to contact physician if symptoms of lactic acidosis or severe hepatomegaly w/ steatosis, depression, or infection occurs. Inform that hepatotoxicity has been reported during treatment. Instruct to immediately stop taking therapy and seek medical attention if patient develops a rash associated w/ any of the following symptoms: fever; blisters; mucosal involvement; eye inflammation (conjunctivitis); severe allergic reaction causing swelling of the face, eyes, lips, mouth, tongue, or throat; and any signs/symptoms of liver problems. Inform that laboratory tests will be performed and appropriate therapy will be initiated if severe rash occurs. Inform that fat redistribution/accumulation, renal impairment, and decreases in BMD may occur. Advise to inform physician if taking any other prescription/nonprescription medications or herbal products (eg, St. John's wort).

COMTAN — entacapone   Rx
Class: COMT inhibitor

ADULT DOSAGE
Parkinson's Disease

Adjunct to levodopa and carbidopa to treat end-of-dose "wearing-off"

Recommended: 200mg w/ each levodopa and carbidopa dose
Max: 1600mg/day

May need to reduce daily levodopa dose or extend the interval between doses

PEDIATRIC DOSAGE
Pediatric use may not have been established

ADMINISTRATION
Oral route

Take w/ or w/o food.
May be combined w/ both immediate- and sustained-release formulations of levodopa and carbidopa.

STORAGE
25°C (77°F); excursions permitted to 15-30°C (59-86°F).

HOW SUPPLIED
Tab: 200mg

CONTRAINDICATIONS
Hypersensitivity to the drug or its ingredients.

WARNINGS/PRECAUTIONS
Falling asleep during activities of daily living and somnolence reported; d/c if daytime sleepiness or episodes of falling asleep during activities that require active participation develop. May impair mental/physical abilities. Orthostatic hypotension/syncope and hallucinations reported. New/worsening mental status and behavioral changes, which may be severe, including psychotic-like behavior, may occur; do not use in patients w/ a major psychotic disorder. Increased sexual urges, intense urges to gamble or spend money, and other intense urges, and the inability to control these urges, may occur; consider dose reduction or discontinuation if such urges develop. Diarrhea and colitis reported; d/c therapy and consider appropriate medical therapy if prolonged diarrhea is suspected to be related to therapy. May cause/exacerbate preexisting dyskinesia. Severe rhabdomyolysis reported. Retroperitoneal fibrosis, pulmonary infiltrates, pleural effusion, and pleural thickening reported w/ ergot-derived dopaminergic agents. May increase risk of developing melanoma. Caution w/ hepatic impairment (eg, biliary obstruction). Rapid withdrawal or abrupt dose reduction may lead to emergence of signs and symptoms of Parkinson's disease, and may lead to hyperpyrexia and confusion, a symptom complex resembling the neuroleptic malignant syndrome (NMS); when discontinuing, closely monitor patients and adjust other dopaminergic treatments prn, and withdraw slowly.

ADVERSE REACTIONS
Dyskinesia, N/V, hyperkinesia, urine discoloration, diarrhea, abdominal pain, dry mouth.

DRUG INTERACTIONS
Avoid w/ nonselective MAOIs (eg, phenelzine, tranylcypromine). Caution w/ drugs metabolized by COMT (eg, isoproterenol, epinephrine, norepinephrine); increased HR, possible arrhythmias, and excessive changes in BP may occur. Caution w/ concomitant use of sedating medications; may increase the risk for drowsiness. Certain medications used to treat psychosis may decrease effectiveness. May potentiate dopaminergic side effects of levodopa. Increased INR w/ warfarin reported; monitor INR when entacapone is initiated or when the dose is increased. Caution w/ drugs known to interfere w/ biliary excretion, glucuronidation, and intestinal β-glucuronidase (eg, probenecid, cholestyramine, erythromycin).

PREGNANCY AND LACTATION
Pregnancy: Category C.
Lactation: It is not known whether entacapone is excreted in human milk. Caution in nursing.

MECHANISM OF ACTION
COMT inhibitor; inhibits COMT and alters the plasma pharmacokinetics of levodopa.

PHARMACOKINETICS
Absorption: Rapid. Absolute bioavailability (35%); C_{max}=1.2mcg/mL; T_{max}=1 hr. **Distribution:** Plasma protein binding (98%); (IV) V_d=20L. **Metabolism:** Isomerization to *cis*-isomer, and direct glucuronidation of the parent drug and *cis*-isomer. **Elimination:** Urine (10%, 0.2% unchanged), feces (90%); $T_{1/2}$=0.4-0.7 hrs (β-phase), 2.4 hrs (gamma-phase).

PATIENT CONSIDERATIONS

Assessment: Assess for hypersensitivity to drug, major psychotic disorder, sleep disorder, dyskinesia, hepatic impairment, biliary obstruction, pregnancy/nursing status, and possible drug interactions.

Monitoring: Monitor for drowsiness/sleepiness, orthostatic hypotension, hallucinations, new/worsening mental status and behavioral changes, psychotic-like behavior, intense urges, diarrhea, dyskinesia, rhabdomyolysis, a symptom complex resembling NMS, retroperitoneal fibrosis, pulmonary infiltrates, pleural effusion, pleural thickening, and other adverse reactions. Monitor for melanomas frequently and on a regular basis; perform periodic skin exams. Monitor INR w/ warfarin.

Counseling: Instruct to take drug only as prescribed. Inform that postural hypotension, hallucinations, psychotic-like behavior, nausea, diarrhea, increased dyskinesia, and change in urine color (brownish orange discoloration) may occur. Caution against rising rapidly after sitting or lying down, especially for prolonged periods, and especially at the initiation of treatment. Instruct not to drive a car or operate other complex machinery until patient is aware of how medication affects mental and/or motor performance. Warn about possibility of sudden onset of sleep during daily activities. Advise to inform physician if unusual urges or behaviors develop. Instruct to notify physician if pregnant/breastfeeding or intending to become pregnant or to breastfeed.

CONCERTA — methylphenidate hydrochloride   CII

Class: CNS stimulant

> Caution w/ history of drug dependence or alcoholism. Chronic abusive use may lead to marked tolerance and psychological dependence w/ varying degrees of abnormal behavior. Frank psychotic episodes may occur, especially w/ parenteral abuse. Careful supervision is required during withdrawal from abusive use since severe depression may occur. Withdrawal following chronic use may unmask symptoms of underlying disorder that may require follow-up.

ADULT DOSAGE
Attention-Deficit Hyperactivity Disorder
18-65 Years:
New to Methylphenidate:
Initial: 18mg or 36mg qam
Range: 18-72mg/day

Currently on Methylphenidate:
Initial:
18mg qam if previous dose 5mg bid-tid
36mg qam if previous dose 10mg bid-tid
54mg qam if previous dose 15mg bid-tid
72mg qam if previous dose 20mg bid-tid
Conversion dosage should not exceed 72mg/day

Titrate: May increase in 18mg increments at weekly intervals if optimal response is not achieved at a lower dose

Max: 72mg/day

Maint/Extended Treatment:
Periodically reevaluate the long-term usefulness of the drug

D/C if no improvement observed after appropriate dosage adjustment over 1 month

PEDIATRIC DOSAGE
Attention-Deficit Hyperactivity Disorder
New to Methylphenidate:
6-12 Years:
Initial: 18mg qam
Range: 18-54mg/day
13-17 Years:
Initial: 18mg qam
Range: 18-72mg/day not to exceed 2mg/kg/day

Currently on Methylphenidate:
≥6 Years:
Initial:
18mg qam if previous dose 5mg bid-tid
36mg qam if previous dose 10mg bid-tid
54mg qam if previous dose 15mg bid-tid
72mg qam if previous dose 20mg bid-tid
Conversion dosage should not exceed 72mg/day

Titrate: May increase in 18mg increments at weekly intervals if optimal response is not achieved at a lower dose

Max:
6-12 Years: 54mg/day
13-17 Years: 72mg/day

Maint/Extended Treatment:
Periodically reevaluate the long-term usefulness of the drug

D/C if no improvement observed after appropriate dosage adjustment over 1 month

---

DOSING CONSIDERATIONS
Adverse Reactions
Reduce dose or, if necessary, d/c if paradoxical aggravation of symptoms or other adverse events occur

ADMINISTRATION
Oral route

Take w/ or w/o food.
Swallow tab whole w/ the aid of liquids; do not chew, divide, or crush.

STORAGE
25°C (77°F); excursions permitted to 15-30°C (59-86°F). Protect from humidity.

HOW SUPPLIED
Tab, Extended-Release: 18mg, 27mg, 36mg, 54mg

CONTRAINDICATIONS
Hypersensitivity to methylphenidate or other components of the medication; marked anxiety, tension, and agitation; glaucoma; motor tics or family history or diagnosis of Tourette's syndrome. Treatment w/ MAOIs or w/in a minimum of 14 days following discontinuation of an MAOI.

WARNINGS/PRECAUTIONS
Avoid w/ known serious structural cardiac abnormalities, cardiomyopathy, serious heart rhythm abnormalities, coronary artery disease, or other serious cardiac problems. Sudden death reported in children and adolescents w/ structural cardiac abnormalities or other serious heart problems. Sudden deaths, stroke, and MI reported in adults. May increase BP and HR; caution w/ conditions that might be compromised by increases in BP/HR (eg, preexisting HTN, heart failure, recent MI, ventricular arrhythmia). Prior to treatment, obtain medical history (including assessment for family history of sudden death or ventricular arrhythmia) and perform physical exam to assess for presence of cardiac disease. Promptly perform cardiac evaluation if symptoms of cardiac disease develop. May exacerbate symptoms of behavior disturbance and thought disorder in patients w/ preexisting psychotic disorder. Caution in patients w/ comorbid bipolar disorder; may induce mixed/manic episode. May cause treatment-emergent psychotic or manic symptoms (eg, hallucinations, delusional thinking, mania) in patients w/o prior history of psychotic illness or mania; consider discontinuation if such symptoms occur. Aggressive behavior or hostility reported. May lower convulsive threshold; d/c if seizures occur. Priapism reported; seek immediate medical attention if abnormally sustained or frequent and painful erections develop. Associated w/ peripheral vasculopathy (eg, Raynaud's phenomenon); carefully observe for digital changes. May cause long-term suppression of growth in children; monitor growth, and may need to interrupt treatment in patients not growing or gaining height or weight as expected. Difficulties w/ accommodation and blurring of vision reported. Tab is nondeformable and does not appreciably change in shape in the GI tract; avoid w/ preexisting severe GI narrowing (pathologic or iatrogenic).

ADVERSE REACTIONS
Children and Adolescents: Upper abdominal pain.
Adults: Decreased appetite, headache, dry mouth, nausea, insomnia, anxiety, dizziness, weight decreased, irritability, hyperhidrosis.

DRUG INTERACTIONS

See Contraindications. Caution w/ vasopressor agents. May inhibit metabolism of coumarin anticoagulants, anticonvulsants (eg, phenobarbital, phenytoin, primidone), and some antidepressants (eg, TCAs, SSRIs); downward dose adjustment and monitoring of plasma drug concentrations (or coagulation times for coumarin) of these drugs may be necessary when initiating or discontinuing methylphenidate.

PREGNANCY AND LACTATION

Pregnancy: Category C.
Lactation: Caution in nursing.

MECHANISM OF ACTION

CNS stimulant. Has not been established; thought to block the reuptake of norepinephrine and dopamine into the presynaptic neuron and increase the release of these monoamines into the extraneuronal space.

PHARMACOKINETICS

Absorption: Readily absorbed. T_{max}=6-10 hrs. (Single-dose [18mg qd]) AUC=41.8ng•hr/mL; C_{max}=3.7ng/mL. **Metabolism:** Via deesterification; α-phenyl-piperidine acetic acid [PPAA] (metabolite). **Elimination:** Urine (90%, approx 80% PPAA); $T_{1/2}$=3.5 hrs.

PATIENT CONSIDERATIONS

Assessment: Assess for hypersensitivity to the drug, marked anxiety, tension, agitation, glaucoma, motor tics, family history or diagnosis of Tourette's syndrome, cardiovascular conditions, history of drug dependence or alcoholism, psychotic disorder, comorbid bipolar disorder, severe GI narrowing, any other conditions where treatment is contraindicated or cautioned, pregnancy/nursing status, and possible drug interactions. Obtain baseline height/weight in children.

Monitoring: Monitor for changes in HR and BP, signs/symptoms of cardiac disease, exacerbation of behavior disturbance and thought disorder, psychosis, mania, appearance of or worsening of aggressive behavior or hostility, seizures, priapism, peripheral vasculopathy (eg, Raynaud's phenomenon), visual disturbances, and other adverse reactions. In pediatric patients, monitor growth. Perform periodic monitoring of CBC, differential, and platelet counts during prolonged therapy. Periodically reevaluate long-term usefulness of drug.

Counseling: Inform about risks, benefits, and appropriate use of the medication. Advise of the possibility of priapism; instruct to seek immediate medical attention in the event of priapism. Inform about the risk of peripheral vasculopathy (eg, Raynaud's phenomenon); instruct to report to physician any new numbness, pain, skin color change, sensitivity to temperature in fingers or toes, or any signs of unexplained wounds appearing on fingers/toes. Advise that the tab shell, along w/ insoluble core components, is eliminated from the body; inform not to be concerned if something that looks like a tab is noticed in the stool. Inform that therapy may impair mental/physical abilities; advise to use caution w/ hazardous tasks (eg, operating machinery, driving).

CONTRAVE — bupropion hydrochloride/naltrexone hydrochloride   Rx

Class: Aminoketone/opioid antagonist

Not approved for use in the treatment of major depressive disorder or other psychiatric disorders. Contains bupropion, the same active ingredient as some other antidepressants (including, but not limited to, Wellbutrin, Wellbutrin SR/XL, and Aplenzin). Antidepressants increased the risk of suicidal thoughts and behavior in children, adolescents, and young adults in short-term trials. Monitor closely for worsening and for the emergence of suicidal thoughts and behaviors. Not approved for use in pediatric patients. Serious neuropsychiatric reactions reported in patients taking bupropion for smoking cessation. Although not approved for smoking cessation, observe all patients for neuropsychiatric reactions.

ADULT DOSAGE

Chronic Weight Management

Adjunct to a reduced-calorie diet and increased physical activity in patients w/ BMI ≥30kg/m², or ≥27kg/m² in the presence of at least 1 weight-related comorbid condition

Week 1: 1 tab qam
Week 2: 1 tab qam and 1 tab qpm
Week 3: 2 tabs qam and 1 tab qpm
Week 4 Onward/Maint: 2 tabs qam and 2 tabs qpm
Max: (32mg/360mg)/day (2 tabs bid)

Evaluate response to therapy after 12 weeks at the maint dose; d/c if patient has not lost at least 5% of baseline weight

Dosing Considerations with MAOIs

Switching to or from an MAOI Antidepressant:

Allow at least 14 days to elapse between discontinuation of an MAOI and initiation of treatment, and conversely allow at least 14 days after discontinuing treatment before starting an MAOI

PEDIATRIC DOSAGE

Pediatric use may not have been established

DOSING CONSIDERATIONS

Concomitant Medications

CYP2B6 Inhibitors:
Max: 2 tabs/day (1 tab qam and qpm)

Renal Impairment

Mild:
There is a lack of adequate information to guide dosing

Moderate/Severe:
Max: 2 tabs/day (1 tab qam and qpm)

ESRD: Not recommended

Hepatic Impairment

Max: 1 tab qam

ADMINISTRATION

Oral route

Take no more than 2 tabs at 1 time.
May take w/ meals; avoid high-fat meals.
Swallow tab whole; do not cut, chew, or crush.

STORAGE

25°C (77°F); excursions permitted to 15-30°C (59-86°F).

HOW SUPPLIED

Tab, Extended-Release: (Naltrexone/Bupropion) 8mg/90mg

CONTRAINDICATIONS

Uncontrolled HTN, seizure disorder or a history of seizures, use of other bupropion-containing products, bulimia or anorexia nervosa, chronic opioid or opiate agonist (eg, methadone) or partial agonists (eg, buprenorphine) use, acute opiate withdrawal, and pregnancy. Undergoing abrupt discontinuation of alcohol, benzodiazepines, barbiturates, and antiepileptic drugs (AEDs). Concomitant administration of MAOIs; allow at least 14 days to elapse between discontinuation of an MAOI and initiation of treatment. Starting treatment in a patient treated w/ reversible MAOIs (eg, linezolid, IV methylene blue). Known allergy to bupropion, naltrexone, or any other component of this medication.

WARNINGS/PRECAUTIONS

Weight loss may increase risk of hypoglycemia in patients w/ type 2 diabetes mellitus (DM) treated w/ insulin and/or insulin secretagogues (eg, sulfonylureas, meglitinides); consider decreasing doses of antidiabetic medications that are non-glucose-dependent to mitigate the risk of hypoglycemia. Appropriate changes should be made to antidiabetic regimen if hypoglycemia develops after starting treatment. Not recommended in patients w/ ESRD. Caution in elderly (>65 yrs of age). **Bupropion:** Dose-related risk of seizures; do not exceed 360mg of bupropion component (4 tabs/day in divided doses [bid]), and escalate dose gradually. D/C and do not restart if seizure occurs while on therapy. Caution w/ predisposing factors that may increase risk of seizure (eg, history of head trauma or prior seizure, severe stroke, arteriovenous malformation, CNS tumor/infection, metabolic disorders [eg, hypoglycemia, hyponatremia, severe hepatic impairment, hypoxia]). May cause an increase in systolic and/or diastolic BP as well as increase in resting HR. Anaphylactoid/anaphylactic reactions reported; d/c treatment if an allergic or anaphylactoid/anaphylactic reaction occurs. Arthralgia, myalgia, fever w/ rash, and other symptoms suggestive of delayed hypersensitivity reported. May precipitate a manic/mixed/hypomanic episode; risk is increased in patients w/ or at risk for bipolar disorder. Pupillary dilation may occur and may trigger an angle-closure attack in a patient w/ anatomically narrow angles who does not have a patent iridectomy. False (+) urine immunoassay screening tests for amphetamines reported. **Naltrexone:** Cases of hepatitis, clinically significant liver dysfunction, and transient, asymptomatic hepatic transaminase elevations reported; d/c in the event of symptoms and/or signs of acute hepatitis.

ADVERSE REACTIONS

N/V, constipation, headache, dizziness, insomnia, dry mouth, diarrhea.

DRUG INTERACTIONS

See Dosage and Contraindications. In patients requiring intermittent opiate treatment, d/c Contrave temporarily and do not increase opioid dose above standard dose; use w/ caution after chronic opioid use has been stopped for 7-10 days to prevent precipitation of withdrawal. May increase levels of drugs transported by the renal organic cation transporter 2 (eg, amantadine, cimetidine, famotidine, metformin); use w/ caution and monitor for adverse effects. **Bupropion:** Increased risk for hypertensive reactions w/ other drugs that inhibit the reuptake of dopamine or norepinephrine, including MAOIs. Caution w/ CYP2D6 substrates (eg, SSRIs, haloperidol, metoprolol, propafenone); initiate the CYP2D6 substrate at the lower end of the dosing range. If Contrave is added to the treatment regimen of a patient already receiving a CYP2D6 substrate, consider the need to decrease the dose of the original medication, particularly for medications w/ a narrow therapeutic index. CYP2B6 inhibitors (eg, ticlopidine, clopidogrel) may increase bupropion exposure but decrease hydroxybupropion exposure. Ritonavir, lopinavir, or efavirenz may decrease bupropion and hydroxybupropion exposure; avoid concomitant use. Extreme caution w/ other drugs that lower the seizure threshold (eg, antipsychotics, antidepressants, theophylline, systemic corticosteroids); use low initial doses and gradually increase dose. CNS toxicity reported w/ levodopa or amantadine; caution and monitor for adverse events when administered concomitantly. Caution w/ excessive use of alcohol or sedatives, addiction to cocaine or stimulants, withdrawal from sedatives, and diabetics treated w/ insulin/oral diabetic medications; may increase risk of seizures. Adverse neuropsychiatric events or reduced alcohol tolerance reported (rarely) w/ alcohol; minimize or avoid alcohol.

PREGNANCY AND LACTATION

Pregnancy: Category X.
Lactation: Not for use in nursing.

MECHANISM OF ACTION
Bupropion: Aminoketone; not established. Weak inhibitor of the neuronal reuptake of norepinephrine and dopamine. **Naltrexone:** Opioid antagonist; not established.

PHARMACOKINETICS
Absorption: Naltrexone: C_{max}=1.4ng/mL, AUC_{0-inf}=8.4ng•hr/mL, T_{max}=2 hrs. Bupropion: C_{max}=168ng/mL, AUC_{0-inf}=1607ng•hr/mL, T_{max}=3 hrs. **Distribution:** Found in breast milk. Naltrexone: V_d=5697L; plasma protein binding (21%). Bupropion: V_d=880L; plasma protein binding (84%). **Metabolism:** Naltrexone: 6-β-naltrexol (major metabolite). Bupropion: Extensive; via CYP2B6; hydroxybupropion, threohydrobupropion, and erythrohydrobupropion (active metabolites). **Elimination:** Naltrexone: Urine (53-79%, <2% unchanged, 43% unchanged and conjugated 6-β-naltrexol), feces (minor); $T_{1/2}$=5 hrs. Bupropion: Urine (87%) feces (10%), (0.5% unchanged); $T_{1/2}$=21 hrs.

PATIENT CONSIDERATIONS
Assessment: Assess for known allergy to drug, uncontrolled HTN, seizure disorder or conditions that may increase risk of seizure, bipolar disorder, susceptibility to angle-closure glaucoma, renal/hepatic impairment, pregnancy/nursing status, any conditions where treatment is contraindicated or cautioned, and possible drug interactions. Measure blood glucose levels in patients w/ type 2 DM. Obtain baseline BP and pulse.

Monitoring: Monitor for clinical worsening, suicidality, or unusual changes in behavior, seizures, neuropsychiatric signs/symptoms, increase in BP and HR, allergic reactions, angle-closure glaucoma, and other adverse reactions. Monitor blood glucose levels in patients w/ type 2 DM. Monitor hepatic/renal function.

Counseling: Inform of benefits/risks of therapy. Advise to take exactly as prescribed. Inform that drug contains the same ingredient found in certain antidepressants and smoking cessation products; instruct not to use in combination w/ other bupropion-containing products. Advise patients and caregivers of need for close observation for clinical worsening and suicidal risks; instruct to immediately report to physician any agitation, hostility, depressed mood, or changes in thinking or behavior that are not typical for them, or if suicidal ideation or behavior develops. Inform that drug may cause mild pupillary dilation, which in susceptible individuals may lead to an episode of angle-closure glaucoma. Inform of the symptoms of hypersensitivity; instruct to d/c therapy if a severe allergic reaction occurs. Instruct to d/c and not restart if a seizure is experienced while on treatment. Inform that excessive use or abrupt discontinuation of alcohol, benzodiazepines, AEDs, or sedatives/hypnotics can increase the risk of seizures. Instruct to minimize or avoid alcohol. Advise patients that they may be more sensitive to lower doses of opioids if they previously used opioids, and may be at risk of accidental overdose should they use opioids after treatment is discontinued or temporarily interrupted. Advise patients that because naltrexone can block the effects of opioids, they will not perceive any effect if they attempt to self-administer any opioid drug in small doses while on therapy and that the attempt to administer large doses of any opioid or to bypass the blockade while on therapy may lead to serious injury, coma, or death. Advise patients not to take medication if they have any symptoms of opioid withdrawal. Advise patients to notify healthcare provider if they experience increased BP or HR. Instruct to notify physician if taking/planning to take any prescription or OTC drugs. Instruct to inform physician if pregnant, intending to become pregnant, or if breastfeeding during therapy. Advise diabetic patients on antidiabetic therapy to monitor their blood glucose levels and to report symptoms of hypoglycemia to physician. If a dose is missed, instruct to wait until the next scheduled dose to resume the regular dosing schedule.

CONZIP — tramadol hydrochloride   CIV
Class: Centrally acting analgesic

ADULT DOSAGE
Moderate to Moderately Severe Pain

Chronic Pain Requiring Around-The-Clock Treatment for an Extended Period:

Not Currently on Tramadol Immediate-Release (IR):
Initial: 100mg qd
Titrate: Increase as necessary by 100mg increments every 5 days to achieve a balance between pain relief and tolerability
Max: 300mg/day

Currently on Tramadol IR:
Initial: Calculate 24-hr tramadol IR dose and initiate total daily dose rounded down to the next lowest 100mg increment
Maint: Individualize according to patient need

PEDIATRIC DOSAGE
Pediatric use may not have been established

DOSING CONSIDERATIONS
Renal Impairment
Severe (CrCl <30mL/min): Do not use

Hepatic Impairment
Severe (Child-Pugh Class C): Do not use

Elderly
≥65 Years:
Initiate dose cautiously; start at lower end of dosing range

>75 Years:
Use greater caution

ADMINISTRATION
Oral route

Administer at the same time every day w/o regard to food
Swallow whole w/ liquid; do not split, chew, dissolve, or crush

STORAGE
25°C (77°F); excursions permitted to 15-30°C (59-86°F).

HOW SUPPLIED
Cap, Extended-Release: 100mg, 200mg, 300mg

CONTRAINDICATIONS
Previous hypersensitivity to tramadol, any other component of drug, or to opioids. Significant respiratory depression, acute/severe bronchial asthma, or hypercapnia in unmonitored settings or absence of resuscitative equipment.

WARNINGS/PRECAUTIONS
Seizures reported; risk increases in patients with epilepsy, history of seizures, risk of seizures (eg, head trauma, metabolic disorders, alcohol/drug withdrawal, CNS infections). Anaphylactoid reactions and potentially life-threatening serotonin syndrome may occur. Avoid in patients who are suicidal or addiction prone and in patients with history of anaphylactoid reactions to codeine and other opioids. Caution in patients with history of misuse and who suffer from emotional disturbances or depression. Caution if at risk for respiratory depression; consider alternative nonopioid analgesic. Caution with increased intracranial pressure (ICP) or head injury, and in elderly. May impair mental/physical abilities. Do not d/c abruptly; withdrawal symptoms may occur. May increase the risk of misuse, abuse, or diversion. May complicate clinical assessment of acute abdominal conditions. Risk of overdosage (eg, CNS/respiratory depression, and death); maintain adequate ventilation with general supportive treatment when treating an overdose. Avoid with severe renal impairment (CrCl <30mL/min) and severe hepatic impairment (Child-Pugh Class C).

ADVERSE REACTIONS
N/V, headache, constipation, somnolence, dizziness, dry mouth, asthenia, pruritus, sweating, anorexia, arthralgia, insomnia.

DRUG INTERACTIONS
Use caution and reduce dose with CNS depressants (eg, alcohol, opioids, anesthetics, narcotics, phenothiazines, tranquilizers, sedative hypnotics); increased risk of CNS/respiratory depression. Avoid alcohol-containing beverages. CYP2D6 inhibitors (eg, quinidine, fluoxetine, paroxetine, amitriptyline) and CYP3A4 inhibitors (eg, ketoconazole, erythromycin) may reduce metabolic clearance and increase risk of serious adverse events (eg, seizures and serotonin syndrome). Increased seizure risk with SSRI/SNRI antidepressants or anorectics, TCAs, other tricyclic compounds (eg, cyclobenzaprine, promethazine), other opioids, MAOIs, neuroleptics, and drugs that reduce seizure threshold. Serotonin syndrome may occur with SSRIs, SNRIs, TCAs, MAOIs, triptans, drugs that impair metabolism of serotonin (eg, MAOI), α_2-adrenergic blockers, or drugs that impair tramadol metabolism (CYP2D6 and CYP3A4 inhibitors). Caution with other drugs that may affect the serotonergic neurotransmitter system (eg, SSRIs, MAOIs, triptans, linezolid, lithium, St. John's wort); monitor carefully, especially during initiation and dose increase. Not recommended with carbamazepine; may decrease analgesic efficacy. Possible digoxin toxicity and altered warfarin effects. May reduce exposure with CYP3A4 inducers (eg, carbamazepine, rifampin, St. John's wort). In drug overdose, naloxone administration may increase the risk of seizure. Use with other tramadol products not recommended.

PREGNANCY AND LACTATION
Category C, not for use in nursing.

MECHANISM OF ACTION
Centrally acting synthetic opioid analgesic; not established. Suspected to be due to binding of parent and M1 metabolite to μ-opioid receptors and weak inhibition of norepinephrine and serotonin reuptake.

PHARMACOKINETICS
Absorption: (Fasted) C_{max}=308ng/mL; AUC=6777ng•hr/mL; T_{max}=10-12 hrs. **Distribution:** (IV) V_d=2.6L/kg (male), 2.9L/kg (female); plasma protein binding (20%); crosses the placenta. **Metabolism:** Extensive via CYP2D6, 3A4 and 2B6; N- and O-demethylation and glucuronidation or sulfation (major pathway); M1 (active metabolite). **Elimination:** Urine (30% unchanged, 60% as metabolites); $T_{1/2}$=10 hrs, 11 hrs (M1).

PATIENT CONSIDERATIONS
Assessment: Assess for previous hypersensitivity to the drug and other opioids, respiratory depression, bronchial asthma, hypercapnia, epilepsy, history of seizures, head trauma, metabolic disorders, alcohol and drug withdrawal, CNS infections, suicidal or addiction proneness, emotional disturbance, depression, increased ICP, pain intensity, drug abuse potential, renal/hepatic impairment, pregnancy/nursing status, and possible drug interactions.

Monitoring: Monitor for anaphylactoid reactions, respiratory/CNS depression, physical dependence/abuse, misuse, seizures, development of serotonin syndrome, elevations in CSF pressure, pupillary changes, withdrawal symptoms, and other adverse reactions.

Counseling: Inform that drug may impair physical/mental abilities; instruct to use caution when driving or operating machinery. Advise that seizures and/or serotonin syndrome may occur with concomitant use of serotonergic agents or drugs that significantly reduce the metabolic clearance of therapy. Instruct not to take drug with alcohol-containing beverages. Tell to use drug with caution when taking tranquilizers, hypnotics, or opiate-containing analgesics. Instruct to notify physician if pregnant/nursing or planning to become pregnant. Educate about single-dose and 24-hr dosing limits and time interval between doses; advise not to exceed the recommended dose. Advise not to abruptly withdraw or d/c therapy.

COPAXONE — glatiramer acetate   Rx

Class: Immunomodulatory agent

ADULT DOSAGE

Multiple Sclerosis

Relapsing Forms:
20mg/mL: Administer SQ qd
40mg/mL: Administer SQ 3X/week and at least 48 hrs apart

20mg/mL and 40mg/mL are not interchangeable

PEDIATRIC DOSAGE

Pediatric use may not have been established

ADMINISTRATION

SQ route

Allow to stand at room temperature for 20 min before administration.
Areas for SQ self-inj include arms, abdomen, hips, and thighs.

STORAGE

2-8°C (36-46°F). If needed, may store at 15-30°C (59-86°F) for up to 1 month, but refrigeration is preferred; avoid exposure to higher temperatures or intense light. Do not freeze; discard if frozen.

HOW SUPPLIED

Inj: 20mg/mL, 40mg/mL

CONTRAINDICATIONS

Known hypersensitivity to glatiramer acetate or mannitol.

WARNINGS/PRECAUTIONS

Immediate post-inj reaction (eg, flushing, chest pain, palpitations, anxiety, dyspnea, throat constriction, urticaria) reported. Transient chest pain reported. Localized lipoatrophy at inj sites and inj-site skin necrosis may occur; follow proper inj technique and rotate inj sites w/ each inj. May interfere w/ immune functions. Continued alteration of cellular immunity due to chronic treatment may result in untoward effects.

ADVERSE REACTIONS

Inj-site reactions, vasodilatation, rash, dyspnea, chest pain.

PREGNANCY AND LACTATION

Pregnancy: Category B.
Lactation: Caution in nursing.

MECHANISM OF ACTION

Immunomodulatory agent; not established. Thought to act by modifying immune processes that are believed to be responsible for the pathogenesis of multiple sclerosis (MS).

PATIENT CONSIDERATIONS

Assessment: Assess for hypersensitivity to drug or mannitol, and pregnancy/nursing status.

Monitoring: Monitor for immediate post-inj reactions, chest pain, lipoatrophy, inj-site skin necrosis, and other adverse reactions.

Counseling: Advise to inform physician if pregnant, planning to become pregnant, or breastfeeding. Inform that drug may cause an immediate post-inj reaction and that symptoms are generally transient and self-limited and do not require specific treatment; inform that these symptoms may occur early or may have their onset several months after treatment initiation. Inform that transient chest pain (either as part of the immediate post-inj reaction or in isolation) may occur; advise to seek medical attention if chest pain of unusual duration or intensity occurs. Instruct to follow proper inj technique and to rotate inj areas and sites w/ each inj to help minimize localized lipoatrophy and inj-site necrosis. Inform that 20mg/mL and 40mg/mL are not interchangeable. Advise to use aseptic technique. Caution against the reuse of needles or syringes. Inform of safe disposal procedures.

CORDARONE — amiodarone hydrochloride   Rx

Class: Class III antiarrhythmic

Use only in patients w/ the indicated life-threatening arrhythmias because of potentially fatal toxicities, including pulmonary toxicity (hypersensitivity pneumonitis or interstitial/alveolar pneumonitis). Liver injury is common, usually mild, and evidenced only by abnormal liver enzymes. Overt liver disease may occur, and has been fatal. May exacerbate arrhythmia. Significant heart block or sinus bradycardia reported. Amiodarone poses major management problems that could be life threatening in a population at risk of sudden death, even in patients at high risk of arrhythmic death in whom the toxicity of amiodarone is an acceptable risk; every effort should be made to utilize alternative agents first. Patients must be hospitalized while LD is given, and a response generally requires at least 1 week, usually 2 or more. Maintenance-dose selection is difficult and may require dosage decrease or discontinuation of treatment.

ADULT DOSAGE

Ventricular Tachycardia

Documented, life-threatening recurrent hemodynamically unstable ventricular arrhythmia that has not responded to documented adequate doses of other available antiarrhythmics or when alternative agents could not be tolerated

LD: 800-1600mg/day for 1-3 weeks (occasionally longer) until initial therapeutic response occurs; give in divided doses w/ meals for total daily dose ≥1000mg or if GI intolerance occurs

Titrate: After control is achieved or w/ prominent side effects, reduce to 600-800mg/day for 1 month
Maint: 400mg/day; up to 600mg/day

Use lowest effective dose

Upon starting therapy, an attempt should be made to gradually d/c prior antiarrhythmic drugs

Ventricular Fibrillation

Documented, life-threatening recurrent ventricular arrhythmia that has not responded to documented adequate doses of other available antiarrhythmics or when alternative agents could not be tolerated

LD: 800-1600mg/day for 1-3 weeks (occasionally longer) until initial therapeutic response occurs; give in divided doses w/ meals for total daily dose ≥1000mg or if GI intolerance occurs

Titrate: After control is achieved or w/ prominent side effects, reduce to 600-800mg/day for 1 month
Maint: 400mg/day; up to 600mg/day

Use lowest effective dose

Upon starting therapy, an attempt should be made to gradually d/c prior antiarrhythmic drugs

PEDIATRIC DOSAGE

Pediatric use may not have been established

DOSING CONSIDERATIONS

Elderly

Start at the lower end of dosing range

Other Important Considerations

Avoid grapefruit juice

ADMINISTRATION

Oral route

Give LD in the hospital.
Administer consistently w/ regard to meals.
May be administered as a single dose, or in patients w/ severe GI intolerance, as a bid dose.

STORAGE

20-25°C (68-77°F). Protect from light.

HOW SUPPLIED

Tab: 200mg* *scored

CONTRAINDICATIONS

Cardiogenic shock; severe sinus-node dysfunction, causing marked sinus bradycardia; 2nd- or 3rd-degree atrioventricular (AV) block; when episodes of bradycardia have caused syncope (except when used w/ a pacemaker); known hypersensitivity to amiodarone or any components of the medication, including iodine.

WARNINGS/PRECAUTIONS

D/C and institute steroid therapy if hypersensitivity pneumonitis occurs. Reduce dose or d/c if interstitial/alveolar pneumonitis occurs and institute appropriate treatment. The risk of arrhythmia exacerbation may be increased when other risk factors are present (eg, electrolytic disorders). Correct hypokalemia, hypomagnesemia, or hypocalcemia whenever possible before initiating therapy; monitor electrolyte and acid-base balance in patients experiencing severe/prolonged diarrhea. Chronic administration w/ implanted defibrillators/pacemakers may affect pacing and defibrillating thresholds. Amiodarone-induced hyperthyroidism may result in thyrotoxicosis and/or the possibility of arrhythmia breakthrough or aggravation. D/C or reduce dose if LFTs are >3X normal or double in patients w/ elevated baseline. Optic neuropathy and/or optic neuritis, usually resulting in visual impairment, reported. May cause fetal harm. May develop reversible corneal microdeposits, photosensitivity, and peripheral neuropathy (rare). May cause hypo/hyperthyroidism and myxedema coma; monitor particularly in elderly and w/ history of thyroid nodules, goiter, or other thyroid dysfunction. Thyroid nodules/cancer reported. Hypotension reported upon discontinuation of cardiopulmonary bypass during open-heart surgery (rare). Adult respiratory distress syndrome (ARDS) reported w/ either cardiac or noncardiac surgery. Lab test interactions may occur. May be contraindicated w/ corneal refractive laser surgery devices. Caution w/ severe left ventricular dysfunction.

ADVERSE REACTIONS

Malaise, fatigue, tremor, involuntary movements, poor coordination and gait, peripheral neuropathy, nausea, vomiting, constipation, anorexia, photosensitivity, visual disturbances, abnormal LFTs, pulmonary inflammation/fibrosis.

DRUG INTERACTIONS

See Dosing Considerations. Symptomatic bradycardia, some requiring pacemaker insertion, reported when ledipasvir/sofosbuvir or sofosbuvir w/ simeprevir were initiated; monitor HR in patients taking or recently discontinuing amiodarone when starting antiviral treatment. Potential for interactions exists not only w/ concomitant medication, but also w/ drugs administered after discontinuation of therapy due to long and variable $T_{1/2}$. The risk of arrhythmia exacerbation may be increased w/ concomitant antiarrhythmics or other interacting drugs. Monitor electrolyte and acid-base balance w/ concomitant diuretics and laxatives, systemic corticosteroids, amphotericin B (IV), or other drugs affecting electrolyte levels. Avoid concomitant use of drugs that prolong the QT interval (eg, Class I and III antiarrhythmics, lithium, certain phenothiazines); increases risk of torsades de pointes. Concomitant use of drugs w/ depressant effects on the sinus and AV node (eg, digoxin, β-blockers, verapamil) can potentiate the electrophysiologic and hemodynamic effects of therapy; monitor HR. May increase sensitivity to myocardial depressant and conduction effects of halogenated inhalation anesthetics. Drugs/substances that inhibit CYP3A (eg, certain protease inhibitors, loratadine, cimetidine, trazodone) may decrease metabolism and increase serum concentrations of therapy. Grapefruit juice may increase levels. Concomitant use of CYP3A inducers (eg, rifampin, St. John's wort) may lead to decreased serum concentrations and loss of efficacy. Consider serial measurement of amiodarone serum concentration during concomitant use of drugs affecting CYP3A activity. Reduced serum levels and $T_{1/2}$ w/ cholestyramine. Inhibits P-gp, CYP1A2, CYP2C9, CYP2D6, and CYP3A and may increase levels of their substrates. Rhabdomyolysis/myopathy reported w/ HMG-CoA reductase inhibitors that are CYP3A substrates; limit simvastatin dose to 20mg/day and lovastatin dose to 40mg/day. Lower initial/maintenance doses of other CYP3A substrates (eg, atorvastatin) may be required. Elevated SrCr reported w/ cyclosporine; monitor cyclosporine drug levels and renal function in patients taking both drugs. May increase levels of cyclosporine, quinidine, and procainamide. May inhibit metabolism of quinidine, procainamide, and flecainide. Initiate any added antiarrhythmic drug at a lower than usual dose w/ monitoring. May increase levels of digoxin; d/c or reduce dose by approx 50% upon amiodarone initiation. May inhibit metabolism of lidocaine, resulting in increased lidocaine levels; sinus bradycardia and seizure reported in patients receiving concomitant lidocaine. Reduce warfarin dose by 1/3-1/2 and monitor PT closely. Ineffective inhibition of platelet aggregation reported w/ clopidogrel. May result in elevated serum levels of dabigatran etexilate. Fentanyl may cause hypotension, bradycardia, and decreased cardiac output. Increased steady-state levels of phenytoin reported; monitor phenytoin levels. May impair metabolism of dextromethorphan, leading to increased serum levels w/ chronic (>2 weeks) amiodarone treatment. Antithyroid drugs' action may be delayed in amiodarone-induced thyrotoxicosis. Radioactive iodine is contraindicated w/ amiodarone-induced hyperthyroidism.

PREGNANCY AND LACTATION
Pregnancy: Fetal exposure may increase the potential for adverse experiences including cardiac, thyroid, neurodevelopmental, neurological, and growth effects in neonate.
Lactation: Not for use in nursing.

MECHANISM OF ACTION
Class III antiarrhythmic; prolongs myocardial cell-action potential duration and refractory period, and causes noncompetitive antagonism of α- and β-adrenoceptors.

PHARMACOKINETICS
Absorption: Slow and variable; bioavailability (approx 50%); T_{max}=3-7 hrs (single dose). **Distribution:** V_d=60L/kg; plasma protein binding (approx 96%); crosses the placenta; found in breast milk. **Metabolism:** Liver via CYP3A, CYP2C8; desethylamiodarone (DEA) (major metabolite). **Elimination:** Bile, urine (negligible); $T_{1/2}$=58 days, 36 days (DEA).

PATIENT CONSIDERATIONS
Assessment: Assess for cardiogenic shock, severe sinus node dysfunction causing marked sinus bradycardia, 2nd- or 3rd-degree AV block, life-threatening arrhythmias, renal/hepatic impairment, thyroid dysfunction, hypersensitivity to the drug (including iodine), pregnancy/nursing status, and possible drug interactions. Assess pacing and defibrillation thresholds in patients w/ implanted defibrillators or pacemakers. Obtain chest x-ray, pulmonary function tests (including diffusion capacity), and physical exam. Correct hypokalemia, hypomagnesemia, or hypocalcemia whenever possible.

Monitoring: Monitor for pulmonary toxicities, worsened arrhythmia, sinus bradycardia, heart block, photosensitivity, and other adverse reactions. Perform history, physical exam, and chest x-ray every 3-6 months. Monitor LFTs and thyroid function tests. Monitor pacing and defibrillation thresholds in patients w/ implanted defibrillators or pacemakers. Peri/postoperative monitoring for patients undergoing general anesthesia and for patients w/ ARDS recommended. Perform regular ophthalmic examination, including funduscopy and slit-lamp examination.

Counseling: Inform about benefits and risks of therapy. Advise to report any adverse reactions to physician. Counsel to take ud and not to take w/ grapefruit juice. Advise to avoid prolonged sunlight exposure and to use sun-barrier cream or protective clothing. Advise that corneal refractive laser surgery is contraindicated w/ therapy. Instruct to notify physician if pregnant/nursing.

COREG CR — carvedilol   Rx
Class: Alpha₁/beta blocker

OTHER BRAND NAMES
Coreg

ADULT DOSAGE
Heart Failure
Tab, Immediate-Release (IR):
Initial: 3.125mg bid for 2 weeks
Titrate: If tolerated, may increase dose to 6.25mg, 12.5mg, and 25mg bid over successive intervals of at least 2 weeks
Max: 50mg bid in patients w/ mild to moderate heart failure (HF) weighing >85kg

PEDIATRIC DOSAGE
Pediatric use may not have been established

Cap, Extended-Release (ER):
Initial: 10mg qd for 2 weeks
Titrate: If tolerated, may increase dose to 20mg, 40mg, and 80mg qd over successive intervals of at least 2 weeks

Left Ventricular Dysfunction Post-Myocardial Infarction
Tab, IR:
Initial: 6.25mg bid
Titrate: Increase after 3-10 days, based on tolerability, to 12.5mg bid, then again to target dose of 25mg bid May use lower starting dose and/or slower titration
Cap, ER:
Initial: 20mg qd
Titrate: Increase after 3-10 days, based on tolerability, to 40mg qd, then again to target dose of 80mg qd May use lower starting dose and/or slower titration

Hypertension
Tab, IR:
Initial: 6.25mg bid
Titrate: If needed, based on blood pressure control, may increase to 12.5mg bid, then to 25mg bid over intervals of 7-14 days
Max: 50mg/day
Cap, ER:
Initial: 20mg qd
Titrate: If needed, based on blood pressure control, may increase to 40mg qd, then to 80mg qd, over intervals of 7-14 days
Max: 80mg/day

Conversions
Daily Dose of IR Tabs to ER Caps:
6.25mg (3.125mg BID): 10mg qd
12.5mg (6.25mg BID): 20mg qd
25mg (12.5mg BID): 40mg qd
50mg (25mg BID): 80mg qd

Elderly/Patients at Increased Risk of Hypotension, Dizziness, or Syncope:
Initial:
Switching from 12.5mg bid IR Tabs: 20mg qd
Switching from 25mg bid IR Tabs: 40mg qd
Titrate: Increase doses, as appropriate, after an interval of at least 2 weeks

---

DOSING CONSIDERATIONS
Hepatic Impairment
Not for use in severe hepatic impairment
ADMINISTRATION
Oral route
Take w/ food.
Cap, ER
Take in am.
Swallow caps whole.
Cap may be opened and beads sprinkled over a spoonful of applesauce and consumed immediately, and may not be stored for future use.
Applesauce should not be warm.
Do not crush, chew, or divide cap and/or its contents.
STORAGE
Cap, ER: 25°C (77°F); excursions permitted to 15-30°C (59-86°F). **Tab:** <30°C (86°F). Protect from moisture.
HOW SUPPLIED
Cap, ER (CR): (Phosphate) 10mg, 20mg, 40mg, 80mg; **Tab:** 3.125mg, 6.25mg, 12.5mg, 25mg
CONTRAINDICATIONS
Bronchial asthma or related bronchospastic conditions, 2nd- or 3rd-degree atrioventricular (AV) block, sick sinus syndrome, severe bradycardia (w/o permanent pacemaker), cardiogenic shock, decompensated HF requiring IV inotropic therapy, severe hepatic impairment, history of serious hypersensitivity reaction (eg, Stevens-Johnson syndrome, anaphylactic reaction, angioedema) to carvedilol or any components of the medication.
WARNINGS/PRECAUTIONS
Minimize fluid retention prior to initiation of treatment. Severe exacerbation of angina and occurrence of MI and ventricular arrhythmias reported in angina patients following abrupt discontinuation; d/c therapy over 1-2 weeks whenever possible. If angina worsens or acute coronary insufficiency develops, promptly reinstitute therapy, at least temporarily. Avoid abrupt discontinuation even in

patients treated only for HTN or HF. Bradycardia reported; reduce dose if HR drops <55 BPM. Hypotension, postural hypotension, and syncope reported; highest risk during the first 30 days of dosing. May impair mental/physical abilities. Worsening HF or fluid retention may occur during up-titration; if such symptoms occur, increase dose of diuretics. If deemed necessary, use w/ caution in patients w/ bronchospastic disease who do not respond to, or cannot tolerate, other antihypertensives. May mask signs of hypoglycemia and hyperthyroidism (eg, tachycardia). May exacerbate symptoms of hyperthyroidism or precipitate thyroid storm w/ abrupt withdrawal. May lead to worsening hyperglycemia in HF patients w/ diabetes. May precipitate or aggravate symptoms of arterial insufficiency in patients w/ peripheral vascular disease. Rarely, use in patients w/ HF resulted in deterioration of renal function; d/c or reduce dosage if worsening of renal function occurs. Chronically administered therapy should not be routinely withdrawn prior to major surgery; may augment risks of general anesthesia and surgical procedures. Caution w/ pheochromocytoma and Prinzmetal's variant angina. Patients w/ history of severe anaphylactic reaction to a variety of allergens may be more reactive to repeated challenge and may be unresponsive to usual doses of epinephrine. Intraoperative floppy iris syndrome observed during cataract surgery.

ADVERSE REACTIONS
Bradycardia, fatigue, hypotension, dizziness, headache, diarrhea, N/V, hyperglycemia, weight increase, increased cough, asthenia.

DRUG INTERACTIONS
Potent CYP2D6 inhibitors (eg, quinidine, fluoxetine, propafenone) may increase levels. Monitor closely for signs of hypotension and/or severe bradycardia w/ drugs that can deplete catecholamines (eg, reserpine, MAOIs). Potentiated BP- and HR-lowering effects w/ clonidine; when coadministration is to be terminated, d/c therapy several days before clonidine is withdrawn. May increase cyclosporine levels; monitor concentrations and adjust dose of cyclosporine as appropriate. Increased risk of bradycardia w/ digitalis glycosides. May increase digoxin levels; monitor digoxin. Rifampin may reduce levels. Cimetidine may increase exposure. Amiodarone and its metabolite desethyl amiodarone, CYP2C9 inhibitors, and P-gp inhibitors may increase levels. Amiodarone or other CYP2C9 inhibitors (eg, fluconazole) may enhance β-blocking properties; monitor for signs of bradycardia or heart block. Conduction disturbance reported w/ diltiazem; monitor ECG and BP w/ calcium channel blockers of the verapamil or diltiazem type. May enhance blood glucose-reducing effect of insulin and oral hypoglycemics; regularly monitor blood glucose. If treatment is to be continued perioperatively, use caution when anesthetic agents that depress myocardial function (eg, ether, cyclopropane, trichloroethylene) are used. Additive effects and exaggerated orthostatic component w/ diuretics.

PREGNANCY AND LACTATION
Pregnancy: Category C.
Lactation: Not for use in nursing.

MECHANISM OF ACTION
Nonselective β-adrenergic and α_1 blocker; not established. (β-adrenoreceptor blocking activity) reduces cardiac output, reduces exercise- and/or isoproterenol-induced tachycardia, and reduces reflex orthostatic tachycardia; (α_1-adrenoreceptor blocking activity) attenuates the pressor effects of phenylephrine, causes vasodilation, and reduces peripheral vascular resistance.

PHARMACOKINETICS
Absorption: (Tab) Rapid and extensive. Absolute bioavailability (25-35%). (Cap, ER) T_{max}=5 hrs. **Distribution:** Plasma protein binding (>98%); V_d=115L. **Metabolism:** Extensive by oxidation and glucuronidation; CYP2D6, 2C9 (primary); CYP3A4, 2C19, 1A2, 2E1 (lesser extent). **Elimination:** Urine (<2% unchanged), feces; $T_{1/2}$=7-10 hrs.

PATIENT CONSIDERATIONS
Assessment: Assess for bronchial asthma, 2nd- or 3rd-degree AV block, sick sinus syndrome, severe bradycardia, cardiogenic shock, hepatic/renal impairment, angina, fluid retention, diabetes, hyperthyroidism, any other conditions where treatment is contraindicated or cautioned, pregnancy/nursing status, and possible drug interactions.

Monitoring: Monitor for bradycardia, worsening HF/fluid retention, masking of signs of hypoglycemia/hyperthyroidism, and other adverse reactions. Monitor BP. Monitor blood glucose during dose initiation, adjustment, or discontinuation. Monitor renal function during up-titration in patients w/ risk factors for renal function deterioration.

Counseling: Instruct not to interrupt or d/c therapy w/o consulting physician. Instruct patients w/ HF to consult physician if signs/symptoms of worsening HF occur. Inform that a drop in BP when standing, resulting in dizziness and, rarely, fainting, may occur; advise to sit or lie down when these symptoms occur. Advise to avoid driving or hazardous tasks if experiencing dizziness or fatigue, and to notify physician if dizziness or faintness occurs. Inform contact lens wearers that decreased lacrimation may be experienced, and diabetic patients to report any changes in blood sugar levels.

CORGARD — nadolol   Rx
Class: Nonselective beta blocker

> Hypersensitivity to catecholamines observed upon withdrawal; exacerbation of angina and, in some cases, myocardial infarction reported after abrupt discontinuation. When discontinuing chronically administered nadolol, particularly in patients w/ ischemic heart disease, reduce dose gradually over a period of 1-2 weeks and monitor carefully. If angina markedly worsens or acute coronary insufficiency develops, administration of therapy should be reinstituted promptly, at least temporarily, and other measures appropriate for the management of unstable angina should be taken. Warn against interruption or discontinuation of therapy w/o the physician's advice. Coronary artery disease (CAD) is common and may be unrecognized; it may be prudent not to d/c therapy abruptly even in patients treated only for HTN.

ADULT DOSAGE
Angina Pectoris
Long-Term Management:
Initial: 40mg qd
Titrate: May gradually increase in 40-80mg increments at 3- to 7-day intervals until optimum response is obtained or there is pronounced slowing of the HR
Usual Maint: 40 or 80mg qd; doses up to 160mg or 240mg qd may be needed

Usefulness and safety of doses exceeding 240mg/day have not been established.
Reduce gradually over a period of 1-2 weeks if treatment is to be discontinued.

Hypertension
Initial: 40mg qd, whether used alone or in addition to diuretic therapy
Titrate: May gradually increase in 40-80mg increments until optimum BP reduction is achieved
Usual Maint: 40 or 80mg qd; doses up to 240mg or 320mg qd may be needed

May be used alone or in combination w/ other antihypertensive agents, especially thiazide-type diuretics

----

DOSING CONSIDERATIONS
Renal Impairment
CrCl >50mL/min/1.73m²: Dose q24h
CrCl 31-50mL/min/1.73m²: Dose q24-36h
CrCl 10-30mL/min/1.73m²: Dose q24-48h
CrCl <10mL/min/1.73m²: Dose q40-60h

ADMINISTRATION
Oral route

May be administered w/o regard to meals.

STORAGE
Room temperature; avoid excessive heat. Protect from light.

HOW SUPPLIED
Tab: 20mg*, 40mg*, 80mg* *scored

CONTRAINDICATIONS
Bronchial asthma, sinus bradycardia and >1st degree conduction block, cardiogenic shock, overt cardiac failure.

WARNINGS/PRECAUTIONS
May precipitate more severe heart failure (HF) in patients w/ congestive heart failure (CHF); caution w/ history of well-compensated HF. In patients w/o a history of HF, continued use of β-blockers can, in some cases, lead to cardiac failure; digitalize and/or treat w/ diuretics at the first sign or symptom of HF and observe response closely or d/c (gradually, if possible). Avoid in patients w/ bronchospastic diseases. Chronically administered therapy should not be routinely withdrawn prior to major surgery; the impaired ability of the heart to respond to reflex adrenergic stimuli may augment the risks of general anesthesia and surgical procedures. May prevent premonitory signs and symptoms of acute hypoglycemia (eg, tachycardia, BP changes). May mask certain clinical signs of hyperthyroidism (eg, tachycardia); carefully manage patients suspected of developing thyrotoxicosis to avoid abrupt withdrawal which might precipitate a thyroid storm. Caution in patients w/ renal impairment. Patients w/ a history of severe anaphylactic reaction to variety of allergens may be more reactive to repeated challenge and may be unresponsive to usual doses of epinephrine.

ADVERSE REACTIONS
Bradycardia, dizziness, fatigue, nausea, diarrhea, anorexia, abdominal discomfort, rash, pruritus, weight gain, blurred vision, peripheral vascular insufficiency, cardiac failure, hypotension, rhythm/conduction disturbances.

DRUG INTERACTIONS
Additive effect w/ catecholamine-depleting drugs (eg, reserpine); monitor closely for hypotension and/or excessive bradycardia. Increased risk of bradycardia w/ digitalis glycosides. Hyperglycemia or hypoglycemia may occur w/ antidiabetic drugs (oral agents and insulin); adjust dose of antidiabetic agents accordingly. May exaggerate hypotension induced by general anesthetics.

PREGNANCY AND LACTATION
Pregnancy: There are no adequate and well-controlled studies in pregnant women. Use during pregnancy only if the potential benefit justifies the potential risk to the fetus.
Lactation: Nadolol is excreted in human milk. Not for use in nursing.

MECHANISM OF ACTION
Nonselective β-blocker; has not been established. Inhibits β_1 and β_2 receptors, inhibiting chronotropic, inotropic, and vasodilator responses to β-adrenergic stimulation.

PHARMACOKINETICS
Absorption: T_{max}=3-4 hrs. **Distribution:** Plasma protein binding (30%); found in breast milk. **Elimination:** Urine (unchanged); $T_{1/2}$=20-24 hrs.

PEDIATRIC DOSAGE
Pediatric use may not have been established

PATIENT CONSIDERATIONS

Assessment: Assess for bronchial asthma, sinus bradycardia, cardiogenic shock, CHF, bronchospastic diseases, CAD, hyperthyroidism, diabetes, renal impairment, hypersensitivity to drug, pregnancy/nursing status, and possible drug interactions.

Monitoring: Monitor for signs/symptoms of CHF, hypoglycemia, thyrotoxicosis, withdrawal symptoms, hypersensitivity reactions, and other adverse reactions.

Counseling: Warn patients, especially those w/ evidence of coronary artery insufficiency, against interruption or discontinuation of therapy w/o consulting physician. Advise to consult physician at 1st sign/symptom of impending cardiac failure. Advise of proper course in the event of an inadvertently missed dose.

CORLANOR — ivabradine   Rx

Class: Hyperpolarization-activated cyclic nucleotide-gated channel blocker

ADULT DOSAGE	PEDIATRIC DOSAGE
Heart Failure	Pediatric use may not have been established
To reduce the risk of hospitalization for worsening heart failure (HF) in patients w/ stable, symptomatic chronic HF w/ left ventricular ejection fraction ≤35%, who are in sinus rhythm w/ resting HR ≥70 bpm and either are on maximally tolerated doses of β-blockers or have a contraindication to β-blocker use	
Initial: 5mg bid	
Titrate: After 2 weeks, assess patient and adjust dose to achieve a resting HR of 50-60 bpm	
Max: 7.5mg bid	
HR <50 bpm or Signs/Symptoms of Bradycardia: Decrease dose by 2.5mg (given bid); if current dose is 2.5mg bid, d/c therapy	
HR 50-60 bpm: Maintain dose	
HR >60 bpm: Increase dose by 2.5mg (given bid) up to a max dose of 7.5mg bid	
Thereafter, adjust dose prn based on resting HR and tolerability	

DOSING CONSIDERATIONS

Hepatic Impairment
Severe (Child-Pugh C): Contraindicated

Other Important Considerations
History of Conduction Defects or Bradycardia Leading to Hemodynamic Compromise:
Initial: 2.5mg bid
Titrate: Increase dose based on HR

ADMINISTRATION
Oral route
Take w/ meals.

STORAGE
25°C (77°F); excursions permitted to 15-30°C (59-86°F).

HOW SUPPLIED
Tab: 5mg*, 7.5mg, *scored

CONTRAINDICATIONS
Acute decompensated HF; BP <90/50mmHg; sick sinus syndrome, sinoatrial block, or 3rd degree atrioventricular (AV) block, unless a functioning demand pacemaker is present; resting HR <60 bpm prior to treatment; severe hepatic impairment; pacemaker dependence (HR maintained exclusively by the pacemaker). Concomitant use of strong CYP3A4 inhibitors.

WARNINGS/PRECAUTIONS
May cause fetal toxicity. Increases the risk of A-fib; d/c if this develops. Bradycardia, sinus arrest, and heart block reported. Risk factors for bradycardia include sinus node dysfunction, conduction defects (eg, 1st/2nd degree AV block, bundle branch block), and ventricular dyssynchrony; avoid use in patients w/ 2nd degree AV block, unless a functioning demand pacemaker is present. Not recommended in patients w/ demand pacemakers set to rates ≥60 bpm.

ADVERSE REACTIONS
Bradycardia, HTN, A-fib.

DRUG INTERACTIONS
See Contraindications. CYP3A4 inhibitors/inducers increase/decrease levels respectively; increased levels may exacerbate bradycardia and conduction disturbances; avoid concomitant use of moderate CYP3A4 inhibitors (eg, diltiazem, verapamil, grapefruit juice) and CYP3A4 inducers (eg, St. John's wort, rifampicin, barbiturates, phenytoin). Increased risk of bradycardia w/ other drugs that slow HR (eg, digoxin, diltiazem, verapamil, amiodarone, β-blockers); monitor HR.

PREGNANCY AND LACTATION
Pregnancy: Fetal harm has been seen in animal studies. Pregnant patients who are started on ivabradine, especially during the 1st trimester, should be followed closely for destabilization of their CHF that could result from HR slowing; monitor pregnant women w/ chronic HF in 3rd trimester of pregnancy for preterm birth.
Lactation: Ivabradine is present in rat milk; not for use in nursing.

Reproductive Potential: Advise females of reproductive potential to use effective contraception during treatment.

MECHANISM OF ACTION
Hyperpolarization-activated cyclic nucleotide-gated channel blocker; blocks the hyperpolarization-activated cyclic nucleotide-gated channel responsible for the cardiac pacemaker I_f current, which regulates HR.

PHARMACOKINETICS
Absorption: Absolute bioavailability (approx 40%); T_{max}=approx 1 hr (fasted).
Distribution: V_d=approx 100L; plasma protein binding (approx 70%). **Metabolism:** Extensively metabolized in the liver and intestines via CYP3A4-mediated oxidation; N-desmethylated derivative (S 18982) (major metabolite). **Elimination:** Urine (4% unchanged), feces. $T_{1/2}$=2 hrs (distribution $T_{1/2}$), approx 6 hrs (effective $T_{1/2}$).

PATIENT CONSIDERATIONS

Assessment: Assess for acute decompensated HF, BP <90/50mmHg, sick sinus syndrome, sinoatrial block, 2nd or 3rd degree AV block, presence of a functioning demand pacemaker, resting HR <60 bpm prior to treatment, severe hepatic impairment, pacemaker dependence, risk factors for bradycardia, history of conduction defects, pregnancy/nursing status, and possible drug interactions.

Monitoring: Monitor for A-fib, bradycardia, sinus arrest, heart block, and other adverse reactions. Monitor cardiac rhythm regularly.

Counseling: Advise pregnant women of the potential risks to a fetus. Advise females of reproductive potential to use effective contraception and to notify their healthcare provider w/ a known/suspected pregnancy. Advise to report significant decreases in HR or symptoms such as dizziness, fatigue, or hypotension. Advise to report symptoms of A-fib (eg, heart palpitations or racing, chest pressure, worsened SOB). Advise about the possible occurrence of luminous phenomena (phosphenes) and that phosphenes may subside spontaneously during continued treatment. Advise to use caution if driving or using machines in situations where sudden changes in light intensity may occur, especially when driving at night. Advise to avoid ingestion of grapefruit juice and St. John's wort.

CORTEF — hydrocortisone   Rx

Class: Glucocorticoid

ADULT DOSAGE	PEDIATRIC DOSAGE
Steroid-Responsive Disorders	**Steroid-Responsive Disorders**
Initial: 20-240mg/day depending on disease	**Initial:** 20-240mg/day depending on disease
Adjust/maintain initial dose until a satisfactory response observed. If no satisfactory clinical response after a reasonable period, D/C and transfer to appropriate therapy	Adjust/maintain initial dose until a satisfactory response observed. If no satisfactory clinical response after a reasonable period, D/C and transfer to appropriate therapy
Maint: Decrease dose by small amounts to lowest effective dose	**Maint:** Decrease dose by small amounts to lowest effective dose
Multiple Sclerosis	**Multiple Sclerosis**
Acute Exacerbations:	**Acute Exacerbations:**
Usual: 200mg/day of prednisolone for 1 week followed by 80mg qod for 1 month (20mg hydrocortisone=5mg prednisolone)	**Usual:** 200mg/day of prednisolone for 1 week followed by 80mg qod for 1 month (20mg hydrocortisone=5mg prednisolone)

DOSING CONSIDERATIONS

Discontinuation
Withdraw gradually after long-term therapy

ADMINISTRATION
Oral route

STORAGE
20-25°C (68-77°F).

HOW SUPPLIED
Tab: 5mg, 10mg, 20mg

CONTRAINDICATIONS
Systemic fungal infections, known hypersensitivity to components.

WARNINGS/PRECAUTIONS
May need to increase dose before, during, and after stressful situations. May mask signs of infection or cause new infections. Prolonged use may produce posterior subcapsular cataract, glaucoma with possible optic nerve damage, may enhance secondary ocular infections. Weigh benefit versus risk in use during pregnancy; may cause hypoadrenalism in infants. May cause elevation of BP, salt/water retention, and increased excretion of K$^+$ and calcium. Dietary salt restriction and K$^+$ supplementation may be necessary. More serious/fatal course of chickenpox and measles reported. Drug-induced secondary adrenocortical insufficiency may be minimized by gradual reduction of dosage. Enhanced effects with hypothyroidism and cirrhosis. Avoid abrupt withdrawal. Psychic derangements may appear and existing emotional instability or psychotic tendencies may be aggravated. Caution with active or latent tuberculosis (TB), *Strongyloides* infestation, ocular herpes simplex, nonspecific ulcerative colitis, diverticulitis, fresh intestinal anastomosis, active or latent peptic ulcer, renal insufficiency, HTN, osteoporosis, and myasthenia gravis. Growth and development of children on prolonged therapy should be monitored. Kaposi's sarcoma reported.

ADVERSE REACTIONS
Fluid and electrolyte disturbances, HTN, osteoporosis, muscle weakness, cushingoid state, menstrual irregularities, impaired wound healing, ulcerative

esophagitis, increased sweating, increased intracranial pressure, carbohydrate intolerance, glaucoma, cataracts.

DRUG INTERACTIONS

Live or live, attenuated vaccines are contraindicated with immunosuppressive doses. May diminish response to killed or inactivated vaccines. Hepatic enzyme inducers (eg, phenobarbital, phenytoin, and rifampin) may decrease levels; may need to increase dose. Troleandomycin and ketoconazole may increase levels. May decrease levels of chronic high dose aspirin; caution with hypoprothrombinemia. Variable effects on oral anticoagulants; monitor coagulation indices. May increase insulin or oral hypoglycemic agents requirements in diabetics.

PREGNANCY AND LACTATION

Safety in pregnancy and nursing not known.

MECHANISM OF ACTION

Glucocorticoid; causes profound and varied metabolic effects and modifies the body's immune responses to diverse stimuli.

PHARMACOKINETICS

Absorption: Readily absorbed from GI tract.

PATIENT CONSIDERATIONS

Assessment: Assess for systemic fungal infections, history/active TB, vaccination history, hypersensitivity to the drug, stress level, *Strongyloides* infestation, ocular herpes simplex, psychotic tendencies, cirrhosis, ulcerative colitis, diverticulitis, intestinal anastomosis, peptic ulcer, renal insufficiency, HTN, osteoporosis, myasthenia gravis, thyroid status, pregnancy/nursing status, and possible drug interactions. Obtain baseline of K^+ and calcium levels, blood sugar, and BP.

Monitoring: Monitor for occurrence of infections, cataracts, glaucoma, ocular infection, reactivation of TB, *Strongyloides* hyperinfection, adrenocortical insufficiency, psychic derangement, psychotic tendencies, myopathy, edema and Kaposi's sarcoma. Monitor for growth and development of children on prolonged therapy. Monitor BP, blood glucose levels, and serum electrolytes.

Counseling: Advise of benefits/risks of therapy. Inform that susceptibility to infections may increase. Advise to avoid exposure to chickenpox and measles; report immediately to physician if exposed. Advise that dietary salt restriction and supplementation of K^+ and calcium may be necessary. Instruct not to d/c therapy abruptly or without medical supervision.

CORTIFOAM — hydrocortisone acetate   Rx

Class: Corticosteroid

ADULT DOSAGE

Ulcerative Proctitis

Adjunctive treatment of ulcerative proctitis of the distal portion of the rectum in patients who cannot retain hydrocortisone or other corticosteroid enemas

Usual: 1 applicatorful rectally qd or bid for 2 or 3 weeks, and every 2nd day thereafter

Maint: After a favorable response is noted, decrease initial dose in small decrements at appropriate time intervals until lowest effective dose is reached

PEDIATRIC DOSAGE

Pediatric use may not have been established

DOSING CONSIDERATIONS

Discontinuation

If drug is to be stopped after long-term therapy, withdraw gradually rather than abruptly

ADMINISTRATION

Rectal route

Directions for Use

1. Shake foam container vigorously for 5-10 sec before each use; do not remove container cap during use of product
2. Hold container upright on a level surface and gently place the tip of the applicator onto the nose of the container cap
3. Pull plunger past the fill line on the applicator barrel
4. To fill applicator barrel, press down firmly on cap flanges, hold for 1-2 sec and release; pause 5-10 sec to allow foam to expand in applicator barrel and repeat until foam reaches fill line
5. Remove applicator from container cap; allow some foam to remain on the applicator tip. A burst of air may come out of container w/ 1st pump
6. Hold applicator firmly by barrel, making sure thumb and middle finger are positioned securely underneath and resting against barrel wings; place index finger over the plunger
7. Gently insert tip into anus; once in place, push plunger to expel foam, then withdraw applicator
8. Do not insert any part of the aerosol container directly into the anus; apply to anus only w/ enclosed applicator

STORAGE

20-25°C (68-77°F). Do not refrigerate.

HOW SUPPLIED

Foam: 10% [15g]

CONTRAINDICATIONS

Hypersensitivity to any components of the medication. Obstruction, abscess, perforation, peritonitis, fresh intestinal anastomoses, extensive fistulas and sinus tracts.

WARNINGS/PRECAUTIONS

Do not insert any part of the aerosol container directly into the anus. Systemic absorption may be greater than from other corticosteroid enema formulations. D/C if no improvement in 2 or 3 weeks, or if condition worsens. Anaphylactoid reactions reported rarely. May cause BP elevation, salt and water retention, increase K^+ and Ca^{2+} excretion. May produce reversible hypothalamic-pituitary-adrenal (HPA) axis suppression w/ the potential for glucocorticosteroid insufficiency after d/c. Decreased metabolic clearance in hypothyroidism and increased in hyperthyroidism; may necessitate dosage adjustment. May mask signs of current infection or increase susceptibility to infections. May exacerbate systemic fungal infections; avoid use in the presence of such infections unless needed to control drug reactions. Latent disease may be activated or intercurrent infections may be exacerbated. Rule out latent or active amebiasis prior to initiation in any patient who spent time in the tropics or w/ unexplained diarrhea. May cause a more serious/fatal course of chickenpox and measles; avoid exposure. May produce posterior subcapsular cataracts, glaucoma w/ possible optic nerve damage, and enhance the establishment of secondary ocular infections. Kaposi's sarcoma reported most often w/ chronic conditions. Drug-induced secondary adrenocortical insufficiency may be minimized by gradual dose reduction. Signs of peritoneal irritation following GI perforation may be minimal or absent. Enhanced effect w/ cirrhosis. May decrease bone formation and increase bone resorption, and may lead to inhibition of bone growth in pediatrics and development of osteoporosis at any age. Acute myopathy observed w/ high doses, especially in patients w/ neuromuscular transmission disorders (eg, myasthenia gravis). Creatinine kinase elevation, psychic derangements, and emotional instability or aggravation of psychotic tendencies may occur. May elevate IOP; monitor IOP if used for >6 weeks. Caution w/ recent MI, *Strongyloides* (threadworm) infestation, active/latent tuberculosis (TB) or tuberculin reactivity, CHF, HTN, renal insufficiency, active or latent peptic ulcers, diverticulitis, fresh intestinal anastomoses, nonspecific ulcerative colitis, and risk of osteoporosis. Avoid w/ cerebral malaria, active ocular herpes simplex, and immediate or early postoperative period following ileorectostomy. May suppress reactions to skin tests.

ADVERSE REACTIONS

Bradycardia, acne, abdominal distention, convulsions, depression, abnormal fat deposits, fluid retention, muscle weakness, pancreatitis, headache, exophthalmos.

DRUG INTERACTIONS

Live or live, attenuated vaccines are contraindicated w/ immunosuppressive doses. May diminish response to toxoids and live or inactivated vaccines. May potentiate replication of some organisms contained in live attenuated vaccines. Aminoglutethimide may lead to a loss of corticosteroid-induced adrenal suppression. K^+-depleting agents (eg, amphotericin B, diuretics) may cause hypokalemia; observe closely. Concomitant amphotericin B may cause cardiac enlargement and CHF. Macrolide antibiotics may decrease clearance. Withdraw anticholinesterase agents at least 24 hrs prior to initiation of therapy. Monitor coagulation indices w/ warfarin. Dosage adjustments of antidiabetic agents may be required. May decrease levels of isoniazid. Convulsions and increased activity of both drugs reported w/ cyclosporine. Cholestyramine may increase clearance. May increase risk of arrhythmias w/ digitalis glycosides. Estrogens and ketoconazole may decrease metabolism. Hepatic enzyme inducers (eg, barbiturates, phenytoin, carbamazepine, rifampin) may enhance metabolism; may need to increase corticosteroid dose. Aspirin (ASA) (or other NSAIDs) may increase risk of GI side effects; use ASA cautiously in hypoprothrombinemia. May increase clearance of salicylates. Acute myopathy reported w/ neuromuscular-blocking drugs (eg, pancuronium).

PREGNANCY AND LACTATION

Pregnancy: Category C.
Lactation: Caution in nursing.

MECHANISM OF ACTION

Corticosteroid; anti-inflammatory.

PHARMACOKINETICS

Distribution: Found in breast milk (systemically administered).

PATIENT CONSIDERATIONS

Assessment: Assess for hypersensitivity to any components of the drug, obstruction, abscess, perforation, peritonitis, fresh intestinal anastomoses, extensive fistulas and sinus tracts, recent MI, thyroid status changes, infections, amebiasis, *Strongyloides* infestation, cerebral malaria, TB, active ocular herpes simplex, CHF, HTN, renal insufficiency, peptic ulcer, diverticulitis, nonspecific ulcerative colitis, recent ileorectostomy, cirrhosis, risk of osteoporosis, emotional instability, psychotic tendencies, pregnancy/nursing status, and possible drug interactions.

Monitoring: Monitor for signs/symptoms of HTN, salt and water retention, increased excretion of K^+, left ventricular free wall rupture (in patients w/ recent MI), glucocorticosteroid insufficiency (upon d/c), infections, reactivation of TB, posterior subcapsular cataracts, glaucoma, Kaposi's sarcoma, acute myopathy, improvement or worsening of condition, and other adverse reactions.

Counseling: Counsel not to d/c abruptly or w/o medical supervision. Advise to inform medical attendants that corticosteroids are being taken. Advise that contents of container are under pressure; do not burn or puncture. Instruct to seek medical advice if fever or other signs of infection develop. Advise to avoid exposure to chickenpox or measles; if exposed, advise to seek medical advice w/o delay.

CORTISPORIN CREAM — hydrocortisone acetate/neomycin sulfate/polymyxin B sulfate   Rx

Class: Antibacterial/corticosteroid combination

ADULT DOSAGE
Dermatoses

Treatment of Corticosteroid Responsive Dermatoses w/ Secondary Infection:
Apply a small quantity bid-qid, as required

PEDIATRIC DOSAGE
Pediatric use may not have been established

DOSING CONSIDERATIONS
Elderly
Start at lower end of dosing range

ADMINISTRATION
Topical route
Gently rub cream into affected areas, if conditions permit.

STORAGE
15-25°C (59-77°F).

HOW SUPPLIED
Cre: (Neomycin/Polymyxin B/Hydrocortisone) (3.5mg/10,000 U/5mg)/g [7.5g]

CONTRAINDICATIONS
Use in eyes or external ear canal if eardrum is perforated. Tuberculous, fungal, or viral lesions of the skin (herpes simplex, vaccinia, varicella). Hypersensitivity to any of the components.

WARNINGS/PRECAUTIONS
Has not been demonstrated to provide greater benefit than the steroid component alone after 7 days of treatment. Should not be used over a wide area or for extended periods of time due to the concern of nephrotoxicity and ototoxicity associated w/ neomycin. Prolonged use may result in overgrowth of nonsusceptible organisms, including fungi; take appropriate measures if this occurs. Caution on infected areas; anti-inflammatory steroids may encourage spread of infection; d/c and use appropriate anti-bacterial drugs if this occurs. Exogenous hyperadrenocorticism, including adrenal suppression, may occur w/ topical corticosteroids. Systemic absorption of topically applied steroids will be increased if extensive BSAs are treated or if occlusive dressings are used; caution when long-term use is anticipated. Sufficient percutaneous absorption of hydrocortisone can occur in pediatric patients during prolonged use to cause growth cessation and other systemic signs/symptoms of hyperadrenocorticism. D/C if redness, irritation, swelling, or pain persists or increases. Caution in elderly.

ADVERSE REACTIONS
Topical Antibiotic Combinations: Allergic sensitization.
Topical Corticosteroids: Burning, itching, irritation, dryness, folliculitis, hypertrichosis, acneiform eruptions, hypopigmentation, perioral dermatitis, allergic contact dermatitis, skin maceration, secondary infection, skin atrophy, striae, miliaria.

PREGNANCY AND LACTATION
Pregnancy: There are no adequate and well-controlled studies in pregnant women. Corticosteroids should be used during pregnancy only if the potential benefit justifies the potential risk to the fetus.
Lactation: Caution in nursing. Hydrocortisone acetate appears in human milk following oral administration; systemic absorption may occur when applied topically.

MECHANISM OF ACTION
Antibacterial/corticosteroid combination. Corticoids suppress inflammatory response to a variety of agents and may delay healing. Since corticoids may inhibit the body's defense mechanism against infection, a concomitant antimicrobial drug may be used when this inhibition is considered to be clinically significant in a particular case.

PHARMACOKINETICS
Distribution: Hydrocortisone appears in breast milk following oral administration.

PATIENT CONSIDERATIONS
Assessment: Assess for perforated eardrum; tuberculous, fungal, or viral skin lesions; and pregnancy/nursing status.

Monitoring: Monitor for nephrotoxicity, ototoxicity, overgrowth of nonsusceptible organisms (eg, fungi), spread of infection, exogenous hyperadrenocorticism (including adrenal suppression), and other adverse reactions.

Counseling: Instruct to use ud. Advise to d/c use and notify physician if redness, irritation, swelling, or pain persists or increases. Instruct to not use in the eyes.

CORVERT — ibutilide fumarate   Rx

Class: Class III antiarrhythmic

May cause potentially fatal arrhythmias, particularly sustained polymorphic ventricular tachycardia, usually in association w/ QT prolongation (torsades de pointes), but sometimes w/o documented QT prolongation. Administer in a setting of continuous ECG monitoring and by personnel trained in identification and treatment of acute ventricular arrhythmias. Patients w/ A-fib of >2-3 days' duration must be adequately anticoagulated, generally for ≥2 weeks. Patients should be carefully selected such that the expected benefits of maintaining sinus rhythm outweigh the immediate and maintenance therapy risks.

ADULT DOSAGE
Atrial Fibrillation/Flutter

Rapid Conversion to Sinus Rhythm in Recent Onset A-Fib/A-Flutter:
Initial:
<60kg: 0.01mg/kg over 10 min
≥60kg: 1mg over 10 min

If arrhythmia still present w/in 10 min after the end of the initial infusion, repeat infusion 10 min after completion of 1st infusion

PEDIATRIC DOSAGE
Pediatric use may not have been established

DOSING CONSIDERATIONS
Elderly
Start at lower end of dosing range

ADMINISTRATION
IV route

Dilution
May be administered undiluted or diluted in 50mL of diluent
May be added to 0.9% NaCl or D5 inj before infusion
The contents of one 10mL vial (0.1mg/mL) may be added to a 50mL infusion bag to form an admixture of approx 0.017mg/mL ibutilide

Compatibility
The following diluents are compatible w/ ibutilide inj (0.1mg/mL):
- D5 inj
- 0.9% NaCl inj

The following IV sol containers are compatible w/ admixtures of ibutilide inj (0.1mg/mL):
- Polyvinyl chloride plastic bags
- Polyolefin bags

STORAGE
Vial: 20-25°C (68-77°F). Admixture: 0.9% NaCl or D5 Inj: Stable at 15-30°C (59-86°F) for 24 hrs and 2-8°C (36-46°F) for 48 hrs in polyvinyl chloride plastic bags or polyolefin bags.

HOW SUPPLIED
Inj: 0.1mg/mL [10mL]

CONTRAINDICATIONS
Previously demonstrated hypersensitivity to ibutilide fumarate or any other components of the medication.

WARNINGS/PRECAUTIONS
May induce/worsen ventricular arrhythmias. Not recommended in patients who have previously demonstrated polymorphic ventricular tachycardia (eg, torsades de pointes). Anticipate proarrhythmic events. Correct hypokalemia and hypomagnesemia before therapy. Reversible heart block reported. Caution in elderly.

ADVERSE REACTIONS
Sustained/nonsustained polymorphic ventricular tachycardia, nonsustained monomorphic ventricular tachycardia, ventricular extrasystoles, headache.

DRUG INTERACTIONS
Avoid Class IA (eg, disopyramide, quinidine, procainamide) and other Class III (eg, amiodarone, sotalol) antiarrhythmics w/ or w/in 4 hrs postinfusion. Increased proarrhythmia potential w/ drugs that prolong the QT interval (eg, phenothiazines, TCAs, tetracyclic antidepressants, antihistamine drugs [H_1-receptor antagonists]). Caution in patients w/ elevated or above the usual therapeutic range of plasma digoxin levels.

PREGNANCY AND LACTATION
Pregnancy: Category C.
Lactation: Not for use in nursing.

MECHANISM OF ACTION
Class III antiarrhythmic agent; prolongs atrial and ventricular action potential duration and refractoriness. Delays repolarization by activation of a slow, inward current, rather than blocking outward K^+ currents.

PHARMACOKINETICS
Distribution: V_d=11L/kg; plasma protein binding (40%). **Metabolism:** Omega-oxidation and β-oxidation. **Elimination:** Urine (82%, 7% unchanged), feces (19%); $T_{1/2}$=6 hrs.

PATIENT CONSIDERATIONS
Assessment: Assess for arrhythmia, bradycardia, polymorphic ventricular tachycardia, electrolyte imbalance, CHF, low ejection fraction, renal/hepatic function, pregnancy/nursing status, and for possible drug interactions. Perform ECG. Obtain baseline QTc.

Monitoring: Monitor for worsening of induction of new ventricular arrhythmia, torsades de pointes (polymorphic ventricular tachycardia), and any arrhythmic activity. Monitor ECG continuously for ≥4 hrs following infusion.

Counseling: Inform about benefits/risks of therapy. Instruct to report any adverse reactions to physician.

PEDIATRIC DOSAGE
Pediatric use may not have been established

COSENTYX — secukinumab   Rx
Class: Monoclonal antibody/IL-17A antagonist

ADULT DOSAGE

Plaque Psoriasis

In Patients Who Are Candidates for Systemic/Phototherapy:

Moderate to Severe:
300mg at Weeks 0, 1, 2, 3, and 4, followed by 300mg every 4 weeks; a dose of 150mg may be acceptable for some patients

Each 300mg dose is given as two 150mg inj

Psoriatic Arthritis

W/ Coexistent Moderate to Severe Plaque Psoriasis:
Use the dosing recommendations for plaque psoriasis

Other Psoriatic Arthritis:
Administer w/ or w/o a LD
W/ a LD: 150mg at Weeks 0, 1, 2, 3, and 4 and every 4 weeks thereafter
W/O a LD: 150mg every 4 weeks
If active psoriatic arthritis continues, consider a dosage of 300mg

May administer w/ or w/o methotrexate

Ankylosing Spondylitis

Administer w/ or w/o a LD

W/ a LD: 150mg at Weeks 0, 1, 2, 3, and 4 and every 4 weeks thereafter
W/O a LD: 150mg every 4 weeks

PEDIATRIC DOSAGE
Pediatric use may not have been established

ADMINISTRATION
SQ route

Administer each inj at a different anatomic location (eg, upper arms, thighs, any quadrant of abdomen) than previous inj.
Do not inject into areas where the skin is tender, bruised, erythematous, indurated, or affected by psoriasis.

Preparation
Pen and Prefilled Syringe:
Before inj, remove from refrigerator and allow to reach room temperature (15-30 min) w/o removing needle cap.
Administer w/in 1 hr after removal from refrigerator and discard any unused product remaining in the pen/prefilled syringe.

Single-Use Vial:
Preparation time from piercing the stopper until end of reconstitution should not exceed 90 min.
1. Remove vial from refrigerator and allow to stand for 15-30 min to reach room temperature; ensure sterile water for inj (SWFI) is at room temperature.
2. Slowly inject 1mL of SWFI into vial.
3. Tilt vial at a 45° angle and gently rotate between fingertips for 1 min; do not shake/invert vial.
4. Allow vial to stand for 10 min at room temperature, then tilt vial at a 45° angle and gently rotate between fingertips for 1 min; do not shake/invert vial.
5. Allow vial to stand undisturbed at room temperature for approx 5 min.
6. Prepare the required number for vials and use immediately or store in refrigerator at 2-8°C (36-46°F) for up to 24 hrs. Do not freeze. After refrigeration, allow reconstituted sol to reach room temperature (15-30 min) before administration; administer w/in 1 hr after removal from 2-8°C (36-46°F) storage.

STORAGE
2-8°C (36-46°F). Protect from light. Do not freeze. To avoid foaming, do not shake.

HOW SUPPLIED
Inj: 150mg/mL [prefilled syringe, Sensoready pen], 150mg [vial]

CONTRAINDICATIONS
Previous serious hypersensitivity reaction to secukinumab or any components of the medication.

WARNINGS/PRECAUTIONS
May increase risk of infections; exercise caution when considering use in patients w/ a chronic infection or a history of recurrent infection. If serious infection develops, closely monitor and d/c until infection resolves. Evaluate for tuberculosis (TB) infection prior to initiating treatment; do not administer to patients w/ active TB infection. Initiate treatment of latent TB prior to administering therapy; consider anti-TB therapy prior to initiation in patients w/ a past history of latent or active TB in whom an adequate course of treatment cannot be confirmed. Caution w/ inflammatory bowel disease; exacerbations and new onset reported. Trend towards greater disease activity and increased adverse events seen w/ active Crohn's disease. Anaphylaxis and urticaria reported; d/c immediately and initiate appropriate therapy if an anaphylactic or other serious allergic reaction occurs. Removable cap of the Sensoready pen and prefilled syringe contains natural rubber latex, which may cause an allergic reaction in latex-sensitive individuals. Prior to initiating therapy, consider completion of all age appropriate immunizations according to current immunization guidelines.

ADVERSE REACTIONS
Ankylosing Spondylitis: Nasopharyngitis, nausea, URTI, infections.
Plaque Psoriasis: Nasopharyngitis, diarrhea, URTI, infections.
Psoriatic Arthritis: Nasopharyngitis, URTI, headache, nausea, hypercholesterolemia, infections.

DRUG INTERACTIONS
Avoid w/ live vaccines. Non-live vaccinations received during a course of therapy may not elicit an immune response sufficient to prevent disease. May normalize formation of CYP450 enzymes; upon initiation or discontinuation of therapy in patients who are receiving concomitant CYP450 substrates, particularly those w/ a narrow therapeutic index, consider monitoring for therapeutic effect (eg, warfarin) or drug concentration (eg, cyclosporine) and consider dosage modification of the CYP450 substrate.

PREGNANCY AND LACTATION
Pregnancy: Category B.
Lactation: Caution in nursing.

MECHANISM OF ACTION
Monoclonal antibody/interleukin-17A (IL-17A) antagonist; selectively binds to the IL-17A cytokine and inhibits its interaction w/ the IL-17 receptor. Inhibits the release of proinflammatory cytokines and chemokines.

PHARMACOKINETICS
Absorption: Bioavailability (55-77%); C_{max}=13.7mcg/mL (150mg), 27.3mcg/mL (300mg); T_{max}=6 days. **Distribution:** V_d=7.10-8.60L (IV). **Elimination:** $T_{1/2}$=22-31 days.

PATIENT CONSIDERATIONS

Assessment: Assess for previous hypersensitivity to the drug, chronic infection or history of recurrent infection, TB infection, inflammatory bowel disease, latex sensitivity, immunization status, pregnancy/nursing status, and possible drug interactions.

Monitoring: Monitor for signs/symptoms of infection, inflammatory bowel disease, anaphylactic/allergic reactions, and other adverse reactions. Monitor for signs/symptoms of active TB during and after treatment.

Counseling: Advise of the potential benefits and risks of therapy. Inform that drug may lower the ability of immune system to fight infections; instruct to contact physician if any symptoms of infection develop. Advise to seek immediate medical attention if any symptoms of a serious hypersensitivity reaction occur. Instruct in inj techniques, as well as proper syringe and needle disposal, and caution against reuse of needles and syringes.

COSOPT — dorzolamide hydrochloride/timolol maleate   Rx
Class: Carbonic anhydrase inhibitor/nonselective beta blocker

OTHER BRAND NAMES
Cosopt PF

ADULT DOSAGE
Elevated Intraocular Pressure
Reduction of elevated IOP in patients w/ open-angle glaucoma or ocular HTN who are insufficiently responsive to β-blockers

1 drop in the affected eye(s) bid

PEDIATRIC DOSAGE
Elevated Intraocular Pressure
Reduction of elevated IOP in patients w/ open-angle glaucoma or ocular HTN who are insufficiently responsive to β-blockers

≥2 Years:
1 drop in the affected eye(s) bid

DOSING CONSIDERATIONS
Concomitant Medications
If >1 topical ophthalmic drug is being used, administer at least 5 min apart

ADMINISTRATION
Ocular route

Cosopt PF
Use the sol from 1 individual unit immediately after opening, and discard the remaining contents immediately after administration.

STORAGE
Cosopt: 15-30°C (59-86°F). Protect from light. **Cosopt PF:** 20-25°C (68-77°F). Do not freeze. Store in original pouch; after pouch is opened, store remaining containers in foil pouch to protect from light. Discard any unused containers 15 days after 1st opening the pouch.

HOW SUPPLIED
Ophthalmic Sol: (Dorzolamide/Timolol) (Cosopt) 2%/0.5% [10mL]; (Cosopt PF) 2%/0.5% [0.2mL, 60^s 180^s]

CONTRAINDICATIONS
Bronchial asthma or history thereof, severe COPD, sinus bradycardia, 2nd- or 3rd-degree atrioventricular (AV) block, overt cardiac failure, cardiogenic shock, hypersensitivity to any component of the medication.

WARNINGS/PRECAUTIONS
Bacterial keratitis associated w/ the use of multiple-dose containers of topical ophthalmic products. **Dorzolamide:** Absorbed systemically. Fatalities reported (rare) due to severe reactions to sulfonamides; sensitization may recur when readministered irrespective of the route of administration. D/C if signs of serious reactions or hypersensitivity occur. Not recommended w/ severe renal impairment (CrCl <30mL/min). Caution w/ hepatic impairment. Increased potential for developing corneal edema in patients w/ low endothelial cell counts. **Timolol:** Absorbed systemically; severe respiratory reactions and rarely death in association w/ cardiac failure reported. Inhibition of sympathetic stimulation may precipitate more severe failure in patients w/ diminished myocardial

contractility; d/c at the first sign/symptom of cardiac failure. Avoid w/ mild or moderate COPD (eg, chronic bronchitis, emphysema), bronchospastic disease, or history of bronchospastic disease. Patients w/ a history of atopy or a history of severe anaphylactic reactions to a variety of allergens may be more reactive to repeated challenge w/ such allergens, and may be unresponsive to usual doses of epinephrine used to treat anaphylactic reactions. May potentiate muscle weakness. May mask signs/symptoms of acute hypoglycemia; caution in patients subject to spontaneous hypoglycemia and in diabetic patients receiving insulin or oral hypoglycemic agents. May mask certain clinical signs of hyperthyroidism (eg, tachycardia); carefully manage patients suspected of developing thyrotoxicosis to avoid abrupt withdrawal that may precipitate a thyroid storm. Withdrawal of therapy prior to major surgery is controversial. β-adrenergic receptor blockade may impair the ability of the heart to respond to β-adrenergically mediated reflex stimuli; gradual withdrawal of β-blocking agents may be recommended in patients undergoing elective surgery.

ADVERSE REACTIONS
Taste perversion, ocular burning and/or stinging, conjunctival hyperemia, blurred vision, superficial punctate keratitis, or eye itching.

DRUG INTERACTIONS
Dorzolamide: Not recommended w/ oral carbonic anhydrase inhibitors. Acid-base and electrolyte disturbances reported w/ oral carbonic anhydrase inhibitors and have, in some instances, resulted in drug interactions; consider potential for such interactions in patients receiving therapy. **Timolol:** Monitor for potential additive effects, both systemic and on IOP, w/ concomitant oral β-blockers; concomitant use of 2 topical β-blocking agents is not recommended. Caution w/ oral or IV calcium antagonists because of possible AV conduction disturbances, left ventricular failure, and hypotension; avoid coadministration in patients w/ impaired cardiac function. Closely observe patients receiving catecholamine-depleting drugs (eg, reserpine) because of possible additive effects and the production of hypotension and/or marked bradycardia. Concomitant use w/ digitalis or calcium antagonists may have additive effects in prolonging AV-conduction time. Potentiated systemic β-blockade (eg, decreased HR, depression) reported w/ concomitant CYP2D6 inhibitors (eg, quinidine, SSRIs). Oral β-blockers may exacerbate the rebound HTN that can follow the withdrawal of clonidine.

PREGNANCY AND LACTATION
Pregnancy: Category C.
Lactation: Not for use in nursing.

MECHANISM OF ACTION
Carbonic anhydrase inhibitor/nonselective β-blocker; decreases elevated IOP, whether or not associated w/ glaucoma, by reducing aqueous humor secretion.

PHARMACOKINETICS
Absorption: Systemically absorbed. Timolol: C_{max}=0.46ng/mL. **Distribution:** Dorzolamide: Plasma protein binding (33%). Timolol: Found in breast milk. **Metabolism:** Dorzolamide: N-desethyl metabolite. **Elimination:** Dorzolamide: Urine (unchanged, metabolite); $T_{1/2}$=4 months.

PATIENT CONSIDERATIONS
Assessment: Assess for hypersensitivity to any component of product or to sulfonamides, bronchial asthma or history thereof, COPD, sinus bradycardia, 2nd- or 3rd-degree AV block, cardiac failure, cardiogenic shock, patients subject to spontaneous hypoglycemia, diabetes, renal/hepatic impairment, any other conditions where the treatment is contraindicated or cautioned, pregnancy/nursing status, and possible drug interactions.

Monitoring: Monitor for respiratory reactions, signs/symptoms of cardiac failure, hypersensitivity reactions, increased reactivity to allergens, muscle weakness, corneal edema, bacterial keratitis, and other adverse reactions.

Counseling: Advise patients w/ bronchial asthma or history thereof, severe COPD, sinus bradycardia, 2nd- or 3rd-degree AV block, or cardiac failure not to take this product. Inform that medication contains dorzolamide (a sulfonamide) and is absorbed systemically; instruct to d/c use and seek physician's advice if serious/unusual reactions or signs of hypersensitivity develop. Advise to immediately contact physician concerning the continued use of the product if undergoing ocular surgery or if an intercurrent ocular condition (eg, trauma, infection) develops. Explain that if >1 topical ophthalmic drug is being used, the drugs should be administered at least 5 min apart. **Cosopt:** Inform that if handled improperly or if the tip of the dispensing container contacts the eye or surrounding structures, the sol can become contaminated. Inform that serious damage to the eye and subsequent loss of vision may result from using contaminated sol. Inform that medication contains benzalkonium chloride, which may be absorbed by soft contact lenses. Instruct to remove contact lenses prior to administration; lenses may be reinserted 15 min following administration. **Cosopt PF:** Inform that drug does not contain a preservative; instruct to use immediately after opening and to discard remaining contents immediately after administration.

COTELLIC — cobimetinib   Rx

Class: Kinase inhibitor

ADULT DOSAGE
Unresectable or Metastatic Melanoma with BRAF V600E or V600K Mutations

- 60mg qd for the first 21 days of each 28-day cycle in combination w/ vemurafenib
- Continue therapy until disease progression or unacceptable toxicity

PEDIATRIC DOSAGE
Pediatric use may not have been established

Missed Dose
If a dose is missed or if vomiting occurs when the dose is taken, resume dosing w/ the next scheduled dose

---

DOSING CONSIDERATIONS
Concomitant Medications
Do not take strong or moderate CYP3A inhibitors. If concurrent short-term (≤14 days) use of moderate CYP3A inhibitors is unavoidable, reduce cobimetinib dose to 20mg; after discontinuation of a moderate CYP3A inhibitor, resume previous dose of cobimetinib 60mg. Use an alternative to a strong or moderate CYP3A inhibitor in patients who are taking a reduced dose of cobimetinib (40 or 20mg daily).

Renal Impairment
Moderate (CrCl 30-89mL/min): Dose adjustment is not recommended
Severe: A recommended dose has not been established

Adverse Reactions
Recommended Dose Reductions for Cobimetinib:
1st Dose Reduction: 40mg qd
2nd Dose Reduction: 20mg qd
Subsequent Modification: Permanently d/c if unable to tolerate 20mg qd

Hemorrhage:
Grade 3: Withhold for ≤4 weeks. If improved to Grade 0 or 1, resume at the next lower dose level. If not improved w/in 4 weeks, permanently d/c.
Grade 4: Permanently d/c

Cardiomyopathy:
Asymptomatic, Absolute Decrease in Left Ventricular Ejection Fraction (LVEF) from Baseline of >10% and <Lower Limit of Normal (LLN): Withhold for 2 weeks; repeat LVEF. Resume at next lower dose if LVEF is ≥LLN and absolute decrease from baseline LVEF is ≤10%. Permanently d/c if LVEF is <LLN or absolute decrease from baseline LVEF is >10%.
Symptomatic LVEF Decrease from Baseline: Withhold for ≤4 weeks; repeat LVEF. Resume at next lower dose if symptoms resolve, LVEF is ≥LLN, and absolute decrease from baseline LVEF is ≤10%. Permanently d/c if symptoms persist, LVEF is <LLN, or absolute decrease from baseline LVEF is >10%.

Dermatologic Reactions:
Grade 2 (Intolerable), Grade 3 or 4: Withhold or reduce dose

Serous Retinopathy or Retinal Vein Occlusion:
Serous Retinopathy: Withhold for ≤4 weeks. If signs and symptoms improve, resume at the next lower dose level. If not improved or symptoms recur at the lower dose w/in 4 weeks, permanently d/c.
Retinal Vein Occlusion: Permanently d/c

Liver Lab Abnormalities and Hepatotoxicity:
1st Occurrence Grade 4: Withhold for ≤4 weeks. If improved to Grade 0 or 1, then resume at the next lower dose level. If not improved to Grade 0 or 1 w/in 4 weeks, permanently d/c.
Recurrent Grade 4: Permanently d/c

Rhabdomyolysis and Creatine Phosphokinase (CPK) Elevations:
Grade 4 CPK Elevation/Any CPK Elevation and Myalgia: Withhold for ≤4 weeks. If improved to Grade 3 or lower, resume at the next lower dose level. If not improved w/in 4 weeks, permanently d/c.

Photosensitivity:
Grade 2 (Intolerable), Grade 3 or Grade 4: Withhold for ≤4 weeks. If improved to Grade 0 or 1, resume at the next lower dose level. If not improved w/in 4 weeks, permanently d/c.

Other:
Grade 2 (Intolerable)/Any Grade 3 Adverse Reactions: Withhold for ≤4 weeks. If improved to Grade 0 or 1, resume at the next lower dose level. If not improved w/in 4 weeks, permanently d/c.
1st Occurrence of Any Grade 4 Adverse Reaction: Withhold until adverse reaction improves to Grade 0 or 1. Then resume at the next lower dose level, or permanently d/c.
Recurrent Grade 4 Adverse Reaction: Permanently d/c

ADMINISTRATION
Oral route

Take w/ or w/o food.

STORAGE
<30°C (86°F).

HOW SUPPLIED
Tab: 20mg

WARNINGS/PRECAUTIONS
See Dosing Considerations. New primary malignancies, cutaneous and non-cutaneous, may occur; monitor patients for signs or symptoms of non-cutaneous malignancies. Perform dermatologic evaluations prior to initiation of therapy and every 2 months during therapy, and monitor for 6 months following discontinuation. Hemorrhage (including major hemorrhages), severe rash and other skin reactions, and photosensitivity (including severe cases) may occur. Cardiomyopathy may occur; evaluate LVEF prior to initiation, 1 month after initiation, and every 3 months thereafter until discontinuation. If restarting treatment after a dose reduction/interruption, evaluate LVEF at approx 2 weeks, 4 weeks, 10 weeks, and 16 weeks, and then as clinically indicated. Ocular toxicities, including serous retinopathy, may occur; perform an ophthalmological evaluation at regular intervals and any time a patient reports new or worsening visual disturbances. Hepatotoxicity may occur; monitor liver lab tests before initiation and monthly during treatment, or more frequently as clinically indicated.

Rhabdomyolysis may occur; obtain baseline serum CPK and creatinine levels prior to initiation, periodically during treatment, and as clinically indicated. May cause fetal harm.

ADVERSE REACTIONS
Diarrhea, photosensitivity reaction, N/V, pyrexia.

DRUG INTERACTIONS
See Dosing Considerations. Strong CYP3A4 inhibitors (itraconazole) may increase systemic exposure. Strong CYP3A inducers may decrease systemic exposure and reduce efficacy; avoid concurrent use w/ strong or moderate CYP3A inducers (eg, carbamazepine, efavirenz, phenytoin).

PREGNANCY AND LACTATION
Pregnancy: Can cause fetal harm when administered to a pregnant woman. **Lactation:** There is no information regarding the presence of cobimetinib in human milk, effects on the breastfed infant, or effects on milk production; advise not to breastfeed during treatment and for 2 weeks after the final dose. **Reproductive Potential:** May reduce fertility in females and males. Females of reproductive potential should use effective contraception during treatment and for 2 weeks after the final dose.

MECHANISM OF ACTION
Kinase inhibitor; reversible inhibitor of mitogen-activated protein kinase/extracellular signal regulated kinase 1 (MEK1) and MEK2, which promotes cellular proliferation. BRAF V600E mutations result in constitutive activation of the BRAF pathway, which includes MEK1 and MEK2. Inhibits tumor cell growth (tumor cell lines expressing BRAF V600E); coadministration w/ vemurafenib resulted in increased apoptosis in vitro and reduced tumor growth. Also prevented vemurafenib-mediated growth enhancement of a wild-type BRAF tumor cell line.

PHARMACOKINETICS
Absorption: Absolute bioavailability (46%); T_{max}=2.4 hrs (median); C_{max}=273ng/mL; AUC_{0-24h}=4340ng•h/mL. **Distribution:** Plasma protein binding (95%); V_d=806L. **Metabolism:** CYP3A oxidation and UGT2B7 glucuronidation. **Elimination:** Feces (76%, 6.6% unchanged), urine (17.8%, 1.6% unchanged); $T_{1/2}$=44 hrs.

PATIENT CONSIDERATIONS

Assessment: Confirm the presence of BRAF V600E or V600K mutation in tumor specimens and evaluate LVEF, liver lab tests, and baseline serum CPK and creatinine levels prior to initiation. Perform dermatologic evaluations. Assess pregnancy/nursing status.

Monitoring: Monitor for signs or symptoms of non-cutaneous malignancies, hemorrhage, photosensitivity, pregnancy, and other adverse reactions. Perform dermatologic evaluations every 2 months during therapy and monitor for 6 months following discontinuation. Monitor LVEF 1 month after initiation, and every 3 months thereafter until discontinuation; if restarting treatment after a dose reduction/interruption, evaluate LVEF at approx 2 weeks, 4 weeks, 10 weeks, and 16 weeks, and then as clinically indicated. Perform ophthalmological evaluations at regular intervals and any time a patient reports new or worsening visual disturbances. Monitor liver lab tests monthly during treatment or as indicated. Obtain serum CPK and creatinine levels periodically.

Counseling: Advise to contact healthcare provider immediately for change in or development of new skin lesions, severe skin changes, any changes in vision, muscle pain or weakness, and any signs/symptoms of unusual severe bleeding/hemorrhage, left ventricular dysfunction, or liver dysfunction. Advise to report any history of cardiac disease and of the requirement for cardiac monitoring prior to and during treatment. Advise that treatment requires monitoring of their liver function. Advise to avoid sun exposure, wear protective clothing, and use broad-spectrum UVA/UVB sunscreen and lip balm (SPF ≥30) when outdoors. Advise females of reproductive potential of the potential risk to a fetus and to use effective contraception during treatment and for at least 2 weeks after the final dose; advise to contact healthcare provider if they become pregnant, or if pregnancy is suspected, during treatment. Advise not to breastfeed during treatment and for 2 weeks after the final dose.

COUMADIN — warfarin sodium   Rx
Class: Vitamin K-dependent coagulation factor inhibitor

> May cause major or fatal bleeding; monitor INR regularly. Drugs, dietary changes, and other factors affect INR levels achieved w/ therapy. Instruct patients about prevention measures to minimize risk of bleeding and to report signs/symptoms of bleeding.

OTHER BRAND NAMES
Jantoven

ADULT DOSAGE

Venous Thromboembolism

Including Deep Vein Thrombosis (DVT) and Pulmonary Embolism (PE): Target INR: 2.5 (INR Range, 2-3) for all treatment durations

Duration of Therapy:
DVT/PE Secondary to Transient Risk Factor: 3 months
Unprovoked DVT/PE: At least 3 months; evaluate risk-benefit ratio of long-term treatment after 3 months of therapy
2 Episodes of Unprovoked DVT/PE: Long-term treatment recommended

PEDIATRIC DOSAGE
General Dosing

Adequate and well-controlled studies have not been conducted in any pediatric population; optimum dosing and safety/efficacy unknown. Pediatric use is based on adult data and recommendations, and available limited pediatric data

Nonvalvular Atrial Fibrillation
Target INR: 2.5 (INR Range, 2-3)
Duration of Therapy:
Persistent/Paroxysmal A-Fib and High Risk of Stroke: Long-term treatment recommended
Persistent/Paroxysmal A-Fib and Intermediate Risk of Ischemic Stroke: Long-term treatment recommended
A-Fib and Mitral Stenosis: Long-term treatment recommended
A-Fib and Prosthetic Heart Valves: Long-term treatment recommended; target INR may be increased and aspirin (ASA) added depending on valve type and position, and on patient factors

Mechanical/Bioprosthetic Heart Valves

Bileaflet Mechanical Valve/Medtronic Hall Tilting Disk Valve in the Aortic Position in Sinus Rhythm and w/o Left Atrial Enlargement: Target INR: 2.5 (INR Range, 2-3)

Tilting Disk Valves and Bileaflet Mechanical Valves in the Mitral Position: Target INR: 3 (INR Range, 2.5-3.5)

Caged Ball or Caged Disk Valves: Target INR: 3 (INR Range, 2.5-3.5)

Bioprosthetic Valve in the Mitral Position: Target INR: 2.5 (INR Range, 2-3) for the first 3 months after valve insertion. If additional risk factors for thromboembolism present, target INR 2.5 (INR Range, 2-3)

Post-Myocardial Infarction
High Risk Patients w/ MI:
Treat w/ combined moderate-intensity (INR, 2-3) warfarin plus low-dose ASA (≤100 mg/day) for at least 3 months after MI

Recurrent Systemic Embolism
Unknown Etiology:
Use a moderate dose regimen (INR, 2-3)

Dosing Based on Genotype Consideration

Expected Maint Daily Doses Based on CYP2C9 and VKORC1 Genotypes:
VKORC1-GG:
CYP2C9 *1/*1: 5-7mg
CYP2C9 *1/*2: 5-7mg
CYP2C9 *1/*3: 3-4mg
CYP2C9 *2/*2: 3-4mg
CYP2C9 *2/*3: 3-4mg
CYP2C9 *3/*3: 0.5-2mg

VKORC1-AG:
CYP2C9 *1/*1: 5-7mg
CYP2C9 *1/*2: 3-4mg
CYP2C9 *1/*3: 3-4mg
CYP2C9 *2/*2: 3-4mg
CYP2C9 *2/*3: 0.5-2mg
CYP2C9 *3/*3: 0.5-2mg

VKORC1-AA:
CYP2C9 *1/*1: 3-4mg
CYP2C9 *1/*2: 3-4mg
CYP2C9 *1/*3: 0.5-2mg
CYP2C9 *2/*2: 0.5-2mg
CYP2C9 *2/*3: 0.5-2mg
CYP2C9 *3/*3: 0.5-2mg

CYP2C9 *1/*3, *2/*2, *2/*3, and *3/*3: May require more prolonged time (>2-4 weeks) to achieve max INR effect

If CYP2C9 and VKORC1 Genotypes Are Unknown:
Initial: 2-5mg qd
Maint: 2-10mg qd

Other Indications

Mitral Stenosis/Valvular Disease Associated w/ A-Fib:
Use a moderate dose regimen (INR, 2-3)

Conversions

From Heparin:

Conversion may begin concomitantly w/ heparin therapy or may be delayed 3-6 days.

Continue full dose heparin therapy and overlap warfarin therapy w/ heparin for 4-5 days; may d/c heparin once warfarin has produced the desired therapeutic response as determined by INR.

Patients receiving both heparin and warfarin should have INR monitoring at least:
- Five hrs after the last IV bolus heparin dose, or
- Four hrs after cessation of continuous IV heparin infusion, or
- Twenty-four hrs after the last SQ heparin inj

Warfarin may increase the aPTT test, even in the absence of heparin; severe elevation (>50 sec) in aPTT w/ INR in desired range has been identified as an indication of increased risk of postoperative hemorrhage

From Other Anticoagulants:

Consult the labeling of other anticoagulants for conversion instructions

DOSING CONSIDERATIONS

Elderly

Elderly/Debilitated: Consider lower initial and maint doses

Other Important Considerations

Asian Patients: Consider lower initial and maint doses
Treatment During Dentistry or Surgery: Some dental or surgical procedures may necessitate an interruption or change in dose. Determine the INR immediately prior to any procedure

ADMINISTRATION

Oral route (Coumadin, Jantoven) or IV route (Coumadin)

Coumadin

IV dose is the same as oral dose.
IV:
Reconstitute vial w/ 2.7mL of sterile water for inj; resulting yield is 2.5mL of a 2mg/mL sol.
After reconstitution, administer as a slow bolus inj into a peripheral vein over 1-2 min.
Reconstituted sol is stable for 4 hrs at room temperature; discard any unused sol.

STORAGE

Tab: (Coumadin) 15-30°C (59-86°F). Protect from light and moisture. (Jantoven) 20-25°C (68-77°F); excursions permitted at 15-30°C (59-86°F). Protect from light and moisture. **Inj:** (Coumadin) 15-30°C (59-86°F). Protect from light. Use reconstituted sol w/in 4 hrs; do not refrigerate. Discard any unused sol.

HOW SUPPLIED

Inj: (Coumadin) 5mg; **Tab:** (Coumadin, Jantoven) 1mg*, 2mg*, 2.5mg*, 3mg*, 4mg*, 5mg*, 6mg*, 7.5mg*, 10mg* *scored

CONTRAINDICATIONS

Pregnancy, except in pregnant women w/ mechanical heart valves, who are at high risk of thromboembolism. Hemorrhagic tendencies or blood dyscrasias. Recent or contemplated surgery of the CNS, eye, or traumatic surgery resulting in large open surfaces. Bleeding tendencies associated w/ active ulceration or overt bleeding of GI/genitourinary/respiratory tract, CNS hemorrhage, cerebral aneurysms, dissecting aorta, pericarditis and pericardial effusions, or bacterial endocarditis. Threatened abortion, eclampsia, and preeclampsia. Unsupervised patients w/ conditions associated w/ potential high level of noncompliance. Spinal puncture and other diagnostic/therapeutic procedures w/ potential for uncontrollable bleeding. Hypersensitivity to warfarin or to any other components of the medication (eg, anaphylaxis). Major regional, lumbar block anesthesia. Malignant HTN.

WARNINGS/PRECAUTIONS

Has no direct effect on established thrombus, nor does it reverse ischemic tissue damage; once a thrombus has occurred, the goals of anticoagulant treatment are to prevent further extension of the formed clot and to prevent secondary thromboembolic complications that may result in serious and possibly fatal sequelae. INR >4 provides no additional therapeutic benefit in most patients and is associated w/ higher risk of bleeding. Bleeding is more likely to occur w/in the 1st month; patients at high risk of bleeding may benefit from more frequent INR monitoring, careful dose adjustment to desired INR, and a shortest duration of therapy. Has a narrow therapeutic range (index) and its action may be affected by endogenous factors, other drugs, and dietary vitamin K. Determine the INR daily after initial dose administration until INR results stabilize in the therapeutic range; after stabilization, perform INR monitoring based on the clinical situation (acceptable interval 1-4 weeks). Risk of necrosis and/or gangrene of skin and other tissues; d/c if necrosis occurs and consider alternative therapy. May enhance the release of atheromatous plaque emboli, and systemic atheroemboli

and cholesterol microemboli may occur. D/C if distinct syndrome resulting from microemboli to the feet ("purple toes syndrome") occurs and consider alternative therapy. Do not use as initial therapy w/ heparin-induced thrombocytopenia (HIT) and w/ heparin-induced thrombocytopenia w/ thrombosis syndrome (HITTS); limb ischemia, necrosis, and gangrene reported when heparin was discontinued and warfarin started or continued. Can cause fetal harm in pregnant women. Increased risks of therapy in patients w/ moderate-severe hepatic impairment, infectious diseases/disturbances of intestinal flora, indwelling catheter, severe/moderate HTN, deficiency in protein C-mediated anticoagulant response, polycythemia vera, vasculitis, or diabetes mellitus, or who are undergoing eye surgery. Caution in elderly. Caution w/ hepatic impairment; can potentiate the response to warfarin.

ADVERSE REACTIONS

Hemorrhage, necrosis of the skin and other tissues, systemic atheroemboli, cholesterol microemboli, hypersensitivity/allergic reactions, vasculitis, hepatitis, elevated liver enzymes, N/V, diarrhea, rash, dermatitis, tracheal/tracheobronchial calcifications, chills.

DRUG INTERACTIONS

Inhibitors of CYP2C9, 1A2, and/or 3A4 may increase effect (increase INR) by increasing exposure of warfarin. Inducers of CYP2C9, 1A2, and/or 3A4 may decrease effect (decrease INR) by decreasing exposure of warfarin. Increased risk of bleeding w/ anticoagulants (argatroban, bivalirudin, heparin), antiplatelet agents (ASA, cilostazol, clopidogrel), NSAIDs (celecoxib, diclofenac, diflunisal), and serotonin reuptake inhibitors (eg, citalopram, desvenlafaxine, duloxetine). Changes in INR reported w/ antibiotics or antifungals; closely monitor INR when starting or stopping any antibiotics or antifungals. Perform more frequent INR monitoring when starting or stopping botanicals; some botanicals (eg, garlic, *Ginkgo biloba*) may cause additive anticoagulant effects, while some botanicals (eg, coenzyme Q10, St. John's wort, ginseng) may decrease effects. Some botanicals and foods can interact w/ warfarin through CYP450 interactions (eg, *echinacea*, grapefruit juice, ginkgo, goldenseal, St. John's wort). Cholestatic hepatitis has been associated w/ coadministration of warfarin and ticlopidine. Perform more frequent INR monitoring when starting or stopping other drugs, including botanicals, or when changing dosages of other drugs, including drugs intended for short-term use (eg, antibiotics, antifungals, corticosteroids).

PREGNANCY AND LACTATION

Pregnancy: Contraindicated in women who are pregnant except in pregnant women w/ mechanical heart valves, who are at high risk of thromboembolism, and for whom benefits may outweigh risks. Can cause fetal harm. Crosses the placenta; concentrations in fetal plasma approach the maternal values.
Lactation: Warfarin was not present in human milk from mothers treated w/ warfarin from a limited published study. Caution in nursing; monitor breastfeeding infants for bruising or bleeding.
Reproductive Potential: Verify pregnancy status of females of reproductive potential prior to initiating therapy. Females of reproductive potential should use effective contraception during treatment and for at least 1 month after the final dose of therapy.

MECHANISM OF ACTION

Vitamin K-dependent coagulation factor inhibitor; inhibits the synthesis of vitamin K-dependent clotting factors, which include Factors II, VII, IX, and X, and the anticoagulant proteins C and S. Thought to interfere w/ clotting factor synthesis by inhibition of the C1 subunit of the vitamin K epoxide reductase enzyme complex, thereby reducing the regeneration of vitamin K1 epoxide.

PHARMACOKINETICS

Absorption: (PO) Complete; T_{max}=4 hrs. **Distribution:** V_d=0.14L/kg; plasma protein binding (99%); crosses placenta. **Metabolism:** Hepatic via CYP2C9, 2C19, 2C8, 2C18, 1A2, 3A4; hydroxylation (major), reduction. **Elimination:** Urine (≤92%, metabolites); $T_{1/2}$=1 week.

PATIENT CONSIDERATIONS

Assessment: Assess for risk factors for bleeding (eg, INR>4, age ≥65 yrs, history of highly variable INR, history of GI bleeding, HTN, cerebrovascular disease, malignancy, anemia, trauma, renal impairment, certain genetic factors, long duration of warfarin therapy), factors affecting INR (eg, diarrhea, hepatic disorders, poor nutritional state, steatorrhea, vitamin K deficiency, increased vitamin K intake, hereditary warfarin resistance), pregnancy/nursing status, other conditions where treatment is contraindicated or cautioned, and possible drug interactions. Assess INR. Obtain platelet counts in patients w/ HIT or HITTS.

Monitoring: Monitor for signs/symptoms of bleeding, necrosis/gangrene of skin and other tissues, systemic atheroemboli, cholesterol microemboli, "purple toes syndrome," and other adverse reactions. For patients receiving long-term anticoagulant treatment, periodically reassess risk-benefit ratio of continuing such treatment. Perform regular INR monitoring.

Counseling: Instruct to inform physician if patient falls often as this may increase risk for complications. Counsel to maintain strict adherence to dosing regimen. Advise not to start or stop other medications, including salicylates (eg, ASA, topical analgesics), OTC drugs, or herbal medications, except on advice of physician. Instruct to inform physician if pregnancy is suspected (to discuss pregnancy planning) or if considering breastfeeding. Counsel to avoid any activity or sport that may result in traumatic injury. Instruct that regular PT tests and visits to physician are required during therapy. Advise patient to carry ID card stating drug is being taken. Instruct to eat a normal, balanced diet to maintain consistent intake of vitamin K and to avoid drastic changes in diet, such as eating large amounts of leafy, green vegetables. Advise to take ud. Advise to immediately report unusual bleeding or symptoms or any serious illness, such as severe diarrhea, infection, or fever. Inform that anticoagulant effects may persist for about 2-5 days after discontinuation.

COVERA-HS — verapamil hydrochloride Rx

Class: Calcium channel blocker (CCB) (nondihydropyridine)

ADULT DOSAGE	PEDIATRIC DOSAGE
Hypertension Individualize dose by titration **Initial:** 180mg qhs **Titrate:** If inadequate response w/ 180mg, increase to 240mg qhs, then 360mg (two 180mg tab) qhs, then 480mg (two 240mg tab) qhs **Angina** Individualize dose by titration **Initial:** 180mg qhs **Titrate:** If inadequate response w/ 180mg, increase to 240mg qhs, then 360mg (two 180mg tab) qhs, then 480mg (two 240mg tab) qhs	Pediatric use may not have been established

DOSING CONSIDERATIONS

Hepatic Impairment
Severe Dysfunction: Give 30% of normal dose

Elderly
Start at lower end of dosing range

ADMINISTRATION
Oral route
Swallow whole; do not chew, break, or crush

STORAGE
20-25°C (68-77°F).

HOW SUPPLIED
Tab, Extended-Release: 180mg, 240mg

CONTRAINDICATIONS
Known hypersensitivity to verapamil, severe left ventricular dysfunction, hypotension or cardiogenic shock, sick sinus syndrome or 2nd/3rd-degree atrioventricular (AV) block (except with functioning artificial ventricular pacemaker), A-fib/flutter with an accessory bypass tract.

WARNINGS/PRECAUTIONS
Has negative inotropic effect; avoid with moderate to severe cardiac failure symptoms or any degree of ventricular dysfunction if taking a β-blocker. Patients with milder ventricular dysfunction should, if possible, be controlled with optimum doses of digitalis and/or diuretics before treatment. May cause CHF, pulmonary edema, hypotension, asymptomatic 1st-degree AV block, transient bradycardia, and PR interval prolongation. Marked 1st-degree block or progressive development to 2nd/3rd-degree AV block requires dose reduction, or discontinuation and institution of appropriate therapy (rare). Elevated transaminases with and without concomitant elevations in alkaline phosphatase and bilirubin reported; periodically monitor LFTs. Sinus bradycardia, 2nd-degree AV block, pulmonary edema, severe hypotension, and sinus arrest reported in patients with hypertrophic cardiomyopathy. Caution with preexisting severe GI narrowing. Caution with hepatic dysfunction; monitor for abnormal PR interval prolongation or other signs of excessive pharmacologic effects. May decrease neuromuscular transmission in patients with Duchenne muscular dystrophy and cause worsening of myasthenia gravis; decrease dose with attenuated neuromuscular transmission. Caution with renal dysfunction; monitor for abnormal PR interval prolongation or other signs of overdosage. Caution in elderly.

ADVERSE REACTIONS
Constipation, dizziness, headache, edema, fatigue, sinus bradycardia, 2nd-degree AV block, upper respiratory infection.

DRUG INTERACTIONS
Increased levels with CYP3A4 inhibitors (eg, erythromycin, ritonavir) and grapefruit juice. Decreased levels with CYP3A4 inducers (eg, rifampin). May cause myopathy/rhabdomyolysis with HMG-CoA reductase inhibitors that are CYP3A4 substrates (eg, atorvastatin) and may increase levels of such drugs; limit dose of simvastatin to 10mg/day or lovastatin to 40mg/day. Increased bleeding times with aspirin. Additive negative effects on HR, AV conduction, and/or cardiac contractility with β-blockers. May produce asymptomatic bradycardia with a wandering pacemaker with timolol eye drops. Decreased metoprolol and propranolol clearance while variable effect with atenolol. Chronic treatment may increase digoxin levels, which may result in digitalis toxicity. May reduce clearance of digitoxin. Additive effect on lowering BP with other antihypertensives (eg, vasodilators, ACE inhibitors, diuretics, β-blockers). Excessive reduction in BP with prazosin. Avoid disopyramide within 48 hrs before or 24 hrs after therapy. Additive negative inotropic effects and AV conduction prolongation with flecainide. Avoid quinidine with hypertrophic cardiomyopathy. Reduced or unchanged clearance with cimetidine. Increased sensitivity to effects of lithium when used concomitantly; monitor carefully. May increase carbamazepine, theophylline, cyclosporine, and alcohol levels. Increased clearance with phenobarbital. Reduced oral bioavailability with rifampin. Titrate carefully with inhalation anesthetics to avoid excessive cardiovascular depression. May potentiate neuromuscular blockers (curare-like and depolarizing); both agents may need dose reduction. May cause hypotension and bradyarrhythmias with telithromycin. Sinus bradycardia resulting in hospitalization and pacemaker insertion with clonidine; monitor HR. Prolonged recovery from neuromuscular blocking agent vecuronium reported.

PREGNANCY AND LACTATION
Category C, not for use in nursing.

MECHANISM OF ACTION
Calcium channel blocker (nondihydropyridine); selectively inhibits transmembrane influx of ionic Ca^{2+} into arterial smooth muscle and in conductile and contractile myocardial cells without altering serum Ca^{2+} concentrations.

PHARMACOKINETICS
Absorption: Administration of variable doses resulted in different pharmacokinetic parameters. T_{max}=11 hrs. (Immediate-release) Bioavailability (33-65%, R-verapamil), (13-34%, S-verapamil). **Distribution:** Plasma protein binding (94% to albumin and 92% to α-1 acid glycoprotein, R-verapamil), (88% to albumin and 86% to α-1 acid glycoprotein, S-verapamil); crosses placenta, found in breast milk. **Metabolism:** Liver (extensive); norverapamil (active metabolite). **Elimination:** Urine (70% metabolites, 3-4% unchanged), feces (≥16%).

PATIENT CONSIDERATIONS
Assessment: Assess for cardiac failure symptoms, ventricular dysfunction, preexisting severe GI narrowing, hypertrophic cardiomyopathy, hepatic/renal function, Duchenne muscular dystrophy, attenuated neuromuscular transmission, any conditions where treatment is contraindicated, pregnancy/nursing status, and possible drug interactions.

Monitoring: Monitor for CHF, hypotension, AV block, abnormal PR interval prolongation, and worsening of myasthenia gravis. Periodically monitor LFTs and renal function.

Counseling: Instruct to swallow tab whole and to not chew, break, or crush. Inform that outer shell of tab does not dissolve and may occasionally be observed in stool. Advise to seek medical attention if any adverse reactions occur. Counsel not to breastfeed and to report immediately if pregnant.

COZAAR — losartan potassium Rx

Class: Angiotensin II receptor blocker (ARB)

> D/C when pregnancy is detected. Drugs that act directly on the renin-angiotensin system (RAS) can cause injury/death to the developing fetus.

ADULT DOSAGE	PEDIATRIC DOSAGE
Hypertension **Initial:** 50mg qd **Max:** 100mg qd **Hypertension with Left Ventricular Hypertrophy** **Reduction in Risk of Stroke:** **Initial:** 50mg qd **Titrate:** Add hydrochlorothiazide (HCTZ) 12.5mg qd and/or increase losartan to 100mg qd, followed by an increase in HCTZ to 25mg qd based on BP response This may not apply to black patients **Diabetic Nephropathy** **Elevated SrCr/Proteinuria (Urinary Albumin to Creatinine Ratio ≥300mg/g) in Patients w/ Type 2 Diabetes and a History of HTN:** **Initial:** 50mg qd **Titrate:** Increase to 100mg qd based on BP response	**Hypertension** **≥6 Years:** **Initial:** 0.7mg/kg qd (up to 50mg total) administered as a tab or sus **Titrate:** Adjust dose according to BP response **Max:** 1.4mg/kg/day (or 100mg/day)

DOSING CONSIDERATIONS
Renal Impairment
Pediatric HTN:
GFR <30mL/min/1.73m²: Not recommended

Hepatic Impairment
Mild-to-Moderate:
Initial: 25mg qd

Other Important Considerations
Adult HTN: Starting dose of 25mg is recommended for patients w/ possible intravascular depletion

ADMINISTRATION
Oral route

Preparation of Sus (for 200mL of a 2.5mg/mL Sus)
1. Add 10mL of purified water to an 8 oz (240mL) amber polyethylene terephthalate (PET) bottle containing ten 50mg Cozaar tabs.
2. Immediately shake for at least 2 min.
3. Let the concentrate stand for 1 hr and then shake for 1 min to disperse the tab contents.
4. Separately prepare a 50/50 volumetric mixture of Ora-Plus and Ora-Sweet SF.
5. Add 190mL of the 50/50 Ora-Plus/Ora-Sweet SF mixture to the tab and water slurry in the PET bottle and shake for 1 min to disperse the ingredients.
6. The sus should be refrigerated at 2-8°C (36-46°F) and can be stored for up to 4 weeks.
7. Shake the sus prior to each use and return promptly to the refrigerator.

STORAGE
(Tab) 25°C (77°F); excursions permitted to 15-30°C (59-86°F). Protect from light. (Sus) 2-8°C (36-46°F) for up to 4 weeks.

HOW SUPPLIED
Tab: 25mg, 50mg*, 100mg *scored

CONTRAINDICATIONS
Hypersensitivity to any component of the medication, coadministration w/ aliskiren in patients w/ diabetes.

WARNINGS/PRECAUTIONS
Symptomatic hypotension may occur in patients w/ an activated RAS (eg, volume- or salt-depleted patients); correct volume or salt depletion prior to administration of therapy. Patients whose renal function may depend in part on the activity of the RAS may be at risk of developing acute renal failure; monitor renal function periodically. Consider withholding or discontinuing therapy in patients who develop a clinically significant decrease in renal function on losartan. Monitor serum K^+ periodically and treat appropriately; dosage reduction or discontinuation of losartan may be required.

ADVERSE REACTIONS
Dizziness, URI, nasal congestion, back pain.

DRUG INTERACTIONS
See Contraindications. Use w/ other drugs that raise serum K^+ may result in hyperkalemia; monitor serum K^+. Increases in serum lithium concentrations and lithium toxicity reported; monitor serum lithium levels during concomitant use. In patients who are elderly, volume-depleted (including those on diuretic therapy), or w/ compromised renal function, coadministration w/ NSAIDs, including selective COX-2 inhibitors, may result in deterioration in renal function, including possible acute renal failure. Antihypertensive effect may be attenuated by NSAIDs, including selective COX-2 inhibitors. Dual blockade of the RAS is associated w/ increased risks of hypotension, syncope, hyperkalemia, and changes in renal function (including acute renal failure); avoid combined use of RAS inhibitors. Closely monitor BP, renal function, and electrolytes w/ concomitant agents that affect the RAS. Avoid w/ aliskiren in patients w/ renal impairment (GFR <60mL/min).

PREGNANCY AND LACTATION
Pregnancy: Category D.
Lactation: Not for use in nursing.

MECHANISM OF ACTION
Angiotensin II receptor antagonist; blocks vasoconstrictor and aldosterone-secreting effects of angiotensin II by selectively blocking the binding of angiotensin II to AT_1 receptor in many tissues (eg, vascular smooth muscle, adrenal gland).

PHARMACOKINETICS
Absorption: Well-absorbed. Systemic bioavailability (33%); T_{max}=1 hr, 3-4 hrs (active metabolite). **Distribution:** V_d=34L, 12L (active metabolite); plasma protein binding (98.7%, 99.8% active metabolite). **Metabolism:** Liver via CYP2C9, 3A4; carboxylic acid (active metabolite). **Elimination:** Urine (35%, 4% unchanged, 6% active metabolite), feces (60%); $T_{1/2}$=2 hrs, 6-9 hrs (active metabolite).

PATIENT CONSIDERATIONS
Assessment: Assess for history of hypersensitivity, volume/salt depletion, CHF, diabetes mellitus, renal artery stenosis, hepatic/renal impairment, pregnancy/nursing status, and possible drug interactions.

Monitoring: Monitor for signs/symptoms of hypotension, changes in renal function, and other adverse reactions. Monitor BP, serum K^+ levels, and renal function periodically.

Counseling: Inform of pregnancy risks and discuss treatment options w/ women planning to become pregnant; instruct to report pregnancy to physician as soon as possible. Instruct not to use K^+ supplements or salt substitutes containing K^+ w/o consulting physician.

CREON — pancrelipase
Rx

Class: Pancreatic enzyme supplement

ADULT DOSAGE
Exocrine Pancreatic Insufficiency

Due to Cystic Fibrosis, Chronic Pancreatitis, Pancreatectomy, or Other Conditions:
Start at the lowest recommended dose and increase gradually
Initial: 500 lipase U/kg/meal
Max: 2500 lipase U/kg/meal (or ≤10,000 lipase U/kg/day) or <4000 lipase U/g fat ingested/day
Half of the dose used for meals should be given w/ each snack

Refer to PI for dosing limitations

PEDIATRIC DOSAGE
Exocrine Pancreatic Insufficiency

Due to Cystic Fibrosis, Chronic Pancreatitis, Pancreatectomy, or Other Conditions:
Start at the lowest recommended dose and increase gradually
≤12 Months:
3000 lipase U/120mL of formula or per breastfeeding; administer immediately prior to each feeding

>12 Months-<4 Years:
Initial: 1000 lipase U/kg/meal
Max: 2500 lipase U/kg/meal (or ≤10,000 lipase U/kg/day) or <4000 lipase U/g fat ingested/day

≥4 Years:
Initial: 500 lipase U/kg/meal
Max: 2500 lipase U/kg/meal (or ≤10,000 lipase U/kg/day) or <4000 lipase U/g fat ingested/day
Half of the dose used for meals should be given w/ each snack

Refer to PI for dosing limitations

DOSING CONSIDERATIONS
Elderly
Reduce dose

ADMINISTRATION
Oral route

Take during meals or snacks, w/ sufficient fluid
Swallow whole; do not crush or chew caps/cap contents
Do not retain in mouth
Do not mix directly into formula or breast milk
For patients who are unable to swallow intact capsules, open the contents and add to a small amount of acidic soft food w/ a pH of 4.5 or less, such as applesauce. The mixture should be swallowed immediately and followed w/ water or juice to ensure complete ingestion

STORAGE
Room temperature up to 25°C (77°F); excursions permitted between 25-40°C (77-104°F) for up to 30 days. Discard if exposed to higher temperature and moisture conditions >70%. Protect from moisture. Store in original container.

HOW SUPPLIED
Cap, Delayed-Release: (Lipase/Protease/Amylase) 3000 U/9500 U/15,000 U; 6000 U/19,000 U/30,000 U; 12,000 U/38,000 U/60,000 U; 24,000 U/76,000 U/120,000 U; 36,000 U/114,000 U/180,000 U

WARNINGS/PRECAUTIONS
Not interchangeable with other pancrelipase products. Fibrosing colonopathy reported; monitor closely for progression to stricture formation. Caution with doses >2500 lipase U/kg/meal (or >10,000 lipase U/kg/day); use only if these doses are documented to be effective by 3-day fecal fat measures indicating significant improvement. Examine patients receiving >6000 lipase U/kg/meal; immediately decrease or titrate dose downward to a lower range. Ensure that no drug is retained in the mouth. Should not be crushed or chewed, or mixed in foods with pH >4.5; may disrupt enteric coating of cap, resulting in early release of enzymes, irritation of oral mucosa, and/or loss of enzyme activity. Caution in patients with gout, renal impairment, or hyperuricemia; may increase blood uric acid levels. Risk for transmission of viral diseases. Caution with known allergy to proteins of porcine origin; severe allergic reactions reported.

ADVERSE REACTIONS
Vomiting, flatulence, abdominal pain, headache, cough, dizziness, frequent bowel movements, abnormal feces, hyperglycemia, hypoglycemia, nasopharyngitis, decreased appetite, irritability.

PREGNANCY AND LACTATION
Category C, caution in nursing.

MECHANISM OF ACTION
Pancreatic enzyme supplement; catalyzes the hydrolysis of fats to monoglyceride, glycerol, and free fatty acids, proteins into peptides and amino acids, and starches into dextrins and short-chain sugars (eg, maltose, maltriose) in the duodenum and proximal small intestine, thereby acting like digestive enzymes physiologically secreted by the pancreas.

PATIENT CONSIDERATIONS
Assessment: Assess for known allergy to porcine proteins, gout, renal impairment, hyperuricemia, and pregnancy/nursing status.

Monitoring: Monitor for fibrosing colonopathy, stricture formation, oral mucosa irritation, viral diseases, and allergic reactions. Monitor serum uric acid levels.

Counseling: Instruct to take ud and with food and fluids. Inform that if a dose is missed, take the next dose with the next meal/snack ud; instruct not to double doses. Inform that cap contents can also be sprinkled on soft acidic foods (eg, applesauce), if necessary. Instruct to notify physician if pregnant/breastfeeding or planning to become pregnant/breastfeed during treatment. Advise to contact physician immediately if allergic reactions develop.

CRESEMBA — isavuconazonium sulfate
Rx

Class: Azole antifungal

ADULT DOSAGE
Aspergillosis

Treatment of invasive aspergillosis

Cap/IV:
LD: 372mg q8h for 6 doses (48 hrs)
Maint: 372mg qd

Start maint doses 12-24 hrs after the last LD

Switching between the IV and oral formulations is acceptable as bioequivalence has been demonstrated; LD is not required when switching between formulations

Mucormycosis

Treatment of invasive mucormycosis

Cap/IV:
LD: 372mg q8h for 6 doses (48 hrs)
Maint: 372mg qd

Start maint doses 12-24 hrs after the last LD

Switching between the IV and oral formulations is acceptable as bioequivalence has been demonstrated; LD is not required when switching between formulations

PEDIATRIC DOSAGE
Pediatric use may not have been established

ADMINISTRATION
Oral/IV route

Cap
- Swallow whole; do not chew, crush, dissolve, or open the cap.
- Take w/ or w/o food.

IV
- Administer via an infusion set w/ an in-line filter (pore size 0.2-1.2 micron).
- Infuse over a minimum of 1 hr in 250mL of a compatible diluent; do not administer as an IV bolus inj.
- Do not infuse w/ other IV medications.
- Flush IV lines w/ 0.9% NaCl inj or D5 inj prior to and after infusion.
- After dilution, avoid unnecessary vibration or vigorous shaking of the sol; do not use a pneumatic transport system.

Reconstitution:
- Reconstitute 1 vial by adding 5mL water for inj to the vial.
- Gently shake to dissolve the powder completely.
- May store at <25°C (77°F) for max 1 hr prior to preparation of infusion sol.

Dilution and Preparation:
- Add 5mL of the reconstituted sol to an infusion bag containing 250mL of a compatible diluent.
- Use gentle mixing or roll bag to minimize the formation of particulates.
- Apply in-line filter w/ a microporous membrane pore size of 0.2-1.2 micron and in-line filter reminder sticker to the infusion bag.
- Complete administration w/in 6 hrs of dilution at room temperature; if not possible, immediately refrigerate (2-8°C [36-46°F]) the infusion sol after dilution and complete the infusion w/in 24 hrs. Do not freeze.

Compatible Diluents:
- 0.9% NaCl inj
- D5 inj

STORAGE
Cap: 20-25°C (68-77°F); excursions permitted between 15-30°C (59-86°F). Store in original container to protect from moisture. **Inj:** Unreconstituted: 2-8°C (36-46°F). Prepared infusion sol should be kept for ≤6 hrs at 20-25°C (68-77°F) or 24 hrs at 2-8°C (36-46°F) prior to use.

HOW SUPPLIED
Cap: 186mg; **Inj:** 372mg

CONTRAINDICATIONS
Known hypersensitivity to isavuconazole. Coadministration of strong CYP3A4 inhibitors (eg, ketoconazole, high-dose ritonavir (RTV) [400mg q12h]) and strong CYP3A4 inducers (eg, rifampin, carbamazepine, St. John's wort, long-acting barbiturates). Familial short QT syndrome.

WARNINGS/PRECAUTIONS
Hepatic adverse drug reactions (eg, elevations in ALT, AST, alkaline phosphate, total bilirubin) reported. Cases of more severe hepatic adverse drug reactions including hepatitis, cholestasis or hepatic failure including death reported in patients w/ serious underlying medical conditions (eg, hematologic malignancy); d/c if clinical signs and symptoms consistent w/ liver disease develop. Infusion-related reactions reported during IV administration; d/c infusion if these reactions occur. Serious hypersensitivity and severe skin reactions such as anaphylaxis or Stevens Johnson syndrome reported during treatment w/ other azole antifungal agents; d/c if a severe cutaneous adverse reaction develops. Caution when prescribing to patients w/ hypersensitivity to other azoles. May cause fetal harm when administered to pregnant woman; use only if the potential benefit to the patient outweighs the risk to the fetus.

ADVERSE REACTIONS
N/V, diarrhea, headache, elevated liver chemistry tests, hypokalemia, constipation, dyspnea, cough, peripheral edema, back pain.

DRUG INTERACTIONS
See Contraindications. CYP3A4 inhibitors/inducers may alter the plasma concentrations of isavuconazole. Ketoconazole may increase isavuconazole exposure. Rifampin may decrease isavuconazole exposure. Caution w/ lopinavir/RTV; coadministration may increase isavuconazole exposure and decrease lopinavir/RTV exposure. May increase atorvastatin exposure; use w/ caution and monitor for adverse reactions that are typical of atorvastatin. May increase cyclosporine, sirolimus, and tacrolimus exposures; use w/ caution and monitor drug concentrations of cyclosporine, sirolimus, and tacrolimus and adjust dose prn. May increase midazolam exposure; use w/ caution and consider dose reduction of midazolam. May decrease bupropion exposure, therefore use w/ caution; may be necessary to increase bupropion dose (do not exceed max recommended dose). May increase mycophenolate mofetil exposure; use w/ caution and monitor for mycophenolic acid-related toxicities. May increase digoxin exposure; use w/ caution and monitor serum digoxin concentrations.

PREGNANCY AND LACTATION
Pregnancy: Category C.
Lactation: Not for use in nursing.

MECHANISM OF ACTION
Azole antifungal; prodrug of isavuconazole. Inhibits the synthesis of ergosterol through the inhibition of CYP450-dependent enzyme lanosterol 14-α-demethylase.

PHARMACOKINETICS
Absorption: (PO) Absolute bioavailability (98%); C_{max}=7499ng/mL (2 caps), 20,028ng/mL (6 caps); T_{max}=3 hrs (2 caps, median), 4 hrs (6 caps, median); AUC=121,402hr•ng/mL (2 caps), 352,805hr•ng/mL (6 caps). **Distribution:** V_d=approx 450L (isavuconazole); plasma protein binding (>99%). **Metabolism:** Rapidly hydrolyzed in blood to isavuconazole by esterases, predominantly by butylcholinesterase. Isavuconazole: CYP3A4, CYP3A5, and subsequently, uridine diphosphate-glucuronosyltransferases. **Elimination:** (PO) Urine (45.5%), feces (46.1%). Isavuconazole: Renal (<1%); $T_{1/2}$=130 hrs.

PATIENT CONSIDERATIONS
Assessment: Assess for hypersensitivity to the drug or to other azole antifungal agents, familial short QT syndrome, serious underlying medical conditions, pregnancy/nursing status, and for possible drug interactions. Evaluate liver-related laboratory tests prior to therapy. Obtain specimens for fungal culture and other relevant laboratory studies in order to identify causative organism(s).

Monitoring: Monitor for hepatic adverse reactions, infusion-related reactions, serious hypersensitivity and severe skin reactions, and other adverse reactions. Monitor liver-related laboratory tests.

Counseling: Inform of benefits/risks of therapy. Advise to inform physician if taking other drugs or before beginning to take other drugs. Advise to inform physician if pregnant, planning to become pregnant, or nursing.

CRESTOR — rosuvastatin calcium   Rx
Class: HMG-CoA reductase inhibitor (statin)

ADULT DOSAGE

Hypercholesterolemia

Hyperlipidemia and Mixed Dyslipidemia/Hypertriglyceridemia/ Primary Dysbetalipoproteinemia (Type III Hyperlipoproteinemia)/ Slowing of the Progression of Atherosclerosis:

General Dose:
Initial: 10-20mg qd
Range: 5-40mg qd

When initiating treatment or switching from another HMG-CoA reductase inhibitor, use the appropriate starting dose 1st, then titrate according to patient's response and individualized goal of therapy

Analyze lipid levels w/in 2-4 weeks and adjust dose accordingly

Use 40mg dose only if LDL goal is not achieved w/ 20mg dose

Homozygous Familial Hypercholesterolemia

Initial: 20mg qd

Prevention of Cardiovascular Disease

Reduce the risk of stroke, MI, and arterial revascularization procedures in patients w/o clinically evident coronary heart disease but w/ an increased risk of cardiovascular disease (CVD) based on age (men ≥50 yrs of age and women ≥60 yrs of age), hsCRP ≥2mg/L, and the presence of at least 1 additional CVD risk factor

PEDIATRIC DOSAGE

Heterozygous Familial Hypercholesterolemia

Individualize dose
8 to <10 Years:
5-10mg qd

10-17 Years:
5-20mg qd

Homozygous Familial Hypercholesterolemia

7-17 Years:
20mg qd

DOSING CONSIDERATIONS
Concomitant Medications
Cyclosporine:
Max: 5mg qd
Atazanavir/Ritonavir, Lopinavir/Ritonavir, or Simeprevir:
Initial: 5mg qd
Max: 10mg qd
Gemfibrozil:
Avoid use; if use cannot be avoided, start at 5mg qd
Max: 10mg qd

Renal Impairment
Severe (CrCl <30mL/min) Not on Hemodialysis:
Initial: 5mg qd
Max: 10mg qd

Hepatic Impairment
Chronic Alcohol Liver Disease: Use w/ caution

Other Important Considerations
Asian Patients:
Initial: 5mg qd

ADMINISTRATION
Oral route

- Take at any time of day, w/ or w/o food.
- Swallow tab whole.
- Do not take 2 doses w/in 12 hrs of each other.

STORAGE
20-25°C (68-77°F). Protect from moisture.

HOW SUPPLIED
Tab: 5mg, 10mg, 20mg, 40mg

CONTRAINDICATIONS
Known hypersensitivity to any component of the medication, active liver disease including unexplained persistent elevations of hepatic transaminase levels, pregnancy, lactation.

WARNINGS/PRECAUTIONS

Myopathy (including immune-mediated necrotizing myopathy [IMNM]) and rhabdomyolysis reported, w/ increased risk at 40mg; caution in patients w/ predisposing factors for myopathy (eg, age ≥65 yrs, inadequately treated hypothyroidism, renal impairment). D/C if markedly elevated creatine phosphokinase (CPK) levels occur or myopathy is diagnosed or suspected. Temporarily withhold in any patient w/ an acute, serious condition suggestive of myopathy or predisposing to the development of renal failure secondary to rhabdomyolysis. Increases in serum transaminases reported. Fatal and nonfatal hepatic failure reported (rare); promptly interrupt therapy if serious liver injury w/ clinical symptoms and/or hyperbilirubinemia or jaundice occurs, and do not restart if no alternate etiology is found. Caution in patients who consume substantial quantities of alcohol and/or have a history of chronic liver disease, or who are elderly. Dipstick-positive proteinuria and microscopic hematuria reported; consider dose reduction for patients w/ unexplained persistent proteinuria and/or hematuria. Increases in HbA1c and FPG levels reported.

ADVERSE REACTIONS

Headache, myalgia, nausea, asthenia, abdominal pain.

DRUG INTERACTIONS

See Dosing Considerations. Cyclosporine, gemfibrozil, lopinavir/ritonavir, atazanavir/ritonavir, and simeprevir may increase levels. Increased risk of myopathy w/ some lipid-lowering therapies (fibrates or niacin), gemfibrozil, cyclosporine, lopinavir/ritonavir, or atazanavir/ritonavir. Caution w/ coumarin anticoagulants. May enhance the risk of skeletal muscle effects w/ ≥1g/day of niacin. Caution w/ drugs that may decrease levels or activity of endogenous steroid hormones (eg, ketoconazole, spironolactone, cimetidine), fenofibrates, or protease inhibitors. Caution w/ colchicine; cases of myopathy, including rhabdomyolysis, reported.

PREGNANCY AND LACTATION

Pregnancy: May cause fetal harm; contraindicated.
Lactation: Present in human milk; contraindicated.
Reproductive Potential: Use effective contraception during treatment.

MECHANISM OF ACTION

HMG-CoA reductase inhibitor; produces lipid-modifying effects by increasing the number of hepatic LDL receptors on the cell surface to enhance uptake and catabolism of LDL and by inhibiting hepatic synthesis of VLDL, which reduces the total number of VLDL and LDL particles.

PHARMACOKINETICS

Absorption: Absolute bioavailability (20%); T_{max}=3-5 hrs. **Distribution:** V_d=134L; plasma protein binding (88%). **Metabolism:** CYP2C9; N-desmethyl rosuvastatin (major metabolite). **Elimination:** Feces (90%); $T_{1/2}$=19 hrs.

PATIENT CONSIDERATIONS

Assessment: Assess for active liver disease (including chronic alcohol liver disease), unexplained persistent elevations in serum transaminases, risk factors for developing myopathy or rhabdomyolysis, pregnancy/nursing status, and possible drug interactions. Obtain baseline lipid profile and LFTs, and evaluate renal function. Check INR w/ coumarin anticoagulants.

Monitoring: Monitor for signs/symptoms of myopathy (including IMNM), rhabdomyolysis, endocrine dysfunction, proteinuria, hematuria, and other adverse reactions. Monitor lipid levels, CPK, and LFTs. Monitor INR w/ coumarin anticoagulants frequently during early therapy.

Counseling: Advise to report promptly any unexplained muscle pain, tenderness, or weakness, particularly if accompanied by malaise or fever or if muscle signs/symptoms persist after discontinuing therapy. Advise to wait at least 2 hrs if taking an antacid containing a combination of aluminum and magnesium hydroxide. Advise females of reproductive potential of the risk to a fetus, to use effective contraception during treatment, and to inform their healthcare provider of a known or suspected pregnancy. Advise women not to breastfeed during treatment. Advise to promptly report any symptoms that may indicate liver injury (eg, fatigue, anorexia, right upper abdominal discomfort, dark urine, jaundice).

CRINONE — progesterone   Rx

Class: Progesterone

ADULT DOSAGE

Assisted Reproductive Technology

For Infertile Women w/ Progesterone Deficiency:

8%:
Women Who Require Progesterone Supplementation:
90mg once daily

Women w/ Partial or Complete Ovarian Failure Who Require Progesterone Replacement:
90mg bid

If pregnancy occurs, may continue treatment until placental autonomy is achieved, up to 10-12 weeks

Secondary Amenorrhea

4%:
Administer qod up to a total of 6 doses

In Women Who Fail to Respond to 4%:
8%:
Administer qod up to a total of 6 doses

PEDIATRIC DOSAGE

Pediatric use may not have been established

ADMINISTRATION

Intravaginal route

STORAGE

20-25°C (68-77°F).

HOW SUPPLIED

Gel: 4% [45mg], 8% [90mg]

CONTRAINDICATIONS

Known sensitivity to this product (progesterone or any of the other ingredients), undiagnosed vaginal bleeding, liver dysfunction or disease, known/suspected malignancy of breast or genital organs, missed abortion, active thrombophlebitis or thromboembolic disorders, history of hormone-associated thrombophlebitis or thromboembolic disorders.

WARNINGS/PRECAUTIONS

A dosage increase from 4% gel can only be accomplished by using the 8% gel; increasing the volume of gel administered does not increase the amount of progesterone absorbed. D/C immediately if signs of thrombotic disorders (eg, thrombophlebitis, cerebrovascular disorders, pulmonary embolism, retinal thrombosis) occur or are suspected. Include special reference to breast and pelvic organs as well as Papanicolaou smear in pretreatment exam. Consider nonfunctional causes in cases of breakthrough bleeding. Adequate diagnostic measures should be taken in cases of undiagnosed vaginal bleeding. May cause fluid retention; carefully observe patients with epilepsy, migraine, asthma, or cardiac/renal dysfunction. Pathologist should be advised of progesterone therapy when relevant specimens are submitted. Caution with history of psychic depression; d/c if depression recurs to a serious degree. May decrease glucose tolerance; carefully observe diabetic patients while on therapy.

ADVERSE REACTIONS

Bloating, abdominal pain/cramps, breast pain, depression, headache, nausea, perineal pain, constipation, diarrhea, arthralgia, libido decreased, nervousness, somnolence, breast enlargement, nocturia.

PREGNANCY AND LACTATION

Safety not known in pregnancy/nursing.

MECHANISM OF ACTION

Progesterone; transforms a proliferative endometrium into a secretory endometrium to increase endometrial receptivity for implantation of embryo. Helps maintain pregnancy.

PHARMACOKINETICS

Absorption: Administration of variable doses resulted in different parameters. **Distribution:** Plasma protein binding (96-99% albumin and corticosteroid binding globulin); found in breast milk. **Metabolism:** (PO) 5β-pregnan-3α, 20α-diol glucuronide (major urinary metabolite); 5β-pregnan-3α-ol-20-one (5β-pregnanolone), 5α-pregnan-3α-ol-20-one (5α-pregnanolone) (plasma metabolites). **Elimination:** Kidney (50-60%, metabolites); bile and feces (10%). Refer to PI for information on additional PK parameters.

PATIENT CONSIDERATIONS

Assessment: Assess for known sensitivity to the product, undiagnosed vaginal bleeding, liver dysfunction or disease, known/suspected malignancy of breast or genital organs, missed abortion, active thrombophlebitis or thromboembolic disorders, history of hormone-associated thrombophlebitis or thromboembolic disorders, epilepsy, migraine, asthma, cardiac/renal dysfunction, history of psychic depression, diabetes, pregnancy/nursing status, and use of other vaginal products. Perform Papanicolaou smear.

Monitoring: Monitor for signs/symptoms of thrombotic disorders, breakthrough bleeding, decrease in glucose tolerance, recurrence of depression, fluid retention, and other adverse reactions.

Counseling: Counsel about risks and benefits of treatment. Instruct not to use with other local intravaginal therapy; if used concurrently, advise that there should be at least a 6-hr period before or after gel administration. Inform that small, white globules may appear as a vaginal discharge possibly due to gel accumulation, even several days after usage.

CRIXIVAN — indinavir sulfate   Rx

Class: Protease inhibitor

ADULT DOSAGE

HIV-1 Infection

Combination w/ Other Antiretrovirals:
800mg q8h

PEDIATRIC DOSAGE

Pediatric use may not have been established

DOSING CONSIDERATIONS
Concomitant Medications
Delavirdine:
Consider dose reduction to 600mg q8h when administering delavirdine 400mg tid
Didanosine:
Administer at least 1 hr apart on an empty stomach
Itraconazole:
Reduce dose to 600mg q8h when administering itraconazole 200mg bid
Ketoconazole:
Reduce dose to 600mg q8h when administering ketoconazole
Rifabutin:
Reduce rifabutin dose to half the standard dose and increase indinavir dose to 1000mg q8h

Hepatic Impairment
Mild-to-Moderate Hepatic Insufficiency Due to Cirrhosis:
Reduce dose to 600mg q8h

Adverse Reactions
Nephrolithiasis/Urolithiasis:
May temporarily interrupt (eg, 1-3 days) or d/c therapy

ADMINISTRATION
Oral route
Administer w/o food but w/ water 1 hr ac or 2 hrs pc.
May administer w/ other liquids (eg, skim milk, juice, coffee, tea) or w/ a light meal.
Drink at least 1.5L of liquids during the course of 24 hrs to ensure adequate hydration.

STORAGE
15-30°C (59-86°F). Protect from moisture.

HOW SUPPLIED
Cap: 200mg, 400mg

CONTRAINDICATIONS
Coadministration w/ CYP3A4 substrates for which elevated concentrations potentially cause serious or life-threatening reactions (eg, alfuzosin, amiodarone, dihydroergotamine, ergonovine, ergotamine, methylergonovine, cisapride, lovastatin, simvastatin, pimozide, sildenafil [for treatment of pulmonary arterial HTN], oral midazolam, triazolam, alprazolam). Clinically significant hypersensitivity to any of its components.

WARNINGS/PRECAUTIONS
Nephrolithiasis/urolithiasis reported. Ensure adequate hydration in all patients. Acute hemolytic anemia, including cases resulting in death, reported; once a diagnosis is apparent, institute appropriate measures, including discontinuation of therapy. Hepatitis, including cases resulting in hepatic failure and death, reported. New onset or exacerbation of diabetes mellitus (DM), hyperglycemia, and diabetic ketoacidosis reported; initiation or dose adjustments of insulin or oral hypoglycemic agents may be required. Indirect hyperbilirubinemia reported frequently during treatment, and infrequently associated w/ increases in serum transaminases. Tubulointerstitial nephritis w/ medullary calcification and cortical atrophy observed in patients w/ asymptomatic severe leukocyturia (>100 cells/high power field); closely follow patients w/ asymptomatic severe leukocyturia and monitor frequently w/ urinalyses. Consider discontinuation of therapy in all patients w/ severe leukocyturia. Immune reconstitution syndrome reported. Autoimmune disorders (eg, Graves' disease, polymyositis, Guillain-Barre syndrome) reported in the setting of immune reconstitution and can occur many months after initiation of treatment. Spontaneous bleeding in patients w/ hemophilia A and B reported. Redistribution/accumulation of body fat reported. Caution in elderly.

ADVERSE REACTIONS
Nephrolithiasis/urolithiasis, hyperbilirubinemia, abdominal pain, headache, N/V, dizziness, pruritus, diarrhea, back pain.

DRUG INTERACTIONS
See Contraindications and Dosing Considerations. Caution w/ atorvastatin, rosuvastatin, parenteral midazolam, sildenafil (for treatment of erectile dysfunction), tadalafil, or vardenafil. Do not coadminister w/ rifampin. Not recommended w/ St. John's wort, atazanavir, salmeterol, or fluticasone (when indinavir is coadministered w/ a potent CYP3A4 inhibitor [eg, ritonavir]). Avoid w/ colchicine in patients w/ renal/hepatic impairment. May increase levels of CYP3A/CYP3A4 substrates, ritonavir, saquinavir, antiarrhythmics, trazodone, colchicine, quetiapine, dihydropyridine calcium channel blockers, clarithromycin, bosentan, atorvastatin, rosuvastatin, immunosuppressants, salmeterol, fluticasone, parenteral midazolam, rifabutin, sildenafil, tadalafil, and vardenafil. CYP3A/CYP3A4 inducers, St. John's wort, efavirenz, nevirapine, anticonvulsants, rifabutin, and venlafaxine may decrease levels. CYP3A/CYP3A4 inhibitors, delavirdine, nelfinavir, ritonavir, clarithromycin, itraconazole, and ketoconazole may increase levels. Refer to PI for dosing modifications when used w/ certain concomitant therapies.

PREGNANCY AND LACTATION
Pregnancy: Category C.
Lactation: Not for use in nursing.

MECHANISM OF ACTION
HIV-1 protease inhibitor; binds to the protease active site and inhibits the activity of the enzyme. This inhibition prevents cleavage of the viral polyproteins resulting in the formation of immature noninfectious viral particles.

PHARMACOKINETICS
Absorption: Rapid (fasted). C_{max}=12,617nM; T_{max}=0.8 hrs; AUC=30,691nM•hr.
Distribution: Plasma protein binding (60%). **Metabolism:** Oxidation (via CYP3A4 [major]) and glucuronide conjugation. **Elimination:** Urine (<20%, unchanged); $T_{1/2}$=1.8 hrs.

PATIENT CONSIDERATIONS
Assessment: Assess for hypersensitivity to drug, hepatic insufficiency, DM, hemophilia, pregnancy/nursing status, and possible drug interactions.
Monitoring: Monitor for nephrolithiasis/urolithiasis, hemolytic anemia, hepatitis, new onset or exacerbation of DM, hyperglycemia, diabetic ketoacidosis, hyperbilirubinemia, serum transaminase elevations, immune reconstitution syndrome, autoimmune disorders, fat redistribution/accumulation, and other adverse reactions. Closely follow patients w/ asymptomatic severe leukocyturia and monitor frequently w/ urinalyses. In patients w/ hemophilia, monitor for bleeding events.

Counseling: Instruct to take drug ud. Inform that drug is not a cure for HIV-1 infection and that illnesses associated w/ HIV may continue. Advise to avoid doing things that can spread HIV to others. Instruct not to modify or d/c therapy w/o consulting physician. Instruct to report the use of any other prescription/nonprescription medication or herbal products (eg, St. John's wort). Inform that fat redistribution/accumulation may occur. Instruct to notify physician if pregnant or nursing.

CUBICIN — daptomycin   Rx

Class: Cyclic lipopeptide

ADULT DOSAGE	PEDIATRIC DOSAGE
Skin and Skin Structure Infections	Pediatric use may not have been established
Caused by susceptible isolates of the following Gram-positive bacteria: *Staphylococcus aureus* (including methicillin-resistant isolates), *Streptococcus pyogenes*, *Streptococcus agalactiae*, *Streptococcus dysgalactiae* subsp. *equisimilis*, and *Enterococcus faecalis* (vancomycin-susceptible isolates only)	
Complicated:	
4mg/kg IV once q24h for 7-14 days	
Bacteremia	
S. aureus bloodstream infections, including those w/ right-sided infective endocarditis, caused by methicillin-susceptible and methicillin-resistant isolates	
6mg/kg IV once q24h for 2-6 weeks; limited safety data for >28 days of use	

DOSING CONSIDERATIONS
Renal Impairment
CrCl <30mL/min, Including Hemodialysis or Continuous Ambulatory Peritoneal Dialysis:
Complicated Skin and Skin Structure Infections (cSSSI): 4mg/kg IV once q48h
S. aureus **Bacteremia:** 6mg/kg IV once q48h

When possible, administer following completion of hemodialysis on hemodialysis days

ADMINISTRATION
IV route

Preparation
Reconstitute 500mg vial to 50mg/mL as follows:
1. Slowly transfer 10mL of 0.9% NaCl inj into daptomycin vial, pointing the transfer needle toward the wall of the vial. A beveled sterile transfer needle that is 21 gauge or smaller in diameter, or a needleless device, is recommended, pointing the transfer needle toward the wall of the vial.
2. Gently rotate vial to ensure that all of the powder is wetted; allow the wetted product to stand undisturbed for 10 min.
3. Gently rotate or swirl vial contents for a few min, prn, to obtain a completely reconstituted sol.
Avoid vigorous agitation or shaking of the vial during or after reconstitution, to minimize foaming.

Administration
Slowly remove reconstituted liquid (50mg/mL) from vial using a beveled sterile needle that is 21 gauge or smaller in diameter.
Administer either by IV inj over 2 min or by IV infusion over 30 min.
IV Inj Over 2 Min: Administer appropriate volume of the reconstituted sol (concentration of 50mg/mL).
IV Infusion Over 30 Min: Further dilute appropriate volume of the reconstituted sol into a 50mL IV infusion bag containing 0.9% NaCl inj.
Discard unused portions.

In-Use Storage Conditions
- Reconstituted sol is stable in the vial for 12 hrs at room temperature and up to 48 hrs if stored under refrigeration at 2-8°C (36-46°F).
- Diluted sol is stable in the infusion bag for 12 hrs at room temperature and 48 hrs if stored under refrigeration.
- The combined storage time (reconstituted sol in vial and diluted sol in infusion bag) should not exceed 12 hrs at room temperature or 48 hrs under refrigeration.

Compatible IV Sol
- 0.9% NaCl inj
- Lactated Ringer's inj

Incompatibilities
- Not compatible w/ dextrose-containing diluents.
- Do not use in conjunction w/ ReadyMED elastomeric infusion pumps.
- Additives and other medications should not be added to daptomycin vials or infusion bags, or infused simultaneously through the same IV line; if the same IV line is used for sequential infusion of different drugs, flush line w/ a compatible IV sol before and after infusion w/ daptomycin.

STORAGE
2-8°C (36-46°F). Avoid excessive heat.

HOW SUPPLIED
Inj: 500mg
CONTRAINDICATIONS
Known hypersensitivity to daptomycin.
WARNINGS/PRECAUTIONS
Not for treatment of pneumonia or of left-sided infective endocarditis due to *S. aureus*. Anaphylaxis/hypersensitivity reactions reported; d/c and institute appropriate therapy if an allergic reaction occurs. Myopathy and rhabdomyolysis (w/ or w/o acute renal failure) reported; do not dose more frequently than qd. Monitor creatine phosphokinase (CPK) levels weekly, and more frequently in patients who received recent prior or concomitant therapy w/ HMG-CoA reductase inhibitor or in whom CPK elevations occur during treatment. Monitor both renal function and CPK more frequently than once weekly in patients w/ renal impairment. D/C in patients w/ unexplained signs/symptoms of myopathy in conjunction w/ CPK elevations to levels >1000 U/L (-5X ULN), and in patients w/o reported symptoms who have marked CPK elevations, w/ levels >2000 U/L (≥10X ULN). Eosinophilic pneumonia reported; d/c therapy immediately and treat w/ systemic steroids if signs and symptoms develop. Peripheral neuropathy reported. Safety and effectiveness not established in pediatric patients; avoid use in pediatric patients <12 months of age due to potential nervous system and/or muscular system effects. *Clostridium difficile*-associated diarrhea (CDAD) reported; may need to d/c if CDAD is suspected or confirmed. Patients w/ persisting or relapsing *S. aureus* bacteremia/endocarditis or poor clinical response should have repeat blood cultures. If a blood culture is positive for *S. aureus*, perform minimum inhibitory concentration susceptibility testing of the isolate and diagnostic evaluation of the patient to rule out sequestered foci of infection; appropriate surgical intervention and/or change in antibacterial regimen may be required. Decreased efficacy in patients w/ moderate baseline renal impairment. Clinically relevant plasma concentrations of daptomycin observed to cause a significant concentration-dependent false prolongation of PT and elevation of INR when certain recombinant thromboplastin reagents are utilized for the assay. May result in bacterial resistance if used in the absence of a proven or suspected bacterial infection; take appropriate measures if superinfection develops.
ADVERSE REACTIONS
cSSSI: Diarrhea, headache, dizziness, rash, abnormal LFTs, elevated CPK, UTIs, hypotension, dyspnea.
***S. aureus* Bacteremia/Endocarditis:** Sepsis, bacteremia, abdominal pain, chest pain, edema, pharyngolaryngeal pain, pruritus, sweating increased, insomnia, CPK increased, HTN.
DRUG INTERACTIONS
Elevated CPK reported in patients who received prior or concomitant treatment w/ HMG-CoA reductase inhibitor; consider suspending use of HMG-CoA reductase inhibitors temporarily in patients receiving daptomycin.
PREGNANCY AND LACTATION
Pregnancy: Category B.
Lactation: Found in breast milk but is poorly bioavailable orally; caution in nursing.
MECHANISM OF ACTION
Cyclic lipopeptide; binds to bacterial cell membranes and causes a rapid depolarization of membrane potential. This loss of membrane potential causes inhibition of DNA, RNA, and protein synthesis, which results in bacterial cell death.
PHARMACOKINETICS
Absorption: (4mg/kg) C_{max}=57.8mcg/mL (over 30 min), 77.7mcg/mL (over 2 min); AUC=494mcg•hr/mL (over 30 min), 475mcg•hr/mL (over 2 min). (6mg/kg) C_{max}=93.9mcg/mL (over 30 min), 116.6mcg/mL (over 2 min); AUC=632mcg•hr/mL (over 30 min), 701mcg•hr/mL (over 2 min). **Distribution:** Plasma protein binding (90-93%); V_d=0.1L/kg; found in breast milk. **Elimination:** Urine (78%), feces (5.7%); $T_{1/2}$=8.1 hrs (4mg/kg over 30 min), 7.9 hrs (6mg/kg over 30 min).

PATIENT CONSIDERATIONS

Assessment: Assess for hypersensitivity to the drug, renal impairment, pregnancy/nursing status, and possible drug interactions.

Monitoring: Monitor for hypersensitivity reactions, myopathy, rhabdomyolysis, eosinophilic pneumonia, peripheral neuropathy, CDAD, superinfection, persisting or relapsing *S. aureus* bacteremia/endocarditis or poor clinical response, and other adverse reactions. Monitor CPK levels weekly, and more frequently in patients who received recent prior or concomitant therapy w/ HMG-CoA reductase inhibitor or in whom CPK elevations occur during treatment. Monitor both renal function and CPK more frequently than once weekly in patients w/ renal impairment. Monitor for muscle pain or weakness, particularly of the distal extremities.

Counseling: Advise that allergic reactions, including serious allergic reactions, can occur and that serious reactions require immediate treatment; instruct to report any previous allergic reactions to the drug. Instruct to report muscle pain/weakness, especially in the forearms and lower legs, as well as tingling/numbness. Advise to report any symptoms of cough, breathlessness, or fever. Advise to contact physician immediately if watery and bloody stools (w/ or w/o stomach cramps and fever) develop, even as late as ≥2 months after the last dose. Inform that therapy should be used to treat bacterial, not viral, infections. Instruct to take exactly ud even if the patient feels better early in the course of therapy; inform that skipping doses or not completing the full course of therapy may decrease effectiveness and increase resistance.

CYCLOBENZAPRINE — cyclobenzaprine hydrochloride   **Rx**

Class: Skeletal muscle relaxant (centrally acting)

OTHER BRAND NAMES
Flexeril (Discontinued)

ADULT DOSAGE	**PEDIATRIC DOSAGE**
Muscle Spasms	**Muscle Spasms**
Adjunct to rest and physical therapy for relief of muscle spasm associated w/ acute, painful musculoskeletal conditions	Adjunct to rest and physical therapy for relief of muscle spasm associated w/ acute, painful musculoskeletal conditions
Usual: 5mg tid **Titrate:** May increase to 10mg tid Use for periods longer than 2 or 3 weeks is not recommended	**≥15 Years:** **Usual:** 5mg tid **Titrate:** May increase to 10mg tid Use for periods longer than 2 or 3 weeks is not recommended

---

DOSING CONSIDERATIONS
Hepatic Impairment
Mild:
Initial: 5mg dose
Titrate: Increase slowly and consider less frequent dosing
Moderate to Severe:
Not recommended
Elderly
Initial: 5mg dose
Titrate: Increase slowly and consider less frequent dosing
ADMINISTRATION
Oral route
STORAGE
20-25°C (68-77°F).
HOW SUPPLIED
Tab: 5mg, 7.5mg, 10mg
CONTRAINDICATIONS
Hypersensitivity to any component of this product, concomitant use of MAOIs or w/in 14 days after their discontinuation. Arrhythmias, heart block or conduction disturbances, CHF, hyperthyroidism, acute recovery phase of MI.
WARNINGS/PRECAUTIONS
Not effective in the treatment of spasticity associated w/ cerebral or spinal cord disease or in children w/ cerebral palsy. May produce arrhythmias, sinus tachycardia, and conduction time prolongation leading to MI and stroke. Caution w/ history of urinary retention, angle-closure glaucoma, increased IOP, mild hepatic impairment, and in elderly. Not recommended w/ moderate to severe hepatic impairment. Consider certain withdrawal symptoms; abrupt cessation after prolonged administration rarely may produce nausea, headache, and malaise.
ADVERSE REACTIONS
Drowsiness, dry mouth, fatigue, headache, dizziness.
DRUG INTERACTIONS
See Contraindications. Serotonin syndrome reported when used w/ SSRIs, SNRIs, TCAs, tramadol, bupropion, meperidine, verapamil, or MAOIs; d/c immediately if this occurs. Observe carefully, particularly during treatment initiation or dose increases, if concomitant use w/ other serotonergic drugs is warranted. May enhance effects of alcohol, barbiturates, and other CNS depressants. Caution w/ anticholinergics. May block the antihypertensive action of guanethidine and similarly acting compounds. May enhance seizure risk w/ tramadol.
PREGNANCY AND LACTATION
Category B, caution in nursing.
MECHANISM OF ACTION
Skeletal muscle relaxant (central-acting); relieves skeletal muscle spasm of local origin w/o interfering w/ muscle function. Reduces tonic somatic motor activity, influencing both gamma and α motor systems.
PHARMACOKINETICS
Absorption: Oral bioavailability (33-55%); C_{max}=25.9ng/mL; AUC=177ng•hr/mL. **Metabolism:** Extensive; N-demethylation via CYP3A4, 1A2, and 2D6. **Elimination:** Kidney (glucuronides); $T_{1/2}$=18 hrs.

PATIENT CONSIDERATIONS

Assessment: Assess for arrhythmias, heart block or conduction disturbances, CHF, hyperthyroidism, acute recovery phase of MI, history of urinary retention, angle-closure glaucoma, increased IOP, hepatic impairment, drug hypersensitivity, pregnancy/nursing status, and possible drug interactions.

Monitoring: Monitor for arrhythmias, sinus tachycardia, conduction time prolongation, stroke, withdrawal symptoms, and other adverse reactions.

Counseling: Inform that the drug, especially when used w/ alcohol or other CNS depressants, may impair mental and/or physical abilities required to perform hazardous tasks (eg, operating machinery, driving). Caution about the risk of serotonin syndrome; instruct to seek medical care immediately if signs/symptoms occur.

CYCLOPHOSPHAMIDE CAPSULES — cyclophosphamide   Rx

Class: Nitrogen mustard alkylating agent

ADULT DOSAGE

Malignant Diseases

Malignant lymphomas (Stages III and IV of the Ann Arbor staging system), Hodgkin's disease, lymphocytic lymphoma (nodular or diffuse), mixed-cell type lymphoma, histiocytic lymphoma, Burkitt's lymphoma; multiple myeloma; chronic lymphocytic leukemia, chronic granulocytic leukemia (usually ineffective in acute blastic crisis), acute myelogenous and monocytic leukemia, acute lymphoblastic (stem-cell) leukemia (cyclophosphamide given during remission is effective in prolonging its duration); mycosis fungoides (advanced disease); neuroblastoma (disseminated disease); adenocarcinoma of the ovary; retinoblastoma; and carcinoma of the breast

1-5mg/kg/day; adjust in accord w/ evidence of antitumor activity and/or leukopenia

As Part of Combined Cytotoxic Regimens:

May be necessary to reduce dose of cyclophosphamide as well as that of the other drugs

PEDIATRIC DOSAGE

Malignant Diseases

Malignant lymphomas (Stages III and IV of the Ann Arbor staging system), Hodgkin's disease, lymphocytic lymphoma (nodular or diffuse), mixed-cell type lymphoma, histiocytic lymphoma, Burkitt's lymphoma; multiple myeloma; chronic lymphocytic leukemia, chronic granulocytic leukemia (usually ineffective in acute blastic crisis), acute myelogenous and monocytic leukemia, acute lymphoblastic (stem-cell) leukemia (cyclophosphamide given during remission is effective in prolonging its duration); mycosis fungoides (advanced disease); neuroblastoma (disseminated disease); adenocarcinoma of the ovary; retinoblastoma; and carcinoma of the breast

1-5mg/kg/day; adjust in accord w/ evidence of antitumor activity and/or leukopenia

As Part of Combined Cytotoxic Regimens:

May be necessary to reduce dose of cyclophosphamide as well as that of the other drugs

Nephrotic Syndrome

Biopsy proven minimal change nephrotic syndrome in patients who failed to adequately respond to or are unable to tolerate adrenocorticosteroid therapy

2mg/kg/day for 8-12 weeks
Max Cumulative Dose: 168mg/kg

DOSING CONSIDERATIONS

Elderly

Start at lower end of dosing range

ADMINISTRATION

Oral route

Take in am; during or immediately after administration, adequate amounts of fluid should be ingested or infused to force diuresis.
Swallow whole; do not open, chew, or crush.

Handling Precautions

Handle and dispose of cyclophosphamide in a manner consistent w/ other cytotoxic drugs.
If contact w/ broken caps occurs, wash hands immediately and thoroughly.

STORAGE

20-25°C (68-77°F).

HOW SUPPLIED

Cap: 25mg, 50mg

CONTRAINDICATIONS

Hypersensitivity to this medication, urinary outflow obstruction.

WARNINGS/PRECAUTIONS

May cause myelosuppression, bone marrow failure, and severe immunosuppression that may lead to serious and sometimes fatal infections. May reactivate latent infections. Do not administer to patients w/ neutrophils ≤1500/mm³ and platelets <50,000/mm³. Treatment may not be indicated, or should be interrupted, or the dose reduced, in patients who have or who develop a serious infection. Granulocyte colony-stimulating factor (G-CSF) may be administered to reduce the risks of neutropenia complications associated w/ cyclophosphamide use. Hemorrhagic cystitis, pyelitis, ureteritis, and hematuria reported; d/c therapy if severe hemorrhagic cystitis occurs. Urotoxicity (bladder ulceration, necrosis, fibrosis, contracture, secondary cancer) may occur and may require interruption of treatment or cystectomy. Exclude or correct any urinary tract obstructions before starting treatment. Caution w/ active UTIs. Myocarditis, myopericarditis, pericardial effusion including cardiac tamponade, CHF, and supraventricular/ventricular arrhythmias reported; caution w/ risk factors for cardiotoxicity and w/ preexisting cardiac disease. Pneumonitis, pulmonary fibrosis, pulmonary veno-occlusive disease (VOD) and other forms of pulmonary toxicity leading to respiratory failure reported during and following treatment. Secondary malignancies (urinary tract cancer, myelodysplasia, acute leukemias, lymphomas, thyroid cancer, sarcomas) reported. Liver VOD, including fatal outcome, reported. May cause fetal harm. Male and female reproductive function and fertility may be impaired. May interfere w/ normal wound healing. Hyponatremia associated w/ increased total body water, acute water intoxication, and a syndrome resembling syndrome of inappropriate secretion of antidiuretic hormone reported. Caution w/ severe renal impairment (CrCl 10-24mL/min). In patients requiring dialysis, consider use of a consistent interval between therapy and dialysis.

ADVERSE REACTIONS

Neutropenia, fever, N/V, anorexia, alopecia, skin pigmentation, changes in nails.

DRUG INTERACTIONS

Severe myelosuppression may be expected particularly in patients pretreated w/ and/or receiving concomitant chemotherapy and/or radiation therapy. Protease inhibitors may increase concentration of cytotoxic metabolites and may increase incidence of infections and neutropenia. Increased hematotoxicity and/or immunosuppression w/ ACE inhibitors, natalizumab, paclitaxel, thiazide diuretics, and zidovudine. Increased cardiotoxicity w/ anthracyclines, cytarabine, pentostatin, radiation therapy of the cardiac region, and trastuzumab. Increased pulmonary toxicity w/ amiodarone and G-CSF or granulocyte macrophage colony-stimulating factor. Increased nephrotoxicity w/ amphotericin B. Acute water intoxication reported w/ indomethacin. Increased risk of hepatotoxicity w/ azathioprine. Increased incidence of liver VOD and mucositis w/ busulfan. Increased incidence of mucositis w/ protease inhibitors. Increased risk of hemorrhagic cystitis w/ past or concomitant radiation treatment. Higher incidence of noncutaneous malignant solid tumors w/ etanercept in patients w/ Wegener's granulomatosis. Acute encephalopathy reported w/ metronidazole. Concomitant use of tamoxifen may increase the risk of thromboembolic complications. Both increased and decreased warfarin effect reported. May lower concentrations of cyclosporine, which may result in an increased incidence of graft-versus-host disease. Prolonged apnea may occur w/ concurrent depolarizing muscle relaxants (eg, succinylcholine); caution if patient has been treated w/in 10 days of general anesthesia.

PREGNANCY AND LACTATION

Pregnancy: Category D. Exposure to cyclophosphamide during pregnancy may cause fetal malformations, miscarriage, fetal growth retardation, and toxic effects in the newborn.
Lactation: Not for use in nursing.
Reproductive Potential: Female patients of reproductive potential should use highly effective contraception during and for up to 1 year after completion of treatment. Male patients who are sexually active w/ female partners who are or may become pregnant should use a condom during and for at least 4 months after treatment. Amenorrhea (transient or permanent) and oligomenorrhea reported in women. Men may develop oligospermia or azoospermia.

MECHANISM OF ACTION

Nitrogen mustard alkylating agent; thought to involve cross-linking of tumor cell DNA.

PHARMACOKINETICS

Absorption: T_{max}=1 hr. **Distribution:** V_d=30-50L; plasma protein binding (20%; >60%, metabolites); found in breast milk. **Metabolism:** Liver to active alkylating metabolites by a mixed function microsomal oxidase system. **Elimination:** (IV) Urine (10-20%, unchanged), bile (4%); $T_{1/2}$=3-12 hrs.

PATIENT CONSIDERATIONS

Assessment: Assess for urinary outflow obstruction, active UTI, infections, risk for neutropenia complications and cardiotoxicity, preexisting cardiac disease, renal impairment, drug hypersensitivity, pregnancy/nursing status, and possible drug interactions. Obtain baseline CBCs.

Monitoring: Monitor for myelosuppression, bone marrow failure, immunosuppression, infections, hemorrhagic cystitis, urinary tract/renal/cardiac/pulmonary toxicity, secondary malignancies, VOD, hyponatremia, and other adverse reactions. Monitor CBCs. Regularly check urinary sediment for presence of erythrocytes and other signs of urotoxicity and/or nephrotoxicity.

Counseling: Inform of the possibility of myelosuppression, immunosuppression, and infections; explain the need for routine blood cell counts. Instruct patients to monitor their temperature frequently and to immediately report any occurrence of fever. Advise to report urinary symptoms and the need for increasing fluid intake and frequent voiding. Advise to contact physician immediately for any of the following; new onset or worsening SOB, cough, swelling of the ankles/legs, palpitations, weight gain of >5 lbs in 24 hrs, dizziness, or loss of consciousness. Advise to report promptly any new or worsening respiratory symptoms. Advise female patients of reproductive potential to use highly effective contraception during treatment and for up to 1 yr after completion of therapy. Advise male patients who are sexually active w/ a female partner who is or may become pregnant to use condoms during treatment and for up to 4 months after completion of therapy. Instruct to immediately contact physician if pregnancy occurs or is suspected. Inform of the possible side effects associated w/ cyclophosphamide administration and of other undesirable effects that could affect the ability to drive or use machines. Instruct patients to swallow cyclophosphamide capsules whole and not to open, chew, or crush the capsules. Advise caregivers to wear gloves when handling containers and caps and to avoid exposure to broken caps; instruct to wash hands immediately and thoroughly if contact w/ broken caps occurs.

CYCLOPHOSPHAMIDE INJECTION — cyclophosphamide   Rx

Class: Nitrogen mustard alkylating agent

ADULT DOSAGE

Malignant Diseases

No Hematologic Deficiency:
IV:
Monotherapy:
Initial: 40-50mg/kg in divided doses over 2-5 days
Other Regimens: 10-15mg/kg every 7-10 days OR 3-5mg/kg twice weekly

PEDIATRIC DOSAGE

Malignant Diseases

No Hematologic Deficiency:
IV:
Monotherapy:
Initial: 40-50mg/kg in divided doses over 2-5 days
Other Regimens: 10-15mg/kg every 7-10 days OR 3-5mg/kg twice weekly

Oral:
Initial/Maint: 1-5mg/kg/day
Adjust IV/Oral doses in accord with evidence of antitumor activity and/or leukopenia

Combined Cytotoxic Regimens:
May need to reduce dose of cyclophosphamide as well as that of the other drugs

Oral:
Initial/Maint: 1-5mg/kg/day
Adjust IV/Oral doses in accord with evidence of antitumor activity and/or leukopenia

Combined Cytotoxic Regimens:
May need to reduce dose of cyclophosphamide as well as that of the other drugs

Nephrotic Syndrome
Biopsy Proven Minimal Change:
Oral:
2 mg/kg/day for 8 to 12 weeks
Max Cumulative Dose: 168mg/kg

DOSING CONSIDERATIONS
Elderly
Start at lower end of dosing range
ADMINISTRATION
IV/Oral route

During or immediately after administration, adequate amounts of fluid should be ingested or infused to force dieresis; administer in the morning

Preparation and Administration
Reconstitution Instructions:
For Direct IV Inj:
500mg: Reconstitute with 25mL 0.9% NaCl
1g: Reconstitute with 50mL 0.9% NaCl
2g: Reconstitute with 100mL 0.9% NaCl
For IV Infusion:
500mg: Reconstitute with 25mL 0.9% NaCl or SWFI
1g: Reconstitute with 50mL 0.9% NaCl or SWFI
2g: Reconstitute with 100mL 0.9% NaCl or SWFI

Dilution Instructions:
Dilute the reconstituted sol to a minimum concentration of 2mg/mL with any of the following:
5% Dextrose Inj
5% Dextrose and 0.9% NaCl Inj
0.45% NaCl Inj

Storage of Reconstituted/Diluted Sol:
Reconstituted Sol (Without Further Dilution):
0.9% NaCl Inj: Up to 24 hrs at room temperature; up to 6 days refrigerated
SWFI: Do not store; use immediately
Diluted Sol:
0.45% NaCl Inj: Up to 24 hrs at room temperature; up to 6 days refrigerated
5% Dextrose Inj: Up to 24 hrs at room temperature; up to 36 hrs refrigerated
5% Dextrose and 0.9% NaCl Inj: Up to 24 hrs at room temperature; up to 36 hrs refrigerated

Use of Reconstituted Sol for Oral Administration:
Prepare by dissolving cyclophosphamide for inj in Aromatic Elixir, National Formulary
Store under refrigeration in glass containers and use within 14 days

STORAGE
≤25°C (77°F).

HOW SUPPLIED
Inj: 500mg, 1g, 2g

CONTRAINDICATIONS
Hypersensitivity to this medication, urinary outflow obstruction.

WARNINGS/PRECAUTIONS
May cause myelosuppression, bone marrow failure, and severe immunosuppression that may lead to serious and sometimes fatal infections. May reactivate latent infections. Do not administer to patients with neutrophils ≤1500/mm^3 and platelets <50,000/mm^3. Interrupt therapy or reduce dose if serious infection develops. Consider primary and secondary prophylaxis with granulocyte colony-stimulating factor (G-CSF) in patients at increased risk for neutropenia complications. Hemorrhagic cystitis, pyelitis, ureteritis, and hematuria reported; d/c therapy if severe hemorrhagic cystitis occurs. Urotoxicity (bladder ulceration, necrosis, fibrosis, contracture, secondary cancer) may require interruption of treatment or cystectomy. Exclude or correct any urinary tract obstructions before starting treatment. Caution with active urinary tract infections (UTIs). Myocarditis, myopericarditis, pericardial effusion including cardiac tamponade, congestive heart failure, and supraventricular/ventricular arrhythmias reported; caution with risk factors for cardiotoxicity and with preexisting cardiac disease. Pneumonitis, pulmonary fibrosis, pulmonary veno-occlusive disease (VOD), and other forms of pulmonary toxicity leading to respiratory failure reported during and following treatment. Secondary malignancies (urinary tract cancer, myelodysplasia, acute leukemias, lymphomas, thyroid cancer, sarcomas) reported. Liver VOD, including fatal outcome, reported. May cause fetal harm. Male and female reproductive function and fertility may be impaired. May interfere with normal wound healing. Hyponatremia associated with increased total body water, acute water intoxication, and a syndrome resembling syndrome of inappropriate secretion of antidiuretic hormone reported. Caution with severe renal impairment (CrCl 10-24mL/min) and in elderly. In patients requiring dialysis, consider use of a consistent interval between therapy and dialysis.

ADVERSE REACTIONS
Neutropenia, N/V, anorexia, alopecia, fever, skin pigmentation, changes in nails.

DRUG INTERACTIONS
Severe myelosuppression may be expected, particularly in patients pretreated with and/or receiving concomitant chemotherapy and/or radiation therapy. Protease inhibitors may increase the concentration of cytotoxic metabolites and may increase the incidence of infections, neutropenia, and mucositis. Increased hematotoxicity and/or immunosuppression with ACE inhibitors, natalizumab, paclitaxel, thiazide diuretics, and zidovudine. Increased cardiotoxicity with anthracyclines, cytarabine, pentostatin, radiation therapy of the cardiac region, and trastuzumab. Increased pulmonary toxicity with amiodarone and G-CSF or granulocyte macrophage colony-stimulating factor. Increased nephrotoxicity with amphotericin B. Acute water intoxication reported with indomethacin. Increased risk of hepatotoxicity with azathioprine. Increased incidence of liver VOD and mucositis with busulfan. Increased risk of hemorrhagic cystitis with past or concomitant radiation treatment. Higher incidence of noncutaneous malignant solid tumors with etanercept in patients with Wegener's granulomatosis. Acute encephalopathy reported with metronidazole. Concomitant use of tamoxifen may increase the risk of thromboembolic complications. Both increased and decreased warfarin effect reported. May lower concentrations of cyclosporine, which may result in an increased incidence of graft-versus-host disease. Prolonged apnea may occur with concurrent depolarizing muscle relaxants (eg, succinylcholine); caution if patient has been treated within 10 days of general anesthesia.

PREGNANCY AND LACTATION
Category D, not for use in nursing.

MECHANISM OF ACTION
Nitrogen mustard alkylating agent; thought to involve cross-linking of tumor cell DNA.

PHARMACOKINETICS
Absorption: (Oral) T_{max}=1 hr. **Distribution:** V_d=30-50L; plasma protein binding (20%; >60%, metabolites); found in breast milk. **Metabolism:** Liver to active alkylating metabolites by a mixed function microsomal oxidase system. **Elimination:** (IV) Urine (10-20%, unchanged); bile (4%); $T_{1/2}$=3-12 hrs.

PATIENT CONSIDERATIONS
Assessment: Assess for urinary outflow obstruction, active UTI, infections, risk for neutropenia complications and cardiotoxicity, preexisting cardiac disease, renal impairment, drug hypersensitivity, pregnancy/nursing status, and possible drug interactions. Obtain baseline CBCs.

Monitoring: Monitor for myelosuppression, bone marrow failure, immunosuppression, infections, hemorrhagic cystitis, urinary tract/renal/cardiac/pulmonary toxicity, secondary malignancies, VOD, hyponatremia, and other adverse reactions. Monitor CBCs. Regularly check urinary sediment for presence of erythrocytes and other signs of urotoxicity and/or nephrotoxicity.

Counseling: Inform of the possibility of myelosuppression, immunosuppression, and infections; explain the need for routine blood cell counts. Instruct patients to monitor their temperature frequently and to immediately report any occurrence of fever. Advise to report urinary symptoms and the need for increasing fluid intake and frequent voiding. Advise to contact physician immediately for any of the following: new onset or worsening SOB, cough, swelling of the ankles/legs, palpitations, weight gain of >5 lbs in 24 hrs, dizziness, or loss of consciousness. Advise to report promptly any new or worsening respiratory symptoms. Advise female patients of reproductive potential to use highly effective contraception during treatment and for up to 1 yr after completion of therapy. Advise male patients who are sexually active with a female partner who is or may become pregnant to use condoms during treatment and for up to 4 months after completion of therapy. Instruct to immediately contact physician if pregnancy occurs or is suspected. Inform of the possible side effects and of other undesirable effects that could affect ability to drive or use machines.

CYCLOPHOSPHAMIDE TABLETS — cyclophosphamide   **Rx**

Class: Nitrogen mustard alkylating agent

ADULT DOSAGE	PEDIATRIC DOSAGE
Malignant Diseases	**Malignant Diseases**
Malignant lymphomas (Stages III and IV of the Ann Arbor staging system), Hodgkin's disease, lymphocytic lymphoma (nodular or diffuse), mixed-cell type lymphoma, histiocytic lymphoma, Burkitt's lymphoma; multiple myeloma; chronic lymphocytic leukemia, chronic granulocytic leukemia (usually ineffective in acute blastic crisis), acute myelogenous and monocytic leukemia, acute lymphoblastic (stem-cell) leukemia in children (cyclophosphamide given during remission is effective in prolonging its duration); mycosis fungoides (advanced disease); neuroblastoma (disseminated disease); adenocarcinoma of the ovary; retinoblastoma; and carcinoma of the breast	Malignant lymphomas (Stages III and IV of the Ann Arbor staging system), Hodgkin's disease, lymphocytic lymphoma (nodular or diffuse), mixed-cell type lymphoma, histiocytic lymphoma, Burkitt's lymphoma; multiple myeloma; chronic lymphocytic leukemia, chronic granulocytic leukemia (usually ineffective in acute blastic crisis), acute myelogenous and monocytic leukemia, acute lymphoblastic (stem-cell) leukemia in children (cyclophosphamide given during remission is effective in prolonging its duration); mycosis fungoides (advanced disease); neuroblastoma (disseminated disease); adenocarcinoma of the ovary; retinoblastoma; and carcinoma of the breast

1-5mg/kg/day; adjust in accord w/ evidence of antitumor activity and/or leukopenia

As Part of Combined Cytotoxic Regimens:
May be necessary to reduce dose of cyclophosphamide as well as that of the other drugs

---

1-5mg/kg/day; adjust in accord w/ evidence of antitumor activity and/or leukopenia

As Part of Combined Cytotoxic Regimens:
May be necessary to reduce dose of cyclophosphamide as well as that of the other drugs

Nephrotic Syndrome
Biopsy proven minimal change nephrotic syndrome in patients whose disease fails to respond adequately to appropriate adrenocorticosteroid therapy or in whom the adrenocorticosteroid therapy produces or threatens to produce intolerable side effects
2.5-3mg/kg/day for 60-90 days
Adrenocorticosteroid therapy may be tapered and discontinued during the course of cyclophosphamide therapy

---

DOSING CONSIDERATIONS
Elderly
Start at lower end of dosing range

ADMINISTRATION
Oral route

STORAGE
≤25°C (77°F); product will withstand brief exposure to temperatures up to 30°C (86°F). Protect from temperatures >30°C (86°F).

HOW SUPPLIED
Tab: 25mg, 50mg

CONTRAINDICATIONS
Severely depressed bone marrow function, prior hypersensitivity to this medication.

WARNINGS/PRECAUTIONS
Second malignancies (eg, urinary bladder, myeloproliferative, lymphoproliferative) reported. May cause fetal harm. Interferes with oogenesis and spermatogenesis. May cause sterility in both sexes; development of sterility appears to depend on the dose, duration of therapy, and the state of gonadal function at the time of treatment. Amenorrhea associated with decreased estrogen and increased gonadotropin secretion reported. Ovarian fibrosis with apparently complete loss of germ cells after prolonged treatment in late prepubescence reported. Testicular atrophy may occur. Hemorrhagic cystitis and/or urinary bladder fibrosis may develop; d/c if severe hemorrhagic cystitis occurs. Cardiac toxicity reported. May cause significant suppression of immune responses. Serious infections may develop in severely immunosuppressed patients; interrupt or reduce dose in patients who have or who develop viral, bacterial, fungal, protozoan, or helminthic infections. Anaphylactic reactions and possible cross-sensitivity with other alkylating agents reported. Caution with leukopenia, thrombocytopenia, tumor cell infiltration of bone marrow, previous x-ray therapy, previous therapy with other cytotoxic agents, and hepatic/renal impairment. May need to adjust dose in adrenalectomized patients. May interfere with normal wound healing. Caution in elderly.

ADVERSE REACTIONS
Leukopenia/neutropenia, N/V, anorexia, alopecia, skin pigmentation, changes in nails, hemorrhagic ureteritis, renal tubular necrosis, syndrome of inappropriate antidiuretic hormone secretion.

DRUG INTERACTIONS
May potentiate doxorubicin-induced cardiotoxicity. Chronic administration of high doses of phenobarbital increases rate of metabolism and leukopenic activity of cyclophosphamide. Potentiates effect of succinylcholine chloride. Caution if patient has been treated with cyclophosphamide within 10 days of general anesthesia.

PREGNANCY AND LACTATION
Category D, not for use in nursing.

MECHANISM OF ACTION
Nitrogen mustard alkylating agent; thought to involve cross-linking of tumor cell DNA.

PHARMACOKINETICS
Absorption: Well absorbed. Bioavailability (>75%). (IV) T_{max}=2-3 hrs (metabolites).
Distribution: Plasma protein binding (>60%, metabolites); found in breast milk.
Metabolism: Liver to active alkylating metabolites by a mixed function microsomal oxidase system. **Elimination:** Urine (5-25%, unchanged); $T_{1/2}$=3-12 hrs.

PATIENT CONSIDERATIONS
Assessment: Assess for bone marrow depression, immunosuppression, infections, hepatic/renal impairment, adrenalectomy, drug hypersensitivity, any other conditions where treatment is cautioned, pregnancy/nursing status, and possible drug interactions.

Monitoring: Monitor for second malignancies, reproductive dysfunction, hemorrhagic cystitis, urinary bladder fibrosis, cardiac dysfunction/toxicity, immunosuppression, infections, anaphylactic reactions, and other adverse reactions. Monitor hematologic profile (particularly neutrophils and platelets), and examine urine for red cells regularly.

Counseling: Inform of the risks and benefits of therapy. Advise women of childbearing potential to avoid becoming pregnant.

CYMBALTA — duloxetine   Rx
Class: Serotonin and norepinephrine reuptake inhibitor (SNRI)

> Antidepressants increased the risk of suicidal thoughts and behavior in children, adolescents, and young adults in short-term studies. Monitor and observe closely for worsening, and for emergence of suicidal thoughts and behaviors in all patients started on antidepressant therapy.

ADULT DOSAGE
Musculoskeletal Pain
Chronic:
Initial: 30mg qd for 1 week before increasing to 60mg qd
Maint: 60mg qd
Max: 60mg/day

Major Depressive Disorder
Initial: 40mg/day (given as 20mg bid) to 60mg/day (given qd or as 30mg bid); may start at 30mg qd for 1 week before increasing to 60mg qd in some patients
Maint: 60mg qd
Max: 120mg/day

Generalized Anxiety Disorder
Initial: 60mg qd; may start at 30mg qd for 1 week before increasing to 60mg qd in some patients
Maint: 60mg qd
Titrate: Dose increases beyond 60mg qd should be in increments of 30mg qd
Max: 120mg/day

Diabetic Peripheral Neuropathy
Initial: 60mg qd. May consider a lower starting dose if tolerability is a concern
Max: 60mg qd

Fibromyalgia
Initial: 30mg qd for 1 week before increasing to 60mg qd; some patients may respond to the starting dose
Maint: 60mg qd
Max: 60mg/day

Dosing Considerations with MAOIs
Switching to/from an MAOI for Psychiatric Disorders:
Allow at least 14 days between discontinuation of an MAOI and initiation of treatment w/ duloxetine, and allow at least 5 days between discontinuation of duloxetine and initiation of an MAOI.

W/ Other MAOIs (eg, Linezolid, IV Methylene Blue):
- Do not start duloxetine in a patient being treated w/ linezolid or IV methylene blue. Consider other interventions (eg, hospitalization) in patients who require more urgent treatment of a psychiatric condition.
- In patients already receiving duloxetine, if acceptable alternatives are not available and benefits outweigh risks, d/c duloxetine promptly and administer linezolid or IV methylene blue; monitor for serotonin syndrome for 5 days or until 24 hrs after the last dose of linezolid or IV methylene blue, whichever comes 1st. May resume duloxetine therapy 24 hrs after the last dose of linezolid or IV methylene blue.

PEDIATRIC DOSAGE
Generalized Anxiety Disorder
7-17 Years:
Initial: 30mg qd for 2 weeks before considering an increase to 60mg
Maint: 30-60mg qd
Titrate: Dose increases beyond 60mg qd should be in increments of 30mg qd
Max: 120mg/day

Dosing Considerations with MAOIs
Switching to/from an MAOI for Psychiatric Disorders:
Allow at least 14 days between discontinuation of an MAOI and initiation of treatment w/ duloxetine, and allow at least 5 days between discontinuation of duloxetine and initiation of an MAOI.

W/ Other MAOIs (eg, Linezolid, IV Methylene Blue):
- Do not start duloxetine in a patient being treated w/ linezolid or IV methylene blue. Consider other interventions (eg, hospitalization) in patients who require more urgent treatment of a psychiatric condition.
- In patients already receiving duloxetine, if acceptable alternatives are not available and benefits outweigh risks, d/c duloxetine promptly and administer linezolid or IV methylene blue; monitor for serotonin syndrome for 5 days or until 24 hrs after the last dose of linezolid or IV methylene blue, whichever comes 1st. May resume duloxetine therapy 24 hrs after the last dose of linezolid or IV methylene blue.

DOSING CONSIDERATIONS
Renal Impairment
Avoid in patients w/ severe renal impairment (GFR <30mL/min)

Diabetic Peripheral Neuropathy:
Consider lower starting dose and gradual increase

Hepatic Impairment
Avoid in patients w/ chronic liver disease or cirrhosis

Elderly
Generalized Anxiety Disorder:
Initial: 30mg qd for 2 weeks before considering increasing to target dose of 60mg

Maint: 60mg qd
Titrate: Dose increases beyond 60mg qd should be in increments of 30mg qd
Max: 120mg/day

Discontinuation
Gradually reduce dose

ADMINISTRATION
Oral route

Swallow cap whole; do not chew, crush, or open to sprinkle on food or mix w/ liquids.
Take w/o regard to meals.

STORAGE
25°C (77°F); excursions permitted to 15-30°C (59-86°F).

HOW SUPPLIED
Cap, Delayed-Release: 20mg, 30mg, 60mg

CONTRAINDICATIONS
Use of an MAOI for psychiatric disorders either concomitantly or w/in 5 days of stopping treatment. Treatment w/in 14 days of stopping an MAOI for psychiatric disorders. Starting treatment in patients being treated w/ other MAOIs (eg, linezolid, IV methylene blue).

WARNINGS/PRECAUTIONS
Not approved for the treatment of bipolar depression; may precipitate mixed/manic episode for those at risk for bipolar disorder. Hepatic failure (sometimes fatal) reported; d/c if jaundice or other evidence of clinically significant hepatic dysfunction develops and do not resume unless another cause can be established. Cases of cholestatic jaundice w/ minimal elevation of transaminase levels and cases of elevated transaminases/bilirubin/alkaline phosphatase in patients w/ chronic liver disease or cirrhosis reported. Avoid w/ substantial alcohol use or evidence of chronic liver disease or cirrhosis. Orthostatic hypotension, falls, and syncope reported; increased risk w/ doses >60mg/day. Consider dose reduction or discontinuation in patients who experience symptomatic orthostatic hypotension, falls, and/or syncope during therapy. Serotonin syndrome reported; d/c immediately if symptoms occur and initiate supportive symptomatic treatment. May increase risk of bleeding events. Severe skin reactions (eg, erythema multiforme, Stevens-Johnson syndrome [SJS]) may occur; d/c at the 1st appearance of blisters, peeling rash, mucosal erosions, or any other signs of hypersensitivity if no other etiology can be identified. Adverse events reported upon discontinuation; avoid abrupt withdrawal. If intolerable symptoms occur following a decrease in the dose or upon discontinuation of treatment, consider resuming the previously prescribed dose; subsequently, may continue decreasing dose but at a more gradual rate. Activation of mania or hypomania reported in patients w/ major depressive disorder; caution w/ history of mania. Pupillary dilation that occurs following use may trigger an angle-closure attack in a patient w/ anatomically narrow angles who does not have a patent iridectomy. Seizures/convulsions reported; caution w/ history of seizure disorder. May increase BP. Hyponatremia may occur; caution in elderly and volume-depleted patients. Consider discontinuation and institute appropriate medical intervention in patients w/ symptomatic hyponatremia. Caution w/ conditions that may slow gastric emptying and w/ diabetes; worsening glycemic control observed in some patients w/ diabetes. Urinary hesitation and retention reported.

ADVERSE REACTIONS
Nausea, dry mouth, somnolence, constipation, decreased appetite, hyperhidrosis.

DRUG INTERACTIONS
See Contraindications. Greater risk of hypotension w/ concomitant use of medications that induce orthostatic hypotension (eg, antihypertensives) and potent CYP1A2 inhibitors. May cause serotonin syndrome w/ other serotonergic drugs (eg, triptans, TCAs, fentanyl) and w/ drugs that impair metabolism of serotonin; immediately d/c therapy and any concomitant serotonergic agent if this occurs. Caution w/ NSAIDs, aspirin (ASA), warfarin, or other drugs that affect coagulation, due to potential increased risk of bleeding. Avoid use w/ thioridazine, potent CYP1A2 inhibitors (eg, fluvoxamine, cimetidine, some quinolone antibiotics), and substantial alcohol use. CYP2D6 inhibitors (eg, paroxetine, fluoxetine, quinidine) may increase levels. Caution w/ drugs metabolized by CYP2D6 having a narrow therapeutic index (eg, TCAs, phenothiazines, type 1C antiarrhythmics); may need to monitor levels/reduce dose of TCA. Caution when combined w/ or substituted for other CNS-acting drugs, including those w/ a similar mechanism of action. Increased risk of hyponatremia w/ diuretics. Potential for interaction w/ drugs that affect gastric acidity. May increase theophylline and desipramine exposure. May increase free concentrations of highly protein-bound drugs.

PREGNANCY AND LACTATION
Pregnancy: Category C. There is a pregnancy registry that monitors the pregnancy outcomes in women exposed to Cymbalta during pregnancy. Neonates exposed during pregnancy to SNRIs or SSRIs have developed complications requiring prolonged hospitalization, respiratory support, and tube feeding which can arise immediately upon delivery. In some cases, the clinical picture is consistent w/ serotonin syndrome.
Lactation: Found in breast milk. Caution in nursing.

MECHANISM OF ACTION
Selective SNRI; not established. Believed to be related to potentiation of serotonergic and noradrenergic activity in the CNS.

PHARMACOKINETICS
Absorption: Well-absorbed; T_{max}=6 hrs. **Distribution:** V_d=1640L; plasma protein binding (>90%); found in breast milk. **Metabolism:** Extensive, hepatic via CYP1A2, 2D6; oxidation and conjugation. **Elimination:** Urine (70% metabolites; <1% unchanged), feces (20%); $T_{1/2}$=12 hrs.

PATIENT CONSIDERATIONS

Assessment: Assess for bipolar disorder risk, history of mania, history of seizures, substantial alcohol use, diseases/conditions that slow gastric emptying (eg, diabetes mellitus), risk factors for hyponatremia, susceptibility to angle-closure glaucoma/urinary retention, hepatic/renal impairment, pregnancy/nursing status, and possible drug interactions. Assess BP.

Monitoring: Monitor for signs/symptoms of clinical worsening (eg, suicidality, unusual changes in behavior), activation of mania/hypomania, serotonin syndrome, hepatotoxicity, bleeding events, skin reactions (eg, erythema multiforme, SJS), hyponatremia, seizures, orthostatic hypotension, falls, worsened glycemic control, urinary hesitation/retention, angle-closure glaucoma, and other adverse reactions. Periodically monitor BP. Carefully monitor patients receiving concomitant warfarin therapy when duloxetine is initiated or discontinued. Periodically reassess need for maintenance treatment and appropriate dose.

Counseling: Inform about benefits, risks, and appropriate use of therapy. Advise to avoid substantial alcohol use. Instruct to seek medical attention for clinical worsening, signs/symptoms of manic episodes, and symptoms of serotonin syndrome. Inform that abnormal bleeding (especially w/ the use of NSAIDs, ASA, warfarin), orthostatic hypotension, falls, syncope, hepatotoxicity, urinary hesitation/retention, seizures, BP increase, or discontinuation symptoms may occur. Caution about risk of angle-closure glaucoma. Advise of the signs/symptoms of hyponatremia. Advise to contact physician immediately if skin blisters, peeling rash, mouth sores, hives, or any other allergic reactions occur. Advise to inform physician if taking/planning to take any prescription or OTC medications, if pregnant, if intending to become pregnant, or if breastfeeding. Inform that therapy may impair judgment, thinking, or motor skills; instruct to use caution when operating hazardous machinery, including automobiles. Inform that improvement may be noticed w/in 1-4 weeks; instruct to continue therapy ud. Advise not to alter dosing regimen or d/c treatment w/o consulting physician.

CYRAMZA — ramucirumab   Rx
Class: Monoclonal antibody/VEGFR2 blocker

> Increased risk of hemorrhage and GI hemorrhage, including severe and sometimes fatal hemorrhagic events; permanently d/c if severe bleeding occurs. May increase risk of GI perforation; permanently d/c if this occurs. Impaired wound healing may occur; d/c therapy in patients w/ impaired wound healing. Withhold therapy prior to surgery and d/c therapy if wound healing complications develop.

ADULT DOSAGE	PEDIATRIC DOSAGE
Advanced or Metastatic, Gastric or Gastroesophageal Junction Adenocarcinoma	Pediatric use may not have been established
W/ Disease Progression on or After Prior Fluoropyrimidine- or Platinum-Containing Chemotherapy: As a Single Agent, or in Combination w/ Paclitaxel:	
Usual: 8mg/kg every 2 weeks administered as an IV infusion over 60 min. Continue until disease progression or unacceptable toxicity	
When given in combination, administer prior to administration of paclitaxel	
Metastatic Non-Small Cell Lung Cancer	
W/ Disease Progression: On or After Platinum-Based Chemotherapy:	
Usual: 10mg/kg IV over 60 min on Day 1 of a 21-day cycle prior to docetaxel infusion. Continue until disease progression or unacceptable toxicity	
Metastatic Colorectal Cancer	
W/ Disease Progression: On or After Prior Therapy w/ Bevacizumab, Oxaliplatin, and a Fluoropyrimidine:	
Usual: 8mg/kg IV over 60 min every 2 weeks prior to FOLFIRI (irinotecan, folinic acid, and 5-fluorouracil) administration. Continue until disease progression or unacceptable toxicity	
Premedication	
Prior to each infusion, premedicate all patients w/ an IV histamine H_1 antagonist (eg, diphenhydramine) For patients who have experienced a Grade 1 or 2 infusion-related reaction, also premedicate w/ dexamethasone (or equivalent) and acetaminophen prior to each infusion	

DOSING CONSIDERATIONS
Adverse Reactions
Infusion Related Reactions (IRRs):
- Reduce infusion rate by 50% for Grade 1 or 2 IRRs
- Permanently d/c for Grade 3 or 4 IRRs

HTN:
- Interrupt for severe HTN until controlled w/ medical management
- Permanently d/c for severe HTN that cannot be controlled w/ antihypertensive therapy

Proteinuria:
- Interrupt for urine protein levels ≥2g/24 hrs
- Reinitiate at a reduced dose (6mg/kg, if initial dose was 8mg/kg; or 8mg/kg, if initial dose was 10mg/kg) once the urine protein level returns to <2g/24 hrs. If protein level ≥2g/24 hrs reoccurs, interrupt and reduce dose (5mg/kg, if initial dose was 8mg/kg; or 6mg/kg, if initial dose was 10mg/kg) once the urine protein level returns to <2g/24 hrs
- Permanently d/c for urine protein level >3g/24 hrs or in the setting of nephrotic syndrome

Wound Healing Complications:
Interrupt prior to scheduled surgery until the wound is fully healed

Arterial Thromboembolic Events, GI Perforation, or Grade 3 or 4 Bleeding:
Permanently d/c

ADMINISTRATION
IV route

Calculate dose and required volume of ramucirumab needed to prepare the infusion sol.
Withdraw required volume of ramucirumab and further dilute w/ only 0.9% NaCl Inj in an IV infusion container to a final volume of 250mL.
Do not use dextrose containing sol.
Gently invert container to ensure adequate mixing.
Do not dilute w/ other sol or coinfuse w/ other electrolytes or medications.
Administer diluted ramucirumab infusion via infusion pump over 60 min through a separate infusion line. Use of a protein sparing 0.22-micron filter is recommended.
Flush line w/ sterile NaCl 0.9% sol for inj at the end of infusion.
Do not administer as an IV push or bolus.
Refer to PI for further administration and preparation instructions.

STORAGE
2-8°C (36-46°F). Protect from light. Do not freeze or shake. **Diluted Sol:** 2-8°C (36-46°F) for no >24 hrs or <25°C (77°F) for 4 hrs. Do not freeze or shake.

HOW SUPPLIED
Inj: 10mg/mL [10mL, 50mL]

WARNINGS/PRECAUTIONS
Serious, sometimes fatal, arterial thromboembolic events (ATEs) (eg, MI, cardiac arrest, cerebrovascular accident) reported. Increased incidence of severe HTN reported; control HTN prior to initiation of treatment. Permanently d/c treatment in patients w/ hypertensive crisis or hypertensive encephalopathy. IRRs reported; monitor during infusion for signs and symptoms of IRRs in a setting w/ available resuscitation equipment. Clinical deterioration, manifested by new onset or worsening encephalopathy, ascites, or hepatorenal syndrome, reported in patients w/ Child-Pugh B or C cirrhosis. Use in patients w/ Child-Pugh B or C cirrhosis only if potential benefits of treatment are judged to outweigh risks of clinical deterioration. Reversible posterior leukoencephalopathy syndrome (RPLS) reported; confirm diagnosis of RPLS w/ MRI and d/c if RPLS develops. Severe proteinuria and hypothyroidism reported. May cause fetal harm.

ADVERSE REACTIONS
Hemorrhage, GI hemorrhage/perforation, impaired wound healing, HTN, diarrhea, hyponatremia, headache, neutropenia, epistaxis, proteinuria, fatigue/asthenia, stomatitis/mucosal inflammation.

PREGNANCY AND LACTATION
Pregnancy: Based on its mechanism of action, ramucirumab can cause fetal harm; animal models link angiogenesis, vascular endothelial growth factor (VEGF) and VEGF Receptor 2 (VEGFR2) to critical aspects of female reproduction, embryofetal development, and postnatal development. Advise pregnant women of the potential risk to a fetus.
Lactation: There is no information on the presence of ramucirumab in human milk; not for use in nursing.
Reproductive Potential: Females of reproductive potential should use effective contraception during treatment and for at least 3 months after the last dose of therapy. May impair fertility of female patients.

MECHANISM OF ACTION
Monoclonal antibody/VEGF receptor 2 antagonist; specifically binds to VEGF receptor 2 and blocks binding of VEGF receptor ligands, VEGF-A, VEGF-C, and VEGF-D. As a result, ramucirumab inhibits ligand-stimulated activation of VEGF receptor 2, thereby inhibiting ligand-induced proliferation, and migration of human endothelial cells.

PHARMACOKINETICS
Elimination: $T_{1/2}$=14 days.

PATIENT CONSIDERATIONS
Assessment: Assess for HTN, presence of wound, upcoming surgery, Child-Pugh B or C cirrhosis, and pregnancy/nursing status.

Monitoring: Monitor for hemorrhage, ATEs, IRRs, GI perforation, wound healing complications, clinical deterioration in patients w/ Child-Pugh B or C cirrhosis patients, RPLS, and other adverse reactions. Monitor BP (every 2 weeks or more frequently as indicated). Monitor proteinuria by urine dipstick and/or urinary protein creatinine ratio for the development of worsening of proteinuria. Monitor thyroid function.

Counseling: Inform of the risks and benefits of therapy. Instruct to contact physician for bleeding or symptoms of bleeding, BP elevation or symptoms of HTN, severe diarrhea, vomiting, or severe abdominal pain. Advise to undergo routine BP monitoring. Inform that drug has the potential to impair wound healing; instruct not to undergo surgery w/o first discussing this potential risk w/ physician. Advise females of reproductive potential regarding potential infertility effects of therapy, and to use effective contraception during treatment and for at least 3 months after the last dose of treatment. Counsel not to breastfeed during treatment.

CYTOTEC — misoprostol   Rx
Class: Prostaglandin E₁ analogue

> Can cause birth defects, abortion, or premature birth. Uterine rupture reported when used to induce labor or induce abortion beyond 8th week of pregnancy. Not for use by pregnant women to reduce risk of NSAID-induced ulcers. Patients must be advised of the abortifacient property and warned not to give the drug to others. Use only in women of childbearing potential if the patient has had a negative serum pregnancy test within 2 weeks of starting therapy, is capable of complying with effective contraceptive measures, has received both oral and written warnings of the hazards of drug use, the risk of contraception failure, and the danger to other women of childbearing potential should the drug be taken by mistake, and will begin therapy only on 2nd or 3rd day of next normal menstrual period.

ADULT DOSAGE	PEDIATRIC DOSAGE
NSAID-Associated Gastric Ulcer	Pediatric use may not have been established
Risk reduction in patients at high risk of complications from gastric ulcer, as well as patients at high risk of developing gastric ulceration	
200mcg qid (last dose of the day should be hs); take for the duration of NSAID therapy. May use 100mcg qid if dose not tolerated	

DOSING CONSIDERATIONS
Renal Impairment
May reduce dose if the 200mcg dose is not tolerated

ADMINISTRATION
Oral route

Take w/ a meal

STORAGE
≤25°C (77°F), in a dry area.

HOW SUPPLIED
Tab: 100mcg, 200mcg

CONTRAINDICATIONS
Pregnant women, history of allergy to prostaglandins.

WARNINGS/PRECAUTIONS
Has not been shown to reduce the risk of duodenal ulcers in patients taking NSAIDs. Caution with preexisting cardiovascular disease (CVD).

ADVERSE REACTIONS
Diarrhea, abdominal pain, nausea.

DRUG INTERACTIONS
May augment the activity of oxytocic agents, especially when given <4 hrs prior to initiating oxytocin treatment; concomitant use is not recommended. Avoid coadministration with Mg²⁺-containing antacids to decrease incidence of diarrhea. Reduced total availability with antacids.

PREGNANCY AND LACTATION
Category X, caution in nursing.

MECHANISM OF ACTION
Synthetic prostaglandin E₁ analogue; has both antisecretory and (in animals) mucosal protective properties. Inhibits basal and nocturnal gastric acid secretion and acid secretion in response to a variety of stimuli (eg, meals, histamine, pentagastrin, coffee).

PHARMACOKINETICS
Absorption: Extensive, rapid. (High Fat Breakfast) C_{max}=303pg/mL, T_{max}=64 min, $AUC_{(0-4)}$=373pg•hr/mL. (Fasting) C_{max}=811pg/mL, T_{max}=14 min, $AUC_{(0-4)}$=417pg•hr/mL. **Distribution:** Plasma protein binding (<90%); found in breast milk. **Metabolism:** De-esterification to its free acid (active metabolite); β-oxidation, omega oxidation. **Elimination:** Urine (80%); $T_{1/2}$=20-40 min.

PATIENT CONSIDERATIONS
Assessment: In women of childbearing potential, assess pregnancy status (negative test within 2 weeks of starting therapy), the ability to comply with effective contraceptive measures, and menstrual cycle. Assess for CVD, risks for gastric ulcer, underlying condition (eg, inflammatory bowel disease), nursing status, previous hypersensitivity to the drug, and possible drug interactions.

Monitoring: Monitor patients with an underlying condition, or those in whom dehydration, were it to occur, would be dangerous.

Counseling: Inform women of childbearing potential that they must not take medication if pregnant and they must use an effective contraception method during therapy. Inform that drug is intended for administration along with NSAIDs, including aspirin, to reduce risk of developing NSAID-induced gastric ulcer. Instruct to take drug only according to directions of physician and contact physician if patient has questions about or problems with the drug. Instruct not to give medication to anyone else.

DAKLINZA — daclatasvir   Rx
Class: HCV NS5A inhibitor

ADULT DOSAGE ·	PEDIATRIC DOSAGE
Chronic Hepatitis C	Pediatric use may not have been established
Indicated for use w/ sofosbuvir, w/ or w/o ribavirin, for the treatment of patients w/ chronic hepatitis C virus (HCV) genotype 1 or genotype 3 infection	
Recommended Daclatasvir Dose: 60mg qd	
Recommended Treatment Regimen and Duration: **Genotype 1:** **W/O Cirrhosis or w/ Compensated (Child-Pugh A) Cirrhosis:** Daclatasvir + sofosbuvir for 12 weeks **Decompensated (Child-Pugh B or C) Cirrhosis or Post-Transplant:** Daclatasvir + sofosbuvir + ribavirin for 12 weeks	
Genotype 3: **W/O Cirrhosis:** Daclatasvir + sofosbuvir for 12 weeks **Compensated (Child-Pugh A) or Decompensated (Child-Pugh B or C) Cirrhosis, or Post-Transplant:** Daclatasvir + sofosbuvir + ribavirin for 12 weeks	
The recommended treatment durations are also applicable to patients w/ HCV/HIV-1 coinfection	
For specific sofosbuvir and ribavirin dosage recommendations, refer to the individual PIs	

DOSING CONSIDERATIONS
Concomitant Medications
Strong CYP3A Inhibitors and Certain HIV Antiviral Agents:
Reduce daclatasvir dose to 30mg qd

Moderate CYP3A Inducers and Nevirapine:
Increase daclatasvir dose to 90mg qd

Discontinuation
D/C daclatasvir if sofosbuvir is permanently discontinued

ADMINISTRATION
Oral route

Take w/ or w/o food.

STORAGE
25°C (77°F); excursions permitted between 15-30°C (59-86°F).

HOW SUPPLIED
Tab: 30mg, 60mg, 90mg

CONTRAINDICATIONS
In combination w/ strong CYP3A inducers (eg, phenytoin, carbamazepine, rifampin, St. John's wort). When used w/ sofosbuvir and ribavirin, refer to the individual PIs.

WARNINGS/PRECAUTIONS
Consider screening for the presence of NS5A polymorphisms at amino acid positions M28, Q30, L31, and Y93 in patients w/ cirrhosis who are infected w/ HCV genotype 1a prior to treatment initiation. Symptomatic bradycardia and cases requiring pacemaker intervention have been reported when amiodarone is coadministered w/ sofosbuvir in combination w/ another chronic HCV direct-acting antiviral, including daclatasvir. Patients also taking β-blockers or those w/ underlying cardiac comorbidities and/or advanced liver disease may be at increased risk for symptomatic bradycardia w/ coadministration of amiodarone. Coadministration of amiodarone w/ daclatasvir in combination w/ sofosbuvir is not recommended; if coadministration is required, cardiac monitoring in an inpatient setting for the first 48 hrs of coadministration is recommended, after which outpatient or self-monitoring of HR should occur on a daily basis through at least the first 2 weeks of treatment. Patients discontinuing amiodarone just prior to starting sofosbuvir in combination w/ daclatasvir should also undergo similar cardiac monitoring. Immediately evaluate patients who develop signs/symptoms of bradycardia. If administered w/ ribavirin, refer to the ribavirin PI for a full list of the warnings and precautions for ribavirin.

ADVERSE REACTIONS
Daclatasvir in Combination w/ Sofosbuvir: Headache, fatigue.
Daclatasvir in Combination w/ Sofosbuvir and Ribavirin: Headache, anemia, fatigue, nausea.

DRUG INTERACTIONS
See Dosing Considerations, Contraindications, and Warnings/Precautions. Strong CYP3A inducers or moderate CYP3A inducers (eg, bosentan, dexamethasone, nafcillin) may decrease levels and therapeutic effect. Strong CYP3A inhibitors (eg, clarithromycin, itraconazole, nefazodone) may increase levels. May increase systemic exposure to medicinal products that are substrates of P-gp, OATP 1B1 or 1B3, or breast cancer resistance protein, which could increase or prolong their therapeutic effect or adverse reactions. HIV protease inhibitors (eg, atazanavir w/ ritonavir, indinavir, nelfinavir, saquinavir) may increase levels; decrease daclatasvir dose to 30mg qd. Cobicistat-containing antiretroviral regimens (eg, atazanavir/cobicistat, elvitegravir/cobicistat/emtricitabine/tenofovir disoproxil fumarate) may increase levels; decrease daclatasvir dose to 30mg qd except w/ darunavir combined w/ cobicistat. Non-nucleoside reverse transcriptase inhibitors (eg, efavirenz, etravirine, nevirapine) may decrease levels; increase daclatasvir dose to 90mg qd. May increase levels of dabigatran. Use w/ dabigatran is not recommended in specific renal impairment groups, depending on the indication; refer to dabigatran PI for specific recommendations. May increase digoxin levels; monitor digoxin levels. May increase levels of HMG-CoA reductase inhibitors (eg, atorvastatin, rosuvastatin, simvastatin); monitor for HMG-CoA reductase inhibitor-associated adverse events (eg, myopathy). May increase levels of buprenorphine and norbuprenorphine; monitor for buprenorphine-associated adverse events. Refer to PI for further information on drug interactions.

PREGNANCY AND LACTATION
Pregnancy: No adequate human data are available to determine whether or not daclatasvir poses a risk to pregnancy outcomes.
Lactation: It is not known whether daclatasvir is present in human milk, affects human milk production, or has effects on the breastfed infant; caution in nursing.

If administered w/ ribavirin, refer to ribavirin PI for additional information.

MECHANISM OF ACTION
HCV NS5A inhibitor; binds to the N-terminus of NS5A and inhibits both viral RNA replication and virion assembly.

PHARMACOKINETICS
Absorption: T_{max}=2 hrs; AUC=10,973ng•hr/mL; absolute bioavailability (67%).
Distribution: Plasma protein binding (approx 99%); V_d=47L. **Metabolism:** Primarily via CYP3A. **Elimination:** Feces (88%, 53% unchanged), urine (6.6%, primarily unchanged); $T_{1/2}$=12-15 hrs.

PATIENT CONSIDERATIONS
Assessment: Assess for hypersensitivity to drug, pregnancy/nursing status, and possible drug interactions. Perform cardiac monitoring in patients discontinuing amiodarone just prior to starting daclatasvir. Consider screening for the presence of NS5A polymorphisms at amino acid positions M28, Q30, L31, and Y93 in patients w/ cirrhosis who are infected w/ HCV genotype 1a prior to treatment initiation.

Monitoring: Monitor for bradycardia if coadministering daclatasvir w/ sofosbuvir and amiodarone. Monitor for other adverse reactions.

Counseling: Inform that therapy may interact w/ other drugs; advise to report to physician the use of any other medication or herbal products. Advise to seek medical evaluation immediately for symptoms of bradycardia (eg, fainting, dizziness, lightheadedness, weakness). Inform that therapy should not be used alone and that it should be used in combination w/ sofosbuvir w/ or w/o ribavirin. Advise to avoid pregnancy during combination treatment w/ daclatasvir and sofosbuvir w/ ribavirin for 6 months after completion of treatment; instruct to notify physician immediately in the event of a pregnancy.

DALIRESP — roflumilast   Rx
Class: Selective phosphodiesterase-4 (PDE-4) inhibitor

ADULT DOSAGE	PEDIATRIC DOSAGE
Chronic Obstructive Pulmonary Disease	Pediatric use may not have been established
Reduce risk of exacerbations in patients w/ severe COPD associated w/ chronic bronchitis and a history of exacerbations	
500mcg qd	

ADMINISTRATION
Oral route

Take w/ or w/o food.

STORAGE
20-25°C (68-77°F); excursions permitted to 15-30°C (59-86°F).

HOW SUPPLIED
Tab: 500mcg

CONTRAINDICATIONS
Moderate to severe liver impairment (Child-Pugh B or C).

WARNINGS/PRECAUTIONS
Not a bronchodilator; not indicated for the relief of acute bronchospasm. Psychiatric adverse reactions, including suicidality, reported; carefully evaluate the risks and benefits of treatment in patients w/ history of depression and/or suicidal thoughts or behavior, and of continuing treatment if such reactions occur. Weight loss reported; evaluate and consider discontinuation if unexplained or clinically significant weight loss occurs. Caution w/ mild liver impairment (Child-Pugh A).

ADVERSE REACTIONS
Diarrhea, weight decreased, nausea, headache, back pain.

DRUG INTERACTIONS
Strong CYP450 inducers (eg, rifampicin, phenobarbital, carbamazepine, phenytoin) decrease exposure and may reduce therapeutic effectiveness; concomitant use is not recommended. CYP3A4 inhibitors or dual inhibitors that inhibit both CYP3A4 and CYP1A2 simultaneously (eg, erythromycin, ketoconazole, fluvoxamine, enoxacin, cimetidine) and oral contraceptives containing gestodene

and ethinyl estradiol may increase exposure and may result in increased adverse reactions; use w/ caution.

PREGNANCY AND LACTATION

Pregnancy: Category C.
Lactation: Excretion of roflumilast and/or its metabolites into human milk is probable; not for use in nursing.

MECHANISM OF ACTION

Selective PDE-4 inhibitor; mechanism not established. Thought to be related to the effects of increased intracellular cAMP in lung cells.

PHARMACOKINETICS

Absorption: Absolute bioavailability (80%); T_{max}=1 hr, 8 hrs (roflumilast N-oxide).
Distribution: V_d=2.9L/kg; plasma protein binding (99%, 97% roflumilast N-oxide). May be found in breast milk. **Metabolism:** Extensive via Phase 1 (CYP450) and Phase 2 (conjugation) reactions; roflumilast N-oxide (major active metabolite).
Elimination: Urine (70%); $T_{1/2}$=17 hrs, 30 hrs (roflumilast N-oxide).

PATIENT CONSIDERATIONS

Assessment: Assess for liver impairment, history of depression and/or suicidal thoughts or behavior, pregnancy/nursing status, and possible drug interactions.

Monitoring: Monitor for psychiatric events (including suicidality) and other adverse reactions. Monitor weight regularly.

Counseling: Inform that drug is not a bronchodilator and should not be used for the relief of acute bronchospasm. Advise of the need to be alert for the emergence or worsening of insomnia, anxiety, depression, suicidal thoughts, or other mood changes; instruct to contact physician if such changes occur. Instruct to monitor weight regularly and to consult physician if unexplained or clinically significant weight loss occurs. Instruct to notify physician of all medications being taken.

DALVANCE — dalbavancin   Rx

Class: Lipoglycopeptide

ADULT DOSAGE	PEDIATRIC DOSAGE
Skin and Skin Structure Infections	Pediatric use may not have been established
Acute Bacterial Infections:	
Single Dose Regimen: 1500mg	
2-Dose Regimen: 1000mg, followed 1 week later by 500mg	
Administer over 30 min by IV infusion	

DOSING CONSIDERATIONS

Renal Impairment
CrCl <30mL/min and Not Receiving Regularly Scheduled Hemodialysis:
Single Dose Regimen: 1125mg
2-Dose Regimen: 750mg, followed 1 week later by 375mg

Patients Receiving Regularly Scheduled Hemodialysis:
No dosage adjustment is recommended and may administer w/o regard to timing of hemodialysis

ADMINISTRATION

IV route

Do not co-infuse w/ other medications or electrolytes.
Do not use saline-based infusion sol.
If a common IV line is being used to administer other drugs in addition to dalbavancin, flush the line before and after each infusion w/ D5 inj.

Reconstitution
1. Reconstitute using 25mL of either sterile water for inj or D5 inj for each 500mg vial.
2. Alternate between gentle swirling and inversion of vial to avoid foaming; do not shake.
3. The reconstituted vial contains 20mg/mL dalbavancin.
4. Store reconstituted vials either at 2-8°C (36-46°F), or at 20-25°C (68-77°F); do not freeze.

Dilution
1. Aseptically transfer the required dose of reconstituted dalbavancin sol from the vial(s) to an IV bag or bottle containing D5 inj.
2. The diluted sol must have a final concentration of 1-5mg/mL.
3. Once diluted into an IV bag or bottle, may store either at 2-8°C (36-46°F), or at 20-25°C (68-77°F); do not freeze.

The total time from reconstitution to dilution to administration should not exceed 48 hrs.

STORAGE

Unreconstituted: 25°C (77°F); excursions permitted to 15-30°C (59-86°F).

HOW SUPPLIED

Inj: 500mg

CONTRAINDICATIONS

Known hypersensitivity to dalbavancin.

WARNINGS/PRECAUTIONS

Serious hypersensitivity (anaphylactic) and skin reactions reported; d/c if an allergic reaction occurs. Caution w/ history of glycopeptide allergy. Rapid IV infusion of therapy can cause reactions that resemble "Red-Man syndrome" (eg, flushing of the upper body, urticaria, pruritus, rash); stopping or slowing infusion may result in cessation of these reactions. ALT elevations reported. *Clostridium difficile*-associated diarrhea (CDAD) reported; may need to d/c if CDAD is

suspected or confirmed. May result in bacterial resistance if used in the absence of proven or suspected bacterial infection. Caution w/ moderate or severe hepatic impairment (Child-Pugh Class B or C) and in elderly.

ADVERSE REACTIONS

Nausea, headache, diarrhea.

PREGNANCY AND LACTATION

Pregnancy: There have been no adequate and well-controlled studies w/ dalbavancin in pregnant women; use during pregnancy only if the benefit justifies risk to the fetus.
Lactation: It is not known whether dalbavancin or its metabolite is excreted in human milk; caution in nursing.

MECHANISM OF ACTION

Semisynthetic lipoglycopeptide antibacterial agent; interferes w/ cell wall synthesis by binding to D-alanyl-D-alanine terminus of the stem pentapeptide in nascent cell wall peptidoglycan, thus preventing cross-linking.

PHARMACOKINETICS

Absorption: C_{max}=287mg/L (1000mg single dose), 423mg/L (1500mg single dose); AUC_{0-inf}=23,443mg•hr/L. **Distribution:** Plasma protein binding (93%). **Elimination:** Urine (33% unchanged, 12% metabolite hydroxy-dalbavancin), feces (20%); $T_{1/2}$=346 hrs.

PATIENT CONSIDERATIONS

Assessment: Assess for hypersensitivity to drug or other glycopeptides, renal/hepatic impairment, and pregnancy/nursing status. Perform culture and susceptibility testing.

Monitoring: Monitor for hypersensitivity reactions, infusion-related reactions, hepatic effects, CDAD, development of drug-resistant bacteria, and other adverse reactions.

Counseling: Advise that allergic reactions may occur and that serious allergic reactions require immediate treatment. Instruct to inform physician about any previous hypersensitivity reactions to dalbavancin, or other glycopeptides. Counsel that therapy should only be used to treat bacterial, not viral, infections. Instruct to take exactly ud, even if the patient feels better early in the course of therapy; inform that skipping doses or not completing full course of therapy may decrease effectiveness of treatment and increase bacterial resistance. Inform that diarrhea is a common problem caused by therapy and usually resolves when therapy is discontinued; instruct to contact physician if severe watery or bloody diarrhea develops.

DARAPRIM — pyrimethamine   Rx

Class: Folic acid antagonist

ADULT DOSAGE	PEDIATRIC DOSAGE
Toxoplasmosis	**Toxoplasmosis**
Initial: 50-75mg/day w/ 1-4g/day of sulfonamide of the sulfapyrimidine type (eg, sulfadoxine); concurrent folinic acid is strongly recommended	1mg/kg/day divided into 2 equal daily doses w/ usual pediatric sulfonamide dose; concurrent folinic acid is strongly recommended
Continue for 1-3 days, depending on the response and tolerance to therapy	After 2-4 days, may reduce dose to 1/2 and continue for approx 1 month
May reduce dose of each drug to 1/2 of previous dose and continue for additional 4-5 weeks	**Malaria**
Malaria	**Monotherapy in Semi-Immune Persons:**
Treatment of Acute Malaria: 25mg/day for 2 days w/ a sulfonamide	**4-10 Years:** 25mg/day for 2 days
Monotherapy in Semi-Immune Persons: 50mg for 2 days	Clinical cure should be followed by once-weekly regimen for chemoprophylaxis. Regimens that include suppression should be extended through any characteristic periods of early recrudescence and late relapse, for at least 10 weeks in each case
Clinical cure should be followed by once-weekly regimen for chemoprophylaxis. Regimens that include suppression should be extended through any characteristic periods of early recrudescence and late relapse, for at least 10 weeks in each case	**Chemoprophylaxis of Malaria:** **<4 Years:** 6.25mg once weekly
Chemoprophylaxis of Malaria: 25mg once weekly	**4-10 Years:** 12.5mg once weekly **>10 Years:** 25mg once weekly

---

DOSING CONSIDERATIONS

Elderly
Start at lower end of dosing range

ADMINISTRATION

Oral route

STORAGE

15-25°C (59-77°F) in a dry place and protect from light.

HOW SUPPLIED

Tab: 25mg* *scored

CONTRAINDICATIONS

Documented megaloblastic anemia due to folate deficiency.

WARNINGS/PRECAUTIONS

Not suitable as a prophylactic agent for travelers to most areas due to pyrimethamine resistance. Not recommended alone in the treatment of acute malaria. Acute malaria treatment is recommended only for patients infected in areas where susceptible plasmodia exist. Dose for toxoplasmosis approaches toxic levels; reduce dose or d/c if signs of folate deficiency develop. Administer folinic acid (leucovorin) 5-15mg/day (PO, IV, or IM) until normal hematopoiesis is restored. May be carcinogenic. Pediatric deaths reported w/ accidental ingestion. Do not exceed recommended dose for chemoprophylaxis of malaria; use small initial dose for toxoplasmosis in patients w/ convulsive disorders to avoid nervous system toxicity. Caution w/ renal/hepatic dysfunction or in patients w/ possible folate deficiency (eg, malabsorption syndrome, alcoholism, pregnancy). Perform semiweekly blood counts, including platelet counts, in patients receiving high dosage, as for the treatment of toxoplasmosis.

ADVERSE REACTIONS

Hypersensitivity reactions, hyperphenylalaninemia, anorexia, vomiting, megaloblastic anemia, leukopenia, thrombocytopenia, pancytopenia, atrophic glossitis, hematuria, cardiac rhythm disorders.

DRUG INTERACTIONS

Caution w/ phenytoin; may affect folate levels. Antifolic drugs or agents associated w/ myelosuppression (eg, sulfonamides or trimethoprim-sulfamethoxazole combinations, proguanil, zidovudine, or cytostatic agents [eg, methotrexate]) may increase the risk of bone marrow suppression. Mild hepatotoxicity reported w/ lorazepam. Hypersensitivity reactions and hyperphenylalaninemia can occur particularly w/ a sulfonamide.

PREGNANCY AND LACTATION

Pregnancy: Category C.
Lactation: Found in breast milk; not for use in nursing.

MECHANISM OF ACTION

Folic acid antagonist; rationale for its therapeutic action is based on the differential requirement between host and parasite for nucleic acid precursors involved in growth. This activity is highly selective against plasmodia and *Toxoplasma gondii*.

PHARMACOKINETICS

Absorption: Well absorbed. T_{max}=2-6 hrs. **Distribution:** Plasma protein binding (87%); found in breast milk. **Elimination:** $T_{1/2}$=96 hrs.

PATIENT CONSIDERATIONS

Assessment: Assess for megaloblastic anemia due to folate deficiency, renal/hepatic dysfunction, folate deficiency, hypersensitivity, pregnancy/nursing status, and possible drug interactions.

Monitoring: Monitor for signs/symptoms of folate deficiency, hypersensitivity reactions, and other adverse effects. Perform semiweekly blood counts, including platelet counts, in patients receiving high dosage, as for the treatment of toxoplasmosis.

Counseling: Instruct to d/c and seek medical attention at the appearance of skin rash (1st appearance), sore throat, pallor, purpura, or glossitis. Inform women of childbearing potential to avoid becoming pregnant. Advise to keep out of reach of children. Advise not to exceed recommended doses. Inform that anorexia and vomiting may be minimized by taking the drug w/ meals. Advise that concurrent administration of folinic acid is strongly recommended when used for the treatment of toxoplasmosis in all patients.

DARZALEX — daratumumab   Rx

Class: Monoclonal antibody/CD38 blocker

ADULT DOSAGE

Multiple Myeloma

Patients w/ multiple myeloma who have received at least 3 prior lines of therapy including a proteasome inhibitor (PI) and an immunomodulatory agent or who are double-refractory to a PI and an immunomodulatory agent

Recommended Dose: 16mg/kg IV
Weeks 1-8: Administer weekly
Weeks 9-24: Administer every 2 weeks
Week 25 Onwards Until Disease Progression: Administer every 4 weeks

Infusion Rates:
1st Infusion:
Dilution Volume: 1000mL
Initial Rate (1st hr): 50mL/hr
Rate Increment: 50mL/hr every hr
Max Rate: 200mL/hr

2nd Infusion:
Dilution Volume: 500mL
Initial Rate (1st hr): 50mL/hr
Rate Increment: 50mL/hr every hr
Max Rate: 200mL/hr

Escalate infusion rate only if there were no Grade 1 or greater infusion

PEDIATRIC DOSAGE

Pediatric use may not have been established

---

reactions during the first 3 hrs of the 1st infusion

Subsequent Infusions:
Dilution Volume: 500mL
Initial Rate (1st hr): 100mL/hr
Rate Increment: 50mL/hr every hr
Max Rate: 200mL/hr

Escalate infusion rate only if there were no Grade 1 or greater infusion reactions during a final infusion rate of ≥100 mL/hr in the first 2 infusions

Premedication

IV corticosteroid (methylprednisolone 100mg, or equivalent dose of an intermediate-acting or long-acting corticosteroid) + oral antipyretics (acetaminophen 650-1000mg) + oral or IV antihistamine (diphenhydramine 25-50mg or equivalent)

Administer to all patients 1 hr prior to every infusion; following 2nd infusion, may reduce the corticosteroid dose (methylprednisolone 60mg IV)

Post-Infusion Medication

Administer to all patients oral corticosteroid (20mg methylprednisolone or equivalent dose of a corticosteroid in accordance w/ local standards) on the 1st and 2nd day after all infusions

For patients w/ a history of obstructive pulmonary disorder, consider prescribing post-infusion medications (eg, short and long-acting bronchodilators, inhaled corticosteroids). Following the first 4 infusions, if patient experiences no major infusion reactions, may d/c additional inhaled post-infusion medications

Missed Dose

If a planned dose is missed, administer the dose as soon as possible and adjust dosing schedule accordingly, maintaining the treatment interval

---

DOSING CONSIDERATIONS

Adverse Reactions

Infusion Reactions:
Immediately interrupt infusion and manage symptoms if an infusion reaction of any grade/severity develops

Grade 1-2: Once reaction symptoms resolve, resume the infusion at no more than 1/2 the rate at which the reaction occurred; may resume infusion rate escalation at increments and intervals as appropriate if patient does not experience any further reaction symptoms

Grade 3: Consider restarting infusion at no more than 1/2 the rate at which the reaction occurred if the intensity of the reaction decreases to Grade 2 or lower. Resume infusion rate escalation if the patient does not experience additional symptoms. Repeat these steps in the event of recurrence of Grade 3 symptoms; permanently d/c upon the 3rd occurrence of a Grade 3 or greater infusion reaction

Grade 4: Permanently d/c treatment

Other Important Considerations

Prophylaxis for Herpes Zoster Reactivation:
Initiate antiviral prophylaxis to prevent herpes zoster reactivation w/in 1 week of starting daratumumab and continue for 3 months following treatment

ADMINISTRATION

IV route

Administer only as an IV infusion after dilution.
Administer diluted sol using an infusion set fitted w/ a flow regulator and w/ an in-line, sterile, non-pyrogenic, low protein-binding polyethersulfone filter (pore size 0.22 or 0.2μm).
Must use polyurethane, polybutadiene, polyvinyl chloride (PVC), polypropylene (PP), or polyethylene (PE) administration sets.
Infusion should be completed w/in 15 hrs.
Do not store any unused portion of the infusion sol for reuse.
Do not infuse concomitantly in the same IV line w/ other agents.

Preparation

1. Calculate the dose (mg), total volume (mL) of daratumumab sol required, and the number of daratumumab vials needed based on patient actual body weight.
2. Aseptically, remove a volume of 0.9% NaCl inj from the infusion bag/container that is equal to the required volume of daratumumab sol.
3. Withdraw the necessary amount of daratumumab sol and dilute to the appropriate volume by adding to the infusion bag/container containing 0.9% NaCl inj; infusion bags/containers must be made of PVC, PP, PE, or polyolefin blend (PE+PP).
4. Gently invert the bag/container to mix the sol; do not shake.

Following dilution, may store the infusion bag/container for up to 24 hrs in a refrigerator at 2-8°C (36-46°F), protected from light; do not freeze. Use immediately after allowing the bag/container to come to room temperature. Diluted sol may develop very small, translucent to white proteinaceous particles; do not use if visibly opaque particles, discoloration, or foreign particles are observed.

STORAGE
2-8°C (36-46°F). Do not freeze or shake. Protect from light.

HOW SUPPLIED
Inj: 20mg/mL [5mL, 20mL]

WARNINGS/PRECAUTIONS
See Dosing Considerations. Should be administered by a healthcare professional, w/ immediate access to emergency equipment and appropriate medical support. Severe infusion reactions (eg, bronchospasm, hypoxia, dyspnea, HTN) reported; interrupt infusion for reactions of any severity and institute medical management as needed. Binds to CD38 on RBCs and results in a positive Indirect Antiglobulin Test (Coombs test); may persist for up to 6 months after the last infusion. Daratumumab bound to RBCs masks detection of antibodies to minor antigens in the patient's serum; determination of a patient's ABO and Rh blood type are not impacted. Notify blood transfusion centers of this interference w/ serological testing and inform blood banks that a patient has received daratumumab. Type and screen patients prior to starting therapy. If an emergency transfusion is required, non-cross-matched ABO/RhD-compatible RBCs can be given per local blood bank practices. Daratumumab may be detected on both, the serum protein electrophoresis and immunofixation assays used for the clinical monitoring of endogenous M-protein; this interference may impact the determination of complete response and of disease progression in some patients w/ IgG kappa myeloma protein; consider other methods to evaluate the depth of response in patients w/ persistent very good partial response.

ADVERSE REACTIONS
Infusion reaction, fatigue, N/V, pyrexia, back pain, cough, URTI, arthralgia, nasal congestion, diarrhea, dyspnea, pain in extremity, nasopharyngitis, decreased appetite, constipation.

PREGNANCY AND LACTATION
Pregnancy: May cause fetal myeloid or lymphoid-cell depletion and decrease bone density; defer administering live vaccines to neonates and infants exposed to daratumumab in utero until a hematology evaluation is completed.
Lactation: Caution in nursing.
Reproductive Potential: Women of reproductive potential should use effective contraception during treatment and for 3 months after cessation of treatment.

MECHANISM OF ACTION
Human CD38-directed monoclonal antibody; binds to CD38 and inhibits the growth of CD38 expressing tumor cells by inducing apoptosis directly through Fc mediated cross linking as well as by immune-mediated tumor cell lysis through complement dependent cytotoxicity, antibody dependent cell mediated cytotoxicity, and antibody dependent cellular phagocytosis.

PHARMACOKINETICS
Absorption: C_{max}=915µg/mL. **Distribution:** V_d=4.7L. **Elimination:** $T_{1/2}$=18 days.

PATIENT CONSIDERATIONS
Assessment: Assess for hypersensitivity to drug, history of an obstructive pulmonary disorder, history of herpes zoster, and pregnancy/nursing status. Type and screen patient's blood.

Monitoring: Monitor for infusion reactions, lab test interactions, and for other adverse reactions.

Counseling: Advise to seek immediate medical attention if any signs/symptoms of an infusion reaction develop. Advise patients to inform healthcare providers including blood transfusion centers/personnel that they are taking daratumumab, in the event of a planned transfusion.

DAYPRO — oxaprozin   Rx
Class: NSAID

> NSAIDs cause an increased risk of serious cardiovascular (CV) thrombotic events, including MI and stroke, which can be fatal. This risk may occur early in treatment and may increase w/ duration of use. Contraindicated in the setting of CABG surgery. NSAIDs cause an increased risk of serious GI adverse events (eg, bleeding, ulceration, stomach/intestinal perforation), which can be fatal and can occur anytime during use and w/o warning symptoms; elderly patients and patients w/ a prior history of peptic ulcer disease and/or GI bleeding are at a greater risk.

ADULT DOSAGE
Osteoarthritis
Initial: 1200mg qd
Titrate: Adjust dose/frequency after observing response to initial therapy
Max: 1800mg/day or 26mg/kg/day (whichever is lower) in divided doses

May start w/ a 1-time LD of 1200-1800mg (not to exceed 26mg/kg) if quick onset of action is needed. Doses >1200mg/day on a chronic basis should be reserved for patients who are >50kg, have normal renal and hepatic function, are at low risk of peptic ulcer, and whose severity of disease justifies maximal therapy.

PEDIATRIC DOSAGE
Juvenile Rheumatoid Arthritis
6-16 Years:
Initial:
22-31kg: 600mg qd
32-54kg: 900mg qd
≥55kg: 1200mg qd
Titrate: Adjust dose/frequency after observing response to initial therapy. Doses >1200mg have not been studied.

Rheumatoid Arthritis
Initial: 1200mg qd
Titrate: Adjust dose/frequency after observing response to initial therapy
Max: 1800mg/day or 26mg/kg/day (whichever is lower) in divided doses

May start w/ a 1-time LD of 1200-1800mg (not to exceed 26mg/kg) if quick onset of action is needed. Doses >1200mg/day on a chronic basis should be reserved for patients who are >50kg, have normal renal and hepatic function, are at low risk of peptic ulcer, and whose severity of disease justifies maximal therapy.

DOSING CONSIDERATIONS
Renal Impairment
Severe/Dialysis:
Initial: 600mg qd
Titrate: May cautiously increase to 1200mg w/ close monitoring if there is insufficient relief of symptoms

Other Important Considerations
Low Body Weight:
Initial: 600mg qd
Titrate: May cautiously increase to 1200mg w/ close monitoring if there is insufficient relief of symptoms

ADMINISTRATION
Oral route

Most patients will tolerate qd dosing; divided doses may be tried in patients unable to tolerate single doses.

STORAGE
20-25°C (68-77°F); excursions permitted to 15-30°C (59-86°F). Protect from light.

HOW SUPPLIED
Tab: 600mg* *scored

CONTRAINDICATIONS
Known hypersensitivity (eg, anaphylactic reactions, serious skin reactions) to oxaprozin or any components of the drug product; history of asthma, urticaria, or allergic-type reactions w/ aspirin (ASA) or other NSAIDs; in the setting of CABG surgery.

WARNINGS/PRECAUTIONS
Use lowest effective dose for the shortest duration possible. Avoid in patients w/ a recent MI unless benefits outweigh the risks of recurrent CV thrombotic events; if used, monitor for signs of cardiac ischemia. Increased risk for GI bleeding w/ longer duration of therapy, older age, poor general health status, and advanced liver disease and/or coagulopathy; avoid use in patients at higher risk unless benefits are expected to outweigh the increased risk and consider alternate therapies. Promptly initiate evaluation and treatment if a serious GI adverse event is suspected; d/c until a serious GI adverse event is ruled out. Hepatotoxicity reported; d/c immediately and perform a clinical evaluation if clinical signs/symptoms consistent w/ liver disease develop, or if systemic manifestations occur. May cause new onset HTN or worsen preexisting HTN. Fluid retention and edema reported. Avoid use in patients w/ severe heart failure (HF) unless benefits outweigh risks; monitor for signs of worsening HF if used. Renal papillary necrosis and other renal injury reported w/ long-term use. Renal toxicity also reported in patients in whom renal prostaglandins have a compensatory role in the maintenance of renal perfusion; increased risk w/ renal/hepatic dysfunction, dehydration, hypovolemia, and HF, and in the elderly. Correct volume status in dehydrated or hypovolemic patients prior to initiating therapy. Avoid use in patients w/ advanced renal disease unless the benefits are expected to outweigh the risk; monitor for signs of worsening renal function if used in patients w/ advanced renal disease. Hyperkalemia reported. Associated w/ anaphylactic reactions. Monitor for changes in the signs/symptoms of asthma in patients w/ preexisting asthma (w/o known ASA sensitivity). May cause serious skin reactions (eg, exfoliative dermatitis, Stevens-Johnson syndrome, toxic epidermal necrolysis); d/c at 1st appearance of skin rash/hypersensitivity. Anemia reported. May increase the risk of bleeding events; coagulation disorders may increase this risk. May mask inflammation and fever. May be associated w/ rash and/or mild photosensitivity. Lab test interactions may occur.

ADVERSE REACTIONS
Constipation, diarrhea, dyspepsia, nausea, rash.

DRUG INTERACTIONS
Drugs that interfere w/ serotonin reuptake may potentiate the risk of bleeding. Synergistic effect on bleeding w/ anticoagulants (eg, warfarin); monitor for signs of bleeding w/ concomitant anticoagulants, antiplatelet agents (eg, ASA), SSRIs, and SNRIs. May increase risk of GI bleeding w/ use of oral corticosteroids, anticoagulants, SSRIs, smoking, and alcohol use. ASA may increase risk of bleeding and serious GI events; concomitant use w/ analgesic doses of ASA is not recommended. Monitor patients more closely for GI bleeding w/ concomitant use of low-dose ASA for cardiac prophylaxis. May diminish antihypertensive effect of ACE inhibitors, ARBs, and β-blockers (eg, propranolol); monitor BP. Coadministration w/ ACE inhibitors or ARBs may result in deterioration of renal function (including possible acute renal failure) in patients who are elderly or volume-depleted (including those on diuretic therapy), or who have renal impairment; monitor for worsening renal function and adequately hydrate patient when these drugs are administered concomitantly. May reduce the natriuretic

effect of loop diuretics (eg, furosemide) and thiazide diuretics; observe for signs of worsening renal function, in addition to assuring diuretic efficacy including antihypertensive effects. May increase digoxin serum concentrations and prolong the $T_{1/2}$ of digoxin; monitor digoxin levels. May elevate plasma lithium levels and reduce renal lithium clearance; monitor for signs of lithium toxicity. May increase the risk for methotrexate (MTX) toxicity; monitor for MTX toxicity. May increase cyclosporine's nephrotoxicity; monitor for signs of worsening renal function. Concomitant use w/ other NSAIDs or salicylates (eg, diflunisal, salsalate) increases the risk of GI toxicity; not recommended w/ other NSAIDs or salicylates. Concomitant use w/ pemetrexed may increase the risk of pemetrexed-associated myelosuppression, renal, and GI toxicity; refer to prescribing information for further information. Monitor blood glucose levels in the beginning phase of concomitant use w/ glyburide.

PREGNANCY AND LACTATION
Pregnancy: Use during the 3rd trimester of pregnancy increases the risk of premature closure of the fetal ductus arteriosus; avoid use in pregnant women starting at 30 weeks of gestation (3rd trimester).
Lactation: It is not known whether Daypro is excreted in human milk; caution in nursing.
Reproductive Potential: Based on the mechanism of action, may delay or prevent rupture of ovarian follicles, which has been associated w/ reversible infertility in some women. Small studies in women treated w/ NSAIDs have also shown a reversible delay in ovulation. Consider withdrawal of therapy in women who have difficulties conceiving or who are undergoing investigation of infertility.

MECHANISM OF ACTION
NSAID; mechanism not completely understood but involves inhibition of COX-1 and COX-2. Mode of action may be due to a decrease of prostaglandins in peripheral tissues; possesses anti-inflammatory, analgesic, and antipyretic activities.

PHARMACOKINETICS
Absorption: Administration of variable doses resulted in different pharmacokinetic parameters. **Distribution:** V_d=11-17L/70kg; plasma protein binding (99%).
Metabolism: Liver via oxidation (65%) and glucuronic acid conjugation (35%).
Elimination: Feces (35% metabolites), urine (5% unchanged, 65% metabolites).

PATIENT CONSIDERATIONS
Assessment: Assess for history of asthma, urticaria, or other allergic-type reactions w/ previous use of ASA or other NSAIDs; asthma; CV disease (CVD) or risk factors for CVD; HTN; history of peptic ulcer disease or GI bleeding; coagulation disorders; renal/hepatic impairment; pregnancy/nursing status; or any other conditions where treatment is contraindicated or cautioned. Assess volume status. Assess for possible drug interactions. Obtain baseline BP, CBC, and chemistry profile.

Monitoring: Monitor for signs/symptoms of CV thrombotic events; cardiac ischemia in patients w/ a recent MI; GI bleeding/ulceration and perforation; hepatotoxicity; new or worsening HTN; HF; edema; renal papillary necrosis and other renal injury; hyperkalemia; anaphylactic reactions; serious skin reactions; anemia; photosensitivity; and other adverse reactions. Monitor BP during initiation of therapy and throughout the course of therapy. Monitor for signs of bleeding in patients on concomitant therapy w/ anticoagulants, antiplatelet agents, SSRIs, or SNRIs. Monitor renal function in patients w/ renal/hepatic impairment, HF, dehydration, or hypovolemia. Monitor CBC and chemistry profiles periodically during long-term treatment.

Counseling: Inform of potential for CV thrombotic events, GI adverse events, and worsening CHF/edema, and advise of symptoms; instruct to report symptoms to healthcare provider if any occur. Inform of the potential for hepatotoxicity, and advise of signs/symptoms; if signs/symptoms occur, instruct to d/c and seek immediate medical therapy. Instruct to seek immediate emergency help if signs of an anaphylactic reaction occur. Advise to d/c immediately if rash develops and to contact healthcare provider as soon as possible. Advise females of reproductive potential who desire pregnancy that therapy may be associated w/ a reversible delay in ovulation. Inform pregnant women to avoid use starting at 30 weeks of gestation. Inform patient to not use other NSAIDs or salicylates concomitantly; notify of the presence of NSAIDs in OTC medications for colds, fever, or insomnia. Inform patient not to use low-dose ASA concomitantly w/o talking to healthcare provider.

DAYTRANA — methylphenidate   CII
Class: CNS stimulant

> Caution w/ history of drug dependence or alcoholism. Chronic abusive use may lead to marked tolerance and psychological dependence w/ varying degrees of abnormal behavior. Frank psychotic episodes may occur, especially w/ parenteral abuse. Careful supervision is required during withdrawal from abusive use, since severe depression may occur. Withdrawal following chronic use may unmask symptoms of underlying disorder that may require follow-up.

PEDIATRIC DOSAGE
Attention-Deficit Hyperactivity Disorder
≥6 Years:
Apply to hip area 2 hrs before effect is needed and remove 9 hrs after application
Titration Schedule:
Week 1: 10mg/9 hrs
Week 2: 15mg/9 hrs
Week 3: 20mg/9 hrs
Week 4: 30mg/9 hrs
Dose/Wear Time Reduction and Discontinuation:
May remove patch earlier than 9 hrs if a shorter duration of effect is desired or late day side effects appear

---

DOSING CONSIDERATIONS
Adverse Reactions
Reduce dose/wear time or, if necessary, d/c drug if aggravation of symptoms or other adverse events occur

ADMINISTRATION
Transdermal route

Apply patch immediately upon removal from the individual protective pouch; press firmly for approx 30 sec.
Apply to clean, dry area of the hip; area should not be oily, damaged, or irritated. Avoid application to waistline.
Alternate sides when applying the next am.
Do not cut patches.
Do not use w/ dressings, tape, or other adhesives.

Refer to PI for further application, removal, and disposal instructions.

STORAGE
25°C (77°F); excursions permitted to 15-30°C (59-86°F). Do not store patches unpouched. Do not refrigerate or freeze patches. Once the sealed tray or outer pouch is opened, use contents w/in 2 months.

HOW SUPPLIED
Patch: 10mg/9 hrs, 15mg/9 hrs, 20mg/9 hrs, 30mg/9 hrs [30^S]

CONTRAINDICATIONS
Known hypersensitivity to methylphenidate or other components of the medication (polyester/ethylene vinyl acetate laminate film backing, acrylic adhesive, silicone adhesive, fluoropolymer-coated polyester); marked anxiety, tension, and agitation; glaucoma; motor tics or family history or diagnosis of Tourette's syndrome. Treatment w/ MAOIs or w/in a minimum of 14 days following discontinuation of an MAOI.

WARNINGS/PRECAUTIONS
Avoid w/ known serious structural cardiac abnormalities, cardiomyopathy, serious heart rhythm abnormalities, coronary artery disease, or other serious cardiac problems. Sudden death reported in children and adolescents w/ structural cardiac abnormalities or other serious heart problems. Sudden deaths, stroke, and MI reported in adults. May increase BP and HR; caution w/ conditions that might be compromised by increases in BP/HR (eg, preexisting HTN, heart failure, recent MI, ventricular arrhythmia). Prior to treatment, obtain medical history (including assessment for family history of sudden death or ventricular arrhythmia) and perform a physical exam to assess for the presence of cardiac disease. Promptly perform cardiac evaluation if symptoms of cardiac disease develop. May exacerbate symptoms of behavior disturbance and thought disorder in patients w/ preexisting psychotic disorder. Caution in patients w/ comorbid bipolar disorder; may induce mixed/manic episode. May cause treatment-emergent psychotic or manic symptoms (eg, hallucinations, delusional thinking, mania) in children and adolescents w/o prior history of psychotic illness or mania; consider discontinuation if such symptoms occur. Aggressive behavior or hostility reported in children and adolescents. May lower convulsive threshold; d/c if seizures occur. Priapism, sometimes requiring surgical intervention, reported. Associated w/ peripheral vasculopathy, including Raynaud's phenomenon; carefully observe for digital changes. May cause long-term suppression of growth in children; monitor growth, and may need to interrupt treatment in patients not growing or gaining height or weight as expected. May result in a persistent loss of skin pigmentation at and around the application site; d/c in patients w/ chemical leukoderma. May lead to contact sensitization; d/c if suspected. Patients who develop contact sensitization to therapy and require oral treatment w/ methylphenidate should be initiated on oral medication under close medical supervision. Difficulties w/ accommodation and blurring of vision reported. Avoid exposing application site to direct external heat sources while wearing the patch; may increase absorption.

ADVERSE REACTIONS
Decreased appetite, headache, insomnia, N/V, decreased weight, irritability, tic, affect lability, anorexia, abdominal pain, dizziness.

DRUG INTERACTIONS
See Contraindications. Caution w/ pressor agents. May decrease effectiveness of drugs used to treat HTN. May inhibit metabolism of coumarin anticoagulants, anticonvulsants (eg, phenobarbital, phenytoin, primidone), and some TCAs (eg, imipramine, clomipramine, desipramine) and SSRIs; downward dose adjustments and monitoring of plasma drug concentrations (or coagulation times for coumarin) of these drugs may be necessary when initiating or discontinuing methylphenidate.

PREGNANCY AND LACTATION
Pregnancy: Category C.
Lactation: Caution in nursing.

MECHANISM OF ACTION
CNS stimulant; has not been established. Thought to block reuptake of norepinephrine and dopamine into presynaptic neuron and increase release of these monoamines into extraneuronal space.

PHARMACOKINETICS
Absorption: T_{max}=10 hrs (single application), 8 hrs (repeated applications). Administration of variable doses resulted in different parameters. **Metabolism:** Via deesterification; α-phenyl-piperidine acetic acid (ritalinic acid) (metabolite). **Elimination:** $T_{1/2}$=approx 4-5 hrs (d-methylphenidate), 1.4-2.9 hrs (l-methylphenidate).

PATIENT CONSIDERATIONS

Assessment: Assess for hypersensitivity to the drug, marked anxiety, tension, agitation, glaucoma, motor tics, family history or diagnosis of Tourette's syndrome, cardiovascular conditions, history of drug dependence or alcoholism, psychotic disorder, comorbid bipolar disorder, any other conditions where treatment is contraindicated or cautioned, pregnancy/nursing status, and possible drug interactions.

Monitoring: Monitor for changes in HR and BP, signs/symptoms of cardiac disease, exacerbation of behavior disturbance and thought disorder, psychosis, mania, appearance of or worsening of aggressive behavior or hostility, seizures, priapism, peripheral vasculopathy (including Raynaud's phenomenon), skin depigmentation, contact sensitization, visual disturbances, and other adverse reactions. In pediatric patients, monitor growth. Perform periodic monitoring of CBC, differential, and platelet counts during prolonged therapy. Periodically reevaluate long-term usefulness of drug.

Counseling: Inform about the benefits and risks of therapy. Counsel on the appropriate use of the medication. Instruct to seek immediate medical attention in the event of priapism. Inform of the risk of peripheral vasculopathy, including Reynaud's syndrome and instruct to contact physician immediately if symptoms occur or w/ any signs of unexplained wounds appearing on fingers or toes while taking the drug. Advise of the possibility of a persistent loss of skin pigmentation at, around, and distant from the application site and to contact physician if this occurs. Advise to avoid exposing application site to direct external heat sources (eg, hair dryers, heating pads, electric blankets, heated water beds) while wearing the patch. Instruct to avoid touching the adhesive side of the patch during application, and to immediately wash hands after application if adhesive side is touched. Advise to take patch off earlier if there is an unacceptable duration of appetite loss or insomnia in the pm. Counsel to not wear the patch and to consult physician if any swelling or blistering occurs. Instruct not to apply hydrocortisone or other sol, cre, oint, or emollients immediately prior to patch application. Caution against operating potentially hazardous machinery or vehicles until accustomed to effects of medication.

DDAVP NASAL — desmopressin acetate   Rx

Class: Synthetic vasopressin analogue

OTHER BRAND NAMES
DDAVP Rhinal Tube

ADULT DOSAGE	PEDIATRIC DOSAGE
Central Cranial Diabetes Insipidus	**Central Cranial Diabetes Insipidus**
Usual: 0.1-0.4mL/day, as single dose or divided into 2 or 3 doses; separately adjust am and pm dose for an adequate diurnal rhythm of water turnover	**3 Months-12 Years:** **Usual:** 0.05-0.3mL/day, as single dose or divided into 2 doses; separately adjust am and pm dose for an adequate diurnal rhythm of water turnover

DOSING CONSIDERATIONS
Elderly
Start at lower end of dosing range

ADMINISTRATION
Intranasal route

Nasal Spray
Pump must be primed prior to 1st use.
To Prime Pump:
1. Press down 4 times.
2. The bottle will now deliver 10mcg/spray.
Discard after 50 sprays.

STORAGE
Nasal Spray: 20-25°C (68-77°F). Store bottle in upright position. **Rhinal Tube:** 2-8°C (36-46°F). When traveling, closed bottles stable for 3 weeks at 20-25°C (68-77°F).

HOW SUPPLIED
Sol: 10mcg/0.1mL [2.5mL (Rhinal Tube), 5mL (Nasal Spray)]

CONTRAINDICATIONS
Known hypersensitivity to desmopressin acetate or any components of the medication, moderate to severe renal impairment (CrCl <50mL/min), hyponatremia, or history of hyponatremia.

WARNINGS/PRECAUTIONS
For intranasal use only. Use only when oral formulations are not feasible. May use inj if intranasal route is compromised. May cause water intoxication and/or hyponatremia; fluid restriction is recommended. May decrease plasma osmolality, resulting in seizures or coma. Caution w/ habitual or psychogenic polydipsia, conditions associated w/ fluid and electrolyte imbalance (eg, cystic fibrosis, heart failure, renal disorders), coronary artery insufficiency, and/or hypertensive cardiovascular disease (CVD). Severe allergic reactions reported (rare). Estimate response by adequate duration of sleep and adequate, not excessive, water turnover. Caution in elderly.

ADVERSE REACTIONS
Headache, rhinitis, epistaxis, dizziness.

DRUG INTERACTIONS
Carefully monitor w/ other pressor agents. Caution w/ drugs that may increase the risk of water intoxication w/ hyponatremia (eg, TCAs, SSRIs, chlorpromazine, opiate analgesics, NSAIDs, lamotrigine, carbamazepine).

PREGNANCY AND LACTATION
Pregnancy: Category B.
Lactation: Caution in nursing.

MECHANISM OF ACTION
Synthetic vasopressin analogue; antidiuretic hormone affecting renal water conservation.

PHARMACOKINETICS
Elimination: Urine; (Inj) $T_{1/2}$=3 hrs.

PATIENT CONSIDERATIONS
Assessment: Assess for renal function, hyponatremia, history of hyponatremia, compromised intranasal route, habitual or psychogenic polydipsia, coronary artery insufficiency, hypertensive CVD, fluid/electrolyte imbalance disorders, hypersensitivity to drug, pregnancy/nursing status, and possible drug interactions.

Monitoring: Monitor for signs/symptoms of hyponatremia, water intoxication, compromised intranasal route, and allergic reactions. Monitor BP, fluid and electrolyte levels, renal function, urine volume and osmolality periodically, and plasma osmolality.

Counseling: Inform that administration in children should be under adult supervision. Instruct to seek medical attention if symptoms of hyponatremia or allergic reactions occur. Instruct to inform physician if symptoms of nasal blockage, discharge, congestion, or other adverse events occur.

DEFITELIO — defibrotide sodium   Rx

Class: Thrombolytic agent

ADULT DOSAGE	PEDIATRIC DOSAGE
Hepatic Veno-Occlusive Disease	**Hepatic Veno-Occlusive Disease**
W/ Renal or Pulmonary Dysfunction Following Hematopoietic Stem-Cell Transplantation (HSCT): 6.25mg/kg q6h for ≥21 days; if signs and symptoms have not resolved, continue until resolution or up to 60 days	**W/ Renal or Pulmonary Dysfunction Following HSCT:** 6.25mg/kg q6h for ≥21 days; if signs and symptoms have not resolved, continue until resolution or up to 60 days

DOSING CONSIDERATIONS
Adverse Reactions
Hypersensitivity Reaction:
Severe/Life-Threatening (Anaphylaxis): D/C permanently; do not resume

Bleeding:
Persistent, Severe or Life-Threatening Bleed: Withhold, treat cause of bleed, and give supportive care. Consider resuming treatment when bleeding has stopped and patient is hemodynamically stable
Recurrent Significant Bleeding: D/C permanently; do not resume

Other Important Considerations
Invasive Procedures: D/C infusion at least 2 hrs prior to an invasive procedure; resume treatment after the procedure, as soon as any procedure-related risk of bleeding is resolved

ADMINISTRATION
IV route

- Must dilute prior to infusion.
- Prior to administration, confirm that patient is not experiencing clinically significant bleeding and is hemodynamically stable on ≤1 vasopressor.
- Administer by constant IV infusion over a 2-hr period.
- Administer diluted sol using an infusion set equipped w/ a 0.2 micron in-line filter. Flush IV administration line (peripheral or central) w/ D5 inj or 0.9% NaCl inj immediately before and after administration.
- Do not coadminister w/ other IV drugs concurrently w/in the same line.

Preparation
1. Determine dose and number of vials based on weight prior to the preparative regimen for HSCT.
2. Withdraw calculated volume and add it to infusion bag containing 0.9% NaCl inj or D5 inj for each dose to make a final concentration of 4-20mg/mL.
3. Gently mix sol for infusion.
4. Use the diluted sol w/in 4 hrs if stored at room temperature or w/in 24 hrs if stored under refrigeration. Up to 4 doses of sol may be prepared at one time, if refrigerated.
5. Discard partially used vials; vials contain no antimicrobial preservatives.

STORAGE
20-25°C (68-77°F); excursions permitted between 15-30°C (59-86°F).

HOW SUPPLIED
Inj: 200mg/2.5mL

CONTRAINDICATIONS
Concomitant administration w/ systemic anticoagulant or fibrinolytic therapy, known hypersensitivity to defibrotide or to any of its excipients.

WARNINGS/PRECAUTIONS
See Dosing Considerations. May increase the risk of bleeding; do not initiate in patients w/ active bleeding. Hypersensitivity reactions reported; monitor for hypersensitivity reactions, especially if there is a history of previous exposure.

ADVERSE REACTIONS
Hypotension, diarrhea, N/V, epistaxis.

DRUG INTERACTIONS

See Contraindications. May enhance the pharmacodynamic activity of antithrombotic/fibrinolytic drugs (eg, heparin, alteplase). Concomitant use w/ a systemic anticoagulant or fibrinolytic therapy (not including use for routine maintenance or reopening of central venous lines) may increase the risk of bleeding; d/c anticoagulants and fibrinolytic agents prior to treatment, and consider delaying start of administration until effects of the anticoagulant have abated.

PREGNANCY AND LACTATION

Pregnancy: Decreased number of implantations and viable fetuses when administered to pregnant rabbits; potential risk of miscarriage.
Lactation: Not for use in nursing.

MECHANISM OF ACTION

Thrombolytic agent; mechanism not fully elucidated. Enhances the enzymatic activity of plasmin to hydrolyze fibrin clots. Increases tissue plasminogen activator and thrombomodulin expression, and decreases von Willebrand factor and plasminogen activator inhibitor-1 expression, thereby reducing endothelial cell (EC) activation and increasing EC-mediated fibrinolysis.

PHARMACOKINETICS

Distribution: V_d=8.1-9.1L; plasma protein binding (93%). **Metabolism:** Nucleases, nucleotidases, nucleosidases, deaminases, and phosphorylases metabolize polynucleotides progressively to oligonucleotides, nucleotides, nucleosides, and then to free 2'-deoxyribose sugar, purine and pyrimidine bases. **Elimination:** (6.25-15mg/kg dose) Urine (5-15%, unchanged).

PATIENT CONSIDERATIONS

Assessment: Assess for known hypersensitivity, active bleeding, pregnancy/nursing status, and for possible drug interactions.

Monitoring: Monitor for hypersensitivity reactions, bleeding, and other adverse reactions.

Counseling: Advise that treatment may increase the risk of bleeding; instruct to immediately report any signs or symptoms suggestive of hemorrhage (eg, unusual bleeding, easy bruising, blood in urine or stool). Advise to notify physician if the patient has been treated w/ defibrotide previously. Instruct on the risk of allergic reactions. Inform about the symptoms of allergic reactions, including anaphylaxis, and instruct to seek medical attention immediately if experiencing such symptoms. Advise pregnant women of the potential risk of miscarriage. Advise that breastfeeding is not recommended.

DELATESTRYL — testosterone enanthate   CIII

Class: Androgen

ADULT DOSAGE	PEDIATRIC DOSAGE
Testosterone Replacement Therapy	**Testosterone Replacement Therapy**
Congenital/Acquired Primary Hypogonadism or Hypogonadotropic Hypogonadism in Males:	**Congenital/Acquired Primary Hypogonadism or Hypogonadotropic Hypogonadism in Males:**
Usual: 50-400mg IM every 2-4 weeks	**Usual:** 50-400mg IM every 2-4 weeks
Metastatic Breast Cancer	**Delayed Puberty in Males**
Used secondarily in women w/ advancing inoperable metastatic (skeletal) mammary cancer who are 1-5 yrs postmenopausal	**Usual:** 50-200mg IM every 2-4 weeks for a limited duration (eg, 4-6 months)
Usual: 200-400mg IM every 2-4 weeks	Consider chronological and skeletal age in determining the initial dose and in adjusting the dose

---

ADMINISTRATION

IM route
Slowly inject deeply into gluteal muscle; avoid intravascular inj

STORAGE

Room temperature. Warming and rotating the vial between the palms of the hands will redissolve any crystals that may have formed during storage at low temperatures.

HOW SUPPLIED

Inj: 200mg/mL [5mL]

CONTRAINDICATIONS

Males w/ carcinomas of the breast or w/ known/suspected carcinomas of the prostate, females who are or may become pregnant, history of hypersensitivity to any component of this medication.

WARNINGS/PRECAUTIONS

May cause hypercalcemia in patients w/ breast cancer or immobilized patients; d/c if this occurs. Peliosis hepatis and hepatic neoplasms, (eg, hepatocellular carcinoma) reported w/ prolonged use of high doses. D/C if cholestatic hepatitis, jaundice, or abnormal LFTs occur. May increase risk of prostatic hypertrophy and prostatic carcinoma in elderly. Venous thromboembolic events reported; evaluate patients who report symptoms of pain, edema, warmth, and erythema in the lower extremity for deep vein thrombosis and those who present w/ acute SOB for pulmonary embolism. D/C treatment and initiate appropriate workup and management if venous thromboembolic event is suspected. Increased risk of major adverse cardiovascular events (MACE) reported. Edema w/ or w/o CHF may be a serious complication in patients w/ preexisting cardiac, renal, or hepatic disease; may require diuretic therapy in addition to discontinuation of therapy. Gynecomastia may develop and persist. Caution in healthy males w/ delayed puberty; monitor bone maturation by assessing bone age of wrist and hand every

6 months. May accelerate bone maturation w/o producing compensatory gain in linear growth in children; compromised adult stature may result. Monitor for signs of virilization in females; d/c therapy at evidence of mild virilism. May alter serum cholesterol concentration; caution w/ history of MI or coronary artery disease. Not indicated in geriatric patients who have age-related hypogonadism only ("andropause"). Rare reports of transient reactions involving urge to cough, coughing fits, and respiratory distress immediately after administration. Caution in women w/ metastatic breast carcinoma as androgen therapy occasionally appears to accelerate the disease.

ADVERSE REACTIONS

(Females) Amenorrhea, menstrual irregularities, inhibition of gonadotropin secretion, virilization. (Males) Gynecomastia, excessive frequency and duration of penile erections, oligospermia (at high doses).

DRUG INTERACTIONS

May decrease oral anticoagulant requirement; close monitoring is required especially when androgens are started or stopped. May decrease blood glucose and insulin requirements in diabetics. ACTH and corticosteroids may enhance edema; use w/ caution especially w/ hepatic/cardiac disease. May increase oxyphenbutazone levels.

PREGNANCY AND LACTATION

Category X, not for use in nursing.

MECHANISM OF ACTION

Androgen; responsible for normal growth and development of male sex organs and for maintenance of secondary sex characteristics.

PHARMACOKINETICS

Absorption: Slow. **Distribution:** Plasma protein binding (98% bound to a specific testosterone-estradiol binding globulin). **Metabolism:** Liver. **Elimination:** Urine (90% [glucuronic and sulfuric acid conjugates]), feces (6% [mostly unconjugated]); $T_{1/2}$=10-100 minutes.

PATIENT CONSIDERATIONS

Assessment: Assess for breast carcinoma in males, prostate carcinoma, cardiac/renal/hepatic disease, pregnancy/nursing status, any other conditions where treatment is contraindicated/cautioned, and possible drug interactions. Confirm diagnosis of hypogonadism by measuring testosterone levels in am on at least 2 separate days prior to initiation.

Monitoring: Monitor for signs/symptoms of hypercalcemia, edema w/ or w/o CHF, prostatic hypertrophy/carcinoma in elderly, virilization in females, venous thromboembolic events, MACE, and other adverse reactions. Periodically monitor urine and serum Ca^{2+} in breast cancer patients, LFTs, and cholesterol levels. Perform periodic (every 6 months) x-ray exam of bone age of prepubertal males. Periodically check Hgb and Hct in patients receiving high androgen doses.

Counseling: Instruct to report to physician any of the following side effects: too frequent or persistent erections of the penis (adult/adolescent males); hoarseness, acne, changes in menstrual period, more facial hair (females); and N/V, changes in skin color, or ankle swelling (all patients). Inform that any male adolescent patients receiving androgens for delayed puberty should have bone development checked every 6 months. Inform of the possible risk of MACE when deciding whether to use or continue to use drug.

DEMEROL INJECTION — meperidine hydrochloride   CII

Class: Opioid analgesic

ADULT DOSAGE	PEDIATRIC DOSAGE
Moderate to Severe Pain	**Moderate to Severe Pain**
Usual: 50-150mg IM/SQ q3-4h prn Adjust dose according to severity of pain and patient's response	**Usual:** 0.5-0.8mg/lb IM/SQ, up to the adult dose, q3-4h prn Adjust dose according to severity of pain and patient's response
Preoperative Medication	**Preoperative Medication**
Usual: 50-100mg IM/SQ 30-90 min before beginning of anesthesia	**Usual:** 0.5-1mg/lb IM/SQ, up to the adult dose, 30-90 min before beginning of anesthesia
Support of Anesthesia	
Use repeated slow IV inj of fractional doses (eg, 10mg/mL) or continuous IV infusion of a more dilute sol (eg, 1mg/mL)	
Titrate: Dependent on the premedication and type of anesthesia being employed, patient characteristics, and nature/duration of operative procedure	
Obstetrical Anesthesia	
Usual: 50-100mg IM/SQ when pain is regular; may repeat at 1- to 3-hr intervals	

DOSING CONSIDERATIONS

Concomitant Medications
Phenothiazines/Other Tranquilizers: Reduce dose by 25-50%

Renal Impairment
Caution; initial dose should be reduced in patients w/ severe renal impairment

Hepatic Impairment
Caution; initial dose should be reduced in patients w/ severe hepatic impairment

Elderly
Start at lower end of dosage range and observe closely

Other Important Considerations
Debilitated/Hypothyroidism/Addison's Disease/Pheochromocytoma/Prostatic
Hypertrophy/Urethral Stricture:
Use w/ caution; initial dose should be reduced

ADMINISTRATION
IM, IV, SQ route

SQ
Suitable for occasional use.

IM
Preferred if repeated doses are required.
Inj should be injected well into the body of a large muscle.

IV
Dosage should be decreased and inj should be made very slowly, preferably
utilizing a diluted sol.

STORAGE
20-25°C (68-77°F).

HOW SUPPLIED
Inj: 25mg/0.5mL [0.5mL, Uni-Amp], 25mg/mL [1mL, Carpuject], 50mg/mL [1mL,
1.5mL, 2mL, Uni-Amp; 30mL, multiple-dose vial; 1mL, Carpuject], 75mg/mL [1mL,
Carpuject], 100mg/mL [1mL, Carpuject; 1mL, Uni-Amp; 20mL, multiple-dose vial]

CONTRAINDICATIONS
Hypersensitivity to meperidine, during or w/in 14 days of MAOI use. Sol of
meperidine and barbiturates are chemically incompatible.

WARNINGS/PRECAUTIONS
May produce drug dependence and tolerance and has potential for abuse;
prescribe and administer w/ caution. Respiratory depressant effects and capacity
to elevate CSF pressure may be markedly exaggerated in the presence of head
injury, other intracranial lesions, or a preexisting increase in intracranial pressure.
May obscure the clinical course of patients w/ head injuries; use w/ extreme
caution and only if deemed essential. Rapid IV inj increases the incidence of
adverse reactions; do not administer IV unless a narcotic antagonist and the
facilities for assisted/controlled respiration are immediately available. Extreme
caution w/ acute asthmatic attack, COPD or cor pulmonale, substantially
decreased respiratory reserve, preexisting respiratory depression, hypoxia, or
hypercapnia. May cause severe hypotension in postoperative patients or any
individual whose ability to maintain BP has been compromised by a depleted
blood volume. May impair mental/physical abilities. May produce orthostatic
hypotension in ambulatory patients. May produce a significant increase in the
ventricular response rate; caution w/ A-flutter and other supraventricular
tachycardias. May aggravate preexisting convulsions in patients w/ convulsive
disorders. Convulsions may occur in individuals w/o a history of convulsive
disorders if dosage is escalated above recommended levels due to tolerance. May
obscure the diagnosis or clinical course in patients w/ acute abdominal conditions.
When used as an obstetrical analgesic, may produce depression of respiration and
psychophysiologic functions in the newborn; resuscitation may be required.

ADVERSE REACTIONS
Lightheadedness, dizziness, sedation, N/V, sweating.

DRUG INTERACTIONS
See Contraindications and Dosing Considerations. Use w/ caution and in reduced
dosage w/ other narcotic analgesics, general anesthetics, phenothiazines, other
tranquilizers, sedative-hypnotics (including barbiturates), TCAs, and other CNS
depressants (eg, alcohol); respiratory depression, hypotension, and profound
sedation or coma may occur.

PREGNANCY AND LACTATION
Pregnancy: Not for use in pregnant women prior to labor, unless potential benefits
outweigh possible hazards.
Lactation: Found in breast milk.

MECHANISM OF ACTION
Narcotic analgesic; has multiple actions qualitatively similar to those of morphine.
Principal actions of therapeutic value are analgesia and sedation.

PHARMACOKINETICS
Distribution: Crosses placenta; found in breast milk.

PATIENT CONSIDERATIONS
Assessment: Assess for level of pain intensity, general condition and medical
status, hypersensitivity to the drug, renal/hepatic impairment, respiratory
depression, pregnancy/nursing status, any other conditions where treatment is
contraindicated or cautioned, and possible drug interactions.

Monitoring: Monitor for respiratory depression, elevations in CSF pressure,
hypotension, convulsions/seizures, drug abuse/tolerance/dependence, and other
adverse reactions.

Counseling: Inform of the risks/benefits of therapy. Inform that medication may
impair mental/physical abilities required to perform hazardous tasks (eg, driving,
operating machinery). Advise about potential for dependence upon repeated
administration. Advise to consult physician if pregnant, planning to become
pregnant, or breastfeeding.

DENAVIR — penciclovir Rx
Class: Nucleoside analogue

ADULT DOSAGE	PEDIATRIC DOSAGE
Herpes Labialis (Cold Sores)	**Herpes Labialis (Cold Sores)**
Recurrent:	**Recurrent:**
Apply q2h during waking hours for a period of 4 days	**≥12 Years:** Apply q2h during waking hours for a period of 4 days
Start treatment as early as possible (eg, during the prodrome or when lesions appear)	Start treatment as early as possible (eg, during the prodrome or when lesions appear)

ADMINISTRATION
Topical route

STORAGE
20-25°C (68-77°F); excursions permitted to 15-30°C (59-86°F).

HOW SUPPLIED
Cre: 1% [1.5g, 5g]

CONTRAINDICATIONS
Known hypersensitivity to this product or any of its components.

WARNINGS/PRECAUTIONS
Should only be used on herpes labialis on the lips and face. Avoid application
in mucous membranes and/or near the eyes. Evaluate for secondary bacterial
infection if lesions worsen or do not improve on therapy. Effect has not been
established in immunocompromised patients.

ADVERSE REACTIONS
Application-site reaction, hypesthesia, local anesthesia, taste perversion, rash
(erythematous).

PREGNANCY AND LACTATION
Category B, not for use in nursing.

MECHANISM OF ACTION
Nucleoside analogue; possesses inhibitory activity against herpes simplex virus
(HSV) types 1 (HSV-1) and 2 (HSV-2). Inhibits HSV polymerase competitively with
deoxyguanosine triphosphate. Consequently, herpes viral DNA synthesis and
replication are selectively inhibited.

PATIENT CONSIDERATIONS
Assessment: Assess for bacterial infection, drug hypersensitivity, and pregnancy/
nursing status.

Monitoring: Monitor for clinical response and improvement of symptoms. Evaluate
for secondary bacterial infection if lesions worsen or do not improve.

Counseling: Inform that drug is not a cure for cold sores and not all patients
respond to treatment. Instruct not to use if allergic to the drug or any of its
ingredients. Instruct to notify physician if pregnant, planning to become pregnant,
or breastfeeding. Instruct to use ud. Instruct to wash hands with soap and water
before and after applying product. Inform that face should be clean and dry.
Instruct to apply a layer to cover only the cold sore area or area of tingling before
the cold sore appears, and to rub in the cre until it disappears. Inform of possible
adverse effects (eg, application-site reactions, local anesthesia, taste perversion,
rash).

DEPAKENE — valproic acid Rx
Class: Carboxylic acid derivative

> Fatal hepatic failure reported, usually during first 6 months of treatment. Serious/fatal hepatotoxicity
> may be preceded by nonspecific symptoms (eg, malaise, weakness, lethargy, facial edema, anorexia,
> vomiting) or a loss of seizure control in patients w/ epilepsy; monitor closely. Increased risk of developing
> fatal hepatotoxicity in children <2 yrs of age, especially if on multiple anticonvulsants, w/ congenital
> metabolic disorders, severe seizure disorders w/ mental retardation, and organic brain disease; use
> w/ extreme caution and as a sole agent in this patient group. Increased risk of drug-induced acute
> liver failure and resultant deaths in patients w/ hereditary neurometabolic syndromes caused by
> DNA mutations of the mitochondrial DNA polymerase gamma (POLG) gene (eg, Alpers-Huttenlocher
> syndrome). Contraindicated in patients known to have mitochondrial disorders caused by POLG mutations
> and children <2 yrs of age who are clinically suspected of having a mitochondrial disorder. In patients >2
> yrs of age who are clinically suspected of having a hereditary mitochondrial disease, drug should only
> be used after other anticonvulsants have failed; closely monitor for the development of acute liver injury.
> May cause major congenital malformations, particularly neural tube defects (eg, spina bifida). May
> cause decreased IQ scores following in utero exposure. Should only be used to treat pregnant women w/
> epilepsy if other medications have failed to control their symptoms or are otherwise unacceptable. Do not
> administer to a woman of childbearing potential unless the drug is essential to the management of her
> medical condition; use effective contraception. Life-threatening pancreatitis reported; d/c if pancreatitis
> is diagnosed and initiate appropriate treatment.

ADULT DOSAGE	PEDIATRIC DOSAGE
Epilepsy	**Epilepsy**
Complex Partial Seizures:	**Complex Partial Seizures:**
Monotherapy/Conversion to Monotherapy/Adjunctive Therapy:	**Monotherapy/Conversion to Monotherapy/Adjunctive Therapy:**
Initial: 10-15mg/kg/day	**≥10 Years:**
Titrate: Increase by 5-10mg/kg/week until optimal response is achieved	**Initial:** 10-15mg/kg/day
Usual Therapeutic Range: 50-100mcg/mL	**Titrate:** Increase by 5-10mg/kg/week until optimal response is achieved
For adjunctive therapy, if total dose	**Usual Therapeutic Range:** 50-100mcg/mL

exceeds 250mg/day, give in divided doses
No recommendation regarding safety at doses >60mg/kg/day

Simple/Complex Absence Seizures:
Initial: 15mg/kg/day
Titrate: Increase weekly by 5-10mg/kg/day until seizures are controlled or side effects preclude further increases
Max: 60mg/kg/day
Usual Therapeutic Range: 50-100mcg/mL
If total dose exceeds 250mg/day, give in divided doses
Refer to PI for initial daily dose guide
Also used for adjunctive therapy for multiple seizure types that include absence seizures

For adjunctive therapy, if total dose exceeds 250mg/day, give in divided doses
No recommendation regarding safety at doses >60mg/kg/day

Simple/Complex Absence Seizures:
Initial: 15mg/kg/day
Titrate: Increase weekly by 5-10mg/kg/day until seizures are controlled or side effects preclude further increases
Max: 60mg/kg/day
Usual Therapeutic Range: 50-100mcg/mL
If total dose exceeds 250mg/day, give in divided doses
Refer to PI for initial daily dose guide
Also used for adjunctive therapy for multiple seizure types that include absence seizures

---

DOSING CONSIDERATIONS
Concomitant Medications
Complex Partial Seizures:
Conversion to Monotherapy from Concomitant Antiepilepsy Drug: Reduce concomitant antiepilepsy drug by approx 25% every 2 weeks (starting at initiation or 1-2 weeks after start of therapy)

Rufinamide: Begin valproate therapy at a low dose and titrate to a clinically effective dose in patients stabilized on rufinamide before being prescribed valproate

Elderly
Reduce initial dose and titrate slowly
Consider dose reduction or discontinuation in patients w/ decreased food or fluid intake or excessive somnolence

Adverse Reactions
Thrombocytopenia: Probability appears to increase significantly at total valproate concentrations of ≥110mcg/mL (females) or ≥135mcg/mL (males)

Discontinuation
Do not abruptly d/c

ADMINISTRATION
Oral route

Swallow caps whole; do not chew.
Take w/ food or slowly build up the dose from an initial low level if experiencing GI irritation.

STORAGE
Cap: 15-25°C (59-77°F). **Oral Sol:** <30°C (86°F).

HOW SUPPLIED
Cap: 250mg; **Oral Sol:** 250mg/5mL

CONTRAINDICATIONS
Hepatic disease, significant hepatic dysfunction, mitochondrial disorders caused by mutations in mitochondrial POLG (eg, Alpers-Huttenlocher syndrome) and children <2 yrs of age who are suspected of having a POLG-related disorder, known hypersensitivity to the medication, known urea cycle disorders (UCDs).

WARNINGS/PRECAUTIONS
Caution w/ prior history of hepatic disease; d/c immediately if significant hepatic dysfunction (suspected or apparent) occurs. Hyperammonemic encephalopathy reported in patients w/ UCDs; d/c and initiate treatment if symptoms develop. Increased risk of suicidal thoughts or behavior reported. Dose-related thrombocytopenia, and decreases in other cell lines and myelodysplasia reported; reduce dose or d/c if hemorrhage, bruising, or a disorder of hemostasis/coagulation occurs. Hyperammonemia reported and may be present despite normal LFTs; consider discontinuation if elevation persists. Measure ammonia levels if unexplained lethargy, vomiting, or mental status changes occur; hyperammonemic encephalopathy should be considered. Hypothermia reported w/ and in the absence of hyperammonemia; consider discontinuation. Drug reaction w/ eosinophilia and systemic symptoms (DRESS), also known as multiorgan hypersensitivity, reported; evaluate immediately if signs/symptoms (eg, fever, lymphadenopathy) are present, and d/c and do not resume if an alternative etiology cannot be established. Altered thyroid function tests and urine ketone tests reported. May stimulate replication of HIV and CMV under certain experimental conditions.

ADVERSE REACTIONS
N/V, headache, asthenia, somnolence, tremor, dizziness, abdominal pain, diplopia, diarrhea, anorexia, amblyopia/blurred vision, flu syndrome, infection, dyspepsia.

DRUG INTERACTIONS
Drugs that affect the level of expression of hepatic enzymes (eg, phenytoin, carbamazepine, phenobarbital), particularly those that elevate levels of glucuronosyltransferases (eg, ritonavir), may increase clearance; monitor valproate and concomitant drug concentrations whenever enzyme-inducing drugs are introduced or withdrawn. Aspirin decreases protein binding and inhibits metabolism; use w/ caution. Carbapenem antibiotics (eg, ertapenem, imipenem, meropenem) may reduce serum concentrations to subtherapeutic levels, resulting in loss of seizure control; monitor serum levels frequently. Cholestyramine decreases levels; delaying cholestyramine administration by 3 hrs may lessen the interaction. Felbamate may increase C_{max}; may require decrease in valproate dosage. Rifampin increases oral clearance; may require valproate

dosage adjustment. Reduces the clearance of amitriptyline and nortriptyline; consider lowering the dose of amitriptyline/nortriptyline. May decrease levels of carbamazepine while increasing carbamazepine-10,11-epoxide serum levels. Use w/ clonazepam may induce absence status in patients w/ absence seizures. Inhibits metabolism of diazepam, ethosuximide, phenobarbital, and phenytoin; monitor drug serum concentrations and adjust dose appropriately. Increased $T_{1/2}$ of lamotrigine, and serious skin reactions reported; reduce lamotrigine dose. Breakthrough seizures reported w/ concomitant phenytoin. Monitor for neurological toxicity w/ concomitant barbiturate therapy. May displace protein-bound drugs (eg, diazepam, phenytoin, tolbutamide, warfarin); monitor coagulation tests when coadministered w/ warfarin. Decreases clearance and increases levels of rufinamide; patients on valproate should begin at a rufinamide dose <10mg/kg/day (pediatric patients) or 400mg/day (adults). May decrease zidovudine clearance in HIV-seropositive patients. Concomitant use w/ topiramate has been associated w/ hypothermia and hyperammonemia, w/ or w/o encephalopathy.

PREGNANCY AND LACTATION
Pregnancy: Category D. Physicians should encourage pregnant patients to enroll in the North American Antiepileptic Drug (NAAED) Pregnancy Registry.
Lactation: Excreted in human milk; caution in nursing.

MECHANISM OF ACTION
Carboxylic acid derivative; has not been established. Suggested that its activity in epilepsy is related to increased brain concentrations of GABA.

PHARMACOKINETICS
Absorption: Depakote: (Tab) T_{max}=4 hrs (fasted), 8 hrs (fed); (Cap) T_{max}=3.3 hrs (fasted), 4.8 hrs (fed). **Distribution:** V_d=11L (total valproate), 92L (free valproate); found in breast milk, CSF. **Metabolism:** Liver (major); mitochondrial β-oxidation (major), glucuronidation. **Elimination:** Urine (30-50% glucuronide conjugate, <3% unchanged); $T_{1/2}$=9-16 hrs (250-1000mg dose).

PATIENT CONSIDERATIONS
Assessment: Assess for hepatic dysfunction, history of hepatic disease, UCDs (especially in high-risk patients [eg, history of unexplained encephalopathy, coma]), pancreatitis, history of hypersensitivity to the drug, mitochondrial disorders caused by mutations in mitochondrial POLG and children <2 yrs of age who are suspected of having a POLG-related disorder, other conditions where treatment is contraindicated or cautioned, pregnancy/nursing status, and possible drug interactions. Assess LFTs, CBCs, and coagulation parameters.

Monitoring: Monitor for hypersensitivity reactions, pancreatitis, hepatotoxicity, hyperammonemia, hypothermia, DRESS, drug-induced acute liver failure, acute liver injury, emergence/worsening of depression, suicidality or unusual changes in behavior, and other adverse reactions. Monitor LFTs frequently, especially during first 6 months. Monitor fluid/nutritional intake and for dehydration, somnolence, and other adverse reactions in the elderly. Monitor ammonia levels, CBCs, and coagulation parameters. Perform periodic plasma concentration determinations of valproate and concomitant drugs during the early course of therapy.

Counseling: Instruct to take ud. Inform pregnant women and women of childbearing potential about the risk in pregnancy (eg, birth defects, decreased IQ); advise to use effective contraception while on therapy and discuss alternative therapeutic options. Instruct to notify physician if pregnant/intending to become pregnant. Encourage patients to enroll in NAAED Pregnancy Registry. Advise to notify physician if depression, suicidal thoughts/behavior, or thoughts about self-harm emerge; instruct to report behaviors of concern. Inform about signs/symptoms of pancreatitis, hepatotoxicity, hyperammonemia, or hyperammonemic encephalopathy; advise to notify physician if any symptoms or adverse effects occur. Advise not to engage in hazardous activities (eg, driving, operating machinery) until the effects of the drug are known. Inform that a fever associated w/ other organ system involvement (eg, rash, lymphadenopathy) may be drug-related; instruct to report to physician.

DEPAKOTE — divalproex sodium   Rx

Class: Carboxylic acid derivative

Fatal hepatic failure reported, usually during first 6 months of treatment. Serious/fatal hepatotoxicity may be preceded by nonspecific symptoms (eg, malaise, weakness, lethargy, facial edema, anorexia, vomiting) or a loss of seizure control in patients w/ epilepsy; monitor closely. Monitor LFTs prior to therapy and at frequent intervals thereafter, especially during first 6 months of treatment. Increased risk of developing fatal hepatotoxicity in children <2 yrs of age, especially if on multiple anticonvulsants or w/ congenital metabolic disorders, severe seizure disorders accompanied by mental retardation, or organic brain disease; use w/ extreme caution and as a sole agent in this patient group. Increased risk of drug-induced acute liver failure and resultant death in patients w/ hereditary neurometabolic syndromes caused by DNA mutations of the mitochondrial DNA polymerase gamma (POLG) gene (eg, Alpers-Huttenlocher syndrome). Contraindicated in patients known to have mitochondrial disorders caused by POLG mutations and in children <2 yrs of age who are clinically suspected of having a mitochondrial disorder. In patients >2 yrs of age who are clinically suspected of having a hereditary mitochondrial disease, drug should only be used after other anticonvulsants have failed; closely monitor for the development of acute liver injury. May cause major congenital malformations, particularly neural tube defects (eg, spina bifida). May cause decreased IQ scores following in utero exposure. Should only be used to treat pregnant women w/ epilepsy or bipolar disorder if other medications have failed to control their symptoms or are otherwise unacceptable. Do not administer to a woman of childbearing potential unless the drug is essential to the management of her medical condition; use effective contraception. Life-threatening pancreatitis reported; d/c if pancreatitis is diagnosed and initiate alternative treatment. **Tab:** Contraindicated in pregnant women treated for migraine prophylaxis.

OTHER BRAND NAMES
Depakote Sprinkle

ADULT DOSAGE

Epilepsy

Monotherapy and Adjunctive Therapy for Complex Partial Seizures and Simple and Complex Absence Seizures; Adjunctive Therapy w/ Multiple Seizure Types (eg, Absence Seizures):

Cap/Tab:

Complex Partial Seizures:
Initial: 10-15mg/kg/day
Titrate: Increase by 5-10mg/kg/week
Usual Therapeutic Range: 50-100mcg/mL
No recommendation regarding safety at doses >60mg/kg/day
For adjunctive therapy, if total dose is >250mg/day, give in divided doses

Simple and Complex Absence Seizures:
Initial: 15mg/kg/day
Titrate: Increase weekly by 5-10mg/kg/day until seizures are controlled or side effects preclude further increases
Max: 60mg/kg/day
Usual Therapeutic Range: 50-100mcg/mL
If daily dose is >250mg/day, give in divided doses

Mania

Associated w/ Bipolar Disorder:
Tab:
Initial: 750mg/day in divided doses
Titrate: Increase dose as rapidly as possible to achieve lowest therapeutic dose
Max: 60mg/kg/day
Trough Plasma Concentration: 50-125mcg/mL

Migraine

Prophylaxis:
Tab:
Initial: 250mg bid
Max: 1000mg/day; no evidence of higher doses leading to greater efficacy

PEDIATRIC DOSAGE

Epilepsy

Monotherapy and Adjunctive Therapy for Complex Partial Seizures and Simple and Complex Absence Seizures; Adjunctive Therapy w/ Multiple Seizure Types (eg, Absence Seizures):

Cap/Tab:

Simple and Complex Absence Seizures:
Initial: 15mg/kg/day
Titrate: Increase weekly by 5-10mg/kg/day until seizures are controlled or side effects preclude further increases
Max: 60mg/kg/day
Usual Therapeutic Range: 50-100mcg/mL
If daily dose is >250mg/day, give in divided doses

Complex Partial Seizures:
≥10 Years:
Initial: 10-15mg/kg/day
Titrate: Increase by 5-10mg/kg/week
Usual Therapeutic Range: 50-100mcg/mL
No recommendation regarding safety at doses >60mg/kg/day
For adjunctive therapy, if total dose is >250mg/day, give in divided doses

DOSING CONSIDERATIONS

Concomitant Medications
Complex Partial Seizures:
Conversion to Monotherapy: Reduce concomitant antiepilepsy drug dosage by approx 25% every 2 weeks; reduction may be started at initiation of divalproex therapy, or delayed by 1-2 weeks if seizures are likely to occur w/ a reduction

Rufinamide: Begin valproate therapy at a low dose and titrate to a clinically effective dose in patients stabilized on rufinamide before being prescribed valproate

Elderly
Reduce initial dose and titrate slowly; consider dose reductions or discontinuation in patients w/ decreased food/fluid intake or excessive somnolence

Adverse Reactions
Thrombocytopenia: Probability appears to increase significantly at total valproate concentrations of ≥110mcg/mL (females) or ≥135mcg/mL (males)

Discontinuation
Do not abruptly d/c

Other Important Considerations
In epileptic patients previously receiving valproic acid, initiate at the same daily dose and frequency; once the patient is stabilized, the frequency of divalproex may be adjusted to bid-tid

ADMINISTRATION
Oral route

Give w/ food or slowly titrate from initial dose in patients w/ GI irritation.

Cap
May be swallowed whole or the contents of the cap may be sprinkled on small amount of soft food.

To Administer w/ Food:
1. Hold the cap so that the end marked "THIS END UP" is straight up and the arrow on the cap is up.
2. To open the cap, gently twist it apart to separate the top from the bottom. It may be helpful to hold the cap over the food to which you will add the sprinkles. If you spill any of the cap contents, start over w/ a new cap and a new portion of food.
3. Place all the sprinkles onto a small amount (about a tsp) of soft food such as applesauce or pudding.
4. Make sure that all of the sprinkle/food mixture is swallowed right away. Do not chew the sprinkle/food mixture.

5. Drinking water right after taking the sprinkle/food mixture will help make sure all sprinkles are swallowed.
6. Throw away any unused sprinkle/food mixture; do not store any for future use.

Tab
Swallow whole; do not crush or chew.

STORAGE
Cap: <25°C (77°F). **Tab:** <30°C (86°F).

HOW SUPPLIED
Cap, Delayed-Release: (Sprinkle) 125mg; **Tab, Delayed-Release:** 125mg, 250mg, 500mg

CONTRAINDICATIONS
Hepatic disease, significant hepatic dysfunction, mitochondrial disorders caused by mutations in mitochondrial DNA POLG (eg, Alpers-Huttenlocher syndrome), children <2 yrs of age who are suspected of having a POLG-related disorder, known hypersensitivity to the medication, known urea cycle disorders (UCDs). **Tab:** Prophylaxis of migraine headaches in pregnant women.

WARNINGS/PRECAUTIONS
Caution w/ prior history of hepatic disease; d/c immediately if significant hepatic dysfunction (suspected or apparent) occurs. Hyperammonemic encephalopathy reported in patients w/ UCDs; d/c and initiate treatment if symptoms develop. Increased risk of suicidal thoughts or behavior reported. Dose-related thrombocytopenia and decreases in other cell lines and myelodysplasia reported; reduce dose or d/c if hemorrhage, bruising, or a disorder of hemostasis/coagulation occurs. Hyperammonemia reported and may be present despite normal LFTs; consider discontinuation if elevation persists. Measure ammonia levels if unexplained lethargy, vomiting, or mental status changes occur; hyperammonemic encephalopathy should be considered. Hypothermia w/ and in absence of hyperammonemia reported; consider discontinuation. Drug reaction w/ eosinophilia and systemic symptoms (DRESS), also known as multiorgan hypersensitivity, reported; evaluate immediately if signs/symptoms (eg, fever, lymphadenopathy) are present, and d/c and do not resume if an alternative etiology cannot be established. Altered thyroid function tests and urine ketone tests reported. May stimulate replication of HIV and CMV under certain experimental conditions. Medication residue in stool reported; check valproate levels and monitor clinical condition, and consider alternative treatment if clinically indicated.

ADVERSE REACTIONS
Epilepsy: N/V, headache, asthenia, somnolence, tremor, dizziness, abdominal pain, diplopia, diarrhea, anorexia, amblyopia/blurred vision, flu syndrome, infection, dyspepsia.
Mania: N/V, somnolence, dizziness, accidental injury, asthenia, abdominal pain, dyspepsia, rash.
Migraine: N/V, asthenia, somnolence, dyspepsia, diarrhea, dizziness, abdominal pain, tremor, weight gain, back pain, alopecia, increased appetite.

DRUG INTERACTIONS
Drugs that affect the level of expression of hepatic enzymes (eg, phenytoin, carbamazepine, phenobarbital), particularly those that elevate levels of glucuronosyltransferases (eg, ritonavir), may increase valproate clearance; monitor valproate and concomitant drug concentrations whenever enzyme-inducing drugs are introduced or withdrawn. Aspirin decreases protein binding and inhibits metabolism; use w/ caution. Carbapenem antibiotics may reduce serum concentrations to subtherapeutic levels, resulting in loss of seizure control; monitor serum levels frequently. Felbamate may increase valproate C_{max}; may require decrease in valproate dosage. Rifampin increases oral clearance; may require valproate dosage adjustment. Reduces the clearance of amitriptyline and nortriptyline; consider lowering the dose of amitriptyline/nortriptyline. May decrease levels of carbamazepine while increasing carbamazepine-10,11-epoxide serum levels. Use w/ clonazepam may induce absence status in patients w/ history of absence seizures. Inhibits metabolism of diazepam, ethosuximide, phenobarbital, and phenytoin; monitor drug serum concentrations and adjust dose appropriately. Monitor for neurological toxicity w/ concomitant barbiturate therapy. Breakthrough seizures reported w/ concomitant use w/ phenytoin. Increased $T_{1/2}$ of lamotrigine, and serious skin reactions reported; reduce lamotrigine dose. May displace protein-bound drugs (eg, diazepam, phenytoin, tolbutamide, warfarin). Monitor coagulation tests when coadministered w/ anticoagulants. Decreases clearance and increases levels of rufinamide; patients on valproate should begin at a rufinamide dose <10mg/kg/day (pediatric patients) or 400mg/day (adults). May decrease zidovudine clearance in HIV-seropositive patients. Concomitant use w/ topiramate has been associated w/ hypothermia and hyperammonemia, w/ or w/o encephalopathy.

PREGNANCY AND LACTATION
Pregnancy: Category D (for epilepsy and for manic episodes w/ bipolar disorder) or X (for prophylaxis of migraine headaches). Physicians should encourage pregnant patients to enroll in the North American Antiepileptic Drug (NAAED) Pregnancy Registry.
Lactation: Excreted in human milk; caution in nursing.

MECHANISM OF ACTION
Valproate compound; has not been established. Disassociates to the valproate ion in the GI tract. Suggested that activity in epilepsy is related to increased brain concentrations of GABA.

PHARMACOKINETICS
Absorption: (Tab) T_{max}=4 hrs (fasted), 8 hrs (fed); (Cap) T_{max}=3.3 (fasted), 4.8 hrs (fed). **Distribution:** V_d=11L (total valproate), 92L (free valproate); found in breast milk, CSF. **Metabolism:** Liver (major); mitochondrial β-oxidation (major), glucuronidation. **Elimination:** Urine (30-50% glucuronide conjugate, <3% unchanged); $T_{1/2}$=9-16 hrs (250-1000mg dose monotherapy).

PATIENT CONSIDERATIONS

Assessment: Assess for hepatic dysfunction, history of hepatic disease, pancreatitis, history of hypersensitivity to the drug, mitochondrial disorders caused by mutations in mitochondrial POLG, children <2 yrs of age who are suspected of having a POLG-related disorder, other conditions where treatment is contraindicated or cautioned, pregnancy/nursing status, and possible drug interactions. Assess LFTs, CBCs, and coagulation parameters. Evaluate for UCDs, especially in high-risk patients (eg, history of unexplained encephalopathy or coma).

Monitoring: Monitor for hypersensitivity reactions, pancreatitis, hepatotoxicity, hyperammonemia, hypothermia, DRESS, drug-induced acute liver failure, acute liver injury, emergence/worsening of depression, suicidality or unusual changes in behavior, medication residue in stool, and other adverse reactions. Monitor LFTs frequently, especially during first 6 months. Monitor fluid/nutritional intake and for dehydration, somnolence, and other adverse reactions in the elderly. Monitor ammonia levels, CBCs, and coagulation parameters. Perform periodic plasma concentration determinations of valproate and concomitant drugs during the early course of therapy.

Counseling: Instruct to take ud. Inform pregnant women and women of childbearing potential about the risk in pregnancy (eg, birth defects, decreased IQ); advise to use effective contraception while on therapy and counsel about alternative therapeutic options. Instruct to notify physician if pregnant/intending to become pregnant. Encourage patients to enroll in the NAAED Pregnancy Registry. Advise to notify physician if depression, suicidal thoughts/behavior, or thoughts about self-harm emerge; instruct to report behaviors of concern. Inform about signs/symptoms of pancreatitis, hepatotoxicity, hyperammonemia, or hyperammonemic encephalopathy; advise to notify physician if any symptoms or adverse effects occur. Advise not to engage in hazardous activities (eg, driving/operating machinery) until the effects of the drug are known. Inform that a fever associated w/ other organ system involvement (eg, rash, lymphadenopathy) may be drug-related; instruct to report to physician. Instruct patients to notify their healthcare provider if they notice medication residue in the stool.

DEPAKOTE ER — divalproex sodium   Rx

Class: Carboxylic acid derivative

Fatal hepatic failure may occur, usually during first 6 months of treatment. Serious/fatal hepatotoxicity may be preceded by nonspecific symptoms (eg, malaise, weakness, lethargy, facial edema, anorexia, vomiting) or loss of seizure control in patients w/ epilepsy; monitor closely. Monitor LFTs prior to therapy and at frequent intervals thereafter, especially during first 6 months of treatment. Increased risk of developing fatal hepatotoxicity in children <2 yrs of age, especially if on multiple anticonvulsants or w/ congenital metabolic disorders, severe seizure disorders w/ mental retardation, or organic brain disease; use w/ extreme caution and as a sole agent. Increased risk of valproate-induced acute liver failure and resultant death in patients w/ hereditary neurometabolic syndromes caused by DNA mutations of the mitochondrial DNA polymerase gamma (POLG) gene (eg, Alpers-Huttenlocher syndrome). Contraindicated in patients known to have mitochondrial disorders caused by POLG mutations and children <2 yrs of age who are clinically suspected of having a mitochondrial disorder. In patients >2 yrs of age who are clinically suspected of having a hereditary mitochondrial disease, drug should only be used after other anticonvulsants have failed; closely monitor for the development of acute liver injury. May cause major congenital malformations, particularly neural tube defects (eg, spina bifida). May cause decreased IQ scores following in utero exposure. Contraindicated in pregnant women treated for prophylaxis of migraine; should only be used to treat pregnant women w/ epilepsy or bipolar disorder if other medications have failed to control their symptoms or are otherwise unacceptable. Do not administer to a woman of childbearing potential unless the drug is essential to the management of her medical condition; use effective contraception. Life-threatening pancreatitis reported; d/c if pancreatitis is diagnosed and initiate alternative treatment for the underlying medical condition as clinically indicated.

ADULT DOSAGE

Mania

Acute Manic/Mixed Episodes Associated w/ Bipolar Disorder:
Initial: 25mg/kg qd
Titrate: May increase as rapidly as possible to achieve lowest dose which produces desired clinical effect or desired range of plasma concentrations
Max: 60mg/kg/day
Trough Plasma Concentration in a Clinical Trial: 85-125mcg/mL

Epilepsy

Monotherapy and Adjunctive Therapy for Complex Partial Seizures and Simple and Complex Absence Seizures; Adjunctive Therapy w/ Multiple Seizure Types that Include Absence Seizures:

Complex Partial Seizures:
Initial: 10-15mg/kg/day
Titrate: Increase by 5-10mg/kg/week to achieve optimal clinical response
Max: 60mg/kg/day
Usual Therapeutic Range: 50-100mcg/mL

Simple/Complex Absence Seizures:
Initial: 15mg/kg/day
Titrate: Increase weekly by 5-10mg/

PEDIATRIC DOSAGE

Epilepsy

Monotherapy and Adjunctive Therapy for Complex Partial Seizures and Simple and Complex Absence Seizures; Adjunctive Therapy w/ Multiple Seizure Types that Include Absence Seizures:

≥10 Years:
Complex Partial Seizures:
Initial: 10-15mg/kg/day
Titrate: Increase by 5-10mg/kg/week to achieve optimal clinical response
Max: 60mg/kg/day
Usual Therapeutic Range: 50-100mcg/mL

Simple/Complex Absence Seizures:
Initial: 15mg/kg/day
Titrate: Increase weekly by 5-10mg/kg/day until seizures are controlled or side effects preclude further treatment
Max: 60mg/kg/day
Usual Therapeutic Range: 50-100mcg/mL

Conversions

≥10 Years:
Conversion from Depakote to Depakote ER:
Administer Depakote ER qd using

kg/day until seizures are controlled or side effects preclude further treatment
Max: 60mg/kg/day
Usual Therapeutic Range: 50-100mcg/mL

Migraine

Prophylaxis:
Initial: 500mg qd for 1 week
Titrate: Increase to 1000mg qd

Use Depakote instead if a patient requires smaller dosage adjustments than that available w/ Depakote ER

Conversions

Conversion from Depakote to Depakote ER in Patients w/ Epilepsy: Administer Depakote ER qd using a dose 8-20% higher than total daily dose of Depakote. If Depakote total daily dose cannot be directly converted to Depakote ER, consider increasing Depakote total daily dose to next higher dose before conversion to appropriate total daily dose of Depakote ER. Refer to PI for additional information.

a dose 8-20% higher than total daily dose of Depakote. If Depakote total daily dose cannot be directly converted to Depakote ER, consider increasing Depakote total daily dose to next higher dose before conversion to appropriate total daily dose of Depakote ER. Refer to PI for additional information.

DOSING CONSIDERATIONS
Concomitant Medications
Complex Partial Seizures:
Conversion to Monotherapy: Reduce concomitant antiepilepsy drugs by 25% every 2 weeks; begin reduction at the initiation of Depakote ER, or delay by 1-2 weeks if seizures are likely to occur w/ a reduction
Rufinamide: Begin valproate therapy at a low dose and titrate to clinically effective dose in patients stabilized on rufinamide before being prescribed valproate

Elderly
Reduce initial dose and titrate more slowly; consider dose reductions/discontinuation in patients w/ decreased food/fluid intake and w/ excessive somnolence

Adverse Reactions
Thrombocytopenia: Probability increases significantly at total valproate concentrations of ≥110mcg/mL (females) or ≥135mcg/mL (males)
GI Irritation: Administer w/ food or slowly build up the dose from an initial low level

Discontinuation
Do not abruptly d/c in patients in whom the drug is administered to prevent major seizures

ADMINISTRATION
Oral route
Swallow tab whole; do not crush or chew.

STORAGE
25°C (77°F); excursions permitted to 15-30°C (59-86°F).

HOW SUPPLIED
Tab, Extended-Release: 250mg, 500mg

CONTRAINDICATIONS
Hepatic disease, significant hepatic dysfunction, mitochondrial disorders caused by mutations in mitochondrial POLG (eg, Alpers-Huttenlocher syndrome) and children <2 yrs of age who are suspected of having a POLG-related disorder, known hypersensitivity to the medication, known urea cycle disorders (UCDs), prophylaxis of migraine headaches in pregnant women.

WARNINGS/PRECAUTIONS
Caution w/ prior history of hepatic disease. D/C immediately if significant hepatic dysfunction (suspected or apparent) occurs. Increased risk of suicidal thoughts or behavior reported. Dose-related thrombocytopenia, inhibition of secondary phase of platelet aggregation, and abnormal coagulation parameters reported; associated w/ decreases in other cell lines and myelodysplasia. Hyperammonemic encephalopathy reported in UCD patients; d/c and initiate treatment if symptoms develop, and evaluate for underlying UCDs. Hyperammonemia reported and may be present despite normal LFTs. Measure ammonia levels if unexplained lethargy, vomiting, or mental status changes occur; consider discontinuation if ammonia elevation persists. Hypothermia reported; consider stopping valproate. Drug reaction w/ eosinophilia and systemic symptoms (DRESS) reported; d/c if signs/symptoms are present. Somnolence in elderly reported; monitor fluid/nutritional intake, and for dehydration, somnolence, and other adverse reactions. Altered thyroid function tests and urine ketone tests reported. May stimulate replication of HIV and CMV; the clinical consequence is unknown, but this should be considered when monitoring HIV and CMV infected patients. Medication residue in stool reported; check valproate levels, monitor clinical condition, and consider alternative treatment if clinically indicated.

ADVERSE REACTIONS
Mania: Somnolence, dyspepsia, N/V, diarrhea, dizziness, pain, abdominal pain, asthenia, pharyngitis.

Epilepsy: N/V, headache, asthenia, somnolence, tremor, dizziness, abdominal pain, diplopia, diarrhea, anorexia, amblyopia/blurred vision, flu syndrome, infection, dyspepsia.
Migraine: N/V, asthenia, somnolence, infection, dyspepsia, diarrhea, dizziness, abdominal pain, tremor, weight gain, back pain, alopecia, increased appetite.

DRUG INTERACTIONS
Drugs that affect the level of expression of hepatic enzymes (eg, phenytoin, carbamazepine, phenobarbital, primidone), particularly those that elevate levels of glucuronosyltransferases (eg, ritonavir), may increase valproate clearance; monitor valproate and concomitant drug concentrations whenever enzyme-inducing drugs are introduced or withdrawn. Aspirin may decrease protein binding and inhibit metabolism of valproate; use w/ caution. Carbapenem antibiotics may reduce serum concentrations to subtherapeutic levels, resulting in loss of seizure control; monitor serum valproic acid concentrations frequently after initiating carbapenem therapy. Felbamate may lead to an increase in valproate C_{max}; may require decrease in valproate dosage. Rifampin increases oral clearance; may require valproate dosage adjustment. Reduces the clearance of amitriptyline and nortriptyline. May decrease levels of carbamazepine while increasing carbamazepine-10,11-epoxide serum levels. Use w/ clonazepam may induce absence status in patients w/ absence seizures. Inhibits metabolism of diazepam, ethosuximide, phenobarbital, and phenytoin; monitor drug serum concentrations and adjust dose appropriately. Increases $T_{1/2}$ of lamotrigine; serious skin reactions reported. Monitor for neurological toxicity w/ barbiturate therapy. Breakthrough seizures reported w/ phenytoin. Decreases clearance and increases levels of rufinamide. May displace protein-bound drugs (eg, diazepam, phenytoin, tolbutamide, warfarin); monitor coagulation tests when coadministered w/ warfarin. May decrease clearance of zidovudine in HIV-seropositive patients. Concomitant use w/ topiramate has been associated w/ hyperammonemia w/ or w/o encephalopathy, and hypothermia. Refer to PI for dosing considerations when used w/ certain concomitant therapies.

PREGNANCY AND LACTATION
Pregnancy: Category D (for epilepsy and for manic episodes w/ bipolar disorder) or X (for prophylaxis of migraine headaches). Physicians should encourage pregnant patients to enroll in the North American Antiepileptic Drug (NAAED) Pregnancy Registry.
Lactation: Excreted in human milk; caution in nursing.

MECHANISM OF ACTION
Valproate compound; has not been established. Dissociates to the valproate ion in the GI tract. It has been suggested its activity in epilepsy is related to increased brain concentrations of GABA.

PHARMACOKINETICS
Absorption: (Fed) Bioavailability (90%); T_{max}=4-17 hrs (median). **Distribution:** Plasma protein binding (concentration dependent; free fraction increases from 10% at 40mcg/mL to 18.5% at 130mcg/mL); V_d=11L/1.73m^2 (total valproate), 92L/1.73m^2 (free valproate); found in breast milk, CSF. **Metabolism:** Liver; mitochondrial β-oxidation (major), glucuronidation. **Elimination:** Urine (30-50% glucuronide conjugate, <3% unchanged); $T_{1/2}$=9-16 hrs.

PATIENT CONSIDERATIONS
Assessment: Assess for hepatic dysfunction, history of hepatic disease, pancreatitis, history of hypersensitivity to the drug, mitochondrial disorders caused by mutations in mitochondrial POLG, children <2 yrs of age who are suspected of having a POLG-related disorder, other conditions where treatment is cautioned, pregnancy/nursing status, and possible drug interactions. Evaluate for UCD in high-risk patients (eg, history of unexplained encephalopathy or coma). Assess LFTs, CBC, and coagulation parameters.

Monitoring: Monitor for hypersensitivity reactions, DRESS, pancreatitis, hepatotoxicity, hyperammonemia, hypothermia, drug-induced acute liver failure, acute liver injury, emergence/worsening of depression, suicidality or unusual changes in behavior, medication residue in stool, and other adverse reactions. Monitor LFTs frequently, especially during first 6 months. Monitor fluid/nutritional intake and for dehydration, somnolence, and other adverse reactions in the elderly. Monitor ammonia levels, CBC, and coagulation parameters. Reevaluate the long-term risk-benefits if used for extended periods for mania.

Counseling: Instruct to take ud. Inform pregnant women and women of childbearing potential about the risk in pregnancy; advise to use effective contraception while on therapy and counsel about alternative therapeutic options. Advise to read the medication guide. Instruct to notify physician if pregnant or intending to become pregnant. Encourage pregnant patients to enroll in NAAED Pregnancy Registry. Advise to notify physician if depression, suicidal thoughts, behavior, or thoughts about self-harm emerge; instruct to report behaviors of concern. Counsel about signs/symptoms of pancreatitis, hepatotoxicity, hyperammonemia, or hyperammonemic encephalopathy; advise to notify physician if any symptoms or adverse effects occur. Advise not to engage in hazardous activities (eg, driving/operating machinery) until the effects of the drug are known. Inform that a fever associated w/ other organ system involvement (eg, rash, lymphadenopathy) may be drug related; instruct to report to physician. Instruct patients to notify their physician if they notice medication residue in the stool.

DEPO-MEDROL — methylprednisolone acetate   Rx
Class: Glucocorticoid

ADULT DOSAGE
Steroid-Responsive Disorders
When Oral Therapy Is Not Feasible:
Initial: 4-120mg depending on disease being treated
Maint: Decrease initial dosage in small decrements at appropriate time intervals until lowest effective dose
Dosage requirements are variable and must be individualized on the basis of the disease under treatment and the response of the patient

Rheumatoid Arthritis
Intra-Articular:
Small Joint: 4-10mg
Medium Joint: 10-40mg
Large Joint: 20-80mg
In chronic cases, may repeat inj at intervals ranging from 1-5 weeks or more, depending on relief

Intramuscular:
Maint: 40-120mg IM weekly

Osteoarthritis
Intra-Articular:
Small Joint: 4-10mg
Medium Joint: 10-40mg
Large Joint: 20-80mg
In chronic cases, may repeat inj at intervals ranging from 1-5 weeks or more, depending on relief

Ganglion/Tendinitis/Epicondylitis
Usual: 4-30mg
May repeat inj if necessary in recurrent or chronic conditions

Dermatologic Conditions
Intralesional:
20-60mg
In large lesions, may distribute 20-40mg dose by repeated inj (usually 1-4 inj)

Intramuscular:
Dermatologic Lesions:
Usual: 40-120mg IM weekly for 1-4 weeks

Acute Severe Dermatitis (Poison Ivy):
80-120mg IM single dose

Chronic Contact Dermatitis: May repeat inj at 5- to 10-day intervals

Seborrheic Dermatitis: 80mg IM weekly

Adrenogenital Syndrome
Single 40mg IM inj every 2 weeks

Multiple Sclerosis
Acute Exacerbations:
160mg/day for 1 week, then 64mg qod for 1 month

Allergic Rhinitis
Usual: 80-120mg IM

Asthma
Usual: 80-120mg IM

PEDIATRIC DOSAGE
Steroid-Responsive Disorders
When Oral Therapy is Not Feasible:
Initial: 0.11-1.6mg/kg/day
Titrate to the lowest effective dose

Dosage requirements are variable and must be individualized on the basis of the disease under treatment and the response of the patient

---

DOSING CONSIDERATIONS
Discontinuation
Withdraw gradually after long-term therapy

ADMINISTRATION
IM/Intra-articular/Soft tissue/Intralesional route

Do not dilute or mix w/ other sol

If signs of stress are associated w/ the condition being treated, the dosage of the sus should be increased
If a rapid hormonal effect of max intensity is required, IV administration of highly soluble methylprednisolone sodium succinate is indicated

STORAGE
20-25°C (68-77°F).

HOW SUPPLIED
Inj: 20mg/mL, 40mg/mL, 80mg/mL

CONTRAINDICATIONS
Known hypersensitivity to this product and its constituents, idiopathic thrombocytopenic purpura (IM preparations), intrathecal administration, systemic

fungal infections (except as an intra-articular inj for localized joint conditions), premature infants (formulations preserved w/ benzyl alcohol).

WARNINGS/PRECAUTIONS

Not for IV administration. Serious neurologic events reported with epidural inj; not approved for epidural administration. Formulations with preservative contain benzyl alcohol, which is potentially toxic to neural tissue. Excessive amounts of benzyl alcohol have been associated with toxicity, particularly in neonates. May result in dermal and/or subdermal changes forming depressions in the skin at inj site. Multiple small inj into the area of lesion should be made whenever possible; caution against inj or leakage into dermis during intra-articular and IM inj. Avoid inj into deltoid muscle or into an infected site/previously infected joint. Anaphylactoid reactions may occur. May need to increase dose before, during, and after stressful situations. High systemic doses should not be used to treat traumatic brain injury. May cause elevation of BP, salt/water retention, and increased excretion of K^+ and Ca^{2+}; dietary salt restriction and K^+ supplementation may be necessary. Caution with recent myocardial infarction (MI). Monitor for hypothalamic-pituitary-adrenal (HPA) axis suppression, Cushing's syndrome, and hyperglycemia with chronic use. May produce reversible HPA-axis suppression with potential for glucocorticosteroid insufficiency after withdrawal of treatment; reduce dose gradually. May increase susceptibility to, mask signs of, or cause new infections; may exacerbate systemic fungal infections. Avoid use intra-articularly, intrabursally, or for intratendinous administration for local effect in the presence of acute local infection. Latent disease due to certain pathogens may be activated or intercurrent infections exacerbated. Rule out latent or active amebiasis before initiating therapy. Caution with *Strongyloides* infestation, active or latent tuberculosis, ocular herpes simplex, HTN, congestive heart failure (CHF), and renal insufficiency. May cause more serious/fatal course of chickenpox and measles. May produce posterior subcapsular cataracts, glaucoma with possible damage to optic nerves, and enhance the establishment of secondary ocular infections; systemic corticosteroids not recommended in the treatment of optic neuritis. Not for use in active ocular herpes simplex or in cerebral malaria. Sensitive to heat; should not be autoclaved when it is desirable to sterilize the exterior of the vial. Kaposi's sarcoma reported. Metabolic clearance is decreased in hypothyroidism and increased in hyperthyroidism; changes in thyroid status may necessitate dose adjustment. Caution with active or latent peptic ulcers, diverticulitis, fresh intestinal anastomoses, and nonspecific ulcerative colitis; may increase risk of perforation. Signs of peritoneal irritation following GI perforation may be minimal/absent. Intra-articularly injected corticosteroids may be systemically absorbed. Enhanced effect in patients with cirrhosis. Appropriate examination of any joint fluid present is necessary to exclude a septic process; institute appropriate antimicrobial therapy if septic arthritis occurs and diagnosis is confirmed. May decrease bone formation and increase bone resorption, and may lead to inhibition of bone growth in pediatric patients and development of osteoporosis at any age; caution with increased risk of osteoporosis. Acute myopathy reported with high doses, most often in patients with disorders of neuromuscular transmission (eg, myasthenia gravis). Elevation of creatine kinase (CK) or intraocular pressure (IOP) may occur; monitor IOP if used >6 weeks. Psychic derangements may appear and existing emotional instability or psychotic tendencies may be aggravated. Caution in elderly. May suppress reactions to skin tests.

ADVERSE REACTIONS

Allergic reactions, bradycardia, cardiac arrest, acne, allergic dermatitis, decreased carbohydrate/glucose tolerance, glycosuria, fluid retention, abdominal distention, bowel/bladder dysfunction, convulsions, depression, exophthalmoses, glaucoma, muscle weakness.

DRUG INTERACTIONS

Aminoglutethimide may lead to a loss of corticosteroid-induced adrenal suppression. Closely monitor for hypokalemia with K^+-depleting agents (eg, amphotericin B, diuretics). Cardiac enlargement and CHF reported following concomitant use of amphotericin B and hydrocortisone. Macrolide antibiotics may decrease clearance and cholestyramine may increase clearance. Concomitant use with anticholinesterase agents may produce severe weakness in patients with myasthenia gravis; d/c anticholinesterase agents at least 24 hrs before initiating therapy. May inhibit response to warfarin; frequently monitor coagulation indices. May increase blood glucose levels; dosage adjustments of antidiabetic agents may be required. May decrease serum levels of isoniazid. Increased activity of both drugs may occur with cyclosporine; convulsions reported with concurrent use. May increase risk of arrhythmias with digitalis glycosides. Estrogens, including oral contraceptives, may decrease hepatic metabolism and enhance effect. Drugs that induce CYP3A4 (eg, barbiturates, phenytoin, carbamazepine) may enhance metabolism and require corticosteroid dosage increase. Drugs that inhibit CYP3A4 (eg, ketoconazole, erythromycin, troleandomycin) may increase plasma levels. Ketoconazole may increase risk of corticosteroid side effects. Aspirin (ASA) or other NSAIDs may increase risk of GI side effects; caution with ASA in hypoprothrombinemia patients. May increase clearance of salicylates. Administration of live or live, attenuated vaccines is contraindicated in patients receiving immunosuppressive doses. Killed or inactivated vaccines may be administered, although response is unpredictable. Acute myopathy reported with neuromuscular blocking drugs (eg, pancuronium).

PREGNANCY AND LACTATION

Category C, not for use in nursing.

MECHANISM OF ACTION

Glucocorticoid; causes profound and varied metabolic effects and modifies the body's immune responses to diverse stimuli.

PHARMACOKINETICS

Distribution: Found in breast milk.

PATIENT CONSIDERATIONS

Assessment: Assess for hypersensitivity to drug, traumatic brain injury, cerebral malaria, ocular herpes simplex, CHF, HTN, recent MI, renal insufficiency, systemic fungal infections, active or latent peptic ulcer, diverticulitis, ulcerative colitis, cirrhosis, any other conditions where treatment is contraindicated or cautioned, pregnancy/nursing status, and possible drug interactions.

Monitoring: Monitor for anaphylactoid reactions, dermal and/or subdermal changes, cataracts, glaucoma, bone growth/development (in pediatric patients), osteoporosis, intestinal perforation, infections, psychic derangements, Kaposi's sarcoma, CK/IOP elevation, and other adverse reactions. Monitor for HPA-axis suppression, Cushing's syndrome, and hyperglycemia with chronic use. Frequently monitor coagulation indices with warfarin.

Counseling: Warn not to d/c abruptly or without medical supervision. Instruct to seek medical advice at once if fever or other signs of infection develop. Warn to avoid exposure to chickenpox or measles; advise to report immediately if exposed.

DEPO-PROVERA — medroxyprogesterone acetate   Rx

Class: Progestogen

ADULT DOSAGE	PEDIATRIC DOSAGE
Inoperable, Recurrent, and Metastatic Endometrial or Renal Carcinoma	Pediatric use may not have been established
Adjunctive Therapy and Palliative Treatment:	
Initial: 400-1000mg/week	
If improvement is noted w/in a few weeks or months and the disease appears stabilized, may be possible to maintain improvement w/ as little as 400mg/month	

ADMINISTRATION

IM route

Cleanse the vial top prior to aspiration of contents of multidose vial.

STORAGE

20-25°C (68-77°F) in upright position.

HOW SUPPLIED

Inj: 400mg/mL [2.5mL]

CONTRAINDICATIONS

Active thrombophlebitis, or current or past history of thromboembolic disorders, or cerebral vascular disease. Known sensitivity to medroxyprogesterone acetate or to any of the other ingredients.

WARNINGS/PRECAUTIONS

D/C if early manifestations of thrombotic disorder (thrombophlebitis, cerebrovascular disorder, pulmonary embolism, retinal thrombosis) occur or are suspected. D/C, pending examination, if there is a sudden partial or complete loss of vision, or a sudden onset of proptosis, diplopia, or migraine. If examination reveals papilledema or retinal vascular lesions, withdraw therapy. Avoid contamination of multidose vials. In cases of undiagnosed, persistent, or recurrent vaginal bleeding, perform adequate diagnostic measures to rule out malignancies. Advise women who have or have had a history of breast cancer against the use of medroxyprogesterone. Perform annual history and physical examination; physical examination should include special reference to BP, breasts, abdomen and pelvic organs, including cervical cytology and relevant lab tests. Carefully monitor women who have a strong family history of breast cancer. May cause fluid retention. Caution w/ history of psychic depression; d/c if depression recurs to a serious degree. May mask the onset of the climacteric. Use w/ estrogen may produce adverse effects on carbohydrate and lipid metabolism. Decrease in glucose tolerance reported in patients on estrogen-progestin combination treatment; caution in diabetic patients. Should not be used by women w/ significant liver disease. Periodically monitor for hepatic dysfunction and temporarily interrupt therapy if hepatic dysfunction develops; do not resume therapy until markers of liver function return to normal. Medroxyprogesterone given as 150mg IM every 3 months reduces serum estrogen levels and is associated w/ loss of bone mineral density (BMD). Some patients may exhibit suppressed adrenal function; medroxyprogesterone may have cortisol-like glucocorticoid activity and provide (-) feedback to the hypothalamus or pituitary; this may result in decreased plasma cortisol levels, decreased cortisol secretion, and low plasma ACTH levels. May produce cushingoid symptoms (eg, weight gain, edema/fluid retention, facial swelling). May change the results of some lab tests (eg, coagulation factors, lipids, glucose tolerance, binding proteins).

ADVERSE REACTIONS

Breakthrough bleeding, change in menstrual flow, changes in cervical erosion and cervical secretions, breast tenderness, headache, dizziness, somnolence, nervousness, euphoria, edema, pyrexia, change in weight, cholestatic jaundice, anaphylactoid reactions.

DRUG INTERACTIONS

Aminoglutethimide may decrease levels. Avoid w/ strong CYP3A inhibitors (eg, ketoconazole, clarithromycin, atazanavir) or strong CYP3A inducers (eg, phenytoin, carbamazepine, St. John's wort).

PREGNANCY AND LACTATION

Pregnancy: Not known whether medroxyprogesterone can cause fetal harm when administered to a pregnant woman; should be given to a pregnant woman only if clearly needed.

Lactation: Caution in nursing.

MECHANISM OF ACTION

Progestogen; inhibits secretion of pituitary gonadotropins, preventing follicular maturation and ovulation. When given parenterally and in recommended doses, transforms proliferative endometrium into secretory endometrium in women w/ adequate endogenous estrogen.

PHARMACOKINETICS

Distribution: Found in breast milk.

PATIENT CONSIDERATIONS

Assessment: Assess for drug hypersensitivity; presence, history, or family history of breast cancer; active thrombophlebitis; current or past history of thromboembolic disorders; and for any other conditions where treatment is contraindicated or cautioned. Assess pregnancy/nursing status and for possible drug interactions.

Monitoring: Monitor for thromboembolic disorders, ocular disorders, breakthrough bleeding, recurrence of depression, fluid retention, hepatic dysfunction, suppressed adrenal function, and other adverse reactions. Perform annual history and physical examination. If undiagnosed, persistent or recurrent abnormal vaginal bleeding occurs, take appropriate measures to rule out malignancy. Monitor BMD. Monitor for adverse effects on carbohydrate and lipid metabolism if used w/ estrogen therapy.

Counseling: Inform of risks/benefits of treatment. Instruct to notify physician if any adverse reactions occur while on therapy.

DEPO-PROVERA CONTRACEPTIVE INJECTION –

medroxyprogesterone acetate   **Rx**

Class: Progestin contraceptive

> May lose significant bone mineral density (BMD); bone loss is greater w/ increasing duration of use and may not be completely reversible. Unknown if use during adolescence or early adulthood will reduce peak bone mass and increase risk for osteoporotic fractures in later life. Should not be used as long-term birth control (eg, >2 yrs) unless other birth control methods are considered inadequate.

ADULT DOSAGE	PEDIATRIC DOSAGE
Contraception	**Contraception**
Usual: 150mg deep IM every 3 months (13 weeks)	Not indicated for use premenarche; refer to adult dosing
Dosage does not need to be adjusted for body weight	
Conversions	
Switching from Other Methods of Contraception:	
Give in a manner that ensures continuous contraceptive coverage based upon the mechanism of action of both methods (eg, switching from oral contraceptives should have the 1st inj on the day after the last active tab or at the latest, on the day following the final inactive tab)	

ADMINISTRATION

IM route

Shake vigorously before use
Administer in the gluteal or deltoid muscle
Give the 1st inj only during the first 5 days of a normal menstrual period, only w/ in the first 5 days postpartum if not breastfeeding, or only at the 6th postpartum week if exclusively nursing
If the interval between inj is >13 weeks, determine that patient is not pregnant before administering

STORAGE

20-25°C (68-77°F). Store vials upright.

HOW SUPPLIED

Inj: 150mg/mL [1mL, vial, prefilled syringe]

CONTRAINDICATIONS

Known or suspected pregnancy or as a diagnostic test for pregnancy, active thrombophlebitis, current or past history of thromboembolic disorders, cerebral vascular disease, known or suspected malignancy of the breast, known hypersensitivity to medroxyprogesterone acetate or any other ingredients in the medication, significant liver disease, undiagnosed vaginal bleeding.

WARNINGS/PRECAUTIONS

May pose additional risk of BMD loss in patients w/ risk factors for osteoporosis (eg, chronic alcohol and/or tobacco use, anorexia nervosa, chronic use of drugs that can reduce bone mass [eg, anticonvulsants, corticosteroids]); consider other birth control methods. Serious thrombotic events reported; d/c if thrombosis develops while on therapy unless there are no other acceptable options for birth control. Do not readminister therapy pending examination if there is sudden partial/complete loss of vision, or sudden onset of proptosis/diplopia/migraine; if examination reveals papilledema or retinal vascular lesions, do not readminister. May increase risk of breast cancer; monitor women w/ strong family history of breast cancer carefully. Be alert to possibility of ectopic pregnancy in patients who become pregnant or complain of severe abdominal pain. Anaphylaxis/anaphylactoid reactions reported; institute emergency medical treatment if an anaphylactic reaction occurs. D/C if jaundice or acute/chronic disturbances of liver function develop; do not resume use until markers of liver function return to normal and medroxyprogesterone acetate causation has been excluded. Convulsions and weight gain reported. Monitor patients who have history of depression; do not readminister if depression recurs. May cause disruption of menstrual bleeding patterns (eg, amenorrhea, irregular or unpredictable bleeding/spotting, prolonged spotting/bleeding, heavy bleeding); rule out possibility of organic pathology if abnormal bleeding persists or is severe, and institute appropriate treatment. Decrease in glucose tolerance reported; monitor diabetic patients carefully. May cause fluid retention. Return to ovulation and fertility after discontinuation of therapy may be delayed. Does not protect against HIV infection and other STDs. May change results of some lab tests (eg, coagulation factors, lipids, glucose tolerance, binding proteins).

ADVERSE REACTIONS

BMD loss, menstrual irregularities, increased weight, abdominal pain/discomfort, dizziness, headache, asthenia/fatigue, nervousness, decreased libido, nausea, leg cramps.

DRUG INTERACTIONS

Drugs or herbal products that induce enzymes, including CYP3A4 that metabolize contraceptive hormones (eg, barbiturates, bosentan, St. John's wort) may decrease levels and effectiveness; use additional contraception or a different method of contraception. HIV protease inhibitors and non-nucleoside reverse transcriptase inhibitors may alter levels. Pregnancy reported w/ antibiotics.

PREGNANCY AND LACTATION

Contraindicated in pregnancy, caution in nursing.

MECHANISM OF ACTION

Progestin contraceptive; inhibits secretion of gonadotropins which, in turn, prevents follicular maturation and ovulation, resulting in endometrial thinning.

PHARMACOKINETICS

Absorption: C_{max}=1-7ng/mL, T_{max}=approx 3 weeks. **Distribution:** Plasma protein binding (86%); found in breast milk. **Metabolism:** Liver (extensive) via CYP450 enzymes; reduction, loss of the acetyl group and hydroxylation. **Elimination:** Urine; $T_{1/2}$=approx 50 days.

PATIENT CONSIDERATIONS

Assessment: Assess for active thrombophlebitis, current/past history of thromboembolic disorders or cerebral vascular disease, known or suspected malignancy of the breast, drug hypersensitivity, significant liver disease, undiagnosed vaginal bleeding, osteoporosis risk factors, family history of breast cancer, history of depression, diabetes mellitus (DM), conditions that may be influenced by fluid retention (eg, epilepsy, migraine, asthma, cardiac/renal dysfunction), pregnancy/nursing status, and possible drug interactions.

Monitoring: Monitor for thrombosis, loss of BMD, breast cancer, sudden/partial loss of vision, proptosis, diplopia, migraine, papilledema, retinal vascular lesions, anaphylaxis/anaphylactoid reactions, jaundice or acute/chronic disturbances in liver function, ectopic pregnancy, convulsions, weight gain, fluid retention, disruption of menstrual bleeding patterns, and other adverse reactions. Monitor patients w/ DM. Monitor for recurrence of depression w/ history of depression. Perform annual exam for a BP check and for other indicated healthcare.

Counseling: Counsel about the risks/benefits of therapy. Advise at the beginning of treatment that the menstrual cycle may be disrupted and that irregular and unpredictable bleeding or spotting may occur; inform that this usually decreases to the point of amenorrhea as treatment continues w/o other therapy being required. Inform about the possible increased risk of breast cancer in women who use the drug. Inform that drug does not protect against HIV infection and other STDs. Counsel to use a back-up method or alternative method of contraception when enzyme inducers are used w/ the drug. Advise to take adequate Ca^{2+} and vitamin D. Advise to have a yearly visit w/ healthcare provider for a BP check and for other indicated healthcare.

DEPO-TESTOSTERONE — testosterone cypionate   **CIII**

Class: Androgen

ADULT DOSAGE	PEDIATRIC DOSAGE
Testosterone Replacement Therapy	**Testosterone Replacement Therapy**
Congenital/Acquired Primary Hypogonadism or Hypogonadotropic Hypogonadism in Males:	**Congenital/Acquired Primary Hypogonadism or Hypogonadotropic Hypogonadism in Males:**
- Individualize dose based on age, sex, and diagnosis	**≥12 Years:**
- 50-400mg every 2-4 weeks	- Individualize dose based on age, sex, and diagnosis
	- 50-400mg every 2-4 weeks

ADMINISTRATION

IM route

Administer deep into gluteal muscle.
Warm and shake the vial to redissolve any crystals that may have formed during storage at temperatures lower than recommended.

STORAGE

20-25°C (68-77°F). Protect from light.

HOW SUPPLIED

Inj: 100mg/mL [10mL], 200mg/mL [1mL, 10mL]

CONTRAINDICATIONS

Known hypersensitivity to the medication. Males w/ carcinoma of the breast or known/suspected carcinoma of the prostate gland. Women who are or may become pregnant. Serious cardiac, hepatic, or renal disease.

WARNINGS/PRECAUTIONS

May cause hypercalcemia in immobilized patients; d/c if this occurs. Peliosis hepatis, hepatocellular carcinoma, and hepatic adenomas reported w/ prolonged use of high doses. May increase risk of prostatic hypertrophy and prostatic carcinoma in elderly. Venous thromboembolic events reported; evaluate patients who report symptoms of pain, edema, warmth, and erythema in the lower extremity for deep vein thrombosis and those who present w/ acute SOB for pulmonary embolism. D/C treatment and initiate appropriate workup and management if venous thromboembolic event is suspected. Increased risk of major adverse cardiovascular events (MACE) reported. Edema w/ or w/o CHF may be a serious complication in patients w/ preexisting cardiac, renal, or hepatic disease. Gynecomastia may develop and persist. Contains benzyl alcohol; has been associated w/ serious adverse events, including gasping syndrome and death, in pediatric patients. Caution in healthy males w/ delayed puberty; monitor bone maturation by assessing bone age of wrist and hand every 6 months. May accelerate bone maturation w/o producing compensatory gain in linear growth in children; compromised adult stature may result. Acute urethral obstruction in patients w/ benign prostatic hypertrophy (BPH), priapism or excessive sexual stimulation, and oligospermia after prolonged use or excessive dosage may develop; if these effects appear d/c therapy and if restarted, use a lower dose. Do not use interchangeably w/ testosterone propionate and for enhancement of athletic performance. May increase serum cholesterol. May decrease levels of thyroxin-binding globulins, resulting in decreased total T4 serum concentrations and increased resin uptake of T3 and T4.

ADVERSE REACTIONS

Gynecomastia, excessive frequency/duration of penile erections, oligospermia (if at high doses), male pattern baldness, increased/decreased libido, hirsutism, acne, MI, stroke, nausea, clotting factor suppression, polycythemia, altered LFTs, headache, anxiety.

DRUG INTERACTIONS

May increase sensitivity to oral anticoagulants; may require dose reduction in anticoagulants. May increase levels of oxyphenbutazone. May decrease blood glucose and insulin requirements in diabetic patients.

PREGNANCY AND LACTATION

Category X, not for use in nursing.

MECHANISM OF ACTION

Endogenous androgen; responsible for normal growth and development of male sex organs and for maintenance of secondary sex characteristics.

PHARMACOKINETICS

Absorption: Slow. **Distribution:** Plasma protein binding (98%, specific testosterone-estradiol binding globulin). **Metabolism:** Liver. **Elimination:** Urine (90% [glucuronic and sulfuric acid conjugates of testosterone]), feces (6%[unconjugated]); $T_{1/2}$=8 days.

PATIENT CONSIDERATIONS

Assessment: Assess for breast carcinoma in males, prostate carcinoma, cardiac/hepatic/renal disease, delayed puberty, BPH, drug hypersensitivity, any other conditions where treatment is contraindicated/cautioned, and possible drug interactions. Confirm diagnosis of hypogonadism by measuring testosterone levels on at least 2 separate days prior to initiation.

Monitoring: Monitor for signs/symptoms of hypercalcemia, edema w/ or w/o CHF, prostatic hypertrophy/carcinoma in elderly, venous thromboembolic events, MACE and other adverse reactions. Monitor bone maturation by assessing bone age of wrist and hand every 6 months. Periodically check Hgb and Hct in patients receiving long-term androgen therapy. Monitor serum cholesterol levels and LFTs.

Counseling: Instruct to report to physician if N/V, changes in skin color, ankle swelling, or too frequent or persistent penile erections occurs. Inform of the possible risk of MACE when deciding whether to use or continue to use drug.

DERMA-SMOOTHE/FS — fluocinolone acetonide   Rx

Class: Corticosteroid

ADULT DOSAGE	PEDIATRIC DOSAGE
Atopic Dermatitis	**Atopic Dermatitis**
Body Oil	**Moderate to Severe:**
Apply as a thin film to the affected area(s) tid	**≥3 Months of Age:**
	Body Oil:
D/C when control is achieved	Moisten skin and apply as a thin film to the affected area(s) bid for up to 4 weeks
Reassess if no improvement seen w/ in 2 weeks	
	D/C when control is achieved
Scalp Psoriasis	
Scalp Oil	
Apply a thin film on the scalp; wet hair and scalp thoroughly	
Massage well and cover scalp w/ supplied shower cap	

ADMINISTRATION
Topical route
Do not apply to diaper area

Body Oil
Apply the least amount needed to cover the affected areas

Scalp Oil
Leave on overnight or for a minimum of 4 hours before washing off
Wash hair w/ regular shampoo and rinse thoroughly

STORAGE
25°C (68°-77°F); excursion permitted to 15-30°C (59-86°F).

HOW SUPPLIED
Oil: 0.01% [4 fl. oz.]

CONTRAINDICATIONS
Scalp Oil: History of hypersensitivity to any components of the medication.

WARNINGS/PRECAUTIONS
May produce reversible hypothalamic-pituitary-adrenal (HPA) axis suppression with potential for glucocorticosteroid insufficiency; when noted, gradually withdraw the drug, reduce frequency of application, or substitute with a less potent steroid. Use over large areas, over prolonged periods, and use with occlusive dressings may increase systemic absorption. May produce Cushing's syndrome, hyperglycemia, and glucosuria. Children may be more susceptible to systemic toxicity due to larger skin surface to body mass ratio. Allergic contact dermatitis may occur; confirm via patch testing. Use appropriate antifungal or antibacterial agent with skin infections; d/c until infection has been adequately treated. Local reactions reported (eg, telangiectasias, burning, itching, dryness, folliculitis, acneiform eruption); may occur with occlusive dressing, prolonged use, or use of higher potency corticosteroids. Not for use on the face, groin, axillae, or eyes. Caution in peanut-sensitive individuals; hypersensitivity or disease exacerbation may occur. Do not apply to the diaper area.

ADVERSE REACTIONS
Telangiectasias, erythema, itching, irritation, hypopigmentation, burning, cough, rhinorrhea, pyrexia, nasopharyngitis, upper respiratory infection, eczema, molluscum, abscess, rash.

PREGNANCY AND LACTATION
Category C, caution in nursing.

MECHANISM OF ACTION
Corticosteroid; not fully established. Possesses anti-inflammatory, antipruritic, and vasoconstrictive properties. Suspected to act by induction of phospholipase A_2 inhibitory proteins called lipocortins, which control biosynthesis of potent mediators of inflammation (eg, prostaglandins, leukotrienes) by inhibiting release of arachidonic acid. Arachidonic acid is released from membrane phospholipids by phospholipase A_2.

PHARMACOKINETICS
Distribution: Systemically administered corticosteroids found in breast milk.
Metabolism: Liver. **Elimination:** Kidney, bile.

PATIENT CONSIDERATIONS
Assessment: Assess for peanut-sensitive individuals, hypersensitivity to corticosteroids, conditions that increase systemic absorption of corticosteroids, concomitant skin infections, and pregnancy/nursing status.

Monitoring: Monitor for HPA-axis suppression, manifestation of Cushing's syndrome, hyperglycemia, glucosuria, skin irritation, allergic contact dermatitis (eg, failure to heal), local adverse reactions, systemic toxicity in children, and skin infections.

Counseling: Instruct to use s/d; for external use only. Inform to avoid contact with eyes; instruct to wash eyes liberally with water in case of contact. Instruct not to use for any disorder other than that for which it was prescribed. Instruct to notify physician if any worsening of skin condition occurs. Instruct not to apply on the face, axillae, groin, or under occlusion, unless directed by physician. Instruct to consult a physician first before using other corticosteroid-containing products. Instruct to d/c when control disease is achieved; contact physician if no improvement is seen within 2 weeks. Instruct not to apply to the diaper area, unless directed by physician.

DESCOVY — emtricitabine/tenofovir alafenamide   Rx

Class: Nucleoside analogue combination

> Lactic acidosis and severe hepatomegaly w/ steatosis, including fatal cases, reported w/ the use of nucleoside analogues in combination w/ other antiretrovirals. Not approved for treatment of chronic hepatitis B virus (HBV). Safety/efficacy not established in patients coinfected w/ HIV-1 and HBV. Severe acute exacerbations of HBV have been reported in patients who are coinfected w/ HIV-1 and HBV and have discontinued products containing emtricitabine (FTC) and/or tenofovir disoproxil fumarate (TDF), and may occur w/ discontinuation of Descovy.

ADULT DOSAGE	PEDIATRIC DOSAGE
HIV-1 Infection	**HIV-1 Infection**
≥35kg and CrCl ≥30mL/min:	**≥12 Years:**
1 tab qd in combination w/ other antiretrovirals	**≥35kg and CrCl ≥30mL/min:**
	1 tab qd in combination w/ other antiretrovirals

DOSING CONSIDERATIONS
Renal Impairment:
CrCl <30mL/min: Not recommended

ADMINISTRATION
Oral route
Take w/ or w/o food.

STORAGE
<30°C (86°F).

HOW SUPPLIED
Tab: (FTC/Tenofovir Alafenamide [TAF]) 200mg/25mg

WARNINGS/PRECAUTIONS
Not indicated for use as pre-exposure prophylaxis to reduce the risk of sexually acquired HIV-1 in adults at high risk. Obesity and prolonged nucleoside exposure may be risk factors for lactic acidosis and severe hepatomegaly w/ steatosis. Caution w/ known risk factors for liver disease. D/C if findings suggestive of lactic acidosis or pronounced hepatotoxicity develop. Test for the presence of chronic HBV before initiating therapy. Closely monitor coinfected patients who d/c Descovy treatment for at least several months after stopping treatment. Redistribution/accumulation of body fat and immune reconstitution syndrome reported. Autoimmune disorders (eg, Graves' disease, polymyositis, Guillain-Barre syndrome) reported in the setting of immune reconstitution and can occur many months after initiation of treatment. **TAF:** Renal impairment (eg, acute renal failure, Fanconi syndrome) reported; d/c if clinically significant decreases in renal function or evidence of Fanconi syndrome develop. Increased risk of renal adverse reactions w/ impaired renal function and in those taking nephrotoxic agents (eg, NSAIDs). Decreased bone mineral density (BMD) and increased biochemical markers of bone metabolism reported. Osteomalacia associated w/ proximal renal tubulopathy reported w/ TDF-containing products.

ADVERSE REACTIONS
Nausea.

DRUG INTERACTIONS
Drugs that reduce renal function or compete for active tubular secretion (eg, acyclovir, gentamicin, high-dose or multiple NSAIDs) may increase concentrations of FTC, tenofovir, and other renally eliminated drugs. **TAF:** Pgp inducers may decrease levels; may lead to development of resistance. Pgp inhibitors may increase levels. Protease inhibitors (eg, tipranavir/ritonavir), anticonvulsants, (eg, carbamazepine, oxcarbazepine, phenobarbital, phenytoin), antimycobacterials (rifabutin, rifampin, rifapentine), and St. John's wort may decrease levels; coadministration is not recommended.

PREGNANCY AND LACTATION
Pregnancy: Insufficient human data on use during pregnancy to inform of a drug-associated risk of birth defects and miscarriage. Physicians are encouraged to register pregnant patients in the Antiretroviral Pregnancy Registry.
Lactation: FTC has been shown to be present in human breast milk; not for use in nursing.

MECHANISM OF ACTION
FTC: Nucleoside analogue of cytidine; inhibits activity of HIV-1 reverse transcriptase (RT) by competing w/ natural substrate deoxycytidine 5'-triphosphate and by being incorporated into nascent viral DNA, which results in chain termination. **TAF:** Phosphonoamidate prodrug of tenofovir; inhibits HIV-1 replication through incorporation into viral DNA by the HIV RT, which results in DNA chain-termination.

PHARMACOKINETICS
Absorption: FTC: C_{max}=2.1mcg/mL; T_{max}=3 hrs; AUC=11.7mcg•hr/mL. TAF: C_{max}=0.16mcg/mL; T_{max}=1 hr; AUC=0.21mcg•hr/mL. **Distribution:** FTC: Found in breast milk. Plasma protein binding (<4%). TAF: Plasma protein binding (~80%). **Metabolism:** FTC: Not significantly metabolized. TAF: Hydrolyzed w/in cells to form tenofovir (major metabolite), which is phosphorylated to tenofovir diphosphate (active metabolite). **Elimination:** FTC: Urine (70%), feces (13.7%); $T_{1/2}$=10 hrs (median), TAF: Urine (<1%), feces (31.7%); $T_{1/2}$=0.51 hrs (median). Refer to PI for more parameters.

PATIENT CONSIDERATIONS
Assessment: Assess for risk factors for lactic acidosis or liver disease, renal dysfunction, HBV infection, pregnancy/nursing status, and possible drug interactions. Assess CrCl, urine glucose, and urine protein. Assess BMD in patients w/ history of pathologic bone fracture or other risk factors for osteoporosis or bone loss.
Monitoring: Monitor for signs/symptoms of lactic acidosis, hepatomegaly w/ steatosis, new onset or worsening renal impairment, bone effects, redistribution/accumulation of body fat, immune reconstitution syndrome, autoimmune disorders, and other adverse reactions. Closely monitor hepatic function w/ both clinical and laboratory follow-up for at least several months in patients coinfected w/ HBV and HIV-1 and who have discontinued therapy. Monitor CrCl, urine glucose, and urine protein periodically. Monitor serum phosphorus in patients w/ chronic kidney disease.
Counseling: Advise to d/c treatment if clinical symptoms suggestive of lactic acidosis or pronounced hepatotoxicity develop. Inform that severe acute exacerbations of hepatitis B have been reported in patients who are coinfected w/ HBV and HIV-1 and have discontinued products containing FTC and/or TDF; advise to not d/c therapy w/o first informing healthcare provider. Inform that redistribution/accumulation of body fat may occur. Advise to inform healthcare provider immediately of any symptoms of infection. Instruct to avoid taking Descovy w/ concurrent or recent use of nephrotoxic agents. Advise that decreases in BMD have been observed. Inform that it is important to take tab on a regular dosing schedule and to avoid missing doses. Inform that there is an antiretroviral pregnancy registry to monitor fetal outcomes of pregnant women exposed to Descovy. Instruct women w/ HIV-1 infection not to breastfeed.

DESLORATADINE — desloratadine   Rx
Class: H₁ antagonist

OTHER BRAND NAMES
Clarinex

ADULT DOSAGE	PEDIATRIC DOSAGE
Seasonal Allergic Rhinitis	**Seasonal Allergic Rhinitis**
Relief of Nasal and Non-Nasal Symptoms:	**Relief of Nasal and Non-Nasal Symptoms:**
Usual: 5mg or 10mL qd	**2-5 Years:** 2.5mL qd
Perennial Allergic Rhinitis	**6-11 Years:** 2.5mg or 5mL qd
Relief of Nasal and Non-Nasal Symptoms:	**≥12 Years:** 5mg or 10mL qd
Usual: 5mg or 10mL qd	**Perennial Allergic Rhinitis**
Chronic Idiopathic Urticaria	**Relief of Nasal And Non-Nasal Symptoms:**
Clarinex Tab/Sol: Relief of pruritus and reduction in number/size of hives	**6-11 Months of Age:** 2mL qd
Usual: 5mg or 10mL qd	**12 Months-5 Years:** 2.5mL qd
	6-11 Years: 2.5mg or 5mL qd
	≥12 Years: 5mg or 10mL qd
	Chronic Idiopathic Urticaria
	Clarinex Tab/Sol: Relief of pruritus and reduction in number/size of hives
	6-11 Months of Age: 2mL qd
	12 Months-5 Years: 2.5mL qd
	6-11 Years: 2.5mg or 5mL qd
	≥12 Years: 5mg or 10mL qd

DOSING CONSIDERATIONS
Renal Impairment
Adults:
Initial: 5mg qod
Hepatic Impairment
Adults:
Initial: 5mg qod

ADMINISTRATION
Oral route
May take w/o regard to meals.
Sol
Administer w/ a measuring dropper or syringe calibrated to deliver 2mL and 2.5mL.
Tab, Disintegrating
Place on tongue and allow to disintegrate before swallowing. Take immediately after opening the blister.
Administer w/ or w/o water.

STORAGE
(Tab/Sol) 25°C (77°F); excursions permitted to 15-30°C (59-86°F). (Tab) Avoid exposure ≥30°C (86°F). (Sol) Protect from light. (Tab, Disintegrating) 20-25°C (68-77°F); excursions permitted to 15-30°C (59-86°F).

HOW SUPPLIED
Tab, Disintegrating: 2.5mg, 5mg; (Clarinex) **Sol:** 0.5mg/mL [4 oz, 16 oz]; **Tab:** 5mg

CONTRAINDICATIONS
Hypersensitivity to this medication or to any of its ingredients or to loratadine.

WARNINGS/PRECAUTIONS
Hypersensitivity reactions reported; d/c therapy if any occur and consider alternative treatment. Caution in elderly.

ADVERSE REACTIONS
Pharyngitis, dry mouth, headache, N/V, fatigue, myalgia, fever, diarrhea, cough, URTI, irritability, somnolence, bronchitis, otitis media, dizziness.

DRUG INTERACTIONS
CYP450 3A4 inhibitors (eg, ketoconazole, erythromycin, azithromycin), fluoxetine, and cimetidine may increase levels.

PREGNANCY AND LACTATION
Category C, not for use in nursing.

MECHANISM OF ACTION
H₁-receptor antagonist; inhibits histamine release from human mast cells in vitro.

PHARMACOKINETICS
Absorption: (5mg tab) T_{max}=3 hrs, C_{max}=4ng/mL, AUC=56.9ng•hr/mL.
Distribution: Plasma protein binding (82-87%, 85-89% active metabolite); found

in breast milk. **Metabolism:** Extensive; glucuronidation; 3-hydroxydesloratadine (active metabolite). **Elimination:** Urine and feces (87%); $T_{1/2}$=27 hrs.

PATIENT CONSIDERATIONS
Assessment: Assess for hypersensitivity to drug, renal/hepatic impairment, pregnancy/nursing status, and possible drug interactions.

Monitoring: Monitor for hypersensitivity reactions and other adverse reactions.

Counseling: Instruct to take ud; advise not to increase dose or dosing frequency. Inform that disintegrating tabs contain phenylalanine.

DESONATE — desonide   Rx
Class: Corticosteroid

ADULT DOSAGE	PEDIATRIC DOSAGE
Atopic Dermatitis	**Atopic Dermatitis**
Mild to Moderate:	**Mild to Moderate:**
Apply thin layer bid to affected area(s)	**≥3 Months of Age:**
D/C when control is achieved	Apply thin layer bid to affected area(s)
If no improvement seen within 4 weeks, reassessment of diagnosis may be necessary	D/C when control is achieved
Max Duration: 4 consecutive weeks	If no improvement seen within 4 weeks, reassessment of diagnosis may be necessary
	Max Duration: 4 consecutive weeks

ADMINISTRATION
Topical route

Rub in gently

Do not use with occlusive dressings

Avoid contact with eyes or other mucous membranes

STORAGE
25°C (77°F), excursions permitted to 15-30°C (59-86°F).

HOW SUPPLIED
Gel: 0.05% [60g]

CONTRAINDICATIONS
History of hypersensitivity to any of the components of the preparation.

WARNINGS/PRECAUTIONS
May produce reversible hypothalamic-pituitary-adrenal (HPA) axis suppression, Cushing's syndrome, hyperglycemia, and may unmask latent diabetes mellitus (DM). Predisposing factors in patients using topical corticosteroids to HPA axis suppression include use of more potent steroids, over large surface areas, over prolonged periods, under occlusion, on an altered skin barrier, and use in patients with liver failure. Periodic evaluation for HPA axis suppression maybe required due to potential absorption. Pediatric patients may be more susceptible to systemic toxicity. Striae, linear growth retardation, delayed weight gain and intracranial hypertension reported in infants and children. Local adverse reactions may be more likely to occur with occlusive dressings, prolonged use or use of higher potency corticosteroids. If concomitant skin infections are present or develop during treatment, appropriate antifungal or antibacterial agent should be used; if favorable response does not occur promptly, d/c until infection is adequately controlled. D/C if skin irritation develops. Not for oral, ophthalmic, or intravaginal use.

ADVERSE REACTIONS
Application-site reactions, adrenal suppression.

DRUG INTERACTIONS
Use of desonide with other corticosteroid-containing products may increase the total systemic exposure.

PREGNANCY AND LACTATION
Category C, caution in nursing.

MECHANISM OF ACTION
Corticosteroid; mechanism not established.

PHARMACOKINETICS
Absorption: Percutaneous. Occlusion, inflammation and/or other disease processes may increase absorption. **Distribution:** Systemically administered corticosteroids appear in breast milk. **Metabolism:** Liver. **Elimination:** Kidneys and bile.

PATIENT CONSIDERATIONS
Assessment: Assess for use with other potent steroids, altered skin barrier, liver failure, DM, infections, hypersensitivity and pregnancy/nursing status.

Monitoring: Monitor for signs/symptoms of HPA-axis suppression, Cushing's syndrome, hyperglycemia, and unmasked latent DM. Perform periodic monitoring for HPA-axis suppression through the cosyntropin or ACTH stimulation test. Monitor for local irritation and allergic dermatitis. In pediatric patients, monitor for systemic toxicity, HPA-axis suppression, Cushing's syndrome, linear growth retardation, delayed weight gain, and intracranial HTN.

Counseling: Advise to use exactly as directed. Inform that medication is for external use only; avoid contact with eyes and other mucous membranes. Instruct not to bandage or cover treated skin area unless directed by a physician. Advise that medication should not be used on underarm or in groin areas unless directed by a physician. Advise not to use in treatment of diaper dermatitis; should not be applied in the diaper area, or with diapers or plastic pants. Instruct to notify physician before using any other corticosteroids, if local adverse effects develop, or if no clinical improvement is seen after 4 weeks of therapy.

DETROL LA — tolterodine tartrate   Rx
Class: Muscarinic antagonist

OTHER BRAND NAMES
Detrol

ADULT DOSAGE	PEDIATRIC DOSAGE
Overactive Bladder	Pediatric use may not have been established
Cap, Extended-Release:	
Usual: 4mg qd; may be lowered to 2mg qd based on response and tolerability	
Tab:	
Usual: 2mg bid; may be lowered to 1mg bid based on response and tolerability	

DOSING CONSIDERATIONS
Concomitant Medications
Potent CYP3A4 Inhibitors:
Cap, ER:
Usual: 2mg qd

Tab:
Usual: 1mg bid

Renal Impairment
Cap, ER:
CrCl 10-30mL/min:
Usual: 2mg qd
CrCl <10mL/min: Not recommended

Tab:
Significantly Reduced Renal Function:
Usual: 1mg bid

Hepatic Impairment
Cap, ER:
Mild to Moderate (Child-Pugh Class A or B):
Usual: 2mg qd
Severe (Child-Pugh Class C): Not recommended

Tab:
Significantly Reduced Hepatic Function:
Usual: 1mg bid

ADMINISTRATION
Oral route

Cap, ER
Take w/ water and swallow whole

STORAGE
(Tab): 25°C (77°F); excursions permitted to 15-30°C (59-86°F). (Cap, ER): 20-25°C (68-77°F); excursions permitted to 15-30°C (59-86°F). Protect from light.

HOW SUPPLIED
Cap, ER: (Detrol LA) 2mg, 4mg; **Tab:** (Detrol) 1mg, 2mg

CONTRAINDICATIONS
Urinary/gastric retention, uncontrolled narrow-angle glaucoma, known hypersensitivity to the drug or its ingredients, or to fesoterodine fumarate extended-release tablets.

WARNINGS/PRECAUTIONS
Anaphylaxis/angioedema requiring hospitalization and emergency treatment occurred with 1st or subsequent doses; d/c and provide appropriate therapy if difficulty in breathing, upper airway obstruction, or fall in BP occurs. Risk of urinary retention; caution in patients with clinically significant bladder outflow obstruction. Risk of gastric retention; caution in patients with GI obstructive disorders (eg, pyloric stenosis). Caution with decreased GI motility (eg, intestinal atony), myasthenia gravis, known history of QT prolongation, hepatic/renal impairment, and in patients being treated for narrow-angle glaucoma. CNS anticholinergic effects (eg, dizziness, somnolence) reported; may impair physical/ mental abilities. Monitor for signs of anticholinergic CNS effects (particularly after beginning treatment and increasing the dose); consider dose reduction or d/c if such effects occur.

ADVERSE REACTIONS
Dry mouth, dizziness, headache, abdominal pain, constipation.

DRUG INTERACTIONS
Caution with Class IA (eg, quinidine, procainamide) or Class III (eg, amiodarone, sotalol) antiarrhythmics. May aggravate dementia symptoms when initiating therapy in patients taking cholinesterase inhibitors. Increased concentrations with ketoconazole or other potent CYP3A4 inhibitors (eg, itraconazole, miconazole, clarithromycin). Increased levels with fluoxetine reported with IR tolterodine. May increase the frequency and/or severity of anticholinergic effects with other anticholinergic (antimuscarinic) agents.

PREGNANCY AND LACTATION
Category C, not for use in nursing.

MECHANISM OF ACTION
Muscarinic receptor antagonist; competitive antagonist of acetylcholine at postganglionic muscarinic receptors mediating urinary bladder contraction and salivation via cholinergic muscarinic receptors.

PHARMACOKINETICS
Absorption: Administration of variable doses resulted in different parameters in extensive metabolizers (EMs) and poor metabolizers (PMs) of CYP2D6. (Tab)

Rapid. **Distribution:** Plasma protein binding (96.3%); (IV) V_d=113L. **Metabolism:** Liver (extensive); oxidation to 5-hydroxymethyl tolterodine (active metabolite) via CYP2D6; dealkylation via CYP3A4 (PMs). **Elimination:** Urine (77%), feces (17%). (Tab) Single Dose: EMs: $T_{1/2}$=2 hrs; PMs: $T_{1/2}$=6.5 hrs. (Cap, ER) Single Dose: EMs: $T_{1/2}$=8.4 hrs.

PATIENT CONSIDERATIONS

Assessment: Assess for hypersensitivity to the drug or fesoterodine fumarate, urinary/gastric retention, bladder outflow obstruction, GI obstructive disorders, decreased GI motility, narrow-angle glaucoma, myasthenia gravis, history of QT prolongation, hepatic/renal impairment, pregnancy/nursing status, and possible drug interactions.

Monitoring: Monitor for anaphylaxis, angioedema, difficulty breathing, upper airway obstruction, fall in BP, urinary retention, gastric retention, CNS anticholinergic effects, QT prolongation, hypersensitivity reactions, and other adverse reactions.

Counseling: Inform patients that drug may produce blurred vision, dizziness, or drowsiness. Advise to exercise caution against potentially dangerous activities until drug's effects have been determined.

DEXAMETHASONE ORAL — dexamethasone   Rx

Class: Glucocorticoid

ADULT DOSAGE
Steroid-Responsive Disorders

Initial: 0.75-9mg/day depending on disease

Maint: Decrease in small amounts at appropriate time intervals to lowest effective dose; may need to increase dose for a period of time in stressful situations

Upon discontinuation after long-term therapy, withdraw gradually

Cushing's Syndrome Test:
1mg at 11 pm; draw blood at 8 am next morning.
Alternately, may give 0.5mg q6h for 48 hrs for greater accuracy.
Obtain 24-hr urine collections.

Test to Distinguish Cushing's Syndrome Due to Pituitary ACTH Excess from Cushing's Syndrome Due to Other Causes:
2mg q6h for 48 hrs; obtain 24-hr urine collections

Elixir:
Less Severe Diseases: <0.75mg may suffice
Severe Diseases: >9mg may be required

D/C and transfer to other therapy if satisfactory clinical response does not occur after a reasonable period of time

Oral Sol/Tab:
Acute Exacerbations of Multiple Sclerosis: 30mg/day for 1 week, then 4-12mg qod for 1 month

Acute, Self-Limited Allergic Disorders/Acute Exacerbations of Chronic Allergic Disorders:
Day 1: 1 or 2mL IM of 4mg/mL dexamethasone sodium phosphate inj
Day 2-3: Four 0.75mg tabs in 2 divided doses
Day 4: Two 0.75mg tabs in 2 divided doses
Day 5-6: One 0.75mg tab/day
Day 7: No treatment
Day 8: Follow-up visit

Palliative Management of Recurrent or Inoperable Brain Tumors:
Maint: 2mg bid or tid

DOSING CONSIDERATIONS
Elderly
Start at lower end of dosing range

ADMINISTRATION
Oral route

Intensol
Mix w/ liquid or semi-solid food (eg, water, juices, soda or soda-like beverages, applesauce, pudding); stir liquid or food gently for a few seconds.
Consume immediately; do not store for future use.
Use only calibrated dropper provided.

PEDIATRIC DOSAGE
Steroid-Responsive Disorders

Oral Sol/Tab:
Initial: 0.02-0.3mg/kg/day in 3 or 4 divided doses (0.6-9mg/m²BSA/day) depending on the disease
Maint: Decrease in small amounts at appropriate time intervals to lowest effective dose; may need to increase dose for a period of time in stressful situations

Upon discontinuation after long-term therapy, withdraw gradually

Cushing's Syndrome Test:
1mg at 11 pm; draw blood at 8 am next morning.
Alternately, may give 0.5mg q6h for 48 hrs for greater accuracy.
Obtain 24-hr urine collections.

Test to Distinguish Cushing's Syndrome Due to Pituitary ACTH Excess from Cushing's Syndrome Due to Other Causes:
2mg q6h for 48 hrs; obtain 24-hr urine collections

Elixir
When large doses are given, may take w/ meals and antacids in between meals to help prevent peptic ulcer.

STORAGE
20-25°C (68-77°F). **Elixir:** Do not freeze. **Intensol:** Do not freeze. Discard opened bottle after 90 days.

HOW SUPPLIED
Elixir: 0.5mg/5mL [237mL]; **Oral Sol:** 0.5mg/5mL [240mL, 500mL], (Intensol) 1mg/mL [30mL]; **Tab:** 0.5mg*, 0.75mg*, 1mg*, 1.5mg*, 2mg*, 4mg*, 6mg* *scored

CONTRAINDICATIONS
Known systemic fungal infections, known hypersensitivity to the medication.

WARNINGS/PRECAUTIONS
May cause BP elevation, salt/water retention, and increased K^+ and Ca^{2+} excretion; dietary salt restriction and K^+ supplementation may be necessary. May cause left ventricular free-wall rupture after a recent MI; use w/ caution. May mask signs of current infection. May increase susceptibility to infections. Rule out latent or active amebiasis before initiating therapy. Use lowest possible dose to control treatment condition; reduce gradually if dosage reduction is possible. Caution w/ active/latent tuberculosis or tuberculin reactivity, active/latent peptic ulcers, diverticulitis, fresh intestinal anastomoses, nonspecific ulcerative colitis, HTN, and renal insufficiency. May have negative effects on pediatric growth; monitor growth and development of pediatric patients on prolonged use. May increase or decrease motility and number of spermatozoa in some patients. Enhanced effect in patients w/ cirrhosis. More serious/fatal course of chickenpox and measles reported; avoid exposure in patients who have not had these diseases. May produce posterior subcapsular cataracts, glaucoma w/ possible optic nerve damage, and enhance establishment of secondary ocular infections. Drug-induced secondary adrenocortical insufficiency may be minimized by gradual dose reduction. Psychic derangements and aggravation of emotional instability or psychotic tendencies may occur. Fat embolism reported. May suppress reactions to skin tests. False (-) dexamethasone suppression test results in patients being treated w/ indomethacin reported. **Elixir:** Prolongation of coma and high incidence of pneumonia and GI bleeding in patients w/ cerebral malaria reported. Enhanced effect in patients w/ hypothyroidism. Caution w/ ocular herpes simplex, osteoporosis, and myasthenia gravis. Withdrawal syndrome reported following prolonged use. May affect the nitroblue-tetrazolium test for bacterial infection and produce false (-) results. **Sol/Tab:** Anaphylactoid reactions may occur. Caution w/ CHF. May produce reversible hypothalamic-pituitary-adrenal axis suppression w/ the potential for corticosteroid insufficiency after withdrawal. Metabolic clearance is decreased in hypothyroid patients and increased in hyperthyroid patients; changes in thyroid status may necessitate dose adjustment. May activate latent disease or exacerbate intercurrent infections. May exacerbate systemic fungal infections; avoid use unless needed to control life-threatening drug reactions. May increase risk of GI perforation w/ certain GI disorders. Caution w/ known or suspected *Strongyloides* infestation. Not for use in cerebral malaria and active ocular herpes simplex. Not recommended in optic neuritis treatment. Kaposi's sarcoma reported. Signs of peritoneal irritation following GI perforation may be minimal/absent. Acute myopathy reported w/ use of high doses. Creatinine kinase elevation may occur. May elevate IOP; monitor IOP if used for >6 weeks.

ADVERSE REACTIONS
Fluid retention, Na^+ retention, muscle weakness, osteoporosis, peptic ulcer, pancreatitis, ulcerative esophagitis, impaired wound healing, headache, psychic disturbances, growth suppression (pediatrics), glaucoma, weight gain, nausea, malaise.

DRUG INTERACTIONS
Live or live, attenuated vaccines are contraindicated w/ immunosuppressive doses. May diminish response to toxoids and live or inactivated vaccines. Observe closely for hypokalemia w/ K^+-depleting agents (eg, amphotericin B, diuretics). Dose adjustment of antidiabetic agents may be required. Barbiturates, phenytoin, and rifampin may enhance metabolism; may need to increase corticosteroid dose. Caution w/ aspirin (ASA) in patients w/ hypoprothrombinemia. Ephedrine may enhance metabolic clearance; may require an increase in corticosteroid dose. **Elixir:** Phenobarbital may enhance the metabolic clearance; may require adjustment of corticosteroid dose. Monitor PT frequently w/ coumarin anticoagulants. **Oral Sol/Tab:** May potentiate replication of some organisms contained in live, attenuated vaccines. D/C anticholinesterase agents at least 24 hrs before start of therapy. Monitor coagulation indices w/ warfarin. Hepatic enzyme inducers (eg, carbamazepine) may enhance metabolism; may need to increase corticosteroid dose. CYP3A4 inhibitors may increase plasma concentrations. May decrease plasma concentrations of CYP3A4 substrates (eg, indinavir). Convulsions and increased activity of both drugs reported w/ cyclosporine. May increase risk of arrhythmias due to hypokalemia w/ digitalis glycosides. Estrogens and ketoconazole may decrease metabolism. ASA or other NSAIDs may increase risk of GI side effects. May increase clearance of salicylates. Acute myopathy reported w/ neuromuscular-blocking drugs (eg, pancuronium). May decrease concentrations of isoniazid. Cholestyramine may increase clearance. Cardiac enlargement and CHF reported when hydrocortisone is used w/ amphotericin B. Aminoglutethimide may diminish adrenal suppression. Macrolide antibiotics may decrease clearance. May increase and decrease levels of phenytoin, leading to alterations in seizure control. Caution w/ thalidomide; toxic epidermal necrolysis reported.

PREGNANCY AND LACTATION
Pregnancy: (Sol/Tab) Category C; (Elixir) Weigh anticipated benefits against possible hazards to the mother and embryo or fetus.
Lactation: Systemically administered corticosteroids appear in human milk and could suppress growth, interfere w/ endogenous corticosteroid production, or cause other untoward effects. Not for use in nursing.

MECHANISM OF ACTION
Glucocorticoid; produces anti-inflammatory effects.

PHARMACOKINETICS
Distribution: Found in breast milk.

PATIENT CONSIDERATIONS
Assessment: Assess for current infections, systemic fungal infections, latent/active amebiasis, cerebral malaria, ocular herpes simplex, cirrhosis, emotional instability or psychotic tendencies, any condition where treatment is cautioned, pregnancy/nursing status, and possible drug interactions. Assess thyroid status and vaccination history.

Monitoring: Monitor for Na+/water retention, infections/secondary ocular infections, changes in thyroid status, posterior subcapsular cataracts, glaucoma, optic nerve damage, Kaposi's sarcoma, development of osteoporosis, acute myopathy, creatinine kinase elevation, psychic derangements, emotional instability or psychotic tendencies aggravation, and other adverse effects. Monitor IOP, BP, and serum K+ and Ca2+ levels. Monitor bone growth and development in pediatric patients.

Counseling: Instruct not to d/c therapy abruptly or w/o medical supervision. Advise to inform any medical attendants about current corticosteroid therapies. Instruct to seek medical advice if an acute illness including fever or other signs of infection develop. Advise to avoid exposure to chickenpox or measles; if exposed, instruct to seek medical advice w/o delay.

DEXEDRINE SPANSULE — dextroamphetamine sulfate   CII
Class: CNS stimulant

> High potential for abuse. Prolonged use may lead to drug dependence and must be avoided. Misuse may cause sudden death and serious cardiovascular (CV) adverse events.

ADULT DOSAGE
Narcolepsy

Individualize dose and administer at the lowest effective dose

Initial: 10mg/day
Titrate: May increase daily dose in increments of 10mg at weekly intervals until optimal response is obtained
Usual: 5-60mg/day in divided doses

PEDIATRIC DOSAGE
Narcolepsy

Individualize dose and administer at the lowest effective dose

Usual: 5-60mg/day in divided doses

6-12 Years:
Initial: 5mg/day
Titrate: May increase daily dose in increments of 5mg at weekly intervals until optimal response is obtained

≥12 Years:
Initial: 10mg/day
Titrate: May increase daily dose in increments of 10mg at weekly intervals until optimal response is obtained

Attention-Deficit Hyperactivity Disorder

Individualize dose and administer at the lowest effective dose

≥6 Years:
Initial: 5mg qd or bid
Titrate: May increase daily dose in increments of 5mg at weekly intervals until optimal response is obtained

Only rarely will it be necessary to exceed 40mg/day

DOSING CONSIDERATIONS
Adverse Reactions
Narcolepsy:
Reduce dose if bothersome adverse reactions appear (eg, insomnia or anorexia)

ADMINISTRATION
Oral route

Avoid late pm doses
May be used for once-a-day dosage wherever appropriate

STORAGE
20-25°C (68-77°F).

HOW SUPPLIED
Cap, Sustained-Release: 5mg, 10mg, 15mg

CONTRAINDICATIONS
Advanced arteriosclerosis, symptomatic CV disease (CVD), moderate to severe HTN, hyperthyroidism, known hypersensitivity or idiosyncrasy to sympathomimetic amines, glaucoma, agitated states, and history of drug abuse. During or w/in 14 days following MAOI use.

WARNINGS/PRECAUTIONS
Avoid w/ known serious structural cardiac abnormalities, cardiomyopathy, serious heart rhythm abnormalities, coronary artery disease, or other serious cardiac problems. Sudden death reported in children and adolescents w/ structural cardiac abnormalities or other serious heart problems. Sudden death, stroke, and MI reported in adults. May cause a modest increase in average BP and HR. Promptly perform cardiac evaluation if symptoms suggestive of cardiac disease develop during treatment. May exacerbate symptoms of behavior disturbance and thought disorder in patients w/ preexisting psychotic disorder. Caution w/ comorbid bipolar disorder; may induce mixed/manic episode. May cause treatment-emergent psychotic or manic symptoms in children and adolescents w/o a prior history of psychotic illness or mania; consider discontinuation if such symptoms occur. Aggressive behavior or hostility reported in children and adolescents w/ ADHD. May cause long-term suppression of growth in children. May lower convulsive threshold; d/c if seizures occur. Associated w/ peripheral vasculopathy, including Raynaud's phenomenon. Difficulties w/ accommodation and blurring of vision reported. May exacerbate motor and phonic tics, and Tourette's syndrome. May significantly elevate plasma corticosteroid levels and interfere w/ urinary steroid determinations. In patients w/ ADHD, where possible, interrupt administration occasionally to determine if there is a recurrence of behavioral symptoms sufficient to require continued therapy.

ADVERSE REACTIONS
Palpitations, tachycardia, BP elevation, dizziness, insomnia, euphoria, dyskinesia, headache, dryness of mouth, diarrhea, constipation, urticaria, impotence, changes in libido, rhabdomyolysis.

DRUG INTERACTIONS
See Contraindications. GI acidifying agents (eg, guanethidine, reserpine, glutamic acid HCl) and urinary acidifying agents (eg, ammonium chloride, sodium acid phosphate) lower blood levels and efficacy. Inhibits adrenergic blockers. GI alkalinizing agents (eg, sodium bicarbonate) and urinary alkalinizing agents (eg, acetazolamide, some thiazides) increase blood levels and therefore potentiate actions. May enhance activity of TCAs or sympathomimetic agents. Desipramine or protriptyline and possibly other TCAs cause striking and sustained increases in the concentration of *d*-amphetamine in the brain; CV effects can be potentiated. May counteract sedative effect of antihistamines. May antagonize hypotensive effects of antihypertensives. Chlorpromazine and haloperidol inhibit central stimulant effects. May delay intestinal absorption of ethosuximide, phenobarbital, and phenytoin; coadministration w/ phenobarbital or phenytoin may produce a synergistic anticonvulsant action. Lithium carbonate may inhibit stimulatory effects. Potentiates analgesic effect of meperidine. Acidifying agents used in methenamine therapy increase urinary excretion and reduce efficacy. Enhances adrenergic effect of norepinephrine. In cases of propoxyphene overdosage, CNS stimulation is potentiated and fatal convulsions can occur. Inhibits hypotensive effect of veratrum alkaloids.

PREGNANCY AND LACTATION
Category C, not for use in nursing.

MECHANISM OF ACTION
Sympathomimetic amine; not established. Has CNS stimulant activity.

PHARMACOKINETICS
Absorption: (15mg cap) C_{max}=23.5ng/mL; T_{max}=8 hrs. **Distribution:** Found in breast milk. **Elimination:** $T_{1/2}$=12 hrs.

PATIENT CONSIDERATIONS
Assessment: Assess for hypersensitivity/idiosyncrasy to sympathomimetic amines, advanced arteriosclerosis, symptomatic CVD, moderate to severe HTN, hyperthyroidism, glaucoma, agitated states, history of drug abuse, tics, Tourette's syndrome, preexisting psychotic disorder, risk for/comorbid bipolar disorder, cardiac disease, medical conditions that might be compromised by increases in BP or HR, family history of sudden death or ventricular arrhythmia, any other conditions where treatment is cautioned, pregnancy/nursing status, and possible drug interactions.

Monitoring: Monitor for changes in HR and BP, signs/symptoms of cardiac disease, exacerbation of behavioral disturbance and thought disorder, psychosis, mania, appearance of or worsening of aggressive behavior or hostility, seizures, peripheral vasculopathy, visual disturbances, exacerbation of motor and phonic tics or Tourette's syndrome, and other adverse reactions. In pediatric patients, monitor growth.

Counseling: Inform about benefits and risks of treatment and counsel about appropriate use. Counsel that drug has high potential for abuse. Caution against engaging in potentially hazardous activities (eg, operating machinery/vehicles). Instruct to report to physician any new numbness, pain, skin color change, or sensitivity to temperature in fingers or toes, and to contact physician immediately w/ any signs of unexplained wounds appearing on fingers or toes while taking the drug.

DEXILANT — dexlansoprazole   Rx
Class: Proton pump inhibitor (PPI)

OTHER BRAND NAMES
Dexilant SoluTab

ADULT DOSAGE
Erosive Esophagitis

Healing:
Cap:
60mg qd for up to 8 weeks

Maint of Healed Erosive Esophagitis (EE) and Relief of Heartburn:
Cap/Tab, Disintegrating:
30mg qd for up to 6 months

Symptomatic Nonerosive Gastroesophageal Reflux Disease

Cap/Tab, Disintegrating:
30mg qd for 4 weeks

PEDIATRIC DOSAGE
Erosive Esophagitis

Healing:
≥12 Years:
Cap:
60mg qd for up to 8 weeks

Maint of Healed EE and Relief of Heartburn:
12-17 Years:
Cap/Tab, Disintegrating:
30mg qd for up to 16 weeks

Symptomatic Nonerosive Gastroesophageal Reflux Disease

≥12 Years:
Cap/Tab, Disintegrating:
30mg qd for 4 weeks

DOSING CONSIDERATIONS
Hepatic Impairment
Healing of EE:
Moderate (Child-Pugh Class B): 30mg qd for up to 8 weeks
Severe (Child-Pugh Class C): Not recommended

ADMINISTRATION
Oral route
Two 30mg orally disintegrating tabs are not interchangeable w/ one 60mg cap.

Cap
Take w/o regard to food.
Swallow cap whole; do not chew.

Administration w/ Applesauce:
1. Open cap and sprinkle intact granules on 1 tbsp of applesauce.
2. Swallow immediately; do not chew granules.
3. Do not save applesauce and granules for later use.

Administration w/ Water in an Oral Syringe:
1. Open the cap and empty granules into 20mL of water.
2. Withdraw entire mixture into a syringe and gently swirl syringe.
3. Administer immediately.
4. Refill syringe 2 more times w/ 10mL of water, swirl gently, and administer.

Administration w/ Water via NG Tube (≥16 French):
1. Open the cap and empty the granules into 20mL of water.
2. Withdraw entire mixture into a catheter-tip syringe.
3. Swirl catheter-tip syringe gently and immediately inject the mixture through the NG tube into the stomach. Do not save water and granule mixture for later use.
4. Refill catheter-tip syringe w/ 10mL of water, swirl gently, and flush the tube.
5. Refill catheter-tip syringe again w/ 10mL of water, swirl gently, and administer.

Tab, Disintegrating
Take at least 30 min before a meal.
Do not break or cut.
Place tab on tongue, allow it to disintegrate, and swallow w/o water; do not chew. May also be swallowed whole w/ water.

Administration w/ Water in an Oral Syringe:
1. Place 1 tab in an oral syringe and draw up 20mL of water.
2. Swirl gently.
3. After tab has dispersed, immediately administer contents into the mouth; do not save water and microgranule mixture for later use.
4. Refill syringe w/ approx 10mL of water, swirl gently, and administer any remaining contents.
5. Refill syringe again w/ approx 10mL of water, swirl gently, and administer any remaining contents.

Administration w/ Water via NG Tube (≥8 French):
1. Place tab in a catheter-tip syringe and draw up 20mL of water.
2. Shake gently.
3. After tab has dispersed, swirl catheter-tip syringe gently, and immediately inject the mixture through the NG tube into the stomach; do not save the water and microgranule mixture for later use.
4. Refill catheter-tip syringe w/ approx 10mL of water, shake gently, and flush the tube.
5. Refill the catheter-tip syringe again w/ 10mL of water, swirl gently, and administer.

STORAGE
20-25°C (68-77°F); excursions permitted to 15-30°C (59-86°F).

HOW SUPPLIED
Cap, Delayed-Release: 30mg, 60mg; **Tab, Disintegrating:** 30mg

CONTRAINDICATIONS
Hypersensitivity to any component of the formulation. Concomitant use w/ rilpivirine-containing products.

WARNINGS/PRECAUTIONS
Symptomatic response does not preclude the presence of gastric malignancy. Acute interstitial nephritis reported; d/c if this develops. Cyanocobalamin (vitamin B12) deficiency may occur due to malabsorption w/ daily long-term treatment (eg, >3 yrs) w/ any acid-suppressing medications. May increase risk of *Clostridium difficile*-associated diarrhea (CDAD), especially in hospitalized patients. May increase risk for osteoporosis-related fractures of the hip, wrist, or spine, especially w/ high-dose and long-term therapy (≥1 yr). Use lowest dose and shortest duration appropriate to the conditions being treated. Hypomagnesemia reported and may require Mg^{2+} replacement and discontinuation of therapy; consider monitoring Mg^{2+} levels prior to and periodically during therapy in patients on prolonged treatment or if taking concomitant drugs such as digoxin or drugs that may cause hypomagnesemia (eg, diuretics). Serum chromogranin A (CgA) levels increase secondary to drug-induced decreases in gastric acidity. Increased CgA level may cause false positive results in diagnostic investigations for neuroendocrine tumors; temporarily stop therapy at least 14 days before assessing CgA levels and consider repeating test if initial CgA levels are high. The same commercial laboratory should be used for testing if serial tests are performed (eg, for monitoring). May interact w/ secretin stimulation test; temporarily stop dexlansoprazole treatment at least 30 days before assessing to allow gastrin levels to return to baseline. False positive urine screening tests for tetrahydrocannabinol reported; consider an alternative confirmatory method to verify positive results.

ADVERSE REACTIONS
Adults: Diarrhea, abdominal pain, N/V, URTI, flatulence.
Pediatrics 12-17 Years: Headache, abdominal pain, diarrhea, nasopharyngitis, oropharyngeal pain.

DRUG INTERACTIONS
See Contraindications. May decrease exposure of some antiretroviral drugs (eg, rilpivirine, atazanavir, nelfinavir) and may reduce antiviral effect and promote the development of drug resistance; avoid use w/ nelfinavir. May increase exposure of some antiretroviral drugs (eg, saquinavir) and may increase toxicity of the antiretroviral drugs; monitor for potential saquinavir toxicities. Concomitant use w/ warfarin may increase INR and PT; monitor INR and PT. Dose adjustment of warfarin may be needed. May elevate and prolong levels of methotrexate (MTX) and/or its metabolite, possibly leading to toxicities; consider temporary withdrawal of dexlansoprazole in some patients receiving high-dose MTX. May increase digoxin exposure; monitor digoxin concentrations. A dose adjustment of digoxin may be needed to maintain therapeutic drug concentrations. May reduce absorption of drugs dependent on gastric pH for absorption (eg, iron salts, erlotinib, dasatinib, nilotinib, mycophenolate mofetil [MMF], ketoconazole, itraconazole). Caution in transplant patients receiving MMF. May increase exposure of tacrolimus, especially in transplant patients who are intermediate or poor metabolizers of CYP2C19; monitor tacrolimus whole blood trough concentrations. A dose adjustment of tacrolimus may be needed. Strong CYP2C19 or CYP3A4 inducers (St. John's wort, rifampin, ritonavir-containing products) may decrease exposure; avoid concomitant use w/ St. John's wort or rifampin. Strong CYP2C19 or CYP3A4 inhibitors (eg, voriconazole) may increase exposure. Alcohol may modify the release rate of dexlansoprazole from the orally disintegrating tab (ODT) and may lead to decreased efficacy; avoid alcoholic beverages when taking the ODT. Refer to the prescribing information of the concomitant medication used w/ dexlansoprazole for further information.

PREGNANCY AND LACTATION
Pregnancy: There are no studies w/ dexlansoprazole use in pregnant women to inform a drug-associated risk.
Lactation: There is no information regarding the presence of dexlansoprazole in human milk, the effects on the breastfed infant, or the effects on milk production; caution in nursing.

MECHANISM OF ACTION
Proton pump inhibitor; suppresses gastric acid secretion by specific inhibition of the (H^+/K^+)-ATPase in the gastric parietal cell. Blocks the final step of acid production.

PHARMACOKINETICS
Absorption: Adults: C_{max}=658ng/mL (30mg cap), 1397ng/mL (60mg cap); AUC_{24}=3275ng•hr/mL (30mg cap), 6529ng•hr/mL (60mg cap); (Cap) T_{max}=1-2 hrs (1st peak), 4-5 hrs (2nd peak); (ODT) C_{max}=688ng/mL; AUC=2866ng•hr/mL; T_{max}=4 hrs (median). Refer to prescribing information for information on pediatric patients. **Distribution:** V_d=40L; plasma protein binding (96-99%). **Metabolism:** Liver (extensive) via CYP3A4 (oxidation) and CYP2C19 (hydroxylation). **Elimination:** Urine (50.7%), feces (47.6%); $T_{1/2}$=1-2 hrs.

PATIENT CONSIDERATIONS
Assessment: Assess for hypersensitivity to the drug, risk for osteoporosis-related fractures, hepatic impairment, pregnancy/nursing status, possible lab test interactions, and for possible drug interactions. Obtain baseline Mg^{2+} levels.

Monitoring: Monitor for signs/symptoms of acute interstitial nephritis, cyanocobalamin deficiency, CDAD, bone fractures, hypersensitivity reactions, and other adverse reactions. Monitor Mg^{2+} levels periodically. Monitor INR and PT when given w/ warfarin.

Counseling: Advise to notify physician if any signs/symptoms consistent w/ a hypersensitivity reaction, acute interstitial nephritis, cyanocobalamin deficiency, CDAD, bone fracture, and/or hypomagnesemia occur. Instruct to notify physician if taking any concomitant medication (eg, high-dose MTX). Instruct how to take cap and ODT.

DIABETA — glyburide   Rx
Class: Sulfonylurea (2nd generation)

ADULT DOSAGE	PEDIATRIC DOSAGE
Type 2 Diabetes Mellitus	Pediatric use may not have been established
Initial: 2.5-5mg qd; 1.25mg qd if more sensitive to hypoglycemic drugs	
Titrate: Increase by ≤2.5mg at weekly intervals	
Maint: 1.25-20mg/day as single dose or in divided doses	
Max: 20mg/day	
Transferring from Other Oral Antidiabetic Agents:	
Initial: 2.5-5mg qd	
No transition period or initial priming dose necessary	
Monitor carefully during 1st two weeks when transitioning from chlorpropamide, due to overlapping drug effects	
Transferring from Insulin:	
Insulin Dose <20 U/Day: 2.5-5mg qd	
Insulin Dose 20-40 U/Day: 5mg qd	

Insulin Dose >40 U/Day:
Decrease insulin dose by 50% and start w/ 5mg qd
Progressively withdraw insulin and increase dose in increments of 1.25-2.5mg every 2-10 days

DOSING CONSIDERATIONS
Concomitant Medications
Colesevelam: Administer at least 4 hrs prior to colesevelam
Renal Impairment
Initial/Maint: Dose conservatively
Hepatic Impairment
Initial/Maint: Dose conservatively
Elderly
Elderly/Debilitated/Malnourished:
Initial/Maint: Dose conservatively

ADMINISTRATION
Oral route
Take w/ breakfast or 1st main meal.

STORAGE
25°C (77°F); excursions permitted to 15-30°C (59-86°F).

HOW SUPPLIED
Tab: 1.25mg*, 2.5mg*, 5mg* *scored

CONTRAINDICATIONS
Known hypersensitivity or allergy to the drug or any of its excipients. Type 1 DM or diabetic ketoacidosis, with or without coma. Coadministration with bosentan.

WARNINGS/PRECAUTIONS
Caution during the first 2 weeks of therapy if transferring from chlorpropamide. May be associated with increased cardiovascular (CV) mortality. May produce severe hypoglycemia; increased risk when caloric intake is deficient, after severe/prolonged exercise, with severe renal/hepatic insufficiency, with adrenal/pituitary insufficiency, or in elderly, debilitated, or malnourished patients. Loss of glycemic control may occur when exposed to stress (eg, fever, trauma, infection, surgery); may be necessary to d/c therapy and administer insulin. Secondary failure may occur over a period of time. May cause hemolytic anemia; caution with G6PD deficiency and consider a non-sulfonylurea alternative. Caution in elderly. Not bioequivalent to Glynase PresTab and therefore not substitutable.

ADVERSE REACTIONS
Hypoglycemia, nausea, epigastric fullness, heartburn, hyponatremia, LFT abnormalities, photosensitivity reactions, leukopenia, agranulocytosis, thrombocytopenia, porphyria cutanea tarda, blurred vision, changes in accommodation, angioedema, arthralgia.

DRUG INTERACTIONS
See Contraindications and Dosage. Hypoglycemic effects may be potentiated by NSAIDs, ACE-inhibitors, disopyramide, fluoxetine, clarithromycin, fluoroquinolones, other highly protein-bound drugs, salicylates, sulfonamides, chloramphenicol, probenecid, MAOIs, and β-adrenergic blocking drugs; monitor closely for hypoglycemia during coadministration and for loss of glycemic control when such drugs are withdrawn. Increased risk of hypoglycemia with alcohol or use of >1 glucose-lowering drug. May be difficult to recognize hypoglycemia with β-adrenergic blocking drugs or other sympatholytics. Potential interaction leading to severe hypoglycemia reported with oral miconazole. Potentiates or weakens effects of coumarin derivatives. Rifampin may worsen glucose control. Thiazides and other diuretics, corticosteroids, phenothiazines, thyroid products, estrogens, oral contraceptives, phenytoin, nicotinic acid, sympathomimetics, calcium channel blockers, and isoniazid may produce hyperglycemia and may lead to loss of glycemic control; monitor closely for loss of control during coadministration and for hypoglycemia when such drugs are withdrawn. May increase cyclosporine plasma levels and toxicity; monitor and adjust dosage of cyclosporine. Colesevelam may decrease levels. Caution with inducers/inhibitors of CYP2C9.

PREGNANCY AND LACTATION
Category C, not for use in nursing.

MECHANISM OF ACTION
Sulfonylurea (2nd generation); acts by stimulating insulin release from functioning pancreatic β-cells.

PHARMACOKINETICS
Absorption: T_{max}=4 hrs. **Distribution:** Plasma protein binding (extensive). **Metabolism:** 4-trans-hydroxy derivative (major metabolite). **Elimination:** Bile (50% metabolites), urine (50% metabolites); $T_{1/2}$=10 hrs.

PATIENT CONSIDERATIONS
Assessment: Assess for previous hypersensitivity to drug or other sulfonamide derivatives, type of DM, risk factors of hypoglycemia, renal/hepatic impairment, G6PD deficiency, pregnancy/nursing status, and possible drug interactions. Obtain baseline FPG and HbA1c levels.

Monitoring: Monitor for CV effects, hypoglycemia, loss of glycemic control when exposed to stress, hypersensitivity reactions, secondary failure, hemolytic anemia, and other adverse reactions. Monitor FPG and HbA1c levels periodically.

Counseling: Inform of the potential risks, benefits, and alternative modes of therapy. Counsel about importance of adherence to dietary instructions, regular exercise program, and regular testing of blood glucose. Inform about the symptoms, treatment, and predisposing conditions of hypoglycemia, as well as primary and secondary failure. During the insulin withdrawal period, instruct patients to test blood glucose and acetone in urine at least tid and report results to physician.

DIAMOX SEQUELS — acetazolamide   Rx
Class: Carbonic anhydrase inhibitor

ADULT DOSAGE
Glaucoma
Chronic Simple (Open-Angle) Glaucoma, Secondary Glaucoma, and Preoperatively in Acute Angle-Closure Glaucoma (Where Delay of Surgery is Desired in Order to Lower IOP):
Adjunctive Treatment:
Usual: 500mg bid (usually in am and in pm)
If adequate control is not obtained by bid administration, the desired control may be established by means of acetazolamide tabs or inj

Acute Mountain Sickness
Prevention/Amelioration of Symptoms Associated w/ Acute Mountain Sickness Despite Gradual Ascent:
Usual: 500-1000mg/day in divided doses; higher dose level of 1000mg is recommended in circumstances of rapid ascent
Initiate dosing 24-48 hrs before ascent and continue for 48 hrs while at high altitude, or longer as necessary

PEDIATRIC DOSAGE
Pediatric use may not have been established

DOSING CONSIDERATIONS
Elderly
Start at lower end of dosing range

ADMINISTRATION
Oral route

STORAGE
20-25°C (68-77°F).

HOW SUPPLIED
Cap, Extended-Release: 500mg

CONTRAINDICATIONS
Hypersensitivity to acetazolamide or any excipients in the formulation, depressed Na^+ and/or K^+ blood serum levels, marked kidney and liver disease/dysfunction, suprarenal gland failure, hyperchloremic acidosis, cirrhosis. (Long-term administration) Chronic noncongestive angle-closure glaucoma.

WARNINGS/PRECAUTIONS
Fatalities reported, although rarely, due to severe reactions to sulfonamides (eg, Stevens-Johnson syndrome, toxic epidermal necrolysis, fulminant hepatic necrosis, anaphylaxis, agranulocytosis, aplastic anemia, other blood dyscrasias); d/c if signs of hypersensitivity or other serious reactions occur. Sensitizations may recur when a sulfonamide is readministered irrespective of the route of administration. Increasing the dose does not increase the diuresis and may increase the incidence of drowsiness and/or paresthesia, and often results in a decrease in diuresis; under certain circumstances, very large doses have been given in conjunction with other diuretics to secure diuresis in complete refractory failure. Increase and decrease in blood glucose may occur; caution with impaired glucose tolerance or diabetes mellitus (DM). May cause electrolyte imbalances (eg, hyponatremia, hypokalemia) and metabolic acidosis; caution with conditions associated with, or that predispose a patient to, electrolyte and acid/base imbalances (eg, renal impairment, DM, impaired alveolar ventilation). Caution in elderly. May impair mental/physical abilities. Lab test interactions may occur. Growth retardation reported in children receiving long-term therapy.

ADVERSE REACTIONS
Headache, malaise, fatigue, fever, GI disturbances, abnormal LFTs, drowsiness, paresthesia, depression, excitement, hearing disturbances, tinnitus, transient myopia, crystalluria, hematuria.

DRUG INTERACTIONS
Caution with high-dose aspirin (ASA); anorexia, tachypnea, lethargy, metabolic acidosis, coma, and death reported. May increase phenytoin levels, which may increase/enhance occurrence of osteomalacia in some patients receiving chronic phenytoin therapy; caution during chronic concomitant therapy. May decrease concentrations of primidone and its metabolites, with a consequent possible decrease in anticonvulsant effect; caution when beginning, discontinuing, or changing the dose of acetazolamide. Possible additive effects with other carbonic anhydrase inhibitors; concomitant use is not advisable. May increase effects of other folic acid antagonists. Decreases urinary excretion of amphetamine and may enhance the magnitude and duration of their effect. Reduces urinary excretion of quinidine and may enhance its effect. May prevent urinary antiseptic effect of methenamine. May decrease lithium levels. Increased risk of renal calculus formation with sodium bicarbonate. May elevate cyclosporine levels.

PREGNANCY AND LACTATION
Category C, not for use in nursing.

MECHANISM OF ACTION

Carbonic anhydrase inhibitor; in the eye, decreases the secretion of aqueous humor and results in a drop in IOP. Diuretic effect is due to its action in the kidney on the reversible reaction involving hydration of carbon dioxide and dehydration of carbonic acid.

PHARMACOKINETICS

Absorption: T_{max}= 3-6 hrs.

PATIENT CONSIDERATIONS

Assessment: Assess for hypersensitivity to drug, sulfonamides, or other sulfonamide derivatives; renal/hepatic impairment; suprarenal gland failure; hyperchloremic acidosis; electrolyte imbalance; any other conditions where treatment is contraindicated or cautioned; pregnancy/nursing status; and possible drug interactions. Obtain baseline CBC and platelet count.

Monitoring: Monitor for signs/symptoms of hypersensitivity or other serious reactions, changes in blood glucose, electrolyte imbalance, and other adverse reactions. Perform periodic monitoring of CBC, platelet count, and serum electrolytes.

Counseling: Inform of the adverse reactions associated with therapy; instruct to promptly report to physician if any signs/symptoms develop. Advise that in order to try to avoid acute mountain sickness, gradual ascent is desirable, but if rapid ascent is undertaken and acetazolamide is used, it should be noted that such use does not obviate the need for prompt descent if severe forms of high altitude sickness occur. Instruct to notify physician of all drugs concurrently being taken (eg, ASA), and if pregnant/breastfeeding. Inform that some adverse reactions, such as drowsiness, fatigue, and myopia, may impair the ability to drive and operate machinery.

DICLEGIS — doxylamine succinate/pyridoxine hydrochloride   Rx

Class: Antihistamine/vitamin B6 analogue

ADULT DOSAGE	PEDIATRIC DOSAGE
Nausea/Vomiting	Pediatric use may not have been established
Treatment of N/V of Pregnancy in Women Who Do Not Respond to Conservative Management:	
Initial: 2 tabs hs (Day 1)	
Titrate: If this dose adequately controls symptoms the next day, continue taking 2 tabs/day hs; if symptoms persist into the afternoon of Day 2, take the usual dose of 2 tabs hs that night then take 3 tabs starting on Day 3 (1 tab in the am and 2 tabs hs)	
If dose adequately controls symptoms on Day 4, continue taking 3 tabs/day; otherwise take 4 tabs starting on Day 4 (1 tab in the am, 1 tab mid-afternoon, and 2 tabs hs)	
Max: 4 tabs/day (1 tab in the am, 1 tab mid-afternoon, and 2 tabs hs)	
Reassess for continued need as pregnancy progresses	

ADMINISTRATION

Oral route

Take on an empty stomach w/ a glass of water
Swallow tab whole; do not crush, chew, or split
Take as a daily prescription and not prn

STORAGE

20-25°C (68-77°F); excursions permitted between 15-30°C (59-86°F). Protect from moisture.

HOW SUPPLIED

Tab, Delayed Release: (Doxylamine/Pyridoxine) 10mg/10mg

CONTRAINDICATIONS

Known hypersensitivity to doxylamine succinate, other ethanolamine derivative antihistamines, pyridoxine HCl, or any inactive ingredient in the formulation. Concomitant MAOIs.

WARNINGS/PRECAUTIONS

Not studied in women with hyperemesis gravidarum. May cause somnolence and impair physical/mental abilities. Caution with asthma, increased intraocular pressure (IOP), narrow-angle glaucoma, stenosing peptic ulcer, pyloroduodenal obstruction, and urinary bladder-neck obstruction.

ADVERSE REACTIONS

Somnolence, dyspnea, vertigo, visual disturbances, abdominal pain, fatigue, dizziness, anxiety, dysuria, pruritus, palpitation, constipation, malaise, paresthesia, rash.

DRUG INTERACTIONS

See Contraindications. Not recommended with alcohol and other CNS depressants (eg, hypnotic sedatives, tranquilizers).

PREGNANCY AND LACTATION

Category A, not for use in nursing.

MECHANISM OF ACTION

Antihistamine and vitamin B6 analog combination; has not been established.

PHARMACOKINETICS

Absorption: GI tract, mainly jejunum. Administration of variable doses resulted in different pharmacokinetic parameters. **Distribution:** Found in breast milk. Pyridoxine: Plasma protein bound (60%). **Metabolism:** Doxylamine: Liver via N-dealkylation; N-desmethyldoxylamine and N, N-didesmethyldoxylamine (principle metabolites). Pyridoxine: Liver; Pyridoxal 5'-phosphate (active metabolite). **Elimination:** Doxylamine: Kidney; $T_{1/2}$=12.5 hrs. Pyridoxine: $T_{1/2}$=0.5 hrs.

PATIENT CONSIDERATIONS

Assessment: Assess for hypersensitivity reaction to the drug or to its components, hyperemesis gravidarum, asthma, IOP, narrow-angle glaucoma, stenosing peptic ulcer, pyloroduodenal obstruction, urinary bladder-neck obstruction, nursing status, and possible drug interactions.

Monitoring: Monitor for somnolence and other adverse reactions. Reassess for continued need as pregnancy progresses.

Counseling: Instruct to avoid engaging in activities requiring complete mental alertness (eg, driving, operating heavy machinery), until cleared to do so. Inform of the importance of not taking the medication with alcohol or sedating medications including other antihistamines, opiates, and sleep aids.

DICYCLOMINE HCL — dicyclomine hydrochloride   Rx

Class: Anticholinergic

OTHER BRAND NAMES

Bentyl

ADULT DOSAGE	PEDIATRIC DOSAGE
Functional Bowel/Irritable Bowel Syndrome	Pediatric use may not have been established
PO:	
Initial: 20mg qid	
Titrate: May increase to 40mg qid after 1 week of initial dose, unless side effects limit dose escalation. D/C if efficacy not achieved w/in 2 weeks or side effects require doses below 80mg/day	
Inj:	
Initial: 10-20mg IM qid for 1-2 days if unable to take oral medication	

DOSING CONSIDERATIONS

Elderly
Start at lower end of dosing range

ADMINISTRATION

Oral, IM route

Aspirate the syringe before injecting to avoid intravascular inj

STORAGE

(Cap/Tab/Inj) Room temperature <30°C (86°F). Sol: 20-25°C (68-77°F). Inj: Protect from freezing. Tab: Avoid exposure to direct sunlight.

HOW SUPPLIED

Oral Sol: 10mg/5mL [473mL]; (Bentyl) **Cap:** 10mg; **Inj:** 10mg/mL; **Tab:** 20mg

CONTRAINDICATIONS

Infants <6 months of age, nursing mothers, unstable cardiovascular status in acute hemorrhage, myasthenia gravis, glaucoma, obstructive uropathy, GI tract obstructive disease, severe ulcerative colitis, reflux esophagitis. **Oral Sol:** Prior hypersensitivity to dicyclomine HCl or other ingredients in the formulation.

WARNINGS/PRECAUTIONS

Caution in conditions characterized by tachyarrhythmia (eg, thyrotoxicosis, CHF, in cardiac surgery). Caution with coronary heart disease; ischemia and infarction may worsen. Peripheral effects (eg, dryness of mouth with difficulty in swallowing/talking) and CNS signs/symptoms (eg, confusional state, disorientation, amnesia) reported. Psychosis and delirium reported in sensitive individuals (eg, elderly patients and/or in patients with mental illness) given anticholinergic drugs. Heat prostration may occur in high environmental temperatures; d/c if symptoms occur and institute supportive measures. May impair mental abilities. Diarrhea may be the early symptom of incomplete intestinal obstruction, especially with ileostomy/colostomy patients; treatment would be inappropriate and possibly harmful. Caution with ulcerative colitis; large doses may suppress intestinal motility and produce paralytic ileus, and use of this drug may precipitate or aggravate the serious complication of toxic megacolon. Caution in patients with HTN, fever, autonomic neuropathy, prostatic enlargement, hepatic/renal impairment, and in the elderly. (Cap/Tab/Inj) Avoid with myasthenia gravis except to reduce adverse muscarinic effects of an anticholinesterase. Ogilvie's syndrome (colonic pseudo-obstruction) rarely reported. Caution with Salmonella dysentery; toxic dilation of intestine and intestinal perforation may occur. (Inj) For IM use only; inadvertent IV use may result in thrombosis, thrombophlebitis, and inj-site reactions. (Sol) Caution with hyperthyroidism and hiatal hernia.

ADVERSE REACTIONS

Dry mouth, dizziness, blurred vision, nausea, somnolence, asthenia, nervousness.

DRUG INTERACTIONS

May antagonize the effect of antiglaucoma agents and drugs that alter GI motility (eg, metoclopramide). Avoid concomitant use with corticosteroids in glaucoma patients. Potentiated by amantadine, Class I antiarrhythmics (eg, quinidine), antihistamines, antipsychotics (eg, phenothiazines), benzodiazepines, MAOIs, narcotic analgesics (eg, meperidine), nitrates/nitrites, sympathomimetics, TCAs, and other drugs with anticholinergic activity. Antacids may interfere with absorption; avoid simultaneous use. May affect GI absorption of various drugs by affecting GI motility; increased serum digoxin concentration may result with slowly dissolving forms of digoxin. Inhibiting effects on gastric hydrochloric acid secretion are antagonized by drugs used to treat achlorhydria and those used to test gastric secretion.

PREGNANCY AND LACTATION

Category B, not for use in nursing.

MECHANISM OF ACTION

Anticholinergic and antispasmodic agent; relieves smooth muscle spasm of the GI tract.

PHARMACOKINETICS

Absorption: Rapid; T_{max}=60-90 min. **Distribution:** (20mg PO) V_d=approximately 3.65L/kg (extensive); found in breast milk. **Elimination:** Urine (79.5%), feces (8.4%); $T_{1/2}$=1.8 hrs.

PATIENT CONSIDERATIONS

Assessment: Assess for cardiovascular conditions, myasthenia gravis, glaucoma, intestinal obstruction, psychosis, ulcerative colitis, tachycardia, or any other conditions where treatment is contraindicated or cautioned. Assess for history of hypersensitivity, pregnancy/nursing status, renal/hepatic dysfunction, and for possible drug interactions.

Monitoring: Monitor for increased HR, worsening of ischemia/infarction, heat prostration, drowsiness, blurred vision, confusion, disorientation, hallucinations, paralytic ileus with large doses, urinary retention, hypersensitivity reactions, and for other adverse reactions. Monitor renal function.

Counseling: Counsel on proper administration. Advise not to breastfeed while on therapy and not to administer to infants <6 months of age. Advise not to engage in activities requiring mental alertness (eg, operating motor vehicle or other machinery) or to perform hazardous work while taking the drug. Inform of risk of heat prostration in high environmental temperature; instruct to d/c if symptoms occur and to consult a physician.

DIFFERIN — adapalene   Rx

Class: Naphthoic acid derivative (retinoid-like)

ADULT DOSAGE	PEDIATRIC DOSAGE
<u>Acne Vulgaris</u>	<u>Acne Vulgaris</u>
Cre: Apply a thin film qpm	**≥12 Years:**
	Cre: Apply a thin film qpm
0.1% Gel: Apply a thin film qpm after washing; therapeutic results should be noticed after 8-12 weeks	**0.1% Gel:** Apply a thin film qpm after washing; therapeutic results should be noticed after 8-12 weeks
0.3% Gel: Apply a thin film qpm after washing	**0.3% Gel:** Apply a thin film qpm after washing
Reevaluate if therapeutic results are not noticed after 12 weeks of treatment	Reevaluate if therapeutic results are not noticed after 12 weeks of treatment
Lot: Apply a thin film (3-4 actuations of the pump) qd after washing	**Lot:** Apply a thin film (3-4 actuations of the pump) qd after washing

ADMINISTRATION

Topical route

Apply enough to cover the entire face or other affected areas completely and lightly.

STORAGE

20-25°C (68-77°F); excursions permitted to 15-30°C (59-86°F). Protect from freezing. **Lot:** Do not refrigerate. Protect from light. Keep away from heat.

HOW SUPPLIED

Cre: 0.1% [45g]; **Gel:** 0.1% [45g], 0.3% [15g, 45g tube; 45g pump]; **Lot:** 0.1% [2 oz]

CONTRAINDICATIONS

Hypersensitivity to adapalene or any components in the vehicle.

WARNINGS/PRECAUTIONS

Not for ophthalmic, oral, or intravaginal use. Avoid exposure to sunlight, including sunlamps; caution in patients w/ high levels of sun exposure and those w/ inherent sensitivity to sun. Extreme weather (eg, wind, cold) may cause irritation. Local skin irritation may be experienced; depending on severity, may use moisturizer, reduce frequency of application, or d/c use. **Cre/Gel:** Apparent exacerbation of acne may occur. **Cre/0.1% Gel:** D/C if reaction suggesting sensitivity or chemical irritation occurs. **Cre/0.3% Gel:** A mild transitory sensation of warmth or light stinging may occur shortly after application. **0.1% Gel:** Avoid in patients w/ sunburn until fully recovered. **0.3% Gel:** Reactions characterized by pruritus, face edema, eyelid edema, and lip swelling, requiring medical treatment reported; d/c use if experiencing allergic or anaphylactoid/anaphylactic reactions during therapy.

ADVERSE REACTIONS

Local cutaneous irritation. **0.3% Gel:** Skin discomfort.

DRUG INTERACTIONS

Caution w/ preparations containing sulfur, resorcinol, or salicylic acid. **Cre/Gel:** Do not start therapy until effects of such preparations in the skin have subsided. Caution w/ other potentially irritating topical products (medicated/abrasive soaps and cleansers, soaps and cosmetics that have a strong drying effect, and products w/ high concentrations of alcohol, astringents, spices, or lime). **Lot:** Caution w/ concomitant topical acne therapy, especially w/ peeling, desquamating, or abrasive agents. Avoid w/ other potentially irritating topical products.

PREGNANCY AND LACTATION

Pregnancy: Category C.

Lactation: It is not known whether adapalene is excreted in human milk; caution in nursing.

MECHANISM OF ACTION

Naphthoic acid derivative; not established. Binds to specific retinoic acid nuclear receptors and modulates cellular differentiation, keratinization, and inflammatory processes.

PHARMACOKINETICS

Absorption: (0.3% Gel, Day 10) C_{max}=0.553ng/mL, AUC_{0-24hr}=8.37ng•hr/mL. (Lot, Day 28) Adolescent; C_{max}=0.128ng/mL, AUC_{0-24hr}=3.07ng•hr/mL. **Elimination:** (Cre/Gel) Bile. (0.3% Gel) $T_{1/2}$=17.2 hrs.

PATIENT CONSIDERATIONS

Assessment: Assess for excessive sun exposure, sun sensitivity, hypersensitivity to any of the components of the drug, pregnancy/nursing status, and for possible drug interactions. Assess for presence of cuts, abrasions, or eczematous or sunburned skin at the treatment site.

Monitoring: Monitor for sensitivity or chemical irritation, cutaneous signs/ symptoms, and other adverse reactions.

Counseling: Advise to cleanse area w/ mild or soapless cleanser before applying the medication. Instruct to minimize or avoid exposure to sunlight and sunlamps. Instruct to use sunscreen products and protective clothing when exposure cannot be avoided. Instruct not to use more than the recommended amount. Instruct to avoid contact w/ eyes, lips, angles of the nose, and mucous membranes. Advise not to apply medication to cuts, abrasions, or eczematous or sunburned skin. Advise to use moisturizers if necessary and to avoid products containing α-hydroxyl or glycolic acids. Instruct to use externally and ud. Inform that an apparent exacerbation of acne may occur during the early weeks of therapy and that it should not be considered a reason for discontinuation. Instruct to contact the physician if signs of allergy or hypersensitivity develop. **Cre/0.3% Gel/Lot:** Avoid waxing as a depilatory method.

DIFICID — fidaxomicin   Rx

Class: Macrolide

ADULT DOSAGE	PEDIATRIC DOSAGE
<u>*Clostridium difficile*-Associated Diarrhea</u>	Pediatric use may not have been established
200mg bid for 10 days	

ADMINISTRATION

Oral route

Take w/ or w/o food

STORAGE

20-25°C (68-77°F); excursions permitted 15-30°C (59-86°F).

HOW SUPPLIED

Tab: 200mg

CONTRAINDICATIONS

Hypersensitivity to fidaxomicin.

WARNINGS/PRECAUTIONS

Not effective for treatment of systemic infections. Acute hypersensitivity reactions (eg, dyspnea, rash, pruritus) reported; d/c therapy if severe hypersensitivity reaction occurs. May increase the risk of the development of drug resistant bacteria when prescribed in the absence of a proven or strongly suspected *C. difficile* infection.

ADVERSE REACTIONS

N/V, abdominal pain, GI hemorrhage.

PREGNANCY AND LACTATION

Category B, caution in nursing.

MECHANISM OF ACTION

Macrolide; bactericidal against *C. difficile*, inhibiting RNA synthesis by RNA polymerases.

PHARMACOKINETICS

Absorption: Minimal; refer to PI for other pharmacokinetic parameters. **Metabolism:** Hydrolysis; OP-1118 (active metabolite). **Elimination:** Urine (0.59% OP-1118), feces (>92% fidaxomicin and OP-1118); (healthy adult males) $T_{1/2}$=11.7 hrs, 11.2 hrs (OP-1118).

PATIENT CONSIDERATIONS

Assessment: Assess for hypersensitivity to the drug, macrolide allergy, and pregnancy/nursing status.

Monitoring: Monitor for development of drug resistant bacteria, hypersensitivity reactions, and other adverse reactions.

Counseling: Inform that drug only treats CDAD infections, not other bacterial or viral infections. Instruct to take exactly ud; inform that skipping doses or not completing full course may decrease effectiveness and increase antibiotic resistance.

DIFLUCAN ORAL — fluconazole   Rx

Class: Azole antifungal

ADULT DOSAGE	PEDIATRIC DOSAGE
Prophylaxis in Bone Marrow Transplant	**Cryptococcal Meningitis**
Decrease Incidence of Candidiasis: 400mg qd	12mg/kg on 1st day, followed by 6mg/kg qd for 10-12 weeks after the CSF becomes culture (-); a dose of 12mg/kg qd may be used (not to exceed 600mg/day)
Start prophylaxis several days before the anticipated onset of neutropenia in patients who are anticipated to have severe granulocytopenia (<500 neutrophils/mm³); continue for 7 days after the neutrophil count rises >1000 cells/mm³	
	Suppression of Cryptococcal Meningitis Relapse in AIDS: 6mg/kg qd
Cryptococcal Meningitis	*Candida* **Infections**
400mg on 1st day, followed by 200mg qd for 10-12 weeks after the CSF becomes culture (-); a dose of 400mg qd may be used	**Systemic:** 6-12mg/kg/day (not to exceed 600mg/day)
Suppression of Cryptococcal Meningitis Relapse in AIDS: 200mg qd	**Esophageal Candidiasis**
Vaginal Candidiasis	6mg/kg on 1st day, followed by 3mg/kg qd for a minimum of 3 weeks and for ≥2 weeks following resolution of symptoms; doses up to 12mg/kg/day may be used (not to exceed 600mg/day)
PO Single Dose: 150mg	
Oropharyngeal Candidiasis	**Oropharyngeal Candidiasis**
200mg on 1st day, followed by 100mg qd for ≥2 weeks	6mg/kg on 1st day, followed by 3mg/kg qd for ≥2 weeks
Esophageal Candidiasis	
200mg on 1st day, followed by 100mg qd for a minimum of 3 weeks and for ≥2 weeks following resolution of symptoms Doses up to 400mg/day may be used	
Candida **Infections**	
Systemic Infections: Max: 400mg qd	
UTIs/Peritonitis: 50-200mg/day	

DOSING CONSIDERATIONS
Renal Impairment
Multiple Doses:
Initial LD: 50-400mg
Maint:
CrCl ≤50mL/min (No Dialysis): Give 50% of recommended dose
Regular Dialysis: Give 100% of recommended dose after each dialysis; on non-dialysis days, administer a reduced dose based on CrCl

ADMINISTRATION
Oral route

Take w/ or w/o food.
Shake sus well before using.
Sus
To reconstitute, add 24mL of distilled or purified water to bottle

STORAGE
Tab: <30°C (86°F). **Sus: Dry Powder:** <30°C (86°F). **Reconstituted:** 5-30°C (41-86°F); discard unused portion after 2 weeks. Protect from freezing.

HOW SUPPLIED
Sus: 10mg/mL, 40mg/mL [35mL]; **Tab:** 50mg, 100mg, 150mg, 200mg

CONTRAINDICATIONS
Hypersensitivity to fluconazole or to any excipients. Coadministration with terfenadine (with multiple doses ≥400mg of fluconazole), other drugs known to prolong the QT interval and that are metabolized via the enzyme CYP3A4 (eg, cisapride, astemizole, erythromycin, pimozide, quinidine).

WARNINGS/PRECAUTIONS
Associated with rare cases of serious hepatic toxicity; monitor for more severe hepatic injury if abnormal LFTs develop. D/C if clinical signs and symptoms consistent with liver disease develop. Anaphylaxis reported (rare). Exfoliative skin disorders reported; closely monitor patients with deep seated fungal infections who develop rashes during treatment and d/c if lesions progress. D/C therapy if rash develops in patients treated for superficial fungal infection. QT prolongation and torsades de pointes reported (rare); caution with potentially proarrhythmic conditions. Caution in elderly or with renal/hepatic dysfunction. May impair mental/physical abilities. (Sus) Contains sucrose; do not use in patients with hereditary fructose, glucose/galactose malabsorption, and sucrase-isomaltase deficiency. (Tab) Consider risk versus benefits of single dose oral tab versus intravaginal agent therapy for the treatment of vaginal yeast infections.

ADVERSE REACTIONS
Headache, N/V, abdominal pain, diarrhea.

DRUG INTERACTIONS
See Contraindications. Carefully monitor coadministration of fluconazole at doses <400mg/day with terfenadine. Avoid with voriconazole. Risk of increased plasma concentration of compounds metabolized by CYP2C9 and CYP3A4; caution when coadministered and monitor patients carefully. May precipitate clinically significant hypoglycemia with oral hypoglycemics; monitor blood glucose and adjust dose of sulfonylurea as necessary. May increase PT with coumarin-type anticoagulants; monitor PT and, if necessary, adjust warfarin dose. May increase levels of phenytoin, cyclosporine, theophylline, rifabutin, oral tacrolimus, triazolam, celecoxib, halofantrine, flurbiprofen, racemic ibuprofen, methadone, saquinavir, sirolimus, and vinca alkaloids (eg, vincristine, vinblastine). May increase exposure of ethinyl estradiol and levonorgestrel. May reduce the metabolism and increase levels of tolbutamide, glyburide, and glipizide. Monitor SrCr with cyclosporine. Rifampin may enhance metabolism. May increase levels and psychomotor effects of oral midazolam; consider dose reduction of short-acting benzodiazepines metabolized by CYP450, and monitor appropriately. May increase systemic exposure to tofacitinib; reduce tofacitinib dose when given concomitantly. HCTZ may increase levels. May reduce clearance/distribution volume and prolong T₁/₂ of alfentanil. May increase effect of amitriptyline and nortriptyline. May increase levels of zidovudine; consider dose reduction. May potentially increase systemic exposure of other NSAIDs that are metabolized by CYP2C9 (eg, naproxen, lornoxicam, meloxicam, diclofenac), and calcium channel antagonists. Risk of carbamazepine toxicity. May increase serum bilirubin and SrCr with cyclophosphamide. May significantly delay elimination of fentanyl, leading to respiratory depression. May increase risk of myopathy and rhabdomyolysis with HMG-CoA reductase inhibitors metabolized through CYP3A4 (eg, atorvastatin, simvastatin) or through CYP2C9 (eg, fluvastatin); monitor for symptoms and d/c statin if a marked increase in creatinine kinase is observed or myopathy/rhabdomyolysis is diagnosed or suspected. May inhibit the metabolism of losartan; monitor BP continuously. Acute adrenal cortex insufficiency reported after discontinuation of a 3-month therapy with fluconazole in a liver-transplanted patient treated with prednisone. CNS-related undesirable effects reported with all-trans-retinoid acid (an acid form of vitamin A).

PREGNANCY AND LACTATION
Category C (single 150mg tab use for vaginal candidiasis) and D (all other indications), caution in nursing.

MECHANISM OF ACTION
Triazole antifungal; selectively inhibits fungal CYP450 dependent enzyme lanosterol 14-α-demethylase, the enzyme that converts lanosterol to ergosterol. Subsequent loss of normal sterol correlates with the accumulation of 14-α-methyl sterols in fungi and may be responsible for the fungistatic activity.

PHARMACOKINETICS
Absorption: Rapid, almost complete. Absolute bioavailability (>90%); C_{max}=6.72mcg/mL (fasted, single 400mg dose); T_{max}=1-2 hrs (fasted).
Distribution: Plasma protein binding (11-12%); found in breast milk. **Elimination:** Urine (80%, unchanged; 11%, metabolites); $T_{1/2}$=30 hrs (fasted). Refer to PI for pediatric and elderly pharmacokinetic parameters.

PATIENT CONSIDERATIONS

Assessment: Assess for hypersensitivity to the drug, renal/hepatic impairment, AIDS, malignancies, risk factors for QT prolongation, any other conditions where treatment is contraindicated or cautioned, pregnancy/nursing status, and possible drug interactions. Obtain specimens for fungal culture and other relevant lab studies (serology, histopathology) to isolate and identify causative organisms. (Sus) Assess for hereditary fructose, glucose/galactose malabsorption, and sucrase-isomaltase deficiency.

Monitoring: Monitor for signs/symptoms of liver disease, rash, and other adverse reactions. Monitor LFTs and renal function. Monitor PT when used with coumarin-type anticoagulants.

Counseling: Inform about risks/benefits of therapy. Advise to notify physician if pregnant/nursing and counsel about potential hazard to the fetus if pregnant or pregnancy occurs. Instruct to inform physician of all medications currently being taken.

DIGOXIN ORAL — digoxin   Rx

Class: Cardiac glycoside

OTHER BRAND NAMES
Lanoxin

ADULT DOSAGE	PEDIATRIC DOSAGE
Atrial Fibrillation	**Heart Failure**
Control of Ventricular Response Rate in Chronic A-Fib:	**Increase Myocardial Contractility:**
Dosing can be either initiated w/ a LD followed by maint dosing if rapid titration is desired or initiated w/ maint dosing w/o a LD	Dosing can be either initiated w/ a LD followed by maint dosing if rapid titration is desired or initiated w/ maint dosing w/o a LD
Sol:	**Sol:**
LD: 10-15mcg/kg	If a LD is needed, administer w/ roughly 1/2 the total given as the 1st dose; additional fractions of the
Maint: 3.0-4.5mcg/kg/dose qd	

Tab:
LD: 10-15mcg/kg; administer 1/2 the total LD initially, then 1/4 the LD q6-8h twice
Maint:
Initial: 3.4-5.1mcg/kg qd
Titrate: May increase dose every 2 weeks according to clinical response, serum drug levels, and toxicity

Heart Failure
Mild to Moderate:
Dosing can be either initiated w/ a LD followed by maint dosing if rapid titration is desired or initiated w/ maint dosing w/o a LD
Sol:
LD: 10-15mcg/kg
Maint: 3.0-4.5mcg/kg/dose qd
Tab:
LD: 10-15mcg/kg; administer 1/2 the total LD initially, then 1/4 the LD q6-8h twice
Maint:
Initial: 3.4-5.1mcg/kg qd
Titrate: May increase dose every 2 weeks according to clinical response, serum drug levels, and toxicity
Where possible, use in combination w/ a diuretic and an ACE inhibitor

Conversions
IV to Oral Conversion:
50mcg inj = 62.5mcg tab
100mcg inj = 125mcg tab
200mcg inj = 250mcg tab
400mcg inj = 500mcg tab

total dose may be given at 4- to 8-hr intervals, w/ careful assessment of clinical response before each additional dose. If the clinical response necessitates a change from the calculated LD, then calculation of the maint dose should be based on the amount actually given as the LD
LD:
Premature Infants: 20-30mcg/kg
Full-Term Infants: 25-35mcg/kg
1-24 Months: 35-60mcg/kg
2-5 Years: 30-45mcg/kg
5-10 Years: 20-35mcg/kg
>10 Years: 10-15mcg/kg
Maint:
Premature Infants: 2.3-3.9mcg/kg/dose bid
Full-Term Infants: 3.8-5.6mcg/kg/dose bid
1-24 Months: 5.6-9.4mcg/kg/dose bid
2-5 Years: 4.7-6.6mcg/kg/dose bid
5-10 Years: 2.8-5.6mcg/kg/dose bid
>10 Years: 3-4.5mcg/kg/dose qd
Tab:
LD:
Administer 1/2 the total LD initially, then 1/4 the LD q6-8h twice
5-10 Years: 20-45mcg/kg
>10 Years: 10-15mcg/kg
Maint:
Initial:
5-10 Years: 3.2-6.4mcg/kg/dose bid
>10 Years: 3.4-5.1mcg/kg qd
Titrate: May increase dose every 2 weeks according to clinical response, serum drug levels, and toxicity

Conversions
IV to Oral Conversion:
50mcg inj = 62.5mcg tab
100mcg inj = 125mcg tab
200mcg inj = 250mcg tab
400mcg inj = 500mcg tab

DOSING CONSIDERATIONS
Renal Impairment
Refer to PI for recommended maint doses based on lean body weight and renal function
ADMINISTRATION
Oral route
Sol
The provided calibrated dropper is not appropriate to measure doses <0.2mL.
STORAGE
25°C (77°F); excursions permitted to 15-30°C (59-86°F). Protect from light. **Tab:** Store in dry place.
HOW SUPPLIED
Sol: 0.05mg/mL [60mL]; (Lanoxin) **Tab:** 62.5mcg, 125mcg*, 187.5mcg, 250mcg* *scored
CONTRAINDICATIONS
Ventricular fibrillation. Known hypersensitivity to digoxin (reactions seen include unexplained rash, swelling of the mouth, lips, or throat or a difficulty in breathing) or to other digitalis preparations.
WARNINGS/PRECAUTIONS
Increased risk of ventricular fibrillation in patients w/ Wolff-Parkinson-White syndrome who develop A-fib. May cause severe sinus bradycardia or sinoatrial block particularly in patients w/ preexisting sinus node disease and may cause advanced or complete heart block in patients w/ preexisting incomplete atrioventricular (AV) block; consider insertion of a pacemaker before treatment. Signs/symptoms of digoxin toxicity may be mistaken for worsening symptoms of heart failure (HF). May be desirable to reduce dose or d/c therapy 1-2 days prior to electrical cardioversion of A-fib. If digitalis toxicity is suspected, delay elective cardioversion, and if it is not prudent to delay cardioversion, select the lowest possible energy level to avoid provoking ventricular arrhythmias. May increase myocardial oxygen demand and lead to ischemia in patients w/ acute MI (AMI). May precipitate vasoconstriction and promote production of pro-inflammatory cytokines in patients w/ myocarditis; avoid use in these patients. Patients w/ certain disorders involving HF associated w/ preserved left ventricular ejection fraction (eg, restrictive cardiomyopathy, constrictive pericarditis, amyloid heart disease, idiopathic hypertrophic subaortic stenosis) may not benefit from treatment and may be particularly susceptible to adverse reactions. Hypercalcemia increased the risk of toxicity, while hypocalcemia may nullify the effects of treatment. Hypothyroidism may reduce the requirements for therapy. HF and/or atrial arrhythmias resulting from hypermetabolic or hyperdynamic states (eg, hyperthyroidism, hypoxia, arteriovenous shunt) are best treated by addressing the underlying condition. Endogenous substances of unknown composition (digoxin-like immunoreactive substances) may interfere

w/ standard radioimmunoassays for digoxin. Caution in the elderly. **Sol:** Toxicity may occur at concentrations w/in therapeutic range in patients w/ hypokalemia or hypomagnesemia; maintain normal K^+ levels and Mg^+ levels while on therapy. May result in potentially detrimental increases in coronary vascular resistance. May prolong the PR interval and depress the ST segment on the ECG. May produce false positive ST-T changes on the ECG during exercise testing that may be indistinguishable from those of ischemia. **Tab:** Patients w/ low body weight, advanced age or impaired renal function, hypokalemia, or hypomagnesemia may be predisposed to digoxin toxicity. Not recommended in patients w/ AMI. Avoid in patients w/ restrictive cardiomyopathy, constrictive pericarditis, amyloid heart disease, acute cor pulmonale, and idiopathic hypertrophic subaortic stenosis. Patients w/ beri beri heart disease may fail to respond adequately to therapy if the underlying thiamine deficiency is not treated concomitantly.
ADVERSE REACTIONS
Cardiac arrhythmias, N/V, abdominal pain, intestinal ischemia, hemorrhagic necrosis of the intestines, headache, weakness, dizziness, apathy, mental disturbances.
DRUG INTERACTIONS
Drugs that induce/inhibit P-gp may alter digoxin pharmacokinetics. Increased levels or exposure w/ amiodarone, captopril, clarithromycin, erythromycin, dronedarone, gentamicin, erythromycin, itraconazole, nitrendipine, propafenone, quinidine, ranolazine, ritonavir, telaprevir, tetracycline, verapamil, atorvastatin, carvedilol, conivaptan, diltiazem, indomethacin, nifedipine, nefazodone, propantheline, quinine, saquinavir, spironolactone, telmisartan, ticagrelor, tolvaptan, trimethoprim, alprazolam, azithromycin, cyclosporine, diclofenac, diphenoxylate, epoprostenol, esomeprazole, ketoconazole, lansoprazole, metformin, omeprazole, and rabeprazole. Decreased levels w/ acarbose, activated charcoal, albuterol, antacids, certain cancer chemotherapy or radiation therapy, cholestyramine, colestipol, exenatide, kaolin-pectin, meals high in bran, metoclopramide, miglitol, neomycin, rifampin, St. John's wort, sucralfate, and sulfasalazine. Proarrhythmic events reported to be more common in patients receiving concomitant therapy w/ sotalol. May increase risk of arrhythmias w/ rapid IV Ca^{2+} administration, sympathomimetics (eg, epinephrine, norepinephrine, dopamine), and succinylcholine. Increased digoxin dose requirement w/ thyroid supplements. Calcium channel blockers and β-adrenergic blockers produce additive effects on AV node conduction, which can result in bradycardia and advanced or complete heart block. Higher rate of torsades de pointes w/ dofetilide. Teriparatide transiently increases serum Ca^{2+}. Refer to PI for dose adjustment information when used w/ certain concomitant therapies. **Sol:** Increased PR interval and QRS duration reported w/ moricizine. **Tab:** Decreased levels w/ penicillamine, and phenytoin. ACE inhibitors, ARBs, NSAIDs, and COX-2 inhibitors may impair digoxin excretion. Sudden death reported to be more common in patients receiving concomitant therapy w/ dronedarone.
PREGNANCY AND LACTATION
Pregnancy: Category C.
Lactation: Caution in nursing.
MECHANISM OF ACTION
Cardiac glycoside; inhibits Na^+-K^+ ATPase, which is responsible for maintaining the intracellular milieu throughout the body by moving Na^+ ions out of and K^+ ions into cells.
PHARMACOKINETICS
Absorption: (Sol) Absolute bioavailability (70-85%); T_{max}=30-90 min. (Tab) Absolute bioavailability (60-80%); T_{max}=1-3 hrs. **Distribution:** V_d=475-500L; plasma protein binding (25%); crosses the blood-brain barrier and placenta; found in breast milk. **Metabolism:** (Sol) 3-β-digoxigenin, 3-keto-digoxigenin, and their glucuronide and sulfate conjugates (metabolites). (Tab) Dihydrodigoxin, digoxigenin bisdigitoxoside, and their glucuronide and sulfate conjugates (metabolites) via hydrolysis, oxidation, and conjugation. **Elimination:** (Healthy, IV) Urine (50-70%, unchanged); $T_{1/2}$=(anuric patients) 3.5-5 days. (Sol) $T_{1/2}$=18-36 hrs (pediatrics), 36-48 hrs (adults). (Tab) $T_{1/2}$=(healthy) 1.5-2 days.

PATIENT CONSIDERATIONS
Assessment: Assess for known hypersensitivity to the drug or other digitalis preparations, ventricular fibrillation, myocarditis, hypermetabolic or hyperdynamic states, sinus node disease, AV block, pregnancy/nursing status, possible drug interactions, and any other conditions where treatment is cautioned. Assess serum electrolytes and renal function. Obtain a baseline digoxin level.

Monitoring: Monitor for signs/symptoms of severe sinus bradycardia, sinoatrial block, advanced or complete heart block, digoxin toxicity, vasoconstriction, and other adverse reactions. Monitor serum electrolytes and renal function periodically. Obtain serum digoxin concentrations just before the next dose or at least 6 hrs after the last dose. Monitor for clinical response.

Counseling: Advise that digoxin is used to treat HF and heart arrhythmias. Advise to inform physician if taking any OTC medications, including herbal medication, or if started on a new prescription. Inform that blood tests will be necessary to ensure the appropriate digoxin dose. Instruct to contact physician if N/V, persistent diarrhea, confusion, weakness, or visual disturbances occur. Advise parents or caregivers that symptoms of having too high doses may be difficult to recognize in infants and pediatric patients; symptoms such as weight loss, failure to thrive in infants, abdominal pain, and behavioral disturbances may be indications of digoxin toxicity. Suggest to monitor and record HR and BP daily. Instruct women of childbearing potential who become or are planning to become pregnant to consult physician prior to initiation or continuing therapy. **Sol:** Instruct to use calibrated dropper to measure the dose and to avoid less precise measuring tools (eg, tsp).

DILANTIN CAPSULES — phenytoin sodium   Rx

Class: Hydantoin

ADULT DOSAGE

Seizures

Tonic-Clonic (Grand Mal) and Psychomotor (Temporal Lobe) Seizures and Prevention/Treatment of Neurosurgery-Associated Seizures:

Divided Daily Dosing:
Initial: (Treatment naive) 100mg tid
Maint: 100mg tid-qid
Titrate: May increase up to 200mg tid, if necessary

QD Dosing:
May consider 300mg qd if seizure is controlled w/ divided doses of three 100mg caps daily

LD (Clinic/Hospital):
In patients who require rapid steady-state serum levels and where IV administration is not desirable
Initial: 1g in 3 divided doses (400mg, 300mg, 300mg) at 2-hr intervals
Maint: Start maint dose 24 hrs after LD

Clinically effective serum level is usually 10-20mcg/mL; do not change dose at intervals <7-10 days

Conversions

May require dose adjustment when switching from product formulated w/ free acid to product formulated w/ Na+ salt and vice versa

PEDIATRIC DOSAGE

Seizures

Tonic-Clonic (Grand Mal) and Psychomotor (Temporal Lobe) Seizures and Prevention/Treatment of Neurosurgery-Associated Seizures:
Initial: 5mg/kg/day in 2 or 3 equally divided doses
Maint: 4-8mg/kg/day
Max: 300mg/day

>6 Years: May require the minimum adult dose (300mg/day)

Clinically effective serum level is usually 10-20mcg/mL; do not change dose at intervals <7-10 days

Conversions

May require dose adjustment when switching from product formulated w/ free acid to product formulated w/ Na+ salt and vice versa

---

DOSING CONSIDERATIONS

Renal Impairment
Caution when interpreting total phenytoin plasma concentrations; unbound phenytoin concentrations may be more useful.
Do not use LD regimen w/ history of renal disease.

Hepatic Impairment
Caution when interpreting total phenytoin plasma concentrations; unbound phenytoin concentrations may be more useful.
Do not use LD regimen w/ history of liver disease.

Elderly
May require lower or less frequent dosing

Other Important Considerations
Hypoalbuminemia:
Caution when interpreting total phenytoin plasma concentrations; unbound phenytoin concentrations may be more useful

ADMINISTRATION
Oral route

STORAGE
20-25°C (68-77°F). Protect from moisture. Preserve in tight, light-resistant containers.

HOW SUPPLIED
Cap, Extended-Release: 30mg, 100mg

CONTRAINDICATIONS
History of hypersensitivity to phenytoin or its inactive ingredients, or other hydantoins. Coadministration w/ delavirdine.

WARNINGS/PRECAUTIONS
Unbound concentration of phenytoin may be elevated in patients w/ hyperbilirubinemia. Avoid abrupt withdrawal; may precipitate status epilepticus. May increase risk of suicidal thoughts/behavior; monitor for emergence/ worsening of depression, suicidal thoughts/behavior, and/or any unusual changes in mood/behavior. Serious and sometimes fatal dermatologic reactions, including toxic epidermal necrolysis (TEN) and Stevens-Johnson syndrome (SJS), reported; d/c at 1st sign of rash, unless the rash is clearly not drug-related. Do not resume therapy, and consider alternative therapy if signs/ symptoms suggest SJS/TEN. Consideration should be given to avoiding use as alternative therapy for carbamazepine in patients positive for HLA-B*1502. Drug reaction w/ eosinophilia and systemic symptoms (DRESS)/multiorgan hypersensitivity reported; evaluate immediately if signs and symptoms (eg, rash, fever, lymphadenopathy) are present and d/c if an alternative etiology cannot be established. Consider alternatives to structurally similar drugs (eg, carboxamides, barbiturates, succinimides, oxazolidinediones) in patients who have experienced phenytoin hypersensitivity. Acute hepatotoxicity (eg, acute hepatic failure) reported; d/c immediately and do not readminister. Hematopoietic complications and lymphadenopathy reported; extended follow-up observation is indicated and every effort should be made to achieve seizure control using alternative antiepileptic drugs in all cases of lymphadenopathy. Decreased bone mineral density and bone fractures reported during chronic use; consider screening and initiating treatment plans as appropriate. Caution w/ porphyria, hepatic

impairment, and in elderly or gravely ill patients. An increase in seizure frequency may occur during pregnancy due to altered phenytoin pharmacokinetics. May cause fetal harm. Bleeding disorder in newborns may occur; give vitamin K to mother before delivery and to neonate after birth. Check plasma levels immediately if early signs of dose-related CNS toxicity develop. Hyperglycemia reported; may increase serum glucose levels in diabetics. Not indicated for seizures due to hypoglycemia or other metabolic causes. Not effective for absence (petit mal) seizures; if tonic-clonic (grand mal) and absence (petit mal) seizures are present, combined drug therapy is needed. Serum levels of phenytoin sustained above the optimal range may produce confusional states or rarely irreversible cerebellar dysfunction and/or cerebellar atrophy; reduce dose if plasma levels are excessive, or d/c if symptoms persist. Lab test interactions may occur. Do not use if discolored.

ADVERSE REACTIONS
Rash, nystagmus, ataxia, slurred speech, decreased coordination, somnolence, mental confusion, dizziness, insomnia, transient nervousness, motor twitching, acute hepatic failure, thrombocytopenia, altered taste sensation, Peyronie's disease.

DRUG INTERACTIONS
See Contraindications. Acute alcohol intake, amiodarone, antiepileptic agents (eg, ethosuximide, felbamate, oxcarbazepine), azoles (eg, fluconazole, ketoconazole, itraconazole), capecitabine, chloramphenicol, chlordiazepoxide, disulfiram, estrogens, fluorouracil, fluoxetine, fluvastatin, fluvoxamine, H2-antagonists (eg, cimetidine), halothane, isoniazid, methylphenidate, omeprazole, phenothiazines, salicylates, sertraline, succinimides, sulfonamides (eg, sulfamethizole, sulfadiazine, sulfamethoxazole-trimethoprim), ticlopidine, tolbutamide, trazodone, and warfarin may increase levels. Anticancer drugs usually in combination (eg, bleomycin, carboplatin, cisplatin), carbamazepine, chronic alcohol abuse, diazepam, diazoxide, folic acid, fosamprenavir, nelfinavir, reserpine, rifampin, ritonavir (RTV), St. John's wort, sucralfate, vigabatrin, and theophylline may decrease levels. Administration w/ preparations that increase gastric pH (eg, supplements or antacids containing calcium carbonate, aluminum hydroxide, and magnesium hydroxide) may affect absorption; do not take at the same time of day. Phenobarbital, sodium valproate, and valproic acid may increase or decrease levels. May impair efficacy of azoles (eg, fluconazole, ketoconazole, itraconazole), corticosteroids, doxycycline, estrogens, furosemide, irinotecan, oral contraceptives, paclitaxel, paroxetine, quinidine, rifampin, sertraline, teniposide, theophylline, and vitamin D. Increased and decreased PT/INR responses reported w/ warfarin. May decrease levels of active metabolites of albendazole, certain HIV antivirals (eg, efavirenz, lopinavir/RTV, indinavir), antiepileptic agents (eg, carbamazepine, felbamate, lamotrigine), atorvastatin, chlorpropamide, clozapine, cyclosporine, digoxin, fluvastatin, folic acid, methadone, mexiletine, nifedipine, nimodipine, nisoldipine, praziquantel, simvastatin, and verapamil. May decrease levels of amprenavir (active metabolite) when given w/ fosamprenavir alone. May increase levels of amprenavir when given w/ the combination of fosamprenavir and RTV. Resistance to the neuromuscular blocking action of pancuronium, vecuronium, rocuronium, and cisatracurium reported in patients chronically administered phenytoin; monitor closely for more rapid recovery from neuromuscular blockade than expected and infusion rate requirements may be higher. Enteral feeding preparations and/or related nutritional supplements may decrease levels; avoid w/ enteral feeding preparations.

PREGNANCY AND LACTATION
Pregnancy: Category D; physicians are advised to recommend that pregnant patients enroll in the North American Antiepileptic Drug (NAAED) Pregnancy Registry.
Lactation: Phenytoin appears to be secreted in low concentrations in human milk; not for use in nursing.

MECHANISM OF ACTION
Hydantoin; inhibits seizure activity by promoting Na+ efflux from neurons, stabilizing the threshold against hyperexcitability caused by excessive stimulation or environmental changes capable of reducing membrane Na+ gradient. Reduces the maximal activity of the brain stem centers responsible for the tonic phase of tonic-clonic (grand mal) seizures.

PHARMACOKINETICS
Absorption: T_{max}=4-12 hrs. **Distribution:** Plasma protein binding (high); crosses the placenta; found in breast milk. **Metabolism:** Liver (hydroxylation). CYP2C9 and CYP2C19. **Elimination:** Urine; $T_{1/2}$=22 hrs.

PATIENT CONSIDERATIONS

Assessment: Assess for hypersensitivity to the drug or other hydantoins, alcohol use, hepatic/renal impairment, porphyria, grave illness, seizures due to hypoglycemia or other metabolic causes, absence seizures, any other conditions where treatment is contraindicated or cautioned, pregnancy/nursing status, and possible drug interactions.

Monitoring: Monitor for hypersensitivity reactions, dermatologic reactions, DRESS/multiorgan hypersensitivity, hepatotoxicity, hematopoietic complications, lymphadenopathy, decreased bone mineral density, bone fractures; exacerbation of porphyria, hyperglycemia, and other adverse reactions. Monitor for emergence/ worsening of depression, suicidal thoughts/behavior, and/or any unusual changes in mood/behavior. Monitor serum levels when switching from Na+ salt to free acid form and vice versa.

Counseling: Instruct to read medication guide and to take ud. Advise of the importance of adhering strictly to the prescribed dosage regimen, and of informing the physician of any clinical condition in which it is not possible to take the drug orally as prescribed (eg, surgery). Inform about the early toxic signs and symptoms of potential hematologic, dermatologic, hypersensitivity, or hepatic reactions; instruct to immediately contact physician if these develop. Caution on the use of other drugs or alcoholic beverages w/o first seeking physician's advice.

Stress the importance of good dental hygiene to minimize the development of gingival hyperplasia and its complications. Advise to notify physician immediately if depression, suicidal thoughts/behavior, or thoughts about self-harm emerge. Encourage patients to enroll in the NAAED Pregnancy Registry if they become pregnant.

DILANTIN INFATABS — phenytoin   Rx

Class: Hydantoin

ADULT DOSAGE

Seizures

Generalized Tonic-Clonic (Grand Mal) and Complex Partial (Psychomotor/Temporal Lobe) Seizures and Prevention/Treatment of Neurosurgery-Associated Seizures:
Initial: (Treatment naive) 100mg (2 tabs) tid
Maint: 300-400mg (6-8 tabs) daily
Titrate: May increase to 600mg (12 tabs) daily, if necessary

Clinically effective serum level usually 10-20mcg/mL; do not change dose at intervals <7-10 days

Conversions

May require dose adjustment when switching from product formulated w/ free acid to product formulated w/ Na+ salt and vice versa

PEDIATRIC DOSAGE

Seizures

Generalized Tonic-Clonic (Grand Mal) and Complex Partial (Psychomotor/Temporal Lobe) Seizures and Prevention/Treatment of Neurosurgery-Associated Seizures:
Initial: 5mg/kg/day in 2 or 3 equally divided doses
Maint: 4-8mg/kg/day
Max: 300mg/day

>6 Years: May require the minimum adult dose (300mg/day)

If daily dose cannot be divided equally, give larger dose hs

Clinically effective serum level usually 10-20mcg/mL; do not change dose at intervals <7-10 days

Conversions

May require dose adjustment when switching from product formulated w/ free acid to product formulated w/ Na+ salt and vice versa

DOSING CONSIDERATIONS

Renal Impairment
Caution when interpreting total phenytoin plasma concentrations; unbound phenytoin concentrations may be more useful

Hepatic Impairment
Caution when interpreting total phenytoin plasma concentrations; unbound phenytoin concentrations may be more useful

Elderly
May require lower or less frequent dosing

Other Important Considerations
Hypoalbuminemia:
Caution when interpreting total phenytoin plasma concentrations; unbound phenytoin concentrations may be more useful

ADMINISTRATION
Oral route

May chew or swallow tab whole.
Not for once-a-day dosing.

STORAGE
20-25°C (68-77°F). Protect from moisture.

HOW SUPPLIED
Tab, Chewable: 50mg* *scored

CONTRAINDICATIONS
History of hypersensitivity to phenytoin or its inactive ingredients, or other hydantoins. Coadministration w/ delavirdine.

WARNINGS/PRECAUTIONS
Unbound concentration of phenytoin may be elevated in patients w/ hyperbilirubinemia. Avoid abrupt withdrawal; may precipitate status epilepticus. May increase risk of suicidal thoughts/behavior; monitor for emergence/worsening of depression, suicidal thoughts/behavior, and/or any unusual changes in mood/behavior. Serious and sometimes fatal dermatologic reactions, including toxic epidermal necrolysis (TEN) and Stevens-Johnson syndrome (SJS), reported; d/c at 1st sign of rash, unless the rash is clearly not drug-related. Do not resume therapy, and consider alternative therapy if signs/symptoms suggest SJS/TEN. Consideration should be given to avoid use as an alternative for carbamazepine in patients positive for HLA-B*1502. Drug reaction w/ eosinophilia and systemic symptoms (DRESS)/multiorgan hypersensitivity reported; evaluate immediately if signs and symptoms (eg, rash, fever, lymphadenopathy) are present and d/c if an alternative etiology cannot be established. Consider alternatives to structurally similar drugs (eg, carboxamides, barbiturates, succinimides, oxazolidinediones) in patients who have experienced phenytoin hypersensitivity. Acute hepatotoxicity (eg, acute hepatic failure) reported; d/c immediately and do not readminister. Hematopoietic complications and lymphadenopathy reported; extended follow-up observation is indicated and every effort should be made to achieve seizure control using alternative antiepileptic drugs in all cases of lymphadenopathy. Decreased bone mineral density and bone fractures reported during chronic use; consider screening and initiating treatment plans as appropriate. Caution w/ porphyria, hepatic impairment, and in elderly or gravely ill patients. An increase in seizure frequency may occur during pregnancy due to altered phenytoin pharmacokinetics. May cause fetal harm. Bleeding disorder in newborns may occur; give vitamin K to mother before delivery and to neonate after birth. Check plasma levels immediately if early signs of dose-related CNS toxicity develop.

Hyperglycemia reported; may increase serum glucose levels in diabetics. Not indicated for seizures due to hypoglycemia or other metabolic causes. Not effective for absence (petit mal) seizures; if tonic-clonic (grand mal) and absence (petit mal) seizures are present, combined drug therapy is needed. Serum levels of phenytoin sustained above the optimal range may produce confusional states or rarely irreversible cerebellar dysfunction and/or cerebellar atrophy; reduce dose if plasma levels are excessive, or d/c if symptoms persist. Lab test interactions may occur.

ADVERSE REACTIONS
Rash, nystagmus, ataxia, slurred speech, decreased coordination, somnolence, mental confusion, dizziness, insomnia, transient nervousness, motor twitching, acute hepatic failure, thrombocytopenia, altered taste sensation, Peyronie's disease.

DRUG INTERACTIONS
See Contraindications. Acute alcohol intake, amiodarone, antiepileptic agents (eg, ethosuximide, felbamate, oxcarbazepine), azoles (eg, fluconazole, ketoconazole, itraconazole), capecitabine, chloramphenicol, chlordiazepoxide, disulfiram, estrogens, fluorouracil, fluoxetine, fluvastatin, fluvoxamine, H2-antagonists (eg, cimetidine), halothane, isoniazid, methylphenidate, omeprazole, phenothiazines, salicylates, sertraline, succinimides, sulfonamides (eg, sulfamethizole, sulfadiazine, sulfamethoxazole-trimethoprim), ticlopidine, tolbutamide, trazodone, and warfarin may increase levels. Anticancer drugs usually in combination (eg, bleomycin, carboplatin, cisplatin), carbamazepine, chronic alcohol abuse, diazepam, diazoxide, folic acid, fosamprenavir, nelfinavir, reserpine, rifampin, ritonavir (RTV), St. John's wort, sucralfate, vigabatrin, and theophylline may decrease levels. Administration w/ preparations that increase gastric pH (eg, supplements or antacids containing calcium carbonate, aluminum hydroxide, and magnesium hydroxide) may affect absorption; do not take at the same time of day. Phenobarbital, sodium valproate, and valproic acid may increase or decrease levels. May impair efficacy of azoles (eg, fluconazole, ketoconazole, itraconazole), corticosteroids, doxycycline, estrogens, furosemide, irinotecan, oral contraceptives, paclitaxel, paroxetine, quinidine, rifampin, sertraline, teniposide, theophylline, and vitamin D. Increased and decreased PT/INR responses reported w/ warfarin. May decrease levels of active metabolites of albendazole, certain HIV antivirals (eg, efavirenz, lopinavir/RTV, indinavir), antiepileptic agents (eg, carbamazepine, felbamate, lamotrigine), atorvastatin, chlorpropamide, clozapine, cyclosporine, digoxin, fluvastatin, folic acid, methadone, mexiletine, nifedipine, nimodipine, nisoldipine, praziquantel, simvastatin, and verapamil. May decrease levels of amprenavir (active metabolite) when given w/ fosamprenavir alone. May increase levels of amprenavir when given w/ the combination of fosamprenavir and RTV. Resistance to the neuromuscular blocking action of pancuronium, vecuronium, rocuronium, and cisatracurium reported in patients chronically administered phenytoin; monitor closely for more rapid recovery from neuromuscular blockade than expected and infusion rate requirements may be higher. Enteral feeding preparations and/or related nutritional supplements may decrease levels; avoid w/ enteral feeding preparations.

PREGNANCY AND LACTATION
Pregnancy: Category D; physicians are advised to recommend that pregnant patients enroll in the North American Antiepileptic Drug (NAAED) Pregnancy Registry.
Lactation: Phenytoin appears to be secreted in low concentrations in human milk; not for use in nursing.

MECHANISM OF ACTION
Hydantoin; inhibits seizure activity by promoting Na+ efflux from neurons, stabilizing the threshold against hyperexcitability caused by excessive stimulation or environmental changes capable of reducing membrane Na+ gradient. Reduces the maximal activity of the brain stem centers responsible for the tonic phase of tonic-clonic (grand mal) seizures.

PHARMACOKINETICS
Absorption: T_{max}=1.5-3 hrs. **Distribution:** Plasma protein binding (high); crosses the placenta; found in breast milk. **Metabolism:** Liver (hydroxylation). CYP2C9 and CYP2C19. **Elimination:** Urine; $T_{1/2}$=14 hrs.

PATIENT CONSIDERATIONS
Assessment: Assess for hypersensitivity to the drug or other hydantoins, alcohol use, hepatic/renal impairment, porphyria, grave illness, seizures due to hypoglycemia or other metabolic causes, absence seizures, any other conditions where treatment is contraindicated or cautioned, pregnancy/nursing status, and possible drug interactions.

Monitoring: Monitor for hypersensitivity reactions, dermatologic reactions, DRESS/multiorgan hypersensitivity, hepatotoxicity, hematopoietic complications, lymphadenopathy, decreased bone mineral density, bone fractures, exacerbation of porphyria, hyperglycemia, and other adverse reactions. Monitor for emergence/worsening of depression, suicidal thoughts/behavior, and/or any unusual changes in mood/behavior. Monitor serum levels when switching from Na+ salt to free acid form and vice versa.

Counseling: Instruct to read medication guide and to take ud. Advise of the importance of adhering strictly to the prescribed dosage regimen, and of informing the physician of any clinical condition in which it is not possible to take the drug orally as prescribed (eg, surgery). Inform about the early toxic signs and symptoms of potential hematologic, dermatologic, hypersensitivity, or hepatic reactions; instruct to immediately contact physician if these develop. Caution on the use of other drugs or alcoholic beverages w/o first seeking physician's advice. Stress the importance of good dental hygiene to minimize the development of gingival hyperplasia and its complications. Advise to notify physician immediately if depression, suicidal thoughts/behavior, or thoughts about self-harm emerge. Encourage patients to enroll in the NAAED Pregnancy Registry if they become pregnant.

DILANTIN-125 — phenytoin

Rx

Class: Hydantoin

ADULT DOSAGE

Seizures

Tonic-Clonic (Grand Mal) and Psychomotor (Temporal Lobe) Seizures:

Initial: (Treatment naive) 125mg (1 tsp) tid

Titrate: May increase to 625mg (5 tsp) daily, if necessary

Clinically effective serum level is usually 10-20mcg/mL; do not change dose at intervals <7-10 days

Conversions

May require dose adjustment when switching from product formulated w/ free acid to product formulated w/ Na+ salt and vice versa

PEDIATRIC DOSAGE

Seizures

Tonic-Clonic (Grand Mal) and Psychomotor (Temporal Lobe) Seizures:

Initial: 5mg/kg/day in 2 or 3 equally divided doses

Maint: 4-8mg/kg/day

Max: 300mg/day

>6 Years: May require the minimum adult dose (300mg/day)

Clinically effective serum level is usually 10-20mcg/mL; do not change dose at intervals <7-10 days

Conversions

May require dose adjustment when switching from product formulated w/ free acid to product formulated w/ Na+ salt and vice versa

DOSING CONSIDERATIONS

Renal Impairment

Caution when interpreting total phenytoin plasma concentrations; unbound phenytoin concentrations may be more useful

Hepatic Impairment

Caution when interpreting total phenytoin plasma concentrations; unbound phenytoin concentrations may be more useful

Elderly

May require lower or less frequent dosing

Other Important Considerations

Hypoalbuminemia:

Caution when interpreting total phenytoin plasma concentrations; unbound phenytoin concentrations may be more useful

ADMINISTRATION

Oral route

Use an accurately calibrated measuring device to ensure accurate dosing.

STORAGE

20-25°C (68-77°F). Protect from freezing and light.

HOW SUPPLIED

Oral Sus: 125mg/5mL [237mL]

CONTRAINDICATIONS

History of hypersensitivity to phenytoin or its inactive ingredients, or other hydantoins. Coadministration w/ delavirdine.

WARNINGS/PRECAUTIONS

Unbound concentration of phenytoin may be elevated in patients w/ hyperbilirubinemia. Avoid abrupt withdrawal; may precipitate status epilepticus. May increase risk of suicidal thoughts/behavior; monitor for emergence/worsening of depression, suicidal thoughts/behavior, and/or any unusual changes in mood/behavior. Serious and sometimes fatal dermatologic reactions, including toxic epidermal necrolysis (TEN) and Stevens-Johnson syndrome (SJS), reported; d/c at 1st sign of rash, unless the rash is clearly not drug-related. Do not resume therapy, and consider alternative therapy if signs/symptoms suggest SJS/TEN. Consideration should be given to avoid use as an alternative for carbamazepine in patients positive for HLA-B*1502. Drug reaction w/ eosinophilia and systemic symptoms (DRESS)/multiorgan hypersensitivity reported; evaluate immediately if signs and symptoms (eg, rash, fever, lymphadenopathy) are present and d/c if an alternative etiology cannot be established. Consider alternatives to structurally similar drugs (eg, carboxamides, barbiturates, succinimides, oxazolidinediones) in patients who have experienced phenytoin hypersensitivity. Acute hepatotoxicity (eg, acute hepatic failure) reported; d/c immediately and do not readminister. Hematopoietic complications and lymphadenopathy reported; extended follow-up observation is indicated and every effort should be made to achieve seizure control using alternative antiepileptic drugs in all cases of lymphadenopathy. Decreased bone mineral density and bone fractures reported during chronic use; consider screening w/ bone-related laboratory and radiological tests as appropriate and initiating treatment plans according to established guidelines. Caution w/ porphyria, hepatic impairment, and in elderly or gravely ill patients. An increase in seizure frequency may occur during pregnancy due to altered phenytoin pharmacokinetics. May cause fetal harm. Bleeding disorder in newborns may occur; give vitamin K to mother before delivery and to neonate after birth. Check plasma levels immediately if early signs of dose-related CNS toxicity develop. Hyperglycemia reported; may increase serum glucose levels in diabetics. Not indicated for seizures due to hypoglycemia or other metabolic causes. Not effective for absence (petit mal) seizures; if tonic-clonic (grand mal) and absence (petit mal) seizures are present, combined drug therapy is needed. Serum levels of phenytoin sustained above the optimal range may produce confusional states or rarely irreversible cerebellar dysfunction and/or cerebellar atrophy; reduce dose if plasma levels are excessive and d/c if symptoms persist. Lab test interactions may occur.

ADVERSE REACTIONS

Rash, nystagmus, ataxia, slurred speech, decreased coordination, somnolence, mental confusion, dizziness, insomnia, transient nervousness, motor twitching, acute hepatic failure, thrombocytopenia, altered taste sensation, Peyronie's disease.

DRUG INTERACTIONS

See Contraindications. Acute alcohol intake, amiodarone, antiepileptic agents (eg, ethosuximide, felbamate, oxcarbazepine), azoles (eg, fluconazole, ketoconazole, itraconazole), capecitabine, chloramphenicol, chlordiazepoxide, disulfiram, estrogens, fluorouracil, fluoxetine, fluvastatin, fluvoxamine, H2-antagonists (eg, cimetidine), halothane, isoniazid, methylphenidate, omeprazole, phenothiazines, salicylates, sertraline, succinimides, sulfonamides (eg, sulfamethizole, sulfadiazine, sulfamethoxazole-trimethoprim), ticlopidine, tolbutamide, trazodone, and warfarin may increase levels. Anticancer drugs usually in combination (eg, bleomycin, carboplatin, cisplatin), carbamazepine, chronic alcohol abuse, diazepam, diazoxide, folic acid, fosamprenavir, nelfinavir, reserpine, rifampin, ritonavir (RTV), St. John's wort, sucralfate, vigabatrin, and theophylline may decrease levels. Administration w/ preparations that increase gastric pH (eg, supplements or antacids containing calcium carbonate, aluminum hydroxide, and magnesium hydroxide) may affect absorption; do not take at the same time of day. Phenobarbital, sodium valproate, and valproic acid may increase or decrease levels. May impair efficacy of azoles (eg, fluconazole, ketoconazole, itraconazole), corticosteroids, doxycycline, estrogens, furosemide, irinotecan, oral contraceptives, paclitaxel, paroxetine, quinidine, rifampin, sertraline, teniposide, theophylline, and vitamin D. Increased and decreased PT/INR responses reported w/ warfarin. May decrease levels of active metabolites of albendazole, certain HIV antivirals (eg, efavirenz, lopinavir/RTV, indinavir), antiepileptic agents (eg, carbamazepine, felbamate, lamotrigine), atorvastatin, chlorpropamide, clozapine, cyclosporine, digoxin, fluvastatin, folic acid, methadone, mexiletine, nifedipine, nimodipine, nisoldipine, praziquantel, simvastatin, and verapamil. May decrease levels of amprenavir (active metabolite) when given w/ fosamprenavir alone. May increase levels of amprenavir when given w/ the combination of fosamprenavir and RTV. Resistance to the neuromuscular blocking action of pancuronium, vecuronium, rocuronium, and cisatracurium reported in patients chronically administered phenytoin; monitor closely for more rapid recovery from neuromuscular blockade than expected and infusion rate requirements may be higher. Enteral feeding preparations and/or related nutritional supplements may decrease levels; avoid w/ enteral feeding preparations.

PREGNANCY AND LACTATION

Pregnancy: Category D; physicians are advised to recommend that pregnant patients enroll in the North American Antiepileptic Drug (NAAED) Pregnancy Registry.

Lactation: Phenytoin appears to be secreted in low concentrations in human milk; not for use in nursing.

MECHANISM OF ACTION

Hydantoin; inhibits seizure activity by promoting Na+ efflux from neurons, stabilizing the threshold against hyperexcitability caused by excessive stimulation or environmental changes capable of reducing membrane Na+ gradient. Reduces the maximal activity of the brain stem centers responsible for the tonic phase of tonic-clonic (grand mal) seizures.

PHARMACOKINETICS

Absorption: T_{max}=1.5-3 hrs. **Distribution:** Plasma protein binding (high); crosses the placenta; found in breast milk. **Metabolism:** Liver (hydroxylation). CYP2C9 and CYP2C19. **Elimination:** Urine; $T_{1/2}$=22 hrs.

PATIENT CONSIDERATIONS

Assessment: Assess for hypersensitivity to the drug or other hydantoins, alcohol use, hepatic/renal impairment, porphyria, grave illness, seizures due to hypoglycemia or other metabolic causes, absence seizures, any other conditions where treatment is contraindicated or cautioned, pregnancy/nursing status, and possible drug interactions.

Monitoring: Monitor for hypersensitivity reactions, dermatologic reactions, DRESS/multiorgan hypersensitivity, hepatotoxicity, hematopoietic complications, lymphadenopathy, decreased bone mineral density, bone fractures, exacerbation of porphyria, hyperglycemia, and other adverse reactions. Monitor for emergence/worsening of depression, suicidal thoughts/behavior, and/or any unusual changes in mood/behavior. Monitor serum levels when switching from Na+ salt to free acid form and vice versa.

Counseling: Instruct to read medication guide and to take ud. Advise of the importance of adhering strictly to the prescribed dosage regimen, and of informing the physician of any clinical condition in which it is not possible to take the drug orally as prescribed (eg, surgery). Inform about the early toxic signs and symptoms of potential hematologic, dermatologic, hypersensitivity, or hepatic reactions; instruct to immediately contact physician if these develop. Caution on the use of other drugs or alcoholic beverages w/o first seeking physician's advice. Stress the importance of good dental hygiene to minimize the development of gingival hyperplasia and its complications. Advise to notify physician immediately if depression, suicidal thoughts/behavior, or thoughts about self-harm emerge. Encourage patients to enroll in the NAAED Pregnancy Registry if they become pregnant.

DILAUDID INJECTION — hydromorphone hydrochloride   CII

Class: Opioid analgesic

> Contains hydromorphone, a Schedule II controlled opioid agonist with an abuse liability similar to other opioid analgesics. May be abused in a manner similar to other opioid agonists, legal or illicit; consider these risks when administering, prescribing, or dispensing in situations where increased risk of misuse, abuse, or diversion is a concern. Has the highest potential for abuse and risk of producing fatal overdose due to respiratory depression. Ethanol, other opioids, and other CNS depressants (eg, sedative-hypnotics, skeletal muscle relaxants) can potentiate the respiratory-depressant effects and increase the risk of adverse outcomes, including death. (HP) A more concentrated sol and is for use in opioid-tolerant patients only; do not confuse with standard parenteral formulations of hydromorphone or other opioids, as overdose and death may result.

OTHER BRAND NAMES
Dilaudid-HP

ADULT DOSAGE

Pain

Dilaudid:
Management of pain where an opioid analgesic is appropriate

SQ/IM:
Initial: 1-2mg q2-3h as necessary
Titrate: Adjust dose according to severity of pain and adverse events, as well as patient's underlying disease and age

IV:
Initial: 0.2-1mg q2-3h, given slowly, over at least 2-3 min, depending on the dose
Titrate: Adjust dose to achieve acceptable analgesia and tolerable adverse events

Dilaudid HP:
Management of moderate to severe pain in opioid-tolerant patients who require higher doses of opioids

Base starting dose on the prior dose of hydromorphone inj or on the prior dose of an alternate opioid; periodically reassess after the initial dosing

Conversions
From Morphine Sulfate: 10mg parenteral or 40-60mg oral
From Hydromorphone HCl: 1.3-2mg parenteral or 6.5-7.5mg oral
From Oxymorphone HCl: 1-1.1mg parenteral or 6.6mg oral
From Levorphanol Tartrate: 2-2.3mg parenteral or 4mg oral
From Meperidine HCl: 75-100mg parenteral or 300-400mg oral
From Methadone HCl: 10mg parenteral or 10-20mg oral
From Nalbuphine HCl: 10-12mg parenteral
From Butorphanol Tartrate: 1.5-2.5mg parenteral

PEDIATRIC DOSAGE
Pediatric use may not have been established

DOSING CONSIDERATIONS
Renal Impairment
Initial: 1/4 to 1/2 the usual starting dose depending on the degree of impairment
Hepatic Impairment
Initial: 1/4 to 1/2 the usual starting dose depending on the extent of impairment
Elderly
Start at lower end of dosing range
ADMINISTRATION
SQ/IM/IV route
Dilaudid Inj and HP Inj are physically compatible/chemically stable for at least 24 hrs at 25°C, protected from light in most large-volume parenteral sol
500mg/50mL Vial
Do not penetrate stopper w/ syringe; remove both flipseal and rubber stopper. Discard any unused portion
Reconstitution of Sterile Lyophilized HP Inj 250mg
Reconstitute immediately prior to use w/ 25mL of SWFI to provide a sol containing 10mg/mL of hydromorphone hydrochloride
STORAGE
20-25°C (68-77°F); excursions permitted to 15-30°C (59-86°F). Protect from light. Diluted Sol: Stable for at least 24 hrs at 25°C (77°F), protected from light in most common large-volume parenteral sol.
HOW SUPPLIED
Inj: 1mg/mL, 2mg/mL, 4mg/mL, (HP) 10mg/mL [1mL, 5mL, ampule; 50mL, vial], 250mg

CONTRAINDICATIONS
Known hypersensitivity to hydromorphone, hydromorphone salts, any other components of the product, or sulfite-containing medications; respiratory depression in the absence of resuscitative equipment or in unmonitored settings; acute or severe bronchial asthma; patients w/, or at risk of developing, GI obstruction, especially paralytic ileus. (HP) Patients who are not opioid-tolerant.

WARNINGS/PRECAUTIONS
Respiratory depression occurs most frequently in elderly, debilitated, and those suffering from upper airway obstruction or conditions accompanied by hypoxia or hypercapnia; extreme caution with chronic obstructive pulmonary disease (COPD) or cor pulmonale, substantially decreased respiratory reserve, hypoxia, hypercapnia, or preexisting respiratory depression. May cause neonatal withdrawal syndrome. Respiratory depressant effects with carbon dioxide retention and secondary elevation of CSF pressure may be markedly exaggerated in the presence of head injury, other intracranial lesions, or preexisting increase in intracranial pressure (ICP). May produce effects on pupillary response and consciousness, which can obscure the clinical course and neurologic signs of further increase ICP in patients with head injuries. May cause severe hypotension, and may produce orthostatic hypotension in ambulatory patients; caution with circulatory shock. Contains sodium metabisulfite, which may cause allergic-type reactions, including anaphylactic symptoms and life-threatening or less severe asthmatic episodes in certain susceptible people. May obscure the diagnosis or clinical course in patients with acute abdominal conditions. May cause spasm of the sphincter of Oddi and diminish biliary and pancreatic secretions; caution with biliary tract disease, including acute pancreatitis. Caution in elderly/debilitated and those with severe pulmonary/hepatic/renal impairment, myxedema/hypothyroidism, adrenocortical insufficiency (eg, Addison's disease), CNS depression or coma, toxic psychoses, prostatic hypertrophy, urethral stricture, acute alcoholism, delirium tremens, or kyphoscoliosis associated with respiratory depression; reduce initial dose. May aggravate preexisting convulsions in patients with convulsive disorders, and may induce or aggravate seizures in some clinical settings. Mild to severe seizures and myoclonus reported in severely compromised patients administered high doses of parenteral hydromorphone. Caution with alcoholism and other drug dependencies. May impair mental/physical abilities. Physical dependence and tolerance may occur. Do not abruptly d/c.

ADVERSE REACTIONS
Respiratory depression, apnea, lightheadedness, dizziness, sedation, N/V, sweating, flushing, dysphoria, euphoria, dry mouth, pruritus.

DRUG INTERACTIONS
See Boxed Warning. Concomitant use with other CNS depressants (eg, general anesthetics, phenothiazines, centrally-acting antiemetics, tranquilizers) increases the risk of hypotension and profound sedation, potentially resulting in coma or death; use with caution and in reduced dosages. May enhance action of neuromuscular blocking agents and produce an increased degree of respiratory depression. May cause severe hypotension with phenothiazines, general anesthetics, or other agents that compromise vasomotor tone. Mixed agonist/antagonist analgesics (pentazocine, nalbuphine, butorphanol, buprenorphine) may reduce the analgesic effect and/or may precipitate withdrawal symptoms; use with caution. MAOIs may potentiate action; allow at least 14 days after discontinuing treatment with MAOIs before starting therapy. Concomitant use with anticholinergics or other medications with anticholinergic activity may increase risk of urinary retention and severe constipation, which may lead to paralytic ileus.

PREGNANCY AND LACTATION
Category C, not for use in nursing.

MECHANISM OF ACTION
Opioid analgesic; μ-opioid receptor agonist. Has not been established. Believed to express pharmacologic effects by combining with specific CNS opiate receptors.

PHARMACOKINETICS
Distribution: Plasma protein binding (8-19%); V_d=302.9L (IV bolus); crosses placenta; found in breast milk. **Metabolism:** Liver (extensive) via glucuronidation; hydromorphone-3-glucuronide (metabolite). **Elimination:** Urine; $T_{1/2}$=2.3 hrs (IV).

PATIENT CONSIDERATIONS
Assessment: Assess for risk factors for drug abuse or addiction, pain type/severity, prior opioid therapy, opioid tolerance, respiratory depression, COPD, cor pulmonale, decreased respiratory reserve, hypoxia, hypercapnia, asthma, GI obstruction, renal/hepatic impairment, pregnancy/nursing status, possible drug interactions, or any other conditions where treatment is contraindicated or cautioned.

Monitoring: Monitor for respiratory depression, increase in ICP, hypotension, spasm of the sphincter of Oddi, aggravation/induction of convulsions/seizures, physical dependence, tolerance, and other adverse reactions. Monitor for signs of misuse, abuse, and addiction.

Counseling: Discuss the risk of respiratory depression. Instruct to report adverse events experienced during therapy. Advise not to adjust dose or combine with alcohol or other CNS depressants without prescriber's consent. Inform that drug may impair mental/physical abilities; instruct to use caution when performing hazardous tasks (eg, operating machinery/driving). Advise to consult physician if pregnant or planning to become pregnant. Inform that drug has potential for abuse; instruct to protect it from theft and never to share with others. Instruct to avoid abrupt withdrawal.

DILAUDID ORAL — hydromorphone hydrochloride   CII
Class: Opioid analgesic

> Contains hydromorphone, a Schedule II controlled opioid agonist with the highest potential for abuse and risk of respiratory depression. Alcohol, other opioids, and CNS depressants (eg, sedative-hypnotics) potentiate respiratory depressant effects, increasing the risk of respiratory depression that may result in death.

ADULT DOSAGE
Pain

Periodically reassess after the initial dosing

Sol:
Usual: 2.5-10mg q3-6h ud by clinical situation

Tab:
Initial: 2-4mg q4-6h
Titrate: May increase gradually if analgesia is inadequate, as tolerance develops, or if pain severity increases

Sol/Tab:
Nonopioid-Tolerant:
Initial: 2-4mg q4h

Taking Opioids:
Base starting dose on prior opioid usage
Give only 1/2 to 2/3 of the estimated dose for the 1st few doses, then increase prn according to response

Chronic Pain:
Administer dose around-the-clock
May give a supplemental dose of 5-15% of the total daily usage q2h prn

Conversions

From Morphine Sulfate: 10mg parenteral or 40-60mg oral
From Hydromorphone HCl: 1.3-2mg parenteral or 6.5-7.5mg oral
From Oxymorphone HCl: 1-1.1mg parenteral or 6.6mg oral
From Levorphanol Tartrate: 2-2.3mg parenteral or 4mg oral
From Meperidine HCl: 75-100mg parenteral or 300-400mg oral
From Methadone HCl: 10mg parenteral or 10-20mg oral

PEDIATRIC DOSAGE
Pediatric use may not have been established

DOSING CONSIDERATIONS
Renal Impairment
Moderate-Severe:
Start on a lower dose and closely monitor during titration
Use oral liquid to adjust the dose

Hepatic Impairment
Moderate:
Start on a lower dose and closely monitor during titration
Use oral liquid to adjust the dose

Elderly
Start at lower end of dosing range

ADMINISTRATION
Oral route

STORAGE
25°C (77°F); excursions permitted to 15-30°C (59-86°F). Protect from light.

HOW SUPPLIED
Sol: 1mg/mL [473mL]; **Tab:** 2mg, 4mg, 8mg* *scored

CONTRAINDICATIONS
Known hypersensitivity to hydromorphone, respiratory depression in the absence of resuscitative equipment, status asthmaticus, obstetrical analgesia.

WARNINGS/PRECAUTIONS
Respiratory depression is more likely to occur in elderly, debilitated, and those suffering from conditions accompanied by hypoxia or hypercapnia; extreme caution with chronic obstructive pulmonary disease (COPD) or cor pulmonale, substantially decreased respiratory reserve, hypoxia, hypercapnia, or preexisting respiratory depression. May cause neonatal withdrawal syndrome. Respiratory depressant effects with carbon dioxide retention and secondary elevation of CSF pressure may be markedly exaggerated in the presence of head injury, other intracranial lesions, or preexisting increase in intracranial pressure (ICP). May produce effects on pupillary response and consciousness, which can obscure the clinical course and neurologic signs of further increase in ICP in patients with head injuries. May cause severe hypotension; caution with circulatory shock. Contains sodium metabisulfite; may cause allergic-type reactions, including anaphylactic symptoms and life-threatening or less severe asthmatic episodes in certain susceptible people. Caution in elderly/debilitated and those with severe pulmonary/hepatic/renal impairment, myxedema/hypothyroidism, adrenocortical insufficiency (eg, Addison's disease), CNS depression or coma, toxic psychoses, prostatic hypertrophy, urethral stricture, gallbladder disease, acute alcoholism, delirium tremens, kyphoscoliosis, or following GI surgery; reduce initial dose. May obscure the diagnosis or clinical course in patients with acute abdominal conditions. May aggravate preexisting convulsions in patients with convulsive disorders. Mild to severe seizures and myoclonus reported in severely compromised patients administered high doses of parenteral hydromorphone. Caution with alcoholism and other drug dependencies. May impair mental/physical abilities. May produce orthostatic hypotension in ambulatory patients. May cause spasm of the sphincter of Oddi; caution in patients about to undergo biliary tract surgery. Physical dependence and tolerance may occur. Do not abruptly d/c.

ADVERSE REACTIONS
Respiratory depression, apnea, lightheadedness, dizziness, sedation, N/V, sweating, flushing, dysphoria, euphoria, dry mouth, pruritus.

DRUG INTERACTIONS
See Boxed Warning. Concomitant use with other CNS depressants (eg, general anesthetics, phenothiazines, tranquilizers) may produce additive depressant effects; use with caution and in reduced dosages. Do not give with alcohol. May enhance action of neuromuscular blocking agents and produce an excessive degree of respiratory depression. May cause severe hypotension with phenothiazines or general anesthetics. Mixed agonist/antagonist analgesics (pentazocine, nalbuphine, butorphanol, buprenorphine) may reduce the analgesic effect and/or may precipitate withdrawal symptoms; use with caution.

PREGNANCY AND LACTATION
Category C, not for use in nursing.

MECHANISM OF ACTION
Opioid analgesic; pure opioid agonist. Has not been established. Believed to express pharmacologic effects by combining with specific CNS opiate receptors.

PHARMACOKINETICS
Absorption: Rapid. (Tab) Bioavailability (24%); C_{max}=5.5ng; T_{max}=0.74 hrs; AUC=23.7ng•hr/mL. (Sol) C_{max}=5.7ng; T_{max}=0.73 hrs; AUC=24.6ng•hr/mL.
Distribution: Plasma protein binding (8-19%); V_d=302.9L (IV bolus); crosses placenta; found in breast milk. **Metabolism:** Liver (extensive) via glucuronidation; hydromorphone-3-glucuronide (metabolite). **Elimination:** Urine; $T_{1/2}$=2.6 hrs (tab), 2.8 hrs (sol).

PATIENT CONSIDERATIONS
Assessment: Assess for risk factors for drug abuse or addiction, pain type/severity, prior opioid therapy, opioid tolerance, respiratory depression, COPD, cor pulmonale, decreased respiratory reserve, hypoxia, hypercapnia, asthma, renal/hepatic impairment, pregnancy/nursing status, possible drug interactions, or any other conditions where treatment is contraindicated or cautioned.

Monitoring: Monitor for respiratory depression, sedation, CNS depression, aggravation/induction of seizures/convulsions, increase in ICP, hypotension, tolerance, physical dependence, and other adverse reactions. Routinely monitor for signs of misuse, abuse, and addiction.

Counseling: Inform that medication may cause severe adverse effects (eg, respiratory depression) if not taken ud. Instruct to report pain and adverse experiences occurring during therapy. Advise not to adjust dose or combine with alcohol or other CNS depressants without prescriber's consent. Inform that drug may impair mental/physical abilities; instruct to use caution when performing hazardous tasks (eg, operating machinery/driving). Advise to consult physician if pregnant or planning to become pregnant. Inform that drug has potential for abuse; instruct to protect it from theft and never to share with others. Advise to avoid abrupt withdrawal if taking medication for more than a few weeks and cessation of therapy is indicated. Instruct to keep drug in a secure place, and to destroy unused tabs by flushing down toilet.

DILTIAZEM TABLETS — diltiazem hydrochloride   Rx
Class: Calcium channel blocker (CCB) (nondihydropyridine)

OTHER BRAND NAMES
Cardizem

ADULT DOSAGE
Angina

Chronic Stable Angina and Angina Due to Coronary Artery Spasm:
Initial: 30mg qid
Titrate: Increase gradually (given in divided doses tid-qid) at 1- to 2-day intervals until optimum response obtained
Usual Range: 180-360mg/day

PEDIATRIC DOSAGE
Pediatric use may not have been established

DOSING CONSIDERATIONS
Concomitant Medications
Sublingual Nitroglycerin: May take as required to abort acute angina attacks during therapy
Prophylactic Nitrate Therapy: May be coadministered w/ short- and long-acting nitrates

Elderly
Start at lower end of dosing range

ADMINISTRATION
Oral route

Take ac and hs.
Swallow tab whole; do not split, crush, or chew.

STORAGE
20-25°C (68-77°F). Protect from light. (Cardizem) 25°C (77°F); excursions permitted to 15-30°C (59-86°F). Avoid excessive humidity.

HOW SUPPLIED
Tab: 90mg*, (Cardizem) 30mg, 60mg*; 120mg* *scored

CONTRAINDICATIONS
Sick sinus syndrome and 2nd- or 3rd-degree atrioventricular (AV) block (except w/ functioning ventricular pacemaker), hypotension (<90mmHg systolic), acute myocardial infarction (MI) and pulmonary congestion documented by x-ray on admission. Hypersensitivity to diltiazem HCl.

WARNINGS/PRECAUTIONS
Prolongs AV node refractory periods w/o significantly prolonging sinus node recovery time, except in patients w/ sick sinus syndrome. Periods of asystole reported in a patient w/ Prinzmetal's angina. Caution w/ renal/hepatic/ventricular impairment. Symptomatic hypotension may occur. Significant elevations in enzymes (eg, alkaline phosphatase, lactate dehydrogenase, AST, ALT) and other phenomena consistent w/ acute hepatic injury noted in rare instances. Transient dermatological events and skin eruptions progressing to erythema multiforme and/or exfoliative dermatitis have been reported; d/c if a dermatologic reaction persists.

ADVERSE REACTIONS
Edema, headache, nausea, dizziness, rash, asthenia.

DRUG INTERACTIONS
Potential additive effects w/ agents known to affect cardiac contractility and/or conduction; caution and careful titration are warranted. Additive effects in prolonging cardiac conduction w/ β-blockers or digitalis. CYP3A4 substrates, inhibitors, or inducers may have a significant impact on the efficacy and side effect profile; substrates, especially in patients w/ renal and/or hepatic impairment, may require dosage adjustment when starting or stopping therapy. May potentiate depression of cardiac contractility, conductivity and automaticity, and vascular dilation associated w/ anesthetics; carefully titrate anesthetics and calcium channel blockers when used concomitantly. May increase levels of midazolam, triazolam, carbamazepine, and lovastatin. May increase exposure and $T_{1/2}$ of quinidine; monitor for adverse effects of quinidine. May increase levels of propranolol; adjustment of the propranolol dose may be warranted during initiation or withdrawal of therapy. May increase levels of buspirone; subsequent dose adjustments may be necessary. Increased levels w/ cimetidine; adjustment of diltiazem dose may be warranted. Sinus bradycardia resulting in hospitalization and pacemaker insertion reported w/ clonidine; monitor HR. Monitor cyclosporine/digoxin concentrations, especially when diltiazem therapy is initiated, adjusted, or discontinued. Rifampin may decrease concentrations; avoid rifampin or any CYP3A4 inducer when possible, and consider alternative therapy. May increase simvastatin exposure; limit daily doses of simvastatin to 10mg and diltiazem to 240mg if coadministration is required. Risk of myopathy/rhabdomyolysis w/ statins metabolized by CYP3A4 may be increased. When possible, use a non-CYP3A4-metabolized statin; otherwise, consider dose adjustments for both agents and closely monitor for signs/symptoms of any statin-related adverse events.

PREGNANCY AND LACTATION
Pregnancy: Embryo and fetal lethality seen in animal studies; use in pregnant women only if the potential benefit justifies the potential risk to the fetus.
Lactation: Found in breast milk; not for use in nursing.

MECHANISM OF ACTION
Calcium channel blocker; inhibits influx of Ca^{2+} ions during membrane depolarization of cardiac and vascular smooth muscle. Angina Due to Coronary Artery Spasm: A potent dilator of coronary arteries both epicardial and subendocardial; inhibits spontaneous and ergonovine-induced coronary artery spasm. Exertional Angina: Produces increases in exercise tolerance by reducing myocardial oxygen demand, accomplished via reduction in HR and systemic BP at submaximal and maximal exercise workloads.

PHARMACOKINETICS
Absorption: Well-absorbed from GI tract. Absolute bioavailability (40%); T_{max}=2-4 hrs. **Distribution:** Plasma protein binding (70-80%); found in breast milk. **Metabolism:** Liver (extensive). **Elimination:** Urine (2-4%, unchanged), bile. $T_{1/2}$ = approx 3-4.5 hrs.

PATIENT CONSIDERATIONS
Assessment: Assess for previous hypersensitivity to the drug, sick sinus syndrome, 2nd- or 3rd-degree AV block, presence of functioning ventricular pacemaker, hypotension, acute MI, pulmonary congestion, ventricular/hepatic/renal impairment, pregnancy/nursing status, and possible drug interactions.

Monitoring: Monitor for bradycardia, AV block, symptomatic hypotension, dermatological reactions, and other adverse reactions. Monitor LFTs and renal function at regular intervals.

Counseling: Inform about benefits/risks of therapy. Counsel to report any adverse reactions to physician and to notify physician if pregnant or nursing.

DIOVAN — valsartan   Rx
Class: Angiotensin II receptor blocker (ARB)

> D/C when pregnancy is detected. Drugs that act directly on the renin-angiotensin system (RAS) can cause injury/death to the developing fetus.

ADULT DOSAGE
Hypertension
Initial: 80mg or 160mg qd
Titrate: May increase to a max of 320mg qd
May add diuretic if BP not controlled

Heart Failure
NYHA Class II-IV
Initial: 40mg bid
Titrate: May increase to 80mg and 160mg bid (use highest dose tolerated)
Max: 320mg/day in divided doses

Post-Myocardial Infarction
Initial: 20mg bid as early as 12 hrs after MI
Titrate: May increase to 40mg bid w/in 7 days, w/ subsequent titrations to 160mg bid as tolerated
Maint: 160mg bid
Consider reducing dose if symptomatic hypotension or renal dysfunction occurs

PEDIATRIC DOSAGE
Hypertension
6-16 Years:
Initial: 1.3mg/kg qd (up to 40mg total)
Titrate: Adjust dose according to BP response
Max: 2.7mg/kg (up to 160mg) qd

DOSING CONSIDERATIONS
Concomitant Medications
Consider reducing concomitant diuretic dose in patients w/ heart failure (HF)

ADMINISTRATION
Oral route
Take w/ or w/o food.
Use of sus is recommended for children who cannot swallow tabs, or if calculated dosage does not correspond to available tab strength.
Adjust dose accordingly when switching dosage forms; exposure w/ sus is 1.6X greater than w/ tab.

Preparation of Sus (for 160mL of a 4mg/mL Sus)
1. Add 80mL of Ora-Plus oral suspending vehicle to an amber glass bottle containing 8 Diovan 80mg tabs, and shake for a minimum of 2 min
2. Allow the sus to stand for a minimum of 1 hr
3. After the standing time, shake the sus for a minimum of 1 additional min
4. Add 80mL of Ora-Sweet SF oral sweetening vehicle to the bottle and shake the sus for at least 10 sec to disperse the ingredients
5. The sus is homogenous and can be stored for either up to 30 days at room temperature (below 30°C/86°F) or up to 75 days at refrigerated conditions (2-8°C/35-46°F) in the glass bottle
6. Shake the bottle well (at least 10 sec) prior to dispensing the sus

STORAGE
(Tab) 25°C (77°F); excursions permitted to 15-30°C (59-86°F). Protect from moisture. (Sus) <30°C (86°F) for up to 30 days or at 2-8°C (35-46°F) for up to 75 days.

HOW SUPPLIED
Tab: 40mg*, 80mg, 160mg, 320mg *scored

CONTRAINDICATIONS
Known hypersensitivity to any component of this medication. Coadministration w/ aliskiren in patients w/ diabetes.

WARNINGS/PRECAUTIONS
Symptomatic hypotension may occur in patients w/ an activated RAS (eg, volume- and/or salt-depleted patients receiving high doses of diuretics); correct this condition prior to therapy. Caution when initiating therapy in patients w/ HF or post-MI. Renal function changes may occur; caution in patients whose renal function depend in part on the activity of the RAS (eg, renal artery stenosis, chronic kidney disease, severe CHF, volume depletion). Consider withholding or discontinuing therapy if clinically significant decrease in renal function develops. Increased K^+ in some patients w/ HF reported, and more likely to occur in patients w/ preexisting renal impairment; dose reduction and/or discontinuation of therapy may be required. Do not readminister to patients who have had angioedema. Caution w/ dosing in patients w/ hepatic or severe renal impairment.

ADVERSE REACTIONS
Headache, abdominal pain, cough, increased BUN, hyperkalemia, dizziness, hypotension, SrCr elevation, viral infection, fatigue, diarrhea, arthralgia, back pain.

DRUG INTERACTIONS
See Contraindications. Dual blockade of the RAS is associated w/ increased risk of hypotension, hyperkalemia, and changes in renal function (including acute renal failure); avoid combined use of RAS inhibitors, or closely monitor BP, renal function, and electrolytes w/ concomitant agents that also affect the RAS. Avoid w/ aliskiren in patients w/ renal impairment (GFR <60mL/min). Inhibitors of the hepatic uptake transporter OATP1B1 (rifampin, cyclosporine) and the hepatic efflux transporter MRP2 (ritonavir) may increase exposure. Other agents that block the RAS, K^+-sparing diuretics, K^+ supplements, salt substitutes containing

K⁺, or other drugs that may increase K⁺ levels (heparin), may increase serum K⁺ levels, and in HF patients may increase serum K⁺ levels. Greater antihypertensive effect w/ atenolol. NSAIDs, including selective COX-2 inhibitors, may result in deterioration of renal function, including possible acute renal failure, and may attenuate antihypertensive effect. Increased lithium levels and lithium toxicity reported; monitor serum lithium levels during concomitant use.

PREGNANCY AND LACTATION
Pregnancy: Category D.
Lactation: Not for use in nursing.

MECHANISM OF ACTION
Angiotensin II receptor blocker; blocks vasoconstrictor and aldosterone-secreting effects of angiotensin II by selectively blocking the binding of angiotensin II to the AT_1 receptor in many tissues (eg, vascular smooth muscle, adrenal gland).

PHARMACOKINETICS
Absorption: Absolute bioavailability (25%); T_{max}=2-4 hrs. **Distribution:** Plasma protein binding (95%); (IV) V_d=17L. **Metabolism:** Via CYP2C9; valeryl 4-hydroxy valsartan (primary metabolite). **Elimination:** (Sol) Feces (83%), urine (13%). (IV) $T_{1/2}$=6 hrs.

PATIENT CONSIDERATIONS
Assessment: Assess for hypersensitivity to the drug and its components, hepatic/renal impairment, volume/salt depletion, renal artery stenosis, HF, pregnancy/nursing status, and possible drug interactions.

Monitoring: Monitor for signs/symptoms of hypotension and other adverse reactions. Monitor electrolytes, BP, and renal function.

Counseling: Counsel about the risk/benefits of therapy and possible adverse effects. Inform of consequences of exposure during pregnancy and discuss treatment options w/ women planning to become pregnant. Instruct to report pregnancies to physician as soon as possible.

DIOVAN HCT — hydrochlorothiazide/valsartan   Rx

Class: Angiotensin II receptor blocker (ARB)/thiazide diuretic

> D/C when pregnancy is detected. Drugs that act directly on the renin-angiotensin system (RAS) can cause injury/death to the developing fetus.

ADULT DOSAGE
Hypertension

Initial: 160mg/12.5mg qd
Titrate: May increase after 1-2 weeks of therapy
Max: 320mg/25mg qd

Add-On Therapy:
Use if not adequately controlled w/ valsartan (or another ARB) alone or HCTZ alone
W/ dose-limiting adverse reactions to either component alone, may switch to therapy containing a lower dose of that component
Titrate: May increase after 3-4 weeks of therapy if BP uncontrolled
Max: 320mg/25mg

Replacement Therapy:
May substitute for titrated components

PEDIATRIC DOSAGE
Pediatric use may not have been established

ADMINISTRATION
Oral route
Take w/ or w/o food.

STORAGE
25°C (77°F); excursions permitted to 15-30°C (59-86°F). Protect from moisture.

HOW SUPPLIED
Tab: (Valsartan/HCTZ) 80mg/12.5mg, 160mg/12.5mg, 160mg/25mg, 320mg/12.5mg, 320mg/25mg

CONTRAINDICATIONS
Anuria, sulfonamide-derived drug hypersensitivity, hypersensitivity to any component of this product. Coadministration w/ aliskiren in patients w/ diabetes.

WARNINGS/PRECAUTIONS
Not for initial therapy w/ intravascular volume depletion. Symptomatic hypotension may occur in patients w/ activated RAS (eg, volume- and/or salt-depleted patients receiving high doses of diuretics); correct this condition prior to therapy. Renal function changes may occur including acute renal failure; caution in patients whose renal function depends in part on the activity of the RAS (eg, renal artery stenosis, chronic kidney disease, severe CHF, volume depletion). Consider withholding or discontinuing therapy if clinically significant decrease in renal function develops. May cause serum electrolyte abnormalities (eg, hyperkalemia, hypokalemia, hyponatremia, hypomagnesemia); correct hypokalemia and any coexisting hypomagnesemia prior to initiation of therapy and monitor periodically. D/C if hypokalemia is accompanied by clinical signs (eg, muscular weakness, paresis, ECG alterations). Increased K⁺ in patients w/ heart failure (HF) reported; dose reduction or discontinuation of therapy may be required. Do not readminister to patients w/ angioedema. **HCTZ:** May cause hypersensitivity reactions and exacerbation or activation of systemic lupus

erythematosus (SLE). May precipitate hepatic coma w/ hepatic impairment or progressive liver disease. May cause idiosyncratic reaction, resulting in acute transient myopia and acute angle-closure glaucoma; d/c as rapidly as possible. May alter glucose tolerance and increase serum cholesterol and TG levels. May cause or exacerbate hyperuricemia and precipitate gout in susceptible patients. May cause hypercalcemia.

ADVERSE REACTIONS
Dizziness, BUN elevations, hypokalemia, angioedema, dry cough, nasopharyngitis.

DRUG INTERACTIONS
See Contraindications. Increased lithium levels and lithium toxicity reported; monitor lithium levels during concomitant use. **Valsartan:** Dual blockade of the RAS is associated w/ increased risk of hypotension, hyperkalemia, and changes in renal function (including acute renal failure); avoid combined use of RAS inhibitors, or closely monitor BP, renal function, and electrolytes w/ concomitant agents that also affect the RAS. Avoid w/ aliskiren in patients w/ renal impairment (GFR <60mL/min). Greater antihypertensive effect w/ atenolol. Inhibitors of the hepatic uptake transporter OATP1B1 (rifampin, cyclosporine) or the hepatic efflux transporter MRP2 (ritonavir) may increase exposure. NSAIDs, including selective COX-2 inhibitors, may result in deterioration of renal function, including possible acute renal failure, and may attenuate antihypertensive effect. Other agents that block the RAS, K⁺-sparing diuretics, K⁺ supplements, salt substitutes containing K⁺, or other drugs that may increase K⁺ levels (heparin), may increase serum K⁺ levels, and in HF patients may increase SrCr; monitor serum K⁺ levels. **HCTZ:** Dosage adjustment of antidiabetic drugs (eg, oral agents, insulin) may be required. May lead to symptomatic hyponatremia w/ carbamazepine. Ion exchange resins (eg, cholestyramine, colestipol) may reduce exposure; space dosing at least 4 hrs before or 4-6 hrs after the administration of ion exchange resins. Cyclosporine may increase risk of hyperuricemia and gout-type complications.

PREGNANCY AND LACTATION
Category D, not for use in nursing.

MECHANISM OF ACTION
Valsartan: Angiotensin II receptor blocker; blocks vasoconstrictor and aldosterone-secreting effects of angiotensin II by selectively blocking binding of angiotensin II to AT_1 receptor in many tissues (eg, vascular smooth muscle, adrenal gland). **HCTZ:** Thiazide diuretic; has not been established. Affects the renal tubular mechanisms of electrolyte reabsorption, directly increasing excretion of Na⁺ and Cl⁻ in approximately equivalent amounts.

PHARMACOKINETICS
Absorption: Valsartan: (Cap) Absolute bioavailability (25%); T_{max}=2-4 hrs. HCTZ: Absolute bioavailability (70%); T_{max}=2-5 hrs. **Distribution:** Valsartan: Plasma protein binding (95%); (IV) V_d=17L. HCTZ: Albumin binding (40-70%); crosses placenta; found in breast milk. **Metabolism:** Valsartan: Via CYP2C9; valeryl 4-hydroxy valsartan (primary metabolite). **Elimination:** Valsartan: (Sol) Feces (83%), urine (13%); (IV) $T_{1/2}$=6 hrs. HCTZ: Urine (70%, unchanged); $T_{1/2}$=10 hrs.

PATIENT CONSIDERATIONS
Assessment: Assess for hypersensitivity to the drug and its components, anuria, history of sulfonamide-derived hypersensitivity or penicillin allergy, renal/hepatic impairment, volume/salt depletion, risk for acute renal failure, SLE, electrolyte imbalances, pregnancy/nursing status, and possible drug interactions.

Monitoring: Monitor for signs/symptoms of hypotension, hypersensitivity/idiosyncratic reactions, exacerbation or activation of SLE, myopia, angle-closure glaucoma, precipitation of gout or hyperuricemia, and other adverse reactions. Monitor BP, serum electrolytes, cholesterol, TG levels, and renal function periodically.

Counseling: Inform about the consequences of exposure during pregnancy and discuss treatment options in women planning to become pregnant. Instruct to report pregnancies to physician as soon as possible. Caution about lightheadedness, especially during the 1st days of therapy; instruct to d/c and consult physician if syncope occurs. Caution that inadequate fluid intake, excessive perspiration, diarrhea, and vomiting may lead to an excessive fall in BP, w/ the same consequences of lightheadedness and possible syncope. Instruct to avoid use of K⁺ supplements or salt substitutes containing K⁺ w/o consulting a physician.

DIPROLENE — betamethasone dipropionate   Rx

Class: Corticosteroid

OTHER BRAND NAMES
Diprolene AF

ADULT DOSAGE
Inflammatory and Pruritic Manifestations of Corticosteroid-Responsive Dermatoses

Lot:
Usual: Apply a few drops to affected skin qd or bid and massage lightly until it disappears
Max: 50mL/week; limit treatment to 2 weeks
D/C when control is achieved; reassess diagnosis if no improvement seen w/in 2 weeks

Oint:
Usual: Apply a thin film to affected skin qd or bid

PEDIATRIC DOSAGE
Inflammatory and Pruritic Manifestations of Corticosteroid-Responsive Dermatoses

≥13 Years:
Lot:
Usual: Apply a few drops to affected skin qd or bid and massage lightly until it disappears
Max: 50mL/week; limit treatment to 2 weeks
D/C when control is achieved; reassess diagnosis if no improvement seen w/in 2 weeks

Oint:
Usual: Apply a thin film to affected skin qd or bid

Max: 50g/week
D/C when control is achieved; reassess diagnosis if no improvement seen w/in 2 weeks

Cre:
Usual: Apply a thin film to affected skin qd or bid
Max: 50g/week
D/C when control is achieved

Max: 50g/week
D/C when control is achieved; reassess diagnosis if no improvement seen w/in 2 weeks

Cre:
Usual: Apply a thin film to affected skin qd or bid
Max: 50g/week
D/C when control is achieved

ADMINISTRATION
Topical route
Avoid use w/ occlusive dressings unless directed

STORAGE
25°C (77°F); excursions permitted to 15-30°C (59-86°F).

HOW SUPPLIED
Cre (AF)/Oint: 0.05% [15g, 50g]; **Lot:** 0.05% [30mL, 60mL]

CONTRAINDICATIONS
Hypersensitivity to betamethasone dipropionate, to other corticosteroids, or to any ingredient in this preparation.

WARNINGS/PRECAUTIONS
Avoid use with occlusive dressings. Avoid use on the face, groin, or axillae or if skin atrophy is present at the treatment site. May produce reversible hypothalamic-pituitary-adrenal (HPA) axis suppression with the potential for glucocorticosteroid insufficiency; may occur during or after withdrawal of treatment. Periodically evaluate for HPA axis suppression and, if noted, gradually withdraw drug, reduce frequency of application, or substitute a less potent corticosteroid. Infrequently, signs/symptoms of steroid withdrawal may occur, requiring supplemental systemic corticosteroids. Cushing's syndrome and hyperglycemia may occur. Pediatric patients may be more susceptible to systemic toxicity. Allergic contact dermatitis reported; confirm by patch testing. D/C and institute appropriate therapy if irritation develops. Not for treatment of diaper dermatitis.

ADVERSE REACTIONS
(Cre) Skin atrophy (telangiectasia, bruising, shininess). (Oint/Lot) Erythema, folliculitis, pruritus, vesiculation.

PREGNANCY AND LACTATION
Category C, caution in nursing.

MECHANISM OF ACTION
Corticosteroid; has not been established. Plays a role in cellular signaling, immune function, inflammation, and protein regulation.

PHARMACOKINETICS
Absorption: Percutaneous; extent of absorption is determined by vehicle, integrity of the epidermal barrier, and use of occlusive dressings. **Distribution:** Bound to plasma proteins in varying degrees; found in breast milk (systemically administered). **Metabolism:** Liver. **Elimination:** Kidneys, bile.

PATIENT CONSIDERATIONS
Assessment: Assess for hypersensitivity to corticosteroids, factors that predispose to HPA axis suppression, pregnancy/nursing status, and possible drug interactions. Evaluate for HPA axis suppression using the adrenocorticotropic hormone (ACTH) stimulation test.

Monitoring: Monitor for signs/symptoms of HPA axis suppression, Cushing's syndrome, hyperglycemia, irritation, and other adverse reactions. Perform periodic monitoring of HPA axis suppression using ACTH stimulation test. Monitor for systemic toxicity in pediatric patients. Monitor response to therapy.

Counseling: Inform to d/c therapy when control is achieved, unless directed otherwise by physician. Counsel to avoid contact with eyes. Instruct not to use on face, underarms, or groin areas unless directed by physician. Instruct not to occlude the treatment area with bandage or other covering, unless directed by the physician. Inform that local reactions and skin atrophy are more likely to occur with occlusive use, prolonged use or use of higher potency corticosteroids. (Lot/Oint) Instruct to use no longer than 2 consecutive weeks.

DITROPAN XL — oxybutynin chloride   Rx
Class: Anticholinergic

ADULT DOSAGE	**PEDIATRIC DOSAGE**
Overactive Bladder	**Detrusor Overactivity**
Initial: 5 or 10mg qd at the same time each day	**Associated w/ a Neurological Condition (eg, Spina Bifida):**
Titrate: May adjust dose in 5mg increments weekly	**≥6 Years:**
Max: 30mg/day	**Initial:** 5mg qd at the same time each day
	Titrate: May adjust dose in 5mg increments
	Max: 20mg/day

ADMINISTRATION
Oral route
May be taken w/ or w/o food
Swallow tab whole w/ aid of liquids; do not chew, divide, or crush

STORAGE
25°C (77°F); excursions permitted to 15-30°C (59-86°F). Protect from moisture and humidity.

HOW SUPPLIED
Tab, Extended-Release: 5mg, 10mg, 15mg

CONTRAINDICATIONS
Urinary retention, gastric retention and other severe decreased GI motility conditions, uncontrolled narrow-angle glaucoma. Hypersensitivity to the drug substance or other components of the product.

WARNINGS/PRECAUTIONS
Angioedema of the face, lips, tongue, and/or larynx reported; d/c promptly and provide appropriate therapy if angioedema occurs. Associated w/ anticholinergic CNS effects; consider dose reduction or discontinuation if any occur. Caution w/ preexisting dementia treated w/ cholinesterase inhibitors, Parkinson's disease, myasthenia gravis, autonomic neuropathy, clinically significant bladder outflow obstruction, GI obstructive disorders, ulcerative colitis, intestinal atony, GERD, and preexisting severe GI narrowing (pathologic or iatrogenic). May decrease GI motility. May impair mental/physical abilities. Not recommended in pediatric patients who cannot swallow tab whole w/o chewing, dividing, or crushing.

ADVERSE REACTIONS
Dry mouth, constipation, diarrhea, headache, somnolence, dizziness, dyspepsia, nausea, blurred vision, dry eyes, insomnia.

DRUG INTERACTIONS
Concomitant use w/ other anticholinergic drugs may increase the frequency and/or severity of anticholinergic-like effects. May alter GI absorption of other drugs due to GI motility effects; caution w/ drugs w/ narrow therapeutic index. May antagonize effects of prokinetic agents (eg, metoclopramide). Increased levels w/ ketoconazole. Caution w/ CYP3A4 inhibitors (eg, antimycotics, macrolides); may alter mean pharmacokinetic parameters. Caution w/ drugs that may cause/exacerbate esophagitis (eg, bisphosphonates).

PREGNANCY AND LACTATION
Category B, caution in nursing.

MECHANISM OF ACTION
Antispasmodic/anticholinergic agent; exerts direct antispasmodic effect on smooth muscle and inhibits muscarinic action of acetylcholine on smooth muscle. Relaxes smooth muscle of bladder.

PHARMACOKINETICS
Absorption: C_{max}=1.0ng/mL (R-oxybutynin), 1.8ng/mL (S-oxybutynin); AUC=21.3ng•hr/mL (R-oxybutynin), 39.5ng•hr/mL (S-oxybutynin); T_{max}=12.7 hrs (R-oxybutynin), 11.8 hrs (S-oxybutynin). Refer to PI for pediatric parameters. **Distribution:** (IV) V_d=193L; plasma protein binding (>99%, >97% metabolites). **Metabolism:** Liver (extensive) via CYP3A4; desethyloxybutynin (active metabolite). **Elimination:** Urine (<0.1% unchanged, <0.1% metabolite); $T_{1/2}$=13.2 hrs (R-oxybutynin), 12.4 hrs (S-oxybutynin).

PATIENT CONSIDERATIONS
Assessment: Assess for urinary/gastric retention, bladder outflow obstruction, GI narrowing/obstructive disorder, GERD, ulcerative colitis, uncontrolled narrow-angle glaucoma, Parkinson's disease, myasthenia gravis, autonomic neuropathy, dementia, hypersensitivity to the drug substance or other components of the product, any other conditions where treatment is contraindicated or cautioned, pregnancy/nursing status, and possible drug interactions.

Monitoring: Monitor for aggravation of myasthenia gravis or autonomic neuropathy, angioedema, hypersensitivity reactions, anticholinergic CNS effects, GI adverse reactions (eg, urinary retention, esophagitis, gastric retention), and other adverse reactions.

Counseling: Inform that angioedema may occur and could result in life-threatening airway obstruction; advise to promptly d/c therapy and seek medical attention if experiencing swelling of the tongue, edema of the laryngopharynx, or difficulty breathing. Inform that heat prostration may occur when administered in high environmental temperature. Inform that drug may produce drowsiness, dizziness, or blurred vision; advise to exercise caution. Inform that alcohol may enhance drowsiness. Advise not to drive or operate heavy machinery until effects have been determined.

DIVIGEL — estradiol   Rx
Class: Estrogen

ADULT DOSAGE	**PEDIATRIC DOSAGE**
Menopausal Vasomotor Symptoms	Pediatric use may not have been established
Moderate to Severe:	
Initial: 0.25g qd applied on skin of right or left upper thigh	
Reevaluate periodically to determine need for treatment	

ADMINISTRATION
Topical route

Application surface area should be about 5 by 7 inches (approx the size of 2 palm prints)

Entire contents of a unit dose pkt should be applied each day

Apply to right or left upper thigh on alternating days to avoid skin irritation

Do not apply on face, breasts, irritated skin, or in or around vagina

Allow gel to dry before dressing

Do not wash the application site w/in 1 hr after application

Contact of gel w/ eyes should be avoided

Wash hands after application

STORAGE
20-25°C (68-77°F); excursions permitted to 15-30°C (59-86°F).

HOW SUPPLIED
Gel: 0.1% [0.25g, 0.5g, 1g pkts]

CONTRAINDICATIONS
Undiagnosed abnormal genital bleeding, known/suspected/history of breast cancer, known/suspected estrogen-dependent neoplasia, active/history of DVT, PE, or arterial thromboembolic disease (eg, stroke, MI), known anaphylactic reaction or angioedema to this medication, liver impairment/disease, protein C/protein S/antithrombin deficiency, or other known thrombophilic disorders, known/suspected pregnancy.

WARNINGS/PRECAUTIONS
D/C immediately if PE, DVT, stroke, or MI occurs or is suspected. Caution in patients w/ risk factors for arterial vascular disease and/or venous thromboembolism (VTE). If feasible, d/c at least 4-6 weeks before surgery of the type associated w/ increased risk of thromboembolism, or during periods of prolonged immobilization. May increase risk of gallbladder disease requiring surgery and ovarian cancer. Consider addition of progestin for women w/ a uterus or w/ residual endometriosis posthysterectomy. May lead to severe hypercalcemia in patients w/ breast cancer and bone metastases; d/c and take appropriate measures if this occurs. Retinal vascular thrombosis reported; d/c therapy pending examination if sudden partial/complete loss of vision, sudden onset of proptosis, diplopia, or migraine occurs. D/C permanently if examination reveals papilledema or retinal vascular lesions. May elevate BP and thyroid-binding globulin levels. May elevate plasma TG levels (w/ preexisting hypertriglyceridemia); consider discontinuation if pancreatitis occurs. Caution w/ history of cholestatic jaundice; d/c in case of recurrence. May cause fluid retention; caution w/ cardiac or renal impairment. Caution w/ hypoparathyroidism; hypocalcemia may occur. May exacerbate symptoms of angioedema in women w/ hereditary angioedema. May exacerbate endometriosis, asthma, diabetes mellitus (DM), epilepsy, migraine, porphyria, systemic lupus erythematosus, and hepatic hemangiomas; use w/ caution. May affect certain endocrine, and blood components in lab tests. Alcohol-based gels are flammable; avoid fire, flame, or smoking until applied dose has dried. Potential for drug transfer following physical contact; cover application site after drying.

ADVERSE REACTIONS
Nasopharyngitis, URTI(s), vaginal mycosis, breast tenderness, metrorrhagia.

DRUG INTERACTIONS
CYP3A4 inducers (eg, St. John's wort, phenobarbital, carbamazepine, rifampin) may decrease levels; may decrease therapeutic effects and/or change uterine bleeding profile. CYP3A4 inhibitors (eg, erythromycin, clarithromycin, ketoconazole) may increase levels; may result in side effects. Patients concomitantly receiving thyroid replacement therapy and estrogens may require increased doses of thyroid replacement therapy. May change systemic exposure w/ sunscreens.

PREGNANCY AND LACTATION
Contraindicated in pregnancy, caution in nursing.

MECHANISM OF ACTION
Estrogen; binds to nuclear receptors in estrogen-responsive tissues. Circulating estrogens modulate pituitary secretion of gonadotropins, luteinizing hormone and follicle-stimulating hormone, through (-) feedback mechanism. Reduces elevated levels of these hormones seen in postmenopausal women.

PHARMACOKINETICS
Absorption: Topical administration of variable doses resulted in different parameters. **Distribution:** Largely bound to sex hormone-binding globulin and albumin; found in breast milk. **Metabolism:** Liver to estrone (metabolite), estriol (major urinary metabolite); sulfate and glucuronide conjugation (liver); hydrolysis (intestine); CYP3A4 (partial metabolism). **Elimination:** Urine; $T_{1/2}$=10 hrs.

PATIENT CONSIDERATIONS
Assessment: Assess for undiagnosed abnormal genital bleeding, liver impairment/disease, presence/history of breast cancer, estrogen-dependent neoplasia, DVT, PE, or arterial thromboembolic disease, pregnancy/nursing status, any other conditions where treatment is contraindicated or cautioned, need for progestin therapy, and possible drug interactions. Assess for protein C, protein S, or antithrombin deficiency, or other known thrombophilic disorders.

Monitoring: Monitor for signs/symptoms of CVD, arterial vascular disease, VTE, malignant neoplasms, dementia, gallbladder disease, hypercalcemia, BP and plasma TG elevations, visual abnormalities, pancreatitis, cholestatic jaundice, hypothyroidism, fluid retention, exacerbation of endometriosis and other adverse reactions. Perform annual breast exam; schedule mammography based on age, risk factors, and prior mammogram results. Monitor thyroid function in patients on thyroid replacement therapy. Perform adequate diagnostic measures (eg, endometrial sampling) in patients w/ undiagnosed persistent or recurrent genital bleeding. Perform periodic evaluation to determine treatment need.

Counseling: Inform postmenopausal women of the importance of reporting vaginal bleeding as soon as possible and of possible serious adverse reactions of therapy and possible less serious but common adverse reactions. Advise to have yearly breast exams by a physician and to perform monthly self-breast exams. Instruct on the proper application and use. Inform that gel contains alcohol that is flammable; instruct to avoid fire, flame, or smoking until the gel has dried. Inform of potential for drug transfer from one individual to the other following physical contact; advise to avoid skin contact w/ other subjects until the gel is completely dried.

DOCEFREZ — docetaxel   Rx
Class: Antimicrotubule agent

> Increased incidence of treatment-related mortality with abnormal liver function, at higher doses, and in patients with non-small cell lung carcinoma (NSCLC) and a history of prior treatment with platinum-based chemotherapy who receive docetaxel as a single agent at 100mg/m². Should not be given to patients with bilirubin >ULN, or with AST/ALT >1.5X ULN concomitant with alkaline phosphatase >2.5X ULN; increased risk of grade 4 neutropenia, febrile neutropenia, infections, severe thrombocytopenia, severe stomatitis, severe skin toxicity, and toxic death. Obtain LFTs prior to each treatment cycle. Should not be given if neutrophils <1500 cells/mm³; perform frequent blood cell counts. Severe hypersensitivity reactions reported in patients who received a 3-day dexamethasone premedication; d/c immediately and administer appropriate therapy. Contraindicated with history of severe hypersensitivity reactions to other drugs formulated with polysorbate 80. Severe fluid retention reported despite dexamethasone premedication.

ADULT DOSAGE
Breast Cancer
Locally advanced or metastatic breast cancer after failure of prior chemotherapy

60-100mg/m² IV over 1 hr every 3 weeks

Non-Small Cell Lung Cancer
Single Agent:
Locally advanced or metastatic non-small cell lung cancer after failure of prior platinum-based chemotherapy

75mg/m² IV over 1 hr every 3 weeks

Combination w/ Cisplatin:
Unresectable, locally advanced or metastatic non-small cell lung cancer in patients who have not previously received chemotherapy for this condition

75mg/m² IV over 1 hr immediately, followed by cisplatin 75mg/m² over 30-60 min every 3 weeks

Metastatic Prostate Cancer
Combination w/ prednisone for androgen independent (hormone refractory) metastatic prostate cancer

75mg/m² IV over 1 hr every 3 weeks + prednisone 5mg PO bid

Premedication
Breast Cancer/Non-Small Cell Lung Cancer:
PO corticosteroids (eg, dexamethasone 8mg bid) for 3 days starting 1 day prior to docetaxel administration

Metastatic Prostate Cancer:
PO dexamethasone 8mg, at 12 hrs, 3 hrs, and 1 hr before docetaxel infusion

PEDIATRIC DOSAGE
Pediatric use may not have been established

DOSING CONSIDERATIONS
Concomitant Medications
Strong CYP3A4 Inhibitors: Avoid concomitant use; if coadministration required, consider a 50% dose reduction

Hepatic Impairment
Bilirubin >ULN: Not recommended for use

AST and/or ALT >1.5X ULN w/ Alkaline Phosphatase >2.5X ULN: Not recommended for use

Adverse Reactions
Breast Cancer:
Initial Dose 100mg/m²:
Experience Febrile Neutropenia, Neutrophils <500 cells/mm³ for >1 Week, or Severe/Cumulative Cutaneous Reactions: Reduce dose to 75mg/m²; if patient continues to experience these reactions, either decrease dose to 55mg/m² or d/c treatment

Initial Dose 60mg/m²:
Do not Experience Febrile Neutropenia, Neutrophils <500 cells/mm³ for >1 Week, Severe/Cumulative Cutaneous Reactions, or Severe Peripheral Neuropathy During Therapy: May tolerate higher doses

Develop ≥Grade 3 Peripheral Neuropathy: D/C treatment

Non-Small Cell Lung Cancer:
Monotherapy:
Experience Febrile Neutropenia, Neutrophils <500 cells/mm³ for >1 Week, Severe/Cumulative Cutaneous Reactions, or Other Grade 3/4 Non-Hematological Toxicities: Withhold treatment until toxicity resolves, then resume at 55mg/m²
Develop ≥Grade 3 Peripheral Neuropathy: D/C treatment

Combination w/ Cisplatin:
Nadir of Platelet Count During Previous Course of Therapy is <25,000 cells/mm³ or Febrile Neutropenia/Serious Non-Hematologic Toxicities Experienced: Reduce dose in subsequent cycles to 65mg/m²; if further dose reduction is required, reduce to 50mg/m²

Prostate Cancer:
Experience Febrile Neutropenia, Neutrophils <500 cells/mm³ for >1 Week, Severe/Cumulative Cutaneous Reactions, or Moderate Neurosensory Signs and/or Symptoms: Reduce dose to 60mg/m²; if patient continues to experience these reactions, d/c treatment

ADMINISTRATION
IV route

Administration Precautions
Contact of reconstituted sol w/ plasticized PVC equipment or devices used to prepare sol for infusion is not recommended; store the infusion sol in bottles (glass, polypropylene) or plastic bags (polypropylene, polyolefin) and administer through polyethylene-lined administration sets

Preparation of Reconstituted Sol
1. Allow the appropriate number of docetaxel vials and diluent (35.4% ethanol in polysorbate 80) vials to stand at room temperature for approx 5 min
2. **For Docetaxel 20:** Use 1mL syringe w/ needle of 18- to 21-gauge, 1 1/2 inch for withdrawing diluent
   For Docetaxel 80: Use 4mL syringe w/ needle of 18- to 21-gauge, 1 1/2 inch for withdrawing diluent
3. **For Docetaxel 20:** Withdraw 1mL from diluent vial into a syringe by partially inverting the vial, and transfer it to the docetaxel vial
   For Docetaxel 80: Withdraw 4mL from diluent vial into a syringe by partially inverting the vial, and transfer it to the docetaxel vial
4. Shake the reconstituted vial well in order to completely dissolve the docetaxel powder present in the vial
   For the 20mg Vial: Resultant concentration is 20mg/0.8mL
   For the 80mg Vial: Resultant concentration is 24mg/mL
5. Some air bubbles may be present in the sol due to the polysorbate 80; allow the sol to stand for a few min to allow any air bubbles to dissipate

Preparation of Infusion Sol
1. Withdraw the required amount of reconstituted docetaxel sol w/ a calibrated syringe and inject into a 250mL infusion bag or bottle of either 0.9% NaCl sol or D5 sol to produce a final concentration of 0.3-0.74mg/mL; if a dose >200mg is required, use a larger volume of the infusion vehicle so that a concentration of 0.74mg/mL is not exceeded
2. Thoroughly mix the infusion by manual rotation
3. Docetaxel reconstituted sol is supersaturated, therefore may crystallize over time; if crystals appear, the sol must no longer be used and shall be discarded

Handling Precautions
If lyophilized powder, reconstituted sol, or infusion sol comes in contact w/ the skin, wash w/ soap and water immediately and thoroughly
If lyophilized powder, reconstituted sol, or infusion sol comes in contact w/ mucosa, wash w/ water immediately and thoroughly

STORAGE
2-8°C (36-46°F). Protect from bright light. Reconstituted Sol: Use immediately or store either in the refrigerator or at room temperature for a max of 8 hrs. Infusion Sol (in either 0.9% NaCl or D5W): Stable at 2-25°C (36-77°F) for 6 hrs; use within 6 hrs including the 1 hr IV administration. Infusion sol is stable in non-PVC bags up to 48 hrs at 2-8°C (36-46°F).

HOW SUPPLIED
Inj: 20mg, 80mg

CONTRAINDICATIONS
History of severe hypersensitivity reactions to docetaxel or to other drugs formulated with polysorbate 80, neutrophils <1500 cells/mm³.

WARNINGS/PRECAUTIONS
Avoid retreatment with subsequent cycles until neutrophils recover to a level >1500 cells/mm³ and platelets recover to a level >100,000 cells/mm³. Fatal GI bleeding associated with severe drug-induced thrombocytopenia reported in BC patients with severe liver impairment. Do not rechallenge patients with a history of severe hypersensitivity reactions to therapy. Monitor from the 1st dose for possible exacerbation of preexisting effusions. Acute myeloid leukemia or myelodysplasia reported in patients given anthracyclines and/or cyclophosphamide, including use in adjuvant therapy for BC. Localized erythema of extremities with edema followed by desquamation reported; adjust dose if severe skin toxicity occurs. Severe neurosensory symptoms (eg, paresthesia, dysesthesia, pain) may develop; adjust dose if symptoms occur and d/c treatment if symptoms persist. Cystoid macular edema (CME) reported; d/c and initiate appropriate treatment if CME is diagnosed, and consider alternative non-taxane cancer treatment. Intoxication reported with some formulations of docetaxel due to the alcohol content. Alcohol content of the drug may affect CNS; caution in whom alcohol intake should be avoided or minimized. Alcohol content of the drug may impair physical/mental abilities. Severe asthenia reported. May cause fetal harm. Caution in elderly.

ADVERSE REACTIONS
Neutropenia, hypersensitivity, fluid retention, asthenia, dysgeusia, thrombocytopenia, constipation, nail disorders, skin reactions, N/V, alopecia, myalgia, neuropathy.

DRUG INTERACTIONS
Avoid with CYP3A4 inhibitors; consider a 50% docetaxel dose reduction if coadministration with a strong CYP3A4 inhibitor (eg, ketoconazole, clarithromycin, atazanavir) cannot be avoided. Protease inhibitors, particularly ritonavir, may increase exposure. CYP3A4 inducers or substrates may alter metabolism.

PREGNANCY AND LACTATION
Category D, not for use in nursing.

MECHANISM OF ACTION
Antimicrotubule agent; acts by disrupting the microtubular network in cells that is essential for mitotic and interphase cellular functions. Binds to free tubulin and promotes assembly of tubulin into stable microtubules while simultaneously inhibiting their disassembly, which results in the inhibition of mitosis in cells.

PHARMACOKINETICS
Distribution: V_d=113L; plasma protein binding (94%). **Metabolism:** Via CYP3A4. **Elimination:** Urine (6%, within 7 days), feces (75%, within 7 days); $T_{1/2}$=11.1 hrs.

PATIENT CONSIDERATIONS
Assessment: Assess for history of severe hypersensitivity reactions to the drug or other drugs formulated with polysorbate 80, preexisting effusion, hepatic impairment, pregnancy/nursing status, and possible drug interactions. Obtain baseline CBC and LFTs. Perform a comprehensive ophthalmologic examination in patients with impaired vision.

Monitoring: Monitor for neutropenia, hypersensitivity reactions, fluid retention, acute myeloid leukemia, hematologic effects, cutaneous reactions, exacerbation of effusions, neurosensory symptoms, asthenia, CME, and other adverse reactions. Monitor CBC frequently and LFTs prior to each cycle of therapy.

Counseling: Inform about risks and benefits of therapy. Inform that drug may cause fetal harm; advise women of childbearing potential to avoid becoming pregnant and use effective contraceptives. Explain the significance of oral corticosteroid administration to help facilitate compliance; instruct to report if not compliant. Instruct to immediately report signs of hypersensitivity reactions, fluid retention, myalgia, or cutaneous/neurologic reactions. Counsel about the side effects associated with the drug. Explain the significance of routine blood cell counts. Instruct to monitor temperature frequently and immediately report any occurrence of fever. Explain about the possible side effects of the alcohol content in the drug, including possible side effects on the CNS. Advise patients in whom alcohol should be avoided or minimized to consider the alcohol content of the drug; inform that alcohol could impair their ability to drive or use machines immediately after infusion.

DOCETAXEL — docetaxel   Rx
Class: Antimicrotubule agent

> Increased incidence of treatment-related mortality reported in patients w/ hepatic dysfunction, in patients receiving higher-doses, and in patients w/ non-small cell lung cancer (NSCLC) and a history of prior treatment w/ platinum-based chemotherapy who receive docetaxel as a single agent at a dose of 100mg/m². Avoid if bilirubin >ULN, or AST/ALT >1.5X ULN concomitant w/ alkaline phosphatase >2.5X ULN; may increase risk for the development of Grade 4 neutropenia, febrile neutropenia, infections, severe thrombocytopenia, severe stomatitis, severe skin toxicity, and toxic death. Patients w/ isolated elevations of transaminase >1.5X ULN reported to have a higher rate of febrile neutropenia Grade 4 but did not have an increased incidence of toxic death. Obtain bilirubin, AST or ALT, and alkaline phosphatase values prior to each cycle. Avoid therapy if neutrophils <1500 cells/mm³. Monitor for the occurrence of neutropenia; perform frequent blood cell counts on all patients. Severe hypersensitivity reactions reported w/ dexamethasone premedication; d/c immediately if symptoms occur. Contraindicated w/ history of severe hypersensitivity reactions to docetaxel or other drugs formulated w/ polysorbate 80. Severe fluid retention may occur despite dexamethasone premedication.

OTHER BRAND NAMES
Taxotere

ADULT DOSAGE	PEDIATRIC DOSAGE
Breast Cancer	Pediatric use may not have been established
Locally advanced or metastatic breast cancer after failure of prior chemotherapy	
60-100mg/m² IV over 1 hr every 3 weeks	
Combination w/ Doxorubicin and Cyclophosphamide:	
Adjuvant treatment of operable node-positive breast cancer	
75mg/m² 1 hr after doxorubicin 50mg/m² and cyclophosphamide 500mg/m² every 3 weeks for 6 courses	
Prophylactic G-CSF may be used to mitigate risk of hematological toxicities	
Non-Small Cell Lung Cancer	
Single Agent:	
Locally advanced or metastatic NSCLC after failure of prior platinum-based chemotherapy	
75mg/m² IV over 1 hr every 3 weeks	
Combination w/ Cisplatin:	
Unresectable, locally advanced or metastatic NSCLC in chemotherapy-naive patients	

75mg/m² IV over 1 hr immediately followed by cisplatin 75mg/m² over 30-60 min every 3 weeks

Metastatic Prostate Cancer

Combination w/ prednisone for androgen-independent (hormone refractory) metastatic prostate cancer

75mg/m² IV over 1 hr every 3 weeks + prednisone 5mg PO bid

Gastric Adenocarcinoma

Combination w/ cisplatin and fluorouracil for advanced gastric adenocarcinoma, including adenocarcinoma of the gastroesophageal junction, in chemotherapy-naive patients

75mg/m² IV over 1 hr, followed by cisplatin 75mg/m² IV over 1-3 hrs (both on Day 1 only), followed by fluorouracil 750mg/m²/day IV over 24 hrs x 5 days, starting at end of cisplatin infusion

Repeat treatment every 3 weeks

Squamous Cell Carcinoma of the Head and Neck

Combination w/ cisplatin and fluorouracil for induction treatment of locally advanced squamous cell carcinoma of the head and neck (SCCHN)

Administer prophylaxis for neutropenic infections

Induction Followed by Radiotherapy:
Locally advanced inoperable SCCHN

75mg/m² IV over 1 hr, followed by cisplatin 75mg/m² IV over 1 hr, on Day 1, followed by fluorouracil as a continuous IV infusion at 750mg/m²/day x 5 days

Administer every 3 weeks for 4 cycles; following chemotherapy, patients should receive radiotherapy

Induction Followed by Chemoradiotherapy:
Locally advanced (unresectable, low surgical cure, or organ preservation) SCCHN

75mg/m² IV over 1 hr on Day 1, followed by cisplatin 100mg/m² IV over 30 min to 3 hrs, followed by fluorouracil 1000mg/m²/day as a continuous IV infusion from Day 1 to Day 4

Administer every 3 weeks for 3 cycles; following chemotherapy, patients should receive chemoradiotherapy

Premedication

All Patients:
Oral corticosteroids (see below for prostate cancer) such as dexamethasone 16mg/day (8mg bid) for 3 days starting 1 day prior to docetaxel administration

Prostate Cancer:
Given the concurrent use of prednisone, the recommended regimen is dexamethasone 8mg PO, at 12 hrs, 3 hrs, and 1 hr before docetaxel infusion

Gastric Adenocarcinoma/Head and Neck Cancer:
Patients must receive antiemetics and appropriate hydration for cisplatin administration

----

DOSING CONSIDERATIONS
Concomitant Medications
Strong CYP3A4 Inhibitors: Avoid use; consider a 50% docetaxel dose reduction if patients require coadministration of a strong CYP3A4 inhibitor

Hepatic Impairment
AST/ALT >2.5 to ≤5X ULN and Alkaline Phosphatase ≤2.5X ULN, or AST/ALT >1.5 to ≤5X ULN and Alkaline Phosphatase >2.5 to ≤5X ULN: Reduce docetaxel dose by 20%
AST/ALT >5X ULN and/or Alkaline Phosphatase >5X ULN: D/C treatment

Adverse Reactions
Breast Cancer:
Initial Dose 100mg/m²:
Experience Febrile Neutropenia, Neutrophils <500 cells/mm³ for >1 Week, or Severe/Cumulative Cutaneous Reactions: Reduce dose to 75mg/m²; if reactions continue, either reduce dose to 55mg/m² or d/c treatment
Initial Dose 60mg/m²:
Do Not Experience Febrile Neutropenia, Neutrophils <500 cells/mm³ for >1 Week, Severe/Cumulative Cutaneous Reactions, or Severe Peripheral Neuropathy: May tolerate higher doses
≥Grade 3 Peripheral Neuropathy: D/C treatment

Combination Therapy in Adjuvant Treatment of Breast Cancer:
Febrile Neutropenia: Administer G-CSF in all subsequent cycles; if reaction continues, continue G-CSF and reduce docetaxel dose to 60mg/m²
Grade 3 or 4 Stomatitis: Reduce docetaxel dose to 60mg/m²
Severe/Cumulative Cutaneous Reactions or Moderate Neurosensory Signs and/or Symptoms: Reduce docetaxel dose to 60mg/m²; if reactions continue at 60mg/m², d/c treatment

NSCLC:
Monotherapy:
Experience Febrile Neutropenia, Neutrophils <500 cells/mm³ for >1 Week, or Severe/Cumulative Cutaneous Reactions, or Other Grade 3-4 Nonhematological Toxicities: Withhold treatment until toxicity resolves, then resume at 55mg/m²
≥Grade 3 Peripheral Neuropathy: D/C treatment

Combination Therapy:
Nadir of Platelet Count During Previous Course of Therapy is <25,000 cells/mm³ w/ Febrile Neutropenia/Serious Nonhematologic Toxicities: Reduce docetaxel dose in subsequent cycles to 65mg/m²; if further dose reduction is required, 50mg/m² is recommended

Prostate Cancer:
Experience Febrile Neutropenia, Neutrophils <500 cells/mm³ for >1 Week, Severe/Cumulative Cutaneous Reactions, or Moderate Neurosensory Signs and/or Symptoms: Reduce docetaxel dose to 60mg/m²; if reactions continue at 60mg/m², d/c treatment

Gastric Adenocarcinoma/Head and Neck Cancer:
Experience Episode of Febrile Neutropenia or Prolonged Neutropenia/Neutropenic Infection Occurs Despite G-CSF Use: Reduce docetaxel dose to 60mg/m²; if subsequent episodes of complicated neutropenia occur, reduce docetaxel dose to 45mg/m². D/C if toxicities persist
Grade 4 Thrombocytopenia: Reduce docetaxel dose to 60mg/m²; do not retreat w/ subsequent cycles until neutrophils recover to >1500 cells/mm³ and platelets recover to >100,000 cells/mm³. D/C if toxicities persist

Toxicities w/ Docetaxel in Combination w/ Cisplatin and Fluorouracil:
Grade 3 Diarrhea:
1st Episode: Reduce fluorouracil dose by 20%
2nd Episode: Reduce docetaxel dose by 20%

Grade 4 Diarrhea:
1st Episode: Reduce docetaxel and fluorouracil doses by 20%
2nd Episode: D/C treatment

Grade 3 Stomatitis/Mucositis:
1st Episode: Reduce fluorouracil dose by 20%
2nd Episode: Stop fluorouracil only, at all subsequent cycles
3rd Episode: Reduce docetaxel dose by 20%

Grade 4 Stomatitis/Mucositis:
1st Episode: Stop fluorouracil only, at all subsequent cycles
2nd Episode: Reduce docetaxel dose by 20%

Refer to PI for cisplatin and fluorouracil dose modifications

ADMINISTRATION
IV route

Administration Precautions
Contact of the docetaxel inj w/ plasticized PVC equipment or devices used to prepare sol for infusion is not recommended; store the final docetaxel dilution for infusion in bottles (glass, polypropylene) or plastic bags (polypropylene, polyolefin) and administer through polyethylene-lined administration sets.

Preparation
Requires no prior dilution w/ a diluent and is ready to add to the infusion sol.

Docetaxel Inj Concentrate (20mg/mL):
Do not use the two-vial formulation (inj concentrate and diluent) w/ the one-vial formulation.

Refer to PI for further administration instructions.

STORAGE
20-25°C (68-77°F), (Taxotere) 2-25°C (36-77°F). Multi-use vials are stable for up to 28 days when stored at 2-8°C (36-46°F) after use. Protect from light. **Reconstituted Sol:** 0.9% NaCl or D5: Stable at 2-25°C (36-77°F) for 4 hrs or (Taxotere) 6 hrs. (Taxotere) Infusion sol is stable in non-PVC bags up to 48 hrs at 2-8°C (36-46°F).

HOW SUPPLIED
Inj: 10mg/mL [2mL, 8mL, 16mL], (Taxotere) 20mg/mL [1mL, 4mL]

CONTRAINDICATIONS
History of severe hypersensitivity reactions to docetaxel or to other drugs formulated w/ polysorbate 80. Neutrophils <1500 cells/mm³.

WARNINGS/PRECAUTIONS
Avoid subsequent cycles until neutrophils recover to level >1500 cells/mm³ and platelets to >100,000 cells/mm³. Severe fluid retention reported; monitor from the 1st dose for possible exacerbation of preexisting effusions. Acute myeloid leukemia or myelodysplasia may occur in adjuvant therapy (eg, adjuvant therapy in breast cancer). Localized erythema of the extremities w/ edema followed

by desquamation reported; adjust dose if severe skin toxicity occurs. Severe neurosensory symptoms (eg, paresthesia, dysesthesia, pain) may develop; adjust dose if symptoms occur and d/c treatment if symptoms persist. Cystoid macular edema (CME) reported; d/c and initiate appropriate treatment if CME is diagnosed, and/or consider alternative non-taxane cancer treatment. Severe asthenia reported. May cause fetal harm. Caution in elderly. Intoxication reported due to alcohol content. Alcohol content of the drug may affect CNS; caution in whom alcohol intake should be avoided or minimized. Alcohol content of the drug may impair physical/mental abilities.

ADVERSE REACTIONS
Infections, neutropenia, anemia, febrile neutropenia, hypersensitivity, thrombocytopenia, neuropathy, dysgeusia, dyspnea, constipation, anorexia, nail disorders, fluid retention, asthenia, pain.

DRUG INTERACTIONS
See Dosing Considerations. Avoid w/ CYP3A4 inhibitors (eg, ketoconazole, clarithromycin, atazanavir); may increase docetaxel exposure. CYP3A4 inducers and substrates may alter metabolism. Protease inhibitors (eg, ritonavir) may increase exposure. Renal insufficiency and renal failure reported w/ concomitant nephrotoxic drugs. Radiation pneumonitis may occur in patients receiving concomitant radiotherapy (rare).

PREGNANCY AND LACTATION
Pregnancy: Category D.
Lactation: Not for use in nursing.

MECHANISM OF ACTION
Antimicrotubule agent; acts by disrupting the microtubular network in cells that is essential for mitotic and interphase cellular functions.

PHARMACOKINETICS
Distribution: V_d=113L; plasma protein binding (94-97%). **Metabolism:** CYP3A4. **Elimination:** Urine (6%), feces (75%); $T_{1/2}$=11.1 hrs.

PATIENT CONSIDERATIONS

Assessment: Assess for history of severe hypersensitivity reactions to the drug or other drugs w/ polysorbate 80, preexisting effusion, hepatic impairment, pregnancy/nursing status, and possible drug interactions. Obtain baseline weight, CBC w/ platelets, and differential count. Obtain bilirubin, AST or ALT, and alkaline phosphatase values prior to each cycle of therapy.

Monitoring: Monitor for fluid retention, acute myeloid leukemia, hematologic effects, skin toxicities, exacerbation of effusions, neurosensory symptoms, hepatic impairment, hypersensitivity reactions, asthenia, CME, and other adverse reactions. Monitor weight, CBC w/ platelets, and differential count. Perform a comprehensive ophthalmologic examination in patients w/ impaired vision.

Counseling: Inform about risks and benefits of therapy. Inform that drug may cause fetal harm; advise to avoid pregnancy and to use effective contraceptives. Explain the significance of oral corticosteroid administration to help facilitate compliance; instruct to report if not compliant. Instruct to report signs of hypersensitivity reactions, fluid retention, myalgia, or cutaneous/neurologic reactions. Counsel about side effects that are associated w/ the drug. Explain the significance of routine blood cell counts. Instruct to monitor temperature frequently and to immediately report any occurrence of fever. Explain about the possible side effects of the alcohol content in the drug, including possible side effects on the CNS. Advise patients in whom alcohol should be avoided or minimized to consider the alcohol content of the drug; inform that alcohol could impair their ability to drive or use machines immediately after infusion.

DOLOPHINE — methadone hydrochloride CII
Class: Opioid analgesic

Exposes patients and other users to the risk of opioid addiction, abuse, and misuse, leading to overdose and death; assess each patient's risk prior to prescribing, and monitor regularly for development of these behaviors/conditions. Serious, life-threatening, or fatal respiratory depression may occur; monitor for respiratory depression, especially during initiation or following a dose increase. Accidental ingestion, especially in children, can result in fatal overdose. QT interval prolongation and serious arrhythmia (torsades de pointes) have occurred during treatment; closely monitor for changes in cardiac rhythm during initiation and titration. Prolonged use during pregnancy can result in neonatal opioid withdrawal syndrome; advise pregnant women of the risk and ensure availability of appropriate treatment. For detoxification and maintenance of opioid dependence, methadone should be administered in accordance w/ treatment standards, including limitations on unsupervised administration.

ADULT DOSAGE
Severe Pain (Daily, Around-the-Clock Management)

Management of pain severe enough to require daily, around-the-clock, long-term opioid treatment and for which alternative treatment options are inadequate

1st Opioid Analgesic: 2.5mg q8-12h
Titration/Maint:
Individually titrate to a dose that provides adequate analgesia and minimizes adverse reactions.
Titrate slowly, w/ dose increases no more frequent than every 3-5 days; some patients may require longer intervals of up to 12 days.
If breakthrough pain is experienced, patient may require a dose increase

PEDIATRIC DOSAGE
Pediatric use may not have been established

or need rescue medication w/ an appropriate dose of an immediate-release medication.
If unacceptable opioid-related adverse reactions are observed, subsequent doses may be reduced and/or the dosing interval adjusted (eg, every 8 or 12 hrs).

Detoxification/Maintenance Treatment of Opioid Addiction

Induction/Initial:
Initial: 20-30mg single dose; use lower initial doses for patients whose tolerance is expected to be low at treatment entry
Max Initial: 30mg
May administer an additional 5-10mg if withdrawal symptoms are not suppressed or if symptoms reappear after 2-4 hrs
Max Total Day 1 Dose: 40mg
Adjust dose over the 1st week of treatment based on control of withdrawal symptoms at the time of expected peak activity (eg, 2-4 hrs after dosing)

Short-Term Detoxification:
Titrate to a total daily dose of 40mg in divided doses to achieve an adequate stabilizing level.
Gradually decrease methadone dose on a daily basis or at 2-day intervals, 2-3 days after stabilization.
Hospitalized patients may tolerate a daily reduction of 20% of the total daily dose; ambulatory patients may need a slower schedule.

Titration and Maint:
Usual: 80-120mg/day

Medically Supervised Withdrawal After a Period of Maint Treatment:
Dose reductions should be <10% of the established tolerance or maint dose w/ 10- to 14-day intervals

Management of Acute Pain During Methadone Maint Treatment:
May require somewhat higher and/or more frequent doses than in nontolerant patients

Conversions

D/C all other around-the-clock opioid drugs when therapy is initiated

From Parenteral Methadone:
Use conversion ratio of 1:2mg for parenteral to oral methadone (eg, 5mg parenteral to 10mg oral)

Conversion Factors to Dolophine:
Use the total daily baseline oral morphine equivalent dose to calculate the estimated daily oral methadone as percent of total daily morphine equivalent dose, as follows:
<100mg: 20-30%
100-300mg: 10-20%
300-600mg: 8-12%
600-1000mg: 5-10%
>1000mg: <5%

Calculation for Estimated Daily Dose for Dolophine:
Always round down, if necessary, to the appropriate Dolophine strength(s) available
On a Single Opioid: Sum the total daily dose of opioid, convert to morphine equivalent dose, then multiply the morphine equivalent dose by the corresponding percentage to calculate approximate daily oral methadone dose
On >1 Opioid: Calculate approximate oral methadone dose for each opioid and sum the totals to obtain approximate daily total methadone dose
On Fixed-Ratio Opioid/Nonopioid Analgesics: Only use the opioid component of these products in the conversion

DOSING CONSIDERATIONS
Renal Impairment
Start on lower dose and w/ longer dosing intervals and titrate slowly
Hepatic Impairment
Start on lower dose and titrate slowly
Pregnancy
May need to increase dose or decrease dosing interval
Elderly
Start at lower end of dosing range
Discontinuation
Avoid abrupt discontinuation; use a gradual downward titration every 2-4 days

ADMINISTRATION
Oral route

STORAGE
20-25°C (68-77°F).

HOW SUPPLIED
Tab: 5mg*, 10mg* *scored

CONTRAINDICATIONS
Significant respiratory depression, acute or severe bronchial asthma in an unmonitored setting or in the absence of resuscitative equipment, known or suspected paralytic ileus, hypersensitivity to methadone.

WARNINGS/PRECAUTIONS
Reserve for use in patients for whom alternative analgesic treatment options (eg, nonopioid or immediate-release opioid analgesics) are ineffective, not tolerated, or would be otherwise inadequate to provide sufficient management of pain. Not indicated as a prn analgesic. Deaths reported during conversion from chronic, high-dose treatment w/ other opioid agonists and during initiation of treatment of addiction in subjects previously abusing high doses of other agonists. Retained in the liver and then slowly released, prolonging the duration of potential toxicity, w/ repeated dosing. Life-threatening respiratory depression is more likely to occur in elderly, cachectic, or debilitated patients; monitor closely when initiating and titrating, and when given w/ drugs that depress respiration. Consider alternative nonopioid analgesics in patients w/ significant COPD or cor pulmonale, and in patients having a substantially decreased respiratory reserve, hypoxia, hypercapnia, or preexisting respiratory depression. May cause severe hypotension including orthostatic hypotension and syncope in ambulatory patients; increased risk in patients w/ compromised ability to maintain BP. Monitor for signs of sedation and respiratory depression in patients susceptible to the intracranial effects of carbon dioxide retention (eg, those w/ increased intracranial pressure or brain tumors). May obscure the clinical course in patients w/ head injury. Avoid w/ GI obstruction and impaired consciousness or coma. May cause spasm of sphincter of Oddi or increase serum amylase. May aggravate convulsions in patients w/ convulsive disorders and may induce or aggravate seizures. May impair mental/physical abilities. Abrupt discontinuation may lead to opioid withdrawal symptoms. Infants born to opioid-dependent mothers may be physically dependent and may exhibit respiratory difficulties and withdrawal symptoms. Lab test interactions may occur.

ADVERSE REACTIONS
Lightheadedness, dizziness, sedation, N/V, sweating.

DRUG INTERACTIONS
Concomitant use w/ other CNS depressants (eg, sedatives, tranquilizers, phenothiazines) may result in hypotension, profound sedation, coma, respiratory depression, and death; reduce dose of one or both drugs when combined therapy is considered. Deaths reported when therapy has been abused in conjunction w/ benzodiazepines. CYP3A4 inhibitors may increase plasma levels and increase or prolong opioid effects; these effects could be more pronounced w/ concomitant use of CYP2C9 and 3A4 inhibitors; monitor for respiratory depression and sedation at frequent intervals and consider dose adjustments until stable drug effects are achieved. CYP3A4 inducers may increase clearance, leading to a decrease in plasma concentrations, lack of efficacy, or possibly, development of a withdrawal syndrome in a patient who had developed physical dependence to therapy; monitor for signs of opioid withdrawal and consider dose adjustments until stable drug effects are achieved. Antiretroviral agents w/ CYP3A4 inhibitory activity (eg, abacavir, darunavir + ritonavir [RTV], efavirenz, lopinavir + RTV) may increase clearance or decrease plasma levels; monitor methadone-maintained patients closely for evidence of withdrawal effects and adjust the methadone dose accordingly. May decrease levels of didanosine and stavudine. May increase zidovudine exposure, which could result in toxic effects. Monitor for cardiac conduction changes w/ drugs known to have potential to prolong the QT interval. Pharmacodynamic interactions may occur w/ potentially arrhythmogenic agents (eg, Class I and III antiarrhythmics, neuroleptics, TCAs, calcium channel blockers). Monitor closely w/ drugs capable of inducing electrolyte disturbances that may prolong the QT interval (eg, diuretics, laxatives, mineralocorticoid hormones). Mixed agonist/antagonist (eg, pentazocine, nalbuphine, butorphanol), and partial agonist (buprenorphine) analgesics may reduce the analgesic effect or precipitate withdrawal symptoms; avoid use. Severe reactions may occur w/ concurrent use or w/in 14 days of MAOI use. May increase levels of desipramine. Anticholinergics may increase risk of urinary retention and/or severe constipation, which may lead to paralytic ileus. Refer to prescribing information for further information on drug interactions.

PREGNANCY AND LACTATION
Pregnancy: Category C.
Lactation: Found in human breast milk. Gradually wean breastfed infants of mothers using methadone in order to prevent development of withdrawal symptoms in the infant.

MECHANISM OF ACTION
Synthetic opioid analgesic; mu-agonist. Produces actions similar to morphine; acts on CNS and organs composed of smooth muscle. May also act as an N-methyl-D-aspartate receptor antagonist.

PHARMACOKINETICS
Absorption: Bioavailability (36-100%); C_{max}=124-1255ng/mL; T_{max}=1-7.5 hrs.
Distribution: V_d=1-8L/kg; plasma protein binding (85-90%). Found in breast milk; crosses placenta. **Metabolism:** Hepatic N-demethylation via CYP3A4, 2B6, 2C19 (major); 2C9, 2D6 (minor). **Elimination:** Urine, feces; $T_{1/2}$=8-59 hrs.

PATIENT CONSIDERATIONS
Assessment: Assess for personal/family history of or risk factors for drug abuse or addiction, general condition and medical status, opioid experience/tolerance, pain type/severity, previous opioid daily dose, type of prior analgesics used, respiratory depression, cardiac conduction abnormalities, COPD or other respiratory complications, GI obstruction, paralytic ileus, hepatic/renal impairment, previous hypersensitivity to drug, pregnancy/nursing status, possible drug interactions, and any other conditions where treatment is contraindicated or cautioned.

Monitoring: Monitor for signs/symptoms of respiratory depression, QT prolongation and arrhythmias, orthostatic hypotension, syncope, symptoms of worsening biliary tract disease, aggravation/induction of seizures, tolerance, physical dependence, mental/physical impairment, withdrawal syndrome, hypersensitivity reactions, and other adverse reactions. Monitor for signs of increased intracranial pressure in patients w/ head injuries. Routinely monitor for signs of misuse, abuse, and addiction.

Counseling: Inform that use of medication, even when taken as recommended, may result in addiction, abuse, and misuse. Instruct not to share w/ others and to take steps to protect from theft or misuse. Inform of the risks of life-threatening respiratory depression; advise how to recognize respiratory depression and to seek medical attention if breathing difficulties develop. Inform that accidental ingestion, especially in children, may result in respiratory depression or death. Instruct to dispose of unused tab by flushing down the toilet. Instruct to seek medical attention immediately if patient experiences symptoms suggestive of an arrhythmia. Inform female patients of reproductive potential that prolonged use of drug during pregnancy may result in neonatal opioid withdrawal syndrome, which may be life threatening if not recognized and treated. Inform that potentially serious additive effects may occur if drug is used w/ alcohol or other CNS depressants, and instruct not to use such drugs unless supervised by a healthcare provider. Advise to use drug exactly ud and not to d/c w/o 1st discussing the need for tapering regimen w/ prescriber. Inform that drug may impair ability to perform potentially hazardous activities (eg, driving a car, operating heavy machinery). Advise about potential for severe constipation, including management instructions and when to seek medical attention. Inform that anaphylaxis may occur; advise how to recognize such a reaction and when to seek medical attention. Instruct nursing mothers to watch for signs of methadone toxicity in their infants (eg, increased sleepiness [more than usual], difficulty breastfeeding, breathing difficulties, limpness); instruct to inform physician immediately if these signs occur.

DONNATAL — atropine sulfate/hyoscyamine sulfate/phenobarbital/scopolamine hydrobromide   Rx

Class: Anticholinergic/barbiturate

ADULT DOSAGE	PEDIATRIC DOSAGE
Irritable Bowel Syndrome	**Irritable Bowel Syndrome**
Adjunctive Therapy:	**Adjunctive Therapy:**
Elixir:	**Elixir:**
1 or 2 tsp tid or qid	**Initial:**
	4.5kg: 0.5mL q4h or 0.75mL q6h
Tab:	**9.1kg:** 1mL q4h or 1.5mL q6h
1 or 2 tabs tid or qid	**13.6kg:** 1.5mL q4h or 2mL q6h
	22.7kg: 2.5mL q4h or 3.75mL q6h
Extentabs:	**34kg:** 3.75mL q4h or 5mL q6h
1 tab q12h. May give 1 tab q8h if indicated	**45.4kg:** 5mL q4h or 7.5mL q6h
Acute Enterocolitis	**Acute Enterocolitis**
Adjunctive Therapy:	**Adjunctive Therapy:**
Elixir:	**Elixir:**
1 or 2 tsp tid or qid	**Initial:**
	4.5kg: 0.5mL q4h or 0.75mL q6h
Tab:	**9.1kg:** 1mL q4h or 1.5mL q6h
1 or 2 tabs tid or qid	**13.6kg:** 1.5mL q4h or 2mL q6h
	22.7kg: 2.5mL q4h or 3.75mL q6h
Extentabs:	**34kg:** 3.75mL q4h or 5mL q6h
1 tab q12h. May give 1 tab q8h if indicated	**45.4kg:** 5mL q4h or 7.5mL q6h
Duodenal Ulcers	**Duodenal Ulcers**
Adjunctive Therapy:	**Adjunctive Therapy:**
Elixir:	**Elixir:**
1 or 2 tsp tid or qid	**Initial:**
	4.5kg: 0.5mL q4h or 0.75mL q6h
Tab:	**9.1kg:** 1mL q4h or 1.5mL q6h
1 or 2 tabs tid or qid	**13.6kg:** 1.5mL q4h or 2mL q6h
	22.7kg: 2.5mL q4h or 3.75mL q6h
Extentabs:	**34kg:** 3.75mL q4h or 5mL q6h
1 tab q12h. May give 1 tab q8h if indicated	**45.4kg:** 5mL q4h or 7.5mL q6h

DOSING CONSIDERATIONS
Hepatic Impairment
Use small initial doses

ADMINISTRATION
Oral route

Elixir
Use pediatric dosing device or oral syringe to measure the dose.

STORAGE
20-25°C (68-77°F). Protect from light and moisture. (Elixir) Avoid freezing.

HOW SUPPLIED
(Atropine/Hyoscyamine/Phenobarbital/Scopolamine) **Elixir:** (0.0194mg/0.1037mg/16.2mg/0.0065mg)/5mL [10mL, 4 fl oz, 1 pint]; **Tab:** 0.0194mg/0.1037mg/16.2mg/0.0065mg; **Tab, Extended-Release:** (Extentabs) 0.0582mg/0.3111mg/48.6mg/0.0195mg

CONTRAINDICATIONS
Glaucoma; obstructive uropathy (eg, bladder-neck obstruction due to prostatic hypertrophy); obstructive GI disease (achalasia, pyloroduodenal stenosis, etc.); paralytic ileus, intestinal atony in elderly/debilitated; unstable cardiovascular status in acute hemorrhage; severe ulcerative colitis (especially if complicated by toxic megacolon); myasthenia gravis; hiatal hernia associated w/ reflux esophagitis; known hypersensitivity to any of the ingredients; acute intermittent porphyria; patients in whom phenobarbital produces restlessness and/or excitement.

WARNINGS/PRECAUTIONS
Heat prostration can occur in high environmental temperatures. Diarrhea may be an early symptom of incomplete intestinal obstruction, especially w/ ileostomy or colostomy; treatment would be inappropriate and possibly harmful. May impair physical/mental abilities. Phenobarbital may be habit forming; avoid in patients prone to addiction or w/ history of physical and/or psychological drug dependence. Caution w/ autonomic neuropathy, renal disease, hyperthyroidism, coronary heart disease, CHF, arrhythmias, tachycardia, and HTN. May delay gastric emptying. Curare-like action may occur w/ overdosage. Abrupt withdrawal may produce delirium or convulsions in patients habituated to barbiturates. Elderly patients may react w/ symptoms of excitement, agitation, drowsiness, and other untoward manifestations to even small doses of the drug. (Elixir/Tab) May cause fetal harm when administered to pregnant women. Do not rely on the use of the drug in the presence of biliary tract disease complications. (Elixir [Mint]) Contains tartrazine, which may cause allergic-type reactions (including bronchial asthma) in certain susceptible persons; frequently seen in patients who also have aspirin sensitivity.

ADVERSE REACTIONS
Xerostomia, urinary hesitancy/retention, blurred vision, tachycardia, mydriasis, cycloplegia, increased ocular tension, loss of taste, headache, nervousness, drowsiness, weakness, dizziness, insomnia.

DRUG INTERACTIONS
Phenobarbital may decrease the effect of anticoagulants; may need larger doses of anticoagulant for optimal effect.

PREGNANCY AND LACTATION
Category D (Elixir/Tab), C (Extentabs); caution in nursing.

MECHANISM OF ACTION
Anticholinergic/barbiturate; provides peripheral anticholinergic/antispasmodic action and mild sedation.

PATIENT CONSIDERATIONS
Assessment: Assess for previous hypersensitivity to the drug or any of its components, diarrhea, ileostomy, colostomy, history of physical and/or psychological drug dependence, biliary tract disease, hepatic dysfunction, pregnancy/nursing status, possible drug interactions, and any other conditions where treatment is contraindicated or cautioned.

Monitoring: Monitor for signs/symptoms of heat prostration, drowsiness, blurred vision, constipation, diarrhea, urinary hesitancy/retention, hypersensitivity reactions, and other adverse reactions.

Counseling: Counsel about possible side effects and advise to notify physician if any occur. Inform that the drug may be habit forming. If drowsiness or blurring of vision occurs, warn patients not to engage in activities requiring mental alertness (eg, operating a motor vehicle or other machinery) and not to perform hazardous work. Inform that treatment may decrease sweating, resulting in heat prostration, fever, or heat strokes. (Elixir/Tab) Advise to notify physician if pregnant or intending to become pregnant during therapy; apprise of the potential hazard to the fetus.

DORAL — quazepam
Class: Benzodiazepine

CIV

ADULT DOSAGE
Insomnia
Treatment of Insomnia Characterized by Difficulty in Falling Asleep, Frequent Nocturnal Awakenings, and/or Early Morning Awakenings:

Initial: 7.5mg
Titrate: May increase to 15mg, if necessary

PEDIATRIC DOSAGE
Pediatric use may not have been established

DOSING CONSIDERATIONS
Elderly
Start on a low dose and observe closely

ADMINISTRATION
Oral route

Split the 15mg tab along the score line to achieve 7.5mg dose

STORAGE
20-25°C (68-77°F).

HOW SUPPLIED
Tab: 15mg* *scored

CONTRAINDICATIONS
Known hypersensitivity to quazepam or other benzodiazepines, established or suspected sleep apnea, pulmonary insufficiency.

WARNINGS/PRECAUTIONS
Prolonged administration is generally not necessary or recommended. May impair daytime function in some patients and impair physical/mental abilities; monitor for excess depressant effects. Withdrawal syndrome may occur following abrupt discontinuation, particularly with higher than recommended doses over an extended time; taper dose gradually. Initiate only after careful evaluation; failure of remission after 7-10 days of treatment may indicate presence of primary psychiatric and/or medical illness. Severe anaphylactic and anaphylactoid reactions reported (eg, dyspnea, throat closing, angioedema involving the tongue, glottis, or larynx); do not rechallenge if angioedema develops. Abnormal thinking and behavior changes (eg, decreased inhibition, bizarre behavior, depersonalization, hallucination) reported. Amnesia and other neuropsychiatric symptoms, and paradoxical reactions may occur. "Sleep-driving" and other complex behaviors (eg, preparing/eating food, making phone calls, or having sex while not fully awake) reported; d/c if "sleep-driving" occurs. May worsen depression; consider limiting the total prescription size and increase monitoring for suicidal ideation. Increased risk of abuse and dependence with addiction-prone individuals; caution with use. May cause confusion and over-sedation in elderly; observe closely. Elderly and debilitated may be more sensitive to benzodiazepines.

ADVERSE REACTIONS
Daytime drowsiness, headache.

DRUG INTERACTIONS
Additive CNS depressant effects with ethanol/alcohol or other CNS depressants (eg, psychotropic medications, anticonvulsants, antihistamines, other benzodiazepines, opioids, TCAs); downward dose adjustments may be necessary because of additive effects. Not recommended for use with other sedative-hypnotics. Avoid use with alcohol. Increased risk of complex behaviors (eg, "sleep-driving") with alcohol and other CNS depressants.

PREGNANCY AND LACTATION
Category C, caution in nursing.

MECHANISM OF ACTION
Benzodiazepine; has not been established. Suspected to bind to stereo-specific receptors at several sites within the CNS.

PHARMACOKINETICS
Absorption: Rapid, well absorbed; C_{max}=20ng/mL; T_{max}=2 hrs. **Distribution:** Plasma protein binding (>95%); found in breast milk. **Metabolism:** Liver (extensive); 2-oxoquazepam and N-desalkyl-2-oxoquazepam (active metabolites). **Elimination:** Urine (31%), feces (23%); $T_{1/2}$=39 hrs (quazepam, 2-oxoquazepam), 73 hrs (N-desalkyl-2-oxoquazepam).

PATIENT CONSIDERATIONS
Assessment: Assess for previous hypersensitivity to the drug or other benzodiazepines, established or suspected sleep apnea, pulmonary insufficiency, primary psychiatric and/or medical illness, depression, history of drug addiction or alcoholism, pregnancy/nursing status, and possible drug interactions.

Monitoring: Monitor for worsening of insomnia, excess depressant effects, emergence of new thinking or behavior abnormalities, complex behaviors, drug tolerance, abuse and dependence, withdrawal syndrome, severe anaphylactic/anaphylactoid reactions, and other adverse reactions. Monitor elderly for confusion and over-sedation.

Counseling: Inform about the benefits and risks of therapy, stressing the importance of use ud. Inform that medication may cause next-day impairment, even in the absence of symptoms, and that daytime impairment may persist for several days following discontinuation. Caution against driving or engaging in other hazardous activities requiring complete mental alertness. Advise to contact physician before discontinuing or decreasing the dose, because withdrawal symptoms can occur. Inform that drug may cause abnormal thinking or behavior change, including "sleep-driving" and other complex behaviors while not fully awake; advise to contact physician if any of these symptoms develop. Advise to seek medical attention if severe allergic reactions occur. Inform that drug can worsen depression, and instruct to immediately report any suicidal thoughts. Advise not to take with alcohol. Instruct to notify physician if pregnant, planning to become pregnant, or if breastfeeding. Advise not to increase dose on their own, and to inform physician if they believe the drug is not working.

DORIBAX — doripenem   Rx

Class: Carbapenem

ADULT DOSAGE

Intra-Abdominal Infections

Complicated Infections:
500mg q8h by IV infusion over 1 hr for 5-14 days

Duration includes a possible switch to an appropriate oral therapy, after at least 3 days of parenteral therapy, once clinical improvement has been demonstrated

Urinary Tract Infections

Complicated UTIs, Including Pyelonephritis:
500mg q8h by IV infusion over 1 hr for 10 days; may extend duration up to 14 days for patients w/ concurrent bacteremia

Duration includes a possible switch to an appropriate oral therapy, after at least 3 days of parenteral therapy, once clinical improvement has been demonstrated

PEDIATRIC DOSAGE

Pediatric use may not have been established

DOSING CONSIDERATIONS

Renal Impairment

CrCl >30 to <50mL/min: 250mg IV (over 1 hr) q8h

CrCl >10 to <30mL/min: 250mg IV (over 1 hr) q12h

ADMINISTRATION

IV route

Do not mix w/ or physically add to sol containing other drugs.

Preparation of Sol

500mg Dose Using the 500mg Vial:
1. Constitute 500mg vial w/ 10mL of sterile water for inj (SWFI) or 0.9% NaCl inj and gently shake to form a sus; resultant concentration is approx 50mg/mL. The constituted sus is not for direct inj.
2. Withdraw sus using a syringe w/ a 21-gauge needle and add to infusion bag containing 100mL of normal saline or D5; gently shake until clear. The final infusion sol concentration is approx 4.5mg/mL.

250mg Dose Using the 250mg Vial:
1. Constitute 250mg vial w/ 10mL of SWFI or 0.9% NaCl inj and gently shake to form a sus; resultant concentration is approx 25mg/mL. The constituted sus is not for direct inj.
2. Withdraw sus using a syringe w/ a 21-gauge needle and add to infusion bag containing either 50mL or 100mL of normal saline or D5; gently shake until clear. The final infusion sol concentration is approx 4.2mg/mL (50mL infusion bag) or approx 2.3mg/mL (100mL infusion bag).

250mg Dose Using the 500mg Vial:
1. Constitute 500mg vial w/ 10mL of SWFI or 0.9% NaCl inj and gently shake to form a sus; resultant concentration is approx 50mg/mL. The constituted sus is not for direct inj.
2. Withdraw sus using a syringe w/ a 21-gauge needle and add to infusion bag containing 100mL of normal saline or D5; gently shake until clear.
3. Remove 55mL of this sol from the bag and discard and infuse remaining sol.
4. Infuse the remaining sol, which contains 250mg (approx 4.5mg/mL).

Storage of Constituted Sol

1. Upon constitution w/ SWFI or 0.9% NaCl inj, doripenem sus in the vial may be held for 1 hr prior to transfer and dilution in the infusion bag.
2. Following dilution of the sus, doripenem infusions prepared in normal saline are stable for 12 hrs at room temperature or for 72 hrs at 2-8°C (36-46°F); doripenem infusions prepared in D5 are stable for 4 hrs at room temperature or for 24 hrs at 2-8°C (36-46°F). Stability times include storage and infusion time.
3. Do not freeze constituted doripenem sus or infusion.

STORAGE

25°C (77°F); excursions permitted to 15-30°C (59-86°F).

HOW SUPPLIED

Inj: 250mg, 500mg

CONTRAINDICATIONS

Known serious hypersensitivity to doripenem or to other drugs in the same class or in patients who have demonstrated anaphylactic reactions to beta-lactams.

WARNINGS/PRECAUTIONS

Not approved for the treatment of ventilator-associated bacterial pneumonia. Serious and occasionally fatal hypersensitivity (anaphylactic) and serious skin reactions reported; d/c if an allergic reaction occurs. Seizures reported; higher risk in patients w/ preexisting CNS disorders (eg, stroke, history of seizures), patients w/ compromised renal function, and patients given doses >500mg q8h. *Clostridium difficile*-associated diarrhea (CDAD) reported; may need to d/c if CDAD is suspected or confirmed. May result in bacterial resistance w/ use in the absence of a proven/strongly suspected bacterial infection. Do not administer via inhalation route; pneumonitis reported. Caution in elderly.

ADVERSE REACTIONS

Headache, nausea, diarrhea, rash, phlebitis, anemia, pruritus, hepatic enzyme elevation, oral candidiasis.

DRUG INTERACTIONS

May reduce serum valproic acid levels to below the therapeutic concentration range, which may increase risk for breakthrough seizures; consider alternative antibacterial therapies for patients receiving valproic acid or sodium valproate, or if treatment w/ the drug is necessary, consider supplemental anticonvulsant therapy. Probenecid may increase levels; coadministration is not recommended.

PREGNANCY AND LACTATION

Pregnancy: Category B.
Lactation: Caution in nursing.

MECHANISM OF ACTION

Carbapenem; exerts bactericidal activity by inhibiting bacterial cell-wall biosynthesis, resulting in cell death.

PHARMACOKINETICS

Absorption: C_{max}=23mcg/mL, AUC=36.3mcg•hr/mL. **Distribution:** V_d=16.8L (median); plasma protein binding (8.1%). **Metabolism:** Via dehydropeptidase-1; doripenem-M1 (inactive ring-opened metabolite). **Elimination:** Urine (71% unchanged, 15% metabolite), feces (<1%); $T_{1/2}$=1 hr.

PATIENT CONSIDERATIONS

Assessment: Assess for ventilator-associated bacterial pneumonia, CNS disorders, renal impairment, pregnancy/nursing status, and possible drug interactions. Carefully assess for previous hypersensitivity reactions to drug, penicillins, cephalosporins, other β-lactams, or other allergens.

Monitoring: Monitor for hypersensitivity reactions, CDAD, seizures, development of drug-resistant bacteria, and other adverse reactions. Monitor renal function in patients w/ moderate or severe renal impairment and in elderly.

Counseling: Advise that allergic reactions could occur and that serious reactions may require immediate treatment. Advise to report any previous hypersensitivity reactions to medications or allergens. Counsel that therapy should only be used to treat bacterial, not viral, infections. Instruct to take exactly ud; inform that skipping doses or not completing the full course of therapy may decrease effectiveness of treatment and increase bacterial resistance. Counsel to inform physician if patient has CNS disorders and if taking valproic acid or sodium valproate.

DORYX — doxycycline hyclate   Rx

Class: Tetracyclines

ADULT DOSAGE

General Dosing

Initial: 100mg q12h on 1st day
Maint: 100mg qd or 50mg q12h

More Severe Infections (eg, Chronic UTIs): 100mg q12h

Streptococcal Infections: Continue therapy for 10 days

Acute Epididymo-Orchitis

Caused by *Chlamydia trachomatis*:
100mg bid for at least 10 days

Malaria

Prophylaxis:
100mg qd beginning 1 or 2 days before travel and continuing daily during travel and for 4 weeks after departure from malarious area

Inhalational Anthrax (Postexposure)

100mg bid for 60 days

Chlamydia trachomatis Infections

Uncomplicated Urethral/ Endocervical/Rectal Infections:
100mg bid for 7 days

Alternate Dosing for Uncomplicated Urethral/Endocervical Infections:
200mg qd for 7 days (Doryx)

Gonococcal Infections

Uncomplicated Infections (Except Anorectal Infections in Men):
100mg bid for 7 days

Alternate Dosing:
Single visit dose of 300mg stat followed in 1 hr by a second 300mg dose

Nongonococcal Urethritis

Caused by *Ureaplasma urealyticum*:
100mg bid for 7 days

Syphilis

Patients Allergic to Penicillin (PCN): Early:
100mg bid for 2 weeks

PEDIATRIC DOSAGE

General Dosing

>8 Years:
≤45kg:
4.4mg/kg divided into 2 doses on 1st day, followed by 2.2mg/kg qd or as 2 divided doses, on subsequent days
More Severe Infections: May use up to 4.4mg/kg

>45kg:
Initial: 100mg q12h on 1st day
Maint: 100mg qd or 50mg q12h
More Severe Infections (eg, Chronic UTIs): 100mg q12h

Streptococcal Infections: Continue therapy for 10 days

Malaria

Prophylaxis:
>8 Years:
2mg/kg qd up to 100mg qd beginning 1 or 2 days before travel and continuing daily during travel and for 4 weeks after departure from malarious area

Inhalational Anthrax (Postexposure)

<45kg:
2.2mg/kg bid for 60 days
≥45kg:
100mg bid for 60 days

>1-Year Duration:
100mg bid for 4 weeks

Other Indications
Rickettsial infections (eg, Rocky Mountain spotted fever, typhus fever and the typhus group, Q fever, rickettsialpox, tick fevers)

Lymphogranuloma venereum
Granuloma inguinale
Chancroid
Respiratory tract infections
Psittacosis (ornithosis)
Relapsing fever
Plague
Tularemia
Cholera
Campylobacter fetus infections
Brucellosis (in conjunction w/ streptomycin)
Bartonellosis
UTIs
Trachoma
Inclusion conjunctivitis
Escherichia coli infections
Enterobacter aerogenes infections
Shigella species infections
Acinetobacter species infections

When PCN is contraindicated, treatment of the following infections: yaws, Vincent's infection, actinomycosis, and infections caused by *Clostridium* species

Adjunctive therapy in acute intestinal amebiasis and severe acne

ADMINISTRATION
Oral route

Administer w/ adequate amounts of fluid.
May be given w/ food or milk if gastric irritation occurs.

Administering w/ Applesauce
May break up tab and sprinkle contents (delayed-release pellets) over a spoonful of applesauce.
Do not crush or damage the pellets when breaking up the tab.
Swallow applesauce/pellet mixture immediately w/o chewing; may follow w/ a glass of water.

STORAGE
25°C (77°F); excursions permitted to 15-30°C (59-86°F). **Generic:** Protect from light.

HOW SUPPLIED
Tab, Delayed-Release: 50mg, 200mg*; (Generic) 75mg*, 100mg*, 150mg* *scored

CONTRAINDICATIONS
Hypersensitivity to any of the tetracyclines.

WARNINGS/PRECAUTIONS
May cause permanent discoloration of the teeth (yellow-gray-brown) if used during tooth development (last 1/2 of pregnancy, infancy, and childhood to 8 yrs of age); do not use in this age group, except for anthrax. Enamel hypoplasia reported. *Clostridium difficile*-associated diarrhea (CDAD) reported; may need to d/c if CDAD is suspected or confirmed. Photosensitivity reported; d/c at the 1st evidence of skin erythema. May result in bacterial resistance if used in the absence of proven or suspected bacterial infection or a prophylactic indication. May result in overgrowth of non-susceptible organisms (including fungi); d/c and institute appropriate therapy if superinfection occurs. Associated w/ intracranial HTN (pseudotumor cerebri); increased risk in women of childbearing age who are overweight or have a history of intracranial HTN. If visual disturbance occurs, prompt ophthalmologic evaluation is warranted. Intracranial pressure can remain elevated for weeks after drug cessation; monitor patients until they stabilize. May decrease fibula growth rate in prematures. May cause an increase in BUN. When used for malaria prophylaxis, patient may still transmit the infection to mosquitoes outside endemic areas. False elevations of urinary catecholamines may occur due to interference w/ the fluorescence test.

ADVERSE REACTIONS
N/V, diarrhea, bacterial vaginitis.

DRUG INTERACTIONS
Avoid concomitant use w/ isotretinoin; may also cause pseudotumor cerebri. Depresses plasma prothrombin activity; may require downward adjustment of anticoagulant dose. May interfere w/ bactericidal action of PCN; avoid concurrent use. Impaired absorption w/ bismuth subsalicylate, antacids containing aluminum, Ca^{2+}, or Mg^{2+}, and iron-containing preparations. May render oral contraceptives less effective. Decreased $T_{1/2}$ w/ barbiturates, carbamazepine, and phenytoin. Fatal renal toxicity reported w/ methoxyflurane.

PREGNANCY AND LACTATION
Pregnancy: Category D.
Lactation: Found in breast milk. Not for use in nursing.

MECHANISM OF ACTION
Tetracycline; has bacteriostatic activity. Inhibits bacterial protein synthesis by binding to the 30S ribosomal subunit.

PHARMACOKINETICS
Absorption: Virtually complete. C_{max}=4.6mcg/mL (200mg single dose), 6.3mcg/mL (200mg multiple dose); T_{max}=3 hrs (median). **Distribution:** Found in breast milk. **Elimination:** Urine (40%/72 hrs w/ CrCl 75mL/min, 1-5%/72 hrs w/ CrCl <10mL/min), feces; $T_{1/2}$=18-22 hrs.

PATIENT CONSIDERATIONS
Assessment: Assess for hypersensitivity to drug or any tetracyclines, pregnancy/nursing status, and possible drug interactions. Perform culture and susceptibility testing.

Monitoring: Monitor for CDAD, photosensitivity, skin erythema, superinfection, intracranial HTN, visual disturbance, and other adverse reactions. In long-term therapy, perform periodic lab evaluation of organ systems, including hematopoietic, renal, and hepatic studies.

Counseling: Apprise of the potential hazard to fetus if used during pregnancy. Inform that therapy does not guarantee protection against malaria; advise to use measures that help avoid contact w/ mosquitoes. Advise to avoid excessive sunlight or artificial UV light and to d/c therapy if phototoxicity (eg, skin eruptions) occurs; advise to consider use of sunscreen or sunblock. Inform that absorption of drug is reduced when taken w/ bismuth subsalicylate, antacids containing aluminum, Ca^{2+}, or Mg^{2+}, iron-containing preparations, and w/ foods, especially those that contain Ca^{2+}. Advise to drink fluids liberally. Inform that drug may increase the incidence of vaginal candidiasis. Inform that diarrhea may be experienced and instruct to immediately contact physician if watery and bloody stools (w/ or w/o stomach cramps and fever) occur, even as late as ≥2 months after the last dose. Inform that therapy should only be used to treat bacterial, not viral, infections. Instruct to take exactly ud even if the patient feels better early in the course of therapy. Inform that skipping doses or not completing the full course of therapy may decrease effectiveness of treatment and increase bacterial resistance.

DOVONEX — calcipotriene   Rx

Class: Vitamin D3 derivative

ADULT DOSAGE	PEDIATRIC DOSAGE
Plaque Psoriasis	Pediatric use may not have been established
Usual: Apply a thin layer to the affected skin bid and rub in gently and completely	
Safety and efficacy demonstrated in patients treated for 8 weeks	

ADMINISTRATION
Topical route

Wash hands thoroughly after use

STORAGE
15-25°C (59-77°F). Do not freeze.

HOW SUPPLIED
Cre: 0.005% [60g, 120g]

CONTRAINDICATIONS
History of hypersensitivity to any components of the preparation, hypercalcemia, evidence of vitamin D toxicity. Do not use on the face.

WARNINGS/PRECAUTIONS
Contact dermatitis, including allergic contact dermatitis, reported. Transient irritation of both lesions and surrounding uninvolved skin may occur; d/c if irritation develops. Reversible elevation of serum Ca^{2+} reported; d/c until normal Ca^{2+} levels are restored. For external use only; not for ophthalmic, oral, or intravaginal use.

ADVERSE REACTIONS
Skin irritation, rash, pruritus, dermatitis, worsening of psoriasis.

PREGNANCY AND LACTATION
Category C, caution in nursing.

MECHANISM OF ACTION
Vitamin D3 derivative.

PHARMACOKINETICS
Metabolism: Liver. **Elimination:** Bile.

PATIENT CONSIDERATIONS
Assessment: Assess for history of hypersensitivity to any of the components of the preparation, hypercalcemia, evidence of vitamin D toxicity, and pregnancy/nursing status.

Monitoring: Monitor for serum Ca^{2+} elevation, irritation, contact dermatitis, and other adverse reactions.

Counseling: Advise to use drug only ud by the physician. Inform that the medication is for external use only; instruct to avoid contact w/ face or eyes. Advise to wash hands after application. Counsel that the drug should not be used for any disorder other than for which it was prescribed. Instruct to report any signs of adverse reactions to the physician. Instruct patients who apply medication to the exposed portions of the body to avoid excessive exposure to either natural or artificial sunlight (eg, tanning booths, sun lamps).

DOXIL — doxorubicin hydrochloride liposome   Rx

Class: Anthracycline

> May cause myocardial damage, including CHF, as the total cumulative dose approaches 550mg/m²; include prior use of other anthracyclines or anthracenediones in total cumulative dose calculations. Risk of cardiomyopathy may be increased at lower cumulative doses w/ prior mediastinal irradiation. Acute infusion-related reactions occurred in patients w/ solid tumors. Serious, life-threatening, and fatal infusion reactions reported.

ADULT DOSAGE

Ovarian Carcinoma

Progressed/Recurred After Platinum-Based Therapy:
50mg/m² IV over 60 min every 28 days until disease progression or unacceptable toxicity

AIDS-Related Kaposi's Sarcoma

After Failure of Prior Systemic Chemotherapy or Intolerance to Such Therapy:
20mg/m² IV over 60 min every 21 days until disease progression or unacceptable toxicity

Multiple Myeloma

In combination w/ bortezomib in patients who have not previously received bortezomib and have received at least 1 prior therapy

30mg/m² IV over 60 min on Day 4 of each 21-day cycle for 8 cycles or until disease progression or unacceptable toxicity

Administer therapy after bortezomib on Day 4 of each cycle

PEDIATRIC DOSAGE

Pediatric use may not have been established

DOSING CONSIDERATIONS

Hepatic Impairment
Serum Bilirubin ≥1.2mg/dL: Reduce dose

Adverse Reactions
Hand-Foot Syndrome (HFS):
Grade 1:
If previous Grade 3 or 4 HFS, delay dose up to 2 weeks, then decrease dose by 25%
Grade 2:
Delay dosing up to 2 weeks or until resolved to Grade 0-1
If resolved to Grade 0-1 w/in 2 weeks, continue treatment at previous dose if no previous Grade 3 or 4 HFS, or decrease dose by 25% if previous Grade 3 or 4 toxicity
D/C if no resolution after 2 weeks
Grade 3 or 4:
Delay dosing up to 2 weeks or until resolved to Grade 0-1, then decrease dose by 25%
D/C if no resolution after 2 weeks

Stomatitis:
Grade 1:
If previous Grade 3 or 4 toxicity, delay dose up to 2 weeks, then decrease by 25%
Grade 2:
Delay dosing up to 2 weeks or until resolved to Grade 0-1
If resolved to Grade 0-1 w/in 2 weeks, resume treatment at previous dose if no previous Grade 3 or 4 stomatitis, or decrease dose by 25% if previous Grade 3 or 4 toxicity
D/C if no resolution after 2 weeks
Grade 3 or 4:
Delay dosing up to 2 weeks or until resolved to Grade 0-1; decrease dose by 25% and return to original dose interval
D/C if no resolution after 2 weeks

Neutropenia/Thrombocytopenia:
Grade 2 or 3:
Delay until ANC ≥1500 and platelet count ≥75,000; resume treatment at previous dose
Grade 4:
Delay until ANC ≥1500 and platelet count ≥75,000; resume at 25% dose reduction or continue previous dose w/ prophylactic granulocyte growth factor

Toxicities When Administered in Combination w/ Bortezomib:
Fever ≥38°C and ANC <1000/mm³: Withhold dose for this cycle if before Day 4; decrease dose by 25% if after Day 4 of previous cycle
On any Day of Administration After Day 1 of Each Cycle:
Platelet Count <25,000/mm³ or Hgb <8g/dL or ANC <500/mm³: Withhold dose for this cycle if before Day 4; decrease dose by 25% if after Day 4 of previous cycle and if bortezomib is reduced for hematologic toxicity
Grade 3 or 4 Nonhematologic Toxicity: Do not dose until recovered to Grade <2, then reduce dose by 25%

Suspected Extravasation:
D/C for burning or stinging sensation or other evidence indicating perivenous infiltration or extravasation

Manage confirmed or suspected extravasation as follows:
1. Do not remove the needle until attempts are made to aspirate extravasated fluid
2. Do not flush the line; avoid applying pressure to the site
3. Apply ice to the site intermittently for 15 min qid for 3 days
4. Elevate extremity if extravasation is in an extremity

ADMINISTRATION
IV route

Do not substitute for doxorubicin HCl inj.
Administer 1st dose at an initial rate of 1mg/min; if no infusion-related adverse reactions are observed, increase infusion rate to complete the administration of the drug over 1 hr.
Do not administer as an undiluted sus or as an IV bolus.
Do not use w/ in-line filters.
Do not rapidly flush the IV line.
Do not mix w/ other drugs.

Preparation
Dilute doses up to 90mg in 250mL of D5 inj prior to administration.
Dilute doses >90mg in 500mL of D5 inj prior to administration.
Refrigerate diluted Doxil at 2-8°C (36-46°F) and administer w/in 24 hrs.

STORAGE
Unopened Vials: 2-8°C (36-46°F). Do not freeze.

HOW SUPPLIED
Inj: 20mg/10mL, 50mg/25mL

CONTRAINDICATIONS
History of severe hypersensitivity reactions, including anaphylaxis, to doxorubicin HCl.

WARNINGS/PRECAUTIONS
Do not substitute for doxorubicin HCl inj. Administer only when potential benefits outweigh the risk in patients w/ a history of cardiovascular disease (CVD). Temporarily stop therapy in the event of an infusion-related reaction until resolution, then resume at a reduced infusion rate; d/c infusion for serious or life-threatening infusion-related reactions. HFS reported; d/c if HFS is severe and debilitating. Secondary oral cancers, primarily squamous cell carcinoma, reported w/ long-term (>1 yr) exposure; malignancies were diagnosed both during treatment and up to 6 yrs after last dose. Examine patients at regular intervals for the presence of oral ulceration or w/ any oral discomfort that may be indicative of secondary oral cancer. May cause fetal harm.

ADVERSE REACTIONS
Asthenia, fatigue, fever, N/V, stomatitis, diarrhea, constipation, anorexia, HFS, rash, neutropenia, thrombocytopenia, anemia.

PREGNANCY AND LACTATION
Pregnancy: Can cause fetal harm.
Lactation: It is not known whether Doxil is present in human milk; not for use in nursing.
Reproductive Potential: May damage spermatozoa and testicular tissue, resulting in possible genetic fetal abnormalities. Females and males w/ female partners of reproductive potential should use effective contraception during and for 6 months after treatment. May cause infertility and result in amenorrhea in females; premature menopause can occur. May result in oligospermia, azoospermia, and permanent loss of fertility in males.

MECHANISM OF ACTION
Anthracycline topoisomerase II inhibitor; suspected to bind DNA and inhibit nucleic acid synthesis.

PHARMACOKINETICS
Absorption: (10mg/m²) C_{max}=4.12mcg/mL, AUC=277mcg/mL•hr. (20mg/m²) C_{max}=8.34mcg/mL, AUC=590mcg/mL•hr. **Distribution:** (10mg/m²) V_d=2.83L/m²; (20mg/m²) V_d=2.72L/m². **Metabolism:** Doxorubicinol (major metabolite). **Elimination:** 1st Phase: $T_{1/2}$=4.7 hrs (10mg/m²), 5.2 hrs (20mg/m²). 2nd Phase: $T_{1/2}$=52.3 hrs (10mg/m²), 55 hrs (20mg/m²).

PATIENT CONSIDERATIONS
Assessment: Assess for drug hypersensitivity, history of CVD, hepatic dysfunction, pregnancy/nursing status. Assess left ventricular cardiac function (eg, multigated acquisition, echocardiogram) prior to initiation of therapy.

Monitoring: Monitor for signs/symptoms of myocardial damage, infusion-related reactions, HFS, secondary oral cancers, and other adverse reactions. Monitor cardiac function.

Counseling: Instruct to contact physician if a new onset of fever, symptoms of an infection, or symptoms of HF develop. Advise about the symptoms of infusion-related reactions and instruct to seek immediate medical attention if any of these symptoms develop. Instruct to notify physician if symptoms of HFS or stomatitis develop. Advise females of reproductive potential of the potential risk to a fetus and to inform physician w/ a known or suspected pregnancy. Advise females and males of reproductive potential to use effective contraception during and for 6 months following treatment, and inform that therapy may cause temporary or permanent infertility. Instruct females not to breastfeed during treatment. Inform that a reddish-orange color may appear in urine and other body fluids.

Doxy 100 — doxycycline

Rx

Class: Tetracyclines

ADULT DOSAGE

General Dosing

Initial: 200mg IV administered in 1 or 2 infusions on 1st day

Maint: 100-200mg/day IV depending on severity of infection, w/ 200mg administered in 1 or 2 infusions

Syphilis

Primary and Secondary Syphilis When Penicillin (PCN) is Contraindicated:
300mg/day IV for at least 10 days

Inhalational Anthrax (Postexposure)

100mg IV bid; institute oral therapy as soon as possible and continue therapy for a total of 60 days

Treatment Duration

Continue therapy for at least 24-48 hrs after symptoms and fever have subsided

Group A β-Hemolytic Streptococci Infections:

Treat for at least 10 days

Infusion Duration:

May vary w/ dose, but is usually 1-4 hrs
Recommended infusion time for 100mg of a 0.5mg/mL sol is 1 hr

Other Indications

Treatment of the Following Infections Caused by Susceptible Organisms:
Rickettsiae infections (eg, Rocky Mountain spotted fever, typhus fever and the typhus group, Q fever, rickettsialpox, tick fevers)
Mycoplasma pneumoniae infections
Psittacosis
Ornithosis
Lymphogranuloma venereum
Granuloma inguinale
Relapsing fever
Chancroid
Yersinia pestis infections
Francisella infections
Bartonella bacilliformis infections
Bacteroides species infections
Vibrio cholera infections
Campylobacter fetus infections
Brucella species (in conjunction w/ streptomycin) infections
Escherichia coli infections
Enterobacter aerogenes infections
Shigella species infections
Acinetobacter species infections
Respiratory infections
Urinary infections
Streptococcus species infections
Skin and soft tissue infections
Trachoma

When PCN is contraindicated, treatment of infections due to *Neisseria gonorrhoeae, Neisseria meningitidis, Treponema pallidum* and *Treponema pertenue* (yaws), *Listeria monocytogenes, Clostridium* species, *Fusobacterium fusiforme* (Vincent's infection), and *Actinomyces* species

Adjunctive therapy in acute intestinal amebiasis

PEDIATRIC DOSAGE

General Dosing

>8 Years:

≤100 lbs:

Initial: 2mg/lb IV administered in 1 or 2 infusions on 1st day

Maint: 1-2mg/lb/day IV given as 1 or 2 infusions, depending on severity of infection

>100 lbs:

Initial: 200mg IV administered in 1 or 2 infusions on 1st day

Maint: 100-200mg/day IV depending on severity of infection, w/ 200mg administered in 1 or 2 infusions

Inhalational Anthrax (Postexposure)

<100 lbs (45kg): 1mg/lb (2.2mg/kg) IV bid; institute oral therapy as soon as possible and continue therapy for a total of 60 days

Treatment Duration

Continue therapy for at least 24-48 hrs after symptoms and fever have subsided

Group A β-Hemolytic Streptococci Infections:

Treat for at least 10 days

Infusion Duration:

May vary w/ dose, but is usually 1-4 hrs
Recommended infusion time for 100mg of a 0.5mg/mL sol is 1 hr

ADMINISTRATION

IV route

Avoid rapid administration.
Do not inject IM or SQ.

Preparation

Reconstitute w/ 10mL (100mg/vial) or 20mL (200mg/vial) of sterile water for inj or any compatible IV sol.
Withdraw entire reconstituted sol from vial and further dilute w/ 100-1000mL of compatible IV sol to achieve desired concentrations of 0.1-1mg/mL.
Concentrations <0.1mg/mL or >1mg/mL not recommended.

Compatible IV Sol

NaCl inj; D5 inj; Ringer's inj; invert sugar, 10% in water; lactated Ringer's inj; D5 in lactated Ringer's; Normosol-M in D5W; Normosol-R in D5W; Plasma-Lyte 56 in D5; or Plasma-Lyte 148 in D5.
Refer to PI for further stability information.

STORAGE

20-25°C (68-77°F). Protect from light. Refer to PI for stability information of reconstituted/diluted sol.

HOW SUPPLIED

Inj: 100mg, 200mg

CONTRAINDICATIONS

Hypersensitivity to any of the tetracyclines.

WARNINGS/PRECAUTIONS

May cause permanent discoloration of the teeth (yellow-gray-brown) if used during tooth development (last 1/2 of pregnancy, infancy, and childhood to 8 yrs of age); do not use in this age group, except for anthrax. Enamel hypoplasia reported. *Clostridium difficile*-associated diarrhea (CDAD) reported; may need to d/c if CDAD is suspected or confirmed. Intracranial hypertension (IH, pseudotumor cerebri) associated w/ use. If visual disturbance occurs during treatment, prompt ophthalmologic evaluation is warranted. Monitor patients until they stabilize since intracranial pressure can remain elevated for weeks after drug cessation. Photosensitivity manifested by an exaggerated sunburn reaction reported; d/c at the 1st evidence of skin erythema. May cause an increase in BUN. May result in bacterial resistance if used in the absence of proven or suspected bacterial infection or a prophylactic indication; take appropriate measures if superinfection develops.

ADVERSE REACTIONS

Anorexia, N/V, diarrhea, glossitis, dysphagia, maculopapular/erythematous rash, urticaria, angioneurotic edema, anaphylaxis, pericarditis, hemolytic anemia, thrombocytopenia, neutropenia, eosinophilia.

DRUG INTERACTIONS

Depresses plasma prothrombin activity; may require downward adjustment of anticoagulant dose. May interfere w/ bactericidal action of PCN; avoid concurrent use. Barbiturates, carbamazepine, and phenytoin decrease the $T_{1/2}$. Concomitant use w/ isotretinoin should be avoided because isotretinoin is known to cause pseudotumor cerebri. Concurrent use of tetracycline and methoxyflurane has been reported to result in fatal renal toxicity. Concurrent use of tetracycline may render oral contraceptives less effective.

PREGNANCY AND LACTATION

Pregnancy: Category D.
Lactation: Not for use in nursing.

MECHANISM OF ACTION

Tetracycline; has bacteriostatic activity and inhibits bacterial protein synthesis by binding to the 30S ribosomal subunit.

PHARMACOKINETICS

Absorption: Readily absorbed. C_{max}=2.5mcg/mL (100mg), 3.6mcg/mL (200mg).
Distribution: Bound to plasma proteins in varying degrees. Found in breast milk.
Elimination: Urine (40%/72 hrs in CrCl 75mL/min, 1-5%/72 hrs in CrCl <10mL/min), feces; $T_{1/2}$=18-22 hrs.

PATIENT CONSIDERATIONS

Assessment: Assess for hypersensitivity to drug or any tetracyclines, pregnancy/nursing status, and possible drug interactions. Perform culture and susceptibility testing. In venereal diseases when coexistent syphilis is suspected, perform a dark-field exam and blood serology.

Monitoring: Monitor for CDAD, photosensitivity, skin erythema, superinfection, discoloration of the teeth, and other adverse reactions. In venereal diseases when coexistent syphilis is suspected, repeat blood serology monthly for at least 4 months. Perform periodic lab evaluation of organ systems, including hematopoietic, renal, and hepatic studies in long-term therapy.

Counseling: Advise patients apt to be exposed to direct sunlight or UV light that photosensitivity manifested by an exaggerated sunburn reaction may occur; instruct to d/c treatment at the 1st evidence of skin erythema. Instruct to notify physician if pregnant/breastfeeding. Inform that therapy should only be used to treat bacterial, not viral, infections. Instruct to take exactly ud even if the patient feels better early in the course of therapy. Inform that skipping doses or not completing the full course of therapy may decrease effectiveness of treatment and increase bacterial resistance. Instruct to immediately contact physician if watery and bloody stools (w/ or w/o stomach cramps and fever) occur, even as late as ≥2 months after the last dose.

Drisdol — ergocalciferol

Rx

Class: Vitamin D analogue

ADULT DOSAGE

Hypoparathyroidism

50,000-200,000 IU daily given concomitantly w/ calcium lactate 4g, 6X/day

Vitamin D Resistant Rickets

12,000-500,000 IU daily

Other Indications

Familial Hypophosphatemia

PEDIATRIC DOSAGE

Hypoparathyroidism

50,000-200,000 IU daily given concomitantly w/ calcium lactate 4g, 6X/day

Vitamin D Resistant Rickets

12,000-500,000 IU daily

Other Indications

Familial Hypophosphatemia

DOSING CONSIDERATIONS
Elderly
Start at lower end of dosing range

ADMINISTRATION
Oral route

STORAGE
25°C (77°F); excursions permitted to 15-30°C (59-86°F). Protect from light.

HOW SUPPLIED
Cap: 1.25mg (50,000 IU vitamin D)

CONTRAINDICATIONS
Hypercalcemia, malabsorption syndrome, abnormal sensitivity to the toxic effects of vitamin D, hypervitaminosis D.

WARNINGS/PRECAUTIONS
Avoid in infants w/ idiopathic hypercalcemia. Readjust the therapeutic dosage as soon as there is clinical improvement. Exercise great care in dose adjustment to prevent serious toxic effects; the range between therapeutic and toxic doses is narrow in vitamin D resistant rickets. IV Ca^{2+}, parathyroid hormone, and/or dihydrotachysterol may be required when treating hypoparathyroidism. Maintain normal serum phosphorus (P) levels (eg, dietary phosphate restriction and/or administration of aluminum gels) when treating hyperphosphatemia to prevent metastatic calcification. Adequate dietary Ca^{2+} is necessary for clinical response to vitamin D therapy. Contains FD&C Yellow No. 5 (tartrazine), which may cause allergic reactions (including bronchial asthma) in susceptible individuals. Avoid excess use of vitamin D during normal pregnancy, unless unique case outweighs the significant hazards.

ADVERSE REACTIONS
Anemia, anorexia, constipation, nausea, stiffness, weakness, calcification of soft tissues, impaired renal function, weight loss.

DRUG INTERACTIONS
Impaired absorption w/ mineral oil. Thiazide diuretics may cause hypercalcemia in hypoparathyroid patients.

PREGNANCY AND LACTATION
Category C, caution in nursing.

MECHANISM OF ACTION
Vitamin D analogue; antirachitic activity. Promote active absorption of Ca^{2+} and P in the small intestine, which then elevates serum Ca^{2+} and phosphate levels sufficiently to permit bone mineralization. Also mobilizes Ca^{2+} and phosphate from bone and increases reabsorption of Ca^{2+} and perhaps also phosphate from renal tubules.

PHARMACOKINETICS
Distribution: (25-hydroxyvitamin D) Found in breast milk. **Metabolism:** Hydroxylation; 25-hydroxyvitamin D in liver and 1,25-dihydroxyvitamin D in kidneys (active major metabolites).

PATIENT CONSIDERATIONS
Assessment: Assess for hypercalcemia, malabsorption syndrome, hypervitaminosis D, sensitivity to tartrazine, hypersensitivity to vitamin D in infants w/ idiopathic hypercalcemia, pregnancy/nursing status, and possible drug interactions. Evaluate vitamin D administration from fortified foods, dietary supplements, self-administered and prescription drug sources.

Monitoring: Monitor for clinical response to therapy and for adverse reactions. Monitor serum Ca^{2+} levels frequently in high doses. Perform monthly bone x-rays until condition is corrected and stabilized. In patients treated for hypoparathyroidism, monitor need for IV Ca^{2+}, parathyroid hormone, and/or dihydrotachysterol, have blood Ca^{2+} and P levels checked every 2 weeks or more frequently if necessary. Monitor serum Ca^{2+} in infants if a nursing mother is given large doses of vitamin D.

Counseling: Inform about risks/benefits of therapy and instruct to take ud. Counsel about signs/symptoms of hypervitaminosis D (eg, hypercalcemia, impaired renal function, calcification of soft tissues).

DUAC — benzoyl peroxide/clindamycin phosphate   Rx

Class: Antibacterial/keratolytic

ADULT DOSAGE	**PEDIATRIC DOSAGE**
Inflammatory Acne Vulgaris	**Inflammatory Acne Vulgaris**
Apply a thin layer to the face qd (pm or ud)	**≥12 Years:**
	Apply a thin layer to the face qd (pm or ud)

- -

ADMINISTRATION
Topical route
Wash skin gently, rinse w/ warm water, and pat dry before application

STORAGE
Do not freeze. Prior to Dispensing: 2-8°C (36-46°F). After Dispensing: Room temperature up to 25°C (77°F). Keep tube tightly closed.

HOW SUPPLIED
Gel: (Clindamycin/Benzoyl Peroxide) 1.2%/5% [45g]

CONTRAINDICATIONS
Hypersensitivity to clindamycin, benzoyl peroxide, any components of the formulation, or lincomycin; history of regional enteritis, ulcerative colitis (UC), pseudomembranous colitis, or antibiotic-associated colitis.

WARNINGS/PRECAUTIONS
Avoid contact w/ the eyes, mouth, lips, mucous membranes, or broken skin areas. Diarrhea, bloody diarrhea, and colitis (including pseudomembranous colitis) reported; d/c if significant diarrhea occurs. Severe colitis, which may result in death, reported following oral or parenteral administration w/ an onset of up to several weeks following cessation of therapy. May cause increased sensitivity to sunlight; minimize sun exposure (including use of tanning beds or sun lamps) following application. Caution in patients who may be required to have considerable sun exposure due to occupation and those w/ inherent sensitivity to sun.

ADVERSE REACTIONS
Facial local skin reactions (eg, erythema, peeling, burning, dryness).

DRUG INTERACTIONS
Avoid w/ erythromycin-containing products. Antiperistaltic agents (eg, opiates, diphenoxylate w/ atropine) may prolong and/or worsen severe colitis. Caution w/ concomitant topical acne therapies (eg, peeling, desquamating, or abrasive agents) because of possible cumulative irritancy effect; if irritancy or dermatitis occurs, reduce frequency of application or temporarily interrupt treatment and resume once the irritation subsides, or d/c treatment if irritation persists. May enhance action of other neuromuscular blocking agents; use w/ caution. May cause skin and facial hair to temporarily change color (yellow/orange) w/ topical sulfone products.

PREGNANCY AND LACTATION
Category C, not for use in nursing.

MECHANISM OF ACTION
Antibacterial/keratolytic. Clindamycin: Lincosamide antibacterial; binds to 50S ribosomal subunits of susceptible bacteria and prevents elongation of peptide chains by interfering w/ peptidyl transfer, thereby suppressing protein synthesis. Benzoyl Peroxide: Oxidizing agent w/ bactericidal and keratolytic effects; has not been established.

PHARMACOKINETICS
Distribution: Clindamycin: (Oral/Parenteral) Found in breast milk. **Metabolism:** Benzoyl Peroxide: Converted to benzoic acid.

PATIENT CONSIDERATIONS
Assessment: Assess for hypersensitivity to drug or lincomycin; history of regional enteritis, UC, pseudomembranous colitis, or antibiotic-associated colitis; pregnancy/nursing status; and possible drug interactions. Assess use in patients who may be required to have considerable sun exposure due to occupation and those w/ inherent sensitivity to the sun.

Monitoring: Monitor for signs/symptoms of diarrhea, colitis, local skin reactions, and other adverse reactions. For colitis, perform stool culture and assay for *Clostridium difficile* toxin.

Counseling: Counsel to d/c use and contact physician immediately if an allergic reaction (eg, severe swelling, SOB) develops. Inform that drug may cause irritation (eg, erythema, scaling, itching, or burning), especially when used in combination w/ other topical acne therapies. Advise to limit exposure to sunlight, wear protective clothing (eg, hat), and use sunscreen. Inform that drug may bleach hair or colored fabric. Inform that drug may cause skin and facial hair to temporarily change color (yellow/orange) when used w/ topical sulfone products.

DUAVEE — bazedoxifene/conjugated estrogens   Rx

Class: Estrogen/estrogen agonist and antagonist

> Do not take additional estrogens. Increased risk of endometrial cancer in a woman w/a uterus who uses unopposed estrogens. Perform adequate diagnostic measures to rule out malignancy in postmenopausal women w/ undiagnosed persistent or recurring abnormal genital bleeding. Should not be used for the prevention of cardiovascular disease (CVD) or dementia. Increased risk of stroke and deep vein thrombosis (DVT) reported in postmenopausal women (50-79 yrs of age) treated w/ daily oral conjugated estrogens (CEs) alone. Increased risk of probable dementia reported in postmenopausal women ≥65 yrs of age treated w/ daily conjugated estrogens alone. Estrogens should be prescribed at the lowest effective dose and for the shortest duration consistent w/ treatment goals and risks.

ADULT DOSAGE	**PEDIATRIC DOSAGE**
Menopausal Vasomotor Symptoms	Pediatric use may not have been established
Moderate to Severe:	
1 tab daily	
Postmenopausal Osteoporosis	
Prevention:	
1 tab daily	
Add supplemental Ca^{2+}/vitamin D if patient has inadequate dietary intake	

- -

DOSING CONSIDERATIONS
Renal Impairment
Use not recommended

Elderly
Not recommended in women >75 years of age

ADMINISTRATION
Oral route
Swallow tab whole; take w/o regard to meals.

STORAGE
20-25°C (68-77°F); excursions permitted to 15-30°C (59-86°F). Protect from moisture; do not place in pill boxes or pill organizers. After opening foil pouch, use w/in 60 days.

HOW SUPPLIED
Tab: (CEs/Bazedoxifene) 0.45mg/20mg

CONTRAINDICATIONS

Undiagnosed abnormal uterine bleeding; known/suspected/history of breast cancer; known/suspected estrogen-dependent neoplasia; active/history of DVT/pulmonary embolism (PE); active/history of arterial thromboembolic disease (eg, stroke, MI); hypersensitivity (eg, anaphylaxis, angioedema) to estrogens, bazedoxifene, or any ingredients; known hepatic impairment or disease; known protein C/protein S/antithrombin deficiency or other known thrombophilic disorders; pregnancy, women who may become pregnant, and nursing mothers.

WARNINGS/PRECAUTIONS

D/C immediately if stroke or DVT occurs or is suspected. If feasible, d/c at least 4-6 weeks before surgery of the type associated w/ an increased risk of thromboembolism, or during periods of prolonged immobilization. Not recommended for use in patients >75 yrs of age or in patients w/ renal impairment. May affect certain endocrine and blood components in lab tests. **CEs:** May increase risk of ovarian cancer and gallbladder disease requiring surgery. Retinal vascular thrombosis reported; d/c therapy pending exam if sudden partial/complete loss of vision, or sudden onset of proptosis, diplopia, or migraine occurs. D/C permanently if exam reveals papilledema or retinal vascular lesions. May elevate BP and thyroid-binding globulin levels. May elevate plasma TGs, leading to pancreatitis in patients w/ preexisting hypertriglyceridemia; consider discontinuation of therapy if pancreatitis occurs. Caution w/ history of cholestatic jaundice associated w/ past estrogen use or w/ pregnancy; d/c in case of recurrence. May cause fluid retention. Caution w/ hypoparathyroidism; hypocalcemia may occur. May exacerbate symptoms of angioedema in women w/ hereditary angioedema. May exacerbate asthma, diabetes mellitus (DM), epilepsy, migraine, porphyria, systemic lupus erythematosus (SLE), and hepatic hemangiomas; caution in women w/ these conditions.

ADVERSE REACTIONS

Muscle spasms, nausea, diarrhea, dyspepsia, upper abdominal pain, oropharyngeal pain, dizziness, neck pain.

DRUG INTERACTIONS

Do not take progestins, additional estrogens, or additional estrogen agonist/antagonists. Itraconazole, a strong CYP3A4 inhibitor, reported to increase bazedoxifene and CE exposure. **CEs:** CYP3A4 inducers (eg, St. John's wort preparations, phenobarbital, carbamazepine) may decrease levels and may decrease therapeutic effects and/or result in changes in the uterine bleeding profile. Women dependent on thyroid hormone replacement therapy who are also receiving estrogens may require increased doses of their thyroid replacement therapy; monitor thyroid function. **Bazedoxifene:** Substances known to induce uridine diphosphate glucuronosyltransferase (eg, rifampin, phenobarbital, carbamazepine) may increase metabolism, decrease exposure, and may be associated w/ an increase in risk of endometrial hyperplasia.

PREGNANCY AND LACTATION

Pregnancy: Category X.
Lactation: Not for use in nursing.

MECHANISM OF ACTION

Estrogen/estrogen agonist and antagonist; binds and activates estrogen receptors (ERs) α and β. Produces a composite effect that is specific to each target tissue. **CEs:** Composed of multiple estrogens and are agonists of ER-α and β. **Bazedoxifene:** Acts as an agonist in some estrogen-sensitive tissues and an antagonist in others (eg, uterus). Reduces the risk of endometrial hyperplasia that can occur w/ the CE component.

PHARMACOKINETICS

Absorption: CE: Well-absorbed; (Estrone) C_{max}=2.6ng/mL, T_{max}=6.5 hrs, AUC=35ng•hr/mL. **Bazedoxifene:** Absolute bioavailability (6%); C_{max}=6.9ng/mL, T_{max}=2.5 hrs, AUC=71ng•hr/mL. **Distribution: CE:** Found in breast milk. Largely bound to sex hormone-binding globulin, and albumin. **Bazedoxifene:** V_d=14.7L/kg (IV, 3mg dose); plasma protein binding (98-99%). **Metabolism: CE:** 17-β estradiol to estrone (metabolite); estriol (major urinary metabolite); sulfate and glucuronide conjugation (liver). **Bazedoxifene:** Extensive; Glucuronidation (major metabolic pathway); bazedoxifene-5-glucuronide (major circulating metabolite). **Elimination: CE:** Urine; $T_{1/2}$=17 hrs. **Bazedoxifene:** Biliary; Feces (85%); Urine (<1%); $T_{1/2}$=30 hrs.

PATIENT CONSIDERATIONS

Assessment: Assess for undiagnosed abnormal uterine bleeding, presence/history of breast cancer, estrogen-dependent neoplasia, active/history of DVT/PE/arterial thromboembolic disease, hepatic impairment/disease, history of cholestatic jaundice, drug hypersensitivity, renal impairment, pregnancy/nursing status, any other conditions where treatment may be contraindicated or cautioned, and possible drug interactions.

Monitoring: Monitor for signs/symptoms of CVD; malignant neoplasms; gallbladder disease; dementia; visual abnormalities; BP and plasma TG elevations; pancreatitis; hypothyroidism; fluid retention; exacerbation of asthma, DM, epilepsy, migraine, porphyria, SLE, and hepatic hemangiomas; and other adverse reactions. Perform annual breast exam; schedule mammography based on age, risk factors, and prior mammogram results. Perform adequate diagnostic measures in patients w/ undiagnosed persistent or recurring genital bleeding. Perform periodic evaluation to determine treatment need.

Counseling: Advise to immediately report to physician any signs/symptoms related to venous thrombosis and thromboembolic events. Inform postmenopausal women of the importance of reporting vaginal bleeding to physician as soon as possible. Inform postmenopausal women of possible serious reactions of therapy (eg, cardiovascular disorders, malignant neoplasms, probable dementia), and possible less serious but common adverse reactions (eg, muscle spasms, nausea, diarrhea). Advise to add supplemental Ca^{2+} and/or vitamin D to the diet if daily intake is inadequate. Instruct to remove only 1 tab from the blister package at the time of use.

DUETACT — glimepiride/pioglitazone   Rx
Class: Sulfonylurea/thiazolidinedione (glitazone)

> Thiazolidinediones, including pioglitazone, cause or exacerbate CHF in some patients. After initiation and dose increases, monitor carefully for signs and symptoms of heart failure (HF); manage accordingly and consider discontinuation or dose reduction if HF develops. Not recommended w/ symptomatic HF. Contraindicated w/ established NYHA Class III or IV HF.

ADULT DOSAGE

Type 2 Diabetes Mellitus

Initial: 30mg/2mg or 30mg/4mg qd

Inadequately Controlled on Glimepiride Monotherapy:
Initial: 30mg/2mg or 30mg/4mg qd

Inadequately Controlled on Pioglitazone Monotherapy:
Initial: 30mg/2mg qd

Titrate: Gradually adjust, prn, after assessing adequacy of response and tolerability

Conversions

Changing from Combination Therapy of Pioglitazone Plus Glimepiride as Separate Tabs:
Initial: Take at doses that are as close as possible to the dose of pioglitazone and glimepiride already being taken

Currently on a Different Sulfonylurea Monotherapy or Switching from Combination Therapy of Pioglitazone Plus a Different Sulfonylurea (eg, Glyburide, Glipizide, Chlorpropamide, Tolbutamide, Acetohexamide):
Initial: 30mg/2mg qd; observe for hypoglycemia for 1-2 weeks due to the potential overlapping drug effect

Titrate: Adjust after assessing adequacy of response

PEDIATRIC DOSAGE

Pediatric use may not have been established

DOSING CONSIDERATIONS

Concomitant Medications

Use w/ an Insulin Secretagogue: Reduce insulin secretagogue dose if hypoglycemia occurs

Use w/ Insulin: Decrease insulin dose by 10-25% if hypoglycemia occurs; further insulin dose adjustments should be individualized based on glycemic response

Use w/ Strong CYP2C8 Inhibitors:
Max: 15mg of pioglitazone qd; switch to individual components of Duetact

Use w/ Colesevelam: Administer at least 4 hrs prior to colesevelam

Renal Impairment
Dose conservatively

Elderly
Dose conservatively

Systolic Dysfunction
Use the lowest approved dose only after titration from 15mg to 30mg of pioglitazone has been safely tolerated

ADMINISTRATION

Oral route

Take qd w/ 1st main meal

STORAGE

25°C (77°F); excursions permitted to 15-30°C (59-86°F). Protect from moisture and humidity.

HOW SUPPLIED

Tab: (Pioglitazone/Glimepiride) 30mg/2mg, 30mg/4mg

CONTRAINDICATIONS

NYHA Class III or IV HF, known hypersensitivity to pioglitazone, glimepiride or any other component of this medication, known history of an allergic reaction to sulfonamide derivatives.

WARNINGS/PRECAUTIONS

Not for use in type 1 DM or for treatment of diabetic ketoacidosis. Caution w/ liver disease. Glimepiride: May cause severe hypoglycemia, which may impair mental/physical abilities; caution in patients predisposed to hypoglycemia. Early warning symptoms of hypoglycemia may be different or less pronounced in patients w/ autonomic neuropathy and in the elderly. Hypersensitivity reactions (eg, anaphylaxis, angioedema, Stevens-Johnson syndrome) reported; if suspected, promptly d/c therapy, assess for other potential causes for the reaction, and institute alternative treatment. Increased risk of cardiovascular mortality. May cause hemolytic anemia; caution w/ G6PD deficiency and consider the use of a non-sulfonylurea alternative. Caution in elderly. Pioglitazone: Fatal and nonfatal hepatic failure reported; caution in patients w/ abnormal LFTs. Measure LFTs promptly in patients who report symptoms that may indicate liver injury. D/C if ALT >3X ULN; do not restart if cause of abnormal LFTs not established or if ALT is >3X ULN w/ total bilirubin >2X ULN w/o alternative etiologies. May use w/

caution in patients w/ lesser elevations of ALT or bilirubin and w/ an alternate probable cause. Not for use in patients w/ active bladder cancer; consider benefits versus risks in patients w/ a prior history of bladder cancer. Dose-related edema reported; caution in patients w/ edema or at risk for CHF. Increased incidence of bone fracture reported in females. Macular edema reported; promptly refer to an ophthalmologist if any visual symptoms occur. May result in ovulation in some premenopausal anovulatory women, which may increase risk for pregnancy; adequate contraception is recommended.

ADVERSE REACTIONS
CHF, hypoglycemia, URTI, weight increased, edema lower limb, headache, UTI, diarrhea, nausea, pain in limb.

DRUG INTERACTIONS
See Dosing Considerations. Glimepiride: Caution w/ other antidiabetic medications. May require dose adjustment of Duetact and close monitoring for hypoglycemia or worsening glycemic control w/ drugs that may increase glucose-lowering effect (eg, ACE inhibitors, fibrates, somatostatin analogues, highly protein-bound drugs), drugs that may reduce glucose-lowering effect (eg, protease inhibitors, corticosteroids, oral contraceptives), or drugs that may either increase or decrease glucose-lowering effect (eg, β-blockers, clonidine, reserpine). Alcohol may potentiate or weaken glucose-lowering action. Signs of hypoglycemia may be reduced or absent w/ sympatholytic drugs (eg, β-blockers, clonidine, guanethidine, reserpine). Potential interaction leading to severe hypoglycemia reported w/ oral miconazole. May interact w/ inhibitors (eg, fluconazole) and inducers (eg, rifampin) of CYP2C9. Colesevelam may reduce levels. Pioglitazone: May cause dose-related fluid retention when used w/ other antidiabetic medications, most commonly w/ insulin. Strong CYP2C8 inhibitors (eg, gemfibrozil) may significantly increase exposure and $T_{1/2}$ of pioglitazone. CYP2C8 inducers (eg, rifampin) may significantly decrease exposure; if a CYP2C8 inducer is started or stopped during treatment, changes in diabetes treatment may be needed based on clinical response.

PREGNANCY AND LACTATION
Category C, not for use in nursing.

MECHANISM OF ACTION
Pioglitazone: Thiazolidinedione; insulin-sensitizing agent that acts primarily by enhancing peripheral glucose utilization. Glimepiride: Sulfonylurea; insulin secretagogue that acts primarily by stimulating release of insulin from functioning pancreatic β cells.

PHARMACOKINETICS
Absorption: Pioglitazone: T_{max}=w/in 2 hrs, 3-4 hrs (w/ food). Glimepiride: T_{max}=2-3 hrs. **Distribution:** Pioglitazone: V_d=0.63L/kg; plasma protein binding (>99%). Glimepiride: (IV) V_d=8.8L; plasma protein binding (>99.5%). **Metabolism:** Pioglitazone: Hydroxylation and oxidation (extensive), CYP2C8, CYP3A4; M-III [keto derivative] and M-IV [hydroxyl derivative] (major active metabolites). Glimepiride: Complete by oxidation; cyclohexyl hydroxy methyl derivative (M1) (via CYP2C9) and carboxyl derivative (M2) (major metabolites). **Elimination:** Pioglitazone: Urine (approx 15-30%), bile and feces; $T_{1/2}$=3-7 hrs, 16-24 hrs (metabolites). Glimepiride: Urine (approx 60%, 80-90% metabolites), feces (approx 40%, 70% metabolites).

PATIENT CONSIDERATIONS
Assessment: Assess for hypersensitivity to drug or sulfonamide derivatives, HF or risk of HF, type of DM, diabetic ketoacidosis, predisposition to hypoglycemia, autonomic neuropathy, G6PD deficiency, active/history of bladder cancer, edema, bone health, any other conditions where treatment is cautioned, pregnancy/nursing status, and possible drug interactions. Obtain baseline LFTs, renal function, and FPG and HbA1c levels.

Monitoring: Monitor for signs/symptoms of HF, hypoglycemia, hypersensitivity reactions, hemolytic anemia, liver injury, edema, fractures, macular edema, and other adverse reactions. Monitor FPG and HbA1c. Periodically monitor LFTs in patients w/ liver disease.

Counseling: Inform of the risks/benefits of therapy. Advise on the importance of adherence to dietary instructions and regular testing of blood glucose and HbA1c. Advise to seek medical advice promptly during periods of stress (eg, fever, trauma, infection, surgery) as medication requirements may change. Instruct to promptly report any signs/symptoms of bladder cancer (eg, macroscopic hematuria, dysuria, urinary urgency), or HF (eg, unusually rapid increase in weight or edema, SOB). Inform about the risk of hypoglycemia, its symptoms and treatment, and conditions that predispose to its development. Instruct to d/c use and seek medical advice promptly if signs/symptoms of hepatotoxicity occur. Counsel premenopausal women to use adequate contraception during treatment. Instruct to take drug ud and that any change in dosing should be made only if directed by physician.

DUEXIS — famotidine/ibuprofen   Rx
Class: H₂ blocker/NSAID

> NSAIDs cause an increased risk of serious cardiovascular (CV) thrombotic events, including MI and stroke, which can be fatal. This risk may occur early in treatment and may increase w/ duration of use. Contraindicated in the setting of CABG surgery. NSAIDs cause an increased risk of serious GI adverse events (eg, bleeding, ulceration, stomach/intestinal perforation), which can be fatal and can occur anytime during use and w/o warning symptoms; elderly patients and patients w/ a prior history of peptic ulcer disease and/or GI bleeding are at a greater risk.

ADULT DOSAGE
Rheumatoid Arthritis
Relief of signs/symptoms of rheumatoid arthritis and to decrease the risk of developing upper GI ulcers (gastric and/or duodenal ulcer) in patients taking ibuprofen for this indication

1 tab tid

Controlled trials do not extend beyond 6 months

Osteoarthritis
Relief of signs/symptoms of osteoarthritis and to decrease the risk of developing upper GI ulcers (gastric and/or duodenal ulcer) in patients taking ibuprofen for this indication

1 tab tid

Controlled trials do not extend beyond 6 months

DOSING CONSIDERATIONS
Renal Impairment
Renal Insufficiency (CrCl <50mL/min): Not recommended
Elderly
If the anticipated benefit outweighs the potential risks, start at lower end of dosing range; monitor for adverse effects

ADMINISTRATION
Oral route

Swallow whole; do not cut to supply a lower dose.
Do not chew, divide, or crush

STORAGE
25°C (77°F); excursions permitted to 15-30°C (59-86°F).

HOW SUPPLIED
Tab: (Ibuprofen/Famotidine) 800mg/26.6mg

CONTRAINDICATIONS
Known hypersensitivity (eg, anaphylactic reactions, serious skin reactions) to ibuprofen, famotidine, or any components of the drug product; history of asthma, urticaria, or allergic-type reactions w/ aspirin (ASA) or other NSAIDs; in the setting of CABG surgery; history of hypersensitivity to other H₂-receptor antagonists.

WARNINGS/PRECAUTIONS
Use lowest effective dose for the shortest duration possible. D/C w/ active and clinically significant bleeding from any source. Periodically monitor Hgb in patients w/ initial Hgb ≤10g receiving long-term therapy. Renal effects of therapy may hasten the progression of renal dysfunction in patients w/ preexisting renal disease. May mask inflammation and fever. Blurred and/or diminished vision, scotomata, and/or changes in color vision reported; d/c and perform an ophthalmologic examination that includes central visual fields and color vision testing, if a patient develops such complaints during therapy. **Ibuprofen:** Increased CV thrombotic risk w/ higher doses reported. Avoid in patients w/ a recent MI unless benefits outweigh the risks of recurrent CV thrombotic events; if used, monitor for signs of cardiac ischemia. Increased risk for GI bleeding w/ longer duration of NSAID therapy, older age, poor general health status, and advanced liver disease and/or coagulopathy; avoid use in patients at higher risk unless benefits are expected to outweigh the increased risk of bleeding. Consider alternate therapies other than NSAIDs for patients at higher risk and patients w/ active GI bleeding. Caution in patients w/ a history of inflammatory bowel disease (ulcerative colitis, Crohn's disease); condition may be exacerbated. Promptly initiate evaluation and treatment if a serious GI adverse event is suspected; d/c until a serious GI adverse event is ruled out. Hepatotoxicity reported; d/c immediately and perform a clinical evaluation if clinical signs/symptoms consistent w/ liver disease develop, or if systemic manifestations occur. May cause new onset HTN or worsen preexisting HTN. Fluid retention and edema reported. Avoid use in patients w/ severe heart failure (HF) unless benefits outweigh risks; monitor for signs of worsening HF if used. Renal papillary necrosis and other renal injury reported w/ long-term use. Renal toxicity also reported in patients in whom renal prostaglandins have a compensatory role in the maintenance of renal perfusion; increased risk w/ renal/hepatic dysfunction, dehydration, hypovolemia, HF, and in the elderly. Correct volume status in dehydrated or hypovolemic patients prior to initiating therapy. Avoid use in patients w/ advanced renal disease unless the benefits are expected to outweigh the risk; monitor for signs of worsening renal function if used in patients w/ advanced renal disease. Hyperkalemia reported. Associated w/ anaphylactic reactions in patients w/ and w/o known hypersensitivity to ibuprofen and in patients w/ ASA-sensitive asthma. Monitor for changes in the signs/symptoms of asthma in patients w/ preexisting asthma (w/o known ASA sensitivity). May cause serious skin reactions (eg, exfoliative dermatitis, Stevens-Johnson syndrome, toxic epidermal necrolysis); d/c at 1st appearance of skin rash/hypersensitivity. May cause premature closure of the fetal ductus arteriosus; avoid use in pregnant women starting at 30 weeks of gestation (3rd trimester). Anemia reported; monitor Hgb or Hct if signs/symptoms of anemia develop. May increase the risk of bleeding events; coagulation disorders may increase this risk. Aseptic meningitis w/ fever and coma observed on rare occasions in patients on ibuprofen. **Famotidine:** CNS adverse effects, including seizures, delirium, and coma, reported w/ moderate (CrCl <50mL/min) and severe (CrCl <10mL/min) renal insufficiency.

PEDIATRIC DOSAGE
Pediatric use may not have been established

ADVERSE REACTIONS
Nausea, diarrhea, constipation, upper abdominal pain, headache.

DRUG INTERACTIONS
May increase cyclosporine's nephrotoxicity; monitor for signs of worsening renal function. Concomitant use w/ pemetrexed may increase the risk of pemetrexed-associated myelosuppression, renal, and GI toxicity; refer to prescribing information for further information. **Ibuprofen:** Synergistic effect on bleeding w/ anticoagulants (eg, warfarin); monitor for signs of bleeding w/ concomitant anticoagulants, antiplatelet agents (eg, ASA), SSRIs, and SNRIs. Drugs that interfere w/ serotonin reuptake may potentiate the risk of bleeding. May increase risk of GI bleeding w/ use of oral corticosteroids, anticoagulants, SSRIs, smoking, and alcohol use. ASA may increase risk of bleeding and serious GI events; concomitant use w/ analgesic doses of ASA is not recommended. Monitor patients more closely for GI bleeding w/ concomitant use of low-dose ASA for cardiac prophylaxis. May diminish antihypertensive effect of ACE inhibitors, ARBs, and β-blockers (eg, propranolol); monitor BP. Coadministration w/ ACE inhibitors or ARBs may result in deterioration of renal function (including possible acute renal failure) in patients who are elderly, volume-depleted (including those on diuretic therapy), or have renal impairment; monitor for worsening renal function when these drugs are administered concomitantly. May reduce the natriuretic effect of loop diuretics (eg, furosemide) and thiazide diuretics; observe for signs of worsening renal function, in addition to assuring diuretic efficacy including antihypertensive effects. May increase digoxin serum concentrations and prolong the $T_{1/2}$ of digoxin; monitor digoxin levels. May elevate plasma lithium levels and reduce renal lithium clearance; monitor for signs of lithium toxicity. May increase the risk for methotrexate (MTX) toxicity; monitor for MTX toxicity. Concomitant use w/ other NSAIDs or salicylates (eg, diflunisal, salsalate) increases the risk of GI toxicity; not recommended w/ other NSAIDs or salicylates. Avoid w/ other ibuprofen-containing products.

PREGNANCY AND LACTATION
Pregnancy: Use of NSAIDs during the 3rd trimester of pregnancy increases the risk of premature closure of the fetal ductus arteriosus. Avoid use in pregnant women starting at 30 weeks of gestation (3rd trimester).
Lactation: Found in breast milk; caution in nursing.
Reproductive Potential: May delay or prevent rupture of ovarian follicles, which has been associated w/ reversible infertility in some women. Small studies in women treated w/ NSAIDs have also shown a reversible delay in ovulation. Consider withdrawal of therapy in women who have difficulties conceiving or who are undergoing investigation of infertility.

MECHANISM OF ACTION
Ibuprofen: NSAID; mechanism not completely understood but involves inhibition of COX-1 and COX-2. Has analgesic, anti-inflammatory, and antipyretic properties.
Famotidine: H_2-receptor blocker; inhibits gastric secretion.

PHARMACOKINETICS
Absorption: Rapid. Ibuprofen: C_{max}=45mcg/mL, T_{max}=1.9 hrs. Famotidine: C_{max}=61ng/mL, T_{max}=2 hrs. **Distribution:** Ibuprofen: Extensively bound to plasma proteins; found in breast milk. Famotidine: Plasma protein binding (15-20%); found in breast milk. **Metabolism:** Famotidine: S-oxide (metabolite). **Elimination:** Ibuprofen: Urine (45-79%, metabolites); $T_{1/2}$=2 hrs. Famotidine: Urine (25-30%, unchanged); $T_{1/2}$=4 hrs.

PATIENT CONSIDERATIONS
Assessment: Assess for history of asthma, urticaria, or other allergic-type reactions w/ previous use of ASA or other NSAIDs; history of hypersensitivity to other H_2-receptor antagonists; preexisting asthma; CV disease (CVD) or risk factors for CVD; HTN; history of peptic ulcer disease or GI bleeding; coagulation disorders; renal/hepatic impairment; pregnancy/nursing status; or any other conditions where treatment is contraindicated or cautioned. Assess volume status. Assess for possible drug interactions. Obtain baseline BP, CBC, and chemistry profile.

Monitoring: Monitor for signs/symptoms of CV thrombotic events; cardiac ischemia in patients w/ a recent MI; GI bleeding/ulceration and perforation; hepatotoxicity; new or worsening HTN; HF; edema; renal papillary necrosis and other renal injury; hyperkalemia; anaphylactic reactions; serious skin reactions; anemia; aseptic meningitis; ophthalmological effects; and other adverse reactions. Monitor BP during initiation of therapy and throughout the course of therapy. Monitor for signs of bleeding in patients on concomitant therapy w/ anticoagulants, antiplatelet agents, SSRIs, or SNRIs. Monitor renal function in patients w/ renal/hepatic impairment, HF, dehydration, or hypovolemia. Monitor CBC and chemistry profiles periodically during long-term treatment.

Counseling: Inform of potential for CV thrombotic events, GI adverse events, and worsening CHF/edema, and advise of symptoms; instruct to report any symptoms to healthcare provider immediately. Inform of the potential for hepatotoxicity, and advise of signs/symptoms; if signs/symptoms occur, instruct to d/c and seek immediate medical therapy. Instruct to seek immediate emergency help if signs of an anaphylactic reaction occur. Advise to d/c immediately if rash develops and to contact healthcare provider as soon as possible. Advise females of reproductive potential who desire pregnancy that therapy may be associated w/ a reversible delay in ovulation. Instruct pregnant women to avoid use starting at 30 weeks of gestation. Advise patient not to use other NSAIDs or salicylates concomitantly; notify of the presence of NSAIDs in OTC medications for colds, fever, or insomnia. Advise patient not to use low-dose ASA concomitantly w/o talking to healthcare provider. Instruct to d/c therapy if nephrotoxicity develops.

DULERA — formoterol fumarate dihydrate/mometasone furoate   Rx
Class: Corticosteroid/long-acting beta₂ agonist (LABA)

> LABAs, such as formoterol, increase the risk of asthma-related death. LABAs may increase the risk of asthma-related hospitalization in pediatric patients and adolescents. Use only for patients not adequately controlled on a long-term asthma control medication (eg, inhaled corticosteroid) or whose disease severity clearly warrants initiation of treatment w/ both an inhaled corticosteroid and LABA. Once asthma control is achieved and maintained, assess the patient at regular intervals and step down therapy if possible w/o loss of asthma control, and maintain the patient on a long-term asthma control medication. Do not use if asthma is adequately controlled on low- or medium-dose inhaled corticosteroids.

ADULT DOSAGE
Asthma
Previously on Inhaled Medium Dose Corticosteroids:
Recommended: 2 inh of 100mcg/5mcg bid (am and pm)
Max: 400mcg/20mcg daily

Previously on Inhaled High Dose Corticosteroids:
Recommended: 2 inh of 200mcg/5mcg bid (am and pm)
Max: 800mcg/20mcg daily

Do not use >2 inh bid of the prescribed strength. If inadequate response after 2 weeks of therapy, higher strength may provide additional asthma control

PEDIATRIC DOSAGE
Asthma
≥12 Years:
Previously on Inhaled Medium Dose Corticosteroids:
Recommended: 2 inh of 100mcg/5mcg bid (am and pm)
Max: 400mcg/20mcg daily

Previously on Inhaled High Dose Corticosteroids:
Recommended: 2 inh of 200mcg/5mcg bid (am and pm)
Max: 800mcg/20mcg daily

Do not use >2 inh bid of the prescribed strength. If inadequate response after 2 weeks of therapy, higher strength may provide additional asthma control

---

ADMINISTRATION
Oral inh route

After each dose, rinse mouth w/ water w/o swallowing.
The Dulera canister should only be used w/ the Dulera actuator.
Shake well prior to each inh.
Refer to PI for proper administration.

Priming
Prime before using for the 1st time by releasing 4 test sprays into the air, away from the face, shaking well before each spray.
In cases where the inhaler has not been used for >5 days, prime the inhaler again.

STORAGE
20-25°C (68-77°F); excursions permitted to 15-30°C (59-86°F). Do not puncture. Do not use or store near heat or open flame. **60-Inhalation Inhaler:** Store w/ the mouthpiece down or in a horizontal position after priming.

HOW SUPPLIED
MDI: (Mometasone/Formoterol) (100mcg/5mcg)/inh, (200mcg/5mcg)/inh [60, 120 inh]

CONTRAINDICATIONS
Primary treatment of status asthmaticus or other acute episodes of asthma where intensive measures are required. Known hypersensitivity to mometasone furoate, formoterol fumarate, or any ingredients in the medication.

WARNINGS/PRECAUTIONS
Not indicated for the relief of acute bronchospasm. Do not initiate during rapidly deteriorating/potentially life-threatening episodes of asthma. D/C regular use of oral/inhaled short-acting β_2-agonists (SABAs) prior to treatment. Inhalation-induced bronchospasm w/ immediate increase in wheezing may occur; d/c immediately and institute alternative therapy. Immediate hypersensitivity reactions may occur. **Formoterol:** Cardiovascular (CV) effects and fatalities reported w/ excessive use; do not use an additional LABA. CV and CNS effects may occur. Caution in elderly and patients w/ CV disorders, aneurysm, pheochromocytoma, convulsive disorders, or thyrotoxicosis and in patients unusually responsive to sympathomimetic amines. May cause changes in blood glucose and serum K^+ levels. **Mometasone:** *Candida albicans* infections of mouth and pharynx reported; treat and, if needed, interrupt therapy. Increased susceptibility to infections. May lead to serious/fatal course of chickenpox or measles; avoid exposure and, if exposed, consider prophylaxis/treatment. Caution w/ active/quiescent tuberculosis (TB); untreated systemic fungal, bacterial, viral, or parasitic infections; or ocular herpes simplex. Deaths due to adrenal insufficiency reported w/ transfer from systemic to inhaled corticosteroids; wean slowly from systemic corticosteroid use after transferring to therapy. Resume oral corticosteroids during periods of stress or a severe asthma attack if patient previously withdrawn from systemic corticosteroid. Transferring from systemic to inhalation therapy may unmask previously suppressed allergic conditions (eg, rhinitis, conjunctivitis, eczema). Observe for systemic corticosteroid withdrawal effects. Reduce dose slowly if hypercorticism and adrenal suppression appear. Decreases in bone mineral density (BMD) reported; caution w/ major risk factors for decreased bone mineral content, including chronic use of drugs that can reduce bone mass (eg, anticonvulsants, corticosteroids). May reduce growth velocity in pediatric patients. Glaucoma, increased IOP, and cataracts reported.

ADVERSE REACTIONS
Nasopharyngitis, sinusitis, headache.

DRUG INTERACTIONS
Formoterol: Do not use w/ other medications containing LABAs. Potentiation of sympathetic effects w/ additional adrenergic drugs; use w/ caution. Potentiation of hypokalemic effect w/ xanthine derivatives and non-K^+-sparing

diuretics. Caution w/ MAOIs, TCAs, macrolides, or drugs known to prolong QTc interval or w/in 2 weeks of discontinuing such agents; effect on CV system may be potentiated. Use w/ β-blockers may block effects and produce severe bronchospasm in asthma patients; if needed, consider cardioselective β-blocker w/ caution. **Mometasone:** Increased plasma concentration w/ ketoconazole; caution w/ long-term ketoconazole and other known strong CYP3A4 inhibitors (eg, ritonavir, clarithromycin, itraconazole). Elevated risk of arrhythmias w/ concomitant anesthesia w/ halogenated hydrocarbons.

PREGNANCY AND LACTATION
Pregnancy: In women w/ poorly/moderately controlled asthma, there is an increased risk of several perinatal adverse outcomes such as preeclampsia in the mother and prematurity, low birth weight, and small for gestational age in the neonate. Closely monitor pregnant women w/ asthma and adjust medication as necessary to maintain optimal asthma control.
Lactation: There are no available data on the presence of Dulera, mometasone furoate, or formoterol fumarate in human milk, the effects on the breastfed child, or the effects on milk production. Caution in nursing.

MECHANISM OF ACTION
Mometasone: Corticosteroid; not established. Shown to have inhibitory effects on multiple cell types (eg, mast cells, eosinophils, neutrophils) and mediators (eg, histamine, eicosanoids, leukotrienes) involved in inflammation and asthmatic response. **Formoterol:** LABA; stimulates intracellular adenyl cyclase, which catalyzes conversion of adenosine triphosphate to cAMP. Increased cAMP levels cause relaxation of bronchial smooth muscle and inhibition of release of mediators of immediate hypersensitivity from cells, especially from mast cells.

PHARMACOKINETICS
Absorption: Mometasone: C_{max}=20pg/mL; AUC=170pg•hr/mL; T_{max}=1-2 hrs. Formoterol: C_{max}=22pmol/L; AUC=125pmol•h/L; T_{max}=0.58-1.97 hrs. **Distribution:** Mometasone: V_d=152L (IV); plasma protein binding (98-99%). Formoterol: Plasma protein binding (61-64%). **Metabolism:** Mometasone: Liver (extensive) via CYP3A4. Formoterol: Direct glucuronidation, O-demethylation (via CYP2D6, 2C19, 2C9, 2A6), and conjugation. **Elimination:** Mometasone: Feces (74%); urine (8%); $T_{1/2}$=25 hrs. Formoterol: Urine (6.2-6.8%, unchanged); $T_{1/2}$=9.1-10.8 hrs (single dose), 9-11 hrs (multidose).

PATIENT CONSIDERATIONS
Assessment: Assess for status asthmaticus, acute asthma episodes, rapidly deteriorating asthma, known hypersensitivity to any drug component, risk factors for decreased bone mineral content, CV or convulsive disorders, thyrotoxicosis, other conditions where treatment is contraindicated or cautioned, pregnancy/nursing status, and possible drug interactions. Obtain baseline BMD and lung function.

Monitoring: Monitor for localized oral *C. albicans* infections, glaucoma, increased IOP, cataracts, CV/CNS effects, hypercorticism, adrenal suppression, inhalation induced bronchospasm, hypokalemia, hyperglycemia, hypersensitivity reactions, signs of increased drug exposure w/ hepatic impairment, and other adverse reactions. Monitor BMD and lung function. Perform regular eye examinations. Monitor growth in pediatric patients routinely.

Counseling: Inform about increased risk of asthma-related hospitalization in pediatric patients/adolescents and asthma-related death. Instruct not to use to relieve acute asthma symptoms; instruct to treat acute symptoms w/ a SABA. Instruct to seek medical attention if symptoms worsen, if lung function decreases, or if more inhalations than usual of a SABA are needed. If a dose is missed, instruct to take next dose at the normal time. Instruct not to d/c or reduce therapy w/o physician's guidance. Instruct not to use w/ other LABAs. Advise to avoid exposure to chickenpox or measles and, if exposed, to consult physician w/o delay. Inform of potential worsening of existing TB, fungal, bacterial, viral, or parasitic infections, or ocular herpes simplex. Inform about risks of hypercorticism and adrenal suppression, decreased BMD, cataracts or glaucoma, and oropharyngeal candidiasis. Inform about the risk of reduced growth velocity in pediatric patients. Inform of adverse events associated w/ β$_2$-agonists. Instruct regarding use of therapy.

DUONEB — albuterol sulfate/ipratropium bromide   Rx
Class: Anticholinergic/short-acting beta$_2$ agonist (SABA)

ADULT DOSAGE	PEDIATRIC DOSAGE
Bronchospasm	Pediatric use may not have been established
Associated w/ COPD:	
3mL qid via nebulizer	
May give up to 2 additional 3mL	
doses/day, prn	

ADMINISTRATION
Inh route
Administer via jet nebulizer connected to an air compressor w/ an adequate air flow, equipped w/ a mouthpiece or suitable face mask

STORAGE
2-25°C (36-77°F). Store in pouch until time of use. Protect from light.

HOW SUPPLIED
Sol, Inhalation: (Ipratropium Bromide/Albuterol Sulfate) (0.5mg/3mg)/3mL

CONTRAINDICATIONS
History of hypersensitivity to any components in the medication, or to atropine and its derivatives.

WARNINGS/PRECAUTIONS
Paradoxical bronchospasm may occur; d/c immediately and institute alternative therapy if occurs. Fatalities reported with excessive use of inhaled products containing sympathomimetic amines and with home use of nebulizers. May produce significant cardiovascular (CV) effects (eg, ECG changes). Immediate hypersensitivity reactions reported. Caution with CV disorders (eg, coronary insufficiency, cardiac arrhythmias, HTN), convulsive disorders, hyperthyroidism, diabetes mellitus (DM), narrow-angle glaucoma, prostatic hypertrophy, bladder neck obstruction, hepatic/renal insufficiency, and in patients unusually responsive to sympathomimetic amines. Aggravation of preexisting DM and ketoacidosis reported with large doses of IV albuterol. May decrease serum K^+.

ADVERSE REACTIONS
Lung disease, pharyngitis, pain, chest pain, diarrhea, dyspepsia, nausea, leg cramps, bronchitis, pneumonia, UTI, constipation, voice alterations.

DRUG INTERACTIONS
Additive effects with other anticholinergic drugs; use with caution. Other sympathomimetic agents may increase risk of adverse CV effects; use with caution. β-blockers and albuterol inhibit the effect of each other; use β-blockers with caution in patients with hyperreactive airways. ECG changes and/or hypokalemia that may result from non-K^+-sparing diuretics (eg, loop or thiazide diuretics) may be worsened by β-agonists; use with caution. Administration with MAOIs or TCAs, or within 2 weeks of discontinuation of such agents may potentiate the action of albuterol on CV system; use with extreme caution.

PREGNANCY AND LACTATION
Category C, not for use in nursing.

MECHANISM OF ACTION
Albuterol: β$_2$-adrenergic bronchodilator; stimulates adenyl cyclase, enzyme that catalyzes formation of cAMP, and the cAMP formed mediates cellular response, resulting in relaxation of bronchial smooth muscle. Ipratropium: Anticholinergic bronchodilator; blocks muscarinic receptors of acetylcholine. Prevents the increases in intracellular concentration of cGMP, resulting from interaction of acetylcholine with the muscarinic receptors of bronchial smooth muscle.

PHARMACOKINETICS
Absorption: Albuterol: C_{max}=4.65mg/mL, T_{max}=0.8 hrs, AUC=24.2ng•hr/mL. **Distribution:** Ipratropium: Plasma protein binding (0-9%). **Metabolism:** Albuterol: Conjugation; albuterol 4'-O-sulfate (metabolite). Ipratropium: Ester hydrolysis. **Elimination:** Albuterol: urine (8.4% unchanged0); $T_{1/2}$=6.7 hrs. Ipratropium: urine (3.9% unchanged).

PATIENT CONSIDERATIONS
Assessment: Assess for history of hypersensitivity to atropine and its derivatives, CV disorders, convulsive disorders, hyperthyroidism, DM, narrow-angle glaucoma, prostatic hypertrophy, bladder neck obstruction, hepatic/renal insufficiency, pregnancy/nursing status, and possible drug interactions. Assess use in patients unusually responsive to sympathomimetic amines.

Monitoring: Monitor for signs/symptoms of hypersensitivity reactions, paradoxical bronchospasm, CV effects, and other adverse reactions. Monitor pulse rate and BP. Reassess therapy if signs of worsening COPD occur.

Counseling: Advise not to exceed recommended dose or frequency without consulting physician. Instruct to contact physician if symptoms worsen. Instruct to avoid exposing eyes to this product as temporary pupillary dilation, blurred vision, eye pain, or precipitation/worsening of narrow-angle glaucoma may occur. Inform that proper nebulizer technique should be assured, particularly if a mask is used. Instruct to contact physician if pregnancy occurs or nursing is started while on therapy.

DUOPA — carbidopa/levodopa   Rx
Class: Dopa-decarboxylase inhibitor/dopamine precursor

ADULT DOSAGE	PEDIATRIC DOSAGE
Parkinson's Disease	Pediatric use may not have been established
Prior to initiation of therapy, convert patient from all other forms of levodopa to oral immediate-release (IR) carbidopa-levodopa (1:4 ratio)	

Initial:
Step 1: Calculate/Administer Morning Dose for Day 1:
a. Determine total amount of levodopa (in mg) in the 1st dose of oral IR carbidopa-levodopa that was taken on the previous day
b. Convert the levodopa dose from mg to mL by multiplying the oral dose by 0.8 and dividing by 20mg/mL (Morning Dose)
c. Add 3mL to the Morning Dose to prime the intestinal tube (Total Morning Dose)
d. Administer Total Morning Dose over 10-30 min
Step 2: Calculate/Administer Continuous Dose for Day 1:
a. Determine amount of oral IR levodopa the patient received from the oral IR carbidopa-levodopa doses

throughout the previous day (16 waking hrs) in mg; do not include doses taken at night when calculating the levodopa amount

b. Subtract 1st oral levodopa dose taken by the patient on the previous day (determined in Step 1 (a)) from total oral levodopa dose (determined in Step 2 (a)) and divide the result by 20mg/mL to get the Continuous Dose (in mL) over 16 hrs

c. The hourly infusion rate (mL/hr) is obtained by dividing the Continuous Dose by 16 (hrs)

d. If persistent/numerous "Off" periods occur during the 16-hr infusion, consider increasing the Continuous Dose or using the Extra Dose function. If dyskinesia/levodopa-related adverse reactions occur, consider decreasing the Continuous Dose or stopping infusion until adverse reactions subside

Titrate:
Morning Dose:
Inadequate Response w/in 1 hr of Morning Dose on Preceding Day:
Morning Dose on Preceding Day <6mL: Increase Morning Dose by 1 mL
Morning Dose on Preceding Day >6mL: Increase Morning Dose by 2mL
Exclude the 3mL to prime tube

Continuous Dose Adjustment:
Consider increasing dose based on clinical response and on the number/volume of Extra Doses that was needed for the previous day

Max: 2g of levodopa component (eg, 1 cassette/day) over 16 hrs

Extra Doses:
Initial: 1mL (20mg of levodopa)
Titrate: Increase in 0.2mL increments
Limit frequency to 1 extra dose q2h

- -

DOSING CONSIDERATIONS
Adverse Reactions
Dyskinesia/Therapy-Related Adverse Reactions on Preceding Day:
Morning Dose: If patient experienced dyskinesias or therapy-related adverse reactions w/in 1 hr of Morning Dose on preceding day, then decrease morning dose by 1mL
Continuous Dose:
Troublesome Adverse Reactions Lasting for a Period of ≥1 hr: Decrease dose by 0.3mL/hr
Troublesome Adverse Reactions Lasting for 2 or More Periods of ≥1 hr: Decrease dose by 0.6mL/hr

Discontinuation
Avoid sudden discontinuation/rapid dose reduction; if patients need to d/c therapy, taper dose or switch to oral IR carbidopa-levodopa tabs.
When using a PEG-J tube, may d/c by withdrawing tube and letting the stoma heal.

ADMINISTRATION
Naso-jejunal/PEG-J route

- Bring to room temperature before administration; 20 min prior to use, take 1 cassette out of the refrigerator/carton.
- Deliver as 16-hr infusion either through a naso-jejunal tube (short-term administration) or through a PEG-J tube (long-term administration).
- Do not use cassettes for longer than 16 hrs; do not reuse an opened cassette.
- At the end of daily infusion, disconnect PEG-J tube from the pump, flush w/ room temperature potable water using a syringe, and take night-time dose of oral IR carbidopa-levodopa.
- Cassettes are specifically designed to be connected to the CADD-Legacy 1400 pump.

Morning of PEG-J Procedure
- Ensure patients take their oral Parkinson's disease medications.
Refer to PI for tubing sets recommendations for long-term and short-term administration.

STORAGE
-20°C (-4°F). Thaw at 2-8°C (36-46°F) prior to dispensing; refer to PI for thawing instructions. Protect from light.

HOW SUPPLIED
Sus: (Carbidopa/Levodopa) (4.63mg/20mg)/mL [100mL]

CONTRAINDICATIONS
Patients who are currently taking a nonselective MAOI (eg, phenelzine, tranylcypromine) or who have recently (w/in 2 weeks) taken a nonselective MAOI.

WARNINGS/PRECAUTIONS
GI complications may occur and may result in serious outcomes (eg, need for surgery, death). Orthostatic hypotension reported; monitor especially after starting or increasing dose. Hallucinations, psychosis, and confusion reported; hallucinations may be responsive to a dose reduction of levodopa. Do not use in patients w/ a major psychotic disorder. Intense urges to gamble, increased sexual urges, intense urges to spend money, binge or compulsive eating, and/or other intense urges, and the inability to control these urges may occur; consider dose reduction or discontinuation if such urges develop. Depression reported. A symptom complex resembling neuroleptic malignant syndrome (hyperpyrexia and confusion) reported in association w/ rapid dose reduction, withdrawal of, or changes in dopaminergic therapy; avoid sudden discontinuation/rapid dose reduction and taper dose if discontinuing therapy. May cause or exacerbate dyskinesias; may require dose reduction of therapy or other medications used to treat Parkinson's disease. Polyneuropathy reported; monitor periodically for signs of neuropathy after starting therapy, especially in patients w/ preexisting neuropathy and in patients taking medications or those who have medical conditions associated w/ neuropathy. MI and arrhythmia reported; monitor for symptoms, especially those w/ a history of MI or cardiac arrhythmias. Perform periodic skin examinations to monitor for melanoma. May increase risk for elevated BUN and CPK. May increase levels of catecholamines and metabolites in plasma and urine, giving false-positive results suggesting the diagnosis of pheochromocytoma. May cause increased IOP in patients w/ glaucoma.
Levodopa: Falling asleep during activities of daily living and somnolence reported; consider discontinuation if significant daytime sleepiness or episodes of falling asleep during activities that require active participation occur.

ADVERSE REACTIONS
Complication of device insertion, nausea, depression, peripheral edema, HTN, URTI, oropharyngeal pain, incision-site erythema, atelectasis.

DRUG INTERACTIONS
See Contraindications. Selective MAO-B inhibitors (eg, rasagiline, selegiline) may be associated w/ orthostatic hypotension; monitor patients. Antihypertensive medications may cause symptomatic postural hypotension; may need a dose reduction of antihypertensive medication after starting or increasing the dose of Duopa. Iron salts or multivitamins containing iron salts may form chelates and may reduce bioavailability; monitor for worsening Parkinson's symptoms.
Levodopa: Caution w/ concomitant use of sedating medications; may increase the risk for somnolence. Dopamine D2 receptor antagonists (eg, phenothiazines, butyrophenones, risperidone, metoclopramide, papaverine) and isoniazid may reduce the effectiveness of levodopa; monitor for worsening Parkinson's symptoms. Absorption may be decreased in patients on a high-protein diet.

PREGNANCY AND LACTATION
Pregnancy: Category C.
Lactation: Caution in nursing.

MECHANISM OF ACTION
Dopa-decarboxylase inhibitor/dopamine precursor. **Carbidopa:** Inhibits decarboxylation of peripheral levodopa, making more levodopa available for delivery to the brain. **Levodopa:** Crosses blood-brain barrier and presumably is converted to dopamine in the brain.

PHARMACOKINETICS
Absorption: Levodopa: Bioavailability (97%); T_{max}=2.5 hrs. **Distribution:** Carbidopa: Plasma protein binding (36%). Levodopa: Plasma protein binding (10-30%); crosses the placenta; found in breast milk. **Metabolism:** Carbidopa: α-methyl-3-methoxy-4-hydroxyphenylpropionic acid and α-methyl-3,4-dihydroxyphenylpropionic acid (main metabolites). Levodopa: Decarboxylation, O-methylation, transamination, and oxidation. **Elimination:** Carbidopa: Urine (30% unchanged); $T_{1/2}$=2 hrs. Levodopa: $T_{1/2}$=1.5 hrs (in the presence of carbidopa).

PATIENT CONSIDERATIONS

Assessment: Assess for major psychotic disorder, risk factors that may increase risk for somnolence (eg, presence of sleep disorders), peripheral neuropathy, history of MI or cardiac arrhythmias, glaucoma, pregnancy/nursing status, and possible drug interactions.

Monitoring: Monitor for GI complications, drowsiness or falling asleep during activities of daily living, orthostatic hypotension, hallucinations/psychosis/confusion, impulse control/compulsive behaviors, depression w/ suicidal tendencies, dyskinesias, neuropathy, ischemic heart disease, arrhythmia, and other adverse reactions. Monitor for hyperpyrexia and confusion if sudden discontinuation or rapid dose reduction occurs. Perform periodic skin examinations to monitor for melanoma. Monitor IOP in patients w/ glaucoma after starting therapy.

Counseling: Inform of risks and benefits of therapy. Instruct to inform physician of any previous surgery in the upper part of the abdomen. Advise that foods that are high in protein may reduce the effectiveness of therapy. Instruct to contact physician if experiencing symptoms of GI complications, depression or worsening of depression, suicidal thoughts, hallucinations, abnormal thinking, psychotic behavior, confusion, new/increased gambling urges, sexual urges, uncontrolled spending, binge/compulsive eating, or other urges, or if any symptoms or features suggesting neuropathy develop. Inform of the potential sedating effects caused by therapy. Advise not to drive a car, operate machinery, or engage in other potentially dangerous activities until effects of therapy are known. Advise of possible additive effects when taking other sedating medications, alcohol, or other CNS depressants in combination w/ therapy. Inform that syncope and hypotension w/ or w/o symptoms may develop; caution against standing rapidly after sitting or lying down, especially if patient has been doing so for prolonged periods and especially at the initiation of treatment. Advise to contact physician before stopping therapy and to notify physician if withdrawal symptoms develop. Inform that therapy may cause or exacerbate preexisting dyskinesia. Advise to have a regular skin examination by a qualified healthcare provider.

DURAGESIC — fentanyl   CII

Class: Opioid analgesic

> Exposes patients and other users to the risk of opioid addiction/abuse/misuse, which may lead to overdose and death; assess risk prior to therapy and monitor all patients regularly for development of these behaviors or conditions. Serious, life-threatening, or fatal respiratory depression may occur; monitor especially during initiation or following a dose increase. Contraindicated for use as a prn analgesic, in nonopioid tolerant patients, in acute pain, and in postoperative pain. Deaths due to fatal overdose have occurred from accidental exposure; strict adherence to handling/disposal instructions is of utmost importance to prevent accidental exposure. Prolonged use during pregnancy may result in neonatal opioid withdrawal syndrome. Concomitant use with all CYP3A4 inhibitors and discontinuation of a concomitantly administered CYP3A4 inducer may increase plasma concentrations and potentially cause fatal respiratory depression; monitor patients during concomitant therapy. Exposure of application site and surrounding area to direct external heat sources may increase absorption and result in fatal overdose and death; patients who develop fever or increased core body temperature due to strenuous exertion are at increased risk and may require dose adjustment.

ADULT DOSAGE

Severe Pain (Daily, Around-the-Clock Management)

Opioid-Tolerant Patients:

D/C or taper all other ER and around-the-clock opioids when beginning therapy

25-300mcg/hr reapplied q72hr; initiate dosing regimen for each patient individually, taking into account the patient's prior analgesic treatment (refer to PI for dose conversions)

Titrate dose based on daily dose of supplemental opioid analgesics required on the 2nd or 3rd day of initial application; use the ratio of 45mg/24 hrs of oral morphine to a 12mcg/hr increase in fentanyl dose

Evaluate for further titration after no less than two 3-day applications before any further increase in dose

A small portion of patients may require systems to be applied q48h; an increase in dose should be evaluated before changing dosing interval

PEDIATRIC DOSAGE

Severe Pain (Daily, Around-the-Clock Management)

Opioid-Tolerant Patients:

≥2 Years:

D/C or taper all other ER and around-the-clock opioids when beginning therapy

25-300mcg/hr reapplied q72hr; initiate dosing regimen for each patient individually, taking into account the patient's prior analgesic treatment (refer to PI for dose conversions)

Titrate dose based on daily dose of supplemental opioid analgesics required on the 2nd or 3rd day of initial application; use the ratio of 45mg/24 hrs of oral morphine to a 12mcg/hr increase in fentanyl dose

Evaluate for further titration after no less than two 3-day applications before any further increase in dose

A small portion of patients may require systems to be applied q48h; an increase in dose should be evaluated before changing dosing interval

DOSING CONSIDERATIONS

Renal Impairment
Mild to Moderate: Start w/ one half of the usual dosage
Severe: Avoid use

Hepatic Impairment
Mild to Moderate: Start w/ one half of the usual dosage
Severe: Avoid use

Discontinuation
Significant amounts of fentanyl continue to be absorbed from the skin for ≥24 hrs after the patch is removed

Converting to Another Opioid:
1. Remove patch and titrate the dose of the new analgesic based upon the patient's report of pain until adequate analgesia has been attained
2. Upon system removal, ≥17 hrs are required for a 50% decrease in serum fentanyl concentrations

Not Converting to Another Opioid:
Use a gradual downward titration (eg, having the dose every 6 days), in order to reduce the possibility of withdrawal symptoms; it is not known at what dose level fentanyl may be discontinued w/o producing the signs and symptoms of opioid withdrawal

Elderly
Start at lower end of the dosing range

ADMINISTRATION
Transdermal route

Application and Handling Instructions
1. Apply to intact, non-irritated, and non-irradiated skin on a flat surface such as the chest, back, flank, or upper arm; in young children and persons w/ cognitive impairment, adhesion should be monitored and the upper back is the preferred location to minimize the potential of inappropriate patch removal
2. Hair at the application site may be clipped (not shaved) prior to system application
3. If the application site must be cleansed prior to application of the patch, do so w/ clear water; do not use soaps, oils, lotions, alcohol, or any other agents that might irritate the skin or alter its characteristics. Allow the skin to dry completely prior to patch application
4. Apply immediately upon removal from the sealed package; the patch must not be altered (eg, cut) in any way prior to application. Do not use if the pouch seal is broken or if the patch is cut or damaged
5. Press the transdermal system firmly in place w/ the palm of the hand for 30 sec, making sure the contact is complete, especially around the edges

6. Each patch may be worn continuously for 72 hrs; the next patch is applied to a different skin site after removal of the previous transdermal system
7. If problems w/ adhesion of the patch occur, the edges of the patch may be taped w/ first aid tape; if adhesion problems persist, the patch may be overlaid w/ a transparent adhesive film dressing
8. If the patch falls off before 72 hrs, dispose of it by folding in 1/2 and flushing down the toilet; a new patch may be applied to a different skin site
9. Patients (or caregivers) should wash their hands immediately w/ soap and water after applying patch
10. Contact w/ unwashed or unclothed application sites can result in secondary exposure and should be avoided

Disposal Instructions
1. Patients should dispose of used patches immediately upon removal by folding the adhesive side of the patch to itself, then flushing down the toilet
2. Unused patches should be removed from their pouches, the protective liners removed, the patches folded so that the adhesive side of the patch adheres to itself, and immediately flushed down the toilet
3. Patients should dispose of any patches remaining from a prescription as soon as they are no longer needed

STORAGE
Up to 25°C (77°F); excursions permitted to 15-30°C (59-86°F). Store in original unopened pouch.

HOW SUPPLIED
Patch: 12mcg/hr, 25mcg/hr, 50mcg/hr, 75mcg/hr, 100mcg/hr [5ˢ]

CONTRAINDICATIONS
Opioid-intolerant patients; management of acute/intermittent pain, or in patients who require opioid analgesia for a short period; management of postoperative pain, including use after outpatient/day surgeries (eg, tonsillectomies); management of mild pain; significant respiratory compromise, especially if adequate monitoring and resuscitative equipment are not readily available; acute or severe bronchial asthma; diagnosis or suspicion of paralytic ileus; known hypersensitivity to fentanyl or any components of the transdermal system.

WARNINGS/PRECAUTIONS
Should be prescribed only by healthcare professionals knowledgeable in the use of potent opioids for the management of chronic pain. Reserve for use in patients for whom alternative treatment options (eg, nonopioid analgesics, immediate-release opioids) are ineffective, not tolerated, or would be otherwise inadequate to provide sufficient management of pain. Do not use as the 1st opioid. Risk of addiction is increased w/ personal/family history of substance abuse or mental illness. Prescribe smallest appropriate quantity. Closely monitor elderly, cachectic, or debilitated patients for respiratory depression. May decrease respiratory drive to the point of apnea in patients with chronic pulmonary disease; consider use of other nonopioid analgesic alternatives if possible. Avoid in patients who may be susceptible to the intracranial effects of CO_2 retention. May obscure clinical course of head injury and may increase intracranial pressure (ICP); monitor patients with brain tumors. May cause severe hypotension, including orthostatic hypotension and syncope, in ambulatory patients; increased risk with reduced blood volume. May produce bradycardia. Avoid use with severe hepatic/renal impairment. May cause spasm of the sphincter of Oddi; monitor patients with biliary tract disease (eg, acute pancreatitis). May cause increases in serum amylase concentration. Tolerance and physical dependence may develop during chronic therapy. May impair mental/physical abilities. Significant absorption from the skin continues for ≥24 hrs after patch removal. Avoid abrupt discontinuation; use a gradual downward dose titration. Not for use in women during and immediately prior to labor.

ADVERSE REACTIONS
Respiratory depression, N/V, constipation, diarrhea, headache, muscle spasms, malaise, palpitations, dizziness, insomnia, somnolence, fatigue, feeling cold, hyperhidrosis, anorexia.

DRUG INTERACTIONS
See Boxed Warning. Monitor respiratory depression when given with other drugs that depress respiration. Concomitant use with CNS depressants (eg, other opioids, sedatives, alcohol) may cause respiratory depression, hypotension, profound sedation, coma, or death; closely monitor and reduce dose of 1 or both agents. Coadministration with CYP3A4 inducers may lead to lack of efficacy of fentanyl or development of withdrawal; monitor for signs of opioid withdrawal and consider dose adjustments until stable drug effects are achieved. Avoid concomitant use with MAOIs or within 14 days of stopping such treatment. Mixed agonist/antagonist (eg, pentazocine, nalbuphine, butorphanol) or partial agonist (buprenorphine) analgesics may reduce analgesic effect or may precipitate withdrawal symptoms; avoid concomitant use. Monitor for signs of urinary retention or reduced GI motility with anticholinergics or other medications with anticholinergic activity.

PREGNANCY AND LACTATION
Category C, not for use in nursing.

MECHANISM OF ACTION
Opioid analgesic; interacts predominantly with the opioid mu-receptor in the brain, spinal cord, and other tissues.

PHARMACOKINETICS
Absorption: T_{max}=20-72 hrs. Transdermal administration of variable doses resulted in different parameters. **Distribution:** V_d=6L/kg; found in breast milk; crosses placenta. **Metabolism:** Liver via CYP3A4; oxidative N-dealkylation to norfentanyl. **Elimination:** (IV) Urine (75%, <10% unchanged), feces (9% primarily metabolites); $T_{1/2}$=7 hrs (IV).

PATIENT CONSIDERATIONS
Assessment: Assess for degree of opioid tolerance, type and severity of pain, risks for opioid abuse, addiction, or misuse, paralytic ileus, acute/severe

bronchial asthma, history of hypersensitivity to drug or any component of patch, debilitation, seizures, biliary tract disease, any other conditions where treatment is contraindicated or cautioned, pregnancy/nursing status, and possible drug interactions.

Monitoring: Monitor for signs/symptoms of respiratory depression, bradycardia, worsening of biliary tract disease, increased ICP, increased serum amylase levels, increased body temperature/fever, abuse, misuse, addiction, tolerance/physical dependence, opioid withdrawal syndrome in neonates born to mothers on prolonged therapy during pregnancy, and other adverse reactions.

Counseling: Inform that use of patch may result in addiction, abuse, and misuse, which may lead to overdose or death; instruct not to share with others and protect from theft, misuse, and from children. Inform of the risk of life-threatening respiratory depression; advise on how to recognize respiratory depression and to seek medical attention. Instruct to avoid accidental contact when holding or caring for children. Instruct to immediately take patch off if it dislodges and accidentally sticks to the skin of another person, wash exposed area with water, and seek medical attention. Advise to never change the dose/number of patches unless instructed. Advise how to safely taper medication and not to stop abruptly. Warn of the potential for temperature-dependent increases in drug release from patch; instruct to avoid strenuous exertion that may increase body temperature and avoid exposing application site and surrounding area to direct external heat sources. Counsel that medication may impair mental and/or physical ability; instruct patients to refrain from potentially hazardous tasks until therapy is established that they have not been adversely affected. Inform of pregnancy risks and advise women of childbearing potential who become/are planning to become pregnant to consult physician prior to initiating or continuing therapy. Advise to notify physician of all medications currently being taken and avoid using other CNS depressants and alcohol. Inform that severe constipation may develop. Instruct to refer to the instructions for use for proper disposal of patch.

DURLAZA — aspirin   Rx

Class: Antiplatelet agent

ADULT DOSAGE

Reduce Risk of Myocardial Infarction

Reduce the risk of death and MI in patients w/ chronic coronary artery disease (eg, history of MI, unstable angina pectoris, chronic stable angina)

Not for use in situations where a rapid onset of action is required (eg, acute treatment of MI or before percutaneous coronary intervention); use immediate-release aspirin.

162.5mg qd

Reduce Risk of Stroke

Reduce the risk of death and recurrent stroke in patients who have had an ischemic stroke or transient ischemic attack

Not for use in situations where a rapid onset of action is required (eg, acute treatment of MI or before percutaneous coronary intervention); use immediate-release aspirin.

162.5mg qd

PEDIATRIC DOSAGE

Pediatric use may not have been established

DOSING CONSIDERATIONS

Renal Impairment

Severe (GFR <10mL/min): Avoid use

Hepatic Impairment

Severe: Avoid use

ADMINISTRATION

Oral route

Do not take 2 hrs before or 1 hr after consuming alcohol.
Take the cap w/ a full glass of water at the same time each day.
Swallow whole; do not cut, crush or chew.

STORAGE

25°C (77°F); excursions permitted to 15-30°C (59-86°F)

HOW SUPPLIED

Cap, Extended Release: 162.5mg

CONTRAINDICATIONS

Hypersensitivity to NSAIDs, syndrome of asthma, rhinitis, and nasal polyps.

WARNINGS/PRECAUTIONS

May cause severe urticaria, angioedema, or bronchospasm. Increases the risk of bleeding. May cause gastric ulceration and bleeding; avoid w/ active peptic ulcer disease. Maternal aspirin (ASA) use during later stages of pregnancy may cause low birth weight, increased incidence for intracranial hemorrhage in premature infants, stillbirths, and neonatal death.

ADVERSE REACTIONS

Dyspepsia, hepatic enzyme elevation, hepatitis, Reye's Syndrome.

DRUG INTERACTIONS

Alcohol may interfere w/ the controlled release properties; do not take 2 hrs before or 1 hr after consuming alcohol. Coadministration w/ inhibitors of the renin-angiotensin system (RAS) may result in deterioration of renal function, including possible acute renal failure, in patients who are elderly, volume depleted, or who have compromised renal function; monitor renal function periodically in patients receiving RAS inhibitors. May also attenuate the antihypertensive effects of RAS inhibitors. Increased risk of bleeding w/ anticoagulants, antiplatelet agents, and other NSAIDs. May decrease total concentration of phenytoin and increase serum valproic acid levels. May inhibit renal clearance of methotrexate, causing bone marrow toxicity, especially in the elderly or renal impaired. Concurrent use w/ other NSAIDs may result in renal impairment. Nonselective NSAIDs (eg, ibuprofen) may interfere w/ the antiplatelet effect of low-dose ASA. Administer a single 400mg dose of ibuprofen ≥2-4 hrs after ingestion of Durlaza; wait 8 hrs after ibuprofen dosing, before giving ASA, to avoid significant interference.

PREGNANCY AND LACTATION

Pregnancy: May cause premature closure of the fetal ductus arteriosus; avoid during 3rd trimester. May cause excessive blood loss at delivery; avoid 1 week prior to and during labor/delivery.
Lactation: Not for use in nursing.

MECHANISM OF ACTION

Salicylate; inhibits prostaglandin synthesis resulting in inhibition of platelet aggregation.

PHARMACOKINETICS

Absorption: T_{max}=2 hrs (median). **Distribution:** V_d=170 mL/kg. **Metabolism:** Rapidly hydrolyzed in the plasma to salicylic acid. Salicylic acid is primarily conjugated in the liver; salicyluric acid, phenolic glucuronide, acyl glucuronide (metabolites). **Elimination:** Urine; $T_{1/2}$=20-60 min.

PATIENT CONSIDERATIONS

Assessment: Assess for hypersensitivity to NSAIDs; syndrome of asthma, rhinitis, and nasal polyps; risk factors for bleeding; active peptic ulcer disease; possible drug interactions; and pregnancy/nursing status.

Monitoring: Monitor renal function periodically in patients receiving RAS inhibitors.

Counseling: Instruct not to d/c therapy w/o notifying physician. Inform that bruising/bleeding may occur more easily and that it may take longer to stop bleeding; instruct to notify physician of any prolonged, unusual, or excessive bleeding and about blood in the stool/urine. Advise to d/c therapy and seek immediate medical attention if any signs/symptoms of a hypersensitivity reaction occur. Inform not to take Durlaza 2 hrs before or 1 hr after consuming alcohol. Advise patients who drink ≥3 alcoholic drinks every day about the risk of bleeding involved in chronic, heavy alcohol use during therapy. Advise to swallow caps whole and not to take ibuprofen around the same time as Durlaza. Advise that ASA containing products may cause fetal harm, especially during the 3rd trimester of pregnancy. Instruct to notify physician if pregnant, intending to become pregnant, breastfeeding, or are considering breastfeeding prior or during treatment.

DUTOPROL — hydrochlorothiazide/metoprolol succinate   Rx

Class: Selective beta₁ blocker/thiazide diuretic

> Exacerbations of angina pectoris and myocardial infarction reported following abrupt discontinuation. When discontinuing chronically administered drug, particularly in patients with ischemic heart disease, gradually reduce dose over a period of 1-2 weeks and monitor patients. Promptly resume therapy, at least temporarily, and take other measures appropriate for the management of unstable angina if angina markedly worsens or acute coronary insufficiency develops. Caution against interruption or discontinuation of therapy without the physician's advice. Coronary artery disease may be unrecognized; avoid abrupt discontinuation of therapy even in patients treated only for HTN.

ADULT DOSAGE

Hypertension

Initial: 25mg-12.5mg qd
Titrate: May titrate at intervals of 2 weeks
Max: 200mg-25mg qd

May be administered with other antihypertensive drugs

PEDIATRIC DOSAGE

Pediatric use may not have been established

ADMINISTRATION

Oral route
Take with or without food

STORAGE

25°C (77°F); excursions permitted to 15-30°C (59-86°F).

HOW SUPPLIED

Tab, Extended-Release: (Metoprolol-HCTZ) 25mg-12.5mg, 50mg-12.5mg, 100mg-12.5mg* *scored

CONTRAINDICATIONS

Cardiogenic shock, decompensated heart failure (HF), sinus bradycardia, sick sinus syndrome, >1st-degree heart block (unless a permanent pacemaker is in place), anuria, hypersensitivity to metoprolol succinate or HCTZ or to other sulfonamide-derived drugs.

WARNINGS/PRECAUTIONS

Bradycardia, including sinus pause, heart block, and cardiac arrest reported; increased risk in patients with 1st-degree atrioventricular (AV) block, sinus node dysfunction, or conduction disorders (eg, Wolff-Parkinson-White). Reduce dose or d/c if severe bradycardia develops. Metoprolol: Worsening cardiac failure may occur during up-titration; if symptoms occur, increase diuretics and restore clinical stability (compensated HF) before advancing the dose of therapy; may need to reduce dose of therapy or temporarily d/c therapy. May cause bronchospasm; avoid with bronchospastic disease, but may use with caution if unresponsive/intolerant to other antihypertensives. Avoid initiation of high-dose regimen in patients with cardiovascular (CV) risk factors undergoing noncardiac surgery; associated with bradycardia, hypotension, stroke and death. Chronically administered therapy should not be routinely withdrawn prior to major surgery; however, may augment risks of general anesthesia and surgical procedures. May mask tachycardia occurring with hypoglycemia. May precipitate or aggravate symptoms of arterial insufficiency in patients with peripheral vascular disease (PVD). Associated with a paradoxical increase in BP in patients with pheochromocytoma; initiate an α-blocker first if used in patients with pheochromocytoma. May mask certain clinical signs of hyperthyroidism (eg, tachycardia); abrupt withdrawal may precipitate thyroid storm. HCTZ: May cause hypokalemia, hyponatremia, and hypomagnesemia. May alter glucose tolerance and increase serum cholesterol and TG levels. Reduces clearance of uric acid; may cause or exacerbate hyperuricemia and precipitate gout. Decreases urinary Ca^{2+} excretion; may cause elevations of serum Ca^{2+}. Increased risk for developing acute renal failure in patients with chronic kidney disease, severe HF, or volume depletion. May cause acute transient myopia and acute angle-closure glaucoma (idiosyncratic reactions); d/c therapy if these symptoms occur and consider prompt medical or surgical treatment if the intraocular pressure remains uncontrolled. May exacerbate or activate systemic lupus erythematosus (SLE). Minor alterations of fluid and electrolyte balance may precipitate hepatic coma in patients with impaired hepatic function or progressive liver disease.

ADVERSE REACTIONS
Nasopharyngitis.

DRUG INTERACTIONS
Metoprolol: Additive effect and increased risk of hypotension or bradycardia with catecholamine-depleting drugs (eg, reserpine, MAOIs). CYP2D6 inhibitors (eg, quinidine, fluoxetine, paroxetine, propafenone) may increase levels. Increased risk of significant bradycardia with nondihydropyridine calcium channel blockers (eg, verapamil, diltiazem), digoxin, or clonidine. If clonidine and Dutoprol are both to be discontinued, withdraw Dutoprol several days before the gradual withdrawal of clonidine to reduce risk of rebound HTN. Delay the introduction of Dutoprol for several days after discontinuation of clonidine if switching to therapy. May decrease responsiveness to epinephrine; consider other medications in patients treated for severe anaphylaxis. HCTZ: Dose adjustment of antidiabetic drugs (eg, oral agents, insulin) may be required. Impaired absorption with anionic exchange resins (eg, cholestyramine and colestipol resins); administer at least 4 hrs before or 4-6 hrs after resin administration. Reduces the renal clearance of lithium and increases the risk of lithium toxicity; monitor serum lithium levels. NSAIDs may reduce diuretic, natriuretic, and antihypertensive effects.

PREGNANCY AND LACTATION
Category C, safety not known in nursing.

MECHANISM OF ACTION
Metoprolol: β_1-selective adrenergic receptor blocker; has not been established. Proposed to competitively antagonize catecholamines at peripheral adrenergic-neuron sites, have central effect leading to reduced sympathetic outflow to periphery, and suppress renin activity. HCTZ: Thiazide diuretic; has not been established. Affects renal tubular mechanism of electrolyte reabsorption and increases excretion of Na^+ and Cl^-.

PHARMACOKINETICS
Absorption: Metoprolol: Complete. Absolute bioavailability (50%) (immediate-release); T_{max}=10-12 hrs. HCTZ: Absolute bioavailability (70%); T_{max}=2-5 hrs. **Distribution:** Metoprolol: Plasma protein binding (12%, albumin); found in breast milk. HCTZ: Plasma protein binding (40-70%, albumin); crosses the placenta; found in breast milk. **Metabolism:** Metoprolol: Liver via CYP2D6. **Elimination:** Metoprolol: Urine (<5% unchanged); $T_{1/2}$=3-7 hrs. HCTZ: Urine (70% unchanged); $T_{1/2}$=10 hrs.

PATIENT CONSIDERATIONS
Assessment: Assess for hypersensitivity to drug or to other sulfonamide-derived drugs, cardiogenic shock, decompensated HF, sinus bradycardia, sick sinus syndrome, AV heart block, presence of pacemaker, anuria, bronchospastic disease, CV risk factors, PVD, pheochromocytoma, history of penicillin allergy, SLE, renal/hepatic impairment, pregnancy/nursing status, any other conditions where treatment is contraindicated or cautioned, and possible drug interactions.

Monitoring: Monitor for signs/symptoms of withdrawal, HF, bronchospasm, bradycardia, hypoglycemia, precipitation/aggravation of symptoms of PVD, paradoxical increase in BP, hyperthyroidism, electrolyte and metabolic effects, idiosyncratic reactions, exacerbation/activation of SLE, and other adverse reactions. Monitor serum electrolytes periodically. Monitor HR and rhythm.

Counseling: Advise to take regularly and continuously, ud. Instruct not to interrupt or d/c therapy without consulting the physician. Inform that therapy may cause bronchospasm; instruct to inform physician if patient starts to wheeze or have difficulty in breathing. Inform that patient may need blood tests to monitor serum electrolytes. Advise to report decreased visual acuity or ocular pain and d/c and to contact physician right away if these symptoms occur. Inform that hypersensitivity reactions may occur. Instruct to inform other physicians that they are taking diuretics.

DYANAVEL XR — amphetamine   CII
Class: CNS stimulant

> High potential for abuse and dependence; assess risk of abuse prior to prescribing and monitor for signs of abuse/dependence while on therapy.

PEDIATRIC DOSAGE
Attention-Deficit Hyperactivity Disorder
≥6 Years:
Initial: 2.5mg or 5mg qam
Titrate: May increase in increments of 2.5-10mg/day every 4-7 days
Max: 20mg/day
Conversions
If switching from other amphetamine products, d/c that treatment, and titrate w/ Dyanavel XR using above titration schedule.
Do not substitute for other amphetamine products on a mg-per-mg basis.

DOSING CONSIDERATIONS
Concomitant Medications
Agents that alter urinary pH can impact urinary excretion and alter blood levels of amphetamine. Acidifying agents (eg, ascorbic acid) decrease blood levels, while alkalinizing agents (eg, sodium bicarbonate) increase blood levels; adjust dose accordingly.

ADMINISTRATION
Oral route
Administer w/ or w/o food.
Shake bottle before use.

STORAGE
20-25°C (68-77°F); excursions permitted from 15-30°C (59-86°F).

HOW SUPPLIED
Oral Sus, Extended-Release: 2.5mg/mL [464mL]

CONTRAINDICATIONS
Known hypersensitivity to amphetamine or other components of this medication. During treatment w/ MAOIs and w/in 14 days following discontinuation of an MAOI.

WARNINGS/PRECAUTIONS
Prior to treatment, assess for the presence of cardiac disease. Sudden death, stroke, and MI reported in adults. Sudden death reported in children and adolescents w/ structural cardiac abnormalities and other serious heart problems. Avoid use in patients w/ known structural cardiac abnormalities, cardiomyopathy, serious heart arrhythmia, coronary artery disease, and other serious heart problems. Further evaluate patients who develop exertional chest pain, unexplained syncope, or arrhythmias during treatment. May increase BP and HR; monitor for tachycardia and HTN. May exacerbate symptoms of behavior disturbance and thought disorder in patients w/ preexisting psychotic disorder. May induce a mixed or manic episode in patients w/ bipolar disorder. Prior to initiation, screen patients for risk factors for developing a manic episode (eg, comorbid/history of depressive symptoms, family history of suicide, bipolar disorder, depression). May cause psychotic or manic symptoms in patients w/o prior history of psychotic illness or mania; consider discontinuing if such symptoms occur. May cause weight loss and slowing of growth rate in children; closely monitor growth (weight and height). Associated w/ peripheral vasculopathy, including Raynaud's phenomenon; signs/symptoms are usually intermittent and mild. Observe carefully for digital changes.

ADVERSE REACTIONS
Epistaxis, allergic rhinitis, upper abdominal pain.

DRUG INTERACTIONS
See Dosing Considerations and Contraindications. GI alkalinizing agents (eg, sodium bicarbonate) and urinary alkalinizing agents (eg, acetazolamide, some thiazides) increase blood levels and potentiate effects; avoid coadministration w/ GI alkalinizing agents. GI acidifying agents (eg, guanethidine, reserpine, glutamic acid HCl) and urinary acidifying agents (eg, ammonium chloride, sodium acid phosphate, methenamine salts) lower blood levels and efficacy. May enhance activity of TCAs (eg, desipramine, protriptyline) or sympathomimetic agents causing increases of d-amphetamine levels in the brain and possibly potentiating cardiovascular (CV) effects; monitor frequently, adjust dose, or use alternative therapy. Proton pump inhibitors (eg, omeprazole) increase T_{max} of amphetamine; monitor for changes in clinical effect and adjust therapy based on clinical response. May cause significant elevations in plasma corticosteroid levels; increase is greatest in evening. May interfere w/ urinary steroid determinations.

PREGNANCY AND LACTATION
Pregnancy: There are limited published data on the use of amphetamines in pregnant women. Adverse pregnancy outcomes, including premature delivery and low birth weight, reported in infants born to mothers dependent on amphetamines.
Lactation: Amphetamine (*d*- or *d, l*-) is present in human milk. Not for use in nursing.

MECHANISM OF ACTION

Sympathomimetic amine w/ CNS stimulant activity; mode of therapeutic action is not known. Thought to block the reuptake of norepinephrine and dopamine into the presynaptic neuron and increase the release of these monoamines into the extraneuronal space.

PHARMACOKINETICS

Absorption: (18.8mg single dose) T_{max}=4 hrs (median). **Distribution:** Found in breast milk. **Metabolism:** CYP2D6 (oxidation); 4-hydroxy-amphetamine and norephedrine (active metabolites). **Elimination:** Urine (30-40%, unchanged; 50%, α-hydroxy-amphetamine derivatives). $T_{1/2}$=12.36 hrs (d-amphetamine), 15.12 hrs (l-amphetamine).

PATIENT CONSIDERATIONS

Assessment: Assess for presence of cardiac disease, risk of abuse, preexisting psychotic disorder, risk factors for developing a manic episode, pregnancy/ nursing status, and possible drug interactions.

Monitoring: Monitor for CV reactions, tachycardia, HTN, psychiatric adverse reactions, peripheral vasculopathy including Raynaud's phenomenon, and other adverse reactions. Monitor growth (weight and height) in children. Periodically reevaluate long-term use of therapy. Monitor for signs of abuse and dependence while on therapy. Monitor infants born to mothers taking amphetamines for symptoms of withdrawal.

Counseling: Inform about benefits and risks of treatment, appropriate administration instructions, and about the potential for abuse/dependence. Advise of serious CV risk and elevations in BP/pulse rate; instruct to contact physician immediately if symptoms such as exertional chest pain, unexplained syncope, or other symptoms suggestive of cardiac disease develop. Advise that at recommended doses, treatment may cause psychotic or manic symptoms, even w/o a prior history of psychotic symptoms or mania. Inform that treatment may cause slowing of growth and weight loss. Inform about the risk of peripheral vasculopathy, including Raynaud's phenomenon; instruct to report to physician any new numbness, pain, skin color change, or sensitivity to temperature in fingers or toes, and to call physician immediately if any signs of unexplained wounds appear on fingers or toes while on therapy. Advise patients of the potential fetal effects from the use of therapy during pregnancy; instruct to notify physician if pregnant/planning to become pregnant during treatment. Advise to avoid breastfeeding. Advise patients to avoid alcohol while taking drug.

DYAZIDE — hydrochlorothiazide/triamterene Rx

Class: Potassium-sparing diuretic/thiazide diuretic

> Abnormal elevation of serum K^+ levels (≥5.5mEq/L) may occur w/ all K^+-sparing diuretic combinations. Hyperkalemia is more likely to occur w/ renal impairment and diabetes (even w/o evidence of renal impairment), and in elderly or severely ill; monitor serum K^+ levels at frequent intervals.

ADULT DOSAGE	PEDIATRIC DOSAGE
Edema	Pediatric use may not have been established
1-2 caps PO qd	
Hypertension	
1-2 caps PO qd	

ADMINISTRATION

Oral route

STORAGE

20-25°C (68-77°F); excursions permitted to 15-30°C (59-86°F). Protect from light. Dispense in a tight, light-resistant container.

HOW SUPPLIED

Cap: (HCTZ-Triamterene) 25mg-37.5mg

CONTRAINDICATIONS

Anuria, acute and chronic renal insufficiency or significant renal impairment, hypersensitivity to the drug or to other sulfonamide-derived drugs, preexisting elevated serum K^+ (hyperkalemia), K^+-sparing agents (eg, spironolactone, amiloride, or other formulations containing triamterene), K^+ salt substitutes, K^+ supplements (except w/ severe hypokalemia).

WARNINGS/PRECAUTIONS

Avoid in severely ill in whom respiratory or metabolic acidosis may occur; if used, frequent evaluations of acid/base balance and serum electrolytes are necessary. May cause idiosyncratic reaction, resulting in acute transient myopia and acute angle-closure glaucoma; d/c as rapidly as possible. Caution w/ diabetes; may cause hyperglycemia and glycosuria. Diabetes mellitus (DM) may become manifest. Caution w/ hepatic impairment; may precipitate hepatic coma w/ severe liver disease. Corrective measures must be taken if hypokalemia develops; d/c and initiate potassium chloride (KCl) supplementation if serious hypokalemia develops (serum K^+ <3.0mEq/L). May potentiate electrolyte imbalance w/ heart failure, renal disease, or cirrhosis of the liver. May cause hypochloremia. Dilutional hyponatremia may occur in edematous patients in hot weather. Caution w/ history of renal stones. May increase BUN and SrCr. May decrease serum PBI levels. Decreased Ca^{2+} excretion reported. Changes in parathyroid glands w/ hypercalcemia and hypophosphatemia reported during prolonged therapy. May interfere w/ the fluorescent measurement of quinidine.

ADVERSE REACTIONS

Muscle cramps, N/V, pancreatitis, weakness, arrhythmia, impotence, dry mouth, jaundice, paresthesia, renal stones, anaphylaxis, acute renal failure, hyperkalemia, hyponatremia.

DRUG INTERACTIONS

See Contraindications. Increased risk of hyperkalemia w/ ACE inhibitors, blood from blood bank, and low-salt milk. Increased risk of severe hyponatremia w/ chlorpropamide. Possible interaction resulting in acute renal failure w/ indomethacin; caution w/ NSAIDs. Avoid w/ lithium due to risk of lithium toxicity. Decreased arterial responsiveness to norepinephrine. Amphotericin B, corticosteroids, and corticotropin may intensify electrolyte imbalance, particularly hypokalemia. Adjust dose of antigout drugs to control hyperuricemia and gout. May decrease effect of oral anticoagulants. May alter insulin requirements. Increased paralyzing effects of nondepolarizing muscle relaxants (eg, tubocurarine). Reduced K^+ levels w/ chronic or overuse of laxatives or use of exchange resins (eg, sodium polystyrene sulfonate). May reduce effectiveness of methenamine. May potentiate action of other antihypertensive drugs (eg, β-blockers).

PREGNANCY AND LACTATION

Category C, not for use in nursing.

MECHANISM OF ACTION

Triamterene: K^+-sparing diuretic; exerts diuretic effect on distal renal tubules to inhibit the reabsorption of Na^+ in exchange for K^+ and hydrogen ions. HCTZ: thiazide diuretic; blocks reabsorption of Na^+ and Cl^- ions and thereby increases the quantity of Na^+ traversing the distal tubule and the volume of water excreted.

PHARMACOKINETICS

Absorption: Well-absorbed. Triamterene: C_{max}=46.4ng/mL; T_{max}=1.1 hrs; AUC=148.7ng•hrs/mL. HCTZ: C_{max}=135.1ng/mL; T_{max}=2 hrs; AUC=834ng•hrs/mL. **Distribution:** Crosses placenta; found in breast milk.

PATIENT CONSIDERATIONS

Assessment: Assess for anuria, renal/hepatic impairment, sulfonamide hypersensitivity, hyperkalemia, diabetes, history of renal stones, pregnancy/ nursing status, and for possible drug interactions. Obtain baseline BUN, SrCr, and serum electrolytes.

Monitoring: Monitor for signs/symptoms of hype/hypokalemia, hyperglycemia, hypochloremia, renal stones, and for electrolyte imbalance. Monitor for hepatic coma in patients w/ severe liver disease. Monitor serum K^+ levels, BUN, SrCr, and serum electrolytes.

Counseling: Inform about risks/benefits of therapy. Advise to seek medical attention if symptoms of hyperkalemia (eg, paresthesias, muscular weakness, fatigue), hypokalemia, hyperglycemia, renal stones, electrolyte imbalance (eg, dry mouth, thirst, weakness), or hypersensitivity reactions occur.

DYLOJECT — diclofenac sodium Rx

Class: NSAID

> NSAIDs cause an increased risk of serious cardiovascular (CV) thrombotic events, including MI and stroke, which can be fatal. This risk may occur early in treatment and may increase w/ duration of use. Contraindicated in the setting of CABG surgery. NSAIDs cause an increased risk of serious GI adverse events (eg, bleeding, ulceration, stomach/intestinal perforation), which can be fatal and can occur anytime during use and w/o warning symptoms; elderly patients and patients w/ a prior history of peptic ulcer disease and/or GI bleeding are at a greater risk.

ADULT DOSAGE	PEDIATRIC DOSAGE
Mild to Moderate Pain	Pediatric use may not have been established
37.5mg IV bolus inj over 15 sec q6h prn	
Titrate: Adjust frequency based on needs; use shortest duration	
Max: 150mg/day	
Moderate to Severe Pain	
37.5mg IV bolus inj over 15 sec q6h prn w/ or w/o opioid analgesics	
Titrate: Adjust frequency based on needs; use shortest duration	
Max: 150mg/day	

DOSING CONSIDERATIONS

Renal Impairment
Moderate to Severe Renal Insufficiency: Not recommended for use

Hepatic Impairment
Moderate to Severe: Not recommended for use

Elderly
Select dose carefully and monitor renal function

ADMINISTRATION

IV route
Must be well hydrated prior to administration.

STORAGE

20-25°C (68-77°F). Do not freeze. Protect from light.

HOW SUPPLIED

Inj: 37.5mg/mL [1mL]

CONTRAINDICATIONS

Known hypersensitivity to diclofenac or any components of the drug product; history of asthma, urticaria, or allergic-type reactions after taking aspirin (ASA) or other NSAIDs; in the setting of CABG surgery; moderate to severe renal insufficiency in the perioperative period and in those at risk for volume depletion.

WARNINGS/PRECAUTIONS

Use lowest effective dose for shortest duration possible. Avoid use w/ recent MI unless benefits outweigh risk of recurrent CV thrombotic events. Monitor for signs of cardiac ischemia if used w/ recent MI. Increased risk for GI bleeding w/ longer duration of use; older age; poor general health status; advanced liver disease and/or coagulopathy. Avoid use in patients at higher risk unless benefits are expected to outweigh the increased risk of bleeding; consider alternate therapies. If a serious GI adverse event is suspected, promptly evaluate, initiate treatment, and d/c until serious GI adverse event is ruled out. Hepatotoxicity reported; d/c immediately and perform a clinical evaluation if clinical signs/symptoms consistent w/ liver disease develop, or if systemic manifestations occur. May lead to new onset of HTN or worsening of preexisting HTN. Fluid retention and edema reported. Avoid use w/ severe heart failure (HF) unless benefits outweigh risks of worsening HF; monitor for signs of worsening HF. Renal papillary necrosis and other renal injury reported w/ long-term use. Renal toxicity also reported in patients in whom renal prostaglandins have a compensatory role in the maintenance of renal perfusion. Increased risk w/ renal/hepatic dysfunction, dehydration, hypovolemia, HF, and in the elderly. Correct volume status if dehydrated or hypovolemic prior to initiating therapy. Monitor renal function w/ renal or hepatic impairment, HF, dehydration, or hypovolemia during use. Avoid use w/ advanced renal disease unless the benefits are expected to outweigh the risk of worsening renal function; monitor for signs of worsening renal function. Increases in K^+, including hyperkalemia, reported. Associated w/ anaphylactic reactions. Monitor for changes in the signs/symptoms of asthma in patients w/ preexisting asthma (w/o known ASA sensitivity). May cause serious skin adverse reactions (eg, exfoliative dermatitis, Stevens-Johnson syndrome, toxic epidermal necrolysis); d/c at the 1st appearance of skin rash or any other sign of hypersensitivity. Anemia reported. May increase the risk of bleeding events; coagulation disorders may increase this risk. May mask inflammation and fever.

ADVERSE REACTIONS

N/V, constipation, headache, infusion site pain, dizziness, flatulence, insomnia.

DRUG INTERACTIONS

Drugs that interfere w/ serotonin reuptake may potentiate the risk of bleeding. Synergistic effect on bleeding w/ anticoagulants (eg, warfarin); monitor for signs of bleeding w/ concomitant anticoagulants, antiplatelet agents, SSRIs, and SNRIs. May increase risk of GI bleeding w/ use of oral corticosteroids, anticoagulants, SSRIs, smoking, and alcohol use. ASA may increase risk of bleeding and serious GI events; concomitant use w/ analgesic doses of ASA is not recommended. Monitor patients more closely for GI bleeding w/ concomitant use of low-dose ASA for cardiac prophylaxis. May diminish antihypertensive effect of ACE inhibitors, ARBs, or β-blockers (eg, propranolol); monitor BP. Coadministration w/ ACE inhibitors or ARBs may result in deterioration of renal function (including possible acute renal failure) in patients who are elderly, volume-depleted (including those on diuretic therapy), or have renal impairment; monitor for worsening renal function. Adequately hydrate and assess renal function at the beginning of the concomitant treatment and periodically thereafter. May reduce natriuretic effect of loop diuretics (eg, furosemide) and thiazide diuretics; observe for signs of worsening renal function, in addition to assuring diuretic efficacy including antihypertensive effects. May increase serum concentration and prolong $T_{1/2}$ of digoxin; monitor serum digoxin levels. May cause elevations in plasma lithium levels and reductions in renal lithium clearance; monitor for signs of lithium toxicity. May increase risk for methotrexate toxicity. May increase cyclosporine's nephrotoxicity; monitor for signs of worsening renal function. Use w/ other NSAIDs or salicylates (eg, diflunisal, salsalate) increases risk of GI toxicity; concomitant use not recommended. May increase the risk of pemetrexed-associated myelosuppression, renal, and GI toxicity; refer to prescribing information for further information. CYP2C9 inhibitors (eg, voriconazole) may enhance exposure and toxicity of diclofenac whereas coadministration w/ CYP2C9 inducers (eg, rifampin) may lead to compromised efficacy of diclofenac; use w/ caution and adjust dose of CYP2C9 inhibitors or inducers if needed.

PREGNANCY AND LACTATION

Pregnancy: Category C, prior to 30 weeks' gestation; Category D, starting at 30 weeks' gestation. Use during the 3rd trimester of pregnancy increases the risk of premature closure of the fetal ductus arteriosus; avoid use in pregnant women starting at 30 weeks of gestation (3rd trimester). **Lactation:** May be present in human milk; caution in nursing. **Reproductive Potential:** May delay or prevent rupture of ovarian follicles. Consider withdrawal of therapy in women who have difficulties conceiving or who are undergoing investigation of infertility.

MECHANISM OF ACTION

NSAID; not established. May involve inhibition of the COX-1 and COX-2 pathways. Mechanism may also be related to inhibition of prostaglandin synthetase. Exhibits anti-inflammatory, analgesic, and antipyretic activities.

PHARMACOKINETICS

Absorption: (Single Dose) C_{max}=6031ng/mL, $AUC_{(inf)}$=1859ng•hr/mL, T_{max}=0.083 hr. (Multiple Dose) C_{max}=5617ng/mL, $AUC_{(0-t)}$=1839ng•hr/mL, T_{max}=0.083 hr. **Distribution:** V_d=40.1L (single dose), 83.4L (multiple dose); plasma protein binding (>99%); crosses placenta, may be found in breast milk. **Metabolism:** 4'-hydroxy-diclofenac (major metabolite). **Elimination:** Urine (approx 65%), bile (approx 35%); $T_{1/2}$=1.44 hrs (single dose), 2.29 hrs (multiple dose).

PATIENT CONSIDERATIONS

Assessment: Assess for hypersensitivity to diclofenac or to any component of this product; history of asthma, urticaria, or other allergic-type reactions after taking ASA or other NSAIDs; asthma; CV disease (CVD) or risk factors for CVD; HTN; history of peptic ulcer disease or GI bleeding; coagulation disorders; renal/hepatic impairment; pregnancy/nursing status; or any other conditions where treatment is contraindicated or cautioned. Assess volume status. Assess for possible drug interactions. Obtain baseline BP, CBC, and chemistry profile.

Monitoring: Monitor for signs/symptoms of CV thrombotic events; cardiac ischemia in patients w/ a recent MI; GI bleeding/ulceration and perforation; hepatotoxicity; new or worsening HTN; HF; edema; renal papillary necrosis and other renal injury; hyperkalemia; anaphylactic reactions; serious skin reactions; anemia; and other adverse reactions. Monitor BP during initiation of therapy and throughout the course of therapy. Monitor for signs of bleeding in patients on concomitant therapy w/ anticoagulants, antiplatelet agents, SSRIs, or SNRIs. Monitor renal function in patients w/ renal/hepatic impairment, HF, dehydration, or hypovolemia. Periodically monitor CBC and chemistry profiles including LFTs in patients receiving long-term treatment.

Counseling: Advise to be alert for the symptoms of CV thrombotic events and to report symptoms immediately. Advise to report symptoms of ulcerations and bleeding. Inform of the increased risk for and the signs and symptoms of GI bleeding w/ ASA. Inform of the warning signs and symptoms of hepatotoxicity; instruct to d/c and seek immediate medical therapy. Advise to be alert for the symptoms of CHF and to contact healthcare provider if such symptoms occur. Inform of the signs of an anaphylactic reaction and instruct to seek immediate emergency help if these occur. Advise to d/c immediately if any type of rash develops, and to contact healthcare provider as soon as possible. Advise females of reproductive potential who desire pregnancy that NSAIDs may be associated w/ a reversible delay in ovulation. Inform pregnant women to avoid use of diclofenac and other NSAIDs starting at 30 weeks' gestation. Inform patients that the concomitant use w/ other NSAIDs or salicylates is not recommended. Alert patients that NSAIDs may be present in OTC medications for treatment of colds, fever, or insomnia. Advise not to use low-dose ASA w/o consultation.

DYMISTA — azelastine hydrochloride/fluticasone propionate Rx

Class: Corticosteroid/H_1 antagonist

ADULT DOSAGE **Seasonal Allergic Rhinitis**	PEDIATRIC DOSAGE **Seasonal Allergic Rhinitis**
1 spray in each nostril bid	**≥6 Years:** 1 spray in each nostril bid

---

DOSING CONSIDERATIONS

Elderly
Dose cautiously; start at lower end of dosing range

ADMINISTRATION

Intranasal route

Shake the bottle gently before each use

Priming
Prime pump before initial use by releasing 6 sprays or until a fine mist appears
Reprime w/ 1 spray or until a fine mist appears if not used for ≥14 days

STORAGE

20-25°C (68-77°F). Store upright w/ dust cap in place. Protect from light. Do not store in the freezer or refrigerator.

HOW SUPPLIED

Spray: (Azelastine/Fluticasone) (137mcg/50mcg)/spray [23g]

WARNINGS/PRECAUTIONS

Somnolence reported; may impair mental/physical abilities. Epistaxis reported. Nasal ulceration and septal perforation reported; avoid w/ recent nasal ulcers, nasal surgery, or nasal trauma. Development of localized infections of the nose and pharynx w/ *Candida albicans* may occur; may require discontinuation and treatment w/ appropriate local therapy if infection develops. Examine periodically for evidence of *Candida* infection or other signs of adverse effects on nasal mucosa if used over several months or longer. D/C slowly if hypercorticism and adrenal suppression occur. Fluticasone: May result in development of glaucoma and/or cataracts; closely monitor patients w/ change in vision or w/ history of increased IOP, glaucoma, and/or cataracts. May increase susceptibility to infections; caution w/ active or quiescent tuberculosis (TB) of the respiratory tract; untreated local or systemic fungal or bacterial infections; systemic viral or parasitic infections; or ocular herpes simplex. Avoid exposure to chickenpox and measles. Risk of adrenal insufficiency and withdrawal symptoms when replacing systemic corticosteroids w/ topical corticosteroids. May cause growth velocity reduction in pediatric patients.

ADVERSE REACTIONS

Dysgeusia, headache, epistaxis, pyrexia, cough, nasal congestion, rhinitis, viral infection, URTI, pharyngitis, pain, diarrhea, N/V, otitis media/externa.

DRUG INTERACTIONS

Avoid w/ alcohol or other CNS depressants. Fluticasone: Ritonavir and other strong CYP3A4 inhibitors may increase exposure; not recommended w/ ritonavir and caution w/ other potent CYP3A4 inhibitors (eg, ketoconazole). Concomitant use of intranasal corticosteroids w/ other inhaled corticosteroids could increase the risk of signs/symptoms of hypercorticism and/or hypothalamic-pituitary-adrenal axis suppression.

PREGNANCY AND LACTATION

Category C, not for use in nursing.

MECHANISM OF ACTION

Azelastine: H_1-receptor antagonist; phthalazinone derivative that exhibits histamine H_1-receptor antagonist activity in isolated tissues, animal models, and humans. Fluticasone: Synthetic trifluorinated corticosteroid; has not been established. Shown to have a wide range of actions on multiple cell types (eg, mast cells, eosinophils, neutrophils, macrophages, lymphocytes) and mediators (eg, histamine, eicosanoids, leukotrienes, cytokines) involved in inflammation.

PHARMACOKINETICS

Absorption: Azelastine: Bioavailability (40%); C_{max}=194.5pg/mL, T_{max}=0.5 hr; AUC=4217pg/mL•hr. Fluticasone: Bioavailability (44-61%); C_{max}=10.3pg/mL, T_{max}=1 hr; AUC=97.7pg/mL•hr. **Distribution:** Azelastine: V_d=14.5L/kg (Oral/IV); plasma protein binding (88%, 97% desmethylazelastine). Fluticasone: V_d=4.2L/kg (IV); plasma protein binding (91%). **Metabolism:** Azelastine: Oxidation via CYP450; desmethylazelastine (major active metabolite). Fluticasone: CYP3A4 pathway. **Elimination:** Azelastine: $T_{1/2}$=25 hrs; (Oral) feces (75%, <10% unchanged). Fluticasone: (IV) $T_{1/2}$=7.8 hrs; (Oral) urine (<5% metabolites), feces (parent drug and metabolites).

PATIENT CONSIDERATIONS

Assessment: Assess for recent nasal ulcers/surgery/trauma, active or quiescent TB, systemic viral/parasitic infections, ocular herpes simplex, untreated fungal/bacterial infections, history of IOP, glaucoma, cataracts, pregnancy/nursing status, and possible drug interactions.

Monitoring: Monitor for somnolence, epistaxis, nasal ulceration, nasal septal perforation, changes in vision, glaucoma, cataracts, hypercorticism, adrenal suppression, and for the development/exacerbation of infections. Routinely monitor growth of pediatric patients.

Counseling: Caution against engaging in hazardous occupations requiring complete mental alertness and motor coordination (eg, driving, operating machinery). Advise to avoid w/ alcohol and other CNS depressants. Instruct to inform physician if a change in vision is noted. Instruct to avoid exposure to chickenpox or measles and, if exposed, to consult physician w/o delay. Inform of potential worsening of existing TB, fungal, bacterial, viral or parasitic infections, or ocular herpes simplex. Counsel that corticosteroids may cause reduction in growth velocity in pediatric patients. Instruct to avoid spraying into eyes; if sprayed in the eyes, instruct to flush eyes w/ water for at least 10 min. Discard the bottle after 120 medicated sprays have been used. Instruct to notify physician of all medications currently taking.

DYNACIN — minocycline hydrochloride
Rx

Class: Tetracyclines

ADULT DOSAGE

General Dosing

Initial: 200mg
Maint: 100mg q12h

Alternate Dosing:

Initial: If more frequent doses are preferred, give two or four 50mg tabs
Maint: One 50mg tab qid

Gonococcal Infections

Uncomplicated Gonococcal Infections Other Than Urethritis and Anorectal Infections in Men:
Initial: 200mg
Maint: 100mg q12h for a minimum of 4 days, w/ post-therapy cultures w/in 2-3 days

Urethral Infections

Uncomplicated Gonococcal Urethritis in Men When Penicillin is Contraindicated:
Usual: 100mg q12h for 5 days

Uncomplicated Infections Caused by Chlamydia trachomatis/Ureaplasma urealyticum:
Usual: 100mg q12h for at least 7 days

Syphilis

When Penicillin is Contraindicated:
Initial: 200mg
Maint: 100mg q12h
Administer for 10-15 days

Meningococcal Carrier State

Usual: 100mg q12h for 5 days

Mycobacterial Infections

Mycobacterium marinum Infections:
Optimal doses have not been established; 100mg q12h for 6-8 weeks have been successfully used

Endocervical Infections

Uncomplicated Infections Caused by Chlamydia trachomatis/Ureaplasma urealyticum:
Usual: 100mg q12h for at least 7 days

Rectal Infections

Uncomplicated Infections Caused by Chlamydia trachomatis/Ureaplasma urealyticum:
Usual: 100mg q12h for at least 7 days

PEDIATRIC DOSAGE

General Dosing

>8 Years:
Initial: 4mg/kg
Maint: 2mg/kg q12h, not to exceed usual adult dose

Other Indications

Rocky Mountain spotted fever
Typhus fever and the typhus group
Q fever
Rickettsialpox
Tick fevers
Respiratory tract infections
Lymphogranuloma venereum
Psittacosis (ornithosis)
Trachoma
Inclusion conjunctivitis
Relapsing fever
Chancroid
Plague
Tularemia
Cholera
Campylobacter fetus infections
Brucellosis (in conjunction w/ streptomycin)
Bartonellosis
Granuloma inguinale
UTIs
Skin and skin structure infections
Escherichia coli infections
Enterobacter aerogenes infections
Shigella species infections
Acinetobacter species infections

When penicillin is contraindicated, treatment of the following infections caused by susceptible microorganisms: infections in women caused by *Neisseria gonorrhoeae*, yaws, listeriosis, anthrax, Vincent's infection, actinomycosis, infections caused by *Clostridium* species

Adjunctive therapy in acute intestinal amebiasis and severe acne

DOSING CONSIDERATIONS

Renal Impairment

CrCl <80mL/min:
Max Dose: 200mg/24 hrs

Elderly

Start at lower end of dosing range

ADMINISTRATION

Oral route

May take w/ or w/o food
Take w/ adequate amounts of fluids

STORAGE

20-25°C (68-77°F). Protect from light, moisture, and excessive heat.

HOW SUPPLIED

Tab: 50mg, 75mg, 100mg

CONTRAINDICATIONS

Hypersensitivity to any of the tetracyclines or to any of the components of the product formulation.

WARNINGS/PRECAUTIONS

May cause fetal harm. May cause permanent discoloration of the teeth (yellow-gray-brown) if used during tooth development (last half of pregnancy, infancy, childhood to 8 yrs of age); do not use during tooth development. Enamel hypoplasia reported. May decrease fibula growth rate in premature infants. Drug rash with eosinophilia and systemic symptoms (DRESS), including fatal cases, reported; d/c immediately if this syndrome is recognized. May cause an increase in BUN; caution with renal impairment. Photosensitivity, manifested by an exaggerated sunburn reaction, reported. CNS side effects reported; may impair mental/physical abilities. *Clostridium difficile*-associated diarrhea (CDAD) reported; d/c if CDAD is suspected or confirmed. May result in bacterial resistance if used in the absence of proven or suspected bacterial infection, or if used in a prophylactic indication; take appropriate measures if superinfection develops. Associated with pseudotumor cerebri (benign intracranial HTN) in adults and bulging fontanels in infants. Hepatotoxicity reported; caution with hepatic dysfunction. Incision and drainage or other surgical procedures should be performed in conjunction with antibiotic therapy when indicated. False elevations of urinary catecholamine levels may occur due to interference with the fluorescence test. Caution in elderly. Not indicated for the treatment of meningococcal infection. Thyroid cancer reported; consider monitoring for signs of thyroid cancer when given over prolonged periods.

ADVERSE REACTIONS

Neutropenia, agranulocytosis, lupus-like syndrome, serum sickness-like syndrome, fever, N/V, diarrhea, increased liver enzymes, cough, anaphylaxis, exfoliative dermatitis, Stevens-Johnson syndrome, skin and mucous membrane pigmentation, headache.

DRUG INTERACTIONS

Caution with other hepatotoxic drugs. Depresses plasma prothrombin activity; may require downward adjustment of anticoagulant dosage. May interfere with bactericidal action of PCN; avoid concurrent use. Impaired absorption with antacids containing aluminum, Ca^{2+}, or Mg^{2+}, and iron-containing preparations. Fatal renal toxicity reported with methoxyflurane. May decrease effectiveness of oral contraceptives. Avoid isotretinoin shortly before, during, and shortly after therapy; each drug alone is associated with pseudotumor cerebri. Increased risk of ergotism with ergot alkaloids or their derivatives.

PREGNANCY AND LACTATION
Category D, not for use in nursing.

MECHANISM OF ACTION
Tetracycline derivative; primarily bacteriostatic and thought to exert antimicrobial effect by inhibition of protein synthesis.

PHARMACOKINETICS
Absorption: Virtually complete. (100mg, Single-dose; Normal fasting adults) C_{max}=758.29ng/mL; T_{max}=1.71 hrs. **Distribution:** Crosses placenta; found in breast milk. **Elimination:** (Normal) Urine, feces; (100mg, Single-dose; Normal fasting adults) $T_{1/2}$=17.03 hrs.

PATIENT CONSIDERATIONS
Assessment: Assess for hypersensitivity to drug or any tetracyclines, hepatic/renal impairment, pregnancy/nursing status, and possible drug interactions. Perform culture and susceptibility tests. In venereal disease when coexistent syphilis is suspected, perform a dark-field examination and blood serology.

Monitoring: Monitor for DRESS, photosensitivity, CNS effects, CDAD, superinfection, benign intracranial HTN in adults, and other adverse reactions. Perform periodic laboratory evaluations of organ systems, including hematopoietic, renal, and hepatic studies. In venereal disease when coexistent syphilis is suspected, repeat blood serology monthly for at least 4 months.

Counseling: Apprise of the potential hazard to fetus if used during pregnancy; instruct to notify physician if pregnant. Inform that diarrhea is a common problem caused by therapy, which usually ends when therapy is discontinued. Instruct to immediately contact physician if watery and bloody stools (with or without stomach cramps and fever) occur, even as late as ≥2 months after having taken the last dose. Advise that photosensitivity manifested by an exaggerated sunburn reaction can occur; instruct to d/c treatment at the 1st evidence of skin erythema. Caution patients who experience CNS symptoms about driving vehicles or using hazardous machinery while on therapy. Inform that drug may render oral contraceptives less effective. Counsel that therapy should only be used to treat bacterial, not viral (eg, common cold), infections. Instruct to take exactly ud, even if patient feels better early in the course of therapy. Inform that skipping doses or not completing the full course of therapy may decrease effectiveness of treatment and increase bacterial resistance.

DYRENIUM — triamterene   Rx

Class: Potassium-sparing diuretic

> Abnormal elevation of serum K^+ levels (≥5.5mEq/L) can occur w/ all K^+-sparing agents, including triamterene. Hyperkalemia is more likely to occur w/ renal impairment and diabetes (even w/o evidence of renal impairment), and in the elderly or severely ill. Monitor serum K^+ at frequent intervals.

ADULT DOSAGE	PEDIATRIC DOSAGE
Edema	Pediatric use may not have been established
Associated w/ CHF, liver cirrhosis, and nephrotic syndrome; steroid-induced edema, idiopathic edema, and edema due to secondary hyperaldosteronism	
Initial: 100mg bid pc, when used alone	
Max: 300mg/day	
When added to other diuretic therapy or switched from other diuretics, all K^+ supplementation should be discontinued	
When combined w/ another diuretic/antihypertensive agent, total daily dose of each agent should be lowered initially and then adjusted to the individual patient's needs	
Other Indications	
Edema during pregnancy that may arise from pathological causes	

ADMINISTRATION
Oral route
Take pc.

STORAGE
25°C (77°F); excursions permitted to 15-30°C (59-86°F).

HOW SUPPLIED
Cap: 50mg, 100mg

CONTRAINDICATIONS
Anuria, severe or progressive kidney disease or dysfunction (except w/ nephrosis), severe hepatic disease, hypersensitivity to triamterene or any components of the medication, hyperkalemia, K^+ supplements, K^+ salts or K^+-containing salt substitutes, K^+-sparing agents (eg, spironolactone, amiloride).

WARNINGS/PRECAUTIONS
Isolated reports of hypersensitivity reactions; monitor for possible occurrence of blood dyscrasias, liver damage, or other idiosyncratic reactions. Check ECG if hyperkalemia occurs; if no widening of the QRS or arrhythmia is present,

d/c therapy and any K^+ supplementation, and substitute a thiazide alone. If a widened QRS complex or arrhythmia is present w/ hyperkalemia, prompt additional therapy is required. May aggravate or cause electrolyte imbalances in CHF, renal disease, or cirrhosis. May cause mild nitrogen retention. May cause a decreasing alkali reserve, w/ the possibility of metabolic acidosis. In cirrhotics w/ splenomegaly may contribute to megaloblastosis in cases where folic stores have been depleted; perform periodic blood studies and observe for exacerbation of liver disease. Caution w/ gouty arthritis; may elevate uric acid levels. Caution w/ history of renal stones. Rebound kaliuresis may occur upon abrupt withdrawal in patients who received intensive therapy or prolonged therapy; gradually withdraw therapy. May interfere w/ fluorescent measurement of quinidine.

ADVERSE REACTIONS
Hypersensitivity reactions, hyper/hypokalemia, azotemia, renal stones, jaundice, thrombocytopenia, megaloblastic anemia, N/V, diarrhea, weakness, dizziness, headache, elevated BUN.

DRUG INTERACTIONS
See Contraindications. May reduce renal clearance and increase lithium levels w/ risk of lithium toxicity; monitor lithium levels and adjust lithium dose if necessary. Indomethacin may cause renal failure; caution w/ NSAIDs. May potentiate nondepolarizing muscle relaxants, antihypertensives, other diuretics, preanesthetics, and anesthetics. Increased risk of hyperkalemia w/ ACE inhibitors. Hyperkalemia may occur when used concomitantly w/ blood from blood bank, low-salt milk, or K^+-containing medications (eg, parenteral penicillin G potassium). May cause hyperglycemia; may need to adjust antidiabetic agents during and/or after therapy. Chlorpropamide may increase risk of severe hyponatremia.

PREGNANCY AND LACTATION
Pregnancy: No evidence of harm to fetus in animal studies; caution in nursing.
Lactation: Not for use in nursing.

MECHANISM OF ACTION
K^+-sparing diuretic; inhibits reabsorption of Na^+ ions in exchange for K^+ and H^+ ions at segment of distal tubule under control of adrenal mineralocorticoids.

PHARMACOKINETICS
Absorption: Rapid; C_{max}=30ng/mL, T_{max}=3 hrs. **Distribution:** Plasma protein binding (67%); crosses placental barrier. **Metabolism:** Hydroxytriamterene (metabolite). **Elimination:** Urine (21%).

PATIENT CONSIDERATIONS
Assessment: Assess for anuria, CHF, diabetes mellitus, gout, hyperkalemia, history of kidney stones, hypersensitivity, liver/renal impairment, pregnancy/nursing status, and for possible drug interactions.

Monitoring: Monitor for signs/symptoms of electrolyte imbalance, exacerbation of gout, hypersensitivity reactions (eg, blood dyscrasias, liver damage), and for liver/renal dysfunction. Monitor for signs/symptoms of hyperkalemia and perform ECG if suspected. Monitor BUN and serum K^+ levels, especially in elderly or diabetes patients. Perform periodic blood studies in cirrhotics w/ splenomegaly.

Counseling: Advise to take pc to avoid stomach upset. Inform that if single dose is prescribed, it may be preferable to take in am to minimize frequency of urination during nighttime sleep. Instruct not to take more than prescribed dose at next dosing interval if a dose is missed. Advise to seek medical attention if symptoms of hyperkalemia, electrolyte imbalance, or hypersensitivity reactions occur.

ECONAZOLE CREAM — econazole nitrate   Rx

Class: Azole antifungal

OTHER BRAND NAMES
Spectazole (Discontinued)

ADULT DOSAGE	PEDIATRIC DOSAGE
Fungal Infections	Pediatric use may not have been established
Cutaneous Candidiasis: Apply bid (am/pm) for 2 weeks	
Tinea Versicolor: Apply qd for 2 weeks	
Tinea Corporis, Tinea Cruris, and Tinea Pedis caused by *Trichophyton rubrum, T. mentagrophytes, T. tonsurans, Microsporum canis, M. audouini, M. gypseum,* and *Epidermophyton floccosum*: Apply qd	
Tinea Corporis and Tinea Cruris: Treat for 2 weeks	
Tinea Pedis: Treat for 4 weeks	
Reevaluate if no improvement after treatment period	

ADMINISTRATION
Topical route

STORAGE
<30°C (86°F).

HOW SUPPLIED
Cre: 1% [15g, 30g, 85g]

CONTRAINDICATIONS
Hypersensitivity to any of the ingredients.

WARNINGS/PRECAUTIONS
D/C if sensitivity or chemical irritation occurs.

ADVERSE REACTIONS
Burning, itching, stinging, erythema.

DRUG INTERACTIONS
Coadministration with warfarin resulted in enhancement of anticoagulation effect; monitoring of INR/PT may be indicated especially in patients who apply the medication to large BSAs, in the genital area, or under occlusion.

PREGNANCY AND LACTATION
Category C, caution in nursing.

MECHANISM OF ACTION
Azole antifungal; exhibits broad-spectrum antifungal activity against susceptible organisms.

PHARMACOKINETICS
Elimination: Urine and feces (<1%).

PATIENT CONSIDERATIONS

Assessment: Assess for hypersensitivity to drug, pregnancy/nursing status, and possible drug interactions.

Monitoring: Monitor for signs/symptoms of sensitivity reaction or chemical irritation, and other adverse reactions. Monitor clinical improvement. May need to monitor INR/PT with warfarin, especially in patients who apply the medication to large BSA, in the genital area, or under occlusion.

Counseling: Counsel that medication is for external use only and to avoid contact with eyes. Instruct to notify physician if any signs of a sensitivity reaction or chemical irritation develop or if signs/symptoms do not improve by end of treatment period.

ECOZA — econazole nitrate   Rx

Class: Azole antifungal

ADULT DOSAGE	**PEDIATRIC DOSAGE**
Fungal Infections	**Fungal Infections**
Interdigital Tinea Pedis Caused by *Trichophyton rubrum*, *Trichophyton mentagrophytes*, and *Epidermophyton floccosum*: Cover the affected areas qd for 4 weeks	**Interdigital Tinea Pedis Caused by *Trichophyton rubrum*, *Trichophyton mentagrophytes*, and *Epidermophyton floccosum*:** **≥12 Years:** Cover the affected areas qd for 4 weeks

ADMINISTRATION
Topical route

STORAGE
20-25°C (68-77°F); excursions permitted between 15-30°C (59-86°F). Do not refrigerate or freeze. Contents under pressure; do not puncture and/or incinerate. Do not expose to heat and/or store at >49°C (120°F) even when empty. Do not store in direct sunlight.

HOW SUPPLIED
Foam: 1% [70g]

WARNINGS/PRECAUTIONS
Not for oral, ophthalmic, or intravaginal use. Flammable; avoid heat, flame, and smoking during and immediately following application.

ADVERSE REACTIONS
Application-site reactions.

DRUG INTERACTIONS
May enhance anticoagulant effect of warfarin; may need to monitor INR and/or PT, especially in patients who apply the medication to large BSA, in the genital area, or under occlusion.

PREGNANCY AND LACTATION
Category C, caution in nursing.

MECHANISM OF ACTION
Azole antifungal; inhibits fungal CYP450-mediated 14 α-lanosterol demethylase enzyme. This enzyme functions to convert lanosterol to ergosterol. The accumulation of 14 α-methyl sterols correlates with the subsequent loss of ergosterol in the fungal cell wall and may be responsible for the fungistatic activity of the drug.

PHARMACOKINETICS
Absorption: (Adults) T_{max}=6.8 hrs; C_{max}=417pg/mL; $AUC_{(0-12)}$=3440pg•hr/mL.

PATIENT CONSIDERATIONS

Assessment: Assess pregnancy/nursing status and for possible drug interactions.

Monitoring: Monitor for application-site reactions and other adverse reactions. May need to monitor INR and/or PT with warfarin, especially in patients who apply the medication to large BSA, in the genital area, or under occlusion.

Counseling: Inform that medication is for topical use only. Instruct to avoid heat, flame, and smoking during and immediately following application. Advise to d/c if a reaction suggesting sensitivity or chemical irritation develops.

EDARBI — azilsartan medoxomil   Rx

Class: Angiotensin II receptor blocker (ARB)

> **D/C when pregnancy is detected. Drugs that act directly on the renin-angiotensin system (RAS) can cause injury/death to the developing fetus.**

ADULT DOSAGE	**PEDIATRIC DOSAGE**
Hypertension	Pediatric use may not have been established
Usual: 80mg qd	
W/ High Dose Diuretics:	
Initial: 40mg qd	

ADMINISTRATION
Oral route
Take w/ or w/o food

STORAGE
25°C (77°F); excursions permitted to 15-30°C (59-86°F). Protect from moisture and light.

HOW SUPPLIED
Tab: 40mg, 80mg

CONTRAINDICATIONS
Coadministration with aliskiren in patients with diabetes.

WARNINGS/PRECAUTIONS
Symptomatic hypotension may occur in patients with an activated RAS (eg, volume- and/or salt-depleted patients receiving high doses of diuretics); correct this condition prior to therapy or start treatment at 40mg. Changes in renal function may occur. Oliguria and/or progressive azotemia and (rarely) acute renal failure and/or death may occur in patients whose renal function is dependent on the RAS (eg, severe CHF, renal artery stenosis, volume depletion). Increases in SrCr or BUN in patients with renal artery stenosis reported.

ADVERSE REACTIONS
Dizziness, postural dizziness, nausea, asthenia, fatigue, muscle spasm, cough, diarrhea.

DRUG INTERACTIONS
See Contraindications. NSAIDs, including selective COX-2 inhibitors, may deteriorate renal function and attenuate the antihypertensive effect. Dual blockade of the RAS is associated with increased risks of hypotension, hyperkalemia, and changes in renal function (including acute renal failure); avoid combined use of RAS inhibitors. Closely monitor BP, renal function, and electrolytes with concomitant agents that also affect the RAS. Avoid with aliskiren in patients with renal impairment (GFR <60mL/min). Increases in lithium levels and lithium toxicity reported; monitor lithium levels. Increases in SrCr may be larger with chlorthalidone or HCTZ.

PREGNANCY AND LACTATION
Category D, not for use in nursing.

MECHANISM OF ACTION
Angiotensin II receptor antagonist; blocks vasoconstrictor and aldosterone-secreting effects of angiotensin II by selectively blocking the binding of angiotensin II to AT_1 receptor in many tissues.

PHARMACOKINETICS
Absorption: Absolute bioavailability (60%); T_{max}=1.5-3 hrs. **Distribution:** V_d=16L; plasma protein binding (>99%). **Metabolism:** Via CYP2C9; O-dealkylation, decarboxylation; azilsartan (active metabolite), M-II (major metabolite), M-I (minor metabolite). **Elimination:** Urine (42%; 15% unchanged), feces (55%); $T_{1/2}$=11 hrs.

PATIENT CONSIDERATIONS

Assessment: Assess for volume/salt depletion, renal impairment, CHF, renal artery stenosis, diabetes, pregnancy/nursing status, and possible drug interactions.

Monitoring: Monitor for signs/symptoms of hypotension and other adverse reactions. Monitor BP and renal function.

Counseling: Inform of pregnancy risks; instruct to notify physician as soon as possible if pregnant/planning to become pregnant. Advise to seek medical attention if symptoms of hypotension or other adverse events occur.

EDARBYCLOR — azilsartan medoxomil/chlorthalidone   Rx

Class: Angiotensin II receptor blocker (ARB)/monosulfamyl diuretic

> **D/C when pregnancy is detected. Drugs that act directly on the renin-angiotensin system (RAS) can cause injury/death to the developing fetus.**

ADULT DOSAGE	**PEDIATRIC DOSAGE**
Hypertension	Pediatric use may not have been established
Initial: 40mg/12.5mg qd	
Titrate: May increase to 40mg/25mg after 2-4 weeks prn to achieve BP goals	
Max: 40mg/25mg	
Add-On Therapy: Use if not adequately controlled on ARBs or diuretic monotherapy	
Replacement Therapy: May receive the corresponding dose of the titrated individual components	
May be administered w/ other antihypertensive agents	

DOSING CONSIDERATIONS
Adverse Reactions
Dose-Limiting Adverse Reaction on Chlorthalidone: Initially give w/ a lower dose of chlorthalidone

ADMINISTRATION
Oral route

Take w/ or w/o food

STORAGE
25°C (77°F); excursions permitted to 15-30°C (59-86°F). Protect from moisture and light.

HOW SUPPLIED
Tab: (Azilsartan/Chlorthalidone) 40mg/12.5mg, 40mg/25mg

CONTRAINDICATIONS
Anuria. Coadministration w/ aliskiren in patients w/ diabetes.

WARNINGS/PRECAUTIONS
Symptomatic hypotension may occur in patients w/ activated RAS (eg, volume- and/or salt-depleted patients receiving high doses of diuretics); correct this condition prior to therapy. Consider withholding or discontinuing therapy if progressive renal impairment becomes evident. Azilsartan: Changes in renal function may occur. Oliguria and/or progressive azotemia and (rarely) acute renal failure and/or death may occur in patients whose renal function is dependent on the RAS (eg, severe CHF). Increases in BUN or SrCr in patients w/ renal artery stenosis reported. May cause hyperkalemia. Chlorthalidone: May cause fetal/neonatal jaundice and thrombocytopenia. May precipitate azotemia w/ renal disease. May cause hyponatremia and hypokalemia. Hyperuricemia may occur or frank gout may be precipitated. May precipitate hepatic coma in patients w/ hepatic dysfunction or progressive liver disease.

ADVERSE REACTIONS
Dizziness, syncope, hypotension, diarrhea, nausea, asthenia, fatigue, muscle spasm, cough, rash, headache, GI upset, elevation of uric acid and cholesterol.

DRUG INTERACTIONS
See Contraindications. May increase risk of symptomatic hypotension w/ high-dose diuretics. May increase risk of lithium toxicity; monitor lithium levels. Azilsartan: NSAIDs, including selective COX-2 inhibitors, may deteriorate renal function and attenuate the antihypertensive effect. Dual blockade of the RAS is associated w/ increased risks of hypotension, hyperkalemia, and changes in renal function, including acute renal failure; avoid combined use of RAS inhibitors. Closely monitor BP, renal function, and electrolytes w/ concomitant agents that affect the RAS. Avoid w/ aliskiren in patients w/ renal impairment (GFR <60mL/min). Chlorthalidone: Coadministration w/ digitalis may exacerbate the adverse effect of hypokalemia.

PREGNANCY AND LACTATION
Category D, not for use in nursing.

MECHANISM OF ACTION
Azilsartan: Angiotensin II receptor antagonist; blocks vasoconstrictor and aldosterone-secreting effects of angiotensin II by selectively blocking binding of angiotensin II to AT_1 receptor in many tissues. Chlorthalidone: Thiazide-like diuretic; has not been established. Produces diuresis w/ increased excretion of Na^+ and Cl^- at the cortical diluting segment of the ascending limb of Henle's loop of the nephron.

PHARMACOKINETICS
Absorption: Azilsartan: Absolute bioavailability (60%), T_{max}=1.5-3 hrs. Chlorthalidone: T_{max}=1 hr. **Distribution:** Azilsartan: V_d=16L; plasma protein binding (>99%). Chlorthalidone: Plasma protein binding (75%); crosses the placenta; found in breast milk. **Metabolism:** Azilsartan: Via CYP2C9; O-dealkylation, decarboxylation; azilsartan (active metabolite), M-II (major metabolite). **Elimination:** Azilsartan: Urine (42%, 15% as azilsartan), feces (55%); $T_{1/2}$=11-12 hrs. Chlorthalidone: Kidney; $T_{1/2}$=45 hrs.

PATIENT CONSIDERATIONS
Assessment: Assess for anuria, volume/salt depletion, CHF, renal/hepatic function, renal artery stenosis, pregnancy/nursing status, and possible drug interactions. Obtain baseline BP.

Monitoring: Monitor for signs/symptoms of hypotension, hyperuricemia, precipitation of frank gout, and other adverse reactions. Monitor BP and hepatic/renal function. Monitor serum electrolytes periodically.

Counseling: Inform about the consequences of exposure during pregnancy and discuss treatment options in women planning to become pregnant. Instruct to report pregnancy to the physician as soon as possible. If a dose is missed, instruct to take it later in the same day; advise not to double the dose on the following day. Instruct to report gout symptoms and lightheadedness; advise to d/c and consult physician if syncope occurs. Inform that dehydration from excessive perspiration, vomiting, and diarrhea may lead to an excessive fall in BP; advise to consult physician if these occur. Advise patients w/ renal impairment to receive periodic blood tests while on therapy.

EDLUAR — zolpidem tartrate   CIV
Class: GABA$_A$ agonist

ADULT DOSAGE	PEDIATRIC DOSAGE
Insomnia	Pediatric use may not have been established
Short-Term Treatment of Insomnia Characterized by Difficulties w/ Sleep Initiation:	
Initial: 5mg (women), and either 5mg or 10mg (men), taken qhs	
Titrate: May increase to 10mg if the 5mg dose is not effective	
Max: 10mg qhs	

DOSING CONSIDERATIONS
Concomitant Medications
Use w/ CNS Depressants: May need to adjust dose of zolpidem
Hepatic Impairment
Hepatic Insufficiency:
Usual: 5mg qhs
Elderly
Elderly/Debilitated:
Usual: 5mg qhs

ADMINISTRATION
SL route

Take immediately before hs w/ at least 7-8 hrs remaining before the planned time of awakening
Do not take w/ or immediately after a meal
Place tab under tongue; do not swallow tab or take w/ water

STORAGE
20-25°C (68-77°F). Protect from light and moisture.

HOW SUPPLIED
Tab, SL: 5mg, 10mg

CONTRAINDICATIONS
Known hypersensitivity to zolpidem

WARNINGS/PRECAUTIONS
Increased risk of next-day psychomotor impairment if taken with less than a full night of sleep remaining (7-8 hrs). May impair mental/physical abilities. Initiate only after careful evaluation; failure of insomnia to remit after 7-10 days of treatment may indicate presence of a primary psychiatric and/or medical illness. Angioedema and anaphylaxis reported; do not rechallenge if such reactions develop. Abnormal thinking, behavior changes, and visual/auditory hallucinations reported. Complex behaviors (eg, sleep-driving) while not fully awake reported; consider discontinuation if a sleep-driving episode occurs. Amnesia, anxiety, and other neuropsychiatric symptoms may occur. Worsening of depression, and suicidal thoughts and actions (including completed suicides) reported primarily in depressed patients; prescribe the least amount of drug that is feasible at a time. Caution with compromised respiratory function; prior to prescribing, consider the risks of respiratory depression in patients with respiratory impairment (eg, sleep apnea, myasthenia gravis). Withdrawal signs and symptoms reported following rapid dose decrease or abrupt discontinuation; monitor for tolerance, abuse, and dependence.

ADVERSE REACTIONS
Drowsiness, dizziness, headache, diarrhea, drugged feeling, lethargy, dry mouth, back pain, pharyngitis, sinusitis, allergy.

DRUG INTERACTIONS
See Dosage. Increased risk of CNS depression and complex behaviors with other CNS depressants (eg, benzodiazepines, opioids, TCAs, alcohol). Use with other sedative-hypnotics (eg, other zolpidem products) at hs or the middle of the night is not recommended. Increased risk of next-day psychomotor impairment with other CNS depressants or drugs that increase zolpidem levels. May decrease peak levels of imipramine. Additive effect of decreased alertness with imipramine or chlorpromazine. Additive adverse effect on psychomotor performance with chlorpromazine or alcohol. Sertraline and CYP3A inhibitors may increase exposure. Fluoxetine may increase $T_{1/2}$. Rifampin (a CYP3A4 inducer) may reduce exposure, pharmacodynamic effects, and efficacy. Ketoconazole (a potent CYP3A4 inhibitor) may increase pharmacodynamic effects; consider lower dose of zolpidem.

PREGNANCY AND LACTATION
Category C, caution in nursing.

MECHANISM OF ACTION
Imidazopyridine, nonbenzodiazepine hypnotic; interacts with a gamma-aminobutyric acid-BZ receptor complex. Binds the BZ_1 receptor preferentially with a high affinity ratio of the α_1/α_5 subunits.

PHARMACOKINETICS
Absorption: Rapid. (10mg) C_{max}=106ng/mL; T_{max}=82 min (median). **Distribution:** Plasma protein binding (92.5%); found in breast milk. **Elimination:** Renal; $T_{1/2}$=2.85 hrs (5mg), 2.65 hrs (10mg).

PATIENT CONSIDERATIONS
Assessment: Assess for physical and/or psychiatric disorder, depression, compromised respiratory function, sleep apnea, myasthenia gravis, hepatic impairment, history of drug/alcohol addiction or abuse, hypersensitivity to the drug, pregnancy/nursing status, and possible drug interactions.

Monitoring: Monitor for angioedema, anaphylaxis, emergence of any new behavioral signs/symptoms of concern, respiratory depression, withdrawal signs/symptoms, tolerance, abuse, dependence, and other adverse reactions.

Counseling: Inform about the benefits and risks of treatment. Instruct to take only as prescribed; advise to wait at least 8 hrs after dosing before driving or engaging in other activities requiring full mental alertness. Instruct to contact physician immediately if any adverse reactions (eg, severe anaphylactic/anaphylactoid reactions, sleep-driving or other complex behaviors, suicidal thoughts) develop. Advise not to use the drug if patient drank alcohol that pm or before bed. Instruct not to increase the dose and to inform physician if it is believed that the drug does not work.

EDURANT — rilpivirine   Rx

Class: Non-nucleoside reverse transcriptase inhibitor (NNRTI)

ADULT DOSAGE	PEDIATRIC DOSAGE
HIV-1 Infection	**HIV-1 Infection**
In combination w/ other antiretrovirals, in antiretroviral treatment-naive patients w/ HIV-1 RNA ≤100,000 copies/mL at the start of therapy	In combination w/ other antiretrovirals, in antiretroviral treatment-naive patients w/ HIV-1 RNA ≤100,000 copies/mL at the start of therapy
25mg qd	**≥12 Years:** **≥35kg:** 25mg qd

DOSING CONSIDERATIONS
Concomitant Medications
W/ Rifabutin: Increase Edurant dose to 50mg qd; when coadministration is stopped, decrease dose to 25mg qd

ADMINISTRATION
Oral route
Take w/ a meal.

STORAGE
25°C (77°F); excursions permitted to 15-30°C (59-86°F). Protect from light.

HOW SUPPLIED
Tab: 25mg

CONTRAINDICATIONS
Concomitant use w/ carbamazepine, oxcarbazepine, phenobarbital, phenytoin, rifampin, rifapentine, proton pump inhibitors (eg, esomeprazole, lansoprazole, omeprazole, pantoprazole, rabeprazole), systemic dexamethasone (more than a single dose), and St. John's wort.

WARNINGS/PRECAUTIONS
Severe skin and hypersensitivity reactions reported, including cases of drug reaction w/ eosinophilia and systemic symptoms; d/c immediately and initiate appropriate therapy if signs/symptoms develop. Depressive disorders reported; immediate medical evaluation is recommended if severe depressive symptoms occur. Hepatotoxicity reported; underlying hepatitis B or C, or marked elevation in transaminases prior to treatment may increase risk for worsening or development of transaminase elevations. Consider liver enzyme monitoring in patients w/o preexisting hepatic dysfunction or other risk factors. Immune reconstitution syndrome, redistribution/accumulation of body fat, and autoimmune disorders (eg, Graves' disease, polymyositis, Guillain-Barre syndrome) in the setting of immune reconstitution reported. Caution w/ severe renal impairment or ESRD; monitor for adverse effects. Caution in elderly.

ADVERSE REACTIONS
Lab abnormalities (increased SrCr, AST/ALT, total bilirubin, total cholesterol, LDL), depressive disorders, insomnia, headache, rash, somnolence, N/V, dizziness, abdominal pain.

DRUG INTERACTIONS
See Dosing Considerations and Contraindications. Caution w/ drugs that may reduce exposure. Coadministration w/ CYP3A inducers or drugs that increase gastric pH may result in decreased levels, loss of virologic response, and possible resistance to rilpivirine or to the class of non-nucleoside reverse transcriptase inhibitors (NNRTIs). CYP3A inhibitors may increase levels. Not recommended w/ delavirdine and other NNRTIs (eg, efavirenz, etravirine, nevirapine). Concomitant didanosine should be given on an empty stomach and at least 2 hrs before or at least 4 hrs after therapy. Darunavir/ritonavir (RTV), lopinavir/RTV, unboosted protease inhibitors (PIs) or other boosted PIs (w/ RTV), may increase levels. Azole antifungals may increase levels; monitor for breakthrough fungal infections w/ azole antifungals. May decrease ketoconazole levels. Clarithromycin, erythromycin, or telithromycin may increase levels; consider alternatives (eg, azithromycin) when possible. Rifabutin may decrease levels. Antacids and H$_2$-receptor antagonists may significantly decrease levels. Administer antacids either at least 2 hrs before or at least 4 hrs after therapy. Administer H$_2$-receptor antagonists at least 12 hrs before or at least 4 hrs after therapy. Clinical monitoring is recommended w/ methadone as methadone maintenance therapy may need to be adjusted in some patients. Caution w/ drugs that have a known risk of torsades de pointes.

PREGNANCY AND LACTATION
Pregnancy: Category B. Physicians are encouraged to register patients in the Antiretroviral Pregnancy Registry.
Lactation: Mothers should be instructed not to breastfeed due to potential for HIV-1 transmission.

MECHANISM OF ACTION
NNRTI; inhibits HIV-1 replication by noncompetitive inhibition of HIV-1 reverse transcriptase.

PHARMACOKINETICS
Absorption: AUC$_{24h}$=2235ng•hr/mL, T$_{max}$=4-5 hrs. **Distribution:** Plasma protein binding (approx 99.7%). **Metabolism:** Liver via CYP3A oxidation. **Elimination:** Feces (85%, 25% unchanged), urine (6.1%, <1% unchanged); T$_{1/2}$=approx 50 hrs.

PATIENT CONSIDERATIONS
Assessment: Assess for severe renal impairment or ESRD, underlying hepatic disease, marked transaminase elevations, pregnancy/nursing status, and possible drug interactions. Perform appropriate lab testing in patients w/ underlying hepatic disease or w/ marked transaminase elevations.
Monitoring: Monitor for severe skin and hypersensitivity reactions, depressive disorders, immune reconstitution syndrome, autoimmune disorders, fat redistribution/accumulation, hepatotoxicity, and other adverse reactions.
Counseling: Inform that product is not a cure for HIV infection; advise that continuous therapy is necessary to control HIV infection and decrease HIV-related illnesses. Advise to continue to practice safer sex and to use latex or polyurethane condoms. Instruct never to reuse or share needles. Inform mothers to avoid nursing to reduce risk of transmission of HIV to their baby. Advise to take medication ud. Advise not to alter the dose or d/c therapy w/o consulting physician. If a dose is missed w/in 12 hrs of the time it is usually taken, instruct to take as soon as possible w/ a meal and then to take the next dose at the regular scheduled time. If dose is missed by >12 hrs of the time it is usually taken, instruct not to take the missed dose, but resume the usual dosing schedule. Advise to report to physician the use of any other prescription/nonprescription or herbal products (eg, St. John's wort). Inform of the signs/symptoms of severe skin and hypersensitivity reactions and instruct to immediately stop taking therapy and seek medical attention if a rash develops associated w/ such symptoms. Inform patients that lab tests will be performed and appropriate therapy will be initiated if severe rash occurs. Instruct to seek medical evaluation if depressive symptoms are experienced. Inform that hepatotoxicity has been reported and redistribution/accumulation of body fat may occur.

EFFEXOR XR — venlafaxine   Rx

Class: Serotonin and norepinephrine reuptake inhibitor (SNRI)

> Antidepressants increased the risk of suicidal thoughts and behavior in children, adolescents, and young adults in short-term studies. Monitor closely for clinical worsening and emergence of suicidal thoughts and behaviors.

ADULT DOSAGE	PEDIATRIC DOSAGE
Major Depressive Disorder	Pediatric use may not have been established
Initial: 75mg/day as a single dose, or 37.5mg/day for 4-7 days and then increase to 75mg/day	
Titrate: May increase by increments of up to 75mg/day at ≥4-day intervals	
Max: 225mg/day	
Anxiety Disorders	
Generalized Anxiety Disorder:	
Initial: 75mg/day as a single dose, or 37.5mg/day for 4-7 days and then increase to 75mg/day	
Titrate: May increase by increments of up to 75mg/day at ≥4-day intervals	
Max: 225mg/day	
Social Anxiety Disorder:	
75mg/day as a single dose	
Panic Disorder	
W/ or w/o Agoraphobia:	
Initial: 37.5mg/day for 7 days	
Titrate: May increase by increments of up to 75mg/day at ≥7-day intervals	
Max: 225mg/day	
Conversions	
Switching from Effexor Immediate-Release (IR) Tabs:	
Depressed patients currently being treated at a therapeutic dose w/ Effexor IR tabs may be switched to Effexor XR at the nearest equivalent dose (mg/day); individual dose adjustments may be necessary	
Dosing Considerations with MAOIs	
Switching to/from an MAOI for Psychiatric Disorders:	
Allow at least 14 days between discontinuation of an MAOI and initiation of treatment, and allow at least 7 days between discontinuation of treatment and initiation of an MAOI	

W/ Other MAOIs (eg, Linezolid, IV Methylene Blue):
Do not start venlafaxine in patients being treated w/ linezolid or IV methylene blue. Consider other interventions (eg, hospitalization) in patients who require more urgent treatment of a psychiatric condition

If acceptable alternatives are not available, d/c venlafaxine and administer linezolid or IV methylene blue. Monitor for serotonin syndrome for 7 days or until 24 hrs after the last dose of linezolid or IV methylene blue, whichever comes 1st. May resume venlafaxine therapy 24 hrs after last dose of linezolid or IV methylene blue

DOSING CONSIDERATIONS
Renal Impairment
Mild (CrCl 60-89mL/min) or Moderate (CrCl 30-59mL/min): Reduce total daily dose by 25-50%
Severe (CrCl <30mL/min) or Hemodialysis: Reduce total daily dose by ≥50%
Hepatic Impairment
Mild (Child-Pugh 5-6) to Moderate (Child-Pugh 7-9): Reduce total daily dose by 50%
Severe (Child-Pugh 10-15) or Hepatic Cirrhosis: May need to reduce by ≥50%
Discontinuation
Gradually reduce dose (eg, reducing daily dose by 75mg at 1-week intervals)

ADMINISTRATION
Oral route

Take w/ food at same time each day, either in am or pm.
Swallow whole w/ fluid and do not divide, crush, chew, or place in water.
May take by carefully opening the cap and sprinkling the entire contents on a spoonful of applesauce; swallow immediately w/o chewing and follow w/ glass of water.

STORAGE
20-25°C (68-77°F).

HOW SUPPLIED
Cap, Extended-Release: 37.5mg, 75mg, 150mg

CONTRAINDICATIONS
Hypersensitivity to venlafaxine HCl, desvenlafaxine succinate, or to any excipients in the formulation. Use of an MAOI for psychiatric disorders either concomitantly or w/in 7 days of discontinuing treatment. Treatment w/in 14 days of discontinuing an MAOI for psychiatric disorders. Starting treatment in patients being treated w/ other MAOIs (eg, linezolid, IV methylene blue).

WARNINGS/PRECAUTIONS
Not approved for the treatment of bipolar depression. Serotonin syndrome reported; d/c immediately and initiate supportive symptomatic treatment. Dose-related increases in systolic and diastolic BP, as well as sustained HTN, reported; control preexisting HTN before initiating treatment and consider dose reduction or discontinuation for patients who experience a sustained increase in BP. May increase the risk of bleeding events. Pupillary dilation that occurs following use may trigger an angle-closure attack in a patient w/ anatomically narrow angles who does not have a patent iridectomy. Mania/hypomania reported. Avoid abrupt discontinuation; gradually reduce dose. Seizures reported; d/c if seizures develop. Hyponatremia may occur; consider discontinuation in patients w/ symptomatic hyponatremia. Interstitial lung disease (ILD) and eosinophilic pneumonia rarely reported; consider discontinuation if symptoms occur. Caution w/ preexisting HTN or cardiovascular (CV) or cerebrovascular conditions that might be compromised by increases in BP, history of mania/hypomania, history of seizures, and in the elderly. False (+) urine immunoassay screening tests for phencyclidine and amphetamines reported.

ADVERSE REACTIONS
Asthenia, sweating, N/V, constipation, anorexia, dry mouth, dizziness, insomnia, nervousness, somnolence, abnormal ejaculation/orgasm, impotence, decreased libido.

DRUG INTERACTIONS
See Contraindications. May cause serotonin syndrome w/ other serotonergic drugs (eg, triptans, TCAs, fentanyl) and w/ drugs that impair metabolism of serotonin; d/c therapy and any concomitant serotonergic agents immediately if this occurs. Not recommended w/ weight-loss agents or tryptophan supplements. Increased risk of hyponatremia w/ diuretics. Increased risk of bleeding w/ aspirin (ASA), NSAIDs, warfarin, and other anticoagulants or other drugs known to affect platelet function. Avoid w/ ethanol. Increased levels w/ cimetidine; use w/ caution in patients w/ HTN, hepatic dysfunction, or in the elderly. Increased levels w/ ketoconazole; use w/ caution. May increase metoprolol levels; use w/ caution and monitor BP. Caution w/ other CNS-active drugs.

PREGNANCY AND LACTATION
Pregnancy: Category C.
Lactation: Not for use in nursing.

MECHANISM OF ACTION
SNRI; exact mechanism of the antidepressant action is unknown, but thought to be related to the potentiation of serotonin and norepinephrine in the CNS, through inhibition of their reuptake.

PHARMACOKINETICS
Absorption: Well-absorbed. Absolute bioavailability (45%); (150mg qd) C_{max}=150ng/mL, T_{max}=5.5 hrs. O-desmethylvenlafaxine (ODV) (metabolite): (150mg qd) C_{max}=260ng/mL, T_{max}=9 hrs. **Distribution:** Plasma protein binding (27% venlafaxine, 30% ODV); found in breast milk. V_d=7.5L/kg (venlafaxine), 5.7L/kg (ODV). **Metabolism:** Extensive. Hepatic via CYP2D6; ODV (major active metabolite). **Elimination:** Urine (87%, 5% unchanged, 29% unconjugated ODV, 26% conjugated ODV); $T_{1/2}$=5 hrs. ODV: $T_{1/2}$=11 hrs.

PATIENT CONSIDERATIONS
Assessment: Assess for history of mania/hypomania, seizures, HTN, susceptibility to angle-closure glaucoma, CV/cerebrovascular conditions, volume depletion, hepatic/renal impairment, hypersensitivity to the drug, pregnancy/nursing status, and possible drug interactions. Perform adequate screening to determine if patient is at risk for bipolar disorder; such screening should include a detailed psychiatric history, including a family history of suicide, bipolar disorder, and depression. Monitor BP before initiating treatment.

Monitoring: Monitor for signs/symptoms of clinical worsening, suicidality, unusual behavior, serotonin syndrome, sustained HTN, abnormal bleeding, angle-closure glaucoma, activation of mania/hypomania, hyponatremia, seizures, ILD, eosinophilic pneumonia, and other adverse reactions. Monitor BP regularly during treatment. If discontinued abruptly, monitor for discontinuation symptoms (eg, dysphoric mood, confusion, agitation). Carefully monitor patients receiving concomitant warfarin therapy when treatment is initiated or discontinued. Periodically reassess to determine the need for maintenance or continued treatment.

Counseling: Inform about the risks and benefits of therapy. Advise to look for emergence of suicidality, worsening of depression, and unusual changes in behavior, especially early during treatment and when the dose is adjusted up or down. Advise not to use concomitantly w/ other venlafaxine- or desvenlafaxine-containing products. Instruct not to take w/ an MAOI or w/in 14 days of stopping an MAOI and to allow 7 days after stopping treatment before starting an MAOI. Caution about the risk of serotonin syndrome. Advise to have regular BP monitoring during therapy. Caution that concomitant use w/ ASA, NSAIDs, warfarin, or other drugs that affect coagulation may increase the risk of bleeding. Inform about the risk of angle-closure glaucoma in susceptible individuals. Advise patients, families, and caregivers to observe for signs of activation of mania/hypomania. Advise that elevations in total cholesterol, LDL, and TGs may occur and that measurement of serum lipids may be considered. Advise not to stop taking medication w/o first talking w/ a healthcare professional; inform that discontinuation effects may occur when stopping treatment. Caution against operating hazardous machinery (including automobiles) until reasonably certain that therapy does not adversely affect ability to engage in such activities. Advise to avoid alcohol while on therapy. Advise to notify physician if allergic phenomena develops, or if pregnant, intending to become pregnant, or if breastfeeding. Inform that spheroids may be passed in the stool or via colostomy.

EFFIENT — prasugrel   Rx
Class: Antiplatelet agent

> May cause significant, sometimes fatal, bleeding; risk factors include <60kg body weight, propensity to bleed, and concomitant use of medications that increase risk of bleeding (eg, warfarin, heparin, fibrinolytic therapy, chronic use of NSAIDs). Do not use in patients w/ active pathological bleeding or a history of transient ischemic attack (TIA) or stroke. Not recommended in patients ≥75 yrs of age, due to increased risk of fatal and intracranial bleeding and uncertain benefit, except in high-risk situations (diabetes or history of prior MI) where the effect appears to be greater and use may be considered. Do not start in patients likely to undergo urgent CABG; d/c at least 7 days prior to any surgery, when possible. Suspect bleeding in any patient who is hypotensive and has recently undergone coronary angiography, percutaneous coronary intervention (PCI), CABG, or other surgical procedures. If possible, manage bleeding w/o discontinuing the drug. Discontinuing therapy, particularly in the 1st few weeks after acute coronary syndrome, increases the risk of subsequent cardiovascular (CV) events.

ADULT DOSAGE
Acute Coronary Syndrome
To reduce the rate of thrombotic CV events (including stent thrombosis) in patients who are to be managed w/ PCI as follows: patients w/ unstable angina or non-ST-elevation MI or patients w/ ST-elevation MI when managed w/ primary or delayed PCI

LD: 60mg as a single dose
Maint: 10mg qd; consider 5mg qd in patients <60kg

Take w/ aspirin (75-325mg/day)

PEDIATRIC DOSAGE
Pediatric use may not have been established

DOSING CONSIDERATIONS
Renal Impairment
No dose adjustment necessary
Hepatic Impairment
Mild to Moderate: No dose adjustment necessary
Severe: Not studied

ADMINISTRATION
Oral route

Take w/ or w/o food.
Do not break the tab.

STORAGE
25°C (77°F); excursions permitted to 15-30°C (59-86°F).

HOW SUPPLIED
Tab: 5mg, 10mg

CONTRAINDICATIONS
Active pathological bleeding (eg, peptic ulcer, intracranial hemorrhage), history of prior TIA or stroke, hypersensitivity (eg, anaphylaxis) to prasugrel or any component of the product.

WARNINGS/PRECAUTIONS
D/C for active bleeding, elective surgery, stroke, or TIA. Those who require premature discontinuation will be at increased risk for cardiac events. Avoid therapy lapses; if temporary discontinuation is needed because of an adverse event(s), restart as soon as possible. Thrombotic thrombocytopenic purpura (TTP) reported; may occur after a brief exposure (<2 weeks) and requires urgent treatment (eg, plasmapheresis). Hypersensitivity including angioedema reported, including in patients w/ a history of hypersensitivity reaction to other thienopyridines. Increased risk for bleeding w/ severe hepatic impairment or moderate to severe renal impairment.

ADVERSE REACTIONS
Bleeding, HTN, hypercholesterolemia/hyperlipidemia, headache, back pain, dyspnea, nausea, dizziness, cough, hypotension, fatigue, noncardiac chest pain.

DRUG INTERACTIONS
See Boxed Warning.

PREGNANCY AND LACTATION
Pregnancy: There are no data w/ prasugrel in pregnant women to inform a drug-associated risk. Due to the mechanism of action, and the associated identified risk of bleeding, consider the benefits and risks when prescribing to a pregnant woman. **Lactation:** There is no information regarding the presence in human milk, the effects on the breastfed infant, or the effects on milk production; caution in nursing.

MECHANISM OF ACTION
Platelet activation and aggregation inhibitor (thienopyridine class); inhibits platelet activation and aggregation through irreversible binding of its active metabolite to the $P2Y_{12}$ class of ADP receptors on platelets.

PHARMACOKINETICS
Absorption: Rapid. T_{max}=30 min (active metabolite). **Distribution:** (Active metabolite) Plasma protein binding (98%, albumin); V_d=44-68L (active metabolite). **Metabolism:** Hydrolysis in the intestine; converted to active metabolite via CYP3A4 and CYP2B6 (primary) and CYP2C9 and CYP2C19; then S-methylation or conjugation w/ cysteine. **Elimination:** Urine (68%, inactive metabolites), feces (27%, inactive metabolites); $T_{1/2}$=7 hrs (active metabolite).

PATIENT CONSIDERATIONS
Assessment: Assess for active pathological bleeding, history of prior TIA or stroke, other risk factors for bleeding, hypersensitivity, pregnancy/nursing status, and possible drug interactions. Assess likelihood of undergoing urgent CABG.

Monitoring: Monitor for signs/symptoms of bleeding, TTP, hypersensitivity, and other adverse reactions.

Counseling: Inform about the benefits and risks of treatment. Instruct to take exactly as prescribed and not to d/c w/o consulting the prescribing physician. Inform that patient may bruise and bleed more easily and that bleeding will take longer than usual to stop. Advise to report to physician any unanticipated, prolonged, or excessive bleeding, or blood in stool/urine. Inform that TTP, a rare but serious condition, has been reported; instruct to seek prompt medical attention if experiencing unexplained fever, weakness, extreme skin paleness, purple skin patches, yellowing of skin/eyes, or neurological changes. Inform that hypersensitivity reactions may occur. Instruct to notify physicians and dentists about therapy before scheduling any invasive procedure, and to inform doctor performing the invasive procedure to talk to the prescribing physician before stopping therapy.

EFUDEX — fluorouracil   Rx

Class: Antimetabolite

ADULT DOSAGE	**PEDIATRIC DOSAGE**
Multiple Actinic or Solar Keratoses	Pediatric use may not have been established
Apply sufficient amount to cover the lesions bid. Continue use until inflammatory response reaches the erosion stage	
Usual Duration: 2-4 weeks; complete healing of the lesions may not be evident for 1-2 months following cessation of therapy	
Superficial Basal Cell Carcinomas	
5%:	
Apply sufficient amount to cover the lesions bid	
Continue treatment for at least 3-6 weeks; therapy may be required for as long as 10-12 weeks before lesions are obliterated	
Use when conventional methods are impractical (eg, w/ multiple lesions or difficult treatment sites)	

ADMINISTRATION
Topical route

Apply preferably w/ a nonmetal applicator or suitable glove. If applied w/ the fingers, wash hands immediately afterward.

STORAGE
25°C (77°F); excursions permitted to 15-30°C (59-86°F).

HOW SUPPLIED
Topical Cre: 5% [40g]; **Topical Sol:** 2%, 5% [10mL, 25mL]

CONTRAINDICATIONS
Women who are or may become pregnant, dihydropyrimidine dehydrogenase (DPD) enzyme deficiency, known hypersensitivity to any of the components.

WARNINGS/PRECAUTIONS
Avoid application to mucous membranes; local inflammation and ulceration may occur. If any occlusive dressing is used in treatment of basal cell carcinoma, there may be an increase in the severity of inflammatory reactions in the adjacent normal skin; a porous gauze dressing may be applied for cosmetic reasons w/o increase in reaction. Minimize exposure to UV rays during and immediately following treatment; intensity of the reaction may be increased. D/C if symptoms of DPD enzyme deficiency develop. Increased absorption may occur through ulcerated or inflamed skin. Not for ophthalmic, oral, or intravaginal use. Solar keratoses which do not respond should be biopsied to confirm the diagnosis; perform follow-up biopsies as indicated in the management of superficial basal cell carcinoma.

ADVERSE REACTIONS
Burning, crusting, allergic contact dermatitis, pruritus, scarring, rash, soreness, ulceration, leukocytosis.

PREGNANCY AND LACTATION
Pregnancy: May cause fetal harm. **Lactation:** Not for use in nursing.

MECHANISM OF ACTION
Antimetabolite; blocks the methylation reaction of deoxyuridylic acid to thymidylic acid, thereby interfering w/ the synthesis of DNA and, to a lesser extent, inhibiting the formation of RNA. Since DNA and RNA are essential for cell division and growth, the effect may be to create a thymine deficiency, which provokes unbalanced growth and death of the cell.

PHARMACOKINETICS
Elimination: Urine (0.76%).

PATIENT CONSIDERATIONS
Assessment: Assess for hypersensitivity to the drug, DPD enzyme deficiency, skin ulceration/inflammation, and pregnancy/nursing status.

Monitoring: Monitor for local reactions and other adverse effects. Biopsy solar keratoses that do not respond to confirm the diagnosis. Perform follow-up biopsies as indicated in the management of superficial basal cell carcinoma.

Counseling: Inform that the reaction in the treated areas may be unsightly during therapy and, usually, for several weeks following cessation of therapy. Instruct to avoid exposure to UV rays during and immediately following treatment. Advise not to apply on the eyelids or directly into the eyes, nose, or mouth.

EGRIFTA — tesamorelin   Rx

Class: Growth hormone (GH)-releasing factor

ADULT DOSAGE	**PEDIATRIC DOSAGE**
Lipodystrophy	Pediatric use may not have been established
Reduction of Excess Abdominal Fat in HIV-Infected Patients:	
2mg SQ in the abdomen qd	

ADMINISTRATION
SQ route

Rotate inj sites to different areas of the abdomen
Do not inject into scar tissue, bruises, or the navel
Administer immediately following reconstitution

Reconstitution
Two vials of tesamorelin must be reconstituted w/ the diluent provided
1. Reconstitute the first vial w/ 2.2mL of diluent
2. Mix by rolling the vial gently in hands for 30 sec; do not shake
3. Reconstitute the second vial w/ the entire sol from the first vial
4. Mix by rolling the vial gently in hands for 30 sec; do not shake

STORAGE
Unreconstituted: 2-8°C (36-46°F). Reconstituted: Do not freeze or refrigerate. Diluent/Syringes/Needles: 20-25°C (68-77°F). Protect from light. Keep in the original box until use.

HOW SUPPLIED
Inj: 1mg

CONTRAINDICATIONS
Pregnancy, newly diagnosed or recurrent active malignancy, disruption of hypothalamic-pituitary axis due to hypophysectomy, hypopituitarism, pituitary tumor/surgery, head irradiation or head trauma, known hypersensitivity to tesamorelin and/or mannitol (an excipient).

WARNINGS/PRECAUTIONS
Carefully consider whether to continue treatment in patients who do not show clear efficacy response. Not indicated for weight loss management (weight neutral effect). Initiate therapy after careful evaluation of the potential benefit

of treatment for patients with history of nonmalignant neoplasms or history of treated and stable malignancies. Carefully consider the increased background risk of malignancies in HIV-positive patients before initiation of therapy. Stimulates growth hormone (GH) production and increases serum insulin growth factor-1 (IGF-1); monitor IGF-1 levels closely and consider discontinuation of therapy in patients with persistent elevations of IGF-1 levels (eg, >3 standard deviation scores), particularly if the efficacy response is not robust. Fluid retention may occur. May cause glucose intolerance and increase the risk for developing diabetes. Hypersensitivity reactions may occur; d/c treatment immediately when suspected. May cause inj-site reactions. Consider discontinuation in critically ill patients; increased mortality in patients with acute critical illness due to complications following open heart surgery, abdominal surgery, or multiple accidental trauma, or those with acute respiratory failure.

ADVERSE REACTIONS
Arthralgia, pain in extremity, peripheral edema, inj-site reactions (eg, erythema, pruritus, pain), myalgia, paresthesia, hypoesthesia, nausea, rash.

DRUG INTERACTIONS
May modulate CYP450 mediated antipyrine clearance; monitor carefully in combination with other drugs known to be metabolized by CYP450 liver enzymes. May require an increase in maintenance or stress doses of glucocorticoids following initiation of therapy, particularly in patients treated with cortisone acetate and prednisone.

PREGNANCY AND LACTATION
Category X, not for use in nursing.

MECHANISM OF ACTION
Human GH-releasing factor synthetic analogue; acts on pituitary somatotroph cells to stimulate the synthesis and pulsatile release of endogenous GH, which is both anabolic and lipolytic. GH exerts its effects by interacting with specific receptors on a variety of target cells, including chondrocytes, osteoblasts, myocytes, hepatocytes, and adipocytes, resulting in a host of pharmacodynamic effects.

PHARMACOKINETICS
Absorption: Absolute bioavailability (<4%); AUC=852.8pg•hr/mL, C_{max}=2822.3pg/mL, T_{max}=0.15 hr. **Distribution:** V_d=10.5L/kg. **Elimination:** $T_{1/2}$=38 min (14 consecutive days of administration).

PATIENT CONSIDERATIONS
Assessment: Assess for hypersensitivity to the drug and/or mannitol, hypothalamic-pituitary axis disruption due to hypophysectomy, hypopituitarism, pituitary tumor/surgery, head irradiation or head trauma, active malignancy, history of nonmalignant neoplasms or treated and stable malignancies, diabetes, acute critical illness, pregnancy/nursing status, and possible drug interactions. Evaluate glucose status.

Monitoring: Monitor for fluid retention, hypersensitivity/inj-site reactions, and other adverse reactions. Monitor for response and IGF-1 levels. Monitor for changes in glucose metabolism periodically in patients who develop impaired glucose tolerance or diabetes and for potential development or worsening of retinopathy in patients with diabetes.

Counseling: Advise that treatment may cause symptoms consistent with fluid retention. Instruct to seek prompt medical attention and to d/c therapy immediately when hypersensitivity reactions occur. Advise to rotate inj site to reduce incidence of inj-site reactions. Counsel not to share syringe with another person, even if the needle is changed. Instruct women to d/c treatment if pregnant and not to breastfeed.

ELAPRASE — idursulfase   Rx
Class: Enzyme

> Life-threatening anaphylactic reactions observed during and up to 24 hrs after infusion. Anaphylaxis, presenting as respiratory distress, hypoxia, hypotension, urticaria, and/or angioedema of throat or tongue reported during and after infusions, regardless of duration of the course of treatment; closely observe patients. Inform patients of the signs/symptoms of anaphylaxis and instruct to seek immediate medical care should symptoms occur. Patients with compromised respiratory function or acute respiratory disease may be at risk of serious acute exacerbation of their respiratory compromise due to hypersensitivity reactions; additional monitoring required.

ADULT DOSAGE
Hunter Syndrome (Mucopolysaccharidosis II)

Usual: 0.5mg/kg once weekly as an IV infusion over 3 hrs; gradually reduce infusion to 1 hr if no hypersensitivity reactions are observed

Patients may require longer infusion times if hypersensitivity reactions occur; however, infusion times should not exceed 8 hrs

Infusion Rate:
Initial: 8mL/hr for the first 15 min
Titrate: May increase rate by 8mL/hr increments every 15 min if well tolerated
Max: 100mL/hr

Infusion rate may be slowed, temporarily stopped, or discontinued for that visit in the event of hypersensitivity reactions

PEDIATRIC DOSAGE
Hunter Syndrome (Mucopolysaccharidosis II)

≥5 Years:
Usual: 0.5mg/kg once weekly as an IV infusion over 3 hrs; gradually reduce infusion to 1 hr if no hypersensitivity reactions are observed

Patients may require longer infusion times if hypersensitivity reactions occur; however, infusion times should not exceed 8 hrs

Infusion Rate:
Initial: 8mL/hr for the first 15 min
Titrate: May increase rate by 8mL/hr increments every 15 min if well tolerated
Max: 100mL/hr

Infusion rate may be slowed, temporarily stopped, or discontinued for that visit in the event of hypersensitivity reactions

ADMINISTRATION
IV Route
Preparation Instructions
1. Determine the total volume of idursulfase to be administered and the number of vials needed based on the patient's weight and the recommended dose; refer to PI for calculation
2. Round up to the next whole vial to determine the total number of vials needed
3. Remove the required number of vials from the refrigerator to allow them to reach room temperature; do not shake the idursulfase sol
4. Withdraw the calculated volume of idursulfase from the appropriate number of vials
5. Add the calculated volume of idursulfase sol to a 100mL bag of 0.9% NaCl inj for IV infusion
6. Mix gently; do not shake the sol

Administration Instructions
Administer the diluted idursulfase sol using a low-protein-binding infusion set equipped w/ a low-protein-binding 0.2μm in-line filter
Do not infuse w/ other products in the infusion tubing

Stability
If immediate use is not possible, store the diluted sol in the refrigerator at 2-8°C (36-46°F) for up to 24 hrs

STORAGE
Vial: 2-8°C (36-46°F). Diluted Sol: 2-8°C (36-46°F) for ≤24 hrs. Protect from light. Do not freeze or shake.

HOW SUPPLIED
Inj: 2mg/mL [3mL]

WARNINGS/PRECAUTIONS
Immediately d/c if anaphylactic or other acute reactions occur and initiate appropriate treatment; medical support should be readily available upon administration. Risk of hypersensitivity, serious adverse reactions, and antibody development in Hunter syndrome patients with severe genetic mutations. Consider delaying infusion in patients with compromised respiratory function or acute febrile or respiratory illness. Caution in patients susceptible to fluid overload, or patients with acute underlying respiratory illness or compromised cardiac and/or respiratory function for whom fluid restriction is indicated; may be at risk of serious exacerbation of cardiac or respiratory status during infusions.

ADVERSE REACTIONS
Anaphylactic/hypersensitivity reactions, rash, urticaria, pruritus, flushing, pyrexia, headache, diarrhea, musculoskeletal pain, cough, fatigue, tachycardia, chills, erythema.

PREGNANCY AND LACTATION
Category C, caution in nursing.

MECHANISM OF ACTION
Hydrolytic lysosomal glycosaminoglycan-specific enzyme; provides exogenous enzyme for uptake into cellular lysosomes.

PHARMACOKINETICS
Absorption: C_{max}=1.5mcg/mL (Week 1), 1.1mcg/mL (Week 27); AUC=206 min•mcg/mL (Week 1), 169 min•mcg/mL (Week 27). **Distribution:** V_d=213mL/kg (Week 1), 254mL/kg (Week 27). **Elimination:** $T_{1/2}$= 44 min (Week 1), 48 min (Week 27).

PATIENT CONSIDERATIONS
Assessment: Assess for compromised respiratory function, genetic mutations, susceptibility to fluid overload, fluid restriction, respiratory/febrile illness, clinical status, and pregnancy/nursing status.

Monitoring: Monitor for anaphylactic/hypersensitivity reactions (eg, respiratory distress, hypoxia, hypotension, urticaria, angioedema of the throat/tongue), respiratory disease exacerbations, and other adverse events.

Counseling: Advise that life-threatening anaphylactic reactions have occurred during and after infusion. Advise that patients who have experienced anaphylactic reactions may require prolonged observation. Inform that patients with compromised respiratory function or acute respiratory disease may be at risk of serious acute exacerbation of their respiratory compromise due to hypersensitivity reactions. Encourage patients to participate in the Hunter Outcome Survey program.

ELIDEL — pimecrolimus   Rx
Class: Calcineurin-inhibitor immunosuppressant

> Rare cases of malignancy (eg, skin and lymphoma) reported with topical calcineurin inhibitors, including pimecrolimus, although causal relationship is not established. Avoid long-term use, and application should be limited to areas of involvement with atopic dermatitis. Not indicated for children <2 yrs of age.

ADULT DOSAGE
Atopic Dermatitis

Short-term/noncontinuous chronic treatment (2nd line) of mild to moderate atopic dermatitis in patients who have failed to respond adequately to other topical treatments, or when those treatments are not advisable

Apply thin layer to the affected skin bid until signs and symptoms resolve

Reexamine if signs and symptoms persist beyond 6 weeks

PEDIATRIC DOSAGE
Atopic Dermatitis

Short-term/noncontinuous chronic treatment (2nd line) of mild to moderate atopic dermatitis in patients who have failed to respond adequately to other topical treatments, or when those treatments are not advisable

≥2 Years:
Apply thin layer to the affected skin bid until signs and symptoms resolve

Reexamine if signs and symptoms persist beyond 6 weeks

ADMINISTRATION
Topical route

STORAGE
25°C (77°F); excursions permitted to 15-30°C (59-86°F). Do not freeze.

HOW SUPPLIED
Cre: 1% [30g, 60g, 100g]

CONTRAINDICATIONS
History of hypersensitivity to pimecrolimus or any components of the medication.

WARNINGS/PRECAUTIONS
Avoid with malignant or premalignant skin conditions, Netherton's syndrome, or other skin diseases that may increase the potential for systemic absorption. Avoid in immunocompromised patients. May cause local symptoms, such as skin burning or pruritus, and may improve as the lesions of atopic dermatitis resolve. Resolve bacterial or viral infections at treatment sites before starting treatment. Increased risk of varicella zoster and herpes simplex virus infection, or eczema herpeticum. Skin papilloma/warts reported; consider discontinuation until complete resolution is achieved if skin papillomas worsen or do not respond to conventional therapy. Lymphadenopathy reported; d/c if lymphadenopathy of uncertain etiology or in the presence of acute infectious mononucleosis. Minimize or avoid natural or artificial sunlight exposure during treatment.

ADVERSE REACTIONS
Application-site burning, application-site reaction, influenza, nasopharyngitis, headache, URTI, sore throat, hypersensitivity, cough, pyrexia, N/V, skin infection, abdominal pain.

DRUG INTERACTIONS
Caution with CYP3A4 inhibitors (eg, erythromycin, ketoconazole, calcium channel blockers) in patients with widespread and/or erythrodermic disease.

PREGNANCY AND LACTATION
Category C, not for use in nursing.

MECHANISM OF ACTION
Macrolactam ascomycin derivative; not established. Demonstrated to bind with high affinity to macrophilin-12 (FKBP-12) and inhibit the Ca^{2+}-dependent phosphatase, calcineurin. Consequently, it inhibits T-cell activation by blocking the transcription of early cytokines. Prevents the release of inflammatory cytokines and mediators from mast cells in vitro after stimulation by antigen/IgE.

PHARMACOKINETICS
Absorption: C_{max}=1.4ng/mL (adults). **Distribution:** Plasma protein binding (99.5%). **Metabolism:** Liver via CYP3A; O-demethylation (metabolites). **Elimination:** Feces (78.4% metabolites, <1% unchanged).

PATIENT CONSIDERATIONS
Assessment: Assess for malignant or premalignant skin conditions, Netherton's syndrome, or other skin diseases that may increase the potential for systemic absorption, immunocompromised state, viral/bacterial skin infections, pregnancy/nursing status, and possible drug interactions.

Monitoring: Monitor for varicella virus infection, herpes simplex virus infection, eczema herpeticum, skin papilloma/warts, lymphomas, lymphadenopathy, skin malignancies, local symptoms, and other adverse reactions.

Counseling: Instruct to use ud. Inform not to use continuously for a long time and to use only on areas of skin with eczema. Instruct not to use sun lamps, tanning beds, or get treatment with UV light therapy. Advise to limit sun exposure, wear loose fitting clothing that protects the treated area from the sun, and not to cover treated skin area with bandages, dressings, or wraps. Inform that the medication is for use on the skin only; instruct to avoid contact with eyes, nose, mouth, vagina, or rectum (mucous membranes). Instruct to wash hands and dry skin before applying cre and not to bathe, shower, or swim after application.

ELIGARD — leuprolide acetate   Rx
Class: Synthetic gonadotropin-releasing hormone (GnRH) analogue

ADULT DOSAGE	PEDIATRIC DOSAGE
Advanced Prostate Cancer	Pediatric use may not have been established
Palliative Treatment:	
7.5mg: 1 inj every month	
22.5mg: 1 inj every 3 months	
30mg: 1 inj every 4 months	
45mg: 1 inj every 6 months	

ADMINISTRATION
SQ route

Inj site should vary periodically; avoid areas w/ brawny or fibrous SQ tissue or locations that could be rubbed or compressed (eg, w/ a belt or clothing waistband). Use gloves during mixing and administration.
Allow the product to reach room temperature before mixing.
Once mixed, administer w/in 30 min; refer to PI for mixing procedure.

Administration Procedure
1. Choose an inj site on the abdomen, upper buttocks, or anywhere w/ adequate amounts of SQ tissue that does not have excessive pigment, nodules, lesions, or hair; choose an area that has not recently been used.
2. Cleanse the inj-site area w/ an alcohol swab.
3. Using the thumb and forefinger of your non-dominant hand, grab and bunch the area of skin around the inj site.
4. Using your dominant hand, insert the needle quickly at a 90° angle to the skin surface; after the needle is inserted, release the skin w/ your non-dominant hand.

5. Inject the drug using a slow, steady push. Press down on the plunger until the syringe is empty.
6. Withdraw the needle quickly at the same 90° angle used for insertion.
7. Immediately following the withdrawal of the needle, activate the safety shield on the needle.

STORAGE
2-8°C (35.6-46.4°F). Once outside the refrigerator, store in its original packaging at 15-30°C (59-86°F) for up to 8 weeks prior to mixing and administration.

HOW SUPPLIED
Inj: 7.5mg, 22.5mg, 30mg, 45mg

CONTRAINDICATIONS
Patients w/ hypersensitivity to GnRH, GnRH agonist analogues, or any of the components of the medication. Women who are or may become pregnant.

WARNINGS/PRECAUTIONS
Transient increase in serum concentrations of testosterone and worsening of symptoms or onset of new signs/symptoms (eg, bone pain, neuropathy, hematuria) during the 1st few weeks of therapy may occur. Cases of ureteral obstruction and/or spinal cord compression reported; institute standard treatment if these complications occur. Closely monitor patients w/ metastatic vertebral lesions and/or urinary tract obstruction during 1st few weeks of therapy. Suppresses pituitary-gonadal system; may affect results of diagnostic tests of pituitary gonadotropic and gonadal functions conducted during and after therapy. Hyperglycemia and increased risk of developing diabetes, MI, sudden cardiac death, and stroke reported. May prolong QT/QTc interval; consider whether the benefits outweigh the potential risks in patients w/ congenital long QT syndrome, CHF, frequent electrolyte abnormalities, and in patients taking drugs known to prolong the QT interval.

ADVERSE REACTIONS
Hot flashes/sweats, inj-site reactions (eg, transient burning/stinging, pain, erythema), malaise/fatigue, testicular atrophy, weakness, gynecomastia, myalgia, arthralgia, dizziness, decreased libido, clamminess, night sweats, nausea.

PREGNANCY AND LACTATION
Pregnancy: Category X.
Lactation: Not for use in nursing.

MECHANISM OF ACTION
Synthetic GnRH analogue; acts as a potent inhibitor of gonadotropin secretion when given continuously.

PHARMACOKINETICS
Absorption: Administration of variable doses resulted in different parameters. **Distribution:** (IV bolus dose) V_d=27L; plasma protein binding (43-49%). **Metabolism:** Pentapeptide (M-1) metabolite (major metabolite). **Elimination:** (1mg IV bolus dose) $T_{1/2}$=3 hrs.

PATIENT CONSIDERATIONS
Assessment: Assess for hypersensitivity to drug, metastatic vertebral lesions, urinary tract obstructions, congenital long QT syndrome, CHF, electrolyte abnormalities, and diabetes mellitus. Obtain baseline serum testosterone levels and prostate specific antigen (PSA) levels. Obtain baseline blood glucose and/or HbA1c levels. Correct electrolyte abnormalities.

Monitoring: Monitor for worsening/occurrence of signs/symptoms of prostate cancer, spinal cord compression, ureteral obstruction, signs/symptoms suggestive of cardiovascular disease development, and other adverse reactions. Periodically monitor blood glucose, HbA1c, testosterone, and PSA levels. Consider periodic monitoring of ECG and electrolytes.

Counseling: Inform that hot flashes may be experienced. Advise that increased bone pain, difficulty in urinating, and onset or aggravation of weakness or paralysis may be experienced during the 1st few weeks of therapy. Instruct to notify physician if new or worsened symptoms develop after beginning treatment. Inform about inj-site related adverse reactions (eg, transient burning/stinging, pain, bruising, redness); instruct to notify physician if such reactions do not resolve. Advise to contact physician immediately if an allergic reaction develops.

ELIMITE — permethrin   Rx
Class: Pyrethroid scabicidal agent

ADULT DOSAGE	PEDIATRIC DOSAGE
Scabies	**Scabies**
Infestation w/ *Sarcoptes scabiei*:	**Infestation w/ *Sarcoptes scabiei*:**
Thoroughly massage into skin from head to soles of feet; remove by washing after 8-14 hrs	**≥2 Months of Age:**
One application is generally curative; retreat if living mites present after 14 days	Thoroughly massage into skin from head to soles of feet (scalp, temple and forehead on infants); remove by washing after 8-14 hrs
Usually 30g is sufficient for an average adult	One application is generally curative; retreat if living mites present after 14 days

ADMINISTRATION
Topical route

STORAGE
20-25°C (68-77°F).

HOW SUPPLIED
Cre: 5% [60g]

WARNINGS/PRECAUTIONS
D/C if hypersensitivity occurs. Scabies infestation is often accompanied by pruritus, edema, and erythema; treatment may temporarily exacerbate these conditions.

ADVERSE REACTIONS
Burning, stinging, pruritus.

PREGNANCY AND LACTATION
Category B, not for use in nursing.

MECHANISM OF ACTION
Pyrethroid scabicidal agent; acts on the nerve cell membrane to disrupt the Na^+ channel current by which the polarization of the membrane is regulated. This disturbance results in delayed repolarization and paralysis of pests.

PHARMACOKINETICS
Metabolism: Rapid via ester hydrolysis. **Elimination:** Urine.

PATIENT CONSIDERATIONS

Assessment: Assess for previous hypersensitivity to the drug or any synthetic pyrethroid or pyrethrin, and pregnancy/nursing status.

Monitoring: Monitor for hypersensitivity, exacerbation of pruritus, edema, or erythema, and other adverse reactions.

Counseling: Inform that itching, mild burning, and/or stinging may occur after application; instruct to consult physician if irritation persists. Advise to avoid contact with eyes during application and to flush with water immediately if medication gets in the eyes.

ELIQUIS — apixaban   Rx
Class: Selective factor Xa inhibitor

> Premature discontinuation increases the risk of thrombotic events. If therapy is discontinued for a reason other than pathological bleeding or completion of a course of therapy, consider coverage w/ another anticoagulant. Epidural or spinal hematomas may occur in patients treated w/ apixaban who are receiving neuraxial anesthesia or undergoing spinal puncture; long-term or permanent paralysis may result. Increased risk of developing epidural/spinal hematomas w/ the use of indwelling epidural catheters, concomitant use of other drugs that affect hemostasis, (eg, NSAIDs, platelet inhibitors, other anticoagulants), history of traumatic or repeated epidural or spinal punctures, history of spinal deformity or spinal surgery, and when optimal timing between the administration of apixaban and neuraxial procedure is not known. Monitor frequently for signs/symptoms of neurologic impairment; urgent treatment is necessary if neurologic compromise is noted. Consider benefits and risks before neuraxial intervention in patients anticoagulated or to be anticoagulated.

ADULT DOSAGE

Reduce Risk of Stroke and Systemic Embolism in Nonvalvular Atrial Fibrillation
5mg bid

Patients w/ at Least 2 of the Following Characteristics:
≥80 Years, ≤60kg, or SrCr ≥1.5mg/dL:
2.5mg bid

Deep Vein Thrombosis/Pulmonary Embolism

Deep Vein Thrombosis (DVT) Prophylaxis Following Hip/Knee Replacement Surgery:
2.5mg bid; give initial dose 12-24 hrs after surgery

Duration:
Hip Replacement Surgery: 35 days
Knee Replacement Surgery: 12 days

DVT/Pulmonary Embolism (PE) Treatment:
10mg bid for the first 7 days, followed by 5mg bid

Risk Reduction of Recurrent DVT/PE:
2.5mg bid after at least 6 months of treatment for DVT/PE

Conversions

Switching from Warfarin:
D/C warfarin and start apixaban when INR <2.0

Switching to Warfarin:
D/C apixaban and begin both a parenteral anticoagulant and warfarin at the time the next dose of apixaban would have been taken; d/c parenteral anticoagulant when INR reaches an acceptable range

Switching from Anticoagulants Other Than Warfarin (Oral or Parenteral):
D/C the anticoagulant and begin apixaban at the usual time of the next dose of the anticoagulant

PEDIATRIC DOSAGE
Pediatric use may not have been established

Switching to Anticoagulants Other Than Warfarin (Oral or Parenteral):
D/C apixaban and begin the new anticoagulant at the usual time of the next dose of apixaban

---

DOSING CONSIDERATIONS
Concomitant Medications
Strong Dual CYP3A4 and P-gp Inhibitors (eg, Ketoconazole, Itraconazole, Ritonavir):
For patients receiving apixaban doses of 5mg or 10mg bid, reduce apixaban dose by 50%; if already taking 2.5mg bid, avoid coadministration w/ strong dual inhibitors of CYP3A4 and P-gp

Hepatic Impairment
Severe (Child-Pugh Class C): Not recommended

Other Important Considerations
Temporary Interruption for Surgery and Other Interventions:
D/C at least 48 hrs prior to elective surgery or invasive procedures w/ a moderate/high risk of unacceptable/clinically significant bleeding, or at least 24 hrs prior w/ a low risk of bleeding or where bleeding would be noncritical in location and easily controlled. Bridging anticoagulation during the 24-48 hrs after discontinuing therapy and prior to the intervention is not generally required. Restart therapy after the surgical or other procedures as soon as adequate hemostasis has been established

ADMINISTRATION
Oral route

Patients Unable to Swallow Tabs Whole
Tabs may be crushed and suspended in 60mL D5W and immediately delivered through a NG tube.

STORAGE
20-25°C (68-77°F); excursions permitted to 15-30°C (59-86°F).

HOW SUPPLIED
Tab: 2.5mg, 5mg

CONTRAINDICATIONS
Active pathological bleeding, severe hypersensitivity reaction to apixaban (eg, anaphylactic reactions).

WARNINGS/PRECAUTIONS
Not recommended in patients w/ prosthetic heart valves. Increases the risk of bleeding and may cause serious, potentially fatal, bleeding; d/c in patients w/ active pathological hemorrhage. Specific antidote for apixaban is not available; activated oral charcoal reduces apixaban absorption. In patients who receive both apixaban and neuraxial anesthesia, removal of indwelling epidural or intrathecal catheters should not be earlier than 24 hrs after the last administration of apixaban; next dose of apixaban should not be administered earlier than 5 hrs after the removal of the catheter. If traumatic spinal/epidural puncture occurs, delay administration of apixaban for 48 hrs. Initiation of apixaban is not recommended as an alternative to unfractionated heparin for the initial treatment of patients w/ PE who present w/ hemodynamic instability or who may receive thrombolysis or pulmonary embolectomy.

ADVERSE REACTIONS
Bleeding.

DRUG INTERACTIONS
See Boxed Warning and Dosing Considerations. CYP3A4 and P-gp inhibitors increase exposure and increase the risk of bleeding. CYP3A4 and P-gp inducers decrease exposure and increase the risk of stroke and other thromboembolic events. Avoid w/ strong dual inducers of CYP3A4 and P-gp (eg, rifampin, carbamazepine, phenytoin, St. John's wort). Increased risk of bleeding w/ drugs affecting hemostasis, including aspirin (ASA) and other antiplatelet agents, other anticoagulants, heparin, thrombolytics, SSRIs, SNRIs, NSAIDs, and fibrinolytics.

PREGNANCY AND LACTATION
Pregnancy: Category B.
Lactation: Not for use in nursing.

MECHANISM OF ACTION
Selective factor Xa (FXa) inhibitor; inhibits free and clot-bound FXa and prothrombinase activity. Has no direct effect on platelet aggregation, but indirectly inhibits platelet aggregation induced by thrombin. By inhibiting FXa, apixaban decreases thrombin generation and thrombus development. Does not require antithrombin III for antithrombotic activity.

PHARMACOKINETICS
Absorption: Absolute bioavailability (approx 50% for doses up to 10mg); T_{max}=3-4 hrs. **Distribution:** V_d=21L; plasma protein binding (approx 87%). **Metabolism:** O-demethylation and hydroxylation mainly via CYP3A4, w/ mild contributions from CYP1A2, 2C8, 2C9, 2C19, and 2J2. **Elimination:** Urine and feces (25% as metabolites); $T_{1/2}$=12 hrs.

PATIENT CONSIDERATIONS
Assessment: Assess for drug hypersensitivity, active pathological bleeding, prosthetic heart valves, PE w/ hemodynamic instability or in patients who may receive thrombolysis or pulmonary embolectomy, hepatic/renal impairment, pregnancy/nursing status, and possible drug interactions.

Monitoring: Monitor for active pathological hemorrhage and other adverse reactions. Monitor for thrombotic events in patients discontinuing therapy. In patients undergoing neuraxial anesthesia or spinal puncture, monitor for epidural or spinal hematomas and neurological impairment.

Counseling: Instruct not to d/c w/o consulting physician. Inform that it may take longer than usual for bleeding to stop, and that bruising/bleeding may occur more easily. Advise on how to recognize bleeding/symptoms of hypovolemia and of the urgent need to report any unusual bleeding to physician. Instruct to inform physicians and dentists of apixaban use, and/or any other product known to affect bleeding (eg, ASA or NSAIDs), before any surgery/medical/dental procedure is scheduled and before any new drug is taken. Advise patients having neuraxial anesthesia or spinal puncture to watch for signs/symptoms of spinal/epidural hematomas (eg, numbness, weakness of legs, bowel/bladder dysfunction); instruct to contact physician immediately if symptoms occur. Advise to inform physician if pregnant/planning to become pregnant, or if breastfeeding/intending to breastfeed during treatment. If a dose is missed, instruct to take it as soon as possible on the same day and that bid administration should be resumed; instruct not to double the dose to make up for a missed dose.

ELLA — ulipristal acetate   Rx

Class: Emergency contraceptive kit

ADULT DOSAGE **Emergency Contraception**	**PEDIATRIC DOSAGE** **Emergency Contraception**
1 tab as soon as possible w/in 120 hrs (5 days) after unprotected intercourse or a known or suspected contraceptive failure Consider repeating the dose if vomiting occurs w/in 3 hrs of intake	**Postpubertal:** 1 tab as soon as possible w/in 120 hrs (5 days) after unprotected intercourse or a known or suspected contraceptive failure Consider repeating the dose if vomiting occurs w/in 3 hrs of intake

---

ADMINISTRATION
Oral route
Can be taken at any time during the menstrual cycle, w/ or w/o food

STORAGE
20-25°C (68-77°F). Keep blister in the outer carton to protect from light.

HOW SUPPLIED
Tab: 30mg

CONTRAINDICATIONS
Known or suspected pregnancy.

WARNINGS/PRECAUTIONS
Not for routine use as a contraceptive. Not indicated for termination of existing pregnancy. Exclude pregnancy prior to prescribing; perform pregnancy test if pregnancy cannot be excluded based on history and/or physical examination. Consider possibility of ectopic pregnancy if lower abdominal pain or pregnancy occurs following use. Repeated use within the same menstrual cycle is not recommended. Rapid return of fertility may occur following treatment; continue or initiate routine contraception as soon as possible following use. After intake, menses sometimes occur earlier or later than expected by a few days; rule out pregnancy if there is a delay in the onset of expected menses beyond 1 week. Intermenstrual bleeding reported. Does not protect against HIV infection (AIDS) or other sexually transmitted infections.

ADVERSE REACTIONS
Headache, abdominal/upper abdominal pain, nausea, dysmenorrhea, fatigue, dizziness.

DRUG INTERACTIONS
Drugs or herbal products that induce CYP3A4 (eg, barbiturates, carbamazepine, St. John's wort) decrease plasma concentrations and may decrease effectiveness; avoid coadministration. CYP3A4 inhibitors (eg, itraconazole, ketoconazole) may increase plasma concentrations. May reduce contraceptive action of regular hormonal contraceptive methods. May increase the concentration of P-glycoprotein (P-gp) substrates (eg, dabigatran etexilate, digoxin) due to inhibition of P-gp at clinically relevant concentrations.

PREGNANCY AND LACTATION
Category X, not for use in nursing.

MECHANISM OF ACTION
Emergency contraceptive kit; synthetic progesterone agonist/antagonist. Postpones follicular rupture when taken immediately before ovulation. Likely primary mechanism of action is inhibition or delay of ovulation; alterations to endometrium that may affect implantation may also contribute to efficacy.

PHARMACOKINETICS
Absorption: (Fasted) C_{max}=176ng/mL, 69ng/mL (monodemethyl-ulipristal acetate); T_{max} (median)=0.9 hr, 1 hr (monodemethyl-ulipristal acetate); AUC_{0-t} =548ng•hr/mL, 240ng•hr/mL (monodemethyl-ulipristal acetate); AUC_{0-inf} =556ng•hr/mL, 246ng•hr/mL (monodemethyl-ulipristal acetate). **Distribution:** Plasma protein binding (>94%); found in breast milk. **Metabolism:** CYP3A4; monodemethyl-ulipristal acetate (active metabolite). **Elimination:** $T_{1/2}$=32.4 hrs, 27 hrs (monodemethyl-ulipristal acetate).

PATIENT CONSIDERATIONS

Assessment: Assess pregnancy/nursing status and for possible drug interactions.

Monitoring: Monitor for ectopic pregnancy and effect on menstrual cycle. Perform follow-up physical/pelvic examination if in doubt concerning general health or pregnancy status.

Counseling: Instruct to take as soon as possible and not >120 hrs after unprotected intercourse or a known or suspected contraceptive failure. Advise not to take if pregnancy is known or suspected and that drug is not indicated for termination of an existing pregnancy. Advise to contact physician immediately if vomiting occurs within 3 hrs of intake, if period is delayed after taking the drug by >1 week beyond expected date, or if experiencing severe lower abdominal pain 3-5 weeks after use. Advise not to use as routine contraception or repeatedly in the same menstrual cycle. Inform that therapy may reduce contraceptive action of regular hormonal contraceptive methods and to use a reliable barrier method of contraception after using medication, for any subsequent acts of intercourse that occur in that same menstrual cycle. Inform that drug does not protect against HIV infection (AIDS) and other sexually transmitted diseases/infections. Instruct not to use if breastfeeding.

ELMIRON — pentosan polysulfate sodium   Rx

Class: Urinary tract analgesic

ADULT DOSAGE **Interstitial Cystitis**	**PEDIATRIC DOSAGE** **Interstitial Cystitis**
Bladder Pain/Discomfort: 100mg tid Reassess patient after 3 months; may continue for another 3 months if no improvement and no limiting adverse events	**Bladder Pain/Discomfort:** **≥16 Years:** 100mg tid Reassess patient after 3 months; may continue for another 3 months if no improvement and no limiting adverse events

---

ADMINISTRATION
Oral route
Take with water ≥1 hr ac or 2 hrs pc

STORAGE
15-30°C (59-86°F).

HOW SUPPLIED
Cap: 100mg

CONTRAINDICATIONS
Known hypersensitivity to the drug, structurally related compounds, or excipients.

WARNINGS/PRECAUTIONS
Rectal hemorrhage, bleeding complications of ecchymosis, epistaxis, gum hemorrhage, and alopecia reported. Evaluate patients undergoing invasive procedures or having signs/symptoms of underlying coagulopathy for hemorrhage. Evaluate patients with aneurysms, thrombocytopenia, hemophilia, GI ulcers, polyps, or diverticula prior to therapy. Caution with history of heparin-induced thrombocytopenia and hepatic impairment. Mildly elevated transaminase, alkaline phosphatase, GGT, and lactic dehydrogenase, and increases in PTT and PT, or thrombocytopenia reported.

ADVERSE REACTIONS
Nausea, diarrhea, alopecia, headache, rash, rectal hemorrhage.

DRUG INTERACTIONS
Coumarin anticoagulants, heparin, tissue plasminogen activator, streptokinase, high-dose aspirin, or NSAIDs may increase risk of bleeding; evaluate for hemorrhage.

PREGNANCY AND LACTATION
Category B, caution in nursing.

MECHANISM OF ACTION
Urinary tract analgesic; has not been established. May act as a buffer in bladder wall mucosal membrane to control cell permeability, preventing irritating solutes in the urine from reaching cells.

PHARMACOKINETICS
Absorption: Bioavailability (6%); T_{max}=0.6-120 hrs. **Metabolism:** Liver and spleen, by partial desulfation; kidney, by partial depolymerization. **Elimination:** Feces [84%, unchanged (300mg); 58%, unchanged (450mg)], urine (6%, mostly as desulfated/depolymerized metabolites; 0.14%, intact); $T_{1/2}$=27 hrs (300mg), 20 hrs (450mg).

PATIENT CONSIDERATIONS

Assessment: Assess for increased risk of bleeding, aneurysms, thrombocytopenia, hemophilia, GI ulcers, polyps, diverticula, history of heparin-induced thrombocytopenia, hepatic impairment, hypersensitivity to drug, pregnancy/nursing status, and possible drug interactions.

Monitoring: Monitor for improvement, bleeding complications, and other adverse reactions.

Counseling: Instruct to take drug as prescribed and no more frequently than prescribed. Inform that drug has a weak anticoagulant effect which may increase bleeding time.

ELOXATIN — oxaliplatin   Rx
Class: Platinum analogue

> Anaphylactic reactions reported, and may occur w/in min of administration. Epinephrine, corticosteroids, and antihistamines have been employed to alleviate symptoms of anaphylaxis.

ADULT DOSAGE
Colon Cancer

Stage III:

In combination w/ 5-fluorouracil (5-FU)/leucovorin (LV) for adjuvant treatment in patients who have undergone complete resection of the primary tumor

Day 1: Oxaliplatin 85mg/m² IV infusion + LV 200mg/m² IV infusion; both given over 120 min at the same time in separate bags using a Y-line, followed by 5-FU 400mg/m² IV bolus given over 2-4 min, followed by 5-FU 600mg/m² IV infusion as a 22-hr continuous infusion

Day 2: LV 200 mg/m² IV infusion over 120 min, followed by 5-FU 400mg/m² IV bolus given over 2-4 min, followed by 5-FU 600 mg/m² IV infusion as a 22-hr continuous infusion

Administer every 2 weeks; treatment is recommended for a total of 6 months (12 cycles)

Advanced Colorectal Cancer

Combination w/ 5-FU/LV:
Day 1: Oxaliplatin 85mg/m² IV infusion + LV 200mg/m² IV infusion; both given over 120 min at the same time in separate bags using a Y-line, followed by 5-FU 400mg/m² IV bolus given over 2-4 min, followed by 5-FU 600mg/m² IV infusion as a 22-hr continuous infusion

Day 2: LV 200 mg/m² IV infusion over 120 min, followed by 5-FU 400mg/m² IV bolus given over 2-4 min, followed by 5-FU 600 mg/m² IV infusion as a 22-hr continuous infusion

Administer every 2 weeks. Continue treatment until disease progression or unacceptable toxicity

Premedication
Antiemetics, including 5-HT₃ blockers w/ or w/o dexamethasone, are recommended

PEDIATRIC DOSAGE
Pediatric use may not have been established

DOSING CONSIDERATIONS
Renal Impairment
Severe:
Initial: 65mg/m²

Adverse Reactions
Adjuvant Therapy in Stage III Colon Cancer:
Persistent Grade 2 Neurosensory Events That Do Not Resolve:
Consider reducing dose to 75mg/m²; 5-FU/LV regimen need not be altered
Persistent Grade 3 Neurosensory Events:
Consider discontinuing; 5-FU/LV regimen need not be altered
After Recovery from Grade 3/4 GI (Despite Prophylactic Treatment), or Grade 4 Neutropenia, or Febrile Neutropenia, or Grade 3/4 Thrombocytopenia:
Reduce oxaliplatin dose to 75mg/m² and 5-FU to 300mg/m² bolus and 500mg/m² 22-hr infusion; delay next dose until neutrophils ≥1.5 x 10⁹/L and platelets ≥75 x 10⁹/L
Advanced Colorectal Cancer (Previously Treated/Untreated):
Persistent Grade 2 Neurosensory Events That Do Not Resolve:
Consider reducing dose to 65mg/m²; 5-FU/LV regimen need not be altered
Persistent Grade 3 Neurosensory Events:
Consider discontinuing therapy; 5-FU/LV regimen need not be altered
After Recovery from Grade 3/4 GI (Despite Prophylactic Treatment), or Grade 4 Neutropenia, or Febrile Neutropenia, or Grade 3/4 Thrombocytopenia:
Reduce oxaliplatin dose to 65mg/m² and 5-FU by 20% (300mg/m² bolus and 500mg/m² 22-hr infusion); delay next dose until neutrophils ≥1.5 x 10⁹/L and platelets ≥75 x 10⁹/L

ADMINISTRATION
IV route

Incompatible in sol w/ alkaline medications or media (eg, basic sol of 5-FU); do not mix w/ these or administer simultaneously through the same infusion line. Flush the infusion line w/ D5 inj prior to administration of any concomitant medication.

Do not use needles or IV administration sets containing aluminum parts to prepare or mix the drug; aluminum has been reported to cause degradation of platinum compounds.
Prolongation of infusion time for oxaliplatin from 2 hrs to 6 hrs may mitigate acute toxicities; infusion times for 5-FU and LV do not need to be changed.

Preparation of Infusion Sol
The sol must be further diluted in an infusion sol of 250-500mL of D5 inj; never perform a final dilution w/ a NaCl sol or other Cl⁻ containing sol.
After dilution, the shelf life is 6 hrs at 20-25°C (68-77°F) or up to 24 hrs at 2-8°C (36-46°F).
After final dilution, protection from light is not required.

STORAGE
25°C (77°F); excursions permitted to 15-30°C (59-86°F). Do not freeze and protect from light (keep in original outer carton).

HOW SUPPLIED
Inj: 5mg/mL [50mg, 100mg]

CONTRAINDICATIONS
History of known allergy to oxaliplatin or other platinum compounds.

WARNINGS/PRECAUTIONS
Should be administered under the supervision of a physician experienced in the use of cancer chemotherapeutic agents. An early onset, acute, reversible, primarily peripheral, sensory neuropathy and a persistent (>14 days), primarily peripheral, sensory neuropathy, reported. Cold temperature/objects may precipitate or exacerbate acute neurological symptoms; avoid ice for mucositis prophylaxis during infusion. Reversible posterior leukoencephalopathy syndrome (RPLS), also known as posterior reversible encephalopathy syndrome (PRES), reported. Grade 3 or 4 neutropenia reported in patients w/ colorectal cancer treated w/ oxaliplatin in combination w/ 5-FU and LV. Sepsis, neutropenic sepsis, and septic shock reported; withhold oxaliplatin for sepsis or septic shock. Potentially fatal pulmonary fibrosis reported. If unexplained respiratory symptoms develop, d/c until further pulmonary investigation excludes interstitial lung disease or pulmonary fibrosis. Hepatotoxicity observed; consider hepatic vascular disorders, and if appropriate, investigate in case of abnormal LFT results or portal HTN, which cannot be explained by liver metastases. QT prolongation and ventricular arrhythmias including fatal torsades de pointes reported; correct hypokalemia or hypomagnesemia prior to initiating therapy and monitor these electrolytes periodically during therapy. Avoid in patients w/ congenital long QT syndrome. ECG monitoring is recommended if therapy is initiated in patients w/ CHF, bradyarrhythmias, drugs known to prolong the QT interval (eg, Class Ia and III antiarrhythmics), and electrolyte abnormalities. Rhabdomyolysis, including fatal cases reported; d/c if any signs/symptoms of rhabdomyolysis occur. May cause fetal harm. Caution w/ renal impairment.

ADVERSE REACTIONS
Peripheral sensory neuropathy, neutropenia, thrombocytopenia, anemia, N/V, increased transaminases/alkaline phosphatase, diarrhea, fatigue, stomatitis, abdominal pain, fever, skin disorder, anorexia, dyspnea.

DRUG INTERACTIONS
Increased 5-FU plasma levels reported w/ doses of 130mg/m² oxaliplatin dosed every 3 weeks. Potentially nephrotoxic agents may decrease clearance. Prolonged PT and INR occasionally associated w/ hemorrhage reported in patients who concomitantly received oxaliplatin plus 5-FU/LV and anticoagulants; monitor patients requiring oral anticoagulants closely.

PREGNANCY AND LACTATION
Pregnancy: Category D.
Lactation: Not for use in nursing.

MECHANISM OF ACTION
Organoplatinum complex; inhibits deoxyribonucleic acid replication and transcription.

PHARMACOKINETICS
Absorption: C_{max}=0.814mcg/mL. **Distribution:** V_d=440L; plasma protein binding (>90%). **Metabolism:** Rapid, extensive nonenzymatic biotransformation. **Elimination:** Urine (54%), feces (2%); $T_{1/2}$=391 hrs.

PATIENT CONSIDERATIONS

Assessment: Assess for history of known allergy to the drug or other platinum compounds, renal impairment, congenital long QT syndrome, hypokalemia, hypomagnesemia, pregnancy/nursing status, and possible drug interactions. Assess LFTs, WBC count w/ differential, Hgb, platelet count, and blood chemistries before each cycle.

Monitoring: Monitor for signs/symptoms of anaphylactic reactions, neurosensory toxicity, pulmonary toxicity, hepatotoxicity, RPLS, neutropenia, sepsis, septic shock, QT prolongation, ventricular arrhythmias, rhabdomyolysis, and other adverse reactions. Monitor patients w/ renal impairment closely and monitor patients requiring oral anticoagulants closely. Monitor Mg²⁺ and K⁺ levels periodically. Perform ECG monitoring in patients w/ CHF, bradyarrhythmias, patients taking drugs known to prolong the QT interval, and in patients w/ electrolyte abnormalities.

Counseling: Inform of pregnancy risks. Advise to expect side effects, particularly neurologic effects, both the acute, reversible effects and the persistent neurosensory toxicity. Inform that acute neurosensory toxicity may be precipitated or exacerbated by exposure to cold or cold objects. Instruct to avoid cold drinks and ice, and to cover exposed skin prior to exposure to cold temperature or cold objects. Inform of the risk of low blood cell counts and to contact physician immediately if fever, particularly if associated w/ persistent diarrhea, or evidence of infection develops. Advise to contact physician if persistent vomiting, diarrhea, fever, signs of dehydration, cough or breathing difficulties, or signs of an allergic reaction occur. Advise of the potential effects of vision abnormalities; instruct to use caution when driving and using machines.

EMBEDA — morphine sulfate/naltrexone hydrochloride

CII

Class: Opioid agonist/opioid antagonist

Exposes users to risks of addiction, abuse, and misuse, which can lead to overdose and death; assess each patient's risk prior to prescribing, and monitor regularly for development of these behaviors/conditions. Serious, life-threatening, or fatal respiratory depression may occur; monitor for respiratory depression, especially during initiation or following a dose increase. Swallow cap whole, or sprinkle contents of cap on applesauce and swallow immediately w/o chewing; crushing, chewing, or dissolving cap can cause rapid release and absorption of potentially fatal dose of morphine. Accidental ingestion, especially in children, can result in a fatal overdose. Prolonged use during pregnancy can result in neonatal opioid withdrawal syndrome, which may be life threatening if not recognized and treated; advise pregnant women of the risk and ensure availability of appropriate treatment. Avoid alcohol consumption or medication that contains alcohol; may result in increased plasma levels and a potentially fatal overdose of morphine.

ADULT DOSAGE

Severe Pain (Daily, Around-the-Clock Management)

Management of Pain Severe Enough to Require Daily, Around-the-Clock, Long-Term Opioid Treatment and for Which Alternative Treatment Options are Inadequate:

Initial:
1st Opioid Analgesic/Not Opioid Tolerant: 20mg/0.8mg q24h

Titration and Maint:
May adjust dose every 1-2 days
Breakthrough pain may require a dose increase or may need a rescue medication w/ an appropriate dose of an immediate-release analgesic
If experiencing inadequate analgesia w/ qd dosing, consider bid regimen
Adjust dose to obtain appropriate balance between management of pain and opioid-related adverse reactions

Discontinuation:
Gradually titrate dose downward every 2-4 days

Conversions

Conversion from Other Opioids:
30mg q24h; d/c all other around-the-clock opioids when therapy is initiated
Conversion from Other Oral Morphine Formulations: Give 1/2 of total daily oral morphine dose as morphine sulfate/naltrexone bid or total daily oral morphine dose as morphine sulfate/naltrexone qd
Conversion from Parenteral Morphine: 2-6mg of oral morphine may be required to provide analgesia equivalent to 1mg of parenteral morphine; a dose of oral morphine that is 3X the daily parenteral morphine requirement is typically sufficient
Conversion from Other Oral/Parenteral Opioids: Specific recommendations are not available because of a lack of systematic evidence for these types of analgesic substitutions. In general, begin w/ 1/2 of estimated daily morphine requirement; manage inadequate analgesia by supplementation w/ immediate-release morphine
Conversion from Methadone: May give 1st dose w/ the last dose of any immediate-release opioid

PEDIATRIC DOSAGE
Pediatric use may not have been established

DOSING CONSIDERATIONS
Adverse Reactions
Unacceptable Opioid-Related Reactions:
Reduce subsequent doses
ADMINISTRATION
Oral route
Administer either qd (q24h) or bid (q12h)
Swallow caps whole or sprinkle contents on applesauce and then swallow immediately w/o chewing; rinse mouth to ensure all pellets have been swallowed
Do not crush, chew, or dissolve pellets in the cap
Do not administer pellets through a NG or gastric tube
STORAGE
25°C (77°F); excursion permitted between 15-30°C (59-86°F).

HOW SUPPLIED
Cap, Extended-Release: (Morphine/Naltrexone) 20mg/0.8mg, 30mg/1.2mg, 50mg/2mg, 60mg/2.4mg, 80mg/3.2mg, 100mg/4mg
CONTRAINDICATIONS
Significant respiratory depression, acute or severe bronchial asthma in an unmonitored setting or in the absence of resuscitative equipment, known or suspected paralytic ileus. Hypersensitivity (eg, anaphylaxis) to morphine or naltrexone.
WARNINGS/PRECAUTIONS
Reserve for use in patients for whom alternative treatment options are ineffective, not tolerated, or would be otherwise inadequate to provide sufficient management of pain. Not for use as prn analgesic. 100mg/4mg caps are only for use in opioid-tolerant patients. Life-threatening respiratory depression is more likely to occur in elderly, cachectic, or debilitated patients. May decrease respiratory drive to the point of apnea in patients w/ significant COPD or cor pulmonale, and patients having a substantially decreased respiratory reserve, hypoxia, hypercapnia, or preexisting respiratory depression; monitor during initiation/titration and consider if possible, alternative nonopioid analgesics. May cause severe hypotension including orthostatic hypotension and syncope in ambulatory patients; increased risk in patients whose ability to maintain BP has already been compromised by a reduced blood volume or concurrent administration of certain CNS depressants. May cause vasodilation that can further reduce cardiac output and BP; avoid use in patients w/ circulatory shock. Monitor for signs of sedation and respiratory depression, particularly when initiating therapy, in patients who may be susceptible to the intracranial effects of carbon dioxide retention (eg, those w/ evidence of increased intracranial pressure or brain tumors). May obscure clinical course in a patient w/ head injury. Avoid w/ impaired consciousness, coma, or GI obstruction. May cause spasm of the sphincter of Oddi; monitor for worsening of symptoms in patients w/ biliary tract disease, including acute pancreatitis. May cause increases in serum amylase. May aggravate convulsions in patients w/ convulsive disorders and may induce/aggravate seizures. Consuming caps altered by crushing, chewing, or dissolving the pellets may release sufficient naltrexone to precipitate withdrawal in opioid-dependent individuals. May impair mental/physical abilities.
ADVERSE REACTIONS
Respiratory depression, constipation, N/V, somnolence, dry mouth, headache, pruritus, dizziness, fatigue, diarrhea, insomnia, hyperhidrosis.
DRUG INTERACTIONS
See Boxed Warning. Concomitant use w/ other CNS depressants (eg, sedatives, hypnotics, general anesthetics) may increase the risk of respiratory depression, profound sedation, coma, and death; if coadministration is considered, reduce dose of one or both agents. Monitor elderly, cachectic, and debilitated patients closely when coadministered w/ other drugs that depress respiration. Mixed agonist/antagonist (eg, pentazocine, nalbuphine, butorphanol) or partial agonist (eg, buprenorphine) analgesics may reduce the analgesic effect and/or precipitate withdrawal symptoms; avoid coadministration. May enhance the neuromuscular blocking action of skeletal muscle relaxants and produce an increased degree of respiratory depression. MAOIs may potentiate effects of morphine; avoid use w/ MAOIs or w/in 14 days of stopping such treatment. Cimetidine may potentiate morphine-induced respiratory depression. May reduce efficacy of diuretics and lead to acute urinary retention. Anticholinergics or other drugs w/ anticholinergic activity may increase risk of urinary retention and/or severe constipation, which may lead to paralytic ileus. P-gp inhibitors (eg, quinidine) may increase absorption/exposure; monitor for signs of respiratory and CNS depression.
PREGNANCY AND LACTATION
Category C, not for use in nursing.
MECHANISM OF ACTION
Morphine: Opioid agonist; binds w/ and activates opioid receptors at sites in the periaqueductal and periventricular grey matter, the ventromedial medulla, and the spinal cord to produce analgesia. Naltrexone: Opioid antagonist; reverses the subjective and analgesic effects of mu-opioid receptor agonists by competitively binding at mu-opioid receptors.
PHARMACOKINETICS
Absorption: Morphine: T_{max}=7.5 hrs (median). **Distribution:** Morphine: V_d=3-4L/kg; plasma protein binding (30-35%); crosses placenta; found in breast milk. **Metabolism:** Morphine: Liver via glucuronidation and sulfation; (metabolites) morphine-3-glucuronide (M3G, about 50%), morphine-6-glucuronide (M6G, about 5-15%), morphine-3-etheral sulfate. Naltrexone: Extensive; 6-β-naltrexol. **Elimination:** Morphine: Urine (M3G/M6G, 10% unchanged), bile; $T_{1/2}$=29 hrs.

PATIENT CONSIDERATIONS
Assessment: Assess for abuse/addiction risk, pain intensity, prior opioid therapy, opioid tolerance, respiratory depression, drug hypersensitivity, COPD or cor pulmonale, history of seizure disorders, pregnancy/nursing status, possible drug interactions, or any other conditions where treatment is contraindicated or cautioned.

Monitoring: Monitor for development of addiction, abuse, or misuse; respiratory depression (especially w/in first 24-72 hrs of initiation); seizures/convulsions; hypotension; syncope; and other adverse reactions. Monitor BP and serum amylase levels. Periodically reassess the continued need for therapy during chronic therapy.

Counseling: Inform that use of drug, even when taken as recommended, can result in addiction, abuse, and misuse, which can lead to overdose or death; instruct not to share w/ others and to take steps to protect from theft or misuse. Inform of the risk of life-threatening respiratory depression; advise how to recognize respiratory depression and to seek medical attention if breathing difficulties develop. Inform that accidental ingestion, especially in children, may result in respiratory depression or death; instruct to take steps to store the drug securely and to dispose unused caps by flushing down the toilet. Inform female patients of reproductive potential that prolonged use during pregnancy may result in neonatal opioid withdrawal syndrome, which may be life threatening if not recognized and treated. Instruct not to consume alcoholic beverages, nor prescription and OTC products that contain alcohol, during treatment. Inform that potentially serious additive effects may occur if used w/ alcohol or other CNS depressants, and advise not to use such drugs unless supervised by a healthcare provider. Instruct about proper administration instructions. Inform that drug may cause orthostatic hypotension and syncope; instruct how to recognize symptoms of low BP and how to reduce the risk of serious consequences should hypotension occur. Inform that drug may impair the ability to perform potentially hazardous activities; advise not to perform such tasks until patients know how they will react to the medication. Advise of potential for severe constipation, including management instructions and when to seek medical attention. Advise how to recognize anaphylaxis and when to seek medical attention. Advise female patients that drug may cause fetal harm; instruct to inform physician if pregnant or planning to become pregnant.

EMEND CAPSULES AND ORAL SUSPENSION —

aprepitant   Rx

Class: Substance P/neurokinin-1 (NK1) receptor antagonist

ADULT DOSAGE

Chemotherapy-Induced Nausea/ Vomiting

Prevention of N/V associated w/ initial and repeat courses of highly emetogenic chemotherapy (HEC) or moderately emetogenic chemotherapy (MEC)

Caps:
Day 1: 125mg, 1 hr prior to chemotherapy
Days 2 and 3: 80mg, 1 hr prior to chemotherapy; administer in the am if no chemotherapy is given on Days 2 and 3

Oral Sus:
Patients Unable to Swallow Caps:
Day 1: 3mg/kg (max dose of 125mg), 1 hr prior to chemotherapy
Days 2 and 3: 2mg/kg (max dose of 80mg), 1 hr prior to chemotherapy; administer in the am if no chemotherapy is given on Days 2 and 3

Administer as part of a regimen that includes a corticosteroid and a 5-HT₃ antagonist; refer to PI

Postoperative Nausea/Vomiting

Prevention:
Caps:
40mg w/in 3 hrs prior to induction of anesthesia

PEDIATRIC DOSAGE

Chemotherapy-Induced Nausea/ Vomiting

Prevention of N/V associated w/ initial and repeat courses of HEC or MEC

Oral Sus:
6 Months to <12 Years of Age or Pediatric Patients Unable to Swallow Caps:
Day 1: 3mg/kg (max dose of 125mg), 1 hr prior to chemotherapy
Days 2 and 3: 2mg/kg (max dose of 80mg), 1 hr prior to chemotherapy; administer in the am if no chemotherapy is given on Days 2 and 3

Caps:
≥12 Years:
Day 1: 125mg, 1 hr prior to chemotherapy
Days 2 and 3: 80mg, 1 hr prior to chemotherapy; administer in the am if no chemotherapy is given on Days 2 and 3

Administer as part of a regimen that includes a corticosteroid and a 5-HT₃ antagonist; refer to PI

DOSING CONSIDERATIONS
Other Important Considerations
Pediatric Patients <6kg: Not recommended

ADMINISTRATION
Oral route
Take w/ or w/o food.
Swallow caps whole.

Oral Sus
Should be prepared by a healthcare provider.
When ready to use, take the cap off the dispenser, place the dispenser in the patient's mouth along the inner cheek on either the right or left side; slowly dispense.
Discard any doses remaining after 72 hrs.

Preparation:
1. Fill the mixing cup w/ room temperature drinking water.
2. Fill the 5mL oral dosing dispenser w/ 4.6mL of water from the mixing cup; make sure no air is in the dispenser.
3. Discard all the unused water remaining in the mixing cup, and then add the 4.6mL of water from the dispenser back into the mixing cup.
4. Shake the pouch and pour the entire contents of the pouch into the 4.6mL of water in the mixing cup and snap the lid shut.
5. Gently swirl 20X; then gently invert the mixing cup 5X.
6. Check for any clumps or foaming and if there are clumps present, repeat step 5 until there are no clumps; if there is foam, wait until it disappears.
7. The final concentration is 25mg/mL; fill the appropriate dispenser w/ the prescribed dose.
8. Place the cap on the dispenser until it clicks.
9. Discard the mixing cup along w/ any remaining sus.

Storage:
Store the pouch at room temperature between 20-25°C (68-77°F).
Store filled dosing dispenser(s) in the refrigerator (2-8°C [36-46°F]) for up to 72 hrs prior to use if the dose is not administered immediately after measuring. When ready to use, mixture may be kept at room temperature (20-25°C [68-77°F]) for up to 3 hours.

STORAGE
Caps: 20-25°C (68-77°F). **Oral Sus:** (Unopened pouch) 20-25°C (68-77°F); excursions permitted at 15-30°C (59-86°F). Do not open until ready for use. (Prepared sus) If not used immediately, refrigerate at 2-8°C (36-46°F) for up to 72 hrs prior to use; when ready to use, mixture can be kept at 20-25°C (68-77°F) for up to 3 hrs.

HOW SUPPLIED
Cap: 40mg, 80mg, 125mg; **Oral Sus:** 125mg

CONTRAINDICATIONS
Hypersensitivity to any component of the product, concomitant use w/ pimozide.

WARNINGS/PRECAUTIONS
Not recommended for chronic continuous use. Additional monitoring for adverse reactions in patients w/ severe hepatic impairment (Child-Pugh score >9) may be warranted. Caution in elderly.

ADVERSE REACTIONS
Prevention of Chemotherapy Induced N/V (CINV): (Adults) Fatigue, diarrhea, asthenia, dyspepsia, abdominal pain, hiccups, decreased WBC count, dehydration, increased alanine aminotransferase. (Pediatrics) Neutropenia, headache, diarrhea, decreased appetite, cough, fatigue, decreased Hgb, dizziness, hiccups.
Prevention of Postoperative N/V (PONV): (Adults) Constipation, hypotension.

DRUG INTERACTIONS
See Contraindications. Use w/ other drugs that are CYP3A4 substrates may result in increased concentration of the concomitant drug. Use w/ strong or moderate CYP3A4 inhibitors (eg, ketoconazole, diltiazem) may increase concentrations and result in increased risk of adverse reactions; avoid concomitant use. Use w/ strong CYP3A4 inducers (eg, rifampin) may reduce concentrations and decrease efficacy; avoid concomitant use. Coadministration w/ warfarin may decrease PT/INR; monitor INR for chronic warfarin therapy in the 2-week period, particularly at 7-10 days, following initiation of aprepitant w/ each chemotherapy cycle, or following single administration for the prevention of PONV. Efficacy of hormonal contraceptives may be reduced; alternative or backup methods of contraception should be used during therapy and for 1 month following the last dose. Increased exposure to midazolam or other benzodiazepines metabolized via CYP3A4 (eg, alprazolam, triazolam); monitor for benzodiazepine-related adverse reactions during use for prevention of CINV and may consider reducing the dose of IV midazolam. Increased dexamethasone exposure; reduce dose of oral dexamethasone by approx 50% during use for prevention of CINV. Increased methylprednisolone exposure; reduce dose of IV methylprednisolone by approx 25% and oral methylprednisolone by approx 50% during use for prevention of CINV. May increase exposure of chemotherapeutic agents metabolized by CYP3A4 (eg, vinblastine, vincristine, ifosfamide); monitor for adverse events.

PREGNANCY AND LACTATION
Pregnancy: There are no available data on aprepitant use in pregnant women to inform the drug associated risk.
Lactation: Lactation studies have not been conducted to assess the presence of aprepitant in human milk, the effects on the breastfed infant, or the effects on milk production; the developmental and health benefits of breastfeeding should be considered along w/ the mother's clinical need and any potential adverse effects on the breastfed infant.
Females and Males of Reproductive Potential: Efficacy of hormonal contraceptives may be reduced. Females using hormonal contraceptives should use an effective alternative or backup nonhormonal contraceptive (eg, condoms, spermicides) during treatment and for 1 month following the last dose.

MECHANISM OF ACTION
Substance P/neurokinin 1 receptor antagonist; augments the antiemetic activity of the 5-HT₃ receptor antagonist ondansetron and the corticosteroid dexamethasone and inhibits both the acute and delayed phases of cisplatin-induced emesis.

PHARMACOKINETICS
Absorption: Administration of variable doses resulted in different parameters.
Distribution: Crosses the blood brain barrier. V_d=70L; plasma protein binding (>95%). **Metabolism:** Liver (extensive) by CYP3A4 (major), 1A2 and 2C19 (minor), via oxidation. **Elimination:** (IV, 100mg dose) Urine (57%), feces (45%). $T_{1/2}$=9-13 hrs.

PATIENT CONSIDERATIONS

Assessment: Assess for hypersensitivity to drug, severe hepatic impairment, ability to swallow caps, pregnancy/nursing status, and possible drug interactions.

Monitoring: Monitor for hypersensitivity reactions and other adverse reactions. Monitor INR closely w/ warfarin.

Counseling: Advise that hypersensitivity reactions, including anaphylaxis, have been reported; instruct to d/c medication and contact physician immediately if an allergic reaction occurs. Advise to inform physician if using any other prescription, nonprescription medication, or herbal products. Inform that drug may reduce efficacy of hormonal contraceptives; advise to use alternative or backup methods of contraception (eg, condoms, spermicides) during therapy and for 1 month after the last dose. Instruct patients on chronic warfarin therapy to follow instructions from physician regarding blood draws to monitor INR.

EMEND FOR INJECTION — fosaprepitant dimeglumine   Rx

Class: Substance P/neurokinin-1 (NK1) receptor antagonist

ADULT DOSAGE

Chemotherapy-Induced Nausea/Vomiting

Prevention of Acute and Delayed N/V Associated w/ Initial and Repeat Courses of Highly Emetogenic Chemotherapy (Including High-Dose Cisplatin):
Emend:
Day 1: 150mg IV over 20-30 min approx 30 min prior to chemotherapy

Dexamethasone:
Day 1: 12mg PO 30 min prior to chemotherapy
Day 2: 8mg PO in am
Day 3: 8mg PO bid (am and pm)
Day 4: 8mg PO bid (am and pm)
50% dose reduction of dexamethasone on Days 1 and 2 recommended to account for a drug interaction w/ Emend

5-HT₃ Antagonist:
Refer to 5-HT₃ antagonist prescribing information

Prevention of Delayed N/V Associated w/ Initial and Repeat Courses of Moderately Emetogenic Chemotherapy:
Emend:
Day 1: 150mg IV over 20-30 min approx 30 min prior to chemotherapy

Dexamethasone:
Day 1: 12mg PO 30 min prior to chemotherapy
50% dose reduction of dexamethasone recommended to account for a drug interaction w/ Emend

5-HT₃ Antagonist:
Day 1: Refer to 5-HT₃ antagonist prescribing information

PEDIATRIC DOSAGE

Pediatric use may not have been established

ADMINISTRATION
IV route

Preparation of 150mg Inj
1. Inject 5mL 0.9% NaCl into the vial. Assure that 0.9% NaCl is added to the vial along the vial wall in order to prevent foaming. Swirl the vial gently; avoid shaking and jetting 0.9% NaCl into the vial.
2. Prepare an infusion bag filled w/ 145mL of 0.9% NaCl.
3. Withdraw entire volume from the vial and transfer into infusion bag containing 145mL of 0.9% NaCl to yield a total volume of 150mL and a final concentration of 1mg/1mL.
4. Gently invert the bag 2-3X.
5. Reconstituted final drug sol is stable for 24 hrs at ≤25°C (77°F).

Do not mix or reconstitute w/ sol for which physical and chemical compatibility have not been established.
Incompatible w/ any sol containing divalent cations (eg, Ca²⁺, Mg²⁺), including lactated Ringer's sol and Hartmann's sol.

STORAGE
2-8°C (36-46°F). **Reconstituted Sol:** Stable for 24 hrs at ≤25°C (77°F).

HOW SUPPLIED
Inj: 150mg

CONTRAINDICATIONS
Hypersensitivity to any component of the product, concomitant use w/ pimozide.

WARNINGS/PRECAUTIONS
Hypersensitivity reactions reported; d/c infusion and administer appropriate medical therapy. Do not reinitiate infusion if hypersensitivity occurs during 1st-time use. Caution w/ severe hepatic impairment (Child-Pugh score >9).

ADVERSE REACTIONS
Fatigue, diarrhea, neutropenia, asthenia, anemia, peripheral neuropathy, leukopenia, dyspepsia, UTI, pain in extremity.

DRUG INTERACTIONS
See Contraindications. May increase concentrations of CYP3A4 substrates (eg, benzodiazepines [midazolam, alprazolam, triazolam], dexamethasone, methylprednisolone, vinblastine, vincristine, ifosfamide or other chemotherapeutic agents, etoposide, vinorelbine, paclitaxel, docetaxel); monitor for adverse reactions. See PI for methylprednisolone dose reductions. Decreased hormonal exposure during administration of and for 28 days after administration of the last dose of Emend; use alternative or backup methods of contraception (eg, condoms, spermicides) during treatment and for 1 month following administration. Coadministration w/ warfarin may decrease PT/INR; in patients on chronic warfarin therapy, closely monitor INR in the 2-week period, particularly at 7-10 days, following initiation of Emend w/ each chemotherapy cycle. Strong CYP3A4 inhibitors (eg, ketoconazole, itraconazole, nefazodone) and moderate CYP3A4 inhibitors (eg, diltiazem) may increase concentrations and may increase the risk of adverse reactions; avoid w/ strong or moderate CYP3A4 inhibitors. Strong CYP3A4 inducers (eg, rifampin, carbamazepine, phenytoin) may decrease concentrations and efficacy; avoid concomitant use.

PREGNANCY AND LACTATION
Pregnancy: Insufficient data on use in pregnant women to inform a drug-associated risk.
Lactation: Lactation studies have not been conducted to assess the presence of aprepitant in human milk, the effects on the breastfed infant, or the effects on milk production; caution in nursing.
Reproductive Potential: Females of reproductive potential using hormonal contraceptives should use an effective alternative or backup non-hormonal contraceptive (eg, condoms, spermicides) during treatment and for 1 month following the last dose.

MECHANISM OF ACTION
Substance P/neurokinin-1 receptor antagonist; prodrug of aprepitant. Augments the antiemetic activity of the 5-HT₃ receptor antagonist ondansetron and the corticosteroid dexamethasone and inhibits both the acute and delayed phases of cisplatin-induced emesis.

PHARMACOKINETICS
Absorption: (Aprepitant, given as 150mg IV fosaprepitant) AUC=37.4mcg•hr/mL, C_{max}=4.2mcg/mL. **Distribution:** (Aprepitant) V_d=70L; plasma protein binding (>95%), crosses blood brain barrier. **Metabolism:** Converted to aprepitant in liver and extrahepatic tissues. (Aprepitant) Liver (extensive) by CYP3A4 (major), 1A2 and 2C19 (minor), via oxidation. **Elimination:** Urine (57%), feces (45%); (Aprepitant) $T_{1/2}$=9-13 hrs.

PATIENT CONSIDERATIONS
Assessment: Assess for hypersensitivity to drug or its components, severe hepatic impairment, pregnancy/nursing status, and possible drug interactions.
Monitoring: Monitor for hypersensitivity reactions and other adverse reactions. Monitor INR closely w/ warfarin.
Counseling: Advise that hypersensitivity reactions, including anaphylaxis, have been reported; instruct to d/c medication and inform physician immediately if experiencing an allergic reaction. Counsel patients who develop an infusion-site reaction on how to care for the local reaction and when to seek further evaluation. Advise to inform physician if using any other prescription, nonprescription medication, or herbal products. Inform that drug may reduce efficacy of hormonal contraceptives; advise to use alternative or backup methods of contraception during therapy and for 1 month after the last dose.

EMLA — lidocaine/prilocaine   Rx

Class: Acetamide local anesthetic

ADULT DOSAGE
Topical Anesthetic

Apply thick layer of cre to intact skin and cover w/ occlusive dressing

Minor Dermal Procedure:
Apply 2.5g over 20-25cm² of skin surface for at least 1 hr

Major Dermal Procedure:
Apply 2g/10cm² of skin for 2 hrs

As an Adjunct Prior to Local Anesthetic Infiltration on Adult Male Genital Skin:
Apply 1g/10cm² of skin surface for 15 min

Minor Procedures on the Female External Genitalia (eg, Removal of Condylomata Acuminata) and Pretreatment for Anesthetic Infiltration:
Apply 5-10g for 5-10 min

PEDIATRIC DOSAGE
Topical Anesthetic

Intact Skin:

0-3 Months of Age:
<5kg:
Max: 1g/10cm² for up to 1 hr

3-12 Months of Age:
>5kg:
Max: 2g/20cm² for up to 4 hrs

1-6 Years:
>10kg:
Max: 10g/100cm² for up to 4 hrs

7-12 Years:
>20kg:
Max: 20g/200cm² for up to 4 hrs

If >3 months and does not meet minimum weight requirement, max dose restricted to corresponding weight

---

ADMINISTRATION
Topical route

Not for ophthalmic use

STORAGE
20-25°C (68-77°F). Keep tightly closed.

HOW SUPPLIED
Cre: (Lidocaine/Prilocaine) 2.5%/2.5%

CONTRAINDICATIONS
Known history of sensitivity to local anesthetics of the amide type or to any other component of the product.

WARNINGS/PRECAUTIONS
Application to larger areas or for longer than recommended times may result in serious adverse effects. Should not be used where penetration or migration beyond the tympanic membrane into the middle ear is possible. Avoid w/ congenital or idiopathic methemoglobinemia and in infants <12 months of age receiving treatment w/ methemoglobin-inducing agents. Very young or

patients w/ G6PD deficiency are more susceptible to methemoglobinemia. Reports of methemoglobinemia in infants and children following excessive applications. Monitor neonates and infants up to 3 months of age for Met-Hb levels before, during, and after application. Repeated doses may increase blood levels; caution in patients who may be more susceptible to systemic effects (eg, acutely ill, debilitated, elderly). Avoid eye contact and application to open wounds. Has been shown to inhibit viral and bacterial growth. Caution w/ severe hepatic disease and in patients w/ drug sensitivities.

ADVERSE REACTIONS
Erythema, edema, abnormal sensations, paleness (pallor or blanching), altered temperature sensations, burning sensation, itching, rash.

DRUG INTERACTIONS
Additive and potentially synergistic toxic effects w/ Class I antiarrhythmic drugs (eg, tocainide, mexiletine). May have additive cardiac effects w/ Class III antiarrhythmic drugs (eg, amiodarone, bretylium, sotalol, dofetilide). Avoid drugs associated w/ drug-induced methemoglobinemia (eg, sulfonamides, acetaminophen, acetanilid, aniline dyes, benzocaine, chloroquine, dapsone, naphthalene, nitrates/nitrites, nitrofurantoin, nitroglycerin, nitroprusside, phenobarbital, phenytoin, primaquine, pamaquine, para-aminosalicylic acid, phenacetin, quinine). Caution w/ other products containing lidocaine/prilocaine; consider the amount absorbed from all formulations.

PREGNANCY AND LACTATION
Category B, caution in nursing.

MECHANISM OF ACTION
Amide-type local anesthetics; stabilizes neuronal membranes by inhibiting ionic fluxes required for initiation and conduction impulses, thereby affecting local anesthetic action.

PHARMACOKINETICS
Absorption: Lidocaine: (3 hrs 400cm²) C_{max}=0.12mcg/mL, T_{max}=4 hrs; (24 hrs 400cm²) C_{max}=0.28mcg/mL, T_{max}=10 hrs. Prilocaine: (3 hrs 400cm²) C_{max}=0.07mcg/mL, T_{max}=4 hrs; (24 hrs 400cm²) C_{max}=0.14mcg/mL, T_{max}=10 hrs. **Distribution:** (IV) V_d=1.5L/kg (lidocaine), 2.6L/kg (prilocaine); (Cre) plasma protein binding 70% (lidocaine), 55% (prilocaine). Crosses placental and blood-brain barrier; found in breast milk. **Metabolism:** Lidocaine: Liver (rapid); monoethylglycinexylidide and glycinexylidide (active metabolites). Prilocaine: Liver and kidneys by amidases; ortho-toluidine and N-n-propylalanine (metabolites). **Elimination:** (IV) Lidocaine: Urine (>98%); $T_{1/2}$=110 min. Prilocaine; $T_{1/2}$=70 min.

PATIENT CONSIDERATIONS
Assessment: Assess for congenital or idiopathic methemoglobinemia, G6PD deficiency, hepatic disease, open wounds, presence of acute illness, presence of debilitation, history of drug sensitivities, pregnancy/nursing status, and for possible drug interactions. In neonates and infants ≤3 months of age, obtain Met-Hb levels prior to application.

Monitoring: Monitor for signs/symptoms of methemoglobinemia, ototoxicity, local skin reactions and for allergic/anaphylactoid reactions. Monitor Met-Hb levels in neonates and infants ≤3 months of age during and after application.

Counseling: Inform about potential risks/benefits of drug. Advise to avoid inadvertent trauma to treated area. Instruct not to apply near eyes or on open wounds. Apply ud by physician. Advise to notify physician if pregnant/nursing or planning to become pregnant. Instruct to remove cre and consult physician if child becomes very dizzy, excessively sleepy, or develops duskiness on the face or lips after application.

EMPLICITI — elotuzumab   Rx
Class: Monoclonal antibody/SLAMF7-directed

ADULT DOSAGE
Multiple Myeloma

Use in combination w/ lenalidomide and dexamethasone for the treatment of patients w/ multiple myeloma who have received 1-3 prior therapies

Recommended Dose: 10mg/kg IV every week for the first 2 cycles and every 2 weeks thereafter; each cycle consists of 28 days

Continue treatment until disease progression or unacceptable toxicity

Dexamethasone:
Administer 28mg PO 3-24 hrs before elotuzumab plus 8mg IV 45-90 min before elotuzumab, on days that elotuzumab is administered.
Administer 40mg PO on days that elotuzumab is not administered but a dose of dexamethasone is scheduled (Days 8 and 22 of cycle 3 and all subsequent cycles).

Lenalidomide:
25mg PO qd on Days 1-21 of a 28-day treatment cycle

PEDIATRIC DOSAGE
Pediatric use may not have been established

Infusion Rate:
Cycle 1, Dose 1:
0-30 min: 0.5mL/min
30-60 min: 1mL/min
≥60 min: 2mL/min
Cycle 1, Dose 2:
0-30 min: 1mL/min
≥30 min: 2mL/min
Cycle 1, Dose 3 and 4 and All Subsequent Cycles:
2mL/min
Max: 2mL/min; 5mL/min in patients who have received 4 cycles of treatment

Premedication
Premedicate w/ the Following 45-90 min Prior to Each Elotuzumab Infusion:
- 8mg IV dexamethasone;
- 25-50mg PO or IV diphenhydramine or equivalent H1 blocker;
- 50mg IV or 150mg oral ranitidine or equivalent H2 blocker;
- 650-1000mg oral acetaminophen

DOSING CONSIDERATIONS
Adverse Reactions
Infusion Reactions:
≥Grade 2: Interrupt elotuzumab infusion and institute appropriate medical/supportive measures. Upon resolution to ≤Grade 1, restart at 0.5mL/min and gradually increase at a rate of 0.5mL/min every 30 min as tolerated to the rate at which the infusion reaction occurred; resume escalation regimen if there is no recurrence of the infusion reaction. Monitor vital signs every 30 min for 2 hrs after end of infusion, in patients who experience an infusion reaction; if infusion reaction recurs, d/c elotuzumab infusion and do not restart on that day
Severe: May require permanent discontinuation and emergency treatment
Other Important Considerations
If the dose of 1 drug in the regimen is delayed, interrupted, or discontinued, treatment w/ the other drugs may continue as scheduled. If dexamethasone is delayed or discontinued, base decision whether to administer elotuzumab on clinical judgment (ie, risk of hypersensitivity)

ADMINISTRATION
IV route

Administer w/ an infusion set and sterile, nonpyrogenic, low-protein-binding filter (w/ a pore size of 0.2-1.2µm) using an automated infusion pump.
Do not mix w/, or administer as an infusion w/, other medicinal products.

Reconstitution
- Reconstitute 300mg vial w/ 13mL sterile water for inj (SWFI) and 400mg vial w/ 17mL SWFI; post-reconstitution concentration is 25mg/mL.
- Use a syringe of adequate size and ≤18-gauge needle.
- Dissolve by swirling/inverting vial; avoid vigorous agitation/shaking. The lyophilized powder should dissolve in <10 min.
- Allow reconstituted sol to stand for 5-10 min.

Dilution
- Once the reconstitution is completed, withdraw necessary volume for calculated dose from each vial, up to a max of 16mL from 400mg vial and 12mL from 300mg vial.
- Further dilute w/ 230mL of either 0.9% NaCl inj or D5 inj into an infusion bag made of polyvinyl chloride or polyolefin.
- Volume of 0.9% NaCl inj or D5 inj can be adjusted so as not to exceed 5mL/kg of patient weight at any given dose.

Complete infusion w/in 24 hrs of reconstitution. If not used immediately, may store at 2-8°C (36-46°F) and protect from light for up to 24 hrs (max of 8 hrs of the total 24 hrs can be at 20-25°C [68-77°F] and room light).

STORAGE
2-8°C (36-46°F). Protect from light. Do not freeze or shake.

HOW SUPPLIED
Inj: 300mg, 400mg

CONTRAINDICATIONS
Refer to the individual monographs for lenalidomide and dexamethasone.

WARNINGS/PRECAUTIONS
See Dosing Considerations. May cause infusion reactions. Infections reported; monitor and treat promptly. Invasive second primary malignancies (SPMs) reported; monitor for development of SPMs. Elevations in liver enzymes consistent w/ hepatotoxicity reported; monitor liver enzymes periodically. D/C treatment upon ≥Grade 3 elevation of liver enzymes; may consider treatment continuation after return to baseline values. Can be detected on both serum protein electrophoresis and immunofixation assays used for the clinical monitoring of endogenous M-protein; may impact determination of complete response and possibly relapse from complete response in patients w/ IgG kappa myeloma protein.

ADVERSE REACTIONS
Fatigue, diarrhea, pyrexia, constipation, cough, peripheral neuropathy, nasopharyngitis, URTI, decreased appetite, pneumonia.

PREGNANCY AND LACTATION
Pregnancy: There are no studies w/ pregnant women to inform any drug-associated risks.
Lactation: Not for use in nursing.

Refer to the individual monographs for lenalidomide and dexamethasone.

MECHANISM OF ACTION

IgG1 monoclonal antibody that specifically targets the SLAMF7 protein. Directly activates natural killer cells through both the SLAMF7 pathway and Fc receptors. Also targets SLAMF7 on myeloma cells and facilitates the interaction w/ natural killer cells to mediate the killing of myeloma cells through antibody-dependent cellular cytotoxicity. The combination of elotuzumab and lenalidomide resulted in enhanced activation of natural killer cells that was greater than the effects of either agent alone and increased anti-tumor activity.

PATIENT CONSIDERATIONS

Assessment: Assess baseline liver enzyme values and pregnancy/nursing status.

Monitoring: Monitor for infusion reactions, infections, SPMs, hepatotoxicity, and other adverse reactions. Monitor liver enzymes periodically.

Counseling: Inform of risks/benefits of therapy. Advise to contact physician if experiencing signs/symptoms of infusion reactions w/in 24 hrs of infusion. Inform that oral premedication is necessary prior to infusion to reduce the risk of infusion reaction. Advise that lenalidomide has the potential to cause fetal harm and has specific requirements regarding contraception, pregnancy testing, blood and sperm donation, and transmission in sperm. Inform of the risk of developing infections and SPMs during treatment; instruct to report any symptoms of infection. Inform of the risk of hepatotoxicity and instruct to report any signs/symptoms associated w/ this event.

Emsam — selegiline   Rx

Class: Monoamine oxidase inhibitor (MAOI) (type B)

> Antidepressants increased the risk of suicidal thoughts and behavior in children, adolescents, and young adults in short-term studies. Monitor closely for clinical worsening and for emergence of suicidal thoughts and behaviors in patients who are started on antidepressant therapy. Contraindicated in patients <12 yrs of age because of an increased risk of hypertensive crisis.

ADULT DOSAGE	PEDIATRIC DOSAGE
Major Depressive Disorder	Pediatric use may not have been established
Initial/Target Dose: 6mg/24 hrs	
Titrate: May increase in increments of 3mg/24 hrs at intervals ≥2 weeks	
Max: 12mg/24 hrs	
Periodically reevaluate long-term usefulness of the drug	

DOSING CONSIDERATIONS
Elderly
≥65 Years:
Usual: 6mg/24 hrs

ADMINISTRATION
Transdermal route

Apply to dry, intact skin on upper torso, upper thigh or outer surface of upper arm q24h

Apply immediately upon removal from the protective pouch

Patients Taking 9mg/24 hrs and 12mg/24 hrs

Avoid tyramine-rich foods and beverages beginning on 1st day of 9mg/24 hrs or 12mg/24 hrs treatment; continue to avoid for 2 weeks after a dose reduction to 6mg/24 hrs or following discontinuation of 9mg/24 hrs or 12mg/24 hrs

STORAGE
20-25°C (68-77°F). Do not store outside of the sealed pouch.

HOW SUPPLIED
Patch: 6mg/24 hrs, 9mg/24 hrs, 12mg/24 hrs [30ˢ]

CONTRAINDICATIONS
Pheochromocytoma, patients <12 yrs of age. Concomitant use with SSRIs (eg, fluoxetine, sertraline, paroxetine), SNRIs (eg, venlafaxine, duloxetine), TCAs (eg, clomipramine, imipramine), opiate analgesics (eg, meperidine, tramadol, methadone, pentazocine, propoxyphene), dextromethorphan, and carbamazepine. After stopping treatment with contraindicated drugs, a time period equal to 4-5 half-lives (approximately 1 week) of the drug or any active metabolite should elapse before starting therapy. At least 5 weeks should elapse between discontinuation of fluoxetine and initiation of treatment. At least 2 weeks should elapse after stopping treatment before starting therapy with any contraindicated drug.

WARNINGS/PRECAUTIONS
May precipitate mixed/manic episode in patients at risk for bipolar disorder; screen for risk for bipolar disorder prior to initiating treatment. Not approved for treatment of bipolar depression. Activation of mania/hypomania may occur; caution with history of mania. External heat may result in an increase in the amount of selegiline absorbed from patch and produce elevated serum levels.

ADVERSE REACTIONS
Headache, diarrhea, dyspepsia, insomnia, dry mouth, pharyngitis, sinusitis, application-site reaction, rash, low standing systolic BP, orthostatic change in BP, weight loss.

DRUG INTERACTIONS
See Contraindications. Serotonin syndrome reported w/ith serotonergic drugs; d/c immediately and initiate treatment if this occurs. Hypertensive crisis can occur with high tyramine-containing foods. Not recommended with alcohol. Use with adrenergic drugs or buspirone may produce substantial increases in BP; monitor

BP if used with buspirone, amphetamines, or cold products or weight-reducing preparations that contain sympathomimetic amines (eg, pseudoephedrine, phenylephrine, phenylpropanolamine, ephedrine).

PREGNANCY AND LACTATION
Category C, not for use in nursing.

MECHANISM OF ACTION
MAOI (Type B); not established. Presumed to be linked to potentiation of monoamine neurotransmitter activity in the CNS resulting from its inhibition of MAO activity.

PHARMACOKINETICS
Distribution: Plasma protein binding (90%). **Metabolism:** Extensive via N-dealkylation or N-depropargylation by CYP2B6, CYP2C9, CYP3A4/5 (major), CYP2A6 (minor); N-desmethylselegiline, R(-)-methamphetamine (metabolites). **Elimination:** Urine (10%, 0.1% unchanged), feces (2%); $T_{1/2}$=18-25 hrs (IV).

PATIENT CONSIDERATIONS

Assessment: Assess for hypersensitivity to the drug or to any component of the transdermal system, pheochromocytoma, risk for bipolar disorder, history of mania, pregnancy/nursing status, and possible drug interactions.

Monitoring: Monitor for clinical worsening, emergence of suicidal thoughts and behaviors, activation of mania/hypomania, and other adverse reactions. Periodically reevaluate long-term usefulness of the drug.

Counseling: Counsel about risks/benefits and appropriate use of therapy. Counsel to be alert for the emergence of suicidal ideation/behavior, especially early during treatment and when the dose is adjusted up or down. Advise to avoid tyramine-containing foods/supplements/beverages; instruct to immediately report occurrence of severe headache, neck stiffness, heart racing or palpitations, or sudden unusual symptoms. Advise to inform physician if taking/planning to take any prescription or OTC medications, including herbals. Inform that medication may potentially impair judgment, thinking, or motor skills; caution about performing hazardous tasks (eg, operating machinery/driving). Inform that concomitant use with alcohol is not recommended. Instruct to use exactly as prescribed and to avoid exposing application site to external sources of direct heat (eg, heating pads, electric blankets). Instruct not to cut patch into smaller portions. Instruct to notify physician if pregnant, planning to become pregnant, or if breastfeeding.

Emtriva — emtricitabine   Rx

Class: Nucleoside reverse transcriptase inhibitor (NRTI)

> Lactic acidosis and severe hepatomegaly with steatosis, including fatal cases, reported with the use of nucleoside analogues alone or in combination with other antiretrovirals. Not approved for the treatment of chronic hepatitis B virus (HBV) infection. Severe acute exacerbations of hepatitis B reported in patients who have discontinued therapy. Closely monitor hepatic function with both clinical and lab follow-up for at least several months in patients who are coinfected with HIV-1 and HBV and d/c therapy. If appropriate, initiation of antihepatitis B therapy may be warranted.

ADULT DOSAGE	PEDIATRIC DOSAGE
HIV-1 Infection	**HIV-1 Infection**
Combination w/ Other Antiretrovirals:	**Combination w/ Other Antiretrovirals**
Cap: 200mg qd	**0-3 Months of Age:**
Sol: 240mg (24mL) qd	**Sol:** 3mg/kg qd
	3 Months-17 Years:
	Cap: >33kg: 200mg qd
	Sol: 6mg/kg qd
	Max: 240mg (24mL) qd

DOSING CONSIDERATIONS
Renal Impairment
CrCl 30-49mL/min:
Cap: 200mg q48h
Sol: 120mg (12mL) q24h

CrCl 15-29mL/min:
Cap: 200mg q72h
Sol: 80mg (8mL) q24h

CrCl <15mL/min or on Hemodialysis:
Cap: 200mg q96h; give dose after dialysis, if dosing on day of dialysis
Sol: 60mg (6mL) q24h; give dose after dialysis, if dosing on day of dialysis

ADMINISTRATION
Oral route

Take w/o regard to food

STORAGE
(Cap) 25°C (77°F); excursions permitted to 15-30°C (59-86°F). (Sol) 2-8°C (36-46°F). Use within 3 months if stored at 25°C (77°F).

HOW SUPPLIED
Cap: 200mg; **Sol:** 10mg/mL [170mL]

CONTRAINDICATIONS
Prior hypersensitivity to any of the components in this product.

WARNINGS/PRECAUTIONS
Obesity and prolonged nucleoside exposure may be risk factors for lactic acidosis and severe hepatomegaly with steatosis. Caution with known risk factors for liver

disease. D/C if lactic acidosis or pronounced hepatotoxicity develops. Test for chronic HBV before initiating therapy. Reduce dose and closely monitor clinical response and renal function with renal impairment. Redistribution/accumulation of body fat and immune reconstitution syndrome reported. Autoimmune disorders (eg, Graves' disease, polymyositis, Guillain-Barre syndrome) in the setting of immune reconstitution reported. Caution in elderly.

ADVERSE REACTIONS
Lactic acidosis, severe hepatomegaly with steatosis, headache, diarrhea, nausea, fatigue, dizziness, depression, insomnia, abnormal dreams, rash, abdominal pain, asthenia, increased cough, rhinitis.

DRUG INTERACTIONS
Do not coadminister with emtricitabine- or lamivudine-containing products.

PREGNANCY AND LACTATION
Category B, not for use in nursing.

MECHANISM OF ACTION
Nucleoside reverse transcriptase inhibitor; inhibits the activity of the HIV-1 reverse transcriptase by competing with the natural substrate deoxycytidine 5'-triphosphate and by being incorporated into nascent viral DNA, which results in chain termination.

PHARMACOKINETICS
Absorption: Rapid and extensive. T_{max}=1-2 hrs. (Cap) Absolute bioavailability (93%); C_{max}=1.8mcg/mL; AUC=10mcg•hr/mL. (Sol) Absolute bioavailability (75%). **Distribution:** Plasma protein binding (<4%); found in breast milk. **Metabolism:** Oxidation and conjugation; 3'-sulfoxide diastereomers and 2'-O-glucuronide (metabolites). **Elimination:** Urine (86%), feces (14%); $T_{1/2}$=10 hrs.

PATIENT CONSIDERATIONS
Assessment: Assess for previous hypersensitivity, risk factors for lactic acidosis and liver disease, HBV infection, renal impairment, pregnancy/nursing status, and possible drug interactions.

Monitoring: Monitor for signs/symptoms of lactic acidosis, severe hepatomegaly with steatosis, hepatotoxicity, redistribution/accumulation of body fat, immune reconstitution syndrome, autoimmune disorders, and other adverse reactions. Closely monitor hepatic function with both clinical and lab follow-up for at least several months in patients who are coinfected with HIV-1 and HBV and d/c therapy. Closely monitor clinical response and renal function with renal impairment.

Counseling: Inform that therapy is not a cure for HIV-1 infection and illnesses associated with HIV-1 infection, including opportunistic infections, may continue. Instruct not to breastfeed, and not to share needles or other injection equipment and personal items that can have blood or body fluids on them (eg, toothbrushes, razor blades). Advise to always practice safer sex by using a latex or polyurethane condom to lower the chance of sexual contact with semen, vaginal secretions, or blood. Inform that it is important to take drug with combination therapy on a regular dosing schedule to avoid missing doses. Instruct to notify physician if symptoms suggestive of lactic acidosis or pronounced hepatotoxicity (eg, N/V, unusual or unexpected stomach discomfort, weakness) develop.

ENABLEX — darifenacin   Rx
Class: Muscarinic antagonist

ADULT DOSAGE	PEDIATRIC DOSAGE
Overactive Bladder	Pediatric use may not have been established
Initial: 7.5mg qd w/ water	
Titrate: May increase to 15mg qd as early as 2 weeks after starting therapy based on individual response	

DOSING CONSIDERATIONS
Concomitant Medications
Potent CYP3A4 Inhibitors:
Max: 7.5mg/day

Hepatic Impairment
Moderate (Child-Pugh B):
Max: 7.5mg/day
Severe (Child-Pugh C): Not recommended

ADMINISTRATION
Oral route
Take w/ or w/o food

STORAGE
25°C (77°F); excursions permitted to 15-30°C (59-86°F). Protect from light.

HOW SUPPLIED
Tab, Extended-Release: 7.5mg, 15mg

CONTRAINDICATIONS
Urinary retention, gastric retention, uncontrolled narrow-angle glaucoma, and in patients at risk for these conditions.

WARNINGS/PRECAUTIONS
Risk of urinary retention; caution with significant bladder outflow obstruction. Risk of gastric retention; caution with GI obstructive disorders. May decrease GI motility; caution with severe constipation, ulcerative colitis, and myasthenia gravis. Caution with moderate hepatic impairment and in patients being treated for narrow-angle glaucoma. Angioedema reported; d/c and institute appropriate therapy if involvement of the tongue, hypopharynx, or larynx occurs. CNS

anticholinergic effects (eg, headache, confusion, hallucinations, somnolence) reported; monitor for signs of anticholinergic CNS effects (particularly after beginning treatment or increasing the dose) and d/c or reduce dose if this occurs.

ADVERSE REACTIONS
Dry mouth, constipation, dyspepsia, abdominal pain, nausea, UTI, headache, flu syndrome.

DRUG INTERACTIONS
Pharmacokinetics may be altered by CYP3A4 inducers and CYP2D6/CYP3A4 inhibitors. Caution with medications metabolized by CYP2D6 and which have a narrow therapeutic window (eg, flecainide, thioridazine, TCAs). May increase the frequency and/or severity of dry mouth, constipation, blurred vision, and other anticholinergic pharmacologic effects with other anticholinergic agents. May alter the absorption of some concomitantly administered drugs due to effects on GI motility. Increased concentration with cimetidine, erythromycin, fluconazole, or ketoconazole. May increase imipramine and desipramine (imipramine active metabolite) concentrations.

PREGNANCY AND LACTATION
Category C, caution in nursing.

MECHANISM OF ACTION
Muscarinic receptor antagonist; inhibits cholinergic muscarinic receptors, which mediate contractions of urinary bladder smooth muscle and stimulation of salivary secretions.

PHARMACOKINETICS
Absorption: Variable doses resulted in different pharmacokinetic parameters in extensive metabolizers and poor metabolizers of CYP2D6. **Distribution:** V_d=163L; plasma protein binding (98%). **Metabolism:** Liver (extensive) via CYP2D6 and 3A4 (monohydroxylation, dihydrobenzofuran ring opening, N-dealkylation). **Elimination:** Urine (60%); feces (40%); unchanged, 3%. $T_{1/2}$=13-19 hrs.

PATIENT CONSIDERATIONS
Assessment: Assess for urinary retention, gastric retention, narrow-angle glaucoma and risk for these conditions, bladder outflow obstruction, GI obstructive disorders, severe constipation, ulcerative colitis, myasthenia gravis, hepatic impairment, pregnancy/nursing status, and possible drug interactions.

Monitoring: Monitor for symptoms of urinary retention, gastric retention, decreased GI motility, and for angioedema (face, lips, tongue, hypopharynx, larynx). Monitor for signs of anticholinergic CNS effects (particularly after beginning treatment or increasing the dose).

Counseling: Advise that dizziness or blurred vision may occur; instruct to exercise caution when engaging in potentially dangerous activities. Instruct to take qd with liquid. Instruct to swallow whole; advise to not chew, divide, or crush. Inform that symptoms of constipation, urinary retention, heat prostration when used in a hot environment, or angioedema may occur. Advise to d/c therapy and seek medical attention if edema of the tongue or laryngopharynx, or difficulty breathing occurs. Advise to read the patient information leaflet before starting therapy.

ENALAPRIL/HCTZ — enalapril maleate/hydrochlorothiazide   Rx
Class: ACE inhibitor/thiazide diuretic

> D/C when pregnancy is detected. Drugs that act directly on the renin-angiotensin system (RAS) can cause injury/death to the developing fetus.

OTHER BRAND NAMES
Vaseretic

ADULT DOSAGE	PEDIATRIC DOSAGE
Hypertension	Pediatric use may not have been established
Uncontrolled BP w/ Either Enalapril or HCTZ Monotherapy:	
5mg/12.5mg or 10mg/25mg qd. Further increases of enalapril, HCTZ or both depend on clinical response; may increase HCTZ dose after 2-3 weeks	
Max: 20mg/50mg qd	
Replacement Therapy: Combination may be substituted for titrated components	

DOSING CONSIDERATIONS
Elderly
Start at lower end of dosing range

Renal Impairment
Severe: Not recommended; loop diuretics preferred

ADMINISTRATION
Oral route

STORAGE
Protect from moisture. **Enalapril/HCTZ:** 20-25°C (68-77°F). **Vaseretic:** 25°C (77°F); excursions permitted to 15-30°C (59-86°F).

HOW SUPPLIED
Tab: (Enalapril/HCTZ) 5mg/12.5mg; (Vaseretic) 10mg/25mg* *scored

CONTRAINDICATIONS
Hypersensitivity to any component of this product, hereditary/idiopathic angioedema, anuria, hypersensitivity to other sulfonamide-derived drugs, history of ACE inhibitor-associated angioedema. Coadministration w/ aliskiren in patients w/ diabetes.

WARNINGS/PRECAUTIONS

Not for initial therapy. Syncope reported. **Enalapril:** Excessive hypotension may occur in salt/volume-depleted patients (eg, patients treated vigorously w/ diuretics or on dialysis). Excessive hypotension reported and may be associated w/ oliguria and/or progressive azotemia, and rarely, w/ acute renal failure and/or death in patients w/ severe CHF; monitor closely during first 2 weeks of therapy and when dose is increased. Caution w/ ischemic heart or cerebrovascular disease in whom an excessive fall in BP could result in a MI or cerebrovascular accident. Head/neck angioedema reported; d/c and administer appropriate therapy. Intestinal angioedema reported. Higher incidence of angioedema in blacks than nonblacks. Patients w/ a history of angioedema unrelated to ACE inhibitor therapy may be at increased risk of angioedema during therapy. Anaphylactoid reactions reported during desensitization w/ hymenoptera venom, dialysis w/ high-flux membranes, and LDL apheresis w/ dextran sulfate absorption. Neutropenia/agranulocytosis may occur; consider monitoring WBCs in patients w/ collagen vascular disease and renal disease. Associated w/ syndrome that starts w/ cholestatic jaundice and progresses to fulminant hepatic necrosis and sometimes death (rare); d/c if jaundice or marked elevations of hepatic enzymes occur. Caution w/ left ventricular outflow obstruction. May cause changes in renal function; may be associated w/ oliguria and/or progressive azotemia and rarely w/ acute renal failure or death in severe CHF patients whose renal function depends on the renin-angiotensin-aldosterone system. May increase BUN/SrCr in patients w/ renal artery stenosis or w/ no preexisting renal vascular disease; may need to reduce dose or d/c therapy. Monitor renal function during the 1st few weeks of therapy in patients w/ renal artery stenosis. Hyperkalemia and persistent nonproductive cough reported. Hypotension may occur w/ major surgery or during anesthesia. **HCTZ:** May precipitate azotemia in patients w/ renal disease. Consider withholding or discontinuing therapy if progressive renal impairment occurs. Caution w/ hepatic impairment or progressive liver disease; may precipitate hepatic coma. Sensitivity reactions may occur. May exacerbate/ activate systemic lupus erythematosus (SLE). May cause idiosyncratic reaction, resulting in acute transient myopia and acute angle-closure glaucoma; d/c as rapidly as possible. Observe for signs of fluid or electrolyte imbalance (eg, hyponatremia, hypochloremic alkalosis, hypokalemia). Hyperuricemia, gout precipitation, hyperglycemia and manifestations of latent diabetes mellitus (DM), hypomagnesemia, hypercalcemia, and increased cholesterol and TG levels may occur. D/C before testing for parathyroid function. Enhanced effects in postsympathectomy patients. Hypokalemia may sensitize or exaggerate the response of the heart to toxic effects of digitalis.

ADVERSE REACTIONS

Dizziness, cough, fatigue, headache.

DRUG INTERACTIONS

See Contraindications. Increased risk of lithium toxicity; avoid w/ lithium. **Enalapril:** Dual blockade of the RAS is associated w/ increased risks of hypotension, hyperkalemia, and changes in renal function (including acute renal failure); in general, avoid combined use of RAS inhibitors, or closely monitor BP, renal function, and electrolytes w/ concomitant agents that affect the RAS. Avoid w/ aliskiren in patients w/ renal impairment (GFR <60mL/min). Hypotension risk and increased BUN and SrCr w/ diuretics. Antihypertensive agents that cause renin release (eg, diuretics) may augment effect. NSAIDs, including selective COX-2 inhibitors, may diminish antihypertensive effect and may cause deterioration of renal function, including possible acute renal failure. Increased risk of hyperkalemia w/ K+-sparing diuretics, K+ supplements, or K+-containing salt substitutes; use w/ caution and monitor serum K+. Nitritoid reactions reported w/ injectable gold. Coadministration w/ mTOR inhibitors (e.g., temsirolimus, sirolimus, everolimus) may increase risk for angioedema. **HCTZ:** Potentiation of orthostatic hypotension may occur w/ alcohol, barbiturates, or narcotics. Dose adjustment of the antidiabetic drug (oral agents and insulin) may be required. Additive effect or potentiation may occur w/ other antihypertensives. Cholestyramine and colestipol resins impair absorption. Corticosteroids and ACTH may intensify electrolyte depletion, particularly hypokalemia. May decrease response to pressor amines (eg, norepinephrine). May increase responsiveness to nondepolarizing skeletal muscle relaxants (eg, tubocurarine). NSAIDs may reduce diuretic effect.

PREGNANCY AND LACTATION

Pregnancy: Category D. Use of drugs that act on the RAS during the 2nd and 3rd trimesters of pregnancy reduces fetal renal function and increases fetal and neonatal morbidity and death. Resulting oligohydramnios can be associated w/ fetal lung hypoplasia and skeletal deformations. When pregnancy is detected, d/c Tekamlo as soon as possible.
Lactation: Enalapril, enalaprilat, and HCTZ have been detected in breast milk. Not for use in nursing.

MECHANISM OF ACTION

Enalapril: ACE inhibitor; decreases plasma angiotensin II, which leads to decreased vasopressor activity and decreased aldosterone secretion. **HCTZ:** Thiazide diuretic; has not been established. Affects distal renal tubular mechanism of electrolyte reabsorption. Increases excretion of Na+ and Cl-.

PHARMACOKINETICS

Absorption: Enalapril: T_{max}=1 hr, 3-4 hrs (enalaprilat). **Distribution:** Found in breast milk. HCTZ: Crosses placenta. **Metabolism:** Enalapril: Hydrolysis to enalaprilat (active metabolite). **Elimination:** Enalapril: Urine and feces (94% as enalapril or enalaprilat); $T_{1/2}$=11 hrs (enalaprilat). HCTZ: Kidneys (at least 61% unchanged); $T_{1/2}$=5.6-14.8 hrs.

PATIENT CONSIDERATIONS

Assessment: Assess for hereditary/idiopathic or history of ACE inhibitor-associated angioedema, anuria, DM, volume/salt depletion, hypersensitivity to the drug or sulfonamide-derived drugs, CHF, left ventricular outflow obstruction, collagen vascular disease, SLE, risk factors for hyperkalemia, renal/hepatic impairment, pregnancy/nursing status, and possible drug interactions.

Monitoring: Monitor for signs/symptoms of angioedema, exacerbation/ activation of SLE, idiosyncratic reaction, latent DM, fluid/electrolyte imbalance, hypercalcemia, hypomagnesemia, hyperuricemia or precipitation of gout, sensitivity reactions, and other adverse reactions. Periodically monitor WBCs in patients w/ collagen vascular disease and renal disease. Monitor BP, serum electrolytes, renal/hepatic function, and cholesterol/TG levels.

Counseling: Inform about fetal risks if taken during pregnancy and discuss treatment options in women planning to become pregnant; instruct to report pregnancy to physician as soon as possible. Instruct to d/c therapy and immediately report any signs/symptoms of angioedema. Instruct to report lightheadedness and to d/c therapy if actual syncope occurs. Inform that excessive perspiration, dehydration, and other causes of volume depletion may lead to an excessive fall in BP. Instruct not to use salt substitutes containing K+ w/o consulting physician, and to report promptly any signs/symptoms of infection.

ENALAPRILAT — enalaprilat   Rx

Class: ACE inhibitor

> ACE inhibitors can cause death/injury to the developing fetus during 2nd and 3rd trimesters. D/C therapy if pregnancy detected.

ADULT DOSAGE	PEDIATRIC DOSAGE
Hypertension	Pediatric use may not have been established
Usual: 1.25mg IV q6h for no longer than 48 hrs	
Max: 20mg/day	
Patients on Diuretic Therapy:	
Initial: 0.625mg IV	
May repeat after 1 hr if response is inadequate. May administer an additional dose of 1.25mg at 6-hr intervals	
Patients at Risk of Excessive Hypotension:	
Initial: 0.625mg IV over 5 min to 1 hr	
Conversions	
Oral to IV: 1.25mg IV q6h.	
IV to Oral:	
Initial: 5mg PO qd w/ subsequent dose adjustments as necessary	
Patients on Diuretic Therapy:	
IV (0.625mg IV q6h) to Oral: 2.5mg PO qd w/ subsequent dose adjustments as necessary	
Renal Impairment:	
CrCl >30mL/min: 5mg PO qd	
CrCl ≤30mL/min: 2.5mg PO qd	
Adjust dose according to BP response	

DOSING CONSIDERATIONS

Renal Impairment

CrCl ≤30mL/min:
Initial: 0.625mg
May repeat after 1 hr if response is inadequate. May administer an additional dose of 1.25mg at 6-hr intervals

Dialysis Patients:
Initial: 0.625mg over 5 min to 1 hr

Elderly

Start at lower end of dose range

ADMINISTRATION

IV route

Administer IV over a 5-min period.

Compatibility and Stability

May administer as provided or may be diluted w/ up to 50mL of a compatible diluent. Stable for up to 24 hrs at room temperature

Compatible Diluents

D5 inj
0.9% NaCl inj
0.9% NaCl inj in D5
D5 in lactated Ringer's inj

STORAGE

Below 30°C (86°F). **Diluted Sol:** Stable for 24 hrs at room temperature.

HOW SUPPLIED

Inj: 1.25mg/mL [1mL, 2mL]

CONTRAINDICATIONS

Hypersensitivity to any component of this product, history of ACE inhibitor-associated angioedema, and hereditary or idiopathic angioedema.

WARNINGS/PRECAUTIONS

Excessive hypotension sometimes associated w/ oliguria or azotemia and (rarely) acute renal failure or death may occur; monitor closely whenever dose is adjusted and/or diuretic increased. May increase risk of angioedema in patients w/ history of angioedema unrelated to ACE inhibitor therapy. Angioedema of the face, extremities, lips, tongue, glottis, and larynx reported; d/c and administer appropriate therapy if this occurs. Higher incidence of angioedema reported in blacks than nonblacks. Anaphylactoid reactions reported during desensitization w/ hymenoptera venom, dialysis w/ high-flux membranes, and LDL apheresis w/ dextran sulfate absorption. Neutropenia or agranulocytosis and bone marrow depression reported; monitor WBCs in patients w/ renal disease and collagen vascular disease. Rarely, a syndrome that starts w/ cholestatic jaundice and progresses to fulminant hepatic necrosis and sometimes death reported; d/c if jaundice or marked elevations of hepatic enzymes develop. Caution w/ left ventricular outflow obstruction. May cause changes in renal function. Increases in BUN and SrCr reported w/ renal artery stenosis; monitor renal function during the 1st few weeks of therapy. Increases in BUN and SrCr reported w/ no preexisting renal vascular disease. Hyperkalemia may occur; risk factors include diabetes mellitus (DM) and renal insufficiency. Persistent nonproductive cough reported. Hypotension may occur w/ major surgery or during anesthesia; may be corrected by volume expansion.

ADVERSE REACTIONS
Hypotension, headache, nausea, angioedema, MI, fatigue, dizziness, fever, rash, constipation, cough.

DRUG INTERACTIONS
Hypotension risk w/ diuretics. May increase BUN and SrCr w/ diuretics; may require dose reduction and/or discontinuation of diuretic and/or therapy. May further decrease renal dysfunction w/ NSAIDs. Increased risk of hyperkalemia w/ K⁺-sparing diuretics, K⁺-containing salt substitutes, or K⁺ supplements. Antihypertensives that cause renin release (eg, thiazides) may augment antihypertensive effect. NSAIDs may diminish antihypertensive effect. Lithium toxicity reported w/ lithium; monitor serum lithium levels frequently. Nitritoid reactions (eg, facial flushing, N/V, hypotension) reported rarely w/ injectable gold.

PREGNANCY AND LACTATION
Pregnancy: Category C (1st trimester) and D (2nd and 3rd trimesters).
Lactation: Not for use in nursing.

MECHANISM OF ACTION
ACE inhibitor; inhibition results in decreased plasma angiotensin II, which leads to decreased vasopressor activity and decreased aldosterone secretion.

PHARMACOKINETICS
Absorption: (Oral) Poorly absorbed. **Distribution:** Crosses placenta (enalapril), found in breast milk. **Elimination:** (Oral) Urine (>90% unchanged), $T_{1/2}$=11 hrs (enalaprilat).

PATIENT CONSIDERATIONS
Assessment: Assess for history of angioedema, renal dysfunction/disease, collagen vascular disease, renal artery stenosis, left ventricular outflow obstruction, DM, pregnancy/nursing status, and possible drug interactions. Obtain baseline BP, WBC count, serum K⁺ levels, and renal function.

Monitoring: Monitor anaphylactoid reaction, angioedema, hypotension, hypersensitivity, and other adverse reactions. Monitor BP, renal function, WBC count, and serum K⁺ levels.

Counseling: Inform about the risks and benefits of therapy.

ENBREL — etanercept   Rx
Class: Tumor necrosis factor (TNF) blocker

> Increased risk for developing serious infections (eg, active tuberculosis [TB], latent TB reactivation, invasive fungal infections, bacterial/viral infections, opportunistic infections) leading to hospitalization or death, mostly w/ concomitant use w/ immunosuppressants (eg, methotrexate [MTX], corticosteroids). D/C if serious infection or sepsis develops. Active/latent reactivation of TB may present w/ disseminated or extrapulmonary disease; test for latent TB before and during therapy and initiate treatment for latent TB prior to therapy. Consider empiric antifungal therapy in patients at risk for invasive fungal infections who develop severe systemic illness. Monitor for development of infection during and after treatment, including development of TB in patients who tested (-) for latent TB infection prior to therapy. Lymphoma and other malignancies, some fatal, reported in children and adolescents.

ADULT DOSAGE
Plaque Psoriasis

Initial: 50mg twice weekly for 3 months; initial doses of 25mg or 50mg/week were also shown to be efficacious
Maint: 50mg once weekly

Rheumatoid Arthritis

50mg weekly
Max: 50mg/week

May continue MTX, glucocorticoids, salicylates, NSAIDs, or analgesics during treatment

Psoriatic Arthritis

50mg weekly
Max: 50mg/week

May continue MTX, glucocorticoids, salicylates, NSAIDs, or analgesics during treatment

Ankylosing Spondylitis

50mg weekly
Max: 50mg/week

May continue MTX, glucocorticoids, salicylates, NSAIDs, or analgesics during treatment

PEDIATRIC DOSAGE
Juvenile Idiopathic Arthritis

Moderately to Severely Active:
≥2 Years:
<63kg: 0.8mg/kg weekly
≥63kg: 50mg weekly

May continue glucocorticoids, NSAIDs, or analgesics during treatment

ADMINISTRATION
SQ route

Do not mix contents of 1 vial of Enbrel sol w/ the contents of another vial of Enbrel.
Do not add any other medications to sol containing Enbrel.
Do not reconstitute Enbrel w/ other diluents.
Do not filter reconstituted sol during preparation or administration.

Preparation Using the Single-Use Prefilled Syringe
Leave at room temperature for about 15-30 min before injecting.
Check to see if the amount of liquid in the prefilled syringe falls between the 2 purple fill level indicator lines; do not use if the syringe does not have the right amount of liquid.

Preparation Using the SureClick Autoinjector
Leave at room temperature for at least 30 min before injecting.

Preparation Using the Multiple-Use Vial
Reconstitute w/ 1mL of sterile bacteriostatic water for inj (0.9% benzyl alcohol).
Do not use vial adaptor if multiple doses are to be withdrawn from the vial; use a 25-gauge needle if the vial will be used for multiple doses.
Reconstituted sol must be refrigerated at 2-8°C (36-46°F) and used w/in 14 days; discard reconstituted sol after 14 days.
Leave at room temperature for about 15-30 min before injecting.

If Using Vial Adapter:
1. Twist adapter onto the diluents syringe.
2. Place vial adapter over Enbrel vial and insert vial adapter into vial stopper.
3. Push down on plunger to inject diluent into Enbrel vial; inject the diluent very slowly into the Enbrel vial if using a 25-gauge needle.
4. Keeping the diluent syringe in place, gently swirl the contents of the Enbrel vial during dissolution.
5. Withdraw the correct dose of reconstituted sol into the syringe.
6. Remove the syringe from the vial adapter or remove the 25-gauge needle from the syringe.
7. Attach a 27-gauge needle to inject Enbrel.

STORAGE
2-8°C (36-46°F). Do not shake. Protect from light or physical damage. Storage at room temperature at 20-25°C (68-77°F) for a max single period of 14 days is permissible, w/ protection from light, sources of heat, and (vial) humidity; once the product has been stored at room temperature, do not place back into the refrigerator. Discard if not used w/in 14 days at room temperature. Do not store in extreme heat or cold. Do not freeze. (Vial) **Reconstituted Sol:** Use immediately or may refrigerate for up to 14 days.

HOW SUPPLIED
Inj: 25mg [multiple-use vial, single-use prefilled syringe], 50mg [single-use prefilled syringe, single-use prefilled SureClick autoinjector]

CONTRAINDICATIONS
Sepsis.

WARNINGS/PRECAUTIONS
Do not initiate in patients w/ an active infection. Increased risk of infection in patients >65 yrs of age and in patients w/ comorbid conditions. New onset or exacerbation of CNS and peripheral nervous system demyelinating disorders, acute and chronic leukemia, new onset and worsening of CHF, melanoma and non-melanoma skin cancer, and Merkel cell carcinoma reported; consider periodic skin examinations for all patients at increased risk for skin cancer. Pancytopenia, including aplastic anemia, reported; consider discontinuation of therapy in patients w/ confirmed significant hematologic abnormalities. Reactivation of hepatitis B in patients who were previously infected w/ hepatitis B virus (HBV) reported; closely monitor for signs of active HBV infection during and for several months after therapy. Consider discontinuing therapy and initiating antiviral therapy w/ appropriate supportive treatment if HBV reactivation develops. Allergic reactions reported; d/c immediately and initiate appropriate therapy if an anaphylactic or other serious allergic reaction occurs. Needle cover of prefilled syringe and needle cover w/in the needle cap of autoinjector contain dry natural rubber; may cause allergic reactions in latex-sensitive individuals. If possible, pediatric patients should be brought up-to-date w/ all immunizations in agreement w/ current immunization guidelines prior to initiating therapy. May result in the formation of autoantibodies and in the development of a lupus-like syndrome or autoimmune hepatitis; d/c and evaluate patient if a lupus-like syndrome or autoimmune hepatitis develops. Caution w/ moderate to severe alcoholic hepatitis and in the elderly. Patients w/ a significant exposure to varicella virus should temporarily d/c therapy and be considered for prophylactic treatment w/ varicella zoster immune globulin.

ADVERSE REACTIONS
Infections, sepsis, malignancies, inj-site reactions, diarrhea, rash, pyrexia, pruritus.

DRUG INTERACTIONS
See Boxed Warning. Avoid w/ live vaccines. Not recommended w/ anakinra or abatacept; may increase risk of serious infections. Not recommended in patients w/ Wegener's granulomatosis receiving immunosuppressive agents; increased incidence of noncutaneous solid malignancies when added to standard therapy (eg, cyclophosphamide). Not recommended w/ cyclophosphamide. Mild decrease in mean neutrophil counts reported w/ sulfasalazine. Hypoglycemia reported following initiation of therapy in patients receiving antidiabetic medication; reduction in antidiabetic medication may be necessary.

PREGNANCY AND LACTATION
Category B, caution in nursing.

MECHANISM OF ACTION
TNF-blocker; inhibits binding of TNF-α and TNF-β (lymphotoxin alpha [LT-α]) to cell surface TNF-receptors, rendering TNF biologically inactive.

PHARMACOKINETICS

Absorption: C_{max}=2.4mcg/mL (50mg once weekly), 2.6mcg/mL (25mg twice weekly); T_{max}=69 hrs (single 25mg dose). **Distribution:** Found in breast milk; crosses the placenta. **Elimination:** $T_{1/2}$=102 hrs (single 25mg dose).

PATIENT CONSIDERATIONS

Assessment: Assess for sepsis, active/chronic/recurrent infection, history of an opportunistic infection, recent travel in areas of endemic TB or endemic mycoses, underlying conditions that may predispose to infection, central or peripheral nervous system demyelinating disorders, CHF, history of significant hematologic abnormalities, latex sensitivity, alcoholic hepatitis, risk for skin cancer, pregnancy/nursing status, and possible drug interactions. Test for latent TB infection and for HBV infection. Assess immunization history in pediatric patients.

Monitoring: Monitor for development of infection during and after treatment. Monitor for sepsis, central or peripheral nervous system demyelinating disorders, malignancies, new or worsening CHF, hematologic abnormalities, allergic reactions, lupus-like syndrome, autoimmune hepatitis, and other adverse reactions. Monitor for active TB and periodically test for latent TB. Monitor for HBV reactivation during therapy and for several months following termination of therapy. Consider periodic skin examinations for all patients at increased risk for skin cancer.

Counseling: Advise of the potential risks and benefits of therapy. Inform that therapy may lower the ability of immune system to fight infections; instruct to contact physician if any symptoms of infection, TB, or HBV develop. Advise to report any signs of new/worsening medical conditions (eg, CNS demyelinating disorders, CHF, autoimmune disorders) or any symptoms suggestive of pancytopenia. Counsel about the risk of lymphoma and other malignancies. Instruct to seek immediate medical attention if any symptoms of a severe allergic reaction develop. Advise that the needle cover of prefilled syringe and the needle cover w/in the needle cap of the autoinjector contain dry natural rubber (a derivative of latex), which may cause allergic reactions in individuals sensitive to latex. Instruct in inj technique, as well as proper syringe and needle disposal, and caution against reuse of needles and syringes. Advise to inform physician if pregnant/breastfeeding.

ENDOMETRIN — progesterone   Rx

Class: Progesterone

ADULT DOSAGE	PEDIATRIC DOSAGE
Assisted Reproductive Technology	Pediatric use may not have been established
To support embryo implantation and early pregnancy by supplementation of corpus luteal function in infertile women	
General Dosing: 100mg vaginally bid or tid starting the day after oocyte retrieval and continuing for up to 10 weeks	

ADMINISTRATION
Intravaginal route

STORAGE
25°C (77°F); excursions permitted to 15-30°C (59-86°F).

HOW SUPPLIED
Vaginal Insert: 100mg [21^s]

CONTRAINDICATIONS
Previous allergic reactions to progesterone or any of the ingredients of the medication; known missed abortion or ectopic pregnancy; liver disease; known/suspected breast cancer; active arterial/venous thromboembolism or severe thrombophlebitis, or a history of these events.

WARNINGS/PRECAUTIONS
D/C if signs/symptoms of MI, cerebrovascular disorders, arterial or venous thromboembolism (venous thromboembolism or pulmonary embolism), thrombophlebitis, or retinal thrombosis suspected. Caution with history of depression; d/c if symptoms of depression worsen.

ADVERSE REACTIONS
Post-oocyte retrieval pain, abdominal pain, N/V, ovarian hyperstimulation syndrome, abdominal distention, headache, uterine spasm, vaginal bleeding.

DRUG INTERACTIONS
Not recommended for use with other vaginal products (eg, antifungals); progesterone release and absorption from vaginal insert may be altered. CYP450 3A4 inducers (eg, rifampin, carbamazepine) may increase elimination.

PREGNANCY AND LACTATION
Safety not known in pregnancy/nursing.

MECHANISM OF ACTION
Progesterone; increases endometrial receptivity for implantation of an embryo and helps maintain pregnancy.

PHARMACOKINETICS
Absorption: Intravaginal administration of different doses resulted in different parameters. **Distribution:** Serum protein binding (96-99%); found in breast milk. **Metabolism:** Liver and gut via reduction, dehydroxylation, and epimerization. **Excretion:** Kidney (50-60%, metabolite), bile and feces (10%).

PATIENT CONSIDERATIONS
Assessment: Assess for known sensitivity to product, known missed or ectopic abortion, liver disease, breast cancer, active/history of arterial/venous

---

thromboembolism, thrombophlebitis, MI, cerebrovascular disorders, depression, use of other vaginal products, pregnancy/nursing status, and possible drug interactions.

Monitoring: Monitor for signs/symptoms of MI, cerebrovascular disorder, arterial/venous thromboembolism, ovarian hyperstimulation syndrome, vaginal bleeding, worsening of depression, and other adverse reactions.

Counseling: Inform of the importance of reporting irregular vaginal bleeding to physician as soon as possible. Counsel about possible side effects (eg, headaches, breast tenderness, bloating, mood swings, irritability, and drowsiness); advise to seek prompt medical attention if any occur. Inform that product is not recommended for use with other vaginal products.

ENGERIX-B — hepatitis B vaccine (recombinant)   Rx

Class: Vaccine

ADULT DOSAGE	PEDIATRIC DOSAGE
Hepatitis B Vaccine	**Hepatitis B Vaccine**
Immunization Against Infection Caused by All Known Subtypes: ≥20 Years:	**Immunization Against Infection Caused by All Known Subtypes: ≤19 Years:**
Primary Immunization: 1mL IM dose as a 3-dose series given on a 0-, 1-, and 6-month schedule	**Primary Immunization:** 0.5mL IM dose as a 3-dose series given on a 0-, 1-, and 6-month schedule
Alternate Schedule: 1mL IM at 0, 1, 2, and 12 months; may be used for specific populations (eg, recent exposure to the virus, travelers to high-risk areas)	**Alternate Schedule:** May be used for specific populations (eg, recent exposure to the virus, travelers to high-risk areas)
Booster: 1mL IM	**Infants Born of HBsAg-Positive Mothers:** 0.5mL IM at 0, 1, 2, and 12 months
Known or Presumed Exposure to Hepatitis B Virus (HBV): Hepatitis B immune globulin should be given in addition to vaccine w/ known or presumed exposure to the HBV	**Birth through 10 Years:** 0.5mL IM at 0, 1, 2, and 12 months
	5-16 Years: 0.5mL IM at 0, 12, and 24 months (for children/adolescents for whom an extended administration schedule is acceptable based on risk of exposure)
	11-19 Years: 1mL IM at 0, 1, and 6 months or at 0, 1, 2, and 12 months
	Booster: **≤10 Years:** 0.5mL IM **≥11 Years:** 1mL IM
	Known or Presumed Exposure to HBV: Hepatitis B immune globulin should be given in addition to vaccine w/ known or presumed exposure to the HBV

DOSING CONSIDERATIONS
Renal Impairment
Hemodialysis:
Adults:
Primary Immunization: 2mL IM dose as a 4-dose series (given as a single 2mL dose or two 1mL doses) on a 0-, 1-, 2-, and 6-month schedule
Booster: 2mL IM dose (given as a single 2mL dose or two 1mL doses) when antibody levels decline <10 mIU/mL

ADMINISTRATION
IM route

Preferred site of administration is the anterolateral aspect of the thigh (<1 yr of age) and deltoid muscle (older children [whose deltoid is large enough for IM inj] and adults); do not administer in the gluteal region.
May give SQ if at risk of hemorrhage (eg, hemophiliacs).
Shake well before use.
Do not dilute to administer.
Do not mix w/ any other vaccine or product in the same syringe or vial.

STORAGE
2-8°C (36-46°F). Do not freeze; discard if product has been frozen.

HOW SUPPLIED
Inj: 10mcg/0.5mL, 20mcg/mL [vial, prefilled syringe]

CONTRAINDICATIONS
Severe allergic reaction (eg, anaphylaxis) after a previous dose of any hepatitis B-containing vaccine, or to any component of Engerix-B, including yeast.

WARNINGS/PRECAUTIONS
Tip caps of prefilled syringes contain natural rubber latex; allergic reactions may occur. Syncope may occur and can be accompanied by transient neurological signs (eg, visual disturbance, paresthesia, tonic-clonic limb movements). Defer vaccine for infants w/ a birth weight <2000g if mother is documented to be HBsAg negative at the time of infant's birth; vaccination can commence at chronological age 1 month or hospital discharge. Infants born weighing <2000g to HBsAg-positive mothers should receive vaccine and hepatitis B immune globulin (HBIG) w/in 12 hrs after birth. Infants born weighing <2000g to mothers of unknown HBsAg status should receive vaccine and HBIG w/in 12 hrs after birth if the mother's HBsAg status cannot be determined w/in the first 12 hrs of life. The birth dose in infants born weighing <2000g should not be counted as the

1st dose in the vaccine series and it should be followed w/ a full 3-dose standard regimen (total of 4 doses). Apnea in premature infants following IM administration observed; decisions about when to administer vaccine should be based on consideration of medical status, and the potential benefits and possible risks of vaccination. Review immunization history for possible vaccine sensitivity and previous vaccination-related adverse reactions; appropriate treatment must be available for possible anaphylactic reactions. Postpone vaccination w/ moderate or severe acute febrile illness unless at immediate risk of hepatitis B infection (eg, infants born of HBsAg-positive mothers). Immunocompromised persons may have a diminished immune response to vaccine. May not prevent hepatitis B infection in individuals who had an unrecognized hepatitis B infection at the time of vaccination. May not prevent infection in individuals who do not achieve protective antibody titers.

ADVERSE REACTIONS
Inj-site soreness, fatigue.

DRUG INTERACTIONS
May diminish immune response w/ immunosuppressant therapy.

PREGNANCY AND LACTATION
Pregnancy: Category C.
Lactation: Caution in nursing.

MECHANISM OF ACTION
Vaccine; may produce immune response for protection against HBV infection.

PATIENT CONSIDERATIONS

Assessment: Assess for hypersensitivity to yeast or latex, moderate or severe acute febrile illness, immunosuppression, unrecognized hepatitis B infection, pregnancy/nursing status, and for possible drug interactions. Review immunization history for possible vaccine sensitivity and previous vaccination-related adverse reactions. If an infant is receiving the vaccine, assess the birth weight.

Monitoring: Monitor for allergic and inj-site reactions, syncope, and other adverse reactions. Monitor immune response. Perform annual antibody testing in hemodialysis patients to assess the need for booster doses.

Counseling: Inform of potential benefits/risks of immunization. Educate about potential side effects and instruct to notify physician if any side effects develop. Inform that vaccine contains noninfectious purified HBsAg and cannot cause hepatitis B infection.

ENJUVIA — synthetic conjugated estrogens, B　　　Rx

Class: Estrogen

> Increased risk of endometrial cancer in a woman w/ a uterus who uses unopposed estrogens. Adding a progestin to estrogen therapy reduces the risk of endometrial hyperplasia. Adequate diagnostic measures should be undertaken to rule out malignancy in postmenopausal women w/ undiagnosed, persistent or recurring abnormal genital bleeding. Should not be used for the prevention of cardiovascular (CV) disease or dementia. Increased risk of stroke and deep vein thrombosis (DVT) reported in postmenopausal women (50-79 yrs of age) treated w/ daily oral conjugated estrogens (CEs) alone and when combined w/ medroxyprogesterone acetate (MPA). Increased risk of developing probable dementia reported in postmenopausal women ≥65 yrs of age treated w/ daily CEs alone and when combined w/ MPA. Increased risks of pulmonary embolism (PE), MI, and invasive breast cancer reported in postmenopausal women (50-79 yrs of age) treated w/ daily oral CEs combined w/ MPA. Should be prescribed at the lowest effective dose and for the shortest duration consistent w/ treatment goals and risks.

ADULT DOSAGE	PEDIATRIC DOSAGE
Menopausal Vasomotor Symptoms	Pediatric use may not have been established
Moderate to Severe:	
Initial: 0.3mg qd	
Titrate: Subsequent dose adjustment may be made based on response	
Use lowest effective dose for the shortest duration; reevaluate at 3- to 6-month intervals	
Menopausal Vulvar/Vaginal Atrophy	
Moderate to Severe Vaginal Dryness and Pain w/ Intercourse: 0.3mg tab qd	
Use lowest effective dose for the shortest duration; reevaluate at 3- to 6-month intervals	

ADMINISTRATION
Oral route

STORAGE
20-25°C (68-77°F); excursions are permitted to 15-30°C (59-86°F).

HOW SUPPLIED
Tab: 0.3mg, 0.45mg, 0.625mg, 0.9mg, 1.25mg

CONTRAINDICATIONS
Undiagnosed abnormal genital bleeding; known/suspected/history of breast cancer; known/suspected estrogen-dependent neoplasia; active or history of DVT/PE; active, recent, or history of arterial thromboembolic disease (eg, stroke, MI); liver impairment or disease; known protein C, protein S, or antithrombin deficiency, or other known thrombophilic disorders; known/suspected pregnancy.

WARNINGS/PRECAUTIONS
D/C immediately if stroke, DVT, PE, or MI occurs or is suspected. If feasible, d/c at least 4-6 weeks before surgery of the type associated w/ an increased risk of thromboembolism, or during prolonged immobilization. May increase risk of gallbladder disease requiring surgery and risk of ovarian cancer. May lead to severe hypercalcemia in patients w/ breast cancer and bone metastases; d/c and take appropriate measures if hypercalcemia occurs. Retinal vascular thrombosis reported; d/c therapy pending examination if sudden partial/complete loss of vision or sudden onset of proptosis, diplopia, or migraine occurs. If examination reveals papilledema or retinal vascular lesions, d/c therapy permanently. May elevate BP and thyroid-binding globulin levels. May be associated w/ elevations of plasma TGs, leading to pancreatitis in patients w/ preexisting hypertriglyceridemia; consider discontinuation if pancreatitis occurs. Caution in patients w/ history of cholestatic jaundice associated w/ past estrogen use or w/ pregnancy; d/c in case of recurrence. May cause fluid retention. Caution in patients w/ hypoparathyroidism; estrogen-induced hypocalcemia may occur. Cases of malignant transformation of residual endometrial implants reported in women treated posthysterectomy w/ estrogen therapy alone; consider addition of progestin for these patients. May exacerbate symptoms of angioedema in women w/ hereditary angioedema. May exacerbate asthma, diabetes mellitus (DM), epilepsy, migraine, porphyria, systemic lupus erythematosus, and hepatic hemangiomas; use w/ caution. May affect certain endocrine function tests, HDL, LDL, TG levels, and blood components in lab tests.

ADVERSE REACTIONS
Abdominal pain, flu syndrome, headache, pain, flatulence, nausea, dizziness, paresthesia, bronchitis, rhinitis, sinusitis, breast pain, dysmenorrhea, vaginitis.

DRUG INTERACTIONS
CYP3A4 inducers (eg, St. John's wort preparations, phenobarbital, carbamazepine) may decrease levels, which may result in a decrease in therapeutic effects and/or changes in the uterine bleeding profile. CYP3A4 inhibitors (eg, erythromycin, ketoconazole, grapefruit juice) may increase levels and may result in side effects. Patients dependent on thyroid hormone replacement therapy who are also receiving estrogens may require increased doses of thyroid replacement therapy; monitor thyroid function.

PREGNANCY AND LACTATION
Contraindicated in pregnancy, not for use in nursing.

MECHANISM OF ACTION
Estrogen; binds to nuclear receptors in estrogen-responsive tissues. Circulating estrogens modulate pituitary secretion of the gonadotropins, luteinizing hormone and follicle-stimulating hormone, through a (-) feedback mechanism. Reduces elevated levels of these hormones in postmenopausal women.

PHARMACOKINETICS
Absorption: Refer to PI for conjugated and unconjugated estrogen parameters.
Distribution: Largely bound to sex hormone-binding globulin and albumin; found in breast milk. **Metabolism:** Liver to estrone (metabolite); estriol (major urinary metabolite); enterohepatic recirculation via sulfate and glucuronide conjugation in the liver, biliary secretion of conjugates into the intestine; hydrolysis in the intestine; reabsorption; CYP3A4 (partial metabolism). **Elimination:** Urine; $T_{1/2}$=14 hrs (estrone), 11 hrs (equilin).

PATIENT CONSIDERATIONS

Assessment: Assess for abnormal genital bleeding, presence/history of breast cancer, estrogen-dependent neoplasia, active/history of DVT/PE/arterial thromboembolic disease, liver impairment/disease, thrombophilic disorders, hypersensitivity to the drug, pregnancy/nursing status, any other conditions where treatment is contraindicated or cautioned, need for progestin therapy, and possible drug interactions.

Monitoring: Monitor for signs/symptoms of CV disorders, malignant neoplasms, dementia, gallbladder disease, hypercalcemia, visual abnormalities, BP and plasma TG elevations, pancreatitis, cholestatic jaundice, hypothyroidism, fluid retention, and other adverse reactions. Perform annual breast exam; schedule mammography based on age, risk factors, and prior mammogram results. Monitor thyroid function in patients on thyroid replacement therapy, and monitor BP. Periodically evaluate (every 3-6 months) to determine need for therapy. If undiagnosed, persistent, or recurring abnormal vaginal bleeding occurs, perform proper diagnostic testing (eg, endometrial sampling) to rule out malignancy.

Counseling: Inform of risks and benefits of therapy. Instruct to use ud. Advise of possible serious adverse reactions of therapy (eg, CV disorders, malignant neoplasms, probable dementia) and of possible less serious, but common adverse reactions of therapy (eg, headaches, breast pain and tenderness, N/V). Instruct to notify physician if vaginal bleeding occurs. Advise to have yearly breast exam by physician and to perform monthly breast self-exams.

ENSTILAR — betamethasone dipropionate/calcipotriene　　　Rx

Class: Corticosteroid/vitamin D3 analogue

ADULT DOSAGE	PEDIATRIC DOSAGE
Plaque Psoriasis	Pediatric use may not have been established
Apply to affected areas qd for up to 4 weeks	
Do not use >60g every 4 days; d/c when control is achieved	

ADMINISTRATION
Topical route

Shake prior to using.
Rub in gently.

Wash hands after applying the product.

Avoid use w/ occlusive dressings unless directed by a physician.

Avoid use on the face, groin, or axillae, or if skin atrophy is present at the treatment site.

STORAGE
20-25°C (68-77°F); excursions permitted between 15-30°C (59-86°F). Do not expose to heat or store at >49°C (120°F). Do not freeze. Use w/in 6 months after it has been opened.

HOW SUPPLIED
Foam: (Calcipotriene/Betamethasone Dipropionate) 0.005%/0.064% [60g]

WARNINGS/PRECAUTIONS
Not for oral, ophthalmic, or intravaginal use. The propellants are flammable; instruct to avoid fire, flame, and smoking during and immediately following application. Hypercalcemia and hypercalciuria observed; d/c until parameters of Ca^{2+} metabolism have normalized. Systemic absorption may produce reversible hypothalamic-pituitary-adrenal (HPA) axis suppression w/ the potential for glucocorticosteroid insufficiency during or upon withdrawal of treatment. Risk factors include the use of high-potency steroids, large treatment surface areas, prolonged use, use of occlusive dressings, altered skin barrier, liver failure, and young age. Gradually withdraw drug, reduce frequency of application, or substitute w/ a less potent corticosteroid if HPA axis suppression is documented. Cushing's syndrome, hyperglycemia, and glucosuria may occur. Pediatric patients may be more susceptible to systemic toxicity. Allergic contact dermatitis may occur. Avoid excessive exposure of treated areas to natural or artificial sunlight; consider limiting or avoiding use of phototherapy.

ADVERSE REACTIONS
Application-site irritation/pruritus, folliculitis, skin hypopigmentation, hypercalcemia, urticaria, exacerbation of psoriasis.

DRUG INTERACTIONS
Use w/ other corticosteroid-containing products at the same time may increase total systemic exposure.

PREGNANCY AND LACTATION
Pregnancy: Category C.

Lactation: It is not known whether topically administered calcipotriene or corticosteroids could result in sufficient systemic absorption to produce detectable quantities in human milk. Caution in nursing. Do not use on the breast when nursing.

MECHANISM OF ACTION
Calcipotriene: Synthetic vitamin D3 analogue. **Betamethasone Dipropionate:** Synthetic corticosteroid. Mechanism not established.

PHARMACOKINETICS
Absorption: Calcipotriene: C_{max}=55.9pg/mL, 24.4pg/mL (MC1080); AUC_{last}=82.5pg•hr/mL, 59.3pg•hr/mL (MC1080). Betamethasone Dipropionate: C_{max}=52.2pg/mL, 147.9pg/mL (betamethasone 17-propionate [B17P]); AUC_{last}=36.5pg•hr/mL, 683.6pg•hr/mL (B17P). **Distribution:** Betamethasone Dipropionate: Found in breast milk (systemically administered). **Metabolism:** Betamethasone Dipropionate: B17P (major metabolite). Calcipotriene: Liver (rapid); MC1080 (major metabolite).

PATIENT CONSIDERATIONS
Assessment: Assess for predisposing factors to HPA axis suppression, treatment-site atrophy, use of phototherapy, pregnancy/nursing status, and possible drug interactions.

Monitoring: Monitor for hypercalcemia, hypercalciuria, HPA axis suppression, Cushing's syndrome, hyperglycemia, glucosuria, allergic contact dermatitis, and other adverse reactions.

Counseling: Instruct to shake before use. Instruct not to use >60g every 4 days, and to d/c therapy when control is achieved. Advise to avoid use on the face, underarms, groin, or eyes; instruct to wash area right away if medicine gets on the face or in the mouth or eyes. Instruct to wash hands after application. Advise not to occlude the treatment area w/ a bandage or other covering unless directed by physician, and not to use other products containing calcipotriene or a corticosteroid during therapy w/o first discussing w/ physician. Instruct patients to avoid excessive exposure to either natural or artificial sunlight (eg, tanning booths, sun lamps). Inform that drug is flammable; advise to avoid heat, flame, or smoking when applying. Inform that the foam can be sprayed holding the can in any orientation except horizontally.

ENTEREG — alvimopan
Class: Opioid antagonist   Rx

> Potential risk of MI w/ long-term use; for short-term hospital use only. Available only through a restricted program for short-term use (15 doses) under a Risk Evaluation and Mitigation Strategy called the Entereg Access Support and Education (E.A.S.E.) Program.

ADULT DOSAGE	PEDIATRIC DOSAGE
Postoperative Gastrointestinal Recovery	Pediatric use may not have been established
To Accelerate the Time to Upper and Lower GI Recovery Following Surgeries that Include Partial Bowel Resection w/ Primary Anastomosis: 12mg given 30 min to 5 hrs prior to surgery followed by 12mg bid beginning the day after surgery until discharge for a max of 7 days	
Max: 15 doses	

DOSING CONSIDERATIONS
Renal Impairment
ESRD: Not recommended

Hepatic Impairment
Severe: Not recommended

ADMINISTRATION
Oral route

STORAGE
25°C (77°F); excursions permitted to 15-30°C (59-86°F).

HOW SUPPLIED
Cap: 12mg

CONTRAINDICATIONS
Patients who have taken therapeutic doses of opioids for >7 consecutive days immediately prior to therapy.

WARNINGS/PRECAUTIONS
Increased sensitivity to therapy and occurrence of GI adverse reactions (eg, abdominal pain, N/V, diarrhea) are expected w/ patients recently exposed to opioids; monitor patients receiving >3 doses of an opioid w/in the week prior to surgery for GI adverse reactions. May be at higher risk of serious adverse reaction in patients w/ severe hepatic impairment. Not recommended for use w/ complete GI obstruction, surgery for correction of complete bowel obstruction, or pancreatic/gastric anastomosis. Closely monitor patients w/ mild to moderate hepatic impairment/mild to severe renal impairment and Japanese patients for possible adverse effects (eg, diarrhea, GI pain, cramping); d/c if adverse events occur.

ADVERSE REACTIONS
Dyspepsia.

DRUG INTERACTIONS
See Contraindications.

PREGNANCY AND LACTATION
Pregnancy: Category B.
Lactation: Caution in nursing.

MECHANISM OF ACTION
Opioid antagonist; selective antagonist of μ-opioid receptor. Antagonizes the peripheral effects of opioids on GI motility and secretion by competitively binding to GI tract μ-opioid receptors.

PHARMACOKINETICS
Absorption: Absolute bioavailability (6%); T_{max}=2 hrs, 36 hrs (median) (metabolite); C_{max}=10.98ng/mL, 35.73ng/mL (metabolite); AUC_{0-12h}=40.2ng•hr/mL. **Distribution:** V_d=30L; plasma protein binding (80%, 94% [metabolite]). **Metabolism:** Intestinal flora; amide hydrolysis compound (active metabolite). **Elimination:** Bile (primary), feces, urine; $T_{1/2}$=10-17 hrs, 10-18 hrs (metabolite).

PATIENT CONSIDERATIONS
Assessment: Assess for hepatic/renal impairment, complete GI obstruction/surgery for correction of complete bowel obstruction, pancreatic/gastric anastomosis, history of opioid use, and pregnancy/nursing status.

Monitoring: Monitor for GI adverse reactions and other adverse effects.

Counseling: Instruct to disclose long-term or intermittent opioid pain therapy, including any use of opioids in the week prior to receiving therapy; inform that recent use of opioids may increase susceptibility to adverse reactions, primarily those limited to the GI tract (eg, abdominal pain, N/V, diarrhea). Advise that therapy is for hospital use only for no more than 7 days after bowel resection surgery. Inform that dyspepsia may occur.

ENTOCORT EC — budesonide
Class: Corticosteroid   Rx

ADULT DOSAGE	PEDIATRIC DOSAGE
Crohn's Disease	**Crohn's Disease**
Mild to Moderate Active Crohn's Disease Involving the Ileum and/or Ascending Colon: 9mg qam for up to 8 weeks; repeated 8-week courses may be given for recurring episodes of active disease	**Mild to Moderate Active Crohn's Disease Involving the Ileum and/or Ascending Colon:** **8-17 Years:** **>25kg:** 9mg qam up to 8 weeks followed by 6mg qam for 2 weeks
Maint of Clinical Remission: 6mg qam for up to 3 months; if symptom control is still maintained at 3 months, attempt to taper to complete cessation	

DOSING CONSIDERATIONS
Concomitant Medications
Avoid consumption of grapefruit juice for the duration of therapy

Hepatic Impairment
Adults:
Moderate (Child-Pugh Class B): Consider reducing the dose to 3mg qam; monitor for increased signs/symptoms of hypercorticism
Severe (Child-Pugh Class C): Avoid use

Elderly
Start at lower end of dosing range

ADMINISTRATION
Oral route

Swallow caps whole; do not chew or break.

STORAGE
25° (77°F); excursions permitted to 15-30°C (59-86°F). Keep container tightly closed.

HOW SUPPLIED
Cap: 3mg

CONTRAINDICATIONS
Hypersensitivity to budesonide or to any of the ingredients of this product.

WARNINGS/PRECAUTIONS
Systemic effects (eg, hypercorticism, adrenal suppression) may occur when used chronically. May reduce response of hypothalamus-pituitary-adrenal axis to stress; supplement w/ a systemic corticosteroid during surgery or other stress situations. Patients w/ moderate/severe hepatic impairment may be at increased risk of hypercorticism and adrenal axis suppression. Monitor if transferred from corticosteroid treatment w/ high systemic effects; withdrawal symptoms may develop. Replacement of systemic glucocorticosteroids may unmask allergies. Increased risk of infection; avoid exposure to chickenpox/measles. Caution w/ active or quiescent tuberculosis (TB), untreated fungal/bacterial/systemic viral/parasitic infections, or ocular herpes simplex. Monitor patients w/ HTN, diabetes mellitus (DM), osteoporosis, peptic ulcer, glaucoma, cataracts, family history of DM or glaucoma or w/ any other condition where corticosteroids may have unwanted effects.

ADVERSE REACTIONS
Headache, respiratory infection, N/V, back pain, dyspepsia, dizziness, abdominal pain, flatulence, fatigue, pain.

DRUG INTERACTIONS
See Dosing Considerations. Avoid use w/ CYP3A4 inhibitors; ketoconazole caused an eight-fold increase of systemic exposure to oral budesonide. Increased levels w/ CYP3A4 inhibitors (eg, ketoconazole, saquinavir, erythromycin, grapefruit juice).

PREGNANCY AND LACTATION
Pregnancy: Limited published studies report on the use in pregnant women; however, the data are insufficient to inform a drug-associated risk for major birth defects and miscarriage. Teratogenic and embryolethal in rabbits and rats. Hypoadrenalism may occur in infants born of mothers receiving corticosteroids during pregnancy; monitor for signs of hypoadrenalism.
Lactation: No information is available on the effects on the breastfed infant or the effects of the drug on milk production.

MECHANISM OF ACTION
Glucocorticosteroid; high glucocorticoid effect and weak mineralocorticoid effect.

PHARMACOKINETICS
Absorption: C_{max}=4nmol/L; T_{max}=30-600 min; AUC=35nmol·hr/L. Oral bioavailability (9-21%). **Distribution:** V_d=2.2-3.9L/kg; plasma protein binding (85-90%). **Metabolism:** Liver (high first pass effect); CYP3A4. **Elimination:** Urine (60%); $T_{1/2}$=2-3.6 hrs.

PATIENT CONSIDERATIONS
Assessment: Assess for hypersensitivity to budesonide or any of the ingredients of this product; history of chickenpox or measles; TB; untreated fungal, bacterial, systemic viral or parasitic infections; ocular herpes simplex; HTN; osteoporosis; peptic ulcers; cataracts; history and/or family history of DM or glaucoma; pregnancy/ nursing status, and possible drug interactions.

Monitoring: Monitor for signs/symptoms of hypercorticism, adrenal axis suppression, infection, hypersensitivity reactions, and any other adverse reaction. Monitor for symptoms of steroid withdrawal in patients transferred from other systemic corticosteroids.

Counseling: Instruct on proper use. Advise that use may cause hypercorticism and adrenal axis suppression and to follow a taper schedule, if transferring to Entocort EC from systemic corticosteroids. Advise that replacement of systemic corticosteroids may unmask allergies (eg, rhinitis, eczema), which were previously controlled by the systemic drug. Advise to avoid exposure to people w/ chickenpox or measles and, if exposed, to consult healthcare provider immediately. Inform that there is an increased risk of developing a variety of infections and instruct to contact healthcare provider if symptoms of infection develop. Advise female patients that use may cause fetal harm and instruct to inform healthcare provider w/ a known or suspected pregnancy.

ENTRESTO — sacubitril/valsartan   Rx
Class: Angiotensin II receptor blocker (ARB)/neprilysin inhibitor

> **D/C when pregnancy is detected. Drugs that act directly on the renin-angiotensin system (RAS) can cause injury/death to the developing fetus.**

ADULT DOSAGE
Heart Failure

Risk reduction of cardiovascular death and hospitalization for heart failure (HF) in patients w/ chronic HF (NYHA Class II-IV) and reduced ejection fraction

Initial: 49mg/51mg bid
Titrate: Double the dose after 2-4

PEDIATRIC DOSAGE
Pediatric use may not have been established

weeks to the target maint dose of 97mg/103mg bid, as tolerated

Patients Not Taking an ACE Inhibitor/ARB or Previously Taking Low Doses of These Agents:
Initial: 24mg/26mg bid
Titrate: Double the dose every 2-4 weeks to the target maint dose of 97mg/103mg bid, as tolerated

Conversions
Switching from an ACE Inhibitor:
Allow a washout period of 36 hrs between administration of the two drugs

DOSING CONSIDERATIONS
Renal Impairment
Severe (eGFR <30mL/min/1.73m²):
Initial: 24mg/26mg bid
Titrate: Double the dose every 2-4 weeks to the target maint dose of 97mg/103mg bid, as tolerated
Hepatic Impairment
Moderate (Child-Pugh B):
Initial: 24mg/26mg bid
Titrate: Double the dose every 2-4 weeks to the target maint dose of 97mg/103mg bid, as tolerated
Severe: Not recommended

ADMINISTRATION
Oral route

Usually administered in conjunction w/ other heart failure therapies, in place of an ACE inhibitor or other ARB.
Take w/ or w/o food.

STORAGE
25°C (77°F); excursions permitted to 15-30°C (59-86°F). Protect from moisture.

HOW SUPPLIED
Tab: (Sacubitril/Valsartan) 24mg/26mg, 49mg/51mg, 97mg/103mg

CONTRAINDICATIONS
Hypersensitivity to any component, history of angioedema related to previous ACE inhibitor or ARB therapy, concomitant use of ACE inhibitors or use w/in 36 hrs of switching from or to an ACE inhibitor, coadministration w/ aliskiren in patients w/ diabetes.

WARNINGS/PRECAUTIONS
May cause angioedema; d/c immediately and do not readminister if angioedema occurs. Associated w/ a higher rate of angioedema in black than in non-black patients. May cause symptomatic hypotension; patients w/ an activated RAS (eg, volume- and/or salt-depleted patients [including those on high doses of diuretics]) are at greater risk. Correct volume or salt depletion prior to therapy or start at a lower dose. If hypotension occurs, consider dose adjustment of diuretics, concomitant antihypertensive drugs, and treatment of other causes of hypotension. If hypotension persists despite such measures, reduce the dosage or temporarily d/c therapy. Decreased renal function may occur; caution w/ patients whose renal function depends upon the activity of the RAS (eg, severe CHF). Closely monitor SrCr, and down-titrate or interrupt therapy in patients who develop a clinically significant decrease in renal function. May increase blood urea and SrCr levels in patients w/ bilateral or unilateral renal artery stenosis. Hyperkalemia may occur; dosage reduction or interruption may be required.

ADVERSE REACTIONS
Hypotension, hyperkalemia, cough, dizziness, renal failure.

DRUG INTERACTIONS
See Contraindications. Avoid use w/ an ARB. Avoid use w/ aliskiren in patients w/ renal impairment (eGFR <60mL/min/1.73m²). Concomitant use of K⁺-sparing diuretics, K⁺ supplements, or salt substitutes containing K⁺ may increase serum K⁺ levels. Concomitant use of NSAIDs, including COX-2 inhibitors, may result in worsening of renal function, including possible acute renal failure, in patients who are elderly, volume-depleted, or w/ compromised renal function; monitor renal function periodically. Increases in lithium levels and lithium toxicity reported during concomitant administration w/ ARBs; monitor serum lithium levels during concomitant use.

PREGNANCY AND LACTATION
Pregnancy: May cause fetal harm; use of drugs that act on the RAS during the 2nd and 3rd trimesters reduces fetal renal function and increases fetal and neonatal morbidity and death. Consider alternative drug treatment and d/c therapy when pregnancy is detected; if there is no appropriate alternative w/ drugs affecting the RAS, and if the drug is considered lifesaving for the mother, advise of the potential risk to the fetus.
Lactation: Not for use in nursing.

MECHANISM OF ACTION
Sacubitril: Neprilysin inhibitor; inhibits neprilysin via LBQ657, the active metabolite of the prodrug sacubitril. Valsartan: ARB; blocks the angiotensin II type-1 receptor. The cardiovascular and renal effects are attributed to the increased levels of peptides that are degraded by neprilysin (eg, natriuretic peptides), by LBQ657, and the simultaneous inhibition of the effects of angiotensin II by valsartan.

PHARMACOKINETICS
Absorption: Sacubitril: T_{max}=0.5 hrs; Absolute bioavailability (≥60%). LBQ657: T_{max}=2 hrs. Valsartan: T_{max}=1.5 hrs. **Distribution:** Sacubitril: Plasma protein binding

(94-97%); V_d=103L. LBQ657: Plasma protein binding (94-97%); crosses blood-brain barrier to a limited extent (0.28%). Valsartan: Plasma protein binding (94-97%); V_d=75L. **Metabolism:** Sacubitril: Readily converted to LBQ657 by esterases. Valsartan: Minimal (20% recovered as metabolites). **Elimination:** Sacubitril: Feces (37-48%; primarily as LBQ657), urine (52-68%; primarily as LBQ657); $T_{1/2}$=1.4 hrs. LBQ657: $T_{1/2}$=11.5 hrs. Valsartan: Feces (86%), urine (about 13%); $T_{1/2}$=9.9 hrs.

PATIENT CONSIDERATIONS

Assessment: Assess for hypersensitivity to any component of the drug, history of angioedema related to previous ACE inhibitor/ARB therapy, diabetes, activated RAS, renal artery stenosis, risk factors for hyperkalemia, renal/hepatic impairment, pregnancy/nursing status, and possible drug interactions.

Monitoring: Monitor for signs/symptoms of angioedema and hypotension. Closely monitor SrCr in patients who develop a clinically significant decrease in renal function. Monitor renal function. Monitor serum K^+ periodically, especially in patients w/ risk factors for hyperkalemia.

Counseling: Advise females of childbearing age about the consequences of exposure to drug during pregnancy. Discuss treatment options w/ women planning to become pregnant. Advise to report pregnancies to physicians as soon as possible. Advise to d/c use of previous ACE inhibitor or ARB and to allow a 36-hr washout period if switching from or to an ACE inhibitor.

ENTYVIO — vedolizumab   **Rx**

Class: Monoclonal antibody/integrin receptor antagonist

ADULT DOSAGE	PEDIATRIC DOSAGE
Ulcerative Colitis	Pediatric use may not have been established
Moderately to Severely Active:	

Moderately to Severely Active:
For inducing/maintaining clinical response and remission, improving endoscopic appearance of the mucosa, and achieving corticosteroid-free remission in patients who have had an inadequate response w/, lost response to, or were intolerant to a TNF blocker or immunomodulator; or had an inadequate response w/, were intolerant to, or demonstrated dependence on corticosteroids

300mg IV infusion over 30 min at 0, 2, and 6 weeks and then every 8 weeks thereafter

D/C if no evidence of therapeutic benefit seen by Week 14

Crohn's Disease
Moderately to Severely Active:
For achieving clinical response and remission, and achieving corticosteroid-free remission in patients who have had an inadequate response w/, lost response to, or were intolerant to a TNF blocker or immunomodulator; or had an inadequate response w/, were intolerant to, or demonstrated dependence on corticosteroids

300mg IV infusion over 30 min at 0, 2, and 6 weeks and then every 8 weeks thereafter

D/C if no evidence of therapeutic benefit seen by Week 14

ADMINISTRATION
IV route

Do not administer as an IV push or bolus.
Lyophilized powder must be reconstituted w/ sterile water for inj (SWFI) and diluted in 250mL of sterile 0.9% NaCl inj prior to administration.
After infusion is complete, flush w/ 30mL of sterile 0.9% NaCl inj.

Reconstitution
1. Reconstitute vial containing lyophilized powder w/ 4.8mL of SWFI using a syringe w/ a 21- to 25- gauge needle.
2. Insert the syringe needle into the vial through the center of the stopper and direct the stream of SWFI to the glass wall of the vial to avoid excessive foaming.
3. Gently swirl vial for at least 15 sec; do not vigorously shake or invert.
4. Allow sol to sit for up to 20 min at room temperature to allow for reconstitution and for any foam to settle; may swirl and inspect for dissolution during this time. If not fully dissolved after 20 min, allow another 10 min for dissolution; do not use vial if the drug product is not dissolved w/in 30 min.
5. Prior to withdrawing the reconstituted sol from vial, gently invert vial 3X.
6. Withdraw 5mL (300mg) of reconstituted sol using a syringe w/ a 21- to 25-gauge needle.

Dilution
Add the 5mL (300mg) of reconstituted sol to 250mL of 0.9% NaCl and gently mix infusion bag; once reconstituted and diluted, use infusion sol as soon as possible.

Do not add other medicinal products to the prepared infusion sol or IV infusion set. May store infusion sol for up to 4 hrs at 2°-8°C (36°-46°F), if necessary; do not freeze.

STORAGE
2-8°C (36-46°F). Protect from light. **Infusion Sol:** 2-8°C (36-46°F) for up to 4 hrs. Do not freeze.

HOW SUPPLIED
Inj: 300mg

CONTRAINDICATIONS
Known serious or severe hypersensitivity reaction to vedolizumab or any of the excipients (eg, dyspnea, bronchospasm, urticaria, flushing, rash, increased HR).

WARNINGS/PRECAUTIONS
Hypersensitivity reactions reported; d/c immediately and initiate appropriate treatment if anaphylaxis or other serious allergic reactions occur. Increased risk for developing infections; not recommended in patients with active, severe infections until the infections are controlled. Consider withholding treatment if a severe infection develops. Consider screening for tuberculosis according to the local practice. Progressive multifocal leukoencephalopathy (PML) may occur; monitor for any new onset, or worsening, of neurological signs and symptoms. If PML is suspected, withhold dosing and refer to a neurologist; if confirmed, d/c dosing permanently. Elevations of transaminase and/or bilirubin reported; d/c if jaundice or other evidence of significant liver injury develops. Prior to initiating treatment, all patients should be brought up to date with all immunizations according to current immunization guidelines.

ADVERSE REACTIONS
Nasopharyngitis, headache, arthralgia, nausea, pyrexia, upper respiratory tract infection, fatigue, cough, bronchitis, influenza, back pain, rash, pruritus, sinusitis, oropharyngeal pain, pain in extremities.

DRUG INTERACTIONS
Avoid with natalizumab; potential for increased risk of PML and other infections. Avoid with TNF blockers; potential for increased risk of infections. Live vaccines may be administered concurrently with therapy only if the benefits outweigh the risks.

PREGNANCY AND LACTATION
Category B, caution in nursing.

MECHANISM OF ACTION
Monoclonal antibody/integrin receptor antagonist; specifically binds to the α4β7 integrin and blocks the interaction of α4β7 integrin with mucosal addressin cell adhesion molecule-1 and inhibits the migration of memory T-lymphocytes across the endothelium into inflamed GI parenchymal tissue.

PHARMACOKINETICS
Distribution: V_d=5L; crosses placenta. **Elimination:** $T_{1/2}$=25 days.

PATIENT CONSIDERATIONS
Assessment: Assess for hypersensitivity to drug, infections, history of recurring severe infections, pregnancy/nursing status, and possible drug interactions. Assess immunization history.

Monitoring: Monitor for infusion/hypersensitivity reactions, infections, PML, liver injury, and other adverse reactions.

Counseling: Instruct to report immediately if symptoms consistent with a hypersensitivity reaction occur during or following infusion. Advise to notify physician if any signs/symptoms of infection develop. Instruct to report immediately any symptoms that may indicate PML (new onset or worsening of neurological signs/symptoms) and/or liver injury (eg, fatigue, anorexia, right upper abdominal discomfort, dark urine, jaundice).

ENULOSE — lactulose   **Rx**

Class: Ammonium detoxicant/osmotic laxative

OTHER BRAND NAMES
Generlac

ADULT DOSAGE	PEDIATRIC DOSAGE
Portal-Systemic Encephalopathy	**Portal-Systemic Encephalopathy**
Including Stages of Hepatic Pre-Coma and Coma:	**Including Stages of Hepatic Pre-Coma and Coma:**
Oral Route:	**Oral Route:**
Usual: 30-45mL (containing 20-30g of lactulose) tid or qid	**Infants:**
Titrate: Adjust dose every day or two, to produce 2 or 3 soft stools daily	**Initial:** 2.5-10mL/day in divided doses, to produce 2-3 soft stools daily
Hourly doses of 30-45mL may be used to induce the rapid laxation indicated in the initial phase of the therapy; when the laxative effect has been achieved, the dose may then be reduced to the recommended daily dose	**Older Children and Adolescents:** 40-90mL/day, to produce 2-3 soft stools daily
Rectal Route:	If initial dose causes diarrhea, reduce dose immediately; if diarrhea persists, d/c lactulose
When the patient is in the impending coma or coma stage and the danger of aspiration exists, or when the necessary endoscopic or intubation procedures physically interfere w/ the administration of the recommended oral doses, lactulose sol may be given as a retention enema via a rectal balloon catheter	

Mix 300mL of lactulose sol w/ 700mL of water or physiologic saline and retain for 30-60 min; may repeat q4-6h

If the enema is inadvertently evacuated too promptly, it may be repeated immediately

Start oral therapy before the enema is stopped entirely

ADMINISTRATION
Oral/Rectal route

STORAGE
Do not freeze. Prolonged exposure >30°C (86°F) or to direct light may cause extreme darkening and turbidity; do not use if this condition develops. Prolonged exposure to freezing temperature may cause change to a semi-solid, too viscous to pour; viscosity will return to normal upon warming to room temperature. **Enulose:** 2-30°C (36-86°F). **Generlac:** 20-25°C (68-77°F).

HOW SUPPLIED
Sol: (Enulose) 10g/15mL [473mL], (Generlac) 10g/15mL [473mL, 1892mL]

CONTRAINDICATIONS
Patients who require a low-galactose diet.

WARNINGS/PRECAUTIONS
Potential explosive reaction with electrocautery procedures during proctoscopy or colonoscopy; patients on therapy undergoing such procedures should have a thorough bowel cleansing with a non-fermentable solution. Contains galactose and lactose; caution with diabetes. May develop hyponatremia and dehydration in infants.

ADVERSE REACTIONS
Flatulence/belching, abdominal discomfort, diarrhea, N/V.

DRUG INTERACTIONS
May interfere the desired degradation and prevent the acidification of colonic contents with neomycin; closely monitor the status of the treated patients. Nonabsorbable antacids may decrease effects. Avoid use with other laxatives, especially during the initial phase of therapy.

PREGNANCY AND LACTATION
Category B, caution in nursing.

MECHANISM OF ACTION
Osmotic laxative; bacterial degradation in the colon acidifies the colonic contents resulting in the retention of ammonia in the colon as ammonium ion; ammonia can be expected to migrate from the blood into the colon to form the ammonium ion; the acid colonic contents convert ammonia to the ammonium ion by trapping and preventing absorption; laxative action of the metabolites then expels the trapped ammonium ion from the colon.

PHARMACOKINETICS
Absorption: Poor. **Elimination:** Urine ($\leq$3%).

PATIENT CONSIDERATIONS
Assessment: Assess for diabetes, patients requiring a low-galactose diet, pregnancy/nursing status, and possible drug interactions. Assess use in electrocautery procedures during proctoscopy or colonoscopy.

Monitoring: Monitor for hyponatremia and dehydration in infants, diarrhea, vomiting, and other adverse reactions.

Counseling: Inform about the risks and benefits of therapy. Instruct to take exactly ud. Advise to report any potential adverse effects.

ENVARSUS XR — tacrolimus   Rx

Class: Calcineurin-inhibitor immunosuppressant

> Increased risk for developing serious infections and malignancies w/ tacrolimus extended-release (ER) or other immunosuppressants that may lead to hospitalization or death.

ADULT DOSAGE
Organ Rejection Prophylaxis
Prophylaxis of organ rejection in kidney transplant patients converted from tacrolimus immediate-release (IR) formulations, in combination w/ other immunosuppressants

Conversion from Tacrolimus IR Formulations:
Administer an Envarsus XR qd dose that is 80% of the total daily dose of the tacrolimus IR product

Monitor tacrolimus whole blood trough concentrations and titrate dose to achieve target whole blood trough concentration ranges of 4-11ng/mL

African-American patients, compared to Caucasian patients, may need to be titrated to higher doses to attain comparable trough concentrations

Therapeutic Drug Monitoring:
Measure tacrolimus whole blood trough concentrations at least 2X on

PEDIATRIC DOSAGE
Pediatric use may not have been established

separate days during the first week after initiation of dosing and after any change in dosage, after a change in coadministration of CYP3A inducers and/or inhibitors, or after a change in renal or hepatic function

When interpreting measured concentrations, consider that the time to achieve tacrolimus steady state is approx 7 days after initiating or changing the dose

Missed Dose
If a dose is missed, the dose should be taken as soon as possible w/in 15 hrs after missing the dose

Beyond the 15-hr time frame, the patient should wait until the usual scheduled time to take the next regular daily dose; it is not recommended to double the next dose to make up for the missed dose

---

DOSING CONSIDERATIONS
Hepatic Impairment
Severe (Child-Pugh >10): May require lower doses

ADMINISTRATION
Oral route

Take on an empty stomach at the same time of the day, preferably in the am. Swallow whole w/ fluid (preferably water); do not chew, divide, or crush. Not interchangeable or substitutable w/ other tacrolimus ER or IR products. Avoid eating grapefruit or drinking grapefruit juice or alcoholic beverages.

STORAGE
25°C (77°F); excursions permitted to 15-30°C (59-86°F).

HOW SUPPLIED
Tab, ER: 0.75mg, 1mg, 4mg

CONTRAINDICATIONS
Known hypersensitivity to tacrolimus.

WARNINGS/PRECAUTIONS
Increases risk of developing lymphomas and other malignancies, particularly of the skin. Post-transplant lymphoproliferative disorder (PTLD), associated w/ Epstein-Barr virus (EBV), has been reported in immunosuppressed organ transplant patients; risk of PTLD appears greatest in those individuals who are EBV seronegative; monitor EBV serology during treatment. Increases risk of developing bacterial, viral (eg, polyomavirus-associated nephropathy, JC virus-associated progressive multifocal leukoencephalopathy, CMV infection), fungal, and protozoal infections, including opportunistic infections; monitor for the development of infection and adjust immunosuppressive regimen to balance the risk of rejection w/ risk of infection. Graft rejection and other serious adverse reactions due to medication errors reported; not interchangeable or substitutable w/ other tacrolimus ER or IR products. New onset diabetes reported after transplant. Can cause acute or chronic nephrotoxicity; consider dosage reduction in patients w/ elevated SrCr and tacrolimus whole blood trough concentrations greater than the recommended range. May cause a spectrum of neurotoxicities; consider dosage reduction or discontinuation if neurotoxicity occurs. Mild to severe hyperkalemia reported. HTN may occur and antihypertensive therapy may be required. May prolong the QT/QTc interval and cause torsades de pointes; avoid in patients w/ congenital long QT syndrome. Consider obtaining ECG and monitoring electrolytes (Mg²⁺, K⁺, Ca²⁺) periodically during treatment in patients w/ CHF, bradyarrhythmias, those taking certain antiarrhythmic medications or other products that lead to QT prolongation, and those w/ electrolyte disturbances. Whenever possible, administer the complete complement of vaccines before transplantation and therapy. Cases of pure red cell aplasia (PRCA) reported; consider discontinuation of therapy if PRCA is diagnosed.

ADVERSE REACTIONS
Diarrhea, increased blood creatinine, UTI, nasopharyngitis, headache, URTI, peripheral edema, HTN.

DRUG INTERACTIONS
See Administration. Risk for nephrotoxicity may increase when concomitantly administered w/ CYP3A inhibitors or drugs associated w/ nephrotoxicity (eg, aminoglycosides, ganciclovir, amphotericin B, cisplatin, protease inhibitors); monitor renal function and consider dosage reduction if nephrotoxicity occurs. Agents associated w/ hyperkalemia (eg, K⁺-sparing diuretics, ACE inhibitors, ARB[s]) may increase risk for hyperkalemia. Avoid use of live attenuated vaccines during treatment. Inactivated vaccines noted to be safe for administration after transplantation may not be sufficiently immunogenic during treatment w/ Envarsus XR. Increases exposure to mycophenolic acid (MPA) products; monitor for MPA associated adverse reactions and reduce dose of concomitantly administered MPA products as needed. Grapefruit or grapefruit juice may increase tacrolimus whole blood trough concentrations and increase risk of serious adverse reactions. Alcohol may modify rate of tacrolimus release. Strong CYP3A inducers (eg, rifampin, phenytoin, St. John's wort) may decrease tacrolimus whole blood trough concentrations and increase risk of rejection; increase Envarsus XR dose and monitor tacrolimus whole blood trough concentrations. Strong CYP3A inhibitors (eg, nelfinavir, telaprevir, voriconazole, posaconazole) may increase tacrolimus whole blood trough concentrations and increase the risk of serious adverse reactions; reduce Envarsus XR (for voriconazole and posaconazole, give 1/3 of the original dose) and adjust dose based on tacrolimus whole blood trough concentrations. Mild or moderate CYP3A inhibitors (eg,

clotrimazole, erythromycin, verapamil, amiodarone) and other drugs (eg, Mg^{2+} and aluminum hydroxide antacids, metoclopramide) may increase tacrolimus whole blood trough concentrations and increase the risk of serious adverse reactions; monitor tacrolimus whole blood trough concentrations and reduce Envarsus XR dose if needed. Mild or moderate CYP3A inducers (eg, methylprednisolone, prednisone) may decrease tacrolimus concentrations; monitor tacrolimus whole blood trough concentrations and adjust Envarsus XR dose if needed.

PREGNANCY AND LACTATION
Pregnancy: Category C.
Lactation: Present in breast milk; not for use in nursing.

MECHANISM OF ACTION
Macrolide immunosuppressant; binds to FKBP-12, forming a complex of tacrolimus-FKBP-12, Ca^{2+}, calmodulin, and calcineurin, and inhibiting phosphatase activity of calcineurin. Inhibits the expression and/or production of several cytokines that include interleukin (IL)-1 beta, IL-2, IL-3, IL-4, IL-5, IL-6, IL-8, IL-10, gamma interferon, TNF-α, and granulocyte macrophage colony stimulating factor. Also inhibits IL-2 receptor expression and nitric oxide release, induces apoptosis and production of transforming growth factor-β that can lead to immunosuppressive activity. Net result is inhibition of T-lymphocyte activation and proliferation as well as T-helper-cell-dependent B-cell response.

PHARMACOKINETICS
Absorption: Administration of variable doses in different populations resulted in different pharmacokinetic parameters. **Distribution:** Plasma protein binding (99%); crosses placenta; found in breast milk. **Metabolism:** Liver (extensive), via CYP3A (demethylation and hydroxylation); 13-demethyl tacrolimus (major metabolite); 31-demethyl metabolite (active metabolite). **Excretion:** Feces (92.6%), urine (2.3%); $T_{1/2}$=31 hrs (2mg qd).

PATIENT CONSIDERATIONS
Assessment: Assess for congenital long QT syndrome, CHF, bradyarrhythmias, electrolyte disturbances, renal/hepatic impairment, hypersensitivity to the drug, pregnancy/nursing status, and possible drug interactions.

Monitoring: Monitor for lymphomas and other malignancies, infections (including opportunistic infections), nephrotoxicity, neurotoxicity, HTN, QT prolongation, PRCA, and for other adverse reactions. Measure tacrolimus whole blood trough concentrations at least 2X on separate days during the first week after initiation of dosing and after any change in dosage, after a change in coadministration of CYP3A inducers and/or inhibitors, or after a change in renal or hepatic function. Monitor serum K^+ and glucose concentrations. Monitor EBV serology. Consider obtaining ECG and monitoring electrolytes (Mg^{2+}, Ca^{2+}) periodically during treatment in patients w/ CHF, bradyarrhythmias, those taking certain antiarrhythmic medications or other products that lead to QT prolongation, and those w/ electrolyte disturbances.

Counseling: Inform of the risks and benefits of therapy. Instruct to inspect the medicine when a new prescription is received and before taking it. Advise to avoid alcohol, grapefruit, or grapefruit juice while on therapy. Instruct to take a missed dose as soon as remembered but not more than 15 hrs after the scheduled time; beyond the 15-hr timeframe, instruct to wait until the usual scheduled time the following am to take the next scheduled dose. Advise to limit exposure to sunlight and UV light by wearing protective clothing and using sunscreen w/ a high protection factor. Instruct to contact physician if any symptoms of infection, frequent urination, increased thirst or hunger, vision changes, delirium, or tremors develop. Inform that therapy can cause high BP that may require treatment w/ antihypertensive therapy. Inform that drug can cause hyperkalemia and that monitoring of K^+ levels may be necessary. Advise that drug can interfere w/ the usual response to immunizations and that patient should avoid live vaccines. Instruct to attend all visits and complete all blood tests ordered by medical team. Instruct to inform physician if planning to become pregnant or to breastfeed, or if starting or stopping any concomitant medications.

EPANED — enalapril   Rx
Class: ACE inhibitor

> **D/C when pregnancy is detected. Drugs that act directly on the renin-angiotensin system (RAS) can cause injury/death to the developing fetus.**

ADULT DOSAGE
Heart Failure

Initial: 2.5mg bid
Titrate: Increase dose as tolerated
Max: 20mg bid

Hyponatremia (Serum Na+ <130mEq/L) or SrCr >1.6mg/dL:
Initial: 2.5mg qd

Diuretic dose may need to be adjusted to minimize hypovolemia and hypotension

Asymptomatic Left Ventricular Dysfunction

Initial: 2.5mg bid
Titrate: Increase dose as tolerated
Max: 10mg bid

May need to adjust diuretic dose

Hypertension

Initial: 5mg qd
Titrate: Increase dose prn
Max: 40mg/day

PEDIATRIC DOSAGE
Hypertension

>1 Month of Age:
Initial: 0.08mg/kg (up to 5mg) qd
Titrate: Adjust dose according to BP response
Max: 0.58mg/kg (or 40mg/day)

Divide dose and administer bid if effect diminishes at the end of the dosing interval

May administer w/ a low dose of diuretic if additional BP reduction is needed

Use w/ Diuretics:
Initial: 2.5mg/day

DOSING CONSIDERATIONS
Renal Impairment
Dialysis Patients:
Adults:
2.5mg on dialysis days; adjust dosage on nondialysis days depending on BP response
Moderate to Severe (CrCl ≤30mL/min): 2.5mg/day
Pediatrics:
GFR <30mL/min: Not recommended

ADMINISTRATION
Oral route

Preparation of Epaned (for 150mL, 1mg/mL Sol)
1. Firmly tap Epaned Powder for Oral Sol bottle on a hard surface 5X.
2. Add 75mL of Ora-Sweet SF diluent to the 150mL Epaned Powder for Oral Sol bottle.
3. Replace cap and shake well for 30 sec.
4. Reopen, and add the remainder of the Ora-Sweet SF diluent to the bottle.
5. Shake well for an additional 30 sec.
6. Discard 60 days from the date of reconstitution.

STORAGE
25°C (77°F); excursions permitted to 15-30°C (59-86°F). Do not freeze. Protect from moisture. Discard 60 days after reconstitution.

HOW SUPPLIED
Sol: 1mg/mL [150mL]

CONTRAINDICATIONS
History of angioedema or hypersensitivity related to previous treatment w/ an ACE inhibitor, hereditary or idiopathic angioedema. Coadministration w/ aliskiren in patients w/ diabetes.

WARNINGS/PRECAUTIONS
Head/neck angioedema reported; d/c and administer appropriate therapy. Higher incidence of angioedema in black patients. Patients w/ history of angioedema unrelated to ACE inhibitor therapy may be at increased risk of angioedema during therapy. Intestinal angioedema reported; monitor for abdominal pain. Anaphylactoid reactions reported during desensitization w/ hymenoptera venom, dialysis w/ high-flux membranes, and LDL apheresis w/ dextran sulfate absorption. May cause symptomatic hypotension, sometimes complicated by oliguria, progressive azotemia, acute renal failure, or death; closely monitor patients at risk of excessive hypotension (eg, those w/ heart failure w/ systolic BP <100mmHg, ischemic heart disease, cerebrovascular disease, hyponatremia, renal dialysis, severe volume and/or salt depletion of any etiology) during first 2 weeks of therapy and whenever dose is increased. Symptomatic hypotension may occur in patients w/ severe aortic stenosis or hypertrophic cardiomyopathy. Hypotension may occur w/ major surgery or during anesthesia; may be corrected by volume expansion. Rarely, a syndrome that starts w/ cholestatic jaundice and progresses to fulminant hepatic necrosis and (sometimes) death reported; d/c if jaundice or marked elevations of hepatic enzymes develop. May cause changes in renal function, including acute renal failure; consider withholding or discontinuing therapy if clinically significant decrease in renal function develops. May cause hyperkalemia; risk factors include renal insufficiency and diabetes mellitus (DM).

ADVERSE REACTIONS
Fatigue, hypotension, dizziness.

DRUG INTERACTIONS
See Contraindications. Hypotension risk w/ high-dose diuretics; closely monitor patients during first 2 weeks of therapy and whenever the dose of enalapril and/or diuretic is increased. NSAIDs, including selective COX-2 inhibitors, may result in deterioration of renal function, including possible acute renal failure; monitor renal function periodically in patients receiving concomitant therapy w/ NSAIDs. NSAIDs may diminish the antihypertensive effect. Dual blockade of the RAS is associated w/ increased risks of hypotension, hyperkalemia, and changes in renal function (including acute renal failure); avoid combined use of RAS inhibitors, or closely monitor BP, renal function, and electrolytes w/ concomitant agents that also affect the RAS. Avoid w/ aliskiren in patients w/ renal impairment (GFR <60mL/min). Increased risk of hyperkalemia w/ K^+-sparing diuretics (eg, spironolactone, triamterene, amiloride), K^+-containing salt substitutes, or K^+ supplements. Lithium toxicity reported; monitor serum lithium levels frequently. Nitritoid reactions reported w/ injectable gold. Coadministration w/ mTOR inhibitors (eg, temsirolimus, sirolimus, everolimus) may increase risk for angioedema.

PREGNANCY AND LACTATION
Pregnancy: Category D.
Lactation: Not for use in nursing.

MECHANISM OF ACTION
ACE inhibitor; decreases plasma angiotensin II, which leads to decreased vasopressor activity and decreased aldosterone secretion.

PHARMACOKINETICS
Absorption: (Tab) T_{max}=1 hr, 3-4 hrs (enalaprilat). **Distribution:** Crosses placenta; found in breast milk. **Metabolism:** Hydrolysis to enalaprilat (active metabolite). **Elimination:** Urine and feces (94% [adults]); urine (68% [pediatric patients]). Enalaprilat: $T_{1/2}$=11 hrs (adults), 14 hrs (pediatric patients).

PATIENT CONSIDERATIONS

Assessment: Assess for hereditary or idiopathic angioedema, DM, risk for excessive hypotension, severe aortic stenosis, hypertrophic cardiomyopathy, risk factors for hyperkalemia, renal impairment, hyponatremia, history of angioedema or hypersensitivity related to previous treatment w/ an ACE inhibitor, pregnancy/nursing status, and possible drug interactions.

Monitoring: Monitor for angioedema, anaphylactoid reactions, and other adverse reactions. Monitor BP, LFTs, renal function, and serum K⁺.

Counseling: Inform about fetal risks if taken during pregnancy and discuss treatment options for women planning to become pregnant; instruct to report pregnancy to physician as soon as possible. Instruct to d/c therapy and to immediately report signs/symptoms of angioedema. Instruct to report lightheadedness, especially during the 1st few days of therapy; advise to d/c and to consult w/ a physician if actual syncope occurs. Inform that excessive perspiration, dehydration, and other causes of volume depletion (eg, vomiting or diarrhea) may lead to an excessive fall in BP; advise to consult w/ physician. Advise not to use salt substitutes containing K⁺ w/o consulting physician.

EPANOVA — omega-3-carboxylic acids　　　Rx

Class: Lipid-regulating agent

ADULT DOSAGE	PEDIATRIC DOSAGE
Hypertriglyceridemia	Pediatric use may not have been established
Adjunct to Diet in Patients w/ Severe (≥500mg/dL) Hypertriglyceridemia: 2g/day (2 caps qd) or 4g/day (4 caps qd)	

DOSING CONSIDERATIONS

Elderly
Start at lower end of dosing range

ADMINISTRATION

Oral route

Take w/o regard to meals.
Swallow caps whole; do not break open, crush, dissolve, or chew.

STORAGE

25°C (77°F); excursions permitted to 15-30°C (59-86°F). Do not freeze.

HOW SUPPLIED

Cap: 1g

CONTRAINDICATIONS

Known hypersensitivity (eg, anaphylactic reaction) to Epanova or any of its components.

WARNINGS/PRECAUTIONS

Attempt to control serum lipids w/ appropriate diet, exercise, weight loss in obese patients, and control of any medical problems that are contributing to the lipid abnormalities (eg, diabetes mellitus, hypothyroidism). D/C or change medications known to exacerbate hypertriglyceridemia (eg, β-blockers, thiazides, estrogens) if possible prior to consideration of TG-lowering drug therapy. May increase LDL levels. Monitor ALT and AST levels periodically during therapy in patients w/ hepatic impairment. Use w/ caution in patients w/ known hypersensitivity to fish and/or shellfish.

ADVERSE REACTIONS

Diarrhea, nausea, abdominal pain/discomfort, eructation.

DRUG INTERACTIONS

Periodically monitor patients receiving concomitant treatment w/ drugs affecting coagulation (eg, antiplatelet agents).

PREGNANCY AND LACTATION

Category C, caution in nursing.

MECHANISM OF ACTION

Lipid-regulating agent; has not been established. Potential mechanisms of action include inhibition of acyl-CoA:1,2-diacylglycerol acyltransferase, increased mitochondrial and peroxisomal β-oxidation in the liver, decreased lipogenesis in the liver, and increased plasma lipoprotein lipase activity.

PHARMACOKINETICS

Absorption: (Repeat dosing w/ 4g/day under low-fat meal conditions) T_{max}=5-8 hrs (total eicosapentaenoic acid [EPA]), 5-9 hrs (total docosahexaenoic acid [DHA]). **Distribution:** Found in breast milk. **Metabolism:** Liver via oxidation. **Elimination:** (Repeat dosing under low-fat meal conditions) $T_{1/2}$=37 hrs (EPA), approx 46 hrs (DHA).

PATIENT CONSIDERATIONS

Assessment: Assess for hypersensitivity to drug, fish, and/or shellfish. Assess for hepatic impairment, pregnancy/nursing status, and possible drug interactions. Attempt to control serum lipids w/ appropriate diet, exercise, weight loss in obese patients, and control of any medical problems (eg, diabetes mellitus, hypothyroidism) that may contribute to lipid abnormalities prior to therapy. Assess lipid levels.

Monitoring: Monitor for allergic reactions and other adverse reactions. Monitor lipid levels. Periodically monitor ALT/AST levels in patients w/ hepatic impairment.

Counseling: Instruct to notify physician if allergic to fish and/or shellfish. Inform that use of lipid-regulating agents does not reduce the importance of adhering to diet. Instruct to take ud. Advise not to alter caps in any way and to ingest intact caps only.

EPCLUSA — sofosbuvir/velpatasvir　　　Rx

Class: HCV NS5A inhibitor/HCV nucleotide analogue NS5B polymerase inhibitor

ADULT DOSAGE	PEDIATRIC DOSAGE
Chronic Hepatitis C	Pediatric use may not have been established
Genotype 1, 2, 3, 4, 5, or 6: **W/O Cirrhosis or w/ Compensated Cirrhosis (Child-Pugh A):** 1 tab qd for 12 weeks	
W/ Decompensated Cirrhosis (Child-Pugh B or C): 1 tab qd + ribavirin for 12 weeks	
For further information on ribavirin dosing and dosing modifications, refer to the ribavirin PI	

DOSING CONSIDERATIONS

Renal Impairment
Mild/Moderate: No dosage adjustment required
Severe (eGFR <30mL/min/1.73m²)/ESRD: No dosage recommendation can be given due to higher exposures of the predominant sofosbuvir metabolite

ADMINISTRATION

Oral route

Take w/ or w/o food.

STORAGE

<30°C (86°F).

HOW SUPPLIED

Tab: (Sofosbuvir/Velpatasvir) 400mg/100mg

CONTRAINDICATIONS

Combination therapy w/ ribavirin is contraindicated in patients for whom ribavirin is contraindicated; refer to ribavirin PI.

WARNINGS/PRECAUTIONS

Serious symptomatic bradycardia reported when amiodarone is coadministered w/ sofosbuvir and another HCV direct-acting antiviral. Fatal cardiac arrest reported in a patient taking amiodarone who was coadministered a sofosbuvir-containing regimen. Patients also taking β-blockers, or those w/ underlying cardiac comorbidities and/or advanced liver disease, may be at increased risk for symptomatic bradycardia w/ coadministration of amiodarone. Not recommended w/ amiodarone. If coadministration is required, cardiac monitoring in an in-patient setting for the first 48 hrs of coadministration is recommended, after which outpatient or self-monitoring of HR should occur on a daily basis through at least the first 2 weeks of therapy. Patients discontinuing amiodarone just prior to starting therapy should also undergo similar cardiac monitoring. P-gp inducers and/or moderate to potent CYP2B6, CYP2C8, or CYP3A4 inducers (eg, rifampin, St. John's wort, carbamazepine) may significantly decrease plasma concentrations; concomitant use not recommended. If administered w/ ribavirin, refer to the ribavirin PI for the warnings and precautions for ribavirin.

ADVERSE REACTIONS

Monotherapy: Headache, fatigue.
W/ Ribavirin: Fatigue, anemia, nausea, headache, insomnia, diarrhea.

DRUG INTERACTIONS

See Warnings/Precautions. May increase topotecan, rosuvastatin, and atorvastatin levels; coadministration w/ topotecan not recommended. Monitor for HMG-CoA reductase inhibitor-associated adverse reactions. May increase digoxin levels; monitor digoxin levels. Do not exceed rosuvastatin dose of 10mg. Decreased levels w/ carbamazepine, phenytoin, phenobarbital, oxcarbazepine, rifabutin, rifampin, rifapentine, tipranavir/ritonavir, and St. John's wort; coadministration not recommended. May increase tenofovir levels when coadministered w/ tenofovir disoproxil fumarate-containing regimens; monitor for tenofovir-associated adverse reactions. **Velpatasvir:** Inhibits drug transporters P-gp, BCRP, OATP1B1, OATP1B3, and OATP2B1; may increase exposure of substrates of these transporters. Decreased concentrations w/ drugs that increase gastric pH (eg, antacids, H₂-receptor antagonists, proton pump inhibitor [PPIs]). Separate antacid administration by 4 hrs. H₂-receptor antagonists may be administered simultaneously w/ or 12 hrs apart from Epclusa at a dose that does not exceed doses comparable to famotidine 40mg bid. Coadministration w/ PPIs not recommended. If necessary, administer Epclusa w/ food 4 hrs before omeprazole 20mg; use w/ other PPIs has not been studied. Decreased levels w/ efavirenz; coadministration w/ efavirenz-containing regimens not recommended. Refer to PI for further dosing modifications when used w/ certain concomitant medications.

PREGNANCY AND LACTATION

Pregnancy: No adequate human data are available to establish whether or not Epclusa poses a risk to pregnancy outcomes.
Lactation: It is not known whether the components of Epclusa and its metabolites are present in human breast milk, affect human milk production, or have effects on the breastfed infant; caution in nursing.

If administered w/ ribavirin, refer to the PI of ribavirin for additional information.

MECHANISM OF ACTION

Sofosbuvir: HCV nucleotide analogue NS5B polymerase inhibitor; undergoes intracellular metabolism to form the pharmacologically active uridine analogue triphosphate (GS-461203), which can be incorporated into HCV RNA by the NS5B polymerase and acts as a chain terminator. **Velpatasvir:** HCV NS5A protein inhibitor; HCV NS5A protein is required for viral replication.

PHARMACOKINETICS

Absorption: Sofosbuvir: T_{max}=0.5-1 hrs. C_{max}=567ng/mL, 898ng/mL (GS-331007). AUC=1268ng•hr/mL, 14,372ng•hr/mL (GS-331007). Velpatasvir: T_{max}=3 hrs. C_{max}=259ng/mL. AUC=2980ng•hr/mL. **Distribution:** Sofosbuvir: Plasma protein binding (61-65% sofosbuvir). Velpatasvir: Plasma protein binding (>99.5% velpatasvir). **Metabolism:** Sofosbuvir: Via Cathepsin A, CES1, and HINT1. Prodrug that undergoes intracellular metabolism to form GS-461203. GS-331007 is the primary circulating metabolite. Velpatasvir: Via CYP2B6, CYP2C8, CYP3A4. **Elimination:** Sofosbuvir: Urine (80%, predominantly as GS-331007), feces (14%); $T_{1/2}$=0.5 hrs, 25 hrs (GS-331007) (median). Velpatasvir: Urine (0.4%), feces (94%); $T_{1/2}$=15 hrs (median).

PATIENT CONSIDERATIONS

Assessment: Assess for hypersensitivity to drug, cardiac comorbidities, renal impairment, pregnancy/nursing status, and for potential drug interactions.

Monitoring: Monitor for bradycardia if coadministering w/ amiodarone or if discontinuing amiodarone just prior to starting therapy; perform cardiac monitoring in an in-patient setting for the first 48 hrs of coadministration, after which outpatient or self-monitoring of the HR should occur on a daily basis through at least the first 2 weeks of treatment. Perform clinical and hepatic lab monitoring for patients w/ decompensated cirrhosis receiving concomitant treatment w/ ribavirin. Monitor for other adverse reactions.

Counseling: Advise to take ud. Inform that it is important not to miss or skip doses and to continue therapy for the recommended duration. Advise to seek medical evaluation immediately for symptoms of bradycardia. Inform that treatment may interact w/ other drugs and advise to report to healthcare provider the use of any other prescription or nonprescription medication or herbal products. Advise to avoid pregnancy during combination treatment w/ ribavirin and for 6 months after completion of treatment. Instruct to notify healthcare provider immediately in the event of a pregnancy.

EPIDUO — adapalene/benzoyl peroxide   Rx

Class: Antibacterial/keratolytic

ADULT DOSAGE	PEDIATRIC DOSAGE
Acne Vulgaris	**Acne Vulgaris**
Apply a thin film to affected areas of the face and/or trunk qd after washing. Use a pea-sized amount for each area of the face (eg, forehead, chin, each cheek)	**≥9 Years:** Apply a thin film to affected areas of the face and/or trunk qd after washing. Use a pea-sized amount for each area of the face (eg, forehead, chin, each cheek)

ADMINISTRATION
Topical route

Apply after washing.
Not for oral, ophthalmic, or intravaginal use.

STORAGE
25°C (77°F); excursions permitted to 15-30°C (59-86°F). Keep tube tightly closed. Protect from light. Keep away from heat.

HOW SUPPLIED
Gel: (Adapalene/Benzoyl Peroxide) 0.1%/2.5% [45g]

WARNINGS/PRECAUTIONS
Minimize exposure to sunlight and sunlamps; use sunscreen and protective apparel if exposure cannot be avoided. Exercise caution in patients w/ high levels of sun exposure and those w/ inherent sensitivity to sun. Extreme weather may cause irritation. Avoid contact w/ the eyes, lips, and mucous membranes. Avoid application to cuts, abrasions, or eczematous or sunburned skin. Erythema, scaling, dryness, stinging/burning, and irritant and allergic contact dermatitis may occur; depending on severity, may apply moisturizer, reduce frequency of application, or d/c use. Avoid waxing as a depilatory method on the treated skin.

ADVERSE REACTIONS
Dry skin, contact dermatitis, application-site burning, application-site irritation, skin irritation.

DRUG INTERACTIONS
Caution w/ concomitant topical acne therapy, especially w/ peeling, desquamating, or abrasive agents. Avoid w/ other potentially irritating topical products (medicated or abrasive soaps and cleansers, soaps and cosmetics that have strong skin-drying effect, and products w/ high concentrations of alcohol, astringents, spices, or limes).

PREGNANCY AND LACTATION
Pregnancy: Category C.
Lactation: Caution in nursing.

MECHANISM OF ACTION
Adapalene: Naphthoic acid derivative; not established. Binds to specific retinoic acid nuclear receptors and modulates cellular differentiation, keratinization, and inflammatory processes. Benzoyl peroxide: Oxidizing agent w/ bactericidal and keratolytic effects.

PHARMACOKINETICS
Absorption: (Adapalene) C_{max}=0.21ng/mL; AUC_{0-24h}=1.99ng•h/mL. **Elimination:** (Adapalene) Bile. (Benzoyl peroxide) Urine.

PATIENT CONSIDERATIONS
Assessment: Assess for presence of cuts, abrasions, or eczematous or sunburned skin at the treatment site. Assess for pregnancy/nursing status and possible drug interactions. Assess if patient has high levels of sun exposure or inherent sensitivity to the sun.

Monitoring: Monitor for irritation, erythema, scaling, dryness, stinging/burning, and other adverse reactions.

Counseling: Advise to cleanse area w/ mild or soapless cleanser and to pat dry. Advise to avoid contact w/ the eyes, lips, and mucous membranes. Instruct not to use more than the recommended amount. Inform that drug may cause irritation and may bleach hair and colored fabric. Instruct to minimize exposure to sunlight and sunlamps. Recommend to use sunscreen products and protective apparel when exposure to sunlight cannot be avoided.

EPIPEN — epinephrine   Rx

Class: Sympathomimetic catecholamine

OTHER BRAND NAMES
EpiPen Jr.

ADULT DOSAGE	PEDIATRIC DOSAGE
Emergency Treatment of Type I Allergic Reactions	**Emergency Treatment of Type I Allergic Reactions**
Including anaphylaxis to stinging and biting insects, allergen immunotherapy, foods, drugs, diagnostic testing substances, and other allergens, as well as idiopathic or exercise-induced anaphylaxis	Including anaphylaxis to stinging and biting insects, allergen immunotherapy, foods, drugs, diagnostic testing substances, and other allergens, as well as idiopathic or exercise-induced anaphylaxis
15-30kg: **EpiPen Jr:** 0.15mg	**15-30kg:** **EpiPen Jr:** 0.15mg
≥30kg: **EpiPen:** 0.3mg	**≥30kg:** **EpiPen:** 0.3mg
Severe Persistent Anaphylaxis: Repeat inj may be necessary	**Severe Persistent Anaphylaxis:** Repeat inj may be necessary

---

ADMINISTRATION
IM/SQ route

- Inject into the anterolateral aspect of the thigh, through clothing if necessary.
- Consider using other forms of injectable epinephrine if doses <0.15mg are deemed necessary.
- Hold uncooperative child's leg firmly in place and limit movement prior to and during an inj.

STORAGE
20-25°C (68-77°F); excursions permitted to 15-30°C (59-86°F). Store in the carrier tube provided. Protect from light. Do not refrigerate.

HOW SUPPLIED
Inj: (EpiPen Jr) 0.15mg/0.3mL; (EpiPen) 0.3mg/0.3mL

WARNINGS/PRECAUTIONS
Intended for immediate administration in patients who are determined to be at increased risk for anaphylaxis, including those w/ a history of anaphylactic reactions. Intended for immediate administration as emergency supportive therapy only and is not a substitute for immediate medical care. More than 2 sequential doses should only be administered under direct medical supervision. Do not inject IV. Large doses or accidental IV inj may result in cerebral hemorrhage due to sharp rise in BP; rapidly acting vasodilators can counteract the marked pressor effects of epinephrine. Do not inject into buttock; may not provide effective treatment of anaphylaxis. Inj into buttock associated w/ Clostridial infections (gas gangrene). Do not inject into digits, hands, or feet; may result in loss of blood flow to the affected area. Rare cases of serious skin and soft tissue infections (eg, necrotizing fasciitis, myonecrosis) caused by Clostridia (gas gangrene), reported at inj site. Contains sodium metabisulfite; may cause allergic-type reactions including anaphylactic symptoms or life-threatening or less severe asthmatic episodes in certain susceptible persons. Caution in patients w/ heart disease, hyperthyroidism, or diabetes mellitus (DM); in patients who are elderly; and in patients who are pregnant. May temporarily worsen symptoms of Parkinson's disease.

ADVERSE REACTIONS
Anxiety, apprehensiveness, restlessness, tremor, weakness, dizziness, sweating, palpitations, pallor, N/V, headache, respiratory difficulties.

DRUG INTERACTIONS
May precipitate/aggravate angina pectoris as well as produce ventricular arrhythmias w/ drugs that may sensitize the heart to arrhythmias; use w/ caution. Monitor for cardiac arrhythmias w/ antiarrhythmics, cardiac glycosides, and diuretics. Effects may be potentiated by TCAs, MAOIs, levothyroxine sodium, and certain antihistamines (notably, chlorpheniramine, tripelennamine, diphenhydramine). Cardiostimulating and bronchodilating effects are antagonized by β-adrenergic blockers (eg, propranolol). Vasoconstricting and hypertensive effects are antagonized by α-adrenergic blockers (eg, phentolamine). Ergot alkaloids may reverse pressor effects.

PREGNANCY AND LACTATION
Pregnancy: Category C.
Lactation: Caution in nursing.

MECHANISM OF ACTION

Sympathomimetic catecholamine; acts on α-adrenergic receptors and lessens the vasodilation and increased vascular permeability that occurs during anaphylaxis. Acts on β-adrenergic receptors, causing bronchial smooth muscle relaxation. Also may alleviate GI and genitourinary symptoms associated w/ anaphylaxis.

PATIENT CONSIDERATIONS

Assessment: Assess for risk of anaphylaxis, heart disease, hyperthyroidism, DM, Parkinson's disease, pregnancy/nursing status, and for possible drug interactions.

Monitoring: Monitor for allergic-type reactions, angina pectoris, ventricular arrhythmias, cerebral hemorrhage, and other adverse reactions. Monitor HR and BP.

Counseling: Advise that therapy may produce signs and symptoms that include increased HR, sensation of more forceful heartbeat, palpitations, sweating, N/V, difficulty breathing, pallor, dizziness, weakness or shakiness, headache, apprehension, nervousness, or anxiety; advise that these signs and symptoms usually subside rapidly, especially w/ rest, quiet, and recumbency. Inform that patients may develop more severe or persistent effects if they have HTN or hyperthyroidism. Inform that patients may experience angina if they have coronary artery disease. Advise that patients may develop increased blood glucose levels following administration if they have DM. Advise that a temporary worsening of symptoms may be noticed if patient has Parkinson's disease. Instruct to seek immediate medical care in case of accidental inj. Advise to seek medical care if signs/symptoms of infection develop at inj site. Instruct caregivers of young, uncooperative children to hold leg firmly in place and limit movement prior to and during an inj.

EPIVIR — lamivudine   Rx

Class: Nucleoside reverse transcriptase inhibitor (NRTI)

> Lactic acidosis and severe hepatomegaly w/ steatosis, including fatal cases, reported w/ nucleoside analogues; d/c treatment if lactic acidosis or pronounced hepatotoxicity occurs. Severe acute exacerbations of hepatitis B reported in patients coinfected w/ hepatitis B virus (HBV) upon discontinuation of therapy; closely monitor hepatic function for at least several months. If appropriate, initiation of antihepatitis B therapy may be warranted. Epivir tabs and oral sol (used to treat HIV-1 infection) contain a higher dose of lamivudine than Epivir-HBV tabs and oral sol (used to treat chronic HBV infection); patients w/ HIV-1 infection should only receive dosage forms appropriate for HIV-1 treatment.

ADULT DOSAGE

HIV-1 Infection

In Combination w/ Other Antiretrovirals:

150mg bid or 300mg qd

If lamivudine is administered to a patient infected w/ HIV-1 and HBV, the dosage indicated for HIV-1 therapy should be used as part of an appropriate combination regimen

PEDIATRIC DOSAGE

HIV-1 Infection

In Combination w/ Other Antiretrovirals:

≥3 Months of Age:
Oral Sol:
4mg/kg bid or 8mg/kg qd
Max: 300mg/day

Tab:
QD Dosing Regimen:
14 to <20kg: 150mg
≥20 to <25kg: 225mg
≥25kg: 300mg

Data regarding the efficacy of qd dosing is limited to subjects who transitioned from bid dosing to qd dosing after 36 weeks of treatment

BID Dosing Regimen (Using Scored 150mg Tab):
14 to <20kg:
AM Dose: 75mg
PM Dose: 75mg
Total Daily Dose: 150mg

≥20 to <25kg:
AM Dose: 75mg
PM Dose: 150mg
Total Daily Dose: 225mg

≥25kg:
AM Dose: 150mg
PM Dose: 150mg
Total Daily Dose: 300mg

DOSING CONSIDERATIONS

Renal Impairment
Adults and Adolescents (≥25kg):
CrCl ≥50mL/min: 150mg bid or 300mg qd
CrCl 30-49mL/min: 150mg qd
CrCl 15-29mL/min: 150mg 1st dose, then 100mg qd
CrCl 5-14mL/min: 150mg 1st dose, then 50mg qd
CrCl <5mL/min: 50mg 1st dose, then 25mg qd

No additional dosing is required after routine (4-hr) hemodialysis or peritoneal dialysis

Pediatric Patients:
Consider dose reduction and/or increase in dosing interval

ADMINISTRATION
Oral route

Take w/ or w/o food.

Pediatric Patients
Epivir scored tab is the preferred formulation for HIV-1 infected pediatric patients who weigh ≥14kg and for whom a solid dosage form is appropriate.
Assess ability to swallow tabs before prescribing; for patients unable to safely and reliably swallow tabs, oral sol should be prescribed.

STORAGE
Tab: 25°C (77°F); excursions permitted to 15-30°C (59-86°F). **Oral Sol:** 25°C (77°F).

HOW SUPPLIED
Oral Sol: 10mg/mL [240mL]; **Tab:** 150mg*, 300mg *scored

CONTRAINDICATIONS
Previous hypersensitivity reaction to lamivudine.

WARNINGS/PRECAUTIONS
Obesity and prolonged nucleoside exposure may be risk factors for lactic acidosis and severe hepatomegaly w/ steatosis. Caution w/ known risk factors for liver disease. Emergence of lamivudine-resistant HBV reported. Caution in pediatric patients w/ a history of prior antiretroviral nucleoside exposure, history of pancreatitis, or other significant risk factors for development of pancreatitis; d/c if pancreatitis develops. Immune reconstitution syndrome reported. Autoimmune disorders (eg, Graves' disease, polymyositis, Guillain-Barre syndrome) reported to occur in the setting of immune reconstitution and can occur many months after initiation of treatment. Redistribution/accumulation of body fat may occur. Lower virologic suppression rates, lower plasma lamivudine exposure, and viral resistance reported more frequently in pediatric patients who received oral sol than those who received tabs; consider more frequent monitoring of HIV-1 viral load w/ oral sol. Consider HIV-1 viral load and CD4+ cell count/percentage when selecting the dosing interval for patients initiating treatment w/ oral sol. Caution in elderly.

ADVERSE REACTIONS
Adults: Headache, nausea, malaise, fatigue, nasal signs/symptoms, diarrhea, cough.
Pediatric Patients: Fever, cough.

DRUG INTERACTIONS
Hepatic decompensation reported in HIV-1/hepatitis C virus coinfected patients receiving antiretroviral therapy for HIV-1 and interferon-alfa w/ or w/o ribavirin; closely monitor for treatment-associated toxicities during coadministration and consider discontinuation of lamivudine as medically appropriate. Possible interaction w/ drugs whose main route of elimination is active renal secretion via the organic cationic transport system (eg, trimethoprim).

PREGNANCY AND LACTATION
Pregnancy: Physicians are encouraged to register patients in the Antiretroviral Pregnancy Registry. Embryonic toxicity produced in rabbits at a dose that produced similar human exposures as the recommended clinical dose; relevance to human pregnancy registry data is unknown.
Lactation: Mothers should be instructed not to breastfeed due to potential for HIV-1 transmission.

MECHANISM OF ACTION
Nucleoside analogue. Lamivudine is phosphorylated to its active 5'-triphosphate metabolite, lamivudine triphosphate (3TC-TP); 3TC-TP inhibits HIV-1 reverse transcriptase via DNA chain termination after incorporation of the nucleotide analogue into viral DNA.

PHARMACOKINETICS
Absorption: Rapid; absolute bioavailability (86% [150mg tab], 87% [oral sol]); $AUC_{(0-12)}$=5.53mcg•h/mL; C_{max}=1.4mcg/mL; T_{max}=0.9 hrs (fasting), 3.2 hrs (fed). **Distribution:** V_d=1.3L/kg (IV); plasma protein binding (<36%); crosses placenta. **Metabolism:** Trans-sulfoxide (metabolite). **Elimination:** Urine (majority unchanged); $T_{1/2}$=5-7 hrs.

PATIENT CONSIDERATIONS

Assessment: Assess for renal impairment, risk factors for lactic acidosis and liver disease, HIV-1 and HBV coinfection, previous hypersensitivity, pregnancy/nursing status, and possible drug interactions. In pediatric patients, assess for a history of prior antiretroviral nucleoside exposure, a history of pancreatitis, or risk factors for pancreatitis. Consider HIV-1 viral load and CD4+ cell count/percentage when selecting the dosing interval for patients initiating treatment w/ oral sol.

Monitoring: Monitor for signs/symptoms of pancreatitis, immune reconstitution syndrome, autoimmune disorders, fat redistribution/accumulation, lactic acidosis, hepatomegaly w/ steatosis, hepatitis B exacerbation, renal dysfunction, and hypersensitivity reactions. Monitor hepatic function closely for several months in patients w/ HIV/HBV coinfection who d/c therapy.

Counseling: Inform about risks/benefits of therapy. Advise that lactic acidosis and severe hepatomegaly w/ steatosis have been reported w/ use of nucleoside analogues; instruct to d/c if symptoms suggestive of lactic acidosis or pronounced hepatotoxicity develop. Advise to discuss any changes in regimen w/ physician. Advise parents/guardians of pediatric patients to monitor for signs and symptoms of pancreatitis. Instruct to inform physician immediately of any signs/symptoms of infection. Inform that redistribution/accumulation of body fat may occur. Advise diabetic patients that each 15mL dose of oral sol contains 3g of sucrose. Advise that there is a pregnancy exposure registry that monitors pregnancy outcomes in women exposed to therapy during pregnancy. Instruct women w/ HIV-1 infection not to breastfeed.

EPIVIR-HBV — lamivudine   Rx

Class: Nucleoside reverse transcriptase inhibitor (NRTI)

> Lactic acidosis and severe hepatomegaly with steatosis, including fatal cases, reported with nucleoside analogues. Suspend treatment if lactic acidosis or pronounced hepatotoxicity occurs. Severe acute exacerbations of hepatitis B reported upon discontinuation of therapy; closely monitor hepatic function for at least several months. If appropriate, initiation of antihepatitis B therapy may be warranted. Not approved for treatment of HIV infection. Lamivudine dosage in Epivir-HBV is subtherapeutic and monotherapy is inappropriate for treatment of HIV infection. HIV-1 resistance may emerge in chronic hepatitis B-infected patients with unrecognized/untreated HIV infection. Offer HIV counseling and testing to all patients prior to therapy and periodically thereafter.

ADULT DOSAGE	**PEDIATRIC DOSAGE**
Chronic Hepatitis B	Chronic Hepatitis B
100mg qd	**2-17 Years:**
	3mg/kg qd
	Max: 100mg/day

DOSING CONSIDERATIONS
Renal Impairment
CrCl 30-49mL/min: 100mg 1st dose, then 50mg qd
CrCl 15-29mL/min: 100mg 1st dose, then 25mg qd
CrCl 5-14mL/min: 35mg 1st dose, then 15mg qd
CrCl <5mL/min: 35mg 1st dose, then 10mg qd

ADMINISTRATION
Oral route

Take w/ or w/o food.
Tabs and oral sol are interchangeable.
Use oral sol for doses <100mg.
Do not use w/ other medications that contain lamivudine or emtricitabine.
Refer to PI for assessing patients during treatment.

STORAGE
Tab: 25°C (77°F); excursions permitted to 15-30°C (59-86°F). **Sol:** 20-25°C (68-77°F); store in tightly closed bottles.

HOW SUPPLIED
Oral Sol: 5mg/mL [240mL]; **Tab:** 100mg

CONTRAINDICATIONS
Previous hypersensitivity reaction (eg, anaphylaxis) to lamivudine or to any component of the tabs or oral sol.

WARNINGS/PRECAUTIONS
Consider initiation of treatment only when use of an alternative antiviral agent with a higher genetic barrier to resistance is not available/appropriate. Obesity and prolonged nucleoside exposure may be risk factors for lactic acidosis and severe hepatomegaly with steatosis. Caution with known risk factors for liver disease. Emergence of resistance-associated HBV substitutions reported; monitor ALT and HBV DNA levels if suspected. Not approved for patients dually infected with HBV and HIV. Epivir HBV contains a lower lamivudine dose than Epivir, Combivir, Epzicom, and Trizivir. If a decision is made to administer lamivudine to such coinfected patients, use the higher dosage indicated for HIV therapy as part of an appropriate combination regimen and refer to PI of such drugs. Caution in elderly patients.

ADVERSE REACTIONS
Lactic acidosis, severe hepatomegaly with steatosis, exacerbations of hepatitis B, ear/nose/throat infections, sore throat, diarrhea, serum lipase increase, CPK increase, ALT increase, thrombocytopenia.

DRUG INTERACTIONS
Avoid with other lamivudine- and emtricitabine-containing products. Possible interaction with other drugs whose main route of elimination is active renal secretion via the organic cationic transport system (eg, trimethoprim).

PREGNANCY AND LACTATION
Category C, not for use in nursing.

MECHANISM OF ACTION
Nucleoside analogue; inhibits HBV reverse transcriptase via DNA chain termination after incorporation of the nucleotide analogue into viral DNA.

PHARMACOKINETICS
Absorption: Absolute bioavailability (86% tab, 87% sol); AUC=4.7mcg•hr/mL (repeated daily doses); C_{max}=1.28mcg/mL; T_{max}=0.5-2.0 hrs. **Distribution:** V_d=1.3L/kg (IV); plasma protein binding (<36%); found in breast milk. **Metabolism:** Trans-sulfoxide (metabolite). **Elimination:** Urine (unchanged); $T_{1/2}$=5-7 hrs.

PATIENT CONSIDERATIONS
Assessment: Assess for hepatic/renal impairment, previous nucleoside exposure, risk factors for liver disease, HIV infection, hypersensitivity to drug, pregnancy/nursing status, and possible drug interactions. Perform HIV counseling and testing. Obtain baseline ALT and HBV DNA levels.

Monitoring: Monitor for renal/hepatic dysfunction, loss of therapeutic response (eg, persistent ALT elevation, increasing HBV DNA levels after an initial decline below assay limit, progression of clinical signs/symptoms of hepatic disease, worsening of hepatic necroinflammatory findings), signs/symptoms of lactic acidosis, hepatomegaly with steatosis, emergence of resistant HIV, hepatitis B exacerbation, and hypersensitivity reactions. Monitor hepatic function closely for several months in patients who d/c therapy.

Counseling: Advise to remain under the care of a physician during therapy and to report any new symptoms or concurrent medications. Inform that drug is not a cure for hepatitis B and that long-term benefits and relationship of initial treatment response to outcomes (eg, hepatocellular carcinoma, decompensated cirrhosis) are unknown. Inform that liver disease deterioration may occur upon discontinuation. Instruct to discuss any changes in regimen with physician. Inform that emergence of resistant HBV and worsening of disease can occur; advise to report any new symptoms to physician. Counsel on importance of HIV testing to avoid inappropriate therapy and development of resistant HIV. Inform that drug contains a lower dose of lamivudine than Epivir, Combivir, Epzicom, and Trizivir; instruct not to take concurrently with these products. Instruct not to take concurrently with emtricitabine-containing products (eg, Atripla, Complera, Emtriva, Stribild, Truvada). Inform that therapy has not been shown to reduce the risk of HBV transmission through sexual contact/blood contamination. Instruct to avoid doing things that can spread HBV infection to others. Inform diabetics that each 20mL dose of oral sol contains 4g of sucrose.

EPOGEN — epoetin alfa   Rx

Class: Erythropoiesis-stimulating agent (ESA)

> Increased risk of death, MI, stroke, venous thromboembolism (VTE), thrombosis of vascular access, and tumor progression or recurrence. Use the lowest dose sufficient to reduce/avoid the need for RBC transfusions. Chronic Kidney Disease (CKD): Greater risks for death, serious adverse cardiovascular (CV) reactions, and stroke when administered to target Hgb level >11g/dL. Cancer: Shortened overall survival and/or increased risk of tumor progression or recurrence in patients with breast, non-small cell lung, head and neck, lymphoid, and cervical cancers. Must enroll in and comply with the ESA APPRISE Oncology Program to prescribe or dispense drug to patients. Use only for anemia from myelosuppressive chemotherapy. Not indicated for patients receiving myelosuppressive chemotherapy when anticipated outcome is cure. D/C following completion of a chemotherapy course. Perisurgery: Due to increased risk of deep venous thrombosis (DVT), DVT prophylaxis is recommended.

ADULT DOSAGE
Anemia
Chronic Kidney Disease Associated Anemia:
Initiate When:
On Dialysis: Hgb <10g/dL
Not On Dialysis: Hgb <10g/dL, the rate of Hgb decline indicates likelihood of requiring a RBC transfusion, and reducing the risk of alloimmunization and/or other RBC transfusion-related risks is a goal
Initial: 50-100 U/kg IV/SQ 3X/week
Titrate:
On Dialysis: When Hgb approaches/exceeds 11g/dL, reduce or interrupt dose
Not On Dialysis: When Hgb approaches/exceeds 10g/dL, reduce or interrupt dose

All Chronic Kidney Disease Patients:
Do not increase dose more frequently than once every 4 weeks; decreases in dose may occur more frequently
If Hgb rises rapidly (eg, >1g/dL in any 2-week period), decrease dose by 25% or more prn to reduce rapid responses
If Hgb has not increased by >1g/dL after 4 weeks, increase dose by 25%
If no response after 12-week escalation period, use lowest dose to maintain sufficient Hgb level to reduce need for RBC transfusions and evaluate other causes of anemia

Zidovudine (≤4200mg) Associated Anemia in HIV-Infected Patients w/ Endogenous Serum Erythropoietin Levels of ≤500 mU/mL:
Initial: 100 U/kg IV/SQ 3X/week
Titrate:
Hgb Does Not Increase After 8 Weeks of Therapy: Increase by 50-100 U/kg at 4- to 8- week intervals until Hgb reaches a level needed to avoid RBC transfusions or 300 U/kg
Hgb >12g/dL: Withhold dose. When Hgb <11g/dL, resume at 25% below the previous dose

D/C if increase in Hgb is not achieved at a dose of 300 U/kg for 8 weeks

Chemotherapy Associated Anemia:
Initiate when Hgb <10g/dL and if there is a minimum of 2 additional months of planned chemotherapy
Initial: 150 U/kg SQ 3X/week or 40,000 U SQ weekly until completion of a chemotherapy course

PEDIATRIC DOSAGE
Anemia
Chronic Kidney Disease Associated Anemia:
1 Month-16 Years:
On Dialysis:
Initial: 50 U/kg IV/SQ 3X weekly
Titrate: When Hgb approaches/exceeds 11g/dL, reduce or interrupt dose
Do not increase dose more frequently than once every 4 weeks; decreases in dose may occur more frequently
If Hgb rises rapidly (eg, >1g/dL in any 2-week period), decrease dose by 25% or more prn to reduce rapid responses
If Hgb has not increased by >1g/dL after 4 weeks, increase dose by 25%
If no response after 12-week escalation period, use lowest dose to maintain sufficient Hgb level to reduce need for RBC transfusions and evaluate other causes of anemia

Chemotherapy Associated Anemia:
5-18 Years:
Initial: 600 U/kg IV weekly until completion of a chemotherapy course
Titrate:
Dose Reduction: Reduce by 25% if Hgb increases >1g/dL in any 2-week period or Hgb reaches a level needed to avoid RBC transfusions. Withhold if Hgb exceeds level needed to avoid RBC transfusions; reinitiate at 25% below previous dose when Hgb approaches a level where RBC transfusions may be required
Dose Increase: If Hgb increases by <1g/dL and remains below 10g/dL after initial 4 weeks, increase dose to 900 U/kg weekly
D/C therapy if there is no response in Hgb levels or if RBC transfusions are still required after 8 weeks
Max: 60,000 U/week

Titrate:
Dose Reduction: Reduce by 25% if Hgb increases >1g/dL in any 2-week period or reaches a level needed to avoid RBC transfusions. Withhold if Hgb exceeds level needed to avoid RBC transfusions; reinitiate at 25% below previous dose when Hgb approaches a level where RBC transfusions may be required
Dose Increase: If Hgb increases by <1g/dL and remains below 10g/dL after initial 4 weeks, increase dose to 300 U/kg 3X/week or 60,000 U/week D/C therapy if there is no response in Hgb levels or if RBC transfusions are still required after 8 weeks

Surgery Patients:
Used to reduce the need for allogeneic RBC transfusions among patients w/ perioperative Hgb >10-≤13g/dL who are at high risk for perioperative blood loss from elective, noncardiac, nonvascular surgery
Usual: 300 U/kg/day SQ qd for 10 days before, on the day of, and for 4 days after surgery; or 600 U/kg SQ in 4 doses administered 21, 14, and 7 days before surgery and on the day of surgery. Deep vein thrombosis prophylaxis is recommended

----

DOSING CONSIDERATIONS
Elderly
Individualize dose selection and adjustment to achieve and maintain target Hgb

ADMINISTRATION
IV/SQ route

IV route is recommended for chronic kidney disease patients on hemodialysis.

Preparation/Administration
Do not shake; do not use if shaken or frozen.
Preservative-free single-use vials may be admixed in a syringe w/ bacteriostatic 0.9% NaCl inj, w/ benzyl alcohol 0.9% in a 1:1 ratio.
Do not dilute or mix w/ other drug sol.
Do not re-enter preservative-free vials; discard unused portions.
Store unused portions of multidose vials at 2-8°C (36-46°F); discard after 21 days after initial entry.

STORAGE
2-8°C (36-46°F). Do not freeze; do not use if it has been frozen. Protect from light. Discard unused portions of multidose vials 21 days after initial entry.

HOW SUPPLIED
Inj: (Single-dose vial) 2000 U/mL, 3000 U/mL, 4000 U/mL, 10,000 U/mL; (multidose vial) 10,000 U/mL [2mL], 20,000 U/mL [1mL]

CONTRAINDICATIONS
Uncontrolled HTN, pure red cell aplasia (PRCA) that begins after treatment with epoetin alfa or other erythropoietin protein drugs, serious allergic reactions to epoetin alfa. **Multidose Vials:** Neonates, infants, pregnant women, and nursing mothers.

WARNINGS/PRECAUTIONS
Not indicated for use in patients with cancer receiving hormonal agents, biologic products, or radiotherapy, unless also receiving concomitant myelosuppressive chemotherapy; in patients scheduled for surgery who are willing to donate autologous blood; in patients undergoing cardiac/vascular surgery; or as a substitute for RBC transfusions in patients requiring immediate correction of anemia. Evaluate transferrin saturation and serum ferritin prior to and during treatment; administer supplemental iron when serum ferritin is <100mcg/L or serum transferrin saturation is <20%. Correct/exclude other causes of anemia (eg, vitamin deficiency, metabolic/chronic inflammatory conditions, bleeding) before initiating therapy. Hypertensive encephalopathy and seizures reported in patients with CKD; increases risk of seizures in CKD patients. Appropriately control HTN prior to initiation of and during treatment; reduce/withhold therapy if BP becomes difficult to control. PRCA and severe anemia, with or without other cytopenias that arise following the development of neutralizing antibodies to erythropoietin, reported. Withhold and evaluate for neutralizing antibodies to erythropoietin if severe anemia and low reticulocyte count develop; d/c permanently if PRCA develops, and do not switch to other erythropoiesis-stimulating agents. Serious allergic reactions may occur; immediately and permanently d/c therapy. Contains albumin; may carry an extremely remote risk for transmission of viral diseases or Creutzfeldt-Jakob disease. Patients may require adjustments in their dialysis prescriptions after initiation of therapy, or require increased anticoagulation with heparin to prevent clotting of extracorporeal circuit during hemodialysis. Multidose vial contains benzyl alcohol; benzyl alcohol is associated with serious adverse events and death, particularly in pediatric patients.

ADVERSE REACTIONS
MI, stroke, VTE, thrombosis of vascular access, tumor progression/recurrence, pyrexia, N/V, HTN, cough, arthralgia, dizziness, pruritus, rash, headache.

PREGNANCY AND LACTATION
Category C, caution in nursing (single-dose vial).

MECHANISM OF ACTION
Erythropoiesis-stimulating glycoprotein; stimulates erythropoiesis by the same mechanism as endogenous erythropoietin.

PHARMACOKINETICS
Absorption: Adults and Pediatrics with CKD: (SQ) T_{max}=5-24 hrs. Anemic Cancer Patients: (SQ) T_{max}=13.3 hrs (150 U/kg 3X weekly), 38 hrs (40,000 U weekly).
Elimination: Adults and Pediatrics with CKD: (IV) $T_{1/2}$=4-13 hrs. Anemic Cancer Patients: (SQ) $T_{1/2}$=16-67 hrs.

PATIENT CONSIDERATIONS
Assessment: Assess for uncontrolled HTN, previous hypersensitivity to the drug, causes of anemia, pregnancy/nursing status, and other conditions where treatment is contraindicated or cautioned. Obtain baseline Hgb levels, transferrin saturation, and serum ferritin.

Monitoring: Monitor for signs/symptoms of an allergic reaction, CV/thromboembolic events, stroke, premonitory neurologic symptoms, PRCA, severe anemia, progression/recurrence of tumor, and other adverse reactions. Monitor BP, transferrin saturation, and serum ferritin. Following initiation of therapy and after each dose adjustment, monitor Hgb weekly until Hgb is stable, then at least monthly, and to maintain Hgb sufficient to minimize need for RBC transfusions.

Counseling: Inform of the risks and benefits of therapy, and of the increased risks of mortality, serious CV reactions, thromboembolic reactions, stroke, and tumor progression. Advise of the need to have regular lab tests for Hgb. Inform cancer patients that they must sign the patient-physician acknowledgment form prior to therapy. Instruct to undergo regular BP monitoring, adhere to prescribed antihypertensive regimen, and follow recommended dietary restrictions. Advise to contact physician for new-onset neurologic symptoms or change in seizure frequency. Instruct regarding proper disposal and caution against reuse of needles, syringes, or unused portions of single-dose vials.

EPZICOM — abacavir sulfate/lamivudine   Rx
Class: Nucleoside reverse transcriptase inhibitor (NRTI) combination

> Lactic acidosis and severe hepatomegaly w/ steatosis, including fatal cases, reported w/ nucleoside analogues and other antiretrovirals; d/c if clinical or laboratory findings suggestive of lactic acidosis or pronounced hepatotoxicity occur. **Abacavir:** Serious and sometimes fatal hypersensitivity reactions w/ multiple organ involvement reported; d/c immediately if a hypersensitivity reaction is suspected and never restart therapy or any other abacavir-containing product because more severe symptoms, including death, can occur w/in hours. Patients who carry the HLA-B*5701 allele are at a higher risk of a hypersensitivity reaction; screen all patients for HLA-B*5701 allele prior to initiating or reinitiating therapy, unless patient has a previously documented HLA-B*5701 allele assessment. **Lamivudine:** Severe acute exacerbations of hepatitis B reported in patients coinfected w/ hepatitis B virus (HBV) and have discontinued therapy; closely monitor hepatic function for at least several months in patients who d/c therapy and are coinfected w/ HBV. If appropriate, initiation of antihepatitis B therapy may be warranted.

ADULT DOSAGE	PEDIATRIC DOSAGE
HIV-1 Infection	**HIV-1 Infection**
Combination w/ Other Antiretrovirals: 1 tab qd	**Combination w/ Other Antiretrovirals:** ≥25kg: 1 tab qd

----

DOSING CONSIDERATIONS
Renal Impairment
CrCl <50mL/min: Not recommended

Hepatic Impairment
Mild (Child-Pugh Class A): Not recommended
Moderate (Child-Pugh Class B) or Severe (Child-Pugh Class C): Contraindicated

ADMINISTRATION
Oral route

Take w/ or w/o food.
Screen for the HLA-B*5701 allele prior to initiating therapy.

STORAGE
25°C (77°F); excursions permitted to 15-30°C (59-86°F).

HOW SUPPLIED
Tab: (Abacavir sulfate/Lamivudine) 600mg/300mg

CONTRAINDICATIONS
Patients w/ HLA-B*5701 allele, prior hypersensitivity reaction to abacavir or lamivudine, moderate or severe hepatic impairment.

WARNINGS/PRECAUTIONS
Immune reconstitution syndrome reported. Autoimmune disorders (eg, Graves' disease, polymyositis, Guillain-Barre syndrome) reported to occur in the setting of immune reconstitution and can occur many months after initiation of treatment. Redistribution/accumulation of body fat reported. Caution in elderly. **Abacavir:** May increase risk of MI. Consider the underlying risk of coronary heart disease when prescribing therapy. **Lamivudine:** Emergence of lamivudine-resistant HBV reported.

ADVERSE REACTIONS
Drug hypersensitivity, insomnia, depression/depressed mood, headache/migraine, fatigue/malaise, dizziness/vertigo, nausea, diarrhea.

DRUG INTERACTIONS
Avoid w/ other abacavir-, lamivudine-, and/or emtricitabine-containing products. **Abacavir:** May increase oral methadone clearance; an increased methadone dose may be required in a small number of patients. **Lamivudine:** Closely monitor for treatment-associated toxicities, especially hepatic decompensation, in patients

receiving interferon alfa w/ or w/o ribavirin and Epzicom; consider discontinuation of Epzicom and dose reduction/discontinuation of interferon alfa, ribavirin, or both.

PREGNANCY AND LACTATION
Pregnancy: Physicians are encouraged to register patients in the Antiretroviral Pregnancy Registry. Fetal harm has been seen in animal studies; relevance to human pregnancy registry data is unknown.
Lactation: Mothers should be instructed not to breastfeed due to potential for HIV-1 transmission.

MECHANISM OF ACTION
Abacavir: Carbocyclic nucleoside analogue; inhibits HIV-1 reverse transcriptase (RT) activity by competing w/ natural substrate dGTP and by its incorporation into viral DNA. **Lamivudine:** Nucleoside analogue; inhibits RT via DNA chain termination after incorporation of the nucleotide analogue.

PHARMACOKINETICS
Absorption: Rapid. Abacavir: Oral bioavailability (86%), C_{max}=4.26mcg/mL, AUC=11.95mcg•hr/mL. Lamivudine: Oral bioavailability (86%), C_{max}=2.04mcg/mL, AUC=8.87mcg•hr/mL. **Distribution:** Abacavir: V_d=0.86L/kg; plasma protein binding (50%). Lamivudine: V_d=1.3L/kg; crosses placenta. **Metabolism:** Abacavir: Via alcohol dehydrogenase and glucuronyl transferase; 5'-carboxylic acid and 5'-glucuronide (metabolites). Lamivudine: Trans-sulfoxide (metabolite). **Elimination:** Abacavir: $T_{1/2}$=1.45 hrs. Lamivudine: Urine (70%, unchanged) (IV); $T_{1/2}$=5-7 hrs.

PATIENT CONSIDERATIONS
Assessment: Assess medical history for prior exposure to any abacavir-containing product. Assess for HBV infection, history of hypersensitivity reactions, HLA-B*5701 status (including patients of unknown HLA-B*5701 status who have previously tolerated abacavir), hepatic/renal impairment, risk factors for coronary heart disease, pregnancy/nursing status, and possible drug interactions.

Monitoring: Monitor for signs/symptoms of hypersensitivity reactions, lactic acidosis, hepatomegaly w/ steatosis, immune reconstitution syndrome, autoimmune disorders, fat redistribution/accumulation, MI, and other adverse reactions. Monitor hepatic/renal function. Closely monitor hepatic function for several months after discontinuing therapy in patients coinfected w/ HIV-1 and HBV.

Counseling: Inform patients regarding hypersensitivity reactions w/ abacavir; instruct to contact physician immediately if symptoms develop and not to restart or replace w/ any other abacavir-containing products w/o medical consultation. Inform that the drug may cause lactic acidosis w/ hepatomegaly. Inform patients coinfected w/ HIV-1 and HBV that worsening of liver disease has occurred in some cases when treatment w/ lamivudine was discontinued; instruct to discuss any changes in regimen w/ the physician. Inform that hepatic decompensation has occurred in HIV-1/hepatitis C virus coinfected patients receiving combination antiretroviral therapy for HIV-1 and interferon alfa w/ or w/o ribavirin. Inform that redistribution/accumulation of body fat may occur. Advise that drug is not a cure for HIV-1 infection and continuous therapy is necessary to control HIV-1 infection and decrease HIV-related illness. Instruct patients to take all HIV medications exactly as prescribed. Advise not to re-use or share needles/other inj equipment and not to share personal items (eg, toothbrush, razor blades), to continue to practice safer sex by using latex or polyurethane condoms, and not to breastfeed.

EQUETRO — carbamazepine   Rx

Class: Carboxamide

> Serious and fatal dermatologic reactions, including toxic epidermal necrolysis (TEN) and Stevens-Johnson syndrome (SJS) reported; increased risk with presence of HLA-B*1502 allele. Screen patients with ancestry in genetically at risk populations for the presence of HLA-B*1502 prior to initiation of therapy. Avoid in patients testing positive for the allele unless the benefit clearly outweighs the risk. D/C therapy if serious dermatologic reaction is suspected. Aplastic anemia and agranulocytosis reported; obtain CBC prior to treatment, and monitor periodically. Consider discontinuing therapy if significant bone marrow depression develops.

ADULT DOSAGE	PEDIATRIC DOSAGE
Bipolar I Disorder	Pediatric use may not have been established
Acute Manic or Mixed Episodes Associated w/ Bipolar I Disorder:	
Initial: 200mg bid	
Titrate: May increase dose by 200mg/day to achieve optimal clinical response	
Max: 1600mg/day	

DOSING CONSIDERATIONS
Elderly
Start at lower end of dosing range

Discontinuation
Reduce dose gradually and avoid abrupt discontinuation when discontinuing treatment

ADMINISTRATION
Oral route

May take orally, or may open and sprinkle beads over food such as a tsp of applesauce
Do not crush or chew caps
Take w/ or w/o meals

STORAGE
25°C (77°F); excursions permitted to 15-30°C (59-86°F). Protect from light and moisture.

HOW SUPPLIED
Cap, Extended-Release: 100mg, 200mg, 300mg

CONTRAINDICATIONS
Bone marrow depression, anaphylactic or serious hypersensitivity reaction to carbamazepine or TCAs (eg, amitriptyline, desipramine, imipramine, protriptyline, and nortriptyline), coadministration w/ delavirdine or other non-nucleoside reverse transcriptase inhibitors (NNRTIs), nefazodone. Concomitant use of an MAOI or w/in 14 days after discontinuing an MAOI.

WARNINGS/PRECAUTIONS
Periodically reevaluate long-term risks and benefits of the drug if used for extended periods. Do not resume treatment if signs/symptoms suggest SJS/TEN. Drug reaction with eosinophilia and systemic symptoms (DRESS), also known as multiorgan hypersensitivity reported; evaluate and d/c therapy if an alternative etiology cannot be established. Hypersensitivity reactions reported. Increased risk of suicidal thoughts or behavior reported. May cause fetal harm. Avoid abrupt discontinuation, especially in patients with seizure disorder; may increase risk of developing seizure and status epilepticus with attendant hypoxia and threat to life. Hyponatremia may occur; consider discontinuing in patients with symptomatic hyponatremia. May impair mental/physical abilities. Avoid in patients with history of hepatic porphyria. Has mild anticholinergic activity; assess intraocular pressure (IOP) prior to therapy and periodically thereafter in patients with history of increased IOP. Consider reducing dose in patients with hepatic impairment. Caution in elderly patients.

ADVERSE REACTIONS
Dizziness, somnolence, N/V, ataxia, constipation, pruritus, dry mouth, rash, blurred vision, speech disorder, HTN, agranulocytosis, aplastic anemia, TEN, SJS.

DRUG INTERACTIONS
See Contraindications. CYP3A4 and/or epoxide hydrolase inhibitors (eg, acetazolamide, cimetidine, clarithromycin, protease inhibitors, valproate) may increase plasma levels. CYP3A4 inducers (eg, cisplatin, phenobarbital, rifampin, theophylline) may decrease plasma levels. May decrease levels of CYP1A2 and CYP3A4 substrates (eg, acetaminophen, bupropion, clonazepam, doxycycline). May increase plasma levels of clomipramine and primidone. May increase/decrease phenytoin plasma levels. May cause contraceptive failure or breakthrough bleeding with oral contraceptives. May reduce anticoagulant effect of warfarin. May increase risk of neurotoxic adverse reactions with lithium. Antimalarial drugs (eg, chloroquine, mefloquine) may antagonize carbamazepine activity. May increase risk of respiratory depression, profound sedation, hypotension, and syncope with other CNS depressants (eg, alcohol, opioid analgesics, benzodiazepines).

PREGNANCY AND LACTATION
Category D, not for use in nursing.

MECHANISM OF ACTION
Carboxamide; not established. Modulates Na^+ and Ca^{2+} ion channels, receptor-mediated neurotransmitters, and intracellular signaling pathways in experimental preparations.

PHARMACOKINETICS
Absorption: C_{max}=1.9mcg/mL (single 200mg dose), 11mcg/mL (multiple 800mg dose), 3.2mcg/mL (400mg dose, fasted), 4.3mcg/mL (400mg dose, fed); T_{max}=19 hrs (single 200mg dose), 5.9 hrs (multiple 800mg dose), 24 hrs (400mg dose, fasted), 14 hrs (400mg dose, fed). **Distribution:** Plasma protein binding (76%); crosses placenta; found in breast milk. **Metabolism:** Liver via CYP3A4; carbamazepine-10,11-epoxide (metabolite). **Elimination:** Urine (72%; 3% unchanged), feces (28%); $T_{1/2}$=35-40 hrs (single dose), 12-17 hrs (multiple doses).

PATIENT CONSIDERATIONS
Assessment: Assess for conditions where treatment is contraindicated or cautioned, pregnancy/nursing status, and possible drug interactions. Screen for HLA-B*1502 allele in suspected population. Obtain CBC, including platelets and differential counts. Assess IOP in patients with increased IOP.

Monitoring: Monitor for dermatological reactions, aplastic anemia, agranulocytosis, bone marrow depression, DRESS, emergence/worsening of depression, suicidal thoughts/behavior, unusual mood/behavior changes, seizures, or hyponatremia. Monitor CBC periodically. Closely monitor patients who exhibit low or decreased WBC or platelet count. Periodically monitor IOP in patients with increased IOP.

Counseling: Inform to take drug as prescribed and to read Medication Guide. Inform about the risk of potentially fatal, serious skin reactions, agranulocytosis, and aplastic anemia; instruct to report immediately if signs and symptoms occur. Inform of the early toxic signs and symptoms of potential hematologic, dermatologic, hypersensitivity, or hepatic reactions. Counsel about the increased risk of suicidal thinking and behavior; advise to report behaviors of concern immediately. Advise women of childbearing potential that drug may cause fetal harm. Advise to notify physician if pregnant or planning to get pregnant; encourage patients to enroll in the North American Antiepileptic Drug Pregnancy Registry. Inform that abrupt discontinuation can cause seizures or an increase in seizure frequency; advise that the drug should be tapered when discontinued. Advise that drug may reduce serum Na^+ concentrations, especially if patient is taking other medications that lower Na^+; report symptoms of low Na^+. Advise to observe caution when operating machinery/automobiles or potentially dangerous tasks. Advise to exercise caution if taking alcohol. Inform to not take with delavirdine, NNRTIs, and any other medications containing carbamazepine.

ERAXIS — anidulafungin   Rx
Class: Echinocandin

ADULT DOSAGE
Candida Infections

Candidemia/Other *Candida* Infections (Intra-Abdominal Abscess and Peritonitis):

>16 Years:
Usual: 200mg LD on Day 1, followed by 100mg/day thereafter

Continue for at least 14 days after last positive culture

Esophageal Candidiasis

>16 Years:
Usual: 100mg LD on Day 1, followed by 50mg/day thereafter

Treat for a minimum of 14 days and for at least 7 days following resolution of symptoms

Due to risk of relapse in patients w/ HIV infection, consider suppressive antifungal therapy after a course of treatment

PEDIATRIC DOSAGE
Pediatric use may not have been established

ADMINISTRATION
IV route

Rate of IV infusion should not exceed 1.1mg/min

Preparation
Reconstitute 50mg or 100mg vial w/ 15mL or 30mL of sterile water for inj, respectively
50mg Dose: Further dilute in 50mL of D5 inj or 0.9% NaCl inj and infuse for a minimum of 45 min
100mg Dose: Further dilute in 100mL of D5 inj or 0.9% NaCl inj and infuse for a minimum of 90 min
200mg Dose: Further dilute in 200mL of D5 inj or 0.9% NaCl inj and infuse for a minimum of 180 min

STORAGE
2-8°C (36-46°F); excursions permitted up to 25°C (77°F) for 96 hrs and can be returned to storage at 2-8°C (36-46°F). Do not freeze. Reconstituted Sol: Up to 25°C (77°F) for up to 24 hrs. Infusion Sol: Up to 25°C (77°F) for up to 48 hrs or stored frozen for at least 72 hrs.

HOW SUPPLIED
Inj: 50mg, 100mg

WARNINGS/PRECAUTIONS
LFTs abnormalities, significant hepatic dysfunction, hepatitis, and hepatic failure reported; monitor for evidence of worsening of hepatic function and evaluate for risk/benefit of continuing therapy. Anaphylactic reactions (eg, shock) reported; d/c if these reactions occur and administer appropriate treatment if any occur. Infusion-related reactions (eg, rash, urticaria, flushing, pruritus, bronchospasm, dyspnea, hypotension), possibly histamine-mediated, reported; do not exceed the infusion rate of 1.1mg/min.

ADVERSE REACTIONS
Diarrhea, hypokalemia, pyrexia, bacteremia, N/V, hypotension, insomnia, UTI, dyspnea, HTN, hypomagnesemia, increased blood alkaline phosphatase, peripheral edema, pleural effusion, dyspepsia.

PREGNANCY AND LACTATION
Category B, caution in nursing.

MECHANISM OF ACTION
Echinocandin; inhibits glucan synthase, which results in inhibition of the formation of 1,3-β-D-glucan, an essential component of fungal cell walls.

PHARMACOKINETICS
Absorption: Administration of variable doses resulted in different parameters.
Distribution: V_d=30-50L; plasma protein binding (>99%). **Elimination:** Urine (<1%), feces (30%, <10% intact drug); $T_{1/2}$=40-50 hrs.

PATIENT CONSIDERATIONS
Assessment: Assess for hypersensitivity to the drug or other echinocandins, hepatic impairment, and pregnancy/nursing status. Obtain specimens for fungal culture and other relevant lab studies (eg, histopathology).

Monitoring: Monitor for hepatic dysfunction, hepatitis or hepatic failure, anaphylactic reactions, infusion-related reactions, and other adverse reactions. Monitor LFTs.

Counseling: Inform about the risk of developing abnormal LFTs and/or hepatic dysfunction; advise that LFTs may be monitored during treatment. Inform that physician may d/c treatment if an anaphylactic reaction (eg, shock) occurs. Instruct to report to physician any symptoms of infusion-related reactions. Advise to notify physician if pregnant, intending to become pregnant, or planning to breastfeed during therapy.

ERBITUX — cetuximab   Rx
Class: Monoclonal antibody/EGFR blocker

> Serious infusion reactions, some fatal, reported; immediately interrupt and permanently d/c infusion if these reactions occur. Cardiopulmonary arrest and/or sudden death occurred in patients w/ squamous cell carcinoma of the head and neck (SCCHN) treated w/ cetuximab in combination w/ radiation therapy or w/ European Union-approved cetuximab in combination w/ platinum-based therapy w/ 5-fluorouracil (5-FU); closely monitor serum electrolytes during and after therapy.

ADULT DOSAGE
Squamous Cell Carcinoma of the Head and Neck

W/ Radiation Therapy for the Initial Treatment of Locally or Regionally Advanced Squamous Cell Carcinoma of the Head and Neck (SCCHN):
Initial: 400mg/m² administered 1 week prior to initiation of a course of radiation therapy as a 120 min IV infusion
Maint: 250mg/m² infused over 60 min weekly for the duration of radiation therapy (6-7 weeks)
Max Infusion Rate: 10mg/min

Complete administration 60 min prior to radiation therapy

W/ Platinum-Based Therapy w/ 5-fluorouracil (5-FU) for the 1st-Line Treatment of Patients w/ Recurrent Locoregional Disease or Metastatic SCCHN:
Initial: 400mg/m² administered on the day of initiation of platinum-based therapy w/ 5-FU as a 120 min IV infusion
Maint: 250mg/m² infused over 60 min weekly until disease progression or unacceptable toxicity
Max Infusion Rate: 10mg/min

Complete administration 60 min prior to platinum-based therapy w/ 5-FU

As Monotherapy in Patients w/ Recurrent/Metastatic SCCHN for Whom Prior Platinum-Based Therapy Failed:
Initial: 400mg/m² administered as a 120 min IV infusion
Maint: 250mg/m² infused over 60 min weekly until disease progression or unacceptable toxicity
Max Infusion Rate: 10mg/min

Metastatic Colorectal Cancer

Treatment of *K-Ras* wild-type, epidermal growth factor receptor-expressing, metastatic colorectal cancer in combination w/ FOLFIRI (irinotecan, 5-fluorouracil, leucovorin) for 1st-line treatment, in combination w/ irinotecan in patients who are refractory to irinotecan-based chemotherapy, and as monotherapy in patients who have failed oxaliplatin- and irinotecan-based chemotherapy or are intolerant to irinotecan

Initial: 400mg/m² administered as a 120-min IV infusion; complete administration 60 min prior to FOLFIRI
Maint: 250mg/m² infused over 60 min weekly until disease progression or unacceptable toxicity; complete administration 60 min prior to FOLFIRI
Max Infusion Rate: 10mg/min

Premedication

H₁-antagonist (eg, 50mg diphenhydramine) IV 30-60 min prior to 1st dose; premedication for subsequent doses should be based on clinical judgment and presence/severity of prior infusion reactions

PEDIATRIC DOSAGE
Pediatric use may not have been established

DOSING CONSIDERATIONS
Adverse Reactions
NCI CTC Grade 1 or 2 and Non-Serious NCI CTC Grade 3 Infusion Reaction:
Reduce infusion rate by 50%; immediately and permanently d/c for serious infusion reactions, requiring medical intervention and/or hospitalization

Severe Acneiform Rash (NCI CTC Grade 3 or 4):
1st Occurrence: Delay infusion 1-2 weeks
W/ Improvement: Continue at 250mg/m^2
No Improvement: D/C treatment

2nd Occurrence: Delay infusion 1-2 weeks
W/ Improvement: Reduce to 200mg/m^2
No Improvement: D/C treatment

3rd Occurrence: Delay infusion 1-2 weeks
W/ Improvement: Reduce to 150mg/m^2
No Improvement: D/C treatment

4th Occurrence: D/C treatment

ADMINISTRATION
IV route
Do not administer as IV push or bolus.
Administer via infusion pump or syringe pump.
Administer through low protein binding 0.22μm in-line filter.
Do not shake or dilute.

STORAGE
Vials: 2-8°C (36-46°F). Do not freeze. **Infusion Containers:** Stable for up to 12 hrs at 2-8°C (36-46°F) and up to 8 hrs at 20-25°C (68-77°F).

HOW SUPPLIED
Inj: 2mg/mL [50mL, 100mL]

WARNINGS/PRECAUTIONS
Caution when used in combination w/ radiation therapy or platinum-based therapy w/ 5-FU in head and neck cancer patients w/ history of coronary artery disease (CAD), CHF, or arrhythmias. Interstitial lung disease (ILD) reported; interrupt for acute onset or worsening of pulmonary symptoms and permanently d/c if ILD is confirmed. Dermatologic toxicities (eg, acneiform rash, skin drying/fissuring, paronychial inflammation, infectious sequelae, hypertrichosis) reported. Life-threatening and fatal bullous mucocutaneous disease w/ blisters, erosions, and skin sloughing has also been observed; limit sun exposure during therapy. Addition of cetuximab to radiation and cisplatin in patients reported to increase incidence of Grade 3-4 mucositis, radiation recall syndrome, acneiform rash, cardiac events, and electrolyte disturbances compared to radiation and cisplatin alone; addition of cetuximab did not improve progression-free survival. Hypomagnesemia and electrolyte abnormalities reported; replete electrolytes as necessary. Do not resume nursing earlier than 60 days following the last dose of therapy if nursing is interrupted. Not indicated for the treatment of *Ras* mutant colorectal cancer or when *Ras* mutation test results are unknown, or for the treatment of patients w/ colorectal cancer that harbor somatic mutations in exon 2 (codons 12 and 13), exon 3 (codons 59 and 61), and exon 4 (codons 117 and 146) of either *K-ras* or *N-ras*.

ADVERSE REACTIONS
Cardiopulmonary arrest, infusion reactions, cutaneous reactions (eg, rash, pruritus, nail changes), headache, diarrhea, infection, sepsis, asthenia, nausea, emesis, fatigue, fever, pain, dyspnea, cough.

PREGNANCY AND LACTATION
Category C, not for use in nursing.

MECHANISM OF ACTION
EGFR antagonist (human/mouse chimeric monoclonal antibody); binds specifically to EGFR on both normal and tumor cells and competitively inhibits the binding of epidermal growth factor and other ligands, such as transforming growth factor-α.

PHARMACOKINETICS
Absorption: C_{max}=168-235mcg/mL. **Distribution:** V_d=2-3L/m^2; may cross the placenta. **Elimination:** $T_{1/2}$=112 hrs.

PATIENT CONSIDERATIONS
Assessment: Assess for history of CAD, CHF, arrhythmias, pulmonary disorders, pregnancy/nursing status, and possible drug interactions. Obtain serum electrolyte levels (including Mg^{2+}, K^+, Ca^{2+}). Determine EGFR-expression status and confirm the absence of a *Ras* mutation in colorectal tumors using FDA-approved tests.

Monitoring: Monitor for signs/symptoms of infusion reactions, cardiopulmonary arrest, acute onset or worsening of pulmonary symptoms, dermatologic toxicities and infectious sequelae, and for other adverse reactions. Monitor patients for 1 hr after infusion in a setting w/ resuscitation equipment and other agents necessary to treat anaphylaxis; monitor longer to confirm resolution of the event in patients requiring treatment for infusion reactions. Periodically monitor for hypomagnesemia, hypocalcemia, and hypokalemia during and for at least 8 weeks after therapy.

Counseling: Advise to report to physician signs/symptoms of infusion reactions. Inform of pregnancy/nursing risks; advise to use adequate contraception during and for 6 months after last dose for both males and females. Inform that nursing is not recommended during and for 2 months following last dose of therapy. Instruct to limit sun exposure (eg, use of sunscreen, wear hats) during and for 2 months after last dose of therapy.

ERIVEDGE — vismodegib   **Rx**
Class: Hedgehog pathway inhibitor

> May cause embryo-fetal death or severe birth defects when administered to pregnant woman. Verify pregnancy status of females of reproductive potential w/in 7 days prior to initiating therapy. Advise females of reproductive potential to use effective contraception during and after therapy. Advise males of the potential risk of exposure through semen and to use condoms w/ a pregnant partner or a female partner of reproductive potential. Advise pregnant women of the potential risks to a fetus.

ADULT DOSAGE
Basal Cell Carcinoma
Metastatic basal cell carcinoma, or locally advanced basal cell carcinoma that has recurred following surgery or in patients who are not candidates for surgery, and who are not candidates for radiation

150mg qd until disease progression or until unacceptable toxicity

PEDIATRIC DOSAGE
Pediatric use may not have been established

ADMINISTRATION
Oral route
Take w/ or w/o food
Swallow caps whole; do not open or crush caps

STORAGE
20-25°C (68-77°F); excursions permitted between 15-30°C (59-86°F).

HOW SUPPLIED
Cap: 150mg

WARNINGS/PRECAUTIONS
Do not donate blood or blood products while on therapy and for 7 months after the final dose. Vismodegib is present is semen; males should not donate semen during and for 3 months after the final dose of therapy.

ADVERSE REACTIONS
Muscle spasm, alopecia, dysgeusia, weight loss, fatigue, N/V, diarrhea, decreased appetite, constipation, arthralgia, ageusia.

PREGNANCY AND LACTATION
Pregnancy: May cause fetal harm.
Lactation: No data are available regarding the presence of vismodegib in human milk. Breastfeeding is not recommended during therapy and for 7 months after the final dose.
Reproductive Potential: Females of reproductive potential should use effective contraception during therapy and for 7 months after the final dose of therapy. Amenorrhea may occur in females of reproductive potential. Vismodegib is present in semen. Males should use condoms, even after vasectomy, to avoid exposure to pregnant partners and female partners of reproductive potential, and should not donate semen, during therapy and for 3 months after the final dose of therapy.

MECHANISM OF ACTION
Hedgehog pathway inhibitor; binds to and inhibits Smoothened, a transmembrane protein involved in Hedgehog signal transduction.

PHARMACOKINETICS
Absorption: Absolute bioavailability (31.8%). **Distribution:** V_d=16.4-26.6L; plasma protein binding (>99%). **Metabolism:** Oxidation, glucuronidation, and pyridine ring cleavage. **Elimination:** Feces (82%), urine (4.4%); $T_{1/2}$=4 days (continuous qd dosing), 12 days (single dose).

PATIENT CONSIDERATIONS
Assessment: Assess pregnancy status w/in 7 days prior to initiating therapy. Assess nursing status and for possible drug interactions.

Monitoring: Monitor for disease progression, toxicities, and other adverse reactions.

Counseling: Inform pregnant women of the potential risk to a fetus; advise females of reproductive potential to use effective contraception during therapy and for 7 months after the final dose of therapy. Advise males, even those w/ prior vasectomy, to use condoms to avoid potential drug exposure in both pregnant partners and female partners of reproductive potential during therapy and for 3 months after the final dose. Advise female patients and female partners of male patients to contact their healthcare provider w/ a known/suspected pregnancy. Advise males not to donate semen during therapy and for 3 months after the final dose. Advise women that breastfeeding is not recommended during therapy and for 7 months after final dose. Advise not to donate blood or blood products while on therapy and for 7 months after the final dose.

ERTACZO — sertaconazole nitrate   Rx
Class: Azole antifungal

ADULT DOSAGE	PEDIATRIC DOSAGE
Fungal Infections	**Fungal Infections**
Interdigital Tinea Pedis Caused by *Trichophyton rubrum*, *T. mentagrophytes*, and *Epidermophyton floccosum*:	**Interdigital Tinea Pedis Caused by *T. rubrum*, *T. mentagrophytes*, and *E. floccosum*:**
Apply sufficient amount to cover both the affected areas between the toes and the immediately surrounding healthy skin bid for 4 weeks	**≥12 Years:** Apply sufficient amount to cover both the affected areas between the toes and the immediately surrounding healthy skin bid for 4 weeks

ADMINISTRATION
Topical route
Wash hands after applying medication.
Dry affected area(s) thoroughly before application if used after bathing.

STORAGE
20-25°C (68-77°F); excursions permitted to 15-30°C (59-86°F).

HOW SUPPLIED
Cre: 2% [60g]

WARNINGS/PRECAUTIONS
D/C and institute appropriate therapy if irritation occurs. Caution in patients sensitive to imidazole antifungals; cross-reactivity may occur.

ADVERSE REACTIONS
Contact dermatitis, dry skin, burning skin, application site skin tenderness.

PREGNANCY AND LACTATION
Category C, caution in nursing.

MECHANISM OF ACTION
Azole antifungal; inhibits fungal CYP450-mediated 14 α-lanosterol demethylase enzyme that converts lanosterol to ergosterol, a key component of fungi cell membranes.

PATIENT CONSIDERATIONS
Assessment: Assess for hypersensitivity to imidazole antifungals and pregnancy/nursing status.
Monitoring: Monitor for irritation and other adverse reactions.
Counseling: Instruct to use externally and ud. Instruct to use medication for the full treatment time, even though symptoms may have improved. Instruct to inform physician if area of application shows signs of increased irritation, redness, itching, burning, blistering, swelling, or oozing. Instruct to avoid the use of occlusive dressings unless directed by physician. Advise not to use for any disorder other than that for which it was prescribed.

ERWINAZE — asparaginase erwinia chrysanthemi   Rx
Class: Enzyme

ADULT DOSAGE	PEDIATRIC DOSAGE
Acute Lymphoblastic Leukemia	**Acute Lymphoblastic Leukemia**
As a component of multiagent chemotherapeutic regimen in patients who have developed hypersensitivity to *Escherichia coli*-derived asparaginase	As a component of multiagent chemotherapeutic regimen in patients who have developed hypersensitivity to *E. coli*-derived asparaginase
To Substitute for a Dose of Pegaspargase: Usual: 25,000 IU/m² IM/IV 3X/week (M/W/F) for 6 doses for each planned pegaspargase dose	**To Substitute for a Dose of Pegaspargase:** Usual: 25,000 IU/m² IM/IV 3X/week (M/W/F) for 6 doses for each planned pegaspargase dose
To Substitute for a Dose of Native *E. coli* Asparaginase: Usual: 25,000 IU/m² IM/IV for each scheduled *E. coli* asparaginase dose	**To Substitute for a Dose of Native *E. coli* Asparaginase:** Usual: 25,000 IU/m² IM/IV for each scheduled *E. coli* asparaginase dose

ADMINISTRATION
IM/IV route

Preparation
Reconstitute the contents of each vial by slowly injecting 1mL or 2mL of preservative free sterile NaCl (0.9%) Inj against the inner vial wall
Dissolve contents by gentle mixing or swirling
Withdraw the volume containing the calculated dose from the vial into a polypropylene syringe w/in 15 min of reconstitution

IM
Limit volume to 2mL/single inj site
If >2mL dose, use multiple inj sites

IV
Slowly inject the reconstituted asparaginase into an IV infusion bag containing 100mL of normal saline acclimatized to room temperature
Do not shake or squeeze the IV bag
Infuse in 100mL of normal saline over 1 hr
Do not infuse other IV drugs through the same IV line while infusing asparaginase

STORAGE
2-8°C (36-46°F). Protect from light. Do not freeze or refrigerate reconstituted sol. Administer w/in 4 hrs or discard.

HOW SUPPLIED
Inj: 10,000 IU

CONTRAINDICATIONS
History of serious hypersensitivity reactions to this medication (eg, anaphylaxis), history of serious thrombosis, pancreatitis, or hemorrhagic events w/ prior L-asparaginase therapy.

WARNINGS/PRECAUTIONS
Grade 3 and 4 hypersensitivity reactions and serious thrombotic events, including sagittal sinus thrombosis and PE, reported; d/c if any of these occur. Pancreatitis reported; d/c for severe or hemorrhagic pancreatitis manifested by abdominal pain >72 hrs and amylase elevation ≥2.0X ULN. W/ mild pancreatitis, hold until signs/symptoms subside and amylase levels return to normal. May resume treatment after resolution of mild pancreatitis or symptoms of thrombotic/hemorrhagic event. Irreversible glucose intolerance may occur. Administer insulin therapy as necessary in patients w/ hyperglycemia. Consider monitoring nadir (predose) serum asparaginase activity (NSAA) levels w/ IV administration and switching to IM administration if desired NSAA levels are not achieved.

ADVERSE REACTIONS
Systemic hypersensitivity, pancreatitis, local reactions, abnormal transaminases, N/V, fever, hyperglycemia.

PREGNANCY AND LACTATION
Category C, not for use in nursing.

MECHANISM OF ACTION
Enzyme; catalyzes the deamidation of asparagine to aspartic acid and ammonia, resulting in a reduction in circulating levels of asparagine. Thought to be based on the inability of leukemic cells to synthesize asparagine, resulting in cytotoxicity specific for leukemic cells that depend on an exogenous source of amino acid asparagine for their protein metabolism and survival.

PATIENT CONSIDERATIONS
Assessment: Assess for history of serious hypersensitivity reactions, pancreatitis, thrombosis, or hemorrhagic events w/ prior L-asparaginase therapy, and pregnancy/nursing status. Obtain baseline serum glucose and coagulation parameters.
Monitoring: Monitor for hypersensitivity reactions, thrombotic or hemorrhagic events, symptoms of pancreatitis, and other adverse reactions. Monitor serum glucose periodically and coagulation parameters. Monitor NSAA levels w/ IV administration.
Counseling: Inform patients of the risk of allergic reactions, pancreatitis, hyperglycemia, glucose intolerance, thrombosis, and hemorrhage, and instruct to seek medical advice immediately if signs/symptoms of these conditions occur. Inform to notify physician if pregnant or nursing.

ERY-TAB — erythromycin   Rx
Class: Macrolide

ADULT DOSAGE	PEDIATRIC DOSAGE
General Dosing	**General Dosing**
Mild to moderate upper/lower respiratory tract and skin and skin structure infections, listeriosis, diphtheria infections, and erythrasma, caused by susceptible strains of microorganisms	30-50mg/kg/day in equally divided doses; may double dose for more severe infections **Max:** 4g/day
250mg qid in equally spaced doses, 333mg q8h, or 500mg q12h; may increase to 4g/day according to severity of infection	**Streptococcal Infections of the Upper Respiratory Tract:** Treat for at least 10 days
When dose is >1g/day, bid dosing is not recommended	**Bacterial Conjunctivitis**
Streptococcal Infections of the Upper Respiratory Tract: Treat for at least 10 days	**Sus:** **Conjunctivitis of the Newborn Caused by *Chlamydia trachomatis*:** 50mg/kg/day in 4 divided doses for at least 2 weeks
Rheumatic Fever	**Pneumonia**
Prevention of Initial Attacks of Rheumatic Fever in Penicillin (PCN)-Allergic Patients: Administer therapeutic dose for 10 days	**Sus:** **Pneumonia of Infancy Caused by *Chlamydia trachomatis*:** 50mg/kg/day in 4 divided doses for at least 3 weeks
Long-Term Prophylaxis of Streptococcal URTIs to Prevent Recurrent Attacks of Rheumatic Fever in Patients Allergic to PCN and Sulfonamides: 250mg bid	**Amebiasis** **Intestinal:** 30-50mg/kg/day in divided doses for 10-14 days
Urogenital Infections	**Pertussis** 40-50mg/kg/day in divided doses for 5-14 days
During Pregnancy Due to *Chlamydia trachomatis*: 500mg qid or two 333mg tab q8h on an empty stomach for at least 7 days; if not tolerated, reduce to 500mg	

q12h, 333mg q8h, or 250mg qid for at least 14 days

Chlamydia trachomatis Infections

Uncomplicated Urethral, Endocervical, or Rectal Infections When Tetracycline is Contraindicated/Not Tolerated:
500mg qid, or two 333mg tabs q8h for at least 7 days

Nongonococcal Urethritis

Caused by *Ureaplasma urealyticum* When Tetracycline is Contraindicated/Not Tolerated:
500mg qid, or two 333mg tabs q8h for at least 7 days

Syphilis

30-40g given in divided doses for 10-15 days

Acute Pelvic Inflammatory Disease

Caused by *Neisseria gonorrhoeae*:
500mg (erythromycin lactobionate) IV q6h for 3 days, followed by 500mg PO q12h or 333mg PO q8h for 7 days

Amebiasis

Intestinal:
500mg q12h, 333mg q8h, or 250mg q6h for 10-14 days

Pertussis

40-50mg/kg/day in divided doses for 5-14 days

Legionnaires' Disease

1-4g/day in divided doses

Prophylaxis of Postoperative Infections

For Elective Colorectal Surgery:
(If proposed surgery time is 8:00 am)
Preop Day 1: Two 500mg tabs, three 333mg tabs, or four 250mg tabs PO at 1:00 pm, 2:00 pm, and 11:00 pm
Refer to PI for additional recommendations

ADMINISTRATION

Oral route

May dose w/o regard to meals; optimal levels are obtained when administered in the fasting state, at least 1/2 hr and preferably 2 hrs ac

STORAGE

<30°C (86°F).

HOW SUPPLIED

Tab, Delayed-Release: 250mg, 333mg, 500mg

CONTRAINDICATIONS

Known hypersensitivity to this antibiotic. Concomitant use of terfenadine, astemizole, cisapride, pimozide, ergotamine, or dihydroergotamine.

WARNINGS/PRECAUTIONS

Hepatic dysfunction, including increased LFTs, and hepatocellular and/or cholestatic hepatitis, with or without jaundice, reported; caution with impaired hepatic function. Associated with QT interval prolongation and arrhythmia (infrequent); cases of torsades de pointes reported. Avoid with known QT interval prolongation and with ongoing proarrhythmic conditions. Cardiovascular malformations reported when used during early pregnancy. Infants born to women treated during pregnancy for early syphilis should be treated with an appropriate PCN regimen. *Clostridium difficile*-associated diarrhea (CDAD) reported; d/c if CDAD is suspected or confirmed. Use in the absence of a proven or strongly suspected bacterial infection or prophylactic indication is unlikely to provide benefit and increases the risk of development of drug-resistant bacteria. Exacerbation of symptoms of myasthenia gravis, new onset of symptoms of myasthenic syndrome, and infantile hypertrophic pyloric stenosis (IHPS) reported. Prolonged and repeated use may result in an overgrowth of nonsusceptible bacteria or fungi; d/c and take appropriate measures if superinfection develops. Lab test interactions may occur. Caution in elderly.

ADVERSE REACTIONS

N/V, abdominal pain, diarrhea, anorexia.

DRUG INTERACTIONS

See Contraindications. Avoid with Class IA (quinidine, procainamide) or Class III (dofetilide, amiodarone, sotalol) antiarrhythmic agents. Serious adverse reactions reported with CYP3A4 substrates such as hypotension with calcium channel blockers (eg, verapamil, amlodipine, diltiazem). Monitor for colchicine toxicity with coadministration; starting dose of colchicine may need to be reduced, and max colchicine dose should be lowered. May increase theophylline levels and potential toxicity with high doses of theophylline; reduce theophylline dose in these cases. Decreased levels with theophylline. Hypotension, bradyarrhythmias, and lactic acidosis observed with verapamil. May elevate digoxin levels. May elevate

concentrations that could increase or prolong both therapeutic and adverse effects of drugs primarily metabolized by CYP3A; closely monitor concentrations and consider dose adjustment. May increase the pharmacological effect of triazolam and midazolam. Increased systemic exposure of sildenafil; consider dose reduction of sildenafil. Increased anticoagulant effects of oral anticoagulants; may be more pronounced in elderly. Increased levels of HMG-CoA reductase inhibitors (eg, lovastatin, simvastatin); rhabdomyolysis (rare) reported. Carefully monitor for creatine kinase and serum transaminase levels with lovastatin. Interactions with drugs metabolized by CYP3A (eg, cyclosporine, carbamazepine, tacrolimus, alfentanil, disopyramide, rifabutin, quinidine, methylprednisolone, cilostazol, vinblastine, bromocriptine), hexobarbital, phenytoin, and valproate reported.

PREGNANCY AND LACTATION

Category B, caution in nursing.

MECHANISM OF ACTION

Macrolide; inhibits protein synthesis by binding 50S ribosomal subunits of susceptible organisms.

PHARMACOKINETICS

Absorption: Readily absorbed. **Distribution:** Largely bound to plasma proteins; crosses placenta, found in breast milk. **Elimination:** Bile, urine (<5%, active form).

PATIENT CONSIDERATIONS

Assessment: Assess for hypersensitivity to drug, hepatic impairment, QT interval prolongation, ongoing proarrhythmic conditions, myasthenia gravis, pregnancy/nursing status, and possible drug interactions. Perform culture and susceptibility tests to confirm diagnosis of causative organism. Perform serologic test for syphilis (if treating gonorrhea) and spinal fluid exam (primary syphilis).

Monitoring: Monitor for hepatic dysfunction, CDAD, QT interval prolongation, arrhythmia, exacerbation of myasthenia gravis symptoms, new onset of symptoms of myasthenic syndrome, IHPS, superinfection, and other adverse reactions. Perform follow-up serologic test for syphilis (after 3 months) and spinal fluid exam (primary syphilis).

Counseling: Inform that therapy should only be used to treat bacterial, not viral, infections. Instruct to take exactly ud. Inform that skipping doses or not completing full course may decrease effectiveness and increase bacterial resistance. Inform that diarrhea is a common problem caused by therapy and will usually end upon discontinuation of therapy. Instruct to immediately contact physician if watery and bloody stools (with or without stomach cramps and fever) occur, even as late as ≥2 months after discontinuation of therapy. Inform caregivers of infant patients to contact physician if vomiting or irritability with feeding occurs.

ESBRIET — pirfenidone   Rx

Class: Pyridone

ADULT DOSAGE	PEDIATRIC DOSAGE
Idiopathic Pulmonary Fibrosis	Pediatric use may not have been established
Days 1-7: 1 cap tid	
Days 8-14: 2 caps tid	
Day 15 Onward: 3 caps tid	
Maint/Max: 2403mg/day (9 caps/day)	

DOSING CONSIDERATIONS

Concomitant Medications
Strong CYP1A2 Inhibitors (eg, Fluvoxamine, Enoxacin):
Reduce to 1 cap tid

Moderate CYP1A2 Inhibitors (eg, Ciprofloxacin 750mg bid):
Reduce to 2 caps tid

Adverse Reactions
Significant (eg, GI, Photosensitivity, Rash):
Consider temporary dosage reductions or interruptions to allow for resolution of symptoms

Elevated Liver Enzymes:
ALT and/or AST >3 but ≤5X ULN w/o Symptoms or Hyperbilirubinemia:
1. D/C confounding medications, exclude other causes, and monitor patient closely
2. Repeat LFTs as clinically indicated
3. Full daily dosage may be maintained, if clinically appropriate, or reduced or interrupted (eg, until LFTs are w/in normal limits) w/ subsequent retitration to full dosage as tolerated

ALT and/or AST >3 but ≤5X ULN w/ Symptoms or Hyperbilirubinemia:
D/C permanently and do not rechallenge

ALT and/or AST >5X ULN:
D/C permanently and do not rechallenge

Other Important Considerations
Treatment Interruption ≥14 Days:
Reinitiate by undergoing the initial 2-week titration regimen up to full maint dose

Treatment Interruption <14 Days:
Resume w/ dosage prior to the interruption

ADMINISTRATION

Oral route

Take at the same time each day w/ food.

STORAGE

25°C (77°F); excursions permitted to 15-30°C (59-86°F).

HOW SUPPLIED
Cap: 267mg

WARNINGS/PRECAUTIONS
Increases in ALT and AST >3X ULN reported; rarely associated w/ concomitant bilirubin elevations. Photosensitivity reactions reported. GI events (eg, N/V, diarrhea, dyspepsia, GERD, abdominal pain) reported. Caution w/ mild (Child-Pugh Class A) to moderate (Child-Pugh Class B) hepatic impairment, or mild (CrCl 50-80mL/min)/moderate (CrCl 30-50mL/min)/severe (CrCl <30mL/min) renal impairment. Not recommended w/ severe (Child-Pugh Class C) hepatic impairment or ESRD requiring dialysis.

ADVERSE REACTIONS
N/V, rash, abdominal pain, URTI, diarrhea, fatigue, headache, dyspepsia, dizziness, anorexia, GERD, sinusitis, insomnia, weight decreased, arthralgia.

DRUG INTERACTIONS
See Dosing Considerations. Fluvoxamine or other strong CYP1A2 inhibitors (eg, enoxacin) significantly increase exposure; d/c use of such agents prior to treatment, and avoid during treatment. If such agents are the only drug of choice, dosage reductions are recommended; monitor for adverse reactions and consider discontinuation of pirfenidone prn. Ciprofloxacin (moderate CYP1A2 inhibitor) moderately increases exposure; if ciprofloxacin at the dosage of 750mg bid cannot be avoided, dosage reductions are recommended. Monitor closely when ciprofloxacin is used at a dosage of 250mg or 500mg qd. Agents or combinations of agents that are moderate or strong inhibitors of both CYP1A2 and ≥1 other CYP isoenzymes involved in the metabolism of pirfenidone (CYP2C9, 2C19, 2D6, 2E1) should be discontinued prior to and avoided during treatment. CYP1A2 inducers may decrease exposure, which may lead to loss of efficacy; d/c use of strong CYP1A2 inducers prior to treatment and avoid concomitant use. Avoid concomitant medications known to cause photosensitivity. Smoking causes decreased exposure, which may alter the efficacy profile; stop smoking prior to treatment and avoid smoking during treatment.

PREGNANCY AND LACTATION
Pregnancy: Category C
Lactation: Not for use in nursing.

MECHANISM OF ACTION
Pyridone; has not been established.

PHARMACOKINETICS
Absorption: C_{max} (median, 801mg single dose)=0.5 hrs. T_{max} (median)=0.5 hrs, 3 hrs (w/ food). **Distribution:** Plasma protein binding (58%); V_d=59-71L. **Metabolism:** Primarily in liver via CYP1A2, CYP2C9, 2C19, 2D6, and 2E1; 5-carboxy-pirfenidone (metabolite). **Elimination:** Urine (80% [approx 99.6% as metabolite]); $T_{1/2}$=3 hrs.

PATIENT CONSIDERATIONS
Assessment: Assess for renal/hepatic impairment, smoking, pregnancy/nursing status, and possible drug interactions. Conduct LFTs.

Monitoring: Monitor for photosensitivity reaction, rash, GI events, and other adverse reactions. Conduct LFTs monthly for the first 6 months and every 3 months thereafter.

Counseling: Inform that periodic monitoring of LFTs may be required. Instruct to immediately report any symptoms of a liver problem, photosensitivity reaction, rash, or persistent GI effects to physician. Advise to avoid or minimize exposure to sunlight (eg, sunlamps) during therapy; instruct to use a sunblock (SPF ≥50) and to wear clothing that protects against sun exposure. Encourage to stop smoking prior to treatment and to avoid smoking while on therapy.

ESTERIFIED ESTROGENS AND METHYLTESTOSTERONE
esterified estrogens/methyltestosterone   **CIII**

Class: Androgen/estrogen

> Estrogens increase the risk of endometrial cancer. Perform adequate diagnostic measures, including endometrial sampling when indicated, to rule out malignancy in all cases of undiagnosed persistent or recurring abnormal vaginal bleeding. Estrogens with or without progestins should not be used for the prevention of cardiovascular disease (CVD). Increased risk of MI, stroke, invasive breast cancer, pulmonary embolism (PE), and deep vein thrombosis (DVT) reported in postmenopausal women (50-79 yrs of age) treated with oral conjugated estrogens combined with medroxyprogesterone acetate. Increased risk of developing probable dementia reported in postmenopausal women ≥65 yrs of age treated with oral conjugated estrogens combined with medroxyprogesterone acetate. Estrogens with or without progestins should be prescribed at the lowest effective dose and for the shortest duration consistent with treatment goals and risks.

ADULT DOSAGE	PEDIATRIC DOSAGE
Menopausal Vasomotor Symptoms	Pediatric use may not have been established
Moderate to Severe Symptoms Not Improved by Estrogens Alone:	
Usual: 1 tab or 1-2 half-strength tabs qd given cyclically (eg, 3 weeks on and 1 week off)	
Short-term use only; attempt to d/c or taper medication at 3- to 6-month intervals	

DOSING CONSIDERATIONS
Elderly
Start at lower end of dosing range

ADMINISTRATION
Oral route

STORAGE
20-25°C (68-77°F); excursions permitted to 15-30°C (59-86°F).

HOW SUPPLIED
Tab: (Esterified Estrogens/Methyltestosterone) 0.625mg/1.25mg (Half Strength), 1.25mg/2.5mg

CONTRAINDICATIONS
Undiagnosed abnormal genital bleeding, known/suspected/history of breast cancer, known/suspected estrogen-dependent neoplasia, active/history of DVT/PE, active/recent (eg, within the past year) arterial thromboembolic disease (eg, stroke, MI), liver dysfunction or disease, known hypersensitivity to the ingredients, known or suspected pregnancy. **Methyltestosterone:** Severe liver damage, breastfeeding mothers.

WARNINGS/PRECAUTIONS
Esterified Estrogens: D/C immediately if an MI, stroke, DVT, or PE occurs or is suspected. If feasible, d/c at least 4-6 weeks before surgery associated with an increased risk of thromboembolism, or during periods of prolonged immobilization. May increase risk of ovarian cancer. Consider addition of a progestin in women with a uterus or in patients with residual endometriosis post-hysterectomy. May increase risk of gallbladder disease requiring surgery. Worsening of glucose tolerance reported; carefully observe diabetic patients during therapy. May lead to severe hypercalcemia in patients with breast cancer and bone metastases; d/c and take appropriate measures if hypercalcemia occurs. Retinal vascular thrombosis reported; d/c therapy pending examination if sudden partial/complete loss of vision, or sudden onset of proptosis, diplopia, or migraine occurs. If examination reveals papilledema or retinal vascular lesions, d/c therapy permanently. May increase BP, thyroid-binding globulin levels, and plasma TG, leading to pancreatitis or other complications. Caution with history of cholestatic jaundice associated with past estrogen use or with pregnancy; d/c in the case of recurrence. May cause fluid retention. Caution with severe hypocalcemia. May exacerbate endometriosis, asthma, DM, epilepsy, migraine or porphyria, systemic lupus erythematosus, and hepatic hemangiomas; use with caution. May affect certain endocrine and blood components in lab tests. **Methyltestosterone:** May cause hypercalcemia in patients with breast cancer; d/c if this occurs. Peliosis hepatis and hepatic neoplasms, including hepatocellular carcinoma, reported with prolonged use of high doses. D/C if cholestatic hepatitis with jaundice appears or if abnormal LFTs occur. Edema with or without heart failure may be a serious complication in patients with preexisting cardiac, renal, or hepatic disease; may require diuretic therapy in addition to discontinuation of therapy. Monitor for signs of virilization; d/c at the time of evidence of mild virilism. Prolonged use may result in sodium and fluid retention; caution with compromised cardiac reserve or renal disease. May decrease protein-bound iodine.

ADVERSE REACTIONS
Amenorrhea, menstrual irregularities, voice deepening, clitoral enlargement, thromboembolism, N/V, chloasma, headache, urticaria, hirsutism, cholestatic jaundice, depression, anxiety, breast tenderness, pruritus.

DRUG INTERACTIONS
Esterified Estrogens: CYP3A4 inducers (eg, St. John's wort preparations, phenobarbital, carbamazepine) may decrease therapeutic effects and/or result in changes in uterine bleeding profile. CYP3A4 inhibitors (eg, erythromycin, ketoconazole, ritonavir) may result in side effects. Patients concomitantly receiving thyroid hormone replacement therapy and estrogens may require increased doses of their thyroid replacement therapy. **Methyltestosterone:** May decrease oral anticoagulant requirement; close monitoring is required, especially when androgens are started or stopped. May increase oxyphenbutazone levels. May decrease blood glucose and insulin requirements in diabetics.

PREGNANCY AND LACTATION
Category X, not for use in nursing.

MECHANISM OF ACTION
Esterified Estrogens: Estrogen; binds to nuclear receptors in estrogen-responsive tissues. Circulating estrogen modulates pituitary secretion of gonadotropins, luteinizing hormone, and follicle-stimulating hormone, through a negative feedback mechanism. Reduces elevated levels of these hormones in postmenopausal women. **Methyltestosterone:** Androgen; responsible for the normal growth and development of the male sex organs and for maintenance of secondary sex characteristics.

PHARMACOKINETICS
Distribution: Esterified Estrogens: Largely bound to sex hormone-binding globulin and albumin; found in breast milk. Methyltestosterone: Plasma protein binding (98% bound to a specific testosterone-estradiol binding globulin). **Metabolism:** Esterified Estrogens: Liver to estrone (metabolite) and estriol (major urinary metabolite); enterohepatic recirculation via sulfate/glucuronide conjugation (liver) and hydrolysis in the gut; CYP3A4 (partial metabolism). Methyltestosterone: Liver. **Elimination:** Esterified Estrogens: Urine (estradiol, estrone, and estriol). Methyltestosterone: Urine (90% [glucuronic and sulfuric acid conjugates]); feces (6% [unconjugated]); $T_{1/2}$=10-100 min.

PATIENT CONSIDERATIONS
Assessment: Assess for undiagnosed abnormal genital bleeding, presence or history of breast cancer, estrogen-dependent neoplasia, active/history deep vein thrombosis, active or recent (within past yr) arterial thromboembolic disease, liver dysfunction, pregnancy/nursing status, any other conditions where treatment is contraindicated or cautioned, need for progestin therapy, and for possible drug interactions.

Monitoring: Monitor for signs/symptoms of hypercalcemia and fluid retention, CVD, malignant neoplasms, gallbladder disease, visual abnormalities, cholestatic jaundice, hypertriglyceridemia, exacerbation of endometriosis, virilization, and for other adverse reactions. In cases of undiagnosed persistent or recurrent vaginal bleeding in women with a uterus, perform adequate diagnostic measures to rule out malignancies. Perform annual breast exam; schedule mammography based on age, risk factors, and prior mammogram results. Periodically monitor BP, thyroid function if on thyroid hormone replacement therapy, and reassess need for therapy every 3-6 months. Monitor LFTs periodically. Frequently monitor urine and serum Ca²⁺ in women with disseminated breast carcinoma. Periodically check Hgb and Hct for polycythemia in patients receiving high doses of androgens.

Counseling: Inform of the risks/benefits of therapy. Inform of the possible adverse reactions of therapy and instruct to contact physician if any adverse reactions occur.

ESTRACE — estradiol   Rx

Class: Estrogen

> Estrogens increase the risk of endometrial cancer. Perform adequate diagnostic measures, including endometrial sampling, to rule out malignancy w/ undiagosed persistent or recurrent abnormal vaginal bleeding. Should not be used for the prevention of cardiovascular disease. Increased risk of MI, stroke, invasive breast cancer, pulmonary embolism (PE), and deep vein thrombosis (DVT) in postmenopausal women (50-79 yrs of age) reported. Increased risk of developing probable dementia in postmenopausal women ≥65 yrs of age reported. Should be prescribed at the lowest effective dose and for the shortest duration consistent w/ treatment goals and risks.

ADULT DOSAGE

Menopausal Vasomotor Symptoms

Moderate to Severe:
Tab:
Initial: 1-2mg/day
Maint: Minimal effective dose should be determined by titration; administer cyclically (eg, 3 weeks on and 1 week off)

Use the lowest effective dose for the shortest duration; reevaluate at 3- to 6-month intervals

Menopausal Vulvar/Vaginal Atrophy

Cre:
Usual: 2-4g/day for 1-2 weeks; then gradually reduce to 1/2 initial dose for a similar period
Maint: 1g 1-3X/week after restoration of the vaginal mucosa

Tab:
Moderate to Severe:
Initial: 1-2mg/day
Maint: Minimal effective dose should be determined by titration; administer cyclically (eg, 3 weeks on and 1 week off)

Use the lowest effective dose for the shortest duration; reevaluate at 3- to 6-month intervals

Hypoestrogenism

Due to Hypogonadism, Castration, or Primary Ovarian Failure:
Tab:
Initial: 1-2mg/day
Titrate: Adjust as necessary to control presenting symptoms
Maint: Minimal effective dose should be determined by titration

Breast Cancer

Palliative Treatment in Appropriately Selected Women and Men w/ Metastatic Disease:
Tab:
10mg tid for at least 3 months

Prostate Carcinoma

Palliative Treatment of Advanced Androgen-Dependent Carcinoma:
Tab:
1-2mg tid

Osteoporosis

Prevention:
Tab:
Consider therapy for women at risk of osteoporosis and for whom non-estrogen medications are not appropriate, when used solely for prevention of postmenopausal osteoporosis

PEDIATRIC DOSAGE

Pediatric use may not have been established

ADMINISTRATION

Cre
Intravaginal route
Tab
Oral route

STORAGE

Cre: Room temperature. Protect from temperatures in excess of 40°C (104°F).
Tab: 20-25°C (68-77°F).

HOW SUPPLIED

Cre: 0.01% [42.5g]; **Tab:** 0.5mg*, 1mg*, 2mg* *scored

CONTRAINDICATIONS

Undiagnosed abnormal genital bleeding, known/suspected/history of breast cancer, known/suspected estrogen-dependent neoplasia, active/history of DVT/PE, active or recent (eg, w/in the past year) arterial thromboembolic disease (eg, stroke, MI), liver dysfunction or disease, known hypersensitivity to the ingredients, known/suspected pregnancy.

WARNINGS/PRECAUTIONS

D/C immediately if stroke, DVT, PE, or MI occurs or is suspected. Caution in patients w/ risk factors for arterial vascular disease and/or venous thromboembolism. If feasible, d/c at least 4-6 weeks before surgery of the type associated w/ an increased risk of thromboembolism, or during periods of prolonged immobilization. May increase the risk of gallbladder disease and ovarian cancer. May lead to severe hypercalcemia in patients w/ breast cancer and bone metastases; d/c and take appropriate measures if hypercalcemia occurs. Retinal vascular thrombosis reported; d/c therapy pending exam if there is a sudden partial/complete loss of vision or a sudden onset of proptosis, diplopia, or migraine. D/C permanently if exam reveals papilledema or retinal vascular lesions. Consider addition of progestin for women w/ a uterus or w/ residual endometriosis post-hysterectomy. May elevate BP and thyroid-binding globulin levels. May elevate plasma TGs leading to pancreatitis in patients w/ preexisting hypertriglyceridemia. Caution w/ impaired liver function, and w/ history of cholestatic jaundice associated w/ past estrogen use or w/ pregnancy; d/c in case of recurrence. May cause fluid retention; caution w/ cardiac/renal impairment. Caution w/ severe hypocalcemia. May exacerbate endometriosis, asthma, diabetes mellitus, epilepsy, migraine, porphyria, systemic lupus erythematosus, and hepatic hemangiomas; use w/ caution. May affect certain endocrine and blood components in lab tests. **Tab:** 2mg tab contains tartrazine, which may cause allergic-type reactions (eg, bronchial asthma) in certain susceptible individuals.

ADVERSE REACTIONS

Vaginal bleeding pattern changes, vaginitis, breast tenderness, breast enlargement, galactorrhea, N/V, thrombophlebitis, melasma, abdominal cramps, headache, mental depression, mood disturbances, weight changes, edema, libido changes.

DRUG INTERACTIONS

CYP3A4 inducers (eg, St. John's wort preparations, phenobarbital, carbamazepine, rifampin) may decrease levels, which may decrease therapeutic effects and/or change uterine bleeding profile. CYP3A4 inhibitors (eg, erythromycin, ketoconazole, ritonavir, grapefruit juice) may increase levels, which may result in side effects. Patients concomitantly receiving thyroid replacement therapy and estrogens may require increased doses of thyroid replacement therapy; monitor thyroid function.

PREGNANCY AND LACTATION

Pregnancy: Contraindicated in pregnancy.
Lactation: Estrogen has been shown to decrease the quantity and quality of milk. Detectable amounts of estrogen have been identified in the milk of mothers receiving this drug. Caution in nursing.

MECHANISM OF ACTION

Estrogen; binds to nuclear receptors in estrogen-responsive tissues. Circulating estrogens modulate pituitary secretion of the gonadotropins, luteinizing hormone and follicle-stimulating hormone, through a (-) feedback mechanism. Reduces elevated levels of these hormones in postmenopausal women.

PHARMACOKINETICS

Absorption: (Cre) Absorbed through skin, mucous membranes, and GI tract.
Distribution: Largely bound to sex hormone-binding globulin and albumin; found in breast milk. **Metabolism:** Liver to estrone (metabolite); estriol (major urinary metabolite); sulfate and glucuronide conjugation (liver); biliary secretion of conjugates into the intestine; hydrolysis (gut); reabsorption; CYP3A4 (partial metabolism). **Elimination:** Urine (parent compound and metabolites).

PATIENT CONSIDERATIONS

Assessment: Assess for undiagnosed abnormal genital bleeding, presence/history of breast cancer, estrogen-dependent neoplasia, active/history of DVT/PE/arterial thromboembolic disease, liver impairment/disease, history of cholestatic jaundice, drug hypersensitivity, pregnancy/nursing status, any other conditions where treatment is contraindicated or cautioned, need for progestin therapy, and possible drug interactions.

Monitoring: Monitor for signs/symptoms of CV events, malignant neoplasms, dementia, gallbladder disease, hypercalcemia, visual abnormalities, BP and serum TG elevations, pancreatitis, fluid retention, cholestatic jaundice, exacerbation of endometriosis and other conditions, and other adverse reactions. Perform annual breast exam; schedule mammography based on age, risk factors, and prior mammogram results. Monitor thyroid function in patients on thyroid hormone replacement therapy. Periodically evaluate (every 3-6 months) to determine need for therapy. In cases of undiagnosed, persistent, or recurrent abnormal vaginal bleeding, perform adequate diagnostic measures (eg, endometrial sampling) to rule out malignancy.

Counseling: Inform of the risks/benefits of therapy. Inform that medication increases risk for breast/uterine cancer. Advise to contact physician if breast lumps, unusual vaginal bleeding, dizziness or faintness, changes in speech, severe headaches, chest pain, SOB, leg pain, visual changes, or vomiting occurs. Advise to have yearly breast exams by a physician and to perform monthly breast self-exams. Advise to notify physician if pregnant/nursing.

ESTRADERM — estradiol   Rx

Class: Estrogen

> Estrogens increase the risk of endometrial cancer. Perform adequate diagnostic measures, including endometrial sampling, to rule out malignancy w/ undiagnosed persistent or recurrent abnormal vaginal bleeding. Should not be used for the prevention of cardiovascular disease (CVD) or dementia. Increased risk of MI, stroke, invasive breast cancer, pulmonary emboli (PE), and deep vein thrombosis (DVT) in postmenopausal women (50-79 yrs of age) reported. Increased risk of developing probable dementia in postmenopausal women ≥65 yrs of age reported. Should be prescribed at the lowest effective dose and for the shortest duration consistent w/ treatment goals and risks.

ADULT DOSAGE

Postmenopausal Osteoporosis

Prevention:

Initial: 0.05mg/day as soon as possible after menopause

Reevaluate treatment need periodically (eg, 3- to 6-month intervals)

Hypoestrogenism

Due to Hypogonadism/Castration/Primary Ovarian Failure:

0.05mg ud

Reevaluate treatment need periodically (eg, 3- to 6-month intervals)

Menopausal Vasomotor Symptoms

Moderate to Severe:

Initial: 0.05mg applied twice weekly

Used lowest effective dose for the shortest duration; reevaluate at 3- to 6-month intervals

Menopausal Vulvar/Vaginal Atrophy

Moderate to Severe:

Initial: 0.05mg applied twice weekly

Used lowest effective dose for the shortest duration; reevaluate at 3- to 6-month intervals

PEDIATRIC DOSAGE

Pediatric use may not have been established

DOSING CONSIDERATIONS

Concomitant Medications

Women Currently on Oral Estrogens: Initiate 1 week after withdrawal of oral hormonal therapy, or sooner if menopausal symptoms reappear in <1 week

Other Important Considerations

Patients w/o Intact Uterus: Administer therapy continuously

Patients w/ Intact Uterus: Administer on a cyclic schedule (eg, 3 weeks on, followed by 1 week off)

ADMINISTRATION

Transdermal route

Place adhesive side on a clean, dry area of skin on trunk of body (including buttocks and abdomen); area selected should not be oily, damaged, or irritated

Site selected should be one that is not exposed to sunlight

Do not apply to breasts and/or waistline

Replace system twice weekly; rotate application sites w/ an interval of at least 1 week allowed between applications to a particular site

Apply immediately after opening pouch and removing the protective liner

Press system firmly in place w/ palm of the hand for about 10 sec

If the system falls off, reapply the same one. If necessary, a new system may be applied; in either case, continue original treatment schedule

STORAGE

Do not store above 30°C (86°F). Do not store unpouched.

HOW SUPPLIED

Patch: 0.05mg/day, 0.1mg/day [8ˢ]

CONTRAINDICATIONS

Undiagnosed abnormal genital bleeding, known/suspected/history of breast cancer, known/suspected estrogen-dependent neoplasia, active or history of DVT/PE, active or recent arterial thromboembolic disease (eg, stroke, MI), liver dysfunction or disease, known/suspected pregnancy, known hypersensitivity to any of the ingredients in this medication.

WARNINGS/PRECAUTIONS

D/C immediately if stroke, DVT, PE, or MI occurs or is suspected. Caution in patients w/ risk factors for arterial vascular disease and/or venous thromboembolism (VTE). If feasible, d/c at least 4-6 weeks before surgery of the type associated w/ an increased risk of thromboembolism, or during periods of prolonged immobilization. May increase risk of breast/ovarian/endometrial cancer and gallbladder disease. Consider addition of progestin for women w/ a uterus or w/ residual endometriosis posthysterectomy. May lead to severe hypercalcemia in patients w/ breast cancer and bone metastases; d/c and take appropriate measures if hypercalcemia occurs. Retinal vascular thrombosis reported; if sudden partial or complete loss of vision, sudden onset of proptosis, diplopia, or migraine occurs, d/c therapy pending examination. If examinations reveal papilledema or retinal vascular lesions, d/c permanently. May elevate BP, thyroid-binding globulin levels, and plasma TG levels leading to pancreatitis and other complications. Caution w/ history of cholestatic jaundice; d/c in case of recurrence. May cause fluid retention; caution w/ cardiac/renal dysfunction. Caution w/ impaired liver function and severe hypocalcemia. May exacerbate endometriosis, asthma, diabetes mellitus (DM), epilepsy, migraine, porphyria, systemic lupus erythematosus (SLE), and hepatic hemangiomas; use w/ caution. May affect certain endocrine and blood components in lab tests.

ADVERSE REACTIONS

Altered vaginal bleeding, vaginal candidiasis, breast tenderness/enlargement, N/V, chloasma, melasma, weight changes, VTE, pulmonary embolism, MI, stroke, application-site redness/irritation.

DRUG INTERACTIONS

CYP3A4 inducers (eg, St. John's wort, phenobarbital, carbamazepine, rifampin) may decrease levels, which may decrease therapeutic effects and/or change uterine bleeding profile. CYP3A4 inhibitors (eg, erythromycin, ketoconazole, ritonavir, grapefruit juice) may increase levels, which may result in side effects. Patients concomitantly receiving thyroid hormone replacement therapy and estrogens may require increased doses of their thyroid replacement therapy.

PREGNANCY AND LACTATION

Contraindicated in pregnancy, caution in nursing.

MECHANISM OF ACTION

Estrogen; binds to nuclear receptors in estrogen-responsive tissues. Circulating estrogen modulates pituitary secretion of gonadotropins, luteinizing hormone and follicle-stimulating hormone, through (-) feedback mechanism. Reduces elevated levels of these hormones in postmenopausal women.

PHARMACOKINETICS

Distribution: Largely bound to sex hormone-binding globulin and albumin; found in breast milk. **Metabolism:** Liver to estrone (metabolite); estriol (major urinary metabolite); sulfate and glucuronide conjugation (liver), gut hydrolysis; CYP3A4 (partial metabolism). **Elimination:** Urine (parent compound and metabolites); $T_{1/2}$=1 hr.

PATIENT CONSIDERATIONS

Assessment: Assess for undiagnosed abnormal genital bleeding, presence/history of breast cancer, estrogen-dependent neoplasia, active or history of DVT/PE, active or recent (w/in past yr) arterial thromboembolic disease, liver dysfunction/disease, known/suspected pregnancy, any other conditions where treatment is contraindicated or cautioned, need for progestin therapy, and possible drug interactions. Assess use in women ≥65 yrs, nursing patients, and those w/ hypertriglyceridemia, hypothyroidism, DM, asthma, epilepsy, migraine or porphyria, SLE, and hepatic hemangiomas.

Monitoring: Monitor for signs/symptoms of CVD, malignant neoplasms, dementia, gallbladder disease, hypercalcemia, visual abnormalities, hypertriglyceridemia, pancreatitis, hypothyroidism, fluid retention, cholestatic jaundice, exacerbation of endometriosis and other conditions. Perform annual breast exam; schedule mammography based on age, risk factors, and prior mammogram results. Regularly monitor BP, thyroid function in patients on thyroid replacement therapy, and periodically evaluate (every 3-6 months) to determine need for therapy. In case of undiagnosed, persistent, or recurrent vaginal bleeding in women w/ uterus, perform adequate diagnostic testing measures (eg, endometrial sampling) to rule out malignancy.

Counseling: Inform that therapy may increase the risk for uterine cancer and may increase chances of getting a heart attack, stroke, breast cancer, blood clots, and dementia. Instruct to report to physician any breast lumps, unusual vaginal bleeding, dizziness and faintness, changes in speech, severe headaches, chest pain, SOB, leg pains, changes in vision, or vomiting. Advise to notify physician if pregnant or nursing. Instruct to have annual breast examination by a physician and perform monthly breast self-examination. Instruct to place medication system on clean, dry skin on the trunk (including buttocks and abdomen); site should not be exposed to sunlight; area should not be oily, damaged, or irritated; and should not be applied on breasts or waistline. Counsel to rotate application sites w/ an interval of 1 week, and to apply immediately after opening pouch. Inform that if medication system falls off, reapply same system or apply new system prn and continue w/ original treatment schedule.

ESTRING — estradiol   Rx

Class: Estrogen

> Increased risk of endometrial cancer in a woman w/ a uterus who uses unopposed estrogens. Adding a progestin to estrogen therapy reduces the risk of endometrial hyperplasia. Adequate diagnostic measures (eg, directed or random endometrial sampling) should be undertaken to rule out malignancy in all cases of undiagnosed, persistent or recurring abnormal genital bleeding. Should not be used for the prevention of cardiovascular (CV) disease or dementia. Increased risk of stroke and deep vein thrombosis (DVT) reported in postmenopausal women (50-79 yrs of age) treated w/ daily oral conjugated estrogens (CE) alone and when combined w/ medroxyprogesterone acetate (MPA). Increased risk of developing probable dementia reported in postmenopausal women ≥65 yrs of age treated w/ daily CE alone and when combined w/ MPA. Increased risks of pulmonary embolism (PE), MI, and invasive breast cancer reported in postmenopausal women (50-79 yrs of age) treated w/ daily oral CE combined w/ MPA. Should be prescribed at the lowest effective dose and for the shortest duration consistent w/ treatment goals and risks.

ADULT DOSAGE

Menopausal Vulvar/Vaginal Atrophy

Moderate to Severe Symptoms:
Insert 1 ring as deeply as possible into the upper 1/3 of the vaginal vault; the ring is to remain in place continuously for 3 months, after which it is to be removed and, if appropriate, replaced by a new ring

Reassess need to continue treatment at 3- or 6-month intervals

PEDIATRIC DOSAGE
Pediatric use may not have been established

ADMINISTRATION
Intravaginal route

Retention of the ring for >90 days does not represent overdosage, but will result in progressively greater underdosage w/ the risk of loss of efficacy and increasing risk of vaginal infections and/or erosions.

Insertion
1. Press ring into an oval and insert into upper 3rd of the vaginal vault; exact position is not critical.
2. If patient feels discomfort, the ring is probably not far enough inside; gently push ring further into the vagina.

Use
The patient should not feel Estring when it is in place and it should not interfere w/ sexual intercourse. Straining at defecation may make Estring move down in the lower part of the vagina; if so, it may be pushed up again w/ a finger. Should the ring be removed or fall out at any time during the 90-day treatment period, it should be rinsed in lukewarm water and re-inserted by the patient (or by a physician/nurse if necessary).

Removal
Remove by hooking a finger through the ring and pulling it out.

STORAGE
15-25°C (59-77°F).

HOW SUPPLIED
Vaginal Ring: 2mg

CONTRAINDICATIONS
Undiagnosed abnormal genital bleeding, known/suspected/history of breast cancer, known/suspected estrogen-dependent neoplasia, active/history of DVT/PE/arterial thromboembolic disease (eg, stroke, MI), known anaphylactic reaction or angioedema or hypersensitivity to the medication, known liver impairment/disease, known protein C/protein S/antithrombin deficiency or other known thrombophilic disorders, known/suspected pregnancy.

WARNINGS/PRECAUTIONS
D/C immediately if stroke, DVT, PE, or MI occurs or is suspected. If feasible, d/c at least 4-6 weeks before surgery of the type associated w/ an increased risk of thromboembolism, or during periods of prolonged immobilization. May increase risk of gallbladder disease requiring surgery and risk of ovarian cancer. May lead to severe hypercalcemia in patients w/ breast cancer and bone metastases; d/c and take appropriate measures if hypercalcemia occurs. Retinal vascular thrombosis reported; d/c therapy pending examination if sudden partial/complete loss of vision, or sudden onset of proptosis, diplopia, or migraine occurs. D/C if exam reveals papilledema or retinal vascular lesions. May exacerbate symptoms of angioedema in women w/ hereditary angioedema. May increase BP and thyroid-binding globulin levels. May be associated w/ elevations of plasma TGs, leading to pancreatitis in patients w/ preexisting hypertriglyceridemia; consider discontinuation if pancreatitis occurs. Caution w/ history of cholestatic jaundice associated w/ past estrogen use or w/ pregnancy; d/c in case of recurrence. Caution w/ hypoparathyroidism; hypocalcemia may occur. May cause fluid retention. Cases of malignant transformation of residual endometrial implants reported in women treated posthysterectomy w/ estrogen-alone therapy; consider addition of progestin for these patients. May exacerbate asthma, diabetes mellitus, epilepsy, migraine, porphyria, systemic lupus erythematosus, and hepatic hemangiomas; use w/ caution. Moving or gliding of Estring w/in vagina may occur; instances of Estring being expelled from vagina in connection w/ moving the bowels, strain, or constipation reported. A narrow vagina, vaginal stenosis, prolapse, or a vaginal infection may make the vagina more susceptible to irritation/ulceration. If a vaginal infection develops, remove and reinsert only after the infection is appropriately treated. May affect certain endocrine and blood components in lab tests.

ADVERSE REACTIONS
Headache, leukorrhea, back pain, genital moniliasis, sinusitis, vaginitis, vaginal discomfort/pain, vaginal hemorrhage, arthritis, insomnia, abdominal pain, upper respiratory tract infection, asymptomatic genital bacterial growth, arthralgia.

DRUG INTERACTIONS
CYP3A4 inducers (eg, St. John's wort preparations, phenobarbital, carbamazepine) may decrease levels, possibly resulting in a decrease in systemic effects and/or changes in the uterine bleeding profile. CYP3A4 inhibitors (eg, erythromycin, ketoconazole, grapefruit juice) may increase levels, and may result in side effects. Patients concomitantly receiving thyroid hormone replacement therapy and estrogens may require increased doses of thyroid replacement therapy; monitor thyroid function.

PREGNANCY AND LACTATION
Pregnancy: Contraindicated in pregnancy.
Lactation: Not for use in nursing. Estrogen administration to nursing women has been shown to decrease the quantity and quality of breast milk. Found in breast milk.

MECHANISM OF ACTION
Estrogen; binds to nuclear receptors in estrogen-responsive tissues. Circulating estrogens modulate the pituitary secretion of the gonadotropins, luteinizing hormone and follicle-stimulating hormone, through a (-) feedback mechanism. Reduces elevated levels of these hormones in postmenopausal women.

PHARMACOKINETICS
Absorption: Well absorbed. C_{max}=63.2pg/mL, 66.3pg/mL (estrone); T_{max}=0.5-1 hr.
Distribution: Largely bound to sex hormone-binding globulin and albumin; found in breast milk. **Metabolism:** Liver to estrone (metabolite) and estriol (major urinary metabolite); enterohepatic recirculation via sulfate and glucuronide conjugation in the liver, biliary secretion of conjugates into the intestine; hydrolysis in the intestine; reabsorption; CYP3A4 (partial metabolism; systemic estrogens).
Elimination: Urine (parent compound and metabolites).

PATIENT CONSIDERATIONS
Assessment: Assess for abnormal genital bleeding, presence/history of breast cancer, estrogen-dependent neoplasia, active/history of DVT/PE/arterial thromboembolic disease, liver impairment/disease, thrombophilic disorders, known anaphylactic reaction or angioedema/hypersensitivity to the drug, pregnancy/nursing status, and any other conditions where treatment is contraindicated or cautioned, need for progestin therapy, and possible drug interactions.

Monitoring: Monitor for signs/symptoms of CV disorders, malignant neoplasms, dementia, gallbladder disease, hypercalcemia, visual abnormalities, BP and plasma TG elevations, pancreatitis, cholestatic jaundice, hypothyroidism, fluid retention, exacerbation of endometriosis or other conditions, vaginal irritation/infection, and other adverse reactions. Perform adequate diagnostic measures (eg, endometrial sampling) in patients w/ undiagnosed, persistent or recurring abnormal genital bleeding. Perform annual breast exam; schedule mammography based on age, risk factors, and prior mammogram results. Monitor thyroid function if on thyroid hormone replacement therapy. Reassess need to continue treatment at 3- or 6-month intervals.

Counseling: Inform of risks and benefits of therapy. Instruct to use ud. Advise of possible serious adverse reactions of therapy (eg, CV disorders, malignant neoplasms, probable dementia). Instruct to notify physician if signs/symptoms of vaginal irritation, abnormal vaginal bleeding, or any adverse reactions occur. Advise to have yearly breast exams by a physician and to perform monthly breast self-exams. Inform that the ring may be expelled from the vagina during bowel movement, straining or w/ constipation; if this occurs, rinse in lukewarm water and reinsert.

EstroGel — estradiol   Rx

Class: Estrogen

> Increased risk of endometrial cancer in women with a uterus who use unopposed estrogens. Adding a progestin to estrogen therapy has been shown to reduce risk of endometrial hyperplasia. Perform adequate diagnostic measures, including endometrial sampling, to rule out malignancy in postmenopausal women with undiagnosed, persistent or recurring abnormal genital bleeding. Should not be used for the prevention of cardiovascular disease (CVD) or dementia. Increased risks of stroke and deep vein thrombosis (DVT) reported in postmenopausal women (50-79 yrs of age) treated with daily oral conjugated estrogens (CE) alone. Increased risk of developing probable dementia in postmenopausal women ≥65 yrs of age reported. Increased risks of DVT, pulmonary embolism (PE), stroke, myocardial infarction (MI), and invasive breast cancer reported in postmenopausal women (50-79 yrs of age) treated with daily oral CE combined with medroxyprogesterone acetate. Should be prescribed at the lowest effective dose and for the shortest duration consistent with treatment goals and risks.

ADULT DOSAGE

Menopausal Vasomotor Symptoms

Moderate to Severe:
Usual: 1.25g/day

Menopausal Vulvar/Vaginal Atrophy

Moderate to Severe:
Usual: 1.25g/day

PEDIATRIC DOSAGE
Pediatric use may not have been established

ADMINISTRATION
Topical route

Priming
Before using the canister for the 1st time, it must be primed
Remove the large canister cover and fully depress the pump 3X
Discard the unused gel by thoroughly rinsing down the sink or placing it in the household trash

Application
Apply a thin layer over the entire arm on the inside and outside from wrist to shoulder

STORAGE
20-25°C (68-77°F); excursions permitted to 15-30°C (59-86°F).

HOW SUPPLIED
Gel: 0.06% [50g]

CONTRAINDICATIONS
Undiagnosed abnormal genital bleeding, known/suspected/history of breast cancer, known/suspected estrogen-dependent neoplasia, active/history of DVT/PE/arterial thromboembolic disease (eg, stroke, MI), known anaphylactic reaction or angioedema to this medication, known liver impairment or disease, known protein C/protein S/antithrombin deficiency or other known thrombophilic disorders, known/suspected pregnancy.

WARNINGS/PRECAUTIONS

D/C immediately if stroke, DVT, PE, or MI occurs or is suspected. Caution in patients with risk factors for arterial vascular disease and/or venous thromboembolism. If feasible, d/c at least 4-6 weeks before surgery of the type associated with an increased risk of thromboembolism, or during periods of prolonged immobilization. May increase risk of ovarian cancer and gallbladder disease. May lead to severe hypercalcemia in patients with breast cancer and bone metastases; d/c and take appropriate measures if hypercalcemia occurs. Retinal vascular thrombosis reported; d/c therapy pending examination if sudden partial/complete loss of vision, or sudden onset of proptosis, diplopia, or migraine occurs. D/C permanently if exam reveals papilledema or retinal vascular lesions. Consider addition of progestin for women with a uterus or with residual endometriosis post-hysterectomy. May increase BP and thyroid-binding globulin levels. May elevate plasma TG levels, leading to pancreatitis in women with preexisting hypertriglyceridemia; consider discontinuation if pancreatitis occurs. Caution with history of cholestatic jaundice associated with past estrogen use or with pregnancy; d/c in case of recurrence. May cause fluid retention; caution with conditions that might be influenced by this factor (eg, cardiac/renal impairment). Caution with hypoparathyroidism as estrogen-induced hypocalcemia may occur. May exacerbate endometriosis, asthma, diabetes mellitus, epilepsy, migraine, porphyria, systemic lupus erythematosus, and hepatic hemangiomas; use with caution. May exacerbate symptoms of angioedema in women with hereditary angioedema. May affect certain endocrine and blood components in lab tests. Use of moisturizing lotion 1 hr after application significantly increased absorption. Alcohol-based gels are flammable; avoid fire, flame, or smoking until the gel has dried.

ADVERSE REACTIONS

Breast pain, headache, flatulence.

DRUG INTERACTIONS

CYP3A4 inducers (eg, St. John's wort preparations, phenobarbital, carbamazepine) may decrease levels, which may decrease therapeutic effects and/or change uterine bleeding profile. CYP3A4 inhibitors (eg, erythromycin, ketoconazole, ritonavir) may increase levels, which may result in side effects. Patients concomitantly receiving thyroid hormone replacement therapy and estrogens may require increased doses of thyroid replacement therapy; monitor thyroid function.

PREGNANCY AND LACTATION

Contraindicated in pregnancy, not for use in nursing.

MECHANISM OF ACTION

Estrogen; binds to nuclear receptors in estrogen-responsive tissues. Circulating estrogens modulate the pituitary secretion of the gonadotropins, luteinizing hormone, and follicle-stimulating hormone through a negative feedback mechanism. Reduces elevated levels of these hormones in postmenopausal women.

PHARMACOKINETICS

Absorption: C_{max}=46.4pg/mL, 64.2pg/mL (estrone). **Distribution:** Largely bound to sex hormone-binding globulin and albumin; found in breast milk. **Metabolism:** Liver to estrone (metabolite); estriol (major urinary metabolite); enterohepatic recirculation via sulfate and glucuronide conjugation (liver); biliary secretion of conjugates into the intestine; hydrolysis (intestine); reabsorption; CYP3A4 (partial metabolism). **Elimination:** Urine (unchanged and metabolites); $T_{1/2}$=36 hrs.

PATIENT CONSIDERATIONS

Assessment: Assess for abnormal genital bleeding, presence/history of breast cancer, estrogen-dependent neoplasia, active/history of DVT/PE/arterial thromboembolic disease, liver impairment/disease, thrombophilic disorders, known anaphylactic reaction or angioedema to the drug, pregnancy/nursing status, any other conditions where treatment is contraindicated or cautioned, need for progestin therapy, and for possible drug interactions.

Monitoring: Monitor for signs/symptoms of CVD, malignant neoplasms, dementia, gallbladder disease, hypercalcemia, visual abnormalities, BP and plasma TG elevations, pancreatitis, cholestatic jaundice, fluid retention, exacerbation of endometriosis and other conditions, and other adverse reactions. Perform adequate diagnostic measures (eg, endometrial sampling) in postmenopausal women with undiagnosed, persistent or recurring genital bleeding. Perform annual breast exam; schedule mammography based on age, risk factors, and prior mammogram results. Reevaluate periodically (eg, 3- to 6-month intervals) to determine if treatment is still necessary. Regularly monitor thyroid function if on thyroid hormone replacement therapy.

Counseling: Inform of the importance of reporting abnormal vaginal bleeding to physician as soon as possible. Advise of possible serious adverse reactions to therapy (eg, CVD, malignant neoplasms, probable dementia) and of possible less serious but common adverse reactions (eg, headache, breast pain and tenderness, N/V). Instruct to have yearly breast exams by a healthcare provider and to perform monthly breast self-exams.

ETODOLAC — etodolac　　　Rx

Class: NSAID

> NSAIDs cause an increased risk of serious cardiovascular (CV) thrombotic events, including MI and stroke, which can be fatal; risk may occur early in treatment and may increase w/ duration of use. Contraindicated in the setting of CABG surgery. NSAIDs cause an increased risk of serious GI adverse events (eg, bleeding, ulceration, perforation of the stomach/intestines), which can be fatal and may occur at any time during use w/o warning symptoms; elderly patients are at greater risk.

OTHER BRAND NAMES

Lodine (Discontinued)

ADULT DOSAGE

Acute Pain

200-400mg q6-8h, up to 1000mg

Doses >1000mg/day have not been adequately evaluated

Osteoarthritis

Acute and Long-Term Management of Signs/Symptoms:

Initial: 300mg bid-tid, or 400mg bid, or 500mg bid

May give a lower dose of 600mg/day for long-term use

Doses >1000mg/day have not been adequately evaluated

Rheumatoid Arthritis

Acute and Long-Term Management of Signs/Symptoms:

Initial: 300mg bid-tid, or 400mg bid, or 500mg bid

May give a lower dose of 600mg/day for long-term use

Doses >1000mg/day have not been adequately evaluated

PEDIATRIC DOSAGE

Pediatric use may not have been established

ADMINISTRATION

Oral route

STORAGE

20-25°C (68-77°F). **Cap:** Protect from moisture.

HOW SUPPLIED

Cap: 200mg, 300mg; **Tab:** 400mg, 500mg

CONTRAINDICATIONS

Known hypersensitivity to etodolac or other ingredients in the medication; asthma, urticaria, or other allergic-type reactions after taking aspirin (ASA) or other NSAIDs; in the setting of CABG surgery.

WARNINGS/PRECAUTIONS

Use lowest effective dose for the shortest duration possible. Increased CV thrombotic risk w/ higher doses reported. Avoid in patients w/ a recent MI unless benefits outweigh the risks; if used, monitor for signs of cardiac ischemia. May cause HTN or worsen preexisting HTN. Fluid retention and edema reported. Avoid use in patients w/ severe heart failure (HF) unless benefits outweigh risk of worsening HF; if used, monitor for signs of worsening HF. Use w/ extreme caution in patients w/ prior history of ulcer disease, GI bleeding, or risk factors for GI bleeding (eg, longer duration of NSAID therapy, older age, poor general health status). D/C if a serious GI adverse event is suspected, until event is ruled out; for high-risk patients, consider alternate therapies that do not involve NSAIDs. Renal papillary necrosis and other renal injury reported after long-term use. Renal toxicity also reported in patients in whom renal prostaglandins have a compensatory role in the maintenance of renal perfusion; increased risk w/ renal/hepatic impairment, HF, and in elderly. Not recommended w/ advanced renal disease; if therapy must be initiated, closely monitor renal function. D/C if renal disease develops. Anaphylactoid reactions may occur; avoid w/ ASA triad. May cause serious skin reactions (eg, exfoliative dermatitis, Stevens-Johnson syndrome, toxic epidermal necrolysis); d/c at 1st appearance of skin rash or any other sign of hypersensitivity. Avoid in late pregnancy; may cause premature closure of ductus arteriosus. Not a substitute for corticosteroids or for the treatment of corticosteroid insufficiency; may mask signs of inflammation and fever. May cause elevations of LFTs or severe hepatic reactions (eg, jaundice, fulminant hepatitis, liver necrosis, hepatic failure); d/c if liver disease develops, systemic manifestations occur, or if abnormal LFTs persist/worsen. Anemia may occur; monitor Hgb/Hct if any signs/symptoms of anemia develop in patients on long-term therapy. May inhibit platelet aggregation and prolong bleeding time; monitor patients w/ coagulation disorders. Caution in debilitated and elderly. Lab test interactions may occur. Caution w/ preexisting asthma.

ADVERSE REACTIONS

Abdominal pain, constipation, diarrhea, dyspepsia, flatulence, heartburn, N/V, GI ulcers, abnormal renal function, anemia, dizziness, headaches, increased bleeding time, pruritus, rashes.

DRUG INTERACTIONS

May diminish the antihypertensive effect of ACE inhibitors. Increased risk of renal toxicity w/ diuretics and ACE inhibitors. May decrease peak concentration w/ antacids. Not recommended w/ ASA due to potential for increased adverse effects. May reduce the natriuretic effect of thiazide and loop diuretics. May increase lithium levels; monitor for lithium toxicity. May increase levels of cyclosporine, digoxin, and methotrexate (MTX), leading to increased toxicity. May enhance nephrotoxicity associated w/ cyclosporine. Avoid use prior to or concomitantly w/ high doses of MTX. May enhance MTX toxicity; caution w/ concomitant use. Increased free fraction of etodolac w/ phenylbutazone; coadministration not recommended. Synergistic effect on GI bleeding w/ warfarin; closely monitor. Increased risk of GI bleeding w/ oral corticosteroids, anticoagulants, smoking, and alcohol use. May blunt the CV effects of several therapeutic agents used to treat fluid retention and edema (eg, diuretics, ACE inhibitors, ARBs).

PREGNANCY AND LACTATION
Pregnancy: Category C.
Lactation: Not for use in nursing.

MECHANISM OF ACTION
NSAID; has not been established. Suspected to inhibit prostaglandin synthetase.

PHARMACOKINETICS
Absorption: Well-absorbed. Systemic bioavailability (100%); C_{max}=14-37mcg/mL, T_{max}=80 min. Administration in various populations resulted in different pharmacokinetic parameters. **Distribution:** Plasma protein binding (>99%); V_d=390mL/kg. **Metabolism:** Liver (extensive); hydroxylation, glucuronidation; 6-, 7-, and 8-hydroxylated-etodolac, etodolac glucuronide (metabolites). **Elimination:** Urine (1% unchanged, 72% parent drug and metabolites), feces (16%); $T_{1/2}$=6.4 hrs.

PATIENT CONSIDERATIONS

Assessment: Assess for history of asthma, urticaria, or allergic-type reactions w/ ASA or other NSAIDs, ASA triad, HTN, recent MI, severe HF, history of ulcer disease or GI bleeding, coagulation disorders, renal/hepatic impairment, pregnancy/nursing status, any other conditions where treatment is contraindicated or cautioned, and possible drug interactions. Obtain baseline BP.

Monitoring: Monitor for GI bleeding/ulceration/perforation, CV thrombotic events, HTN, fluid retention, edema, serious skin reactions, anaphylactoid reactions, and other adverse reactions. Monitor BP, CBC, bleeding time, LFTs, renal function, and chemistry profile periodically.

Counseling: Instruct to seek medical advice if symptoms of CV events, GI ulceration/bleeding, skin/hypersensitivity reactions, congestive HF, hepatotoxicity, or anaphylactoid reactions occur. Inform that medication should be avoided in late pregnancy.

ETODOLAC EXTENDED-RELEASE — etodolac   Rx
Class: NSAID

> NSAIDs cause an increased risk of serious cardiovascular (CV) thrombotic events, including MI and stroke, which can be fatal; risk may occur early in treatment and may increase w/ duration of use. NSAIDs cause an increased risk of serious GI adverse events (eg, bleeding, ulceration, stomach/intestinal perforation) that can be fatal and occur anytime during use w/o warning symptoms; elderly patients are at greater risk for serious GI events. Contraindicated in the setting of CABG surgery.

OTHER BRAND NAMES
Lodine XL (Discontinued)

ADULT DOSAGE	**PEDIATRIC DOSAGE**
Rheumatoid Arthritis	**Juvenile Rheumatoid Arthritis**
Initial: 400-1000mg qd	**6-16 Years:**
Titrate: Use lowest effective dose	**20-30kg:** 400mg qd
	31-45kg: 600mg qd
Osteoarthritis	**46-60kg:** 800mg qd
Initial: 400-1000mg qd	**>60kg:** 1000mg qd
Titrate: Use lowest effective dose	

ADMINISTRATION
Oral route

STORAGE
20-25°C (68-77°F). Protect from excessive heat and humidity.

HOW SUPPLIED
Tab, Extended-Release: 400mg, 500mg, 600mg

CONTRAINDICATIONS
Known hypersensitivity to etodolac. History of asthma, urticaria, or allergic-type reactions w/ aspirin (ASA) or other NSAIDs. In the setting of CABG surgery.

WARNINGS/PRECAUTIONS
Use lowest effective dose for the shortest duration possible. Increased CV thrombotic risk w/ higher doses reported. Avoid in patients w/ a recent MI unless benefits outweigh the risks; if used, monitor for signs of cardiac ischemia. May cause HTN or worsen preexisting HTN. Fluid retention and edema reported. Avoid use in patients w/ severe heart failure (HF) unless benefits outweigh risk of worsening HF; if used, monitor for signs of worsening HF. Use extreme caution in patients w/ history of ulcer disease or GI bleeding, or risk factors for GI bleeding (eg, longer duration of NSAID therapy, older age, poor general health status). D/C if a serious GI adverse event is suspected, until event is ruled out; for high risk patients, consider alternate therapies that do not involve NSAIDs. Renal papillary necrosis and other renal injury reported after long-term use; increased risk w/ renal/hepatic impairment, HF, and in elderly. Not recommended for use w/ advanced renal disease; if therapy must be initiated, monitor renal function closely. D/C if renal disease develops. Anaphylactoid reactions may occur; avoid w/ ASA triad. May cause serious skin adverse events; d/c at 1st appearance of skin rash or any other sign of hypersensitivity. Avoid in late pregnancy; may cause premature closure of ductus arteriosus. Not a substitute for corticosteroids or to treat corticosteroid insufficiency. May mask signs of inflammation and fever. May cause elevations of LFTs or severe hepatic reactions; d/c if liver disease develops, systemic manifestations occur, or abnormal LFTs persist/worsen. Anemia may occur; monitor Hgb/Hct if signs/symptoms of anemia develop w/ long-term use. May inhibit platelet aggregation and prolong bleeding time; monitor patients w/ coagulation disorders. Caution w/ preexisting asthma. Lab test interactions may occur. Caution in elderly/debilitated.

ADVERSE REACTIONS
Dyspepsia, abdominal pain, diarrhea, flatulence, N/V, constipation, rash, dizziness, pharyngitis, rhinitis, headache, infection, HTN, asthenia, pruritus.

DRUG INTERACTIONS
May diminish antihypertensive effects of ACE inhibitors. Increased risk of renal toxicity w/ diuretics and ACE inhibitors; monitor renal function. Not recommended w/ ASA due to potential for increased adverse effects. May elevate serum levels of digoxin, lithium, and cyclosporine; monitor for signs of toxicity. May enhance nephrotoxicity w/ cyclosporine. May enhance methotrexate toxicity; caution w/ concomitant use. Not recommended w/ phenylbutazone. May reduce the natriuretic effect of thiazide and loop diuretics. Increased risk of GI bleeding w/ anticoagulants (eg, warfarin), oral corticosteroids, smoking, and alcohol. May blunt the CV effects of several therapeutic agents used to treat fluid retention and edema (eg, diuretics, ACE inhibitors, ARBs).

PREGNANCY AND LACTATION
Pregnancy: Category C.
Lactation: Not for use in nursing.

MECHANISM OF ACTION
NSAID; mechanism not established. Thought to inhibit prostaglandin synthetase.

PHARMACOKINETICS
Absorption: Systemic bioavailability (≥80%); T_{max}=6.7 hrs. **Distribution:** V_d=566mL/kg; plasma protein binding (>99%). **Metabolism:** Hydroxylation, glucuronidation. **Elimination:** Urine (72% unchanged and metabolites, 1% unchanged), feces (16%); $T_{1/2}$=8.4 hrs.

PATIENT CONSIDERATIONS

Assessment: Confirm that use is not in the setting of CABG surgery. Assess for history of asthma, urticaria, or allergic reactions to ASA or other NSAIDs, ASA triad, hypersensitivity to drug, severe HF, HTN, hepatic/renal impairment, history of ulcer disease, history of/risk factors for GI bleeding, general health status, pregnancy/nursing status, and possible drug interactions.

Monitoring: Monitor for hypersensitivity reactions, CV thrombotic events, MI, stroke, GI bleeding/ulceration/perforation, HF, HTN, fluid retention, asthma, skin reactions, and other adverse reactions. Monitor BP, LFTs, renal function, coagulation profile, CBC w/ differential, and platelet count.

Counseling: Instruct to seek medical advice if symptoms of CV thrombotic events, GI ulceration/bleeding, skin/hypersensitivity reactions, congestive HF, hepatotoxicity, or anaphylactoid reactions occur. Advise to d/c therapy and to contact physician if any type of rash or signs/symptoms of hepatotoxicity occur. Inform that medication should be avoided in late pregnancy.

EVAMIST — estradiol   Rx
Class: Estrogen

> Increased risk of endometrial cancer in a woman with a uterus who uses unopposed estrogens. Adding a progestin to estrogen therapy has been shown to reduce risk of endometrial hyperplasia. Adequate diagnostic measures should be undertaken to rule out malignancy in all cases of undiagnosed persistent or recurring abnormal genital bleeding. Should not be used for the prevention of cardiovascular disease (CVD) or dementia. Increased risk of stroke and deep vein thrombosis (DVT) reported in postmenopausal women (50-79 yrs of age) treated with daily oral conjugated estrogens (CEs) alone and when combined with medroxyprogesterone acetate (MPA). Increased risk of developing probable dementia reported in postmenopausal women ≥65 yrs of age treated with daily CEs alone and when combined with MPA. Increased risks of pulmonary embolism (PE), myocardial infarction (MI), and invasive breast cancer reported in postmenopausal women (50-79 yrs of age) treated with daily oral CEs combined with MPA. Should be prescribed at the lowest effective dose for the shortest duration consistent with treatment goals and risks. Breast budding and breast masses in prepubertal females and gynecomastia and breast masses in prepubertal males reported following unintentional secondary exposure to therapy by women using this product. Women should ensure that children do not come into contact with the site(s) where product is applied.

ADULT DOSAGE	**PEDIATRIC DOSAGE**
Menopausal Vasomotor Symptoms	Pediatric use may not have been established
Moderate to Severe:	
Initial: 1 spray/day	
Titrate: Adjust dose based on clinical response	
Usual: 1-3 sprays qam	

ADMINISTRATION
Topical route

Priming
Before applying the 1st dose, prime the pump by spraying 3 sprays w/ the cover on
Hold container upright and vertical when spraying

Application
Apply spray(s) each morning to adjacent, non-overlapping areas on the inner surface of the forearm, starting near the elbow
Allow sprays to dry for approx 2 min before covering the site w/ clothing
Do not wash the site for ≥1 hr
Do not apply to skin surfaces other than the forearm

STORAGE
20-25°C (68-77°F); excursions permitted to 15-30°C (59-86°F). Do not freeze.

HOW SUPPLIED
Spray: 1.53mg/spray [8.1mL]

CONTRAINDICATIONS
Undiagnosed abnormal genital bleeding, known/suspected/history of breast cancer, known/suspected estrogen-dependent neoplasia, active/history of DVT/PE/arterial thromboembolic disease (eg, stroke, MI), known liver impairment/

disease, known protein C/protein S/antithrombin deficiency or other known thrombophilic disorders, known/suspected pregnancy.

WARNINGS/PRECAUTIONS

D/C immediately if PE, DVT, stroke, or MI occurs or is suspected. If feasible, d/c at least 4-6 weeks before surgery of the type associated with an increased risk of thromboembolism, or during periods of prolonged immobilization. May increase risk of gallbladder disease requiring surgery and risk of ovarian cancer. Application site should be covered with clothing if another person may come into contact with the site. May lead to severe hypercalcemia in women with breast cancer and bone metastases; d/c and take appropriate measures if hypercalcemia occurs. Retinal vascular thrombosis reported; d/c therapy pending exam if sudden partial/complete loss of vision or sudden onset of proptosis, diplopia, or migraine occurs. D/C permanently if exam reveals papilledema or retinal vascular lesions. May increase BP and thyroid-binding globulin levels. May be associated with elevations of plasma TGs leading to pancreatitis in patients with preexisting hypertriglyceridemia; consider discontinuation if pancreatitis occurs. Caution with history of cholestatic jaundice associated with past estrogen use or with pregnancy; d/c in case of recurrence. May cause fluid retention. Caution with hypoparathyroidism; hypocalcemia may occur. Cases of malignant transformation of residual endometrial implants reported in women treated posthysterectomy with estrogen therapy alone; consider addition of progestin for patients known to have residual endometriosis posthysterectomy. May exacerbate symptoms of angioedema in women with hereditary angioedema. May exacerbate asthma, diabetes mellitus, epilepsy, migraine, porphyria, systemic lupus erythematosus, and hepatic hemangiomas. Consider addition of progestin for women with residual endometriosis posthysterectomy. Flammable; avoid fire, flame, or smoking until spray has dried. Decreased absorption with sunscreen applied 1 hr after estradiol application. May affect certain endocrine and blood components in lab tests.

ADVERSE REACTIONS

Headache, breast tenderness, nipple pain, nausea, back pain, nasopharyngitis, arthralgia.

DRUG INTERACTIONS

CYP3A4 inducers (eg, St. John's wort preparations, phenobarbital, carbamazepine) may decrease levels, which may decrease therapeutic effects and/or changes in the uterine bleeding profile. CYP3A4 inhibitors (eg, erythromycin, ketoconazole, grapefruit juice) may increase levels, which may result in side effects. Patients concomitantly receiving thyroid hormone replacement therapy and estrogens may require increased doses of thyroid replacement therapy; monitor thyroid function.

PREGNANCY AND LACTATION

Contraindicated in pregnancy, not for use in nursing.

MECHANISM OF ACTION

Estrogen; binds to nuclear receptors in estrogen-responsive tissues. Circulating estrogens modulate pituitary secretion of the gonadotropins, luteinizing hormone and follicle-stimulating hormone, through a (-) feedback mechanism. Reduces elevated levels of these hormones in postmenopausal women.

PHARMACOKINETICS

Absorption: Topical administration of various doses resulted in different parameters. **Distribution:** Largely bound to sex hormone-binding globulin and albumin; found in breast milk. **Metabolism:** Liver to estrone (metabolite) and estriol (major urinary metabolite); enterohepatic recirculation via sulfate and glucuronide conjugation in the liver; biliary secretion of conjugates into the intestine; hydrolysis in the intestine; reabsorption; CYP3A4 (partial metabolism). **Elimination:** Urine (parent compound and metabolites).

PATIENT CONSIDERATIONS

Assessment: Assess for abnormal genital bleeding, presence/history of breast cancer, estrogen-dependent neoplasia, active/history of DVT/PE/arterial thromboembolic disease, liver impairment/disease, thrombophilic disorders, known anaphylactic reaction to the drug, hereditary or angioedema, pregnancy/nursing status, and for any other conditions where treatment is contraindicated or cautioned. Assess for possible drug interactions.

Monitoring: Monitor for signs/symptoms of CVD, malignant neoplasms, dementia, gallbladder disease, hypercalcemia, visual abnormalities, BP and plasma TG elevations, pancreatitis, cholestatic jaundice, hypothyroidism, fluid retention, exacerbation of endometriosis, and other adverse reactions. Perform adequate diagnostic measures (eg, endometrial sampling) in patients with undiagnosed, persistent or recurring abnormal genital bleeding. Perform annual breast exam; schedule mammography based on patient's age, risk factors, and prior mammogram results. Monitor thyroid function if on thyroid hormone replacement therapy. Perform periodic evaluation to determine treatment need.

Counseling: Inform of the importance of reporting unusual vaginal bleeding to physician as soon as possible. Instruct to apply therapy ud and keep children from contacting exposed application site(s); advise to thoroughly wash the contact area with soap and water if direct contact with the application site occurs. Inform about risk of unintentional secondary exposure; advise to have children evaluated by a physician if signs of unintentional secondary exposure are noticed and to d/c therapy until cause is identified if a child under patient's care has any unexpected sexual development. Advise of possible serious adverse reactions to therapy (eg, CVD, malignant neoplasms, probable dementia) and of possible less serious but common adverse reactions (eg, headache, breast pain and tenderness, N/V). Instruct to have yearly breast exams by a physician and to perform monthly breast self-exams.

EVEKEO — amphetamine sulfate CII

Class: CNS stimulant

> High potential for abuse; prolonged use may lead to drug dependence and must be avoided. Misuse may cause sudden death and serious cardiovascular (CV) adverse events.

ADULT DOSAGE

Narcolepsy

Initial: 10mg/day
Titrate: May increase in increments of 10mg at weekly intervals until optimal response is obtained
Usual: 5-60mg/day in divided doses

Give 1st dose on awakening; additional doses (5 or 10mg) at intervals of 4-6 hrs

Obesity

Management of exogenous obesity as a short-term (few weeks) adjunct in a regimen of weight reduction based on caloric restriction, for patients refractory to alternative therapy

Usual: Up to 30mg/day in divided doses of 5-10mg, 30-60 min ac

PEDIATRIC DOSAGE

Narcolepsy

Usual: 5-60mg/day in divided doses

Give 1st dose on awakening; additional doses (5 or 10mg) at intervals of 4-6 hrs

6-12 Years:
Initial: 5mg/day
Titrate: May increase in increments of 5mg at weekly intervals until optimal response is obtained

≥12 Years:
Initial: 10mg/day
Titrate: May increase in increments of 10mg at weekly intervals until optimal response is obtained

Attention-Deficit Hyperactivity Disorder

3-5 Years:
Initial: 2.5mg/day
Titrate: May increase in increments of 2.5mg at weekly intervals until optimal response is obtained

≥6 Years:
Initial: 5mg qd or bid
Titrate: May increase in increments of 5mg at weekly intervals until optimal response is obtained
Only in rare cases will it be necessary to exceed a total of 40mg/day

Give 1st dose on awakening; additional doses (1-2 tabs) at intervals of 4-6 hrs

Where possible, interrupt therapy occasionally to determine if there is a recurrence of behavioral symptoms sufficient to require continued therapy

Obesity

Management of exogenous obesity as a short-term (few weeks) adjunct in a regimen of weight reduction based on caloric restriction, for patients refractory to alternative therapy

≥12 Years:
Usual: Up to 30mg/day in divided doses of 5-10mg, 30-60 min ac

---

DOSING CONSIDERATIONS

Adverse Reactions
Narcolepsy:
Reduce dose if bothersome adverse reactions (eg, insomnia, anorexia) appear

ADMINISTRATION

Oral route

Avoid late pm dosing.

STORAGE

20-25°C (68-77°F).

HOW SUPPLIED

Tab: 5mg*, 10mg* *scored

CONTRAINDICATIONS

Advanced arteriosclerosis, symptomatic cardiovascular disease (CVD), moderate to severe HTN, hyperthyroidism, agitated states, history of drug abuse, during or w/in 14 days following MAOI use, known hypersensitivity or idiosyncrasy to the sympathomimetic amines.

WARNINGS/PRECAUTIONS

Sudden death reported in children and adolescents w/ structural cardiac abnormalities or other serious heart problems. Sudden deaths, stroke, and MI reported in adults. Avoid w/ serious structural cardiac abnormalities, cardiomyopathy, serious heart rhythm abnormalities, coronary artery disease, or other serious cardiac problems. May cause modest increase in average BP and HR; caution w/ underlying medical conditions that may be compromised (eg, preexisting HTN, heart failure, recent MI). Perform prompt cardiac evaluation when symptoms suggestive of cardiac disease develop. May exacerbate symptoms of behavior disturbance and thought disorder in patients w/ preexisting psychotic disorder. Caution in patients w/ comorbid bipolar disorder; may induce mixed/manic episodes. May cause treatment-emergent psychotic/manic symptoms (eg, hallucinations, delusional thinking, mania) in children and adolescents w/o prior history of psychotic illness or mania; consider discontinuation if such symptoms occur. Aggressive behavior or hostility reported in children and adolescents w/ ADHD. May cause suppression of growth in children; may need to interrupt treatment in patients not growing or gaining weight as expected. May lower convulsive threshold; d/c if seizures develop. Associated w/ peripheral vasculopathy, including Raynaud's phenomenon. Difficulties w/ accommodation and blurring of vision reported. Caution w/ even mild HTN. May exacerbate motor and phonic tics and Tourette's syndrome. May cause a significant elevation in plasma corticosteroid levels and interfere w/ urinary steroid determinations.

ADVERSE REACTIONS
Palpitations, tachycardia, elevation of BP, overstimulation, restlessness, dizziness, insomnia, euphoria, dryness of the mouth, unpleasant taste, diarrhea, urticaria, impotence, changes in libido, rhabdomyolysis.

DRUG INTERACTIONS
See Contraindications. GI acidifying agents (eg, guanethidine, reserpine, glutamic acid HCl) and urinary acidifying agents (eg, ammonium chloride, sodium acid phosphate) lower blood levels and efficacy. Inhibits adrenergic blockers. GI alkalinizing agents (eg, sodium bicarbonate) and urinary alkalinizing agents (eg, acetazolamide, some thiazides) increase blood levels and potentiate action of amphetamines. May enhance activity of TCAs or sympathomimetic agents. Desipramine or protriptyline and possibly other TCAs cause striking and sustained increases in the concentration of d-amphetamine in the brain; CV effects can be potentiated. May counteract sedative effect of antihistamines. May antagonize the hypotensive effects of antihypertensives. Chlorpromazine and haloperidol block dopamine and norepinephrine reuptake, thus inhibiting the central stimulant effects. Lithium carbonate may inhibit the antiobesity and stimulatory effects. Potentiates the analgesic effect of meperidine. Acidifying agents used in methenamine therapy increase urinary excretion and reduce efficacy. Enhances adrenergic effect of norepinephrine. May delay intestinal absorption of ethosuximide, phenobarbital, and phenytoin; may produce a synergistic anticonvulsant action if coadministered w/ phenobarbital or phenytoin. In cases of propoxyphene overdosage, CNS stimulation and fatal convulsions may occur. Inhibits the hypotensive effect of veratrum alkaloids.

PREGNANCY AND LACTATION
Pregnancy: Category C. Infants born to mothers dependent on amphetamines have an increased risk of premature delivery and low birth weight; these infants may experience withdrawal symptoms.
Lactation: Excreted in human milk; not for use in nursing.

MECHANISM OF ACTION
Sympathomimetic amines; not been established. Has CNS stimulant activity.

PHARMACOKINETICS
Distribution: Found in breast milk.

PATIENT CONSIDERATIONS
Assessment: Assess for hypersensitivity/idiosyncrasy to sympathomimetic amines, structural cardiac abnormalities, advanced arteriosclerosis, symptomatic CVD, HTN, hyperthyroidism, history of drug abuse, tics, Tourette's syndrome, psychotic disorder, any other conditions where treatment is contraindicated or cautioned, pregnancy/nursing status, and possible drug interactions. Adequately screen patients w/ comorbid depressive symptoms to determine if they are at risk for bipolar disorder.

Monitoring: Monitor for changes in HR and BP, signs/symptoms of cardiac disease, exacerbation of symptoms of behavior disturbance and thought disorder, psychosis, mania, appearance of or worsening of aggressive behavior or hostility, seizures, peripheral vasculopathy (eg, digital changes), visual disturbances, exacerbation of motor and phonic tics or Tourette's syndrome, and other adverse reactions. In pediatric patients, monitor growth.

Counseling: Inform about benefits and risks of treatment. Advise that drug has high potential for abuse. Caution that therapy may impair the ability to engage in potentially hazardous activities (eg, operating machinery or vehicles). Inform about the risk of peripheral vasculopathy (eg, Raynaud's phenomenon); instruct to report to physician any numbness, pain, skin color change, or sensitivity to temperature in fingers or toes and to call physician immediately if any signs of unexplained wounds appearing on fingers or toes while on therapy. Advise to avoid breastfeeding and to notify physician if pregnant/planning to become pregnant.

EVISTA — raloxifene hydrochloride   Rx
Class: Selective estrogen receptor modulator

> Increased risk of deep vein thrombosis (DVT) and pulmonary embolism (PE) reported. Avoid use in women with active or past history of venous thromboembolism (VTE). Increased risk of death due to stroke in postmenopausal women with documented coronary heart disease or at increased risk for major coronary events; consider risk-benefit balance in women at risk for stroke.

ADULT DOSAGE
Osteoporosis

Treatment and Prevention in Postmenopausal Women:
60mg qd

Reduction in Risk of Invasive Breast Cancer

Postmenopausal Women w/ Osteoporosis/Postmenopausal Women at High Risk for Invasive Breast Cancer:
60mg qd

PEDIATRIC DOSAGE
Pediatric use may not have been established

DOSING CONSIDERATIONS
Other Important Considerations
Ca²⁺ and Vitamin D Supplementation:
Total Daily Ca²⁺ Requirement: 1500mg/day
Total Daily Vitamin D: 400-800 IU/day

ADMINISTRATION
Oral route
May be given at any time of day w/o regard to meals.

STORAGE
20-25°C (68-77°F); excursions permitted to 15-30°C (59-86°F).

HOW SUPPLIED
Tab: 60mg

CONTRAINDICATIONS
Active/past history of VTE (eg, DVT, PE, retinal vein thrombosis), pregnancy, women who may become pregnant, nursing mothers.

WARNINGS/PRECAUTIONS
VTE events, including superficial venous thrombophlebitis, reported. D/C at least 72 hrs prior to and during prolonged immobilization (eg, postsurgical recovery, prolonged bed rest); resume therapy only after patient is fully ambulatory. Caution in women at risk of thromboembolic disease for other reasons (eg, CHF, superficial thrombophlebitis, active malignancy). Should not be used for primary or secondary prevention of cardiovascular disease (CVD). Avoid use in premenopausal women. Monitor serum TG levels in women with history of hypertriglyceridemia in response to treatment with estrogen or estrogen plus progestin. Use in women with history of breast cancer has not been adequately studied. Caution with hepatic impairment or with moderate or severe renal impairment. Not recommended for use in men. Monitor for unexplained uterine bleeding and breast abnormalities.

ADVERSE REACTIONS
DVT, PE, hot flashes, leg cramps, infection, flu syndrome, headache, N/V, diarrhea, peripheral edema, arthralgia, vaginal bleeding, pharyngitis, sinusitis, cough increased.

DRUG INTERACTIONS
Avoid concomitant administration with cholestyramine, other anion exchange resins, and systemic estrogens. Monitor PT with warfarin and other warfarin derivatives. Caution with certain other highly protein-bound drugs (eg, diazepam, diazoxide, lidocaine).

PREGNANCY AND LACTATION
Category X, not for use in nursing.

MECHANISM OF ACTION
Selective estrogen receptor modulator; binds to estrogen receptors. Binding results in activation of estrogenic pathways in some tissues and blockade of estrogenic pathways in others, depending on extent of recruitment of coactivators and corepressors to estrogen receptor target gene promoters. Acts as an estrogen agonist in bone; decreases bone resorption and bone turnover, increases bone mineral density, and decreases fracture incidence.

PHARMACOKINETICS
Absorption: Rapid; absolute bioavailability (2%). Single dose: C_{max}=0.5(ng/mL)/(mg/kg); AUC=27.2(ng•hr/mL)/(mg/kg). Multiple doses: C_{max}=1.36(ng/mL)/(mg/kg); AUC=24.2(ng•hr/mL)/(mg/kg). **Distribution:** V_d=2348L/kg (single dose), 2853L/kg (multiple doses); plasma protein binding (95%). **Metabolism:** Extensive; glucuronidation; raloxifene-4'-glucuronide, raloxifene-6-glucuronide, raloxifene-6',4'-diglucuronide (metabolites). **Elimination:** Feces (primary), urine (<0.2% unchanged); $T_{1/2}$=27.7 hrs (single dose), 32.5 hrs (multiple doses).

PATIENT CONSIDERATIONS
Assessment: Assess for active or history of VTE (eg, DVT, PE, retinal vein thrombosis), CVD, risk factors for stroke, history of breast cancer, history of hypertriglyceridemia, prolonged immobilization, renal/hepatic impairment, pregnancy/nursing status, and for possible drug interactions. Perform breast exams and mammograms prior to treatment.

Monitoring: Monitor for VTE (eg, DVT, PE, retinal vein thrombosis), stroke, unexplained uterine bleeding, breast abnormalities, and other adverse reactions. Monitor serum TG levels with history of hypertriglyceridemia. Monitor PT with warfarin and other warfarin derivatives. Perform regular breast exams and mammograms after initial treatment.

Counseling: For osteoporosis treatment/prevention, instruct to take supplemental Ca²⁺ and/or vitamin D if intake is inadequate. Counsel on weight-bearing exercise and modification of certain behavioral factors (eg, smoking, excessive alcohol consumption) for osteoporosis treatment/prevention. Advise to d/c therapy at least 72 hrs prior to and during prolonged immobilization. Instruct to avoid prolonged restrictions of movement during travel. Counsel that therapy may increase incidence of hot flashes or hot flashes may occur upon initiation of therapy. Inform that regular breast exams and mammography should be done before initiation of therapy and should continue during therapy.

EVOCLIN — clindamycin phosphate   Rx

Class: Lincomycin derivative

ADULT DOSAGE

Acne Vulgaris

Apply enough to cover entire affected area(s) qd

D/C if no improvement after 6-8 weeks or if condition worsens

PEDIATRIC DOSAGE

Acne Vulgaris

≥12 Years:

Apply enough to cover entire affected area(s) qd

D/C if no improvement after 6-8 weeks or if condition worsens

ADMINISTRATION

Topical route

Not for oral, ophthalmic, or intravaginal use

Wash skin w/ mild soap and allow to fully dry before application

STORAGE

20-25°C (68-77°F). Do not expose to heat or store at >49°C (120°F). Contents under pressure; do not puncture or incinerate.

HOW SUPPLIED

Foam: 1% [50g, 100g]

CONTRAINDICATIONS

History of regional enteritis, ulcerative colitis, or antibiotic-associated colitis (including pseudomembranous colitis).

WARNINGS/PRECAUTIONS

Diarrhea, bloody diarrhea, and colitis (including pseudomembranous colitis) reported; d/c if significant diarrhea occurs. May cause irritation; d/c if irritation or dermatitis occurs. Avoid contact w/ eyes, mouth, lips, other mucous membranes, or areas of broken skin; rinse thoroughly w/ water if contact occurs. Caution in atopic individuals.

ADVERSE REACTIONS

Diarrhea, bloody diarrhea, colitis, headache, application-site burning.

DRUG INTERACTIONS

Antiperistaltic agents (eg, opiates, diphenoxylate w/ atropine) may prolong and/or worsen severe colitis. Avoid w/ topical/oral erythromycin-containing products due to possible antagonism to clindamycin. May enhance the action of other neuromuscular blockers; use w/ caution. Caution w/ concomitant topical acne therapy (eg, peeling, desquamating, abrasive agents) due to possible cumulative irritancy effect.

PREGNANCY AND LACTATION

Category B, not for use in nursing.

MECHANISM OF ACTION

Lincomycin derivative; not established. Binds to the 50S ribosomal subunits of susceptible bacteria and prevents elongation of peptide chains by interfering w/ peptidyl transfer, thereby suppressing protein synthesis. Shown to have in vitro activity against *Propionibacterium acnes*, which is associated w/ acne vulgaris.

PHARMACOKINETICS

Distribution: Orally and parenterally administered clindamycin found in breast milk. **Elimination:** Urine (<0.024% unchanged).

PATIENT CONSIDERATIONS

Assessment: Assess for history of regional enteritis/ulcerative colitis or antibiotic-associated colitis (including pseudomembranous colitis), pregnancy/nursing status, and possible drug interactions. Assess use in atopic individuals.

Monitoring: Monitor for significant diarrhea, colitis, and irritation/dermatitis. For colitis, perform stool culture and assay for *Clostridium difficile* toxin.

Counseling: Instruct to dispense foam directly into cap or onto cool surface, then apply enough to cover the face. Instruct to wash hands after application, and to avoid contact w/ eyes, mouth, lips, other mucous membranes, or areas of broken skin; instruct to rinse thoroughly w/ water if contact occurs. Inform that irritation (eg, erythema, scaling, itching, burning, stinging) may occur; advise to d/c if excessive irritancy or dermatitis occurs. Instruct to d/c and contact physician if experiencing severe diarrhea or GI discomfort. Inform that medication is flammable; avoid fire, flame, and/or smoking during and immediately following application.

EVOMELA — melphalan   Rx

Class: Alkylating agent

> Severe bone marrow suppression w/ resulting infection/bleeding may occur; monitor hematologic lab parameters. IV melphalan has shown more myelosuppression than oral melphalan. Hypersensitivity reactions (eg, anaphylaxis) reported; d/c treatment for serious hypersensitivity reactions. Produces chromosomal aberrations and should be considered potentially leukemogenic.

ADULT DOSAGE

Multiple Myeloma

High-dose Conditioning Treatment Prior to Hematopoietic Progenitor (Stem) Cell Transplantation:
100mg/m² /day IV for 2 consecutive days (Day 3 and Day 2) prior to autologous stem cell transplantation (ASCT, Day 0); administer prophylactic antiemetics

PEDIATRIC DOSAGE

Pediatric use may not have been established

For patients weighing >130% of their ideal body weight, body surface area should be calculated based on adjusted ideal body weight

Palliative Treatment When Oral Therapy Is Not Appropriate:
16mg/m² IV at 2-week intervals for 4 doses, then, after adequate recovery from toxicity, at 4-week intervals; administer prophylactic antiemetics

DOSING CONSIDERATIONS

Renal Impairment

Conditioning Treatment: No dose adjustment is necessary

Palliative Treatment (BUN ≥30mg/dL): Consider dose reduction of up to 50%

ADMINISTRATION

IV route

Cytotoxic drug; follow applicable special handling and disposal procedures. Do not mix w/ other melphalan for inj drug products.

Reconstitution/Infusion

1. Use 8.6mL of normal saline to reconstitute and make a 50mg/10mL (5mg/mL) nominal concentration.
2. Calculate the required volume needed for dose and withdraw from vial.
3. Add required volume to appropriate volume of 0.9% NaCl inj to a final concentration of 0.45mg/mL.
4. Infuse over 30 min (conditioning treatment) or as a single IV infusion over 15-20 min (palliative treatment). May cause local tissue damage should extravasation occur; do not administer by direct inj into a peripheral vein. Administer by injecting slowly into a fast-running IV infusion via a central venous access line.

Stability

- Reconstituted drug product is stable for 24 hrs at 5°C w/o any precipitation, due to high solubility.
- Reconstituted drug product is stable for 1 hr at room temperature.
- Admixture sol is stable for 4 hrs at room temperature in addition to the 1 hr following reconstitution.

STORAGE

25°C (77°F); excursions permitted between 15-30°C (59-86°F). Protect from light; retain in original carton until use.

HOW SUPPLIED

Inj: 50mg

CONTRAINDICATIONS

History of serious allergic reaction to melphalan.

WARNINGS/PRECAUTIONS

Hepatic disorders (eg, abnormal LFTs, hepatitis, jaundice) and hepatic veno-occlusive disease reported; monitor liver chemistries. Acute hypersensitivity reactions, (eg, anaphylaxis) reported; d/c treatment for serious hypersensitivity reactions. Chromatid or chromosome damage and secondary malignancies (eg, myeloproliferative syndrome or acute leukemia) reported; consider potential benefit against possible risk. May cause fetal harm. May cause reversible/irreversible testicular suppression or suppression of ovarian function in premenopausal women. **Conditioning Regimen:** Myeloablation occurs in all patients receiving conditioning treatment; do not begin if a stem cell product is not available for rescue. Monitor CBC, and provide supportive care for infections, anemia, and thrombocytopenia until there is adequate hematopoietic recovery. May cause N/V, mucositis, and diarrhea; provide supportive care. Provide nutritional support and analgesics for patients w/ severe mucositis. **Palliative Treatment:** Risk of severe myelosuppression is increased in patients w/ compromised bone marrow (by prior irradiation, prior chemotherapy, or recovering from chemotherapy); perform periodic CBC during course of treatment and provide supportive care for infections, bleeding, and symptomatic anemia. N/V, diarrhea, and oral ulceration may occur; provide supportive care.

ADVERSE REACTIONS

Diarrhea, N/V, fatigue, hypokalemia, anemia, decrease in neutrophil, WBC, lymphocyte, and platelet counts.

DRUG INTERACTIONS

Severe renal impairment reported w/ oral cyclosporine. May reduce the threshold for BCNU lung toxicity. Nalidixic acid may increase incidence of severe hemorrhagic necrotic enterocolitis in pediatric patients.

PREGNANCY AND LACTATION

Pregnancy: Can cause fetal harm.

Lactation: It is not known whether melphalan is present in human milk. Not for use in nursing.

Reproductive Potential: Avoid pregnancy; females of reproductive potential should use effective contraception methods during and after treatment. May damage spermatozoa and testicular tissue, resulting in possible genetic fetal abnormalities; males w/ female sexual partners of reproductive potential should use effective contraception during and after treatment.

MECHANISM OF ACTION

Alkylating agent; cytotoxicity appears to be related to the extent of its interstrand cross-linking w/ DNA, probably by binding at the N^7 position of guanine. Active against both resting and rapidly dividing tumor cells.

PHARMACOKINETICS

Absorption: C_{max}=1.2mcg/mL (10mg/m²), 2.8mcg/mL (20mg/m²). **Distribution:** V_d=0.5L/kg; plasma protein binding (50-90%). **Metabolism:** Hydrolysis. **Elimination:** $T_{1/2}$=75 min. Urine (5.8-21.3%).

PATIENT CONSIDERATIONS

Assessment: Assess for prior irradiation or chemotherapy, renal impairment, pregnancy/nursing status, drug hypersensitivity, and possible drug interactions. Obtain baseline hematological parameters.

Monitoring: Monitor for GI toxicity, hepatotoxicity, induction of a second malignancy, amenorrhea, testicular suppression, bone marrow suppression, hypersensitivity reactions, and other adverse events. Monitor CBC and other hematologic lab parameters.

Counseling: Advise to report any signs or symptoms of thrombocytopenia, leukopenia, and anemia; inform of the need for routine blood counts. Inform of signs/symptoms of mucositis; instruct on ways to reduce risk of development, and on ways to maintain nutrition and control discomfort if it occurs. Advise to report symptoms of N/V and diarrhea. Advise to immediately report symptoms of hypersensitivity reactions. Inform of the potential long-term risks related to secondary malignancy. Advise of the potential risk to a fetus. Advise females of reproductive potential to avoid pregnancy, which may include use of effective contraception during and after treatment. Advise females to contact their healthcare provider if they become pregnant, or if pregnancy is suspected. Inform about the risk for infertility. Advise not to breastfeed. Advise males w/ female sexual partners of reproductive potential that effective contraception should be used during and after treatment.

EVOTAZ — atazanavir/cobicistat   Rx

Class: CYP3A inhibitor/protease inhibitor

ADULT DOSAGE	PEDIATRIC DOSAGE
HIV-1 Infection	Pediatric use may not have been established
In Combination w/ Other Antiretroviral Agents in Treatment Naive/Experienced Patients: 1 tab qd	

DOSING CONSIDERATIONS

Concomitant Medications
Dose separation may be required when coadministered w/ H_2-receptor antagonists (H_2RAs) or proton-pump inhibitors (PPIs)

Renal Impairment
CrCl <70mL/min: Coadministration w/ tenofovir disoproxil fumarate (TDF) is not recommended
ESRD on Hemodialysis (Treatment-Experienced Patients): Not recommended

Hepatic Impairment
Not recommended

ADMINISTRATION
Oral route
Take w/ food.

STORAGE
25°C (77°F); excursions permitted to 15-30°C (59-86°F).

HOW SUPPLIED
Tab: (Atazanavir [ATV]/Cobicistat) 300mg/150mg

CONTRAINDICATIONS
Prior significant hypersensitivity (eg, Stevens-Johnson syndrome, erythema multiforme, or toxic skin eruptions) to any of the components of this product. Coadministration w/ drugs that are highly dependent on CYP3A or UGT1A1 for clearance, and for which elevated plasma concentrations of the interacting drugs are associated w/ serious and/or life-threatening events, and w/ strong CYP3A inducers that may lead to lower exposure and loss of efficacy of therapy (alfuzosin, ranolazine, dronedarone, carbamazepine, phenobarbital, phenytoin, colchicine, rifampin, irinotecan, lurasidone, triazolam, oral midazolam, dihydroergotamine, ergotamine, methylergonovine, cisapride, St. John's wort, lovastatin, simvastatin, pimozide, nevirapine, sildenafil [when used for the treatment of pulmonary HTN], indinavir).

WARNINGS/PRECAUTIONS
Use in treatment-experienced patients should be guided by the number of baseline primary protease inhibitor resistance substitutions. Patients w/ underlying hepatitis B or C infections or marked elevations in transaminases may be at increased risk for developing further transaminase elevations or hepatic decompensation. Redistribution/accumulation of body fat reported. Caution in elderly. **ATV:** May prolong the PR interval. 2nd-degree atrioventricular block and other conduction abnormalities reported; consider ECG monitoring in patients w/ preexisting conduction system disease. Cases of Stevens-Johnson syndrome, erythema multiforme, mild-to-moderate maculopapular skin eruptions, and toxic skin eruptions, including drug rash eosinophilia and systemic symptoms (DRESS) syndrome, reported; d/c if severe rash develops. Cases of nephrolithiasis and/or cholelithiasis reported; consider temporary interruption or discontinuation of therapy if signs/symptoms occur. Asymptomatic elevations in indirect (unconjugated) bilirubin may occur. Hepatic transaminase elevations that occur w/ hyperbilirubinemia should be evaluated for alternative etiologies. Consider alternative therapy if jaundice or scleral icterus associated w/ bilirubin elevations presents cosmetic concerns for patients. Immune reconstitution syndrome and autoimmune disorders (eg, Graves' disease, polymyositis, Guillain-Barre syndrome) in the setting of immune reconstitution reported. New-onset or exacerbation of diabetes mellitus (DM), hyperglycemia, and diabetic ketoacidosis reported; may require either initiation or dose adjustments of insulin or oral hypoglycemic agents. Increased bleeding in patients w/ hemophilia A and

B reported. **Cobicistat:** Decreases estimated CrCl w/o affecting actual renal glomerular function; consider effect when interpreting changes in estimated CrCl in patients initiating therapy, particularly w/ medical conditions or receiving drugs needing monitoring w/ estimated CrCl. Closely monitor patients w/ confirmed increase in SrCr >0.4mg/dL from baseline for renal safety. Consider alternative medications that do not require dosage adjustments in patients w/ renal impairment.

ADVERSE REACTIONS
Jaundice, ocular icterus, nausea.

DRUG INTERACTIONS
See Dosing Considerations and Contraindications. Coadministration of therapy w/ TDF in combination w/ concomitant or recent use of a nephrotoxic agent is not recommended. Not recommended w/ products containing the individual components of Evotaz, ritonavir (RTV) or products containing RTV, other antiretroviral drugs that require CYP3A inhibition to achieve adequate exposures (eg, other HIV protease inhibitors, elvitegravir), efavirenz, etravirine, boceprevir, telaprevir, simeprevir, voriconazole, apixaban, rivaroxaban, dabigatran etexilate (in specific renal impairment groups), salmeterol, inhaled/nasal corticosteroids that are metabolized by CYP3A, or avanafil. Not recommended w/ drugs highly dependent on CYP2C8 for clearance w/ narrow therapeutic indices (eg, paclitaxel, repaglinide). Coadministration w/ TDF and H_2RA in treatment-experienced patients is not recommended; administer either at the same time or at a minimum of 10 hrs after H_2RA dose. Coadministration w/ PPIs in treatment-experienced patients is not recommended; give therapy a minimum of 12 hrs after PPI administration in treatment-naive patients. CYP3A4 inhibitors may increase levels. Clarithromycin, erythromycin, telithromycin, ketoconazole, and itraconazole may increase levels; consider alternative antibiotics. Bosentan may decrease levels. CYP3A4 inducers may decrease levels and reduce the therapeutic effect leading to development of resistance to ATV. Anticonvulsants that induce CYP3A (eg, oxcarbazepine) may decrease levels; consider alternative anticonvulsant or antiretroviral therapy, if coadministration is necessary, monitor for lack/loss of virologic response and clinical monitoring of anticonvulsants is recommended. May increase levels of maraviroc, antiarrhythmics, digoxin, clarithromycin, erythromycin, telithromycin, dasatinib, nilotinib, vinblastine, vincristine, anticonvulsants metabolized by CYP3A (eg, clonazepam), TCAs, trazodone, ketoconazole, itraconazole, colchicine, rifabutin, quetiapine, β-blockers, calcium channel blockers, corticosteroids, bosentan, atorvastatin, fluvastatin, pravastatin, rosuvastatin, immunosuppressants (eg, cyclosporine, everolimus, sirolimus, tacrolimus), fentanyl, tramadol, neuroleptics, PDE-5 inhibitors, and sedatives/hypnotics (eg, buspirone, diazepam, zolpidem). May increase levels of drugs that are primarily metabolized by CYP3A, UGT1A1 and/or CYP2D6 or substrates of P-gp, BCRP, OATP1B1, and/or OATP1B3, increasing/prolonging their therapeutic effects and adverse reactions, and requiring dose adjustments and/or additional monitoring of these drugs. Monitor for tenofovir-associated adverse reactions w/ TDF. Monitor INR w/ warfarin. Caution w/ antidepressants (eg, SSRIs, TCAs) and w/ narcotics used for treatment of opioid dependence (buprenorphine, naloxone, methadone). Coadministration w/ corticosteroids that are metabolized by CYP3A, particularly long-term use, may increase the risk for development of systemic corticosteroid effects. Coadministration w/ dexamethasone or other corticosteroids that induce CYP3A may result in loss of therapeutic effect and development of resistance to ATV. Consider alternative nonhormonal forms of contraception if taking hormonal contraceptives. Coadministration w/ parenteral midazolam should be done in a setting that ensures close clinical monitoring and appropriate medical management in case of respiratory depression and/or prolonged sedation. **ATV:** Reduced levels w/ PPIs, antacids, buffered medications, or H_2RAs. Administer a minimum of 2 hrs apart w/ concomitant use of antacids. Coadministration w/ didanosine buffered tabs may decrease atazanavir exposure. Simultaneous coadministration w/ didanosine enteric coated caps and atazanavir w/ food, may decrease didanosine exposure. **Cobicistat:** Renal impairment, including cases of acute renal failure and Fanconi syndrome, reported when used in an antiretroviral regimen containing TDF. Refer to PI for further detailed information on drug interactions, including dosing modifications required when used w/ certain concomitant therapies.

PREGNANCY AND LACTATION
Pregnancy: Category B. Do not use in treatment-experienced pregnant patients taking an H_2RA and/or TDF during the 2nd or 3rd trimester. Physicians are encouraged to register patients who become pregnant in the Antiretroviral Pregnancy Registry.
Lactation: Mothers should be instructed not to breastfeed due to potential for HIV-1 transmission.

MECHANISM OF ACTION
ATV: Protease inhibitor; selectively inhibits the virus-specific processing of viral Gag and Gag-Pol polyproteins in HIV-1 infected cells, thus preventing formation of mature virions. **Cobicistat:** CYP3A inhibitor; increases the systemic exposure of the CYP3A substrate ATV by inhibiting its metabolism.

PHARMACOKINETICS
Absorption: ATV: Rapid. T_{max}=3.5 hrs (median). Cobicistat: (Fed) C_{max}=1.5µg/mL, AUC_{tau}=11.1µg•hr/mL, T_{max}=3 hrs (median). **Distribution:** ATV: Plasma protein binding (86%). Cobicistat: Plasma protein binding (97-98%). **Metabolism:** ATV: Extensive via CYP3A; glucuronidation, N-dealkylation, hydrolysis, and oxygenation w/ dehydrogenation (minor). Cobicistat: CYP3A, CYP2D6 (minor). **Elimination:** ATV: $T_{1/2}$=approx 7.5 hrs (w/ light meal). Cobicistat: Feces (86.2%), urine (8.2%); $T_{1/2}$=approx 3-4 hrs (median).

PATIENT CONSIDERATIONS
Assessment: Assess for previous hypersensitivity to the drug, preexisting conduction system disease, hemophilia, preexisting DM, renal/hepatic impairment, pregnancy/nursing status, and possible drug interactions. Assess estimated

CrCl. Assess for primary protease inhibitor resistance substitutions in treatment-experienced patients. When coadministering w/ TDF, assess estimated CrCl, urine glucose, and urine protein at baseline. Perform baseline hepatic laboratory testing in patients w/ underlying hepatitis B or C infections or marked transaminase elevations.

Monitoring: Monitor for fat redistribution/accumulation, cardiac conduction abnormalities, rash, Stevens-Johnson syndrome, DRESS syndrome, nephrolithiasis, cholelithiasis, hyperbilirubinemia, new onset or exacerbation of DM, hyperglycemia, diabetic ketoacidosis, immune reconstitution syndrome, autoimmune disorders, and other adverse reactions. Monitor for bleeding in patients w/ hemophilia. Perform routine monitoring of estimated CrCl, urine glucose, and urine protein when used w/ TDF. Monitor serum phosphorus levels in patients at risk for renal impairment when used w/ TDF. Perform hepatic laboratory testing in patients w/ underlying hepatitis B or C infections or marked transaminase elevations.

Counseling: Inform that therapy is not a cure for HIV and that illnesses associated w/ HIV may continue. Advise to remain under the care of a physician during therapy. Advise to avoid activities that can spread HIV infection to others. Instruct to take ud and not to d/c therapy w/o consulting physician. Advise not to miss a dose, but if a dose is missed by ≤12 hrs, instruct to take the missed dose right away and take next dose at the usual time, or if missed by >12 hrs, instruct to wait and take next dose at the usual time and not to double next dose. Inform of the potential for serious drug interactions, and explain that some drugs should not be taken concomitantly, or some drugs may need a change in dose. Advise to report use of any prescription/nonprescription medication or herbal products, particularly St. John's wort. Instruct patients receiving hormonal contraceptives to use additional or alternative nonhormonal contraceptive measures during therapy. Inform that therapy may produce ECG changes; advise to consult physician if symptoms (eg, dizziness, lightheadedness) are experienced. Inform that mild rashes w/o other symptoms and severe skin reactions have been reported; advise to immediately contact physician if signs/symptoms of severe skin/hypersensitivity reactions develop. Inform that kidney stones and/or gallstones, and fat redistribution/accumulation have been reported. Inform that asymptomatic elevations in indirect bilirubin accompanied by yellowing of the skin or whites of the eyes have occurred and that alternative antiretroviral therapy may be considered if patients have cosmetic concerns.

Evzio — naloxone hydrochloride   Rx

Class: Opioid antagonist

ADULT DOSAGE	**PEDIATRIC DOSAGE**
Opioid Overdose	**Opioid Overdose**
Emergency treatment of known or suspected opioid overdose, as manifested by respiratory and/or CNS depression	Emergency treatment of known or suspected opioid overdose, as manifested by respiratory and/or CNS depression
Administer initial dose (0.4mg) IM/SQ into the anterolateral aspect of the thigh, through clothing if necessary, and seek emergency medical assistance	Administer initial dose (0.4mg) IM/SQ into the anterolateral aspect of the thigh, through clothing if necessary, and seek emergency medical assistance
If desired response is not obtained after 2 or 3 min, may administer another dose; if there is still no response and additional doses are available, may administer additional doses every 2-3 min until emergency medical assistance arrives	If desired response is not obtained after 2 or 3 min, may administer another dose; if there is still no response and additional doses are available, may administer additional doses every 2-3 min until emergency medical assistance arrives
Reversal of respiratory depression by partial agonists or mixed agonists/antagonists (eg, buprenorphine, pentazocine) may be incomplete or require higher doses of naloxone	Reversal of respiratory depression by partial agonists or mixed agonists/antagonists (eg, buprenorphine, pentazocine) may be incomplete or require higher doses of naloxone

ADMINISTRATION
IM/SQ route

For single use only; do not attempt to reuse
If voice instruction system does not operate properly, device will still deliver intended dose when properly administered
Once the red safety guard is removed, use immediately or dispose properly; do not attempt to replace the red safety guard once it is removed
Upon actuation, the needle is automatically inserted and delivers 0.4mg naloxone inj, then the needle is fully retracted into its housing

Pediatrics
<1 Year: Caregiver should pinch the thigh muscle while administering the treatment

STORAGE
15-25°C (59-77°F); excursions permitted between 4-40°C (39-104°F).

HOW SUPPLIED
Inj: 0.4mg/0.4mL

CONTRAINDICATIONS
Known hypersensitivity to naloxone HCl or to any of the other ingredients.

WARNINGS/PRECAUTIONS
Not a substitute for emergency medical care. May precipitate an acute abstinence syndrome in patients who are opioid dependent. In neonates, opioid withdrawal

may be life-threatening if not recognized and properly treated; signs and symptoms may include convulsions, excessive crying, and hyperactive reflexes. Abrupt postoperative reversal of opioid depression may result in N/V, sweating, tremulousness, tachycardia, hypotension, HTN, seizures, ventricular tachycardia and fibrillation, pulmonary edema, and cardiac arrest; caution in patients w/ preexisting cardiac disease or who have received medications w/ potential adverse cardiovascular effects.

ADVERSE REACTIONS
Hypotension, HTN, ventricular tachycardia and fibrillation, dyspnea, pulmonary edema, cardiac arrest.

PREGNANCY AND LACTATION
Category B, caution in nursing.

MECHANISM OF ACTION
Opioid antagonist; antagonizes opioid effects by competing for the same receptor sites.

PHARMACOKINETICS
Absorption: T_{max}=15 min (median); C_{max}=1.24ng/mL. **Distribution:** Crosses placenta. **Metabolism:** Liver, primarily by glucuronide conjugation; naloxone-3-glucuronide (major metabolite). **Elimination:** Urine (25-40% metabolites w/ in 6 hrs, 50% in 24 hrs, 60-70% in 72 hrs) (PO/IV); $T_{1/2}$=1.28 hrs (adults), 3.1 hrs (neonates).

PATIENT CONSIDERATIONS

Assessment: Assess for hypersensitivity to drug, opioid dependence, cardiac disease, and pregnancy/nursing status.

Monitoring: Monitor for precipitation of opioid withdrawal and for other adverse reactions.

Counseling: Instruct patients, family members, and caregivers on how to recognize the signs/symptoms of an opioid overdose requiring the use of drug, and how to properly use it. Instruct to seek emergency medical assistance after administering the 1st dose. Advise that the reversal of respiratory depression by partial agonists or mixed agonist/antagonists may be incomplete. Inform that use in patients who are opioid dependent may precipitate an acute abstinence syndrome.

Exalgo — hydromorphone hydrochloride   CII

Class: Opioid analgesic

> Exposes patients and other users to the risks of opioid addiction, abuse, and misuse, potentially leading to overdose and death; assess each patient's risk prior to prescribing, and monitor regularly for development of these behaviors/conditions. Serious, life-threatening, or fatal respiratory depression may occur; monitor for occurrence, especially during initiation or following a dose increase. Crushing, dissolving, or chewing tabs can cause rapid release and absorption of potentially fatal dose; instruct to swallow tabs whole. Accidental ingestion, especially in children, can result in a fatal overdose. Prolonged use during pregnancy can result in neonatal opioid withdrawal syndrome.

ADULT DOSAGE	**PEDIATRIC DOSAGE**
Severe Pain (Daily, Around-the-Clock Management)	Pediatric use may not have been established
Opioid-Tolerant:	
>17 Years:	
D/C or taper all other extended-release opioids	
Conversion from Other Oral Hydromorphone Formulations to Exalgo:	
Initial: Administer starting dose equivalent to patient's total daily oral hydromorphone dose, given once daily	
Conversion from Other Oral Opioids to Exalgo:	
Initial: 50% of the calculated estimate of daily hydromorphone requirement using the appropriate conversion factor	
On a Single Opioid: Sum the current total daily dose of the opioid, then multiply the total daily dose by the conversion factor to calculate the approx oral hydromorphone daily dose	
On Regimen of >1 Opioid: Calculate the approx oral hydromorphone dose for each opioid and sum the totals to obtain the approx total hydromorphone daily dose	
On Regimen of Fixed-Ratio Opioid/Nonopioid Analgesic Products: Use only the opioid component of these products in the conversion	
Approx Oral Conversion Factor to Exalgo:	
Always round the dose down, if necessary to appropriate Exalgo strengths available	
Prior Oral Opioid: Approx Oral Conversion Factor	
Hydromorphone: 1	
Codeine: 0.06	

Hydrocodone: 0.4
Methadone: 0.6
Morphine: 0.2
Oxycodone: 0.4
Oxymorphone: 0.6

Close observation and frequent titration are warranted until pain management is stable on the new opioid

From Transdermal Fentanyl:
Initiate treatment 18 hrs following removal of transdermal fentanyl patch
Calculate 24-hr hydromorphone dose by using a conversion factor of 25mcg/hr fentanyl transdermal patch to 12mg of hydromorphone, then reduce dose by 50%

- -

DOSING CONSIDERATIONS
Renal Impairment
Moderate: Start w/ 50% of dose
Severe: Start w/ 25% of dose; consider use of an alternate analgesic that may permit more flexibility w/ dosing interval
Closely monitor for respiratory and CNS depression during initiation and dose titration

Hepatic Impairment
Moderate: Start w/ 25% of dose; closely monitor for respiratory and CNS depression during initiation and dose titration
Severe: Use of alternate analgesics is recommended

Discontinuation
Taper dose gradually by 25-50% every 2-3 days down to a dose of 8mg before discontinuation of therapy to prevent signs and symptoms of withdrawal

ADMINISTRATION
Oral route

Swallow tabs whole; do not crush, dissolve, or chew
May be administered w/o regard to meals

Disposal
Flush all remaining tabs down the toilet or remit to authorities at a certified drug take-back program

STORAGE
25°C (77°F); excursions permitted to 15-30°C (59-86°F).

HOW SUPPLIED
Tab, Extended-Release (ER): 8mg, 12mg, 16mg, 32mg

CONTRAINDICATIONS
Opioid nontolerant patients, significant respiratory depression, acute or severe bronchial asthma in unmonitored settings or in the absence of resuscitative equipment, known or suspected paralytic ileus, previous surgical procedures and/or underlying disease resulting in narrowing of the GI tract, or "blind loops" of the GI tract or GI obstruction, hypersensitivity (eg, anaphylaxis) to hydromorphone or sulfite-containing medications.

WARNINGS/PRECAUTIONS
Reserve use in patients for whom alternative treatment options are ineffective, not tolerated, or would be otherwise inadequate to provide sufficient management of pain. Should only be prescribed by healthcare professionals knowledgeable in the use of potent opioids for the management of chronic pain. Do not begin as the 1st opioid. Not indicated as a PRN analgesic. Overestimating the dose when converting from another opioid product may result in fatal overdose with the 1st dose. Life-threatening respiratory depression is more likely to occur in elderly, cachectic, or debilitated patients. Consider alternative nonopioid analgesics in patients with significant chronic obstructive pulmonary disease (COPD) or cor pulmonale, and in patients having a substantially decreased respiratory reserve, hypoxia, hypercapnia, or preexisting respiratory depression. May cause severe hypotension including orthostatic hypotension and syncope in ambulatory patients; increased risk in patients whose ability to maintain BP has already been compromised. Monitor for signs of sedation and respiratory depression in patients who may be susceptible to the intracranial effects of carbon dioxide retention (eg, those with increased intracranial pressure [ICP] or brain tumors). May obscure clinical course in patients with head injury. Avoid with impaired consciousness or coma. May cause spasm of the sphincter of Oddi; monitor for worsening of symptoms in patients with biliary tract disease, including acute pancreatitis. Contains sodium metabisulfite; may cause allergic-type reactions in certain susceptible people. May aggravate convulsions with convulsive disorders, and may induce or aggravate seizures; monitor for worsened seizure control in patients with history of seizure disorders. Avoid abrupt discontinuation; taper dose gradually. May impair mental/physical abilities. Not for use during and immediately prior to labor. Caution in elderly.

ADVERSE REACTIONS
Respiratory depression, constipation, N/V, somnolence, headache, asthenia, dizziness, diarrhea, pruritus, insomnia, anorexia, hyperhidrosis, dry mouth, peripheral edema, abdominal pain.

DRUG INTERACTIONS
Concomitant use with alcohol and other CNS depressants (eg, sedatives, hypnotics, neuroleptics, general anesthetics) may increase the risk of respiratory depression, hypotension, profound sedation, coma, and death; reduce dose of one or both drugs when combined therapy is considered. Monitor elderly, cachectic, and debilitated patients closely when coadministered with other drugs that depress respiration. Mixed agonist/antagonist (eg, pentazocine, nalbuphine, butorphanol) and partial agonist (eg, buprenorphine) analgesics may reduce the analgesic effect or precipitate withdrawal symptoms; avoid coadministration. Not recommended for use in patients who have received MAOIs within 14 days; if concurrent therapy is unavoidable, monitor patients for increased respiratory and CNS depression. Anticholinergics or other medications with anticholinergic activity may increase risk of urinary retention and/or severe constipation, which may lead to paralytic ileus.

PREGNANCY AND LACTATION
Category C, not for use in nursing.

MECHANISM OF ACTION
Opioid analgesic; has not been established. Thought to be mediated through opioid-specific receptors located predominantly in the CNS.

PHARMACOKINETICS
Absorption: Administration of variable doses resulted in different parameters. **Distribution:** Plasma protein binding (27%); (IV) V_d=2.9L/kg; crosses placenta, found in breast milk. **Metabolism:** Liver (extensive) via glucuronidation; hydromorphone-3-glucuronide (metabolite). **Elimination:** Urine (75%, 7% unchanged), feces (1% unchanged); $T_{1/2}$ varies based on dosing; refer to PI for further information.

PATIENT CONSIDERATIONS

Assessment: Assess for abuse/addiction risk, opioid tolerance, prior opioid therapy, drug hypersensitivity, increased ICP, brain tumor, respiratory depression, COPD or other respiratory complications, GI obstruction, paralytic ileus, history of seizures, renal/hepatic impairment, pregnancy/nursing status, possible drug interactions, and any other conditions where treatment is contraindicated or cautioned.

Monitoring: Monitor for signs/symptoms of respiratory depression (especially within first 24-72 hrs of initiation), physical dependence, tolerance, hypotension, syncope, aggravation/induction of seizures, symptoms of worsening biliary tract disease, mental/physical impairment, and other adverse reactions. Routinely monitor for signs of addiction, abuse, or misuse. Periodically reassess the continued need for therapy.

Counseling: Inform that use of drug may result in addiction, abuse, and misuse; instruct not to share with others and to take steps to protect from theft or misuse. Inform of the risk of life-threatening respiratory depression; advise how to recognize respiratory depression and to seek medical attention if experiencing breathing difficulties. Inform that accidental ingestion, especially in children, may result in respiratory depression or death; instruct to store securely and dispose unused tab by flushing down the toilet. Inform female patients of reproductive potential that prolonged use of drug during pregnancy may result in neonatal opioid withdrawal syndrome and instruct to inform physician if pregnant or planning to become pregnant. Inform that potentially serious additive effects may occur if drug is used with alcohol or other CNS depressants, and advise not to use such drugs unless supervised by a healthcare provider. Inform of the proper administration instructions. Advise that patients with certain stomach or intestinal problems may be at higher risk of developing a blockage; instruct to contact healthcare provider immediately if symptoms develop. Inform that drug may cause orthostatic hypotension and syncope; instruct how to recognize symptoms of low BP and how to reduce the risk of serious consequences should hypotension occur. Inform that drug may impair the ability to perform potentially hazardous activities; advise not to perform such tasks until they know how they will react to the medication. Advise of potential for severe constipation, including management instructions. Advise how to recognize anaphylaxis and when to seek medical attention.

- -

EXELDERM — sulconazole nitrate   **Rx**

Class: Azole antifungal

ADULT DOSAGE	PEDIATRIC DOSAGE
Fungal Infections	Pediatric use may not have been established
Tinea Cruris, Tinea Corporis, and Tinea Versicolor:	
Gently massage a small amount into the affected and surrounding skin areas qd or bid for 3 weeks	
Tinea Pedis:	
Cre:	
Gently massage a small amount into the affected and surrounding skin areas bid for 4 weeks	
Consider an alternate diagnosis if significant clinical improvement is not seen after 4 weeks of treatment (sol) or 4-6 weeks of treatment (cre)	

- -

ADMINISTRATION
Topical route

STORAGE
Avoid excessive heat, >40°C (104°F). **Sol:** Protect from light.

HOW SUPPLIED
Cre: 1% [15g, 30g, 60g]; **Sol:** 1% [30mL]

CONTRAINDICATIONS
History of hypersensitivity to any of the ingredients in the medication.

WARNINGS/PRECAUTIONS
Not for ophthalmic use. For external use only. Avoid contact w/ eyes. D/C and institute appropriate therapy if irritation develops.

ADVERSE REACTIONS
Itching, burning, stinging.

PREGNANCY AND LACTATION
Pregnancy: Category C.
Lactation: Caution in nursing.

MECHANISM OF ACTION
Imidazole derivative; broad-spectrum antifungal agent that inhibits the growth of the common pathogenic dermatophytes. Also inhibits the organism responsible for tinea versicolor, *Malassezia furfur*.

PATIENT CONSIDERATIONS
Assessment: Assess for history of hypersensitivity to drug and pregnancy/nursing status.

Monitoring: Monitor for irritation and other adverse reactions. Consider an alternate diagnosis if no significant clinical improvement is seen after 4 weeks (sol) or 4-6 weeks (cre) of therapy.

Counseling: Instruct to use externally ud and to avoid contact w/ eyes. Advise to d/c use and notify physician if irritation develops.

EXELON — rivastigmine　　　Rx
Class: Acetylcholinesterase (AChE) inhibitor

ADULT DOSAGE

Alzheimer's Disease

Cap/Sol:
Mild to Moderate Dementia:
Initial: 1.5mg bid
Titrate: May increase to 3mg bid after at least 2 weeks; subsequent increases to 4.5mg bid and 6mg bid should be attempted after a minimum of 2 weeks at the previous dose
Usual: 6-12mg/day (3-6mg bid)
Max: 12mg/day (6mg bid)

Patch:
Mild to Moderate Dementia:
Initial: Apply one 4.6mg/24 hrs patch qd
Titrate: Increase dose only after a minimum of 4 weeks at the previous dose
Maint: 9.5mg/24 hrs qd or 13.3mg/24 hrs qd
Max: 13.3mg/24 hrs

Severe Dementia:
Initial: Apply one 4.6mg/24 hrs patch qd
Titrate: Increase dose only after a minimum of 4 weeks at the previous dose
Maint: 13.3mg/24 hrs qd
Max: 13.3mg/24 hrs

Parkinson's Disease

Mild to Moderate Dementia:
Cap/Sol:
Initial: 1.5mg bid
Titrate: May increase to 3mg bid after at least 4 weeks; subsequent increases to 4.5mg bid and 6mg bid should be attempted after a minimum of 4 weeks at the previous dose
Max: 12mg/day (6mg bid)

Patch:
Initial: Apply one 4.6mg/24 hrs patch qd
Titrate: Increase dose only after a minimum of 4 weeks at the previous dose
Maint: 9.5mg/24 hrs qd or 13.3mg/24 hrs qd
Max: 13.3mg/24 hrs

Conversions
Switching to Patch from Cap/Sol:
Total Daily PO Dose <6mg: 4.6mg/24 hrs patch
Total Daily PO Dose 6-12mg: 9.5mg/24 hrs patch

Apply 1st patch on the day following the last oral dose

PEDIATRIC DOSAGE
Pediatric use may not have been established

DOSING CONSIDERATIONS
Renal Impairment
Moderate to Severe:
Cap/Sol: May only be able to tolerate lower doses

Hepatic Impairment
Mild to Moderate (Child-Pugh 5-9):
Cap/Sol: May only be able to tolerate lower doses
Patch: Consider using the 4.6mg/24 hrs patch as both initial and maint dose

Adverse Reactions
Treatment Interruption w/ Adverse Reactions:
Cap/Sol:
≤3-Day Interruption: Restart treatment w/ same or lower dose
>3-Day Interruption: Restart treatment w/ 1.5mg bid and titrate
Patch:
≤3-Day Interruption: Restart w/ same or lower strength patch
>3-Day Interruption: Restart w/ 4.6mg/24 hrs patch and titrate

Other Important Considerations
Low Body Weight (<50kg):
Cap/Sol: Consider reducing dose if toxicities develop
Patch: Consider reducing maint dose to the 4.6mg/24 hrs patch if toxicities develop

ADMINISTRATION
Oral/Transdermal route

Oral
Take w/ meals in divided doses in am and pm.
Cap and sol may be interchanged at equal doses.

Oral Sol Administration Instructions:
Remove the oral dosing syringe provided in its protective case, and using the provided syringe, withdraw the prescribed amount of sol from container.
Each dose of sol may be swallowed directly from the syringe or 1st mixed w/ a small glass of water, cold fruit juice, or soda.

Patch
Do not use the patch if the pouch seal is broken or the patch is cut, damaged, or changed in any way.
Apply once a day; press down firmly for 30 sec until the edges stick well when applying to clean, dry, hairless, intact, healthy skin in a place that will not be rubbed against by tight clothing.
Use the upper or lower back as the site of application. If sites on the back are not accessible, apply the patch to the upper arm or chest; do not apply to a skin area where cre, lotion, or powder has recently been applied.
Do not apply to skin that is red, irritated, or cut.
Replace w/ a new patch every 24 hrs. Instruct patients to only wear 1 patch at a time. If a patch falls off or if a dose is missed, apply a new patch immediately and then replace this patch the following day at the usual application time.
Change the site of patch application daily, although a new patch can be applied to the same general area (eg, another spot on the upper back) on consecutive days.
Do not apply a new patch to the same location for at least 14 days.
Patch may be worn during bathing and in hot weather; avoid long exposure to external heat sources (excessive sunlight, saunas, solariums).
Place used patches in the previously saved pouch and discard in the trash, away from pets or children.

STORAGE
25°C (77°F); excursions permitted to 15-30°C (59-86°F). **Oral Sol:** Store in upright position and protect from freezing. Stable for up to 4 hrs at room temperature if combined w/ cold fruit juice or soda. **Patch:** Keep in sealed pouch until use.

HOW SUPPLIED
Cap: 1.5mg, 3mg, 4.5mg, 6mg; **Oral Sol:** 2mg/mL [120mL]; **Patch:** 4.6mg/24 hrs, 9.5mg/24 hrs, 13.3mg/24 hrs [30^S]

CONTRAINDICATIONS
Known hypersensitivity to rivastigmine, other carbamate derivatives, or other components of the formulation. Previous history of application-site reactions w/ rivastigmine transdermal patch suggestive of allergic contact dermatitis. **Oral:** In the absence of negative allergy testing.

WARNINGS/PRECAUTIONS
May cause dose-related GI adverse reactions (eg, significant N/V, diarrhea, anorexia/decreased appetite, and weight loss). Disseminated allergic dermatitis irrespective of route of administration reported; d/c if these occur. In patients who develop application-site reactions to patch suggestive of allergic contact dermatitis and who still require therapy, switch to oral therapy only after negative allergy testing and under close medical supervision. May increase gastric acid secretion; monitor for symptoms of active/occult bleeding. Caution in those at increased risk of developing ulcers. May have vagotonic effects on HR (eg, bradycardia), which may be particularly important in sick sinus syndrome or supraventricular cardiac conduction conditions. May cause urinary obstruction and seizures. Caution in patients w/ asthma and obstructive pulmonary disease. May exacerbate or induce extrapyramidal symptoms and impair mental/physical abilities. Caution in patients w/ low or high body weights. **Oral:** Syncopal episodes reported. Worsening of parkinsonian symptoms, particularly tremor, observed in patients treated w/ cap. **Patch:** Skin application-site reactions may occur. Allergic contact dermatitis should be suspected if application-site reactions spread beyond the patch size; d/c treatment if there is evidence of more intense local reaction (eg, increasing erythema, edema, papules), and if symptoms do not significantly improve w/in 48 hrs after patch removal.

ADVERSE REACTIONS
N/V, anxiety, decreased weight, anorexia, headache, dizziness, fatigue, diarrhea, depression, asthenia, tremor, dyspepsia. **Oral:** Abdominal pain.

DRUG INTERACTIONS

Increased risk of additive extrapyramidal adverse reactions w/ metoclopramide; avoid concomitant use. May increase cholinergic effects of other cholinomimetics and may interfere w/ the activity of anticholinergics (eg, oxybutynin, tolterodine); avoid concomitant use unless clinically necessary. Additive bradycardic effects resulting in syncope may occur w/ β-blockers, especially cardioselective β-blockers (eg, atenolol); avoid concomitant use. May exaggerate succinylcholine-type muscle relaxation during anesthesia. Caution w/ NSAIDs; monitor for symptoms of active/occult bleeding.

PREGNANCY AND LACTATION

Category B, not for use in nursing.

MECHANISM OF ACTION

Reversible cholinesterase inhibitor; has not been established, but suspected to enhance cholinergic function by increasing concentration of acetylcholine through reversible inhibition of its hydrolysis by cholinesterase.

PHARMACOKINETICS

Absorption: (Patch) T_{max}=8-16 hrs. (Oral) Rapid, complete; absolute bioavailability (36%) (3mg); T_{max}=1 hr. **Distribution:** V_d=1.8-2.7L/kg; plasma protein binding (40%). **Metabolism:** Rapid and extensive; cholinesterase-mediated hydrolysis. **Elimination:** (Oral) Urine (97%, 40% sulfate conjugate of decarbamylated metabolite), feces (0.4%); $T_{1/2}$=1.5 hrs. (Patch) Urine (>90%), feces (<1%); $T_{1/2}$=3 hrs after patch removal.

PATIENT CONSIDERATIONS

Assessment: Assess for hypersensitivity to drug, history of GI ulcer disease, sick sinus syndrome, supraventricular cardiac conduction conditions, asthma or obstructive pulmonary disease, pregnancy/nursing status, and possible drug interactions. Assess body weight, for history of application-site reactions w/ rivastigmine patch suggestive of allergic contact dermatitis, and hepatic impairment. **Oral:** Assess for renal impairment.

Monitoring: Monitor for signs/symptoms of active or occult GI bleeding, hypersensitivity reactions, extrapyramidal symptoms, urinary obstruction, seizures, GI adverse events, cardiac conduction effects, and other adverse reactions. Closely monitor patients w/ high or low body weight. Monitor for toxicities (eg, excessive N/V) in patients w/ low body weight. **Patch:** Monitor for skin reactions (allergic contact dermatitis).

Counseling: Instruct caregivers to monitor for GI adverse reactions and to inform physician if these occur. Inform that allergic skin reactions have been reported regardless of formulation; instruct to consult physician immediately in case of skin reaction while on therapy. Instruct to d/c if disseminated skin hypersensitivity reaction occurs. Advise that therapy may exacerbate or induce extrapyramidal symptoms. **Patch:** Instruct to rotate application site, not to use the same site w/in 14 days, to replace patch q24h at consistent time of day, and to wear only 1 patch at a time. Instruct to avoid exposure to external heat for long periods. Instruct on proper usage and discarding of patch. In case of accidental contact w/ eyes or if eyes become red after handling the patch, instruct to rinse immediately w/ plenty of water and seek medical advice if symptoms do not resolve. Advise not to take rivastigmine cap or oral sol, or other drugs w/ cholinergic effects while wearing patch. Instruct to inform physician if application-site reactions spread beyond the patch size, if there is evidence of more intense local reaction, and if symptoms do not significantly improve w/in 48 hrs after patch removal.

EXFORGE — amlodipine/valsartan   Rx

Class: Angiotensin II receptor blocker (ARB)/calcium channel blocker (CCB) (dihydropyridine)

> D/C therapy as soon as possible when pregnancy is detected. Drugs that act directly on the renin-angiotensin system (RAS) can cause injury/death to the developing fetus.

ADULT DOSAGE
Hypertension

Initial Therapy:

Initial: 5mg/160mg qd in patients who are not volume-depleted
Titrate: May increase after 1-2 weeks
Max: 10mg/320mg qd

Add-On Therapy:
May be used if BP is not adequately controlled w/ amlodipine (or another dihydropyridine calcium channel blocker) or valsartan (or another ARB) alone. Patients w/ dose-limiting adverse reactions to either component alone may be switched to therapy containing a lower dose of that component in combination w/ the other to achieve similar BP reductions.
Titrate: May increase dose if BP remains uncontrolled after 3-4 weeks
Max: 10mg/320mg qd

Replacement Therapy:
May substitute for individually titrated components

May be administered w/ other antihypertensive agents

PEDIATRIC DOSAGE
Pediatric use may not have been established

DOSING CONSIDERATIONS
Hepatic Impairment
Initial: 2.5mg of amlodipine
Elderly
Initial: 2.5mg of amlodipine

ADMINISTRATION
Oral route
Take w/ or w/o food.

STORAGE
25°C (77°F); excursions permitted to 15-30°C (59-86°F). Protect from moisture.

HOW SUPPLIED
Tab: (Amlodipine/Valsartan) 5mg/160mg, 10mg/160mg, 5mg/320mg, 10mg/320mg

CONTRAINDICATIONS
Known hypersensitivity to any component, coadministration w/ aliskiren in patients w/ diabetes.

WARNINGS/PRECAUTIONS
Excessive hypotension reported. Symptomatic hypotension may occur in patients w/ an activated RAS (eg, volume- and/or salt-depleted patients receiving high doses of diuretics); correct volume depletion prior to therapy. Initiate therapy cautiously in patients w/ heart failure (HF) or recent MI, and in patients undergoing surgery/dialysis. Changes in renal function may occur; consider withholding or discontinuing therapy if clinically significant decrease in renal function develops. Patients whose renal function may depend in part on the activity of the RAS (eg, patients w/ renal artery stenosis, chronic kidney disease, severe CHF, volume depletion) may be at particular risk of developing acute renal failure; periodically monitor renal function in these patients. Hyperkalemia may occur; dose reduction and/or discontinuation of therapy may be required. **Amlodipine:** Acute hypotension reported (rare); caution w/ severe aortic stenosis. Worsening angina and acute MI may develop after starting or increasing dose, particularly w/ severe obstructive coronary artery disease (CAD). **Valsartan:** Increases in K^+ reported in some patients w/ HF; more likely to occur in patients w/ preexisting renal impairment.

ADVERSE REACTIONS
Peripheral edema, nasopharyngitis, URTI, dizziness.

DRUG INTERACTIONS
See Contraindications. **Amlodipine:** CYP3A inhibitors (moderate and strong) increased systemic exposure and may require dose reduction; monitor for symptoms of hypotension and edema to determine the need for dose adjustment. Monitor BP closely when coadministered w/ CYP3A inducers. Monitor for hypotension when coadministered w/ sildenafil. Increases systemic exposure of simvastatin; limit simvastatin dose to 20mg/day. May increase systemic exposure of cyclosporine or tacrolimus; frequently monitor trough levels of cyclosporine and tacrolimus and adjust dose when appropriate. **Valsartan:** NSAIDs, including selective COX-2 inhibitors, may attenuate antihypertensive effect and result in deterioration of renal function, including possible acute renal failure; monitor renal function periodically. Concomitant use w/ other agents that block the RAS, K^+-sparing diuretics (eg, spironolactone, triamterene, amiloride), K^+ supplements, salt substitutes containing K^+, or other drugs that may increase K^+ levels (eg, heparin) may lead to increases in serum K^+, and in HF patients to increases in SrCr; monitor serum K^+ if comedication is necessary. Inhibitors of the hepatic uptake transporter OATP1B1 (rifampin, cyclosporine) or the hepatic efflux transporter MRP2 (ritonavir) may increase systemic exposure. Dual blockade of the RAS is associated w/ increased risks of hypotension, hyperkalemia, and changes in renal function (including acute renal failure); in general, avoid combined use of RAS inhibitors, or closely monitor BP, renal function, and electrolytes w/ concomitant agents that affect the RAS. Avoid w/ aliskiren in patients w/ renal impairment (GFR <60mL/min). Increases in lithium levels and lithium toxicity reported; monitor serum lithium levels during concomitant use.

PREGNANCY AND LACTATION
Pregnancy: Category D.
Lactation: Not for use in nursing.

MECHANISM OF ACTION
Amlodipine: Dihydropyridine CCB; inhibits Ca^{2+} ion influx across cell membranes selectively, w/ a greater effect on vascular smooth muscle cells than on cardiac muscle cells. Peripheral arterial vasodilator that acts directly on vascular smooth muscle to cause a reduction in peripheral vascular resistance and reduction in BP. **Valsartan:** ARB; blocks the vasoconstrictor and aldosterone-secreting effects of angiotensin II by selectively blocking the binding of angiotensin II to the AT_1 receptor in many tissues (eg, vascular smooth muscle, adrenal gland).

PHARMACOKINETICS
Absorption: Amlodipine: Absolute bioavailability (64-90%); T_{max}=6-12 hrs. Valsartan: Absolute bioavailability (25%); T_{max}=2-4 hrs. **Distribution:** Amlodipine: V_d=21L/kg; plasma protein binding (93%). Valsartan: (IV) V_d=17L; plasma protein binding (95%). **Metabolism:** Amlodipine: Hepatic (extensive). Valsartan: Via CYP2C9; valeryl 4-hydroxy valsartan (primary metabolite). **Elimination:** Amlodipine: Urine (10% unchanged, 60% metabolites); $T_{1/2}$=30-50 hrs. Valsartan: (Oral Sol) Feces (83%), urine (13%); (IV) $T_{1/2}$=6 hrs.

PATIENT CONSIDERATIONS
Assessment: Assess for hypersensitivity to any component of the drug, volume/salt depletion, HF, recent MI, renal artery stenosis, severe aortic stenosis, severe obstructive CAD, renal/hepatic impairment, pregnancy/nursing status, and possible drug interactions.

Monitoring: Monitor for signs/symptoms of hypotension, hyperkalemia, hypersensitivity reactions, and other adverse reactions. Monitor for symptoms of angina or MI, particularly in patients w/ severe obstructive CAD, after initiation of therapy or dose increase. Monitor BP, serum electrolytes, and renal function.

Counseling: Counsel about risks/benefits of therapy. Inform females of childbearing age about the consequences of exposure to therapy during pregnancy; discuss treatment options w/ women planning to become pregnant. Instruct to report pregnancies to physician as soon as possible.

EXFORGE HCT — amlodipine/hydrochlorothiazide/valsartan   Rx

Class: Angiotensin II receptor blocker (ARB)/calcium channel blocker (CCB) (dihydropyridine)/ thiazide diuretic

> D/C therapy as soon as possible when pregnancy is detected. Drugs that act directly on the renin-angiotensin system (RAS) can cause injury/death to the developing fetus.

ADULT DOSAGE

Hypertension
Usual: Dose qd
Titrate: May increase dose after 2 weeks
Max: 10mg/320mg/25mg qd

Add-On/Switch Therapy:
May use for patients not adequately controlled on any 2 of the following classes: CCBs, ARBs, and diuretics. Patients w/ dose-limiting adverse reactions to an individual component while on any dual combination of the components of therapy may be switched to therapy containing a lower dose of that component

Replacement Therapy:
May substitute for individually titrated components

May be administered w/ other antihypertensive agents

PEDIATRIC DOSAGE
Pediatric use may not have been established

DOSING CONSIDERATIONS
Hepatic Impairment
Initial: 2.5mg of amlodipine

Elderly
Initial: 2.5mg of amlodipine

ADMINISTRATION
Oral route
Take w/ or w/o food.

STORAGE
25°C (77°F); excursions permitted to 15-30°C (59-86°F). Protect from moisture.

HOW SUPPLIED
Tab: (Amlodipine/Valsartan/Hydrochlorothiazide [HCTZ]) 5mg/160mg/12.5mg, 5mg/160mg/25mg, 10mg/160mg/12.5mg, 10mg/160mg/25mg, 10mg/320mg/25mg

CONTRAINDICATIONS
Anuria, sulfonamide-derived drug hypersensitivity, hypersensitivity to any component of the product, coadministration w/ aliskiren in patients w/ diabetes.

WARNINGS/PRECAUTIONS
This fixed combination drug is not indicated for initial therapy of HTN. Excessive hypotension, including orthostatic hypotension, reported. Symptomatic hypotension may occur in patients w/ an activated RAS (eg, volume- and/or salt-depleted patients receiving high doses of diuretics); correct this condition prior to therapy. Avoid w/ aortic or mitral stenosis or obstructive hypertrophic cardiomyopathy. Changes in renal function, including acute renal failure, may occur; consider withholding or discontinuing therapy if clinically significant decrease in renal function develops. Patients whose renal function may depend in part on the activity of the RAS (eg, patients w/ renal artery stenosis, chronic kidney disease, severe CHF, volume depletion) may be at particular risk of developing acute renal failure; periodically monitor renal function in these patients. Hyperkalemia may occur. HCTZ may cause hypokalemia, hyponatremia, and hypomagnesemia. D/C therapy if hypokalemia is accompanied by clinical signs (eg, muscular weakness, paresis, ECG alterations); correct hypokalemia and any coexisting hypomagnesemia prior to the initiation of thiazides.
Amlodipine: Worsening angina and acute MI may develop after starting or increasing dose, particularly in patients w/ severe obstructive coronary artery disease (CAD). **Valsartan:** Increases in K+ reported in some patients w/ heart failure (HF), and are more likely to occur in patients w/ preexisting renal impairment; dose reduction and/or discontinuation of diuretic and/or valsartan may be required. **HCTZ:** May cause hypersensitivity reactions and exacerbation/ activation of systemic lupus erythematosus (SLE). May alter glucose tolerance and increase serum cholesterol and TG levels. May cause or exacerbate hyperuricemia and precipitate gout in susceptible patients. Decreases urinary Ca^{2+} excretion and may cause elevations of serum Ca^{2+}; monitor Ca^{2+} levels in patients w/ hypercalcemia. May cause idiosyncratic reaction, resulting in acute transient myopia and acute angle-closure glaucoma; d/c as rapidly as possible. Minor alterations of fluid and electrolyte balance may precipitate hepatic coma in patients w/ impaired hepatic function or progressive liver disease.

ADVERSE REACTIONS
Dizziness, edema, headache, dyspepsia, fatigue, muscle spasms, back pain, nausea, nasopharyngitis.

DRUG INTERACTIONS
See Contraindications. **Amlodipine:** CYP3A inhibitors (moderate and strong) increased systemic exposure and may require dose reduction; monitor for symptoms of hypotension and edema to determine the need for dose adjustment. Monitor BP closely when coadministered w/ CYP3A inducers. Monitor for hypotension when coadministered w/ sildenafil. Increases systemic exposure of simvastatin; limit simvastatin dose to 20mg/day. May increase systemic exposure of cyclosporine or tacrolimus; frequently monitor trough levels of cyclosporine and tacrolimus and adjust dose when appropriate. **Valsartan:** Concomitant use w/ other agents that block the RAS, K+-sparing diuretics (eg, spironolactone, triamterene, amiloride), K+ supplements, salt substitutes containing K+, or other drugs that may increase K+ levels (eg, heparin) may lead to increases in serum K+, and in HF patients to increases in SrCr; monitor serum K+ levels if comedication is necessary. NSAIDs, including selective COX-2 inhibitors, may attenuate antihypertensive effect and result in deterioration of renal function, including possible acute renal failure; monitor renal function periodically. Dual blockade of the RAS is associated w/ increased risks of hypotension, hyperkalemia, and changes in renal function (including acute renal failure); in general, avoid combined use of RAS inhibitors, or closely monitor BP, renal function, and electrolytes w/ concomitant agents that affect the RAS. Avoid w/ aliskiren in patients w/ renal impairment (GFR <60mL/min). **HCTZ:** Dosage adjustment of antidiabetic drugs (eg, oral agents, insulin) may be required. When used concomitantly w/ NSAIDs, monitor closely to determine if the desired effect of diuretic is obtained. May lead to symptomatic hyponatremia w/ carbamazepine. Staggering the dose of HCTZ and ion exchange resins (eg, cholestyramine, colestipol) such that HCTZ is administered at least 4 hrs before or 4-6 hrs after the administration of resins would potentially minimize the interaction. Cyclosporine may increase risk of hyperuricemia and gout-type complications. **Valsartan and HCTZ:** Increases in lithium levels and lithium toxicity reported; monitor serum lithium levels during concomitant use.

PREGNANCY AND LACTATION
Pregnancy: Category D.
Lactation: Not for use in nursing.

MECHANISM OF ACTION
Amlodipine: Dihydropyridine CCB; inhibits Ca^{2+} ion influx across cell membranes selectively, w/ a greater effect on vascular smooth muscle cells than on cardiac muscle cells. Peripheral arterial vasodilator that acts directly on vascular smooth muscle to cause a reduction in peripheral vascular resistance and reduction in BP. **Valsartan:** ARB; blocks the vasoconstrictor and aldosterone-secreting effects of angiotensin II by selectively blocking the binding of angiotensin II to AT_1 receptor in many tissues (eg, vascular smooth muscle, adrenal gland). **HCTZ:** Thiazide diuretic; mechanism not established. Affects renal tubular mechanisms of electrolyte reabsorption, directly increasing excretion of Na^+ and Cl^- in approximately equivalent amounts and indirectly reduces plasma volume.

PHARMACOKINETICS
Absorption: Amlodipine: Absolute bioavailability (64-90%); T_{max}=6-12 hrs. Valsartan: Absolute bioavailability (25%); T_{max}=2-4 hrs. HCTZ: Absolute bioavailability (70%); T_{max}=2-5 hrs. **Distribution:** Amlodipine: V_d=21L/kg; plasma protein binding (93%). Valsartan: (IV) V_d=17L; plasma protein binding (95%). HCTZ: Plasma protein binding (40-70%); crosses placenta; found in breast milk. **Metabolism:** Amlodipine: Hepatic (extensive). Valsartan: Via CYP2C9; valeryl-4-hydroxy valsartan (primary metabolite). **Elimination:** Amlodipine: Urine (10% unchanged, 60% metabolites), $T_{1/2}$=30-50 hrs. Valsartan: (Oral Sol) Feces (83%), urine (13%); (IV) $T_{1/2}$=6 hrs. HCTZ: Urine (70% unchanged), $T_{1/2}$=10 hrs.

PATIENT CONSIDERATIONS
Assessment: Assess for hypersensitivity to the drug and its components, anuria, sulfonamide-derived drug or penicillin hypersensitivity, renal/hepatic impairment, HF, aortic or mitral stenosis, renal artery stenosis, obstructive hypertrophic cardiomyopathy, SLE, volume/salt depletion, electrolyte imbalances, CAD, pregnancy/nursing status, and possible drug interactions.

Monitoring: Monitor for signs/symptoms of hypotension, hypersensitivity/ idiosyncratic reactions, metabolic disturbances, myopia and angle-closure glaucoma, worsening angina or acute MI, fluid imbalance, exacerbation or activation of SLE, hyperglycemia, hyperuricemia or precipitation of gout, increases in cholesterol and TG levels, and other adverse reactions. Monitor BP, serum electrolytes, and renal function.

Counseling: Counsel about risks/benefits of therapy. Inform females of childbearing age about the consequences of exposure to therapy during pregnancy; discuss treatment options w/ women planning to become pregnant. Instruct to report pregnancies to physician as soon as possible. Caution that lightheadedness may occur, especially during the 1st days of therapy, and that it should be reported to physician. Instruct to d/c therapy until the physician has been consulted if syncope occurs. Caution that inadequate fluid intake, excessive perspiration, diarrhea, or vomiting may lead to an excessive fall in BP, w/ the same consequences of lightheadedness and possible syncope. Instruct patients not to use K+ supplements or salt substitutes containing K+ w/o consulting prescribing physician.

EXTAVIA — interferon beta-1b

Rx

Class: Biological response modifier

ADULT DOSAGE

Multiple Sclerosis

Relapsing Forms:

Initial: 0.0625mg (0.25mL) SQ qod

Titrate: Increase over a 6-week period to 0.25mg (1mL) SQ qod

Titration Schedule:

Weeks 1-2: 0.0625mg (0.25mL) qod

Weeks 3-4: 0.125mg (0.5mL) qod

Weeks 5-6: 0.1875mg (0.75mL) qod

Week 7 and After: 0.25mg (1mL) qod

Premedication

For Flu-Like Symptoms:

Concurrent use of analgesics and/or antipyretics on treatment days may help ameliorate flu-like symptoms

Missed Dose

Take it as soon as possible; do not take therapy on 2 consecutive days. The next inj should be taken about 48 hrs (2 days) after that dose

PEDIATRIC DOSAGE

Pediatric use may not have been established

ADMINISTRATION

SQ route

Rotate inj sites.

Do not reuse needles or syringes.

After reconstitution, if not used immediately, refrigerate reconstituted sol at 2-8°C (35-46°F) and use w/in 3 hrs; do not freeze.

Reconstitution

1. Attach the prefilled syringe containing the diluent (NaCl, 0.54% sol) to vial using the vial adapter. The removable rubber cap of the diluent prefilled syringe contains natural latex, which may cause allergic reactions and should not be handled by latex-sensitive individuals.
2. Slowly inject 1.2mL of diluent into vial.
3. Gently swirl vial to dissolve drug completely; do not shake. If foaming occurs, allow the vial to sit undisturbed until the foam settles.
4. Keeping syringe and vial adapter in place, turn assembly over so that vial is on top; withdraw appropriate dose.
5. Remove the vial from the vial adapter before injecting.

STORAGE

20-25°C (68-77°F); excursions of 15-30°C (59-86°F) are permitted for up to 3 months. After reconstitution, if not used immediately, refrigerate and use w/in 3 hrs. Do not freeze.

HOW SUPPLIED

Inj: 0.3mg

CONTRAINDICATIONS

Hypersensitivity to natural or recombinant interferon beta, albumin (human), mannitol, or any other component of the formulation.

WARNINGS/PRECAUTIONS

Severe hepatic injury including hepatic failure (rare) and asymptomatic elevation of serum transaminases reported; consider discontinuing therapy if serum transaminase levels significantly increase, or if associated w/ clinical symptoms (eg, jaundice). Anaphylaxis (rare) and other allergic reactions reported; d/c if anaphylaxis occurs. The removable rubber cap of the diluent prefilled syringe contains natural rubber latex, which may cause allergic reactions and should not be handled by latex-sensitive individuals. Depression and suicide reported; consider discontinuation of therapy if depression develops. CHF, cardiomyopathy, and cardiomyopathy w/ CHF reported; monitor for worsening of cardiac condition during initiation of and continued treatment in patients w/ preexisting CHF. Consider discontinuation of therapy if worsening of CHF occurs w/ no other etiology. Inj-site necrosis/reactions reported; avoid administration into affected area until fully healed in patients who continue therapy after inj-site necrosis has occurred. If multiple lesions occur, d/c until healed. Leukopenia reported; patients w/ myelosuppression may require more intensive monitoring of CBC, w/ differential and platelet counts. Cases of thrombotic microangiopathy (TMA), including thrombotic thrombocytopenic purpura and hemolytic uremic syndrome, reported; d/c if clinical symptoms and lab findings consistent w/ TMA occur and manage as clinically indicated. May cause seizures. Drug-induced lupus erythematosus reported; d/c therapy in patients developing new signs/symptoms characteristic of this syndrome.

ADVERSE REACTIONS

Inj-site reaction, lymphopenia, flu-like symptoms, myalgia, leukopenia, neutropenia, increased liver enzymes, headache, hypertonia, pain, rash, insomnia, abdominal pain, asthenia.

DRUG INTERACTIONS

Potential risk for hepatic injury w/ known hepatotoxic drugs or other products (eg, alcohol).

PREGNANCY AND LACTATION

Pregnancy: Category C. Spontaneous abortions while on treatment were reported in four patients participating in the interferon beta-1b RRMS clinical trial.

Lactation: Not for use in nursing.

MECHANISM OF ACTION

Biological response modifier; has not been established. Believed that interferon β-1b receptor binding induces expression of proteins that are responsible for pleiotropic bioactivities. Immunomodulatory effects include the enhancement of suppressor T-cell activity, reduction of proinflammatory cytokine production, down-regulation of antigen presentation, and inhibition of lymphocyte trafficking into the CNS.

PHARMACOKINETICS

Absorption: (0.5mg, SQ) Bioavailability (50%); C_{max}=40 IU/mL; T_{max}=1-8 hrs.

Distribution: (0.006-2mg, IV) V_d=0.25-2.88L/kg. **Elimination:** (0.006-2mg, IV) $T_{1/2}$=8 min-4.3 hrs.

PATIENT CONSIDERATIONS

Assessment: Assess for hypersensitivity to the drug or human albumin, preexisting CHF, myelosuppression, latex sensitivity, pregnancy/nursing status, and possible drug interactions. Obtain baseline CBC, differential WBC counts, platelet counts, and blood chemistries, including LFTs.

Monitoring: Monitor for hepatic injury, anaphylaxis, depression, suicidal ideation, worsening of CHF, inj-site necrosis/reactions, leukopenia, TMA, flu-like symptom complex, seizures, drug-induced lupus erythematosus, and other adverse reactions. Monitor CBC and differential WBC count, platelet counts, and blood chemistries, including LFTs, at regular intervals (1, 3, and 6 months) following introduction, and then periodically thereafter in the absence of clinical symptoms. Periodically evaluate patient understanding and use of aseptic self-inj techniques and procedures, particularly if inj-site necrosis occurred.

Counseling: Instruct on proper aseptic technique and procedures. Advise not to reuse needles/syringes and instruct on safe disposal procedures. Inform of the importance of rotating inj sites w/ each dose. Instruct to notify physician if pregnant, planning to become pregnant, or if any adverse reactions (eg, hepatic dysfunction, allergic reactions, anaphylaxis, worsening of cardiac condition, inj-site necrosis, seizures, drug-induced lupus erythematosus) occur. Inform latex-sensitive individuals that the removable rubber cap of the diluent prefilled syringe contains natural rubber latex. Inform that symptoms of depression or suicidal ideation may occur and instruct to notify physician immediately if these occur. Inform that flu-like symptoms are common following initiation of therapy. Instruct to take missed dose as soon as possible, but not to take on 2 consecutive days.

EXTINA — ketoconazole

Rx

Class: Azole antifungal

ADULT DOSAGE

Seborrheic Dermatitis

Apply to affected area(s) bid for 4 weeks

PEDIATRIC DOSAGE

Seborrheic Dermatitis

≥12 Years:

Apply to affected area(s) bid for 4 weeks

ADMINISTRATION

Topical route

1. Hold the container upright, and dispense foam into the cap of the can or other cool surface in an amount sufficient to cover the affected area(s)
2. Dispensing directly onto hands is not recommended, as the foam will begin to melt immediately upon contact with warm skin
3. Pick up small amounts of foam with the fingertips, and gently massage into the affected area(s) until the foam disappears
4. For hair-bearing areas, part the hair, so that foam may be applied directly to the skin (rather than on the hair)

STORAGE

20-25°C (68-77°F). Do not store under refrigerated conditions or in direct sunlight. Do not expose containers to heat or store at temperatures above 49°C (120°F). Do not puncture and/or incinerate container.

HOW SUPPLIED

Foam: 2% [50g, 100g]

WARNINGS/PRECAUTIONS

Not for ophthalmic, oral, or intravaginal use. Safety and efficacy for the treatment of fungal infections not established. May cause contact sensitization, including photoallergenicity. Contents are flammable; avoid fire, flame, and/or smoking during and immediately following application. Hepatitis, lowered testosterone, and adrenocorticotropic hormone-induced corticosteroid serum levels reported with orally administered ketoconazole; not seen with topical ketoconazole.

ADVERSE REACTIONS

Application-site burning, application-site reactions (eg, dryness, erythema, irritation, paresthesia, pruritus, rash, warmth), photoallergenicity, contact sensitization.

PREGNANCY AND LACTATION

Category C, caution in nursing.

MECHANISM OF ACTION

Azole antifungal; not established. Inhibits the synthesis of ergosterol, a key sterol in the cell membrane of *Malassezia furfur*.

PATIENT CONSIDERATIONS

Assessment: Assess pregnancy/nursing status.

Monitoring: Monitor for contact sensitization and application-site reactions.

Counseling: Instruct to use ud. Instruct to avoid fire, flame, and/or smoking during and immediately following application. Instruct not to apply directly to hands;

apply to affected areas using the fingertips. Inform that skin irritation and contact sensitization may occur; instruct to inform a physician if the area shows signs of increased irritation, and to report any signs of adverse reactions. Instruct to wash hands after application.

EYLEA — aflibercept   Rx
Class: Vascular endothelial growth factor (VEGF) inhibitor

ADULT DOSAGE	PEDIATRIC DOSAGE
Neovascular (Wet) Age-Related Macular Degeneration	Pediatric use may not have been established
2mg (0.05mL) every 4 weeks for first 12 weeks, followed by 2mg once every 8 weeks; some patients may need every 4 week dosing after the first 12 weeks	
Macular Edema	
Following Retinal Vein Occlusion:	
2mg (0.05mL) once every 4 weeks	
Diabetic Macular Edema	
2mg (0.05mL) every 4 weeks for first 5 inj, followed by 2mg once every 8 weeks; some patients may need every 4 week dosing after the first 20 weeks (5 months)	
Diabetic Retinopathy	
In Patients w/ Diabetic Macular Edema:	
2mg (0.05mL) every 4 weeks for first 5 inj, followed by 2mg once every 8 weeks; some patients may need every 4 week dosing after the first 20 weeks (5 months)	

ADMINISTRATION
Intravitreal route

Intravitreal inj should be performed w/ a 30-gauge x 1/2-inch inj needle.

Preparation for Administration
1. Attach the 19-gauge x 1.5-inch, 5-micron, filter needle to the 1-mL syringe.
2. Push the filter needle into the center of the vial stopper until the needle is completely inserted into the vial and the tip touches the bottom or bottom edge of the vial.
3. Withdraw all of the vial contents into the syringe, keeping the vial in an upright position, slightly inclined to ease complete withdrawal. To deter the introduction of air, ensure the bevel of the filter needle is submerged into the liquid. Continue to tilt the vial during withdrawal keeping the bevel of the filter needle submerged in the liquid.
4. Ensure that the plunger rod is drawn sufficiently back when emptying the vial in order to completely empty the filter needle.
5. Remove the filter needle from the syringe and properly dispose of the filter needle; do not use the filter needle for intravitreal inj.
6. Attach the 30-gauge x 1/2-inch inj needle to the syringe.
7. Holding the syringe w/ the needle pointing up, check for bubbles. If there are bubbles, gently tap the syringe w/ finger until the bubbles rise to the top.
8. To eliminate all of the bubbles and to expel excess drug, slowly depress plunger so that the plunger tip aligns w/ the line that marks 0.05mL on the syringe.

Injection Procedure
Adequate anesthesia and a topical broad-spectrum microbicide should be given prior to the inj.
Each vial should only be used for the treatment of a single eye; if the contralateral eye requires treatment, use a new vial and change the sterile field, syringe, gloves, drapes, eyelid speculum, filter, and inj needles before administering to the other eye.
After inj, discard any unused product.

STORAGE
2-8°C (36-46°F). Do not freeze. Protect from light.

HOW SUPPLIED
Inj: 40mg/mL [0.05mL]

CONTRAINDICATIONS
Ocular/periocular infections, active intraocular inflammation. Known hypersensitivity to aflibercept or any of the excipients in this medication.

WARNINGS/PRECAUTIONS
Endophthalmitis and retinal detachments may occur. Acute increases in IOP noted w/in 60 min of inj. Sustained increases in IOP reported after repeated dosing. Monitor IOP and perfusion of the optic nerve head and manage appropriately. Potential risk of arterial thromboembolic events (ATEs) (nonfatal stroke, nonfatal MI, vascular death).

ADVERSE REACTIONS
Conjunctival hemorrhage, eye pain, cataract, vitreous floaters, intraocular pressure increased, vitreous detachment.

PREGNANCY AND LACTATION
Pregnancy: Category C.
Lactation: Not for use in nursing.

Reproductive Potential: Females of reproductive potential should use effective contraception prior to the initial dose, during treatment, and for at least 3 months after the last inj.

MECHANISM OF ACTION
VEGF inhibitor; acts as a soluble decoy receptor that binds VEGF-A and placental growth factor, and thereby can inhibit the binding and activation of these cognate VEGF receptors.

PHARMACOKINETICS
Absorption: C_{max}=0.02mcg/mL (wet age-related macular degeneration), 0.05mcg/mL (retinal vein occlusion), 0.03mcg/mL (diabetic macular edema); T_{max}=1-3 days. **Distribution:** (IV) V_d=6L. **Metabolism:** Proteolysis. **Elimination:** (IV, 2-4mg/kg) $T_{1/2}$=5-6 days.

PATIENT CONSIDERATIONS
Assessment: Assess for hypersensitivity to the drug, ocular/periocular infections, active intraocular inflammation, and pregnancy/nursing status.

Monitoring: Monitor for signs/symptoms of endophthalmitis, retinal detachment, ATEs, and other adverse reactions. Monitor IOP and perfusion of the optic nerve head.

Counseling: Advise to seek immediate care from an ophthalmologist if eye becomes red, sensitive to light, painful, or patient develops a change in vision in the days following administration. Inform that temporary visual disturbances may be experienced after inj and the associated eye examinations; advise not to drive or use machinery until visual function has recovered sufficiently.

FABIOR — tazarotene   Rx
Class: Retinoid

ADULT DOSAGE	PEDIATRIC DOSAGE
Acne Vulgaris	**Acne Vulgaris**
Lightly cover affected area w/ thin layer qpm	**≥12 Years:** Lightly cover affected area w/ thin layer qpm

ADMINISTRATION
Topical route
1. Shake can before use
2. Clean and dry affected area
3. Dispense a small amount of foam into the palm of hand
4. Gently massage the foam into skin until foam disappears
5. Wash hands after application

STORAGE
20-25°C (68-77°F); excursions permitted to 15-30°C (59-86°F). Protect from freezing. Do not expose to heat or store at >49°C (120°F).

HOW SUPPLIED
Foam: 0.1% [50g, 100g]

CONTRAINDICATIONS
Pregnancy.

WARNINGS/PRECAUTIONS
Females of childbearing potential should use adequate birth-control measures during treatment. Obtain negative pregnancy test result (sensitivity down to at least 25 mIU/mL for human chorionic gonadotropin [hCG]) w/in 2 weeks prior to therapy; initiate therapy during normal menstrual period. Caution w/ history of local tolerability reactions or local hypersensitivity. May cause severe irritation; do not use on abraded or eczematous skin. Avoid contact w/ mouth, eyes, and mucous membranes; rinse well w/ water in case of accidental contact. May cause skin redness, peeling, burning or excessive pruritus; d/c therapy until integrity of skin is restored, or reduce dosing interval to an interval the patient can tolerate. Weather extremes (eg, wind, cold) may be more irritating. Avoid exposure to sunlight (eg, sunlamps); use sunscreens and protective clothing if exposure is necessary. Avoid w/ sunburn. Caution w/ personal or family history of skin cancer. Propellant in drug is flammable; avoid fire, flame, and/or smoking during and immediately following application.

ADVERSE REACTIONS
Application-site irritation/dryness/erythema/exfoliation.

DRUG INTERACTIONS
Avoid w/ dermatologic medications and cosmetics that have a strong drying effect. Oxidizing agents (eg, benzoyl peroxide) may cause degradation and may reduce clinical efficacy; if combination therapy is required, apply at different times of the day. Cumulative irritant effect may occur w/ topical acne therapy; use w/ caution; reduce frequency of application or temporarily interrupt treatment if irritancy or dermatitis occurs; resume once the irritation subsides and d/c if irritation persists. Possibility of augmented photosensitivity increased w/ photosensitizers (eg, thiazides, tetracyclines, fluoroquinolones, phenothiazines, sulfonamides); use w/ caution.

PREGNANCY AND LACTATION
Category X, not for use in nursing.

MECHANISM OF ACTION
Retinoid; not established. May be due to anti-hyperproliferative, normalizing-of-differentiation, and anti-inflammatory effects.

PHARMACOKINETICS
Absorption: Tazarotenic Acid: C_{max}=0.43ng/mL; T_{max}=6 hrs (median); $AUC_{0-24hrs}$=6.98ng•hr/mL. **Distribution:** Tazarotenic Acid: Plasma protein binding (>99%).
Metabolism: Esterase hydrolysis to form tazarotenic acid (active metabolite).
Elimination: Urine, feces; $T_{1/2}$=8.1 hrs, 21.7 hrs (tazarotenic acid).

PATIENT CONSIDERATIONS

Assessment: Assess for hypersensitivity, eczematous skin, sunburn, considerable sun exposure due to occupation, sunlight sensitivity, personal or family history of skin cancer, nursing status, and possible drug interactions. In females of childbearing potential, perform a pregnancy test having a sensitivity down to at least 25 mIU/mL for hCG w/in 2 weeks prior to therapy.

Monitoring: Monitor for local irritation (skin redness, peeling, burning or excessive pruritus) and other adverse reactions.

Counseling: Advise to use effective method of contraception during treatment to avoid pregnancy; instruct to d/c medication and contact physician if pregnancy occurs. Advise to reduce application frequency or temporarily interrupt treatment if undue irritation (redness, peeling, discomfort) occurs; inform that treatment may be resumed once irritation subsides. Instruct to avoid exposure of treated areas to either natural or artificial sunlight (eg, tanning beds, sunlamps). Instruct to avoid contact w/ the eyes; rinse well w/ water in case of accidental contact. Instruct to avoid fire, flame, or smoking during and immediately following application since foam is flammable. Instruct to wash hands after application.

FACTIVE — gemifloxacin mesylate   Rx

Class: Fluoroquinolone

> Fluoroquinolones have been associated w/ disabling and potentially irreversible serious adverse reactions that have occurred together, including tendinitis and tendon rupture, peripheral neuropathy, CNS effects; d/c immediately and avoid fluoroquinolone use in patients who experience any of these serious adverse reactions. May exacerbate muscle weakness in patients w/ myasthenia gravis; avoid w/ known history of myasthenia gravis. Because fluoroquinolones have been associated w/ serious adverse reactions, reserve gemifloxacin for use in patients who have no alternative treatment options for acute bacterial exacerbation of chronic bronchitis.

ADULT DOSAGE	PEDIATRIC DOSAGE
Acute Bacterial Exacerbation of Chronic Bronchitis	Pediatric use may not have been established
320mg qd for 5 days	
Community-Acquired Pneumonia	
Mild to Moderate Severity:	
Due to *Streptococcus pneumoniae, Haemophilus influenzae, Mycoplasma pneumoniae,* or *Chlamydia pneumoniae*:	
320mg qd for 5 days	
Due to Multidrug Resistant *S. pneumoniae, Klebsiella pneumoniae,* or *Moraxella catarrhalis*:	
320mg qd for 7 days	

DOSING CONSIDERATIONS
Renal Impairment
CrCl ≤40mL/min or Dialysis: 160mg q24h
ADMINISTRATION
Oral route
Take w/ or w/o food; swallow whole w/ a liberal amount of liquid.
STORAGE
25°C (77°F); excursions permitted to 15-30°C (59-86°F). Protect from light.
HOW SUPPLIED
Tab: 320mg* *scored
CONTRAINDICATIONS
History of hypersensitivity to gemifloxacin, fluoroquinolone antibiotic agents, or any of the product components.
WARNINGS/PRECAUTIONS
Tendinitis or tendon rupture can occur w/in hours or days of starting therapy or as long as several months after completion of therapy and may occur bilaterally; increased risk in patients >60 yrs and in patients w/ kidney, heart, or lung transplants. Avoid in patients who have a history of tendon disorders or who have experienced tendinitis or tendon rupture. Cases of sensory or sensorimotor axonal polyneuropathy resulting in paresthesias, hypoesthesias, dysesthesias, and weakness reported; symptoms may occur soon after initiation of therapy and may be irreversible in some patients. Caution in patients w/ CNS diseases (eg, epilepsy) or in patients predisposed to convulsions. May prolong the QT interval; avoid w/ history of QTc interval prolongation or in patients w/ uncorrected electrolyte disorders (hypokalemia or hypomagnesemia). Caution w/ proarrhythmic conditions. Serious hypersensitivity and/or anaphylactic reactions and other serious and sometimes fatal adverse reactions reported; d/c immediately and institute supportive measures at the 1st appearance of a skin rash, jaundice, or any other sign of hypersensitivity. *Clostridium difficile*-associated diarrhea (CDAD) reported; may need to d/c if CDAD is suspected or confirmed. May cause moderate to severe photosensitivity/phototoxicity reactions; d/c if phototoxicity occurs. Avoid excessive exposure to sun/UV light. Liver enzyme elevations reported; do not exceed the recommended dose of 320mg qd and do not exceed the recommended length of therapy. Caution in elderly and w/ renal impairment. Maintain adequate hydration. May result in bacterial resistance if used in the absence of a proven/strongly suspected bacterial infection.
ADVERSE REACTIONS
Diarrhea, rash, N/V, headache, abdominal pain, dizziness.

DRUG INTERACTIONS

Absorption of gemifloxacin is significantly reduced by the concomitant administration of an antacid containing aluminum and Mg^{2+}; avoid Mg^{2+}- and/or aluminum-containing antacids, products containing ferrous sulfate (iron), multivitamin preparations containing zinc or other metal cations, or Videx (didanosine) chewable/buffered tab or pediatric powder for oral sol, w/in 3 hrs before or 2 hrs after therapy. Avoid sucralfate w/in 2 hrs of therapy. Increased levels w/ probenecid. Avoid Class IA (eg, quinidine, procainamide) or Class III (eg, amiodarone, sotalol) antiarrhythmics. Caution w/ drugs that prolong the QTc interval (eg, erythromycin, antipsychotics, TCAs). Increased INR, or PT and/or clinical episodes of bleeding reported w/ warfarin or its derivatives; closely monitor PT, INR, or other suitable coagulation test. Increased risk of developing fluoroquinolone-associated tendinitis and tendon rupture in patients taking corticosteroid drugs.

PREGNANCY AND LACTATION
Pregnancy: Category C.
Lactation: Not for use in nursing unless the potential benefit to the mother outweighs the risk.

MECHANISM OF ACTION
Fluoroquinolone; inhibits DNA synthesis through inhibition of both DNA gyrase and topoisomerase IV, which are essential for bacterial growth.

PHARMACOKINETICS
Absorption: Rapid. Absolute bioavailability (71%); T_{max}=0.5-2 hrs; (Healthy) AUC=9.93μg•hr/mL, C_{max}=1.61μg/mL. **Distribution:** V_d=4.18L/kg; (Healthy) plasma protein binding (60-70%). **Metabolism:** Liver (limited). **Elimination:** (Healthy) Feces (61%, unchanged and metabolites), urine (36%, unchanged and metabolites); $T_{1/2}$=7 hrs.

PATIENT CONSIDERATIONS

Assessment: Assess for history of hypersensitivity to gemifloxacin, fluoroquinolone antibiotic agents, or any of this product's components; risk factors for developing tendinitis and tendon rupture; history of myasthenia gravis, tendon disorders, or peripheral neuropathy; CNS diseases; history of QTc interval prolongation; uncorrected electrolyte disorders (hypokalemia or hypomagnesemia); pregnancy/nursing status; and possible drug interactions. Obtain baseline culture and susceptibility tests. Obtain baseline renal function and LFTs.

Monitoring: Monitor for signs/symptoms of tendinitis or tendon rupture, peripheral neuropathy, CNS effects, exacerbation of muscle weakness in patients w/ myasthenia gravis, QT interval prolongation, hypersensitivity/anaphylactic reactions, CDAD, photosensitivity/phototoxicity reactions, and other adverse reactions. Monitor renal function and LFTs. Monitor PT, INR, or other suitable coagulation test if administered concomitantly w/ warfarin or its derivatives.

Counseling: Inform about benefits/risks of therapy. Advise to d/c if an adverse reaction is experienced and to call physician for advice on completing the full course of treatment w/ another antibacterial drug. Advise about the disabling and potentially irreversible serious adverse reactions that may occur together if using gemifloxacin (eg, tendinitis and tendon rupture, peripheral neuropathies, CNS effects). Instruct to d/c and contact physician if pain, swelling, or inflammation of a tendon, or weakness or inability to use joints is experienced; advise to rest and refrain from exercise. Instruct to d/c immediately and contact physician if symptoms of peripheral neuropathy (eg, pain, burning, tingling, numbness, and/or weakness) develop. Advise to inform physician if patient has history of convulsions, seizures, or epilepsy. Inform that therapy may cause dizziness; instruct not to operate an automobile or machinery or engage in activities requiring mental alertness or coordination if dizziness occurs. Inform that therapy may cause worsening of myasthenia gravis symptoms; advise to notify physician if symptoms of muscle weakness or breathing problems develop. Inform that therapy may cause a hypersensitivity reaction; instruct to immediately d/c therapy at the sign of a rash or other allergic reaction and to seek medical care. Inform that diarrhea is a common problem; instruct to notify physician if experiencing watery and bloody stools (w/ or w/o stomach cramps/fever) even as late as ≥2 months after having taken the last dose of treatment. Inform that QT interval prolongation may occur; instruct to inform physician of any personal or family history of QT prolongation or proarrhythmic conditions. Advise to minimize or avoid exposure to natural or artificial light (eg, tanning beds or UVA/B treatment); instruct to contact physician if a sunburn-like reaction or skin eruption occurs. Inform physician of any other medications that the patient is concurrently taking. Inform that drug treats only bacterial, not viral, infections. Instruct to take exactly ud and to swallow tab whole w/ a liberal amount of liquid. Advise that skipping doses or not completing full course may decrease effectiveness and increase bacterial resistance. Instruct to avoid taking Mg^{2+}- and/or aluminum-containing antacids, products containing ferrous sulfate (iron), multivitamin preparations containing zinc or other metal cations, or Videx (didanosine) chewable/buffered tab or pediatric powder for oral sol, w/in 3 hrs before or 2 hrs after therapy. Advise to avoid sucralfate w/in 2 hrs of therapy.

FAMOTIDINE — famotidine   Rx

Class: H_2 blocker

OTHER BRAND NAMES
Pepcid

ADULT DOSAGE	PEDIATRIC DOSAGE
Active Duodenal Ulcer	**Peptic Ulcer**
Inj:	**1-16 Years:**
20mg q12h	**Oral Sus/Tab:**
Oral Sus/Tab:	**Initial:** 0.5mg/kg/day qhs or divided bid
Acute Therapy:	**Max:** 40mg/day
20mg bid or 40mg qhs for 4-8 weeks	

Maint Therapy:
20mg qhs

Gastroesophageal Reflux Disease

Short-Term Treatment of GERD:
20mg bid for up to 6 weeks

Short-Term Treatment of GERD w/ Esophagitis:
20 or 40mg bid for up to 12 weeks

Pathological Hypersecretory Conditions

Treatment of Pathological Hypersecretory Conditions (eg, Zollinger-Ellison Syndrome, Multiple Endocrine Adenomas):
Oral Sus/Tab:
Initial: 20mg q6h
Titrate: Adjust dose to individual patient needs and continue as long as clinically indicated

Oral doses up to 160mg q6h have been administered to some patients w/ severe Zollinger-Ellison syndrome

Inj:
Initial: 20mg q12h
Titrate: Adjust dose to individual patient needs and continue as long as clinically indicated

Gastric Ulcers

Acute Therapy for Active Benign Gastric Ulcer:
Oral Sus/Tab:
40mg qhs

Inj:
20mg q12h

Inj:
Initial: 0.25mg/kg IV over ≥2 min or as 15-min infusion q12h
Max: 40mg/day

Individualize dose based on response and/or gastric/esophageal pH determination and endoscopy

Gastroesophageal Reflux Disease

Oral Sus:
<3 Months of Age:
0.5mg/kg/dose qd for up to 8 weeks
3 Months of Age to <1 Year:
0.5mg/kg/dose bid
GERD w/ or w/o Esophagitis:
1-16 Years:
Oral Sus/Tab:
Initial: 1mg/kg/day divided bid
Max: 40mg bid

Individualize dose based on response and/or gastric/esophageal pH determination and endoscopy

DOSING CONSIDERATIONS
Renal Impairment
Moderate (CrCl <50mL/min) or Severe (CrCl <10mL/min): May reduce to 1/2 dose, or prolong dosing interval to 36-48 hrs

ADMINISTRATION
IV/Oral route

May take w/ antacids if needed.

Preparation
IV Sol:
- Dilute 2mL of famotidine inj w/ 0.9% NaCl or other compatible IV sol to a total volume of either 5mL or 10mL and inject over a period of not less than 2 min.

IV Infusion Sol:
- Dilute 2mL of famotidine inj w/ 100mL of D5W or other compatible sol, and infuse over 15-30 min.

Oral Sus Preparation:
- Slowly add 46mL of purified water and shake vigorously for 5-10 sec immediately after adding the water and immediately before use.
- Discard after 30 days.

Stability
- When added to or diluted w/ water for inj, 0.9% NaCl, D5W and D10W, or lactated Ringer's inj, diluted famotidine inj is physically and chemically stable for 7 days at room temperature.
- When added to or diluted w/ sodium bicarbonate inj 5%, famotidine inj at a concentration of 0.2mg/mL is physically and chemically stable for 7 days at room temperature.

STORAGE
Inj: 2-8°C (36-46°F). Bring to room temperature if sol freezes. **Diluted Sol:** Stable at room temperature for 7 days. Refrigeration and use w/in 48 hrs is recommended if not used immediately after preparation. **Sus:** 25°C (77°F); excursions permitted to 15-30°C (59-86°F). Protect from freezing. Discard unused suspension after 30 days. **Tab:** 20-25°C (68-77°F).

HOW SUPPLIED
Inj: 10mg/mL [2mL, 4mL, 20mL]; **Oral Sus:** (Pepcid) 40mg/5mL [50mL]; **Tab:** (Pepcid) 20mg, 40mg

CONTRAINDICATIONS
Hypersensitivity to any component of famotidine, history of hypersensitivity to other H₂-receptor antagonists.

WARNINGS/PRECAUTIONS
See Dosing Considerations. Symptomatic response to therapy does not preclude presence of gastric malignancy. CNS adverse effects reported w/ moderate and severe renal insufficiency; may need to prolong dosing intervals or lower dose. Caution in elderly. **Tab:** Very rarely, prolonged QT interval reported in patients w/ impaired renal function whose dose/dosing interval may not have been adjusted appropriately.

ADVERSE REACTIONS
Headache, agitation.

PREGNANCY AND LACTATION
Pregnancy: Category B.
Lactation: Not for use in nursing.

MECHANISM OF ACTION
Histamine H_2-receptor antagonist; inhibits both acid concentration and volume of gastric secretion.

PHARMACOKINETICS
Absorption: (PO) Incomplete; bioavailability (40-45%); T_{max}=1-3 hrs. **Distribution:** Plasma protein binding (15-20%); found in breast milk. **Metabolism:** S-oxide (metabolite). **Elimination:** Renal (65-70%; 25-30% unchanged [PO], 65-70% unchanged [IV]), metabolic (30-35%); $T_{1/2}$=2.5-3.5 hrs. Refer to PI for pediatric parameters.

PATIENT CONSIDERATIONS
Assessment: Assess for hypersensitivity to the drug or to other H_2-receptor antagonists, renal insufficiency, gastric malignancy, pregnancy/nursing status, and possible drug interactions.

Monitoring: Monitor for hypersensitivity reactions and other adverse reactions. Monitor renal function in the elderly.

Counseling: Inform of risks/benefits of therapy. Instruct to contact physician if hypersensitivity or other adverse reactions develop. Advise to avoid nursing while on medication.

FAMVIR — famciclovir   Rx

Class: Nucleoside analogue

ADULT DOSAGE
Herpes Zoster
500mg q8h for 7 days
Initiate as soon as diagnosed

Herpes
Orolabial/Genital:
Recurrent in HIV-Infected Patients:
500mg bid for 7 days
Initiate at 1st sign/symptom

Herpes Labialis (Cold Sores)
Recurrent:
1500mg single dose
Initiate at 1st sign/symptom

Genital Herpes
Recurrent Episodes:
1000mg bid for 1 day
Initiate at 1st sign/symptom
Suppressive Therapy:
250mg bid

PEDIATRIC DOSAGE
Pediatric use may not have been established

DOSING CONSIDERATIONS
Renal Impairment
Recurrent Herpes Labialis:
CrCl 40-59mL/min: 750mg single dose
CrCl 20-39mL/min: 500mg single dose
CrCl <20mL/min: 250mg single dose
Hemodialysis: 250mg single dose following dialysis

Recurrent Genital Herpes:
CrCl 40-59mL/min: 500mg q12h for 1 day
CrCl 20-39mL/min: 500mg single dose
CrCl <20mL/min: 250mg single dose
Hemodialysis: 250mg single dose following dialysis

Suppression of Recurrent Genital Herpes:
CrCl 20-39mL/min: 125mg q12h
CrCl <20mL/min: 125mg q24h
Hemodialysis: 125mg following each dialysis

Herpes Zoster:
CrCl 40-59mL/min: 500mg q12h
CrCl 20-39mL/min: 500mg q24h
CrCl <20mL/min: 250mg q24h
Hemodialysis: 250mg following each dialysis

Recurrent Orolabial/Genital Herpes in HIV-Infected Patients:
CrCl 20-39mL/min: 500mg q24h
CrCl <20mL/min: 250mg q24h
Hemodialysis: 250mg following each dialysis

ADMINISTRATION
Oral route

Take w/ or w/o food.

STORAGE
25°C (77°F); excursions permitted to 15-30°C (59-86°F).

HOW SUPPLIED
Tab: 125mg, 250mg, 500mg

CONTRAINDICATIONS
Known hypersensitivity to the product, its components, or penciclovir.

WARNINGS/PRECAUTIONS
Acute renal failure reported in patients with underlying renal disease who have received inappropriately high doses. Caution in elderly and with renal impairment.

ADVERSE REACTIONS
Headache, N/V, diarrhea, elevated lipase, ALT elevation, fatigue, flatulence, pruritus, rash, neutropenia, abdominal pain, dysmenorrhea, migraine.

DRUG INTERACTIONS
Probenecid or other drugs significantly eliminated by active renal tubular secretion may increase levels of penciclovir. Potential interaction with drugs metabolized by and/or inhibiting aldehyde oxidase. Raloxifene may decrease formation of penciclovir.

PREGNANCY AND LACTATION
Category B, not for use in nursing.

MECHANISM OF ACTION
Nucleoside analogue; prodrug of penciclovir, which has demonstrated inhibitory activity against herpes simplex virus types 1 and 2 and varicella zoster virus.

PHARMACOKINETICS
Absorption: Penciclovir: Absolute bioavailability (77%). Oral administration of variable doses resulted in different parameters. **Distribution:** Penciclovir: (IV) V_d=1.08L/kg; plasma protein binding (<20%). **Metabolism:** Deacetylation and oxidation; famciclovir (prodrug) converted to penciclovir. **Elimination:** Urine (73%, 82% penciclovir, 7% 6-deoxy penciclovir), feces (27%); $T_{1/2}$=2.8 hrs (single dose, herpes zoster patients), 2.7 hrs (repeated doses, herpes zoster patients).

PATIENT CONSIDERATIONS
Assessment: Assess for hypersensitivity to the drug, renal impairment, pregnancy/nursing status, and possible drug interactions.

Monitoring: Monitor renal function and for adverse reactions.

Counseling: Inform to take exactly ud. Advise to initiate treatment at earliest signs/symptoms of recurrence of cold sores, at the 1st sign/symptom of recurrent genital herpes if episodic therapy is indicated, and as soon as possible after a diagnosis of herpes zoster. Inform that drug is not a cure for cold sores or genital herpes. Advise to avoid contact with lesions or intercourse when lesions and/or symptoms are present to avoid infecting partners. Counsel to use safer sex practices. Instruct to refrain from driving or operating machinery if dizziness, somnolence, confusion, or other CNS disturbances occur. Inform that drug contains lactose; instruct to notify physician if with rare hereditary problems of galactose intolerance, a severe lactase deficiency, or glucose-galactose malabsorption.

FANAPT — iloperidone

Rx

Class: Atypical antipsychotic

> Elderly patients w/ dementia-related psychosis treated w/ antipsychotic drugs are at an increased risk of death. Not approved for the treatment of patients w/ dementia-related psychosis.

ADULT DOSAGE
Schizophrenia

Initial: 1mg bid

Titrate: Dose increases may be made w/ daily dosage adjustments not to exceed 2mg bid (4mg/day) to reach the target range of 6-12mg bid (12-24mg/day)

Max: 12mg bid (24mg/day) Periodically reassess need for maint treatment

Reinitiation of Treatment:
Follow initiation titration schedule if patients have had an interval off therapy for >3 days

PEDIATRIC DOSAGE
Pediatric use may not have been established

DOSING CONSIDERATIONS
Concomitant Medications
Strong CYP2D6 Inhibitors or Strong CYP3A4 Inhibitors:
Reduce dose by 50%; increase to previous iloperidone dose upon withdrawal of strong CYP2D6/CYP3A4 inhibitors

Hepatic Impairment
Moderate: May require dose reduction
Severe: Not recommended

Other Important Considerations
Poor CYP2D6 Metabolizers:
Reduce dose by 50%

ADMINISTRATION
Oral route
Take w/o regard to meals.

STORAGE
25°C (77°F); excursions permitted to 15-30°C (59-86°F). Protect from light and moisture.

HOW SUPPLIED
Tab: 1mg, 2mg, 4mg, 6mg, 8mg, 10mg, 12mg

CONTRAINDICATIONS
Known hypersensitivity reaction to the product.

WARNINGS/PRECAUTIONS
QT prolongation reported; avoid w/ congenital long QT syndrome, history of cardiac arrhythmias, or history of significant cardiovascular (CV) illnesses. D/C if persistent QTc measurements are >500 msec. Obtain baseline measurements and periodically monitor K+ and Mg2+ levels in patients at risk of electrolyte disturbances. Risk of tardive dyskinesia (TD), especially in the elderly; consider discontinuation if signs/symptoms develop. Neuroleptic malignant syndrome (NMS) reported; immediately d/c and treat. May cause metabolic changes (eg, hyperglycemia, dyslipidemia, weight gain) that may increase CV and cerebrovascular risk. Hyperglycemia, in some cases extreme and associated w/ ketoacidosis or hyperosmolar coma or death, reported; monitor for worsening of glucose control, and perform FPG testing at the beginning of therapy and periodically in patients at risk for diabetes mellitus (DM). Caution w/ a history of seizures, conditions that lower the seizure threshold, or patients w/ reduced CYP2D6 activity. May induce orthostatic hypotension; caution w/ CV disease (CVD), cerebrovascular disease, or conditions that predispose to hypotension. Leukopenia, neutropenia, and agranulocytosis reported; d/c in cases of severe neutropenia (ANC <1000/mm^3). Monitor CBC and d/c at 1st sign of decline in WBC count if w/ preexisting low WBC count or history of drug-induced leukopenia/neutropenia and in the absence of other causative factors. May elevate prolactin levels. May disrupt body's ability to reduce core body temperature. Esophageal dysmotility and aspiration reported; caution in patients at risk of aspiration pneumonia. Closely supervise high-risk patients for suicide attempt. Priapism reported. May impair mental/physical abilities. Evaluate for history of drug abuse; monitor for drug misuse/abuse in these patients.

ADVERSE REACTIONS
Dizziness, dry mouth, fatigue, nasal congestion, orthostatic hypotension, somnolence, tachycardia, increased weight.

DRUG INTERACTIONS
See Dosing Considerations. Caution w/ CYP3A4 (eg, ketoconazole, clarithromycin) or CYP2D6 (eg, fluoxetine, paroxetine) inhibitors; may increase levels and may augment effect on the QTc interval. May increase total exposure of dextromethorphan w/ concomitant use. Avoid w/ Class IA (eg, quinidine, procainamide) or Class III (eg, amiodarone, sotalol) antiarrhythmics, antipsychotics (eg, chlorpromazine, thioridazine), antibiotics (eg, gatifloxacin, moxifloxacin), or other drugs known to prolong the QTc interval (eg, pentamidine, levomethadyl acetate, methadone). Caution w/ other centrally acting drugs and alcohol. May enhance hypotensive effects of antihypertensive agents. Concomitant use w/ medications w/ anticholinergic activity may contribute to an elevation in core body temperature. May increase levels of drugs that are predominantly eliminated by CYP3A4.

PREGNANCY AND LACTATION
Pregnancy: There is a pregnancy exposure registry that monitors pregnancy outcomes in women exposed to iloperidone during pregnancy. Neonates exposed to antipsychotic drugs during the 3rd trimester of pregnancy are at risk for extrapyramidal and/or withdrawal symptoms. **Lactation:** There is no information regarding the presence of iloperidone or its metabolites in human milk, the effects on a breastfed child, nor the effects on human milk production; not for use in nursing.

MECHANISM OF ACTION
Piperidinyl-benzisoxazole derivative; not established. Proposed to be mediated through a combination of dopamine type 2 and serotonin type 2 antagonisms.

PHARMACOKINETICS
Absorption: Well-absorbed; T_{max}=2-4 hrs. **Distribution:** V_d=1340-2800L; plasma protein binding (97%, 92% metabolite). **Metabolism:** Liver via carbonyl reduction, hydroxylation (CYP2D6), O-demethylation (CYP3A4); P88, P95 (major metabolites). **Elimination:** Urine (58.2% extensive metabolizers [EM], 45.1% poor metabolizers [PM]), feces (19.9% EM, 22.1% PM); $T_{1/2}$= EM: 18 hrs (iloperidone), 26 hrs (P88), 23 hrs (P95); PM: 33 hrs (iloperidone), 37 hrs (P88), 31 hrs (P95).

PATIENT CONSIDERATIONS
Assessment: Assess for known hypersensitivity to the drug, dementia-related psychosis, hepatic impairment, DM, risk factors for DM, CVD, cerebrovascular disease, congenital long QT syndrome, history of cardiac arrhythmias, conditions that predispose to hypotension, conditions that may contribute to an elevation in core body temperature, history of low WBC counts or drug-induced leukopenia/neutropenia, history of seizures, conditions that lower the seizure threshold, history of drug abuse, poor metabolizers of CYP2D6, risk for aspiration pneumonia, risk for suicide, pregnancy/nursing status, and possible drug interactions. Obtain baseline FPG in patients w/ DM or w/ risk factors for DM. Obtain baseline CBC, orthostatic vital signs, and serum K+ and Mg2+ levels.

Monitoring: Monitor for TD, NMS, hyperprolactinemia, priapism, extrapyramidal symptoms, esophageal dysmotility, aspiration, orthostatic hypotension, body temperature lability, seizures, weight gain, dyslipidemia, QT prolongation, cognitive/motor impairment, and other adverse effects. Monitor for signs of hyperglycemia; monitor FPG levels in patients w/ DM or at risk for DM. Monitor for suicide attempts, and for drug misuse/abuse in patients w/ a history of drug misuse/abuse. Monitor for signs/symptoms of leukopenia, neutropenia, and agranulocytosis; frequently monitor CBC in patients w/ risk factors for leukopenia/neutropenia. Monitor serum K+ and Mg2+ levels, and orthostatic vital signs.

Counseling: Advise to inform physician immediately if feeling faint, or if loss of consciousness or heart palpitations occur. Advise to avoid drugs that cause QT interval prolongation and instruct to inform physician of all medications patient is taking or planning to take (prescription or OTC drugs). Inform about the signs/symptoms of NMS, hyperglycemia, and DM. Explain that weight gain may occur during treatment. Advise of risk of orthostatic hypotension, particularly during initiation/reinitiation/dose increases. Inform that the drug may impair judgment, thinking, or motor skills; advise to use caution when driving or operating hazardous machinery. Advise that 3rd trimester use may cause extrapyramidal and/or withdrawal symptoms in a neonate. Instruct to notify physician of known/suspected pregnancy. Explain that there is a pregnancy exposure registry that monitors pregnancy outcomes in women exposed to iloperidone during pregnancy. Advise not to breastfeed. Advise to avoid alcohol during treatment. Counsel about appropriate care to avoid overheating and dehydration.

FARXIGA — dapagliflozin   Rx

Class: Sodium-glucose cotransporter 2 (SGLT2) inhibitor

ADULT DOSAGE	PEDIATRIC DOSAGE
Type 2 Diabetes Mellitus	Pediatric use may not have been established
Initial: 5mg qam	
Titrate: May increase to 10mg qd in patients tolerating 5mg qd who require additional glycemic control	

DOSING CONSIDERATIONS
Renal Impairment
eGFR <60mL/min/1.73m^2: Initiation of therapy not recommended
eGFR ≥60mL/min/1.73m^2: No dose adjustment needed
eGFR Persistently Between 30 and <60mL/min/1.73m^2: Use not recommended
eGFR <30mL/min/1.73m^2: Contraindicated

Other Important Considerations
Patients w/ Volume Depletion:
Correct this condition before initiating treatment

ADMINISTRATION
Oral route

Take w/ or w/o food.

STORAGE
20-25°C (68-77°F); excursions permitted between 15-30°C (59-86°F).

HOW SUPPLIED
Tab: 5mg, 10mg

CONTRAINDICATIONS
History of a serious hypersensitivity reaction to dapagliflozin. Severe renal impairment (eGFR <30mL/min/1.73m^2), ESRD, or patients on dialysis.

WARNINGS/PRECAUTIONS
Not recommended for type 1 diabetes mellitus (DM) or for treatment of diabetic ketoacidosis. Causes intravascular volume contraction. Symptomatic hypotension may occur after initiating therapy, particularly in patients w/ renal impairment (eGFR <60mL/min/1.73m^2), elderly patients, or patients on loop diuretics; assess and correct volume status before initiating treatment in patients w/ ≥1 of these characteristics. Ketoacidosis (including fatal cases) reported; if suspected, d/c and institute prompt treatment. Assess for ketoacidosis in patients presenting w/ signs/symptoms consistent w/ severe metabolic acidosis regardless of presenting blood glucose levels. Consider temporarily discontinuing therapy in clinical situations known to predispose to ketoacidosis (eg, prolonged fasting due to acute illness or surgery). Can cause intravascular volume contraction and renal impairment. Acute kidney injury reported; consider factors that may predispose to acute kidney injury before initiating therapy. Consider temporarily discontinuing therapy in any setting of reduced oral intake or fluid losses. D/C therapy promptly and institute treatment if acute kidney injury occurs. Increases SrCr and decreases eGFR; caution in elderly patients and patients w/ renal impairment. Adverse reactions related to renal function may occur. Serious UTIs (eg, urosepsis, pyelonephritis), requiring hospitalization, reported; evaluate for signs/symptoms of UTIs and treat promptly, if indicated. Increases risk of genital mycotic infections; monitor and treat appropriately. Increases in LDL levels reported. Newly diagnosed cases of bladder cancer reported; do not use in patients w/ active bladder cancer and caution in patients w/ prior history of bladder cancer. Caution in patients w/ severe hepatic impairment. Monitoring glycemic control w/ urine glucose tests or 1,5-anhydroglucitol assay is not recommended.

ADVERSE REACTIONS
Genital mycotic infections, nasopharyngitis, UTIs, back pain, increased urination.

DRUG INTERACTIONS
May increase risk of hypoglycemia when combined w/ insulin or an insulin secretagogue; a lower dose of insulin or insulin secretagogue may be required.

PREGNANCY AND LACTATION
Pregnancy: Category C. Based on animal studies, dapagliflozin may affect renal development and maturation. During pregnancy, consider appropriate alternative therapies, especially during the 2nd and 3rd trimesters.
Lactation: Not for use in nursing.

MECHANISM OF ACTION
SGLT2 inhibitor; reduces reabsorption of filtered glucose and lowers the renal threshold for glucose, and thereby increases urinary glucose excretion.

PHARMACOKINETICS
Absorption: Absolute oral bioavailability (78%) (10mg); T_{max}=2 hrs. **Distribution:** Plasma protein binding (91%). **Metabolism:** Primarily mediated by UGT1A9; CYP-mediated metabolism (minor). **Elimination:** (Single 50mg dose) Urine (75%, <2% unchanged), feces (21%, 15% unchanged). $T_{1/2}$=12.9 hrs (10mg).

PATIENT CONSIDERATIONS
Assessment: Assess for diabetic ketoacidosis, type of DM, volume depletion, history of genital mycotic infections, active/history of bladder cancer, drug hypersensitivity, predisposition to ketoacidosis, hypovolemia, chronic renal insufficiency, CHF, pregnancy/nursing status, and possible drug interactions. Assess baseline renal/hepatic function, LDL levels, and BP.

Monitoring: Monitor for signs/symptoms of hypotension, ketoacidosis, UTIs, genital mycotic infections, and other adverse reactions. Monitor renal function and LDL levels.

Counseling: Inform of the risks, benefits, and alternative modes of therapy. Advise about the importance of adherence to dietary instructions, regular physical activity, periodic blood glucose monitoring and HbA1c testing, recognition and management of hypo/hyperglycemia, and assessment of diabetes complications. Instruct to seek medical advice promptly during periods of stress (eg, fever, trauma, infection, surgery) as medication requirements may change. Instruct to immediately inform physician if pregnant, breastfeeding, planning to become pregnant or to breastfeed, or if experiencing signs/symptoms of hypotension or bladder cancer. Inform of the most common adverse reactions associated w/ therapy. Instruct to have adequate fluid intake. Instruct to d/c and seek medical advice immediately if symptoms of ketoacidosis occur. Counsel on the signs/symptoms of vaginal yeast infections, UTIs, balanitis, and balanoposthitis; inform of treatment options and when to seek medical advice. Instruct to d/c therapy and consult physician if any signs/symptoms suggesting an allergic reaction or angioedema develop. Inform to seek medical advice immediately if experiencing reduced oral intake (due to acute illness or fasting) or increased fluid losses (due to vomiting, diarrhea, or excessive heat exposure).

FARYDAK — panobinostat   Rx

Class: Histone deacetylase (HDAC) inhibitor

> Severe diarrhea reported; monitor for symptoms, institute antidiarrheal treatment, interrupt panobinostat, and then reduce dose or d/c panobinostat. Severe and fatal cardiac ischemic events, severe arrhythmias, and ECG changes reported. Arrhythmias may be exacerbated by electrolyte abnormalities. Obtain ECG and electrolytes at baseline and periodically during treatment as clinically indicated.

ADULT DOSAGE	PEDIATRIC DOSAGE
Multiple Myeloma	Pediatric use may not have been established
In combination w/ bortezomib (BTZ) and dexamethasone for the treatment of patients w/ multiple myeloma who have received at least 2 prior regimens, including BTZ and an immunomodulatory agent	
Initial: 20mg once qod for 3 doses/week in Weeks 1 and 2 of each 21-day cycle for up to 8 cycles	
Consider continuing treatment for an additional 8 cycles for patients w/ clinical benefit who do not experience unresolved severe or medically significant toxicity; total duration of treatment may be up to 16 cycles (48 weeks)	
Recommended Dosing Schedule w/ BTZ and Dexamethasone:	
Cycles 1-8:	
- Panobinostat on Days 1, 3, 5, 8, 10, 12, and then rest for 1 week	
- BTZ (1.3mg/m^2 inj) on Days 1, 4, 8, 11, and then rest for 1 week	
- Dexamethasone (20mg PO) on Days 1, 2, 4, 5, 8, 9, 11, 12, and then rest for 1 week	
Cycles 9-16:	
- Panobinostat on Days 1, 3, 5, 8, 10, 12, and then rest for 1 week	
- BTZ (1.3mg/m^2 inj) on Days 1, 8, and then rest for 1 week	
- Dexamethasone (20mg PO) on Days 1, 2, 8, 9, and then rest for 1 week	
Missed Dose	
- If a dose is missed it can be taken up to 12 hrs after the specified time	
- If vomiting occurs, patient should not repeat the dose but should take the next usual scheduled dose	

DOSING CONSIDERATIONS
Concomitant Medications
Strong CYP3A Inhibitors:
Reduce starting dose to 10mg

Hepatic Impairment
Mild: Reduce starting dose to 15mg
Moderate: Reduce starting dose to 10mg
Severe: Avoid use

Adverse Reactions
Management of adverse reactions may require treatment interruption and/or dose reductions.
If dose reduction is required, the dose of panobinostat should be reduced in increments of 5mg.
If the dosing of panobinostat is reduced <10mg given 3X per week, d/c panobinostat. Keep the same treatment schedule (3-week treatment cycle) when reducing dose.

Thrombocytopenia:
Platelets <50 x 10^9/L (CTCAE Grade 3): Maintain panobinostat dose; monitor platelet counts at least weekly.
Maintain BTZ dose.
Platelets <50 x 10^9/L w/ Bleeding (CTCAE Grade 3) or Platelets <25 x 10^9/L (CTCAE Grade 4): Interrupt panobinostat; monitor platelet counts at least weekly until ≥50 x 10^9/L, then restart at reduced dose.

Interrupt BTZ until thrombocytopenia resolves to ≥50 x 10⁹/L.
If only 1 dose was omitted prior to correction to these levels, restart BTZ at same dose.
If ≥2 doses were omitted consecutively, or w/in the same cycle, BTZ should be restarted at a reduced dose.

Neutropenia:
ANC 0.75-1.0 x 10⁹/L (CTCAE Grade 3): Maintain panobinostat dose. Maintain BTZ dose.
ANC 0.5-0.75 x 10⁹/L (CTCAE Grade 3) (2 or More Occurrences): Interrupt panobinostat until ANC ≥1.0 x 10⁹/L, then restart at same dose. Maintain BTZ dose.
ANC <1.0 x 10⁹/L (CTCAE Grade 3) w/ Febrile Neutropenia (Any Grade): Interrupt panobinostat until febrile neutropenia resolves and ANC ≥1.0 x 10⁹/L, then restart at reduced dose.
Interrupt BTZ until febrile neutropenia resolves and ANC ≥1.0 x 10⁹/L.
If only 1 dose was omitted prior to correction to these levels, restart BTZ at same dose.
If ≥2 doses were omitted consecutively, or w/in the same cycle, BTZ should be restarted at a reduced dose.
ANC <0.5 x 10⁹/L (CTCAE Grade 4): Interrupt panobinostat until ANC ≥1.0 x 10⁹/L, then restart at reduced dose.
Interrupt BTZ until febrile neutropenia resolves and ANC ≥1.0 x 10⁹/L.
If only 1 dose was omitted prior to correction to these levels, restart BTZ at same dose.
If ≥2 doses were omitted consecutively, or w/in the same cycle, BTZ should be restarted at a reduced dose.

Anemia:
Hgb <8g/dL (CTCAE Grade 3): Interrupt panobinostat until Hgb ≥10g/dL. Restart at reduced dose.

Diarrhea:
Moderate Diarrhea, 4-6 Stools/Day (CTCAE Grade 2): Interrupt panobinostat until resolved, then restart at same dose.
Consider interruption of BTZ until resolved; restart at same dose.
Severe Diarrhea (≥7 Stools/Day) IV Fluids or Hospitalization Required (CTCAE Grade 3): Interrupt panobinostat until resolved, then restart at reduced dose. Interrupt BTZ until resolved, then restart at reduced dose.
Life-Threatening Diarrhea (CTCAE Grade 4): Permanently d/c panobinostat. Permanently d/c BTZ.

N/V:
Severe Nausea (CTCAE Grade 3/4) or Severe/Life-Threatening Vomiting (CTCAE Grade 3/4): Interrupt panobinostat until resolved, then restart at reduced dose

Myelosuppression:
Interrupt or reduce dose of panobinostat in patients who have thrombocytopenia, neutropenia, or anemia according to instructions listed above.
Consider platelet transfusions in patients w/ severe thrombocytopenia.
D/C panobinostat treatment if thrombocytopenia does not improve despite the recommended treatment modifications or if repeated platelet transfusions are required.
Consider dose reduction and/or use of growth factors (eg, granulocyte colony-stimulating factor) in the event of Grade 3 or 4 neutropenia.
D/C panobinostat if neutropenia does not improve despite dose modifications, colony-stimulating factors, or in case of severe infection.

GI Toxicity:
May require treatment interruption or dose reduction if diarrhea, nausea, or vomiting occurs.
Treat w/ antidiarrheal medication (eg, loperamide) at 1st sign of abdominal cramping, loose stools, or onset of diarrhea.
Consider and administer prophylactic antiemetics as clinically indicated.

Other Adverse Drug Reactions:
Patients Experiencing Grade 3/4 Adverse Drug Reactions Other Than Thrombocytopenia, Neutropenia, or GI Toxicity:
CTC Grade 2 Toxicity Recurrence and CTC Grade 3 and 4: Omit dose until recovery to CTC ≤Grade 1 and restart treatment at a reduced dose
CTC Grade 3 or 4 Toxicity Recurrence: May consider further dose reduction once the adverse events have resolved to CTC ≤Grade 1

ADMINISTRATION
Oral route

Take on each scheduled day at about the same time, either w/ or w/o food.
Swallow cap whole w/ a cup of water; do not open, crush, or chew.
Direct contact of the powder in cap w/ skin or mucous membranes should be avoided; wash thoroughly if such contact occurs.

STORAGE
20-25°C (68-77°F); excursions permitted between 15-30°C (59-86°F). Protect from light.

HOW SUPPLIED
Cap: 10mg, 15mg, 20mg

WARNINGS/PRECAUTIONS
Do not initiate in patients w/ history of recent MI or unstable angina. May prolong cardiac ventricular repolarization (QT interval); do not initiate in patients w/ a QTcF >450 msec or clinically significant baseline ST-segment or T-wave abnormalities. If during therapy the QTcF increases to ≥480 msec, interrupt therapy. If QT prolongation does not resolve, d/c therapy permanently. Fatal and serious hemorrhage reported. Myelosuppression (eg, severe thrombocytopenia, neutropenia, anemia) may occur. Localized and systemic infections (eg, pneumonia, bacterial infections, invasive fungal infections, viral infections) reported; if diagnosis of infection is made, institute appropriate anti-infective treatment promptly and consider interruption or discontinuation of therapy. Should not be initiated in patients w/ active infections. Hepatic dysfunction

reported; if abnormal LFTs are observed, may consider dose adjustment until values return to normal or pretreatment levels. May cause fetal harm.

ADVERSE REACTIONS
Diarrhea, fatigue, N/V, peripheral edema, decreased appetite, pyrexia, hypophosphatemia, hypokalemia, hyponatremia, increased creatinine, thrombocytopenia, lymphopenia, leukopenia, neutropenia, anemia.

DRUG INTERACTIONS
See Dosing Considerations. Avoid w/ strong CYP3A inducers. Increased levels w/ strong CYP3A inhibitors; avoid star fruit, pomegranate or pomegranate juice, and grapefruit or grapefruit juice. Avoid coadministration w/ sensitive CYP2D6 substrates (eg, atomoxetine, metoprolol, venlafaxine) or CYP2D6 substrates that have a narrow therapeutic index (eg, thioridazine, pimozide); if concomitant use of CYP2D6 substrates is unavoidable, monitor patients frequently for adverse reactions. Not recommended w/ antiarrhythmics (eg, amiodarone, disopyramide, procainamide) and other drugs known to prolong the QT interval (eg, chloroquine, halofantrine, clarithromycin). Antiemetic drugs w/ known QT prolonging risk (eg, dolasetron, ondansetron, tropisetron) can be used w/ frequent ECG monitoring.

PREGNANCY AND LACTATION
Pregnancy: May cause fetal harm.
Lactation: It is not known if panobinostat is present in human milk; not for use in nursing.
Reproductive Potential: Females of reproductive potential should avoid becoming pregnant while on therapy. Sexually active females of reproductive potential should use effective contraception while taking therapy and for at least 3 months after the last dose of therapy. Sexually active men should use condoms while on treatment and for 6 months after last dose of therapy.

MECHANISM OF ACTION
Histone deacetylase inhibitor (HDAC); inhibits the enzymatic activity of HDACs at nanomolar concentrations, resulting in increased acetylation of histone proteins, an epigenetic alteration that results in a relaxing of chromatin and leads to transcriptional activation.

PHARMACOKINETICS
Absorption: Absolute bioavailability (approx 21%); T_{max}=2 hrs. Distribution: Plasma protein binding (90%). Metabolism: Extensive; reduction, hydrolysis, oxidation, and glucuronidation; CYP3A; 2D6, 2C19 (minor). Elimination: Urine (29-51%, <2.5% unchanged), feces (44-77%, <3.5% unchanged); $T_{1/2}$=37 hrs.

PATIENT CONSIDERATIONS

Assessment: Assess for history of recent MI or unstable angina, active infection, pregnancy/nursing status, and possible drug interactions. Obtain baseline CBC, LFTs, ECG, and electrolyte levels (including K^+, Mg^{2+}, and phosphate). Assess hydration status.

Monitoring: Monitor for signs/symptoms of diarrhea, cardiac ischemic events, arrhythmias, hemorrhage, infection, and other adverse reactions. Monitor ECG periodically as clinically indicated. Monitor CBC, hydration status, and electrolyte blood levels weekly (or more frequently if clinically indicated). Monitor LFTs regularly. Monitor for toxicity more frequently in patients >65 yrs of age, especially for GI toxicity, myelosuppression, and cardiac toxicity.

Counseling: Instruct to take exactly ud. If a dose is missed, advise to take dose as soon as possible and up to 12 hrs after the specified dose time. If vomiting occurs, advise not to repeat dose, but to take the next usual prescribed dose on schedule. Instruct to avoid star fruit, pomegranate/pomegranate juice, and grapefruit/grapefruit juice while on therapy. Advise to report to physician if any signs/symptoms of a heart problem develop while on therapy (eg, chest pain/discomfort, changes in heartbeat, palpitations). Inform about risk of thrombocytopenia; advise to contact physician right away if any signs of bleeding occur. Explain the need to perform laboratory tests prior to start of therapy and while on therapy. Inform about the risk of neutropenia and severe, life-threatening infections; instruct to contact physician immediately if fever and/or any sign of infection develops. Inform that drug may cause severe N/V and diarrhea that may require medication for treatment; advise to contact physician at the start of diarrhea, if persistent vomiting develops, or if any signs of dehydration develop. Instruct to consult w/ physician prior to using medications w/ laxative properties. Inform that drug may cause fetal harm. Advise women of reproductive potential to use effective contraception while taking therapy and for at least 3 months after the last dose of the drug. Counsel sexually active men to use condoms while receiving therapy and for at least 6 months following the last dose of the drug. Instruct not to breastfeed during therapy.

FAZACLO — clozapine   Rx
Class: Atypical antipsychotic

> Severe neutropenia, defined as an ANC <500/μL, reported; may lead to serious infection and death. Prior to initiating treatment, a baseline ANC must be ≥1500/μL for the general population, and ≥1000/μL for patients w/ documented benign ethnic neutropenia (BEN). Regularly monitor ANC during treatment. Available only through a restricted program under a Risk Evaluation Mitigation Strategy (REMS) called the Clozapine REMS program. Orthostatic hypotension, bradycardia, syncope, and cardiac arrest reported; risk is highest during the initial titration period, particularly w/ rapid dose escalation. Caution w/ cardiovascular (CV)/cerebrovascular disease or conditions predisposing to hypotension (eg, dehydration, use of antihypertensives). Seizures reported and risk is dose related; caution w/ history of seizures or other predisposing risk factors for seizure (eg, CNS pathology, medications that lower seizure threshold, alcohol abuse). Fatal myocarditis and cardiomyopathy reported; d/c and obtain cardiac evaluation upon suspicion of these reactions. Do not rechallenge patients w/ clozapine-related myocarditis or cardiomyopathy. Elderly patients w/ dementia-related psychosis treated w/ antipsychotic drugs are at an increased risk of death. Not approved for the treatment of dementia-related psychosis.

ADULT DOSAGE

Schizophrenia

Treatment of severely ill patients w/ schizophrenia who fail to respond adequately to standard antipsychotic treatment. Risk reduction of recurrent suicidal behavior in patients w/ schizophrenia or schizoaffective disorder who are judged to be at chronic risk for reexperiencing suicidal behavior

Initial: 12.5mg qd or bid
Titrate: May increase total daily dose in increments of 25-50mg/day, if well tolerated
Target Dose: 300-450mg/day (in divided doses) by the end of 2 weeks. Subsequently, may increase dose once weekly or twice weekly, in increments of up to 100mg
Max: 900mg/day

Patients responding to treatment should generally continue maint treatment on their effective dose beyond the acute episode

Reinitiation of Treatment:

When restarting in patients who have discontinued clozapine (≥2 days since last dose), reinitiate w/ 12.5mg qd or bid; if well tolerated, may increase to previous therapeutic dose more quickly than recommended for initial treatment

---

DOSING CONSIDERATIONS
Concomitant Medications
Strong CYP1A2 Inhibitors:
During coadministration, use 1/3 of clozapine dose; when discontinuing comedication, increase clozapine dose based on clinical response

Moderate or Weak CYP1A2 Inhibitors:
During coadministration, monitor for adverse reactions and consider reducing clozapine dose if necessary; when discontinuing comedication, monitor for lack of effectiveness and consider increasing clozapine dose if necessary

CYP2D6 or CYP3A4 Inhibitors:
During coadministration, monitor for adverse reactions and consider reducing clozapine dose if necessary; when discontinuing comedication, monitor for lack of effectiveness and consider increasing clozapine dose if necessary

Strong CYP3A4 Inducers:
Concomitant use is not recommended; however, if the inducer is necessary, may need to increase clozapine dose and monitor for decreased effectiveness. When discontinuing comedication, reduce clozapine dose based on clinical response

Moderate or Weak CYP1A2 or CYP3A4 Inducers:
During coadministration, monitor for decreased effectiveness and consider increasing clozapine dose if necessary; when discontinuing comedication, monitor for adverse reactions and consider reducing clozapine dose if necessary

Renal Impairment
May need to reduce dose w/ significant renal impairment

Hepatic Impairment
May need to reduce dose w/ significant hepatic impairment

Discontinuation
Method of treatment discontinuation will vary depending on patient's last ANC:
1. If abrupt treatment discontinuation is necessary due to moderate-severe neutropenia, refer to PI for appropriate ANC monitoring based on the level of neutropenia
2. If termination of therapy is planned and there is no evidence of moderate-severe neutropenia, reduce dose gradually over 1-2 weeks
3. For abrupt discontinuation for a reason unrelated to neutropenia, continue existing ANC monitoring for general population patients until ANC is ≥1500/μL and for BEN patients until ANC is ≥1000/μL or above baseline
4. During the 2 weeks after discontinuation, additional ANC monitoring is required for any patient reporting onset of fever (temperature of ≥38.5°C [≥101.3°F])

Other Important Considerations
CYP2D6 Poor Metabolizers:
May need to reduce dose

ADMINISTRATION
Oral route

Administer in divided doses.
May be taken w/ or w/o food.
Immediately place tabs in mouth after removing from the blister pack or bottle. Tabs may be allowed to disintegrate, or may be chewed.
May swallow tabs w/ saliva; no water is necessary for administration.
Leave in the unopened blister until time of use. Just prior to use, peel the foil from the blister and gently remove tab; do not push through the foil.

STORAGE
20-25°C (68-77°F); excursions permitted to 15-30°C (59-86°F). Protect from moisture.

PEDIATRIC DOSAGE
Pediatric use may not have been established

HOW SUPPLIED
Tab, Disintegrating: 12.5mg, 25mg, 100mg, 150mg, 200mg

CONTRAINDICATIONS
History of serious hypersensitivity to clozapine (eg, photosensitivity, vasculitis, erythema multiforme, or Stevens-Johnson Syndrome) or any other component of this medication.

WARNINGS/PRECAUTIONS
In general, do not rechallenge patients who develop severe neutropenia w/ clozapine; for some patients, the risk of serious psychiatric illness from discontinuing treatment may be greater than the risk of rechallenge. Eosinophilia may occur and may be associated w/ myocarditis, pancreatitis, hepatitis, colitis, and nephritis. Evaluate promptly for signs/symptoms of systemic reactions if eosinophilia develops and d/c immediately if clozapine-related systemic disease is suspected. QT prolongation, torsades de pointes, and other life-threatening ventricular arrhythmias, cardiac arrest, and sudden death reported. D/C if QTc interval exceeds 500 msec or symptoms consistent w/ torsades de pointes or other arrhythmias develop. Caution in patients at risk for significant electrolyte disturbance, particularly hypokalemia; correct electrolyte abnormalities before initiating treatment. Associated w/ metabolic changes (eg, hyperglycemia sometimes associated w/ ketoacidosis or hyperosmolar coma, dyslipidemia, weight gain) that may increase CV and cerebrovascular risk. Neuroleptic malignant syndrome (NMS) reported; d/c therapy immediately and institute symptomatic treatment. Transient fever may occur and may necessitate discontinuing treatment; carefully evaluate patients to rule out severe neutropenia or infection, and consider the possibility of NMS. Pulmonary embolism (PE), deep vein thrombosis (DVT), and tardive dyskinesia (TD) reported; consider discontinuation if TD occurs. Has potent anticholinergic effects; may result in CNS and peripheral anticholinergic toxicity. Caution w/ narrow-angle glaucoma, prostatic hypertrophy, or other conditions in which anticholinergic effects can lead to significant adverse reactions. May result in GI adverse reactions (eg, constipation, intestinal obstruction, fecal impaction, paralytic ileus). May impair mental/physical abilities. Consider dose reduction if sedation, or impairment of cognitive/motor performance occurs. Caution in patients w/ risk factors for cerebrovascular adverse reactions. If abrupt discontinuation is necessary, monitor carefully for the recurrence of psychotic symptoms and adverse reactions related to cholinergic rebound (eg, profuse sweating, headache, N/V, diarrhea). Contains phenylalanine (a component of aspartame); caution w/ phenylketonurics. Caution in elderly. Refer to PI for treatment recommendations based on ANC monitoring for the general patient population and for patients w/ BEN.

ADVERSE REACTIONS
CNS reactions (eg, sedation, dizziness/vertigo, headache, tremor), CV reactions (eg, tachycardia, hypotension, syncope), autonomic nervous system reactions (eg, hypersalivation, sweating, dry mouth, visual disturbances), GI reactions (eg, constipation, nausea), fever.

DRUG INTERACTIONS
See Boxed Warning and Dosing Considerations. Caution w/ drugs that are inducers or inhibitors of CYP1A2, CYP3A4, and CYP2D6. CYP1A2 inhibitors (eg, fluvoxamine, ciprofloxacin, oral contraceptives), CYP2D6 or CYP3A4 inhibitors (eg, cimetidine, escitalopram, erythromycin) may increase levels, potentially resulting in adverse reactions. CYP1A2 (eg, tobacco) or CYP3A4 inducers (eg, carbamazepine, phenytoin, St. John's wort) may decrease levels, resulting in decreased effectiveness. Caution w/ medications that prolong the QT interval (eg, ziprasidone, erythromycin, quinidine) or inhibit the metabolism of clozapine. Use caution when coadministering w/ other drugs metabolized by CYP2D6 (eg, phenothiazines, carbamazepine, propafenone) and may be necessary to use lower doses of such drugs; concomitant use may increase levels these CYP2D6 substrates. Caution w/ anticholinergic medications. NMS reported w/ CNS-active medications, including lithium. If used concurrently w/ an agent known to cause neutropenia (eg, some chemotherapeutic agents), consider monitoring more closely than the treatment guidelines.

PREGNANCY AND LACTATION
Pregnancy: Category B.
Lactation: Not for use in nursing.

MECHANISM OF ACTION
Atypical antipsychotic; tricyclic dibenzodiazepine derivative. Has not been established. Efficacy proposed to be mediated through antagonism of the dopamine type 2 and the serotonin type 2A receptors. Also acts as an antagonist at adrenergic, cholinergic, histaminergic, and other dopaminergic and serotonergic receptors.

PHARMACOKINETICS
Absorption: (100mg bid) C_{max}=413ng/mL; T_{max}=2.3 hrs. **Distribution:** Plasma protein binding (97%); found in breast milk. **Metabolism:** CYP1A2, CYP2D6, CYP3A4; demethylation, hydroxylation, N-oxidation. Norclozapine (limited activity); **Elimination:** Urine (50%), feces (30%); $T_{1/2}$=8 hrs (75mg single dose), 12 hrs (100mg bid).

PATIENT CONSIDERATIONS
Assessment: Assess for hypersensitivity to drug, history of seizures or other predisposing factors for seizure, risk factors for QT prolongation and serious CV reactions, narrow-angle glaucoma, prostatic hypertrophy, renal/hepatic impairment, any other conditions where treatment is cautioned, pregnancy/nursing status, and possible drug interactions. Obtain baseline ANC, lipid evaluations, ECG, and serum chemistry panel (K^+ and Mg^{2+}). Obtain baseline FPG in patients w/ diabetes mellitus (DM) or at risk for DM.

Monitoring: Monitor for signs/symptoms of severe neutropenia, orthostatic hypotension, bradycardia, syncope, cardiac arrest, seizures, myocarditis, cardiomyopathy, cognitive/motor impairment, eosinophilia, NMS, recurrence of psychosis and cholinergic rebound after abrupt discontinuation, metabolic changes (hyperglycemia, DM, dyslipidemia, weight gain), QT interval prolongation, fever, PE, DVT, TD, cerebrovascular adverse reactions, and other adverse reactions. Monitor serum electrolyte levels, glucose control in patients w/ DM and periodic FPG levels if at risk for hyperglycemia. Monitor ANC regularly to continue treatment; refer to PI for monitoring frequency.

Counseling: Inform about benefits/risks of therapy. Advise about risk of developing severe neutropenia and infection. Instruct to immediately report any sign/symptom of infection occurring at any time during therapy. Inform that drug is available only through a restricted program called the Clozapine REMS Program designed to ensure the required blood monitoring; advise of the importance of having blood tested ud. Inform about risks of orthostatic hypotension and syncope, especially during the period of initial dose titration; instruct to strictly follow the instructions of the physician for dosage and administration. Advise to consult physician immediately if patients feel faint, lose consciousness, or have signs/symptoms suggestive of bradycardia or arrhythmia. Inform about significant risk of seizure during therapy; caution about driving and any other potentially hazardous activity while taking treatment. Instruct to inform physician if taking clozapine before any new drug. Educate about the risk of metabolic changes and the need for specific monitoring. If dose was missed for >2 days, instruct not to restart medication at same dose but to contact physician for dosing instructions. Advise to notify physician if taking/planning to take any prescription or OTC drugs. Instruct to notify physician if pregnant/intending to become pregnant during therapy. Advise not to breastfeed if taking the drug. Inform that drug contains phenylalanine.

FELDENE — piroxicam   Rx
Class: NSAID

> NSAIDs cause an increased risk of serious cardiovascular (CV) thrombotic events, including MI and stroke, which can be fatal. This risk may occur early in treatment and may increase w/ duration of use. Contraindicated in the setting of CABG surgery. NSAIDs cause an increased risk of serious GI adverse events (eg, bleeding, ulceration, stomach/intestinal perforation), which can be fatal and can occur anytime during use and w/o warning symptoms; elderly patients and patients w/ a prior history of peptic ulcer disease and/or GI bleeding are at a greater risk.

ADULT DOSAGE	PEDIATRIC DOSAGE
Rheumatoid Arthritis	Pediatric use may not have been established
20mg qd; may divide daily dose	
Adjust dose and frequency after observing response to initial therapy. Use lowest effective dose for shortest duration consistent w/ individual patient treatment goals.	
Osteoarthritis	
20mg qd; may divide daily dose	
Adjust dose and frequency after observing response to initial therapy. Use lowest effective dose for shortest duration consistent w/ individual patient treatment goals.	

DOSING CONSIDERATIONS
Elderly
Use caution; start at lower end of dosing range

ADMINISTRATION
Oral route

STORAGE
20-25°C (68-77°F); excursions permitted between 15-30°C (59-86°F).

HOW SUPPLIED
Cap: 10mg, 20mg

CONTRAINDICATIONS
Known hypersensitivity to piroxicam or any components of the drug product; history of asthma, urticaria, or other allergic-type reactions after taking aspirin (ASA) or other NSAIDs; in the setting of CABG surgery.

WARNINGS/PRECAUTIONS
Avoid use w/ recent MI unless benefits are expected to outweigh risk of recurrent CV thrombotic events; if used w/ recent MI, monitor for signs of cardiac ischemia. Increased risk of GI bleed w/ longer duration of therapy; older age; poor general health status; advanced liver disease and/or coagulopathy. Avoid use in patients at higher risk unless benefits are expected to outweigh the increased risk of bleeding; consider alternate therapies other than NSAIDs. Consider alternate therapies other than NSAIDs in patients w/ active GI bleeding. If serious GI adverse event is suspected, promptly evaluate, initiate treatment, and d/c until serious GI adverse event is ruled out. Hepatotoxicity reported; d/c immediately and perform a clinical evaluation if clinical signs/symptoms consistent w/ liver disease develop, or if systemic manifestations occur. May lead to new onset of HTN or worsening of preexisting HTN. Fluid retention and edema reported. Avoid use w/ severe heart failure (HF) unless benefits outweigh risks of worsening HF; monitor for signs of worsening HF if used in patients w/ severe HF. Renal papillary necrosis and other renal injury reported w/ long-term use. Renal toxicity also reported in patients in whom renal prostaglandins have a compensatory role in the maintenance of renal perfusion; increased risk w/ renal/hepatic dysfunction, dehydration, hypovolemia, HF, and in the elderly. Correct volume status if dehydrated or hypovolemic prior to initiating therapy. Monitor renal function w/ renal or hepatic impairment, HF, dehydration, or hypovolemia during use. Avoid use w/ advanced renal

disease unless the benefits are expected to outweigh the risk of worsening renal function; monitor for signs of worsening renal function. Increases in K+, including hyperkalemia, reported. Associated w/ anaphylactic reactions. Monitor for changes in the signs/symptoms of asthma in patients w/ preexisting asthma (w/o known ASA sensitivity). May cause serious skin adverse reactions (eg, exfoliative dermatitis, Stevens-Johnson syndrome, toxic epidermal necrolysis); d/c at the 1st appearance of skin rash or any other sign of hypersensitivity. Anemia reported. May increase risk of bleeding events; coagulation disorders may increase this risk. May mask inflammation and fever. Adverse eye findings reported; perform ophthalmic evaluations in patients who develop visual complaints.

ADVERSE REACTIONS
Nausea, constipation, flatulence, abdominal pain, diarrhea, headache, dizziness, edema, rash.

DRUG INTERACTIONS
Drugs that interfere w/ serotonin reuptake may potentiate the risk of bleeding. Synergistic effect on bleeding w/ anticoagulants (eg, warfarin); monitor for signs of bleeding w/ concomitant anticoagulants, antiplatelet agents, SSRIs, and SNRIs. May increase risk of GI bleeding w/ use of oral corticosteroids, anticoagulants, SSRIs, smoking, and alcohol use. ASA may increase risk of bleeding and serious GI events; concomitant use w/ analgesic doses of ASA is not recommended. May diminish antihypertensive effect of ACE inhibitors, ARBs, or β-blockers (eg, propranolol); monitor BP. Coadministration w/ ACE inhibitors or ARBs may result in deterioration of renal function (including possible acute renal failure) in patients who are elderly, or volume-depleted (including those on diuretic therapy), or who have renal impairment; monitor for worsening renal function. Adequately hydrate and assess renal function at the beginning of the concomitant treatment and periodically thereafter. May reduce natriuretic effect of loop diuretics (eg, furosemide) and thiazide diuretics; observe for signs of worsening renal function, in addition to assuring diuretic efficacy including antihypertensive effects. May increase serum concentration and prolong $T_{1/2}$ of digoxin; monitor serum digoxin levels. May cause elevations in plasma lithium levels and reductions in renal lithium clearance; monitor for signs of lithium toxicity. May increase risk for methotrexate toxicity. May increase cyclosporine's nephrotoxicity; monitor for signs of worsening renal function. Use w/ other NSAIDs or salicylates (eg, diflunisal, salsalate) increases risk of GI toxicity; concomitant use not recommended. May increase the risk of pemetrexed-associated myelosuppression, renal, and GI toxicity; refer to prescribing information for further information. Expected to displace other protein bound drugs; closely monitor for a change in dosage requirements. Corticosteroids may increase risk of GI ulceration or bleeding; monitor for signs of bleeding.

PREGNANCY AND LACTATION
Pregnancy: Category C, prior to 30 weeks' gestation; Category D, starting 30 weeks' gestation. Use during the 3rd trimester of pregnancy increases the risk of premature closure of the fetal ductus arteriosus; avoid use in pregnant women starting at 30 weeks of gestation (3rd trimester).
Lactation: May be present in human milk; caution in nursing.
Reproductive Potential: May delay or prevent rupture of ovarian follicles. Consider withdrawal in women who have difficulties conceiving or who are undergoing investigation of infertility.

MECHANISM OF ACTION
NSAID; not established. Involves inhibition of COX-1 and COX-2 and has analgesic, anti-inflammatory, and antipyretic properties.

PHARMACOKINETICS
Absorption: Well absorbed. C_{max}=1.5-2mcg/mL (single dose), 3-8mcg/mL (multiple doses); T_{max}=3-5 hrs. **Distribution:** V_d=0.14L/kg; plasma protein binding (99%); found in breast milk. **Metabolism:** Hydroxylation via CYP2C9, conjugation, cyclodehydration, hydrolysis, decarboxylation, ring contraction, and N-demethylation; 5'-hydroxy-piroxicam (major metabolite). **Elimination:** Urine and feces (5% unchanged); $T_{1/2}$=50 hrs.

PATIENT CONSIDERATIONS

Assessment: Assess for hypersensitivity to piroxicam or to any component of this product; history of asthma, urticaria, or other allergic-type reactions after taking ASA or other NSAIDs; asthma; CV disease (CVD) or risk factors for CVD; HTN; history of peptic ulcer disease or GI bleeding; coagulation disorders; renal/hepatic impairment; pregnancy/nursing status; or any other conditions where treatment is contraindicated or cautioned. Assess volume status. Assess for possible drug interactions. Obtain baseline BP, CBC, and chemistry profile.

Monitoring: Monitor for signs/symptoms of CV thrombotic events; cardiac ischemia in patients w/ a recent MI; GI bleeding/ulceration and perforation; hepatotoxicity; new or worsening HTN; HF; edema; renal papillary necrosis and other renal injury; hyperkalemia; anaphylactic reactions; serious skin reactions; anemia; ophthalmologic effects; and other adverse reactions. Monitor BP during initiation of therapy and throughout the course of therapy. Monitor for signs of bleeding in patients on concomitant therapy w/ anticoagulants, antiplatelet agents, SSRIs, or SNRIs. Monitor renal function in patients w/ renal/hepatic impairment, HF, dehydration, or hypovolemia. Periodically monitor CBC and chemistry profiles in patients receiving long-term treatment. Monitor LFTs.

Counseling: Advise to be alert for the symptoms of CV thrombotic events and to report symptoms immediately. Advise to report symptoms of ulcerations and bleeding. Inform of the increased risk for and the signs and symptoms of GI bleeding w/ ASA. Inform of the warning signs and symptoms of hepatotoxicity; instruct to d/c and seek immediate medical therapy. Advise to be alert for the symptoms of CHF and to contact healthcare provider if such symptoms occur. Inform of the signs of an anaphylactic reaction and advise to seek immediate emergency help if these occur. Advise to d/c immediately if any type of rash develops, and to contact their healthcare provider as soon as possible. Advise females of reproductive potential who desire pregnancy that NSAIDs may be associated w/ a reversible delay in ovulation. Inform pregnant women to avoid use of piroxicam and other NSAIDs starting at 30 weeks' gestation. Inform patients that the concomitant use w/ other NSAIDs or salicylates is not recommended. Alert patients that NSAIDs may be present in OTC medications for treatment of colds, fever, or insomnia. Inform not to use low-dose ASA w/o consultation.

FELODIPINE ER — felodipine   Rx

Class: Calcium channel blocker (CCB) (dihydropyridine)

OTHER BRAND NAMES
Plendil (Discontinued)

ADULT DOSAGE
Hypertension
Initial: 5mg qd
Titrate: May decrease to 2.5mg qd or increase to 10mg qd at intervals of not <2 weeks, depending on the patient's response
Range: 2.5-10mg qd

PEDIATRIC DOSAGE
Pediatric use may not have been established

DOSING CONSIDERATIONS
Hepatic Impairment
Initial: 2.5mg qd
Elderly
Initial: 2.5mg qd

ADMINISTRATION
Oral route
Take regularly either w/o food or w/ a light meal. Swallow whole; do not crush or chew.

STORAGE
20-25°C (68-77°F). Protect from light.

HOW SUPPLIED
Tab, Extended-Release: 2.5mg, 5mg, 10mg

CONTRAINDICATIONS
Hypersensitivity to this product.

WARNINGS/PRECAUTIONS
May occasionally precipitate significant hypotension and, rarely, syncope. May lead to reflex tachycardia, which may precipitate angina pectoris. Caution with heart failure (HF) or compromised ventricular function, particularly in combination with a β-blocker. Closely monitor BP during dose adjustment in patients with hepatic impairment and in elderly. Peripheral edema reported. Caution in elderly.

ADVERSE REACTIONS
Peripheral edema, headache, asthenia, dyspepsia, dizziness, upper respiratory infection, flushing.

DRUG INTERACTIONS
CYP3A4 inhibitors (eg, ketoconazole, erythromycin, grapefruit juice, cimetidine) may increase plasma levels by several-fold. Decreased levels with long-term anticonvulsant therapy (eg, phenytoin, carbamazepine, phenobarbital); consider alternative antihypertensive therapy. May increase metoprolol and tacrolimus levels; monitor tacrolimus blood concentration and adjust tacrolimus dose if needed.

PREGNANCY AND LACTATION
Category C, not for use in nursing.

MECHANISM OF ACTION
Calcium channel blocker (dihydropyridine); reversibly competes with nitrendipine and/or other calcium channel blockers for dihydropyridine binding sites and blocks voltage-dependent Ca^{2+} currents in vascular smooth muscle.

PHARMACOKINETICS
Absorption: Almost complete. Systemic bioavailability (20%); C_{max}=23nmol/L (20mg); T_{max}=2.5-5 hrs. **Distribution:** V_d=10L/kg; plasma protein binding (>99%). **Metabolism:** Extensive 1st-pass. **Elimination:** Urine (70%), feces (10%); $T_{1/2}$=11-16 hrs (immediate-release).

PATIENT CONSIDERATIONS
Assessment: Assess for hypersensitivity to the drug, HF, compromised ventricular function, hepatic impairment, pregnancy/nursing status, and possible drug interactions.
Monitoring: Monitor for syncope, angina pectoris, peripheral edema, and other adverse reactions. Monitor BP.
Counseling: Inform that mild gingival hyperplasia (gum swelling) has been reported and that good dental hygiene decreases its incidence and severity.

FEMARA — letrozole   Rx

Class: Nonsteroidal aromatase inhibitor

ADULT DOSAGE
Breast Cancer
Adjuvant Treatment of Postmenopausal Women w/ Hormone Receptor Positive Early Breast Cancer:
2.5mg qd; d/c at relapse

PEDIATRIC DOSAGE
Pediatric use may not have been established

Extended Adjuvant Treatment of Early Breast Cancer in Postmenopausal Women, Who Have Received 5 Years of Adjuvant Tamoxifen Therapy:
2.5mg qd; d/c at tumor relapse
1st-Line Treatment of Postmenopausal Women w/ Hormone Receptor Positive or Unknown, Locally Advanced or Metastatic Breast Cancer; Treatment of Advanced Breast Cancer in Postmenopausal Women w/ Disease Progression Following Antiestrogen Therapy:
2.5mg qd; continue until tumor progression is evident

DOSING CONSIDERATIONS
Hepatic Impairment
Cirrhosis/Severe Hepatic Dysfunction: 2.5mg qod

ADMINISTRATION
Oral route
Take w/o regard to meals

STORAGE
25°C (77°F); excursions permitted to 15-30°C (59-86°F).

HOW SUPPLIED
Tab: 2.5mg

CONTRAINDICATIONS
Women who are or may become pregnant.

WARNINGS/PRECAUTIONS
May decrease bone mineral density (BMD); consider monitoring BMD. Bone fractures and osteoporosis reported. Hypercholesterolemia reported; consider monitoring serum cholesterol levels. Reduce dose by 50% with cirrhosis and severe hepatic impairment. May impair physical/mental abilities. Moderate decreases in lymphocyte counts and thrombocytopenia reported.

ADVERSE REACTIONS
Hypercholesterolemia, hot flushes, fatigue, edema, arthralgia/arthritis, myalgia, headache, dizziness, night sweats, nausea, back pain, bone fractures, weight increase, depression, osteopenia.

DRUG INTERACTIONS
Reduced plasma levels with coadministered tamoxifen.

PREGNANCY AND LACTATION
Category X, not for use in nursing.

MECHANISM OF ACTION
Nonsteroidal aromatase inhibitor; inhibits the conversion of androgens to estrogens. Inhibits the aromatase enzyme by competitively binding to the heme of the CYP450 subunit of the enzyme, resulting in a reduction of estrogen biosynthesis in all tissues.

PHARMACOKINETICS
Absorption: Rapid and complete. **Distribution:** V_d=1.9L/kg. **Metabolism:** Liver via CYP3A4, CYP2A6. **Elimination:** Urine (75%, glucuronide of carbinol metabolite; 9%, unidentified metabolites; 6%, unchanged); $T_{1/2}$=2 days.

PATIENT CONSIDERATIONS
Assessment: Assess for premenopausal endocrine status, cirrhosis or hepatic impairment, pregnancy/nursing status, and possible drug interactions.
Monitoring: Monitor for bone fractures, osteoporosis, fatigue, dizziness, somnolence, and other adverse reactions. Monitor BMD and serum cholesterol levels.
Counseling: Inform that the drug is contraindicated in pregnant women and women of premenopausal endocrine status. Counsel perimenopausal and recently postmenopausal women to use contraception until postmenopausal status is fully established. Advise about possible fatigue, dizziness, and somnolence; caution against operating machinery/driving. Advise that BMD may be monitored while on therapy.

FEMRING — estradiol acetate   Rx

Class: Estrogen

> Increased risk of endometrial cancer in a woman w/ a uterus who uses unopposed estrogens. Adding a progestin to estrogen therapy reduces the risk of endometrial hyperplasia. Adequate diagnostic measures (eg, directed or random endometrial sampling) should be undertaken to rule out malignancy in postmenopausal women w/ undiagnosed, persistent or recurring abnormal genital bleeding. Should not be used for the prevention of cardiovascular (CV) disease or dementia. Increased risk of stroke and deep vein thrombosis (DVT) reported in postmenopausal women (50-79 yrs of age) treated w/ daily oral conjugated estrogens (CE) alone and when combined w/ medroxyprogesterone acetate (MPA). Increased risk of developing probable dementia reported in postmenopausal women ≥65 yrs of age treated w/ daily CE alone and when combined w/ MPA. Increased risks of pulmonary embolism (PE), MI, and invasive breast cancer reported in postmenopausal women (50-79 yrs of age) treated w/ daily oral CE combined w/ MPA. Should be prescribed at the lowest effective dose and for the shortest duration consistent w/ treatment goals and risks.

ADULT DOSAGE

Menopausal Vasomotor Symptoms
Moderate to Severe:
Initial: 0.05mg/day
Titrate: Adjust dose based on clinical response

Ring should remain in place for 3 months; attempts to taper or d/c therapy should be made at 3- to 6-month intervals

Menopausal Vulvar/Vaginal Atrophy
Moderate to Severe:
Initial: 0.05mg/day
Titrate: Adjust dose based on clinical response

Ring should remain in place for 3 months; attempts to taper or d/c therapy should be made at 3- to 6-month intervals

----

DOSING CONSIDERATIONS
Renal Impairment
Has not been studied

Hepatic Impairment
Has not been studied

ADMINISTRATION
Intravaginal route

Insert immediately upon removal from protective pouch.
Refer to PI for further instructions on proper insertion, use, and removal.

STORAGE
25°C (77°F); excursions permitted to 15-30°C (59-86°F). Do not store unpouched.

HOW SUPPLIED
Vaginal Ring: 0.05mg/day, 0.10mg/day

CONTRAINDICATIONS
Undiagnosed abnormal genital bleeding, known/suspected/history of breast cancer, known/suspected estrogen-dependent neoplasia, active/history of DVT/PE, active/history of arterial thromboembolic disease (eg, stroke, MI), known anaphylactic reaction or angioedema to Femring, known liver impairment or disease, known protein C/protein S/antithrombin deficiency or other known thrombophilic disorders, known/suspected pregnancy.

WARNINGS/PRECAUTIONS
D/C immediately if stroke, DVT, PE, or MI occurs or is suspected. If feasible, d/c at least 4-6 weeks before surgery of the type associated w/ an increased risk of thromboembolism, or during periods of prolonged immobilization. May increase risk of ovarian cancer and of gallbladder disease requiring surgery. May lead to severe hypercalcemia in women w/ breast cancer and bone metastases; d/c and take appropriate measures if hypercalcemia occurs. Retinal vascular thrombosis reported; d/c therapy pending examination if sudden partial/complete loss of vision or sudden onset of proptosis, diplopia, or migraine occurs. D/C permanently if exam reveals papilledema or retinal vascular lesions. May elevate BP and thyroid-binding globulin levels. May elevate plasma TGs leading to pancreatitis in women w/ preexisting hypertriglyceridemia; consider discontinuation if pancreatitis occurs. Caution w/ history of cholestatic jaundice associated w/ past estrogen use or w/ pregnancy; d/c in case of recurrence. May cause fluid retention; caution w/ cardiac/renal impairment. Caution w/ hypoparathyroidism as estrogen-induced hypocalcemia may occur. Cases of malignant transformation of residual endometrial implants reported in women treated post-hysterectomy w/ estrogen therapy alone; consider addition of progestin for patients known to have residual endometriosis post-hysterectomy. May exacerbate symptoms of angioedema in women w/ hereditary angioedema. May exacerbate asthma, diabetes mellitus, epilepsy, migraine, porphyria, systemic lupus erythematosus, and hepatic hemangiomas; use w/ caution. May not be suitable w/ conditions that make the vagina more susceptible to vaginal irritation or ulceration, or make expulsions more likely (eg, narrow vagina, vaginal stenosis/infection, cervical prolapse, rectoceles, cystoceles). May affect certain endocrine and blood components in lab tests.

ADVERSE REACTIONS
Headache, intermenstrual bleeding, vaginal candidiasis, breast tenderness, back pain, abdominal distension, sinusitis, uterine pain, UTI.

DRUG INTERACTIONS
CYP3A4 inducers (eg, St. John's wort preparations, phenobarbital, carbamazepine) may decrease levels and may decrease therapeutic effects and/or changes in the uterine bleeding profile. CYP3A4 inhibitors (eg, erythromycin, clarithromycin, ketoconazole) may increase levels and may result in side effects. Patients concomitantly receiving thyroid replacement therapy and estrogens may require increased doses of their thyroid replacement therapy; monitor thyroid function.

PREGNANCY AND LACTATION
Pregnancy: Contraindicated in pregnancy.
Lactation: Not for use in nursing.

MECHANISM OF ACTION
Estrogen; binds to nuclear receptors in estrogen-responsive tissues. Circulating estrogens modulate pituitary secretion of the gonadotropins, luteinizing hormone and follicle-stimulating hormone, through negative feedback mechanism. Reduces elevated levels of these hormones in postmenopausal women.

PEDIATRIC DOSAGE
Pediatric use may not have been established

PHARMACOKINETICS
Absorption: (0.05mg/day) C_{max}=1129pg/mL, 141pg/mL (estrone), 2365pg/mL (estrone sulfate); T_{max}=0.9 hr, 6.2 hrs (estrone), 9.3 hrs (estrone sulfate). (0.10mg/day) C_{max}=1665pg/mL; T_{max}=0.7 hr. **Distribution:** Largely bound to sex hormone-binding globulin and albumin; found in breast milk. **Metabolism:** Liver to estrone (metabolite) and estriol (major urinary metabolite); enterohepatic recirculation via sulfate and glucuronide conjugation in the liver, biliary secretion of conjugates into the intestine, and hydrolysis in the intestine followed by reabsorption. **Elimination:** Urine; $T_{1/2}$=21-26 hrs.

PATIENT CONSIDERATIONS
Assessment: Assess for undiagnosed abnormal genital bleeding, presence/history of breast cancer, estrogen-dependent neoplasia, active or history of DVT/PE/arterial thromboembolic disease, liver impairment/disease, thrombophilic disorders, drug hypersensitivity, pregnancy/nursing status, any other conditions where treatment is contraindicated or cautioned, need for progestin therapy, and possible drug interactions.

Monitoring: Monitor for signs/symptoms of CV disorders, malignant neoplasms, dementia, gallbladder disease, hypercalcemia, visual abnormalities, BP and plasma TG elevations, cholestatic jaundice, fluid retention, angioedema, exacerbation of endometriosis and other conditions, and other adverse reactions. Perform annual breast exam; schedule mammography based on age, risk factors, and prior mammogram results. Periodically reevaluate to determine need for therapy. Perform adequate diagnostic measures (eg, endometrial sampling) to rule out malignancy in case of undiagnosed persistent or recurring abnormal genital bleeding. Regularly monitor thyroid function if on thyroid hormone replacement therapy.

Counseling: Inform of the importance of reporting abnormal vaginal bleeding to physician as soon as possible. Inform of possible serious adverse reactions of therapy (eg, CV disorders, malignant neoplasms, probable dementia) and of possible less serious but common adverse reactions (eg, headache, breast pain and tenderness, N/V). Inform that contact w/ blood may cause discoloration of Femring during use and that this does not affect the release rate of the drug. Instruct to have yearly breast exams by a healthcare provider and to perform monthly breast self-exams.

FENTORA — fentanyl   CII
Class: Opioid analgesic

> Fatal respiratory depression may occur. Contraindicated in the management of acute or postoperative pain (eg, headache/migraine) and in opioid-nontolerant patients. Keep out of reach of children. Concomitant use with CYP3A4 inhibitors may increase plasma levels, and may cause fatal respiratory depression. Do not convert patients on a mcg-per-mcg basis from any other fentanyl products to Fentora. Do not substitute for any other fentanyl products; may result in fatal overdose. Contains fentanyl with abuse liability similar to other opioid analgesics. Available only through a restricted program called Transmucosal Immediate Release Fentanyl Risk Evaluation Mitigation Strategy (TIRF REMS) Access program due to risk of misuse, abuse, addiction, and overdose. Outpatients, healthcare professionals who prescribe to outpatients, pharmacies, and distributors must enroll in this program.

ADULT DOSAGE
Cancer Pain
Breakthrough Pain:
Initial: 100mcg
Max: 2 doses/episode of breakthrough pain
Titrate:
If higher dose is needed, may give two 100mcg tabs (1 on each side of the mouth) w/ their next breakthrough pain episode
May titrate to two 100mcg tabs on each side of mouth (total of four 100mcg tabs), if pain is not adequately controlled
For doses >400mcg, titrate using multiples of 200mcg tabs
Do not use >4 tabs simultaneously
Maint:
Once titrated to effective dose, use only 1 tab of the appropriate strength per breakthrough pain episode
If breakthrough pain is not relieved after 30 min, may give only 1 additional dose of the same strength for that episode; wait at least 4 hrs before treating another breakthrough pain episode
If >4 episodes/day are experienced, dose of the around-the-clock opioid should be reevaluated

Conversions
Initial Fentora Dose Based on Current Actiq Dose:
200mcg of Actiq: 100mcg
400mcg of Actiq: 100mcg
600mcg of Actiq: 200mcg
800mcg of Actiq: 200mcg
1200mcg of Actiq: 2 x 200mcg tabs
1600mcg of Actiq: 2 x 200mcg tabs

Titrate to effective dose

PEDIATRIC DOSAGE
Pediatric use may not have been established

DOSING CONSIDERATIONS
Discontinuation
Gradual downward titration is recommended

ADMINISTRATION
Buccal/SL route

Do not split, crush, suck, chew, or swallow whole
Do not attempt to push tab through the blister as this may cause damage to the tab
Immediately place entire tab in the buccal cavity (above a rear molar, between the upper cheek and gum)
Once effective dose is determined during titration, an alternate route is SL
Leave tab in place until it has disintegrated (usually about 14-25 min)
If remnants from the tab remain after 30 min, may swallow w/ a glass of water
Alternate sides of the mouth when administering subsequent doses in the buccal cavity

STORAGE
20-25°C (68-77°F); excursions permitted to 15-30°C (59-86°F). Protect from freezing and moisture.

HOW SUPPLIED
Tab, Buccal: 100mcg, 200mcg, 400mcg, 600mcg, 800mcg

CONTRAINDICATIONS
Opioid-nontolerant patients, management of acute or postoperative pain, including headache/migraine and dental pain, known intolerance or hypersensitivity to fentanyl or any of the components in this medication.

WARNINGS/PRECAUTIONS
Increased risk of respiratory depression in patients with underlying respiratory disorders and in elderly/debilitated. May impair mental and/or physical abilities. Caution with chronic obstructive pulmonary disease or preexisting medical conditions predisposing to respiratory depression; may further decrease respiratory drive to the point of respiratory failure. May obscure clinical course of head injuries; use extreme caution in patients who may be susceptible to the intracranial effects of carbon dioxide retention (eg, with evidence of increased intracranial pressure or impaired consciousness). Application-site reactions (paresthesia, ulceration, bleeding) reported. Avoid use during labor and delivery. Caution with renal/hepatic impairment, bradyarrhythmias, and in elderly.

ADVERSE REACTIONS
Respiratory depression, headache, N/V, constipation, dizziness, dyspnea, somnolence, fatigue, anemia, asthenia, abdominal pain, dehydration, peripheral edema, diarrhea, anorexia.

DRUG INTERACTIONS
See Boxed Warning. CYP3A4 inducers (eg, carbamazepine, efavirenz, modafinil, phenobarbital, pioglitazone, rifampin, St. John's wort) may decrease levels. Respiratory depression is more likely to occur when given with other drugs that depress respiration. Increased depressant effects with other CNS depressants (eg, sedatives, hypnotics, tranquilizers, skeletal muscle relaxants, sedating antihistamines, alcohol); consider adjusting fentanyl dose if warranted. Not recommended for use in patients who have received MAOIs within 14 days.

PREGNANCY AND LACTATION
Category C, not for use in nursing.

MECHANISM OF ACTION
Opioid analgesic; has not been established. Known to be μ-opioid receptor agonist; specific CNS opioid receptors for endogenous compounds with opioid-like activity have been identified throughout the brain and spinal cord and play a role in analgesic effects.

PHARMACOKINETICS
Absorption: Readily absorbed. Absolute bioavailability (65%). Administration of variable doses resulted in different pharmacokinetic parameters. **Distribution:** V_d=25.4L/kg; plasma protein binding (80-85%); found in breast milk; crosses placenta. **Metabolism:** Liver and intestinal mucosa via CYP3A4; norfentanyl (metabolite). **Elimination:** Urine (<7%, unchanged), feces (1%, unchanged). $T_{1/2}$=2.63 hrs (100mcg), 4.43 hrs (200mcg), 11.09 hrs (400mcg), 11.7 hrs (800mcg).

PATIENT CONSIDERATIONS
Assessment: Assess for degree of opioid tolerance, previous opioid dose, type and severity of pain, general condition and medical status, and any other conditions where treatment is contraindicated or cautioned. Assess for hypersensitivity to the drug, renal/hepatic impairment, pregnancy/nursing status, and possible drug interactions.

Monitoring: Monitor for signs/symptoms of respiratory depression, impairment of mental/physical abilities, application-site reactions, bradycardia, drug abuse/addiction, and other adverse reactions.

Counseling: Instruct outpatients to enroll in the TIRF REMS Access program. Instruct to keep drug out of reach of children. Advise to take ud and to not share it with anyone else. Instruct to notify physician if breakthrough pain is not alleviated or worsens after taking the drug. Inform that drug may impair mental/physical abilities; caution against performing activities that require high level of attention (eg, operating machinery/driving). Advise not to combine with alcohol, sleep aids, or tranquilizers except by order of prescribing physician. Instruct to notify physician if pregnant or planning to become pregnant. Inform of proper storage, administration, and disposal.

FERRALET 90 — docusate sodium/iron (carbonyl iron, ferrous gluconate)/vitamin B9 (folic acid)/vitamin B12 (cyanocobalamin)/ vitamin C (ascorbic acid)   **Rx**

Class: Iron/mineral/vitamin

> Accidental overdose of iron-containing products is a leading cause of fatal poisoning in children <6 yrs; keep out of reach of children. In case of accidental overdose, call a physician or poison control center immediately.

ADULT DOSAGE	**PEDIATRIC DOSAGE**
Anemia	Pediatric use may not have been established
Anemias responsive to oral iron therapy (eg, hypochromic anemia associated w/ pregnancy, chronic and/or acute blood loss, metabolic disease, postsurgical convalescence, dietary needs)	
1 tab qd or ud	

DOSING CONSIDERATIONS
Elderly
Start at lower end of dosing range

ADMINISTRATION
Oral route

Do not chew tab.
Take 2 hrs pc.

STORAGE
25°C (77°F); excursions permitted to 15-30°C (59-86°F). Avoid moisture.

HOW SUPPLIED
Tab: Iron 90mg/Folic Acid 1mg/Vitamin B12 12mcg/Vitamin C 120mg/Docusate 50mg

CONTRAINDICATIONS
Hypersensitivity to any of the ingredients; hemolytic anemia, hemochromatosis, and hemosiderosis.

WARNINGS/PRECAUTIONS
Folic acid alone is improper therapy in the treatment of pernicious anemia and other megaloblastic anemias where vitamin B12 is deficient. D/C use if symptoms of intolerance appear. Determine type of anemia and underlying causes before starting therapy. Determine Hgb, Hct, and reticulocyte counts before starting therapy and periodically thereafter during prolonged treatment. Periodically review therapy to determine if it needs to be continued without change or if a dose change is indicated. Contains FD&C Yellow No. 5 (tartrazine), which may cause allergic-type reactions (including bronchial asthma). Folic acid in doses >0.1mg/day may obscure pernicious anemia; hematologic remission may occur while neurological manifestations remain progressive. Exclude pernicious anemia before use. Caution in elderly.

ADVERSE REACTIONS
GI irritation, constipation, diarrhea, N/V, dark stools, allergic sensitization.

DRUG INTERACTIONS
Iron may interact with antacids, tetracyclines, or fluoroquinolones.

PREGNANCY AND LACTATION
Safety not known in nursing.

MECHANISM OF ACTION
Iron/vitamin/mineral.

PATIENT CONSIDERATIONS
Assessment: Assess for hemolytic anemia, hemochromatosis, hemosiderosis, type of anemia, underlying causes of anemia, hypersensitivity to drug, nursing status, and possible drug interactions. Determine Hgb, Hct, and reticulocyte counts.

Monitoring: Monitor for symptoms of intolerance, allergic-type reactions, and masking of pernicious anemia. Determine Hgb, Hct, and reticulocyte counts periodically during prolonged therapy. Periodically review therapy to determine if it needs to be continued without change or if a dose change is indicated.

Counseling: Instruct to use qd or ud, and to d/c use and consult physician if symptoms of intolerance appear. Advise to keep drug out of reach of children, and to immediately call a doctor or poison control center in case of accidental overdose.

FETZIMA — levomilnacipran   **Rx**

Class: Serotonin and norepinephrine reuptake inhibitor (SNRI)

> Antidepressants increased the risk of suicidal thoughts and behavior in children, adolescents, and young adults in short-term studies. Monitor and observe closely for worsening, and for emergence of suicidal thoughts and behaviors. Not approved for use in pediatric patients.

ADULT DOSAGE	**PEDIATRIC DOSAGE**
Major Depressive Disorder	Pediatric use may not have been established
Initial: 20mg qd for 2 days	
Titrate: Increase to 40mg qd. Based on efficacy and tolerability, may then be increased in increments of 40mg at intervals of ≥2 days	

Range: 40-120mg qd
Max: 120mg qd

Periodically reassess need for maint treatment and the appropriate dose

Dosing Considerations with MAOIs

Switching to/from an MAOI for Psychiatric Disorders:
Allow at least 14 days between discontinuation of an MAOI and initiation of treatment, and allow at least 7 days between discontinuation of treatment and initiation of an MAOI

W/ Other MAOIs (eg, Linezolid, IV Methylene Blue):
Do not start levomilnacipran in patients being treated w/ linezolid or IV methylene blue
In patients already receiving levomilnacipran, if acceptable alternatives are not available and benefits outweigh risks, d/c levomilnacipran and administer linezolid or IV methylene blue; monitor for serotonin syndrome for 2 weeks or until 24 hrs after the last dose of linezolid or IV methylene blue, whichever comes 1st. May resume levomilnacipran therapy 24 hrs after the last dose of linezolid or IV methylene blue

---

DOSING CONSIDERATIONS
Concomitant Medications
Use w/ Strong CYP3A4 Inhibitors:
Max: 80mg qd
Renal Impairment
Moderate (CrCl 30-59mL/min):
Max Maint: 80mg qd
Severe (CrCl 15-29mL/min):
Max Maint: 40mg qd

ESRD: Not recommended

Discontinuation
Gradually reduce dose, whenever possible; if intolerable symptoms occur following a dose decrease or upon discontinuation of treatment, consider resuming previously prescribed dose and decreasing the dose at a more gradual rate

ADMINISTRATION
Oral route

Take at the same time each day, w/ or w/o food.
Swallow cap whole; do not open, chew, or crush.

STORAGE
25°C (77°F); excursions permitted between 15-30°C (59-86°F).

HOW SUPPLIED
Cap, Extended-Release: 20mg, 40mg, 80mg, 120mg; (Titration Pack) 20mg [2s], 40mg [26s]

CONTRAINDICATIONS
Hypersensitivity to levomilnacipran, milnacipran HCl, or to any excipient in the formulation. Use of MAOIs intended to treat psychiatric disorders w/ levomilnacipran or w/in 7 days of stopping treatment w/ levomilnacipran. Use of levomilnacipran w/in 14 days of stopping an MAOI intended to treat psychiatric disorders. Starting levomilnacipran in a patient who is being treated w/ MAOIs (eg, linezolid or IV methylene blue).

WARNINGS/PRECAUTIONS
Not recommended for patients with end-stage renal disease. Not approved for the treatment of bipolar depression. Serotonin syndrome reported; d/c immediately if symptoms occur and initiate supportive symptomatic treatment. Associated with increases in BP and HR; control preexisting HTN or treat preexisting tachyarrhythmias and other cardiac disease before initiating treatment. Caution with preexisting HTN, cardiovascular (CV) or cerebrovascular conditions that might be compromised by increases in BP. Consider discontinuation or other appropriate medical intervention if sustained increase in BP or HR occurs. May increase risk of bleeding events. Pupillary dilation that occurs following therapy may trigger an angle-closure attack in a patient with anatomically narrow angles who does not have a patent iridectomy. May affect urethral resistance; caution in patients prone to obstructive urinary disorders. If symptoms of urinary hesitation, urinary retention, or dysuria develop, consider discontinuation or other appropriate medical intervention. Activation of mania/hypomania reported; caution with history or family history of bipolar disorder, mania, or hypomania. Seizures reported; caution in patients with a seizure disorder. Discontinuation symptoms may occur. Avoid abrupt discontinuation; reduce dose gradually whenever possible. Hyponatremia may occur; elderly and volume-depleted patients may be at greater risk. D/C in patients with symptomatic hyponatremia and institute appropriate medical intervention.

ADVERSE REACTIONS
N/V, constipation, hyperhidrosis, HR/BP increased, erectile dysfunction, tachycardia, palpitations, testicular pain, ejaculation disorder, urinary hesitation, hot flush, hypotension, HTN, decreased appetite.

DRUG INTERACTIONS
See Contraindications and Dosage. May cause serotonin syndrome with other serotonergic drugs (eg, triptans, TCAs, fentanyl, lithium, St. John's wort) and with drugs that impair metabolism of serotonin; d/c immediately if serotonin syndrome occurs. Caution with NSAIDs, aspirin (ASA), warfarin, and other drugs that affect coagulation or bleeding due to potential increased risk of bleeding. Increased exposure with CYP3A4 inhibitor ketoconazole. Caution with other CNS-active drugs, including those with a similar mechanism of action. Do not give with alcohol; pronounced accelerated drug release may occur. Caution with drugs that increase BP and HR. Increased risk of hyponatremia with diuretics.

PREGNANCY AND LACTATION
Category C, not for use in nursing.

MECHANISM OF ACTION
SNRI; has not been established. Thought to be related to the potentiation of serotonin and norepinephrine in the CNS, through inhibition of reuptake at serotonin and norepinephrine transporters.

PHARMACOKINETICS
Absorption: C_{max}=341ng/mL; AUC=5196ng•hr/mL; T_{max}=6-8 hrs (median).
Distribution: V_d=387-473L; plasma protein binding (22%). **Metabolism:** Desethylation (primarily via CYP3A4 with minor contribution by CYP2C8, 2C19, 2D6, and 2J2) and hydroxylation; further conjugation with glucuronide. **Elimination:** Urine (58% unchanged, 18% N-desethyl levomilnacipran); $T_{1/2}$=12 hrs.

PATIENT CONSIDERATIONS

Assessment: Assess for risk for bipolar disorder, HTN, CV/cerebrovascular conditions, tachyarrhythmias, susceptibility to angle-closure glaucoma/obstructive urinary disorders, history of mania/hypomania, seizure disorder, volume depletion, hypersensitivity to the drug, renal impairment, pregnancy/nursing status, and possible drug interactions.

Monitoring: Monitor for signs/symptoms of clinical worsening, suicidality, unusual changes in behavior, serotonin syndrome, bleeding events, angle-closure glaucoma, urinary hesitation/retention, dysuria, activation of mania/hypomania, seizures, discontinuation symptoms, hyponatremia, and other adverse reactions. Monitor BP and HR periodically. Periodically reassess the need for maintenance treatment and the appropriate dose.

Counseling: Advise about the benefits and risks of therapy and counsel on its appropriate use. Counsel to look for the emergence of suicidality, especially early during treatment and when the dose is adjusted up or down. Caution about the risk of serotonin syndrome, particularly with the concomitant use with other serotonergic agents. Inform that concomitant use with ASA, NSAIDs, warfarin, or other drugs that affect coagulation may increase the risk of abnormal bleeding. Inform that drug can cause mild pupillary dilation, which in susceptible individuals, can lead to an episode of angle-closure glaucoma. Advise to have BP and HR monitored regularly, to observe for signs of activation of mania/hypomania, to avoid alcohol consumption, and not to d/c therapy without notifying physician. Caution against operating hazardous machinery until reasonably certain that therapy does not adversely affect ability to engage in such activities. Advise to notify physician if allergic reactions develop, if pregnant/intending to become pregnant, or if breastfeeding.

FIBRICOR — fenofibric acid   Rx

Class: Fibric acid derivative

ADULT DOSAGE	PEDIATRIC DOSAGE
Severe Hypertriglyceridemia	Pediatric use may not have been established
Initial: 35-105mg/day	
Titrate: Adjust dose if necessary following repeat lipid determinations at 4- to 8-week intervals; may consider reducing dose if lipid levels fall significantly below targeted range	
Max: 105mg qd	
D/C if no adequate response after 2 months of treatment with max dose	
Primary Hypercholesterolemia/Mixed Dyslipidemia	
Usual/Max: 105mg/day	
Titrate: May consider reducing dose if lipid levels fall significantly below targeted range	
D/C if no adequate response after 2 months of treatment with max dose	

DOSING CONSIDERATIONS
Renal Impairment
Mild to Moderate:
Initial: 35mg qd
Titrate: Increase only after evaluation of effects on renal function and lipid levels
ADMINISTRATION
Oral route

May be taken without regard to meals
Swallow tab whole; do not crush, dissolve, or chew

STORAGE
20-25°C (68-77°F).

HOW SUPPLIED
Tab: 35mg, 105mg

CONTRAINDICATIONS
Severe renal impairment (including dialysis), active liver disease (including primary biliary cirrhosis and unexplained persistent liver function abnormalities), preexisting gallbladder disease, hypersensitivity to fenofibric acid or fenofibrate, nursing mothers.

WARNINGS/PRECAUTIONS
Not shown to reduce coronary heart disease morbidity and mortality in patients with type 2 diabetes mellitus. Increased risk of myopathy and rhabdomyolysis; risk increased with diabetes, renal failure, hypothyroidism, and in elderly. D/C if marked CPK elevation occurs or myopathy/myositis is suspected or diagnosed. Increases in serum transaminases, hepatocellular, chronic active, and cholestatic hepatitis, and cirrhosis (rare) reported; perform baseline and regular periodic monitoring of LFTs, and d/c therapy if enzyme levels persist >3X the normal limit. Elevations in SrCr reported; monitor renal function in patients with renal impairment or at risk for renal insufficiency. May cause cholelithiasis; d/c if gallstones are found. Acute hypersensitivity reactions and pancreatitis reported. Mild to moderate decreases in Hgb, Hct, and WBCs, thrombocytopenia, and agranulocytosis reported; periodically monitor RBC and WBC counts during the first 12 months of therapy. May cause venothromboembolic disease. Severe decreases in HDL levels reported; check HDL levels within the 1st few months after initiation of therapy. If a severely depressed HDL level is detected, withdraw therapy, monitor HDL level until it has returned to baseline, and do not reinitiate therapy. Estrogen therapy, thiazide diuretics, and β-blockers may be associated with massive rises in plasma TGs; discontinuation of these drugs may obviate the need for specific drug therapy of hypertriglyceridemia.

ADVERSE REACTIONS
Abdominal pain, back pain, headache, abnormal LFTs, increased ALT/AST/CPK, respiratory disorder.

DRUG INTERACTIONS
Increased risk of rhabdomyolysis with HMG-CoA reductase inhibitors (statins); avoid combination unless benefit outweighs risk. May potentiate anticoagulant effects of coumarin anticoagulants; use with caution, reduce anticoagulant dosage, and monitor PT/INR frequently. Bile acid-binding resins may bind other drugs given concurrently; take at least 1 hr before or 4-6 hrs after the bile acid-binding resin. Immunosuppressants (eg, cyclosporine, tacrolimus) may produce nephrotoxicity; consider benefits and risks, use lowest effective dose, and monitor renal function with immunosuppressants and other potentially nephrotoxic agents. Cases of myopathy, including rhabdomyolysis, reported when coadministered with colchicine; caution when prescribing with colchicine.

PREGNANCY AND LACTATION
Category C, not for use in nursing.

MECHANISM OF ACTION
Fibric acid derivative; activates peroxisome proliferator-activated receptor α. Increases lipolysis and elimination of TG-rich particles from plasma by activating lipoprotein lipase and reducing production of apoprotein C-III (lipoprotein lipase activity inhibitor). Also, induces an increase in the synthesis of apoproteins A-I, A-II, and HDL.

PHARMACOKINETICS
Absorption: T_{max}=2.5 hrs (median). **Distribution:** Plasma protein binding (99%). **Metabolism:** Conjugation with glucuronic acid. **Elimination:** Urine; $T_{1/2}$=20 hrs.

PATIENT CONSIDERATIONS

Assessment: Assess for renal impairment, active liver disease, gallbladder disease, other medical conditions (eg, diabetes, hypothyroidism), hypersensitivity to the drug, pregnancy/nursing status, and possible drug interactions. Obtain baseline LFTs.

Monitoring: Monitor for myopathy, myositis, or rhabdomyolysis; measure CPK levels in patients reporting such symptoms. Monitor for cholelithiasis, pancreatitis, hypersensitivity reactions, pulmonary embolus, and deep vein thrombosis. Monitor renal function, LFTs, CBC, and lipid levels. Monitor PT/INR frequently with coumarin anticoagulants.

Counseling: Advise of potential benefits and risks of therapy, and of medications to avoid during treatment. Instruct to follow appropriate lipid-modifying diet during therapy, and to take ud. Instruct to inform physician of all medications, supplements, and herbal preparations being taken, any changes in medical condition, development of muscle pain, tenderness, or weakness, and onset of abdominal pain or any other new symptoms. Advise to return for routine monitoring.

Finacea Foam — azelaic acid   Rx
Class: Dicarboxylic acid antimicrobial

ADULT DOSAGE	**PEDIATRIC DOSAGE**
Rosacea	Pediatric use may not have been established
Inflammatory Papules/Pustules of Mild to Moderate Rosacea: Apply a thin layer to the entire facial area (cheeks, chin, forehead, and nose) bid (am and pm)	
Use continuously over 12 weeks; reassess if no improvement is observed upon completing 12 weeks of therapy	

ADMINISTRATION
Topical route
Shake well before use.
Cosmetics may be applied after the application of foam has dried.
Avoid the use of occlusive dressings or wrappings.

STORAGE
25°C (77°F); excursions permitted between 15-30°C (59-86°F). Product is flammable; avoid fire, flame, or smoking during and immediately following application. Do not puncture or incinerate drug container, expose to heat, or store at temperatures >49°C (120°F).

HOW SUPPLIED
Foam: 15% [50g]

WARNINGS/PRECAUTIONS
Hypopigmentation reported; monitor patients w/ dark complexion for early signs of hypopigmentation. Irritation of the eyes reported; avoid contact w/ the eyes, mouth, and other mucous membranes. Propellant in foam is flammable; avoid fire, flame, and smoking during and immediately following application. Caution in elderly.

ADVERSE REACTIONS
Application-site pain.

PREGNANCY AND LACTATION
Pregnancy: Category B.
Lactation: Not for use in nursing.

MECHANISM OF ACTION
Dicarboxylic acid antimicrobial; has not been established.

PHARMACOKINETICS
Absorption: C_{max}=51.8ng/mL (azelaic acid), 5ng/mL (pimelic acid); AUC=442ng·hr/mL (azelaic acid), 43.4ng·hr/mL (pimelic acid). **Metabolism:** β-oxidation to shorter chain dicarboxylic acids; pimelic acid (metabolite). **Elimination:** Urine (mainly unchanged).

PATIENT CONSIDERATIONS

Assessment: Assess hypersensitivity to drug and pregnancy/nursing status.

Monitoring: Monitor for skin reactions; eyes, mouth, and other mucous membranes irritation; and for other adverse reactions. Monitor for early signs of hypopigmentation in patients w/ dark complexion. Monitor response to therapy; reassess if no improvement is observed upon completing 12 weeks of therapy.

Counseling: Advise to cleanse affected area(s) w/ a very mild soap or a soapless cleansing lotion and pat dry w/ a soft towel. Instruct to avoid use of alcoholic cleansers, tinctures and astringents, abrasives, and peeling agents. Instruct to avoid contact w/ the eyes, mouth, and other mucous membranes explaining that if contact w/ the eyes occurs, patient should wash eyes w/ large amounts of water and consult physician if eye irritation persists. Instruct to d/c use and consult physician if an allergic reaction occurs. Advise to wash hands immediately following application of the foam. Inform that cosmetics may be applied after the application of foam has dried. Advise to avoid the use of occlusive dressings and wrappings. Instruct to avoid any triggers that may provoke erythema, flushing, and blushing (eg, spicy and thermally hot food and drinks, alcoholic beverages). Inform that the propellant in the foam is flammable; instruct to avoid fire, flame, or smoking during and immediately following application. Instruct to discard the product 8 weeks after opening.

Finacea Gel — azelaic acid   Rx
Class: Dicarboxylic acid antimicrobial

ADULT DOSAGE	**PEDIATRIC DOSAGE**
Rosacea	Pediatric use may not have been established
Inflammatory Papules/Pustules of Mild to Moderate Rosacea: Apply and gently massage thin layer into affected areas on the face bid (am and pm)	
Reassess if no improvement observed upon completing 12 weeks of therapy	

ADMINISTRATION
Topical route

- Cleanse affected area w/ very mild soaps or soapless cleansing lotion and pat dry w/ soft towel before application.
- Cosmetics may be applied after the application of gel has dried.
- Avoid the use of occlusive dressings or wrappings.
- Avoid spicy foods, thermally hot foods and drinks, and alcoholic beverages.

STORAGE
25°C (77°F); excursions permitted to 15-30°C (59-86°F). Discard pump after 8 weeks after opening.

HOW SUPPLIED
Gel: 15% [45g pump, 50g tube]

WARNINGS/PRECAUTIONS
Hypersensitivity reactions reported; avoid use w/ known hypersensitivity. D/C if hypersensitivity develops and institute appropriate therapy. Skin irritation (eg, pruritus, burning, stinging) may occur during 1st few weeks of treatment; d/c if sensitivity or severe irritation develops/persists and institute appropriate therapy. Hypopigmentation reported. Avoid contact w/ eyes, mouth, and other mucous membranes. Worsening of asthma reported.

ADVERSE REACTIONS

Burning/stinging/tingling, pruritus, scaling/dry skin/xerosis, erythema/irritation.

PREGNANCY AND LACTATION

Pregnancy: Category B.

Lactation: Not for use in nursing.

MECHANISM OF ACTION

Dicarboxylic acid antimicrobial; has not been established.

PHARMACOKINETICS

Metabolism: β-oxidation to shorter chain dicarboxylic acids. **Elimination:** Urine (mainly unchanged).

PATIENT CONSIDERATIONS

Assessment: Assess for previous hypersensitivity and pregnancy/nursing status.

Monitoring: Monitor for sensitivity reactions or skin irritation/reaction and other adverse reactions. Monitor for early signs of hypopigmentation in patients w/ dark complexion.

Counseling: Inform that medication is for external use only. Instruct to avoid contact w/ eyes, mouth, and other mucous membranes; if contact w/ eyes occurs, instruct to wash eyes w/ large amounts of water and to consult physician if eye irritation persists. Advise to avoid alcoholic cleansers, tinctures and astringents, abrasives, and peeling agents. Instruct to wash hands immediately after application. Inform that cosmetics may be applied after application of gel has dried. Instruct to avoid using occlusive dressings or wrappings and to avoid eating spicy foods, alcoholic beverages, and thermally hot food and drinks. Inform that skin irritation may occur, usually during 1st few weeks of treatment; if irritation is excessive or persists, or allergic reactions occur, instruct to d/c therapy and consult a physician. Instruct to report abnormal changes in skin color. Instruct on how to properly use pump. Instruct to d/c and consult healthcare provider if allergic reaction occurs. Advise to inform of worsening asthma.

FIORINAL — aspirin/butalbital/caffeine CIII

Class: Analgesic/barbiturate

ADULT DOSAGE	PEDIATRIC DOSAGE
Tension Headache	Pediatric use may not have been established
1-2 caps q4h	
Max: 6 caps/day	

ADMINISTRATION

Oral route

STORAGE

Below 25°C (77°F); tight container. Protect from moisture.

HOW SUPPLIED

Cap: (Butalbital/Aspirin [ASA]/Caffeine) 50mg/325mg/40mg

CONTRAINDICATIONS

Hypersensitivity or intolerance to ASA, caffeine, or butalbital; hemorrhagic diathesis (eg, hemophilia, hypoprothrombinemia, von Willebrand's disease, the thrombocytopenias, thrombasthenia and other ill-defined hereditary platelet dysfunctions, severe vitamin K deficiency and severe liver damage); syndrome of nasal polyps, angioedema, and bronchospastic reactivity to ASA or other NSAIDs; peptic ulcer or other serious GI lesions; porphyria.

WARNINGS/PRECAUTIONS

Not for extended and repeated use. May be habit-forming. Caution in elderly, debilitated, with severe renal/hepatic impairment, hypothyroidism, urethral stricture, head injuries, elevated intracranial pressure, acute abdominal conditions, Addison's disease, prostatic hypertrophy, presence of peptic ulcer, and coagulation disorders. Therapeutic doses of ASA can lead to anaphylactic shock and severe allergic reactions. Significant bleeding possible with peptic ulcers, GI lesions, or bleeding disorders. Caution in children, including teenagers, with chickenpox or flu. Preoperative ASA may prolong bleeding time.

ADVERSE REACTIONS

Drowsiness, lightheadedness, dizziness, N/V, flatulence.

DRUG INTERACTIONS

Caution with anticoagulant therapy; may enhance bleeding. CNS effects enhanced by MAOIs. Additive CNS depression with alcohol, other narcotic analgesics, general anesthetics, tranquilizers (eg, chlordiazepoxide), sedatives/hypnotics, other CNS depressants. May cause hypoglycemia with oral antidiabetic agents and insulin. May cause bone marrow toxicity and blood dyscrasias with 6-mercaptopurine and methotrexate. Increased risk of peptic ulceration and bleeding with NSAIDs. Decreased effects of uricosuric agents (eg, probenecid, sulfinpyrazone). Withdrawal of corticosteroids may cause salicylism with chronic ASA use.

PREGNANCY AND LACTATION

Category C, not for use in nursing.

MECHANISM OF ACTION

Butalbital: Short- to intermediate-acting barbiturate. ASA: Analgesic, antipyretic, and anti-inflammatory. Caffeine: CNS stimulant. Combines analgesic properties of ASA with anxiolytic and muscle relaxant properties of butalbital.

PHARMACOKINETICS

Absorption: ASA: (650mg dose) T_{max}=40 min, C_{max}=8.8mcg/mL. Butalbital: Well-absorbed; (100mg dose) C_{max}=2020ng/mL, T_{max}=1.5 hrs. Caffeine: Rapid; (80mg dose) C_{max}=1660ng/mL, T_{max}=<1 hr. **Distribution:** ASA: Found in fetal tissue, breast milk; Plasma protein binding (50-80%). Butalbital: Crosses placenta,

found in breast milk; Plasma protein binding (45%). Caffeine: Found in fetal tissue, breast milk. **Metabolism:** ASA: Liver; salicyluric acid, phenolic/acyl glucuronides of salicylate, gentisic and gentisuric acid (major metabolites). Caffeine: Liver; 1-methylxanthine and 1-methyluric acid (metabolites). **Elimination:** ASA: Urine; $T_{1/2}$=12 min (ASA), 3 hrs (salicylic acid/total salicylates). Butalbital: Urine (59-88%); $T_{1/2}$=35 hrs. Caffeine: Urine (70%, 3% unchanged); $T_{1/2}$=3 hrs.

PATIENT CONSIDERATIONS

Assessment: Assess for previous hypersensitivity to drug, renal/hepatic function, porphyria, peptic ulcer, other serious GI lesions, bleeding disorders, or any other conditions where treatment is cautioned or contraindicated. Assess for pregnancy/nursing status and possible drug interactions.

Monitoring: Serial monitoring of LFTs and/or renal function with severe hepatic/renal disease. Monitor for anaphylactoid/hypersensitivity reactions, drug abuse/dependence and bleeding.

Counseling: Advise not to take if patient has ASA allergy. Instruct to take exactly as prescribed; instruct to avoid coadministration with alcohol or other CNS depressants. Advise to avoid hazardous tasks (eg, operating machinery/driving) while on therapy. Counsel that drug may be habit-forming.

FLAGYL — metronidazole Rx

Class: Nitroimidazole

> Shown to be carcinogenic in mice and rats. Avoid unnecessary use. Should be reserved for the conditions for which it is indicated.

ADULT DOSAGE	PEDIATRIC DOSAGE
Anaerobic Bacterial Infections	**Amebiasis**
IV metronidazole is usually administered initially in the treatment of most serious infections	**Cap/Tab:** 35-50mg/kg/24 hrs, divided into 3 doses, for 10 days
Cap/Tab:	
Usual: 7.5mg/kg q6h	
Max: 4g/24 hrs	
Duration: 7-10 days; bone and joint, lower respiratory tract, and endocardium infections may require longer treatment	
Trichomoniasis	
Female:	
7-Day Course of Treatment:	
Cap: 375mg bid for 7 consecutive days	
Tab: 250mg tid for 7 consecutive days	
1-Day Treatment:	
Tab: 2g given as a single dose or in 2 divided doses of 1g each, given in the same day	
When repeat courses are required, allow an interval of 4-6 weeks between courses, and reconfirm presence of the trichomonad	
Male:	
Individualize treatment as it is for the female	
Amebiasis	
Acute Intestinal Amebiasis (Acute Amebic Dysentery):	
Cap/Tab:	
750mg tid for 5-10 days	
Amebic Liver Abscess:	
Cap:	
750mg tid for 5-10 days	
Tab:	
500mg or 750mg tid for 5-10 days	

DOSING CONSIDERATIONS

Renal Impairment

Hemodialysis: If administration cannot be separated from hemodialysis session, consider supplementation of metronidazole dosage following hemodialysis session

Hepatic Impairment

Severe (Child-Pugh C):

Cap:

Amebiasis: 375mg q8h for 5-10 days

Trichomoniasis: 375mg q24h for 7 days

Tab:

Reduce dosage by 50%

ADMINISTRATION

Oral route

STORAGE

Cap: 15-25°C (59-77°F). **Tab:** <25°C (77°F). Protect from light.

HOW SUPPLIED
Cap: 375mg; **Tab:** 250mg, 500mg

CONTRAINDICATIONS
Prior history of hypersensitivity to metronidazole or other nitroimidazole derivatives. Disulfiram use w/in the last 2 weeks. Consumption of alcohol or products containing propylene glycol during and for at least 3 days after therapy w/ metronidazole. Use during the 1st trimester of pregnancy in trichomoniasis patients.

WARNINGS/PRECAUTIONS
Cases of encephalopathy and peripheral neuropathy (including optic neuropathy), convulsive seizures, and aseptic meningitis reported; promptly evaluate benefit/risk ratio of the continuation of therapy if abnormal neurologic signs/symptoms appear. Known or previously unrecognized candidiasis may present more prominent symptoms during therapy and requires treatment w/ a candidacidal agent. Caution w/ hepatic/renal impairment, evidence of or history of blood dyscrasia, and in the elderly. Mild leukopenia reported; monitor total and differential leukocyte counts before and after therapy. May result in bacterial/parasitic resistance if used in the absence of proven or suspected bacterial/parasitic infection, or a prophylactic indication. Lab test interactions may occur. **Tab:** In pregnant patients for whom alternative treatment has been inadequate, the 1-day course of therapy should not be used for trichomoniasis.

ADVERSE REACTIONS
Headache, syncope, dizziness, vertigo, incoordination, nausea, diarrhea, epigastric distress, abdominal cramping, constipation, unpleasant metallic taste, erythematous rash, pruritus, urticaria, dysuria.

DRUG INTERACTIONS
See Contraindications. May potentiate anticoagulant effect of warfarin and other oral coumarin anticoagulants, resulting in PT prolongation; carefully monitor PT and INR. May increase serum lithium, and may cause lithium toxicity; obtain serum lithium and serum creatinine levels several days after beginning metronidazole. May increase busulfan levels, which may increase risk for serious busulfan toxicity; avoid concomitant use, or, if coadministration is medically needed, frequently monitor busulfan concentration and adjust busulfan dose accordingly. Simultaneous administration of drugs that decrease microsomal liver enzyme activity (eg, cimetidine) may prolong $T_{1/2}$ and decrease clearance. Simultaneous administration of drugs that induce microsomal liver enzymes (eg, phenytoin, phenobarbital) may accelerate elimination, resulting in reduced levels. Impaired clearance of phenytoin reported.

PREGNANCY AND LACTATION
Pregnancy: Category B.
Lactation: Not for use in nursing.

MECHANISM OF ACTION
Nitroimidazole antimicrobial; exerts antibacterial effects in an anaerobic environment. Upon entering the organism, the drug is reduced by intracellular electron transport proteins, transfer of an electron to the nitro group, and formation of a short-lived nitroso free radical. Because of this alteration, a concentration gradient is maintained, promoting intracellular transport. The reduced metronidazole and free radicals interact w/ DNA, leading to inhibition of DNA synthesis and DNA degradation, leading to death of the bacteria.

PHARMACOKINETICS
Absorption: Well-absorbed. Administration of multiple doses resulted in different parameters. **Distribution:** Plasma protein binding (<20%); found in breast milk; crosses the placenta. **Metabolism:** Side-chain oxidation and glucuronide conjugation; 1-(β-hydroxyethyl)-2-hydroxymethyl-5-nitroimidazole and 2-methyl-5-nitroimidazole-1-yl-acetic acid (metabolites). **Elimination:** Urine (60-80%, 20% unchanged), feces (6-15%); (Healthy) $T_{1/2}$=8 hrs.

PATIENT CONSIDERATIONS
Assessment: Assess for candidiasis, alcohol use, hepatic/renal impairment, evidence/history of blood dyscrasia, hypersensitivity to drug or other nitroimidazole derivatives, pregnancy/nursing status, and possible drug interactions. Obtain total and differential leukocyte counts.

Monitoring: Monitor for abnormal neurologic signs/symptoms, candidiasis, and other adverse reactions. Monitor total and differential leukocyte counts after therapy. Monitor PT and INR w/ oral coumarin anticoagulants (eg, warfarin).

Counseling: Instruct to d/c consumption of alcoholic beverages or products containing propylene glycol while taking the drug and for at least 3 days afterward. Inform that therapy should only be used to treat bacterial and parasitic, not viral, infections. Instruct to take exactly ud. Inform that skipping doses or not completing the full course of therapy may decrease effectiveness of treatment and increase bacterial resistance.

FLAGYL ER — metronidazole   Rx
Class: Nitroimidazole

> Shown to be carcinogenic in mice and rats. Avoid unnecessary use. Should be reserved for the conditions for which it is indicated.

ADULT DOSAGE	PEDIATRIC DOSAGE
Bacterial Vaginosis	**Bacterial Vaginosis**
Nonpregnant Women: 750mg qd for 7 consecutive days	**Post-Menarche/Nonpregnant Females:** 750mg qd for 7 consecutive days

---

DOSING CONSIDERATIONS
Renal Impairment
Hemodialysis: If administration cannot be separated from hemodialysis session, consider supplementation of dosage following the session, depending on patient's clinical situation

Elderly
May need to adjust dose based on serum levels

ADMINISTRATION
Oral route

Take at least 1 hr ac or 2 hrs pc
Do not split, chew, or crush

STORAGE
25°C (77°F); excursions permitted to 15-30°C (59-86°F). Store in a dry place.

HOW SUPPLIED
Tab, Extended-Release: 750mg

CONTRAINDICATIONS
Prior history of hypersensitivity to metronidazole or other nitroimidazole derivatives, disulfiram use w/in the last 2 weeks, consumption of alcohol or products containing propylene glycol during and for at least 3 days after therapy.

WARNINGS/PRECAUTIONS
Cases of encephalopathy and peripheral neuropathy (including optic neuropathy), convulsive seizures, and aseptic meningitis reported; promptly evaluate benefit/risk ratio of the continuation of therapy if abnormal neurologic signs/symptoms appear. Known or previously unrecognized candidiasis may present more prominent symptoms during therapy and requires treatment with a candidacidal agent. Do not administer to patients with severe (Child-Pugh C) hepatic impairment unless benefits outweigh risks. Caution with hepatic/renal impairment, evidence of or history of blood dyscrasia, and in the elderly. Mild leukopenia reported; monitor total and differential leukocyte counts before and after therapy. May result in bacterial resistance if used in the absence of proven or suspected bacterial infection, or a prophylactic indication. Lab test interactions may occur.

ADVERSE REACTIONS
Headache, vaginitis, nausea, metallic taste, bacterial infection, influenza-like symptoms, genital pruritus, abdominal pain, dizziness, diarrhea, upper respiratory tract infection, rhinitis, sinusitis, pharyngitis, dysmenorrhea.

DRUG INTERACTIONS
See Contraindications. May potentiate anticoagulant effect of warfarin and other oral coumarin anticoagulants, resulting in PT prolongation; carefully monitor PT and INR. May increase serum lithium, and may cause lithium toxicity; obtain serum lithium and SrCr levels several days after beginning metronidazole. May increase busulfan concentrations, which can result in increased risk for serious busulfan toxicity; avoid concomitant use, or, if coadministration is medically needed, frequently monitor busulfan concentration and adjust busulfan dose accordingly. Simultaneous administration of drugs that decrease microsomal liver enzyme activity (eg, cimetidine) may prolong $T_{1/2}$ and decrease clearance. Simultaneous administration of drugs that induce microsomal liver enzymes (eg, phenytoin, phenobarbital) may accelerate elimination, resulting in reduced levels. Impaired clearance of phenytoin reported.

PREGNANCY AND LACTATION
Category B, not for use in nursing.

MECHANISM OF ACTION
Nitroimidazole antimicrobial; exerts antibacterial effects in an anaerobic environment. Upon entering the organism, the drug is reduced by intracellular electron transport proteins. Because of this alteration, a concentration gradient is maintained which promotes the drug's intracellular transport. Presumably, free radicals are formed which, in turn, react with cellular components, resulting in death of the bacteria.

PHARMACOKINETICS
Absorption: (Healthy adults) C_{max}=19.4mcg/mL (fed), 12.5mcg/mL (fasted); T_{max}=4.6 hrs (fed), 6.8 hrs (fasted); AUC=211mcg•hr/mL (fed), 198mcg•hr/mL (fasted). **Distribution:** Plasma protein binding (<20%); found in breast milk; crosses the placenta. **Metabolism:** Side-chain oxidation and glucuronide conjugation; 1-(β-hydroxyethyl)-2-hydroxymethyl-5-nitroimidazole and 2-methyl-5-nitroimidazole-1-yl-acetic acid (metabolites). **Elimination:** Urine (60-80%, 20% unchanged), feces (6-15%); (Healthy adults) $T_{1/2}$=7.4 hrs (fed), 8.7 hrs (fasted).

PATIENT CONSIDERATIONS
Assessment: Assess for candidiasis, alcohol use, hepatic/renal impairment, evidence/history of blood dyscrasia, hypersensitivity to drug or other nitroimidazole derivatives, pregnancy/nursing status, and possible drug interactions. Obtain total and differential leukocyte counts.

Monitoring: Monitor for abnormal neurologic signs/symptoms, candidiasis, and other adverse reactions. Monitor total and differential leukocyte counts after therapy. Monitor PT and INR with oral coumarin anticoagulants (eg, warfarin).

Counseling: Instruct to d/c consumption of alcoholic beverages or products containing propylene glycol while taking the drug and for at least 3 days afterward. Counsel that therapy should only be used to treat bacterial, not viral (eg, common cold), infections. Instruct to take exactly ud. Inform that skipping doses or not completing full course of therapy may decrease effectiveness of treatment and increase bacterial resistance.

FLAREX — fluorometholone acetate   Rx

Class: Corticosteroid

ADULT DOSAGE

Steroid-Responsive Inflammatory Ocular Conditions

Treatment of Steroid Responsive Inflammatory Conditions of the Palpebral and Bulbar Conjunctiva, Cornea, and Anterior Segment of Eye:
Instill 1-2 drops into the conjunctival sac(s) qid; may increase to 2 drops q2h during initial 24-48 hrs

PEDIATRIC DOSAGE
Pediatric use may not have been established

ADMINISTRATION
Ocular route
Shake well before using.

STORAGE
Store upright between 2-25°C (36-77°F). Protect from freezing.

HOW SUPPLIED
Ophthalmic Sus: 0.1% [5mL]

CONTRAINDICATIONS
Acute superficial herpes simplex keratitis, vaccinia, varicella, viral diseases of cornea and conjunctiva, tuberculosis, fungal diseases, acute purulent untreated infections, known hypersensitivity to any component of this preparation.

WARNINGS/PRECAUTIONS
Caution in herpes simplex infection. Prolonged use may result in glaucoma, optic nerve damage, defect in visual acuity and visual field, cataract formation, and/or may aid in the establishment of secondary ocular infections from pathogens due to suppression of host response. May mask or exacerbate acute purulent infections of the eye. In those diseases causing thinning of the cornea or sclera, perforation may occur w/ chronic use; frequently check IOP. Fungal infections of the cornea may develop during long-term therapy; fungus invasion must be considered in any persistent corneal ulceration where a steroid has been used or is in use.

ADVERSE REACTIONS
Glaucoma w/ optic nerve damage, visual acuity and field defects, cataract formation, secondary ocular infection, and perforation of the globe.

PREGNANCY AND LACTATION
Pregnancy: Category C.
Lactation: It is not known whether topical administration of corticosteroids could result in sufficient systemic absorption to produce detectable quantities in human milk. Caution in nursing.

MECHANISM OF ACTION
Corticosteroid; suppress the inflammatory response to inciting mechanical, chemical, or immunological agents.

PATIENT CONSIDERATIONS

Assessment: Assess for acute superficial herpes simplex keratitis, vaccinia, varicella, viral diseases of cornea and conjunctiva, tuberculosis, fungal diseases, acute purulent untreated infections, and pregnancy/nursing status. Assess IOP.

Monitoring: Monitor for glaucoma, optic nerve damage, visual acuity and field defects, cataract formation, secondary ocular infection, and perforation of the globe. Monitor IOP.

Counseling: Instruct patients not to touch dropper tip at any surface, as this may contaminate the medication. Inform that the preservative, benzalkonium chloride, may be absorbed by soft contact lenses; instruct not to administer while wearing soft contact lenses.

FLECAINIDE — flecainide acetate   Rx

Class: Class IC antiarrhythmic

> Excessive mortality or nonfatal cardiac arrest rate reported in patients w/ asymptomatic non-life-threatening ventricular arrhythmias who had MI >6 days but <2 yrs previously. It is prudent to consider the risks of Class IC agents, coupled w/ the lack of any evidence of improved survival, generally unacceptable in patients w/o life-threatening ventricular arrhythmias, even if patients are experiencing unpleasant, but not life-threatening, symptoms or signs. Ventricular tachycardia (VT) reported in patients treated for paroxysmal A-fib/A-flutter. Use not recommended in patients w/ chronic A-fib. Case reports of ventricular proarrhythmic effects in patients treated for A-fib/A-flutter have included increased premature ventricular contractions (PVCs), VT, ventricular fibrillation (VF), and death. Patients treated for A-flutter have been reported w/ 1:1 atrioventricular (AV) conduction due to slowing the atrial rate. A paradoxical increase in ventricular rate also may occur in patients w/ A-fib. Concomitant negative chronotropic therapy (eg, digoxin, β-blockers) may lower the risk of this complication.

OTHER BRAND NAMES
Tambocor (Discontinued)

ADULT DOSAGE

Paroxysmal Supraventricular Tachycardia

Prevention of paroxysmal supraventricular tachycardias, including atrioventricular nodal reentrant tachycardia, atrioventricular reentrant tachycardia, and other supraventricular tachycardias of unspecified mechanism associated w/ disabling symptoms in patients w/o structural heart disease

Initial: 50mg q12h
Titrate: May increase in increments of 50mg bid every 4 days until efficacy is achieved
Max: 300mg/day
A patient not adequately controlled by (or intolerant to) a dose given at 12-hr intervals may be dosed at 8-hr intervals

Paroxysmal Atrial Fibrillation/Flutter
Prevention of paroxysmal A-fib/A-flutter associated w/ disabling symptoms in patients w/o structural heart disease

Initial: 50mg q12h
Titrate: May increase in increments of 50mg bid every 4 days until efficacy is achieved

A patient not adequately controlled by (or intolerant to) a dose given at 12-hr intervals may be dosed at 8-hr intervals

Ventricular Arrhythmias
Prevention of documented ventricular arrhythmias (life-threatening)

Sustained VT:
Initial: 100mg q12h
Titrate: May increase in increments of 50mg bid every 4 days until efficacy is achieved
Max: 400mg/day; most patients do not require >150mg q12h (300mg/day)

Initiate therapy in the hospital w/ rhythm monitoring

A patient not adequately controlled by (or intolerant to) a dose given at 12-hr intervals may be dosed at 8-hr intervals

Conversions
Transferring from Another Antiarrhythmic Drug:
Allow at least 2-4 plasma half-lives to elapse for the drug being discontinued before starting flecainide at the usual dosage. In patients where withdrawal of a previous antiarrhythmic agent is likely to produce life-threatening arrhythmias, consider hospitalizing the patient.

PEDIATRIC DOSAGE
Arrhythmias
<6 Months of Age:
Initial: 50mg/m²/day divided into 2 or 3 equally spaced doses

>6 Months of Age:
Initial: 100mg/m²/day divided into 2 or 3 equally spaced doses

Max: 200mg/m²/day
Initiate therapy in the hospital w/ rhythm monitoring

DOSING CONSIDERATIONS
Concomitant Medications
Amiodarone: Reduce flecainide dose by 50%
Renal Impairment
Less Severe Renal Disease:
Initial: 100mg q12h
Severe (CrCl ≤35mL/min):
Initial: 100mg qd or 50mg bid
Hepatic Impairment
Significant Impairment: Flecainide should not be used unless the potential benefits clearly outweigh the risks
Other Important Considerations
Once adequate control of arrhythmia is achieved, it may be possible to reduce the dose as necessary in some patients. Evaluate efficacy at lower dose in these patients
Plasma Level Monitoring:
The large majority of patients successfully treated w/ flecainide were found to have trough plasma levels between 0.2 and 1mcg/mL. Periodic monitoring of trough plasma levels may be useful in patient management. Plasma level monitoring is required in patients w/ severe renal failure or severe hepatic disease. Monitoring of plasma levels is strongly recommended in patients on concurrent amiodarone therapy and may also be helpful in patients w/ CHF or moderate renal disease.

ADMINISTRATION
Oral route

STORAGE
20-25°C (68-77°F).

HOW SUPPLIED
Tab: 50mg, 100mg*, 150mg* *scored

CONTRAINDICATIONS
Preexisting 2nd- or 3rd-degree AV block, or right bundle branch block when associated w/ a left hemiblock (bifascicular block), unless a pacemaker is present to sustain the cardiac rhythm should complete heart block occur. Presence of cardiogenic shock or known hypersensitivity to the drug.

WARNINGS/PRECAUTIONS

May cause new or worsened supraventricular or ventricular arrhythmias. May cause or worsen CHF; caution w/ history of CHF or myocardial dysfunction. Close attention must be given to maintenance of cardiac function. Slows cardiac conduction, producing dose-related increases in PR, QRS, and QT intervals; may consider dose reduction. Rare cases of torsades de pointes-type arrhythmia reported. Conduction changes (eg, sinus pause, sinus arrest, symptomatic bradycardia, 2nd- or 3rd-degree AV block) reported; manage on the lowest effective dose. D/C therapy if 2nd- or 3rd-degree AV block or right bundle branch block associated w/ a left hemiblock occurs, unless a temporary or implanted ventricular pacemaker is in place to ensure an adequate ventricular rate. Extreme caution in patients w/ sick sinus syndrome. Known to increase endocardial pacing thresholds and may suppress ventricular escape rhythms; caution in patients w/ permanent pacemakers or temporary pacing electrodes. Should not be administered to patients w/ existing poor thresholds or nonprogrammable pacemakers unless suitable pacing rescue is available. Hypokalemia/hyperkalemia may alter effects; correct preexisting hypokalemia/hyperkalemia before administration of flecainide.

ADVERSE REACTIONS

Cardiac arrest, dizziness, visual disturbances, dyspnea, headache, nausea, fatigue, palpitation, chest pain, asthenia, tremor, constipation, edema, abdominal pain.

DRUG INTERACTIONS

Coadministration may increase digoxin levels. Additive negative inotropic effects w/ β-blockers (eg, propranolol). Concomitant enzyme inducers (phenytoin, phenobarbital, carbamazepine) may increase the rate of elimination. Cimetidine may increase levels and $T_{1/2}$. CYP2D6 inhibitors (eg, quinidine) may increase levels in patients that are on chronic flecainide therapy, especially if these patients are extensive metabolizers. Amiodarone may increase levels if flecainide dosage is not reduced. Avoid w/ disopyramide, verapamil, nifedipine, or diltiazem. Milk may inhibit absorption in infants; consider a reduction in flecainide dosage when milk is removed from diet of infants.

PREGNANCY AND LACTATION

Pregnancy: Category C.
Lactation: Found in breast milk.

MECHANISM OF ACTION

Class IC antiarrhythmic agent w/ local anesthetic activity; decreases intracardiac conduction in all parts of the heart w/ greatest effect on His-Purkinje system (H-V conduction).

PHARMACOKINETICS

Absorption: Nearly complete; T_{max}=3 hrs. **Distribution:** Plasma protein binding (40%); found in breast milk. **Metabolism:** Extensive via CYP2D6 conjugation; meta-O-dealkylated flecainide (major, active urinary metabolite), meta-O-dealkylated lactam of flecainide (major, non-active urinary metabolite). **Elimination:** Urine (30% unchanged), feces (5%); $T_{1/2}$=19 hrs (NYHA Class III CHF patients), 20 hrs (PVC patients), 29 hrs (at birth), 11-12 hrs (3 months of age, 12-15 yrs of age), 6 hrs (1 yr of age), 8 hrs (1-12 yrs of age).

PATIENT CONSIDERATIONS

Assessment: Assess for preexisting 2nd- or 3rd-degree AV block, right bundle branch block associated w/ a left hemiblock, implanted pacemaker, asymptomatic non-life-threatening ventricular arrhythmia, A-fib/A-flutter, cardiogenic shock, MI, cardiomyopathy, preexisting CHF or low ejection fractions (<30%), sick sinus syndrome, hypersensitivity, pregnancy/nursing status, renal/hepatic impairment, and possible drug interactions. Correct preexisting hypokalemia or hyperkalemia prior to therapy. Determine pacing threshold in patients w/ pacemaker.

Monitoring: Monitor for paradoxical increase in ventricular rate, new or worsened supraventricular/ventricular arrhythmias, worsening of CHF, effects on cardiac conduction, bradycardia, hypersensitivity reactions, and other adverse reactions. Monitor for plasma trough levels and monitor ECGs either after initiation or change in dose, whether the dose was increased for lack of effectiveness, or increased growth of pediatric patient. Periodically monitor plasma levels w/ renal/hepatic impairment, CHF, and/or if on concurrent amiodarone therapy. Determine pacing threshold in patients w/ pacemakers after 1 week and at regular intervals thereafter.

Counseling: Inform about risks/benefits of therapy and instruct to report any adverse reactions to physician.

FLECTOR — diclofenac epolamine   Rx

Class: NSAID

> NSAIDs cause an increased risk of serious cardiovascular (CV) thrombotic events, including MI and stroke, which can be fatal. This risk may occur early in treatment and may increase w/ duration of use. Contraindicated in the setting of CABG surgery. NSAIDs cause an increased risk of serious GI adverse events (eg, bleeding, ulceration, stomach/intestinal perforation), which can be fatal and can occur anytime during use and w/o warning symptoms; elderly patients and patients w/ a prior history of peptic ulcer disease and/or GI bleeding are at a greater risk.

ADULT DOSAGE
Acute Pain

Due to Minor Strains, Sprains, and Contusions:
Apply 1 patch to most painful area bid

PEDIATRIC DOSAGE
Pediatric use may not have been established

DOSING CONSIDERATIONS
Elderly
If the anticipated benefit outweighs the potential risks, start at lower end of dosing range; monitor for adverse effects

Concomitant Medications
Do not use in combination therapy w/ an oral NSAID unless benefit outweighs risk; conduct periodic lab evaluations

ADMINISTRATION
Transdermal route

- Do not apply to non-intact or damaged skin resulting from any etiology (eg, exudative dermatitis, eczema, infected lesion, burns, wounds).
- Do not wear patch when bathing or showering.
- Wash hands after applying, handling, or removing patch.
- Avoid eye contact.

STORAGE
20-25°C (68-77°F); excursions permitted between 15-30°C (59-86°F).

HOW SUPPLIED
Patch: 180mg (1.3%) [5s]

CONTRAINDICATIONS
Known hypersensitivity to diclofenac or any component of the drug product; history of asthma, urticaria, or other allergic-type reactions after taking aspirin (ASA) or other NSAIDs; in the setting of CABG surgery; use on non-intact or damaged skin.

WARNINGS/PRECAUTIONS
Use the lowest effective dose for the shortest duration possible. Avoid in patients w/ a recent MI unless benefits outweigh the risks of recurrent CV thrombotic events; if used, monitor for signs of cardiac ischemia. Increased risk for GI bleeding w/ longer duration of therapy, older age, poor general health status, advanced liver disease, and/or coagulopathy; avoid use in patients at higher risk unless benefits are expected to outweigh the increased risk. Consider alternate therapies other than NSAIDs for patients at higher risk and patients w/ active GI bleeding. Promptly initiate evaluation and treatment if a serious GI adverse event is suspected; d/c until a serious GI adverse event is ruled out. Hepatotoxicity reported; d/c immediately and perform a clinical evaluation if clinical signs/symptoms consistent w/ liver disease develop, if systemic manifestations occur, or if abnormal liver tests persist/worsen. May cause new onset HTN or worsen preexisting HTN. Fluid retention and edema reported. Avoid use in patients w/ severe heart failure (HF) unless benefits outweigh risks; monitor for signs of worsening HF if used. Renal papillary necrosis and other renal injury reported w/ long-term use. Renal toxicity also reported in patients in whom renal prostaglandins have a compensatory role in the maintenance of renal perfusion; increased risk w/ renal/hepatic dysfunction, dehydration, hypovolemia, and HF, and in the elderly. Correct volume status in dehydrated or hypovolemic patients prior to initiating therapy. Avoid use in patients w/ advanced renal disease unless the benefits are expected to outweigh the risk; monitor for signs of worsening renal function if used in patients w/ advanced renal disease. Hyperkalemia reported. Associated w/ anaphylactic reactions. Monitor for changes in the signs/symptoms of asthma in patients w/ preexisting asthma (w/o known ASA sensitivity). May cause serious skin reactions (eg, exfoliative dermatitis, Stevens-Johnson syndrome, toxic epidermal necrolysis); d/c at 1st appearance of skin rash/hypersensitivity. Anemia reported. May increase the risk of bleeding events; coagulation disorders may increase this risk. Monitor for signs of bleeding. May mask inflammation and fever. Avoid contact w/ eyes and mucosa.

ADVERSE REACTIONS
Application-site reactions.

DRUG INTERACTIONS
See Dosing Considerations. Drugs that interfere w/ serotonin reuptake may potentiate the risk of bleeding. Synergistic effect on bleeding w/ anticoagulants (eg, warfarin); monitor for signs of bleeding w/ concomitant anticoagulants, antiplatelet agents, SSRIs, and SNRIs. May increase risk of GI bleeding w/ use of oral corticosteroids, anticoagulants, w/ SSRIs; smoking; and alcohol use. ASA may increase risk of bleeding and serious GI events; concomitant use w/ analgesic doses of ASA is not recommended. Monitor patients more closely for GI bleeding w/ concomitant use of low-dose ASA for cardiac prophylaxis. May diminish antihypertensive effect of ACE inhibitors, ARBs, and β-blockers (eg, propranolol); monitor BP. Coadministration w/ ACE inhibitors or ARBs may result in deterioration of renal function (including possible acute renal failure) in patients who are elderly or volume-depleted (including those on diuretic therapy), or who have renal impairment; monitor for worsening renal function and adequately hydrate patient when these drugs are administered concomitantly. May reduce the natriuretic effect of loop diuretics (eg, furosemide) and thiazide diuretics; observe for signs of worsening renal function, in addition to assuring diuretic efficacy including antihypertensive effects. May increase digoxin serum concentrations and prolong the $T_{1/2}$ of digoxin; monitor digoxin levels. May elevate plasma lithium levels and reduce renal lithium clearance; monitor for signs of lithium toxicity. May increase the risk for methotrexate (MTX) toxicity; monitor for MTX toxicity. May increase cyclosporine's nephrotoxicity; monitor for signs of worsening renal function. Concomitant use w/ other NSAIDs or salicylates (eg, diflunisal, salsalate) increases the risk of GI toxicity; not recommended w/ other NSAIDs or salicylates. Concomitant use w/ pemetrexed may increase the risk of pemetrexed-associated myelosuppression, renal, and GI toxicity; refer to prescribing information for further information. Caution w/ drugs that are known to be potentially hepatotoxic (eg, acetaminophen, antibiotics, anti-epileptics).

PREGNANCY AND LACTATION
Pregnancy: Category C, prior to 30 weeks' gestation; Category D, starting at 30 weeks' gestation. Use during the 3rd trimester of pregnancy increases the risk of premature closure of the fetal ductus arteriosus; avoid use in pregnant women starting at 30 weeks of gestation (3rd trimester).
Lactation: Maybe be present in human milk; caution in nursing.
Reproductive Potential: May delay or prevent rupture of ovarian follicles, which has been associated w/ reversible infertility in some women. Small studies in

women treated w/ NSAIDs have also shown a reversible delay in ovulation. Consider withdrawal of therapy in women who have difficulties conceiving or who are undergoing investigation of infertility.

MECHANISM OF ACTION
NSAID; mechanism not completely understood but involves inhibition of COX-1 and COX-2. Has analgesic, anti-inflammatory, and antipyretic properties. Mode of action may be due to a decrease of prostaglandins in peripheral tissues.

PHARMACOKINETICS
Absorption: C_{max}=0.7-6ng/mL, T_{max}=10-20 hrs. **Distribution:** Serum albumin binding (>99%). **Metabolism:** CYP2C9, CYP2C8, CYP3A4, and UGT2B7; glucuronidation and sulfation; 4'-hydroxy-diclofenac (major metabolite). **Elimination:** Urine (65%), bile (35%); $T_{1/2}$=12 hrs.

PATIENT CONSIDERATIONS

Assessment: Assess for history of hypersensitivity to diclofenac or to any component of this product; history of asthma, urticaria, other allergic-type reactions w/ ASA or other NSAIDs; asthma; CV disease (CVD) or risk factors for CVD; HTN; history of peptic ulcer disease or GI bleeding; coagulation disorders; renal/hepatic impairment; pregnancy/nursing status; or any other conditions where treatment is contraindicated or cautioned. Assess volume status. Assess for possible drug interactions. Obtain baseline LFTs, BP, CBC, and chemistry profile.

Monitoring: Monitor for signs/symptoms of CV thrombotic events; cardiac ischemia in patients w/ a recent MI; GI bleeding/ulceration and perforation; hepatotoxicity; new or worsening HTN; HF; edema; renal papillary necrosis and other renal injury; hyperkalemia; anaphylactic reactions; serious skin reactions; anemia; and other adverse reactions. Monitor BP during initiation of therapy and throughout the course of therapy. Monitor for signs of bleeding in patients on concomitant therapy w/ anticoagulants, antiplatelet agents, SSRIs, or SNRIs. Monitor renal function in patients w/ renal/hepatic impairment, HF, dehydration, or hypovolemia. Monitor LFTs, CBC, and chemistry profiles periodically during long-term treatment.

Counseling: Instruct on proper application. Inform that, if patch begins to peel-off, edges may be taped down; instruct to overlay patch w/ non-occlusive mesh netting sleeve, where appropriate (eg, to secure patches applied to ankles, knees, or elbows), if problems w/ adhesion persist. Inform of potential for CV thrombotic events, GI adverse events, hepatotoxicity, and worsening CHF/edema, and advise of symptoms; instruct to report symptoms to healthcare provider if any occur. Instruct to seek immediate emergency help if signs of an anaphylactic reaction occur. Advise to d/c immediately if rash develops and to contact healthcare provider as soon as possible. Advise females of reproductive potential who desire pregnancy that therapy may be associated w/ a reversible delay in ovulation. Instruct pregnant women to avoid use starting at 30 weeks of gestation. Instruct patient not to use other NSAIDs or salicylates concomitantly; notify of the presence of NSAIDs in OTC medications for colds, fever, or insomnia. Inform patient not to use low-dose ASA concomitantly w/o talking to healthcare provider. Instruct to avoid contact w/ the eyes and mucosa; explain that if contact occurs, to immediately wash eye w/ water or saline and consult physician if irritation persists for >1 hr.

FLO-PRED — prednisolone acetate   Rx

Class: Glucocorticoid

ADULT DOSAGE
Steroid-Responsive Disorders

Initial: 5-60mg/day depending on disease and response
Maintain or adjust dose until response is satisfactory. If no satisfactory clinical response after a reasonable period, D/C and transfer to appropriate therapy

Maint: Decrease dose by small amounts to lowest effective dose at appropriate time intervals
May need to increase dose for a period of time in stressful situations

D/C if period of spontaneous remission occurs in a chronic condition

Multiple Sclerosis
Acute Exacerbations:
Usual: 200mg qd for 1 week, followed by 80mg qod for 1 month

PEDIATRIC DOSAGE
Steroid-Responsive Disorders

Initial: 0.14-2mg/kg/day in 3 or 4 divided doses (4-60mg/m2/day) depending on disease and response

Nephrotic Syndrome
>2 Years:
Usual: 60mg/m2/day in 3 divided doses for 4 weeks, followed by 4 weeks of single-dose alternate-day therapy at 40mg/m2/day

Asthma
Uncontrolled by Inhaled Corticosteroids and Long-Acting Bronchodilators:
Usual: 1-2mg/kg/day in single or divided doses; continue short course ("burst" therapy) until peak expiratory flow rate of 80% of personal best is achieved or symptoms resolve (usually 3-10 days)

DOSING CONSIDERATIONS
Elderly
Start at low end of dosing range

Discontinuation
Withdraw gradually after long-term therapy

ADMINISTRATION
Oral route
May take w/ food to avoid GI irritation.

STORAGE
20-25°C (68-77°F). Do not refrigerate.

HOW SUPPLIED
Sus: 15mg/5mL [37mL, 52mL, 65mL]

CONTRAINDICATIONS
Hypersensitivity to corticosteroids (eg, prednisolone), or any components of this product.

WARNINGS/PRECAUTIONS
May cause hypothalamic-pituitary-adrenal (HPA) axis suppression, Cushing's syndrome, and hyperglycemia; monitor patients and taper doses gradually. May cause reversible HPA axis suppression with potential for glucocorticosteroid insufficiency after withdrawal. May impair mineralocorticoid secretion; administer salt and/or mineralocorticoid concurrently. Changes in thyroid status may necessitate dose adjustment; clearance may be decreased in hypothyroidism and increased in hyperthyroidism. May mask/exacerbate infections, reduce resistance to new infections, increase risk of disseminated infection, increase risk of reactivation/exacerbation of latent infection. Avoid exposure to chickenpox and measles. Caution in patients with known or suspected *Strongyloides* infestation, active/latent tuberculosis or tuberculin reactivity, active/latent peptic ulcers, diverticulitis, and fresh intestinal anastomoses. Avoid with systemic fungal infections unless needed to control drug reactions. Rule out latent/active amebiasis before initiating therapy. Not for use in cerebral malaria and active ocular herpes simplex. May cause BP elevation, salt/water retention, and increase excretion of K^+ and calcium; caution with HTN, congestive heart failure (CHF), or renal insufficiency. May cause left ventricular free wall rupture after recent myocardial infarction; use caution. May increase risk of GI perforation with certain GI disorders. May be associated with CNS effects (eg, euphoria, insomnia, mood swings, personality changes, severe depression, frank psychotic manifestations). Emotional instability or psychotic tendency aggravation may occur. May inhibit bone growth in pediatrics and adolescents and cause osteoporosis at any age. Caution in patients at risk for osteoporosis. May produce posterior subcapsular cataracts, glaucoma with possible optic nerve damage, and enhance establishment of secondary ocular infections. Not recommended in optic neuritis treatment. May elevate intraocular pressure (IOP); monitor IOP if used for >6 weeks. May have negative effect on growth and development in children; monitor growth and development with prolonged therapy. May cause fetal harm. Acute myopathy reported with use of high doses. Creatine kinase elevation may occur. Kaposi's sarcoma reported. May suppress reaction to skin tests.

ADVERSE REACTIONS
Fluid retention, alteration in glucose tolerance, elevation in BP, behavioral and mood changes, increased appetite, weight gain.

DRUG INTERACTIONS
May lead to a loss of corticosteroid-induced adrenal suppression with aminoglutethimide. May develop hypokalemia with K^+-depleting agents (eg, amphotericin B, diuretics). Cases of cardiac enlargement and CHF with amphotericin B reported. Anticholinesterase agents may produce severe weakness in patients with myasthenia gravis; d/c anticholinesterase agents at least 24 hours before start of therapy. May inhibit response to warfarin; frequently monitor coagulation indices. May require dose adjustments of antidiabetic agents. May decrease isoniazid levels. Cholestyramine may increase clearance. Convulsions and increased activity of both drugs reported with cyclosporine. May increase risk of arrhythmias with digitalis glycosides. Estrogens, including oral contraceptives, may decrease hepatic metabolism and enhance effect. May enhance metabolism and require dosage increase with CYP3A4 inducers (eg, barbiturates, phenytoin, carbamazepine, rifampin). May decrease metabolism and increase risk of corticosteroid side effects with CYP3A4 inhibitors (eg, ketoconazole). May increase risk of GI side effects with aspirin (ASA) or other NSAIDs. Caution with ASA in patients with hypoprothrombinemia. May increase clearance of salicylates. Live or live, attenuated vaccines is contraindicated in patients receiving immunosuppressive doses. Killed or inactivated vaccines may be administered, although response is unpredictable. May diminish response to toxoids and live or inactivated vaccines. May potentiate replication of some organisms contained in live attenuated vaccines. Acute myopathy reported with neuromuscular blocking drugs (eg, pancuronium).

PREGNANCY AND LACTATION
Category D, caution in nursing.

MECHANISM OF ACTION
Glucocorticoid; causes profound and varied metabolic effects and modifies the body's immune response to diverse stimuli.

PHARMACOKINETICS
Absorption: T_{max}=1-2 hrs. **Distribution:** V_d=0.22-0.7L/kg; plasma protein binding (70-90%); found in breast milk. **Metabolism:** Liver. **Elimination:** Urine (sulfate and glucuronide conjugates); $T_{1/2}$=2-3 hrs.

PATIENT CONSIDERATIONS

Assessment: Assess for vaccination history, current infections, systemic fungal infections, thyroid status, latent/active amebiasis, cerebral malaria, active ocular herpes simplex, emotional instability or psychotic tendencies, any condition where treatment is cautioned, pregnancy/nursing status, and possible drug interactions.

Monitoring: Monitor for salt/water retention, infections/secondary ocular infections, changes in thyroid status, posterior subcapsular cataracts, glaucoma, optic nerve damage, Kaposi's sarcoma, development of osteoporosis, acute myopathy, creatine kinase elevation, and emotional instability or psychotic tendencies aggravation. Monitor IOP, BP, body weight, routine laboratory studies, including two-hour postprandial blood glucose and serum K^+, chest x-ray, bone density, and bone growth and development in pediatrics. Obtain upper GI x-rays with known/suspected peptic ulcer disease.

Counseling: Advise not to d/c abruptly or without medical supervision, to inform any medical attendants about therapy, and to seek medical advice at once if fever or other signs of infection develop. Instruct to notify physician if had recent or ongoing infection or have recently received a vaccine. Counsel to avoid exposure to chickenpox or measles; instruct to immediately report if exposed. Inform of possibility of developing fluid retention, alteration in glucose tolerance, elevation in BP, behavioral and mood changes, increased appetite and weight gain. Advise that if a dose is missed, to take it as soon as remember, if it is almost time for next dose, skip the missed dose and take it at the next regular scheduled time, and not to take an extra dose to make up for the missed dose. Advise to take with food. Instruct to notify physician if using other Rx/OTC medications, dietary supplements, or herbal products.

FLOMAX — tamsulosin hydrochloride Rx

Class: Alpha₁ antagonist

ADULT DOSAGE
Benign Prostatic Hyperplasia
0.4mg qd 30 min after the same meal each day

Titrate: May increase to 0.8mg qd after 2-4 weeks if response is inadequate

If therapy is discontinued or interrupted for several days at either the 0.4mg or 0.8mg dose, restart w/ 0.4mg qd

PEDIATRIC DOSAGE
Pediatric use may not have been established

DOSING CONSIDERATIONS
Concomitant Medications
Do not combine w/ strong CYP3A4 (eg, ketoconazole)

ADMINISTRATION
Oral route
Do not crush, chew, or open cap.

STORAGE
25°C (77°F); excursions permitted to 15-30°C (59-86°F).

HOW SUPPLIED
Cap: 0.4mg

CONTRAINDICATIONS
Hypersensitivity to tamsulosin HCl or any component of this product.

WARNINGS/PRECAUTIONS
Orthostasis/syncope may occur; caution to avoid situations in which injury could result should syncope occur. May cause priapism. Prostate cancer and BPH frequently coexist; screen patients for the presence of prostate cancer prior to treatment and at regular intervals afterwards. Intraoperative floppy iris syndrome (IFIS) observed during cataract and glaucoma surgery; initiation of therapy in patients who are scheduled for cataract or glaucoma surgery is not recommended. Allergic reaction reported (rare) in patients w/ sulfa allergy. Caution in patients known to be CYP2D6 poor metabolizers particularly at a dose >0.4mg.

ADVERSE REACTIONS
Headache, dizziness, rhinitis, infection, abnormal ejaculation, asthenia, back pain, diarrhea, pharyngitis, chest pain, cough increased, somnolence, insomnia, sinusitis, nausea.

DRUG INTERACTIONS
See Dosing Considerations. Ketoconazole (a strong CYP3A4 inhibitor) and paroxetine (a strong CYP2D6 inhibitor) increased levels. Potential for significant increase in exposure when tamsulosin 0.4mg is coadministered w/ a combination of both CYP3A4 and CYP2D6 inhibitors. Caution w/ moderate CYP3A4 inhibitors (eg, erythromycin), and w/ strong (eg, paroxetine) or moderate (eg, terbinafine) CYP2D6 inhibitors. Cimetidine increased exposure; caution w/ cimetidine, particularly at a tamsulosin dose >0.4mg. Avoid w/ other α-adrenergic blockers. Caution w/ PDE-5 inhibitors; concomitant use may cause symptomatic hypotension. Caution w/ warfarin.

PREGNANCY AND LACTATION
Not indicated for use in women.
Pregnancy: Category B.

MECHANISM OF ACTION
α₁-antagonist; selective blockade of α₁ receptors in the prostate results in relaxation of the smooth muscles of the bladder neck and prostate, improving urine flow and reducing symptoms.

PHARMACOKINETICS
Absorption: Essentially complete (>90%). Administration of variable doses w/ light breakfast, high-fat breakfast, or fasted conditions resulted in different pharmacokinetic parameters. **Distribution:** (IV) V_d=16L; plasma protein binding (94-99%). **Metabolism:** Liver (extensive) mainly by CYP3A4 and CYP2D6. **Elimination:** Urine (76%, <10% unchanged), feces (21%); $T_{1/2}$=14-15 hrs.

PATIENT CONSIDERATIONS
Assessment: Assess for known hypersensitivity to the drug, sulfa allergy, and possible drug interactions. Assess if patient is planning to undergo cataract/glaucoma surgery. Screen for the presence of prostate cancer.
Monitoring: Monitor for signs/symptoms of orthostasis, syncope, priapism, IFIS, allergic reactions, and other adverse reactions. Monitor for the presence of prostate cancer at regular intervals.

Counseling: Advise patient about the possible occurrence of symptoms related to orthostatic hypotension; caution about driving, operating machinery, or performing hazardous tasks. Advise that therapy should not be used in combination w/ strong inhibitors of CYP3A4. Advise about the possibility of priapism as a result of treatment and instruct to seek immediate medical attention if it occurs. Inform of the importance of screening for prostate cancer prior to therapy and at regular intervals afterwards. Advise to inform ophthalmologist of drug use if considering cataract or glaucoma surgery.

FLOVENT DISKUS — fluticasone propionate Rx

Class: Corticosteroid

ADULT DOSAGE
Asthma
Maintenance Treatment
Previous Therapy:
Bronchodilators Alone:
Initial: 100mcg bid
Max: 500mcg bid
Inhaled Corticosteroids:
Initial: 100-250mcg bid
Max: 500mcg bid
May consider starting doses >100mcg bid with poorer asthma control or previous high-dose inhaled corticosteroid requirement

Oral Corticosteroids:
Initial: 500-1000mcg bid
Max: 1000mcg bid
Reduce oral prednisone no faster than 2.5-5mg/day on a weekly basis beginning after at least 1 week of fluticasone therapy
Titrate: Reduce to lowest effective dose once asthma stability is achieved. Higher dosages may provide additional asthma control if response to initial dose is inadequate after 2 weeks

PEDIATRIC DOSAGE
Asthma
Maintenance Treatment
4-11 Years:
Previous Therapy:
Oral Corticosteroids:
Initial: 50mcg bid
May consider starting doses >50mcg bid with poorer asthma control or previous high-dose inhaled corticosteroid requirement
Max: 100mcg bid

≥12 Years:
Previous Therapy:
Bronchodilators Alone:
Initial: 100mcg bid
Max: 500mcg bid
Inhaled Corticosteroids:
Initial: 100-250mcg bid
May consider starting doses >100mcg bid with poorer asthma control or previous high-dose inhaled corticosteroid requirement
Max: 500mcg bid

Oral Corticosteroids:
Initial: 500-1000mcg bid
Max: 1000mcg bid
Reduce oral prednisone no faster than 2.5-5mg/day on a weekly basis beginning after at least 1 week of fluticasone therapy
Titrate: Reduce to lowest effective dose once asthma stability is achieved. Higher dosages may provide additional asthma control if response to initial dose is inadequate after 2 weeks

ADMINISTRATION
Orally inhaled powder
Rinse mouth after inhalation.

STORAGE
20-25°C (68-77°F); excursions permitted from 15-30°C (59-86°F). Store in a dry place away from direct heat or sunlight. Store inside unopened moisture-protective pouch and only remove immediately before initial use. Discard 6 weeks (50-mcg strength) or 2 months (100-mcg and 250-mcg strengths) after opening the foil pouch or when counter reads "0," whichever comes 1st.

HOW SUPPLIED
Disk: 50mcg/inh [60 blisters]; 100mcg/inh, 250mcg/inh [28, 60 blisters]

CONTRAINDICATIONS
Primary treatment of status asthmaticus or other acute episodes of asthma where intensive measures are required. Milk protein hypersensitivity.

WARNINGS/PRECAUTIONS
Not indicated for acute bronchospasm relief. *Candida albicans* infections of mouth and pharynx reported; treat and/or interrupt therapy if needed. Increased susceptibility to infections. May lead to serious/fatal course of chickenpox or measles; avoid exposure and, if exposed, consider prophylaxis/treatment. Caution with active/quiescent tuberculosis (TB), systemic fungal/bacterial/viral/parasitic infections, or ocular herpes simplex. Deaths due to adrenal insufficiency reported during and after transfer from systemic to inhaled corticosteroids; wean slowly from systemic corticosteroid use after transferring to therapy. Resume oral corticosteroids during periods of stress or a severe asthma attack in patients previously withdrawn from systemic corticosteroids. Transfer from systemic to inhaled corticosteroids may unmask allergic conditions previously suppressed by systemic therapy (eg, rhinitis, conjunctivitis, eczema). Monitor for systemic corticosteroid effects. Reduce dose slowly if hypercorticism and adrenal suppression/crisis occur. Immediate hypersensitivity reactions may occur. Decreases in bone mineral density (BMD) reported with long-term use; caution with major risk factors for decreased bone mineral content, including chronic use of drugs that can reduce bone mass (eg, anticonvulsants, oral corticosteroids). May cause reduction in growth velocity in pediatric patients; routinely monitor growth. Glaucoma, increased intraocular pressure (IOP), and cataracts reported

with long-term use. Systemic eosinophilic conditions and vasculitis consistent with Churg-Strauss syndrome may occur. Paradoxical bronchospasm with immediate increase in wheezing may occur; treat immediately with an inhaled, short-acting bronchodilator; d/c and institute alternative therapy. Closely monitor patients with hepatic disease.

ADVERSE REACTIONS
Upper respiratory tract infection, throat irritation, headache, sinusitis, N/V, rhinitis, cough, muscle pain, oral candidiasis, arthralgia, fatigue, fever, nasal congestion, bronchitis, GI discomfort.

DRUG INTERACTIONS
Not recommended with strong CYP3A4 inhibitors (eg, ritonavir, clarithromycin, itraconazole); increased systemic corticosteroid adverse effects may occur. Ritonavir and ketoconazole may increase levels and reduce cortisol levels.

PREGNANCY AND LACTATION
Category C, caution in nursing.

MECHANISM OF ACTION
Corticosteroid; shown to have a wide range of actions on multiple cell types (eg, mast cells, eosinophils, neutrophils, macrophages, lymphocytes) and mediators (eg, histamine, eicosanoids, leukotrienes, cytokines) involved in inflammation.

PHARMACOKINETICS
Absorption: Absolute bioavailability (7.8%). **Distribution:** (IV) V_d=4.2L/kg; plasma protein binding (99%). **Metabolism:** Liver via CYP3A4; 17β-carboxylic acid derivative (metabolite). **Elimination:** Urine (<5% metabolites), feces (unchanged and metabolites); (IV) $T_{1/2}$=7.8 hrs.

PATIENT CONSIDERATIONS

Assessment: Assess for hypersensitivity to drug or to milk proteins, status asthmaticus, acute bronchospasm, risk factors for decreased bone mineral content, history of increased IOP, glaucoma, cataracts, active/quiescent TB, ocular herpes simplex, systemic infections, hepatic impairment, pregnancy/nursing status, and possible drug interactions.

Monitoring: Monitor for signs of infections, systemic corticosteroid effects (eg, hypercorticism, adrenal suppression), hypersensitivity reactions, decreased BMD, glaucoma, increased IOP, cataracts, paradoxical bronchospasm, eosinophilic conditions, asthma instability, and other adverse reactions. Monitor growth of pediatric patients routinely. Closely monitor patients with hepatic disease.

Counseling: Advise to contact physician if oropharyngeal candidiasis develops. Inform that product is not a bronchodilator and not intended for use as rescue medication for acute asthma exacerbations; instruct to contact physician immediately if deterioration of asthma occurs. Instruct to avoid exposure to chickenpox or measles and to consult physician without delay if exposed. Inform about risks of immunosuppression, hypercorticism, adrenal suppression, reduction in BMD, reduced growth velocity in pediatric patients, and ocular effects. Instruct to d/c therapy if immediate hypersensitivity reaction occurs. Instruct to use at regular intervals ud and not to stop use abruptly; advise to contact physician immediately if use is discontinued.

FLOVENT HFA — fluticasone propionate   Rx

Class: Corticosteroid

ADULT DOSAGE

Asthma

Prophylactic Maint Treatment:

Previous Therapy:

Bronchodilators Alone:
Initial: 88mcg bid
Max: 440mcg bid

Inhaled Corticosteroids:
Initial: 88-220mcg bid
Max: 440mcg bid

Oral Corticosteroids:
Initial: 440mcg bid
Max: 880mcg bid

Reduce oral prednisone no faster than 2.5-5mg/day on a weekly basis beginning after at least 1 week of fluticasone therapy; reduce fluticasone dosage to the lowest effective dose once prednisone reduction is complete

Titrate:
Reduce to lowest effective dose once asthma stability is achieved. Higher dosages may provide additional asthma control if response to initial dose is inadequate after 2 weeks

PEDIATRIC DOSAGE

Asthma

Prophylactic Maint Treatment:

4-11 Years:
Initial/Max: 88mcg bid

≥12 Years:
Previous Therapy:

Bronchodilators Alone:
Initial: 88mcg bid
Max: 440mcg bid

Inhaled Corticosteroids:
Initial: 88-220mcg bid
Max: 440mcg bid

Oral Corticosteroids:
Initial: 440mcg bid
Max: 880mcg bid

Reduce oral prednisone no faster than 2.5-5mg/day on a weekly basis beginning after at least 1 week of fluticasone therapy; reduce fluticasone dosage to the lowest effective dose once prednisone reduction is complete

Titrate:
Reduce to lowest effective dose once asthma stability is achieved. Higher dosages may provide additional asthma control if response to initial dose is inadequate after 2 weeks

ADMINISTRATION
Oral inh route
Rinse mouth w/ water w/o swallowing after inh.
Shake well before each spray.
May use a valved holding chamber and mask to deliver medicine to young patients.

Priming
Prime the inhaler before using for the first time by releasing 4 sprays into the air away from the face, shaking well for 5 sec before each spray.
If the inhaler has not been used for more than 7 days or has been dropped, prime inhaler by shaking well for 5 sec and releasing 1 spray into the air away from the face.

STORAGE
20-25°C (68-77°F); excursions permitted to 15-30°C (59-86°F). Store w/ mouthpiece down. Do not puncture, use/store near heat or open flame, or throw canister into fire/incinerator. Exposure to temperatures >49°C (120°F) may cause bursting. Discard when counter reads 000.

HOW SUPPLIED
MDI: 44mcg/inh, 110mcg/inh, 220mcg/inh [120 inhalations]

CONTRAINDICATIONS
Primary treatment of status asthmaticus or other acute episodes of asthma where intensive measures are required, hypersensitivity to any of the ingredients.

WARNINGS/PRECAUTIONS
Not indicated for acute bronchospasm relief. *Candida albicans* infections of mouth and pharynx reported; treat and/or interrupt therapy if needed. Increased susceptibility to infections. May lead to serious/fatal course of chickenpox or measles in children; avoid exposure, and if exposed, consider prophylaxis/treatment. Caution w/ active/quiescent tuberculosis (TB), systemic fungal/bacterial/viral/parasitic infections, or ocular herpes simplex. Deaths due to adrenal insufficiency reported during and after transfer from systemic to inhaled corticosteroids; wean slowly from systemic corticosteroid use after transferring to therapy. Resume oral corticosteroids during periods of stress or a severe asthma attack in patients previously withdrawn from systemic corticosteroids. Transfer from systemic to inhaled corticosteroids may unmask allergic conditions previously suppressed by systemic therapy (eg, rhinitis, conjunctivitis, eczema). Monitor for systemic corticosteroid effects. Reduce dose slowly and consider other treatments if hypercorticism and adrenal suppression/crisis occur. Immediate hypersensitivity reactions may occur. Decreases in bone mineral density (BMD) reported w/ long-term use; caution w/ major risk factors for decreased bone mineral content, including chronic use of drugs that can reduce bone mass (eg, anticonvulsants, oral corticosteroids). May cause reduction in growth velocity in pediatric patients; routinely monitor growth. Glaucoma, increased intraocular pressure (IOP), and cataracts reported w/ long-term use. Systemic eosinophilic conditions, and vasculitis consistent w/ Churg-Strauss syndrome may occur. Paradoxical bronchospasm w/ immediate increase in wheezing may occur; treat immediately w/ an inhaled short-acting bronchodilator; d/c and institute alternative therapy. Closely monitor patients w/ hepatic disease.

ADVERSE REACTIONS
Upper respiratory tract infection/inflammation, throat irritation, sinusitis/sinus infection, hoarseness/dysphonia, candidiasis, cough, bronchitis, headache.

DRUG INTERACTIONS
Not recommended w/ strong CYP3A4 inhibitors (eg, ritonavir [RTV], atazanavir, clarithromycin); increased systemic corticosteroid adverse effects may occur. RTV and ketoconazole may increase exposure and reduce cortisol levels.

PREGNANCY AND LACTATION
Pregnancy: There are no randomized clinical studies of Flovent HFA in pregnant women. In women w/ poorly or moderately controlled asthma, there is an increased risk of several perinatal adverse outcomes such as preeclampsia in the mother and prematurity, low birth weight, and small for gestational age in the neonate. Closely monitor and adjust medication as necessary to maintain optimal asthma control.
Lactation: There are no available data on the presence of fluticasone propionate in human milk, the effects on the breastfed child, or the effects on milk production. However, fluticasone propionate concentrations in plasma after inhaled therapeutic doses are low and therefore concentrations in human breast milk are likely to be correspondingly low. Caution in nursing.

MECHANISM OF ACTION
Corticosteroid; shown to have a wide range of actions on multiple cell types (eg, mast cells, eosinophils, neutrophils, macrophages, lymphocytes) and mediators (eg, histamine, eicosanoids, leukotrienes, cytokines) involved in inflammation.

PHARMACOKINETICS
Distribution: (IV) V_d=4.2L/kg; plasma protein binding (99%). **Metabolism:** Liver via CYP3A4; 17β-carboxylic acid derivative (metabolite). **Elimination:** Urine (<5% metabolites), feces (unchanged and metabolites). (IV) $T_{1/2}$=7.8 hrs.

PATIENT CONSIDERATIONS
Assessment: Assess for hypersensitivity to drug, status asthmaticus, acute bronchospasm, active/quiescent TB, ocular herpes simplex, systemic infections, risk factors for decreased bone mineral content, history of increased IOP, glaucoma, cataracts, hepatic impairment, pregnancy/nursing status, and possible drug interactions.

Monitoring: Monitor for signs of infection, systemic corticosteroid effects (eg, hypercorticism, adrenal suppression), hypersensitivity reactions, decreased BMD, glaucoma, increased IOP, cataracts, paradoxical bronchospasm, eosinophilic conditions, asthma instability, and other adverse reactions. Monitor growth in pediatric patients routinely. Closely monitor patients w/ hepatic disease.

Counseling: Advise to contact physician if oropharyngeal candidiasis develops. Advise to rinse the mouth w/ water w/o swallowing after inh to help reduce the risk of thrush. Inform that product is not a bronchodilator and not intended for use as rescue medicine for acute asthma exacerbations; instruct to contact physician immediately if deterioration of asthma occurs. Instruct to avoid exposure to chickenpox or measles and to consult physician w/o delay if exposed. Inform about risks of immunosuppression, hypercorticism, adrenal suppression, reduction in BMD, reduced growth velocity in pediatric patients, and ocular effects. Instruct to d/c therapy if immediate hypersensitivity reactions occur. Instruct to use at regular intervals ud and not to stop use abruptly; advise to contact physician immediately if use is discontinued. Instruct to avoid spraying in eyes. Advise women to contact physician if they become pregnant while on therapy.

FLUARIX — influenza vaccine   Rx

Class: Vaccine

OTHER BRAND NAMES
Fluarix Quadrivalent

ADULT DOSAGE	**PEDIATRIC DOSAGE**
Influenza	**Influenza**
Active Immunization Against Influenza A Subtype Viruses and Type B Virus:	**Active Immunization Against Influenza A Subtype Viruses and Type B Virus:**
One 0.5mL dose	**3-8 Years:**
	Not Previously Vaccinated: Two doses (0.5mL each) at least 4 weeks apart
	Vaccinated in a Previous Season: One or two doses (0.5mL each); if two doses, administer each dose at least 4 weeks apart
	≥9 Years:
	One 0.5mL dose

ADMINISTRATION
IM route

1. Shake well before administration
2. Attach a sterile needle to the prefilled syringe and administer; preferred inj site is the deltoid muscle of upper arm (do not inject in gluteal area or areas where there may be a major nerve trunk)
3. Do not mix w/ any other vaccine in the same syringe or vial; when concomitant administration of other vaccines is required, the vaccines should be administered at different inj sites

STORAGE
2-8°C (36-46°F). Do not freeze; discard if frozen. Protect from light.

HOW SUPPLIED
Inj: 0.5mL

CONTRAINDICATIONS
History of severe allergic reactions (eg, anaphylaxis) to egg proteins or following a previous administration of any influenza vaccine.

WARNINGS/PRECAUTIONS
Caution if Guillain-Barre syndrome (GBS) has occurred w/in 6 weeks of receipt of a prior influenza vaccine. Syncope may occur and may be accompanied by transient neurological signs. Review immunization history for possible vaccine sensitivity and previous vaccination-related adverse reactions; appropriate treatment and supervision must be available for possible anaphylactic reactions. Immunosuppressed persons may have a lower immune response than immunocompetent persons. May not protect all susceptible individuals. Caution in patients w/ bleeding disorders (eg, hemophilia) and in patients on anticoagulant therapy, to avoid the risk of hematoma following inj. (Fluarix) Tip caps may contain natural rubber latex; may cause allergic reactions in latex-sensitive individuals.

ADVERSE REACTIONS
Inj-site reactions (eg, pain, redness, swelling), muscle aches, fatigue, headache, irritability, loss of appetite, drowsiness, GI symptoms.

DRUG INTERACTIONS
Immunosuppressive therapies, including irradiation, antimetabolites, alkylating agents, cytotoxic drugs, and corticosteroids (used in greater than physiological doses), may reduce immune response to vaccine.

PREGNANCY AND LACTATION
Category B, caution in nursing.

MECHANISM OF ACTION
Vaccine; elicits the formation of antibodies that may protect against influenza A subtype viruses and type B virus.

PATIENT CONSIDERATIONS
Assessment: Assess for history of severe allergic reactions to any component of the vaccine (eg, egg protein, latex sensitivity [Fluarix]), immunosuppression, bleeding disorders, development of GBS following a prior dose of influenza vaccine, pregnancy/nursing status, and for possible drug interactions. Review current health/medical status and immunization history.
Monitoring: Monitor for signs/symptoms of GBS, allergic reactions, local inj-site reactions, syncope, and other adverse reactions.

Counseling: Inform of potential benefits/risks of immunization. Educate regarding potential side effects. Inform that vaccine contains noninfectious killed viruses and cannot cause influenza. Advise that vaccine is intended to provide protection against illness due to influenza viruses only and cannot provide protection against all respiratory illnesses. Instruct to notify physician if pregnant. Encourage pregnant women receiving the vaccine to enroll in the pregnancy registry. Inform that annual revaccination is recommended. Instruct to report any adverse events to physician.

FLUDROCORTISONE — fludrocortisone acetate   Rx

Class: Corticosteroid

OTHER BRAND NAMES
Florinef (Discontinued)

ADULT DOSAGE	**PEDIATRIC DOSAGE**
Addison's Disease	Pediatric use may not have been established
Primary and Secondary Adrenocortical Insufficiency:	
Usual: 0.1mg/day	
Range: 0.1mg 3X weekly to 0.2mg/day	
Preferably administered w/ cortisone (10-37.5mg/day in divided doses) or hydrocortisone (10-30mg/day in divided doses)	
Salt-Losing Adrenogenital Syndrome	
0.1-0.2mg/day	

DOSING CONSIDERATIONS
Adverse Reactions
Addison's Disease:
Transient HTN: Reduce dose to 0.05mg/day

ADMINISTRATION
Oral route

STORAGE
15-30°C (59-86°F). Avoid excessive heat.

HOW SUPPLIED
Tab: 0.1mg* *scored

CONTRAINDICATIONS
Systemic fungal infections, history of possible or known hypersensitivity to these agents.

WARNINGS/PRECAUTIONS
May mask signs of infection, and new infections may appear during therapy. There may be decreased resistance and inability to localize infection; promptly control infection with suitable antimicrobial therapy. Prolonged use may produce posterior subcapsular cataracts, glaucoma with possible damage to optic nerves, and secondary ocular infections due to fungi or viruses. May cause elevation of BP, salt and water retention, and increased K⁺ excretion; carefully monitor dosage and salt intake to avoid HTN, edema, or weight gain. Periodic serum electrolyte monitoring is advisable during prolonged therapy; dietary salt restriction and K⁺ supplementation may be necessary. May increase Ca²⁺ excretion. Use in patients with active tuberculosis (TB) should be restricted to fulminating or disseminated cases in conjunction with an appropriate antituberculous regimen. Reactivation of TB may occur; caution in patients with latent TB or tuberculin reactivity; patients on prolonged therapy should receive chemoprophylaxis. Avoid exposure to chickenpox or measles. Adverse effects may occur by too rapid withdrawal or by continued use of large doses. Enhanced effects with hypothyroidism and cirrhosis. To avoid drug-induced adrenal insufficiency, supportive dosage may be required in times of stress (eg, trauma, surgery, severe illness) both during treatment and for a yr afterwards. Use lowest possible dose; gradually reduce dosage when possible. Caution with ocular herpes simplex, nonspecific ulcerative colitis, HTN, diverticulitis, fresh intestinal anastomoses, active/latent peptic ulcer, renal insufficiency, osteoporosis, and myasthenia gravis. Psychic derangements may appear and existing emotional instability or psychotic tendencies may be aggravated. Lab test interactions may occur.

ADVERSE REACTIONS
HTN, CHF, edema, cardiac enlargement, K⁺ loss, hypokalemic alkalosis.

DRUG INTERACTIONS
Decreased pharmacologic effect and increased ulcerogenic effect of aspirin (ASA); monitor salicylate levels or therapeutic effect of ASA and adjust salicylate dosage accordingly if effect is altered. Caution with ASA in patients with hypoprothrombinemia. Enhanced hypokalemia with amphotericin B or K⁺-depleting diuretics (eg, benzothiadiazines, furosemide, ethacrynic acid) and enhanced possibility of arrhythmias or digitalis toxicity associated with hypokalemia with digitalis glycosides; monitor serum K⁺ levels and use K⁺ supplements if necessary. Rifampin, barbiturates, or phenytoin may diminish steroid effect; increase steroid dosage accordingly. Decreased PT response with oral anticoagulants; monitor prothrombin levels and adjust anticoagulant dosage accordingly. Diminished effect of oral hypoglycemics and insulin; monitor for symptoms of hyperglycemia and adjust dosage of antidiabetic drug upward if necessary. Enhanced tendency toward edema with anabolic steroids (particularly C-17 alkylated androgens [eg, oxymetholone, methandrostenolone, norethandrolone]); use with caution especially in patients with hepatic/cardiac disease. May require a reduction of corticosteroid dose when estrogen therapy is initiated, and may require increased amounts when estrogen is terminated. Avoid

smallpox vaccination and other immunizations; possible hazards of neurologic complications and a lack of antibody response.

PREGNANCY AND LACTATION
Category C, caution in nursing.

MECHANISM OF ACTION
Corticosteroid; acts on the distal tubules of the kidney to enhance reabsorption of Na$^+$ ions from tubular fluid into the plasma and increase urinary excretion of both K$^+$ and hydrogen ions.

PHARMACOKINETICS
Distribution: Found in breast milk. **Elimination:** $T_{1/2}$=18-36 hrs.

PATIENT CONSIDERATIONS

Assessment: Assess for hypersensitivity to drug, systemic fungal infections, active/latent TB, HTN, renal insufficiency, psychotic tendencies, hypothyroidism, osteoporosis, myasthenia gravis, peptic ulcer, fresh intestinal anastomoses, ocular herpes simplex, diverticulitis, ulcerative colitis, other conditions where treatment is cautioned, pregnancy/nursing status, and possible drug interactions.

Monitoring: Monitor for infections, edema, weight gain, psychic derangement, cataracts, latent TB reactivation, and other adverse reactions. Monitor dosage, salt intake, serum electrolytes, and BP. Monitor for remission or exacerbations of disease and stress (surgery, infection, trauma). Monitor prothrombin levels if used with oral anticoagulants.

Counseling: Advise to report any medical history of heart disease, high BP, and kidney/liver disease, and to report current use of any medicines. Instruct to avoid exposure to chickenpox or measles and, if exposed, to obtain medical advice. Inform of steroid-dependent status and of increased dosage requirement with stress; advise to carry medical identification indicating this dependence and, if necessary, instruct to carry an adequate supply of medication for emergency use. Inform of the importance of regular follow-up visits and the need to promptly notify physician of dizziness, severe or continuing headaches, swelling of feet or lower legs, or unusual weight gain. Instruct to take only ud, to take a missed dose as soon as possible, unless it is almost time for next dose, and not to double next dose.

FLUMIST QUADRIVALENT — influenza vaccine live, intranasal
Class: Vaccine   **Rx**

ADULT DOSAGE	**PEDIATRIC DOSAGE**
Influenza	**Influenza**
Active Immunization Against Influenza A Subtype Viruses and Type B Viruses:	**Active Immunization Against Influenza A Subtype Viruses and Type B Viruses:**
≤49 Years:	**2-8 Years:**
One 0.2mL dose (0.1mL/nostril)	One or two 0.2mL doses (0.1mL/nostril), depending on vaccination history. If 2 doses, administer at least 1 month apart
	≥9 Years:
	One 0.2mL dose (0.1mL/nostril)

ADMINISTRATION
Intranasal route

For administration by a healthcare provider.
Each sprayer contains a single dose (0.2mL); administer approx 1/2 of the contents of the single-dose intranasal sprayer into each nostril.

STORAGE
2-8°C (35-46°F). Do not freeze. Keep sprayer in outer carton in order to protect from light. A single temperature excursion up to 25°C (77°F) for 12 hrs permitted. After a temperature excursion, the vaccine should be returned immediately to the recommended storage condition and used as soon as feasible. Subsequent excursions are not permitted.

HOW SUPPLIED
Intranasal Spray: 0.2mL [10^s]

CONTRAINDICATIONS
Severe allergic reaction (eg, anaphylaxis) to egg protein, or after a previous dose of any influenza vaccine. Children and adolescents through 17 yrs of age who are receiving aspirin (ASA) or ASA-containing therapy.

WARNINGS/PRECAUTIONS
Increased risk of hospitalization and wheezing in children <2 yrs of age. Children <5 yrs of age w/ recurrent wheezing and persons of any age w/ asthma may be at increased risk of wheezing following administration of vaccine. Caution if Guillain-Barre syndrome (GBS) has occurred w/in 6 weeks of any prior influenza vaccination. Appropriate treatment and supervision must be available to manage possible anaphylactic reactions. May not protect all individuals receiving the vaccine.

ADVERSE REACTIONS
Runny nose/nasal congestion, headache, lethargy, sore throat, decreased appetite, muscle aches, fever, cough.

DRUG INTERACTIONS
See Contraindications. Avoid ASA-containing therapy in children and adolescents (through 17 yrs of age) during the first 4 weeks after vaccination unless clearly needed. Antiviral drugs that are active against influenza A and/or B viruses may reduce the effectiveness of vaccine if administered w/in 48 hrs before, or w/in 2

weeks after vaccination; consider revaccination when appropriate if administered concomitantly w/ antiviral agents.

PREGNANCY AND LACTATION
Pregnancy: Category B.
Lactation: Caution in nursing.

MECHANISM OF ACTION
Vaccine. Immune mechanisms conferring protection against influenza following receipt of vaccine are not fully understood; serum antibodies, mucosal antibodies, and influenza-specific T cells may play a role. Contains live attenuated influenza viruses that must infect and replicate in cells lining the nasopharynx of the recipient to induce immunity.

PATIENT CONSIDERATIONS

Assessment: Assess for history of severe allergic reaction to any component of the vaccine (eg, egg protein) or after a previous dose of any influenza vaccination, history of asthma, recurrent wheezing in children <5 yrs of age, development of GBS following a prior dose of influenza vaccine, pregnancy/nursing status, and possible drug interactions. Review current health/medical status and immunization history.

Monitoring: Monitor for signs/symptoms of GBS, acute allergic reactions, and other adverse reactions.

Counseling: Inform vaccinee/caregivers of benefits/risks and the need for 2 doses at least 1 month apart in children 2-8 yrs of age, depending on vaccination history. Inform that the vaccine is an attenuated live virus vaccine and has the potential for transmission to immunocompromised household contacts. Inform vaccinee/caregiver that there may be an increased risk of wheezing associated w/ vaccine in persons <5 yrs of age w/ recurrent wheezing and persons of any age w/ asthma. Instruct to inform physician if adverse reactions occur.

FLUPHENAZINE DECANOATE — fluphenazine decanoate   **Rx**
Class: Piperazine phenothiazine

OTHER BRAND NAMES
Prolixin Decanoate (Discontinued)

ADULT DOSAGE	**PEDIATRIC DOSAGE**
Psychotic Disorders	Pediatric use may not have been established
Management of Patients Requiring Prolonged Parenteral Neuroleptic Therapy (eg, Chronic Schizophrenics):	
Initial: 12.5-25mg IM/SQ	
Titrate: Determine subsequent inj and dose interval based on response; single inj given as maint therapy may be effective for up to 4-6 weeks. If doses >50mg are necessary, cautiously increase next and succeeding doses in increments of 12.5mg	
Max: 100mg/dose	
Phenothiazine-Naive: Treat initially w/ shorter-acting form of fluphenazine before administering decanoate to determine response and establish appropriate dose	
Severely Agitated Patients: May treat initially w/ rapid-acting phenothiazine (eg, fluphenazine HCl), then give 25mg of fluphenazine decanoate when acute symptoms subside; adjust subsequent doses as necessary	
"Poor Risk" Patients: May initiate therapy cautiously w/ PO or parenteral fluphenazine HCl, then administer equivalent dose of fluphenazine decanoate when pharmacologic effects and appropriate dose are apparent; adjust subsequent dose according to response	
Stabilized on a Fixed Daily Dosage of Fluphenazine HCl Tab/Elixir: Conversion from these short-acting oral forms to the long-acting fluphenazine decanoate inj may be indicated; approximate conversion ratio of 12.5mg of decanoate every 3 weeks for every 10mg/day of fluphenazine HCl. Carefully monitor and adjust dose appropriately at the time of each inj	

ADMINISTRATION
IM/SQ route
Use a dry syringe and needle of at least 21 gauge.

STORAGE
20-25°C (68-77°F). Protect from light.

HOW SUPPLIED
Inj: 25mg/mL [5mL]

CONTRAINDICATIONS
Suspected or established subcortical brain damage, patients receiving large doses of hypnotics, comatose or severely depressed states, presence of blood dyscrasia or liver damage, children <12 yrs of age, hypersensitivity to fluphenazine.

WARNINGS/PRECAUTIONS
May develop tardive dyskinesia (TD); consider discontinuation if signs/symptoms develop. Neuroleptic malignant syndrome (NMS) reported; d/c therapy immediately and institute symptomatic treatment. May impair mental/physical abilities. Leukopenia, neutropenia, and agranulocytosis reported; d/c with severe neutropenia (absolute neutrophil count <1000/mm^3). D/C at 1st sign of WBC decline in absence of other causative factors in patients with preexisting low WBC or history of drug induced leukopenia/neutropenia. Monitor for fever or other signs/symptoms of infections in patients with neutropenia; treat promptly if such signs/symptoms occur. Caution in patients who developed cholestatic jaundice, dermatoses, or other allergic reactions to phenothiazine derivatives. May cause hypotension phenomena in patients on large doses undergoing surgery. Caution in patients exposed to extreme heat, with mitral insufficiency or other cardiovascular disease (CVD), and pheochromocytoma. Caution with history of convulsive disorders; grand mal convulsions reported. May develop liver damage, pigmentary retinopathy, lenticular and corneal deposits, and irreversible dyskinesia with prolonged therapy. Monitor renal function with long-term therapy; d/c if BUN becomes abnormal. May develop "silent pneumonias". May elevate prolactin levels; galactorrhea, amenorrhea, gynecomastia, and impotence reported.

ADVERSE REACTIONS
Extrapyramidal symptoms, TD, HTN, hypotension, allergic reactions, nausea, loss of appetite, dry mouth, constipation, perspiration, salivation, liver damage, fever, muscle rigidity, blood dyscrasias.

DRUG INTERACTIONS
See Contraindications. May potentiate the effects of CNS depressants (eg, opiates, analgesics, antihistamines, barbiturates, alcohol) and atropine. Avoid epinephrine in treating severe hypotension caused by phenothiazine derivatives; reversal of action, resulting in further lowering of BP, may occur. Dose of anesthetics or CNS depressants may need to be reduced. Caution with phosphorus insecticides.

PREGNANCY AND LACTATION
Safety not known in pregnancy/nursing.

MECHANISM OF ACTION
Trifluoromethyl phenothiazine derivative; not established. Suspected to have activity at all levels of the CNS as well as on multiple organ systems.

PATIENT CONSIDERATIONS
Assessment: Assess for previous hypersensitivity to the drug or cross-sensitivity to phenothiazine derivatives, subcortical brain damage, comatose or severely depressed states, current use of hypnotics, blood dyscrasias, liver damage, history of convulsive disorders, mitral insufficiency or other CVD, pheochromocytoma, renal/hepatic impairment, any conditions where treatment is contraindicated or cautioned, pregnancy/nursing status, and possible drug interactions.

Monitoring: Monitor for signs/symptoms of TD, NMS, grand mal convulsions, liver damage, pigmentary retinopathy, lenticular and corneal deposits, irreversible dyskinesia, elevated prolactin levels, infection, and other adverse reactions. Monitor for hypotensive phenomena in patients undergoing surgery. Monitor CBC, hepatic and renal function periodically. Frequently monitor CBC during 1st few months of therapy in patients with preexisting low WBC or history of drug induced leukopenia/neutropenia. Periodically reassess the need for continued treatment.

Counseling: Inform about the risks and benefits of therapy. Inform that therapy may impair mental and physical abilities.

FLUVIRIN — influenza virus vaccine   Rx

Class: Vaccine

ADULT DOSAGE	PEDIATRIC DOSAGE
Influenza	**Influenza**
Immunization Against Influenza Virus Subtypes A And Type B: One 0.5mL dose	**Immunization Against Influenza Virus Subtypes A And Type B:** **4-8 Years:** One or two doses (0.5mL each); if two doses, administer at least 1 month apart **≥9 Years:** One 0.5mL dose

---

ADMINISTRATION
IM route
Shake well before administration.

Multidose Vial
1. Shake each time before withdrawing a dose.

2. Between uses, return to the recommended storage conditions; do not freeze (discard if vaccine has been frozen).
3. A separate sterile syringe and needle must be used for each inj.
4. Use small syringes (0.5mL to 1mL) to minimize any product loss.

Pediatrics
Needle size may range from 7/8 to 1 1/4 inches, depending on the size of the child's deltoid muscle, and should be of sufficient length to penetrate the muscle tissue.
The anterolateral thigh can be used, but the needle should be longer, usually 1 inch.

Adults
Use a needle of ≥1 inch; preferred site for inj is the deltoid muscle of the upper arm (do not inject in the gluteal region or areas where there may be a major nerve trunk).

STORAGE
2-8°C (36-46°F). Do not freeze; discard if has been frozen. Protect from light. Return multidose vial to the recommended storage conditions between uses.

HOW SUPPLIED
Inj: 0.5mL [prefilled syringe], 5mL [multidose vial]

CONTRAINDICATIONS
History of severe allergic reactions (eg, anaphylaxis) to egg proteins (eggs or egg products) or any component of Fluvirin or has had a life-threatening reaction to previous influenza vaccinations.

WARNINGS/PRECAUTIONS
Caution if Guillain-Barre syndrome (GBS) occurred w/in 6 weeks of receipt of prior influenza vaccine. Expected immune response may not be obtained in immunocompromised persons. Review immunization history for possible adverse events prior to administration; appropriate treatment and supervision must be available to manage possible anaphylactic reactions. Tip caps of prefilled syringes may contain rubber latex, which may cause allergic reactions in latex-sensitive individuals. May not protect all individuals. Syncope can occur and can be accompanied by transient neurological signs (eg, visual disturbance, paresthesia, tonic-clonic limb movements); procedures should be in place to avoid falling injury and to restore cerebral perfusion following syncope by maintaining a supine or Trendelenburg position.

ADVERSE REACTIONS
Inj-site reactions (eg, pain, erythema, mass, induration, swelling), headache, malaise, myalgia, fatigue.

DRUG INTERACTIONS
Do not mix w/ any other vaccine in the same syringe or vial; when concomitant administration of other vaccines is required, the vaccines should be administered at different inj sites. Immunosuppressive therapies, including irradiation, antimetabolites, alkylating agents, cytotoxic drugs, and corticosteroids (used in greater than physiological doses), may reduce immune response.

PREGNANCY AND LACTATION
Pregnancy: Category B; this vaccine should be used during pregnancy only if clearly needed.
Lactation: It is not known whether influenza virus vaccine is excreted in human milk; caution in nursing.

MECHANISM OF ACTION
Vaccine; elicits the formation of antibodies that may protect against influenza virus subtypes A and type B.

PATIENT CONSIDERATIONS
Assessment: Assess for history of severe allergic reactions to egg proteins or life-threatening reactions to previous influenza vaccination, hypersensitivity to latex, development of GBS following a prior dose of influenza vaccine, pregnancy/nursing status, and possible drug interactions. Review immunization history, current health/medical status (eg, immunosuppression), and existence of any contraindication to immunization.

Monitoring: Monitor for signs/symptoms of GBS, allergic reactions, local inj-site reactions, and other adverse reactions.

Counseling: Inform of potential benefits and risks of immunization. Educate about the potential side effects and instruct to report to the physician if any severe or unusual adverse reactions occur. Inform that vaccine contains noninfectious particles and cannot cause influenza. Advise that vaccine provides protection against illness due to influenza viruses only and not against all respiratory illness. Inform that annual vaccination is recommended.

FML — fluorometholone   Rx

Class: Corticosteroid

OTHER BRAND NAMES
FML Forte

ADULT DOSAGE	PEDIATRIC DOSAGE
Steroid-Responsive Inflammatory Ocular Conditions	**Steroid-Responsive Inflammatory Ocular Conditions**
Treatment of Palpebral and Bulbar Conjunctiva, Cornea, and Anterior Segment of Globe: **Oint:** Apply a small amount (approximately 1/2 inch ribbon) to the conjunctival sac qd-tid	**Treatment of Palpebral and Bulbar Conjunctiva, Cornea, and Anterior Segment of Globe:** **≥2 Years:** **Oint:** Apply a small amount (approximately 1/2 inch ribbon) to the conjunctival sac qd-tid

Sus:
1 drop into the conjunctival sac bid-qid

Oint/Sus:
May increase frequency to 1 application q4h during the initial 24-48 hrs

Reevaluate if signs/symptoms fail to improve after 2 days

In chronic conditions, withdraw treatment by gradually decreasing frequency of applications

Sus:
1 drop into the conjunctival sac bid-qid

Oint/Sus:
May increase frequency to 1 application q4h during the initial 24-48 hrs

Reevaluate if signs/symptoms fail to improve after 2 days

In chronic conditions, withdraw treatment by gradually decreasing frequency of applications

---

ADMINISTRATION
Ocular route

Sus
Shake well before using

STORAGE
(Oint) 15-25°C (59-77°F). Avoid exposure to temperatures >40°C (104°F). (Sus) 2-25°C (36-77°F). Protect from freezing. Store in an upright position.

HOW SUPPLIED
Oint: 0.1% [3.5g]; **Sus:** 0.1% [5mL, 10mL], (Forte) 0.25% [5mL, 10mL]

CONTRAINDICATIONS
Most viral diseases of the cornea and conjunctiva (eg, epithelial herpes simplex keratitis [dendritic keratitis], vaccinia, and varicella), mycobacterial infection of the eye, fungal diseases of ocular structures, known or suspected hypersensitivity to any of the ingredients of this preparation and to other corticosteroids.

WARNINGS/PRECAUTIONS
Prolonged use may increase intraocular pressure (IOP) in susceptible individuals, resulting in glaucoma with damage to the optic nerve, defects in visual acuity and fields of vision, and in posterior subcapsular cataract formation. Prolonged use may suppress the host immune response and increase the hazard of secondary ocular infections. Use in the presence of thin corneal or scleral tissue, which may be caused by various ocular diseases or long-term use of topical corticosteroids, may lead to perforation. Acute purulent infections of the eye may be masked or activity enhanced. Routinely monitor IOP if used for ≥10 days. Caution with glaucoma; check IOP frequently. Use after cataract surgery may delay healing and increase incidence of bleb formation. May prolong the course and may exacerbate the severity of many viral infections of the eye (including herpes simplex). Extreme caution with history of herpes simplex; frequent slit lamp microscopy is recommended. Initial prescription and renewal of the medication order beyond 8g of oint or 20mL of sus should be made only after examination of the patient with the aid of magnification (eg, slit lamp biomicroscopy) and where appropriate, fluorescein staining. Fungal infections of the cornea may develop coincidentally with long-term use; suspect fungal invasion in any persistent corneal ulceration. May reduce dose, but caution not to d/c therapy prematurely. (Oint) May retard corneal healing.

ADVERSE REACTIONS
Acute anterior uveitis, globe perforation, keratitis, conjunctivitis, corneal ulcers, mydriasis, conjunctival hyperemia, loss of accommodation, ptosis, transient ocular burning/stinging upon instillation, allergic reactions, foreign body sensation, erythema of the eyelid, eyelid edema.

PREGNANCY AND LACTATION
Category C, not for use in nursing.

MECHANISM OF ACTION
Corticosteroid; not established. Thought to act by induction of phospholipase A_2 inhibitory proteins called lipocortins, which control the biosynthesis of potent mediators of inflammation (eg, prostaglandins, leukotrienes) by inhibiting the release of their precursor, arachidonic acid.

PHARMACOKINETICS
Distribution: Found in breast milk (systemic use).

PATIENT CONSIDERATIONS

Assessment: Assess for viral diseases of the cornea and conjunctiva, mycobacterial infection of the eye, fungal diseases of ocular structures, hypersensitivity to drug or to other corticosteroids, thin corneal or scleral tissue, glaucoma, recent cataract surgery, history of herpes simplex, and pregnancy/nursing status.

Monitoring: Monitor for glaucoma, optic nerve damage, visual acuity and fields of vision defects, posterior subcapsular cataracts, secondary ocular infections, perforation of the cornea/sclera, exacerbation of viral infections of the eye, fungal invasion, and other adverse reactions. Routinely monitor IOP if used for ≥10 days. Monitor for improvement of signs/symptoms.

Counseling: Advise to d/c use and consult physician if inflammation or pain persists >48 hrs or becomes aggravated. Instruct to use caution to avoid touching the tube/bottle tip to eyelids or to any other surface to prevent contamination. Advise that the use of the tube/bottle by more than 1 person may spread infection. Inform that the preservative in sus, benzalkonium chloride, may be absorbed by soft contact lenses; instruct those wearing soft contact lenses to wait at least 15 min after instilling sus to insert soft contact lenses.

FOCALIN — dexmethylphenidate hydrochloride CII
Class: CNS stimulant

> Caution w/ history of drug dependence or alcoholism. Chronic, abusive use may lead to marked tolerance and psychological dependence w/ varying degrees of abnormal behavior may occur w/ chronic abusive use. Frank psychotic episodes may occur, especially w/ parenteral abuse. Careful supervision is required during withdrawal from abusive use, since severe depression may occur. Withdrawal following chronic use may unmask symptoms of underlying disorder that may require follow-up.

ADULT DOSAGE
Attention-Deficit Hyperactivity Disorder
Refer to pediatric dosing

PEDIATRIC DOSAGE
Attention-Deficit Hyperactivity Disorder
≥6 Years:
Methylphenidate-Naive:
Initial: 5mg/day (2.5mg bid)
Titrate: May adjust weekly in 2.5-5mg increments
Max: 20mg/day (10mg bid)

Currently on Methylphenidate:
Initial: 1/2 the dose of racemic methylphenidate
Max: 20mg/day (10mg bid)

DOSING CONSIDERATIONS
Adverse Reactions
Reduce dose or d/c if paradoxical aggravation of symptoms or other adverse events occur
D/C if no improvement seen after appropriate dosage adjustment over 1 month

ADMINISTRATION
Oral route

Take w/ or w/o food.
Administer bid, at least 4 hrs apart.

STORAGE
25°C (77°F); excursions permitted to 15-30°C (59-86°F). Protect from light and moisture.

HOW SUPPLIED
Tab: 2.5mg, 5mg, 10mg

CONTRAINDICATIONS
Marked anxiety, tension, and agitation; hypersensitivity to methylphenidate or other components of the product; glaucoma; motor tics or family history or diagnosis of Tourette's syndrome; during treatment w/ MAOIs, and w/in a minimum of 14 days following discontinuation of an MAOI.

WARNINGS/PRECAUTIONS
Avoid in patients w/ known serious structural cardiac abnormalities, cardiomyopathy, serious heart rhythm abnormalities, coronary artery disease, or other serious cardiac problems. Sudden death reported in children and adolescents w/ structural cardiac abnormalities or other serious heart problems. Sudden death, stroke, and myocardial infarction (MI) reported in adults. May cause modest increase in average BP and HR; caution in patients whose underlying medical conditions might be compromised by increases in BP or HR. Prior to treatment, perform medical history (including assessment for family history of sudden death or ventricular arrhythmia) and physical exam to assess for presence of cardiac disease. Promptly perform cardiac evaluation if symptoms of cardiac disease develop during treatment. May exacerbate symptoms of behavior disturbance and thought disorder in patients w/ a preexisting psychotic disorder. May induce mixed/manic episode in patients w/ comorbid bipolar disorder. May cause treatment-emergent psychotic or manic symptoms at usual doses in children and adolescents w/o a prior history of psychotic illness or mania; discontinuation may be appropriate if such symptoms occur. Aggressive behavior or hostility reported in children and adolescents. May cause long-term suppression of growth in children; may need to interrupt treatment in patients not growing or gaining height or weight as expected. May lower convulsive threshold; d/c in the presence of seizures. Priapism reported; immediate medical attention should be sought if abnormally sustained or frequent and painful erections develop. Associated w/ peripheral vasculopathy, including Raynaud's phenomenon; monitor for digital changes. Difficulties w/ accommodation and blurring of vision reported. Periodically monitor CBC, differential, and platelet counts during prolonged therapy.

ADVERSE REACTIONS
Abdominal pain, fever, anorexia, nausea.

DRUG INTERACTIONS
See Contraindications. May decrease the effectiveness of drugs used to treat HTN. Caution w/ pressor agents. May inhibit metabolism of coumarin anticoagulants, anticonvulsants (eg, phenobarbital, phenytoin, primidone) and some antidepressants (eg, TCAs, SSRIs); downward dose adjustments and monitoring of plasma drug concentration (or coagulation times for coumarin) of these drugs may be necessary when initiating or discontinuing dexmethylphenidate.

PREGNANCY AND LACTATION
Category C, caution in nursing.

MECHANISM OF ACTION
Sympathomimetic amine; CNS stimulant. Mechanism in ADHD has not been established; suspected to block the reuptake of norepinephrine and dopamine into the presynaptic neuron and increase the release of these monoamines into the extraneuronal space.

PHARMACOKINETICS

Absorption: Readily absorbed; T_{max}=2.9 hrs (fed), 1-1.5 hrs (fasted). **Metabolism:** Deesterification; d-ritalinic acid (primary metabolite). **Elimination:** Urine (90%, primarily as metabolite); $T_{1/2}$=2.2 hrs.

PATIENT CONSIDERATIONS

Assessment: Assess for previous hypersensitivity to the drug, history of drug dependence or alcoholism, marked anxiety, agitation, tension, glaucoma, motor tics, family history or diagnosis of Tourette's syndrome, preexisting psychotic disorder, comorbid bipolar disorder, history of seizures, medical conditions that might be compromised by increases in BP or HR, any other conditions where treatment is contraindicated or cautioned, pregnancy/nursing status, and possible drug interactions. Perform a careful history (including assessment for a family history of sudden death or ventricular arrhythmia) and physical exam to assess for the presence of cardiac disease, and perform further cardiac evaluation if findings suggest such disease (eg, ECG, echocardiogram). Adequately screen patients w/ comorbid depressive symptoms to determine if they are at risk for bipolar disorder (eg, detailed psychiatric history, including a family history of suicide, bipolar disorder, and depression).

Monitoring: Monitor for signs/symptoms of cardiac disease, exacerbation of behavioral disturbance and thought disorder, psychosis, mania, appearance of or worsening of aggressive behavior or hostility, seizures, priapism, digital changes, visual disturbances, and other adverse reactions. Monitor BP and HR. During prolonged use, periodically evaluate usefulness of therapy and monitor CBC, differential, and platelet counts. In pediatric patients, monitor growth.

Counseling: Inform about risks and benefits of treatment. Counsel on the appropriate use of the medication. Advise of the possibility of priapism; instruct to seek immediate medical attention in the event of priapism. Instruct to report to physician any new numbness, pain, skin color change, sensitivity to temperature in fingers or toes, or any signs of unexplained wounds appearing on the fingers or toes.

FOCALIN XR — dexmethylphenidate hydrochloride   CII

Class: CNS stimulant

> Caution w/ history of drug dependence or alcoholism. Marked tolerance and psychological dependence w/ varying degrees of abnormal behavior may occur w/ chronic abusive use. Frank psychotic episodes may occur, especially w/ parenteral abuse. Careful supervision is required during withdrawal from abusive use, since severe depression may occur. Withdrawal following chronic therapeutic use may unmask symptoms of underlying disorder that may require follow-up.

ADULT DOSAGE	PEDIATRIC DOSAGE
Attention-Deficit Hyperactivity Disorder	**Attention-Deficit Hyperactivity Disorder**
	≥6 Years:
New to Methylphenidate:	**New to Methylphenidate:**
Initial: 10mg qam	**Initial:** 5mg qam
Titrate: May adjust weekly in 10mg increments	**Titrate:** May adjust weekly in 5mg increments
Max: 40mg/day	**Max:** 30mg/day
Currently on Methylphenidate:	**Currently on Methylphenidate:**
Initial: 1/2 of methylphenidate total daily dose	**Initial:** 1/2 of methylphenidate total daily dose
Currently on Dexmethylphenidate Immediate-Release:	**Currently on Dexmethylphenidate Immediate-Release:**
May switch to the same daily dose of the extended-release	May switch to the same daily dose of the extended-release
D/C if no improvement seen after appropriate dosage adjustment over 1 month	D/C if no improvement seen after appropriate dosage adjustment over 1 month

DOSING CONSIDERATIONS

Adverse Reactions
Reduce dose or d/c if paradoxical aggravation of symptoms or other adverse events occur

ADMINISTRATION
Oral route
Swallow caps whole or sprinkle contents on a spoonful of applesauce.
Do not crush, chew, or divide.
Consume drug and applesauce mixture immediately; do not store for future use.

STORAGE
25°C (77°F); excursions permitted to 15-30°C (59-86°F).

HOW SUPPLIED
Cap, Extended-Release: 5mg, 10mg, 15mg, 20mg, 25mg, 30mg, 35mg, 40mg

CONTRAINDICATIONS
Marked anxiety, tension, and agitation; hypersensitivity to methylphenidate or other components of the product; glaucoma; motor tics or family history or diagnosis of Tourette's syndrome; during treatment w/ MAOIs, and w/in a minimum of 14 days following discontinuation of an MAOI.

WARNINGS/PRECAUTIONS
Avoid in patients w/ known serious structural cardiac abnormalities, cardiomyopathy, serious heart rhythm abnormalities, coronary artery disease, or other serious cardiac problems. Sudden death reported in children and adolescents w/ structural cardiac abnormalities or other serious heart problems. Sudden death, stroke, MI reported in adults. May cause modest increase in average BP and HR; caution w/ HTN, heart failure, recent MI, or ventricular arrhythmia. Promptly perform cardiac evaluation if symptoms of cardiac disease develop during treatment. May exacerbate symptoms of behavior disturbance and thought disorder in patients w/ preexisting psychotic disorder. Caution in patients w/ comorbid bipolar disorder; may induce mixed/manic episodes. May cause treatment-emergent psychotic or manic symptoms (eg, hallucinations, delusional thinking, mania) in children and adolescents w/o prior history of psychotic illness or mania; discontinuation may be appropriate if such symptoms occur. Aggressive behavior or hostility reported in children and adolescents. May cause long-term suppression of growth in children; monitor growth, and may need to interrupt treatment in patients not growing or gaining height or weight as expected. May lower convulsive threshold; d/c in the presence of seizures. Priapism reported; seek immediate medical attention if abnormally sustained or frequent and painful erections develop. Associated w/ peripheral vasculopathy, including Raynaud's phenomenon; monitor for digital changes. Difficulties w/ accommodation and blurring of vision reported.

ADVERSE REACTIONS
Dyspepsia, headache, anxiety, insomnia, anorexia, dry mouth, pharyngolaryngeal pain, feeling jittery, dizziness, decreased appetite, vomiting.

DRUG INTERACTIONS
See Contraindications. Caution w/ pressor agents. May decrease the effectiveness of drugs used to treat HTN. May inhibit metabolism of coumarin anticoagulants, anticonvulsants (eg, phenobarbital, phenytoin, primidone), and tricyclic drugs (eg, imipramine, clomipramine, desipramine); downward dose adjustments and monitoring of plasma drug concentration (or coagulation times for coumarin) of these drugs may be necessary when initiating or discontinuing therapy. Antacids or acid suppressants could alter drug release.

PREGNANCY AND LACTATION
Category C, caution in nursing.

MECHANISM OF ACTION
Sympathomimetic amine; CNS stimulant. Mechanism in ADHD has not been established; suspected to block the reuptake of norepinephrine and dopamine into the presynaptic neuron and increase the release of these monoamines into the extraneuronal space.

PHARMACOKINETICS
Absorption: Absolute bioavailability (22-25%); T_{max}=1.5 hrs (1st peak), 6.5 hrs (2nd peak). **Distribution:** Plasma protein binding (12-15%, racemic methylphenidate); V_d=2.65L/kg. **Metabolism:** Deesterification; d-ritalinic acid (primary metabolite). **Elimination:** Urine (90%, racemic methylphenidate); (IV) $T_{1/2}$=2-4.5 hrs (healthy adults), 2-3 hrs (children).

PATIENT CONSIDERATIONS
Assessment: Assess for previous hypersensitivity to the drug, history of drug dependence or alcoholism, marked anxiety, tension, agitation, glaucoma, motor tics, family history or diagnosis of Tourette's syndrome, preexisting psychotic disorder, comorbid bipolar disorder, cardiac disease, medical conditions that might be compromised by increases in BP and HR, any other conditions where treatment is cautioned, pregnancy/nursing status, and possible drug interactions.

Monitoring: Monitor BP, HR, and for signs/symptoms of cardiac disease (eg, exertional chest pain, unexplained syncope), exacerbation of behavioral disturbance and thought disorder, psychosis, mania, appearance of or worsening of aggressive behavior or hostility, seizures, priapism, digital changes, visual disturbances, and other adverse reactions. During prolonged use, periodically reevaluate usefulness of therapy and monitor CBC, differential, and platelet counts. In pediatric patients, monitor growth.

Counseling: Inform about benefits and risks of treatment. Counsel on the appropriate use of the medication. Advise of the possibility of priapism; instruct to seek immediate medical attention in the event of priapism. Instruct to report to physician any new numbness, pain, skin color change, sensitivity to temperature in fingers or toes, or any signs of unexplained wounds appearing on fingers or toes.

FOLIC ACID — folic acid   Rx

Class: Erythropoiesis agent

ADULT DOSAGE	PEDIATRIC DOSAGE
Anemia	**Anemia**
Megaloblastic Anemias (Due to Folic Acid Deficiency)/Anemias of Nutritional Origin, Pregnancy, Infancy, or Childhood:	**Megaloblastic Anemias (Due to Folic Acid Deficiency)/Anemias of Nutritional Origin, Pregnancy, Infancy, or Childhood:**
Usual: Up to 1mg/day. Resistant cases may require larger doses	**Usual:** Up to 1mg/day. Resistant cases may require larger doses
Maint: 0.4mg	**Maint:**
Pregnant and Lactating Women: 0.8mg	**Infants:** 0.1mg
Minimum: 0.1mg/day	**<4 Years:** Up to 0.3mg
	>4 Years: 0.4mg
	Minimum: 0.1mg/day
May need to increase maint level in the presence of alcoholism, hemolytic anemia, anticonvulsant therapy, or chronic infection	May need to increase maint level in the presence of alcoholism, hemolytic anemia, anticonvulsant therapy, or chronic infection

ADMINISTRATION
Oral route

STORAGE
20-25°C (68-77°F).

HOW SUPPLIED
Tab: 1mg* *scored

WARNINGS/PRECAUTIONS
Folic acid alone is improper therapy for pernicious anemia and other megaloblastic anemias in which vitamin B12 is deficient. Folic acid >0.1mg/day may obscure pernicious anemia in that hematologic remission may occur while neurologic manifestations remain progressive; potential danger exists in administering folic acid to patients w/ undiagnosed anemia.

ADVERSE REACTIONS
Allergic sensitization.

DRUG INTERACTIONS
Antagonizes anticonvulsant action of phenytoin; increased doses may be required in a patient whose epilepsy is completely controlled by phenytoin. False low serum and red cell folate levels may occur w/ antibiotics (eg, tetracycline), which suppress the growth of *Lactobacillus casei*.

PREGNANCY AND LACTATION
Category A, safe in nursing.

MECHANISM OF ACTION
Erythropoiesis agent; acts on megaloblastic bone marrow to produce normoblastic marrow. Required for nucleoprotein synthesis and maintenance of normal erythropoiesis. Precursor of tetrahydrofolic acid, which is involved as a cofactor for transformylation reactions in the biosynthesis of purines and thymidylates of nucleic acids.

PHARMACOKINETICS
Absorption: Rapid (small intestine). T_{max}=1 hr. **Distribution:** Found in breast milk. **Metabolism:** Liver via reduced diphosphopyridine nucleotide and folate reductase. **Elimination:** Urine, feces.

PATIENT CONSIDERATIONS
Assessment: Assess for alcoholism, hemolytic anemia, chronic infection, pernicious anemia and other megaloblastic anemias, previous intolerance to the drug, pregnancy/nursing status, and possible drug interactions.

Monitoring: Monitor for allergic sensitization, and obtain CBC.

Counseling: Inform of risks and benefits of therapy.

FOLLISTIM AQ — follitropin beta   Rx

Class: Follicle-stimulating hormone (FSH)

ADULT DOSAGE

Ovulation Induction

Induction of ovulation and pregnancy in anovulatory infertile women in whom the cause of infertility is functional and not due to primary ovarian failure

Vial:
Initial: 75 IU qd for at least the first 7 days
Titrate: Make subsequent dose adjustments at weekly intervals based on ovarian response; if needed, increase dose by 25-50 IU at weekly intervals until follicular growth and/or serum estradiol levels indicate adequate ovarian response
Max: 300 IU/day

Cartridge:
Initial: 50 IU qd for at least the first 7 days
Titrate: Make subsequent dose adjustments at weekly intervals based on ovarian response; if needed, increase dose by 25-50 IU at weekly intervals until follicular growth and/or serum estradiol levels indicate adequate ovarian response
Max: 250 IU/day

Continue treatment until ultrasonic visualizations/serum estradiol determinations approximate pre-ovulatory conditions seen in normal individuals

Ovarian Stimulation

Pregnancy in normal ovulatory women undergoing controlled ovarian stimulation as part of an in vitro fertilization or intracytoplasmic sperm inj cycle

Cartridge:
Initial: 200 IU qd for at least the first 7 days of treatment

Titrate: Adjust subsequent doses up or down based on ovarian response
Dose reduction in high responders can be considered from the 6th day onward
Maint:
Normal Responders: Daily starting dose can be continued until pre-ovulatory conditions are achieved (7-12 days)
Low or Poor Responders: Increase daily dose according to ovarian response; max of 500 IU/day
High Responders (At Risk of Abnormal Ovarian Enlargement and/or Ovarian Hyperstimulation Syndrome): Decrease or temporarily d/c the daily dose or d/c the cycle, depending on response

Perform oocyte retrieval 34-36 hrs following human chorionic gonadotropin administration

Assisted Reproductive Technology

Development of multiple follicles in ovulatory women

Vial:
Initial: 150-225 IU qd for at least the first 4 days of treatment
Titrate: Adjust subsequent dosing based on ovarian response
Maint:
Normal Responders: Daily starting dose can be continued until pre-ovulatory conditions are achieved (6-12 days)
Low or Poor Responders: Increase daily dose according to ovarian response; max of 600 IU/day
High Responders (At Risk of Abnormal Ovarian Enlargement and/or Ovarian Hyperstimulation Syndrome): Decrease or temporarily d/c the daily dose or d/c the cycle, depending on response

Perform oocyte retrieval 34-36 hrs following human chorionic gonadotropin administration

Induction of Spermatogenesis

In men w/ primary and secondary hypogonadotropic hypogonadism in whom the cause of infertility is not due to primary testicular failure

Pretreatment w/ human chorionic gonadotropin (hCG) is required
Usual: 450 IU/week (given as 225 IU twice weekly or 150 IU 3X/week) w/ hCG; consider lower dose w/ Follistim AQ cartridge
Continue concomitant therapy for at least 3-4 months before any improvement can be expected

Conversions

When administering Follistim AQ Cartridge, a lower starting dose and lower dose adjustments (as compared to reconstituted Follistim) should be considered

Follistim AQ Cartridge w/ the pen injector device delivers on average an 18% higher amount of follitropin beta when compared to reconstituted Follistim delivered w/ a conventional syringe and needle; refer to PI for conversion chart

---

PEDIATRIC DOSAGE
Pediatric use may not have been established

ADMINISTRATION
(Cartridge) SQ route, (Vial) SQ/IM route

Cartridge
Do not add any other medicines into the cartridge

Vial
Do not mix w/ any other medicines in the same vial or in the same syringe

STORAGE
2-8°C (36-46°F). Upon Dispensing: 2-8°C (36-46°F) until expiration date, or 25°C (77°F) (cartridge)/≤25°C (77°F) (vial) for 3 months or until expiration date, whichever occurs 1st. Protect from light. Do not freeze. (Cartridge) Once Used: 2-25°C (36-77°F) for a max of 28 days.

HOW SUPPLIED
Inj: (Cartridge) 150 IU, 300 IU, 600 IU, 900 IU; (Vial) 75 IU/0.5mL, 150 IU/0.5mL.

CONTRAINDICATIONS
Prior hypersensitivity to recombinant FSH products, FSH levels indicating primary gonadal failure, presence of uncontrolled nongonadal endocrinopathies (eg, thyroid, adrenal, or pituitary disorders), tumor of the ovary, breast, uterus, testis, hypothalamus, or pituitary gland, pregnancy, heavy or irregular vaginal bleeding of undetermined origin, ovarian cysts or enlargement not due to polycystic ovary syndrome. Hypersensitivity to streptomycin or neomycin.

WARNINGS/PRECAUTIONS
Should be used only by physicians experienced in infertility treatment. May cause ovarian hyperstimulation syndrome (OHSS) with or without pulmonary/vascular complications and multiple births. Use lowest effective dose to minimize hazards associated with abnormal ovarian enlargement. Do not administer HCG if ovaries are abnormally enlarged on the last day of therapy; prohibit intercourse with significant ovarian enlargement after ovulation. Hepatic dysfunction reported in association with OHSS. Withhold HCG if there is a risk for OHSS evident prior to HCG administration. Monitor for OHSS development for at least 2 weeks after HCG administration; d/c therapy, including HCG, and consider hospitalization if serious OHSS occurs. OHSS increases the risk of injury to the ovary; avoid pelvic examination. Serious pulmonary conditions (eg, atelectasis, acute respiratory distress syndrome), thromboembolic reactions (both in association with, and separate from, OHSS), ovarian torsion, multifetal gestation and births, ectopic pregnancies, ovarian neoplasms, and increased risk of spontaneous abortions reported. Incidence of congenital malformations after IVF/ICSI or ART may be slightly higher than after spontaneous conception. Increased risk of venous/arterial thromboembolic events in women with recognized risk factors for thrombosis; caution in such patients. Women who are undergoing ovulation induction should be encouraged with their partners to have intercourse daily, beginning on the day prior to the administration of hCG and until ovulation becomes apparent. (Cartridge) Not recommended for the blind or visually impaired without the assistance of an individual with good vision who is trained in the proper use of the inj device.

ADVERSE REACTIONS
Headache, OHSS, inj-site reaction/pain, dermoid cyst, acne, rash, gynecomastia, pelvic pain.

PREGNANCY AND LACTATION
Category X, not for use in nursing.

MECHANISM OF ACTION
FSH; stimulates ovarian follicular growth in women who do not have primary ovarian failure. Stimulates spermatogenesis in men with hypogonadotropic hypogonadism when administered with HCG.

PHARMACOKINETICS
Absorption: Administration of variable doses resulted in different parameters. **Distribution:** (IV) V_d=8L. **Elimination:** (IM, Single 300 IU Dose): $T_{1/2}$=43.9 hrs. 7-Day Treatment: $T_{1/2}$=26.9 hrs (75 IU), 30.1 hrs (150 IU), 28.9 hrs (225 IU). (SQ, Cartridge, Single 150 IU Dose): $T_{1/2}$=33.4 hrs.

PATIENT CONSIDERATIONS
Assessment: Assess for hypersensitivity to drug or to streptomycin or neomycin, high FSH levels indicating primary gonadal failure, uncontrolled nongonadal endocrinopathies, heavy/irregular vaginal bleeding, ovarian cysts/enlargement, pregnancy/nursing status, risk factors for thrombosis, and tumors of the ovary, breast, uterus, testis, hypothalamus, or pituitary gland. Obtain complete gynecologic, medical, and endocrinologic evaluation. Evaluate the fertility status of the female or male partner.

Monitoring: Monitor for OHSS, abnormal ovarian enlargement, pulmonary/vascular complications, ovarian torsion, and other adverse reactions. Monitor for ovulation and spermatogenesis. Monitor for signs of excessive ovarian stimulation at least qod during treatment and during a 2-week post-treatment period.

Counseling: Prior to beginning therapy, inform about the time commitment and monitoring procedures necessary to undergo treatment. Counsel about risk of multifetal gestations, OHSS, and other possible side effects. Inform not to double the next dose if a dose is missed and to contact physician for further dosing instructions.

FORADIL — formoterol fumarate   Rx
Class: Long-acting beta₂ agonist (LABA)

Long-acting β_2-adrenergic agonists (LABAs) may increase the risk of asthma-related death. Contraindicated in asthma without use of a long-term asthma control medication (eg, inhaled corticosteroid). Do not use if asthma is adequately controlled on low- or medium-dose inhaled corticosteroids. LABAs may increase risk of asthma-related hospitalization in pediatric patients and adolescents; ensure adherence with both long-term asthma control medication and LABAs.

ADULT DOSAGE

Asthma

Combination w/ Long-Term Asthma Control Medication:
Usual: One 12mcg cap q12h
Max: 24mcg/day

Exercise-Induced Bronchospasm

Acute Prevention:
Usual: One 12mcg cap at least 15 min before exercise prn; additional doses should not be used for 12 hrs after administration

PEDIATRIC DOSAGE

Asthma

Combination w/ Long-Term Asthma Control Medication:
≥5 Years:
Usual: One 12mcg cap q12h
Max: 24mcg/day

Exercise-Induced Bronchospasm

Acute Prevention:
≥5 Years:
Usual: One 12mcg cap at least 15 min before exercise prn; additional doses should not be used for 12 hrs after administration
Additional dose should not be used for prevention of exercise-induced bronchospasm if already receiving bid dosing for asthma

Chronic Obstructive Pulmonary Disease

Maint Treatment of Bronchoconstriction:
Usual: One 12mcg cap q12h
Max: 24mcg/day

should not be used for 12 hrs after administration
Additional doses should not be used for prevention of exercise-induced bronchospasm if already receiving bid dosing for asthma

ADMINISTRATION
Oral inh route
Administer caps only using the Aerolizer Inhaler; caps should not be swallowed
Only remove caps from blister immediately before use

STORAGE
Prior to Dispensing: 2-8°C (36-46°F). After Dispensing: 20-25°C (68-77°F). Protect from heat and moisture. Always store caps in blister and only remove from blister immediately before use.

HOW SUPPLIED
Cap, Inh: 12mcg [12ˢ, 60ˢ]

CONTRAINDICATIONS
Treatment of asthma without concomitant use of long-term asthma control medication (eg, inhaled corticosteroid). Primary treatment of status asthmaticus or other acute episodes of asthma or COPD where intensive measures are required. History of hypersensitivity to milk proteins, formoterol fumarate, or any components of this product.

WARNINGS/PRECAUTIONS
Not indicated for the relief of acute bronchospasm. Should not be initiated with significantly worsening, acutely deteriorating, or potentially life-threatening episodes of asthma or COPD. D/C regular use of inhaled, short-acting β_2-agonists (SABAs) when beginning treatment; use only for relief of acute asthma symptoms. Not a substitute for oral/inhaled corticosteroids. Do not use more often or at doses higher than recommended or with other LABAs (eg, salmeterol xinafoate, arformoterol tartrate). D/C if paradoxical bronchospasm or clinically significant cardiovascular (CV) effects occur. Caution in patients with CV disorders (eg, coronary insufficiency, cardiac arrhythmias, HTN, aneurysm, pheochromocytoma), convulsive disorders, thyrotoxicosis, preexisting diabetes mellitus (DM), and ketoacidosis. Caution in patients who are unusually responsive to sympathomimetic amines. ECG changes, immediate hypersensitivity reactions, significant hypokalemia, and changes in blood glucose may occur. Contains lactose; may cause allergic reactions in patients with severe milk protein allergy.

ADVERSE REACTIONS
Viral infection, URTI, CV events, asthma exacerbations, bronchitis, back pain, pharyngitis, chest pain.

DRUG INTERACTIONS
Adrenergic drugs may potentiate sympathetic effects; use with caution. Xanthine derivatives or systemic corticosteroids may potentiate any hypokalemic effect. ECG changes or hypokalemia that may result from non-K⁺-sparing diuretics (eg, loop/thiazide diuretics) can be acutely worsened; use with caution. MAOIs, TCAs, macrolides, and drugs known to prolong the QTc interval may potentiate effect on CV system; use with extreme caution. Drugs known to prolong the QTc interval have an increased risk of ventricular arrhythmias. Use with β-blockers may block effects and produce severe bronchospasm in asthmatic patients; if needed, consider cardioselective β-blocker with caution. Elevated risk of arrhythmias with concomitant anesthesia with halogenated hydrocarbons.

PREGNANCY AND LACTATION
Category C, caution in nursing.

MECHANISM OF ACTION
LABA; acts as a bronchodilator, stimulates intracellular adenyl cyclase, and increases cAMP levels, causing relaxation of bronchial smooth muscle and inhibition of release of mediators of immediate hypersensitivity from cells, especially from mast cells.

PHARMACOKINETICS
Absorption: Rapid; C_{max}=92pg/mL, T_{max}=5 min. **Distribution:** Plasma protein binding (61-64%). **Metabolism:** Direct glucuronidation, O-demethylation via CYP2D6, 2C19, 2C9, 2A6. **Elimination:** With Asthma: Urine (10%, unchanged; 15-18%, conjugates). With COPD: Urine (7%, unchanged; 6-9%, conjugates). $T_{1/2}$=10 hrs.

PATIENT CONSIDERATIONS
Assessment: Assess for previous hypersensitivity to the drug or milk proteins, CV disorders, convulsive disorders, thyrotoxicosis, DM, ketoacidosis, pregnancy/nursing status, and possible drug interactions. Assess use in patients unusually responsive to sympathomimetic amines. Obtain baseline serum K⁺ and blood glucose levels. In patients with asthma, assess for status asthmaticus or presence of an acute asthma episode and assess for use of long-term asthma control medication. In patients with COPD, assess for presence of an acute COPD episode.

Monitoring: Monitor for paradoxical bronchospasm, signs of worsening asthma, CV effects, hypersensitivity reactions, aggravation of DM, and ketoacidosis. Monitor pulse rate, BP, ECG changes, and serum K⁺ and blood glucose levels.

Counseling: Inform of the risks and benefits of therapy. Instruct not to use to relieve acute asthma symptoms or exacerbations of COPD. Advise to seek medical attention if symptoms worsen, if treatment becomes less effective, or if more than usual inhalations of SABA are needed. Instruct not to exceed prescribed dose, d/c, or reduce dose without 1st contacting physician. Inform that treatment may lead to palpitations, chest pain, rapid HR, tremor, or nervousness. Advise to administer only via the Aerolizer device, to always use the new device that comes with each refill, and not to use the device for other medications. Instruct not to use with a spacer and never to exhale into the device. Advise to avoid exposing caps to moisture and to handle with dry hands. Advise to strictly follow storage conditions, remove cap from blister only immediately before use, and pierce caps only once. Advise to contact physician if patient is pregnant/nursing or if patient has severe milk protein allergy.

FORFIVO XL — bupropion hydrochloride   Rx

Class: Aminoketone

> Antidepressants increased the risk of suicidal thoughts and behavior in children, adolescents, and young adults in short-term trials. In patients of all ages who are started on antidepressant therapy, monitor closely for worsening and for emergence of suicidal thoughts/behaviors. Not approved for use in pediatric patients. Serious neuropsychiatric reactions reported in patients taking bupropion for smoking cessation; observe all patients for neuropsychiatric reactions. Not approved for smoking cessation.

ADULT DOSAGE

Major Depressive Disorder

1 tab (450mg) qd

Do not initiate treatment w/ Forfivo XL; use another bupropion formulation for initial dose titration

May be used in patients who are receiving 300mg/day of another bupropion formulation for at least 2 weeks, and require a dosage of 450mg/day

Patients currently being treated w/ other bupropion products at 450mg/day may be switched to equivalent dose of Forfivo XL qd

Dosing Considerations with MAOIs

Switching to/from an MAOI Antidepressant:
Allow at least 14 days between discontinuation of an MAOI intended to treat depression and initiation of treatment w/ Forfivo XL; allow at least 14 days between discontinuation of treatment and initiation of an MAOI antidepressant

W/ Reversible MAOIs (eg, Linezolid, IV Methylene Blue):
Do not start Forfivo XL in a patient being treated w/ a reversible MAOI. In patients already receiving Forfivo XL, if acceptable alternatives to linezolid or IV methylene blue treatment are not available and benefits outweigh risks, d/c Forfivo XL promptly and administer linezolid or IV methylene blue; monitor for 2 weeks or until 24 hrs after the last dose of linezolid or IV methylene blue, whichever comes 1st.
May resume Forfivo XL therapy 24 hrs after the last dose of linezolid or IV methylene blue.

PEDIATRIC DOSAGE
Pediatric use may not have been established

DOSING CONSIDERATIONS

Renal Impairment
Not recommended

Hepatic Impairment
Not recommended

Discontinuation
Use another bupropion formulation for tapering dose prior to discontinuation

ADMINISTRATION
Oral route

Take w/o regard to meals.
Swallow whole; do not crush, divide, or chew.

STORAGE
20-25°C (68-77°F).

HOW SUPPLIED
Tab, Extended-Release: 450mg

CONTRAINDICATIONS
Seizure disorder; current treatment w/ other bupropion products; current or prior diagnosis of bulimia or anorexia nervosa; undergoing abrupt discontinuation of alcohol, benzodiazepines, barbiturates, and antiepileptic drugs; known hypersensitivity to bupropion or other ingredients of the medication. Use of MAOIs (intended to treat psychiatric disorders) concomitantly or w/in 14 days of discontinuing treatment. Treatment w/in 14 days of discontinuing an MAOI.

Starting treatment in a patient treated w/ reversible MAOIs such as linezolid or IV methylene blue.

WARNINGS/PRECAUTIONS
May cause seizures; risk is dose related. D/C and do not restart treatment in patients who experience a seizure while on treatment. Contraindicated in patients w/ conditions that increase the risk of seizure (eg, severe head injury, arteriovenous malformation, CNS tumor or infection, severe stroke). Metabolic disorders (eg, hypoglycemia, hyponatremia, severe hepatic impairment, hypoxia) may also increase the risk of seizure. May result in elevated BP and HTN. May precipitate a manic, mixed, or hypomanic manic episode; increased risk in patients w/ bipolar disorder or who have risk factors for bipolar disorder. Not approved for the treatment of bipolar depression. Neuropsychiatric signs and symptoms (eg, delusions, hallucinations, psychosis, concentration disturbance) reported; d/c if these reactions occur. Pupillary dilation that occurs following use may trigger an angle-closure attack in a patient w/ anatomically narrow angles who does not have a patent iridectomy. Anaphylactoid/anaphylactic reactions reported; d/c treatment if allergic or anaphylactoid/anaphylactic reactions occur. Arthralgia, myalgia, fever w/ rash, and other symptoms of serum sickness suggestive of delayed hypersensitivity reported. False (+) urine immunoassay screening tests for amphetamines reported.

ADVERSE REACTIONS
Dry mouth, nausea, insomnia, dizziness, pharyngitis, abdominal pain, agitation, anxiety, tremor, palpitation, sweating, tinnitus, myalgia, anorexia, urinary frequency.

DRUG INTERACTIONS
See Dosage and Contraindications. Potential interaction w/ CYP2B6 inhibitors or inducers. Ticlopidine and clopidogrel may increase bupropion exposure but decrease hydroxybupropion exposure; coadministration w/ ticlopidine or clopidogrel is not recommended. Ritonavir, lopinavir, or efavirenz may decrease exposure; may need to increase bupropion dose but not to exceed max dose. Carbamazepine, phenytoin, and phenobarbital may induce metabolism and decrease exposure. If used concomitantly w/ a CYP inducer, may need to increase the dose of bupropion, but not to exceed the max dose. May increase exposure of CYP2D6 substrates (eg, venlafaxine, nortriptyline, haloperidol, metoprolol, propafenone); may need to decrease the dose of CYP2D6 substrates, particularly for drugs w/ a narrow therapeutic index. May reduce efficacy of drugs that require metabolic activation by CYP2D6 to be effective (eg, tamoxifen); may require increased doses of such drugs. Extreme caution w/ drugs that lower seizure threshold (eg, other bupropion products, antipsychotics, antidepressants, theophylline, systemic corticosteroids). CNS toxicity reported when coadministered w/ levodopa or amantadine; use w/ caution. Adverse neuropsychiatric events or reduced alcohol tolerance reported (rarely) w/ alcohol; avoid alcohol consumption during treatment. Increased risk of seizure w/ use of illicit drugs (eg, cocaine), abuse or misuse of prescription drugs (eg, CNS stimulants), use of oral hypoglycemic drugs or insulin, use of anorectic drugs, excessive use of alcohol, and use of benzodiazepines, sedative/hypnotics, or opiates. Monitor BP w/ nicotine replacement therapy. Increased risk of HTN w/ MAOIs or other drugs that increase dopaminergic or noradrenergic activity.

PREGNANCY AND LACTATION
Pregnancy: Category C.
Lactation: Bupropion and its metabolites are present in human milk; caution in nursing.

MECHANISM OF ACTION
Aminoketone antidepressant; has not been established. Presumed that action is mediated by noradrenergic and/or dopaminergic mechanisms. Weak inhibitor of the neuronal uptake of norepinephrine and dopamine, and does not inhibit monoamine oxidase or the reuptake of serotonin.

PHARMACOKINETICS
Absorption: C_{max}=207.46ng/mL, AUC=2147.53ng•hr/mL; T_{max}=5 hrs (median, fasted), 12 hrs (fed). **Distribution:** Plasma protein binding (84%); found in breast milk. **Metabolism:** Extensive; via hydroxylation (CYP2B6) and reduction of carbonyl group; hydroxybupropion, threohydrobupropion, and erythrohydrobupropion (active metabolites). **Elimination:** Feces (10%), urine (87%), (0.5% unchanged); $T_{1/2}$=14.44 hrs, 20 hrs (hydroxybupropion), 33 hrs (erythrohydrobupropion), 37 hrs (threohydrobupropion).

PATIENT CONSIDERATIONS

Assessment: Assess for history of bipolar disorder or presence of risk factors for bipolar disorder, hepatic/renal impairment, seizure disorders or conditions that may increase risk of seizure, susceptibility to angle-closure glaucoma, hypersensitivity to the drug, any other conditions where treatment is contraindicated or cautioned, pregnancy/nursing status, and for possible drug interactions. Assess BP.

Monitoring: Monitor for clinical worsening, suicidality, unusual changes in behavior, neuropsychiatric symptoms, seizures, HTN, activation of mania or hypomania, psychosis and other neuropsychiatric reactions, angle-closure glaucoma, anaphylactoid/anaphylactic reactions, delayed hypersensitivity, and other adverse reactions. Monitor BP periodically. Periodically reassess the need for maint treatment.

Counseling: Inform of the benefits/risks of therapy. Advise patients and caregivers of need for close observation for clinical worsening, suicidality, or unusual changes in behavior. Instruct to contact physician if neuropsychiatric reactions occur. Educate on the symptoms of hypersensitivity and instruct to d/c if a severe allergic reaction occurs. Instruct to d/c and not to restart if seizure occurs while on therapy. Inform that excessive use or abrupt discontinuation of alcohol, benzodiazepines, antiepileptic drugs, or sedatives/hypnotics can increase the risk of seizure; advise to avoid the use of alcohol. Caution about the risk of angle-closure glaucoma in susceptible patients. Inform that product contains same active ingredient found in Zyban; instruct not to use in combination w/ Zyban or any other medications that contain bupropion. Inform that therapy may impair mental/physical abilities; advise to refrain from operating hazardous machinery/driving until effects of therapy are known. Instruct to notify physician if taking/planning to take any prescription or OTC medications. Advise to contact physician if pregnant or intending to become pregnant during therapy. Instruct to take ud.

FORTAMET — metformin hydrochloride   Rx

Class: Biguanide

> Lactic acidosis reported (rare). May occur in association w/ other conditions such as diabetes mellitus (DM) w/ significant renal insufficiency, CHF, and conditions w/ risk of hypoperfusion and hypoxemia. Risk increases w/ the degree of renal dysfunction and age. Avoid in patients ≥80 yrs unless renal function is normal. Avoid w/ clinical/lab evidence of hepatic disease. Temporarily d/c prior to IV radiocontrast studies or surgical procedures. Caution against excessive alcohol intake; may potentiate effects of metformin on lactate metabolism. Withhold in the presence of any condition associated w/ hypoxemia, dehydration, or sepsis. Regularly monitor renal function and use minimum effective dose to decrease risk. If lactic acidosis is suspected, immediately d/c and institute general supportive measures.

ADULT DOSAGE
Type 2 Diabetes Mellitus
≥17 Years:
Initial: 500-1000mg qd
Titrate: May increase in increments of 500mg weekly
Max: 2500mg/day

Transfer from Other Antidiabetic Therapy:
From Standard Oral Hypoglycemic Agents Other Than Chlorpropamide:
No transition period necessary
From Chlorpropamide: Exercise care during first 2 weeks for overlapping drug effects and possible hypoglycemia

PEDIATRIC DOSAGE
Pediatric use may not have been established

DOSING CONSIDERATIONS
Concomitant Medications
Oral Sulfonylurea Therapy:
If unresponsive to 4 weeks of max dose of metformin HCl extended-release (ER) monotherapy, consider gradual addition of an oral sulfonylurea while continuing metformin HCl ER at max dose
If patients have not satisfactorily responded to 1-3 months of concomitant therapy (max dose of metformin HCl ER and max dose of an oral sulfonylurea), consider therapeutic alternatives (eg, switching to insulin w/ or w/o metformin HCl ER)

Insulin Therapy:
Initial: 500mg qd while continuing current insulin dose
Titrate: May increase by 500mg after approx 1 week and by 500mg every week thereafter
Max: 2500mg/day
Decrease insulin dose by 10-25% if FPG <120mg/dL

Elderly
Initial/Maint: Use conservative dosing
Do not titrate to max dose

Other Important Considerations
Debilitated/Malnourished Patients:
Do not titrate to max dose

ADMINISTRATION
Oral route
Take w/ a full glass of water w/ pm meal.

STORAGE
20-25°C (68-77°F); excursions permitted to 15-30°C (59-86°F). Keep tightly closed. Protect from light and moisture. Avoid excessive heat and humidity.

HOW SUPPLIED
Tab, ER: 500mg, 1000mg

CONTRAINDICATIONS
Renal disease/dysfunction (eg, SrCr ≥1.5mg/dL [males], ≥1.4mg/dL [females], or abnormal CrCl); known hypersensitivity to metformin; acute or chronic metabolic acidosis, including diabetic ketoacidosis, w/ or w/o coma.

WARNINGS/PRECAUTIONS
Lactic acidosis may be suspected in diabetic patients w/ metabolic acidosis lacking evidence of ketoacidosis (ketonuria and ketonemia). Caution w/ concomitant medications that may affect renal function, result in significant hemodynamic change, or interfere w/ the disposition of metformin. Temporarily d/c prior to surgical procedures associated w/ restricted oral intake. Temporarily withhold drug before, during, and 48 hrs after radiologic studies w/ IV iodinated contrast materials; reinstitute only when renal function is normal. D/C in hypoxic states (eg, shock, CHF, acute myocardial infarction [MI]), dehydration, and sepsis. Avoid w/ clinical or lab evidence of hepatic disease. May decrease vitamin B12 levels. Increased risk of hypoglycemia in elderly, debilitated/malnourished, adrenal or pituitary insufficiency, or alcohol intoxication. Temporarily withhold metformin and administer insulin if loss of glycemic control occurs due to stress; reinstitute metformin after acute episode is resolved.

ADVERSE REACTIONS
Lactic acidosis, infection, diarrhea, nausea, headache, dyspepsia, rhinitis, flatulence, abdominal pain.

DRUG INTERACTIONS
Furosemide, nifedipine, cimetidine, and cationic drugs (eg, amiloride, digoxin, morphine) may increase metformin levels. Thiazides, other diuretics, corticosteroids, phenothiazines, thyroid products, estrogens, oral contraceptives, phenytoin, nicotinic acid, sympathomimetics, calcium channel blockers, and isoniazid may cause hyperglycemia and loss of glycemic control. May decrease furosemide levels.

PREGNANCY AND LACTATION
Category B, not for use in pregnancy or nursing.

MECHANISM OF ACTION
Biguanide; decreases hepatic production and intestinal absorption of glucose, and improves insulin sensitivity by increasing peripheral glucose uptake and utilization.

PHARMACOKINETICS
Absorption: C_{max}=2849ng/mL, T_{max}=6 hrs, AUC=26811ng•hr/mL. **Elimination:** Urine (90%); $T_{1/2}$=6.2 hrs (plasma), 17.6 hrs (blood).

PATIENT CONSIDERATIONS
Assessment: Assess for hypoxic states (eg, acute CHF, acute MI, cardiovascular collapse), septicemia, acute/chronic metabolic acidosis, adrenal/pituitary insufficiency, alcoholism, pregnancy/nursing status, and possible drug interactions. Evaluate for other medical conditions, and for any IV radiocontrast study or surgical procedure. Assess FPG, HbA1c, renal function, LFTs, and hematologic parameters (eg, Hgb/Hct, RBC indices).

Monitoring: Monitor for lactic acidosis, hypoglycemia, prerenal azotemia, hypoxic states, hypersensitivity reactions, and other adverse reactions. Monitor FPG, HbA1c, renal function (eg, SrCr), LFTs, and hematologic parameters (eg, Hgb/Hct, RBC indices).

Counseling: Inform of the potential risks, benefits, and alternative modes of therapy. Inform about the importance of adherence to dietary instructions, regular exercise programs, and regular testing of blood glucose, HbA1c, renal function, and hematologic parameters. Inform of the risk of lactic acidosis w/ therapy and to contact physician if unexplained hyperventilation, myalgia, malaise, unusual somnolence, or other nonspecific symptoms occur. Counsel against excessive alcohol intake. Explain risks, symptoms, and conditions that predispose to the development of hypoglycemia when initiating combination therapy. Instruct that drug must be taken w/ food, swallowed whole w/ a full glass of water and should not be chewed, cut, or crushed, and that inactive ingredients may be eliminated in the feces as a soft mass.

FORTAZ — ceftazidime   Rx

Class: Cephalosporin (3rd generation)

ADULT DOSAGE
General Dosing
Usual: 1g IM/IV q8-12h

Life-Threatening Infections:
2g IV q8h

Continue therapy for 2 days after signs and symptoms of infection have disappeared; complicated infections may require longer duration of therapy

Urinary Tract Infections
Uncomplicated: 250mg IM/IV q12h
Complicated: 500mg IM/IV q8-12h

Bone/Joint Infections
2g IV q12h

Pneumonia
Uncomplicated:
500mg-1g IM/IV q8h

Skin and Skin Structure Infections
Mild:
500mg-1g IM/IV q8h

Gynecologic Infections
Serious:
2g IV q8h

Intra-Abdominal Infections
Serious:
2g IV q8h

Meningitis
2g IV q8h

Lung Infection
Caused by *Pseudomonas* spp. in Cystic Fibrosis:
30-50mg/kg IV q8h
Max: 6g/day

Treatment Duration
Continue for 2 days after signs/symptoms of infection disappear;

PEDIATRIC DOSAGE
General Dosing
Neonates (0-4 Weeks of Age):
30mg/kg IV q12h

Infants and Children (1 Month-12 Years):
30-50mg/kg IV q8h
Max: 6g/day

Use higher doses for immunocompromised patients w/ cystic fibrosis or meningitis

Continue for 2 days after signs/symptoms of infection disappear; may require longer therapy w/ complicated infections

may require longer therapy w/ complicated infections

Other Indications
Treatment of the Following Infections Caused by Susceptible Strains of microorganisms:
Lower respiratory tract
CNS infections
Bacterial septicemia
Sepsis

DOSING CONSIDERATIONS
Renal Impairment
If normal recommended dose is lower than recommended dose for renal impairment, the lower dose should be used
CrCl 31-50mL/min: 1g q12h
CrCl 16-30mL/min: 1g q24h
CrCl 6-15mL/min: 500mg q24h
CrCl <5mL/min: 500mg q48h
Hemodialysis: May receive 1g LD, followed by 1g after each hemodialysis period
Intraperitoneal/Continuous Peritoneal Dialysis: May receive 1g LD, followed by 500mg q24h
May include ceftazidime inj in dialysis fluid at a concentration of 250mg/2L dialysis fluid

ADMINISTRATION
IM/IV route
Avoid intra-arterial administration

IM
Administer into large muscle mass (eg, upper outer quadrant of gluteus maximus or lateral part of thigh)
Reconstitute 500mg vial or 1g vial w/ 1.5mL or 3mL (respectively) of appropriate diluent (eg, sterile water for inj [SWFI], bacteriostatic water for inj, or 0.5% or 1% lidocaine HCl inj)

IV
Do not use plastic containers in series connections
Add 5.3mL of diluent to 500mg IV vial, 10mL of diluent to 1g or 2g IV vial, or 26mL of diluent to 6g pharmacy bulk package vial; constitute w/ SWFI
Direct Intermittent IV Administration: Slowly inject directly into the vein over 3-5 min, or give through tubing of administration set while patient is also receiving one of the compatible IV fluids
IV Infusion: Constitute 500mg, 1g, or 2g vial and withdraw 5mL, 10mL, or 11.5mL (respectively) to IV container w/ a compatible IV fluid
Intermittent IV Infusion w/ Y-Type Administration Set: Administer w/ compatible solutions; do not infuse w/ sol containing ceftazidime

Compatible IV Fluid for Solutions w/ Concentrations Between 1-40mg/mL
0.9% NaCl inj
1/6 M sodium lactate inj
5% dextrose inj
5% dextrose and 0.225% NaCl inj
5% dextrose and 0.45% NaCl inj
5% dextrose and 0.9% NaCl inj
10% dextrose inj
Ringer's inj
Lactated Ringer's inj
10% invert sugar in water for inj
Normosol-M in 5% dextrose inj

Refer to PI for additional administration instructions

STORAGE
15-30°C (59-86°F), in dry state. Protect from light. Frozen as premixed sol should not be stored above -20°C.

HOW SUPPLIED
Inj: 500mg, 1g, 2g; 1g, 2g [ADD-Vantage]; 1g/50mL, 2g/50mL [Galaxy]

CONTRAINDICATIONS
Hypersensitivity to ceftazidime or the cephalosporin group of antibiotics.

WARNINGS/PRECAUTIONS
Cross hypersensitivity among β-lactam antibiotics reported; caution with penicillin (PCN) sensitivity. D/C if allergic reaction occurs. *Clostridium difficile*-associated diarrhea (CDAD) reported. May result in bacterial resistance with prolonged use or use in the absence of a proven/suspected bacterial infection or a prophylactic indication; take appropriate measures if superinfection develops. Elevated levels with renal insufficiency may lead to seizures, encephalopathy, coma, asterixis, myoclonia, and neuromuscular excitability. Associated with fall in prothrombin activity; caution with renal/hepatic impairment, poor nutritional state, and protracted course of antimicrobial therapy. Caution with colitis, history of GI disease, and elderly. Distal necrosis may occur after inadvertent intra-arterial administration. Lab test interactions may occur.

ADVERSE REACTIONS
Allergic reactions, increased ALT/AST/GGT/LDH, eosinophilia, local/GI reactions.

DRUG INTERACTIONS
Nephrotoxicity reported with aminoglycosides or potent diuretics (eg, furosemide). Avoid with chloramphenicol. May reduce efficacy of combined oral estrogen/progesterone contraceptives.

PREGNANCY AND LACTATION
Category B, caution in nursing.

MECHANISM OF ACTION
Cephalosporin (3rd generation); bactericidal, inhibits enzymes responsible for bacterial cell-wall synthesis.

PHARMACOKINETICS
Absorption: (IV/IM) Administration of variable doses resulted in different parameters. **Distribution:** Plasma protein binding (<10%); found in breast milk. **Elimination:** Urine (80-90%, unchanged); $T_{1/2}$=1.9 hrs (IV), 2 hrs (IM).

PATIENT CONSIDERATIONS
Assessment: Assess for history of hypersensitivity to cephalosporins/PCNs, history of GI disease, colitis, renal/hepatic impairment, nursing status, and for possible drug interactions.

Monitoring: Monitor for signs and symptoms of hypersensitivity reactions, CDAD, LDH, LFTs, renal function, PT, hemolytic anemia, and for superinfection. Monitor for seizures, encephalopathy, coma, asterixis, neuromuscular excitability, and myoclonia with renal impairment. Perform periodic susceptibility testing.

Counseling: Inform that therapy only treats bacterial, not viral, infections. Instruct to take exactly ud; explain that skipping doses or not completing full course may decrease effectiveness and increase resistance. Advise that patient may experience diarrhea; instruct to notify physician if watery/bloody stools (with/without stomach cramps and fever) occur.

FORTEO — teriparatide (rDNA origin)   Rx
Class: Recombinant human parathyroid hormone

> Increased incidence of osteosarcoma seen in animal studies; prescribe only when benefits outweigh risks. Do not prescribe for patients who are at increased baseline risk for osteosarcoma (including those w/ Paget's disease of bone or unexplained alkaline phosphatase elevations, pediatric and young adult patients w/ open epiphyses, or prior external beam or implant radiation therapy involving the skeleton).

ADULT DOSAGE	PEDIATRIC DOSAGE
Osteoporosis	Pediatric use may not have been established
High Risk for Fracture:	
Postmenopausal Women w/ Osteoporosis: 20mcg qd	
Primary or Hypogonadal Osteoporosis in Men: 20mcg qd	
Glucocorticoid-Induced Osteoporosis in Men and Women: 20mcg qd	
Use for >2 yrs during a patient's lifetime is not recommended	

ADMINISTRATION
SQ route

Inject into the thigh or abdominal wall.
Administer initially under circumstances where the patient can sit or lie down if symptoms of orthostatic hypotension occur.

STORAGE
2-8°C (36-46°F). Recap pen when not in use. Minimize time out of the refrigerator during the use period; may deliver dose immediately following removal from the refrigerator. Do not freeze; do not use if it has been frozen. Discard after the 28-day use period.

HOW SUPPLIED
Inj: 20mcg/dose [28 doses]

CONTRAINDICATIONS
Hypersensitivity to teriparatide or to any of its excipients.

WARNINGS/PRECAUTIONS
Use for >2 yrs during a patient's lifetime is not recommended. Do not give in patients w/ bone metastases or history of skeletal malignancies, metabolic bone diseases other than osteoporosis, preexisting hypercalcemia, or underlying hypercalcemic disorder (eg, primary hyperparathyroidism). Transiently increases serum Ca^{2+}. Consider measurement of urinary Ca^{2+} excretion if active urolithiasis or preexisting hypercalciuria are suspected; caution w/ active or recent urolithiasis. Transient episodes of symptomatic orthostatic hypotension reported w/ administration of initial doses; administer initially under circumstances where the patient can sit or lie down if symptoms of orthostatic hypotension occur.

ADVERSE REACTIONS
Pain, arthralgia, rhinitis, asthenia, N/V, dizziness, headache, HTN, increased cough, pharyngitis, constipation, dyspepsia, diarrhea, rash, insomnia.

DRUG INTERACTIONS
Hypercalcemia may predispose to digitalis toxicity; caution if taking digoxin concomitantly.

PREGNANCY AND LACTATION
Category C, not for use in nursing.

MECHANISM OF ACTION
Recombinant human parathyroid hormone; binds to specific high-affinity cell-surface receptors. Stimulates new bone formation on trabecular and cortical (periosteal and/or endosteal) bone surfaces by preferential stimulation of osteoblastic activity over osteoclastic activity. Produces an increase in skeletal mass, markers of bone formation and resorption, and bone strength.

PHARMACOKINETICS

Absorption: Rapid. Absolute bioavailability (approx 95%); T_{max}=30 min. **Distribution:** (IV) V_d=approx 0.12L/kg. **Metabolism:** Liver (nonspecific enzymatic mechanisms). **Elimination:** Kidneys; $T_{1/2}$=approx 1 hr.

PATIENT CONSIDERATIONS

Assessment: Assess for increased baseline risk for osteosarcoma, bone metastases or history of skeletal malignancies, metabolic bone disease other than osteoporosis, hypercalcemia, hypercalcemic disorder, hypercalciuria, active or recent urolithiasis, hypersensitivity to drug, pregnancy/nursing status, and possible drug interactions. Consider measurement of urinary Ca^{2+} excretion if active urolithiasis or preexisting hypercalciuria are suspected.

Monitoring: Monitor for signs/symptoms of osteosarcoma, orthostatic hypotension, and other adverse reactions.

Counseling: Inform of potential risk of osteosarcoma and encourage to enroll in the voluntary Forteo Patient Registry. Instruct to sit or lie down if lightheadedness or palpitations following inj develop; if symptoms persist or worsen, advise to consult physician before continuing treatment. Instruct to contact physician if persistent symptoms of hypercalcemia (eg, N/V, constipation, lethargy, muscle weakness) develop. Counsel on roles of supplemental Ca^{2+} and/or vitamin D, weight-bearing exercise, and modification of certain behavioral factors (eg, smoking, alcohol consumption). Instruct on proper use of delivery device (pen) and proper disposal of needles; advise not to share pen w/ other patients and not to transfer contents to a syringe.

FORTESTA — testosterone   CIII

Class: Androgen

> Virilization reported in children secondarily exposed to testosterone gel. Children should avoid contact w/ unwashed or unclothed application sites in men using testosterone gel. Advise patients to strictly adhere to recommended instructions for use.

ADULT DOSAGE	PEDIATRIC DOSAGE
Testosterone Replacement Therapy	Pediatric use may not have been established
Congenital/Acquired Primary Hypogonadism or Hypogonadotropic Hypogonadism in Males:	
Initial: Apply 40mg qam	
Titrate: May adjust between 10-70mg based on serum testosterone concentration from a single blood draw 2 hrs after application at approx 14 days and 35 days after starting treatment or following dose adjustment	
Max: 70mg	
Dose Adjustment Based on Total Serum Testosterone Concentration 2 Hrs Post Application:	
<500ng/dL: Increase daily dose by 10mg	
≥500-<1250ng/dL: Continue on current dose	
≥1250-<2500ng/dL: Decrease daily dose by 10mg	
≥2500ng/dL: Decrease daily dose by 20mg	

ADMINISTRATION
Topical route

Apply to clean, dry, intact skin of the front and inner thighs; do not apply to genitals or other parts of the body
Avoid swimming, showering, or washing the administration site for a minimum of 2 hrs after application
Prime canister pump in upright position; slowly and fully depress the actuator 8X prior to 1st use
Wash hands immediately w/ soap and water after application
Refer to PI for further application instructions

STORAGE
20-25°C (68-77°F); excursions permitted to 15-30°C (59-86°F). Do not freeze, Discard used canisters in household trash in a manner that prevents accidental application or ingestion by children or pets.

HOW SUPPLIED
Gel: 10mg/actuation [120 actuations]

CONTRAINDICATIONS
Breast carcinoma or known/suspected prostate carcinoma in men; women who are or may become pregnant, or are breastfeeding.

WARNINGS/PRECAUTIONS
Application site and dose are not interchangeable w/ other topical testosterone products. Patients w/ BPH and geriatric patients may be at increased risk of worsening of signs/symptoms of BPH. May increase risk for prostate cancer. Risk of virilization in women due to secondary exposure; d/c until cause is identified. Not indicated for use in women. Increases in Hct/RBC mass may increase risk for thromboembolic events; may require dose reduction or discontinuation of therapy until Hct decreases to an acceptable concentration. Venous thromboembolic events (VTEs), including deep vein thrombosis and pulmonary embolism, reported; d/c treatment and initiate workup and management if venous thromboembolic event is suspected. Increased risk of major adverse cardiovascular events (MACE) reported. Suppression of spermatogenesis may occur w/ large doses. Hepatic adverse effects reported w/ prolonged use of high doses of orally active 17-α-alkyl androgens and long-term therapy w/ IM testosterone enanthate. Risk of edema w/ or w/o CHF in patients w/ preexisting cardiac, renal, or hepatic disease. Gynecomastia may develop and persist. May potentiate sleep apnea. Changes in serum lipid profile may require dose adjustment or discontinuation of therapy. Caution in cancer patients at risk of hypercalcemia and associated hypercalciuria. May decrease levels of thyroxin-binding globulins, resulting in decreased total T4 serum levels and increased resin uptake of T3 and T4. Flammable; avoid fire, flame, or smoking until the gel has dried.

ADVERSE REACTIONS
Application-site skin reactions.

DRUG INTERACTIONS
Changes in insulin sensitivity or glycemic control may occur; may decrease blood glucose and, therefore, decrease insulin requirements in diabetic patients. Adrenocorticotropic hormone or corticosteroids may increase fluid retention; caution in patients w/ cardiac, renal, or hepatic disease. Changes in anticoagulant activity may occur; frequently monitor INR and PT in patients taking anticoagulants, especially at initiation and termination of androgen therapy.

PREGNANCY AND LACTATION
Category X, not for use in nursing.

MECHANISM OF ACTION
Androgen; responsible for normal growth and development of male sex organs and for maintenance of secondary sex characteristics.

PHARMACOKINETICS
Distribution: Plasma protein binding (98%; approx 40% bound to sex hormone-binding globulin). **Metabolism:** Estradiol and dihydrotestosterone (major active metabolites). **Elimination:** (IM) Urine (90% glucuronic and sulfuric acid conjugates), feces (6% mostly unconjugated); $T_{1/2}$=10-100 min.

PATIENT CONSIDERATIONS
Assessment: Assess for BPH, prostate cancer, cardiac/renal/hepatic disease, obesity, chronic lung disease, conditions where treatment is contraindicated or cautioned, and for possible drug interactions. Check Hct prior to therapy. Confirm diagnosis of hypogonadism by measuring testosterone levels in am on at least 2 separate days prior to initiation.

Monitoring: Monitor for prostate carcinoma, edema w/ or w/o CHF, gynecomastia, worsening of signs/symptoms of BPH, sleep apnea, VTEs, MACE, and other adverse reactions. Perform periodic monitoring of Hgb, LFTs, prostate-specific antigen, and serum lipid profile. Obtain serum testosterone levels 14 days and 35 days after initiation of therapy or following dose adjustment. In cancer patients at risk for hypercalcemia, regularly monitor serum Ca^{2+} levels. Reevaluate Hct 3-6 months after start of therapy, then annually.

Counseling: Inform that men w/ known or suspected prostate/breast cancer should not use androgen therapy. Advise to report signs/symptoms of secondary exposure in children and in women to the physician. Inform that children and women should avoid contact w/ unwashed or unclothed application sites of men using testosterone gel. Instruct to apply ud; instruct to cover application site w/ clothing after gel dries, and wash application site w/ soap and water prior to direct skin-to-skin contact w/ others. Inform about possible adverse reactions. Inform that drug is flammable; instruct to avoid fire, flame, or smoking until the gel has dried. Advise not to share the medication w/ anyone. Instruct to adhere to all the recommended monitoring, to wait 2 hrs before swimming or washing following application, and to report changes in their state of health.

FORTICAL — calcitonin-salmon (rDNA origin)   Rx

Class: Hormonal bone resorption inhibitor

ADULT DOSAGE	PEDIATRIC DOSAGE
Postmenopausal Osteoporosis	Pediatric use may not have been established
In Women >5 Years Postmenopause:	
1 spray qd intranasally, alternating nostrils daily	
Calcium and Vitamin D Supplementation:	
Patients should receive adequate Ca^{2+} (≥1000mg elemental Ca^{2+}/day) and vitamin D (≥400 IU/day)	
Periodically reevaluate the need for continued therapy	

ADMINISTRATION
Intranasal route

Wait until the bottle has reached room temperature before using the 1st dose.
To prime the pump before it is used for the 1st time, hold the bottle upright and depress the 2 white side arms of the pump toward the bottle at least 5 times until a full spray is produced; the pump is primed once the 1st full spray is emitted.
To administer, carefully place the nozzle into the nostril w/ the patient's head in the upright position, then firmly depress the pump toward the bottle.
Do not prime the pump before each daily use.

STORAGE

Unopened: 2-8°C (36-46°F). Protect from freezing. Opened: 20-25°C (68-77°F); excursions permitted to 15-30°C (59-86°F). Discard after 30 doses have been used.

HOW SUPPLIED

Spray: 200 IU/spray [3.7mL]

CONTRAINDICATIONS

Hypersensitivity to calcitonin-salmon or any of the excipients.

WARNINGS/PRECAUTIONS

Reserve for patients for whom alternative treatments are not suitable. Serious hypersensitivity reactions reported; usual provisions should be made for emergency treatment if such a reaction occurs. Consider skin testing prior to treatment for patients w/ suspected hypersensitivity to drug. Hypocalcemia associated w/ tetany and seizure activity reported. Correct hypocalcemia and treat other disorders affecting mineral metabolism (eg, vitamin D deficiency) before initiating therapy. Adequate intake of Ca^{2+} and vitamin D is recommended. Nasal adverse reactions (eg, rhinitis, epistaxis) reported, and development of mucosal alterations may occur; perform periodic nasal exams prior to start of treatment and during therapy, and at any time nasal symptoms occur. D/C if severe ulceration of the nasal mucosa occurs; d/c temporarily until healing occurs in patients w/ smaller ulcers. Increased risk of malignancies; carefully consider benefits against possible risks. Consider possibility of antibody formation in any patient w/ an initial response to therapy who later stops responding to treatment. Urine sediment abnormalities may occur; consider periodic exam of urine sediment.

ADVERSE REACTIONS

Rhinitis, nasal symptoms, back pain, arthralgia, epistaxis, headache.

DRUG INTERACTIONS

May reduce lithium concentrations; dose of lithium may require adjustment.

PREGNANCY AND LACTATION

Category C, caution in nursing.

MECHANISM OF ACTION

Hormonal bone resorption inhibitor; calcitonin receptor agonist. Actions on bone have not been fully established. Causes inhibition of the ongoing bone resorptive process. Prolonged use causes a smaller decrease in the rate of bone resorption, which is associated w/ a decreased number of osteoclasts as well as a decrease in their resorptive activity.

PHARMACOKINETICS

Absorption: Rapid. T_{max}=10 min. Elimination: $T_{1/2}$=23 min.

PATIENT CONSIDERATIONS

Assessment: Assess for hypersensitivity to drug, hypocalcemia or other disorders affecting mineral metabolism, pregnancy/nursing status, and possible drug interactions. Consider skin testing for patients w/ suspected hypersensitivity to drug. Perform baseline nasal exam.

Monitoring: Monitor for signs/symptoms of hypersensitivity reactions, hypocalcemia, nasal adverse reactions, malignancy, antibody formation, and other adverse reactions. Perform nasal exams periodically during therapy and at any time nasal symptoms occur. Perform periodic exams of urine sediment. Periodically reevaluate the need for continued therapy.

Counseling: Instruct on pump assembly, priming of the pump, and nasal introduction of medication. Advise to notify physician if significant nasal irritation develops. Inform of the potential increase in risk of malignancy. Advise to maintain an adequate Ca^{2+} and vitamin D intake. Instruct to seek emergency medical help if any signs/symptoms of a serious allergic reaction develop.

FOSAMAX PLUS D — alendronate sodium/cholecalciferol   Rx

Class: Bisphosphonate/vitamin D analogue

ADULT DOSAGE	PEDIATRIC DOSAGE
Osteoporosis **Treatment of Osteoporosis in Postmenopausal Women/Treatment to Increase Bone Mass in Men w/ Osteoporosis:** 1 tab (70mg/2800 IU or 70mg/5600 IU) once weekly For most osteoporotic women/men, appropriate dose is 70mg/5600 IU once weekly **Missed Dose** If once-weekly dose is missed, administer 1 tab on am after patient remembers; do not take 2 tabs on same day, but return to taking 1 tab once a week, as originally scheduled on chosen day	Pediatric use may not have been established

DOSING CONSIDERATIONS

Renal Impairment
CrCl <35mL/min: Not recommended

ADMINISTRATION

Oral route

Take upon arising for the day.
Swallow tabs w/ full glass of water (6-8 oz); do not chew or suck on the tab. Take at least 1/2 hr before the 1st food, beverage, or medication of the day w/ plain water only.
Do not lie down for at least 30 min and until after 1st food of the day.

STORAGE

20-25°C (68-77°F); excursions permitted to 15-30°C (59-86°F). Protect from moisture and light.

HOW SUPPLIED

Tab: (Alendronate/Cholecalciferol) 70mg/2800 IU, 70mg/5600 IU

CONTRAINDICATIONS

Esophageal abnormalities that delay esophageal emptying (eg, stricture, achalasia), inability to stand or sit upright for at least 30 min, hypocalcemia. Hypersensitivity to any component of this product.

WARNINGS/PRECAUTIONS

Do not use alone to treat vitamin D deficiency. Consider discontinuation after 3-5 yrs of use in patients at low-risk for fracture; periodically reevaluate risk for fracture in patients who d/c therapy. May cause local irritation of the upper GI mucosa; caution w/ active upper GI problems (eg, Barrett's esophagus, dysphagia, other esophageal diseases, gastritis, duodenitis, ulcers). Esophageal reactions (eg, esophagitis, esophageal ulcers/erosions) reported; d/c and seek medical attention if dysphagia, odynophagia, retrosternal pain, or new/worsening heartburn develops. Use under appropriate supervision in patients who cannot comply w/ dosing instructions due to mental disability. Gastric and duodenal ulcers reported. Treat hypocalcemia or other disorders affecting mineral metabolism (eg, vitamin D deficiency) prior to therapy. Asymptomatic decreases in serum Ca^{2+} and phosphate may occur. Severe and occasionally incapacitating bone, joint, and/or muscle pain reported; d/c if severe symptoms develop. Osteonecrosis of the jaw (ONJ) reported; risk may increase w/ duration of exposure to drug. If invasive dental procedures are required, discontinuation of treatment may reduce risk for ONJ. Consider discontinuation if ONJ develops. Atypical, low-energy, or low trauma fractures of the femoral shaft reported; evaluate any patient w/ a history of bisphosphonate exposure who presents w/ thigh/groin pain to rule out incomplete femur fracture, and consider interruption of therapy. Vitamin D3 supplementation may worsen hypercalcemia and/or hypercalciuria in patients w/ diseases associated w/ unregulated overproduction of 1,25-dihydroxyvitamin D (eg, leukemia, lymphoma, sarcoidosis).

ADVERSE REACTIONS

Abdominal pain, musculoskeletal pain, nausea, dyspepsia, constipation, diarrhea.

DRUG INTERACTIONS

Ca^{2+} supplements, antacids, or oral medications containing multivalent cations will interfere w/ absorption of alendronate; wait at least 1/2 hr after dosing before taking any other oral medications. NSAID use is associated w/ GI irritation; use w/ caution. Alendronate: Increased incidence of upper GI adverse events in patients receiving concomitant therapy w/ daily doses of alendronate >10mg and aspirin-containing products. Cholecalciferol: Olestra, mineral oils, orlistat, and bile acid sequestrants (eg, cholestyramine, colestipol) may impair absorption; consider additional supplementation. Anticonvulsants, cimetidine, and thiazides may increase catabolism; consider additional supplementation.

PREGNANCY AND LACTATION

Pregnancy: Category C.
Lactation: Caution in nursing.

MECHANISM OF ACTION

Alendronate: Bisphosphonate; binds to hydroxyapatite found in bone and specifically inhibits the osteoclast-mediated bone-resorption. Cholecalciferol: Vitamin D analog; increases intestinal absorption of both Ca^{2+} and phosphate. Regulates serum Ca^{2+}, renal Ca^{2+} and phosphate excretion, bone formation and bone resorption.

PHARMACOKINETICS

Absorption: Alendronate: Absolute bioavailability (0.64% in women), (0.59% in men). Cholecalciferol: (2800 IU) C_{max}=4ng/mL, T_{max}=10.6 hrs, $AUC_{0-120\ hrs}$=120.7ng•hr/mL. Refer to PI for further information. Distribution: Alendronate: V_d=at least 28L; plasma protein binding (78%). Cholecalciferol: Found in breast milk. Metabolism: Cholecalciferol: Liver (rapid) via hydroxylation to 25-hydroxyvitamin D3; subsequently metabolized in the kidney to 1,25-dihydroxyvitamin D3 (active metabolite). Elimination: Alendronate: (IV) Urine (50%); $T_{1/2}$ >10 yrs. Cholecalciferol: (IV) Urine (2.4%), feces (4.9%); (Oral) $T_{1/2}$=14 hrs.

PATIENT CONSIDERATIONS

Assessment: Assess for esophageal abnormalities, ability to stand or sit upright for at least 30 min, hypocalcemia, risk for ONJ, active upper GI problems, mental disability, renal impairment, drug hypersensitivity, any other conditions where treatment is contraindicated or cautioned, pregnancy/nursing status, and possible drug interactions.

Monitoring: Monitor for signs/symptoms of ONJ, atypical fractures, esophageal reactions, musculoskeletal pain, hypocalcemia, and other adverse events. Monitor urine and serum Ca^{2+} in patients w/ diseases associated w/ unregulated overproduction of 1,25-dihydroxyvitamin D. Periodically reevaluate the need for continued therapy.

Counseling: Instruct to take supplemental Ca^{2+} and vitamin D if dietary intake is inadequate. Counsel to consider weight-bearing exercise along w/ the modification of certain behavioral factors (eg, cigarette smoking, excessive alcohol consumption), if these factors exist. Instruct to take upon arising for the day and at least 1/2 hr before the 1st food, beverage, or other medication of the day w/ plain water only; advise to swallow tab w/ 6-8 oz of water. Advise to avoid lying down for at least 30 min after taking the drug and until after 1st food of the day. Instruct to follow all dosing instructions and inform that failure to follow them may increase risk of esophageal problems. Advise to d/c and consult physician if symptoms of esophageal disease develop. Instruct that if a once-weekly dose is missed, to take 1 dose on the am after patient remembers and to return to taking 1 dose once a week, as originally scheduled on patient's chosen day; instruct not to take 2 doses on the same day.

FOSINOPRIL — fosinopril sodium   Rx

Class: ACE inhibitor

> May cause injury and even death to the developing fetus during the 2nd and 3rd trimesters of pregnancy. D/C when pregnancy is detected.

OTHER BRAND NAMES
Monopril (Discontinued)

ADULT DOSAGE
Hypertension
Initial: 10mg qd
Titrate: May adjust dosage based on BP response at peak and trough levels
Usual: 20-40mg qd, but some may respond to 80mg

Divide daily dose if trough response is inadequate
Diuretic may be added if BP is not adequately controlled w/ therapy alone

Currently Treated w/ Diuretic:
D/C diuretic 2-3 days prior to initiating therapy, if possible. May resume diuretic therapy if BP is not controlled w/ therapy alone
Initial: 10mg qd w/ careful monitoring until BP is stabilized if diuretic cannot be discontinued

Heart Failure
Adjunct to Diuretics w/ or w/o Digitalis:
Initial: 10mg qd; observe for at least 2 hrs for hypotension/orthostasis
Titrate: Increase over several weeks as tolerated
Usual: 20-40mg qd
Max: 40mg qd

PEDIATRIC DOSAGE
Hypertension
≥6 Years:
>50kg: 5-10mg qd as monotherapy

DOSING CONSIDERATIONS
Renal Impairment
Heart Failure (HF):
Moderate to Severe Renal Failure/Vigorous Diuresis:
Initial: 5mg

Elderly
Start at lower end of dosing range

ADMINISTRATION
Oral route

STORAGE
20-25°C (68-77°F). Protect from moisture.

HOW SUPPLIED
Tab: 10mg*, 20mg, 40mg *scored

CONTRAINDICATIONS
Hypersensitivity to this product or to any other ACE inhibitor (eg, angioedema).

WARNINGS/PRECAUTIONS
Head and neck angioedema reported; d/c and administer appropriate therapy if laryngeal stridor or angioedema of the face, lips, tongue, mucous membranes, glottis, or extremities occurs. More reports of angioedema in blacks than nonblacks. Intestinal angioedema reported; monitor for abdominal pain. Anaphylactoid reactions reported during desensitization w/ hymenoptera venom, dialysis w/ high-flux membranes, and LDL apheresis w/ dextran sulfate absorption. Symptomatic hypotension may occur, most likely in patients w/ volume and/or salt depletion; correct depletion prior to therapy. Excessive hypotension associated w/ oliguria, azotemia, and rarely acute renal failure and death may occur in patients w/ HF, w/ or w/o associated renal insufficiency; monitor closely during the first 2 weeks of treatment and whenever dose of therapy or diuretic is increased. Therapy may usually be continued following restoration of blood pressure and volume. May cause agranulocytosis and bone marrow depression; consider monitoring of WBC counts in patients w/ collagen-vascular disease, especially w/ renal impairment. Rarely, associated w/ syndrome that starts w/ cholestatic jaundice and progresses to fulminant hepatic necrosis and sometimes death; d/c if jaundice or marked elevation of hepatic enzymes occur. May cause renal function changes. May increase BUN and SrCr levels w/ renal artery stenosis or w/ no preexisting renal vascular disease; may need to reduce dose of therapy and/or d/c diuretic. Hyperkalemia reported; risk factors include diabetes mellitus (DM) and renal insufficiency. Hypotension may occur w/ surgery or during anesthesia. Persistent nonproductive cough reported. Caution in elderly.

ADVERSE REACTIONS
HTN: Cough, dizziness, N/V.
HF: Dizziness, cough, hypotension, musculoskeletal pain.

DRUG INTERACTIONS
May increase lithium levels and symptoms of lithium toxicity; frequently monitor serum lithium levels. Hypotension risk w/ diuretics. Increased risk of hyperkalemia w/ K+-sparing diuretics (eg, spironolactone, amiloride, triamterene), K+-containing salt substitutes, or K+ supplements; use w/ caution. Antacids may impair absorption; separate doses by 2 hrs. Nitritoid reactions reported rarely w/ injectable gold (sodium aurothiomalate). May cause false low measurement of serum digoxin levels w/ certain lab tests.

PREGNANCY AND LACTATION
Pregnancy: Category C (1st trimester) and D (2nd and 3rd trimesters).
Lactation: Detectable levels of fosinoprilat reported in breast milk; not for use in nursing.

MECHANISM OF ACTION
ACE inhibitor; fosinopril sodium (prodrug) is hydrolyzed to the pharmacologically active form, fosinoprilat. Therapeutic effects believed to be primarily by the suppression of the renin-angiotensin-aldosterone system. Decreases plasma angiotensin II, which leads to decreased vasopressor activity and decreased aldosterone secretion.

PHARMACOKINETICS
Absorption: Slow (prodrug). T_{max}=3 hrs (fosinoprilat). **Distribution:** (Fosinoprilat) Plasma protein binding (99.4%); found in breast milk. **Metabolism:** Hepatic; glucuronidation; fosinoprilat (active form). **Elimination:** Urine (50% of the absorbed dose), feces. (Fosinoprilat) $T_{1/2}$=11.5 hrs (HTN), 14 hrs (HF).

PATIENT CONSIDERATIONS
Assessment: Assess for history of angioedema, hypersensitivity to drug, volume/salt depletion, collagen vascular disease, DM, renal artery stenosis, HF, renal impairment, pregnancy/nursing status, and possible drug interactions.
Monitoring: Monitor for signs/symptoms of hypotension, anaphylactoid or hypersensitivity reactions, head/neck/intestinal angioedema, agranulocytosis, neutropenia, bone marrow depression, hyperkalemia, and other adverse reactions. Monitor BP and renal/hepatic function. Consider monitoring WBC counts in patients w/ collagen vascular disease, especially if w/ renal impairment.
Counseling: Instruct to d/c therapy and immediately report signs/symptoms of angioedema. Caution about lightheadedness, especially during the 1st days of therapy; advise to d/c therapy and consult physician if syncope occurs. Caution that inadequate fluid intake or excessive perspiration, diarrhea, or vomiting may lead to an excessive fall in BP resulting in lightheadedness or syncope. Instruct to avoid using K+ supplements or salt substitutes-containing K+ w/o consulting physician. Advise to report any symptoms of infection. Inform of pregnancy risks during the 2nd or 3rd trimesters and instruct to report to physician as soon as possible if pregnant.

FOSINOPRIL/HCTZ — fosinopril sodium/hydrochlorothiazide   Rx

Class: ACE inhibitor/thiazide diuretic

> D/C when pregnancy is detected. Drugs that act directly on the renin-angiotensin system (RAS) can cause injury/death to developing fetus.

OTHER BRAND NAMES
Monopril-HCT (Discontinued)

ADULT DOSAGE
Hypertension
Not Controlled w/ Fosinopril/HCTZ Monotherapy:
10mg/12.5mg tab or 20mg/12.5mg tab qd
Titrate: Dosage must be guided by clinical response

PEDIATRIC DOSAGE
Pediatric use may not have been established

DOSING CONSIDERATIONS
Elderly
Start at lower end of dosing range

ADMINISTRATION
Oral route

STORAGE
20-25°C (68-77°F). Protect from moisture.

HOW SUPPLIED
Tab: (Fosinopril/HCTZ) 10mg/12.5mg, 20mg/12.5mg* *scored

CONTRAINDICATIONS
Anuria; hypersensitivity to fosinopril, to any other ACE inhibitor, to hydrochlorothiazide, or other sulfonamide-derived drugs, or any other ingredient or component in the formulation.

WARNINGS/PRECAUTIONS
Not indicated for initial therapy. Caution in elderly and w/ severe renal disease. Avoid if CrCl <30mL/min. Caution w/ impaired hepatic function or progressive liver disease; may precipitate hepatic coma. **Fosinopril:** Angioedema reported; d/c and administer appropriate therapy if laryngeal stridor or angioedema of the face, tongue, or glottis occurs. Higher rate of angioedema in blacks than nonblacks. Intestinal angioedema reported; monitor for abdominal pain. Anaphylactoid reactions reported during desensitization

Add furosemide inj to NaCl inj, D5, or lactated Ringer's inj after pH has been adjusted to above 5.5.
Administer as a controlled IV infusion at a rate no greater than 4mg/min.
Care must be taken to ensure that the pH of the prepared infusion sol is in the weakly alkaline to neutral range.
Acid sol, including other parenteral medications (eg, labetalol, ciprofloxacin, amrinone, milrinone), must not be administered concurrently in the same infusion because they may cause precipitation of the furosemide; furosemide inj should not be added to a running IV line containing any of these acidic products.

STORAGE
Protect from light. **Inj/Sol:** 20-25°C (68-77°F). **Lasix:** 25°C (77°F); excursions permitted to 15-30°C (59-86°F).

HOW SUPPLIED
Inj: 10mg/mL [2mL, 4mL, 10mL]; **Sol:** 10mg/mL [60mL, 120mL], 40mg/5mL [500mL]; **Tab:** (Lasix) 20mg, 40mg*, 80mg *scored

CONTRAINDICATIONS
Anuria, history of hypersensitivity to furosemide.

WARNINGS/PRECAUTIONS
Initiate therapy in hospital w/ hepatic cirrhosis and ascites. Do not institute therapy until basic condition is improved in patients w/ hepatic coma and in states of electrolyte depletion. D/C if increasing azotemia and oliguria occur during treatment of severe progressive renal disease. Tinnitus, reversible or irreversible hearing impairment, and deafness reported. Ototoxicity is associated w/ rapid inj, severe renal impairment, use of higher than recommended doses, hypoproteinemia, or concomitant use w/ aminoglycoside antibiotics, ethacrynic acid, or other ototoxic drugs; control IV infusion rate if using high-dose parenteral therapy. Excessive diuresis may cause dehydration, blood volume reduction w/ circulatory collapse, vascular thrombosis, and embolism, particularly in elderly. Monitor for fluid/electrolyte imbalance (hyponatremia, hypochloremic alkalosis, hypokalemia, hypomagnesemia, or hypocalcemia), liver/kidney damage, blood dyscrasias, or other idiosyncratic reactions. Increases in blood glucose and alterations in glucose tolerance tests, and rarely, precipitation of diabetes mellitus (DM) reported. May cause acute urinary retention in patients w/ severe symptoms of urinary retention; monitor carefully, especially during the initial stages of treatment. May lead to a higher incidence of deterioration in renal function after receiving radiocontrast in patients at high risk for radiocontrast nephropathy. May potentiate ototoxicity and effect of therapy may be weakened in patients w/ hypoproteinemia. Asymptomatic hyperuricemia may occur and gout may rarely be precipitated. Caution in patients w/ sulfonamide allergy. May activate/exacerbate systemic lupus erythematosus (SLE). May precipitate nephrocalcinosis/nephrolithiasis in premature infants and children <4 yrs of age w/ no history of prematurity; monitor renal function and consider renal ultrasonography. May increase risk of persistence of patent ductus arteriosus if administered to premature infants during the 1st weeks of life. Caution in elderly. (Inj) Use only in patients unable to take oral medication or in emergency situations; replace w/ oral therapy as soon as practical. Premature infants w/ post conceptual age (gestational plus postnatal) <31 weeks receiving doses >1mg/kg/24 hrs may develop plasma levels which could be associated w/ potential toxic effects. May cause hearing loss in neonates.

ADVERSE REACTIONS
Pancreatitis, jaundice, increased liver enzymes, anorexia, severe anaphylactic/anaphylactoid reactions, systemic vasculitis, tinnitus/hearing loss, paresthesias, aplastic anemia, thrombocytopenia, toxic epidermal necrolysis, orthostatic hypotension, hyperglycemia.

DRUG INTERACTIONS
See Dosing Considerations. May increase ototoxic potential of aminoglycoside antibiotics, especially in the presence of impaired renal function; avoid this combination, except in life-threatening situations. Avoid w/ ethacrynic acid and lithium. Patients receiving high doses of salicylates concomitantly w/ furosemide may experience salicylate toxicity at lower doses because of competitive renal excretory sites. Risk of ototoxic effects if given concomitantly w/ cisplatin. Nephrotoxicity of nephrotoxic drugs such as cisplatin may be enhanced if furosemide is not given in lower doses and w/ positive fluid balance when used to achieve forced diuresis during cisplatin treatment. May antagonize skeletal muscle relaxing effect of tubocurarine. May potentiate action of succinylcholine. Concomitant use w/ ACE inhibitors or ARBs may lead to severe hypotension and deterioration in renal function, including renal failure; an interruption or reduction in the dosage of furosemide, ACE inhibitors, or ARBs may be necessary. Potentiation occurs w/ ganglionic or peripheral adrenergic blockers. May decrease arterial responsiveness to norepinephrine. Reduced CrCl in patients w/ chronic renal insufficiency w/ acetylsalicylic acid. Increased BUN, SrCr, and K^+ levels, and weight gain reported w/ NSAIDs. Hypokalemia may develop w/ adrenocorticotropic hormone and corticosteroids. Reduced natriuretic and antihypertensive effects w/ indomethacin. Indomethacin may affect plasma renin levels, aldosterone excretion, and renin profile evaluation. Digitalis may exaggerate metabolic effects of hypokalemia. Avoid w/ chloral hydrate. Phenytoin interferes w/ renal action of furosemide. Methotrexate and other drugs that undergo significant renal tubular secretion may reduce the effect of furosemide. May decrease renal elimination of other drugs that undergo tubular secretion; high-dose treatment of both furosemide and these other drugs may result in elevated serum levels of these drugs and may potentiate their toxicity as well as the toxicity of furosemide. May increase the risk of cephalosporin-induced nephrotoxicity. Increased risk of gouty arthritis w/ cyclosporine. High doses (>80mg) may inhibit binding of thyroid hormones to carrier proteins; may result in transient increase in free thyroid hormones, followed by overall decrease in total thyroid hormone levels. Hypokalemia may develop w/ licorice in large amounts or w/ prolonged use of laxatives. May add to or potentiate the therapeutic effect of other antihypertensive drugs. Phenytoin may decrease levels. **Tab/Sol:** Reduced natriuretic and antihypertensive effects w/ sucralfate; separate intake by at least 2 hrs.

PREGNANCY AND LACTATION
Pregnancy: Category C.
Lactation: Caution in nursing.

MECHANISM OF ACTION
Loop diuretic; primarily inhibits the absorption of Na^+ and Cl^- not only in the proximal and distal tubules but also in the loop of Henle.

PHARMACOKINETICS
Absorption: Bioavailability (64% tab), (60% sol). **Distribution:** Plasma protein binding (91-99%); found in breast milk. **Metabolism:** Biotransformation; furosemide glucuronide (major metabolite). **Elimination:** Urine; $T_{1/2}$=2 hrs.

PATIENT CONSIDERATIONS
Assessment: Assess for anuria, sulfonamide/drug hypersensitivity, SLE, hepatic/renal impairment, hypoproteinemia, pregnancy/nursing status, and possible drug interactions.

Monitoring: Monitor for signs/symptoms of fluid/electrolyte imbalance, blood dyscrasias, hyperglycemia, hyperuricemia, precipitation of gout or DM, ototoxicity, dehydration, activation or exacerbation of SLE, blood volume reduction w/ circulatory collapse, vascular thrombosis and embolism, liver or kidney damage, and other adverse reactions. Monitor serum electrolytes, carbon dioxide, creatinine, and BUN frequently during 1st few months of therapy, then periodically thereafter. Monitor urine and blood glucose periodically in diabetics. Periodically monitor Mg^{2+} and Ca^{2+} levels. Monitor renal function and perform renal ultrasonography in pediatric patients. Carefully monitor patients w/ severe symptoms of urinary retention, especially during the initial stages of treatment.

Counseling: Advise that patient may experience symptoms from excessive fluid and/or electrolyte losses. Advise that postural hypotension can be managed by getting up slowly. Inform patients w/ DM that drug may increase blood glucose levels and affect urine glucose tests. Advise that skin may be more sensitive to sunlight during therapy. Advise hypertensive patients to avoid medications that may increase BP, including OTC products for appetite suppression and cold symptoms.

FYCOMPA — perampanel

CIII

Class: AMPA glutamate receptor antagonist (non-competitive)

Serious or life-threatening psychiatric and behavioral adverse reactions including aggression, hostility, irritability, anger, and homicidal ideation and threats reported; monitor these reactions as well as changes in mood, behavior, or personality that are not typical for the patient, particularly during the titration period and at higher doses. Reduce dose if these symptoms occur and d/c immediately if symptoms are severe or are worsening.

ADULT DOSAGE

Partial Onset Seizures

Adjunctive therapy in patients w/ or w/o secondarily generalized seizures w/ epilepsy

Not Receiving Concomitant Enzyme-Inducing Antiepileptic Drugs (AEDs):
Initial: 2mg qhs
Titrate: Increase by increments of 2mg qd no more frequently than at weekly intervals
Maint: 8-12mg qd in the absence of enzyme-inducing AEDs; some may respond to a dose of 4mg qd

Tonic-Clonic Seizures

Adjunctive therapy for the treatment of primary generalized tonic-clonic seizures w/ epilepsy

Not Receiving Concomitant Enzyme-Inducing AEDs:
Initial: 2mg qhs
Titrate: Increase by increments of 2mg qd no more frequently than at weekly intervals
Maint: 8mg qhs; may increase up to 12mg qd if 8mg qd is tolerated but further reduction is needed

PEDIATRIC DOSAGE

Partial Onset Seizures

Adjunctive therapy in patients w/ or w/o secondarily generalized seizures w/ epilepsy

≥12 Years:
Not Receiving Concomitant Enzyme-Inducing AEDs:
Initial: 2mg qhs
Titrate: Increase by increments of 2mg qd no more frequently than at weekly intervals
Maint: 8-12mg qd in the absence of enzyme-inducing AEDs; some may respond to a dose of 4mg qd

Tonic-Clonic Seizures

Adjunctive therapy for the treatment of primary generalized tonic-clonic seizures w/ epilepsy

≥12 Years:
Not Receiving Concomitant Enzyme-Inducing AEDs:
Initial: 2mg qhs
Titrate: Increase by increments of 2mg qd no more frequently than at weekly intervals
Maint: 8mg qhs; may increase up to 12mg qd if 8mg qd is tolerated but further reduction is needed

DOSING CONSIDERATIONS

Concomitant Medications

Enzyme-Inducing AEDs (eg, Phenytoin, Carbamazepine, Oxcarbazepine):
Initial: 4mg qhs
Titrate: Increase by increments of 2mg qd no more frequently than at weekly intervals

Renal Impairment

Moderate: Monitor closely and titrate slowly
Severe/Undergoing Hemodialysis: Not recommended

w/ hymenoptera venom, dialysis w/ high-flux membranes, and LDL apheresis w/ dextran sulfate absorption. Symptomatic hypotension may occur, most likely in patients w/ volume and/or salt depletion; correct volume and/or salt depletion prior to therapy. Excessive hypotension associated w/ oliguria, azotemia, and rarely acute renal failure and/or death may occur in patients w/ CHF; monitor closely during the first 2 weeks of treatment and when dose is increased. May cause changes in renal function. May increase BUN and SrCr levels w/ renal artery stenosis and w/ no preexisting renal vascular disease; monitor renal function during 1st few weeks of therapy in patients w/ renal artery stenosis. May cause agranulocytosis and bone marrow depression; consider monitoring of WBCs in patients w/ collagen vascular disease and renal disease. Rarely, associated w/ syndrome that starts w/ cholestatic jaundice and progresses to fulminant necrosis and sometimes death; d/c if jaundice or marked hepatic enzyme elevations occur. Hyperkalemia and persistent nonproductive cough reported. Hypotension may occur w/ surgery or during anesthesia. **HCTZ:** May precipitate azotemia w/ severe renal disease. May exacerbate or activate systemic lupus erythematosus (SLE). Dilutional hyponatremia may occur in edematous patients; institute appropriate therapy of water restriction rather than salt administration, except for life-threatening hyponatremia. May increase cholesterol, TGs, uric acid levels, and decrease glucose tolerance. Hyponatremia, hypokalemia, and hypochloremic alkalosis reported. Hypokalemia may sensitize or exaggerate the response of the heart to toxic effects of digitalis. Pathological changes in the parathyroid glands, w/ hypercalcemia and hypophosphatemia observed w/ prolonged therapy. May enhance effects in postsympathectomy patients. Neutropenia/agranulocytosis reported. Lab test interactions may occur.

ADVERSE REACTIONS
Headache, cough, fatigue, dizziness.

DRUG INTERACTIONS
Dual blockade of the RAS is associated w/ increased risks of hypotension, hyperkalemia, and changes in renal function (including acute renal failure); closely monitor BP, renal function, and electrolytes w/ concomitant agents that also affect the RAS. Avoid concomitant use of aliskiren in patients w/ diabetes and w/ renal impairment (GFR <60mL/min). Increased risk of hyperkalemia w/ K^+-sparing diuretics, K^+ supplements, or K^+-containing salt substitutes; use w/ caution and monitor serum K+ frequently. Caution w/ other antihypertensives. May alter insulin requirements in diabetic patients. May increase lithium levels and risk of toxicity; use w/ caution and monitor serum lithium levels frequently. Nitritoid reactions reported rarely w/ injectable gold (eg, sodium aurothiomalate). **Fosinopril:** Antacids (aluminum hydroxide, magnesium hydroxide, simethicone) may impair absorption; separate doses by 2 hrs. **HCTZ:** May potentiate action of other antihypertensives, especially ganglionic or peripheral adrenergic-blocking drugs. May decrease effectiveness of methenamine. May increase responsiveness to tubocurarine. May decrease arterial responsiveness to norepinephrine. NSAIDs may decrease diuretic, natriuretic, and antihypertensive effects. Cholestyramine or colestipol resins reduce absorption. Increased risk of hypokalemia w/ corticosteroids and adrenocorticotropic hormone.

PREGNANCY AND LACTATION
Category D, not for use in nursing.

MECHANISM OF ACTION
Fosinopril: ACE inhibitor; decreases plasma angiotensin II, which leads to decreased vasopressor activity and decreased aldosterone secretion. HCTZ: Thiazide diuretic; affects renal tubular mechanism of electrolyte reabsorption directly increasing excretion of Na^+ and Cl^- and indirectly reducing plasma volume.

PHARMACOKINETICS
Absorption: Fosinoprilat: T_{max}=3 hrs; HCTZ: T_{max}=1-2.5 hrs. **Distribution:** Found in breast milk. Fosinoprilat: Plasma protein binding (95%). HCTZ: V_d=3.6-7.8L/kg; plasma protein binding (67.9%), crosses placenta. **Metabolism:** Fosinopril: Hepatic, glucuronidation; fosinoprilat (active metabolite). **Elimination:** Fosinoprilat: Urine, feces, $T_{1/2}$=11.5 hrs. HCTZ: Renal; $T_{1/2}$=5-15 hrs.

PATIENT CONSIDERATIONS
Assessment: Assess for anuria, history of allergy or bronchial asthma, hypersensitivity to drug or to sulfonamides, volume/salt depletion, CHF, SLE, renal/hepatic function, collagen vascular disease, risk factors for hyperkalemia, pregnancy/nursing status, and possible drug interactions.

Monitoring: Monitor for signs/symptoms of angioedema, agranulocytosis, anaphylactoid/hypersensitivity reactions, hypotension, exacerbation/activation of SLE, and other adverse reactions. Monitor BP, serum electrolytes, serum uric acid levels, hepatic/renal function, cholesterol/TG levels, and glucose tolerance. Monitor WBCs in patients w/ collagen vascular disease and renal impairment.

Counseling: Inform females of childbearing age of the consequences of exposure during pregnancy and of the treatment options for women planning to become pregnant; report pregnancy to physician as soon as possible. Instruct to d/c therapy and immediately report signs/symptoms of angioedema (eg, swelling of face, eyes, lips, tongue, difficulty breathing). Caution that lightheadedness can occur, especially during the 1st days of therapy and advise to report to physician; instruct to d/c therapy and consult physician if syncope occurs. Caution that inadequate fluid intake, excessive perspiration, diarrhea, or vomiting can lead to excessive fall in BP, resulting in lightheadedness or syncope. Instruct not to use salt substitutes containing K^+ or K^+ supplements w/o consulting physician. Instruct to promptly report any indication of infection (eg, sore throat, fever).

FRAGMIN — dalteparin sodium

Rx

Class: Low molecular weight heparin (LMWH)

Epidural or spinal hematomas may occur in patients who are anticoagulated w/ LMWHs or heparinoids and are receiving neuraxial anesthesia or undergoing spinal puncture; may result in long-term or permanent paralysis. Consider these risks when scheduling patients for spinal procedures. Factors that can increase the risk of developing epidural or spinal hematomas in these patients include: use of indwelling epidural catheters, concomitant use of other drugs that affect hemostasis (eg, NSAIDs, platelet inhibitors, other anticoagulants), history of traumatic or repeated epidural or spinal punctures, or history of spinal deformity or spinal surgery. Optimal timing between administration of Fragmin and neuraxial procedures is not known. Monitor frequently for signs/symptoms of neurologic impairment; if neurologic compromise is noted, urgent treatment is necessary. Consider benefits and risks before neuraxial intervention in patients anticoagulated or to be anticoagulated for thromboprophylaxis.

ADULT DOSAGE

Unstable Angina

Prophylaxis of Ischemic Complications:
120 IU/kg (but not more than 10,000 IU) q12h w/ oral aspirin (ASA) therapy (75-165mg qd) until clinically stabilized
Usual Duration: 5-8 days

Refer to PI for quantity and volume to be administered based on patient weight

Non-Q-Wave Myocardial Infarction

Prophylaxis of Ischemic Complications:
120 IU/kg (but not more than 10,000 IU) q12h w/ oral ASA therapy (75-165mg qd) until clinically stabilized
Usual Duration: 5-8 days

Refer to PI for quantity and volume to be administered based on patient weight

Deep Vein Thrombosis

Prophylaxis Following Hip Replacement Surgery:
Postoperative Start: 2500 IU 4-8 hrs after surgery (or later, if hemostasis has not been achieved), followed by 5000 IU qd in the postop period (at least 6 hrs after previous dose)
Preoperative Start:
Day of Surgery: 2500 IU w/in 2 hrs before surgery, then 2500 IU 4-8 hrs after surgery (or later, if hemostasis has not been achieved), followed by 5000 IU qd in the postop period (at least 6 hrs after previous dose)
Evening Before Surgery: 5000 IU 10-14 hrs before surgery, then 5000 IU 4-8 hrs after surgery (or later, if hemostasis has not been achieved), followed by 5000 IU qd in the postop period. Allow approx 24 hrs between doses.
Usual Duration: 5-10 days postoperatively; up to 14 days of treatment have been well tolerated in clinical trials

Prophylaxis in Patients Undergoing Abdominal Surgery:
W/ a Risk of Thromboembolic Complications:
2500 IU qd, starting 1-2 hrs prior to surgery and repeated qd postoperatively
Associated w/ a High Risk of Thromboembolic Complications (eg, Malignant Disorder):
5000 IU the evening before surgery, then qd postoperatively. Alternatively, in patients w/ malignancy, 2500 IU can be administered 1-2 hrs before surgery followed by 2500 IU 12 hrs later, and then 5000 IU qd postoperatively
Usual Duration: 5-10 days postoperatively

Prophylaxis in Medical Patients at Risk For Thromboembolic Complications Due to Severely Restricted Mobility During Acute Illness:
5000 IU qd for 12-14 days

PEDIATRIC DOSAGE

Pediatric use may not have been established

<u>Venous Thromboembolism</u>

Extended Treatment of Symptomatic Venous Thromboembolism (VTE) to Reduce Recurrence in Patients w/ Cancer:
Month 1 (First 30 Days of Treatment): 200 IU/kg qd (should not exceed 18,000 IU/day)
Months 2-6: 150 IU/kg qd (should not exceed 18,000 IU/day)Refer to PI for dose to be administered based on patient weight.
Safety and efficacy beyond 6 months have not been evaluated.

DOSING CONSIDERATIONS
<u>Renal Impairment</u>
Extended Treatment of Acute Symptomatic VTE in Cancer Patients:
Severe (CrCl <30mL/min): Monitor anti-Factor Xa levels to determine appropriate dose; target anti-Xa range is 0.5-1.5 IU/mL. When monitoring anti-Xa levels, perform sampling 4-6 hrs after dosing and only after the patient has received 3-4 doses
<u>Adverse Reactions</u>
Thrombocytopenia:
In Patients w/ Cancer and Acute Symptomatic VTE:
Platelet Count <50,000/mm³: D/C therapy until platelet count recovers to >50,000/mm³
Platelet Count 50,000-100,000/mm³: Reduce daily dose by 2500 IU until platelet count recovers to ≥100,000/mm³

ADMINISTRATION
SQ route
Do not mix w/ other inj or infusions unless compatible.
<u>SQ Inj Technique</u>
- Patients should be sitting or lying down; administer by deep SQ inj.
- May be injected in a U-shape area around the navel, the upper outer side of the thigh, or the upper outer quadrangle of the buttock; vary inj site daily.
- When the area around the navel or the thigh is used, use the thumb and forefinger to lift up a fold of skin while injecting; entire length of the needle should be inserted at a 45-90° angle.
- After 1st penetration of the rubber stopper, store the multiple-dose vials at room temperature for up to 2 weeks; discard any unused sol after 2 weeks.

Refer to PI for instructions for using the prefilled single-dose syringes preassembled w/ needle guard devices.

STORAGE
20-25°C (68-77°F); excursion permitted between 15-30°C (59-86°F). **Multiple-Dose Vials:** Room temperature for up to 2 weeks after 1st penetration of the rubber stopper.

HOW SUPPLIED
Inj: 2500 IU/0.2mL, 5000 IU/0.2mL, 7500 IU/0.3mL, 12,500 IU/0.5mL, 15,000 IU/0.6mL, 18,000 IU/0.72mL [single-dose prefilled syringe]; 10,000 IU/mL [single-dose graduated syringe]; 25,000 IU/mL [3.8mL, multiple-dose vial]

CONTRAINDICATIONS
Active major bleeding, history of heparin-induced thrombocytopenia or heparin-induced thrombocytopenia w/ thrombosis, hypersensitivity to dalteparin sodium (eg, pruritus, rash, anaphylactic reactions), as treatment for unstable angina/non-Q-wave MI and for prolonged VTE prophylaxis in patients undergoing epidural/neuraxial anesthesia, and hypersensitivity to heparin or to pork products.

WARNINGS/PRECAUTIONS
Not indicated for acute treatment of VTE. Consider pharmacokinetic profile of dalteparin to reduce the potential risk of bleeding associated w/ concurrent use w/ epidural or spinal anesthesia/analgesia or spinal puncture. Placement or removal of catheter should be delayed for at least 12 hrs after administration of 2500 IU qd, at least 15 hrs after administration of 5000 IU qd, and at least 24 hrs after administration of higher doses (200 IU/kg qd, 120 IU/kg bid) of therapy. For patients w/ CrCl <30mL/min, consider doubling the timing of removal of catheter, at least 24 hrs for the lower prescribed dose and at least 48 hrs for the higher dose. Extreme caution in patients w/ increased risk of hemorrhage (eg, severe uncontrolled HTN; bacterial endocarditis; hemorrhagic stroke; shortly after brain, spinal, or ophthalmological surgery). May enhance the risk of bleeding in patients w/ thrombocytopenia or platelet defects, severe liver/kidney insufficiency, hypertensive or diabetic retinopathy, and recent GI bleeding. Bleeding may occur at any site during therapy. Heparin-induced thrombocytopenia may occur. Serious and fatal adverse reactions including "gasping syndrome" can occur in neonates and low-birth weight infants treated w/ medications that contain the preservative benzyl alcohol. Benzyl alcohol may cross placenta; caution when administering Fragmin preserved w/ benzyl alcohol to pregnant women and if anticoagulation is needed during pregnancy, use preservative-free formulations, where possible. When administered at recommended prophylaxis doses, routine coagulation tests (eg, prothrombin time, activated partial thromboplastin time) are relatively insensitive measures of Fragmin activity and, therefore, unsuitable for monitoring the anticoagulant effect. Anti-Factor Xa may be used to monitor the anticoagulant effect (eg, patients w/ severe renal impairment or if abnormal coagulation parameters or bleeding occurs during therapy). Caution in elderly, particularly w/ low body weight (<45kg) and those predisposed to decreased renal function.

ADVERSE REACTIONS
Inj-site hematoma.

DRUG INTERACTIONS
See Boxed Warning. Caution w/ oral anticoagulants, platelet inhibitors, and thrombolytic agents due to increased risk of bleeding.

PREGNANCY AND LACTATION
Pregnancy: Category B.
Lactation: Minimally excreted in human milk. Caution in nursing.

MECHANISM OF ACTION
LMWH; enhances inhibition of Factor Xa and thrombin by antithrombin, while only slightly affecting the activated PTT.

PHARMACOKINETICS
Absorption: Absolute bioavailability (87%); (Peak levels of plasma anti-Factor Xa activity) C_{max}=0.19 IU/mL (2500 IU), 0.41 IU/mL (5000 IU), 0.82 IU/mL (10,000 IU); T_{max}=4 hrs. **Distribution:** V_d=40-60mL/kg; minimally excreted in breast milk. **Elimination:** $T_{1/2}$=3-5 hrs.

PATIENT CONSIDERATIONS
Assessment: Assess for hypersensitivity reaction to drug/heparin or pork products, conditions that increase risk of hematomas/hemorrhage, renal/hepatic impairment, any other conditions where treatment is contraindicated or cautioned, pregnancy/nursing status, and possible drug interactions.
Monitoring: Monitor for bleeding, thrombocytopenia, hypersensitivity reactions, and other adverse reactions. Monitor for signs/symptoms of spinal or epidural hematomas and neurologic impairment in patients receiving neuraxial anesthesia or undergoing spinal puncture. Perform periodic CBCs w/ platelet count, blood chemistry, and stool occult blood tests. Monitor anti-Factor Xa levels in patients w/ severe renal impairment or if abnormal coagulation parameters or bleeding occurs.
Counseling: Inform patients who had neuraxial anesthesia/spinal puncture, particularly if taking concomitant NSAIDs, platelet inhibitors, or other anticoagulants, to watch for signs/symptoms of spinal/epidural hematoma (eg, tingling, numbness [especially in the lower limbs], muscular weakness); instruct to notify physician immediately if any of these symptoms occur. Instruct to d/c use of ASA or other NSAIDs prior to therapy whenever possible. Inform about injecting instructions if therapy is to continue after discharge from hospital. Inform that it will take longer than usual to stop bleeding and that the patient may bruise and/or bleed more easily while on therapy. Instruct to report to physician any unusual bleeding, bruising, or signs of thrombocytopenia. Advise to inform physicians and dentists that the patient takes dalteparin and/or any other product known to affect bleeding before any surgery is scheduled, or before any new drug is taken. Instruct to inform physicians and dentists of all medications being taken, including those obtained w/o prescription.

FROVA — frovatriptan succinate Rx

Class: $5\text{-}HT_{1B/1D}$ agonist (triptans)

ADULT DOSAGE
<u>Migraine</u>
W/ or w/o Aura:
2.5mg w/ fluids
May administer 2nd dose 2 hrs after 1st dose if migraine recurs after initial relief
Max: 7.5mg/day
Safety of treating >4 migraines/30 days not known

PEDIATRIC DOSAGE
Pediatric use may not have been established

ADMINISTRATION
Oral route

STORAGE
25°C (77°F); excursions permitted to 15-30°C (59-86°F). Protect from moisture.

HOW SUPPLIED
Tab: 2.5mg

CONTRAINDICATIONS
Ischemic coronary artery disease (CAD) (eg, angina pectoris, history of MI, or documented silent ischemia), or coronary artery vasospasm, including Prinzmetal's angina; Wolff-Parkinson-White syndrome or arrhythmias associated w/ other cardiac accessory conduction pathway disorders; history of stroke, transient ischemic attack, or history of hemiplegic or basilar migraine; peripheral vascular disease; ischemic bowel disease; uncontrolled HTN; recent use (w/in 24 hours) of another 5-HT1 agonist or an ergotamine containing or ergot-type medication (eg, dihydroergotamine or methysergide); hypersensitivity to frovatriptan succinate.

WARNINGS/PRECAUTIONS
Use only if a clear diagnosis of migraine has been established. If no treatment response for the 1st migraine attack, reconsider diagnosis before treating any subsequent attacks. Not indicated for prevention of migraine attacks. Serious cardiac adverse reactions, including acute MI, reported. May cause coronary artery vasospasm (Prinzmetal's angina). Perform cardiovascular (CV) evaluation in triptan-naive patients who have multiple CV risk factors prior to therapy; consider administering 1st dose in a medically supervised setting and perform ECG immediately following administration in patients with a negative CV evaluation. Consider periodic CV evaluation in intermittent long-term users who have CV risk factors. Life-threatening cardiac rhythm disturbances (eg, ventricular tachycardia/fibrillation leading to death) reported; d/c if these occur. Sensations of pain, tightness, pressure, and heaviness reported in the chest, throat, neck, and jaw after treatment and are usually noncardiac in origin; perform a cardiac evaluation if at high cardiac risk. Cerebral/subarachnoid hemorrhage, stroke, and other cerebrovascular events reported. Care should be taken to exclude other potentially serious neurological conditions before treatment. May cause noncoronary vasospastic reactions (eg, peripheral vascular ischemia, GI vascular ischemia and infarction [presenting with abdominal pain and bloody diarrhea], splenic infarction, Raynaud's syndrome); rule out vasospastic reaction before using if experiencing signs/symptoms suggestive of noncoronary vasospasm reaction. Transient and permanent blindness and significant partial vision loss reported. Overuse of acute migraine drugs may lead to exacerbation of headache (medication overuse headache); detoxification, including withdrawal of the overused drugs, and treatment of withdrawal symptoms may be necessary. Serotonin syndrome may occur; d/c if serotonin syndrome is suspected. Significant elevation in BP, including hypertensive crisis with acute impairment of organ systems, reported; monitor BP. Anaphylaxis, anaphylactoid, and hypersensitivity reactions including angioedema reported; more likely to occur in patients with history of sensitivity to multiple allergens. Caution with severe hepatic impairment.

ADVERSE REACTIONS
Dizziness, fatigue, headache, paresthesia, flushing, dry mouth, hot or cold sensation, skeletal pain.

DRUG INTERACTIONS
See Contraindications. Serotonin syndrome reported with SSRIs, SNRIs, TCAs, and MAOIs.

PREGNANCY AND LACTATION
Category C, not for use in nursing.

MECHANISM OF ACTION
$5\text{-}HT_{1B/1D}$agonist; binds with high affinity to $5\text{-}HT_{1B/1D}$ receptors. Thought to be due to the agonist effects at the $5\text{-}HT_{1B/1D}$ receptors on intracranial blood vessels (including the arteriovenous anastomoses) and sensory nerves of the trigeminal system, resulting in cranial vessel constriction and inhibition of proinflammatory neuropeptide release.

PHARMACOKINETICS
Absorption: Absolute bioavailability: (20%) male, (30%) female; T_{max}=2-4 hrs. **Distribution:** V_d=(IV) 4.2L/kg (male), 3L/kg (female); plasma protein binding (15%). **Metabolism:** Via CYP1A2. **Elimination:** Feces (62%), urine (32%); $T_{1/2}$=26 hrs.

PATIENT CONSIDERATIONS
Assessment: Assess for ischemic CAD, coronary artery vasospasm, uncontrolled HTN, neurological conditions, hepatic impairment, history of sensitivity to multiple allergens, drug hypersensitivity, any conditions where treatment is cautioned or contraindicated, pregnancy/nursing status, and possible drug interactions. Perform CV evaluation in triptan-naive patients prior to therapy who have multiple CV risk factors.
Monitoring: Monitor for cardiac adverse reactions, coronary artery vasospasm, cardiac rhythm disturbances, cerebrovascular events, noncoronary vasospastic reactions, serotonin syndrome, BP elevation, exacerbation of headache, anaphylactic/hypersensitivity reactions, ophthalmic changes, and other adverse events. Consider periodic CV evaluation in intermittent long-term users who have CV risk factors. Perform ECG immediately following administration in patients with a negative CV evaluation.
Counseling: Inform that drug may cause serious CV side effects, to be alert for the signs/symptoms of chest pain, SOB, weakness, and slurring of speech, and to ask for medical advice when observing any indicative signs/symptoms. Inform that anaphylactic/anaphylactoid reactions have occurred and that they are more likely to occur in patients with history of sensitivity to multiple allergens. Inform that overuse (≥10 days/month) may lead to exacerbation of headache; encourage to record headache frequency and drug use. Caution about the risk of serotonin syndrome. Advise to notify physician if pregnant/nursing or planning to become pregnant.

FULYZAQ — crofelemer Rx

Class: Antidiarrheal

ADULT DOSAGE
<u>Noninfectious Diarrhea</u>
Symptomatic Relief in Patients w/ HIV/AIDS on Antiretroviral Therapy
125mg bid

PEDIATRIC DOSAGE
Pediatric use may not have been established

ADMINISTRATION
Oral route
Take w/ or w/o food.
Swallow whole; do not crush or chew.

STORAGE
20-25°C (68-77°F); excursions permitted between 15-30°C (59-86°F).

HOW SUPPLIED
Tab, Delayed-Release: 125mg

WARNINGS/PRECAUTIONS
Not indicated for the treatment of infectious diarrhea; rule out infectious etiologies of diarrhea before initiating therapy.

ADVERSE REACTIONS
URTI, bronchitis, cough, flatulence, increased bilirubin.

PREGNANCY AND LACTATION
Pregnancy: Category C.
Lactation: Not for use in nursing.

MECHANISM OF ACTION
Antidiarrheal; an inhibitor of both the cAMP-stimulated cystic fibrosis transmembrane conductance regulator Cl^- channel, and the Ca^{2+}-activated Cl^- channels at the luminal membrane of enterocytes. Blocks Cl^- secretion an[d] accompanying high volume water loss in diarrhea, normalizing the flow of Cl^- water in the GI tract.

PATIENT CONSIDERATIONS
Assessment: Assess etiology of diarrhea and pregnancy/nursing status.
Monitoring: Monitor for adverse reactions.
Counseling: Instruct to take ud.

FUROSEMIDE — furosemide Rx

Class: Loop diuretic

May lead to profound diuresis w/ water and electrolyte depletion if given in excessive amounts; careful medical supervision required and dose and dose schedule must be adjusted to individual patient's needs.

OTHER BRAND NAMES
Lasix

ADULT DOSAGE
<u>Edema</u>
Associated w/ CHF, Liver Cirrhosis, and Renal Disease (Nephrotic Syndrome):
Oral:
Initial: 20-80mg as a single dose
Titrate: May repeat the same dose if needed or increase dose by 20mg or 40mg. Give dose no sooner than 6-8 hrs after the previous dose until desired diuretic effect has been obtained; give individually determined single dose qd or bid
Severe Edematous States: May carefully titrate dose up to 600mg/day
Consider giving on 2-4 consecutive days each week
Closely monitor when exceeding 80mg/day for prolonged periods
Inj:
Initial: 20-40mg as a single dose IV/IM; give IV dose slowly (1-2 min)
Titrate: May repeat the same dose if needed or increase by 20mg no sooner than 2 hrs after the previous dose; give individually determined single dose qd or bid
Closely monitor when given for prolonged periods
<u>Hypertension</u>
Oral:
Initial: 40mg bid
Titrate: Adjust dose according to response
Add other antihypertensive agents if response is not satisfactory
<u>Acute Pulmonary Edema</u>
Inj:
Initial: 40mg IV slowly (over 1-2 min)
Titrate: May increase to 80mg IV slowly (over 1-2 min), if satisfactory response does not occur w/in 1 hr
Additional therapy (eg, digitalis, oxygen) may be administered concomitantly if necessary

PEDIATRIC DOSAGE
<u>Edema</u>
Associated w/ CHF, Liver Cirrhosis, and Renal Disease (Nephrotic Syndrome):
Oral:
Initial: 2mg/kg as a single dose
Titrate: May increase by 1 or 2mg/kg no sooner than 6-8 hrs after the previous dose, if diuretic response is not satisfactory after the initial dose
Maint: Adjust to the minimum effective level
Max: 6mg/kg
Inj:
Initial: 1mg/kg IV/IM
Titrate: If response is not satisfactory, may increase by 1mg/kg no sooner than 2 hrs after the previous dose, until the desired diuretic effect has been obtained
Max: 6mg/kg
Premature Infants: Max: 1mg/kg/day

DOSING CONSIDERATIONS
<u>Concomitant Medications</u>
Antihypertensives:
Oral:
Reduce dose of other agents by at least 50%
May further reduce dose or d/c therapy of other antihypertensive drugs as BP falls
<u>Elderly</u>
Oral/Inj:
Start at lower end of dosing range

ADMINISTRATION
Oral/IV/IM route

Hepatic Impairment
Mild and Moderate:
Initial: 2mg qd
Titrate: Increase by increments of 2mg qd no more frequently than every 2 weeks
Max: 6mg/day (mild), 4mg/day (moderate)
Severe: Not recommended

Elderly
Increase dose no more frequently than every 2 weeks during titration

ADMINISTRATION
Oral route

- Shake sus well before every administration.
- Use provided adapter and graduated dosing syringe; do not use spoon.
- Discard unused sus after 90 from opening the bottle.

STORAGE
20-25°C (68-77°F); excursions permitted to 15-30°C (59-86°F).

HOW SUPPLIED
Sus: 0.5mg/mL; **Tab:** 2mg, 4mg, 6mg, 8mg, 10mg, 12mg

WARNINGS/PRECAUTIONS
Increased risk of suicidal thoughts or behavior. May increase dose-related events related to dizziness, disturbance in gait/coordination, somnolence, and fatigue. May impair mental and physical abilities. Increased risk of falls. Potential of increased seizure frequency w/ abrupt withdrawal; gradual withdrawal generally recommended.

ADVERSE REACTIONS
Dizziness, somnolence, fatigue, irritability, falls, N/V, ataxia, balance disorder, gait disturbance, vertigo, weight gain, URTI, headache, abdominal pain.

DRUG INTERACTIONS
See Dosing Considerations. Concomitant use w/ contraceptives containing levonorgestrel may render them less effective due to reduced exposure; additional non-hormonal forms of contraception recommended. CYP450 inducers (eg, carbamazepine, phenytoin, oxcarbazepine) may decrease levels; monitor closely for clinical response and tolerability. Not recommended w/ other strong CYP3A inducers (eg, rifampin, St. John's wort). CNS depressants (eg, benzodiazepines, narcotics, barbiturates, sedating antihistamines) including alcohol may increase CNS depression; use caution when administering w/ these agents.

PREGNANCY AND LACTATION
Pregnancy: In animal studies, perampanel induced developmental toxicity in pregnant rat and rabbit at clinically relevant doses.
Lactation: No data on the presence of perampanel in human milk, the effects on the breastfed child, or the effects of the drug on milk production; present in rat milk.
Females and Males of Reproductive Potential: May reduce the efficacy of hormonal contraceptives containing levonorgestrel; use an additional non-hormonal form of contraception while on therapy and for a month after discontinuation.

MECHANISM OF ACTION
Non-competitive AMPA glutamate receptor antagonist; has not been established.

PHARMACOKINETICS
Absorption: Rapid and complete. T_{max}=0.5-2.5 hrs (fasted, median). **Distribution:** Plasma protein binding (95-96%). **Metabolism:** Liver (extensive); primary oxidation and sequential glucuronidation via CYP3A4, CYP3A5, CYP1A2, CYP2B6. **Elimination:** Urine (22%), feces (48%); $T_{1/2}$=105 hrs.

PATIENT CONSIDERATIONS
Assessment: Assess for psychiatric history, behavioral problems, hepatic/renal impairment, pregnancy/nursing status, and possible drug interactions.

Monitoring: Monitor for signs/symptoms of psychiatric and behavioral reactions, suicidal behavior and ideation, dizziness, gait disturbance, somnolence, worsening of depression, clinical response and tolerability, fatigue, falls, and other adverse reactions.

Counseling: Advise on proper use of sus. Inform about the risks and benefits of therapy. Explain the need to monitor for the emergence of anger, aggression, hostility, unusual changes in mood/personality/behavior, and other behavioral symptoms; advise to report any such symptoms immediately to physician. Counsel patients, caregivers, and families that therapy may increase risk of suicidal thinking and behavior. Inform that therapy may cause dizziness, gait disturbance, somnolence, and fatigue; advise not to drive, operate complex machinery, or engage in hazardous activities until accustomed to any such effects associated w/ therapy. Explain that therapy may cause falls and injuries. Inform that therapy may decrease efficacy of contraceptives containing levonorgestrel, and may enhance the impairment effects of alcohol and other CNS depressants. Explain that abrupt discontinuation of therapy may increase seizure frequency. Inform that therapy is a controlled substance that can be misused and abused. Encourage pregnant patients to enroll in the North American Antiepileptic Drug Pregnancy Registry. Advise females of reproductive potential to use an additional non-hormonal form of contraception while on therapy and for a month after discontinuation.

GARDASIL — human papillomavirus quadrivalent (types 6, 11, 16, and 18) vaccine, recombinant   **Rx**
Class: Vaccine

ADULT DOSAGE
Human Papillomavirus

Vaccination of girls and women 9-26 yrs of age for the prevention of cervical, vulvar, vaginal, and anal cancer caused by human papillomavirus (HPV) types 16 and 18; genital warts (condyloma acuminata) caused by HPV types 6 and 11; and cervical intraepithelial neoplasia (CIN) grade 2/3 and cervical adenocarcinoma in situ, CIN grade 1, vulvar intraepithelial neoplasia grades 2 and 3, vaginal intraepithelial neoplasia grades 2 and 3, and anal intraepithelial neoplasia (AIN) grades 1, 2, and 3 caused by HPV types 6, 11, 16, and 18. Vaccination of boys and men 9-26 yrs of age for the prevention of anal cancer caused by HPV types 16 and 18; genital warts (condyloma acuminata) caused by HPV types 6 and 11; and AIN grades 1, 2, and 3 caused by HPV types 6, 11, 16, and 18

9-26 Years:
0.5mL dose at the following schedule: 0, 2, and 6 months

PEDIATRIC DOSAGE
Human Papillomavirus

Vaccination of girls and women 9-26 yrs of age for the prevention of cervical, vulvar, vaginal, and anal cancer caused by human papillomavirus (HPV) types 16 and 18; genital warts (condyloma acuminata) caused by HPV types 6 and 11; and cervical intraepithelial neoplasia (CIN) grade 2/3 and cervical adenocarcinoma in situ, CIN grade 1, vulvar intraepithelial neoplasia grades 2 and 3, vaginal intraepithelial neoplasia grades 2 and 3, and anal intraepithelial neoplasia (AIN) grades 1, 2, and 3 caused by HPV types 6, 11, 16, and 18. Vaccination of boys and men 9-26 yrs of age for the prevention of anal cancer caused by HPV types 16 and 18; genital warts (condyloma acuminata) caused by HPV types 6 and 11; and AIN grades 1, 2, and 3 caused by HPV types 6, 11, 16, and 18

9-26 Years:
0.5mL dose at the following schedule: 0, 2, and 6 months

ADMINISTRATION
IM route

Shake well before use.
Administer in the deltoid region of the upper arm or in the higher anterolateral area of the thigh.
Do not dilute or mix w/ other vaccines.
Administer as soon as possible after being removed from refrigeration; can be out of refrigeration (≤25°C [77°F]) for a total time of not more than 72 hrs.

Single-Dose Vial
Withdraw the 0.5mL dose of vaccine using a sterile needle and syringe and use promptly.

Prefilled Syringe
Attach needle by twisting in clockwise direction until needle fits securely on syringe; administer entire dose as per standard protocol.

STORAGE
2-8°C (36-46°F). Do not freeze. Protect from light.

HOW SUPPLIED
Inj: 0.5mL [prefilled syringe, vial]

CONTRAINDICATIONS
Hypersensitivity to Gardasil or any of its components (eg, severe allergic reactions to yeast), or after a previous dose of Gardasil.

WARNINGS/PRECAUTIONS
Syncope may occur; observe for 15 min after administration. Appropriate medical treatment and supervision must be readily available in case of anaphylactic reactions. Women should continue to undergo cervical cancer screening. Recipients should not d/c anal cancer screening if it has been recommended by healthcare provider. Does not protect against disease from vaccine and non-vaccine HPV types to which a person has previously been exposed through sexual activity. Not intended for treatment of active external genital lesions; cervical, vulvar, vaginal, and anal cancers; CIN; VIN; VaIN; or AIN. Vaccination may not result in protection in all vaccine recipients. Response to vaccine may be diminished in immunocompromised individuals.

ADVERSE REACTIONS
Inj-site pain/swelling/erythema/pruritus, pyrexia, nausea, dizziness, diarrhea, headache.

DRUG INTERACTIONS
Immunosuppressive therapies, including irradiation, antimetabolites, alkylating agents, cytotoxic drugs, and corticosteroids (used in greater than physiologic doses), may reduce the immune responses to vaccines.

PREGNANCY AND LACTATION
Category B, caution in nursing.

MECHANISM OF ACTION
Vaccine; not established. May involve the development of humoral immune response.

PATIENT CONSIDERATIONS
Assessment: Assess for hypersensitivity to yeast or the vaccine, immunocompromised conditions, pregnancy/nursing status, and possible drug interactions.

Monitoring: Monitor for syncope, anaphylactic reactions, and other adverse reactions.

Counseling: Inform about benefits and risks associated w/ vaccine. Instruct women to continue to undergo cervical cancer screening per standard of care. Advise not to d/c anal cancer screening if recommended by physician. Inform that vaccine does not provide protection against disease from vaccine and non-vaccine HPV types to which a person has previously been exposed through sexual activity. Inform that syncope may occur following vaccination. Advise that vaccine is not recommended during pregnancy. Counsel about the importance of completing the immunization series unless contraindicated. Instruct to report any adverse reactions to physician.

GARDASIL 9 — human papillomavirus 9-valent vaccine, recombinant   Rx

Class: Vaccine

ADULT DOSAGE
Human Papillomavirus

Vaccination of females 9-26 yrs of age for the prevention of cervical, vulvar, vaginal, and anal cancer caused by human papillomavirus (HPV) types 16, 18, 31, 33, 45, 52, and 58; genital warts (condyloma acuminata) caused by HPV types 6 and 11; and cervical intraepithelial neoplasia (CIN) grade 2/3 and cervical adenocarcinoma in situ, CIN grade 1, vulvar intraepithelial neoplasia (VIN) grades 2 and 3, vaginal intraepithelial neoplasia (VaIN) grades 2 and 3, and anal intraepithelial neoplasia (AIN) grades 1, 2, and 3 caused by HPV types 6, 11, 16, 18, 31, 33, 45, 52, and 58

Vaccination of males 9-26 yrs of age for the prevention of anal cancer caused by HPV types 16, 18, 31, 33, 45, 52, and 58; genital warts (condyloma acuminata) caused by HPV types 6 and 11; and AIN grades 1, 2, and 3 caused by HPV types 6, 11, 16, 18, 31, 33, 45, 52, and 58

9-26 Years:
0.5mL dose at the following schedule: 0, 2, and 6 months

PEDIATRIC DOSAGE
Human Papillomavirus

Vaccination of females 9-26 yrs of age for the prevention of cervical, vulvar, vaginal, and anal cancer caused by HPV types 16, 18, 31, 33, 45, 52, and 58; genital warts (condyloma acuminata) caused by HPV types 6 and 11; and CIN grade 2/3 and cervical adenocarcinoma in situ, CIN grade 1, VIN grades 2 and 3, VaIN grades 2 and 3, and AIN grades 1, 2, and 3 caused by HPV types 6, 11, 16, 18, 31, 33, 45, 52, and 58

Vaccination of males 9-26 yrs of age for the prevention of anal cancer caused by HPV types 16, 18, 31, 33, 45, 52, and 58; genital warts (condyloma acuminata) caused by HPV types 6 and 11; and AIN grades 1, 2, and 3 caused by HPV types 6, 11, 16, 18, 31, 33, 45, 52, and 58

9-26 Years:
0.5mL dose at the following schedule: 0, 2, and 6 months

ADMINISTRATION
IM route

Shake well before use.
Administer in the deltoid region of the upper arm or in the higher anterolateral area of the thigh.
Do not dilute or mix w/ other vaccines.
Administer as soon as possible after being removed from refrigeration; cumulative multiple excursions out of refrigeration (8-25°C [46-77°F]) or between 0-2°C (32-36°F) are permitted for a total time of not more than 72 hrs.

STORAGE
2-8°C (36-46°F). Do not freeze. Protect from light.

HOW SUPPLIED
Inj: 0.5mL [prefilled syringe, single-dose vial]

CONTRAINDICATIONS
Hypersensitivity, including severe allergic reactions to yeast (a vaccine component), or after a previous dose of this vaccine or to Gardasil.

WARNINGS/PRECAUTIONS
Women should continue to undergo cervical cancer screening per standard of care. Recipients should not d/c anal cancer screening if it has been recommended by healthcare provider. Has not been demonstrated to provide protection against disease from vaccine HPV types to which a person has previously been exposed through sexual activity. Not a treatment for external genital lesions; cervical, vulvar, vaginal, and anal cancers; CIN; VIN; VaIN; or AIN. Vaccination may not result in protection in all vaccine recipients. Syncope may occur; observe for 15 min after administration. Appropriate medical treatment and supervision must be readily available in case of anaphylactic reactions following administration. Response to vaccine may be diminished in immunocompromised individuals.

ADVERSE REACTIONS
Females 9-15 Years: Inj-site pain/swelling/erythema, headache, pyrexia, nausea.
Females 16-26 Years: Inj-site pain/swelling/erythema, headache, pyrexia, nausea, dizziness.
Males 9-15 Years: Inj-site pain/swelling/erythema, headache, pyrexia.
Males 16-26 Years: Inj-site pain/swelling/erythema, headache.

DRUG INTERACTIONS
Immunosuppressive therapies, including irradiation, antimetabolites, alkylating agents, cytotoxic drugs, and corticosteroids (used in greater than physiologic doses), may reduce the immune responses to vaccines.

PREGNANCY AND LACTATION
Pregnancy: Category B. A pregnancy registry is available.
Lactation: Caution in nursing.

MECHANISM OF ACTION
Vaccine; exact mechanism of protection is unknown. Efficacy of vaccine is thought to be mediated by humoral immune responses induced by the vaccine.

PATIENT CONSIDERATIONS
Assessment: Assess for hypersensitivity to yeast or the vaccine, immunocompromised conditions, pregnancy/nursing status, and possible drug interactions.
Monitoring: Monitor for syncope, anaphylactic reactions, and other adverse reactions.
Counseling: Inform about benefits and risks associated w/ vaccine. Instruct women to continue to undergo cervical cancer screening per standard of care. Advise not to d/c anal cancer screening if recommended by healthcare provider. Inform that vaccine has not been demonstrated to provide protection against disease from vaccine and non-vaccine HPV types to which a person has previously been exposed through sexual activity. Inform that syncope may occur following vaccination. Instruct female patients to notify physician if pregnant or nursing; encourage women exposed to vaccine around time of conception or during pregnancy to register. Counsel about the importance of completing the immunization series unless contraindicated. Instruct to report any adverse reactions to physician.

GAZYVA — obinutuzumab   Rx

Class: Monoclonal antibody/CD20 blocker

> Hepatitis B virus (HBV) reactivation may occur, in some cases resulting in fulminant hepatitis, hepatic failure, and death; screen all patients for HBV infection before treatment initiation. Monitor HBV-positive patients during and after treatment. D/C therapy and concomitant medications in the event of HBV reactivation. Progressive multifocal leukoencephalopathy (PML), including fatal PML, may occur.

ADULT DOSAGE
Chronic Lymphocytic Leukemia

In combination w/ chlorambucil for the treatment of patients w/ previously untreated chronic lymphocytic leukemia (CLL)

Recommended Dose: Each dose is 1000mg IV, w/ the exception of the 1st infusions in Cycle 1, which are administered on Day 1 (100mg) and Day 2 (900mg)

Dose to Be Administered During 6 Treatment Cycles, Each of 28 Days Duration:
Cycle 1 (LD):
Day 1: 100mg administered at 25mg/hr over 4 hrs; do not increase the infusion rate
Day 2: 900mg administered at 50mg/hr; may escalate infusion rate in increments of 50mg/hr every 30 min to a max rate of 400mg/hr
Days 8 and 15: 1000mg; if no infusion reaction occurred during the previous infusion and the final infusion rate was 100mg/hr or faster, infusions can be started at a rate of 100mg/hr and increased by 100mg/hr increments every 30 min to a max of 400mg/hr

Cycles 2-6:
Day 1: 1000mg; if no infusion reaction occurred during the previous infusion and the final infusion rate was 100mg/hr or faster, infusions can be started at a rate of 100mg/hr and increased by 100mg/hr increments every 30 min to a max of 400mg/hr

Follicular Lymphoma

In combination w/ bendamustine followed by obinutuzumab monotherapy for the treatment of patients w/ follicular lymphoma who relapsed after, or are refractory to, a rituximab-containing regimen

Recommended Dose: 1000mg IV

Dose to Be Administered During 6 Treatment Cycles, Each of 28 Days Duration, Followed by Obinutuzumab Monotherapy:
Cycle 1 (LD):
Day 1: 1000mg administered at 50mg/hr; may escalate in 50mg/hr increments every 30 min to a max of 400mg/hr

PEDIATRIC DOSAGE
Pediatric use may not have been established

Days 8 and 15: 1000mg. If no infusion reaction occurred during the previous infusion and the final infusion rate was 100mg/hr or faster, infusions can be started at a rate of 100mg/hr and increased by 100mg/hr increments every 30 min to a max of 400mg/hr

Cycles 2-6:
Day 1: 1000mg. If no infusion reaction occurred during the previous infusion and the final infusion rate was 100mg/hr or faster, infusions can be started at a rate of 100mg/hr and increased by 100mg/hr increments every 30 min to a max of 400mg/hr

Monotherapy:
1000mg every 2 months for 2 years. If no infusion reaction occurred during the previous infusion and the final infusion rate was 100mg/hr or faster, infusions can be started at a rate of 100mg/hr and increased by 100mg/hr increments every 30 min to a max of 400mg/hr

Premedication
Tumor Lysis Syndrome (TLS):
Patients w/ high tumor burden, high circulating absolute lymphocyte counts (>25 x 10⁹/L), or renal impairment are considered at risk of TLS and should receive prophylaxis. Premedicate w/ antihyperuricemics (eg, allopurinol or rasburicase) and ensure adequate hydration prior to start of therapy; continue prophylaxis prior to each subsequent infusion, prn.

Infusion Related Reactions (IRR):
Cycle 1:
CLL Days 1 and 2; Follicular Lymphoma (FL) Day 1:
All Patients: 20mg IV dexamethasone or 80mg IV methylprednisolone completed at least 1 hr before obinutuzumab infusion, 650-1000mg acetaminophen and an antihistamine (eg, 50mg diphenhydramine) at least 30 min before obinutuzumab infusion

All Subsequent Infusions:
All Patients: 650-1000mg acetaminophen at least 30 min before obinutuzumab infusion.

Patients w/ IRR (Grade 1-2) w/ Previous Infusion: 650-1000mg acetaminophen and an antihistamine (eg, 50mg diphenhydramine) at least 30 min before obinutuzumab infusion.

Patients w/ Grade 3 IRR w/ Previous Infusion or Lymphocyte Count >25 x 10⁹/L Prior to Next Treatment: 20mg IV dexamethasone or 80mg IV methylprednisolone completed at least 1 hr prior to obinutuzumab infusion, and 650-1000mg acetaminophen and an antihistamine (eg, 50mg diphenhydramine) at least 30 min before obinutuzumab infusion

Antimicrobial Prophylaxis:
Patients w/ Grade 3-4 neutropenia lasting >1 week are strongly recommended to receive antimicrobial prophylaxis until resolution of neutropenia to Grade 1 or 2. Consider antiviral and antifungal prophylaxis

Missed Dose
If a planned dose is missed, administer as soon as possible

CLL: Adjust dosing schedule accordingly. If appropriate, patients who do not complete the Day 1 Cycle 1 dose may proceed to the Day 2 Cycle 1 dose

FL: During Gazyva and bendamustine treatment, adjust the dosing schedule accordingly. During monotherapy, maintain the original dosing schedule for subsequent doses

DOSING CONSIDERATIONS
Adverse Reactions
Infusion Reaction:
Grade 1-2 (Mild to Moderate):
Reduce infusion rate or interrupt infusion and treat symptoms; once symptoms resolve, continue/resume infusion.
If no further symptoms, infusion rate escalation may resume at the increments and intervals as appropriate for the treatment cycle dose.
CLL Patients Only: Day 1 infusion rate may be increased back up to 25mg/hr after 1 hr but not increased further

Grade 3 (Severe):
Interrupt infusion and manage symptoms; once symptoms resolve, consider restarting infusion at no more than 1/2 the previous rate.
If no further symptoms, infusion rate escalation may resume at the increments and intervals as appropriate for the treatment cycle dose.
Permanently d/c treatment if a Grade 3 infusion-related symptom occurs at re-challenge.
CLL Patients Only: Day 1 infusion rate may be increased back up to 25mg/hr after 1 hr but not increased further

Grade 4 (Life Threatening):
Stop infusion immediately and permanently d/c therapy
Interruption for Toxicity:
Infection, Grade 3 or 4 Cytopenia, or a ≥Grade 2 Nonhematologic Toxicity:
Consider treatment interruption

ADMINISTRATION
IV route
Administer only as an IV infusion through a dedicated line.
Do not administer as IV push or bolus.
Do not mix w/ other drugs.
Should only be administered by a healthcare professional w/ appropriate medical support to manage severe infusion reactions.

Preparation
Dilute into a 0.9% NaCl PVC or non-PVC polyolefin infusion bag; do not use other diluents (eg, D5).
Mix diluted sol by gentle inversion.
Do not shake or freeze.
CLL:
Preparation of Sol for Infusion on Day 1/Day 2 of Cycle 1:
1. Withdraw 40mL of obinutuzumab sol and dilute 4mL into a 100mL infusion bag for immediate administration.
2. Dilute remaining 36mL into a 250mL infusion bag at the same time for use on Day 2. Store at 2-8°C (36-46°F) for up to 24 hrs. Use immediately once the diluted bag comes to room temperature.

Preparation of Sol for Infusion on Day 8/Day 15 of Cycle 1 and Day 1 of Cycles 2-6:
Withdraw 40mL of obinutuzumab sol and dilute into a 250mL infusion bag.
FL:
Preparation of Sol for Infusion:
Withdraw 40mL of obinutuzumab sol and dilute 40mL into a 250mL infusion bag.
Can be administered at final concentration of 0.4-4mg/mL.

Stability
Use diluted infusion sol immediately.
If not used immediately, store in refrigerator at 2-8°C (36-46°F) for up to 24 hrs prior to use.

STORAGE
2-8°C (36-46°F). Protect from light. Do not freeze. **Diluted Sol:** Stable in 0.9% NaCl at 0.4-20mg/mL for 24 hrs at 2-8°C (36-46°F) followed by 48 hrs (including infusion time) at room temperature ≤30°C (86°F).

HOW SUPPLIED
Inj: 1000mg/40mL

WARNINGS/PRECAUTIONS
See Dosing Considerations. Consider diagnosis of PML in any patient presenting w/ new onset or changes to preexisting neurologic manifestations; d/c therapy and consider discontinuation or reduction of any concomitant chemotherapy or immunosuppressive therapy in patients who develop PML. May cause severe and life-threatening infusion reactions; institute medical management for infusion reactions prn. Monitor patients w/ preexisting cardiac/pulmonary conditions more frequently throughout infusion and postinfusion period. Hypotension may occur as part of an infusion reaction; consider withholding antihypertensive treatments for 12 hrs prior to and during each infusion, and for the 1st hr after administration until BP is stable. TLS, including fatal cases, reported; monitor lab parameters of patients at risk for TLS, during the initial days of treatment. Correct electrolyte abnormalities, monitor renal function and fluid balance, and administer supportive care to treat TLS. Serious bacterial, fungal, and new/reactivated viral infections may occur during and following therapy; fatal infections reported. Do not administer to patients w/ active infection; patients w/ a history of recurring/chronic infections may be at increased risk of infection. Severe, life-threatening neutropenia (eg, febrile neutropenia) reported; consider granulocyte colony-stimulating factors or dose delays w/ Grade 3 or 4 neutropenia. Severe and life-threatening thrombocytopenia and fatal hemorrhagic events reported; monitor for thrombocytopenia and hemorrhagic events, especially during the 1st cycle. Monitor platelet counts more frequently in patients w/ Grade 3 or 4 thrombocytopenia until resolution and consider subsequent dose delays of obinutuzumab and chemotherapy or dose reductions of chemotherapy.

ADVERSE REACTIONS
CLL: Infusion reactions, neutropenia, thrombocytopenia, anemia, pyrexia, cough, nausea, diarrhea.
Non-Hodgkin Lymphoma: Cough, URTIs, neutropenia, sinusitis, diarrhea, infusion related reactions, nausea, fatigue, bronchitis, arthralgia, pyrexia, nasopharyngitis, UTIs.

DRUG INTERACTIONS
Immunization w/ live virus vaccines is not recommended during treatment and until B-cell recovery. Consider withholding concomitant medications, which may increase bleeding risk (platelet inhibitors, anticoagulants), especially during the 1st cycle.

PREGNANCY AND LACTATION
Pregnancy: Likely to cause fetal B-cell depletion based on findings from animal studies and the drug's mechanism of action. Avoid administering live vaccines to neonates and infants exposed to therapy in utero until B-cell recovery occurs.
Lactation: There is no information regarding the presence of obinutuzumab in human milk, the effects on the breastfed infant, or the effects on milk production; caution in nursing.

MECHANISM OF ACTION
Monoclonal antibody/CD20-blocker; binds to CD20 antigen expressed on the surface of pre B- and mature B-lymphocytes, mediating B-cell lysis through engagement of immune effector cells, by directly activating intracellular death signaling pathways, and/or activation of the complement cascade.

PHARMACOKINETICS
Distribution: V_d=4.1L (CLL). V_d=4.3L (Non-Hodgkin Lymphoma). Crosses placenta.
Elimination: $T_{1/2}$=26.4 days (CLL). $T_{1/2}$=36.8 days (Non-Hodgkin Lymphoma).

PATIENT CONSIDERATIONS
Assessment: Assess for active/history of chronic/recurring infection, preexisting cardiac/pulmonary conditions, preexisting neurologic manifestations, any other conditions where treatment is cautioned, pregnancy/nursing status, and possible drug interactions. Assess for HBV infection by measuring HBsAg and anti-HBc. Obtain baseline blood counts.

Monitoring: Monitor for signs/symptoms of bacterial/fungal/viral infections, PML, infusion reactions, TLS, neutropenia, thrombocytopenia, hemorrhagic events, and other adverse reactions. Monitor blood counts at regular intervals. Closely monitor patients during entire infusion. Monitor patients w/ evidence of current or prior HBV infection for clinical and lab signs of hepatitis or HBV reactivation during and for several months following treatment. Monitor patients w/ preexisting cardiac/pulmonary conditions more frequently throughout the infusion and the postinfusion period. Monitor renal function and fluid balance in patients w/ TLS.

Counseling: Instruct to seek immediate medical attention for signs/symptoms of infusion reactions, symptoms of TLS, signs of infections, symptoms of hepatitis, and new or changes in neurological symptoms. Advise of the need for periodic monitoring of blood counts and instruct to avoid vaccination w/ live viral vaccines. Inform patients w/ a history of HBV infection that they should be monitored and sometimes treated for their hepatitis. Advise pregnant women of potential fetal B-cell depletion.

GELNIQUE — oxybutynin   Rx
Class: Muscarinic antagonist

ADULT DOSAGE	PEDIATRIC DOSAGE
Overactive Bladder	Pediatric use may not have been established
3% Gel:	
Apply 3 pumps (84mg/day) qd	
10% Gel:	
Apply contents of 1 sachet qd	

ADMINISTRATION
Topical route

Apply to clean, dry, intact skin on the abdomen, upper arms/shoulders, or thighs.
Apply immediately after actuating the dose (3% Gel), or after the sachets are opened and contents expelled (10% Gel).
Rotate application sites; avoid use of same site on consecutive days.
Wash hands immediately after application.

STORAGE
Protect from moisture and humidity. Discard used sachets/pump dispensers in a manner that prevents accidental application or ingestion by children, pets, or others. (3% Gel) 25°C (77°F); excursions permitted to 15-30°C (59-86°F). (10% Gel) 20-25°C (68-77°F).

HOW SUPPLIED
Gel: 3% [92g], (Chloride) 10% [1g, 30^s]

CONTRAINDICATIONS
Urinary/gastric retention, uncontrolled narrow-angle glaucoma, hypersensitivity reaction to oxybutynin or to any of the components of this medication.

WARNINGS/PRECAUTIONS
Flammable; avoid open fire or smoking until gel has dried. Caution w/ bladder outflow obstruction, GI obstructive disorders, gastroesophageal reflux, and myasthenia gravis. May decrease GI motility; caution w/ conditions such as ulcerative colitis or intestinal atony. Angioedema reported w/ oral oxybutynin; d/c and promptly provide appropriate therapy if this occurs. Skin transference may occur; cover application site w/ clothing after gel has dried. CNS anticholinergic effects (eg, headache, dizziness, somnolence) reported; consider discontinuation

---

if these effects occur. May impair mental/physical abilities. (3% Gel) Caution in patients being treated for narrow-angle glaucoma. (10% Gel) Skin hypersensitivity may occur; d/c if hypersensitivity develops.

ADVERSE REACTIONS
Dry mouth, application-site reactions (eg, erythema, rash), UTI, nasopharyngitis, (3% Gel) conjunctivitis, (10% Gel) URTIs.

DRUG INTERACTIONS
Caution w/ drugs (eg, bisphosphonates) that may cause or exacerbate esophagitis. Concomitant use w/ other anticholinergic (antimuscarinic) agents may increase the frequency and/or severity of dry mouth, constipation, blurred vision, somnolence, and other anticholinergic pharmacological effects.

PREGNANCY AND LACTATION
Category B, caution in nursing.

MECHANISM OF ACTION
Antispasmodic, antimuscarinic agent; acts as competitive antagonist of acetylcholine at postganglionic muscarinic receptors, resulting in relaxation of bladder smooth muscle.

PHARMACOKINETICS
Absorption: (3% Gel) Abdomen: AUC=284.1ng•hr/mL, C_{max}=6.3ng/mL, T_{max}=24 hrs. Thigh: AUC=286.9ng•hr/mL, C_{max}=5.8ng/mL, T_{max}=36 hrs. Upper Arm/Shoulder: AUC=329.1ng•hr/mL, C_{max}=8.8ng/mL, T_{max}=24 hrs. (10% Gel) Abdomen: AUC=112.7ng•hr/mL, C_{max}=6.8ng/mL. Upper Arm/Shoulder: AUC=133.8ng•hr/mL, C_{max}=8.3ng/mL. Thigh: AUC=125.1ng•hr/mL, C_{max}=7ng/mL. **Distribution:** (IV) V_d=193L. **Metabolism:** Liver (extensive) by CYP3A4; N-desethyloxybutynin (active metabolite). **Elimination:** Urine (<0.1% unchanged, <0.1% N-desethyloxybutynin); $T_{1/2}$=30 hrs (3% Gel), 64 hrs (10% Gel), 2 hrs (IV).

PATIENT CONSIDERATIONS
Assessment: Assess for urinary/gastric retention, uncontrolled narrow-angle glaucoma, bladder outflow obstruction, GI obstructive disorders, ulcerative colitis or intestinal atony, gastroesophageal reflux, myasthenia gravis, pregnancy/nursing status, and for possible drug interactions.

Monitoring: Monitor for signs/symptoms of urinary retention, gastric retention, esophagitis, angioedema, CNS effects, and other adverse reactions.

Counseling: Advise that therapy is for topical application only and should not be ingested. Instruct not to apply to recently shaved skin surfaces. Advise to avoid showering or water immersion for 1 hr after application. Counsel to avoid open fire or smoking until gel has dried. Counsel to cover treated sites w/ clothing if close skin-to-skin contact is anticipated. Instruct to avoid open fire or smoking until gel has dried. Advise that adverse reactions related to anticholinergic pharmacological activity may occur. Inform that heat prostration may occur in hot environment. Advise to exercise caution in engaging in potentially dangerous activities until effects have been determined. Inform that alcohol may enhance drowsiness. Instruct to avoid skin w/ open sores, wounds, irritation, scars, and tattoos. Advise to thoroughly rinse eyes right away with warm, clean water if gel gets in the eyes and to seek medical attention if needed. (3% Gel) Instruct not to use any gel that comes out while priming.

GENERESS FE — ethinyl estradiol/ferrous fumarate/norethindrone   Rx
Class: Estrogen/progestogen combination

> Cigarette smoking increases the risk of serious cardiovascular (CV) events from combination oral contraceptive (COC) use. Risk increases with age (>35 yrs of age) and with the number of cigarettes smoked. Should not be used by women who are >35 yrs of age and smoke.

ADULT DOSAGE	PEDIATRIC DOSAGE
Contraception	**Contraception**
1 tab qd for 28 days, then repeat	Not indicated for use premenarche; refer to adult dosing
Start on 1st day of menses	
Conversions	
Switching from Combination Hormonal Method:	
Another Pill: Start on same day that new pack of the previous oral contraceptive would have been started	
Vaginal Ring/Patch: Start on same day that the ring/patch would have been restarted	
Switching from Progestin-Only Method (eg, Progestin-Only Pill, Implant, Intrauterine System, Inj): Start on same day that next progestin-only pill/inj would have been taken/administered, or on the day that implant/intrauterine system is removed	
Use a nonhormonal backup method (eg, condom, spermicide) for the first 7 days	

DOSING CONSIDERATIONS
Adverse Reactions
GI Disturbances: If vomiting/diarrhea occurs w/in 3-4 hrs after taking active tab, may regard as missed dose

Other Important Considerations
Postpartum Women Who Do Not Breastfeed/After Second Trimester Abortion: May start therapy no earlier than 4 weeks postpartum; use nonhormonal contraceptive during first 7 days

ADMINISTRATION
Oral route

May be administered w/o regard to meals
Chew and swallow tab without water at the same time every day
Take tabs in the order directed on the blister pack
Do not skip or take tabs at intervals exceeding 24 hrs
Use a nonhormonal contraceptive as backup during the first 7 days if therapy is not started on the 1st day of the menstrual cycle

STORAGE
20-25°C (68-77°F).

HOW SUPPLIED
Tab, Chewable: (Norethindrone-Ethinyl Estradiol [EE]) 0.8mg-0.025mg; **Tab, Chewable:** (Ferrous Fumarate) 75mg

CONTRAINDICATIONS
High risk of arterial/venous thrombotic disease (eg, smoking if >35 yrs of age, history/presence of deep vein thrombosis/pulmonary embolism, cerebrovascular disease, coronary artery disease, thrombogenic valvular or thrombogenic rhythm diseases of the heart [eg, subacute bacterial endocarditis with valvular disease, or atrial fibrillation], inherited/acquired hypercoagulopathies, uncontrolled HTN, diabetes with vascular disease, headaches with focal neurological symptoms or migraine with/without aura if >35 yrs of age), history/presence of breast or other estrogen-/progestin-sensitive cancer, benign/malignant liver tumors, liver disease, undiagnosed abnormal uterine bleeding, pregnancy.

WARNINGS/PRECAUTIONS
Increased risk of venous thromboembolism and arterial thrombosis (eg, stroke, myocardial infarction); d/c if an arterial/deep venous thrombotic event occurs. D/C at least 4 weeks before and through 2 weeks after major surgery or other surgeries known to have an elevated risk of thromboembolism. Start therapy no earlier than 4 weeks postpartum in women who do not breastfeed. Caution with CV disease (CVD) risk factors. D/C if there is unexplained loss of vision, proptosis, diplopia, papilledema, or retinal vascular lesions; evaluate for retinal vein thrombosis immediately. May increase risk of breast and cervical cancer, intraepithelial neoplasia, and gallbladder disease. Hepatic adenoma and increased risk of hepatocellular carcinoma reported; d/c if jaundice or acute/chronic disturbances of liver function occur. Cholestasis may occur with history of pregnancy-related cholestasis. Increased BP reported; d/c if BP rises significantly. May decrease glucose tolerance; monitor prediabetic and diabetic women. Consider alternative contraception with uncontrolled dyslipidemia. Increased risk of pancreatitis with hypertriglyceridemia or family history thereof. May increase frequency/severity of migraine; d/c if new headaches that are recurrent, persistent, or severe develop. Unscheduled bleeding and spotting may occur; rule out pregnancy or malignancies. Caution with history of depression; d/c if depression recurs to serious degree. May change results of lab tests (eg, coagulation factors, lipids, glucose tolerance, binding proteins). May induce/exacerbate angioedema in patients with hereditary angioedema. Chloasma may occur; women with chloasma should avoid sun exposure or UV radiation. Absorption may not be complete in case of severe vomiting or diarrhea; if vomiting or diarrhea occurs within 3-4 hrs after tab-taking, regard this as a missed tab.

ADVERSE REACTIONS
N/V, headaches/migraine, depression/mood complaints, dysmenorrhea, acne, anxiety symptoms, breast pain/tenderness, increased weight.

DRUG INTERACTIONS
Agents that induce certain enzymes, including CYP3A4 (eg, barbiturates, bosentan, carbamazepine, felbamate, griseofulvin, oxcarbazepine, phenytoin, rifampin, St. John's wort, topiramate), may decrease COC efficacy or increase breakthrough bleeding; consider additional or alternative contraceptive method. Significant changes (increase or decrease) in plasma estrogen and progestin levels reported with HIV protease inhibitors or non-nucleoside reverse transcriptase inhibitors. Pregnancy reported with antibiotics. Atorvastatin, ascorbic acid, acetaminophen, and CYP3A4 inhibitors (eg, itraconazole, ketoconazole) may increase plasma hormone levels. May decrease concentrations of lamotrigine and reduce seizure control; dose adjustment of lamotrigine may be needed. Increases thyroid-binding globulin; may need to increase dose of thyroid hormone in patients on thyroid hormone replacement therapy.

PREGNANCY AND LACTATION
Contraindicated in pregnancy, not for use in nursing.

MECHANISM OF ACTION
Estrogen/progestogen combination oral contraceptive; acts by suppressing ovulation. Also causes cervical mucus changes that inhibit sperm penetration and endometrial changes that reduce the likelihood of implantation.

PHARMACOKINETICS
Absorption: Norethindrone: Absolute bioavailability (64%). EE: Absolute bioavailability (43%). Refer to PI for different parameters. **Distribution:** V_d=2-4L/kg; plasma protein binding (>95%); found in breast milk. **Metabolism:** Norethindrone: Extensive, primarily via reduction, followed by sulfate and glucuronide conjugation. EE: Extensive, by oxidation and by conjugation with sulfate and glucuronide; 2-hydroxy EE (primary metabolite, formed via CYP3A4). **Elimination:** Urine, feces. Norethindrone: $T_{1/2}$=11 hrs. EE: $T_{1/2}$=17 hrs.

PATIENT CONSIDERATIONS
Assessment: Assess for abnormal uterine bleeding, liver disease, pregnancy, and other conditions where treatment is cautioned or contraindicated. Assess use in women who are >35 yrs of age and smoke, and/or who have CVD and arterial/venous thrombosis risk factors, pregnancy-related cholestasis, HTN, diabetes, uncontrolled dyslipidemia, history of hypertriglyceridemia, history of depression, hereditary angioedema, or history of chloasma. Assess for possible drug interactions.

Monitoring: Monitor for bleeding irregularities, venous/arterial thrombotic and thromboembolic events, cervical cancer or intraepithelial neoplasia, retinal vein thrombosis or any other ophthalmic changes, jaundice, acute/chronic disturbances in liver function, new/worsening headaches or migraines, serious depression, gallbladder disease, cholestasis with history of pregnancy-related cholestasis, and pancreatitis. Monitor thyroid function if receiving thyroid replacement therapy, glucose levels in diabetic or prediabetic women, lipids with dyslipidemia, and check BP annually.

Counseling: Counsel that cigarette smoking increases the risk of serious CV events from COC use, and that women who are >35 yrs of age and smoke should not use COCs. Inform that drug does not protect against HIV infection and other sexually transmitted diseases. Instruct on what to do if pills are missed; inform that if vomiting/diarrhea occurs within 3-4 hrs after tab-taking, this is regarded as a missed tab. Inform that COCs may reduce breast milk production. Inform that amenorrhea may occur and pregnancy should be ruled out if amenorrhea occurs in ≥2 consecutive cycles. Advise to inform physician of preexisting medical conditions and/or drugs currently being taken. Counsel women who start COCs postpartum, and who have not yet had a period, to use an additional method of contraception until after the first 7 consecutive days of administration. Instruct to d/c if pregnancy occurs during treatment.

GENGRAF — cyclosporine   Rx
Class: Calcineurin-inhibitor immunosuppressant

> Should only be prescribed by physicians experienced in the management of systemic immunosuppressive therapy for indicated diseases. Manage patients in facilities equipped and staffed w/ adequate lab and supportive medical resources. Increased susceptibility to infection and development of neoplasia (eg, lymphoma) may result from immunosuppression. May be coadministered w/ other immunosuppressive agents in kidney, liver, and heart transplant patients. Not bioequivalent to Sandimmune and cannot be used interchangeably w/o physician supervision. Caution in switching from Sandimmune. Monitor cyclosporine blood levels in transplant and rheumatoid arthritis (RA) patients to avoid toxicity due to high levels. Dose adjustments should be made in transplant patients to minimize possible organ rejection due to low levels. (Psoriasis) Increased risk of developing skin malignancies in psoriasis patients previously treated w/ PUVA, methotrexate (MTX) or other immunosuppressive agents, UVB, coal tar, or radiation therapy. May cause systemic HTN and nephrotoxicity; risk increases w/ increasing dose and duration. Monitor for renal dysfunction, including structural kidney damage, during therapy.

ADULT DOSAGE
Organ Rejection Prophylaxis

Kidney, Liver, and Heart Allogeneic Transplants:
Newly Transplanted Patients:
Initial dose may be given 4-12 hrs prior to transplant or postoperatively; dose varies depending on transplanted organ and other immunosuppressive agents included in protocol

Suggested Initial Doses:
Renal Transplant: 9mg/kg/day ± 3mg/kg/day
Liver Transplant: 8mg/kg/day ± 4mg/kg/day
Heart Transplant: 7mg/kg/day ± 3mg/kg/day

Always administer daily dose in 2 divided doses (bid) and adjust subsequent dose to achieve a predefined cyclosporine blood concentration

Adjunct therapy w/ adrenal corticosteroids is recommended initially

Conversion from Sandimmune:
Start w/ the same daily dose as was previously used w/ Sandimmune (1:1 dose conversion); dose should subsequently be adjusted to attain the pre-conversion blood trough concentration

It is strongly recommended that the blood trough concentration be monitored every 4-7 days after conversion to Gengraf, until the blood trough concentration attains the pre-conversion value

Patients w/ Poor Absorption of Sandimmune:
Due to the increase in bioavailability of cyclosporine following conversion

PEDIATRIC DOSAGE
Organ Rejection Prophylaxis

Kidney, Liver, and Heart Allogeneic Transplants:
Transplant recipients as young as 1 year of age have received cyclosporine (MODIFIED) w/ no unusual adverse effects

to Gengraf, the blood trough concentration may exceed the target range; caution when converting patients at doses >10mg/kg/day

Titrate dose individually based on trough levels, tolerability, and clinical response; measure blood trough concentrations more frequently, at least 2X a week (daily, if initial dose >10mg/kg/day) until the concentration stabilizes w/in the desired range

Has been used in combination w/ azathioprine and corticosteroids

Rheumatoid Arthritis

Severe active rheumatoid arthritis where the disease has not adequately responded to MTX

Initial: 2.5mg/kg/day, taken in 2 divided doses
Titrate: May increase by 0.5-0.75mg/kg/day after 8 weeks and again after 12 weeks
Max: 4mg/kg/day

Salicylates, NSAIDs, and oral corticosteroids may be continued

D/C if no benefit is seen by 16 weeks of therapy

Combination w/ MTX:

Use same initial dose and dosage range; most patients can be treated w/ Gengraf doses of ≤3mg/kg/day when combined w/ MTX doses of up to 15mg/week

Plaque Psoriasis

In immunocompetent patients w/ severe, recalcitrant, plaque psoriasis who failed to respond to at least 1 systemic therapy (eg, PUVA, retinoids, MTX) or in patients for whom other systemic therapies are contraindicated, or cannot be tolerated

Initial: 2.5mg/kg/day, taken in 2 divided doses for at least 4 weeks
Titrate: If significant clinical improvement does not occur, increase the dose at 2-week intervals by approx 0.5mg/kg/day
Max: 4mg/kg/day

D/C if satisfactory response cannot be achieved after 6 weeks at 4mg/kg/day or the patient's max tolerated dose

Once a patient is adequately controlled and appears stable, the dose should be lowered, and the patient treated w/ the lowest dose that maintains an adequate response

----

DOSING CONSIDERATIONS
Renal Impairment
In Kidney, Liver, and Heart Transplant: Reduce dose if indicated
In Rheumatoid Arthritis/Psoriasis: Not recommended for use

Hepatic Impairment
Severe: Dose reduction may be necessary

Elderly
Start at lower end of dosing range

Adverse Reactions
Rheumatoid Arthritis/Psoriasis: Decrease dose by 25-50% at any time to control adverse events or clinically significant lab abnormalities; d/c if dose reduction is not effective in controlling abnormalities or if the adverse event or abnormality is severe

Other Important Considerations
Avoid consumption of grapefruit or grapefruit juice during therapy

ADMINISTRATION
Oral route

Always administer daily dose in 2 divided doses (bid).
Administer on a consistent schedule w/ regard to time of day and relation to meals.

Sol
To make the sol more palatable, dilute w/ room temperature orange or apple juice; avoid switching diluents frequently.

Instructions:
1. Take the prescribed amount of sol from the container using the dosing syringe supplied, and transfer the sol to a glass of orange or apple juice; use a glass container, not plastic.
2. Stir well and drink at once; do not allow diluted sol to stand before drinking.
3. Rinse the glass w/ more diluent to ensure that the total dose is consumed.
4. After use, dry the outside of the dosing syringe w/ a clean towel and store in a clean, dry place; do not rinse the dosing syringe w/ water or other cleaning agents.
5. If the syringe requires cleaning, it must be completely dry before resuming use.

STORAGE
20-25°C (68-77°F). **Sol:** Do not refrigerate. Use w/in 2 months once opened. May form gel at <20°C (68°F); light flocculation, or formation of light sediment may occur. Allow to warm to 25°C (77°F) to reverse these changes.

HOW SUPPLIED
Cap: 25mg, 50mg, 100mg; **Sol:** 100mg/mL [50mL]

CONTRAINDICATIONS
Hypersensitivity to cyclosporine or to any components of the medication. **RA/Psoriasis:** Abnormal renal function, uncontrolled HTN, malignancies. **Psoriasis:** Concomitant PUVA or UVB therapy, MTX or other immunosuppressants, coal tar or radiation therapy.

WARNINGS/PRECAUTIONS
Elevations in SrCr and BUN may occur and reflect a reduction in GFR; impaired renal function at any time requires close monitoring, and frequent dose adjustment may be indicated. Elevations in SrCr and BUN levels in renal transplant patients do not necessarily indicate rejection; evaluate patient before initiating dose adjustment. Thrombocytopenia and microangiopathic hemolytic anemia, resulting in graft failure, reported. Significant hyperkalemia (sometimes associated w/ hyperchloremic metabolic acidosis) and hyperuricemia reported. May cause hepatotoxicity and liver injury (eg, cholestasis, jaundice, hepatitis, liver failure). Avoid excessive UV light exposure. Oversuppression of the immune system may result in an increased risk of infection/malignancy; caution when using a treatment regimen containing multiple immunosuppressants. Increased risk of developing bacterial, viral, fungal, protozoal, and opportunistic infections (eg, polyoma virus infections). JC virus-associated progressive multifocal leukoencephalopathy and polyomavirus-associated nephropathy, especially due to BK virus infection, reported; consider reduction in immunosuppression if either develops. Convulsions and encephalopathy including posterior reversible encephalopathy syndrome, and rarely, optic disc edema, reported. HTN may occur and persist, and may require antihypertensive therapy. **Cap:** Consider the alcohol content of the drug when giving to patients in whom alcohol intake should be avoided or minimized (eg, pregnant or breastfeeding women, patients presenting w/ liver disease or epilepsy, alcoholic patients, pediatric patients).

ADVERSE REACTIONS
Kidney, Liver, and Heart Transplantation: Renal dysfunction, tremor, hirsutism, HTN, gum hyperplasia.
RA: Renal dysfunction, HTN, headache, GI disturbances, hirsutism/hypertrichosis.
Psoriasis: Renal dysfunction, headache, HTN, hypertriglyceridemia, hirsutism/hypertrichosis, paresthesia/hyperesthesia, influenza-like symptoms, N/V, diarrhea, abdominal discomfort, lethargy, musculoskeletal/joint pain.

DRUG INTERACTIONS
See Boxed Warning, Dosing Considerations, and Contraindications. Avoid w/ K+-sparing diuretics, aliskiren, bosentan, dabigatran, and compounds that decrease drug absorption (eg, orlistat). Vaccination may be less effective; avoid live vaccines during therapy. Caution w/ rifabutin, nephrotoxic drugs, HIV protease inhibitors, K+-sparing drugs (eg, ACE inhibitors, ARBs), K+-containing drugs, and K+-rich diet. Ciprofloxacin, gentamicin, tobramycin, vancomycin, trimethoprim w/ sulfamethoxazole, melphalan, amphotericin B, ketoconazole, azapropazone, colchicine, diclofenac, naproxen, sulindac, cimetidine, ranitidine, tacrolimus, fibric acid derivatives (eg, bezafibrate, fenofibrate), MTX, and NSAIDs may potentiate renal dysfunction; closely monitor renal function and reduce dose of coadministered drug or consider alternative treatment if a significant impairment of renal function occurs. CYP3A4 and/or P-gp inducers/inhibitors may alter levels; adjust cyclosporine dose appropriately. Diltiazem, nicardipine, verapamil, fluconazole, itraconazole, ketoconazole, voriconazole, azithromycin, clarithromycin, erythromycin, quinupristin/dalfopristin, methylprednisolone, allopurinol, amiodarone, bromocriptine, colchicine, danazol, imatinib, metoclopramide, nefazodone, oral contraceptives, HIV protease inhibitors, grapefruit, grapefruit juice, boceprevir, and telaprevir may increase levels. St. John's wort, nafcillin, rifampin, carbamazepine, oxcarbazepine, phenobarbital, phenytoin, bosentan, octreotide, sulfinpyrazone, terbinafine, and ticlopidine may decrease levels. May increase plasma levels of bosentan, dabigatran, and substrates of CYP3A4, P-gp, or organic anion transporter proteins. May increase levels of ambrisentan; do not titrate ambrisentan dose to the recommended max daily dose when coadministering w/ cyclosporine. May reduce clearance of digoxin, colchicine, prednisolone, HMG-CoA reductase inhibitors (statins), aliskiren, bosentan, dabigatran, repaglinide, NSAIDs, sirolimus, and etoposide. Digitalis toxicity reported; monitor digoxin levels. May increase levels and enhance toxic effects of colchicine; reduce colchicine dose. Myotoxicity cases seen w/ statins; temporarily withhold or d/c statin therapy if signs of myopathy develop or w/ risk factors predisposing to severe renal injury. May increase levels of repaglinide and thereby increase the risk of hypoglycemia; closely monitor blood glucose levels. High doses of cyclosporine may increase the exposure to anthracycline antibiotics (eg, doxorubicin, mitoxantrone, daunorubicin) in cancer patients. May double diclofenac blood levels; dose of diclofenac should be in the lower end of the therapeutic range. May increase MTX levels and decrease levels of MTX metabolite. Concomitant use w/ sirolimus increases levels of sirolimus and causes elevations of SrCr; give sirolimus 4 hrs after cyclosporine. Frequent

gingival hyperplasia reported w/ nifedipine; avoid concomitant use w/ nifedipine in patients in whom gingival hyperplasia develops as a side effect of cyclosporine. Convulsions reported w/ high-dose methylprednisolone. Calcium antagonists may interfere w/ cyclosporine metabolism.

PREGNANCY AND LACTATION
Pregnancy: Category C.
Lactation: Not for use in nursing.

MECHANISM OF ACTION
Cyclic polypeptide immunosuppressant; specific and reversible inhibition of immunocompetent lymphocytes in the G_0- and G_1-phase of the cell cycle. T-lymphocytes are preferentially inhibited w/ T-helper cell as main target, although T-suppressor cell may also be suppressed. Also inhibits lymphokine production and release (eg, interleukin-2).

PHARMACOKINETICS
Absorption: Incomplete; T_{max}=1.5-2 hrs. Pharmacokinetic parameters varied w/ different indications (renal/liver transplant, RA, and/or psoriasis). **Distribution:** V_d=3-5L/kg (IV, solid organ transplant recipients); plasma protein binding (90%); found in breast milk. **Metabolism:** (Extensive) Liver via CYP3A and less in the GI tract and kidneys. Oxidation and demethylation pathways; M1, M9, M4N (major metabolites). **Elimination:** Bile (primary), urine (6%, 0.1% unchanged); $T_{1/2}$=8.4 hrs.

PATIENT CONSIDERATIONS
Assessment: Assess for hypersensitivity to the drug, renal dysfunction, uncontrolled HTN, presence of malignancies, pregnancy/nursing status, and for possible drug interactions. **RA:** Before initiating treatment, assess BP (on at least 2 occasions) and obtain 2 SrCr levels. **Psoriasis:** Prior to treatment, perform a dermatological and physical examination, including measuring BP (on at least 2 occasions). Assess for presence of occult infection and for the presence of tumors. Assess for atypical skin lesions and biopsy them. Obtain baseline SrCr (on 2 occasions), BUN, CBC, Mg^{2+}, K^+, uric acid, and lipid levels.

Monitoring: Monitor for signs/symptoms of hepatotoxicity, liver injury, nephrotoxicity, thrombocytopenia, microangiopathic hemolytic anemia, HTN, hyperkalemia, lymphomas and other malignancies, serious/opportunistic/polyomavirus infections, convulsions and other neurotoxicities, and other adverse reactions. Monitor cyclosporine blood levels routinely in transplant patients and periodically in RA patients. **RA:** Monitor BP and SrCr every 2 weeks during the initial 3 months of therapy and then monthly if patient is stable. Monitor SrCr and BP after an increase of the dose of NSAIDs and after initiation of new NSAID therapy. If coadministered w/ MTX, monitor CBC and LFTs monthly. **Psoriasis:** Monitor for occult infection and for the presence of tumors. Monitor SrCr, BUN, BP, CBC, uric acid, K^+, lipids, and Mg^{2+} every 2 weeks during first 3 months of treatment, then monthly if stable, or more frequently during dose adjustments.

Counseling: Instruct to contact physician before changing formulations of cyclosporine, which may require dose changes. Inform that repeated lab tests are required while on therapy. Advise of the potential risks if used during pregnancy and inform of the increased risk of neoplasia, HTN, and renal dysfunction. Inform that vaccinations may be less effective and instruct to avoid live vaccines during therapy. Advise to avoid grapefruit/grapefruit juice and excessive sun exposure.

GENTAMICIN INJECTION — gentamicin sulfate   Rx

Class: Aminoglycoside

> Potential for nephrotoxicity, neurotoxicity, and ototoxicity; adjust dose or d/c on evidence of ototoxicity/nephrotoxicity. Risk of nephrotoxicity is greater w/ impaired renal function and in those who receive high dosage or prolonged therapy. Neurotoxicity (eg, vestibular and auditory ototoxicity) can occur w/ preexisting renal damage or w/ normal renal function treated at higher doses and/or longer treatment periods than recommended. Closely monitor renal and 8th cranial nerve function, especially in patients w/ known or suspected reduced renal function at onset of therapy and also in those whose renal function is initially normal but who develop signs of renal dysfunction during therapy. Examine urine for decreased specific gravity, increased protein excretion, and presence of cells/casts. Monitor BUN, SrCr, or CrCl periodically. Obtain serial audiograms in patients old enough to be tested, particularly high-risk patients, when feasible. Periodically monitor peak and trough serum concentrations to assure adequate levels and to avoid toxicity. Dose should be adjusted when monitoring peak and trough concentrations; avoid prolonged peak levels >12mcg/mL and trough levels >2mcg/mL. Hemodialysis may aid in the removal of gentamicin from the blood, especially if renal function is or becomes compromised. Consider exchange transfusions in the newborn infant. Avoid concurrent and/or sequential systemic or topical use of other potentially neurotoxic and/or nephrotoxic drugs (eg, cisplatin, cephaloridine, kanamycin, amikacin, neomycin, polymyxin B, colistin, paromomycin, streptomycin, tobramycin, vancomycin, viomycin). Advanced age and dehydration may increase risk of toxicity. Avoid w/ potent diuretics (eg, ethacrynic acid, furosemide). May cause fetal harm.

OTHER BRAND NAMES
Gentamicin in 0.9% Sodium Chloride

ADULT DOSAGE
General Dosing
Treatment of bacterial neonatal sepsis, bacterial septicemia, and infections of the CNS (meningitis), urinary tract, respiratory tract, GI tract (including peritonitis), skin, bone, and soft tissue (including burns) caused by susceptible strains of microorganisms; for initial therapy in suspected/confirmed gram-negative infections or as initial therapy in conjunction w/ a penicillin (PCN)-type or cephalosporin-type drug in

PEDIATRIC DOSAGE
General Dosing
Use concomitantly w/ PCN-type drug in neonates w/ suspected bacterial sepsis or staphylococcal pneumonia

Premature or Full-Term Neonates ≤1 Week of Age:
5mg/kg/day (2.5mg/kg q12h)
Infants and Neonates:
7.5mg/kg/day (2.5mg/kg q8h)
Children:
6-7.5mg/kg/day (2-2.5mg/kg q8h)

serious infections when the causative organisms are unknown; for treatment of life-threatening infections caused by *Pseudomonas aeruginosa* in combination w/ carbenicillin, and endocarditis caused by group D streptococci in combination w/ a PCN-type drug; in treatment of serious staphylococcal infections; and for treatment of mixed infections caused by susceptible strains of staphylococci and gram-negative infections

Serious Infections: 3mg/kg/day given in 3 equal doses q8h
Life-Threatening Infections: 5mg/kg/day in 3 or 4 equal doses; reduce to 3mg/kg/day as soon as clinically indicated

Treat for 7-10 days; may need longer course in difficult and complicated infections. Reduce dose if clinically indicated

Treat for 7-10 days; may need longer course in difficult and complicated infections. Reduce dose if clinically indicated.

DOSING CONSIDERATIONS
Renal Impairment
Increasing Intervals:
Multiply SrCr level (mg/100mL) by 8 (eg, SrCr of 2mg/100mL x 8 = q16h)
Reducing Dosage at 8-Hour Intervals After Initial Dose:
CrCl 70-100mL/min: 80% of usual dose
CrCl 55-70mL/min: 65% of usual dose
CrCl 45-55mL/min: 55% of usual dose
CrCl 40-45mL/min: 50% of usual dose
CrCl 35-40mL/min: 40% of usual dose
CrCl 30-35mL/min: 35% of usual dose
CrCl 25-30mL/min: 30% of usual dose
CrCl 20-25mL/min: 25% of usual dose
CrCl 15-20mL/min: 20% of usual dose
CrCl 10-15mL/min: 15% of usual dose
CrCl <10mL/min: 10% of usual dose
Hemodialysis:
Adults: 1-1.7mg/kg at the end of each dialysis period, depending on the severity of infection
Pediatrics: May administer 2mg/kg

Other Important Considerations
Obese Patients:
Base dose on estimate of lean body mass
Extensive Burns:
Adjust dose based on serum concentrations

ADMINISTRATION
IM/IV route

Do not physically premix w/ other drugs; administer separately.
IV route may be preferred w/ bacterial septicemia, CHF, hematologic disorders, severe burns, reduced muscle mass, or those in shock.
Infuse over a period of 1/2 to 2 hrs.

0.9% NaCl
No dilution or buffering required.
If administration is controlled by a pumping device, use caution when discontinuing pumping action before container runs dry.
Intended for use only as an IV secondary medication unit.
Do not use in plastic containers in series connection.

Intermittent IV Administration
10mg/mL: May dilute a single-dose in 0.9% NaCl or in D5 inj.
40mg/mL: May dilute in 50-200mL of sterile isotonic saline sol or in a sterile sol of D5W; in infants and children, the volume of diluent should be less.
0.9% NaCl: Single dose of gentamicin sulfate may be administered according to individual requirements from appropriate premixed container.

STORAGE
(10mg/mL, 40mg/mL) 20-25°C (68-77°F). (0.9% NaCl) 25°C (77°F); brief exposure up to 40°C (104°F) does not adversely affect the product. Avoid excessive heat.

HOW SUPPLIED
Inj: 10mg/mL [2mL], 40mg/mL [2mL, 20mL]; (0.9% NaCl) 60mg [50mL], 80mg, 100mg [50mL, 100mL], 120mg [100mL]

CONTRAINDICATIONS
Hypersensitivity to gentamicin, history of hypersensitivity or serious toxic reactions to aminoglycosides.

WARNINGS/PRECAUTIONS
Neuromuscular blockade, respiratory paralysis, ototoxicity, and nephrotoxicity may occur after local irrigation or topical application of neurotoxic and nephrotoxic antibiotics during surgical procedures. Caution w/ neuromuscular disorders (eg, myasthenia gravis, parkinsonism); may aggravate muscle weakness. During or following therapy, paresthesia, tetany, mental confusion, and positive Chvostek and Trousseau signs have been described in patients w/ hypomagnesemia, hypocalcemia, and hypokalemia; appropriate corrective electrolyte therapy is required. Fanconi-like syndrome w/ aminoaciduria and metabolic acidosis reported. Cross-allergenicity among aminoglycosides

demonstrated. Maintain adequate hydration. May result in overgrowth of nonsusceptible organisms; take appropriate measures if this occurs. Not for uncomplicated initial episodes of UTI unless the causative organisms are susceptible and are not susceptible to antibiotics having less potential for toxicity. (40mg/mL, 0.9% NaCl) Caution in elderly. (40mg/mL) Contains sodium metabisulfite; allergic-type reactions may occur more frequently in asthmatics. (0.9% NaCl) Contains Na⁺; caution w/ CHF, severe renal insufficiency, and edema w/ Na⁺ retention.

ADVERSE REACTIONS
Peripheral neuropathy, encephalopathy, respiratory depression, lethargy, confusion, depression, visual disturbances, decreased appetite, weight loss, hypo/hypertension, rash, N/V, fever, headache.

DRUG INTERACTIONS
See Boxed Warning. Increased nephrotoxicity w/ cephalosporins. Neuromuscular blockade and respiratory paralysis may occur in anesthetized patients, those receiving neuromuscular blockers (eg, succinylcholine, tubocurarine, decamethonium), or those receiving massive transfusions of citrate-anticoagulated blood. May increase risk of toxicity w/ previous exposure to ototoxic drugs. Rapid and significant inactivation of gentamicin w/ carbenicillin in vitro; concomitant use w/ carbenicillin in patients w/ severe renal impairment reported a reduction in gentamicin serum $T_{1/2}$.

PREGNANCY AND LACTATION
Pregnancy: Category D.
Lactation: (0.9% NaCl) Not for use in nursing.

MECHANISM OF ACTION
Aminoglycoside antibiotic; inhibits normal protein synthesis in susceptible microorganisms.

PHARMACOKINETICS
Absorption: (IM) T_{max}=30-60 min. Administration of different doses resulted in different parameters. **Distribution:** Plasma protein binding (0-30%); crosses the placenta. **Elimination:** Urine (70% [40mg/mL, 0.9% NaCl]), bile. (10mg/mL) $T_{1/2}$=3-3.5 hrs (1 week-6 months of age), 5.5 hrs (full-term and large premature infants <1 week old), 11.5 hrs (premature infants <1500g), 8 hrs (premature infants 1500-2000g), 5 hrs (premature infants >2000g).

PATIENT CONSIDERATIONS
Assessment: Obtain pretreatment body weight for calculation of correct dosage. Assess and document bacterial infection using culture and susceptibility techniques. Assess for history of hypersensitivity to drug, other aminoglycosides, or to sulfites. Assess for CHF, hypomagnesemia, hypocalcemia, hypokalemia, neuromuscular disorders, pregnancy/nursing status, and for possible drug interactions. Assess renal function.

Monitoring: Monitor for signs/symptoms of ototoxicity, neurotoxicity, nephrotoxicity, hypersensitivity reactions, Fanconi-like syndrome w/ aminoaciduria and metabolic acidosis, and other adverse reactions. Monitor hydration status, LFTs, BUN, SrCr, CrCl, CBC, and serum electrolytes. Monitor peak and trough serum levels of gentamicin periodically. Repeat culture and susceptibility test.

Counseling: Inform that drug only treats bacterial, not viral, infections. Instruct to take up; inform that skipping doses or not completing full course may decrease effectiveness and may increase likelihood of bacterial resistance. Advise to keep well hydrated during treatment. Instruct to inform physician if pregnant/breastfeeding.

GENVOYA — cobicistat/elvitegravir/emtricitabine/tenofovir alafenamide
Rx

Class: CYP3A inhibitor/HIV integrase strand transfer inhibitor/nucleoside reverse transcriptase inhibitor (NRTI) combination

> Lactic acidosis and severe hepatomegaly w/ steatosis, including fatal cases, reported w/ the use of nucleoside analogues in combination w/ other antiretrovirals. Not approved for the treatment of chronic hepatitis B virus (HBV) infection. Severe acute exacerbations of hepatitis B reported in patients who are coinfected w/ HBV and HIV-1 and have discontinued products containing emtricitabine and/or tenofovir disoproxil fumarate (TDF); closely monitor hepatic function w/ both clinical and lab follow-up for at least several months in patients who are coinfected w/ HIV-1 and HBV and d/c therapy. If appropriate, initiation of anti-hepatitis B therapy may be warranted.

ADULT DOSAGE
HIV-1 Infection

For use as a complete regimen in adults who have no antiretroviral treatment history or to replace the current antiretroviral regimen in those who are virologically-suppressed (HIV-1 RNA <50 copies/mL) on a stable antiretroviral regimen for at least 6 months w/ no history of treatment failure and no known substitutions associated w/ resistance to the individual components of the drug

≥35kg:
1 tab qd

PEDIATRIC DOSAGE
HIV-1 Infection

For use as a complete regimen in pediatrics who have no antiretroviral treatment history or to replace the current antiretroviral regimen in those who are virologically-suppressed (HIV-1 RNA <50 copies/mL) on a stable antiretroviral regimen for at least 6 months w/ no history of treatment failure and no known substitutions associated w/ resistance to the individual components of the drug

≥12 Years and ≥35kg:
1 tab qd

DOSING CONSIDERATIONS
Renal Impairment
CrCl <30mL/min: Not recommended for use

Hepatic Impairment
Severe (Child-Pugh Class C): Not recommended for use

ADMINISTRATION
Oral route
Take w/ food.

STORAGE
<30°C (86°F).

HOW SUPPLIED
Tab: (Cobicistat/Elvitegravir/Emtricitabine/Tenofovir Alafenamide [TAF]) 150mg/150mg/200mg/10mg

CONTRAINDICATIONS
Concomitant use w/ drugs that are highly dependent on CYP3A for clearance and for which elevated plasma concentrations are associated w/ serious and/or life-threatening events (eg, alfuzosin, carbamazepine, phenobarbital, phenytoin, rifampin, dihydroergotamine, ergotamine, methylergonovine, cisapride, St. John's wort, lovastatin, simvastatin, pimozide, sildenafil [when dosed as Revatio for the treatment of pulmonary arterial HTN], triazolam, oral midazolam).

WARNINGS/PRECAUTIONS
Test for HBV infection prior to initiation of therapy. Redistribution/accumulation of body fat reported. Not recommended in patients w/ estimated CrCl <30mL/min. **Emtricitabine and TAF:** Obesity and prolonged nucleoside exposure may be risk factors for lactic acidosis and severe hepatomegaly. Caution in any patient w/ known risk factors for liver disease. **Emtricitabine:** Immune reconstitution syndrome and autoimmune disorders (eg, Graves' disease, polymyositis, Guillain-Barre syndrome) in the setting of immune reconstitution reported. **TAF:** Renal impairment, including cases of acute renal failure and Fanconi syndrome, reported w/ tenofovir prodrugs; d/c in patients who develop clinically significant decreases in renal function or evidence of Fanconi syndrome. Decreased bone mineral density (BMD) and increased biochemical markers of bone metabolism reported. Osteomalacia associated w/ proximal renal tubulopathy reported in association w/ the use of TDF-containing products. Hypophosphatemia and osteomalacia secondary to proximal renal tubulopathy have occurred in patients at risk of renal dysfunction who present w/ persistent or worsening bone or muscle symptoms while receiving products containing TDF. **Cobicistat:** May produce elevations of SrCr.

ADVERSE REACTIONS
Nausea.

DRUG INTERACTIONS
See Contraindications. Avoid w/ elvitegravir, cobicistat, emtricitabine, TDF, lamivudine, adefovir dipivoxil, ritonavir, other antiretrovirals, rifabutin, rifapentine, or salmeterol. CYP3A inducers may decrease plasma concentration of cobicistat, elvitegravir, and TAF and may lead to loss of therapeutic effect and development of resistance. Coadministration w/ drugs that reduce renal function or compete for active tubular secretion (eg, acyclovir, cidofovir, ganciclovir, valacyclovir, valganciclovir, aminoglycosides [eg, gentamicin]) may increase concentrations of emtricitabine, tenofovir, and other renally eliminated drugs and this may increase the risk of adverse reactions. May increase levels of antiarrhythmics (eg, digoxin), itraconazole, ketoconazole, voriconazole, colchicine, quetiapine, ethosuximide, β-blockers, calcium channel blockers, inhaled or nasal fluticasone, bosentan, atorvastatin, immunosuppressants, salmeterol, neuroleptics, PDE-5 inhibitors, and sedatives/hypnotics. May increase levels of clarithromycin and telithromycin; reduce clarithromycin dose by 50% in patients w/ CrCl 50-60mL/min. Monitor INR upon coadministration w/ warfarin. Ethosuximide and oxcarbazepine may decrease elvitegravir, cobicistat, and TAF levels; consider alternative anticonvulsants w/ oxcarbazepine and monitor upon coadministration w/ ethosuximide. May increase levels of antidepressants (eg, SSRIs [except sertraline], TCAs, trazodone); carefully titrate antidepressant dose and monitor response. Ketoconazole, itraconazole, and voriconazole may increase levels of elvitegravir and cobicistat. Avoid w/ colchicine in patients w/ renal or hepatic impairment. Rifabutin and rifapentine may decrease elvitegravir, cobicistat, and TAF levels. Consider alternative antiretroviral therapy w/ quetiapine if initiating therapy while on quetiapine. Dexamethasone may decrease elvitegravir and cobicistat levels; consider an alternative corticosteroid. May increase levels of diazepam and parenterally administered midazolam; consider dose reduction for midazolam. May increase norgestimate and decrease ethinyl estradiol levels; consider alternative (nonhormonal) methods of contraception. Cyclosporine may increase elvitegravir and cobicistat levels. May increase levels of buprenorphine and norbuprenorphine and may decrease levels of naloxone. **TAF:** Patients taking nephrotoxic agents (eg, NSAIDs) are at increased risk of developing renal-related adverse reactions. P-gp inducers may decrease levels. **Cobicistat:** May increase levels of CYP3A substrates or CYP2D6 substrates, and substrates of P-gp, BCRP, OATP1B1, or OATP1B3. CYP3A inhibitors may increase levels. Clarithromycin and telithromycin may increase levels. **Elvitegravir:** May decrease plasma levels of CYP2C9 substrates. Antacids (eg, aluminum and magnesium hydroxide) may decrease levels; separate administration by at least 2 hrs. Refer to PI for dosing modifications when used w/ certain concomitant therapies.

PREGNANCY AND LACTATION
Pregnancy: Category B. An antiretroviral pregnancy registry has been established to monitor fetal outcomes of pregnant women.
Lactation: Emtricitabine is secreted in human milk. Not for use in nursing.

MECHANISM OF ACTION
Elvitegravir: HIV-1 integrase strand inhibitor; inhibits the strand transfer activity of HIV-1 integrase, preventing the integration of HIV-1 DNA into host genomic DNA, blocking the formation of HIV-1 provirus and propagation of the viral infection.
Cobicistat: CYP3A inhibitor; inhibits CYP3A-mediated metabolism that leads to enhancement of systemic exposure of CYP3A substrates (eg, elvitegravir).

Emtricitabine: Nucleoside analogue of cytidine; inhibits the activity of HIV-1 reverse transcriptase by competing w/ the natural substrate deoxycytidine 5'-triphosphate and by being incorporated into nascent viral DNA, resulting in chain termination. **TAF:** Acyclic nucleoside phosphonate (nucleotide) analogue of adenosine 5'-monophosphate; inhibits HIV replication through incorporation into viral DNA by the HIV reverse transcriptase, which results in DNA chain-termination.

PHARMACOKINETICS

Absorption: Elvitegravir: C_{max}=2.1mcg/mL, AUC=22.8mcg•hr/mL, T_{max}=4 hrs. Cobicistat: C_{max}=1.5mcg/mL, AUC=9.5mcg•hr/mL, T_{max}=3 hrs. Emtricitabine: C_{max}=2.1mcg/mL, AUC=11.7mcg•hr/mL, T_{max}=3 hrs. TAF: C_{max}=0.16mcg/mL, AUC=0.21mcg•hr/mL, T_{max}=1 hr. **Distribution:** Elvitegravir: Plasma protein binding (99%). Cobicistat: Plasma protein binding (98%). Emtricitabine: Plasma protein binding (<4%); found in breast milk. TAF: Plasma protein binding (80%). **Metabolism:** Elvitegravir: CYP3A (major); UGT1A1/3 (minor). Cobicistat: CYP3A (major), CYP2D6 (minor). TAF: Hydrolysis, tenofovir (major metabolite), phosphorylation, tenofovir diphosphate (active metabolite). **Elimination:** Elvitegravir: Feces (94.8%), urine (6.7%); $T_{1/2}$=12.9 hrs (median). Cobicistat: Feces (86.2%), urine (8.2%); $T_{1/2}$=3.5 hrs (median). Emtricitabine: Urine (70%), feces (13.7%); $T_{1/2}$=10 hrs (median). TAF: Feces (31.7%), urine (<1%); $T_{1/2}$=0.51 hrs (median).

PATIENT CONSIDERATIONS

Assessment: Assess for obesity, prolonged nucleoside exposure, risk factors for liver disease, renal/hepatic impairment, pregnancy/nursing status, and possible drug interactions. Assess BMD in patients who have a history of pathological bone fracture or w/ other risk factors for osteoporosis or bone loss. Obtain baseline estimated CrCl, urine glucose, urine protein, and SrCr. Perform test for HBV infection prior to therapy.

Monitoring: Monitor for signs/symptoms of lactic acidosis, severe hepatomegaly w/ steatosis, new onset/worsening renal impairment, immune reconstitution syndrome, autoimmune disorders, fat redistribution/accumulation, decreased BMD, increased biochemical markers for bone metabolism, osteomalacia, and other adverse reactions. Monitor for exacerbations of hepatitis B in patients w/ coinfection for at least several months upon discontinuation of therapy. Monitor BMD, estimated CrCl, urine glucose, urine protein, and SrCr. Monitor serum phosphorus levels in patients w/ chronic kidney disease. Monitor INR upon coadministration w/ warfarin.

Counseling: Instruct to take on a regular dosing schedule w/ food and to avoid missing doses. Advise to report use of any prescription or nonprescription medication or herbal products, including St. John's wort. Instruct to contact physician if symptoms of lactic acidosis/pronounced hepatotoxicity or any symptoms of infection occur. Inform that hepatitis B testing is recommended prior to initiating therapy. Advise that fat redistribution/accumulation, renal impairment, and decreases in BMD may occur. Inform that there is an antiretroviral pregnancy registry to monitor fetal outcomes of pregnant women exposed to the drug. Instruct mothers not to breastfeed.

GEODON — ziprasidone hydrochloride; ziprasidone mesylate　　Rx

Class: Atypical antipsychotic

> Elderly patients w/ dementia-related psychosis treated w/ antipsychotic drugs are at an increased risk of death; most deaths appeared to be cardiovascular (CV) (eg, heart failure [HF], sudden death) or infectious (eg, pneumonia) in nature. Not approved for treatment of dementia-related psychosis.

ADULT DOSAGE

Schizophrenia

Cap:
Initial: 20mg bid
Titrate: May adjust up to 80mg bid at intervals of not <2 days
Max: 80mg bid

Maint Treatment: No additional benefit demonstrated for doses >20mg bid

Acute Agitation in Schizophrenia:
IM:
10mg (may give q2h) to 20mg (may give q4h)
Max: 40mg/day

IM administration for >3 consecutive days has not been studied; if long-term therapy is indicated, replace w/ oral formulation as soon as possible

Bipolar I Disorder

Mixed or Manic Episodes:
Cap:
Acute (Monotherapy):
Initial: 40mg bid
Titrate: May increase to 60mg or 80mg bid on 2nd day of treatment, and subsequently adjust based on tolerance and efficacy w/in the range 40-80mg bid

Maint (Adjunct to Lithium or Valproate):
Continue treatment at the same dose on which the patient was initially stabilized, w/in the range of 40-80mg bid

PEDIATRIC DOSAGE

Pediatric use may not have been established

DOSING CONSIDERATIONS
Elderly
Start at lower end of dosing range

ADMINISTRATION
Oral/IM route

Cap
Take w/ food.

IM
Add 1.2mL of sterile water for inj (SWFI) to vial and shake vigorously until all the drug is dissolved.
Draw up 0.5mL of reconstituted sol to administer a 10mg dose; draw up 1mL of reconstituted sol to administer a 20mg dose.
Do not mix w/ other medicinal products or solvents other than SWFI.

STORAGE
25°C (77°F); excursions permitted to 15-30°C (59-86°F). **Inj:** Protect from light.
Reconstituted Sol: 15-30°C (59-86°F) for up to 24 hrs when protected from light, or at 2-8°C (36-46°F) for up to 7 days.

HOW SUPPLIED
Cap: 20mg, 40mg, 60mg, 80mg; **Inj:** 20mg/mL

CONTRAINDICATIONS
Known history of QT prolongation (including congenital long QT syndrome); recent acute MI; uncompensated HF; concomitant use w/ dofetilide, sotalol, quinidine, other Class Ia and III antiarrhythmics, mesoridazine, thioridazine, chlorpromazine, droperidol, pimozide, sparfloxacin, gatifloxacin, moxifloxacin, halofantrine, mefloquine, pentamidine, arsenic trioxide, levomethadyl acetate, dolasetron mesylate, probucol or tacrolimus, or other drugs that have demonstrated QT prolongation; known hypersensitivity to the product.

WARNINGS/PRECAUTIONS
Avoid in patients w/ history of cardiac arrhythmias. D/C in patients w/ persistent QTc measurements >500 msec. Hypokalemia and/or hypomagnesemia may increase risk of QT prolongation and arrhythmia; replete those electrolytes before treatment. Initiate further evaluation if symptoms of torsades de pointes occur. Neuroleptic malignant syndrome (NMS) reported; d/c therapy and institute symptomatic treatment. Drug reaction w/ eosinophilia and systemic symptoms (DRESS) and other severe cutaneous reactions reported; d/c if suspected. May cause tardive dyskinesia (TD), especially in the elderly; consider discontinuation if this occurs. Associated w/ metabolic changes (eg, hyperglycemia, dyslipidemia, weight gain) that may increase CV/cerebrovascular risk. Rash and/or urticaria reported; d/c upon appearance of rash. May induce orthostatic hypotension and syncope; caution w/ CV disease, cerebrovascular disease, or conditions that predispose to hypotension. Leukopenia, neutropenia, and agranulocytosis reported; d/c in patients w/ severe neutropenia (ANC <1000/mm^3) or at 1st sign of decline in WBCs in patients w/ preexisting low WBC count or history of drug-induced leukopenia/neutropenia. Seizures reported. May cause esophageal dysmotility and aspiration; caution in patients at risk for aspiration pneumonia. May elevate prolactin levels. May impair physical/mental abilities. Somnolence and priapism reported. May disrupt the body's ability to reduce core body temperature. Caution in cardiac patients and in those at risk for suicide. Caution w/ renal impairment when administered IM. Concomitant use of IM and oral preparations in schizophrenic patients is not recommended.

ADVERSE REACTIONS
Schizophrenia: Somnolence, respiratory tract infection.
Bipolar I Disorder: Somnolence, extrapyramidal symptoms, dizziness, akathisia, abnormal vision, asthenia, vomiting.
IM: Headache, nausea, somnolence.

DRUG INTERACTIONS
See Contraindications. Caution w/ centrally acting drugs and medications w/ anticholinergic activity. May enhance effects of certain antihypertensives. May antagonize effects of levodopa and dopamine agonists. Decreased exposure w/ carbamazepine. Increased levels w/ CYP3A4 inhibitors (eg, ketoconazole). Periodically monitor serum electrolytes w/ diuretics.

PREGNANCY AND LACTATION
Pregnancy: Category C.
Lactation: Not for use in nursing.

MECHANISM OF ACTION
Atypical antipsychotic; mechanism not established. Proposed that efficacy in schizophrenia is mediated through a combination of dopamine type 2 and serotonin type 2 antagonism.

PHARMACOKINETICS
Absorption: (Oral) Well-absorbed. Absolute bioavailability (approx 60%); T_{max}=6-8 hrs. (IM) Absolute bioavailability (100%); T_{max}=60 min. **Distribution:** (Oral) V_d=1.5L/kg; plasma protein binding (>99%). **Metabolism:** (Oral) Liver (extensive) via aldehyde oxidase (primary), CYP3A4 and CYP1A2; benzisothiazole (BITP) sulphoxide, BITP-sulphone, ziprasidone sulphoxide, and S-methyldihydroziprasidone (major metabolites). **Elimination:** (Oral) Urine (20%, <1% unchanged), feces (66%, <4% unchanged); $T_{1/2}$=7 hrs. (IM) $T_{1/2}$=2-5 hrs.

PATIENT CONSIDERATIONS
Assessment: Assess for drug hypersensitivity, history of QT prolongation, recent acute MI, uncompensated HF, dementia-related psychosis, history of seizures/conditions that lower seizure threshold, other conditions where treatment is contraindicated or cautioned, pregnancy/nursing status, and possible drug interactions. Obtain baseline serum electrolytes (K^+, Mg^{2+}) in patients at risk for significant electrolyte disturbances. Obtain baseline FPG in patients w/ diabetes mellitus (DM) or at risk for DM. Obtain baseline CBC if at risk for leukopenia/neutropenia.

Monitoring: Monitor for QT prolongation, torsades de pointes, NMS, DRESS and other severe cutaneous reactions, TD, metabolic changes, rash, orthostatic hypotension, seizures, esophageal dysmotility, aspiration, suicidal ideation, hypokalemia, hypomagnesemia, and other adverse reactions. Monitor CBC frequently during the 1st few months of therapy in patients w/ preexisting low WBCs or history of drug-induced leukopenia/neutropenia. Monitor for fever or other signs/symptoms of infection in patients w/ neutropenia. Monitor for worsening of glucose control in patients w/ DM and monitor FPG in patients at risk for DM. Reassess periodically to determine need for maintenance treatment.

Counseling: Inform of the risks and benefits of therapy. Advise to inform physician of any history of QT prolongation, recent acute MI, uncompensated HF, risk for electrolyte abnormalities, history of cardiac arrhythmia, or if taking other QT-prolonging drugs. Instruct to report conditions that increase risk for electrolyte disturbances (eg, hypokalemia, taking diuretics, prolonged diarrhea) and if dizziness, palpitations, or syncope occurs. Instruct to report to physician at the earliest onset any signs/symptoms that may be associated w/ DRESS or w/ severe cutaneous reactions (eg, Stevens-Johnson syndrome).

GIAZO — balsalazide disodium   Rx

Class: 5-aminosalicylic acid derivative

ADULT DOSAGE	PEDIATRIC DOSAGE
Ulcerative Colitis	Pediatric use may not have been
Mildly to Moderately Active:	established
Males: 3 tabs bid (6.6g/day) for up to 8 weeks	

ADMINISTRATION
Oral route
Take w/ or w/o food.

STORAGE
20-25°C (68-77°F); excursions permitted between 15-30°C (59-86°F).

HOW SUPPLIED
Tab: 1.1g

CONTRAINDICATIONS
Hypersensitivity to salicylates, aminosalicylates, or their metabolites, or to any of the components of this medication.

WARNINGS/PRECAUTIONS
Associated w/ acute intolerance syndrome (eg, cramping, acute abdominal pain and bloody diarrhea, fever, headache, and rash) that may be difficult to distinguish from exacerbation of ulcerative colitis; observe closely for worsening of symptoms and d/c therapy if acute intolerance syndrome is suspected. Renal impairment, including minimal change nephropathy, acute/chronic interstitial nephritis, and renal failure, reported; evaluate renal function prior to initiation and periodically while on therapy. Caution w/ known renal dysfunction or history of renal disease. Hepatic failure reported in patients w/ preexisting liver disease; use caution and consider LFTs in patients w/ liver disease. Caution in elderly; closely monitor blood cell counts during therapy.

ADVERSE REACTIONS
Headache, nasopharyngitis, anemia, diarrhea, fatigue, pharyngolaryngeal pain, urinary tract infection, GI disorders.

PREGNANCY AND LACTATION
Category B, caution in nursing.

MECHANISM OF ACTION
5-aminosalicylic acid (5-ASA) derivative; has not been established. Prodrug of mesalamine; action appears to be local to the colonic mucosa rather than systemic. Suspected to diminish inflammation by blocking production of arachidonic acid metabolites in the colon.

PHARMACOKINETICS
Absorption: Different dosing conditions (fed/fasted, single/repeated doses) resulted in different parameters. **Distribution:** Plasma protein binding (≥99% balsalazide, 43% 5-ASA, 78% N-Ac-5-ASA); crosses placenta. **Metabolism:** Bacterial azoreduction and acetylation; 5-ASA, N-Ac-5-ASA (metabolites). **Elimination:** Urine (23%, 0.16% unchanged); $T_{1/2}$=1.9 hrs (balsalazide), 9.5 hrs (5-ASA), 10.5 hrs (N-Ac-5-ASA).

PATIENT CONSIDERATIONS
Assessment: Assess for hypersensitivity to salicylates, aminosalicylates, or their metabolites, and renal/hepatic function.

Monitoring: Monitor for signs/symptoms of acute intolerance syndrome, renal/hepatic impairment, and other adverse reactions. Monitor blood cell counts in elderly.

Counseling: Instruct not to take drug if hypersensitive to salicylates (eg, aspirin). Advise patients who need to control Na+ intake that the recommended dosing of 6.6g/day provides about 756mg of Na+/day. Instruct to contact physician if worsening of ulcerative colitis symptoms is experienced. Instruct to inform physician if they have or are later diagnosed w/ renal dysfunction and/or liver disease.

GILENYA — fingolimod   Rx

Class: Sphingosine 1-phosphate receptor modulator

ADULT DOSAGE	PEDIATRIC DOSAGE
Multiple Sclerosis	Pediatric use may not have been
Treatment of relapsing forms of multiple sclerosis (MS) to reduce the frequency of clinical exacerbations and to delay the accumulation of physical disability	established
0.5mg qd	

ADMINISTRATION
Oral route

Take w/ or w/o food.
Patients who initiate therapy and those who reinitiate treatment after discontinuation for >14 days require 1st dose monitoring.

First Dose Monitoring
Administer the 1st dose in a setting in which resources to appropriately manage symptomatic bradycardia are available. Observe all patients for 6 hrs for signs/symptoms of bradycardia w/ hourly pulse and BP measurement. Obtain an ECG prior to dosing and at the end of the observation period.

Additional observation should be instituted until the finding has resolved in the following situations:
1. HR 6 hrs post-dose is <45 bpm.
2. HR 6 hrs post-dose is at the lowest value post-dose (suggesting that the max pharmacodynamic effect on the heart may not have occurred).
3. ECG 6 hrs post-dose shows new onset 2nd degree or higher atrioventricular (AV) block.

Should post-dose symptomatic bradycardia occur, initiate appropriate management, begin continuous ECG monitoring, and continue observation until the symptoms have resolved.

Should a patient require pharmacologic intervention for symptomatic bradycardia, continuous overnight ECG monitoring in a medical facility should be instituted, and the 1st dose monitoring strategy should be repeated after the 2nd dose.

Reinitiation of Therapy Following Discontinuation
If therapy is discontinued for >14 days, after the 1st month of treatment, the same precautions (1st dose monitoring) as for initial dosing should apply. W/in the first 2 weeks of treatment, 1st dose procedures are recommended after interruption of ≥1 day; during weeks 3 and 4 of treatment, 1st dose procedures are recommended after treatment interruption of >7 days.

STORAGE
25°C (77°F); excursions permitted to 15-30°C (59-86°F). Protect from moisture.

HOW SUPPLIED
Cap: 0.5mg

CONTRAINDICATIONS
Patients who in the last 6 months experienced MI, unstable angina, stroke, transient ischemic attack (TIA), decompensated heart failure (HF) requiring hospitalization, or Class III/IV HF. History/presence of Mobitz Type II 2nd- or 3rd-degree AV block or sick sinus syndrome (unless w/ functioning pacemaker), baseline QTc interval ≥500 msec, treatment w/ Class IA/III anti-arrhythmic drugs, hypersensitivity reaction to fingolimod or any of the excipients of the formulation.

WARNINGS/PRECAUTIONS
Bradyarrhythmia and AV blocks may occur; monitor during treatment initiation. Cases of syncope reported after 1st dose. May increase risk of infections; consider suspending treatment if a serious infection develops. Do not start treatment in patients w/ active acute/chronic infections until the infection(s) is resolved. Include disseminated herpetic infections in the differential diagnosis of patients receiving therapy and present w/ an atypical MS relapse or multiorgan failure. Cases of Kaposi's sarcoma reported. Cryptococcal infections reported; initiate prompt diagnostic evaluation and treatment if signs/symptoms occur. Caution when switching to fingolimod from immune-modulating or immunosuppressive medications to avoid unintended additive effects. Test for antibodies to varicella zoster virus (VZV) prior to commencing treatment in patients w/o a healthcare professional confirmed history of chickenpox or w/o a documentation of a full course of vaccination against VZV. Give VZV vaccination to antibody-negative patients; initiate therapy 1 month after vaccination. Progressive multifocal leukoencephalopathy (PML) reported; withhold therapy and perform appropriate diagnostic evaluation at the 1st sign/symptom suggestive of PML. May increase risk of macular edema; patients w/ history of uveitis or w/ diabetes mellitus (DM) are at increased risk. Posterior reversible encephalopathy syndrome (PRES) reported rarely; d/c if suspected. Dose-dependent reductions in forced expiratory volume over 1 sec and diffusion lung capacity for carbon monoxide (DLCO) reported. Liver transaminase elevations and liver injury w/ hepatocellular and/or cholestatic hepatitis reported; d/c if significant liver injury confirmed. May cause fetal harm; women of childbearing potential should use effective contraception during and for 2 months after stopping therapy. May cause HTN and decreased lymphocyte counts. Basal cell carcinoma associated w/ therapy; promptly evaluate suspicious skin lesions. Hypersensitivity reactions (eg, rash, urticaria, angioedema) reported. Caution w/ severe hepatic impairment and in elderly.

ADVERSE REACTIONS
Headache, liver transaminase elevations, influenza, abdominal/back pain, diarrhea, cough, pain in extremity, sinusitis.

DRUG INTERACTIONS
See Contraindications. Monitor patients on QT prolonging drugs w/ known risk of torsades de pointes (eg, citalopram, methadone, erythromycin) overnight w/

continuous ECG in a medical facility. Severe bradycardia or heart block may occur w/ drugs that slow the HR or AV conduction (eg, β-blockers, digoxin, HR-slowing calcium channel blockers). Increased blood levels w/ ketoconazole. May reduce the immune response to vaccination. Vaccination may be less effective during and for up to 2 months after discontinuation of treatment; avoid live attenuated vaccines during and for 2 months after treatment. Antineoplastic, immune-modulating, or immunosuppressive therapies (eg, corticosteroids) may increase the risk of immunosuppression; consider the risk of additive immune system effects if these therapies are coadministered w/ fingolimod. Consider the duration and mode of action when switching from drugs w/ prolonged immune effects (eg, natalizumab, teriflunomide, mitoxantrone) to avoid unintended additive immunosuppressive effects.

PREGNANCY AND LACTATION
Pregnancy: Category C. A pregnancy registry has been established to collect information about the effect of this drug during pregnancy.
Lactation: It is not known whether this drug is excreted in human milk. Not for use in nursing.

MECHANISM OF ACTION
Sphingosine 1-phosphate receptor modulator. Fingolimod is metabolized to the active metabolite, fingolimod-phosphate. Fingolimod-phosphate binds w/ high affinity to sphingosine 1-phosphate receptors 1, 3, 4, and 5 and blocks the capacity of lymphocytes to egress from lymph nodes, reducing the number of lymphocytes in peripheral blood. The mechanism by which fingolimod exerts its effects in MS is unknown, but may involve reduction of lymphocyte migration into the CNS.

PHARMACOKINETICS
Absorption: Absolute oral bioavailability (93%); T_{max}=12-16 hrs. **Distribution:** V_d=1200L; protein binding (>99.7%). **Metabolism:** Reversible stereoselective phosphorylation; oxidative biotransformation catalyzed by CYP4F2 and possibly other CYP4F isoenzymes; formation of inactive non-polar ceramide analogues. **Elimination:** Urine (81%, inactive metabolites), feces (<2.5%, parent drug and fingolimod-phosphate); $T_{1/2}$=6-9 days.

PATIENT CONSIDERATIONS
Assessment: Assess if MI, unstable angina, stroke, TIA, decompensated HF requiring hospitalization, or Class III/IV HF was experienced in the last 6 months. Assess for history or presence of Mobitz Type II 2nd- or 3rd-degree AV block or sick sinus syndrome, pregnancy/nursing status, any other conditions where treatment is cautioned or contraindicated, and for drug interactions. Assess ECG, CBC, and LFTs. Perform an examination of the fundus including the macula.

Monitoring: Monitor for signs/symptoms of bradyarrhythmia, AV blocks, hepatic dysfunction, infection, PML, macular edema, PRES, and other adverse reactions. Monitor BP and lymphocyte counts. Perform spirometric evaluation of respiratory function and evaluation of DLCO if clinically indicated. Perform an examination of the fundus including the macula 3-4 months after starting therapy, at any time after a patient reports visual disturbances while on therapy, and regularly in patients w/ DM or history of uveitis.

Counseling: Instruct not to d/c w/o 1st consulting the prescribing physician. Advise to contact physician if patient accidently takes more drug than prescribed. Advise that decreased HR may occur upon initiation of treatment and that observation in the clinic or other facility for at least 6 hrs after the 1st dose will be required. Instruct to contact physician if symptoms of infection, new onset/worsening of dyspnea, unexplained N/V, abdominal pain, fatigue, anorexia, jaundice, dark urine, and/or any changes in vision develop. Instruct to delay treatment w/ fingolimod until after VZV vaccination if patient has not had chickenpox or a previous VZV vaccination. Inform on the importance of contacting the physician if symptoms suggestive of PML develop; explain that typical symptoms are diverse, progress over days to weeks, and include progressive weakness on one side of the body or clumsiness of limbs, disturbance of vision, and changes in thinking, memory, and orientation leading to confusion and personality changes. Advise women of childbearing age to use effective contraception during and for 2 months after stopping treatment. Inform that drug remains in the blood and continues to have effects for up to 2 months following the last dose. Advise that basal cell carcinoma is associated w/ therapy, and that suspicious skin lesions should be promptly evaluated. Advise that drug may cause hypersensitivity reactions, and to contact physician if any symptoms occur.

GILOTRIF — afatinib   Rx
Class: Kinase inhibitor

ADULT DOSAGE
Metastatic Non-Small Cell Lung Cancer

1st-line Treatment for Tumors Which Have Epidermal Growth Factor Receptor (EGFR) Exon 19 Deletions or Exon 21 (L858R) Substitution Mutations:
40mg qd until disease progression or no longer tolerated

Metastatic Squamous Non-Small Cell Lung Cancer (NSCLC) Progressing After Platinum-Based Chemotherapy:
40mg qd until disease progression or no longer tolerated

Missed Dose

Do not take a missed dose w/in 12 hrs of the next dose

PEDIATRIC DOSAGE
Pediatric use may not have been established

DOSING CONSIDERATIONS
Concomitant Medications
If P-gp Inhibitor is Required:
Reduce afatinib daily dose by 10mg if not tolerated; resume previous dose after discontinuation of the P-gp inhibitor as tolerated

If Chronic Therapy w/ a P-gp Inducer is Required:
Increase afatinib daily dose by 10mg as tolerated; resume previous dose 2-3 days after discontinuation of the P-gp inducer

Renal Impairment
Severe (GFR 15-29mL/min/1.73m²):
Initial: 30mg qd

Hepatic Impairment
Severe (Child-Pugh C): Closely monitor and adjust dose if not tolerated

Adverse Reactions
Withhold for Any Adverse Reactions Of:
1. NCI CTCAE Grade ≥3
2. Diarrhea of Grade ≥2 persisting for ≥2 consecutive days while taking antidiarrheal medication
3. Cutaneous reactions of Grade 2 that are prolonged (lasting >7 days) or intolerable
4. Renal impairment of ≥Grade 2
Resume treatment when adverse reaction fully resolves, returns to baseline, or improves to Grade 1; reinstitute at a reduced dose (eg, 10mg/day less than the dose at which the adverse reaction occurred)

Permanently D/C For:
1. Life-threatening bullous, blistering, or exfoliative skin lesions
2. Confirmed interstitial lung disease (ILD)
3. Severe drug-induced hepatic impairment
4. Persistent ulcerative keratitis
5. Symptomatic left ventricular dysfunction
6. Severe or intolerable adverse reaction occurring at a dose of 20mg/day

ADMINISTRATION
Oral route

Take at least 1 hr ac or 2 hrs pc.

STORAGE
25°C (77°F); excursions permitted to 15-30°C (59-86°F). Protect from exposure to high humidity and light.

HOW SUPPLIED
Tab: 20mg, 30mg, 40mg

WARNINGS/PRECAUTIONS
See Dosing Considerations. Select patients for first-line treatment of metastatic NSCLC based on the presence of EGFR exon 19 deletions or exon 21 (L858R) substitution mutations in tumor specimens. May cause diarrhea that results in dehydration w/ or w/o renal impairment; provide an antidiarrheal agent (eg, loperamide) for administration at onset of diarrhea and continue anti-diarrheal therapy until loose bowel movements cease for 12 hrs. Bullous and exfoliative skin disorders (eg, toxic epidermal necrolysis, Stevens-Johnson syndrome) reported. ILD or ILD-like adverse reactions (eg, lung infiltration, pneumonitis, acute respiratory distress syndrome) reported; withhold therapy during evaluation of patients w/ suspected ILD and d/c in patients w/ confirmed ILD. Liver test abnormalities reported; withhold therapy in patients who develop worsening liver function and d/c in patients who develop severe hepatic impairment while on therapy. Keratitis reported; withhold during evaluation of patients w/ suspected keratitis. Interrupt or d/c therapy if diagnosis of ulcerative keratitis is confirmed. Caution w/ a history of keratitis, ulcerative keratitis, or severe dry eye. May cause fetal harm.

ADVERSE REACTIONS
Diarrhea, rash/acneiform dermatitis, stomatitis, paronychia, dry skin, decreased appetite, N/V, pruritus.

DRUG INTERACTIONS
See Dosing Considerations. P-gp inhibitors (eg, ritonavir, ketoconazole, verapamil) may increase exposure. P-gp inducers (eg, rifampicin, carbamazepine, phenytoin) may decrease exposure.

PREGNANCY AND LACTATION
Pregnancy: May cause fetal harm.
Lactation: Lactating woman should not breastfeed during treatment and for 2 weeks after the final dose.
Reproductive Potential: Females of reproductive potential should use effective contraception during treatment and for at least 2 weeks after the last dose. May reduce fertility in females and males of reproductive potential.

MECHANISM OF ACTION
Tyrosine kinase inhibitor; covalently binds to the kinase domains of EGFR (ErbB1), HER2 (ErbB2), and HER4 (ErbB4) and irreversibly inhibits tyrosine kinase autophosphorylation, resulting in downregulation of ErbB signaling.

PHARMACOKINETICS
Absorption: T_{max}=2-5 hrs. **Distribution:** Plasma protein binding (approx 95%). **Metabolism:** Covalent adducts to proteins (major circulating metabolites); enzymatic metabolism (minimal). **Elimination:** Feces (85%), urine (4%); $T_{1/2}$=37 hrs.

PATIENT CONSIDERATIONS
Assessment: Assess for history of keratitis, ulcerative keratitis, severe dry eye, renal/hepatic impairment, pregnancy/nursing status, and possible drug interactions. Assess for presence of EGFR exon 19 deletions or exon 21 (L858R) substitution mutations in tumor specimens in patients receiving treatment for EGFR mutation-positive metastatic NSCLC.

Monitoring: Monitor for diarrhea, cutaneous reactions, renal dysfunction, ILD, hepatic toxicity, keratitis, symptomatic left ventricular dysfunction, and other adverse reactions. Obtain periodic liver testing during treatment.

Counseling: Advise to notify physician if diarrhea develops and instruct to seek medical attention promptly for severe/persistent diarrhea. Advise to minimize sun exposure w/ protective clothing and to use sunscreen while taking therapy. Instruct to immediately report any new/worsening lung symptoms, or any combination of the following symptoms: trouble breathing or SOB, cough, or fever. Advise to immediately report any symptoms of a liver problem, eye problems, and for any of the following: new onset or worsening SOB or exercise intolerance, cough, fatigue, swelling of the ankles/legs, palpitations, or sudden weight gain. Advise not to take a missed dose w/in 12 hrs of the next dose. Advise females of reproductive potential to use highly effective contraception during treatment, and for at least 2 weeks after taking the last dose. Advise to d/c nursing while taking therapy and for 2 weeks after the last dose.

GLEEVEC — imatinib mesylate   Rx

Class: Kinase inhibitor

ADULT DOSAGE

Hypereosinophilic Syndrome/Chronic Eosinophilic Leukemia

In patients who have the FIP1L1-PDGFRα fusion kinase (mutational analysis or FISH demonstration of CHIC2 allele deletion) and for patients who are FIP1L1-PDGFRα fusion kinase negative or unknown

400mg/day

Demonstrated FIP1L1-PDGFRα Fusion Kinase:
Initial: 100mg qd
Titrate: May increase to 400mg qd in the absence of adverse reactions if response is insufficient

Dermatofibrosarcoma Protuberans

Unresectable, Recurrent, and/or Metastatic:
800mg/day (as 400mg bid)

Kit (CD117)-Positive Gastrointestinal Stromal Tumors

Unresectable and/or Metastatic Malignant:
400mg qd
Titrate: May increase up to 800mg/day (as 400mg bid) as clinically indicated

Adjuvant Treatment Following Complete Gross Resection:
400mg qd; optimal treatment duration unknown

Ph+ Chronic Myeloid Leukemia

Newly diagnosed patients in chronic phase and patients in blast crisis, accelerated phase, or in chronic phase after failure of interferon-alpha therapy

Chronic Phase:
400mg qd
Titrate: May increase to 600mg qd

Accelerated Phase/Blast Crisis:
600mg qd
Titrate: May increase to 800mg/day (as 400mg bid)

A dose increase may be considered in the absence of severe adverse reaction and severe non-leukemia related neutropenia or thrombocytopenia in the following circumstances: disease progression (at any time), failure to achieve a satisfactory hematologic response after at least 3 months of treatment, failure to achieve a cytogenetic response after 6-12 months of treatment, or loss of a previously achieved hematologic or cytogenetic response

Ph+ Acute Lymphoblastic Leukemia

Relapsed/Refractory:
600mg qd

Myelodysplastic/Myeloproliferative Diseases

PEDIATRIC DOSAGE

Ph+ Chronic Myeloid Leukemia

Newly Diagnosed Patients in Chronic Phase:
≥1 Year:
340mg/m²/day
Max: 600mg/day

Dose can be given qd or split in 2 (am and pm)

Ph+ Acute Lymphoblastic Leukemia

In Combination w/ Chemotherapy for Newly Diagnosed Patients:
≥1 Year:
340mg/m² qd
Max: 600mg qd

Associated w/ PDGFR Gene Re-Arrangements:
400mg qd

Determine PDGFRb gene rearrangements status prior to initiating treatment w/ an FDA-approved test

Aggressive Systemic Mastocytosis

Determine D816V c-Kit mutation status prior to initiating treatment w/ an FDA-approved test

W/O D816V c-Kit Mutation:
400mg qd

c-Kit Mutational Status Unknown/Unavailable:
400mg qd may be considered for patients not responding satisfactorily to other therapies

Associated w/ Eosinophilia:
Initial: 100mg qd
Titrate: May increase to 400mg qd in the absence of adverse reactions if response is insufficient

DOSING CONSIDERATIONS
Concomitant Medications
Strong CYP3A4 Inducers: Avoid use; if necessary, increase imatinib dose by at least 50% and carefully monitor clinical response

Renal Impairment
Mild (CrCl 40-59mL/min):
Max: 600mg

Moderate (CrCl 20-39mL/min):
Initial: Reduce dose by 50%; future doses can be increased as tolerated
Max: 400mg

Severe (CrCl <20mL/min): Use w/ caution; a dose of 100mg/day was tolerated in 2 patients w/ severe renal impairment

Hepatic Impairment
Mild and Moderate: Dose adjustment is not required
Severe: Reduce dose by 25%

Adverse Reactions
Bilirubin >3X Institutional ULN (IULN) or Liver Transaminases >5X IULN:
1. Withhold therapy until bilirubin levels return to <1.5X IULN and transaminase levels to <2.5X IULN
2. Continue treatment at a reduced daily dose:
Adults: 400mg to 300mg, 600mg to 400mg, or 800mg to 600mg
Pediatrics: 340mg/m²/day to 260mg/m²/day

Severe Nonhematologic (eg, Severe Hepatotoxicity, Severe Fluid Retention):
Withhold therapy until the event has resolved; resume treatment as appropriate depending on initial severity of event

Neutropenia/Thrombocytopenia:
ANC <1.0 x 10⁹/L and/or Platelets <50 x 10⁹/L:
Adults:

Initial Dose 100mg:
1. Withhold treatment until ANC ≥1.5 x 10⁹/L and platelets ≥75 x 10⁹/L
2. Resume treatment at previous dose (dose before severe adverse reaction)

Initial Dose 400mg:
1. Withhold treatment until ANC ≥1.5 x 10⁹/L and platelets ≥75 x 10⁹/L
2. Resume treatment at the original starting dose of 400mg
3. If recurrence of ANC <1.0 x 10⁹/L and/or platelets <50 x 10⁹/L, repeat step 1 and resume at a reduced dose of 300mg

Initial Dose 800mg:
1. Withhold treatment until ANC ≥1.5 x 10⁹/L and platelets ≥75 x 10⁹/L
2. Resume treatment at 600mg
3. In the event of recurrence of ANC <1.0 x 10⁹/L and/or platelets <50 x 10⁹/L, repeat step 1 and resume at reduced dose of 400mg

Pediatrics:
Initial Dose 340mg/m²:
1. Withhold treatment until ANC ≥1.5 x 10⁹/L and platelets ≥75 x 10⁹/L
2. Resume treatment at previous dose (dose before severe adverse reaction)
3. In the event of recurrence of ANC <1.0 x 10⁹/L and/or platelets <50 x 10⁹/L, repeat step 1 and resume at reduced dose of 260mg/m²

ANC <0.5 x 10⁹/L and/or Platelets <10 x 10⁹/L:
Adults:
Initial Dose 600mg:
1. Check if cytopenia is related to leukemia (marrow aspirate or biopsy)
2. If cytopenia is unrelated to leukemia, reduce dose to 400mg
3. If cytopenia persists 2 weeks, reduce further to 300mg
4. If cytopenia persists 4 weeks and is still unrelated to leukemia, withhold treatment until ANC ≥1 x 10⁹/L and platelets ≥20 x 10⁹/L and then resume treatment at 300mg

ADMINISTRATION
Oral route

Take w/ a meal and a large glass of water.
Do not crush tabs.

Doses of 400mg or 600mg should be administered qd, whereas a dose of 800mg should be administered as 400mg bid. Doses ≥800mg/day should be accomplished using the 400mg tab to reduce iron exposure.
Treatment may be continued as long as there is no evidence of progressive disease or unacceptable toxicity.

Patients Unable to Swallow Tabs
1. Disperse tabs in a glass of water or apple juice.
2. Required number of tabs should be placed in the appropriate volume of beverage (approx 50mL for a 100mg tab and 200mL for a 400mg tab).
3. Stir w/ a spoon and administer immediately after complete disintegration of tab.

STORAGE
25°C (77°F); excursions permitted to 15-30°C (59-86°F). Protect from moisture.

HOW SUPPLIED
Tab: 100mg*, 400mg* *scored

WARNINGS/PRECAUTIONS
Edema and serious fluid retention reported. Hematologic toxicity (eg, anemia/neutropenia/thrombocytopenia) reported; perform CBCs weekly for the 1st month, biweekly for the 2nd month, and periodically thereafter as clinically indicated (eg, every 2-3 months). CHF and left ventricular dysfunction reported; carefully monitor patients w/ cardiac disease or risk factors for cardiac failure or history of renal failure, and evaluate/treat any patient w/ cardiac or renal failure. Hepatotoxicity may occur. Cases of fatal liver failure and severe liver injury requiring liver transplants reported. Grade 3/4 hemorrhages in clinical studies in patients w/ newly diagnosed CML and w/ GIST reported. GI tumor sites may be the source of GI hemorrhages; GI hemorrhage in patients w/ newly diagnosed Ph+ CML reported, and gastric antral vascular ectasia reported. GI irritation/perforation reported. In patients w/ HES w/ occult infiltration of HES cells w/in the myocardium, cases of cardiogenic shock/left ventricular dysfunction have been associated w/ HES cell degranulation upon initiation of therapy; reversible w/ administration of systemic steroids, circulatory support measures, and temporarily withholding treatment. Consider echocardiogram and determination of serum troponin in patients w/ HES/CEL, MDS/MPD, or ASM associated w/ high eosinophil levels; if either is abnormal, consider prophylactic use of systemic steroids (1-2mg/kg) for 1-2 weeks concomitantly at initiation of therapy. Bullous dermatologic reactions, including erythema multiforme and Stevens-Johnson syndrome, reported. May cause fetal harm; sexually active female patients of reproductive potential should use highly effective contraception during treatment and for 14 days after stopping therapy. Growth retardation reported in children and preadolescents; closely monitor growth. Tumor lysis syndrome (TLS) reported in patients w/ CML, GIST, ALL, and eosinophilic leukemia; caution in patients at risk of TLS (those w/ tumors w/ high proliferative rate or high tumor burden prior to treatment), and correct dehydration and treat high uric acid levels prior to initiation of treatment. May impair mental/physical abilities.

ADVERSE REACTIONS
N/V, edema, muscle cramps, musculoskeletal pain, diarrhea, rash, fatigue, headache, abdominal pain.

DRUG INTERACTIONS
See Dosing Considerations. Concomitant administration w/ strong CYP3A4 inducers may reduce total exposure of imatinib; consider alternative agents. Concomitant administration w/ strong CYP3A4 inhibitors may significantly increase imatinib levels. Grapefruit juice may increase levels; avoid grapefruit juice. Imatinib will increase levels of CYP3A4 substrates (eg, triazolo-benzodiazepines, dihydropyridine calcium channel blockers, certain HMG-CoA reductase inhibitors); caution when administering w/ CYP3A4 substrates that have a narrow therapeutic window. Because warfarin is metabolized by CYP2C9 and CYP3A4, use low-molecular weight or standard heparin instead of warfarin in patients who require anticoagulation. Use caution when administering w/ CYP2D6 substrates that have a narrow therapeutic window. When concomitantly used w/ chemotherapy, liver toxicity reported; monitor hepatic function. Hypothyroidism reported in thyroidectomy patients undergoing levothyroxine replacement; closely monitor TSH levels.

PREGNANCY AND LACTATION
Pregnancy: May cause fetal harm when administered to a pregnant woman. Women should avoid pregnancy during therapy.
Lactation: Imatinib and its active metabolite are excreted into human milk. Not for use in nursing.
Reproductive Potential: Test pregnancy status in females w/ reproductive potential prior to the initiation of treatment. Females of reproductive potential should use effective contraception (methods that result in <1% pregnancy rates) during treatment and for 14 days after stopping treatment.

MECHANISM OF ACTION
Protein-tyrosine kinase inhibitor; inhibits the BCR-ABL tyrosine kinase, the constitutive abnormal tyrosine kinase created by the Philadelphia chromosome abnormality in CML. Inhibits proliferation and induces apoptosis in BCR-ABL positive cell lines as well as fresh leukemic cells from Ph+ CML. Inhibits the receptor tyrosine kinases for PDGF and SCF, c-Kit, and inhibits PDGF- and SCF-mediated cellular events. Inhibits proliferation and induces apoptosis in GIST cells, which express an activating c-Kit mutation, in vitro.

PHARMACOKINETICS
Absorption: Well-absorbed. Absolute bioavailability (98%); T_{max}=2-4 hrs.
Distribution: Plasma protein binding (95%); found in breast milk. **Metabolism:** Liver via CYP3A4 (major), CYP1A2, CYP2D6, CYP2C9, CYP2C19 (minor); N-demethylated piperazine derivative (major active metabolite). **Elimination:** Feces (68%, 20% unchanged), urine (13%, 5% unchanged); $T_{1/2}$=18 hrs (imatinib), 40 hrs (active metabolite).

PATIENT CONSIDERATIONS
Assessment: Assess for cardiac disease, renal impairment, dehydration, high uric acid levels, pregnancy/nursing status, and possible drug interactions. Perform echocardiogram and determine troponin levels in patients w/ HES/CEL and w/ MDS/MPD or ASM associated w/ high eosinophil levels. Obtain baseline CBC and LFTs.
Monitoring: Monitor for signs and symptoms of fluid retention, CHF, left ventricular dysfunction, hemorrhage, GI disorders, TLS, bullous dermatologic reactions, and other adverse events. Perform CBCs weekly for the 1st month, biweekly for the 2nd month, and periodically thereafter. Monitor LFTs monthly or as clinically indicated. Monitor growth in children, and TSH levels in thyroidectomy patients undergoing levothyroxine replacement.
Counseling: Instruct to take drug exactly as prescribed and not to change the dose or to stop taking the medication unless told to do so by physician. Inform of the possibility of developing edema and fluid retention; instruct to contact physician if unexpected rapid weight gain occurs. Inform of the possibility of developing liver function abnormalities and serious hepatic toxicity; instruct to immediately contact physician if signs of liver failure occur (eg, jaundice, anorexia, bleeding, bruising). Advise women of reproductive potential to avoid becoming pregnant and instruct to notify physician if pregnant. Instruct females of reproductive potential to use highly effective contraception during treatment and for 14 days after stopping treatment. Instruct to avoid breastfeeding during treatment and for 1 month after the last dose. Inform that the drug and certain other medicines can interact w/ each other; advise to inform physician if taking/planning to take iron supplements. Inform to avoid grapefruit juice and other foods known to inhibit CYP3A4 while on therapy. Advise that growth retardation has been reported in children and preadolescents, and that growth should be monitored. Caution about driving a car or operating machinery.

GLEOSTINE — lomustine ⬛ Rx
Class: Nitrosourea alkylating agent

> Causes myelosuppression including fatal myelosuppression. Myelosuppression is delayed, dose-related, cumulative and may occur 4-6 weeks after administration and persist for 1-2 weeks. Cumulative myelosuppression is manifested by greater severity and longer duration of cytopenias. Monitor blood counts for ≥6 weeks after each dose. Do not give more frequently than one dose every 6 weeks. Prescribe, dispense, and administer only enough caps for one dose; fatal toxicity occurs w/ overdosage.

OTHER BRAND NAMES
CeeNU (Discontinued)

ADULT DOSAGE	PEDIATRIC DOSAGE
Brain Tumors	**Brain Tumors**
For both primary and metastatic tumors, in patients who have already received appropriate surgical and/or radiotherapeutic procedures	For both primary and metastatic tumors, in patients who have already received appropriate surgical and/or radiotherapeutic procedures
130mg/m² single dose every 6 weeks; round doses to nearest 5mg	130mg/m² single dose every 6 weeks; round doses to nearest 5mg
Compromised Bone Marrow Function: Reduce dose to 100mg/m² every 6 weeks	**Compromised Bone Marrow Function:** Reduce dose to 100mg/m² every 6 weeks
Hodgkin's Disease	**Hodgkin's Disease**
Combination chemotherapy for the treatment of patients w/ Hodgkin's lymphoma whose disease has progressed following initial chemotherapy.	As secondary therapy in combination w/ other approved drugs in patients who relapse while being treated w/ primary therapy, or who fail to respond to primary therapy
130mg/m² single dose every 6 weeks; round doses to nearest 5mg	130mg/m² single dose every 6 weeks; round doses to nearest 5mg
Compromised Bone Marrow Function: Reduce dose to 100mg/m² every 6 weeks	**Compromised Bone Marrow Function:** Reduce dose to 100mg/m² every 6 weeks

DOSING CONSIDERATIONS
Concomitant Medications
Myelosuppressive Drugs: Reduce dose accordingly

Adverse Reactions
Perform weekly CBC and withhold each subsequent dose for >6 weeks if needed until platelet counts recover to ≥100,000/mm³ and leukocytes recover to ≥4000/mm³
Dose Adjustments Based on Nadir After Previous Dose:
Leukocytes 2000-2999/mm³, Platelets 25,000-74,999/mm³: Reduce dose by 30%
Leukocytes <2000/mm³, Platelets <25,000/mm³: Reduce dose by 50%

ADMINISTRATION
Oral route

STORAGE
25°C (77°F); excursions permitted to 15-30°C (59-86°F). Avoid temperatures >40°C (104°F). Cytotoxic drug; follow special handling/disposal procedures.

HOW SUPPLIED
Cap: 5mg, 10mg, 40mg, 100mg

WARNINGS/PRECAUTIONS

Pulmonary toxicity characterized by pulmonary infiltrates and/or fibrosis reported; increased risk w/ baseline <70% of the predicted forced vital capacity or carbon monoxide diffusing capacity. Onset of pulmonary toxicity occurs after an interval of ≥6 months from the start of therapy, w/ cumulative doses >1100mg/m^2. Obtain baseline pulmonary function tests and repeat frequently during treatment. Permanently d/c w/ pulmonary fibrosis. Secondary malignancies (eg, acute leukemia, myelodysplasia) reported w/ long-term use. Hepatic toxicity, manifested by increased levels of transaminases, alkaline phosphatase, and bilirubin reported. Progressive renal failure w/ a decrease in kidney size reported; monitor renal function. May cause fetal harm. Caution in elderly.

ADVERSE REACTIONS

Delayed myelosuppression, N/V, stomatitis, alopecia.

PREGNANCY AND LACTATION

Pregnancy: May cause fetal harm.
Lactation: Do not breastfeed during treatment and for 2 weeks after the final dose.
Females and Males of Reproductive Potential: Females of reproductive potential should use effective contraception during treatment and for 2 weeks after final dose. Males w/ female partners of reproductive potential should use effective contraception during treatment and for 3.5 months after final dose. May reduce fertility in males and females of reproductive potential.

MECHANISM OF ACTION

Nitrosourea alkylating agent; alkylates DNA and RNA. May also inhibit several key enzymatic processes by carbamoylation of amino acids in proteins.

PHARMACOKINETICS

Distribution: Crosses blood-brain barrier. **Elimination:** Urine (50%, metabolites). $T_{1/2}$=16-48 hrs (metabolites).

PATIENT CONSIDERATIONS

Assessment: Assess for pregnancy/nursing status, and for possible drug interactions. Obtain baseline CBC, renal/hepatic function, and pulmonary function.

Monitoring: Monitor for myelosuppression, pulmonary toxicity, secondary malignancies, and for other adverse reactions. Monitor LFTs and renal function tests periodically, pulmonary function tests frequently, and blood counts weekly for ≥6 weeks after a dose.

Counseling: Advise that periodic assessment of blood counts are required; advise to contact healthcare provider for new onset of bleeding or fever or symptoms of infection. Advise that toxicity including fatal toxicity occurs w/ overdosage; advise to take as a single oral dose that will not be repeated for 6 weeks. Inform that there may be ≥2 different strengths and colors of caps. Advise to contact healthcare provider for new or worsening cough, chest pain, or shortness of breath. Inform that treatment can cause hepatotoxicity and that liver function monitoring during treatment is necessary. Inform that treatment can cause nephrotoxicity and that renal function and electrolyte monitoring during treatment is necessary. Advise females of reproductive potential of the potential risk to a fetus and instruct to inform their healthcare provider of a known or suspected pregnancy. Advise females of reproductive potential to use effective contraception during treatment and for at least 2 weeks after final dose. Advise male patients w/ female partners of reproductive potential to use condoms during treatment and for 4 months after the final dose. Advise not to breastfeed during treatment and for 2 weeks after the final dose. Advise females and males of reproductive potential of the potential for reduced fertility.

GLIMEPIRIDE — glimepiride   Rx

Class: Sulfonylurea (2nd generation)

OTHER BRAND NAMES

Amaryl

ADULT DOSAGE

Type 2 Diabetes Mellitus

Initial: 1mg or 2mg qd
Titrate: After reaching 2mg/day, may further increase dose in increments of 1mg or 2mg based on glycemic response, not more frequently than every 1-2 weeks
Max: 8mg qd

PEDIATRIC DOSAGE

Pediatric use may not have been established

DOSING CONSIDERATIONS

Concomitant Medications

Colesevelam: Administer at least 4 hrs prior to colesevelam

Renal Impairment

Initial: 1mg qd
Titrate: Adjust conservatively
Max: 8mg qd

Elderly

Initial: 1mg qd
Titrate: Adjust conservatively
Max: 8mg qd

ADMINISTRATION

Oral route

Administer w/ breakfast or the 1st main meal of the day.

STORAGE

20-25°C (68-77°F). (Amaryl) 25°C (77°F); excursions permitted to 20-25°C (68-77°F).

HOW SUPPLIED

Tab: 3mg*, 6mg*, 8mg*; (Amaryl) 1mg*, 2mg*, 4mg* *scored

CONTRAINDICATIONS

History of a hypersensitivity reaction to glimepiride or any of the product's ingredients, history of an allergic reaction to sulfonamide derivatives.

WARNINGS/PRECAUTIONS

Not for treatment of type 1 DM or diabetic ketoacidosis. Patients being transferred from longer $T_{1/2}$ sulfonylureas (eg, chlorpropamide) may have overlapping drug effect for 1-2 weeks; monitor for hypoglycemia. May cause severe hypoglycemia, which may impair mental/physical abilities; caution in patients predisposed to hypoglycemia. Early warning symptoms of hypoglycemia may be different/less pronounced in patients w/ autonomic neuropathy and in the elderly. Hypersensitivity reactions (eg, anaphylaxis, angioedema, Stevens-Johnson syndrome) reported; if suspected, promptly d/c therapy, assess for other potential causes for the reaction, and institute alternative treatment. May cause hemolytic anemia; caution w/ G6PD deficiency and consider the use of a non-sulfonylurea alternative. Increased risk of cardiovascular mortality. Caution in elderly.

ADVERSE REACTIONS

Dizziness, nausea, asthenia, headache, hypoglycemia, flu syndrome.

DRUG INTERACTIONS

See Dosage. Oral antidiabetic medications, pramlintide acetate, insulin, ACE inhibitors, H$_2$-receptor antagonists, fibrates, propoxyphene, pentoxifylline, somatostatin analogues, anabolic steroids and androgens, cyclophosphamide, phenyramidol, guanethidine, fluconazole, sulfinpyrazone, tetracyclines, clarithromycin, disopyramide, quinolones, and drugs that are highly protein-bound (eg, fluoxetine, NSAIDs, salicylates, sulfonamides, chloramphenicol, coumarins, probenecid, MAOIs) may increase glucose-lowering effect; monitor for hypoglycemia during coadministration and for worsening glycemic control during withdrawal of these drugs. Danazol, glucagon, somatropin, protease inhibitors, atypical antipsychotics (eg, olanzapine, clozapine), barbiturates, diazoxide, laxatives, rifampin, thiazides and other diuretics, corticosteroids, phenothiazines, thyroid hormones, estrogens, oral contraceptives, phenytoin, nicotinic acid, sympathomimetics (eg, epinephrine, albuterol, terbutaline), and isoniazid may reduce glucose-lowering effect; monitor for worsening glycemic control during coadministration and for hypoglycemia during withdrawal of these drugs. β-blockers, clonidine, reserpine, and alcohol intake may potentiate or weaken glucose-lowering effect. Signs of hypoglycemia may be reduced or absent w/ sympatholytic drugs (eg, β-blockers, clonidine, guanethidine, reserpine). Potential interaction leading to severe hypoglycemia reported w/ oral miconazole. May interact w/ inhibitors (eg, fluconazole) and inducers (eg, rifampin) of CYP2C9. Colesevelam may reduce levels.

PREGNANCY AND LACTATION

Category C, not for use in nursing.

MECHANISM OF ACTION

Sulfonylurea (2nd generation); lowers blood glucose by stimulating insulin release from pancreatic β cells.

PHARMACOKINETICS

Absorption: T_{max}=2-3 hrs. **Distribution:** (IV) V_d=8.8L; plasma protein binding (>99.5%). **Metabolism:** Complete by oxidation; cyclohexyl hydroxy methyl derivative (M1) (via CYP2C9) and carboxyl derivative (M2) (major metabolites). **Elimination:** Urine (60%, 80-90% metabolites), feces (40%, 70% metabolites).

PATIENT CONSIDERATIONS

Assessment: Assess for hypersensitivity to drug or sulfonamide derivatives, predisposition to hypoglycemia, autonomic neuropathy, G6PD deficiency, pregnancy/nursing status, and possible drug interactions.

Monitoring: Monitor for hypoglycemia, hypersensitivity reactions, hemolytic anemia, and other adverse reactions.

Counseling: Inform about importance of adherence to dietary instructions, a regular exercise program, and regular testing of blood glucose. Advise about potential side effects (eg, hypoglycemia, weight gain). Inform about the symptoms and treatment of hypoglycemia, and the conditions that predispose to it. Inform that ability to concentrate and react may be impaired as a result of hypoglycemia; caution when driving/operating machinery. Advise to inform physician if pregnant/breastfeeding or contemplating pregnancy/breastfeeding.

GLIPIZIDE/METFORMIN — glipizide/metformin hydrochloride Rx

Class: Biguanide/sulfonylurea

> Cases of metformin-associated lactic acidosis resulting in death, hypothermia, hypotension, and resistant bradyarrhythmias reported; risk factors include renal impairment, concomitant use of certain drugs (eg, cationic drugs such as topiramate), age ≥65 years, having a radiological study w/ contrast, surgery and other procedures, hypoxic states (eg, acute CHF), excessive alcohol intake, and hepatic impairment. D/C therapy immediately and institute general supportive measures in a hospital setting if metformin-associated lactic acidosis is suspected.

OTHER BRAND NAMES

Metaglip (Discontinued)

ADULT DOSAGE
Type 2 Diabetes Mellitus
Inadequate Glycemic Control on Diet and Exercise Alone:
Initial: 2.5mg/250mg qd w/ a meal; may consider an initial dose of 2.5mg/500mg bid if FPG is 280-320mg/dL
Titrate: Increase by 1 tab/day every 2 weeks
Max: (10mg/2000mg)/day in divided doses

Inadequately Controlled on Glipizide (or another Sulfonylurea) and/or Metformin:
Initial: 2.5mg/500mg or 5mg/500mg bid w/ am and pm meals; starting dose should not exceed the daily doses of the individual components already being taken
Titrate: Increase by no more than (5mg/500mg)/day
Max: (20mg/2000mg)/day

DOSING CONSIDERATIONS
Concomitant Medications
Colesevelam: Administer at least 4 hrs prior to colesevelam

Renal Impairment
eGFR 30-45mL/min/1.73m²: Initiation of therapy is not recommended
eGFR <30mL/min/1.73m²: Contraindicated
If eGFR Falls <45mL/min/1.73m² During Therapy: Assess benefit/risk of continuing therapy
If eGFR Falls <30mL/min/1.73m² During Therapy: D/C

Hepatic Impairment
Not recommended

Pregnancy
Not recommended for use during pregnancy

Elderly
Elderly/Debilitated/Malnourished:
Initial/Maint: Dose conservatively; do not titrate to max dose

Other Important Considerations
Iodinated Contrast Imaging Procedures:
D/C therapy at the time of, or prior to, an iodinated contrast imaging procedure in patients w/ an eGFR 30-60mL/min/1.73m²; in patients w/ a history of liver disease, alcoholism, or heart failure; or in patients who will be administered intra-arterial iodinated contrast. Reevaluate eGFR 48 hrs after the imaging procedure and restart therapy if renal function is stable

ADMINISTRATION
Oral route

Take w/ meals.

STORAGE
20-25°C (68-77°F).

HOW SUPPLIED
Tab: (Glipizide/Metformin) 2.5mg/250mg, 2.5mg/500mg, 5mg/500mg

CONTRAINDICATIONS
Severe renal impairment (eGFR <30mL/min/1.73m²); known hypersensitivity to glipizide or metformin HCl; acute or chronic metabolic acidosis, including diabetic ketoacidosis, w/ or w/o coma.

WARNINGS/PRECAUTIONS
See Dosing Considerations. May be associated w/ increased cardiovascular (CV) mortality. May cause hypoglycemia; increased risk when caloric intake is deficient, when strenuous exercise is not compensated by caloric supplementation, w/ renal/hepatic or adrenal/pituitary insufficiency, w/ alcohol intoxication, and in elderly, debilitated, or malnourished patients. Hypoglycemia may be difficult to recognize in the elderly. Use not recommended during pregnancy. **Glipizide:** May cause hemolytic anemia; caution w/ G6PD deficiency and consider a non-sulfonylurea alternative. **Metformin:** Temporarily d/c while patient has restricted food and fluid intake. Prompt hemodialysis is recommended in patients w/ a diagnosis or strong suspicion of lactic acidosis. D/C if a condition associated w/ hypoxemia occurs (eg, cardiovascular collapse, acute MI, sepsis). May decrease vitamin B12 levels; monitor hematologic parameters annually.

ADVERSE REACTIONS
URI, HTN, headache, diarrhea, dizziness, musculoskeletal pain, N/V, abdominal pain.

DRUG INTERACTIONS
See Boxed Warning and Dosing Considerations. Increased risk of hypoglycemia w/ other glucose-lowering agents or ethanol. May be difficult to recognize hypoglycemia w/ β-blockers. Thiazides and other diuretics, corticosteroids, phenothiazines, thyroid products, estrogens, oral contraceptives, phenytoin, nicotinic acid, sympathomimetics, calcium channel blockers, and isoniazid may produce hyperglycemia and may lead to loss of blood glucose control; monitor closely for loss of control during coadministration and for hypoglycemia during withdrawal of these drugs. **Glipizide:** Hypoglycemic action may be potentiated by NSAIDs, some azoles, other highly protein-bound drugs, salicylates, sulfonamides, chloramphenicol, probenecid, coumarins, MAOIs, and β-blockers;

PEDIATRIC DOSAGE
Pediatric use may not have been established

----

monitor closely for hypoglycemia during coadministration and for loss of blood glucose control during withdrawal of these drugs. Potential interaction leading to severe hypoglycemia reported w/ oral miconazole. Fluconazole may increase exposure. Colesevelam may reduce levels. **Metformin:** Furosemide, nifedipine, and cimetidine may increase levels. May decrease furosemide levels and may decrease furosemide $T_{1/2}$. Drugs that are eliminated by renal tubular secretion, drugs that impair renal function, drugs that result in significant hemodynamic change, drugs that interfere w/ acid-base balance, or drugs that increase metformin accumulation may increase the risk of metformin-associated lactic acidosis; consider more frequent monitoring of these patients. Avoid excessive alcohol intake. Carbonic anhydrase inhibitors (eg, zonisamide, acetazolamide, dichlorphenamide) may increase the risk of lactic acidosis; consider more frequent monitoring of these patients.

PREGNANCY AND LACTATION
Pregnancy: Category C. Prolonged severe hypoglycemia (4-10 days) reported in neonates born to mothers who were receiving a sulfonylurea drug at the time of delivery. Use not recommended during pregnancy; however, if used, d/c at least 1 month before the expected delivery date.
Lactation: Not for use in nursing.

MECHANISM OF ACTION
Glipizide: Sulfonylurea; lowers blood glucose acutely by stimulating the release of insulin from the pancreas. **Metformin:** Biguanide; decreases hepatic glucose production, decreases intestinal absorption of glucose, and improves insulin sensitivity by increasing peripheral glucose uptake and utilization.

PHARMACOKINETICS
Absorption: Glipizide: Rapid, complete. T_{max}=1-3 hrs. Metformin: Absolute bioavailability (50-60%) (500mg); C_{max}=1.48mcg/mL (850mg single dose); T_{max}=3.32 hrs (850mg single dose). **Distribution:** Glipizide: Plasma protein binding (98-99%); V_d=11L (IV). Metformin: V_d=654L (850mg single dose). **Metabolism:** Glipizide: Liver (extensive). **Elimination:** Glipizide: Urine (<10% unchanged); $T_{1/2}$=2-4 hrs. Metformin: Urine (90%); $T_{1/2}$=6.2 hrs (plasma), 17.6 hrs (blood).

PATIENT CONSIDERATIONS
Assessment: Assess for acute/chronic metabolic acidosis (including diabetic ketoacidosis), type of diabetes mellitus, risk factors for lactic acidosis, renal/hepatic impairment, predisposition to developing subnormal vitamin B12 levels, G6PD deficiency, previous hypersensitivity to the drug, any other conditions where treatment is cautioned, pregnancy/nursing status, and possible drug interactions. Assess if patient is planning to undergo any surgical procedure. Obtain baseline FPG, HbA1c, eGFR, and hematologic parameters.

Monitoring: Monitor for signs/symptoms of lactic acidosis, CV effects, hypoglycemia, hemolytic anemia, and other adverse reactions. Monitor eGFR at least annually; monitor more frequently in patients at risk of developing renal impairment. Monitor FPG, HbA1c, and hepatic function periodically. Monitor hematological parameters annually. Perform routine serum vitamin B12 measurements at 2- to 3-yr intervals in patients predisposed to developing subnormal vitamin B12 levels.

Counseling: Inform of the potential risks, benefits, and alternative modes of therapy. Advise on the importance of adherence to dietary instructions, regular exercise program, and regular testing of blood glucose, HbA1c, renal function, and hematologic parameters. Inform of the risk of lactic acidosis, its symptoms, and conditions that predispose to its development; instruct to d/c therapy immediately and to notify physician if unexplained hyperventilation, myalgia, malaise, unusual somnolence, or other nonspecific symptoms occur. Inform of the risk of hypoglycemia. Counsel against excessive alcohol intake.

GLUCAGON — glucagon (rDNA origin)   Rx

Class: Glucagon

ADULT DOSAGE	PEDIATRIC DOSAGE
Hypoglycemia	**Hypoglycemia**
Severe:	**Severe:**
>20kg:	**<20kg:**
1mg (1 U) SQ/IM/IV	0.5mg (0.5 U) or a dose equivalent to 20-30mcg/kg
Diagnostic Aid	**>20kg:**
Relaxation of the Stomach:	1mg (1 U) SQ/IM/IV
IV:	
0.5mg (0.5 U)	
IM:	
2mg (2 U)	
Relaxation of Duodenum/Small Bowel:	
IV:	
0.25-0.5mg (0.25-0.5 U) or 2mg (2 U)	
IM:	
1mg (1 U) or 2mg (2 U)	
Relaxation of the Colon:	
IM:	
2mg (2 U) 10 min prior to procedure	

DOSING CONSIDERATIONS
Elderly
Start at lower end of dosing range

ADMINISTRATION
IM/IV/SQ routes

The diluent is provided for use only in the preparation of glucagon for parenteral inj

Do not use at concentrations >1mg/mL (1 U/mL)

Use reconstituted glucagon immediately; discard any unused portion

Severe Hypoglycemia
1. Treat initially w/ IV glucose if possible; if parenteral glucose cannot be used, dissolve the lyophilized glucagon using the accompanying diluting sol and use immediately
2. An unconscious patient will usually awaken w/in 15 min following the glucagon inj. If the response is delayed, there is no contraindication to the administration of an additional dose of glucagon; however, emergency aid should be sought so that parenteral glucose can be given
3. After the patient responds, supplemental carbohydrate should be given to restore liver glycogen and to prevent secondary hypoglycemia

Diagnostic Aid
1. Dissolve the lyophilized glucagon using the accompanying diluting sol and use immediately
2. Select dose depending on the onset and duration of effect required for the examination; refer to PI

STORAGE
Before reconstitution: 20-25°C (68-77°F); excursions allowed between 15-30°C (59-86°F).

HOW SUPPLIED
Inj: 1mg/mL (1 U/mL)

CONTRAINDICATIONS
Pheochromocytoma, hypersensitivity to this product.

WARNINGS/PRECAUTIONS
Caution with a history suggestive of insulinoma and/or pheochromocytoma. In patients with insulinoma, IV glucagon may produce an initial increase in blood glucose and then subsequently cause hypoglycemia. In the presence of pheochromocytoma, may cause the tumor to release catecholamines, which may result in a sudden and marked increase in BP. Generalized allergic reactions (eg, urticaria, respiratory distress, and hypotension) reported. Effective in treating hypoglycemia only if sufficient liver glycogen is present. Little or no help in states of starvation, adrenal insufficiency, or chronic hypoglycemia; treat with glucose.

ADVERSE REACTIONS
N/V, allergic reactions, urticaria, respiratory distress, hypotension.

DRUG INTERACTIONS
Addition of an anticholinergic during diagnostic examination may increase side effects.

PREGNANCY AND LACTATION
Category B, caution in nursing.

MECHANISM OF ACTION
Glucagon; polypeptide hormone that increases blood glucose levels and relaxes smooth muscle of the GI tract.

PHARMACOKINETICS
Absorption: (SQ) C_{max}=7.9ng/mL, T_{max}=20 min; (IM) C_{max}=6.9ng/mL, T_{max}=13 min. **Distribution:** V_d=0.25L/kg (1mg dose). **Metabolism:** Extensively degraded in liver, kidneys, plasma. **Elimination:** $T_{1/2}$=8-18 min (1mg dose).

PATIENT CONSIDERATIONS
Assessment: Assess if patient is in state of starvation, has adrenal insufficiency or chronic hypoglycemia. Assess for history suggestive of insulinoma and/or pheochromocytoma, pregnancy/nursing status, and possible drug interactions.

Monitoring: Monitor for signs/symptoms of an allergic reaction, HTN, and hypoglycemia. Monitor blood glucose levels in patients with hypoglycemia until asymptomatic.

Counseling: Instruct patient and family members in event of emergency how to properly prepare and administer glucagon. Inform about measures to prevent hypoglycemia, including following a uniform regimen on a regular basis, careful adjustment of the insulin program, frequent testing of blood or urine for glucose, and routinely carrying hyperglycemic agents to quickly elevate blood glucose levels (eg, sugar, candy, readily absorbed carbohydrates). Inform about symptoms of hypoglycemia and how to treat it appropriately. Inform caregivers that if patient is hypoglycemic, they should be kept alert and hypoglycemia should be treated as quickly as possible to prevent CNS damage. Advise to inform physician when hypoglycemia occurs.

GLUCOPHAGE XR — metformin hydrochloride   **Rx**

Class: Biguanide

> Lactic acidosis reported (rare); increased risk w/ increased age, renal dysfunction, or CHF. Risk of lactic acidosis may be significantly decreased by regular monitoring of renal function and by use of the minimum effective dose of metformin. Avoid use in patients ≥80 yrs of age unless renal function is normal. Withhold therapy in the presence of any condition associated w/ hypoxemia, dehydration, or sepsis. Avoid w/ clinical or lab evidence of hepatic disease. Caution against excessive alcohol intake; may potentiate the effects of metformin on lactate metabolism. Temporarily d/c prior to any IV radiocontrast study and for any surgical procedure. Lactic acidosis should be suspected in any diabetic patient w/ metabolic acidosis lacking evidence of ketoacidosis (ketonuria and ketonemia). D/C use and institute appropriate therapy if lactic acidosis occurs.

OTHER BRAND NAMES
Glucophage

ADULT DOSAGE
Type 2 Diabetes Mellitus
Tab:
Initial: 500mg bid or 850mg qd w/ meals
Titrate: Increase by 500mg/week or 850mg every 2 weeks, up to a total of 2000mg/day, given in divided doses; may also titrate from 500mg bid to 850mg bid after 2 weeks
Max: 2550mg/day; doses >2000mg/day may be better tolerated given tid

Tab, Extended-Release (ER):
Initial: 500mg qd w/ pm meal
Titrate: Increase by 500mg/week
Max: 2000mg/day; consider 1000mg bid if unable to achieve glycemic control on 2000mg qd

PEDIATRIC DOSAGE
Type 2 Diabetes Mellitus
10-16 Years:
Tab:
Initial: 500mg bid w/ meals
Titrate: Increase by 500mg/week
Max: 2000mg/day

DOSING CONSIDERATIONS
Concomitant Medications
Insulin Therapy in Adults:
Initial: 500mg qd while continuing current insulin dose
Titrate: Increase by 500mg/week; decrease insulin dose by 10-25% when FPG <120mg/dL
Max: 2500mg/day (tab) and 2000mg/day (tab, extended-release [ER])

Oral Sulfonylurea Therapy in Adults:
Consider gradual addition of an oral sulfonylurea if unresponsive to 4 weeks of max dose of Glucophage or Glucophage XR monotherapy; if patient has not satisfactorily responded to 1-3 months of concomitant therapy w/ the max dose of Glucophage or Glucophage XR and the max dose of an oral sulfonylurea, consider therapeutic alternatives (eg, switching to insulin w/ or w/o Glucophage or Glucophage XR)

Elderly
Dose conservatively; do not titrate to max dose

Other Important Considerations
Transferring Patients from Chlorpropamide: Exercise care during the first 2 weeks because of the prolonged retention of chlorpropamide in the body
Debilitated/Malnourished: Do not titrate to max dose

ADMINISTRATION
Oral route

Tab
Give in divided doses w/ meals.

Tab, ER
Give qd w/ the pm meal.
Must be swallowed whole; do not crush or chew.

STORAGE
20-25°C (68-77°F); excursions permitted to 15-30°C (59-86°F).

HOW SUPPLIED
Tab: (Glucophage) 500mg, 850mg, 1000mg; **Tab, ER:** (Glucophage XR) 500mg, 750mg

CONTRAINDICATIONS
Renal disease or dysfunction (eg, SrCr ≥1.5mg/dL [males], ≥1.4mg/dL [females] or abnormal CrCl); known hypersensitivity to metformin HCl; acute or chronic metabolic acidosis, including diabetic ketoacidosis, w/ or w/o coma.

WARNINGS/PRECAUTIONS
D/C therapy if conditions associated w/ lactic acidosis and characterized by hypoxemia states (eg, acute CHF, cardiovascular [CV] collapse, acute MI), or prerenal azotemia develop. Temporary loss of glycemic control may occur when a patient stabilized on a diabetic regimen is exposed to stress (eg, fever, trauma, infection, surgery); may be necessary to withhold metformin and temporarily administer insulin; may reinstitute metformin after acute episode is resolved. May decrease serum vitamin B12 levels. Increased risk of hypoglycemia in elderly, debilitated/malnourished or w/ adrenal or pituitary insufficiency or alcohol intoxication. Consider therapeutic alternatives, including initiation of insulin, if secondary failure w/ combined metformin/sulfonylurea therapy occurs. Hypoglycemia may be difficult to recognize in the elderly; caution in elderly.

ADVERSE REACTIONS
Diarrhea, N/V, flatulence, asthenia, indigestion, abdominal discomfort, headache.

DRUG INTERACTIONS
See Boxed Warning and Contraindications. Furosemide, nifedipine, cimetidine, and cationic drugs that are eliminated by renal tubular secretion (eg, digoxin, amiloride, procainamide, quinidine, quinine, ranitidine, trimethoprim, vancomycin, triamterene, morphine) may increase levels. Observe for loss of glycemic control w/ thiazides, other diuretics, corticosteroids, phenothiazines, thyroid products, estrogens, oral contraceptives, phenytoin, nicotinic acid, sympathomimetics, calcium channel blockers, and isoniazid. May interact w/ highly protein-bound drugs (eg, salicylates, sulfonamides, chloramphenicol, probenecid). May decrease furosemide or glyburide levels. Caution w/ drugs that may affect renal function or result in significant hemodynamic change or may interfere w/ the disposition of metformin (eg, cationic drugs that are eliminated by renal tubular secretion). Hypoglycemia may occur w/ concomitant use of other glucose-lowering agents (eg, sulfonylureas, insulin) or ethanol. Hypoglycemia may be difficult to recognize w/ β-adrenergic blocking drugs.

PREGNANCY AND LACTATION
Pregnancy: There are no adequate and well-controlled studies in pregnant women w/ metformin; metformin should not be used during pregnancy unless clearly needed.
Lactation: Not for use in nursing.

MECHANISM OF ACTION
Biguanide; decreases hepatic glucose production and intestinal absorption of glucose, and improves insulin sensitivity by increasing peripheral glucose uptake and utilization.

PHARMACOKINETICS
Absorption: (Tab) Absolute bioavailability (50-60%); (Tab, ER) T_{max}=7 hrs (median). Administration of different doses resulted in different parameters.
Distribution: (Tab) V_d=654L. **Elimination:** Urine (90%); $T_{1/2}$=6.2 hrs (plasma), 17.6 hrs (blood).

PATIENT CONSIDERATIONS
Assessment: Assess for renal disease or renal dysfunction, hepatic impairment, acute/chronic metabolic acidosis, presence of a hypoxic state (eg, acute CHF, acute MI, CV collapse), dehydration, sepsis, alcoholism, nutritional status, adrenal/pituitary insufficiency, pregnancy/nursing status, or any other conditions where treatment is contraindicated or cautioned. Assess for possible drug interactions. Assess baseline renal function, FPG, HbA1c, and hematological parameters (eg, Hct, Hgb, RBC indices).

Monitoring: Monitor for lactic acidosis, hypoglycemia, hypoxemia (eg, CV collapse, acute CHF, acute MI), prerenal azotemia, decreases in vitamin B12 levels, and for any other adverse reactions. Monitor FPG, HbA1c, renal function, and hematological parameters (eg, Hgb, Hct, RBC indices).

Counseling: Inform of the potential risks/benefits of therapy. Inform about the importance of adherence to dietary instructions, a regular exercise program, and of regular testing of blood glucose, HbA1c, renal function, and hematologic parameters. Inform of the risk of developing lactic acidosis during therapy; advise to d/c therapy immediately and contact physician if unexplained hyperventilation, myalgia, malaise, unusual somnolence, or other nonspecific symptoms occur. Instruct to avoid excessive alcohol intake. Counsel to take tab w/ meals and ER tab w/ pm meal. Instruct that ER tab must be swallowed whole and not crushed or chewed.

GLUCOTROL — glipizide   Rx

Class: Sulfonylurea (2nd generation)

ADULT DOSAGE
Type 2 Diabetes Mellitus

Initial: 5mg qd
Titrate: Increase by 2.5-5mg every several days; may divide dose if response to single dose is not satisfactory
Max qd Dose: 15mg
Max Total Daily Dose: 40mg

Doses >15mg/day should be divided

Switching from Insulin:
Daily Insulin Requirement:
≤20 U/day: D/C insulin and begin glipizide at usual dose
>20 U/day: Reduce insulin dose by 50% and begin glipizide at usual dose; subsequent insulin reductions should depend on individual patient response

Switching from Longer Half-Life Sulfonylureas (eg, Chlorpropamide): Observe patient carefully for 1-2 weeks

PEDIATRIC DOSAGE
Pediatric use may not have been established

DOSING CONSIDERATIONS
Concomitant Medications
Colesevelam: Administer glipizide at least 4 hrs prior to colesevelam

Renal Impairment
Initial/Maint: Dose conservatively

Hepatic Impairment
Initial: 2.5mg qd
Maint: Dose conservatively

Elderly
Initial: 2.5mg qd
Maint: Dose conservatively

Other Important Considerations
Debilitated/Malnourished Patients:
Initial/Maint: Dose conservatively

ADMINISTRATION
Oral route

Administer approx 30 min ac.

STORAGE
<30°C (86°F).

HOW SUPPLIED
Tab: 5mg*, 10mg* *scored

CONTRAINDICATIONS
Known hypersensitivity to the drug; type 1 diabetes mellitus; diabetic ketoacidosis, w/ or w/o coma.

WARNINGS/PRECAUTIONS
Caution during first 1-2 weeks of therapy if transferring from longer $T_{1/2}$ sulfonylureas (eg, chlorpropamide). Consider hospitalization during the insulin withdrawal period if patient has been receiving >40 U/day of insulin. May be associated with increased risk of cardiovascular mortality. May produce severe hypoglycemia; increased risk in elderly, debilitated, or malnourished patients; with renal/hepatic impairment, or adrenal/pituitary insufficiency; when caloric intake is deficient; or after severe/prolonged exercise. Loss of glycemic control may occur when exposed to stress (eg, fever, trauma, infection, surgery); may be necessary to d/c therapy and administer insulin. Secondary failure may occur over time. May cause hemolytic anemia; caution with G6PD deficiency and consider a non-sulfonylurea alternative. Caution in elderly.

ADVERSE REACTIONS
Hypoglycemia, GI disturbances, dizziness, drowsiness, headache, porphyria cutanea tarda, photosensitivity reactions, leukopenia, agranulocytosis, thrombocytopenia, hemolytic anemia.

DRUG INTERACTIONS
See Dosage. Hypoglycemic effects may be potentiated by NSAIDs, some azoles, other highly protein-bound drugs, salicylates, sulfonamides, chloramphenicol, probenecid, coumarins, MAOIs, and β-blockers; monitor closely for hypoglycemia during coadministration and for loss of glycemic control when such drugs are withdrawn. Potential interaction leading to severe hypoglycemia reported with oral miconazole. Fluconazole may increase levels. Thiazides and other diuretics, corticosteroids, phenothiazines, thyroid products, estrogens, oral contraceptives, phenytoin, nicotinic acid, sympathomimetics, calcium channel blockers, and isoniazid may produce hyperglycemia and may lead to loss of glycemic control; monitor closely for loss of control during coadministration and for hypoglycemia when such drugs are withdrawn. Increased likelihood of hypoglycemia with alcohol and use of >1 glucose-lowering drug. May be difficult to recognize hypoglycemia with β-blockers. Caution with salicylate or dicumarol. Colesevelam may reduce levels.

PREGNANCY AND LACTATION
Category C, not for use in nursing.

MECHANISM OF ACTION
Sulfonylurea (2nd generation); lowers blood glucose acutely by stimulating insulin release from pancreatic β cells.

PHARMACOKINETICS
Absorption: Rapid and complete. T_{max}=1-3 hrs. **Distribution:** Plasma protein binding (98-99%); (IV) V_d=11L. **Metabolism:** Liver (extensive). **Elimination:** Urine (<10% unchanged); $T_{1/2}$=2-4 hrs.

PATIENT CONSIDERATIONS
Assessment: Assess for previous hypersensitivity to drug, renal/hepatic impairment, type of DM, diabetic ketoacidosis, risk factors for hypoglycemia, G6PD deficiency, pregnancy/nursing status, and possible drug interactions. Obtain baseline FPG and HbA1c levels.

Monitoring: Monitor for hypoglycemia, loss of glycemic control when exposed to stress, hypersensitivity reactions, secondary failure, hemolytic anemia, and other adverse reactions. Monitor blood/urine glucose and HbA1c levels periodically.

Counseling: Inform of the risks, benefits, and alternative modes of therapy. Counsel about the importance of adherence to dietary instructions, regular exercise program, and regular testing of urine and/or blood glucose. Inform about the symptoms, treatment, and predisposing conditions of hypoglycemia, as well as primary and secondary failure. During the insulin withdrawal period, instruct to test for sugar and ketone bodies in urine at least tid and to contact physician immediately if these tests are abnormal.

GLUCOTROL XL — glipizide   Rx

Class: Sulfonylurea (2nd generation)

ADULT DOSAGE
Type 2 Diabetes Mellitus

Initial: 5mg qd; start at 2.5mg qd if at increased risk of hypoglycemia
Titrate: Adjust dose based on patient's glycemic control
Max: 20mg qd

Switching from Immediate-Release Glipizide:
May give qd dose at the nearest equivalent total daily dose

PEDIATRIC DOSAGE
Pediatric use may not have been established

DOSING CONSIDERATIONS
Concomitant Medications
Other Blood-Glucose-Lowering Agents: Initiate Glucotrol XL at 5mg qd; start at lower dose if at increased risk for hypoglycemia
Colesevelam: Administer at least 4 hrs prior to colesevelam

Renal Impairment
Initial: 2.5mg qd

Hepatic Impairment
Initial: 2.5mg qd
Dose conservatively

Elderly
Initial: 2.5mg qd
Dose conservatively

Other Important Considerations
Debilitated/Malnourished/Adrenal Impairment/Pituitary Impairment:
Initial: 2.5mg qd

ADMINISTRATION
Oral route

Administer w/ breakfast or the first main meal of the day.
Swallow tab whole; do not chew, divide, or crush.

STORAGE
20-25°C (68-77°F); excursions permitted between 15-30°C (59-86°F). Protect from moisture and humidity.

HOW SUPPLIED
Tab, Extended-Release (ER): 2.5mg, 5mg, 10mg

CONTRAINDICATIONS
Known hypersensitivity to glipizide or any components of the medication, hypersensitivity to sulfonamide derivatives.

WARNINGS/PRECAUTIONS
Not recommended for the treatment of type 1 diabetes mellitus (DM) or diabetic ketoacidosis. May produce severe hypoglycemia. There is an increased risk for hypoglycemia w/ debilitated or malnourished patients; adrenal, pituitary, or hepatic impairment; deficient caloric intake; or after severe/prolonged exercise. May cause hemolytic anemia; avoid in patients w/ G6PD deficiency. May be associated w/ increased risk of cardiovascular mortality. Obstructive symptoms reported in patients w/ known strictures in association w/ ingestion of another drug w/ non-dissolvable ER formulation; avoid in patients w/ preexisting severe GI narrowing (pathologic or iatrogenic).

ADVERSE REACTIONS
Hypoglycemia, dizziness, diarrhea, nervousness, tremor, flatulence.

DRUG INTERACTIONS
See Dosing Considerations. Ingestion of alcohol may increase likelihood of hypoglycemia. Potential interaction leading to severe hypoglycemia reported w/ oral miconazole; monitor for hypoglycemia. Fluconazole may increase levels which may lead to hypoglycemia; monitor for hypoglycemia. Colesevelam may reduce max plasma concentration and total exposure of glipizide. Concomitant use w/ other anti-diabetic medications may increase the risk of hypoglycemia; a lower dose of glipizide may be required. Early warning symptoms of hypoglycemia may be different or less pronounced in patients who are taking β-adrenergic blocking medications or other sympatholytic agents.

PREGNANCY AND LACTATION
Pregnancy: Category C.
Lactation: Not for use in nursing.

MECHANISM OF ACTION
Sulfonylurea (2nd generation); primarily lowers blood glucose by stimulating insulin release from the pancreas. Binds to the sulfonylurea receptor in the pancreatic β-cell plasma membrane, leading to closure of the ATP-sensitive potassium channel, thereby stimulating the release of insulin.

PHARMACOKINETICS
Absorption: (Single dose) Absolute bioavailability (100%); T_{max}=6-12 hrs.
Distribution: V_d=10L; plasma protein binding (98-99%). **Metabolism:** Liver (primary); aromatic hydroxylation products (inactive, major metabolites); acetylamino-ethyl benzene derivative (active minor metabolite). **Elimination:** Urine (80%, <10% unchanged), feces (10%, <10% unchanged); $T_{1/2}$=2-5 hrs.

PATIENT CONSIDERATIONS
Assessment: Assess for hypersensitivity to glipizide or any components of the medication, hypersensitivity to sulfonamide derivatives, renal/hepatic impairment, type of DM, diabetic ketoacidosis, risk factors for hypoglycemia, G6PD deficiency, severe GI narrowing (pathologic or iatrogenic), pregnancy/nursing status, and for possible drug interactions. Obtain baseline FPG and HbA1c levels.

Monitoring: Monitor for hypoglycemia, hypersensitivity reactions, secondary failure, hemolytic anemia, and other adverse reactions. Periodically monitor blood glucose levels and HbA1c levels.

Counseling: Advise of the risks and benefits of therapy. Inform about the risk of hypoglycemia, its symptoms and treatment, and conditions that predispose to its development. Counsel about the importance of adherence to dietary instructions, of a regular exercise program, and of regular testing of glycemic control. Advise patients that they may occasionally notice something that looks like a tablet in their stool. Advise to inform healthcare provider if pregnant, contemplating pregnancy, breastfeeding, or contemplating breastfeeding.

GLUCOVANCE — glyburide/metformin hydrochloride   Rx
Class: Biguanide/sulfonylurea

Lactic acidosis may occur due to metformin accumulation; risk increases w/ CHF, degree of renal dysfunction, and patient's age. Regularly monitor renal function and use the minimum effective dose of metformin. Do not initiate in patients ≥80 yrs of age unless measurement of CrCl demonstrates that renal function is not reduced. Promptly withhold therapy in the presence of any condition associated w/ hypoxemia, dehydration, or sepsis. Avoid w/ clinical or lab evidence of hepatic disease. Caution against excessive alcohol intake; alcohol potentiates the effects of metformin on lactate metabolism. Temporarily d/c therapy prior to any intravascular radiocontrast study and for any surgical procedure. D/C use immediately and promptly institute general supportive measures if lactic acidosis occurs. Prompt hemodialysis is recommended to correct the acidosis and remove the accumulated metformin.

ADULT DOSAGE
Type 2 Diabetes Mellitus
Currently on Diet and Exercise:
Initial: 1.25mg/250mg qd w/ a meal; may use 1.25mg/250mg bid w/ the am and pm meals if baseline HbA1c >9% or FPG >200mg/dL
Titrate: Increase by 1.25mg/250mg/day every 2 weeks
Max: 20mg/2000mg/day

Currently on a Sulfonylurea and/or Metformin:
Initial: 2.5mg/500mg or 5mg/500mg bid w/ the am and pm meals; starting dose should not exceed daily doses of the sulfonylurea or metformin already being taken.
Titrate: Increase by no more than 5mg/500mg/day
Max: 20mg/2000mg/day

Addition of Thiazolidinediones:
Continue current dose of Glucovance and initiate thiazolidinedione at its recommended starting dose

DOSING CONSIDERATIONS
Concomitant Medications
Colesevelam: Administer Glucovance at least 4 hrs prior to colesevelam
Elderly
Initial/Maint: Dose conservatively; do not titrate to max dose
Adverse Reactions
Hypoglycemia w/ Glucovance/Thiazolidinedione Combination: Consider reducing the dose of the glyburide component; consider adjusting the dosages of the other components of the regimen as clinically warranted
Other Important Considerations
Debilitated/Malnourished Patients: Do not titrate to max dose

ADMINISTRATION
Oral route

STORAGE
Up to 25°C (77°F).

HOW SUPPLIED
Tab: (Glyburide/Metformin) 1.25mg/250mg, 2.5mg/500mg, 5mg/500mg

CONTRAINDICATIONS
Renal disease or dysfunction (eg, SrCr ≥1.5mg/dL [males], ≥1.4mg/dL [females], or abnormal CrCl); known hypersensitivity to metformin HCl or glyburide; acute or chronic metabolic acidosis, including diabetic ketoacidosis, w/ or w/o coma; concomitant administration of bosentan.

WARNINGS/PRECAUTIONS
May be associated w/ increased cardiovascular (CV) mortality. May cause hypoglycemia; increased risk when caloric intake is deficient; when strenuous exercise is not compensated by caloric supplementation; w/ renal/hepatic insufficiency, adrenal/pituitary insufficiency, alcohol intoxication; or in elderly, debilitated, or malnourished patients. Not recommended during pregnancy. Caution in elderly. Glyburide: May cause hemolytic anemia; caution w/ G6PD deficiency. Metformin: Assess renal function before initiation of therapy and at least annually thereafter; d/c w/ evidence of renal impairment. Temporarily d/c at the time of or prior to radiologic studies involving the use of intravascular iodinated contrast materials, withhold for 48 hrs subsequent to the procedure, and reinstitute only if renal function is normal. D/C promptly if CV collapse (shock), acute MI and other conditions characterized by hypoxemia occur. Temporarily suspend for any surgical procedure (except minor procedures not associated w/ restricted intake of food and fluids); restart when oral intake is resumed and renal function is normal. May decrease serum vitamin B12 levels; monitor hematologic parameters annually. Caution in patients predisposed to developing subnormal vitamin B12 levels (eg, those w/ inadequate vitamin B12 or Ca²⁺ intake or absorption). Evaluate patients previously well controlled on therapy who develop lab abnormalities or clinical illness for evidence of ketoacidosis or lactic acidosis; d/c if acidosis occurs.

ADVERSE REACTIONS
Lactic acidosis, upper respiratory infection, N/V, abdominal pain, headache, dizziness, diarrhea.

DRUG INTERACTIONS
See Boxed Warning, Dosage, Dosing Considerations, and Contraindications. Increased risk of hypoglycemia w/ other glucose-lowering agents or ethanol. May be difficult to recognize hypoglycemia w/ β-blockers. Thiazides and other diuretics, corticosteroids, phenothiazines, thyroid products, estrogens, oral contraceptives, phenytoin, nicotinic acid, sympathomimetics, calcium channel blockers, and isoniazid may produce hyperglycemia and may lead to loss of glycemic control; monitor closely for loss of control during coadministration and for hypoglycemia during withdrawal of these drugs. Weight gain observed w/ the addition of rosiglitazone to therapy. Monitor LFTs during coadministration w/ a thiazolidinedione. Metformin: Caution w/ drugs that may affect renal function or result in significant hemodynamic change or may interfere w/ the disposition of metformin (eg, cationic drugs eliminated by renal tubular secretion). Furosemide, nifedipine, and cimetidine may increase levels. May decrease furosemide levels. Cationic drugs that are eliminated by renal tubular secretion (eg, cimetidine,

PEDIATRIC DOSAGE
Pediatric use may not have been established

amiloride, digoxin, morphine, quinidine, vancomycin) may potentially produce an interaction; monitor and adjust dose of therapy and/or the interfering drug. Glyburide: Hypoglycemic effects may be potentiated by NSAIDs and other highly protein-bound drugs, salicylates, sulfonamides, chloramphenicol, probenecid, coumarins, MAOIs, and β-blockers; monitor closely for hypoglycemia during coadministration and for loss of glycemic control during withdrawal of these drugs. Possible interaction w/ ciprofloxacin (a fluoroquinolone antibiotic), resulting in potentiation of hypoglycemic action. Potential interaction leading to severe hypoglycemia reported w/ oral miconazole. Colesevelam may reduce levels.

PREGNANCY AND LACTATION
Pregnancy: Category B.
Lactation: Not for use in nursing.

MECHANISM OF ACTION
Glyburide: Sulfonylurea; lower blood glucose acutely by stimulating release of insulin from the pancreas. **Metformin:** Biguanide; decreases hepatic glucose production, decreases intestinal absorption of glucose, and improves insulin sensitivity by increasing peripheral glucose uptake and utilization.

PHARMACOKINETICS
Absorption: Glyburide: T_{max}=4 hrs. Metformin: Absolute bioavailability (50-60%) (500mg); C_{max}=1.48mcg/mL (850mg single-dose); T_{max}=3.32 hrs (850mg single-dose). **Distribution:** Glyburide: plasma protein binding (extensive). Metformin: V_d=654L (850mg single-dose). **Metabolism:** Glyburide: metabolites: 4-trans-hydroxy derivative (major) and 3-cis hydroxy derivative. **Elimination:** Glyburide: Bile (50%, metabolites), urine (50%, metabolites); $T_{1/2}$=10 hrs. Metformin: Urine (90%); $T_{1/2}$=6.2 hrs (plasma), 17.6 hrs (blood).

PATIENT CONSIDERATIONS
Assessment: Assess for metabolic acidosis, diabetic ketoacidosis, risk factors for lactic acidosis, renal/hepatic impairment, presence of malnourishment or debilitation, adrenal/pituitary insufficiency, alcoholism, G6PD deficiency, hypoxemia, inadequate vitamin B12 or Ca^{2+} intake/absorption, previous hypersensitivity to the drug, pregnancy/nursing status, and possible drug interactions. Assess if patient is planning to undergo any surgical procedure, or radiologic studies involving the use of intravascular iodinated contrast materials. Obtain baseline FPG and HbA1c levels, and hematologic parameters.

Monitoring: Monitor for signs/symptoms of lactic acidosis, CV effects, hypoglycemia, hemolytic anemia, and other adverse reactions. Monitor for changes in clinical status. Monitor renal function, especially in elderly, at least annually. Monitor hematologic parameters annually. Perform routine serum vitamin B12 measurements at 2- to 3-yr intervals in patients predisposed to developing subnormal vitamin B12 levels. Monitor FPG and HbA1c levels periodically.

Counseling: Inform of the risks, benefits, and alternative modes of therapy. Advise on the importance of adherence to dietary instructions, regular exercise program, and regular testing of blood glucose, HbA1c, renal function, and hematologic parameters. Inform of the risk of lactic acidosis; instruct to d/c therapy immediately and notify physician if unexplained hyperventilation, myalgia, malaise, unusual somnolence, or other nonspecific symptoms occur. Inform of the risk of hypoglycemia. Counsel against excessive alcohol intake.

GLUMETZA — metformin hydrochloride   Rx
Class: Biguanide

Cases of metformin-associated lactic acidosis resulting in death, hypothermia, hypotension, and resistant bradyarrhythmias reported; risk factors include renal impairment, concomitant use of certain drugs (eg, cationic drugs such as topiramate), age ≥65 years, having a radiological study w/ contrast, surgery and other procedures, hypoxic states (eg, acute CHF), excessive alcohol intake, and hepatic impairment. D/C therapy immediately and institute general supportive measures in a hospital setting if metformin-associated lactic acidosis is suspected. Prompt hemodialysis is recommended.

ADULT DOSAGE
Type 2 Diabetes Mellitus
Not Currently Taking Metformin:
Initial: 500mg qd w/ evening meal
Titrate: Increase dose in 500mg increments every 1-2 weeks if higher dose is needed and there are no GI adverse reactions
Max: 2000mg/day

Switching from Immediate-Release Metformin:
Initiate Glumetza qd at the same total dose, up to 2000mg qd

PEDIATRIC DOSAGE
Pediatric use may not have been established

DOSING CONSIDERATIONS
Renal Impairment
eGFR 30-45mL/min/1.73m²: Initiation of therapy is not recommended
eGFR <30mL/min/1.73m²: Contraindicated

If eGFR Falls <45mL/min/1.73m² During Therapy: Assess benefit/risk of continuing therapy
If eGFR Falls <30mL/min/1.73m² During Therapy: D/C

Hepatic Impairment
Not recommended

Elderly
Start at lower end of dosing range

Other Important Considerations
Iodinated Contrast Imaging Procedures:
D/C therapy at the time of, or prior to, an iodinated contrast imaging procedure in patients w/ an eGFR 30-60mL/min/1.73m²; in patients w/ a history of liver disease, alcoholism, or heart failure; or in patients who will be administered intra-arterial iodinated contrast. Reevaluate eGFR 48 hrs after the imaging procedure and restart therapy if renal function is stable

ADMINISTRATION
Oral route

Take w/ evening meal.
Swallow whole; do not split, crush, or chew.

STORAGE
20-25°C (68-77°F); excursions permitted to 15-30°C (59-86°F).

HOW SUPPLIED
Tab, Extended-Release: 500mg, 1000mg

CONTRAINDICATIONS
Severe renal impairment (eGFR <30mL/min/1.73m²); known hypersensitivity to metformin hydrochloride; acute or chronic metabolic acidosis, including diabetic ketoacidosis.

WARNINGS/PRECAUTIONS
See Dosing Considerations. Not for treatment of type 1 diabetes or diabetic ketoacidosis. Temporarily d/c while patient has restricted food and fluid intake (eg, during surgical or other procedures). D/C if a condition associated w/ hypoxemia occurs (eg, cardiovascular collapse, acute MI, sepsis). May decrease vitamin B12 levels; monitor hematologic parameters annually. Hypoglycemia may occur when caloric intake is deficient or when strenuous exercise is not compensated by caloric supplementation; elderly, debilitated, or malnourished patients and those w/ adrenal or pituitary insufficiency or alcohol intoxication are particularly susceptible to hypoglycemic effects. Hypoglycemia may be difficult to recognize in the elderly.

ADVERSE REACTIONS
Hypoglycemia, diarrhea, nausea.

DRUG INTERACTIONS
See Boxed Warning. Hypoglycemia may occur w/ other glucose-lowering agents (eg, sulfonylureas, insulin) or ethanol; may require lower doses of insulin secretagogues (eg, sulfonylurea) or insulin. Hypoglycemia may be difficult to recognize w/ β-adrenergic blocking drugs. Topiramate or other carbonic anhydrase inhibitors (eg, zonisamide, acetazolamide, dichlorphenamide) may increase the risk of lactic acidosis; consider more frequent monitoring of these patients. Drugs that are eliminated by renal tubular secretion, drugs that impair renal function, drugs that result in significant hemodynamic change, drugs that interfere w/ acid-base balance, or drugs that increase metformin accumulation may increase the risk of metformin-associated lactic acidosis; consider more frequent monitoring of these patients. Avoid excessive alcohol intake. Thiazides and other diuretics, corticosteroids, phenothiazines, thyroid products, estrogens, oral contraceptives, phenytoin, nicotinic acid, sympathomimetics, calcium channel blockers, and isoniazid may produce hyperglycemia and lead to loss of glycemic control; observe closely for loss of blood glucose control when such drugs are administered and observe closely for hypoglycemia when such drugs are withdrawn.

PREGNANCY AND LACTATION
Pregnancy: Category B.
Lactation: Potential for hypoglycemia in nursing infants.

MECHANISM OF ACTION
Biguanide; decreases hepatic glucose production, decreases intestinal absorption of glucose, and improves insulin sensitivity by increasing peripheral glucose uptake and utilization.

PHARMACOKINETICS
Absorption: T_{max}=7-8 hrs (1000mg, single dose). **Distribution:** V_d=654L (850mg immediate-release, single dose). **Elimination:** Urine (90%, unchanged); $T_{1/2}$=6.2 hrs (plasma), 17.6 hrs (blood).

PATIENT CONSIDERATIONS
Assessment: Assess for acute/chronic metabolic acidosis (including diabetic ketoacidosis), type of diabetes mellitus, risk factors for lactic acidosis, renal/hepatic impairment, previous hypersensitivity to the drug, predisposition to developing subnormal vitamin B12 levels, pregnancy/nursing status, and possible drug interactions. Assess if patient is planning to undergo any surgical procedure. Obtain baseline FPG, HbA1c, eGFR, and hematologic parameters.

Monitoring: Monitor for lactic acidosis, hypoxic states, decreases in vitamin B12 levels, and other adverse reactions. Monitor eGFR at least annually; monitor more frequently in patients at risk of developing renal impairment. Monitor FPG, HbA1c, and hepatic function periodically. Monitor hematologic parameters annually. Perform routine serum vitamin B12 measurements at 2- to 3-yr intervals in patients predisposed to developing subnormal vitamin B12 levels.

Counseling: Inform of the potential risks/benefits of therapy and of alternative modes of therapy. Advise to take ud. Inform about the importance of adherence to dietary instructions, regular exercise program, and regular testing of blood glucose and HbA1c. Advise to seek medical advice during periods of stress (eg, fever, trauma, infection, surgery). Advise about the risks of lactic acidosis, its symptoms, and conditions that predispose to its development; instruct to d/c therapy immediately and to contact physician if unexplained hyperventilation, myalgia, malaise, unusual somnolence, or other nonspecific symptoms occur. Inform about the importance of regular testing of renal function and hematological parameters. Counsel against excessive alcohol intake, either acute or chronic, while on therapy. Inform that hypoglycemia may occur when used in conjunction w/ insulin secretagogues (eg, sulfonylureas) and insulin. Advise that inactive ingredients may occasionally be eliminated in the feces as soft mass resembling the original tab.

GLYXAMBI — empagliflozin/linagliptin   Rx

Class: Dipeptidyl peptidase-4 (DPP-4) inhibitor/sodium-glucose cotransporter 2 (SGLT2) inhibitor

ADULT DOSAGE	PEDIATRIC DOSAGE
Type 2 Diabetes Mellitus	Pediatric use may not have been established
Recommended Dose: 10mg/5mg qam	
Titrate: May increase to 25mg/5mg qd in patients tolerating therapy	

DOSING CONSIDERATIONS

Renal Impairment

eGFR ≥45mL/min/1.73m²: No dose adjustment needed

eGFR <45mL/min/1.73m²: Do not initiate treatment

eGFR Persistently <45mL/min/1.73m²: D/C therapy

Other Important Considerations

Patients w/ Volume Depletion:
Correct this condition prior to initiating therapy

ADMINISTRATION

Oral route

Take w/ or w/o food.

STORAGE

25°C (77°F); excursions permitted to 15-30°C (59-86°F).

HOW SUPPLIED

Tab: (Empagliflozin/Linagliptin) 10mg/5mg, 25mg/5mg

CONTRAINDICATIONS

History of hypersensitivity reaction (eg, anaphylaxis, angioedema, exfoliative skin conditions, urticaria, bronchial hyperreactivity) to linagliptin; history of serious hypersensitivity reaction to empagliflozin. Severe renal impairment, ESRD, dialysis.

WARNINGS/PRECAUTIONS

Not recommended w/ type 1 diabetes mellitus (DM) or for treatment of diabetic ketoacidosis. **Empagliflozin:** May cause intravascular volume contraction. Symptomatic hypotension may occur, particularly w/ renal impairment, the elderly, patients w/ low systolic BP, and in patients on diuretics. Ketoacidosis, including fatal cases, reported; if suspected, d/c and institute prompt treatment. Assess for ketoacidosis in patients presenting w/ signs/symptoms consistent w/ severe metabolic acidosis regardless of presenting blood glucose levels. Consider temporarily discontinuing therapy in clinical situations known to predispose to ketoacidosis (eg, prolonged fasting due to acute illness or surgery). May increase SrCr and decrease eGFR; risk of impaired renal function is increased in elderly and in patients w/ moderate renal impairment. Serious UTIs (eg, urosepsis, pyelonephritis), requiring hospitalization, reported; evaluate for signs/symptoms of UTIs and treat promptly, if indicated. Increases risk for genital mycotic infections and UTIs; monitor and treat as appropriate. Increases in LDL may occur; monitor and treat as appropriate. Monitoring glycemic control w/ urine glucose tests or 1,5-anhydroglucitol assay is not recommended. **Linagliptin:** Acute pancreatitis, including fatal pancreatitis, reported; d/c therapy and initiate appropriate management if pancreatitis is suspected. Serious hypersensitivity reactions reported; if suspected, d/c therapy, assess for other potential causes, and institute alternative treatment for DM. Caution in patients w/ history of angioedema to another DPP-4 inhibitor. Severe and disabling arthralgia may occur; consider as a possible cause for severe joint pain and d/c therapy if appropriate.

ADVERSE REACTIONS

UTI, URTI, nasopharyngitis.

DRUG INTERACTIONS

Use in combination w/ an insulin secretagogue (eg, sulfonylurea) or insulin may be associated w/ a higher rate of hypoglycemia; may require a lower dose of insulin secretagogue or insulin. **Empagliflozin:** Coadministration w/ diuretics resulted in increased urine volume and frequency of voids; may enhance potential for volume depletion. **Linagliptin:** Rifampin decreased exposure. Strong P-gp or CYP3A4 inducers may reduce linagliptin efficacy; use of alternative treatments is strongly recommended.

PREGNANCY AND LACTATION

Pregnancy: Category C.

Lactation: Not for use in nursing.

MECHANISM OF ACTION

Empagliflozin: SGLT2 inhibitor; reduces renal reabsorption of filtered glucose and lowers the renal threshold for glucose, thereby increasing urinary glucose excretion. **Linagliptin:** DPP-4 inhibitor; increases the concentrations of active incretin hormones, stimulating the release of insulin in a glucose-dependent manner and decreasing the levels of glucagon in the circulation.

PHARMACOKINETICS

Absorption: Empagliflozin: C_{max}=259nmol/L (10mg), 687nmol/L (25mg); AUC=1870nmol•hr/L (10mg), 4740nmol•hr/L (25mg); T_{max}=1.5 hrs. Linagliptin: Absolute bioavailability (30%). **Distribution:** Empagliflozin: V_d=73.8L; plasma protein binding (86.2%). Linagliptin: V_d=1110L (IV); plasma protein binding (concentration-dependent). **Metabolism:** Empagliflozin: Glucuronidation (primary) by the uridine 5'-diphospho-glucuronosyltransferases UGT2B7, UGT1A3, UGT1A8, and UGT1A9; 2-O-, 3-O-, and 6-O-glucuronide (metabolites). **Elimination:**

Empagliflozin: Urine (54.4%), feces (41.2%); $T_{1/2}$=12.4 hrs. Linagliptin: Enterohepatic (80%), urine (5%).

PATIENT CONSIDERATIONS

Assessment: Assess for history of hypersensitivity to either drug, type of DM, diabetic ketoacidosis, renal impairment, history of chronic or recurrent genital mycotic infections, history of angioedema w/ another DPP-4 inhibitor, pregnancy/nursing status, and possible drug interactions. Obtain baseline FPG and HbA1c levels. Assess for volume contraction and correct volume status if indicated.

Monitoring: Monitor for signs/symptoms of pancreatitis, hypotension, ketoacidosis, genital mycotic infections, UTIs, hypersensitivity reactions, LDL increase, severe joint pain, and other adverse reactions. Monitor FPG, HbA1c levels, and renal function periodically.

Counseling: Inform of the potential risks and benefits of therapy, alternative modes of therapy, importance of adherence to dietary instructions, regular physical activity, periodic blood glucose monitoring and HbA1c testing, recognition/management of hypo/hyperglycemia, and assessment of diabetes complications. Advise to seek medical advice promptly during periods of stress (eg, fever, trauma, infection), as medication requirements may change. Instruct to immediately report to physician if pregnant/nursing, if experiencing symptoms of hypotension, if any unusual symptom develops, or if any known symptom persists or worsens. Instruct to d/c use and notify physician if signs/symptoms of pancreatitis (eg, severe abdominal pain) or allergic reactions (eg, rash) occur. Instruct to d/c and seek medical advice immediately if symptoms of ketoacidosis occur. Inform that dehydration may increase the risk for hypotension, and to have adequate fluid intake. Advise on the signs/symptoms of UTIs, vaginal yeast infections, balanitis, and balanoposthitis; explain of treatment options and when to seek medical advice. Inform that severe and disabling joint pain may occur and to seek medical advice if this occurs.

GoLYTELY — polyethylene glycol 3350/potassium chloride/sodium bicarbonate/sodium chloride/sodium sulfate   Rx

Class: Bowel cleanser

ADULT DOSAGE	PEDIATRIC DOSAGE
Bowel Cleansing	Pediatric use may not have been established
Prior to Colonoscopy and Barium Enema X-Ray Examination:	
PO:	
240mL (8 oz) every 10 min until 4L consumed or rectal effluent is clear	
NG Tube:	
20-30mL/min (1.2-1.8L/hr)	

ADMINISTRATION

Oral/NG tube route

Must be reconstituted w/ water before use; not for direct ingestion.

May consume water or clear liquids during bowel preparation and after completion of bowel preparation up until 2 hrs before the time of colonoscopy; sol is more palatable if chilled prior to administration.

Rapid drinking of each portion is preferred to drinking small amounts continuously.

First bowel movements should occur approx 1 hr after the start of administration.

Administration Instructions Prior to Dosage

On the day prior to the colonoscopy, instruct patients to:

1. Take only clear liquids; avoid red and purple liquids. Patients may consume a light breakfast.

2. Early in the pm prior to colonoscopy, fill the supplied container containing powder w/ lukewarm water to the 4L fill line; sol is clear and colorless when reconstituted.

3. Shake vigorously several times to ensure that the ingredients are dissolved; use w/in 48 hrs when reconstituted.

STORAGE

15-30°C (59-86°F). Reconstituted Sol: Keep refrigerated. Use w/in 48 hrs.

HOW SUPPLIED

Sol (Powder): (Polyethylene Glycol (PEG) 3350/Sodium Sulfate/ Sodium Bicarbonate/Sodium Chloride/Potassium Chloride) 236g/22.74g/6.74g/5.86g/2.97g [4L], 227.1g/21.5g/6.36g/5.53g/2.82g [1 gallon]

CONTRAINDICATIONS

GI obstruction, ileus, or gastric retention; bowel perforation; toxic colitis or toxic megacolon; known allergy or hypersensitivity to any component of this product.

WARNINGS/PRECAUTIONS

Adequately hydrate before, during, and after use; caution w/ congestive heart failure when replacing fluids. Consider performing postcolonoscopy lab tests (electrolytes, SrCr, BUN) and treat accordingly if significant vomiting or signs of dehydration develop. Correct fluid and electrolyte abnormalities before treatment. Caution w/ conditions that increase risk for fluid and electrolyte disturbances or may increase risk of adverse events (eg, seizures, arrhythmias, and renal impairment). Serious arrhythmias reported rarely; caution in patients at increased risk of arrhythmias and consider predose and postcolonoscopy ECGs. Generalized tonic-clonic seizures and/or loss of consciousness reported; caution in patients w/ a history of or at increased risk of seizures (eg, w/ known/suspected hyponatremia). Caution w/ impaired renal function; consider performing baseline and postcolonoscopy lab tests. May produce colonic mucosal aphthous ulcerations; consider this when interpreting colonoscopy findings in patients w/

known/suspected inflammatory bowel disease. Serious cases of ischemic colitis reported. Slow administration or temporarily d/c if severe bloating, distention, or abdominal pain develops; caution w/ severe ulcerative colitis. Caution in patients w/ impaired gag reflex, unconscious or semiconscious patients, and patients prone to regurgitation or aspiration; observe during administration especially if administered via NG tube. Not for direct ingestion; direct ingestion of undissolved powder may increase risk of N/V, dehydration, and electrolyte disturbances.

ADVERSE REACTIONS
Nausea, abdominal fullness/bloating.

DRUG INTERACTIONS
Caution w/ medications that increase risk for fluid and electrolyte disturbances or may increase risk of adverse events (eg, seizures, arrhythmias, prolonged QT, renal impairment). Caution w/ drugs that lower seizure threshold (eg, TCAs) and in patients withdrawing from alcohol or benzodiazepines. Caution w/ drugs that may affect renal function (eg, diuretics, ACE inhibitors, ARBs, NSAIDs). Oral medication administered w/in 1 hr of start of administration may be flushed from GI tract and may not be absorbed properly. Avoid w/ stimulant laxatives (eg, bisacodyl, sodium picosulfate); may increase the risk of mucosal ulceration or ischemic colitis.

PREGNANCY AND LACTATION
Category C, caution in nursing.

MECHANISM OF ACTION
Osmotic laxative; primary mode of action is thought to be through the osmotic effect of PEG 3350 which causes water to be retained in the colon and produces a watery stool.

PHARMACOKINETICS
Absorption: Poor (Oral PEG 3350).

PATIENT CONSIDERATIONS
Assessment: Assess for drug hypersensitivity, GI obstruction, gastric retention, bowel perforation, ileus, toxic colitis, toxic megacolon, fluid and electrolyte abnormalities, renal impairment, any other conditions where treatment is cautioned, pregnancy/nursing status, and possible drug interactions. Consider predose ECG in patients at increased risk of serious cardiac arrhythmias.

Monitoring: Monitor for arrhythmias, generalized tonic-clonic seizures, loss of consciousness, colonic mucosal aphthous ulceration, ischemic colitis, and other adverse reactions. Monitor patients w/ impaired gag reflex, unconscious or semiconscious patients, and patients prone to regurgitation or aspiration, especially if administered via NG tube. Consider performing postcolonoscopy lab tests (electrolytes, SrCr, BUN) in patients w/ dehydration or renal impairment.

Counseling: Inform that sol is more palatable if chilled. Instruct to inform physician if have trouble swallowing or are prone to regurgitation or aspiration. Instruct not to take other laxatives. Instruct to consume water or clear liquids during the bowel preparation and after completion of the bowel preparation up until 2 hrs before the time of the colonoscopy. If severe bloating, distention, or abdominal pain occur, instruct to slow or temporarily d/c administration until symptoms abate; advise to report these events to physician. Instruct to d/c and contact physician if hives, rashes, or any allergic reaction develop. Instruct to notify physician if signs/symptoms of dehydration develop. Inform that oral medication administered w/in 1 hr of the start of administration may be flushed from the GI tract and the medication may not be absorbed completely. Counsel that rapid drinking of each portion is preferred rather than drinking small amounts continuously. Inform that the 1st bowel movement should occur approximately 1 hr after start of administration and to continue drinking until the watery stool is clear and free of solid matter.

GONAL-F RFF — follitropin alfa   Rx
Class: Follicle-stimulating hormone (FSH)

ADULT DOSAGE
Ovulation Induction

Infertile Women w/ Oligo-Anovulation:
Initial: 75 IU/day for 1st cycle
Titrate: Incremental adjustments of up to 37.5 IU may be considered after 14 days; may further increase dose, if necessary, every 7 days
Treatment duration should not exceed 35 days unless E2 rise indicates imminent follicular development
Administer human chorionic gonadotropin (hCG) after the last dose of follitropin alfa; withhold if serum estradiol is >2000pg/mL
Do not administer hCG and d/c therapy if ovaries are abnormally enlarged or abdominal pain occurs
Max: 300 IU/day

Assisted Reproductive Technology
For development of multiple follicles in ovulatory women

Initial: 150 IU/day starting in the early follicular phase (cycle day 2 or 3) until sufficient follicular development is attained (should not exceed 10 days)

<35 Years w/ Suppressed Endogenous Gonadotropin Levels:
Initial: 150 IU/day
≥35 Years w/ Suppressed Endogenous Gonadotropin Levels:
Initial: 225 IU/day
Continue treatment until adequate follicular development is indicated

Titrate: Adjust dose after 5 days based on response; do not adjust more frequently than every 3-5 days and by no more than 75-150 IU additionally at each adjustment
Max: 450 IU/day

Administer human chorionic gonadotropin once adequate follicular development is evident; withhold in cases where ovaries are abnormally enlarged on the last day of therapy

PEDIATRIC DOSAGE
Pediatric use may not have been established

ADMINISTRATION
SQ route

Pen
Administer SQ in the abdomen

Inj
Dissolve contents of ≥1 single-dose vials in 1mL of sterile water for inj; concentration should not exceed 450 IU/mL
Administer SQ immediately
Discard any unused reconstituted material

STORAGE
Pen: Prior To Dispensing: 2-8°C (36-46°F). Upon Dispensing: 2-8°C (36-46°F) until expiration date or 20-25°C (68-77°F) for up to 3 months or until expiration date, whichever comes first. After 1st Inj: 2-8°C (36-46°F) or 20-25°C (68-77°F) for up to 28 days. Protect from light. Do not freeze. Discard unused material after 28 days. Vial: 2-25°C (36-77°F). Protect from light. Use immediately after reconstitution. Discard unused material.

HOW SUPPLIED
Inj: 75 IU [vial]; 300 IU/0.5mL, 450 IU/0.75mL, 900 IU/1.5mL [prefilled pen]

CONTRAINDICATIONS
High follicle-stimulating hormone (FSH) levels indicating primary gonadal failure, uncontrolled thyroid or adrenal dysfunction, sex-hormone-dependent tumors of the reproductive tract and accessory organs, organic intracranial lesion (eg, pituitary tumor), abnormal uterine bleeding of undetermined origin, ovarian cyst or enlargement of undetermined origin, pregnancy.

WARNINGS/PRECAUTIONS
Should only be used by physicians thoroughly familiar with infertility problems and their management. Uncomplicated ovarian enlargement with abdominal distention and/or abdominal pain may occur; d/c treatment, do not administer hCG, and advise patient not to have intercourse. May cause ovarian hyperstimulation syndrome (OHSS) with or without pulmonary or vascular complications. Hepatic dysfunction reported in association with OHSS. Withhold hCG if evidence of OHSS develops prior to hCG administration. Monitor patients for at least 2 weeks after hCG administration; d/c treatment and hospitalize patient if severe OHSS occurs. Serious pulmonary conditions (eg, atelectasis, acute respiratory distress syndrome, and exacerbation of asthma), thromboembolic events (both associated with and separate from OHSS), and multiple births reported. In infertile patients with oligo-anovulation, the couple should be encouraged to have intercourse daily, beginning on the day prior to administration of hCG until ovulation becomes apparent from the indices employed for determination of progestational activity. Patients with tubal obstruction should receive therapy only if enrolled in an in vitro fertilization program. Evaluation of partner's fertility potential must be conducted prior to initiation of therapy.

ADVERSE REACTIONS
Vaginal hemorrhage, abdomen enlargement, ovarian cyst, ovarian hyperstimulation, abdominal pain, breast pain, diarrhea, flatulence, headache, pharyngitis, rhinitis, sinusitis, nausea, inj-site bruising/pain.

PREGNANCY AND LACTATION
Category X, not for use in nursing.

MECHANISM OF ACTION
FSH; stimulates ovarian follicular growth in women who do not have primary ovarian failure.

PHARMACOKINETICS
Absorption: C_{max}=9.83 IU/L; T_{max}=15.5 hrs; AUC=884 IU•hr/L. **Elimination:** $T_{1/2}$=53 hrs.

PATIENT CONSIDERATIONS
Assessment: Assess for prior hypersensitivity to drug, primary gonadal failure, uncontrolled thyroid or adrenal dysfunction, sex-hormone-dependent tumors of the reproductive tract and accessory organs, organic intracranial lesions, abnormal uterine bleeding or other signs of endometrial abnormalities, ovarian cysts or enlargement, tubal obstruction, and for any other conditions where treatment is contraindicated or cautioned. Assess pregnancy/nursing status and partner's fertility potential. Perform thorough gynecologic/endocrinologic evaluation, including pelvic anatomy assessment. Obtain baseline FSH and gonadotropin levels.

Monitoring: Monitor for OHSS, pulmonary/vascular complications, ovarian enlargement, abdominal pain, and other adverse reactions. Monitor ovarian response with serum estradiol and vaginal ultrasound regularly. In infertile patients with oligo-anovulation, conduct a follow-up visit in the luteal phase. Confirm ovulation by direct and indirect indices of progesterone production and by sonographic visualization of the ovaries.

Counseling: Inform about duration of treatment and the required monitoring of the condition. Counsel about possibility of multiple births, risk of OHSS, and other adverse reactions. In infertile patients with oligo-anovulation, encourage to have intercourse daily, beginning on the day prior to administration of hCG until ovulation becomes apparent. If ovaries become abnormally enlarged or abdominal pain occurs, advise patient not to have intercourse and to consult physician.

GRALISE — gabapentin   Rx

Class: GABA analogue

ADULT DOSAGE
Postherpetic Neuralgia
Recommended Titration Schedule:
Day 1: 300mg qd
Day 2: 600mg qd
Days 3-6: 900mg qd
Days 7-10: 1200mg qd
Days 11-14: 1500mg qd
Day 15: 1800mg qd

Dose reduction or substitution w/ an alternative medication should be done gradually over ≥1 week

PEDIATRIC DOSAGE
Pediatric use may not have been established

DOSING CONSIDERATIONS
Renal Impairment
Initial: 300mg qd
Titrate: Refer to Adult Dosage
CrCl ≥60mL/min: 1800mg qd
CrCl 30-60mL/min: 600-1800mg qd
CrCl <30mL/min or Hemodialysis: Do not administer

Discontinuation
D/C gradually over ≥1 week

ADMINISTRATION
Oral route

Take w/ pm meal
Swallow tabs whole; do not split, crush, or chew

STORAGE
25°C (77°F); excursions permitted to 15-30°C (59-86°F).

HOW SUPPLIED
Tab: 300mg, 600mg

CONTRAINDICATIONS
Hypersensitivity to gabapentin or to any of the ingredients in this medication.

WARNINGS/PRECAUTIONS
Not interchangeable w/ other gabapentin products. Increased risk of suicidal thoughts or behavior. May have tumorigenic potential. Drug reaction w/ eosinophilia and systemic symptoms (DRESS)/multiorgan hypersensitivity reported; evaluate immediately if signs/symptoms are present, and d/c therapy if an alternative etiology cannot be established. Lab test interactions may occur.

ADVERSE REACTIONS
Dizziness, somnolence, headache, peripheral edema, diarrhea.

DRUG INTERACTIONS
Naproxen may increase absorption. May reduce levels of hydrocodone. Hydrocodone and morphine may increase AUC. Cimetidine may decrease oral clearance and CrCl. Reduced bioavailability w/ an antacid containing aluminum hydroxide and magnesium hydroxide; take at least 2 hrs following the antacid.

PREGNANCY AND LACTATION
Category C, caution in nursing.

MECHANISM OF ACTION
Gamma-aminobutyric acid analogue; not established. Hypothesized to antagonize thrombospondin binding to α2delta-1 as a receptor involved in excitatory synapse formation. May function therapeutically by blocking new synapse formation.

PHARMACOKINETICS
Absorption: (1800mg qd) C_{max}=9585ng/mL; T_{max}=8 hrs; AUC_{0-24}=132,808ng•hr/mL. **Distribution:** Plasma protein binding (<3%); found in breast milk; (150mg IV) V_d=58L. **Elimination:** Renal (unchanged); (1200-3000mg/day) $T_{1/2}$=5-7 hrs.

PATIENT CONSIDERATIONS

Assessment: Assess for preexisting tumors, depression, hypersensitivity to drug, renal function, pregnancy/nursing status, and possible drug interactions.

Monitoring: Monitor for emergence or worsening of depression, suicidal thoughts/behavior, and/or any unusual changes in mood/behavior, new or worsening tumors, DRESS, and other adverse reactions.

Counseling: Advise that drug is not interchangeable w/ other formulations of gabapentin, and to take only as prescribed. Inform that drug may cause dizziness, somnolence, and other signs and symptoms of CNS depression; advise not to

drive or operate machinery until sufficient experience on therapy is gained. Advise that if a dose is missed, to take drug w/ food as soon as remembered, or, if it is almost time for the next dose, to just skip the missed dose and take the next dose at the regular time; instruct not to take 2 doses at the same time. Inform that drug may increase the risk of suicidal thoughts and behavior; advise to report to physician any behaviors of concern.

GRANISETRON — granisetron hydrochloride   Rx

Class: 5-HT$_3$ receptor antagonist

OTHER BRAND NAMES
Kytril (Discontinued)

ADULT DOSAGE
Chemotherapy-Induced Nausea/Vomiting

Prevention of N/V Associated w/ Initial and Repeat Courses of Cancer Therapy (eg, High Dose Cisplatin):
PO:
2mg qd up to 1 hr before chemotherapy or 1mg bid up to 1 hr before chemotherapy and 12 hrs later
IV:
10mcg/kg w/in 30 min before initiation of chemotherapy

Radiotherapy Associated Nausea/Vomiting

Prevention of N/V Associated w/ Radiation (Total Body Irradiation and Fractionated Abdominal Radiation):
PO:
2mg qd w/in 1 hr of radiation

PEDIATRIC DOSAGE
Chemotherapy-Induced Nausea/Vomiting

Prevention of N/V Associated w/ Initial and Repeat Courses of Cancer Therapy (eg, High Dose Cisplatin):
2-16 Years:
10mcg/kg IV w/in 30 min before initiation of chemotherapy

ADMINISTRATION
Oral, IV route

Give only on the days chemotherapy is given
May be administered IV either undiluted over 30 sec, or diluted w/ 0.9% NaCl or D5W and infused over 5 min
Stable for at least 24 hrs when diluted in 0.9% NaCl or D5W and stored at room temperature under normal lighting conditions
Do not mix in sol w/ other drugs

STORAGE
20-25°C (68-77°F). Protect from light. (Inj) Excursions permitted to 15-30°C (59-86°F). Do not freeze. Once the multidose vial is penetrated, use w/in 30 days.

HOW SUPPLIED
Inj: 0.1mg/mL [1mL], 1mg/mL [1mL, 4mL]; **Tab:** 1mg

CONTRAINDICATIONS
Known hypersensitivity to granisetron or any of the components in this product.

WARNINGS/PRECAUTIONS
Does not stimulate gastric or intestinal peristalsis; do not use instead of NG suction. Use in patients following abdominal surgery or w/ chemotherapy-induced N/V may mask a progressive ileus and/or gastric distention. QT prolongation reported; caution w/ preexisting arrhythmias or cardiac conduction disorders. Serotonin syndrome reported; d/c and initiate supportive treatment if symptoms occur. (Inj) Hypersensitivity reactions may occur in patients w/ known hypersensitivity to other selective 5-HT$_3$ receptor antagonists.

ADVERSE REACTIONS
Headache, constipation, fever, AST/ALT elevation. (Tab) Asthenia, diarrhea, abdominal pain, dyspepsia, dizziness, leukopenia, decreased appetite, insomnia, anemia, alopecia.

DRUG INTERACTIONS
Hepatic CYP450 enzyme inducers or inhibitors may change the clearance and $T_{1/2}$. Caution w/ cardiotoxic chemotherapy, drugs known to prolong QT interval and/or arrhythmogenic drugs. Serotonin syndrome reported w/ concomitant use of other serotonergic drugs (eg, SSRIs, SNRIs, MAOIs); d/c and initiate supportive treatment if symptoms occur.

PREGNANCY AND LACTATION
Category B, caution in nursing.

MECHANISM OF ACTION
5-HT$_3$ receptor antagonist; blocks serotonin stimulation and subsequent vomiting after emetogenic stimuli.

PHARMACOKINETICS
Absorption: C_{max}=63.8ng/mL (IV, 40mcg/kg), 5.99ng/mL (median) (Oral). **Distribution:** Plasma protein binding (65%). V_d=3.07L/kg (IV, 40mcg/kg). **Metabolism:** CYP3A; N-demethylation, aromatic ring oxidation, conjugation. **Elimination:** (Oral) Urine (11% unchanged, 48% metabolites), feces (38% metabolites). (IV) Urine (12% unchanged, 49% metabolites), feces (34% metabolites); $T_{1/2}$=8.95 hrs (IV, 40mcg/kg).

PATIENT CONSIDERATIONS

Assessment: Assess for preexisting arrhythmias, cardiac conduction disorders, cardiac disease, electrolyte abnormalities, previous hypersensitivity to drug, pregnancy/nursing status, and possible drug interactions.

Monitoring: Monitor for masking of progressive ileus and gastric distention, QT prolongation, serotonin syndrome, hypersensitivity reactions, and other adverse reactions.

Counseling: Inform about risks/benefits of therapy. Advise to report any adverse events to physician. Instruct to seek immediate medical attention if symptoms of serotonin syndrome occur.

GRANISOL — granisetron hydrochloride Rx

Class: 5-HT$_3$ receptor antagonist

ADULT DOSAGE	PEDIATRIC DOSAGE
Chemotherapy-Induced Nausea/Vomiting	Pediatric use may not have been established
Prevention of N/V Associated w/ Initial and Repeat Courses of Emetogenic Cancer Therapy (Including High-Dose Cisplatin): 2mg qd given up to 1 hr before chemotherapy or 1mg bid given up to 1 hr before chemotherapy and 12 hrs later	
Radiotherapy Associated Nausea/Vomiting	
Prevention of N/V Associated w/ Radiation (Including Total Body Irradiation and Fractionated Abdominal Radiation): 2mg qd w/in 1 hr of radiation	

ADMINISTRATION
Oral route

STORAGE
20-25°C (68-77°F); excursions permitted to 15-30°C (59-86°F). Store upright. Keep tightly closed. Protect from light.

HOW SUPPLIED
Sol: 2mg/10mL [30mL]

CONTRAINDICATIONS
Known hypersensitivity to the drug or any of its components.

WARNINGS/PRECAUTIONS
Does not stimulate gastric or intestinal peristalsis; do not use instead of nasogastric suction. May mask progressive ileus or gastric distention. QT prolongation reported; caution with preexisting arrhythmias, cardiac conduction disorders, cardiac disease, and electrolyte abnormalities.

ADVERSE REACTIONS
Headache, constipation, asthenia, diarrhea, abdominal pain, dyspepsia, dizziness, insomnia, fever, leukopenia, decreased appetite, anemia, alopecia.

DRUG INTERACTIONS
Hepatic CYP450 enzyme inducers or inhibitors may alter clearance and T$_{1/2}$. Caution with cardiotoxic chemotherapy; drugs known to prolong QT interval and/or arrhythmogenic drugs. May inhibit metabolism with ketoconazole. (IV) Increased total plasma clearance with phenobarbital.

PREGNANCY AND LACTATION
Category B, caution in nursing.

MECHANISM OF ACTION
5-HT$_3$ receptor antagonist; blocks serotonin stimulation and subsequent vomiting after emetogenic stimuli.

PHARMACOKINETICS
Absorption: C_{max}=5.99ng/mL (1mg bid), 3.63ng/mL (1mg single dose).
Distribution: Plasma protein binding (65%); V_d=3.94L/kg (1mg single dose).
Metabolism: CYP3A; N-demethylation, aromatic ring oxidation, then conjugation.
Elimination: Urine (11% unchanged, 48% metabolites), feces (38% metabolites); T$_{1/2}$=6.23 hrs (1mg single dose).

PATIENT CONSIDERATIONS
Assessment: Assess for preexisting arrhythmias, cardiac conduction disorders, cardiac disease, electrolyte abnormalities, hypersensitivity to drug, pregnancy/nursing status, and possible drug interactions.

Monitoring: Monitor for masking of progressive ileus and gastric distention, QT prolongation, and hypersensitivity reactions.

Counseling: Inform about risks/benefits of therapy. Advise patients to report any adverse events to their healthcare provider.

GRANIX — tbo-filgrastim Rx

Class: Granulocyte colony-stimulating factor (G-CSF)

ADULT DOSAGE	PEDIATRIC DOSAGE
Chemotherapy-Associated Neutropenia	Pediatric use may not have been established
Reducing the Duration of Severe Neutropenia in Patients w/ Non-Myeloid Malignancies Receiving Myelosuppressive Anticancer Drugs: 5mcg/kg/day SQ	

Continue daily dosing until the expected neutrophil nadir is passed and the neutrophil count has recovered to the normal range

ADMINISTRATION
SQ route
Administer the 1st dose no earlier than 24 hrs following myelosuppressive chemotherapy; do not administer w/in 24 hrs prior to chemotherapy.
Prefilled syringes are for single use only; discard unused portions.
Recommended sites of administration include abdomen (except for the 2-inch area around the navel), the front of the middle thighs, the upper outer areas of the buttocks, or the upper back portion of the upper arms.
Vary inj site daily.
Do not inject into an area that is tender, red, bruised, hard, or that has scars or stretch marks.
Avoid shaking syringe.

STORAGE
2-8°C (36-46°F). Protect from light. May be removed from 2-8°C (36-46°F) storage for a single period of up to 5 days between 23-27°C (73-81°F); if not used w/in 5 days, may be returned to 2-8°C (36-46°F).

HOW SUPPLIED
Inj: 300mcg/0.5mL, 480mcg/0.8mL

WARNINGS/PRECAUTIONS
May be administered by either a healthcare professional or by a patient/caregiver; before a decision is made to allow therapy to be administered by a patient/caregiver, ensure that the patient is an appropriate candidate for self-administration or administration by a caregiver. Splenic rupture, including fatal cases, may occur; d/c therapy and evaluate for an enlarged spleen or splenic rupture if upper abdominal or shoulder pain occurs. Acute respiratory distress syndrome (ARDS) may occur; evaluate for ARDS if fever and lung infiltrates or respiratory distress develops, and d/c if ARDS occurs. Serious allergic reactions may occur; permanently d/c if such reactions occur. Severe and sometimes fatal sickle cell crises may occur in patients w/ sickle cell disease; d/c in patients undergoing a sickle cell crisis. Capillary leak syndrome (CLS) may occur; closely monitor and give standard symptomatic treatment if symptoms develop. May act as a growth factor for any tumor type. Increased hematopoietic activity of the bone marrow in response to therapy has been associated w/ transient positive bone imaging changes; consider this when interpreting bone-imaging results.

ADVERSE REACTIONS
Bone pain.

DRUG INTERACTIONS
Caution w/ drugs that may potentiate the release of neutrophils (eg, lithium).

PREGNANCY AND LACTATION
Pregnancy: Category C.
Lactation: Caution in nursing.

MECHANISM OF ACTION
Granulocyte colony-stimulating factor (G-CSF); binds to G-CSF receptors and stimulates proliferation of neutrophils. Known to stimulate differentiation commitment and some end-cell functional activation, which increases neutrophil counts and activity.

PHARMACOKINETICS
Absorption: Absolute bioavailability (33%); T_{max}=4-6 hrs (median). **Elimination:** $T_{1/2}$=3.2-3.8 hrs (median).

PATIENT CONSIDERATIONS
Assessment: Assess for history of hypersensitivity to the drug, history of serious allergic reactions to filgrastim or pegfilgrastim, sickle cell disease, pregnancy/nursing status, and possible drug interactions. Assess CBC prior to chemotherapy.

Monitoring: Monitor for enlarged spleen/splenic rupture, ARDS, serious allergic reactions, sickle cell crisis (in patients w/ sickle cell disease), CLS, and other adverse reactions. Monitor CBC twice per week until recovery.

Counseling: Instruct patient or caregivers on the proper storage, preparation, and administration technique once it is determined that a patient is an appropriate candidate for self-administration or administration by a caregiver. Instruct to report any symptoms of adverse reactions to physician. Inform that bone pain is common and analgesics may be necessary. Counsel to be alert for signs of infection and to report these findings to physician immediately. Inform not to become pregnant while on therapy; advise of the possibility of fetal harm if pregnancy occurs.

GRISEOFULVIN — griseofulvin Rx

Class: *Penicillium*-derived antifungal

OTHER BRAND NAMES
Grifulvin V

ADULT DOSAGE	PEDIATRIC DOSAGE
Tinea Infections	**Tinea Infections**
Treatment of dermatophyte infections of the skin not adequately treated by topical therapy, hair and nails, namely: tinea corporis, tinea pedis, tinea cruris,	Treatment of dermatophyte infections of the skin not adequately treated by topical therapy, hair and nails, namely: tinea corporis, tinea pedis, tinea cruris,

tinea barbae, tinea capitis; and tinea unguium caused by *Epidermophyton floccosum, Microsporum audouinii, M. canis, M. gypseum, Trichophyton crateriform, T. gallinae, T. interdigitalis, T. megnini, T. mentagrophytes, T. rubrum, T. schoenleini, T. sulphureum, T. tonsurans,* and *T. verrucosum*

Sus/Tab:
500mg/day (125mg qid, 250mg bid, or 500mg/day)

Widespread Lesions:
Tab:
Initial: 0.75-1g/day; may reduce gradually to ≤0.5g after a response has been noted

Infections Difficult to Eradicate (eg, Tinea Pedis/Tinea Unguium):
Sus:
1g/day

Treatment Duration

Tinea Capitis:
4-6 weeks
Tinea Corporis:
2-4 weeks
Tinea Pedis:
4-8 weeks
Tinea Unguium:
≥4 months (fingernails) or ≥6 months (toenails), depending on rate of growth

---

ADMINISTRATION
Oral route
STORAGE
20-25°C (68-77°F).
HOW SUPPLIED
Sus: 125mg/5mL [120mL]; **Tab:** (Grifulvin V) 500mg* *scored
CONTRAINDICATIONS
Porphyria, hepatocellular failure, women who are or may become pregnant, history of hypersensitivity to griseofulvin.
WARNINGS/PRECAUTIONS
Serious skin reactions (eg, Stevens-Johnson syndrome, toxic epidermal necrolysis) and erythema multiforme reported; d/c if these occur. Elevations in AST, ALT, bilirubin, and jaundice reported; monitor for hepatic adverse events and consider discontinuation if warranted. Possibility of cross-sensitivity with penicillin (PCN) exists. Lupus erythematosus, lupus-like syndromes or exacerbation of existing lupus erythematosus reported. Photosensitivity reactions reported; avoid exposure to intense or prolonged natural/artificial sunlight. D/C if granulocytopenia occurs. Male patients should wait at least 6 months after completing therapy before fathering a child. Concomitant use of appropriate topical agents is usually required (particularly in tinea pedis).
ADVERSE REACTIONS
Skin rash, urticaria.
DRUG INTERACTIONS
Decreases activity of warfarin-type anticoagulants; may require dosage adjustment of the anticoagulant during and after therapy. May reduce the effectiveness of estrogen-containing oral contraceptives and cause menstrual irregularities; an alternate or 2nd form of birth control may be indicated during periods of concurrent use. May reduce cyclosporine and serum salicylate levels. Barbiturates may decrease plasma levels; coadministration may require dosage adjustment of the antifungal agent. N/V, flushing, tachycardia, and severe hypotension reported following alcohol ingestion during therapy.
PREGNANCY AND LACTATION
Category X, not for use in nursing.
MECHANISM OF ACTION
Penicillium-derived antifungal; binds to microtubular proteins, which are required for mitosis.
PHARMACOKINETICS
Absorption: Primarily absorbed in the duodenum. (Fasted, 0.5g dose) C_{max}=0.5-2mcg/mL; T_{max}=4 hrs. **Metabolism:** Liver via glucuronidation; 6-desmethylgriseofulvin (metabolite). **Elimination:** Feces (1/3 of dose within 5 days), urine (30% within 24 hrs, 50% within 5 days, <1% unchanged), perspiration; $T_{1/2}$=9-24 hrs.

PATIENT CONSIDERATIONS

Assessment: Assess for porphyria, hepatocellular failure, lupus erythematosus, PCN sensitivity, history of hypersensitivity to the drug, pregnancy/nursing status, and possible drug interactions. Obtain specimens for lab testing (potassium hydroxide preparation, fungal culture, or nail biopsy) to confirm diagnosis. Obtain baseline LFTs.

Monitoring: Monitor for photosensitivity reactions, lupus erythematosus or exacerbation of lupus erythematosus, lupus-like syndrome, granulocytopenia, serious skin reactions, jaundice, and other adverse reactions. Periodically monitor renal, hepatic, and hematopoietic functions with prolonged therapy.

tinea barbae, tinea capitis; and tinea unguium caused by *Epidermophyton floccosum, Microsporum audouinii, M. canis, M. gypseum, Trichophyton crateriform, T. gallinae, T. interdigitalis, T. megnini, T. mentagrophytes, T. rubrum, T. schoenleini, T. sulphureum, T. tonsurans,* and *T. verrucosum*

>2 Years:
10mg/kg/day (approx 5mg/lb/day)
30-50 lbs:
125-250mg/day
>50 lbs:
250-500mg/day in divided doses

Counseling: Inform of benefits and risks of therapy. Instruct to avoid exposure to intense or prolonged natural/artificial sunlight. Instruct to inform physician if pregnant, intending to become pregnant, or planning to breastfeed. Counsel male patients to wait at least 6 months after completing therapy before fathering a child. Instruct to contact physician if any adverse reactions occur.

HALAVEN — eribulin mesylate   Rx

Class: Antimicrotubule agent

ADULT DOSAGE	**PEDIATRIC DOSAGE**

ADULT DOSAGE

Metastatic Breast Cancer
Treatment of patients who have previously received at least 2 chemotherapeutic regimens (anthracycline and a taxane in adjuvant/metastatic setting) for the treatment of metastatic disease

Recommended: 1.4mg/m²
Administer IV over 2-5 min on Days 1 and 8 of a 21-day cycle

Unresectable or Metastatic Liposarcoma
Treatment of patients who have received a prior anthracycline-containing regimen

Recommended: 1.4mg/m²
Administer IV over 2-5 min on Days 1 and 8 of a 21-day cycle

PEDIATRIC DOSAGE
Pediatric use may not have been established

DOSING CONSIDERATIONS
Renal Impairment
Moderate to Severe (CrCl 15-49mL/min):
1.1mg/m²

Hepatic Impairment
Mild (Child-Pugh A):
1.1mg/m²

Moderate (Child-Pugh B):
0.7mg/m²

Adverse Reactions
Do Not Administer on Day 1 or Day 8 for Any of the Following:
ANC <1000/mm³
Platelets <75,000/mm³
Grade 3 or 4 nonhematological toxicities

The Day 8 Dose May Be Delayed for a Maximum of 1 Week:
If toxicities do not resolve or improve to ≤Grade 2 severity by Day 15, omit the dose.
If toxicities resolve or improve to ≤Grade 2 severity by Day 15, administer at a reduced dose and initiate the next cycle no sooner than 2 weeks later.

Permanently Reduce to 1.1mg/m² for Any of the Following:
ANC <500/mm³ for >7 days
ANC <1000/mm³ w/ fever or infection
Platelets <25,000/mm³
Platelets <50,000/mm³ requiring transfusion
Nonhematologic Grade 3 or 4 toxicities
Omission or delay of Day 8 dose in previous cycle for toxicity

Reduce to 0.7mg/m² If:
Occurrence of any event requiring permanent dose reduction while receiving 1.1mg/m²

D/C If:
Occurrence of any event requiring permanent dose reduction while receiving 0.7mg/m²
If a dose has been delayed for toxicity and toxicities have recovered to ≤Grade 2, resume at a reduced dose.
Do not re-escalate dose after it has been reduced.

ADMINISTRATION
IV route
Withdraw required amount of eribulin from the single use vial and administer undiluted or diluted in 100mL of 0.9% NaCl inj.
Do not dilute in or administer through an IV line containing sol w/ dextrose.
Do not administer in the same IV line concurrent w/ other medicinal products.
Store undiluted eribulin in the syringe for up to 4 hrs at room temperature or for up to 24 hrs under refrigeration (4°C [40°F]).
Store diluted sol of eribulin for up to 4 hrs at room temperature or up to 24 hrs under refrigeration.
STORAGE
25°C (77°F); excursions permitted to 15-30°C (59-86°F). Do not freeze.
HOW SUPPLIED
Inj: 0.5mg/mL [2mL]
WARNINGS/PRECAUTIONS
See Dosing Considerations. Severe neutropenia (ANC <500/mm³) reported. Peripheral neuropathy reported. Can cause fetal harm. QT prolongation reported; monitor ECG in patients w/ CHF, bradyarrhythmias, and electrolyte abnormalities.

Correct hypokalemia or hypomagnesemia prior to therapy. Avoid w/ congenital long QT syndrome.

ADVERSE REACTIONS
Metastatic Breast Cancer: Neutropenia, anemia, asthenia/fatigue, alopecia, peripheral neuropathy, nausea, constipation.
Liposarcoma: Fatigue, nausea, alopecia, constipation, peripheral neuropathy, abdominal pain, pyrexia.

DRUG INTERACTIONS
Monitor ECG w/ drugs known to prolong the QT interval (eg, Class IA and III antiarrhythmics).

PREGNANCY AND LACTATION
Pregnancy: Can cause fetal harm based on findings from an animal reproduction study and mechanism of action. Advise pregnant women of the potential risk to fetus.
Lactation: There is no information regarding the presence of eribulin or its metabolites in human milk, the effects on the breastfed infant, or the effects on milk production. Advise women not to breastfeed during treatment and for 2 weeks after the final dose.
Reproductive Potential: Advise females of reproductive potential to use effective contraception during treatment and for at least 2 weeks following the final dose. Advise males w/ female partners of reproductive potential to use effective contraception during treatment and for 3.5 months following the final dose. May result in damage to male reproductive tissues leading to impaired fertility of unknown duration.

MECHANISM OF ACTION
Antimicrotubule agent; inhibits the growth phase of microtubules via a tubulin-based antimitotic mechanism leading to G_2/M cell-cycle block, disruption of mitotic spindles, and, ultimately, apoptotic cell death after prolonged mitotic blockage.

PHARMACOKINETICS
Distribution: V_d=43-114L/m^2; plasma protein binding (49-65%). **Elimination:** Urine (9%, 91% unchanged), feces (82%, 88% unchanged); $T_{1/2}$=40 hrs.

PATIENT CONSIDERATIONS
Assessment: Assess for renal/hepatic impairment, CHF, bradyarrhythmias, congenital long QT syndrome, electrolyte abnormalities, pregnancy/nursing status, and possible drug interactions. Correct hypokalemia or hypomagnesemia prior to initiating therapy. Assess for peripheral neuropathy and obtain CBC prior to each dose.
Monitoring: Monitor for severe neutropenia, peripheral motor and sensory neuropathy, and other adverse reactions. Monitor ECG in patients w/ CHF, bradyarrhythmias, and electrolyte abnormalities. Monitor K$^+$ and Mg^{2+} levels periodically. Increase frequency of CBC monitoring if Grade 3 or 4 cytopenias develop.
Counseling: Advise to contact physician for a fever ≥38.1°C (100.5°F) or other signs/symptoms of infection (eg, chills, cough, burning/pain on urination). Advise to inform physician of new/worsening numbness, tingling, and pain in the extremities. Advise females of reproductive potential of the potential risk to a fetus, to inform physician of known/suspected pregnancy, and to use effective contraception during treatment and for at least 2 weeks after the final dose. Advise males w/ female partners of reproductive potential to use effective contraception during treatment and for 3.5 months following the final dose. Advise women not to breastfeed during treatment and for 2 weeks after the final dose.

HALCION — triazolam   CIV
Class: Benzodiazepine

ADULT DOSAGE	PEDIATRIC DOSAGE
Insomnia	Pediatric use may not have been established
Short-Term Treatment (Generally 7-10 Days): 0.25mg qhs; 0.125mg may be sufficient for some patients (eg, low body weight) **Max:** 0.5mg	

DOSING CONSIDERATIONS
Elderly
Elderly/Debilitated:
Initial: 0.125mg
Max: 0.25mg

ADMINISTRATION
Oral route

STORAGE
20-25°C (68-77°F).

HOW SUPPLIED
Tab: 0.25mg* *scored

CONTRAINDICATIONS
Known hypersensitivity to this drug or other benzodiazepines; pregnancy; concomitant use w/ medications that significantly impair the oxidative metabolism mediated by CYP3A (eg, ketoconazole, itraconazole, nefazodone, HIV protease inhibitors).

WARNINGS/PRECAUTIONS
Initiate only after careful evaluation; failure of insomnia to remit after 7-10 days of treatment may indicate presence of a primary psychiatric and/or medical illness.

Use lowest effective dose, especially in elderly. Complex behaviors (eg, sleep-driving, preparing/eating food, making phone calls, having sex) reported; consider discontinuation if sleep-driving occurs. Severe anaphylactic and anaphylactoid reactions reported; do not rechallenge if angioedema develops. Increased daytime anxiety reported; may d/c if observed. Abnormal thinking, behavior changes, anterograde amnesia, paradoxical reactions, traveler's amnesia, and dose-related side effects (eg, drowsiness, dizziness, lightheadedness, amnesia) reported. Worsening of depression, including suicidal thinking, reported in primarily depressed patients. May impair mental/physical abilities. Respiratory depression and apnea reported in patients with compromised respiratory function. Caution in patients with signs or symptoms of depression that could be intensified by hypnotic drugs, renal/hepatic impairment, chronic pulmonary insufficiency, and sleep apnea. Dependence and tolerance to drug may develop; caution with history of alcoholism, drug abuse, or with marked personality disorders, due to increased risk of dependence. Withdrawal symptoms reported following abrupt discontinuation; avoid abrupt discontinuation, and taper dose gradually in any patient taking more than the lowest dose for more than a few weeks or with history of seizure.

ADVERSE REACTIONS
Drowsiness, dizziness, lightheadedness, headache, nervousness, coordination disorders/ataxia, N/V.

DRUG INTERACTIONS
See Contraindications. Avoid with very potent CYP3A inhibitors (eg, azole-type antifungals). Caution and consider triazolam dose reduction with drugs inhibiting CYP3A to a lesser but significant degree. Macrolide antibiotics (eg, erythromycin, clarithromycin) and cimetidine may increase levels; use with caution and consider triazolam dose reduction. Isoniazid, oral contraceptives, grapefruit juice, and ranitidine may increase levels; use with caution. Additive CNS depressant effects with psychotropic medications, anticonvulsants, antihistamines, ethanol, and other CNS depressants. Increased risk of complex behaviors with alcohol and other CNS depressants. Caution with fluvoxamine, diltiazem, verapamil, sertraline, paroxetine, ergotamine, cyclosporine, amiodarone, nicardipine, and nifedipine.

PREGNANCY AND LACTATION
Category X, not for use in nursing.

MECHANISM OF ACTION
Triazolobenzodiazepine hypnotic agent.

PHARMACOKINETICS
Absorption: C_{max}=1-6ng/mL; T_{max}=2 hrs. **Metabolism:** Hydroxylation via CYP3A.
Elimination: Urine (79.9% metabolites); $T_{1/2}$=1.5-5.5 hrs.

PATIENT CONSIDERATIONS
Assessment: Assess for physical and/or psychiatric disorder, depression, compromised respiratory function, renal/hepatic impairment, chronic pulmonary insufficiency, sleep apnea, history of seizures, alcoholism or drug abuse, marked personality disorders, hypersensitivity to the drug, pregnancy/nursing status, and possible drug interactions.
Monitoring: Monitor for complex behaviors, anaphylactic/anaphylactoid reactions, increased daytime anxiety, emergence of any new behavioral signs/symptoms of concern, tolerance, dependence, withdrawal symptoms, and other adverse reactions.
Counseling: Inform of the risks and benefits of therapy. Caution against engaging in hazardous activities requiring complete mental alertness (eg, operating machinery, driving). Instruct to immediately report to physician if any adverse reactions (eg, sleep-driving, other complex behaviors) develop. Caution about the concomitant ingestion of alcohol and other CNS depressant drugs during treatment. Instruct to notify physician if pregnant, planning to become pregnant, or if nursing.

HALOPERIDOL — haloperidol   Rx
Class: Butyrophenone

> Elderly patients w/ dementia-related psychosis treated w/ antipsychotic drugs are at an increased risk of death; most deaths appeared to be cardiovascular (CV) (eg, heart failure, sudden death) or infectious (eg, pneumonia) in nature. Not approved for the treatment of patients w/ dementia-related psychosis.

OTHER BRAND NAMES
Haldol

ADULT DOSAGE	PEDIATRIC DOSAGE
Psychosis	**Psychosis**
Sol/Tab:	**Sol/Tab:**
Initial:	**3-12 Years (15-40kg):**
Moderate Symptoms: 0.5-2mg bid or tid	**Initial:** 0.5mg/day
Severe Symptoms/Chronic or Resistant Patients: 3-5mg bid or tid	**Titrate:** Increase by 0.5mg increments at 5- to 7-day intervals
Remain Severely Disturbed/ Inadequately Controlled: May need up to 100mg/day; >100mg/day has been used for severely resistant patients but safety of prolonged use not demonstrated	**Maint:** Gradually reduce to lowest effective dose; 0.05-0.15mg/kg/day Severely disturbed psychotic children may require higher doses
Maint: Gradually reduce to lowest effective dose	Total dose may be given bid or tid
	Behavioral Problems
	Failed Response to Psychotherapy/ Non-Antipsychotic Medications:
	Sol/Tab:
	3-12 Years (15-40kg):

Schizophrenia

Inj:
Acutely Agitated:
Moderately Severe to Very Severe Symptoms: 2-5mg
Subsequent Doses: May give as often as every hr; 4- to 8-hr intervals may be satisfactory
Max: 20mg/day

Tourette's Disorder
Sol/Tab:
Initial:
Moderate Symptoms:
0.5-2mg bid or tid
Severe Symptoms/Chronic or Resistant Patients:
3-5mg bid or tid
Remain Severely Disturbed/ Inadequately Controlled:
May need up to 100mg/day; >100mg/day has been used for severely resistant patients but safety of prolonged use not demonstrated
Maint:
Gradually reduce to lowest effective dose

Conversions
From IM to Oral Formulations:
For the initial approximation of the total daily dose required, the parenteral dose administered in the preceding 24 hrs should be used w/in 12-24 hrs following the last parenteral dose

Monitor clinical signs and symptoms periodically for the 1st several days

---

Initial: 0.5mg/day
Titrate: Increase by 0.5mg increments at 5- to 7-day intervals
Maint: Gradually reduce to lowest effective dose; 0.05-0.075mg/kg/day

Short-term treatment may suffice for severely disturbed, nonpsychotic/ hyperactive children w/ conduct disorders

There is no evidence establishing a max effective dose; little evidence exists that behavior improvement is further enhanced in dosages beyond 6mg/day

Total dose may be given bid or tid

Tourette's Disorder
Sol/Tab:
3-12 Years (15-40kg):
Initial: 0.5mg/day
Titrate: Increase by 0.5mg increments at 5- to 7-day intervals
Maint: Gradually reduce to lowest effective dose; 0.05-0.075mg/kg/day

Total dose may be given bid or tid

DOSING CONSIDERATIONS
Elderly
Inj:
Initial: May require lower dose
Sol/Tab:
Initial: 0.5-2mg bid or tid

Other Important Considerations
Debilitated Patients:
Inj:
Initial: May require lower dose
Sol/Tab:
Initial: 0.5-2mg bid or tid

History of Adverse Reactions to Antipsychotic Drugs:
Inj:
Initial: May require lower dose

ADMINISTRATION
Oral/IM route

STORAGE
Protect from light. **Tab/Sol:** 20-25°C (68-77°F). **Inj:** 15-30°C (59-86°F). **Inj/Sol:** Do not freeze.

HOW SUPPLIED
Inj: (Haldol) 5mg/mL; **Sol:** 2mg/mL [15mL, 120mL]; **Tab:** 0.5mg*, 1mg*, 2mg*, 5mg*, 10mg*, 20mg* *scored

CONTRAINDICATIONS
Severe toxic CNS depression or comatose states, Parkinson's disease, hypersensitivity to haloperidol.

WARNINGS/PRECAUTIONS
Risk of tardive dyskinesia (TD), especially in the elderly; consider discontinuation if signs/symptoms develop. Neuroleptic malignant syndrome (NMS) reported; d/c immediately, institute symptomatic treatment, and monitor. Hyperpyrexia, heat stroke, and bronchopneumonia reported. Dehydration, hemoconcentration, and reduced pulmonary ventilation may develop; institute prompt remedial therapy if signs/symptoms appear. Decreased serum cholesterol and/or cutaneous and ocular changes reported in patients receiving chemically related drugs. Leukopenia, neutropenia, and agranulocytosis reported; d/c if severe neutropenia (ANC <1000/mm^3) develops. Monitor CBC frequently during the 1st few months of therapy and consider discontinuation at 1st sign of clinically significant decline in WBCs in the absence of other causative factors if history of clinically significant preexisting low WBCs or drug-induced leukopenia/neutropenia exists. Caution w/ severe CV disease (CVD), in the elderly, and in patients w/ known/history of allergic reactions to drugs. May cause transient hypotension and/or precipitation of anginal pain in patients w/ severe CV disorders. If hypotension occurs and a vasopressor is required, treat w/ metaraminol, phenylephrine, or norepinephrine. There may be a rapid mood swing to depression when haloperidol is used to control mania in cyclic disorders. Severe neurotoxicity may occur in patients w/ thyrotoxicosis. May increase prolactin levels. May impair mental/physical abilities. May lower convulsive threshold; caution w/ history of seizures or EEG abnormalities. **Inj/Tab:** Sudden death, QT prolongation, and torsades de pointes

reported. Caution w/ other QT-prolonging conditions (eg, electrolyte imbalance, underlying cardiac abnormalities, hypothyroidism, familial long QT syndrome).

ADVERSE REACTIONS
Extrapyramidal symptoms, TD, dystonia, ECG changes, insomnia, restlessness, tachycardia, hypotension, HTN, N/V, constipation, diarrhea, dry mouth, blurred vision, urinary retention.

DRUG INTERACTIONS
Encephalopathic syndrome followed by irreversible brain damage may occur w/ lithium; monitor closely for early evidence of neurological toxicity and promptly d/c treatment if such signs appear. Caution w/ anticonvulsants and anticoagulants (eg, phenindione). Anticholinergics, including antiparkinson agents, may increase IOP. If an antiparkinson medication is discontinued simultaneously w/ haloperidol, extrapyramidal symptoms may occur. May potentiate CNS depressants (eg, alcohol, anesthetics, opiates); avoid w/ alcohol. Avoid w/ epinephrine for hypotension treatment; vasopressor activity may be blocked and paradoxical further lowering of BP may occur. **Inj/Tab:** Caution w/ drugs known to prolong the QT interval or cause electrolyte imbalance. Rifampin may decrease levels. **Inj:** Ketoconazole (400mg/day) and paroxetine (20mg/day) may increase QTc. Potential increased levels and risk of certain adverse events w/ inhibitors of CYP450 or glucuronidation. CYP3A4 or CYP2D6 substrates/inhibitors (eg, itraconazole, nefazodone, buspirone, venlafaxine) may increase levels. A significant reduction of haloperidol plasma levels may occur when prolonged treatment (1-2 weeks) w/ enzyme-inducing drugs (eg, carbamazepine) is added to haloperidol; carefully monitor clinical status when enzyme inducing drugs are administered or discontinued; haloperidol dose may need to be adjusted during concomitant use; may be necessary to reduce the haloperidol dose after discontinuation of such drugs.

PREGNANCY AND LACTATION
Pregnancy: Neonates exposed to antipsychotic drugs during the third trimester of pregnancy are at risk for extrapyramidal and/or withdrawal symptoms following delivery; agitation, hypertonia, hypotonia, tremor, somnolence, respiratory distress, and feeding disorder have been reported in these neonates. Haloperidol should be used during pregnancy only if the potential benefit justifies the potential risk to the fetus.
Lactation: Infants should not be nursed during drug treatment.

MECHANISM OF ACTION
Butyrophenone; not established.

PHARMACOKINETICS
Distribution: (Inj) Found in breast milk.

PATIENT CONSIDERATIONS
Assessment: Assess for severe toxic CNS depression or comatose states, Parkinson's disease, CVD, history of seizures, EEG abnormalities, hypersensitivity to drug, pregnancy/nursing status, and for any other conditions where treatment is contraindicated or cautioned. Assess for possible drug interactions.

Monitoring: Monitor for signs/symptoms of NMS, TD, bronchopneumonia, hyperpyrexia, heat stroke, QT prolongation, torsades de pointes, leukopenia, neutropenia, agranulocytosis, and for other adverse reactions. Monitor for neurotoxicity in patients w/ thyrotoxicosis. Monitor CBC frequently during the first few months of therapy in patients w/ a preexisting low WBC count or a history of drug-induced leukopenia/neutropenia. Carefully monitor for fever or other symptoms or signs of infection in patients w/ neutropenia. Monitor vital signs, ECG, EEG, serum electrolytes, and cholesterol levels.

Counseling: Inform about risks/benefits of therapy. Instruct to use caution when performing hazardous tasks (eg, operating machinery/driving). Instruct to avoid alcohol due to possible additive effects and hypotension. Advise to inform physician if nursing, pregnant, or planning to get pregnant.

HARVONI — ledipasvir/sofosbuvir Rx

Class: HCV NS5A inhibitor/HCV nucleotide analogue NS5B polymerase inhibitor

ADULT DOSAGE
Chronic Hepatitis C

Chronic HCV Genotype 1, 4, 5, or 6 Infection:
1 tab qd w/ or w/o ribavirin

Treatment Duration:

Genotype 1:
Treatment-Naive w/o Cirrhosis or w/ Compensated Cirrhosis (Child-Pugh A): 12 weeks; may consider treatment duration of 8 weeks in patients w/o cirrhosis who have pre-treatment HCV RNA <6 mIU/mL
Treatment-Experienced w/o Cirrhosis: 12 weeks
Treatment-Experienced w/ Compensated Cirrhosis: 24 weeks; may consider Harvoni + ribavirin for 12 weeks in patients w/ cirrhosis who are eligible for ribavirin
Treatment-Naive and Treatment-Experienced w/ Decompensated Cirrhosis (Child-Pugh B or C): Harvoni + ribavirin for 12 weeks

PEDIATRIC DOSAGE
Pediatric use may not have been established

Genotype 1 or 4:
Treatment-Naïve and Treatment-Experienced Liver Transplant Recipients w/o Cirrhosis, or w/ Compensated Cirrhosis: Harvoni + ribavirin for 12 weeks

Genotype 4, 5, or 6:
Treatment-Naïve and Treatment-Experienced w/o Cirrhosis or w/ Compensated Cirrhosis: 12 weeks

The recommended treatment durations are also applicable to patients w/ HCV/HIV-1 coinfection

For further information on ribavirin dosing and dosing modifications, refer to the ribavirin PI

DOSING CONSIDERATIONS
Renal Impairment
Mild/Moderate: No dosage adjustment required
Severe/ESRD: No dosage recommendation can be given due to higher exposures of the predominant sofosbuvir metabolite

ADMINISTRATION
Oral route

Take w/ or w/o food.

STORAGE
Room temperature <30°C (86°F).

HOW SUPPLIED
Tab: (Ledipasvir/Sofosbuvir) 90mg/400mg

CONTRAINDICATIONS
If administered w/ ribavirin, refer to the ribavirin prescribing information for a list of contraindications for ribavirin.

WARNINGS/PRECAUTIONS
Symptomatic bradycardia, as well as fatal cardiac arrest and cases requiring pacemaker intervention, reported when coadministered w/ amiodarone. Patients also taking β-blockers, or those w/ underlying cardiac comorbidities and/or advanced liver disease, may be at increased risk for symptomatic bradycardia w/ coadministration of amiodarone. Not recommended w/ amiodarone. If coadministration is required, cardiac monitoring in an in-patient setting for the first 48 hrs of coadministration is recommended, after which outpatient or self-monitoring of HR should occur on a daily basis through at least the first 2 weeks of therapy. Patients discontinuing amiodarone just prior to starting therapy should also undergo similar cardiac monitoring. P-gp inducers (eg, rifampin, St. John's wort) may decrease levels and may lead to a reduced therapeutic effect; not recommended w/ P-gp inducers. Not recommended w/ other products containing sofosbuvir. If administered w/ ribavirin, refer to the ribavirin prescribing information for the warnings and precautions for ribavirin.

ADVERSE REACTIONS
Fatigue, headache, asthenia.

DRUG INTERACTIONS
See Warnings/Precautions. Not recommended w/ carbamazepine, phenytoin, phenobarbital, oxcarbazepine, rifabutin, rifapentine, or tipranavir/ritonavir (RTV); may decrease levels. Not recommended w/ rosuvastatin; may increase rosuvastatin levels and consequently increase risk of myopathy, including rhabdomyolysis. May increase digoxin levels; monitor digoxin levels. Monitor for tenofovir-associated adverse reactions in patients receiving concomitant therapy w/ a regimen containing tenofovir disoproxil fumarate (TDF) w/o an HIV protease inhibitor/RTV or cobicistat. Coadministration w/ regimens containing TDF and an HIV protease inhibitor/RTV or cobicistat may increase tenofovir levels; consider alternative HCV or antiretroviral therapy to avoid increases in tenofovir exposures; if coadministration is necessary, monitor for tenofovir-associated adverse reactions. Coadministration w/ combination of elvitegravir, cobicistat, emtricitabine, and TDF is not recommended; may increase tenofovir levels. **Ledipasvir:** May increase intestinal absorption of coadministered substrates of P-gp or breast cancer resistance protein. Drugs that increase gastric pH may decrease levels. Separate administration w/ antacids by 4 hrs. May administer H2-receptor antagonists (eg, famotidine) simultaneously or 12 hrs apart from Harvoni at a dose that does not exceed doses comparable to famotidine 40mg bid. Proton-pump inhibitor doses comparable to omeprazole ≤20mg can be administered simultaneously under fasted conditions. Not recommended w/ simeprevir; may increase levels. Refer to PI for further information on drug interactions.

PREGNANCY AND LACTATION
Pregnancy: No adequate human data are available to establish whether or not Harvoni poses a risk to pregnancy outcomes.
Lactation: It is not known whether Harvoni and its metabolites are present in human breast milk, affect human milk production, or have effects on the breastfed infant; caution in nursing.

If administered w/ ribavirin, refer to the prescribing information of ribavirin for additional information.

MECHANISM OF ACTION
Ledipasvir: Inhibits HCV NS5A protein, which is required for viral replication.
Sofosbuvir: Inhibits HCV NS5B RNA-dependent RNA polymerase, which is required for viral replication.

PHARMACOKINETICS
Absorption: Ledipasvir: C_{max}=323ng/mL; T_{max}=4-4.5 hrs (median); AUC_{0-24}=7290ng•hr/mL. Sofosbuvir: C_{max}=618ng/mL, 707ng/mL (GS-331007); T_{max}=0.8-1 hr (median), 3.5-4 hrs (GS-331007); AUC_{0-24}=1320ng•hr/mL, 12,000ng•hr/mL (GS-331007). **Distribution:** Ledipasvir: Plasma protein binding (>99.8%). Sofosbuvir: Plasma protein binding (61-65%). **Metabolism:** Ledipasvir: Slow oxidative metabolism via an unknown mechanism. Sofosbuvir: Liver (extensive) to pharmacologically active nucleoside analogue triphosphate GS-461203; dephosphorylation to GS-331007 (inactive metabolite). **Elimination:** Ledipasvir: Urine (1%), feces (86%; 70% unchanged, 2.2% metabolite); $T_{1/2}$=47 hrs (median). Sofosbuvir: Urine (80%; 78% GS-331007, 3.5% unchanged), feces (14%), expired air (2.5%); $T_{1/2}$=0.5 hr (median), 27 hrs (GS-331007, median).

PATIENT CONSIDERATIONS
Assessment: Assess for hypersensitivity to drug, pregnancy/nursing status, and possible drug interactions.

Monitoring: Monitor for bradycardia if coadministering w/ amiodarone or if discontinuing amiodarone just prior to starting therapy; perform cardiac monitoring in an in-patient setting for the first 48 hrs of coadministration, after which outpatient or self-monitoring of the HR should occur on a daily basis through at least the first 2 weeks of treatment. Perform clinical and hepatic lab monitoring for patients w/ decompensated cirrhosis receiving concomitant treatment w/ ribavirin. Monitor for other adverse reactions.

Counseling: Advise to seek medical evaluation immediately for symptoms of bradycardia. Inform that therapy may interact w/ other drugs; advise to report to physician the use of any other medication or herbal products. Advise to avoid pregnancy during combination treatment w/ ribavirin and for 6 months after completion of treatment; instruct to notify physician immediately in the event of a pregnancy. Advise to take therapy at the regularly scheduled time w/ or w/o food.

HAVRIX — hepatitis A vaccine   Rx
Class: Vaccine

ADULT DOSAGE	PEDIATRIC DOSAGE
Hepatitis A Vaccine	**Hepatitis A Vaccine**
Active Immunization:	**Active Immunization:**
Single 1mL dose, then 1mL booster dose anytime between 6-12 months later	**≥12 Months of Age:** Single 0.5mL dose, then 0.5mL booster dose anytime between 6-12 months later

---

ADMINISTRATION
IM route

Administer primary immunization at least 2 weeks prior to expected exposure to hepatitis A virus (HAV).

Preparation
- Shake well before use.
- For the prefilled syringes, attach a sterile needle and administer IM.
- For the vials, use a sterile needle and sterile syringe to withdraw the vaccine dose and administer IM.
- Changing needles between drawing vaccine from a vial and injecting it into a recipient is not necessary unless the needle has been damaged or contaminated.
- Use a separate sterile needle and syringe for each individual.
- Do not dilute to administer.

Administration
- Administer in the anterolateral aspect of the thigh in young children or in deltoid muscle of the upper arm in older children and adults; do not administer in the gluteal region.
- When concomitant administration of other vaccines or immune globulin is required, administer w/ different syringes and at different inj sites.
- Do not mix w/ any other vaccine or product in the same syringe or vial.

STORAGE
2-8°C (36-46°F). Do not freeze; discard if vaccine has been frozen.

HOW SUPPLIED
Inj: 720 EL.U./0.5mL, 1440 EL.U./mL [vial, prefilled syringe]

CONTRAINDICATIONS
Severe allergic reaction (eg, anaphylaxis) after a previous dose of any hepatitis A-containing vaccine, or to any component of Havrix, including neomycin.

WARNINGS/PRECAUTIONS
Tip caps of prefilled syringes contain natural rubber latex; may cause allergic reactions. Syncope may occur and can be accompanied by transient neurological signs (eg, visual disturbance, paresthesia, tonic-clonic limb movements); procedures should be in place to avoid falling injury and to restore cerebral perfusion following syncope. Appropriate treatment and supervision must be available for possible anaphylactic reactions. Immunocompromised persons may have a diminished immune response to vaccine. May not prevent hepatitis A infection in individuals who have an unrecognized hepatitis A infection at the time of vaccination. May not protect all individuals. Lower antibody response reported in patients w/ chronic liver disease.

ADVERSE REACTIONS
Inj-site reactions (eg, soreness, redness, swelling, induration), headache, fever, fatigue, malaise, anorexia, nausea.

DRUG INTERACTIONS
Immunosuppressive therapies, including irradiation, antimetabolites, alkylating agents, cytotoxic drugs, and corticosteroids (used in greater than physiologic doses), may reduce the immune response to vaccine.

PREGNANCY AND LACTATION
Pregnancy: Category C.
Lactation: It is not known whether the vaccine is excreted in human milk; caution in nursing.

MECHANISM OF ACTION
Vaccine; presence of antibodies to HAV confers protection against hepatitis A infection.

PATIENT CONSIDERATIONS
Assessment: Assess for history of severe allergic reaction to hepatitis A vaccine or neomycin. Assess for latex sensitivity, immunosuppression, chronic liver disease, unrecognized hepatitis A infection, immunization status/vaccination history, pregnancy/nursing status, and possible drug interactions.

Monitoring: Monitor for allergic reactions, syncope, neurological signs, and other adverse reactions. Monitor immune response to vaccine.

Counseling: Inform of the potential benefits and risks of immunization. Advise about potential side effects and emphasize that the vaccine contains noninfectious killed viruses and cannot cause hepatitis A infection. Instruct to report any adverse events to physician.

HEMANGEOL — propranolol hydrochloride   Rx
Class: Nonselective beta blocker

PEDIATRIC DOSAGE
Infantile Hemangioma

Proliferating Infantile Hemangioma Requiring Systemic Therapy:
Initiate treatment at ages 5 weeks to 5 months

Initial: 0.15mL/kg (0.6mg/kg) bid, taken at least 9 hrs apart

Titrate: After 1 week, increase daily dose to 0.3mL/kg (1.1mg/kg) bid. After 2 weeks, increase dose to 0.4mL/kg (1.7mg/kg) bid for 6 months

Readjust dose periodically as child's weight increases

May reinitiate treatment if hemangiomas recur

ADMINISTRATION
Oral route

Administer during or right after a feeding to reduce risk of hypoglycemia. Administer directly into the child's mouth; if necessary, may be diluted in a small quantity of milk or fruit juice, given in a baby's bottle.

STORAGE
25°C (77°F); excursions permitted from 15-30°C (59-86°F). Do not freeze. Do not shake bottle before use. Stable for 2 months after 1st opening.

HOW SUPPLIED
Sol: 4.28mg/mL [120mL]

CONTRAINDICATIONS
Premature infants w/ corrected age <5 weeks, infants weighing <2 kg, known hypersensitivity to propranolol or any of the excipients, asthma or history of bronchospasm, HR <80 beats/min, >1st degree heart block, decompensated heart failure (HF), BP <50/30mmHg, pheochromocytoma.

WARNINGS/PRECAUTIONS
May mask the adrenergic warning signs of hypoglycemia, particularly tachycardia, palpitations, and sweating. May cause hypoglycemia in children, especially when not feeding regularly or are vomiting; withhold the dose under these conditions. May cause or worsen bradycardia or hypotension; d/c treatment if severe (<80 beats/min) or symptomatic bradycardia or hypotension (systolic BP <50mmHg) occurs. May cause bronchospasm; interrupt treatment in the event of a lower respiratory tract infection associated with dyspnea and wheezing. Sympathetic stimulation supports circulatory function in patients with congestive heart failure; β blockade may precipitate more severe failure. By dropping BP, may increase the risk of stroke in PHACE syndrome patients with severe cerebrovascular anomalies. β-blockers will interfere with epinephrine used to treat serious anaphylaxis.

ADVERSE REACTIONS
Sleep disorder, bronchitis, peripheral coldness, agitation, diarrhea, somnolence, nightmare, irritability, decreased appetite, abdominal pain.

DRUG INTERACTIONS
CYP2D6, CYP1A2, or CYP2C19 inhibitors increase plasma levels. CYP1A2 inducers (phenytoin, phenobarbital) or CYP2C19 inducers (rifampin) decrease plasma levels. Concomitant treatment with corticosteroids may increase the risk of hypoglycemia; monitor for signs of hypoglycemia. Prolongation of 1st dose hypotension and syncope reported with α-blockers (prazosin). May exacerbate hypotensive effect of MAOIs and TCAs. May attenuate antihypertensive effect of β-adrenoreceptor blocking agents; monitor BP.

PREGNANCY AND LACTATION
Category C, not for use in nursing.

MECHANISM OF ACTION
Nonselective β-adrenergic receptor blocker; has not been established. Blockade of cardiac β1-adrenergic receptors leads to a decrease in the activity of both normal and ectopic pacemaker cells and a decrease in A-V nodal conduction velocity. Blockade of cardiac β1-adrenergic receptors also decreases the myocardial force of contraction and may provoke cardiac decompensation in patients with minimal cardiac reserve. Blockade of β2-adrenergic receptors results in constriction.

PHARMACOKINETICS
Absorption: (Adults) Almost complete; (Infants) T_{max}=2 hrs. **Distribution:** (Adults) V_d=4L/kg; plasma protein binding (90%); found in breast milk, crosses placenta. **Metabolism:** (Adults) Extensive 1st-pass metabolism by the liver; aromatic hydroxylation, N-dealkylation followed by further side-chain oxidation, and direct glucuronidation; CYP2D6, CYP1A2, and CYP2C19 (lesser extent); propranolol glucuronide, naphthyloxylactic acid and glucuronic acid, and sulfate conjugates of 4-hydroxy propranolol (major metabolites). **Elimination:** (Adults) Urine (<1% unchanged); (Infants) $T_{1/2}$=3.5 hrs.

PATIENT CONSIDERATIONS
Assessment: Assess for known hypersensitivity to drug or any of its excipients, asthma or history of bronchospasm, heart block, decompensated HF, pheochromocytoma, and possible drug interactions. Assess for potential arteriopathy associated with PHACE syndrome in infants with large facial infantile hemangioma. Assess BP, HR, weight, and in premature infants, corrected age.

Monitoring: Monitor for hypoglycemia, bradycardia, hypotension, bronchospasm, exacerbation of lower respiratory tract infections, worsening of HF, and other adverse reactions. Monitor HR and BP for 2 hrs after treatment initiation or increase in dose. Monitor for stroke in PHACE syndrome patients with severe cerebrovascular anomalies.

Counseling: Instruct parents/caregivers on the use of the oral dosing syringe. Inform that there is a risk of hypoglycemia when medication is given to infants who are not feeding regularly or who are vomiting; instruct to skip dosing under such conditions. Instruct on how to recognize the signs of hypoglycemia and to d/c and call physician immediately or take the child to the emergency room in case of suspected hypoglycemia. Advise that there is a potential risk for bradycardia, aggravation of preexisting conduction disorders, and hypotension associated with use of drug; instruct to contact physician in case of fatigue, pallor, slow or uneven heart beats, peripheral coldness, or fainting. Inform that drug carries risk of bronchospasm or exacerbation of lower respiratory tract infections; instruct to contact physician or go to the nearest emergency room if child has breathing problems or wheezing during treatment. Inform that changes in sleep patterns may occur. Instruct to inform physician of all the medications the parents/caregivers are administering to the child, including prescription/OTC medicines, vitamins, and herbal supplements. Instruct breastfeeding mothers to inform physician of all medications they are currently taking, as these may pass into the milk.

HEPAGAM B — hepatitis B immune globulin
intravenous (human)   Rx
Class: Immune globulin

ADULT DOSAGE
Prevention of Hepatitis B Recurrence Following Liver Transplantation

In HBsAg-Positive Patients:
Usual: 20,000 IU/dose IV according to the following regimen
Infusion Rate: 2mL/min

Dosing Regimen:
Anhepatic Phase: 1st dose
Week 1 Postoperative: Daily from Day 1-7
Weeks 2-12 Postoperative: Every 2 weeks from Day 14
Month 4 Onwards: Monthly

May need to adjust dose if anti-HBs levels of 500 IU/L are not reached w/ in 1st week post-liver transplantation

Postexposure Prophylaxis

Acute Exposure to Blood Containing HBsAg:
0.06mL/kg IM as soon as possible after exposure.
Give 2nd dose 1 month after the 1st dose in patients who refuse hepatitis B vaccine or are known non-responders to vaccine

Sexual Exposure to HBsAg-Positive Persons:
0.06mL/kg IM + hepatitis B vaccine series; give w/in 14 days of sexual contact or if sexual contact w/ infected person will continue

Household Exposure to Person w/ Acute Hepatitis B Virus Infection:
Prophylaxis not indicated unless there is an identifiable blood exposure to

PEDIATRIC DOSAGE
Postexposure Prophylaxis

Perinatal Exposure of Infants Born to HBsAg-Positive Mothers:
0.5mL IM administered after physiologic stabilization of infant and preferably w/in 12 hrs of birth. Administer concurrently w/ hepatitis B vaccine

Household Exposure to Person w/ Acute Hepatitis B Virus Infection:
<12 Months of Age:
0.5mL IM + hepatitis B vaccine

≥12 Months of Age:
Prophylaxis not indicated unless there is an identifiable blood exposure to the index patient (eg, by sharing toothbrushes/razors); treat such exposures like sexual exposures

the index patient (eg, by sharing toothbrushes/razors); treat such exposures like sexual exposures

DOSING CONSIDERATIONS
Elderly
Start at lower end of dosing range

Adverse Reactions
Prevention of Hepatitis B Recurrence Following Liver Transplantation:
If discomfort or infusion-related adverse reaction develops, decrease to 1mL/min or slower

Other Important Considerations
Prevention of Hepatitis B Recurrence Following Liver Transplantation: Surgical Bleeding, Abdominal Fluid Drainage (>500mL), or Undergoing Plasmapheresis:
May increase to 1/2 dose IV (10,000 IU) q6h until the target anti-HBs is reached

ADMINISTRATION
IV/IM route
May be administered at the same time (but at a different site), or ≤1 month preceding hepatitis B vaccination
Do not shake vials during preparation
Promptly use any vial that has been entered; do not reuse or save for future use
For IV administration, administer through a separate IV line using an infusion pump
Use normal saline as diluent if dilution is preferred prior to IV administration; do not use D5W

STORAGE
2-8°C (36-46°F). Do not freeze. Use within 6 hrs after vial has been entered.

HOW SUPPLIED
Inj: >312 IU/mL [1mL, 5mL]

CONTRAINDICATIONS
Immunoglobulin A (IgA) deficient patients with the potential to develop anti-IgA antibodies and have an anaphylactoid reaction. Patients with severe thrombocytopenia or any coagulation disorder that would contraindicate IM inj.

WARNINGS/PRECAUTIONS
Severe hypersensitivity reactions may occur; d/c infusion immediately and begin appropriate emergency treatment. Administer in a setting with appropriate equipment, medication, and personnel trained in the management of hypersensitivity, anaphylaxis, and shock. Contains maltose that may interfere with some types of blood glucose monitoring systems (eg, those based on the glucose dehydrogenase pyrroloquinoline quinone method); may result in falsely elevated glucose readings and, consequently, inappropriate administration of insulin, resulting in life-threatening hypoglycemia. Monitor liver transplant patients regularly for serum anti-HBs antibody levels using a quantitative assay to ensure that adequate protective levels are maintained. Monitor for any symptoms of an infusion reaction throughout the infusion period and immediately following an infusion; follow recommended infusion rate closely. Made from human plasma; may carry a risk of transmitting infectious agents (eg, viruses, Creutzfeldt-Jakob disease agent). Thrombotic events may occur during or following treatment; caution with a history of atherosclerosis, multiple cardiovascular (CV) risk factors, advanced age, impaired cardiac output, coagulation disorders, prolonged periods of immobilization, and/or known/suspected hyperviscosity. Consider baseline assessment of blood viscosity in patients at risk for hyperviscosity, including those with cryoglobulins, fasting chylomicronemia/markedly high triglycerides, or monoclonal gammopathies. Administer at the min rate of infusion practicable in patients at risk of thrombotic events. May interfere with some serological tests. Caution in elderly.

ADVERSE REACTIONS
Hypotension, nausea.

DRUG INTERACTIONS
May impair efficacy of live attenuated virus vaccines (eg, measles, rubella, mumps, varicella); if patient received hepatitis B immune globulin <14 days after live virus vaccination, revaccinate 3 months after administration of the immune globulin, unless serologic test results indicate that antibodies were produced.

PREGNANCY AND LACTATION
Category C, caution in nursing.

MECHANISM OF ACTION
Immune globulin; provides passive immunization for individuals exposed to HBV, by binding to the surface antigen and reducing the rate of hepatitis B infection.

PHARMACOKINETICS
Absorption: (IM) T_{max}=4-5 days (healthy). **Distribution:** (IM) V_d=7.5L (healthy). **Elimination:** (IM) $T_{1/2}$=22-25 days (healthy).

PATIENT CONSIDERATIONS
Assessment: Assess for history of anaphylactic or severe systemic reactions to parenteral administration of human globulin preparations, IgA deficiency, thrombocytopenia or any coagulation disorder, risk factors for thrombotic events (eg, history of atherosclerosis, multiple CV risk factors, advanced age, impaired cardiac output, prolonged periods of immobilization, hyperviscosity), any other conditions where treatment is contraindicated or cautioned, pregnancy/nursing status, and for possible drug interactions. Consider baseline assessment of blood viscosity in patients at risk for hyperviscosity.

Monitoring: Monitor for hypersensitivity reactions, infection, thrombotic events, and for other adverse reactions. Monitor for infusion reactions throughout the infusion period and immediately following an infusion. Monitor serum anti-HBs antibody levels regularly in liver transplant patients.

Counseling: Inform about the risks and benefits of treatment. Inform that the drug may contain infectious agents such as viruses that may cause disease. Inform that persons known to have severe, life-threatening reactions to human globulin products should not receive the drug. Instruct to notify physician immediately if any signs or symptoms of an allergic reaction develop. Advise liver transplant patients about the potential interference with non-glucose specific monitoring systems.

HEPARIN SODIUM IN 5% DEXTROSE —
heparin sodium　　　　　　　　　　　　　　　**Rx**

Class: Glycosaminoglycan

ADULT DOSAGE
General Dosing
Although dose must be adjusted according to the results of suitable lab tests, the following dose schedules may be used as guidelines:

Intermittent IV Inj:
Initial: 10,000 U
Maint: 5000-10,000 U q4-6h

Continuous IV Infusion:
Initial: 5000 U by IV inj
Maint: 20,000-40,000 U/24 hrs
Recommended dose is based on 150 lb (68kg) patient

Heart and Blood Vessel Surgery
Prevention of Clotting in Arterial/Cardiac Surgery:
Patients undergoing total body perfusion for open-heart surgery should receive an initial dose ≥150 U/kg; frequently, a dose of 300 U/kg is used for procedures estimated to last <60 min, or 400 U/kg for those estimated to last >60 min

Conversions
Converting to Warfarin:
Continue full heparin therapy for several days until INR (PT) has reached a stable therapeutic range; heparin therapy may then be discontinued w/o tapering

Converting to Oral Anticoagulants Other Than Warfarin:
For patients currently receiving IV heparin, stop IV infusion immediately after administering first dose of oral anticoagulant; for intermittent IV administration of heparin sodium, start oral anticoagulant 0-2 hrs before the time that the next dose of heparin was to have been administered

Extracorporeal Dialysis
25-30 U/kg followed by an infusion rate of 1500-2000 U/hr is suggested if specific manufacturers' recommendations are not available

Other Indications
- Prophylaxis and treatment of venous thrombosis and pulmonary embolism
- Prophylaxis and treatment of thromboembolic complications associated w/ atrial fibrillation
- Treatment of acute and chronic consumption coagulopathies (disseminated intravascular coagulation)
- Prophylaxis and treatment of peripheral arterial embolism
- Anticoagulant use in blood transfusions, extracorporeal circulation, and dialysis procedures

PEDIATRIC DOSAGE
General Dosing
There are no adequate and well-controlled studies on heparin use in pediatric patients. Dosing recommendations are based on clinical experience. The following dose schedule may be used as a guideline:

Initial: 75-100 U/kg (IV bolus over 10 min)
Maint:
Infants: 25-30 U/kg/hr; infants <2 months of age have the highest requirements (average 28 U/kg/hr)
Children >1 Year: 18-20 U/kg/hr; older children may require less heparin, similar to weight-adjusted adult dose

Adjust to maintain APTT of 60-85 sec, assuming this reflects an anti-Factor Xa level of 0.35-0.70

DOSING CONSIDERATIONS
Elderly
>60 Years: May require lower doses of heparin

ADMINISTRATION
IV route

- Confirm selection of the correct formulation and strength prior to administration of the drug.
- Do not use heparin sodium in 5% dextrose inj as a "catheter lock flush" product.
- Do not admix w/ other drugs.
- Do not use plastic containers in series connection.
- Do not infuse under pressure.

STORAGE
25°C (77°F); brief exposure up to 40°C (104°F) does not adversely affect product. Avoid excessive heat. Protect from freezing.

HOW SUPPLIED
Inj: 40 U/mL [500mL], 50 U/mL [500mL], 100 U/mL [250mL]

CONTRAINDICATIONS
History of heparin-induced thrombocytopenia (HIT) w/ or w/o thrombosis; known hypersensitivity to heparin or pork products (eg, anaphylactoid reactions); in patients whom suitable blood coagulation tests (eg, the whole blood clotting time, PTT) cannot be performed at appropriate intervals.

WARNINGS/PRECAUTIONS
Fatal medication errors reported; carefully examine all heparin products to confirm the correct container choice prior to administration. Hemorrhage, including fatal events, reported; avoid use in the presence of major bleeding, except when benefits outweigh risks. Hemorrhage may occur at virtually any site; use w/ caution in disease states w/ increased danger of hemorrhage. Higher incidence of bleeding reported in women >60 years. Thrombocytopenia and HIT (w/ or w/o thrombosis) reported; promptly d/c if platelet count falls <100,000/mm^3 or recurrent thrombosis develops, evaluate for HIT, and, if necessary, administer alternative anticoagulant. D/C promptly if coagulation tests are unduly prolonged or if hemorrhage occurs. Periodic platelet counts, hematocrits are recommended during the entire course of therapy. Increased heparin resistance w/ fever, thrombosis, thrombophlebitis, infections w/ thrombosing tendencies, MI, cancer, in postsurgical patients, and in patients w/ antithrombin III deficiency; dose adjustment based on anti-Factor Xa levels may be warranted. Patients w/ documented hypersensitivity to heparin should be given the drug only in clearly life-threatening situations; monitor for signs/symptoms of hypersensitivity when it is used in patients w/ a history of allergy. Contains sodium metabisulfite; may cause allergic-type reactions including anaphylactic symptoms and life-threatening or less severe asthmatic episodes in certain susceptible people. May prolong one-stage PT.

ADVERSE REACTIONS
Hemorrhage, thrombocytopenia, HIT (w/ or w/o thrombosis), hypersensitivity reactions, elevations of aminotransferase levels.

DRUG INTERACTIONS
When taken w/ dicumarol or warfarin sodium, wait at least 5 hrs after last IV heparin dose or 24 hrs after last SQ heparin dose if a valid PT is to be obtained. Platelet inhibitors (eg, acetylsalicylic acid, dextran, phenylbutazone) may induce bleeding; use w/ caution. Digitalis, tetracyclines, nicotine, antihistamines, or IV nitroglycerin may partially counteract the anticoagulant action. IV nitroglycerin administered to heparinized patients may result in a decrease of the PTT w/ subsequent rebound effect upon discontinuation of nitroglycerin; carefully monitor PTT and adjust heparin dose w/ concurrent use.

PREGNANCY AND LACTATION
Pregnancy: Exposure during pregnancy did not show evidence of an increased risk of adverse maternal or fetal outcomes in humans. Consider benefits and risks of use in pregnant women and possible risks to the fetus when prescribing.
Lactation: There is no information regarding presence in human milk, the effects on the breastfed infant, or the effects on milk production. Heparin is not likely to be excreted in human milk, and any heparin in milk would not be orally absorbed by a nursing infant. Caution in nursing.

MECHANISM OF ACTION
Glycosaminoglycan; inhibits reactions that lead to the clotting of blood and the formation of fibrin clots. Acts at multiple sites in the normal coagulation system. Small amounts in combination w/ antithrombin III (heparin cofactor) can inhibit thrombosis by inactivating activated Factor X and inhibiting the conversion of prothrombin to thrombin. Once active thrombosis has developed, larger amounts of heparin can inhibit further coagulation by inactivating thrombin and preventing the conversion of fibrinogen to fibrin. Also prevents the formation of a stable fibrin clot by inhibiting activation of fibrin stabilizing factor.

PHARMACOKINETICS
Absorption: (SQ) T_{max}=2-4 hrs. **Metabolism:** Liver and reticuloendothelial system. **Elimination:** $T_{1/2}$=10 min.

PATIENT CONSIDERATIONS
Assessment: Assess for hypersensitivity to heparin, pork products, or sulfites; thrombocytopenia; history of HIT; active bleeding; pregnancy/nursing status; and for any other conditions where treatment is contraindicated or cautioned. Assess for possible drug interactions. Obtain baseline platelet counts and Hct levels.

Monitoring: Monitor for signs/symptoms of hemorrhage, HIT, thrombocytopenia, heparin resistance, hypersensitivity reactions, and other adverse reactions. Perform periodic monitoring of platelet counts, Hct, tests for occult blood in stool during entire therapy course, and frequent blood coagulation tests. If given by continuous IV infusion, monitor coagulation time q4h in early stages of treatment. If given intermittently by IV inj, perform coagulation tests before each inj during the early stages of treatment and then at appropriate intervals thereafter.

Counseling: Inform that it may take longer than usual to stop bleeding and that bruising and/or bleeding may occur more easily. Instruct to report any unusual bleeding or bruising to physician. Advise patients to inform physicians and dentists that they are receiving heparin before any surgery is scheduled. Inform of the risk of HIT and that generalized hypersensitivity reactions have been reported. Instruct to inform physicians and dentists of all medications being taking, including non-prescription medications, and before starting any new medication.

HERCEPTIN — trastuzumab
Rx

Class: Monoclonal antibody/HER2 blocker

> May result in cardiac failure; incidence and severity were highest w/ anthracycline-containing chemotherapy regimens. Evaluate left ventricular function prior to and during treatment; d/c in patients receiving adjuvant therapy and withhold in patients w/ metastatic disease for clinically significant decrease in left ventricular function. May result in serious and fatal infusion reactions and pulmonary toxicity; interrupt infusion for dyspnea or clinically significant hypotension, and monitor until symptoms completely resolve. D/C for anaphylaxis, angioedema, interstitial pneumonitis, or acute respiratory distress syndrome. Exposure during pregnancy may result in oligohydramnios and oligohydramnios sequence manifesting as pulmonary hypoplasia, skeletal abnormalities, and neonatal death.

ADULT DOSAGE

HER2 Overexpressing Node Positive or Node Negative Breast Cancer

Adjuvant Treatment:
During and Following Paclitaxel, Docetaxel, or Docetaxel/Carboplatin:
Initial: 4mg/kg IV infusion over 90 min, then at 2mg/kg IV infusion over 30 min weekly during chemotherapy for the first 12 weeks (paclitaxel or docetaxel) or 18 weeks (docetaxel/carboplatin)
Subsequent Doses: 1 week following the last weekly dose, give 6mg/kg IV infusion over 30-90 min every 3 weeks

Single Agent w/in 3 Weeks Following Completion of Multimodality Anthracycline-Based Chemotherapy Regimens:
Initial: 8mg/kg IV infusion over 90 min
Subsequent Doses: 6mg/kg IV infusion over 30-90 min every 3 weeks

Administer for a total of 52 weeks; extending adjuvant treatment >1 yr is not recommended

HER2 Overexpressing Metastatic Breast Cancer

Alone or in Combination w/ Paclitaxel:
Initial: 4mg/kg IV infusion over 90 min
Subsequent Doses: 2mg/kg IV infusion over 30 min once a week until disease progression

HER2 Overexpressing Metastatic Gastric or Gastroesophageal Junction Adenocarcinoma

Patients Who Have Not Received Prior Treatment for Metastatic Disease:
Initial: 8mg/kg IV infusion over 90 min
Subsequent Doses: 6mg/kg IV infusion over 30-90 min every 3 weeks until disease progression

Give in combination w/ cisplatin and capecitabine or 5-fluorouracil

Missed Dose

Dose Missed by ≤1 Week:
- Administer the usual maint dose (weekly schedule: 2mg/kg; 3-weekly schedule: 6mg/kg) as soon as possible; do not wait until the next planned cycle
- Administer subsequent maint doses 7 days or 21 days later according to the weekly or 3-weekly schedules, respectively

Dose Missed by >1 Week:
- Administer a reloading dose over approx 90 min (weekly schedule: 4mg/kg; 3-weekly schedule: 8mg/kg) as soon as possible
- Administer subsequent maint doses (weekly schedule: 2mg/kg; 3-weekly schedule: 6mg/kg) 7 days or 21 days later according to the weekly or 3-weekly schedules, respectively

PEDIATRIC DOSAGE
Pediatric use may not have been established

DOSING CONSIDERATIONS
Adverse Reactions
Infusion Reactions:
Mild or Moderate: Decrease rate of infusion
Dyspnea/Clinically Significant Hypotension: Interrupt infusion
Severe/Life-threatening: D/C therapy
Cardiomyopathy:
Withhold Therapy for at Least 4 Weeks for Either of the Following:
1. ≥16% absolute decrease in left ventricular ejection fraction (LVEF) from pretreatment values
2. LVEF below institutional limits of normal and ≥10% absolute decrease in LVEF from pretreatment values
May Resume Therapy If:
LVEF returns to normal limits and absolute decrease from baseline is ≤15% w/in 4-8 weeks
Permanently D/C Therapy For:
Persistent (>8 weeks) LVEF decline or for suspension of dosing on more than 3 occasions for cardiomyopathy

ADMINISTRATION
IV route

Do not administer as IV push or bolus.
Do not mix w/ other drugs.
Do not substitute for or w/ ado-trastuzumab emtansine.

Reconstitution
Reconstitute each 440mg vial w/ 20mL of bacteriostatic water for inj, containing 1.1% benzyl alcohol as a preservative to yield a multidose sol containing 21mg/mL.
In patients w/ known hypersensitivity to benzyl alcohol, reconstitute w/ 20mL of sterile water for inj (SWFI) w/o preservative to yield a single-use sol.
Swirl vial gently; do not shake.
Allow vial to stand undisturbed for approx 5 min after reconstitution.
If reconstituted w/ SWFI w/o preservative, use immediately and discard any unused portion.
Store reconstituted product at 2-8°C (36-46°F); discard any unused product after 28 days.

Dilution
1. Determine the dose (mg) and calculate the volume of the 21mg/mL reconstituted sol needed.
2. Withdraw this amount from the vial and add it to an infusion bag containing 250mL of 0.9% NaCl inj; do not use D5 sol.
3. Gently invert the bag to mix the sol.

STORAGE
2-8°C (36-46°F). Do not freeze following reconstitution/dilution. **Diluted in Polyvinylchloride or Polyethylene Bags Containing 0.9% NaCl Inj:** 2-8°C (36-46°F) for no more than 24 hrs prior to use.

HOW SUPPLIED
Inj: 440mg

WARNINGS/PRECAUTIONS
See Dosing Considerations. Patients w/ symptomatic intrinsic lung disease or extensive tumor involvement of the lungs, resulting in dyspnea at rest, may have more severe pulmonary toxicity. Detection of HER2 protein overexpression is necessary for appropriate patient selection; use FDA-approved tests for the specific tumor type to assess HER2 protein overexpression and HER2 gene amplification.

ADVERSE REACTIONS
Adjuvant and Metastatic Breast Cancer: Fever, N/V, infusion reactions, diarrhea, infections, increased cough, headache, fatigue, dyspnea, rash, neutropenia, anemia, myalgia.
Metastatic Gastric Cancer: Neutropenia, diarrhea, fatigue, anemia, stomatitis, weight loss, URTIs, fever, thrombocytopenia, mucosal inflammation, nasopharyngitis, dysgeusia.

DRUG INTERACTIONS
See Boxed Warning. Higher incidence of neutropenia w/ myelosuppressive chemotherapy. Increased risk of cardiac dysfunction in patients who receive anthracycline after stopping trastuzumab; if possible, avoid anthracycline-based therapy for up to 7 months after stopping trastuzumab, but if anthracyclines are used, carefully monitor cardiac function.

PREGNANCY AND LACTATION
Pregnancy: May cause fetal harm; cases of oligohydramnios and of oligohydramnios sequence reported. Monitor women who received trastuzumab during pregnancy or w/in 7 months prior to conception for oligohydramnios. There is a pregnancy exposure registry and a pregnancy pharmacovigilance program for women who become pregnant during treatment or w/in 7 months following the last dose.
Lactation: It is not known if trastuzumab is excreted in human milk; caution in nursing.
Reproductive Potential: Verify the pregnancy status of females of reproductive potential prior to the initiation of therapy. Advise females of reproductive potential to use effective contraception during treatment and for 7 months following the last dose of trastuzumab.

MECHANISM OF ACTION
Monoclonal antibody (IgG1 kappa)/HER2 blocker; inhibits proliferation of human tumor cells that overexpress HER2.

PHARMACOKINETICS
Absorption: Administration of various doses resulted in different pharmacokinetic parameters.

PATIENT CONSIDERATIONS
Assessment: Assess cardiac function, including baseline LVEF. Assess HER2 protein overexpression and HER2 gene amplification. Assess for symptomatic intrinsic lung disease or extensive tumor involvement of lungs, pregnancy/nursing status, and possible drug interactions.

Monitoring: Monitor for infusion reactions, pulmonary toxicity, neutropenia, and other adverse reactions. Monitor LVEF every 3 months during and upon completion of therapy, and every 6 months for at least 2 yrs following completion of therapy as a component of adjuvant therapy. Repeat LVEF measurement at 4-week intervals if therapy is withheld for significant left ventricular cardiac dysfunction.

Counseling: Advise to contact physician immediately for any symptoms of cardiomyopathy (eg, new onset/worsening SOB, cough, swelling of ankles/legs). Advise women that exposure to trastuzumab during pregnancy or w/in 7 months prior to conception may result in fetal harm. Advise to contact physician w/ a known/suspected pregnancy. Advise women who may be exposed to therapy during pregnancy or w/in 7 months of conception to enroll in the MotHER Pregnancy Registry and to report pregnancy to manufacturer. Advise females of reproductive potential to use effective contraception during treatment and for at least 7 months following the last dose of therapy.

HETLIOZ — tasimelteon   Rx
Class: Melatonin receptor agonist

ADULT DOSAGE	PEDIATRIC DOSAGE
Non-24-Hour Sleep-Wake Disorder 20mg/day before hs, at the same time every night	Pediatric use may not have been established

DOSING CONSIDERATIONS
Hepatic Impairment
Severe (Child-Pugh Class C): Not recommended

ADMINISTRATION
Oral route

Take w/o food.
Swallow cap whole.

STORAGE
25°C (77°F); excursions permitted to 15-30°C (59-86°F). Protect from exposure to light and moisture.

HOW SUPPLIED
Cap: 20mg

WARNINGS/PRECAUTIONS
Effects of therapy may not occur for weeks or months because of individual differences in circadian rhythms. May cause somnolence; limit activity before going to bed. May impair mental/physical abilities. Not recommended w/ severe hepatic impairment.

ADVERSE REACTIONS
Headache, increased ALT, nightmare/abnormal dreams, URTI, UTI.

DRUG INTERACTIONS
Large increase in exposure w/ fluvoxamine or other strong CYP1A2 inhibitors; avoid concomitant use. Decreased exposure w/ reduced efficacy w/ rifampin or other CYP3A4 inducers; avoid concomitant use. Efficacy may be reduced in smokers due to induction of CYP1A2 levels.

PREGNANCY AND LACTATION
Category C, caution in nursing.

MECHANISM OF ACTION
Melatonin receptor agonist; not established. Activity at MT_1 and MT_2 receptors thought to be involved in the control of circadian rhythms.

PHARMACOKINETICS
Absorption: Absolute bioavailability (38.3%); T_{max}=0.5-3 hrs (fasted).
Distribution: V_d=59-126L; plasma protein binding (90%). **Metabolism:** Extensive. Oxidation at multiples sites and oxidative dealkylation via CYP1A2 and CYP3A4. Phenolic glucuronidation (major phase II metabolic route).
Elimination: Urine (80%, <1% unchanged), feces (4%); $T_{1/2}$=1.3 hrs, 1.3-3.7 hrs (metabolites).

PATIENT CONSIDERATIONS
Assessment: Assess for severe hepatic impairment, smoking, pregnancy/nursing status, and possible drug interactions.

Monitoring: Monitor for somnolence, impairment of mental/physical abilities, and other adverse reactions.

Counseling: Inform about the potential risks and benefits of therapy. Advise to take therapy before hs at the same time every night; advise to skip dose if unable to take at scheduled time. Instruct to limit activity before going to bed after taking drug. Inform that daily use for several weeks or months may be necessary before benefit from therapy is observed.

HIBERIX — haemophilus b conjugate vaccine (tetanus toxoid conjugate)

Rx

Class: Vaccine

PEDIATRIC DOSAGE
Haemophilus influenza **Type B**
Active Immunization for Prevention of Invasive Disease:
6 Weeks-4 Years (Prior to 5th Birthday):
0.5mL IM single dose
Administer as a 4-dose series; series consists of a primary immunization course of 3 doses administered at 2, 4, and 6 months of age, followed by a booster dose administered at 15-18 months of age. May give first dose as early as 6 weeks of age

ADMINISTRATION
IM route

Administer into anterolateral aspect of thigh or deltoid.
Do not mix w/ any other vaccine in the same syringe or vial.
Administer other vaccines at different inj sites.

Reconstitution
1. Withdraw 0.6mL of saline diluent from accompanying vial; reconstitute only w/ accompanying saline diluent.
2. Transfer 0.6mL saline diluent into lyophilized vaccine vial; shake the vial well.
3. Withdraw 0.5mL of reconstituted vaccine and administer.

Administer immediately after reconstitution or store refrigerated between 2-8°C (35- 46°F) and administer w/in 24 hrs; if not administered immediately, shake sol well again before administration.

STORAGE
2-8°C (36-46°F). Protect from light. **Diluent:** 2-25°C (36-77°F). Do not freeze.
After Reconstitution: 2-8°C (36-46°F). Do not freeze. Discard if not used w/in 24 hrs or if has been frozen.

HOW SUPPLIED
Inj: 0.5mL

CONTRAINDICATIONS
Severe allergic reaction (eg, anaphylaxis) after a previous dose of any *Haemophilus influenzae* type b- or tetanus toxoid-containing vaccine or any component of the vaccine.

WARNINGS/PRECAUTIONS
Evaluate potential benefits and risks if Guillain-Barre syndrome has occurred w/in 6 weeks of receipt of a prior tetanus toxoid-containing vaccine. Syncope may occur and can be accompanied by transient neurological signs. Apnea following IM vaccination reported in some infants born prematurely; decision on when to administer to premature infants should be based on the individual infant's medical status, and the potential benefits and possible risks of vaccination. Review immunization history for possible vaccine hypersensitivity; epinephrine and other appropriate agents must be immediately available if an anaphylactic reaction occurs. Expected immune response may not be obtained in immunosuppressed children. Urine antigen detection may not have a diagnostic value in suspected disease due to *H. influenzae* type b w/in 1-2 weeks after receipt of vaccine. Not a substitute for routine tetanus immunization.

ADVERSE REACTIONS
Pain and redness at inj site, irritability, drowsiness, fever, loss of appetite, fussiness, restlessness.

DRUG INTERACTIONS
Immunosuppressive therapies, including irradiation, antimetabolites, alkylating agents, cytotoxic drugs, and corticosteroids (used in greater than physiologic doses) may reduce immune response to vaccine.

PREGNANCY AND LACTATION
Pregnancy: Category C.
Lactation: Safety not known in nursing.

MECHANISM OF ACTION
Vaccine; protects against invasive disease due to *H. influenzae* type b.

PATIENT CONSIDERATIONS
Assessment: Assess for history of a severe allergic reaction to previous dose of any *H. influenzae* type b vaccination, tetanus toxoid-containing vaccine, or any component of the vaccine; history of Guillain-Barre syndrome w/in 6 weeks of receipt of a prior vaccine containing tetanus toxoid; immunosuppression; and for possible drug interactions. Review immunization history.

Monitoring: Monitor for allergic reactions, signs/symptoms of Guillain-Barre syndrome, inj-site reactions (eg, pain, redness, swelling), syncope, apnea in premature infants, and for any other possible adverse events. Monitor immune response.

Counseling: Inform patient's parents/guardians about benefits/risks of immunization. Counsel about the potential for adverse reactions; instruct to notify physician if any adverse reactions occur.

HORIZANT — gabapentin enacarbil

Rx

Class: GABA analogue

ADULT DOSAGE
Restless Legs Syndrome
Moderate-Severe Primary Restless Legs Syndrome:
Usual: 600mg qd at about 5 pm
If dose is not taken at the recommended time, the next dose should be taken the following day as prescribed
Postherpetic Neuralgia
Initial: 600mg qam for 3 days
Titrate: Increase to 600mg bid (1200mg/day) on Day 4
Usual: 600mg bid

PEDIATRIC DOSAGE
Pediatric use may not have been established

DOSING CONSIDERATIONS
Renal Impairment
Restless Leg Syndrome:
CrCl ≥60mL/min:
600mg/day
CrCl 30-59mL/min:
Initial: 300mg/day
Titrate: Increase to 600mg prn
CrCl 15-29mL/min:
300mg/day
CrCl <15mL/min:
300mg qod
CrCl <15mL/min on Hemodialysis:
Not recommended
Postherpetic Neuralgia:
CrCl ≥60mL/min:
Titration: 600mg qam for 3 days
Maint: 600mg bid
Tapering: 600mg qam for 1 week
CrCl 30-59mL/min:
Titration: 300mg qam for 3 days
Maint: 300mg bid; increase to 600mg bid if needed based on tolerability and efficacy
Tapering: Reduce current maint dose to qd in am for 1 week
CrCl 15-29mL/min:
Titration: 300mg qam on Day 1 and Day 3
Maint: 300mg qam; increase to 300mg bid if needed based on tolerability and efficacy
Tapering: If taking 300mg bid, reduce to 300mg qd in am for 1 week. If taking 300mg qd, no taper needed
CrCl <15mL/min:
Maint: 300mg qod in am; increase to 300mg qd in am if needed based on tolerability and efficacy
CrCl <15mL/min on Hemodialysis:
Maint: 300mg following every dialysis; increase to 600mg following every dialysis if needed based on tolerability and efficacy

ADMINISTRATION
Oral route

Take w/ food.
Swallow tab whole; do not cut, crush, or chew.

STORAGE
25°C (77°F); excursions permitted to 15-30°C (59-86°F). Protect from moisture.

HOW SUPPLIED
Tab, Extended-Release: 300mg, 600mg

WARNINGS/PRECAUTIONS
Not recommended for patients who are required to sleep during the day and remain awake at night or in restless legs syndrome patients w/ CrCl <15mL/min on hemodialysis. May cause significant driving impairment, somnolence/sedation, and dizziness. Not interchangeable w/ other gabapentin products. Increases the risk of suicidal thoughts or behavior; monitor for the emergence or worsening of depression, suicidal thoughts/behavior, and/or any unusual changes in mood or behavior. Drug reaction w/ eosinophilia and systemic symptoms (DRESS)/ multiorgan hypersensitivity reported; evaluate immediately if signs/symptoms (eg, hypersensitivity, fever, lymphadenopathy) are present and d/c if alternative etiology cannot be established. For RLS patients, if recommended daily dose is exceeded, reduce dose to 600mg daily for 1 week prior to discontinuation to minimize potential for withdrawal seizure. For postherpetic neuralgia patients receiving bid dose, reduce dose to qd for 1 week prior to discontinuation to minimize potential for withdrawal seizure. May have tumorigenic potential. Caution in elderly and w/ renal impairment.

ADVERSE REACTIONS
Somnolence/sedation, dizziness, headache, nausea, dry mouth, flatulence, fatigue, insomnia, irritability, feeling drunk/abnormal, peripheral edema, weight increase, vertigo.

DRUG INTERACTIONS
Drug is released faster from extended-release tab in the presence of alcohol; avoid alcohol consumption. Increased somnolence/sedation, dizziness, and nausea when taken in conjunction w/ morphine.

PREGNANCY AND LACTATION
Category C, not for use in nursing.

MECHANISM OF ACTION
Gamma-aminobutyric acid analog; not established. Prodrug of gabapentin; binds w/ high affinity to the α2delta subunit of voltage-activated calcium channels.

PHARMACOKINETICS
Absorption: (PHN: 600mg bid) C_{max}=5.35µg/mL, AUC_{24}=109µg•hr/mL; bioavailability (75% [fed], 42-65% [fasted]); T_{max}=5 hrs (fasted), 7.3 hrs (fed). **Distribution:** Plasma protein binding (<3%); V_d=76L. **Metabolism:** Extensive 1st-pass hydrolysis to gabapentin (active form). **Elimination:** Kidney (unchanged); urine (94%), feces (5%); $T_{1/2}$=5.1-6 hrs.

PATIENT CONSIDERATIONS
Assessment: Assess for preexisting tumors, history of depression, pregnancy/nursing status, renal function (CrCl), and possible drug interactions.

Monitoring: Monitor for withdrawal seizures w/ discontinuation, somnolence/sedation, dizziness, emergence or worsening of depression, suicidal thoughts/behavior, and/or any unusual changes in mood/behavior, DRESS, development or worsening of tumors, renal function, and hypersensitivity reactions.

Counseling: Inform that therapy may cause significant driving impairment, somnolence, and dizziness; advise not to drive or operate dangerous machinery until sufficient experience on therapy is gained. Counsel that treatment may increase the risk of suicidal thoughts and behavior; advise to report to physician any behaviors of concern. Advise that multiorgan hypersensitivity reactions may occur; instruct to contact physician if experiencing any signs or symptoms of this condition. Advise not to interchange w/ other gabapentin products. If the dose is missed, instruct to take the next dose at the time of the next scheduled dose. Instruct about how to d/c therapy. Advise to avoid alcohol when taking the drug.

HUMALOG — insulin lispro   Rx

Class: Insulin (rapid-acting)

ADULT DOSAGE	PEDIATRIC DOSAGE
Diabetes Mellitus	**Type 1 Diabetes Mellitus**
IV/SQ:	**≥3 Years:**
Individualize and adjust dose based on route of administration, metabolic needs, blood glucose monitoring results, and glycemic control goal	**SQ (Humalog U-100):** Individualize and adjust dose based on metabolic needs, blood glucose monitoring results, and glycemic control goal

DOSING CONSIDERATIONS
Renal Impairment
May require more frequent dose adjustment

Hepatic Impairment
May require more frequent dose adjustment

Other Important Considerations
May require dose adjustments w/ changes in physical activity/meal patterns, or during acute illness

ADMINISTRATION
IV/SQ route

Do not transfer Humalog U-200 from the KwikPen to a syringe for administration.
Do not perform dose conversion when using either Humalog U-100 or Humalog U-200 KwikPens.
Do not mix Humalog U-200 w/ any other insulins.

SQ (Humalog U-100 or U-200)
Administer w/in 15 min ac or immediately pc by inj into the SQ tissue of the abdominal wall, thigh, upper arm, or buttocks; rotate inj sites w/in the same region
Generally used w/ an intermediate- or long-acting insulin

Continuous SQ Infusion (Insulin Pump); Humalog U-100 Only
Administer into the SQ tissue of the abdominal wall; rotate infusion sites w/in the same region
Do not dilute or mix w/ other insulins
Change Humalog U-100 in the pump reservoir at least every 7 days; change infusion sets and infusion set insertion site at least every 3 days
Do not expose Humalog U-100 in the pump reservoir to temperatures >37°C (98.6°F)
Use Humalog U-100 in pump systems suitable for insulin infusion

IV (Humalog U-100 Only)
Dilute to concentrations from 0.1 U/mL to 1.0 U/mL using 0.9% NaCl

Instructions for Mixing Humalog U-100 w/ Other Insulins
SQ:
May be mixed w/ NPH insulin preparations only; draw insulin lispro into syringe 1st and inject immediately after mixing

STORAGE
Unused: 2-8°C (36-46°F) until expiration date. Do not freeze; do not use if it has been frozen. **Opened:** <30°C (86°F) for up to 28 days. Protect from direct heat and light. (Vials) May refrigerate. (Cartridge/KwikPen) Do not refrigerate. Discard cartridge used in the D-Tron pumps after 7 days, even if it still contains the drug. **Diluted Humalog U-100 for SQ Inj:** 5°C (41°F) for 28 days or 30°C (86°F) for 14 days. Do not dilute drug contained in a cartridge or drug used in an external insulin pump. **IV Admixture:** 2-8°C (36-46°F) for 48 hrs; may be used at room temperature for up to an additional 48 hrs.

HOW SUPPLIED
Inj: 100 U/mL [3mL, cartridge, KwikPen, vial; 10mL, vial], 200 U/mL [3mL, KwikPen]

CONTRAINDICATIONS
During episodes of hypoglycemia. Hypersensitivity to Humalog or to any of its excipients.

WARNINGS/PRECAUTIONS
KwikPen, cartridges, reusable pens, and syringes must never be shared between patients, even if needle is changed; may carry a risk for transmission of blood-borne pathogens. Changes in strength, manufacturer, type, or method of administration may affect glycemic control and predispose to hypo/hyperglycemia; these changes should be made cautiously and under close medical supervision and the frequency of blood glucose monitoring should be increased. Hypoglycemia may occur; increase frequency of blood glucose monitoring in patients at higher risk for hypoglycemia and patients who have reduced symptomatic awareness of hypoglycemia. Hypoglycemia may impair concentration ability and reaction time. Accidental mix-ups between insulin products and other insulins, particularly rapid-acting insulins, reported. Severe, life-threatening, generalized allergy, including anaphylaxis, may occur; if hypersensitivity reactions occur, d/c therapy, treat per standard of care, and monitor until symptoms and signs resolve. Hypokalemia may occur. Malfunction of the insulin pump or infusion set or insulin degradation can rapidly lead to hyperglycemia and ketoacidosis; prompt identification and correction of the cause is necessary. Train patients using continuous SQ infusion pump therapy to administer by inj and have alternate insulin therapy available in case of pump failure. IV administration should be under medical supervision w/ close monitoring of blood glucose and K⁺ levels. More frequent glucose monitoring may be necessary w/ renal/hepatic impairment.

ADVERSE REACTIONS
Flu syndrome, pharyngitis, rhinitis, headache, pain, cough increased, infection, diarrhea, nausea, fever, abdominal pain, asthenia, bronchitis, myalgia, UTI.

DRUG INTERACTIONS
Dose adjustment and increased frequency of glucose monitoring may be required w/ drugs that may increase the risk of hypoglycemia (eg, salicylates, sulfonamide antibiotics, MAOIs, ACE inhibitors, somatostatin analogues [eg, octreotide]), drugs that may decrease blood glucose-lowering effect (eg, corticosteroids, oral contraceptives, sympathomimetic agents [eg, epinephrine, albuterol, terbutaline], atypical antipsychotics, protease inhibitors), or drugs that may increase or decrease blood glucose-lowering effect (eg, β-blockers, clonidine, lithium salts, alcohol). Pentamidine may cause hypoglycemia, sometimes followed by hyperglycemia. Signs and symptoms of hypoglycemia may be blunted w/ β-blockers, clonidine, guanethidine, and reserpine. Monitor K⁺ levels w/ K⁺-lowering medications or medications sensitive to serum K⁺ concentrations. Observe for signs/symptoms of heart failure (HF) if treated concomitantly w/ a peroxisome proliferator-activated receptor (PPAR)-gamma agonist (eg, thiazolidinedione); consider discontinuation or dose reduction of the PPAR-gamma agonist if HF develops.

PREGNANCY AND LACTATION
Category B, caution in nursing.

MECHANISM OF ACTION
Insulin lispro (rDNA origin); regulates glucose metabolism. Lowers blood glucose by stimulating peripheral glucose uptake by skeletal muscle and fat, and by inhibiting hepatic glucose production. Inhibits lipolysis and proteolysis, and enhances protein synthesis.

PHARMACOKINETICS
Absorption: (SQ, 0.1-0.2 U/kg) Absolute bioavailability (55-77%). Administration of variable doses resulted in different pharmacokinetic parameters. **Distribution:** (IV) V_d=1.55L/kg (0.1 U/kg), 0.72L/kg (0.2 U/kg). **Elimination:** (IV) $T_{1/2}$=0.85 hrs (0.1 U/kg), 0.92 hrs (0.2 U/kg); (SQ) $T_{1/2}$=1 hr.

PATIENT CONSIDERATIONS
Assessment: Assess for predisposition to hypoglycemia, risk for hypokalemia, hypersensitivity, renal/hepatic impairment, pregnancy/nursing status, and possible drug interactions. Obtain baseline blood glucose and HbA1c levels.

Monitoring: Monitor for signs/symptoms of hypoglycemia, hypokalemia, hypersensitivity reactions, and other adverse effects. Monitor blood glucose, HbA1c, K⁺ levels, and renal/hepatic function.

Counseling: Advise to never share KwikPen, cartridge, reusable pen, or syringe w/ another person, even if needle is changed. Instruct on self-management procedures (eg, glucose monitoring, proper inj technique, management of hypo/hyperglycemia), especially at initiation of therapy. Advise on handling of special situations, such as intercurrent conditions (eg, illness, stress, emotional disturbances), inadequate or skipped doses, inadvertent administration of an increased dose, inadequate food intake, and skipped meals. Inform that the ability to concentrate and react may be impaired as a result of hypoglycemia; advise patients who have frequent hypoglycemia or reduced/absent warning signs of hypoglycemia to use caution when driving/operating machinery. Advise that hypersensitivity reactions may occur; inform about the symptoms of hypersensitivity reactions. Instruct to always check the label before each inj to avoid mix-ups between insulin products. Advise females of reproductive potential w/ diabetes to inform physician if pregnant or contemplating pregnancy. Instruct on how to use external infusion pump, and to follow healthcare provider recommendations when setting basal and meal time infusion rate.

HUMALOG MIX 50/50 — insulin lispro protamine (rDNA origin)/insulin lispro (rDNA origin)
Rx

Class: Insulin (combination)

ADULT DOSAGE	PEDIATRIC DOSAGE
Diabetes Mellitus	Pediatric use may not have been established
Individualize dose	

DOSING CONSIDERATIONS
Renal Impairment
Dose adjustments may be necessary

Hepatic Impairment
Dose adjustments may be necessary

ADMINISTRATION
SQ route

Inject w/in 15 min ac.

STORAGE
Unopened: 2-8°C (36-46°F) until expiration date, or at room temperature (<30°C [86°F]) for 28 days (vial) or 10 days (KwikPen). Do not freeze; do not use if it has been frozen. **Opened:** <30°C (86°F) for 28 days (vial) or 10 days (KwikPen). Do not refrigerate KwikPen. Protect from direct heat and light.

HOW SUPPLIED
Inj: (Insulin Lispro Protamine/Insulin Lispro) (50 U/50 U)/mL [3mL, KwikPen; 10mL, vial]

CONTRAINDICATIONS
During episodes of hypoglycemia. Sensitivity to insulin lispro or any of the excipients contained in the formulation.

WARNINGS/PRECAUTIONS
KwikPens and syringes must never be shared between patients, even if needle is changed; may carry a risk for transmission of blood-borne pathogens. Any change of insulin should be made cautiously and only under medical supervision. Changes in strength, manufacturer, type, species, or method of manufacture may result in the need for a change in dosage. Hypoglycemia and hypokalemia may occur; caution in patients in whom such potential side effects may be clinically relevant (eg, patients w/ autonomic neuropathy). Lipodystrophy and hypersensitivity may occur. Dosage adjustment may be necessary if patient changes physical activity or usual meal plan. Illness, emotional disturbances, or other stress may alter insulin requirements. Careful glucose monitoring and insulin dose adjustment may be necessary w/ hepatic/ renal impairment. Inj-site redness/swelling/itching and severe, life-threatening, generalized allergy may occur. Contains cresol as excipient; localized reactions and generalized myalgias reported. Antibody production reported. Caution in elderly.

ADVERSE REACTIONS
Hypoglycemia, allergic reactions, inj-site reactions, lipodystrophy, pruritus, rash.

DRUG INTERACTIONS
Drugs w/ hyperglycemic activity (eg, corticosteroids, certain lipid-lowering drugs [eg, niacin], oral contraceptives, phenothiazines, thyroid replacement therapy) may increase insulin requirements. Drugs that increase insulin sensitivity or have hypoglycemic activity (eg, salicylates, sulfa antibiotics, MAOIs, ACE inhibitors, inhibitors of pancreatic function [eg, octreotide]) may decrease insulin requirements. β-blockers may mask symptoms of hypoglycemia. Caution w/ K+-lowering drugs or drugs sensitive to serum K+ levels. Observe for signs/symptoms of heart failure (HF) if treated concomitantly w/ a peroxisome proliferator-activated receptor (PPAR)-gamma agonist (eg, thiazolidinedione); consider discontinuation or dose reduction of the PPAR-gamma agonist if HF develops.

PREGNANCY AND LACTATION
Category B, caution in nursing.

MECHANISM OF ACTION
Insulin; regulates glucose metabolism. In muscle and other tissues (except the brain), causes rapid transport of glucose and amino acids intracellularly, promotes anabolism, and inhibits protein catabolism. In the liver, promotes the uptake and storage of glucose in the form of glycogen, inhibits gluconeogenesis, and promotes the conversion of excess glucose into fat.

PHARMACOKINETICS
Absorption: T_{max}=45-120 min (0.3 U/kg). **Distribution:** V_d=0.26-0.36L/kg (insulin lispro).

PATIENT CONSIDERATIONS
Assessment: Assess for presence of hypoglycemia or hypokalemia and for conditions where such potential side effects might be clinically relevant. Assess for hypersensitivity, renal/hepatic impairment, pregnancy/nursing status, and possible drug interactions. Obtain baseline blood glucose and HbA1c levels.

Monitoring: Monitor for signs/symptoms of hypoglycemia, hypokalemia, lipodystrophy, allergic reactions, antibody production, and other adverse effects. Monitor blood glucose, HbA1c, K+ levels, and renal/hepatic function.

Counseling: Inform of the potential risks and advantages of therapy and alternative therapies. Instruct not to mix drug w/ any other insulin. Inform of the importance of proper insulin storage, inj technique, timing of dosage, adherence to meal planning, regular physical activity, regular blood glucose monitoring, periodic HbA1c testing, recognition and management of hypo/hyperglycemia, and periodic assessment for diabetes complications. Advise to inform physician if pregnant or planning to become pregnant. Instruct patients using insulin pen delivery device on how to properly use the delivery device, prime the pen to a stream of insulin, and properly dispose of needles. Advise not to share insulin pen w/ others.

HUMALOG MIX 75/25 — insulin lispro protamine (rDNA origin)/insulin lispro (rDNA origin)
Rx

Class: Insulin (combination)

ADULT DOSAGE	PEDIATRIC DOSAGE
Diabetes Mellitus	Pediatric use may not have been established
Individualize dose	

DOSING CONSIDERATIONS
Renal Impairment
Dose adjustments may be necessary

Hepatic Impairment
Dose adjustments may be necessary

ADMINISTRATION
SQ route

Inject w/in 15 min ac.

STORAGE
Unopened: 2-8°C (36-46°F) until expiration date, or room temperature (<30°C [86°F]) for 28 days (vial) or 10 days (KwikPen). Do not freeze; do not use if it has been frozen. **Opened:** <30°C (86°F) for 28 days (vial) or 10 days (KwikPen). Do not refrigerate KwikPen. Protect from direct heat and light.

HOW SUPPLIED
Inj: (Insulin Lispro Protamine/Insulin Lispro) (75 U/25 U)/mL [3mL, KwikPen; 10mL, vial]

CONTRAINDICATIONS
During episodes of hypoglycemia. Sensitivity to insulin lispro or any of the excipients contained in the formulation.

WARNINGS/PRECAUTIONS
KwikPens and syringes must never be shared between patients, even if needle is changed; may carry a risk for transmission of blood-borne pathogens. Any change of insulin should be made cautiously and only under medical supervision. Changes in strength, manufacturer, type, species, or method of manufacture may result in the need for a change in dosage. Hypoglycemia and hypokalemia may occur; caution in patients in whom such potential side effects might be clinically relevant (eg, patients w/ autonomic neuropathy). Lipodystrophy and hypersensitivity may occur. Dosage adjustment may be necessary if patient changes physical activity or usual meal plan. Illness, emotional disturbances, or other stress may alter insulin requirements. Careful glucose monitoring and insulin dose adjustment may be necessary w/ hepatic/ renal impairment. Inj-site redness/swelling/itching, and severe, life-threatening, generalized allergy may occur. Contains cresol as excipient; localized reactions and generalized myalgias reported. Antibody production reported. Caution in elderly.

ADVERSE REACTIONS
Hypoglycemia, allergic reactions, inj-site reactions, lipodystrophy, pruritus, rash.

DRUG INTERACTIONS
Drugs w/ hyperglycemic activity (eg, corticosteroids, certain lipid-lowering drugs [eg, niacin], oral contraceptives, phenothiazines, thyroid replacement therapy) may increase insulin requirements. Drugs that increase insulin sensitivity or have hypoglycemic activity (eg, salicylates, sulfa antibiotics, MAOIs, ACE inhibitors, inhibitors of pancreatic function [eg, octreotide]) may decrease insulin requirements. β-blockers may mask symptoms of hypoglycemia. Caution w/ K+-lowering drugs or drugs sensitive to serum K+ levels. Observe for signs/symptoms of heart failure (HF) if treated concomitantly w/ a peroxisome proliferator-activated receptor (PPAR)-gamma agonist (eg, thiazolidinedione); consider discontinuation or dose reduction of the PPAR-gamma agonist if HF develops.

PREGNANCY AND LACTATION
Category B, caution in nursing.

MECHANISM OF ACTION
Insulin; regulates glucose metabolism. In muscle and other tissues (except the brain), causes rapid transport of glucose and amino acids intracellularly, promotes anabolism, and inhibits protein catabolism. In the liver, promotes the uptake and storage of glucose in the form of glycogen, inhibits gluconeogenesis, and promotes the conversion of excess glucose into fat.

PHARMACOKINETICS
Absorption: T_{max}=30-240 min (0.3 U/kg). **Distribution:** V_d=0.26-0.36L/kg (insulin lispro).

PATIENT CONSIDERATIONS
Assessment: Assess for presence of hypoglycemia or hypokalemia and for conditions where such potential side effects might be clinically relevant. Assess for hypersensitivity, renal/hepatic impairment, pregnancy/nursing status, and possible drug interactions. Obtain baseline blood glucose and HbA1c levels.

Monitoring: Monitor for signs/symptoms of hypoglycemia, hypokalemia, lipodystrophy, allergic reactions, antibody production, and other adverse effects. Monitor blood glucose, HbA1c, K+ levels, and renal/hepatic function.

Counseling: Inform of the potential risks and advantages of therapy and alternative therapies. Instruct not to mix drug w/ any other insulin. Inform of the importance of proper insulin storage, inj technique, timing of dosage, adherence to meal planning, regular physical activity, regular blood glucose monitoring, periodic HbA1c testing, recognition and management of hypo/hyperglycemia, and periodic assessment for diabetes complications. Advise to inform physician if pregnant/ planning to become pregnant. Instruct patients using insulin pen delivery device on how to properly use delivery device, prime the pen to a stream of insulin, and properly dispose of needles. Advise not to share insulin pen w/ others.

HUMATROPE — somatropin (rDNA origin)   Rx

Class: Recombinant human growth hormone (hGH)

ADULT DOSAGE

Growth Hormone Deficiency

Adult or Childhood-Onset Etiology:
Non-Weight Based:
Initial: 0.2mg/day SQ (range, 0.15-0.30mg/day)
Titrate: May increase gradually every 1-2 months by increments of 0.1-0.2mg/day based on clinical response and serum insulin-like growth factor-I (IGF-I) concentrations
Maint: Individualize dose

Weight-Based:
Initial: ≤0.006mg/kg/day SQ
Titrate: May increase based on individual requirements
Max: 0.0125mg/kg/day

Clinical response, side effects, and determination of age- and gender-adjusted serum IGF-I concentrations should be used as guidance in dose titration

PEDIATRIC DOSAGE

Growth Hormone Deficiency

Due to an inadequate secretion of endogenous growth hormone

Individualize dose
Usual: 0.026-0.043mg/kg/day SQ (0.18-0.30mg/kg/week)

The calculated weekly dose should be divided into equal doses given either 6 or 7 days/week

Turner Syndrome

Treatment of short stature associated w/ Turner syndrome

Individualize dose
Usual: Up to 0.054mg/kg/day SQ (0.375mg/kg/week)

The calculated weekly dose should be divided into equal doses given either 6 or 7 days/week

Idiopathic Short Stature

Treatment of idiopathic short stature defined by height standard deviation score (SDS) ≤-2.25 and associated w/ growth rates unlikely to permit attainment of adult height in the normal range, in pediatric patients for whom diagnostic evaluation excludes other causes of short stature that should be observed or treated by other means

Individualize dose
Usual: Up to 0.053mg/kg/day SQ (0.37mg/kg/week)

The calculated weekly dose should be divided into equal doses given either 6 or 7 days/week

Small for Gestational Age

Treatment of growth failure in children born small for gestational age (SGA) who fail to demonstrate catch-up growth by age 2-4 yrs

Individualize dose
Usual: Up to 0.067mg/kg/day SQ (0.47mg/kg/week)

The calculated weekly dose should be divided into equal doses given either 6 or 7 days/week

Short Stature Homeobox-Containing Gene (SHOX) Deficiency

Individualize dose
Usual: 0.050mg/kg/day SQ (0.35mg/kg/week)
The calculated weekly dose should be divided into equal doses given either 6 or 7 days/week

DOSING CONSIDERATIONS

Concomitant Medications

Oral Estrogen: May increase the dose requirements in women

Elderly

Consider lower starting dose and smaller dose increments

ADMINISTRATION

SQ route

Rotate inj sites to avoid lipoatrophy.
For pediatric patients, the calculated weekly dosage should be divided into equal doses given either 6 or 7 days/week.
For adult patients, the prescribed dose should be administered daily.

Reconstitution

Vial:
1. Each 5mg vial should be reconstituted w/ 1.5-5mL of diluent
2. Following reconstitution, swirl the vial w/ a gentle rotary motion until contents are completely dissolved; do not shake, and use it only if it is clear
3. If sensitivity to the diluent occurs, may reconstitute w/ bacteriostatic water for inj (benzyl alcohol preserved), or sterile water for inj; the reconstituted sol should be used immediately and any unused sol should be discarded
4. If it is reconstituted w/ bacteriostatic water for inj, the sol should be kept refrigerated at 36-46°F (2-8°C) and used w/in 14 days
5. When administered to a newborn infant, it should be reconstituted w/ the diluent provided or, if the infant is sensitive to the diluent, sterile water for inj
6. When reconstituted w/ sterile water for inj, the sol should be kept refrigerated at 36-46°F (2-8°C) and used w/in 24 hrs

Cartridge:
1. The cartridge has been designed for use only w/ the Humatrope inj device
2. Each cartridge should be reconstituted using only the diluent syringe that accompanies the cartridge and should not be reconstituted w/ the diluent for Humatrope provided w/ the vials
3. The reconstituted sol should be clear. If the sol is cloudy or contains particulate matter, the contents must not be injected
4. Cartridges should not be used if the patient is allergic to metacresol or glycerin

STORAGE

2-8°C (36-46°F). Avoid freezing diluent. (Vial) After Reconstitution with Diluent for Humatrope or Bacteriostatic Water for Inj: 2-8°C (36-46°F) for up to 14 days. Avoid freezing. After Reconstitution with Sterile Water: 2-8°C (36-46°F); used within 24 hrs. Discard unused portion. (Cartridge) After Reconstitution with Diluent for Humatrope: 2-8°C (36-46°F) for up to 28 days. Avoid freezing.

HOW SUPPLIED

Inj: 5mg [vial]; 6mg, 12mg, 24mg [cartridge]

CONTRAINDICATIONS

Acute critical illness due to complications following open heart surgery, abdominal surgery, multiple accidental trauma, or w/ acute respiratory failure. Pediatric patients w/ Prader-Willi syndrome (PWS) who are severely obese, have a history of upper airway obstruction or sleep apnea, or have severe respiratory impairment. Pediatric patients who have growth failure due to genetically confirmed PWS. Active malignancy or evidence of progression or recurrence of an underlying intracranial tumor. Active proliferative or severe nonproliferative diabetic retinopathy. Growth promotion in pediatric patients w/ closed epiphyses. Known hypersensitivity to somatropin or diluent.

WARNINGS/PRECAUTIONS

Reevaluate adults who were treated with somatropin for GHD in childhood and whose epiphyses are closed. Implement effective weight control in patients with PWS and treat respiratory infections aggressively. Increased risk of a second neoplasm in childhood cancer survivors reported. Increased risk of developing malignancies in children with certain rare genetic causes of short stature; monitor for development of neoplasms if treatment is initiated. Monitor for increased growth, or potential malignant changes, of preexisting nevi. Undiagnosed impaired glucose tolerance and overt diabetes mellitus (DM) may be unmasked, and new onset type 2 DM reported. Intracranial HTN with papilledema, visual changes, headache, N/V reported; d/c if papilledema occurs. Fluid retention in adults may occur. Monitor other hormonal replacement treatments in patients with hypopituitarism. Undiagnosed/untreated hypothyroidism may prevent optimal response. Hypothyroidism may become evident or worsen. Slipped capital femoral epiphysis (SCFE) and progression of scoliosis may occur in pediatric patients. Increased risk of ear/hearing disorders and cardiovascular (CV) disorders in TS patients. Pancreatitis reported rarely. Tissue atrophy may occur; rotate inj site. Allergic reactions may occur. Serum levels of inorganic phosphorus, alkaline phosphatase, parathyroid hormone, and IGF-I may increase. Obese individuals are more likely to manifest adverse effects when treated w/ a weight-based regimen. Estrogen replete women may need higher doses than men. Caution in the elderly.

ADVERSE REACTIONS

Otitis media, ear disorder, arthrosis, pain, edema, arthralgia, myalgia, HTN, paresthesia, gynecomastia, scoliosis, hyperlipidemia, rhinitis, flu syndrome, AST increased.

DRUG INTERACTIONS

May inhibit 11β-hydroxysteroid dehydrogenase type 1, resulting in reduced serum cortisol concentrations; may need glucocorticoid replacement or dose adjustments of glucocorticoid therapy. Glucocorticoid therapy may attenuate growth-promoting effects in children; carefully adjust glucocorticoid replacement dosing. May increase clearance of antipyrine. May alter clearance of compounds metabolized by CYP450 liver enzymes (eg, corticosteroids, sex steroids, anticonvulsants, cyclosporine); monitor carefully. May require greater dose with oral estrogen replacement. May need to adjust dose of insulin and/or other hypoglycemic agents, and thyroid hormone replacement therapy.

PREGNANCY AND LACTATION

Category C, caution in nursing.

MECHANISM OF ACTION

Recombinant human GH; binds to dimeric GH receptors located within the cell membranes of target tissue cells, resulting in intracellular signal transduction and subsequent induction of transcription and translation of GH-dependent proteins, including IGF-I, IGF BP-3, and acid labile subunit.

PHARMACOKINETICS

Absorption: Absolute bioavailability (75%); C_{max}=63.3ng/mL; AUC=585ng•hr/mL.
Distribution: V_d=0.957L/kg. **Metabolism:** Liver and kidneys (protein catabolism).
Elimination: Urine; $T_{1/2}$=3.81 hrs.

PATIENT CONSIDERATIONS

Assessment: Assess for PWS, preexisting DM or impaired glucose tolerance, hypothyroidism, hypopituitarism, history of scoliosis, hypersensitivity to drug or diluent, pregnancy/nursing status, any other conditions where treatment is contraindicated or cautioned, and possible drug interactions. Perform funduscopic exam.

Monitoring: Monitor for SCFE and progression of scoliosis in pediatric patients (eg, onset of limp, hip or knee pain), growth, clinical response, compliance, neoplasm, increased growth or malignant changes of preexisting nevi, intracranial HTN, pancreatitis, fluid retention, allergic reactions, and other adverse reactions. In patients with PWS, monitor weight as well as for signs of respiratory infection, sleep apnea, and upper airway obstruction. Monitor patients with a history of

GHD secondary to an intracranial neoplasm for progression/recurrence of the tumor. Perform periodic thyroid function tests, funduscopic exam, and monitoring glucose levels. In patients with TS, monitor for ear/CV disorders.

Counseling: Inform of the potential benefits and risks of therapy, proper administration, and usage and disposal. Caution against any reuse of needles and syringes.

HUMIRA — adalimumab   Rx

Class: Monoclonal antibody/TNF blocker

> Increased risk of serious infections (eg, active tuberculosis [TB], including latent TB reactivation; invasive fungal infections; and bacterial, viral, and other infections due to opportunistic pathogens) that may lead to hospitalization or death, mostly w/ concomitant use of immunosuppressants (eg, methotrexate [MTX], corticosteroids). D/C if serious infection or sepsis develops. TB patients have frequently presented w/ disseminated or extrapulmonary disease; test for latent TB before and during therapy and initiate treatment for latent TB prior to adalimumab use. Consider empiric antifungal therapy in patients at risk for invasive fungal infections who develop severe systemic illness. Monitor patients closely for development of infection during and after treatment, including development of TB in patients who tested negative for latent TB infection prior to therapy. Lymphoma and other malignancies, some fatal, reported in children and adolescents. Postmarketing cases of aggressive and fatal hepatosplenic T-cell lymphoma reported; the majority of cases occurred in patients w/ Crohn's disease (CD) or ulcerative colitis (UC) and the majority were in adolescent and young adult males. Almost all of these patients were treated concomitantly w/ azathioprine or 6-mercaptopurine.

ADULT DOSAGE

Rheumatoid Arthritis

To reduce signs/symptoms, induce major clinical response, inhibit progression of structural damage, and improve physical function in patients w/ moderately to severely active rheumatoid arthritis

40mg every other week; may increase to 40mg every week in patients not taking concomitant MTX

May be used alone or in combination w/ MTX or other nonbiologic DMARDs

Psoriatic Arthritis

To reduce signs/symptoms, inhibit progression of structural damage, and improve physical function in patients w/ active psoriatic arthritis

40mg every other week

May be used alone or in combination w/ nonbiologic disease-modifying anti-rheumatic drugs

Ankylosing Spondylitis

To reduce signs/symptoms in patients w/ active ankylosing spondylitis

40mg every other week

Crohn's Disease

To reduce signs/symptoms and induce/maintain clinical remission in patients w/ moderately to severely active CD who have had an inadequate response to conventional therapy and/or lost response to or are intolerant to infliximab

Day 1: 160mg (given as four 40mg inj in 1 day or as two 40mg inj/day for 2 consecutive days)
Day 15: 80mg
Day 29 and Onward: 40mg every other week

Use beyond 1 year has not been evaluated

Plaque Psoriasis

Treatment of moderate to severe chronic plaque psoriasis in candidates for systemic therapy or phototherapy when other systemic therapies are medically less appropriate

Initial: 80mg
Maint: 40mg every other week starting 1 week after initial dose

Ulcerative Colitis

To induce and sustain clinical remission in patients w/ moderately to severely active UC who have had an inadequate response to immunosuppressants

Day 1: 160mg (given as four 40mg inj in 1 day or as two 40mg inj/day for 2 consecutive days)

PEDIATRIC DOSAGE

Juvenile Idiopathic Arthritis

To reduce signs/symptoms of moderately to severely active polyarticular juvenile idiopathic arthritis

≥2 Years:
10 to <15kg: 10mg every other week
15 to <30kg: 20mg every other week
≥30kg: 40mg every other week

May be used alone or in combination w/ MTX

Crohn's Disease

To reduce signs/symptoms and induce/maintain clinical remission in patients w/ moderately to severely active CD who have had an inadequate response to corticosteroids or immunomodulators

≥6 Years:
17 to <40kg:
Day 1: 80mg (given as two 40mg inj in 1 day)
Day 15: 40mg
Day 29 and Onward: 20mg every other week
≥40kg:
Day 1: 160mg (given as four 40mg inj in 1 day or as two 40mg inj/day for 2 consecutive days)
Day 15: 80mg (given as two 40mg inj in 1 day)
Day 29 and Onward: 40mg every other week

Day 15: 80mg
Day 29 and Onward: 40mg every other week

Only continue if clinical remission is evident by 8 weeks (Day 57) of therapy

Hidradenitis Suppurativa

Treatment of moderate to severe hidradenitis suppurativa

Day 1: 160mg (given as four 40mg inj on Day 1 or as two 40mg inj/day for 2 consecutive days)
Day 15: 80mg
Day 29 and Onward: 40mg every week

Uveitis

Treatment of non-infectious intermediate, posterior and panuveitis

Initial: 80mg
Maint: 40mg every other week starting 1 week after initial dose

---

ADMINISTRATION

SQ route

May be left at room temperature for about 15-30 min before injecting; do not remove the cap or cover while allowing it to reach room temperature.
Inject at separate sites in the thigh or abdomen. Rotate inj sites; avoid areas where skin is tender, bruised, red, or hard.

STORAGE

2-8°C (36-46°F). Do not freeze; do not use if frozen, even if it has been thawed. Store in original carton until time of administration to protect from light. May be stored up to a max of 25°C (77°F) for up to 14 days, if needed. Do not store in extreme heat or cold.

HOW SUPPLIED

Inj: 10mg/0.2mL, 20mg/0.4mL [prefilled syringe]; 40mg/0.4mL, 40mg/0.8mL [prefilled syringe, prefilled pen]; 40mg/0.8mL [vial]

WARNINGS/PRECAUTIONS

Do not initiate in patients w/ an active infection. Increased risk of infection in patients >65 yrs of age and in patients w/ comorbid conditions. Malignancies, including acute and chronic leukemia, lymphoma, and nonmelanoma skin cancer (NMSC), reported in adults. Anaphylaxis and angioneurotic edema reported; d/c immediately and institute appropriate therapy if an anaphylactic or other serious allergic reaction occurs. May increase risk of HBV reactivation in chronic carriers; closely monitor for signs of active HBV infection during and for several months after therapy termination. D/C if HBV reactivation develops and start effective antiviral therapy w/ appropriate supportive treatment. Caution in considering the use in patients w/ new onset or exacerbation of central or peripheral nervous system demyelinating disorders; D/C if these disorders develop. New or worsening congestive heart failure (CHF), and hematologic system adverse reactions, including significant cytopenia (eg, thrombocytopenia, leukopenia), reported. May result in the formation of autoantibodies and development of a lupus-like syndrome; d/c if symptoms suggestive of a lupus-like syndrome develop. If possible, pediatric patients should be brought up to date w/ all immunizations in agreement w/ current immunization guidelines prior to initiating therapy. Avoid having latex-sensitive patients handle the needle cover of the prefilled syringe; it contains dry rubber (latex). Caution in elderly.

ADVERSE REACTIONS

URTI, sinusitis, inj-site reactions, headache, rash, nausea, flu syndrome, abdominal pain, hyperlipidemia, hypercholesterolemia, back pain, hematuria, increased alkaline phosphatase, UTI, HTN.

DRUG INTERACTIONS

See Boxed Warning. Reduced clearance w/ MTX. Concomitant administration w/ other biologic DMARDs (eg, anakinra, abatacept) or other TNF blockers is not recommended due to possible increased risk for infections and other potential pharmacological interactions. Avoid w/ live vaccines. Upon initiation or discontinuation of adalimumab in patients being treated w/ CYP450 substrates w/ a narrow therapeutic index, monitor therapeutic effect (eg, warfarin) or drug concentration (eg, cyclosporine, theophylline) and adjust individual dose of the drug product prn.

PREGNANCY AND LACTATION

Pregnancy: Limited clinical data available from the Humira Pregnancy Registry. Monoclonal antibodies are increasingly transported across the placenta as pregnancy progresses w/ the largest amount transferred during the 3rd trimester. Consider risks and benefits prior to administering live or live-attenuated vaccines to infants exposed to Humira in utero.
Lactation: Low amount (0.1-1%) found in human milk. No reports of adverse effects on infant and no effects on milk production. Caution in nursing.

MECHANISM OF ACTION

Monoclonal antibody/TNF-α receptor blocker; binds specifically to TNF-α and blocks its interaction w/ the p55 and p75 cell surface TNF receptors. Also lyses surface TNF-expressing cells in vitro in the presence of complement.

PHARMACOKINETICS

Absorption: (40mg SQ single dose) Absolute bioavailability (64%), C_{max}=4.7mcg/mL, T_{max}=131 hrs. **Distribution:** Found in breast milk; (0.25-10mg/kg IV dose) V_d=4.7-6L. **Elimination:** (0.25-10mg/kg IV dose) $T_{1/2}$=2 weeks.

PATIENT CONSIDERATIONS

Assessment: Assess for active/chronic/recurrent infection, history of an opportunistic infection, recent travel in areas of endemic TB or endemic mycoses, underlying conditions that may predispose to infection, central or peripheral nervous system demyelinating disorders, CHF, latex sensitivity, drug hypersensitivity, pregnancy/nursing status, and for possible drug interactions. Test for latent TB infection and for HBV infection. Assess immunization history in pediatric patients. Perform a skin examination, particularly in patients w/ a medical history of prior prolonged immunosuppressant therapy or in psoriasis patients w/ a history of psoralen plus ultraviolet light (PUVA) treatment for the presence of NMSC.

Monitoring: Monitor for development of infection during and after treatment. Monitor for malignancies, hypersensitivity reactions, neurological reactions, hematological reactions, worsening/new-onset CHF, lupus-like syndrome, and other adverse reactions. Monitor for active TB and periodically test for latent TB. Monitor for HBV reactivation during therapy and for several months following termination of therapy. Perform periodic skin examinations, particularly in patients w/ a medical history of prior prolonged immunosuppressant therapy or in psoriasis patients w/ a history of PUVA treatment for the presence of NMSC.

Counseling: Inform about the potential benefits/risks of therapy. Inform that therapy may lower the ability of the immune system to fight infections; instruct to contact physician if any symptoms of infection, including TB, invasive fungal infections, or reactivation of HBV infections, develop. Counsel about the risk of malignancies. Advise to seek immediate medical attention if any symptoms of a severe allergic reaction develop. Advise latex-sensitive patients that the needle cap of the prefilled syringe contains latex. Advise to report to physician any signs of new/worsening medical conditions (eg, CHF, neurological disease, autoimmune disorders) or any symptoms suggestive of a cytopenia (eg, bleeding, bruising, persistent fever). Instruct on proper inj technique, as well as proper syringe and needle disposal.

HUMULIN 70/30 — NPH, human insulin isophane (rDNA origin)/regular, human insulin (rDNA origin)   OTC

Class: Insulin (combination)

ADULT DOSAGE	PEDIATRIC DOSAGE
Diabetes Mellitus	Pediatric use may not have been established
Individualize dose	
May need to adjust dosage based on metabolic needs, blood glucose monitoring results, and glycemic control goal	
Administer SQ approx 30-45 min ac	

DOSING CONSIDERATIONS
Renal Impairment
May require more frequent dose adjustment

Hepatic Impairment
May require more frequent dose adjustment

Other Important Considerations
May require dose adjustments w/ changes in physical activity/meal patterns, or during acute illness

ADMINISTRATION
SQ route
Should appear uniformly cloudy after mixing; do not use if particulate matter is seen.
Do not mix w/ any other insulins/diluents.
Administer in the abdominal wall, thigh, upper arm, or buttocks; rotate the inj site w/in the same region from 1 inj to the next.
Do not use in an insulin infusion pump.

STORAGE
Protect from heat and light. Do not freeze; do not use if it has been frozen. **Vial: Unopened:** 2-8°C (36-46°F) until expiration date, or room temperature <30°C (86°F) for 31 days. **Opened:** 2-8°C (36-46°F) or room temperature <30°C (86°F) for 31 days. **Pen/KwikPen: Unopened:** 2-8°C (36-46°F) until expiration date, or room temperature <30°C (86°F) for 10 days. **Opened:** Room temperature <30°C (86°F) for 10 days. Do not refrigerate.

HOW SUPPLIED
Inj: (Insulin Isophane/Regular) (70 U/30 U)/mL [3mL, vial, pen, KwikPen; 10mL, vial]

CONTRAINDICATIONS
During episodes of hypoglycemia. Hypersensitivity reactions to Humulin 70/30 or any of its excipients.

WARNINGS/PRECAUTIONS
Pens and KwikPens must never be shared between patients, even if the needle is changed; may carry a risk for transmission of blood-borne pathogens. Changes in strength, manufacturer, type, or method of administration may affect glycemic control and predispose to hypo/hyperglycemia; these changes should be made cautiously and under close medical supervision and the frequency of blood glucose monitoring should be increased. Hypoglycemia may occur; increase frequency of blood glucose monitoring in patients at higher risk for hypoglycemia and patients who have reduced symptomatic awareness of hypoglycemia. Hypoglycemia may impair concentration ability and reaction time. Severe, life-threatening, generalized allergy, including anaphylaxis, may occur;

if hypersensitivity reactions occur, d/c therapy, treat per standard of care, and monitor until symptoms and signs resolve. May cause hypokalemia.

ADVERSE REACTIONS
Hypoglycemia, allergic reactions, peripheral edema, lipodystrophy, weight gain, immunogenicity.

DRUG INTERACTIONS
May require dose adjustment and increased frequency of glucose monitoring w/ drugs that may increase the risk of hypoglycemia (eg, antidiabetic agents, salicylates, sulfonamide antibiotics), drugs that may decrease the glucose-lowering effect (eg, corticosteroids, isoniazid, niacin), or drugs that may increase or decrease glucose-lowering effect (eg, β-blockers, clonidine, lithium salts, alcohol). Pentamidine may cause hypoglycemia, sometimes followed by hyperglycemia. Signs and symptoms of hypoglycemia may be blunted w/ β-blockers, clonidine, guanethidine, and reserpine. Monitor K$^+$ levels w/ K$^+$-lowering medications or medications sensitive to serum K$^+$ concentrations. Observe for signs/symptoms of heart failure (HF) if treated concomitantly w/ a peroxisome proliferator-activated receptor (PPAR)-gamma agonist (eg, thiazolidinedione); consider discontinuation or dose reduction of the PPAR-gamma agonist if HF develops.

PREGNANCY AND LACTATION
Pregnancy: Category B.
Lactation: Women w/ diabetes who are lactating may require adjustments in their insulin dose.

MECHANISM OF ACTION
Insulin; lowers blood glucose by stimulating peripheral glucose uptake by skeletal muscle and fat, and by inhibiting hepatic glucose production. Inhibits lipolysis and proteolysis, and enhances protein synthesis.

PHARMACOKINETICS
Absorption: T_{max}=2.2 hrs. **Metabolism:** Liver, kidney, muscle, and adipocytes.

PATIENT CONSIDERATIONS
Assessment: Assess for risk of hypoglycemia or hypokalemia, hypersensitivity, renal/hepatic impairment, pregnancy/nursing status, and possible drug interactions. Obtain baseline FPG and HbA1c.

Monitoring: Monitor for signs and symptoms of hypoglycemia, hypokalemia, hypersensitivity reactions, and other adverse reactions. Monitor FPG, HbA1c, and renal/hepatic function.

Counseling: Advise never to share a pen or KwikPen w/ another person, even if the needle is changed. Instruct on self-management procedures, including glucose monitoring, proper inj technique, and management of hypo/hyperglycemia, and on handling of special situations, such as intercurrent conditions, inadequate or skipped insulin dose, inadvertent administration of an increased insulin dose, inadequate food intake, and skipped meals. Inform that hypoglycemia may impair ability to concentrate and react; advise to use caution when driving or operating machinery. Instruct to always check the label before each inj to avoid medication errors/accidental mix-ups. Inform on the symptoms of hypersensitivity reactions. Advise to inform physician if pregnant/contemplating pregnancy. Advise to use only if product contains no particulate matter and appears uniformly cloudy after mixing.

HUMULIN N — NPH, human insulin isophane (rDNA origin)   OTC

Class: Insulin (intermediate-acting)

ADULT DOSAGE	PEDIATRIC DOSAGE
Diabetes Mellitus	**Diabetes Mellitus**
Individualize dose	Individualize dose
May need to adjust dosage based on metabolic needs, blood glucose monitoring results, and glycemic control goal	May need to adjust dosage based on metabolic needs, blood glucose monitoring results, and glycemic control goal

DOSING CONSIDERATIONS
Renal Impairment
May require more frequent dose adjustment

Hepatic Impairment
May require more frequent dose adjustment

Other Important Considerations
May require dose adjustments w/ changes in physical activity/meal patterns, or during acute illness

ADMINISTRATION
SQ route
Should appear uniformly cloudy after mixing; do not use if particulate matter is seen.
Administer in the abdominal wall, thigh, upper arm, or buttocks; rotate the inj site w/in the same region from 1 inj to the next.
Do not administer IV/IM and do not use in an insulin infusion pump.

Mixing w/ Other Insulins
If Humulin N is mixed w/ Humulin R or Humalog, draw Humulin R or Humalog into syringe 1st; inject immediately after mixing.

STORAGE
Protect from heat and light. Do not freeze; do not use if it has been frozen. **Vial:** (Unopened) 2-8°C (36-46°F) until expiration date, or room temperature <30°C (86°F) for 31 days. (Opened) 2-8°C (36-46°F) or room temperature <30°C (86°F) for 31 days. **Pen/KwikPen:** (Unopened) 2-8°C (36-46°F) until expiration date, or

room temperature <30°C (86°F) for 14 days. (Opened) Room temperature <30°C (86°F) for 14 days. Do not refrigerate.

HOW SUPPLIED
Inj: 100 U/mL [3mL, vial, pen, KwikPen; 10mL, vial]

CONTRAINDICATIONS
During episodes of hypoglycemia. Hypersensitivity reactions to Humulin N or any of its excipients.

WARNINGS/PRECAUTIONS
Pens and KwikPens must never be shared between patients, even if needle is changed; may carry a risk for transmission of blood-borne pathogens. Changes in strength, manufacturer, type, or method of administration may affect glycemic control and predispose to hypo/hyperglycemia; these changes should be made cautiously and under close medical supervision and the frequency of blood glucose monitoring should be increased. Hypoglycemia may occur; increase frequency of blood glucose monitoring in patients at higher risk for hypoglycemia and in patients who have reduced symptomatic awareness of hypoglycemia. Hypoglycemia may impair concentration ability and reaction time. Severe, life-threatening, generalized allergy, including anaphylaxis, may occur; if hypersensitivity reactions occur, d/c therapy, treat per standard of care, and monitor until symptoms and signs resolve. May cause hypokalemia. May require more frequent glucose monitoring w/ hepatic/renal impairment.

ADVERSE REACTIONS
Hypoglycemia, allergic reactions, peripheral edema, lipodystrophy, weight gain, immunogenicity.

DRUG INTERACTIONS
May require dose adjustment and increased frequency of glucose monitoring w/ drugs that may increase the risk of hypoglycemia (eg, antidiabetic agents, salicylates, sulfonamide antibiotics), drugs that may decrease the glucose-lowering effect (eg, corticosteroids, isoniazid, niacin), or drugs that may increase or decrease glucose-lowering effect (eg, β-blockers, clonidine, lithium salts, alcohol). Pentamidine may cause hypoglycemia, sometimes followed by hyperglycemia. Signs and symptoms of hypoglycemia may be blunted w/ β-blockers, clonidine, guanethidine, and reserpine. Monitor K^+ levels w/ K^+-lowering medications or medications sensitive to serum K^+ concentrations. Observe for signs/symptoms of heart failure (HF) if treated concomitantly w/ a peroxisome proliferator-activated receptor (PPAR)-gamma agonist (eg, thiazolidinedione); consider discontinuation or dose reduction of the PPAR-gamma agonist if HF develops.

PREGNANCY AND LACTATION
Pregnancy: Category B.
Lactation: Women w/ diabetes who are lactating may require adjustments in their insulin dose.

MECHANISM OF ACTION
Insulin; lowers blood glucose by stimulating peripheral glucose uptake by skeletal muscle and fat, and by inhibiting hepatic glucose production. Inhibits lipolysis and proteolysis, and enhances protein synthesis.

PHARMACOKINETICS
Absorption: T_{max}=approx 4 hrs (median). **Metabolism:** Liver, kidney, muscle, and adipocytes. **Elimination:** $T_{1/2}$=approx 4.4 hrs.

PATIENT CONSIDERATIONS
Assessment: Assess for risk of hypoglycemia or hypokalemia, hypersensitivity, renal/hepatic impairment, pregnancy/nursing status, and possible drug interactions. Obtain baseline FPG and HbA1c.

Monitoring: Monitor for signs and symptoms of hypoglycemia, hypokalemia, hypersensitivity reactions, and other adverse reactions. Monitor FPG, HbA1c, and renal/hepatic function.

Counseling: Advise never to share a pen or KwikPen w/ another person even if needle is changed. Instruct on self-management procedures, including glucose monitoring, proper inj technique, management of hypo/hyperglycemia, and on handling of special situations such as intercurrent conditions, inadequate or skipped insulin dose, inadvertent administration of an increased insulin dose, inadequate food intake, and skipped meals. Inform that hypoglycemia may impair ability to concentrate and react; advise to use caution when driving or operating machinery. Instruct to always check the label before each inj to avoid medication errors/accidental mix-ups. Educate on the symptoms of hypersensitivity reactions. Advise to inform physician if pregnant/contemplating pregnancy. Advise to use only if product contains no particulate matter and appears uniformly cloudy after mixing.

HUMULIN R — regular, human insulin (rDNA origin)   OTC
Class: Insulin (short-acting)

ADULT DOSAGE
Diabetes Mellitus
Initial: 0.2-0.4 U/kg/day
Maint:
Total Daily Insulin Requirement:
0.5-1 U/kg/day; requirement may be substantially higher in insulin-resistant patients

PEDIATRIC DOSAGE
Diabetes Mellitus
Initial: 0.2-0.4 U/kg/day
Maint:
Total Daily Insulin Requirement:
0.5-1 U/kg/day; requirement may be substantially higher in insulin-resistant patients
Prepubertal Children: Average total daily insulin requirement varies from 0.7-1 U/kg/day, but may be much lower during the period of partial remission

DOSING CONSIDERATIONS
Renal Impairment
May require frequent dose reduction

Hepatic Impairment
May require frequent dose reduction

ADMINISTRATION
SQ/IV route

May be used in combination w/ oral antihyperglycemics or longer-acting insulin products.

SQ
Usually given ≥3X daily ac.
Inj should be followed by a meal w/in approx 30 min.
Inject in the abdominal wall, thigh, gluteal region, or upper arm; rotate inj sites w/in the same region.

IV
Use at concentrations from 0.1-1 U/mL in infusion systems w/ the infusion fluids 0.9% NaCl using polyvinyl chloride infusion bags.

Mixing of Insulins
Humulin R is often used in combination w/ intermediate- or long-acting insulins; when mixed w/ an intermediate-acting insulin (eg, NPH insulin isophane sus), draw Humulin R into the syringe first.
A U-100 insulin syringe should always be used.

STORAGE
Do not use if it has been frozen. **Unopened:** 2-8°C (36-46°F). Do not freeze. **Opened:** <30°C (86°F). Protect from heat and light. Use w/in 31 days. **Admixture:** 2-8°C (36-46°F) for 48 hrs, then may use at room temperature for up to an additional 48 hrs.

HOW SUPPLIED
Inj: 100 U/mL [3mL, 10mL]

CONTRAINDICATIONS
During episodes of hypoglycemia. Hypersensitivity to Humulin R U-100 or any of its excipients.

WARNINGS/PRECAUTIONS
Needles or syringes must never be reused or shared between patients; may carry a risk for transmission of blood-borne pathogens. Any change in insulin should be made cautiously and only under medical supervision. Changes in strength, manufacturer, type, species, or method of administration may result in the need for a change in dosage. May require dosage adjustments w/ change in physical activity or usual meal plan. Stress, illness, or emotional disturbances may alter insulin requirements. Hypoglycemia may occur and may impair ability to concentrate and react; caution in patients w/ hypoglycemia unawareness and those predisposed to hypoglycemia (eg, pediatric population, those who fast or have erratic food intake). Hyperglycemia, diabetic ketoacidosis, or hyperosmolar coma may develop if taken less than needed. Hypokalemia may occur. Severe, life-threatening, generalized allergy, including anaphylaxis, may occur. Contains metacresol as excipient; localized reactions and generalized myalgias reported. Frequent glucose monitoring and dose reduction may be required w/ hepatic/renal impairment. May be administered IV under medical supervision; close monitoring of blood glucose and K^+ is required.

ADVERSE REACTIONS
Hypoglycemia, lipodystrophy, weight gain, peripheral edema.

DRUG INTERACTIONS
May require dose adjustment and close monitoring w/ drugs that may increase blood-glucose-lowering effect and susceptibility to hypoglycemia (eg, oral antihyperglycemics, salicylates, sulfa antibiotics), drugs that may reduce blood-glucose-lowering effect (eg, corticosteroids, isoniazid, certain lipid-lowering drugs [eg, niacin]), or drugs that may increase or decrease blood-glucose-lowering effect (eg, β-blockers, clonidine, lithium salts, alcohol). Pentamidine may cause hypoglycemia, which may sometimes be followed by hyperglycemia. β-blockers, clonidine, guanethidine, and reserpine may mask the signs of hypoglycemia. Caution w/ K^+-lowering medications or medications sensitive to serum K^+ concentrations. Observe for signs/symptoms of heart failure (HF) if treated concomitantly w/ a peroxisome proliferator-activated receptor (PPAR)-gamma agonist (eg, thiazolidinedione); consider discontinuation or dose reduction of the PPAR-gamma agonist if HF develops.

PREGNANCY AND LACTATION
Category B, caution in nursing.

MECHANISM OF ACTION
Insulin; regulates glucose metabolism. Lowers blood glucose by stimulating peripheral glucose uptake by skeletal muscle and fat, and by inhibiting hepatic glucose production. Inhibits lipolysis, proteolysis, and gluconeogenesis, and enhances protein synthesis and conversion of excess glucose into fat.

PATIENT CONSIDERATIONS
Assessment: Assess for risk of hypoglycemia or hypokalemia, hypersensitivity, renal/hepatic impairment, pregnancy/nursing status, and possible drug interactions. Obtain baseline FPG and HbA1c.

Monitoring: Monitor for signs and symptoms of hypoglycemia, hypokalemia, allergic reactions, and other adverse reactions. Monitor FPG, HbA1c, and renal/hepatic function.

Counseling: Instruct not to share syringes w/ other people, even if the needle has been changed. Instruct to always carry a quick source of sugar (eg, hard candy or glucose tabs). Counsel about proper dose preparation, administration technique, signs/symptoms of hypoglycemia, importance of frequent monitoring of blood glucose levels, and need for a balanced diet and regular exercise. Advise to always keep an extra supply of insulin as well as a spare syringe and needle on hand, and to always wear diabetic identification. Instruct to exercise caution when driving or operating machinery. Instruct to notify physician if pregnant/nursing, planning to become pregnant, or taking any other medications.

HUMULIN R U-500 — insulin human   Rx

Class: Insulin (short-acting)

ADULT DOSAGE	PEDIATRIC DOSAGE
Diabetes Mellitus	**Diabetes Mellitus**
To improve glycemic control in patients w/ diabetes mellitus (DM) requiring >200 U of insulin per day	To improve glycemic control in patients w/ DM requiring >200 U of insulin per day
Give bid-tid approx 30 min ac	Give bid-tid approx 30 min ac
Individualize and titrate dose based on the patient's metabolic needs, blood glucose monitoring results, and glycemic control goal	Individualize and titrate dose based on the patient's metabolic needs, blood glucose monitoring results, and glycemic control goal

DOSING CONSIDERATIONS
Renal Impairment
May require frequent glucose monitoring and insulin dose reduction

Hepatic Impairment
May require frequent glucose monitoring and insulin dose reduction

Other Important Considerations
May require dose adjustments w/ changes in physical activity/meal patterns/medications, or during acute illness

ADMINISTRATION
SQ route
Vial prescribed must be the U-500 insulin syringe to avoid medication errors. Inject into the thigh, upper arm, abdomen, or buttocks; rotate inj sites w/in the same region.
Do not dilute or mix w/ any other insulin products or sol.
Do not administer IV or IM.

Delivery of Humulin R U-500 Using the Humulin R U-500 Disposable Prefilled KwikPen Device
Do not perform dose conversion when using the Humulin R U-500 KwikPen; dose window of the Humulin R U-500 KwikPen shows the number of units of Humulin R U-500 to be injected.
Do not transfer Humulin R U-500 from the Humulin R U-500 KwikPen into a syringe for administration as overdose and severe hypoglycemia can occur. Humulin R U-500 KwikPen is for single patient use only.

Delivery of Humulin R U-500 Using the Vial Presentation and the U-500 Insulin Syringe
Do not perform dose conversion when using a U-500 insulin syringe. The markings on the U-500 insulin syringe show the number of units of Humulin R U-500 to be injected. Each marking on the syringe represents 5 U of insulin.
Prescribe patients a U-500 insulin syringe to administer Humulin R U-500 from the vial to avoid administration errors. Do not use any other type of syringe.

STORAGE
Protect from heat and light. Do not freeze; do not use if it has been frozen. Do not shake the vial. **KwikPen:** (Unopened) 2-8°C (36-46°F); or <30°C (86°F) for 28 days. (Opened) <30°C (86°F) for 28 days. Do not refrigerate. **Vial:** (Unopened) 2-8°C (36-46°F); or <30°C (86°F) for 40 days. (Opened) 2-8°C (36-46°F) for 40 days; or <30°C (86°F) for 40 days.

HOW SUPPLIED
Inj: 500 U/mL [3mL, KwikPen; 20mL, vial]

CONTRAINDICATIONS
Episodes of hypoglycemia. Hypersensitivity to Humulin R U-500 or any of its excipients.

WARNINGS/PRECAUTIONS
Medication errors in dispensing, prescribing, and administration have occurred and resulted in patients experiencing hyperglycemia, hypoglycemia, or death. Prescribe U-500 insulin syringes; the prescribed dose should always be expressed in insulin units. Never share a KwikPen or syringe between patients; may carry a risk for transmission of blood-borne pathogens. Changes in insulin, manufacturer, type, or method of administration may affect glycemic control and predispose to hypoglycemia or hyperglycemia; changes should be made cautiously and only under medical supervision w/ increased frequency of blood glucose monitoring. Patients w/ type 2 DM who have a change in their insulin regimen may require adjustments in concomitant oral anti-diabetic treatment. Hypoglycemia may occur and may impair concentration ability and reaction time. Severe hypoglycemia may develop as long as 18-24 hrs after the original inj and may cause seizures, be life threatening, or cause death. Symptomatic awareness of hypoglycemia may be less pronounced in patients w/ longstanding diabetes, in patients w/ diabetic nerve disease, in patients using medications that block the sympathetic nervous system, or in patients who experience recurrent hypoglycemia. Monitor blood glucose levels more frequently in patients at higher risk for hypoglycemia, and in patients who have reduced symptomatic awareness of hypoglycemia. Severe, life-threatening, generalized allergy, including anaphylaxis, may occur; d/c and treat appropriately and monitor until signs and symptoms resolve. Hypokalemia may occur; caution in patients who may be at risk for hypokalemia.

ADVERSE REACTIONS
Hypoglycemia, allergic reactions, lipodystrophy, inj-site reactions, weight gain, peripheral edema.

DRUG INTERACTIONS
May require dose adjustment and increased frequency of glucose monitoring w/ drugs that may increase the risk of hypoglycemia (eg, antidiabetic agents, ACE inhibitors, disopyramide, fibrates, fluoxetine, MAOIs, pentoxifylline, pramlintide, propoxyphene, somatostatin analogues, salicylates, sulfonamide antibiotics), drugs that may decrease the glucose-lowering effect (eg, atypical antipsychotics (eg, olanzapine, clozapine), corticosteroids, danazol, diuretics, estrogens, glucagon, isoniazid, niacin, oral contraceptives, phenothiazines, progestogens, protease inhibitors, somatropin, sympathomimetic agents (eg, albuterol) and thyroid hormones), or drugs that may increase or decrease glucose-lowering effect (eg, alcohol, β-blockers, clonidine, lithium salts). Signs/symptoms of hypoglycemia may be blunted w/ β-blockers, clonidine, guanethidine, and reserpine. Caution w/ K$^+$-lowering medications or medications sensitive to serum K$^+$ concentrations. Observe for signs/symptoms of heart failure (HF) if treated concomitantly w/ a peroxisome proliferator-activated receptor (PPAR)-gamma agonist (eg, thiazolidinedione); consider discontinuation or dose reduction of the PPAR-gamma agonist if HF develops.

PREGNANCY AND LACTATION
Pregnancy: Category B.
Lactation: Women w/ diabetes who are lactating may require adjustments in their insulin dose.

MECHANISM OF ACTION
Insulin; lowers blood glucose by stimulating peripheral glucose uptake by skeletal muscle and fat, and by inhibiting hepatic glucose production. Inhibits lipolysis and proteolysis, and enhances protein synthesis.

PHARMACOKINETICS
Absorption: T_{max}(healthy, obese)=4 hrs (median, 50 U), 8 hrs (median, 100 U). **Metabolism:** Liver, kidney, muscle, and adipocytes. **Elimination:** $T_{1/2}$(healthy, obese)=4.5 hrs (50 U and 100 U)

PATIENT CONSIDERATIONS
Assessment: Assess for risk of hypoglycemia or hypokalemia, hypersensitivity, renal/hepatic impairment, pregnancy/nursing status, and possible drug interactions. Obtain baseline FPG and HbA1c.

Monitoring: Monitor for signs and symptoms of hypoglycemia, hypokalemia, hypersensitivity reactions, and other adverse reactions. Monitor FPG, HbA1c, and renal/hepatic function.

Counseling: Inform that this formulation is concentrated and that extreme caution must be observed in the measurement of dosage because inadvertent overdose may result in serious adverse reaction or life-threatening hypoglycemia. Instruct to always check the label before each inj to avoid medication errors/accidental mix-ups. If using the KwikPen, counsel to dial and dose the prescribed number of units of insulin. When using the insulin from a vial, use only a U-500 insulin syringe to avoid administration errors. Instruct on self-management procedures, including glucose monitoring, proper inj technique, management of hypo/hyperglycemia, and handling of special situations (eg, intercurrent conditions, inadequate or skipped insulin dose, inadvertent administration of an increased insulin dose, inadequate food intake, skipped meals). Advise to inform physician if pregnant/contemplating pregnancy.

HYCAMTIN CAPSULES — topotecan   Rx

Class: Topoisomerase I inhibitor

> May cause severe myelosuppression. Administer only to patients with neutrophil counts of ≥1500 cells/mm^3 and platelet counts ≥100,000 cells/mm^3. Monitor blood cell counts.

ADULT DOSAGE	PEDIATRIC DOSAGE
Relapsed Small Cell Lung Cancer	Pediatric use may not have been established
In patients w/ a prior complete or partial response and who are ≥45 days from the end of 1st-line chemotherapy	
2.3mg/m^2/day qd for 5 consecutive days, repeated every 21 days	
Round dose to nearest 0.25mg, and prescribe the minimum number of 1mg and 0.25mg caps; prescribe the same number of caps for each of the 5 dosing days	

DOSING CONSIDERATIONS
Renal Impairment
Moderate (CrCl 30-49mL/min): 1.5mg/m^2/day
Severe (CrCl <30mL/min): 0.6mg/m^2/day

Dose can be increased after the 1st course by 0.4mg/m^2/day if no severe hematologic or GI toxicities occur

Adverse Reactions
Diarrhea
Grade 3 or 4: Do not administer
After Recovery ≤Grade 1: Reduce dose by 0.4mg/m^2/day for subsequent courses

Hematologic Toxicities:
Do not administer subsequent courses until neutrophils recover to >1000 cells/mm^3, platelets recover to >100,000 cells/mm^3, Hgb levels recover to ≥9.0g/dL (w/ transfusion if necessary)

Reduce Dose by 0.4mg/m^2/day for:
1. Neutrophil counts <500 cells/mm^3 associated w/ fever or infection or lasting for ≥7 days
2. Neutrophil counts 500-1000 cells/mm^3 lasting beyond Day 21 of the treatment course
3. Platelet counts <25,000 cells/mm^3

ADMINISTRATION
Oral route

Take w/ or w/o food
Swallow whole; do not chew, crush, or divide
Do not prescribe a replacement dose for emesis

STORAGE
2-8°C (36-46°F). Protect from light.

HOW SUPPLIED
Cap: 0.25mg, 1mg

CONTRAINDICATIONS
History of severe hypersensitivity reactions to topotecan.

WARNINGS/PRECAUTIONS
Do not give a replacement dose for emesis. May cause fatal typhlitis (neutropenic enterocolitis); consider the possibility of typhlitis in patients presenting with fever, neutropenia, and abdominal pain. Diarrhea, including severe and life-threatening diarrhea requiring hospitalization reported; manage diarrhea aggressively and avoid with Grade 3 or 4 diarrhea. Interstitial lung disease (ILD), including fatalities, reported; monitor for pulmonary symptoms indicative of ILD (eg, cough, fever, dyspnea, and/or hypoxia) and d/c therapy if a new diagnosis of ILD is confirmed. May cause fetal harm during pregnancy. May have acute and long-term effects on fertility in females. May damage spermatozoa in males, resulting in possible genetic and fetal abnormalities.

ADVERSE REACTIONS
Severe myelosuppression, anemia, neutropenia, thrombocytopenia, N/V, diarrhea, alopecia, fatigue, anorexia, pyrexia, asthenia.

DRUG INTERACTIONS
P-glycoprotein inhibitors (eg, azithromycin, ketoconazole, ritonavir) and breast cancer resistance protein inhibitors (eg, cyclosporine, eltrombopag) may increase the systemic exposure to oral topotecan; avoid concomitant use.

PREGNANCY AND LACTATION
Category D, not for use in nursing.

MECHANISM OF ACTION
Topoisomerase I inhibitor; binds to the topoisomerase I-DNA complex and prevents religation of these single strand breaks.

PHARMACOKINETICS
Absorption: Rapid. T_{max}=1-2 hrs; oral bioavailability (40%). **Distribution:** Plasma protein binding (35%). **Metabolism:** Reversible pH dependent hydrolysis; N-desmethyl topotecan (metabolite). **Elimination:** Urine (20%, 2% N-desmethyl topotecan), feces (33%, 1.5% N-desmethyl topotecan); $T_{1/2}$=3-6 hrs.

PATIENT CONSIDERATIONS
Assessment: Assess for history of severe hypersensitivity reactions to drug, Grade 3 or 4 diarrhea, risk factors for ILD, pregnancy/nursing status, renal impairment, and possible drug interactions. Assess baseline neutrophil and platelet counts.

Monitoring: Monitor for signs/symptoms of myelosuppression, typhlitis, ILD, diarrhea, and other adverse reactions. Monitor peripheral blood cell counts frequently.

Counseling: Inform that therapy decreases blood cell counts and frequent blood tests will be performed while on therapy to monitor for bone marrow suppression. Instruct to notify physician promptly if fever or other signs of infection develop. Advise patients on pregnancy planning and prevention. Advise females of reproductive potential to use highly effective contraception during therapy and for 1 month following treatment and for men with female sexual partners of reproductive potential to use effective contraception during therapy and for 3 months following therapy. Advise to d/c nursing during treatment. Advise male and female patients of the potential risk for impaired fertility and possible family planning options. Inform that therapy may cause diarrhea, which may be severe and life-threatening; instruct patients how to manage and/or prevent diarrhea and to inform physician if severe diarrhea occurs during treatment.

Hydrochlorothiazide Tablets –

hydrochlorothiazide   Rx

Class: Thiazide diuretic

ADULT DOSAGE
Edema

For edema due to renal dysfunction (eg, nephrotic syndrome, acute glomerulonephritis, chronic renal failure), edema in pregnancy due to pathologic causes and adjunctive therapy for edema associated w/ congestive heart failure, hepatic cirrhosis, and corticosteroid and estrogen therapy

PEDIATRIC DOSAGE
Diuresis

Usual: 1-2mg/kg/day in single or 2 divided doses
Max:
<6 Months: 3mg/kg/day in 2 divided doses
Infants up to 2 Years: 37.5mg/day
2-12 Years: 100mg/day

Usual: 25-100mg/day as a single or divided dose. May give qod or 3-5 days/week

Hypertension

Initial: 25mg qd
Titrate: May increase to 50mg/day as a single or 2 divided doses

ADMINISTRATION
Oral route

STORAGE
20-25°C (68-77°F).

HOW SUPPLIED
Tab: 12.5mg, 25mg*, 50mg* *scored

CONTRAINDICATIONS
Anuria, hypersensitivity to this product or to other sulfonamide-derived drugs.

WARNINGS/PRECAUTIONS
Caution with severe renal disease; may precipitate azotemia. Caution with hepatic impairment or progressive liver disease; may precipitate hepatic coma. Sensitivity reactions may occur in patients with or without a history of allergy or bronchial asthma. Possibility of exacerbation/activation of systemic lupus erythematosus (SLE) reported. May cause idiosyncratic reaction, resulting in acute transient myopia and acute angle-closure glaucoma; d/c as rapidly as possible. Observe for evidence of fluid/electrolyte imbalance (eg, hyponatremia, hypochloremic alkalosis, hypokalemia). Hypokalemia may sensitize or exaggerate the response of the heart to toxic effects of digitalis. Hyperuricemia or precipitation of acute gout, hyperglycemia, manifestations of latent diabetes mellitus (DM), hypomagnesemia, hypercalcemia, and increases in cholesterol and TG levels may occur. Enhanced antihypertensive effects in postsympathectomy patients. Consider withholding or discontinuing therapy if progressive renal impairment becomes evident. D/C before testing for parathyroid function.

ADVERSE REACTIONS
Weakness, hypotension, pancreatitis, jaundice, diarrhea, aplastic anemia, agranulocytosis, anaphylactic reactions, muscle spasm, vertigo, paresthesia, renal failure, erythema multiforme, transient blurred vision, impotence.

DRUG INTERACTIONS
Potentiation of orthostatic hypotension may occur with alcohol, barbiturates, or narcotics. Dosage adjustment of antidiabetic drugs (oral agents and insulin) may be required. Additive effect or potentiation with other antihypertensives. Anionic exchange resins (eg, cholestyramine, colestipol) may impair absorption. Corticosteroids and adrenocorticotropic hormone may intensify electrolyte depletion, particularly hypokalemia. May decrease response to pressor amines (eg, norepinephrine). May increase responsiveness to nondepolarizing skeletal muscle relaxants (eg, tubocurarine). May increase risk of lithium toxicity; avoid concomitant use. NSAIDs may reduce diuretic, natriuretic, and antihypertensive effects.

PREGNANCY AND LACTATION
Category B, not for use in nursing.

MECHANISM OF ACTION
Thiazide diuretic; has not been established. Affects distal renal tubular mechanism of electrolyte reabsorption. Increases excretion of Na$^+$ and Cl$^-$ in approximately equivalent amounts.

PHARMACOKINETICS
Distribution: Crosses placenta; found in breast milk. **Elimination:** Kidney (≥61% unchanged); $T_{1/2}$=5.6-14.8 hrs.

PATIENT CONSIDERATIONS
Assessment: Assess for anuria, hypersensitivity to drug or sulfonamide-derived drugs, renal/hepatic impairment, history of allergy or bronchial asthma, SLE, DM, postsympathectomy status, pregnancy/nursing status, and possible drug interactions.

Monitoring: Monitor for signs/symptoms of fluid/electrolyte imbalance, sensitivity reactions, exacerbation/activation of SLE, idiosyncratic reaction, hyperuricemia or precipitation of acute gout, hyperglycemia, latent DM, increases in cholesterol and TG levels, and other adverse reactions. Monitor serum electrolytes.

Counseling: Inform of the risks and benefits of therapy. Advise to report to physician any adverse reactions.

Hypertension

Usual: 1-2mg/kg/day in single or 2 divided doses
Max:
<6 Months: 3mg/kg/day in 2 divided doses
Infants up to 2 Years: 37.5mg/day
2-12 Years: 100mg/day

Hydrocortisone – hydrocortisone   Rx

Class: Corticosteroid

OTHER BRAND NAMES
Anusol-HC Cream, Proctozone-HC,

ADULT DOSAGE
Inflammatory and Pruritic Manifestations of Corticosteroid-Responsive Dermatoses

Apply a thin film to the affected area bid-qid depending on the severity of the condition

PEDIATRIC DOSAGE
Inflammatory and Pruritic Manifestations of Corticosteroid-Responsive Dermatoses

Apply a thin film to the affected area bid-qid depending on the severity of the condition

Use least effective amount

ADMINISTRATION
Topical route

May use occlusive dressings for the management of psoriasis or recalcitrant conditions; d/c use of occlusive dressings and institute appropriate antimicrobial therapy if an infection develops.

Lot
Shake well before use.

STORAGE
Lot/Oint: 15-30°C (59-86°F). **Cre:** (Anusol) 20-25°C (68-77°F). Store away from heat. Protect from freezing. (Proctozone) 20-25°C (68-77°F); excursion permitted to 15-30°C (59-86°F).

HOW SUPPLIED
Cre: (Proctozone/Anusol) 2.5% [30g]; **Lot:** 2.5% [59mL]; **Oint:** 2.5% [28.35g, 453.6g]

CONTRAINDICATIONS
History of hypersensitivity to any of the components of the preparation.

WARNINGS/PRECAUTIONS
Systemic absorption may produce reversible hypothalamic-pituitary-adrenal (HPA) axis suppression, manifestations of Cushing's syndrome, hyperglycemia, and glucosuria. Application of more potent steroids, use over large surface areas, prolonged use, and the addition of occlusive dressings may augment systemic absorption. Periodically evaluate for evidence of HPA axis suppression when a large dose of a potent topical steroid is applied to a large surface area and under an occlusive dressing; if noted, withdraw treatment, reduce frequency of application, or substitute w/ a less potent steroid. Infrequently, signs/symptoms of steroid withdrawal may occur requiring supplemental systemic corticosteroids. D/C and institute appropriate therapy if irritation occurs. Use appropriate antifungal or antibacterial agent in the presence of dermatological infections; if favorable response does not occur promptly, d/c until infection is controlled. Children may be more susceptible to systemic toxicity. Chronic therapy may interfere w/ growth and development of children.

ADVERSE REACTIONS
Burning, itching, irritation, dryness, folliculitis, hypertrichosis, acneiform eruptions, hypopigmentation, perioral dermatitis, allergic contact dermatitis, maceration of the skin, secondary infection, skin atrophy, striae, miliaria.

PREGNANCY AND LACTATION
Pregnancy: Category C.
Lactation: Caution in nursing.

MECHANISM OF ACTION
Corticosteroid; possesses anti-inflammatory, antipruritic, and vasoconstrictive actions. Mechanism of anti-inflammatory activity is unclear.

PHARMACOKINETICS
Absorption: Extent of percutaneous absorption is determined by many factors (eg, vehicle, integrity of epidermal barrier, use of occlusive dressings). **Distribution:** Bound to plasma proteins in varying degrees; found in breast milk (systemically administered). **Metabolism:** Liver. **Elimination:** Kidneys, bile.

PATIENT CONSIDERATIONS
Assessment: Assess for previous hypersensitivity to any of the components of the drug, dermatological infections, conditions that augment systemic absorption, and pregnancy/nursing status.

Monitoring: Monitor for signs/symptoms of reversible HPA axis suppression, Cushing's syndrome, hyperglycemia, glucosuria, skin irritation, systemic toxicity in children, hypersensitivity reactions, steroid withdrawal, and other adverse reactions. When a large dose is applied to a large surface area or under occlusive dressings, monitor for HPA axis suppression by using urinary free cortisol and adrenocorticotropic hormone stimulation tests.

Counseling: Instruct to use externally ud and to avoid contact w/ eyes. Advise not to use for any disorder other than for which it was prescribed. Instruct not to bandage, cover, or wrap treated skin area, unless directed by physician. Advise to report any signs of local adverse reactions, especially under occlusive dressing. Instruct not to use tight-fitting diapers or plastic pants on a child being treated in the diaper area, as these garments may constitute occlusive dressings.

HYDROMET — homatropine methylbromide/hydrocodone bitartrate
CII

Class: Opioid antitussive

OTHER BRAND NAMES
Tussigon

ADULT DOSAGE	PEDIATRIC DOSAGE
Cough	**Cough**
Hydromet:	**6-12 Years:**
1 tsp (5mL) q4-6h prn	**Hydromet:**
Max: 6 tsp (30mL)/24 hrs	1/2 tsp (2.5mL) q4-6h prn
	Max: 3 tsp (15mL)/24 hrs
Tussigon:	**Tussigon:**
1 tab q4-6h prn	1/2 tab q4-6h prn
Max: 6 tabs/24 hrs	**Max:** 3 tabs/24 hrs

ADMINISTRATION
Oral route

STORAGE
15-30°C (59-86°F).

HOW SUPPLIED
(Hydrocodone/Homatropine) Syrup: (Hydromet) (5mg/1.5mg)/5mL [473mL]; **Tab:** (Tussigon) 5mg/1.5mg* *scored

CONTRAINDICATIONS
Hypersensitivity to hydrocodone or homatropine methylbromide.

WARNINGS/PRECAUTIONS
May be habit forming and has potential for abuse. Psychic/physical dependence and tolerance may develop upon repeated administration; use w/ caution. May produce dose-related respiratory depression; may be antagonized by the use of naloxone HCl and other supportive measures when indicated. Respiratory depression effects and the capacity to elevate CSF pressure may be markedly exaggerated in the presence of head injury, other intracranial lesions, or preexisting increased intracranial pressure (ICP). May obscure clinical course of head injuries and acute abdominal conditions. Carefully consider benefit to risk ratio, especially in pediatric patients w/ respiratory embarrassment (eg, croup). Before prescribing medication to suppress/modify cough, it is important to ascertain the underlying cause of cough, that the modification of cough does not increase the risk of clinical or physiological complications, and that appropriate therapy for the primary disease is provided. Caution in elderly, debilitated, severe hepatic/renal impairment, hypothyroidism, Addison's disease, prostatic hypertrophy or urethral stricture, asthma, and narrow-angle glaucoma.

ADVERSE REACTIONS
Sedation, drowsiness, lethargy, mental/physical impairment, anxiety, fear, dizziness, psychic dependence, N/V, ureteral spasm, urinary retention, respiratory depression, skin rash, pruritus.

DRUG INTERACTIONS
May exhibit additive CNS depression w/ other narcotics, antihistamines, antipsychotics, antianxiety agents, or other CNS depressants (including alcohol); reduce dose of 1 or both agents. May increase effects of either antidepressants or hydrocodone w/ MAOIs or TCAs.

PREGNANCY AND LACTATION
Pregnancy: Category C.
Lactation: Not for use in nursing.

MECHANISM OF ACTION
Hydrocodone: Narcotic antitussive and analgesic; has not been established, but believed to act directly on the cough center.

PHARMACOKINETICS
Absorption: Hydrocodone: C_{max}=23.6ng/mL, T_{max}=1.3 hrs. **Metabolism:** Hydrocodone: O-demethylation, N-demethylation, and 6-keto reduction; 6-α- and 6-β-hydroxymetabolites (metabolites). **Elimination:** Hydrocodone: $T_{1/2}$=3.8 hrs.

PATIENT CONSIDERATIONS
Assessment: Assess for drug hypersensitivity, cough cause, head injury, intracranial lesions, preexisting increased ICP, acute abdominal conditions, respiratory embarrassment in pediatric patients, presence of debilitation, hepatic/renal impairment, hypothyroidism, Addison's disease, prostatic hypertrophy or urethral stricture, asthma, narrow-angle glaucoma, pregnancy/nursing status, and possible drug interactions.

Monitoring: Monitor for drug abuse/dependence, respiratory depression, and other adverse reactions.

Counseling: Inform about risks and benefits of therapy. Advise to take caution w/ hazardous activities (eg, operating machinery/driving); inform that medication may impair mental and physical abilities.

HYDROXYZINE HCL — hydroxyzine hydrochloride
Rx

Class: Piperazine antihistamine

OTHER BRAND NAMES
Vistaril Injection (Discontinued)

ADULT DOSAGE	PEDIATRIC DOSAGE
Pruritus	**Pruritus**
Management of pruritus due to allergic conditions (eg, chronic urticaria, atopic/contact dermatoses) and histamine-mediated pruritus	Management of pruritus due to allergic conditions (eg, chronic urticaria, atopic/contact dermatoses) and histamine-mediated pruritus
Syrup/Tab:	**Syrup/Tab:**
25mg tid or qid	**<6 Years:**
	50mg/day in divided doses
Sedation	**>6 Years:**
As premedication and following general anesthesia	50-100mg/day in divided doses
Syrup/Tab:	**Sedation**
50-100mg	As premedication and following general anesthesia
Nausea/Vomiting	**Syrup/Tab:**
Excluding N/V of pregnancy	0.6mg/kg
IM:	**Nausea/Vomiting**
25-100mg	Excluding N/V of pregnancy
Surgery	**IM:**
As pre- and postoperative adjunctive medication to permit reduction in narcotic dosage, allay anxiety, and control emesis	0.5mg/lb
IM:	**Surgery**
25-100mg	As pre- and postoperative adjunctive medication to permit reduction in narcotic dosage, allay anxiety, and control emesis

Anxiety

Syrup/Tab:
Symptomatic relief of anxiety and tension associated w/ psychoneurosis and as an adjunct in organic disease states

50-100mg qid

IM:
Management of anxiety, tension, and psychomotor agitation in conditions of emotional stress. Useful in alleviating manifestations of anxiety/tension as in the preparation for dental procedures and in acute emotional problems. Management of anxiety associated w/ organic disturbances and as adjunctive therapy in alcoholism and allergic conditions w/ strong emotional overlay (eg, asthma, chronic urticaria, pruritus). Treatment of acutely disturbed or hysterical patient and acute/chronic alcoholic w/ anxiety withdrawal symptoms or delirium tremens

50-100mg immediately, and q4-6h prn

Pregnancy

As pre- and postpartum adjunctive medication to permit reduction in narcotic dosage, allay anxiety, and control emesis

IM:
25-100mg

IM:
0.5mg/lb

Anxiety

Symptomatic relief of anxiety and tension associated w/ psychoneurosis and as an adjunct in organic disease states

Syrup/Tab:

<6 Years:
50mg/day in divided doses

>6 Years:
50-100mg/day in divided doses

DOSING CONSIDERATIONS

Elderly
Start at lower end of dosing range

ADMINISTRATION
Oral/IM route

Adjust dose according to response.
When treatment is initiated by IM route, subsequent doses may be administered orally.

IM
May be administered w/o further dilution.
Inject well w/in the body of a relatively large muscle; preferred site in adults is the upper outer quadrant of the buttock or midlateral thigh and in children is the midlateral thigh.

STORAGE
20-25°C (68-77°F). **Inj:** Excursions permitted to 15-30°C (59-86°F). **Syrup:** Protect from freezing. **Inj/Syrup:** Protect from light.

HOW SUPPLIED
Inj: 25mg/mL [1mL], 50mg/mL [1mL, 2mL, 10mL]; **Syrup:** 10mg/5mL [118mL, 473mL]; **Tab:** 10mg, 25mg, 50mg

CONTRAINDICATIONS
Prolonged QT interval, known hypersensitivity to hydroxyzine HCl, early pregnancy. **Inj:** SQ, intra-arterial, or IV administration. **Syrup/Tab:** Known hypersensitivity to cetirizine or levocetirizine.

WARNINGS/PRECAUTIONS
Patients may be started on IM therapy when indicated and should be maintained on oral therapy whenever this route is practicable. QT prolongation and torsades de pointes reported; caution in patients w/ risk factors for QT prolongation, congenital long QT syndrome, a family history of long QT syndrome, other conditions that predispose to QT prolongation, ventricular arrhythmia, recent MI, uncompensated heart failure, and bradyarrhythmias. Drowsiness may occur. May impair mental/physical abilities. Caution in elderly. **Inj:** Should not be used as sole treatment of psychosis or for clearly demonstrated cases of depression. Inadvertent SQ inj may result in significant tissue damage. IM inj may result in severe inj-site reactions requiring surgical intervention. Inj into the deltoid area should be used only if well developed (eg, certain adults and older children), and then only w/ caution to avoid radial nerve injury. In infants and small children, inj into the periphery of the upper outer quadrant of the gluteal region should be used only when necessary, in order to minimize the possibility of damage to the sciatic nerve. IM inj in children should not be made into the lower and mid-third of the upper arm.

ADVERSE REACTIONS
Dry mouth, drowsiness, involuntary motor activity.

DRUG INTERACTIONS
May potentiate CNS depressants (eg, narcotics, non-narcotic analgesics and barbiturates, alcohol); reduce dose of CNS depressants when administered concomitantly. Modify use of meperidine and barbiturates, on an individual basis, when used in preanesthetic adjunctive therapy. Caution during the concomitant use of drugs known to prolong the QT interval (eg, quinidine, amiodarone, sotalol, ziprasidone, clozapine, quetiapine, chlorpromazine, fluoxetine, azithromycin, erythromycin, moxifloxacin, pentamidine, methadone, ondansetron, droperidol).

Inj: Cardiac arrests and death reported when combined w/ other CNS depressants. Administration of meperidine may result in severe hypotension in the postoperative patient or any individual whose ability to maintain BP has been compromised by a depleted blood volume. Use meperidine w/ great caution and in reduced dosage in patients who are receiving other pre- and/or postoperative medications and in whom there is a risk of respiratory depression, hypotension, and profound sedation or coma occurring.

PREGNANCY AND LACTATION
Pregnancy: Contraindicated in early pregnancy.
Lactation: (Syrup/Tab) Not for use in nursing; (Inj) Safety not known in nursing.

MECHANISM OF ACTION
Piperazine antihistamine; believed to suppress activity in certain key regions of the subcortical area of the CNS and shown to have primary skeletal muscle relaxation and antihistaminic effects. (PO) Shown to have bronchodilator activity and analgesic effects. (Inj) Shown to have antispasmodic and antiemetic effects.

PHARMACOKINETICS
Absorption: (PO) Rapid.

PATIENT CONSIDERATIONS
Assessment: Assess for hypersensitivity to drug, QT prolongation, risk factors for QT prolongation, pregnancy/nursing status, and for possible drug interactions. (Syrup/Tab) Assess for hypersensitivity to cetirizine or levocetirizine.

Monitoring: Monitor for hypersensitivity reactions, QT prolongation, torsades de pointes, drowsiness, and other adverse reactions. Periodically reassess the usefulness of therapy.

Counseling: Inform about risks/benefits of therapy. Inform that drowsiness may occur; instruct to use caution when driving or operating heavy machinery. Instruct to notify physician if pregnant, nursing, or taking any other concomitant therapy.

HYDROXYZINE PAMOATE — hydroxyzine pamoate   Rx
Class: Piperazine antihistamine

OTHER BRAND NAMES
Vistaril

ADULT DOSAGE

Anxiety
Symptomatic relief of anxiety and tension associated w/ psychoneurosis and as an adjunct in organic disease states

50-100mg qid

Pruritus
Management of pruritus due to allergic conditions (eg, chronic urticaria, atopic/contact dermatoses) and in histamine-mediated pruritus

25mg tid or qid

Sedation
As premedication and following general anesthesia

50-100mg

PEDIATRIC DOSAGE

Anxiety
Symptomatic relief of anxiety and tension associated w/ psychoneurosis and as an adjunct in organic disease states

<6 Years:
50mg/day in divided doses
>6 Years:
50-100mg/day in divided doses

Pruritus
Management of pruritus due to allergic conditions (eg, chronic urticaria, atopic/contact dermatoses) and in histamine-mediated pruritus

<6 Years:
50mg/day in divided doses
>6 Years:
50-100mg/day in divided doses

Sedation
As premedication and following general anesthesia

0.6mg/kg

DOSING CONSIDERATIONS
Elderly
Start at lower end of dosing range

ADMINISTRATION
Oral route

When treatment is initiated by IM route, subsequent doses may be administered orally.

Sus
Shake vigorously until completely resuspended.

STORAGE
20-25°C (68-77°F). **Vistaril:** <30°C (86°F).

HOW SUPPLIED
Cap: 100mg, (Vistaril) 25mg, 50mg; **Sus:** (Vistaril) 25mg/5mL [120mL, 473mL]

CONTRAINDICATIONS
Early pregnancy. In patients w/ a prolonged QT interval. Previous hypersensitivity to any component of the medication.

WARNINGS/PRECAUTIONS
Drowsiness may occur. May impair mental/physical abilities. Cases of QT prolongation and torsades de pointes reported; caution in patients w/ risk factors for QT prolongation, congenital long QT syndrome, family history of long QT syndrome, other conditions that predispose to QT prolongation and ventricular arrhythmia, recent MI, uncompensated heart failure, and bradyarrhythmias. Caution in elderly.

ADVERSE REACTIONS
Dry mouth, drowsiness, headache, hallucination, pruritus, rash, urticaria.

DRUG INTERACTIONS
May potentiate CNS depressants (eg, narcotics, non-narcotic analgesics, barbiturates, alcohol); reduce dose of CNS depressants when administered concomitantly. Modify use of meperidine and barbiturates, on an individualized basis, when used in preanesthetic adjunctive therapy. Caution w/ drugs known to prolong the QT interval, including Class IA (eg, quinidine, procainamide) or Class III (eg, amiodarone, sotalol) antiarrhythmics, certain antipsychotics (eg, ziprasidone, iloperidone, chlorpromazine), certain antidepressants (eg, citalopram, fluoxetine), certain antibiotics (eg, azithromycin, gatifloxacin, moxifloxacin), and others (eg, pentamidine, methadone, ondansetron).

PREGNANCY AND LACTATION
Pregnancy: Contraindicated in early pregnancy.
Lactation: Not for use in nursing.

MECHANISM OF ACTION
Piperazine antihistamine; believed to suppress activity in certain key regions of the subcortical area of the CNS and shown to have primary skeletal muscle relaxation, bronchodilator activity, antihistaminic, antiemetic, and analgesic effects.

PHARMACOKINETICS
Absorption: Rapid.

PATIENT CONSIDERATIONS
Assessment: Assess for hypersensitivity to the drug, QT prolongation or risk factors for QT prolongation and torsades de pointes, pregnancy/nursing status, and possible drug interactions.

Monitoring: Monitor for drowsiness, QT prolongation, torsades de pointes, and other adverse reactions. Periodically reassess the usefulness of therapy.

Counseling: Inform about risks/benefits of therapy. Caution that the effect of alcohol may be increased. Advise that drowsiness may occur; caution against driving a car or operating heavy machinery. Instruct to notify physician if pregnant, nursing, or if taking any other concomitant therapy.

HYOSYNE — hyoscyamine sulfate   Rx
Class: Anticholinergic

ADULT DOSAGE
General Dosing
Elixir:
1-2 tsp q4h or prn
Max: 12 tsp/24 hrs

Sol:
1-2mL q4h or prn
Max: 12mL/24 hrs

Other Indications
Adjunctive therapy in the treatment of peptic ulcer, irritable bowel syndrome (irritable colon, spastic colon, mucous colitis), functional GI disorders, neurogenic bladder, neurogenic bowel disturbances (eg, splenic flexure syndrome, neurogenic colon)

To control gastric secretion, visceral spasm and hypermotility in spastic colitis, spastic bladder, cystitis, pylorospasm, and associated abdominal cramps

To reduce symptoms (eg, those seen in mild dysenteries, diverticulitis, and acute enterocolitis) in functional intestinal disorders

Treatment of infant colic

Along w/ morphine or other narcotics in symptomatic relief of biliary and renal colic

As a "drying agent" in the relief of symptoms of acute rhinitis

To reduce rigidity and tremors and to control associated sialorrhea and hyperhidrosis in the therapy of parkinsonism

May be used in the therapy of poisoning by anticholinesterase agents

PEDIATRIC DOSAGE
General Dosing
Sol:
<2 Years:
3.4kg:
Usual: 4 drops q4h or prn
Max: 24 drops/24 hrs

5kg:
Usual: 5 drops q4h or prn
Max: 30 drops/24 hrs

7kg:
Usual: 6 drops q4h or prn
Max: 36 drops/24 hrs

10kg:
Usual: 8 drops q4h or prn
Max: 48 drops/24 hrs

2-<12 Years:
1/4-1mL q4h or prn
Max: 6mL/24 hrs

≥12 Years:
1-2mL q4h or prn
Max: 12mL/24 hrs

Elixir:
2-<12 Years:
10kg:
Usual: 1/4 tsp (1.25mL) q4h or prn
Max: 6 tsp/24 hrs

20kg:
Usual: 1/2 tsp (2.5mL) q4h or prn
Max: 6 tsp/24 hrs

40kg:
Usual: 3/4 tsp (3.75mL) q4h or prn
Max: 6 tsp/24 hrs

50kg:
Usual: 1 tsp (5mL) q4h or prn
Max: 6 tsp/24 hrs

≥12 Years:
1-2 tsp q4h or prn
Max: 12 tsp/24 hrs

Other Indications
Adjunctive therapy in the treatment of peptic ulcer, irritable bowel syndrome (irritable colon, spastic colon, mucous colitis), functional GI disorders, neurogenic bladder, neurogenic bowel disturbances (eg, splenic flexure syndrome, neurogenic colon)

To control gastric secretion, visceral spasm and hypermotility in spastic colitis, spastic bladder, cystitis, pylorospasm, and associated abdominal cramps

To reduce symptoms (eg, those seen in mild dysenteries, diverticulitis, and acute enterocolitis) in functional intestinal disorders

Treatment of infant colic

Along w/ morphine or other narcotics in symptomatic relief of biliary and renal colic

As a "drying agent" in the relief of symptoms of acute rhinitis

To reduce rigidity and tremors and to control associated sialorrhea and hyperhidrosis in the therapy of parkinsonism

May be used in the therapy of poisoning by anticholinesterase agents

---

DOSING CONSIDERATIONS
Elderly
Start at lower end of dosing range

ADMINISTRATION
Oral route
Sol
Refer to PI for approximate equivalent amount of drops (mL) to mg

STORAGE
20-25°C (68-77°F); excursions permitted to 15-30°C (59-86°F).

HOW SUPPLIED
Elixir: 0.125mg/5mL [473mL]; **Sol:** 0.125mg/mL [15mL]

CONTRAINDICATIONS
Glaucoma, obstructive uropathy (eg, bladder neck obstruction due to prostatic hypertrophy), obstructive GI tract disease (achalasia, pyloroduodenal stenosis), paralytic ileus, intestinal atony of elderly/debilitated, unstable cardiovascular status in acute hemorrhage, severe ulcerative colitis, toxic megacolon complicating ulcerative colitis, myasthenia gravis.

WARNINGS/PRECAUTIONS
Heat prostration can occur with high environmental temperature. Diarrhea may be an early symptom of incomplete intestinal obstruction, especially with ileostomy or colostomy; treatment would be inappropriate and possibly harmful. May impair physical/mental abilities. Psychosis reported in sensitive patients. Caution with autonomic neuropathy, hyperthyroidism, coronary heart disease, congestive heart failure, cardiac arrhythmias, HTN, renal disease, and hiatal hernia associated with reflux esophagitis. May increase HR; investigate any tachycardia prior to initiation. Caution in elderly.

ADVERSE REACTIONS
Dry mouth, urinary hesitancy, blurred vision, tachycardia, palpitations, mydriasis, increased ocular tension, loss of taste, headache, nervousness, drowsiness, weakness, fatigue, dizziness, N/V.

DRUG INTERACTIONS
Additive adverse effects resulting from cholinergic blockade may occur with other antimuscarinics, amantadine, haloperidol, phenothiazines, MAOIs, TCAs, or some antihistamines. Antacids may interfere with absorption; administer hyoscyamine ac and antacids pc.

PREGNANCY AND LACTATION
Category C, caution in nursing.

MECHANISM OF ACTION
Belladonna alkaloid; inhibits action of acetylcholine on structures innervated by postganglionic cholinergic nerves and on smooth muscles that respond to acetylcholine but lack cholinergic innervation, inhibiting GI propulsive motility, decreasing gastric acid secretion, and controlling excess pharyngeal, tracheal, and bronchial secretions.

PHARMACOKINETICS
Absorption: Complete. **Distribution:** Crosses placenta; found in breast milk. **Metabolism:** Partial hydrolysis; tropic acid, tropine (metabolites). **Elimination:** Urine (unchanged); $T_{1/2}$=2-3.5 hrs.

PATIENT CONSIDERATIONS
Assessment: Assess for diarrhea, ileostomy, colostomy, sensitivity towards anticholinergic drugs, tachycardia, pregnancy/nursing status, possible drug interactions, and any other conditions where treatment is contraindicated or cautioned.

Monitoring: Monitor for signs/symptoms of heat prostration, incomplete intestinal obstruction, blurred vision, psychosis, CNS events, diarrhea, and other adverse reactions. Monitor renal function particularly in elderly.

Counseling: If drowsiness, dizziness, or blurring of vision occurs, warn patients not to engage in activities requiring mental alertness (eg, operating a motor vehicle or other machinery) and not to perform hazardous work. Inform that treatment may decrease sweating resulting in heat prostration, fever, or heat stroke; advise to use caution if febrile or exposed to elevated environmental temperatures.

HYSINGLA ER — hydrocodone bitartrate   CII

Class: Opioid analgesic

> Exposes users to risks of addiction, abuse, and misuse, which can lead to overdose and death; assess each patient's risk prior to prescribing, and monitor regularly for development of these behaviors/conditions. Serious, life-threatening, or fatal respiratory depression may occur; monitor for respiratory depression, especially during initiation or following a dose increase. Swallow tab whole; crushing, chewing, or dissolving tab can cause rapid release and absorption of a potentially fatal dose. Accidental ingestion of even 1 dose, especially by children, can result in a fatal overdose. Prolonged use during pregnancy can result in neonatal opioid withdrawal syndrome, which may be life threatening if not recognized and treated, and requires management according to protocols developed by neonatology experts; advise pregnant women of the risk and ensure availability of appropriate treatment. Concomitant use w/ all CYP3A4 inhibitors may result in an increase in plasma concentrations, which could increase or prolong adverse drug effects and may cause potentially fatal respiratory depression. Discontinuation of a concomitantly used CYP3A4 inducer may result in an increase in plasma concentrations. Monitor patients receiving concomitant therapy w/ any CYP3A4 inhibitor or inducer.

ADULT DOSAGE

Chronic Pain

Management of Pain Severe Enough to Require Daily, Around-the-Clock, Long-Term Opioid Treatment and for Which Alternative Treatment Options are Inadequate:

Initial Dosing:
1st Opioid Analgesic/Opioid Intolerant: 20mg q24h

Titration and Maint of Therapy:
Adjust in increments of 10-20mg every 3-5 days prn.
Patients who experience breakthrough pain may require a dose increase, or may need rescue medication w/ an appropriate dose of an immediate-release analgesic. If level of pain increases after dose stabilization, attempt to identify source of increased pain before increasing dose.

If unacceptable opioid-related adverse reactions are observed, next daily dose may be reduced.

Daily doses ≥80mg are only for use in opioid-tolerant patients

Conversions

Initial Dosing:
From Oral Hydrocodone Formulations:
Administer patient's total daily oral hydrocodone dose as extended-release hydrocodone qd

From Other Oral Opioids:
D/C all other around-the-clock opioids when extended-release hydrocodone is initiated

Conversion Factors from Other Oral Opioids (Previous Oral Opioid: Approximate Oral Conversion Factor):
Codeine 133mg: 0.15
Hydromorphone 5mg: 4
Methadone 13.3mg: 1.5
Morphine 40mg: 0.5
Oxycodone 20mg: 1
Oxymorphone 10mg: 2
Tramadol 200mg: 0.1

Calculation of Estimated Total Hydrocodone Daily Dose:
On Single Opioid: Sum current total daily dose of opioid, then multiply the total daily dose by the approximate oral conversion factor
On >1 Opioid: Calculate approximate oral hydrocodone dose for each opioid and sum the totals to obtain the approximate oral hydrocodone daily dose
On Fixed-Ratio Opioid/Nonopioid Analgesic Products: Use only the opioid component of these products in the conversion.
Reduce calculated daily oral hydrocodone dose by 25%

From Methadone:
Close monitoring is of particular importance. Ratio between methadone and other opioid agonists

PEDIATRIC DOSAGE

Pediatric use may not have been established

---

may vary widely as a function of previous dose exposure. Methadone has a long $T_{1/2}$ and can accumulate in the plasma

From Transdermal Fentanyl:
May initiate 18 hrs following removal of patch; for each 25mcg/hr fentanyl transdermal patch, a dose of 20mg q24h represents a conservative initial dose

From Transdermal Buprenorphine:
All patients receiving transdermal buprenorphine (≤20mcg/hr) should initiate w/ 20mg q24h

Refer to PI for further conversion information

DOSING CONSIDERATIONS

Renal Impairment
Moderate to Severe Impairment and ESRD:
Initial: 1/2 initial dose and monitor closely for respiratory depression and sedation

Hepatic Impairment
Severe Impairment:
Initial: 1/2 initial dose and monitor closely for respiratory depression and sedation

Elderly
Start on low doses and monitor closely for adverse events (eg, respiratory depression, sedation, confusion)

Discontinuation
Gradually reduce dose every 2-4 days; next dose should be at least 50% of the prior dose
After reaching 20mg dose for 2-4 days, may d/c

ADMINISTRATION

Oral route

Take whole, w/ enough water to ensure complete swallowing immediately after placing in the mouth.
Do not crush, chew, or dissolve.
Do not pre-soak, lick or otherwise wet tab prior to placing in mouth.

STORAGE
25°C (77°F); excursions permitted between 15-30°C (59-86°F).

HOW SUPPLIED
Tab, Extended-Release: 20mg, 30mg, 40mg, 60mg, 80mg, 100mg, 120mg

CONTRAINDICATIONS
Significant respiratory depression, acute or severe bronchial asthma in an unmonitored setting or in the absence of resuscitative equipment, known/suspected paralytic ileus and GI obstruction, hypersensitivity to any component of this medication or the active ingredient, hydrocodone bitartrate.

WARNINGS/PRECAUTIONS
Reserve for use in patients for whom alternative treatment options are ineffective, not tolerated, or would be otherwise inadequate to provide sufficient management of pain. Should be prescribed only by healthcare professionals knowledgeable in the use of potent opioids for the management of chronic pain. Overestimating the dose when converting from another opioid product may result in fatal overdose w/ the 1st dose. Life-threatening respiratory depression is more likely to occur in elderly, cachectic, or debilitated patients. Consider alternative nonopioid analgesics in patients w/ significant COPD or cor pulmonale, and in patients having a substantially decreased respiratory reserve, hypoxia, hypercapnia, or preexisting respiratory depression. Respiratory depressant effects and elevation of CSF pressure (resulting from vasodilation following carbon dioxide retention) may be markedly exaggerated in the presence of head injury, intracranial lesions, or preexisting increase in intracranial pressure (ICP). May produce effects on pupillary response and consciousness, which can obscure neurologic signs of further increases in ICP in patients w/ head injuries. Monitor patients closely who may be susceptible to intracranial effects of carbon dioxide retention. May obscure clinical course of a patient w/ a head injury. Avoid w/ impaired consciousness, coma, or circulatory shock. May cause severe hypotension, including orthostatic hypotension and syncope in ambulatory patients; increased risk in patients whose ability to maintain BP has been compromised by depleted blood volume, or after concurrent administration w/ drugs such as phenothiazines or other agents that compromise vasomotor tone. Esophageal obstruction, dysphagia, and choking reported; consider use of an alternative analgesic in patients who have difficulty swallowing and patients at risk for underlying GI disorders resulting in a small GI lumen. Diminishes propulsive peristaltic waves in the GI tract and decreases bowel motility. May obscure diagnosis or clinical course in patients w/ acute abdominal conditions. May cause spasm of the sphincter of Oddi; monitor patients w/ biliary tract disease, including acute pancreatitis. May impair mental/physical abilities. QTc prolongation reported following daily doses of 160mg; consider this in making clinical decisions regarding patient monitoring when prescribing in patients w/ CHF, bradyarrhythmias, electrolyte abnormalities, or who are taking medications that are known to prolong the QTc interval. Avoid in patients w/ congenital long QT syndrome; consider reducing dose by 33-50% or changing to an alternate analgesic in patients who develop QTc prolongation. Caution w/ severe hepatic impairment, moderate or severe renal impairment or ESRD, and in elderly.

ADVERSE REACTIONS
Respiratory depression, constipation, N/V, fatigue, URTI, dizziness, headache, somnolence, pruritus, insomnia, influenza.

DRUG INTERACTIONS

See Boxed Warning. Caution when initiating treatment in patients currently taking, or discontinuing, CYP3A4 inhibitors or inducers; evaluate at frequent intervals and consider dose adjustments until stable drug effects are achieved. Concomitant use w/ alcohol or other CNS depressants (eg, sedatives, hypnotics, tranquilizers, general anesthetics, phenothiazines, other opioids) may increase the risk of respiratory depression, profound sedation, coma, and death; if coadministration is considered, reduce dose of 1 or both agents. Monitor use in elderly, cachectic, and debilitated patients when given concomitantly w/ other drugs that depress respiration. Mixed agonist/antagonist (eg, pentazocine, nalbuphine, butorphanol) and partial agonist (buprenorphine) analgesics may reduce analgesic effect or precipitate withdrawal symptoms; avoid use. Severe and unpredictable potentiation by MAOIs reported; not recommended for use in patients who have received MAOIs w/in 14 days. Anticholinergics or other drugs w/ anticholinergic activity may increase the risk of urinary retention or severe constipation, which may lead to paralytic ileus; monitor for signs of urinary retention and constipation in addition to respiratory and CNS depression when used concurrently. Strong laxatives (eg, lactulose) that rapidly increase GI motility may decrease hydrocodone absorption and result in decreased plasma levels; closely monitor for development of adverse events and changing analgesic requirements.

PREGNANCY AND LACTATION

Category C, not for use in nursing.

MECHANISM OF ACTION

Opioid analgesic; semi-synthetic opioid agonist w/ relative selectivity for the μ-opioid receptor, although it can interact w/ other opioid receptors at higher doses. Acts as an agonist binding to and activating opioid receptors in the brain and spinal cord, which are coupled to G-protein complexes and modulate synaptic transmission through adenylate cyclase.

PHARMACOKINETICS

Absorption: T_{max}=14-16 hrs (median). Administration of variable doses resulted in different pharmacokinetic parameters. **Distribution:** Plasma protein binding (36%); V_d=402L; crosses placenta; found in breast milk. **Metabolism:** N-demethylation (CYP3A4, CYP2B6, CYP2C19), O-demethylation (CYP2D6, CYP2B6, CYP2C19), and 6-keto reduction; hydromorphone (metabolite). **Elimination:** Urine (6.5% unchanged); $T_{1/2}$=7-9 hrs.

PATIENT CONSIDERATIONS

Assessment: Assess for abuse/addiction risk, pain type/severity, prior opioid therapy, opioid tolerance, respiratory depression, COPD or other respiratory complications, head injury, paralytic ileus, drug hypersensitivity, pregnancy/nursing status, possible drug interactions, and any other conditions where treatment is contraindicated or cautioned.

Monitoring: Monitor for respiratory depression (especially w/in the first 24-72 hrs of initiating therapy), hypotension, decreased bowel motility in postoperative patients, QTc prolongation, and other adverse reactions. Monitor for development of addiction, abuse, or misuse. Periodically reassess the continued need for therapy.

Counseling: Inform that use of drug can result in addiction, abuse, and misuse; instruct not to share w/ others and to take steps to protect from theft or misuse. Inform of the risk of life-threatening respiratory depression; advise how to recognize respiratory depression and to seek medical attention if experiencing breathing difficulties. Inform that accidental exposure, especially in children, may result in respiratory depression or death. Advise to store securely and to dispose of unused tabs in accordance w/ local state guidelines and/or regulations. Inform female patients of reproductive potential that use during pregnancy may cause fetal harm; instruct to notify physician if pregnant/planning to become pregnant. Inform that potentially serious additive effects may occur if used w/ alcohol or other CNS depressants, and not to use such drugs unless supervised by a healthcare provider. Instruct how to properly take the drug. Inform that drug may cause orthostatic hypotension and syncope; instruct how to recognize symptoms of low BP and how to reduce risk of serious consequences should hypotension occur. Inform that drug may impair the ability to perform potentially hazardous activities; advise not to perform such tasks until patients know how they will react to the medication. Advise of potential for severe constipation, including management instructions and when to seek medical attention; instruct to monitor analgesic response following the use of strong laxatives and to contact the prescriber if changes are noted. Instruct patients w/ a history of CHF or bradyarrhythmias, and patients at risk for electrolyte abnormalities or who are taking other medications known to prolong QT interval that periodic monitoring of ECGs and electrolytes may be necessary during therapy. Advise how to recognize anaphylaxis and when to seek medical attention.

HYZAAR — hydrochlorothiazide/losartan potassium   Rx

Class: Angiotensin II receptor blocker (ARB)/thiazide diuretic

> D/C when pregnancy is detected. Drugs that act directly on the renin-angiotensin system (RAS) can cause injury/death to the developing fetus.

ADULT DOSAGE

Hypertension

Initial: 50mg/12.5mg qd
Titrate: May increase after 3 weeks
Max: 100mg/25mg qd

BP Not Adequately Controlled w/ Losartan 50mg Monotherapy:
Initial: 50mg/12.5mg qd

Titrate: May increase after 3 weeks to 100mg/25mg qd

BP Not Adequately Controlled w/ Losartan 100mg Monotherapy:
Initial: 100mg/12.5mg qd
Titrate: May increase after 3 weeks to 100mg/25mg qd

BP Not Adequately Controlled w/ Hydrochlorothiazide (HCTZ) 25mg QD/Hypokalemia Develops w/ HCTZ 25mg QD:
Initial: 50mg/12.5mg qd
Titrate: May increase after 3 weeks to 100mg/25mg qd

Hypertension with Left Ventricular Hypertrophy

Reduction in Risk of Stroke:
Initial (BP Uncontrolled on Losartan 50mg QD): 50mg/12.5mg
Titrate: Increase to 100mg/12.5mg, followed by 100mg/25mg; add other antihypertensives for further reduction

This benefit may not apply to black patients

PEDIATRIC DOSAGE

Pediatric use may not have been established

DOSING CONSIDERATIONS

Renal Impairment
Consider withholding or discontinuing therapy in patients who develop a clinically significant decrease in renal function

ADMINISTRATION

Oral route

STORAGE

25°C (77°F); excursions permitted to 15-30°C (59-86°F). Protect from light.

HOW SUPPLIED

Tab: (Losartan/HCTZ) 50mg/12.5mg, 100mg/12.5mg, 100mg/25mg

CONTRAINDICATIONS

Hypersensitivity to any component, anuria, coadministration w/ aliskiren in patients w/ diabetes.

WARNINGS/PRECAUTIONS

Not indicated for initial therapy of HTN except when HTN is severe enough that the value of achieving prompt BP control exceeds the risk of initiating combination therapy. Symptomatic hypotension may occur in patients w/ an activated RAS (eg, volume- or salt-depleted patients); do not use as initial therapy in patients w/ intravascular volume depletion. Correct volume or salt depletion prior to administration of therapy. Patients whose renal function may depend in part on the activity of the RAS may be at risk of developing acute renal failure; monitor renal function periodically. Can cause hypokalemia, hyponatremia, and hypomagnesemia; monitor serum electrolytes periodically. The antihypertensive effects of the drug may be enhanced in the postsympathectomy patient. Initiation not recommended for patients w/ hepatic impairment. **HCTZ:** Hypersensitivity reactions may occur; more likely to occur in patients w/ history of allergy or bronchial asthma. May alter glucose tolerance and raise serum levels of cholesterol and TGs. Decreases urinary calcium excretion and may cause elevations of serum calcium; monitor calcium levels. May cause idiosyncratic reaction, resulting in acute transient myopia and acute angle-closure glaucoma; d/c as rapidly as possible. May cause exacerbation or activation of systemic lupus erythematosus (SLE). May cause hyperuricemia or frank gout may be precipitated.

ADVERSE REACTIONS

Dizziness, URI, cough, back pain.

DRUG INTERACTIONS

See Contraindications. Increases in serum lithium concentrations and lithium toxicity reported; monitor serum lithium levels during concomitant use. NSAIDs, including selective COX-2 inhibitors, may decrease effects of diuretics and ARBs and may deteriorate renal function (possible acute renal failure). Avoid w/ aliskiren in patients w/ renal impairment (GFR <60mL/min). **Losartan:** Use w/ other drugs that raise serum K+ may result in hyperkalemia; monitor serum K+. Dual blockade of the RAS is associated w/ increased risks of hypotension, syncope, hyperkalemia, and changes in renal function (including acute renal failure); closely monitor BP, renal function, and electrolytes w/ concomitant agents that affect the RAS. **HCTZ:** Dose adjustment of antidiabetic drugs (oral agents, insulin) may be required. Anionic exchange resins (eg, cholestyramine, colestipol) may impair absorption; stagger the dose of HCTZ and the resin such that HCTZ is administered at least 4 hrs before or 4-6 hrs after the administration of the resin.

PREGNANCY AND LACTATION

Pregnancy: Category D.
Lactation: Not for use in nursing.

MECHANISM OF ACTION

Losartan: Angiotensin II receptor antagonist; blocks the vasoconstrictor and aldosterone-secreting effects of angiotensin II by selectively blocking the binding of angiotensin II to AT_1 receptor found in many tissues (eg, vascular smooth muscle, adrenal gland). **HCTZ:** Thiazide diuretic; has not been established. Affects the renal tubular mechanisms of electrolyte reabsorption, directly increasing excretion of Na+ and Cl- in approximately equivalent amounts.

PHARMACOKINETICS

Absorption: Losartan: Well-absorbed. Systemic bioavailability (33%); T_{max}=1 hr, 3-4 hrs (active metabolite). **Distribution:** Losartan: V_d=34L, 12L (active metabolite); plasma protein binding (98.7%, 99.8% active metabolite). HCTZ: Crosses placenta; found in breast milk. **Metabolism:** Losartan: CYP2C9, 3A4; carboxylic acid (active metabolite). **Elimination:** Losartan: Urine (35%, 4% unchanged, 6% active metabolite), feces (60%); $T_{1/2}$=2 hrs, 6-9 hrs (active metabolite). HCTZ: Kidney ($\geq$61% unchanged); $T_{1/2}$=5.6-14.8 hrs.

PATIENT CONSIDERATIONS

Assessment: Assess for hypersensitivity to drugs and their components, anuria, history of sulfonamide or penicillin allergy, volume/salt depletion, SLE, diabetes, hepatic/renal impairment, postsympathectomy status, pregnancy/nursing status, and possible drug interactions. Obtain baseline BP.

Monitoring: Monitor for signs/symptoms of fluid/electrolyte imbalance, exacerbation/activation of SLE, idiosyncratic reaction, precipitation of gout, hypersensitivity reactions, and other adverse reactions. Monitor BP, serum electrolytes, renal/hepatic function, Ca^{2+} levels, cholesterol, and TG levels periodically.

Counseling: Inform females of childbearing potential of the consequences of exposure during pregnancy and of the treatment options for women planning to become pregnant. Instruct to report pregnancy to the physician as soon as possible. Counsel that lightheadedness may occur, especially during the 1st days of therapy; instruct to report to physician. Instruct to consult physician if syncope occurs. Inform that dehydration from inadequate fluid intake, excessive perspiration, vomiting, or diarrhea may lead to an excessive fall in blood pressure. Instruct not to use K^+ supplements or salt substitutes containing K^+ w/o consulting physician. Advise to d/c and seek immediate medical attention if experiencing symptoms of acute myopia or secondary angle closure glaucoma.

IBRANCE — palbociclib   Rx

Class: Kinase inhibitor

ADULT DOSAGE	PEDIATRIC DOSAGE
HR Positive, HER2 Negative Advanced or Metastatic Breast Cancer	Pediatric use may not have been established
Initial Endocrine-Based Therapy in Postmenopausal Women: 125mg qd for 21 consecutive days followed by 7 days off treatment + 2.5mg letrozole qd continuously throughout the 28-day cycle	
Women w/ Disease Progression Following Endocrine Therapy: 125mg qd for 21 consecutive days followed by 7 days off treatment + 500mg fulvestrant on Days 1, 15, 29, and once monthly thereafter	
Pre/perimenopausal should be treated w/ luteinizing hormone-releasing hormone agonists according to current clinical practice standards	
Missed Dose If patient vomits/misses dose, patient should not take an additional dose that day; patient should take next prescribed dose at usual time	

- -

DOSING CONSIDERATIONS
Concomitant Medications:
Strong CYP3A Inhibitors:
Avoid concomitant use and consider alternative concomitant medication w/ no or minimal CYP3A inhibition
If Concomitant Use Cannot Be Avoided: Reduce palbociclib dose to 75mg qd. If strong inhibitor is discontinued, increase dose (after 3-5 half lives of the inhibitor) to the dose used prior to initiating the strong inhibitor

Adverse Reactions
Recommended Starting Dose: 125mg/day
1st Dose Reduction: 100mg/day
2nd Dose Reduction: 75mg/day
If further dose reduction below 75mg/day is required, d/c treatment
Hematologic Toxicities (Except Lymphopenia Unless Associated w/ Clinical Events):
Monitor CBC prior to start of therapy, at the beginning of each cycle, as well as on Day 14 of the first 2 cycles, and as clinically indicated
Grade 1 or 2: No dose adjustment required
Grade 3:
Day 1 of Cycle:
Withhold, repeat CBC monitoring w/in 1 week. When recovered to Grade $\leq$2, start the next cycle at the same dose
Day 14 of First 2 Cycles:
Continue at current dose to complete cycle. Repeat CBC on Day 21
Consider dose reduction in cases of prolonged (>1 week) recovery from Grade 3 neutropenia or recurrent Grade 3 neutropenia in subsequent cycles
Grade 3 Neutropenia w/ Fever $\geq$38.5°C and/or Infection:
Withhold until recovery to Grade $\leq$2; resume at the next lower dose

Grade 4:
Withhold until recovery to Grade $\leq$2; resume at the next lower dose
Nonhematologic Toxicities:
Grade 1 or 2: No dose adjustment required
Grade $\geq$3: If persisting despite medical treatment, withhold until symptoms resolve to Grade $\leq$1 or Grade $\leq$2 (if not considered a safety risk for patient). Resume at next lower dose

ADMINISTRATION
Oral route

Take w/ food at the same time each day.
Swallow whole; do not chew, crush, or open prior to swallowing.
STORAGE
20-25°C (68-77°F); excursions permitted between 15-30°C (59-86°F).
HOW SUPPLIED
Cap: 75mg, 100mg, 125mg
WARNINGS/PRECAUTIONS
Decreased neutrophil counts and febrile neutropenia reported; dose interruption, reduction, or delay in starting treatment cycles is recommended for patients who develop Grade 3 or 4 neutropenia. Pulmonary embolism (PE) reported; monitor and treat as medically appropriate. May cause fetal harm.

ADVERSE REACTIONS
Neutropenia, leukopenia, infections, fatigue, nausea, anemia, stomatitis, headache, diarrhea, thrombocytopenia, constipation, alopecia, vomiting, rash, decreased appetite.

DRUG INTERACTIONS
See Dosing Considerations. Increased plasma exposure w/ strong CYP3A inhibitors (itraconazole). Avoid grapefruit or grapefruit juice. Decreased plasma exposure w/ strong CYP3A inducers (eg, rifampin); avoid concomitant use w/ strong CYP3A inducers (eg, phenytoin, carbamazepine, St John's wort). Multiple doses increased midazolam plasma exposure. May need to reduce dose of sensitive CYP3A substrate w/ a narrow therapeutic index (eg, alfentanil, cyclosporine, ergotamine) as therapy may increase their exposure.

PREGNANCY AND LACTATION
Pregnancy: Can cause fetal harm.
Lactation: It is not known if palbociclib is present in human milk; not for use in nursing.
Reproductive Potential: Females of reproductive potential should use effective contraception during and for at least 3 weeks after last dose. Male fertility may be compromised.

MECHANISM OF ACTION
Kinase inhibitor; reduces cellular proliferation of estrogen receptor-positive breast cancer cell lines by blocking progression of the cell from G1 into S phase of the cell cycle.

PHARMACOKINETICS
Absorption: Absolute bioavailability (46%) (125mg); T_{max}=6-12 hrs. **Distribution:** Plasma protein binding (approx 85%); V_d=2583L. **Metabolism:** Hepatic (extensive); oxidation, sulfonation, acylation, glucuronidation; glucuronide conjugate (major circulating metabolite). **Elimination:** Feces (2.3% unchanged, 26% [sulfamic acid conjugate]), urine (6.9% unchanged); $T_{1/2}$=29 hrs.

PATIENT CONSIDERATIONS
Assessment: Assess for pregnancy/nursing status and possible drug interactions. Obtain baseline CBC.

Monitoring: Monitor for signs/symptoms of PE, and other adverse reactions. Monitor CBC at the beginning of each cycle, as well as on Day 14 of the first 2 cycles, and as clinically indicated.

Counseling: Advise to immediately report any signs/symptoms of myelosuppression/infection, or PE. Instruct not to consume grapefruit products while on therapy. Inform patients to avoid strong CYP3A inhibitors/inducers. Advise to inform physician of all concomitant medications, including prescription medicines, OTC drugs, vitamins, and herbal products. Instruct not to take additional dose if the patient vomits or misses a dose and to take the next dose at the usual time. Advise females of reproductive potential to use effective contraception during therapy and for at least 3 weeks after the last dose. Advise women not to breastfeed during treatment and for 3 weeks after the last dose. Advise to contact physician if patient becomes pregnant, or if pregnancy is suspected, during treatment.

ICLUSIG — ponatinib   Rx

Class: Kinase inhibitor

> Arterial and venous thrombosis and occlusions, including fatal MI, stroke, stenosis of large arterial vessels of the brain, severe peripheral vascular disease, and the need for urgent revascularization procedures, reported; monitor for evidence of thromboembolism and vascular occlusion, and interrupt or d/c immediately for vascular occlusion. Heart failure (HF), including fatalities, reported; monitor cardiac function and interrupt or d/c therapy for new/worsening HF. Hepatotoxicity, liver failure, and death reported; monitor hepatic function and interrupt therapy if hepatotoxicity is suspected.

ADULT DOSAGE	PEDIATRIC DOSAGE
Chronic Myeloid Leukemia	Pediatric use may not have been established
Chronic/Accelerated/Blast Phase: In Patients for Whom No Other Tyrosine Kinase Inhibitor is Indicated or Who are T315I-Positive: **Initial:** 45mg qd	

Titrate: Consider dose reduction for patients in chronic or accelerated phase who have achieved a major cytogenetic response

Chronic Myeloid Leukemia
Chronic/Accelerated/Blast Phase: In Patients for Whom No Other Tyrosine Kinase Inhibitor is Indicated or Who are T315I-Positive:
Initial: 45mg qd
Titrate: Consider dose reduction for patients in chronic or accelerated phase who have achieved a major cytogenetic response

Ph+ Acute Lymphoblastic Leukemia
In Patients for Whom No Other Tyrosine Kinase Inhibitor is Indicated or Who are T315I-Positive:
Initial: 45mg qd

Ph+ Acute Lymphoblastic Leukemia
In Patients for Whom No Other Tyrosine Kinase Inhibitor is Indicated or Who are T315I-Positive:
Initial: 45mg qd

DOSING CONSIDERATIONS
Concomitant Medications
Strong CYP3A Inhibitors: Reduce ponatinib dose to 30mg qd

Hepatic Impairment
Child-Pugh A, B, or C:
Initial: 30mg qd

Adverse Reactions
Myelosuppression:
ANC <1 x 10⁹/L or Platelet Count <50 x 10⁹/L:

ANC $<1 \times 10^9$/L or Platelet Count $<50 \times 10^9$/L:
First Occurrence:
Interrupt therapy and resume at 45mg after recovery to ANC $\geq1.5 \times 10^9$/L and platelet $\geq75 \times 10^9$/L
Second Occurrence:
Interrupt therapy and resume at 30mg after recovery to ANC $\geq1.5 \times 10^9$/L and platelet $\geq75 \times 10^9$/L
Third Occurrence:
Interrupt therapy and resume at 15mg after recovery to ANC $\geq1.5 \times 10^9$/L and platelet $\geq75 \times 10^9$/L

Serious Non-Hematologic:
Modify the dose or interrupt treatment
Arterial/Venous Occlusion:
Do not restart unless the potential benefit outweighs the risk of recurrence and the patient has no other treatment options
Reactions Other Than Arterial/Venous Occlusion:
Do not restart until the serious event has resolved or the potential benefit of resuming therapy outweighs the risk

Hepatic Toxicity:
Liver Transaminase >3X ULN (≥Grade 2):
Occurrence at 45mg:
Interrupt therapy and resume at 30mg after recovery to ≤Grade 1 (<3X ULN)
Occurrence at 30mg:
Interrupt therapy and resume at 15mg after recovery to ≤Grade 1
Occurrence at 15mg:
D/C therapy
AST/ALT ≥3X ULN w/ Bilirubin >2X ULN and Alkaline Phosphatase <2X ULN:
D/C therapy

Pancreatitis/Lipase Elevation:
Asymptomatic Grade 1 or 2 Lipase Elevation:
Consider therapy interruption or dose reduction

Asymptomatic Grade 3 or 4 Lipase Elevation (>2X ULN)/Asymptomatic Radiologic Pancreatitis (Grade 2 Pancreatitis):
Occurrence at 45mg:
Interrupt therapy and resume at 30mg after recovery to ≤Grade 1 (<1.5X ULN)
Occurrence at 30mg:
Interrupt therapy and resume at 15mg after recovery to ≤Grade 1
Occurrence at 15mg:
D/C therapy

Symptomatic Grade 3 Pancreatitis:
Occurrence at 45mg:
Interrupt therapy and resume at 30mg after complete resolution of symptoms and recovery of lipase elevation to ≤Grade 1
Occurrence at 30mg:
Interrupt therapy and resume at 15mg after complete resolution of symptoms and recovery of lipase elevation to ≤Grade 1
Occurrence at 15mg:
D/C therapy

Grade 4 Pancreatitis:
D/C therapy

Discontinuation
Consider if response has not occurred by 3 months of therapy

ADMINISTRATION
Oral route
Take w/ or w/o food.
Swallow whole; do not crush or dissolve.

STORAGE
20-25°C (68-77°F); excursions permitted to 15-30°C (59-86°F).

HOW SUPPLIED
Tab: 15mg, 30mg, 45mg

WARNINGS/PRECAUTIONS
Not indicated and not recommended for the treatment of patients w/ newly diagnosed chronic phase chronic myeloid leukemia. Venous thromboembolic events reported; consider dose modification or discontinuation if serious venous thromboembolism (VTE) develops. HTN reported; interrupt, reduce dose, or d/c therapy if HTN is not medically controlled. Interrupt treatment and consider evaluating for renal artery stenosis in the event of significant worsening, labile, or treatment-resistant HTN. Pancreatitis reported; check serum lipase every 2 weeks for the first 2 months and then monthly thereafter or as clinically indicated. Consider additional serum lipase monitoring in patients w/ a history of pancreatitis or alcohol abuse. Peripheral and cranial neuropathy reported; consider interrupting therapy and evaluate if neuropathy is suspected. Serious ocular toxicities leading to blindness or blurred vision reported. Serious bleeding events reported; interrupt therapy for serious or severe hemorrhage and evaluate. Fluid retention reported; interrupt, reduce, or d/c therapy as clinically indicated. Symptomatic bradyarrhythmias and supraventricular tachyarrhythmias reported; interrupt therapy and evaluate. Severe (Grade 3 or 4) myelosuppression reported; adjust the dose as recommended. Tumor lysis syndrome may occur in patients w/ advanced disease; ensure adequate hydration and treat high uric acid levels prior to initiating therapy. May compromise wound healing. Serious GI perforation (fistula) reported in 1 patient 38 days postcholecystectomy. Interrupt therapy for at least 1 week prior to major surgery; base decision when to resume therapy after surgery on clinical judgment of adequate wound healing. May cause fetal harm. Caution in elderly.

ADVERSE REACTIONS
HTN, rash, abdominal pain, fatigue, headache, dry skin, constipation, arthralgia, nausea, pyrexia, thrombocytopenia, neutropenia, leukopenia, anemia, lymphopenia.

DRUG INTERACTIONS
See Dosing Considerations. Ketoconazole may increase levels; reduce ponatinib starting dose when administering w/ strong CYP3A inhibitors (eg, boceprevir, clarithromycin, conivaptan, grapefruit juice). Avoid w/ strong CYP3A inducers (eg, carbamazepine, phenytoin, rifampin, St. John's wort) unless the benefit outweighs the risk of decreased ponatinib exposure; monitor for reduced efficacy. Lansoprazole may decrease exposure minimally.

PREGNANCY AND LACTATION
Pregnancy: Category D. Based on its mechanism of action and findings in animals, ponatinib can cause fetal harm when administered to a pregnant woman; pregnancy should be avoided while taking therapy.
Lactation: Not for use in nursing.

MECHANISM OF ACTION
Kinase inhibitor; inhibits the tyrosine kinase activity of ABL and T315I mutant ABL. Inhibits the activity of additional kinases including members of the VEGFR, PDGFR, FGFR, EPH receptors and SRC families of kinases, and KIT, RET, TIE2, and FLT3. Inhibits the viability of cells expressing native or mutant BCR-ABL, including T315I.

PHARMACOKINETICS
Absorption: C_{max}=73ng/mL; AUC=1253ng•hr/mL; T_{max}=6 hrs. **Distribution:** V_d=1223L; plasma protein binding (>99%). **Metabolism:** Phase I (via CYP3A4, and to a lesser extent CYP2C8, CYP2D6, and CYP3A5) and phase II; also by esterases and/or amidases. **Elimination:** Feces (87%), urine (5%); $T_{1/2}$=24 hrs.

PATIENT CONSIDERATIONS
Assessment: Assess for history of pancreatitis or alcohol abuse, upcoming surgery, pregnancy/nursing status, and possible drug interactions. Assess hydration status and uric acid levels. Obtain baseline LFTs. Conduct comprehensive eye exams at baseline.

Monitoring: Monitor for signs/symptoms of thromboembolism, vascular occlusion, HF, hepatotoxicity, VTE, HTN, pancreatitis, neuropathy, ocular toxicity, hemorrhage, fluid retention, cardiac arrhythmias, myelosuppression, tumor lysis syndrome, compromised wound healing, GI perforation, and other adverse reactions. Monitor cardiac function. Monitor LFTs at least monthly or as clinically indicated. Monitor serum lipase every 2 weeks for the first 2 months and then monthly thereafter or as clinically indicated. Conduct comprehensive eye exams periodically. Monitor CBC every 2 weeks for the first 3 months and then monthly or as clinically indicated.

Counseling: Inform of the risks and benefits of therapy. Instruct to immediately contact physician w/ any signs/symptoms suggestive of a blood clot, HF, slow/fast HR, liver failure, HTN, pancreatitis, neuropathy, ocular toxicity, hemorrhage, fluid retention, or if fever develops, particularly in association w/ any suggestion of infection. Advise to inform physician if patient is planning to undergo or recently had a surgical procedure. Inform that cases of GI perforation have been reported. Advise women of the potential hazard to a fetus and to avoid becoming pregnant. Instruct to take drug exactly as prescribed and not to change dose or stop taking the drug w/o physician's advice. Inform that drug contains 121mg of lactose monohydrate in a 45mg daily dose.

ILARIS — canakinumab   Rx

Class: Monoclonal antibody/interleukin-1 (IL-1) beta blocker

ADULT DOSAGE	PEDIATRIC DOSAGE
Cryopyrin-Associated Periodic Syndromes	**Cryopyrin-Associated Periodic Syndromes**
Including familial cold autoinflammatory syndrome and Muckle-Wells syndrome	Including familial cold autoinflammatory syndrome and Muckle-Wells syndrome
15-40kg: 2mg/kg	**≥4 Years:**
>40kg: 150mg	**15-40kg:** 2mg/kg; may increase to 3mg/kg if response is inadequate
Administer every 8 weeks as a single dose via SQ inj	**>40kg:** 150mg
	Administer every 8 weeks as a single dose via SQ inj
	Systemic Juvenile Idiopathic Arthritis
	≥2 Years:
	≥7.5kg: 4mg/kg SQ every 4 weeks
	Max: 300mg/dose

ADMINISTRATION

SQ route

Supplied in a single-use vial; discard any unused product or waste material. Avoid inj into scar tissue as this may result in insufficient exposure.

Preparation and Administration

1. Reconstitute each vial by slowly injecting 1mL of preservative-free sterile water for inj w/ a 1mL syringe and an 18-gauge x 2-inch needle.
2. Swirl the vial slowly at an angle of about 45° for approx 1 min and allow to stand for 5 min; do not shake. Then gently turn the vial upside down and back again 10X.
3. Allow to stand for about 15 min at room temperature to obtain a clear sol. The reconstituted sol has a final concentration of 150mg/mL. Tap the side of the vial to remove any residual liquid from the stopper; the reconstituted sol should be essentially free from particulates, and clear to opalescent. The sol should be colorless or may have a slight brownish-yellow tint; if the sol has a distinctly brown discoloration it should not be used. Slight foaming of the product upon reconstitution is not unusual.
4. Using a sterile syringe and needle, carefully withdraw the required volume depending on the dose to be administered (0.2-1mL) and SQ inject using a 27-gauge x 0.5-inch needle.

STORAGE

2-8°C (36-46°F). Do not freeze. Protect from light. **Reconstituted Sol:** Room temperature if used w/in 60 min of reconstitution, or 2-8°C (36-46°F) and use w/in 4 hrs of reconstitution. Protect from light.

HOW SUPPLIED

Inj: 180mg

CONTRAINDICATIONS

Confirmed hypersensitivity to the active substance or to any of the excipients.

WARNINGS/PRECAUTIONS

Associated w/ an increased risk of serious infections; caution in patients w/ infections or history of recurring infections or underlying conditions that may predispose to infections, and do not administer during an active infection requiring medical intervention. D/C if serious infection develops. May increase risk of tuberculosis (TB) reactivation or of opportunistic infections (eg, aspergillosis, atypical mycobacterial infections, cytomegalovirus). Evaluate for active and latent TB infection prior to treatment initiation; perform appropriate screening tests in all patients, and treat those testing positive according to standard medical practice prior to therapy. May increase risk of malignancies. Hypersensitivity reactions reported. Prior to initiation of therapy, patients should receive all recommended vaccinations, as appropriate, including pneumococcal vaccine and inactivated influenza vaccine. Macrophage activation syndrome (MAS) reported in systemic juvenile idiopathic arthritis (SJIA) patients.

ADVERSE REACTIONS

Cryopyrin-Associated Periodic Syndromes (CAPS): Nasopharyngitis, diarrhea, influenza, headache, nausea.
SJIA: Infections (nasopharyngitis and URTI), abdominal pain, inj-site reactions.

DRUG INTERACTIONS

Increased risk of serious infections w/ TNF inhibitors; coadministration is not recommended. Not recommended w/ other agents that block interleukin-1 (IL-1) or its receptors. Do not give w/ live vaccines. May alter effect or concentration of drugs metabolized by CYP450 enzymes; monitor effect or concentration and adjust dose of CYP450 substrates w/ a narrow therapeutic index (eg, warfarin) as needed.

PREGNANCY AND LACTATION

Pregnancy: The limited human data from postmarketing reports are not sufficient to inform a drug-associated risk. Transported across the placenta in a linear fashion as pregnancy progresses; therefore, potential fetal exposure is likely to be greater during the 2nd and 3rd trimesters.
Lactation: There is no information regarding the presence of canakinumab in human milk, the effects on the breastfed infant, or the effects on milk production. Caution in nursing.

MECHANISM OF ACTION

Monoclonal anti-human IL-1β antibody of the IgG1/kappa isotype; binds to human IL-1β and neutralizes its activity by blocking its interaction w/ IL-1 receptors.

PHARMACOKINETICS

Absorption: Adults w/ CAPS: Absolute bioavailability (66%); C_{max}=16mcg/mL; T_{max}=7 days. Pediatric Patients w/ CAPS: T_{max}=2-7 days. **Distribution:** CAPS, 70kg Patients: V_d=6.01L. SJIA, 33kg Patients: V_d=3.2L. **Elimination:** Adults w/ CAPS: $T_{1/2}$=26 days. Pediatric Patients w/ CAPS: $T_{1/2}$=22.9-25.7 days.

PATIENT CONSIDERATIONS

Assessment: Assess for drug hypersensitivity, infections, history of recurring infections or underlying conditions that may predispose to infections, active/latent TB, vaccination history, pregnancy/nursing status, and possible drug interactions.

Monitoring: Monitor for serious infections, signs/symptoms of TB, malignancies, hypersensitivity reactions, MAS or triggers for MAS, and other adverse reactions.

Counseling: Advise of the potential benefits and risks of therapy. Advise that healthcare providers should perform administration of drug. Instruct to immediately contact physician if an infection, signs of an allergic reaction, persistent inj-site reaction, or signs/symptoms or high-risk exposure suggestive of TB (eg, persistent cough, weight loss, subfebrile temperature) develop. Advise female patients of the potential risk to a fetus.

ILEVRO — nepafenac   Rx

Class: NSAID

ADULT DOSAGE	PEDIATRIC DOSAGE
Ocular Pain and Inflammation	**Ocular Pain and Inflammation**
1 drop to the affected eye qd, beginning 1 day prior to cataract surgery, continued on the day of surgery, and through the first 2 weeks of postoperative period	**≥10 Years:**
	1 drop to the affected eye qd, beginning 1 day prior to cataract surgery, continued on the day of surgery, and through the first 2 weeks of postoperative period
Administer additional drop 30-120 min prior to surgery	Administer additional drop 30-120 min prior to surgery

DOSING CONSIDERATIONS

Concomitant Medications

Space dosing ≥5 min apart w/ other topical ophthalmic medications

ADMINISTRATION

Ocular route

Shake well before use.

STORAGE

2-25°C (36-77°F). Protect from light.

HOW SUPPLIED

Sus: 0.3% [1.7mL, 3mL]

CONTRAINDICATIONS

Previously demonstrated hypersensitivity to any of the ingredients in the formula or to other NSAIDs.

WARNINGS/PRECAUTIONS

Potential for increased bleeding time due to interference w/ thrombocyte aggregation. Increased bleeding of ocular tissues (eg, hyphemas) reported in conjunction w/ ocular surgery; caution w/ known bleeding tendencies. May slow or delay healing, or result in keratitis. Continued use may result in sight threatening epithelial breakdown, corneal thinning/erosion/ulceration/perforation; d/c if evidence of corneal epithelial breakdown occurs and monitor for corneal health. Caution w/ complicated ocular surgeries, corneal denervation, corneal epithelial defects, diabetes mellitus (DM), ocular surface diseases (eg, dry eye syndrome), rheumatoid arthritis (RA), or repeat ocular surgeries w/in a short period of time. Use >1 day prior to surgery or beyond 14 days post-surgery may increase risk and severity of corneal adverse events. Avoid use w/ contact lenses and during late pregnancy.

ADVERSE REACTIONS

Capsular opacity, decreased visual acuity, foreign body sensation, IOP, sticky sensation, conjunctival edema, corneal edema, dry eye, lid margin crusting, ocular discomfort, ocular hyperemia/pain/pruritus, photophobia, tearing, vitreous detachment.

DRUG INTERACTIONS

May increase potential for healing problems w/ topical steroids. Caution w/ agents that may prolong bleeding time.

PREGNANCY AND LACTATION

Pregnancy: Category C.
Lactation: Caution in nursing.

MECHANISM OF ACTION

NSAID; thought to inhibit the action of prostaglandin H synthase (cyclooxygenase), an enzyme required for prostaglandin production.

PHARMACOKINETICS

Absorption: C_{max}=0.847ng/mL (nepafenac), 1.13ng/mL (amfenac); T_{max}=0.5 hr (nepafenac), 0.75 hr (amfenac). **Metabolism:** Hydrolysis via ocular tissue hydrolases to amfenac (metabolite).

PATIENT CONSIDERATIONS

Assessment: Assess for previous hypersensitivity to the drug, bleeding tendencies, complicated or repeated ocular surgeries, corneal denervation, corneal epithelial defects, DM, ocular surface diseases, RA, contact lens use, pregnancy/nursing status, and possible drug interactions.

Monitoring: Monitor for hypersensitivity reactions, wound healing problems, keratitis, increased bleeding time, bleeding of ocular tissues in conjunction w/ ocular surgery, epithelial breakdown, corneal thinning/erosion/ulceration/perforation, and other adverse reactions.

Counseling: Inform of possibility that slow or delayed healing may occur. Instruct to avoid allowing the tip of the container to contact the eye or surrounding structures. Advise that use of the same bottle for both eyes is not recommended. Instruct not to use while wearing contact lens. Advise to notify physician if an intercurrent ocular condition (eg, trauma or infection) develops or if undergoing ocular surgery.

ILUVIEN — fluocinolone acetonide Rx

Class: Corticosteroid

ADULT DOSAGE
Diabetic Macular Edema
Previously Treated with Corticosteroids without a Significant Rise in Intraocular Pressure:
0.19mg (1 implant) in the affected eye

PEDIATRIC DOSAGE
Pediatric use may not have been established

ADMINISTRATION
Intravitreal route

Inj Procedure
1. Remove the applicator from the tray with sterile gloved hands touching only the sterile interior tray surface and applicator
2. Prior to injection, the applicator tip must be kept above the horizontal plane to ensure that the implant is properly positioned within the applicator
3. Before inserting the needle into the eye, push the applicator button down and slide it to the first stop (at the curved black marks alongside the button track). At the first stop, release the button and it should move to the UP position. If the button does not rise to the UP position, do not proceed with this unit
4. Optimal placement of the implant is inferior to the optic disc and posterior to the equator of the eye
5. Measure 4 millimeters inferotemporal from the limbus with the aid of calipers for point of entry into the sclera
6. Remove the protective cap from the needle and inspect the tip to ensure it is not bent
7. Gently displace the conjunctiva so that after withdrawing the needle, the conjunctival and scleral needle entry sites will not align
8. Insert the needle through the conjunctiva and sclera. To release the implant, while the button is in the UP position, advance the button by sliding it forward to the end of the button track and remove the needle. Ensure that the button reaches the end of the track before removing the needle

STORAGE
15-30°C (59-86°F).

HOW SUPPLIED
Implant: 0.19mg

CONTRAINDICATIONS
Glaucoma w/ cup to disc ratios of >0.8; active or suspected ocular or periocular infections including most viral diseases of the cornea and conjunctiva, including active epithelial herpes simplex keratitis (dendritic keratitis), vaccinia, varicella, mycobacterial infections, and fungal diseases; known hypersensitivity to any components of this product.

WARNINGS/PRECAUTIONS
Intravitreal inj has been associated with endophthalmitis, eye inflammation, increased IOP, and retinal detachments. May produce posterior subcapsular cataracts, increased IOP, and glaucoma, and may enhance the establishment of secondary ocular infections due to bacteria, fungi, or viruses. Not recommended in patients with history of ocular herpes simplex; potential for reactivation of the viral infection. Risk of implant migration into the anterior chamber in patients whose posterior lens capsule is absent or has a tear.

ADVERSE REACTIONS
Cataract, myodesopsia, eye pain, conjunctival hemorrhage, posterior capsule opacification, eye irritation, conjunctivitis, corneal edema, foreign body sensation in eyes, eye pruritus, ocular hyperemia, anemia, headache, renal failure, pneumonia.

PREGNANCY AND LACTATION
Category C, caution in nursing.

MECHANISM OF ACTION
Corticosteroid; inhibits inflammatory responses to a variety of inciting agents. Inhibits edema, fibrin deposition, capillary dilation, leukocyte migration, capillary proliferation, fibroblast proliferation, deposition of collagen, and scar formation associated with inflammation.

PHARMACOKINETICS
Distribution: Found in breast milk (systemically administered).

PATIENT CONSIDERATIONS
Assessment: Assess for hypersensitivity to product components, glaucoma with cup to disc ratios of >0.8, active or suspected ocular or periocular infections, history of ocular herpes simplex, absent or torn posterior lens capsule, and pregnancy/nursing status.

Monitoring: Monitor for eye inflammation, retinal detachment, posterior subcapsular cataracts, glaucoma, secondary ocular infections, and other adverse reactions. Monitor for elevation of IOP and for endophthalmitis by checking for

perfusion of the optic nerve head immediately after inj, tonometry within 30 min following inj, and biomicroscopy between 2-7 days after inj.

Counseling: Advise that a cataract may occur after treatment; if this occurs, inform that vision will decrease and that an operation to remove the cataract and restore vision will be needed. Advise that increased IOP may develop, which may need to be managed with eye drops or surgery. Inform that in the days following intravitreal inj, patients are at risk for potential complications including development of endophthalmitis or elevated IOP; instruct to report any symptoms suggestive of endophthalmitis without delay. Advise to seek immediate care from an ophthalmologist if the eye becomes red, sensitive to light, painful, or if a change in vision develops. Inform that temporary visual blurring after receiving an intravitreal inj may be experienced; instruct to avoid driving/using machines until this has resolved.

IMBRUVICA — ibrutinib Rx

Class: Kinase inhibitor

ADULT DOSAGE
Mantle Cell Lymphoma
Patients Who Have Received at Least 1 Prior Therapy:
560mg qd until disease progression or unacceptable toxicity occurs

Chronic Lymphocytic Leukemia/Small Lymphocytic Lymphoma
Patients w/ or w/o 17p Deletion:
420mg qd until disease progression or unacceptable toxicity occurs

Combination w/ Bendamustine and Rituximab:
Bendamustine and rituximab administered every 28 days for up to 6 cycles + 420mg ibrutinib qd until disease progression or unacceptable toxicity occurs

Waldenstrom's Macroglobulinemia
420mg qd until disease progression or unacceptable toxicity occurs

Missed Dose
If a dose is not taken at the scheduled time, it can be taken as soon as possible on the same day w/ a return to the normal schedule the following day; extra capsules of ibrutinib should not be taken to make up for the missed dose

PEDIATRIC DOSAGE
Pediatric use may not have been established

DOSING CONSIDERATIONS
Concomitant Medications
Avoid coadministration w/ strong or moderate CYP3A inhibitors and consider alternative agents w/ less CYP3A inhibition

Strong CYP3A Inhibitors Taken Chronically (eg, Ritonavir, Indinavir, Nelfinavir): Concomitant use is not recommended
Short-term Use (for ≤7 Days) of Strong CYP3A Inhibitors (eg, Antifungals, Antibiotics): Consider interrupting ibrutinib therapy until the CYP3A inhibitor is no longer needed
If Moderate CYP3A Inhibitor (eg, Fluconazole, Darunavir, Erythromycin) Is Necessary: Reduce ibrutinib dose to 140mg
Hepatic Impairment
Mild (Child-Pugh Class A): 140mg qd
Moderate or Severe (Child-Pugh Classes B and C): Avoid use
Adverse Reactions
Interrupt Therapy For:
- Any Grade ≥3 nonhematological toxicities
- Grade ≥3 neutropenia w/ infection or fever
- Grade 4 hematological toxicities

1st Toxicity Occurrence:
Mantle Cell Lymphoma (MCL): Restart at 560mg qd once symptoms of the toxicity have resolved to Grade 1 or baseline (recovery)
Chronic Lymphocytic Leukemia (CLL), Small Lymphocytic Lymphoma (SLL) and Waldenstrom's Macroglobulinemia (WM): Restart at 420mg qd after recovery
2nd Toxicity Occurrence:
MCL: Restart at 420mg qd after recovery
CLL, SLL and WM: Restart at 280mg qd after recovery
3rd Toxicity Occurrence:
MCL: Restart at 280mg qd after recovery
CLL, SLL and WM: Restart at 140mg qd after recovery
4th Toxicity Occurrence:
MCL, CLL, SLL, and WM: D/C ibrutinib
ADMINISTRATION
Oral route

Take at approx the same time each day.
Swallow caps whole w/ water; do not open, break, or chew.

STORAGE
20-25°C (68-77°F); excursions permitted between 15-30°C (59-86°F). Retain in original package until dispensing.

HOW SUPPLIED
Cap: 140mg

WARNINGS/PRECAUTIONS
See Dosing Considerations. Fatal and ≥Grade 3 bleeding events reported. Consider the benefit-risk of withholding therapy for at least 3-7 days pre- and post-surgery depending upon the type of surgery and the risk of bleeding. Fatal and nonfatal infections reported. Cases of progressive multifocal leukoencephalopathy (PML) reported. Evaluate patients for fever and infections and treat appropriately. Treatment-emergent Grade 3 or 4 cytopenias reported; monitor CBC monthly. A-fib and A-flutter reported, particularly in patients w/ cardiac risk factors, HTN, acute infections, and a previous history of A-fib; perform ECG if arrhythmic symptoms (eg, palpitations, lightheadedness) or new onset dyspnea develop. Manage A-fib appropriately and if it persists, consider the risks and benefits of treatment and follow dose modification guidelines. HTN reported; monitor for new onset HTN or HTN that is not adequately controlled after starting therapy. Secondary primary malignancies (eg, nonmelanoma skin cancer, non-skin carcinomas) reported. Tumor lysis syndrome (TLS) reported. Assess baseline risk (eg, high tumor burden) and take appropriate precautions; monitor patients closely and treat as appropriate. May cause fetal harm. Management of hyperviscosity in patients w/ WM may include plasmapheresis before and during treatment; modifications to ibrutinib dosing are not required.

ADVERSE REACTIONS
Neutropenia, thrombocytopenia, diarrhea, anemia, musculoskeletal pain, rash, nausea, bruising, fatigue, hemorrhage, pyrexia.

DRUG INTERACTIONS
See Dosing Considerations. Risk of bleeding may be increased in patients receiving antiplatelet or anticoagulant therapies. Ketoconazole (a strong CYP3A inhibitor) increased levels. Closely monitor patients taking concomitant strong or moderate CYP3A inhibitors for signs of ibrutinib toxicity. Avoid grapefruit and Seville oranges during treatment. Rifampin (a strong CYP3A inducer) decreased levels; avoid use w/ strong CYP3A inducers (eg, carbamazepine, rifampin, St. John's wort) and consider alternative agents w/ less CYP3A induction.

PREGNANCY AND LACTATION
Pregnancy: Can cause fetal harm based on findings from animal studies. **Lactation:** There is no information regarding the presence of ibrutinib or its metabolites in human milk, the effects on the breastfed infant, or the effects on milk production. Caution in nursing. **Reproductive Potential:** Verify the pregnancy status of females of reproductive potential prior to initiating therapy. Females of reproductive potential should avoid pregnancy while taking ibrutinib and for up to 1 month after ending treatment. Men should avoid fathering a child while receiving ibrutinib, and for 1 month following the last dose of therapy.

MECHANISM OF ACTION
Bruton's tyrosine kinase (BTK) inhibitor; forms a covalent bond w/ a cysteine residue in the BTK active site, leading to inhibition of BTK enzymatic activity. BTK is a signaling molecule of the B-cell antigen receptor and cytokine receptor pathways. BTK's role in signaling through the B-cell surface receptors results in activation of pathways necessary for B-cell trafficking, chemotaxis, and adhesion.

PHARMACOKINETICS
Absorption: Absolute bioavailability (2.9%, fasted condition); T_{max}=1-2 hrs (median); AUC=953ng•hr/mL (560mg), 680ng•hr/mL (420mg). **Distribution:** Plasma protein binding (97.3%); V_d=10,000L. **Metabolism:** Liver via CYP3A (primary), CYP2D6 (minor); PCI-45227 (a dihydrodiol metabolite) (active). **Elimination:** Feces (80%, 1% unchanged), urine (<10%); $T_{1/2}$=4-6 hrs.

PATIENT CONSIDERATIONS
Assessment: Assess for cardiac risk factors, acute infections, HTN, history of A-fib, planned/recent surgery, hepatic impairment, pregnancy/nursing status, and possible drug interactions.

Monitoring: Monitor for signs of bleeding, fever, infections, PML, A-fib, HTN, secondary primary malignancies, TLS, and other adverse reactions. Monitor CBC monthly. Perform ECG in patients who develop arrhythmic symptoms (eg, palpitations, lightheadedness) or new onset dyspnea.

Counseling: Inform of the possibility of bleeding, and instruct to report any signs/symptoms of bleeding (eg, blood in stools or urine, prolonged or uncontrolled bleeding) to physician. Advise that therapy may need to be interrupted for medical or dental procedures. Inform of the possibility of serious infection, and instruct to report any signs/symptoms of infection (eg, fever, chills, weakness, confusion) to physician. Counsel to report any signs of A-Fib (eg, palpitations, lightheadedness, fainting, SOB, chest discomfort) to physician. Inform that high blood pressure may occur, which may require treatment w/ anti-hypertensive therapy. Inform that other malignancies (eg, skin cancers) may occur. Advise of the potential risk of TLS and instruct to report any signs/symptoms associated w/ this event to physician. Inform women of the potential hazard of therapy to a fetus and instruct to avoid becoming pregnant during treatment and for 1 month after the last dose. Inform of the common side effects associated w/ therapy. Advise to inform physician of all concomitant medications, including prescription medicines, OTC drugs, vitamins, and herbal products. Inform that loose stools or diarrhea may occur and instruct to contact physician if diarrhea persists. Counsel to maintain adequate hydration.

IMDUR — isosorbide mononitrate   Rx
Class: Nitrate vasodilator

ADULT DOSAGE	PEDIATRIC DOSAGE
Angina Pectoris	Pediatric use may not have been established
Prevention:	
Initial: 30mg or 60mg qam	
Titrate: Increase to 120mg qam after several days; rarely, 240mg qam may be required	

DOSING CONSIDERATIONS
Elderly
Start at lower end of dosing range

ADMINISTRATION
Oral route

Take qam on arising.
Swallow tab whole w/ a half-glassful of fluid; do not crush or chew.
Do not break 30mg tab.

STORAGE
20-25°C (68-77°F).

HOW SUPPLIED
Tab, Extended-Release: 30mg*, 60mg*, 120mg *scored

CONTRAINDICATIONS
Hypersensitivity or idiosyncratic reactions to other nitrates or nitrites.

WARNINGS/PRECAUTIONS
Not useful in aborting acute anginal episode. Not recommended for use in patients w/ acute MI or congestive heart failure; perform careful clinical or hemodynamic monitoring if used in these conditions. Severe hypotension, particularly w/ upright posture, may occur; caution in volume depleted, hypotensive, or elderly patients. Nitrate-induced hypotension may be accompanied by paradoxical bradycardia and increased angina pectoris. May aggravate angina caused by hypertrophic cardiomyopathy. May develop tolerance. Chest pain, acute MI, and sudden death reported during temporary withdrawal.

ADVERSE REACTIONS
Headache, dizziness, dry mouth, asthenia, cardiac failure, abdominal pain, earache, arrhythmia, hyperuricemia, arthralgia, purpura, anxiety, hypochromic anemia, atrophic vaginitis, bacterial infection.

DRUG INTERACTIONS
Sildenafil amplifies vasodilatory effects that can result in severe hypotension. Additive vasodilating effects w/ other vasodilators (eg, alcohol). Marked symptomatic orthostatic hypotension reported w/ calcium channel blockers; dose adjustments of either class of agents may be necessary.

PREGNANCY AND LACTATION
Category B, caution in nursing.

MECHANISM OF ACTION
Nitrate vasodilator; relaxes vascular smooth muscle, producing dilatation of peripheral arteries and veins, especially the latter. Dilatation of the veins leads to reducing the left ventricular end-diastolic pressure and pulmonary capillary wedge pressure (preload). Arteriolar relaxation reduces systemic vascular resistance, systolic arterial pressure, and mean arterial pressure (afterload). It also dilates the coronary artery.

PHARMACOKINETICS
Absorption: Single Dose (60mg): C_{max}=424-541ng/mL, T_{max}=3.1-4.5 hrs, AUC=5990-7452ng•hr/mL. Multiple Dose: C_{max}=557-572ng/mL (60mg), 1151-1180ng/mL (120mg); T_{max}=2.9-4.2 hrs (60mg), 3.1-3.2 hrs (120mg); AUC=6625-7555ng•hr/mL (60mg), 14,241-16,800ng•hr/mL (120mg). **Distribution:** V_d=0.6-0.7L/kg (IV); plasma protein binding (5%). **Metabolism:** Liver; denitration and glucuronidation. **Elimination:** Urine (96%, 2% unchanged), feces (1%); $T_{1/2}$=6.3-6.6 hrs (60mg single dose), 6.2-6.3 hrs (60mg multiple dose), 6.2-6.4 hrs (120mg multiple dose).

PATIENT CONSIDERATIONS
Assessment: Assess for drug hypersensitivity, hypotension, volume depletion, angina caused by hypertrophic cardiomyopathy, pregnancy/nursing status, possible drug interactions, and any other conditions where treatment is cautioned or contraindicated.

Monitoring: Monitor for hypotension w/ paradoxical bradycardia and increased angina pectoris, tachycardia, aggravation of angina caused by hypertrophic cardiomyopathy, tolerance, manifestations of true physical dependence (eg, chest pain, acute MI), and other adverse reactions.

Counseling: Inform about the risks and benefits of therapy. Counsel to carefully follow the prescribed schedule of dosing. Advise that daily headaches may accompany treatment and instruct to avoid altering schedule of treatment as the headaches are a marker of the activity of the medication and loss of headache may be associated w/ loss of antianginal efficacy. Inform that treatment may be associated w/ lightheadedness on standing, especially just after rising from a recumbent/seated position and may be more frequent w/ alcohol consumption.

IMITREX — sumatriptan

Rx

Class: 5-HT$_{1B/1D}$ agonist (triptans)

ADULT DOSAGE

Cluster Headache

Inj:
Max Single Dose: 6mg SQ
Max Dose/24 Hrs: Two 6mg inj separated by at least 1 hr; consider a 2nd dose only if some response to 1st inj was observed

Migraine

W/ or w/o Aura:
May use lower doses (1-5mg) if side effects are dose limiting

Inj:
Max Single Dose: 6mg SQ
Max Dose/24 hrs: Two 6mg inj separated by at least 1 hr; consider a 2nd dose only if some response to 1st inj was observed

Spray:
5mg, 10mg, or 20mg
Additional Dose: May administer 1 additional dose at least 2 hrs after 1st dose if migraine has not resolved or returns after transient improvement
Max: 40mg/24 hrs
The 5mg and 20mg doses are given as a single spray in 1 nostril; 10mg dose may be achieved by administering a single 5mg dose in each nostril

Tab:
25mg, 50mg, or 100mg
Additional Dose: May administer a 2nd dose at least 2 hrs after 1st dose if migraine has not resolved or returns after transient improvement
Use After Inj: If migraine returns after initial treatment w/ inj, may give additional single tab (up to 100mg/day), w/ an interval of at least 2 hrs between tab doses
Max: 200mg/24 hrs

PEDIATRIC DOSAGE

Pediatric use may not have been established

DOSING CONSIDERATIONS

Hepatic Impairment
Mild to Moderate:
Max Tab Single Dose: 50mg

Elderly
Start at lower end of dosing range

ADMINISTRATION
Oral/SQ/Nasal route

SQ
Use the 6mg single dose vial for patients receiving doses other than 4mg or 6mg; do not use autoinjector.
Avoid IM or intravascular delivery.

STORAGE
2-30°C (36-86°F). **Spray/Inj:** Protect from light.

HOW SUPPLIED
Inj: 4mg, 6mg [prefilled syringe], 6mg/0.5mL [vial]; **Spray:** 5mg, 20mg [6^s]; **Tab:** 25mg, 50mg, 100mg

CONTRAINDICATIONS
Ischemic coronary artery disease (CAD) (eg, angina pectoris, history of MI, documented silent ischemia), coronary artery vasospasm (eg, Prinzmetal's angina), Wolff-Parkinson-White syndrome or arrhythmias associated w/ other cardiac accessory conduction pathway disorders, history of stroke or transient ischemic attack, history of hemiplegic/basilar migraine, peripheral vascular disease, ischemic bowel disease, uncontrolled HTN, hypersensitivity to sumatriptan, and severe hepatic impairment. Recent use (w/in 24 hrs) of another 5-HT$_1$ agonist, or of an ergotamine-containing or ergot-type medication (eg, dihydroergotamine, methysergide). Concurrent administration or recent use (w/in 2 weeks) of an MAO-A inhibitor.

WARNINGS/PRECAUTIONS
Use only where a clear diagnosis of migraine headache or (Inj) cluster headache has been established. Reconsider diagnosis of migraine or (Inj) cluster headache before treating any subsequent attacks if patient does not respond to the 1st dose of therapy. Serious cardiac adverse reactions (eg, acute MI) reported. May cause coronary artery vasospasm. Perform cardiovascular (CV) evaluation in triptan-naive patients w/ multiple CV risk factors (eg, increased age, diabetes, HTN, smoking, obesity, strong family history of CAD) prior to therapy; if negative, consider administering 1st dose under medical supervision and perform an ECG immediately following administration. Consider periodic CV evaluation in intermittent long-term users w/ multiple CV risk factors. Sensations of tightness, pain, pressure, and heaviness in the precordium, throat, neck, and jaw, usually noncardiac in origin, reported; perform cardiac evaluation if at high cardiac risk. Life-threatening cardiac rhythm disturbances (eg, ventricular tachycardia, ventricular fibrillation leading to death) reported; d/c if these occur. Cerebral/subarachnoid hemorrhage and stroke reported; d/c therapy if a cerebrovascular event occurs. Patients w/ migraine may be at increased risk of certain cerebrovascular events. Exclude other potentially serious neurological conditions prior to therapy in patients not previously diagnosed w/ migraine or (Inj) cluster headache or in patients who present w/ atypical symptoms. May cause noncoronary vasospastic reactions (eg, peripheral vascular ischemia, GI vascular ischemia/infarction, splenic infarction, Raynaud's syndrome); rule out therapy-related vasospastic reactions before additional therapy is given. May cause transient/permanent blindness and significant partial vision loss. Overuse of acute migraine drugs may lead to exacerbation of headache; detoxification, including drug withdrawal, and treatment of withdrawal symptoms may be necessary. Serotonin syndrome may occur; d/c if suspected. Significant elevation in BP, including hypertensive crisis w/ acute impairment of organ systems, reported. Anaphylactic/anaphylactoid reactions may occur. Seizures reported; caution w/ history of epilepsy or conditions associated w/ a lowered seizure threshold. **Spray/Tab:** Safety of treating >4 headaches/30 days not known. **Spray:** Local irritative symptoms reported.

ADVERSE REACTIONS
Inj: Tingling, warm/hot/burning/pressure sensation, feeling of heaviness, tightness, numbness, flushing, chest/throat discomfort, inj-site reaction, weakness, neck pain/stiffness, dizziness/vertigo, drowsiness/sedation.
Spray: Disorder/discomfort of nasal cavity/sinuses, N/V, bad/unusual taste.
Tab: Paresthesia, warm/cold sensation, chest/neck/throat/jaw pain and other pressure sensations, malaise/fatigue.

DRUG INTERACTIONS
See Contraindications. Serotonin syndrome reported w/ SSRIs, SNRIs, TCAs, or MAOIs.

PREGNANCY AND LACTATION
Pregnancy: Category C.
Lactation: Excreted in human milk (Inj); avoid breastfeeding for 12 hrs after administration.

MECHANISM OF ACTION
Selective 5-HT$_{1B/1D}$ receptor agonist; thought to be due to the agonist effects at the 5-HT$_{1B/1D}$ receptors on intracranial blood vessels and sensory nerves of the trigeminal system, which result in cranial vessel constriction and inhibition of proinflammatory neuropeptide release.

PHARMACOKINETICS
Absorption: Spray: Bioavailability (approx 17%); C_{max}=5ng/mL (5mg), 16ng/mL (20mg). Tab: Bioavailability (approx 15%); C_{max}=18ng/mL (25mg), 51ng/mL (100mg). Inj: Bioavailability (97%); C_{max}=74ng/mL (manual inj, deltoid), 61ng/mL (manual inj, thigh), 52ng/mL (autoinjector, thigh); T_{max}=12 min (manual inj, deltoid). **Distribution:** V_d=2.7L/kg (spray/tab), 50L (Inj); plasma protein binding (approx 14-21%); found in breast milk (Inj). **Metabolism:** Via MAO-A; indole acetic acid (IAA) (major metabolite). **Elimination:** Spray: Urine (3% unchanged, 42% IAA); $T_{1/2}$=2 hrs. Tab: Urine (60%, mostly IAA or the IAA glucuronide), feces (40%); $T_{1/2}$=2.5 hrs. Inj: Urine (22% unchanged, 38% IAA); $T_{1/2}$=115 min.

PATIENT CONSIDERATIONS
Assessment: Confirm diagnosis of migraine or (Inj) cluster headache and exclude other potentially serious neurologic conditions and noncoronary vasospastic reactions prior to therapy. Assess for CV disease, HTN, hemiplegic/basilar migraine, hypersensitivity to drug, and any other conditions where treatment is cautioned or contraindicated. Assess hepatic function, pregnancy/nursing status, and for possible drug interactions. Perform CV evaluation in triptan-naive patients w/ multiple CV risk factors.

Monitoring: Monitor for signs/symptoms of cardiac events, cerebrovascular events, peripheral vascular ischemia, GI vascular ischemia/infarction, serotonin syndrome, hypersensitivity reactions, BP, and other adverse reactions. Perform periodic CV evaluation in intermittent long-term users w/ risk factors for CAD.

Counseling: Inform that therapy may cause CV side effects and anaphylactic/anaphylactoid reactions. Instruct to seek medical attention if such signs/symptoms occur. Inform that use of acute migraine drugs for ≥10 days/month may lead to an exacerbation of headache; encourage to record headache frequency and drug use (eg, by keeping a headache diary). Inform about the risk of serotonin syndrome. Inform that drug may cause somnolence and dizziness; instruct to evaluate ability to perform complex tasks after administration of drug. Inform that medication should not be used during pregnancy unless the potential benefit justifies the potential risk to the fetus; instruct to notify physician if breastfeeding or planning to breastfeed.
Inj: Instruct to read instructions prior to use and advise on proper use, storage, and disposal of inj. Advise to avoid IM or intravascular delivery, and to use inj sites w/ adequate skin and SQ thickness to accommodate length of needle. **Spray:** Inform that local irritation of the nose and throat may occur and that symptoms will generally resolve in <2 hrs. Instruct on proper use of spray and caution to avoid spraying in eyes.

IMLYGIC — talimogene laherparepvec

Rx

Class: Oncolytic viral therapy

ADULT DOSAGE
Melanoma
Local treatment of unresectable cutaneous, subcutaneous, and nodal lesions in patients w/ melanoma recurrent after initial surgery

PEDIATRIC DOSAGE
Pediatric use may not have been established

The total inj volume for each treatment visit should not exceed 4mL for all injected lesions combined

Initial Treatment:
Up to 4mL at a concentration of 10^6 (1 million) plaque-forming units (PFU)/mL

Second Treatment (3 Weeks After Initial Treatment):
Up to 4mL at a concentration of 10^8 (100 million) PFU/mL

All Subsequent Treatments Including Reinitiation (2 Weeks After Previous Treatment):
Up to 4mL at a concentration of 10^8 (100 million) PFU/mL

Continue treatment for at least 6 months unless other treatment is required or until there are no injectable lesions to treat

Reinitiate treatment if new unresectable cutaneous, subcutaneous, or nodal lesions appear after a complete response

ADMINISTRATION
Intralesional route

Administer by inj into cutaneous, subcutaneous, and/or nodal lesions that are visible, palpable, or detectable by ultrasound guidance.

Prioritization of Lesions to be Injected
Initial Treatment:
-Inject largest lesion(s) first.
-Prioritize inj of remaining lesion(s) based on lesion size until max inj volume is reached or until all injectable lesion(s) have been treated.

Second and All Subsequent Treatments:
-Inject any new lesion(s) (lesions that have developed since initial or previous treatment) first.
-Prioritize inj of remaining lesion(s) based on lesion size until max inj volume is reached or until all injectable lesion(s) have been treated.

Inj Volume Determination (Per Lesion)
>5cm Lesion: Up to 4mL inj
>2.5-5cm Lesion: Up to 2mL inj
>1.5-2.5cm Lesion: Up to 1mL inj
>0.5-1.5cm Lesion: Up to 0.5mL inj
≤0.5cm Lesion: Up to 0.1mL inj

When lesions are clustered together, inject them as a single lesion according to above.

Preparation and Handling
Healthcare providers who are immunocompromised or pregnant should not prepare or administer talimogene laherparepvec and should not come into direct contact w/ the inj sites, dressings, or body fluids of treated patients.
Avoid accidental exposure and follow universal biohazard precautions for preparation, administration, and handling.

1. Determine the total volume required for inj, up to 4mL.
2. Thaw frozen vials at room temperature (20-25°C [68-77°F]) until talimogene laherparepvec is liquid (approx 30 min). Do not expose the vial to higher temperatures. Keep the vial in original carton during thawing.
3. Swirl gently. Do not shake.
4. After thawing, administer immediately or store in original vial and carton, protected from light in a refrigerator (2-8°C [36-46°F]) for no longer than the following:
10^6 (1 million) PFU/mL: 12 hrs
10^8 (100 million) PFU/mL: 48 hrs
NOTE: Do not refreeze after thawing. Discard any vial left in the refrigerator longer than the specified times.
5. Prepare sterile syringes and needles. A detachable needle of 18-26G may be used for withdrawal and a detachable needle of 22-26G may be used for inj. Small unit syringes (eg, 0.5mL insulin syringes) are recommended for better inj control.
6. Using aseptic technique, remove the vial cap and withdraw the product from the vial into the syringe(s), noting the total volume. Avoid generating aerosols when loading syringes w/ product, and use a biologic safety cabinet if available.

Administration
1. Treat the inj site w/ a topical or local anesthetic agent, if necessary. Do not inject anesthetic agent directly into the lesion. Inject anesthetic agent around the periphery of the lesion.
2. Using a single insertion point, inject talimogene laherparepvec along multiple tracks as far as the radial reach of the needle allows w/in the lesion to achieve even and complete dispersion. Multiple insertion points may be used if a lesion is larger than the radial reach of the needle.
3. Inject talimogene laherparepvec evenly and completely w/in the lesion by pulling the needle back w/o exiting the lesion. Redirect the needle as many times as necessary while injecting the remainder of the dose. Continue until the full dose is evenly and completely dispersed.
4. When removing the needle, withdraw it from the lesion slowly to avoid leakage of talimogene laherparepvec at the insertion point.
5. Repeat steps 1-4 for other lesions to be injected.

6. Use a new needle any time the needle is completely removed from a lesion and each time a different lesion is injected.

Post-Inj
1. Apply pressure to the inj site(s) w/ sterile gauze for at least 30 sec.
2. Swab the inj site(s) and surrounding area w/ alcohol.
3. Change gloves and cover the injected lesion(s) w/ an absorbent pad and dry occlusive dressing.
4. Wipe the exterior of occlusive dressing w/ alcohol.
5. Advise patients to:
-Keep the inj site(s) covered for at least the 1st week after each treatment visit or longer if the inj site is weeping or oozing.
-Replace the dressing if it falls off.

STORAGE
Store at -90 to -70°C (-130 to -94°F). Protect from light and store in the carton until use.

HOW SUPPLIED
Inj: 10^6 (1 million) PFU/mL, 10^8 (100 million) PFU/mL [1mL]

CONTRAINDICATIONS
Immunocompromised patients, including those w/ a history of primary or acquired immunodeficient states, leukemia, lymphoma, AIDS or other clinical manifestations of infection w/ HIV, and those on immunosuppressive therapy. Pregnant patients.

WARNINGS/PRECAUTIONS
Accidental exposure may lead to transmission of talimogene laherparepvec and herpetic infection. Healthcare providers, close contacts (household members, caregivers, sex partners, or persons sharing the same bed), pregnant women, and newborns should avoid direct contact w/ injected lesions, dressings, or body fluids of treated patients. Caregivers should wear protective gloves when assisting patients in applying or changing occlusive dressings and observe safety precautions for disposal of used dressings, gloves, and cleaning materials. In the event of an accidental exposure, exposed individuals should clean the affected area thoroughly w/ soap and water and/or a disinfectant. If signs or symptoms of herpetic infection develop, the exposed individuals should contact their healthcare provider for appropriate treatment. Patients should avoid touching or scratching inj sites or their occlusive dressings. Patients who develop suspicious herpes-like lesions should follow standard hygienic practices to prevent viral transmission. Patients or close contacts w/ suspected herpetic infections should also contact their healthcare provider to evaluate the lesions. Necrosis or ulceration of tumor tissue may occur; careful wound care and infection precautions are recommended, particularly if tissue necrosis results in open wounds. Impaired healing at the inj site reported. May increase the risk of impaired healing in patients w/ underlying risk factors (eg, previous radiation at the inj site or lesions in poorly vascularized areas); consider risks and benefits of continuing treatment if there is persistent infection or delayed healing of the inj site(s). Immune-mediated events, including glomerulonephritis, vasculitis, pneumonitis, worsening psoriasis, and vitiligo, reported; consider risks and benefits before initiating treatment in patients who have underlying autoimmune disease or before continuing treatment in patients who develop immune-mediated events. Plasmacytoma reported in proximity to the inj site after administration in a patient w/ smoldering multiple myeloma. Consider risks and benefits of treatment in patients w/ multiple myeloma or in whom plasmacytoma develops during treatment.

ADVERSE REACTIONS
Fatigue, chills, pyrexia, nausea, influenza-like illness, inj-site pain.

DRUG INTERACTIONS
Acyclovir or other antiherpetic viral agents may interfere w/ effectiveness; consider the risks and benefits before administering antiviral agents to manage herpetic infection.

PREGNANCY AND LACTATION
Pregnancy: Women of childbearing potential should use an effective method of contraception to prevent pregnancy during treatment. If a pregnant woman has an infection w/ wild-type herpes simplex virus type 1 (primary or reactivation), there is potential for the virus to cross the placental barrier and also a risk of transmission during birth due to viral shedding. While there are no clinical data to date on talimogene laherparepvec infections in pregnant women, there could be a risk to the fetus or neonate if this drug were to act in the same manner.
Lactation: There is no information regarding the presence in human milk, the effects on the breastfed infant, or the effects on milk production. Not for use in nursing.

MECHANISM OF ACTION
Genetically modified oncolytic viral therapy; replicates w/in tumors to produce the immune stimulatory protein GM-CSF. Causes lysis of tumors, followed by release of tumor-derived antigens, which together w/ virally derived GM-CSF may promote an antitumor immune response; exact mechanism is unknown.

PATIENT CONSIDERATIONS
Assessment: Assess for history of primary or acquired immunodeficient states, leukemia, lymphoma, AIDS or other clinical manifestations of infection w/ HIV, immunosuppressive therapy, underlying autoimmune disease, multiple myeloma, pregnancy/nursing status, and possible drug interactions.

Monitoring: Monitor for accidental exposure, herpetic infection, inj-site complications, immune-mediated events, and plasmacytoma at the inj site.

Counseling: Advise to avoid direct contact w/ inj sites, dressings, or body fluids; wear gloves when changing dressing; and avoid touching or scratching inj sites. Advise to keep inj sites covered for at least the first week after each treatment visit or longer if the inj site is weeping or oozing. Advise to dispose of used dressings and cleaning materials in household waste in a sealed plastic bag. Instruct females of childbearing potential to use an effective method of contraception during treatment. Advise that close contacts who are pregnant or immunocompromised should not change dressings or clean inj sites. In case of accidental exposure, instruct to clean the exposed area w/ soap and water and/ or a disinfectant.

effective contraception during therapy if vomiting and/or diarrhea occurs. Advise nursing mothers not to breastfeed during therapy and for 5 months after therapy is completed. Inform that drug may cause reproductive effects (eg, impaired fertility).

IMPAVIDO — miltefosine   Rx
Class: Antileishmanial agent

> May cause fetal harm; do not administer to pregnant women. Obtain a serum or urine pregnancy test in females of reproductive potential prior to prescribing therapy; advise to use effective contraception during therapy and for 5 months after therapy.

ADULT DOSAGE	PEDIATRIC DOSAGE
Leishmaniasis	**Leishmaniasis**
Treatment of visceral, cutaneous, and mucosal leishmaniasis caused by susceptible *Leishmania* species	Treatment of visceral, cutaneous, and mucosal leishmaniasis caused by susceptible *Leishmania* species
30-44kg: 50mg bid w/ food (breakfast and dinner)	**≥12 Years:** **30-44kg:** 50mg bid w/ food (breakfast and dinner)
≥45kg: 50mg tid w/ food (breakfast, lunch, and dinner)	**≥45kg:** 50mg tid w/ food (breakfast, lunch, and dinner)
Treat for 28 consecutive days	Treat for 28 consecutive days

ADMINISTRATION
Oral route

Take w/ food to ameliorate GI adverse reactions.
Swallow caps whole; do not chew or break.

STORAGE
20-25°C (68-77°F); excursions permitted to 15-30°C (59-86°F). Protect from light.

HOW SUPPLIED
Cap: 50mg

CONTRAINDICATIONS
Pregnancy, Sjogren-Larsson syndrome, hypersensitivity to miltefosine or any of its excipients.

WARNINGS/PRECAUTIONS
Leishmania species studied in clinical trials were based on epidemiologic data. There may be geographic variation in clinical response of the same *Leishmania* species to therapy. May cause reproductive effects (eg, impaired fertility). Scrotal pain and decreased/absent ejaculation during therapy reported. Elevations of SrCr reported. Elevations in liver transaminases (ALT, AST) and bilirubin reported in the treatment of visceral leishmaniasis. Vomiting and/or diarrhea commonly occur during administration and may result in volume depletion; encourage fluid intake. Vomiting and/or diarrhea occurring during therapy may affect absorption of oral contraceptives, and therefore compromise their efficacy; additional nonhormonal or alternative method(s) of effective contraception should be used if vomiting and/or diarrhea occur. Thrombocytopenia reported in patients treated for visceral leishmaniasis. Stevens-Johnson syndrome (SJS) reported; d/c if an exfoliative or bullous rash is noted. Avoid breastfeeding for 5 months after therapy.

ADVERSE REACTIONS
N/V, decreased appetite, diarrhea, asthenia, motion sickness, headache, dizziness, abdominal pain, lymphangitis, pruritus, malaise, pyrexia, somnolence.

PREGNANCY AND LACTATION
Category D, not for use in nursing.

MECHANISM OF ACTION
Antileishmanial agent; has not been established. Likely to involve interaction w/ lipids (phospholipids and sterols), including membrane lipids, inhibition of cytochrome c oxidase (mitochondrial function), and apoptosis-like cell death.

PHARMACOKINETICS
Absorption: Administration of multiple doses resulted in different parameters. **Distribution:** Plasma protein binding (98%). **Metabolism:** Slow metabolic breakdown, resulting in the release of choline by phospholipase D-like cleavage; fatty alcohol-containing fragment of miltefosine can enter the metabolism of fatty acids after being oxidized to palmitic acid. **Elimination:** Urine (<0.2%) (visceral leishmaniasis patients).

PATIENT CONSIDERATIONS
Assessment: Assess for drug hypersensitivity, Sjogren-Larsson syndrome, pregnancy/nursing status, and possible drug interactions. Obtain a serum or urine pregnancy test in females of reproductive potential.

Monitoring: Monitor for reproductive effects, vomiting/diarrhea, volume depletion, SJS, and other adverse reactions. Monitor renal function weekly during therapy and for 4 weeks after end of therapy. Monitor liver transaminases and bilirubin. Monitor platelet count during therapy for visceral leishmaniasis.

Counseling: Instruct to complete the full course of therapy. Inform that abdominal pain, N/V, and diarrhea are common side effects of therapy and instruct to inform physician if these GI side effects are severe or persistent. Instruct to consume sufficient fluids to avoid dehydration and, consequently, the risk of kidney injury. Advise women of reproductive potential to use effective contraception during therapy and for 5 months after therapy ends. Advise women who use oral contraceptives to use additional nonhormonal or alternative method(s) of

IMURAN — azathioprine   Rx
Class: Purine antagonist antimetabolite

> Increased risk of malignancy w/ chronic immunosuppression. Malignancy (eg, post-transplant lymphoma, hepatosplenic T-cell lymphoma) reported in patients w/ inflammatory bowel disease. Physician should be familiar w/ this risk as well as mutagenic potential to both men and women and possible hematologic toxicities.

OTHER BRAND NAMES
Azasan

ADULT DOSAGE	PEDIATRIC DOSAGE
Renal Transplant	Pediatric use may not have been established
Adjunct Therapy for Prevention of Rejection in Renal Homotransplantation:	
Initial: 3-5mg/kg/day, beginning at the time of transplant	
Usually given as a single daily dose on the day of, and in a minority of cases 1-3 days before, transplantation	
Maint: 1-3mg/kg/day	
Discontinuation may be necessary for severe hematologic or other toxicity, even if rejection of the homograft may be a consequence of drug withdrawal	
Rheumatoid Arthritis	
Treatment of Active Rheumatoid Arthritis (RA) to Reduce Signs/ Symptoms:	
Initial: 1mg/kg/day (50-100mg) given qd or bid	
Titrate: May increase dose by 0.5mg/ kg/day increments beginning at 6-8 weeks and thereafter by steps at 4-week intervals	
Max: 2.5mg/kg/day	
May be considered refractory if no improvement after 12 weeks	
Maint Therapy:	
Use lowest effective dose; decrease by 0.5mg/kg/day or 25mg/day every 4 weeks to lowest effective dose while other therapy is kept constant	
During treatment, may continue aspirin, NSAIDs, and/or low dose glucocorticoids	

DOSING CONSIDERATIONS
Renal Impairment
Oliguric patients may have delayed clearance; give lower doses

ADMINISTRATION
Oral route

STORAGE
20-25°C (68-77°F). Store in a dry place and protect from light.

HOW SUPPLIED
Tab: 50mg*, (Azasan) 75mg*, 100mg* *scored

CONTRAINDICATIONS
Hypersensitivity to the drug. RA: Pregnancy, patients previously treated w/ alkylating agents (eg, cyclophosphamide, chlorambucil, melphalan).

WARNINGS/PRECAUTIONS
Renal transplant patients are known to have an increased risk of malignancy, predominantly skin cancer and reticulum cell or lymphomatous tumors. Risk of post-transplant lymphomas may be increased w/ aggressive immunosuppressive treatment; maintain therapy at the lowest effective levels. Acute myelogenous leukemia as well as solid tumors reported in patients w/ RA. Severe leukopenia, thrombocytopenia, anemias (eg, macrocytic anemia, pancytopenia), and severe bone marrow suppression may occur. Hematologic toxicities are dose-related and may be more severe in renal transplant patients whose homograft is undergoing rejection. Monitor CBCs, including platelet counts, weekly during the 1st month, twice monthly for the 2nd and 3rd months of therapy, then monthly or more frequently if dose/therapy changes are necessary. Delayed hematologic suppression may occur. Prompt dose reduction or temporary drug withdrawal may be necessary if there is a rapid fall in or persistently low leukocyte count, or other evidence of bone marrow depression. Increased risk for bacterial, viral, fungal, protozoal, and opportunistic infections, including reactivation of latent infections that may lead to serious, including fatal, outcomes. JC virus-associated infection resulting in progressive multifocal leukoencephalopathy (PML) reported; consider reducing the amount of immunosuppression in patients who develop PML. May cause fetal harm. GI hypersensitivity reaction characterized by severe

N/V reported. Myelotoxicity risk may be increased in patients w/ intermediate thiopurine S-methyl transferase (TPMT) activity. Increased risk of severe, life-threatening myelotoxicity in patients w/ low or absent TPMT activity; consider alternative therapies. Caution in patients having one non-functional allele who are at risk for reduced TPMT activity; dose reduction is recommended in patients w/ reduced TPMT activity. TPMT testing cannot be a substitute for CBC monitoring. Consider early drug discontinuation in patients w/ abnormal CBC results that do not respond to dose reduction.

ADVERSE REACTIONS
Hematologic toxicities, infections, N/V.

DRUG INTERACTIONS
See Contraindications. Combined use w/ disease-modifying antirheumatic drugs cannot be recommended. Caution w/ concomitant aminosalicylate derivatives (eg, sulfasalazine, mesalazine, olsalazine); may inhibit TPMT enzyme. Allopurinol inhibits one of the inactivation pathways; reduce azathioprine dose to approx 1/3-1/4 of the usual dose and consider further dose reduction or alternative therapies for patients w/ low or absent TPMT activity. Drugs that may affect leukocyte production (eg, co-trimoxazole) may lead to exaggerated leukopenia, especially in renal transplant recipients. ACE inhibitors may induce anemia and severe leukopenia. May inhibit anticoagulant effect of warfarin. Use of ribavirin for hepatitis C has been reported to induce severe pancytopenia and may increase the risk of azathioprine-related myelotoxicity.

PREGNANCY AND LACTATION
Pregnancy: Category D.
Lactation: Not for use in nursing. Azathioprine or its metabolites are transferred at low levels, both transplacentally and in breast milk.

MECHANISM OF ACTION
Purine antagonist antimetabolite; an imidazolyl derivative of 6-mercaptopurine (6-MP). In homograft survival, it suppresses hypersensitivities of the cell-mediated type and causes variable alterations in antibody production. Immuno-inflammatory response mechanisms not established; suppresses disease manifestation and underlying pathology in autoimmune disease.

PHARMACOKINETICS
Absorption: Well-absorbed; T_{max}=1-2 hrs. **Distribution:** Plasma protein binding (30%); crosses placenta, found in breast milk. **Metabolism:** Liver and erythrocytes (extensive); 6-MP activated to 6-thioguanine nucleotides (major metabolites); 6-MP inactivated via thiol methylation by TPMT and oxidation by xanthine oxidase. **Elimination:** Urine; $T_{1/2}$=5 hrs (decay rate for all S-containing metabolites of azathioprine).

PATIENT CONSIDERATIONS
Assessment: Assess for drug hypersensitivity, renal/hepatic dysfunction, previous treatment of RA w/ alkylating agents, pregnancy/nursing status, and for possible drug interactions. Conduct TPMT genotyping/phenotyping to identify absent or reduced TPMT activity.

Monitoring: Monitor for signs/symptoms of cytopenias, malignancies, infections, GI hypersensitivity reactions, and other adverse reactions. Monitor CBCs, including platelet counts, weekly during the 1st month, twice monthly for the 2nd and 3rd months of therapy, then monthly or more frequently if dose/therapy changes are necessary. Periodically monitor serum transaminases, alkaline phosphatase, and bilirubin levels. Consider TPMT testing in patients w/ abnormal CBC results unresponsive to dose reduction.

Counseling: Inform about necessity of periodic blood counts while on therapy and risks of malignancy and infection. Instruct to report to physician any unusual bleeding/bruising or signs/symptoms of infections. Educate about proper dosage instructions, especially w/ impaired renal function or concomitant use w/ allopurinol. Inform of the potential risks during pregnancy and nursing; advise to notify physician if pregnant or nursing. Instruct patients w/ increased risk for skin cancer to limit exposure to sunlight and UV light (eg, wearing protective clothing, using a sunscreen).

INCRUSE ELLIPTA — umeclidinium   Rx

Class: Anticholinergic

ADULT DOSAGE	PEDIATRIC DOSAGE
Chronic Obstructive Pulmonary Disease	Pediatric use may not have been established
Long-Term Maint Treatment of Airflow Obstruction: 1 inh qd at the same time every day; do not use >1 time q24h	

DOSING CONSIDERATIONS
Hepatic Impairment
Severe: Not studied

ADMINISTRATION
Oral inh route

STORAGE
20-25°C (68-77°F); excursions permitted from 15-30°C (59-86°F). Store in a dry place away from direct heat or sunlight. Store inside the unopened moisture-protective foil tray and only remove from the tray immediately before initial use. Discard 6 weeks after opening the foil tray or when the counter reads "0" (after all blisters have been used), whichever comes 1st.

HOW SUPPLIED
Powder, Inh: 62.5mcg/blister [7, 30 blisters]

CONTRAINDICATIONS
Severe hypersensitivity to milk proteins, hypersensitivity to umeclidinium or any of the excipients.

WARNINGS/PRECAUTIONS
Do not initiate during rapidly deteriorating or potentially life-threatening episodes of COPD. Not for relief of acute symptoms. May produce paradoxical bronchospasm; treat immediately w/ an inhaled, short-acting bronchodilator; d/c umeclidinium and institute alternative therapy. Hypersensitivity reactions may occur. Caution w/ narrow-angle glaucoma and urinary retention. Monitor for signs and symptoms of acute narrow-angle glaucoma and urinary retention (especially in those w/ prostatic hyperplasia or bladder neck obstruction).

ADVERSE REACTIONS
Nasopharyngitis, URTI, cough.

DRUG INTERACTIONS
Avoid w/ other anticholinergic-containing drugs; may increase anticholinergic adverse effects.

PREGNANCY AND LACTATION
Pregnancy: Category C.
Lactation: Not for use in nursing.

MECHANISM OF ACTION
Anticholinergic (long-acting) bronchodilator; exhibits effects through inhibition of M3 receptor at the smooth muscle, leading to bronchodilation.

PHARMACOKINETICS
Absorption: Lung; T_{max}=5-15 min. **Distribution:** V_d=86L (IV); plasma protein binding (89%). **Metabolism:** Via CYP2D6; hydroxylation, O-dealkylation followed by glucuronidation. **Elimination:** Feces (92%), urine (<1%); $T_{1/2}$=11 hrs.

PATIENT CONSIDERATIONS
Assessment: Assess for hypersensitivity to drug or to milk proteins, COPD status, narrow-angle glaucoma, urinary retention, prostatic hyperplasia, bladder neck obstruction, pregnancy/nursing status, and possible drug interactions.

Monitoring: Monitor for deteriorating disease, paradoxical bronchospasm, hypersensitivity reactions, narrow-angle glaucoma, urinary retention, and other adverse reactions.

Counseling: Inform that drug is not meant to relieve acute symptoms of COPD. Advise that acute symptoms should be treated w/ a rescue inhaler (eg, albuterol). Instruct to seek medical attention immediately if experiencing worsening of symptoms, decreased effectiveness of the rescue inhaler, or a need for more inhalations than usual of the rescue inhaler. Advise not to d/c therapy w/o physician guidance. Instruct to d/c therapy if paradoxical bronchospasm occurs. Inform about risk of worsening narrow-angle glaucoma and urinary retention; instruct to consult physician immediately if any signs/symptoms develop. Advise to contact physician if pregnancy occurs while on therapy. Inform that the inhaler is not reusable and advise not to take the inhaler apart.

INDERAL LA — propranolol hydrochloride   Rx

Class: Nonselective beta blocker

ADULT DOSAGE	PEDIATRIC DOSAGE
Hypertension	Pediatric use may not have been established
Initial: 80mg qd	
Titrate: May increase to 120mg qd or higher until adequate BP control is achieved	
Maint: 120-160mg qd; 640mg/day may be required	
Angina Pectoris	
To decrease angina frequency and increase exercise tolerance	
Initial: 80mg qd	
Titrate: Increase gradually at 3- to 7-day intervals until optimal response is obtained	
Maint: 160mg qd	
Max: 320mg qd	
Reduce dose gradually over a period of a few weeks if therapy is to be discontinued	
Migraine	
For Prophylaxis:	
Initial: 80mg qd; may increase gradually to achieve optimal response	
Usual: 160-240mg qd	
D/C gradually over a period of several weeks if a satisfactory response is not obtained w/in 4-6 weeks after reaching maximal dose	
Hypertrophic Subaortic Stenosis	
Usual: 80-160mg qd	

DOSING CONSIDERATIONS
Elderly
Start at lower end of dosing range

ADMINISTRATION
Oral route

STORAGE
20-25°C (68-77°F); excursions permitted to 15-30°C (59-86°F). Protect from light, moisture, freezing, and excessive heat.

HOW SUPPLIED
Cap, Extended-Release: 60mg, 80mg, 120mg, 160mg

CONTRAINDICATIONS
Cardiogenic shock, sinus bradycardia and greater than 1st-degree block, bronchial asthma, known hypersensitivity to propranolol HCl.

WARNINGS/PRECAUTIONS
Exacerbation of angina and MI following abrupt discontinuation reported; when discontinuation is planned, reduce dose gradually over at least a few weeks. Reinstitute therapy if exacerbation of angina occurs upon interruption and take other measures for management of angina pectoris; follow same procedure in patients at risk of occult atherosclerotic heart disease who are given propranolol for other indications since coronary artery disease may be unrecognized. Hypersensitivity reactions (eg, anaphylactic/anaphylactoid reactions) and cutaneous reactions (eg, Stevens-Johnson syndrome, toxic epidermal necrolysis, exfoliative dermatitis) reported. May precipitate more severe failure in patients w/ CHF; avoid w/ overt CHF and caution in patients w/ history of heart failure (HF) who are well compensated and are receiving diuretics prn. Continued use in patients w/o history of HF may cause cardiac failure. Caution w/ bronchospastic lung disease; may provoke a bronchial asthmatic attack. Chronically administered therapy should not be routinely withdrawn prior to major surgery; however, may augment risks of general anesthesia and surgical procedures. May prevent the appearance of signs/symptoms of acute hypoglycemia, especially w/ labile insulin-dependent diabetics; may be more difficult to adjust insulin dose. Hypoglycemia reported. May mask certain clinical signs of hyperthyroidism; abrupt withdrawal may be followed by an exacerbation of symptoms of hyperthyroidism, including thyroid storm. Associated w/ severe bradycardia requiring treatment w/ a pacemaker in patients w/ Wolff-Parkinson-White (WPW) syndrome and tachycardia. Caution w/ hepatic/renal impairment. May reduce IOP. Patients w/ history of severe anaphylactic reaction to a variety of allergens may be more reactive to repeated accidental/diagnostic/therapeutic challenge; may be unresponsive to usual doses of epinephrine. Lab test interactions may occur (eg, changes to thyroid function tests). Not for treatment of hypertensive emergencies. Inderal LA should not be considered a simple mg-for-mg substitute for Inderal.

ADVERSE REACTIONS
Bradycardia, CHF, hypotension, lightheadedness, mental depression, N/V, agranulocytosis, bronchospasm, urticaria, alopecia.

DRUG INTERACTIONS
Caution w/ drugs that have an effect on CYP2D6, 1A2, or 2C19 metabolic pathways; may lead to clinically relevant drug interactions and changes on its efficacy and/or toxicity. Alcohol may increase levels. Propafenone and amiodarone may cause additive effects. Quinidine may increase levels and may cause postural hypotension. Reduced clearance of lidocaine and lidocaine toxicity reported following coadministration. Caution w/ drugs that slow atrioventricular (AV) nodal conduction (eg, digitalis, lidocaine, calcium channel blocker); increased risk of bradycardia w/ digitalis. Bradycardia, HF, and cardiovascular collapse reported w/ verapamil. Bradycardia, hypotension, high-degree heart block, and HF reported w/ diltiazem. ACE inhibitors may cause hypotension, particularly in the setting of acute MI. May antagonize effects of clonidine; administer cautiously to patients withdrawing from clonidine. May prolong 1st dose hypotension w/ prazosin. Postural hypotension reported w/ terazosin or doxazosin. May cause excessive reduction of resting sympathetic nervous activity w/ catecholamine-depleting drugs (eg, reserpine). May experience uncontrolled HTN w/ epinephrine. Effects can be reversed by β-receptor agonists (eg, dobutamine, isoproterenol). May reduce sensitivity to dobutamine stress echocardiography in patients undergoing evaluation for myocardial ischemia. Indomethacin may reduce efficacy and NSAIDs may blunt antihypertensive effects. May exacerbate hypotensive effects of MAOIs or TCAs. May depress myocardial contractility w/ methoxyflurane and trichloroethylene. May increase levels of warfarin; monitor PT. Hypotension and cardiac arrest reported w/ haloperidol. May lower T3 concentration w/ thyroxine.

PREGNANCY AND LACTATION
Pregnancy: Category C.
Lactation: Excreted in human milk; caution in nursing.

MECHANISM OF ACTION
Nonselective β-adrenergic receptor blocker; has not been established. Thought to decrease cardiac output, inhibit renin release by the kidneys, and lessen tonic sympathetic nerve outflow from vasomotor centers in the brain.

PHARMACOKINETICS
Absorption: Almost complete; T_{max}=6 hrs. **Distribution:** V_d=4L/kg; plasma protein binding (90%); crosses blood brain barrier and placenta; found in breast milk. **Metabolism:** Liver (extensive); CYP2D6 (hydroxylation), CYP1A2, 2D6 (oxidation), N-dealkylation, glucuronidation; propranolol glucuronide, naphthyloxylactic acid, glucuronic acid, sulfate conjugates of 4-hydroxylpropranolol (major metabolites). **Elimination:** $T_{1/2}$=10 hrs.

PATIENT CONSIDERATIONS
Assessment: Assess for cardiogenic shock, sinus bradycardia, AV heart block, bronchial asthma, CHF, bronchospastic lung disease, hyperthyroidism, diabetes, WPW syndrome, tachycardia, hepatic/renal impairment, history of HF, risk for occult atherosclerotic heart disease, hypersensitivity to drug, pregnancy/nursing status, and possible drug interactions.
Monitoring: Monitor for signs/symptoms of cardiac failure, hypoglycemia, decreased IOP, hyperthyroidism, withdrawal symptoms, hypersensitivity reactions, and other adverse reactions. Monitor PT w/ warfarin.
Counseling: Inform of the risks/benefits of therapy. Instruct not to interrupt or d/c therapy w/o consulting physician. Inform that therapy may interfere w/ glaucoma screening test.

INDOMETHACIN — indomethacin   Rx
Class: NSAID

> NSAIDs cause an increased risk of serious cardiovascular (CV) thrombotic events, including MI and stroke, which can be fatal. This risk may occur early in treatment and may increase w/ duration of use. Contraindicated in the setting of CABG surgery. NSAIDs cause an increased risk of serious GI adverse events (eg, bleeding, ulceration, stomach/intestinal perforation), which can be fatal and can occur at any time during use and w/o warning symptoms; elderly patients and patients w/ a prior history of peptic ulcer disease and/or GI bleeding are at a greater risk.

OTHER BRAND NAMES
Indocin

ADULT DOSAGE
Ankylosing Spondylitis
Moderate to Severe Active Stages:
Initial: 25mg (5mL) bid-tid
Titrate: May increase by 25mg (5mL) or 50mg (10mL) at weekly intervals
Max: 150-200mg (30-40mL)/day

May give a large portion (up to a max of 100mg [20mL]) of the total daily dose hs in patients who have persistent night pain and/or morning stiffness

Rheumatoid Arthritis
Moderate to Severe Active Stages (Including Acute Flares of Chronic Disease):
Initial: 25mg (5mL) bid-tid
Titrate: May increase by 25mg (5mL) or 50mg (10mL) at weekly intervals
Max: 150-200mg (30-40mL)/day

May give a large portion (up to a max of 100mg [20mL]) of the total daily dose hs in patients who have persistent night pain and/or morning stiffness

Osteoarthritis
Moderate to Severe Active Stages:
Initial: 25mg (5mL) bid-tid
Titrate: May increase by 25mg (5mL) or 50mg (10mL) at weekly intervals
Max: 150-200mg (30-40mL)/day

May give a large portion (up to a max of 100mg [20mL]) of the total daily dose hs in patients who have persistent night pain and/or morning stiffness

Bursitis/Tendinitis
Acute Painful Shoulder:
Active Stages:
75-150mg (15-30mL)/day given in 3 or 4 divided doses; d/c after signs/symptoms of inflammation have been controlled for several days
Usual Duration: 7-14 days

Acute Gouty Arthritis
Active Stages:
50mg (10mL) tid until pain is tolerable, then rapidly reduce dose to complete cessation of therapy

PEDIATRIC DOSAGE
General Dosing
Safety and effectiveness in patients ≤14 yrs of age has not been established and should not be prescribed unless toxicity or lack of efficacy associated w/ other drugs warrants the risk

≥2 Years:
Suggested Dose:
Initial: 1-2mg/kg/day given in divided doses
Max: 3mg/kg/day or 150-200mg/day, whichever is less

As symptoms subside, reduce the total daily dose to the lowest level required to control symptoms, or d/c drug

----

DOSING CONSIDERATIONS
Elderly
If the anticipated benefit outweighs the potential risks, start at lower end of dosing range; monitor for adverse effects

Adverse Reactions
If minor adverse effects develop as the dose is increased, reduce dose rapidly to a tolerated dose and observe closely.
If severe adverse reactions occur, d/c therapy; after the acute phase of the disease is under control, attempt to reduce the daily dose repeatedly until the patient is receiving the smallest effective dose or the drug is discontinued.

ADMINISTRATION
Oral route

STORAGE
Cap: 20-25°C (68-77°F). Protect from light. **Oral Sus:** <30°C (86°F); avoid temperatures >50°C (122°F). Do not freeze.

HOW SUPPLIED
Cap: 25mg, 50mg; **Oral Sus:** (Indocin) 25mg/5mL [237mL]

CONTRAINDICATIONS
Known hypersensitivity (eg, anaphylactic reactions, serious skin reactions) to indomethacin or any components of the drug product; history of asthma, urticaria, or allergic-type reactions w/ aspirin (ASA) or other NSAIDs; in the setting of CABG surgery.

WARNINGS/PRECAUTIONS
Use the lowest effective dose for the shortest duration possible. Increased CV thrombotic risk at higher doses reported. Avoid use in patients w/ a recent MI unless benefits outweigh the risks of recurrent CV thrombotic events; if used, monitor for signs of cardiac ischemia. Increased risk for GI bleeding w/ longer duration of NSAID therapy, older age, poor general health status, and advanced liver disease and/or coagulopathy; avoid use in patients at higher risk unless benefits are expected to outweigh the increased risk of bleeding. Consider alternate therapies other than NSAIDs for patients at higher risk and patients w/ active GI bleeding. Promptly initiate evaluation and treatment if a serious GI adverse event is suspected; d/c until a serious GI adverse event is ruled out. Hepatotoxicity reported; d/c immediately and perform a clinical evaluation if clinical signs/symptoms consistent w/ liver disease develop, or if systemic manifestations occur. May cause new onset HTN or worsen preexisting HTN. Fluid retention and edema reported. Avoid use in patients w/ severe heart failure (HF) unless benefits outweigh risks; monitor for signs of worsening HF if used. Renal papillary necrosis and other renal injury reported w/ long-term use. Renal toxicity also reported in patients in whom renal prostaglandins have a compensatory role in the maintenance of renal perfusion; increased risk w/ renal/hepatic dysfunction, dehydration, hypovolemia, and HF, and in the elderly. Correct volume status in dehydrated or hypovolemic patients prior to initiating therapy. Avoid use in patients w/ advanced renal disease unless the benefits are expected to outweigh the risk; monitor for signs of worsening renal function if used in patients w/ advanced renal disease. Hyperkalemia reported. Associated w/ anaphylactic reactions in patients w/ and w/o known hypersensitivity to indomethacin and in patients w/ ASA-sensitive asthma. Monitor for changes in the signs/symptoms of asthma in patients w/ preexisting asthma (w/o known ASA sensitivity). May cause serious skin reactions (eg, exfoliative dermatitis, Stevens-Johnson syndrome, toxic epidermal necrolysis); d/c at 1st appearance of skin rash/hypersensitivity. Anemia reported; monitor Hgb or Hct if signs/symptoms of anemia develop. May increase the risk of bleeding events; coagulation disorders may increase this risk. May mask inflammation and fever. May aggravate depression or other psychiatric disturbances, epilepsy, and parkinsonism; use w/ caution. D/C if severe CNS adverse reactions develop. May impair mental/physical abilities. Corneal deposits and retinal disturbances, including those of the macula, reported w/ prolonged therapy; d/c if such changes are observed. Perform ophthalmologic examination at periodic intervals in patients receiving prolonged therapy. Not indicated for long-term treatment. Lab test interactions may occur.

ADVERSE REACTIONS
Headache, dizziness, nausea, dyspepsia.

DRUG INTERACTIONS
Drugs that interfere w/ serotonin reuptake may potentiate the risk of bleeding. Synergistic effect on bleeding w/ anticoagulants (eg, warfarin); monitor for signs of bleeding w/ concomitant anticoagulants, antiplatelet agents (eg, ASA), SSRIs, and SNRIs. May increase risk of GI bleeding w/ use of oral corticosteroids, anticoagulants, and SSRIs; smoking; and alcohol use. ASA may increase risk of bleeding and serious GI events; concomitant use w/ analgesic doses of ASA is not recommended. Monitor patients more closely for GI bleeding w/ concomitant use of low-dose ASA for cardiac prophylaxis. May diminish antihypertensive effect of ACE inhibitors, ARBs, and β-blockers (eg, propranolol); monitor BP. Coadministration w/ ACE inhibitors or ARBs may result in deterioration of renal function (including possible acute renal failure) in patients who are elderly or volume-depleted (including those on diuretic therapy), or who have renal impairment; monitor for worsening renal function and ensure adequate hydration when these drugs are administered concomitantly. May reduce the natriuretic effect of loop diuretics (eg, furosemide) and thiazide diuretics; observe for signs of worsening renal function, in addition to assuring diuretic efficacy including antihypertensive effects. The addition of triamterene to a maintenance schedule of indomethacin resulted in reversible acute renal failure; indomethacin and triamterene should not be administered together. Consider potential effects of indomethacin and potassium-sparing diuretics on K^+ levels and renal function when administered concurrently. May increase digoxin serum concentrations and prolong the $T_{1/2}$ of digoxin; monitor digoxin levels. May elevate plasma lithium levels and reduce renal lithium clearance; monitor for signs of lithium toxicity. May increase the risk for methotrexate (MTX) toxicity; monitor for MTX toxicity. May increase cyclosporine's nephrotoxicity; monitor for signs of worsening renal function. Concomitant use w/ other NSAIDs or salicylates (eg, diflunisal, salsalate) increases the risk of GI toxicity. Combined use w/ diflunisal may be particularly hazardous; diflunisal causes significantly higher plasma levels of indomethacin and was associated w/ fatal GI hemorrhage in some patients. Concomitant use w/ other NSAIDs or salicylates, especially diflunisal, is not recommended. Concomitant use w/ pemetrexed may increase the risk of pemetrexed-associated myelosuppression, renal, and GI toxicity; refer to prescribing information for further information. Probenecid may increase plasma levels; use lower total daily dose of indomethacin during concomitant use and when increases in the dose of indomethacin are made, increase cautiously and in small increments.

PREGNANCY AND LACTATION
Pregnancy: Use of NSAIDs during the 3rd trimester of pregnancy increases the risk of premature closure of the fetal ductus arteriosus. Avoid use in pregnant women starting at 30 weeks of gestation (3rd trimester).
Lactation: Based on available published clinical data, indomethacin may be present in human milk. Caution in nursing.
Reproductive Potential: May delay or prevent rupture of ovarian follicles, which has been associated w/ reversible infertility in some women. Small studies in women treated w/ NSAIDs have also shown a reversible delay in ovulation. Consider withdrawal of therapy in women who have difficulties conceiving or who are undergoing investigation of infertility.

MECHANISM OF ACTION
NSAID; mechanism not completely understood but involves inhibition of COX-1 and COX-2. Has analgesic, anti-inflammatory, and antipyretic properties. Mode of action may be due to a decrease of prostaglandins in peripheral tissues.

PHARMACOKINETICS
Absorption: Readily absorbed. (Cap) Bioavailability (100%); C_{max}=1-2mcg/mL; T_{max}=2 hrs. **Distribution:** Plasma protein binding (99%); crosses blood-brain barrier and placenta; found in breast milk. **Metabolism:** Desmethyl, desbenzoyl, desmethyldesbenzoyl (metabolites). **Elimination:** Urine (60%), feces (33%, 1.5% unchanged); $T_{1/2}$=4.5 hrs.

PATIENT CONSIDERATIONS
Assessment: Assess for history of asthma, urticaria, or other allergic-type reactions w/ previous use of ASA or other NSAIDs; preexisting asthma; CV disease (CVD) or risk factors for CVD; HTN; history of peptic ulcer disease or GI bleeding; coagulation disorders; renal/hepatic impairment; pregnancy/nursing status; or any other conditions where treatment is contraindicated or cautioned. Assess volume status. Assess for possible drug interactions. Obtain baseline BP, CBC, and chemistry profile.

Monitoring: Monitor for signs/symptoms of CV thrombotic events; cardiac ischemia in patients w/ a recent MI; GI bleeding/ulceration and perforation; hepatotoxicity; new or worsening HTN; HF; edema; renal papillary necrosis and other renal injury; hyperkalemia; anaphylactic reactions; serious skin reactions; anemia; ocular/CNS effects; and other adverse reactions. Monitor BP during initiation of therapy and throughout the course of therapy. Monitor for signs of bleeding in patients on concomitant therapy w/ anticoagulants, antiplatelet agents, SSRIs, or SNRIs. Monitor renal function in patients w/ renal/hepatic impairment, HF, dehydration, or hypovolemia. Monitor CBC and chemistry profiles periodically during long-term treatment.

Counseling: Inform of the benefits/risks of therapy. Inform of potential for CV thrombotic events, GI adverse events, and worsening CHF/edema, and advise of symptoms; instruct to report any symptoms to healthcare provider immediately. Inform of the potential for hepatotoxicity, and advise of signs/symptoms; if signs/symptoms occur, instruct to d/c and seek immediate medical therapy. Instruct to seek immediate emergency help if signs of an anaphylactic reaction occur. Advise to d/c immediately if any type of rash develops and to contact healthcare provider as soon as possible. Advise females of reproductive potential who desire pregnancy that therapy may be associated w/ a reversible delay in ovulation. Instruct pregnant women to avoid use starting at 30 weeks of gestation. Advise patient not to use other NSAIDs or salicylates (eg, diflunisal, salsalate) concomitantly; notify of the presence of NSAIDs in OTC medications for colds, fever, or insomnia. Advise patient not to use low-dose ASA concomitantly w/o talking to healthcare provider.

INDOMETHACIN EXTENDED-RELEASE – indomethacin Rx

Class: NSAID

> NSAIDs may cause an increased risk of serious cardiovascular (CV) thrombotic events, including MI and stroke, which may be fatal; increased risk w/ duration of use. Increased risk of serious GI adverse events, including bleeding, ulceration, and perforation of the stomach or intestines; elderly patients are at a greater risk. Contraindicated in the setting of CABG surgery.

OTHER BRAND NAMES
Indocin SR (Discontinued)

ADULT DOSAGE
Rheumatoid Arthritis

Moderate to Severe, Including Acute Flares of Chronic Disease:
Initial: 75mg/day
Titrate: May increase to 150mg/day (given as 75mg bid)
Max: 150mg/day

Ankylosing Spondylitis

Moderate to Severe:
Initial: 75mg/day
Titrate: May increase to 150mg/day (given as 75mg bid)
Max: 150mg/day

Osteoarthritis

Moderate to Severe:
Initial: 75mg/day
Titrate: May increase to 150mg/day (given as 75mg bid)
Max: 150mg/day

PEDIATRIC DOSAGE
General Dosing

Safety and effectiveness in patients <14 yrs of age have not been established

>14 Years:
Initial: 75mg/day
Titrate: May increase to 150mg/day (given as 75mg bid)
Max: 150mg/day

Bursitis/Tendinitis
Acute Painful Shoulder:
Initial: 75-150mg/day for 7-14 days
Titrate: May increase to 150mg/day (given as 75mg bid)
D/C after signs/symptoms of inflammation have been controlled for several days

----

DOSING CONSIDERATIONS
Adverse Reactions
Minor: Reduce dose rapidly to a tolerated dose and monitor closely
Severe: Stop therapy; repeatedly attempt to reduce daily dose after acute phase of disease is under control, until smallest effective dose or therapy is discontinued

ADMINISTRATION
Oral route

Take w/ food, immediately after meals, or w/ antacids.

STORAGE
20-25°C (68-77°F). Protect from moisture.

HOW SUPPLIED
Cap, Extended-Release: 75mg

CONTRAINDICATIONS
Known hypersensitivity to indomethacin; history of asthma, urticaria, or allergic-type reactions w/ aspirin (ASA) or other NSAIDs; treatment in the setting of CABG surgery.

WARNINGS/PRECAUTIONS
May be substituted for all indications of indomethacin cap except acute gouty arthritis. Use lowest effective dose for the shortest duration possible. Increased CV thrombotic risk at higher doses reported. Avoid use in patients w/ a recent MI unless benefits outweigh the risks; if used, monitor for signs of cardiac ischemia. May lead to onset of new HTN or worsening of preexisting HTN; monitor BP closely. Avoid use in patients w/ severe heart failure (HF) unless benefits outweigh the risks; if used, monitor for signs of worsening HF. Fluid retention and edema reported. Extreme caution w/ a prior history of ulcer disease or GI bleeding. Increased risk of GI bleeding w/ prolonged NSAID therapy, smoking, alcohol use, older age, and poor general health status; d/c if serious GI adverse event occurs. Renal papillary necrosis and other renal injury reported w/ long-term use. Renal toxicity reported; increased risk w/ renal/hepatic impairment, HF, and elderly. Not recommended w/ advanced renal disease; if therapy must be initiated, closely monitor renal function. Anaphylactoid reactions may occur; avoid in patients w/ ASA triad. May cause serious skin adverse events (eg, exfoliative dermatitis, Stevens-Johnson syndrome, toxic epidermal necrolysis); d/c at the 1st appearance of skin rash or any other signs of hypersensitivity. Avoid in late pregnancy; may cause premature closure of ductus arteriosus. Not a substitute for corticosteroid or treatment for corticosteroid insufficiency. May mask signs of inflammation and fever. Contains tartrazine, which may cause allergic type reactions (including bronchial asthma) in susceptible patients. May cause elevations of LFTs or severe hepatic reactions (eg, jaundice, fulminant hepatitis, liver necrosis, hepatic failure); d/c if abnormal LFTs persist or worsen, or liver disease or systemic manifestations occur. Anemia may occur; w/ long-term use, monitor Hgb/Hct if signs or symptoms of anemia develop. May inhibit platelet aggregation and prolong bleeding time; carefully monitor patients w/ coagulation disorders. Caution w/ preexisting asthma and avoid w/ ASA-sensitive asthma. Caution in elderly or debilitated patients.

ADVERSE REACTIONS
Headache, dizziness, N/V, dyspepsia.

DRUG INTERACTIONS
Avoid w/ ASA and other salicylates; may increase risk of GI side effects. Risk of renal toxicity w/ diuretics and ACE inhibitors. Coadministration may decrease efficacy and reduce natriuretic effect of thiazides or loop diuretics; monitor for signs of renal failure and diuretic efficacy. May diminish antihypertensive effect of ACE inhibitors. May decrease lithium clearance; monitor for toxicity. May enhance methotrexate toxicity; caution w/ concomitant use. Synergistic effect on GI bleeding w/ warfarin. May increase risk of serious GI bleeding when used concomitantly w/ oral corticosteroids or anticoagulants, alcohol, or smoking; carefully monitor patients receiving anticoagulants.

PREGNANCY AND LACTATION
Pregnancy: Category C.
Lactation: Not for use in nursing.

MECHANISM OF ACTION
NSAID; has not been established; exhibits antipyretic, analgesic, and anti-inflammatory properties. Suspected to inhibit prostaglandin synthesis.

PHARMACOKINETICS
Distribution: Plasma protein binding (99%); crosses blood-brain barrier and placenta. **Metabolism:** Desmethyl, desbenzoyl, desmethyl-desbenzoyl (metabolites). **Elimination:** Urine (60%), feces (33%); $T_{1/2}$=4.5 hrs.

PATIENT CONSIDERATIONS
Assessment: Confirm use is not in the setting of CABG surgery. Assess for history of asthma, urticaria or allergic-type reactions after previous use of ASA or other NSAIDs, CV disorders, HTN, HF, history of ulcer disease or GI bleeding, ASA triad, anemia, renal/hepatic impairment, pregnancy/nursing status, coagulation disorders, tobacco/alcohol use, and possible drug interactions. Obtain baseline BP.

Monitoring: Monitor for signs/symptoms of GI events, CV thrombotic events, HTN, allergic or skin reactions, hematological effects (eg, anemia, prolongation of

bleeding time), renal injury/toxicity, hepatotoxicity, and other adverse reactions. Monitor BP, CBC, and chemistry profile periodically.

Counseling: Inform of potential serious side effects. Advise to seek medical attention if signs and symptoms of CV events, GI tract ulcerations or bleeding, skin reactions, CHF, hepatotoxicity, or anaphylactoid reactions occur. Inform of risks if used during pregnancy.

INLYTA — axitinib
Class: Kinase inhibitor

Rx

ADULT DOSAGE	PEDIATRIC DOSAGE
Advanced Renal Cell Carcinoma	Pediatric use may not have been established
Initial: 5mg bid (q12h)	

DOSING CONSIDERATIONS
Concomitant Medications
Strong CYP3A4/5 Inhibitors:
Avoid coadministration, but if needed, decrease dose by half and increase or decrease subsequent doses based on individual safety and tolerability
Strong CYP3A4/5 Inhibitors Discontinuation:
Allow 3-5 half-lives of CYP3A4/5 inhibitor to elapse after discontinuation before returning to dose used prior to coadministration

Hepatic Impairment
Moderate (Child-Pugh Class B): Reduce dose by half
Titrate: Increase or decrease dose based on individual safety and tolerability

Adverse Reactions
May require temporary interruption or permanent discontinuation, and/or dose reduction to 3mg bid
May further reduce to 2mg bid if needed

Other Important Considerations
Normotensive/No Concomitant Antihypertensive/Tolerated for ≥2 Consecutive Weeks w/ No Adverse Reaction >Grade 2:
May increase to 7mg bid, and further to 10mg bid (using the same criteria)

ADMINISTRATION
Oral route

Take w/ or w/o food
Swallow whole w/ a glass of water

STORAGE
20-25°C (68-77°F); excursions permitted to 15-30°C (59-86°F).

HOW SUPPLIED
Tab: 1mg, 5mg

WARNINGS/PRECAUTIONS
HTN/Hypertensive crisis reported; treat prn with standard antihypertensive therapy. Reduce dose if persistent HTN occurs despite antihypertensive therapy; d/c if HTN is severe and persistent or if hypertensive crisis develops. Arterial/venous thromboembolic events reported; caution with history of or risk for arterial/venous thromboembolic events. Hemorrhagic events reported; do not use in patients with evidence of untreated brain metastasis or recent active GI bleeding. Temporarily interrupt treatment if any bleeding requiring medical intervention occurs. Cardiac failure reported; management may require permanent discontinuation of therapy. GI perforation/fistulas, hypothyroidism, and hyperthyroidism reported. Treat thyroid dysfunction according to standard medical practice to maintain euthyroid state. D/C treatment at least 24 hrs prior to surgery; resume therapy after surgery based on clinical judgment of adequate wound healing. D/C if reversible posterior leukoencephalopathy (RPLS) occurs. Proteinuria reported; reduce dose or interrupt temporarily if moderate to severe proteinuria develops. Increased ALT reported. Caution with moderate hepatic impairment and with end-stage renal disease (CrCl <15mL/min). May cause fetal harm.

ADVERSE REACTIONS
Diarrhea, HTN, fatigue, decreased appetite, N/V, dysphonia, palmar-plantar erythrodysesthesia syndrome, weight decrease, asthenia, constipation, hypothyroidism, cough, mucosal inflammation, arthralgia, stomatitis.

DRUG INTERACTIONS
See Dosing Considerations. Avoid with grapefruit, grapefruit juice, and strong CYP3A4/5 inducers (eg, rifampin, dexamethasone, phenytoin, St. John's wort). Moderate CYP3A4/5 inducers (eg, bosentan, efavirenz, etravirine) may reduce exposure; avoid use if possible.

PREGNANCY AND LACTATION
Category D, not for use in nursing.

MECHANISM OF ACTION
Kinase inhibitor; inhibits receptor tyrosine kinases, including vascular endothelial growth factor receptors (VEGFR)-1, VEGFR-2, and VEGFR-3, resulting in inhibition of VEGF-mediated endothelial cell proliferation, cell survival, and tumor growth.

PHARMACOKINETICS
Absorption: (Single 5mg dose) Absolute bioavailability (58%); C_{max}=27.8ng/mL, AUC=265ng•hr/mL, T_{max}=2.5-4.1 hrs (median). **Distribution:** V_d=160L; plasma protein binding (>99%). **Metabolism:** Liver via CYP3A4/5 (primary), CYP1A2, 2C19, and UGT1A1 (lesser extent). **Elimination:** Feces (41%, 12% unchanged), urine (23%, metabolites); $T_{1/2}$=2.5-6.1 hrs.

PATIENT CONSIDERATIONS
Assessment: Assess for HTN, risk for/history of arterial/venous thromboembolic events, untreated brain metastasis, recent active GI bleeding, thyroid dysfunction,

proteinuria, renal/hepatic impairment, pregnancy/nursing status, and possible drug interactions. Obtain baseline AST, ALT, and bilirubin levels. Control BP prior to initiation of treatment.

Monitoring: Monitor for HTN/hypertensive crisis, thromboembolic events, hemorrhage, symptoms of GI perforation/fistula, thyroid dysfunction, RPLS, proteinuria, signs/symptoms of cardiac failure, and other adverse events. Monitor AST, ALT, and bilirubin levels periodically.

Counseling: Inform about benefits/risks of therapy. Inform that HTN may develop; instruct to have BP monitored regularly during treatment. Instruct to inform physician if experiencing symptoms suggestive of thromboembolic events, abnormal thyroid function, any bleeding episodes, or persistent/severe abdominal pain. Advise that cardiac failure may develop during therapy and that signs/symptoms should be monitored regularly during treatment. Advise to inform physician if patient has an unhealed wound or has surgery scheduled. Advise to inform physician if patient has worsening of neurological function consistent with RPLS (eg, headache, seizure, lethargy, confusion, blindness, other visual and neurologic disturbances). Advise to avoid becoming pregnant while on therapy and counsel both male and female patients to use effective birth control. Instruct female patients not to breastfeed while receiving treatment. Advise to inform physician about all concomitant medications, vitamins, or dietary and herbal supplements. Instruct not to take additional dose if the patient vomits or misses a dose and to take the next dose at the usual time.

InnoPran XL — propranolol hydrochloride   Rx

Class: Nonselective beta blocker

> Exacerbation of angina pectoris and myocardial infarction (MI) reported following abrupt discontinuation. When discontinuing chronically administered drug, particularly in ischemic heart disease, gradually reduce dose over a period of 1-2 weeks and monitor patients. Promptly resume therapy at least temporarily and take other measures appropriate for the management of unstable angina if angina markedly worsens or acute coronary insufficiency develops. Caution against interruption or discontinuation of therapy without a physician's advice. Coronary artery disease (CAD) may be unrecognized; avoid abrupt discontinuation of therapy even in patient treated only for HTN.

ADULT DOSAGE
Hypertension

Initial: 80mg qhs taken consistently, either on empty stomach or with food
Titrate: May titrate to 120mg qhs prn for BP control
Max: 120mg qhs

PEDIATRIC DOSAGE
Pediatric use may not have been established

DOSING CONSIDERATIONS
Elderly
Start at lower end of dosing range

ADMINISTRATION
Oral route

STORAGE
25°C (77°F); excursions permitted to 15-30°C (59-86°F).

HOW SUPPLIED
Cap, Extended-Release: 80mg, 120mg

CONTRAINDICATIONS
Cardiogenic shock or decompensated heart failure (HF), sinus bradycardia, sick sinus syndrome and >1st-degree heart block (unless a permanent pacemaker is in place), bronchial asthma. Known hypersensitivity (eg, anaphylactic reaction) to propranolol hydrochloride or any components of this medication.

WARNINGS/PRECAUTIONS
May cause depression of myocardial contractility and precipitate HF and cardiogenic shock; may be necessary to lower dose or d/c therapy. Avoid routine withdrawal prior to surgery. May mask tachycardia occurring with hypoglycemia and hyperthyroidism. Abrupt withdrawal may precipitate thyroid storm. Bradycardia including sinus pause, heart block, and cardiac arrest reported. Increased risk in patients with 1st-degree AV block, sinus node dysfunction, and conduction disorders (eg, Wolff-Parkinson-White). D/C or reduce dose if severe bradycardia occurs. Patients treated for severe anaphylactic reaction may be unresponsive to usual doses of epinephrine; consider other medications (eg, IV fluids, glucagon). Caution in elderly.

ADVERSE REACTIONS
Fatigue, dizziness, constipation.

DRUG INTERACTIONS
Increased concentrations with warfarin; monitor PT. Increased concentrations with propafenone. Increase levels with CYP2D6 inhibitors (eg, bupropion, fluoxetine, paroxetine, quinidine), CYP1A2 inhibitors (eg, ciprofloxacin, enoxamine, fluvoxamine), and CYP2C19 inhibitors (eg, fluconazole, fluvoxamine, ticlopidine). Decreased levels with CYP1A2 inducers (eg, phenytoin, montelukast, smoking) and CYP2C19 inducers (eg, rifampin), and cholestyramine and colestipol, leading to loss of efficacy. May antagonize antihypertensive effects of clonidine; may result to rebound HTN if withdrawn abruptly. May prolong 1st dose hypotension and syncope with prazosin. May reduce sensitivity to dobutamine stress echocardiography in patients undergoing evaluation for myocardial ischemia. May exacerbate hypotensive effects of MAOIs or TCAs. NSAIDs may attenuate the antihypertensive effect of β-adrenoreceptor blocking agents. Increased risk of significant bradycardia with non-dihydropyridine calcium-channel blockers (eg, verapamil, diltiazem), digoxin, or clonidine.

PREGNANCY AND LACTATION
Category C, caution in nursing.

MECHANISM OF ACTION
Nonselective β-adrenergic receptor blocker; has not been established. Thought to decrease cardiac output, inhibit renin release by the kidneys, and diminish tonic sympathetic nerve outflow from vasomotor centers in the brain.

PHARMACOKINETICS
Absorption: Almost complete; T_{max}=12-14 hrs (fasted). **Distribution:** V_d=4L; plasma protein binding (90%); found in breast milk. **Metabolism:** Liver (extensive); CYP2D6 (aromatic hydroxylation), CYP1A2, 2D6 (oxidation), N-dealkylation, glucuronidation. Propranolol glucuronide, naphthyloxylactic acid, and glucuronic acid and sulfate conjugates of 4-hydroxy propranolol (major metabolites). **Elimination:** $T_{1/2}$=8 hrs.

PATIENT CONSIDERATIONS
Assessment: Assess for cardiogenic shock, decompensated HF, sinus bradycardia, sick sinus syndrome, AV heart block, presence of pacemaker, bronchial asthma, hepatic or renal impairment, hyperthyroidism, hypoglycemia, history of anaphylactic reactions, possible drug interactions, and pregnancy/nursing status.

Monitoring: Monitor for signs/symptoms of HF, hyperthyroidism, hypoglycemia, anaphylactic reactions, and other adverse reactions. Monitor HR and PT.

Counseling: Inform about risks and benefits of therapy. Instruct not to interrupt or d/c therapy without a physician's advice. Advise to contact physician if signs/symptoms of HF worsens (eg, weight gain or increasing SOB).

Inspra — eplerenone   Rx

Class: Aldosterone blocker

ADULT DOSAGE
Congestive Heart Failure Post-Myocardial Infarction

To improve survival of stable patients w/ left ventricular systolic dysfunction (ejection fraction ≤40%) and clinical evidence of CHF after an acute MI

Initial: 25mg qd
Titrate: Increase to the recommended dose preferably w/in 4 weeks as tolerated
Recommended Dose: 50mg qd
Dose Adjustment Based on Serum K⁺ Level:
Serum K⁺ <5mEq/L:
Increase from 25mg qod to 25mg qd
Increase from 25mg qd to 50mg qd
Serum K⁺ 5-5.4mEq/L:
No adjustment
Serum K⁺ 5.5-5.9mEq/L:
Decrease from 50mg qd to 25mg qd
Decrease from 25mg qd to 25mg qod
Adjust from 25mg qod to withhold
Serum K⁺ ≥6mEq/L:
Withhold and restart at 25mg qod when serum K⁺ falls to <5.5mEq/L

Hypertension

Initial: 50mg qd
Titrate: Increase to 50mg bid if BP response is inadequate
Max: 100mg/day
May be used alone or in combination w/ other antihypertensive agents

PEDIATRIC DOSAGE
Pediatric use may not have been established

DOSING CONSIDERATIONS
Concomitant Medications
Moderate CYP3A Inhibitors (eg, Erythromycin, Saquinavir, Verapamil):
CHF Post-MI:
Max: 25mg qd
HTN:
Initial: 25mg qd
Max: 25mg bid

ADMINISTRATION
Oral route

STORAGE
25°C (77°F); excursions permitted to 15-30°C (59-86°F).

HOW SUPPLIED
Tab: 25mg, 50mg

CONTRAINDICATIONS
All Patients: Serum K⁺ >5.5mEq/L at initiation, CrCl ≤30mL/min, concomitant administration of strong CYP3A inhibitors (eg, ketoconazole, itraconazole, nefazodone, troleandomycin, clarithromycin, ritonavir, nelfinavir).
Patients Treated for HTN: Type 2 diabetes w/ microalbuminuria, SrCr >2mg/dL (males) or >1.8mg/dL (females), CrCl <50mL/min, concomitant administration of K⁺ supplements or K⁺-sparing diuretics (eg, amiloride, spironolactone, triamterene).

WARNINGS/PRECAUTIONS

Hyperkalemia risk is higher in patients w/ renal impairment, proteinuria, and diabetes; minimize risk w/ proper patient selection and monitoring. Monitor for hyperkalemia until effect of therapy is established. Patients who develop hyperkalemia (5.5-5.9mEq/L) may continue therapy w/ proper dose adjustment.

ADVERSE REACTIONS

CHF Post-MI: Hyperkalemia, increased SrCr.

DRUG INTERACTIONS

See Contraindications and Dosing Considerations. Monitor serum K^+ and SrCr w/in 3-7 days of a patient initiating a moderate CYP3A4 inhibitor, ACE inhibitor, ARB, or NSAID. Increased risk of hyperkalemia w/ an ACE inhibitor and/or an ARB; closely monitor serum K^+ and renal function, especially in patients at risk for impaired renal function (eg, elderly). Monitor serum lithium levels frequently if coadministered w/ lithium. Increased risk of hyperkalemia w/ NSAIDs; monitor BP and serum K^+ levels w/ NSAIDs.

PREGNANCY AND LACTATION

Pregnancy: Category B.
Lactation: Not for use in nursing.

MECHANISM OF ACTION

Aldosterone blocker; binds to mineralocorticoid receptor and blocks the binding of aldosterone, a component of the renin-angiotensin-aldosterone-system.

PHARMACOKINETICS

Absorption: Absolute bioavailability (69%) (100mg tab); T_{max}=1.5-2 hrs.
Distribution: V_d=42-90L; plasma protein binding (50%). **Metabolism:** Via CYP3A4.
Elimination: Urine (67%), feces (32%), <5% unchanged in urine and feces; $T_{1/2}$=3-6 hrs.

PATIENT CONSIDERATIONS

Assessment: Assess for type 2 diabetes w/ microalbuminuria/proteinuria, pregnancy/nursing status, and possible drug interactions. Assess serum K^+ levels and renal function (eg, CrCl, SrCr).

Monitoring: Monitor for signs/symptoms of hyperkalemia and other adverse reactions. Monitor serum K^+ w/in the 1st week of therapy, at 1 month after start of treatment or dose adjustment, and periodically thereafter. Monitor BP and renal function.

Counseling: Advise not to use K^+ supplements or salt substitutes containing K^+ w/o consulting the prescribing physician. Instruct to contact physician if dizziness, diarrhea, vomiting, rapid or irregular heartbeat, lower extremity edema, or difficulty breathing occurs.

INTEGRILIN — eptifibatide   Rx

Class: Glycoprotein IIb/IIIa inhibitor

ADULT DOSAGE
Acute Coronary Syndrome

To decrease the rate of a combined endpoint of death or new MI in patients w/ acute coronary syndrome, including patients who are to be managed medically and those undergoing percutaneous coronary intervention (PCI)

Usual: 180mcg/kg IV bolus as soon as possible after diagnosis, followed by continuous infusion of 2mcg/kg/min

Continue infusion until discharge or initiation of CABG surgery, up to 72 hrs; if a patient is to undergo PCI, continue infusion until discharge or for up to 18-24 hrs after procedure, whichever comes 1st, allowing up to 96 hrs of therapy

Give aspirin 160-325mg/day

Concomitant Heparin Administration:
During Medical Management:
Target APTT: 50-70 sec
≥70kg: 5000 U bolus, followed by infusion of 1000 U/hr
<70kg: 60 U/kg bolus, followed by infusion of 12 U/kg/hr

During PCI:
Target ACT: 200-300 sec
If heparin is initiated prior to PCI, administer additional boluses during PCI to maintain ACT w/in target; infusion after the PCI is discouraged

Percutaneous Coronary Intervention

To decrease the rate of a combined endpoint of death, new MI, or need for urgent intervention in patients undergoing percutaneous coronary intervention (PCI), including those undergoing intracoronary stenting

Usual: 180mcg/kg IV bolus immediately before PCI followed by

PEDIATRIC DOSAGE
Pediatric use may not have been established

---

continuous infusion of 2mcg/kg/min and a 2nd bolus of 180mcg/kg (given 10 min after 1st bolus)

Continue infusion until discharge or for up to 18-24 hrs, whichever comes 1st (minimum of 12 hrs of infusion is recommended); in patients who undergo CABG surgery, d/c infusion prior to surgery

Give aspirin 160-325mg 1-24 hrs prior to PCI and daily thereafter

Concomitant Heparin Administration:
Target ACT: 200-300 sec
Administer 60 U/kg bolus initially in patients not treated w/ heparin w/in 6 hrs prior to PCI. Administer boluses during PCI to maintain ACT w/in target; infusion after the PCI is strongly discouraged

---

DOSING CONSIDERATIONS
Renal Impairment
CrCl <50mL/min:
Acute Coronary Syndrome: 180mcg/kg IV bolus as soon as possible after diagnosis, followed by continuous infusion of 1mcg/kg/min
PCI: 180mcg/kg IV bolus immediately before PCI, followed by continuous infusion of 1mcg/kg/min and a 2nd bolus of 180mcg/kg (given 10 min after 1st bolus)

ADMINISTRATION
IV route

Administration Instructions
1. May be administered in the same IV line as alteplase, atropine, dobutamine, heparin, lidocaine, meperidine, metoprolol, midazolam, morphine, nitroglycerin, or verapamil. Do not administer through the same IV line as furosemide
2. May be administered in the same IV line w/ 0.9% NaCl or 0.9% NaCl/D5; w/ either vehicle, the infusion may also contain up to 60mEq/L of KCl
3. Withdraw the bolus dose(s) from the 10mL vial into a syringe and administer by IV push
4. Immediately following bolus dose administration, initiate a continuous infusion
5. When using an IV infusion pump, administer Integrilin undiluted directly from the 100mL vial. Spike the 100mL vial w/ a vented infusion set. Center the spike w/ in the circle on the stopper top
6. Discard any unused portion left in the vial

STORAGE
2-8°C (36-46°F). May store at 25°C (77°F) for ≤2 months with excursions permitted to 15-30°C (59-86°F).

HOW SUPPLIED
Inj: 0.75mg/mL [100mL vial], 2mg/mL [10mL, 100mL vial]

CONTRAINDICATIONS
History of bleeding diathesis or evidence of active abnormal bleeding within the previous 30 days, severe HTN (systolic BP >200mmHg or diastolic BP >110mmHg) not adequately controlled on antihypertensives, major surgery within preceding 6 weeks, history of stroke within 30 days or any history of hemorrhagic stroke, current or planned administration of another parenteral glycoprotein (GP) IIb/IIIa inhibitor, and renal dialysis dependency. Hypersensitivity to eptifibatide or any component of the product.

WARNINGS/PRECAUTIONS
Maintain activated PTT (aPTT) between 50-70 sec unless PCI is to be performed. Associated with an increase in major and minor bleeding. Minimize the use of arterial and venous punctures, IM inj, urinary catheters, nasotracheal intubation, and NG tubes. Avoid noncompressible sites (eg, subclavian or jugular veins) when obtaining IV access. Caution in patients undergoing PCI; d/c infusion and heparin immediately if bleeding at access site cannot be controlled with pressure. Both infusion and heparin should be discontinued and sheath hemostasis should be achieved at least 2-4 hrs before hospital discharge. Thrombocytopenia (immune-mediated and non-immune mediated) reported. D/C infusion and heparin if acute profound thrombocytopenia occurs or platelet count decreases to <100,000/mm³; monitor serial platelet counts, assess the presence of drug-dependent antibodies, and treat as appropriate.

ADVERSE REACTIONS
Bleeding, hypotension.

DRUG INTERACTIONS
See Contraindications. Increased risk of bleeding with antiplatelet agents, thrombolytics, heparin, ASA, chronic NSAID use, oral anticoagulants, and $P2Y_{12}$ inhibitors; monitor aPTT and activated clotting time (ACT) with heparin.

PREGNANCY AND LACTATION
Category B, caution in nursing.

MECHANISM OF ACTION
GP IIb/IIIa inhibitor; reversibly inhibits platelet aggregation by preventing the binding of fibrinogen, von Willebrand factor, and other adhesive ligands to GP IIb/IIIa.

PHARMACOKINETICS
Distribution: Plasma protein binding (25%). **Elimination:** Urine; $T_{1/2}$=2.5 hrs.

PATIENT CONSIDERATIONS
Assessment: Assess for drug hypersensitivity, history of bleeding diathesis or stroke, active abnormal bleeding within previous 30 days, severe HTN, major

surgery within preceding 6 weeks, history of hemorrhagic stroke, dependency on renal dialysis, renal insufficiency, pregnancy/nursing status, and possible drug interactions. Obtain baseline Hgb, Hct, platelet count, SrCr, and PT/aPTT to identify preexisting hemostatic abnormalities. Measure ACT in patients undergoing PCI.

Monitoring: Monitor for signs/symptoms of bleeding, thrombocytopenia, and hypersensitivity reactions. Monitor platelet count in patients with low platelet counts.

Counseling: Inform about the risks and benefits of therapy. Instruct to inform physician about any medical conditions, medications, and allergies.

INTELENCE — etravirine   Rx

Class: Non-nucleoside reverse transcriptase inhibitor (NNRTI)

ADULT DOSAGE	PEDIATRIC DOSAGE
HIV-1 Infection	**HIV-1 Infection**
Combination w/ Other Antiretrovirals Treatment-Experienced: Evidence of Viral Replication and HIV-1 Strains Resistant to an NNRTI and Other Antiretrovirals: 200mg bid	**Combination w/ Other Antiretrovirals Treatment-Experienced:** Evidence of Viral Replication and HIV-1 Strains Resistant to an NNRTI and Other Antiretrovirals: **6 to <18 Years:** ≥16 to <20kg: 100mg bid ≥20 to <25kg: 125mg bid ≥25 to <30kg: 150mg bid ≥30kg: 200mg bid

---

ADMINISTRATION
Oral route

Take after a meal.
Swallow whole w/ liquid.
May be dispersed in a glass of water if unable to swallow whole.

Dispersion Instructions
- Place the tablet(s) in 5mL (1 tsp) of water, or at least enough liquid to cover the medication, stir well until the water looks milky.
- If desired, add more water or alternatively orange juice or milk (Do not place the tablets in orange juice or milk w/out first adding water). The use of grapefruit juice or warm (>40°C) or carbonated beverages should be avoided.
- Drink it immediately, rinse the glass several times w/ water, orange juice, or milk and completely swallow the rinse each time to takes the entire dose.

STORAGE
25°C (77°F); excursions permitted to 15-30°C (59-86°F). Store in the original bottle. Protect from moisture.

HOW SUPPLIED
Tab: 25mg*, 100mg, 200mg *scored

WARNINGS/PRECAUTIONS
Severe, potentially life-threatening, and fatal skin reactions (eg, erythema multiforme, toxic epidermal necrolysis, Stevens-Johnson syndrome), and hypersensitivity reactions including drug rash with eosinophilia and systemic symptoms reported; d/c immediately if these occur and initiate appropriate therapy. Immune reconstitution syndrome, autoimmune disorders (eg, Graves' disease, polymyositis, Guillain-Barre syndrome) in the setting of immune reconstitution, and redistribution/accumulation of body fat reported. Caution in elderly.

ADVERSE REACTIONS
Rash, peripheral neuropathy.

DRUG INTERACTIONS
May alter therapeutic effect and adverse reaction profile with drugs that induce, inhibit, or are substrates of CYP3A, CYP2C9, and CYP2C19, or are transported by P-glycoprotein. Avoid with other NNRTIs, delavirdine, rilpivirine, atazanavir (ATV) without low-dose ritonavir (RTV), fosamprenavir (FPV) without low-dose RTV, FPV/RTV, tipranavir/RTV, indinavir without low-dose RTV, nelfinavir without low-dose RTV, RTV (600mg bid), carbamazepine, phenobarbital, phenytoin, rifampin, rifapentine, and St. John's wort. Coadministration with boceprevir is not recommended in the presence of other drugs which may further decrease etravirine exposure (eg, darunavir/RTV, lopinavir/RTV, saquinavir/RTV, tenofovir disoproxil fumarate, or rifabutin). Caution with digoxin; use lowest dose initially. May increase levels of nelfinavir without RTV, digoxin, warfarin (monitor INR), anticoagulants, 14-OH-clarithromycin, voriconazole, diazepam, boceprevir, fluvastatin, and pitavastatin. May increase maraviroc levels in the presence of a potent CYP3A inhibitor (eg, RTV boosted protease inhibitor). May decrease levels of maraviroc, antiarrhythmics, itraconazole, ketoconazole, rifabutin, telaprevir, atorvastatin, lovastatin, simvastatin, immunosuppressant, and clopidogrel (active) metabolite. May decrease dolutegravir levels; should only be used with dolutegravir when coadministered with ATV/RTV, darunavir/RTV, or lopinavir/RTV. Fluconazole and voriconazole may increase exposure. May decrease Posaconazole, itraconazole, or ketoconazole may increase levels. May decrease clarithromycin exposure. Caution with artemether/lumefantrine. Efavirenz, nevirapine, rifabutin, systemic dexamethasone, and boceprevir may decrease levels. Darunavir/RTV, lopinavir/RTV, and saquinavir/RTV may decrease exposure. Consider alternatives to clarithromycin, such as azithromycin, for treatment/ment of *Mycobacterium avium* complex. Monitor for withdrawal symptoms when coadministered with methadone, buprenorphine, buprenorphine/naloxone. May need to alter sildenafil dose. Refer to PI for additional drug interaction information.

PREGNANCY AND LACTATION
Category B, not for use in nursing.

MECHANISM OF ACTION
NNRTI; binds directly to reverse transcriptase and blocks the RNA-dependent and DNA-dependent DNA polymerase activities by causing a disruption of the enzyme's catalytic site.

PHARMACOKINETICS
Absorption: T_{max}=2.5-4 hrs; AUC_{12h}=4522ng•hr/mL (adults), 3742ng•hr/mL (pediatric patients). **Distribution:** Plasma protein binding (99.9%). **Metabolism:** Liver via CYP3A, CYP2C9, and CYP2C19; methyl hydroxylation. **Elimination:** Feces (93.7%, 81.2-86.4% unchanged), urine (1.2%); $T_{1/2}$=41 hrs.

PATIENT CONSIDERATIONS
Assessment: Assess treatment history, pregnancy/nursing status, and for possible drug interactions. Perform resistance testing where possible.

Monitoring: Monitor for signs/symptoms of severe skin/hypersensitivity reactions, body fat redistribution/accumulation, immune reconstitution syndrome (eg, opportunistic infections), autoimmune disorders, and other adverse reactions. Monitor clinical status, including liver transaminases. Monitor INR when combined with warfarin.

Counseling: Inform that product is not a cure for HIV infection and patients may continue to develop opportunistic infections and other complications associated with HIV disease. Advise to avoid doing things that can spread HIV-1 infection to others. Advise to take medication ud. Instruct to always use in combination with other antiretrovirals. Advise not to alter dose or d/c therapy without consulting physician. If a dose is missed within 6 hrs of time usually taken, instruct to take as soon as possible following a meal. If scheduled time exceeds 6 hrs, instruct not to take the missed dose and resume the usual dosing schedule. Advise to report to physician the use of any other prescription/nonprescription or herbal products (eg, St. John's wort). Counsel to d/c and notify physician if severe rash develops. Advise that redistribution or accumulation of body fat may occur.

INTERMEZZO — zolpidem tartrate   CIV

Class: GABA$_A$ agonist

ADULT DOSAGE	PEDIATRIC DOSAGE
Insomnia	Pediatric use may not have been established
PRN treatment when a middle-of-the-night awakening is followed by difficulty returning to sleep	
Recommended/Max: 1.75mg (women), 3.5mg (men) once per night prn	

DOSING CONSIDERATIONS
Concomitant Medications
CNS Depressants: Recommended zolpidem dose is 1.75mg; dose adjustment of CNS depressants may also be necessary
Other Sedative-Hypnotics (eg, Other Zolpidem Products): Not recommended

Hepatic Impairment
Recommended: 1.75mg, once per night if needed

Elderly
1.75mg, once per night if needed

ADMINISTRATION
SL route

Take in bed only if ≥4 hrs of bedtime remain before planned time of waking. Place under tongue and allow to disintegrate completely before swallowing; do not swallow whole.
Do not administer w/ or immediately after a meal.
Remove tab from pouch just prior to dosing.

STORAGE
20-25°C (68-77°F); excursions permitted between 15-30°C (59-86°F). Protect from moisture. Do not remove tab from unit-dose pouch until time of use.

HOW SUPPLIED
Tab, SL: 1.75mg, 3.5mg

CONTRAINDICATIONS
Known hypersensitivity to zolpidem.

WARNINGS/PRECAUTIONS
Not indicated for treatment of middle-of-the-night insomnia when patient has fewer than 4 hrs of bedtime remaining before planned time of waking. Has CNS depressant effects; may be at risk for next-day driving and psychomotor impairment if taken with <4 hrs of bedtime remaining or if higher than recommended dose is taken. Initiate only after careful evaluation; failure of insomnia to remit after 7-10 days of treatment may indicate presence of a primary psychiatric and/or medical illness. Angioedema reported; do not rechallenge if angioedema or anaphylaxis develops. Abnormal thinking, behavior changes, and visual/auditory hallucinations reported. Complex behaviors (eg, sleep-driving) reported; consider discontinuation if a "sleep-driving" episode occurs. Amnesia, anxiety, and other neuropsychiatric symptoms may occur. Worsening of depression, and suicidal thoughts and actions (including complete suicide) reported in primarily depressed patients; prescribe the lowest number of tabs feasible at any one time. Caution w/ compromised respiratory function, including sleep apnea and myasthenia gravis. Withdrawal signs/symptoms reported

following rapid dose decrease or abrupt discontinuation; monitor for tolerance, abuse, and dependence.

ADVERSE REACTIONS
Nausea, fatigue, headache.

DRUG INTERACTIONS
See Dosing Considerations. May increase risk of CNS depression w/ other CNS depressants (eg, benzodiazepines, opioids, TCAs, alcohol). Increased risk of next-day driving impairment and psychomotor impairment w/ other CNS depressants or other drugs that increase blood levels of zolpidem. Increased risk of complex behaviors w/ alcohol and other CNS depressants. May have additive effects of decreased alertness and psychomotor performance w/ imipramine, chlorpromazine, and alcohol. Caution w/ chronic haloperidol administration. Sertraline may increase exposure and increase pharmacodynamic effect. CYP3A inhibitors may increase exposure. May increase $T_{1/2}$ w/ multiple doses of fluoxetine. Rifampin may reduce exposure and decrease efficacy. Increased pharmacodynamic effects w/ ketoconazole; consider using a lower dose of zolpidem.

PREGNANCY AND LACTATION
Pregnancy: Category C.
Lactation: Effect on nursing infant not known.

MECHANISM OF ACTION
Imidazopyridine hypnotic; interacts w/ GABA-BZ complex. Binds the BZ_1 receptor w/ a high affinity ratio of $\alpha1/\alpha5$ subunits.

PHARMACOKINETICS
Absorption: Rapid. T_{max}=35-75 min. Women: (3.5mg) C_{max}=77ng/mL, AUC=296ng•hr/mL. (1.75mg) C_{max}=37ng/mL, AUC=151ng•hr/mL. Men: (3.5mg) C_{max}=53ng/mL, AUC=198ng•hr/mL. **Distribution:** Plasma protein binding (93%); found in breast milk. **Elimination:** Urine (inactive metabolites); (3.5mg) $T_{1/2}$=2.5 hrs.

PATIENT CONSIDERATIONS
Assessment: Assess for psychiatric and/or medical illness, respiratory impairment, myasthenia gravis, hepatic impairment, hypersensitivity to the drug, pregnancy/nursing status, and possible drug interactions.

Monitoring: Monitor for signs/symptoms CNS depression, respiratory depression, abnormal thinking, behavioral changes, visual/auditory hallucinations, complex behaviors, worsening of depression, suicidal thoughts/actions, angioedema/anaphylaxis, and other adverse reactions. Monitor for withdrawal signs/symptoms following rapid dose decrease or abrupt discontinuation.

Counseling: Inform about the benefits and risks of treatment. Instruct patient to take as prescribed. Advise that medication has the potential to cause next-day impairment, and the risk is increased if dosing instructions are not carefully followed. Advise to wait at least 4 hrs after dosing and until they feel fully awake before driving or engaging in other activities requiring mental alertness. Inform that severe anaphylactic and anaphylactoid reactions may occur; instruct to notify physician immediately if signs/symptoms occur. Instruct to inform families that therapy has been associated w/ "sleep-driving" and other complex behaviors while not being fully awake; instruct to call healthcare provider immediately if symptoms develop. Instruct to report immediately any suicidal thoughts. Advise not to take medication if alcohol has been consumed on that day or before going to bed.

INTUNIV — guanfacine

Rx

Class: Alpha$_{2A}$ agonist

PEDIATRIC DOSAGE
Attention-Deficit Hyperactivity Disorder

Monotherapy/Adjunctive Therapy to Stimulant Medications:

6-17 Years:
Initial: 1mg/day
Titrate: Adjust in increments of no more than 1mg/week
Target Dose Range: 0.05-0.12mg/kg/day (total daily dose 1-7mg), depending on clinical response and tolerability
Max: Doses above 4mg/day in children 6-12 yrs of age and doses above 7mg/day in adolescents 13-17 yrs of age have not been evaluated

Weight-Based Target Dose Range:
25-33.9kg: 2-3mg/day
34-41.4kg: 2-4mg/day
41.5-49.4kg: 3-5mg/day
49.5-58.4kg: 3-6mg/day
58.5-91kg: 4-7mg/day
>91kg: 5-7mg/day

Maint Treatment:
Periodically reevaluate the long-term use of the drug and adjust weight-based dose prn

Missed Dose
When reinitiating to the previous maint dose after ≥2 missed consecutive doses, consider titration based on tolerability

Conversions
Switching from Immediate-Release (IR):
D/C IR, and titrate w/ extended-release following the recommended schedule
Do not substitute for IR tabs on a mg-per-mg basis

DOSING CONSIDERATIONS
Concomitant Medications
Strong and Moderate CYP3A4 Inhibitors:
(Based on Weight-Based Target Dose Range)
Continue CYP3A4 Inhibitor/Initiate Guanfacine: Decrease guanfacine dose by 1/2
Continue Guanfacine/Initiate CYP3A4 Inhibitor: Decrease guanfacine dose by 1/2
Stop CYP3A4 Inhibitor/Continue Guanfacine: Increase guanfacine to recommended level

Strong and Moderate CYP3A4 Inducers:
(Based on Weight-Based Target Dose Range)
Continue CYP3A4 Inducer/Initiate Guanfacine: Consider increasing guanfacine up to twice the recommended dose
Continue Guanfacine/Initiate CYP3A4 Inducer: Consider increasing guanfacine up to twice the recommended dose over 1-2 weeks
Stop CYP3A4 Inducer/Continue Guanfacine: Decrease guanfacine dose to recommended level over 1-2 weeks

Renal Impairment
Significant Impairment: May need to reduce dose

Hepatic Impairment
Significant Impairment: May need to reduce dose

Discontinuation
Taper dose in decrements of no more than 1mg every 3-7 days

ADMINISTRATION
Oral route

Take either in am or pm, at approx same time each day.
Swallow tabs whole w/ water, milk, or other liquid; do not crush, chew, or break.
Do not administer w/ high-fat meals.

STORAGE
20-25°C (68-77°F); excursions permitted to 15-30°C (59-86°F).

HOW SUPPLIED
Tab, Extended-Release: 1mg, 2mg, 3mg, 4mg

CONTRAINDICATIONS
History of a hypersensitivity reaction to Intuniv or its inactive ingredients, or other products containing guanfacine.

WARNINGS/PRECAUTIONS
May experience increase in BP and HR following discontinuation of therapy. May cause dose-dependent decreases in BP and HR. Orthostatic hypotension and syncope reported. Titrate slowly in patients w/ a history of hypotension, and those w/ underlying conditions that may be worsened by hypotension and bradycardia (eg, heart block, cardiovascular disease, vascular disease). In patients who have a history of syncope or may have a condition that predisposes to syncope (eg, hypotension, orthostatic hypotension, bradycardia), avoid dehydration or overheating. Somnolence and sedation commonly reported. May impair mental/physical abilities. May worsen sinus node dysfunction and atrioventricular (AV) block; titrate slowly and monitor vital signs frequently in patients w/ cardiac conduction abnormalities.

ADVERSE REACTIONS
Fixed-Dose Monotherapy ADHD Trials in Children & Adolescents (6-17 yrs):
Hypotension, somnolence, fatigue, nausea, lethargy.
Flexible Dose-Optimization ADHD Trials in Children (6-12 yrs) & Adolescents (13-17 yrs): Somnolence, hypotension, abdominal pain, insomnia, fatigue, dizziness, dry mouth, irritability, N/V, bradycardia.
Adjunctive Treatment to Psychostimulant ADHD Trial in Children & Adolescents (6-17 yrs): Somnolence, fatigue, insomnia, dizziness, abdominal pain.

DRUG INTERACTIONS
See Dosing Considerations. Strong and moderate CYP3A4 inhibitors (eg, ketoconazole) may increase exposure. Strong and moderate CYP3A4 inducers (eg, rifampin) may decrease exposure. Monitor BP and HR, and adjust dosages accordingly w/ antihypertensives or other drugs that can reduce BP/HR or increase the risk of syncope. Consider the potential for additive sedative effects before using w/ other centrally active depressants. Avoid w/ alcohol. May worsen sinus node dysfunction and AV block, especially w/ other sympatholytic drugs; titrate slowly and monitor vital signs frequently w/ other sympatholytic drugs.

PREGNANCY AND LACTATION
Pregnancy: Category B.
Lactation: Caution in nursing; observe human milk-fed infants for sedation and somnolence.

MECHANISM OF ACTION
Central alpha$_{2A}$-adrenergic agonist; has not been established. Reduces sympathetic nerve impulses from the vasomotor center to the heart and blood vessels, resulting in decreased peripheral vascular resistance and reduction in HR.

PHARMACOKINETICS

Absorption: Readily absorbed. Children (6-12 yrs of age): C_{max}=10ng/mL; AUC=162ng•hr/mL. Adolescents (13-17 yrs of age): C_{max}=7ng/mL; AUC=116ng•hr/mL. Children and Adolescents: T_{max}=5 hrs. **Distribution:** Plasma protein binding (70%). **Metabolism:** CYP3A4. **Elimination:** $T_{1/2}$=18 hrs (1mg qd, adults).

PATIENT CONSIDERATIONS

Assessment: Assess for history of hypotension, underlying conditions that may be worsened by hypotension and bradycardia, history of syncope, condition that predisposes to syncope, cardiac conduction abnormalities, hypersensitivity to drug, renal/hepatic impairment, pregnancy/nursing status, and possible drug interactions. Assess HR and BP.

Monitoring: Monitor for hypotension, bradycardia, syncope, somnolence, sedation, cardiac conduction abnormalities, and other adverse reactions. Monitor HR and BP following dose increases, and periodically while on therapy. Monitor BP and pulse when reducing the dose or discontinuing the drug. Observe human milk-fed infants for sedation and somnolence. Monitor vital signs frequently in patients w/ cardiac conduction abnormalities. Periodically reevaluate the long term use of the drug.

Counseling: Instruct caregiver to supervise the child or adolescent taking the drug. Counsel on how to properly taper the medication, if the physician decides to d/c treatment. Instruct patients not to d/c therapy w/o consulting their physician. Inform of the adverse reactions (eg, sedation, headache, abdominal pain) that may occur; advise to consult physician if any of these symptoms persist or other symptoms occur. Caution patients against operating heavy equipment or driving until accustomed to effects of medication. Advise to avoid becoming dehydrated or overheated, and to avoid use w/ alcohol.

INVANZ — ertapenem   Rx

Class: Carbapenem

ADULT DOSAGE

Intra-Abdominal Infections

Complicated:
1g qd IV/IM for 5-14 days

Skin and Skin Structure Infections

Complicated Infections, Including Diabetic Foot Infections:
1g qd IV/IM for 7-14 days; patients w/ diabetic foot infections received up to 28 days of treatment (parenteral or parenteral + oral switch therapy)

Community-Acquired Pneumonia

1g qd IV/IM for 10-14 days (duration includes a possible switch to oral therapy, after at least 3 days of parenteral therapy, once clinical improvement has been demonstrated)

Urinary Tract Infections

Complicated UTIs, Including Pyelonephritis:
1g qd IV/IM for 10-14 days (duration includes a possible switch to oral therapy, after at least 3 days of parenteral therapy, once clinical improvement has been demonstrated)

Acute Pelvic Infections

Including Postpartum Endomyometritis, Septic Abortion, and Postsurgical Gynecological Infections:
1g qd IV/IM for 3-10 days

Prophylaxis of Postoperative Infections

Prophylaxis of Surgical-Site Infection, Following Colorectal Surgery:
1g as a single IV dose given 1 hr prior to surgical incision

PEDIATRIC DOSAGE

Intra-Abdominal Infections

Complicated:
3 Months-12 Years:
15mg/kg IV/IM bid for 5-14 days; not to exceed 1g/day
≥13 Years:
1g qd IV/IM for 5-14 days

Skin and Skin Structure Infections

Complicated Infections, Including Diabetic Foot Infections:
3 Months-12 Years:
15mg/kg IV/IM bid for 7-14 days; not to exceed 1g/day
≥13 Years:
1g qd IV/IM for 7-14 days

Community-Acquired Pneumonia

3 Months-12 Years:
15mg/kg IV/IM bid for 10-14 days; not to exceed 1g/day
≥13 Years:
1g qd IV/IM for 10-14 days
Duration includes a possible switch to oral therapy, after at least 3 days of parenteral therapy, once clinical improvement has been demonstrated

Urinary Tract Infections

Complicated UTIs, Including Pyelonephritis:
3 Months-12 Years:
15mg/kg IV/IM bid for 10-14 days; not to exceed 1g/day
≥13 Years:
1g qd IV/IM for 10-14 days
Duration includes a possible switch to oral therapy, after at least 3 days of parenteral therapy, once clinical improvement has been demonstrated

Acute Pelvic Infections

3 Months-12 Years:
15mg/kg IV/IM bid for 3-10 days; not to exceed 1g/day
≥13 Years:
1g qd IV/IM for 3-10 days

DOSING CONSIDERATIONS

Renal Impairment

Adults:
Severe Impairment (CrCl ≤30mL/min)/ESRD (CrCl ≤10mL/min): 500mg/day
Hemodialysis: 500mg/day; if administered w/in 6 hrs prior to hemodialysis, give 150mg supplementary dose following hemodialysis session

ADMINISTRATION

IV/IM route

Do not mix or coinfuse w/ other medications
Do not use diluents containing dextrose

IV

Reconstitute and then dilute prior to administration
Complete infusion w/in 6 hrs of reconstitution; infuse over a period of 30 min
May administer by IV infusion for up to 14 days
Preparation:
Reconstitute 1g vial w/ 10mL of water for inj, 0.9% NaCl for inj, or bacteriostatic water for inj; shake well
3 Months-12 Years: Withdraw volume equal to 15mg/kg of body weight (not to exceed 1g/day) and dilute in 0.9% NaCl inj to a final concentration of 20mg/mL or less
≥13 Years: Immediately transfer reconstituted sol to 50mL of 0.9% NaCl inj

IM

Reconstitute prior to administration
Use reconstituted sol w/in 1 hr after preparation
May administer by IM inj for up to 7 days
Preparation:
Reconstitute 1g vial w/ 3.2mL of 1% lidocaine HCl inj (w/o epinephrine); shake thoroughly
Immediately withdraw appropriate dose and administer by deep IM inj into a large muscle mass (eg, gluteal muscles or lateral part of thigh)

Refer to PI for ADD-Vantage Vial Instructions

STORAGE

≤25°C (77°F). Reconstituted and Infusion Sol: 25°C (77°F) and use within 6 hrs, or 5°C (41°F) for 24 hrs and use within 4 hrs after removal from refrigeration. Do not freeze sol.

HOW SUPPLIED

Inj: 1g

CONTRAINDICATIONS

(IM) Hypersensitivity to amide-type local anesthetic. Known hypersensitivity to any component of this product or to other drugs in the same class or in patients who have demonstrated anaphylactic reactions to beta-lactams.

WARNINGS/PRECAUTIONS

Serious and occasionally fatal hypersensitivity (anaphylactic) reactions reported; d/c immediately if an allergic reaction occurs. Seizures and other CNS adverse experiences reported; caution with known factors that predispose to convulsive activity, and continue anticonvulsant therapy with known seizure disorders. If focal tremors, myoclonus, or seizures occur, evaluate neurologically, place on anticonvulsant therapy if not already instituted, and reexamine dosage to determine whether it should be decreased or discontinued. *Clostridium difficile*-associated diarrhea (CDAD) reported; d/c if CDAD is suspected or confirmed. Use caution when administering IM to avoid inadvertent inj into a blood vessel. May result in bacterial resistance with prolonged use in the absence of proven or suspected bacterial infection, or a prophylactic indication; take appropriate measures if superinfection develops. Caution in elderly.

ADVERSE REACTIONS

Diarrhea, infused vein complication, N/V, anemia, headache, edema/swelling, fever, abdominal pain, constipation, altered mental status, insomnia, vaginitis, infusion-site pain, infusion-site erythema.

DRUG INTERACTIONS

Increased plasma concentrations with probenecid; coadministration is not recommended. May reduce concentrations of valproic acid, thereby increasing the risk of breakthrough seizures; concomitant use with valproic acid/divalproex sodium is generally not recommended, but if necessary, consider supplemental anticonvulsant therapy.

PREGNANCY AND LACTATION

Category B, caution in nursing.

MECHANISM OF ACTION

Carbapenem; bactericidal activity results from the inhibition of cell-wall synthesis and is mediated through ertapenem binding to penicillin (PCN)-binding proteins.

PHARMACOKINETICS

Absorption: (IM) Almost complete. Bioavailability (90%); T_{max}=2.3 hrs. **Distribution:** V_d=0.12L/kg (adults), 0.16L/kg (13-17 yrs of age), 0.2L/kg (3 months-12 yrs of age); plasma protein binding (85% [300mcg/mL plasma concentration], 95% [<100mcg/mL plasma concentration]); found in breast milk. **Metabolism:** Hydrolysis of the β-lactam ring; inactive ring-opened derivative (major metabolite). **Elimination:** (IV) Urine (80% [38% unchanged, 37% metabolite]), feces (10%); $T_{1/2}$=4 hrs (≥13 yrs of age), 2.5 hrs (3 months-12 yrs of age).

PATIENT CONSIDERATIONS

Assessment: Assess for factors that predispose to convulsive activity, seizure disorders, renal impairment, pregnancy/nursing status, and possible drug interactions. Carefully assess for previous hypersensitivity reactions to drug, PCN, cephalosporins, other β-lactams, and other allergens. (IM) Assess for hypersensitivity to amide-type local anesthetics.

Monitoring: Monitor for hypersensitivity (anaphylactic) reactions, CNS effects (eg, focal tremors, myoclonus, seizures), CDAD, superinfection, and other adverse reactions. Periodically monitor organ system function (eg, renal, hepatic, hematopoietic) during prolonged therapy.

Counseling: Advise that allergic reactions, including serious allergic reactions, could occur, and that serious reactions may require immediate treatment. Advise to report any previous hypersensitivity reactions to the medication, other β-lactams, or other allergens. Counsel to inform physician if taking valproic acid or divalproex sodium. Counsel that therapy should only be used to treat bacterial, not viral, infections. Instruct to take exactly ud even if the patient feels better early in the course of therapy. Inform that skipping doses or not completing the full course of therapy may decrease effectiveness of treatment and increase bacterial resistance. Inform that diarrhea is a common problem caused by therapy that usually ends when therapy is discontinued. Instruct to immediately contact physician if watery and bloody stools (with or without stomach cramps and fever) occur, even as late as ≥2 months after the last dose.

INVEGA — paliperidone   Rx

Class: Atypical antipsychotic

> Elderly patients w/ dementia-related psychosis treated w/ antipsychotic drugs are at an increased risk of death; most deaths appeared to be cardiovascular (CV) (eg, heart failure, sudden death) or infectious (eg, pneumonia) in nature. Not approved for the treatment of patients w/ dementia-related psychosis.

ADULT DOSAGE
Schizophrenia
6mg qd; a lower dose of 3mg qd may be sufficient
Titrate: If indicated, may increase by 3mg/day; dose increases >6mg/day should be made at intervals >5 days
Max: 12mg/day

Schizoaffective Disorder
Monotherapy or Adjunct to Mood Stabilizers and/or Antidepressants:
6mg qd
Range: 3-12mg qd
Titrate: If indicated, may increase by 3mg/day at intervals of >4 days
Max: 12mg/day

PEDIATRIC DOSAGE
Schizophrenia
12-17 Years:
Initial: 3mg qd
Titrate: If indicated, may increase by 3mg/day at intervals of >5 days

DOSING CONSIDERATIONS
Renal Impairment
CrCl ≥50 to <80mL/min (Mild):
Initial: 3mg qd
Max: 6mg qd
CrCl ≥10 to <50mL/min (Moderate to Severe):
Initial: 1.5mg qd
Max: 3mg qd
CrCl <10mL/min: Has not been studied; not recommended

Hepatic Impairment
Mild to Moderate (Child-Pugh Class A and B): No dose adjustment needed
Severe: Has not been studied

Elderly
Adjust dose according to renal function

ADMINISTRATION
Oral route

Take w/ or w/o food.
Swallow whole w/ liquids; do not crush, divide, or chew.

STORAGE
Up to 25°C (77°F); excursions permitted to 15-30°C (59-86°F). Protect from moisture.

HOW SUPPLIED
Tab, Extended-Release: 1.5mg, 3mg, 6mg, 9mg

CONTRAINDICATIONS
Known hypersensitivity to either paliperidone or risperidone, or to any of the excipients in this medication.

WARNINGS/PRECAUTIONS
Neuroleptic malignant syndrome (NMS) reported; immediately d/c if this occurs. May increase QTc interval; avoid w/ congenital long QT syndrome and history of cardiac arrhythmias. Tardive dyskinesia (TD) may develop; consider discontinuation if signs/symptoms of TD appear. Hyperglycemia and diabetes mellitus (DM), in some cases extreme and associated w/ ketoacidosis or hyperosmolar coma or death, reported. Undesirable alterations in lipids and weight gain reported. May elevate prolactin levels. Avoid w/ preexisting severe GI narrowing. May induce orthostatic hypotension and syncope; caution w/ known CV disease, cerebrovascular disease, or conditions that predispose to hypotension. Leukopenia, neutropenia, and agranulocytosis reported; d/c in cases of severe neutropenia (ANC <1000/mm³). Consider discontinuation at the 1st sign of a clinically significant decline in WBC count in the absence of other causative factors in patients w/ a history of a clinically significant low WBC count or a drug-induced leukopenia/neutropenia. Somnolence reported. May impair mental/physical abilities. Seizures reported; caution w/ history of seizures or conditions that lower the seizure threshold. May cause esophageal dysmotility and aspiration; caution w/ risk of aspiration pneumonia. May induce priapism; severe cases may require surgical intervention. May disrupt body's ability to reduce core body temperature; caution w/ conditions that may contribute to an elevated core body temperature. May have an antiemetic effect that may mask signs/symptoms of overdosage w/ certain drugs or of conditions (eg, intestinal obstruction, Reye's syndrome, brain tumor). Patients w/ Parkinson's disease or dementia w/ Lewy bodies may have an increased sensitivity to therapy. Caution in patients who are high-risk for suicide.

ADVERSE REACTIONS
Schizophrenia: (Adults) Extrapyramidal symptoms (EPS), tachycardia, akathisia. (Adolescents) Somnolence, EPS, akathisia, headache, vomiting, weight gain,

anxiety, tachycardia, salivary hypersecretion, dizziness, amenorrhea, asthenia, fatigue, nasopharyngitis, lethargy.
Schizoaffective Disorder: EPS, somnolence, dyspepsia, constipation, weight gain, nasopharyngitis.

DRUG INTERACTIONS
Consider additive exposure w/ risperidone. Avoid w/ other drugs known to prolong QTc interval, including Class 1A (eg, quinidine, procainamide) or Class III (eg, amiodarone, sotalol) antiarrhythmics, antipsychotics (eg, chlorpromazine, thioridazine), and antibiotics (eg, gatifloxacin, moxifloxacin). Caution w/ other centrally acting drugs, alcohol, and drugs w/ anticholinergic activity. May antagonize the effect of levodopa and other dopamine agonists. Additive effect may be observed w/ other agents that cause orthostatic hypotension. Carbamazepine may decrease levels; reevaluate doses, if necessary. Paroxetine may increase exposure in CYP2D6 extensive metabolizers. Divalproex sodium may increase levels; consider dose reduction w/ valproate.

PREGNANCY AND LACTATION
Pregnancy: Category C. Neonates exposed to antipsychotic drugs during the 3rd trimester of pregnancy are at risk for extrapyramidal and/or withdrawal symptoms following delivery.
Lactation: Excreted in human breast milk; not for use in nursing.

MECHANISM OF ACTION
Benzisoxazole derivative; has not been established. Active metabolite of risperidone; proposed to be mediated through a combination of central dopamine type 2 and $5HT_{2A}$ receptor antagonism.

PHARMACOKINETICS
Absorption: Absolute bioavailability (28%); T_{max}=24 hrs. **Distribution:** Plasma protein binding (74%); V_d=487L; found in breast milk. **Metabolism:** CYP2D6, 3A4 (limited); (IR) dealkylation, hydroxylation, dehydrogenation, and benzisoxazole scission. **Elimination:** (IR) Urine (80%; 59% unchanged), feces (11%); $T_{1/2}$=23 hrs.

PATIENT CONSIDERATIONS
Assessment: Assess for hypersensitivity to drug, dementia-related psychosis, congenital long QT syndrome, history of cardiac arrhythmias, DM, risk factors for DM, severe GI narrowing, history of clinically significant low WBCs or drug-induced leukopenia/neutropenia, Parkinson's disease, dementia w/ Lewy bodies, renal/hepatic impairment, any other conditions where treatment is contraindicated or cautioned, pregnancy/nursing status, and possible drug interactions. Obtain baseline FPG in patients at risk for DM.

Monitoring: Monitor for NMS, TD, QT prolongation, hyperprolactinemia, orthostatic hypotension, syncope, cognitive and motor impairment, seizures, esophageal dysmotility, aspiration, priapism, disruption of body temperature, and other adverse reactions. Monitor for signs of hyperglycemia; perform periodic monitoring of FPG levels in patients w/ DM or at risk for DM. Monitor for signs/symptoms of leukopenia/neutropenia; frequently monitor CBC in patients w/ a history of clinically significant low WBC count or drug-induced leukopenia/neutropenia. Monitor weight and renal function. Periodically reevaluate long-term usefulness of therapy.

Counseling: Inform of the risk of orthostatic hypotension during initiation/reinitiation or dose increases. Inform that therapy has the potential to impair judgment, thinking, or motor skills; advise to use caution when operating hazardous machinery (eg, automobiles). Advise to avoid alcohol during therapy. Instruct to notify physician of all prescription and nonprescription drugs currently taking, and if pregnant, intending to become pregnant, or breastfeeding. Advise regarding appropriate care in avoiding overheating and dehydration. Advise that the tab shell, along w/ insoluble core components, may be found in stool.

INVEGA SUSTENNA — paliperidone palmitate   Rx

Class: Atypical antipsychotic

> Elderly patients w/ dementia-related psychosis treated w/ antipsychotic drugs are at an increased risk of death. Not approved for use in patients w/ dementia-related psychosis.

ADULT DOSAGE
Schizophrenia
Initial: 234mg on Day 1, then 156mg on Day 8 (both in deltoid muscle)
Maint: 117mg/month (in deltoid/gluteal muscle), administer 5 weeks after 1st inj; some may benefit from lower or higher dose w/in the available strengths (39-234mg)
Max: 234mg/month

Establish tolerability w/ oral paliperidone/risperidone prior to initiating therapy in oral paliperidone- or oral/injectable risperidone-naive patients

Schizoaffective Disorder
Monotherapy and Adjunctive Therapy to Mood Stabilizers/Antidepressants:
Initial: 234mg on Day 1, then 156mg on Day 8 (both in deltoid muscle)
Maint: 78-234mg/month (in deltoid/gluteal muscle), administer 5 weeks

PEDIATRIC DOSAGE
Pediatric use may not have been established

after 1st inj; adjust maint dose monthly based on tolerability and/or efficacy using available strengths
Max: 234mg/month

Establish tolerability w/ oral paliperidone/risperidone prior to initiating therapy in oral paliperidone- or oral/injectable risperidone-naive patients

Conversions

Switching from Oral Antipsychotics:
Gradually d/c oral antipsychotics at the time of initiation of therapy

Tab, Extended-Release to Inj Maint Dose Conversion:
3mg PO qd: 39-78mg IM every 4 weeks
6mg PO qd: 117mg IM every 4 weeks
12mg PO qd: 234mg IM every 4 weeks

Switching from Long-Acting Injectable Antipsychotics:
Initiate therapy in place of the next scheduled inj and continue w/ monthly maint dose; the 1-week initiation dosing regimen is not required

Missed Dose

Avoiding Missed Doses:
May give 2nd initiation dose 4 days before/after the 1-week time point. May give 3rd and subsequent monthly inj up to 7 days before/after the monthly time point

Management of a Missed 2nd Initiation Dose:
<4 Weeks Since 1st Inj:
Administer 2nd inj (156mg) as soon as possible. A 3rd inj (117mg) is recommended 5 weeks after 1st inj (regardless of timing of 2nd inj), followed thereafter by normal monthly inj
4-7 Weeks Since 1st Inj:
Resume dosing w/ 2 inj of 156mg, administered in the deltoid 1 week apart, then resume usual monthly inj cycle
>7 Weeks Since 1st Inj:
Restart therapy

Management of a Missed Maint Dose:
4-6 Weeks Since Last Inj:
Resume regular monthly dosing as soon as possible at previously stabilized dose, followed by inj at monthly intervals
>6 Weeks to 6 Months Since Last Inj:
Resume the same previously stabilized dose as soon as possible into the deltoid, followed by another deltoid inj at the same dose 1 week later. Resume monthly dosing thereafter. If previous stabilized dose was 234mg, then 1st two inj should be 156mg each
>6 Months Since Last Inj:
Restart therapy

- - -

DOSING CONSIDERATIONS
Concomitant Medications
Strong CYP3A4/P-gp Inducers:
May need to increase dose; may need to decrease the dose when the strong inducer is discontinued
Risperidone/Oral Paliperidone:
Caution when coadministered for extended periods of time

Renal Impairment
Mild (CrCl 50 to <80mL/min):
Initial: 156mg on Day 1, then 117mg 1 week later (both in the deltoid muscle)
Maint: 78mg/month (in deltoid or gluteal muscle)
Moderate or Severe (CrCl <50mL/min): Not recommended

ADMINISTRATION
IM route

Inject slowly, deep into muscle.
Administer as a single inj; do not administer dose in divided inj.
Avoid inadvertent inj into a blood vessel.

Deltoid Muscle Inj
Alternate deltoid inj between the 2 deltoid muscles.

Needle Size Recommendations:
<90kg: 1-inch, 23-gauge needle
≥90kg: 1.5-inch, 22-gauge needle

Gluteal Muscle Inj
Administer into the upper outer quadrant of gluteal muscle; alternate gluteal inj between the 2 gluteal muscles.
Needle Size Recommendations:
1.5-inch, 22-gauge needle size regardless of weight

STORAGE
25°C (77°F); excursions permitted to 15-30°C (59-86°F).

HOW SUPPLIED
Inj, Extended-Release: 39mg, 78mg, 117mg, 156mg, 234mg

CONTRAINDICATIONS
Known hypersensitivity to either paliperidone or risperidone, or to any of the excipients in this formulation.

WARNINGS/PRECAUTIONS
Neuroleptic malignant syndrome (NMS) reported; d/c immediately if this occurs. May increase QTc interval; avoid w/ congenital long QT syndrome and history of cardiac arrhythmias. May develop tardive dyskinesia (TD); consider discontinuing if this occurs. Hyperglycemia and diabetes mellitus (DM), in some cases extreme and associated w/ ketoacidosis or hyperosmolar coma or death, reported. Dyslipidemia, weight gain, and hyperprolactinemia reported. May induce orthostatic hypotension and syncope; caution w/ known cardiovascular/cerebrovascular disease or conditions that predispose the patient to hypotension. Leukopenia, neutropenia, and agranulocytosis reported; d/c in cases of severe neutropenia (ANC <1000/mm^3). Somnolence, sedation, and dizziness reported. May impair mental/physical abilities. Seizures reported; caution w/ history of seizures or conditions that potentially lower the seizure threshold. May cause esophageal dysmotility and aspiration; use w/ caution in patients w/ a risk of aspiration pneumonia. May induce priapism; severe cases may require surgical intervention. May disrupt body's ability to reduce core body temperature; caution w/ conditions that may contribute to an elevated core body temperature. Patients w/ Parkinson's disease or dementia w/ Lewy bodies may have increased sensitivity to therapy. Caution in elderly.

ADVERSE REACTIONS
N/V, inj-site reactions, nasopharyngitis, weight gain, dizziness, akathisia, extrapyramidal disorder, headache, somnolence/sedation, agitation, anxiety, pyrexia, hyperprolactinemia.

DRUG INTERACTIONS
See Dosing Considerations. May antagonize the effect of levodopa and other dopamine agonists. An additive effect may occur w/ other agents that also cause orthostatic hypotension. Avoid w/ other drugs known to prolong QTc interval, including Class 1A (eg, quinidine, procainamide) or Class III (eg, amiodarone, sotalol) antiarrhythmics, antipsychotics (eg, chlorpromazine, thioridazine), or antibiotics (eg, gatifloxacin, moxifloxacin). Caution w/ anticholinergics; may contribute to an elevated body temperature.

PREGNANCY AND LACTATION
Category C, not for use in nursing.

MECHANISM OF ACTION
Atypical antipsychotic; has not been established. Proposed to be mediated through a combination of central dopamine type 2 and 5HT$_{2A}$ receptor antagonism.

PHARMACOKINETICS
Absorption: T_{max}=13 days. **Distribution:** V_d=391L; plasma protein binding (74%); found in breast milk. **Metabolism:** (PO) Dealkylation, hydroxylation, dehydrogenation, and benzisoxazole scission; CYP2D6, CYP3A4 (limited). **Elimination:** (39-234mg IM single-dose) $T_{1/2}$=25-49 days.

PATIENT CONSIDERATIONS

Assessment: Assess for known hypersensitivity to drug/risperidone/any of the excipients, dementia-related psychosis, congenital long QT syndrome, history of cardiac arrhythmias, DM, risk factors for DM, history of clinically significant low WBC counts or drug-induced leukopenia/neutropenia, Parkinson's disease, dementia w/ Lewy bodies, renal impairment, any other conditions where treatment is contraindicated or cautioned, pregnancy/nursing status, and possible drug interactions. Obtain baseline FPG in patients at risk for DM.

Monitoring: Monitor for hypersensitivity reactions, NMS, QT prolongation, TD, hyperprolactinemia, orthostatic hypotension, syncope, seizures, aspiration, priapism, disruption of body temperature, and other adverse reactions. Monitor for signs of hyperglycemia; perform periodic monitoring of FPG levels in patients w/ DM or at risk for DM. Monitor for signs/symptoms of leukopenia/neutropenia; frequently monitor CBC in patients w/ a history of clinically significant low WBC counts or drug-induced leukopenia/neutropenia. Monitor weight and renal function. Reassess periodically to determine need for continued treatment.

Counseling: Advise patients on risk of orthostatic hypotension. Caution about operating machinery/driving until certain that therapy does not affect the patient adversely. Advise to avoid overheating and becoming dehydrated. Instruct to inform physician about any concomitant prescription or OTC medications. Advise to notify physician if pregnancy occurs or is intended. Instruct not to breastfeed.

INVEGA TRINZA — paliperidone palmitate

Class: Atypical antipsychotic

Rx

> Elderly patients w/ dementia-related psychosis treated w/ antipsychotic drugs are at an increased risk of death. Not approved for use in patients w/ dementia-related psychosis.

ADULT DOSAGE

Schizophrenia

3-month inj for the treatment of schizophrenia in patients after they have been adequately treated w/ Invega Sustenna (1-month paliperidone palmitate ER injectable sus) for at least 4 months

Initiate when the next 1-month paliperidone dose is scheduled w/ an Invega Trinza dose based on the previous 1-month inj dose, using the equivalent 3.5-fold higher dose; refer to initial Invega Trinza dose listed below

Administer up to 7 days before or after the monthly time point of the next scheduled paliperidone 1-month dose

Initial Invega Trinza Dose Based on Last Dose of Invega Sustenna:
Invega Sustenna 78mg: 273mg Invega Trinza every 3 months
Invega Sustenna 117mg: 410mg Invega Trinza every 3 months
Invega Sustenna 156mg: 546mg Invega Trinza every 3 months
Invega Sustenna 234mg: 819mg Invega Trinza every 3 months

If needed, dose adjustment can be made every 3 months in increments w/in the range of 273-819mg based on individual patient tolerability and/ or efficacy

In order to establish a consistent maint dose, it is recommended that the last 2 doses of Invega Sustenna be the same dosage strength before starting Invega Trinza

Missed Dose

Dosing Window:
Avoid missing doses; may give the inj up to 2 weeks before or after the 3-month time point if necessary

Missed Dose 3.5-4 Months Since Last Inj:
Administer the previously administered dose as soon as possible, then continue w/ the 3-month inj following this dose

Missed Dose 4-9 Months Since Last Inj:
Do not administer the next dose; refer to PI for reinitiation regimen

Missed Dose Longer Than 9 Months Since Last Inj:
Reinitiate treatment w/ the 1-month paliperidone ER injectable sus; may resume Invega Trinza after the patient has been adequately treated w/ the 1-month paliperidone ER injectable sus for at least 4 months

Conversions

Switching from Invega Trinza (Last Dose) to Invega Sustenna (1-Month Paliperidone ER Injectable Sus):
Invega Trinza 273mg: Initiate 78mg Invega Sustenna 3 months later
Invega Trinza 410mg: Initiate 117mg Invega Sustenna 3 months later
Invega Trinza 546mg: Initiate 156mg Invega Sustenna 3 months later
Invega Trinza 819mg: Initiate 234mg Invega Sustenna 3 months later

The 1-month paliperidone ER injectable sus should then continue, dosed at monthly intervals

PEDIATRIC DOSAGE

Pediatric use may not have been established

Switching from Invega Trinza to Oral Paliperidone ER Tabs:
Daily dosing of the paliperidone ER tabs should start 3 months after the last Invega Trinza dose and be transitioned over the next several months following the last Invega Trinza dose; refer to PI for Invega Trinza doses and once daily paliperidone ER conversion regimens needed to attain similar paliperidone exposures

----

DOSING CONSIDERATIONS

Concomitant Medications

Use w/ Risperidone or w/ Oral Paliperidone: Use w/ caution when coadministered for extended periods of time

Renal Impairment

Mild (CrCl ≥50 to <80mL/min): Adjust dose and stabilize the patient using the 1-month paliperidone ER injectable sus, then transition to Invega Trinza
Moderate/Severe (CrCl <50mL/min): Not recommended

ADMINISTRATION

IM route

Administer once every 3 months.
Each inj must be administered only by a healthcare professional.
Shake syringe vigorously for at least 15 sec; inject w/in 5 min of shaking vigorously to ensure a homogeneous sus and ensure needle does not get clogged during inj.
Avoid inadvertent inj into a blood vessel.
Administer as a single inj; do not administer dose in divided inj.
Inject slowly, deep into the deltoid or gluteal muscle.
Administer using only the thin wall needles that are provided in the pack; do not use needles from the 1-month paliperidone ER injectable sus pack or other commercially-available needles.
Do not re-inject dose remaining in the syringe and do not administer another dose in the event of an incompletely administered dose.

Needle Size Recommendations

Deltoid Muscle:
<90kg: 1-inch, 22-gauge needle
≥90kg: 1.5-inch, 22-gauge needle
Gluteal Muscle:
1.5-inch, 22-gauge needle size, regardless of weight

STORAGE

20-25°C (68-77°F); excursions permitted between 15-30°C (59-86°F).

HOW SUPPLIED

Inj, ER: 273mg, 410mg, 546mg, 819mg

CONTRAINDICATIONS

Known hypersensitivity to either paliperidone or risperidone, or to any of the excipients in this formulation.

WARNINGS/PRECAUTIONS

Neuroleptic malignant syndrome (NMS) reported; d/c therapy and institute symptomatic treatment. May increase QTc interval; avoid in patients w/ congenital long QT syndrome and in patients w/ history of cardiac arrhythmias. May cause tardive dyskinesia (TD), especially in the elderly; consider discontinuation if this occurs. Hyperglycemia and diabetes mellitus (DM), in some cases extreme and associated w/ ketoacidosis or hyperosmolar coma or death, reported. Dyslipidemia, weight gain, and hyperprolactinemia reported. May induce orthostatic hypotension and syncope; caution w/ known cardiovascular/ cerebrovascular disease or conditions that predispose to hypotension. Leukopenia, neutropenia, and agranulocytosis reported; consider discontinuation at 1st sign of a clinically significant decline in WBC count in the absence of other causative factors in patients w/ a history of a clinically significant low WBC count/ANC or a drug-induced leukopenia/neutropenia. D/C therapy and follow WBC count until recovery in patients w/ severe neutropenia (ANC <1000/mm^3). Somnolence, sedation, and dizziness reported. May impair mental/physical abilities. Caution w/ history of seizures or other conditions that potentially lower the seizure threshold. May cause esophageal dysmotility and aspiration; caution in patients at risk for aspiration pneumonia. May induce priapism; severe cases may require surgical intervention. May disrupt body's ability to reduce core body temperature; caution w/ conditions that may contribute to an elevated core body temperature. Patients w/ Parkinson's disease or dementia w/ Lewy bodies may experience increased sensitivity to therapy.

ADVERSE REACTIONS

Inj-site reaction, URTI, weight increase, akathisia, headache, parkinsonism, UTI.

DRUG INTERACTIONS

Avoid in combination w/ other drugs that are known to prolong QTc interval including Class 1A (eg, quinidine, procainamide) or Class III (eg, amiodarone, sotalol) antiarrhythmics, antipsychotics (eg, chlorpromazine, thioridazine), antibiotics (eg, gatifloxacin, moxifloxacin), and any other class of medications known to prolong the QTc interval. An additive effect may occur w/ drugs that have potential for inducing orthostatic hypotension; monitor orthostatic vital signs in patients who are vulnerable to hypotension. Strong inducers of CYP3A4 and P-gp (eg, carbamazepine, rifampin, St. John's wort) may decrease exposure; avoid using CYP3A4 and/or P-gp inducers during the 3-month dosing interval, if possible, and consider managing the patient using paliperidone ER tabs if administering a strong inducer is necessary. Caution if receiving a concomitant medication w/ anticholinergic activity. May antagonize the effect of levodopa and other dopamine agonists; monitor and manage patients as clinically appropriate.

PREGNANCY AND LACTATION

Pregnancy: There is a pregnancy exposure registry that monitors pregnancy outcomes in women exposed to paliperidone during pregnancy. Neonates exposed to antipsychotic drugs during the 3rd trimester of pregnancy are at risk for extrapyramidal and/or withdrawal symptoms following delivery; monitor and manage symptoms appropriately.
Lactation: Found in breast milk and has been detected in plasma at very low levels up to 18 months after a single-dose administration; safety not known in nursing.

MECHANISM OF ACTION

Atypical antipsychotic; has not been established. Proposed to be mediated through a combination of central dopamine type 2 and $5HT_{2A}$ receptor antagonism.

PHARMACOKINETICS

Absorption: T_{max}=30-33 days (median). **Distribution:** V_d=1960L; plasma protein binding (74%); found in breast milk. **Metabolism:** Dealkylation, hydroxylation, dehydrogenation, and benzisoxazole scission; CYP2D6, CYP3A4 (limited). **Elimination:** Urine (approx 80%, approx 59% unchanged), feces (11%); $T_{1/2}$ (median)=(273-819mg) 84-95 days following deltoid inj, 118-139 days following gluteal inj.

PATIENT CONSIDERATIONS

Assessment: Assess for known hypersensitivity to the drug, dementia-related psychosis, congenital long QT syndrome, history of cardiac arrhythmias, DM, history of clinically significant low WBCs or drug-induced leukopenia/neutropenia, renal impairment, any other conditions where treatment is contraindicated or cautioned, pregnancy/nursing status, and possible drug interactions. Obtain baseline FPG in patients at risk for DM.

Monitoring: Monitor for hypersensitivity reactions, NMS, QT prolongation, TD, hyperglycemia, weight gain, dyslipidemia, orthostatic hypotension, syncope, seizures, esophageal dysmotility, aspiration, priapism, cognitive and motor impairment, disruption of body temperature, and other adverse reactions. Monitor CBC frequently in patients w/ a history of a clinically significant low WBC count/ANC or drug-induced leukopenia/neutropenia. Monitor for fever or other signs/symptoms of infection in patients w/ neutropenia. Monitor for worsening of glucose control in patients w/ DM. Monitor FPG levels in patients at risk for DM periodically during therapy. Reassess periodically to determine need for continued treatment.

Counseling: Inform of the risks/benefits of therapy. Inform about risk of developing NMS and explain its signs and symptoms. Counsel on the signs and symptoms of TD and advise to contact physician if these abnormal movements occur. Counsel about the risk of metabolic changes, how to recognize symptoms of hyperglycemia and DM, and the need for specific monitoring. Inform about risk of orthostatic hypotension, particularly at the time of initiating treatment, reinitiating treatment, or increasing the dose. Advise patients w/ preexisting low WBC counts or history of drug-induced leukopenia/neutropenia to have their CBC monitored. Counsel on signs and symptoms of hyperprolactinemia that may be associated w/ chronic use; advise to seek medical attention if a female patient experiences amenorrhea or galactorrhea or if a male patient experiences erectile dysfunction or gynecomastia. Caution about operating hazardous machinery, including automobiles. Advise of the possibility of painful or prolonged penile erections; instruct to seek immediate medical attention in the event of priapism. Counsel on the importance of avoiding overheating and dehydration. Advise to inform physician if taking/planning to take any prescription or OTC drugs. Advise female patients to notify physician if pregnancy occurs or is intended during treatment. Advise that there is a pregnancy registry that monitors pregnancy outcomes in women exposed to paliperidone during pregnancy.

INVOKAMET — canagliflozin/metformin hydrochloride   Rx

Class: Biguanide/sodium-glucose cotransporter 2 (SGLT2) inhibitor

> Cases of metformin-associated lactic acidosis resulting in death, hypothermia, hypotension, and resistant bradyarrhythmias reported. Risk factors include renal impairment; concomitant use of certain drugs (eg, cationic drugs such as topiramate); age ≥65 years; having a radiological study w/ contrast, surgery, and other procedures; hypoxic states (eg, acute CHF); excessive alcohol intake; and hepatic impairment. D/C therapy immediately and institute general supportive measures in a hospital setting if metformin-associated lactic acidosis is suspected. Prompt hemodialysis is recommended.

ADULT DOSAGE

Type 2 Diabetes Mellitus

When treatment w/ both canagliflozin and metformin is appropriate

Patients Currently Not Treated w/ Either Canagliflozin or Metformin:
Initiate therapy w/ Invokamet containing canagliflozin 50mg and metformin 500mg

Patients on Metformin:
Switch to Invokamet containing canagliflozin 50mg and the same, or nearest appropriate, daily dose of metformin

Patients on Canagliflozin:
Switch to Invokamet containing metformin 500mg w/ the same daily dose of canagliflozin

PEDIATRIC DOSAGE

Pediatric use may not have been established

Patients Already Treated w/ Canagliflozin and Metformin:
Switch to Invokamet containing the same daily dose of canagliflozin and the same, or nearest appropriate, daily dose of metformin

eGFR of ≥60mL/min/1.73m²:
Titrate: May increase dose for the canagliflozin component to 150mg bid, w/ gradual metformin dose escalation to reduce the GI side effects due to metformin, in patients tolerating canagliflozin 50mg bid who require additional glycemic control
Max: (300mg/2000mg)/day

Take 1 tab bid w/ meals

DOSING CONSIDERATIONS

Concomitant Medications
UDP-Glucuronosyl Transferase Enzyme Inducers (eg, Rifampin, Phenytoin, Phenobarbital, Ritonavir):
eGFR ≥60mL/min/1.73m²: Consider increasing canagliflozin dose to 150mg bid in patients currently tolerating 50mg bid and requiring additional glycemic control
eGFR 45 to <60mL/min/1.73m²: Consider another antihyperglycemic agent

Renal Impairment
Moderate (eGFR 45 to <60mL/min/1.73m²): Limit canagliflozin dose to 50mg bid
eGFR <45mL/min/1.73m²: Contraindicated

Hepatic Impairment
Not recommended

Other Important Considerations
Patients w/ Volume-Depletion Not Previously Treated w/ Canagliflozin: Correct this condition before initiating treatment

Iodinated Contrast Imaging Procedures:
D/C therapy at the time of, or prior to, an iodinated contrast imaging procedure in patients w/ an eGFR 45-60mL/min/1.73m²; in patients w/ a history of liver disease, alcoholism, or HF; or in patients who will be administered intra-arterial iodinated contrast. Reevaluate eGFR 48 hrs after the imaging procedure and restart therapy if renal function is stable

ADMINISTRATION
Oral route

STORAGE
20-25°C (68-77°F); excursions permitted between 15-30°C (59-86°F). Store in original container.

HOW SUPPLIED
Tab: (Canagliflozin/Metformin) 50mg/500mg, 50mg/1000mg, 150mg/500mg, 150mg/1000mg

CONTRAINDICATIONS
Moderate to severe renal impairment (eGFR <45mL/min/1.73m²), ESRD, or patients on dialysis. Acute or chronic metabolic acidosis, including diabetic ketoacidosis. History of a serious hypersensitivity reaction to canagliflozin or metformin (eg, anaphylaxis, angioedema).

WARNINGS/PRECAUTIONS
See Dosing Considerations. Not recommended in patients w/ type 1 diabetes mellitus (DM) or for treatment of diabetic ketoacidosis. **Canagliflozin:** Symptomatic hypotension may occur after initiating therapy, particularly in patients w/ eGFR <60mL/min/1.73m², elderly patients, patients on either diuretics or medications that interfere w/ the renin-angiotensin-aldosterone system (RAAS), or patients w/ low systolic BP; assess and correct volume status before initiating treatment in patients w/ ≥1 of these characteristics who were not already on canagliflozin. Ketoacidosis reported; if suspected, d/c and institute prompt treatment. Assess for ketoacidosis in patients presenting w/ signs/symptoms consistent w/ severe metabolic acidosis regardless of presenting blood glucose levels. Consider temporarily discontinuing therapy in clinical situations known to predispose to ketoacidosis (eg, prolonged fasting due to acute illness or surgery). Causes intravascular volume contraction and can cause renal impairment. Consider temporarily discontinuing in any setting of reduced oral intake or fluid losses. D/C and institute treatment if acute kidney injury occurs. Increases SrCr and decreases eGFR; patients w/ hypovolemia may be more susceptible. Renal function abnormalities may occur; monitor renal function more frequently in patients w/ an eGFR <60mL/min/1.73m². May lead to hyperkalemia; increased risk in patients w/ moderate renal impairment who are taking medications that interfere w/ K+ excretion or medications that interfere w/ the RAAS. Serious UTIs (eg, urosepsis, pyelonephritis), requiring hospitalization, reported; evaluate for signs/symptoms of UTIs and treat promptly, if indicated. Increases risk of genital mycotic infections; increased risk w/ a history of genital mycotic infections and uncircumcised males. Hypersensitivity reactions (eg, angioedema, anaphylaxis) reported; d/c and treat if this occurs, and monitor until signs/symptoms resolve. Increased risk of bone fractures reported; consider factors that contribute to fracture risk prior to initiating therapy. Dose-related increases in LDL levels reported. Monitoring glycemic control w/ urine glucose tests or 1,5-anhydroglucitol assay is not recommended. **Metformin:** Withholding of food and fluids during surgical or other procedures may increase the risk for volume depletion, hypotension, and renal impairment; temporarily d/c while patient has restricted food and fluid intake. D/C if a condition associated w/ hypoxemia occurs (eg, cardiovascular collapse, acute MI, sepsis). May decrease vitamin B12 levels to subnormal levels; monitor hematologic parameters annually. Hypoglycemia may occur when caloric intake is deficient

or when strenuous exercise is not compensated by caloric supplementation; elderly, debilitated, or malnourished patients and those w/ adrenal or pituitary insufficiency or alcohol intoxication are particularly susceptible to hypoglycemic effects. Hypoglycemia may be difficult to recognize in the elderly.

ADVERSE REACTIONS
Canagliflozin: Female genital mycotic infections, UTIs, increased urination. **Metformin:** Diarrhea, N/V, flatulence, asthenia, indigestion, abdominal discomfort, headache.

DRUG INTERACTIONS
See Boxed Warning and Dosing Considerations. **Canagliflozin:** May increase the risk of hypoglycemia when combined w/ insulin or an insulin secretagogue; a lower dose of insulin or insulin secretagogue may be required to minimize the risk of hypoglycemia. Rifampin lowered exposure, which may reduce efficacy. Increased digoxin exposure; monitor for a need to adjust dose of either drug. **Metformin:** Topiramate and other carbonic anhydrase inhibitors (eg, zonisamide, acetazolamide, dichlorphenamide) may increase the risk of lactic acidosis; consider more frequent monitoring of these patients. Drugs that are eliminated by renal tubular secretion, drugs that impair renal function, drugs that result in significant hemodynamic change, drugs that interfere w/ acid-base balance, or drugs that increase metformin accumulation may increase the risk of metformin-associated lactic acidosis; consider more frequent monitoring of these patients. Avoid excessive alcohol intake; alcohol is known to potentiate the effect of metformin on lactate metabolism. Thiazides and other diuretics, corticosteroids, phenothiazines, thyroid products, estrogens, oral contraceptives, phenytoin, nicotinic acid, sympathomimetics, calcium channel blockers, and isoniazid may produce hyperglycemia and lead to loss of glycemic control; monitor for loss of blood glucose control when such drugs are administered and monitor for hypoglycemia when such drugs are withdrawn. Hypoglycemia may occur during concomitant use w/ other glucose-lowering agents (eg, sulfonylureas, insulin) or ethanol. Hypoglycemia may be difficult to recognize w/ β-adrenergic blocking drugs.

PREGNANCY AND LACTATION
Pregnancy: Based on animal data showing adverse renal effects, not recommended during the 2nd and 3rd trimesters of pregnancy. **Lactation:** Not for use in nursing. **Reproductive Potential:** Discuss the potential for unintended pregnancy w/ premenopausal women as therapy w/ metformin may result in ovulation in some anovulatory women.

MECHANISM OF ACTION
Canagliflozin: SGLT2 inhibitor; reduces reabsorption of filtered glucose and lowers the renal threshold for glucose, and thereby increases urinary glucose excretion. **Metformin:** Biguanide; decreases hepatic glucose production, decreases intestinal absorption of glucose, and improves insulin sensitivity by increasing peripheral glucose uptake and utilization.

PHARMACOKINETICS
Absorption: Canagliflozin: Absolute oral bioavailability (65%); T_{max}=1-2 hrs (median). Metformin: Absolute bioavailability (50-60%) (500mg, fasted). **Distribution:** Canagliflozin: Plasma protein binding (99%); (IV) V_d=83.5L. Metformin: V_d=654L (850mg). **Metabolism:** Canagliflozin: O-glucuronidation (major) by UGT1A9 and UGT2B4; oxidation (minor) via CYP3A4. **Elimination:** Canagliflozin: Feces (41.5% unchanged, 7% hydroxylated metabolite, 3.2% O-glucuronide metabolite), urine (33%; <1% unchanged, 30.5% O-glucuronide metabolite); $T_{1/2}$=10.6 hrs (100mg), 13.1 hrs (300mg). Metformin: Urine (90%); $T_{1/2}$=6.2 hrs (plasma), 17.6 hrs (blood).

PATIENT CONSIDERATIONS
Assessment: Assess for acute/chronic metabolic acidosis (including diabetic ketoacidosis); drug hypersensitivity; risk for lactic acidosis, genital mycotic infections, or fractures; type of DM; predisposition to developing subnormal vitamin B12 levels, ketoacidosis, hyperkalemia, or acute kidney injury; renal/hepatic impairment; volume status; alcoholism; hypoxemia; adrenal/pituitary insufficiency; any other conditions where treatment is contraindicated or cautioned; pregnancy/nursing status; and possible drug interactions. Assess if patient is planning to undergo any surgical procedure. Obtain baseline LFTs, FPG, HbA1c, eGFR, and hematologic parameters.

Monitoring: Monitor for signs/symptoms of lactic acidosis, hypotension, ketoacidosis, UTIs, genital mycotic infections, hypersensitivity reactions, bone fractures, and other adverse reactions. Monitor eGFR at least annually; monitor more frequently in patients at risk of developing renal impairment. Monitor hematologic parameters annually. Perform routine serum vitamin B12 measurements at 2- to 3-yr intervals in patients predisposed to developing subnormal vitamin B12 levels. Monitor FPG, HbA1c, and LDL levels. Periodically monitor serum K^+ levels in patients w/ impaired renal function and in patients predisposed to hyperkalemia due to medications or other medical conditions.

Counseling: Inform of the risks of lactic acidosis, its symptoms, and conditions that predispose to its development; instruct to d/c immediately and notify physician if unexplained hyperventilation, myalgias, malaise, unusual somnolence, or other nonspecific symptoms occur. Counsel against excessive alcohol intake. Inform about the importance of regular testing of renal function and hematological parameters while on therapy. Instruct to seek medical advice promptly during periods of stress (eg, fever, trauma, infection) as medication requirements may change. Instruct to take only as prescribed and inform not to put in pill boxes or pill organizers. Instruct to report to physician if pregnant, nursing, or experiencing symptoms of hypotension. Instruct to have adequate fluid intake. Instruct to d/c and seek medical advice immediately if symptoms of ketoacidosis occur. Advise to seek medical advice if patient has reduced oral intake or increased fluid losses. Counsel on the signs/symptoms of UTI, vaginal

yeast infection, balanitis, and balanoposthitis; inform of treatment options and when to seek medical advice. Inform that serious hypersensitivity reactions have been reported; advise to report any signs or symptoms suggesting an allergic reaction, and to d/c therapy until they have consulted their prescribing physicians. Inform that bone fractures have been reported and provide information on factors that may contribute to fracture risk. Advise patients that they will test positive for glucose in their urine while on therapy. Inform females that treatment may result in ovulation in some premenopausal anovulatory women, which may lead to unintended pregnancy.

INVOKANA — canagliflozin
Rx

Class: Sodium-glucose cotransporter 2 (SGLT2) inhibitor

ADULT DOSAGE	PEDIATRIC DOSAGE
Type 2 Diabetes Mellitus	Pediatric use may not have been established
Initial: 100mg qd before the 1st meal of the day	
Titrate: May increase to 300mg qd in patients tolerating 100mg qd who have an eGFR ≥60mL/min/1.73m² and require additional glycemic control	

DOSING CONSIDERATIONS
Concomitant Medications
UDP-Glucuronosyl Transferase Enzyme Inducers (eg, Rifampin, Phenytoin, Phenobarbital, Ritonavir):
eGFR ≥60mL/min/1.73m²: Consider increasing canagliflozin dose to 300mg qd in patients tolerating 100mg qd and requiring additional glycemic control
eGFR 45 to <60mL/min/1.73m²: Consider another antihyperglycemic agent

Renal Impairment
Moderate (eGFR 45 to <60mL/min/1.73m²): Limit dose to 100mg qd
eGFR <45mL/min/1.73m²: Treatment initiation is not recommended
Not recommended when eGFR is persistently <45mL/min/1.73m²

Hepatic Impairment
Severe: Not recommended

Other Important Considerations
Patients w/ Volume-Depletion:
Correct this condition before initiating treatment

ADMINISTRATION
Oral route

Take w/ or w/o food.

STORAGE
25°C (77°F); excursions permitted to 15-30°C (59-86°F).

HOW SUPPLIED
Tab: 100mg, 300mg

CONTRAINDICATIONS
History of a serious hypersensitivity reaction to canagliflozin (eg, anaphylaxis, angioedema). Severe renal impairment (eGFR <30mL/min/1.73m²), ESRD, patients on dialysis.

WARNINGS/PRECAUTIONS
Not recommended w/ type 1 diabetes mellitus (DM) or for treatment of diabetic ketoacidosis. Symptomatic hypotension may occur, particularly in patients w/ renal impairment (eGFR <60mL/min/1.73m²), elderly patients, patients on either diuretics or medications that interfere w/ the renin-angiotensin-aldosterone system (RAAS), or patients w/ low systolic BP; assess and correct volume status before initiating treatment in patients w/ ≥1 of these characteristics. Ketoacidosis reported; if suspected, d/c and institute prompt treatment. Assess for ketoacidosis in patients presenting w/ signs/symptoms consistent w/ severe metabolic acidosis regardless of presenting blood glucose levels. Consider temporarily discontinuing therapy in clinical situations known to predispose to ketoacidosis (eg, prolonged fasting due to acute illness or surgery). Causes intravascular volume contraction and can cause renal impairment. Consider temporarily discontinuing in any setting of reduced oral intake or fluid losses. D/C and institute treatment if acute kidney injury occurs. Increases SrCr and decreases eGFR; patients w/ hypovolemia may be more susceptible. Renal function abnormalities may occur; monitor renal function more frequently in patients w/ an eGFR <60mL/min/1.73m². May lead to hyperkalemia; increased risk in patients w/ moderate renal impairment who are taking medications that interfere w/ K^+ excretion or medications that interfere w/ the RAAS. Serious UTIs (eg, urosepsis, pyelonephritis), requiring hospitalization, reported; evaluate for signs/symptoms of UTIs and treat promptly, if indicated. Increases risk of genital mycotic infections; increased risk w/ a history of genital mycotic infections and uncircumcised males. Hypersensitivity reactions (eg, angioedema, anaphylaxis) reported; d/c and treat if this occurs and monitor until signs/symptoms resolve. Increased risk of bone fractures observed; consider factors that contribute to fracture risk prior to initiation. Dose-related increases in LDL levels reported. Monitoring glycemic control w/ urine glucose tests or 1,5-anhydroglucitol assay is not recommended.

ADVERSE REACTIONS
Female genital mycotic infections, UTIs, increased urination.

DRUG INTERACTIONS
See Dosing Considerations. Rifampin decreases exposure. Increases levels of digoxin; monitor appropriately. May increase risk of hypoglycemia when combined w/ insulin or an insulin secretagogue; lower dose of insulin or insulin secretagogue may be required.

PREGNANCY AND LACTATION
Pregnancy: Based on animal data showing adverse renal effects, not recommended during the 2nd and 3rd trimesters of pregnancy.
Lactation: Not for use in nursing.

MECHANISM OF ACTION
SGLT2 inhibitor; reduces reabsorption of filtered glucose and lowers the renal threshold for glucose, and thereby increases urinary glucose excretion.

PHARMACOKINETICS
Absorption: Absolute oral bioavailability (65%); T_{max}=1-2 hrs (median).
Distribution: Plasma protein binding (99%); (IV) V_d=83.5L. **Metabolism:** O-glucuronidation (major) by UGT1A9 and UGT2B4; oxidation (minor) via CYP3A4.
Elimination: Feces (41.5% unchanged, 7% hydroxylated metabolite, 3.2% O-glucuronide metabolite), urine (33%; <1% unchanged, 30.5% O-glucuronide metabolite); $T_{1/2}$=10.6 hrs (100mg), 13.1 hrs (300mg).

PATIENT CONSIDERATIONS
Assessment: Assess for diabetic ketoacidosis; type of DM; volume status; predisposition to ketoacidosis, acute kidney injury, or hyperkalemia; risk for genital mycotic infections or fractures; drug hypersensitivity; pregnancy/nursing status; and possible drug interactions. Assess baseline renal/hepatic function, LDL levels, and BP.

Monitoring: Monitor for signs/symptoms of hypotension, ketoacidosis, UTIs, genital mycotic infections, hypersensitivity reactions, bone fractures, and other adverse reactions. Monitor renal function and LDL levels. Monitor serum K^+ levels w/ impaired renal function and in patients predisposed to hyperkalemia.

Counseling: Inform of the risks, benefits, and alternative modes of therapy. Advise about the importance of adherence to dietary instructions, regular physical activity, periodic blood glucose monitoring and HbA1c testing, recognition and management of hypo/hyperglycemia, and assessment for diabetes complications. Instruct to seek medical advice promptly during periods of stress (eg, fever, trauma, infection, surgery) as medication requirements may change. Instruct to report to physician if pregnant, nursing, or experiencing symptoms of hypotension. Instruct to have adequate fluid intake. Instruct to d/c and seek medical advice immediately if symptoms of ketoacidosis occur. Advise to seek medical advice if patient has reduced oral intake or increased fluid losses. Counsel on the signs/symptoms of UTI, vaginal yeast infection, balanitis, and balanoposthitis; inform of treatment options and when to seek medical advice. Inform that serious hypersensitivity reactions have been reported; advise to report any signs or symptoms suggesting an allergic reaction, and to d/c therapy until they have consulted their prescribing physicians. Inform that bone fractures have been reported and provide information on factors that may contribute to fracture risk.

IRESSA — gefitinib   Rx

Class: Kinase inhibitor

ADULT DOSAGE
Metastatic Non-Small Cell Lung Cancer
1st-line treatment of patients whose tumors have EGFR exon 19 deletions or exon 21 (L858R) substitution mutations as detected by an FDA-approved test
250mg qd until disease progression or unacceptable toxicity

Missed Dose
Do not take a missed dose w/in 12 hrs of the next dose

PEDIATRIC DOSAGE
Pediatric use may not have been established

DOSING CONSIDERATIONS
Concomitant Medications
Strong CYP3A4 Inducers:
Increase Iressa to 500mg/day in the absence of severe adverse drug reaction; resume at 250mg seven days after discontinuation of the strong CYP3A4 inducer

Adverse Reactions
Withhold Therapy (for up to 14 Days) for Any of the Following:
1. Acute onset or worsening of pulmonary symptoms (dyspnea, cough, fever)
2. NCI CTCAE ≥Grade 2 in ALT and/or AST elevations
3. NCI CTCAE ≥Grade 3 diarrhea
4. Signs/symptoms of severe or worsening ocular disorders including keratitis
5. NCI CTCAE ≥Grade 3 skin reactions

Resume treatment when the adverse reaction fully resolves or improves to NCI CTCAE Grade 1

Permanently D/C for:
1. Confirmed interstitial lung disease (ILD)
2. Severe hepatic impairment
3. GI perforation
4. Persistent ulcerative keratitis

ADMINISTRATION
Oral route
Take w/ or w/o food.

Patients w/ Difficulty Swallowing Solids
1. Immerse tabs in 4-8 oz of water by dropping the tab in water, and stir for approx 15 min.

2. Immediately drink the liquid or administer through a NG tube.
3. Rinse the container w/ 4-8 oz of water and immediately drink or administer through the NG tube.

STORAGE
20-25°C (68-77°F).

HOW SUPPLIED
Tab: 250mg

WARNINGS/PRECAUTIONS
Select patients for treatment based on the presence of EGFR exon 19 deletion or exon 21 (L858R) substitution mutations in their tumor. ILD or ILD-like adverse reactions reported; withhold therapy and promptly investigate in any patient w/ worsening of respiratory symptoms, and permanently d/c therapy if ILD is confirmed. Liver test abnormalities reported; withhold therapy in patients w/ worsening liver function and d/c in patients w/ severe hepatic impairment. GI perforation reported; permanently d/c therapy if GI perforation occurs. Grade 3 or 4 diarrhea reported; withhold therapy for severe/persistent (up to 14 days) diarrhea. Ocular disorders including keratitis reported; interrupt or d/c therapy for severe/worsening ocular disorders. Bullous conditions including toxic epidermal necrolysis, Stevens-Johnson syndrome, and erythema multiforme reported; interrupt or d/c therapy if the patient develops severe bullous, blistering, or exfoliating conditions. May cause fetal harm.

ADVERSE REACTIONS
Skin reactions, diarrhea, decreased appetite, N/V, asthenia, pyrexia, stomatitis, conjunctivitis/blepharitis/dry eye, nail disorders, alopecia, hemorrhage (including epistaxis and hematuria).

DRUG INTERACTIONS
See Dosing Considerations. Strong CYP3A4 inducers (eg, rifampicin, phenytoin, TCA) increase metabolism and decrease levels of gefitinib. Strong CYP3A4 inhibitors (eg, ketoconazole, itraconazole) decrease metabolism and increase levels of gefitinib; monitor adverse reactions during coadmination. Drugs that elevate gastric pH may reduce gefitinib levels; avoid concomitant use w/ PPIs, if possible. If treatment w/ a PPI is required, take gefitinib 12 hrs after the last dose or 12 hrs before the next dose of the PPI. Take gefitinib 6 hrs after or 6 hrs before an H₂-receptor antagonist or an antacid. INR elevations and/or hemorrhage reported during coadmination w/ warfarin; regularly monitor patients taking warfarin for changes in prothrombin time or INR.

PREGNANCY AND LACTATION
Pregnancy: May cause fetal harm.
Lactation: Not for use in nursing.
Reproductive Potential: Females of reproductive potential should use effective contraception during treatment, and for at least 2 weeks following completion of therapy. Therapy may result in reduced fertility in females of reproductive potential.

MECHANISM OF ACTION
Kinase inhibitor; reversibly inhibits the kinase activity of wild-type and certain activating mutations of EGFR, preventing autophosphorylation of tyrosine residues associated w/ the receptor, thereby inhibiting further downstream signaling and blocking EGFR-dependent proliferation.

PHARMACOKINETICS
Absorption: Bioavailability (60%); T_{max}=3-7 hrs. **Distribution:** V_d=1400L (IV); plasma protein binding (90%; albumin and α1-acid glycoprotein). **Metabolism:** Extensive via CYP3A4; O-desmethyl gefitinib (major active component) produced by CYP2D6. **Elimination:** Feces (86%), urine (<4%); (IV) $T_{1/2}$=48 hrs.

PATIENT CONSIDERATIONS
Assessment: Assess for hepatic impairment, pregnancy/nursing status, and possible drug interactions. Assess for presence of EGFR exon 19 deletions or exon 21 (L858R) substitution mutations in tumors.

Monitoring: Monitor for ILD, hepatotoxicity, GI perforation, diarrhea, ocular disorders, bullous and exfoliative skin disorders, and other adverse reactions. Obtain periodic liver function testing.

Counseling: Advise to immediately contact physician for new onset/worsening of pulmonary symptoms. Instruct to contact physician to report any new symptoms indicating hepatic toxicity. Advise that therapy can increase the risk of GI perforation and to seek immediate medical attention for severe abdominal pain. Instruct to contact physician for severe/persistent diarrhea. Counsel to promptly contact physician if eye symptoms, lacrimation, light sensitivity, blurred vision, eye pain, red eye, or changes in vision develop. Advise that therapy can increase the risk of bullous and exfoliative skin disorders and to seek immediately medical attention for severe skin reactions. Inform pregnant women of the potential risk to a fetus or potential risk for loss of the pregnancy. Advise females of reproductive potential to use effective contraception during treatment, and for at least 2 weeks following completion of therapy. Advise to d/c nursing during treatment.

ISENTRESS — raltegravir   Rx

Class: HIV-integrase strand transfer inhibitor

ADULT DOSAGE
HIV-1 Infection

Combination w/ Other Antiretrovirals:
Tab:
400mg bid

In Combination w/ Rifampin:
800mg bid

PEDIATRIC DOSAGE
HIV-1 Infection

Combination w/ Other Antiretrovirals:
≥4 Weeks of Age:
Tab:
≥25kg: 400mg bid

Tab, Chewable:
11-<14kg: 75mg bid
14-<20kg: 100mg bid
20-<28kg: 150mg bid
28-<40kg: 200mg bid
≥40kg: 300mg bid
Max: 300mg bid

Sus:
3-<4kg: 1mL (20mg) bid
4-<6kg: 1.5mL (30mg) bid
6-<8kg: 2mL (40mg) bid
8-<11kg: 3mL (60mg) bid
11-<14kg: 4mL (80mg) bid
14-<20kg: 5mL (100mg) bid
Max: 100mg bid

ADMINISTRATION
Oral route

Take w/ or w/o food.

Tab
Swallow whole.

Tab, Chewable
Chew or swallow whole.

Sus
1. Pour sus pack contents into mixing cup, add 5mL of water, and mix.
2. To mix, swirl mixing cup w/ a gentle circular motion for 30-60 sec; do not turn mixing cup upside down.
3. Measure the recommended dose w/ provided syringe and administer w/in 30 min of mixing.
4. Discard any remaining sus.

STORAGE
20-25°C (68-77°F); excursions permitted to 15-30°C (59-86°F). **Tab, Chewable:** Protect from moisture. **Sus:** Do not open foil pkt until ready for use.

HOW SUPPLIED
Sus (Powder): 100mg/pkt; **Tab:** 400mg; **Tab, Chewable:** 25mg, 100mg* *scored

WARNINGS/PRECAUTIONS
Do not substitute chewable tabs or oral sus for the 400mg film-coated tab; not bioequivalent. Severe, potentially life-threatening, and fatal skin reactions (eg, Stevens-Johnson syndrome, toxic epidermal necrolysis), and hypersensitivity reactions reported; d/c therapy and other suspect agents immediately if signs/ symptoms develop. Immune reconstitution syndrome reported. Autoimmune disorders (eg, Graves' disease, polymyositis, Guillain-Barre syndrome) reported in the setting of immune reconstitution and can occur many months after initiation of treatment. Caution in patients at increased risk of myopathy or rhabdomyolysis and in elderly. Avoid dosing before a dialysis session. **Tab, Chewable:** Contains phenylalanine.

ADVERSE REACTIONS
Insomnia, headache, nausea, hyperglycemia, ALT/AST elevation, hyperbilirubinemia, low ANC, serum lipase/creatine kinase/pancreatic amylase increase, thrombocytopenia.

DRUG INTERACTIONS
See Dosage. UGT1A1 inhibitors may increase levels. UGT1A1 inducers (eg, rifampin) may decrease levels. Coadministration or staggered administration w/ aluminum- and/or magnesium hydroxide-containing antacids is not recommended.

PREGNANCY AND LACTATION
Category C, not for use in nursing.

MECHANISM OF ACTION
HIV-1 integrase strand transfer inhibitor; inhibits the catalytic activity of HIV-1 integrase thus preventing the formation of HIV-1 provirus, resulting in the prevention of propagation of the viral infection.

PHARMACOKINETICS
Absorption: Adults: (Tab) T_{max}=3 hrs (fasted); AUC_{0-12h}=14.3μM•hr. Pediatrics: AUC_{0-12h}=14.1μM•hr (tab), 22.1μM•hr (tab, chewable; ≥25kg patient), 18.6μM•hr (tab, chewable; 11-<25kg patient), 24.5μM•hr (sus). **Distribution:** Adults: Plasma protein binding (83%). **Metabolism:** Glucuronidation via UGT1A1; raltegravir-glucuronide (metabolite). **Elimination:** Adults: Urine (9% unchanged, 23% raltegravir-glucuronide), feces (51% unchanged); $T_{1/2}$=9 hrs.

PATIENT CONSIDERATIONS
Assessment: Assess for risk of myopathy or rhabdomyolysis, previous hypersensitivity to the drug, pregnancy/nursing status, and possible drug interactions. Assess if patient is undergoing dialysis session. **Tab, Chewable:** Assess for phenylketonuria.

Monitoring: Monitor for signs/symptoms of severe skin/hypersensitivity reactions, immune reconstitution syndrome, autoimmune disorders, and other adverse reactions. If a severe skin reaction or hypersensitivity reaction develops, monitor clinical status, including liver aminotransferases.

Counseling: Instruct to inform physician if any unusual symptom develops, or if any known symptom persists or worsens. Inform that drug is not a cure for HIV-1 infection and that illnesses associated w/ HIV-1 may still be experienced. Advise to avoid doing things that can spread HIV-1 to others. Instruct to always practice safe sex by using a latex or polyurethane condom. Instruct to immediately d/c therapy and seek medical attention if rash develops w/ signs/symptoms of a more serious skin reaction. Instruct to immediately report to physician if any unexplained muscle pain, tenderness, or weakness occurs. Instruct to avoid taking

aluminum- and/or magnesium hydroxide-containing antacids. **Tab, Chewable:** Inform patients w/ phenylketonuria that product contains phenylalanine. **Sus:** Instruct to administer w/in 30 min of mixing.

ISONIAZID — isoniazid

Class: Isonicotinic acid hydrazide

Rx

> Severe and sometimes fatal hepatitis associated w/ isoniazid (INH) therapy reported and may develop even after many months of treatment. The risk of developing hepatitis is age related and is increased w/ daily alcohol consumption. Carefully monitor and interview at monthly intervals. Measure hepatic enzymes prior to starting therapy and periodically throughout treatment in addition to monthly symptom reviews in patients ≥35 years old. Strongly consider discontinuation if abnormalities of liver function exceed 3-5X ULN. D/C drug promptly if signs and symptoms of hepatic damage occur. Patients w/ tuberculosis (TB) who have INH-induced hepatitis should be given appropriate treatment w/ alternative drugs. If INH must be reinstituted, do so only after symptoms and lab abnormalities have cleared. Restart in very small and gradually increasing doses and withdraw immediately if there is any indication of recurrent liver involvement. Defer preventive treatment in persons w/ acute hepatic disease.

ADULT DOSAGE
Tuberculosis

In conjunction w/ other effective antituberculous agents

Treatment:
Usual: 5mg/kg (up to 300mg/day) in a single dose; or 15mg/kg (up to 900mg/day) 2 or 3X/week

Patients w/ Pulmonary TB w/o HIV Infection:
Option 1: Daily INH + rifampin + pyrazinamide for 8 weeks followed by 16 weeks of INH + rifampin daily or 2-3X/week; ethambutol or streptomycin should be added to the initial regimen until sensitivity to INH and rifampin is demonstrated. Addition of a 4th drug is optional if the relative prevalence of INH-resistant *Mycobacterium tuberculosis* isolates in the community is ≤4%.

Option 2: Daily INH + rifampin + pyrazinamide + streptomycin or ethambutol for 2 weeks followed by 2X/week administration of the same drugs for 6 weeks, subsequently 2X/week INH + rifampin for 16 weeks

Option 3: INH + rifampin + pyrazinamide + ethambutol or streptomycin 3X/week for 6 months

All regimens given 2 or 3X/week should be administered by directly observed therapy

Prevention:
>30kg: 300mg/day as a single dose

Concomitant Administration of Pyridoxine (B6):
Recommended in malnourished patients and in those predisposed to neuropathy (eg, alcoholics and diabetics)

Refer to PI for additional information (eg, treatment of patients w/ pulmonary TB and HIV infection, extrapulmonary TB, pregnant women w/ TB, multi-drug resistant TB)

PEDIATRIC DOSAGE
Tuberculosis

In conjunction w/ other effective antituberculous agents

Treatment:
Usual: 10-15mg/kg (up to 300mg/day) as a single dose; or 20-40mg/kg (up to 900mg/day), 2 or 3X/week

Patients w/ Pulmonary TB w/o HIV Infection:
Option 1: Daily INH + rifampin + pyrazinamide for 8 weeks followed by 16 weeks of INH + rifampin, daily or 2-3X/week; ethambutol or streptomycin should be added to the initial regimen until sensitivity to INH and rifampin is demonstrated. Addition of a 4th drug is optional if the relative prevalence of INH-resistant *M. tuberculosis* isolates in the community is ≤4%.

Option 2: Daily INH + rifampin + pyrazinamide + streptomycin or ethambutol for 2 weeks followed by 2X/week administration of the same drugs for 6 weeks, subsequently 2X/week INH + rifampin for 16 weeks

Option 3: INH + rifampin + pyrazinamide + ethambutol or streptomycin 3X/week for 6 months

All regimens given 2 or 3X/week should be administered by directly observed therapy

Prevention:
10mg/kg (up to 300mg/day) as a single dose or 20-30mg/kg (not to exceed 900mg/day) 2X/week, under the direct observation of a healthcare worker at the time of administration

Concomitant Administration of Pyridoxine (B6):
Recommended in malnourished patients and in those predisposed to neuropathy (eg, alcoholics and diabetics)

Refer to PI for additional information (eg, treatment of patients w/ pulmonary TB and HIV infection, extrapulmonary TB, multi-drug resistant TB)

ADMINISTRATION
Oral and IM routes

Do not administer w/ food.
IM administration is intended for use whenever oral administration is not possible.

STORAGE
Tab: 20-25°C (68-77°F). Protect from light and moisture. **Sol:** 15-30°C (59-86°F). Protect from light. **Inj:** 20-25°C (68-77°F). Protect from light. If vial contents crystallize, warm vial to room temperature to redissolve crystals before use.

HOW SUPPLIED
Inj: 100mg/mL [10mL]; **Sol:** 50mg/5mL [473mL]; **Tab:** 100mg*, 300mg* *scored

CONTRAINDICATIONS
Severe hypersensitivity reactions, including drug-induced hepatitis, previous INH-associated hepatic injury, severe adverse effects to INH (eg, drug fever, chills, arthritis), acute liver disease of any etiology.

WARNINGS/PRECAUTIONS
D/C all drugs and evaluate patient at 1st sign of a hypersensitivity reaction. Carefully monitor w/ daily alcohol use, active chronic liver disease, severe renal dysfunction, age >35, concurrent use of any chronically administered medication, history of previous discontinuation of INH, peripheral neuropathy or conditions predisposing to neuropathy, pregnancy, inj drug use, women belonging to minority groups (particularly in the postpartum period), and HIV-seropositive patients. **Inj:** Periodic ophthalmologic examinations during therapy are recommended when visual symptoms occur.

ADVERSE REACTIONS
Peripheral neuropathy, elevated serum transaminases, bilirubinemia, bilirubinuria, jaundice, hepatitis.

DRUG INTERACTIONS
Severe acetaminophen toxicity reported. Known to increase levels of carbamazepine; determine carbamazepine levels prior to concurrent INH administration, monitor for signs/symptoms of carbamazepine toxicity, and appropriately adjust dose of the anticonvulsant. Decreased ketoconazole exposure when given in combination w/ INH and rifampin. May increase levels of phenytoin; appropriately adjust dose of the anticonvulsant. May increase levels of theophylline and valproate; monitor levels and appropriately adjust dose of theophylline/valproate. Theophylline may cause a slight decrease in INH elimination. **Inj/Tab:** Avoid tyramine- and histamine-containing foods.

PREGNANCY AND LACTATION
Pregnancy: Category C. Should be used as treatment for active TB during pregnancy because the benefit justifies the potential risk to fetus. Preventive therapy generally should be started after delivery to prevent putting fetus at risk of exposure. **Lactation:** Small concentrations of INH in breast milk do not produce toxicity in nursing newborn; therefore, breastfeeding should not be discouraged.

MECHANISM OF ACTION
Isonicotinic acid hydrazide; inhibits the synthesis of mycolic acids, an essential component of the bacterial cell wall. Bactericidal against actively growing intracellular and extracellular *M. tuberculosis* organisms.

PHARMACOKINETICS
Absorption: T_{max}=1-2 hrs (oral administration). **Distribution:** Crosses placenta, found in breast milk. **Metabolism:** Acetylation and dehydrazination. **Elimination:** Urine (50-70%).

PATIENT CONSIDERATIONS
Assessment: Assess for severe hypersensitivity reactions, previous INH-associated hepatic injury, severe adverse reactions to INH, acute/active chronic liver disease, daily alcohol use, severe renal dysfunction, peripheral neuropathy or conditions predisposing to neuropathy, any other conditions where treatment is contraindicated or cautioned, and possible drug interactions. Assess age, pregnancy/nursing status, and HIV status. Measure hepatic enzymes prior to therapy.

Monitoring: Monitor for hepatitis, hypersensitivity reactions, and other adverse reactions. Measure hepatic enzymes periodically or monthly in >35 years of age, daily alcohol use, chronic liver disease, inj drug use, and women belonging to minority groups.

Counseling: Instruct to immediately report signs/symptoms consistent w/ liver damage or other adverse events (unexplained anorexia, N/V, dark urine). Instruct to take drug w/o food.

ISOSORBIDE DINITRATE — isosorbide dinitrate   Rx
Class: Nitrate vasodilator

OTHER BRAND NAMES
Isordil Titradose

ADULT DOSAGE
Angina Pectoris
Due to Coronary Artery Disease:
Prevention:
Tab/Isordil Titradose:
Initial: 5-20mg bid-tid
Maint: 10-40mg bid-tid
Allow a dose-free interval of ≥14 hrs

Tab, Extended Release (ER):
Refer to PI for dosing based on clinical trials

Tab, SL:
Prevention: 1 tab (2.5mg-5mg) 15 min before activity
Treatment: Use to abort acute angina episode recommended only in patients who fail to respond to SL nitroglycerin
Must provide a daily dose-free interval; 1 of the daily dose-free intervals must be somewhat >14 hrs

PEDIATRIC DOSAGE
Pediatric use may not have been established

DOSING CONSIDERATIONS
Elderly
Start at lower end of dosing range

ADMINISTRATION
Oral/SL route

STORAGE
Tab: 25°C (77°F); (Isordil Titradose) excursions permitted to 15-30°C (59-86°F). Protect from light. **Tab, SL/Tab, ER:** 20-25°C (68-77°F). **Tab, SL:** Protect from light and moisture.

HOW SUPPLIED
Tab, ER: 40mg*; **Tab, SL:** 2.5mg, 5mg; **Tab:** 10mg*, 20mg*, 30mg*, (Isordil Titradose) 5mg*, 40mg* *scored

CONTRAINDICATIONS
Allergic to isosorbide dinitrate or any of its other ingredients. **Tab:** Coadministration w/ certain drugs for erectile dysfunction (PDE inhibitors) (eg, sildenafil, tadalafil, or vardenafil); concomitant use w/ the soluble guanylate cyclase stimulator riociguat.

WARNINGS/PRECAUTIONS
Severe hypotension, particularly w/ upright posture, may occur. Perform careful clinical or hemodynamic monitoring if used in patients w/ acute MI or CHF to avoid the hazards of hypotension and tachycardia. Hypotension may be accompanied by paradoxical bradycardia and increased angina pectoris. May aggravate angina caused by hypertrophic cardiomyopathy. Caution w/ volume depletion and hypotension. May develop tolerance. Chest pain, acute MI, and sudden death reported during temporary withdrawal in patients w/ long term exposure to therapy. **Tab, SL:** Not the 1st drug of choice for abortion of acute anginal episode.

ADVERSE REACTIONS
Headache, lightheadedness, hypotension, syncope, crescendo angina, rebound HTN.

DRUG INTERACTIONS
See Contraindications. Additive vasodilation w/ other vasodilators (eg, alcohol).

PREGNANCY AND LACTATION
Category C, caution in nursing.

MECHANISM OF ACTION
Nitrate vasodilator; relaxes vascular smooth muscle and dilates peripheral arteries and veins; venous dilatation reduces left ventricular end diastolic pressure and pulmonary capillary wedge pressure (preload); arteriolar relaxation reduces systemic vascular resistance, systolic arterial pressure, and mean arterial pressure (afterload); dilates the coronary artery.

PHARMACOKINETICS
Absorption: (Tab) Nearly complete; bioavailability (10-90%); T_{max}=1 hr. (Tab, SL) Bioavailability (40-50%); T_{max}=10-15 min. **Distribution:** V_d=2-4L/kg. **Metabolism:** Liver (extensive 1st-pass) (tab); 2-mononitrate, 5-mononitrate (active metabolites). **Elimination:** $T_{1/2}$=1 hr, 5 hrs (5-mononitrate), 2 hrs (2-mononitrate).

PATIENT CONSIDERATIONS
Assessment: Assess for drug hypersensitivity, hypotension, acute MI, CHF, volume depletion, hypertrophic cardiomyopathy, alcohol intake, pregnancy/nursing status, and possible drug interactions.

Monitoring: Monitor for paradoxical bradycardia, increased angina pectoris, hypotension, hemodynamic rebound, decreased exercise tolerance, chest pain, acute MI, and other adverse reactions. In patients w/ MI or CHF, perform careful clinical or hemodynamic monitoring.

Counseling: Counsel to carefully follow prescribed dosing regimen. Inform that headaches sometimes accompany therapy and are markers of drug activity; instruct not to alter schedule of therapy since loss of headache may be associated w/ simultaneous loss of antianginal efficacy. Inform that lightheadedness on standing may occur, which may be more frequent w/ alcohol consumption.

ISTODAX — romidepsin   Rx
Class: Histone deacetylase (HDAC) inhibitor

ADULT DOSAGE
Cutaneous T-Cell Lymphoma
Use in patients that have received at least 1 prior systemic therapy
14mg/m² over 4 hrs on Days 1, 8, and 15 of a 28-day cycle
Repeat cycle every 28 days provided that patient continues to benefit from and tolerates the drug

Peripheral T-Cell Lymphoma
Use in patients that have received at least 1 prior therapy
14mg/m² over 4 hrs on Days 1, 8, and 15 of a 28-day cycle
Repeat cycle every 28 days provided that patient continues to benefit from and tolerates the drug

PEDIATRIC DOSAGE
Pediatric use may not have been established

DOSING CONSIDERATIONS
Renal Impairment
ESRD: Use w/ caution

Hepatic Impairment
Moderate/Severe: Use w/ caution

Adverse Reactions
Nonhematologic Toxicities (Except Alopecia):
Grade 2 or 3: Delay treatment until toxicity returns to ≤Grade 1 or baseline, then restart at 14mg/m². If Grade 3 toxicity recurs, delay treatment until toxicity returns to ≤Grade 1 or baseline, then permanently reduce dose to 10mg/m²
Grade 4: Delay treatment until toxicity returns to ≤Grade 1 or baseline, then permanently reduce dose to 10mg/m²
Recurrence of Grade 3 or 4 Toxicities After Dose Reduction: D/C therapy
Hematologic Toxicities:
Grade 3 or 4 Neutropenia or Thrombocytopenia: Delay treatment until specific cytopenia returns to ANC ≥1.5 x 10⁹/L and platelet count ≥75 x 10⁹/L or baseline, then restart at 14mg/m²
Grade 4 Febrile (≥38.5°C [101.3°F]) Neutropenia or Thrombocytopenia Requiring Platelet Transfusion: Delay treatment until specific cytopenia returns to ≤Grade 1 or baseline, then permanently reduce dose to 10mg/m²

ADMINISTRATION
IV route

Preparation and Administration
1. Withdraw 2.2mL from the supplied diluent vial, and slowly inject it into the 10mg single-use vial. The reconstituted sol will contain 5mg/mL and is stable for up to 8 hrs at room temperature.
2. Before infusion, further dilute romidepsin in 500mL 0.9% NaCl inj.
3. Infuse over 4 hrs.

The diluted sol is compatible w/ polyvinyl chloride, ethylene vinyl acetate, and polyethylene infusion bags as well as glass bottles, and is chemically stable for up to 24 hrs at room temperature. However, it should be administered as soon after dilution as possible

STORAGE
Carton: 20-25°C (68-77°F); excursions permitted between 15-30°C (59-86°F).

HOW SUPPLIED
Inj: 10mg

WARNINGS/PRECAUTIONS
May cause thrombocytopenia, leukopenia (neutropenia/lymphopenia), and anemia. Serious/fatal infections (eg, pneumonia, sepsis, and viral reactivation, including Epstein Barr and hepatitis B viruses) reported; increased risk w/ history of prior treatment w/ monoclonal antibodies directed against lymphocyte antigens and in patients w/ disease involvement of the bone marrow. Consider monitoring for reactivation and antiviral prophylaxis in patients w/ evidence of prior hepatitis B infection. ECG changes reported; caution w/ congenital long QT syndrome and history of significant cardiovascular disease (CVD). Confirm that K⁺/Mg²⁺ levels are w/in the normal range prior to administration. Tumor lysis syndrome (TLS) reported; increased risk in patients w/ advanced stage disease and/or high tumor burden. May cause fetal harm.

ADVERSE REACTIONS
Neutropenia, lymphopenia, thrombocytopenia, infections, N/V, fatigue, anorexia, anemia, ECG T-wave changes.

DRUG INTERACTIONS
Avoid w/ rifampin and other potent CYP3A4 inducers (eg, dexamethasone, phenytoin, rifapentine, St. John's wort). Caution w/ antiarrhythmics or drugs that prolong QT. Strong CYP3A4 inhibitors (eg, ketoconazole, clarithromycin, indinavir, nelfinavir) may increase concentrations. Prolongation of PT and elevation of INR w/ warfarin; monitor PT and INR more frequently w/ warfarin. Caution w/ P-gp inhibitors; may increase levels of romidepsin.

PREGNANCY AND LACTATION
Pregnancy: Category D.
Lactation: Not for use in nursing.

MECHANISM OF ACTION
Histone deacetylase inhibitor; catalyzes the removal of acetyl groups from acetylated lysine residues in histones, resulting in the modulation of gene expression.

PHARMACOKINETICS
Absorption: C_{max}=377ng/mL; AUC_{0-inf}=1549ng•hr/mL. **Distribution:** Plasma protein binding (92-94%). **Metabolism:** Extensive. CYP3A4 (primary); CYP3A5, CYP1A1, CYP2B6, and CYP2C19 (minor). **Elimination:** $T_{1/2}$=3 hrs.

PATIENT CONSIDERATIONS
Assessment: Assess for normal K⁺/Mg²⁺ levels, history of hepatitis B, history of prior treatment w/ monoclonal antibodies directed against lymphocyte antigens, disease involvement of the bone marrow, hepatic/renal function, congenital long QT syndrome/history of CVD, pregnancy/nursing status, and possible drug interactions. Obtain baseline ECG.

Monitoring: Monitor for myelosuppression, infections, reactivation of viral infection, and other adverse reactions. Closely monitor for TLS w/ advanced stage disease and/or high tumor burden. Monitor PT/INR w/ warfarin. Perform ECGs periodically and monitor blood counts regularly.

Counseling: Inform that N/V, low blood counts, and infections may occur; instruct to report symptoms of N/V, fever or other signs of infection, significant fatigue, SOB, bleeding, cough, burning on urination, flu-like symptoms, muscle aches, or worsening skin problems. Advise to report any previous history of hepatitis B prior to therapy. Advise of the risk of TLS (especially those w/ advanced stage disease and/or high tumor burden) and to maintain high fluid intake for at least 72 hrs after each dose. Advise to seek medical counseling if pregnancy occurs during treatment.

ISUPREL — isoproterenol hydrochloride   Rx
Class: Nonselective beta-adrenergic agonist

ADULT DOSAGE	PEDIATRIC DOSAGE

ADULT DOSAGE

Heart Block/Adams-Stokes Attack/Cardiac Arrest
IV Bolus:
Initial: 0.02-0.06mg (1-3mL)
Subsequent Range: 0.01-0.2mg
IV:
Initial: 5mcg/min (1.25mL/min)
IM:
Initial: 0.2mg (1mL)
Subsequent Range: 0.02-1mg (0.1-5mL)
SQ:
Initial: 0.2mg (1mL)
Subsequent Range: 0.15-0.2mg (0.75-1mL)
Intracardiac:
Initial: 0.02mg (0.1mL)
Start at the lowest recommended dose and increase rate gradually with careful monitoring of patient

Shock and Hypoperfusion States
IV
0.5-5mcg/min (0.25-2.5mL)
Advanced Stages of Shock: Rates >30mcg/min have been used. Adjust infusion rate based on HR, central venous pressure, systemic BP, and urine flow. May decrease or temporarily d/c if HR>110 beats/min.

Adjunct to fluid/electrolyte replacement therapy, and use of other drugs and procedures

Bronchospasm
Bronchospasm During Anesthesia:
IV Bolus:
Initial: 0.01-0.02mg (0.5-1mL)
Subsequent Dose: May repeat initial dose when necessary

PEDIATRIC DOSAGE
Pediatric use may not have been established

DOSING CONSIDERATIONS
Elderly
Start at lower end of dosing range
ADMINISTRATION
IV/IM/SQ/Intracardiac route

Initial therapy by IM or SQ inj is preferred if time is not of the utmost importance
May administer by intracardiac inj in dire emergencies
Usual route of administration is by IV infusion or bolus IV inj
IM/SQ/intracardiac inj are administered undiluted

Preparation of Dilution
IV Bolus: Dilute 1mL (0.2mg) in 9mL of NaCl inj or 5% dextrose inj
IV Infusion: Dilute 10mL (2mg) [Arrhythmias] or 5mL (1mg) [Hypoperfusion States] in 500mL of 5% dextrose inj
STORAGE
20-25°C (68-77°F). Protect from light.
HOW SUPPLIED
Inj: 0.2 mg/mL [1mL, 5mL]
CONTRAINDICATIONS
Tachyarrhythmias, tachycardia or heart block caused by digitalis intoxication, ventricular arrhythmias which require inotropic therapy, and angina pectoris.
WARNINGS/PRECAUTIONS
May have deleterious effect on the injured/failing heart by increasing myocardial oxygen requirements while decreasing effective coronary perfusion. Use as the initial agent in treating cardiogenic shock following myocardial infarction is discouraged; may, however, produce beneficial hemodynamic/metabolic effects when a low arterial pressure has been elevated by other means. Paradoxical worsening of heart block or precipitation of Adams-Stokes attacks during normal sinus rhythm or transient heart block reported in a few patients, presumably with organic disease of the AV node and its branches. Doses sufficient to increase HR to >130 beats/min may increase likelihood of inducing ventricular arrhythmias and will also tend to increase cardiac work and oxygen requirements, which may adversely affect the failing heart or the heart with a significant degree of arteriosclerosis. If HR exceeds 110 beats/min, it may be advisable to decrease the infusion rate or temporarily d/c infusion. Take appropriate measures to ensure adequate ventilation. Pay attention to acid-base balance and correct electrolyte disturbances.
ADVERSE REACTIONS
Nervousness, headache, dizziness, nausea, visual blurring, tachycardia, palpitations, angina, Adams-Stokes attacks, pulmonary edema, HTN, hypotension, dyspnea, flushing of the skin.

DRUG INTERACTIONS

Do not administer simultaneously with epinephrine because combined effects may induce serious arrhythmias; may administer alternately provided a proper interval has elapsed between doses. Avoid use with potent inhalational anesthetics (eg, halothane) because of the potential to sensitize the myocardium to effects of sympathomimetic amines.

PREGNANCY AND LACTATION

Category C, caution in nursing.

MECHANISM OF ACTION

Nonselective β-adrenergic agonist; relaxes almost all varieties of smooth muscle when tone is high but is most pronounced on bronchial and GI smooth muscle.

PHARMACOKINETICS

Metabolism: Liver (primary) and other tissues by catechol-O-methyltransferase.

PATIENT CONSIDERATIONS

Assessment: Assess for tachyarrhythmias, tachycardia or heart block caused by digitalis intoxication, ventricular arrhythmias requiring inotropic therapy, angina pectoris, organic disease of the AV node and its branches, arteriosclerosis, pregnancy/nursing status, and for possible drug interactions. Obtain baseline BP, serum electrolytes, and ECG.

Monitoring: Monitor for paradoxical worsening of heart block or precipitation of Adam-Stokes attacks, ventricular arrhythmia, and other adverse reactions. Monitor response to therapy by frequent determination of the central venous pressure and blood gases. Routinely monitor BP, HR, urine flow, serum electrolytes, and ECG. Closely observe patients in shock during administration.

Counseling: Inform of the benefits and risks of therapy. Advise to report any adverse reactions.

IXEMPRA — ixabepilone   **Rx**

Class: Antimicrotubule agent

> In combination with capecitabine, contraindicated in patients with AST/ALT >2.5X ULN or bilirubin >1X ULN due to increased risk of toxicity and neutropenia-related death.

ADULT DOSAGE

Breast Cancer

Combination w/ Capecitabine:
Metastatic or locally advanced breast cancer resistant to treatment w/ an anthracycline and a taxane, or in patients whose cancer is taxane resistant and for whom further anthracycline therapy is contraindicated

40mg/m² IV over 3 hrs every 3 weeks
BSA >2.2m²: Calculate dose based on 2.2m²

Monotherapy:
Metastatic or locally advanced breast cancer in patients whose tumors are resistant or refractory to anthracyclines, taxanes, and capecitabine

40mg/m² IV over 3 hrs every 3 weeks
BSA >2.2m²: Calculate dose based on 2.2m²

Retreatment Criteria:
Do not begin a new cycle of treatment unless neutrophil count is ≥1500 cells/mm³, platelet count is ≥100,000 cells/mm³, and nonhematologic toxicities have improved to Grade 1 (mild) or resolved

Premedication

All patients must be premedicated approx 1 hr before infusion w/:

An H₁ antagonist (eg, diphenhydramine 50mg PO or equivalent) and an H₂ antagonist (eg, ranitidine 150-300mg PO or equivalent)

Patients who experienced a hypersensitivity reaction require premedication w/ corticosteroids (eg, dexamethasone 20mg IV, 30 min before infusion or PO, 60 min before infusion) in addition to pretreatment w/ H₁ and H₂ antagonists

PEDIATRIC DOSAGE

Pediatric use may not have been established

DOSING CONSIDERATIONS

Concomitant Medications

Strong CYP3A4 Inhibitors (Including Grapefruit Juice): Avoid concomitant use; if coadministration is necessary, reduce dose to 20mg/m². If the strong inhibitor is discontinued, allow a washout period of approx 1 week before adjusting the dose upward to the indicated dose

Strong CYP3A4 Inducers: Avoid concomitant use; if coadministration is necessary, gradually increase dose to 60mg/m² once patient has been maintained on a strong CYP3A4 inducer. If the strong inducer is discontinued, return to the dose used prior to initiation of the strong inducer

Hepatic Impairment

Monotherapy:
AST and ALT ≤10X ULN and Bilirubin ≤1.5X ULN: 32mg/m²
AST and ALT ≤10X ULN and Bilirubin >1.5-≤3X ULN: 20-30mg/m²

Recommendations are for 1st course of therapy; further decreases in subsequent courses should be based on individual tolerance

Adverse Reactions

Monotherapy or Combination Therapy:
Nonhematologic Toxicities:
Grade 2 Neuropathy (Moderate) Lasting ≥7 Days: Decrease dose by 20%
Grade 3 Neuropathy (Severe) Lasting <7 Days: Decrease dose by 20%
Grade 3 Neuropathy (Severe) Lasting ≥7 Days or Disabling Neuropathy: D/C treatment
Any Grade 3 Toxicity (Severe) Other Than Neuropathy: Decrease dose by 20%
Any Grade 4 Toxicity (Disabling): D/C treatment

Hematologic Toxicities:
Neutrophil <500 cells/mm³ for ≥7 Days: Decrease dose by 20%
Febrile Neutropenia: Decrease dose by 20%
Platelets <25,000/mm³ or Platelets <50,000/mm³ w/ Bleeding: Decrease dose by 20%

Refer to PI for capecitabine dose modifications

ADMINISTRATION

IV route

Preparation and Administration

Prior to constituting ixabepilone for inj, remove the kit from the refrigerator and allowed to stand at room temperature for approx 30 min. When the vials are 1st removed from the refrigerator, a white precipitate may be observed in the diluents vial. This precipitate will dissolve to form a clear sol once the diluents warms to room temperature. After constituting w/ the diluent, the concentration of ixabepilone is 2mg/mL

To Constitute:
1. W/ a suitable syringe, withdraw the diluents and slowly inject it into the ixabepilone for inj vial:
15mg Ixempra: Constitute w/ 8mL of diluent
45mg Ixempra: Constitute w/ 23.5mL of diluent
2. Gently swirl and invert the vial until the powder is completely dissolved

To Dilute:
Before administration, the constituted sol must be further diluted w/ 1 of the specified infusion fluids listed below. The infusion must be prepared in a DEHP [di-(2-ethylhexyl) phthalate] free bag
The following infusion fluids have been qualified for use:
1. Lactated Ringer's inj
2. 0.9% NaCl inj (pH adjusted w/ sodium bicarbonate inj)
When using a 250mL or a 500mL bag of 0.9% NaCl inj to prepare the infusion, the pH must be adjusted to a pH between 6.0 and 9.0 by adding 2mEq (eg, 2mL of an 8.4% w/v sol or 4mL of a 4.2% w/v sol) of sodium bicarbonate inj, prior to the addition of the constituted sol
3. PLASMA-LYTE A inj pH 7.4

For most doses, a 250mL bag of infusion fluid is sufficient. However, it is necessary to check the final infusion concentration of each dose based on the volume of infusion fluid to be used. The final concentration for infusion must be between 0.2mg/mL and 0.6mg/mL; refer to PI for how to calculate the final infusion concentration

1. Withdraw the appropriate volume of constituted sol containing 2mg/mL
2. Transfer to an IV bag containing an appropriate volume of infusion fluid to achieve the final desired concentration
3. Thoroughly mix the infusion bag by manual rotation

The infusion sol must be administered through an appropriate in-line filter w/ a microporous membrane of 0.2-1.2μm. DEHP-free infusion containers and administration sets must be used. Any remaining sol should be discarded according to institutional procedures for antineoplastics

STORAGE

2-8°C (36-46°F). Protect from light. Constituted Sol: Dilute as soon as possible or store in the vial (not the syringe) for a max of 1 hr at room temperature and room light. Diluted with Infusion Fluid: Stable at room temperature and room light for a max of 6 hrs.

HOW SUPPLIED

Inj: 15mg, 45mg

CONTRAINDICATIONS

History of a severe (CTC Grade 3/4) hypersensitivity reaction to agents containing Cremophor EL or its derivatives (eg, polyoxyethylated castor oil). Neutrophil count <1500 cells/mm³ or platelet count <100,000 cells/mm³. In combination with capecitabine, patients with AST/ALT >2.5X ULN or bilirubin >1X ULN.

WARNINGS/PRECAUTIONS

Peripheral neuropathy reported; caution with diabetes mellitus (DM) or preexisting peripheral neuropathy. Myelosuppression, which is dose-dependent and primarily manifested as neutropenia, reported; frequently monitor peripheral blood cell counts. Monotherapy is not recommended in patients with AST/ALT >10X ULN or bilirubin >3X ULN, and should be used with caution in patients with AST/ALT >5X ULN. Observe for hypersensitivity reactions; d/c infusion and start aggressive supportive treatment if severe hypersensitivity reactions occur. May cause fetal harm. Cardiac adverse reactions (eg, myocardial ischemia, ventricular dysfunction) reported during combination therapy; caution with history of cardiac disease, and consider discontinuation of ixabepilone if cardiac ischemia or impaired cardiac function develops. Contains dehydrated alcohol USP; consider possibility of CNS and other effects of alcohol.

ADVERSE REACTIONS
Peripheral sensory neuropathy, fatigue/asthenia, myalgia/arthralgia, alopecia, N/V, stomatitis/mucositis, diarrhea, musculoskeletal pain, palmar-plantar erythrodysesthesia (hand-foot) syndrome, anorexia, abdominal pain, nail disorder, constipation, hematologic abnormalities.

DRUG INTERACTIONS
Strong CYP3A4 inhibitors (eg, ketoconazole, itraconazole, clarithromycin, atazanavir, grapefruit juice) may increase levels; avoid, or if must be coadministered, reduce dose of ixabepilone. Caution with mild/moderate CYP3A4 inhibitors (eg, erythromycin, fluconazole, verapamil). Monitor closely for acute toxicities in patients receiving CYP3A4 inhibitors during treatment. Strong CYP3A4 inducers (eg, rifampin, dexamethasone) may decrease levels; avoid, or if must be coadministered, consider gradual dose adjustment of ixabepilone. St. John's wort may decrease levels unpredictably; avoid concomitant use.

PREGNANCY AND LACTATION
Category D, not for use in nursing.

MECHANISM OF ACTION
Microtubule inhibitor; semi-synthetic analog of epothilone B. Binds directly to β-tubulin subunits on microtubules, leading to suppression of microtubule dynamics. Blocks cells in the mitotic phase of the cell division cycle, leading to cell death.

PHARMACOKINETICS
Absorption: C_{max}=252ng/mL; T_{max}=3 hrs; AUC=2143ng•hr/mL. **Distribution:** V_d>1000L; plasma protein binding (67-77%). **Metabolism:** Liver (extensive); oxidation via CYP3A4. **Elimination:** Feces (65%, 1.6% unchanged), urine (21%, 5.6% unchanged); $T_{1/2}$=52 hrs.

PATIENT CONSIDERATIONS
Assessment: Assess for history of a severe hypersensitivity reaction to Cremophor EL or its derivatives (eg, polyoxyethylated castor oil), DM, preexisting peripheral neuropathy, history of cardiac disease, pregnancy/nursing status, and possible drug interactions. Obtain CBC and LFTs.

Monitoring: Monitor for signs/symptoms of neuropathy, myelosuppression, hypersensitivity reactions, cardiac ischemia/impairment, and other adverse reactions. Perform periodic clinical observation and lab tests (eg, CBC, LFTs).

Counseling: Advise to report to physician any numbness and tingling of the hands or feet, chest pain, difficulty breathing, palpitations, or unusual weight gain. Instruct to contact physician if a fever of ≥100.5°F or other evidence of potential infection (eg, chills, cough, burning or pain on urination) develops, or if experiencing urticaria, pruritus, rash, flushing, swelling, dyspnea, chest tightness, or other hypersensitivity-related symptoms following an infusion. Advise to use effective contraceptive measures to prevent pregnancy and to avoid nursing during treatment.

Izba — travoprost
Class: Prostaglandin analogue

Rx

ADULT DOSAGE
Elevated Intraocular Pressure
Open-Angle Glaucoma/Ocular HTN:
1 drop in the affected eye(s) qpm

PEDIATRIC DOSAGE
Elevated Intraocular Pressure
Open-Angle Glaucoma/Ocular HTN:
≥16 Years:
1 drop in the affected eye(s) qpm

DOSING CONSIDERATIONS
Concomitant Medications
Space dosing by at least 5 min if using >1 topical ophthalmic drug

ADMINISTRATION
Ocular route

STORAGE
2-25°C (36-77°F).

HOW SUPPLIED
Sol: 0.003% [2.5mL, 5mL]

WARNINGS/PRECAUTIONS
May cause changes to pigmented tissues (eg, increased pigmentation of the iris [may be permanent], periorbital tissue, and eyelashes [may be reversible]); regularly examine patients who develop noticeably increased iris pigmentation. May gradually change eyelashes and vellus hair in the treated eye. Caution with active intraocular inflammation (eg, uveitis); inflammation may be exacerbated. Macular edema, including cystoid macular edema, reported; caution in aphakic patients, pseudophakic patients with a torn posterior lens capsule, or patients with known risk factors for macular edema. Bacterial keratitis associated with the use of multiple-dose containers reported. Contact lenses should be removed prior to instillation and may be reinserted 15 min following administration.

ADVERSE REACTIONS
Ocular hyperemia, decreased visual acuity, eye discomfort, foreign body sensation, pain, pruritus.

PREGNANCY AND LACTATION
Category C, caution in nursing.

MECHANISM OF ACTION
Prostaglandin analog; not established. Selective FP prostanoid receptor agonist that is believed to reduce IOP by increasing uveoscleral outflow.

PHARMACOKINETICS
Absorption: C_{max}=0.018ng/mL; T_{max}=30 min. **Metabolism:** Cornea; hydrolyzed by esterases to active free acid. **Elimination:** Urine (<2%, travoprost free acid); $T_{1/2}$=45 min.

PATIENT CONSIDERATIONS
Assessment: Assess for active intraocular inflammation, aphakia, pseudophakia with a torn posterior lens capsule, risk factors for macular edema, and pregnancy/nursing status.

Monitoring: Monitor for increased iris/eyelid/eyelash pigmentation, changes in eyelashes/vellus hair in the treated eye, macular edema, bacterial keratitis, and other adverse reactions.

Counseling: Inform of the possibility of increased brown pigmentation of the iris, eyelid skin darkening, and eyelash and vellus hair changes in the treated eye. Instruct to avoid allowing the tip of the dispensing container to contact the eye, surrounding structures, fingers, or any other surface to avoid contamination. Advise to immediately consult physician about the continued use of treatment if an intercurrent ocular condition (eg, trauma, infection) develops, if undergoing ocular surgery, or if any ocular reactions, particularly conjunctivitis and eyelid reactions, develop. Advise that contact lenses should be removed prior to instillation and may be reinserted 15 min following administration. Instruct that if using >1 topical ophthalmic drug, to administer the drugs at least 5 min apart.

JADENU — deferasirox
Class: Iron-chelating agent

Rx

> May cause acute renal failure and death, particularly in patients w/ comorbidities and those in the advanced stages of their hematologic disorders. Measure SrCr and determine CrCl in duplicate prior to initiation of therapy and monitor renal function at least monthly thereafter. Monitor creatinine weekly for the 1st month, then at least monthly for patients w/ baseline renal impairment or increased risk of acute renal failure. Consider dose reduction, interruption, or discontinuation based on increases in SrCr. May cause hepatic injury, including hepatic failure and death. Measure serum transaminases and bilirubin prior to initiating treatment, every 2 weeks during the 1st month, and at least monthly thereafter. Avoid in patients w/ severe (Child-Pugh C) hepatic impairment and reduce dose w/ moderate (Child-Pugh B) hepatic impairment. May cause GI hemorrhages, which may be fatal, especially in elderly who have advanced hematologic malignancies and/or low platelet counts. Monitor patients and d/c therapy if GI ulceration or hemorrhage is suspected.

ADULT DOSAGE
Chronic Iron Overload

Transfusional Iron Overload:
Only consider when a patient has evidence of chronic transfusional iron overload, which should include the transfusion of at least 100mL/kg of packed RBCs (eg, at least 20 U of packed RBCs for a 40kg person or more in individuals weighing >40kg), and a serum ferritin consistently >1000mcg/L

Initial: 14mg/kg qd; calculate doses (mg/kg/day) to the nearest whole tab
Maint: May adjust dose every 3-6 months based on serum ferritin trends. Make dose adjustments in steps of 3.5 or 7mg/kg and tailor adjustments to individual response and therapeutic goals. If inadequately controlled w/ doses of 21mg/kg (eg, serum ferritin levels persistently >2500mcg/L and not showing a decreasing trend over time), doses of up to 28mg/kg may be considered. Consider temporarily interrupting therapy if serum ferritin falls consistently <500mcg/L.
Max: 28mg/kg

In Non-Transfusion-Dependent Thalassemia (NTDT) Syndromes:
Only consider in a patient w/ a liver iron concentration (LIC) of at least 5mg of iron per gram of liver dry weight (mg Fe/g dw) and a serum ferritin >300mcg/L

Initial: 7mg/kg qd; calculate doses (mg/kg/day) to the nearest whole tab. Consider increasing dose to 14mg/kg/day after 4 weeks if baseline LIC is >15mg Fe/g dw.
Maint: Interrupt treatment when serum ferritin is <300mcg/L and obtain an LIC to determine whether LIC has fallen to <3mg Fe/g dw. After 6 months of therapy, if LIC remains >7mg Fe/g dw, increase dose to a max of 14mg/kg/day. If after 6 months of therapy, LIC is 3-7mg

PEDIATRIC DOSAGE
Chronic Iron Overload

Transfusional Iron Overload:
Only consider when a patient has evidence of chronic transfusional iron overload, which should include the transfusion of at least 100mL/kg of packed RBCs (eg, at least 20 U of packed RBCs for a 40kg person or more in individuals weighing >40kg), and a serum ferritin consistently >1000mcg/L

≥2 Years:
Initial: 14mg/kg qd; calculate doses (mg/kg/day) to the nearest whole tab
Maint: May adjust dose every 3-6 months based on serum ferritin trends. Make dose adjustments in steps of 3.5 or 7mg/kg and tailor adjustments to individual response and therapeutic goals. If inadequately controlled w/ doses of 21mg/kg (eg, serum ferritin levels persistently >2500mcg/L and not showing a decreasing trend over time), doses of up to 28mg/kg may be considered. Consider temporarily interrupting therapy if serum ferritin falls consistently <500mcg/L.
Max: 28mg/kg

In NTDT Syndromes:
Only consider in a patient w/ an LIC of at least 5mg Fe/g dw and a serum ferritin >300mcg/L

≥10 Years:
Initial: 7mg/kg qd; calculate doses (mg/kg/day) to the nearest whole tab. Consider increasing dose to 14mg/kg/day after 4 weeks if baseline LIC is >15mg Fe/g dw.
Maint: Interrupt treatment when serum ferritin is <300mcg/L and obtain an LIC to determine whether LIC has fallen to <3mg Fe/g dw. After 6 months of therapy, if LIC remains >7mg Fe/g dw, increase dose to a max of 14mg/kg/day. If after 6 months of therapy, LIC is 3-7mg Fe/g dw, continue treatment at no

Fe/g dw, continue treatment at no more than 7mg/kg/day. When LIC is <3mg Fe/g dw, interrupt treatment and continue to monitor LIC. Restart treatment when LIC rises again to >5mg Fe/g dw.
Max: 14mg/kg/day

Conversions
Converting from Exjade to Jadenu: Jadenu dose should be about 30% lower, rounded to nearest whole tab

Transfusion-Dependent Iron Overload:
Initial: 14mg/kg/day (for 20mg/kg/day Exjade)
Titration Increments: 3.5-7mg/kg (for 5-10mg/kg Exjade)
Max: 28mg/kg/day (for 40mg/kg/day Exjade)

NTDT Syndromes:
Initial: 7mg/kg/day (for 10mg/kg/day Exjade)
Titration Increments: 3.5-7mg/kg (for 5-10mg/kg Exjade)
Max: 14mg/kg/day (for 20mg/kg/day Exjade)

more than 7mg/kg/day. When LIC is <3mg Fe/g dw, interrupt treatment and continue to monitor LIC. Restart treatment when LIC rises again to >5mg Fe/g dw.
Max: 14mg/kg/day

Conversions
Converting from Exjade to Jadenu: Jadenu dose should be about 30% lower, rounded to nearest whole tab

Transfusion-Dependent Iron Overload:
Initial: 14mg/kg/day (for 20mg/kg/day Exjade)
Titration Increments: 3.5-7mg/kg (for 5-10mg/kg Exjade)
Max: 28mg/kg/day (for 40mg/kg/day Exjade)

NTDT Syndromes:
Initial: 7mg/kg/day (for 10mg/kg/day Exjade)
Titration Increments: 3.5-7mg/kg (for 5-10mg/kg Exjade)
Max: 14mg/kg/day (for 20mg/kg/day Exjade)

DOSING CONSIDERATIONS
Concomitant Medications
Bile Acid Sequestrants/Potent UDP-Glucuronosyltransferase (UGT) Inducers: Avoid w/ bile acid sequestrants (eg, cholestyramine, colesevelam, colestipol) or potent UGT inducers (eg, rifampicin, phenytoin, phenobarbital, ritonavir). If concomitant use is necessary w/ 1 of these agents, consider increasing initial deferasirox dose by 50%, and monitor serum ferritin levels and clinical responses for further dose modification.

Renal Impairment
Baseline Renal Impairment:
CrCl 40-60mL/min: Reduce initial dose by 50%
SrCr >2X ULN or CrCl <40mL/min: Contraindicated

Increases in SrCr During Therapy:
All Patients: D/C therapy for SrCr >2X the age-appropriate ULN or for CrCl <40mL/min

Transfusional Iron Overload:
2-15 Years: Reduce dose by 7mg/kg if SrCr increases to >33% above the average baseline measurement and greater than the age-appropriate ULN
≥16 Years: If SrCr increases by ≥33% above the average baseline measurement, repeat SrCr w/in 1 week, and if still elevated by ≥33%, reduce dose by 7mg/kg

NTDT Syndromes:
10-15 Years: Reduce dose by 3.5mg/kg if SrCr increases to >33% above the average baseline measurement and greater than the age-appropriate ULN
≥16 Years: If SrCr increases by ≥33% above the average baseline measurement, repeat SrCr w/in 1 week, and if still elevated by ≥33%, interrupt therapy if the dose is 3.5mg/kg, or reduce by 50% if the dose is 7 or 14mg/kg

Hepatic Impairment
Baseline Hepatic Impairment:
Mild (Child-Pugh A): No dose adjustment necessary
Moderate (Child-Pugh B): Reduce initial dose by 50%
Severe (Child-Pugh C): Avoid therapy

Elderly
Start at lower end of dosing range

ADMINISTRATION
Oral route

Swallow tab w/ water or other liquids, preferably at the same time each day. May be taken on an empty stomach or w/ a light meal (containing <7% fat content and approx 250 calories).

For patients who have difficulty swallowing whole tabs, may crush tabs and mix w/ soft foods (eg, yogurt, applesauce) immediately prior to use; dose should be immediately and completely consumed and not stored for future use. Avoid commercial crushers w/ serrated surfaces for crushing a single 90mg tab.

STORAGE
25°C (77°F); excursions permitted to 15-30°C (59-86°F). Protect from moisture.

HOW SUPPLIED
Tab: 90mg, 180mg, 360mg

CONTRAINDICATIONS
SrCr >2X the age-appropriate ULN or CrCl <40mL/min, poor performance status, high-risk myelodysplastic syndrome (MDS), advanced malignancies, platelet counts <50 x 10⁹/L, known hypersensitivity to deferasirox or any component of this medication.

WARNINGS/PRECAUTIONS
Renal tubular damage including Fanconi's syndrome reported, most commonly in children and adolescents w/ β-thalassemia and serum ferritin levels <1500mcg/L. Intermittent proteinuria reported; monitor for proteinuria monthly. Hepatic toxicity appears to be more common in patients >55 yrs of age. Hepatic failure was more common in patients w/ significant comorbidities, including liver cirrhosis and multiorgan failure. Consider dose modifications or interruption of

treatment for severe or persistent elevations in serum transaminases and bilirubin. Patients w/ mild (Child-Pugh A) or moderate (Child-Pugh B) hepatic impairment may be at higher risk for hepatic toxicity. Nonfatal upper GI irritation, ulceration, and hemorrhage reported. There have been reports of ulcers complicated w/ GI perforation (including fatal outcome). Neutropenia, agranulocytosis, worsening anemia, and thrombocytopenia, including fatal events, reported; risk may increase w/ preexisting hematologic disorders. Interrupt treatment in patients who develop cytopenias until the cause has been determined. Increased risk of toxicity in elderly; monitor more frequently. May cause serious hypersensitivity reactions (eg, anaphylaxis, angioedema); d/c and institute appropriate medical intervention if reactions are severe. Do not reintroduce in patients who have experienced previous hypersensitivity reactions on deferasirox products. Severe skin reactions, including Stevens-Johnson syndrome (SJS), toxic epidermal necrolysis (TEN), and erythema multiforme, reported. Cannot exclude risk of other skin reactions (eg, drug reaction w/ eosinophilia and systemic symptoms). D/C immediately and do not reintroduce if severe skin reactions are suspected. Rashes may occur; interrupt treatment in severe cases and may consider reintroduction at a lower dose w/ escalation after resolution of rash. Auditory and ocular disturbances reported. Perform auditory and ophthalmic testing every 12 months; monitor more frequently if disturbances are noted and consider dose reduction or interruption. Measure serum ferritin monthly for possible overchelation of iron for patients w/ transfusional iron overload. For patients w/ NTDT, measure serum ferritin monthly and measure LIC by liver biopsy or by using an FDA-cleared/approved method for monitoring patients receiving therapy every 6 months on treatment.

ADVERSE REACTIONS
Transfusional Iron Overload: Abdominal pain, N/V, diarrhea, skin rashes, increases in SrCr.
NTDT Syndromes: Nausea, rash, diarrhea.

DRUG INTERACTIONS
See Dosing Considerations. Avoid w/ aluminum-containing antacid preparations. May induce CYP3A4, resulting in a decrease in CYP3A4 substrate concentration; closely monitor for signs of reduced effectiveness w/ drugs metabolized by CYP3A4 (eg, cyclosporine, fentanyl, quetiapine). Inhibits CYP2C8 and CYP1A2, resulting in an increase in CYP2C8 (eg, repaglinide, paclitaxel) and CYP1A2 (eg, duloxetine, theophylline, tizanidine) substrate concentration; closely monitor for signs of exposure-related toxicity. Consider decreasing the dose of repaglinide and monitor blood glucose levels carefully. Avoid w/ theophylline or other CYP1A2 substrates w/ a narrow therapeutic index (eg, tizanidine); monitor theophylline concentrations and consider theophylline dose modification if theophylline must be coadministered. Increased risk of GI hemorrhage w/ drugs that have ulcerogenic or hemorrhagic potential (eg, NSAIDs, corticosteroids, oral bisphosphonates, anticoagulants).

PREGNANCY AND LACTATION
Pregnancy: There are no adequate or well-controlled studies in pregnant women. Administration to animals during pregnancy and lactation resulted in decreased offspring viability and an increase in renal anomalies in male offspring at exposures that were less than the recommended human exposure. Use during pregnancy only if potential benefit justifies the potential risk to the fetus.
Lactation: Not for use in nursing.

MECHANISM OF ACTION
Iron-chelating agent; a tridentate ligand that binds iron w/ high affinity in a 2:1 ratio.

PHARMACOKINETICS
Absorption: Absolute bioavailability (tab for oral sus: 70%, tab: 36% greater than tab for oral sus); T_{max}=1.5-4 hrs (median). **Distribution:** V_d=14.37L (adults); plasma protein binding (99%). **Metabolism:** Glucuronidation via UGT1A1 (major) and UGT1A3 (minor) followed by deconjugation in the intestine and reabsorption (enterohepatic recycling); oxidation via CYP450 (minor). **Elimination:** Feces (84%), urine (8%); $T_{1/2}$=8-16 hrs.

PATIENT CONSIDERATIONS
Assessment: Assess for high-risk MDS, performance status, renal/hepatic impairment, advanced malignancies, hematological disorders, comorbidities, hypersensitivity to the drug, pregnancy/nursing status, and possible drug interactions. Perform baseline auditory and ophthalmic examinations. Obtain baseline SrCr in duplicate, serum transaminases, bilirubin, and blood counts. Determine CrCl (Cockcroft-Gault method). In patients w/ transfusional iron overload, obtain baseline serum ferritin level. In patients w/ iron overload in NTDT syndromes, obtain LIC by liver biopsy or by an FDA-cleared/approved method for identifying patients for treatment w/ deferasirox therapy, and obtain baseline serum ferritin level on at least 2 measurements 1 month apart.

Monitoring: Monitor for acute renal failure, hepatic failure, GI ulceration/hemorrhage, neutropenia, agranulocytosis, worsening anemia, thrombocytopenia, hypersensitivity reactions, rashes, SJS, TEN, erythema multiforme, and other adverse reactions. Monitor blood counts. Perform auditory and ophthalmic tests every 12 months. Monitor closely for efficacy and adverse reactions that may require dose titration in patients w/ mild or moderate hepatic impairment. Monitor serum transaminases and bilirubin every 2 weeks during the 1st month of therapy and at least monthly thereafter. Monitor SrCr weekly during the 1st month after initiation or modification of therapy and at least monthly thereafter. Monitor SrCr and/or CrCl more frequently if creatinine levels are increasing. Monitor serum ferritin and for proteinuria monthly. In patients w/ iron overload in NTDT syndromes, monitor LIC every 6 months. Monitor elderly more frequently for toxicity.

Counseling: Instruct to take ud. Instruct not to take the medication simultaneously w/ aluminum-containing antacids. Inform of the importance of auditory and ophthalmic testing before starting treatment and thereafter at regular intervals. Caution patients experiencing dizziness to avoid driving or operating machinery.

Inform about drug interactions including potential for GI ulcers/bleeding and loss of effectiveness due to drug interactions. Advise that blood tests will be performed every month or more frequently if patient is at increased risk of complications. Inform that severe kidney and liver problems, blood disorders, stomach hemorrhage, and death have been reported. Inform that skin rash and serious allergic reactions have been reported; advise to d/c therapy and contact physician immediately if severe reactions occur.

JAKAFI — ruxolitinib   Rx
Class: Kinase inhibitor

ADULT DOSAGE	PEDIATRIC DOSAGE
Intermediate or High-Risk Myelofibrosis	Pediatric use may not have been established

Including Primary Myelofibrosis, Post-Polycythemia Vera Myelofibrosis, Post-Essential Thrombocythemia Myelofibrosis:

Initial:
Platelet Count >200 x 10⁹/L: 20mg bid
Platelet Count 100-200 x 10⁹/L: 15mg bid
Platelet Count 50 to <100 x 10⁹/L: 5mg bid
Titrate: Based on safety and efficacy

Polycythemia Vera

In Patients Who Have Had an Inadequate Response to or Are Intolerant of Hydroxyurea:

Initial: 10mg bid
Titrate: Based on safety and efficacy

DOSING CONSIDERATIONS
Dose Reductions
Myelofibrosis:
Starting Treatment w/ Platelet Count of 50 to <100 x 10⁹/L:
Platelet Count <25 x 10⁹/L or ANC <0.5 x 10⁹/L: Interrupt treatment; may restart after recovery of platelet count to >35 x 10⁹/L and ANC to >0.75 x 10⁹/L
Starting Treatment w/ Platelet Count of ≥100 x 10⁹/L:
Platelet Count <50 x 10⁹/L or ANC <0.5 x 10⁹/L: Interrupt treatment and may restart after recovery of platelet count to >50 x 10⁹/L and ANC to >0.75 x 10⁹/L
Refer to PI for further information on restarting treatment

Polycythemia Vera:
Hgb <8g/dL or Platelet Count <50 x 10⁹/L or ANC <1.0 x 10⁹/L: Interrupt dosing; may restart after recovery of hematologic parameters to acceptable levels
Hgb 8 to <10g/dL or Platelet Count 50 to <75 x 10⁹/L: Reduce dose by 5mg bid; if on 5mg bid, decrease to 5mg qd
Hgb 10 to <12g/dL and Platelet Count 75 to <100 x 10⁹/L: Consider dose reductions w/ the goal of avoiding dose interruptions for anemia and thrombocytopenia
Refer to PI for further information on restarting treatment

Concomitant Medications
Strong CYP3A4 Inhibitors or Fluconazole Doses ≤200mg:
Initial Dose:

Myelofibrosis:
Platelet Count 50 to <100 x 10⁹/L: 5mg qd
Platelet Count ≥100 x 10⁹/L: 10mg bid

Polycythemia Vera: 5mg bid

Maint Dose:
5mg QD: Avoid concomitant use or interrupt treatment for the duration of strong CYP3A4 inhibitor or fluconazole use
5mg BID: Reduce to 5mg qd
≥10mg BID: Reduce dose by 50% (round up to the closest available tab strength)
Daily Fluconazole Doses >200mg: Avoid concomitant use
Renal Impairment
Initial Dose:

Myelofibrosis w/ Moderate or Severe (CrCl 15-59mL/min) Impairment:
Platelet Count <50 x 10⁹/L: Avoid use
Platelet Count 50 to <100 x 10⁹/L: 5mg/day
Platelet Count 100-150 x 10⁹/L: 10mg bid
ESRD on Dialysis:
Platelet Count 100-200 x 10⁹/L: 15mg once after a dialysis session
Platelet Count >200 x 10⁹/L: 20mg once after a dialysis session

Polycythemia Vera w/ Moderate or Severe (CrCl 15-59mL/min) Impairment:
Any Platelet Count: 5mg bid
ESRD on Dialysis: 10mg

Hepatic Impairment
Initial Dose:

Myelofibrosis w/ Mild, Moderate, or Severe (Child-Pugh Categories A, B, C) Impairment:
Platelet Count <50 x 10⁹/L: Avoid use
Platelet Count 50 to <100 x 10⁹/L: 5mg/day
Platelet Count 100-150 x 10⁹/L: 10mg bid

Polycythemia Vera w/ Mild, Moderate, or Severe (Child-Pugh Categories A, B, C) Impairment:
Any Platelet Count: 5mg bid
Adverse Reactions
Hematologic Toxicity and Thrombocytopenia:
Refer to PI for further modifications for myelofibrosis and polycythemia vera

Bleeding:
- Interrupt treatment for bleeding requiring intervention regardless of platelet count
- Once bleeding event has resolved, consider resuming treatment at prior dose if underlying cause of bleeding has been controlled
- If bleeding event has resolved but underlying cause persists, consider resuming treatment at a lower dose
Discontinuation
When discontinuing for reasons other than thrombocytopenia, consider gradual tapering (eg, 5mg bid each week)
Other Important Considerations
Insufficient Response:
- Doses should not be increased during the first 4 weeks of therapy and not more frequently than every 2 weeks
- D/C if no spleen size reduction or symptom improvement after 6 months of therapy
Myelofibrosis:
Starting Treatment w/ Platelet Count 50 to <100 x 10⁹/L:
May increase by increments of 5mg/day to a max of 10mg bid if:
1. Platelet count has remained at least 40 x 10⁹/L, and
2. Platelet count has not fallen by more than 20% in the prior 4 weeks, and
3. ANC is >1 x 10⁹/L, and
4. Dose has not been reduced or interrupted for an adverse event or hematological toxicity in the prior 4 weeks
Continuation of treatment for >6 months should be limited to when the benefits outweigh the potential risks

Starting Treatment w/ Platelet Count ≥100 x 10⁹/L:
If platelet and neutrophil counts are adequate, may increase in 5mg bid increments to a max of 25mg bid if:
1. Failure to achieve a reduction from pretreatment baseline in either palpable spleen length of 50% or a 35% reduction in spleen volume measured by CT or MRI;
2. Platelet count >125 x 10⁹/L at 4 weeks and platelet count never <100 x 10⁹/L;
3. ANC levels >0.75 x 10⁹/L

Long-term maintenance at 5mg bid should be limited to when the benefits outweigh the potential risks

Polycythemia Vera:
If platelet, Hgb, and neutrophil counts are adequate, may increase in 5mg bid increments to a max of 25mg bid if:
1. Inadequate efficacy demonstrated by one or more of the following:
a. Continued need for phlebotomy
b. WBC count greater than ULN range
c. Platelet count greater than ULN range
d. Palpable spleen that is reduced by <25% from baseline
2. Platelet count ≥140 x 10⁹/L
3. Hgb ≥12g/dL
4. ANC ≥1.5 x 10⁹/L
ADMINISTRATION
Oral route

Take w/ or w/o food.

NG Tube (8 French or Greater) Alternative
Use if unable to ingest tabs.
Suspend one tab in approx 40mL of water w/ stirring for approx 10 min. W/IN 6 hrs after tab has dispersed, the sus can be administered using an appropriate syringe.
STORAGE
20-25°C (68-77°F); excursions permitted between 15-30°C (59-86°F).
HOW SUPPLIED
Tab: 5mg, 10mg, 15mg, 20mg, 25mg
WARNINGS/PRECAUTIONS
See Dosing Considerations. Avoid in ESRD (CrCl <15mL/min) not requiring dialysis. May cause thrombocytopenia, anemia, and neutropenia. Manage thrombocytopenia by reducing the dose or temporarily interrupting treatment; platelet transfusions may be necessary. May require blood transfusions and/ or dose modifications in patients developing anemia. Withhold treatment until recovery of severe neutropenia (ANC <0.5 x 10⁹/L). Serious bacterial, mycobacterial, fungal, and viral infections may occur; active serious infections should be resolved before starting therapy. Tuberculosis (TB) reported; test for latent infection in those at higher risk prior to treatment initiation. Observe for signs/symptoms of active TB and manage promptly. Progressive multifocal leukoencephalopathy (PML) reported; d/c and evaluate if PML is suspected. Hepatitis B viral load (HBV-DNA titer) increases, w/ or w/o associated elevations in ALT and AST reported in patients w/ chronic HBV infections; patients w/ chronic HBV infection should be treated and monitored according to clinical guidelines. Symptoms from myeloproliferative neoplasms may return to pretreatment levels over a period of 1 week following discontinuation of therapy. Fever, respiratory distress, hypotension, disseminated intravascular coagulation, or multiorgan failure may occur after discontinuation; evaluate for and treat any intercurrent illness and consider restarting or increasing dose if one or more of these adverse events occur. Non-melanoma skin cancers (eg, basal cell, squamous cell, Merkel cell carcinoma) reported. Increases in lipid parameters including total

cholesterol, LDL cholesterol, and TGs reported; assess lipid parameters approx 8-12 weeks following initiation of therapy and monitor and treat according to clinical guidelines.

ADVERSE REACTIONS
Bruising, dizziness, headache, UTIs, weight gain, flatulence, thrombocytopenia, anemia, neutropenia, ALT/AST/cholesterol elevations, abdominal pain, diarrhea, fatigue, pruritus.

DRUG INTERACTIONS
See Dosing Considerations. Strong CYP3A4 inhibitor ketoconazole may increase levels and exposure. Concomitant use w/ combined CYP3A4 and CYP2C9 inhibitor fluconazole at doses of 100-400mg qd may increase exposure of ruxolitinib. Strong CYP3A4 inducer rifampin may decrease levels and exposure; monitor patients frequently and adjust ruxolitinib dose based on safety and efficacy.

PREGNANCY AND LACTATION
Pregnancy: Category C.
Lactation: Not for use in nursing.

MECHANISM OF ACTION
Kinase inhibitor; inhibits Janus associated kinases (JAKs) JAK1 and JAK2 which mediate the signaling of a number of cytokines and growth factors that are important for hematopoiesis and immune function.

PHARMACOKINETICS
Absorption: Rapid; T_{max}=1-2 hrs. **Distribution:** V_d=72L (myelofibrosis), 75L (polycythemia vera); plasma protein binding (97%). **Metabolism:** Via CYP3A4 and CYP2C9 (lesser extent). **Elimination:** Urine (74%), feces (22%); $T_{1/2}$=3 hrs (ruxolitinib), 5.8 hrs (ruxolitinib and metabolites).

PATIENT CONSIDERATIONS
Assessment: Assess for risk factors for TB, renal/hepatic impairment, pregnancy/nursing status, and possible drug interactions. Resolve active serious infections prior to therapy. Perform CBC and platelet count before initiating therapy. Assess baseline lipid levels.

Monitoring: Monitor for thrombocytopenia, anemia, neutropenia, infections, PML, TB, exacerbation of symptoms from myeloproliferative neoplasms following discontinuation of therapy, non-melanoma skin cancers, and other adverse reactions. Monitor CBCs and platelet counts every 2-4 weeks until doses are stabilized, and then as clinically indicated. Perform periodic skin examinations. Monitor HBV-DNA titer levels in patients w/ HBV. Monitor lipid levels approx 8-12 weeks following initiation of therapy.

Counseling: Inform that therapy is associated w/ thrombocytopenia, anemia, and neutropenia and of the need to monitor CBC before and during treatment; advise to observe for and report bleeding to the physician. Inform of the signs/symptoms of infection, herpes zoster, and PML; instruct to report and seek medical advice if such symptoms are observed. Inform that after discontinuation of therapy, signs/symptoms from myeloproliferative neoplasms are expected to return; instruct not to interrupt or d/c therapy w/o consulting physician. Inform that drug may increase the risk of certain non-melanoma skin cancers; advise to inform physician if patient has have ever had any type of skin cancer or if the patient observes any new or changing skin lesions. Inform that therapy may increase blood cholesterol, and advise of the need to monitor blood cholesterol levels. Advise to inform physician of all medications, including OTC medications, herbal products, and dietary supplements, that are being taken. Instruct patients on dialysis to not take their dose before dialysis but only following dialysis. Advise patients to continue taking the medication every day ud and not to change the dose or stop therapy w/o consulting their physician.

JALYN — dutasteride/tamsulosin hydrochloride   Rx
Class: 5-alpha-reductase inhibitor (5-ARI)/alpha antagonist

ADULT DOSAGE	PEDIATRIC DOSAGE
Benign Prostatic Hyperplasia 1 cap qd, 30 min after the same meal each day	Pediatric use may not have been established

ADMINISTRATION
Oral route
Swallow cap whole; do not chew, crush, or open.

STORAGE
25°C (77°F); excursions permitted to 15-30°C (59-86°F).

HOW SUPPLIED
Cap: (Dutasteride/Tamsulosin) 0.5mg/0.4mg

CONTRAINDICATIONS
Pregnancy, women of childbearing potential, pediatric patients. Previously demonstrated, clinically significant hypersensitivity (eg, serious skin reactions, angioedema, urticaria, pruritus, respiratory symptoms) to dutasteride, other 5-alpha-reductase inhibitors, tamsulosin, or any other component of Jalyn.

WARNINGS/PRECAUTIONS
Not approved for the prevention of prostate cancer. Orthostatic hypotension/syncope may occur; avoid situations where syncope may result in an injury. May reduce serum prostate specific antigen (PSA) concentration during therapy; establish a new baseline PSA at least 3 months after starting therapy and monitor PSA periodically thereafter. Any confirmed increase from the lowest PSA value during treatment may signal the presence of prostate cancer and should be evaluated. May increase the risk of high-grade prostate cancer. Prior to initiating

treatment, consideration should be given to other urological conditions that may cause similar symptoms; BPH and prostate cancer may coexist. Risk to male fetus; cap should not be handled by pregnant women or women who may become pregnant. May cause priapism; may lead to permanent impotence if not properly treated. Avoid blood donation until at least 6 months following the last dose. Intraoperative floppy iris syndrome (IFIS) reported during cataract surgery; initiation of therapy is not recommended in patients for whom cataract surgery is scheduled. Caution w/ sulfa allergy; allergic reaction rarely reported. Reduced total sperm count, semen volume, and sperm motility reported.

ADVERSE REACTIONS
Ejaculation disorders, impotence, decreased libido, breast disorders, dizziness.

DRUG INTERACTIONS
Avoid w/ strong CYP3A4 inhibitors (eg, ketoconazole); may increase tamsulosin exposure. Caution w/ potent, chronic CYP3A4 inhibitors (eg, ritonavir), moderate CYP3A4 inhibitors (eg, erythromycin), strong (eg, paroxetine) or moderate (eg, terbinafine) CYP2D6 inhibitors; potential for significant increase in tamsulosin exposure. Potential for significant increase in tamsulosin exposure when coadministered w/ a combination of both CYP3A4 and CYP2D6 inhibitors. Caution w/ cimetidine and warfarin. Avoid w/ other α-adrenergic antagonists; may increase the risk of symptomatic hypotension. Caution w/ PDE-5 inhibitors; may cause symptomatic hypotension.

PREGNANCY AND LACTATION
Category X, not for use in nursing.

MECHANISM OF ACTION
Dutasteride: Selective type I and II 5α-reductase inhibitor; inhibits conversion of testosterone to dihydrotestosterone, the androgen primarily responsible for the initial development and subsequent enlargement of the prostate gland. Tamsulosin: $α_{1A}$ antagonist; selective blockade of $α_1$ adrenoceptors in the prostate results in relaxation of the smooth muscles of the bladder neck and prostate, improving urine flow rate and reducing BPH symptoms.

PHARMACOKINETICS
Absorption: (Fed) Dutasteride: Absolute bioavailability (60%); C_{max}=2.14ng/mL, T_{max}=3 hrs, AUC=39.6ng•hr/mL. Tamsulosin: Complete; C_{max}=11.3ng/mL, T_{max}=6 hrs, AUC=187.2ng•hr/mL. **Distribution:** Dutasteride: V_d=300-500L, plasma protein binding (99% albumin, 96.6% α-1 acid glycoprotein). Tamsulosin: Plasma protein binding (94-99%); (IV) V_d=16L. **Metabolism:** Dutasteride: Extensive. CYP3A4/3A5; 4'-hydroxydutasteride, 1,2-dihydroxydutasteride, 6-hydroxydutasteride (major metabolites). Tamsulosin: Liver (extensive); CYP3A4, CYP2D6. **Elimination:** Dutasteride: Urine (<1% unchanged), feces (5% unchanged, 40% metabolites); $T_{1/2}$=5 weeks. Tamsulosin: Urine (76%, <10% unchanged), feces (21%); $T_{1/2}$=14-15 hrs, 9-13 hrs.

PATIENT CONSIDERATIONS
Assessment: Assess for urological conditions that may cause similar symptoms, previous hypersensitivity to the drug, sulfa allergy, and possible drug interactions. Assess if patient is planning to undergo cataract surgery.

Monitoring: Monitor for signs/symptoms of prostate cancer, other urological diseases, orthostatic hypotension, syncope, priapism, IFIS, and allergic reactions. Obtain new baseline PSA at least 3 months after starting treatment and monitor PSA periodically thereafter.

Counseling: Inform about the possible occurrence of symptoms related to orthostatic hypotension and the potential risk of syncope; instruct to avoid situations where injury may result if syncope occurs. Inform that an increase in high-grade prostate cancer was reported. Inform females who are pregnant or who may become pregnant not to handle the drug due to potential risk to the fetus. Instruct that if a pregnant woman or woman of childbearing potential comes in contact w/ a leaking cap to wash the area immediately w/ soap and water. Inform that cap may become deformed and/or discolored if kept at high temperatures; instruct to avoid use if this occurs. Advise about the possibility of priapism (rare) that may lead to permanent erectile dysfunction if not brought to immediate medical attention. Advise not to donate blood for at least 6 months following the last dose. Instruct to inform ophthalmologist of drug if considering cataract surgery.

JANUMET — metformin hydrochloride/sitagliptin   Rx
Class: Biguanide/dipeptidyl peptidase-4 (DPP-4) inhibitor

> Lactic acidosis may occur due to metformin accumulation; risk increases w/ conditions such as sepsis, dehydration, excess alcohol intake, hepatic/renal impairment, and acute CHF. If acidosis is suspected, d/c therapy and hospitalize patient immediately.

ADULT DOSAGE	PEDIATRIC DOSAGE
Type 2 Diabetes Mellitus Adjunct to diet and exercise to improve glycemic control when treatment w/ both sitagliptin and metformin is appropriate **Initial:** **Not Currently on Metformin:** 50mg/500mg bid **Currently on Metformin:** 50mg bid of sitagliptin + current metformin dose **Currently on Metformin 850mg bid:** 50mg/1000mg bid **Titrate:** Gradually escalate dose to reduce GI side effects **Max:** (100mg/2000mg)/day	Pediatric use may not have been established

DOSING CONSIDERATIONS
Concomitant Medications
Insulin Secretagogue (eg, Sulfonylurea)/Insulin: May require lower doses of insulin secretagogue or insulin

ADMINISTRATION
Oral route

Take bid w/ meals.
Do not split or divide tab before swallowing.

STORAGE
20-25°C (68-77°F); excursions permitted to 15-30°C (59-86°F).

HOW SUPPLIED
Tab: (Sitagliptin/Metformin) 50mg/500mg, 50mg/1000mg

CONTRAINDICATIONS
Renal impairment (eg, SrCr ≥1.5mg/dL [men], ≥1.4mg/dL [women], or abnormal CrCl), acute or chronic metabolic acidosis, including diabetic ketoacidosis. Hypersensitivity to metformin HCl, history of a serious hypersensitivity reaction to Janumet or sitagliptin (eg, anaphylaxis or angioedema).

WARNINGS/PRECAUTIONS
Not for use in type 1 diabetes mellitus (DM) or for treatment of diabetic ketoacidosis. Acute pancreatitis, including fatal and nonfatal hemorrhagic or necrotizing pancreatitis, reported; d/c if pancreatitis is suspected and initiate appropriate management. Avoid in patients w/ clinical or lab evidence of hepatic disease. Worsening renal function, including acute renal failure, reported. Assess renal function before initiation of therapy and at least annually thereafter; d/c w/ evidence of renal impairment. Temporarily d/c for any surgical procedure (except minor procedures not associated w/ restricted food and fluid intake); restart when oral intake is resumed and renal function is evaluated as normal. Evaluate patients previously well controlled on therapy who develop lab abnormalities or clinical illness for evidence of ketoacidosis or lactic acidosis; d/c if acidosis of either form occurs. Promptly d/c in the event of cardiovascular collapse (shock) from whatever cause, acute CHF, acute MI, and other conditions characterized by hypoxemia. Temporary loss of glycemic control may occur when a patient is exposed to stress (eg, fever, trauma, infection, surgery); may be necessary to withhold therapy and temporarily administer insulin. Caution in elderly. **Sitagliptin:** Serious hypersensitivity reactions reported; d/c if suspected, assess for other potential causes, and institute alternative treatment for DM. Caution in patients w/ history of angioedema to another DPP-4 inhibitor. Severe and disabling arthralgia reported in patients taking DPP-4 inhibitors; d/c if appropriate. **Metformin:** May decrease serum vitamin B12 levels; monitor hematologic parameters annually. Elderly, debilitated, or malnourished patients, and those w/ adrenal/pituitary insufficiency or alcohol intoxication are particularly susceptible to hypoglycemic effects. Temporarily d/c at the time of or prior to radiologic studies involving the use of intravascular iodinated contrast materials, withhold for 48 hrs subsequent to the procedure, and reinstitute only after renal function is confirmed to be normal.

ADVERSE REACTIONS
Diarrhea, URTI, headache, nausea, abdominal pain.

DRUG INTERACTIONS
See Dosing Considerations. **Sitagliptin:** Incidence of hypoglycemia is increased when used in combination w/ insulin secretagogues (eg, sulfonylurea) or insulin. **Metformin:** Hypoglycemia may occur during concomitant use w/ other glucose-lowering agents (eg, sulfonylureas, insulin) or ethanol. Hypoglycemia may be difficult to recognize w/ β-adrenergic blocking drugs. Alcohol potentiates the effect of metformin on lactate metabolism; avoid excessive alcohol intake. Caution w/ drugs that may affect renal function or result in significant hemodynamic change or may interfere w/ the disposition of metformin. Topiramate or other carbonic anhydrase inhibitors (eg, zonisamide, acetazolamide, dichlorphenamide) may induce metabolic acidosis; use w/ caution. Cationic drugs (eg, cimetidine, amiloride, digoxin) that are eliminated by renal tubular secretion may interact w/ metformin; monitor and adjust dose of Janumet and/or the interfering drug. Thiazides and other diuretics, corticosteroids, phenothiazines, thyroid products, estrogens, oral contraceptives, phenytoin, nicotinic acid, sympathomimetics, calcium channel blockers, and isoniazid tend to produce hyperglycemia and may lead to loss of glycemic control; observe closely when such drugs are administered.

PREGNANCY AND LACTATION
Pregnancy: Category B. A pregnancy registry is available.
Lactation: Caution in nursing.

MECHANISM OF ACTION
Sitagliptin: DPP-4 inhibitor; slows inactivation of incretin hormones, thereby increasing insulin release and decreasing glucagon levels in the circulation in a glucose-dependent manner. **Metformin:** Biguanide; decreases hepatic glucose production, decreases intestinal absorption of glucose, and improves insulin sensitivity by increasing peripheral glucose uptake and utilization.

PHARMACOKINETICS
Absorption: Sitagliptin: Absolute bioavailability (87%). Metformin: Absolute bioavailability (50-60%) (fasted). **Distribution:** Sitagliptin: (IV) V_d=198L; plasma protein binding (38%). Metformin: V_d=654L. **Metabolism:** Sitagliptin: Via CYP3A4 (primary) and CYP2C8. **Elimination:** Sitagliptin: Feces (13%), urine (87%, 79% unchanged); $T_{1/2}$=12.4 hrs. Metformin: Urine (90%); $T_{1/2}$=6.2 hrs (plasma), 17.6 hrs (blood).

PATIENT CONSIDERATIONS
Assessment: Assess for previous hypersensitivity to the drug, metabolic acidosis including diabetic ketoacidosis, risk factors for lactic acidosis, renal/hepatic impairment, history of pancreatitis, inadequate vitamin B12 or Ca^{2+} absorption, type of DM, alcoholism, hypoxemia, presence of malnourishment or debilitation,

adrenal/pituitary insufficiency, history of angioedema w/ another DPP-4 inhibitor, pregnancy/nursing status, and possible drug interactions. Assess if patient is planning to undergo any surgical procedure, radiologic studies involving the use of intravascular iodinated contrast materials, or is under any form of stress. Obtain baseline FPG and HbA1c levels, and hematologic parameters.

Monitoring: Monitor for signs/symptoms of lactic acidosis, pancreatitis, hypoxic states, hypersensitivity reactions, severe and disabling arthralgia, and other adverse reactions. Monitor for changes in clinical status. Monitor renal function, especially in elderly, at least annually. Monitor hematologic parameters annually. Perform routine serum vitamin B12 measurements at 2- to 3-yr intervals in patients predisposed to developing subnormal vitamin B12 levels. Monitor FPG and HbA1c levels, and hepatic function periodically.

Counseling: Inform of the risks, benefits, and alternative modes of therapy. Advise on the importance of adherence to dietary instructions, regular physical activity, periodic blood glucose monitoring and HbA1c testing, recognition/management of hypo/hyperglycemia, and assessment of diabetic complications. Instruct to seek medical advice during periods of stress (eg, fever, trauma, infection, surgery) as medication needs may change. Inform of the risk of lactic acidosis; instruct to d/c therapy immediately and contact physician if unexplained hyperventilation, myalgia, malaise, unusual somnolence, dizziness, slow or irregular heartbeat, sensation of feeling cold (especially in the extremities), or other nonspecific symptoms occur. Counsel against excessive alcohol intake. Inform that GI symptoms and acute pancreatitis may occur; instruct to d/c therapy promptly and contact physician if persistent severe abdominal pain occurs. Inform that allergic reactions may occur; instruct to d/c therapy and seek medical advice promptly if symptoms occur. Inform that severe and disabling joint pain may occur. Instruct not to split or divide the tabs before swallowing. Instruct to inform physician if any bothersome or unusual symptoms develop, or if any symptoms persist or worsen.

JANUMET XR — metformin hydrochloride/sitagliptin   Rx
Class: Biguanide/dipeptidyl peptidase-4 (DPP-4) inhibitor

> Lactic acidosis may occur due to metformin accumulation; risk increases w/ conditions such as sepsis, dehydration, excess alcohol intake, hepatic/renal impairment, and acute CHF. If acidosis is suspected, d/c therapy and hospitalize patient immediately.

ADULT DOSAGE	PEDIATRIC DOSAGE
Type 2 Diabetes Mellitus	Pediatric use may not have been established
Adjunct to diet and exercise to improve glycemic control when treatment w/ both sitagliptin and metformin extended-release (ER) is appropriate	
Initial:	
Not Currently on Metformin: (100mg/1000mg)/day	
Currently on Metformin: 100mg/day of sitagliptin + current metformin dose	
Currently on Metformin Immediate-Release 850mg bid or 1000mg bid: Two 50mg/1000mg tabs qd	
Changing Between Janumet and Janumet XR: Maintain the same total daily dose of sitagliptin and metformin	
Titrate: If metformin dose is inadequate to achieve glycemic control, gradually titrate dose to reduce GI side effects	
Max: (100mg/2000mg)/day	

DOSING CONSIDERATIONS
Concomitant Medications
Insulin Secretagogue (eg, Sulfonylurea)/Insulin: May require lower doses of insulin secretagogue or insulin

ADMINISTRATION
Oral route

Take qd w/ a meal, preferably in pm.
Swallow tab whole; do not split, crush, or chew.
Patients taking 2 tabs should take the 2 tabs together qd.
Reports of incompletely dissolved tabs being eliminated in the feces; assess adequacy of glycemic control if patient reports repeatedly seeing tabs in feces.

STORAGE
20-25°C (68-77°F); excursions permitted to 15-30°C (59-86°F). Store in a dry place.

HOW SUPPLIED
Tab, ER: (Sitagliptin/Metformin ER) 50mg/500mg, 50mg/1000mg, 100mg/1000mg

CONTRAINDICATIONS
Renal impairment (eg, SrCr ≥1.5 mg/dL [men], ≥1.4mg/dL [women] or abnormal CrCl); hypersensitivity to metformin HCl; acute or chronic metabolic acidosis, including diabetic ketoacidosis; history of a serious hypersensitivity reaction to Janumet XR or sitagliptin (eg, anaphylaxis or angioedema).

WARNINGS/PRECAUTIONS

Not for use in type 1 diabetes mellitus or for treatment of diabetic ketoacidosis. Acute pancreatitis, including fatal and nonfatal hemorrhagic or necrotizing pancreatitis, reported; d/c if pancreatitis is suspected and initiate appropriate management. Avoid in patients w/ clinical or lab evidence of hepatic disease. Worsening renal function, including acute renal failure, reported. Assess renal function before initiation of therapy and at least annually thereafter; d/c w/ evidence of renal impairment. Temporarily suspend for any surgical procedure (except minor procedures not associated w/ restricted food and fluid intake); restart when oral intake is resumed and renal function is normal. Evaluate patients previously controlled on therapy who develop lab abnormalities or clinical illness for evidence of ketoacidosis or lactic acidosis; d/c if acidosis occurs. Promptly d/c in the event of cardiovascular collapse (shock) from whatever cause, acute CHF, acute MI, and other conditions characterized by hypoxemia. Temporary loss of glycemic control may occur when exposed to stress (eg, fever, trauma, infection, surgery); may be necessary to withhold therapy and temporarily administer insulin. Caution in elderly. **Sitagliptin:** Serious hypersensitivity reactions reported; if suspected, d/c therapy, assess for other potential causes, and institute alternative treatment for DM. Caution in patients w/ history of angioedema w/ another DPP-4 inhibitor. Severe and disabling arthralgia reported w/ DPP-4 inhibitors; d/c if appropriate. **Metformin:** May decrease vitamin B12 levels; monitor hematologic parameters annually. Elderly or debilitated/malnourished patients, and those w/ adrenal/pituitary insufficiency or alcohol intoxication are particularly susceptible to hypoglycemic effects. Temporarily d/c at the time of or prior to radiologic studies involving the use of intravascular iodinated contrast materials, withhold for 48 hrs subsequent to the procedure, and reinstitute only if renal function is normal.

ADVERSE REACTIONS

Diarrhea, URTI, headache, nausea, abdominal pain.

DRUG INTERACTIONS

See Dosing Considerations. **Sitagliptin:** Incidence of hypoglycemia is increased when used in combination w/ insulin secretagogues (eg, sulfonylurea) or insulin. **Metformin:** Hypoglycemia may occur during concomitant use w/ other glucose-lowering agents (eg, sulfonylureas, insulin) or ethanol. May be difficult to recognize hypoglycemia w/ β-adrenergic blocking drugs. Alcohol potentiates the effects of metformin on lactate metabolism; avoid excessive alcohol intake. Caution w/ drugs that may affect renal function or result in significant hemodynamic change or may interfere w/ the disposition of metformin. Topiramate or other carbonic anhydrase inhibitors (eg, zonisamide, acetazolamide, dichlorphenamide) may induce metabolic acidosis; use w/ caution as risk of lactic acidosis may increase. Cationic drugs (eg, cimetidine, amiloride, digoxin) that are eliminated by renal tubular secretion may potentially produce an interaction; monitor and adjust dose of Janumet XR and/or the interfering drug. Thiazides and other diuretics, corticosteroids, phenothiazines, thyroid products, estrogens, oral contraceptives, phenytoin, nicotinic acid, sympathomimetics, calcium channel blockers, and isoniazid may produce hyperglycemia and lead to loss of glycemic control; observe closely when such drugs are administered.

PREGNANCY AND LACTATION

Pregnancy: Category B. A pregnancy registry is available.
Lactation: Caution in nursing.

MECHANISM OF ACTION

Sitagliptin: DPP-4 inhibitor; slows the inactivation of incretin hormones, thereby increasing insulin release and decreasing glucagon levels in the circulation in a glucose-dependent manner. **Metformin:** Biguanide; decreases hepatic glucose production, decreases intestinal absorption of glucose, and improves insulin sensitivity by increasing peripheral glucose uptake and utilization.

PHARMACOKINETICS

Absorption: Sitagliptin: Absolute bioavailability (87%); T_{max}=3 hrs (median). Metformin ER: T_{max}=8 hrs (median). **Distribution:** Sitagliptin: (IV) V_d=198L; plasma protein binding (38%). Metformin IR: V_d=654L. **Metabolism:** Sitagliptin: Via CYP3A4 (primary) and CYP2C8. **Elimination:** Sitagliptin: Feces (13%), urine (87%, 79% unchanged); $T_{1/2}$=12.4 hrs. Metformin: Urine (90%); $T_{1/2}$=6.2 hrs (plasma), 17.6 hrs (blood).

PATIENT CONSIDERATIONS

Assessment: Assess for metabolic acidosis including diabetic ketoacidosis, risk factors for lactic acidosis, renal/hepatic impairment, previous hypersensitivity to the drug, history of pancreatitis, inadequate vitamin B12 or Ca^{2+} intake/absorption, type of DM, alcoholism, hypoxemia, presence of malnourishment or debilitation, adrenal/pituitary insufficiency, history of angioedema w/ another DPP-4 inhibitor, pregnancy/nursing status, and possible drug interactions. Assess if patient is planning to undergo any surgical procedure, radiologic studies involving the use of intravascular iodinated contrast materials, or is under any form of stress. Obtain baseline FPG and HbA1c levels, and hematologic parameters.

Monitoring: Monitor for signs/symptoms of lactic acidosis, pancreatitis, hypoxic states, hypersensitivity reactions, severe and disabling arthralgia, and other adverse reactions. Monitor for changes in clinical status. Monitor renal function, especially in elderly, at least annually. Monitor hematologic parameters annually. Perform routine serum vitamin B12 measurements at 2- to 3-yr intervals in patients predisposed to developing subnormal vitamin B12 levels. Monitor FPG and HbA1c levels, and hepatic function periodically.

Counseling: Inform of the risks, benefits, and alternative modes of therapy. Advise on the importance of adherence to dietary instructions, regular physical activity, periodic blood glucose monitoring and HbA1c testing, regular testing of renal function and hematologic parameters, recognition/management of hypo/hyperglycemia, and assessment of diabetes complications. Instruct to seek medical advice during periods of stress (eg, fever, trauma, infection, surgery) as medication needs may change. Inform of the risk of lactic acidosis; instruct to d/c

therapy immediately and notify physician if unexplained hyperventilation, myalgia, malaise, unusual somnolence, dizziness, slow or irregular heartbeat, sensation of feeling cold (especially in the extremities), or other nonspecific symptoms occur. Counsel against excessive alcohol intake. Inform that GI symptoms may occur. Inform that acute pancreatitis may occur; instruct to d/c therapy promptly and contact physician if persistent severe abdominal pain occurs. Inform that allergic reactions may occur; instruct to d/c therapy and seek medical advice promptly if symptoms occur. Inform that severe and disabling joint pain may occur. Inform that incompletely dissolved tabs may be eliminated in the feces; advise to report to physician if patient repeatedly sees tabs in feces. Instruct to inform physician if any bothersome or unusual symptom develops, or if any known symptom persists or worsens.

JANUVIA — sitagliptin   Rx

Class: Dipeptidyl peptidase-4 (DPP-4) inhibitor

ADULT DOSAGE	PEDIATRIC DOSAGE
Type 2 Diabetes Mellitus 100mg qd	Pediatric use may not have been established

DOSING CONSIDERATIONS

Concomitant Medications
Insulin Secretagogue (eg, Sulfonylurea)/Insulin: May require lower dose of insulin secretagogue or insulin

Renal Impairment
Moderate (CrCl ≥30 to <50mL/min): 50mg qd
Severe (CrCl <30mL/min): 25mg qd
ESRD Requiring Hemodialysis/Peritoneal Dialysis: 25mg qd; administer w/o regard to timing of dialysis

ADMINISTRATION

Oral route

May be taken w/ or w/o food.

STORAGE

20-25°C (68-77°F); excursions permitted to 15-30°C (59-86°F).

HOW SUPPLIED

Tab: 25mg, 50mg, 100mg

CONTRAINDICATIONS

History of a serious hypersensitivity reaction to sitagliptin (eg, anaphylaxis or angioedema).

WARNINGS/PRECAUTIONS

Not for use w/ type 1 diabetes mellitus (DM) or for treatment of diabetic ketoacidosis. Acute pancreatitis reported; d/c if pancreatitis is suspected. Worsening renal function, including acute renal failure, reported. Severe and disabling arthralgia reported in patients taking DPP-4 inhibitors. Serious hypersensitivity reactions reported; if suspected, d/c therapy, assess for other potential causes, and institute alternative treatment. Caution in patients w/ a history of angioedema w/ another DPP-4 inhibitor and in the elderly.

ADVERSE REACTIONS

Nasopharyngitis, URTI, headache.

DRUG INTERACTIONS

See Dosing Considerations. May slightly increase digoxin levels; monitor appropriately.

PREGNANCY AND LACTATION

Pregnancy: Category B.
Lactation: Caution in nursing.

MECHANISM OF ACTION

DPP-4 inhibitor; slows inactivation of incretin hormones, thereby increasing insulin release and decreasing glucagon levels in the circulation in a glucose-dependent manner.

PHARMACOKINETICS

Absorption: Rapid. Absolute bioavailability (87%); T_{max}=1-4 hrs (median); AUC=8.52μM•hr; C_{max}=950nM. **Distribution:** (IV) V_d=198L; plasma protein binding (38%). **Metabolism:** Via CYP3A4 and CYP2C8. **Elimination:** Feces (13%), urine (87%, 79% unchanged); $T_{1/2}$=12.4 hrs.

PATIENT CONSIDERATIONS

Assessment: Assess for previous hypersensitivity to the drug, type of DM, diabetic ketoacidosis, history of pancreatitis, history of angioedema w/ another DPP-4 inhibitor, pregnancy/nursing status, and possible drug interactions. Obtain baseline renal function, FPG, and HbA1c levels.

Monitoring: Monitor for pancreatitis, hypersensitivity reactions, and other adverse reactions. Monitor FPG, HbA1c, and renal function periodically.

Counseling: Inform of risks, benefits, and alternative modes of therapy. Advise on the importance of adherence to dietary instructions, regular physical activity, periodic blood glucose monitoring, HbA1c testing, recognition/management of hypo/hyperglycemia, and assessment of diabetic complications. Instruct to seek medical advice during periods of stress as medication requirements may change. Instruct to d/c use and notify physician if signs and symptoms of pancreatitis or allergic reactions occur. Instruct to inform physician if any unusual symptom develops, or if any known symptom persists or worsens. Inform patients that severe and disabling joint pain may occur and to seek medical advice if severe joint pain occurs.

JARDIANCE — empagliflozin

Rx

Class: Sodium-glucose cotransporter 2 (SGLT2) inhibitor

ADULT DOSAGE	PEDIATRIC DOSAGE
Type 2 Diabetes Mellitus	Pediatric use may not have been established
Recommended Dose: 10mg qam	
Titrate: May increase to 25mg in patients tolerating therapy	

DOSING CONSIDERATIONS
Renal Impairment
Baseline eGFR <45mL/min/1.73m²: Do not initiate treatment
eGFR Persistently <45mL/min/1.73m²: D/C treatment
Other Important Considerations
Patients w/ Volume Depletion: Correct this condition prior to initiating therapy

ADMINISTRATION
Oral route

Take w/ or w/o food.

STORAGE
25°C (77°F); excursions permitted to 15-30°C (59-86°F).

HOW SUPPLIED
Tab: 10mg, 25mg

CONTRAINDICATIONS
History of serious hypersensitivity reaction to empagliflozin, severe renal impairment, ESRD, dialysis.

WARNINGS/PRECAUTIONS
Not recommended w/ type 1 diabetes mellitus (DM) or for treatment of diabetic ketoacidosis. Causes intravascular volume contraction. Symptomatic hypotension may occur, particularly in patients w/ renal impairment, the elderly, in patients w/ low systolic BP, and in patients on diuretics; assess for volume contraction and correct volume status before initiating treatment, if indicated. Monitor for signs/symptoms of hypotension after initiating therapy and increase monitoring in clinical situations where volume contraction is expected. Ketoacidosis reported; if suspected, d/c and institute prompt treatment. Assess for ketoacidosis in patients presenting w/ signs/symptoms consistent w/ severe metabolic acidosis regardless of presenting blood glucose levels. Consider temporarily discontinuing therapy in clinical situations known to predispose to ketoacidosis (eg, prolonged fasting due to acute illness or surgery). Increases SrCr and decreases eGFR; risk of impaired renal function is increased in elderly patients and patients w/ moderate renal impairment. Serious UTIs (eg, urosepsis, pyelonephritis), requiring hospitalization, reported; evaluate for signs/symptoms of UTIs and treat promptly, if indicated. Increases risk for genital mycotic infections; monitor and treat as appropriate. Increases in LDL levels may occur. Monitoring glycemic control w/ urine glucose tests or 1,5-anhydroglucitol assay is not recommended; use alternative methods to monitor glycemic control.

ADVERSE REACTIONS
UTIs, genital mycotic infections, dyslipidemia, increased urination, URTI.

DRUG INTERACTIONS
Increased risk of hypoglycemia w/ insulin secretagogues (eg, sulfonylurea) or insulin; a lower dose of the insulin secretagogue or insulin may be required. Coadministration w/ diuretics resulted in increased urine volume and frequency of voids, which might enhance the potential for volume depletion.

PREGNANCY AND LACTATION
Pregnancy: Category C. Based on results from animal studies, empagliflozin may affect renal development and maturation. During pregnancy, consider appropriate alternative therapies, especially during the 2nd and 3rd trimesters.
Lactation: Not for use in nursing.

MECHANISM OF ACTION
SGLT2 inhibitor; reduces renal reabsorption of filtered glucose and lowers the renal threshold for glucose, and thereby increases urinary glucose excretion.

PHARMACOKINETICS
Absorption: T_{max}=1.5 hrs; AUC=1870nmol•h/L (10mg), 4740nmol•h/L (25mg); C_{max}=259nmol/L (10mg), 687nmol/L (25mg). **Distribution:** Plasma protein binding (86.2%); V_d=73.8L. **Metabolism:** Glucuronidation (primary) by the uridine 5'-diphospho-glucuronosyltransferases UGT2B7, UGT1A3, UGT1A8, and UGT1A9. **Elimination:** Feces (41.2%), urine (54.4%); $T_{1/2}$=12.4 hrs.

PATIENT CONSIDERATIONS
Assessment: Assess type of DM, and for diabetic ketoacidosis, volume contraction, history of chronic/recurrent genital mycotic infections, drug hypersensitivity, predisposition to ketoacidosis, pregnancy/nursing status, and possible drug interactions. Assess baseline renal function, LDL levels, and BP.

Monitoring: Monitor for signs/symptoms of hypotension, ketoacidosis, genital mycotic infections, UTIs, and other adverse reactions. Monitor renal function and LDL levels.

Counseling: Inform of the risks, benefits, and alternative modes of therapy. Advise about the importance of adherence to dietary instructions, regular physical activity, periodic blood glucose monitoring and HbA1c testing, recognition and management of hypoglycemia and hyperglycemia, and assessment for diabetes complications. Instruct to seek medical advice promptly during periods of stress (eg, fever, trauma, infection), as medication requirements may change. Inform that the most common adverse reactions associated w/ therapy are UTIs and mycotic genital infections. Instruct to inform physician if pregnant/nursing, if experiencing symptoms of hypotension, if any unusual symptom develops, or if any known symptom persists or worsens. Instruct to have adequate fluid intake. Inform that ketoacidosis is a serious life threatening condition. Instruct to d/c and seek medical advice immediately if symptoms of ketoacidosis (eg, N/V, abdominal pain, tiredness, labored breathing) occur. Counsel on the signs/symptoms of UTIs, vaginal yeast infections, balanitis, and balanoposthitis; inform of treatment options and when to seek medical advice.

JENTADUETO — linagliptin/metformin hydrochloride

Rx

Class: Biguanide/dipeptidyl peptidase-4 (DPP-4) inhibitor

> Lactic acidosis may occur due to metformin accumulation; risk increases w/ conditions such as sepsis, dehydration, excess alcohol intake, hepatic/renal impairment, and acute CHF. If acidosis is suspected, d/c therapy and hospitalize patient immediately.

ADULT DOSAGE	PEDIATRIC DOSAGE
Type 2 Diabetes Mellitus	Pediatric use may not have been established
Initial Dose:	
Not Currently on Metformin: 2.5mg/500mg bid	
Currently on Metformin: 2.5mg linagliptin + current metformin dose taken at each of the 2 daily meals (eg, a patient on metformin 1000mg bid would be started on 2.5mg/1000mg bid)	
Currently on Linagliptin and Metformin Individually: Switch to Jentadueto containing the same doses of each component	
Titrate: Dose escalation should be gradual to reduce the GI side effects associated w/ metformin use	
Max: 2.5mg/1000mg bid	

DOSING CONSIDERATIONS
Concomitant Medications
Insulin Secretagogue (eg, Sulfonylurea)/Insulin: May require lower dose of insulin secretagogue or insulin

ADMINISTRATION
Oral route

Take w/ meals.

STORAGE
25°C (77°F); excursions permitted to 15-30°C (59-86°F). Protect from exposure to high humidity.

HOW SUPPLIED
Tab: (Linagliptin/Metformin) 2.5mg/500mg, 2.5mg/850mg, 2.5mg/1000mg

CONTRAINDICATIONS
Renal impairment (eg, SrCr ≥1.5mg/dL [men], ≥1.4mg/dL [women], or abnormal CrCl); acute or chronic metabolic acidosis, including diabetic ketoacidosis; history of hypersensitivity reaction to linagliptin (eg, anaphylaxis, angioedema, exfoliative skin conditions, urticaria, or bronchial hyperreactivity); hypersensitivity to metformin.

WARNINGS/PRECAUTIONS
Not for use in type 1 diabetes mellitus (DM) or for treatment of diabetic ketoacidosis. Promptly d/c in the event of cardiovascular collapse (shock) from whatever cause (eg, acute CHF, acute MI, other conditions characterized by hypoxemia). Caution in elderly. **Linagliptin:** Acute pancreatitis, including fatal pancreatitis, reported; d/c if suspected and initiate appropriate management. If therapy is discontinued due to renal impairment, may continue linagliptin as a single entity tab. Serious hypersensitivity reactions reported; d/c if suspected, assess for other potential causes, and institute alternative treatment for DM. Caution in patients w/ history of angioedema to another DPP-4 inhibitor. Severe and disabling arthralgia reported; d/c if therapy is a possible cause for severe joint pain. **Metformin:** D/C if evidence of renal impairment is present. Temporarily d/c at the time of or prior to radiologic studies involving the use of intravascular iodinated contrast materials, withhold for 48 hrs subsequent to the procedure, and reinstitute only after renal function is confirmed to be normal. Temporarily d/c for any surgical procedure (except minor procedures not associated w/ restricted food and fluid intake); restart when oral intake is resumed and renal function is evaluated as normal. Avoid in patients w/ clinical or lab evidence of hepatic disease. Elderly, debilitated, or malnourished patients, and those w/ adrenal/pituitary insufficiency or alcohol intoxication are particularly susceptible to hypoglycemic effects. May decrease serum vitamin B12 to subnormal levels; monitor hematologic parameters annually.

ADVERSE REACTIONS
Nasopharyngitis, diarrhea, hypoglycemia.

DRUG INTERACTIONS
See Dosing Considerations. Thiazides and other diuretics, corticosteroids, phenothiazines, thyroid products, estrogens, oral contraceptives, phenytoin, nicotinic acid, sympathomimetics, calcium channel blockers, and isoniazid tend to produce hyperglycemia and may lead to loss of glycemic control; observe closely for hypoglycemia when such drugs are withdrawn. **Linagliptin:** Increased risk of hypoglycemia w/ insulin or insulin secretagogue (eg, sulfonylurea); may require lower dose of insulin or insulin secretagogue. Rifampin decreased linagliptin exposure, suggesting that strong P-gp or CYP3A4 inducers may reduce efficacy;

use alternative treatments (not containing linagliptin) when a strong P-gp or CYP3A4 inducer is necessary. **Metformin:** Caution w/ drugs that may affect renal function, result in significant hemodynamic change, or interfere w/ the disposition of metformin. Hypoglycemia may occur w/ other glucose-lowering agents (eg, sulfonylureas, insulin) or ethanol. Hypoglycemia may be difficult to recognize w/ β-adrenergic blocking drugs. Alcohol potentiates the effect of metformin on lactate metabolism; avoid excessive alcohol intake. Cationic drugs (eg, cimetidine, amiloride, digoxin) that are eliminated by renal tubular secretion may potentially produce an interaction; monitor and adjust dose of Jentadueto and/or the interfering drug. Topiramate or other carbonic anhydrase inhibitors (eg, zonisamide, acetazolamide, dichlorphenamide) may induce metabolic acidosis; use w/ caution.

PREGNANCY AND LACTATION
Pregnancy: Category B.
Lactation: Not for use in nursing.

MECHANISM OF ACTION
Linagliptin: DPP-4 inhibitor; increases the concentrations of active incretin hormones, stimulating the release of insulin in a glucose-dependent manner and decreasing the levels of glucagon in the circulation. **Metformin:** Biguanide; decreases hepatic glucose production, decreases intestinal absorption of glucose, and improves insulin sensitivity by increasing peripheral glucose uptake and utilization.

PHARMACOKINETICS
Absorption: Linagliptin: Absolute bioavailability (30%). Metformin: Absolute bioavailability (50-60%) (500mg, fasted). **Distribution:** Linagliptin: V_d=1110L (IV); plasma protein binding (concentration-dependent). Metformin: V_d=654L (850mg); crosses placenta; found in breast milk in low concentrations. **Elimination:** Linagliptin: Enterohepatic (80%), urine (5%); $T_{1/2}$=12 hrs. Metformin: Urine (90%); $T_{1/2}$=6.2 hrs (plasma), 17.6 hrs (blood).

PATIENT CONSIDERATIONS
Assessment: Assess for metabolic acidosis, risk factors for lactic acidosis, renal/hepatic impairment, previous hypersensitivity to the drug, history of pancreatitis, inadequate vitamin B12 or Ca^{2+} intake/absorption, type of DM, diabetic ketoacidosis, alcoholism, hypoxemia, presence of malnourishment or debilitation, adrenal/pituitary insufficiency, history of angioedema w/ another DPP-4 inhibitor, pregnancy/nursing status, and possible drug interactions. Assess if patient is planning to undergo any surgical procedure, radiologic studies involving the use of intravascular iodinated contrast materials, or is under any form of stress. Obtain baseline FPG and HbA1c levels, and hematologic parameters.

Monitoring: Monitor for signs/symptoms of lactic acidosis, pancreatitis, hypoxic states, hypersensitivity reactions, severe joint pain, and other adverse reactions. Monitor renal function, especially in elderly, at least annually. Monitor hematologic parameters annually. Perform routine serum vitamin B12 measurement at 2- to 3-yr intervals in patients predisposed to developing subnormal vitamin B12 levels. Monitor FPG and HbA1c levels and hepatic function periodically.

Counseling: Inform of the risks and benefits of therapy. Advise on the importance of adherence to dietary instructions, regular physical activity, periodic blood glucose monitoring and HbA1c testing, recognition/management of hypo/hyperglycemia, and assessment for diabetes complications. Instruct to seek medical advice promptly during periods of stress as medication needs may change. Inform of the risk of lactic acidosis; instruct to d/c therapy immediately and contact physician if unexplained hyperventilation, malaise, myalgia, unusual somnolence, slow or irregular heartbeat, sensation of feeling cold (especially in the extremities), or other nonspecific symptoms occur. Inform that GI symptoms and acute pancreatitis may occur; instruct to d/c therapy promptly and contact physician if persistent severe abdominal pain occurs. Instruct to inform of Jentadueto use prior to any surgical or radiological procedure. Inform that allergic reactions may occur; instruct to d/c therapy and seek medical advice promptly if symptoms occur. Advise against excessive alcohol intake. Inform that severe and disabling joint pain may occur; instruct to seek medical advice if this occurs.

JENTADUETO XR — linagliptin/metformin hydrochloride   Rx
Class: Biguanide/dipeptidyl peptidase-4 (DPP-4) inhibitor

> Cases of metformin-associated lactic acidosis resulting in death, hypothermia, hypotension, and resistant bradyarrhythmias reported; risk factors include renal impairment, concomitant use of certain drugs (eg, cationic drugs such as topiramate), age ≥65 years, having a radiological study w/ contrast, surgery and other procedures, hypoxic states (eg, acute CHF), excessive alcohol intake, and hepatic impairment. D/C therapy immediately and institute general supportive measures in a hospital setting if metformin-associated lactic acidosis is suspected. Prompt hemodialysis is recommended.

ADULT DOSAGE
Type 2 Diabetes Mellitus

When treatment w/ both alogliptin and metformin is appropriate

Initial:
Not Currently on Metformin:
5mg/1000mg qd
Currently on Metformin or Already Treated w/ Linagliptin and Metformin or Jentadueto: 5mg linagliptin + similar total daily dose of metformin qd
Max: 5mg/2000mg qd

PEDIATRIC DOSAGE
Pediatric use may not have been established

DOSING CONSIDERATIONS
Renal Impairment
Initiation of Therapy:
eGFR 30-45mL/min/1.73m²: Not recommended
eGFR <30mL/min/1.73m²: Contraindicated
Currently Taking Jentadueto XR:
eGFR Falls to <45mL/min/1.73m²: Assess benefits and risks of continuing therapy
eGFR Falls to <30mL/min/1.73m²: D/C use
Hepatic Impairment
Not recommended
Other Important Considerations
Iodinated Contrast Imaging Procedures:
D/C therapy at the time of, or prior to, an iodinated contrast imaging procedure in patients w/ an eGFR 30-60mL/min/1.73m²; in patients w/ a history of liver disease, alcoholism, or heart failure (HF); or in patients who will be administered intra-arterial iodinated contrast. Reevaluate eGFR 48 hrs after the imaging procedure and restart therapy if renal function is stable

ADMINISTRATION
Oral route

Swallow tab whole; do not split, crush, dissolve, or chew before swallowing. Take w/ a meal.

STORAGE
25°C (77°F); excursions permitted to 15-30°C (59-86°F). Protect from exposure to high humidity.

HOW SUPPLIED
Tab, Extended-Release: (Linagliptin/Metformin) 2.5mg/1000mg, 5mg/1000mg

CONTRAINDICATIONS
Severe renal impairment (eGFR <30mL/min/1.73m²); acute or chronic metabolic acidosis, including diabetic ketoacidosis; history of hypersensitivity to linagliptin; hypersensitivity to metformin.

WARNINGS/PRECAUTIONS
See Dosing Considerations. Not for use in type 1 diabetes mellitus (DM) or for treatment of diabetic ketoacidosis. **Linagliptin:** Acute pancreatitis, including fatal pancreatitis, reported; d/c if suspected and initiate appropriate management. Serious hypersensitivity reactions reported; d/c if suspected, assess for other potential causes, and institute alternative treatment for DM. Caution in patients w/ history of angioedema to another DPP-4 inhibitor. Severe and disabling arthralgia reported; d/c if appropriate. **Metformin:** Assess renal function more frequently in elderly patients. Temporarily d/c while patient has restricted food and fluid intake. D/C if a condition associated w/ hypoxemia occurs (eg, cardiovascular collapse, acute MI, sepsis). Elderly, debilitated, or malnourished patients, and those w/ adrenal/pituitary insufficiency or alcohol intoxication are particularly susceptible to hypoglycemic effects. Hypoglycemia may be difficult to recognize in the elderly. May decrease serum vitamin B12 to subnormal levels; monitor hematologic parameters annually.

ADVERSE REACTIONS
Nasopharyngitis, diarrhea.

DRUG INTERACTIONS
See Boxed Warning. Thiazides and other diuretics, corticosteroids, phenothiazines, thyroid products, estrogens, oral contraceptives, phenytoin, nicotinic acid, sympathomimetics, calcium channel blockers, and isoniazid tend to produce hyperglycemia and may lead to loss of glycemic control; observe closely for hypoglycemia when such drugs are withdrawn. **Linagliptin:** Rifampin decreased linagliptin exposure, suggesting that strong P-gp or CYP3A4 inducers may reduce efficacy; use alternative treatments (not containing linagliptin) when a strong P-gp or CYP3A4 inducer is necessary. Increased risk of hypoglycemia w/ insulin or insulin secretagogue (eg, sulfonylurea); may require a lower dose of insulin or insulin secretagogue. **Metformin:** Drugs that impair renal function, drugs that result in significant hemodynamic change, drugs that interfere w/ acid-base balance, or drugs that increase metformin accumulation may increase the risk of metformin-associated lactic acidosis; consider more frequent monitoring of these patients. Alcohol potentiates the effect of metformin on lactate metabolism; avoid excessive alcohol intake. Hypoglycemia may be difficult to recognize w/ β-adrenergic blocking drugs. Topiramate or other carbonic anhydrase inhibitors (eg, zonisamide, acetazolamide, dichlorphenamide) may increase the risk of lactic acidosis; consider more frequent monitoring of these patients. Drugs that are eliminated by renal tubular secretion (eg, cationic drugs such as cimetidine) have the potential for interaction w/ metformin by competing for common renal tubular transport systems, and may increase the accumulation of metformin and the risk for lactic acidosis; consider more frequent monitoring of these patients.

PREGNANCY AND LACTATION
Pregnancy: The limited data w/ Jentadueto XR and linagliptin use in pregnant women are not sufficient to inform of a drug-associated risk for major birth defects and miscarriage. Studies w/ metformin use during pregnancy have not reported a clear association w/ metformin and major birth defect or miscarriage risk.
Lactation: There is no information regarding the presence of Jentadueto XR in human milk or linagliptin in human milk, the effects on the breastfed infant, or the effects on milk production. Limited published studies report that metformin is present in human milk; caution in nursing.
Reproductive Potential: Use w/ metformin may result in ovulation in some anovulatory women.

MECHANISM OF ACTION
Linagliptin: DPP-4 inhibitor; increases the concentrations of active incretin hormones, stimulating the release of insulin in a glucose-dependent manner

and decreasing the levels of glucagon in the circulation. **Metformin:** Biguanide; decreases hepatic glucose production, decreases intestinal absorption of glucose, and improves insulin sensitivity by increasing peripheral glucose uptake and utilization.

PHARMACOKINETICS

Absorption: Linagliptin: Absolute bioavailability (30%). Metformin: T_{max}=7-8 hrs.
Distribution: Linagliptin: V_d=1110L (IV); plasma protein binding (concentration-dependent). Metformin: V_d=654L (850mg, immediate-release); found in breast milk. **Elimination:** Linagliptin: Enterohepatic (80%), urine (5%); $T_{1/2}$= >100 hrs. Metformin: Urine (90%); $T_{1/2}$=6.2 hrs (plasma), 17.6 hrs (blood).

PATIENT CONSIDERATIONS

Assessment: Assess for acute/chronic metabolic acidosis (including diabetic ketoacidosis), history of hypersensitivity to linagliptin or metformin, type of DM, risk factors for lactic acidosis, renal/hepatic impairment, HF or risk factors for HF, history of pancreatitis, predisposition to developing subnormal vitamin B12 levels, history of angioedema w/ another DPP-4 inhibitor, pregnancy/nursing status, and possible drug interactions. Assess if patient is planning to undergo any surgical procedure. Obtain baseline FPG, HbA1c, eGFR, and hematologic parameters.

Monitoring: Monitor for signs/symptoms of lactic acidosis, pancreatitis, hypoxic states, hypersensitivity reactions, severe and disabling arthralgia, and other adverse reactions. Monitor renal function, especially in elderly, at least annually. Monitor hematologic parameters annually. Perform routine serum vitamin B12 measurement at 2- to 3-yr intervals in patients predisposed to developing subnormal vitamin B12 levels. Monitor FPG and HbA1c levels and hepatic function periodically.

Counseling: Inform of the risks and benefits of therapy. Advise on the importance of adherence to dietary instructions, regular physical activity, periodic blood glucose monitoring and HbA1c testing, recognition/management of hypo/hyperglycemia, and assessment for diabetes complications. Instruct to seek medical advice promptly during periods of stress as medication needs may change. Inform of the risk of lactic acidosis; instruct to d/c therapy immediately and contact physician if unexplained hyperventilation, malaise, myalgia, unusual somnolence, slow or irregular heartbeat, sensation of feeling cold (especially in the extremities), or if other nonspecific symptoms occur. Inform that GI symptoms may occur during initiation of therapy; instruct to notify physician if GI symptoms develop after stabilization of therapy. Advise that acute pancreatitis may occur; instruct to d/c therapy promptly and contact physician if persistent severe abdominal pain occurs. Inform of the importance of regular testing of renal function and hematological parameters when receiving therapy. Instruct patients to inform their physician that they are taking Jentadueto XR prior to any surgical or radiological procedure. Inform that serious allergic reactions may occur; instruct to d/c therapy and seek medical advice promptly if symptoms occur. Advise against excessive alcohol intake. Inform that severe and disabling joint pain may occur; instruct to seek medical advice if this occurs. Instruct patients to notify physician if they see tabs in their feces. Inform females that therapy w/ metformin may result in an unintended pregnancy in some premenopausal anovulatory females.

JETREA — ocriplasmin

Class: Enzyme

Rx

ADULT DOSAGE
Vitreomacular Adhesion
Symptomatic:
0.125mg (0.1mL of the diluted sol) by intravitreal inj to the affected eye once as a single dose

PEDIATRIC DOSAGE
Pediatric use may not have been established

ADMINISTRATION
Intravitreal route

Must dilute before use.
Adequate anesthesia and broad spectrum microbiocide should be administered. Insert inj needle 3.5-4mm posterior to limbus aiming towards center of vitreous cavity, avoiding horizontal meridian; inj volume of 0.1mL is then delivered into mid-vitreous.
Each vial should only be used to provide a single inj for a single eye. If contralateral eye requires treatment, use new vial; treatment of the other eye is not recommended w/in 7 days of the initial inj.
Repeated administration in the same eye is not recommended.

Preparation
1. Remove vial from freezer and allow to thaw at room temperature (w/in a few min).
2. Add 0.2mL of 0.9% w/v NaCl inj (sterile, preservative-free) into vial and gently swirl until mixed.
3. Withdraw all of diluted sol using a sterile #19 gauge needle and discard needle after withdrawal of vial contents; do not use this needle for intravitreal inj.
4. Replace the needle w/ a sterile #30 gauge needle, carefully expel air bubbles and excess drug from syringe and adjust dose to the 0.1mL mark on syringe; use sol immediately.

STORAGE
Store frozen at ≤-20°C (-4°F). Protect from light.
HOW SUPPLIED
Inj: 2.5mg/mL [0.2mL]

WARNINGS/PRECAUTIONS
Must only be administered by a qualified physician. Monitor for IOP elevation immediately following inj. Decreased vision reported; majority were due to progression of the condition w/ traction and many required surgical intervention. Intraocular inflammation/infection/hemorrhage, increased IOP, retinal detachment/tear, and dyschromatopsia (electroretinographic changes reported in approx half of these cases) reported; monitor appropriately. Lens subluxation reported in a premature infant who received a dose 1.4X higher than the recommended dose.

ADVERSE REACTIONS
Vitreous floaters, conjunctival hemorrhage, eye pain, photopsia, blurred vision, macular hole, reduced visual acuity, visual impairment, retinal edema.

PREGNANCY AND LACTATION
Pregnancy: Category C.
Lactation: Not known if excreted in human milk; caution in nursing.
MECHANISM OF ACTION
Proteolytic enzyme; has proteolytic activity against protein components of the vitreous body and the vitreoretinal interface (eg, laminin, fibronectin, collagen), thereby dissolving the protein matrix responsible for the vitreomacular adhesion.

PATIENT CONSIDERATIONS
Assessment: Assess pregnancy/nursing status.

Monitoring: Monitor for decreased vision, increased IOP (eg, check for perfusion of the optic nerve head, tonometry), lens subluxation, retinal detachment/tear, dyschromatopsia, and other adverse reactions.

Counseling: Advise to seek immediate care from an ophthalmologist if the eye becomes red, sensitive to light, painful, or develops a change in vision. Inform that temporary visual impairment may be experienced; instruct patients not to drive or operate heavy machinery until visual impairment has resolved, and advise to seek care from an ophthalmologist if visual impairment persists or decreases further.

JEVTANA — cabazitaxel

Class: Antimicrotubule agent

Rx

> Neutropenic deaths reported. Perform frequent blood cell counts to monitor for neutropenia. Contraindicated in patients w/ neutrophil counts of ≤1500 cells/mm³. Severe hypersensitivity reactions may occur; may include generalized rash/erythema, hypotension, and bronchospasm. D/C infusion immediately if a severe hypersensitivity reaction occurs and administer appropriate therapy. Patients should receive premedication. Contraindicated in patients who have a history of severe hypersensitivity reactions to cabazitaxel or other drugs formulated w/ polysorbate 80.

ADULT DOSAGE
Metastatic Prostate Cancer
Treatment of patients w/ hormone-refractory metastatic prostate cancer previously treated w/ a docetaxel-containing treatment regimen

25mg/m² as a 1-hr IV infusion every 3 weeks in combination w/ oral prednisone 10mg administered daily throughout treatment

Premedication
Premedicate at least 30 min prior to each dose w/ the following IV medications:
Antihistamine: Dexchlorpheniramine 5mg, diphenhydramine 25mg, or equivalent
Corticosteroid: Dexamethasone 8mg or equivalent
H₂ Antagonist: Ranitidine 50mg or equivalent

Antiemetic prophylaxis is recommended and may be given PO or IV prn

PEDIATRIC DOSAGE
Pediatric use may not have been established

DOSING CONSIDERATIONS
Concomitant Medications
Strong CYP3A Inhibitors: Avoid coadministration w/ these drugs; if coadministration is required, consider a 25% cabazitaxel dose reduction
Hepatic Impairment
Mild (Total Bilirubin >1 to ≤1.5X ULN or AST >1.5X ULN): Reduce dose to 20mg/m²
Moderate (Total Bilirubin >1.5 to ≤3X ULN and AST=Any): Reduce dose to 15mg/m²
Adverse Reactions
Prolonged Grade ≥3 Neutropenia (>1 Week) Despite Appropriate Medication (Including G-CSF): Delay treatment until neutrophil count is >1500 cells/mm³, then reduce dose to 20mg/m²; use G-CSF for secondary prophylaxis
Febrile Neutropenia/Neutropenic Infections: Delay treatment until improvement or resolution, and until neutrophil count is >1500 cells/mm³, then reduce dose to 20mg/m²; use G-CSF for secondary prophylaxis
Grade ≥3 Diarrhea or Persisting Diarrhea Despite Appropriate Medication, Fluid, and Electrolyte Replacement: Delay treatment until improvement or resolution, then reduce dose to 20mg/m²

Grade 2 Peripheral Neuropathy: Delay treatment until improvement or resolution, then reduce dose to $20mg/m^2$
Grade ≥3 Peripheral Neuropathy: D/C therapy

D/C therapy if patient continues to experience any of the above reactions at $20mg/m^2$

ADMINISTRATION
IV route

Do not mix w/ any other drugs
Do not use PVC infusion containers or polyurethane infusion sets for preparation and administration of infusion sol
Use an in-line filter of 0.22μm nominal pore size (also referred to as 0.2μm) during administration

Preparation Instructions
Cabazitaxel requires 2 dilutions prior to administration

Step 1 - First Dilution:
1. Mix each vial of cabazitaxel 60mg/1.5mL w/ entire contents of supplied diluent; once reconstituted, the resultant sol contains 10mg/mL cabazitaxel
2. When transferring the diluent, direct the needle onto the inside wall of cabazitaxel vial and inject slowly to limit foaming
3. Remove syringe/needle and gently mix the initial diluted sol by repeated inversions for at least 45 sec to assure full mixing of drug and diluent; do not shake
4. Let the sol stand for a few min to allow any foam to dissipate, and check that the sol is homogeneous and contains no visible particulate matter; it is not required that all foam dissipate prior to continuing the preparation process
5. The resulting initial diluted sol (cabazitaxel 10mg/mL) requires further dilution before administration; the 2nd dilution should be done immediately (w/in 30 min) to obtain the final infusion

Step 2 - Second (Final) Dilution:
1. Withdraw the recommended dose from the cabazitaxel sol containing 10mg/mL using a calibrated syringe and further dilute into a sterile 250mL PVC-free container of either 0.9% NaCl sol or D5 sol for infusion; if a dose >65mg of cabazitaxel is required, use a larger volume of the infusion vehicle so that a concentration of 0.26mg/mL is not exceeded
2. The concentration of final infusion sol should be between 0.10mg/mL and 0.26mg/mL
3. Remove syringe and thoroughly mix the final infusion sol by gently inverting the bag or bottle
4. As the final infusion sol is supersaturated, it may crystallize over time; do not use if this occurs and discard

Fully prepared cabazitaxel infusion sol (in either 0.9% NaCl sol or D5 sol) should be used w/in 8 hrs at ambient temperature (including the 1-hr infusion), or for a total of 24 hrs under refrigeration (including the 1-hr infusion)

If cabazitaxel 1st diluted sol, or 2nd (final) dilution for IV infusion should come into contact w/ skin or mucosae, immediately and thoroughly wash w/ soap and water

STORAGE
25°C (77°F); excursions permitted to 15-30°C (59-86°F). Do not refrigerate.

HOW SUPPLIED
Inj: 60mg/1.5mL

CONTRAINDICATIONS
Neutrophil counts ≤1500/mm³, severe hepatic impairment (total bilirubin >3X ULN), history of severe hypersensitivity reactions to cabazitaxel or to other drugs formulated with polysorbate 80.

WARNINGS/PRECAUTIONS
Bone marrow suppression manifested as neutropenia, anemia, thrombocytopenia, and/or pancytopenia may occur. G-CSF may be administered to reduce risks of neutropenia complications; consider primary prophylaxis w/ G-CSF in patients w/ high-risk clinical features (eg, >65 yrs of age, poor performance status, previous episodes of febrile neutropenia, extensive prior radiation ports, poor nutritional status, or other serious comorbidities) that predispose them to increased complications from prolonged neutropenia. Caution in patients w/ Hgb <10g/dL. Observe patients closely for hypersensitivity reactions, especially during the 1st and 2nd infusions. N/V and severe diarrhea may occur. Death related to diarrhea and electrolyte imbalance reported; intensive measures may be required for severe diarrhea and electrolyte imbalance. GI hemorrhage and perforation, ileus, enterocolitis, neutropenic enterocolitis, including fatal outcome, reported; risk may be increased w/ neutropenia, age, steroid use, concomitant use of NSAIDs, antiplatelet therapy, or anticoagulants, and prior history of pelvic radiotherapy, adhesions, ulceration, and GI bleeding. Abdominal pain/tenderness, fever, persistent constipation, diarrhea (w/ or w/o neutropenia), may be early manifestations of serious GI toxicity and should be evaluated and treated promptly; treatment delay or discontinuation may be necessary. Renal failure, including cases w/ fatal outcome, reported; identify causes and treat aggressively. Carefully monitor patients w/ ESRD (CrCl <15mL/min). Caution in elderly. Not indicated for use in female patients; may cause fetal harm when administered to a pregnant woman.

ADVERSE REACTIONS
Hypersensitivity reactions, neutropenia, anemia, leukopenia, thrombocytopenia, diarrhea, fatigue, N/V, constipation, asthenia, abdominal pain, anorexia, back pain, hematuria, dyspnea.

DRUG INTERACTIONS
See Dosing Considerations. Strong CYP3A inhibitors (eg, ketoconazole, clarithromycin, atazanavir) may increase levels.

PREGNANCY AND LACTATION
Category D, not for use in nursing.

MECHANISM OF ACTION
Antimicrotubule agent; binds to tubulin and promotes its assembly into microtubules while simultaneously inhibiting disassembly, which results in the inhibition of mitotic and interphase cellular functions.

PHARMACOKINETICS
Absorption: C_{max}=226ng/mL; AUC=991ng•hr/mL; T_{max}=1 hr. **Distribution:** V_d=4864L; plasma protein binding (89-92%). **Metabolism:** Liver (extensive) via CYP3A4/5, and to a lesser extent, CYP2C8. **Elimination:** Urine (3.7%, 2.3% unchanged), feces (76%); $T_{1/2}$=95 hrs.

PATIENT CONSIDERATIONS
Assessment: Assess for history of hypersensitivity to drug or to other drugs formulated w/ polysorbate 80, hepatic/renal impairment, risk of developing GI complications, pregnancy/nursing status, and possible drug interactions. Assess for high-risk clinical features that may predispose to increased complications from prolonged neutropenia. Obtain baseline CBC, including neutrophil count.

Monitoring: Monitor for signs/symptoms of neutropenia, infections, hypersensitivity reactions, severe diarrhea, dehydration, N/V, electrolyte imbalance, renal failure, serious GI toxicity, and other adverse reactions. Monitor CBCs, including neutrophil count, on a weekly basis during cycle 1 and before each treatment cycle thereafter.

Counseling: Counsel about the risk of potential hypersensitivity; instruct to immediately report signs of a hypersensitivity reaction. Inform that drug decreases blood count (eg, WBCs, platelets, and RBCs), and thus it is important that periodic assessment of their blood count be performed to detect the development of neutropenia, thrombocytopenia, anemia, and/or pancytopenia. Instruct to frequently monitor temperature and to immediately report any occurrence of fever to physician. Explain that it is important to take the oral prednisone as prescribed; instruct to report to physician if not compliant w/ oral corticosteroid regimen. Instruct to immediately report to physician any occurrence of fever, significant vomiting or diarrhea, decreased urinary output, or hematuria. Counsel about side effects associated w/ exposure, such as severe and fatal infections, dehydration, and renal failure. Inform about importance of providing a list of prescription and non-prescription drugs to physician. Inform elderly patients that certain side effects may be more frequent or severe.

JUBLIA — efinaconazole   Rx

Class: Azole antifungal

ADULT DOSAGE	PEDIATRIC DOSAGE
Fungal Infections	Pediatric use may not have been established
Onychomycosis of the Toenail(s) Due to *Trichophyton rubrum* and *Trichophyton mentagrophytes*: Apply to affected toenails qd for 48 weeks	

ADMINISTRATION
Topical route

Apply using the integrated flow-through brush applicator.
When applying, ensure toenail, toenail folds, toenail bed, hyponychium, and undersurface of toenail plate are completely covered.

STORAGE
20-25°C (68-77°F); excursions permitted to 15-30°C (59-86°F). Store in upright position. Flammable; keep away from heat or flame. Protect from freezing.

HOW SUPPLIED
Sol: 10% [4mL, 8mL]

WARNINGS/PRECAUTIONS
Not for oral, ophthalmic, or intravaginal use.

ADVERSE REACTIONS
Ingrown toenail, application-site dermatitis/vesicles/pain.

PREGNANCY AND LACTATION
Pregnancy: Category C.
Lactation: Not known whether efinaconazole is excreted in human milk; caution in nursing.

MECHANISM OF ACTION
Azole antifungal; inhibits fungal lanosterol 14α-demethylase involved in the biosynthesis of ergosterol, a constituent of fungal cell membranes.

PHARMACOKINETICS
Absorption: C_{max}=0.67ng/mL (Day 28); AUC=12.15ng•hr/mL. **Elimination:** $T_{1/2}$=29.9 hrs.

PATIENT CONSIDERATIONS
Assessment: Assess pregnancy/nursing status.

Monitoring: Monitor for adverse reactions.

Counseling: Inform that therapy is for use on toenails and immediately adjacent skin only. Instruct to use ud to clean dry toenails and to wait for at least 10 min after showering, bathing, or washing before applying. Advise to inform physician if the area of application shows signs of persistent irritation (eg, redness, itching, swelling). Inform that the impact of nail polish or other cosmetic nail products on the efficacy of therapy has not been evaluated. Advise to avoid using near heat or open flame.

JUXTAPID — lomitapide

Class: Lipid-regulating agent

Rx

> May cause elevations in transaminases; measure ALT, AST, alkaline phosphatase, and total bilirubin prior to therapy, and then ALT/AST regularly as recommended. Adjust dose if ALT/AST is ≥3X ULN. D/C for clinically significant liver toxicity. May increase hepatic fat w/ or w/o increases in transaminases. Hepatic steatosis associated w/ lomitapide treatment may be a risk factor for progressive liver disease, including steatohepatitis and cirrhosis. Available only through a restricted program under a Risk Evaluation and Mitigation Strategy (REMS) because of the risk of hepatotoxicity. Prescribe only to patients w/ a clinical or laboratory diagnosis consistent w/ homozygous familial hypercholesterolemia.

ADULT DOSAGE

Homozygous Familial Hypercholesterolemia

Prior to treatment, initiate a low-fat diet supplying <20% of energy from fat

Initial: 5mg qd
Titrate: After ≥2 weeks, may increase dose to 10mg qd; and then at ≥4-week intervals, may increase to 20mg qd, then 40mg qd, and then up to a max of 60mg qd
Max: 60mg qd

PEDIATRIC DOSAGE

Pediatric use may not have been established

DOSING CONSIDERATIONS

Concomitant Medications

W/ Moderate and Strong CYP3A4 Inhibitors: Contraindicated

W/ Weak CYP3A4 Inhibitors:
Max: 30mg/day

W/ Oral Contraceptives:
Max: 40mg/day

Initiating Weak CYP3A4 Inhibitor in Patients Already Taking Lomitapide 10mg qd or More:
Decrease dose of lomitapide by half; patients taking lomitapide 5mg qd may continue w/ same dosage. May carefully titrate to a max of 30mg qd except when coadministered w/ oral contraceptives, in which case the max recommended lomitapide dosage is 40mg qd

Renal Impairment
ESRD Receiving Dialysis:
Max: 40mg/day

Hepatic Impairment
Mild (Child-Pugh A):
Max: 40mg/day

Adverse Reactions
ALT/AST ≥3X and <5X ULN:
- Confirm elevation w/ repeat measurement w/in 1 week.
- If confirmed, reduce dose and obtain additional liver-related tests if not already measured (eg, alkaline phosphatase, total bilirubin, INR).
- Repeat tests weekly and withhold dosing if signs of abnormal liver function (increase in bilirubin/INR) are present, if transaminase levels rise above 5X ULN, or if transaminase levels do not fall below 3X ULN w/in approx 4 weeks; investigate to identify probable cause in these cases of persistent or worsening abnormalities.
- Consider reducing dose and monitor liver-related tests more frequently if resuming therapy after transaminases resolve to <3X ULN.

ALT/AST ≥5X ULN:
- Withhold dosing, obtain additional liver-related tests if not already measured (eg, alkaline phosphatase, total bilirubin, INR), and investigate to identify probable cause.
- Reduce dose and monitor liver-related tests more frequently if resuming therapy after transaminases resolve to <3X ULN.

If transaminase elevations are accompanied by clinical symptoms of liver injury, increases in bilirubin ≥2X ULN, or active liver disease, d/c treatment and investigate to identify probable cause

ADMINISTRATION
Oral route

Take qd w/ a glass of water, w/o food, at least 2 hrs after pm meal.
Swallow cap whole; do not open, crush, dissolve, or chew.
Take daily supplements containing 400 IU vitamin E and at least 200mg linoleic acid, 210mg α-linolenic acid, 110mg eicosapentaenoic acid, and 80mg docosahexaenoic acid.

STORAGE
20-25°C (68-77°F); excursions permitted to 15-30°C (59-86°F). May tolerate brief exposure up to 40°C (104°F), provided the mean kinetic temperature does not exceed 25°C (77°F); however, such exposure should be minimized. Protect from moisture.

HOW SUPPLIED
Cap: 5mg, 10mg, 20mg, 30mg, 40mg, 60mg

CONTRAINDICATIONS
Pregnancy, moderate or severe hepatic impairment (based on Child-Pugh category B or C), active liver disease including unexplained persistent elevations of serum transaminases, concomitant moderate or strong CYP3A4 inhibitors.

WARNINGS/PRECAUTIONS
See Contraindications and Dosing Considerations. If baseline LFTs are abnormal, consider initiating therapy after an appropriate work-up and the baseline abnormalities are explained or resolved. May cause fetal harm. May reduce absorption of fat-soluble nutrients, especially in patients w/ chronic bowel or pancreatic diseases that predispose to malabsorption. GI adverse reactions reported; absorption of concomitant oral medications may be affected in patients who develop diarrhea or vomiting. Severe diarrhea reported; monitor patients who are more susceptible to complications from diarrhea and consider reducing the dose or suspending therapy. Avoid in patients w/ rare hereditary problems of galactose intolerance, Lapp lactase deficiency, or glucose-galactose malabsorption; may result in diarrhea and malabsorption. Caution in elderly.

ADVERSE REACTIONS
Diarrhea, N/V, dyspepsia, abdominal pain.

DRUG INTERACTIONS
See Dosing Considerations and Contraindications. Not recommended w/ other LDL-lowering agents that can increase hepatic fat. Avoid grapefruit juice. Alcohol may increase levels of hepatic fat and induce/exacerbate liver injury; avoid consumption of >1 alcoholic drink/day. Caution w/ other medications known to have potential for hepatotoxicity (eg, isotretinoin, amiodarone, acetaminophen [>4g/day for ≥3 days/week]). Increased exposure w/ weak CYP3A4 inhibitors (eg, alprazolam, atorvastatin, cimetidine). May increase INR and plasma concentrations of both R(+)-warfarin and S(-)-warfarin; regularly monitor INR (particularly after any changes in lomitapide dosage) and adjust dose of warfarin as clinically indicated. May double the exposure of simvastatin; refer to simvastatin PI for dosing recommendations. May increase the exposure of lovastatin; consider reducing dose of lovastatin when initiating therapy. May increase the absorption of P-gp substrates (eg, aliskiren, colchicine, digoxin); consider dose reduction of the P-gp substrate. Separate dosing by at least 4 hrs w/ bile acid sequestrants.

PREGNANCY AND LACTATION
Pregnancy: Category X. There is a pregnancy exposure registry that monitors pregnancy outcomes in women exposed to drug during pregnancy.
Lactation: Not for use in nursing.
Reproductive Potential: Females of reproductive potential should have a negative pregnancy test before starting therapy, and should use effective contraception during therapy.

MECHANISM OF ACTION
Lipid-regulating agent; directly binds and inhibits microsomal TG transfer protein, which resides in the lumen of the endoplasmic reticulum, thereby preventing the assembly of apolipoprotein B-containing lipoproteins in enterocytes and hepatocytes. This inhibits the synthesis of chylomicrons and VLDL. The inhibition of the synthesis of VLDL leads to reduced levels of plasma LDL.

PHARMACOKINETICS
Absorption: Absolute bioavailability (7%); T_{max}=6 hrs. **Distribution:** V_d=985-1292L; plasma protein binding (99.8%). **Metabolism:** Liver (extensive) via oxidation, oxidative N-dealkylation, glucuronide conjugation, piperidine ring opening. CYP3A4; M1 and M3 (major metabolites). **Elimination:** Feces (33.4-35.1%, mostly unchanged), urine (52.9-59.5%, mostly M1); $T_{1/2}$=39.7 hrs.

PATIENT CONSIDERATIONS

Assessment: Assess for active liver disease, including unexplained persistent elevations of serum transaminases, bowel/pancreatic disease, galactose intolerance, renal dysfunction, pregnancy/nursing status, and possible drug interactions. Measure ALT/AST, alkaline phosphatase, and serum bilirubin prior to therapy.

Monitoring: Monitor for hepatic steatosis, hepatotoxicity, and GI and other adverse reactions. Monitor renal/hepatic function. During the 1st yr, perform hepatic-related tests (eg, ALT, AST) prior to each increase in dose or monthly, whichever occurs 1st. After the 1st yr, perform these tests at least every 3 months and before any dose increase. Monitor INR w/ warfarin.

Counseling: Inform to take ud. Encourage to participate in the registry to monitor/evaluate long-term effects and inform that participation is voluntary. Advise that medication is only available from certified pharmacies enrolled in the REMS program. Discuss the importance of liver-related tests before initiation, prior to each dose escalation, and periodically thereafter. Advise of the potential for increased risk of liver injury if alcohol is consumed and instruct to limit alcohol consumption to not >1 drink/day. Advise to report any symptoms of possible liver injury (eg, fever, jaundice, lethargy, flu-like symptoms). Advise females of reproductive potential to have a negative pregnancy test before starting treatment and to use effective contraception while on therapy. Discuss the importance of taking daily supplements. Inform that GI adverse reactions are common and that strict adherence to a low-fat diet (<20% of total calories from fat) may reduce these reactions. Instruct to d/c therapy and contact physician if severe diarrhea occurs or if symptoms such as lightheadedness, decreased urine output, or tiredness occur. Inform that absorption of oral medications may be affected in patients who develop diarrhea or vomiting; instruct to seek physician's advice if symptoms develop. Instruct to omit grapefruit juice from diet; advise to inform physician about all medications, nutritional supplements, and vitamins taken. If a dose is missed, instruct to take the normal dose at the usual time the next day; if dose is interrupted for more than a week, advise to contact physician before restarting treatment.

K-Phos No. 2 — potassium acid phosphate/sodium acid phosphate anhydrous   Rx

Class: Urinary acidifier

ADULT DOSAGE

Urinary Acidification

For use in patients w/ elevated urinary pH. Helps keep Ca^{2+} soluble and reduces odor and rash caused by ammoniacal urine. Increases the antibacterial activity of methenamine mandelate and methenamine hippurate by acidifying the urine

Usual: 1 tab qid; when urine is difficult to acidify, administer 1 tab q2h

Max: 8 tabs in a 24-hr period

PEDIATRIC DOSAGE

Pediatric use may not have been established

ADMINISTRATION

Oral route

Take w/ a full glass of water

STORAGE

20-25°C (68-77°F).

HOW SUPPLIED

Tab: (Potassium Acid Phosphate/Sodium Acid Phosphate Anhydrous) 305mg/700mg* *scored

CONTRAINDICATIONS

Infected phosphate stones, severely impaired renal function (<30% of normal), and hyperphosphatemia.

WARNINGS/PRECAUTIONS

Contains K^+ and Na^+; caution if regulation of these elements is desired. May experience a mild laxative effect during the 1st few days of therapy; if laxation persists to an unpleasant degree, reduce daily dose until effect subsides or, if necessary, d/c therapy. Caution with cardiac disease (particularly in digitalized patients), Addison's disease, acute dehydration, extensive tissue breakdown, myotonia congenita, cardiac failure, cirrhosis of the liver or severe hepatic disease, peripheral/pulmonary edema, hypernatremia, HTN, toxemia of pregnancy, hypoparathyroidism, acute pancreatitis, and rickets. High serum phosphate levels may increase extra-skeletal calcification risk.

ADVERSE REACTIONS

GI upset, bone and joint pain, headache, dizziness, mental confusion, seizures, weakness or heaviness of legs, unusual tiredness or weakness, muscle cramps, fast or irregular heartbeat, SOB or troubled breathing, swelling of feet or lower legs, unusual weight gain, low urine output, unusual thirst.

DRUG INTERACTIONS

Antacids containing Mg^{+2}, aluminum, or Ca^{+2} in conjunction with phosphate preparations may bind the phosphate and prevent its absorption. Concurrent use of antihypertensives, especially diazoxide, guanethidine, hydralazine, methyldopa, or rauwolfia alkaloid; or corticosteroids, especially mineralocorticoids or corticotropin, with sodium phosphate may result in hypernatremia. K^+-containing medications or K^+-sparing diuretics may cause hyperkalemia; monitor serum K^+ level periodically. May increase plasma salicylate levels; administration of monobasic phosphates to patients stabilized on salicylates may lead to toxic salicylate levels.

PREGNANCY AND LACTATION

Category C, caution in nursing.

MECHANISM OF ACTION

Urinary acidifier; plays key role in osteoblastic and osteoclastic activities; plays vital role in metabolism of carbohydrate, lipid, and protein; plays role in modifying steady-state tissue concentrations of Ca^{2+}. Phosphate ions are important buffers of the intracellular fluid, and also play a primary role in the renal excretion of hydrogen ion.

PHARMACOKINETICS

Elimination: Urine.

PATIENT CONSIDERATIONS

Assessment: Assess for infected phosphate stones, severely impaired renal function (<30% of normal), hyperphosphatemia, and other conditions where treatment is cautioned or contraindicated. Assess pregnancy/nursing status and for possible drug interactions.

Monitoring: Monitor renal function and serum Ca^{2+}, phosphorus, K^+, and Na^+ periodically. Monitor for laxative effects, extra-skeletal calcification, and other adverse reactions.

Counseling: Warn patients with kidney stones about the possibility of passing old stones when therapy is started. Advise to avoid the use of antacids containing aluminum, Mg^{+2}, or Ca^{+2}, which may prevent the absorption of phosphate.

KADCYLA — ado-trastuzumab emtansine   Rx

Class: Monoclonal antibody/HER2 blocker/antimicrotubule agent

Do not substitute for or w/ trastuzumab. Serious hepatotoxicity, including liver failure and death, reported; monitor serum transaminases and bilirubin prior to initiation of therapy and prior to each dose. Reduce dose or d/c as appropriate in cases of increased serum transaminases/total bilirubin. May lead to reductions in left ventricular ejection fraction (LVEF). Evaluate left ventricular function prior to and during treatment; withhold treatment for clinically significant decrease in left ventricular function. Exposure during pregnancy may result in embryo-fetal harm; advise patients of these risks and the need for effective contraception.

ADULT DOSAGE

HER2-Positive Metastatic Breast Cancer

As a single agent for patients who previously received trastuzumab and a taxane, separately or in combination; patients should have either received prior therapy for metastatic disease, or developed disease recurrence during or w/in 6 months of completing adjuvant therapy

3.6mg/kg IV infusion every 3 weeks (21-day cycle) until disease progression or unacceptable toxicity

Max: 3.6mg/kg/dose

1st Infusion: Administer over 90 min; observe during infusion and for at least 90 min following the initial dose

Subsequent Infusions: Administer over 30 min if prior infusions were well tolerated; observe during infusion and for at least 30 min after infusion

Missed Dose

If a planned dose is delayed or missed, administer as soon as possible; do not wait until the next planned cycle. Adjust the schedule of administration to maintain a 3-week interval between doses; administer at the dose and rate the patient tolerated in the most recent infusion.

DOSING CONSIDERATIONS

Renal Impairment

Mild (CrCl 60-89mL/min): Dose adjustment not needed

Moderate (CrCl 30-59mL/min): Dose adjustment not needed

Severe (CrCl <30mL/min): Limited data available; no dose adjustment can be recommended

Hepatic Impairment

Mild or Moderate: No adjustment to the starting dose is required

Severe: Not studied

Adverse Reactions

Infusion-Related Reactions: Slow or interrupt infusion rate

Life-Threatening Infusion-Related Reactions: Permanently d/c

Dose Reduction Schedule:

1st Reduction: 3mg/kg

2nd Reduction: 2.4mg/kg

Requirement for Further Reduction: D/C treatment

Do not re-escalate after a dose reduction is made

Increased Serum Transaminases (AST/ALT):

Grade 2 (>2.5 to ≤5X ULN): Treat at same dose level

Grade 3 (>5 to ≤20X ULN): Do not administer until AST/ALT recovers to Grade ≤2, then reduce 1 dose level

Grade 4 (>20X ULN): Permanently d/c treatment

Hyperbilirubinemia:

Grade 2 (>1.5 to <3X ULN): Do not administer until total bilirubin recovers to Grade ≤1, then treat at same dose level

Grade 3 (>3 to ≤10X ULN): Do not administer until total bilirubin recovers to Grade ≤1, then reduce 1 dose level

Grade 4 (>10X ULN): Permanently d/c treatment

Serum Transaminases >3X ULN w/ Total Bilirubin >2X ULN: Permanently d/c treatment

Nodular Regenerative Hyperplasia: Permanently d/c treatment

Left Ventricular Dysfunction:

Symptomatic CHF: D/C treatment

LVEF <40%: Do not administer. Repeat LVEF assessment w/in 3 weeks; if LVEF <40% is confirmed, d/c treatment

LVEF 40% to ≤45% and Decrease is ≥10% Points from Baseline: Do not administer. Repeat LVEF assessment w/in 3 weeks; if LVEF has not recovered to w/in 10% points from baseline, d/c treatment

LVEF 40% to ≤45% and Decrease is <10% Points from Baseline: Continue treatment and repeat LVEF assessment w/in 3 weeks

LVEF >45%: Continue treatment

Thrombocytopenia:

Grade 3 (Platelets 25,000/mm³ to <50,000/mm³): Do not administer until platelet count recovers to ≤Grade 1 (≥75,000/mm³), then treat at same dose level

Grade 4 (Platelets <25,000/mm³): Do not administer until platelet count recovers to ≤Grade 1, then reduce 1 dose level

Pulmonary Toxicity: Permanently d/c in patients diagnosed w/ interstitial lung disease or pneumonitis

Peripheral Neuropathy: Temporarily d/c w/ Grade 3 or 4 until resolution to ≤Grade 2

ADMINISTRATION

IV route

PEDIATRIC DOSAGE

Pediatric use may not have been established

Do not substitute for or w/ trastuzumab.
Do not administer as an IV push or bolus.
Do not mix or administer as an infusion w/ other medicinal products.
Administer as an IV infusion only w/ a 0.2 or 0.22 micron in-line polyethersulfone filter.
Reconstituted product contains no preservative and is intended for single use only.

Reconstitution
1. Slowly inject 5mL of sterile water for inj (SWFI) into the 100mg vial, or 8mL of SWFI into the 160mg vial to yield a sol containing 20mg/mL.
2. Swirl the vial gently until completely dissolved; do not shake.
3. The reconstituted lyophilized vials should be used immediately following reconstitution; if not used immediately, may store the reconstituted vials for up to 24 hrs at 2-8°C (36-46°F). Discard unused reconstituted vials after 24 hrs. Do not freeze.

Dilution
1. Calculate the volume of the 20mg/mL reconstituted sol needed.
2. Withdraw this amount from the vial and add it to an infusion bag containing 250mL of 0.9% NaCl inj; do not use D5 inj.
3. Gently invert the bag to mix the sol; do not shake.
4. The diluted infusion sol should be used immediately; if not used immediately, may store at 2-8°C (36-46°F) for up to 24 hrs prior to use (this storage time is additional to the time allowed for the reconstituted vials). Do not freeze or shake.

STORAGE
2-8°C (36-46°F) until time of reconstitution. Do not freeze or shake.

HOW SUPPLIED
Inj: 100mg, 160mg

WARNINGS/PRECAUTIONS
See Dosing Considerations. Serious hepatobiliary disorders and nodular regenerative hyperplasia of the liver reported. Increased risk of developing left ventricular dysfunction. Cases of interstitial lung disease, including pneumonitis, some leading to acute respiratory distress syndrome or fatal outcome, reported. Patients w/ dyspnea at rest due to complications of advanced malignancy and co-morbidities may be at increased risk of pulmonary toxicity. Not recommended for patients who had trastuzumab permanently discontinued due to infusion-related reactions and/or hypersensitivity. Infusion-related reactions reported. Serious, allergic/anaphylactic-like reaction reported; medications/emergency equipment should be available for immediate use. Cases of hemorrhagic events, including CNS, respiratory, and GI hemorrhage, reported. Thrombocytopenia and peripheral neuropathy reported. Detection of HER2 protein overexpression or gene amplification is necessary for selection of patients appropriate for therapy; assessment of HER2 status should be performed by laboratories w/ demonstrated proficiency in the specific technology being utilized. Reactions secondary to extravasation reported; closely monitor the infusion site for possible subcutaneous infiltration during drug administration. May cause fetal harm.

ADVERSE REACTIONS
Fatigue, nausea, musculoskeletal pain, hemorrhage, thrombocytopenia, headache, increased transaminases, constipation, epistaxis.

DRUG INTERACTIONS
Avoid w/ strong CYP3A4 inhibitors (eg, ketoconazole, clarithromycin, atazanavir) due to the potential for increase in exposure and toxicity; consider alternate medication w/ no or minimal potential to inhibit CYP3A4. If unavoidable, consider delaying treatment until the strong CYP3A4 inhibitors have cleared from circulation. If a strong CYP3A4 inhibitor is coadministered and treatment cannot be delayed, closely monitor for adverse reactions. Caution w/ anticoagulant or antiplatelet therapy; consider additional monitoring when concomitant use is medically necessary.

PREGNANCY AND LACTATION
Pregnancy: Can cause fetal harm when administered to a pregnant woman. Monitor women who received Kadcyla during pregnancy or w/in 7 months prior to conception for oligohydramnios; if oligohydramnios occurs, perform fetal testing that is appropriate for gestational age and consistent w/ community standards of care. There is a pregnancy exposure registry that monitors pregnancy outcomes in women exposed to Kadcyla during pregnancy; women who received Kadcyla during pregnancy or w/in 7 months prior to conception should enroll in the MotHER Pregnancy Registry. In addition, there is a pregnancy pharmacovigilance program; if Kadcyla is administered during pregnancy, or if a patient becomes pregnant while receiving Kadcyla or w/in 7 months following the last dose of Kadcyla, immediately report exposure to Genentech.
Lactation: There is no information regarding the presence of Kadcyla in human milk, the effects on the breastfed infant, or the effects on milk production. DM1, the cytotoxic component of Kadcyla, may cause serious adverse reactions in breastfed infants based on its mechanism of action. Avoid breastfeeding during treatment and for 7 months following the last dose of Kadcyla.
Reproductive Potential: Females of reproductive potential should use effective contraception during treatment and for 7 months following the last dose. Verify pregnancy status prior to initiation of therapy. Male patients w/ female partners of reproductive potential should use effective contraception during treatment and for 4 months following the last dose. May impair fertility in females and males of reproductive potential.

MECHANISM OF ACTION
Monoclonal antibody (IgG1)/HER2 blocker/Antimicrotubule agent (DM1); the HER2-targeted antibody-drug conjugate binds to HER2 receptor and intracellularly releases DM1-containing cytotoxic catabolites. Binding of DM1 to tubulin disrupts microtubule networks, resulting in cell cycle arrest and apoptotic death. Also inhibits HER2 receptor signaling, mediates antibody-dependent cell-mediated cytotoxicity, and inhibits shedding of the HER2 extracellular domain in human breast cancer cells that overexpress HER2.

PHARMACOKINETICS
Absorption: C_{max}=83.4mg/mL (ado-trastuzumab emtansine conjugate [ADC]); 4.61ng/mL (DM1). **Distribution:** ADC: V_d=3.13L. DM1: Plasma protein binding (93%). **Metabolism:** DM1: Liver via CYP3A4/5. **Elimination:** $T_{1/2}$=4 days (ADC).

PATIENT CONSIDERATIONS
Assessment: Assess for history of trastuzumab-induced infusion-related reactions, left ventricular dysfunction, dyspnea at rest, pregnancy/nursing status, and for possible drug interactions. Assess HER2 status. Assess LVEF prior to initiation of therapy. Assess platelet counts, serum transaminases, and bilirubin at baseline.

Monitoring: Monitor for signs/symptoms of neurotoxicity, hepatotoxicity, nodular regenerative hyperplasia, left ventricular dysfunction, interstitial lung disease (eg, pneumonitis), peripheral neuropathy, hemorrhage, thrombocytopenia, infusion-related reactions, allergic/anaphylactic reactions, and other adverse reactions. Monitor LVEF at regular intervals (eg, every 3 months). Repeat LVEF assessment w/in approx 3 weeks in patients whose treatment was withheld due to significant decrease in left ventricular function. Monitor platelet counts, serum transaminases, and bilirubin prior to each dose.

Counseling: Inform of the possibility of severe liver injury and advise to immediately seek medical attention if symptoms of acute hepatitis occur. Advise to contact physician immediately if new onset/worsening SOB, cough, ankles/legs swelling, weight gain (>5 lbs in 24 hrs), dizziness, loss of consciousness, or palpitations occur. Inform pregnant women/females of reproductive potential that drug exposure during pregnancy or w/in 7 months prior to conception can result in fetal harm; advise to use effective contraception during therapy and for 7 months following last dose. Advise women exposed to therapy during pregnancy or who become pregnant w/in 7 months following last dose that there is a pregnancy exposure registry and a pregnancy pharmacovigilance program that monitors pregnancy outcomes. Advise to enroll in the MotHER Pregnancy Registry and report pregnancy to Genentech. Advise male patients w/ female partners of reproductive potential to use effective contraception during treatment and for 4 months following the last dose. Advise women not to breastfeed during treatment and for 7 months after the last dose.

KALETRA — lopinavir/ritonavir

Class: Protease inhibitor

Rx

ADULT DOSAGE	PEDIATRIC DOSAGE
HIV-1 Infection	**HIV-1 Infection**
In Combination w/ Other Antiretrovirals:	**In Combination w/ Other Antiretrovirals:**
<3 Lopinavir Resistance-Associated Substitutions:	**14 Days-6 Months of Age:**
400mg/100mg bid or 800mg/200mg qd	**Sol:**
	Weight-Based: (16mg/4mg)/kg bid
≥3 Resistance-Associated Substitutions:	**BSA-Based:** (300mg/75mg)/m² bid
400mg/100mg bid	Therapy is not recommended in combination w/ efavirenz, nevirapine, or nelfinavir in patients <6 months or age
	6 Months-18 Years:
	W/O Concomitant Efavirenz, Nevirapine, or Nelfinavir:
	Sol:
	Weight-Based:
	<15kg: (12mg/3mg)/kg bid
	≥15-40kg: (10mg/2.5mg)/kg bid
	Max: 400mg/100mg bid
	BSA-Based: (230mg/57.5mg)/m² bid
	Max: 400mg/100mg bid
	Tab:
	Weight-Based:
	15-25kg: 200mg/50mg bid
	>25-35kg: 300mg/75mg bid
	>35kg: 400mg/100mg bid
	BSA-Based:
	≥0.6 to <0.9m²: 200mg/50mg bid
	≥0.9 to <1.4m²: 300mg/75mg bid
	≥1.4m²: 400mg/100mg bid

DOSING CONSIDERATIONS
Concomitant Medications
Combination w/ Efavirenz/Nevirapine/Nelfinavir:
6 Months-18 Years:
Sol:
Weight-Based:
<15kg: (13mg/3.25mg)/kg bid
>15-45kg: (11mg/2.75mg)/kg bid
Max: 533mg/133mg bid
BSA-Based: Increase dose to (300mg/75mg)/m² bid
Max: 533mg/133mg bid

Tab:
Weight-Based:
15-20kg: 200mg/50mg bid
>20-30kg: 300mg/75mg bid
>30-45kg: 400mg/100mg bid
>45kg: 500mg/125mg bid

BSA-Based:
≥0.6 to <0.8m²: 200mg/50mg bid
≥0.8 to <1.2m²: 300mg/75mg bid
≥1.2 to <1.7m²: 400mg/100mg bid
≥1.7m²: 500mg/125mg bid

Adults:
Increase dose to 500mg/125mg bid

ADMINISTRATION
Oral route

Tab
Take w/ or w/o food.
Swallow whole; do not crush, break, or chew.

Sol
Take w/ food.

STORAGE
Tab: 20-25°C (68-77°F); excursions permitted to 15-30°C (59-86°F). **Sol:** 2-8°C (36-46°F). Avoid exposure to excessive heat. If stored at room temperature up to 25°C (77°F), sol should be used w/in 2 months.

HOW SUPPLIED
(Lopinavir/Ritonavir) **Sol:** (80mg/20mg)/mL [160mL]; **Tab:** 100mg/25mg, 200mg/50mg

CONTRAINDICATIONS
Previously demonstrated clinically significant hypersensitivity (eg, toxic epidermal necrolysis, Stevens-Johnson syndrome, erythema multiforme, urticaria, angioedema) to Kaletra or any of its components. Coadministration w/ CYP3A substrates for which elevated plasma concentrations are associated w/ serious and/or life-threatening reactions and w/ potent CYP3A inducers where significantly reduced lopinavir levels may be associated w/ the potential for loss of virologic response and possible resistance and cross-resistance (eg, alfuzosin, rifampin, dihydroergotamine, ergotamine, methylergonovine, St. John's wort, cisapride, lovastatin, simvastatin, sildenafil [when used to treat pulmonary arterial HTN], pimozide, triazolam, oral midazolam).

WARNINGS/PRECAUTIONS
Pancreatitis, including marked TG elevations, reported; evaluate and suspend therapy if clinically appropriate. Patients w/ underlying hepatitis B or C or marked serum transaminase elevations prior to treatment may be at increased risk for developing or worsening of transaminase elevations or hepatic decompensation; conduct appropriate lab testing prior to therapy and monitor closely during treatment. PR and QT interval prolongation, torsades de pointes, and cases of 2nd- and 3rd-degree atrioventricular block reported; caution w/ underlying structural heart disease, preexisting conduction system abnormalities, ischemic heart disease, or cardiomyopathies. Avoid use w/ congenital long QT syndrome or hypokalemia and w/ other drugs that prolong QT interval. New onset or exacerbation of diabetes mellitus (DM), hyperglycemia, diabetic ketoacidosis, immune reconstitution syndrome, autoimmune disorders (eg, Graves' disease, polymyositis, Guillain-Barre syndrome) in the setting of immune reconstitution, redistribution/accumulation of body fat, lipid elevations, and increased bleeding w/ hemophilia A and B reported. QD regimen is not recommended for adults w/ ≥3 lopinavir resistance-associated substitutions or in pediatric patients <18 yrs. Caution w/ hepatic impairment and in elderly. **Sol:** Contains alcohol and propylene glycol. Avoid sol in preterm neonates in the immediate postnatal period; preterm neonates may be at increased risk of propylene glycol-associated adverse events and other toxicities. If benefit of treating infants immediately after birth outweighs potential risk, monitor closely for increases in serum osmolality and SrCr, and for drug-related toxicity.

ADVERSE REACTIONS
Diarrhea, N/V, hypertriglyceridemia and hypercholesterolemia, dysgeusia, rash, decreased weight, insomnia.

DRUG INTERACTIONS
See Contraindications and Dosing Considerations. Caution w/ drugs that prolong the PR interval (eg, calcium channel blockers [CCBs], β-adrenergic blockers, digoxin, atazanavir). Avoid w/ colchicine in patients w/ renal/hepatic impairment, tadalafil during initiation, tipranavir/ritonavir combination, and drugs that prolong the QT interval. Not recommended w/ voriconazole, high doses of itraconazole or ketoconazole, boceprevir, avanafil, salmeterol, and simeprevir. Not recommended w/ fluticasone or other glucocorticoids that are metabolized by CYP3A unless benefit outweighs the risk of systemic corticosteroid effects. May increase levels of CYP3A substrates, colchicine, fentanyl, tenofovir, indinavir, nelfinavir, saquinavir, maraviroc, antiarrhythmics, vincristine, vinblastine, dasatinib, nilotinib, trazodone, itraconazole, ketoconazole, bedaquiline, rifabutin and rifabutin metabolite, clarithromycin in patients w/ renal impairment, IV midazolam, dihydropyridine CCBs, bosentan, atorvastatin, rosuvastatin, immunosuppressants, salmeterol, rivaroxaban, glucocorticoids, sildenafil, tadalafil, vardenafil, rilpivirine, simeprevir, and quetiapine. May decrease levels of methadone, phenytoin, bupropion, atovaquone, ethinyl estradiol, abacavir, zidovudine, lamotrigine, valproate, voriconazole, boceprevir, amprenavir, and etravirine. Delavirdine and CYP3A inhibitors may increase levels. May alter concentrations of warfarin; monitor INR. Efavirenz, nevirapine, nelfinavir, carbamazepine, phenobarbital, and phenytoin may decrease levels; not for qd dosing regimen. Rifampin, fosamprenavir/ritonavir, systemic corticosteroids, and CYP3A inducers may decrease levels. May require initiation or dose adjustments of insulin or oral hypoglycemics for treatment of DM. **Sol:** Contains alcohol; may produce disulfiram-like reactions w/ disulfiram or metronidazole. Didanosine should be given 1 hr before or 2 hrs after sol. Refer to PI for further information and dosing modifications when used w/ certain concomitant therapies.

PREGNANCY AND LACTATION
Pregnancy: Physicians are encouraged to register patients in the Antiretroviral Pregnancy Registry. There are insufficient data to recommend dosing for pregnant patients w/ lopinavir-associated resistance substitutions. QD dosing is not recommended in pregnancy. Avoid use of oral sol during pregnancy due to alcohol content.
Lactation: Not for use in nursing.

MECHANISM OF ACTION
Lopinavir: HIV-1 protease inhibitor; prevents cleavage of the Gag-Pol polyprotein, resulting in the production of immature, noninfectious viral particles. **Ritonavir:** HIV-1 protease inhibitor; CYP3A inhibitor that inhibits metabolism of lopinavir, increasing its plasma levels.

PHARMACOKINETICS
Absorption: Lopinavir: (400mg/100mg bid) C_{max}=9.8μg/mL, T_{max}=4 hrs, AUC=92.6μg•h/mL. Refer to PI for pediatric parameters. **Distribution:** Lopinavir: Plasma protein binding (98-99%). **Metabolism:** Lopinavir: Hepatic via CYP3A (extensive). Ritonavir: Induces own metabolism. **Elimination:** Unchanged Lopinavir: Urine (2.2%), feces (19.8%).

PATIENT CONSIDERATIONS
Assessment: Assess for history of hypersensitivity reactions, history of pancreatitis, hepatitis B or C, cirrhosis, DM or hyperglycemia, dyslipidemia, hemophilia type A or B, structural heart disease, preexisting conduction system abnormalities, ischemic heart disease or cardiomyopathies, congenital long QT syndrome, hypokalemia, renal/hepatic impairment, pregnancy/nursing status, and for possible drug interactions. Assess children for the ability to swallow intact tab.

Monitoring: Monitor for signs/symptoms of pancreatitis, hyperglycemia, hepatic dysfunction, immune reconstitution syndrome, autoimmune disorders, fat redistribution/accumulation, hypersensitivity reactions, and other adverse reactions. Monitor lipid profile, glucose levels, total bilirubin levels, ECG changes, serum lipase levels, and serum amylase levels. Monitor infants for increase in serum osmolality, SrCr, and other toxicities.

Counseling: Instruct to take prescribed dose ud. Advise to inform physician if weight changes in children occur. Inform that if a dose is missed, a dose should be taken as soon as possible and to return to normal schedule; instruct not to double the next dose. Advise that therapy is not a cure for HIV; opportunistic infections may still occur. Instruct to avoid doing things that can spread HIV-1 infection to others. Instruct not to have any kind of sex w/o protection; advise to practice safe sex by always using a latex or polyurethane condom to lower the chance of sexual contact w/ semen, vaginal secretions, or blood. Instruct to notify physician if using other prescription/OTC or herbal products, particularly St. John's wort. Inform that skin rashes, liver function changes, ECG changes, redistribution/accumulation of body fat, new onset or worsening of preexisting diabetes, and hyperglycemia may occur. Instruct to seek medical attention if symptoms of worsening liver disease (eg, loss of appetite, abdominal pain, jaundice, itchy skin), dizziness, abnormal heart rhythm, loss of consciousness, or any other adverse reactions develop.

KALYDECO — ivacaftor   **Rx**

Class: CFTR potentiator

ADULT DOSAGE
Cystic Fibrosis

W/ G551D, G1244E, G1349D, G178R, G551S, S1251N, S1255P, S549N, S549R, or R117H mutation in the cystic fibrosis transmembrane conductance regulator gene

Usual: 150mg tab q12h

PEDIATRIC DOSAGE
Cystic Fibrosis

W/ G551D, G1244E, G1349D, G178R, G551S, S1251N, S1255P, S549N, S549R, or R117H mutation in the cystic fibrosis transmembrane conductance regulator gene

Granules:
2-<6 Years:
<14kg:
Usual: 50mg pkt q12h
≥14kg:
Usual: 75mg pkt q12h

Tab:
≥6 Years:
Usual: 150mg tab q12h

- -

DOSING CONSIDERATIONS
Concomitant Medications
Moderate CYP3A Inhibitors: Reduce dose to 1 tab or 1 pkt of granules qd
Strong CYP3A Inhibitors: Reduce dose to 1 tab or 1 pkt of granules 2X/week
Avoid food containing grapefruit or Seville oranges

Hepatic Impairment
Moderate (Child-Pugh Class B): Reduce dose to 1 tab or 1 pkt of granules qd
Severe (Child-Pugh Class C): Use w/ caution at 1 tab or 1 pkt of granules qd or less frequently

ADMINISTRATION
Oral route

Take w/ fat-containing food (eg, eggs, butter, whole-milk dairy products)

Granules
Mix the entire contents of each pkt w/ 1 tsp (5mL) of age-appropriate soft food or liquid (eg, pureed fruits or vegetables, yogurt, applesauce, water, milk, juice) and consume completely.
Food or liquid should be at or below room temperature.
Once mixed, the product has been shown to be stable for 1 hr, and therefore should be consumed during this period.
Administer each dose just before or just after fat-containing food.

STORAGE
20-25°C (68-77°F); excursions permitted to 15-30°C (59-86°F).

HOW SUPPLIED
Granules: 50mg/pkt, 75mg/pkt; **Tab:** 150mg

WARNINGS/PRECAUTIONS
Elevated transaminases reported. Monitor closely if increased transaminase levels develop until abnormalities resolve and interrupt dosing w/ ALT or AST >5X ULN; consider benefits and risks of resuming dosing. Consider more frequent monitoring of LFTs w/ history of transaminase elevations. Caution w/ severe renal impairment (CrCl ≤30mL/min), or ESRD. Non-congenital lens opacities/cataracts reported in pediatric patients. Use FDA-cleared CF mutation test to detect the presence of CFTR mutation followed by verification w/ bidirectional sequencing when recommended by the mutation test instructions for use if patient's genotype is unknown. Not effective in patients w/ CF who are homozygous for the F508del mutation in the CFTR gene.

ADVERSE REACTIONS
Headache, oropharyngeal pain, URTI, nasal congestion, abdominal pain, nasopharyngitis, diarrhea, rash, nausea, dizziness, rhinitis, arthralgia, bacteria in sputum, wheezing, acne.

DRUG INTERACTIONS
See Dosing Considerations. Not recommended w/ strong CYP3A inducers (eg, rifampin, phenytoin, St. John's wort); these drugs may substantially decrease exposure. Strong CYP3A inhibitors (eg, ketoconazole, itraconazole, clarithromycin), moderate CYP3A inhibitors (eg, fluconazole, erythromycin), and grapefruit juice may increase levels. May increase levels of sensitive CYP3A substrates (eg, midazolam) and/or P-gp substrates (eg, digoxin, cyclosporine, tacrolimus); use w/ caution and monitor appropriately.

PREGNANCY AND LACTATION
Category B, caution in nursing.

MECHANISM OF ACTION
CFTR potentiator; facilitates increased Cl⁻ transport by potentiating the channel-open probability (or gating) of the CFTR protein.

PHARMACOKINETICS
Absorption: Administration of variable doses resulted in different parameters in pediatric patients. (150mg) C_{max}=768ng/mL, AUC=10,600ng•hr/mL, T_{max}=approx 4 hrs (median). **Distribution:** V_d=353L (150mg); plasma protein binding (approx 99%); likely found in breast milk. **Metabolism:** Extensive via CYP3A; M1 and M6 (major metabolites). **Elimination:** Feces (87.8%, approx 65% metabolites), urine (negligible as unchanged drug); $T_{1/2}$=approx 12 hrs.

PATIENT CONSIDERATIONS

Assessment: Assess for history of transaminase elevations, renal/hepatic impairment, patients who are homozygous for the F508del mutation in the CFTR gene, pregnancy/nursing status, and possible drug interactions. If genotype is unknown, perform FDA-cleared CF mutation test to detect the presence of the CFTR mutation followed by verification w/ bidirectional sequencing when recommended by the mutation test instructions for use. Obtain baseline ophthalmological examinations in pediatric patients.

Monitoring: Monitor for adverse reactions. Monitor ALT/AST levels every 3 months during the 1st yr of therapy and annually thereafter. Perform follow-up ophthalmological examinations in pediatric patients.

Counseling: Inform that elevation in liver tests have occurred and LFTs will be performed prior to initiating therapy, every 3 months during the 1st yr, and annually thereafter. Instruct to inform physician of all medications that are currently being taken, including any herbal supplements or vitamins. Instruct to avoid food containing grapefruit or Seville oranges. Instruct to take exactly ud. In case a dose of drug is missed w/in 6 hrs of the time it is usually taken, instruct to take the prescribed dose w/ fat-containing food as soon as possible. If >6 hrs have passed since drug is usually taken, instruct not to take the missed dose, and to resume the usual dosing schedule. Advise to contact physician if patients have questions about missed dose. Inform that abnormality of the eye lens has been noted in children and adolescents receiving therapy.

KANUMA — sebelipase alfa

Rx

Class: Enzyme

ADULT DOSAGE
Lysosomal Acid Lipase Deficiency

1mg/kg IV infusion once every other week

PEDIATRIC DOSAGE
Lysosomal Acid Lipase Deficiency

Rapidly Progressive Lysosomal Acid Lipase (LAL) Deficiency Presenting w/in First 6 Months of Life:
Initial: 1mg/kg IV infusion once weekly

Titrate: Increase to 3mg/kg once weekly if optimal response is not achieved

Pediatric Patients w/ LAL Deficiency:
1mg/kg IV infusion once every other week

ADMINISTRATION
IV route

Vials are for single-use only; discard any unused product.
Use immediately after dilution; if immediate use is not possible, store ≤24 hrs at

2-8°C (36-46°F).
Do not freeze or shake.
Protect from light.

Preparation
1. Determine the number of vials needed based on the patient's weight and the recommended dose of 1mg/kg or 3mg/kg.
2. Round to the next whole vial and remove required number of vials from refrigerator and allow to reach room temperature.
3. Mix gently by inversion; do not shake vials or prepared infusion.

Administration
Administer sol as an IV infusion using a low-protein binding infusion set w/ an in-line, low-protein binding 0.2 micron filter.
Infuse over ≥2 hrs; consider further prolonging the infusion time for patients receiving 3mg/kg dose or those who have experienced hypersensitivity reactions. A 1-hr infusion may be considered for patients receiving 1mg/kg dose who tolerate the infusion.

STORAGE
2-8°C (36-46°F) in original carton to protect from light. Do not shake or freeze vials.

HOW SUPPLIED
Inj: 20mg/10mL

WARNINGS/PRECAUTIONS
Hypersensitivity reactions, including anaphylaxis, reported; immediately d/c infusion and initiate appropriate medical treatment if anaphylaxis occurs. Management of hypersensitivity reactions should be based on severity of the reaction and may include temporarily interrupting infusion, lowering infusion rate, and/or treatment w/ antihistamines, antipyretics, and/or corticosteroids. If interrupted, infusion may resume at a slower rate w/ increases as tolerated. Pretreatment w/ antipyretics and/or antihistamines may prevent subsequent reactions. Immediately d/c infusion and initiate appropriate medical treatment if a severe hypersensitivity reaction occurs; consider risks/benefits of readministration following a severe reaction. Observe closely during and after infusion. Produced in the egg whites of genetically engineered chickens; caution w/ known systemic hypersensitivity reactions to eggs or egg products.

ADVERSE REACTIONS
Rapidly Progressive Disease Presenting w/in First 6 Months of Life: Diarrhea, vomiting, fever, rhinitis, anemia, cough, nasopharyngitis, urticaria.
Pediatrics and Adults: Headache, fever, oropharyngeal pain, nasopharyngitis, asthenia, constipation, nausea.

PREGNANCY AND LACTATION
Pregnancy: There are no available data on sebelipase alfa in pregnant women to inform any drug-associated risk.
Lactation: There are no data on the presence of sebelipase alfa in human milk, the effects on the breastfed infant, or the effects on milk production; caution in nursing.

MECHANISM OF ACTION
Recombinant human LAL; binds to cell surface receptors via glycans expressed on the protein and is subsequently internalized into lysosomes. Catalyzes the lysosomal hydrolysis of cholesteryl esters and triglycerides to free cholesterol, glycerol, and free fatty acids.

PHARMACOKINETICS
Absorption: AUC=942ng•hr/mL (4-11 yrs), 1454ng•hr/mL (12-17 yrs), 1861ng•hr/mL (≥18 yrs); C_{max}=490ng/mL (4-11 yrs), 784ng/mL (12-17 yrs), 957ng/mL (≥18 yrs); T_{max}=1.3 hr (4-11 yrs), 1.1 hr (12-17 yrs), 1.3 hr (≥18 yrs). **Distribution:** 3.6L (4-11 yrs), 5.4L (12-17 yrs), 5.3L (≥18 yrs). **Elimination:** $T_{1/2}$=5.4 min (4-11 yrs), 6.6 min (12-17 yrs), 6.6 min (≥18 yrs).

PATIENT CONSIDERATIONS

Assessment: Assess for known systemic hypersensitivity reactions to eggs or egg products.

Monitoring: Monitor for hypersensitivity/anaphylactic reactions.

Counseling: Advise that hypersensitivity/anaphylactic reactions may occur during and after treatment. Inform of the signs/symptoms of anaphylaxis/hypersensitivity reactions, and advise to seek immediate medical care should signs/symptoms occur.

KAPVAY — clonidine hydrochloride

Rx

Class: Alpha₂ agonist

PEDIATRIC DOSAGE
Attention-Deficit Hyperactivity Disorder

Monotherapy or Adjunctive Therapy to Stimulant Medications:
6-17 Years:
Initial: 0.1mg hs

Titrate: Adjust daily dose in increments of 0.1mg/day at weekly intervals until desired response is achieved; doses should be taken bid, w/ either an equal or higher split dosage being given hs

Doses >0.4mg/day were not evaluated in clinical trials for ADHD and are not recommended

Dosing Guidance:
Total Daily Dose of 0.1mg: 0.1mg qhs
Total Daily Dose of 0.2mg: 0.1mg qam and 0.1mg qhs
Total Daily Dose of 0.3mg: 0.1mg qam and 0.2mg qhs
Total Daily Dose of 0.4mg: 0.2mg qam and 0.2mg qhs

Missed Dose

If a dose is missed, skip that dose and take the next dose as scheduled; do not take more than the prescribed total daily amount in any 24-hr period

DOSING CONSIDERATIONS
Concomitant Medications
Concomitant Psychostimulant: Adjust psychostimulant dose depending on response to clonidine

Renal Impairment
Give initial dosage based on degree of impairment; titrate to higher doses cautiously

Discontinuation
Taper total daily dose in decrements of no more than 0.1mg every 3-7 days

ADMINISTRATION
Oral route
Take w/ or w/o food.
Swallow tabs whole; do not crush, chew, or break.

STORAGE
20-25°C (68-77°F).

HOW SUPPLIED
Tab, Extended-Release: 0.1mg, 0.2mg

CONTRAINDICATIONS
History of a hypersensitivity reaction to clonidine.

WARNINGS/PRECAUTIONS
Substitution for other clonidine products on mg-per-mg basis is not recommended. May cause dose-related decreases in BP and HR. Titrate slowly in patients w/ history of hypotension and those w/ underlying conditions that may be worsened by hypotension and bradycardia (eg, heart block, bradycardia, cardiovascular/vascular/cerebrovascular disease, chronic renal failure). Caution w/ a history of syncope or w/ a condition that predisposes to syncope (eg, hypotension, orthostatic hypotension, bradycardia, dehydration); avoid becoming dehydrated or overheated. Somnolence and sedation reported. May impair mental/physical abilities. Abrupt discontinuation may cause rebound HTN; gradually reduce dose when discontinuing therapy. May elicit allergic reactions (eg, generalized rash, urticaria, angioedema) in patients who develop an allergic reaction from clonidine transdermal system. May worsen sinus node dysfunction and atrioventricular (AV) block; titrate slowly and monitor vital signs frequently in patients w/ cardiac conduction abnormalities.

ADVERSE REACTIONS
Monotherapy: Somnolence, fatigue, irritability, insomnia, nightmare, constipation, dry mouth.
Adjunctive Therapy: Somnolence, fatigue, decreased appetite, dizziness.

DRUG INTERACTIONS
TCAs increase BP and may counteract hypotensive effects, while antihypertensives potentiate hypotensive effect; monitor BP and adjust dose prn. Avoid w/ CNS depressants; may potentiate sedating effects. Avoid w/ drugs that affect sinus node function or AV node conduction (eg, digitalis, calcium channel blockers, β-blockers); may potentiate bradycardia and risk of AV block. Monitor BP and HR, and adjust dosages accordingly in patients treated concomitantly w/ antihypertensives or other drugs that can reduce BP/HR or increase risk of syncope. Consider the potential for additive sedative effects w/ other centrally active depressants (eg, phenothiazines, barbiturates, benzodiazepines). Titrate slowly and monitor vital signs frequently w/ other sympatholytics. Avoid use w/ alcohol.

PREGNANCY AND LACTATION
Pregnancy: Category C.
Lactation: Present in human milk. Caution in nursing.

MECHANISM OF ACTION
α_2-agonist; not established. Stimulates α_2-adrenergic receptors in the brain.

PHARMACOKINETICS
Absorption: (Adults) C_{max}=235pg/mL (fed), 258pg/mL (fasted); AUC=6505pg•hr/mL (fed), 6729pg•hr/mL (fasted); T_{max}=6.80 hrs (fed), 6.50 hrs (fasted).
Distribution: Found in breast milk. **Elimination:** (Adults) $T_{1/2}$=12.67 hrs (fed), 12.65 hrs (fasted).

PATIENT CONSIDERATIONS
Assessment: Assess for drug hypersensitivity, history of hypotension, underlying conditions that may be worsened by hypotension and bradycardia, history of syncope or conditions that predispose to syncope, cardiac conduction abnormalities, renal impairment, pregnancy/nursing status, and for possible drug interactions. Obtain baseline HR and BP.

Monitoring: Monitor for somnolence, sedation, hypotension, bradycardia, allergic reactions, dehydration, overheating, and for other adverse reactions. Monitor BP and HR following dose increases and periodically while on therapy. Monitor vital signs frequently in patients w/ cardiac conduction abnormalities.

Counseling: Inform about risks/benefits of therapy and instruct to take ud. If a dose is missed, instruct to skip that dose and take the next dose as scheduled; advise not to take more than the prescribed total daily amount in any 24-hr period. Advise patients w/ a history of syncope or who may have a condition that predisposes them to syncope (eg, hypotension, orthostatic hypotension, bradycardia, dehydration) to avoid becoming dehydrated or overheated. Instruct to use caution when driving or operating hazardous machinery until they know how they will respond to treatment. Advise to avoid use of therapy w/ other centrally active depressants and w/ alcohol. Advise not to d/c therapy abruptly. Instruct to d/c therapy and seek immediate medical attention if any signs/symptoms of a hypersensitivity reaction (eg, generalized rash, urticaria, angioedema) occur.

KAZANO — alogliptin/metformin hydrochloride   Rx
Class: Biguanide/dipeptidyl peptidase-4 (DPP-4) inhibitor

> Cases of metformin-associated lactic acidosis resulting in death, hypothermia, hypotension, and resistant bradyarrhythmias reported; risk factors include renal impairment, concomitant use of certain drugs (eg, cationic drugs such as topiramate), age ≥65 years, having a radiological study w/ contrast, surgery and other procedures, hypoxic states (eg, acute CHF), excessive alcohol intake, and hepatic impairment. D/C therapy immediately and institute general supportive measures in a hospital setting if metformin-associated lactic acidosis is suspected. Prompt hemodialysis is recommended.

ADULT DOSAGE
Type 2 Diabetes Mellitus
When treatment w/ both alogliptin and metformin is appropriate
Initial: Individualize based on current regimen; dose bid w/ gradual dose escalation to reduce GI side effects due to metformin
Titrate: May adjust dose based on effectiveness/tolerability
Max: (25mg/2000mg)/day

PEDIATRIC DOSAGE
Pediatric use may not have been established

DOSING CONSIDERATIONS
Renal Impairment
eGFR 30-60mL/min/1.73m²: Not recommended
eGFR <30mL/min/1.73m²: Contraindicated

Hepatic Impairment
Not recommended

Other Important Considerations
Iodinated Contrast Imaging Procedures:
D/C therapy at the time of, or prior to, an iodinated contrast imaging procedure in patients w/ an eGFR 30-60mL/min/1.73m²; in patients w/ a history of liver disease, alcoholism or heart failure (HF); or in patients who will be administered intra-arterial iodinated contrast. Reevaluate eGFR 48 hrs after the imaging procedure and restart therapy if renal function is stable

ADMINISTRATION
Oral route
Take bid w/ food.
Do not split tab before swallowing.

STORAGE
25°C (77°F); excursions permitted to 15-30°C (59-86°F). Keep container tightly closed.

HOW SUPPLIED
Tab: (Alogliptin/Metformin) 12.5mg/500mg, 12.5mg/1000mg

CONTRAINDICATIONS
Severe renal impairment (eGFR <30mL/min/1.73m²); acute or chronic metabolic acidosis, including diabetic ketoacidosis; history of a serious hypersensitivity reaction to alogliptin or metformin (eg, anaphylaxis, angioedema, severe cutaneous adverse reactions).

WARNINGS/PRECAUTIONS
See Dosing Considerations. Not for the treatment of type 1 diabetes mellitus (DM) or diabetic ketoacidosis. **Alogliptin:** Acute pancreatitis reported; promptly d/c if suspected and initiate appropriate management. Hospitalization for CHF reported in patients w/ recent acute coronary syndrome; evaluate and manage accordingly and consider discontinuation if HF develops. Consider the risks and benefits of therapy prior to initiating treatment in patients at risk for HF. Serious hypersensitivity reactions reported; d/c if suspected, assess for other potential causes, and institute alternative treatment for DM. Caution w/ history of angioedema to another DPP-4 inhibitor. Fatal and nonfatal hepatic failure and serum ALT >3X ULN reported; measure liver tests promptly in patients who report symptoms that may indicate liver injury. Interrupt treatment and investigate the cause if clinically significant liver enzyme elevations exist and if abnormal liver tests persist or worsen; do not restart w/o another explanation for abnormal LFTs. Severe and disabling arthralgia reported; consider DPP-4 inhibitors as a possible cause and d/c therapy if appropriate. **Metformin:** Temporarily d/c in patient has restricted food and fluid intake. D/C if a condition associated w/ hypoxemia occurs (eg, cardiovascular collapse, acute MI, sepsis). May decrease vitamin B12 levels; monitor hematologic parameters annually. Hypoglycemia may occur when caloric intake is deficient or when strenuous exercise is not compensated by caloric supplementation; elderly, debilitated or malnourished patients and those w/ adrenal or pituitary insufficiency or alcohol intoxication are particularly susceptible to hypoglycemic effects. Hypoglycemia may be difficult to recognize in the elderly.

ADVERSE REACTIONS

URTI, nasopharyngitis, diarrhea, HTN, headache, back pain, UTI.

DRUG INTERACTIONS

See Boxed Warning. When used w/ an insulin secretagogue (eg, sulfonylurea) or w/ insulin, a lower dose of the insulin secretagogue or insulin may be required to reduce the risk of hypoglycemia. **Metformin:** Hypoglycemia may occur during concomitant use w/ other glucose-lowering agents (eg, sulfonylureas, insulin) or ethanol. Hypoglycemia may be difficult to recognize w/ β-adrenergic blocking drugs. Carbonic anhydrase inhibitors (eg, zonisamide, acetazolamide, dichlorphenamide) may increase the risk of lactic acidosis; consider more frequent monitoring of these patients. Drugs that are eliminated by renal tubular secretion, drugs that impair renal function, drugs that result in significant hemodynamic change, drugs that interfere w/ acid-base balance, or drugs that increase metformin accumulation may increase the risk of metformin-associated lactic acidosis; consider more frequent monitoring of these patients. Patient should avoid excessive alcohol intake. Thiazides and other diuretics, corticosteroids, phenothiazines, thyroid products, estrogens, oral contraceptives, phenytoin, nicotinic acid, sympathomimetics, calcium channel blockers, and isoniazid may produce hyperglycemia and lead to loss of glycemic control; observe closely for loss of blood glucose control when such drugs are administered and observe closely for hypoglycemia when such drugs are withdrawn.

PREGNANCY AND LACTATION

Pregnancy: Category B.
Lactation: Caution in nursing.

MECHANISM OF ACTION

Alogliptin: DPP-4 inhibitor; slows inactivation of incretin hormones, thereby increasing their bloodstream concentrations and reducing fasting and postprandial glucose concentrations in a glucose-dependent manner. **Metformin:** Biguanide; decreases hepatic glucose production, decreases intestinal absorption of glucose, and improves insulin sensitivity by increasing peripheral glucose uptake and utilization.

PHARMACOKINETICS

Absorption: Alogliptin: Absolute bioavailability (approx 100%). Metformin: Absolute bioavailability (approx 50-60%) (fasting). **Distribution:** Alogliptin: V_d=417L (IV); plasma protein binding (20%). Metformin: V_d=654L. **Metabolism:** Alogliptin: CYP3A4 and CYP2D6 contribute to the limited metabolism of alogliptin; N-demethylated alogliptin, M-I (minor, active metabolite). **Elimination:** Alogliptin: Feces (13%), urine (76%, 60-71% unchanged). Metformin: Urine (90%); $T_{1/2}$=6.2 hrs (plasma), 17.6 hrs (blood).

PATIENT CONSIDERATIONS

Assessment: Assess for acute/chronic metabolic acidosis (including diabetic ketoacidosis), type of DM, risk factors for lactic acidosis, renal/hepatic impairment, previous hypersensitivity to the drug, HF or risk factors for HF, history of pancreatitis, predisposition to developing subnormal vitamin B12 levels, history of angioedema w/ another DPP-4 inhibitor, pregnancy/nursing status, and possible drug interactions. Assess if patient is planning to undergo any surgical procedure. Obtain baseline FPG, HbA1c, eGFR, and hematologic parameters.

Monitoring: Monitor for lactic acidosis, pancreatitis, HF, hypoxic states, decreases in vitamin B12 levels, hypersensitivity reactions, severe and disabling arthralgia, and other adverse reactions. Monitor eGFR at least annually; monitor more frequently in patients at risk of developing renal impairment. Monitor FPG, HbA1c, and hepatic function periodically. Monitor hematologic parameters annually. Perform routine serum vitamin B12 measurements at 2- to 3-yr intervals in patients predisposed to developing subnormal vitamin B12 levels.

Counseling: Inform of risks/benefits of therapy and instruct to take ud. Advise of the risks of lactic acidosis, its symptoms, and conditions that predispose to its development; instruct to d/c therapy immediately and contact physician if unexplained hyperventilation, myalgia, malaise, unusual somnolence, or other nonspecific symptoms occur. Inform that acute pancreatitis may occur; instruct to promptly d/c therapy and contact physician if persistent severe abdominal pain occurs. Advise about the signs/symptoms of HF; instruct to contact physician as soon as possible if symptoms of HF (eg, increasing SOB, rapid increase in weight, swelling of the feet) are experienced. Inform that allergic reactions may occur; instruct to d/c and promptly seek medical advice if symptoms of allergic reactions occur. Inform about risk of liver injury; instruct to d/c and promptly seek medical advice if signs/symptoms of liver injury occur. Inform about the importance of regular testing of renal function and hematological parameters during treatment. Counsel against excessive alcohol intake. Inform that hypoglycemia can occur, particularly when used in combination w/ an insulin secretagogue or insulin. Inform that severe and disabling joint pain may occur; advise to seek medical advice if severe joint pain occurs.

KENALOG-10 — triamcinolone acetonide   Rx

Class: Corticosteroid

ADULT DOSAGE
Dermatoses
Intralesional:

For alopecia areata; discoid lupus erythematosus; keloids; localized hypertrophic, infiltrated, inflammatory lesions of granuloma annulare, lichen planus, lichen simplex chronicus (neurodermatitis), and psoriatic plaques; necrobiosis lipoidica

PEDIATRIC DOSAGE
General Dosing
Initial: 0.11-1.6mg/kg/day (3.2-48mg/m²/day) in 3 or 4 divided doses depending on disease being treated
Titrate: Adjust to the lowest effective dose
Upon discontinuation after long-term therapy, withdraw gradually

diabeticorum; and cystic tumors of an aponeurosis or tendon (ganglia)
Initial: Varies depending on the specific disease and lesion being treated; multiple sites separated by 1cm or more may be injected. May be repeated at weekly or less frequent intervals if necessary
Maint: After a favorable response is noted, decrease initial dose in small decrements at appropriate time intervals until lowest dosage achieves adequate clinical response

Arthritic Disorders
Intra-articular/Soft Tissue:
Adjunctive therapy for short-term administration in acute gouty arthritis, acute/subacute bursitis, acute nonspecific tenosynovitis, epicondylitis, rheumatoid arthritis, synovitis, or osteoarthritis

Initial:
Smaller Joints: 2.5-5mg depending on disease being treated
Larger Joints: 5-15mg depending on disease being treated
Single inj into several joints, up to a total of 20mg or more, have been given

Maint: After a favorable response is noted, decrease initial dose in small decrements at appropriate time intervals until lowest dosage achieves adequate clinical response

---

DOSING CONSIDERATIONS
Other Important Considerations
Localization of Doses:
Lower initial dosage ranges of triamcinolone may produce the desired effect when administered to provide a localized concentration.
Carefully consider the site and volume of the inj when triamcinolone acetonide is administered for this purpose.

ADMINISTRATION
Intra-articular/Soft Tissue/Intralesional route

Inj Technique
Joints: If an excessive amount of synovial fluid is present in the joint, some, but not all, should be aspirated to aid in the relief of pain and to prevent undue dilution of the steroid.
Intra-articular: Carefully inject, particularly in the deltoid region, to avoid injecting sus into the tissues surrounding the site; may lead to tissue atrophy.
Acute Nonspecific Tenosynovitis: Ensure that inj is made into the tendon sheath rather than the tendon substance.
Epicondylitis: Infiltrate the preparation into the area of greatest tenderness.
Intralesional: For accuracy of dosage measurement and ease of administration, it is preferable to employ a tuberculin syringe and a small-bore needle (23-25 gauge). Ethyl chloride spray may be used to alleviate the discomfort of the inj.
Dermal Lesions: Inj directly into the lesion (intradermally or subcutaneously).

STORAGE
20-25°C (68-77°F), avoid freezing and protect from light. Do not refrigerate.

HOW SUPPLIED
Inj: 10mg/mL [5mL]

CONTRAINDICATIONS
Hypersensitivity to any components of the medication.

WARNINGS/PRECAUTIONS
Serious neurologic events reported w/ epidural inj; not approved for epidural administration. Not for use in neonates; contains benzyl alcohol, which has been associated w/ gasping syndrome in neonates, and increased incidence of kernicterus in small preterm infants. Anaphylaxis may occur. Not suitable for use in acute stressful situations. High systemic doses should not be used to treat traumatic brain injury. May cause BP elevation, salt/water retention, and increased K^+ and Ca^{2+} excretion; dietary salt restriction and K^+ supplementation may be necessary. Caution w/ a recent MI. May produce reversible hypothalamic-pituitary-adrenal (HPA) axis suppression w/ potential for glucocorticosteroid insufficiency after withdrawal. Drug-induced secondary adrenocortical insufficiency may be minimized by gradual dose reduction. Metabolic clearance is decreased in hypothyroidism and increased in hyperthyroidism; changes in thyroid status may necessitate dose adjustment. May increase susceptibility to infections, mask signs of current infection, activate latent disease, or exacerbate intercurrent infections/systemic fungal infections. Avoid use in the presence of systemic fungal infections unless needed to control drug reactions. Rule out latent or active amebiasis before initiating therapy. Caution w/ *Strongyloides* infestation, active or latent tuberculosis (TB), congestive heart failure (CHF), HTN, and renal insufficiency. Not for use in cerebral malaria or active ocular herpes simplex. May cause more

serious/fatal course of chickenpox and measles; avoid exposure. Reports of severe medical events have been associated w/ the intrathecal route of administration; avoid intrathecal administration. May produce posterior subcapsular cataracts, glaucoma w/ possible damage to the optic nerves, and enhance the establishment of secondary ocular infections; not recommended in the treatment of optic neuritis. Endophthalmitis, eye inflammation, increased intraocular pressure (IOP), and visual disturbances including vision loss reported w/ intravitreal administration. Administration intraocularly or into the nasal turbinates is not recommended. Sensitive to heat; should not be autoclaved when it is desirable to sterilize the exterior of the vial. Kaposi's sarcoma reported. Caution w/ active or latent peptic ulcers, diverticulitis, fresh intestinal anastomoses, and nonspecific ulcerative colitis; may increase risk of perforation. Signs of peritoneal irritation following GI perforation may be minimal/absent. Enhanced effect in patients w/ cirrhosis. May decrease bone formation and increase bone resorption and may lead to inhibition of bone growth in pediatric patients and development of osteoporosis at any age; caution w/ increased risk of osteoporosis. Acute myopathy reported w/ high doses, most often in patients w/ neuromuscular transmission disorders (eg, myasthenia gravis). Elevation of creatine kinase (CK) or IOP may occur; monitor IOP if used for >6 weeks. Psychiatric derangements may appear and existing emotional instability or psychotic tendencies may be aggravated. May suppress reactions to skin tests. **Intra-articular/Soft Tissue Administration:** Intra-articularly injected corticosteroids may be systemically absorbed. Appropriate examination of any joint fluid present is necessary to exclude a septic process; institute appropriate antimicrobial therapy if septic arthritis occurs and diagnosis is confirmed. Avoid inj into an infected site/previously infected joint or into unstable joints. Intra-articular inj may result in damage to joint tissues.

ADVERSE REACTIONS
Bradycardia, HTN, edema, allergic dermatitis, impaired wound healing, urticaria, glycosuria, hirsutism, abdominal distention, ulcerative esophagitis, negative nitrogen balance, muscle weakness, osteoporosis, convulsions, depression.

DRUG INTERACTIONS
Administration of live or live, attenuated vaccines is contraindicated in patients receiving immunosuppressive doses. Killed or inactivated vaccines may be administered, although response is unpredictable; if possible, routine vaccine/toxoid administration should be deferred until therapy is discontinued. Aminoglutethimide may lead to loss of corticosteroid-induced adrenal suppression. Closely monitor for hypokalemia w/ K⁺-depleting agents (eg, amphotericin B, diuretics). Cardiac enlargement and CHF following concomitant use of amphotericin B and hydrocortisone reported. Macrolide antibiotics may decrease clearance and cholestyramine may increase clearance. Concomitant use w/ anticholinesterase agents may produce severe weakness in patients w/ myasthenia gravis; d/c anticholinesterase agents at least 24 hrs before initiating therapy. May inhibit response to warfarin; frequently monitor coagulation indices. May increase blood glucose levels; dosage adjustments of antidiabetic agents may be required. May decrease serum concentrations of isoniazid. Increased activity of both drugs may occur w/ cyclosporine; convulsions reported w/ concurrent use. May increase risk of arrhythmias w/ digitalis glycosides. Estrogens, including oral contraceptives, may decrease hepatic metabolism and enhance effect. Hepatic enzyme inducers (eg, barbiturates, phenytoin, carbamazepine, rifampin) may enhance metabolism and require corticosteroid dosage increase. Ketoconazole may increase risk of corticosteroid side effects. Aspirin (ASA) or other NSAIDs may increase the risk of GI side effects; caution w/ ASA in hypoprothrombinemia patients. May increase clearance of salicylates. Acute myopathy reported w/ neuromuscular blocking drugs (eg, pancuronium).

PREGNANCY AND LACTATION
Pregnancy: Category C. Carefully observe infants born to mothers who received corticosteroids during pregnancy for signs of hypoadrenalism.
Lactation: Systemically administered corticosteroids appear in human milk and may suppress growth, interfere w/ endogenous corticosteroid production, or cause other untoward effects; caution in nursing.

MECHANISM OF ACTION
Corticosteroid; synthetic glucocorticoid analogue w/ anti-inflammatory effects.

PHARMACOKINETICS
Absorption: Readily absorbed from GI tract. **Distribution:** Found in breast milk (systemic administration).

PATIENT CONSIDERATIONS
Assessment: Assess for hypersensitivity to drug, unusual stress, recent MI, systemic fungal infections, other current infections, active/latent TB, cerebral malaria, ocular herpes simplex, CHF, HTN, renal insufficiency, traumatic brain injury, diverticulitis, intestinal anastomoses, ulcerative colitis, psychotic tendencies, cirrhosis, myasthenia gravis, any other conditions where treatment is contraindicated or cautioned, pregnancy/nursing status, and possible drug interactions.
Monitoring: Monitor for anaphylaxis, HPA axis suppression, Kaposi's sarcoma, acute myopathy, infections, psychiatric derangements, intestinal perforation, cataracts, glaucoma, growth/development (in pediatric patients), osteoporosis, and other adverse reactions. Monitor BP, serum electrolytes, CK, and IOP. Frequently monitor coagulation indices w/ warfarin.
Counseling: Instruct not to d/c abruptly or use w/o medical supervision. Instruct to inform any medical attendants of intake of corticosteroids and to seek medical advice at once if fever or signs of infection develop. Advise to avoid exposure to chickenpox or measles; instruct to seek medical advice w/o delay if exposed.

KENGREAL — cangrelor   Rx
Class: Antiplatelet agent

ADULT DOSAGE
Percutaneous Coronary Intervention
Adjunct to percutaneous coronary intervention (PCI) to reduce the risk of periprocedural MI, repeat coronary revascularization, and stent thrombosis in patients who have not been treated w/ a P2Y₁₂ platelet inhibitor and are not being given a glycoprotein IIb/IIIa inhibitor

30mcg/kg IV bolus followed immediately by a 4mcg/kg/min infusion

Initiate the bolus prior to PCI. Maint infusion should be continued for at least 2 hrs or for the duration of PCI, whichever is longer

Conversions
Transitioning to Oral P2Y₁₂ Therapy:
Ticagrelor: 180mg at any time during infusion or immediately after discontinuation
Prasugrel: 60mg immediately after discontinuation
Clopidogrel: 600mg immediately after discontinuation

PEDIATRIC DOSAGE
Pediatric use may not have been established

ADMINISTRATION
IV route
Administer via a dedicated IV line.
Administer the bolus volume rapidly (<1 min), from the diluted bag via manual IV push or pump. Ensure the bolus is completely administered before the start of PCI. Start the infusion immediately after administration of the bolus.

Preparation
Reconstitute 50mg vial by adding 5mL of sterile water for inj. Swirl gently until all material is dissolved; avoid vigorous mixing and allow any foam to settle. Ensure that reconstituted material is a clear, colorless to pale yellow sol. Reconstitute the vial prior to dilution in a bag.

Do not use w/o dilution. Before administration, each reconstituted vial must be diluted further w/ NaCl 0.9% inj or D5W. Withdraw the contents from 1 reconstituted vial and add to one 250mL saline bag. Mix the bag thoroughly; this dilution will result in a concentration of 200mcg/mL and should be sufficient for at least 2 hrs of dosing. Patients ≥100kg will require a minimum of 2 bags.

Reconstituted vial should be diluted immediately. Diluted sol is stable for up to 12 hrs in D5W and 24 hrs in normal saline at room temperature.

STORAGE
20-25°C (68-77°F) w/ excursions between 15-30°C (59-86°F).

HOW SUPPLIED
Inj: 50mg [10mL]

CONTRAINDICATIONS
Significant active bleeding, known hypersensitivity (eg, anaphylaxis) to cangrelor or any component of the product.

WARNINGS/PRECAUTIONS
Increased risk of bleeding; after discontinuation, there is no antiplatelet effect after an hr. Worsening renal function reported in patients w/ severe renal impairment (CrCl <30mL/min).

ADVERSE REACTIONS
Bleeding.

DRUG INTERACTIONS
If clopidogrel or prasugrel is administered during cangrelor infusion, it will have no antiplatelet effect until the next dose is administered; do not administer until infusion is discontinued.

PREGNANCY AND LACTATION
Category C, safety not known in nursing.

MECHANISM OF ACTION
Direct-acting P2Y₁₂ platelet receptor inhibitor; blocks ADP-induced platelet activation and aggregation. Binds selectively and reversibly to the P2Y₁₂ receptor to prevent further signaling and platelet activation.

PHARMACOKINETICS
Absorption: T_{max}=2 min. **Distribution:** V_d=3.9L. Plasma protein binding (97-98%). **Metabolism:** Rapidly deactivated via dephosphorylation to primary metabolite, a nucleoside. **Elimination:** Urine (58%), feces (35%). $T_{1/2}$=3-6 min.

PATIENT CONSIDERATIONS
Assessment: Assess for hypersensitivity, active bleeding, renal impairment, pregnancy/nursing status, and possible drug interactions.
Monitoring: Monitor for bleeding and other adverse reactions.
Counseling: Inform of the risks and benefits of therapy. Instruct to contact physician if hypersensitivity reactions (eg, anaphylaxis) or unusual bleeding develops.

KEPPRA — levetiracetam

Rx

Class: Pyrrolidine derivative

ADULT DOSAGE

Partial Onset Seizures

Adjunctive Therapy for Patients w/ Epilepsy:
≥16 Years:
Initial: 500mg bid
Titrate: May increase by 1000mg/day every 2 weeks
Max: 3000mg/day

Myoclonic Seizures

Adjunctive Therapy for Patients w/ Juvenile Myoclonic Epilepsy:
Initial: 500mg bid
Titrate: Increase by 1000mg/day every 2 weeks to recommended dose of 3000mg/day

Tonic-Clonic Seizures

Adjunctive Therapy in the Treatment of Primary Generalized Tonic-Clonic Seizures w/ Idiopathic Generalized Epilepsy:
≥16 Years:
Initial: 500mg bid
Titrate: Increase by 1000mg/day every 2 weeks to recommended dose of 3000mg/day

Conversions

Switching from Oral Dosing:
Initial total daily IV dose should be equivalent to the total daily dose and frequency of oral formulation

Switching to Oral Dosing:
At the end of IV treatment period, switch at equivalent daily dose and frequency of IV administration

PEDIATRIC DOSAGE

Partial Onset Seizures

Adjunctive Therapy for Patients w/ Epilepsy:
1-<6 Months of Age:
Initial: 7mg/kg bid
Titrate: Increase by 14mg/kg/day every 2 weeks to recommended dose of 21mg/kg bid
6 Months-<4 Years:
Initial: 10mg/kg bid
Titrate: Increase by 20mg/kg/day in 2 weeks to recommended dose of 25mg/kg bid; may reduce dose if 50mg/kg/day cannot be tolerated
4-<16 Years:
Initial: 10mg/kg bid
Titrate: Increase by 20mg/kg/day every 2 weeks to recommended dose of 30mg/kg bid; may reduce dose if 60mg/kg/day cannot be tolerated
Max: 3000mg/day
Tab:
20-40kg:
Initial: 250mg bid
Titrate: Increase by 500mg/day every 2 weeks
Max: 750mg bid
>40kg:
Initial: 500mg bid
Titrate: Increase by 1000mg/day every 2 weeks
Max: 1500mg bid

Myoclonic Seizures

Adjunctive Therapy for Patients w/ Juvenile Myoclonic Epilepsy:
≥12 Years:
Initial: 500mg bid
Titrate: Increase by 1000mg/day every 2 weeks to recommended dose of 3000mg/day

Tonic-Clonic Seizures

Adjunctive Therapy in the Treatment of Primary Generalized Tonic-Clonic Seizures w/ Idiopathic Generalized Epilepsy:
6-<16 Years:
Initial: 10mg/kg bid
Titrate: Increase by 20mg/kg/day every 2 weeks to recommended dose of 30mg/kg bid

Conversions

Switching from Oral Dosing:
Initial total daily IV dose should be equivalent to the total daily dose and frequency of oral formulation

Switching to Oral Dosing:
At the end of IV treatment period, switch at equivalent daily dose and frequency of IV administration

DOSING CONSIDERATIONS

Renal Impairment

Adults:
Mild (CrCl 50-80mL/min): 500-1000mg q12h
Moderate (CrCl 30-50mL/min): 250-750mg q12h
Severe (CrCl <30mL/min): 250-500mg q12h
ESRD Using Dialysis: 500-1000mg q24h
Following dialysis, a supplemental dose of 250-500mg is recommended

ADMINISTRATION

Oral/IV route

Oral

Take w/ or w/o food.
Prescribe oral sol for pediatric patients ≤20kg.
Prescribe oral sol or tabs for pediatric patients >20kg.
Tab:
Swallow whole; do not crush or chew.
Sol:
Dosing is weight-based using a calibrated measuring device.

IV

Use only as an alternative for patients when oral administration is temporarily not feasible.
Administer as a 15-min IV infusion following dilution.
Dilute in 100mL of a compatible diluent; if smaller volume is required, amount of diluent should be calculated to not exceed a max. levetiracetam concentration of 15mg/mL of diluted sol.
Consider total daily fluid intake of patient.
May be stored in polyvinyl chloride bags.
Diluted sol should not be stored for >4 hrs at 15-30°C (59-86°F).

Compatible Diluents:
0.9% NaCl inj
Lactated Ringer's inj
D5 inj

Compatible Antiepileptic Drugs:
Lorazepam
Diazepam
Valproate sodium

IV/Sol

Refer to PI for weight-based dosing calculation

STORAGE

25°C (77°F); excursions permitted to 15-30°C (59-86°F).

HOW SUPPLIED

Inj: 100mg/mL [5mL]; **Sol:** 100mg/mL [16 fl oz]; **Tab:** 250mg*, 500mg*, 750mg*, 1000mg* *scored

WARNINGS/PRECAUTIONS

May cause behavioral abnormalities, psychotic symptoms, somnolence, fatigue, and coordination difficulties. May impair mental/physical abilities. May increase risk of suicidal thoughts/behavior. Serious dermatological reactions (eg, Stevens-Johnson syndrome [SJS], toxic epidermal necrolysis [TEN]), and recurrence of serious skin reactions following rechallenge reported; d/c at the 1st sign of rash, unless the rash is clearly not drug-related. Do not resume, and consider alternative therapy if signs/symptoms suggest SJS/TEN. Withdraw gradually to minimize the potential of increased seizure frequency. Hematologic abnormalities reported. Increased diastolic BP reported w/ an oral formulation of Keppra in patients 1 month to <4 years of age. Physiological changes may decrease plasma levels of levetiracetam throughout pregnancy; monitor patients during pregnancy and through the postpartum period, especially if the dose was changed during pregnancy. Caution in elderly.

ADVERSE REACTIONS

Adults: Somnolence, asthenia, infection, dizziness.
Pediatrics: Fatigue, aggression, nasal congestion, decreased appetite, irritability.

PREGNANCY AND LACTATION

Pregnancy: Category C; physicians are advised to recommend that pregnant patients enroll in the North American Antiepileptic Drug (NAAED) Pregnancy Registry.
Lactation: Levetiracetam is excreted in human milk; not for use in nursing.

MECHANISM OF ACTION

Pyrrolidine derivative; has not been established. Inhibits burst firing w/o affecting normal neuronal excitability, suggesting that it may selectively prevent hypersynchronization of epileptiform burst firing and propagation of seizure activity.

PHARMACOKINETICS

Absorption: (Oral) Rapid and almost complete. Oral bioavailability (100%); T_{max}=1 hr (fasting). **Distribution:** Plasma protein binding (<10%); found in breast milk. **Metabolism:** Enzymatic hydrolysis of acetamide group; ucb L057 (metabolite). **Elimination:** Renal (66%, unchanged); $T_{1/2}$=7 hrs.

PATIENT CONSIDERATIONS

Assessment: Assess for renal impairment, depression, suicidal thoughts/behavior, and pregnancy/nursing status.

Monitoring: Monitor for behavioral abnormalities, psychotic symptoms, suicidal behavior/ideation, somnolence, fatigue, coordination difficulties, serious dermatological reactions, hematologic abnormalities, and other adverse reactions. Monitor patients during pregnancy and continue close monitoring through the postpartum period, especially if the dose was changed during pregnancy. Monitor for increase in diastolic BP in patients 1 month to <4 yrs of age.

Counseling: Advise patients and their caregivers that the drug may cause behavioral changes and psychotic symptoms. Inform that the drug may increase the risk of suicidal thoughts and behavior; advise to be alert for the emergence or worsening of symptoms of depression, unusual changes in mood/behavior, or the emergence of suicidal thoughts, behavior, or thoughts about self-harm. Instruct to immediately report behaviors of concern to physician. Inform that dizziness and somnolence may occur; advise not to drive, operate heavy machinery, or engage in other hazardous activities until patients have gained sufficient experience to gauge whether it adversely affects their performance of these activities. Inform that serious dermatological adverse reactions have been reported; advise to notify physician if a rash develops. Advise to notify physician if patient becomes pregnant or intends to become pregnant; encourage to enroll in the NAAED pregnancy registry.

KEPPRA XR — levetiracetam

Rx

Class: Pyrrolidine derivative

ADULT DOSAGE

Partial Onset Seizures

Adjunctive Therapy in Patients w/ Epilepsy:
Initial: 1000mg qd
Titrate: Adjust dose in increments of 1000mg every 2 weeks
Max: 3000mg/day

PEDIATRIC DOSAGE

Partial Onset Seizures

Adjunctive Therapy in Patients w/ Epilepsy:
≥12 Years:
Initial: 1000mg qd
Titrate: Adjust dose in increments of 1000mg every 2 weeks
Max: 3000mg/day

DOSING CONSIDERATIONS

Renal Impairment

Adults:
Mild (CrCl 50-80mL/min): 1000-2000mg q24h
Moderate (CrCl 30-50mL/min): 500-1500mg q24h
Severe (CrCl <30mL/min): 500-1000mg q24h
ESRD on Dialysis: Use immediate-release formulation

ADMINISTRATION

Oral route

Swallow tabs whole; do not chew, break, or crush.

STORAGE

25°C (77°F); excursions permitted to 15-30°C (59-86°F).

HOW SUPPLIED

Tab, Extended-Release: 500mg, 750mg

WARNINGS/PRECAUTIONS

May cause behavioral abnormalities, psychotic symptoms, somnolence, fatigue, and coordination difficulties. Increased risk of suicidal thoughts/behavior. May impair mental/physical abilities. Serious dermatological reactions (eg, Stevens-Johnson syndrome [SJS], toxic epidermal necrolysis [TEN]) and recurrence of serious skin reactions following rechallenge reported; d/c at the 1st sign of rash, unless the rash is clearly not drug-related. If signs/symptoms suggest SJS/TEN, do not resume therapy and consider alternative therapy. Withdraw gradually to minimize the potential of increased seizure frequency. Hematologic abnormalities reported. Physiological changes may decrease plasma levels of levetiracetam throughout pregnancy; carefully monitor during pregnancy and continue close monitoring through the postpartum period especially if the dose was changed during pregnancy. Caution in elderly.

ADVERSE REACTIONS

Somnolence, irritability.

PREGNANCY AND LACTATION

Pregnancy: Category C; physicians are advised to recommend that pregnant patients enroll in the North American Antiepileptic Drug (NAAED) Pregnancy Registry.
Lactation: Levetiracetam is excreted in human milk; not for use in nursing.

MECHANISM OF ACTION

Pyrrolidine derivative; not established. Inhibits burst firing w/o affecting normal neuronal excitability, suggesting that it may selectively prevent hypersynchronization of epileptiform burst firing and propagation of seizure activity.

PHARMACOKINETICS

Absorption: Almost complete; T_{max}=4 hrs. **Distribution:** Plasma protein binding (<10%); found in breast milk. **Metabolism:** Enzymatic hydrolysis of acetamide group; ucb L057 (metabolite). **Elimination:** Renal (66%, unchanged); $T_{1/2}$=7 hrs.

PATIENT CONSIDERATIONS

Assessment: Assess for renal impairment, depression, suicidal thoughts/behavior, and pregnancy/nursing status.

Monitoring: Monitor for behavioral abnormalities, psychotic symptoms, suicidal behavior/ideation, somnolence, fatigue, coordination difficulties, serious dermatological reactions, hematologic abnormalities, and other adverse reactions. Monitor patients during pregnancy and continue close monitoring through the postpartum period, especially if the dose was changed during pregnancy.

Counseling: Inform that the drug may increase the risk of suicidal thoughts/behavior; instruct to immediately report the emergence or worsening of symptoms of depression, any unusual changes in mood/behavior, or suicidal thoughts, behavior, or thoughts about self-harm to physician. Counsel that medication may cause changes in behavior (eg, irritability and aggression). Inform that dizziness and somnolence may occur; advise not to drive or operate heavy machinery or engage in other hazardous activities until patients have gained sufficient experience to gauge whether it adversely affects their performance of these activities. Advise that serious dermatological adverse reactions may occur; instruct to notify physician immediately if rash develops. Instruct to take as directed. Inform patients that they should not be concerned if they occasionally notice something that looks like swollen pieces of the original tablet in their stool. Advise to notify physician if patient becomes pregnant or intends to become pregnant; encourage to enroll in the NAAED pregnancy registry.

KERYDIN — tavaborole

Rx

Class: Antifungal agent

ADULT DOSAGE

Onychomycosis

Onychomycosis of the Toenails Due to *Trichophyton rubrum*/*Trichophyton mentagrophytes*:

Apply to affected toenails qd for 48 weeks

PEDIATRIC DOSAGE

Pediatric use may not have been established

ADMINISTRATION

Topical route

Apply to the entire toenail surface and under the tip of each toenail being treated

STORAGE

20-25°C (68-77°F); excursions permitted to 15-30°C (59-86°F). Flammable; keep away from heat and flame. Discard w/in 3 months after insertion of the dropper.

HOW SUPPLIED

Sol: 5% [4mL, 10mL]

ADVERSE REACTIONS

Application-site exfoliation/erythema/dermatitis, ingrown toenail.

PREGNANCY AND LACTATION

Category C, caution in nursing.

MECHANISM OF ACTION

Oxaborole antifungal; inhibits fungal protein synthesis by inhibition of an aminoacyl-transfer ribonucleic acid synthetase.

PHARMACOKINETICS

Absorption: (Single dose) C_{max}=3.54ng/mL; AUC=44.4ng•hr/mL. (Multiple dose) C_{max}=5.17ng/mL; AUC=75.8ng•hr/mL. **Metabolism:** Extensive. **Elimination:** Urine.

PATIENT CONSIDERATIONS

Assessment: Assess pregnancy/nursing status.

Monitoring: Monitor for adverse reactions.

Counseling: Instruct to use ud, and to avoid contact w/ eyes, mouth, or vagina. Advise to avoid contact w/ skin other than that immediately surrounding the treated nail(s); instruct to wipe away excess sol from surrounding skin. Instruct to clean and dry nails prior to use. Advise to allow sol to dry following application. Inform that the impact of nail polish or other cosmetic nail products on the efficacy of therapy has not been evaluated. Instruct to inform physician if the area of application shows signs of persistent irritation (eg, redness, itching, swelling). Advise not to use for any disorder other than that for which it is prescribed.

KETEK — telithromycin

Rx

Class: Ketolide antibiotic

> Contraindicated w/ myasthenia gravis. Fatal and life-threatening respiratory failure reported in patients w/ myasthenia gravis.

ADULT DOSAGE

Community-Acquired Pneumonia

Mild to Moderate:
800mg qd for 7-10 days

PEDIATRIC DOSAGE

Pediatric use may not have been established

DOSING CONSIDERATIONS

Renal Impairment

Severe (CrCl <30mL/min)/Hemodialysis: 600mg qd; give after dialysis session on dialysis days if undergoing hemodialysis
Severe Impairment (CrCl <30mL/min) w/ Hepatic Impairment: 400mg qd

ADMINISTRATION

Oral route

Take w/ or w/o food.

STORAGE

25°C (77°F); excursions permitted to 15-30°C (59-86°F).

HOW SUPPLIED

Tab: 300mg, 400mg

CONTRAINDICATIONS

Myasthenia gravis; history of hepatitis and/or jaundice associated w/ use of telithromycin or any macrolide antibacterial; history of hypersensitivity to telithromycin, any components of this medication, or any macrolide antibacterial; concomitant use w/ cisapride or pimozide; and concomitant use w/ colchicine in patients w/ renal or hepatic impairment.

WARNINGS/PRECAUTIONS

Acute hepatic failure and severe liver injury, including fulminant hepatitis and hepatic necrosis, reported; d/c if any signs/symptoms of hepatitis occur. Permanently d/c if clinical hepatitis or transaminase elevations combined w/ systemic symptoms occur. Less severe hepatic dysfunction w/ increased liver enzymes, hepatitis, and jaundice reported. May prolong QTc interval leading to increased risk for ventricular arrhythmias, including ventricular tachycardia and torsades de pointes; avoid in patients w/ congenital prolongation of QTc interval, w/ ongoing proarrhythmic conditions (eg, uncorrected hypokalemia/hypomagnesemia), or w/ clinically significant bradycardia. May cause visual disturbances or loss of consciousness; avoid hazardous activities (eg, driving, operating heavy machinery) if these symptoms occur. *Clostridium difficile*-associated diarrhea (CDAD) reported; may need to d/c if CDAD is suspected or confirmed. May result in bacterial resistance if used in the absence of a proven or suspected bacterial infection.

ADVERSE REACTIONS
Diarrhea, nausea.

DRUG INTERACTIONS
See Contraindications. If coadministration w/ colchicine is necessary in patients w/ normal renal/hepatic function, reduce colchicine dose and monitor for symptoms of colchicine toxicity. CYP3A4 inducers/inhibitors may affect levels, resulting in diminished efficacy or an increase or prolongation of effects; dose adjustments may be necessary for these drugs. Avoid w/ simvastatin, lovastatin, atorvastatin, ergot alkaloid derivatives (eg, ergotamine, dihydroergotamine), Class IA (eg, quinidine, procainamide) or Class III (eg, dofetilide) antiarrhythmics, rifampin and other CYP3A4 inducers (phenytoin, carbamazepine, phenobarbital), itraconazole, and ketoconazole. Hypotension, bradyarrhythmia, and loss of consciousness reported w/ calcium channel blockers (CCBs) that are CYP3A4 substrates (eg, verapamil, amlodipine, diltiazem); monitor for these adverse reactions and toxicity related to CCBs and adjust CCB dosage as necessary. Monitor for benzodiazepine-related adverse reactions and adjust midazolam dosage if necessary; caution w/ other benzodiazepines, which are metabolized by CYP3A4 and undergo a high 1st-pass effect (eg, triazolam). Caution w/ other drugs metabolized by the CYP3A4 (eg, cyclosporine, tacrolimus, sirolimus, hexobarbital); increases or prolongation of effects of these drugs may be observed. Coadministration w/ metoprolol in patients w/ heart failure may lead to metoprolol toxicity; monitor for metoprolol toxicity and adjust metoprolol dosage. Caution w/ digoxin; monitor for digoxin side effects or serum levels. Theophylline may worsen GI side effects, especially in females; administer 1 hr apart to decrease likelihood of GI side effects. May potentiate the effects of oral anticoagulants; consider monitoring PT/INR.

PREGNANCY AND LACTATION
Pregnancy: Category C.
Lactation: May be excreted in human milk; caution in nursing.

MECHANISM OF ACTION
Ketolide antibiotic; blocks protein synthesis by binding to domains II and V of 23S rRNA of 50S ribosomal subunit and may also inhibit assembly of nascent ribosomal units.

PHARMACOKINETICS
Absorption: Absolute bioavailability (57%); C_{max}=1.9mcg/mL (single dose), 2.27mcg/mL (multiple dose); T_{max}=1 hr (median); $AUC_{(0-24)}$=8.25mcg•hr/mL (single dose), 12.5mcg•hr/mL (multiple dose). **Distribution:** V_d=2.9L/kg (IV); plasma protein binding (60-70%). **Metabolism:** Via CYP3A4 dependent and independent pathways. **Elimination:** Urine (13% unchanged), feces (7% unchanged); $T_{1/2}$=7.16 hrs (single dose), 9.81 hrs (multiple dose).

PATIENT CONSIDERATIONS
Assessment: Assess for myasthenia gravis, history of hepatitis and/or jaundice associated w/ the use of telithromycin or any macrolides, history of hypersensitivity to telithromycin or any macrolides, renal/hepatic impairment, risk for QTc prolongation, pregnancy/nursing status, and possible drug interactions. Perform culture and susceptibility testing.

Monitoring: Monitor for signs/symptoms of hepatitis, QTc prolongation, ventricular arrhythmias, visual disturbances, loss of consciousness, CDAD, and other adverse reactions. Monitor LFTs in patients w/ signs and symptoms of hepatitis. Consider monitoring PT/INR w/ oral anticoagulants.

Counseling: Inform that therapy treats only bacterial, not viral, infections. Instruct to take exactly ud even if the patient feels better early in the course of therapy; inform that skipping doses or not completing full course may decrease effectiveness and may increase likelihood of bacterial resistance. Instruct to d/c and seek medical attention immediately if signs/symptoms of liver injury occur. Advise to report any fainting or palpitations occurring during treatment. Counsel on problems w/ vision and loss of consciousness. Advise to minimize engaging in hazardous activities (eg, driving, operating machinery) and to seek physician's advice before taking another dose if visual difficulties, loss of consciousness/fainting, confusion, or hallucination occurs. Advise to inform physician of any other medications concurrently being taken, including OTC products and dietary supplements. Inform that diarrhea is a common problem caused by therapy; instruct to contact physician as soon as possible if watery and bloody stools (w/ or w/o stomach cramps and fever) occur, even as late as ≥2 months after taking last dose.

KETOPROFEN — ketoprofen
Class: NSAID

Rx

> NSAIDs cause an increased risk of serious cardiovascular (CV) thrombotic events (eg, MI, stroke), which can be fatal; risk may occur early in treatment and may increase w/ duration of use. Contraindicated in the setting of CABG surgery. NSAIDs cause an increased risk of serious GI adverse events (eg, bleeding, ulceration, perforation of the stomach/intestines), which can be fatal and can occur at any time during use and w/o warning symptoms; elderly patients are at greater risk.

OTHER BRAND NAMES
Orudis (Discontinued)

ADULT DOSAGE
Osteoarthritis
Initial: 75mg tid or 50mg qid
Max: 300mg/day

PEDIATRIC DOSAGE
Pediatric use may not have been established

Rheumatoid Arthritis
Initial: 75mg tid or 50mg qid
Max: 300mg/day
Mild to Moderate Pain
Usual: 25-50mg q6-8h prn; doses >75mg not shown to give added analgesia
Max: 300mg/day
Primary Dysmenorrhea
Usual: 25-50mg q6-8h prn; doses >75mg not shown to give added analgesia
Max: 300mg/day

DOSING CONSIDERATIONS
Renal Impairment
Mild:
Max: 150mg/day
Severe (GFR <25mL/min/1.73m² or End-Stage Renal Impairment):
Max: 100mg/day
Hypoalbuminemia and Reduced Renal Function: Start on lower dose
Hepatic Impairment
Impaired Liver Function and Serum Albumin <3.5g/dL:
Max Initial: 100mg/day
Elderly
≥75 Years: Reduce initial dose
Other Important Considerations
Smaller Individuals/Debilitated: Reduce initial dose

ADMINISTRATION
Oral route

May take w/ antacids, food, or milk to reduce GI effects.
Concomitant use of ketoprofen immediate-release caps and ketoprofen extended-release caps is not recommended.

STORAGE
20-25°C (68-77°F). Protect from direct light and excessive heat and humidity.

HOW SUPPLIED
Cap: 50mg, 75mg

CONTRAINDICATIONS
Hypersensitivity to ketoprofen; asthma, urticaria, or allergic-type reactions after taking aspirin (ASA) or other NSAIDs; treatment in the setting of CABG surgery.

WARNINGS/PRECAUTIONS
Use lowest effective dose for the shortest duration possible. Increased CV thrombotic risk reported at higher doses. Avoid in patients w/ a recent MI unless benefits outweigh the risks; if used, monitor for signs of cardiac ischemia. May cause HTN or worsen preexisting HTN. Fluid retention and edema reported. Avoid in patients w/ severe heart failure (HF) unless benefits outweigh the risks; if used, monitor for signs of worsening HF. Use w/ extreme caution in patients w/ history of ulcer disease or GI bleeding, or risk factors for GI bleeding (eg, longer duration of NSAID therapy, older age, poor general health status). D/C if a serious GI adverse event is suspected, until event is ruled out; for high-risk patients, consider alternate therapies that do not involve NSAIDs. Renal papillary necrosis and other renal injury reported w/ long-term use. Renal toxicity also reported in patients in whom renal prostaglandins have a compensatory role in the maintenance of renal perfusion; increased risk w/ renal/hepatic impairment, HF, and in elderly. Not recommended w/ advanced renal disease; if therapy must be initiated, closely monitor renal function. Interstitial nephritis or nephrotic syndrome reported (rare). Anaphylactoid reactions may occur; avoid w/ ASA triad. May cause serious skin reactions (eg, exfoliative dermatitis, Stevens-Johnson syndrome, toxic epidermal necrolysis); d/c at 1st appearance of skin rash or any other sign of hypersensitivity. Avoid in late pregnancy; may cause premature closure of ductus arteriosus. Not a substitute for corticosteroids or for the treatment of corticosteroid insufficiency. May mask signs of inflammation and fever. May cause elevation of LFTs or severe hepatic reactions (eg, jaundice, fatal fulminant hepatitis, liver necrosis, hepatic failure); d/c if liver disease develops, systemic manifestations occur, or abnormal LFTs persist/worsen. Anemia may occur; monitor Hgb/Hct if anemia develops. May inhibit platelet aggregation and prolong bleeding time; carefully monitor patients w/ coagulation disorders. Caution w/ preexisting asthma.

ADVERSE REACTIONS
Dyspepsia, nausea, abdominal pain, diarrhea, constipation, flatulence, headache, CNS inhibition or excitation.

DRUG INTERACTIONS
May diminish the antihypertensive effect of ACE inhibitors. Increased risk of renal toxicity w/ diuretics and ACE inhibitors. Not recommended w/ ASA due to potential for increased adverse effects. May reduce the natriuretic effect of thiazide and loop diuretics. May increase lithium levels; monitor for lithium toxicity. May enhance methotrexate toxicity; caution w/ concomitant use. Probenecid increases both free and bound ketoprofen; combination not recommended. Synergistic effect on GI bleeding w/ warfarin. Monitor patients receiving anticoagulants. Increased risk of GI bleeding w/ oral corticosteroids, anticoagulants, smoking, and alcohol use. May blunt the CV effects of several therapeutic agents used to treat fluid retention and edema (eg, diuretics, ACE inhibitors, ARBs).

PREGNANCY AND LACTATION
Pregnancy: Category C.
Lactation: Not for use in nursing.

MECHANISM OF ACTION

NSAID; has not been established. Has anti-inflammatory, analgesic, and antipyretic properties. Shown to have inhibitory effects on prostaglandin and leukotriene synthesis, to have antibradykinin activity, as well as to have lysosomal membrane-stabilizing action.

PHARMACOKINETICS

Absorption: Rapid and well-absorbed; bioavailability (approx 90%); C_{max}=3.9mg/L (fasted), 2.4mg/L (fed), T_{max}=1.2 hrs (fasted), 2 hrs (fed). AUC_{0-24h}=32.1mg•h/L (fasted), 36.6mg•h/L (fed). **Distribution:** Plasma protein binding (>99%). **Metabolism:** Glucuronide conjugation. **Elimination:** Urine (80% primarily as the glucuronide metabolite); $T_{1/2}$=2.1 hrs.

PATIENT CONSIDERATIONS

Assessment: Assess for history of asthma, urticaria, or allergic-type reactions w/ ASA or other NSAIDs, ASA triad, HTN, recent MI, severe HF, history of ulcer disease or GI bleeding, coagulation disorders, renal/hepatic impairment, pregnancy/nursing status, any other conditions where treatment is contraindicated or cautioned, and possible drug interactions. Obtain baseline BP.

Monitoring: Monitor for GI bleeding/ulceration/perforation, CV thrombotic events, MI, stroke, HTN, fluid retention, edema, serious skin reactions, anaphylactoid reactions, and other adverse reactions. Monitor BP, CBC, bleeding time, LFTs, renal function, and chemistry profile periodically.

Counseling: Instruct to notify physician immediately if symptoms of CV thrombotic events, GI ulceration/bleeding, skin/hypersensitivity reactions, CHF, hepatotoxicity, or anaphylactoid reactions occur. Instruct to avoid in late pregnancy.

KETOPROFEN EXTENDED-RELEASE – ketoprofen Rx

Class: NSAID

> NSAIDs cause an increased risk of serious cardiovascular (CV) thrombotic events (eg, MI, stroke), which can be fatal; risk may occur early in treatment and may increase w/ duration of use. Contraindicated in the setting of CABG surgery. NSAIDs cause an increased risk of serious GI adverse events (eg, bleeding, ulceration, perforation of the stomach/intestines), which can be fatal and can occur at any time during use and w/o warning symptoms; elderly patients are at greater risk.

OTHER BRAND NAMES

Oruvail (Discontinued)

ADULT DOSAGE

Osteoarthritis

Initial: 200mg qd
Max: 200mg/day

Rheumatoid Arthritis

Initial: 200mg qd
Max: 200mg/day

PEDIATRIC DOSAGE

Pediatric use may not have been established

DOSING CONSIDERATIONS

Renal Impairment
Mild:
Max: 150mg/day
Severe (GFR <25mL/min/1.73m² or End-Stage Renal Impairment):
Max: 100mg/day

Hypoalbuminemia and Reduced Renal Function: Start on lower dose

Hepatic Impairment
Impaired Liver Function and Serum Albumin <3.5g/dL:
Max Initial: 100mg/day

Elderly
≥75 Years: Reduce initial dose

Other Important Considerations
Smaller Individuals/Debilitated: Reduce initial dose

ADMINISTRATION

Oral route

May take w/ antacids, food, or milk to reduce GI effects.
Concomitant use of ketoprofen immediate-release caps and ketoprofen extended-release caps is not recommended.

STORAGE

20-25°C (68-77°F). Protect from direct light and excessive heat and humidity.

HOW SUPPLIED

Cap, Extended-Release: 200mg

CONTRAINDICATIONS

Hypersensitivity to ketoprofen; asthma, urticaria, or allergic-type reactions after taking aspirin (ASA) or other NSAIDs; treatment in the setting of CABG surgery.

WARNINGS/PRECAUTIONS

Not recommended for treatment of acute pain. Use lowest effective dose for the shortest duration possible. Increased CV thrombotic risk reported at higher doses. Avoid in patients w/ a recent MI unless benefits outweigh the risks; if used, monitor for signs of cardiac ischemia. May cause HTN or worsen preexisting HTN. Fluid retention and edema reported. Avoid in patients w/ severe heart failure (HF) unless benefits outweigh the risks; if used, monitor for signs of worsening HF. Use w/ extreme caution in patients w/ history of ulcer disease or GI bleeding, or risk factors for GI bleeding (eg, longer duration of NSAID therapy, older age, poor general health status). D/C if a serious GI adverse event is suspected, until event is ruled out; for high-risk patients, consider alternate therapies that do not involve NSAIDs. Renal papillary necrosis and other renal injury reported w/ long-term use. Renal toxicity also reported in patients in whom renal prostaglandins have a compensatory role in the maintenance of renal perfusion; increased risk w/ renal/hepatic impairment, HF, and in elderly. Not recommended w/ advanced renal disease; if therapy must be initiated, closely monitor renal function. Interstitial nephritis or nephrotic syndrome reported (rare). D/C if renal disease develops. Anaphylactoid reactions may occur; avoid w/ ASA triad. May cause serious skin reactions (eg, exfoliative dermatitis, Stevens-Johnson syndrome, toxic epidermal necrolysis); d/c at 1st appearance of skin rash or any other sign of hypersensitivity. Avoid in late pregnancy; may cause premature closure of ductus arteriosus. Not a substitute for corticosteroids or for the treatment of corticosteroid insufficiency. May mask signs of inflammation and fever. May cause elevation of LFTs or severe hepatic reactions (eg, jaundice, fatal fulminant hepatitis, liver necrosis, hepatic failure); d/c if liver disease develops, systemic manifestations occur, or abnormal LFTs persist/worsen. Anemia may occur; monitor Hgb/Hct if anemia develops. May inhibit platelet aggregation and prolong bleeding time; carefully monitor patients w/ coagulation disorders. Caution w/ preexisting asthma.

ADVERSE REACTIONS

Dyspepsia, nausea, abdominal pain, diarrhea, constipation, flatulence, headache, CNS inhibition or excitation.

DRUG INTERACTIONS

May diminish the antihypertensive effect of ACE inhibitors. Increased risk of renal toxicity w/ diuretics and ACE inhibitors. Not recommended w/ ASA due to potential for increased adverse effects. May reduce the natriuretic effect of thiazide and loop diuretics. May increase lithium levels; monitor for lithium toxicity. May enhance methotrexate toxicity; caution w/ concomitant use. Probenecid increases both free and bound ketoprofen; combination not recommended. Synergistic effect on GI bleeding w/ warfarin. Monitor patients receiving anticoagulants. Increased risk of GI bleeding w/ oral corticosteroids, anticoagulants, smoking, and alcohol use. May blunt the CV effects of several therapeutic agents used to treat fluid retention and edema (eg, diuretics, ACE inhibitors, ARBs).

PREGNANCY AND LACTATION

Pregnancy: Category C.
Lactation: Not for use in nursing.

MECHANISM OF ACTION

NSAID; has not been established. Has anti-inflammatory, analgesic, and antipyretic properties. Shown to have inhibitory effects on prostaglandin and leukotriene synthesis, to have antibradykinin activity, as well as to have lysosomal membrane-stabilizing action.

PHARMACOKINETICS

Absorption: Well-absorbed; bioavailability (approx 90%); C_{max}=3.1mg/L (fasted), 3.4mg/L (fed); T_{max}=6.8 hrs (fasted), 9.2 hrs (fed); AUC_{0-24h}=30.1mg•h/L (fasted), 31.3mg•h/L (fed). **Distribution:** Plasma protein binding (>99%). **Metabolism:** Glucuronide conjugation. **Elimination:** Urine (80% primarily as the glucuronide metabolite); $T_{1/2}$=5.4 hrs.

PATIENT CONSIDERATIONS

Assessment: Assess for history of asthma, urticaria, or allergic-type reactions w/ ASA or other NSAIDs, ASA triad, HTN, recent MI, severe HF, history of ulcer disease or GI bleeding, coagulation disorders, renal/hepatic impairment, pregnancy/nursing status, any other conditions where treatment is contraindicated or cautioned, and possible drug interactions. Obtain baseline BP.

Monitoring: Monitor for GI bleeding/ulceration/perforation, CV thrombotic events, MI, stroke, HTN, fluid retention, edema, serious skin reactions, anaphylactoid reactions, and other adverse reactions. Monitor BP, CBC, bleeding time, LFTs, renal function, and chemistry profile periodically.

Counseling: Instruct to notify physician immediately if symptoms of CV thrombotic events, GI ulceration/bleeding, skin/hypersensitivity reactions, congestive HF, hepatotoxicity, or anaphylactoid reactions occur. Instruct to avoid in late pregnancy.

KETOROLAC – ketorolac tromethamine Rx

Class: NSAID

> For short-term (up to 5 days in adults) use only; total combined duration of oral and inj use should not exceed 5 days. Use tab only as continuation therapy following IV/IM dosing, if necessary. Not indicated for use in pediatric patients and not indicated for minor or chronic painful conditions. Increasing the dose beyond the label recommendations will not provide better efficacy but will increase risk of developing serious adverse events. May cause peptic ulcers, GI bleeding, and/or perforation of the stomach or intestines; contraindicated w/ active peptic ulcer disease, recent GI bleeding or perforation, and in patients w/ a history of peptic ulcer disease or GI bleeding. The elderly are at greater risk for serious GI events. May increase risk of serious cardiovascular (CV) thrombotic events, including MI and stroke; risk may increase w/ duration of use. Contraindicated in the setting of CABG surgery, as prophylactic analgesic before any major surgery, w/ advanced renal impairment, in patients at risk for renal failure due to volume depletion, w/ suspected or confirmed cerebrovascular bleeding, w/ hemorrhagic diathesis, incomplete hemostasis, and in those at high-risk of bleeding, in labor and delivery, and in patients currently receiving aspirin (ASA) or NSAIDs. Adjust dosage for patients ≥65 yrs of age, <50kg (110 lbs), and w/ moderately elevated SrCr; doses of inj are not to exceed 60mg/day in these patients. (Inj) Hypersensitivity reactions reported and appropriate counteractive measures must be available when administering the 1st dose. Contraindicated in patients w/ previously demonstrated allergic manifestations to ASA or other NSAIDs, for intrathecal/epidural administration, and in nursing mothers.

OTHER BRAND NAMES

Toradol (Discontinued)

ADULT DOSAGE
Acute Pain

Short-Term (≤5 Days) Management of Moderately Severe Acute Pain:

Single-Dose Treatment:
IM Dosing:
<65 Years: One 60mg dose
≥65 Years: One 30mg dose
IV Dosing:
<65 Years: One 30mg dose
≥65 Years: One 15mg dose

Multiple-Dose Treatment (IV or IM):
<65 Years: 30mg q6h
Max: 120mg/day
≥65 Years: 15mg q6h
Max: 60mg/day

Breakthrough Pain:
Do not increase the dose or frequency of ketorolac; consider supplementing these regimens w/ low doses of opioids prn unless otherwise contraindicated

Oral (Following IV or IM Dosing):
17-64 Years: 20mg once, then 10mg q4-6h prn
≥65 Years: 10mg once, then 10mg q4-6h prn
Max: 40mg/day

PEDIATRIC DOSAGE
Pediatric use may not have been established

DOSING CONSIDERATIONS
Renal Impairment
Single-Dose Treatment:
IM Dosing: One 30mg dose
IV Dosing: One 15mg dose

Multiple-Dose Treatment (IV or IM):
15mg q6h
Max: 60mg/day

Oral (Following IV or IM Dosing):
10mg once, then 10mg q4-6h prn
Max: 40mg/day

Other Important Considerations
Patients <50kg (110 lbs):
Single-Dose Treatment:
IM Dosing: One 30mg dose
IV Dosing: One 15mg dose

Multiple-Dose Treatment (IV or IM):
15mg q6h
Max: 60mg/day

Oral (Following IV or IM Dosing):
10mg once, then 10mg q4-6h prn
Max: 40mg/day

ADMINISTRATION
IM/IV/Oral route

Combined duration of use of IV or IM dosing of ketorolac and ketorolac tabs is not to exceed 5 days.

Inj
IV bolus must be given over ≥15 sec.
IM administration should be given slowly and deeply into muscle.
Do not mix in a small volume (eg, in a syringe) w/ morphine sulfate, meperidine HCl, promethazine HCl, or hydroxyzine HCl; this will result in precipitation of ketorolac from sol.

Tab
Do not administer as initial dose; use is only indicated as continuation therapy to IV or IM dosing.
Do not shorten dosing interval of 4-6 hrs.

STORAGE
20-25°C (68-77°F). Protect from light.

HOW SUPPLIED
Inj: 15mg/mL [1mL], 30mg/mL [1mL, 2mL, 10mL]; **Tab:** 10mg

CONTRAINDICATIONS
Hypersensitivity to ketorolac tromethamine, active/history of peptic ulcer disease, recent/history of GI bleeding, recent GI perforation, advanced renal impairment or risk of renal failure due to volume depletion, labor and delivery, cerebrovascular bleeding, hemorrhagic diathesis, incomplete hemostasis, patients at high risk of bleeding. Patients who have experienced asthma, urticaria, or allergic reactions after taking ASA or other NSAIDs. Prophylactic analgesic before major surgery. Use in the setting of CABG surgery. Current ASA or NSAID use. Concomitant use of probenecid and pentoxifylline. (Inj) Neuraxial (epidural or intrathecal) administration. Nursing mothers.

WARNINGS/PRECAUTIONS
Do not give oral formulation as an initial dose. Use lowest effective dose for the shortest duration possible. Increased risk for GI bleeding w/ increased dose and duration of NSAID therapy, older age, and poor general health status. D/C and promptly initiate additional evaluation and treatment if a serious GI adverse event is suspected; consider alternate therapy that does not involve NSAIDs for high risk patients. May exacerbate inflammatory bowel disease (eg, ulcerative colitis, Crohn's disease). Renal papillary necrosis and other renal injury reported w/ long-term use. Renal toxicity reported; increased risk w/ renal/hepatic impairment, heart failure (HF), and in the elderly. Acute renal failure, interstitial nephritis, and nephrotic syndrome reported. Caution w/ impaired renal function or history of kidney disease. May cause anaphylactoid reactions and serious skin adverse events (eg, exfoliative dermatitis, Stevens-Johnson syndrome, toxic epidermal necrolysis); d/c at 1st appearance of skin rash or any other signs of hypersensitivity. Increased CV thrombotic risk w/ higher doses. Avoid use w/ a recent MI unless benefits outweigh the risks; if used w/ a recent MI, monitor for signs of cardiac ischemia. May lead to onset of new HTN or worsening of preexisting HTN; caution in patients w/ HTN. NSAID use may increase risk of MI, hospitalization, and death in patients w/ HF. Avoid use w/ severe HF unless benefits outweigh the risks; if used w/ severe HF, monitor for signs of worsening HF. Fluid retention and edema reported. Avoid in late pregnancy; may cause premature closure of the ductus arteriosus. Not a substitute for corticosteroids or for the treatment of corticosteroid insufficiency. May mask signs of inflammation. Caution w/ impaired hepatic function or history of liver disease; rare cases of severe hepatic reactions (eg, jaundice, fatal fulminant hepatitis, liver necrosis, hepatic failure) reported. Evaluate patients w/ signs/symptoms suggesting liver dysfunction, or w/ abnormal LFTs, for development of a more severe hepatic reaction; d/c if signs/symptoms of liver disease develop or systemic manifestations (eg, eosinophilia, rash) occur. Anemia may occur; monitor Hgb or Hct if signs/symptoms of anemia develop w/ long-term use. May inhibit platelet aggregation and prolong bleeding time; caution w/ coagulation disorders and in postoperative setting when hemostasis is critical. Caution w/ preexisting asthma and avoid w/ ASA-sensitive asthma. Use w/ extreme caution in the elderly. Caution in debilitated patients. (Inj) Correct hypovolemia prior to administration.

ADVERSE REACTIONS
Hypersensitivity reactions, nausea, headache, dyspepsia, abdominal pain, edema, drowsiness, dizziness, abnormal renal function.

DRUG INTERACTIONS
See Boxed Warning and Contraindications. Binding reduced w/ concomitant use w/ salicylate. May increase risk of bleeding w/ drugs affecting hemostasis (eg, warfarin, dicumarol derivatives, heparin, dextrans). May increase risk of serious GI bleeding w/ oral corticosteroids, anticoagulants, SSRIs, smoking, and alcohol. May reduce natriuretic effect of furosemide and thiazide diuretics; observe closely for signs of renal failure and diuretic efficacy. May elevate plasma lithium levels and reduce renal lithium clearance; monitor for lithium toxicity. May enhance methotrexate toxicity; caution w/ concomitant use. Caution w/ ACE inhibitors and/or ARBs; may increase risk of renal impairment and diminish antihypertensive effect of ACE inhibitors and/or ARBs. Sporadic cases of seizures reported w/ concomitant use w/ antiepileptic drugs (eg, phenytoin, carbamazepine). Hallucinations reported w/ psychoactive drugs (eg, fluoxetine, thiothixene, alprazolam). (Inj) Apnea reported w/ nondepolarizing muscle relaxants.

PREGNANCY AND LACTATION
Category C, (Inj) not for use in nursing, (Tab) caution in nursing.

MECHANISM OF ACTION
NSAID; has not been established. Suspected to inhibit prostaglandin synthetase.

PHARMACOKINETICS
Absorption: Absolute bioavailability (100%). Administration of variable doses/routes and in different populations resulted in different parameters. **Distribution:** V_d=13L; plasma protein binding (99%); found in breast milk. **Metabolism:** Liver; hydroxylation, conjugation. **Elimination:** Urine (92%; 40% metabolites, 60% unchanged), feces (6%); $T_{1/2}$=5-6 hrs (racemate), 2.5 hrs (S-enantiomer), 5 hrs (R-enantiomer).

PATIENT CONSIDERATIONS
Assessment: Confirm that use is not for CABG surgery. Assess for previous hypersensitivity to drug, history of asthma, urticaria, or allergic-type reactions w/ ASA or other NSAIDs, CV disease, risk factors for GI events, active/history of peptic ulcer disease, recent/history of GI bleeding, recent GI perforation, cerebrovascular bleeding, hemorrhagic diathesis, incomplete hemostasis, high risk of bleeding, renal/hepatic impairment, severe HF, any other conditions where therapy is cautioned or contraindicated, pregnancy/nursing status, and for possible drug interactions. Obtain baseline BP.

Monitoring: Monitor for GI events, anaphylactoid/skin/hypersensitivity reactions, CV events, fluid retention, edema, hematological effects, and other adverse reactions. Monitor BP, LFTs, and renal function. Monitor CBC and chemistry profile periodically during long-term use.

Counseling: Inform about potential risks/benefits of therapy. Advise not to give tab to other family members and to discard any unused drug. Instruct that the duration of use should not exceed 5 days. Inform that therapy is not indicated for use in pediatric patients. Instruct to seek medical attention for signs/symptoms of GI ulceration/bleeding, CV events, hepatotoxicity, skin reactions, anaphylactoid reaction, or congestive HF. Instruct to avoid use in late pregnancy.

KEVEYIS — dichlorphenamide   Rx

Class: Carbonic anhydrase inhibitor

ADULT DOSAGE

Periodic Paralysis

Primary Hyperkalemic Periodic Paralysis, Primary Hypokalemic Periodic Paralysis, and Related Variants:

Initial: 50mg bid
Titrate: Increase or decrease at weekly intervals based on response
Max: 200mg/day

Evaluate therapy after 2 months of treatment

PEDIATRIC DOSAGE

Pediatric use may not have been established

ADMINISTRATION
Oral route

STORAGE
20-25°C (68-77°F).

HOW SUPPLIED
Tab: 50mg* *scored

CONTRAINDICATIONS
Hypersensitivity to dichlorphenamide or other sulfonamides; hepatic insufficiency; severe pulmonary disease, limiting compensation to metabolic acidosis caused by dichlorphenamide; and concomitant use w/ high-dose aspirin (ASA).

WARNINGS/PRECAUTIONS
Fatalities associated w/ sulfonamides have occurred due to adverse reactions (eg, Stevens-Johnson syndrome, toxic epidermal necrolysis, fulminant hepatic necrosis, agranulocytosis, aplastic anemia, other blood dyscrasias); d/c at first appearance of skin rash or any sign of immune-mediated or idiosyncratic adverse reaction. Increases K^+ excretion and can cause hypokalemia; risk is greater when given to patients w/ conditions associated w/ hypokalemia, and in patients receiving other drugs that may cause hypokalemia. May cause hyperchloremic non-anion gap metabolic acidosis; concomitant use w/ other drugs that cause metabolic acidosis may increase the severity of metabolic acidosis. Baseline and periodic measurement of serum K^+ and serum bicarbonate are recommended. If hypokalemia or metabolic acidosis develops/persists, consider reducing dose or discontinuing dichlorphenamide. Increases risk of falls; risk is greater in elderly and w/ higher doses. Consider dose reduction/discontinuation in patients who experience falls while on therapy.

ADVERSE REACTIONS
Paresthesia, cognitive disorder, dysgeusia, confusional state, headache, hypoesthesia, lethargy, fatigue, muscle spasms, rash, diarrhea, nausea, malaise, decreased weight, dyspnea.

DRUG INTERACTIONS
See Contraindications. Anorexia, tachypnea, lethargy, and coma reported w/ high-dose ASA. Caution w/ low-dose ASA.

PREGNANCY AND LACTATION
Pregnancy: Category C.
Lactation: Caution in nursing.

MECHANISM OF ACTION
Carbonic anhydrase inhibitor; precise mechanism unknown.

PATIENT CONSIDERATIONS

Assessment: Assess for hypersensitivity to drug or other sulfonamides, hepatic insufficiency, severe pulmonary disease, conditions associated w/ hypokalemia, ASA use, and pregnancy/nursing status. Obtain baseline serum K^+ and serum bicarbonate levels.

Monitoring: Monitor for skin rash or any sign of immune-mediated or idiosyncratic adverse reaction. Evaluate patient's response to therapy after 2 months of treatment. Monitor serum K^+ and serum bicarbonate levels.

Counseling: Advise to notify physician if experiencing worsening symptoms of periodic paralysis. Inform that treatment may cause drowsiness/fatigue and may impair ability to drive and operate machinery.

KEYTRUDA — pembrolizumab   Rx

Class: Monoclonal antibody/programmed death receptor-1 (PD-1) blocker

ADULT DOSAGE

Unresectable or Metastatic Melanoma

2mg/kg every 3 weeks until disease progression or unacceptable toxicity

Metastatic Non-Small Cell Lung Cancer

Treatment of metastatic non-small cell lung cancer (NSCLC) in patients whose tumors express PD-L1 as determined by an FDA-approved test w/ disease progression on or after platinum-containing chemotherapy

Patients w/ epidermal growth factor

PEDIATRIC DOSAGE

Pediatric use may not have been established

receptor or anaplastic lymphoma kinase genomic tumor aberrations should have disease progression on FDA-approved therapy for these aberrations prior to receiving pembrolizumab

2mg/kg every 3 weeks until disease progression or unacceptable toxicity

Squamous Cell Carcinoma of the Head and Neck

Treatment of recurrent or metastatic head and neck squamous cell carcinoma (HNSCC) w/ disease progression on or after platinum-containing chemotherapy

200mg every 3 weeks until disease progression, unacceptable toxicity, or up to 24 months in patients w/o disease progression

---

DOSING CONSIDERATIONS

Adverse Reactions

Withhold for the Following:
- Grade 2 pneumonitis
- Grade 2 or 3 colitis
- Grade 3 or 4 endocrinopathies
- Grade 2 nephritis
- AST/ALT >3 and up to 5X ULN or total bilirubin >1.5 and up to 3X ULN
- Any other severe or Grade 3 treatment-related adverse reaction

Resume Therapy:
In patients whose adverse reactions recover to Grade 0-1

Permanently D/C for the Following:
- Any life-threatening adverse reaction (excluding endocrinopathies controlled w/ hormone replacement therapy)
- Grade 3 or 4 pneumonitis or recurrent pneumonitis of Grade 2 severity
- Grade 3 or 4 nephritis
- AST/ALT >5X ULN or total bilirubin >3X ULN; for patients w/ liver metastasis who begin treatment w/ Grade 2 AST/ALT, if AST/ALT increases by ≥50% relative to baseline and lasts for at least 1 week
- Grade 3 or 4 infusion-related reactions
- Inability to reduce corticosteroid dose to ≤10mg/day of prednisone (or equivalent) w/in 12 weeks
- Persistent Grade 2 or 3 adverse reactions (excluding endocrinopathies controlled w/ hormone replacement therapy) that do not recover to Grade 0-1 w/in 12 weeks after last dose of therapy
- Any severe or Grade 3 treatment-related adverse reaction that recurs

ADMINISTRATION
IV route

Administer as an IV infusion over 30 min through an IV line containing a sterile, non-pyrogenic, low-protein binding 0.2-5 micron in-line/add-on filter. Do not coadminister other drugs through the same infusion line.

Preparation
- Add 2.3mL of sterile water for inj for a resulting concentration of 25mg/mL; inject the water along the walls of the vial, not directly on lyophilized powder.
- Slowly swirl vial and allow up to 5 min for bubbles to clear; do not shake.
- Dilute inj sol or reconstituted powder prior to IV administration by withdrawing required volume from vial(s) and transferring into an IV bag containing 0.9% NaCl inj or D5 inj.
- Mix diluted sol by gentle inversion; final concentration should be 1-10mg/mL.

Reconstituted/Diluted Sol from 50mg Vial
Store at room temperature for ≤6 hrs from the time of reconstitution, or at 2-8°C (36-46°F) for ≤24 hrs from the time of reconstitution. If refrigerated, allow the diluted sol to come to room temperature prior to administration. Do not freeze.

Diluted Sol from 25mg/mL Vial
Store at room temperature for ≤6 hrs from the time of dilution, or at 2-8°C (36-46°F) for ≤24 hrs from the time of dilution. If refrigerated, allow the diluted sol to come to room temperature prior to administration. Do not freeze.

STORAGE
2-8°C (36-46°F). **Sol:** Protect from light. Do not freeze. Do not shake.

HOW SUPPLIED
Inj: (Powder) 50mg; (Sol) 25mg/mL [4mL]

WARNINGS/PRECAUTIONS
Immune-mediated pneumonitis, colitis, hepatitis, and nephritis reported; administer corticosteroids for ≥Grade 2. Hypophysitis reported; administer corticosteroids and hormone replacement as clinically indicated. Thyroid disorders can occur at any time during treatment. Administer replacement hormones for hypothyroidism and manage hyperthyroidism w/ thionamides and beta-blockers as appropriate. Type 1 diabetes mellitus (DM), including diabetic ketoacidosis, reported; administer insulin for type 1 DM, and withhold therapy and administer antihyperglycemics in patients w/ severe hyperglycemia. Other clinically important immune-mediated reactions may occur; evaluate and administer corticosteroids based on severity of the adverse reaction. Upon improvement to ≤Grade 1, initiate corticosteroid taper and continue to taper over at least 1 month. Severe and life-threatening infusion-related reactions reported. Can cause fetal harm.

ADVERSE REACTIONS

Melanoma: Fatigue, diarrhea.
NSCLC: Fatigue; decreased appetite, dyspnea, cough.
HNSCC: Fatigue, decreased appetite, dyspnea.

PREGNANCY AND LACTATION

Pregnancy: Can cause fetal harm based on its mechanism of action.
Lactation: D/C nursing during treatment and for 4 months after the final dose.
Reproductive Potential: Females of reproductive potential should use effective contraception during treatment and for at least 4 months following the final dose.

MECHANISM OF ACTION

Human PD-1-blocking antibody; binds to PD-1 receptor on T cells and blocks its interaction w/ PD-L1 and PD-L2, releasing PD-1 pathway-mediated inhibition of the immune response, including the anti-tumor immune response.

PHARMACOKINETICS

Distribution: V_d=7.38L. **Elimination:** $T_{1/2}$=27 days.

PATIENT CONSIDERATIONS

Assessment: Assess pregnancy/nursing status. Obtain baseline liver/renal/thyroid function.

Monitoring: Monitor for signs/symptoms of pneumonitis, colitis, hypophysitis, changes in liver/renal function, hyperglycemia/type 1 DM, infusion-related reactions, and other adverse reactions. Evaluate patients w/ suspected pneumonitis w/ radiographic imaging. Monitor for changes in thyroid function (periodically during treatment, and as indicated based on clinical evaluation) and for signs/symptoms of thyroid disorders. Monitor for immune-mediated adverse reactions; ensure adequate evaluation to confirm etiology or exclude other causes.

Counseling: Inform of the risk of immune-mediated adverse reactions that may require corticosteroid treatment and interruption or discontinuation of therapy (eg, pneumonitis, colitis, hepatitis, hypophysitis, nephritis, hyper/hypothyroidism, type 1 DM); instruct to immediately contact physician if signs/symptoms of an immune-mediated adverse reaction occur. Advise to contact physician immediately for signs/symptoms of infusion-related reactions. Advise of the importance of keeping scheduled appointments for blood work or other lab tests. Advise women that drug may cause fetal harm; instruct women of reproductive potential to use highly effective contraception during and for 4 months after the last dose of therapy. Advise nursing mothers not to breastfeed while taking therapy.

KHEDEZLA — desvenlafaxine   Rx

Class: Serotonin and norepinephrine reuptake inhibitor (SNRI)

> Antidepressants increased the risk of suicidal thoughts and behavior in children, adolescents, and young adults in short-term studies. Monitor and observe closely for worsening, and emergence of suicidal thoughts and behaviors. Not approved for use in pediatric patients.

ADULT DOSAGE

Major Depressive Disorder

50mg qd

Doses up to 400mg/day were effective but w/ no additional benefit; more frequent adverse reactions reported at higher doses

Periodically reassess need for continued treatment

Conversions

Switching from Other Antidepressants:
May need to taper the initial antidepressant to minimize discontinuation symptoms

Dosing Considerations with MAOIs

Switching to/from an MAOI for Psychiatric Disorders:
Allow at least 14 days between discontinuation of an MAOI and initiation of treatment, and conversely allow at least 7 days between discontinuing treatment and initiation of an MAOI

W/ Other MAOIs (eg, Linezolid, IV Methylene Blue):
Do not start desvenlafaxine in patients being treated w/ linezolid or IV methylene blue
In patients already receiving desvenlafaxine, if acceptable alternatives are not available and benefits outweigh risks, d/c desvenlafaxine and administer linezolid or IV methylene blue; monitor for serotonin syndrome for 7 days or until 24 hrs after the last dose of linezolid or IV methylene blue, whichever comes 1st. May resume desvenlafaxine therapy 24 hrs after the last dose of linezolid or IV methylene blue

PEDIATRIC DOSAGE

Pediatric use may not have been established

DOSING CONSIDERATIONS

Renal Impairment
Moderate (CrCl 30-50mL/min):
Max: 50mg/day

Severe (CrCl <30mL/min)/ESRD:
Max: 50mg qod. Do not give supplemental doses after dialysis

Hepatic Impairment
Moderate-Severe: 50mg/day
Max: 100mg/day

Discontinuation
Gradually reduce dose whenever possible
If intolerable symptoms occur following a decrease in dose or upon discontinuation of treatment, may consider resuming the previously prescribed dose; subsequently, may continue decreasing dose, but at a more gradual rate

ADMINISTRATION
Oral route

Take at the same time each day, w/ or w/o food.
Swallow tab whole w/ fluid; do not divide, crush, chew, or dissolve.

STORAGE
20-25°C (68-77°F); excursions permitted to 15-30°C (59-86°F).

HOW SUPPLIED
Tab, Extended-Release: 50mg, 100mg

CONTRAINDICATIONS
Hypersensitivity to desvenlafaxine succinate, venlafaxine hydrochloride or to any excipients in this formulation; use of an MAOI intended to treat psychiatric disorders either concomitantly or w/in 7 days of stopping treatment; treatment w/in 14 days of stopping an MAOI intended to treat psychiatric disorders. Starting treatment in patients being treated w/ other MAOIs (eg, linezolid, IV methylene blue).

WARNINGS/PRECAUTIONS
Not approved for the treatment of bipolar depression; screen patients to determine risk for bipolar disorder prior to initiating therapy. Serotonin syndrome reported; d/c immediately if symptoms occur and initiate supportive symptomatic treatment. May increase BP; caution w/ preexisting HTN, cardiovascular (CV), or cerebrovascular conditions that might be compromised by increases in BP. Consider dose reduction or discontinuation of therapy if sustained increases in BP occur. May increase risk of bleeding events. Pupillary dilation that occurs following use may trigger an angle-closure attack in a patient w/ anatomically narrow angles who does not have a patent iridectomy. Activation of mania/hypomania reported; caution w/ history or family history of mania/hypomania. Discontinuation symptoms reported. Avoid abrupt discontinuation; gradually reduce dose whenever possible. Seizures reported. Hyponatremia may occur; caution in elderly and volume-depleted patients. Consider discontinuation in patients w/ symptomatic hyponatremia and institute appropriate medical intervention. Interstitial lung disease and eosinophilic pneumonia may occur; consider this diagnosis in patients w/ progressive dyspnea, cough, or chest discomfort, and consider discontinuing therapy.

ADVERSE REACTIONS
Nausea, dizziness, insomnia, hyperhidrosis, constipation, somnolence, decreased appetite, anxiety, specific male sexual function disorders.

DRUG INTERACTIONS
See Contraindications. Avoid w/ other desvenlafaxine-containing products or venlafaxine products; may increase levels and increase dose-related adverse reactions. Avoid alcohol consumption. May increase risk of serotonin syndrome when used concomitantly w/ other serotonergic drugs (eg, triptans, TCAs, fentanyl) and w/ drugs that impair metabolism of serotonin; d/c desvenlafaxine and any concomitant serotonergic agent immediately and initiate supportive symptomatic treatment if serotonin syndrome occurs. Caution w/ NSAIDs, aspirin, warfarin, and other drugs that affect coagulation or bleeding, due to increased risk of bleeding. May increase risk of hyponatremia w/ diuretics. Potent CYP3A4 inhibitors (eg, ketoconazole) may increase levels. CYP2D6 substrates (eg, desipramine, atomoxetine, dextromethorphan) should be dosed at the original level when coadministered w/ 100mg desvenlafaxine or lower; reduce dose of these substrates by 1/2 if coadministered w/ 400mg of desvenlafaxine; increase substrate dose to original level when 400mg of desvenlafaxine is discontinued.

PREGNANCY AND LACTATION
Pregnancy: Category C.
Lactation: Found in breast milk; not for use in nursing.

MECHANISM OF ACTION
SNRI; has not been established. Thought to be related to the potentiation of serotonin and norepinephrine in the CNS through inhibition of their reuptake.

PHARMACOKINETICS
Absorption: Absolute bioavailability (80%). (50mg dose) T_{max}=6 hrs (median).
Distribution: Plasma protein binding (30%); V_d=3.4L/kg (IV); found in breast milk.
Metabolism: Conjugation via UGT isoforms (primary) and N-demethylation via CYP3A4 (minor). **Elimination:** Urine (45% unchanged, 19% glucuronide metabolite, <5% oxidative metabolite). $T_{1/2}$=9.5 hrs.

PATIENT CONSIDERATIONS
Assessment: Assess for risk for bipolar disorder, history of mania/hypomania, seizure disorders, HTN, CV/cerebrovascular conditions, susceptibility to angle-closure glaucoma, volume depletion, hypersensitivity to the drug, hepatic/renal impairment, pregnancy/nursing status, and possible drug interactions.
Monitoring: Monitor for signs/symptoms of clinical worsening (eg, suicidality, unusual changes in behavior), serotonin syndrome, abnormal bleeding, angle-closure glaucoma, activation of mania/hypomania, seizures, hyponatremia,

interstitial lung disease, eosinophilic pneumonia, and other adverse reactions. Monitor BP, LFTs, and renal function. Monitor for discontinuation symptoms (eg, dysphoric mood, irritability, agitation) when discontinuing therapy. Carefully monitor patients receiving concomitant warfarin therapy when treatment w/ desvenlafaxine is initiated or discontinued. Periodically reassess to determine the need for continued treatment.

Counseling: Advise patients, families, and caregivers about the benefits and risks of treatment and counsel on its appropriate use. Counsel patients, families, and caregivers to look for the emergence of suicidality, especially early during treatment and when the dose is adjusted up or down. Caution about the risk of serotonin syndrome, particularly w/ the concomitant use w/ other serotonergic agents. Inform that concomitant use w/ ASA, NSAIDs, warfarin, or other drugs that affect coagulation may increase the risk of bleeding. Advise to monitor BP regularly, to observe for signs/symptoms of activation of mania/hypomania, to avoid alcohol, and not to d/c therapy w/o notifying physician. Inform that discontinuation effects may occur when stopping treatment. Caution about risk of angle-closure glaucoma. Caution against operating hazardous machinery (including automobiles) until reasonably certain that therapy does not adversely affect ability to engage in such activities. Advise to notify physician if allergic phenomena develops, if pregnant, intending to become pregnant, or if breastfeeding. Inform that an inert matrix tab may pass in the stool or via colostomy.

KINRIX — diphtheria and tetanus toxoids and acellular pertussis adsorbed and inactivated poliovirus vaccine

Rx

Class: Toxoid/vaccine combination

PEDIATRIC DOSAGE
Active Immunization Against Diphtheria, Tetanus, Pertussis, and Poliomyelitis
For use as the 5th dose in the diphtheria, tetanus, and acellular pertussis (DTaP) vaccine series and 4th dose in the inactivated poliovirus vaccine series in patients whose previous DTaP vaccine doses have been w/ Infanrix and/or Pediarix for the first 3 doses and Infanrix for the 4th dose

4-6 Years:
0.5mL dose IM

ADMINISTRATION
IM route
- The preferred site of administration is the deltoid muscle of the upper arm.
- Do not mix w/ any other vaccine in the same syringe or vial.

Preparation
- Shake vigorously; do not use if resuspension does not occur w/ vigorous shaking.
- For prefilled syringes, attach a sterile needle and administer IM.
- For vials, use a sterile needle and sterile syringe to withdraw dose and administer IM; not necessary to change needles between drawing vaccine from a vial and injecting into recipient, unless needle has been damaged or contaminated.

STORAGE
2-8°C (36-46°F). Do not freeze; discard if vaccine has been frozen.

HOW SUPPLIED
Inj: 0.5mL [vial, prefilled syringe]

CONTRAINDICATIONS
Severe allergic reaction (eg, anaphylaxis) after a previous dose of any diphtheria toxoid-, tetanus toxoid-, pertussis-, or poliovirus-containing vaccine, or to any component of Kinrix, including neomycin and polymyxin B; encephalopathy (eg, coma, decreased level of consciousness, prolonged seizures) w/in 7 days of administration of a previous dose of a pertussis-containing vaccine that is not attributable to another identifiable cause; progressive neurologic disorder, including infantile spasms, uncontrolled epilepsy, or progressive encephalopathy.

WARNINGS/PRECAUTIONS
Evaluate potential benefits and risks of vaccine administration if Guillain-Barre syndrome occurs w/in 6 weeks of receipt of a prior tetanus toxoid-containing vaccine. Tip caps of prefilled syringes may contain natural rubber latex; may cause allergic reactions. Syncope may occur and can be accompanied by transient neurological signs. Evaluate the potential benefits and risks of vaccine administration if any of the following events occur in temporal relation to receipt of a pertussis-containing vaccine: temperature ≥40.5°C (105°F) w/in 48 hrs not due to another identifiable cause; collapse or shock-like state w/in 48 hrs; persistent, inconsolable crying lasting ≥3 hrs, occurring w/in 48 hrs; or seizures w/ or w/o fever occurring w/in 3 days. May administer an antipyretic at the time of vaccination and for the ensuing 24 hrs in children at higher risk for seizures. Review immunization history for possible vaccine sensitivity and previous vaccination-related adverse reactions; epinephrine and other appropriate agents must be immediately available should an acute anaphylactic reaction occur.

ADVERSE REACTIONS
Local inj-site reactions (eg, pain, redness, arm circumference increase, swelling), drowsiness, fever, loss of appetite.

DRUG INTERACTIONS
Immunosuppressive therapies, including irradiation, antimetabolites, alkylating agents, cytotoxic drugs, and corticosteroids (used in greater than physiologic doses), may reduce immune response to vaccine.

PREGNANCY AND LACTATION
Pregnancy: Category C.
Lactation: Safety not known in nursing.

MECHANISM OF ACTION
Toxoid/vaccine combination; produces neutralizing antibodies that protect against diphtheria, tetanus, pertussis, and poliomyelitis disease.

PATIENT CONSIDERATIONS
Assessment: Assess for history of encephalopathy, development of Guillain-Barre syndrome following a prior tetanus toxoid-containing vaccine, progressive neurologic disorder, immunosuppression, risk for seizures, possible drug interactions, and hypersensitivity to latex, neomycin, or polymyxin B. Review immunization history for possible vaccine sensitivity and previous vaccination-related adverse reactions.

Monitoring: Monitor for signs/symptoms of Guillain-Barre syndrome, allergic reactions, syncope, neurological signs, and other adverse reactions.

Counseling: Inform parents/guardians of the potential benefits and risks of immunization, and about the potential for adverse reactions.

KITABIS PAK — tobramycin

Rx

Class: Aminoglycoside

ADULT DOSAGE
Cystic Fibrosis
Patients w/ *Pseudomonas aeruginosa*:
1 single-use ampule (300mg/5mL) bid by oral inh in alternating periods of 28 days on drug followed by 28 days off drug

PEDIATRIC DOSAGE
Cystic Fibrosis
Patients w/ *Pseudomonas aeruginosa*:
>6 Years:
1 single-use ampule (300mg/5mL) bid by oral inh in alternating periods of 28 days on drug followed by 28 days off drug

---

ADMINISTRATION
Oral inh route

Take doses as close to 12 hrs apart as possible; not <6 hrs apart.
Administer using only the Pari LC Plus Reusable Nebulizer with a DeVilbiss Pulmo-Aide air compressor.
Entire treatment should take approximately 15 min to complete; continue treatment until all inh sol has been delivered and there is no longer any mist being produced.
Do not dilute/mix inh sol with other drugs in the nebulizer, including dornase alfa.

STORAGE
2-8°C (36-46°F). Upon removal from the refrigerator, or if refrigeration is unavailable, may be stored at room temperature (up to 25°C [77°F]) for up to 28 days. Do not expose to intense light.

HOW SUPPLIED
Sol, Inhalation: 300mg/5mL

CONTRAINDICATIONS
Known hypersensitivity to any aminoglycoside.

WARNINGS/PRECAUTIONS
Bronchospasm, ototoxicity (eg, tinnitus), and nephrotoxicity may occur. If ototoxicity is noted, or nephrotoxicity develops, patient should be managed as medically appropriate, including potentially discontinuing tobramycin inh sol. May aggravate muscle weakness because of a potential curare-like effect on neuromuscular function. If neuromuscular blockade occurs, it may be reversed by administration of Ca^{2+} salts but mechanical assistance may be necessary. May cause fetal harm.

ADVERSE REACTIONS
Cough, pharyngitis, increased sputum, dyspnea, hemoptysis, decreased lung function, voice alteration, taste perversion, rash.

DRUG INTERACTIONS
Avoid concurrent and/or sequential use with other drugs with neurotoxic, nephrotoxic, or ototoxic potential. Some diuretics may enhance aminoglycoside toxicity by altering aminoglycoside concentrations in serum and tissue; do not administer with ethacrynic acid, furosemide, urea, or IV mannitol. Monitor for toxicities associated with aminoglycosides if used concomitantly with parenteral aminoglycosides; monitor serum tobramycin levels.

PREGNANCY AND LACTATION
Category D, not for use in nursing.

MECHANISM OF ACTION
Aminoglycoside; acts primarily by disrupting protein synthesis, leading to altered cell membrane permeability, progressive disruption of the cell envelope, and eventual cell death.

PHARMACOKINETICS
Distribution: Crosses placenta. **Elimination:** Expectorated sputum (Unabsorbed); $T_{1/2}$=2 hrs (IV).

PATIENT CONSIDERATIONS
Assessment: Assess for auditory or vestibular dysfunction, renal dysfunction, neuromuscular disorders, drug hypersensitivity, pregnancy/nursing status, and possible drug interactions.

Monitoring: Monitor for bronchospasm, ototoxicity, nephrotoxicity, neuromuscular effects, and other adverse reactions.

Counseling: Advise to inform physician if SOB or wheezing occurs soon after administration, or if ringing in the ears, dizziness, or any changes in hearing develop. Instruct to notify physician if planning to become pregnant or if nursing. Instruct patients on multiple therapies to take their medications prior to inhaling the tobramycin inh sol, or ud by physician.

KLOR-CON M — potassium chloride

Rx

Class: Potassium supplement

OTHER BRAND NAMES
Klor-Con

ADULT DOSAGE
Hypokalemia

Prevention:
20mEq/day

Treatment:
≥40-100mEq/day or more; divide dose so that no more than 20mEq is given in a single dose

PEDIATRIC DOSAGE
Pediatric use may not have been established

DOSING CONSIDERATIONS
Elderly
Start at lower end of dosing range

ADMINISTRATION
Oral route

Take w/ meals and w/ a glass of water or other liquid

Klor-Con
Swallow tab whole; do not crush, chew, or suck

Klor-Con M
If Unable to Swallow Whole Tab:
A) Break tab in 1/2 and take each half separately w/ a glass of water, or
B) Prepare an aqueous sus

Aqueous Sus Preparation:
1. Place whole tab in approx 4 fl oz of water
2. Allow 2 min for tab to disintegrate
3. Stir for 30 sec after tab has disintegrated
4. Swirl sus and consume entire contents of the glass immediately by drinking or using a straw
5. Add another 1 fl oz of water, swirl, and consume immediately
6. Then, add an additional 1 fl oz of water, swirl, and consume immediately

STORAGE
Klor-Con: 15-30°C (59-86°F). Klor-Con M: 20-25°C (68-77°F); excursions permitted to 15-30°C (59-86°F).

HOW SUPPLIED
Tab, Extended-Release (ER): (Klor-Con M) 10mEq, 15mEq, 20mEq; (Klor-Con) 8mEq, 10mEq

CONTRAINDICATIONS
Hyperkalemia. ER formulations should not be used in certain cardiac patients w/ esophageal compression due to an enlarged left atrium; if indicated, give as liquid preparation or aqueous sus. **Solid Dosage Forms:** Structural, pathological (eg, diabetic gastroparesis), or pharmacologic (use of anticholinergic agents or other agents w/ anticholinergic properties) cause for arrest or delay in tab passage through the GI tract.

WARNINGS/PRECAUTIONS
Potentially fatal hyperkalemia and cardiac arrest may occur; monitor serum K⁺ levels and adjust dose appropriately. Extreme caution with acidosis and cardiac and renal disease; monitor ECG and electrolytes. Hypokalemia with metabolic acidosis should be treated with an alkalinizing K⁺ salt (eg, potassium bicarbonate, potassium citrate, potassium acetate, potassium gluconate). Solid oral dosage forms may produce ulcerative and/or stenotic lesions of the GI tract; d/c use if severe vomiting, abdominal pain, distention, or GI bleeding occurs. Reserve use for those who cannot tolerate, cannot comply, or refuse to take liquid or effervescent preparations. Caution in elderly.

ADVERSE REACTIONS
Hyperkalemia, GI effects (eg, obstruction, bleeding, ulceration), N/V, abdominal pain/discomfort, flatulence, diarrhea.

DRUG INTERACTIONS
See Contraindications. Risk of hyperkalemia with ACE inhibitors (eg, captopril, enalapril). Risk of hyperkalemia with K⁺-sparing diuretics (eg, spironolactone, triamterene, amiloride).

PREGNANCY AND LACTATION
Category C, safety not known in nursing.

MECHANISM OF ACTION
K⁺ supplement (electrolyte replenisher); participates in a number of essential physiological processes, including the maintenance of intracellular tonicity, the transmission of nerve impulses, the contraction of cardiac, skeletal, and smooth muscle, and the maintenance of normal renal function.

PHARMACOKINETICS
Absorption: (Klor-Con) GI tract. **Elimination:** Urine.

PATIENT CONSIDERATIONS

Assessment: Assess for hyperkalemia, chronic renal failure, systemic acidosis, cardiac patients, if patient cannot tolerate, refuses to take, or cannot comply with taking liquid or effervescent K⁺ preparations prior to administration of an ER tab formulation. Obtain baseline ECG, serum electrolyte levels, and renal function.

Monitoring: Monitor for signs/symptoms of hyperkalemia and other adverse events that may occur. In patients taking solid oral dosage forms, monitor for signs/symptoms of GI lesions. In patients with cardiac disease, acidosis, or renal disease, monitor acid-base balance and perform appropriate monitoring of serum electrolytes, ECG, renal function, and the clinical status of the patient.

Counseling: Inform about benefits and risks of therapy. Instruct to report to physician if patient develops any type of GI symptoms (eg, tarry stools or other evidence of GI bleeding, vomiting, abdominal pain/distention) or if other adverse events occur. Instruct to contact physician if difficulty in swallowing develops or if the tabs are sticking in the throat. (Klor-Con): Instruct to swallow tabs whole and to take with meals and full glass of water or other liquid. Follow the frequency and amount prescribed by the physician, especially if also taking diuretics and/or digitalis preparations. (Klor-Con M): Instruct to take each dose with meals and with full glass of water or other liquid. Inform that patient may break tabs in half or make an oral aqueous sus with tabs and 4 fl oz of water (see PI for proper preparation). Inform that aqueous sus not taken immediately should be discarded and use of other liquids for suspending is not recommended.

KOMBIGLYZE XR — metformin hydrochloride/saxagliptin

Rx

Class: Biguanide/dipeptidyl peptidase-4 (DPP-4) inhibitor

> Lactic acidosis may occur due to metformin accumulation; risk increases w/ conditions such as sepsis, dehydration, excess alcohol intake, hepatic impairment, renal impairment, and acute CHF. If acidosis is suspected, d/c and hospitalize patient immediately.

ADULT DOSAGE
Type 2 Diabetes Mellitus

Adjunct to diet and exercise to improve glycemic control when treatment w/ both saxagliptin and metformin is appropriate

Patients Requiring 5mg of Saxagliptin:
Not Currently Treated w/ Metformin:
Initial: 5mg/500mg qd
Patients Treated w/ Metformin:
Dose should provide metformin at the dose already being taken, or the nearest therapeutically appropriate dose

Patients Requiring 2.5mg of Saxagliptin:
Currently on Metformin Extended-Release (ER): 2.5mg/1000mg qd
Metformin Naive/Requiring >1000mg Metformin: Use individual components

Max: (5mg/2000mg)/day

PEDIATRIC DOSAGE
Pediatric use may not have been established

DOSING CONSIDERATIONS
Concomitant Medications
Strong CYP3A4/5 Inhibitors:
Max: 2.5mg/1000mg qd

Insulin Secretagogue (eg, Sulfonylurea)/Insulin:
May require lower doses of insulin secretagogue or insulin

ADMINISTRATION
Oral route

Swallow tab whole; do not cut, crush, or chew.
Take qd w/ pm meal.

STORAGE
20-25°C (68-77°F); excursions permitted to 15-30°C (59-86°F).

HOW SUPPLIED
Tab, Extended-Release: (Saxagliptin/Metformin ER) 5mg/500mg, 5mg/1000mg, 2.5mg/1000mg

CONTRAINDICATIONS
Renal impairment (eg, SrCr ≥1.5mg/dL [men], ≥1.4mg/dL [women], or abnormal CrCl); hypersensitivity to metformin HCl; acute or chronic metabolic acidosis, including diabetic ketoacidosis; history of a serious hypersensitivity reaction to Kombiglyze XR or saxagliptin (eg, anaphylaxis, angioedema, or exfoliative skin conditions).

WARNINGS/PRECAUTIONS
Not for treatment of type 1 diabetes mellitus (DM) or diabetic ketoacidosis. Assess renal function before initiation of therapy and at least annually thereafter; d/c w/ evidence of renal impairment. Temporarily suspend for any surgical procedure (except minor procedures not associated w/ restricted intake of foods and fluids); restart when oral intake is resumed and renal function is normal. Evaluate patients previously well controlled on therapy who develop lab abnormalities or clinical illness for evidence of ketoacidosis or lactic acidosis; d/c if acidosis occurs. Promptly d/c in the event of cardiovascular collapse (shock), acute CHF,

acute MI, and other conditions characterized by hypoxemia. Caution in elderly. **Metformin:** Avoid in patients w/ clinical or lab evidence of hepatic disease. Do not initiate in patients ≥80 yrs of age unless renal function is not reduced. May decrease vitamin B12 levels; monitor hematological parameters annually. Elderly or debilitated/malnourished patients and those w/ adrenal/pituitary insufficiency or alcohol intoxication are particularly susceptible to hypoglycemic effects. Temporarily d/c at time of or prior to intravascular contrast studies w/ iodinated materials, withhold for 48 hrs subsequent to the procedure, and reinstitute only if renal function is normal. **Saxagliptin:** Acute pancreatitis reported; promptly d/c if pancreatitis is suspected and initiate appropriate management. Serious hypersensitivity reactions reported; d/c if suspected, assess for other potential causes, and institute alternative treatment for DM. Increased incidence of hospitalization for heart failure (HF) reported in patients w/ established atherosclerotic cardiovascular disease (ASCVD) or multiple risk factors for ASCVD; consider the risks and benefits of therapy prior to initiating treatment in patients at a higher risk for HF. Evaluate and manage according to current standards of care and consider discontinuation of therapy if HF develops. Caution in patients w/ history of angioedema to another DPP-4 inhibitor. Severe and disabling arthralgia reported w/ DPP-4 inhibitors; d/c if appropriate.

ADVERSE REACTIONS
Metformin ER: Diarrhea, N/V.
Saxagliptin: URTI, UTI, headache.
Saxagliptin and Metformin Immediate-Release (IR): Headache, nasopharyngitis.

DRUG INTERACTIONS
See Dosing Considerations. **Metformin:** Hypoglycemia may occur during concomitant use w/ other glucose-lowering agents (eg, sulfonylureas, insulin) or ethanol. Cationic drugs that are eliminated by renal tubular secretion (eg, cimetidine, amiloride, digoxin) may potentially produce an interaction; monitor and adjust dose of Kombiglyze XR and/or the interfering drug. Thiazides and other diuretics, corticosteroids, phenothiazines, thyroid products, estrogens, oral contraceptives, phenytoin, nicotinic acid, sympathomimetics, calcium channel blockers, and isoniazid may predispose to hyperglycemia and may lead to loss of glycemic control; observe closely when such drugs are administered. Alcohol may potentiate the effect of metformin on lactate metabolism; avoid excessive alcohol intake. Caution w/ drugs that may affect renal function or result in significant hemodynamic change or may interfere w/ the disposition of metformin. May be difficult to recognize hypoglycemia w/ β-adrenergic blocking drugs. **Saxagliptin:** Incidence of hypoglycemia is increased when used in combination w/ insulin secretagogues (eg, sulfonylurea) or insulin. Ketoconazole and other strong CYP3A4/5 inhibitors (eg, atazanavir, clarithromycin, itraconazole) may significantly increase plasma concentrations.

PREGNANCY AND LACTATION
Pregnancy: Category B.
Lactation: Caution in nursing.

MECHANISM OF ACTION
Metformin: Biguanide; decreases hepatic glucose production, decreases intestinal absorption of glucose, and improves insulin sensitivity by increasing peripheral glucose uptake and utilization. **Saxagliptin:** DPP-4 inhibitor; slows the inactivation of the incretin hormones, thereby increasing their bloodstream concentrations and reducing fasting and postprandial glucose concentrations in a glucose-dependent manner.

PHARMACOKINETICS
Absorption: Saxagliptin: C_{max}=24ng/mL; AUC=78ng•hr/mL; T_{max}=2 hrs (median). 5-hydroxy saxagliptin: C_{max}=47ng/mL; AUC=214ng•hr/mL; T_{max}=4 hrs (median). Metformin: T_{max}=7 hrs (median). **Distribution:** Metformin IR: V_d=654L. **Metabolism:** Saxagliptin: Via CYP3A4/5; 5-hydroxy saxagliptin (active metabolite). **Elimination:** Saxagliptin: Feces (22%), urine (24% unchanged, 36% active metabolite); $T_{1/2}$=2.5 hrs (saxagliptin), 3.1 hrs (5-hydroxy saxagliptin). Metformin: Urine (90%); $T_{1/2}$=6.2 hrs (plasma), 17.6 hrs (blood).

PATIENT CONSIDERATIONS
Assessment: Assess for metabolic acidosis (including diabetic ketoacidosis), risk factors for lactic acidosis, renal/hepatic impairment, previous hypersensitivity to the drug, history of pancreatitis, HF or risk for HF, inadequate vitamin B12 or Ca^{2+} absorption, type of DM, history of angioedema w/ another DPP-4 inhibitor, pregnancy/nursing status, and possible drug interactions. Assess if patient is planning to undergo any surgical procedure or radiologic studies involving the use of intravascular iodinated contrast materials. Obtain baseline FPG and HbA1c levels, and hematological parameters.

Monitoring: Monitor for signs/symptoms of lactic acidosis, pancreatitis, HF, hypoxic states, hypoglycemia, hypersensitivity reactions, severe and disabling arthralgia, and other adverse reactions. Monitor for changes in clinical status. Monitor renal function, especially in elderly, at least annually. Monitor hematologic parameters annually. Perform routine serum vitamin B12 measurements at 2- to 3-yr intervals in patients predisposed to develop subnormal vitamin B12 levels. Monitor FPG and HbA1c levels. Monitor hepatic function periodically.

Counseling: Inform of the risks, benefits, and alternative modes of therapy. Advise on the importance of adherence to dietary instructions, regular physical activity, periodic blood glucose monitoring and HbA1c testing, recognition/management of hypo/hyperglycemia, and assessment of diabetes complications. Instruct to seek medical advice promptly during periods of stress as medication needs may change. Inform of the risk of lactic acidosis; instruct to d/c therapy immediately and notify physician if unexplained hyperventilation, myalgia, malaise, unusual somnolence, dizziness, slow or irregular heartbeat, sensation of feeling cold (especially in the extremities), or other nonspecific symptoms occur. Counsel against excessive alcohol intake. Inform that acute pancreatitis may occur; instruct to d/c therapy promptly and contact physician if persistent severe abdominal pain occurs. Inform about the signs/symptoms of HF; instruct to contact physician as soon as possible if the patient experiences symptoms of HF (eg, increasing SOB,

rapid increase in weight, swelling of the feet). Inform that allergic reactions may occur; instruct to d/c therapy and seek medical advice promptly if symptoms occur. Inform about the importance of regular testing of renal function and hematological parameters when receiving treatment. Inform that severe and disabling joint pain may occur; instruct to seek medical advice if severe joint pain occurs. Inform that inactive ingredients may occasionally be eliminated in the feces as a soft mass that may resemble the original tab.

KORLYM — mifepristone   Rx
Class: Glucocorticoid receptor antagonist

> A potent antagonist of progesterone and cortisol. Antiprogestational effect will result in termination of pregnancy; pregnancy must be excluded before initiation of treatment and prevented during treatment and for 1 month after stopping treatment by the use of a nonhormonal medically acceptable method of contraception, unless patient has had surgical sterilization. Pregnancy must be excluded if treatment is interrupted for >14 days in females of reproductive potential.

ADULT DOSAGE	PEDIATRIC DOSAGE
Hyperglycemia Secondary to Hypercortisolism In patients w/ endogenous Cushing's syndrome who have type 2 diabetes mellitus or glucose intolerance and have failed surgery or are not candidates for surgery **Initial:** 300mg qd **Titrate:** May increase dose by 300mg/day; do not increase dose more frequently than once every 2-4 weeks **Max:** 1200mg qd (not to exceed 20mg/kg/day) **If Treatment is Interrupted:** Reinitiate at lowest dose (300mg); if interrupted because of adverse reactions, titration should aim for a dose lower than the one that resulted in treatment interruption	Pediatric use may not have been established

DOSING CONSIDERATIONS
Renal Impairment
Max: 600mg/day

Hepatic Impairment
Mild to Moderate:
Max: 600mg/day

ADMINISTRATION
Oral route

Take as a single daily dose w/ a meal
Swallow tab whole; do not split, crush, or chew

STORAGE
25°C (77°F); excursions permitted to 15-30°C (59-86°F).

HOW SUPPLIED
Tab: 300mg

CONTRAINDICATIONS
Pregnancy, endometrial hyperplasia w/ atypia or endometrial carcinoma, or history of unexplained vaginal bleeding. Concomitant simvastatin, lovastatin, CYP3A substrates w/ narrow therapeutic ranges (eg, cyclosporine, dihydroergotamine, ergotamine, fentanyl, pimozide, quinidine, sirolimus, tacrolimus), or systemic corticosteroids for serious medical conditions/illnesses (eg, immunosuppression after organ transplantation), prior hypersensitivity reactions to mifepristone or to any of the product components.

WARNINGS/PRECAUTIONS
May experience adrenal insufficiency; if suspected, d/c immediately and administer glucocorticoids without delay. Hypokalemia reported; correct hypokalemia prior to treatment. Treat hypokalemia with IV/PO K⁺-supplementation based on severity; consider adding mineralocorticoid antagonists if hypokalemia persists. May cause vaginal bleeding and endometrial changes; caution with hemorrhagic disorders or if receiving concurrent anticoagulant therapy. Refer to a gynecologist if vaginal bleeding occurs. May prolong QT interval; always use the lowest effective dose. Risk for opportunistic infections (eg, *Pneumocystis jiroveci* pneumonia); perform appropriate diagnostic tests and consider treatment for *P. jiroveci*. Caution in patients with underlying heart conditions (eg, heart failure, coronary vascular disease). Avoid with severe hepatic impairment.

ADVERSE REACTIONS
N/V, fatigue, headache, decreased blood K⁺, arthralgia, peripheral edema, HTN, dizziness, decreased appetite, endometrial hypertrophy, vaginal bleeding, dry mouth, diarrhea, myalgia.

DRUG INTERACTIONS
See Contraindications. Avoid with CYP3A inducers (eg, rifampin, rifabutin, rifapentine, phenobarbital, phenytoin, carbamazepine, St. John's wort). Increases levels of drugs whose metabolism is largely or solely mediated by CYP3A; discontinuation/dose reduction or therapeutic drug monitoring may be necessary. Increased levels with ketoconazole and other strong CYP3A inhibitors (eg, itraconazole, nefazodone, ritonavir, nelfinavir, indinavir, atazanavir, amprenavir, fosamprenavir, boceprevir, clarithromycin, conivaptan, lopinavir, mibefradil, posaconazole, saquinavir, telaprevir, telithromycin, voriconazole); when use is necessary, use extreme caution and limit

dose of mifepristone to 300mg/day. Caution with moderate CYP3A inhibitors (eg, amprenavir, aprepitant, atazanavir, ciprofloxacin, darunavir/ritonavir, diltiazem, erythromycin, fluconazole, fosamprenavir, grapefruit juice, imatinib, verapamil). May increase levels of CYP2C8/2C9 substrates (eg, NSAIDs, warfarin, repaglinide); use the smallest recommended dose of these drugs and closely monitor for adverse effects. May significantly increase fluvastatin exposure. Caution with drugs that are metabolized by CYP2B6 (eg, bupropion, efavirenz); may significantly increase exposure of these drugs. May interfere with the effectiveness of hormonal contraceptives; use nonhormonal contraceptive methods. Use in patients who receive corticosteroids for other conditions (eg, autoimmune disorders) may lead to exacerbation or deterioration of such conditions; antagonizes the desired effects of glucocorticoid in these clinical settings. Use lowest effective dose with other QT prolonging drugs or K+-channel variants resulting in a long QT interval.

PREGNANCY AND LACTATION
Category X, not for use in nursing.

MECHANISM OF ACTION
Glucocorticoid receptor antagonist; selective antagonist of progesterone receptor at low doses and blocks glucocorticoid receptor at higher doses.

PHARMACOKINETICS
Absorption: T_{max}=1-2 hrs (single dose), 1-4 hrs (multiple 600mg doses). **Distribution:** Plasma protein binding (99.2%); found in breast milk. **Metabolism:** Liver; demethylation and hydroxylation; CYP3A4. **Elimination:** Feces (90%); $T_{1/2}$=85 hrs (multiple 600mg doses).

PATIENT CONSIDERATIONS
Assessment: Assess for drug hypersensitivity, immunosuppression after organ transplant and autoimmune disorders treated with corticosteroids, history of unexplained vaginal bleeding and endometrial hyperplasia with atypia or endometrial carcinoma, women with hemorrhagic disorders, underlying heart conditions, renal/hepatic impairment, pregnancy/nursing status, and for possible drug interactions. Evaluate for precipitating causes of hypoadrenalism (eg, infection, trauma).

Monitoring: Monitor for adrenal insufficiency, hypokalemia, vaginal bleeding, endometrial changes, QT interval prolongation, infection, hypersensitivity reactions, and other adverse reactions. Monitor serum K+ 1-2 weeks after starting or increasing dose and periodically thereafter.

Counseling: Advise females of reproductive potential that drug will cause termination of pregnancy; counsel regarding pregnancy prevention and planning with a nonhormonal contraceptive prior to therapy and up to 1 month after the end of treatment. Instruct to contact physician immediately if pregnancy is suspected or confirmed.

KOVALTRY — antihemophilic factor (recombinant)   Rx

Class: Antihemophilic factor (recombinant)

ADULT DOSAGE	PEDIATRIC DOSAGE
Congenital Hemophilia A	**Congenital Hemophilia A**
Dose:	**Dose:**
Required dose (IU) = body weight (kg) x desired Factor VIII (FVIII) rise (% of normal or IU/dL) x reciprocal of expected/observed recovery (eg, 0.5 for a recovery of 2 IU/dL per IU/kg)	Required dose (IU) = body weight (kg) x desired FVIII rise (% of normal or IU/dL) x reciprocal of expected/observed recovery (eg, 0.5 for a recovery of 2 IU/dL per IU/kg)
Treatment/Control of Bleeding Episodes:	**Treatment/Control of Bleeding Episodes:**
Minor Bleed:	**Minor Bleed:**
Required FVIII Level 20-40 IU/dL: Repeat q12-24h for at least 1 day, until bleeding episode as indicated by pain is resolved or healing is achieved	**Required FVIII Level 20-40 IU/dL:** Repeat q12-24h for at least 1 day, until bleeding episode as indicated by pain is resolved or healing is achieved
Moderate Bleed:	**Moderate Bleed:**
Required FVIII Level 30-60 IU/dL: Repeat q12-24h for 3-4 days or more until pain and acute disability are resolved	**Required FVIII Level 30-60 IU/dL:** Repeat q12-24h for 3-4 days or more until pain and acute disability are resolved
Major Bleed:	**Major Bleed:**
Required FVIII Level 60-100 IU/dL: Repeat q8-24h until bleeding is resolved	**Required FVIII Level 60-100 IU/dL:** Repeat q8-24h until bleeding is resolved
Perioperative Management:	**Perioperative Management:**
Minor Surgery:	**Minor Surgery:**
Required FVIII Level 30-60 IU/dL (Pre- and Post-Operative): Repeat q24h for at least 1 day until healing is achieved	**Required FVIII Level 30-60 IU/dL (Pre- and Post-Operative):** Repeat q24h for at least 1 day until healing is achieved
Major Surgery:	**Major Surgery:**
Required FVIII Level 80-100 IU/dL (Pre- and Post-Operative): Repeat q8-24h until adequate wound healing is complete, then continue therapy for at least another 7 days to maintain FVIII activity of 30-60 IU/dL	**Required FVIII Level 80-100 IU/dL (Pre- and Post-Operative):** Repeat q8-24h until adequate wound healing is complete, then continue therapy for at least another 7 days to maintain FVIII activity of 30-60 IU/dL
Routine Prophylaxis:	**Routine Prophylaxis:**
20-40 IU/kg IV 2-3X/week; adjust dose based on response	**Adolescents:** 20-40 IU/kg 2-3X/week; adjust dose based on response
	≤12 Years: 25-50 IU/kg 2-3X/week or qod according to individual requirements

ADMINISTRATION
IV route
- Refer to PI for reconstitution instructions.
- Administer as soon as possible; if not, store at room temperature for <3 hrs.
- Infuse IV over a period of 1-15 min; adapt rate of administration to response of each individual patient.

STORAGE
2-8°C (36-46°F) for up to 30 months from the date of manufacture; may be stored for a single period of up to 12 months at temperatures up to 25°C (77°F). Do not freeze. Record starting date of room temperature storage on the unopened product carton. Once stored at room temperature, do not return to refrigerator. Protect from extreme light exposure. Store vial w/ lyophilized powder in carton prior to use.

HOW SUPPLIED
Inj: 250 IU, 500 IU, 1000 IU, 2000 IU, 3000 IU

CONTRAINDICATIONS
History of hypersensitivity reactions to the active substance, to any of the excipients, or to mouse or hamster proteins.

WARNINGS/PRECAUTIONS
Not indicated for the treatment of von Willebrand disease. Hypersensitivity reactions, including anaphylaxis, are possible w/ treatment; d/c if symptoms occur and seek emergency treatment. Formation of neutralizing antibodies (inhibitors) can occur; greater risk in previously untreated patients. Carefully monitor for development of FVIII inhibitors. If expected plasma FVIII activity levels are not attained, or if bleeding is not controlled as expected w/ administered dose, perform Bethesda assay that measures FVIII inhibitor concentration. Hemophilic patients w/ cardiovascular (CV) risk factors/diseases may be at the same risk to develop CV events as non-hemophilic patients when clotting has been normalized by treatment. Catheter-related infections may be observed when administered via central venous access devices. Monitor plasma FVIII activity levels using a validated test to confirm that adequate FVIII levels have been achieved and maintained.

ADVERSE REACTIONS
Headache, pyrexia, pruritus.

PREGNANCY AND LACTATION
Pregnancy: There are no data for use in pregnant women to inform on drug-associated risk.
Lactation: There is no information regarding the presence of drug in human milk, the effects on the breastfed infant, or the effects on milk production; caution in nursing.

MECHANISM OF ACTION
Antihemophilic factor (recombinant); temporarily replaces the missing coagulation FVIII that is needed for effective hemostasis.

PHARMACOKINETICS
Absorption: C_{max}=99.7 IU/dL; AUC=1601.3 IU•h/dL. **Distribution:** V_d=0.63dL/kg. **Elimination:** $T_{1/2}$=14.3 hrs. Refer to PI for pediatric parameters.

PATIENT CONSIDERATIONS
Assessment: Assess for hypersensitivity reactions including anaphylaxis to mouse/hamster protein or other constituents of the product, location and extent of bleeding, patient's clinical condition, and pregnancy/nursing status. Assess FVIII activity levels.

Monitoring: Monitor for signs/symptoms of hypersensitivity reactions and other adverse reactions. Monitor plasma FVIII activity levels, clinical response, and development of FVIII inhibitors.

Counseling: Warn of the early signs of hypersensitivity reaction; advise to d/c use and seek immediate emergency treatment if symptoms occur. Advise to contact physician or treatment center for further treatment and/or assessment if experiencing a lack of clinical response, as this may be a manifestation of an inhibitor. Advise to discard all equipment, including any unused product, in an appropriate container. Advise to consult w/ healthcare provider prior to travel; advise to bring an adequate supply while traveling based on current regimen.

KRISTALOSE — lactulose   Rx

Class: Osmotic laxative

ADULT DOSAGE	PEDIATRIC DOSAGE
Constipation	Pediatric use may not have been established
Usual: 10-20g/day	
Max: 40g/day	
24-48 hrs may be required to produce a normal bowel movement	

ADMINISTRATION
Oral route

Dissolve contents of pkt in 4 oz of water

STORAGE
15-30°C (59-86°F).

HOW SUPPLIED
Sol (Powder): 10g/pkt, 20g/pkt [1ˢ, 30ˢ]

CONTRAINDICATIONS
Patients who require a low galactose diet.

WARNINGS/PRECAUTIONS

Caution in diabetes mellitus (DM) due to galactose and lactose content. Monitor electrolytes periodically in elderly or debilitated if used for >6 months. Potential for explosive reaction with electrocautery procedures during proctoscopy or colonoscopy.

ADVERSE REACTIONS

Flatulence, intestinal cramps, diarrhea, N/V.

DRUG INTERACTIONS

Nonabsorbable antacids may decrease effects.

PREGNANCY AND LACTATION

Category B, caution in nursing.

MECHANISM OF ACTION

Osmotic laxative; increases osmotic pressure and slight acidification of the colonic contents.

PHARMACOKINETICS

Absorption: Poorly absorbed from GI tract. **Elimination:** Urine (≤3%).

PATIENT CONSIDERATIONS

Assessment: Assess for DM, patients requiring a low-galactose diet, pregnancy/nursing status, and possible drug interactions.

Monitoring: Monitor serum electrolytes (K^+, Na^+, Cl^-, carbon dioxide). Monitor for diarrhea, vomiting, and other adverse reactions.

Counseling: Advise to report any potential adverse effects.

KRYSTEXXA — pegloticase   Rx

Class: Recombinant urate-oxidase enzyme

> Anaphylaxis and infusion reactions reported during and after administration. Anaphylaxis may occur w/ any infusion, including a 1st infusion, and generally manifests w/in 2 hrs of infusion; delayed-type hypersensitivity reactions also reported. Should be administered in a healthcare setting by a healthcare provider prepared to manage anaphylaxis and infusion reactions. Premedicate w/ antihistamines and corticosteroids. Closely monitor for an appropriate period of time for anaphylaxis after administration. Monitor serum uric acid levels prior to infusions and consider discontinuing treatment if levels increase to >6mg/dL, particularly when 2 consecutive levels >6mg/dL are observed.

ADULT DOSAGE

Chronic Gout

In Patients Refractory to Conventional Therapy:
8mg given as an IV infusion every 2 weeks

Premedication

Patients should receive pre-infusion medications (eg, antihistamines, corticosteroids) to minimize the risk of anaphylaxis and infusion reactions

PEDIATRIC DOSAGE
Pediatric use may not have been established

DOSING CONSIDERATIONS

Concomitant Medications

Oral Urate-Lowering Medications: Before starting pegloticase, d/c oral urate-lowering medications and do not institute therapy w/ oral urate-lowering agents while patient is receiving pegloticase therapy

Adverse Reactions

If an infusion reaction occurs during administration, the infusion may be slowed, or stopped and restarted at a slower rate

ADMINISTRATION

IV route

Preparation

1. Withdraw 1mL of pegloticase from the vial into a sterile syringe; discard any unused portion of product remaining in the 2mL vial.
2. Inject into a single 250mL bag of 0.9% NaCl inj or 0.45% NaCl inj for IV infusion; do not mix or dilute w/ other drugs.
3. Invert the infusion bag containing the dilute pegloticase sol a number of times to ensure thorough mixing; do not shake.
4. Pegloticase diluted in infusion bags is stable for 4 hrs at 2-8°C (36-46°F) and at 20-25°C (68-77°F); however, recommended to be stored under refrigeration, not frozen, protected from light, and used w/in 4 hrs of dilution.
5. Before administration, allow diluted sol to reach room temperature; never subject pegloticase in a vial or in an IV infusion fluid to artificial heating (eg, hot water, microwave).

Administration

Use diluted sol w/in 4 hrs of dilution.
Administer only by IV infusion over no less than 120 min via gravity feed, syringe-type pump, or infusion pump.
Do not administer as an IV push or bolus.
Consider observing patients for approx 1 hr post-infusion, since infusion reactions may occur after completion of infusion.

STORAGE

2-8°C (36-46°F). Protect from light. Do not shake or freeze.

HOW SUPPLIED

Inj: 8mg/mL

CONTRAINDICATIONS

G6PD deficiency.

WARNINGS/PRECAUTIONS

Not recommended for the treatment of asymptomatic hyperuricemia. Gout flares may occur after initiation of therapy; gout flare prophylaxis w/ an NSAID or colchicine is recommended starting at least 1 week before initiation of therapy and lasting at least 6 months, unless medically contraindicated or not tolerated. Therapy does not need to be discontinued because of a gout flare; manage the gout flare concurrently as appropriate for the individual patient. CHF exacerbation reported; caution w/ CHF and monitor closely following infusion. Risk of anaphylaxis and infusion reactions may increase during retreatment due to immunogenicity; carefully monitor patients receiving retreatment after a drug-free interval.

ADVERSE REACTIONS

Anaphylaxis, infusion reactions, gout flares, N/V, contusion/ecchymosis, nasopharyngitis, constipation, chest pain.

DRUG INTERACTIONS

See Dosing Considerations. Potential for anti-PEG antibody development that may bind to other pegylated drugs; impact on response to other PEG-containing therapeutics is unknown.

PREGNANCY AND LACTATION

Pregnancy: Category C.
Lactation: Not for use in nursing unless clear benefit can overcome unknown risk.

MECHANISM OF ACTION

Recombinant urate-oxidase enzyme; catalyzes the oxidation of uric acid to allantoin, thereby lowering serum uric acid.

PATIENT CONSIDERATIONS

Assessment: Assess for G6PD deficiency, CHF, and pregnancy/nursing status. Assess serum uric acid levels prior to infusion.

Monitoring: Monitor for signs/symptoms of anaphylaxis, infusion reactions, gout flares, CHF exacerbation, and other adverse reactions.

Counseling: Inform that anaphylaxis and infusion reactions may occur at any infusion while on therapy; counsel on the importance of adhering to any prescribed medications to help prevent or lessen the severity of these reactions. Advise to seek medical care immediately if patient experiences any symptoms of an allergic reaction during or at any time after infusion. Advise to d/c any oral urate-lowering agents before therapy and not to take any oral urate-lowering agents while on therapy. Inform that gout flares may initially increase when starting therapy, and that medications to help reduce flares may need to be taken regularly for the 1st few months after therapy is started; advise not stop therapy if a flare occurs.

KYBELLA — deoxycholic acid   Rx

Class: Cytolytic agent

ADULT DOSAGE

Submental Fat

Improvement in appearance of moderate to severe convexity or fullness associated w/ submental fat

Inject using an area-adjusted dose of 2mg/cm²

Single treatment consists of up to a max of 50 inj, 0.2mL each (up to a total of 10mL), spaced 1cm apart

Up to 6 single treatments may be administered at intervals no <1 month apart

PEDIATRIC DOSAGE
Pediatric use may not have been established

DOSING CONSIDERATIONS

Elderly

Start at the lower end of dosing range

ADMINISTRATION

SQ route

Do not dilute
Inject into SQ fat tissue in the submental area
Refer to PI for inj technique

STORAGE

20-25°C (68-77°F); excursions permitted between 15-30°C (59-86°F).

HOW SUPPLIED

Inj: 10mg/mL [2mL]

CONTRAINDICATIONS

Presence of infection at the inj sites.

WARNINGS/PRECAUTIONS

Give careful consideration to the use of drug in patients w/ excessive skin laxity, prominent platysmal bands, or other conditions for which reduction of submental fat may result in an aesthetically undesirable outcome. Caution in patients who have had prior surgical or aesthetic treatment of the submental area. Changes in anatomy/landmarks or the presence of scar tissue may impact the ability to safely administer drug or to obtain the desired aesthetic result. Cases of marginal mandibular nerve injury, manifested as an asymmetric smile or facial muscle weakness (paresis), reported. To avoid potential for nerve injury, do not inject into or in close proximity to the marginal mandibular branch of the facial nerve. Dysphagia may occur; avoid use in patients w/

current or prior history of dysphagia. Inj-site hematoma/bruising reported; caution w/ bleeding abnormalities, as excessive bleeding or bruising in the treatment area may occur. To avoid potential tissue damage, do not inject into or in close proximity (1-1.5cm) to salivary glands, lymph nodes, and muscles.

ADVERSE REACTIONS
Inj-site reactions, headache, oropharyngeal pain, HTN.

DRUG INTERACTIONS
Caution in patients who are currently being treated w/ antiplatelet or anticoagulant therapy.

PREGNANCY AND LACTATION
Pregnancy: In animal reproduction studies, no fetal harm was observed w/ the administration of doses greater than the max recommended human dose.
Lactation: There is no information regarding the presence of synthetic deoxycholic acid in human milk; caution in nursing.

MECHANISM OF ACTION
Cytolytic agent; when injected into tissue, physically destroys the cell membrane, causing lysis.

PHARMACOKINETICS
Absorption: Rapid. T_{max}=18 min (median), C_{max}=1024ng/mL, AUC_{0-24}=7896ng•hr/mL. **Distribution:** Plasma protein binding (98%). **Elimination:** Feces.

PATIENT CONSIDERATIONS
Assessment: Assess for presence of infection at the inj site, current or prior history of dysphagia, bleeding abnormalities, any other conditions where treatment is contraindicated or cautioned, pregnancy/nursing status, and for possible drug interactions. Screen for other potential causes of submental convexity/fullness (eg, thyromegaly, cervical lymphadenopathy).

Monitoring: Monitor for marginal mandibular nerve injury, dysphagia, inj-site hematoma/bruising, and other adverse reactions.

Counseling: Advise to inform physician if signs of marginal mandibular nerve paresis (eg, asymmetric smile, facial muscle weakness) or difficulty swallowing develops, or if any existing symptom worsens.

KYNAMRO — mipomersen sodium
Class: Lipid-regulating agent

Rx

> May cause elevations in transaminases; measure ALT, AST, alkaline phosphatase, and total bilirubin prior to therapy, and then ALT/AST regularly as recommended. Withhold dose if ALT/AST is ≥3X ULN. D/C for clinically significant liver toxicity. May increase hepatic fat, w/ or w/o concomitant increases in transaminases. Available only through a restricted program under a Risk Evaluation and Mitigation Strategy (REMS) because of the risk of hepatotoxicity. Prescribe only to patients w/ a clinical or laboratory diagnosis consistent w/ homozygous familial hypercholesterolemia.

ADULT DOSAGE	PEDIATRIC DOSAGE
Homozygous Familial Hypercholesterolemia	Pediatric use may not have been established
200mg SQ once weekly; give on the same day every week, but if dose is missed, give at least 3 days from the next weekly dose	

DOSING CONSIDERATIONS
Renal Impairment
W/ Severe Renal Impairment, Clinically Significant Proteinuria, or On Renal Dialysis: Not recommended
Hepatic Impairment
Moderate or Severe (Child-Pugh B or C) or Active Liver Disease (eg, Unexplained Persistent Elevations of Serum Transaminases): Contraindicated
Adverse Reactions
Transaminase Elevations:
ALT/AST ≥3X and <5X ULN:
- Confirm elevation w/ repeat measurement w/in 1 week
- If confirmed, withhold dosing, and obtain additional liver-related tests if not already measured (eg, total bilirubin, alkaline phosphatase, INR) and investigate to identify probable cause
- If resuming therapy after transaminases resolve to <3X ULN, consider monitoring liver-related tests more frequently

ALT/AST ≥5X ULN:
- Withhold dosing, obtain additional liver-related tests if not already measured (eg, total bilirubin, alkaline phosphatase, INR) and investigate to identify probable cause
- If resuming therapy after transaminases resolve to <3X ULN, monitor liver-related tests more frequently

If transaminase elevations are accompanied by clinical symptoms of liver injury, increases in bilirubin ≥2X ULN, or active liver disease, d/c therapy and investigate to identify probable cause

ADMINISTRATION
SQ route

Remove from refrigerated storage and allow to reach room temperature for at least 30 min prior to administration.
Inject into abdomen, thigh region, or outer area of the upper arm.
Do not inject in areas of active skin disease or injury; avoid areas of tattooed skin and scarring.

STORAGE
2-8°C (36-46°F). Protect from light and keep in the original carton until time of use. If refrigeration is unavailable, may store at ≤30°C (86°F), away from heat sources, for up to 14 days.

HOW SUPPLIED
Inj: 200mg/mL [1mL]

CONTRAINDICATIONS
Moderate or severe hepatic impairment (Child-Pugh B or C); active liver disease, including unexplained persistent elevations of serum transaminases; known hypersensitivity to any component of this product.

WARNINGS/PRECAUTIONS
See Dosing Considerations and Contraindications. Not recommended as an adjunct to LDL apheresis. If baseline LFTs are abnormal, consider initiating therapy after an appropriate work-up and the baseline abnormalities are explained or resolved. During the 1st year, measure liver-related tests monthly; after the 1st year, measure liver-related tests at least every 3 months. At any time during treatment, d/c for persistent/clinically significant elevations. Inj-site reactions (eg, erythema, pain, tenderness) reported; follow proper technique for SQ administration. Flu-like symptoms (eg, influenza-like illness, pyrexia, chills) reported.

ADVERSE REACTIONS
Inj-site reactions, flu-like symptoms, nausea, headache, elevations in serum transaminases (specifically ALT).

DRUG INTERACTIONS
Not recommended w/ other LDL-lowering agents that can increase hepatic fat. Alcohol may increase levels of hepatic fat and induce/exacerbate liver injury; avoid consumption of >1 alcoholic drink/day. Caution w/ other medications known to have potential for hepatotoxicity (eg, isotretinoin, amiodarone, acetaminophen [>4g/day for ≥3 days/week], methotrexate, tetracyclines, tamoxifen); more frequent monitoring of liver-related tests may be warranted.

PREGNANCY AND LACTATION
Pregnancy: Category B. May cause fetal harm.
Lactation: Not for use in nursing.
Reproductive Potential: Females of reproductive potential should use effective contraception during therapy.

MECHANISM OF ACTION
Lipid-regulating agent; an antisense oligonucleotide targeted to human messenger ribonucleic acid (mRNA) for Apo B-100, the principal apolipoprotein of LDL and its metabolic precursor, VLDL. Complementary to the coding region of the mRNA for Apo B-100, and binds by Watson and Crick base pairing. The hybridization to the cognate mRNA results in RNase H-mediated degradation of the cognate mRNA, thus inhibiting translation of the Apo B-100 protein.

PHARMACOKINETICS
Absorption: T_{max}=3-4 hrs. **Distribution:** Plasma protein binding (≥90%). **Metabolism:** In tissues via endonucleases to form shorter oligonucleotides that are then substrates for additional metabolism by exonucleases. **Elimination:** Urine (<4%); $T_{1/2}$=1-2 months.

PATIENT CONSIDERATIONS
Assessment: Assess for hepatic/renal impairment, drug hypersensitivity, pregnancy/nursing status, and possible drug interactions. Obtain baseline lipid levels, ALT/AST, alkaline phosphatase, and total bilirubin.

Monitoring: Monitor for inj-site reactions, flu-like symptoms, and other adverse reactions. Monitor LFTs monthly during 1st yr and at least every 3 months after 1st yr of therapy. Monitor lipid levels at least every 3 months for the 1st yr of therapy. Evaluate LDL level after 6 months to determine if LDL reduction achieved is sufficiently robust to warrant the potential risk of liver toxicity.

Counseling: Inform that transaminase elevations and hepatic steatosis may occur; inform of the importance of monitoring LFTs prior to therapy and periodically thereafter. Advise of the potential for increased risk of liver injury if alcohol is consumed; instruct to limit alcohol consumption to ≤1 drink/day. Advise to report any symptoms of possible liver injury (eg, N/V, fever, anorexia). Inform that inj-site reactions and flu-like symptoms have been reported. Instruct patient or caregiver on the proper technique of administration and safe disposal procedures. Instruct females of reproductive potential to use effective contraception during therapy.

KYPROLIS — carfilzomib
Class: Proteasome inhibitor

Rx

ADULT DOSAGE	PEDIATRIC DOSAGE
Relapsed or Refractory Multiple Myeloma	Pediatric use may not have been established
In Combination w/ Lenalidomide + Dexamethasone in Patients Who Have Received 1-3 Lines of Therapy: Each 28-day period is considered 1 treatment cycle; treatment may be continued until disease progression or unacceptable toxicity occurs	
Lenalidomide: 25mg PO on Days 1-21 of each cycle	
Dexamethasone: 40mg PO or IV on Days 1, 8, 15, and 22 of each cycle	

Cycle 1:
Administer 20mg/m^2 carfilzomib on Days 1 and 2. If tolerated, escalate to a target dose of 27mg/m^2 on Day 8; continue w/ tolerated dose on Days 9, 15, and 16

Cycles 2-12:
Administer 27mg/m^2 carfilzomib on Days 1, 2, 8, 9, 15, and 16

Cycles 13 and Thereafter:
Administer 27mg/m^2 carfilzomib on Days 1, 2, 15, and 16. D/C carfilzomib after Cycle 18

In Combination w/ Dexamethasone in Patients Who Have Received 1-3 Lines of Therapy:
Each 28-day period is considered 1 treatment cycle; treatment may be continued until disease progression or unacceptable toxicity occurs

Dexamethasone: 20mg PO or IV on Days 1, 2, 8, 9, 15, 16, 22, and 23 of each cycle

Cycle 1:
Administer 20mg/m^2 carfilzomib on Days 1 and 2. If tolerated, escalate to a target dose of 56mg/m^2 starting on Day 8; continue w/ tolerated dose on Days 9, 15, and 16

Cycles 2 and Thereafter:
Administer 56mg/m^2 carfilzomib on Days 1, 2, 8, 9, 15, and 16

Single Agent in Patients Who Have Received ≥1 Line of Therapy:
Each 28-day period is considered 1 treatment cycle; treatment may be continued until disease progression or unacceptable toxicity occurs

20/27mg/m^2 Regimen:
Cycle 1:
Administer 20mg/m^2 carfilzomib on Days 1 and 2. If tolerated, escalate to a target dose of 27mg/m^2 starting on Day 8; continue w/ tolerated dose on Days 9, 15, and 16

Cycles 2-12:
Administer 27mg/m^2 carfilzomib on Days 1, 2, 8, 9, 15, and 16

Cycles 13 and Thereafter:
Administer 27mg/m^2 carfilzomib on Days 1, 2, 15, and 16

20/56mg/m^2 Regimen:
Cycle 1:
Administer 20mg/m^2 carfilzomib on Days 1 and 2. If tolerated, escalate to a target dose of 56mg/m^2 starting on Day 8; continue w/ tolerated dose on Days 9, 15, and 16

Cycles 2-12:
Administer 56mg/m^2 carfilzomib on Days 1, 2, 8, 9, 15, and 16

Cycles 13 and Thereafter:
Administer 56mg/m^2 carfilzomib on Days 1, 2, 15, and 16

Premedication

Hydration and Fluid Monitoring:
Prior to Each Dose in Cycle 1: Give both oral (30mL/kg at least 48 hrs before Cycle 1, Day 1) and IV fluids (250-500mL of appropriate IV fluid prior to each dose in Cycle 1); if needed, give an additional 250-500mL of IV fluids following administration
Subsequent Cycles: Continue oral and/or IV hydration prn

Dexamethasone:
Administer recommended dexamethasone 30 min to 4 hrs prior to all doses of carfilzomib during Cycle 1 to reduce the incidence and severity of infusion reactions; reinstate dexamethasone premedication if these symptoms occur during subsequent cycles

20/27mg/m^2 Regimen: 4mg PO or IV
20/56mg/m^2 Regimen: 8mg PO or IV
Thromboprophylaxis:
Recommended for patients being treated w/ combination of carfilzomib w/ dexamethasone or w/ lenalidomide + dexamethasone; base regimen on underlying risks

Infection Prophylaxis:
Consider antiviral prophylaxis to decrease the risk of herpes zoster reactivation

----

DOSING CONSIDERATIONS
Adverse Reactions
Dose Level Reductions:

27mg/m^2 Dose:
First Dose Reduction: 20mg/m^2
Second Dose Reduction: 15mg/m^2; d/c if toxicity persists

56mg/m^2 Dose:
First Dose Reduction: 45mg/m^2
Second Dose Reduction: 36mg/m^2
Third Dose Reduction: 27mg/m^2; d/c if toxicity persists

Hematologic Toxicity:
ANC <0.5 x 10^9/L:
- Withhold dose
- If recovered to ≥0.5 x 10^9/L, continue at same dose level
- For subsequent drops to <0.5 x 10^9/L, follow same recommendations as above and consider 1 dose level reduction when restarting carfilzomib

Febrile Neutropenia (ANC <0.5 x 10^9/L and an Oral Temperature >38.5°C (101.3°F) or 2 Consecutive Readings of >38.0°C (100.4°F) for 2 Hrs):
- Withhold dose
- If ANC returns to baseline grade and fever resolves, resume at the same dose level

Platelets <10 x 10^9/L or Evidence of Bleeding w/ Thrombocytopenia:
- Withhold dose; if recovered to ≥10 x 10^9/L and/or bleeding is controlled, continue at same dose level
- For subsequent drops to <10 x 10^9/L, follow the same recommendations as above and consider 1 dose level reduction when restarting carfilzomib

Renal Toxicity:
SrCr ≥2X Baseline, or CrCl <15mL/min or CrCl Decreases to ≤50% of Baseline, or Need for Dialysis:
- Withhold dose and continue monitoring renal function (SrCr or CrCl)
- If attributable to carfilzomib, resume when renal function has recovered to w/in 25% of baseline; start at 1 dose level reduction
- If not attributable to carfilzomib, dosing may be resumed at the discretion of the physician
- For patients on dialysis, administer the dose after dialysis

Other Non-Hematologic Toxicity:
All Other Severe or Life-Threatening (CTCAE Grades 3 and 4) Non-Hematological Toxicities:
- Withhold until resolved or returned to baseline
- Consider restarting the next scheduled treatment at 1 dose level reduction

ADMINISTRATION
IV route
- Calculate dose based on actual BSA at baseline; patients w/ BSA >2.2m^2 should receive a dose based on a BSA of 2.2m^2.
- Dose does not need to be adjusted for weight change of ≤20%.
- Do not mix w/ or administer as an infusion w/ other medicinal products.
- Flush IV line w/ normal saline or D5 inj immediately before and after administration.
- Do not administer as a bolus.

Infusion Times
W/ Lenalidomide and Dexamethasone: 10 min
W/ Dexamethasone: 30 min
20/27mg/m^2 Monotherapy Regimen: 10 min
20/56mg/m^2 Monotherapy Regimen: 30 min

Reconstitution/Preparation
1. Slowly inject 29mL (for 60mg vial) or 15mL (for 30mg vial) of sterile water for inj, directing the sol onto the inside wall of the vial to minimize foaming.
2. Gently swirl and/or invert vial slowly for about 1 min, or until complete dissolution; do not shake. If foaming occurs, allow sol to settle in the vial until foaming subsides (approx 5 min) and the sol is clear.
3. When administering in an IV bag, withdraw calculated dose from vial and dilute into 50mL or 100mL D5 inj IV bag.
4. Discard any unused portion left in the vial; do not administer more than one dose from a vial.

Stability of Reconstituted Carfilzomib
Total time from reconstitution to administration should not exceed 24 hrs.
Stable for 24 hrs at 2-8°C (36-46°F).
Stable for 4 hrs at 15-30°C (59-86°F).

STORAGE
Unopened Vials: 2-8°C (36-46°F). Protect from light.

HOW SUPPLIED
Inj: 30mg, 60mg

WARNINGS/PRECAUTIONS

See Dosing Considerations. New onset/worsening of preexisting cardiac failure, restrictive cardiomyopathy, myocardial ischemia, and MI including fatalities reported following administration. Death due to cardiac arrest has occurred w/in a day of administration. Renal insufficiency adverse events reported; acute renal failure was reported more frequently in patients w/ advanced relapsed and refractory multiple myeloma who received carfilzomib monotherapy. Cases of tumor lysis syndrome (TLS), including fatal outcomes, reported; monitor for evidence of TLS during treatment and manage promptly, including interruption of therapy until TLS is resolved. Consider uric acid-lowering drugs in patients at risk for TLS. Acute respiratory distress syndrome, acute respiratory failure, and acute diffuse infiltrative pulmonary disease reported; d/c in the event of drug-induced pulmonary toxicity. Pulmonary arterial HTN (PAH) reported; withhold therapy until resolved or returned to baseline and consider whether to restart therapy based on a benefit/risk assessment. Dyspnea reported; evaluate dyspnea to exclude cardiopulmonary conditions. HTN, including hypertensive crisis and hypertensive emergency, reported; withhold carfilzomib and evaluate if HTN cannot be adequately controlled. Venous thromboembolic events (eg, deep venous thrombosis, pulmonary embolism) reported; consider an alternative method of contraception during treatment w/ carfilzomib in combination w/ dexamethasone or lenalidomide + dexamethasone in patients using oral contraceptives or a hormonal method of contraception associated w/ a risk of thrombosis. Infusion reactions may occur immediately following or up to 24 hrs after treatment. Fatal or serious cases of hemorrhage, including GI, pulmonary, and intracranial hemorrhage and epistaxis, have been reported; promptly evaluate signs/symptoms of blood loss and reduce or withhold dose as appropriate. Thrombocytopenia reported; reduce or withhold dose as appropriate. Hepatic failure, including fatal cases, reported. May increase serum transaminases; reduce or withhold dose as appropriate. Thrombotic microangiopathy, including thrombotic thrombocytopenic purpura/hemolytic uremic syndrome (TTP/HUS), reported; if diagnosis is suspected, d/c therapy and evaluate. If diagnosis of TTP/HUS is excluded, therapy can be restarted. Posterior reversible encephalopathy syndrome (PRES) reported; d/c if suspected and evaluate. May cause fetal harm.

ADVERSE REACTIONS

Monotherapy: Anemia, fatigue, thrombocytopenia, nausea, pyrexia, dyspnea, diarrhea, headache, cough, peripheral edema.
Combination Therapy: Anemia, neutropenia, diarrhea, dyspnea, fatigue, thrombocytopenia, pyrexia, insomnia, muscle spasm, cough, URTI, hypokalemia.

PREGNANCY AND LACTATION

Pregnancy: Can cause fetal harm based on animal studies and the drug's mechanism of action.
Lactation: There is no information regarding the presence of carfilzomib in human milk, the effects on the breastfed infant, or the effects on milk production; caution in nursing.
Females and Males of Reproductive Potential: Females of reproductive potential should use effective contraceptive measures or abstain from sexual activity to prevent pregnancy during therapy and for at least 30 days following completion of therapy. Males of reproductive potential should use effective contraceptive measures or abstain from sexual activity to prevent pregnancy during therapy and for at least 90 days following completion of therapy.

MECHANISM OF ACTION

Proteasome inhibitor; irreversibly binds to the N-terminal threonine-containing active sites of the 20S proteasome, the proteolytic core particle w/in the 26S proteasome.

PHARMACOKINETICS

Absorption: (27mg/m² single dose) AUC=379ng•hr/mL; C_{max}=4232ng/mL; (56mg/m² single dose) AUC=948ng•hr/mL; C_{max}=2079ng/mL. **Distribution:** (20mg/m²) V_d=28L; plasma protein binding (97%). **Metabolism:** Rapid and extensive; peptidase cleavage and epoxide hydrolysis (major); CYP450 (minor). **Elimination:** (Doses ≥15mg/m²) $T_{1/2}$≤1 hr.

PATIENT CONSIDERATIONS

Assessment: Assess for dehydration, hypersensitivity to drug, preexisting cardiac failure, hepatic dysfunction, renal impairment, and pregnancy/nursing status. Obtain baseline CBC, LFTs, SrCr, and weight. Consider antiviral prophylaxis therapy.

Monitoring: Monitor for signs/symptoms of cardiac toxicities, acute renal failure, TLS, dehydration, pulmonary toxicity, PAH, dyspnea, HTN, venous thromboembolic events, infusion reactions, hemorrhage, TTP/HUS, PRES, hepatic failure, and other adverse reactions. Monitor CBC, LFTs, and SrCr.

Counseling: Inform of the risks and symptoms of cardiac failure and ischemia. Advise on appropriate measures to take to avoid dehydration and instruct to notify physician if dehydration symptoms develop. Inform that patient may experience cough or SOB and instruct to contact physician if SOB occurs. Inform of the risk of venous thromboembolism and counsel on the options for prophylaxis. Advise to seek immediate medical attention for symptoms of venous thrombosis or embolism. Inform about the common signs/symptoms of infusion reactions. Advise patients that they may bruise or bleed more easily or that it may take longer to stop bleeding; inform of the signs of occult bleeding and instruct to report to physician any prolonged, unusual, or excessive bleeding. Inform about the risk of developing hepatic failure and advise to contact physician if jaundice develops. Instruct to contact physician if neurologic symptoms (eg, headaches, confusion, seizures, visual loss) develop. Instruct not to drive or operate machinery if fatigue, dizziness, fainting, and/or drop in BP are experienced. Advise females of reproductive potential to use effective contraceptive measures to prevent pregnancy during and for at least 30 days after treatment and instruct to inform physician immediately if pregnant. Advise males of reproductive potential to use effective contraceptive measures to prevent pregnancy during and for at least 90 days after treatment. Instruct not to breastfeed while on therapy. Advise to notify physician if using or planning to take other prescription or OTC drugs.

LABETALOL INJECTION — labetalol hydrochloride   Rx

Class: Alpha₁ blocker/nonselective beta blocker

OTHER BRAND NAMES

Trandate Injection (Discontinued)

ADULT DOSAGE

Severe Hypertension

Repeated IV Inj:
Initial: 20mg slow IV inj over 2 min; measure supine BP immediately before and at 5 and 10 min after inj to evaluate response
Titrate: May give additional 40mg or 80mg inj at 10-min intervals until desired supine BP is achieved or a total of 300mg has been injected

Slow Continuous Infusion:
2mg/min
Titrate: May adjust infusion rate according to BP response
Effective Dose Range: 50-200mg
Max: 300mg
When a satisfactory response is obtained, d/c and start oral labetalol

Initiation of Dosing w/ Labetalol Tabs:
Begin when supine diastolic BP has begun to rise
Initial: 200mg, followed by an additional 200mg or 400mg 6-12 hrs later, depending on BP response

Thereafter, inpatient titration w/ labetalol tabs may proceed as follows: 200mg bid (400mg/day), 400mg bid (800mg/day), 800mg bid (1600mg/day), 1200mg bid (2400mg/day)
If needed, total daily dose may be given in 3 divided doses.
While in hospital, may increase dose of tabs at 1-day intervals to achieve the desired BP reduction.

PEDIATRIC DOSAGE

Pediatric use may not have been established

ADMINISTRATION

IV route

Administer in supine position.

Slow Continuous Infusion

Refer to PI for examples of methods of preparing the infusion sol.

Compatibility

Compatible w/ and stable (for 24 hrs refrigerated or at room temperature) in mixtures with the following solutions:
Ringers inj
Lactated Ringers inj
D5 and Ringers inj
5% lactated Ringers and D5 inj
D5 inj
0.9% NaCl inj
D5 and 0.2% NaCl inj
2.5% Dextrose and 0.45% NaCl inj
D5 and 0.9% NaCl inj
D5 and 0.33% NaCl inj

Incompatibility

5% Sodium bicarbonate inj
Care should be taken when administering alkaline drugs, including furosemide, in combination w/ labetalol.

STORAGE

20-25°C (68-77°F). Protect from freezing and light.

HOW SUPPLIED

Inj: 5mg/mL [20mL, 40mL]

CONTRAINDICATIONS

Bronchial asthma, overt cardiac failure, >1st-degree heart block, cardiogenic shock, severe bradycardia, other conditions associated w/ severe and prolonged hypotension, history of hypersensitivity to any component of the product, and history of obstructive airway disease.

WARNINGS/PRECAUTIONS

For IV use in hospitalized patients. Severe hepatocellular injury (rare) reported. Caution w/ hepatic impairment. Perform appropriate lab testing at the 1st symptom/sign of liver dysfunction. D/C and do not restart if patient has jaundice or lab evidence of liver injury. May precipitate more severe failure in patients w/ congestive heart failure (CHF); avoid w/ overt CHF and caution w/ history of well-compensated heart failure (HF). May lead to cardiac failure in patients w/o a history of HF; digitalize and/or treat w/ a diuretic at the 1st sign/symptom of HF and observe carefully. D/C (gradually, if possible) if cardiac failure continues. Exacerbation of angina and, in some cases, myocardial infarction reported after abrupt discontinuation. If angina markedly worsens or acute coronary insufficiency develops, reinstitute therapy promptly, at least temporarily, and take other appropriate measures for the management of unstable angina. Avoid in patients w/ nonallergic bronchospastic disease. Caution w/ pheochromocytoma; paradoxical hypertensive responses reported. May prevent appearance of premonitory signs/symptoms of acute hypoglycemia (eg, tachycardia). Chronically administered therapy should not be routinely withdrawn prior to major surgery. Several deaths have occurred during surgery (including when used in cases to control bleeding). Caution when reducing severely elevated BP; cerebral infarction, optic nerve infarction, angina, and ECG ischemic changes reported w/ other agents. Avoid rapid/excessive falls in BP; achieve desired BP lowering over as long a period of time as is compatible w/ patient status. Symptomatic postural hypotension may occur if patients are tilted or allowed to assume upright position w/in 3 hrs of administration; establish patient's ability to tolerate an upright position before permitting any ambulation. Intraoperative floppy iris syndrome (IFIS) observed during cataract surgery. Avoid in patients w/ low cardiac indices and elevated systemic vascular resistance. Hypotension or bradycardia reported w/ administration of up to 3g/day as an infusion for up to 2-3 days. Patients w/ a history of severe anaphylactic reactions to a variety of allergens may be more reactive to repeated challenge and may be unresponsive to usual doses of epinephrine. Lab test interactions may occur.

ADVERSE REACTIONS
Symptomatic postural hypotension, dizziness, N/V, somnolence/yawning, increased sweating, tingling of scalp/skin, transient BUN/SrCr increase.

DRUG INTERACTIONS
Tremors reported w/ oral labetalol in combination w/ TCAs. May blunt the bronchodilator effect of β-agonists in patients w/ bronchospasm; doses greater than the normal antiasthmatic dose may be required. Cimetidine may increase bioavailability of oral labetalol; caution in establishing required dose for BP control in patients w/ conditions that enhance absorption or alter hepatic metabolism. Synergistic effect w/ halothane; do not use ≥3% halothane during controlled hypotensive anesthesia. Additional antihypertensive effects w/ nitroglycerin. Caution w/ calcium antagonists of the verapamil type. May need to adjust dose of antidiabetic drugs. White precipitate noted when administered in combination w/ drug products that are alkaline (eg, furosemide); avoid administration in the same infusion line.

PREGNANCY AND LACTATION
Pregnancy: Category C. Hypotension, bradycardia, hypoglycemia, and respiratory depression reported in infants of mothers who were treated with labetalol for HTN during pregnancy.
Lactation: Small amounts of labetalol are excreted in human milk. Caution in nursing.

MECHANISM OF ACTION
α_1-blocker/nonselective β-blocker; produces dose-related falls in BP w/o reflex tachycardia and significant reduction in HR.

PHARMACOKINETICS
Distribution: Plasma protein binding (50%); found in breast milk; crosses placenta.
Metabolism: Conjugation to glucuronide metabolites. **Elimination:** Urine (55-60%, unchanged or conjugates), feces; $T_{1/2}$=5.5 hrs.

PATIENT CONSIDERATIONS
Assessment: Assess for hypersensitivity to the drug, bronchospastic disease, heart block, severe bradycardia, cardiogenic shock, overt cardiac failure, diabetes mellitus, pheochromocytoma, ischemic heart disease, hepatic/renal impairment, any other conditions where treatment is contraindicated or cautioned, pregnancy/nursing status, and possible drug interactions. Obtain baseline BP.

Monitoring: Monitor BP. Monitor LFTs periodically. In patients w/ concomitant illnesses (eg, renal impairment), monitor these conditions. Monitor for signs/symptoms of HF, postural hypotension, exacerbation of ischemic heart disease following abrupt withdrawal, hypersensitivity reactions, IFIS during cataract surgery, and other adverse reactions. Monitor patient when discontinuing therapy.

Counseling: Instruct to remain supine during and immediately following (for up to 3 hrs) inj; advise on how to proceed gradually to become ambulatory. Instruct to consult physician at any sign/symptom of impending HF or hepatic dysfunction. Instruct on appropriate directions for titration of dosage when started on labetalol tabs following adequate BP control w/ labetalol inj. Inform that transient scalp tingling may occur when treatment w/ tabs is initiated. Instruct patients being treated w/ labetalol tabs not to interrupt or d/c therapy w/o physician's advice. Advise to limit physical activity when discontinuing therapy.

LABETALOL TABLETS — labetalol hydrochloride   Rx

Class: Alpha₁ blocker/nonselective beta blocker

OTHER BRAND NAMES
Trandate Tablets

ADULT DOSAGE
Hypertension
Initial: 100mg bid
Titrate: After 2-3 days, may be titrated in increments of 100mg bid q2-3 days
Maint: 200-400mg bid
Severe HTN:
1200-2400mg/day given bid w/ or w/o diuretics
Titration increments should not exceed 200mg bid

PEDIATRIC DOSAGE
Pediatric use may not have been established

Should side effects (eg, N/V) occur, same total daily dose administered tid may improve tolerability and facilitate further titration

---

DOSING CONSIDERATIONS
Elderly
Usual Maint: 100-200mg bid
Concomitant Medications
W/ Diuretic: Dosage adjustment of labetalol may be necessary

ADMINISTRATION
Oral route

STORAGE
20-25°C (68-77°F).

HOW SUPPLIED
Tab: 100mg*, 200mg*, 300mg *scored

CONTRAINDICATIONS
Bronchial asthma, overt cardiac failure, greater than 1st-degree heart block, cardiogenic shock, severe bradycardia, other conditions associated w/ severe and prolonged hypotension, history of hypersensitivity to any component of the product, history of obstructive airway disease.

WARNINGS/PRECAUTIONS
Severe hepatocellular injury (rare) reported. Caution with hepatic impairment. Perform appropriate lab testing at the 1st symptom/sign of liver dysfunction. D/C and do not restart with lab evidence of liver injury or jaundice. May precipitate more severe failure in patients with congestive heart failure (CHF); avoid with overt CHF and caution with history of well-compensated heart failure (HF). May lead to cardiac failure in patients without a history of HF; digitalize and/or treat with a diuretic at the 1st sign/symptom of HF and observe carefully; d/c (gradually, if possible) if cardiac failure continues. Hypersensitivity to catecholamines observed upon withdrawal; exacerbation of angina, and in some cases, myocardial infarction reported after abrupt discontinuation. When discontinuing chronically administered labetalol, particularly in patients with ischemic heart disease, reduce dose over a period of 1-2 weeks and monitor carefully. If angina markedly worsens or acute coronary insufficiency develops, reinstitute therapy promptly, at least temporarily, and other appropriate measures for the management of unstable angina should be taken. Avoid in patients with bronchospastic disease but may use with caution in those who do not respond to, or cannot tolerate, other antihypertensive agents; smallest effective dose should be used. Caution with pheochromocytoma; paradoxical hypertensive responses reported. May prevent appearance of premonitory signs/symptoms of acute hypoglycemia (eg, tachycardia). Chronically administered therapy should not be routinely withdrawn prior to major surgery. Intraoperative floppy iris syndrome (IFIS) observed during cataract surgery. Patients with a history of severe anaphylactic reaction to a variety of allergens may be more reactive to repeated challenge and may be unresponsive to usual doses of epinephrine. Lab test interactions may occur. Caution in elderly.

ADVERSE REACTIONS
Fatigue, dizziness, dyspepsia, nausea, nasal stuffiness, ejaculation failure, impotence.

DRUG INTERACTIONS
Tremors reported with TCAs. May blunt the bronchodilator effect of β-agonists in patients with bronchospasm; doses greater than the normal antiasthmatic dose may be required. Increased bioavailability with cimetidine; caution in establishing required dose for BP control in patients with conditions that enhance absorption or alter hepatic metabolism. Synergistic effects with halothane and IV labetalol reported; do not use ≥3% halothane during controlled hypotensive anesthesia. Additional antihypertensive effect with nitroglycerin. Caution with calcium antagonists of the verapamil type. Concomitant use of digitalis glycosides may increase risk of bradycardia. May need to adjust dose of antidiabetic drugs.

PREGNANCY AND LACTATION
Category C, caution in nursing.

MECHANISM OF ACTION
α1 blocker/nonselective β-blocker; produces dose-related falls in BP without reflex tachycardia and without significant reduction in HR.

PHARMACOKINETICS
Absorption: Complete; T_{max}=1-2 hrs. Absolute bioavailability (25%). **Distribution:** Plasma protein binding (50%); found in breast milk; crosses placenta. **Metabolism:** Conjugation to glucuronide metabolites. **Elimination:** Urine (55%-60%, glucuronide conjugates or unchanged), feces; $T_{1/2}$=6-8 hrs.

PATIENT CONSIDERATIONS
Assessment: Assess for hypersensitivity to drug, bronchospastic disease, heart block, severe bradycardia, cardiogenic shock, overt cardiac failure, diabetes mellitus, pheochromocytoma, ischemic heart disease, hepatic/renal impairment, any other conditions where treatment is contraindicated or cautioned, pregnancy/nursing status, and possible drug interactions. Obtain baseline BP.

Monitoring: Monitor BP. Monitor LFTs periodically. In patients with concomitant illnesses (eg, renal impairment), monitor these conditions. Monitor for signs/symptoms of HF, exacerbation of ischemic heart disease following abrupt withdrawal, hypersensitivity reactions, IFIS during cataract surgery, and other adverse reactions.

Counseling: Instruct not to interrupt or d/c therapy without physician's advice. Instruct to consult a physician at any signs/symptoms of HF or hepatic dysfunction (eg, pruritus, dark urine, persistent anorexia, jaundice). Inform that transient scalp itching may occur, usually when treatment is initiated.

LAMICTAL — lamotrigine

Class: Phenyltriazine

Rx

> Serious life-threatening rashes, including Stevens-Johnson syndrome, toxic epidermal necrolysis, and/or rash-related death reported. Serious rash occurs more often in pediatric patients than in adults. D/C at 1st sign of rash, unless rash is clearly not drug related. Potential increased risk w/ concomitant valproate (including valproic acid and divalproex sodium) or exceeding the recommended initial dose/dose escalation.

OTHER BRAND NAMES
Lamictal ODT

ADULT DOSAGE

Epilepsy

Adjunctive Therapy for Partial-Onset, Primary Generalized Tonic-Clonic Seizures, or Generalized Seizures of Lennox-Gastaut Syndrome:

Taking Valproate:
Weeks 1 and 2: 25mg qod
Weeks 3 and 4: 25mg/day
Week 5 Onward: Increase every 1-2 weeks by 25-50mg/day
Maint: 100-200mg/day w/ valproate alone or 100-400mg/day w/ valproate and other drugs inducing glucuronidation in 1 or 2 divided doses

Not Taking Carbamazepine, Phenytoin, Phenobarbital, Primidone, or Valproate:
Weeks 1 and 2: 25mg qd
Weeks 3 and 4: 50mg/day
Week 5 Onward: Increase every 1-2 weeks by 50mg/day
Maint: 225-375mg/day in 2 divided doses

Taking Carbamazepine, Phenytoin, Phenobarbital, or Primidone, w/o Valproate:
Weeks 1 and 2: 50mg/day
Weeks 3 and 4: 100mg/day in 2 divided doses
Week 5 Onward: Increase every 1-2 weeks by 100mg/day
Maint: 300-500mg/day in 2 divided doses

Bipolar I Disorder

Maint Treatment to Delay the Time to Occurrence of Mood Episodes in Patients Treated for Acute Mood Episodes w/ Standard Therapy:

Taking Valproate:
Weeks 1 and 2: 25mg qod
Weeks 3 and 4: 25mg/day
Week 5: 50mg/day
Weeks 6 and 7: 100mg/day

Not Taking Carbamazepine, Phenytoin, Phenobarbital, Primidone, or Valproate:
Weeks 1 and 2: 25mg/day
Weeks 3 and 4: 50mg/day
Week 5: 100mg/day
Weeks 6 and 7: 200mg/day

Taking Carbamazepine, Phenytoin, Phenobarbital, or Primidone, w/o Valproate:
Weeks 1 and 2: 50mg/day
Weeks 3 and 4: 100mg/day
Week 5: 200mg/day
Week 6: 300mg/day
Week 7: Up to 400mg/day
Weeks 3-7: Take in divided doses

Conversions

Conversion from Adjunctive Therapy to Monotherapy:
≥16 Years:
Monotherapy Maint: 500mg/day in 2 divided doses

From Adjunctive Therapy w/ Carbamazepine, Phenytoin, Phenobarbital, or Primidone:
After achieving a dose of 500mg/day of lamotrigine, withdraw concomitant antiepileptic drug by 20% decrements each week over a 4-week period

PEDIATRIC DOSAGE

Epilepsy

Adjunctive Therapy for Partial-Onset, Primary Generalized Tonic-Clonic Seizures, or Generalized Seizures of Lennox-Gastaut Syndrome:

2-12 Years:
Round dose down to the nearest whole tab; give in 1-2 divided doses

Taking Valproate:
Initial Weight-Based Dosing Guide (Weeks 1-4): Refer to PI
Weeks 1 and 2: 0.15mg/kg/day
Weeks 3 and 4: 0.3mg/kg/day
Week 5 Onward: Increase every 1-2 weeks by 0.3mg/kg/day
Maint: 1-5mg/kg/day (max 200mg/day) or 1-3mg/kg/day w/ valproate alone

Not Taking Carbamazepine, Phenytoin, Phenobarbital, Primidone, or Valproate:
Weeks 1 and 2: 0.3mg/kg/day
Weeks 3 and 4: 0.6mg/kg/day
Week 5 Onward: Increase every 1-2 weeks by 0.6mg/kg/day
Maint: 4.5-7.5mg/kg/day
Max: 300mg/day in 2 divided doses

Taking Carbamazepine, Phenytoin, Phenobarbital, or Primidone, w/o Valproate:
Weeks 1 and 2: 0.6mg/kg/day
Weeks 3 and 4: 1.2mg/kg/day
Week 5 Onward: Increase every 1-2 weeks by 1.2mg/kg/day
Maint: 5-15mg/kg/day
Max: 400mg/day in 2 divided doses

>12 Years:
Taking Valproate:
Weeks 1 and 2: 25mg qod
Weeks 3 and 4: 25mg/day
Week 5 Onward: Increase every 1-2 weeks by 25-50mg/day
Maint: 100-200mg/day w/ valproate alone or 100-400mg/day w/ valproate and other drugs inducing glucuronidation in 1 or 2 divided doses

Not Taking Carbamazepine, Phenytoin, Phenobarbital, Primidone, or Valproate:
Weeks 1 and 2: 25mg qd
Weeks 3 and 4: 50mg/day
Week 5 Onward: Increase every 1-2 weeks by 50mg/day
Maint: 225-375mg/day in 2 divided doses

Taking Carbamazepine, Phenytoin, Phenobarbital, or Primidone, w/o Valproate:
Weeks 1 and 2: 50mg/day
Weeks 3 and 4: 100mg/day in 2 divided doses
Week 5 Onward: Increase every 1-2 weeks by 100mg/day
Maint: 300-500mg/day in 2 divided doses

From Adjunctive Therapy w/ Valproate:
1. Maintain lamotrigine at 200mg/day and decrease valproate by decrements no >500mg/day/week to 500mg/day and then maintain for 1 week
2. Increase lamotrigine to 300mg/day and maintain for 1 week; simultaneously decrease valproate to 250mg/day and maintain for 1 week
3. Increase lamotrigine by 100mg/day every week to achieve maint dose of 500mg/day; d/c valproate

- -

DOSING CONSIDERATIONS

Concomitant Medications

Taking Estrogen-Containing Oral Contraceptives w/o Other Drugs Known to Induce Glucuronidation:
May need to increase maint dose of lamotrigine by as much as 2-fold

Starting Estrogen-Containing Oral Contraceptives w/o Other Drugs Known to Induce Glucuronidation:
May need to increase maint dose of lamotrigine by as much as 2-fold. Increase lamotrigine dose at the same time the oral contraceptive is introduced; no more than 50-100mg/day every week.
If adverse reactions occur during the pill-free week due to lamotrigine, may need to adjust overall maint dose; dose adjustments limited to pill-free week not recommended

Stopping Estrogen-Containing Oral Contraceptives w/o Other Drugs Known to Induce Glucuronidation:
May need to decrease maint dose of lamotrigine by as much as 50%; decreases should not exceed 25% of total daily dose/week over a 2-week period, unless clinical response or lamotrigine plasma levels indicate otherwise

Taking Atazanavir/Ritonavir But Not Taking Other Glucuronidation Inducers:
Lamotrigine may need to be increased if atazanavir/ritonavir is added or decreased if atazanavir/ritonavir is discontinued

Bipolar Disorder:
Discontinuation of Psychotropic Drugs Excluding Valproate, Carbamazepine, Phenytoin, Phenobarbital, or Primidone:
Maintain current dose of lamotrigine
After Discontinuation of Valproate w/ Current dose of 100mg/day Lamotrigine:
Week 1: 150mg/day
Week 2 Onward: 200mg/day
After Discontinuation of Carbamazepine, Phenytoin, Phenobarbital, or Primidone w/ Current Dose of 400mg/day Lamotrigine:
Week 1: 400mg/day
Week 2: 300mg/day
Week 3 Onward: 200mg/day

Renal Impairment
Significant: Reduce maint doses

Hepatic Impairment
Moderate/Severe w/o Ascites: Reduce initial, escalation, and maint doses by approx 25%
Severe w/ Ascites: Reduce initial, escalation, and maint doses by 50%
Adjust maint and escalation doses based on clinical response

Elderly
Start at lower end of dosing range

Discontinuation
A step-wise reduction over at least 2 weeks (approx 50% per week) is recommended unless safety concerns require a more rapid withdrawal

Other Important Considerations
<30kg: Maint dose may need to be increased by as much as 50%, based on clinical response

ADMINISTRATION
Oral route

Tab, Chewable
May swallow whole, chewed, or dispersed in water or diluted fruit juice.
If tabs are chewed, consume a small amount of water or diluted fruit juice to aid in swallowing.
To disperse chewable tabs, add tabs to a small amount of liquid (1 tsp, or enough to cover the medication); approx 1 min later when tabs are completely dispersed, swirl sol and consume entire quantity immediately.

Tab, Orally Disintegrating
Place onto the tongue and move around in the mouth
Can be swallowed w/ or w/o water and taken w/ or w/ food

STORAGE
(Tab/Tab, Chewable) 25°C (77°F); excursions permitted to 15-30°C (59-86°F) in a dry place. (Tab) Protect from light. (Tab, Disintegrating) 20-25°C (68-77°F); excursions permitted between 15-30°C (59-86°F).

HOW SUPPLIED
Tab: 25mg*, 100mg*, 150mg*, 200mg*; **Tab, Chewable:** 2mg, 5mg, 25mg; **Tab, Disintegrating:** (ODT) 25mg, 50mg, 100mg, 200mg *scored

CONTRAINDICATIONS
Hypersensitivity (eg, rash, angioedema, acute urticaria, extensive pruritus, mucosal ulceration) to the drug or its ingredients.

WARNINGS/PRECAUTIONS

Not recommended for treatment of acute manic/mixed episodes. Drug reaction w/ eosinophilia and systemic symptoms (DRESS), also known as multiorgan hypersensitivity reactions, reported. Fatalities from acute multiorgan failure and various degrees of hepatic failure reported. Isolated liver failure w/o rash or involvement of other organs reported. D/C if alternative etiology for signs/symptoms of early manifestations of hypersensitivity cannot be established. Blood dyscrasias (eg, neutropenia, leukopenia) reported. Increased risk of suicidal thoughts or behavior. Increases risk of developing aseptic meningitis; evaluate for other causes of aseptic meningitis and treat appropriately. Avoid abrupt withdrawal due to risk of withdrawal seizures. Treatment-emergent status epilepticus and sudden unexplained death in epilepsy reported. May cause toxicity in the eyes and other melanin-rich tissues due to melanin binding. Medication errors reported. Do not restart therapy in patients who discontinued due to rash associated w/ prior treatment, unless potential benefits outweigh the risks. If restarting after discontinuation, assess the need to restart w/ initial dosing recommendations. May interfere w/ assay used in some rapid urine screens, which can result in false-positive readings, particularly for phencyclidine; use a more specific analytical method to confirm a positive result.

ADVERSE REACTIONS

Rash, dizziness, diplopia, infection, headache, ataxia, blurred vision, N/V, somnolence, fever, pharyngitis, rhinitis, diarrhea, abdominal pain, tremor.

DRUG INTERACTIONS

See Boxed Warning and Dosing Considerations. Estrogen-containing oral contraceptives, carbamazepine, lopinavir/ritonavir, phenobarbital/primidone, and phenytoin decreased levels. Atazanavir/ritonavir and rifampin decreased exposure. May decrease levels of levonorgestrel. Valproate may increase levels. May increase carbamazepine epoxide levels. Drugs known to induce or inhibit glucuronidation may affect clearance. May increase plasma levels of drugs substantially excreted via organic cationic transporter 2 (OCT2) proteins; avoid w/ OCT2 substrates w/ a narrow therapeutic index (eg, dofetilide).

PREGNANCY AND LACTATION

Category C, caution in nursing.

MECHANISM OF ACTION

Phenyltriazine; has not been established. Suspected to inhibit voltage-sensitive Na$^+$ channels, thereby stabilizing neuronal membranes and consequently modulating presynaptic transmitter release of excitatory amino acids (eg, glutamate, aspartate).

PHARMACOKINETICS

Absorption: Rapid and complete. Absolute bioavailability (98%); T_{max}=1.4-4.8 hrs. **Distribution:** V_d=0.9-1.3L/kg; plasma protein binding (55%); found in breast milk. **Metabolism:** Liver via glucuronic acid conjugation; 2-N-glucuronide conjugate (major metabolite, inactive). **Elimination:** Urine (94%; 10% unchanged, 76% 2-N-glucuronide), feces (2%). Refer to PI for variable parameters w/ concomitant AEDs.

PATIENT CONSIDERATIONS

Assessment: Assess for history of allergy/rash to other AEDs, renal/hepatic impairment, depression, systemic lupus erythematosus or other autoimmune diseases, hypersensitivity to drug, pregnancy/nursing status, and possible drug interactions.

Monitoring: Monitor for signs/symptoms of rash, DRESS, multiorgan failure, status epilepticus, blood dyscrasias, emergence/worsening of depression, suicidal thoughts or behavior, unusual mood/behavior changes, aseptic meningitis, ophthalmologic effects, and other adverse reactions. Periodically reassess patients w/ bipolar disorder taking lamotrigine for >16 weeks to determine need for maintenance treatment.

Counseling: Inform that a rash or other signs/symptoms of hypersensitivity may herald a serious medical event; instruct to report such symptoms to healthcare providers immediately; instruct to notify healthcare providers immediately if blood dyscrasias, DRESS, acute multiorgan failure, or aseptic meningitis occur. Inform about increased risk of suicidal thoughts and behavior; instruct to be alert for emergence/worsening of symptoms of depression, any unusual changes in mood/behavior, suicidal thoughts/behavior, or thoughts about self-harm. Instruct to immediately report behaviors of concern to healthcare providers. Instruct to notify healthcare providers if worsening of seizure control occurs. Inform that CNS depression may occur; instruct to avoid operating machinery/driving until effects of the drug are known. Instruct to notify healthcare providers if pregnant, intending to become pregnant, or if breastfeeding. Encourage patients to enroll in the North American Antiepileptic Drug Pregnancy Registry. Instruct women to notify healthcare providers if they plan to start/stop use of oral contraceptives or other hormonal preparations. Instruct to promptly notify healthcare providers of changes in menstrual pattern and adverse reactions. Instruct to notify healthcare providers if medication is discontinued and not to resume therapy w/o consulting healthcare providers. Strongly advise to visually inspect tab to verify if correct drug/formulation was dispensed each time prescription is filled.

LAMICTAL XR — lamotrigine   Rx

Class: Phenyltriazine

ADULT DOSAGE

Seizures

Adjunctive Therapy for Primary Generalized Tonic-Clonic Seizures

PEDIATRIC DOSAGE

Seizures

Adjunctive Therapy for Primary Generalized Tonic-Clonic Seizures

---

and Partial-Onset Seizures w/ or w/o Secondary Generalization:

Taking Valproate:
Weeks 1 and 2: 25mg qod
Weeks 3 and 4: 25mg qd
Week 5: 50mg qd
Week 6: 100mg qd
Week 7: 150mg qd
Week 8 Onward (Maint): 200-250mg qd

Not Taking Carbamazepine, Phenytoin, Phenobarbital, Primidone, or Valproate:
Weeks 1 and 2: 25mg qd
Weeks 3 and 4: 50mg qd
Week 5: 100mg qd
Week 6: 150mg qd
Week 7: 200mg qd
Week 8 Onward (Maint): 300-400mg qd

Taking Carbamazepine, Phenytoin, Phenobarbital, or Primidone, w/o Valproate:
Weeks 1 and 2: 50mg qd
Weeks 3 and 4: 100mg qd
Week 5: 200mg qd
Week 6: 300mg qd
Week 7: 400mg qd
Week 8 Onward (Maint): 400-600mg qd

Dose increases at week 8 or later should not exceed 100mg/day at weekly intervals

Conversions

Conversion from Adjunctive Therapy to Monotherapy:
Monotherapy Maint: 250-300mg qd

From Adjunctive Therapy w/ Carbamazepine, Phenytoin, Phenobarbital, or Primidone:
1. After achieving 500mg/day Lamictal XR, withdraw concomitant antiepileptic drug by 20% decrements/week over a 4-week period
2. Two weeks after withdrawal of the antiepileptic drug, Lamictal XR may be decreased no faster than 100mg/day each week to achieve monotherapy maint dosage range of 250-300mg/day

From Adjunctive Therapy w/ Valproate:
1. Achieve dose of 150mg/day of Lamictal XR; maintain established stable valproate dose
2. Maintain dose of Lamictal XR at 150mg/day; decrease valproate by decrements no >500mg/day/week to 500mg/day and maintain for 1 week
3. Increase Lamictal XR to 200mg/day; simultaneously decrease valproate to 250mg/day and maintain for 1 week
4. Increase Lamictal XR to 250 or 300mg/day; d/c valproate

From Adjunctive Therapy w/ Antiepileptic Drugs Other than Carbamazepine, Phenytoin, Phenobarbital, Primidone, or Valproate:
After achieving 250-300mg/day of Lamictal XR, withdraw concomitant antiepileptic drug by 20% decrements each week over a 4-week period

Conversion from Immediate Release (IR) to Extended Release Tabs:
Initial dose of therapy should match the total daily dose of IR lamotrigine

---

and Partial-Onset Seizures w/ or w/o Secondary Generalization:
≥13 Years:

Taking Valproate:
Weeks 1 and 2: 25mg qod
Weeks 3 and 4: 25mg qd
Week 5: 50mg qd
Week 6: 100mg qd
Week 7: 150mg qd
Week 8 Onward (Maint): 200-250mg qd

Not Taking Carbamazepine, Phenytoin, Phenobarbital, Primidone, or Valproate:
Weeks 1 and 2: 25mg qd
Weeks 3 and 4: 50mg qd
Week 5: 100mg qd
Week 6: 150mg qd
Week 7: 200mg qd
Week 8 Onward (Maint): 300-400mg qd

Taking Carbamazepine, Phenytoin, Phenobarbital, or Primidone, w/o Valproate:
Weeks 1 and 2: 50mg qd
Weeks 3 and 4: 100mg qd
Week 5: 200mg qd
Week 6: 300mg qd
Week 7: 400mg qd
Week 8 Onward (Maint): 400-600mg qd

Dose increases at week 8 or later should not exceed 100mg/day at weekly intervals

Conversions

≥13 Years:

Conversion from Adjunctive Therapy to Monotherapy:
Monotherapy Maint: 250-300mg qd

From Adjunctive Therapy w/ Carbamazepine, Phenytoin, Phenobarbital, or Primidone:
1. After achieving 500mg/day of Lamictal XR, withdraw concomitant antiepileptic drug by 20% decrements/week over a 4-week period
2. Two weeks after withdrawal of the antiepileptic drug, Lamictal XR may be decreased no faster than 100mg/day each week to monotherapy maint dosage range of 250-300mg/day.

From Adjunctive Therapy w/ Valproate:
1. Achieve dose of 150mg/day of Lamictal XR; maintain established stable valproate dose
2. Maintain dose of Lamictal XR at 150mg/day; decrease valproate by decrements no >500mg/day/week to 500mg/day and maintain for 1 week
3. Increase Lamictal XR to 200mg/day; simultaneously decrease valproate to 250mg/day and maintain for 1 week
4. Increase Lamictal XR to 250 or 300mg/day; d/c valproate

From Adjunctive Therapy w/ Antiepileptic Drugs Other than Carbamazepine, Phenytoin, Phenobarbital, Primidone, or Valproate:
After achieving 250-300mg/day of Lamictal XR, withdraw concomitant antiepileptic drug by 20% decrements each week over a 4-week period

Conversion from Immediate Release (IR) to Extended Release Tabs:
Initial dose of therapy should match the total daily dose of IR lamotrigine

---

DOSING CONSIDERATIONS

Concomitant Medications
Taking Estrogen-Containing Oral Contraceptives w/o Other Drugs Known to Induce Glucuronidation:
May need to increase maint dose by as much as 2-fold

Starting Estrogen-Containing Oral Contraceptives w/o Other Drugs Known to Induce Glucuronidation:

May need to increase maint dose by as much as 2-fold
Increase at the same time the oral contraceptive is introduced and continue no more rapidly than 50-100mg/day every week
If adverse reactions occur during the pill-free week, may need to adjust overall maint dose; dose adjustments limited to pill-free week are not recommended

Stopping Estrogen-Containing Oral Contraceptives w/o Other Drugs Known to Induce Glucuronidation:
May need to decrease maint dose by as much as 50%; decreases should not exceed 25% of the total daily dose/week over a 2-week period, unless clinical response or lamotrigine plasma levels indicate otherwise

Atazanavir/Ritonavir Not Taking Other Glucuronidation Inducers:
May need to increase dose if atazanavir/ritonavir is added, or decrease if atazanavir/ritonavir is discontinued

Renal Impairment
Significant: Reduce maint doses

Hepatic Impairment
Moderate/Severe w/o Ascites: Reduce initial, escalation, and maint doses by 25%
Severe w/ Ascites: Reduce initial, escalation, and maint doses by 50%
Adjust maint and escalation doses based on clinical response

Elderly
Start at lower end of dosing range

Discontinuation
A step-wise reduction of dose over at least 2 weeks (approx 50% per week) is recommended unless safety concerns require a more rapid withdrawal

ADMINISTRATION
Oral route

May take w/ or w/o food
Swallow whole; do not chew, crush, or divide

STORAGE
25°C (77°F); excursions permitted to 15-30°C (59-86°F).

HOW SUPPLIED
Tab, Extended Release (ER): 25mg, 50mg, 100mg, 200mg, 250mg, 300mg

CONTRAINDICATIONS
Hypersensitivity (eg, rash, angioedema, acute urticaria, extensive pruritus, mucosal ulceration) to the drug or its ingredients.

WARNINGS/PRECAUTIONS
Drug reaction w/ eosinophilia and systemic symptoms (DRESS), also known as multiorgan hypersensitivity reactions, reported. Fatalities from acute multiorgan failure and various degrees of hepatic failure reported. Isolated liver failure w/o rash or involvement of other organs reported. D/C if alternative etiology for signs/symptoms of early manifestations of hypersensitivity cannot be established. Blood dyscrasias (eg, neutropenia, leukopenia) w/ the IR formulation reported. Increased risk of suicidal thoughts or behavior. Increases risk of developing aseptic meningitis; evaluate for other causes of aseptic meningitis and treat appropriately. Avoid abrupt withdrawal due to risk of withdrawal seizures. Treatment-emergent status epilepticus and sudden unexplained death in epilepsy reported w/ IR formulation. May cause toxicity in the eyes and other melanin-rich tissues due to melanin binding. Medication errors including errors due to product name confusion, reported. Caution w/ significant renal impairment, moderate/severe hepatic impairment, and in the elderly. Do not restart therapy in patients who discontinued due to rash associated w/ prior treatment, unless potential benefits outweigh the risks. If restarting after discontinuation, assess the need to restart w/ initial dosing recommendations. May interfere w/ assay used in some rapid urine screens, which can result in false-positive readings, particularly for phencyclidine; use a more specific analytical method to confirm a positive result. May increase incidence of subnormal values in some hematology analytes (eg, total WBC, monocytes).

ADVERSE REACTIONS
Rash, dizziness, N/V, tremor, asthenia, somnolence, diplopia, diarrhea, vertigo, depression, anxiety, blurred vision, anorexia, pharyngolaryngeal pain, cerebellar coordination and balance disorder.

DRUG INTERACTIONS
See Boxed Warning and Dosing Considerations. Estrogen-containing oral contraceptives, carbamazepine, lopinavir/ritonavir, phenobarbital/primidone, and phenytoin may decrease levels. Atazanavir/ritonavir and rifampin may decrease exposure. May decrease levels of levonorgestrel. Valproate may increase levels. May increase carbamazepine epoxide levels. Drugs known to induce or inhibit glucuronidation may affect clearance. May increase plasma levels of drugs substantially excreted via organic cationic transporter 2 (OCT2) proteins; avoid w/ OCT2 substrates w/ a narrow therapeutic index (eg, dofetilide).

PREGNANCY AND LACTATION
Category C, caution in nursing.

MECHANISM OF ACTION
Phenyltriazine; has not been established. Suspected to inhibit voltage-sensitive Na⁺ channels, thereby stabilizing neuronal membranes and consequently modulating presynaptic transmitter release of excitatory amino acids (eg, glutamate, aspartate).

PHARMACOKINETICS
Absorption: T_{max}(median)=4-6 hrs (w/ carbamazepine, phenytoin, phenobarbital, or primidone), 9-11 hrs (w/ valproate), 6-10 hrs (w/ other antiepileptic drugs [AEDs]).
Distribution: V_d=0.9-1.3L/kg; plasma protein binding (55%); found in breast milk.
Metabolism: Liver via glucuronic acid conjugation; 2-N-glucuronide conjugate (major metabolite, inactive). **Elimination:** Urine (94%; 10% unchanged, 76% 2-N-glucuronide), feces (2%). Refer to PI for further Reference on elimination parameters.

PATIENT CONSIDERATIONS
Assessment: Assess for history of allergy/rash to other AEDs, renal/hepatic impairment, depression, hypersensitivity to drug, pregnancy/nursing status, and possible drug interactions.

Monitoring: Monitor for signs/symptoms of rash, DRESS, multiorgan failure, status epilepticus, blood dyscrasias, emergence/worsening of depression, suicidal thoughts or behavior, unusual mood/behavior changes, aseptic meningitis, ophthalmologic effects, and other adverse reactions. Monitor for seizure control following conversion to ER, especially those on drugs that induce lamotrigine glucuronidation. If indicated, monitor plasma levels of lamotrigine and concomitant medications, particularly during dosage adjustments.

Counseling: Inform that a rash or other signs/symptoms of hypersensitivity may herald a serious medical event; instruct to report such symptoms to healthcare provider immediately. Instruct to notify healthcare provider immediately if blood dyscrasias, DRESS, acute multiorgan failure, or aseptic meningitis occur. Inform about increased risk of suicidal thoughts and behavior; instruct to be alert for emergence/worsening of signs/symptoms of depression, any unusual changes in mood/behavior, suicidal thoughts/behavior, or thoughts about self-harm. Instruct to immediately report behaviors of concern to healthcare provider. Instruct to notify healthcare provider if worsening of seizure control occurs. Inform that CNS depression may occur; instruct to avoid operating machinery/driving until effects of the drug are known. Advise to notify healthcare provider if pregnant/intending to become pregnant, or breastfeeding. Encourage patients to enroll in the North American Antiepileptic Drug Pregnancy Registry if they become pregnant. Instruct women to notify healthcare provider if they plan to start/stop oral contraceptives or other hormonal preparations. Instruct to promptly notify healthcare provider of changes in menstrual pattern and adverse reactions. Instruct to notify healthcare provider if medication is discontinued and not to resume therapy w/o consulting healthcare provider. Strongly advise to visually inspect tab to verify if correct drug/formulation is dispensed each time prescription is filled.

LAMISIL — terbinafine hydrochloride

Class: Allylamine antifungal

Rx

ADULT DOSAGE	PEDIATRIC DOSAGE
Tinea Capitis	**Tinea Capitis**
Granules:	**≥4 Years:**
<25kg: 125mg/day qd	**Granules:**
25-35kg: 187.5mg/day qd	**<25kg:** 125mg/day
>35kg: 250mg/day qd	**25-35kg:** 187.5mg/day
Treatment Duration: 6 weeks	**>35kg:** 250mg/day
Onychomycosis	**Treatment Duration:** 6 weeks
Due to Dermatophytes (Tinea Unguium):	
Tab:	
Fingernail: 250mg qd for 6 weeks	
Toenail: 250mg qd for 12 weeks	

DOSING CONSIDERATIONS
Elderly
Tab:
Start at lower end of dosing range

ADMINISTRATION
Oral route

Granules
Take w/ food
Sprinkle contents of 1 pkt on a spoonful of pudding or other soft, nonacidic food (eg, mashed potatoes), and swallow entire spoonful (w/o chewing); do not use applesauce or fruit-based foods
Either the contents of both pkts may be sprinkled on 1 spoonful, or the contents of both pkts may be sprinkled on 2 spoonfuls of nonacidic food if 2 pkts are required/dose

Tab
Take w/ or w/o food

STORAGE
Tab: <25°C (77°F); in a tight container. Protect from light. **Granules:** 25°C (77°F); excursions permitted to 15-30°C (59-86°F).

HOW SUPPLIED
Granules: 125mg/pkt, 187.5mg/pkt; **Tab:** 250mg

CONTRAINDICATIONS
History of allergic reaction to oral terbinafine.

WARNINGS/PRECAUTIONS
Cases of liver failure, some leading to liver transplant or death, reported in individuals with and without preexisting liver disease; d/c therapy if evidence of liver injury develops. Hepatotoxicity may occur. Not recommended for patients with chronic or active liver disease; perform LFTs prior to initiating therapy and periodically thereafter. D/C immediately in case of LFTs elevation or if any symptoms of persistent N/V, anorexia, fatigue, right upper abdominal pain, jaundice, dark urine, or pale stools occur. Taste/smell disturbance reported; d/c if symptoms occur. Depressive symptoms reported. Transient decreases in absolute lymphocyte counts and severe neutropenia reported; d/c and start supportive management if neutrophil count is ≤1000 cells/mm³. Consider monitoring CBCs in patients with known or suspected immunodeficiency if treatment continues for >6 weeks. Serious skin/hypersensitivity reactions (eg, Stevens-Johnson syndrome, toxic epidermal necrolysis, erythema multiforme, exfoliative/bullous dermatitis, drug reaction with eosinophilia and systemic symptoms (DRESS) syndrome) reported; d/c if progressive skin rash or signs/symptoms of DRESS occur.

Precipitation and exacerbation of cutaneous and systemic lupus erythematosus reported; d/c in patients with clinical signs/symptoms suggestive of lupus erythematosus.

ADVERSE REACTIONS

Headache, diarrhea. (Granules) Nasopharyngitis, pyrexia, cough, vomiting, URTI, upper abdominal pain. (Tab) Dyspepsia, nausea, rash, liver enzyme abnormalities, pruritus, taste disturbances.

DRUG INTERACTIONS

Coadministration with drugs predominantly metabolized by CYP2D6 (eg, TCAs, β-blockers, SSRIs, antiarrhythmics class 1C [eg, flecainide, propafenone], MAOIs type B, dextromethorphan) should be done with careful monitoring; may require dose reduction of the CYP2D6-metabolized drug. Increased dextromethorphan/ dextrorphan metabolite ratio in urine in patients who are extensive metabolizers of dextromethorphan; may convert extensive CYP2D6 metabolizers to poor metabolizer status. Increased levels/exposure of desipramine. Increased clearance of cyclosporine. Decreased clearance of caffeine. Fluconazole may increase levels and exposure. May increase systemic exposure with other inhibitors of both CYP2C9 and CYP3A4 (eg, ketoconazole, amiodarone). Clearance increased by rifampin and decreased by cimetidine. Increased or decreased PT with warfarin.

PREGNANCY AND LACTATION

Category B, not for use in nursing.

MECHANISM OF ACTION

Allylamine antifungal; acts by inhibiting squalene epoxidase, thus blocking biosynthesis of ergosterol, an essential component of fungal cell membrane.

PHARMACOKINETICS

Absorption: (Tab) Well-absorbed; bioavailability (40%); (250mg single dose) C_{max}=1mcg/mL, T_{max}=2 hrs, AUC=4.56mcg•hr/mL. **Distribution:** Plasma protein binding (>99%); found in breast milk. **Metabolism:** Extensive, (Granules) rapid. CYP2C9, CYP1A2, CYP3A4, CYP2C8, CYP2C19 (major). **Elimination:** Urine (70%). (Tab) $T_{1/2}$=200-400 hrs; (Granules) $T_{1/2}$=26.7 hrs (125mg dose), 30.5 hrs (187.5mg dose).

PATIENT CONSIDERATIONS

Assessment: Assess for known hypersensitivity to the drug, active/chronic liver disease, immunodeficiency, lupus erythematosus, pregnancy/nursing status, and possible drug interactions. Confirm diagnosis of onychomycosis (potassium hydroxide preparation, fungal culture, or nail biopsy). Obtain baseline LFTs.

Monitoring: Monitor for signs/symptoms of hepatotoxicity, taste/smell disturbances, progressive skin rash, DRESS, depressive symptoms, lupus erythematosus, and other adverse reactions. Monitor CBC in patients with known or suspected immunodeficiency if therapy continues for >6 weeks, or if signs/ symptoms of secondary infection occur. Monitor LFTs periodically.

Counseling: Advise to d/c treatment and report immediately to physician if N/V, right upper abdominal pain, jaundice, dark urine, pale stools, taste/smell disturbance, anorexia, fatigue, depressive symptoms, hives, mouth sores, blistering and peeling of skin, swelling of face, lips, tongue, or throat, difficulty breathing/ swallowing, fever, skin eruption, erythema, scaling, loss of pigment, unusual photosensitivity that can result in a rash, and lymph node enlargement occur. Instruct to minimize exposure to natural and artificial sunlight (tanning beds or UVA/B treatment) while on therapy. Advise to call physician if too many doses have been taken. If a dose is missed, advise to take tab as soon as remembered, unless it is <4 hrs before the next dose is due.

LANOXIN INJECTION — digoxin

Rx

Class: Cardiac glycoside

ADULT DOSAGE

Heart Failure

Mild to Moderate:
Dosing can be either initiated w/ a LD followed by maint dosing if rapid titration is desired or initiated w/ maint dosing w/o a LD

LD: 8-12mcg/kg; administer 1/2 the total LD initially, then 1/4 the LD q6-8h twice

Maint:
Initial: 2.4-3.6mcg/kg qd
Titrate: May increase dose every 2 weeks according to clinical response, serum drug levels, and toxicity
Max: 500mcg in a single site

Atrial Fibrillation

Control of Ventricular Response Rate in Chronic A-Fib:
Dosing can be either initiated w/ a LD followed by maint dosing if rapid titration is desired or initiated w/ maint dosing w/o a LD

LD: 8-12mcg/kg; administer 1/2 the total LD initially, then 1/4 the LD q6-8h twice

Maint:
Initial: 2.4-3.6mcg/kg qd

PEDIATRIC DOSAGE

Heart Failure

Increase Myocardial Contractility:
Dosing can be either initiated w/ a LD followed by maint dosing if rapid titration is desired or initiated w/ maint dosing w/o a LD

LD:
Administer 1/2 the total LD initially, then 1/4 the LD q6-8h twice
Premature Infants: 15-25mcg/kg
Full-Term Infants: 20-30mcg/kg
1-24 Months: 30-50mcg/kg
2-5 Years: 25-35mcg/kg
5-10 Years: 15-30mcg/kg
>10 Years: 8-12mcg/kg

Maint:
Initial:
Premature Infants: 1.9-3.1mcg/kg/ dose bid
Full-Term: 3.0-4.5mcg/kg/dose bid
1-24 Months: 4.5-7.5mcg/kg/dose bid
2-5 Years: 3.8-5.3mcg/kg/dose bid
5-10 Years: 2.3-4.5mcg/kg/dose bid
>10 Years: 2.4-3.6mcg/kg qd; may be increased every 2 weeks according to clinical response, serum drug levels, and toxicity

Max: 200mcg in a single site

Titrate: May increase dose every 2 weeks according to clinical response, serum drug levels, and toxicity
Max: 500mcg in a single site

Conversions
IV to Oral Conversion:
50mcg inj = 62.5mcg tab
100mcg inj = 125mcg tab
200mcg inj = 250mcg tab
400mcg inj = 500mcg tab

Conversions
IV to Oral Conversion:
50mcg inj = 62.5mcg tab
100mcg inj = 125mcg tab
200mcg inj = 250mcg tab
400mcg inj = 500mcg tab

DOSING CONSIDERATIONS
Renal Impairment
Refer to PI for recommended maint doses based on lean body weight and renal function

ADMINISTRATION
IV/IM route
Parenteral administration should be used only when the need for rapid digitalization is urgent or when the drug cannot be taken orally.
IV route is preferred; if IM route is necessary, inject deep into the muscle and follow w/ massage.
Administer over a period of ≥5 min; avoid bolus administration.
May be administered undiluted or diluted w/ a ≥4-fold volume of SWFI, 0.9% NaCl inj, or D5 inj; use of <4-fold volume of diluent could lead to precipitation of digoxin.
Used diluted sol immediately.
Do not mix w/ other drugs in the same container or administer simultaneously in the same IV line.

STORAGE
25°C (77°F); excursions permitted to 15-30°C (59-86°F). Protect from light.

HOW SUPPLIED
Inj: (Lanoxin) 0.25mg/mL, (Lanoxin Pediatric) 0.1mg/mL

CONTRAINDICATIONS
Ventricular fibrillation. Known hypersensitivity to digoxin (reactions seen include unexplained rash, swelling of the mouth, lips, or throat or a difficulty in breathing) or to other digitalis preparations.

WARNINGS/PRECAUTIONS
Increased risk of ventricular fibrillation in patients w/ Wolff-Parkinson-White syndrome who develop A-fib. May cause severe sinus bradycardia or sinoatrial block particularly in patients w/ preexisting sinus node disease and may cause advanced or complete heart block in patients w/ preexisting incomplete atrioventricular (AV) block; consider insertion of a pacemaker before treatment. Patients w/ low body weight, advanced age or impaired renal function, hypokalemia, hypercalcemia, or hypomagnesemia may be predisposed to digoxin toxicity. Signs/symptoms of digoxin toxicity may be mistaken for worsening symptoms of heart failure (HF). May be desirable to reduce dose or d/c therapy 1-2 days prior to electrical cardioversion of A-fib. If digitalis toxicity is suspected, delay elective cardioversion, and if it is not prudent to delay cardioversion, select the lowest possible energy level to avoid provoking ventricular arrhythmias. May increase myocardial oxygen demand and lead to ischemia in patients w/ acute MI; not recommended in these patients. May precipitate vasoconstriction and promote production of pro-inflammatory cytokines in patients w/ myocarditis; avoid use in these patients. Avoid in patients w/ HF associated w/ preserved left ventricular ejection fraction (eg, restrictive cardiomyopathy, constrictive pericarditis, amyloid heart disease, acute cor pulmonale) and patients w/ idiopathic hypertrophic subaortic stenosis. Hypocalcemia may nullify the effects of treatment. Hypothyroidism may reduce the requirements for therapy. HF and/ or atrial arrhythmias resulting from hypermetabolic or hyperdynamic states (eg, hyperthyroidism, hypoxia, arteriovenous shunt) are best treated by addressing the underlying condition. Patients w/ beri beri heart disease may fail to respond adequately to therapy if the underlying thiamine deficiency is not treated concomitantly. Endogenous substances of unknown composition (digoxin-like immunoreactive substances) may interfere w/ standard radioimmunoassays for digoxin. Caution in the elderly.

ADVERSE REACTIONS
Cardiac arrhythmias, N/V, abdominal pain, intestinal ischemia, hemorrhagic necrosis of the intestines, headache, weakness, dizziness, apathy, mental disturbances.

DRUG INTERACTIONS
Drugs that induce/inhibit P-gp may alter digoxin pharmacokinetics. Increased levels w/ quinidine, ritonavir, amiodarone, propafenone, quinine, spironolactone, and verapamil; refer to PI for recommendations to reduce digoxin concentrations. Drugs that affect renal function (eg, ACE inhibitors, ARBs, NSAIDs, COX-2 inhibitors) may impair excretion. Higher rate of torsades de pointes w/ dofetilide. Proarrhythmic events were more common w/ concomitant sotalol. Sudden death was more common w/ concomitant dronedarone. Teriparatide transiently increases serum calcium. Thyroid supplements may increase digoxin dose requirement. Increased risk of arrhythmias w/ epinephrine, norepinephrine, dopamine, and succinylcholine. Rapid IV calcium administration can produce serious arrhythmias in digitalized patients. Additive effects on AV node conduction w/ β-adrenergic blockers and calcium channel blockers.

PREGNANCY AND LACTATION
Pregnancy: Category C.
Lactation: The estimated exposure of a nursing infant to digoxin is far below the usual infant maintenance dose; this amount should have no pharmacologic effect on the infant.

MECHANISM OF ACTION

Cardiac glycoside; inhibits Na^+-K^+ ATPase, which is responsible for maintaining the intracellular milieu throughout the body by moving Na^+ ions out of and K^+ ions into cells.

PHARMACOKINETICS

Absorption: Absolute bioavailability (100%). **Distribution:** V_d=475-500L. Plasma protein binding (25%); crosses the blood-brain barrier and placenta; found in breast milk. **Metabolism:** Dihydrodigoxin, digoxigenin bisdigitoxoside, and their glucuronide and sulfate conjugates (metabolites) via hydrolysis, oxidation, and conjugation. **Elimination:** (Healthy, IV) Urine (50-70%, unchanged); $T_{1/2}$=(healthy) 1.5-2 days, (anuric patients) 3.5-5 days.

PATIENT CONSIDERATIONS

Assessment: Assess for known hypersensitivity to the drug or other digitalis preparations, ventricular fibrillation, myocarditis, hypermetabolic or hyperdynamic states, sinus node disease, AV block, pregnancy/nursing status, possible drug interactions, and any other conditions where treatment is cautioned. Assess serum electrolytes and renal function. Obtain a baseline digoxin level; serum digoxin concentrations may be falsely elevated by endogenous digoxin-like substances.

Monitoring: Monitor for signs/symptoms of severe sinus bradycardia, sinoatrial block, advanced or complete heart block, digoxin toxicity, vasoconstriction, and other adverse reactions. Monitor serum electrolytes and renal function periodically. Obtain serum digoxin concentrations just before the next dose or at least 6 hrs after the last dose. Monitor for clinical response.

Counseling: Advise that digoxin is used to treat HF and heart arrhythmias. Advise to inform physician if taking any OTC medications, including herbal medication, or if started on a new prescription. Inform that blood tests will be necessary to ensure the appropriate digoxin dose. Instruct to contact physician if N/V, persistent diarrhea, confusion, weakness, or visual disturbances occur. Advise parents or caregivers that symptoms of having too high doses may be difficult to recognize in infants and pediatric patients; inform that symptoms such as weight loss, failure to thrive in infants, abdominal pain, and behavioral disturbances may be indications of digoxin toxicity. Suggest to monitor and record HR and BP daily. Instruct women of childbearing potential who become or are planning to become pregnant to consult physician prior to initiating or continuing therapy.

LANTUS — insulin glargine

Class: Insulin (long-acting)

Rx

ADULT DOSAGE

Type 1 Diabetes Mellitus

Initial: Approx 1/3 of total daily insulin requirements
Titrate: Based on individual's metabolic needs, blood glucose monitoring results, and glycemic control goal

Use short-acting, premeal insulin to satisfy remainder of the daily insulin requirements

Type 2 Diabetes Mellitus

Not Currently Treated w/ Insulin:
Initial: 0.2 U/kg or up to 10 U qd
Titrate: Based on individual's metabolic needs, blood glucose monitoring results, and glycemic control goal

Conversions

From QD Toujeo 300 U/mL:
Initial Lantus dose is 80% of Toujeo that is being discontinued

From Intermediate- or Long-Acting Insulin:
Change in basal insulin dose may be required and amount and timing of the shorter-acting insulins and doses of any oral antidiabetic drugs may need to be adjusted

From QD NPH Insulin:
Initial Lantus dose is the same as the dose of NPH that is being discontinued

From BID NPH Insulin:
Initial Lantus dose is 80% of total NPH dose that is being discontinued

PEDIATRIC DOSAGE

Type 1 Diabetes Mellitus

≥6 Years:
Initial: Approx 1/3 of total daily insulin requirements
Titrate: Based on individual's metabolic needs, blood glucose monitoring results, and glycemic control goal

Use short-acting, premeal insulin to satisfy remainder of the daily insulin requirements

Conversions

From QD Toujeo 300 U/mL:
Initial Lantus dose is 80% of Toujeo that is being discontinued

From Intermediate- or Long-Acting Insulin:
Change in basal insulin dose may be required and amount and timing of the shorter-acting insulins and doses of any oral antidiabetic drugs may need to be adjusted

From QD NPH Insulin:
Initial Lantus dose is the same as the dose of NPH that is being discontinued

From BID NPH Insulin:
Initial Lantus dose is 80% of total NPH dose that is being discontinued

DOSING CONSIDERATIONS

Concomitant Medications

For patients w/ type 2 diabetes, may need to adjust dosage of concomitant oral antidiabetic products

Renal Impairment

Frequent glucose monitoring and dose adjustments may be necessary

Hepatic Impairment

Frequent glucose monitoring and dose adjustments may be necessary

Elderly

Dose conservatively

Other Important Considerations

Dosage adjustments may be needed w/ changes in physical activity, changes in meal patterns (eg, macronutrient content, timing of food intake), changes in hepatic/renal function, or during acute illness

ADMINISTRATION

SQ route

Inject into the abdominal area, thigh, or deltoid, and rotate inj sites w/in the same region from 1 inj to the next.
Inject qd at the same time every day.
Must be used w/ short-acting insulin in patients w/ type 1 diabetes mellitus.
Do not administer IV or via an insulin pump.
Do not dilute or mix w/ any other insulin or sol.
Refrigerate unused (unopened) vials and SoloStar prefilled pens.

SoloStar Prefilled Pen

For single patient use only.

STORAGE

Do not freeze; discard if drug has been frozen. **Unopened:** 2-8°C (36-46°F) until expiration date or <30°C (86°F) for 28 days. **Open (In-Use):** 2-8°C (36-46°F) or <30°C (86°F) for vials and <30°C (86°F) for SoloStar. Discard after 28 days. Protect from direct heat and light.

HOW SUPPLIED

Inj: 100 U/mL [3mL SoloStar, 10mL vial]

CONTRAINDICATIONS

During episodes of hypoglycemia; hypersensitivity to Lantus or one of its excipients.

WARNINGS/PRECAUTIONS

Not recommended for the treatment of diabetic ketoacidosis. Insulin pens, syringes, or needles must never be shared between patients, even if the needle is changed; may carry a risk for transmission of blood-borne pathogens. Changes in insulin strength, manufacturer, type, or method of administration may affect glycemic control and predispose to hypo/hyperglycemia. Hypoglycemia may occur and may impair concentration ability and reaction time. Symptomatic awareness of hypoglycemia may be less pronounced in patients w/ longstanding diabetes, diabetic nerve disease, w/ medications that block the sympathetic nervous system (eg, β-blockers), or in patients who experience recurrent hypoglycemia. The long-acting effect of insulin glargine may delay recovery from hypoglycemia. Accidental mix-ups among insulin products reported. Severe, life-threatening, generalized allergy, including anaphylaxis, may occur. If hypersensitivity reactions occur, d/c therapy; treat per standard of care and monitor until signs/symptoms resolve. May cause hypokalemia; monitor K^+ levels in patients at risk for hypokalemia (eg, patients using K^+-lowering medications or medications sensitive to serum K^+ concentrations) if indicated.

ADVERSE REACTIONS

Hypoglycemia, URTI, peripheral edema, HTN, influenza, sinusitis, cataract, bronchitis, arthralgia, infection, pain in extremities, back pain, cough, UTI, diarrhea.

DRUG INTERACTIONS

See Dosing Considerations. Dose adjustments and increased frequency of glucose monitoring may be required w/ drugs that may increase the risk of hypoglycemia (eg, ACE inhibitors, ARBs, disopyramide, fibrates, fluoxetine, MAOIs, pentoxifylline, pramlintide, propoxyphene, salicylates, somatostatin analogues [eg, octreotide], sulfonamide antibiotics), drugs that may decrease blood glucose-lowering effect (eg, atypical antipsychotics [eg, olanzapine, clozapine], corticosteroids, danazol, diuretics, estrogens, glucagon, isoniazid, niacin, oral contraceptives, phenothiazines, progestogens [eg, in oral contraceptives], protease inhibitors, somatropin, sympathomimetic agents [eg, albuterol, epinephrine, terbutaline], thyroid hormones), or drugs that may increase/decrease blood glucose-lowering effect (eg, alcohol, β-blockers, clonidine, lithium salts, pentamidine). Signs/symptoms of hypoglycemia may be blunted w/ β-blockers, clonidine, guanethidine, or reserpine. Observe for signs/symptoms of heart failure (HF) if treated concomitantly w/ a peroxisome proliferator-activated receptor (PPAR)-gamma agonist (eg, thiazolidinediones); consider discontinuation or dose reduction of the PPAR-gamma agonist if HF develops.

PREGNANCY AND LACTATION

Pregnancy: There are no well-controlled clinical studies in pregnant women; use during pregnancy only if potential benefit justifies potential risk to the fetus.
Lactation: It is not known if insulin glargine is excreted in human milk; caution in nursing. Use is compatible w/ breastfeeding, but women may require adjustments of insulin doses.

MECHANISM OF ACTION

Insulin glargine; regulates glucose metabolism. Lowers blood glucose by stimulating peripheral glucose uptake and by inhibiting hepatic glucose production. Inhibits lipolysis and proteolysis, and enhances protein synthesis.

PHARMACOKINETICS

Metabolism: M1 (21^A-Gly-insulin) and M2 (21^A-Gly-des-30^B-Thr-insulin) (active metabolites).

PATIENT CONSIDERATIONS

Assessment: Assess for diabetic ketoacidosis, predisposition to hypoglycemia, risk factors for hypokalemia, hypersensitivity, renal/hepatic impairment, pregnancy/nursing status, and possible drug interactions. Obtain baseline blood glucose and HbA1c levels.

Monitoring: Monitor for signs/symptoms of hypoglycemia, allergic reactions, and other adverse reactions. Monitor blood glucose and HbA1c levels, and renal/hepatic function. Monitor K^+ levels in patients at risk for hypokalemia if indicated.

Counseling: Advise to never share SoloStar pen w/ another person, even if needle is changed. Instruct not to reuse or share needles or syringes. Inform of hypoglycemia symptoms, including impairment of the ability to concentrate and react; advise to use caution when driving/operating machinery. Advise that changes in insulin regimen can predispose to hypo/hyperglycemia and that changes should be made under close medical supervision. Instruct to always check the label before each inj to avoid medication errors and to not dilute or mix w/ any other insulin or sol. Instruct on self-management procedures, including glucose monitoring, proper inj technique, management of hypo/hyperglycemia, and on handling of special situations (eg, intercurrent conditions, inadequate or skipped dose, inadvertent administration of increased insulin dose, inadequate food intake, skipped meals). Advise to inform physician if pregnant or contemplating pregnancy.

LASTACAFT — alcaftadine
Rx

Class: H₁ antagonist

ADULT DOSAGE
Allergic Conjunctivitis

Prevention of Itching:
1 drop in ou qd

PEDIATRIC DOSAGE
Allergic Conjunctivitis

Prevention of Itching:
≥2 Years:
1 drop in ou qd

DOSING CONSIDERATIONS
Concomitant Medications
Space dosing by at least 5 min if using >1 topical ophthalmic drug

ADMINISTRATION
Ocular route

STORAGE
15-25°C (59-77°F). Keep bottle tightly closed when not in use.

HOW SUPPLIED
Ophthalmic Sol: 0.25% [3mL]

CONTRAINDICATIONS
Hypersensitivity to any component in the product.

WARNINGS/PRECAUTIONS
Caution not to touch the dropper tip to eyelids or surrounding areas to minimize eye injury and contamination. Do not wear contact lens if the eye is red. Not for treatment of contact lens-related irritation. Do not instill while wearing contact lenses; may reinsert lenses after 10 min following administration.

ADVERSE REACTIONS
Eye irritation, burning and/or stinging upon instillation, eye redness, eye pruritus, nasopharyngitis, headache.

PREGNANCY AND LACTATION
Pregnancy: Category B.
Lactation: Caution in nursing.

MECHANISM OF ACTION
H₁-receptor antagonist; inhibits release of histamine from mast cells, decreases chemotaxis, and inhibits eosinophil activation.

PHARMACOKINETICS
Absorption: C_{max}=60pg/mL, 3ng/mL (active metabolite); T_{max}=15 min (median), 1 hr after dosing (active metabolite). **Distribution:** Plasma protein binding (39.2%), (62.7%, active metabolite). **Metabolism:** Non-CYP450 cytosolic enzymes; carboxylic acid metabolite (active metabolite). **Excretion:** Urine (unchanged); $T_{1/2}$=2 hrs (active metabolite).

PATIENT CONSIDERATIONS
Assessment: Assess for hypersensitivity to the drug, contact lens-related irritation, and pregnancy/nursing status.

Monitoring: Monitor for possible adverse reactions.

Counseling: Advise to avoid touching the eyelids or surrounding areas w/ the dropper tip to minimize eye injury and contamination of the dropper tip and sol. Instruct to administer ≥5 min apart if >1 topical ophthalmic drug is being used. Advise not to wear contact lenses if the eye is red. Advise not to use to treat contact lens-related irritation. Advise to remove contact lenses prior to instillation; lenses may be reinserted after 10 min following administration.

LATISSE — bimatoprost
Rx

Class: Prostaglandin analogue

ADULT DOSAGE
Hypotrichosis of the Eyelashes

Apply 1 drop qpm

PEDIATRIC DOSAGE
Hypotrichosis of the Eyelashes

≥5 Years:
Apply 1 drop qpm

ADMINISTRATION
Topical route

1. Ensure face is clean, and that makeup and contact lenses are removed.
2. Place one drop on disposable sterile applicator and apply evenly along the skin of the upper eyelid margin at the base of eyelashes; do not apply to lower eyelash line.
3. Upper lid margin in area of lash growth should feel lightly moist w/o runoff; blot

any excess sol runoff outside upper eyelid margin w/ a tissue or other absorbent cloth.
4. Dispose of applicator after one use; repeat for the opposite eyelid margin using a new sterile applicator.
5. Do not reuse applicators and do not use any other brush/applicator to apply sol.

STORAGE
2-25°C (36-77°F).

HOW SUPPLIED
Sol: 0.03% [3mL, 5mL]

WARNINGS/PRECAUTIONS
May lower intraocular pressure (IOP) when instilled directly to the eye. Increased iris pigmentation reported; may continue therapy in patients who develop noticeably increased iris pigmentation. May cause pigment changes (darkening) to periorbital pigmented tissues and eyelashes. May cause hair growth to occur in areas where sol comes in repeated contact with skin surface. Caution with active intraocular inflammation (eg, uveitis); inflammation may be exacerbated. Macular edema (eg, cystoid macular edema) reported during treatment of elevated IOP; caution in aphakic patients, pseudophakic patients with a torn posterior lens capsule, or in patients at risk for macular edema. Do not allow the bottle tip to contact any other surface. Use the accompanying sterile applicators on 1 eye and then discard; reuse of applicators increases the potential for contamination and infections. Bacterial keratitis associated with the use of multiple-dose containers reported. Contains benzalkonium chloride, which may be absorbed by and cause discoloration of soft contact lenses; contact lenses should be removed prior to application and may be reinserted 15 min following administration.

ADVERSE REACTIONS
Eye pruritus, conjunctival hyperemia, skin hyperpigmentation, ocular irritation, dry eye symptoms, periorbital erythema.

DRUG INTERACTIONS
May interfere with the desired reduction in IOP when given with other prostaglandin analogues for the treatment of elevated IOP.

PREGNANCY AND LACTATION
Category C, caution in nursing.

MECHANISM OF ACTION
Prostaglandin analogue; not established. Growth of eyelashes is believed to occur by increasing the percent of hairs in, and the duration of the anagen or growth phase.

PHARMACOKINETICS
Absorption: C_{max}=0.08ng/mL; AUC=0.09ng•hr/mL; T_{max}=10 min. **Distribution:** V_d=0.67L/kg. **Metabolism:** Oxidation, N-deethylation, and glucuronidation. **Elimination:** (IV) Urine (up to 67%), feces (25%); $T_{1/2}$=45 min.

PATIENT CONSIDERATIONS
Assessment: Assess for active intraocular inflammation, aphakia, pseudophakia with a torn posterior lens capsule, risk for macular edema, pregnancy/nursing status, and possible drug interactions.

Monitoring: Monitor for IOP changes, increased iris pigmentation, pigment changes (darkening) to periorbital pigmented tissues and eyelashes, macular edema, bacterial keratitis, and other adverse reactions.

Counseling: Instruct to apply medication ud. Counsel that if any sol gets into the eye proper, it will not cause harm, and the eye should not be rinsed. Counsel that the effect is not permanent and can be expected to gradually return to original level upon discontinuation. Instruct that the bottle must be maintained intact and to avoid contaminating the bottle tip or applicator. Advise that serious infections may result from using contaminated sol or applicators. Instruct to consult physician before use if using prostaglandin analogues for IOP reduction. Inform about the possibility of eyelid skin darkening, increased brown iris pigmentation (may be permanent), hair growth outside of the target treatment area, and disparity between eyes in length, thickness, pigmentation, number of eyelashes or vellus hairs, and/or direction of eyelash growth. Advise to consult physician if patient has ocular surgery, develops a new ocular condition (eg, trauma, infection), experiences a sudden decrease in visual acuity, or if any ocular reactions (eg, conjunctivitis, eyelid reactions) develop. Advise that contact lenses should be removed prior to application, and may be reinserted 15 min following administration.

LATUDA — lurasidone hydrochloride
Rx

Class: Atypical antipsychotic

> Elderly patients with dementia-related psychosis treated with antipsychotic drugs are at an increased risk of death. Not approved for use in patients with dementia-related psychosis. Antidepressants increased the risk of suicidal thoughts and behavior in children, adolescents, and young adults in short-term studies. Monitor closely for worsening, and for emergence of suicidal thoughts and behaviors in patients who are started on antidepressant therapy.

ADULT DOSAGE
Schizophrenia

Initial: 40mg qd
Range: 40-160mg/day
Max: 160mg/day
Periodically reevaluate long-term usefulness of therapy for individual patient

Bipolar I Disorder

Treatment of major depressive episodes as monotherapy or as

PEDIATRIC DOSAGE
Pediatric use may not have been established

adjunctive therapy w/ either lithium or valproate
Initial: 20mg qd
Range: 20-120mg/day
Max: 120mg/day
Periodically reevaluate long-term usefulness of therapy for individual patient

----

DOSING CONSIDERATIONS
Concomitant Medications
Moderate CYP3A4 Inhibitors (eg, Diltiazem, Atazanavir, Erythromycin, Fluconazole, Verapamil):
Moderate CYP3A4 Inhibitor Added to Current Therapy w/ Lurasidone: Reduce lurasidone dose to 1/2 of the original dose level
Lurasidone Added to Current Therapy w/ a Moderate CYP3A4 Inhibitor:
Initial: 20mg/day
Max: 80mg/day
Moderate CYP3A4 Inducers:
May need to increase lurasidone dose after chronic treatment (≥7 days) w/ the CYP3A4 inducer

Renal Impairment
Moderate (CrCl 30-<50mL/min) and Severe (CrCl <30mL/min):
Initial: 20mg/day
Max: 80mg/day

Hepatic Impairment
Moderate (Child-Pugh Score 7-9):
Initial: 20mg/day
Max: 80mg/day
Severe (Child-Pugh Score 10-15):
Initial: 20mg/day
Max: 40mg/day

ADMINISTRATION
Oral route
Take w/ food (at least 350 calories)

STORAGE
25°C (77°F); excursions permitted to 15-30°C (59-86°F).

HOW SUPPLIED
Tab: 20mg, 40mg, 60mg, 80mg, 120mg

CONTRAINDICATIONS
Known hypersensitivity to lurasidone HCl or any components in the formulation; concomitant use w/ strong CYP3A4 inhibitors (eg, ketoconazole, clarithromycin, ritonavir, voriconazole, mibefradil) or strong CYP3A4 inducers (eg, rifampin, avasimibe, St. John's wort, phenytoin, carbamazepine).

WARNINGS/PRECAUTIONS
Neuroleptic malignant syndrome (NMS) reported; d/c immediately and institute symptomatic treatment. May cause tardive dyskinesia (TD), especially in the elderly; d/c if this occurs. May cause metabolic changes (eg, hyperglycemia, dyslipidemia, weight gain) that may increase cardiovascular (CV)/cerebrovascular risk. Hyperglycemia, in some cases extreme and associated with ketoacidosis or hyperosmolar coma or death, reported; monitor glucose control regularly in patients with diabetes mellitus (DM) and FPG in patients at risk for DM. May elevate prolactin levels. Leukopenia, neutropenia, and agranulocytosis may occur; monitor CBC frequently during the 1st few months in patients with preexisting low WBCs or history of drug-induced leukopenia/neutropenia, and d/c at 1st sign of decline in WBCs without other causative factors. D/C therapy and follow WBCs until recovery in patients with severe neutropenia (absolute neutrophil count <1000/mm³). May cause orthostatic hypotension and syncope; consider using a lower starting dose/slower titration and monitor orthostatic vital signs in patients at increased risk of these reactions or at increased risk of developing complications from hypotension (eg, dehydration, hypovolemia, treatment with antihypertensives, history of CV/cerebrovascular disease, antipsychotic-naive patients). Caution with history of seizures or with conditions that lower the seizure threshold. May impair mental/physical abilities. May disrupt body's ability to reduce core body temperature; caution when prescribing for patients who will be experiencing conditions that may contribute to an elevation in core body temperature (eg, concomitant anticholinergics). Closely supervise patients at high risk of suicide. May increase risk of developing a manic or hypomanic episode, particularly in patients with bipolar disorder. May cause esophageal dysmotility and aspiration; caution in patients at risk for aspiration pneumonia. Increased sensitivity reported in patients with Parkinson's disease or dementia with Lewy bodies. Evaluate for history of drug abuse; observe for drug misuse/abuse in these patients.

ADVERSE REACTIONS
Somnolence, akathisia, N/V, extrapyramidal symptoms, agitation, dyspepsia, back pain, dizziness, insomnia, anxiety, restlessness, diarrhea, dry mouth, nasopharyngitis.

DRUG INTERACTIONS
See Contraindications. Grapefruit/grapefruit juice may inhibit CYP3A4 and alter concentrations; avoid concomitant use. Adjust lurasidone dose when used in combination with moderate CYP3A4 inhibitors/inducers.

PREGNANCY AND LACTATION
Category B, not for use in nursing.

MECHANISM OF ACTION
Benzisothiazol derivative; not established. Efficacy could be mediated through a combination of central dopamine type 2 and serotonin type 2 receptor antagonism.

PHARMACOKINETICS
Absorption: T_{max}=1-3 hrs. **Distribution:** (40mg) V_d=6173L; plasma protein binding (~99%). **Metabolism:** Mainly via CYP3A4; oxidative N-dealkylation, hydroxylation of norbornane ring, and S-oxidation; ID-14283 and ID-14326 (active metabolites), ID-20219 and ID-20220 (major metabolites). **Elimination:** Urine (9%), feces (80%); (40mg) $T_{1/2}$=18 hrs.

PATIENT CONSIDERATIONS
Assessment: Assess for dementia-related psychosis, DM, renal/hepatic impairment, drug hypersensitivity, any other conditions where treatment is cautioned, pregnancy/nursing status, and possible drug interactions. Obtain baseline FPG in patients with DM or at risk for DM. Obtain baseline CBC if at risk for leukopenia/neutropenia.

Monitoring: Monitor for signs/symptoms of clinical worsening, suicidality, unusual changes in behavior, NMS, TD, hyperglycemia, hyperprolactinemia, orthostatic hypotension/syncope, cognitive/motor impairment, seizures, disruption of body temperature, manic/hypomanic episodes, esophageal dysmotility, aspiration, and other adverse reactions. Monitor FPG in patients with DM or at risk for DM, lipid profile, and weight. Monitor CBC frequently during the 1st few months in patients with preexisting low WBCs or history of drug-induced leukopenia/neutropenia. Monitor for fever or other signs/symptoms of infection in patients with neutropenia. Periodically reevaluate long-term usefulness for individual patient.

Counseling: Advise to monitor for the emergence of suicidal thoughts and behavior, manic/hypomanic symptoms, irritability, agitation, or unusual changes in behavior and to report such symptoms to physician. Counsel about signs/symptoms of NMS (eg, hyperpyrexia, muscle rigidity, altered mental status, autonomic instability), hyperglycemia, and DM. Advise of the risk of dyslipidemia, weight gain, CV reactions, and orthostatic hypotension. Advise patients with preexisting low WBCs or history of drug-induced leukopenia/neutropenia to have their CBC monitored. Instruct to use caution when performing activities requiring mental alertness (eg, operating hazardous machinery, driving) until patients are reasonably certain that therapy does not affect them adversely. Instruct to notify physician if pregnant/intending to become pregnant, or if taking/planning to take any other medications. Advise to avoid alcohol while on treatment. Counsel regarding appropriate care in avoiding overheating and dehydration.

LAZANDA — fentanyl

Class: Opioid analgesic

CII

> Fatal respiratory depression may occur. Contraindicated in the management of acute or postoperative pain (eg, headache/migraine) and in opioid-nontolerant patients. Keep out of reach of children. Concomitant use with CYP3A4 inhibitors may increase plasma levels, and may cause fatal respiratory depression. Do not convert patients on a mcg-per-mcg basis from any other fentanyl products to Lazanda. Do not substitute for any other fentanyl products; may result in fatal overdose. Contains fentanyl with abuse liability similar to other opioid analgesics. Available only through a restricted program called Transmucosal Immediate Release Fentanyl Risk Evaluation Mitigation Strategy (TIRF REMS) Access program, due to risk of misuse, abuse, addiction, and overdose. Outpatients, healthcare professionals who prescribe to outpatients, pharmacies, and distributors must enroll in this program.

ADULT DOSAGE
Pain

Management of Breakthrough Pain in Cancer Patients Already Receiving and Tolerant to Opioid Therapy for Underlying Persistent Cancer Pain:
≥18 Years:
Initial (Including Switching from Another Fentanyl Product):
One 100mcg spray (1 spray in 1 nostril); if adequate analgesia is obtained w/in 30 min, treat subsequent episodes w/ this dose
Titrate:
If adequate analgesia is not achieved w/ the first 100mcg dose, escalate dose in a step-wise manner over consecutive episodes until adequate analgesia w/ tolerable side effects is achieved
100mcg/dose: 1 x 100mcg spray
200mcg/dose: 2 x 100mcg spray (1 in each nostril)
400mcg/dose: 4 x 100mcg spray (2 in each nostril) or 1 x 400mcg spray
800mcg/dose: 2 x 400mcg spray (1 in each nostril)
Confirm dose w/ a 2nd episode of breakthrough pain and review experience if dose is appropriate or further adjustment is warranted
Wait at least 2 hrs before treating another episode of breakthrough cancer pain
Maint:
Use the established dose for each subsequent episode; limit to ≤4 doses/day and wait at least 2 hrs before treating another episode

PEDIATRIC DOSAGE
Pediatric use may not have been established

May use rescue medication if pain relief is inadequate after 30 min following dosing or if a separate episode occurs before the next dose is permitted
Max: 800mcg

DOSING CONSIDERATIONS
Renal Impairment
Severe: Use w/ caution; titrate to clinical effect

Hepatic Impairment
Severe: Use w/ caution; titrate to clinical effect

Discontinuation
No Longer Requires Opioid Therapy: Consider discontinuation along w/ a gradual downward titration of other opioids
Continuing to Take Chronic Opioid Therapy but No Longer Requires Treatment for Breakthrough Pain: Therapy can be discontinued immediately

Other Important Considerations
Dose Readjustment:
Response (Analgesia or Adverse Reactions) to Titrated Dose Markedly Changes: An adjustment may be necessary
>4 Episodes of Breakthrough Pain/Day: Reevaluate the dose of the long-acting opioid used; if the long-acting opioid or dose of long-acting opioid is changed, reevaluate and retitrate the Lazanda dose as necessary

ADMINISTRATION
Intranasal route

Prime device before use by spraying into the pouch (4 sprays total).
If not used for 5 days, reprime by spraying once.
Insert nozzle of the bottle a short distance (about 1/2 inch or 1cm) into nose and point towards bridge of nose, tilting bottle slightly.
Press down firmly on the finger grips until a click is heard and the number in the counting window advances by 1.
Fine mist spray is not always felt; rely on audible click and dose counter to confirm a spray has been administered.
Refer to PI for further priming and disposal instructions.

STORAGE
Up to 25°C (77°F). Do not freeze. Protect from light.

HOW SUPPLIED
Spray: 100mcg/spray, 400mcg/spray

CONTRAINDICATIONS
Opioid non-tolerant patients; management of acute or postoperative pain, including headache/migraine, or dental pain; known intolerance or hypersensitivity to any of its components or the drug fentanyl.

WARNINGS/PRECAUTIONS
Increased risk of respiratory depression in patients with underlying respiratory disorders and in elderly/debilitated. May impair mental and/or physical abilities. Caution with COPD or preexisting medical conditions predisposing to respiratory depression; may further decrease respiratory drive to the point of respiratory failure. Extreme caution in patients who may be susceptible to intracranial effects of CO_2 retention (eg, with evidence of increased intracranial pressure or impaired consciousness). May obscure the clinical course of head injuries. May produce bradycardia; caution with bradyarrhythmias. Avoid use during labor and delivery. Caution in the elderly.

ADVERSE REACTIONS
Respiratory depression, N/V, somnolence, dizziness, headache, constipation, pyrexia.

DRUG INTERACTIONS
See Boxed Warning. Increase dose conservatively when beginning therapy with or increasing dose of CYP3A4 inhibitors. Not recommended with MAOIs or within 14 days of discontinuation of MAOIs. Increased depressant effects with other CNS depressants (eg, other opioids, sedatives/hypnotics, skeletal muscle relaxants); may require adjustment of Lazanda dose. CYP3A4 inducers (eg, barbiturates, carbamazepine, efavirenz) may decrease levels; adjust dose of Lazanda accordingly. Vasoconstrictive nasal decongestants such as oxymetazoline may decrease efficacy; avoid titration while patient is experiencing an acute episode of rhinitis as it could lead to incorrect dose identification. Respiratory depression reported with other drugs that depress respiration.

PREGNANCY AND LACTATION
Category C, not for use in nursing.

MECHANISM OF ACTION
Opioid analgesic; has not been established. Known to be μ-opioid receptor agonist; specific CNS opioid receptors for endogenous compounds with opioid-like activity have been identified throughout the brain and spinal cord and play a role in analgesic effects.

PHARMACOKINETICS
Absorption: Administration of various doses resulted in different parameters.
Distribution: V_d=4L/kg; plasma protein binding (80-85%); crosses placenta; found in breast milk. **Metabolism:** Liver and intestinal mucosa via CYP3A4; norfentanyl (metabolite). **Elimination:** Urine (<7%, unchanged), feces (1%, unchanged); $T_{1/2}$=21.9 hrs (100mcg), 24.9 hrs (200mcg and 800mcg), 15 hrs (400mcg).

PATIENT CONSIDERATIONS
Assessment: Assess for degree of opioid tolerance, previous opioid dose, level of pain intensity, type of pain, patient's general condition and medical status, and any other conditions where treatment is contraindicated or cautioned. Assess for

hypersensitivity to the drug, renal/hepatic impairment, pregnancy/nursing status, and possible drug interactions.
Monitoring: Monitor for signs/symptoms of respiratory depression, impairment of mental/physical abilities, drug abuse/addiction, bradycardia, hypersensitivity reactions, and other adverse reactions.
Counseling: Inform outpatients to enroll in the TIRF REMS Access program. Explain that therapy may be fatal in children, in individuals for whom it was not prescribed, and in those who are not opioid tolerant. Counsel on proper administration and disposal. Advise to take drug as prescribed and to avoid sharing it with anyone else. Instruct not to take medication for acute or postoperative pain, pain from injuries, headache, migraine, or any other short-term pain. Instruct to notify physician if breakthrough pain is not alleviated or worsens after taking the drug. Inform that drug may impair mental/physical abilities; caution against performing activities that require high level of attention (eg, driving/using heavy machinery). Advise not to combine with alcohol, sleep aids, or tranquilizers, except if ordered by the physician. Instruct to notify physician if pregnant or planning to become pregnant.

LEMTRADA — alemtuzumab   Rx
Class: Monoclonal antibody/CD52 blocker

> May cause serious, sometimes fatal, autoimmune conditions such as immune thrombocytopenia (ITP) and anti-glomerular basement membrane disease; monitor CBCs with differential, SrCr levels, and urinalysis with urine cell counts at periodic intervals for 48 months after the last dose. May cause serious and life threatening infusion reactions; administer in a setting with appropriate equipment and personnel to manage anaphylaxis or serious infusion reactions. Monitor patients for 2 hrs after each infusion. Serious infusion reactions can also occur after the 2-hr monitoring period. May cause an increased risk of malignancies, including thyroid cancer, melanoma, and lymphoproliferative disorders; perform baseline and yearly skin exams. Available only through a restricted distribution program, Lemtrada Risk Evaluation Mitigation Strategy (REMS).

ADULT DOSAGE	PEDIATRIC DOSAGE
Multiple Sclerosis	Pediatric use may not have been established
Relapsing Forms:	
Usual: 12mg/day for 2 treatment courses	
First Treatment Course: 12mg/day on 5 consecutive days (60mg total dose)	
Second Treatment Course: 12mg/day on 3 consecutive days (36mg total dose) administered 12 months after the first treatment course	
Corticosteroids: Premedicate with high dose corticosteroids (1000mg methylprednisolone or equivalent) immediately prior to infusion and for the first 3 days of each treatment course	
Herpes Prophylaxis: Administer antiviral prophylaxis for herpetic viral infections starting on the first day of each treatment course and continue for at least 2 months following treatment or until CD4+ lymphocyte count is ≥200 cells/μL, whichever occurs later	

ADMINISTRATION
IV route

Preparation and Infusion
Withdraw 1.2mL from the vial into a syringe and inject into a 100mL bag of 0.9% NaCl or D5W.
Invert the bag to mix the sol.
Infuse Lemtrada over 4 hrs starting within 8 hrs after dilution.
Do not add or simultaneously infuse other drug substances through the same IV line.
Do not give as an IV push or bolus.

STORAGE
2-8°C (36-46°F). Do not freeze or shake. Store in original carton to protect from light. Diluted Sol: Store for as long as 8 hrs either at 15-25°C (59-77°F) or at 2-8°C (36-46°F). Protect from light.

HOW SUPPLIED
Inj: 10mg/mL

CONTRAINDICATIONS
Human immunodeficiency virus (HIV).

WARNINGS/PRECAUTIONS
Reserve for patients who have had an inadequate response to two or more drugs indicated for the treatment of MS. Determine whether patient has a history of varicella or if has been vaccinated for varicella zoster virus (VZV) prior to treatment; if not, test patient for antibodies to VZV and consider vaccination for those who are antibody-negative. Complete any necessary immunizations

at least 6 weeks prior to treatment. Therapy can result in the formation of autoantibodies; autoantibodies may be transferred from the mother to the fetus during pregnancy. Case of transplacental transfer of anti-thyrotropin receptor antibodies resulting in neonatal Graves' disease occurred after alemtuzumab treatment in the mother. May cause cytokinase release syndrome resulting in infusion reactions; consider pretreatment with antihistamines and/or antipyretics prior to therapy. Caution when initiating therapy in patients with preexisting or ongoing malignancies. Immediately obtain CBC if ITP is suspected and promptly initiate appropriate medical intervention if confirmed. Glomerular nephropathies reported. Perform further evaluation for nephropathies if significant changes from baseline in SrCr, unexplained hematuria, or proteinuria are observed. Autoimmune thyroid disorders reported; administer only if potential benefit justifies potential risks in patients with an ongoing thyroid disorder. Autoimmune cytopenias such as neutropenia, hemolytic anemia, and pancytopenia reported; use CBC results to monitor for cytopenias and prompt medical intervention is indicated if a cytopenia is confirmed. Infections (eg, urinary tract infection, appendicitis, gastroenteritis, pneumonia, tooth infection) reported. Consider delaying administration in patients with active infection until the infection is fully controlled. Herpes viral infection, cervical human papilloma virus (HPV) (eg, cervical dysplasia) infection, active/latent tuberculosis (TB), fungal infections (oral and vaginal candidiasis), and Listeria meningitis reported. Avoid or adequately heat foods that are potential sources of *Listeria monocytogenes*. Caution in patients identified as carriers of hepatitis B virus (HBV) and/or hepatitis C virus (HCV) as these patients may be at risk of irreversible liver damage relative to a potential virus reactivation as a consequence of their preexisting status. Hypersensitivity pneumonitis and pneumonitis with fibrosis reported. Contains same active ingredient (alemtuzumab) found in Campath; exercise increased vigilance for additive and long-lasting effects on the immune system if use is considered in a patient who has previously received Campath.

ADVERSE REACTIONS
Autoimmune conditions, infusion reactions, malignancies, rash, headache, pyrexia, nasopharyngitis, N/V, urinary tract infection, fatigue, insomnia, upper respiratory tract infection, herpes viral infection, urticaria, pruritus.

DRUG INTERACTIONS
Do not administer live viral vaccines following a course of therapy; may increase the risk of infection. Concomitant use with antineoplastic or immunosuppressive therapies could increase risk of immunosuppression.

PREGNANCY AND LACTATION
Category C, not for use in nursing.

MECHANISM OF ACTION
Monoclonal antibody/CD52-blocker; has not been established. Presumed to involve binding to CD52. Following cell surface binding to T and B lymphocytes, results in antibody-dependent cellular cytolysis and complement-mediated lysis.

PHARMACOKINETICS
Absorption: C_{max}=3014ng/mL (Day 5, 1st treatment course), 2276ng/mL (Day 3, 2nd treatment course). **Distribution:** V_d= 14.1 L. **Elimination:** $T_{1/2}$= 2 weeks.

PATIENT CONSIDERATIONS
Assessment: Assess for HIV, history of varicella, thyroid disorder, HBV, HBC, any other conditions where treatment is cautioned, pregnancy/nursing status, and possible drug interactions. Obtain CBC with differential, SrCr levels, and urinalysis with urine cell counts. Perform a test of thyroid function (eg, thyroid-stimulating hormone level). Perform TB screening according to local guidelines. Perform baseline skin examination. Assess vital signs and immunization history.

Monitoring: Monitor for autoimmune conditions (eg, ITP, anti-glomerular basement membrane disease), malignancies (eg, thyroid cancer, melanoma, lymphoproliferative disorders, lymphoma), glomerular nephropathies, infusion reactions, thyroid disorders, autoimmune cytopenias, infections, TB, and other adverse reactions. Monitor CBCs with differential, SrCr levels, and urinalysis with urine cell counts monthly for 48 months after the last dose; perform testing after 48 months based on clinical findings. Monitor vital signs periodically during infusion. Monitor for infusion reactions during and for at least 2 hrs after each infusion. Perform thyroid function test every 3 months until 48 months after the last infusion; continue to test thyroid function after 48 months if clinically indicated. Consider additional monitoring in patients with medical conditions that may predispose to cardiovascular or pulmonary compromise. Perform yearly skin examination. Perform annual HPV screening in female patients.

Counseling: Inform of benefits and risks of therapy. Instruct to contact physician promptly if experience any symptoms of potential autoimmune disease (eg, bleeding, easy bruising, petechiae). Advise of the importance of monthly blood and urine tests for 48 months following the last course of therapy; inform that monitoring may need to continue past 48 months if there are signs/symptoms of autoimmunity. Instruct to contact physician if experience symptoms reflective of a potential thyroid disorder. Inform that infusion reactions can occur after patient leaves the infusion center; instruct to report symptoms that occur during and after each infusion to physician. Inform that must enroll in the Lemtrada REMS Program. Instruct to carry the Lemtrada REMS patient safety information card in case of an emergency. Advise of the risk of malignancies, including thyroid cancer and melanoma; instruct to have yearly skin examinations. Instruct to take prescribed medication for herpes prophylaxis ud. Advise that yearly screening for HPV is recommended. Advise to avoid, or adequately heat foods that are potential sources of *L. monocytogenes* if have had a recent course of therapy. Instruct to notify physician if pregnant, breastfeeding, or if any adverse reactions develop. Instruct patients to inform physician if they have taken Campath.

LENVIMA — lenvatinib
Class: Kinase inhibitor

Rx

ADULT DOSAGE
Differentiated Thyroid Carcinoma
Locally Recurrent or Metastatic, Progressive, Radioactive Iodine-Refractory Differentiated Thyroid Cancer (DTC):
24mg (two 10mg caps and one 4mg cap) qd

Continue until disease progression or until unacceptable toxicity

Advanced Renal Cell Carcinoma
In Combination w/ Everolimus for the Treatment of Advanced Renal Cell Carcinoma (RCC) Following 1 Prior Anti-Angiogenic Therapy:
18mg (one 10mg cap and two 4mg caps) in combination w/ 5mg everolimus qd

Continue lenvatinib plus everolimus until disease progression or until unacceptable toxicity

Missed Dose
If a dose is missed and cannot be taken w/in 12 hrs, skip that dose and take the next dose at the usual time of administration

PEDIATRIC DOSAGE
Pediatric use may not have been established

DOSING CONSIDERATIONS
Renal Impairment
Severe (CrCl <30mL/min):
DTC: 14mg qd
RCC: 10mg qd

Mild or Moderate: No dose adjustment is recommended
ESRD: Not studied

Hepatic Impairment
Severe (Child-Pugh C):
DTC: 14mg qd
RCC: 10mg qd

Mild or Moderate: No dose adjustment is recommended

Adverse Reactions
HTN:
- **Grade 3 (Despite Optimal Antihypertensive Therapy):** Withhold; resume at a reduced dose after resolution to Grade 0, 1, or 2
- **Grade 4:** D/C therapy; do not resume

Cardiac Dysfunction:
- **Grade 3:** Withhold; resume at a reduced dose after resolution to Grade 0, 1, or baseline
- **Grade 4:** D/C therapy; do not resume

Arterial Thrombotic Event:
- **Any Grade:** D/C therapy; do not resume

Hepatotoxicity:
- **Grade 3 or 4:** Withhold or d/c; consider resuming at reduced dose if resolves to Grade 0-1 or baseline

Hepatic Failure:
- **Grade 3 or 4:** D/C therapy; do not resume

Proteinuria:
- **Greater Than or Equal to 2g/24 hrs:** Withhold; resume at reduced dose after resolution to <2g/24 hrs

Nephrotic Syndrome:
D/C therapy; do not resume

Nausea, Vomiting, and Diarrhea:
- **Grade 3:** Withhold; resume at reduced dose after resolution to Grade 0, 1, or baseline. Initiate prompt medical management for N/V or diarrhea

Vomiting and Diarrhea:
- **Grade 4 (Despite Medical Management):** D/C therapy; do not resume

Renal Failure or Impairment:
- **Grade 3 or 4:** Withhold or d/c; consider resuming at reduced dose if resolves to Grade 0-1 or baseline

GI Perforation:
- **Any Grade:** D/C therapy; do not resume

Fistula:
- **Grade 3 or 4:** D/C therapy; do not resume

QTc Prolongation:
- **Greater Than 500 ms:** Withhold; resume at reduced dose after resolution to <480 ms or baseline

Reversible Posterior Leukoencephalopathy Syndrome (RPLS):
- **Any Grade:** Withhold or d/c; consider resuming at reduced dose if resolves to Grade 0 to 1

Hemorrhage:
- **Grade 3:** Withhold; resume at reduced dose after resolution to Grade 0 to 1
- **Grade 4:** D/C therapy; do not resume

Manage other adverse reactions according to the instructions below for DTC or RCC.

Persistent and Intolerable Grade 2 or 3 Adverse Reactions or Grade 4 Lab Abnormalities in DTC:
1st Occurrence: Interrupt until resolved to Grade 0-1 or baseline; decrease dose to 20mg (two 10mg caps) qd
2nd Occurrence: Interrupt until resolved to Grade 0-1 or baseline; decrease dose to 14mg (one 10mg cap + one 4mg cap) qd
3rd Occurrence: Interrupt until resolved to Grade 0-1 or baseline; decrease dose to 10mg (one 10mg cap) qd
- Initiate medical management for N/V or diarrhea prior to interruption or dose reduction
- Reduce dose in succession based on the previous daily dose level (24mg/day, 20mg/day, or 14mg/day)
- 2nd or 3rd occurrence may refer to either the same or a different adverse reaction that requires dose modification

Persistent and Intolerable Grade 2 or 3 Adverse Reactions or Grade 4 Lab Abnormalities in RCC:
1st Occurrence: Interrupt until resolved to Grade 0-1 or baseline; decrease dose to 14mg (one 10mg cap + one 4mg cap) qd
2nd Occurrence: Interrupt until resolved to Grade 0-1 or baseline; decrease dose to 10mg (one 10mg cap) qd
3rd Occurrence: Interrupt until resolved to Grade 0-1 or baseline; decrease dose to 8mg (two 4 mg cap) qd
- Initiate medical management for N/V or diarrhea prior to interruption or dose reduction
- Reduce dose in succession based on the previous daily dose level (18mg/day, 14mg/day, 10mg/day, or 8mg/day)
- 2nd or 3rd occurrence may refer to either the same or a different adverse reaction that requires dose modification

Refer to the full prescribing information for everolimus for recommended dose modifications. For toxicities thought to be related to everolimus alone, d/c, interrupt, or use alternate day dosing. For toxicities thought to be related to both lenvatinib and everolimus, 1st reduce lenvatinib and then everolimus

ADMINISTRATION
Oral route

Take w/ or w/o food.
Take at the same time each day.
Swallow caps whole.
Alternatively, may dissolve caps in a small glass of liquid.
- Measure 1 tbsp of water or apple juice and put caps into the liquid w/o breaking or crushing them.
- Leave caps in the liquid for at least 10 min, stir for at least 3 min, and then drink mixture.
- After drinking, add the same amount (1 tbsp) of water or apple juice to the glass, swirl the contents a few times, and then swallow the additional liquid.

STORAGE
25°C (77°F); excursions permitted to 15-30°C (59-86°F).

HOW SUPPLIED
Cap: 4mg, 10mg

WARNINGS/PRECAUTIONS
See Dosing Considerations. HTN, cardiac dysfunction, arterial thromboembolic events, increases in AST/ALT, hepatic failure (including fatal events), acute hepatitis, renal failure/impairment, GI perforation or fistula, and RPLS reported. Proteinuria reported; obtain a 24-hr urine protein if urine dipstick proteinuria $\geq 2+$ is detected. Diarrhea reported; initiate prompt medical management for the development of diarrhea and monitor for dehydration. QT interval prolongation reported; monitor ECG in patients w/ congenital long QT syndrome, CHF, bradyarrhythmias, or in patients taking drugs known to prolong the QT interval (eg, Class Ia and III antiarrhythmics). Hypocalcemia reported; monitor blood Ca^{2+} levels at least monthly and replace Ca^{2+} as necessary. Hemorrhagic events including fatal events and serious tumor related bleeds reported; consider the risk of severe or fatal hemorrhage associated w/ tumor invasion/infiltration of major blood vessels (eg, carotid artery). Impairment of exogenous thyroid suppression and thyroid dysfunction may occur; monitor thyroid function before initiation of, and at least monthly throughout, treatment. Treat hypothyroidism accordingly to maintain a euthyroid state. May cause fetal harm.

ADVERSE REACTIONS
DTC: HTN, fatigue, diarrhea, arthralgia/myalgia, decreased appetite, weight decreased, N/V, stomatitis, headache, proteinuria, palmar-plantar erythrodysesthesia syndrome, abdominal pain, dysphonia.
RCC: Diarrhea, fatigue, arthralgia/myalgia, decreased appetite, N/V, stomatitis/oral inflammation, HTN, peripheral edema, cough, abdominal pain, dyspnea, rash, weight decreased, hemorrhagic events, proteinuria.

PREGNANCY AND LACTATION
Pregnancy: May cause fetal harm.
Lactation: Not for use in nursing.
Reproductive Potential: Females of reproductive potential should use effective contraception during treatment and for at least 2 weeks following completion of therapy. May result in reduced fertility in females of reproductive potential. May result in damage to male reproductive tissues leading to reduced fertility of unknown duration.

MECHANISM OF ACTION
Kinase inhibitor; inhibits the kinase activities of vascular endothelial growth factor (VEGF) receptors VEGFR1 (FLT1), VEGFR2 (KDR), and VEGFR3 (FLT4). Also inhibits other receptor tyrosine kinases that have been implicated in pathogenic angiogenesis, tumor growth, and cancer progression in addition to their normal cellular functions, including fibroblast growth factor (FGF) receptors FGFR 1, 2, 3, and 4; the platelet derived growth factor receptor alpha, KIT, and RET.

PHARMACOKINETICS
Absorption: T_{max}=1-4 hrs. **Distribution:** Plasma protein binding (98-99%).
Metabolism: Enzymatic (CYP3A and aldehyde oxidase) and non-enzymatic processes. **Elimination:** Feces (64%), urine (25%); $T_{1/2}$=28 hrs.

PATIENT CONSIDERATIONS
Assessment: Assess for proteinuria, congenital long QT syndrome, CHF, bradyarrhythmias, electrolyte abnormalities, renal/hepatic impairment, pregnancy/nursing status, and if taking drugs known to prolong the QT interval. Assess BP and control prior to treatment.

Monitoring: Monitor for signs/symptoms of cardiac decompensation, arterial thromboembolic events, renal failure/impairment, GI perforation and fistula formation, proteinuria, diarrhea, RPLS, hemorrhagic events, QT interval prolongation, and other adverse reactions. Monitor BP after 1 week, then every 2 weeks for the first 2 months, and then at least monthly thereafter. Monitor LFTs every 2 weeks for the first 2 months, and at least monthly thereafter. Monitor and correct electrolyte abnormalities. Monitor ECG in patients w/ congenital long QT syndrome, CHF, bradyarrhythmias, and in patients taking drugs known to prolong QT interval. Monitor blood Ca^{2+} levels at least monthly. Monitor thyroid function at least monthly.

Counseling: Advise to undergo regular BP monitoring and to contact physician if BP is elevated. Inform that therapy may cause cardiac dysfunction; instruct to immediately contact physician if any clinical symptoms of cardiac dysfunction are experienced. Advise to seek immediate medical attention for new onset chest pain or acute neurologic symptoms consistent w/ MI or stroke. Inform of the need to undergo lab tests to monitor for kidney function, protein in the urine, and liver function; instruct to report any new symptoms indicating hepatic toxicity or failure. Advise when to start standard anti-diarrheal therapy and to maintain adequate hydration; instruct to contact physician if unable to maintain adequate hydration. Advise that therapy may increase the risk of GI perforation or fistula; instruct to seek immediate medical attention for severe abdominal pain. Inform patients who are at risk for QTc prolongation that they will need to undergo regular ECGs; advise all patients of the need to undergo laboratory tests to monitor electrolytes. Explain that therapy may increase the risk of bleeding; instruct to contact physician for bleeding or symptoms of severe bleeding. Inform females of reproductive potential of the potential risk to a fetus and instruct to inform physician of a known or suspected pregnancy. Instruct females of reproductive potential to use effective contraception during treatment and for at least 2 weeks following completion of therapy. Advise nursing women to d/c breastfeeding during treatment.

LETAIRIS — ambrisentan   Rx

Class: Endothelin receptor antagonist

> Do not administer to a pregnant female; may cause serious birth defects. Exclude pregnancy before initiation of treatment. Females of reproductive potential must use acceptable methods of contraception during and for 1 month after treatment; obtain monthly pregnancy tests during and 1 month after discontinuation of treatment. Females can only receive the drug through a restricted program called the Letairis Risk Evaluation and Mitigation Strategy (REMS) program.

ADULT DOSAGE	PEDIATRIC DOSAGE
Pulmonary Arterial Hypertension	Pediatric use may not have been established
Treatment of pulmonary arterial HTN (PAH) (WHO Group 1) to improve exercise ability and delay clinical worsening; can be used w/ tadalafil to reduce the risks of disease progression and hospitalization for worsening PAH, and to improve exercise ability	
Initial: 5mg qd w/ or w/o tadalafil 20mg qd	
Titrate: At 4-wk intervals, either dose of ambrisentan or tadalafil can be increased to ambrisentan 10mg or tadalafil 40mg	

DOSING CONSIDERATIONS
Hepatic Impairment
Elevation of Liver Transaminases:
D/C if elevations of ALT/AST >5X ULN or if elevations are accompanied by bilirubin >2X ULN, or by signs/symptoms of liver dysfunction and other causes are excluded

ADMINISTRATION
Oral route

Do not split, crush, or chew tabs.

STORAGE
25°C (77°F); excursions permitted to 15-30°C (59-86°F).

HOW SUPPLIED
Tab: 5mg, 10mg

CONTRAINDICATIONS
Pregnancy, idiopathic pulmonary fibrosis (IPF), including IPF patients w/ pulmonary HTN (WHO Group 3).

WARNINGS/PRECAUTIONS

May cause peripheral edema; more common w/ concomitant tadalafil and in the elderly. If clinically significant fluid retention develops, evaluate further to determine the cause and the possible need for specific treatment or discontinuation of therapy. If acute pulmonary edema develops during initiation of therapy, consider the possibility of pulmonary veno-occlusive disease (PVOD); d/c if confirmed. May decrease sperm counts. Decreases in Hgb concentration and Hct reported and may result in anemia requiring transfusion. Initiation of therapy is not recommended w/ clinically significant anemia. Consider discontinuation if a clinically significant Hgb decrease is observed and other causes have been excluded. Avoid w/ preexisting moderate/severe hepatic impairment. Fully investigate the cause of liver injury if hepatic impairment develops.

ADVERSE REACTIONS

W/O Tadalafil: peripheral edema, nasal congestion, flushing, sinusitis.
W/ Tadalafil: peripheral edema, headache, nasal congestion, cough, anemia, dyspepsia, bronchitis.

DRUG INTERACTIONS

Cyclosporine may increase exposure; limit dose of ambrisentan to 5mg qd when coadministered w/ cyclosporine.

PREGNANCY AND LACTATION

Pregnancy: Category X.
Lactation: Not for use in nursing.

MECHANISM OF ACTION

Endothelin receptor antagonist; highly selective for endothelin type-A (ET_A) receptor versus endothelin type-B (ET_B) receptor. ET_A and ET_B help mediate effects of endothelin-1 (ET-1) in the vascular smooth muscle and endothelium. Primary actions of ET_A are vasoconstriction and cell proliferation. Predominant actions of ET_B are vasodilation, antiproliferation, and ET-1 clearance.

PHARMACOKINETICS

Absorption: T_{max}=2 hrs. **Distribution:** Plasma protein binding (99%). **Metabolism:** Liver via CYP3A, 2C19, and UGTs 1A9S, 2B7S, and 1A3S. **Elimination:** $T_{1/2}$=9 hrs.

PATIENT CONSIDERATIONS

Assessment: Assess for IPF, anemia, hepatic impairment, pregnancy/nursing status, and possible drug interactions. Obtain baseline Hgb level.
Monitoring: Monitor for fluid retention, pulmonary edema, PVOD, hepatic impairment, and other adverse reactions. Obtain monthly pregnancy tests in females of reproductive potential during therapy and 1 month after discontinuation of treatment. Measure Hgb at 1 month after initiating therapy and periodically thereafter.
Counseling: Instruct on the risk of fetal harm when used in pregnancy and instruct to immediately contact physician if pregnancy is suspected. Inform female patients that drug is only available through a restricted program called the Letairis REMS program. Inform female patients that they must sign an enrollment form and that female patients of reproductive potential must comply w/ pregnancy testing and contraception requirements. Educate and counsel females of reproductive potential on the use of emergency contraception in the event of unprotected sex or known or suspected contraceptive failure. Advise prepubertal females to immediately report to physician any reproductive status changes. Instruct to contact physician if any symptoms of liver injury occur. Advise of the importance of Hgb testing and of other risks associated w/ therapy (eg, decreases in Hgb, Hct, and sperm count; fluid overload).

LEUCOVORIN INJECTION — leucovorin calcium   Rx

Class: Cytoprotective agent

ADULT DOSAGE

Rescue Therapy

After High Dose Methotrexate (MTX) Therapy in Osteosarcoma:

Normal MTX Elimination:
15mg (10mg/m^2) q6h for 10 doses starting 24 hrs after the beginning of MTX infusion

Delayed Late MTX Elimination:
Continue 15mg PO/IM/IV q6h until MTX level is <0.05µm

Delayed Early MTX and/or Evidence of Acute Renal Injury:
150mg IV q3h until MTX level is <1µm, then 15mg IV q3h until MTX level is <0.05µm. Continue therapy, hydration, and urinary alkalization (pH of ≥7) until MTX level is <0.05µm

If significant clinical toxicity w/ less severe abnormalities in MTX elimination/renal function is observed, extend rescue therapy for an additional 24 hrs in subsequent courses of therapy

Methotrexate Toxicity

Used to diminish the toxicity and counteract the effects of impaired MTX elimination and of inadvertent overdosage of folic acid antagonists

PEDIATRIC DOSAGE

Pediatric use may not have been established

Initial: 10mg/m^2 IV/IM/PO q6h until serum MTX level is <10^{-8} M
Titrate: Increase to 100mg/m^2 IV q3h until MTX level is <10^{-8} M if 24-hr SrCr has increased 50% over baseline, or if 24-hr MTX level is >5 x 10^{-6} M, or the 48-hr level is >9 x 10^{-7} M

Employ concurrent hydration (3L/day) and urinary alkalinization w/ sodium bicarbonate; adjust bicarbonate dose to maintain urine pH at ≥7

Begin rescue therapy as soon as possible after an inadvertent overdosage and w/in 24 hrs of MTX administration when there is delayed excretion

Advanced Colorectal Cancer

Palliative Treatment in Combination w/ 5-Fluorouracil (5-FU):
Usual: 200mg/m^2 slow IV over a minimum of 3 min, followed by 370mg/m^2 5-FU IV, daily for 5 days,
or
20mg/m^2 IV, followed by 425mg/m^2 5-FU IV, daily for 5 days

May repeat at 4-week intervals for 2 courses, then at 4- to 5-week intervals provided that the patient has completely recovered from the toxic effects of the prior treatment course

May increase 5-FU dose by 10% if no toxicity. Reduce 5-FU daily dose by 20% w/ moderate GI/hematologic toxicity and by 30% w/ severe toxicity

Megaloblastic Anemia

Usual: Up to 1mg/day

ADMINISTRATION

IM/IV route

Do not mix in same infusion as 5-FU; may form precipitate.
Do not administer intrathecally.
Reconstitute 50mg, 100mg, and 200mg vials w/ 5mL, 10mL, and 20mL, respectively, of bacteriostatic water for inj (benzyl alcohol preserved) or sterile water for inj.
Reconstitute 350mg vial w/ 17.5mL of bacteriostatic water for inj (benzyl alcohol preserved) or sterile water for inj (SWFI).
Must use sol reconstituted w/ bacteriostatic water for inj w/in 7 days; must use sol reconstituted w/ SWFI immediately and discard any unused portion.
When doses >10mg/m^2 are administered, reconstitute w/ SWFI and use immediately.
No more than 160mg/min should be injected IV (16mL/min of 10mg/mL sol, or 8mL/min of 20mg/mL sol).

STORAGE

Sol: 2-8°C (36-46°F). Protect from light. **Powder:** 20-25°C (68-77°F). Protect from light. **Reconstitution w/ Bacteriostatic Water for Inj:** Use within 7 days. **Reconstitution w/ Sterile Water for Inj:** Use immediately.

HOW SUPPLIED

Inj: 10mg/mL [50mL], 50mg, 100mg, 200mg, 350mg

CONTRAINDICATIONS

Pernicious anemia and other megaloblastic anemias secondary to lack of vitamin B12.

WARNINGS/PRECAUTIONS

Do not administer intrathecally; may be harmful or fatal. Monitor serum MTX to determine the optimal dose and duration of treatment. Delayed MTX excretion may be caused by 3rd space fluid accumulation (eg, ascites, pleural effusion), renal insufficiency, or inadequate hydration; higher doses or prolonged administration may be indicated. Bacteriostatic water for inj diluent contains benzyl alcohol; when doses >10mg/m^2 are administered, reconstitute with sterile water for inj and use immediately. Sol contains Ca^{2+}; no more than 160mg should be injected IV per min (16mL of a 10mg/mL, or 8mL of a 20mg/mL sol per min). Do not initiate or continue therapy with leucovorin and 5-FU in patients with symptoms of GI toxicity until symptoms have completely resolved; caution in elderly and/or debilitated patients. Monitor patients with diarrhea until it has resolved, as rapid clinical deterioration leading to death can occur. Seizures and/or syncope reported rarely in cancer patients, most commonly in those with CNS metastases or other predisposing factors. Leucovorin/5-FU combination therapy for advanced colorectal cancer should be administered under supervision of a physician experienced in the use of antimetabolite cancer chemotherapy. Defer 5-FU/leucovorin treatment until WBCs are 4000/mm^3 and platelets 130,000/mm^3; d/c if blood counts do not reach these levels within 2 weeks. Follow up with physical exam prior to each treatment course and appropriate radiological exam as needed. D/C when there is clear evidence of tumor progression.

ADVERSE REACTIONS

Allergic sensitization (eg, anaphylactoid reactions, urticaria), stomatitis, N/V, leukopenia, diarrhea, alopecia, dermatitis, thrombocytopenia, infection, lethargy/malaise/fatigue, anorexia, constipation.

DRUG INTERACTIONS

May enhance 5-FU toxicity. Seizures and/or syncope reported with fluoropyrimidine. Use with trimethoprim-sulfamethoxazole for the acute treatment of *Pneumocystis carinii* pneumonia in patients with HIV infection reported to be associated with increased rates of treatment failure and morbidity. Folic acid in large amounts may counteract antiepileptic effect of phenobarbital, phenytoin, and primidone, and increase seizure frequency in susceptible pediatric patients. High doses may reduce efficacy of intrathecally administered MTX.

PREGNANCY AND LACTATION

Category C, caution in nursing.

MECHANISM OF ACTION

Folic acid derivative; counteracts the therapeutic and toxic effects of folic acid antagonists (eg, MTX), which act by inhibiting dihydrofolate reductase. Enhances therapeutic effects of fluoropyrimidines used in cancer therapy (eg, 5-FU).

PHARMACOKINETICS

Absorption: Administration via different routes resulted in different parameters of both the parent drug and metabolite. **Metabolism:** 5-methyltetrahydrofolate (5-methyl-THF) (active metabolite). **Elimination:** (IV) Urine (83%, biologically active IV dose; 31%, 5-methyl-THF). Refer to PI for $T_{1/2}$.

PATIENT CONSIDERATIONS

Assessment: Assess for pernicious anemia and other megaloblastic anemias secondary to lack of vitamin B12, 3rd space fluid accumulation, renal impairment, inadequate hydration, GI toxicity, CNS metastases, pregnancy/nursing status, and possible drug interactions. (Leucovorin/5-FU Combination) Obtain CBC with differential and platelets prior to each treatment. Check electrolytes and LFTs prior to each treatment for the first 3 cycles, then prior to every other cycle.

Monitoring: Monitor for GI toxicity, seizures, syncope, and other adverse reactions. Monitor patients with diarrhea until it has resolved. Monitor fluid and electrolyte status in patients with abnormalities in MTX elimination. Monitor SrCr and MTX levels at least qd. (Leucovorin/5-FU Combination) Monitor CBC with differential and platelets weekly during the first 2 courses, and thereafter once each cycle at the time of anticipated WBC nadir. Perform physical exam prior to each treatment course and appropriate radiological exam as needed.

Counseling: Inform about risks and benefits of therapy. Instruct to notify physician if any adverse reactions occur. Instruct to inform physician if pregnant/nursing.

LEUPROLIDE PEDIATRIC — leuprolide acetate   Rx

Class: Synthetic gonadotropin-releasing hormone (GnRH) analogue

OTHER BRAND NAMES

Lupron (Discontinued)

PEDIATRIC DOSAGE
Central Precocious Puberty

Confirm clinical diagnosis prior to initiation of therapy

Initial: 50mcg/kg/day, administered as a single SQ inj
Titrate: Increase by 10mcg/kg/day if total downregulation is not achieved; this dose will be considered the maint dose

---

DOSING CONSIDERATIONS
Discontinuation
Consider before age 11 for females and age 12 for males

ADMINISTRATION
SQ route

Rotate inj site periodically

STORAGE
<25°C (77°F). Do not freeze. Protect from light.

HOW SUPPLIED
Inj: 5mg/mL [2.8mL]

CONTRAINDICATIONS
Known hypersensitivity to GnRH, GnRH agonist analogs, or any of the excipients in leuprolide acetate inj; women who are or may become pregnant.

WARNINGS/PRECAUTIONS
Anaphylactic reactions reported. An increase in clinical signs and symptoms may be observed during the early phase of therapy. Noncompliance/inadequate dosing may result in inadequate control of the pubertal process and the return of pubertal signs (eg, menses, breast development, testicular growth). Long-term consequences of inadequate control may include a further compromise of adult stature. Suppresses pituitary-gonadal system at therapeutic dose. Contains benzyl alcohol; monitor for symptoms of hypersensitivity, usually local, at the inj site.

ADVERSE REACTIONS
Inj-site reactions including abscess, emotional lability, vaginitis/vaginal bleeding/vaginal discharge, acne/seborrhea, general pain, rash including erythema multiforme, headache, vasodilation.

PREGNANCY AND LACTATION
Category X, not for use in nursing.

MECHANISM OF ACTION

Synthetic GnRH agonist; potent inhibitor of gonadotropin secretion. Following an initial stimulation of gonadotropins, chronic administration results in suppression of ovarian and testicular steroidogenesis.

PHARMACOKINETICS

Distribution: V_d=27L (IV bolus, adult male); plasma protein binding (43-49%). (M-1) T_{max}=2-6 hrs. **Metabolism:** M-I (major metabolite). **Elimination:** (3.75mg Depot Sus) Urine (<5% as parent and M-I) (adults); (1mg IV Bolus) $T_{1/2}$=3 hrs (adult male).

PATIENT CONSIDERATIONS

Assessment: Assess for previous hypersensitivity to drug and for hypersensitivity to benzyl alcohol. Assess pregnancy status. Confirm clinical diagnosis of CPP by a pubertal response to a GnRH stimulation test and bone age advanced 1 yr beyond the chronological age. Obtain baseline height and weight, sex steroid levels, adrenal steroid level, β human chorionic gonadotropin level, pelvic/adrenal/testicular ultrasound, and computerized tomography of the head.

Monitoring: Monitor for signs/symptoms of noncompliance. Monitor for signs/symptoms of a hypersensitivity reaction and for other adverse reactions.

Counseling: Instruct to notify physician if any type of a hypersensitivity reaction occurs. Inform parent/guardian of the importance of continuous therapy and that irregular dosing could restart the maturation process. Inform that a female patient may experience menses/spotting during the first 2 months of therapy and instruct to notify the physician immediately if bleeding continues beyond the 2nd month. Instruct to report any unusual signs/symptoms (eg, continued pubertal changes, substantial mood swings, behavioral changes).

LEVAQUIN — levofloxacin   Rx

Class: Fluoroquinolone

> Fluoroquinolones have been associated w/ disabling and potentially irreversible serious adverse reactions that have occurred together, including tendinitis and tendon rupture, peripheral neuropathy, CNS effects; d/c immediately and avoid fluoroquinolone use in patients who experience any of these serious adverse reactions. May exacerbate muscle weakness in patients w/ myasthenia gravis; avoid w/ known history of myasthenia gravis. Because fluoroquinolones have been associated w/ serious adverse reactions, reserve levofloxacin for use in patients who have no alternative treatment options for the following indications: uncomplicated UTI, acute bacterial exacerbation of chronic bronchitis, and acute bacterial sinusitis.

ADULT DOSAGE
Pneumonia

Oral/IV:
Nosocomial Pneumonia: 750mg q24h for 7-14 days
Community-Acquired Pneumonia:
Due to methicillin-susceptible *Staphylococcus aureus*, *Streptococcus pneumoniae* (including multi-drug-resistant isolates), *Haemophilus influenzae*, *Haemophilus parainfluenzae*, *Klebsiella pneumoniae*, *Moraxella catarrhalis*, *Chlamydophila pneumoniae*, *Legionella pneumophila*, or *Mycoplasma pneumoniae*:

500mg q24h for 7-14 days

Due to *S. pneumoniae* (excluding multi-drug-resistant isolates), *H. influenzae*, *H. parainfluenzae*, *M. pneumoniae*, or *C. pneumoniae*:
750mg q24h for 5 days

Acute Bacterial Sinusitis

Oral/IV:
750mg q24h for 5 days or 500mg q24h for 10-14 days

Acute Bacterial Exacerbation of Chronic Bronchitis

Oral/IV:
500mg q24h for 7 days

Skin and Skin Structure Infections

Oral/IV:
Complicated: 750mg q24h for 7-14 days
Uncomplicated: 500mg q24h for 7-10 days

Chronic Bacterial Prostatitis

Oral/IV:
500mg q24h for 28 days

Urinary Tract Infections

Oral/IV:
Complicated UTI (cUTI) due to *Escherichia coli, K. pneumoniae, Proteus mirabilis /* **Acute Pyelonephritis (AP) Due to** *E. coli,* **Including Cases w/ Concurrent Bacteremia:**
750mg q24h for 5 days

PEDIATRIC DOSAGE
Inhalational Anthrax (Postexposure)

Oral/IV:
≥6 Months of Age:
<50kg: 8mg/kg q12h for 60 days
Max: 250mg/dose
>50kg: 500mg q24h for 60 days

Plague

Oral/IV:
Pneumonic/Septicemic Plague and Prophylaxis:
≥6 Months of Age:
<50kg: 8mg/kg q12h for 10-14 days
Max: 250mg/dose
>50kg: 500mg q24h for 10-14 days

cUTI Due to *Enterococcus faecalis, Enterobacter cloacae, E. coli, K. pneumoniae, P. mirabilis, Pseudomonas aeruginosa* / AP Due to *E. coli:*

250mg q24h for 10 days

Uncomplicated: 250mg q24h for 3 days

Inhalational Anthrax (Postexposure)
Oral/IV:
>50kg: 500mg q24h for 60 days

Plague
Pneumonic/Septicemic Plague and Prophylaxis:
Oral/IV:
500mg q24h for 10-14 days

DOSING CONSIDERATIONS
Concomitant Medications
Take antacids, metal cations, and multivitamins at least 2 hrs before or 2 hrs after oral administration

Renal Impairment
750mg q24h:
CrCl 20-49mL/min: 750mg q48h
CrCl 10-19mL/min or Hemodialysis/Chronic Ambulatory Peritoneal Dialysis (CAPD): 750mg initial dose, then 500mg q48h

500mg q24h:
CrCl 20-49mL/min: 500mg initial dose, then 250mg q24h
CrCl 10-19mL/min or Hemodialysis/CAPD: 500mg initial dose, then 250mg q48h

250mg q24h:
CrCl 20-49mL/min: No dose adjustment
CrCl 10-19mL/min: 250mg q48h; if treating uncomplicated UTI, no dose adjustment required
Hemodialysis/CAPD: No information on dose adjustment available

ADMINISTRATION
IV/Oral route

Drink fluids liberally; maintain adequate hydration.

Oral
- Take at the same time each day.
Tab: Take w/ or w/o food.
Sol: Take 1 hr before or 2 hrs after eating.

IV
- Not for rapid or bolus IV infusion.
- Do not coadminister w/ any sol containing multivalent cations through the same IV line.
- Infuse over 60 min (250-500mg) or over 90 min (750mg).
- Refer to PI for administration, preparation, stability, compatibility, and thawing instructions.

STORAGE
Tab: 15-30°C (59-86°F). **Sol:** 25°C (77°F); excursions permitted to 15-30°C (59-86°F). **Inj:** ≤25°C (77°F); brief exposure to ≤40°C (104°F) does not adversely affect product. Avoid excessive heat and protect from freezing and light.

HOW SUPPLIED
Inj: 5mg/mL in D5W [50mL, 100mL, 150mL]; **Sol:** 25mg/mL [480mL]; **Tab:** 250mg, 500mg, 750mg

CONTRAINDICATIONS
Known hypersensitivity to levofloxacin, or other quinolone antibacterials.

WARNINGS/PRECAUTIONS
Tendinitis or tendon rupture can occur w/in hours or days of starting therapy or as long as several months after completion of therapy and may occur bilaterally; increased risk in patients >60 yrs and in patients w/ kidney, heart, or lung transplants. Avoid in patients who have a history of tendon disorders or tendon rupture. Cases of sensory or sensorimotor axonal polyneuropathy, resulting in paresthesias, hypoesthesias, dysesthesias, and weakness reported; symptoms may occur soon after initiation of therapy and may be irreversible in some patients. Avoid in patients who have previously experienced peripheral neuropathy. Caution in patients w/ a known or suspected CNS disorder (eg, severe cerebral arteriosclerosis, epilepsy) or in the presence of other risk factors that may predispose to seizures or lower the seizure threshold (eg, certain drug therapy, renal dysfunction). Serious anaphylactic reactions and other serious and sometimes fatal adverse reactions reported; d/c immediately and institute supportive measures at the 1st appearance of a skin rash, jaundice, or any other sign of hypersensitivity. Severe hepatotoxicity, including acute hepatitis and fatal events, reported; d/c immediately if signs and symptoms of hepatitis occur. *Clostridium difficile*-associated diarrhea (CDAD) reported; may need to d/c if CDAD is suspected or confirmed. May prolong the QT interval; avoid w/ known QT interval prolongation or uncorrected hypokalemia. Increased incidence of musculoskeletal disorders in pediatric patients. Blood glucose disturbances (eg, symptomatic hyper/hypoglycemia) reported, usually in diabetic patients receiving concomitant treatment w/ an oral hypoglycemic agent (eg, glyburide) or w/ insulin; d/c and initiate appropriate therapy if a hypoglycemic reaction occurs. May cause moderate to severe photosensitivity/phototoxicity reactions; d/c if photosensitivity/phototoxicity occurs. Avoid excessive exposure to sun/UV light. May increase risk of bacterial resistance if used in the absence of a proven/suspected bacterial infection or a prophylactic indication. Crystalluria and cylindruria reported; maintain adequate hydration. May produce false-positive urine screening results for opiates. Caution in elderly and w/ renal impairment.

ADVERSE REACTIONS
Nausea, headache, diarrhea, insomnia, constipation, dizziness.

DRUG INTERACTIONS
Increased risk of developing fluoroquinolone-associated tendinitis and tendon rupture in patients taking corticosteroid drugs. Avoid w/ Class IA (eg, quinidine, procainamide) and Class III (eg, amiodarone, sotalol) antiarrhythmics. Caution w/ drugs that may lower the seizure threshold. May enhance effects of warfarin; monitor for evidence of bleeding and closely monitor PT, INR, or other suitable anticoagulation tests. Disturbances of blood glucose in diabetic patients receiving a concomitant antidiabetic agent reported; monitor glucose levels. NSAIDs may increase risk of CNS stimulation and convulsive seizures. May prolong theophylline $T_{1/2}$ and increase theophylline levels/risk of theophylline-related adverse reactions; monitor theophylline levels closely and adjust dose appropriately. Probenecid or cimetidine may increase exposure and $T_{1/2}$, and reduce renal clearance. **Tab/Sol:** Antacids containing Mg^{2+} or aluminum, sucralfate, metal cations (eg, iron), multivitamin preparations w/ zinc, or didanosine chewable/buffered tab or pediatric powder for oral sol may substantially interfere w/ the GI absorption of levofloxacin and lower systemic concentrations; take at least 2 hrs before or 2 hrs after oral levofloxacin.

PREGNANCY AND LACTATION
Pregnancy: Category C.
Lactation: May be excreted in human milk; not for use in nursing.

MECHANISM OF ACTION
Fluoroquinolone; inhibits bacterial topoisomerase IV and DNA gyrase (both of which are type II topoisomerases), enzymes required for DNA replication, transcription, repair, and recombination.

PHARMACOKINETICS
Absorption: Administration of variable doses resulted in different parameters. (PO) Rapid and complete. (Tab: 500mg, 750mg) Absolute bioavailability (99%).
Distribution: V_d=74-112L (500mg, 750mg); plasma protein binding (24-38%).
Metabolism: Limited. **Elimination:** (PO) Urine (87% unchanged, <5% desmethyl and N-oxide metabolites), feces (<4%). Refer to PI for additional pharmacokinetic information.

PATIENT CONSIDERATIONS
Assessment: Assess for risk factors for developing tendinitis and tendon rupture, history of myasthenia gravis, tendon disorders, or peripheral neuropathy, drug hypersensitivity, CNS disorders or risk factors that may predispose to seizures or lower seizure threshold, QT interval prolongation, uncorrected hypokalemia, renal/hepatic impairment, pregnancy/nursing status, and possible drug interactions.

Monitoring: Monitor for tendinitis, tendon rupture, peripheral neuropathy, CNS effects, exacerbation of myasthenia gravis, hypersensitivity reactions, hepatotoxicity, CDAD, QT prolongation, arrhythmias, musculoskeletal disorders (pediatric patients), photosensitivity/phototoxicity reactions, and other adverse reactions. Monitor hydration status, blood glucose levels, and renal function. Monitor for evidence of bleeding, PT, and INR if administered w/ warfarin.

Counseling: Inform about benefits/risks of therapy. Advise to d/c if an adverse reaction is experienced and to call physician for advice on completing the full course of treatment w/ another antibacterial drug. Inform about the risks of tendinitis and tendon rupture, peripheral neuropathies, CNS effects, exacerbation of myasthenia gravis, and QT interval prolongation. Instruct to d/c and contact physician if pain, swelling, or inflammation of a tendon or weakness or inability to use joints is experienced; advise to rest and refrain from exercise. Instruct to d/c immediately and contact physician if symptoms of peripheral neuropathy (eg, pain, burning, tingling, numbness and/or weakness) develop. Advise to inform physician if patient has history of convulsions or myasthenia gravis. Instruct to notify physician if persistent headache w/ or w/o blurred vision occurs. Inform patients that they should know how they react to therapy before operating an automobile or machinery or engaging in other activities requiring mental alertness/coordination. Advise to notify physician if symptoms of muscle weakness, including respiratory difficulties, are experienced. Instruct to d/c at the 1st sign of a skin rash, hives, or other skin reactions; a rapid heartbeat; difficulty in swallowing or breathing; any swelling suggesting angioedema; or other symptoms of an allergic reaction. Advise to notify physician if experiencing any signs or symptoms of liver injury. Inform that diarrhea is a common problem; instruct to notify physician if experiencing watery and bloody stools (w/ or w/o stomach cramps/fever) even as late as ≥2 months after having taken the last dose of treatment. Instruct to inform physician of any personal or family history of QT prolongation or proarrhythmic conditions. Advise to minimize or avoid exposure to natural or artificial light (eg, tanning beds or UVA/B treatment); instruct to contact physician if a sunburn-like reaction or skin eruption occurs. Instruct diabetic patients being treated w/ insulin or an oral hypoglycemic agent to d/c therapy and notify physician if hypoglycemia occurs. Inform that drug treats only bacterial, not viral, infections. Instruct to take exactly ud; inform that skipping doses or not completing full course may decrease effectiveness and increase bacterial resistance. Inform that antacids (containing Mg^{2+} or aluminum), sucralfate, metal cations (eg, iron), multivitamin preparations w/ zinc, or didanosine should be taken at least 2 hrs before or 2 hrs after oral levofloxacin.

LEVBID — hyoscyamine sulfate   Rx

Class: Anticholinergic

ADULT DOSAGE	PEDIATRIC DOSAGE
General Dosing	**General Dosing**
1-2 tabs q12h	**≥12 Years:**
Max: 4 tabs/24 hrs	1-2 tabs q12h
Other Indications	**Max:** 4 tabs/24 hrs
Adjunctive therapy in the treatment of peptic ulcer, irritable bowel syndrome (irritable colon, spastic colon, mucous colitis), functional GI disorders, neurogenic bladder, neurogenic bowel disturbances (eg, splenic flexure syndrome, neurogenic colon)	**Other Indications**
	Adjunctive therapy in the treatment of peptic ulcer, irritable bowel syndrome (irritable colon, spastic colon, mucous colitis), functional GI disorders, neurogenic bladder, neurogenic bowel disturbances (eg, splenic flexure syndrome, neurogenic colon)
May be used to control gastric secretion, visceral spasm and hypermotility in spastic colitis, spastic bladder, cystitis, pylorospasm, and associated abdominal cramps	May be used to control gastric secretion, visceral spasm and hypermotility in spastic colitis, spastic bladder, cystitis, pylorospasm, and associated abdominal cramps
May be used to reduce symptoms in functional intestinal disorders (eg, mild dysenteries, diverticulitis, acute enterocolitis)	May be used to reduce symptoms in functional intestinal disorders (eg, mild dysenteries, diverticulitis, acute enterocolitis)
Along w/ morphine or other narcotics in symptomatic relief of biliary and renal colic	Along w/ morphine or other narcotics in symptomatic relief of biliary and renal colic
As a "drying agent" in the relief of symptoms of acute rhinitis	As a "drying agent" in the relief of symptoms of acute rhinitis
To reduce rigidity and tremors and to control associated sialorrhea and hyperhidrosis in the therapy of parkinsonism	To reduce rigidity and tremors and to control associated sialorrhea and hyperhidrosis in the therapy of parkinsonism
May be used in the therapy of poisoning by anticholinesterase agents	May be used in the therapy of poisoning by anticholinesterase agents

DOSING CONSIDERATIONS
Elderly
Start at lower end of dosing range

ADMINISTRATION
Oral route

Do not crush or chew.

STORAGE
20-25°C (68-77°F); excursions permitted to 15-30°C (59-86°F).

HOW SUPPLIED
Tab, Extended-Release: 0.375mg

CONTRAINDICATIONS
Glaucoma; obstructive uropathy (eg, bladder neck obstruction due to prostatic hypertrophy); obstructive disease of the GI tract (as in achalasia, pyloroduodenal stenosis); paralytic ileus, intestinal atony of elderly/debilitated patients; unstable cardiovascular status in acute hemorrhage; severe ulcerative colitis; toxic megacolon complicating ulcerative colitis; myasthenia gravis.

WARNINGS/PRECAUTIONS
Heat prostration may occur w/ high environmental temperature. Diarrhea may be an early symptom of incomplete intestinal obstruction, especially in patients w/ ileostomy or colostomy; in this instance, treatment would be inappropriate and possibly harmful. May impair physical/mental abilities. Psychosis reported in sensitive individuals. CNS signs/symptoms usually resolve w/in 12-48 hrs after discontinuation of the drug. Caution w/ autonomic neuropathy, hyperthyroidism, coronary heart disease, CHF, cardiac arrhythmias, HTN, renal disease, and hiatal hernia associated w/ reflux esophagitis. May increase HR; investigate any tachycardia prior to therapy.

ADVERSE REACTIONS
Dry mouth, urinary hesitancy/retention, blurred vision, tachycardia, palpitations, mydriasis, increased ocular tension, loss of taste, headache, nervousness, drowsiness, weakness, fatigue, dizziness, N/V.

DRUG INTERACTIONS
Additive adverse effects resulting from cholinergic blockade may occur when administered concomitantly w/ other antimuscarinics, amantadine, haloperidol, phenothiazines, MAOIs, TCAs, or some antihistamines. Antacids may interfere w/ absorption.

PREGNANCY AND LACTATION
Category C, caution in nursing.

MECHANISM OF ACTION
Anticholinergic/antispasmodic; inhibits action of acetylcholine on structures innervated by postganglionic cholinergic nerves and on smooth muscles that respond to acetylcholine but lack cholinergic innervation, inhibits GI propulsive motility, decreases gastric acid secretion, and controls excess pharyngeal, tracheal, and bronchial secretions.

PHARMACOKINETICS
Absorption: Complete; T_{max}=4.2 hrs. **Distribution:** Crosses blood-brain barrier and placenta; trace amounts found in breast milk. **Metabolism:** Partial hydrolysis; tropic acid, tropine (metabolites). **Elimination:** Urine (unchanged); $T_{1/2}$=7.47 hrs.

PATIENT CONSIDERATIONS
Assessment: Assess for glaucoma, obstructive uropathy, GI obstruction, paralytic ileus, sensitivity towards anticholinergic drugs, tachycardia, any other conditions where treatment is contraindicated or cautioned, pregnancy/nursing status, and possible drug interactions.

Monitoring: Monitor for signs/symptoms of heat prostration, drowsiness, dizziness, blurred vision, psychosis, CNS signs/symptoms, diarrhea, and other adverse reactions.

Counseling: Inform that drug may produce drowsiness, dizziness, or blurred vision; warn not to engage in activities requiring mental alertness (eg, operating a motor vehicle or other machinery) and not to perform hazardous work while taking drug. Advise that treatment may decrease sweating, resulting in heat prostration, fever or heat stroke; instruct to use caution if febrile or exposed to elevated environmental temperatures.

LEVEMIR — insulin detemir (rDNA origin)   Rx

Class: Insulin (long-acting)

ADULT DOSAGE	PEDIATRIC DOSAGE
Type 1 Diabetes Mellitus	**Type 1 Diabetes Mellitus**
Initial: Approx 1/3 of total daily insulin requirements	**≥2 Years:**
Titrate: Adjust dose based on blood glucose measurements	**Initial:** Approx 1/3 of total daily insulin requirements
	Titrate: Adjust dose based on blood glucose measurements
Use rapid-acting or short-acting, premeal insulin to satisfy the remainder of the daily insulin requirements	Use rapid-acting or short-acting, premeal insulin to satisfy the remainder of the daily insulin requirements
Type 2 Diabetes Mellitus	**Conversions**
Inadequately Controlled on Oral Antidiabetics:	**From Insulin Glargine/NPH Insulin:**
Initial: 10 U (or 0.1-0.2 U/kg) qpm or divided bid	Convert on a unit-to-unit basis
Titrate: Adjust dose based on blood glucose measurements	In converting from NPH insulin, some type 2 diabetes mellitus patients may require more units of therapy than NPH insulin
Inadequately Controlled on Glucagon-Like Peptide (GLP)-1 Receptor Agonist:	
Initial: 10 U qpm	
Titrate: Adjust dose based on blood glucose measurements	
Administer as separate inj when using w/ a GLP-1 receptor agonist	
Conversions	
From Insulin Glargine/NPH Insulin:	
Convert on a unit-to-unit basis	
In converting from NPH insulin, some type 2 diabetes mellitus patients may require more units of therapy than NPH insulin	

DOSING CONSIDERATIONS
Elderly
Dose conservatively

ADMINISTRATION
SQ route

Rotate inj sites w/in the same region (abdomen, thigh, or deltoid) from 1 inj to the next

Do not dilute or mix w/ any other insulin or sol

QD Dosing
Administer dose w/ pm meal or hs

BID Dosing
Administer pm dose w/ pm meal, hs, or 12 hrs after am dose

STORAGE
Unopened: 2-8°C (36-46°F) until expiration date. If refrigeration is not possible, may be kept at room temperature <30°C (86°F) for 42 days. Do not freeze. Protect from direct heat and light. **Opened: Vial:** 2-8°C (36-46°F) or room temperature <30°C (86°F). Discard refrigerated vials 42 days after initial use and discard unrefrigerated vials 42 days after they are 1st kept out of the refrigerator. Do not freeze. Protect from direct heat and light. **FlexTouch:** Room temperature <30°C (86°F) for 42 days; do not refrigerate after initial use or store w/ the needle in place. Protect from direct heat and light. Always remove the needle after each inj and use a new needle for each inj.

HOW SUPPLIED
Inj: 100 U/mL [3mL, FlexTouch; 10mL, vial]

CONTRAINDICATIONS
Hypersensitivity to Levemir or any of its excipients.

WARNINGS/PRECAUTIONS
Not recommended for treatment of diabetic ketoacidosis. Do not share insulin device between patients, even if the needle is changed; may carry a risk for

transmission of blood-borne pathogens. Changes to an insulin regimen should be made cautiously and only under medical supervision. Changes in strength, manufacturer, type, or method of administration may result in the need for a change in dose or an adjustment of concomitant antidiabetic treatment. Not for IV/IM use or use in insulin infusion pumps. Hypoglycemia may occur; caution in patients w/ hypoglycemia unawareness and patients predisposed to hypoglycemia. Hypoglycemia may impair ability to concentrate and react. Severe, life-threatening, generalized allergy, including anaphylaxis, may occur. Caution in renal/hepatic impairment.

ADVERSE REACTIONS
Hypoglycemia, URTI, headache, pharyngitis, influenza-like illness, abdominal pain, back pain, gastroenteritis, bronchitis, pyrexia, cough, viral infection, N/V, rhinitis.

DRUG INTERACTIONS
May require insulin dose adjustment and close monitoring w/ drugs that may increase blood-glucose-lowering effect and susceptibility to hypoglycemia (eg, oral antidiabetic drugs, pramlintide acetate, ACE inhibitors), drugs that may reduce blood-glucose-lowering effect (eg, corticosteroids, niacin, danazol), or drugs that may either increase or decrease blood-glucose-lowering effect (eg, β-blockers, clonidine, lithium salts, alcohol). Pentamidine may cause hypoglycemia, sometimes followed by hyperglycemia. Signs of hypoglycemia may be reduced or absent w/ antiadrenergic drugs (eg, β-blockers, clonidine, guanethidine, reserpine). May need to lower or more conservatively titrate dose when used w/ a GLP-1 receptor agonist to minimize risk of hypoglycemia. Observe for signs/symptoms of heart failure (HF) if treated concomitantly w/ a peroxisome proliferator-activated receptor (PPAR)-gamma agonist (eg, thiazolidinedione); consider discontinuation or dose reduction of the PPAR-gamma agonist if HF develops.

PREGNANCY AND LACTATION
Category B, caution in nursing.

MECHANISM OF ACTION
Insulin detemir (rDNA origin); regulates glucose metabolism. Lowers blood glucose by facilitating cellular uptake of glucose into skeletal muscle and adipose tissue and by inhibiting the output of glucose from the liver. Inhibits lipolysis in the adipocyte, inhibits proteolysis, and enhances protein synthesis.

PHARMACOKINETICS
Absorption: Absolute bioavailability (approx 60%); T_{max}=6-8 hrs. **Distribution:** Plasma protein binding (>98%); V_d=0.1L/kg. **Elimination:** $T_{1/2}$=5-7 hrs (type 1 diabetes).

PATIENT CONSIDERATIONS
Assessment: Assess for diabetic ketoacidosis, predisposition to hypoglycemia, hypersensitivity, renal/hepatic impairment, pregnancy/nursing status, and possible drug interactions. Obtain baseline blood glucose and HbA1c levels.

Monitoring: Monitor for signs/symptoms of hypoglycemia, allergic reactions, and other adverse reactions. Monitor blood glucose and HbA1c levels, and renal/hepatic function.

Counseling: Inform about the potential side effects, including hypoglycemia, weight gain, lipodystrophy, and allergic reactions. Inform that hypoglycemia may impair ability to concentrate and react; advise to use caution when driving or operating machinery. Instruct to always check the label before each inj to avoid medication errors/accidental mix-ups. Advise to use only if sol is clear and colorless w/ no particles visible. Instruct on self-management procedures, including glucose monitoring, proper inj technique, and management of hypoglycemia and hyperglycemia, and on handling of special situations (eg, intercurrent conditions, inadequate or skipped insulin dose, inadequate food intake). Advise to inform physician if pregnant/contemplating pregnancy. Counsel to never share insulin device w/ another person, even if the needle is changed.

LEVITRA — vardenafil hydrochloride   Rx

Class: Phosphodiesterase-5 (PDE-5) inhibitor

ADULT DOSAGE
Erectile Dysfunction
Initial: 10mg prn, 60 min prior to sexual activity
Titrate: May decrease to 5mg or increase to max of 20mg based on efficacy and side effects
Max: 1 dose/day

PEDIATRIC DOSAGE
Pediatric use may not have been established

DOSING CONSIDERATIONS
Concomitant Medications
Ritonavir:
Max: 2.5mg/72 hrs

Indinavir/Saquinavir/Atazanavir/Clarithromycin/Ketoconazole (400mg/day)/Itraconazole (400mg/day):
Max: 2.5mg/24 hrs

Ketoconazole (200mg/day)/Itraconazole (200mg/day)/Erythromycin:
Max: 5mg/24 hrs

Stable on α-Blocker:
Initial: 5mg; 2.5mg when used w/ certain CYP3A4 inhibitors
Consider a time interval between dosing

Renal Impairment
Dialysis: Avoid use

Hepatic Impairment
Moderate (Child-Pugh B):
Initial: 5mg
Max: 10mg
Severe (Child-Pugh C): Avoid use
Elderly
≥65 Years:
Initial: 5mg

ADMINISTRATION
Oral route
Take w/ or w/o food.

STORAGE
25°C (77°F); excursions permitted to 15-30°C (59-86°F).

HOW SUPPLIED
Tab: 2.5mg, 5mg, 10mg, 20mg

CONTRAINDICATIONS
Concomitant use w/ guanylate cyclase stimulators and regular or intermittent use w/ nitrates and nitric oxide donors.

WARNINGS/PRECAUTIONS
Avoid if sexual activity is not recommended due to underlying cardiovascular (CV) status, or if w/ severe hepatic impairment (Child-Pugh C)/congenital QT prolongation, or if on renal dialysis. Patients w/ left ventricular outflow obstruction (eg, aortic stenosis, idiopathic hypertrophic subaortic stenosis) may be sensitive to vasodilation. Has vasodilatory properties resulting in transient decreases in supine BP. Not recommended w/ unstable angina, hypotension (resting systolic BP <90mmHg), uncontrolled HTN (>170/110mmHg), recent history of stroke, life-threatening arrhythmia, or MI (w/in last 6 months), severe cardiac failure, or hereditary degenerative retinal disorders, including retinitis pigmentosa. Rare reports of prolonged erections >4 hrs and priapism. Caution w/ bleeding disorders, significant active peptic ulceration, anatomical deformation of the penis (eg, angulation, cavernosal fibrosis, Peyronie's disease) or conditions that predispose to priapism (eg, sickle cell anemia, multiple myeloma, leukemia). Non-arteritic anterior ischemic optic neuropathy (NAION) reported (rare); d/c if sudden loss of vision occurs. Caution in patients w/ underlying NAION risk factors; increased risk w/ previous history of NAION and individuals w/ "crowded" optic disc. Sudden decrease or loss of hearing accompanied by tinnitus and dizziness reported; d/c if this occurs. QT prolongation may occur.

ADVERSE REACTIONS
Headache, flushing, rhinitis, dyspepsia, sinusitis, flu syndrome.

DRUG INTERACTIONS
See Contraindications. Avoid w/ Class IA (eg, quinidine, procainamide) or Class III (eg, amiodarone, sotalol) antiarrhythmics and other agents for ED. Caution w/ medications known to prolong QT interval. Increased levels w/ CYP3A4 inhibitors (eg, ritonavir, ketoconazole, clarithromycin). Caution when coadministering α-blockers; additive effect on BP may be anticipated. CYP3A4/5 or CYP2C9 inhibitors may reduce clearance.

PREGNANCY AND LACTATION
Pregnancy: Category B.
Lactation: Not for use in nursing.

MECHANISM OF ACTION
PDE-5 inhibitor; increases the amount of cGMP, triggering smooth muscle relaxation and allowing increased blood flow into the penis.

PHARMACOKINETICS
Absorption: Rapid. Absolute bioavailability (15%); (20mg dose, fasted) T_{max}=30 min-2 hrs. **Distribution:** V_d=208L; plasma protein binding (95%). **Metabolism:** Liver via CYP3A4, CYP3A5, CYP2C. M1 (major metabolite). **Elimination:** Feces (91-95%), urine (2-6%); $T_{1/2}$=4-5 hrs.

PATIENT CONSIDERATIONS
Assessment: Assess for CV disease, left ventricular outflow obstruction, congenital or history of QT prolongation, hereditary degenerative retinal disorders, bleeding disorders, active peptic ulceration, anatomical deformation of the penis, conditions that predispose to priapism, renal/hepatic impairment, potential underlying causes of ED, risk for NAION, and for possible drug interactions. Obtain baseline BP.

Monitoring: Monitor for priapism, changes in vision/hearing, QT prolongation, and other adverse reactions.

Counseling: Instruct to take ud. Inform that regular and/or intermittent use of nitrates may cause BP to suddenly drop to an unsafe level. Inform that use is contraindicated w/ guanylate cyclase stimulators (eg, riociguat). Inform patients w/ preexisting CV risk factors of the potential cardiac risk of sexual activity. Inform that concomitant use of α-blockers may lower BP significantly. Instruct to contact physician for dose modification if not satisfied w/ quality of sexual performance or in case of an unwanted effect. Instruct to seek immediate medical assistance if erection persists >4 hrs; inform that penile tissue damage and permanent loss of potency may result. Instruct to d/c and seek medical attention in the event of sudden loss of vision in 1 or both eyes; inform of the increased risk of NAION w/ history of NAION in 1 eye and in patients w/ a "crowded" optic disc. Instruct to d/c treatment and seek prompt medical attention in the event of sudden decrease or loss of hearing that may be accompanied by tinnitus and dizziness. Counsel about protective measures necessary to guard against STDs, including HIV; inform that drug does not protect against STDs.

LEVOPHED — norepinephrine bitartrate **Rx**

Class: Alpha-adrenergic agonist

> To prevent sloughing and necrosis in area of extravasation, area should be infiltrated w/ 10-15mL saline sol containing 5-10mg of Regitine (brand of phentolamine), an adrenergic blocking agent. Sympathetic blockade w/ phentolamine causes immediate and conspicuous local hyperemic changes if infiltrated w/in 12 hrs. Give phentolamine as soon as possible after the extravasation is noted.

ADULT DOSAGE

Acute Hypotension

For BP control in certain acute hypotensive states (eg, pheochromocytomectomy, sympathectomy, poliomyelitis, spinal anesthesia, MI, septicemia, blood transfusion, and drug reactions)

Average Dosage:
Initial: 8-12mcg/min (2-3mL) as IV infusion until low normal BP (80-100mmHg systolic) is established and maintained by adjusting rate of flow
Maint: 2-4mcg/min (0.5-1mL)

High Dosage:
Individualize dose (as high as 68mg/day)
Continue infusion until adequate BP and tissue perfusion are maintained w/o therapy
Reduce dose gradually, avoiding abrupt withdrawal

Adjunct Treatment of Cardiac Arrest and Profound Hypotension:
Average Dosage:
Initial: 8-12mcg/min (2-3mL) as IV infusion until low normal BP (80-100mmHg systolic) is established and maintained by adjusting rate of flow
Maint: 2-4mcg/min (0.5-1mL)

PEDIATRIC DOSAGE
Pediatric use may not have been established

DOSING CONSIDERATIONS
Elderly
Start at lower end of dosing range

ADMINISTRATION
IV route

Inj is a concentrated, potent drug that must be diluted in dextrose containing sol prior to infusion.
An infusion should be given into a large vein.
Avoid contact w/ iron salts, alkalis, or oxidizing agents.

Diluent
Dilute in D5 inj or D5 and NaCl inj.
Whole blood or plasma, if indicated to increase blood volume, should be administered separately (eg, Y-tube and individual containers if given simultaneously).

STORAGE
20-25°C (68-77°F); (vial) excursions permitted to 15-30° (59-86°F). Protect from light.

HOW SUPPLIED
Inj: 4mg/4mL

CONTRAINDICATIONS
Hypotension from blood volume deficits, except as an emergency measure to maintain coronary and cerebral artery perfusion until blood volume replacement therapy can be completed, mesenteric or peripheral vascular thrombosis (unless administration is necessary as a life-saving procedure in the opinion of the attending physician), profound hypoxia or hypercarbia, concomitant use of cyclopropane and halothane anesthetics.

WARNINGS/PRECAUTIONS
Contains sodium metabisulfite; may cause allergic-type reactions (eg, anaphylactic symptoms, life-threatening or less severe asthmatic episodes). May produce dangerously high BP w/ overdoses due to potency and varying response; monitor BP every 2 min from initial administration until desired BP is obtained, then every 5 min if administration is to be continued. Headache may be a symptom of HTN due to overdosage; monitor rate of flow constantly. Infusions should be given into a large vein, particularly an antecubital vein whenever possible. Avoid a catheter tie-in technique if possible. Occlusive vascular diseases (eg, atherosclerosis, arteriosclerosis, diabetic endarteritis, Buerger's disease) more likely to occur in the lower than in the upper extremity; avoid leg veins in elderly or in those suffering from such disorders. Gangrene in lower extremity reported when given in an ankle vein. Check infusion site frequently for free flow. Avoid extravasation into the tissues; local necrosis might ensue. Blanching may occur; consider changing the infusion site at intervals to allow effects of local vasoconstriction to subside. Caution in elderly.

ADVERSE REACTIONS
Ischemic injury, bradycardia, arrhythmias, anxiety, headache, respiratory difficulty, extravasation necrosis at inj site.

DRUG INTERACTIONS
See Contraindications. Caution w/ MAOI or triptyline/imipramine antidepressants; severe, prolonged HTN may result.

PREGNANCY AND LACTATION
Category C, caution in nursing.

MECHANISM OF ACTION
Alpha-adrenergic agonist; peripheral vasoconstrictor (α-adrenergic action) and inotropic stimulator of the heart and dilator of coronary arteries (β-adrenergic action).

PATIENT CONSIDERATIONS
Assessment: Assess hypotension and need for blood volume replacement. Assess use as emergency measure or life-saving procedure (eg, hypotension from blood volume deficits to maintain coronary and cerebral artery perfusion until blood volume replacement therapy can be completed, mesenteric or peripheral vascular thrombosis). Assess for profound hypoxia or hypercarbia, sulfite sensitivity, pregnancy/nursing status, and possible drug interactions. Assess use in elderly and occlusive vascular diseases. Obtain baseline BP.

Monitoring: Monitor for HTN, headache, gangrene, extravasation, blanching, and hypersensitivity/allergic reactions. Monitor infusion site, rate of flow, BP, and central venous pressure.

Counseling: Inform of risks/benefits of therapy. Advise to inform physician if headache occurs.

LEVORPHANOL — levorphanol tartrate **CII**

Class: Opioid analgesic

OTHER BRAND NAMES
Levo-Dromoran (Discontinued)

ADULT DOSAGE

Moderate to Severe Pain

Initial: 2mg; may repeat in 6-8 hrs prn
Titrate: If necessary, may increase up to 3mg q6-8h after adequate evaluation of patient's response
Opioid Tolerant:
Higher doses may be appropriate
Opioid Intolerant:
Doses >6-12mg/day not recommended as starting dose; lower total daily doses may be appropriate

Conversions

From Morphine:
Total daily dose should begin at approx 1/15 to 1/12 of the total daily dose of oral morphine
Titrate: Adjust based on clinical response

If patient is on fixed-schedule (round-the-clock) dosing, allow adequate time after each dose change (approx 72 hrs)

PEDIATRIC DOSAGE
Pediatric use may not have been established

DOSING CONSIDERATIONS
Elderly
Reduce initial dose by ≥50%

Other Important Considerations
Patients w/ Condition Affecting Respiratory Reserve/Concomitant Drugs Affecting Respiration: Reduce initial dose by ≥50%

ADMINISTRATION
Oral route

STORAGE
20-25°C (68-77°F).

HOW SUPPLIED
Tab: 2mg* *scored

CONTRAINDICATIONS
Hypersensitivity to levorphanol tartrate.

WARNINGS/PRECAUTIONS
May produce serious/fatal respiratory depression if given in excessive dose, too frequently, or if given in full dosage to compromised/vulnerable patients; individualize dose. Caution with impaired respiratory reserve or respiratory depression from some other cause (eg, from other medication, uremia, severe infection, obstructive respiratory conditions). Not recommended in acute/severe bronchial asthma or for use in biliary surgery. Respiratory depressant effects with carbon dioxide retention and secondary elevation of CSF pressure may be markedly exaggerated in the presence of head injury, other intracranial lesions or preexisting increase in intracranial pressure. May obscure neurological signs of head injuries and diagnosis/clinical course of acute abdominal conditions. Limit use in acute myocardial infarction, myocardial dysfunction, or coronary insufficiency. May cause severe hypotension in postoperative patients or individuals whose ability to maintain BP has been compromised by a depleted blood volume or by administration of drugs (eg, phenothiazines, general anesthetics). May cause orthostatic hypotension, dizziness, and syncope in

ambulatory patients. Caution with extensive liver disease. Potential for abuse. Caution and reduce initial dose in elderly or debilitated, severe renal/hepatic impairment, hypothyroidism, Addison's disease, toxic psychosis, prostatic hypertrophy or urethral stricture, acute alcoholism, or delirium tremens. May impair mental/physical abilities.

ADVERSE REACTIONS
N/V, altered mood and mentation, pruritus, flushing, difficulties in urination, constipation, biliary spasm, abdominal pain, cardiac arrest, coma, suicide attempt, apnea, cyanosis, abnormal vision.

DRUG INTERACTIONS
Avoid with MAOIs and mixed agonist/antagonist analgesics (eg, pentazocine, nalbuphine, butorphanol). Additive CNS depressant effect with CNS depressants (eg, alcohol, sedatives, general anesthetics, TCAs); reduce dose of one or both agents.

PREGNANCY AND LACTATION
Category C, not for use in nursing.

MECHANISM OF ACTION
Opioid analgesic; believed to act at receptors in the periventricular and periaqueductal gray matter in both the brain and spinal cord to alter the transmission and perception of pain.

PHARMACOKINETICS
Absorption: Well-absorbed; T_{max}=1 hr. **Distribution:** V_d=10-13 L/kg (IV). Plasma protein binding (40%). **Elimination:** $T_{1/2}$=11-16 hrs (IV).

PATIENT CONSIDERATIONS

Assessment: Assess for degree of opioid tolerance, level of pain intensity, type of pain, and patient's general condition and medical status. Assess for previous hypersensitivity to the drug, preexisting pulmonary disease, head injury, increase in intracranial pressure, myocardial dysfunction or coronary insufficiency, hepatic/renal impairment, history of alcohol or drug dependence, pregnancy/nursing status, and any other conditions where treatment is cautioned. Assess for possible drug interactions.

Monitoring: Monitor for signs/symptoms of respiratory depression, hypotension, and other adverse reactions.

Counseling: Advise to use caution against performing hazardous tasks requiring complete mental alertness (eg, operating machinery/driving). Inform about the risk of orthostatic hypotension, dizziness, and syncope. Inform that concomitant use with CNS depressants (eg, alcohol, other analgesics) may result in additive CNS depressant effects.

LEVOXYL — levothyroxine sodium

Rx

Class: Thyroid replacement hormone

> Do not use for the treatment of obesity or weight loss; doses within range of daily hormonal requirements are ineffective for weight reduction in euthyroid patients. Serious or life-threatening manifestations of toxicity may occur when given in larger doses, particularly when given in association with sympathomimetic amines.

ADULT DOSAGE
Hypothyroidism

Replacement/supplemental therapy in hypothyroidism of any etiology, except transient hypothyroidism during the recovery phase of subacute thyroiditis

Adjust dose based on periodic assessment of patient's clinical response and lab parameters

Usual: 1.7mcg/kg/day; >200mcg/day seldom required

Severe Hypothyroidism:
Initial: 12.5-25mcg/day
Titrate: Increase by 25mcg/day every 2-4 weeks until TSH level normalized

Secondary (Pituitary)/Tertiary (Hypothalamic) Hypothyroidism: Titrate until euthyroid and serum free-T4 level is restored to the upper 1/2 of the normal range

Subclinical Hypothyroidism: Lower doses may be adequate to normalize TSH level (eg, 1mcg/kg/day)

Pituitary TSH Suppressant

Used to treat/prevent various types of euthyroid goiters (eg, thyroid nodules, subacute or chronic lymphocytic thyroiditis, multinodular goiter) and to manage thyroid cancer

Well-Differentiated (Papillary and Follicular) Thyroid Cancer:

Usual: >2mcg/kg/day, w/ target TSH level <0.1 mU/L
High-Risk Tumors: Target TSH level <0.01 mU/L

PEDIATRIC DOSAGE
Hypothyroidism

Replacement/supplemental therapy in hypothyroidism of any etiology, except transient hypothyroidism during the recovery phase of subacute thyroiditis

Adjust dose based on periodic assessment of patient's clinical response and lab parameters

Usual:

0-3 Months of Age: 10-15mcg/kg/day
3-6 Months of Age: 8-10mcg/kg/day
6-12 Months of Age: 6-8mcg/kg/day
1-5 Years: 5-6mcg/kg/day
6-12 Years: 4-5mcg/kg/day
>12 Years: 2-3mcg/kg/day
Growth/Puberty Complete: 1.7mcg/kg/day

Infants w/ Serum T4 <5mcg/dL or Undetectable T4:
Initial: 50mcg/day

Chronic/Severe Hypothyroidism: Children:
Initial: 25mcg/day
Titrate: Increase by 25mcg increments every 2-4 weeks until desired effect is achieved

Benign Nodules and Nontoxic Multinodular Goiter:
Suppressed to a higher TSH target than that used for treatment of thyroid cancer (eg, 0.1-0.5 mU/L for nodules, 0.5-1.0 mU/L for multinodular goiter)

DOSING CONSIDERATIONS
Pregnancy
May increase levothyroxine requirements

Elderly
Hypothyroidism:
>50 Years:
Initial: 25-50mcg/day
Titrate: Increase by 12.5-25mcg increments every 6-8 weeks prn

W/ Underlying Cardiac Disease:
Initial: 12.5-25mcg/day
Titrate: Increase by 12.5-25mg increments every 4-6 weeks

Adverse Reactions
Minimize Hyperactivity in Older Children:
Initial: Give 1/4 of full replacement dose
Titrate: Increase on a weekly basis by 1/4 the full recommended replacement dose until the full recommended replacement dose is reached

Other Important Considerations
Hypothyroidism w/ Underlying Cardiac Disease:

Infants (Risk for Cardiac Failure):
Initial: Consider lower dose (eg, 25mcg/day)
Titrate: Increase dose in 4-6 weeks prn
<50 Years:
Initial: 25-50mcg/day
Titrate: Increase by 12.5-25mcg increments every 6-8 weeks prn

ADMINISTRATION
Oral route

Take in the am on an empty stomach at least 30 min before food
Take w/ water
Take at least 4 hrs apart from drugs that are known to interfere w/ its absorption
Pediatrics
May crush tab and mix w/ 5-10mL of water

STORAGE
20-25°C (68-77°F); excursions permitted to 15-30°C (59-86°F). Store away from heat, moisture, and light.

HOW SUPPLIED
Tab: 25mcg, 50mcg, 75mcg, 88mcg, 100mcg, 112mcg, 125mcg, 137mcg, 150mcg, 175mcg, 200mcg

CONTRAINDICATIONS
Untreated subclinical (suppressed serum TSH level w/ normal T3 and T4 levels) or overt thyrotoxicosis of any etiology, acute MI, uncorrected adrenal insufficiency, hypersensitivity to any of the inactive ingredients in the formulation.

WARNINGS/PRECAUTIONS
Should not be used in the treatment of male or female infertility unless associated with hypothyroidism. Contraindicated in patients with nontoxic diffuse goiter or nodular thyroid disease, particularly in elderly or with underlying cardiovascular (CV) disease if serum TSH level is already suppressed; use with caution if TSH level is not suppressed and carefully monitor thyroid function. Has narrow therapeutic index; carefully titrate dose to avoid over- or under-treatment. May decrease bone mineral density (BMD) with long term use; give minimum dose necessary to achieve desired clinical and biochemical response. Caution with CV disorders and the elderly. If cardiac symptoms develop or worsen, reduce or withhold dose for 1 week and then restart at lower dose. Overtreatment may produce CV effects (eg, increase in HR, increase in cardiac wall thickness, increase in cardiac contractility, precipitation of angina or arrhythmias). Monitor patients with coronary artery disease (CAD) closely during surgical procedures; may precipitate cardiac arrhythmias. Caution in patients with diabetes mellitus (DM). Patients with concomitant adrenal insufficiency should be treated with replacement glucocorticoids prior to therapy.

ADVERSE REACTIONS
Fatigue, increased appetite, weight loss, heat intolerance, headache, hyperactivity, irritability, insomnia, palpitations, arrhythmias, dyspnea, hair loss, menstrual irregularities. **Children:** pseudotumor cerebri, slipped capital femoral epiphysis.

DRUG INTERACTIONS
Concurrent sympathomimetics may increase effects of sympathomimetics or thyroid hormone; may increase risk of coronary insufficiency with CAD. Upward dose adjustments may be needed for insulin and oral hypoglycemic agents. May decrease absorption with soybean flour, cottonseed meal, walnuts, and dietary fiber. May increase oral anticoagulant activity; adjust dose of anticoagulant and monitor PT. May decrease levels and effects of digitalis glycosides. Transient reduction in TSH secretion with dopamine/dopamine agonists, glucocorticoids, octreotide. Decreased thyroid hormone secretion with aminoglutethimide, amiodarone, iodide (including iodine-containing radiographic contrast agents), lithium, methimazole, propylthiouracil (PTU), sulfonamides, and tolbutamide. May increase thyroid hormone secretion with amiodarone and iodide. May decrease T4 absorption with antacids (aluminum and magnesium hydroxides), simethicone, bile acid sequestrants (cholestyramine, colestipol), calcium carbonate, cation exchange resins (kayexalate), ferrous sulfate, orlistat, and sucralfate; administer at least 4 hrs apart. May increase serum thyroxine-binding globulin (TBG)

concentrations with clofibrate, estrogen-containing oral contraceptives, oral estrogens, heroin/methadone, 5-fluorouracil, mitotane, and tamoxifen. May decrease serum TBG concentrations with androgens/anabolic steroids, asparaginase, glucocorticoids, and slow-release nicotinic acid. May cause protein-binding site displacement with furosemide (>80mg IV), heparin, hydantoins, NSAIDs (fenamates, phenylbutazone), and salicylates (>2g/day). May alter T4 and T3 metabolism with carbamazepine, hydantoins, phenobarbital, and rifampin. May decrease T4 5'-deiodinase activity with amiodarone, β-adrenergic antagonists (eg, propranolol >160mg/day), glucocorticoids (eg, dexamethasone >4mg/day), and PTU. Concurrent use with tricyclic (eg, amitriptyline) and tetracyclic (eg, maprotiline) antidepressants may increase the therapeutic and toxic effects of both drugs. Coadministration with sertraline in patients stabilized on levothyroxine may result in increased levothyroxine requirements. Interferon-α may cause development of antithyroid microsomal antibodies and transient hypothyroidism, hyperthyroidism, or both. Interleukin-2 has been associated with transient painless thyroiditis. Excessive use with growth hormones (eg, somatropin, somatrem) may accelerate epiphyseal closure. Ketamine may produce marked HTN and tachycardia. May reduce uptake of radiographic agents. Decreased theophylline clearance may occur in hypothyroid patients. Altered levels of thyroid hormone and/or TSH levels with choral hydrate, diazepam, ethionamide, lovastatin, metoclopramide, 6-mercaptopurine, nitroprusside, para-aminosalicylate sodium, perphenazine, resorcinol (excessive topical use), and thiazide diuretics.

PREGNANCY AND LACTATION
Category A, caution in nursing.

MECHANISM OF ACTION
Thyroid replacement hormone; mechanism not established. Suspected that principal effects are exerted through control of DNA transcription and protein synthesis.

PHARMACOKINETICS
Absorption: Majority absorbed from jejunum and upper ileum. **Distribution:** Plasma protein binding (>99%); found in breast milk. **Metabolism:** Sequential deiodination and conjugation in liver (mainly), kidneys, and other tissues. **Elimination:** Urine, feces (approximately 20% unchanged); $T_{1/2}$=6-7 days (T4), ≤2 days (T3).

PATIENT CONSIDERATIONS
Assessment: Assess for untreated subclinical or overt thyrotoxicosis, acute MI, uncorrected adrenal insufficiency, CAD, CV disorders, nontoxic diffuse goiter, nodular thyroid disease, DM, hypersensitivity, pregnancy/nursing status, and possible drug interactions. In patients with secondary or tertiary hypothyroidism, assess for additional hypothalamic/pituitary hormone deficiencies. Assess TSH levels. In infants with congenital hypothyroidism, assess for other congenital anomalies.

Monitoring: Monitor for CV effects. In patients on long-term therapy, monitor for signs/symptoms of decreased BMD. In patients with nontoxic diffuse goiter or nodular thyroid disease, monitor for precipitation of thyrotoxicosis. In adults with primary hypothyroidism, perform periodic monitoring of serum TSH levels. In pediatric patients with congenital hypothyroidism, perform periodic monitoring of serum TSH levels and total or free T4 levels. In patients with secondary and tertiary hypothyroidism, perform periodic monitoring of serum free T4 levels. Refer to PI for TSH and T4 monitoring parameters. Closely monitor PT if coadministered with an oral anticoagulant.

Counseling: Instruct to notify physician if allergic to any foods or medicines, pregnant or plan to become pregnant, breastfeeding or taking any other drugs, including prescriptions and OTC preparations. Instruct to notify physician of any other medical conditions, particularly heart disease, diabetes, clotting disorders, and adrenal or pituitary gland problems. Instruct not to stop or change dose unless directed by physician. Instruct to take on empty stomach, at least 1/2 hr before eating any food. Advise that partial hair loss may occur during the 1st few months of therapy, but is usually temporary. Instruct to notify physician or dentist prior to surgery about levothyroxine therapy. Inform that drug should not be used for weight control. Inform patients that tabs may rapidly swell and disintegrate, resulting in choking, gagging, tab getting stuck in throat, or difficulty swallowing; advise to take with a full glass of water. Instruct to notify physician if rapid or irregular heartbeat, chest pain, SOB, leg cramps, headache, or any other unusual medical event occurs. Inform that dose may be increased during pregnancy. Inform that drug should not be administered within 4 hrs of agents such as iron/calcium supplements and antacids.

LEXAPRO — escitalopram oxalate   Rx
Class: Selective serotonin reuptake inhibitor (SSRI)

> Antidepressants increased the risk of suicidal thinking and behavior (suicidality) in children, adolescents, and young adults in short-term studies of major depressive disorder (MDD) and other psychiatric disorders. Monitor and observe closely for clinical worsening, suicidality, or unusual changes in behavior in patients who are started on antidepressant therapy. Advise families and caregivers of the need for close observation and communication with the prescriber. Not approved for use in pediatric patients <12 yrs of age.

ADULT DOSAGE
Major Depressive Disorder
Initial: 10mg qd
Titrate: May increase to 20mg after a minimum of 1 week
Generalized Anxiety Disorder
Initial: 10mg qd

PEDIATRIC DOSAGE
Major Depressive Disorder
≥12 Years:
Initial: 10mg qd
Titrate: May increase to 20mg after a minimum of 3 weeks

Titrate: May increase to 20mg after a minimum of 1 week

Dosing Considerations with MAOIs
Switching to/from an MAOI for Psychiatric Disorders:
Allow at least 14 days between discontinuation of an MAOI and initiation of treatment, and allow at least 14 days between discontinuation of treatment and initiation of an MAOI

W/ Other MAOIs (eg, Linezolid, IV Methylene Blue):
Do not start escitalopram in a patient being treated w/ linezolid or IV methylene blue
In patients already receiving escitalopram, if acceptable alternatives are not available and benefits outweigh risks, d/c escitalopram and administer linezolid or IV methylene blue; monitor for serotonin syndrome for 2 weeks or until 24 hrs after the last dose of linezolid or IV methylene blue, whichever comes 1st. May resume escitalopram therapy 24 hrs after the last dose of linezolid or IV methylene blue

Dosing Considerations with MAOIs
Switching to/from an MAOI for Psychiatric Disorders:
Allow at least 14 days between discontinuation of an MAOI and initiation of treatment, and allow at least 14 days between discontinuation of treatment and initiation of an MAOI

W/ Other MAOIs (eg, Linezolid, IV Methylene Blue):
Do not start escitalopram in a patient being treated w/ linezolid or IV methylene blue
In patients already receiving escitalopram, if acceptable alternatives are not available and benefits outweigh risks, d/c escitalopram and administer linezolid or IV methylene blue; monitor for serotonin syndrome for 2 weeks or until 24 hrs after the last dose of linezolid or IV methylene blue, whichever comes 1st. May resume escitalopram therapy 24 hrs after the last dose of linezolid or IV methylene blue

---

DOSING CONSIDERATIONS
Hepatic Impairment
10mg/day

Elderly
10mg/day

Discontinuation
Gradually reduce dose; if intolerable symptoms occur following a decrease in dose or upon discontinuation, consider resuming previously prescribed dose or continue decreasing dose at a more gradual rate

ADMINISTRATION
Oral route
Administer in the am or pm, w/ or w/o food.

STORAGE
25°C (77°F); excursions permitted to 15-30°C (59-86°F).

HOW SUPPLIED
Sol: 5mg/5mL [240mL]; **Tab:** 5mg, 10mg*, 20mg*. *scored

CONTRAINDICATIONS
Use of MAOIs intended to treat psychiatric disorders w/ escitalopram oxalate or w/in 14 days of stopping treatment w/ escitalopram oxalate. Use of escitalopram oxalate w/in 14 days of stopping an MAOI intended to treat psychiatric disorders. Starting escitalopram oxalate in a patient being treated w/ MAOIs (eg, linezolid or IV methylene blue). Concomitant use w/ pimozide. Hypersensitivity to escitalopram, citalopram, or any of the inactive ingredients in this product.

WARNINGS/PRECAUTIONS
Not approved for the treatment of bipolar depression. Serotonin syndrome reported; d/c immediately and initiate supportive symptomatic treatment. Avoid abrupt discontinuation; gradual dose reduction is recommended whenever possible. Convulsions reported; caution with history of seizure disorder. Activation of mania/hypomania reported; caution with history of mania. Hyponatremia may occur; caution in elderly and volume-depleted patients. Consider discontinuation in patients with symptomatic hyponatremia and institute appropriate medical intervention. May increase the risk of bleeding events. May impair mental/physical abilities. Pupillary dilation that occurs following use may trigger an angle-closure attack in a patient with anatomically narrow angles who does not have a patent iridectomy. May precipitate mixed/manic episode in patients at risk for bipolar disorder; screen for risk for bipolar disorder prior to initiating treatment. Caution with diseases/conditions that produce altered metabolism or hemodynamic responses, and with severe renal impairment.

ADVERSE REACTIONS
N/V, insomnia, ejaculation disorder, increased sweating, somnolence, fatigue, diarrhea, dry mouth, headache, constipation, decreased appetite, neck/shoulder pain, decreased libido, anorgasmia.

DRUG INTERACTIONS
See Contraindications. Not recommended for use with alcohol. May cause serotonin syndrome with other serotonergic drugs (eg, triptans, TCAs, fentanyl) and with drugs that impair metabolism of serotonin; d/c immediately if this occurs. Caution with other centrally acting drugs, and drugs metabolized by CYP2D6 (eg, desipramine). Increased risk of bleeding with aspirin, NSAIDs, warfarin, and other drugs that affect coagulation. May increase levels with cimetidine. Rare reports of weakness, hyperreflexia, and incoordination with sumatriptan. Possible increased clearance with carbamazepine. May decrease levels of ketoconazole. May increase levels of metoprolol. Increased risk of hyponatremia with diuretics. Monitor lithium levels and adjust its dose appropriately.

PREGNANCY AND LACTATION
Category C, caution in nursing.

MECHANISM OF ACTION

SSRI; presumed to be linked to potentiation of serotonergic activity in the CNS resulting from its inhibition of CNS neuronal reuptake of serotonin.

PHARMACOKINETICS

Absorption: (20mg single dose) T_{max}=5 hrs. **Distribution:** Plasma protein binding (56%); found in breast milk. **Metabolism:** Liver; N-demethylation via CYP3A4, CYP2C19. **Elimination:** Urine (8% unchanged); $T_{1/2}$=27-32 hrs.

PATIENT CONSIDERATIONS

Assessment: Assess for drug hypersensitivity, risk for bipolar disorder, history of seizure disorder, history of mania, volume depletion, diseases/conditions that produce altered metabolism or hemodynamic response, susceptibility to angle-closure glaucoma, hepatic/renal impairment, pregnancy/nursing status, and possible drug interactions. Obtain detailed psychiatric history.

Monitoring: Monitor for signs/symptoms of clinical worsening, serotonin syndrome, bleeding events, hyponatremia, seizures, cognitive and motor impairment, activation of mania/hypomania, angle-closure glaucoma, and other adverse reactions. If therapy is abruptly discontinued, monitor for discontinuation symptoms. Regularly monitor weight and growth in pediatrics. Periodically reassess the need for maintenance treatment.

Counseling: Inform about the benefits and risks of therapy. Counsel on the appropriate use of the drug. Advise to look for emergence of symptoms associated with an increased risk for suicidal thinking and behavior; instruct to report such symptoms, especially if severe, abrupt in onset, or not part of presenting symptoms. Caution about risk of serotonin syndrome with other serotonergic agents (eg, triptans, buspirone, St. John's wort) and about risk of bleeding with ASA, warfarin, or other drugs that affect coagulation. Caution about risk of angle-closure glaucoma. Instruct to notify physician if taking or planning to take any prescription or OTC drugs. Inform that improvement may be noticed in 1-4 weeks; instruct to continue therapy ud. Caution about operating hazardous machinery, including automobiles. Instruct to avoid alcohol. Instruct to notify physician if pregnant, intending to become pregnant, or if breastfeeding. Inform of the need for comprehensive treatment program.

LIALDA — mesalamine

Class: 5-aminosalicylic acid derivative

Rx

ADULT DOSAGE	**PEDIATRIC DOSAGE**
Ulcerative Colitis	Pediatric use may not have been established
Induction of Remission:	
Active, Mild to Moderate: 2-4 tabs qd	
Maint of Remission:	
2 tabs qd	

DOSING CONSIDERATIONS

Elderly
Start at lower end of dosing range.

ADMINISTRATION

Oral route

Take w/ a meal.
Swallow tab whole.

STORAGE

15-25°C (59-77°F); excursions permitted to 30°C (86°F).

HOW SUPPLIED

Tab, Delayed-Release: 1.2g

CONTRAINDICATIONS

Known hypersensitivity to salicylates or aminosalicylates or to any of the ingredients in this product.

WARNINGS/PRECAUTIONS

Renal impairment, including minimal change nephropathy, acute/chronic interstitial nephritis, and, rarely, renal failure reported; evaluate renal function prior to therapy and periodically thereafter. Caution with known renal impairment or history of renal disease. Has been associated with an acute intolerance syndrome that may be difficult to distinguish from an exacerbation of ulcerative colitis (UC); observe closely for worsening of symptoms and d/c therapy if acute intolerance syndrome is suspected. Patients with sulfasalazine hypersensitivity may have similar reaction to therapy. Mesalamine-induced cardiac hypersensitivity reactions (eg, myocarditis, pericarditis) reported; caution with conditions that predispose to the development of myocarditis or pericarditis. Hepatic failure reported in patients with preexisting liver disease; caution with liver disease. Pyloric stenosis or other organic/functional obstruction in the upper GI tract may cause prolonged gastric retention of therapy, which could delay drug release in the colon. Caution with sulfasalazine hypersensitivity and in elderly. May interfere with lab tests.

ADVERSE REACTIONS

Headache, flatulence, UC, abnormal LFTs, abdominal pain.

DRUG INTERACTIONS

Nephrotoxic agents, including NSAIDs, may increase risk of renal reactions. Azathioprine or 6-mercaptopurine may increase risk for blood disorders.

PREGNANCY AND LACTATION

Category B, caution in nursing.

MECHANISM OF ACTION

5-aminosalicylic acid (5-ASA) derivative; has not been established. Suspected to diminish inflammation by blocking cyclooxygenase and inhibiting prostaglandin production in the colon.

PHARMACOKINETICS

Absorption: Administration of variable doses and different populations resulted in different parameters. **Distribution:** Plasma protein binding (43%); found in breast milk; crosses placenta. **Metabolism:** Liver and intestinal mucosa (acetylation); N-acetyl-5-ASA (major metabolite). **Elimination:** Urine (<8% unchanged, >13% N-acetyl-5-ASA); $T_{1/2}$=7-9 hrs (2.4g), 8-12 hrs (4.8g).

PATIENT CONSIDERATIONS

Assessment: Assess for hypersensitivity to the drug, salicylates/aminosalicylates, or sulfasalazine, conditions that predispose to the development of myocarditis or pericarditis, pyloric stenosis or other organic/functional upper GI tract obstruction, hepatic impairment, pregnancy/nursing status, and possible drug interactions. Evaluate renal function prior to initiation of therapy.

Monitoring: Monitor for acute intolerance syndrome, hypersensitivity reactions, hepatic failure, and other adverse reactions. Perform periodic monitoring of renal function. Monitor blood cell counts in elderly.

Counseling: Instruct not to take drug if hypersensitive to salicylates (eg, aspirin) or other mesalamines. Inform to notify physician of all medications being taken and if pregnant, planning to become pregnant, or breastfeeding. Instruct to inform physician if allergic to sulfasalazine, if taking NSAIDs or other nephrotoxic agents, azathioprine, or 6-mercaptopurine, and if experiencing cramping, abdominal pain, bloody diarrhea, fever, headache, or rash. Inform to notify physician of history of myocarditis/pericarditis or stomach blockage, and if patient has kidney/liver disease.

LIBRAX — chlordiazepoxide hydrochloride/clidinium bromide

Class: Anticholinergic/benzodiazepine

Rx

ADULT DOSAGE	**PEDIATRIC DOSAGE**
Acute Enterocolitis	Pediatric use may not have been established
Adjunctive Therapy:	
Maint: 1-2 caps tid-qid ac and hs	
Peptic Ulcer	
Adjunctive Therapy:	
Maint: 1-2 caps tid-qid ac and hs	
Irritable Bowel Syndrome	
Adjunctive Therapy:	
Maint: 1-2 caps tid-qid ac and hs	

DOSING CONSIDERATIONS

Elderly/Debilitated
Initial: Not more than 2 caps/day
Titrate: Increase gradually prn and as tolerated

ADMINISTRATION

Oral route

STORAGE

25°C (77°F); excursions permitted to 15-30°C (59-86°F).

HOW SUPPLIED

Cap: (Chlordiazepoxide/Clidinium) 5mg/2.5mg

CONTRAINDICATIONS

Glaucoma, prostatic hypertrophy, benign bladder neck obstruction, known hypersensitivity to chlordiazepoxide HCl and/or clidinium bromide.

WARNINGS/PRECAUTIONS

Use lowest effective dose in debilitated patients. May impair mental/physical abilities. Caution with renal/hepatic impairment and in elderly. Chlordiazepoxide: Increased risk of congenital malformations during 1st trimester of pregnancy; avoid use. Paradoxical reactions (eg, excitement, stimulation, acute rage) reported in psychiatric patients. Caution in the treatment of anxiety states with evidence of impending depression; suicidal tendencies may be present. Avoid abrupt withdrawal after extended therapy; withdrawal symptoms reported following discontinuation. Clidinium: Inhibition of lactation may occur.

ADVERSE REACTIONS

Drowsiness, ataxia, confusion, skin eruptions, edema, extrapyramidal symptoms, dry mouth, nausea, constipation, altered libido, blood dyscrasias, jaundice, hepatic dysfunction, blurred vision, urinary hesitancy.

DRUG INTERACTIONS

Additive effects with alcohol and other CNS depressants. Coadministration with other psychotropic agents is not recommended; caution with MAOIs and phenothiazines. Constipation has occurred more often when coadministered with other spasmolytic agents. Chlordiazepoxide: Altered coagulation effects reported with oral anticoagulants.

PREGNANCY AND LACTATION

Not for use in pregnancy; safety not known in nursing.

MECHANISM OF ACTION

Chlordiazepoxide: Benzodiazepine; antianxiety agent. Clidinium: Anticholinergic; shown to have a pronounced antispasmodic and antisecretory effect on the GI tract.

PATIENT CONSIDERATIONS

Assessment: Assess for glaucoma, prostatic hypertrophy, benign bladder neck obstruction, anxiety, renal/hepatic dysfunction, alcohol intake, history of drug abuse, drug hypersensitivity, pregnancy/nursing status, and possible drug interactions.

Monitoring: Monitor for ataxia, oversedation, drowsiness, confusion, and other adverse reactions. Monitor for paradoxical reactions (eg, excitement, stimulation, acute rage) in psychiatric patients. Periodic blood counts and LFTs are advisable when treatment is protracted. Monitor for signs of impending depression, or any suicidal tendencies.

Counseling: Inform that psychological and physical dependence may develop, and advise to consult physician before increasing dose or discontinuing abruptly. Advise to observe caution when performing hazardous tasks (eg, operating machinery/driving). Advise to notify physician if pregnant/breastfeeding or planning to become pregnant. Inform of potential additive effects with alcohol and other CNS depressants.

LIBRIUM — chlordiazepoxide hydrochloride   CIV

Class: Benzodiazepine

ADULT DOSAGE
Anxiety Disorders

Management of anxiety disorders or for short-term relief of anxiety symptoms

Relief of Mild and Moderate Anxiety Disorders and Symptoms of Anxiety:
Usual: 5-10mg tid-qid

Relief of Severe Anxiety Disorders and Symptoms of Anxiety:
Usual: 20-25mg tid-qid

Preoperative Medication

Preoperative Apprehension and Anxiety:
5-10mg tid-qid on days preceding surgery
If used as preoperative medication, 50-100mg IM 1 hr prior to surgery

Alcohol Withdrawal

Relief of Withdrawal Symptoms of Acute Alcoholism:
Initial: 50-100mg, followed by repeated doses prn until agitation is controlled
Max: 300mg/day

PEDIATRIC DOSAGE
Anxiety Disorders

Management of anxiety disorders or for short-term relief of anxiety symptoms

≥6 Years:
Usual: 5mg bid-qid; may increase to 10mg bid-tid in some patients

DOSING CONSIDERATIONS
Elderly
Elderly/Debilitated:
Usual: 5mg bid-qid

ADMINISTRATION
Oral route

STORAGE
25°C (77°F); excursions permitted to 15-30°C (59-86°F).

HOW SUPPLIED
Cap: 5mg, 10mg, 25mg

CONTRAINDICATIONS
Known hypersensitivity to the drug.

WARNINGS/PRECAUTIONS
May impair mental/physical abilities, including mental alertness in children. Risk of congenital malformations during 1st trimester of pregnancy; avoid use. Paradoxical reactions (eg, excitement, stimulation, and acute rage) reported in psychiatric patients, and in hyperactive aggressive pediatric patients. Caution in treatment of anxiety states with evidence of impending depression; suicidal tendencies may be present. Caution with porphyria, renal or hepatic dysfunction. Use lowest effective dose in elderly and debilitated patients. Avoid abrupt withdrawal after extended therapy; withdrawal symptoms reported following discontinuation.

ADVERSE REACTIONS
Drowsiness, ataxia, confusion, skin eruptions, edema, nausea, constipation, extrapyramidal symptoms, libido changes, EEG changes.

DRUG INTERACTIONS
Additive effects with CNS depressants and alcohol. Coadministration with other psychotropic agents not recommended; caution with MAOIs and phenothiazines. Altered coagulation effects reported with oral anticoagulants.

PREGNANCY AND LACTATION
Not for use in pregnancy, safety not known in nursing.

MECHANISM OF ACTION
Benzodiazepine; not established. Has antianxiety, sedative, appetite stimulating, and weak analgesic actions; blocks EEG arousal from stimulation of brain stem reticular formation.

PHARMACOKINETICS
Elimination: Urine (1-2% unchanged, 3-6% conjugates); $T_{1/2}$=24-48 hrs.

PATIENT CONSIDERATIONS
Assessment: Assess for pregnancy status, hepatic/renal function, and possible drug interactions.

Monitoring: Monitor elderly/debilitated patients for ataxia and oversedation, drowsiness, confusion. Monitor for paradoxical reactions in psychiatric patients and in hyperactive aggressive pediatric patients. Periodic blood counts and LFTs are advisable when treatment is protracted. Monitor for signs of impending depression or any suicidal tendencies.

Counseling: Inform that psychological/physical dependence may occur; advise to consult physician prior to increasing dose or abruptly discontinuing therapy. Advise to notify physician if patient becomes pregnant or plans to become pregnant. May impair mental/physical abilities; caution while operating machinery/driving. May impair mental alertness in children. Avoid alcohol and other CNS depressant drugs.

LIDODERM PATCH — lidocaine   Rx

Class: Acetamide local anesthetic

ADULT DOSAGE
Postherpetic Neuralgia

Relief of Pain:
Apply to intact skin to cover the most painful area
Apply up to 3 patches, only once for up to 12 hrs w/in 24-hr period

PEDIATRIC DOSAGE
Pediatric use may not have been established

DOSING CONSIDERATIONS
Concomitant Medications
Consider total amount absorbed from all formulations when used concomitantly w/ other local anesthetics

Adverse Reactions
Remove patch if irritation or burning occurs; may reapply when irritation subsides

Other Important Considerations
Debilitated/Impaired Elimination:
Treat smaller areas

ADMINISTRATION
Transdermal route

May cut patches into smaller sizes before removal of the release liner.
Avoid contact with water (eg, bathing, swimming, or showering).
Wash hands after handling and avoid eye contact.
Apply immediately after removal from protective envelope.
May wear clothing over the area of application.
Fold used patches and discard patches or pieces of patches.

STORAGE
Store at 25°C (77°F); excursions permitted to 15-30°C (59-86°F).

HOW SUPPLIED
Patch: 5% [30^s]

CONTRAINDICATIONS
Known history of sensitivity to local anesthetics of the amide type, or to any other component of the product.

WARNINGS/PRECAUTIONS
Serious adverse events may occur in children or pets if ingested; keep out of reach. Excessive dosing by applying to larger areas or for longer than the recommended wearing time may result in serious adverse effects. Increased risk of toxicity in patients with severe hepatic disease. Caution with history of drug sensitivities, smaller patients, and patients with impaired elimination. Avoid broken or inflamed skin, placement of external heat (eg, heating pads, electric blankets) and eye contact.

ADVERSE REACTIONS
Application-site reactions (eg, erythema, edema, bruising, papules, vesicles, discoloration, depigmentation, burning sensation, pruritus, dermatitis, petechia, blisters, exfoliation, abnormal sensation).

DRUG INTERACTIONS
Additive toxic effects with concomitant Class I antiarrhythmics (eg, tocainide, mexiletine); use caution. Consider total amount absorbed from all formulations containing other local anesthetics.

PREGNANCY AND LACTATION
Category B, caution in nursing.

MECHANISM OF ACTION
Local anesthetic; stabilizes neuronal membranes by inhibiting ionic fluxes required for initiation and conduction of impulses.

PHARMACOKINETICS
Absorption: C_{max}=0.13mcg/mL; T_{max}=11 hrs. **Distribution:** V_d=0.7-2.7L/kg (IV); plasma protein binding (70%). Crosses placenta; found in breast milk. **Metabolism:** Liver (rapid); monoethylglycinexylidide, glycinexylidide (active metabolites). **Elimination:** Urine (<10%, unchanged); $T_{1/2}$=81-149 min (IV).

PATIENT CONSIDERATIONS
Assessment: Assess for history of drug sensitivities to local anesthetics of the amide type and para-aminobenzoic acid derivatives, hepatic disease, pregnancy/nursing status, and for possible drug interactions.

Monitoring: Monitor for local skin reactions, allergic/anaphylactoid reactions, liver function, pain intensity, pain relief (periodically), and other adverse reactions.

Counseling: Instruct to remove patch if irritation or burning sensation occurs during application and not to reapply until irritation subsides. If eye contact occurs, instruct to immediately wash with water or saline and protect eye until sensation returns. Counsel to avoid application to larger areas and for longer than recommended wearing time. Advise to avoid applying to broken or inflamed skin. Instruct to wash hands after handling patch and to fold used patches so adhesive side sticks to itself. Instruct to keep out of reach of children and pets.

LILETTA — levonorgestrel

Class: Progestin contraceptive

Rx

ADULT DOSAGE

Contraception

Not Currently Using Hormonal/ Intrauterine Contraception:
Insert any time during the first 7 days of menstrual cycle.
If not inserted during the first 7 days, use a barrier method of contraception (eg, condoms and spermicide) or abstain from vaginal intercourse for 7 days

Conversions

Switching from an Oral, Transdermal, or Vaginal Hormonal Contraceptive:
May be inserted at any time.
May be inserted during the hormone-free interval of the previous method.
If inserted during active use of previous method, continue previous method after insertion for 7 days or until end of current cycle.
If using continuous hormonal contraception, d/c the method 7 days after insertion

Switching from an Injectable Progestin Contraceptive:
May be inserted at any time; a barrier method of contraception (eg, condoms and spermicide) should also be used for 7 days if inserted as instructed >3 months (13 weeks) after last inj

Switching from a Contraceptive Implant or Another Intrauterine System (IUS):
Insert on same day the implant or IUS is removed.
May insert at any time during menstrual cycle

Switching to a Different Birth Control Method:
Regular Cycle:
Remove device during first 7 days of menstrual cycle and start new method, or start new method at least 7 days prior to removing device if removal is to occur at other times during the cycle
Irregular Cycle/Amenorrhea:
Start new method at least 7 days before removal

PEDIATRIC DOSAGE

Contraception

Not indicated for use premenarche; refer to adult dosing

DOSING CONSIDERATIONS
Other Important Considerations
1st Trimester Abortion or Miscarriage: May be inserted immediately
After Childbirth/2nd Trimester Abortion or Miscarriage: Do not insert until a minimum of 6 weeks or until the uterus is fully involuted. May then be inserted any time healthcare provider can be reasonably certain woman is not pregnant. Use a barrier method of contraception or abstain from vaginal intercourse for 7 days if not inserted during first 7 days of the menstrual cycle

ADMINISTRATION
Intrauterine route

May remove device at any time but must be removed by end of 3rd yr; may be replaced at time of removal w/ a new device if continued contraceptive protection is desired.
If removed but no other contraceptive method has already been started, new contraceptive method can be started on day device is removed; patient should use a backup barrier method of contraception or abstain from vaginal intercourse for 7 days to prevent pregnancy.
Refer to PI for insertion and additional removal instructions.

STORAGE
20-25°C (68-77°F); excursions permitted to 15-30°C (59-86°F). Do not resterilize. Protect from light.

HOW SUPPLIED
Intrauterine Insert: 52mg

CONTRAINDICATIONS
Pregnancy or suspected pregnancy, for use as post-coital contraception (emergency contraception), congenital or acquired uterine anomaly (including fibroids that distort the uterine cavity), acute or history of pelvic inflammatory disease (PID) (unless there has been a subsequent intrauterine pregnancy), postpartum endometritis or infected abortion in the past 3 months, known/suspected uterine or cervical neoplasia, known/suspected or history of breast cancer or other progestin-sensitive cancer, uterine bleeding of unknown etiology, untreated acute cervicitis or vaginitis (including bacterial vaginosis, known chlamydial or gonococcal cervical infection, or other lower genital tract infections, until infection is controlled), acute liver disease or liver tumor (benign or malignant), conditions associated w/ increased susceptibility to pelvic infections, previously inserted intrauterine system (IUS) that has not been removed, hypersensitivity to any component of this product.

WARNINGS/PRECAUTIONS
Should only be inserted by a trained healthcare provider. Evaluate for ectopic pregnancy if patient becomes pregnant w/ device in place; remove device if ectopic pregnancy is confirmed. If pregnancy occurs while using device, determine if device is in the uterus; attempt to remove device if it is in the uterus. Increased risk of septic abortion, miscarriage, sepsis, and premature delivery/labor if pregnancy occurs and device is left in place. Severe infection or sepsis, including Group A streptococcal sepsis may occur; aseptic technique is essential during insertion of device. Associated w/ increased risk of PID or endometritis and actinomycosis. Perforation may occur and may reduce contraceptive effectiveness; risk increased if device is inserted in lactating women and may be increased if device is inserted when the uterus is fixed retroverted or not completely involuted during the postpartum period. Partial or complete expulsion may occur, resulting in the loss of contraceptive protection. If expulsion has occurred, a new device may be inserted w/in 7 days after the onset of a menstrual period after pregnancy has been ruled out. Ovarian cysts reported. May alter bleeding pattern and result in spotting, irregular bleeding, heavy bleeding, oligomenorrhea, and amenorrhea; perform appropriate diagnostic measures to rule out endometrial pathology if significant change in bleeding develops during prolonged use. Consider possibility of pregnancy if menstruation does not occur w/in 6 weeks of the onset of a previous menstruation. Breast cancer reported w/ another levonorgestrel-releasing IUS. Caution in patients w/ coagulopathy or receiving anticoagulants, migraine, focal migraine w/ asymmetrical visual loss or other symptoms indicating transient cerebral ischemia, exceptionally severe headache, marked increase of BP, and in patients w/ severe arterial disease. Consider removing device if uterine/cervical malignancy or jaundice arises during use. If the threads are not visible or are significantly shortened, they may have broken or retracted into the cervical canal or uterus; consider possibility that the IUS may have been displaced; exclude pregnancy and verify location of device. Remove device if it is displaced. Device is magnetic resonance (MR) safe.

ADVERSE REACTIONS
Vaginal infections, vulvovaginal infections, acne, headache/migraine, N/V, dyspareunia, abdominal discomfort/pain, breast tenderness/pain, pelvic discomfort/pain, depression/depressed mood, mood changes.

PREGNANCY AND LACTATION
Contraindicated in pregnancy, caution in nursing.

MECHANISM OF ACTION
Progestin contraceptive; has not been established. Thickens cervical mucus, which inhibits sperm passage through the cervix, inhibits sperm mobility and function (capacitation), and alters endometrium.

PHARMACOKINETICS
Distribution: Plasma protein binding (98.9%); V_d=approx 1.8L/kg; found in breast milk. **Metabolism:** Conjugation; sulfate and glucuronide (lesser extent) conjugates (metabolites). **Elimination:** Urine (45%), feces (32%, glucuronide conjugates); $T_{1/2}$=approx 13.9 hrs (oral).

PATIENT CONSIDERATIONS

Assessment: Assess for drug hypersensitivity, congenital or acquired uterine anomaly, acute or history of PID, known/suspected or history of breast cancer or other progestin-sensitive cancer, acute liver disease or liver tumor, pregnancy/nursing status, and any other conditions where treatment is contraindicated or cautioned. Perform a complete medical and social history and if indicated, a physical examination and appropriate tests for genital or sexually transmitted infections (STIs).

Monitoring: Monitor for intrauterine/ectopic pregnancy, sepsis, PID or endometritis, actinomycosis, bleeding pattern alterations, perforation, migraine/exceptionally severe headache, jaundice, marked BP increase, and other adverse reactions. Reexamine and evaluate 4-6 weeks after insertion and once a yr thereafter, or more frequently if clinically indicated. Monitor if thread is still visible and length of thread. Evaluate persistent ovarian cysts. Perform a pelvic examination promptly to evaluate for possible pelvic infection if patient develops lower abdominal or pelvic pain, odorous discharge, unexplained bleeding, fever, or genital lesions or sores.

Counseling: Inform that product does not protect against HIV infection (AIDS) and other STIs. Inform of the risk of ectopic pregnancy, including loss of fertility; instruct to promptly report any symptoms of ectopic pregnancy to physician. Explain that if pregnancy occurs while using device, the device will likely need to be removed because leaving it in place may increase risk of spontaneous abortion and preterm labor but that removal of device or probing of the uterus may also result in spontaneous abortion. Explain that if pregnancy occurs while using device, septic abortion may occur; warn that if device cannot be removed or patient chooses not to have it removed, there may be an increased risk of miscarriage, sepsis, premature labor/delivery. Inform that severe infection or sepsis may occur w/in 1st few days after device is inserted; instruct to immediately contact physician if severe pain or fever develops shortly after device is inserted. Inform of the possibility of PID or endometritis; instruct to promptly notify physician if any symptoms of PID develop. Inform that perforation may occur; explain that if perforation occurs, device will have to be located and removed, surgery may be required, and that delayed detection or removal in case of perforation may result in migration of the IUS outside the uterine cavity, adhesions, peritonitis, intestinal perforations/obstruction, abscesses, and erosion of adjacent viscera. Explain how to check if the device's threads still protrude from the cervix and instruct not to pull on the threads. Inform that there is no contraceptive protection if device is displaced or expelled. Discuss the risk of ovarian cysts and that cysts may cause clinical symptoms and infrequently will need surgery. Advise that irregular/prolonged bleeding and spotting, and/or cramps may occur during the first 3-6 months after insertion; instruct to report to physician if symptoms continue or are severe. Inform that it is safe for patient to have MR imaging w/ device in place. Instruct to contact physician if any adverse reactions develop, if pregnancy is suspected or occurs, if patient or patient's partner becomes HIV positive, or if possible exposure to STIs occurs.

LINZESS — linaclotide   Rx

Class: Guanylate cyclase-C (GC-C) agonist

> Contraindicated in pediatric patients up to 6 yrs of age. Avoid use in pediatric patients 6-17 yrs of age; safety and efficacy has not been established in pediatric patients <18 yrs of age.

ADULT DOSAGE

Irritable Bowel Syndrome with Constipation
290mcg qd

Chronic Idiopathic Constipation
145mcg qd

PEDIATRIC DOSAGE

Pediatric use may not have been established

ADMINISTRATION
Oral route

Take PO on an empty stomach, at least 30 min prior to 1st meal of the day.
Swallow cap whole; do not crush or chew cap or contents.
For patients w/ swallowing difficulties, administer w/ applesauce or water.

Administration in Applesauce:
1. Place one tsp of applesauce at room temperature into a clean container.
2. Open cap and sprinkle entire contents in applesauce.
3. Consume entire contents immediately; do not chew beads.
4. Do not store the applesauce and beads for later use.

Administration in Water:
1. Pour approx 30mL of bottled water at room temperature into a clean cup.
2. Open cap and sprinkle entire contents into water.
3. Gently swirl beads and water for at least 10 sec.
4. Swallow entire mixture of beads and water immediately.
5. Add another 30mL of water to any beads remaining in cup, swirl for 10 sec, and swallow immediately; it is not necessary to consume all beads to deliver complete dose.
6. Do not store the bead-water mixture for future use.

NG or Gastric Feeding Tube:
1. Open the cap and empty the beads into a clean container w/ 30mL of room temperature bottled water.
2. Mix by gently swirling beads for at least 10 sec.
3. Draw-up the beads and water mixture to an appropriately sized catheter-tipped syringe and apply rapid and steady pressure (10mL/10 sec) to dispense the syringe contents into the tube.
4. After administering the bead-water mixture, flush NG/gastric tube w/ a min of 10mL of water; it is not necessary to flush all the beads through to deliver the complete dose.

STORAGE
25°C (77°F); excursions permitted between 15-30°C (59-86°F). Keep caps in the original container. Do not subdivide or repackage. Protect from moisture. Do not remove desiccant from the container.

HOW SUPPLIED
Cap: 145mcg, 290mcg

CONTRAINDICATIONS
Pediatric patients <6 yrs of age, known or suspected mechanical GI obstruction.

WARNINGS/PRECAUTIONS
Diarrhea commonly reported; consider dose suspension and rehydration if severe diarrhea occurs.

ADVERSE REACTIONS
Diarrhea, abdominal pain, flatulence, abdominal distension, viral gastroenteritis, headache, URTI, sinusitis.

PREGNANCY AND LACTATION
Pregnancy: Category C.
Lactation: It is not known whether linaclotide is excreted in human milk; however, linaclotide and its active metabolite are not measurable in plasma following administration of the recommended clinical doses. Caution in nursing.

MECHANISM OF ACTION
GC-C agonist; acts locally on the luminal surface of the intestinal epithelium by binding to and activating GC-C, resulting in an increase in both intracellular and extracellular cGMP levels. Elevation in intracellular cGMP stimulates secretion of

---

Cl⁻ and bicarbonate into the intestinal lumen, resulting in increased intestinal fluid and accelerated transit.

PHARMACOKINETICS
Absorption: Minimal. **Metabolism:** GI tract. **Elimination:** Feces (5% [fasted], 3% [fed]).

PATIENT CONSIDERATIONS
Assessment: Assess for known or suspected mechanical GI obstruction and pregnancy/nursing status.

Monitoring: Monitor for diarrhea and other adverse reactions.

Counseling: Advise to seek medical attention if experiencing unusual or severe abdominal pain and/or severe diarrhea, especially if in combination w/ hematochezia or melena; instruct to d/c treatment and contact physician if severe diarrhea occurs. Instruct to skip dose if the dose is missed, and take next dose at the regular time; advise not to take 2 doses at the same time.

LIPITOR — atorvastatin calcium   Rx

Class: HMG-CoA reductase inhibitor (statin)

ADULT DOSAGE

Hyperlipidemia/Mixed Dyslipidemia

Initial: 10mg or 20mg qd (or 40mg qd for LDL reduction >45%)
Range: 10-80mg qd

After initiation and/or upon titration, analyze lipid levels w/in 2-4 weeks and adjust dose accordingly

Homozygous Familial Hypercholesterolemia
10-80mg qd

Prevention of Cardiovascular Disease
Dose based on current clinical practice

PEDIATRIC DOSAGE

Heterozygous Familial Hypercholesterolemia

10-17 Years (Boys and Postmenarchal Girls):
Initial: 10mg/day
Titrate: Adjust dose at intervals of ≥4 weeks
Max: 20mg/day

DOSING CONSIDERATIONS
Concomitant Medications
Cyclosporine/Tipranavir plus Ritonavir/Telaprevir:
Avoid use

Lopinavir plus Ritonavir:
Use lowest dose necessary

Clarithromycin/Itraconazole/Fosamprenavir/Ritonavir plus Saquinavir, Darunavir, or Fosamprenavir:
Limit to 20mg/day; use lowest dose necessary

Nelfinavir or Boceprevir:
Limit to 40mg/day; use lowest dose necessary

ADMINISTRATION
Oral route
Take as a single dose at any time of the day, w/ or w/o food.

STORAGE
20-25°C (68-77°F).

HOW SUPPLIED
Tab: 10mg, 20mg, 40mg, 80mg

CONTRAINDICATIONS
Active liver disease, which may include unexplained persistent elevations in hepatic transaminase levels; hypersensitivity to any component of this medication; women who are pregnant or may become pregnant; nursing mothers.

WARNINGS/PRECAUTIONS
Has not been studied in conditions where the major lipoprotein abnormality is elevation of chylomicrons (Fredrickson Types I and V). Rare cases of rhabdomyolysis w/ acute renal failure secondary to myoglobinuria reported. Increased risk of rhabdomyolysis w/ history of renal impairment; closely monitor for skeletal muscle effects. May cause myopathy (including immune-mediated necrotizing myopathy [IMNM]); d/c if markedly elevated CPK levels occur or if myopathy is diagnosed or suspected. Temporarily withhold or d/c in any patient w/ an acute, serious condition suggestive of myopathy or having a risk factor predisposing to development of renal failure secondary to rhabdomyolysis. Persistent increases in serum transaminases reported. Fatal and nonfatal hepatic failure reported (rare); promptly interrupt therapy if serious liver injury w/ clinical symptoms and/or hyperbilirubinemia or jaundice occurs and do not restart if no alternate etiology found. Caution in patients who consume substantial quantities of alcohol and/or have history of liver disease. Increases in HbA1c and FPG levels reported. May blunt adrenal and/or gonadal steroid production. Increased risk of hemorrhagic stroke in patients w/ recent stroke or transient ischemic attack (TIA). Caution in elderly.

ADVERSE REACTIONS
Nasopharyngitis, arthralgia, diarrhea, pain in extremity, UTI, dyspepsia, nausea, musculoskeletal pain, muscle spasms, myalgia, insomnia.

DRUG INTERACTIONS
See Dosing Considerations. Avoid w/ gemfibrozil. Caution w/ fibrates and drugs that decrease levels or activity of endogenous steroid hormones (eg, ketoconazole, spironolactone, cimetidine). Increased risk of myopathy w/ fibric acid derivatives, erythromycin, lipid-modifying doses of niacin, strong

CYP3A4 inhibitors (eg, clarithromycin, HIV protease inhibitors), and azole antifungals; consider lower initial and maintenance doses. Strong CYP3A4 inhibitors and grapefruit juice may increase levels. CYP3A4 inducers (eg, efavirenz, rifampin) may decrease levels. Delayed atorvastatin administration after rifampin administration associated w/ a significant reduction in atorvastatin levels; simultaneous coadministration w/ rifampin is recommended. May increase digoxin levels; monitor appropriately. May increase exposure for norethindrone and ethinyl estradiol; consider such increases when selecting an oral contraceptive for a woman taking atorvastatin. Myopathy, including rhabdomyolysis, reported w/ colchicine; use w/ caution. OATP1B1 inhibitors (eg, cyclosporine) may increase bioavailability.

PREGNANCY AND LACTATION
Category X, not for use in nursing.

MECHANISM OF ACTION
HMG-CoA reductase inhibitor; inhibits conversion of HMG-CoA to mevalonate (precursor of sterols, including cholesterol).

PHARMACOKINETICS
Absorption: Rapid; absolute bioavailability (14%); T_{max}=1-2 hrs. **Distribution:** V_d=381L; plasma protein binding (≥98%). **Metabolism:** Extensive via CYP3A4; ortho- and parahydroxylated derivatives (active metabolites). **Elimination:** Bile (major), urine (<2%); $T_{1/2}$=14 hrs (atorvastatin), 20-30 hrs (active metabolites).

PATIENT CONSIDERATIONS
Assessment: Assess for active or history of liver disease, unexplained and persistent elevations in serum transaminase levels, pregnancy/nursing status, history of renal impairment, risk factors predisposing to the development of renal failure secondary to rhabdomyolysis, alcohol intake, recent stroke or TIA, hypersensitivity to the drug, and possible drug interactions. Obtain baseline LFTs.

Monitoring: Monitor for signs/symptoms of rhabdomyolysis and myopathy (including IMNM). Monitor lipid profile and CPK levels. Perform LFTs as clinically indicated.

Counseling: Advise to adhere to the National Cholesterol Education Program-recommended diet, a regular exercise program, and periodic testing of a fasting lipid panel. Inform of the substances that should not be taken concomitantly w/ the drug. Advise to inform other healthcare professionals that they are taking the drug. Inform of the risk of myopathy; instruct to report promptly any unexplained muscle pain, tenderness, or weakness, particularly if accompanied by malaise or fever or if these muscle signs or symptoms persist after discontinuation. Inform that liver function will be checked prior to initiation and if signs or symptoms of liver injury occur; instruct to report promptly any symptoms that may indicate liver injury. Instruct women of childbearing age to use effective method of birth control to prevent pregnancy. Advise to d/c therapy and contact physician if pregnancy occurs. Instruct not to use the drug if breastfeeding.

LIPTRUZET — atorvastatin/ezetimibe
Rx

Class: Cholesterol absorption inhibitor/HMG-CoA reductase inhibitor (statin)

ADULT DOSAGE
Primary Hyperlipidemia/Mixed Hyperlipidemia
Initial: 10mg/10mg/day or 10mg/20mg/day as a single dose at any time of the day
Range: 10mg/10mg to 10mg/80mg qd
Titrate: After initiation and/or upon titration, analyze lipid levels w/in ≥2 weeks and adjust dose, if needed

Patients Requiring Larger LDL Reduction (>55%):
Initial: 10mg/40mg/day

Homozygous Familial Hypercholesterolemia
10mg/40mg/day or 10mg/80mg/day

PEDIATRIC DOSAGE
Pediatric use may not have been established

DOSING CONSIDERATIONS
Concomitant Medications
Bile Acid Sequestrants: Take either ≥2 hrs before or ≥4 hrs after bile acid sequestrant
Cyclosporine, Tipranavir Plus Ritonavir (RTV), Telaprevir, Gemfibrozil: Avoid therapy w/ Liptruzet
Lopinavir Plus RTV: Use caution; use lowest dose of Liptruzet necessary
Clarithromycin, Itraconazole, Saquinavir Plus RTV, Darunavir Plus RTV, Fosamprenavir, Fosamprenavir Plus RTV:
Max: 10mg/20mg/day
Nelfinavir, Boceprevir:
Max: 10mg/40mg/day

ADMINISTRATION
Oral route

Take w/ or w/o food
Swallow tab whole; do not crush, dissolve, or chew

STORAGE
20-25°C (68-77°F); excursions permitted to 15-30°C (59-86°F). Store in foil pouch until use. Protect from moisture and light and store in a dry place after the foil pouch is opened. Once a tab is removed, slide blister card back into case. Discard any unused tab 30 days after pouch is opened.

HOW SUPPLIED
Tab: (Ezetimibe/Atorvastatin) 10mg/10mg, 10mg/20mg, 10mg/40mg, 10mg/80mg

CONTRAINDICATIONS
Active liver disease or unexplained persistent elevations in hepatic transaminase levels, hypersensitivity to any component of this product, women who are or may become pregnant, nursing mothers.

WARNINGS/PRECAUTIONS
Has not been studied in Fredrickson type I, III, IV, and V dyslipidemias. Myopathy (including immune-mediated necrotizing myopathy [IMNM]) and rhabdomyolysis reported; d/c if markedly elevated CPK levels occur or myopathy is diagnosed or suspected. Temporarily withhold or d/c therapy in any patient w/ an acute, serious condition suggestive of a myopathy or having a risk factor predisposing to development of renal failure secondary to rhabdomyolysis (eg, severe acute infection, hypotension, major surgery, trauma, severe metabolic/endocrine/electrolyte disorders, uncontrolled seizures). Liver enzyme elevations and fatal and nonfatal hepatic failure (rare) reported; obtain LFTs prior to initiating therapy and repeat as clinically indicated; promptly interrupt therapy if serious liver injury w/ clinical symptoms and/or hyperbilirubinemia or jaundice occurs and do not restart if no alternative etiology found. Caution in patients who consume substantial quantities of alcohol and/or have a history of liver disease. Increases in HbA1c and FPG levels reported. May blunt adrenal and/or gonadal steroid production. Increased risk of hemorrhagic stroke in patients w/ recent stroke or transient ischemic attack (TIA). Caution in elderly.

ADVERSE REACTIONS
Increased ALT/AST, musculoskeletal pain, abdominal pain, nausea, arthralgia.

DRUG INTERACTIONS
See Dosing Considerations. Caution w/ drugs that decrease levels or activity of endogenous steroid hormones (eg, ketoconazole, spironolactone, cimetidine). Increased risk of myopathy w/ fibric acid derivatives, erythromycin, lipid-modifying doses of niacin, strong CYP3A4 inhibitors (eg, clarithromycin, HIV protease inhibitors), and azole antifungals; consider lower initial and maint doses. Monitor INR levels when used w/ warfarin. Atorvastatin: Strong CYP3A4 inhibitors, grapefruit juice, saquinavir plus ritonavir, diltiazem, and amlodipine may increase levels. Itraconazole may increase exposure. Myopathy, including rhabdomyolysis, reported w/ colchicine; use w/ caution. OATP1B1 inhibitors may increase bioavailability. May increase levels of digoxin; monitor appropriately. May increase exposure of norethindrone and ethinyl estradiol. CYP3A4 inducers (eg, efavirenz, rifampin) may decrease levels; simultaneous coadministration w/ rifampin is recommended. Ezetimibe: Cholestyramine may decrease exposure of total ezetimibe.

PREGNANCY AND LACTATION
Category X, not for use in nursing.

MECHANISM OF ACTION
Atorvastatin: HMG-CoA reductase inhibitor; lowers plasma cholesterol and lipoprotein levels by inhibiting HMG-CoA reductase and cholesterol synthesis in the liver and by increasing the number of hepatic LDL receptors on the cell-surface to enhance uptake and catabolism of LDL; also reduces LDL production and the number of LDL particles. Ezetimibe: Cholesterol absorption inhibitor; localizes at the brush border of the small intestine and inhibits absorption of cholesterol and decreases intestinal cholesterol delivery to the liver.

PHARMACOKINETICS
Absorption: Atorvastatin: Absolute bioavailability (14%); T_{max}=1-2 hrs. **Distribution:** Atorvastatin: V_d=381L; plasma protein binding (≥98%). Ezetimibe: Plasma protein binding (>90%). **Metabolism:** Atorvastatin: CYP3A4 (extensive); ortho- and parahydroxylated derivatives (metabolites). Ezetimibe: Small intestine and liver via glucuronide conjugation; ezetimibe-glucuronide (active metabolite). **Elimination:** Atorvastatin: Bile (major), urine (<2%); $T_{1/2}$=approx 14 hrs. Ezetimibe: Feces (78%, 69% unchanged drug), urine (11%, 9% metabolite); $T_{1/2}$=approx 22 hrs.

PATIENT CONSIDERATIONS
Assessment: Assess for history of or active liver disease, unexplained persistent elevations in hepatic transaminases, risk factors for developing myopathy (eg, advanced age, hypothyroidism, renal impairment), recent stroke or TIA, hypersensitivity to the drug, pregnancy/nursing status, and possible drug interactions. Assess use in patients who consume substantial quantities of alcohol. Obtain baseline lipid profile (total-C, LDL, HDL, TGs) and LFTs (eg, AST, ALT).

Monitoring: Monitor for signs/symptoms of myopathy, rhabdomyolysis, liver dysfunction, and other adverse reactions. Analyze lipid levels w/in 2 or more weeks after initiation and/or upon titration. Monitor LFTs as clinically indicated, and for increases in HbA1c and FPG levels.

Counseling: Advise to adhere to the National Cholesterol Education Program recommended diet, a regular exercise program, and periodic testing of a fasting lipid panel. Counsel about risk of myopathy and inform that consuming large quantities (>1L) of grapefruit juice may increase this risk. Advise to discuss w/ physician all medications, both prescription and OTC, currently taking. Instruct to report to physician any unexplained muscle pain, tenderness, or weakness, particularly if accompanied by malaise or fever, or if signs/symptoms persist after discontinuing therapy. Advise to report promptly any signs of liver injury, including fatigue, anorexia, right upper abdominal discomfort, dark urine, or jaundice. Counsel women of childbearing age to use an effective method of birth control while using the drug and to discuss future pregnancy plans; instruct to d/c therapy and contact physician if pregnancy occurs. Advise not to breastfeed during treatment.

LITHIUM 450MG ER TABLETS — lithium carbonate   Rx

Class: Antimanic agent

> Lithium toxicity is closely related to serum levels, and can occur at doses close to therapeutic levels. Facilities for prompt and accurate serum lithium determinations should be available before initiating therapy.

ADULT DOSAGE
Manic-Depressive Illness
Individualize dose according to serum levels and clinical response

Acute Mania:
1800mg/day in divided doses to achieve desired serum levels of 1-1.5mEq/L

Monitor serum levels 2X/week during the acute phase, and until serum level and clinical condition have been stabilized

Long-Term Control:
Desirable serum lithium levels are 0.6-1.2mEq/L; dose will vary, but usually 900-1200mg/day in divided doses will maintain this level

Serum lithium levels in uncomplicated cases receiving maint therapy during remission should be monitored at least every 2 months

Patients unusually sensitive to lithium may exhibit toxic signs at serum levels <1mEq/L

Conversions
Switching from Immediate-Release (IR) Caps to Extended-Release (ER) Tabs:
Give the same total daily dose when possible

When previous dosage of IR lithium is not a multiple of 450mg (eg, 1500mg), initiate ER tab at the multiple of 450mg nearest to, but below, the original daily dose (eg, 1350mg)

When the 2 doses are unequal, give larger dose in pm (eg, 1350mg/day [450mg am and 900mg pm]); if desired, give total daily dose tid (eg, 1350mg/day [450mg tid])

Monitor at 1- to 2-week intervals and adjust dose if necessary, until stable and satisfactory serum levels and clinical state achieved

When closer titration is required than that available w/ doses of ER tabs in increments of 450mg, use IR caps

Most patients on maint therapy are stabilized on 900mg daily (eg, 450mg bid ER tab)

PEDIATRIC DOSAGE
Manic-Depressive Illness
≥12 Years:
Individualize dose according to serum levels and clinical response

Acute Mania:
1800mg/day in divided doses to achieve desired serum levels of 1-1.5mEq/L

Monitor serum levels 2X/week during the acute phase, and until serum level and clinical condition have been stabilized

Long-Term Control:
Desirable serum lithium levels are 0.6-1.2mEq/L; dose will vary, but usually 900-1200mg/day in divided doses will maintain this level

Serum lithium levels in uncomplicated cases receiving maint therapy during remission should be monitored at least every 2 months

Patients unusually sensitive to lithium may exhibit toxic signs at serum levels <1mEq/L

Conversions
Switching from IR Caps to ER Tabs:
Give the same total daily dose when possible

When previous dosage of IR lithium is not a multiple of 450mg (eg, 1500mg), initiate ER tab at the multiple of 450mg nearest to, but below, the original daily dose (eg, 1350mg)

When the 2 doses are unequal, give larger dose in pm (eg, 1350mg/day [450mg am and 900mg pm]); if desired, give total daily dose tid (eg, 1350mg/day [450mg tid])

Monitor at 1- to 2-week intervals and adjust dose if necessary, until stable and satisfactory serum levels and clinical state achieved

When closer titration is required than that available w/ doses of ER tabs in increments of 450mg, use IR caps

Most patients on maint therapy are stabilized on 900mg daily (eg, 450mg bid ER tab)

DOSING CONSIDERATIONS
Elderly
May respond to reduced dose and may exhibit signs of toxicity at serum levels ordinarily tolerated by other patients

Other Important Considerations
Blood samples for serum lithium determinations should be drawn immediately prior to next dose when lithium concentrations are relatively stable (eg, 8-12 hrs after previous dose)

ADMINISTRATION
Oral route

Doses are usually given bid (approx 12-hr intervals).

STORAGE
20-25°C (68-77°F). Protect from moisture.

HOW SUPPLIED
Tab, ER: 450mg* *scored

WARNINGS/PRECAUTIONS
Avoid w/ significant renal or cardiovascular (CV) disease, severe debilitation/dehydration, or Na+ depletion; if the psychiatric indication is life-threatening, and if patient fails to respond to other measures, lithium treatment may be undertaken w/ extreme caution (including daily serum lithium determinations, adjustment to the usually low doses ordinarily tolerated). May be associated w/ the unmasking of Brugada syndrome; avoid w/ known or suspected Brugada syndrome. Chronic therapy may be associated w/ diminution of renal concentrating ability; carefully manage to avoid dehydration w/ resulting lithium retention and toxicity.

Morphologic changes w/ glomerular and interstitial fibrosis and nephron atrophy reported in patients on chronic therapy. Assess kidney function prior to and during therapy. During lithium therapy, progressive or sudden changes in renal function, even w/in the normal range, indicate the need for reevaluation of treatment. May decrease Na+ reabsorption, which could lead to Na+ depletion; maintain normal diet, including salt, and an adequate fluid intake at least during the initial stabilization period. Decreased tolerance reported to ensue from protracted sweating or diarrhea; if this occurs, administer supplemental fluid and salt. Sweating, diarrhea, and concomitant infection w/ elevated temperatures may necessitate a temporary reduction or cessation of medication. If hypothyroidism preexists, carefully monitor thyroid function during lithium stabilization and maintenance. If hypothyroidism occurs during lithium stabilization and maintenance, supplemental thyroid treatment may be used. May impair mental/physical abilities.

ADVERSE REACTIONS
Fine hand tremor, polyuria, mild thirst, general discomfort, diarrhea, N/V, drowsiness, lithium toxicity, blackout spells, ataxia, dry mouth, alopecia, oliguria, albuminuria.

DRUG INTERACTIONS
Encephalopathic syndrome followed by irreversible brain damage reported w/ neuroleptics; monitor for evidence of neurological toxicity and d/c therapy if such signs appear. May prolong effects of neuromuscular blockers; use w/ caution. Diuretics may increase serum lithium levels; use w/ caution, monitor lithium levels, and adjust lithium dose if necessary. Caution w/ calcium channel blockers; may increase risk of neurotoxicity. Increased levels w/ indomethacin, piroxicam, and other NSAIDs (eg, selective COX-2 inhibitors); monitor levels closely when initiating or discontinuing NSAID use. Acetazolamide, urea, xanthine preparations, and alkalinizing agents (eg, sodium bicarbonate) may decrease levels. May provoke lithium toxicity w/ metronidazole; monitor closely. Risk of lithium toxicity w/ ACE inhibitors (eg, enalapril, captopril) and angiotensin II receptor antagonists (eg, losartan); may need to reduce lithium dose and monitor lithium levels more often. Caution w/ SSRIs. May interact w/ methyldopa, phenytoin, and carbamazepine.

PREGNANCY AND LACTATION
Pregnancy: May cause fetal harm.
Lactation: Excreted in human milk; not for use in nursing except in rare and unusual circumstances where the potential benefits to the mother outweigh possible hazards to the child.

MECHANISM OF ACTION
Antimanic agent; not established. Alters Na+ transport in nerve and muscle cells and effects a shift toward intraneuronal metabolism of catecholamines.

PHARMACOKINETICS
Distribution: Found in breast milk. **Elimination:** Urine (primary); $T_{1/2}$=approx 24 hrs.

PATIENT CONSIDERATIONS
Assessment: Assess for significant renal or CV disease, severe debilitation, dehydration, Na+ depletion, thyroid disorders, Brugada syndrome or risk factors, pregnancy/nursing status, and for possible drug interactions. Assess baseline renal function.

Monitoring: Monitor for unmasking of Brugada syndrome, renal effects, decreased tolerance to therapy, decreased Na+ reabsorption, signs of lithium toxicity, and other adverse reactions. Monitor renal function. In patients w/ preexisting hypothyroidism, monitor thyroid function during therapy stabilization and maintenance. Monitor patient's clinical state and serum lithium levels regularly.

Counseling: Inform of the risks and benefits of therapy. Counsel about clinical signs of lithium toxicity (eg, diarrhea, vomiting, tremor); advise to d/c therapy and notify physician if any of these signs occur. Advise to seek immediate emergency assistance if fainting, lightheadedness, abnormal heartbeats, SOB, or other adverse reactions develop. Advise to use caution w/ activities requiring alertness.

LITHOBID — lithium carbonate   Rx

Class: Antimanic agent

> Lithium toxicity is closely related to serum levels, and can occur at doses close to therapeutic levels. Facilities for prompt and accurate serum lithium determinations should be available before initiating therapy.

ADULT DOSAGE
Bipolar Disorder
Acute Mania:
AM Dose: 3 tabs (900mg)
PM Dose: 3 tabs (900mg)
May also be administered on 600mg tid dosing interval

Such doses will normally produce an effective serum level of 1-1.5 mEq/L; individualize according to serum levels and clinical response.
Monitor serum levels 2X/week during acute phase, and until serum level and clinical condition have been stabilized

Long-Term Control:
AM Dose: 2 tabs (600mg)
PM Dose: 2 tabs (600mg)

PEDIATRIC DOSAGE
Bipolar Disorder
≥12 Years:
Acute Mania:
AM Dose: 3 tabs (900mg)
PM Dose: 3 tabs (900mg)
May also be administered on 600mg tid dosing interval

Such doses will normally produce an effective serum level of 1-1.5 mEq/L; individualize according to serum levels and clinical response.
Monitor serum levels 2X/week during acute phase, and until serum level and clinical condition have been stabilized

Long-Term Control:
AM Dose: 2 tabs (600mg)

May administer on tid dosing interval up to 1200mg/day

Desirable serum lithium concentrations are 0.6-1.2 mEq/L, which can usually be achieved w/ 900-1200mg/day

Serum lithium concentrations in uncomplicated cases receiving maint therapy during remission should be monitored at least every 2 months

Patients abnormally sensitive to lithium may exhibit toxic signs at serum levels of 1-1.5mEq/L

PM Dose: 2 tabs (600mg)
May administer on tid dosing interval up to 1200mg/day

Desirable serum lithium concentrations are 0.6-1.2 mEq/L, which can usually be achieved w/ 900-1200mg/day

Serum lithium concentrations in uncomplicated cases receiving maint therapy during remission should be monitored at least every 2 months

Patients abnormally sensitive to lithium may exhibit toxic signs at serum levels of 1-1.5mEq/L

DOSING CONSIDERATIONS
Elderly
Start at lower end of dosing range

Other Important Considerations
Blood samples for serum lithium determinations should be drawn immediately prior to next dose when lithium concentrations are relatively stable (eg, 8-12 hrs after previous dose)

ADMINISTRATION
Oral route
Swallow tab whole; do not chew or crush.

STORAGE
15-30°C (59-86°F). Protect from moisture.

HOW SUPPLIED
Tab, Extended-Release: 300mg

WARNINGS/PRECAUTIONS
Increased risk of lithium toxicity in patients w/ significant renal or cardiovascular (CV) disease, severe debilitation or dehydration, or Na⁺ depletion; consider starting w/ lower doses and titrating slowly while frequently monitoring serum lithium levels and signs of lithium toxicity. May be associated w/ the unmasking of Brugada syndrome; avoid in patients w/ known/suspected Brugada syndrome. Chronic therapy may be associated w/ diminution of renal concentrating ability; carefully manage to avoid dehydration w/ resulting lithium retention and toxicity. Cases consistent w/ nephrotic syndrome reported; d/c therapy in patients w/ nephrotic syndrome. During lithium therapy, progressive or sudden changes in renal function, even w/in the normal range, indicate the need for reevaluation of treatment. Morphologic changes w/ glomerular and interstitial fibrosis and nephron atrophy reported during chronic therapy. Monitor patients w/ organic brain syndrome or other CNS impairment closely for early evidence of neurologic toxicity; d/c promptly if such signs appear. May cause fetal harm. May decrease Na⁺ reabsorption, which could lead to Na⁺ depletion; maintain normal diet, including salt, and an adequate fluid intake (2500-3500mL) at least during initial stabilization period. Decreased tolerance to lithium reported to ensue from protracted sweating or diarrhea; if this occurs, administer supplemental fluid and salt under careful medical supervision and reduce or suspend lithium intake until the condition is resolved. Concomitant infection w/ elevated temperatures may necessitate a temporary reduction or cessation of lithium. If hypothyroidism preexists, carefully monitor thyroid function during lithium stabilization and maintenance. If hypothyroidism occurs during lithium stabilization and maintenance, supplemental thyroid treatment may be used. May impair mental/physical abilities.

ADVERSE REACTIONS
Fine hand tremor, polyuria, muscle hyperirritability, mild thirst, cardiac arrhythmia, general discomfort, diarrhea, N/V, ataxia, tinnitus, blurred vision, hypertonicity, hypotension, glycosuria, drying and thinning of hair.

DRUG INTERACTIONS
Encephalopathic syndrome followed by irreversible brain damage w/ haloperidol and other neuroleptics reported; monitor for evidence of neurologic toxicity and d/c therapy promptly if such signs appear. May prolong effects of neuromuscular blockers; use w/ caution. May increase risk of neurotoxic effects w/ calcium channel blockers or carbamazepine. Increased levels w/ indomethacin, piroxicam, and other NSAIDs (eg, COX-2 inhibitors); monitor levels closely when initiating or discontinuing NSAID use. Acetazolamide, urea, xanthine preparations, and alkalinizing agents (eg, sodium bicarbonate) may decrease levels. May produce hypothyroidism w/ extended use of iodide preparations, especially potassium iodide. May provoke lithium toxicity w/ metronidazole; monitor closely. Fluoxetine may increase and decrease lithium levels; monitor closely. Increased risk of lithium toxicity in patients receiving prescribed medications that may affect kidney function (eg, ACE inhibitors, ARBs, diuretics [loops and thiazides], NSAIDs); consider starting w/ lower doses of lithium and titrating slowly while frequently monitoring serum lithium levels and signs of lithium toxicity.

PREGNANCY AND LACTATION
Pregnancy: Category D.
Lactation: Excreted in human milk; not for use in nursing.

MECHANISM OF ACTION
Antimanic agent; not established. Alters Na⁺ transport in nerve and muscle cells and effects a shift toward intraneuronal metabolism of catecholamines.

PHARMACOKINETICS
Distribution: Found in breast milk. **Elimination:** Urine (primary). T₁/₂=approx 24 hrs.

PATIENT CONSIDERATIONS
Assessment: Assess for significant renal or CV disease, severe debilitation, dehydration, Na⁺ depletion, thyroid disorder, Brugada syndrome or risk factors for Brugada syndrome, pregnancy/nursing status, and for possible drug interactions. Assess baseline renal function.

Monitoring: Monitor for diminution of renal concentrating ability, glomerular and interstitial fibrosis, nephron atrophy, decreased tolerance to therapy, mental/physical ability impairment, decreased Na⁺ reabsorption, signs of lithium toxicity, unmasking of Brugada syndrome, and other adverse reactions. Monitor renal function. In patients w/ preexisting hypothyroidism, monitor thyroid function during therapy stabilization and maintenance. Monitor patient's clinical state and serum lithium levels regularly.

Counseling: Inform of risks and benefits of therapy. Counsel about clinical signs of lithium toxicity (eg, diarrhea, vomiting, tremor); advise to d/c therapy and notify physician if any of these signs occur. Advise to seek immediate emergency assistance if fainting, lightheadedness, abnormal heartbeats, SOB, or other adverse reactions develop. Inform that lithium may impair mental/physical abilities; advise to use caution w/ activities requiring alertness.

LIVALO — pitavastatin
Class: HMG-CoA reductase inhibitor (statin)

Rx

ADULT DOSAGE	PEDIATRIC DOSAGE
Primary Hypercholesterolemia/Mixed Dyslipidemia	Pediatric use may not have been established
Initial: 2mg qd	
Range: 1-4mg qd	
Max: 4mg qd	
After initiation or upon titration, analyze lipid levels after 4 weeks and adjust dose accordingly	

DOSING CONSIDERATIONS
Concomitant Medications
Erythromycin:
Max: 1mg qd

Rifampin:
Max: 2mg qd

Renal Impairment
Moderate/Severe (GFR 30-59mL/min/1.73m² and GFR 15-29mL/min/1.73m² Not Receiving Hemodialysis, Respectively)/ESRD Receiving Hemodialysis:
Initial: 1mg qd
Max: 2mg qd

ADMINISTRATION
Oral route
Take PO at any time of the day w/ or w/o food

STORAGE
15-30°C (59-86°F). Protect from light.

HOW SUPPLIED
Tab: 1mg, 2mg, 4mg

CONTRAINDICATIONS
Active liver disease, including unexplained persistent elevations of hepatic transaminase levels, women who are pregnant or may become pregnant, nursing mothers, and coadministration with cyclosporine. Known hypersensitivity to any component of this product.

WARNINGS/PRECAUTIONS
Increased risk for severe myopathy with doses >4mg qd. Myopathy (including immune-mediated necrotizing myopathy [IMNM]) and rhabdomyolysis with acute renal failure secondary to myoglobinuria reported. Caution with predisposing factors for myopathy (eg, advanced age [≥65 yrs], renal impairment, and inadequately treated hypothyroidism). D/C if markedly elevated creatine kinase (CK) levels occur or myopathy is diagnosed/suspected and temporarily withhold in any patient experiencing an acute or serious condition suggestive of myopathy or predisposing to the development of renal failure secondary to rhabdomyolysis (eg, sepsis, hypotension, dehydration). Increases in serum transaminases (eg, AST, ALT) reported; perform LFTs before the initiation of treatment and if signs or symptoms of liver injury occur. Fatal and nonfatal hepatic failure reported (rare); promptly interrupt therapy if serious liver injury with clinical symptoms and/or hyperbilirubinemia or jaundice occurs; do not restart if no alternative etiology found. Increases in HbA1c and fasting serum glucose levels reported. Caution with substantial alcohol consumption.

ADVERSE REACTIONS
Back pain, constipation, myalgia.

DRUG INTERACTIONS
See Contraindications. Erythromycin and rifampin may increase exposure. Due to an increased risk of myopathy/rhabdomyolysis, avoid coadministration with gemfibrozil and use caution when coadministered with fibrates and colchicine. May enhance risk of skeletal muscle effects with niacin; consider dose reduction with lipid-modifying doses of niacin. Monitor PT and INR with warfarin.

PREGNANCY AND LACTATION
Category X, not for use in nursing.

MECHANISM OF ACTION
HMG-CoA reductase inhibitor; inhibits the rate-determining enzyme involved with biosynthesis of cholesterol so that it inhibits cholesterol synthesis in the liver.

PHARMACOKINETICS

Absorption: (Oral Sol) Absolute bioavailability (51%); T_{max}=1 hr. **Distribution:** Plasma protein binding (>99%); V_d=148L. **Metabolism:** CYP2C9, 2C8; lactone (major metabolite) via glucuronide conjugate by uridine 5'-diphosphate glucuronosyltransferase (UGT1A3 and UGT2B7). **Elimination:** Urine (15%), feces (79%); $T_{1/2}$=12 hrs.

PATIENT CONSIDERATIONS

Assessment: Assess for hepatic/renal impairment, inadequately treated hypothyroidism, substantial alcohol consumption, pregnancy/nursing status, possible drug interactions, and other conditions where treatment is cautioned/contraindicated. Obtain baseline lipid profile.

Monitoring: Monitor signs/symptoms of myopathy, rhabdomyolysis, IMNM, acute renal failure, hypersensitivity reactions, and other adverse reactions. Monitor for increases in HbA1c and fasting serum glucose levels. Perform periodic monitoring of lipid profile and CK levels. Analyze lipid levels 4 weeks after initiation/titration. Perform LFTs with signs or symptoms of liver injury. Monitor PT and INR when using warfarin.

Counseling: Advise to promptly notify physician of any unexplained muscle pain, tenderness, or weakness, particularly if accompanied by malaise or fever, or if these muscle signs/symptoms persist after discontinuing treatment. Advise to discuss all medications, both prescription and OTC, with physician. Counsel women of childbearing age to use effective method of birth control to prevent pregnancy during therapy. Instruct pregnant or breastfeeding women to d/c therapy and consult physician. Inform that liver enzymes will be checked before therapy and if signs/symptoms of liver injury occur (eg, fatigue, anorexia, right upper abdominal discomfort, dark urine, or jaundice). Advise to report promptly any symptoms that may indicate liver injury.

Lo/Ovral-28 — ethinyl estradiol/norgestrel

Class: Estrogen/progestogen combination

Rx

> **Cigarette smoking increases the risk of serious cardiovascular side effects. Risk increases with age (>35 yrs of age) and extent of smoking (≥15 cigarettes/day). Women who use oral contraceptives should be strongly advised not to smoke.**

OTHER BRAND NAMES

Low-Ogestrel, Cryselle

ADULT DOSAGE

Contraception

1 tab qd at the same time each day for 28 days, then repeat

Start 1st Sunday after menses begin or on 1st day of menses

Conversions

Lo/Ovral:

Switching from 21-Day Regimen:
Wait 7 days after last tab before starting therapy

Switching from 28-Day Regimen:
Start therapy on the day after her last tab; do not wait any days between packs

Switching from Progestin-Only Pill:
Start therapy next day; use a nonhormonal backup method of birth control for first 7 days of therapy

Switching from an Implant or Inj:
Start therapy on the day of implant removal or day the next inj is due; use a nonhormonal backup method of birth control for first 7 days of therapy

Missed Dose

Cryselle:
If ≥2 white tabs are missed, another method of contraception should be used until a white tab is taken for 7 consecutive days.
If ≥1 light-green tabs are missed, no other method of contraception is needed.

PEDIATRIC DOSAGE

Contraception

Not indicated for use premenarche; refer to adult dosing

DOSING CONSIDERATIONS

Other Important Considerations

Lo/Ovral:
Postpartum Women Who Do Not Breastfeed/After 2nd Trimester Abortion: Start therapy no earlier than 28 days postpartum; advise to use a nonhormonal backup method for the first 7 days of therapy

1st Trimester Abortion/Miscarriage: May be initiated immediately; backup contraception is not needed if therapy started immediately

Cryselle:
Nonlactating Mother: May initiate postpartum

Lo-Ogestrel:
Postpartum Women After Full-Term Delivery: Do not initiate earlier than 4-6 weeks postpartum

Termination of Pregnancy in the First 12 Weeks: Start therapy immediately or w/ in 7 days
Termination of Pregnancy After 12 Weeks: Start therapy after 2 weeks

ADMINISTRATION

Oral route

Take dose at intervals not exceeding 24 hrs

Cryselle: Take preferably after pm meal or at hs

STORAGE

20-25°C (68-77°F). **Low-Ogestrel:** 15-25°C (59-77°F).

HOW SUPPLIED

Tab: (Ethinyl Estradiol [EE]/Norgestrel) 0.03mg/0.3mg

CONTRAINDICATIONS

Thrombophlebitis, thromboembolic disorders, history of deep vein thrombophlebitis/thromboembolic disorders, cerebrovascular disease or coronary artery disease (CAD), known or suspected carcinoma of the breast, carcinoma of the endometrium or other known or suspected estrogen-dependent neoplasia, undiagnosed abnormal genital bleeding, cholestatic jaundice of pregnancy or jaundice with prior pill use, known or suspected pregnancy, hepatic adenomas or carcinomas or (Low-Ogestrel) benign liver tumors. **Lo/Ovral:** Past history of cerebrovascular disease or CAD, active liver disease, valvular heart disease with thrombogenic complications, thrombogenic rhythm disorders, hereditary or acquired thrombophilias, major surgery with prolonged immobilization, diabetes with vascular involvement, headaches with focal neurological symptoms, uncontrolled HTN, personal history of breast cancer, hypersensitivity to any of the components of the product.

WARNINGS/PRECAUTIONS

Increased risk of myocardial infarction (MI), vascular disease, thromboembolism, stroke, hepatic neoplasia, and gallbladder disease. Increased risk of morbidity and mortality if other risk factors (eg, certain inherited or acquired thrombophilia, HTN, hyperlipidemia, obesity, diabetes) are present. If feasible, d/c at least 4 weeks prior to and for 2 weeks after elective surgery of a type associated with an increased risk of thromboembolism and during and following prolonged immobilization. Start use no earlier than 4-6 weeks after delivery in women who elect not to breastfeed, or a midtrimester pregnancy termination. May increase risk of breast cancer and cancer of the reproductive organs. Retinal thrombosis reported; d/c if there is unexplained partial or complete loss of vision; onset of proptosis or diplopia; papilledema; or if retinal vascular lesions develop. Contact lens wearers who develop visual changes or changes in lens tolerance should be assessed by an ophthalmologist. Should not be used to induce withdrawal bleeding as a test for pregnancy, nor to treat threatened or habitual abortion during pregnancy. Rule out pregnancy if 2 consecutive periods are missed. May cause glucose intolerance; monitor prediabetic and diabetic patients. May elevate serum TG and LDL levels and may render the control of hyperlipidemias more difficult. Elevations of plasma TGs may lead to pancreatitis and other complications. May elevate BP; monitor closely and d/c use if significant BP elevation occurs. New onset/exacerbation of migraine or recurrent, persistent, severe headache may develop; d/c and evaluate the cause if this occurs. Women with migraine may be at increased risk of stroke. Breakthrough bleeding and spotting reported; rule out malignancy or pregnancy. Post-pill amenorrhea or oligomenorrhea may occur. D/C if jaundice develops. May cause fluid retention. Caution with history of depression; d/c if depression recurs to serious degree. Diarrhea and/or vomiting may reduce hormone absorption. May affect certain endocrine function tests, LFTs, and blood components in lab tests. **Lo/Ovral:** Ectopic and intrauterine pregnancy may occur in contraceptive failures. If using Sunday Start method, during the first cycle, contraceptive reliance should not be placed on therapy until a white tab has been taken daily for 7 consecutive days. **Low-Ogestrel:** Use an additional method of protection until after the first 7 days of administration in the initial cycle. **Cryselle:** During the first cycle, contraceptive reliance should not be placed on therapy until a white tab has been taken daily for 7 consecutive days.

ADVERSE REACTIONS

N/V, breakthrough bleeding, spotting, amenorrhea, migraine, depression, vaginal candidiasis, edema, weight changes, change in cervical erosion and secretion, menstrual flow changes, GI symptoms (eg, abdominal pain, cramps, bloating), rash (allergic).

DRUG INTERACTIONS

Lo/Ovral: Reduced effects resulting in pregnancy or breakthrough bleeding may occur with antibiotics, anticonvulsants, and other drugs that increase the metabolism of contraceptive steroids (eg, rifabutin, primidone, dexamethasone, modafinil); consider back up nonhormonal method of birth control. Significant changes (increase or decrease) in estrogen and progestin levels noted in some cases with anti-HIV protease inhibitors. Herbal products containing St. John's wort may induce hepatic enzymes (cytochrome P450) and p-glycoprotein transporter and may reduce the effectiveness of contraceptive steroids, and may also result in breakthrough bleeding. Atorvastatin increases EE exposure; ascorbic acid and acetaminophen (APAP) increases EE bioavailability. CYP3A4 inhibitors (eg, indinavir, itraconazole, ketoconazole) increase levels. Troleandomycin may increase risk of intrahepatic cholestasis. Increased plasma concentrations of cyclosporine, prednisolone and other corticosteroids, and theophylline. Decreased plasma concentrations of APAP. Increased clearance of temazepam, salicylic acid, morphine, and clofibric acid. **Cryselle/Low-Ogestrel:** Reduced efficacy and increased incidence of breakthrough bleeding and menstrual irregularities with rifampin, barbiturates, phenylbutazone, phenytoin sodium, and possibly with griseofulvin, ampicillin, and tetracyclines.

PREGNANCY AND LACTATION

Category X, not for use in nursing.

MECHANISM OF ACTION

Estrogen/progestogen oral contraceptive; acts by suppression of gonadotropins, primarily inhibiting ovulation and causing other alterations, including changes in the cervical mucus (increases difficulty of sperm entry into uterus) and the endometrium (reduces likelihood of implantation).

PHARMACOKINETICS
Distribution: Found in breast milk.

PATIENT CONSIDERATIONS

Assessment: Assess for hypersensitivity to drug, breast cancer, estrogen-dependent neoplasia, abnormal genital bleeding, thrombophlebitis, thromboembolic disorders, past history of deep vein thrombophlebitis or thromboembolic disorders, cerebrovascular disease or CAD, known/suspected pregnancy, or any other conditions where treatment is cautioned/contraindicated. Assess nursing status and for possible drug interactions.

Monitoring: Monitor for MI, stroke, hepatic neoplasia, bleeding irregularities, thromboembolism, onset or exacerbation of headaches or migraines, and other adverse reactions. Monitor serum glucose levels in diabetic and prediabetic patients, BP with history of HTN, lipid levels with history of hyperlipidemia, and for signs of worsening depression with previous history of the disorder. Monitor liver function. Monitor women with strong family history of breast cancer or with breast nodules. Refer contact lens wearers to an ophthalmologist if visual changes develop. Perform periodic medical history and physical exam.

Counseling: Inform of the benefits and risks of therapy. Inform that drug does not protect against HIV infection (AIDS) and other sexually transmitted diseases. Advise to avoid smoking. Instruct to take exactly ud at intervals not exceeding 24 hrs. Advise about risks of pregnancy if dose is missed. Instruct that if one dose is missed, to take as soon as possible and take next pill at regular scheduled time. Inform that spotting, light bleeding, or nausea may occur during the first 1-3 packs of pills; advise not to d/c medication and if symptoms persist, to notify physician. Instruct to d/c if pregnancy is confirmed/suspected. Inform that certain drugs may make therapy less effective and the possible need to use additional contraception. Instruct to notify physician if breastfeeding. If scheduled for any lab test, advise patient to inform physician that taking birth control pills.

LOESTRIN 21 — ethinyl estradiol/norethindrone acetate   Rx

Class: Estrogen/progestogen combination

> Cigarette smoking increases the risk of serious cardiovascular (CV) side effects. Risk increases w/ age and w/ heavy smoking (≥15 cigarettes/day) and is quite marked in women >35 yrs of age. Women who use oral contraceptives are strongly advised not to smoke.

OTHER BRAND NAMES
Junel 1.5/30, Gildess 1/20, Junel 1/20, Microgestin 1.5/30, Gildess 1.5/30, Microgestin 1/20, Loestrin 21 1.5/30, Loestrin 21 1/20

ADULT DOSAGE
Contraception

1 tab qd for 21 days, stop for 7 days, and then repeat

Start 1st Sunday after menses begin or 1st day of menses

Missed Dose

Miss 1 Tab: Take as soon as dose is remembered; take next tab at regular time

Miss 2 Consecutive Tabs in Week 1 or 2: Take 2 tabs as soon as remembered and 2 tabs the next day; use another birth control method for 7 days following the missed tabs

Miss 2 Consecutive Tabs in Week 3 or Miss ≥3 Consecutive Tabs: (Sunday Start) Take 1 tab qd until Sunday, then discard remaining tabs and start a new pack of tabs immediately on Sunday. (Day 1 Start) Throw out rest of the pack and start new pack that same day. (Sunday/Day 1 Start) Use another birth control method for 7 days following missed tabs

PEDIATRIC DOSAGE
Contraception

Not indicated for use premenarche; refer to adult dosing

ADMINISTRATION
Oral route

Take regularly w/ a meal or hs
Take exactly ud at intervals not exceeding 24 hrs
Use an additional method of protection until after the 1st week of administration in the initial cycle when utilizing the Sunday Start regimen

STORAGE
20-25°C (68-77°F).

HOW SUPPLIED
Tab: (Norethindrone-Ethinyl Estradiol [EE]) (1/20) 1mg-0.02mg, (1.5/30) 1.5mg-0.03mg

CONTRAINDICATIONS
Thrombophlebitis, thromboembolic disorders, past history of deep vein thrombophlebitis or thromboembolic disorders, cerebral vascular or coronary artery disease, known or suspected carcinoma of the breast, carcinoma of the endometrium or other known or suspected estrogen-dependent neoplasia, undiagnosed abnormal genital bleeding, cholestatic jaundice of pregnancy or jaundice w/ prior pill use, hepatic adenomas or carcinomas, known/suspected pregnancy.

WARNINGS/PRECAUTIONS
Increased risk of MI, thromboembolism, stroke, hepatic neoplasia, gallbladder disease, and vascular disease. If feasible, d/c at least 4 weeks prior to and for 2 weeks after elective surgery of a type associated w/ an increased risk of thromboembolism, and during and following prolonged immobilization. Start use no earlier than 4-6 weeks after delivery in women who elect not to breastfeed. May increase risk of breast cancer and increase the risk of cervical intraepithelial neoplasia. Retinal thrombosis reported; d/c if unexplained partial or complete loss of vision occurs, or if onset of proptosis or diplopia, papilledema, or retinal vascular lesions develop. Rule out pregnancy before continuing therapy in any patient who has missed 2 consecutive periods; consider possibility of pregnancy at the first missed period if patient has not adhered to the prescribed dosing schedule. May cause glucose intolerance; monitor prediabetic and diabetic patients. May elevate serum TG and LDL levels and may render the control of hyperlipidemias more difficult. May cause increased BP and fluid retention; monitor closely and d/c use if significant BP elevation occurs. D/C and evaluate the cause if onset/exacerbation of a migraine or development of a headache w/ a new pattern which is recurrent, persistent, or severe develops. Breakthrough bleeding and spotting reported; rule out malignancy or pregnancy. Post-pill amenorrhea or oligomenorrhea may occur. D/C if jaundice develops. Carefully observe women w/ history of depression; d/c if depression recurs to a serious degree. Contact lens wearers who develop visual changes or changes in lens tolerance should be assessed by an ophthalmologist. May affect certain endocrine function tests, LFTs, and blood components in lab tests.

ADVERSE REACTIONS
N/V, GI symptoms, breakthrough bleeding, spotting, amenorrhea, migraine, mental depression, vaginal candidiasis, edema, weight changes, menstrual flow changes, melasma, breast changes, changes in cervical erosion and secretion, rash (allergic).

DRUG INTERACTIONS
Reduced effects, increased breakthrough bleeding, and menstrual irregularities w/ rifampin. Increased metabolism and possibly reduced contraceptive effectiveness w/ anticonvulsants (eg, phenobarbital, phenytoin, carbamazepine). Reduced plasma levels w/ troglitazone, resulting in possible reduced contraceptive effectiveness. Pregnancy reported w/ antimicrobials (eg, ampicillin, tetracycline, griseofulvin). Atorvastatin may increase norethindrone and EE exposure. Ascorbic acid and acetaminophen (APAP) may increase EE levels. Increased plasma levels of cyclosporine, prednisolone, and theophylline reported w/ concomitant use. Decreased levels of APAP and increased clearance of temazepam, salicylic acid, morphine, and clofibric acid reported w/ concomitant use. A reduction in contraceptive effectiveness and increased incidence of breakthrough bleeding may occur w/ phenylbutazone.

PREGNANCY AND LACTATION
Category X, not for use in nursing.

MECHANISM OF ACTION
Estrogen/progestogen oral contraceptive; acts by suppressing gonadotropins, primarily inhibiting ovulation, and causing other alterations, including changes in cervical mucus (increases difficulty of sperm entry into the uterus) and the endometrium (reduces likelihood of implantation).

PHARMACOKINETICS
Absorption: EE: Absolute bioavailability (43%). Norethindrone: Absolute bioavailability (64%). **Distribution:** V_d=2-4L/kg; plasma protein binding (>95%); found in breast milk. **Metabolism:** EE: Extensive via CYP3A4; oxidation, sulfate and glucuronide conjugation; 2-hydroxy ethinyl estradiol (primary oxidative metabolite). Norethindrone: Extensive; reduction, sulfate and glucuronide conjugation. **Elimination:** Urine, feces.

PATIENT CONSIDERATIONS

Assessment: Assess for hypersensitivity to drug, thrombophlebitis or thromboembolic disorders, HTN, hyperlipidemia, diabetes, breast cancer, endometrial cancer or other estrogen-dependent neoplasia, undiagnosed abnormal genital bleeding, cholestatic jaundice of pregnancy or jaundice w/ prior pill use, pregnancy/nursing status, and for any other conditions where treatment is contraindicated/cautioned. Assess for possible drug interactions.

Monitoring: Monitor for MI, thromboembolism, stroke, hepatic neoplasia, and other adverse effects. Monitor BP w/ history of HTN, serum glucose levels in diabetic or prediabetic patients, lipid levels w/ hyperlipidemia, and for signs of worsening depression w/ previous history. Monitor liver function. Monitor women who have breast nodules or a strong family history of breast cancer. Perform annual history and physical exam including special reference to BP, breasts, abdomen and pelvic organs, including cervical cytology, and relevant laboratory tests.

Counseling: Counsel about potential adverse effects. Inform that drug does not protect against HIV infection (AIDS) and other sexually transmitted diseases. Counsel that cigarette smoking increases the risk of serious CV effects and that women who use oral contraceptives should not smoke. Instruct to take exactly ud and at intervals not exceeding 24 hrs. Instruct on what to do if pills are missed. Instruct to use additional method of protection until after the 1st week of administration in the initial cycle when utilizing the Sunday Start regimen. Inform that spotting or breakthrough bleeding may occur; advise not to d/c medication and instruct to notify physician if symptoms persist. Instruct to d/c if pregnancy is confirmed/suspected during treatment. If scheduled for any lab test, advise to inform physician of use of birth control pills. Instruct to notify physician if breastfeeding. Inform that certain drugs may make therapy less effective and that additional contraception may be needed.

LOMOTIL — atropine sulfate/diphenoxylate hydrochloride   CV

Class: Anticholinergic/opioid

ADULT DOSAGE	PEDIATRIC DOSAGE
Diarrhea	**Diarrhea**
Adjunctive Therapy:	**Adjunctive Therapy:**
Initial: 2 tabs or 10mL qid	**2-12 Years:**
Titrate: Reduce dose after symptoms are controlled	**Initial:** 0.3-0.4mg/kg/day of sol in four divided doses
Maint: 2 tabs or 10mL qd	**Titrate:** Reduce dose after symptoms are controlled
Max: 20mg/day diphenoxylate	**Maint:** May be as low as 25% of initial dose
D/C if symptoms not controlled after 10 days at max dose of 20mg/day (diphenoxylate)	D/C if no improvement w/in 48 hrs

ADMINISTRATION
Oral route

Plastic dropper should be used when measuring liquid for administration to children

STORAGE
Dispense liquids in original container.

HOW SUPPLIED
(Diphenoxylate/Atropine) **Sol:** 2.5mg/0.025mg/5mL [60mL]; **Tab:** 2.5mg/0.025mg

CONTRAINDICATIONS
Known hypersensitivity to diphenoxylate or atropine, obstructive jaundice, diarrhea associated w/ pseudomembranous enterocolitis or enterotoxin-producing bacteria.

WARNINGS/PRECAUTIONS
Avoid in children <2 yrs. Overdosage may result in severe respiratory depression and coma, leading to brain damage or death. Avoid use with severe dehydration or electrolyte imbalance until corrective therapy is initiated. May induce toxic megacolon with acute ulcerative colitis; d/c if abdominal distention occurs or untoward symptoms develop. May cause intestinal fluid retention. Avoid with diarrhea associated with organisms that penetrate the intestinal mucosa, and with pseudomembranous enterocolitis. Extreme caution with advanced hepatorenal disease and liver dysfunction. Caution in pediatrics, especially with Down's syndrome.

ADVERSE REACTIONS
Numbness of extremities, dizziness, anaphylaxis, drowsiness, toxic megacolon, N/V, urticaria, pruritus, anorexia, pancreatitis, paralytic ileus, euphoria, malaise/lethargy.

DRUG INTERACTIONS
MAOIs may precipitate hypertensive crisis. (Diphenoxylate) May potentiate barbiturates, tranquilizers, and alcohol. Potential to prolong $T_{1/2}$ of drugs for which the rate of elimination is dependent on the microsomal drug metabolizing enzyme system.

PREGNANCY AND LACTATION
Category C, caution in nursing.

MECHANISM OF ACTION
Diphenoxylate: Antidiarrheal. Atropine: Anticholinergic.

PHARMACOKINETICS
Absorption: (4 tabs) C_{max}=163ng/mL; T_{max}=2 hrs. **Metabolism:** Rapid and extensive metabolism through ester hydrolysis to diphenoxylic acid (major metabolite). **Elimination:** Urine (14%), feces (49%). $T_{1/2}$=12-14 hrs (diphenoxylic acid).

PATIENT CONSIDERATIONS
Assessment: Assess for hypersensitivity, obstructive jaundice, diarrhea associated with pseudomembranous enterocolitis or enterotoxin-producing bacteria, severe dehydration, electrolyte imbalance, hepatic dysfunction, hepatorenal disease, ulcerative colitis, Down's syndrome, diarrhea (caused by *Escherichia coli*, *Salmonella*, *Shigella*), pregnancy/nursing status, and possible drug interactions.

Monitoring: Monitor for severe dehydration, electrolyte imbalance, renal function, toxic megacolon in ulcerative colitis, abdominal distention, signs of atropinism, and other adverse reactions.

Counseling: Instruct to take ud and not to exceed the recommended dosage. Inform of consequences of overdosage, including severe respiratory depression and coma, possibly leading to permanent brain damage or death. Instruct to exercise caution while operating machinery/driving. Advise to avoid alcohol and other CNS depressants. Advise to keep medicines out of reach of children. Inform patient that drowsiness or dizziness may occur.

LONSURF — tipiracil/trifluridine   Rx

Class: Thymidine phosphorylase inhibitor/nucleoside metabolic inhibitor

ADULT DOSAGE	PEDIATRIC DOSAGE
Metastatic Colorectal Cancer	Pediatric use may not have been established
Treatment of patients who have been previously treated w/ fluoropyrimidine-, oxaliplatin- and irinotecan-based chemotherapy, an anti-VEGF biological therapy, and if RAS wild-type, an anti-EGFR therapy	

Initial: 35mg/m²/dose bid on Days 1-5 and Days 8-12 of each 28-day cycle until disease progression or unacceptable toxicity
Max: 80mg/dose (based on the trifluridine component)
Round dose to the nearest 5mg increment

DOSING CONSIDERATIONS
Obtain CBC counts prior to and on Day 15 of each cycle

Do Not Initiate the Cycle Until:
ANC ≥1500/mm³ or febrile neutropenia is resolved
Platelets are ≥75,000/mm³
Grade 3 or 4 nonhematological adverse reactions are resolved to Grade 0 or 1

W/in a Treatment Cycle, Withhold for Any of the Following:
ANC <500/mm³ or febrile neutropenia
Platelets <50,000/mm³
Grade 3 or 4 nonhematological adverse reactions

After Recovery, Resume Therapy After Reducing the Dose by 5mg/m²/dose from the Previous Dose Level, if the Following Occur:
Febrile neutropenia
Uncomplicated Grade 4 neutropenia (which has recovered to ≥1500/mm³) or thrombocytopenia (which has recovered to ≥75,000/mm³) that results in >1 week delay in start of next cycle
Nonhematologic Grade 3 or Grade 4 adverse reaction except for Grade 3 nausea and/or vomiting controlled by antiemetic therapy or Grade 3 diarrhea responsive to antidiarrheal medication

Max of 3 dose reductions are permitted to a minimum dose of 20mg/m² bid. Do not escalate dose after it has been reduced.

ADMINISTRATION
Oral route
Take w/in 1 hr of completion of morning and evening meals.

STORAGE
20-25°C (68-77°F); excursions permitted to 15-30°C (59-86°F). If stored outside original bottle, discard after 30 days.

HOW SUPPLIED
Tab: (Trifluridine/Tipiracil) 15mg/6.14mg, 20mg/8.19mg

WARNINGS/PRECAUTIONS
Severe and life-threatening myelosuppression consisting of anemia, neutropenia, thrombocytopenia, and febrile neutropenia reported; obtain CBC counts prior to and on Day 15 of each cycle of therapy and more frequently as clinically indicated. May cause fetal harm. Females of reproductive potential should use effective contraception during treatment.

ADVERSE REACTIONS
Anemia, neutropenia, asthenia/fatigue, N/V, thrombocytopenia, decreased appetite, diarrhea, abdominal pain, pyrexia.

PREGNANCY AND LACTATION
Pregnancy: Based on animal data and the drug's mechanism of action, therapy may cause fetal harm.
Lactation: There are no data to assess effects of drug or its metabolites on the breastfed infant or the effects on milk production. Due to the potential for serious adverse reactions in breastfeeding infants, women should not breastfeed during treatment and for 1 day following the final dose.
Reproductive Potential: Females of reproductive potential should use effective contraception during treatment. Males w/ female partners of reproductive potential should use condoms during treatment and for at least 3 months after the final dose.

MECHANISM OF ACTION
Tipiracil: Thymidine phosphorylase inhibitor; increases trifluridine exposure by inhibiting its metabolism by thymidine phosphorylase. **Trifluridine:** Nucleoside metabolic inhibitor; following uptake into cancer cells, trifluridine is incorporated into DNA, interferes w/ DNA synthesis and inhibits cell proliferation.

PHARMACOKINETICS
Absorption: Trifluridine: T_{max}=2 hrs. **Distribution:** Trifluridine: Plasma protein binding (>96%). Tipiracil: Plasma protein binding (<8%). **Metabolism:** Trifluridine: Mainly via thymidine phosphorylase. **Elimination:** Trifluridine: Urine (1.5% unchanged, 19.2% metabolite); $T_{1/2}$=2.1 hrs. Tipiracil: Urine (29.3% unchanged); $T_{1/2}$=2.4 hrs.

PATIENT CONSIDERATIONS
Assessment: Assess pregnancy/nursing status. Obtain CBC counts prior to each cycle.
Monitoring: Monitor for adverse reactions. Obtain CBC counts on Day 15 of each cycle and more frequently as clinically indicated.
Counseling: Advise to immediately contact healthcare provider if patients experience signs/symptoms of infection and advise to keep all appointments for blood tests. Advise not to take additional doses to make up for missed or held doses. Instruct to contact healthcare provider for severe or persistent N/V, diarrhea, or abdominal pain. Instruct to take w/in 1 hr after eating am and pm meals. Inform patient that anyone else who handles the medication should wear gloves. Advise pregnant women of the potential risk to the fetus. Instruct females of reproductive potential to use effective contraception during treatment. Instruct males w/ female partners of reproductive potential to use condoms during treatment and for at least 3 months after the final dose. Advise women not to breastfeed during treatment and for 1 day following the final dose.

LOPERAMIDE HCL — loperamide hydrochloride

Rx

Class: Antidiarrheal

ADULT DOSAGE

Diarrhea

Control and symptomatic relief of diarrhea associated w/ inflammatory bowel disease. Also indicated for reducing the volume of discharge from ileostomies

Acute Nonspecific Diarrhea:
Initial: 4mg then 2mg after each unformed stool
Max: 16mg/day

Chronic Diarrhea:
4mg then 2mg after each unformed stool until diarrhea is controlled; reduce dose to meet the individual requirements. When optimal daily dosage has been established, may give as single or divided doses.
Maint: 4-8mg. If no clinical improvements after 16mg/day for at least 10 days, symptoms are unlikely to be controlled by further administration

May continue administration if diarrhea cannot be adequately controlled w/ diet or specific treatment

PEDIATRIC DOSAGE

Diarrhea

Control and symptomatic relief of diarrhea associated w/ inflammatory bowel disease. Also indicated for reducing the volume of discharge from ileostomies

Acute Diarrhea:
1st Day Dosage Schedule:
2-5 Years:
13-20kg: Use OTC liquid formulation
6-8 Years:
20-30kg:
Initial: 2mg bid
Max: 4mg/day
8-12 Years:
>30kg:
Initial: 2mg tid
Max: 6mg/day
Subsequent Daily Dosage:
After 1st treatment day, give subsequent doses (1mg/10kg) only after a loose stool

ADMINISTRATION

Oral route

STORAGE

20-25°C (68-77°F).

HOW SUPPLIED

Cap: 2mg

CONTRAINDICATIONS

Known hypersensitivity to loperamide HCl or to any of the excipients, abdominal pain in the absence of diarrhea, infants <24 months of age. As primary therapy for acute dysentery (characterized by blood in stool and high fever), acute ulcerative colitis, bacterial enterocolitis caused by invasive organism (including *Salmonella*, *Shigella*, *Campylobacter*), pseudomembranous colitis associated with broad-spectrum antibiotics.

WARNINGS/PRECAUTIONS

Use of drug does not preclude the need for appropriate fluid and electrolyte therapy. Do not use when inhibition of peristalsis is to be avoided due to possible risk of significant sequelae, including ileus, megacolon, and toxic megacolon. D/C promptly if constipation, abdominal distention, or ileus develop. Symptomatic treatment only; determine underlying etiology and treat when appropriate/indicated. AIDS patients treated for diarrhea should d/c therapy at earliest signs of abdominal distention; toxic megacolon reported with infectious colitis from viral/bacterial pathogens. Caution in young children; dehydration may influence variability of response to the drug. Extremely rare allergic reactions, including anaphylaxis and anaphylactic shock, reported. In acute diarrhea, d/c therapy if no improvement is observed in 48 hrs. Caution with hepatic impairment; monitor closely for signs of CNS toxicity.

ADVERSE REACTIONS

Constipation, nausea, abdominal cramps.

DRUG INTERACTIONS

Increased plasma levels with quinidine or ritonavir; caution when coadministered with P-gp inhibitors. Decreased saquinavir exposure; monitor closely for therapeutic efficacy of saquinavir.

PREGNANCY AND LACTATION

Category C, not for use in nursing.

MECHANISM OF ACTION

Antidiarrheal; prolongs the transit time of intestinal contents. Reduces the daily fecal volume, increases the viscosity and bulk density, and diminishes the loss of fluid and electrolytes.

PHARMACOKINETICS

Distribution: Found in breast milk. **Metabolism:** Oxidative N-demethylation (CYP2C8 and CYP3A4). **Elimination:** Feces; $T_{1/2}$=10.8 hrs.

PATIENT CONSIDERATIONS

Assessment: Assess for known hypersensitivity, abdominal pain in absence of diarrhea, acute dysentery, acute ulcerative colitis, bacterial enterocolitis, pseudomembranous colitis, fluid and electrolyte depletion, hepatic dysfunction, pregnancy/nursing status, and possible drug interactions.

Monitoring: Monitor for allergic reactions, constipation, abdominal distention, ileus, megacolon, and other adverse reactions.

Counseling: Counsel patient to notify physician if diarrhea does not improve in 48 hrs, has blood in stool, or if fever or abdominal distention develops. Advise that tiredness, dizziness, or drowsiness may occur in the setting of diarrheal syndromes; use caution when driving or operating machinery.

LOPID — gemfibrozil

Rx

Class: Fibric acid derivative

ADULT DOSAGE

Coronary Heart Disease

Adjunctive therapy to diet to reduce risk of developing coronary heart disease only in Type IIb patients w/o history of or symptoms of existing coronary heart disease who have had an inadequate response to weight loss, dietary therapy, exercise, and other pharmacologic agents and who have the triad of low HDL, elevated LDL, and elevated TG levels

1200mg in 2 divided doses 30 min before am and pm meals

Hypertriglyceridemia

Adjunctive therapy to diet for treatment of adults w/ very high elevations of serum TG levels (Types IV and V hyperlipidemia) who present a risk of pancreatitis and who do not respond adequately to diet

1200mg in 2 divided doses 30 min before am and pm meals

PEDIATRIC DOSAGE

Pediatric use may not have been established

ADMINISTRATION

Oral route

Take 30 min before am and pm meals.

STORAGE

20-25°C (68-77°F). Protect from light and humidity.

HOW SUPPLIED

Tab: 600mg* *scored

CONTRAINDICATIONS

Hepatic or severe renal dysfunction, including primary biliary cirrhosis; preexisting gallbladder disease; hypersensitivity to gemfibrozil; combination therapy w/ repaglinide, dasabuvir, or simvastatin.

WARNINGS/PRECAUTIONS

Cholelithiasis reported; perform gallbladder studies if cholelithiasis is suspected and d/c therapy if gallstones are found. May be associated w/ myositis; d/c if myositis is suspected/diagnosed. Control any medical problems (eg, diabetes mellitus [DM], hypothyroidism) that contribute to lipid abnormalities before initiating therapy. D/C if lipid response is inadequate after 3 months of therapy. Mild Hgb, Hct, and WBC count decreases, and severe anemia, leukopenia, thrombocytopenia, and bone marrow hypoplasia reported; periodically monitor blood counts during the first 12 months of therapy. Abnormal LFTs reported; periodically monitor LFTs and d/c if abnormalities persist. Worsening renal insufficiency reported upon the addition of therapy in patients w/ baseline plasma creatinine >2mg/dL. Estrogen therapy is associated w/ massive rises in plasma TGs; discontinuation of estrogen therapy may obviate the need for specific drug therapy of hypertriglyceridemia.

ADVERSE REACTIONS

Dyspepsia, abdominal pain, diarrhea, fatigue.

DRUG INTERACTIONS

See Contraindications. Caution w/ anticoagulants; reduce anticoagulant dose and frequently monitor prothrombin until it has been definitely determined that prothrombin level has stabilized. Increased risk of myopathy and rhabdomyolysis w/ HMG-CoA reductase inhibitors. Reduced exposure w/ resin-granule drugs (eg, colestipol); administer ≥2 hrs apart. May potentiate myopathy w/ colchicine; caution when prescribing w/ colchicine, especially in elderly patients or patients w/ renal dysfunction. May increase exposure of CYP2C8 or OATP1B1 substrates; dose reduction of substrates may be required.

PREGNANCY AND LACTATION

Pregnancy: Category C.
Lactation: Not for use in nursing.

MECHANISM OF ACTION

Fibric acid derivative; not established. Inhibits peripheral lipolysis and decreases hepatic extraction of free fatty acids, thus reducing hepatic TG production. Inhibits synthesis and increases clearance of VLDL carrier apolipoprotein B, leading to a decrease in VLDL production.

PHARMACOKINETICS

Absorption: Complete. T_{max}=1-2 hrs. **Distribution:** Plasma protein binding (highly bound). **Metabolism:** Oxidation to form a hydroxymethyl and a carboxyl metabolite. **Elimination:** Urine (70%, <2% unchanged), feces (6%).

PATIENT CONSIDERATIONS

Assessment: Assess for hepatic/renal dysfunction, gallbladder disease, other medical conditions (eg, DM, hypothyroidism), hypersensitivity to drug, pregnancy/nursing status, and possible drug interactions. Obtain lipid levels.

Monitoring: Monitor for signs/symptoms of cholelithiasis, myositis, worsening renal insufficiency, and other adverse reactions. Periodically monitor serum lipids levels, CBC, and LFTs. Frequently monitor prothrombin w/ anticoagulants. Closely observe patients w/ significantly elevated TGs during therapy.

Counseling: Inform about potential risks/benefits of therapy. Advise to report to physician any muscle pain/tenderness/weakness, or other adverse reactions. Instruct to notify physician if pregnant/nursing or planning to become pregnant.

LORAZEPAM ORAL — lorazepam   CIV

Class: Benzodiazepine

OTHER BRAND NAMES
Ativan

ADULT DOSAGE
Anxiety Disorders

Anxiety Disorders or Short-Term Relief of Symptoms of Anxiety or Anxiety Associated w/ Depressive Symptoms:
Initial: 2-3mg/day given bid or tid
Usual: 2-6mg/day in divided doses; take largest dose before hs
Dosage Range: 1-10mg/day

Increase dose gradually prn; when higher dosage is indicated, increase pm dose before daytime doses

Insomnia Due to Anxiety or Transient Situational Stress:
2-4mg as a single daily dose qhs

PEDIATRIC DOSAGE
Anxiety Disorders

Anxiety Disorders or Short-Term Relief of Symptoms of Anxiety or Anxiety Associated w/ Depressive Symptoms:
≥12 Years:
Initial: 2-3mg/day given bid or tid
Usual: 2-6mg/day in divided doses; take largest dose before hs
Dosage Range: 1-10mg/day

Increase dose gradually prn; when higher dosage is indicated, increase pm dose before daytime doses

Insomnia Due to Anxiety or Transient Situational Stress:
2-4mg as a single daily dose qhs

DOSING CONSIDERATIONS
Elderly
Elderly/Debilitated:
Initial: 1-2mg/day in divided doses; adjust prn and as tolerated

ADMINISTRATION
Oral route

Sol
Dispense only in the bottle and only w/ the calibrated dropper provided. Mix w/ liquid or semi-solid food for a few sec; Intensol formulation blends quickly and completely.
Entire amount of mixture, of drug and liquid or drug and food, should be consumed immediately.

STORAGE
(Sol) 2-8°C (36-46°F). Protect from light. Discard opened bottle after 90 days.
(Tab) 25°C (77°F); excursions permitted to 15-30°C (59-86°F).

HOW SUPPLIED
Sol: 2mg/mL; **Tab:** (Ativan) 0.5mg, 1mg*, 2mg* *scored

CONTRAINDICATIONS
Hypersensitivity to benzodiazepines or to any components of the formulation, acute narrow-angle glaucoma.

WARNINGS/PRECAUTIONS
Effectiveness in long-term use (>4 months) has not been assessed; prescribe for short periods only (eg, 2-4 weeks) and periodically reassess usefulness of drug. Continuous long-term use is not recommended. Preexisting depression may emerge or worsen; not for use with primary depressive disorder or psychosis. May lead to potentially fatal respiratory depression. May impair mental/physical abilities. Use may lead to physical and psychological dependence; increased risk with higher doses, longer term use, and in patients with history of alcoholism/drug abuse, or with significant personality disorders. Withdrawal symptoms reported; avoid abrupt d/c and follow a gradual dosage-tapering schedule after extended therapy. May develop tolerance to sedative effects. Paradoxical reactions reported; d/c if these occur. May have abuse potential, especially with a history of drug and/or alcohol abuse. Possible suicide in patients with depression; do not use in such patients without adequate antidepressant therapy. Caution with compromised respiratory function (eg, COPD, sleep apnea syndrome), impaired renal/hepatic function, hepatic encephalopathy, in elderly, and in debilitated patients. May worsen hepatic encephalopathy. Adjust dose with severe hepatic insufficiency; lower doses may be sufficient. Monitor frequently for symptoms of upper GI disease. Leukopenia and elevations of lactate dehydrogenase reported; perform periodic blood counts and LFTs with long-term therapy.

ADVERSE REACTIONS
Sedation, dizziness, weakness, unsteadiness.

DRUG INTERACTIONS
Increased CNS-depressant effects with other CNS depressants (eg, alcohol, barbiturates, antipsychotics, sedative/hypnotics, anxiolytics, antidepressants, narcotic analgesics, sedative antihistamines, anticonvulsants, anesthetics); may lead to potentially fatal respiratory depression. Concomitant use with clozapine may produce marked sedation, excessive salivation, hypotension, ataxia, delirium, and respiratory arrest. Increased plasma concentrations with valproate and more rapid onset or prolonged effect with probenecid; reduce dose by 50%. Decreased sedative effects with theophylline or aminophylline.

PREGNANCY AND LACTATION
Not for use in pregnancy/nursing.

MECHANISM OF ACTION
Benzodiazepine; has a tranquilizing action on the CNS with no appreciable effect on the respiratory or cardiovascular systems.

PHARMACOKINETICS
Absorption: Readily absorbed. Absolute bioavailability (90%); (2mg) C_{max}=20ng/mL; T_{max}=2 hrs. **Distribution:** Plasma protein binding (85%); found in breast milk. **Metabolism:** Glucuronidation. **Elimination:** Urine; $T_{1/2}$=12 hrs.

PATIENT CONSIDERATIONS
Assessment: Assess for acute narrow-angle glaucoma, primary depressive disorder, psychosis, personality disorders, compromised respiratory function, impaired renal/hepatic function, hepatic encephalopathy, history of alcohol/drug abuse, previous hypersensitivity to the drug, pregnancy/nursing status, and possible drug interactions.

Monitoring: Monitor for respiratory depression, physical/psychological dependence, withdrawal symptoms, tolerance, abuse, suicidal thinking, paradoxical reactions, symptoms of upper GI disease, and emergence/worsening of depression. Reassess usefulness of drug periodically. Monitor elderly/debilitated frequently and addiction-prone individuals carefully. Perform periodic blood counts and LFTs with long-term therapy.

Counseling: Inform that psychological/physical dependence may occur; instruct to consult physician before increasing dose or abruptly d/c drug. Warn not to operate dangerous machinery or motor vehicles and that tolerance for alcohol and other CNS depressants will be diminished. Advise to consult physician if pregnancy occurs.

LORCET — acetaminophen/hydrocodone bitartrate   CII

Class: Opioid analgesic

> Associated with cases of acute liver failure, at times resulting in liver transplant and death. Most cases of liver injury are associated with acetaminophen (APAP) use at doses >4000 mg/day and often involve >1 APAP-containing product.

OTHER BRAND NAMES
Lorcet Plus, Lorcet HD

ADULT DOSAGE
Moderate to Moderately Severe Pain

Lorcet 5mg/325mg:
Usual: 1-2 tabs q4-6h
Max: 12 tabs/day

Lorcet Plus 7.5mg/325mg:
Usual: 1 tab q4-6h
Max: 6 tabs/day

Lorcet HD 10mg/325mg:
Usual: 1 tab q4-6h
Max: 6 tabs/day

Adjust dose according to the severity of pain and response of the patient

PEDIATRIC DOSAGE
Pediatric use may not have been established

ADMINISTRATION
Oral route

STORAGE
20-25°C (68-77°F).

HOW SUPPLIED
Tab: (Hydrocodone/APAP) 5mg/325mg*, (Plus) 7.5mg/325mg*, (HD) 10mg/325mg* *scored

CONTRAINDICATIONS
Prior hypersensitivity to hydrocodone or acetaminophen; known hypersensitivity to other opioids.

WARNINGS/PRECAUTIONS
Increased risk of acute liver failure in patients with underlying liver disease. May cause serious skin reactions (eg, acute generalized exanthematous pustulosis, Stevens-Johnson syndrome, toxic epidermal necrolysis), which can be fatal; d/c at the 1st appearance of skin rash or any other sign of hypersensitivity. Hypersensitivity and anaphylaxis reported; d/c immediately if signs/symptoms occur. May produce dose-related respiratory depression at high doses and irregular/periodic breathing. Respiratory depressant effects and CSF pressure elevation capacity may be markedly exaggerated in the presence of head injury, other intracranial lesions, or a preexisting increase in intracranial pressure. May obscure diagnosis or clinical course of acute abdominal conditions or head injuries. Caution in with severe hepatic/renal impairment, hypothyroidism, Addison's disease, prostatic hypertrophy, urethral stricture, or in elderly/debilitated. Suppresses the cough reflex; caution with pulmonary disease and in postoperative use. Physical dependence and tolerance may develop. Lab test interactions may occur.

ADVERSE REACTIONS
Acute liver failure, dizziness, lightheadedness, sedation, N/V.

DRUG INTERACTIONS
Additive CNS depression with other narcotics, antianxiety agents, antihistamines, antipsychotics, other CNS depressants (eg, alcohol); reduce dose of one or both agents. Concomitant use with MAOIs or TCAs may increase the effect of either the antidepressant or hydrocodone. Increased risk of acute liver failure with alcohol ingestion.

PREGNANCY AND LACTATION
Category C, not for use in nursing.

MECHANISM OF ACTION

Hydrocodone: Opioid analgesic; has not been established. Suspected to relate to existence of opiate receptors in the CNS. APAP: Nonopiate, nonsalicylate analgesic and antipyretic; has not been established. Antipyretic activity is mediated through hypothalamic heat regulating centers; inhibits prostaglandin synthetase.

PHARMACOKINETICS

Absorption: Hydrocodone: (10mg) C_{max}=23.6ng/mL; T_{max}=1.3 hrs. APAP: Rapid. **Distribution:** APAP: Found in breast milk. **Metabolism:** Hydrocodone: O-demethylation, N-demethylation, and 6-keto reduction. APAP: Liver (conjugation). **Elimination:** Hydrocodone: (10mg) $T_{1/2}$=3.8 hrs. APAP: Urine (85%); $T_{1/2}$=1.25-3 hrs.

PATIENT CONSIDERATIONS

Assessment: Assess for level of pain intensity, type of pain, patient's general condition and medical status, or any other conditions where treatment is contraindicated or cautioned. Assess for history of hypersensitivity, pregnancy/nursing status, renal/hepatic dysfunction, and possible drug interactions.

Monitoring: Monitor for acute liver failure, skin/hypersensitivity/anaphylactic reactions, respiratory depression, elevations in CSF pressure, drug dependence, tolerance, and drug abuse. In patients with severe hepatic/renal disease, monitor serial hepatic and/or renal function tests.

Counseling: Advise to d/c and contact physician if signs of allergy develop. Instruct to look for APAP on package labels and not to use >1 APAP-containing product. Instruct to seek immediate medical attention upon ingestion of >4000mg/day of APAP, even if feeling well. Inform that drug may impair mental/physical abilities, and to use caution if performing potentially hazardous tasks (eg, driving, operating machinery). Instruct to avoid alcohol and other CNS depressants. Inform that drug may be habit-forming; instruct to take only ud.

LORTAB — acetaminophen/hydrocodone bitartrate

Class: Opioid analgesic

CII

> Associated w/ cases of acute liver failure, at times resulting in liver transplant and death. Most cases of liver injury are associated w/ acetaminophen (APAP) use at doses >4000mg/day and often involve >1 APAP-containing product.

OTHER BRAND NAMES

Hycet

ADULT DOSAGE

Moderate to Moderately Severe Pain

Hycet:
Usual: 1 tbsp q4-6h prn
Max: 6 tbsp/day

Lortab Elixir:
Usual: 11.25mL q4-6h prn
Max: 67.5mL/day

Lortab Tab:
5mg/325mg Strength:
Usual: 1 or 2 tabs q4-6h prn
Max: 12 tabs/day

7.5mg/325mg or 10mg/325mg Strengths:
Usual: 1 tab q4-6h prn
Max: 6 tabs/day

PEDIATRIC DOSAGE

Moderate to Moderately Severe Pain

Hycet:
12-15kg (2-3 Years):
3.75mL q4-6h prn
Max: 22.5mL/day

16-22kg (4-6 Years):
5mL q4-6h prn
Max: 30mL/day

23-31kg (7-9 Years):
7.5mL q4-6h prn
Max: 45mL/day

32-45kg (10-13 Years):
10mL q4-6h prn
Max: 60mL/day

≥46kg (≥14 Years):
15mL q4-6h prn
Max: 90mL/day

Lortab Elixir:
12-15kg (2-3 Years):
2.8mL q4-6h prn
Max: 16.8mL/day

16-22kg (4-6 Years):
3.75mL q4-6h prn
Max: 22.5mL/day

23-31kg (7-9 Years):
5.6mL q4-6h prn
Max: 33.6mL/day

32-45kg (10-13 Years):
7.5mL q4-6h prn
Max: 45mL/day

≥46kg (≥14 Years):
11.25mL q4-6h prn
Max: 67.5mL/day

DOSING CONSIDERATIONS

Elderly
Start at lower end of dosing range

ADMINISTRATION

Oral route

Hycet/Lortab Elixir
Administer using a calibrated measuring device

STORAGE

(Sol) 20-25°C (68-77°F). (Tab) 25°C (77°F); excursions permitted to 15-30°C (59-86°F).

HOW SUPPLIED

(Hydrocodone/APAP) Sol: (Hycet) (7.5mg/325mg)/15mL [473mL], (Lortab Elixir) (10mg/300mg)/15mL [473mL]; **Tab:** (Lortab) 5mg/325mg*, 7.5mg/325mg*, 10mg/325mg* *scored

CONTRAINDICATIONS

Prior hypersensitivity to hydrocodone, acetaminophen, or any other component of this product and known hypersensitivity to other opioids.

WARNINGS/PRECAUTIONS

Caution w/ severe hepatic/renal impairment, hypothyroidism, Addison's disease, prostatic hypertrophy, urethral stricture, or in the elderly/debilitated. APAP: Increased risk of acute liver failure in patients w/ underlying liver disease. Hypersensitivity and anaphylaxis reported; d/c if signs/symptoms occur. May cause serious skin reactions (eg, acute generalized exanthematous pustulosis, Stevens-Johnson syndrome, toxic epidermal necrolysis); d/c at the 1st appearance of skin rash or any other sign of hypersensitivity. Lab test interactions may occur. Hydrocodone: May produce dose-related respiratory depression and irregular/periodic breathing. Respiratory depressant effects and CSF pressure elevation capacity may be exaggerated in the presence of head injury, other intracranial lesions, or preexisting increase in intracranial pressure. May obscure diagnosis or clinical course of acute abdominal conditions and clinical course of head injuries. Suppresses cough reflex; caution w/ pulmonary disease and in postoperative use. May be habit-forming. Physical dependence and tolerance may develop. Potential for abuse. Infants may have increased sensitivity to respiratory depressant effects of opioids; if use is contemplated, administer cautiously, in substantially reduced initial doses, by personnel experienced in administering opioids to infants, and w/ intensive monitoring.

ADVERSE REACTIONS

Acute liver failure, bradycardia, dizziness, sedation, N/V.

DRUG INTERACTIONS

Additive CNS depression w/ other narcotics, antihistamines, antipsychotics, antianxiety agents, or other CNS depressants (eg, alcohol); reduce dose of 1 or both agents. Hydrocodone: Concomitant use w/ MAOIs or TCAs may increase the effect of either the antidepressant or hydrocodone. APAP: Increased risk of acute liver failure w/ alcohol.

PREGNANCY AND LACTATION

Category C, not for use in nursing.

MECHANISM OF ACTION

Hydrocodone: Opioid analgesic and antitussive; has not been established. Action believed to be related to the existence of opiate receptors in CNS. APAP: Nonopiate, nonsalicylate analgesic and antipyretic; has not been established. Antipyretic activity is mediated through hypothalamic heat-regulating centers; inhibits prostaglandin synthetase.

PHARMACOKINETICS

Absorption: Hydrocodone: (10mg) C_{max}=23.6ng/mL; T_{max}=1.3 hrs. APAP: Rapid. **Distribution:** Hydrocodone: Crosses the placenta. APAP: Found in breast milk. **Metabolism:** Hydrocodone: O-demethylation, N-demethylation, and 6-keto reduction. APAP: Liver (conjugation). **Elimination:** Hydrocodone: $T_{1/2}$=3.8 hrs. APAP: Urine (85%); $T_{1/2}$=1.25-3 hrs.

PATIENT CONSIDERATIONS

Assessment: Assess for history of hypersensitivity to drug, level of pain intensity, type of pain, patient's general condition and medical status, renal/hepatic impairment, pregnancy/nursing status, any other conditions where treatment is contraindicated or cautioned, and possible drug interactions.

Monitoring: Monitor for signs/symptoms of hypersensitivity or anaphylaxis, serious skin reactions, respiratory depression, elevations in CSF pressure, drug dependence, tolerance, abuse, and other adverse reactions. In patients w/ severe hepatic/renal disease, monitor effects w/ serial hepatic and/or renal function tests.

Counseling: Instruct to look for APAP on package labels and not to use >1 APAP-containing product. Instruct to seek medical attention immediately upon ingestion of >4000mg/day APAP, even if feeling well. Advise to d/c and contact physician if signs of allergy develop. Inform that drug may impair mental/physical abilities; instruct to avoid potentially hazardous tasks (eg, operating machinery, driving). Instruct to avoid alcohol and other CNS depressants. Inform that drug may be habit-forming; instruct to take only ud.

LORZONE — chlorzoxazone

Class: Muscular analgesic (centrally acting)

Rx

ADULT DOSAGE

Musculoskeletal Conditions

Adjunct to rest, physical therapy, and other measures for relief of discomfort associated w/ acute, painful musculoskeletal conditions

375mg Tab:
Usual: 1 tab tid or qid
Titrate: May increase to 2 tabs (750mg) tid or qid if adequate response is not obtained

Dosage can be reduced as improvement occurs

PEDIATRIC DOSAGE

Pediatric use may not have been established

750mg Tab:
Usual: 1/3 tab (250mg) tid or qid. Give 2/3 tab (500mg) tid or qid for painful musculoskeletal conditions
Titrate: May increase to 1 tab (750mg) tid or qid if adequate response is not obtained

Dosage can be reduced as improvement occurs

ADMINISTRATION
Oral route

STORAGE
20-25°C (68-77°F).

HOW SUPPLIED
Tab: 375mg, 750mg

CONTRAINDICATIONS
Known intolerance to the drug.

WARNINGS/PRECAUTIONS
Serious (including fatal) hepatocellular toxicity reported rarely; d/c immediately if any signs/symptoms of hepatotoxicity or abnormal liver enzymes develop. Caution w/ known allergies or w/ history of allergic reactions to drugs; d/c if a sensitivity reaction occurs.

ADVERSE REACTIONS
Drowsiness, dizziness, lightheadedness, malaise, overstimulation.

DRUG INTERACTIONS
May have additive effect w/ alcohol or other CNS depressants.

PREGNANCY AND LACTATION
Safety not known in pregnancy/nursing.

MECHANISM OF ACTION
Muscular analgesic (centrally acting); acts primarily at the level of the spinal cord and subcortical areas of the brain where it inhibits multisynaptic reflex arcs involved in producing and maintaining skeletal muscle spasm of varied etiology.

PHARMACOKINETICS
Absorption: T_{max}=1-2 hrs. **Metabolism:** Rapid; glucuronidation. **Elimination:** Urine (<1% unchanged).

PATIENT CONSIDERATIONS
Assessment: Assess for intolerance to chlorzoxazone, known allergies or history of allergic reactions to drugs, hepatic impairment, pregnancy/nursing status, and possible drug interactions.

Monitoring: Monitor for signs/symptoms of hepatotoxicity, sensitivity reactions, and other adverse reactions. Monitor LFTs.

Counseling: Inform of the risks and benefits of therapy. Instruct to d/c immediately and contact physician if signs/symptoms of hepatotoxicity (eg, fever, rash, right upper quadrant pain, dark urine) or a sensitivity reaction (eg, urticaria, redness, itching of the skin) occur.

LOTEMAX GEL AND OINTMENT — loteprednol etabonate Rx

Class: Corticosteroid

ADULT DOSAGE
Ocular Pain and Inflammation

Gel:
Apply 1-2 drops into the conjunctival sac of affected eye qid, beginning the day after surgery and continuing throughout the first 2 weeks of postoperative period

Oint:
Apply a small amount (1/2-inch ribbon) into the conjunctival sac(s) qid, beginning 24 hrs after surgery and continuing throughout the first 2 weeks of postoperative period

PEDIATRIC DOSAGE
Pediatric use may not have been established

ADMINISTRATION
Ocular route

Gel
Invert closed bottle and shake once to fill tip before instilling drops

STORAGE
15-25°C (59-77°F). (Gel) Store upright.

HOW SUPPLIED
Gel: 0.5% [5g] **Oint:** 0.5% [3.5g]

CONTRAINDICATIONS
Most viral diseases of the cornea and conjunctiva (eg, epithelial herpes simplex keratitis [dendritic keratitis], vaccinia, varicella), mycobacterial infection of the eye and fungal diseases of ocular structures.

WARNINGS/PRECAUTIONS
Prolonged use may result in glaucoma with optic nerve damage, defects in visual acuity, and fields of vision. Monitor intraocular pressure (IOP) if used for ≥10 days. May result in posterior subcapsular cataract formation. May delay healing and increase the incidence of bleb formation after cataract surgery. Perforations reported with diseases causing thinning of cornea/sclera. Initial prescription and renewal of medication order should only be made after examination of the patient with aid of magnification (eg, slit lamp biomicroscopy) and, where appropriate, fluorescein staining. Prolonged use may suppress host response and increase hazard of secondary ocular infections. May mask or enhance existing infection in acute purulent conditions of the eye. Caution with history of herpes simplex; may prolong course and exacerbate severity of many viral infections of the eye. Fungal infections of the cornea may develop coincidentally with long-term use; consider fungal invasion in any persistent corneal ulceration and take fungal cultures when appropriate. Avoid wearing contact lenses. Caution with glaucoma. (Oint) Reevaluate if signs and symptoms fail to improve after 2 days. Not to be used in children following ocular surgery; may interfere with amblyopia treatment. Not for intraocular administration.

ADVERSE REACTIONS
Anterior chamber inflammation, eye pain. (Gel) Foreign body sensation. (Oint) Conjunctival hyperemia, corneal edema.

PREGNANCY AND LACTATION
Category C, caution in nursing.

MECHANISM OF ACTION
Corticosteroid; inhibits inflammatory response to a variety of inciting agents and probably delays or slows healing. Thought to inhibit prostaglandin production through several independent mechanisms

PHARMACOKINETICS
Metabolism: (Gel) Extensive.

PATIENT CONSIDERATIONS
Assessment: Assess for viral diseases of cornea and conjunctiva, mycobacterial infection of the eye, fungal diseases of ocular structures, history of herpes simplex, thinning of the cornea/sclera, cataract surgery, glaucoma, and pregnancy/nursing status. Perform examination of patient with the aid of magnification (eg, slit lamp biomicroscopy, fluorescein staining).

Monitoring: Monitor for glaucoma with damage to the optic nerve, defects in visual acuity and fields of vision, posterior subcapsular cataract formation, perforation of cornea/sclera, secondary ocular infections, fungal infections, masking of existing infections, and other adverse reactions. Monitor IOP during prolonged use (≥10 days). Perform examination with the aid of magnification before renewal of order (Oint) beyond 14 days. (Oint) Reevaluate if signs/symptoms fail to improve after 2 days.

Counseling: Advise not to wear contact lenses during therapy and to consult physician if pain develops, or if redness, itching, or inflammation becomes aggravated. (Oint) Advise not to touch the eyelid or surrounding areas with the tip of the tube; instruct to keep cap on the tube when not in use. Advise to wash hands prior to use. (Gel) Instruct to invert closed bottle and to shake once to fill tip before instilling drops. Advise not to allow the dropper tip to touch any surface, as this may contaminate the gel.

LOTEMAX SUSPENSION — loteprednol etabonate Rx

Class: Corticosteroid

ADULT DOSAGE
Steroid-Responsive Inflammatory Ocular Conditions

Treatment of palpebral and bulbar conjunctiva, cornea, and anterior segment of the globe, such as allergic conjunctivitis, acne rosacea, superficial punctate keratitis, herpes zoster keratitis, iritis, cyclitis, and selected infective conjunctivitides

Apply 1-2 drops into the conjunctival sac of the affected eye(s) qid; may increase up to 1 drop qh, if necessary, during initial treatment w/in the 1st week

Reevaluate if signs/symptoms fail to improve after 2 days

Postoperative Inflammation

Apply 1-2 drops into the conjunctival sac of the operated eye(s) qid beginning 24 hrs after surgery, and continuing throughout the first 2 weeks of the postoperative period

PEDIATRIC DOSAGE
Pediatric use may not have been established

ADMINISTRATION
Ocular route

Shake vigorously before use

STORAGE
15-25°C (59-77°F); store upright. Do not freeze.

HOW SUPPLIED
Sus: 0.5% [5mL, 10mL, 15mL]

CONTRAINDICATIONS
Most viral diseases of the cornea and conjunctiva (eg, epithelial herpes simplex keratitis [dendritic keratitis], vaccinia, varicella), mycobacterial infection of the

eye, fungal diseases of ocular structures, known or suspected hypersensitivity to any of the ingredients of this preparation and to other corticosteroids.

WARNINGS/PRECAUTIONS

For ophthalmic use only. Prolonged use may result in glaucoma with damage to the optic nerve, defects in visual acuity and fields of vision, and in posterior subcapsular cataract formation; caution with glaucoma. Prolonged use may suppress host response and increase hazard of secondary ocular infections. Perforations reported with diseases causing thinning of cornea/sclera. May mask or enhance existing infection in acute purulent conditions of the eye. Caution with history of herpes simplex; may prolong course and exacerbate severity of many viral infections of the eye. May delay healing and increase incidence of bleb formation after cataract surgery. Initial prescription and renewal of medication order beyond 14 days should only be made after examination of the patient with aid of magnification (eg, slit-lamp biomicroscopy) and, where appropriate, fluorescein staining. Monitor IOP if used for ≥10 days. Fungal infections of the cornea may develop coincidentally with long-term use; consider fungal invasion in any persistent corneal ulceration and take fungal cultures when appropriate. For steroid-responsive diseases, caution not to d/c therapy prematurely. Should not be used for acute anterior uveitis in patients who require a more potent corticosteroid.

ADVERSE REACTIONS

Abnormal vision/blurring, burning on instillation, chemosis, discharge, dry eyes, epiphora, foreign body sensation, itching, photophobia, headache, rhinitis, pharyngitis.

PREGNANCY AND LACTATION

Category C, caution in nursing.

MECHANISM OF ACTION

Corticosteroid; mechanism not been established. Thought to act by the induction of phospholipase A$_2$ inhibitory proteins, which control the biosynthesis of potent mediators of inflammation such as prostaglandins and leukotrienes.

PATIENT CONSIDERATIONS

Assessment: Assess for previous drug hypersensitivity, viral diseases of the cornea and conjunctiva, mycobacterial infection of the eye, fungal diseases of ocular structures, glaucoma, thinning of the cornea/sclera, history of herpes simplex, and pregnancy/nursing status. Perform examination of patient with the aid of magnification (eg, slit-lamp biomicroscopy, fluorescein staining). Assess use in patients who have undergone recent cataract surgery.

Monitoring: Monitor for glaucoma and its complications, defects in visual acuity and fields of vision, posterior subcapsular cataract formation, perforation of the cornea/sclera, secondary ocular infections, fungal infections, masking of existing infections, and other adverse reactions. Reevaluate if signs/symptoms fail to improve after 2 days. Monitor IOP during prolonged use (≥10 days). Perform examination of patient with the aid of magnification (eg, slit-lamp biomicroscopy, fluorescein staining) before renewal of medication order beyond 14 days.

Counseling: Advise not to allow dropper tip to touch any surface to avoid contamination of sus. Instruct to consult physician if pain develops or if redness, itching, or inflammation becomes aggravated. Inform not to wear soft contact lenses during treatment.

LOTENSIN HCT — benazepril hydrochloride/ hydrochlorothiazide

Class: ACE inhibitor/thiazide diuretic

Rx

> D/C when pregnancy is detected. Drugs that act directly on the renin-angiotensin system (RAS) can cause injury/death to the developing fetus.

ADULT DOSAGE

Hypertension

Uncontrolled BP on Benazepril or HCTZ Alone:
Initial: 10mg/12.5mg qd
Titrate: May increase after 2-3 weeks prn to help achieve BP goals
Max: 20mg/25mg
Replacement Therapy: May be substituted for the titrated individual components

PEDIATRIC DOSAGE

Pediatric use may not have been established

ADMINISTRATION

Oral route

STORAGE

≤30°C (86°F). Protect from moisture and light.

HOW SUPPLIED

Tab: (Benazepril/HCTZ) 5mg/6.25mg*, 10mg/12.5mg*, 20mg/12.5mg*, 20mg/25mg* *scored

CONTRAINDICATIONS

Anuria; hypersensitivity to benazepril, to any other ACE inhibitor, to hydrochlorothiazide, or to other sulfonamide-derived drugs; history of angioedema w/ or w/o previous ACE inhibitor treatment. Coadministration w/ aliskiren in patients w/ diabetes.

WARNINGS/PRECAUTIONS

Not for initial therapy of HTN. Head/neck angioedema reported; d/c and institute appropriate therapy immediately. Higher incidence of angioedema in blacks than nonblacks. Intestinal angioedema reported; monitor for abdominal pain. Anaphylactoid reactions reported during desensitization with hymenoptera venom, dialysis with high-flux membranes, and LDL apheresis with dextran sulfate absorption. Symptomatic hypotension may occur, most likely in patients with volume and/or salt depletion; correct depletion before initiating therapy. Enhanced effects in postsympathectomy patients. Excessive hypotension, which may be associated with oliguria, azotemia, and (rarely) with acute renal failure and death, may occur in patients with CHF; monitor closely during first 2 weeks of therapy and whenever dose is increased. May cause changes in renal function, including renal failure; consider withholding or discontinuing therapy if clinically significant decrease in renal function develops. May increase BUN or SrCr in patients with renal artery stenosis. May cause agranulocytosis and bone marrow depression. Associated with syndrome that starts with cholestatic jaundice and progresses to fulminant hepatic necrosis and sometimes death (rare); d/c if jaundice or marked hepatic enzyme elevations develop. May cause exacerbation or activation of systemic lupus erythematosus (SLE). May cause idiosyncratic reaction, resulting in acute transient myopia and acute angle-closure glaucoma; d/c as rapidly as possible. May cause serum electrolyte abnormalities. Persistent nonproductive cough reported. Hypotension may occur with surgery or during anesthesia. May decrease serum protein-bound iodine levels without signs of thyroid disturbance. D/C before testing for parathyroid function. **HCTZ:** May alter glucose tolerance and raise serum cholesterol and TG levels. May cause or exacerbate hyperuricemia and precipitate gout. May elevate serum Ca^{2+}; avoid with hypercalcemia. May precipitate hepatic coma in patients with hepatic impairment or progressive liver disease.

ADVERSE REACTIONS

Dizziness, fatigue, postural dizziness, headache.

DRUG INTERACTIONS

See Contraindications. Caution with other antihypertensives. May affect K$^+$ levels with K$^+$ supplements and K$^+$-sparing diuretics; monitor K$^+$ periodically. Increased lithium levels and lithium toxicity reported; monitor lithium levels. Dual blockade of the RAS is associated with increased risks of hypotension, hyperkalemia, and changes in renal function (including acute renal failure); closely monitor BP, renal function, and electrolytes with concomitant agents that also affect the RAS. Avoid aliskiren in patients with renal impairment (GFR <60mL/min). NSAIDs, including selective COX-2 inhibitors, may attenuate antihypertensive effect and may cause deterioration of renal function. **Benazepril:** Nitritoid reactions reported with injectable gold. **HCTZ:** May potentiate action of other antihypertensives, especially ganglionic/peripheral adrenergic-blocking drugs. Cholestyramine and colestipol resins reduce absorption from GI tract; administer at least 4 hrs before or 4-6 hrs after administration of resins. Drug-induced hypokalemia or hypomagnesemia may predispose patient to digoxin toxicity. May increase responsiveness to skeletal muscle relaxants (eg, curare derivatives). Dosage adjustment of antidiabetic drugs may be required. May reduce renal excretion of cytotoxic agents (eg, cyclophosphamide, methotrexate) and enhance their myelosuppressive effects. Anticholinergics (eg, atropine, biperiden) may increase bioavailability due to decrease in GI motility and stomach emptying rate. Prokinetic drugs may decrease bioavailability. Increased risk of hyperuricemia and gout-type complications with cyclosporine. May potentiate orthostatic hypotension with alcohol, barbiturates, or narcotics. May reduce response to pressor amines (eg, noradrenaline).

PREGNANCY AND LACTATION

Category D, not for use in nursing.

MECHANISM OF ACTION

Benazepril: ACE inhibitor; decreases plasma angiotensin II, which leads to decreased vasopressor activity and aldosterone secretion. HCTZ: Thiazide diuretic; has not been established. Affects renal tubular mechanisms of electrolyte reabsorption, directly increasing excretion of Na$^+$ and Cl$^-$.

PHARMACOKINETICS

Absorption: Benazepril: T$_{max}$=0.5-1 hr, 1-2 hrs (benazeprilat, fasting), 2-4 hrs (benazeprilat, nonfasting). HCTZ: Absolute bioavailability (70%); T$_{max}$=2-5 hrs.
Distribution: Found in breast milk; crosses placenta. Benazepril: Plasma protein binding (96.7%, 95.3% benazeprilat). HCTZ: Plasma protein binding (40-70%).
Metabolism: Benazepril: Liver, cleavage of ester group; benazeprilat (active metabolite). **Elimination:** Benazepril: Urine (trace amounts, unchanged; 20%, benazeprilat), bile (11-12%, benazeprilat); T$_{1/2}$=10-11 hrs (benazeprilat). HCTZ: Urine (70%, unchanged); T$_{1/2}$=10 hrs.

PATIENT CONSIDERATIONS

Assessment: Assess for anuria, sulfonamide-derived drug hypersensitivity, history of angioedema/allergy/asthma, risk factors for angle-closure glaucoma, volume/salt depletion, CHF, collagen vascular diseases, SLE, hypercalcemia, diabetes, renal/hepatic impairment, postsympathectomy status, pregnancy/nursing status, and possible drug interactions.

Monitoring: Monitor for angioedema, anaphylactoid reactions, exacerbation/activation of SLE, myopia, angle-closure glaucoma, hyperuricemia or precipitation of gout, and other adverse reactions. Monitor BP, LFTs, renal function, serum electrolytes, cholesterol, and TG levels. Monitor WBCs in patients with collagen vascular disease and renal impairment.

Counseling: Inform about fetal risks if taken during pregnancy and discuss treatment options in women planning to become pregnant; instruct to report pregnancy as soon as possible. Instruct to d/c therapy and to immediately report signs/symptoms of angioedema. Instruct to report lightheadedness, especially during the 1st days of therapy; advise to d/c and consult with a physician if syncope occurs. Inform that inadequate fluid intake, excessive perspiration, diarrhea, or vomiting may lead to excessive fall in BP, with the same consequences of lightheadedness and possible syncope. Advise not to use K$^+$ supplements or salt substitutes containing K$^+$ without consulting physician. Advise to promptly report any indication of infection.

LOTREL — amlodipine besylate/benazepril hydrochloride   Rx

Class: ACE inhibitor/calcium channel blocker (CCB) (dihydropyridine)

> D/C when pregnancy is detected. Drugs that act directly on the renin-angiotensin system (RAS) can cause injury/death to the developing fetus.

ADULT DOSAGE

Hypertension

Not Adequately Controlled on Monotherapy w/ Either Agent:
Initial: 2.5mg/10mg qd
Titrate: May increase up to 10mg/40mg qd if BP remains uncontrolled

Replacement Therapy: May substitute for titrated components

PEDIATRIC DOSAGE
Pediatric use may not have been established

DOSING CONSIDERATIONS
Renal Impairment
CrCl ≤30mL/min: Not recommended for use

Hepatic Impairment
Consider using lower doses

Elderly
Consider lower initial doses

ADMINISTRATION
Oral route

STORAGE
25°C (77°F); excursions permitted to 15-30°C (59-86°F). Protect from moisture.

HOW SUPPLIED
Cap: (Amlodipine/Benazepril) 2.5mg/10mg, 5mg/10mg, 5mg/20mg, 5mg/40mg, 10mg/20mg, 10mg/40mg

CONTRAINDICATIONS
Coadministration w/ aliskiren in patients w/ diabetes. History of angioedema, w/ or w/o previous ACE inhibitor treatment; hypersensitivity to benazepril, to any other ACE inhibitor, to amlodipine, or to any of the excipients of this product.

WARNINGS/PRECAUTIONS
Symptomatic hypotension may occur, most likely in patients w/ volume- or salt-depletion; correct volume and/or salt depletion before starting therapy. Symptomatic hypotension may occur in patients w/ severe aortic stenosis. Benazepril: Head and neck angioedema reported; d/c and treat immediately if laryngeal stridor or angioedema of face/tongue/glottis occurs. Black patients have a higher incidence of angioedema compared to nonblacks. Intestinal angioedema reported; monitor for abdominal pain. Anaphylactoid reactions reported during desensitization w/ hymenoptera (wasp sting) venom, in patients dialyzed w/ high-flux membranes, and in patients undergoing LDL apheresis w/ dextran sulfate absorption. Excessive hypotension, which may be associated w/ oliguria, azotemia, and (rarely) acute renal failure and death, may occur in CHF patients; monitor patients during first 2 weeks of therapy and whenever dose is increased or a diuretic is added or its dose increased. Cholestatic hepatitis and acute liver failure reported rarely; d/c if jaundice or marked elevation of hepatic enzymes develops. May cause changes in renal function, including acute renal failure; patients whose renal function depends on the RAS (eg, renal artery stenosis, severe heart failure, post MI) may be at particular risk; consider withholding or discontinuing therapy if clinically significant decrease in renal function develops. Hyperkalemia and persistent nonproductive cough reported. Hypotension may occur w/ surgery or during anesthesia. Amlodipine: Worsening angina and acute MI (AMI) may develop after starting or increasing the dose, particularly in patients w/ severe obstructive coronary artery disease (CAD). Caution w/ aortic/mitral stenosis, or obstructive hypertrophic cardiomyopathy.

ADVERSE REACTIONS
Cough, headache, dizziness, edema, angioedema.

DRUG INTERACTIONS
See Contraindications. **Benazepril:** Increased risk for angioedema w/ mammalian target of rapamycin inhibitor (eg, temsirolimus, sirolimus, everolimus). Coadministration w/ NSAIDs, including selective COX-2 inhibitors, may result in deterioration of renal function and attenuation of antihypertensive effect. Diabetic patients receiving concomitant insulin or oral antidiabetics may develop hypoglycemia. Dual blockade of the RAS is associated w/ increased risks of hypotension, hyperkalemia, and changes in renal function (including acute renal failure); avoid combined use of RAS inhibitors, and closely monitor BP, renal function, and electrolytes w/ concomitant agents that also block the RAS. Avoid w/ aliskiren in patients w/ renal impairment (GFR <60mL/min). K⁺ supplements, K⁺-sparing diuretics (eg, spironolactone, amiloride, triamterene), or K⁺-containing salt substitutes may increase risk of hyperkalemia; frequently monitor serum K⁺. May attenuate K⁺ loss caused by thiazide diuretics. Increased lithium levels and symptoms of lithium toxicity reported; frequently monitor lithium levels. Nitritoid reactions (eg, facial flushing, N/V, hypotension) reported w/ injectable gold. **Amlodipine:** May increase exposure of simvastatin; limit dose of simvastatin to 20mg daily. Increased systemic exposure w/ moderate and strong CYP3A inhibitors; monitor for symptoms of hypotension and edema. Monitor BP when coadministered w/ CYP3A4 inducers.

PREGNANCY AND LACTATION
Category D, not for use in nursing.

MECHANISM OF ACTION
Amlodipine: Calcium channel blocker (dihydropyridine); inhibits transmembrane influx of Ca^{2+} ions into vascular smooth muscle and cardiac muscle. Acts directly on vascular smooth muscle to cause a reduction in peripheral vascular resistance and reduction in BP. Benazepril: ACE inhibitor; inhibition results in decreased plasma angiotensin II, which leads to decreased vasopressor activity and decreased aldosterone secretion.

PHARMACOKINETICS
Absorption: Amlodipine: Absolute bioavailability (64-90%); T_{max}=6-12 hrs. Benazepril: Bioavailability (≥37%); T_{max}=0.5-2 hrs, 1.5-4 hrs (benazeprilat). **Distribution:** Amlodipine: V_d=21L/kg; plasma protein binding (approx 93%). Benazepril: V_d=0.7L/kg (benazeprilat); crosses the placenta; found in breast milk. **Metabolism:** Amlodipine: Liver (extensive). Benazepril: Liver (extensive) by enzymatic hydrolysis to benazeprilat (active metabolite). **Elimination:** Amlodipine: Urine (10% unchanged, 60% metabolites); $T_{1/2}$=approx 30-50 hrs. Benazepril: Urine (<1% unchanged, 20% benazeprilat), bile; $T_{1/2}$=22 hrs (benazeprilat).

PATIENT CONSIDERATIONS
Assessment: Assess for history of angioedema, diabetes, hypersensitivity to drug, aortic/mitral stenosis, obstructive hypertrophic cardiomyopathy, CHF, severe obstructive CAD, volume/salt depletion, hepatic/renal impairment, pregnancy/nursing status, and possible drug interactions.

Monitoring: Monitor for signs/symptoms of hypotension, anaphylactoid or hypersensitivity reactions, head/neck and intestinal angioedema, worsening angina or AMI, and other adverse reactions. Monitor BP, hepatic/renal function, and serum K⁺ levels.

Counseling: Inform of the consequences of exposure to the medication during pregnancy and of treatment options in women planning to become pregnant. Advise to report pregnancies as soon as possible. Advise diabetic patients about the possibility of hypoglycemic reactions when drug is used concomitantly w/ insulin or oral antidiabetics. Advise to seek medical attention if symptoms of hypotension, anaphylactoid or hypersensitivity reactions, angioedema, infection, trouble swallowing, breathing problems, or hepatic dysfunction occurs

LOTRISONE — betamethasone dipropionate/clotrimazole   Rx

Class: Azole antifungal/corticosteroid

ADULT DOSAGE
Tinea Corporis (Ringworm)

≥17 Years:
Apply a thin film into affected skin areas bid for 1 week
Max: 45g/week

Reevaluate if no improvement seen after 1 week; do not use for >2 weeks

Tinea Cruris (Jock Itch)

≥17 Years:
Apply a thin film into affected skin areas bid for 1 week
Max: 45g/week

Reevaluate if no improvement seen after 1 week; do not use for >2 weeks

Tinea Pedis (Athlete's Foot)

≥17 Years:
Gently massage sufficient amount into affected skin areas bid for 2 weeks
Max: 45g/week

Reevaluate if no improvement seen after 2 weeks; do not use for >4 weeks

PEDIATRIC DOSAGE
Pediatric use may not have been established

ADMINISTRATION
Topical route

Do not use w/ occlusive dressings unless directed by a physician.

STORAGE
20-25°C (68-77°F); excursions permitted to 15-30°C (59-86°F).

HOW SUPPLIED
Cre: (Betamethasone/Clotrimazole) 0.05%/1% [15g, 45g]

WARNINGS/PRECAUTIONS
Not for oral, ophthalmic, or intravaginal use. Avoid use with occlusive dressings. May cause reversible hypothalamic-pituitary-adrenal (HPA) axis suppression with the potential for glucocorticosteroid insufficiency during and after withdrawal of treatment. Cushing's syndrome and hyperglycemia may occur. Factors predisposing to HPA axis suppression include use of high-potency steroids, large treatment surface areas, prolonged use, use of occlusive dressings, altered skin barrier, liver failure, and young age. Evaluate periodically for evidence of HPA axis suppression. Gradually withdraw drug, reduce frequency of application, or substitute a less potent corticosteroid if HPA axis suppression is documented. Pediatric patients may be more susceptible to systemic toxicity. Not recommended for treatment of diaper dermatitis. Caution in elderly.

ADVERSE REACTIONS
Paresthesia, rash, edema, secondary infection.

PREGNANCY AND LACTATION
Category C, caution in nursing.

MECHANISM OF ACTION
Azole antifungal agent/corticosteroid. Betamethasone: Corticosteroid; has not been established. Plays a role in cellular signaling, immune function, inflammation, and protein regulation. Clotrimazole: Imidazole antifungal agent; inhibits 14-α-demethylation of lanosterol in fungi by binding to one of the CYP450 enzymes. This leads to accumulation of 14-α-methylsterols and reduced concentrations of ergosterol. Methylsterols may affect the electron transport system, thereby inhibiting growth of fungi.

PHARMACOKINETICS
Absorption: Betamethasone: Percutaneous; extent of absorption is determined by vehicle, integrity of epidermal barrier, and use of occlusive dressings. **Distribution:** Betamethasone: Bound to plasma proteins in varying degrees; found in breast milk (systemically absorbed). **Metabolism:** Betamethasone: Liver. **Elimination:** Betamethasone: Kidney, bile.

PATIENT CONSIDERATIONS
Assessment: Assess for hypersensitivity to drug, predisposing factors to HPA axis suppression, and pregnancy/nursing status.

Monitoring: Monitor for signs/symptoms of HPA axis suppression, Cushing's syndrome, hyperglycemia, and other adverse reactions. Perform periodic monitoring for HPA axis suppression using adrenocorticotropic hormone stimulation test. Review diagnosis if no clinical improvement seen after 1 week of treatment for tinea corporis or tinea cruris, and 2 weeks for tinea pedis.

Counseling: Inform to use externally ud. Advise to avoid intravaginal contact or contact with the eyes or mouth. Advise not to use on the face or underarms. When using in the groin area, counsel to use only for 2 weeks and apply the cream sparingly; advise to wear loose-fitting clothing and to notify physician if condition persists after 2 weeks. Instruct not to bandage, cover, or wrap the treatment area unless directed by physician. Advise to avoid use in the diaper area. Instruct to report any signs of local adverse reactions to physician. Instruct to notify physician if no improvement seen after 1 week of treatment for tinea cruris or tinea corporis, or 2 weeks for tinea pedis.

LOTRONEX — alosetron hydrochloride
Class: 5-HT₃ receptor antagonist

Rx

> Infrequent but serious GI adverse reactions (eg, ischemic colitis, serious constipation complications) resulting in hospitalization, and rarely, blood transfusion, surgery, and death, reported. Indicated only for women w/ severe diarrhea-predominant irritable bowel syndrome (IBS) who have not responded adequately to conventional therapy. D/C immediately if constipation or symptoms of ischemic colitis develop; do not resume therapy in patients who develop ischemic colitis. Patients who have constipation should immediately contact prescriber if it does not resolve after therapy is discontinued. Patients w/ resolved constipation should resume therapy only on the advice of prescriber.

ADULT DOSAGE
Irritable Bowel Syndrome

Treatment of women w/ severe diarrhea-predominant IBS who have chronic symptoms (generally lasting ≥6 months), had anatomic or biochemical abnormalities of GI tract excluded, and have not responded adequately to conventional therapy

Initial: 0.5mg bid
Titrate: If after 4 weeks the dose is well tolerated but does not adequately control symptoms, may increase up to 1mg bid; d/c if symptoms are not adequately controlled after 4 weeks of treatment w/ 1mg bid

PEDIATRIC DOSAGE
Pediatric use may not have been established

DOSING CONSIDERATIONS
Adverse Reactions
Constipation:
Patients who become constipated at initial dosage should d/c drug until constipation resolves; may restart at 0.5mg qd. If constipation recurs at the lower dose, d/c immediately

Ischemic Colitis:
D/C immediately in patients who develop signs of ischemic colitis; do not restart

ADMINISTRATION
Oral route

May take w/ or w/o food.

STORAGE
20-25°C (68-77°F). Protect from light and moisture.

HOW SUPPLIED
Tab: 0.5mg, 1mg

CONTRAINDICATIONS
Constipation. History of chronic/severe constipation or sequelae from constipation, intestinal obstruction, stricture, toxic megacolon, GI perforation, and/or adhesions, ischemic colitis, impaired intestinal circulation, thrombophlebitis, or hypercoagulable state, Crohn's disease or ulcerative colitis, diverticulitis, severe hepatic impairment. Concomitant administration w/ fluvoxamine.

WARNINGS/PRECAUTIONS
Indicated only in those patients for whom the benefit-to-risk balance is most favorable. Caution in elderly and debilitated patients; may be at greater risk for complications of constipation. Caution w/ mild or moderate hepatic impairment.

ADVERSE REACTIONS
Constipation, abdominal/GI discomfort and pain, nausea.

DRUG INTERACTIONS
See Contraindications. Increased risk of serious complications of constipation w/ medications that decrease GI motility. CYP1A2, CYP3A4 or CYP2C9 inducers or inhibitors may alter clearance. Avoid w/ moderate CYP1A2 inhibitors (eg, quinolone antibiotics, cimetidine) unless clinically necessary. Caution w/ strong CYP3A4 inhibitors (eg, ketoconazole, clarithromycin, protease inhibitors, voriconazole).

PREGNANCY AND LACTATION
Pregnancy: Category B.
Lactation: It is not known whether alosetron is excreted in human milk; caution in nursing.

MECHANISM OF ACTION
5-HT₃ receptor antagonist; inhibits activation of nonselective cation channels, which results in the modulation of the enteric nervous system.

PHARMACOKINETICS
Absorption: Rapid. Absolute bioavailability (50-60%). C_{max}=9ng/mL, T_{max}=1 hr. **Distribution:** V_d=65-95L; plasma protein binding (82%). **Metabolism:** Liver (extensive) via CYP2C9, 3A4, and 1A2. **Elimination:** Urine (74%, 13% unchanged), feces (11%, <1% unchanged); $T_{1/2}$=1.5 hrs.

PATIENT CONSIDERATIONS
Assessment: Assess for constipation; history of chronic or severe constipation or sequelae from constipation, intestinal obstruction or stricture, toxic megacolon, GI perforation or adhesion, ischemic colitis, impaired intestinal circulation, thrombophlebitis or hypercoagulable state, Crohn's disease or ulcerative colitis, diverticulitis; hepatic impairment or history thereof, debilitation, pregnancy/nursing status, and possible drug interactions.

Monitoring: Monitor for signs/symptoms of ischemic colitis, serious complications of constipation, GI perforation, and other adverse reactions. Monitor LFTs w/ mild/moderate hepatic impairment.

Counseling: Inform of the risks and benefits of therapy and discuss the impact of IBS symptoms on patient's life. Instruct to read the medication guide before starting therapy and each time prescription is refilled. Instruct not to start taking medication if constipated, and to immediately d/c and contact prescriber if constipation or symptoms of ischemic colitis (eg, new/worsening abdominal pain, bloody diarrhea, blood in stool) develop, to contact prescriber again if constipation does not resolve after discontinuation of therapy, and to resume therapy only if constipation has resolved and after discussion w/ and the agreement of treating prescriber. Instruct to stop taking medication and contact prescriber if therapy does not adequately control IBS symptoms after 4 weeks of taking 1mg bid.

LOVASTATIN — lovastatin
Class: HMG-CoA reductase inhibitor (statin)

Rx

OTHER BRAND NAMES
Mevacor (Discontinued)

ADULT DOSAGE
Primary Hypercholesterolemia
Initial: 20mg qd w/ pm meal (LDL reductions of ≥20%); may consider 10mg if smaller reductions required
Range: 10-80mg/day in single or 2 divided doses
Titrate: Adjust at ≥4-week intervals
Max: 80mg/day

Consider dose reduction if cholesterol levels fall significantly below the targeted range

Coronary Artery Disease
Primary prevention of coronary heart disease. Slow progression of coronary atherosclerosis in patients w/ coronary heart disease

Dose based on current clinical practice

PEDIATRIC DOSAGE
Heterozygous Familial Hypercholesterolemia
Treatment of adolescents w/ the following findings: LDL remains >189mg/dL, or LDL remains >160mg/dL and there is a positive family history of premature cardiovascular disease or 2 or more other cardiovascular disease risk factors are present

10-17 Years (at Least 1 Year Postmenarche):
Initial: 20mg/day (LDL reductions of ≥20%); may consider 10mg if smaller reductions required
Range: 10-40mg/day
Titrate: Adjust at ≥4-week intervals
Max: 40mg/day

DOSING CONSIDERATIONS
Concomitant Medications
W/ Amiodarone:
Max: 40mg/day

W/ Danazol, Diltiazem, Dronedarone, or Verapamil:
Initial: 10mg/day
Max: 20mg/day

Renal Impairment
Severe (CrCl <30mL/min): Carefully consider dosage increases above 20mg/day; give cautiously if deemed necessary

ADMINISTRATION
Oral route

Take w/ meals

STORAGE
20-25°C (68-77°F). Protect from light.

HOW SUPPLIED
Tab: 10mg, 20mg, 40mg

CONTRAINDICATIONS
Hypersensitivity to any component of this medication, active liver disease or unexplained persistent elevations of serum transaminases, pregnancy, women of childbearing age who may become pregnant, and nursing mothers. Concomitant administration w/ strong CYP3A4 inhibitors (eg, itraconazole, ketoconazole, posaconazole, voriconazole, HIV protease inhibitors, boceprevir, telaprevir, erythromycin, clarithromycin, telithromycin, nefazodone, cobicistat-containing products).

WARNINGS/PRECAUTIONS
Myopathy (including immune-mediated necrotizing myopathy [IMNM]) and rhabdomyolysis reported; d/c if markedly elevated CPK levels occur or myopathy is diagnosed/suspected, and temporarily withhold in any patient experiencing acute or serious condition predisposing to development of renal failure secondary to rhabdomyolysis. Risk of myopathy/rhabdomyolysis is dose related. Persistent increases in serum transaminases reported; obtain LFTs prior to initiation and repeat as clinically indicated. Fatal and nonfatal hepatic failure (rare) reported; promptly interrupt therapy if serious liver injury with clinical symptoms and/or hyperbilirubinemia or jaundice occurs and do not restart if no alternate etiology found. Caution in patients who consume substantial quantities of alcohol and/or have history of liver disease. Increases in HbA1c and FPG levels reported. Evaluate patients who develop endocrine dysfunction. Caution in the elderly.

ADVERSE REACTIONS
Headache, constipation, flatulence, myalgia.

DRUG INTERACTIONS
See Contraindications and Dosing Considerations. Ranolazine may increase risk of myopathy/rhabdomyolysis; consider dose adjustment of lovastatin. Due to the risk of myopathy, avoid with gemfibrozil, cyclosporine, and grapefruit juice, and caution with fibrates, lipid-lowering doses (≥1g/day) of niacin, colchicine, danazol, diltiazem, dronedarone, verapamil, and amiodarone. Determine PT before initiation and frequently during therapy with coumarin anticoagulants. Caution with drugs that may decrease the levels or activity of endogenous steroid hormones (eg, spironolactone, cimetidine).

PREGNANCY AND LACTATION
Category X, not for use in nursing.

MECHANISM OF ACTION
HMG-CoA reductase inhibitor; may involve both reduction of VLDL concentration and induction of LDL receptor, leading to reduced production and/or increased catabolism of LDL.

PHARMACOKINETICS
Absorption: T_{max}=2-4 hrs. **Distribution:** Plasma protein binding (>95%). **Metabolism:** Liver (extensive 1st pass), by hydrolysis via CYP3A4; β-hydroxyacid and 6'-hydroxy derivative (major active metabolites). **Elimination:** Feces (83%), urine (10%).

PATIENT CONSIDERATIONS
Assessment: Assess for history of or active liver disease, unexplained persistent serum transaminase elevations, secondary causes for hypercholesterolemia, alcohol consumption, diabetes, drug hypersensitivity, pregnancy/nursing status, and possible drug interactions. Assess lipid profile, LFTs, and renal function.

Monitoring: Monitor for signs/symptoms of myopathy (including IMNM), rhabdomyolysis, liver/renal/endocrine dysfunction, increases in HbA1c and FPG levels, and other adverse reactions. Monitor lipid profile, creatine kinase, and LFTs. Check PT frequently with coumarin anticoagulants.

Counseling: Advise about substances to be avoided and to report promptly any unexplained muscle pain, tenderness, or weakness, particularly if accompanied by malaise or fever or if muscle signs and symptoms persist after discontinuation. Inform that liver function will be checked prior to therapy and if signs/symptoms of liver injury occur; instruct to report promptly any symptoms that may indicate liver injury (eg, right upper abdominal discomfort, dark urine, jaundice). Instruct women of childbearing age to use an effective method of birth control, to stop taking drug if they become pregnant, and not to breastfeed while on therapy. Advise patients to inform other physicians prescribing a new medication, that they are taking lovastatin.

LOVAZA — omega-3-acid ethyl esters   Rx

Class: Lipid-regulating agent

ADULT DOSAGE
Severe Hypertriglyceridemia (≥500mg/dL)

4g/day (4 caps qd or 2 caps bid)

PEDIATRIC DOSAGE
Pediatric use may not have been established

ADMINISTRATION
Oral route

Swallow caps whole; do not break open, crush, dissolve, or chew

STORAGE
25°C (77°F); excursions permitted to 15-30°C (59-86°F). Do not freeze.

HOW SUPPLIED
Cap: 1g

CONTRAINDICATIONS
Known hypersensitivity (eg, anaphylactic reaction) to Lovaza or any of its components.

WARNINGS/PRECAUTIONS
Increases in ALT levels without a concurrent increase in AST levels reported. May increase LDL levels; monitor LDL levels periodically during therapy. Contains ethyl esters of omega-3 fatty acids (eicosapentaenoic acid [EPA] and docosahexaenoic acid [DHA]), obtained from oil of several fish sources; caution with known hypersensitivity to fish and/or shellfish. Recurrent symptomatic atrial fibrillation/flutter (A-fib/flutter) reported in patients with paroxysmal or persistent A-fib, particularly within the first 2-3 months of initiating therapy. Assess TG levels carefully before initiating therapy and monitor TG levels periodically during therapy.

ADVERSE REACTIONS
Eructation, taste perversion, dyspepsia.

DRUG INTERACTIONS
Periodically monitor patients receiving concomitant treatment with an anticoagulant or other drugs affecting coagulation (eg, antiplatelet agents). D/C or change medications known to exacerbate hypertriglyceridemia (eg, β-blockers, thiazides, estrogens), if possible, prior to consideration of therapy.

PREGNANCY AND LACTATION
Category C, caution in nursing.

MECHANISM OF ACTION
Lipid-regulating agent; not established. Potential mechanisms of action include inhibition of acyl-CoA: 1,2-diacylglycerol acyltransferase, increased mitochondrial and peroxisomal β-oxidation in the liver, decreased lipogenesis in the liver, and increased plasma lipoprotein lipase activity. May reduce the synthesis of TGs in the liver because EPA and DHA are poor substrates for the enzymes responsible for TG synthesis, and EPA and DHA inhibit esterification of other fatty acids.

PHARMACOKINETICS
Distribution: Found in breast milk.

PATIENT CONSIDERATIONS
Assessment: Assess for hypersensitivity to drug, fish and/or shellfish; hepatic impairment; A-fib/flutter; pregnancy/nursing status; and possible drug interactions. Attempt to control serum lipids with appropriate diet, exercise, weight loss in obese patients, and control of any medical problems that are contributing to lipid abnormalities (eg, diabetes mellitus, hypothyroidism). Assess TG and LDL levels.

Monitoring: Monitor for recurrent symptomatic A-fib/flutter in patients with paroxysmal or persistent A-fib. Monitor for allergic reactions and other adverse reactions. Periodically monitor ALT and AST levels in patients with hepatic impairment. Periodically monitor LDL and TG levels.

Counseling: Instruct to notify physician if allergic to fish and/or shellfish. Advise that the use of lipid-regulating agents does not reduce the importance of adhering to diet. Advise not to alter caps in any way and to ingest intact caps only. Instruct to take as prescribed.

LOVENOX — enoxaparin sodium   Rx

Class: Low molecular weight heparin (LMWH)

> Epidural or spinal hematomas resulting in long-term or permanent paralysis may occur in patients anticoagulated with low molecular weight heparins (LMWHs) or heparinoids and are receiving neuraxial anesthesia or undergoing spinal puncture. Increased risk with indwelling epidural catheters, concomitant use of other drugs that affect hemostasis (eg, NSAIDs, platelet inhibitors, other anticoagulants), history of traumatic or repeated epidural or spinal punctures, a history of spinal deformity or spinal surgery, or when optimal timing between the administration of enoxaparin and neuraxial procedures is not known. Monitor frequently for signs/symptoms of neurological impairment; if neurological compromise noted, urgent treatment is necessary. Consider benefit and risks before neuraxial intervention in patients anticoagulated or to be anticoagulated for thromboprophylaxis.

ADULT DOSAGE
Deep Vein Thrombosis

Prophylaxis:
Abdominal Surgery:
40mg SQ qd w/ initial dose given 2 hrs prior to surgery for 7-10 days (up to 12 days in clinical trials)

Hip Replacement Surgery:
Twice-Daily Dosing: 30mg SQ q12h w/ initial dose given 12-24 hrs after surgery for 7-10 days (up to 14 days in clinical trials)

Once-Daily Dosing: 40mg SQ qd w/ initial dose given 12 hrs prior to surgery for 7-10 days (up to 14 days in clinical trials)

PEDIATRIC DOSAGE
Pediatric use may not have been established

Continue prophylaxis w/ 40mg SQ qd for 3 weeks following initial phase

Knee Replacement Surgery:
30mg SQ q12h w/ initial dose given 12-24 hrs after surgery for 7-10 days (up to 14 days in clinical trials)

Acute Illness w/ Severely Restricted Mobility:
40mg SQ qd for 6-11 days (up to 14 days in clinical trials)

Acute Treatment:
Outpatient (w/o Pulmonary Embolism):
1mg/kg SQ q12h for 7 days (up to 17 days in clinical trials)

Inpatient (w/ or w/o Pulmonary Embolism):
1mg/kg SQ q12h, or 1.5mg/kg SQ qd at the same time every day for 7 days (up to 17 days in clinical trials)

Outpatient and Inpatient Treatments:
Initiate warfarin therapy when appropriate (usually w/in 72 hrs of enoxaparin); continue enoxaparin for at least 5 days and until therapeutic oral anticoagulant effect has been achieved

Unstable Angina
Prophylaxis:
1mg/kg SQ q12h in conjunction w/ oral aspirin therapy (100-325mg qd) for 2-8 days (up to 12.5 days in clinical trials)

Myocardial Infarction
Non-Q-Wave:
Prophylaxis:
1mg/kg SQ q12h in conjunction w/ oral aspirin therapy (100-325mg qd) for 2-8 days (up to 12.5 days in clinical trials)

Acute ST- Segment Elevation:
Treatment:
<75 Years:
Initial: 30mg single IV bolus plus a 1mg/kg SQ dose, followed by 1mg/kg SQ q12h
Max: 100mg for the first 2 SQ doses only

All patients should receive aspirin (75-325mg qd) as soon as they are identified as having ST-segment elevation MI unless contraindicated

Concomitant Thrombolytic (Fibrin-Specific or Non-Fibrin Specific):
Administer enoxaparin between 15 min before and 30 min after the start of fibrinolytic therapy

Percutaneous Coronary Intervention:
Last SQ Enoxaparin Dose Given <8 hrs Before Balloon Inflation: No additional dosing needed
Last SQ Enoxaparin Dose Given >8 hrs Before Balloon Inflation:
Administer 0.3mg/kg IV bolus

DOSING CONSIDERATIONS
Renal Impairment
Severe (CrCl <30mL/min):
Prophylaxis in Abdominal Surgery: 30mg SQ qd
Prophylaxis in Hip/Knee Replacement Surgery: 30mg SQ qd
Prophylaxis in Acute Illness: 30mg SQ qd
Outpatient Treatment of Acute DVT w/o Pulmonary Embolism (w/ Warfarin): 1mg/kg SQ qd
Inpatient Treatment of Acute DVT w/ or w/o Pulmonary Embolism (w/ Warfarin): 1mg/kg SQ qd
Ischemic Prophylaxis in Unstable Angina/Non-Q-Wave MI (w/ Aspirin): 1mg/kg SQ qd
Treatment of Acute ST-Segment Elevation MI in Patients <75 Years (w/ Aspirin): 30mg single IV bolus plus a 1mg/kg SQ dose, followed by 1mg/kg SQ qd
Treatment of Acute ST-Segment Elevation MI in Patients ≥75 Years (w/ Aspirin): 1mg/kg SQ qd (no initial bolus)

Elderly
≥75 Years:
Acute ST-Segment Elevation MI:
Do not use initial IV bolus

Initial: 0.75mg/kg SQ q12h
Max: 75mg for the first 2 doses only

ADMINISTRATION
SQ or IV (for multidose vial) route

Use tuberculin syringe or equivalent when using multidose vials.
Prefilled syringes and graduated prefilled syringes are for single, one-time use only and are available w/ a system that shields the needle after inj.

SQ Inj Technique
Remove the prefilled syringe from the blister packaging by peeling at the arrow as directed on the blister; do not remove by pulling on the plunger as this may damage the syringe.
Patients should be lying down and enoxaparin administered by deep SQ inj.
Do not expel the air bubble from the prefilled syringe before the inj.
Administration should be alternated between the left and right anterolateral and left and right posterolateral abdominal wall.
The whole length of the needle should be introduced into a skin fold held between the thumb and forefinger; the skin fold should be held throughout the inj.
Do not rub the inj site after completion of the inj.

IV (Bolus) Inj
Use multiple-dose vial and administer through an IV line.
Do not mix or coadminister w/ other medications.
Flush the chosen IV access w/ a sufficient amount of saline or dextrose sol prior to and following the IV bolus administration of enoxaparin to clear the port of drug; enoxaparin may be safely administered w/ normal saline sol (0.9%) or D5W.

STORAGE
25°C (77°F); excursions permitted to 15-30°C (59-86°F). Do not store multidose vials for >28 days after first use.

HOW SUPPLIED
Inj: (Multidose Vial) 300mg/3mL; (Prefilled Syringe) 30mg/0.3mL, 40mg/0.4mL, 60mg/0.6mL, 80mg/0.8mL, 100mg/mL, 120mg/0.8mL, 150mg/mL

CONTRAINDICATIONS
Active major bleeding, thrombocytopenia associated with a positive in vitro test for antiplatelet antibody in the presence of enoxaparin sodium, hypersensitivity to heparin or pork products, hypersensitivity to benzyl alcohol (only with the multidose formulation), Known hypersensitivity to enoxaparin sodium (eg, pruritus, urticaria, anaphylactic/anaphylactoid reactions).

WARNINGS/PRECAUTIONS
Consider pharmacokinetic profile of enoxaparin to reduce the potential risk of bleeding associated with concurrent use with epidural or spinal anesthesia/analgesia or spinal puncture. Placement or removal of catheter should be delayed for at least 12 hrs after administration of lower doses and at least 24 hrs after higher doses. Extreme caution with increased risk of hemorrhage (eg, bacterial endocarditis, congenital or acquired bleeding disorders) and with history of heparin-induced thrombocytopenia. Major hemorrhages, including retroperitoneal and intracranial bleeding, reported. To minimize the risk of bleeding following vascular instrumentation during treatment of unstable angina, non-Q-wave MI, and acute STEMI, adhere precisely to the intervals recommended between doses. Observe for signs of bleeding or hematoma formation at the site of the procedure. Caution in patients with bleeding diathesis, uncontrolled arterial HTN or history of recent GI ulceration, diabetic retinopathy, renal dysfunction, and hemorrhage. Thrombocytopenia reported; d/c if platelet count <100,000/mm³. Cannot be used interchangeably (unit for unit) with heparin or other LMWH. Pregnant women with mechanical prosthetic heart valves may be at higher risk for thromboembolism and have a higher rate of fetal loss; monitor anti-factor Xa levels, and adjust dosage prn. Multidose vial contains benzyl alcohol that crosses the placenta and has been associated with fatal "gasping syndrome" in premature neonates; use with caution or only when clearly needed in pregnant women. Periodic CBC, including platelet count and stool occult blood tests are recommended during course of treatment. Anti-factor Xa may be used to monitor anticoagulant activity in patients with significant renal impairment or if abnormal coagulation parameters or bleeding occurs. Hyperkalemia reported in patients with renal failure. Increase in exposure with prophylactic dosages (non-weight adjusted) observed in low-weight women (<45kg) and low-weight men (<57kg). Higher risk for thromboembolism in obese patients; observe for signs/symptoms of thromboembolism. Caution with hepatic impairment.

ADVERSE REACTIONS
Epidural or spinal hematoma, hemorrhage, ecchymosis, anemia, peripheral edema, fever, dyspnea, nausea, ALT/AST elevations.

DRUG INTERACTIONS
See Boxed Warning. D/C agents that may enhance the risk of hemorrhage prior to therapy (eg, anticoagulants, platelet inhibitors, such as acetylsalicylic acid, salicylates, NSAIDs [including ketorolac tromethamine], dipyridamole, or sulfinpyrazone). If coadministration is essential, conduct close monitoring. May increase risk of hyperkalemia with K⁺-sparing drugs, and administration of K⁺.

PREGNANCY AND LACTATION
Category B, not for use in nursing.

MECHANISM OF ACTION
LMWH; has antithrombotic properties.

PHARMACOKINETICS
Absorption: (SQ) Administration of variable doses resulted in different parameters. Absolute bioavailability (100%). (Anti-factor Xa/Antithrombin [Anti-factor IIa]) Max activity=3-5 hrs. **Distribution:** (Anti-factor Xa activity) V_d=4.3L. **Metabolism:** Liver; via desulfation and/or depolymerization. **Elimination:** Urine; (Anti-factor Xa activity) $T_{1/2}$=4.5-7 hrs.

PATIENT CONSIDERATIONS

Assessment: Assess for presence of active major bleeding, thrombocytopenia, hypersensitivity to heparin or pork products, hypersensitivity to benzyl alcohol, renal dysfunction, obesity, any other conditions where treatment is cautioned, nursing/pregnancy status, and for possible drug interactions.

Monitoring: Monitor for signs/symptoms of hemorrhage, thrombocytopenia, hyperkalemia, thromboembolism, and other adverse reactions. Monitor for epidural or spinal hematomas, and for neurological impairment if used concomitantly with spinal/epidural anesthesia or spinal puncture. Periodically monitor CBC, including platelet count, and stool occult blood tests. If bleeding occurs, monitor anti-factor Xa levels.

Counseling: Inform of the benefits and risks of therapy. Instruct to watch for signs/symptoms of spinal or epidural hematoma (tingling, numbness, muscular weakness) if patients have had neuraxial anesthesia or spinal puncture, particularly, if they are taking concomitant NSAIDs, platelet inhibitors, or other anticoagulants; instruct to contact physician if these occur. Advise to seek medical attention if unusual bleeding, bruising, signs of thrombocytopenia, or allergic reactions develop. Counsel that it will take longer than usual to stop bleeding; explain that patient may bruise and/or bleed more easily when treated with enoxaparin. Inform of administration instructions if therapy is to continue after discharge. Instruct to notify physicians and dentists of enoxaparin therapy prior to surgery or taking a new drug.

LUCENTIS — ranibizumab

Rx

Class: Monoclonal antibody/vascular endothelial growth factor (VEGF)-A blocker

ADULT DOSAGE
Neovascular (Wet) Age-Related Macular Degeneration

0.5mg (0.05mL of 10mg/mL sol) once a month (approx 28 days)

May administer 3 monthly doses followed by less frequent dosing (eg, 4-5 doses on average in 9 months)

May also administer 1 dose every 3 months after 4 monthly doses

Macular Edema
Following Retinal Vein Occlusion:
0.5mg (0.05mL of 10mg/mL sol) once a month (approx 28 days)

Diabetic Macular Edema
0.3mg (0.05mL of 6mg/mL sol) once a month (approx 28 days)

Diabetic Retinopathy
Non-Proliferative/Proliferative Diabetic Retinopathy w/ Diabetic Macular Edema:
0.3mg (0.05mL of 6mg/mL sol) once a month (approx 28 days)

PEDIATRIC DOSAGE
Pediatric use may not have been established

ADMINISTRATION
Intravitreal route

Preparation
1. All of vial contents are withdrawn through a 5-micron, 19-gauge filter needle attached to a 1-cc tuberculin syringe.
2. Discard filter needle after withdrawal of the vial contents and do not use for intravitreal inj.
3. Replace filter needle w/ a sterile 30-gauge x 1/2-inch needle for intravitreal inj.
4. Contents should be expelled until plunger tip is aligned w/ line that marks 0.05mL on the syringe.

Administration
1. Adequate anesthesia and a broad-spectrum microbicide should be given prior to inj.
2. Each vial should only be used for treatment of a single eye; if contralateral eye requires treatment, a new vial should be used and the sterile field, syringe, gloves, drapes, eyelid speculum, filter, and inj needles should be changed before administration to other eye.

STORAGE
2-8°C (36-46°F). Do not freeze. Protect from light. Store in the original carton until time of use.

HOW SUPPLIED
Inj: 6mg/mL, 10mg/mL

CONTRAINDICATIONS
Ocular or periocular infections. Known hypersensitivity to ranibizumab or any of the excipients in the medication.

WARNINGS/PRECAUTIONS
Endophthalmitis and retinal detachments may occur; always use proper aseptic inj technique. Increases in IOP reported both preinj and postinj (at 60 min); monitor IOP prior to/following inj and manage appropriately. Potential risk of arterial thromboembolic events (ATEs) (eg, nonfatal stroke, nonfatal MI, vascular death). Fatal events may occur in patients w/ DME and DR at baseline.

ADVERSE REACTIONS
Conjunctival hemorrhage, eye pain, vitreous floaters/detachment, increased IOP, intraocular inflammation, cataract, nasopharyngitis, foreign body sensation in eyes, eye irritation, lacrimation increased, visual disturbance/vision blurred, ocular hyperemia, dry eye, influenza, headache.

DRUG INTERACTIONS
Serious intraocular inflammation may develop when used adjunctively w/ verteporfin photodynamic therapy (PDT); incidence reported when drug was administered 7 days after verteporfin PDT.

PREGNANCY AND LACTATION
Pregnancy: Fetal harm has been seen in animal studies. Treatment may pose a risk to embryo-fetal development and reproductive capacity. Give to a pregnant woman only if clearly needed.
Lactation: It is not known if ranibizumab is present in human milk; caution in nursing.

MECHANISM OF ACTION
Monoclonal antibody/human vascular endothelial growth factor A (VEGF-A) blocker; binds to receptor-binding site of VEGF-A and prevents the interaction of VEGF-A w/ its receptors (VEGFR1 and VEGFR2) on the surface of endothelial cells, reducing endothelial cell proliferation, vascular leakage, and new blood vessel formation.

PHARMACOKINETICS
Absorption: (Neovascular Age-Related Macular Degeneration) C_{max}=1.7ng/mL, T_{max}=1 day. **Elimination:** $T_{1/2}$=9 days.

PATIENT CONSIDERATIONS
Assessment: Assess for ocular or periocular infections, hypersensitivity to the drug, pregnancy/nursing status, and possible drug interactions.

Monitoring: Monitor for signs/symptoms of endophthalmitis, retinal detachments, ATEs, hypersensitivity reactions, and other adverse reactions. Monitor IOP prior to and 30 min following inj using tonometry. Check for perfusion of the optic nerve head immediately after inj. Monitor following inj to permit early treatment should an infection occur.

Counseling: Inform about the risk of developing endophthalmitis following administration. Instruct to seek immediate care from an ophthalmologist if the eye becomes red, sensitive to light, painful, or develops a change in vision.

LUMIGAN — bimatoprost

Rx

Class: Prostaglandin analogue

ADULT DOSAGE
Elevated Intraocular Pressure
Open-Angle Glaucoma/Ocular HTN:
1 drop in the affected eye(s) qpm

PEDIATRIC DOSAGE
Elevated Intraocular Pressure
Open-Angle Glaucoma/Ocular HTN:
≥16 Years:
1 drop in the affected eye(s) qpm

DOSING CONSIDERATIONS
Concomitant Medications
Space dosing by at least 5 min if using >1 topical ophthalmic drug

ADMINISTRATION
Ocular route

STORAGE
2-25°C (36-77°F).

HOW SUPPLIED
Sol: 0.01% [2.5mL, 5mL, 7.5mL]

WARNINGS/PRECAUTIONS
Changes to pigmented tissues, including increased pigmentation of iris (may be permanent), eyelid, and eyelashes (may be reversible) reported. Regularly examine patients with noticeably increased iris pigmentation. May cause changes to eyelashes and vellus hair in the treated eye. Intraocular inflammation reported; caution with active intraocular inflammation (eg, uveitis). Macular edema, including cystoid macular edema, reported; caution with aphakic patients, pseudophakic patients with a torn posterior lens capsule, or patients at risk of macular edema. Bacterial keratitis reported with multidose containers. Remove contact lenses prior to instillation; may reinsert 15 min after administration.

ADVERSE REACTIONS
Conjunctival hyperemia/edema/hemorrhage, eye irritation/pain/pruritus, reduced visual acuity, blurred vision, skin hyperpigmentation, eyelid erythema/pruritus, growth of eyelashes, hypertrichosis, instillation site irritation, punctate keratitis.

PREGNANCY AND LACTATION
Category C, caution in nursing.

MECHANISM OF ACTION
Prostaglandin analogue; selectively mimics the effects of naturally occurring substances, prostamides. Believed to lower IOP by increasing outflow of aqueous humor through both the trabecular meshwork and uveoscleral routes.

PHARMACOKINETICS
Absorption: (0.03%) C_{max}=0.08ng/mL, T_{max}=10 min, AUC=0.09ng•hr/mL.
Distribution: V_d=0.67L/kg. **Metabolism:** Via oxidation, N-deethylation, and glucuronidation. **Elimination:** (IV) Urine (≤67%), feces (25%); $T_{1/2}$=45 min.

PATIENT CONSIDERATIONS
Assessment: Assess for active intraocular inflammation, risk of macular edema, contact lens use, and pregnancy/nursing status. Assess use in aphakic patients, and in pseudophakic patients with a torn posterior lens capsule.

Monitoring: Monitor for changes to pigmented tissue, changes in eyelashes and vellus hair, intraocular inflammation, exacerbation of intraocular inflammation, macular edema, bacterial keratitis, and other adverse reactions.

Counseling: Advise about the potential for increased brown pigmentation of iris (may be permanent) and the possibility of darkening of eyelid skin (may be reversible after discontinuation). Inform about the possibility of eyelash and vellus hair changes in the treated eye during treatment. Instruct to avoid touching tip of dispensing container to the eye, surrounding structures, fingers, or any other surface in order to avoid contamination of the sol. Advise to consult physician if having ocular surgery, if an intercurrent ocular condition (eg, trauma or infection) develops, or if any ocular reactions develop. Instruct to remove contact lenses prior to instillation and reinsert 15 min after administration. Instruct to administer at least 5 min apart if using more than 1 topical ophthalmic drug.

LUNESTA — eszopiclone

CIV

Class: Nonbenzodiazepine hypnotic agent

ADULT DOSAGE
Insomnia

Initial: 1mg immediately hs
Titrate: May increase to 2mg or 3mg if clinically indicated
Max: 3mg qd immediately hs
Use lowest effective dose

PEDIATRIC DOSAGE
Pediatric use may not have been established

DOSING CONSIDERATIONS
Concomitant Medications
Potent CYP3A4 Inhibitors:
Max: 2mg

Concomitant CNS Depressants: Dose adjustments may be necessary

Hepatic Impairment
Severe:
Max: 2mg

Elderly
Elderly/Debilitated:
Max: 2mg

ADMINISTRATION
Oral route

Take immediately hs with at least 7-8 hrs remaining before planned time of awakening.
Do not administer with or immediately after a meal.

STORAGE
25°C (77°F); excursions permitted to 15-30°C (59-86°F).

HOW SUPPLIED
Tab: 1mg, 2mg, 3mg

CONTRAINDICATIONS
Known hypersensitivity to eszopiclone.

WARNINGS/PRECAUTIONS
May impair daytime function at the higher dose (2mg or 3mg), even when used as prescribed; monitor for excess depressant effects. May impair physical/mental abilities. Increased risk of next-day psychomotor impairment if taken with less than a full night of sleep remaining (7-8 hrs) or if higher than recommended dose is taken. Initiate only after careful evaluation; failure of insomnia to remit after 7-10 days of treatment may indicate presence of a primary psychiatric and/or medical illness. Use the lowest possible effective dose, especially in elderly. Severe anaphylactic/anaphylactoid reactions reported; do not rechallenge if angioedema develops. Abnormal thinking and behavioral changes (eg, bizarre behavior, agitation, hallucinations, depersonalization) reported. Amnesia and other neuropsychiatric symptoms may occur unpredictably. Worsening of depression, including suicidal thoughts and actions (including completed suicides), reported in primarily depressed patients. Complex behaviors (eg, sleep-driving) reported; consider discontinuation if a sleep-driving episode occurs. Withdrawal signs/symptoms reported following rapid dose decrease or abrupt discontinuation. Should be taken immediately hs; taking medication while still up and about may result in short-term memory impairment, hallucinations, impaired coordination, dizziness, and lightheadedness. Caution with severe hepatic impairment, elderly/debilitated patients, patients with diseases/conditions that could affect metabolism/hemodynamic responses, compromised respiratory function, history of alcohol/drug abuse, history of psychiatric disorders, and in patients exhibiting signs and symptoms of depression.

ADVERSE REACTIONS
Headache, unpleasant taste, somnolence, dry mouth, dizziness, infection, rash, pain, N/V, diarrhea, hallucinations, dyspepsia, nervousness, depression, anxiety.

DRUG INTERACTIONS
See Dosing Considerations. Not recommended with other sedative-hypnotics hs or in the middle of the night. Additive effects may occur with other CNS depressants (eg, benzodiazepines, opioids, TCAs, alcohol), including daytime use; consider downward dose adjustment of both drugs. Increased risk of next-day psychomotor impairment if coadministered with other CNS depressants and other drugs that increase blood levels of eszopiclone. Increased risk of complex behaviors with alcohol and other CNS depressants. May produce additive effect on psychomotor performance with ethanol. Decreased digit symbol substitution test scores with olanzapine. Decreased exposure and effects with CYP3A4 inducers (eg, rifampicin). Increased exposure with ketoconazole and other strong CYP3A4 inhibitors (eg, clarithromycin, nefazodone, ritonavir); dose reduction needed.

PREGNANCY AND LACTATION
Category C, safety not known in nursing.

MECHANISM OF ACTION
Nonbenzodiazepine hypnotic agent; has not been established. Effects believed to result from its interaction with GABA-receptor complexes at binding domains located close to or allosterically coupled to benzodiazepine receptors.

PHARMACOKINETICS
Absorption: Rapid. T_{max}=1 hr. **Distribution:** Plasma protein binding (52-59%). **Metabolism:** Liver (extensive) via oxidation and demethylation pathways; CYP3A4 and CYP2E1. (S)-zopiclone-N-oxide and (S)-N-desmethyl zopiclone (primary metabolites). **Elimination:** Urine (75% metabolites, <10% parent drug); $T_{1/2}$=6 hrs.

PATIENT CONSIDERATIONS
Assessment: Assess for psychiatric or physical disorder, depression, severe hepatic impairment, diseases/conditions that could affect metabolism/hemodynamic responses, compromised respiratory function, history of alcohol/drug abuse, history of psychiatric disorders, drug hypersensitivity, pregnancy/nursing status, and possible drug interactions.

Monitoring: Monitor for excessive depressant effects, anaphylactic/anaphylactoid reactions, emergence of any new behavioral signs/symptoms, withdrawal symptoms, abnormal thinking, and other adverse reactions.

Counseling: Inform of the risks and benefits of therapy. Inform that therapy may cause next-day impairment even when used as prescribed. Caution patients taking the 3mg dose against driving and other activities requiring complete mental alertness the day after use; inform that impairment may be present despite feeling fully awake. Advise to seek medical attention immediately if any adverse reactions (eg, severe anaphylactic/anaphylactoid reactions, sleep-driving, other complex behaviors) develop. Advise to immediately report any suicidal thoughts. Advise not to use therapy if patient drank alcohol that pm or hs.

LUPRON DEPOT-PED — leuprolide acetate

Rx

Class: Synthetic gonadotropin-releasing hormone (GnRH) analogue

PEDIATRIC DOSAGE
Central Precocious Puberty
≥2 Years:
Confirm clinical diagnosis prior to initiation of therapy

1-Month Administration:
Administer as a single IM inj once a month
≤25kg: 7.5mg
>25-≤37.5kg: 11.25mg
>37.5kg: 15mg

Titrate: Increase to the next available higher dose (eg, 11.25mg or 15mg at the next monthly inj) if adequate suppression is not achieved w/ the starting dose. Similarly, the dose may be adjusted w/ changes in body weight

Maint: Once a dose that results in adequate hormonal suppression is found, it can often be maintained for the duration of therapy in most children

3-Month Administration:
11.25mg or 30mg, as a single IM inj once every 3 months (12 weeks)

DOSING CONSIDERATIONS
Discontinuation
D/C at the appropriate age of onset of puberty

ADMINISTRATION
IM route

Rotate inj site periodically
Do not use partial syringes or a combination of syringes to achieve a particular dose

Reconstitution and Administration Instructions
1. Do not use the syringe if clumping or caking is evident; a thin layer of powder on the wall of the syringe is considered normal prior to mixing w/ the diluent
2. To prepare for inj, screw the white plunger into the end stopper until the stopper begins to turn
3. Hold the syringe upright and release the diluent by slowly pushing (6-8 sec) the plunger until the 1st stopper is at the blue line in the middle of the barrel
4. Keeping the syringe upright, mix the microspheres (powder) thoroughly by gently shaking the syringe until the powder forms a uniform sus; the sus will appear milky
5. If the powder adheres to the stopper or caking/clumping is present, tap the syringe w/ your finger to disperse; do not use if any of the powder has not gone into sus
6. Hold the syringe upright and pull the needle cap upward w/o twisting using the opposite hand
7. Keep the syringe upright and advance the plunger to expel the air from the syringe; now the syringe is ready for inj
8. Insert the needle at a 90° angle into the gluteal area, anterior thigh, or shoulder; alternate inj sites

NOTE: If a blood vessel is accidentally penetrated, aspirated blood would be visible just below the luer lock connection and can be seen through the transparent LuproLoc safety device; if blood is present, remove the needle immediately and do not inject the medication

9. Inject the entire contents of the syringe IM at the time of reconstitution. The sus settles very quickly following reconstitution; therefore, it should be mixed and used immediately

10. Once the syringe has been withdrawn, activate immediately the LuproLoc safety device by pushing the arrow on the lock upward towards the needle tip w/ the thumb or finger until the needle cover of the safety device is fully extended over the needle and a click is heard or felt

STORAGE
25°C (77°F); excursions permitted to 15-30°C (59-86°F). Reconstituted Sus: Discard if not used within 2 hrs.

HOW SUPPLIED
Inj: (1-Month) 7.5mg, 11.25mg, 15mg; (3-Month) 11.25mg, 30mg

CONTRAINDICATIONS
Women who are or may become pregnant. Known hypersensitivity to GnRH, GnRH agonist analogues, or any of the excipients in leuprolide acetate inj.

WARNINGS/PRECAUTIONS
Increase in clinical signs and symptoms of puberty may occur during the early phase of therapy due to initial rise in gonadotropins and sex steroids. Convulsions reported in patients with and without a history of seizures, epilepsy, cerebrovascular disorders, CNS anomalies or tumors, and in patients on concomitant medications that have been associated with convulsions (eg, bupropion, SSRIs). If noncompliant with drug regimen or dose is inadequate, gonadotropins and/or sex steroids may increase or rise above prepubertal levels. Suppresses pituitary-gonadal system; may affect diagnostic tests of pituitary gonadotropic and gonadal functions conducted during treatment and up to 6 months after discontinuation. Do not use partial syringes or combination of syringes to achieve a particular dose; each formulation and strength have different release characteristics.

ADVERSE REACTIONS
Inj-site reactions/pain, general pain, headache, acne/seborrhea, rash including erythema multiforme, emotional lability, vaginal bleeding/discharge/vaginitis, weight increase, mood altered.

PREGNANCY AND LACTATION
Category X, not for use in nursing.

MECHANISM OF ACTION
Synthetic gonadotropin-releasing hormone (GnRH) analog; potent inhibitor of gonadotropin secretion. Following an initial stimulation of gonadotropins, chronic stimulation results in suppression or "downregulation" of these hormones and consequent suppression of ovarian and testicular steroidogenesis.

PHARMACOKINETICS
Absorption: (7.5mg in adults) C_{max}=20ng/mL, T_{max}=4 hrs; (11.25mg) C_{max}=19.1ng/mL; (30mg) C_{max}=52.5ng/mL; (11.5mg and 30mg) T_{max}=1 hr. **Distribution:** Plasma protein binding (43-49%), V_d=27L (IV). **Metabolism:** M-I (major metabolite). **Elimination:** (3.75mg) Urine (<5% as parent and M-1 metabolite); $T_{1/2}$=3 hrs (1mg IV).

PATIENT CONSIDERATIONS
Assessment: Assess for history of seizures, cerebrovascular disorders, CNS anomalies or tumors. Assess for drug hypersensitivity and pregnancy status. Confirm clinical diagnosis of CPP by measuring blood concentrations of luteinizing hormone (LH) (basal or stimulated with a GnRH analog), sex steroids, and assessment of bone age versus chronological age. Obtain baseline evaluations of height and weight measurements, diagnostic imaging of the brain, pelvic/testicular/adrenal ultrasound, human chorionic gonadotropin levels, and adrenal steroid measurements to exclude congenital adrenal hyperplasia.

Monitoring: Monitor for convulsions and other adverse reactions. Monitor response with a GnRH stimulation test, basal LH or serum concentration of sex steroid levels; (1-Month) beginning 1-2 months following initiation of therapy, with changing doses, or potentially during therapy in order to confirm maintenance of efficacy or (3-Month) at months 2-3, month 6 and further as judged clinically appropriate, to ensure adequate suppression. (1-Month) Measure bone age for advancement every 6-12 months. (3-Month) Monitor height and bone age every 6-12 months.

Counseling: Counsel about the potential risk to the fetus if inadvertently used during pregnancy, or if patient becomes pregnant while taking the drug. Counsel about the importance of continuous therapy and adherence to drug administration schedule. Inform that signs of puberty (eg, vaginal bleeding) may occur during 1st few weeks of therapy; instruct to notify physician if symptoms continue beyond 2nd month. Inform about the most common side effects related to treatment. Advise that some pain and irritation is expected after inj; instruct to report if more severe or any unusual signs or symptoms occur. Advise parents/caregivers to notify physician if new or worsened symptoms develop after beginning treatment.

Luvox CR — fluvoxamine maleate   Rx

Class: Selective serotonin reuptake inhibitor (SSRI)

ADULT DOSAGE
Obsessive Compulsive Disorder

Initial: 100mg qhs
Titrate: Increase by 50mg every week, as tolerated, until max therapeutic benefit is achieved
Max: 300mg/day

Maint/Continuation of Extended Treatment:
Adjust to lowest effective dose; periodically reassess need for continued treatment

Dosing Considerations with MAOIs

Switching to/from an MAOI for Psychiatric Disorders:
Allow at least 14 days between discontinuation of an MAOI and initiation of treatment, and allow at least 14 days between discontinuation of treatment and initiation of an MAOI

W/ Other MAOIs (eg, Linezolid, IV Methylene Blue):
Do not start fluvoxamine in patients being treated w/ linezolid or IV methylene blue
In patients already receiving fluvoxamine, if acceptable alternatives are not available and benefits outweigh risks, d/c fluvoxamine and administer linezolid or IV methylene blue; monitor for serotonin syndrome for 2 weeks or until 24 hrs after the last dose of linezolid or IV methylene blue, whichever comes 1st. May resume fluvoxamine therapy 24 hrs after the last dose of linezolid or IV methylene blue

---

DOSING CONSIDERATIONS
Hepatic Impairment
Titrate slowly

Elderly
Titrate slowly

Discontinuation
Gradually reduce dose whenever possible
If intolerable symptoms occur following a decrease in dose or upon discontinuation of treatment, may resume the previously prescribed dose; subsequently, may continue decreasing dose but at a more gradual rate

ADMINISTRATION
Oral route

Do not crush or chew caps

STORAGE
Store at 25°C (77°F); excursions permitted to 15-30°C (59-86°F). Avoid exposure to >30°C (86°F). Protect from high humidity.

HOW SUPPLIED
Cap, Extended-Release: 100mg, 150mg

CONTRAINDICATIONS
Use of an MAOI for psychiatric disorders either concomitantly or within 14 days of stopping treatment. Treatment within 14 days of stopping an MAOI for psychiatric disorders. Starting treatment in patients being treated with MAOIs (eg, linezolid, IV methylene blue). Concomitant use of thioridazine, tizanidine, pimozide, alosetron, or ramelteon.

WARNINGS/PRECAUTIONS
Not approved for the treatment of bipolar depression. May precipitate mixed/manic episode in patients at risk for bipolar disorder; screen for risk of bipolar disorder prior to initiating therapy. Serotonin syndrome reported; d/c immediately and initiate supportive symptomatic treatment. Pupillary dilation that occurs following use may trigger an angle-closure attack in a patient with anatomically narrow angles who does not have a patent iridectomy. Adverse events reported upon discontinuation; gradually reduce dose. May increase risk of bleeding events. Activation of mania/hypomania reported. Avoid with unstable epilepsy and monitor patients with controlled epilepsy; d/c if seizures occur or seizure frequency increases. Hyponatremia may occur; caution in the elderly, volume-depleted patients, and patients taking a diuretic. Consider discontinuation in patients with symptomatic hyponatremia and institute appropriate medical intervention. Caution with diseases/conditions that affect metabolism or hemodynamic responses, and in pregnancy (3rd trimester).

ADVERSE REACTIONS
Insomnia, N/V, headache, somnolence, asthenia, diarrhea, anorexia, dizziness, abnormal ejaculation, dry mouth, dyspepsia, sweating, anxiety, tremor, decreased libido.

DRUG INTERACTIONS
See Contraindications. Inhibits several CYP450 enzymes that are known to be involved in metabolism of other drugs, such as CYP1A2 (eg, theophylline, propranolol, tizanidine), CYP3A4 (eg, alprazolam), CYP2C9 (eg, warfarin), and

PEDIATRIC DOSAGE
Pediatric use may not have been established

CYP2C19 (eg, omeprazole). Caution with CYP450 inhibitors (eg, quinidine), and in patients with reduced levels of CYP2D6 activity. Clinically significant interactions possible with drugs that have a narrow therapeutic ratio (eg, pimozide, omeprazole, phenytoin). Avoid with alcohol and diazepam. May increase levels of TCAs, carbamazepine, warfarin, clozapine, methadone, tacrine, propranolol, amitriptyline, clomipramine, or imipramine. Bradycardia reported with diltiazem. Orthostatic hypotension, hypotension, and bradycardia reported with metoprolol. May reduce clearance of mexiletine, theophylline, and benzodiazepines metabolized by hepatic oxidation (eg, alprazolam, midazolam, triazolam). Increased risk of bleeding with aspirin, NSAIDs, and other drugs that affect coagulation. May increase PT with warfarin; monitor PT and adjust dose of oral anticoagulants. Caution with lithium; may enhance serotonergic effects and cause seizures. May cause serotonin syndrome with other serotonergic drugs (eg, triptans, TCAs, fentanyl, tryptophan) and with drugs that impair metabolism of serotonin; d/c immediately if this occurs. Smoking increases metabolism. Refer to PI for dosing modifications when used with certain concomitant therapies.

PREGNANCY AND LACTATION
Category C, not for use in nursing.

MECHANISM OF ACTION
SSRI; presumed to be linked to its inhibition of CNS neuronal uptake of serotonin.

PHARMACOKINETICS
Absorption: C_{max} (at doses 100mg, 200mg, 300mg) =47ng/mL, 161ng/mL, 319ng/mL. **Distribution:** V_d =25L/kg; plasma protein binding (80%); found in breast milk. **Metabolism:** Liver (extensive) via oxidative demethylation and deamination. **Elimination:** Urine (2% unchanged); $T_{1/2}$ =16.3 hrs.

PATIENT CONSIDERATIONS
Assessment: Assess for susceptibility to angle-closure glaucoma, risk/presence of bipolar disorder, volume depletion, history of mania, seizures, history of drug abuse, disease/condition that affects metabolism or hemodynamic response, hepatic impairment, pregnancy/nursing status, and possible drug interactions.

Monitoring: Monitor for signs/symptoms of clinical worsening, suicidality, unusual changes in behavior, serotonin syndrome, angle-closure glaucoma, bleeding events, hyponatremia, seizures, activation of mania/hypomania, discontinuation symptoms, hepatic dysfunction, and other adverse reactions. Monitor height and weight periodically in children. Monitor PT with warfarin and other oral anticoagulants. Periodically reassess the need for continued treatment.

Counseling: Inform of risks, benefits, and appropriate use of therapy. Counsel to be alert for the emergence of suicidality, unusual changes in behavior, or worsening of depression, especially early during treatment and when the dose is adjusted up or down; instruct to report such symptoms especially if severe, abrupt in onset, or not part of presenting symptoms. Advise to inform physician if taking or planning to take any prescription or OTC drugs. Advise that drug may increase the risk of bleeding events. Inform that drug may cause mild pupillary dilation, which in susceptible individuals, may lead to an episode of angle-closure glaucoma. Caution about operating hazardous machinery. Instruct to notify physician if pregnant, intending to become pregnant, or breastfeeding. Instruct to avoid alcohol. Advise to notify physician if allergic reactions develop during therapy.

LUXIQ — betamethasone valerate
Rx

Class: Corticosteroid

ADULT DOSAGE	PEDIATRIC DOSAGE
Inflammatory and Pruritic Manifestations of Corticosteroid-Responsive Dermatoses Apply small amounts to affected scalp area bid (am and pm) D/C when control is achieved Reassess diagnosis if no improvement w/in 2 weeks	Pediatric use may not have been established

ADMINISTRATION
Topical route

Avoid use w/ occlusive dressing unless directed.

Application
Invert can and dispense a small amount of foam onto a saucer or other cool surface; do not dispense directly onto hands as foam will begin to melt immediately upon contact w/ warm skin.
Pick up small amounts of foam w/ fingers and gently massage into affected area until foam disappears.
Repeat until entire affected scalp area is treated.

STORAGE
20-25°C (68-77°F). Do not expose to heat or store at >49°C (120°F).

HOW SUPPLIED
Foam: 0.12% [50g, 100g]

CONTRAINDICATIONS
Hypersensitivity to betamethasone valerate, other corticosteroids, or to any ingredient in the preparation.

WARNINGS/PRECAUTIONS
Systemic absorption may produce reversible hypothalamic-pituitary-adrenal (HPA) axis suppression, manifestations of Cushing's syndrome, hyperglycemia, and glucosuria. Evaluate periodically for evidence of HPA axis suppression when applying to large surface area or to areas under occlusion; d/c treatment, reduce frequency of application, or substitute a less potent steroid if HPA axis suppression is noted. D/C and institute appropriate therapy if irritation develops. Use appropriate antifungal or antibacterial agent in the presence of dermatological infections; if favorable response does not occur promptly, d/c until infection is controlled. Pediatric patients may be more susceptible to systemic toxicity from equivalent doses.

ADVERSE REACTIONS
Application-site burning/itching/stinging.

PREGNANCY AND LACTATION
Category C, caution in nursing.

MECHANISM OF ACTION
Corticosteroid; possesses anti-inflammatory, antipruritic, and vasoconstrictive properties. Anti-inflammatory activity not established; thought to induce phospholipase A_2 inhibitory proteins, lipocortins, which control biosynthesis of potent mediators of inflammation (eg, prostaglandins, leukotrienes) by inhibiting release of their precursor, arachidonic acid.

PHARMACOKINETICS
Absorption: Percutaneous; occlusion, inflammation, and/or other disease processes in the skin may increase absorption. **Distribution:** Found in breast milk (systemically administered). **Metabolism:** Liver. **Elimination:** Kidney (major), bile.

PATIENT CONSIDERATIONS
Assessment: Assess for hypersensitivity to the drug, dermatological infections, and pregnancy/nursing status.

Monitoring: Monitor for signs/symptoms of HPA axis suppression, Cushing's syndrome, hyperglycemia, glucosuria, skin irritation, allergic contact dermatitis, and other adverse reactions. Monitor for signs of glucocorticosteroid insufficiency after withdrawal. Monitor clinical improvement; if no improvement seen within 2 weeks, reassess diagnosis.

Counseling: Advise to use externally and ud, to avoid contact with eyes, and not to use for any disorder other than that for which it was prescribed. Instruct not to bandage, cover, or wrap treated scalp area unless directed by physician. Advise to report any signs of local adverse reactions to physician. Advise to d/c use when control is achieved, and to notify physician if no improvement is seen within 2 weeks. Instruct to avoid fire, flame, or smoking during and immediately following application.

LUZU — luliconazole
Rx

Class: Azole antifungal

ADULT DOSAGE	PEDIATRIC DOSAGE
Fungal Infections **Caused by *Trichophyton rubrum* and *Epidermophyton floccosum*:** **Interdigital Tinea Pedis:** Apply a thin layer to affected area and approx 1 inch of the immediate surrounding area(s) qd for 2 weeks **Tinea Cruris/Tinea Corporis:** Apply to the affected area and approx 1 inch of the immediate surrounding area(s) qd for 1 week	Pediatric use may not have been established

ADMINISTRATION
Topical route

STORAGE
20-25°C (68-77°F); excursions permitted from 15-30°C (59-86°F).

HOW SUPPLIED
Cre: 1% [60g]

ADVERSE REACTIONS
Application-site reactions.

DRUG INTERACTIONS
May inhibit the activity of CYP2C19 and CYP3A4.

PREGNANCY AND LACTATION
Category C, caution in nursing.

MECHANISM OF ACTION
Azole antifungal; has not been established. Appears to inhibit ergosterol synthesis by inhibiting the enzyme lanosterol demethylase. Inhibition results in decreased amounts of ergosterol, a constituent of fungal cell membranes, and a corresponding accumulation of lanosterol.

PHARMACOKINETICS
Absorption: (Tinea pedis) AUC_{0-24}=6.88ng•hr/mL (1st dose), 18.74ng•hr/mL (final dose); C_{max}=0.40ng/mL (1st dose), 0.93ng/mL (final dose); T_{max}=16.9 hrs (1st dose), 5.8 hrs (final dose). (Tinea cruris) AUC_{0-24}=85.1ng•hr/mL (1st dose), 121.74ng•hr/mL (final dose); C_{max}=4.91ng/mL (1st dose), 7.36ng/mL (final dose); T_{max}=21 hrs (1st dose), 6.5 hrs (final dose). **Distribution:** Plasma protein binding (>99%).

PATIENT CONSIDERATIONS
Assessment: Assess pregnancy/nursing status and for possible drug interactions.
Monitoring: Monitor for application-site reactions and other adverse reactions.
Counseling: Instruct to use ud. Inform that the product is for topical use only and not intended for intravaginal or ophthalmic use.

LYNPARZA — olaparib   Rx
Class: PARP inhibitor

ADULT DOSAGE
Advanced Ovarian Cancer
Monotherapy in Patients w/ Deleterious/Suspected Deleterious Germline BRCA Mutation Who Have Been Treated w/ ≥3 Prior Lines of Chemotherapy:
Usual: 400mg bid; continue until disease progression or unacceptable toxicity

Missed Dose
If patient misses a dose, instruct to take next dose at its scheduled time

PEDIATRIC DOSAGE
Pediatric use may not have been established

DOSING CONSIDERATIONS
Concomitant Medications
CYP3A Inhibitors:
Avoid concomitant use of strong/moderate inhibitors and consider alternatives w/ less CYP3A inhibition.
If Inhibitor Cannot Be Avoided:
Strong CYP3A Inhibitor: Reduce dose to 150mg bid
Moderate CYP3A Inhibitor: Reduce dose to 200mg bid

Adverse Reactions
To manage adverse reactions, consider dose interruption of treatment or dose reduction
Usual: 200mg bid; may reduce to 100mg bid if further dose reduction is required

ADMINISTRATION
Oral route
Swallow whole; do not chew, dissolve, or open.
Do not take if cap appears deformed or shows evidence of leakage.

STORAGE
25°C (77°F); excursions permitted to 15-30°C (59-86°F). Do not expose to >40°C (104°F); do not take the drug if it is suspected of having been exposed to >40°C (104°F).

HOW SUPPLIED
Cap: 50mg

WARNINGS/PRECAUTIONS
Myelodysplastic syndrome/acute myeloid leukemia (MDS/AML) reported. Do not start therapy until patients have recovered from hematological toxicity caused by previous chemotherapy (≤CTCAE Grade 1). For prolonged hematological toxicities, interrupt therapy and monitor blood counts weekly until recovery; if the levels have not recovered to ≤CTCAE Grade 1 after 4 weeks, refer to a hematologist for further investigations. D/C if MDS/AML is confirmed. Pneumonitis (including fatal cases) reported; interrupt treatment and initiate prompt investigation if new or worsening respiratory symptoms (eg, dyspnea, fever, cough, wheezing, radiological abnormality) occur. D/C if pneumonitis is confirmed. May cause fetal harm; avoid pregnancy while taking therapy. If contraceptive methods are being considered, use highly effective contraception during treatment and for at least 1 month following the last dose of therapy.

ADVERSE REACTIONS
Anemia, N/V, dyspepsia, abdominal pain/discomfort, decreased appetite, diarrhea, fatigue/asthenia, nasopharyngitis/URI, arthralgia/musculoskeletal pain, myalgia, lab abnormalities.

DRUG INTERACTIONS
Potentiation and prolongation of myelosuppressive toxicity w/ other myelosuppressive anticancer agents, including DNA damaging agents. Avoid w/ strong CYP3A inhibitors (eg, itraconazole, telithromycin, clarithromycin) and moderate CYP3A inhibitors (eg, amprenavir, ciprofloxacin, imatinib); if strong or moderate CYP3A inhibitors must be coadministered, reduce dose of olaparib. Avoid grapefruit and Seville oranges. Avoid w/ strong CYP3A inducers (eg, phenytoin, carbamazepine, St. John's wort) and moderate CYP3A4 inducers (eg, bosentan, efavirenz, modafinil); if a moderate CYP3A inducer cannot be avoided, be aware of a potential for decreased efficacy of olaparib.

PREGNANCY AND LACTATION
Category D, not for use in nursing.

MECHANISM OF ACTION
Poly (ADP-ribose) polymerase (PARP) inhibitor; inhibits PARP enzymes, including PARP1, PARP2, and PARP3, which are involved in normal cellular homeostasis (eg, DNA transcription, cell cycle regulation, DNA repair).

PHARMACOKINETICS
Absorption: Rapid. T_{max}=1-3 hrs. **Distribution:** V_d=167L; plasma protein binding (82%). **Metabolism:** Extensive; CYP3A4 (primary); oxidation (major) and glucuronide or sulfate conjugation. **Elimination:** Urine (44%, 15% unchanged), feces (42%, 6% unchanged); $T_{1/2}$=11.9 hrs.

PATIENT CONSIDERATIONS
Assessment: Assess pregnancy/nursing status, and for possible drug interactions. Assess for presence of deleterious or suspected deleterious germline BRCA-mutations. Obtain baseline CBC.

Monitoring: Monitor for MDS/AML, pneumonitis, and for other adverse reactions. For prolonged hematological toxicities, monitor blood counts weekly until recovery. Monitor CBC monthly.

Counseling: Instruct to take ud and to not take w/ grapefruit or Seville oranges. Advise to contact physician if experiencing any new or worsening respiratory symptoms, or signs of hematological toxicity or MDS/AML. Instruct to inform physician if patient is pregnant or becomes pregnant. Inform female patients of the risk to a fetus and potential loss of pregnancy. Advise females of reproductive potential to use effective contraception during therapy and for at least 1 month after receiving the last dose. Advise not to breastfeed while on therapy. Counsel that mild or moderate N/V is very common in patients receiving olaparib and that patients should contact their physician who will advise on available antiemetic treatment options.

LYRICA — pregabalin   CV
Class: GABA analogue

ADULT DOSAGE
Neuropathic Pain
Associated w/ Diabetic Peripheral Neuropathy:
Initial: 50mg tid (150mg/day)
Titrate: May increase to 300mg/day w/in 1 week prn
Max: 100mg tid (300mg/day)

Associated w/ Spinal Cord Injury:
Initial: 75mg bid
Titrate: May increase to 150mg bid (300mg/day) w/in 1 week prn
Max: 300mg bid (600mg/day) if no sufficient pain relief experienced following 2-3 weeks of treatment w/ 150mg bid

Postherpetic Neuralgia
Initial: 75mg bid or 50mg tid (150mg/day)
Titrate: May increase to 300mg/day w/in 1 week prn
Max: 600mg/day divided bid or tid if no sufficient pain relief experienced following 2-4 weeks of treatment w/ 300mg/day

Partial Onset Seizures
Adjunctive Therapy:
Initial: 150mg/day divided bid-tid
Titrate: May increase up to max dose of 600mg/day

Fibromyalgia
Initial: 75mg bid
Titrate: May increase to 150mg bid (300mg/day) w/in 1 week prn
Max: 225mg bid (450mg/day)

PEDIATRIC DOSAGE
Pediatric use may not have been established

DOSING CONSIDERATIONS
Renal Impairment
Recommended Dose of 150mg/day BID or TID w/ Normal Renal Function:
CrCl 30-60mL/min: 75mg/day bid or tid
CrCl 15-30mL/min: 25-50mg/day qd or bid
CrCl <15mL/min: 25mg/day qd

Recommended Dose of 300mg/day BID or TID w/ Normal Renal Function:
CrCl 30-60mL/min: 150mg/day bid or tid
CrCl 15-30mL/min: 75mg/day qd or bid
CrCl <15mL/min: 25-50mg/day qd

Recommended Dose of 450mg/day BID or TID w/ Normal Renal Function:
CrCl 30-60mL/min: 225mg/day bid or tid
CrCl 15-30mL/min: 100-150mg/day qd or bid
CrCl <15mL/min: 50-75mg/day qd

Recommended Dose of 600mg/day BID or TID w/ Normal Renal Function:
CrCl 30-60mL/min: 300mg/day bid or tid
CrCl 15-30mL/min: 150mg/day qd or bid
CrCl <15mL/min: 75mg/day qd

Hemodialysis:
25mg QD Regimen: Take 1 supplemental dose of 25mg or 50mg
25-50mg QD Regimen: Take 1 supplemental dose of 50mg or 75mg
50-75mg QD Regimen: Take 1 supplemental dose of 75mg or 100mg
75mg QD Regimen: Take 1 supplemental dose of 100mg or 150mg

Discontinuation
Taper over minimum of 1 week

ADMINISTRATION
Oral route

STORAGE
25°C (77°F); excursions permitted to 15-30°C (59-86°F).

HOW SUPPLIED
Cap: 25mg, 50mg, 75mg, 100mg, 150mg, 200mg, 225mg, 300mg; Sol: 20mg/mL [16 fl oz]

CONTRAINDICATIONS
Known hypersensitivity to pregabalin or any of its components.

WARNINGS/PRECAUTIONS
Angioedema reported; d/c immediately if symptoms of angioedema w/ respiratory compromise occur. Caution in patients who had a previous episode of angioedema. Hypersensitivity reactions reported; d/c immediately if symptoms occur. Avoid abrupt withdrawal; gradually taper over a minimum of 1 week. Increased risk of suicidal thoughts/behavior; monitor for emergence or worsening of depression, suicidal thoughts/behavior, and/or unusual changes in mood/behavior. May cause weight gain and peripheral edema; caution w/ CHF. May cause dizziness and somnolence; may impair physical/mental abilities. New or worsening of preexisting tumors reported. Blurred vision, decreased visual acuity, visual field changes, and funduscopic changes reported. Creatine kinase (CK) elevations and rhabdomyolysis reported; d/c if myopathy is diagnosed or suspected or if markedly elevated CK levels occur. Associated w/ a decrease in platelet counts and PR interval prolongation. Caution in patients w/ renal impairment.

ADVERSE REACTIONS
Somnolence, dizziness, peripheral edema, ataxia, weight gain, dry mouth, fatigue, asthenia, blurred vision, diplopia, edema, nasopharyngitis, constipation, abnormal thinking, tremor.

DRUG INTERACTIONS
May increase risk of angioedema w/ other drugs associated w/ angioedema (eg, ACE inhibitors). Additive effects on cognitive and gross motor functioning w/ oxycodone, lorazepam, and ethanol. Caution w/ thiazolidinedione class of antidiabetic drugs; higher frequencies of weight gain and peripheral edema reported. Gabapentin reported to cause a small reduction in absorption rate. Reduced lower GI tract function (eg, intestinal obstruction, paralytic ileus, constipation) reported w/ medications that have the potential to produce constipation, such as opioid analgesics.

PREGNANCY AND LACTATION
Pregnancy: There is a pregnancy exposure registry that monitors pregnancy outcomes in women exposed to Lyrica during pregnancy. Increased incidences of fetal structural abnormalities and other manifestations of developmental toxicity, (eg, skeletal malformations, retarded ossification, decreased fetal body weight) reported in animal studies.
Lactation: Found in breast milk; not for use in nursing.

MECHANISM OF ACTION
Gamma-aminobutyric acid derivative; not fully established; binds w/ high affinity to the α_2-delta site (an auxiliary subunit of voltage-gated calcium channels) in CNS tissues.

PHARMACOKINETICS
Absorption: Well-absorbed; T_{max}=1.5 hrs (fasting), 3 hrs (fed). **Distribution:** V_d=0.5L/kg. **Metabolism:** Negligible metabolism. N-methylated derivative (major metabolite). **Elimination:** Urine (90% unchanged); $T_{1/2}$=6.3 hrs.

PATIENT CONSIDERATIONS
Assessment: Assess for hypersensitivity, renal impairment, preexisting tumors, history of drug abuse, history of depression, previous episode of angioedema, CHF, pregnancy/nursing status, and possible drug interactions. Obtain baseline weight.

Monitoring: Monitor for angioedema, hypersensitivity reactions, peripheral edema, weight gain, new tumors or worsening of preexisting tumors, ophthalmological effects, rhabdomyolysis, dizziness, somnolence, emergence or worsening of depression, suicidal thoughts or behavior, and/or changes in behavior. Monitor CK levels and platelet counts. Monitor ECG for PR interval prolongation.

Counseling: Instruct to d/c therapy and seek medical attention if hypersensitivity reactions or symptoms of angioedema occur. Advise patients and caregivers to be alert for the emergence or worsening of depression, unusual changes in mood or behavior, or the emergence of suicidal thoughts or behavior; instruct to report behaviors of concern to physician immediately. Explain that dizziness, somnolence, blurred vision, and other CNS signs and symptoms may occur; advise to use caution when operating machinery/driving. Inform that weight gain and edema may occur. Instruct not to abruptly/rapidly d/c therapy. Instruct to report unexplained muscle pain, tenderness, or weakness, particularly if accompanied by malaise or fever, to physician. Instruct not to consume alcohol while on therapy. Advise pregnant women of the potential risk to fetus. Advise that breastfeeding is not recommended during treatment. Inform men on therapy who plan to father a child of the potential risk of male-mediated teratogenicity. Instruct diabetic patients to pay attention to skin integrity while on therapy.

LYSTEDA — tranexamic acid   Rx
Class: Antifibrinolytic agent

ADULT DOSAGE	PEDIATRIC DOSAGE
Cyclic Heavy Menstrual Bleeding	**Cyclic Heavy Menstrual Bleeding**
2 tabs tid (3900mg/day) for a max of 5 days during monthly menstruation	**Adolescents (Postmenarchal):** 2 tabs tid (3900mg/day) for a max of 5 days during monthly menstruation

DOSING CONSIDERATIONS
Renal Impairment
SrCr >1.4 to ≤2.8mg/dL: 2 tabs bid (2600mg/day) for a max of 5 days during menstruation
SrCr >2.8 to ≤5.7mg/dL: 2 tabs qd (1300mg/day) for a max of 5 days during menstruation
SrCr >5.7mg/dL: 1 tab qd (650mg/day) for a max of 5 days during menstruation

ADMINISTRATION
Oral route

May be administered w/o regard to meals.
Swallow whole; do not chew or break apart.

STORAGE
25°C (77°F); excursions permitted to 15-30°C (59-86°F).

HOW SUPPLIED
Tab: 650mg

CONTRAINDICATIONS
Concomitant use of combination hormonal contraception. Active thromboembolic disease (eg, deep vein thrombosis, pulmonary embolism, cerebral thrombosis); history of thrombosis or thromboembolism (including retinal vein or artery occlusion); intrinsic risk of thrombosis or thromboembolism (eg, thrombogenic valvular disease, thrombogenic cardiac rhythm disease, or hypercoagulopathy); or known hypersensitivity to tranexamic acid.

WARNINGS/PRECAUTIONS
Exclude endometrial pathology that can be associated w/ heavy menstrual bleeding prior to prescribing. Venous and arterial thrombosis or thromboembolism reported. Retinal venous and arterial occlusion reported; if visual and ocular symptoms occur, d/c immediately and refer to an ophthalmologist for a complete ophthalmic evaluation, including dilated retinal examination, to exclude the possibility of retinal venous or arterial occlusion. A case of severe allergic reaction reported, involving dyspnea, throat tightening, and facial flushing that required medical treatment. A case of anaphylactic shock reported w/ IV bolus administration of the drug. Cerebral edema and cerebral infarction may occur in women w/ subarachnoid hemorrhage. Ligneous conjunctivitis reported. Not intended for use in premenarcheal girls or postmenopausal women.

ADVERSE REACTIONS
Headache, nasal and sinus symptoms, back pain, abdominal pain, musculoskeletal pain, arthralgia, muscle cramps and spasms, migraine, anemia, fatigue.

DRUG INTERACTIONS
See Contraindications. Not recommended w/ Factor IX complex concentrates or anti-inhibitor coagulant concentrates; risk of thrombosis may be increased. Caution w/ all-trans retinoic acid for remission induction of acute promyelocytic leukemia; may exacerbate the procoagulant effect of all-trans retinoic acid. Concomitant therapy w/ tissue plasminogen activators may decrease efficacy of both drugs; use w/ caution.

PREGNANCY AND LACTATION
Pregnancy: Category B. Not indicated for use in pregnant women.
Lactation: Found in breast milk; caution in nursing.

MECHANISM OF ACTION
Antifibrinolytic agent; synthetic lysine amino acid derivative, which diminishes the dissolution of hemostatic fibrin by plasmin. In the presence of tranexamic acid, the lysine receptor binding sites of plasmin for fibrin are occupied, preventing binding to fibrin monomers, thus preserving and stabilizing fibrin's matrix structure.

PHARMACOKINETICS
Absorption: Absolute bioavailability (45%); C_{max}=13.83mcg/mL (single dose), 16.41mcg/mL (multiple dose); T_{max}=2.5 hrs (median); AUC_{inf}=80.19mcg•hr/mL (single dose). **Distribution:** V_d=0.18L/kg (initial), 0.39L/kg (steady-state); plasma protein binding (3%); crosses placenta; found in breast milk. **Elimination:** Urine (>95% unchanged); $T_{1/2}$=11.08 hrs (single dose).

PATIENT CONSIDERATIONS
Assessment: Assess for active thromboembolic disease, history or intrinsic risk of thrombosis or thromboembolism, renal impairment, subarachnoid hemorrhage, drug hypersensitivity, pregnancy/nursing status, and possible drug interactions. Exclude endometrial pathology that can be associated w/ heavy menstrual bleeding prior to prescribing.

Monitoring: Monitor for venous and arterial thrombosis or thromboembolism, visual and ocular symptoms, allergic reactions, and other adverse reactions.

Counseling: Instruct to take as prescribed. Instruct to immediately d/c if any eye symptoms or change in vision is noticed; instruct to promptly notify physician and follow-up w/ an ophthalmologist for a complete ophthalmic evaluation, including dilated retinal examination of the retina. Advise to d/c and seek immediate medical attention if symptoms of a severe allergic reaction (eg, SOB, throat tightening) are noticed. Inform that common side effects of therapy include headache, sinus and nasal symptoms, back pain, abdominal pain, musculoskeletal pain, joint pain, muscle cramps, migraine, anemia, and fatigue. Advise to contact physician if heavy menstrual bleeding symptoms persist or worsen.

M-M-R II — measles, mumps, and rubella virus vaccine live   Rx
Class: Vaccine

ADULT DOSAGE	PEDIATRIC DOSAGE
Measles, Mumps, and Rubella Vaccine	**Measles, Mumps, and Rubella Vaccine**
0.5mL SQ	**≥12 Months of Age:**
Refer to PI for vaccination considerations	0.5mL SQ; recommended age for primary vaccination is 12-15 months; revaccinate prior to elementary school entry
	If vaccinated when <12 months of age, give another dose between 12-15 months of age followed by revaccination before elementary school entry
	Refer to PI for measles outbreak schedule and other vaccination considerations

ADMINISTRATION
SQ route

Inject preferably into the outer aspect of upper arm.
A 25-gauge, 5/8" needle is recommended.

Reconstitution
1. Use only diluent supplied.
2. Withdraw entire volume of diluent into syringe to be used for reconstitution.
3. Inject all diluent in syringe into vial of lyophilized vaccine; agitate to mix thoroughly.
4. Withdraw entire contents into a syringe and inject total volume of restored vaccine SQ.

STORAGE
Protect from light. **Unreconstituted Vaccine:** -50 to +8°C (-58 to +46°F). **Before Reconstitution:** 2-8°C (36-46°F). May refrigerate diluent or store separately at room temperature; do not freeze diluent. **Reconstituted Vaccine:** 2-8°C (36-46°F) in a dark place; discard if not used w/in 8 hrs.

HOW SUPPLIED
Inj: 0.5mL

CONTRAINDICATIONS
Hypersensitivity to any component of the vaccine (including gelatin), pregnancy, anaphylactic/anaphylactoid reactions to neomycin, febrile respiratory illness or other active febrile infection, immunosuppressive therapy (except corticosteroids as replacement therapy), blood dyscrasias, leukemia, lymphomas of any type, malignant neoplasms affecting bone marrow or lymphatic systems, primary and acquired immunodeficiency states (including immunosuppression associated w/ AIDS or other clinical manifestations of HIV infection, cellular immune deficiencies, hypogammaglobulinemic and dysgammaglobulinemic states), family history of congenital or hereditary immunodeficiency.

WARNINGS/PRECAUTIONS
Caution w/ history of cerebral injury, individual or family histories of convulsions or any other condition in which stress due to fever should be avoided. Extreme caution w/ history of anaphylactic/anaphylactoid, or other immediate reactions (eg, hives, swelling of mouth and throat, difficulty breathing, hypotension, shock) subsequent to egg ingestion; may be at an enhanced risk of immediate-type hypersensitivity reactions. Neomycin allergy often manifests as a contact dermatitis; a history of contact dermatitis to neomycin is not a contraindication. Severe thrombocytopenia may develop in individuals w/ current thrombocytopenia; individuals who experienced thrombocytopenia w/ 1st dose may also develop thrombocytopenia w/ repeat doses. Evaluate serologic status to determine need for additional doses. Have adequate treatment provisions, including epinephrine inj (1:1000), available for immediate use should an anaphylactic/anaphylactoid reaction occur. HIV infected children and young adults who are not immunosuppressed may be vaccinated, but vaccine may be less effective than for uninfected persons; monitor closely for vaccine-preventable diseases. Ensure that inj does not enter a blood vessel. Excretion of small amounts of the live attenuated rubella virus from the nose or throat 7-28 days after vaccination reported. Avoid w/ active untreated tuberculosis (TB). May not result in protection in 100% of vaccinees. Persons vaccinated w/ inactivated vaccine followed w/in 3 months by live vaccine should be revaccinated w/ 2 doses of live vaccine. May result in temporary depression of tuberculin skin sensitivity; administer tuberculin test either before or simultaneously w/ vaccine.

ADVERSE REACTIONS
Panniculitis, atypical measles, fever, syncope, headache, dizziness, malaise, diarrhea, N/V, irritability, arthralgia, arthritis, pneumonia, sore throat, Stevens-Johnson syndrome.

DRUG INTERACTIONS
See Contraindications. Do not give w/ immune globulin (IG); may interfere w/ expected immune response. Give vaccine 1 month before or after administration of other live viral vaccines. Defer vaccination for ≥3 months following administration of IG (human), or blood/plasma transfusions. Concurrent administration w/ diphtheria, tetanus, pertussis (DTP), and/or oral poliovirus vaccines is not recommended.

PREGNANCY AND LACTATION
Pregnancy: Category C. The vaccine should not be administered to pregnant females, and pregnancy should be avoided for 3 months following vaccination. **Lactation:** Caution in nursing.

MECHANISM OF ACTION
Vaccine; may induce antibodies that protect against measles, mumps, and rubella.

PHARMACOKINETICS
Distribution: Live Attenuated Rubella Vaccine: Found in breast milk.

PATIENT CONSIDERATIONS
Assessment: Assess for hypersensitivity to any component of the vaccine, current health/medical status, vaccination history, thrombocytopenia, active untreated TB, any other conditions where treatment is contraindicated or cautioned, pregnancy/nursing status, and possible drug interactions.

Monitoring: Monitor for anaphylactic/anaphylactoid reactions, thrombocytopenia, vaccine-preventable diseases in HIV patients, and other adverse reactions.

Counseling: Inform of benefits/risks of vaccination. Instruct to report any serious adverse reactions. Instruct to avoid pregnancy for 3 months after vaccination and inform of the reasons for this precaution.

MACROBID — nitrofurantoin macrocrystals/ nitrofurantoin monohydrate   **Rx**

Class: Imidazolidinedione antibacterial

ADULT DOSAGE	PEDIATRIC DOSAGE
Urinary Tract Infections	**Urinary Tract Infections**
Caused by susceptible strains of *Escherichia coli* or *Staphylococcus saprophyticus*	Caused by susceptible strains of *Escherichia coli* or *Staphylococcus saprophyticus*
Acute Uncomplicated (Acute Cystitis): 100mg q12h for 7 days	**>12 Years:** **Acute Uncomplicated (Acute Cystitis):** 100mg q12h for 7 days

ADMINISTRATION
Oral route

Take with food

STORAGE
15-30°C (59-86°F).

HOW SUPPLIED
Cap: 100mg

CONTRAINDICATIONS
Anuria, oliguria, significant impairment of renal function (CrCl <60mL/min or clinically significant elevated SrCr), pregnancy at term (38-42 weeks' gestation), during labor and delivery or when onset of labor is imminent, and neonates <1 month of age, previous history of cholestatic jaundice/hepatic dysfunction associated w/ nitrofurantoin, known hypersensitivity to nitrofurantoin.

WARNINGS/PRECAUTIONS
Not for treatment of pyelonephritis or perinephric abscesses. Many patients who undergo treatment are predisposed to persistence/reappearance of bacteriuria; if this occurs after treatment, select other therapeutic agents with broader tissue distribution. Acute, subacute, or chronic pulmonary reactions (diffuse interstitial pneumonitis, pulmonary fibrosis, or both) reported; d/c and take appropriate measures if these occur. Closely monitor pulmonary condition if on long-term therapy. Hepatic reactions (eg, hepatitis, cholestatic jaundice, chronic active hepatitis, hepatic necrosis) occur rarely. Monitor periodically for changes in biochemical tests that would indicate liver injury; withdraw immediately and take appropriate measures if hepatitis occurs. Peripheral neuropathy, which may become severe or irreversible, reported; risk may be enhanced with renal impairment, anemia, diabetes mellitus (DM), electrolyte imbalance, vitamin B deficiency, and debilitating disease. Monitor periodically for renal function changes with long-term therapy. Optic neuritis reported rarely. May induce hemolytic anemia of the primaquine-sensitivity type; d/c therapy if hemolysis occurs. *Clostridium difficile*-associated diarrhea (CDAD) reported; d/c therapy is CDAD is suspected/confirmed. Use in the absence of a proven or strongly suspected bacterial infection or prophylactic indication is unlikely to provide benefit and increases the risk of the development of drug-resistant bacteria. Lab test interactions may occur. Caution with impaired renal function and in elderly.

ADVERSE REACTIONS
Nausea, headache.

DRUG INTERACTIONS
Antacids containing magnesium trisilicate reduce both the rate and extent of absorption. Uricosuric drugs (eg, probenecid, sulfinpyrazone) may inhibit renal tubular secretion of nitrofurantoin; resulting increased nitrofurantoin serum levels may increase toxicity, and the decreased urinary levels could lessen its efficacy.

PREGNANCY AND LACTATION
Category B, not for use in nursing.

MECHANISM OF ACTION
Imidazolidinedione/nitrofuran antimicrobial agent; inhibits the vital biochemical processes of protein synthesis, aerobic energy metabolism, and DNA, RNA, and cell-wall synthesis.

PHARMACOKINETICS
Absorption: C_{max}=<1mcg/mL. **Distribution:** Found in breast milk. **Elimination:** Urine (20-25% unchanged).

PATIENT CONSIDERATIONS
Assessment: Assess for anuria, oliguria, significant renal impairment, history of cholestatic jaundice/hepatic dysfunction associated with nitrofurantoin, G6PD deficiency, DM, anemia, electrolyte imbalance, vitamin B deficiency, debilitating disease, drug hypersensitivity, pregnancy/nursing status, and possible drug interactions. Obtain urine specimens for culture and susceptibility testing prior to therapy.

Monitoring: Monitor for persistence or reappearance of bacteriuria, acute/ subacute/chronic pulmonary reactions, hepatic reactions, peripheral neuropathy, optic neuritis, hematologic manifestations, and CDAD. Monitor LFTs periodically. Monitor renal and pulmonary function periodically during long-term therapy. Obtain urine specimens for culture and susceptibility testing after completion of therapy.

Counseling: Inform of the potential risks and benefits of therapy. Advise to take with food (ideally breakfast and dinner) to further enhance tolerance and improve drug absorption. Instruct to complete the full course of therapy and advise to contact physician if any unusual symptoms occur during therapy. Advise not to take antacids containing magnesium trisilicate while on therapy. Inform that therapy treats bacterial, not viral, infections. Advise to take exactly ud; skipping doses or not completing full course may decrease effectiveness and increase drug resistance. Inform that diarrhea is a common problem that usually ends when antibiotic is discontinued. Inform that watery and bloody stools (with/without stomach cramps and fever) may develop even as late as 2 or more months after having taken the last dose; instruct to contact physician as soon as possible if this occurs.

MACRODANTIN — nitrofurantoin macrocrystals   Rx

Class: Imidazolidinedione antibacterial

ADULT DOSAGE
Urinary Tract Infections

Due to susceptible *Escherichia coli*, enterococci, *Staphylococcus aureus*, and certain susceptible *Klebsiella* and *Enterobacter* species

50-100mg qid for 1 week or for at least 3 days after sterility of the urine obtained

Long-Term Suppressive Therapy:
Reduce dose to 50-100mg qhs

PEDIATRIC DOSAGE
Urinary Tract Infections

Due to susceptible *Escherichia coli*, enterococci, *Staphylococcus aureus*, and certain susceptible *Klebsiella* and *Enterobacter* species

≥1 Month of Age:
5-7mg/kg/day given in 4 divided doses for 1 week or for at least 3 days after sterility of the urine obtained

Long-Term Suppressive Therapy:
1mg/kg/day given in a single dose or in 2 divided doses

ADMINISTRATION
Oral route

Take with food

STORAGE
20-25°C (68-77°F).

HOW SUPPLIED
Cap: 25mg, 50mg, 100mg

CONTRAINDICATIONS
Anuria, oliguria, significant impairment of renal function (CrCl <60mL/min or clinically significant elevated SrCr), pregnancy at term (38-42 weeks' gestation), during labor and delivery, or when the onset of labor is imminent, neonates <1 month of age, previous history of cholestatic jaundice/hepatic dysfunction associated w/ nitrofurantoin, known hypersensitivity to nitrofurantoin.

WARNINGS/PRECAUTIONS
Not for the treatment of pyelonephritis or perinephric abscesses. Many patients who undergo treatment are predisposed to persistence/reappearance of bacteriuria; if this occurs after treatment, select other therapeutic agents with broader tissue distribution. Acute, subacute, or chronic pulmonary reactions (diffuse interstitial pneumonitis, pulmonary fibrosis, or both) reported; d/c and take appropriate measures if these occur. Closely monitor pulmonary condition if on long-term therapy. Hepatic reactions (eg, hepatitis, cholestatic jaundice, chronic active hepatitis, hepatic necrosis) occur rarely. Monitor periodically for changes in biochemical tests that would indicate liver injury; withdraw immediately and take appropriate measures if hepatitis occurs. Peripheral neuropathy, which may become severe or irreversible, reported; risk may be enhanced with renal impairment, anemia, diabetes mellitus (DM), electrolyte imbalance, vitamin B deficiency, and debilitating disease. Monitor periodically for renal function changes with long-term therapy. Optic neuritis reported rarely. May induced hemolytic anemia of the primaquine-sensitivity type; d/c therapy if hemolysis occurs. *Clostridium difficile*-associated diarrhea (CDAD) reported; d/c therapy if CDAD is suspected/confirmed. Use in the absence of a proven or strongly suspected bacterial infection or prophylactic indication is unlikely to provide benefit and increases the risk of the development of drug-resistant bacteria. Lab test interactions may occur. Caution with impaired renal function and in elderly.

ADVERSE REACTIONS
Pulmonary hypersensitivity reactions, hepatic reactions, peripheral neuropathy, exfoliative dermatitis, erythema multiforme, lupus-like syndrome, nausea, emesis, anorexia, asthenia, vertigo, nystagmus, dizziness, headache, drowsiness.

DRUG INTERACTIONS
Antacids containing magnesium trisilicate reduce both the rate and extent of absorption. Uricosuric drugs (eg, probenecid, sulfinpyrazone) may inhibit renal tubular secretion of nitrofurantoin; resulting increased nitrofurantoin serum levels may increase toxicity, and the decreased urinary levels could lessen its efficacy.

PREGNANCY AND LACTATION
Category B, not for use in nursing.

MECHANISM OF ACTION
Imidazolidinedione antibacterial. Nitrofuran antimicrobial agent; inhibits the vital biochemical processes of protein synthesis, aerobic energy metabolism, and DNA, RNA, and cell-wall synthesis.

PHARMACOKINETICS
Distribution: Found in breast milk. **Elimination:** Urine (100mg qid for 7 days: Day 1: 37.9%; Day 7: 35%).

PATIENT CONSIDERATIONS
Assessment: Assess for anuria, oliguria, significant renal impairment, history of cholestatic jaundice/hepatic dysfunction associated with nitrofurantoin, G6PD deficiency, DM, anemia, electrolyte imbalance, vitamin B deficiency, debilitating disease, drug hypersensitivity, pregnancy/nursing status, and possible drug interactions. Obtain urine specimen for culture and susceptibility testing prior to therapy.

Monitoring: Monitor for persistence or reappearance of bacteriuria, acute/subacute/chronic pulmonary reactions, hepatic reactions, peripheral neuropathy, optic neuritis, hematologic manifestations, and CDAD. Monitor LFTs periodically. Monitor renal and pulmonary function periodically during long-term therapy. Obtain urine specimens for culture and susceptibility testing after completion of therapy.

Counseling: Inform of the potential risks and benefits of therapy. Advise to take with food to further enhance tolerance and improve drug absorption. Instruct to complete full course of therapy and advise to contact physician if any unusual symptoms occur during therapy. Advise not to take antacid preparations containing magnesium trisilicate while on therapy. Inform that therapy treats bacterial, not viral, infections. Advise to take exactly ud; skipping doses or not completing full course may decrease effectiveness and increase drug resistance. Inform that diarrhea is a common problem that usually ends when antibiotic is discontinued. Inform that watery and bloody stools (with/without stomach cramps and fever) may develop even as late as ≥2 months after having taken the last dose; instruct to contact physician as soon as possible if this occurs.

MAKENA — hydroxyprogesterone caproate   Rx

Class: Progestogen

ADULT DOSAGE
Preterm Birth

To reduce the risk of preterm birth in women w/ a singleton pregnancy who have a history of singleton spontaneous preterm birth

≥16 Years:
250mg (1mL) IM once weekly (every 7 days); inject slowly (over ≥1 min)

Begin treatment between 16 weeks, 0 days and 20 weeks, 6 days of gestation; continue administration once weekly until Week 37 (through 36 weeks, 6 days) of gestation or delivery, whichever occurs 1st

PEDIATRIC DOSAGE
Pediatric use may not have been established

ADMINISTRATION
IM route

Must be administered by a healthcare provider.

Instructions for Administration
1. Draw up 1mL of drug into a 3mL syringe w/ an 18-gauge needle.
2. Change the needle to a 21-gauge 1 1/2-inch needle.
3. Inject slowly (over ≥1 min) in the upper outer quadrant of the gluteus maximus; sol is viscous and oily.
4. Applying pressure to the inj site may minimize bruising and swelling.

If the 5mL multidose vial is used, discard any unused product 5 weeks after 1st use.

STORAGE
15-30°C (59-86°F). Protect from light. Store upright. **Multidose Vial:** Use w/in 5 weeks after 1st use.

HOW SUPPLIED
Inj: 250mg/mL [1mL, 5mL]

CONTRAINDICATIONS
Current/history of thrombosis or thromboembolic disorders, known/suspected/history of breast cancer or other hormone-sensitive cancer, undiagnosed abnormal vaginal bleeding unrelated to pregnancy, cholestatic jaundice of pregnancy, liver tumors (benign or malignant), active liver disease, uncontrolled HTN.

WARNINGS/PRECAUTIONS
Not intended for use in women w/ multiple gestations or other risk factors for preterm birth. D/C if an arterial/deep venous thrombotic or thromboembolic event occurs. Allergic reactions reported; consider discontinuation if such reactions occur. Decreased glucose tolerance observed; carefully monitor prediabetic/diabetic women. May cause fluid retention; carefully monitor women w/ conditions that might be influenced by this effect (eg, preeclampsia, epilepsy, migraine, asthma, cardiac/renal dysfunction). Monitor women who have a history of clinical depression; d/c if clinical depression recurs. Carefully monitor women who develop jaundice or HTN during treatment; consider whether the benefit of use warrants continuation. Not intended for use to stop active preterm labor.

ADVERSE REACTIONS
Inj-site pain/swelling/pruritus/nodule, urticaria, pruritus, nausea, diarrhea.

PREGNANCY AND LACTATION
Pregnancy: Category B.
Lactation: D/C at 37 weeks of gestation or upon delivery. Detectable amounts of progestins have been identified in the milk of mothers receiving progestin treatment.

MECHANISM OF ACTION
Synthetic progestin; has not been established.

PHARMACOKINETICS
Absorption: (Single 1000mg in non-pregnant females) C_{max}=27.8ng/mL; T_{max}=4.6 days. **Distribution:** Found in breast milk; extensive plasma protein binding. **Metabolism:** Extensive reduction, hydroxylation and conjugation via CYP3A4 and CYP3A5. **Elimination:** Feces (50%), urine (30%); (single 1000mg in non-pregnant females) $T_{1/2}$=7.8 days.

PATIENT CONSIDERATIONS

Assessment: Assess for multiple gestations or other risk factors for preterm birth, prediabetes/diabetes, conditions that might be influenced by fluid retention, history of clinical depression, and for other conditions where treatment is contraindicated or cautioned. Assess nursing status.

Monitoring: Monitor for arterial/deep venous thrombotic or thromboembolic events, allergic reactions, fluid retention, clinical depression, jaundice, HTN, and other adverse reactions. Monitor glucose levels in prediabetic and diabetic women.

Counseling: Explain that inj may cause pain, soreness, swelling, itching, or bruising. Instruct to contact physician if patient notices increased discomfort over time, oozing of blood or fluid, or if inflammatory reactions at the inj site occur.

MALARONE — atovaquone/proguanil hydrochloride   Rx

Class: Antiprotozoal agent/dihydrofolate reductase inhibitor

OTHER BRAND NAMES
Malarone Pediatric

ADULT DOSAGE

Malaria

Prophylaxis of *Plasmodium falciparum* Malaria, Including in Areas Resistant to Chloroquine:
1 adult strength tab (250mg/100mg) qd; start 1 or 2 days before entering a malaria-endemic area and continue daily during stay and for 7 days after return

Treatment of Acute, Uncomplicated *P. falciparum* Malaria:
4 adult strength tabs (1g/400mg) qd for 3 consecutive days

PEDIATRIC DOSAGE

Malaria

Prophylaxis of *Plasmodium falciparum* Malaria, Including in Areas Resistant to Chloroquine:
11-20kg:
1 pediatric tab (62.5mg/25mg) qd
21-30kg:
2 pediatric tabs (125mg/50mg) qd
31-40kg:
3 pediatric tabs (187.5mg/75mg) qd
>40kg:
1 adult strength tab (250mg/100mg) qd

Start 1 or 2 days before entering a malaria-endemic area and continue daily during stay and for 7 days after return

Treatment of Acute, Uncomplicated *P. falciparum* Malaria:
5-8kg:
2 pediatric tabs (125mg/50mg) qd
9-10kg:
3 pediatric tabs (187.5mg/75mg) qd
11-20kg:
1 adult strength tab (250mg/100mg) qd
21-30kg:
2 adult strength tabs (500mg/200mg) qd
31-40kg:
3 adult strength tabs (750mg/300mg) qd
>40kg:
4 adult strength tabs (1g/400mg) qd
Treat for 3 consecutive days

ADMINISTRATION
Oral route
Take at the same time each day w/ food or a milky drink.
Repeat dose in the event of vomiting w/in 1 hr after dosing.
May crush and mix w/ condensed milk just prior to administration for patients who may have difficulty swallowing tabs.

STORAGE
25°C (77°F); excursions permitted to 15-30°C (59-86°F).

HOW SUPPLIED
Tab: (Atovaquone/Proguanil) 250mg/100mg (adult), 62.5mg/25mg (pediatric)

CONTRAINDICATIONS
Known hypersensitivity reactions to atovaquone or proguanil hydrochloride or any component of the formulation. For prophylaxis in patients w/ severe renal impairment (CrCl <30mL/min).

WARNINGS/PRECAUTIONS
Reduced atovaquone absorption in patients with diarrhea or vomiting; monitor for parasitemia and consider use of an antiemetic if vomiting occurs. Alternative antimalarial therapy may be required in patients with severe or persistent diarrhea or vomiting. In mixed *P. falciparum* and *Plasmodium vivax* infections, *P. vivax* parasite relapse occurred commonly when patients were treated with atovaquone-proguanil alone. Treat with a different blood schizonticide in the event of recrudescent *P. falciparum* infections after treatment or failure of chemoprophylaxis. Elevated liver lab tests and cases of hepatitis and hepatic failure requiring liver transplantation reported with prophylactic use. Patients with severe malaria are not candidates for oral therapy. Caution for the treatment of malaria in patients with severe renal impairment. Caution in elderly.

ADVERSE REACTIONS
Abdominal pain, headache, N/V, diarrhea, asthenia, anorexia, dizziness, dreams, insomnia, oral ulcers, cough, pruritus.

DRUG INTERACTIONS
Atovaquone: Decreased levels with rifampin or rifabutin; not recommended with rifampin or rifabutin. Decreased levels with tetracycline; monitor for parasitemia. Reduced bioavailability with metoclopramide; use only if other antiemetics are not available. Decreased indinavir trough concentrations; use caution. **Proguanil:** May potentiate anticoagulant effect of warfarin and other coumarin-based anticoagulants; use caution when initiating or withdrawing in patients on continuous treatment with coumarin-based anticoagulants, and closely monitor coagulation tests with concomitant use.

PREGNANCY AND LACTATION
Category C, caution in nursing.

MECHANISM OF ACTION
Atovaquone: Antiprotozoal; selective inhibitor of parasite mitochondrial electron transport. **Proguanil:** Dihydrofolate reductase inhibitor; disrupts deoxythymidylate synthesis.

PHARMACOKINETICS
Absorption: Atovaquone: Absolute bioavailability (23% with food). **Distribution:** Atovaquone: V_d=8.8L/kg; plasma protein binding (>99%). Proguanil: V_d=1617-2502L (patients >15 yrs of age with body weight 31-110kg), 462-966L (pediatric patients ≤15 yrs of age with body weight 11-56kg); plasma protein binding (75%); found in breast milk. **Metabolism:** Proguanil: via CYP2C19; cycloguanil and 4-chlorophenylbiguanide (metabolites). **Elimination:** Atovaquone: Feces (>94% unchanged), urine (<0.6%); $T_{1/2}$=2-3 days (adults), 1-2 days (pediatrics). Proguanil: Urine (40-60%); $T_{1/2}$=12-21 hrs (adults and pediatrics).

PATIENT CONSIDERATIONS
Assessment: Assess for severity of malaria, drug hypersensitivity, renal dysfunction, diarrhea, vomiting, pregnancy/nursing status, and possible drug interactions.

Monitoring: Monitor for clinical response, N/V, diarrhea, hepatic/renal dysfunction, hypersensitivity, and other adverse reactions. Monitor parasitemia in patients who are vomiting. Monitor for relapse of infection when patients are treated with atovaquone-proguanil alone. Closely monitor coagulation tests when concomitant use with warfarin and other coumarin-based anticoagulants.

Counseling: Instruct that if a dose is missed, to take a dose as soon as possible and then to return to normal dosing schedule. Advise not to double the next dose if a dose is skipped. Counsel about serious adverse events associated with therapy (eg, hepatitis, severe skin reactions, neurological and hematological events). Instruct to consult physician regarding alternative forms of prophylaxis if prophylaxis is prematurely discontinued for any reason. Inform that protective clothing, insect repellents, and bednets are important components of malaria prophylaxis. Instruct to seek medical attention for any febrile illness that occurs during or after return from a malaria-endemic area. Discuss with pregnant women anticipating travel to malarious areas about the risks/benefits of such travel.

MARQIBO — vincristine sulfate liposome   Rx

Class: Vinca alkaloid

> For IV use only; fatal if given by other routes. Death has occurred with intrathecal administration. Has different dosage recommendations than vincristine sulfate injection; verify drug name and dose prior to preparation and administration to avoid overdosage.

ADULT DOSAGE

Acute Lymphoblastic Leukemia

Philadelphia Chromosome-Negative:
In ≥2nd relapse or if disease has progressed following ≥2 antileukemia therapies
2.25mg/m² over 1 hr once every 7 days

PEDIATRIC DOSAGE
Pediatric use may not have been established

DOSING CONSIDERATIONS
Adverse Reactions
Peripheral Neuropathy:
Grade 3 or Persistent Grade 2:
Interrupt therapy
D/C therapy if peripheral neuropathy remains at Grade 3 or 4
Reduce dose to 2mg/m² if peripheral neuropathy recovers to Grade 1 or 2

Persistent Grade 2 After 1st Dose Reduction to 2mg/m²:
Interrupt therapy for up to 7 days
D/C therapy if peripheral neuropathy increases to Grade 3 or 4
Reduce dose to 1.825mg/m² if peripheral neuropathy recovers to Grade 1

Persistent Grade 2 After 2nd Dose Reduction to 1.825mg/m²:
Interrupt therapy for up to 7 days
D/C therapy if peripheral neuropathy increases to Grade 3 or 4
Reduce dose to 1.5mg/m² if peripheral neuropathy recovers to Grade 1

ADMINISTRATION
IV route
Do not use w/ in-line filters
Do not mix w/ other drugs

Preparation Instructions
1. Fill a water bath w/ water to a level of at least 8cm (3.2 inches) measured from the bottom and maintain this minimum water level throughout the procedure; water bath must remain outside of the sterile area

2. Place a calibrated thermometer in the water bath to monitor water temperature and leave it in the water bath until the procedure has been completed

3. Preheat water bath to 63-67°C; maintain this temperature until completion of the procedure using the calibrated thermometer

4. Vent the sodium phosphate inj vial w/ a sterile venting needle equipped w/ a sterile 0.2 micron filter or other suitable venting device in the biological safety cabinet; always position venting needle point well above liquid level before adding sphingomyelin/cholesterol liposome inj and vincristine sulfate inj

5. Withdraw 1mL of sphingomyelin/cholesterol liposome inj

6. Inject 1mL of sphingomyelin/cholesterol liposome inj into the sodium phosphate inj vial

7. Withdraw 5mL of vincristine sulfate inj

8. Inject 5mL of vincristine sulfate inj into the sodium phosphate inj vial

9. Remove the venting needle and gently invert the sodium phosphate inj vial 5 times to mix; do not shake

10. Fit flotation ring around the neck of the sodium phosphate inj vial

11. Confirm that the water bath temperature is at 63-67°C using the calibrated thermometer

12. Remove the sodium phosphate inj vial containing vincristine sulfate inj, sphingomyelin/cholesterol liposome inj, and sodium phosphate inj from the biological safety cabinet and place into the water bath for 10 min using the calibrated electronic timer. Monitor the temperature to ensure it is maintained at 63-67°C

13. Immediately after placing the sodium phosphate inj vial into the water bath, record the constitution start time and water temperature on the overlabel

14. At the end of the 10 min, confirm that the water temperature is 63-67°C using the calibrated thermometer and remove the vial from the water bath (use tongs to prevent burns) and remove the flotation ring

15. Record the final constitution time and the water temperature on the overlabel

16. Dry the exterior of the sodium phosphate inj vial w/ a clean paper towel, affix overlabel, and gently invert 5 times to mix; do not shake

17. Permit the constituted vial contents to equilibrate for at least 30 min to controlled room temperature

18. Vial now contains 5mg/31mL (0.16mg/mL) vincristine sulfate; return the vial back into the biological safety cabinet

19. Calculate the patient's dose based on the patient's actual BSA and remove the volume corresponding to the patient's dose from an infusion bag containing 100mL of D5 inj or 0.9% NaCl inj

20. Inject the dose into the infusion bag to result in a final volume of 100mL

21. Complete the information required on the infusion bag label and apply to the infusion bag

22. Finish administration of the diluted product w/in 12 hrs of the initiation of preparation

23. Empty, clean, and dry the water bath after each use

24. Deviations in temperature, time, and preparation procedures may fail to ensure proper encapsulation of vincristine sulfate into the liposomes. In the event that the preparation deviates from the instructions in the above steps, the components of the kit should be discarded and a new kit should be used to prepare the dose

STORAGE
2-8°C (36-46°F). Do not freeze.

HOW SUPPLIED
Inj: 5mg/31mL

CONTRAINDICATIONS
Demyelinating conditions including Charcot-Marie-Tooth syndrome, hypersensitivity to vincristine sulfate or any of the other components of this product, intrathecal administration.

WARNINGS/PRECAUTIONS
For IV use only. Administer through a secure and free-flowing venous access line only. May cause extravasation tissue injury; d/c immediately and consider local treatment measures. Sensory/motor neuropathies and orthostatic hypotension may occur; delay dose, reduce or d/c if worsening neuropathy occurs. Risk of neurologic toxicity is greater with preexisting neuromuscular disorders or when other drugs with risk of neurologic toxicity are given. Dose delay, reduction, or d/c may be necessary when severe fatigue develops. May cause myelosuppression; consider dose modification/reduction and supportive care measures if Grade 3 or 4 neutropenia, thrombocytopenia, or anemia develops. Tumor lysis syndrome reported; anticipate, monitor, and manage. Ileus, bowel obstruction, and colonic pseudo-obstruction reported; institute prophylactic bowel regimen and consider additional treatments. Fatal liver toxicity and elevated AST reported; reduce/interrupt therapy if toxicity occurs. Avoid use in pregnancy; may cause fetal harm. Caution with elderly.

ADVERSE REACTIONS
Constipation, nausea, pyrexia, fatigue, peripheral neuropathy, febrile neutropenia, diarrhea, anemia, decreased appetite, insomnia.

DRUG INTERACTIONS
Simultaneous administration of PO or IV phenytoin and antineoplastic chemotherapy combinations that include non-liposomal vincristine sulfate may reduce levels of phenytoin and increase seizure activity. Vincristine sulfate is a CYP3A and P-glycoprotein (P-gp) substrate. Avoid concomitant use with strong CYP3A inhibitors/inducers and potent P-gp inhibitors/inducers. Effect of concomitant use with potent P-gp inhibitors/inducers has not been investigated; it is likely that pharmacokinetics or pharmacodynamics will be altered.

PREGNANCY AND LACTATION
Category D, not for use in nursing.

MECHANISM OF ACTION
Vinca alkaloid; non-liposomal vincristine sulfate binds to tubulin, altering the tubulin polymerization equilibrium, resulting in altered microtubule structure and function; stabilizes spindle apparatus, preventing chromosome segregation, triggering metaphase arrest and inhibition of mitosis.

PHARMACOKINETICS
Absorption: C_{max}=1220ng/mL; AUC=14,566h•ng/mL. **Elimination:** Feces (69%, non-liposomal vincristine sulfate), urine (<8%).

PATIENT CONSIDERATIONS
Assessment: Assess for drug hypersensitivity, demyelinating conditions including Charcot-Marie-Tooth syndrome, preexisting neuromuscular disorders, hepatic dysfunction, pregnancy/nursing status, and possible drug interactions.

Monitoring: Monitor for symptoms of neuropathy (eg, hypoesthesia, hyperesthesia, paresthesia, hyporeflexia, areflexia, neuralgia, jaw pain, decreased vibratory sense), tumor lysis syndrome, CBC prior to each dose, LFTs, and other adverse reactions.

Counseling: Inform of the risks and benefits of therapy. Advise to report immediately any burning or local irritation during/after infusion. Instruct not to drive or operate machinery if fatigue and peripheral neuropathy are experienced. May cause constipation; advise to take with diet high in bulk fiber, fruits and vegetables, and adequate fluid intake as well as stool softener use (eg, docusate). Notify physician if constipation symptoms, fever, productive cough, decreased appetite, new or worsening symptoms of peripheral neuropathy are experienced. Advise women of childbearing potential to use effective contraceptive measures to prevent pregnancy; report immediately to physician if pregnant. Inform not to receive treatment while pregnant or breastfeeding; if wishes to restart breastfeeding after treatment, instruct to discuss appropriate timing with physician. Counsel to inform any current medications.

MATULANE — procarbazine hydrochloride   Rx
Class: Hydrazine derivative

> Administer only by or under the supervision of a physician experienced in the use of potent antineoplastic drugs. Adequate clinical and laboratory facilities should be available for proper monitoring of treatment.

ADULT DOSAGE
Hodgkin Lymphoma

Stage III/IV Hodgkin's Disease in Combination w/ other Anticancer Drugs:
Initial: 2-4mg/kg/day as single or divided doses for 1st week (to minimize N/V), then 4-6mg/kg/day until max response is achieved or until WBC falls <4000/cmm or platelets fall <100,000/cmm
Maint: 1-2mg/kg/day when max response is achieved; d/c upon evidence of hematologic or other toxicity
May resume at 1-2mg/kg/day after toxic side effects subside based on clinical evaluation and appropriate laboratory studies

MOPP (Nitrogen Nustard, Vincristine, Procarbazine, Prednisone) Regimen:
100mg/m² daily for 14 days

PEDIATRIC DOSAGE
Hodgkin Lymphoma

Stage III/IV Hodgkin's Disease in Combination with Other Anticancer Drugs:
Initial: 50mg/m²/day for the 1st week, then 100mg/m²/day until max response is achieved or until leukopenia or thrombocytopenia occurs
Maint: 50mg/m²/day when max response is achieved; d/c upon evidence of hematologic or other toxicity
May resume therapy after toxic side effects have subsided

ADMINISTRATION
Oral route

STORAGE
15-30°C (59-86°F).

HOW SUPPLIED
Cap: 50mg

CONTRAINDICATIONS
Known hypersensitivity to procarbazine, inadequate marrow reserve as demonstrated by bone marrow aspiration.

WARNINGS/PRECAUTIONS
Hemolysis and appearance of Heinz-Ehrlich inclusion bodies in erythrocytes may occur. May cause fetal harm. Risks of secondary lung cancer may be multiplied by tobacco use. Allow an interval of ≥1 month without radiation/chemotherapeutic agent known to have marrow-depressant activity (determined by evidence of bone marrow recovery based on successive bone marrow studies) to elapse before initiating therapy. Undue toxicity may occur in patients with renal and/or hepatic impairment; consider hospitalization for the initial course of therapy when appropriate. Few cases of undue toxicity (eg, tremors, coma, convulsions) reported in pediatric patients. D/C promptly if CNS signs/symptoms (eg, paresthesia, neuropathies, confusion), leukopenia (WBC <4000/cmm), thrombocytopenia (platelets <100,000/cmm), hypersensitivity reaction, stomatitis, diarrhea, hemorrhage or bleeding tendencies occur. Bone marrow depression often occurs 2-8 weeks after start of therapy. If leukopenia occurs, hospitalization may be needed to prevent systemic infection.

ADVERSE REACTIONS
Leukopenia, anemia, thrombopenia, N/V.

DRUG INTERACTIONS
Avoid sympathomimetics, TCAs (eg, amitriptyline, imipramine), and other high tyramine-containing drugs/foods (eg, wine, yogurt, ripe cheese and bananas). Avoid with ethyl alcohol; Antabuse (disulfiram)-like reaction may occur. Caution with barbiturates, antihistamines, narcotics, hypotensive agents or phenothiazines

to minimize CNS depression and possible potentiation. Second nonlymphoid malignancies reported with other chemotherapy and/or radiation. Azoospermia and antifertility effects reported with other chemotherapeutic agents for treating Hodgkin's disease.

PREGNANCY AND LACTATION
Category D, not for use in nursing.

MECHANISM OF ACTION
Hydrazine derivative; not established. May act by inhibition of protein, RNA, and DNA synthesis. May inhibit transmethylation of methyl groups of methionine into t-RNA. May also directly damage DNA.

PHARMACOKINETICS
Absorption: Rapid and complete; (30mg) T_{max}=60 min. **Metabolism:** Liver and kidney; oxidation, isomerization, hydrolysis; N-isopropylterephthalamic acid (metabolite). **Elimination:** (PO/IV) Urine (70% metabolite). $T_{1/2}$=10 min (IV).

PATIENT CONSIDERATIONS
Assessment: Assess for hypersensitivity to drug, leukopenia, thrombocytopenia, anemia, history of radiation or use of chemotherapeutic agent known to have marrow-depressant activity (<1 month prior to treatment initiation), pregnancy/nursing status, and possible drug interactions. Evaluate hepatic/renal function and perform bone marrow aspiration before initiating therapy.

Monitoring: Monitor for CNS signs/symptoms, leukopenia, thrombocytopenia, anemia, hypersensitivity reaction, stomatitis, diarrhea, hemorrhage or bleeding tendencies, toxicity, and other adverse reactions. Closely monitor pediatric patients for tremors, coma or convulsions. Closely monitor hematologic status (eg, Hgb, Hct, WBC, differential, reticulocytes and platelets) at least every 3 or 4 days. Repeat urinalysis, transaminase, alkaline phosphatase, and BUN tests at least weekly.

Counseling: Instruct to avoid alcoholic beverages while on therapy; inform that Antabuse (disulfiram)-like reaction may occur. Advise to avoid foods with known high tyramine content (eg, wine, yogurt, ripe cheese and bananas). Instruct to avoid OTC drugs containing antihistamines or sympathomimetics. Warn against use of prescription drugs without the knowledge and consent of physician. Advise to d/c tobacco use.

MAVIK — trandolapril   Rx
Class: ACE inhibitor

> D/C when pregnancy is detected. Drugs that act directly on the renin-angiotensin system (RAS) can cause injury/death to the developing fetus.

ADULT DOSAGE
Hypertension
Not Receiving Diuretics:
Initial:
1mg qd in nonblack patients
2mg qd in black patients
Titrate: Adjust dose at intervals of at least 1 week based on BP response
Usual: 2-4mg qd

May treat w/ bid dosing if inadequately treated w/ 4mg qd
May add diuretic if not adequately controlled

Receiving Diuretics:
If possible, d/c diuretic 2-3 days prior to therapy to avoid hypotension. If BP is not controlled w/ trandolapril alone, then diuretic therapy should be resumed
Initial: 0.5mg
Titrate: Adjust to the optimal response

Heart Failure Post-Myocardial Infarction
Initial: 1mg qd
Titrate: Increase to target dose of 4mg qd as tolerated
If not tolerated, continue w/ the greatest tolerated dose

Left Ventricular Dysfunction Post-Myocardial Infarction
Initial: 1mg qd
Titrate: Increase to target dose of 4mg qd as tolerated
If not tolerated, continue w/ the greatest tolerated dose

PEDIATRIC DOSAGE
Pediatric use may not have been established

DOSING CONSIDERATIONS
Renal Impairment
CrCl <30mL/min:
Initial: 0.5mg qd
Titrate: Adjust to optimal response

Hepatic Impairment
Cirrhosis:
Initial: 0.5mg qd
Titrate: Adjust to optimal response

ADMINISTRATION
Oral route

STORAGE
20-25°C (68-77°F).

HOW SUPPLIED
Tab: 1mg*, 2mg, 4mg *scored

CONTRAINDICATIONS
Hypersensitivity to this product, hereditary/idiopathic angioedema, history of ACE inhibitor-associated angioedema. Coadministration w/ aliskiren in patients w/ diabetes.

WARNINGS/PRECAUTIONS
Anaphylactoid reactions reported during desensitization w/ hymenoptera venom, dialysis w/ high-flux membranes, and LDL apheresis w/ dextran sulfate absorption. Angioedema reported; d/c, treat appropriately, and monitor until swelling disappears if laryngeal stridor or angioedema of the face, tongue, or glottis occurs. Intestinal angioedema reported; monitor for abdominal pain. Higher rate of angioedema in blacks than nonblacks. Symptomatic hypotension may occur w/ volume and/or salt depletion, major surgery, or during anesthesia. Excessive hypotension associated w/ oliguria and/or azotemia, and rarely w/ acute renal failure and/or death, may occur in patients w/ CHF; monitor during first 2 weeks of therapy and w/ dosage increases. Caution w/ ischemic heart disease, aortic stenosis, or cerebrovascular disease; avoid hypotension. Consider lower doses of drug or concomitant diuretic if transient hypotension occurs. May cause agranulocytosis and bone marrow depression; consider periodic monitoring of WBCs in patients w/ collagen vascular disease (eg, systemic lupus erythematosus, scleroderma) and/or renal disease. Rarely associated w/ syndrome of cholestatic jaundice, fulminant hepatic necrosis, and death; d/c if jaundice develops. May cause changes in renal function. Increases in BUN and SrCr reported; dosage reduction and/or discontinuation may be required. Hyperkalemia reported; caution w/ renal insufficiency and diabetes mellitus (DM). Persistent nonproductive cough reported.

ADVERSE REACTIONS
Cough, dizziness, hypotension, elevated serum uric acid, elevated BUN, dyspepsia, syncope, hyperkalemia, bradycardia, hypocalcemia, myalgia, elevated creatinine, gastritis, cardiogenic shock, intermittent claudication.

DRUG INTERACTIONS
See Contraindications. Dual blockade of the RAS is associated w/ increased risks of hypotension, hyperkalemia, and changes in renal function (including acute renal failure); closely monitor BP, renal function, and electrolytes w/ concomitant agents that also affect the RAS. Avoid combined use of RAS inhibitors. Avoid w/ aliskiren in patients w/ renal impairment (GFR <60mL/min). Excessive BP reduction reported w/ diuretics. K^+-sparing diuretics (spironolactone, triamterene, amiloride), K^+ supplements, or K^+-containing salt substitutes may increase risk of hyperkalemia; use w/ caution and monitor serum K^+. May increase blood glucose lowering effect of antidiabetic medications (insulin, oral hypoglycemic agents). Increased lithium levels and symptoms of lithium toxicity reported; use w/ caution and frequently monitor serum lithium levels. Increased risk of lithium toxicity if a diuretic is also used. Coadministration w/ NSAIDs, including selective COX-2 inhibitors, may result in deterioration of renal function; monitor renal function periodically. Antihypertensive effect may be attenuated by NSAIDs. Nitritoid reactions (eg, facial flushing, N/V, hypotension) reported rarely w/ injectable gold. May enhance hypotensive effect of certain inhalation anesthetics. Concomitant mTOR inhibitor therapy may increase risk for angioedema.

PREGNANCY AND LACTATION
Pregnancy: Category D.
Lactation: Not for use in nursing.

MECHANISM OF ACTION
ACE inhibitor; reduces angiotensin II formation, decreases vasoconstriction and aldosterone secretion, and increases plasma renin.

PHARMACOKINETICS
Absorption: Trandolapril: Absolute bioavailability (10%); T_{max}=1 hr. Trandolaprilat: Absolute bioavailability (70%); T_{max}=4-10 hrs. **Distribution:** V_d=18L; plasma protein binding (80% trandolapril; 65-94% trandolaprilat). **Metabolism:** Liver via glucuronidation and deesterification; trandolaprilat (active metabolite). **Elimination:** Urine (33%), feces (66%); $T_{1/2}$=6 hrs (trandolapril), 22.5 hrs (trandolaprilat).

PATIENT CONSIDERATIONS
Assessment: Assess for hereditary/idiopathic angioedema, history of ACE inhibitor-associated angioedema, volume/salt depletion, CHF, ischemic heart disease, aortic stenosis, cerebrovascular disease, collagen vascular disease, DM, renal/hepatic impairment, hypersensitivity to the drug, pregnancy/nursing status, and possible drug interactions.

Monitoring: Monitor for anaphylactoid reactions, angioedema, hypotension, jaundice, hyperkalemia, cough, and other adverse reactions. Consider periodic monitoring of WBCs in patients w/ collagen vascular disease and/or renal disease. Monitor BP and renal/hepatic function.

Counseling: Advise to d/c and to consult physician if any signs/symptoms of angioedema develop (eg, swelling of the face, extremities, eyes, lips, or tongue, or difficulty in swallowing or breathing) or if syncope occurs. Inform that lightheadedness may occur, especially during the 1st days of therapy; instruct to report to physician if this occurs. Inform that inadequate fluid intake, excessive perspiration, diarrhea, or vomiting may lead to an excessive fall in BP w/ the same consequences of lightheadedness and possible syncope. Advise to inform physician of therapy prior to surgery and/or anesthesia. Advise not to use K⁺ supplements or salt substitutes containing K⁺ w/o consulting physician. Instruct to immediately report any signs/symptoms of infection (eg, sore throat, fever). Inform females of childbearing age about the consequences of exposure during pregnancy. Instruct to report pregnancy to physician as soon as possible.

MAXALT — rizatriptan benzoate   Rx

Class: 5-HT$_{1B/1D}$ agonist (triptans)

OTHER BRAND NAMES
Maxalt-MLT

ADULT DOSAGE
Migraine

W/ or w/o Aura:
Initial: 5mg or 10mg single dose; separate repeat doses by at least 2 hrs if migraine returns
Max: 30mg/24 hrs

PEDIATRIC DOSAGE
Migraine

W/ or w/o Aura:
6-17 Years:
<40kg: 5mg single dose
≥40kg: 10mg single dose

DOSING CONSIDERATIONS
Concomitant Medications
Propranolol:
6-17 Years:
≥40kg:
5mg single dose
Max: 5mg/24 hrs
≥18 Years:
5mg single dose
Max: 3 doses/24 hrs

Elderly
Start at lower end of dosing range

ADMINISTRATION
Oral route

Tab, Disintegrating
Do not remove blister from outer pouch until just prior to dosing.
Peel open w/ dry hands and place tab on tongue, where it will dissolve and be swallowed w/ saliva.

STORAGE
15-30°C (59-86°F).

HOW SUPPLIED
Tab: 5mg, 10mg; **Tab, Disintegrating:** (MLT) 5mg, 10mg

CONTRAINDICATIONS
Ischemic coronary artery disease (CAD) (angina pectoris, history of MI, or documented silent ischemia) or other significant underlying cardiovascular (CV) disease, coronary artery vasospasm (eg, Prinzmetal's angina), history of stroke or transient ischemic attack (TIA), peripheral vascular disease (PVD), ischemic bowel disease, uncontrolled HTN, hemiplegic/basilar migraine. Recent use (w/in 24 hrs) of another 5-HT$_1$ agonist or ergotamine-containing/ergot-type medication (eg, dihydroergotamine, methysergide). Concurrent use or recent discontinuation (w/in 2 weeks) of an MAO-A inhibitor. Hypersensitivity to rizatriptan benzoate.

WARNINGS/PRECAUTIONS
Use only when diagnosis of migraine has been clearly established. If no response after the 1st migraine attack, reconsider diagnosis before treating subsequent attacks. Not indicated for prevention of migraine attacks. Serious cardiac adverse reactions, including acute MI, reported. May cause coronary artery vasospasm (Prinzmetal's angina). Perform CV evaluation prior to therapy with multiple CV risk factors; consider administering 1st dose in a medically supervised setting and perform ECG immediately following administration in patients with a negative CV evaluation. Consider periodic CV evaluation in intermittent long-term users who have CV risk factors. Life-threatening cardiac rhythm disturbances (eg, ventricular tachycardia/fibrillation leading to death) reported; d/c if these occur. Sensations of tightness, pain, pressure, and heaviness in precordium, throat, neck, and jaw, usually of noncardiac origin, commonly occur after treatment; evaluate if cardiac origin is suspected. Cerebral/subarachnoid hemorrhage and stroke reported; d/c if cerebrovascular event occurs. Evaluate for other potentially serious neurological conditions before treatment. May cause noncoronary vasospastic reactions (eg, peripheral vascular ischemia, GI vascular ischemia, splenic infarction, Raynaud's syndrome); rule out before administering additional doses if experiencing signs/symptoms of noncoronary vasospasms. Transient and permanent blindness and significant partial vision loss reported. Overuse of acute migraine drugs may lead to exacerbation of headache (medication overuse headache); detoxification, including withdrawal of the overused drugs, and treatment of withdrawal symptoms may be necessary. Serotonin syndrome may occur; d/c if serotonin syndrome is suspected. Significant elevation in BP, including hypertensive crisis with acute impairment of organ systems, reported. Caution in elderly. **Tab, Disintegrating:** Contains phenylalanine.

ADVERSE REACTIONS
Paresthesia, dry mouth, nausea, dizziness, somnolence, asthenia/fatigue, pain/pressure sensation.

DRUG INTERACTIONS
See Contraindications. Increased plasma area under the curve with propranolol; adjust dose. Serotonin syndrome reported with SSRIs, SNRIs, and TCAs.

PREGNANCY AND LACTATION
Category C, caution in nursing.

MECHANISM OF ACTION
5-HT$_{1B/1D}$ receptor agonist; binds with high affinity to human cloned 5-HT$_{1B/1D}$ receptors located on intracranial blood vessels and sensory nerves of the trigeminal system.

PHARMACOKINETICS
Absorption: Complete. Absolute bioavailability (45%) (tab); T_{max}=1-1.5 hrs (tab), delayed by up to 0.7 hr (tab, disintegrating). **Distribution:** V_d=140L (male), 110L (female); plasma protein binding (14%). **Metabolism:** Oxidative deamination by MAO-A; N-monodesmethyl-rizatriptan (active metabolite). **Elimination:** Urine (82%; 14% unchanged, 51% indole acetic acid metabolite), feces (12%); $T_{1/2}$=2-3 hrs.

PATIENT CONSIDERATIONS
Assessment: Assess for ischemic CAD or other significant underlying CV disease, history of stroke or TIA, PVD, ischemic bowel disease, uncontrolled HTN, hemiplegic/basilar migraine, neurological conditions, phenylketonuria, drug hypersensitivity, pregnancy/nursing status, and possible drug interactions. Perform CV evaluation with multiple CV risk factors.

Monitoring: Monitor for coronary artery vasospasm, cardiac rhythm disturbances, cerebrovascular event, noncoronary vasospastic reactions, serotonin syndrome, BP elevation, and other adverse reactions. Consider periodic CV evaluation in intermittent long-term users who have CV risk factors.

Counseling: Inform of possible serious CV side effects, including chest pain, SOB, weakness, and slurring of speech, and to seek medical advice in the presence of such symptoms. Caution about the risk of serotonin syndrome. Advise to notify physician if pregnant, breastfeeding, or planning to breastfeed. Instruct to evaluate their ability to perform complex tasks during migraine attacks and after administration. Inform that overuse (≥10 days/month) may lead to exacerbation of headache; encourage to record headache frequency and drug use. **Tab, Disintegrating:** Inform phenylketonuric patients that tab contains phenylalanine.

MAXIDEX — dexamethasone   Rx

Class: Corticosteroid

ADULT DOSAGE
Steroid-Responsive Inflammatory Ocular Conditions

Treatment of steroid responsive inflammatory conditions of the palpebral and bulbar conjunctiva, cornea, and anterior segment of globe, such as allergic conjunctivitis, acne rosacea, superficial punctate keratitis, herpes zoster keratitis, iritis, cyclitis, or selected infective conjunctivitides

1-2 drops in the conjunctival sac(s)

Mild:
Drops may be used up to 4-6X daily

Severe:
Drops may be used qh, being tapered to discontinuation as inflammation subsides

Corneal Injury

Chemical, Radiation, or Thermal Burns, or Penetration of Foreign Bodies:

1-2 drops in the conjunctival sac(s)

Mild:
Drops may be used up to 4-6X daily

Severe:
Drops may be used qh, being tapered to discontinuation as inflammation subsides

PEDIATRIC DOSAGE
Pediatric use may not have been established

ADMINISTRATION
Ocular route

Shake well before using.

STORAGE
8-25°C (46-77°F). Store upright.

HOW SUPPLIED
Ophthalmic Sus: 0.1% [5mL]

CONTRAINDICATIONS
Epithelial herpes simplex (dendritic keratitis), vaccinia, varicella, and most other viral diseases of the cornea and conjunctiva, tuberculosis of the eye, fungal diseases of ocular structures, hypersensitivity to any component of this preparation.

WARNINGS/PRECAUTIONS
Prolonged use may result in ocular HTN and/or glaucoma, w/ damage to the optic nerve, defects in visual acuity and fields of vision, and posterior subcapsular cataract formation. Prolonged use may suppress the host response and thus increase the hazard of secondary ocular infections. May cause perforations in

diseases causing thinning of the cornea or sclera. May mask infection or enhance existing infection in acute purulent conditions of the eye. Routinely monitor IOP if used for ≥10 days. Caution w/ herpes simplex; periodic slit-lamp microscopy is essential. Consider the possibility of persistent fungal infections of the cornea after prolonged dosing.

ADVERSE REACTIONS
Glaucoma w/ optic nerve damage, visual acuity and field defects, cataract formation, secondary ocular infection, globe perforation.

PREGNANCY AND LACTATION
Pregnancy: Category C.
Lactation: It is not known whether topical administration of corticosteroids could result in sufficient systemic absorption to produce detectable quantities in human milk. Caution in nursing.

MECHANISM OF ACTION
Corticosteroid; suppresses the inflammatory response to a variety of agents and probably delays or slows healing.

PATIENT CONSIDERATIONS
Assessment: Assess for hypersensitivity, diseases causing thinning of the cornea/sclera, acute purulent conditions of the eye, herpes simplex, pregnancy/nursing status, and any other conditions where treatment is contraindicated or cautioned.

Monitoring: Monitor for ocular HTN, glaucoma, optic nerve damage, defects in visual acuity and fields of vision, cataract formation, secondary ocular infections, fungal infections, and other adverse reactions. Routinely monitor IOP if used for ≥10 days.

Counseling: Instruct not to touch dropper tip to any surface, as this may contaminate the sus. Instruct not to administer the drug while wearing soft contact lenses.

MAXIPIME — cefepime hydrochloride   **Rx**

Class: Cephalosporin (4th generation)

ADULT DOSAGE

Pneumonia
Pneumonia due to *Streptococcus pneumoniae* (including cases associated w/ concurrent bacteremia), *Klebsiella pneumoniae*, or *Enterobacter* species

Moderate to Severe: 1-2g IV q8-12h for 10 days

Pseudomonas aeruginosa Infections: 2g IV q8h

Febrile Neutropenia
Empiric Therapy:
2g IV q8h for 7 days or until neutropenia resolves

Frequently reevaluate the need for continued antimicrobial therapy in patients whose fever resolves but remain neutropenic for >7 days

Urinary Tract Infections
Uncomplicated or Complicated Infections, Including Pyelonephritis and Cases Associated w/ Concurrent Bacteremia:

Mild to Moderate Infections Due to *Escherichia coli*, *Klebsiella pneumoniae*, or *Proteus mirabilis*:
0.5-1g IM/IV q12h for 7-10 days
IM administration is only for infections due to *E. coli* when IM route is considered more appropriate

Severe Infections Due to *E. coli* or *K. pneumoniae*:
2g IV q12h for 10 days

Skin and Skin Structure Infections
Uncomplicated Infections Due to *Staphylococcus aureus* or *Streptococcus pyogenes*:
Moderate to Severe:
2g IV q12h for 10 days

Intra-Abdominal Infections
Complicated infections due to *E. coli*, viridans group streptococci, *K. pneumoniae*, *Enterobacter* species, or *Bacteroides fragilis*

2g IV q8-12h for 7-10 days in combination w/ metronidazole

P. aeruginosa Infections: 2g IV q8h

PEDIATRIC DOSAGE

Urinary Tract Infections
Uncomplicated or Complicated Infections, Including Pyelonephritis and Cases Associated w/ Concurrent Bacteremia:
2 Months-16 Years:
Up to 40kg:
Mild to Moderate Infections Due to *E. coli*, *K. pneumoniae*, or *P. mirabilis*:
50mg/kg q12h IV/IM for 7-10 days
IM administration is only for infections due to *E. coli* when IM route is considered more appropriate
Severe Infections Due to *E. coli* or *K. pneumoniae*: 50mg/kg q12h IV for 10 days
Max: Do not exceed the recommended adult dose

Skin and Skin Structure Infections
Uncomplicated Infections Due to *S. aureus* or *S. pyogenes*:
2 Months-16 Years:
Up to 40kg:
Moderate to Severe: 50mg/kg q12h for 10 days
Max: Do not exceed the recommended adult dose

Pneumonia
Pneumonia due to *S. pneumoniae* (including cases associated w/ concurrent bacteremia), *K. pneumoniae*, or *Enterobacter* species
2 Months-16 Years:
Up to 40kg:
Moderate to Severe: 50mg/kg/dose q12h for 10 days
P. aeruginosa Infections: 50mg/kg/dose q8h for 10 days
Max: Do not exceed the recommended adult dose

Febrile Neutropenia
Empiric Therapy:
2 Months-16 Years:
Up to 40kg:
50mg/kg q8h for 7 days or until neutropenia resolves
Max: Do not exceed the recommended adult dose

Frequently reevaluate the need for continued antimicrobial therapy in patients whose fever resolves but remain neutropenic for >7 days

DOSING CONSIDERATIONS
Renal Impairment
Adults:
Recommended Maint Dose of 500mg q12h:
CrCl 11-60mL/min: 500mg q24h
CrCl <11mL/min: 250mg q24h
Recommended Maint Dose of 1g q12h:
CrCl 30-60mL/min: 1g q24h
CrCl 11-29mL/min: 500mg q24h
CrCl <11mL/min: 250mg q24h
Recommended Maint Dose of 2g q12h:
CrCl 30-60mL/min: 2g q24h
CrCl 11-29mL/min: 1g q24h
CrCl <11mL/min: 500mg q24h
Recommended Maint Dose of 2g q8h:
CrCl 30-60mL/min: 2g q12h
CrCl 11-29mL/min: 2g q24h
CrCl <11mL/min: 1g q24h

Continuous Ambulatory Peritoneal Dialysis: Receive normal recommended doses q48h

Hemodialysis:
Administer at the same time each day and following the completion of hemodialysis on hemodialysis days
All Infections Except Febrile Neutropenia: 1g on Day 1, then 500mg q24h thereafter
Febrile Neutropenia: 1g q24h
Pediatrics:
Changes in dosing regimen proportional to those in adults are recommended

ADMINISTRATION
IV/IM route

Preparation
- Reconstitute 500mg single-dose vial w/ 5mL (for IV administration) or 1.3mL (for IM administration) of diluent.
- Reconstitute 1g single dose vial w/ 10mL (for IV administration) or 2.4mL (for IM administration) of diluent.
- Reconstitute 2g single vial dose w/ 10mL (for IV administration) of diluent.
- Reconstitute ADD-Vantage vials only w/ 50mL or 100mL of D5 inj or 0.9% NaCl inj in ADD-Vantage flexible diluent containers.

IV
Dilute w/ suitable parenteral vehicle and administer resulting sol approx over 30 min; compatible at concentrations between 1-40mg/mL w/ the following:
- 0.9% NaCl
- D5 and D10 inj
- M/6 sodium lactate inj
- D5 and 0.9% NaCl inj
- Lactated Ringer's and D5 inj
- Normosol-R
- Normosol-M in D5 inj

May administer intermittent IV infusion w/ a Y-type administration set w/ compatible sol; however, desirable to d/c other sol when infusing sol containing cefepime.
May store up to 24 hrs at room temperature (20-25°C [68-77°F]) or 7 days in a refrigerator (2-8°C [36-46°F]).
ADD-Vantage vials are stable at concentrations between 10-40mg/mL in D5 inj or 0.9% NaCl inj for 24 hrs at room temperature (20-25°C [68-77°F]) or 7 days in a refrigerator (2-8°C [36-46°F]).

IM
Constituted sol is stable for 24 hrs at room temperature (20-25°C [68-77°F]) or 7 days in a refrigerator (2-8°C [36-46°F]) w/ the following diluents:
- Sterile water for inj
- 0.9% NaCl
- D5 inj
- 0.5% or 1% lidocaine HCl
- Sterile bacteriostatic water for inj (w/ parabens or benzyl alcohol)

Refer to PI for admixture compatibility/incompatibility and instructions for use.

STORAGE
Dry State: 20-25°C (68-77°F). Protect from light.

HOW SUPPLIED
Inj: 500mg [vial], 1g, 2g [vial, ADD-Vantage]

CONTRAINDICATIONS
Hypersensitivity to cefepime or the cephalosporin class of antibiotics, penicillins (PCNs) or other β-lactam antibiotics.

WARNINGS/PRECAUTIONS
Cross-hypersensitivity among β-lactam antibiotics reported; caution in PCN-sensitive patients. D/C if an allergic reaction occurs. Serious adverse reactions reported including life-threatening or fatal occurrences of encephalopathy, aphasia, myoclonus, seizures, and nonconvulsive status epilepticus. If neurotoxicity associated w/ therapy occurs, d/c and institute appropriate supportive measures. *Clostridium difficile*-associated diarrhea (CDAD) reported; d/c if CDAD is suspected or confirmed. May result in overgrowth of nonsusceptible organisms w/ prolonged use; take appropriate measures if superinfection develops. Use in the absence of a proven or strongly suspected bacterial infection is unlikely to provide benefit and increases the risk of development of drug-resistant bacteria. May be associated w/ a fall in prothrombin activity; monitor PT in patients at risk (eg, patients w/ renal/hepatic impairment, poor nutritional state, receiving a protracted course of antimicrobial therapy) and administer exogenous vitamin K as indicated. Caution in elderly. Lab test interactions may occur.

ADVERSE REACTIONS

Local reactions, (+) Coombs' test, decreased phosphorous, increased ALT and AST, increased PT and PTT, rash.

DRUG INTERACTIONS

Monitor renal function if aminoglycosides are to be administered w/ cefepime because of the increased potential of nephrotoxicity and ototoxicity of aminoglycosides. Nephrotoxicity reported w/ potent diuretics (eg, furosemide); monitor renal function.

PREGNANCY AND LACTATION

Pregnancy: Category B.
Lactation: Caution in nursing.

MECHANISM OF ACTION

Cephalosporin (4th generation); bactericidal agent that acts by inhibiting cell-wall synthesis.

PHARMACOKINETICS

Absorption: Complete (IM). (IV/IM) Administration of variable doses resulted in different parameters. **Distribution:** V_d=18L; plasma protein binding (20%); found in breast milk. **Metabolism:** Metabolized to N-methylpyrrolidine (NMP), which is rapidly converted to the N-oxide (NMP-N-oxide). **Elimination:** Urine (85% unchanged, <1% NMP, 6.8% NMP-N-oxide, 2.5% epimer of cefepime); $T_{1/2}$=2 hrs.

PATIENT CONSIDERATIONS

Assessment: Assess for hypersensitivity to drug, cephalosporins, PCNs, or other β-lactam antibiotics, poor nutritional status, renal/hepatic impairment, pregnancy/nursing status, and possible drug interactions. Perform culture and susceptibility testing.

Monitoring: Monitor for signs/symptoms of hypersensitivity reactions, CDAD, superinfection, encephalopathy, myoclonus, seizures, nonconvulsive status epilepticus, and other adverse reactions. Monitor PT in patients w/ renal/hepatic impairment, poor nutritional state, or who are receiving a protracted course of antimicrobial therapy.

Counseling: Advise that therapy should only be used to treat bacterial, not viral, infections. Instruct to take exactly ud; inform that skipping doses or not completing the full course of therapy may decrease effectiveness of immediate treatment and increase bacterial resistance. Inform that diarrhea may occur and will usually end when therapy is discontinued. Instruct to contact physician as soon as possible if watery/bloody stools (w/ or w/o stomach cramps, fever) develop even as late as 2 or more months after the last dose. Advise that neurological adverse events may occur; instruct to inform physician at once of any neurological signs or symptoms that develop.

MAXITROL — dexamethasone/neomycin sulfate/
polymyxin B sulfate   Rx

Class: Antibacterial/corticosteroid combination

ADULT DOSAGE	**PEDIATRIC DOSAGE**
Steroid-Responsive Inflammatory Ocular Conditions	**Steroid-Responsive Inflammatory Ocular Conditions**
For which a corticosteroid is indicated and where bacterial infection or risk of bacterial infection exists	For which a corticosteroid is indicated and where bacterial infection or risk of bacterial infection exists
Oint:	**Sus:**
Apply small amount (1/2 inch) in conjunctival sac(s) up to 3-4X daily	**≥2 Years:**
Not more than 8g should be prescribed initially	Instill 1-2 drops in conjunctival sac(s) up to 4-6X daily in mild disease and hourly in severe disease; taper to d/c as inflammation subsides
Sus:	Not more than 20mL should be prescribed initially
Instill 1-2 drops in conjunctival sac(s) up to 4-6X daily in mild disease and hourly in severe disease; taper to d/c as inflammation subsides	
Not more than 20mL should be prescribed initially	

ADMINISTRATION

Ocular route

Oint

Tilt head back. Place finger on cheek just under the eye and gently pull down until a "V" pocket is formed between eyeball and lower lid. Place small amount of oint in the "V" pocket. Look downward before closing eye

STORAGE

Oint: 2-25°C (36-77°F). **Sus:** 8-27°C (46-80°F). Store upright.

HOW SUPPLIED

Oint: (Dexamethasone/Neomycin Sulfate/Polymyxin Sulfate) (0.1%/3.5mg/10,000 U)/g [3.5g]; **Sus:** (Dexamethasone/Neomycin Sulfate/Polymyxin Sulfate) (0.1%/3.5mg/10,000 U)/mL [5mL]

CONTRAINDICATIONS

Epithelial herpes simplex keratitis (dendritic keratitis), vaccinia, varicella, and other viral diseases of the cornea and conjunctiva; mycobacterial infection of the eye; fungal diseases of ocular structures; known or suspected hypersensitivity to any of the ingredients of this preparation and to other corticosteroids.

WARNINGS/PRECAUTIONS

For topical ophthalmic use only. Prolonged use may cause glaucoma with damage to the optic nerve, defects in visual acuity and fields of vision, posterior subcapsular cataract formation, suppressed host response, increased risk of secondary ocular infections, or persistent corneal fungal infections. May cause perforations when used with diseases causing thinning of cornea or sclera. May mask infection or enhance existing infection in acute purulent conditions of the eye. Monitor intraocular pressure (IOP) if used for ≥10 days. May cause cutaneous sensitization. Caution in the treatment of herpes simplex. Perform eye exam prior to therapy and renewal of medication. **Sus:** Usage after cataract surgery may delay healing and increase incidence of bleb formation. May prolong course and exacerbate severity of ocular viral infections (eg, herpes simplex). Do not inject subconjunctivally, nor directly introduce into anterior chamber of the eye. Reevaluate patient if no improvement seen after 2 days. Suspect fungal invasion in any persistent corneal ulceration during or after therapy; take fungal cultures when appropriate.

ADVERSE REACTIONS

Allergic sensitizations, elevated IOP, posterior subcapsular cataract formation, delayed wound healing, secondary infections.

PREGNANCY AND LACTATION

Category C, caution in nursing.

MECHANISM OF ACTION

Antibacterial/corticosteroid combination. Dexamethasone: Corticosteroid; suppresses the inflammatory response to a variety of agents. May inhibit the body's defense mechanism against infection.

PHARMACOKINETICS

Distribution: (Systemically administered) found in breast milk.

PATIENT CONSIDERATIONS

Assessment: Assess for active viral diseases of the cornea and conjunctiva, epithelial herpes simplex keratitis, vaccinia, varicella, mycobacterial infection of the eye, fungal disease of ocular structures, diseases causing thinning of sclera or cornea, acute purulent conditions, history of cataract surgery, hypersensitivity to the drug or its components, and pregnancy/nursing status. Perform eye exam (eg, slit-lamp biomicroscopy, fluorescein staining) prior to therapy.

Monitoring: Monitor for signs/symptoms of glaucoma, optic nerve damage, visual acuity and visual field defects, subcapsular cataract, ocular/corneal perforations, cutaneous sensitizations, and for bacterial, viral, and fungal infections. Monitor IOP and perform eye exams (eg, slit-lamp biomicroscopy, fluorescein staining) prior to renewal of medication. **Sus:** Monitor use after cataract surgery. Perform fungal cultures when fungal invasion is suspected.

Counseling: Advise not to touch dropper tip to any surface; may contaminate drug. Instruct to keep out of reach of children. Instruct to use medication as prescribed. Inform that medication is for topical ophthalmic use only. Instruct to inform physician if pregnant or breastfeeding. **Oint:** Advise not to wear contact lenses if signs and symptoms of bacterial ocular infection are present. Instruct not to use product if the imprinted carton seals have been damaged or removed. **Sus:** Advise to d/c and consult physician if inflammation or pain persists >48 hrs or becomes aggravated. Warn that use of the same bottle by more than one person may spread infection. Instruct to shake well before use and keep bottle tightly closed when not in use.

MAXZIDE — hydrochlorothiazide/triamterene   Rx

Class: Potassium-sparing diuretic/thiazide diuretic

> Abnormal elevation of serum K⁺ levels (≥5.5mEq/L) may occur with all K⁺-sparing diuretic combinations. Hyperkalemia is more likely to occur with renal impairment and diabetes (even without evidence of renal impairment), and in elderly or severely ill; monitor serum K⁺ levels at frequent intervals.

OTHER BRAND NAMES

Maxzide-25

ADULT DOSAGE	**PEDIATRIC DOSAGE**
Hypertension	Pediatric use may not have been established
Treatment when hypokalemia occurs on hydrochlorothiazide (HCTZ) alone, or when a thiazide diuretic is required and cannot risk hypokalemia	
Maxzide-25:	
1-2 tabs qd, given as a single dose	
Maxzide:	
1 tab qd	
Edema	
Treatment when hypokalemia occurs on HCTZ alone, or when a thiazide diuretic is required and cannot risk hypokalemia	
Maxzide-25:	
1-2 tabs qd, given as a single dose	
Maxzide:	
1 tab qd	

ADMINISTRATION

Oral route

STORAGE

20-25°C (68-77°F). Protect from light.

HOW SUPPLIED

Tab: (Triamterene/HCTZ) (Maxzide) 75mg/50mg*, (Maxzide-25) 37.5mg/25mg*
*scored

CONTRAINDICATIONS

Elevated serum K^+ (≥5.5mEq/L); anuria, acute or chronic renal insufficiency or significant renal impairment; concomitant K^+-sparing agents (eg, spironolactone, amiloride, or other formulations containing triamterene), K^+ supplements, K^+ salt substitutes, K^+-enriched diets; hypersensitivity to triamterene, HCTZ, or other sulfonamide-derived drugs.

WARNINGS/PRECAUTIONS

Obtain ECG if hyperkalemia is suspected. Avoid in severely ill in whom respiratory or metabolic acidosis may occur; if used, frequent evaluations of acid/base balance and serum electrolytes are necessary. May cause idiosyncratic reaction, resulting in acute transient myopia and acute angle-closure glaucoma; d/c as rapidly as possible. Monitor for fluid/electrolyte imbalances. May manifest latent diabetes mellitus (DM). Caution with hepatic impairment or progressive liver disease; minor alterations in fluid and electrolyte balance may precipitate hepatic coma. May cause hypochloremia. Dilutional hyponatremia may occur in edematous patients in hot weather. Caution with history of renal lithiasis. May increase BUN and SrCr; d/c if azotemia increases. May contribute to megaloblastosis in folic acid deficiency. Hyperuricemia may occur or acute gout may be precipitated. May decrease serum PBI levels. Decreased Ca^{2+} excretion reported. Changes in parathyroid glands with hypercalcemia and hypophosphatemia reported during prolonged use. Sensitivity reactions may occur. May exacerbate or activate systemic lupus erythematosus (SLE). May interfere with the fluorescent measurement of quinidine.

ADVERSE REACTIONS

Hyperkalemia, jaundice, pancreatitis, N/V, taste alteration, drowsiness, dry mouth, depression, anxiety, tachycardia, fluid/electrolyte imbalances.

DRUG INTERACTIONS

See Contraindications. Increased risk of hyperkalemia with ACE inhibitors. Hypokalemia may develop with corticosteroids, adrenocorticotropic hormone, or amphotericin B. Insulin requirements may be increased, decreased, or unchanged. May potentiate other antihypertensives (eg, β-blockers); dosage adjustments may be necessary. Avoid with lithium due to risk of lithium toxicity. Acute renal failure reported with indomethacin; caution with NSAIDs. May increase responsiveness to tubocurarine. May decrease arterial responsiveness to norepinephrine. Alcohol, barbiturates, or narcotics may aggravate orthostatic hypotension. May cause hypokalemia, which can sensitize or exaggerate the response of the heart to the toxic effects of digitalis (eg, increased ventricular irritability).

PREGNANCY AND LACTATION

Category C; not for use in nursing.

MECHANISM OF ACTION

Triamterene: K^+-sparing diuretic; exerts diuretic effect on distal renal tubule to inhibit the reabsorption of Na^+ in exchange for K^+ and H^+. HCTZ: Thiazide diuretic; blocks renal tubular absorption of Na^+ and Cl^- ions. This natriuresis and diuresis is accompanied by a secondary loss of K^+ and bicarbonate.

PHARMACOKINETICS

Absorption: Well-absorbed. HCTZ: T_{max}=2 hrs. Triamterene: Rapid, T_{max}=1 hr. **Distribution:** Crosses placenta; found in breast milk. **Metabolism:** Triamterene: Sulfate conjugation; hydroxytriamterene (metabolite). **Elimination:** HCTZ: Urine (unchanged).

PATIENT CONSIDERATIONS

Assessment: Assess for conditions where treatment is contraindicated or cautioned, DM, risk for respiratory or metabolic acidosis, SLE, pregnancy/nursing status, and for possible drug interactions. Obtain baseline BUN, SrCr, and serum electrolytes.

Monitoring: Monitor for signs/symptoms of hyperkalemia, idiosyncratic reaction, hypokalemia, azotemia, renal stones, hepatic coma, and for fluid/electrolyte imbalances. Monitor BUN, SrCr, and serum K^+ and folic acid levels. Monitor serum and urine electrolytes if vomiting or receiving parenteral fluids.

Counseling: Inform about risks/benefits of therapy. Advise to seek medical attention if symptoms of hyperkalemia, hypokalemia, renal stones, electrolyte imbalance, or hypersensitivity reactions occur. Instruct to notify physician if pregnant/nursing.

MECLOFENAMATE — meclofenamate sodium   Rx

Class: NSAID

> NSAIDs may increase risk of serious cardiovascular (CV) thrombotic events, including MI and stroke; increased risk w/ duration of use. Contraindicated in the setting of CABG surgery. Increased risk of serious GI adverse events (eg, bleeding, ulceration, stomach/intestinal perforation) that can be fatal and occur anytime during use and w/o warning symptoms; elderly patients are at greater risk.

OTHER BRAND NAMES

Meclomen (Discontinued)

ADULT DOSAGE

Mild to Moderate Pain

Usual: 50mg q4-6h; doses of 100mg may be needed in some patients for optimal relief
Max: 400mg/day

Rheumatoid Arthritis

Including acute exacerbations of chronic disease

Usual: 200-400mg/day, given in 3-4 equal doses

PEDIATRIC DOSAGE

Juvenile Arthritis

Safety and effectiveness in pediatric patients <14 yrs of age have not been established

Titrate: Adjust as needed to improve clinical response
Max: 400mg/day

Osteoarthritis

Including acute exacerbations of chronic disease

Usual: 200-400mg/day, given in 3-4 equal doses
Titrate: Adjust as needed to improve clinical response
Max: 400mg/day

Primary Dysmenorrhea

Usual: 100mg tid for up to 6 days, starting at onset of menstrual flow

Idiopathic Heavy Menstrual Blood Loss

Usual: 100mg tid for up to 6 days, starting at onset of menstrual flow

Other Indications

Fever
Ankylosing spondylitis
Acute subacromial bursitis/ Supraspinatus tendinitis
Acute gouty arthritis

ADMINISTRATION

Oral route

Administer w/ meals or w/ milk if GI complaints occur.

STORAGE

20-25°C (68-77°F). Protect from light and moisture.

HOW SUPPLIED

Cap: 50mg, 100mg

CONTRAINDICATIONS

Known hypersensitivity to meclofenamate sodium; patients who have experienced asthma, urticaria, or allergic-type reactions w/ aspirin (ASA) or other NSAIDs; in the setting of CABG surgery.

WARNINGS/PRECAUTIONS

Use the lowest effective dose for the shortest duration possible. Increased CV thrombotic risk at higher doses reported. Avoid use in patients w/ a recent MI unless benefits outweigh risks; if used, monitor for signs of cardiac ischemia. Avoid use in patients w/ severe heart failure (HF) unless benefits outweigh risks; if used, monitor for signs of worsening HF. Fluid retention and edema reported. May lead to onset of new or worsening of preexisting HTN. Extreme caution w/ history of ulcer disease or GI bleeding, or risk factors for GI bleeding (eg, smoking, prolonged NSAID therapy, older age, poor general health status); monitor for GI ulceration/ bleeding, and d/c if serious GI adverse event occurs. Renal papillary necrosis and other renal injury reported w/ long-term use. Renal toxicity reported in patients in whom renal prostaglandins have a compensatory role in the maintenance of renal perfusion; increased risk w/ renal/hepatic impairment, HF, and in elderly. Not recommended w/ advanced renal disease; if therapy must be initiated, closely monitor renal function. D/C if clinical signs and symptoms consistent w/ renal disease develop. Anaphylactoid reactions may occur; avoid w/ ASA triad. May cause serious skin adverse events (eg, exfoliative dermatitis, Stevens-Johnson syndrome); d/c at 1st appearance of skin rash or any other sign of hypersensitivity. Avoid in late pregnancy; may cause premature closure of ductus arteriosus. Not a substitute for corticosteroids or for the treatment of corticosteroid insufficiency. May mask signs of inflammation and fever. May cause elevation of LFTs or severe hepatic reactions; d/c if liver disease develops, systemic manifestations occur, or abnormal LFTs persist/worsen. Anemia may occur; monitor Hgb/Hct if signs/ symptoms of anemia occur w/ prolonged use. May inhibit platelet aggregation and prolong bleeding time. Caution w/ preexisting asthma, and in elderly/debilitated.

ADVERSE REACTIONS

Diarrhea, nausea, GI disorders, abdominal pain, pyrosis, flatulence, rash, headache, dizziness.

DRUG INTERACTIONS

May diminish antihypertensive effect of ACE inhibitors. Not recommended w/ ASA due to potential for increased adverse effects. May impair response of thiazides or loop diuretics. May reduce the natriuretic effect of furosemide and thiazides. May increase lithium levels and reduce lithium clearance; monitor for toxicity. May enhance methotrexate toxicity; use w/ caution. Enhanced synergistic effects w/ warfarin on GI bleeding. Increased risk of GI bleeding w/ oral corticosteroids, anticoagulants (eg, warfarin), smoking, or alcohol. Increased risk of renal toxicity w/ diuretics and ACE inhibitors.

PREGNANCY AND LACTATION

Category C; not for use in nursing.

MECHANISM OF ACTION

NSAID; has not been established. Inhibits human leukocyte 5-lipoxygenase activity.

PHARMACOKINETICS

Absorption: Rapid. C_{max}=4.8mcg/mL, 1mcg/mL (3-hydroxymethyl metabolite); T_{max}=0.9 hr, 2.4 hrs (3-hydroxymethyl metabolite). **Distribution:** V_d=23.3L; plasma protein binding (>99%); trace amounts found in breast milk. **Metabolism:** Extensive; 3-hydroxymethyl metabolite (active metabolite). **Elimination:** Urine (70%; 8-35% conjugates of meclofenamic acid and active metabolite, 35-62% other metabolites), feces (30%); $T_{1/2}$=1.3 hrs, 15.3 hrs (3-hydroxymethyl metabolite).

PATIENT CONSIDERATIONS

Assessment: Confirm that use is not in the setting of CABG surgery. Assess for CV disorders, HTN, history of hypersensitivity reactions to ASA or other NSAIDs, history of ulcer disease or GI bleeding, coagulation disorders, renal/hepatic impairment, hypersensitivity to the drug, pregnancy/nursing status, possible drug interactions, or any other conditions where treatment is contraindicated or cautioned.

Monitoring: Monitor for signs/symptoms of CV thrombotic events, GI events, anaphylactoid/hypersensitivity/skin reactions, hematological effects, and other adverse reactions. Monitor BP, LFTs, renal function, CBC, and chemistry profiles.

Counseling: Inform of the benefits/risks of therapy. Instruct to seek medical advice if symptoms of CV events, GI ulceration/bleeding, skin/hypersensitivity reactions, congestive HF, hepatotoxicity, or anaphylactoid reactions occur. Advise to d/c drug immediately if any type of rash or signs/symptoms of hepatotoxicity occur. Instruct to avoid therapy in late pregnancy.

MEDROL — methylprednisolone   Rx

Class: Glucocorticoid

ADULT DOSAGE	PEDIATRIC DOSAGE
Steroid-Responsive Disorders	**Steroid-Responsive Disorders**
Initial: 4-48mg/day, depending on disease and response	**Initial:** 4-48mg/day, depending on disease and response
Maint: Decrease dose by small amounts to lowest effective dose. Withdraw gradually after long-term therapy	**Maint:** Decrease dose by small amounts to lowest effective dose. Withdraw gradually after long-term therapy
Acute Exacerbations of Multiple Sclerosis: 200mg/day for 1 week followed by 80mg qod for 1 month	**Acute Exacerbations of Multiple Sclerosis:** 200mg/day for 1 week followed by 80mg qod for 1 month
Alternate Day Therapy (ADT): Twice the usual daily dose administered every other am Refer to PI for detailed information on ADT	**ADT:** Twice the usual daily dose administered every other am Refer to PI for detailed information on ADT

ADMINISTRATION
Oral route

STORAGE
20-25°C (68-77°F).

HOW SUPPLIED
Tab: 2mg*, 4mg*, 8mg*, 16mg*, 32mg*; (Dose-Pak) 4mg* [21§] *scored

CONTRAINDICATIONS
Systemic fungal infections, known hypersensitivity to components.

WARNINGS/PRECAUTIONS
May need to increase dose before, during, and after stressful situations. May mask signs of infection or cause new infections. Possible benefits should be weighed against potential hazards if used during pregnancy/nursing. Prolonged use may produce glaucoma, optic nerve damage, and secondary ocular infections. May cause BP elevation, increased K^+ excretion, and salt/water retention. More severe/fatal course of infections reported with chickenpox and measles. Caution with *Strongyloides*, latent tuberculosis (TB), hypothyroidism, cirrhosis, ocular herpes simplex, HTN, diverticulitis, fresh intestinal anastomoses, ulcerative colitis, osteoporosis, myasthenia gravis, renal insufficiency, and peptic ulcer disease. Kaposi's sarcoma reported. Growth and development of children on prolonged therapy should be monitored. Monitor for psychic disturbances. Avoid abrupt withdrawal.

ADVERSE REACTIONS
Fluid and electrolyte disturbances, HTN, osteoporosis, muscle weakness, cushingoid state, menstrual irregularities, impaired wound healing, convulsions, ulcerative esophagitis, excessive sweating, increased intracranial pressure, glaucoma, abdominal distention, headache, decreased carbohydrate tolerance.

DRUG INTERACTIONS
Reduced efficacy with hepatic enzyme inducers (eg, phenobarbital, phenytoin, rifampin). Increases clearance of chronic high-dose aspirin (ASA). Caution with ASA in hypoprothrombinemia. Effects on oral anticoagulants are variable; monitor PT. Increased insulin and oral hypoglycemic requirements in diabetics. Avoid live vaccines with immunosuppressive doses. Possible decreased vaccine response with killed or inactivated vaccines with immunosuppressive doses. Mutual inhibition of metabolism with cyclosporine; convulsions reported. Potentiated by ketoconazole and troleandomycin. Concomitant administration with immunosuppressive agents may be associated with development of infections.

PREGNANCY AND LACTATION
Safety in pregnancy and nursing not known.

MECHANISM OF ACTION
Anti-inflammatory glucocorticoid; causes profound and varied metabolic effects and modifies the body's immune responses to diverse stimuli.

PHARMACOKINETICS
Absorption: Readily absorbed from GI tract.

PATIENT CONSIDERATIONS
Assessment: Assess for systemic fungal infections, current infections, active TB, vaccination history, ulcerative colitis, diverticulitis, peptic ulcer with impending

---

perforation, renal/hepatic insufficiency, septic arthritis/unstable joint, HTN, osteoporosis, myasthenia gravis, thyroid status, psychotic tendencies, drug hypersensitivity, and possible drug interactions.

Monitoring: Monitor for adrenocortical insufficiency, occurrence of infection, psychic derangement, cataracts, acute myopathy, Kaposi's sarcoma, and fluid retention. Monitor serum electrolytes, TSH, LFTs, intraocular pressure, and BP. Monitor urinalysis, blood sugar, weight, chest x-ray, and upper GI x-ray (if ulcer history) regularly during prolonged therapy. Monitor growth and development of infants and children on prolonged corticosteroids therapy.

Counseling: Advise not to d/c abruptly or without medical supervision. Inform that susceptibility to infections may increase. Instruct to avoid exposure to chickenpox or measles and to seek medical advice immediately if exposed. Recommend dietary salt restriction and K^+ supplementation.

MEGACE ES — megestrol acetate   Rx

Class: Progesterone

OTHER BRAND NAMES
Megace

ADULT DOSAGE	PEDIATRIC DOSAGE
Weight Loss	Pediatric use may not have been established
Anorexia, Cachexia or Unexplained Significant Weight Loss in AIDS Patients:	
Megace ES: **Initial:** 625mg/day (5mL/day)	
Megace: **Initial:** 800mg/day (20mL/day); Daily doses of 400mg/day and 800mg/day found to be effective	

DOSING CONSIDERATIONS
Elderly
Start at lower end of dosing range

ADMINISTRATION
Oral route

Shake well before use

STORAGE
15-25°C (59-77°F). Protect from heat.

HOW SUPPLIED
Sus: (ES) 125mg/mL [150mL]; (Megace) 40mg/mL [240mL]

CONTRAINDICATIONS
History of hypersensitivity to megestrol acetate or any component of the formulation, known or suspected pregnancy.

WARNINGS/PRECAUTIONS
Institute only after treatable causes of weight loss are sought and addressed. 125mg/mL strength is not substitutable with other strengths (eg, 40mg/mL). Overt Cushing's syndrome and asymptomatic pituitary-adrenal suppression reported with chronic use. Adrenal insufficiency reported in patients receiving or being withdrawn from chronic therapy; consider use of replacement or stress doses of a rapidly acting glucocorticoid. New onset diabetes mellitus (DM) and exacerbation of preexisting DM reported with chronic use. Breakthrough bleeding reported in women. Caution with history of thromboembolic disease and in elderly.

ADVERSE REACTIONS
Diarrhea, rash, flatulence, N/V, HTN, headache, pain, asthenia, insomnia, anemia, fever, decreased libido, impotence, hyperglycemia.

DRUG INTERACTIONS
(ES) May decrease exposure of indinavir; consider higher dose of indinavir.

PREGNANCY AND LACTATION
Category X, not for use in nursing.

MECHANISM OF ACTION
Progesterone; has not been established. Has appetite-enhancing property.

PHARMACOKINETICS
Absorption: (800mg qd) C_{max}=753ng/mL; AUC=10,476ng•hr/mL; T_{max}=5 hrs (median). (750mg qd) C_{max}=490ng/mL; AUC=6779ng•hr/mL; T_{max}=3 hrs (median). **Elimination:** Urine (66.4%, 5-8% metabolites); feces (19.8%); (ES) $T_{1/2}$=20-50 hrs.

PATIENT CONSIDERATIONS
Assessment: Assess for preexisting DM, history of thromboembolic disease, hypersensitivity to drug, pregnancy/nursing status, and possible drug interactions.

Monitoring: Monitor for adrenal insufficiency, new onset/exacerbation of DM, vaginal bleeding, and other adverse reactions.

Counseling: Inform about product differences to avoid overdosing or underdosing. Instruct to use ud. Advise to report any adverse reactions. Advise women of childbearing potential to use contraception while on therapy, and to notify physician if pregnancy occurs.

MEKINIST — trametinib   Rx
Class: Kinase inhibitor

ADULT DOSAGE

Unresectable or Metastatic Melanoma with BRAF V600E or V600K Mutations

2mg qd, at the same time each day, as a single agent or in combination w/ dabrafenib until disease progression or unacceptable toxicity occurs

Missed Dose

Do not take a missed dose w/in 12 hrs of the next dose

PEDIATRIC DOSAGE

- Pediatric use may not have been established

DOSING CONSIDERATIONS

Adverse Reactions
Dose Reductions for Trametinib:
First Dose Reduction: 1.5mg qd
Second Dose Reduction: 1mg qd
Subsequent Modification: Permanently d/c if unable to tolerate 1mg qd

Febrile Drug Reaction:
Fever >104°F or Fever Complicated by Rigors, Hypotension, Dehydration, or Renal Failure: Withhold until fever resolves, then resume at same or lower dose level

Cutaneous:
Grade 3 or 4 Skin Toxicity or Intolerable Grade 2 Skin Toxicity: Withhold for up to 3 weeks; resume at a lower dose level if improved or permanently d/c if not improved

Cardiac:
Asymptomatic, Absolute Decrease in Left Ventricular Ejection Fraction (LVEF) of 10% or Greater from Baseline and Below Lower Limits of Normal (LLN) from Pretreatment Value: Withhold for up to 4 weeks. If improved to normal LVEF value, resume at a lower dose level. If not improved to normal LVEF value, permanently d/c
Symptomatic CHF/Absolute Decrease in LVEF >20% from Baseline that is Below LLN: Permanently d/c

Venous Thromboembolism (VTE):
Uncomplicated Deep Vein Thrombosis (DVT) or Pulmonary Embolism (PE): Withhold for up to 3 weeks; resume at a lower dose level if improved to Grade 0-1 or permanently d/c if not improved
Life-Threatening PE: Permanently d/c

Ocular Toxicities:
Retinal Pigment Epithelial Detachments: Withhold for up to 3 weeks. If improved, resume at same or lower dose level. If not improved, d/c or resume at a lower dose
Retinal Vein Occlusion (RVO): Permanently d/c

Pulmonary:
Interstitial Lung Disease (ILD)/Pneumonitis: Permanently d/c

Other:
Any Grade 3 Adverse Reactions or Intolerable Grade 2 Adverse Reactions: Withhold; resume at a lower dose level if improved to Grade 0-1 or permanently d/c if not improved
First Occurrence of Any Grade 4 Adverse Reaction: Withhold until adverse reaction improves to Grade 0-1, then resume at a lower dose level; or permanently d/c
Recurrent Grade 4 Adverse Reaction: Permanently d/c

Refer to dabrafenib PI for recommended dose modifications

ADMINISTRATION
Oral route

Take at least 1 hr ac or 2 hrs pc.

STORAGE
2-8°C (36-46°F). Do not freeze. Protect from moisture and light. Do not place in pill boxes.

HOW SUPPLIED
Tab: 0.5mg, 2mg

WARNINGS/PRECAUTIONS
See Dosing Considerations. Not indicated for treatment of patients who have received prior BRAF-inhibitor therapy. New primary malignancies, cutaneous and noncutaneous, may occur when therapy is administered w/ dabrafenib. Perform dermatologic evaluations prior to initiation of therapy when used w/ dabrafenib, every 2 months while on therapy, and for up to 6 months following discontinuation of the combination. Hemorrhages (eg, major hemorrhages defined as symptomatic bleeding in a critical area or organ) and VTE may occur. Cardiomyopathy, including cardiac failure, may occur; assess LVEF by echocardiogram or multigated acquisition (MUGA) scan before initiation of therapy as a single agent or w/ dabrafenib, 1 month after initiation, and then at 2- to 3-month intervals while on treatment. RVO reported and may lead to macular edema, decreased visual function, neovascularization, and glaucoma; urgently (w/in 24 hrs), perform ophthalmological evaluation for patient-reported loss of vision or other visual disturbances. Retinal pigment epithelial detachments may occur; retinal detachments may be bilateral and multifocal, occurring in the central macular region of the retina or elsewhere in the retina. Perform ophthalmological evaluation periodically and at any time a patient reports

visual disturbances. ILD or pneumonitis reported; withhold therapy in patients presenting w/ new/progressive pulmonary symptoms and findings (eg, cough, dyspnea, hypoxia, pleural effusion, infiltrates) pending clinical investigations. Serious febrile reactions and fever of any severity accompanied by hypotension, rigors or chills, dehydration, or renal failure may occur when therapy is administered w/ dabrafenib. Monitor SrCr and other evidence of renal function during and following severe pyrexia. Administer antipyretics as secondary prophylaxis when resuming therapy if patient had a prior episode of severe febrile reaction or fever associated w/ complications. Administer corticosteroids (eg, prednisone 10mg daily) for at least 5 days for second or subsequent pyrexia if temperature does not return to baseline w/in 3 days of onset of pyrexia, or for pyrexia associated w/ complications (eg, dehydration, hypotension, renal failure, severe chills/rigors), and there is no evidence of active infection. Serious skin toxicity may occur. Hyperglycemia may occur when therapy is administered w/ dabrafenib; monitor serum glucose levels upon initiation and as clinically appropriate in patients w/ preexisting diabetes or hyperglycemia. May cause fetal harm.

ADVERSE REACTIONS
Single Agent Trametinib: Rash, diarrhea, lymphedema, acneiform dermatitis, dry skin, pruritus, paronychia, stomatitis, abdominal pain, HTN, hemorrhage.
W/ Dabrafenib: Pyrexia, N/V, rash, chills, diarrhea, HTN, and peripheral edema.

PREGNANCY AND LACTATION
Pregnancy: May cause fetal harm.
Lactation: Advise women not to breastfeed during treatment and for 4 months following the last dose.
Reproductive Potential: Females of reproductive potential should use effective contraception during treatment and for 4 months after the last dose. May impair fertility in females of reproductive potential.

MECHANISM OF ACTION
Kinase inhibitor; reversible inhibitor of mitogen-activated extracellular signal regulated kinase 1 (MEK1) and MEK2 activation and of MEK1 and MEK2 kinase activity, which promote cellular proliferation. BRAF V600E mutations result in constitutive activation of the BRAF pathway, which includes MEK1 and MEK2. Inhibits BRAF V600 mutation-positive melanoma cell growth in vitro and in vivo. Use of trametinib and dabrafenib in combination resulted in greater growth inhibition of BRAF V600 mutation-positive melanoma cell lines in vitro and prolonged inhibition of tumor growth in BRAF V600 mutation positive melanoma xenografts compared w/ either drug alone.

PHARMACOKINETICS
Absorption: Absolute bioavailability (72%) (single 2mg dose); T_{max}=1.5 hrs (median). **Distribution:** Plasma protein binding (97.4%); V_d=214L. **Metabolism:** Predominantly via deacetylation alone or w/ mono-oxygenation or in combination w/ glucuronidation biotransformation pathways. Deacetylation is mediated by carboxylesterases and may also be mediated by other hydrolytic enzymes. **Elimination:** Feces (>80%), urine (<20%, <0.1% parent drug); $T_{1/2}$=3.9-4.8 days.

PATIENT CONSIDERATIONS
Assessment: Assess for diabetes, hyperglycemia, and pregnancy/nursing status. Confirm the presence of BRAF V600E or V600K mutation in tumor specimens. Assess if patient has received prior BRAF-inhibitor therapy. Perform dermatologic evaluations prior to initiation of therapy when used w/ dabrafenib. Assess LVEF by echocardiogram or MUGA scan before initiation of therapy as a single agent or w/ dabrafenib.

Monitoring: Monitor for new primary malignancies, hemorrhagic events, VTE, cardiomyopathy, retinal pigment epithelial detachment, RVO, ILD, pneumonitis, febrile reactions, skin toxicity, and other adverse reactions. When used w/ dabrafenib, perform dermatologic evaluations every 2 months while on therapy, and for up to 6 months following discontinuation of the combination. When therapy is given as a single agent or w/ dabrafenib, assess LVEF by echocardiogram or MUGA scan 1 month after initiation, and then at 2- to 3-month intervals while on treatment. Perform ophthalmological evaluation periodically and at any time a patient reports visual disturbances. Monitor serum glucose levels when therapy is used in combination w/ dabrafenib upon initiation and as clinically appropriate in patients w/ preexisting diabetes or hyperglycemia.

Counseling: Inform that evidence of BRAF V600E or V600K mutation w/in the tumor specimen is necessary to identify patients for whom treatment is indicated. Inform that combined use w/ dabrafenib may result in development of new primary cutaneous and noncutaneous malignancies, increase risk of intracranial and GI hemorrhage, increase risk of PE/DVT, and cause serious febrile reactions; advise to contact physician for signs/symptoms of malignancies, unusual bleeding/hemorrhage, venous thrombosis, or if fever develops. Advise to immediately report any signs/symptoms of heart failure, visual changes, cough or dyspnea, progressive or intolerable rash, and severe diarrhea. Advise of the need to undergo BP monitoring and to notify physician if symptoms of HTN develop. Inform of the risk of fetal harm if taken during pregnancy; instruct females of reproductive potential to use highly effective contraception during treatment and for 4 months after the last dose. Advise to contact physician if patient becomes pregnant, or if pregnancy is suspected. Instruct not to breastfeed during treatment and for 4 months after the last dose. Inform of the potential risk for impaired fertility. Instruct to take ud.

MENACTRA — meningococcal (groups A, C, Y and W-135) polysaccharide diphtheria toxoid conjugate vaccine   Rx
Class: Vaccine

ADULT DOSAGE	PEDIATRIC DOSAGE
Meningococcal Vaccine	**Meningococcal Vaccine**
Active Immunization to Prevent Invasive Disease Caused By *Neisseria meningitidis* Serogroups A, C, Y and W-135:	**Active Immunization to Prevent Invasive Disease Caused By *Neisseria meningitidis* Serogroups A, C, Y and W-135:**
≤55 Years:	**Primary Vaccination:**
Primary Vaccination:	**9-23 Months of Age:**
0.5mL IM dose single dose	0.5mL IM dose given as a 2-dose series 3 months apart
Booster Vaccination:	**≥2 Years:**
A single booster dose may be given to individuals at continued risk for meningococcal disease, if at least 4 yrs have elapsed since prior dose	0.5mL IM single dose
	Booster Vaccination:
	≥15 Years:
	A single booster dose may be given to individuals at continued risk for meningococcal disease, if at least 4 yrs have elapsed since prior dose

ADMINISTRATION
IM route
Do not mix w/ any other vaccine in the same syringe

STORAGE
2-8°C (35-46°F). Do not freeze.

HOW SUPPLIED
Inj: 0.5mL

WARNINGS/PRECAUTIONS
Guillain-Barre syndrome (GBS) reported; may be at increased risk if previously diagnosed with GBS. Review immunization history for possible vaccine hypersensitivity and previous vaccination-related adverse reactions. Epinephrine and other appropriate agents must be immediately available for possible acute anaphylactic reactions. Immunocompromised persons may have diminished immune response to therapy. May not protect all recipients. Syncope (fainting) reported; procedures should be in place to prevent falling injury and manage syncopal reactions.

ADVERSE REACTIONS
Inj-site reactions, headache, fatigue, malaise, arthralgia, anorexia, chills, fever, diarrhea, drowsiness, irritability, rash, vomiting.

DRUG INTERACTIONS
Immunosuppressive therapies (eg, irradiation, antimetabolites, alkylating agents, cytotoxic drugs, and corticosteroids [used in greater than physiologic doses]) may reduce immune response to vaccine. Pneumococcal antibody responses to some serotypes in pneumococcal conjugate vaccine 7 (PCV7) were decreased following coadministration with PCV7.

PREGNANCY AND LACTATION
Category C, caution in nursing.

MECHANISM OF ACTION
Vaccine; leads to production of bactericidal antibodies specific to the capsular polysaccharides of serogroups A, C, Y, and W-135.

PATIENT CONSIDERATIONS
Assessment: Assess current health and immune status, for history of GBS, pregnancy/nursing status, and possible drug interactions. Review immunization history for possible vaccine sensitivity and previous vaccination-related adverse reactions.

Monitoring: Monitor for GBS, allergic/anaphylactic reactions, syncope, and other potential adverse effects.

Counseling: Inform of the potential benefits/risks of immunization therapy. Instruct to report any adverse reactions to physician.

MENHIBRIX — meningococcal groups C and Y and haemophilus b tetanus toxoid conjugate vaccine   Rx
Class: Toxoid/vaccine combination

PEDIATRIC DOSAGE
Active Immunization to Prevent Invasive Disease Caused by *Neisseria meningitidis* Serogroups C and Y, and *Haemophilus influenzae* Type B
6 Weeks-18 Months of Age:
0.5mL given IM as a 4-dose series at 2, 4, 6, and 12-15 months of age; may give 1st dose as early as 6 weeks of age and 4th dose may be given as late as 18 months of age

ADMINISTRATION
IM route
The preferred administration site is the anterolateral aspect of the thigh for most infants <1 yr of age; in older children, the deltoid muscle is usually large enough for an IM inj
Do not mix w/ any other vaccine in the same syringe or vial
Administer immediately after reconstitution

Reconstitution
Reconstitute only w/ accompanying saline diluent
1. Cleanse both vial stoppers
2. Withdraw 0.6mL of saline from diluent vial and transfer into lyophilized vaccine vial
3. Shake vial well
4. After reconstitution, withdraw 0.5mL of reconstituted vaccine and administer IM

STORAGE
2-8°C (36-46°F). Protect from light. Diluent: 2-25°C (36-77°F). Do not freeze. After Reconstitution: Administer immediately. Do not freeze; discard if frozen.

HOW SUPPLIED
Inj: 0.5mL

WARNINGS/PRECAUTIONS
Caution if Guillain-Barre syndrome occurs within 6 weeks of receipt of a prior tetanus toxoid-containing vaccine. Syncope may occur and can be accompanied by transient neurological signs. Apnea in premature infants following IM administration observed; decision about timing of administration should be based on individual's medical status, potential benefits, and possible risks. Review immunization history for possible vaccine hypersensitivity; appropriate treatment should be available for possible allergic reactions. Expected immune response may not be obtained in immunosuppressed children. Not a substitute for routine tetanus immunization. Urine antigen detection may not have a diagnostic value in suspected disease due to *H. influenzae* type b within 1-2 weeks after receipt of vaccine.

ADVERSE REACTIONS
Local inj-site reactions (eg, redness, pain, swelling), irritability, drowsiness, loss of appetite, fever.

DRUG INTERACTIONS
Immunosuppressive therapies, including irradiation, antimetabolites, alkylating agents, cytotoxic drugs, and corticosteroids (used in greater than physiologic doses), may reduce immune response to vaccine.

PREGNANCY AND LACTATION
Category C, safety not known in nursing.

MECHANISM OF ACTION
Vaccine/toxoid combination: *N. meningitidis*; induces production of bactericidal antibodies specific to the capsular polysaccharides of serogroups C and Y. *H. influenzae*; protects against invasive disease due to *H. influenzae* type b.

PATIENT CONSIDERATIONS
Assessment: Review immunization history, current health/medical status (eg, immunosuppression), and previous sensitivity/vaccination-related adverse reactions. Assess use in premature infants and for possible drug interactions.

Monitoring: Monitor for signs/symptoms of Guillain-Barre syndrome, syncope, allergic reactions, and other possible adverse events. Monitor immune response. Monitor for apnea in premature infants.

Counseling: Inform patient's parents/guardians of potential benefits and risks of immunization, and of the importance of completing the immunization series. Counsel about potential adverse reactions; instruct to report any adverse events to healthcare provider.

MENOMUNE-A/C/Y/W-135 — meningococcal polysaccharide vaccine, groups A, C, Y and W-135 combined   Rx
Class: Vaccine

ADULT DOSAGE	PEDIATRIC DOSAGE
Meningococcal Vaccine	**Meningococcal Vaccine**
Active Immunization for the Prevention of Invasive Disease Caused By *Neisseria meningitidis* Serogroups A, C, Y, and W-135:	**Active Immunization for the Prevention of Invasive Disease Caused By *Neisseria meningitidis* Serogroups A, C, Y, and W-135:**
Primary Immunization:	**≥2 Years:**
0.5mL SQ single dose	**Primary Immunization:**
Revaccination (Persons at High Risk Who Were Previously Vaccinated):	0.5mL SQ single dose
0.5mL SQ	**Revaccination (Persons at High Risk Who Were Previously Vaccinated):**
	0.5mL SQ

ADMINISTRATION
SQ route
Preferred site of administration is deltoid region.
Do not combine through reconstitution or mix w/ any other vaccine.
Use separate inj sites/syringes in case of concomitant administration.

Reconstitution
After removing "flip-off" caps, cleanse vaccine and diluent vial stoppers w/ a suitable germicide; do not remove vial stoppers or metal seals holding them in place.

Withdraw supplied diluent (0.6mL for single-dose presentation and 6mL for multidose presentation) and inject into vial containing lyophilized vaccine. Swirl vial until vaccine is thoroughly dissolved.

Use single-dose presentation immediately after reconstitution; multidose presentation may be used for up to 35 days after reconstitution if stored at 2-8°C.

STORAGE
2-8°C (35-46°F). Do not freeze. Use single dose vials immediately after reconstitution. Discard remainder of multidose vials within 35 days after reconstitution.

HOW SUPPLIED
Inj: 0.6mL, 6mL

CONTRAINDICATIONS
History of a severe allergic reaction (eg, anaphylaxis) to this vaccine.

WARNINGS/PRECAUTIONS
Does not prevent *N. meningitidis* serogroup B disease. Stoppers to the vials of lyophilized vaccine and diluent contain dry natural latex rubber that may cause allergic reactions in latex-sensitive persons. Appropriate treatment must be available to manage possible anaphylactic reactions. Postpone vaccination in persons with moderate or severe acute illness to avoid diagnostic confusion between manifestations of acute illness and possible vaccine adverse effects. May not protect all recipients. Immunosuppressed persons may have a diminished immune response to vaccine.

ADVERSE REACTIONS
Inj-site reactions (pain, redness, induration, swelling), anorexia, diarrhea, drowsiness, irritability, arthralgia, fatigue, headache, malaise, chills, fever, rash.

DRUG INTERACTIONS
Immunosuppressive therapies may reduce immune response to vaccine.

PREGNANCY AND LACTATION
Category C, caution in nursing.

MECHANISM OF ACTION
Vaccine; induces the production of bactericidal antibodies specific to the capsular polysaccharides of serogroups A, C, Y, and W-135.

PATIENT CONSIDERATIONS
Assessment: Assess for hypersensitivity to drug, latex sensitivity, current health status, immunization history, moderate or severe acute illness, pregnancy/nursing status, and possible drug interactions.
Monitoring: Monitor for anaphylactic reactions and for other potential adverse reactions.
Counseling: Inform patients, parents, or guardians of the potential benefits/risks of immunization. Instruct to report any adverse reactions to physician.

MENTAX — butenafine hydrochloride   Rx
Class: Benzylamine antifungal

ADULT DOSAGE	PEDIATRIC DOSAGE
Tinea Versicolor	**Tinea Versicolor**
Apply to affected areas and immediate surrounding skin of affected areas qd for 2 weeks	**≥12 Years:** Apply to affected areas and immediate surrounding skin of affected areas qd for 2 weeks
If no improvement following treatment period, review diagnosis and therapy	If no improvement following treatment period, review diagnosis and therapy

ADMINISTRATION
Topical route

STORAGE
5-30°C (41-86°F).

HOW SUPPLIED
Cre: 1% [15g, 30g]

CONTRAINDICATIONS
Known or suspected sensitivity to this product or any of its components.

WARNINGS/PRECAUTIONS
Not for ophthalmic, oral or intravaginal use. D/C if irritation or sensitivity develops. Confirm diagnosis by culture or direct microscopic examination. Caution if sensitive to allylamine antifungals.

ADVERSE REACTIONS
Burning, stinging, itching, contact dermatitis, irritation, erythema, worsening of condition.

PREGNANCY AND LACTATION
Category C, caution in nursing.

MECHANISM OF ACTION
Benzylamine antifungal; inhibits epoxidation of squalene, thus blocking the biosynthesis of ergosterol, which is an essential component of fungal cell membranes.

PHARMACOKINETICS
Absorption: (6g) C_{max}=1.4ng/mL; T_{max}=15 hrs; AUC_{0-24}=23.9ng•hr/mL. (20g) C_{max}=5.0ng/mL; T_{max}=6 hrs; AUC_{0-24}=87.8ng•hr/mL. **Metabolism:** Hydroxylation. **Elimination:** Urine; $T_{1/2}$= (6g) 35 hrs; (20g) >150 hrs.

PATIENT CONSIDERATIONS
Assessment: Assess for proper diagnosis of causative organisms (eg, culture, direct microscopic exam), hypersensitivity to allylamine antifungals and pregnancy/nursing status.

Monitoring: Monitor for signs/symptoms of skin irritation or sensitivity. Monitor response to therapy.
Counseling: Instruct to use exactly as directed. Advise to wash hands following application of medication. Instruct to avoid contact of medication with eyes, nose, mouth and other mucous membranes. Counsel to dry application site thoroughly prior to administration. Advise to use for full treatment time recommended by physician even if symptoms improve. Instruct to notify physician if application-site reactions occur (eg, increased irritation, redness, itching, burning, blistering, swelling), the condition worsens or no improvement is seen. Instruct to avoid using occlusive dressings on treatment site unless otherwise directed by physician.

MENVEO — meningococcal (groups A, C, Y and W-135) oligosaccharide diphtheria CRM197 conjugate vaccine   Rx
Class: Vaccine

ADULT DOSAGE	PEDIATRIC DOSAGE
Meningococcal Vaccine	**Meningococcal Vaccine**
Active Immunization to Prevent Invasive Disease Caused by *Neisseria meningitidis* Serogroups A, C, Y and W-135:	**Active Immunization to Prevent Invasive Disease Caused by *Neisseria meningitidis* Serogroups A, C, Y and W-135:**
≤55 Years: Single 0.5mL IM dose	**2 Months of Age:** 0.5mL IM dose as a 4-dose series at 2, 4, 6, and 12 months of age
	7-23 Months of Age: 0.5mL IM dose as a 2-dose series w/ the 2nd dose administered in 2nd yr of life and at least 3 months after 1st dose
	2-10 Years: Single 0.5mL IM dose; may administer a 2nd dose 2 months after 1st dose for children 2-5 yrs of age at continued high risk of meningococcal disease
	≥11 Years: Single 0.5mL IM dose

ADMINISTRATION
IM route
Administer preferably into the anterolateral aspect of the thigh in infants or into the deltoid muscle (upper arm) in toddlers, adolescents, and adults. Do not mix w/ any other vaccine or diluent in the same syringe or vial.

Reconstitution
Supplied in 2 vials that must be combined prior to administration; prepare for administration by reconstituting the MenA lyophilized conjugate vaccine component w/ the MenCYW-135 liquid conjugate vaccine component. Using a graduated syringe, withdraw entire contents of the vial of MenCYW-135 liquid conjugate component and inject into the MenA lyophilized conjugate component vial; invert vial and shake well until vaccine is dissolved and then withdraw 0.5mL of reconstituted product. Use reconstituted vaccine immediately, but may be held at or below 77°F (25°C) for up to 8 hrs.

STORAGE
2-8°C (36-46°F); maintain at 2-8°C (36-46°F) during transport. Do not freeze or use frozen/previously frozen product. Protect from light. Use reconstituted vaccine immediately, but may be held at or below 25°C (77°F) for up to 8 hrs.

HOW SUPPLIED
Inj: 0.5mL

WARNINGS/PRECAUTIONS
Appropriate medical treatment must be available should an acute allergic reaction, including an anaphylactic reaction, occur. Syncope resulting in falling injury associated with seizure-like movements reported; observe for at least 15 min after administration to prevent and manage syncopal reactions. Expected immune response may not be obtained in immunocompromised persons. Guillain-Barre syndrome (GBS) reported; caution with history of GBS. Apnea reported in premature infants; consider individual infant's medical status, and the potential benefits and possible risks.

ADVERSE REACTIONS
Inj-site reactions (eg, pain, tenderness, erythema, induration), irritability, sleepiness, change in eating, diarrhea, headache, myalgia, malaise, N/V, rash, fever, chills.

DRUG INTERACTIONS
Immunosuppressive therapies (eg, irradiation, antimetabolites, alkylating agents, cytotoxic drugs, and corticosteroids [used in greater than physiologic doses]) may reduce immune response to vaccine. Lower geometric mean antibody concentrations for antibodies to the pertussis antigens filamentous hemagglutinin and pertactin observed when coadministered with Tdap and HPV as compared with Tdap alone.

PREGNANCY AND LACTATION
Category B, caution in nursing.

MECHANISM OF ACTION
Vaccine; leads to production of bactericidal antibodies directed against the capsular polysaccharides of serogroups A, C, Y, and W-135.

PATIENT CONSIDERATIONS

Assessment: Assess for previous hypersensitivity to vaccine or other vaccines containing similar components, immune system status, *N. meningitidis* serogroup B infections, history of GBS, infant's medical status, pregnancy/nursing status, and possible drug interactions. Assess children 2-5 yrs of age for continued high risk of meningococcal disease. Review immunization history for possible vaccine sensitivity and previous vaccination-related adverse reactions.

Monitoring: Monitor for allergic reactions, syncope, seizure-like activity, GBS, apnea in premature infants, and other adverse reactions. Monitor immune response.

Counseling: Inform about the potential benefits/risks of immunization therapy, importance of completing the immunization series, and potential adverse reactions temporally associated with the vaccine. Instruct to report any side effects to the physician. Inform about the pregnancy registry, as appropriate.

MEPERIDINE INJECTION (10MG/ML) —

meperidine hydrochloride

Class: Opioid analgesic   **CII**

> Exposes patients and other users to the risks of opioid addiction, abuse, and misuse, potentially leading to overdose and death; assess risk prior to prescribing, and monitor regularly for development of these behaviors/conditions. Serious, life-threatening, or fatal respiratory depression may occur; monitor for occurrence, especially during initiation or following dose increase. Prolonged use during pregnancy can result in neonatal opioid withdrawal syndrome, which may be life-threatening if not recognized and treated; advise of the risk and ensure availability of appropriate treatment if opioid use is required for a prolonged period in a pregnant woman.

ADULT DOSAGE

Moderate to Severe Pain

Management of moderate to pain severe enough to require an opioid and for which alternative treatments are inadequate

≥19 Years:
Initial: 10mg, w/ a range of 1-5mg/ incremental dose
Lockout Interval: 6-10 min
Minimum Lockout Interval: 5 min
Titrate/Maint: May adjust dose or lockout interval, depending on response. Individually titrate to a dose that provides adequate analgesia and minimizes adverse reactions; continually reevaluate to assess the maintenance of pain control and the relative incidence of adverse reactions, as well as monitoring for the development of addiction, abuse, or misuse. Attempt to identify the source of increased pain before increasing the dose if the level of pain increases after dose stabilization.
Continuous Infusion: 15-35mg/hr

PEDIATRIC DOSAGE

Pediatric use may not have been established

DOSING CONSIDERATIONS

Concomitant Medications
CNS Depressants: Reduced dosage is indicated

Renal Impairment
Reduced dosage is indicated

Hepatic Impairment
Reduced dosage is indicated

Elderly
Start at lower end of dosing range and titrate slowly; use w/ caution

Adverse Reactions
Unacceptable Opioid-Related Adverse Reactions: Consider reducing dose

Discontinuation
Use a gradual downward titration; do not d/c abruptly

Other Important Considerations
Poor-Risk/Very Young or Old Patients: Reduced dosage is indicated
Surgical Patients: Base dose on response, other premedication and concomitant medications, the anesthetic being used and the nature and duration of the operation

ADMINISTRATION
IV route
- Administer by very slow IV inj.
- Use only w/ a compatible Hospira PCA pump set w/ injector and a compatible Hospira infusion device.
- When administered parenterally, especially IV, patient should be lying down.
- Each vial is for single dose only; discard unused portion in appropriate manner.
- Do not autoclave.

Incompatibility
- Soluble barbiturates
- Aminophylline
- Heparin
- Morphine sulfate
- Methicillin
- Phenytoin
- Sodium bicarbonate
- Iodide
- Sulfadiazine
- Sulfisoxazole

STORAGE
20-25°C (68-77°F).

HOW SUPPLIED
Inj: 10mg/mL [30mL]

CONTRAINDICATIONS
Significant respiratory depression, acute or severe bronchial asthma in an unmonitored setting or in the absence of resuscitative equipment, hypersensitivity to meperidine, during or w/in 14 days of MAOI use.

WARNINGS/PRECAUTIONS
Reserve for use in patients for whom alternative treatment options have not been tolerated, are not expected to be tolerated, have not provided adequate analgesia, or are not expected to provide adequate analgesia. Respiratory depressant effects and its capacity to elevate CSF pressure may be markedly exaggerated in the presence of head injury, other intracranial lesions, or a preexisting increase in intracranial pressure; use w/ extreme caution and only if its use is deemed essential. May obscure clinical course of patients w/ head injuries. May cause severe hypotension in the postoperative patient or when ability to maintain BP has been compromised by a depleted blood volume. May impair mental/physical abilities. May produce orthostatic hypotension in ambulatory patients. Not for use in pregnant women prior to the labor period, unless potential benefits outweigh possible hazards. When used as obstetrical analgesia, meperidine crosses placental barrier and can produce depression of respiration and psychophysiologic functions in newborn. Increased risk of decreased respiratory drive in patients w/ significant COPD or cor pulmonale, and those w/ a substantially decreased respiratory reserve, hypoxia, hypercapnia, or preexisting respiratory depression. Life-threatening respiratory depression is more likely to occur in elderly, cachectic, or debilitated patients; monitor closely (particularly when initiating and titrating and when given concomitantly w/ other drugs that depress respiration) and alternatively, consider use of non-opioid analgesics. Adrenal insufficiency reported w/ opioid use, more often following >1 month of use; if suspected, confirm w/ diagnostic testing as soon as possible. If diagnosed, treat w/ physiologic replacement doses of corticosteroids; wean off the opioid and continue corticosteroid treatment until adrenal function recovers. Caution w/ A-flutter and other supraventricular tachycardias; may produce a significant increase in the ventricular response rate. May aggravate convulsions w/ convulsive disorders; convulsive potential may be increased w/ prolonged infusions or repeated doses. May obscure the diagnosis or clinical course in patients w/ acute abdominal conditions. Caution and reduce initial dose w/ elderly/debilitated, hypothyroidism, Addison's disease, prostatic hypertrophy or urethral stricture, and severe renal/hepatic impairment.

ADVERSE REACTIONS
Light-headedness, dizziness, sedation, N/V, sweating.

DRUG INTERACTIONS
See Dosing Considerations and Contraindications. Increased risk of hypotension, profound sedation, respiratory depression, coma, and death w/ CNS depressants (eg, alcohol, sedatives/hypnotics, general anesthetics); start w/ a lower dosage of meperidine, monitor for signs of respiratory depression, sedation, and hypotension, and consider using a lower dose of the concomitant CNS depressant. Concomitant use w/ other drugs that affect the serotonergic neurotransmitter system (eg, SSRIs, SNRIs, TCAs, MAOIs), may cause serotonin syndrome; carefully observe, particularly during treatment initiation and dose adjustment. D/C if serotonin syndrome is suspected.

PREGNANCY AND LACTATION
Pregnancy: Prolonged use of opioid analgesics during pregnancy can result in physical dependence in the neonate and neonatal opioid withdrawal syndrome shortly after birth; observe newborns for symptoms of neonatal opioid withdrawal syndrome and manage accordingly. Not recommended during or immediately prior to labor, when other analgesic techniques are more appropriate; monitor exposed neonates during labor for excess sedation and respiratory depression.
Lactation: Monitor infants exposed to meperidine through breast milk for excess sedation and respiratory depression. Withdrawal symptoms can occur in breastfed infants when maternal administration of an opioid analgesic is stopped, or when breastfeeding is stopped. Caution in nursing.
Reproductive Potential: Chronic use may cause reduced fertility.

MECHANISM OF ACTION
Narcotic analgesic; has multiple actions qualitatively similar to those of morphine. Principal actions of therapeutic value are analgesia and sedation.

PHARMACOKINETICS
Distribution: Crosses placenta; found in breast milk. **Metabolism:** Biotransformation; normeperidine (active metabolite). **Elimination:** $T_{1/2}$=3-8 hrs, 20.6 hrs (normeperidine).

PATIENT CONSIDERATIONS
Assessment: Assess for level of pain intensity, risk of addiction/abuse/misuse, patient's general condition and medical status, renal/hepatic impairment, significant respiratory depression, acute or severe bronchial asthma, hypersensitivity, any other conditions where treatment is contraindicated or cautioned, pregnancy/nursing status, and for possible drug interactions.

Monitoring: Monitor for addiction/abuse/misuse, respiratory depression (especially w/in the first 24-72 hrs of initiation and following a dose increase), elevations in CSF pressure, hypotension, convulsions, and other adverse reactions.

Counseling: Inform that use, even when taken as recommended, can result in addiction, abuse, and misuse. Instruct not to share w/ others and to take steps to protect from theft or misuse. Inform of the risk of life-threatening respiratory depression; advise on how to recognize respiratory depression and to seek medical attention if breathing difficulties develop. Inform that potentially serious additive effects may occur if used w/ CNS depressants and to seek medical attention if experiencing increased sedation or difficulty breathing. Warn of the symptoms of serotonin syndrome and to seek medical attention right away if symptoms develop. Instruct to inform physicians if taking or planning to take serotonergic medications. Inform that prolonged use during pregnancy may result in neonatal opioid withdrawal syndrome. Inform female patients of reproductive potential that use can cause fetal harm and advise to inform prescriber of a known or suspected pregnancy. Advise nursing mothers to monitor infants for increased sleepiness (more than usual), breathing difficulties, or limpness; instruct to seek immediate medical care if they notice these signs.

MEPERIDINE ORAL — meperidine hydrochloride

CII

Class: Opioid analgesic

OTHER BRAND NAMES
Demerol

ADULT DOSAGE
Moderate to Severe Pain

Usual: 50-150mg q3-4h prn

Adjust dose according to severity of pain and patient's response

PEDIATRIC DOSAGE
Moderate to Severe Pain

Usual: 1.1-1.8mg/kg, up to the adult dose, q3-4h prn

Adjust dose according to severity of pain and patient's response

---

DOSING CONSIDERATIONS
Concomitant Medications
Phenothiazines/Other Tranquilizers: Proportionately reduce meperidine dose (usually by 25-50%)

Elderly
Reduction in total daily dose is recommended

ADMINISTRATION
Oral route

Oral Sol
Each dose of the oral sol should be taken in 1/2 glass of water; it may exert a slight topical anesthetic effect on mucous membranes if taken undiluted.

STORAGE
25°C (77°F); excursions permitted to 15-30°C (59-86°F).

HOW SUPPLIED
Oral Sol: 50mg/5mL [500mL]; (Demerol) **Tab:** 50mg*, 100mg *scored

CONTRAINDICATIONS
Hypersensitivity to meperidine or to any ingredient; during or w/in 14 days of MAOI use; severe respiratory insufficiency.

WARNINGS/PRECAUTIONS
May be habit forming. Not for treatment of chronic pain; prolonged use may increase risk of toxicity (eg, seizures) from the accumulation of the meperidine metabolite, normeperidine. May be abused in a manner similar to other opioid agonists; abuse by crushing, chewing, snorting, or injecting the dissolved product will pose a significant risk that could result in overdose or death. Respiratory depressant effects and capacity to elevate CSF pressure may be markedly exaggerated in the presence of head injury, other intracranial lesions, or a preexisting increase in intracranial pressure; use w/ extreme caution and only if deemed essential. May obscure the clinical course of patients w/ head injuries. Use w/ extreme caution w/ acute asthmatic attack; COPD or cor pulmonale; substantially decreased respiratory reserve; and preexisting respiratory depression, hypoxia, or hypercapnia. May cause severe hypotension in postoperative patients or any individual whose ability to maintain BP has been compromised by a depleted blood volume. May impair mental/physical abilities. May produce orthostatic hypotension in ambulatory patients. Not recommended during labor. Caution and consider reducing initial dose w/ sickle cell anemia, pheochromocytoma, acute alcoholism, adrenocortical insufficiency (eg, Addison's disease), CNS depression/coma, delirium tremens, kyphoscoliosis associated w/ respiratory depression, myxedema/hypothyroidism, prostatic hypertrophy/ urethral stricture, hepatic/pulmonary/renal impairment and toxic psychosis, and in elderly/debilitated. May obscure the diagnosis or clinical course in patients w/ acute abdominal conditions. May aggravate preexisting convulsions in patients w/ convulsive disorders and may induce or aggravate seizures in some clinical settings. Convulsions may occur in individuals w/o a history of convulsive disorders if dosage is escalated above recommended levels due to tolerance. Caution w/ a-flutter and other supraventricular tachycardias; may produce a significant increase in the ventricular response rate. May produce tolerance and drug dependence; caution w/ alcoholism or other drug dependencies. Avoid abrupt discontinuation. May provoke HTN in patients w/ pheochromocytoma. Meperidine may have a slower elimination rate in neonates and young infants; use w/ caution.

ADVERSE REACTIONS
Lightheadedness, dizziness, sedation, N/V, sweating.

DRUG INTERACTIONS
See Contraindications and Dosing Considerations. Respiratory depression, hypotension, profound sedation, coma, or death may occur w/ other CNS depressants (eg, sedatives/hypnotics, general anesthetics, phenothiazines, tranquilizers, alcohol, other opioids); use meperidine w/ caution and consider starting w/ a reduced dose. Mixed agonist/antagonist analgesics (pentazocine, nalbuphine, butorphanol, buprenorphine) may reduce analgesic effect and/or may precipitate withdrawal symptoms; use w/ caution. Acyclovir may increase levels; use w/ caution. Cimetidine may reduce clearance and V_d and also the formation of the metabolite, normeperidine; use w/ caution. Phenytoin may enhance hepatic metabolism, and may increase levels of normeperidine; use w/ caution. Ritonavir may increase levels of the active metabolite normeperidine; avoid coadministration. Serotonin syndrome reported w/ serotonergic drugs (eg, SSRIs, SNRIs, St. John's wort); avoid coadministration. May enhance neuromuscular-blocking action of skeletal muscle relaxants and increase respiratory depression.

PREGNANCY AND LACTATION
Pregnancy: Category C. Crosses placenta and can produce depression of respiration and psychophysiologic functions in the newborn; not recommended during labor.
Lactation: Found in breast milk; not for use in nursing.

MECHANISM OF ACTION
Opioid analgesic; has multiple actions qualitatively similar to those of morphine (the most prominent of these involve the CNS and organs composed of smooth muscle). Principal actions of therapeutic value are analgesia and sedation.

PHARMACOKINETICS
Distribution: Crosses placenta; found in breast milk. **Metabolism:** Liver; normeperidine (active metabolite).

PATIENT CONSIDERATIONS
Assessment: Assess for level of pain intensity, risk of addiction/abuse/misuse, patient's general condition and medical status, renal/hepatic impairment, severe respiratory insufficiency, asthmatic attack, COPD, hypersensitivity, any other conditions where treatment is contraindicated or cautioned, pregnancy/nursing status, and for possible drug interactions.

Monitoring: Monitor for addiction/abuse/misuse, respiratory depression, elevations in CSF pressure, hypotension, convulsions/seizures, and other adverse reactions.

Counseling: Advise to report pain and adverse experiences occurring during therapy. Instruct not to adjust dose w/o consulting physician and not to abruptly d/c if on treatment for more than a few weeks. Inform that drug may impair mental/physical abilities required to perform hazardous tasks (eg, driving, operating heavy machinery). Instruct not to combine w/ alcohol or other CNS depressants. Advise to consult physician if pregnant, planning to become pregnant, or breastfeeding. Inform that drug has potential for abuse and should be protected from theft. Advise to destroy unused tabs by flushing down the toilet.

MERREM — meropenem

Rx

Class: Carbapenem

ADULT DOSAGE
Skin and Skin Structure Infections

Complicated:
500mg q8h

Caused by *Pseudomonas aeruginosa*:
1g q8h

Useful as presumptive therapy prior to identification of causative organisms

Intra-Abdominal Infections
Complicated Appendicitis and Peritonitis:
1g q8h

Useful as presumptive therapy prior to identification of causative organisms

PEDIATRIC DOSAGE
Skin and Skin Structure Infections

Complicated:
≥3 Months of Age:
10mg/kg q8h or 500mg q8h if >50kg
Max: 500mg q8h

Caused by *P. aeruginosa*:
20mg/kg (or 1g if >50kg) q8h

Useful as presumptive therapy prior to identification of causative organisms

Intra-Abdominal Infections
Complicated Appendicitis and Peritonitis:

<3 Months of Age:
<32 Weeks Gestational Age (GA) and <2 Weeks Postnatal Age (PNA):
20mg/kg q12h
<32 Weeks GA and ≥2 Weeks PNA:
20mg/kg q8h
≥32 Weeks GA and <2 Weeks PNA:
20mg/kg q8h
≥32 Weeks GA and ≥2 Weeks PNA:
30mg/kg q8h

≥3 Months of Age:
20mg/kg q8h or 1g q8h if >50kg
Max: 1g q8h

Useful as presumptive therapy prior to identification of causative organisms

Bacterial Meningitis
≥3 Months of Age:
40mg/kg q8h or 2g q8h if >50kg
Max: 2g q8h

Useful as presumptive therapy prior to identification of causative organisms

DOSING CONSIDERATIONS
Renal Impairment
Adults:
CrCl >25-50mL/min: Give recommended dose q12h
CrCl 10-25mL/min: Give 1/2 recommended dose q12h
CrCl <10mL/min: Give 1/2 recommended dose q24h

ADMINISTRATION
IV route

Administer by IV infusion over approx 15-30 min; doses of 1g may also be given as an IV bolus inj (5-20mL) over approx 3-5 min.

IV Bolus
Add 10mL sterile water for inj (SWFI) to 500mg vial size (20mL for 1g vial size).

IV Infusion
May be directly constituted w/ a compatible infusion fluid.
Alternatively, may constitute inj vial and add resulting sol to an IV container and further dilute w/ an appropriate infusion fluid.

Compatibility and Stability
Do not mix w/ or physically add to sol containing other drugs.
Sol should not be frozen.
Inj vials reconstituted w/ SWFI for bolus administration (up to 50mg/mL) may be stored for up to 3 hrs at up to 25°C (77°F) or for 13 hrs at up to 5°C (41°F).
Sol prepared for infusion (concentrations ranging from 1-20mg/mL) constituted w/ NaCl inj 0.9% may be stored for 1 hr at up to 25°C (77°F) or 15 hrs at up to 5°C (41°F).
Use sol constituted w/ D5 inj immediately.

STORAGE
20-25°C (68-77°F).

HOW SUPPLIED
Inj: 500mg, 1g

CONTRAINDICATIONS
Known hypersensitivity to any component of this product or to other drugs in the same class or in patients who have demonstrated anaphylactic reactions to β-lactams.

WARNINGS/PRECAUTIONS
Serious and occasionally fatal hypersensitivity (anaphylactic) reactions reported w/ β-lactams; d/c immediately if an allergic reaction occurs. Increased risk w/ a history of sensitivity to multiple allergens. Seizures and other adverse CNS effects reported; caution in patients w/ CNS disorders (eg, brain lesions, history of seizures) or w/ bacterial meningitis and/or compromised renal function. Continue anticonvulsant therapy in patients w/ known seizure disorders. If focal tremors, myoclonus, or seizures occur, evaluate neurologically, place on anticonvulsant therapy if not already instituted, and reexamine dosage to determine whether it should be decreased or discontinued. *Clostridium difficile*-associated diarrhea (CDAD) reported; may need to d/c if CDAD is suspected or confirmed. May result in bacterial resistance if used in the absence of proven or suspected bacterial infection, or a prophylactic indication; take appropriate measures if superinfection develops. Thrombocytopenia reported in patients w/ renal impairment. Inadequate information on use in patients on hemodialysis or peritoneal dialysis. May impair mental/physical abilities. Caution in elderly.

ADVERSE REACTIONS
Adults: Diarrhea, N/V, headache, constipation, diarrhea, anemia, pain.
Pediatrics: Diarrhea, rash, N/V, convulsion, hyperbilirubinemia.

DRUG INTERACTIONS
Increased plasma concentrations w/ probenecid; coadministration is not recommended. May reduce concentrations of valproic acid, thereby increasing the risk of breakthrough seizures; concomitant use w/ valproic acid or divalproex sodium is generally not recommended, but if necessary, consider supplemental anticonvulsant therapy.

PREGNANCY AND LACTATION
Pregnancy: Category B.
Lactation: Reported to be excreted in human milk; caution in nursing.

MECHANISM OF ACTION
Carbapenem; bactericidal activity results from the inhibition of cell wall synthesis.

PHARMACOKINETICS
Absorption: 30-min IV Infusion (Single Dose): C_{max}=23mcg/mL (500mg), 49mcg/mL (1g). 5-min IV Bolus Inj: C_{max}=45mcg/mL (500mg), 112mcg/mL (1g).
Distribution: Plasma protein binding (2%); found in breast milk. **Elimination:** Urine (70% unchanged), feces (2%); $T_{1/2}$=1 hr, 1.5 hrs (pediatric patients 3 months-2 yrs of age).

PATIENT CONSIDERATIONS
Assessment: Assess for CNS/seizure disorders, factors that predispose to convulsive activity, renal impairment, pregnancy/nursing status, and possible drug interactions. Carefully assess for previous hypersensitivity reactions to drug, penicillins, cephalosporins, other β-lactams, and other allergens.

Monitoring: Monitor for hypersensitivity reactions, CNS effects (eg, focal tremors, myoclonus, seizures), CDAD, superinfection, and other adverse reactions. Periodically monitor organ system functions including renal, hepatic, and hematopoietic, during prolonged therapy.

Counseling: Inform that therapy should only be used to treat bacterial, not viral, infections. Instruct to take exactly ud, even if patient feels better early in the course of therapy. Inform that skipping doses or not completing the full course of therapy may decrease effectiveness of treatment and increase bacterial resistance. Inform that diarrhea is a common problem caused by therapy, which usually ends when therapy is discontinued. Instruct to immediately contact

physician if watery and bloody stools (w/ or w/o stomach cramp and fever) occur, even as late as ≥2 months after the last dose. Advise to inform physician if taking valproic acid or divalproex sodium. Advise that adverse events (eg, seizures, headaches, and/or paresthesias) may develop that could interfere w/ mental alertness and/or cause motor impairment; instruct not to operate machinery or motorized vehicles until it is reasonably well established that therapy is well tolerated.

METADATE CD — methylphenidate hydrochloride   CII
Class: CNS stimulant

> Caution with history of drug dependence or alcoholism. Chronic abuse may lead to marked tolerance and psychological dependence with varying degrees of abnormal behavior. Frank psychotic episodes may occur, especially with parenteral abuse. Careful supervision is required during withdrawal from abusive use since severe depression may occur. Withdrawal following chronic use may unmask symptoms of underlying disorder that may require follow-up.

ADULT DOSAGE **Attention-Deficit Hyperactivity Disorder**	PEDIATRIC DOSAGE **Attention-Deficit Hyperactivity Disorder**
Refer to pediatric dosing	**≥6 Years:** **Initial:** 20mg qam **Titrate:** May adjust in weekly 10-20mg increments, depending upon tolerability and degree of efficacy observed **Max:** 60mg/day

DOSING CONSIDERATIONS
Adverse Reactions
Reduce dose or d/c if paradoxical aggravation of symptoms or other adverse events occur
D/C if no improvement seen after appropriate dosage adjustment over 1 month

ADMINISTRATION
Oral route

Administer qam before breakfast
May be swallowed whole w/ the aid of liquids, or alternatively, may open caps and sprinkle contents onto a small amount (tbsp) of applesauce and consume immediately
Drinking some fluids (eg, water) should follow the intake of sprinkles w/ applesauce
Do not crush or chew cap or cap contents

STORAGE
25°C (77°F); excursions permitted to 15-30°C (59-86°F).

HOW SUPPLIED
Cap, Extended-Release: 10mg, 20mg, 30mg, 40mg, 50mg, 60mg

CONTRAINDICATIONS
Marked anxiety, tension, agitation, glaucoma, motor tics, family history or diagnosis of Tourette's syndrome, severe HTN, angina pectoris, cardiac arrhythmias, heart failure, recent myocardial infarction (MI), hyperthyroidism, or thyrotoxicosis. Known hypersensitivity to methylphenidate or other components of the product. Rare hereditary problems of fructose intolerance, glucose-galactose malabsorption, or sucrase-isomaltase insufficiency. On the day of surgery. Treatment w/ MAOIs or w/in a minimum of 14 days following discontinuation of an MAOI.

WARNINGS/PRECAUTIONS
Avoid with known serious structural cardiac abnormalities, cardiomyopathy, serious heart rhythm abnormalities, coronary artery disease, or other serious cardiac problems. Sudden death reported in children and adolescents with structural cardiac abnormalities or other serious heart problems. Sudden deaths, stroke, and MI reported in adults. May increase BP and HR; caution with conditions that might be compromised by increases in BP/HR. Prior to treatment, obtain medical history (including assessment for family history of sudden death or ventricular arrhythmia) and perform physical exam to assess for presence of cardiac disease. Promptly perform cardiac evaluation if symptoms of cardiac disease develop. May exacerbate symptoms of behavior disturbance and thought disorder in patients with preexisting psychotic disorder. Caution in patients with comorbid bipolar disorder; may induce mixed/manic episodes. May cause treatment-emergent psychotic or manic symptoms (eg, hallucinations, delusional thinking, mania) in children and adolescents without prior history of psychotic illness or mania; consider discontinuation if such symptoms occur. Aggressive behavior or hostility reported in children and adolescents. May cause long-term suppression of growth in children; monitor growth, and may need to interrupt treatment in patients not growing or gaining height or weight as expected. May lower convulsive threshold; d/c if seizures occur. Priapism, sometimes requiring surgical intervention, reported. Associated with peripheral vasculopathy, including Raynaud's phenomenon; carefully observe for digital changes. Difficulties with accommodation and blurring of vision reported. May produce a positive result during drug testing.

ADVERSE REACTIONS
Headache, abdominal pain, anorexia, insomnia.

DRUG INTERACTIONS
See Contraindications. Caution with pressor agents. May inhibit metabolism of coumarin anticoagulants, anticonvulsants (eg, phenobarbital, phenytoin, primidone), phenylbutazone, and some antidepressants (eg, TCAs, SSRIs);

downward dose adjustment and monitoring of plasma drug concentrations (or coagulation times for coumarin) of these drugs may be necessary when initiating or discontinuing methylphenidate. Clearance might be affected by urinary pH, either being increased with acidifying agents or decreased with alkalinizing agents; caution with agents that alter urinary pH. Avoid with alcohol.

PREGNANCY AND LACTATION
Category C, caution in nursing.

MECHANISM OF ACTION
Sympathomimetic amine; CNS stimulant. Has not been established; thought to block reuptake of norepinephrine and dopamine into presynaptic neuron and increase release of these monoamines into extraneuronal space.

PHARMACOKINETICS
Absorption: Readily absorbed. Administration of variable doses resulted in different parameters. **Metabolism:** Via deesterification; α-phenyl-piperidine acetic acid (ritalinic acid) (metabolite). **Elimination:** (Healthy) $T_{1/2}$=6.8 hrs.

PATIENT CONSIDERATIONS
Assessment: Assess for hypersensitivity to the drug, hereditary problems of fructose intolerance, glucose-galactose malabsorption, or sucrase-isomaltase insufficiency, marked anxiety, tension, agitation, glaucoma, motor tics, family history or diagnosis of Tourette's syndrome, cardiovascular conditions, history of drug dependence or alcoholism, psychotic disorder, comorbid bipolar disorder, any other conditions where treatment is contraindicated or cautioned, pregnancy/nursing status, and possible drug interactions.

Monitoring: Monitor for changes in HR and BP, signs/symptoms of cardiac disease, exacerbation of behavior disturbance and thought disorder, psychosis, mania, appearance of or worsening of aggressive behavior or hostility, seizures, priapism, peripheral vasculopathy (including Raynaud's phenomenon), visual disturbances, and other adverse reactions. In pediatric patients, monitor growth. Perform periodic monitoring of CBC, differential, and platelet counts during prolonged therapy. Periodically reevaluate long-term usefulness of drug.

Counseling: Advise to avoid alcohol while taking the drug. Inform about the benefits and risks of therapy. Counsel on the appropriate use of the medication. Instruct to seek immediate medical attention in the event of priapism. Instruct to report to physician any new numbness, pain, skin color change, or sensitivity to temperature in fingers or toes; instruct to contact physician immediately with any signs of unexplained wounds appearing on fingers or toes while taking the drug.

METADATE ER — methylphenidate hydrochloride   CII

Class: CNS stimulant

> Caution with history of drug dependence or alcoholism. Chronic abuse may lead to marked tolerance and psychological dependence with varying degrees of abnormal behavior. Frank psychotic episodes may occur, especially with parenteral abuse. Careful supervision is required during withdrawal from abusive use since severe depression may occur. Withdrawal following chronic use may unmask symptoms of underlying disorder that may require follow-up.

ADULT DOSAGE
Attention Deficit Disorders
Immediate-Release (IR)
Methylphenidate Tabs:
10-60mg/day given in divided doses bid-tid

Tab, Extended-Release (ER):
May be used in place of the IR tabs when the 8-hr dosage of ER tabs corresponds to the titrated 8-hr dosage of the IR tabs

Narcolepsy
Immediate-Release (IR)
Methylphenidate Tabs:
10-60mg/day given in divided doses bid-tid

Tab, Extended-Release (ER):
May be used in place of the IR tabs when the 8-hr dosage of ER tabs corresponds to the titrated 8-hr dosage of the IR tabs

PEDIATRIC DOSAGE
Attention Deficit Disorders
≥6 Years:
Immediate-Release (IR)
Methylphenidate Tabs:
Initial: 5mg bid before breakfast and lunch
Titrate: Increase gradually in increments of 5-10mg weekly
Max: 60mg/day

Tab, Extended-Release (ER):
May be used in place of the IR tabs when the 8-hr dosage of ER tabs corresponds to the titrated 8-hr dosage of the IR tabs

D/C periodically to assess the child's condition; therapy should not be indefinite

Narcolepsy
≥6 Years:
Immediate-Release (IR)
Methylphenidate Tabs:
Initial: 5mg bid before breakfast and lunch
Titrate: Increase gradually in increments of 5-10mg weekly
Max: 60mg/day

Tab, Extended-Release (ER):
May be used in place of the IR tabs when the 8-hr dosage of ER tabs corresponds to the titrated 8-hr dosage of the IR tabs

D/C periodically to assess the child's condition; therapy should not be indefinite

DOSING CONSIDERATIONS
Adverse Reactions
Children ≥6 Years:
Reduce dose or d/c if paradoxical aggravation of symptoms or other adverse effects occur
D/C if no improvement seen after appropriate dosage adjustment over 1-month period

ADMINISTRATION
Oral route

Tab, ER
Swallow tabs whole; do not crush or chew

IR Methylphenidate Tabs
Administer in divided doses bid-tid, preferably 30-45 min ac
Patients who are unable to sleep if medication is taken late in the day should take last dose before 6pm

STORAGE
20-25°C (68-77°F); excursions permitted to 15-30°C (59-86°F). Protect from moisture.

HOW SUPPLIED
Tab, ER: 20mg

CONTRAINDICATIONS
Marked anxiety, tension, agitation, glaucoma, motor tics, family history or diagnosis of Tourette's syndrome, severe HTN, angina pectoris, cardiac arrhythmias, heart failure, recent myocardial infarction (MI), hyperthyroidism, or thyrotoxicosis. Known hypersensitivity to methylphenidate or other components of the product. Rare hereditary problems of galactose intolerance, the Lapp lactase deficiency, or glucose-galactose malabsorption. On the day of surgery. Treatment w/ MAOIs or w/in a minimum of 14 days following discontinuation of an MAOI.

WARNINGS/PRECAUTIONS
Avoid with known serious structural cardiac abnormalities, cardiomyopathy, serious heart rhythm abnormalities, coronary artery disease, or other serious cardiac problems. Sudden death reported in children and adolescents with structural cardiac abnormalities or other serious heart problems. Sudden deaths, stroke, and MI reported in adults. May increase BP and HR; caution with conditions that might be compromised by increases in BP/HR. Prior to treatment, obtain medical history (including assessment for family history of sudden death or ventricular arrhythmia) and perform physical exam to assess for presence of cardiac disease. Promptly perform cardiac evaluation if symptoms of cardiac disease develop. May exacerbate symptoms of behavior disturbance and thought disorder in patients with preexisting psychotic disorder. Caution in patients with comorbid bipolar disorder; may induce mixed/manic episodes. May cause treatment-emergent psychotic or manic symptoms (eg, hallucinations, delusional thinking, mania) in children and adolescents without prior history of psychotic illness or mania; consider discontinuation if such symptoms occur. Aggressive behavior or hostility reported in children and adolescents. May cause long-term suppression of growth in children; monitor growth, and may need to interrupt treatment in patients not growing or gaining height or weight as expected. May lower convulsive threshold; d/c if seizures occur. Priapism, sometimes requiring surgical intervention, reported. Associated with peripheral vasculopathy, including Raynaud's phenomenon; carefully observe for digital changes. Difficulties with accommodation and blurring of vision reported. Patients with an element of agitation may react adversely; d/c if necessary. May produce a positive result during drug testing.

ADVERSE REACTIONS
Nervousness, insomnia, hypersensitivity reactions, anorexia, nausea, dizziness, palpitations, headache, dyskinesia, drowsiness, BP and pulse changes, tachycardia, angina, cardiac arrhythmia, abdominal pain.

DRUG INTERACTIONS
See Contraindications. Caution with pressor agents. May decrease effectiveness of drugs used to treat HTN. May inhibit metabolism of coumarin anticoagulants, anticonvulsants (eg, phenobarbital, phenytoin, primidone), phenylbutazone, and TCAs (eg, imipramine, clomipramine, desipramine); downward dose adjustment and monitoring of plasma drug concentration (or coagulation times for coumarin) of these drugs may be necessary when initiating or discontinuing methylphenidate. Clearance might be affected by urinary pH, either being increased with acidifying agents or decreased with alkalinizing agents; caution with agents that alter urinary pH.

PREGNANCY AND LACTATION
Category C, caution in nursing.

MECHANISM OF ACTION
Sympathomimetic amine; mild CNS stimulant. Has not been established; suspected to activate the brain stem arousal system and cortex to produce its stimulant effect.

PHARMACOKINETICS
Absorption: (Children) T_{max}=4.7 hrs (sustained-release tab), 1.9 hrs (IR tab).

PATIENT CONSIDERATIONS
Assessment: Assess for hypersensitivity to the drug, hereditary problems of galactose intolerance, the Lapp lactase deficiency, or glucose-galactose malabsorption, marked anxiety, tension, agitation, glaucoma, motor tics, family history or diagnosis of Tourette's syndrome, cardiovascular conditions, history of drug dependence or alcoholism, psychotic disorder, comorbid bipolar disorder, any other conditions where treatment is contraindicated or cautioned, pregnancy/nursing status, and possible drug interactions.

Monitoring: Monitor for changes in HR and BP, signs/symptoms of cardiac disease, exacerbation of behavior disturbance and thought disorder, psychosis, mania, appearance of or worsening of aggressive behavior or hostility, seizures, priapism, peripheral vasculopathy (including Raynaud's phenomenon), visual disturbances, and other adverse reactions. In pediatric patients, monitor growth. Perform periodic monitoring of CBC, differential, and platelet counts during prolonged therapy.

Counseling: Inform about the benefits and risks of therapy. Counsel on the appropriate use of the medication. Instruct to seek immediate medical attention in the event of priapism. Instruct to report to physician any new numbness, pain, skin color change, or sensitivity to temperature in fingers or toes; instruct to contact physician immediately with any signs of unexplained wounds appearing on fingers or toes while taking the drug.

METAXALONE — *metaxalone*　　Rx

Class: Muscular analgesic (centrally acting)

OTHER BRAND NAMES
Skelaxin

ADULT DOSAGE
Musculoskeletal Pain

Relief of Discomforts Associated w/ Acute Conditions:
800mg tid-qid

PEDIATRIC DOSAGE
Musculoskeletal Pain

Relief of Discomforts Associated w/ Acute Conditions:
>12 Years:
800mg tid-qid

ADMINISTRATION
Oral route
Taking w/ food may enhance general CNS depression.

STORAGE
20-25°C (68-77°F). **Skelaxin:** 15-30°C (59-86°F).

HOW SUPPLIED
Tab: 400mg*, (Skelaxin) 800mg* *scored

CONTRAINDICATIONS
Known hypersensitivity to any components of this product; known tendency to drug-induced, hemolytic, and other anemias; significantly impaired renal or hepatic function.

WARNINGS/PRECAUTIONS
Serotonin syndrome (SS) reported; reports generally occurred when used concomitantly w/ serotonergic drugs or when used at doses higher than the recommended dose. Caution w/ preexisting liver damage; perform serial liver function studies in these patients. False (+) Benedict's tests reported; glucose-specific test will differentiate findings. Taking w/ food may enhance general CNS depression; elderly patients may be especially susceptible to this CNS effect.

ADVERSE REACTIONS
Drowsiness, dizziness, headache, nervousness, irritability, N/V, GI upset.

DRUG INTERACTIONS
Additive sedative effects may occur w/ other CNS depressants (eg, alcohol, benzodiazepines, opioids, TCAs); use w/ caution if taking >1 CNS depressant simultaneously. Caution w/ drugs that may affect the serotonergic neurotransmitter systems (eg, tramadol, SSRIs).

PREGNANCY AND LACTATION
Pregnancy: Should not be used in women who are or may become pregnant and particularly during early pregnancy unless, in the judgment of the physician, the potential benefits outweigh the possible hazards.
Lactation: It is not known whether metaxalone is secreted in human milk; not for use in nursing.

MECHANISM OF ACTION
Muscular analgesic (central-acting); has not been established. Activity may be due to general depression of CNS. Has no direct action on the contractile mechanism of striated muscle, the motor end plate, or the nerve fiber.

PHARMACOKINETICS
Absorption: (400mg) C_{max}=983ng/mL, T_{max}=3.3 hrs; AUC=7479ng•hr/mL. (800mg) C_{max}=1816ng/mL, T_{max}=3 hrs; AUC=15,044ng•hr/mL. **Distribution:** V_d=800L. **Metabolism:** Liver; via CYP1A2, 2D6, 2E1, 3A4, and to a lesser extent CYP2C8, 2C9, C19. **Elimination:** Urine (metabolites); $T_{1/2}$=9 hrs (400mg), 8 hrs (800mg).

PATIENT CONSIDERATIONS

Assessment: Assess for known tendency to drug-induced, hemolytic, or other anemias, significant renal/hepatic impairment, hypersensitivity to the drug, pregnancy/nursing status, and possible drug interactions.

Monitoring: Monitor for signs/symptoms of SS, CNS depression, and any other adverse reaction. Perform serial liver function studies in patients w/ preexisting liver damage.

Counseling: Inform that drug may impair mental and/or physical abilities required to perform hazardous tasks, especially when used w/ alcohol or other CNS depressants.

METHADONE HCL INTENSOL ORAL CONCENTRATE — *methadone hydrochloride*　　CII

Class: Opioid analgesic

> Exposes patients and other users to the risks of opioid addiction, abuse, and misuse, leading to overdose and death; assess each patient's risk prior to prescribing, and monitor all patients regularly for the development of these behaviors/conditions. Serious, life-threatening, or fatal respiratory depression may occur; monitor for respiratory depression, especially during initiation or following a dose increase. Accidental ingestion, especially by children, can result in fatal overdose. QT interval prolongation and serious arrhythmia (torsades de pointes) reported; closely monitor for changes in cardiac rhythm during initiation and titration. Prolonged use during pregnancy can result in neonatal opioid withdrawal syndrome; advise pregnant women of the risk and ensure availability of appropriate treatment. For detoxification and maintenance of opioid dependence, methadone should be administered in accordance w/ treatment standards, including limitations on unsupervised administration.

ADULT DOSAGE
Severe Pain (Daily, Around-the-Clock Management)

Requiring long-term opioid treatment for which alternative treatment options are inadequate

1st Opioid Analgesic:
Initial: 2.5mg q8-12h
Titration and Maint:
Individually titrate to a dose that provides adequate analgesia and minimizes adverse reactions
Titrate slowly, w/ dose increases no more frequent than every 3-5 days; some patients may require longer intervals of up to 12 days
If breakthrough pain is experienced, patient may require a dose increase or need rescue medication w/ an appropriate dose of an immediate-release medication

Conversions
D/C all other around-the-clock opioid drugs when therapy is initiated

From Parenteral Methadone:
Use conversion ratio of 1:2mg for parenteral to oral methadone (eg, 5mg parenteral to 10mg oral)

Conversion Factors to Methadone:
Use the total daily baseline oral morphine equivalent dose to calculate the estimated daily oral methadone as percent of morphine equivalent dose, as follows:
<100mg: 20-30%
100-300mg: 10-20%
300-600mg: 8-12%
600-1000mg: 5-10%
>1000mg: <5%

Calculation for Estimated Daily Dose for Oral Methadone:
Always round down, if necessary, to the appropriate methadone strength(s) available
On a Single Opioid: Sum the total daily dose of opioid, convert to morphine equivalent dose, then multiply the morphine equivalent dose by the corresponding percentage to calculate approximate daily oral methadone dose
On >1 Opioid: Calculate approximate oral methadone dose for each opioid and sum the totals to obtain approximate daily total methadone dose
On Fixed-Ratio Opioid/Nonopioid Analgesics: Only use the opioid component of these products in the conversion

Detoxification/Maintenance Treatment of Opioid Addiction

Induction/Initial:
Initial: 20-30mg single dose; use lower initial doses for patients whose tolerance is expected to be low at treatment entry
Max Initial: 30mg
May administer an additional 5-10mg if withdrawal symptoms are not suppressed or if symptoms reappear

PEDIATRIC DOSAGE
Pediatric use may not have been established

Max Total Day 1 Dose: 40mg
Adjust dose over the 1st week of treatment based on control of withdrawal symptoms at the time of expected peak activity (eg, 2-4 hrs after dosing)

Short-Term Detoxification:
Titrate to a total daily dose of 40mg in divided doses to achieve an adequate stabilizing level
Gradually decrease methadone dose on a daily basis or at 2-day intervals, 2-3 days after stabilization
Hospitalized patients may tolerate a daily reduction of 20% of the total daily dose; ambulatory patients may need a slower schedule

Titration and Maint:
Usual: 80-120mg/day

Medically Supervised Withdrawal After a Period of Maint Treatment:
Dose reductions should be <10% of the established tolerance or maint dose w/ 10- to 14-day intervals

Management of Acute Pain During Methadone Maint Treatment:
May require somewhat higher and/or more frequent doses than in nontolerant patients

----

DOSING CONSIDERATIONS
Renal Impairment
Start on lower dose and w/ longer dosing intervals and titrate slowly
Hepatic Impairment
Start on lower dose and w/ longer dosing intervals and titrate slowly
Pregnancy
May need to increase dose or decrease dosing interval
Elderly
Start at lower end of dosing range
Discontinuation
Gradually taper dose; avoid abrupt discontinuation

ADMINISTRATION
Oral route

STORAGE
20-25°C (68-77°F). Protect from light. Discard open bottle after 90 days.

HOW SUPPLIED
Oral Concentrate: 10mg/mL [30mL]

CONTRAINDICATIONS
Significant respiratory depression, acute or severe bronchial asthma in unmonitored setting or in the absence of resuscitative equipment, known or suspected paralytic ileus, hypersensitivity (eg, anaphylaxis) to methadone.

WARNINGS/PRECAUTIONS
Reserve for use in patients for whom alternative analgesic treatment options (eg, nonopioid or immediate-release opioid analgesics) are ineffective, not tolerated, or would be otherwise inadequate to provide sufficient management of pain. Not indicated as a prn analgesic. Deaths reported during conversion from chronic, high-dose treatment w/ other opioid agonists and during initiation of treatment of addiction in subjects previously abusing high doses of other agonists. Retained in the liver and then slowly released, prolonging the duration of potential toxicity w/ repeated dosing. Abuse or misuse of drug by crushing, chewing, snorting, or injecting the dissolved product will result in uncontrolled delivery and can result in overdose and death. Carbon dioxide retention may exacerbate the sedating effects of opioids. Dysrhythmias reported w/ high doses. Life-threatening respiratory depression is more likely to occur in elderly, cachectic, or debilitated patients; monitor closely when initiating and titrating, and when giving w/ drugs that depress respiration. May decrease respiratory drive to the point of apnea, even at therapeutic doses, in patients w/ significant COPD or cor pulmonale, and in patients having a substantially decreased respiratory reserve, hypoxia, hypercapnia, or preexisting respiratory depression; monitor for respiratory depression and consider alternative nonopioid analgesic. May cause severe hypotension including orthostatic hypotension and syncope in ambulatory patients; increased risk in patients w/ compromised ability to maintain BP. Monitor for signs of sedation and respiratory depression in patients susceptible to the intracranial effects of carbon dioxide retention (eg, those w/ increased intracranial pressure, brain tumors). May obscure clinical course in patients w/ head injury. Avoid w/ GI obstruction and impaired consciousness or coma. May cause spasm of the sphincter of Oddi or may increase serum amylase. May aggravate convulsions in patients w/ convulsive disorders and may induce or aggravate seizures. May impair mental/physical abilities. Lab-test interactions may occur. Abrupt discontinuation may lead to opioid withdrawal symptoms. Infants born to opioid-dependent mothers may be physically dependent and may exhibit respiratory difficulties and withdrawal symptoms.

ADVERSE REACTIONS
Respiratory depression, QT prolongation, arrhythmia, systemic hypotension, lightheadedness, dizziness, sedation, N/V, sweating.

DRUG INTERACTIONS
Concomitant use w/ other CNS depressants including sedatives, hypnotics, tranquilizers, general anesthetics, phenothiazines, other opioids, and alcohol may increase the risk of respiratory depression, profound sedation, coma, and death; reduce dose of one or both drugs when combined therapy is considered. Deaths reported when methadone has been abused in conjunction w/ benzodiazepines. CYP3A4 inhibitors may cause decreased clearance, leading to an increase in plasma levels and increased or prolonged opioid effects; these effects could be more pronounced w/ concomitant use of CYP2C9 and 3A4 inhibitors. CYP3A4 inducers may induce metabolism and, therefore, may increase clearance, leading to a decrease in plasma concentrations, lack of efficacy, or (possibly) development of a withdrawal syndrome in a patient who had developed physical dependence to therapy. Antiretroviral drugs (eg, abacavir, amprenavir, darunavir + ritonavir (RTV), efavirenz, nelfinavir, nevirapine, RTV, telaprevir, lopinavir + RTV, saquinavir + RTV, tipranavir + RTV) may increase clearance or decrease plasma levels. May decrease levels of didanosine and stavudine. May increase AUC of zidovudine. Monitor for cardiac conduction changes w/ drugs known to have potential to prolong QT interval. Pharmacodynamic interactions may occur w/ potentially arrhythmogenic agents (eg, Class I and III antiarrhythmics, neuroleptics, TCAs, calcium channel blockers). Monitor closely w/ drugs capable of inducing electrolyte imbalance that may prolong QT interval, including diuretics, laxatives, mineralocorticoid hormones, and medications affecting cardiac conduction. Mixed agonist/antagonist (eg, pentazocine, nalbuphine, butorphanol), and partial agonist (buprenorphine) analgesics may reduce the analgesic effect or precipitate withdrawal symptoms; avoid use. Meperidine w/ or w/in 14 days of MAOI use may precipitate severe reactions; if use of methadone w/ an MAOI is necessary, a sensitivity test should be performed. May increase levels of desipramine. Anticholinergics may increase risk of urinary retention and/or severe constipation, which may lead to paralytic ileus.

PREGNANCY AND LACTATION
Category C, caution in nursing.

MECHANISM OF ACTION
Synthetic opioid analgesic; mu-agonist. Produces actions similar to morphine; acts on CNS and organs composed of smooth muscle. May also act as an N-methyl-D-aspartate receptor antagonist.

PHARMACOKINETICS
Absorption: Bioavailability (36-100%); C_{max}=124-1255ng/mL; T_{max}=1-7.5 hrs.
Distribution: V_d=1-8L/kg; plasma protein binding (85-90%); found in breast milk.
Metabolism: Hepatic N-demethylation via CYP3A4, 2B6, 2C19 (major); 2C9, 2D6 (minor). **Elimination:** Urine, feces; $T_{1/2}$=8-59 hrs.

PATIENT CONSIDERATIONS
Assessment: Assess for personal/family history of or risk factors for drug abuse or addiction, general condition and medical status, opioid experience/tolerance, pain type/severity, previous opioid daily dose, potency and type of prior analgesics used, respiratory depression, cardiac conduction abnormalities, COPD or other respiratory complications, GI obstruction, paralytic ileus, hepatic/renal impairment, previous hypersensitivity to drug, pregnancy/nursing status, possible drug interactions, and any other conditions where treatment is contraindicated or cautioned.

Monitoring: Monitor for respiratory depression (especially w/in the first 24-72 hrs), QT prolongation and arrhythmias, orthostatic hypotension, syncope, symptoms of worsening biliary tract disease, aggravation/induction of seizure, tolerance, physical dependence, mental/physical impairment, withdrawal syndrome, hypersensitivity reactions, and other adverse reactions. Monitor for signs of misuse, abuse, and addiction. Periodically reassess the continued need for therapy during chronic therapy.

Counseling: Inform that use of medication, even when taken as recommended, may result in addiction, abuse, and misuse. Inform that drug may cause orthostatic hypotension and syncope; instruct how to recognize symptoms of low BP and how to reduce the risk of serious consequences should hypotension occur (eg, sit or lie down, carefully rise from a sitting or lying position). Instruct not to share drug w/ others and to take steps to protect from theft or misuse. Inform of the risks of life-threatening respiratory depression; advise how to recognize respiratory depression and to seek medical attention if breathing difficulties develop. Inform that accidental ingestion, especially in children, may result in respiratory depression or death. Instruct to dispose of unused methadone by flushing the drug down the toilet. Instruct to seek medical attention immediately if patient experiences symptoms suggestive of an arrhythmia. Inform female patients of reproductive potential that prolonged use of drug during pregnancy may result in neonatal opioid withdrawal syndrome, which may be life threatening if not recognized and treated. Inform that potentially severe additive effects may occur if drug is used w/ alcohol or other CNS depressants, and instruct not to use such drugs unless supervised by a healthcare provider. Advise to use drug exactly ud and not to d/c w/o 1st discussing the need for a tapering regimen w/ prescriber. Inform that drug may impair ability to perform potentially hazardous activities (eg, driving a car, operating heavy machinery). Inform that severe constipation or anaphylaxis may occur, and advise when to seek medical attention. Instruct nursing mothers to watch for signs of methadone toxicity in their infants; instruct to inform physician immediately if these signs occur.

METHADONE INJECTION — methadone hydrochloride   CII

Class: Opioid analgesic

> Cases of QT prolongation and serious arrhythmia (torsades de pointes) commonly associated with higher dose treatment (>200mg/day) observed. Only certified/approved opioid treatment programs can dispense oral methadone for treatment of opioid addiction in detoxification or maint programs.

ADULT DOSAGE

Moderate to Severe Pain

Not Responsive to Non-Narcotic Analgesics:
Opioid Nontolerant:
Initial: 2.5-10mg q8-12h, slowly titrated to effect; more frequent administration may be required to maintain adequate analgesia

Conversions

Equianalgesic methadone dosing varies between patients and w/in the same patient, depending on baseline morphine dose; always individualize methadone conversion and dose titration methods

From Oral Methadone:
Initial: Use 2:1 dose ratio (eg, 10mg oral methadone to 5mg parenteral methadone)

From Baseline Oral Morphine to Daily IV Methadone:
<100mg: 10-15% of total daily morphine
100-300mg: 5-10% of total daily morphine
300-600mg: 4-6% of total daily morphine
600-1000mg: 3-5% of total daily morphine
>1000mg: <3% of total daily morphine

From Baseline Parenteral Morphine to Daily IV Methadone:
10-30mg: 40-66% of total daily morphine
30-50mg: 27-66% of total daily morphine dose
50-100mg: 22-50% of total daily morphine dose
100-200mg: 15-34% of total daily morphine dose
200-500mg: 10-20% of total daily morphine dose

Opioid Dependence

Temporary Treatment in Patients Unable to Take Oral Medication:
Use 2:1 dose ratio (eg, 10mg oral methadone to 5mg parenteral methadone)

PEDIATRIC DOSAGE

Pediatric use may not have been established

DOSING CONSIDERATIONS

Pregnancy
May need to increase dose or decrease dosing interval

Elderly
Start at the low end of the dosing range

ADMINISTRATION
IV, IM, SQ routes

STORAGE
25°C (77°F); excursions permitted to 15-30°C (59-86°F). Protect from light.

HOW SUPPLIED
Inj: 10mg/mL [20mL]

CONTRAINDICATIONS
Known hypersensitivity to methadone hydrochloride or any other ingredient in this medication; in any situation where opioids are contraindicated, such as respiratory depression (in the absence of resuscitative equipment or in unmonitored settings), acute bronchial asthma, or hypercarbia.

WARNINGS/PRECAUTIONS
Not approved for outpatient treatment of opioid dependence. Used only for patients unable to take oral medication (eg, hospitalized patients). Caution in patients with risk of prolonged QT interval; monitor CV status, including QT prolongation and dysrhythmias. Methadone given on fixed-dose schedule or use as analgesia in acute or chronic pain should be initiated only if benefits outweigh risks. May cause respiratory depression; caution with hypoxia, hypercapnia, or decreased respiratory reserve. Respiratory depressant effects and CSF pressure elevation may be markedly exaggerated in the presence of head injury, intracranial lesions, or preexisting increased intracranial pressure (ICP). May obscure diagnosis/clinical course of acute abdominal conditions or the clinical course of head injuries. Patients tolerant to other opioids may be incompletely tolerant to methadone. Deaths reported in opioid-tolerant patients during conversion to methadone. Drug tolerance, misuse, abuse, diversion, and physical dependence may occur; abstinence syndrome may occur if d/c abruptly in physically dependent patient. Abrupt d/c may lead to opioid withdrawal symptoms. May produce hypotension. Ineffective in relieving anxiety. Higher and/or more frequent doses for acute pain required in maint patients on stable dose of methadone. Infants born to opioid-dependent mothers may exhibit decreased fetal growth with reduce birth weight, mild but persistent deficits in performance on psychometric and behavioral tests, respiratory depression, or withdrawal symptoms. Caution in elderly, debilitated, severe hepatic or renal impairment, hypothyroidism, Addison's disease, prostatic hypertrophy, or urethral stricture; reduce initial dose.

ADVERSE REACTIONS
Respiratory depression, lightheadedness, dizziness, sedation, N/V, sweating.

DRUG INTERACTIONS
Concomitant use with other opioid analgesics, general anesthesia, phenothiazines, tranquilizers, sedatives, hypnotics, and other CNS depressants (including alcohol) may precipitate respiratory depression, hypotension, profound sedation, or coma. Additive effects with alcohol, other opioids, or illicit drugs that cause CNS depression. Deaths reported when abused in conjunction with benzodiazepines. May decrease effects with CYP450 inducers (eg, rifampin, phenytoin) while CYP450 inhibitors (eg, azole antifungals such as ketoconazole, macrolide antibiotics such as erythromycin, SSRIs such as sertraline and fluvoxamine) may potentiate effects. CYP3A4 inducers (eg, rifampin, phenytoin, St. John's wort, phenobarbital, carbamazepine), opioid antagonists, mixed agonist/antagonist, and partial agonists may precipitate withdrawal symptoms. Avoid with agonist/antagonist analgesics (eg, pentazocine, nalbuphine, butorphanol, buprenorphine). MAOIs may cause severe reactions. Caution with drugs known to prolong QT interval (eg, diuretics) and concomitant medications that may predispose to dysrhythmia. Pharmacodynamic interaction may occur with Class I and III antiarrhythmics, some neuroleptics, TCAs, and calcium channel blockers. Caution with drugs capable of inducing electrolyte imbalance (eg, diuretics, laxatives, mineralocorticoids). Monitor patients taking medications affecting cardiac conduction. Antiretrovirals (eg, nevirapine, efavirenz, ritonavir, ritonavir/lopinavir, didanosine, stavudine) may decrease levels. May increase levels of zidovudine and desipramine.

PREGNANCY AND LACTATION
Category C, not for use in nursing.

MECHANISM OF ACTION
Opioid analgesic; μ-agonist. Produces actions similar to morphine; acts on CNS and organs composed of smooth muscle. May also act as an N-methyl-D-aspartate (NMDA) receptor antagonist.

PHARMACOKINETICS
Distribution: V_d=2-6L/kg; plasma protein binding (85-90%); found breast milk.
Metabolism: Hepatic N-demethylation via CYP3A4 (primary), 2D6. **Elimination:** Urine, feces; $T_{1/2}$=8-59 hrs.

PATIENT CONSIDERATIONS

Assessment: Assess for respiratory depression, history of acute bronchial asthma, hypercarbia, CNS depression, cardiac conduction abnormalities, increased intracranial pressure, acute abdominal conditions, renal/hepatic impairment, or any other conditions where treatment is contraindicated or cautioned. Assess hypersensitivity to drug, pregnancy/nursing status, and possible drug interactions.

Monitoring: Monitor for signs/symptoms of respiratory depression, QT prolongation and arrhythmias (eg, torsades de pointes); misuse or abuse of medication, physical dependence and tolerance, withdrawal symptoms, elevations in CSF pressure, orthostatic hypotension, and hypersensitivity reactions.

Counseling: Inform that drug may impair mental/physical abilities; instruct to use caution when performing hazardous tasks (eg, operating machinery/driving). Advise that drug may produce orthostatic hypotension. Counsel to avoid use of other CNS depressants and alcohol during therapy. Instruct to seek medical attention if symptoms suggestive of arrhythmia (eg, palpitations, dizziness, lightheadedness, syncope) develop. Counsel to take drug as prescribed and avoid abrupt withdrawal.

METHADONE ORAL SOLUTION —
methadone hydrochloride   CII

Class: Opioid analgesic

> Exposes patients and other users to the risk of opioid addiction, abuse, and misuse, leading to overdose and death; assess each patient's risk prior to prescribing and monitor all patients regularly for the development of these behaviors/conditions. Serious, life-threatening, or fatal respiratory depression may occur; monitor for respiratory depression, especially during initiation or following a dose increase. Accidental ingestion, especially in children, can result in fatal overdose. QT interval prolongation and serious arrhythmia (torsades de pointes) reported; closely monitor for changes in cardiac rhythm during initiation and titration. Prolonged use during pregnancy can result in neonatal opioid withdrawal syndrome; advise pregnant women of the risk and ensure availability of appropriate treatment. For detoxification and maintenance of opioid dependence, methadone should be administered in accordance w/ treatment standards, including limitations on unsupervised administration.

ADULT DOSAGE
Severe Pain (Daily, Around-the-Clock Management)

Requiring long-term opioid treatment for which alternative treatment options are inadequate

1st Opioid Analgesic:
Initial: 2.5mg q8-12h

Titration and Maint:
Individually titrate to a dose that provides adequate analgesia and minimizes adverse reactions

PEDIATRIC DOSAGE
Pediatric use may not have been established

Titrate slowly, with dose increases no more frequent than every 3-5 days; some patients may require longer intervals of up to 12 days
If breakthrough pain is experienced, patient may require a dose increase or need rescue medication w/ an appropriate dose of an immediate-release medication

Conversions
D/C all other around-the-clock opioid drugs when therapy is initiated

From Parenteral Methadone:
Use conversion ratio of 1:2mg for parenteral to oral methadone (eg, 5mg parenteral to 10mg oral)

Conversion Factors to Methadone: Total Daily Baseline Oral Morphine Equivalent Dose: Estimated Daily Oral Methadone as Percent of Morphine Equivalent Dose
<100mg: 20-30%
100-300mg: 10-20%
300-600mg: 8-12%
600-1000mg: 5-10%
>1000mg: <5%

Calculation for Estimated Daily Dose for Oral Methadone:
Always round down, if necessary, to the appropriate methadone strength(s) available
On a Single Opioid: Sum the total daily dose of opioid, convert to morphine equivalent dose, then multiply the morphine equivalent dose by the corresponding percentage to calculate approximate daily oral methadone dose
On >1 Opioid: Calculate approximate oral methadone dose for each opioid and sum the totals to obtain approximate daily total methadone dose
On Fixed-Ratio Opioid/Nonopioid Analgesics: Only use the opioid component of these products in the conversion

Detoxification/Maintenance Treatment of Opioid Addiction
Induction/Initial:
Initial: 20-30mg single dose; use lower initial doses for patients whose tolerance is expected to be low at treatment entry
Max Initial: 30mg
May administer an additional 5-10mg if withdrawal symptoms are not suppressed or if symptoms reappear
Max Total Day 1 Dose: 40mg
Adjust dose over the 1st week of treatment based on control of withdrawal symptoms at the time of expected peak activity (eg, 2-4 hrs after dosing)

Short-Term Detoxification:
Titrate to a total daily dose of 40mg in divided doses to achieve an adequate stabilizing level
Gradually decrease methadone dose on a daily basis or at 2-day intervals, 2-3 days after stabilization
Hospitalized patients may tolerate a daily reduction of 20% of the total daily dose; ambulatory patients may need a slower schedule

Titration and Maint:
Usual: 80-120mg/day

Medically Supervised Withdrawal After a Period of Maint Treatment:
Dose reductions should be <10% of the established tolerance or maint dose w/ 10- to 14-day intervals

Management of Acute Pain During Methadone Maint Treatment:
May require somewhat higher and/or more frequent doses than in nontolerant patients

DOSING CONSIDERATIONS
Renal Impairment
Start on lower dose and w/ longer dosing intervals and titrate slowly
Hepatic Impairment
Start on lower dose and titrate slowly
Pregnancy
May need to increase dose or decrease dosing interval
Elderly
Start at lower end of dosing range
Discontinuation
Avoid abrupt discontinuation; use a gradual downward titration every 2-4 days

ADMINISTRATION
Oral route

STORAGE
20-25°C (68-77°F).

HOW SUPPLIED
Sol: 5mg/5mL, 10mg/5mL [500mL]

CONTRAINDICATIONS
Significant respiratory depression, acute or severe bronchial asthma in unmonitored setting or in the absence of resuscitative equipment, known or suspected paralytic ileus, hypersensitivity (eg, anaphylaxis) to methadone.

WARNINGS/PRECAUTIONS
Reserve for use in patients for whom alternative analgesic treatment options (eg, nonopioid or IR opioid analgesics) are ineffective, not tolerated, or would be otherwise inadequate to provide sufficient management of pain. Not indicated as a prn analgesic. Deaths reported during conversion from chronic, high dose treatment w/ other opioid agonists and during initiation of treatment of addiction in subjects previously abusing high doses of other agonists. Retained in the liver and then slowly released, prolonging the duration of potential toxicity, w/ repeated dosing. Life-threatening respiratory depression is more likely to occur in elderly, cachectic, or debilitated patients; monitor closely when initiating and titrating, and when given w/ drugs that depress respiration. May decrease respiratory drive to the point of apnea, even at therapeutic doses, in patients w/ significant COPD or cor pulmonale, and in patients having a substantially decreased respiratory reserve, hypoxia, hypercapnia, or preexisting respiratory depression; monitor for respiratory depression and consider alternative nonopioid analgesics. May cause severe hypotension including orthostatic hypotension and syncope in ambulatory patients; increased risk in patients w/ compromised ability to maintain BP. Monitor for signs of sedation and respiratory depression in patients susceptible to the intracranial effects of carbon dioxide retention (eg, those w/ increased intracranial pressure, or brain tumors). May obscure clinical course in patients w/ head injury. Avoid w/ GI obstruction and impaired consciousness or coma. May cause spasm of the sphincter of Oddi or increase serum amylase. May aggravate convulsions in patients w/ convulsive disorders and may induce or aggravate seizures. May impair mental/physical abilities. Abrupt discontinuation may lead to opioid withdrawal symptoms. Infants born to opioid-dependent mothers may be physically dependent and may exhibit respiratory difficulties and withdrawal symptoms.

ADVERSE REACTIONS
Respiratory depression, QT prolongation, arrhythmia, systemic hypotension, lightheadedness, dizziness, sedation, N/V, sweating.

DRUG INTERACTIONS
Concomitant use w/ other CNS depressants (eg, sedatives, tranquilizers, phenothiazines) may result in hypotension, profound sedation, coma, respiratory depression, and death; reduce dose of one or both drugs when combined therapy is considered. Deaths reported when therapy has been abused in conjunction w/ benzodiazepines. CYP3A4 inhibitors may cause decreased clearance, leading to an increase in plasma levels and increased or prolonged opioid effects; these effects could be more pronounced w/ concomitant use of CYP2C9 and 3A4 inhibitors. CYP3A4 inducers may induce metabolism and, therefore, may increase clearance, leading to a decrease in plasma concentrations, lack of efficacy, or (possibly) development of a withdrawal syndrome in a patient who had developed physical dependence to therapy. Antiretroviral agents w/ CYP3A4 inhibitory activity (eg, abacavir, darunavir + ritonavir [RTV], efavirenz, lopinavir + RTV) may increase clearance or decrease plasma levels. May decrease levels of didanosine and stavudine. May increase AUC of zidovudine. Monitor for cardiac conduction changes w/ drugs known to have potential to prolong QT interval. Pharmacodynamic interactions may occur w/ potentially arrhythmogenic agents (eg, Class I and III antiarrhythmics, neuroleptics, TCAs, calcium channel blockers). Monitor closely w/ drugs capable of inducing electrolyte disturbances that may prolong QT interval, including diuretics, laxatives, mineralocorticoid hormones. Mixed agonist/antagonist (eg, pentazocine, nalbuphine, butorphanol), and partial agonist (buprenorphine) analgesics may reduce the analgesic effect or precipitate withdrawal symptoms; avoid use. Meperidine w/ or w/in 14 days of MAOI use may precipitate severe reactions; if use of methadone w/ an MAOI is necessary, a sensitivity test should be performed. May increase levels of desipramine. Anticholinergics may increase risk of urinary retention and/or severe constipation, which may lead to paralytic ileus.

PREGNANCY AND LACTATION
Category C, caution in nursing.

MECHANISM OF ACTION
Synthetic opioid analgesic; mu-agonist. Produces actions similar to morphine; acts on CNS and organs composed of smooth muscle. May also act as an N-methyl-D-aspartate receptor antagonist.

PHARMACOKINETICS
Absorption: Bioavailability (36-100%); C_{max}=124-1255ng/mL; T_{max}=1-7.5 hrs.
Distribution: V_d=1-8L/kg; plasma protein binding (85-90%); found in breast milk.

Metabolism: Hepatic N-demethylation via CYP3A4, 2B6, 2C19 (major); 2C9, 2D6 (minor). **Elimination:** Urine, feces; $T_{1/2}$=8-59 hrs.

PATIENT CONSIDERATIONS

Assessment: Assess for personal/family history or risk factors for drug abuse or addiction, general condition and medical status, opioid/experience/tolerance, pain type/severity, previous opioid daily dose, potency, and type of prior analgesics used, respiratory depression, cardiac conduction abnormalities, COPD or other respiratory complications, GI obstruction, paralytic ileus, hepatic/renal impairment, previous hypersensitivity to drug, pregnancy/nursing status, possible drug interactions, and any other conditions where treatment is contraindicated or cautioned.

Monitoring: Monitor for respiratory depression (especially w/in the first 24-72 hrs), QT prolongation and arrhythmias, orthostatic hypotension, syncope, symptoms of worsening biliary tract disease, aggravation/induction of seizure, tolerance, physical dependence, mental/physical impairment, withdrawal syndrome, hypersensitivity reactions, and other adverse reactions. Monitor for signs of misuse, abuse, and addiction. Periodically reassess the continued need for therapy during chronic therapy.

Counseling: Inform that use of medication, even when taken as recommended, may result in addiction, abuse, and misuse. Instruct not to share w/ others and to take steps to protect from theft or misuse. Inform of the risks of life-threatening respiratory depression; advise how to recognize respiratory depression and to seek medical attention if breathing difficulties develop. Inform that accidental ingestion, especially in children, may result in respiratory depression or death. Instruct to dispose of unused methadone by flushing the drug down the toilet. Instruct to seek medical attention immediately if patient experiences symptoms suggestive of an arrhythmia. Inform female patients of reproductive potential that prolonged use of drug during pregnancy may result in neonatal opioid withdrawal syndrome, which may be life threatening if not recognized and treated. Inform that potentially severe additive effects may occur if drug is used w/ alcohol or other CNS depressants, and instruct not to use such drug unless supervised by a healthcare provider. Advise to use drug exactly and not to d/c w/o 1st discussing the need for tapering regimen w/ prescriber. Inform that drug may impair ability to perform potentially hazardous activities (eg, driving a car, operating heavy machinery). Advise about potential for severe constipation, including management instructions and when to seek medical attention. Inform that anaphylaxis may occur; advise how to recognize such a reaction and when to seek medical attention. Instruct nursing mothers to watch for signs of methadone toxicity in their infants (eg, increased sleepiness [more than usual], difficulty breastfeeding, breathing difficulties, limpness); instruct to inform physician immediately if these signs occur.

METHYCLOTHIAZIDE — methyclothiazide Rx

Class: Thiazide diuretic

OTHER BRAND NAMES
Enduron (Discontinued)

ADULT DOSAGE	PEDIATRIC DOSAGE
Edema	Pediatric use may not have been established
Usual: 2.5-10mg qd	
Max: 10mg qd	
Hypertension	
Usual: 2.5-5mg qd	
If BP control is not satisfactory after 8-12 weeks of therapy with 5mg qd, add another antihypertensive drug	

ADMINISTRATION
Oral route

STORAGE
20-25°C (68-77°F). Protect from light and moisture.

HOW SUPPLIED
Tab: 5mg* *scored

CONTRAINDICATIONS
Anuria, hypersensitivity to this medication or other sulfonamide-derived drugs.

WARNINGS/PRECAUTIONS
Caution with renal disease or significant renal impairment; may precipitate azotemia. Caution with hepatic impairment or progressive liver disease; may precipitate hepatic coma. Sensitivity reactions may occur in patients with history of allergy or bronchial asthma. Possibility of exacerbation/activation of systemic lupus erythematosus (SLE) reported. Observe for clinical signs of electrolyte imbalances (eg, hyponatremia, hypochloremic alkalosis, hypokalemia). Hypokalemia may sensitize or exaggerate the response of the heart to toxic effects of digitalis. Hyperuricemia or precipitation of frank gout, manifestation of latent diabetes mellitus (DM), and hypercalcemia may occur. Enhanced antihypertensive effects in postsympathectomy patients. Consider withholding or discontinuing therapy if progressive renal impairment becomes evident. D/C before testing for parathyroid function. May cause increased concentrations of total serum cholesterol, total TG, and LDL; caution with moderate or high cholesterol concentrations, and elevated TG levels.

ADVERSE REACTIONS
Headache, cramping, orthostatic hypotension, pancreatitis, jaundice, sialadenitis, aplastic anemia, hemolytic anemia, anaphylactic reactions, hyperglycemia, vertigo, dizziness, transient blurred vision, xanthopsia, glycosuria.

DRUG INTERACTIONS
Hypokalemia may develop during concomitant use of steroids or adrenocorticotropic hormone. Adjustment of insulin requirements in diabetic patients may be required. May decrease arterial responsiveness to norepinephrine. May increase responsiveness of tubocurarine. May reduce lithium clearance and increase risk of lithium toxicity. May add to or potentiate the action of other antihypertensives. Potentiation occurs with ganglionic or peripheral adrenergic blocking drugs; give ganglionic blocking agents at only 1/2 the usual dose. Alcohol, barbiturates, or narcotics may potentiate orthostatic hypotension.

PREGNANCY AND LACTATION
Category B, not for use in nursing.

MECHANISM OF ACTION
Thiazide diuretic; has not been established. Inhibits renal tubular reabsorption of electrolytes. Enhances excretion of Na^+ and Cl^-; K^+ excretion is also enhanced to a variable degree.

PHARMACOKINETICS
Absorption: Rapid. **Distribution:** Crosses the placenta; found in breast milk. **Elimination:** Kidneys.

PATIENT CONSIDERATIONS
Assessment: Assess for anuria, hypersensitivity to drug or sulfonamide-derived drugs, hepatic/renal impairment, history of allergy or bronchial asthma, SLE, DM, postsympathectomy status, pregnancy/nursing status, and possible drug interactions. Assess serum electrolytes, cholesterol, and TG levels.

Monitoring: Monitor for signs/symptoms of fluid/electrolyte imbalance, sensitivity reactions, exacerbation/activation of SLE, hyperuricemia or precipitation of frank gout, latent DM, and other adverse reactions. Monitor serum electrolytes, cholesterol, TG, and LDL levels.

Counseling: Inform of possible side effects and instruct to report any symptoms of electrolyte imbalance to physician. Advise to take drug ud, and inform that drinking alcohol may increase the chance of dizziness.

METHYLDOPA — methyldopa Rx

Class: Alpha-adrenergic agonist

ADULT DOSAGE	PEDIATRIC DOSAGE
Hypertension	**Hypertension**
Initial: 250mg bid-tid for first 48 hrs	**Initial:** 10mg/kg/day given bid-qid
Titrate: Adjust dose at intervals of not less than 2 days until adequate response is achieved	**Titrate:** May increase or decrease until adequate response is achieved
Maint: 500mg-2g/day given bid-qid	**Max:** 65mg/kg/day or 3g/day, whichever is less
Max: 3g/day	

DOSING CONSIDERATIONS
Concomitant Medications
Antihypertensives (Other Than Thiazides):
Initial: Limit to 500mg/day in divided doses

Renal Impairment
May lower dose

Elderly
May lower dose

ADMINISTRATION
Oral route

STORAGE
20-25°C (68-77°F).

HOW SUPPLIED
Tab: 250mg, 500mg

CONTRAINDICATIONS
Active hepatic disease (eg, acute hepatitis, active cirrhosis), liver disorders previously associated w/ methyldopa, hypersensitivity to any component of this product, concomitant MAOIs.

WARNINGS/PRECAUTIONS
Positive Coombs' test may occur. D/C and do not reinstitute if Coombs'-positive hemolytic anemia occurs (rare). Obtain blood count at baseline and periodically during therapy. May perform direct Coombs' test before therapy and at 6 and 12 months after start of therapy. Caution with history of liver disease/dysfunction. Findings consistent with cholestasis, hepatitis, or hepatocellular injury (eg, fever associated with eosinophilia or LFT abnormalities, jaundice) may occur. D/C and do not reinstitute if fever, LFT abnormalities, or jaundice appear. Rare cases of liver disorders (eg, fatal hepatic necrosis), reversible reduction of WBC with a primary effect on granulocytes, granulocytopenia, and reversible thrombocytopenia reported. Clinical edema or weight gain may occur; d/c if edema progresses or signs of heart failure appear. HTN may recur after dialysis. Involuntary choreoathetotic movements observed rarely with severe bilateral cerebrovascular disease; d/c if these occur. Interferes with diagnosis of pheochromocytoma; not recommended with pheochromocytoma. Caution in elderly.

ADVERSE REACTIONS
Aggravation of angina pectoris, congestive heart failure, pancreatitis, hyperprolactinemia, bone marrow depression, liver disorders, myocarditis, parkinsonism, rise in BUN, arthralgia, nasal stuffiness, toxic epidermal necrolysis, rash, amenorrhea, breast enlargement.

DRUG INTERACTIONS

See Contraindications. May potentiate other antihypertensives. Anesthetics may need dose reduction. Monitor for lithium toxicity with concomitant lithium. Not recommended with ferrous sulfate/gluconate.

PREGNANCY AND LACTATION

Category B, caution in nursing.

MECHANISM OF ACTION

Aromatic-amino-acid decarboxylase inhibitor; not established. Metabolized to α-methylnorepinephrine, which is suspected to lower arterial pressure by stimulating central inhibitory α-adrenergic receptors, false neurotransmission, and/or reduction of plasma renin activity.

PHARMACOKINETICS

Distribution: Crosses placenta, found in breast milk. **Metabolism:** Extensive. **Elimination:** Urine (70%, parent and mono-O-sulfate conjugate); $T_{1/2}$=105 min.

PATIENT CONSIDERATIONS

Assessment: Assess for hypersensitivity to drug and its components, active hepatic disease, previous liver disorders, pheochromocytoma, severe bilateral cerebrovascular disease, pregnancy/nursing status, and possible drug interactions. Obtain baseline BP, blood count (Hct, Hgb, RBC), direct Coombs' test, LFTs, and hepatic/renal function.

Monitoring: Monitor for signs/symptoms of hemolytic anemia, progressive edema, heart failure, hypersensitivity reactions, hepatic dysfunction, and other adverse events. Perform direct Coombs' test 6 and 12 months after the start of therapy and monitor hepatic function during the first 6-12 weeks or whenever an unexplained fever occurs. Perform periodic blood counts.

Counseling: Advise to contact physician if any adverse events occur. Advise to inform physician if pregnant/breastfeeding.

METHYLDOPA/HCTZ — hydrochlorothiazide/methyldopa   **Rx**

Class: Alpha agonist/thiazide diuretic

Fixed combination drug is not indicated for initial therapy of HTN.

ADULT DOSAGE	**PEDIATRIC DOSAGE**
Hypertension	Pediatric use may not have been established
Dose determined by titration of individual components	
Initial: 250mg-15mg tab bid-tid or 250mg-25mg tab bid	
Alternatively, 500mg/30mg qd or 500mg/50mg qd	
Max:	
HCTZ: 50mg/day	
Methyldopa: 3g/day	

DOSING CONSIDERATIONS

Concomitant Medications

Concomitant Antihypertensives Other than Thiazides:

Initial:

Methyldopa: 500mg/day in divided doses

Renal Impairment

May lower dose

Elderly

Start at lower end of dosing range

ADMINISTRATION

Oral route

STORAGE

20-25°C (68-77°F). Protect from light.

HOW SUPPLIED

Tab: (Methyldopa-HCTZ) 250mg-15mg, 250mg-25mg

CONTRAINDICATIONS

Active hepatic disease (eg, acute hepatitis, active cirrhosis); liver disorders previously associated w/ methyldopa; anuria; hypersensitivity to methyldopa, HCTZ, or other sulfonamide-derived drugs; concomitant MAOIs.

WARNINGS/PRECAUTIONS

Methyldopa: Positive Coombs' test may occur. D/C and do not reinstitute if Coombs'-positive hemolytic anemia occurs (rare). Obtain blood count at baseline and periodically during therapy. May perform direct Coombs' test before therapy and at 6 and 12 months after start of therapy. Caution with history of liver disease/dysfunction. D/C and do not reinstitute if fever, LFT abnormalities, or jaundice appear. Rare cases of liver disorders (eg, fatal hepatic necrosis), reversible reduction of WBC with a primary effect on granulocytes, granulocytopenia, and reversible thrombocytopenia reported. Clinical edema or weight gain may occur; d/c if edema progresses or signs of heart failure appear. HTN may recur after dialysis. Involuntary choreoathetotic movements observed rarely with severe bilateral cerebrovascular disease; d/c if these occur. Interferes with diagnosis of pheochromocytoma; not recommended with pheochromocytoma. HCTZ: Caution with severe renal disease. May precipitate azotemia with renal disease. Caution with hepatic impairment or progressive liver disease; may precipitate hepatic coma. Sensitivity reactions may occur. May exacerbate or activate systemic lupus erythematosus (SLE). Observe for signs of fluid/electrolyte imbalance (eg, hyponatremia, hypochloremic alkalosis, hypokalemia). Hyperuricemia or gout

precipitation may occur. Hyperglycemia, hypomagnesemia, and hypercalcemia may occur. Withhold or d/c if progressive renal impairment becomes evident. D/C before testing for parathyroid function. Enhanced effects in postsympathectomy patients. Increased cholesterol, TG levels reported. Caution with elderly.

ADVERSE REACTIONS

Aggravation of angina pectoris, pancreatitis, hyperprolactinemia, bone marrow depression, liver disorders, myocarditis, parkinsonism, toxic epidermal necrolysis, amenorrhea, weakness, hypotension, aplastic anemia, anaphylactic reactions, electrolyte imbalance, renal failure.

DRUG INTERACTIONS

See Contraindications. Avoid with lithium. May potentiate other antihypertensives. Methyldopa: Not recommended with ferrous sulfate/gluconate. Anesthetics may need dose reduction. HCTZ: Potentiates orthostatic hypotension with alcohol, barbiturates, or narcotics. Adjust dose of antidiabetic drugs (eg, oral agents and insulin). Cholestyramine and colestipol resins impair absorption. Corticosteroids and adrenocorticotropic hormone may intensify electrolyte depletion, particularly hypokalemia. May decrease response to pressor amines (eg, norepinephrine). Possible increased responsiveness to nondepolarizing skeletal muscle relaxants (eg, tubocurarine). May reduce efficacy with NSAIDs; observe if desired effect is obtained.

PREGNANCY AND LACTATION

Category C, not for use in nursing.

MECHANISM OF ACTION

Methyldopa: Aromatic-amino-acid decarboxylase inhibitor; not established. Metabolized to α-methylnorepinephrine, which is suspected to lower arterial pressure by stimulating central inhibitory α-adrenergic receptors, false neurotransmission, and/or reduction of plasma renin activity. HCTZ: Thiazide diuretic; affects distal renal tubular mechanism of electrolyte reabsorption, increasing excretion of Na and Cl.

PHARMACOKINETICS

Distribution: Crosses placenta, found in breast milk. **Metabolism:** Methyldopa: Extensive. **Elimination:** Methyldopa: Urine (70%); $T_{1/2}$=105 min. HCTZ: Urine (≥61% unchanged); $T_{1/2}$=5.6-14.8 hrs.

PATIENT CONSIDERATIONS

Assessment: Assess for hypersensitivity to drugs and its components, active hepatic disease, liver disorders, anuria, diabetes mellitus (DM), SLE, pregnancy/nursing status, and possible drug interactions. Assess blood count, direct Coombs' test, LFTs, PT, bilirubin, serum electrolytes, and hepatic/renal functions. Obtain baseline BP.

Monitoring: Monitor for signs/symptoms of fluid/electrolyte imbalance, exacerbation/activation of SLE, hypotension, latent DM, hyperglycemia, hypomagnesemia, hypercalcemia, hyperuricemia or precipitation of gout, hypersensitivity reactions, and other adverse effects. Monitor BP, serum electrolytes, renal function, lipid profiles, blood count, LFTs, bilirubin, PT, BUN. Perform direct Coombs' test 6 and 12 months after the start of therapy and monitor hepatic function during the first 6-12 weeks or whenever an unexplained fever occurs.

Counseling: Advise to contact physician if any adverse events occur.

METHYLIN — methylphenidate hydrochloride   **CII**

Class: CNS stimulant

Caution w/ history of drug dependence or alcoholism. Chronic abuse may lead to marked tolerance and physiological dependence w/ varying degrees of abnormal behavior. Frank psychotic episodes may occur, especially w/ parenteral abuse. Careful supervision is required during withdrawal from abusive use, since severe depression may occur. Withdrawal following chronic use may unmask symptoms of the underlying disorder that may require follow-up.

ADULT DOSAGE	**PEDIATRIC DOSAGE**
Attention Deficit Disorders	**Attention Deficit Disorders**
20-30mg/day given in divided doses bid or tid 30-45 min ac; some may require 40-60mg/day or for others, 10-15mg/day may be adequate	**≥6 Years:** **Initial:** 5mg bid before breakfast and lunch
Take last dose before 6 pm if unable to sleep as a result of taking medication late in the day	**Titrate:** Increase gradually in increments of 5-10mg weekly **Max:** 60mg/day
Narcolepsy	D/C if no improvement seen after appropriate dosage adjustment over 1 month
20-30mg/day given in divided doses bid or tid 30-45 min ac; some may require 40-60mg/day or for others, 10-15mg/day may be adequate	D/C periodically to assess the child's condition; therapy should not be indefinite
Take last dose before 6 pm if unable to sleep as a result of taking medication late in the day	**Narcolepsy** **≥6 Years:** **Initial:** 5mg bid before breakfast and lunch
	Titrate: Increase gradually in increments of 5-10mg weekly **Max:** 60mg/day
	D/C if no improvement seen after appropriate dosage adjustment over 1 month
	D/C periodically to assess the child's condition; therapy should not be indefinite

DOSING CONSIDERATIONS

Adverse Reactions

Children ≥6 Years:
Reduce dose or d/c if paradoxical aggravation of symptoms or other adverse effects occur

ADMINISTRATION

Oral route

Tab, Chewable

Take w/ at least 8 oz (full glass) of water or other fluid.

STORAGE

20-25°C (68-77°F). **Tab, Chewable:** Protect from moisture.

HOW SUPPLIED

Oral Sol: 5mg/5mL [500mL], 10mg/5mL [500mL]; **Tab, Chewable:** 2.5mg, 5mg, 10mg* *scored

CONTRAINDICATIONS

Marked anxiety, tension, agitation, known hypersensitivity to drug, glaucoma, motor tics, or family history or diagnosis of Tourette's syndrome. Treatment w/ MAOIs or w/in a minimum of 14 days following discontinuation of an MAOI.

WARNINGS/PRECAUTIONS

Avoid w/ known serious structural cardiac abnormalities, cardiomyopathy, serious heart rhythm abnormalities, coronary artery disease, or other serious cardiac problems. Sudden death reported in children and adolescents w/ structural cardiac abnormalities or other serious heart problems. Sudden death, stroke, and MI reported in adults. May increase BP and HR; caution w/ conditions that might be compromised by increases in BP/HR (eg, preexisting HTN, heart failure, recent MI, ventricular arrhythmias). Prior to treatment, obtain medical history (including assessment for family history of sudden death or ventricular arrhythmia) and perform physical exam to assess for presence of cardiac disease. Promptly perform cardiac evaluation if symptoms suggestive of cardiac disease develop. May exacerbate symptoms of behavior disturbance and thought disorder in patients w/ a preexisting psychotic disorder. Caution in patients w/ comorbid bipolar disorder; may induce mixed/manic episode. May cause treatment-emergent psychotic or manic symptoms (eg, hallucinations, delusional thinking, mania) in children and adolescents w/o prior history of psychotic illness or mania; discontinuation may be appropriate if such symptoms occur. Aggressive behavior or hostility reported in children and adolescents. May lower convulsive threshold; d/c if seizures occur. Priapism, sometimes requiring surgical intervention, reported. May cause long-term suppression of growth in children; monitor growth and may need to interrupt treatment in patients not growing or gaining height or weight as expected. Associated w/ peripheral vasculopathy, including Raynaud's phenomenon; monitor for digital changes. Difficulties w/ accommodation and blurring of vision reported. Patients w/ an element of agitation may react adversely; d/c therapy if necessary. Not indicated in all cases of this behavioral syndrome, and in symptoms associated w/ acute stress reactions. Long-term effects in children not well established.

ADVERSE REACTIONS

Nervousness, insomnia, hypersensitivity, anorexia, nausea, dizziness, palpitations, headache, dyskinesia, drowsiness, BP and pulse changes, tachycardia, weight loss, abdominal pain, loss of appetite.

DRUG INTERACTIONS

See Contraindications. May decrease hypotensive effect of guanethidine. Caution w/ pressor agents. May inhibit metabolism of coumarin anticoagulants, anticonvulsants (eg, phenobarbital, diphenylhydantoin, primidone), phenylbutazone, and TCAs (eg, imipramine, clomipramine, desipramine); may require downward dose adjustments of these drugs.

PREGNANCY AND LACTATION

Pregnancy: Should not be prescribed for women of childbearing age unless benefits outweigh the possible risks.
Lactation: Safety not known in nursing.

MECHANISM OF ACTION

CNS stimulant; has not been established. Thought to block the reuptake of norepinephrine and dopamine into the presynaptic neuron and increase the release of monoamines into the extraneuronal space. Presumably activates the brain stem arousal system and cortex to produce stimulant effect.

PHARMACOKINETICS

Absorption: T_{max}=1-2 hrs. C_{max}=10ng/mL (20mg tab, chewable), 9ng/mL (20mg oral sol). **Metabolism:** Deesterification to α-phenyl-piperidine acetic acid (major metabolite). **Elimination:** Urine (90%; 80% metabolite). $T_{1/2}$=2.7 hrs (20mg oral sol), 3 hrs (20mg tab, chewable).

PATIENT CONSIDERATIONS

Assessment: Assess for previous hypersensitivity to the drug, history of drug dependence or alcoholism, marked anxiety, tension, agitation, glaucoma, motor tics, family history or diagnosis of Tourette's syndrome, preexisting psychotic disorder, comorbid bipolar disorder, cardiac disease, any other conditions where treatment is cautioned or contraindicated, pregnancy/nursing status, and possible drug interactions.

Monitoring: Monitor BP/HR, signs/symptoms of cardiac disease, exacerbations of behavior disturbances and thought disorders, psychosis, mania, appearance of or worsening of aggressive behavior or hostility, seizures, priapism, digital changes, visual disturbances, and other adverse reactions. Monitor growth in children. Perform periodic monitoring of CBC, differential, and platelet counts during prolonged therapy.

Counseling: Inform patients/families/caregivers about risks, benefits, and appropriate use of treatment. Instruct to seek immediate medical attention in the event of priapism. Inform of the risk of peripheral vasculopathy, including Reynaud's phenomenon and instruct to report to physician if symptoms occur. **Tab, Chewable:** Advise not to take the drug if patient has difficulty swallowing. Seek immediate medical attention if experience chest pain, vomiting, or difficulty in swallowing or breathing after taking the drug. Inform that drug contains phenylalanine.

METOCLOPRAMIDE — metoclopramide   Rx

Class: Dopamine antagonist/prokinetic

> May cause tardive dyskinesia (TD); risk increases w/ duration of treatment and total cumulative dose. D/C if signs/symptoms of TD develop. Avoid treatment w/ metoclopramide for >12 weeks unless benefit outweighs risk.

OTHER BRAND NAMES

Reglan

ADULT DOSAGE

Gastroesophageal Reflux Disease

Short-term (4-12 weeks) therapy for patients w/ symptomatic, documented gastroesophageal reflux who fail to respond to conventional therapy

Oral:
10-15mg up to qid 30 min ac and hs; if symptoms occur only intermittently or at specific times of the day, use single doses up to 20mg prior to the provoking situation

Esophageal Erosions/Ulcerations:
15mg/dose qid Therapy should not exceed 12 weeks in duration

Diabetic Gastroparesis

Relief of Acute and Recurrent Symptoms:
Initial route of administration should be determined by the severity of the presenting symptoms

Oral:
10mg 30 min ac and hs for 2-8 weeks; therapy should not exceed 12 weeks in duration

Inj:
Begin therapy w/ IM/IV if severe symptoms are present; doses of 10mg IV may be administered slowly over 1-2 min
Administration of inj up to 10 days may be required before symptoms subside, at which time oral administration may be instituted
Reinstitute metoclopramide at the earliest manifestation

Postoperative Nausea/Vomiting

Prophylaxis in Circumstances Where NG Suction is Undesirable:
Inj:
Usual: 10mg IM near end of surgery; doses of 20mg may be used

Chemotherapy-Induced Nausea/Vomiting

Prophylaxis:
Inj:
IV infusions should be made slowly over at least 15 min, 30 min before chemotherapy and repeated q2h for two doses, then q3h for 3 doses

Initial Two Doses:
Highly Emetogenic Drugs (eg, Cisplatin, Dacarbazine): 2mg/kg
Less Emetogenic Regimens: 1mg/kg

Small Bowel Intubation

Inj:
10mg single dose (undiluted) IV over 1-2 min if the tube has not passed the pylorus w/ conventional maneuvers in 10 min

Aid in Radiological Exam

To stimulate gastric emptying and intestinal transit of barium in cases where delayed emptying interferes w/ radiological examination of the stomach and/or small intestine

Inj:
10mg single dose (undiluted) IV over 1-2 min

PEDIATRIC DOSAGE

Small Bowel Intubation

Inj:
Administer as a single dose (undiluted) IV over 1-2 min if the tube has not passed the pylorus w/ conventional maneuvers in 10 min

<6 Years: 0.1mg/kg
6-14 Years: 2.5-5mg
>14 Years: 10mg

DOSING CONSIDERATIONS
Renal Impairment
Oral/Inj:
CrCl <40mL/min:
Initial: 1/2 the recommended dose; adjust dose as appropriate
Elderly
Oral: 5mg/dose
Adverse Reactions
Inj:
Acute Dystonic Reactions: Inject 50mg diphenhydramine IM

ADMINISTRATION
Oral, IV, IM route
Inj
Doses >10mg: Dilute in 50mL of a parenteral sol.
The preferred parenteral sol is NaCl; if diluted w/ NaCl, may be stored frozen for up to 4 weeks.
If diluted in NaCl, D5W, D5 in 0.45% NaCl, Ringer's inj, or lactated Ringer's inj, may be stored up to 48 hrs (w/o freezing) after preparation if protected from light. All dilutions may be stored unprotected from light under normal light conditions up to 24 hrs after preparation.
Refer to PI for admixture compatibilities and incompatibilities.

STORAGE
20-25°C (68-77°F). **Inj:** Protect from light.

HOW SUPPLIED
Inj: 5mg/mL [2mL]; **Oral Sol:** 5mg/5mL [473mL]; **Tab:** (Reglan) 5mg, 10mg* *scored

CONTRAINDICATIONS
When GI motility stimulation is dangerous (eg, GI hemorrhage, mechanical obstruction, perforation), pheochromocytoma, known sensitivity or intolerance to the drug, epilepsy, concomitant drugs that cause extrapyramidal reactions.

WARNINGS/PRECAUTIONS
Mental depression reported; caution w/ prior history of depression. Extrapyramidal symptoms (EPS), primarily as acute dystonic reactions, may occur; usually seen during the first 24-48 hrs of treatment. May cause parkinsonism-like symptoms; caution w/ preexisting Parkinson's disease. May suppress signs of TD; do not use for symptomatic control of TD. Neuroleptic malignant syndrome (NMS) reported (rare); d/c and institute intensive symptomatic treatment and medical monitoring if NMS occurs. Risk of developing fluid retention and volume overload in patients w/ cirrhosis or CHF; d/c if these occur. Caution w/ HTN, renal impairment, and/or in elderly. May increase risk of developing methemoglobinemia and/or sulfhemoglobinemia in patients w/ NADH-cytochrome b_5 reductase deficiency.
Oral: May experience withdrawal symptoms after discontinuation. **Inj:** IV inj of undiluted metoclopramide should be given slowly allowing 1-2 min for 10mg since rapid administration may cause anxiety, restlessness, and drowsiness. IV administration of metoclopramide diluted in a parenteral sol should be made slowly over a period of not less than 15 min. May increase pressure on suture lines after a gut anastomosis or closure; use caution w/ PONV.

ADVERSE REACTIONS
Restlessness, drowsiness, fatigue, lassitude.

DRUG INTERACTIONS
See Contraindications. GI motility effect antagonized by anticholinergics and narcotic analgesics. Additive sedative effects can occur w/ alcohol, sedatives, hypnotics, narcotics, or tranquilizers. Caution w/ MAOIs. May diminish absorption of drugs from stomach (eg, digoxin) and increase rate and/or extent of absorption of drugs from small bowel (eg, acetaminophen, tetracycline, levodopa, ethanol, cyclosporine). Insulin dose or timing of dose may require adjustment.

PREGNANCY AND LACTATION
Pregnancy: Category B.
Lactation: Metoclopramide is excreted in human milk. Caution in nursing.

MECHANISM OF ACTION
Dopamine antagonist/prokinetic; not established. Appears to sensitize tissues to the action of acetylcholine; stimulates motility of upper GI tract w/o stimulating gastric, biliary, or pancreatic secretions and accelerates gastric emptying and intestinal transit. Also increases resting tone of the lower esophageal sphincter. Antiemetic; antagonizes central and peripheral dopamine receptors, thereby blocking stimulation of chemoreceptor trigger zone.

PHARMACOKINETICS
Absorption: Rapid and well-absorbed; (PO) absolute bioavailability (80%); (PO) T_{max}=1-2 hrs; IV administration in pediatric patients resulted in varying parameters.
Distribution: Plasma protein binding (30%); V_d=3.5L/kg; found in breast milk.
Elimination: (PO) Urine (85%; about half is present as free or conjugated); $T_{1/2}$=5-6 hrs.

PATIENT CONSIDERATIONS
Assessment: Assess for conditions when GI motility stimulation is dangerous, pheochromocytoma, epilepsy, sensitivity or tolerance to the drug, CHF, cirrhosis, history of depression, Parkinson's disease, HTN, NADH-cytochrome b_5 reductase deficiency, renal impairment, pregnancy/nursing status, and possible drug interactions.
Monitoring: Monitor for signs/symptoms of depression, EPS, parkinsonian-like symptoms, TD, NMS, HTN, fluid retention/volume overload, withdrawal symptoms, hypersensitivity reactions, and other adverse reactions.
Counseling: Inform that drug may impair mental and physical abilities; advise to use caution while operating machinery/driving. Discuss the risks and benefits of treatment.

METOLAZONE — metolazone   Rx
Class: Quinazoline diuretic

OTHER BRAND NAMES
Zaroxolyn

ADULT DOSAGE	PEDIATRIC DOSAGE
Edema	Pediatric use may not have been established
Accompanying Congestive Heart Failure/Renal Disease (Nephrotic Syndrome and States of Diminished Renal Function):	
Initial: 5-20mg qd	
May be advisable to give a larger dose for patients who experience paroxysmal nocturnal dyspnea	
Hypertension	
Mild-Moderate:	
Initial: 2.5-5mg qd	
Adjust dose at appropriate intervals to achieve max therapeutic effect	

ADMINISTRATION
Oral route

STORAGE
25°C (77°F); excursions permitted to 15-30°C (59-86°F). Protect from light.

HOW SUPPLIED
Tab: 10mg; (Zaroxolyn) 2.5mg, 5mg

CONTRAINDICATIONS
Anuria, hepatic coma or precoma, known allergy or hypersensitivity to metolazone.

WARNINGS/PRECAUTIONS
Do not interchange metolazone tabs, Zaroxolyn tabs, and other formulations of metolazone that share their slow/incomplete bioavailability and are not therapeutically equivalent at the same doses to Mykrox tabs, a more rapidly available and completely bioavailable metolazone product. Formulations bioequivalent to Zaroxolyn or to Mykrox should not be interchanged for one another. May cause rapid onset of severe hyponatremia and/or hypokalemia following initial doses; d/c and initiate supportive measures immediately when symptoms of severe electrolyte imbalance appear rapidly. Monitor serum K^+ at regular and appropriate intervals, and institute dose reduction, K^+ supplementation, or addition of a K^+-sparing diuretic whenever indicated. Cross-allergy may occur in patients allergic to sulfonamide-derived drugs, thiazides, or quinethazone. Sensitivity reactions (eg, angioedema, bronchospasm) may occur with 1st dose. Observe for signs of fluid and/or electrolyte imbalance (eg, hyponatremia, hypochloremic alkalosis, hypokalemia). May produce low-salt syndrome in patients with severe edema accompanying cardiac failure or renal disease, especially with hot weather and a low-salt diet. Monitor serum and urine electrolytes in patients with protracted vomiting, severe diarrhea, or who are receiving parenteral fluids. Increased risk of hypokalemia with rapid diuresis, severe liver disease, inadequate oral intake, or when excess K^+ is being lost extrarenally. May increase urinary excretion of Mg^{2+}, which may result in hypomagnesemia. May cause hyperglycemia and glycosuria in patients with diabetes or latent diabetes. Increases serum uric acid and may occasionally precipitate gouty attacks. May precipitate azotemia; d/c if azotemia and oliguria worsen during treatment in patients with severe renal disease. Caution with severe renal impairment and in elderly. Orthostatic hypotension may occur. Hypercalcemia may occur, especially in patients with high bone turnover states, and may signify hidden hyperparathyroidism; d/c before tests for parathyroid function are performed. May exacerbate/activate systemic lupus erythematosus (SLE).

ADVERSE REACTIONS
Chest pain, orthostatic hypotension, syncope, neuropathy, toxic epidermal necrolysis, Stevens-Johnson syndrome, necrotizing angiitis, hepatitis, intrahepatic cholestatic jaundice, pancreatitis, joint pain, aplastic anemia, blurred vision, chills, dry mouth.

DRUG INTERACTIONS
Concomitant administration with furosemide and other loop diuretics may result in unusually large/prolonged fluid and electrolyte losses. Caution to avoid excessive reduction of BP, especially during initial therapy with other antihypertensives; dose adjustments of other antihypertensives may be necessary. Orthostatic hypotension may be potentiated with alcohol, barbiturates, narcotics, or other antihypertensives. Drug-induced hypokalemia may increase sensitivity of myocardium to digitalis. May reduce lithium clearance and increase risk of its toxicity; avoid concomitant use. Hypercalcemia may occur with high doses of vitamin D. Corticosteroids or adrenocorticotropic hormone may increase salt/water retention and increase risk of hypokalemia. Drug-induced hypokalemia may enhance neuromuscular blocking effects of curariform drugs (eg, tubocurarine); may be advisable to d/c metolazone 3 days before elective surgery. Salicylates or other NSAIDs may decrease antihypertensive effects. May decrease arterial responsiveness to norepinephrine. May decrease methenamine efficacy. May affect hypoprothrombinemic response to anticoagulants; dose adjustments may be necessary.

PREGNANCY AND LACTATION
Category B, not for use in nursing.

MECHANISM OF ACTION
Quinazoline diuretic; inhibits Na⁺ reabsorption at cortical diluting site and, to a lesser extent, in proximal convoluted tubule.

PHARMACOKINETICS
Absorption: T_{max}=8 hrs. **Distribution:** Found in breast milk; crosses placenta. **Elimination:** Urine (mostly unchanged).

PATIENT CONSIDERATIONS
Assessment: Assess for hypersensitivity to drug, thiazides, quinethazone, or sulfonamide-derived drugs. Assess for anuria, hepatic coma or precoma, diabetes, high bone turnover states, hepatic/renal impairment, any other conditions where treatment is cautioned, pregnancy/nursing status, and possible drug interactions.

Monitoring: Monitor for exacerbation or activation of SLE, hyperglycemia, glycosuria, hyperuricemia or precipitation of gout, hypersensitivity reactions, orthostatic hypotension, azotemia, and other adverse reactions. Monitor serum electrolytes periodically.

Counseling: Advise to take ud. Inform of possible adverse effects; advise to promptly report any adverse reactions to physician.

METOPROLOL — metoprolol tartrate   Rx

Class: Selective beta₁ blocker

> Do not abruptly d/c therapy in patients w/ coronary artery disease (CAD). Severe exacerbation of angina, MI, and ventricular arrhythmias reported in patients w/ CAD following abrupt discontinuation of therapy w/ β-blockers. When discontinuing chronically administered metoprolol, particularly in patients w/ CAD, gradually reduce dose over a period of 1-2 weeks w/ careful monitoring. If angina markedly worsens or acute CAD develops, promptly reinstate metoprolol administration, at least temporarily, and take other measures appropriate for management of unstable angina. CAD may be unrecognized; may be prudent not to d/c therapy abruptly even in patients treated only for HTN.

OTHER BRAND NAMES
Lopressor

ADULT DOSAGE
Hypertension
Tab:
Initial: 100mg/day PO in single or divided doses, whether used alone or added to a diuretic
Titrate: May increase at weekly (or longer) intervals until optimum BP reduction is achieved
Effective Range: 100-450mg/day

Doses >450mg/day not studied. May be used alone or in combination w/ other antihypertensive agents. Lower doses (especially 100mg) may not maintain full effect at the end of 24-hr period, and larger more frequent daily doses may be required.

Angina Pectoris
Long-Term Treatment:
Tab:
Initial: 100mg/day PO in 2 divided doses
Titrate: Gradually increase at weekly intervals until optimum clinical response is achieved or there is pronounced slowing of HR
Effective Range: 100-400mg/day

Doses >400mg/day not studied. If treatment is to be discontinued, gradually decrease dose over 1-2 weeks.

Myocardial Infarction
Treatment of hemodynamically stable patients w/ definite or suspected acute MI to reduce cardiovascular mortality; oral tabs can be initiated after IV therapy or, alternatively, oral treatment can begin w/in 3-10 days of the acute event

Early Phase:
5mg IV bolus every 2 min for 3 doses (monitor BP, HR, and ECG); initiate treatment as soon as possible after patient's arrival in the hospital
In Patients Who Tolerate Full IV Dose (15mg): Initiate tabs, 50mg q6h, 15 min after last IV dose and continue for 48 hrs; thereafter, maint dose is 100mg bid
In Patients Who Cannot Tolerate Full IV Dose: Initiate tabs, either 25mg or 50mg q6h (depending on the degree

PEDIATRIC DOSAGE
Pediatric use may not have been established

of intolerance) 15 min after the last IV dose or as soon as clinical condition allows; d/c w/ severe intolerance

Late Phase:
Initiate tabs, 100mg bid, as soon as clinical condition allows, for ≥3 months; start in patients w/ contraindications to early phase treatment, patients intolerant to the full early treatment, and patients in whom the physician wishes to delay therapy for any other reason

---

DOSING CONSIDERATIONS
Hepatic Impairment
Initiate at low doses w/ cautious gradual dose titration according to clinical response

Elderly
>65 Years: Start at lower end of dosing range

ADMINISTRATION
Oral/IV route

Tab
Swallow unchewed w/ a glass of water. Always take in standardized relation w/ meals; continue taking w/ the same schedule during the course of therapy.

Inj
Parenteral administration should be done in a setting w/ intensive monitoring.

STORAGE
20-25°C (68-77°F). Protect from moisture. (Lopressor) 25°C (77°F); excursions permitted to 15-30°C (59-86°F). **Tab:** Protect from moisture and heat. **Inj:** Protect from light and heat.

HOW SUPPLIED
Tab: 25mg*, 37.5mg*, 75mg*; (Lopressor) 50mg*, 100mg*; **Inj:** (Lopressor) 5mg/5mL *scored

CONTRAINDICATIONS
Hypersensitivity to metoprolol tartrate and related derivatives, to any of the excipients, or to other β-blockers. **MI:** HR <45 beats/min, 2nd- and 3rd-degree heart block, significant 1st-degree heart block (PR interval ≥0.24 sec), systolic BP <100mmHg, moderate to severe cardiac failure. **HTN and Angina:** Sinus bradycardia, >1st-degree heart block, cardiogenic shock, overt cardiac failure, sick sinus syndrome, severe peripheral arterial circulatory disorders.

WARNINGS/PRECAUTIONS
May cause depression of myocardial contractility and may precipitate heart failure (HF) and cardiogenic shock. May be necessary to lower the dose or d/c if signs/symptoms of HF develop. Chronically administered therapy should not be routinely withdrawn prior to major surgery; however, may augment risks of general anesthesia and surgical procedures. Bradycardia, including sinus pause, heart block, and cardiac arrest reported; increased risk in patients w/ 1st degree atrioventricular block, sinus node dysfunction, or conduction disorders. Reduce dose or d/c if severe bradycardia develops. Avoid w/ bronchospastic diseases; may be used in patients w/ bronchospastic disease who do not respond to or cannot tolerate other antihypertensive treatment. May mask tachycardia occurring w/ hypoglycemia; other manifestations (eg, dizziness, sweating) may not be significantly affected. If used in the setting of pheochromocytoma, should be given in combination w/ an α-blocker, and only after the α-blocker has been initiated; may cause a paradoxical increase in BP if administered alone. May mask certain clinical signs (eg, tachycardia) of hyperthyroidism and may precipitate thyroid storm w/ abrupt withdrawal. Patients w/ a history of severe anaphylactic reaction to a variety of allergens may be more reactive to repeated challenge and may be unresponsive to usual doses of epinephrine.

ADVERSE REACTIONS
HTN/Angina: Bradycardia, tiredness, dizziness, depression, SOB, diarrhea, vomiting, pruritus, rash.
MI: Hypotension, bradycardia, 2nd- or 3rd-degree heart block, 1st-degree heart block.

DRUG INTERACTIONS
Additive effects w/ catecholamine-depleting drugs (eg, reserpine). May increase risk of bradycardia w/ digitalis glycosides; monitor HR and PR interval. May produce an additive reduction in myocardial contractility w/ calcium channel blockers. Potent CYP2D6 inhibitors (eg, fluvoxamine, chlorpromazine, quinidine) may increase levels. Hydralazine may inhibit presystemic metabolism, leading to increased levels. May potentiate antihypertensive effects of α-blockers (eg, guanethidine, betanidine, reserpine). May potentiate the postural hypotensive effect of 1st dose of prazosin. May potentiate hypertensive response to withdrawal of clonidine; when given concomitantly w/ clonidine, d/c several days before clonidine is withdrawn. May enhance vasoconstrictive action of ergot alkaloids. Withhold therapy before dipyridamole testing, w/ careful monitoring of HR following the dipyridamole inj. **Inj:** Some inhalational anesthetics may enhance cardiodepressant effect.

PREGNANCY AND LACTATION
Pregnancy: Category C.
Lactation: Excreted in breast milk in a very small quantity. An infant consuming 1L of breast milk daily would receive a dose of <1mg of the drug.

MECHANISM OF ACTION
Selective β₁-blocker; has not been established. Possible mechanisms proposed include competitive antagonism of catecholamines at peripheral (especially

cardiac) adrenergic neuron sites, leading to decreased cardiac output; a central effect leading to reduced sympathetic outflow to the periphery; and suppression of renin activity. In angina pectoris, reduces oxygen requirements of the heart.

PHARMACOKINETICS

Absorption: (Immediate-Release) Oral bioavailability (50%). **Distribution:** V_d=3.2-5.6L/kg. Plasma serum binding (10% to albumin); crosses placenta and blood brain barrier; found in breast milk. **Metabolism:** Liver via CYP2D6. **Elimination:** Urine (95%; [PO] <5% unchanged, [IV] <10% unchanged, [poor metabolizers] 30% or 40% unchanged); $T_{1/2}$=3-4 hrs, 7-9 hrs (poor CYP2D6 metabolizers).

PATIENT CONSIDERATIONS

Assessment: Assess for hypersensitivity to the drug, sinus bradycardia, heart block, cardiogenic shock, HF, CAD, bronchospastic diseases, hypoglycemia, hyperthyroidism, hepatic impairment, any other conditions where treatment is contraindicated or cautioned, pregnancy/nursing status, and possible drug interactions. Obtain baseline ECG.

Monitoring: Monitor for signs/symptoms of HF, cardiogenic shock, bradycardia, thyroid storm, hypersensitivity reactions, and other adverse reactions. Monitor BP, HR, ECG, and hemodynamic status.

Counseling: Advise to take tabs regularly and continuously, ud, w/ or immediately following meals. Warn against interruption or discontinuation of therapy w/o physician's advice. Advise to avoid operating automobiles and machinery or engaging in other tasks requiring alertness until response to therapy has been determined. Instruct to contact physician if difficulty in breathing or other adverse reactions occur, and to inform physician/dentist of therapy before undergoing any type of surgery.

METOPROLOL TARTRATE/HCTZ –

hydrochlorothiazide/metoprolol tartrate   **Rx**

Class: Selective beta₁ blocker/thiazide diuretic

> Exacerbation of angina and, in some cases, myocardial infarction (MI) reported following abrupt discontinuation. When discontinuing therapy, avoid abrupt withdrawal even without overt angina pectoris. Caution patients against interruption of therapy without physician's advice.

OTHER BRAND NAMES
Lopressor HCT

ADULT DOSAGE	PEDIATRIC DOSAGE
Hypertension	Pediatric use may not have been established
If fixed combination represents dose titrated to patient's needs; therapy with combination may be more convenient than with separate components	
Combination Therapy: 100-200mg of metoprolol and hydrochlorothiazide (HCTZ) 25-50mg per day given qd or in divided doses **Max HCTZ:** 50mg/day	
May gradually add another antihypertensive when necessary, beginning with 50% of the usual recommended starting dose	

DOSING CONSIDERATIONS
Elderly
Start at lower end of dosing range

ADMINISTRATION
Oral route

STORAGE
(Lopressor HCT) 25°C (77°F); excursions permitted to 15-30°C (59-86°F). (Metoprolol/HCTZ) 20-25°C (68-77°F). Protect from moisture.

HOW SUPPLIED
Tab: (Metoprolol/HCTZ) 50mg/25mg*, 100mg/25mg*, 100mg/50mg*; (Lopressor HCT) 50mg/25mg*, 100mg/25mg* *scored

CONTRAINDICATIONS
Metoprolol Tartrate: Sinus bradycardia; >1st-degree heart block; cardiogenic shock; overt cardiac failure; hypersensitivity to metoprolol tartrate and related derivatives, any of the excipients, or to other β-blockers; sick sinus syndrome; severe peripheral arterial circulatory disorders. **HCTZ:** Anuria, hypersensitivity to HCTZ or sulfonamide-derived drugs.

WARNINGS/PRECAUTIONS
Not for initial therapy. Caution with hepatic dysfunction and in elderly. Metoprolol: May cause/precipitate heart failure; d/c if cardiac failure continues despite adequate treatment. Avoid with bronchospastic diseases, but may use with caution if unresponsive to/intolerant of other antihypertensives. Avoid withdrawal of chronically administered therapy prior to major surgery; however, may augment risks of general anesthesia and surgical procedures. Caution with diabetic patients; may mask tachycardia occurring with hypoglycemia. Paradoxical BP increase reported with pheochromocytoma; give in combination with and only after initiating α-blocker therapy. May mask hyperthyroidism. Avoid abrupt withdrawal in suspected thyrotoxicosis; may precipitate thyroid storm. HCTZ: Caution with severe renal disease; may precipitate azotemia. If progressive renal impairment

becomes evident, d/c therapy. May precipitate hepatic coma in patients with liver dysfunction/disease. Sensitivity reactions are more likely to occur with history of allergy or bronchial asthma. May exacerbate/activate systemic lupus erythematosus (SLE). May cause idiosyncratic reaction, resulting in acute transient myopia and acute angle-closure glaucoma; d/c HCTZ as rapidly as possible. Fluid/electrolyte imbalance (eg, hyponatremia, hypochloremic alkalosis, hypokalemia) may develop. May cause hyperuricemia and precipitation of frank gout. Latent diabetes mellitus (DM) may manifest during therapy. Enhanced effects seen in postsympathectomy patients. D/C prior to parathyroid function test. Decreased Ca^{2+} excretion observed. Altered parathyroid gland, with hypercalcemia and hypophosphatemia observed with prolonged therapy. May increase urinary excretion of Mg^{2+}, resulting in hypomagnesemia.

ADVERSE REACTIONS
Fatigue, lethargy, dizziness, vertigo, flu syndrome, drowsiness, somnolence, hypokalemia, headache, bradycardia.

DRUG INTERACTIONS
Metoprolol: May exhibit additive effect with catecholamine-depleting drugs (eg, reserpine). Digitalis glycosides may increase risk of bradycardia. Some inhalation anesthetics may enhance cardiodepressant effect. May be unresponsive to usual doses of epinephrine. Potent CYP2D6 inhibitors (eg, certain antidepressants, antipsychotics, antiarrhythmics, antiretrovirals, antihistamines, antimalarials, antifungals, stomach ulcer drugs) may increase levels. Increased risk for rebound HTN following clonidine withdrawal; d/c metoprolol several days before withdrawing clonidine. Effects can be reversed by β-agonists (eg, dobutamine, isoproterenol). HCTZ: Hypokalemia can sensitize/exaggerate cardiac response to toxic effects of digitalis. Risk of hypokalemia with steroids or adrenocorticotropic hormone. Insulin requirements may change in diabetic patients. May decrease arterial responsiveness to norepinephrine. May increase responsiveness to tubocurarine. May increase risk of lithium toxicity. Rare reports of hemolytic anemia with methyldopa. NSAIDs may reduce diuretic, natriuretic, and antihypertensive effects. Impaired absorption reported with cholestyramine and colestipol. Alcohol, barbiturates, and narcotics may potentiate orthostatic hypotension. May potentiate other antihypertensive drugs (eg, ganglionic or peripheral adrenergic-blocking drugs).

PREGNANCY AND LACTATION
Category C, not for use in nursing.

MECHANISM OF ACTION
Metoprolol: β₁-adrenergic receptor blocker; not established. Proposed to competitively antagonize catecholamines at peripheral adrenergic-neuron sites, have central effect leading to reduced sympathetic outflow to periphery, and suppress renin activity. HCTZ: Thiazide diuretic; not established. Affects renal tubular mechanism of electrolyte reabsorption and increases excretion of Na^+ and Cl^-.

PHARMACOKINETICS
Absorption: Metoprolol: Rapid and complete. HCTZ: Rapid; T_{max}=1-2.5 hrs. **Distribution:** Found in breast milk. Metoprolol: Plasma protein binding (12%); found in CSF. HCTZ: V_d=3.6-7.8L/kg; plasma protein binding (67.9%); crosses the placenta. **Metabolism:** Metoprolol: Liver (extensive) via CYP2D6 (oxidation). **Elimination:** Metoprolol: Urine (<5%, unchanged); $T_{1/2}$=2.8 hrs (extensive metabolizers), 7.5 hrs (poor metabolizers). HCTZ: Urine (72-97%); $T_{1/2}$=10-17 hrs.

PATIENT CONSIDERATIONS
Assessment: Assess for history of heart failure, sulfonamide hypersensitivity, SLE, hyperthyroidism, DM, pheochromocytoma, hepatic/renal impairment, any other conditions where treatment is contraindicated/cautioned, pregnancy/nursing status, and possible drug interactions. Obtain baseline serum electrolytes.

Monitoring: Monitor for signs/symptoms of cardiac failure, hypoglycemia, thyrotoxicosis, electrolyte imbalance, exacerbation/activation of SLE, hyperuricemia or precipitation of gout, hypersensitivity reactions, hepatic/renal dysfunction, myopia, angle-closure glaucoma, and other adverse reactions. Monitor serum electrolytes.

Counseling: Instruct to take regularly and continuously, ud, with or immediately following meals. If dose is missed, instruct to take next dose at scheduled time (without doubling the dose) and not to d/c without consulting physician. Instruct to avoid driving, operating machinery, or engaging in tasks requiring alertness until response to therapy is determined. Advise to contact physician if difficulty in breathing or other adverse reactions occur, and to inform physician/dentist of drug therapy before undergoing any type of surgery.

METOZOLV ODT — metoclopramide hydrochloride   **Rx**

Class: Dopamine antagonist/prokinetic

> May cause tardive dyskinesia (TD); d/c if signs/symptoms of TD develop. Avoid use for >12 weeks of therapy unless benefit outweighs risk.

ADULT DOSAGE	PEDIATRIC DOSAGE
Gastroesophageal Reflux Disease	Pediatric use may not have been established
Short-Term (4-12 Weeks) Therapy for Patients w/ Symptomatic, Documented GERD Who Fail to Respond to Conventional Therapy: 10-15mg up to qid	
Intermittent Symptoms: Single doses up to 20mg prior to the symptoms	

Esophageal Erosions/Ulcerations:
15mg/dose qid

Therapy should not exceed 12 weeks in duration

Diabetic Gastroparesis

Acute/Recurrent:
10mg up to qid for 2-8 weeks

Therapy should not exceed 12 weeks in duration

Initial route of administration should be determined by the severity of the presenting symptoms; if severe symptoms are present, begin w/ inj. Inj administration may require up to 10 days before symptoms subside, at which time PO administration may be instituted

----

DOSING CONSIDERATIONS
Renal Impairment
CrCl <40mL/min:
Initial: 1/2 the recommended dose; adjust dose as appropriate

Elderly
Start at lower end of dosing range

ADMINISTRATION
Oral route

Take on an empty stomach at least 30 min ac and hs.
Do not repeat dose if inadvertently taken w/ food.
Only remove each dose from packaging just prior to taking.
Handle tab w/ dry hands and place on tongue; if tab breaks or crumbles while handling, discard and remove a new tab.
Disintegrates on tongue in approx 1 min.
Take w/o liquid.

STORAGE
20-25°C (68-77°F).

HOW SUPPLIED
Tab, Disintegrating: 5mg, 10mg

CONTRAINDICATIONS
When GI motility stimulation is dangerous (eg, GI hemorrhage, mechanical obstruction, or perforation), pheochromocytoma, known sensitivity or intolerance to the drug, epilepsy, and concomitant drugs that cause extrapyramidal reactions.

WARNINGS/PRECAUTIONS
May cause extrapyramidal symptoms (EPS); usually seen during the 1st 24-48 hrs of treatment. May cause drug-induced parkinsonism; symptoms generally subside within 2-3 months following d/c. Caution with history of Parkinson's disease. Neuroleptic malignant syndrome (NMS) reported; d/c and institute intensive symptomatic treatment and medical monitoring if NMS occurs. Depression may occur; caution with history of depression. Caution with HTN, renal impairment, and in the elderly. May increase risk of developing methemoglobinemia and/or sulfhemoglobinemia with NADH-cytochrome b5 reductase deficiency. Risk of developing fluid retention and volume overload in patients with cirrhosis or congestive heart failure (CHF); d/c if these occur. May experience withdrawal symptoms (eg, dizziness, nervousness, headaches) after d/c.

ADVERSE REACTIONS
N/V, fatigue, somnolence, headache.

DRUG INTERACTIONS
See Contraindications. GI motility effect antagonized by anticholinergics and narcotic analgesics. Additive sedation may occur with alcohol, sedatives, hypnotics, narcotics, or tranquilizers. Caution with MAOIs. May decrease gastric absorption of some drugs (eg, digoxin) and increase intestinal absorption of others (eg, acetaminophen, tetracycline, levodopa, ethanol, cyclosporine). Insulin dose or timing of dose may need adjustment to prevent hypoglycemia. Avoid with antidepressants, antipsychotics, and/or neuroleptics associated with TD or NMS. Rare cases of hepatotoxicity with drugs with hepatotoxic potential. Inhibits the central and peripheral effects of apomorphine.

PREGNANCY AND LACTATION
Category B, not for use in nursing.

MECHANISM OF ACTION
Dopamine antagonist/promotility agent; not established. Appears to sensitize tissues to the action of acetylcholine; accelerates gastric emptying and intestinal transit, and stimulates motility of upper GI tract without stimulating gastric, biliary, or pancreatic secretions; increases resting tone of lower esophageal sphincter. Antiemetic; antagonizes central and peripheral dopamine receptors, thereby blocking stimulation of chemoreceptor trigger zone.

PHARMACOKINETICS
Absorption: Rapid and well absorbed. T_{max}=1-2 hrs. **Distribution:** Plasma protein binding (30%); V_d=3.5L/kg; found in breast milk. **Elimination:** Urine (85%; 50% free or conjugated); $T_{1/2}$=5-6 hrs.

PATIENT CONSIDERATIONS
Assessment: Assess for conditions where treatment is contraindicated or cautioned, pregnancy/nursing status, and for possible drug interactions.

Monitoring: Monitor for signs/symptoms of depression, EPS, Parkinsonism, TD, NMS, HTN, fluid retention/volume overload, withdrawal symptoms, and other adverse reactions.

Counseling: Advise to take drug at least 30 min ac and hs. Inform that drug may impair mental and physical abilities. Inform of serious and potential issues associated with treatment (during and after treatment) and advise to inform physician if symptoms occur.

MetroCream — metronidazole   **Rx**
Class: Imidazole antibiotic

ADULT DOSAGE	PEDIATRIC DOSAGE
Rosacea	Pediatric use may not have been established
Inflammatory Papules/Pustules: Apply and rub a thin layer to entire affected area(s) bid, am and pm	

ADMINISTRATION
Topical route

Wash affected area before application
May use cosmetics after application

STORAGE
20-25°C (68-77°F).

HOW SUPPLIED
Cre: 0.75% [45g]

CONTRAINDICATIONS
History of hypersensitivity to metronidazole, or other ingredients of the formulation.

WARNINGS/PRECAUTIONS
Avoid eye contact; tearing of the eyes reported. Decrease frequency of use or d/c if skin irritation occurs. Caution with evidence or history of blood dyscrasia.

ADVERSE REACTIONS
Skin discomfort (eg, burning, stinging), irritation, erythema, pruritus, worsening of rosacea, dryness, transient redness, metallic taste, tingling or numbness of extremities, nausea.

DRUG INTERACTIONS
Oral metronidazole may potentiate warfarin and coumarin anticoagulants resulting in prothrombin time prolongation; unknown effect with topical formulation.

PREGNANCY AND LACTATION
Category B, not for use in nursing.

MECHANISM OF ACTION
Imidazole antibiotic; action in the treatment of rosacea unknown, but appears to include an anti-inflammatory effect.

PATIENT CONSIDERATIONS
Assessment: Assess pregnancy/nursing status, evidence/history of blood dyscrasias, and for possible drug interactions.

Monitoring: Monitor for irritation and other adverse reactions.

Counseling: Instruct to use medication exactly as directed (for external use only). Instruct to avoid contact with eyes, and cleanse affected area(s) before applying. Advise to report adverse reactions, and use less frequently or d/c if local skin irritation develops. Inform that patients may use cosmetics following application.

MetroGel-Vaginal — metronidazole   **Rx**
Class: Nitroimidazole

ADULT DOSAGE	PEDIATRIC DOSAGE
Bacterial Vaginosis	Pediatric use may not have been established
1 applicatorful (5g) intravaginally qd or bid for 5 days	

ADMINISTRATION
Intravaginal route

Administer hs for qd dosing
Refer to PI for administration instructions

STORAGE
15-30°C (59-86°F). Protect from freezing.

HOW SUPPLIED
Gel: 0.75% [70g]

CONTRAINDICATIONS
Prior history of hypersensitivity to metronidazole, parabens, other ingredients of the formulation, or other nitroimidazole derivatives.

WARNINGS/PRECAUTIONS
Not for ophthalmic, dermal, or PO use. Convulsive seizures and peripheral neuropathy reported; d/c promptly if abnormal neurologic signs appear. Caution with CNS diseases and severe hepatic disease. Known or previously unrecognized vaginal candidiasis may present more prominent symptoms during therapy. May develop symptomatic *Candida* vaginitis during or immediately after therapy. Contains ingredients that may cause burning and irritation of the eye; rinse with copious amounts of cool tap water in the event of accidental contact. May interfere with certain types of serum chemistry values (eg, AST, ALT, LDH, TG, glucose hexokinase).

ADVERSE REACTIONS

Symptomatic *Candida* cervicitis/vaginitis, vaginal discharge, pelvic discomfort, N/V, headache, vulva/vaginal irritation, GI discomfort.

DRUG INTERACTIONS

May potentiate anticoagulant effect of warfarin and other coumarin anticoagulants, resulting in prolongation of PT. Elevation of serum lithium levels and signs of lithium toxicity may occur in short-term therapy with high doses of lithium. Cimetidine may prolong $T_{1/2}$ and decrease plasma clearance. May cause disulfiram-like reaction with alcohol. May cause psychotic reactions in alcoholic patients using disulfiram concurrently; do not administer within 2 weeks of discontinuation of disulfiram.

PREGNANCY AND LACTATION

Category B, not for use in nursing.

MECHANISM OF ACTION

Nitroimidazole; intracellular targets of action on anaerobes unknown. Reduced by metabolically active anaerobes and the reduced form of the drug interacts with bacterial DNA.

PHARMACOKINETICS

Absorption: C_{max}=214ng/mL (Day 1), 294ng/mL (Day 5); T_{max}=6-12 hrs; AUC=4977ng•hr/mL. **Distribution:** Found in breast milk (PO); crosses the placenta.

PATIENT CONSIDERATIONS

Assessment: Assess for hypersensitivity to drug, CNS/severe hepatic diseases, vaginal candidiasis, alcohol intake, nursing status, and possible drug interactions. Assess for clinical diagnosis of bacterial vaginosis.

Monitoring: Monitor for convulsive seizures, peripheral neuropathy, *Candida* vaginitis, and other adverse reactions.

Counseling: Caution about drinking alcohol while on therapy. Instruct not to engage in vaginal intercourse during treatment. Inform to avoid contact with eyes and instruct to rinse with copious amounts of cool tap water in the event of accidental contact.

METRONIDAZOLE INJECTION — metronidazole   Rx

Class: Nitroimidazole

> Shown to be carcinogenic in mice and rats. Avoid unnecessary use. Should be reserved for the conditions for which it is indicated.

OTHER BRAND NAMES

Flagyl I.V. (Discontinued)

ADULT DOSAGE

General Dosing

LD: 15mg/kg IV infusion over 1 hr (approx 1g for a 70kg adult)
Maint: 7.5mg/kg IV infusion over 1 hr q6h (approx 500mg for a 70kg adult), starting 6 hrs after LD initiation
Max: 4g/24 hrs
Usual Duration: 7-10 days; infections of the bone and joint, lower respiratory tract, and endocardium may require longer treatment

May change to oral metronidazole when conditions warrant, based on severity of disease and response

Prophylaxis of Postoperative Infections

In Contaminated or Potentially Contaminated Colorectal Surgery:

15mg/kg IV infusion over 30-60 min (complete 1 hr before surgery), then 7.5mg/kg IV infusion over 30-60 min at 6 and 12 hrs after initial dose

D/C w/in 12 hrs after surgery

Other Indications

Treatment of the Following Infections Caused by Susceptible Organisms (Anaerobic Bacteria):

Intra-abdominal infections
Skin and skin structure infections
Gynecologic infections
Bone/joint infections (as adjunctive therapy)
CNS infections
Lower respiratory tract infections
Bacterial septicemia
Endocarditis caused by susceptible strains of microorganisms (anaerobic bacteria)

Effective in *Bacteroides fragilis* infections resistant to clindamycin, chloramphenicol, and penicillin

PEDIATRIC DOSAGE

Pediatric use may not have been established

DOSING CONSIDERATIONS

Renal Impairment

Hemodialysis: If administration cannot be separated from hemodialysis session, consider supplementation of dosage following the session, depending on patient's clinical situation

Hepatic Impairment

Severe (Child-Pugh C): Reduce dose by 50%

ADMINISTRATION

IV route

No dilution/buffering required.
Administer by slow IV drip infusion only (either as continuous or intermittent infusion).
Do not introduce additives into drug sol.
If used w/ a primary IV fluid system, the primary sol should be discontinued during metronidazole infusion.
Do not use equipment containing aluminum (eg, needles, cannulae) that would come in contact w/ the drug sol.

Refer to PI for additional preparation and administration instructions.

STORAGE

25°C (77°F). Protect from light. Do not remove unit from overwrap until ready for use.

HOW SUPPLIED

Inj: 5mg/mL [100mL]

CONTRAINDICATIONS

Prior history of hypersensitivity to metronidazole or other nitroimidazole derivatives, disulfiram use w/in the last 2 weeks, consumption of alcohol or products containing propylene glycol during and for at least 3 days after therapy.

WARNINGS/PRECAUTIONS

Encephalopathy and peripheral neuropathy (including optic neuropathy), convulsive seizures, and aseptic meningitis reported; promptly evaluate benefit/risk ratio of the continuation of therapy if abnormal neurologic signs/symptoms appear. Known or previously unrecognized candidiasis may present more prominent symptoms during therapy and requires treatment w/ a candicidal agent. Caution w/ hepatic/renal impairment, evidence of or history of blood dyscrasia, and in the elderly. Mild leukopenia reported; monitor total and differential leukocyte counts before, during, and after prolonged or repeated courses of therapy. May cause Na^+ retention due to Na^+ content; caution in patients receiving corticosteroids or predisposed to edema. May result in bacterial resistance if used in the absence of proven or suspected bacterial infection, or a prophylactic indication. Lab test interactions may occur.

ADVERSE REACTIONS

Headache, syncope, dizziness, vertigo, incoordination, N/V, diarrhea, epigastric distress, abdominal cramping, constipation, unpleasant metallic taste, erythematous rash, pruritus, urticaria.

DRUG INTERACTIONS

See Contraindications. May potentiate anticoagulant effect of warfarin and other oral coumarin anticoagulants, resulting in PT prolongation; carefully monitor PT and INR. May increase serum lithium, and may cause lithium toxicity; obtain serum lithium and SrCr levels several days after beginning metronidazole. May increase busulfan concentrations, which can result in increased risk for serious busulfan toxicity; avoid concomitant use or, if coadministration is medically needed, frequently monitor busulfan concentration and adjust busulfan dose accordingly. Simultaneous administration of drugs that decrease microsomal liver enzyme activity (eg, cimetidine) may prolong $T_{1/2}$ and decrease clearance. Simultaneous administration of drugs that induce microsomal liver enzyme activity (eg, phenytoin, phenobarbital) may accelerate elimination, resulting in reduced levels. Impaired clearance of phenytoin reported.

PREGNANCY AND LACTATION

Pregnancy: Category B.
Lactation: Not for use in nursing.

MECHANISM OF ACTION

Nitroimidazole antibacterial; precise mechanism is unclear. Exerts antibacterial effects in an anaerobic environment. Upon entering the organism, the drug is reduced by intracellular electron transport proteins and free radicals are formed. Because of this alteration, a concentration gradient is created and maintained that promotes the drug's intracellular transport. The reduced form of metronidazole and free radicals interact w/ DNA, leading to inhibition of DNA synthesis and DNA degradation, resulting in the death of bacteria.

PHARMACOKINETICS

Absorption: C_{max}=25mcg/mL. **Distribution:** Plasma protein binding (<20%); found in breast milk; crosses the placenta. **Metabolism:** Side-chain oxidation and glucuronide conjugation; 1-(β-hydroxyethyl)-2-hydroxymethyl-5-nitroimidazole and 2-methyl-5-nitroimidazole-1-yl-acetic acid (metabolites). **Elimination:** Urine (60-80%, 20% unchanged), feces (6-15%); $T_{1/2}$=8 hrs.

PATIENT CONSIDERATIONS

Assessment: Assess for candidiasis, alcohol use, hepatic/renal impairment, evidence/history of blood dyscrasia, predisposition to edema, hypersensitivity to drug or other nitroimidazole derivatives, pregnancy/nursing status, and possible drug interactions. Obtain total and differential leukocyte counts before prolonged/repeated courses of therapy.

Monitoring: Monitor for abnormal neurologic signs/symptoms, candidiasis, Na^+ retention, and other adverse reactions. Monitor total and differential leukocyte counts during and after prolonged or repeated courses of therapy. Monitor PT and INR w/ oral coumarin anticoagulants (eg, warfarin).

Counseling: Instruct to d/c consumption of alcoholic beverages or products containing propylene glycol while taking the drug and for at least 3 days afterward. Counsel that therapy should only be used to treat bacterial, not viral, infections. Instruct to take exactly ud even if the patient feels better early in the course of therapy. Inform that skipping doses or not completing the full course of therapy may decrease effectiveness of treatment and increase bacterial resistance.

MIACALCIN — calcitonin-salmon   Rx

Class: Hormonal bone resorption inhibitor

ADULT DOSAGE	**PEDIATRIC DOSAGE**
Paget's Disease	Pediatric use may not have been established
Moderate to Severe Symptomatic Disease:	
Inj:	
100 IU (0.5mL) SQ/IM qd	
Hypercalcemia	
Early treatment of hypercalcemic emergencies, along w/ other appropriate agents, when a rapid decrease in serum Ca^{2+} is required, until more specific treatment of the underlying disease can be accomplished	
Inj:	
Initial: 4 IU/kg SQ/IM q12h	
Titrate: If response is not satisfactory after 1 or 2 days, dose may be increased to 8 IU/kg q12h; if response remains unsatisfactory after 2 more days, dose may be further increased to a max of 8 IU/kg q6h	
Postmenopausal Osteoporosis	
In Women >5 Years Postmenopause:	
Inj:	
100 IU (0.5mL) SQ/IM qd	
Spray:	
1 spray (200 IU) qd intranasally, alternating nostrils daily	

DOSING CONSIDERATIONS
Other Important Considerations
Postmenopausal Osteoporosis:
Calcium and Vitamin D Supplementation: Patients should receive adequate Ca^{2+} (≥1000mg elemental Ca^{2+}/day) and vitamin D (≥400 IU/day)

ADMINISTRATION
(Inj) IM/SQ route; (Spray) Intranasal route

Inj
If volume to be injected is >2mL, IM inj is preferable and total dose should be distributed across multiple inj sites

Nasal Spray
Wait until the bottle has reached room temperature before using the 1st dose
To prime the pump before it is used for the 1st time, hold the bottle upright and depress the 2 white side arms of the pump toward the bottle until a full spray is released; the pump is primed once the 1st full spray is emitted
To administer, carefully place the nozzle into the nostril w/ the patient's head in the upright position, then firmly depress the pump toward the bottle
Do not prime the pump before each daily use

STORAGE
(Spray) Unopened: 2-8°C (36-46°F). Protect from freezing. In Use: 15-30°C (59-86°F) in an upright position for up to 35 days. Discard after 30 doses. (Inj) 2-8°C (36-46°F).

HOW SUPPLIED
Inj: 200 IU/mL [2mL]; **Spray:** 200 IU/actuation [3.7mL]

CONTRAINDICATIONS
Hypersensitivity to calcitonin-salmon or any of the excipients.

WARNINGS/PRECAUTIONS
Serious hypersensitivity reactions reported; appropriate medical support and monitoring measures should be readily available. Consider skin testing prior to treatment with suspected sensitivity to therapy. Hypocalcemia associated with tetany and seizure activity reported. Correct hypocalcemia and treat other disorders affecting mineral metabolism (eg, vitamin D deficiency) before initiating therapy. Provisions for parenteral Ca^{2+} administration should be available during the 1st several administrations of therapy in patients at risk for hypocalcemia. Adequate intake of Ca^{2+} and vitamin D is recommended in patients treated for Paget's disease or postmenopausal osteoporosis. Increased risk of malignancies; carefully consider benefits against possible risks. Consider possibility of antibody formation in any patient with an initial response to therapy who later stops responding to treatment. Urinary casts reported; consider periodic exam of urine sediment. (Spray) Nasal adverse reactions (eg, rhinitis, epistaxis) reported; dhevelopment of mucosal referations may occur. Periodic nasal exams are recommended prior to start of treatment, periodically during therapy, and at any time nasal symptoms occur. D/C if severe ulceration of the nasal mucosa occurs; d/c temporarily until healing occurs in patients with smaller ulcers.

ADVERSE REACTIONS
Nausea, flushing, malignancy. (Inj) Inj-site local inflammatory reactions, vomiting. (Spray) Nasal symptoms, rhinitis, back pain, epistaxis, headache, arthralgia.

DRUG INTERACTIONS
May reduce plasma lithium concentrations; lithium dose may require adjustment.

PREGNANCY AND LACTATION
Category C, caution in nursing.

MECHANISM OF ACTION
Hormonal bone resorption inhibitor; calcitonin receptor agonist. Actions on bone have not been fully established. Causes inhibition of the ongoing bone resorptive process. Prolonged use causes a smaller decrease in the rate of bone resorption, which is associated with a decreased number of osteoclasts as well as a decrease in their resorptive activity.

PHARMACOKINETICS
Absorption: (Inj) Absolute bioavailability (66% IM), (71% SQ); T_{max}=23 min (SQ). (Spray) Rapid; T_{max}=13 min. **Distribution:** (Inj) V_d=0.15-0.3L/kg. **Elimination:** (Inj) $T_{1/2}$=58 min (IM), $T_{1/2}$=59-64 min (SQ). (Spray) $T_{1/2}$=18 min.

PATIENT CONSIDERATIONS
Assessment: Assess for hypersensitivity to drug or any of the excipients, hypocalcemia or other disorders affecting mineral metabolism, pregnancy/nursing status, and possible drug interactions. Consider skin testing for patients with suspected sensitivity to therapy. (Spray) Perform baseline nasal exam.

Monitoring: Monitor for signs/symptoms of serious hypersensitivity reactions, malignancy, hypocalcemia associated with tetany and seizure activity, antibody formation, and other adverse reactions. Periodically assess need for continued therapy. Perform periodic exams of urine sediment. (Spray) Perform periodic nasal exams during therapy and when nasal symptoms occur.

Counseling: Inform of the potential increase in risk of malignancy. Advise patients with postmenopausal osteoporosis or Paget's disease of bone to maintain an adequate Ca^{2+} and vitamin D intake. Instruct to seek emergency medical help if any sign/symptoms of a serious allergic reaction develop. (Inj) Instruct about sterile inj technique and to dispose of needles properly. (Spray) Instruct on pump assembly, priming of pump, and nasal introduction of medication. Advise to notify physician if significant nasal irritation develops.

MICARDIS — telmisartan   Rx

Class: Angiotensin II receptor blocker (ARB)

> **D/C when pregnancy is detected. Drugs that act directly on the renin-angiotensin system (RAS) can cause injury/death to the developing fetus.**

ADULT DOSAGE	**PEDIATRIC DOSAGE**
Hypertension	Pediatric use may not have been established
Initial: 40mg qd	
Range: 40-80mg/day	
May add diuretic if BP not controlled w/ 80mg	
Risk Reduction of Myocardial Infarction, Stroke, Cardiovascular Death	
For use in patients ≥55 years of age at high risk of developing major CV events who are unable to take ACE inhibitors	
80mg qd	

DOSING CONSIDERATIONS
Hepatic Impairment
Including Biliary Obstructive Disorders:
Start at low doses and titrate slowly

ADMINISTRATION
Oral route

Take w/ or w/o food

STORAGE
25°C (77°F); excursions permitted to 15-30°C (59-86°F).

HOW SUPPLIED
Tab: 20mg, 40mg, 80mg

CONTRAINDICATIONS
Known hypersensitivity (eg, anaphylaxis, angioedema) to telmisartan or any other component of this product, coadministration w/ aliskiren in patients w/ diabetes.

WARNINGS/PRECAUTIONS
May develop orthostatic hypotension in patients on dialysis. Symptomatic hypotension may occur in patients with an activated RAS (eg, volume- and/or salt-depleted patients receiving high doses of diuretics); correct this condition before therapy or monitor closely. Hyperkalemia may occur, particularly in patients with advanced renal impairment, HF, and on renal replacement therapy; monitor serum electrolytes periodically. Caution in patients with hepatic impairment (eg, biliary obstructive disorders); reduced clearance may be expected. Oliguria and/or progressive azotemia and (rarely) acute renal failure and/or death may occur in patients whose renal function is dependent on the RAS (eg, severe CHF). May increase SrCr/BUN in patients with renal artery stenosis.

ADVERSE REACTIONS

URTI, back pain, sinusitis, diarrhea, intermittent claudication, skin ulcer.

DRUG INTERACTIONS

See Contraindications. Dual blockade of the RAS is associated with increased risk of hypotension, hyperkalemia, and changes in renal function (eg, acute renal failure); avoid combined use of RAS inhibitors. Closely monitor BP, renal function, and electrolytes with concomitant agents that also affect the RAS. Avoid with aliskiren in patients with renal impairment (GFR <60mL/min). Avoid with an ACE inhibitor. Coadministration with ramipril may increase ramipril/ ramiprilat levels and decrease telmisartan levels; not recommended with ramipril. Hyperkalemia may occur with K^+ supplements, K^+-sparing diuretics, K^+-containing salt substitutes, or other drugs that increase K^+ levels. May increase digoxin levels; monitor digoxin levels upon initiating, adjusting, and discontinuing therapy. May increase serum lithium levels/toxicity; monitor lithium levels during concomitant use. NSAIDs, including selective COX-2 inhibitors, may attenuate antihypertensive effect and may deteriorate renal function; monitor renal function periodically.

PREGNANCY AND LACTATION

Category D, not for use in nursing.

MECHANISM OF ACTION

Angiotensin II receptor antagonist; blocks the vasoconstrictor and aldosterone-secreting effects of angiotensin II by selectively blocking the binding of angiotensin II to the AT_1 receptor in many tissues.

PHARMACOKINETICS

Absorption: Absolute bioavailability: 40mg (42%), 160mg (58%); T_{max}=0.5-1 hr. **Distribution:** V_d=500L; plasma protein binding (>99.5%). **Metabolism:** Conjugation. **Elimination:** Feces (>97%, unchanged), urine (0.49%); $T_{1/2}$=24 hrs.

PATIENT CONSIDERATIONS

Assessment: Assess for known hypersensitivity to drug, biliary obstructive disorders, CHF, renal artery stenosis, hepatic/renal impairment, volume/ salt depletion, dialysis patients, pregnancy/nursing status, and possible drug interactions.

Monitoring: Monitor for symptomatic hypotension and other adverse reactions. Monitor BP, ECG, renal function, and serum electrolytes.

Counseling: Inform women of childbearing age about the consequences of exposure to the medication during pregnancy. Discuss treatment options with women planning to become pregnant. Instruct to report pregnancies to the physician as soon as possible.

MICARDIS HCT — hydrochlorothiazide/telmisartan   Rx

Class: Angiotensin II receptor blocker (ARB)/thiazide diuretic

> D/C when pregnancy is detected. Drugs that act directly on the renin-angiotensin system (RAS) can cause injury/death to the developing fetus.

ADULT DOSAGE	PEDIATRIC DOSAGE
Hypertension	Pediatric use may not have been established
Patients whose BP is not adequately controlled w/ telmisartan monotherapy 80mg, or is not adequately controlled by 25mg qd hydrochlorothiazide (HCTZ), or is controlled but experience hypokalemia	
Initial: 80mg/12.5mg qd	
Titrate: May increase up to 160mg/25mg after 2-4 weeks	
Patients titrated to the individual components may instead receive the corresponding dose of Micardis HCT	

DOSING CONSIDERATIONS

Renal Impairment
Severe (CrCl ≤30mL/min): Not recommended

Hepatic Impairment
Severe: Not recommended

Biliary Obstructive Disorders/Hepatic Insufficiency:
Initial: 40mg/12.5mg qd under close medical supervision

Elderly
Start at lower end of dosing range

ADMINISTRATION

Oral route

Do not remove tab from blister until immediately before administration. May be administered w/ other antihypertensive drugs.

STORAGE

25°C (77°F); excursions permitted to 15-30°C (59-86°F).

HOW SUPPLIED

Tab: (Telmisartan/HCTZ) 40mg/12.5mg, 80mg/12.5mg, 80mg/25mg

CONTRAINDICATIONS

Hypersensitivity to any component of the medication, anuria, coadministration w/ aliskiren in patients w/ diabetes.

WARNINGS/PRECAUTIONS

Not for initial therapy. Symptomatic hypotension may occur in patients w/ an activated RAS (eg, volume- or salt-depleted patients). Correct volume or salt depletion prior to administration of therapy. Changes in renal function (eg, acute renal failure) may occur. Patients whose renal function may depend in part on the activity of the RAS may be at risk of developing oliguria, progressive azotemia, or acute renal failure. Consider withholding or discontinuing therapy in patients who develop a clinically significant decrease in renal function. **HCTZ:** May cause hypokalemia, hyponatremia, and hypomagnesemia. Decreases urinary calcium excretion and may cause elevations of serum calcium. May alter glucose tolerance and raise serum levels of cholesterol and TGs. Hyperuricemia may occur or frank gout may be precipitated. Hypersensitivity reactions may occur; more likely to occur in patients w/ history of allergy or bronchial asthma. May cause an idiosyncratic reaction, resulting in acute transient myopia and acute angle-closure glaucoma; d/c as rapidly as possible. May cause exacerbation or activation of systemic lupus erythematosus (SLE). The antihypertensive effects of the drug may be enhanced in the postsympathectomy patient. **Telmisartan:** May cause hyperkalemia, particularly in patients w/ renal insufficiency or diabetes.

ADVERSE REACTIONS

URTI, dizziness, sinusitis, fatigue, diarrhea.

DRUG INTERACTIONS

See Contraindications. Increases in serum lithium concentrations and lithium toxicity reported; monitor serum lithium levels during concomitant use. NSAIDs, including selective COX-2 inhibitors, may decrease effects of diuretics and ARBs and may deteriorate renal function (possible acute renal failure). Avoid w/ aliskiren in patients w/ renal impairment (GFR <60mL/min). **HCTZ:** Dosage adjustment of antidiabetic drugs (eg, oral agents, insulin) may be required. Anionic exchange resins (eg, cholestyramine, colestipol) may impair absorption; stagger the dose of HCTZ and the resin such that HCTZ is administered at least 4 hrs before or 4-6 hrs after the administration of the resin. **Telmisartan:** Use w/ other drugs that raise serum K^+ may result in hyperkalemia; monitor serum K^+. Dual blockade of the RAS is associated w/ increased risks of hypotension, hyperkalemia, and renal impairment; avoid combined use of RAS inhibitors. Closely monitor BP, renal function, and electrolytes in patients on concomitant agents that affect the RAS. May increase digoxin peak plasma concentration and digoxin trough concentrations; monitor digoxin levels.

PREGNANCY AND LACTATION

Pregnancy: Category D.
Lactation: Thiazides appear in breast milk. Not for use in nursing.

MECHANISM OF ACTION

Telmisartan: ARB; blocks the vasoconstrictor and aldosterone-secreting effects of angiotensin II by selectively blocking the binding of angiotensin II to the AT_1 receptor in many tissues. **HCTZ:** Thiazide diuretic; has not been established. Affects the renal tubular mechanisms of electrolyte reabsorption, directly increasing excretion of Na^+ salt and Cl^- in approximately equivalent amounts.

PHARMACOKINETICS

Absorption: Telmisartan: Absolute bioavailability: 42% (40mg), 58% (160mg); T_{max}=0.5-1 hr. **Distribution:** Telmisartan: V_d=500L; plasma protein binding (>99.5%). HCTZ: Crosses placenta; found in breast milk. **Metabolism:** Telmisartan: Conjugation. **Elimination:** Telmisartan: Feces (>97%, unchanged), urine (0.49%); $T_{1/2}$=24 hrs. HCTZ: Urine (61%, unchanged); $T_{1/2}$=5.6-14.8 hrs.

PATIENT CONSIDERATIONS

Assessment: Assess for hypersensitivity to the drugs and their components, anuria, sulfonamide-derived hypersensitivity, history of penicillin allergy, volume/ salt depletion, SLE, diabetes, CHF, hepatic/renal impairment, biliary obstructive disorder, renal artery stenosis, postsympathectomy status, pregnancy/nursing status, and possible drug interactions. Obtain baseline BP.

Monitoring: Monitor for signs/symptoms of fluid/electrolyte imbalance, exacerbation/activation of SLE, idiosyncratic reaction, precipitation of gout, hypersensitivity reactions, and other adverse reactions. Monitor BP, serum electrolytes, renal/hepatic function, Ca^{2+} levels, cholesterol, and TG levels periodically.

Counseling: Inform women of childbearing age about the consequences of exposure to the medication during pregnancy. Discuss treatment options w/ women planning to become pregnant. Instruct to report pregnancies to the physician as soon as possible. Caution that lightheadedness may occur, especially during the 1st days of therapy. Inform that inadequate fluid intake, excessive perspiration, diarrhea, or vomiting can lead to an excessive fall in BP, w/ the same consequences of lightheadedness and possible syncope. Instruct to contact physician if syncope occurs. Advise not to use K^+ supplements or salt substitutes that contain K^+ w/o consulting physician. Advise to d/c therapy and seek immediate medical attention if the patient experiences symptoms of acute myopia or secondary angle-closure glaucoma.

MICRO-K — potassium chloride   Rx

Class: Potassium supplement

ADULT DOSAGE	PEDIATRIC DOSAGE
Hypokalemia	Pediatric use may not have been established
Prevention: 20mEq/day	
Treatment: 40-100mEq/day or more	
Divide dose if >20mEq/day is given such that no more than 20mEq is given in a single dose	

DOSING CONSIDERATIONS
Elderly
Start at lower end of dosing range

ADMINISTRATION
Oral route

Take w/ meals and a full glass of water or other liquid
May sprinkle on a spoonful of soft food (eg, applesauce, pudding) in patients who have difficulty swallowing caps; swallow immediately w/o chewing and follow w/ a glass of cool water or juice

STORAGE
20-25°C (68-77°F).

HOW SUPPLIED
Cap, Extended-Release: 8mEq, 10mEq

CONTRAINDICATIONS
Hyperkalemia, esophageal ulceration, delay in GI passage (from structural, pathological, pharmacologic causes [eg, anticholinergic agents]), cardiac patients with esophageal compression due to enlarged left atrium.

WARNINGS/PRECAUTIONS
Potentially fatal hyperkalemia may occur. Extreme caution with acidosis, cardiac, and renal disease; monitor ECG and electrolytes. Hypokalemia with metabolic acidosis should be treated with an alkalinizing potassium salt (eg, potassium bicarbonate, potassium citrate). May produce ulcerative or stenotic GI lesions.

ADVERSE REACTIONS
Hyperkalemia, GI effects (obstruction, bleeding, ulceration), N/V, abdominal pain, diarrhea.

DRUG INTERACTIONS
See Contraindications. Risk of hyperkalemia with ACE inhibitors (eg, captopril, enalapril), K^+-sparing diuretics, and K^+ supplements.

PREGNANCY AND LACTATION
Category C, safe for use in nursing.

MECHANISM OF ACTION
K^+ supplement; helps in maintenance of intracellular tonicity, transmission of nerve impulses, contraction of cardiac, skeletal, and smooth muscle, and maintenance of normal renal function.

PATIENT CONSIDERATIONS
Assessment: Assess for conditions that impair excretion of K^+, hyperkalemia, esophageal compression due to enlarged left atrium, conditions causing arrest or delay in passage through GI, renal insufficiency, diabetes mellitus, and possible drug interactions.

Monitoring: Monitor serum K^+ levels regularly; renal function, ECG, and acid-base balance. Monitor for GI ulceration/obstruction/perforation, hyperkalemia, renal dysfunction, and hypersensitivity reactions.

Counseling: Instruct to take with meals; swallow with full glass of water or other suitable liquid. Instruct to not crush, chew, or suck. Instruct to seek medical attention if symptoms of GI ulceration, obstruction, perforation (vomiting, abdominal pain, distention, GI bleeding), hyperkalemia, or hypersensitivity reactions occur.

MICROZIDE — hydrochlorothiazide   Rx

Class: Thiazide diuretic

ADULT DOSAGE	PEDIATRIC DOSAGE
Hypertension	Pediatric use may not have been established
Initial: 12.5mg qd	
Max: 50mg/day	

DOSING CONSIDERATIONS
Elderly
Start at lower end of dosing range, utilizing 12.5mg increments for further titration

ADMINISTRATION
Oral route

STORAGE
20-25°C (68-77°F). Protect from light, moisture, freezing, -20°C (-4°F). Keep container tightly closed.

HOW SUPPLIED
Cap: 12.5mg

CONTRAINDICATIONS
Anuria, hypersensitivity to this product or other sulfonamide-derived drugs.

WARNINGS/PRECAUTIONS
May cause idiosyncratic reaction, resulting in acute transient myopia and acute angle-closure glaucoma; d/c as rapidly as possible. May manifest latent diabetes mellitus (DM). May precipitate azotemia with renal impairment. Hypokalemia reported; monitor serum electrolytes and for sign/symptoms of fluid/electrolyte disturbances. Dilutional hyponatremia may occur in edematous patients in hot weather. Hyperuricemia or acute gout may be precipitated. Caution with hepatic impairment; hepatic coma may occur with severe liver disease. Decreased Ca^{2+} excretion and changes in parathyroid glands with hypercalcemia and hypophosphatemia reported during prolonged use. D/C prior to parathyroid test.

ADVERSE REACTIONS
Weakness, hypotension, pancreatitis, jaundice, diarrhea, vomiting, hematologic abnormalities, anaphylactic reactions, electrolyte imbalance, muscle spasm, vertigo, renal failure, erythema multiforme, transient blurred vision, impotence.

DRUG INTERACTIONS
Potentiation of orthostatic hypotension with alcohol, barbiturates, narcotics. Additive effect or potentiation with antihypertensive drugs. Dose adjustment of antidiabetic drugs (oral agents or insulin) may be required. Reduced absorption with cholestyramine or colestipol. Increased risk of electrolyte depletion (eg, hypokalemia) with corticosteroids and adrenocorticotropic hormone. May decrease response to pressor amines (eg, norepinephrine). May increase responsiveness to nondepolarizing skeletal muscle relaxants (eg, tubocurarine). Increased risk of lithium toxicity; avoid with lithium. NSAIDs may reduce diuretic, natriuretic, and antihypertensive effects. May cause hypokalemia, which can sensitize or exaggerate the response of the heart to the toxic effects of digitalis.

PREGNANCY AND LACTATION
Category B, not for use in nursing.

MECHANISM OF ACTION
Thiazide diuretic; blocks reabsorption of Na^+ and Cl^- ions, thereby increasing the quantity of Na^+ traversing the distal tubule and the volume of water excreted. Also decreases the excretion of Ca^{2+} and uric acid, may increase the excretion of iodide, and may reduce GFR.

PHARMACOKINETICS
Absorption: Well-absorbed; C_{max}=70-490ng/mL; T_{max}=1-5 hrs. **Distribution:** Plasma protein binding (40-68%); crosses placenta; found in breast milk. **Elimination:** Urine (55-77%, >95% unchanged); $T_{1/2}$=6-15 hrs.

PATIENT CONSIDERATIONS
Assessment: Assess for anuria, known hypersensitivity to sulfonamide-derived drugs, history of penicillin allergy, DM, risk for developing hypokalemia, impaired renal/hepatic function, edema, pregnancy/nursing status, and for possible drug interactions. Obtain baseline serum electrolytes.

Monitoring: Monitor for signs/symptoms of decreased visual acuity, ocular pain, azotemia, hypokalemia, fluid/electrolyte disturbances, dilutional hyponatremia, hyperuricemia or acute gout, and hepatic coma. Periodically monitor serum electrolytes in patients with risk for developing hypokalemia.

Counseling: Counsel about signs/symptoms of fluid and electrolyte imbalance and advise to seek prompt medical attention.

MINASTRIN 24 FE — ethinyl estradiol/ferrous fumarate/norethindrone acetate   Rx

Class: Estrogen/progestogen combination

> Cigarette smoking increases the risk of serious cardiovascular (CV) events. Risk increases with age (>35 yrs of age) and with the number of cigarettes smoked. Should not be used by women who are >35 yrs of age and smoke.

ADULT DOSAGE	PEDIATRIC DOSAGE
Contraception	**Contraception**
1 tab qd for 28 days at the same time each day, then repeat	Not indicated for use premenarche; refer to adult dosing
Start 1st Sunday after menses begins or 1st day of menses	
Conversions	
Switching from Combination Hormonal Method:	
Another Pill: Start on the day the next combination oral contraceptive pill would have been taken; do not continue previous birth control pack and do not skip any days between packs	
Vaginal Ring/Patch: Start on the day previous product would have been resumed	
Switching from Progestin-Only Method (eg, Progestin-Only Pill, Implant, Intrauterine System, Inj): May switch any day from progestin-only pill; start on day that next progestin-only pill would have been taken and use a nonhormonal method of contraception for 7 consecutive days If switching from implant/inj, start on the day next inj would have been administered, or on the day of implant removal If switching from intrauterine device, may need backup contraception depending on the timing of removal	

DOSING CONSIDERATIONS
Adverse Reactions
GI Disturbances: If vomiting/diarrhea occurs w/in 3-4 hrs after administration of white tab, follow missed dose instructions

Other Important Considerations
Postpartum Women Who Do Not Breastfeed/After Second Trimester Abortion: Initiate therapy no earlier than 4 weeks postpartum; if patient has not yet had a

period, she should use additional method of contraception until she has taken tabs for 7 consecutive days

First Trimester Abortion/Miscarriage:
May initiate immediately; if patient starts immediately, additional contraceptive measures are not needed

ADMINISTRATION
Oral route

Take w/o regard to meals
Chew and swallow tab; drink full glass (8 oz) of water immediately after chewing/swallowing white tabs
Take in the order directed on the blister pack
Do not skip or take at intervals exceeding 24 hrs

Day 1 Start
Use a nonhormonal contraceptive as backup during the first 7 days of initiating therapy if patient begins on a day other than the 1st day of menstrual cycle

Sunday Start
Do not consider as effective contraception until after first 7 consecutive days of product administration; instruct to use a nonhormonal contraceptive as backup during the first 7 days
Anytime a subsequent cycle is started later than the day following administration of the last brown tab, use another method of contraception until white tab has been taken daily for 7 consecutive days

STORAGE
20-25°C (68-77°F); excursions permitted to 15-30°C (59-86°F).

HOW SUPPLIED
Tab, Chewable: (Ethinyl Estradiol [EE]-Norethindrone) 20mcg-1mg; **Tab:** (Ferrous Fumarate) 75mg

CONTRAINDICATIONS
High risk for arterial/venous thrombotic diseases (eg, smoking if >35 yrs of age, history/presence of deep vein thrombosis [DVT]/pulmonary embolism [PE], cerebrovascular disease, coronary artery disease [CAD], thrombogenic valvular/thrombogenic rhythm diseases of the heart, inherited/acquired hypercoagulopathies, uncontrolled HTN, diabetes mellitus with vascular disease, headaches with focal neurological symptoms or migraine headaches with aura, if >35 yrs of age with migraine headaches), benign/malignant liver tumors, liver disease, undiagnosed abnormal uterine bleeding, pregnancy, history/presence of breast cancer or other estrogen/progestin-sensitive cancer.

WARNINGS/PRECAUTIONS
Efficacy of therapy in women with a BMI of >35kg/m^2 has not been evaluated. Use a nonhormonal contraceptive as backup during the first 7 days if starting therapy on a day other than the first day of menstrual cycle. For postpartum women who do not breastfeed or after a second trimester abortion, start therapy no earlier than 4 weeks postpartum. May be initiated immediately after a first-trimester abortion or miscarriage; if starting therapy immediately, additional contraception is not needed. Increased risk of venous thrombotic event (VTE) and arterial thrombosis (eg, stroke, myocardial infarction); d/c if an arterial or deep VTE occurs. D/C if unexplained loss of vision, proptosis, diplopia, papilledema, or retinal vascular lesions occur; evaluate for retinal vein thrombosis immediately. If feasible, d/c at least 4 weeks before and through 2 weeks after major surgery or other surgeries known to have an elevated risk of VTE. D/C if jaundice develops. Hepatic adenoma and increased risk of hepatocellular carcinoma reported. Increased BP reported; monitor BP and d/c if BP rises significantly. May increase risk of cervical cancer, intraepithelial neoplasia, or gallbladder disease. May increase risk of cholestasis in those with history of pregnancy-related cholestasis. May decrease glucose tolerance; monitor prediabetic and diabetic women. Consider alternative contraception with uncontrolled dyslipidemias. May increase risk of pancreatitis with hypertriglyceridemia or family history thereof. Evaluate cause and d/c if indicated, if new headaches that are recurrent, persistent, or severe develop. Consider discontinuation of therapy in the case of an increased frequency or severity of migraine headaches. Unscheduled bleeding and spotting may occur; rule out pregnancy and malignancies. May cause amenorrhea; some may experience post-pill amenorrhea or oligomenorrhea. Rule out pregnancy if prescribed regimen adhered to and two consecutive periods are missed. Administration to induce withdrawal bleeding should not be used as a test for pregnancy. Carefully monitor with history of depression and d/c if depression recurs to a serious degree. May raise the serum concentrations of sex hormone-binding globulin. May influence the results of certain lab tests (eg, coagulation factors, lipids, glucose tolerance, binding proteins). In women with hereditary angioedema, may induce or exacerbate symptoms of angioedema. Chloasma may occur, especially with history of chloasma gravidarum; avoid sun exposure or UV radiation in women at risk.

ADVERSE REACTIONS
Nausea, headache, vaginal candidiasis, menstrual cramps, breast tenderness, bacterial vaginitis, abnormal cervical smear.

DRUG INTERACTIONS
May decrease effectiveness or increase breakthrough bleeding when used concomitantly with drugs or herbal products that induce certain enzymes, including CYP3A4 (eg, phenytoin, barbiturates, carbamazepine); use an alternative or backup method of contraception and continue backup contraception for 28 days after discontinuing the enzyme inducer. Atorvastatin may increase EE exposure; ascorbic acid and acetaminophen may increase EE levels. CYP3A4 inhibitors (eg, itraconazole, ketoconazole) may increase levels. Significant level changes (increase or decrease) in estrogen and progestin levels noted with HIV/HCV protease inhibitors or with non-nucleoside reverse transcriptase inhibitors. Pregnancy reported while taking hormonal contraceptives and antibiotics. May inhibit metabolism of other compounds. May significantly decrease levels of lamotrigine and may reduce seizure control; dosage adjustment of lamotrigine

may be needed. May increase serum levels of thyroid-binding globulin and cortisol-binding globulin; dose of replacement thyroid hormones or cortisol therapy may need to be increased.

PREGNANCY AND LACTATION
Contraindicated in pregnancy, not for use in nursing.

MECHANISM OF ACTION
Estrogen/progestogen oral contraceptive; acts by primarily suppressing ovulation. Other possible mechanisms may include changes in cervical mucus (inhibiting sperm penetration) and endometrial changes (reducing likelihood of implantation).

PHARMACOKINETICS
Absorption: EE: Absolute bioavailability (43%); T_{max}=1.3 hrs. Norethindrone: Absolute bioavailability (64%); T_{max}=1 hr. **Distribution:** V_d=2-4L/kg; plasma protein binding (>95%); found in breast milk. **Metabolism:** EE: Extensive via CYP3A4; oxidation, sulfate and glucuronide conjugation; 2-hydroxy ethinyl estradiol (primary oxidative metabolite). Norethindrone: Extensive; reduction, sulfate and glucuronide conjugation. **Elimination:** Urine, feces. EE: $T_{1/2}$=14 hrs. Norethindrone: $T_{1/2}$=8 hrs.

PATIENT CONSIDERATIONS
Assessment: Assess for hypersensitivity to therapy, risk of arterial/venous thrombotic diseases (eg, smoking at >35 yrs of age, history or presence of DVT/PE, cerebrovascular disease, CAD), CV risk factors, pregnancy/nursing status, or any other condition where treatment is contraindicated or cautioned. Assess for possible drug interactions.

Monitoring: Monitor for VTE, arterial thromboses, hepatocellular carcinoma, gallbladder disease, bleeding irregularities, new headaches or increased migraine headaches, signs of liver dysfunction (eg, jaundice), signs of depression if with history thereof, and other adverse effects. Monitor serum glucose levels in diabetic and prediabetic patients, and lipid levels with history of hyperlipidemia. Conduct a yearly visit for a BP check and for other indicated healthcare.

Counseling: Inform that drug does not protect against HIV infection (AIDS) and other sexually transmitted infections. Advise that cigarette smoking increases the risk of serious CV events and women who are >35 yrs of age and smoke should not use combination oral contraceptives (COCs). Instruct to take medication by mouth at the same time every day, and explain what to do in the event pills are missed. Counsel to use backup or alternative method of contraception when enzyme inducers are used concomitantly. Inform that COCs may reduce breast milk production. Counsel any patient who uses COCs postpartum, and has not yet had a period, to use an additional method of contraception until taking a white tab for 7 consecutive days. Advise that amenorrhea may occur; inform that pregnancy should be ruled out in the event of amenorrhea in 2 or more consecutive cycles.

MINIPRESS — *prazosin hydrochloride*   **Rx**
Class: Alpha$_1$ blocker (quinazoline)

ADULT DOSAGE	PEDIATRIC DOSAGE
Hypertension	Pediatric use may not have been established
Initial: 1mg bid-tid	
Titrate: May slowly increase to a total of 20mg/day in divided doses	
Maint: 6-15mg/day in divided doses Doses >20mg usually do not increase efficacy; however, some may benefit from further increases up to 40mg/day in divided doses May maintain adequately on a bid dose regimen	

DOSING CONSIDERATIONS
Concomitant Medications
Use w/ a Diuretic or Other Antihypertensive Agent:
Reduce to 1mg or 2mg tid, then retitrate

Use w/ a PDE-5 Inhibitor:
Initiate PDE-5 inhibitor at the lowest dose

ADMINISTRATION
Oral route

STORAGE
<30°C (86°F).

HOW SUPPLIED
Cap: 1mg, 2mg, 5mg

CONTRAINDICATIONS
Known sensitivity to quinazolines, prazosin, or any of the inert ingredients.

WARNINGS/PRECAUTIONS
May cause syncope w/ sudden loss of consciousness; minimize syncopal episodes by limiting initial dose to 1mg, by subsequently increasing the dose slowly, and by introducing any additional antihypertensive w/ caution. Prolonged erections and priapism reported; penile tissue damage and permanent loss of potency may result if priapism is not treated immediately. Intraoperative floppy iris syndrome observed during cataract surgery. False (+) results may occur in screening tests for pheochromocytoma; d/c w/ elevated urinary vanillylmandelic acid levels and retest after 1 month.

ADVERSE REACTIONS
Dizziness, headache, drowsiness, lack of energy, weakness, palpitations, N/V, edema, orthostatic hypotension, dyspnea, syncope, depression, urinary frequency, diarrhea.

DRUG INTERACTIONS
See Dosing Considerations. Additive hypotensive effects w/ diuretics, β-blockers (eg, propranolol), or other antihypertensives. Additive BP-lowering effects and symptomatic hypotension w/ PDE-5 inhibitors.

PREGNANCY AND LACTATION
Category C, caution in nursing.

MECHANISM OF ACTION
α_1-blocker (quinazoline derivative); has not been established. Causes a decrease in total peripheral resistance and thought to have a direct relaxant action on vascular smooth muscle.

PHARMACOKINETICS
Absorption: T_{max}=3 hrs. **Distribution:** Plasma protein binding (highly bound); found in breast milk. **Metabolism:** Extensive. Primarily by demethylation and conjugation. **Elimination:** Bile and feces; $T_{1/2}$=2-3 hrs.

PATIENT CONSIDERATIONS
Assessment: Assess for previous hypersensitivity to drug/quinazolines, pregnancy/nursing status, and for possible drug interactions. Obtain baseline BP.

Monitoring: Monitor for signs/symptoms of hypotension, dizziness, lightheadedness, syncope, priapism, and other adverse reactions.

Counseling: Inform that dizziness or drowsiness may occur after 1st dose; instruct to avoid driving or performing hazardous tasks for first 24 hrs after taking the drug or when dose is increased. Advise that dizziness, lightheadedness, or fainting may occur, especially when rising from a lying or sitting position; inform that getting up slowly may lessen these problems. Inform that these problems may also occur if taking alcohol, standing for long periods, exercising, or during hot weather, and advise caution during these situations. Instruct to seek immediate medical attention if an erection persists >4 hrs.

Minivelle — estradiol   Rx

Class: Estrogen

> Increased risk of endometrial cancer in a woman with a uterus who uses unopposed estrogens. Adding a progestin to estrogen therapy has been shown to reduce risk of endometrial hyperplasia. Adequate diagnostic measures should be undertaken to rule out malignancy in postmenopausal women with undiagnosed persistent or recurring abnormal genital bleeding. Should not be used for the prevention of cardiovascular (CV) disease or dementia. Increased risk of stroke and deep vein thrombosis (DVT) reported in postmenopausal women (50-79 yrs of age) treated with daily oral conjugated estrogens (CEs) alone and when combined with medroxyprogesterone acetate (MPA). Increased risk of developing probable dementia reported in postmenopausal women ≥65 yrs of age treated with daily CEs alone and when combined with MPA. Increased risks of pulmonary embolism (PE), myocardial infarction (MI), and invasive breast cancer reported in postmenopausal women (50-79 yrs of age) treated with daily oral CEs combined with MPA. Should be prescribed at the lowest effective dose and for the shortest duration consistent with treatment goals and risks.

ADULT DOSAGE
Postmenopausal Osteoporosis
Prevention:
Initial: 0.025mg/day 2X weekly
Titrate: Adjust dose as necessary
Menopausal Vasomotor Symptoms
Moderate to Severe:
Initial: 0.0375mg/day 2X weekly
Titrate: Adjust dose based on response. Attempts to taper or d/c therapy should be made at 3- to 6-month intervals

PEDIATRIC DOSAGE
Pediatric use may not have been established

ADMINISTRATION
Transdermal route

Patch Application Instructions
Place adhesive side on a clean, dry area on the lower abdomen (below the umbilicus) or buttocks
Replace 2X weekly (every 3-4 days)
Rotate application sites, with an interval of at least 1 week allowed between applications to a particular site
Refer to PI for further application instructions

STORAGE
20-25°C (68-77°F); excursions permitted between 15-30°C (59-86°F). Do not store unpouched; apply immediately upon removal from the protective pouch.

HOW SUPPLIED
Patch: 0.025mg/day, 0.0375mg/day, 0.05mg/day, 0.075mg/day, 0.1mg/day [8^s]

CONTRAINDICATIONS
Undiagnosed abnormal genital bleeding, known/suspected/history of breast cancer, known/suspected estrogen-dependent neoplasia, active/history of DVT/PE/arterial thromboembolic disease (eg, stroke, MI), known anaphylactic reaction/angioedema/hypersensitivity w/ estradiol, known liver impairment/disease, known protein C/protein S/antithrombin deficiency or other known thrombophilic disorders, known/suspected pregnancy.

WARNINGS/PRECAUTIONS
D/C immediately if PE, DVT, stroke, or MI occurs or is suspected. If feasible, d/c at least 4-6 weeks before surgery of the type associated with an increased risk of thromboembolism, or during periods of prolonged immobilization. May increase risk of gallbladder disease requiring surgery and risk of ovarian cancer.

May lead to severe hypercalcemia in patients with breast cancer and bone metastases; d/c and take appropriate measures if hypercalcemia occurs. Retinal vascular thrombosis reported; d/c therapy pending exam if sudden partial/complete loss of vision, or sudden onset of proptosis, diplopia, or migraine occurs. D/C permanently if exam reveals papilledema or retinal vascular lesions. May increase BP and thyroid-binding globulin levels. May be associated with elevations of plasma TGs leading to pancreatitis in patients with preexisting hypertriglyceridemia; consider discontinuation if pancreatitis occurs. Caution with history of cholestatic jaundice associated with past estrogen use or with pregnancy; d/c in case of recurrence. May cause fluid retention. Caution with hypoparathyroidism; hypocalcemia may occur. Cases of malignant transformation of residual endometrial implants reported in women treated posthysterectomy with estrogen therapy alone; consider addition of progestin for patients known to have residual endometriosis posthysterectomy. Anaphylactic/anaphylactoid reactions, and angioedema involving eye/eyelid, face, larynx, pharynx, tongue, and extremity with or without urticaria requiring medical intervention reported; do not reapply in patients who develop angioedema anytime during the course of treatment. May exacerbate symptoms of angioedema in women with hereditary angioedema. May exacerbate asthma, diabetes mellitus, epilepsy, migraines, porphyria, systemic lupus erythematosus, and hepatic hemangiomas. May affect certain endocrine and blood components in lab tests.

ADVERSE REACTIONS
Constipation, dyspepsia, nausea, influenza-like illness, pain, nasopharyngitis, sinusitis, upper respiratory tract infection, back pain, headache, depression, insomnia, breast tenderness, intermenstrual bleeding, sinus congestion.

DRUG INTERACTIONS
CYP3A4 inducers (eg, St. John's wort preparations, phenobarbital, carbamazepine) may decrease levels, possibly resulting in a decrease in therapeutic effects and/or changes in the uterine bleeding profile. CYP3A4 inhibitors (eg, erythromycin, ketoconazole, grapefruit juice) may increase levels, and may result in side effects. Patients concomitantly receiving thyroid hormone replacement therapy and estrogens may require increased doses of thyroid replacement therapy; monitor thyroid function.

PREGNANCY AND LACTATION
Contraindicated in pregnancy, not for use in nursing.

MECHANISM OF ACTION
Estrogen; binds to nuclear receptors in estrogen-responsive tissues. Circulating estrogen modulates pituitary secretion of gonadotropins, luteinizing hormone, and follicle-stimulating hormone, through a negative feedback mechanism. Reduces elevated concentrations of these hormones in postmenopausal women.

PHARMACOKINETICS
Absorption: Transdermal administration of various doses resulted in different parameters. **Distribution:** Largely bound to sex hormone-binding globulin and albumin; found in breast milk. **Metabolism:** Liver to estrone (metabolite) and estriol (major urinary metabolite); enterohepatic recirculation via sulfate and glucuronide conjugation in the liver; biliary secretion of conjugates into the intestine; hydrolysis in the intestine; reabsorption; CYP3A4 (partial metabolism). **Elimination:** Urine (parent compound and metabolites); $T_{1/2}$=6.2-7.9 hrs.

PATIENT CONSIDERATIONS
Assessment: Assess for abnormal genital bleeding, presence/history of breast cancer, estrogen-dependent neoplasia, active/history of DVT/PE/arterial thromboembolic disease, liver impairment/disease, thrombophilic disorders, known anaphylactic reaction or angioedema/hypersensitivity to the drug, pregnancy/nursing status, any other conditions where treatment is contraindicated or cautioned, need for progestin therapy, and for possible drug interactions.

Monitoring: Monitor for signs/symptoms of CV disorders, malignant neoplasms, dementia, gallbladder disease, hypercalcemia, visual abnormalities, BP and plasma TG elevations, pancreatitis, cholestatic jaundice, hypothyroidism, fluid retention, exacerbation of endometriosis, anaphylactic/anaphylactoid reactions, angioedema, and other adverse reactions. Perform adequate diagnostic measures (eg, endometrial sampling) in patients with undiagnosed, persistent or recurring abnormal genital bleeding. Perform annual breast exam; schedule mammography based on patient's age, risk factors, and prior mammogram results. Monitor thyroid function if on thyroid hormone replacement therapy. Perform periodic evaluation to determine treatment need.

Counseling: Inform of the importance of reporting unusual vaginal bleeding to physician as soon as possible. Inform of possible serious adverse reactions of therapy (eg, CV disorders, malignant neoplasms, probable dementia) and of possible less serious but common adverse reactions (eg, headache, breast pain and tenderness, N/V). Instruct to have yearly breast exams by a physician and to perform monthly breast self-exams.

Minocin — minocycline   Rx

Class: Tetracyclines

ADULT DOSAGE
General Dosing

Cap:
Initial: 200mg
Maint: 100mg q12h
Alternate Dosing:
Initial: If more frequent doses are preferred, give two or four 50mg caps

PEDIATRIC DOSAGE
General Dosing

>8 Years:
Cap/Inj:
Initial: 4mg/kg
Maint: 2mg/kg q12h, not to exceed usual adult dose

Maint: One 50mg cap qid

Inj:
Initial: 200mg
Maint: 100mg q12h
Max: 400mg/24 hrs

Parenteral therapy is indicated only when oral therapy is not adequate or tolerated; institute oral therapy as soon as possible

Gonococcal Infections

Uncomplicated Infections Other Than Urethritis and Anorectal Infections in Men:
Cap:
Initial: 200mg
Maint: 100mg q12h for a minimum of 4 days, w/ post-therapy cultures w/in 2-3 days

Urethral Infections

Cap:
Uncomplicated Gonococcal Urethritis in Men When Penicillin is Contraindicated:
100mg q12h for 5 days

Uncomplicated Infections Caused by *Chlamydia trachomatis/Ureaplasma urealyticum*:
100mg q12h for at least 7 days

Syphilis

When Penicillin is Contraindicated:
Cap:
Initial: 200mg
Maint: 100mg q12h over a period of 10-15 days

Meningococcal Carrier State

Cap:
Usual: 100mg q12h for 5 days

Mycobacterial Infections

***Mycobacterium marinum* Infections:**
Cap:
Optimal doses have not been established; 100mg q12h for 6-8 weeks have been successfully used

Endocervical Infections

Uncomplicated Infections Caused by *Chlamydia trachomatis/Ureaplasma urealyticum*:
Cap:
100mg q12h for at least 7 days

Rectal Infections

Uncomplicated Infections Caused by *Chlamydia trachomatis/Ureaplasma urealyticum*:
Cap:
100mg q12h for at least 7 days

Other Indications

Treatment of the Following Infections Caused by Susceptible Microorganisms:
Rocky Mountain spotted fever
Typhus fever and the typhus group
Q fever
Rickettsialpox
Tick fevers
Respiratory tract infections
Lymphogranuloma venereum
Psittacosis (ornithosis)
Trachoma
Inclusion conjunctivitis
Relapsing fever
Chancroid (cap)
Plague
Tularemia
Cholera
Campylobacter fetus infections
Brucellosis (in conjunction w/ streptomycin)
Bartonellosis
Granuloma inguinale
UTIs
Skin and skin structure infections

Treatment of Infections Caused by Susceptible Strains:
Escherichia coli
Enterobacter aerogenes
Shigella species
Acinetobacter species

Treatment of the following infections caused by susceptible microorganisms When Penicillin is Contraindicated:
Infections in women caused by *Neisseria gonorrhoeae* (cap)
Meningitis (inj)
Yaws
Listeriosis
Anthrax
Vincent's infection
Actinomycosis
Clostridium species infection

Adjunctive therapy in acute intestinal amebiasis and severe acne

---

DOSING CONSIDERATIONS

Renal Impairment
CrCl <80mL/min:
Max Dose: 200mg/24 hrs

Elderly
Start at lower end of dosing range

ADMINISTRATION
Oral/IV routes

Cap
Take w/ or w/o food
Swallow whole w/ adequate amounts of fluids

IV
Administer as an IV infusion over 60 min
Avoid rapid administration

Reconstitution:
Reconstitute w/ 5mL of sterile water for inj and immediately further dilute in 100-1000mL w/ NaCl inj, dextrose inj, or dextrose and NaCl inj, or in 250-1000mL lactated Ringer's inj, but not w/ other sol containing Ca^{2+}

Incompatibilities:
Do not add additives or other medications or infuse simultaneously through the same IV line including Y-connectors; if the same IV line is used for sequential infusion of additional medications, the line should be flushed before and after infusion of minocycline w/ NaCl inj, dextrose inj, dextrose and NaCl inj, or lactated Ringer's inj

STORAGE
20-25°C (68-77°F). (Cap) Protect from light, moisture, and excessive heat. (Inj) Once diluted into an IV bag, store either at room temperature for up to 4 hrs or refrigerated at 2-8°C (36-46°F) for up to 24 hrs; discard any unused portions after that period.

HOW SUPPLIED
Cap: 50mg, 75mg, 100mg; **Inj:** 100mg

CONTRAINDICATIONS
Hypersensitivity to any of the tetracyclines or to any of the components of the product formulation.

WARNINGS/PRECAUTIONS
May cause fetal harm. May cause permanent discoloration of the teeth (yellow-gray-brown) if used during tooth development (last 1/2 of pregnancy, infancy, and childhood to 8 yrs of age); do not use during tooth development. Enamel hypoplasia reported. May decrease fibula growth rate in premature infants. Drug rash w/ eosinophilia and systemic symptoms (DRESS), including fatal cases, reported; d/c immediately if this syndrome is recognized. May cause an increase in BUN; w/ significant impaired renal function, high levels of therapy may lead to azotemia, hyperphosphatemia, and acidosis. Photosensitivity manifested by an exaggerated sunburn reaction reported. CNS side effects reported; may impair mental/physical abilities. *Clostridium difficile*-associated diarrhea (CDAD) reported; may need to d/c if CDAD is suspected or confirmed. Associated w/ intracranial HTN (pseudotumor cerebri); increased risk in women of childbearing age who are overweight or have a history of intracranial HTN. If visual disturbance occurs, prompt ophthalmologic evaluation is warranted. Intracranial pressure can remain elevated for weeks after drug cessation; monitor patients until they stabilize. May result in bacterial resistance if used in the absence of proven or suspected bacterial infection, or a prophylactic indication; take appropriate measures if superinfection develops. Hepatotoxicity reported. False elevations of urinary catecholamine levels may occur due to interference w/ the fluorescence test. (Cap) Not indicated for the treatment of meningococcal infection; reserve prophylactic use for situations in which the risk of meningococcal meningitis is high. (Inj) Contains magnesium sulfate heptahydrate; caution in patients w/ heart block or myocardial damage.

ADVERSE REACTIONS
Neutropenia, agranulocytosis, lupus-like syndrome, serum sickness-like syndrome, fever, N/V, diarrhea, increased liver enzymes, thyroid cancer, anaphylaxis, exfoliative dermatitis, Stevens-Johnson syndrome, skin and mucous membrane pigmentation, headache.

DRUG INTERACTIONS
Caution w/ other hepatotoxic drugs. Depresses plasma prothrombin activity; may require downward adjustment of anticoagulant dosage. May interfere w/ bactericidal action of PCN; avoid concurrent use. Fatal renal toxicity reported w/ methoxyflurane. May decrease effectiveness of oral contraceptives. Avoid

isotretinoin shortly before, during, and after therapy; each drug alone is associated w/ pseudotumor cerebri. Increased risk of ergotism w/ ergot alkaloids or their derivatives. (Cap) Impaired absorption w/ antacids containing aluminum, Ca^{2+}, or Mg^{2+}, and iron-containing preparations. (Inj) Potentially serious drug interactions may occur when IV magnesium sulfate heptahydrate is given concomitantly w/ CNS depressants, neuromuscular blocking agents, and cardiac glycosides.

PREGNANCY AND LACTATION
Category D, not for use in nursing.

MECHANISM OF ACTION
Tetracycline; primarily bacteriostatic and thought to exert antimicrobial effect by inhibition of protein synthesis.

PHARMACOKINETICS
Absorption: (Cap) C_{max}=3.5mcg/mL; T_{max}=2.1 hrs. **Distribution:** Crosses placenta; found in breast milk. **Elimination:** (Cap) Urine, feces; $T_{1/2}$=15.5 hrs. (IV) $T_{1/2}$=15-23 hrs.

PATIENT CONSIDERATIONS

Assessment: Assess for hypersensitivity to drug, risk for intracranial HTN, hepatic/renal impairment, pregnancy/nursing status, and possible drug interactions. Perform culture and susceptibility tests. (Cap) In venereal disease when coexistent syphilis is suspected, perform a dark-field examination and blood serology. (Inj) Assess for heart block or myocardial damage. Perform serologic test for syphilis (if treating gonorrhea). Obtain baseline serum Mg^{2+} levels in patients w/ renal impairment.

Monitoring: Monitor for DRESS, photosensitivity, CNS effects, CDAD, intracranial HTN, superinfection, and other adverse reactions. Perform periodic lab evaluations of organ systems, including hematopoietic, renal, and hepatic studies. (Cap) In venereal disease when coexistent syphilis is suspected, repeat blood serology monthly for at least 4 months. (Inj) In patients w/ gonorrhea, perform a follow-up serologic test for syphilis after 3 months. Monitor serum Mg^{2+} levels in patients w/ renal impairment. Closely monitor patients w/ heart block or myocardial damage.

Counseling: Apprise of the potential hazard to fetus if used during pregnancy; instruct to notify physician if pregnant. Counsel that therapy should only be used to treat bacterial, not viral, infections. Instruct to take exactly ud even if the patient feels better early in the course of therapy. Inform that skipping doses or not completing the full course of therapy may decrease effectiveness of treatment and increase bacterial resistance. Inform that diarrhea may be experienced; instruct to immediately contact physician if watery and bloody stools (w/ or w/o stomach cramps and fever) occur, even as late as ≥2 months after the last dose. Advise that photosensitivity manifested by an exaggerated sunburn reaction may occur; instruct to d/c treatment at the 1st evidence of skin erythema. Caution patients who experience CNS symptoms about driving vehicles or using hazardous machinery while on therapy. Inform that drug may render oral contraceptives less effective.

MINOCYCLINE EXTENDED-RELEASE TABLETS —
minocycline hydrochloride   **Rx**

Class: Tetracyclines

OTHER BRAND NAMES
Solodyn

ADULT DOSAGE
Acne Vulgaris

Treatment of Inflammatory Lesions of Non-Nodular Moderate to Severe Acne:

1mg/kg qd for 12 weeks

Body Weight and Strength to Achieve Approximately 1mg/kg:
45-49kg: 45mg (1-0.92mg/kg)
50-59kg: 55mg (1.10-0.93mg/kg)
60-71kg: 65mg (1.08-0.92mg/kg)
72-84kg: 80mg (1.11-0.95mg/kg)
85-96kg: 90mg (1.06-0.94mg/kg)
97-110kg: 105mg (1.08-0.95mg/kg)
111-125kg: 115mg (1.04-0.92mg/kg)
126-136kg: 135mg (1.07-0.99mg/kg)

PEDIATRIC DOSAGE
Acne Vulgaris

Treatment of Inflammatory Lesions of Non-Nodular Moderate to Severe Acne:
≥12 Years:
1mg/kg qd for 12 weeks

Body Weight and Strength to Achieve Approximately 1mg/kg:
45-49kg: 45mg (1-0.92mg/kg)
50-59kg: 55mg (1.10-0.93mg/kg)
60-71kg: 65mg (1.08-0.92mg/kg)
72-84kg: 80mg (1.11-0.95mg/kg)
85-96kg: 90mg (1.06-0.94mg/kg)
97-110kg: 105mg (1.08-0.95mg/kg)
111-125kg: 115mg (1.04-0.92mg/kg)
126-136kg: 135mg (1.07-0.99mg/kg)

DOSING CONSIDERATIONS
Renal Impairment
Decrease total dosage by either reducing the recommended individual doses and/or by extending time intervals between doses

Elderly
Start at lower end of dosing range

ADMINISTRATION
Oral route
Swallow tab whole; do not chew, crush, or split.
May take w/ or w/o food; ingestion w/ food may help reduce the risk of esophageal irritation and ulceration.

STORAGE
20-25°C (68-77°F). Protect from light, moisture, and excessive heat. **Solodyn:** 25°C (77°F); excursions permitted to 15-30°C (59-86°F). Protect from light, moisture, and excessive heat.

HOW SUPPLIED
Tab, Extended-Release: 45mg, 90mg, 135mg; (Solodyn) 55mg, 65mg, 80mg, 105mg, 115mg

CONTRAINDICATIONS
Hypersensitivity to any of the tetracyclines.

WARNINGS/PRECAUTIONS
Higher doses may be associated w/ more acute vestibular side effects. May cause fetal harm; avoid use during pregnancy or by individuals of either gender who are attempting to conceive a child. Avoid use during tooth development (last 1/2 of pregnancy, infancy, childhood up to 8 yrs of age); may cause permanent discoloration (yellow-gray-brown) of the teeth. Enamel hypoplasia reported. May decrease fibula growth rate in premature infants. *Clostridium difficile* associated diarrhea (CDAD) reported; may need to d/c if CDAD is suspected or confirmed. Serious liver injury, including irreversible drug-induced hepatitis and fulminant hepatic failure (sometimes fatal) reported. May cause an increase in BUN; w/ significant renal impairment, higher levels of therapy may lead to azotemia, hyperphosphatemia, and acidosis. CNS side effects reported; may impair mental/physical abilities. Pseudotumor cerebri (benign intracranial HTN) reported; if visual disturbance occurs during treatment, check for papilledema. Associated w/ development of autoimmune syndromes; d/c immediately and perform LFTs, antinuclear antibody (ANA) test, CBC, and other appropriate tests. Photosensitivity manifested by an exaggerated sunburn reaction reported. Cases of anaphylaxis, serious skin reactions (eg, Stevens-Johnson syndrome), erythema multiforme, and drug rash w/ eosinophilia and systemic symptoms (DRESS) syndrome reported; d/c immediately if DRESS occurs. May induce hyperpigmentation in many organs. Drug-resistant bacteria may develop; use only as indicated. May result in overgrowth of nonsusceptible organisms, including fungi; d/c and institute appropriate therapy if superinfection occurs. False elevations of urinary catecholamine levels may occur due to interference with the fluorescence test.

ADVERSE REACTIONS
Headache, fatigue, dizziness, pruritus, malaise, mood alteration.

DRUG INTERACTIONS
Avoid w/ isotretinoin; may also cause pseudotumor cerebri. Depresses plasma prothrombin activity; may require downward adjustment of anticoagulant dosage. May interfere w/ bactericidal action of penicillin; avoid concomitant use. Fatal renal toxicity reported w/ methoxyflurane. Antacids containing aluminum, Ca^{2+}, or Mg^{2+}, and iron-containing preparations may impair absorption. May cause changes in estradiol, progestinic hormone, follicle-stimulating hormone and luteinizing hormone levels, of breakthrough bleeding, or of contraceptive failure w/ low dose oral contraceptives.

PREGNANCY AND LACTATION
Pregnancy: Category D. Should not be used during pregnancy; crosses placenta and may cause fetal harm when administered to a pregnant woman.
Lactation: Tetracycline-class antibiotics are excreted in human milk. Not for use in nursing.

MECHANISM OF ACTION
Semi-synthetic tetracycline derivative; not established.

PHARMACOKINETICS
Absorption: C_{max}=2.63mcg/mL; T_{max}=3.5-4 hrs; AUC_{0-24}=33.32mcg•hr/mL.
Distribution: Crosses placenta, found in breast milk.

PATIENT CONSIDERATIONS

Assessment: Assess for renal impairment, visual disturbances, hypersensitivity to any tetracyclines, pregnancy/nursing status, and possible drug interactions.

Monitoring: Monitor for signs/symptoms of CDAD, hepatotoxicity, superinfection, pseudotumor cerebri, visual disturbance, papilledema, DRESS syndrome, CNS side effects, autoimmune syndrome, photosensitivity, and other adverse reactions. Periodically monitor hematopoietic/renal/hepatic function. Perform LFTs, ANA test, and CBC in patients showing symptoms of an autoimmune syndrome. Perform drug serum level determinations w/ prolonged therapy in patients w/ renal impairment.

Counseling: Instruct to avoid use if pregnant, or if planning to conceive a child (patients of either gender). Inform that pseudomembranous colitis may occur; instruct to seek medical attention if watery/bloody stools develop. Inform of the possibility of hepatotoxicity; instruct to seek medical advice if loss of appetite, tiredness, diarrhea, skin turning yellow, bleeding easily, confusion, or sleepiness occurs. Instruct patients who experience CNS symptoms to use caution in driving or operating machinery and advise to seek medical help for persistent headaches/blurred vision. Inform that drug may render oral contraceptives less effective; advise to use 2nd form of contraception during therapy. Inform that autoimmune syndromes may occur; instruct to d/c immediately and seek medical help if symptoms (eg, arthralgia, fever, rash, malaise) are experienced. Counsel about discoloration of skin, scars, teeth, or gums that may arise from therapy. Inform that photosensitivity reactions may occur; advise to minimize/avoid exposure to natural/artificial sunlight (tanning beds, UVA/B treatment), to wear loose-fitting clothes when outdoors, and to d/c at 1st evidence of skin erythema. Instruct to take exactly ud; inform that skipping doses or not completing full course of therapy may decrease effectiveness and increase likelihood of bacterial resistance.

MIRAPEX — pramipexole dihydrochloride   Rx

Class: Dopamine receptor agonist

ADULT DOSAGE

Parkinson's Disease

Initial: 0.375mg/day given in 3 divided doses

Titrate: May increase gradually not more frequently than every 5-7 days

Maint: 1.5-4.5mg/day administered in equally divided doses tid w/ or w/o levodopa; consider reduction of levodopa dose when used in combination w/ pramipexole

Suggested Ascending Dosage Schedule:

Week 1: 0.125mg tid
Week 2: 0.25mg tid
Week 3: 0.5mg tid
Week 4: 0.75mg tid
Week 5: 1mg tid
Week 6: 1.25mg tid
Week 7: 1.5mg tid

If a significant interruption in therapy has occurred, retitration may be warranted

Restless Legs Syndrome

Moderate to Severe Primary Restless Legs Syndrome (RLS):

Initial: 0.125mg qd

Titrate: If additional symptomatic relief is required, may increase dose every 4-7 days; no evidence that the 0.75mg dose provides additional benefit beyond the 0.5mg dose

Ascending Dosage Schedule:

Titration Step 1: 0.125mg qd
Titration Step 2 (If Needed): 0.25mg qd
Titration Step 3 (If Needed): 0.5mg qd

Administer 2-3 hrs before hs

If a significant interruption in therapy has occurred, retitration may be warranted

PEDIATRIC DOSAGE

Pediatric use may not have been established

DOSING CONSIDERATIONS

Renal Impairment

Parkinson's Disease:

Mild (CrCl >50mL/min):
Initial: 0.125mg tid
Max: 1.5mg tid

Moderate (CrCl 30-50mL/min):
Initial: 0.125mg bid
Max: 0.75mg tid

Severe (CrCl 15 to <30mL/min):
Initial: 0.125mg qd
Max: 1.5mg qd

Very Severe (CrCl <15mL/min and Hemodialysis Patients):
Has not been adequately studied in this group of patients

RLS:

Moderate and Severe Renal Impairment (CrCl 20-60mL/min):
Increase duration between titration steps to 14 days

Discontinuation

Parkinson's Disease:
May be tapered off at a rate of 0.75mg/day until daily dose has been reduced to 0.75mg; thereafter, may reduce dose by 0.375mg/day

RLS:
Worsening of symptom severity reported in a clinical trial w/ sudden withdrawal; see Warnings/Precautions

ADMINISTRATION

Oral route

Take w/ or w/o food.

STORAGE

25°C (77°F); excursions permitted to 15-30°C (59-86°F). Protect from light.

HOW SUPPLIED

Tab: 0.125mg, 0.25mg*, 0.5mg*, 0.75mg, 1mg*, 1.5mg* *scored

WARNINGS/PRECAUTIONS

Falling asleep during activities of daily living and somnolence reported; should ordinarily be discontinued if significant daytime sleepiness or episodes of falling asleep during activities that require active participation develop. May impair mental/physical abilities. May cause orthostatic hypotension; monitor for signs/symptoms, especially during dose escalation. May cause intense urges (eg, to gamble/spend money, increased sexual urges, binge eating) and patients may experience the inability to control these urges while on therapy; consider dose reduction or discontinuation of therapy. Hallucinations reported; risk appears to increase w/ age. May experience new or worsening mental status and behavioral changes, which may be severe, including psychotic-like behavior during treatment or after starting/increasing the dose. Avoid w/ major psychotic disorder. May cause or exacerbate preexisting dyskinesia. Rhabdomyolysis and retinal deterioration may occur. Symptom complex resembling the neuroleptic malignant syndrome reported w/ rapid dose reduction, withdrawal of, or changes in dopaminergic therapy; if possible, avoid sudden discontinuation/rapid dose reduction, and if a decision is made to d/c therapy, taper to reduce the risk of hyperpyrexia and confusion. May cause fibrotic complications (eg, retroperitoneal fibrosis, pulmonary infiltrates, pleural effusion, pleural thickening, pericarditis, cardiac valvulopathy). Monitor for melanomas frequently and regularly; perform periodic skin examinations. Rebound and augmentation in RLS reported.

ADVERSE REACTIONS

Early Parkinson's Disease (w/o Levodopa): Nausea, dizziness, somnolence, insomnia, constipation, asthenia, hallucinations.

Advanced Parkinson's Disease (w/ Levodopa): Postural (orthostatic) hypotension, dyskinesia, extrapyramidal syndrome, insomnia, dizziness, hallucinations, dream abnormalities, confusion, constipation, asthenia, somnolence, dystonia, gait abnormality, hypertonia, dry mouth, amnesia, urinary frequency.

RLS: Nausea, somnolence.

DRUG INTERACTIONS

Sedating medications or alcohol, and medications that increase plasma levels of pramipexole (eg, cimetidine) may increase risk for somnolence. Dopamine antagonists (eg, neuroleptics [phenothiazines, butyrophenones, thioxanthenes] or metoclopramide) may diminish effectiveness. May potentiate dopaminergic side effects of levodopa.

PREGNANCY AND LACTATION

Pregnancy: There are no adequate data on the developmental risk associated w/ use in pregnant women.

Lactation: There are no data on the presence in human milk, the effects on the breastfed infant, or the effects on milk production. Inhibition of lactation is expected because pramipexole inhibits prolactin secretion. Consider the developmental and health benefits of breastfeeding along w/ the mother's clinical need for pramipexole and any potential adverse effects on the breastfed infant from pramipexole or from the underlying maternal condition.

MECHANISM OF ACTION

Non-ergot dopamine agonist; has not been established. In Parkinson's disease, suspected to be related to its ability to stimulate dopamine receptors in the striatum.

PHARMACOKINETICS

Absorption: Rapid. Absolute bioavailability (>90%); T_{max}=approx 2 hrs.

Distribution: V_d=500L; plasma protein binding (15%). **Elimination:** Urine (90%, unchanged); $T_{1/2}$=8 hrs (healthy), 12 hrs (elderly).

PATIENT CONSIDERATIONS

Assessment: Assess for preexisting dyskinesia, major psychotic disorder, sleep disorders, renal impairment, pregnancy/nursing status, and possible drug interactions.

Monitoring: Monitor for drowsiness or sleepiness, orthostatic hypotension, impulse control/compulsive behaviors, hallucinations, new/worsening mental status and behavioral changes, dyskinesia, signs/symptoms of rhabdomyolysis, retinal deterioration, fibrotic complications, melanomas (perform periodic skin exams), and other adverse reactions.

Counseling: Instruct to take as prescribed. If a dose is missed, advise not to double the next dose. Advise that the occurrence of nausea may be reduced if taken w/ food. Instruct not to take both immediate-release pramipexole and extended-release pramipexole. Alert patient about the potential sedating effects, including somnolence and the possibility of falling asleep while engaged in activities of daily living; instruct not to drive a car or engage in other potentially dangerous activities until the patient has gained sufficient experience w/ pramipexole tabs to gauge whether or not it affects the patient's mental and/or motor performance adversely. Advise to inform physician if taking alcohol or other sedating medications. Inform of the possibility to experience intense urges and the inability to control these urges. Inform that hallucinations and other psychotic-like behavior may occur. Advise that postural (orthostatic) hypotension may develop w/ or w/o symptoms. Advise to monitor for melanomas frequently and regularly. Instruct to notify physician if pregnant/intending to become pregnant during therapy or if breastfeeding/intending to breastfeed.

MIRAPEX ER — pramipexole dihydrochloride   Rx

Class: Dopamine receptor agonist

ADULT DOSAGE

Parkinson's Disease

Initial: 0.375mg qd

Titrate: Based on efficacy and tolerability, may increase gradually not more frequently than every 5-7 days, 1st to 0.75mg/day and then by 0.75mg increments

Max: 4.5mg/day

If a significant interruption in therapy occurs, retitration may be warranted

PEDIATRIC DOSAGE

Pediatric use may not have been established

Conversions

Switching from Immediate-Release (IR) Pramipexole Tabs to Extended-Release (ER) Pramipexole Tabs:
May switch overnight at the same daily dose; monitor to determine if dosage adjustment is necessary

DOSING CONSIDERATIONS

Renal Impairment
Mild (CrCl >50mL/min):
No dose adjustment required

Moderate (CrCl 30-50mL/min):
Initial: Administer qod
Titrate: Use caution and carefully assess therapeutic response and tolerability before increasing to daily dosing after 1 week, and before any additional titration in 0.375mg increments. Dose adjustment should occur no more frequently than at weekly intervals.
Max: 2.25mg/day

Severe (CrCl <30mL/min)/Hemodialysis:
Not recommended

Discontinuation
May taper off at a rate of 0.75mg/day until daily dose has been reduced to 0.75mg; thereafter, may reduce dose by 0.375mg/day

ADMINISTRATION
Oral route
Take w/ or w/o food.
Swallow whole; do not chew, crush, or divide tab.

STORAGE
25°C (77°F); excursions permitted to 15-30°C (59-86°F). Protect from exposure to high humidity.

HOW SUPPLIED
Tab, ER: 0.375mg, 0.75mg, 1.5mg, 2.25mg, 3mg, 3.75mg, 4.5mg

WARNINGS/PRECAUTIONS
Falling asleep during activities of daily living and somnolence reported; should ordinarily be discontinued if significant daytime sleepiness or episodes of falling asleep during activities that require active participation develop. May impair mental/physical abilities. May cause orthostatic hypotension; monitor for signs/symptoms, especially during dose escalation. May cause intense urges (eg, to gamble/spend money, increased sexual urges, binge eating) and patients may experience the inability to control these urges while on therapy; consider dose reduction or discontinuation of therapy. Hallucinations (visual, auditory, or mixed) reported; risk appears to increase w/ age. May experience new or worsening mental status and behavioral changes, which may be severe, including psychotic-like behavior during treatment or after starting/increasing the dose. Avoid w/ major psychotic disorder. May cause or exacerbate preexisting dyskinesia. Rhabdomyolysis and retinal deterioration may occur. Symptom complex resembling the neuroleptic malignant syndrome may occur w/ rapid dose reduction, withdrawal of, or changes in dopaminergic therapy; if possible, avoid sudden discontinuation/rapid dose reduction, and if a decision is made to d/c therapy, taper to reduce the risk of hyperpyrexia and confusion. May cause fibrotic complications (eg, retroperitoneal fibrosis, pulmonary infiltrates, pleural effusion, pleural thickening, pericarditis, cardiac valvulopathy). Monitor for melanomas frequently and regularly; perform periodic skin examinations.

ADVERSE REACTIONS
Early Parkinson's Disease (w/o Levodopa): Somnolence, nausea, constipation, dizziness, fatigue, hallucinations, dry mouth, muscle spasms, peripheral edema.
Advanced Parkinson's Disease (w/ Levodopa): Dyskinesia, nausea, constipation, hallucinations, headache, anorexia.

DRUG INTERACTIONS
Sedating medications or alcohol, and medications that increase plasma levels of pramipexole (eg, cimetidine) may increase risk for somnolence. May potentiate dopaminergic side effects of levodopa. Dopamine antagonists (eg, neuroleptics [phenothiazines, butyrophenones, thioxanthenes] or metoclopramide) may diminish effectiveness.

PREGNANCY AND LACTATION
Pregnancy: There are no adequate data on the developmental risk associated w/ use in pregnant women.
Lactation: There are no data on the presence in human milk, the effects on the breastfed infant, or the effects on milk production. Inhibition of lactation is expected because pramipexole inhibits prolactin secretion. Consider the developmental and health benefits of breastfeeding along w/ the mother's clinical need for pramipexole and any potential adverse effects on the breastfed infant from pramipexole or from the underlying maternal condition.

MECHANISM OF ACTION
Non-ergot dopamine agonist; has not been established. Suspected to be related to its ability to stimulate dopamine receptors in the striatum.

PHARMACOKINETICS
Absorption: Well-absorbed. Absolute bioavailability (>90%); T_{max}=6 hrs.
Distribution: V_d=500L; plasma protein binding (15%). **Elimination:** Urine (90%, unchanged).

PATIENT CONSIDERATIONS
Assessment: Assess for preexisting dyskinesia, major psychotic disorder, renal impairment, sleep disorders, pregnancy/nursing status, and possible drug interactions.

Monitoring: Monitor for drowsiness or sleepiness, orthostatic hypotension, impulse control/compulsive behaviors, hallucinations, new or worsening mental status and behavioral changes, dyskinesia, signs/symptoms of rhabdomyolysis, melanomas (perform periodic skin exams), fibrotic complications, retinal deterioration, and other adverse reactions. Monitor therapeutic response/tolerability at a minimal interval of 5 days or longer after each dose increment.

Counseling: Instruct to take therapy as prescribed. Advise that if a dose is missed, to take it as soon as possible, but no later than 12 hrs after the regularly scheduled time. Instruct that if 12 hrs have passed, to skip the missed dose and take the next dose on the following day at the regularly scheduled time. Advise that nausea may be reduced if taken w/ food. Inform that there may be residue in the stool that may resemble a swollen original tab or swollen pieces of the original tab; instruct to contact physician if this occurs. Instruct not to take both IR and ER pramipexole. Alert patient about the potential sedating effects; instruct not to drive a car or engage in other dangerous activities until gaining sufficient experience w/ therapy to gauge whether or not it affects the patient's mental and/or motor performance adversely. Advise to inform physician if taking alcohol or other sedating medications. Inform of the possibility to experience intense urges and the inability to control these urges. Inform that hallucinations and other psychotic-like behavior may occur. Advise that postural (orthostatic) hypotension may develop w/ or w/o symptoms. Advise to monitor for melanomas frequently and regularly. Advise to contact physician if any unexplained muscle pain, tenderness, or weakness is experienced. Instruct to notify physician if pregnant/intending to be pregnant during therapy or if breastfeeding/intending to breastfeed.

MIRCETTE — desogestrel/ethinyl estradiol   **Rx**

Class: Estrogen/progestogen combination

> Cigarette smoking increases the risk of serious cardiovascular (CV) side effects. Risk increases with age and with heavy smoking (≥15 cigarettes/day) and is quite marked in women >35 yrs. Women who use oral contraceptives should be strongly advised not to smoke.

OTHER BRAND NAMES
Kariva

ADULT DOSAGE
Contraception
1 tab qd for 28 days, then repeat
Start 1st Sunday after menses begins or 1st day of menses

Missed Dose
Miss 1 Active Tab: Take missed tab as soon as remembered
Miss 2 Consecutive Active Tabs in Week 1 or 2: Take 2 tabs the day remembered and 2 tabs the next day; thereafter, resume taking 1 tab qd until pack is finished. Use backup method of birth control if having intercourse in the 7 days after missing pills
Miss 2 Consecutive Active Tabs in Week 3 or Miss ≥3 Active Tabs in a Row at Any Time: (Sunday Start) Continue to take 1 tab qd until Sunday, then throw out the rest of the pack and start a new pack of pills that same day. (Day 1 Start) Throw out rest of the pack and start new pack the same day. (Sunday/Day 1 Start) Use backup method of birth control if having intercourse in the 7 days after missing pills

Conversions
Switching from a Sunday Start Oral Contraceptive:
Sunday Start:
Take 1st tab on the 2nd Sunday after last tab of a 21-day regimen or take on the 1st Sunday after last inactive tab of a 28-day regimen

Switching Directly from Another Oral Contraceptive:
Day 1 Start:
Take 1st tab on the 1st day of menstruation which begins after last active tab of previous product

PEDIATRIC DOSAGE
Contraception
Not indicated for use premenarche; refer to adult dosing

ADMINISTRATION
Oral route
Take exactly ud and at intervals not exceeding 24 hrs
Use another method of contraception until after the first 7 consecutive days of administration when initiating a Sunday Start regimen

STORAGE
20-25°C (68-77°F).

HOW SUPPLIED
Tab: (Ethinyl Estradiol-Desogestrel) 0.02mg-0.15mg, (Ethinyl Estradiol) 0.01mg

CONTRAINDICATIONS
Thrombophlebitis or past history of deep vein thrombophlebitis, thromboembolic disorders (current or past history), suspected/known pregnancy, cerebral vascular or coronary artery disease, undiagnosed abnormal genital bleeding, cholestatic jaundice of pregnancy or jaundice with prior pill use, known/suspected breast carcinoma, carcinoma of the endometrium or other known/suspected estrogen-dependent neoplasia, hepatic adenomas or carcinomas.

WARNINGS/PRECAUTIONS
Increased risk of MI, vascular disease, thromboembolism, stroke, hepatic neoplasia, and gallbladder disease. Increased risk of morbidity and mortality with HTN, hyperlipidemias, obesity, and diabetes mellitus (DM). D/C at least 4 weeks prior to and for 2 weeks after elective surgery associated with an increased risk of thromboembolism and during and following prolonged immobilization, if feasible. Start use no earlier than 4 weeks after delivery in women who elect not to breastfeed. Caution in women with CV disease risk factors. May develop visual changes or changes in lens tolerance in contact lens wearers. Retinal thrombosis reported; d/c if unexplained partial or complete loss of vision, onset of proptosis or diplopia, papilledema, or retinal vascular lesions develop. Should not be used to induce withdrawal bleeding as a test for pregnancy, or to treat threatened or habitual abortion during pregnancy. May decrease glucose tolerance; monitor prediabetic and diabetic patients. May elevate BP; monitor closely and d/c use if significant BP elevation occurs. New onset/exacerbation of migraine, or recurrent, persistent, severe headache may develop; d/c if these occur. Breakthrough bleeding and spotting reported; rule out malignancy or pregnancy. D/C if jaundice develops. May be poorly metabolized in patients with impaired liver function. May cause fluid retention; caution with conditions that aggravate fluid retention. Caution with history of depression; d/c if depression recurs to a serious degree. Does not protect against HIV infection (AIDS) and other STDs. Perform annual history/physical exam; monitor women with history of breast cancer. Not for use before menarche. May affect certain endocrine, LFTs, and blood components in laboratory tests.

ADVERSE REACTIONS
N/V, breakthrough bleeding, spotting, amenorrhea, migraine, mental depression, vaginal candidiasis, edema, weight changes, abdominal cramps/bloating, menstrual flow changes, pulmonary embolism, MI, HTN.

DRUG INTERACTIONS
Reduced efficacy and increased breakthrough bleeding and menstrual irregularities with rifampin, barbiturates, phenylbutazone, phenytoin sodium, carbamazepine, and possibly with griseofulvin, ampicillin, and tetracyclines. May decrease lamotrigine levels; dosage adjustment of lamotrigine may be necessary.

PREGNANCY AND LACTATION
Category X, not for use in nursing.

MECHANISM OF ACTION
Estrogen/progestogen combination; acts by suppressing gonadotropins, primarily inhibiting ovulation, and causing other alterations, including changes in cervical mucus (increases difficulty of sperm entry into uterus) and endometrium (reduces likelihood of implantation).

PHARMACOKINETICS
Absorption: Rapid and almost complete. Relative bioavailability 100% (Desogestrel), 93-99% (Ethinyl estradiol). Oral administration on various days during dosing led to altered parameters; refer to PI. **Distribution:** Found in breast milk. Etonogestrel: Plasma protein binding (99%), sex hormone-binding globulin (primary). Ethinyl estradiol: Plasma albumin binding (98.3%). **Metabolism:** Desogestrel: Etonogestrel (active metabolite). Liver and intestinal mucosa via hydroxylation, glucuronidation, and sulfate conjugation. Ethinyl estradiol: Conjugation. **Elimination:** Urine, bile, feces. Etonogestrel: $T_{1/2}$=27.8 hrs. Ethinyl estradiol: $T_{1/2}$=23.9 hrs (combination), 18.9 hrs (0.01mg).

PATIENT CONSIDERATIONS
Assessment: Assess for current or history of thrombophlebitis or thromboembolic disorders, history of HTN, hyperlipidemia, DM, obesity, breast cancer, nursing status, or any other conditions where treatment is contraindicated/cautioned, and possible drug interactions.

Monitoring: Monitor for MI, thromboembolism, stroke, hepatic neoplasia, and other adverse effects. Monitor BP with history of HTN, serum glucose levels in diabetic or prediabetic patients, lipid levels with hyperlipidemia, and for signs of worsening depression with previous history. Refer contact lens wearer to ophthalmologist if ocular changes develop. Perform annual history and physical exam. Monitor women with strong family history of breast cancer or who have breast nodules. Monitor LFTs, PT, thyroxine binding-globulin, T3 and T4, and serum folate levels.

Counseling: Counsel about potential adverse effects, and to avoid smoking while on therapy. Inform that drug does not protect against HIV infection and other STDs. Inform about pregnancy risk if pills are missed. Instruct to take at the same time every day and that intervals between doses should not exceed 24 hrs. Instruct that when initiating a Sunday Start regimen, to use another method of contraception until after first 7 consecutive days of administration. Instruct if one "active" pill is missed to take as soon as remembered, and take next pill at regular time.

MIRENA — levonorgestrel

Rx

Class: Progestin contraceptive

ADULT DOSAGE

Contraception

Recommended for females who have had at least 1 child

Contraception for Up to 5 Years:
Insert into the uterine cavity during the first 7 days of the menstrual cycle

Following 1st Trimester Abortion:
Insert immediately after a 1st trimester abortion

Following 2nd Trimester Abortion/Postpartum: Postpone insertion by a minimum of 6 weeks or until the uterus is fully involuted; wait until involution is complete before insertion

Timing of Removal:
Should not remain in the uterus after 5 yrs.
If pregnancy is not desired, removal should be carried out during menstruation, provided the woman is still experiencing regular menses.
If removal will occur at other times during the cycle, consider starting a new contraceptive method a week prior to removal.

Heavy Menstrual Bleeding

Recommended for females who have had at least 1 child

In Women Who Choose to Use Intrauterine Contraception as their Method of Contraception:
Insert into the uterine cavity during the first 7 days of the menstrual cycle

Following 1st Trimester Abortion:
Insert immediately after a 1st trimester abortion

Following 2nd Trimester Abortion/Postpartum: Postpone insertion by a minimum of 6 weeks or until the uterus is fully involuted; wait until involution is complete before insertion

Timing of Removal:
Should not remain in the uterus after 5 yrs.
If pregnancy is not desired, removal should be carried out during menstruation, provided the woman is still experiencing regular menses.
If removal will occur at other times during the cycle, consider starting a new contraceptive method a week prior to removal.

Conversions

Switching to a Different Birth Control Method:

Patients w/ Regular Cycles:
Time removal and initiation of new method to ensure continuous contraception. Either remove Mirena during the first 7 days of the menstrual cycle and start the new method immediately, or start the new method at least 7 days prior if removal is to occur at other times during the cycle

Patients w/ Irregular Cycles/Amenorrhea:
Start the new method at least 7 days before removal

PEDIATRIC DOSAGE

Contraception

Not indicated for use premenarche; refer to adult dosing

Heavy Menstrual Bleeding

Not indicated for use premenarche; refer to adult dosing

ADMINISTRATION
Intrauterine route

Should be inserted by a trained healthcare provider.
Back-up contraception is not needed if inserted as directed.
Consider administering analgesics prior to insertion.
Remove Mirena if it is not positioned completely w/in the uterus; do not reinsert once it is removed.
Must be removed by the end of the 5th year.
Refer to PI for additional insertion and removal instructions.

STORAGE
25°C (77°F); excursions permitted to 15-30°C (59-86°F).

HOW SUPPLIED
Intrauterine Insert: 52mg

CONTRAINDICATIONS
Pregnancy or suspicion of pregnancy, congenital or acquired uterine anomaly (including fibroids if they distort the uterine cavity), acute or history of pelvic inflammatory disease (PID) (unless there has been a subsequent intrauterine pregnancy), postpartum endometritis or infected abortion in the past 3 months, known/suspected uterine or cervical neoplasia, known/suspected or history of breast cancer or other progestin-sensitive cancer, uterine bleeding of unknown etiology, untreated acute cervicitis or vaginitis (including bacterial vaginosis or other lower genital tract infections until infection is controlled), acute liver disease or liver tumor (benign or malignant), conditions associated w/ increased susceptibility to pelvic infections, and previously inserted IUD that has not been removed. Hypersensitivity to any component of this product.

WARNINGS/PRECAUTIONS
Not for post-coital contraception. Should be inserted by a trained healthcare provider. Evaluate for ectopic pregnancy and remove device if pregnancy occurs. Increased risk of septic abortion, miscarriage, sepsis, premature delivery/labor, and possible congenital anomalies if pregnancy occurs and device is left in place. Severe infection or sepsis, including Group A streptococcal sepsis (GAS) reported; use aseptic technique during insertion of device. Associated w/ increased risk of PID and actinomycosis. May alter bleeding pattern and result in spotting, irregular bleeding, heavy bleeding, oligomenorrhea, and amenorrhea; perform appropriate diagnostic measures to rule out endometrial pathology if bleeding irregularities develop during prolonged use. Perforation may occur and may reduce contraceptive effectiveness; risk increased if inserted in lactating women and may be increased if inserted when the uterus is fixed retroverted or not completely involuted during postpartum. Partial or complete expulsion may occur; may be replaced w/in 7 days after the onset of a menstrual period after ruling out pregnancy. Ovarian cysts and breast cancer reported. Caution in patients w/ coagulopathy, migraine, focal migraine w/ asymmetrical visual loss or other symptoms indicating transient cerebral ischemia, exceptionally severe headache, marked increase in BP, and in patients w/ severe arterial disease. Consider removing device if uterine/cervical malignancy or jaundice arises during use. Consider possibility that device may have been displaced (eg, expelled or perforated the uterus) if the threads are not visible or are significantly shortened; exclude pregnancy and verify location of device. If device is displaced, remove it.

ADVERSE REACTIONS
Alterations of menstrual bleeding patterns (eg, unscheduled uterine bleeding, decreased uterine bleeding, increased scheduled uterine bleeding, female genital tract bleeding), abdominal/pelvic pain, amenorrhea, headache/migraine, genital discharge, vulvovaginitis.

DRUG INTERACTIONS
Drugs or herbal products that induce enzymes, including CYP3A4, that metabolize progestins (eg, barbiturates, bosentan, carbamazepine) may decrease levels. HIV protease inhibitors or non-nucleoside reverse transcriptase inhibitors may significantly increase or decrease plasma levels. CYP3A4 inhibitors (eg, itraconazole, ketoconazole) may increase plasma hormone levels. Caution w/ use of anticoagulants.

PREGNANCY AND LACTATION
Pregnancy: Contraindicated in pregnancy.
Lactation: Caution in nursing; small amounts of progestins were observed to pass into breast milk, resulting in detectable steroid levels in infant serum.

MECHANISM OF ACTION
Progestogen; mechanism not established. Thickens cervical mucus (preventing passage of sperm into uterus), inhibits sperm capacitation or survival, and alters endometrium.

PHARMACOKINETICS
Distribution: V_d=1.8L/kg; plasma protein binding (97.5-99%); found in breast milk. **Metabolism:** Conjugation; sulfate and glucuronide (lesser extent) conjugates (metabolites). **Elimination:** Urine (45%), feces (32%); (PO) $T_{1/2}$=17 hrs.

PATIENT CONSIDERATIONS
Assessment: Assess for congenital or acquired uterine anomaly, acute or history of PID, known/suspected or history of breast cancer or other progestin-sensitive cancer, acute liver disease or liver tumor, pregnancy/nursing status, any other conditions where treatment is contraindicated or cautioned, and for possible drug interactions. Perform a complete medical and social history and if indicated, a physical examination, and appropriate tests for any forms of genital or other STIs.

Monitoring: Monitor for intrauterine/ectopic pregnancy, severe infection/sepsis, GAS, PID, actinomycosis, bleeding pattern alterations, perforation, expulsion, migraine/exceptionally severe headache, jaundice, marked BP increase, and other adverse reactions. Reexamine and evaluate 4-6 weeks after insertion and once a yr thereafter, or more frequently if clinically indicated. Monitor if threads are still visible and for length of threads.

Counseling: Inform that product does not protect against HIV infection (AIDS) and other STIs. Explain the risks/benefits/side effects of the device. Inform of the risk of ectopic pregnancy, including loss of fertility; instruct to promptly report symptoms of ectopic pregnancy to physician. Inform of the possibility of PID and of its symptoms; instruct to promptly notify physician if any symptoms of PID develop. Inform that irregular/prolonged bleeding and spotting, and/or cramps may occur during the 1st few weeks after insertion; instruct to report to physician if symptoms continue or are severe. Instruct on how to check if the device's threads still protrude from the cervix and caution not to pull on the threads and displace device. Inform that no contraceptive protection exists if device is displaced or expelled. Instruct to contact physician if any adverse reactions develop, if pregnancy is suspected or occurs, if HIV positive seroconversion occurs in the patient or her partner, or if possible exposure to STIs occurs.

MIRTAZAPINE — mirtazapine   Rx
Class: Alpha$_2$ antagonist

> Antidepressants increased the risk of suicidal thinking and behavior (suicidality) in children, adolescents, and young adults in short-term studies of major depressive disorder and other psychiatric disorders. Monitor and observe closely for clinical worsening, suicidality, or unusual changes in behavior in patients who are started on antidepressant therapy. Not approved for use in pediatric patients.

OTHER BRAND NAMES
RemeronSolTab, Remeron

ADULT DOSAGE
Major Depressive Disorder
Initial: 15mg qhs
Titrate: Dose changes should not be made at intervals of <1-2 weeks
Max: 45mg/day
Periodically reassess to determine the need for maint treatment and the appropriate dose for such treatment

Dosing Considerations with MAOIs
Switching to/from an MAOI for Psychiatric Disorders:
Allow at least 14 days between discontinuation of an MAOI and initiation of mirtazapine, and allow at least 14 days between discontinuation of mirtazapine and initiation of an MAOI

W/ Other MAOIs (eg, Linezolid, IV Methylene Blue):
Do not start mirtazapine in patients being treated w/ linezolid or IV methylene blue.
In patients already receiving mirtazapine, if acceptable alternatives are not available and benefits outweigh risks, d/c mirtazapine promptly and administer linezolid or IV methylene blue; monitor for serotonin syndrome for 2 weeks or until 24 hrs after the last dose of linezolid or IV methylene blue, whichever comes 1st. May resume mirtazapine therapy 24 hrs after the last dose of linezolid or IV methylene blue

PEDIATRIC DOSAGE
Pediatric use may not have been established

DOSING CONSIDERATIONS
Discontinuation
Gradually reduce dose over several weeks whenever possible

ADMINISTRATION
Oral route

RemeronSolTab
Open blister pack w/ dry hands and place tab on the tongue.
Use immediately after removal from blister; once removed, it cannot be stored.
Tab will disintegrate rapidly on the tongue and can be swallowed w/ saliva; no water is needed.
Do not split the tab.

STORAGE
20-25°C (68-77°F); excursions permitted to 15-30°C (59-86°F). Protect from light and moisture.

HOW SUPPLIED
Tab: 7.5mg; (Remeron) 15mg*, 30mg*, 45mg; **Tab, Disintegrating:** (RemeronSolTab) 15mg, 30mg, 45mg *scored

CONTRAINDICATIONS
Known hypersensitivity to mirtazapine or to any of the excipients. Use of an MAOI for psychiatric disorders either concomitantly or w/in 14 days of stopping treatment w/ mirtazapine. Use of mirtazapine w/in 14 days of stopping an MAOI for psychiatric disorders. Starting mirtazapine in patients being treated w/ other MAOIs (eg, linezolid, IV methylene blue).

WARNINGS/PRECAUTIONS
Not approved for treatment of bipolar depression. May precipitate a mixed/manic episode in patients at risk for bipolar disorder; screen for risk of bipolar disorder prior to initiating treatment. Agranulocytosis and severe neutropenia reported; d/c if sore throat, fever, stomatitis, or other signs of infection develop, along w/ low WBC counts. Serotonin syndrome reported; d/c immediately if symptoms occur and initiate supportive symptomatic treatment. Pupillary dilation that occurs following use may trigger an angle-closure attack in a patient w/ anatomically narrow angles who does not have a patent iridectomy. Cases of QT prolongation, torsades de pointes, ventricular tachycardia, and sudden death, have been reported. Caution when prescribed in patients w/ known cardiovascular (CV) disease or family history of QT prolongation, and in concomitant use w/ other medications thought to prolong the QTc interval. Akathisia/psychomotor restlessness reported; increasing the dose may be detrimental in patients who develop these symptoms. May impair mental/physical abilities. Hyponatremia,

mania/hypomania, somnolence, dizziness, increased appetite, weight gain, and elevation in cholesterol/TG/ALT levels reported. May cause seizures. Caution w/ hepatic/renal impairment, diseases/conditions affecting metabolism or hemodynamic responses, and the elderly. May cause orthostatic hypotension; caution w/ CV or cerebrovascular disease that could be exacerbated by hypotension and conditions that predispose to hypotension. Decreased clearance in elderly patients and in patients w/ moderate to severe renal or hepatic impairment.

ADVERSE REACTIONS

Somnolence, increased appetite, weight gain, dizziness, dry mouth, constipation, asthenia, flu syndrome, abnormal dreams, abnormal thinking.

DRUG INTERACTIONS

See Dosing Considerations and Contraindications. May cause serotonin syndrome w/ other serotonergic drugs (eg, triptans, TCAs, fentanyl) and w/ drugs that impair metabolism of serotonin; d/c immediately if this occurs. Caution w/ antihypertensives and drugs known to cause hyponatremia. Phenytoin, carbamazepine, and other hepatic metabolism inducers (eg, rifampicin) may decrease levels; may need to increase mirtazapine dose or if such inducers are discontinued, may need to reduce mirtazapine. Cimetidine and ketoconazole may increase levels; may need to decrease mirtazapine dose when concomitant treatment w/ cimetidine is started, or increase dose when cimetidine treatment is discontinued. Avoid alcohol and diazepam or drugs similar to diazepam while on therapy. Caution w/ potent CYP3A4 inhibitors, HIV protease inhibitors, azole antifungals, erythromycin, or nefazodone. Increased INR w/ warfarin; monitor INR. Risk of QT prolongation and/or ventricular arrhythmias may be increased w/ concomitant use of medicines which prolong the QTc interval (eg, some antipsychotics, antibiotics).

PREGNANCY AND LACTATION

Pregnancy: Category C.
Lactation: May be excreted in breast milk; caution in nursing.

MECHANISM OF ACTION

Alpha$_2$ antagonist; not established. Acts as an antagonist at central presynaptic α_2-adrenergic inhibitory autoreceptors and heteroreceptors, an action that is postulated to result in an increase in central noradrenergic and serotonergic activity.

PHARMACOKINETICS

Absorption: Rapid and complete. Absolute bioavailability (50%); T_{max}=2 hrs. **Distribution:** Plasma protein binding (approx 85%); may be found in breast milk. **Metabolism:** Extensive; demethylation and hydroxylation via CYP2D6, CYP1A2, and CYP3A followed by glucuronide conjugation. **Elimination:** Urine (75%), feces (15%); $T_{1/2}$=approx 20-40 hrs.

PATIENT CONSIDERATIONS

Assessment: Assess for risk of bipolar disorder or hyponatremia, susceptibility to angle-closure glaucoma, CV or cerebrovascular diseases, family history of QT prolongation, history of mania/hypomania/seizure, conditions that predispose to hypotension, renal/hepatic impairment, diseases/conditions affecting metabolism or hemodynamic response, hypersensitivity to drug, pregnancy/nursing status, and possible drug interactions.

Monitoring: Monitor for signs/symptoms of clinical worsening, suicidality, unusual changes in behavior, agranulocytosis, neutropenia, serotonin syndrome, angle-closure glaucoma, akathisia, somnolence, dizziness, increased appetite, weight gain, elevation in cholesterol/TG/ALT levels, hyponatremia, seizures, orthostatic hypotension, and other adverse reactions. Monitor INR w/ warfarin. Periodically reevaluate long-term usefulness of the drug.

Counseling: Inform about the risks, benefits, and appropriate use of therapy. Advise families and caregivers of the need for close observation for signs of clinical worsening and suicidal risks and to report such signs to physician. Warn about risk of developing agranulocytosis and instruct to contact physician if signs of infection (eg, fever, chills, sore throat) develop. Advise to use caution when engaging in hazardous activities. Advise that improvement may be noticed in 1-4 weeks of therapy; instruct to continue therapy ud. Advise to inform physician if taking or intending to take any prescription or OTC drugs. Instruct to avoid alcohol while on therapy. Instruct to notify physician if pregnant, intending to become pregnant, or breastfeeding. Caution about the risk of angle-closure glaucoma. **RemeronSolTab:** Inform phenylketonuric patients that the tab contains phenylalanine.

MIRVASO — brimonidine   Rx

Class: Selective alpha$_2$ agonist

ADULT DOSAGE	PEDIATRIC DOSAGE
Rosacea	Pediatric use may not have been established
Persistent (Nontransient) Erythema: Apply a pea-sized amount qd to each of the 5 areas of the face: central forehead, chin, nose, each cheek	

ADMINISTRATION

Topical route

Apply gel smoothly and evenly as a thin layer across the entire face, avoiding eyes and lips.
Wash hands after application.

STORAGE

20-25°C (68-77°F); excursions permitted between 15-30°C (59-86°F).

HOW SUPPLIED

Gel: 0.33% [30g, 45g]

CONTRAINDICATIONS

Hypersensitivity reaction to any component.

WARNINGS/PRECAUTIONS

Not for oral, ophthalmic, or intravaginal use. Caution w/ depression, cerebral/coronary insufficiency, Raynaud's phenomenon, orthostatic hypotension, thromboangiitis obliterans, scleroderma, or Sjogren's syndrome. May lower BP; caution w/ severe/unstable/uncontrolled cardiovascular disease (CVD). Serious adverse reactions reported following oral ingestion. Bradycardia, hypotension (including orthostatic hypotension), and dizziness reported; avoid application to irritated skin or open wounds. Erythema and flushing reported. Pallor or excessive whitening at or outside the application site reported. Allergic contact dermatitis, angioedema, throat tightening, tongue swelling, and urticaria reported; d/c brimonidine and institute appropriate therapy if clinically significant hypersensitivity reaction occurs.

ADVERSE REACTIONS

Erythema, flushing, skin burning sensation, contact dermatitis.

DRUG INTERACTIONS

Caution w/ β-blockers, antihypertensives, and/or cardiac glycosides. Possible additive or potentiating effect w/ CNS depressants (alcohol, barbiturates, opiates, sedatives, or anesthetics). MAOIs may theoretically interfere w/ metabolism and potentially increase systemic side effects (eg, hypotension); use w/ caution.

PREGNANCY AND LACTATION

Pregnancy: Category B.
Lactation: Not for use in nursing.

MECHANISM OF ACTION

Relatively selective α_2 adrenergic agonist; may reduce erythema through direct vasoconstriction.

PHARMACOKINETICS

Absorption: (Day 15) C_{max}=46pg/mL; AUC=417pg•hr/mL. **Metabolism:** Liver (extensive). **Elimination:** Urine (major).

PATIENT CONSIDERATIONS

Assessment: Assess for hypersensitivity, depression, cerebral/coronary insufficiency, Raynaud's phenomenon, orthostatic hypotension, thromboangiitis obliterans, scleroderma, Sjogren's syndrome, severe/unstable/uncontrolled CVD, pregnancy/nursing status, and possible drug interactions.

Monitoring: Monitor for bradycardia, hypotension, dizziness, erythema, flushing, excessive whitening, and hypersensitivity reactions.

Counseling: Instruct to use externally and ud, not to apply to irritated skin or open wounds, to wash hands immediately after application, and to report any adverse reactions to physician. Inform that erythema, flushing, or excessive whitening may be experienced.

MITIGARE — colchicine   Rx

Class: Miscellaneous gout agent

ADULT DOSAGE	PEDIATRIC DOSAGE
Gout Flares	Pediatric use may not have been established
Prophylaxis: 0.6mg qd or bid **Max:** 1.2mg/day	

DOSING CONSIDERATIONS

Concomitant Medications

CYP3A4 or P-gp Inhibitors: If concomitant use cannot be avoided, reduce daily dose or frequency and monitor for colchicine toxicity

Renal Impairment

Severe: Consider dose reduction or alternative therapy
Hemodialysis: Monitor carefully for colchicine toxicity

Hepatic Impairment

Severe: Consider dose reduction or alternative therapy

Elderly

Consider dose reduction

ADMINISTRATION

Oral route

Take w/o regard to meals.

STORAGE

20-25°C (68-77°F). Protect from light and moisture.

HOW SUPPLIED

Cap: 0.6mg

CONTRAINDICATIONS

Concomitant use w/ drugs that inhibit both P-gp and CYP3A4 inhibitors in patients w/ renal or hepatic impairment. Patients w/ both renal and hepatic impairment.

WARNINGS/PRECAUTIONS

Not an analgesic medication and should not be used to treat pain from other causes. Fatal overdoses reported. Myelosuppression, leukopenia, granulocytopenia, thrombocytopenia, pancytopenia, and aplastic anemia reported. Neuromuscular toxicity and rhabdomyolysis reported w/ chronic use; increased risk w/ drugs known to cause these effects and in patients w/ impaired renal function and in the elderly.

ADVERSE REACTIONS

Abdominal pain, diarrhea, N/V.

DRUG INTERACTIONS
See Contraindications and Dosing Considerations. Inhibition of both CYP3A4 and P-gp by dual inhibitors (eg, clarithromycin) reported to produce life-threatening or fatal colchicine toxicity. Toxicities reported w/ CYP3A4 inhibitors (eg, grapefruit juice, erythromycin, verapamil) or P-gp inhibitors (eg, cyclosporine); avoid use. May increase risk of myopathy w/ HMG-CoA reductase inhibitors and fibrates.

PREGNANCY AND LACTATION
Pregnancy: Category C.
Lactation: Caution in nursing.

MECHANISM OF ACTION
Alkaloid; blocks neutrophil-mediated inflammatory responses induced by monosodium urate crystals in synovial fluid; disrupts the polymerization of β-tubulin into microtubules, thereby preventing the activation, degranulation, and migration of neutrophils to sites of inflammation; and interferes w/ the inflammasome complex found in neutrophils and monocytes that mediates interleukin-1β activation.

PHARMACOKINETICS
Absorption: Absolute bioavailability (45%); C_{max}=3ng/mL; T_{max}=1.3 hrs.
Distribution: V_d=5-8L/kg; plasma protein binding (39%). Crosses placenta; found in breast milk. **Metabolism:** Via CYP3A4 to 2-O-demethylcolchicine and 3-O-demethylcolchicine. **Elimination:** Urine (40-65%, unchanged); $T_{1/2}$=31 hrs.

PATIENT CONSIDERATIONS

Assessment: Assess for renal/hepatic impairment, pregnancy/nursing status, and possible drug interactions.

Monitoring: Monitor for myelosuppression, leukopenia, granulocytopenia, thrombocytopenia, pancytopenia, aplastic anemia, neuromuscular toxicity, rhabdomyolysis, and other adverse reactions. Monitor patients on hemodialysis for colchicine toxicity.

Counseling: If a dose is missed, advise to take dose as soon as possible and return to normal dosing schedule; advise not to double the next dose if a dose is skipped. Advise that fatal overdoses have been reported; instruct to keep out of the reach of children. Advise that bone marrow depression w/ agranulocytosis, aplastic anemia, and thrombocytopenia may occur. Advise that many drugs or other substances may interact w/ treatment; instruct to provide all healthcare providers w/ a list of current medications (including nonprescription medications or herbal products) patients are taking and to check w/ healthcare provider before starting new medications. Advise to avoid grapefruit and grapefruit juice. Advise patients that muscle pain or weakness, tingling or numbness in fingers or toes may occur; instruct to d/c and seek medical evaluation immediately.

MITOMYCIN — mitomycin   Rx

Class: DNA synthesis inhibitor

> Administer under the supervision of a physician experienced in the use of cancer chemotherapeutic agents. Adequate diagnostic and treatment facilities should be readily available. Bone marrow suppression (eg, thrombocytopenia, leukopenia) is the most common and severe of the toxic effects. Hemolytic uremic syndrome (HUS) reported and may occur at any time during systemic therapy with mitomycin as a single agent or in combination with other cytotoxic drugs, mostly at doses ≥60mg of mitomycin. Blood product transfusion may exacerbate associated symptoms.

ADULT DOSAGE
Stomach/Pancreas Disseminated Adenocarcinoma

Combination w/ other approved chemotherapeutic agents and as palliative treatment when other modalities have failed

After Full Hematological Recovery from Any Previous Chemotherapy:
20mg/m² IV as a single dose via a functioning IV catheter at 6- to 8-week intervals
Max: 20mg/m²

Dose Adjustment Based on Nadir After Prior Dose:
Leukocytes 2000-2999/mm³ and Platelets 25,000-74,999/mm³: Administer 70% of prior dose
Leukocytes <2000/mm³ and Platelets <25,000/mm³: Administer 50% of prior dose

Do not repeat dose until leukocyte count has returned to 4000/mm³ and platelet count to 100,000/mm³

D/C therapy if disease continues to progress after 2 courses

PEDIATRIC DOSAGE
Pediatric use may not have been established

ADMINISTRATION
IV route

Preparation
1. Each vial contains either mitomycin 5mg and mannitol 10mg, mitomycin 20mg and mannitol 40mg, or mitomycin 40mg and mannitol 80mg; to administer, add sterile water for inj, 10mL, 40mL or 80mL respectively

2. Shake to dissolve; if product does not dissolve immediately, allow to stand at room temperature until sol is obtained

STORAGE
Dry Powder: 25°C (77°F); excursion permitted between 15-30°C (59-86°F). Protect from light. Avoid excessive heat >40°C (104°F). Reconstituted Sol: 2-8°C (36-46°F); discard after 14 days if refrigerated or after 7 days if unrefrigerated. Protect from light.

HOW SUPPLIED
Inj: 5mg, 20mg, 40mg

CONTRAINDICATIONS
Prior hypersensitivity or idiosyncratic reaction to this medication, thrombocytopenia, coagulation disorder, or an increase in bleeding tendency due to other causes.

WARNINGS/PRECAUTIONS
Not recommended as single-agent, primary therapy, or to replace appropriate surgery and/or radiotherapy. Avoid extravasation; cellulitis, ulceration, slough, and necrosis may result. Observe patient carefully and frequently during and after therapy. Monitor platelet count, WBC, differential count, and Hgb during therapy and for at least 8 weeks following therapy; if platelet count <100,000/mm³, WBC <4000/mm³, or progressive decline is seen in either, withhold further therapy until blood counts have recovered above these levels. Deaths due to septicemia as a result of leukopenia reported. Observe for evidence of renal toxicity; do not give with SrCr >1.7mg percent. Adult respiratory distress syndrome reported when given in combination with other chemotherapy and maintained at FIO_2 concentrations >50% perioperatively; exercise caution, using only enough oxygen to provide adequate arterial saturation. Monitor fluid balance; avoid overhydration. Bladder fibrosis/contraction reported with intravesical administration. Caution in elderly.

ADVERSE REACTIONS
Bone marrow suppression, HUS, inj site cellulitis, stomatitis, alopecia, fever, anorexia, N/V.

DRUG INTERACTIONS
See Boxed Warning. Acute SOB and severe bronchospasm reported following administration of vinca alkaloids in patients who had previously or simultaneously received mitomycin.

PREGNANCY AND LACTATION
Safety not known in pregnancy, not for use in nursing.

MECHANISM OF ACTION
DNA synthesis inhibitor; selectively inhibits DNA synthesis. At high concentrations, cellular RNA and protein synthesis are also suppressed.

PHARMACOKINETICS
Absorption: C_{max}=2.4mcg/mL (30mg), 1.7mcg/mL (20mg), 0.52mcg/mL (10mg).
Metabolism: Liver. **Elimination:** Urine (10% unchanged); $T_{1/2}$=17 min (30mg).

PATIENT CONSIDERATIONS

Assessment: Assess for previous hypersensitivity/idiosyncratic reaction to the drug, thrombocytopenia, coagulation disorder, increase in bleeding tendency due to other causes, renal impairment, pregnancy/nursing status, and possible drug interactions. Obtain baseline platelet count, WBC count, differential, and Hgb.

Monitoring: Monitor for bone marrow suppression, HUS, renal toxicity, adult respiratory distress syndrome, and other adverse reactions. Monitor platelet count, WBC count, differential count and Hgb during therapy and for 8 weeks following therapy. Monitor fluid balance and hydration status.

Counseling: Inform about the risks and benefits of therapy. Advise of the potential toxicities of the drug, particularly bone marrow suppression. Instruct to notify physician if pregnant/nursing. Advise to contact physician if any adverse reactions develop while on therapy.

MOBIC — meloxicam   Rx

Class: NSAID

> NSAIDs cause an increased risk of serious cardiovascular (CV) thrombotic events, including MI and stroke, which can be fatal. This risk may occur early in treatment and may increase w/ duration of use. Contraindicated in the setting of CABG surgery. NSAIDs cause an increased risk of serious GI adverse events (eg, bleeding, ulceration, stomach/intestinal perforation), which can be fatal and can occur anytime during use and w/o warning symptoms; elderly patients and patients w/ a prior history of peptic ulcer disease and/or GI bleeding are at a greater risk.

ADULT DOSAGE
Osteoarthritis

Initial/Maint: 7.5mg qd
Max: 15mg/day

Rheumatoid Arthritis

Initial/Maint: 7.5mg qd
Max: 15mg/day

PEDIATRIC DOSAGE
Juvenile Rheumatoid Arthritis

Pauciarticular or Polyarticular Course:
≥60kg:
Recommended: 7.5mg qd
Max: 7.5mg/day

DOSING CONSIDERATIONS
Renal Impairment
Mild to Moderate: No dose adjustment necessary
Severe: Not recommended
Hemodialysis:
Max: 7.5mg/day

Hepatic Impairment
Mild to Moderate: No dose adjustment necessary
Severe: Not adequately studied
Elderly
If the anticipated benefit outweighs the potential risks, start at lower end of dosing range; monitor for adverse effects

ADMINISTRATION
Oral route

May be taken w/o regard to timing of meals.
Not interchangeable w/ other formulations of oral meloxicam product even if the total mg strength is the same; do not substitute similar dose strengths of Mobic tabs w/ other formulations of oral meloxicam product.

STORAGE
25°C (77°F); excursions permitted to 15-30°C (59-86°F). Keep tabs in a dry place.

HOW SUPPLIED
Tab: 7.5mg, 15mg

CONTRAINDICATIONS
Known hypersensitivity (eg, anaphylactic reactions, serious skin reactions) to meloxicam or any components of the drug product; history of asthma, urticaria, or allergic-type reactions after taking aspirin (ASA) or other NSAIDs; in the setting of CABG surgery.

WARNINGS/PRECAUTIONS
Use lowest effective dose for the shortest duration possible. Avoid in patients w/ a recent MI unless benefits outweigh the risks of recurrent CV thrombotic events; if used, monitor for signs of cardiac ischemia. Increased risk for GI bleeding w/ longer duration of NSAID therapy, older age, poor general health status, and advanced liver disease and/or coagulopathy; avoid use in patients at higher risk unless benefits are expected to outweigh the increased risk of bleeding. Consider alternate therapies other than NSAIDs for patients at higher risk and patients w/ active GI bleeding. Promptly initiate evaluation and treatment if a serious GI adverse event is suspected; d/c until a serious GI adverse event is ruled out. Hepatotoxicity reported; d/c immediately and perform a clinical evaluation if clinical signs/symptoms consistent w/ liver disease develop, or if systemic manifestations occur. May cause new onset HTN or worsen preexisting HTN. Fluid retention and edema reported. Avoid use in patients w/ severe heart failure (HF) unless benefits outweigh risks; monitor for signs of worsening HF if used. Renal papillary necrosis, renal insufficiency, acute renal failure, and other renal injury w/ long-term use. Renal toxicity also reported in patients in whom renal prostaglandins have a compensatory role in the maintenance of renal perfusion; increased risk w/ renal/hepatic dysfunction, dehydration, hypovolemia, and HF, and in the elderly. Renal effects of therapy may hasten the progression of renal dysfunction in patients w/ preexisting renal disease. Correct volume status in dehydrated or hypovolemic patients prior to initiating therapy. Avoid use in patients w/ advanced renal disease unless the benefits are expected to outweigh the risk; monitor for signs of worsening renal function if used in patients w/ advanced renal disease. Hyperkalemia reported. Associated w/ anaphylactic reactions. Monitor for changes in the signs/symptoms of asthma in patients w/ preexisting asthma (w/o known ASA sensitivity). May cause serious skin reactions (eg, exfoliative dermatitis, Stevens-Johnson syndrome, toxic epidermal necrolysis); d/c at 1st appearance of skin rash/hypersensitivity. Anemia reported. May increase the risk of bleeding events; coagulation disorders may increase this risk. May mask inflammation and fever.

ADVERSE REACTIONS
Adults: Abdominal pain, diarrhea, dyspepsia, nausea, headache, URTI, dizziness, pharyngitis, edema, influenza-like symptoms.
Pediatric Patients: Abdominal pain, vomiting, diarrhea, headache, pyrexia.

DRUG INTERACTIONS
Drugs that interfere w/ serotonin reuptake may potentiate the risk of bleeding. Synergistic effect on bleeding w/ anticoagulants (eg, warfarin); monitor for signs of bleeding w/ concomitant anticoagulants, antiplatelet agents, SSRIs, and SNRIs. May increase risk of GI bleeding w/ use of oral corticosteroids, anticoagulants, or SSRIs; smoking; and alcohol use. ASA may increase risk of bleeding and serious GI events; concomitant use of low-dose ASA or analgesic doses of ASA is not recommended. Monitor patients more closely for GI bleeding w/ concomitant use of low-dose ASA for cardiac prophylaxis. May diminish antihypertensive effect of ACE inhibitors, ARBs, and β-blockers (eg, propranolol); monitor BP. Coadministration w/ ACE inhibitors or ARBs may result in deterioration of renal function (including possible acute renal failure) in patients who are elderly or volume-depleted (including those on diuretic therapy), or who have renal impairment; monitor for worsening renal function and adequately hydrate patients when these drugs are administered concomitantly. May reduce natriuretic effect of loop diuretics (eg, furosemide) and thiazide diuretics; observe for signs of worsening renal function, in addition to assuring diuretic efficacy including antihypertensive effects during concomitant use w/ diuretics. May elevate plasma lithium levels and reduce renal lithium clearance; monitor for signs of lithium toxicity. May increase the risk for methotrexate toxicity. May increase cyclosporine's nephrotoxicity; monitor for signs of worsening renal function. Concomitant use w/ other NSAIDs or salicylates (eg, diflunisal, salsalate) increases the risk of GI toxicity; not recommended w/ other NSAIDs or salicylates. Concomitant use w/ pemetrexed may increase the risk of pemetrexed-associated myelosuppression, renal, and GI toxicity; refer to prescribing information for further information.

PREGNANCY AND LACTATION
Pregnancy: Use during the 3rd trimester of pregnancy increases the risk of premature closure of the fetal ductus arteriosus; avoid use in pregnant women starting at 30 weeks of gestation (3rd trimester).
Lactation: There are no human data available on whether meloxicam is present in human milk, on the effects on breastfed infants, or on milk production; caution in nursing.
Reproductive Potential: Based on the mechanism of action, may delay or prevent rupture of ovarian follicles, which has been associated w/ reversible infertility in some women. Small studies in women treated w/ NSAIDs have also shown a reversible delay in ovulation. Consider withdrawal of therapy in women who have difficulties conceiving or who are undergoing investigation of infertility.

MECHANISM OF ACTION
NSAID; mechanism not completely understood but involves inhibition of COX-1 and COX-2. Has analgesic, anti-inflammatory, and antipyretic properties. Meloxicam is a potent inhibitor of prostaglandin synthesis.

PHARMACOKINETICS
Absorption: Administration of variable doses in different populations resulted in different parameters. Absolute bioavailability (89%). **Distribution:** V_d=10L, plasma protein binding (99.4%). **Metabolism:** Liver (extensive); oxidation via CYP2C9 (major), CYP3A4 (minor). **Elimination:** Urine (0.2% unchanged), feces (1.6% unchanged); $T_{1/2}$=15-20 hrs.

PATIENT CONSIDERATIONS
Assessment: Assess for hypersensitivity to meloxicam or to any component of this product; history of asthma, urticaria, or other allergic-type reactions after taking ASA or other NSAIDs; asthma; CV disease (CVD) or risk factors for CVD; HTN; history of peptic ulcer disease or GI bleeding; coagulation disorders; renal/hepatic impairment; pregnancy/nursing status; or any other conditions where treatment is contraindicated or cautioned. Assess volume status. Assess for possible drug interactions. Obtain baseline BP, CBC, and chemistry profile.

Monitoring: Monitor for signs/symptoms of CV thrombotic events; cardiac ischemia in patients w/ a recent MI; GI bleeding/ulceration and perforation; hepatotoxicity; new or worsening HTN; HF; edema; renal papillary necrosis and other renal injury; hyperkalemia; anaphylactic reactions; serious skin reactions; anemia; and other adverse reactions. Monitor BP during initiation of therapy and throughout the course of therapy. Monitor for signs of bleeding in patients on concomitant therapy w/ anticoagulants, antiplatelet agents, SSRIs, or SNRIs. Monitor renal function in patients w/ renal/hepatic impairment, HF, dehydration, or hypovolemia. Periodically monitor CBC and chemistry profiles including LFTs in patients receiving long-term treatment.

Counseling: Inform of potential for CV thrombotic events, GI adverse events, and worsening CHF/edema, and advise of symptoms; instruct to report any symptoms to healthcare provider immediately. Inform of the potential for hepatotoxicity, and advise of signs/symptoms; if signs/symptoms occur, instruct to d/c and seek immediate medical therapy. Instruct to seek immediate emergency help if signs of an anaphylactic reaction occur. Advise to d/c immediately if rash develops and to contact healthcare provider as soon as possible. Advise females of reproductive potential who desire pregnancy that therapy may be associated w/ a reversible delay in ovulation. Advise pregnant women to avoid use starting at 30 weeks of gestation. Advise not to use other NSAIDs or salicylates concomitantly; notify of the presence of NSAIDs in OTC medications for colds, fever, or insomnia. Advise not to use low-dose ASA concomitantly w/o talking to healthcare provider.

MODERIBA — ribavirin   Rx
Class: Nucleoside analogue

> Not for monotherapy treatment of chronic hepatitis C (CHC) virus infection. Primary toxicity is hemolytic anemia. Anemia associated w/ therapy may result in worsening of cardiac disease and lead to fatal and nonfatal MIs. Avoid w/ history of significant/unstable cardiac disease. Contraindicated in women who are pregnant and in male partners of pregnant women. Extreme care must be taken to avoid pregnancy during therapy and for 6 months after completion of therapy in both female patients and in female partners of male patients who are taking therapy. Use at least 2 reliable forms of effective contraception during treatment and for 6 months after discontinuation.

ADULT DOSAGE
Chronic Hepatitis C with Compensated Liver Disease

Combination w/ Peginterferon Alfa-2a:
Not Previously Treated w/ Interferon Alpha:
Monoinfection:
Genotypes 1, 4:
<75kg: 1000mg/day in 2 divided doses
≥75kg: 1200mg/day in 2 divided doses
Treatment Duration: 48 weeks

Genotypes 2, 3:
800mg/day in 2 divided doses
Treatment Duration: 24 weeks

HIV Coinfection:
800mg/day
Treatment Duration: 48 weeks (regardless of genotype)

PEDIATRIC DOSAGE
Chronic Hepatitis C with Compensated Liver Disease

Combination w/ Peginterferon Alfa-2a:
Not Previously Treated w/ Interferon Alpha:
Monoinfection:
5-17 Years:
23-33kg: 200mg qam and 200mg qpm
34-46kg: 200mg qam and 400mg qpm
47-59kg: 400mg qam and 400mg qpm
60-74kg: 400mg qam and 600mg qpm
≥75kg: 600mg qam and 600 mg qpm

Patients who reach their 18th birthday while receiving combination therapy should remain on the pediatric dosing regimen through the completion of therapy

Treatment Duration:
Genotypes 2, 3: 24 weeks
Other Genotypes: 48 weeks

DOSING CONSIDERATIONS

Renal Impairment

Adults:

CrCl 30-50mL/min: Alternating doses, 200mg and 400mg qod

CrCl<30mL/min or Hemodialysis: 200mg/day

Adverse Reactions

W/O Cardiac Disease:

Hgb <10g/dL:

Adults: 200mg qam and 400mg qpm

Pediatrics:

23-33kg: 200mg qam

34-46kg: 200mg qam and 200mg qpm

47-59kg: 200mg qam and 200mg qpm

60-74kg: 200mg qam and 400mg qpm

≥75kg: 200mg qam and 400mg qpm

Hgb <8.5g/dL:

Adults and Pediatrics: D/C ribavirin

W/ History of Stable Cardiac Disease:

Hgb Decrease of ≥2g/dL During any 4-Week Treatment Period:

Adults: 200mg qam and 400mg qpm

Pediatrics:

23-33kg: 200mg qam

34-46kg: 200mg qam and 200mg qpm

47-59kg: 200mg qam and 200mg qpm

60-74kg: 200mg qam and 400mg qpm

≥75kg: 200mg qam and 400mg qpm

Hgb <12g/dL After 4 Weeks at Reduced Dose:

Adults and Pediatrics: D/C ribavirin

Adults:

If ribavirin has been withheld due to either a lab abnormality or clinical adverse reaction, may attempt to restart at 600mg/day and further increase to 800mg/day; not recommended to increase to the original assigned dose (1000-1200mg)

Pediatrics:

Upon resolution of a lab abnormality or clinical adverse reaction, may attempt to increase ribavirin dose to the original dose. If ribavirin has been withheld due to a lab abnormality or clinical adverse reaction, may make attempt to restart ribavirin at 1/2 the full dose

Discontinuation

Consider if at least a 2 $\log_{10}$ HCV RNA reduction from baseline by Week 12 is not achieved

Consider if HCV RNA levels remain detectable after treatment Week 24

D/C if hepatic decompensation develops during treatment

ADMINISTRATION

Oral route

Take w/ food

Refer to peginterferon alfa-2a labeling for dosage and administration instructions

STORAGE

25°C (77°F); excursions permitted between 15-30°C (59-86°F).

HOW SUPPLIED

Tab: 200mg, 400mg, 600mg

CONTRAINDICATIONS

Women who are or may become pregnant, men whose female partners are pregnant, hemoglobinopathies (eg, thalassemia major, sickle cell anemia), and in combination w/ didanosine. When used w/ peginterferon alfa-2a, refer to the individual monograph.

WARNINGS/PRECAUTIONS

Combination therapy is associated w/ significant adverse reactions (eg, severe depression and suicidal ideation, hemolytic anemia, suppression of bone marrow function, autoimmune/infectious/ophthalmologic/cerebrovascular disorders, pulmonary dysfunction, colitis, pancreatitis, diabetes). Do not start therapy unless a negative pregnancy test has been obtained immediately prior to therapy. Caution w/ baseline risk of severe anemia (eg, spherocytosis, history of GI bleeding). Caution w/ preexisting cardiac disease; suspend or d/c therapy if cardiovascular status deteriorates. Risk of hepatic decompensation and death in CHC patients w/ cirrhosis. Severe acute hypersensitivity reactions and serious skin reactions reported. D/C w/ hepatic decompensation, confirmed pancreatitis, severe hypersensitivity, or if signs/symptoms of severe skin reactions develop. Pulmonary disorders (eg, dyspnea, pulmonary infiltrates, pneumonitis, pulmonary HTN, pneumonia) reported. Closely monitor if pulmonary infiltrates/function impairment develop and d/c if appropriate. Decreases in height and weight reported in pediatric patients.

ADVERSE REACTIONS

Hemolytic anemia, fatigue/asthenia, neutropenia, headache, pyrexia, myalgia, irritability/anxiety/nervousness, insomnia, alopecia, rigors, N/V, anorexia.

DRUG INTERACTIONS

See Contraindications. Closely monitor for treatment associated toxicities (eg, hepatic decompensation) w/ nucleoside reverse transcriptase inhibitors; consider dose reduction or discontinuation of peginterferon alfa-2a and/or ribavirin. Severe neutropenia and severe anemia reported w/ zidovudine; consider discontinuation of zidovudine if appropriate. Severe pancytopenia and bone marrow suppression reported w/ azathioprine; monitor CBC, including platelet counts, weekly for the 1st month, twice monthly for the 2nd and 3rd months of treatment, then monthly or more frequently if dosage or other therapy changes are necessary; d/c peginterferon alfa-2a, ribavirin, and azathioprine if pancytopenia develops.

PREGNANCY AND LACTATION

Category X, not for use in nursing.

MECHANISM OF ACTION

Nucleoside analogue; not established. Has direct antiviral activity in tissue culture against many RNA viruses; increases mutation frequency in the genomes of several RNA viruses and ribavirin triphosphate inhibits HCV polymerase in a biochemical reaction.

PHARMACOKINETICS

Absorption: C_{max}=2748ng/mL; T_{max}=2 hrs; AUC=25,361ng•hr/mL. **Elimination:** $T_{1/2}$=120-170 hrs.

PATIENT CONSIDERATIONS

Assessment: Assess for hemoglobinopathies, autoimmune hepatitis, hepatic decompensation, baseline risk of severe anemia, history of or preexisting cardiac disease, nursing status, and possible drug interactions. Conduct pregnancy test (including in female partners of male patients), standard hematological and biochemical lab tests, ECG in patients w/ preexisting cardiac abnormalities, renal/thyroid function test, and CD4 count in HIV patients. Assess baseline height and weight in pediatric patients.

Monitoring: Monitor for hemolytic anemia, hepatic decompensation, pancreatitis, hypersensitivity/skin reactions, pulmonary infiltrates/function impairment, and other adverse reactions. Monitor cardiac status, TSH, and HCV RNA. Perform hematological tests at Weeks 2 and 4 and biochemical tests at Week 4; perform additional testing periodically. Perform pregnancy testing monthly and for 6 months after discontinuation (including female partners of male patients). Monitor height and weight in pediatric patients. In patients on concomitant therapy w/ azathioprine, monitor CBC, including platelet counts, weekly for the 1st month, twice monthly for the 2nd and 3rd months of treatment, then monthly or more frequently if dosage or other therapy changes are necessary.

Counseling: Counsel on risks/benefits associated w/ treatment. Inform of pregnancy risks; instruct to use at least 2 forms of effective contraception during therapy and for 6 months after discontinuation of therapy (including female partners of male patients). Advise to notify physician immediately in the event of pregnancy. Advise that lab evaluations are required prior to starting therapy and periodically thereafter. Advise to be well-hydrated, especially during the initial stages of treatment. Caution to avoid driving/operating machinery if dizziness, confusion, somnolence, or fatigue develops. Instruct not to drink alcohol; inform that alcohol may exacerbate CHC infection. Inform to take appropriate precautions to prevent HCV transmission.

MONODOX — doxycycline monohydrate   Rx

Class: Tetracyclines

ADULT DOSAGE

General Dosing

Initial: 100mg q12h or 50mg q6h on 1st day

Maint: 100mg qd or 50mg q12h

More Severe Infections (eg, Chronic UTIs):

100mg q12h

Streptococcal Infections:

Continue therapy for 10 days

Gonococcal Infections

Uncomplicated Infections (Except Anorectal Infections in Men):

100mg bid for 7 days

Alternate Dosing:

Single visit dose of 300mg stat followed in 1 hr by a second 300mg dose

Acute Epididymo-Orchitis

Caused by *Neisseria gonorrhoeae*/*Chlamydia trachomatis*:

100mg bid for at least 10 days

Syphilis

Primary and Secondary:

300mg/day in divided doses for at least 10 days

***Chlamydia trachomatis* Infections**

Uncomplicated Urethral/Endocervical/Rectal Infections:

100mg bid for at least 7 days

Nongonococcal Urethritis

Caused by *Chlamydia trachomatis* and *Ureaplasma urealyticum*:

100mg bid for at least 7 days

Inhalational Anthrax (Postexposure)

100mg bid for 60 days

Other Indications

Treatment of the Following Infections Caused by Susceptible

PEDIATRIC DOSAGE

General Dosing

>8 Years:

≤100 lbs:

2mg/lb divided into 2 doses on 1st day, followed by 1mg/lb qd or as 2 divided doses, on subsequent days

More Severe Infections: Up to 2mg/lb

>100 lbs:

Initial: 100mg q12h or 50mg q6h on 1st day

Maint: 100mg qd or 50mg q12h

More Severe Infections (eg, Chronic UTIs): 100mg q12h

Streptococcal Infections:

Continue therapy for 10 days

Inhalational Anthrax (Postexposure)

<100 lbs:

1mg/lb bid for 60 days

≥100 lbs:

100mg bid for 60 days

Microorganisms:
Rocky Mountain spotted fever
Typhus fever and the typhus group
Q fever
Rickettsialpox
Tick fevers
Respiratory tract infections
Lymphogranuloma venereum
Psittacosis (ornithosis)
Trachoma
Inclusion conjunctivitis
Relapsing fever
Chancroid
Plague
Tularemia
Cholera
Campylobacter fetus infections
Brucellosis (in conjunction w/ streptomycin)
Bartonellosis
Granuloma inguinale
UTIs

Treatment of Infections Caused by the Following Susceptible Strains:
Escherichia coli
Enterobacter aerogenes
Shigella species
Acinetobacter species

Treatment of the Following Infections Caused by Susceptible Microorganisms When Penicillin is Contraindicated:
Uncomplicated gonorrhea
Yaws
Listeriosis
Vincent's infection
Actinomycosis
Clostridium species
Adjunctive therapy in acute intestinal amebiasis and severe acne

ADMINISTRATION
Oral route
Administer w/ adequate amounts of fluid.
May be given w/ food if gastric irritation occurs.

STORAGE
20-25°C (68-77°F); excursions permitted to 15-30°C (59-86°F).

HOW SUPPLIED
Cap: 50mg, 75mg, 100mg

CONTRAINDICATIONS
Hypersensitivity to any of the tetracyclines.

WARNINGS/PRECAUTIONS
May cause permanent discoloration of the teeth (yellow-gray-brown) if used during tooth development (last 1/2 of pregnancy, infancy, and childhood to 8 yrs of age); do not use in this age group, except for anthrax. Enamel hypoplasia reported. *Clostridium difficile*-associated diarrhea (CDAD) reported; d/c if CDAD is suspected or confirmed. May decrease fibula growth rate in prematures. May cause an increase in BUN. Photosensitivity, manifested by an exaggerated sunburn reaction, reported; d/c at the 1st evidence of skin erythema. May result in bacterial resistance if used in the absence of proven or suspected bacterial infection, or a prophylactic indication; take appropriate measures if superinfection develops. Associated w/ intracranial HTN (pseudotumor cerebri); increased risk in women of childbearing age who are overweight or have a history of intracranial HTN. If visual disturbance occurs, prompt ophthalmologic evaluation is warranted. Intracranial pressure can remain elevated for weeks after drug cessation; monitor patients until they stabilize. Incision and drainage or other surgical procedures should be performed in conjunction w/ antibacterial therapy when indicated. False elevations of urinary catecholamine levels may occur due to interference w/ the fluorescence test.

ADVERSE REACTIONS
Diarrhea, hepatotoxicity, maculopapular/erythematous rash, Stevens-Johnson syndrome, toxic epidermal necrolysis, anorexia, N/V, urticaria, serum sickness, pericarditis, hemolytic anemia, thrombocytopenia, neutropenia, eosinophilia.

DRUG INTERACTIONS
Avoid concomitant use w/ isotretinoin; may increase risk of intracranial HTN. Depresses plasma prothrombin activity; may require downward adjustment of anticoagulant dose. May interfere w/ bactericidal action of PCN; avoid concurrent use. Impaired absorption w/ antacids containing aluminum, Ca^{2+}, or Mg^{2+}, and iron-containing preparations. Decreased $T_{1/2}$ w/ barbiturates, carbamazepine, and phenytoin. Fatal renal toxicity reported w/ methoxyflurane. May render oral contraceptives less effective.

PREGNANCY AND LACTATION
Category D, not for use in nursing.

MECHANISM OF ACTION
Tetracycline; has bacteriostatic activity. Inhibits bacterial protein synthesis by binding to the 30S ribosomal subunit.

PHARMACOKINETICS
Absorption: Readily absorbed; virtually complete. (200mg) C_{max}=3.61mcg/mL; T_{max}=2.6 hrs. **Distribution:** Found in breast milk. **Elimination:** Urine (40%/72 hrs in CrCl 75mL/min, 1-5%/72 hrs in CrCl <10mL/min), feces; (200mg) $T_{1/2}$=16.33 hrs.

PATIENT CONSIDERATIONS
Assessment: Assess for hypersensitivity to drug or any tetracyclines, risk for intracranial HTN, pregnancy/nursing status, and possible drug interactions. Perform culture and susceptibility tests. In venereal disease when coexistent syphilis is suspected, perform a dark-field examination and blood serology.

Monitoring: Monitor for CDAD, photosensitivity, skin erythema, superinfection, intracranial HTN, visual disturbance, and other adverse reactions. In long-term therapy, perform periodic lab evaluations of organ systems, including hematopoietic, renal, and hepatic studies. In venereal disease when coexistent syphilis is suspected, repeat blood serology monthly for at least 4 months.

Counseling: Apprise of the potential hazard to fetus if used during pregnancy. Advise to avoid excessive sunlight or artificial UV light, and to d/c therapy if phototoxicity (eg, skin eruptions) occurs; advise to consider use of sunscreen or sunblock. Inform that absorption of drug is reduced when taken w/ bismuth subsalicylate, or w/ foods, especially those that contain Ca^{2+}. Inform that drug may increase incidence of vaginal candidiasis. Inform that diarrhea is a common problem caused by therapy, which usually ends when therapy is discontinued. Instruct to immediately contact physician if watery and bloody stools (w/ or w/o stomach cramps and fever) occur, even as late as ≥2 months after the last dose. Counsel that therapy should only be used to treat bacterial, not viral, infections. Instruct to take exactly ud, even if patient feels better early in the course of therapy. Inform that skipping doses or not completing the full course of therapy may decrease effectiveness of treatment and increase bacterial resistance.

MORPHABOND — morphine sulfate   CII
Class: Opioid analgesic

> Risk of opioid addiction, abuse, and misuse, which can lead to overdose and death; assess risk prior to prescribing and monitor regularly for development of these behaviors or conditions. Serious, life-threatening, or fatal respiratory depression may occur; monitor for respiratory depression, especially during initiation or following dose increase. Swallow whole; crushing, chewing, or dissolving tab can cause rapid release and absorption of a potentially fatal dose of morphine. Accidental ingestion of even one dose, especially by children, can result in fatal overdose. Prolonged use during pregnancy can result in life-threatening neonatal opioid withdrawal syndrome; advise patient of the risk of neonatal opioid withdrawal syndrome and ensure that appropriate treatment will be available if use is required.

ADULT DOSAGE	PEDIATRIC DOSAGE
Severe Pain (Daily, Around-the-Clock Management)	Pediatric use may not have been established
Initial:	
As First Opioid or in Opioid-Naive Patients: 15mg q12h	
Titration: Titrate to a dose that provides adequate analgesia and minimizes adverse reactions; dose adjustments may be done every 1-2 days. If level of pain increases after dose stabilization, attempt to identify source of increased pain before increasing dose	
Breakthrough Pain: May require dose increase or rescue medication	
Conversions	
Initial:	
From Other Oral Morphine: Half of 24-hr requirement q12h	
From Other Opioids: D/C other opioid and initiate w/ 15mg q12h	
Parenteral Morphine to Oral Morphine Ratio: Between 2-6mg of oral morphine may be required to provide analgesia equivalent to 1mg of parenteral morphine; typically, a dose that is approx 3X the previous daily parenteral morphine requirement is sufficient	
Other Parenteral or Oral Non-Morphine Opioids to Oral Morphine: Specific recommendations are not available. In general, begin w/ half of the estimated daily morphine requirement as the initial dose, managing inadequate analgesia by supplementation w/ immediate-release morphine	
From Methadone: Close monitoring is required; ratio may vary widely due to previous dose exposure	

DOSING CONSIDERATIONS
Adverse Reactions
Unacceptable Opioid-Related Reactions: May reduce subsequent doses; adjust the dosage to obtain an appropriate balance between management of pain and adverse reactions

Discontinuation
Use a gradual downward titration of the dose; do not abruptly d/c

ADMINISTRATION
Oral route
- 100mg tabs, a single dose >60mg, or a total daily dose >120mg, are only for use in opioid-tolerant patients.
- Take whole; do not crush, chew, or dissolve.
- Administer PO q12h.

STORAGE
25°C (77°F); excursions permitted between 15-30°C (59-86°F). Protect from light.

HOW SUPPLIED
Tab, Extended-Release: 15mg, 30mg, 60mg, 100mg

CONTRAINDICATIONS
Significant respiratory depression; acute or severe bronchial asthma in an unmonitored setting or in the absence of resuscitative equipment; known or suspected GI obstruction, including paralytic ileus; hypersensitivity (eg, anaphylaxis) to morphine.

WARNINGS/PRECAUTIONS
Reserve for use in patients for whom alternative treatment options are ineffective, not tolerated, or would be otherwise inadequate to provide sufficient management of pain. Closely monitor patients for respiratory depression, especially w/in the first 24-72 hrs of initiating therapy and following dose increases. Risk for respiratory depression is greatest during the initiation of therapy or following a dose increase and is more likely to occur in elderly, cachectic, or debilitated patients. Caution and consider alternative nonopioid analgesics w/ COPD or cor pulmonale, and in patients having substantially decreased respiratory reserve, hypoxia, hypercapnia, or preexisting respiratory depression. May cause severe hypotension including orthostatic hypotension and syncope in ambulatory patients; increased risk in patients whose ability to maintain BP has already been compromised by a reduced blood volume or concurrent administration of certain CNS depressant drugs (eg, phenothiazines, general anesthetics). Avoid w/ circulatory shock. May reduce respiratory drive and the resultant CO_2 retention may further increase intracranial pressure in patients who may be susceptible to the intracranial effects of CO_2 retention; monitor for signs of sedation and respiratory depression. May obscure clinical course in patients w/ a head injury. Avoid w/ impaired consciousness or coma. May cause spasm of the sphincter of Oddi. May cause increases in serum amylase; monitor patients w/ biliary tract disease for worsening of symptoms. May increase the frequency of seizures in patients w/ seizure disorders, and may increase risk of seizures occurring in other clinical settings associated w/ seizures; monitor for worsened seizure control. May impair mental/physical abilities.

ADVERSE REACTIONS
Constipation, dizziness, sedation, N/V, sweating, dysphoria, euphoric mood.

DRUG INTERACTIONS
Concomitant use of CNS depressants (eg, alcohol, sedatives, tranquilizers) may increase risk of hypotension, respiratory depression, profound sedation, coma, and death; reduce dose and consider using a lower dose of CNS depressant. Mixed agonist/antagonist (eg, pentazocine, nalbuphine, butorphanol) and partial agonist (eg, buprenorphine) opioid analgesics may reduce analgesic effect and/or precipitate withdrawal symptoms; avoid concomitant use. May enhance neuromuscular blocking action of skeletal muscle relaxants and produce increased degree of respiratory depression; monitor for signs of respiratory depression that may be greater than otherwise expected and decrease the dose of morphine and/or the muscle relaxant as necessary. MAOIs may potentiate effects and increase risk of hypotension, respiratory depression, profound sedation, coma, and death; avoid concomitant use w/ an MAOI or w/in 14 days of stopping such treatment. Cimetidine may potentiate morphine effects and increase risk of hypotension, respiratory depression, profound sedation, coma, and death; monitor for signs of respiratory depression that may be greater than otherwise expected and decrease the dose of morphine and/or cimetidine as necessary. May reduce the efficacy of diuretics; monitor for signs of diminished diuresis and/or effects on BP and increase dose of the diuretic as needed. Anticholinergics may increase risk of urinary retention and/or severe constipation, which may lead to paralytic ileus; monitor patients for signs of urinary retention or reduced gastric motility. PGP-inhibitors may increase exposure to morphine and increase risk of hypotension, respiratory depression, profound sedation, coma, and death; monitor for signs of respiratory depression that may be greater than otherwise expected and decrease dose of morphine and/or the PGP-inhibitor as necessary.

PREGNANCY AND LACTATION
Pregnancy: Category C.
Labor and Delivery: Not recommended for use in women during and immediately prior to labor. Crosses the placenta and may produce respiratory depression and psychophysiologic effects in neonates; opioid antagonist (eg, naloxone) should be available for reversal of opioid-induced respiratory depression in the neonate.
Lactation: Excreted in breast milk; withdrawal symptoms may occur in breastfeeding infants when maternal administration is stopped. Not for use in nursing.

MECHANISM OF ACTION
Opioid analgesic; interacts w/ one or more classes of specific opioid receptors located throughout the body. Acts as a full agonist, binding w/ and activating opioid receptors at sites in the peri-aqueductal and peri-ventricular grey matter, the ventro-medial medulla, and spinal cord to produce analgesia.

PHARMACOKINETICS
Absorption: Oral bioavailability (20-40%). **Distribution:** V_d=3-4L; plasma protein binding (30-35%); crosses placenta, found in breast milk. **Metabolism:** Liver via glucuronidation, sulfation, and oxidation; morphine-6-glucuronide (active analgesic), morphine-3-glucuronide (inactive as analgesic). **Elimination:** Urine (10% unchanged); $T_{1/2}$=2-4 hrs (IV).

PATIENT CONSIDERATIONS
Assessment: Assess for hypersensitivity to the drug or to any components of the product, drug abuse/addiction risk, prior opioid therapy, opioid tolerance, respiratory depression, any other conditions where treatment is contraindicated or cautioned, pregnancy/nursing status, and for possible drug interactions.

Monitoring: Monitor for respiratory depression, increased intracranial pressure, orthostatic hypotension, syncope, worsened seizure control, and other adverse reactions. During chronic therapy, periodically reassess the continued need for use of therapy.

Counseling: Instruct on how to properly take drug. Inform that use can result in addiction, abuse, and misuse, which can lead to overdose and death. Instruct not to share w/ others and to take steps to protect from theft or misuse. Inform of the risk of life-threatening respiratory depression, and that risk is greatest when starting or when dose is increased. Advise how to recognize respiratory depression and to seek medical attention if breathing difficulties develop. Inform that accidental ingestion, especially by children, may result in respiratory depression or death. Instruct to take steps to store securely and to dispose of unused tabs by flushing them down toilet. Inform that potentially serious additive effects may occur w/ alcohol or other CNS depressants, and to avoid such drugs unless supervised by a healthcare provider. Inform that treatment may cause orthostatic hypotension and syncope. Instruct on how to recognize symptoms of low BP and how to reduce the risk of serious consequences. Inform that treatment may impair the ability to perform potentially hazardous activities (eg, driving a car, operating heavy machinery); advise not to perform such tasks until they know how they will react to treatment. Advise of the potential for severe constipation, including management instructions and when to seek medical attention. Inform that anaphylaxis has been reported; advise patients how to recognize such a reaction and when to seek medical attention. Inform that prolonged use during pregnancy may result in neonatal opioid withdrawal syndrome. Inform female patients of reproductive potential that treatment may cause fetal harm and instruct to inform the prescriber of a known or suspected pregnancy.

MORPHINE ORAL SOLUTION AND TABLETS — morphine sulfate

CII

Class: Opioid analgesic

> Oral sol is available in 10mg/5mL, 20mg/5mL, and 100mg/5mL concentrations. The 100mg/5mL (20mg/mL) concentration is indicated for use in opioid-tolerant patients only. Use caution when prescribing and administering to avoid dosing errors due to confusion between different concentrations and between mg and mL, which could result in accidental overdose and death. Ensure the proper dose is communicated and dispensed. Keep sol out of reach of children. Seek emergency medical help immediately in case of accidental ingestion.

ADULT DOSAGE	PEDIATRIC DOSAGE
Moderate to Severe Pain	Pediatric use may not have been established
Acute and Chronic:	
Opioid-Naive Patients:	
Initial: 10-20mg (sol) or 15-30mg (tab) q4h prn	
Titrate: Adjust dose based on response to the initial dose	
Opioid-Tolerant Patients:	
Use the 100mg/5mL sol only for patients who have already been titrated to a stable analgesic regimen using lower strengths of morphine sulfate and who can benefit from use of a smaller volume of sol	
Conversions	
From Parenteral Morphine to Oral Morphine Sulfate:	
Anywhere from 3-6mg of oral morphine sulfate may be required to provide pain relief equivalent to 1mg of parenteral morphine	
From Parenteral/Oral Non-Morphine Opioids to Oral Morphine Sulfate:	
Adjust based on response to oral morphine sulfate; refer to published relative potency information	
From Controlled-Release Oral Morphine to Oral Morphine Sulfate:	
The same total amount of morphine sulfate is available from oral sol, tabs, and controlled-release and extended-release capsules; the extended duration of release of morphine sulfate results in reduced	

maximum and increased minimum plasma concentrations as compared to shorter acting morphine sulfate products. Dosage adjustment w/ close observation is necessary

DOSING CONSIDERATIONS
Renal Impairment
Start w/ lower doses and titrate slowly
Hepatic Impairment
Start w/ lower doses and titrate slowly
Elderly
Start at lower end of dosing range
Discontinuation
Gradually taper dose
ADMINISTRATION
Oral route
100mg/5mL Sol
Always use the enclosed calibrated oral syringe
STORAGE
20-25°C (68-77°F). Protect from moisture.
HOW SUPPLIED
Sol: 10mg/5mL [15mL, 100mL, 500mL], 20mg/5mL [100mL, 500mL], 100mg/5mL [15mL, 30mL, 120mL]; **Tab:** 15mg*, 30mg* *scored
CONTRAINDICATIONS
Known hypersensitivity to morphine, morphine salts, or any components of the product; respiratory depression in absence of resuscitative equipment; acute or severe bronchial asthma or hypercarbia; confirmed/suspected paralytic ileus.
WARNINGS/PRECAUTIONS
Respiratory depression occurs more frequently in elderly or debilitated patients and in those w/ conditions accompanied by hypoxia, hypercapnia, or upper airway obstruction. Caution and consider alternative nonopioid analgesics w/ COPD or cor pulmonale, and in patients having substantially decreased respiratory reserve (eg, severe kyphoscoliosis), hypoxia, hypercapnia, or preexisting respiratory depression; use only under careful medical supervision at the lowest effective dose. High potential for abuse; is subject to misuse, abuse, or diversion. Possible respiratory depressant effects and potential to elevate CSF pressure may be markedly exaggerated in the presence of head injury, intracranial lesions, or a preexisting increase in intracranial pressure (ICP); may produce effects on pupillary response and consciousness which may obscure neurologic signs of further increases in ICP in patients w/head injuries. May cause severe hypotension in patients whose ability to maintain BP has already been compromised by a depleted blood volume or concurrent administration of drugs (eg, phenothiazines, general anesthetics). May produce orthostatic hypotension and syncope in ambulatory patients. Caution w/ circulatory shock. Avoid w/GI obstruction, especially paralytic ileus; may prolong the obstruction. May obscure diagnosis or clinical course w/ acute abdominal conditions. Caution w/ biliary tract disease, including acute pancreatitis; may cause spasm of the sphincter of Oddi and diminish biliary and pancreatic secretions. Caution w/and reduce dose in patients w/ severe renal or hepatic impairment, Addison's disease, hypothyroidism, prostatic hypertrophy, or urethral stricture, and in elderly or debilitated patients. Caution w/ CNS depression, toxic psychosis, acute alcoholism, and delirium tremens. May aggravate convulsions in patients w/ convulsive disorders and may induce/aggravate seizures. May impair mental/physical abilities. (100mg/5mL Sol) May cause fatal respiratory depression when administered to patients who are not tolerant to the respiratory depressant effects of opioids. Use only for patients who have already been titrated to a stable analgesic regimen using lower strengths and who can benefit from use of a smaller volume of oral sol.
ADVERSE REACTIONS
Respiratory depression, apnea, circulatory depression, respiratory arrest, shock, cardiac arrest, lightheadedness, dizziness, sedation, N/V, sweating, constipation, somnolence.
DRUG INTERACTIONS
Caution w/ CNS depressants (eg, sedatives, hypnotics, general anesthetics, antiemetics, phenothiazines, alcohol); may increase risk of respiratory depression, hypotension, profound sedation, or coma. May enhance neuromuscular-blocking action of skeletal muscle relaxants and produce an increased degree of respiratory depression. Do not administer mixed agonist/antagonist analgesics (eg, pentazocine, nalbuphine, butorphanol) to patients who have received or are receiving a course of therapy w/ morphine; may reduce analgesic effect and/or may precipitate withdrawal symptoms. Apnea, confusion, and muscle twitching reported w/ cimetidine; monitor for increased respiratory and CNS depression. MAOIs potentiate action of morphine; allow at least 14 days after stopping MAOIs before initiating treatment. Anticholinergics or other medications w/ anticholinergic activity may increase risk of urinary retention and/or severe constipation, which may lead to paralytic ileus. Absorption/exposure may be increased w/ P-gp inhibitors (eg, quinidine); use w/ caution.
PREGNANCY AND LACTATION
Category C, not for use in nursing.
MECHANISM OF ACTION
Opioid analgesic; not established. Specific CNS opiate receptors and endogenous compounds w/ morphine-like activity have been identified throughout the brain and spinal cord and are likely to play a role in the expression and perception of analgesic effects. Causes respiratory depression, in part by a direct effect on the brainstem respiratory centers, and depresses cough reflex by direct effect on the cough center in the medulla.

PHARMACOKINETICS
Absorption: Bioavailability (<40%); C_{max}=78ng/mL (tab), 58ng/mL (sol). **Distribution:** V_d=1-6L/kg; plasma protein binding (20-35%); crosses placenta, found in breast milk. **Metabolism:** Liver via conjugation; morphine-6-glucuronide (active analgesic), morphine-3-glucuronide (M3G) (inactive as analgesic). **Elimination:** Urine (10% unchanged), feces (7-10%); $T_{1/2}$=2 hrs (IV).
PATIENT CONSIDERATIONS
Assessment: Assess for hypersensitivity to the drug or to any components of the product, drug abuse/addiction risk, prior opioid therapy, opioid tolerance, respiratory depression, or any other conditions where treatment is contraindicated or cautioned, pregnancy/nursing status, and for possible drug interactions.

Monitoring: Monitor for respiratory depression, CSF pressure elevation, orthostatic hypotension, syncope, aggravation of convulsions/seizures, and other adverse reactions. During chronic therapy, especially for noncancer-related pain, periodically reassess the continued need for the use of therapy.

Counseling: Advise to take only ud and not to adjust dose w/o consulting a physician. Inform that the drug may impair the ability to perform potentially hazardous activities (eg, operating machinery/driving); advise to refrain from any potentially dangerous activity until it is established that patient is not adversely affected. Advise to avoid CNS depressants except by the orders of the prescribing physician, and to avoid alcohol during therapy. Instruct women of childbearing potential who become or are planning to become pregnant to consult physician prior to therapy; advise that prolonged use during pregnancy may cause fetal-neonatal physical dependence and neonatal withdrawal may also occur. Counsel on the importance of safely tapering the dose if patient has been receiving therapy for more than a few weeks and cessation of therapy is indicated. Inform that drug has a potential for abuse and should be protected from theft and never be given to anyone other than for whom it was prescribed. Instruct to keep in a secure place out of reach of children, and that when no longer needed, destroy the unused sol/tabs by flushing down the toilet. Inform of the most common adverse events that may occur during therapy and the potential for severe constipation.

MOVANTIK — naloxegol   **Rx**

Class: Opioid antagonist

ADULT DOSAGE	PEDIATRIC DOSAGE
Opioid-Induced Constipation **In Patients W/ Chronic Non-Cancer Pain:** **Usual:** 25mg qd in am; reduce dose to 12.5mg qd if not tolerated D/C all maint laxative therapy prior to initiation of therapy Laxative(s) can be used prn, if suboptimal response to therapy after 3 days	Pediatric use may not have been established

DOSING CONSIDERATIONS
Concomitant Medications
Moderate CYP3A4 Inhibitors: Avoid use; reduce dose to 12.5mg qd and monitor for adverse reactions if use is unavoidable
Renal Impairment
CrCl <60mL/min:
Initial: 12.5mg qd
Titrate: If dosage is well tolerated but opioid-induced constipation symptoms continue, may increase dose to 25mg qd taking into consideration potential for markedly increased exposures in some patients w/ renal impairment and increased risk of adverse reactions w/ higher exposures
Hepatic Impairment
Severe (Child-Pugh Class C): Avoid use
Discontinuation
D/C therapy if treatment w/ the opioid pain medication is also discontinued
Other Important Considerations
Shown to be efficacious in patients who have taken opioids for at least 4 weeks
Avoid consumption of grapefruit or grapefruit juice during treatment
ADMINISTRATION
Oral route
Take on an empty stomach at least 1 hr prior to or 2 hrs after the 1st meal of the day
Swallow tab whole, do not crush or chew
STORAGE
20-25°C (68-77°F); excursions permitted to 15-30°C (59-86°F).
HOW SUPPLIED
Tab: 12.5mg, 25mg
CONTRAINDICATIONS
Known/suspected GI obstruction and patients at increased risk of recurrent obstruction, concomitant use of strong CYP3A4 inhibitors (eg, clarithromycin, ketoconazole), known serious or severe hypersensitivity reaction to naloxegol or any of its excipients.
WARNINGS/PRECAUTIONS
GI perforation may occur in patients w/ conditions that may be associated w/ localized or diffuse reduction of structural integrity in the wall of the GI tract

(eg, peptic ulcer disease, Ogilvie's syndrome, diverticular disease, infiltrative GI tract malignancies); caution in patients w/ these conditions and in patients w/ other conditions which might result in impaired integrity of the GI tract wall (eg, Crohn's disease). D/C in patients who develop severe, persistent, or worsening abdominal pain. Clusters of symptoms consistent w/ opioid withdrawal (eg, hyperhidrosis, chills, diarrhea) reported. Patients receiving methadone as therapy for pain were reported to have higher frequency of GI adverse reactions that may have been related to opioid withdrawal than patients receiving other opioids. May be at increased risk for opioid withdrawal or reduced analgesia in patients w/ disruptions to the blood-brain barrier; use w/ caution.

ADVERSE REACTIONS
Abdominal pain, diarrhea, N/V, flatulence, headache, hyperhidrosis.

DRUG INTERACTIONS
See Dosing Considerations and Contraindications. Potential for additive effect of opioid receptor antagonism and increased risk of opioid withdrawal w/ other opioid antagonists; avoid use w/ another opioid antagonist. Strong CYP3A4 inducers (eg, rifampin, carbamazepine, St. John's wort) may significantly decrease plasma levels and efficacy; not recommended for use w/ strong CYP3A4 inducers. Grapefruit or grapefruit juice may increase plasma levels.

PREGNANCY AND LACTATION
Category C, not for use in nursing.

MECHANISM OF ACTION
Opioid antagonist; antagonist of opioid binding at the mu-opioid receptor. Peripherally acts as mu-opioid receptor antagonist in tissues such as the GI tract, thereby decreasing the constipating effects of opioids.

PHARMACOKINETICS
Absorption: T_{max}<2 hrs. **Distribution:** V_d=968-2140L; plasma protein binding (4.2%). **Metabolism:** CYP3A; N-dealkylation, O-demethylation, oxidation, and partial loss of the PEG chain. **Elimination:** Feces (68%, approx 16% unchanged), urine (16%, <6% parent); $T_{1/2}$= 6-11 hrs.

PATIENT CONSIDERATIONS

Assessment: Assess for serious/severe hypersensitivity reaction to the drug or any of its excipients, GI obstruction, increased risk of recurrent GI obstruction, conditions associated w/ localized or diffuse reduction of structural integrity in the wall of the GI tract, conditions which might result in impaired integrity of GI tract wall, disruptions to the blood-brain barrier, renal/hepatic impairment, pregnancy/nursing status, and other possible drug interactions.

Monitoring: Monitor for signs/symptoms of GI perforation, severe/persistent/ worsening abdominal pain, opioid withdrawal symptoms, and other adverse reactions.

Counseling: Advise to take exactly ud. Counsel to inform physician when starting or stopping any concomitant medication. Advise to d/c therapy and to promptly seek medical attention if unusually severe, persistent, or worsening abdominal pain develops. Inform that clusters of symptoms consistent w/ opioid withdrawal may occur while taking therapy. Counsel that taking methadone as therapy for pain condition may increase likelihood of having GI adverse reactions that may be related to opioid withdrawal. Advise females of reproductive potential that the use of drug during pregnancy may precipitate opioid withdrawal in a fetus. Advise females who are nursing against breastfeeding during treatment due to potential for opioid withdrawal in nursing infants.

MoviPrep — ascorbic acid/polyethylene glycol 3350/potassium chloride/sodium ascorbate/sodium chloride/sodium sulfate   Rx

Class: Bowel cleanser

ADULT DOSAGE
Bowel Cleansing

Prior to Colonoscopy:
Split-Dose (2-Day) Regimen (Preferred Method):
Take Dose 1 the pm before the colonoscopy (10-12 hrs before Dose 2) and then take Dose 2 the next morning on the day of the colonoscopy, starting at least 3.5 hrs prior to colonoscopy

Evening-Only (1-Day) Regimen (Alternative Method):
Take Dose 1 at least 3.5 hrs before hs the pm before the colonoscopy and then take Dose 2 about 1.5 hrs after starting Dose 1 on the pm before the colonoscopy

PEDIATRIC DOSAGE
Pediatric use may not have been established

ADMINISTRATION
Oral route
- Take 2 separate doses in conjunction w/ fluids.
- Drink only clear liquids up to 2 hrs before the colonoscopy or as prescribed by healthcare provider and then stop drinking liquids until after the colonoscopy.
- Take w/in 24 hrs after it is mixed in water; do not add other ingredients to the sol.

Split-Dose (2-Day) Regimen (Preferred Method)
Dose 1:
1. Empty the contents of 1 Pouch A and 1 Pouch B into the container.
2. Add lukewarm water to the fill line on the container and mix.

3. Drink one 8-oz glass (240mL) every 15 min; be sure to drink all of the sol. This should take about 1 hr.
4. Fill the container w/ 16 oz (two 8-oz glasses) of clear liquid and drink all of this liquid before going to bed.
Dose 2:
1. Repeat steps 1-3 from Dose 1 instructions.
2. Fill the container w/ 16 oz (two 8-oz glasses) of clear liquid and drink all of this liquid at least 2 hrs before the colonoscopy.

Evening-Only (1-Day) Regimen (Alternative Method)
Dose 1:
1. Empty the contents of 1 Pouch A and 1 Pouch B into the container.
2. Add lukewarm water to the fill line on the container and mix.
3. Drink one 8-oz glass (240mL) every 15 min; be sure to drink all of the sol. This should take about 1 hr.
Dose 2:
1. Repeat steps 1-3 from Dose 1 instructions.
2. Fill the container again to the fill line w/ clear liquid and drink all of this liquid before going to bed.

STORAGE
20-25°C (68-77°F); excursions permitted to 15-30°C (59-86°F). **Reconstituted Sol:** Store upright and keep refrigerated. Use w/in 24 hrs.

HOW SUPPLIED
Sol (Powder): Pouch A (Polyethylene Glycol 3350/Sodium Sulfate/Sodium Chloride/Potassium Chloride) 100g/7.5g/2.691g/1.015g; Pouch B (Ascorbic Acid/Sodium Ascorbate) 4.7g/5.9g

CONTRAINDICATIONS
GI obstruction, bowel perforation, gastric retention, ileus, toxic colitis, toxic megacolon, hypersensitivity to any components of MoviPrep.

WARNINGS/PRECAUTIONS
Consume only clear liquids (no solid food) from the start of treatment until after the colonoscopy. Do not consume any clear liquids at least 2 hrs before the colonoscopy. Adequately hydrate before, during, and after use. If significant vomiting or signs of dehydration develop, consider performing postcolonoscopy lab tests (electrolytes, SrCr, and BUN). Correct electrolyte abnormalities before treatment. Consider performing predose and postcolonoscopy lab tests in patients w/ known or suspected hyponatremia. Serious arrhythmias reported (rare); use w/ caution and consider predose and postcolonoscopy ECGs in patients at increased risk of serious cardiac arrhythmias. Generalized tonic-clonic seizures and/or loss of consciousness reported (rare); caution in patients w/ a history of or at increased risk of seizures (eg, w/ known/suspected hyponatremia). Caution w/ impaired renal function. May produce colonic mucosal aphthous ulcerations; consider this when interpreting colonoscopy findings in patients w/ known/suspected inflammatory bowel disease. Serious cases of ischemic colitis reported. If severe bloating, abdominal distention/pain occurs, slow administration or temporarily d/c until symptoms abate. Caution w/ severe ulcerative colitis; w/ impaired gag reflex; in patients prone to regurgitation/aspiration; or w/ G6PD deficiency, especially in G6PD-deficient patients w/ an active infection, history of hemolysis, or taking concomitant medications known to precipitate hemolytic reactions. Contains phenylalanine.

ADVERSE REACTIONS
Split Dosing: Malaise, N/V, abdominal pain, upper abdominal pain.
Evening Only Dosing: Abdominal distension, anal discomfort, thirst, nausea, abdominal pain, sleep disorder, rigors, hunger, malaise, vomiting, dizziness.

DRUG INTERACTIONS
Increased risk of colonic mucosal aphthous ulcerations w/ stimulant laxatives; concurrent use not recommended. Caution w/ drugs that increase risk of electrolyte abnormalities (eg, diuretics, ACE inhibitors, ARBs) or affect renal function (eg, NSAIDs). Caution w/ drugs that lower seizure threshold (eg, TCAs) and in patients withdrawing from alcohol or benzodiazepines. Caution w/ drugs that increase the risk of arrhythmias and prolonged QT in the setting of fluid and electrolyte abnormalities. Consider additional patient evaluations as appropriate. Oral medication administered w/in 1 hr of the start of administration may be flushed from GI tract and may not be absorbed.

PREGNANCY AND LACTATION
Pregnancy: Category C.
Lactation: Caution in nursing.

MECHANISM OF ACTION
Bowel cleanser; action thought to be through the osmotic effect that causes water to be retained in the colon and produces a watery stool.

PATIENT CONSIDERATIONS

Assessment: Assess for GI obstruction, bowel perforation, gastric retention, ileus, toxic colitis, toxic megacolon, electrolyte abnormalities, G6PD deficiency, renal impairment, drug hypersensitivity, any other conditions where treatment is cautioned, pregnancy/nursing status, and possible drug interactions. Consider performing predose lab tests (electrolytes, SrCr, and BUN) in patients w/ electrolyte abnormalities or renal impairment. Consider predose ECGs in patients at increased risk of serious cardiac arrhythmias.

Monitoring: Monitor for arrhythmias, generalized tonic-clonic seizures, loss of consciousness, colonic mucosal aphthous ulceration, ischemic colitis, bloating, abdominal distention/pain, and other adverse reactions. Monitor patients w/ impaired gag reflex and patients prone to regurgitation/aspiration. Consider performing postcolonoscopy lab tests (electrolytes, SrCr, BUN) in patients who develop significant vomiting or signs of dehydration after taking therapy, in patients w/ electrolyte abnormalities, and in patients w/ renal impairment. Consider postcolonoscopy ECGs in patients at increased risk of serious cardiac arrhythmias.

Counseling: Inform patients who require a low phenylalanine diet that the product contains a max of 233mg aspartame/treatment (provides 131mg phenylalanine). Instruct to inform physician if patient has trouble swallowing or is prone to regurgitation/aspiration. Inform that each pouch needs to be diluted in water before ingestion and instruct to drink additional clear liquid. Inform that oral medications may not be absorbed properly if taken w/in 1 hr of starting each dose of MoviPrep. Instruct not to take other laxatives during therapy. Advise to adequately hydrate before, during, and after use. Explain that clear soup and/or plain yogurt may be taken for dinner, finishing at least 1 hr prior to treatment. Inform that the 1st bowel movement may occur 1 hr after the start of administration, and abdominal bloating and distention may occur before the 1st bowel movement. If severe abdominal discomfort or distention occurs, advise to stop treatment temporarily or drink each portion at longer intervals until symptoms diminish; if severe symptoms persist, instruct to notify physician. Instruct to consume only clear liquids (no solid food) from the start of treatment until after the colonoscopy. Instruct not to consume any clear liquids at least 2 hrs before the colonoscopy.

MOXATAG — amoxicillin   Rx

Class: Semisynthetic ampicillin derivative

ADULT DOSAGE	PEDIATRIC DOSAGE
Tonsillitis and/or Pharyngitis	**Tonsillitis and/or Pharyngitis**
Secondary to *Streptococcus pyogenes*:	**Secondary to *Streptococcus pyogenes*:**
775mg qd for 10 days	**≥12 Years:**
	775mg qd for 10 days

DOSING CONSIDERATIONS
Renal Impairment
Severe (CrCl <30mL/min)/Hemodialysis: Not recommended

ADMINISTRATION
Oral route
Take w/in 1 hr of finishing a meal
Do not chew or crush

STORAGE
25°C (77°F); excursions permitted to 15-30°C (59-86°).

HOW SUPPLIED
Tab, Extended-Release: 775mg

CONTRAINDICATIONS
Known serious hypersensitivity to amoxicillin or to other drugs in the same class or anaphylactic reactions to β-lactams.

WARNINGS/PRECAUTIONS
Serious, occasionally fatal, hypersensitivity (anaphylactic) reactions may occur; increased risk w/ a history of penicillin hypersensitivity and/or history of sensitivity to multiple allergens. D/C if allergic reaction occurs and institute appropriate therapy. *Clostridium difficile*-associated diarrhea (CDAD) reported; may need to d/c if CDAD is suspected or confirmed. May result in bacterial resistance w/ use in the absence of a proven/suspected bacterial infection or a prophylactic indication; d/c and institute appropriate therapy if superinfection develops. Avoid w/ mononucleosis; may cause erythematous skin rash. Lab test interactions may occur. Caution in elderly.

ADVERSE REACTIONS
Vulvovaginal mycotic infection, diarrhea, N/V, abdominal pain, headache.

DRUG INTERACTIONS
Concurrent use w/ probenecid may increase/prolong levels; decreases renal tubular secretion of amoxicillin. Chloramphenicol, macrolides, sulfonamides, and tetracyclines may interfere w/ bactericidal effects. Lowers estrogen reabsorption and potentially reduces efficacy of combined oral estrogen/progesterone contraceptives.

PREGNANCY AND LACTATION
Category B, caution in nursing.

MECHANISM OF ACTION
Ampicillin analogue; has bactericidal action against susceptible organisms during the stage of multiplication. Acts through the inhibition of cell wall biosynthesis that leads to the death of the bacteria.

PHARMACOKINETICS
Absorption: C_{max}=6.6mcg/mL. T_{max}=3.1 hrs. AUC=29.8mcg·h/mL. **Distribution:** Plasma protein binding (20%). **Elimination:** Urine [60% unchanged (immediate release)]; $T_{1/2}$=1.5 hrs.

PATIENT CONSIDERATIONS
Assessment: Assess for known serious hypersensitivity reactions to the drug or to other drugs in the same class, anaphylactic reactions to β-lactams, mononucleosis, renal impairment, pregnancy/nursing status, and for possible drug interactions.

Monitoring: Monitor for serious anaphylactic and hypersensitivity reactions, erythematous skin rash, development of drug resistance or superinfection, signs/symptoms of CDAD, and other adverse reactions. Monitor renal function, particularly in elderly.

Counseling: Instruct to take w/in 1 hr of finishing a meal and at approx the same time every day. Instruct not to chew or crush tab. Inform that no other forms of immediate-release amoxicillin can be substituted for this therapy. Instruct to take exactly ud; explain that skipping doses or not completing full course may decrease effectiveness and increase resistance. Advise to notify physician immediately if serious hypersensitivity reactions occur. Instruct to notify physician as soon as possible if watery and bloody stools (w/ or w/o stomach cramps and fever) develop, even as late as 2 or more months after the last dose of therapy.

MOXEZA — moxifloxacin hydrochloride   Rx

Class: Fluoroquinolone

ADULT DOSAGE	PEDIATRIC DOSAGE
Bacterial Conjunctivitis	**Bacterial Conjunctivitis**
1 drop in the affected eye(s) bid for 7 days	**≥4 Months of Age:**
	1 drop in the affected eye(s) bid for 7 days

ADMINISTRATION
Ocular route

STORAGE
2-25°C (36-77°F).

HOW SUPPLIED
Sol: 0.5% [3mL]

WARNINGS/PRECAUTIONS
For topical ophthalmic use only; should not be injected subconjunctivally or introduced directly into the anterior chamber of the eye. Serious and sometimes fatal hypersensitivity reactions reported w/ systemic use; d/c and institute appropriate therapy if allergic reaction occurs. Prolonged use may cause overgrowth of nonsusceptible organisms, including fungi. D/C use and consider alternative therapy if superinfection occurs. Avoid wearing contact lenses when signs/symptoms of bacterial conjunctivitis are present.

ADVERSE REACTIONS
Eye irritation, pyrexia, conjunctivitis.

PREGNANCY AND LACTATION
Category C, caution in nursing.

MECHANISM OF ACTION
Fluoroquinolone antibiotic; inhibition of topoisomerase II (DNA gyrase) and topoisomerase IV.

PHARMACOKINETICS
Absorption: AUC=8.17ng·hr/mL. **Distribution:** Presumed to be excreted in breast milk.

PATIENT CONSIDERATIONS
Assessment: Assess severity of infection, symptoms, and pregnancy/nursing status.

Monitoring: Monitor for signs/symptoms of hypersensitivity/anaphylactic reactions and other adverse reactions. Monitor for overgrowth of nonsusceptible organisms and superinfection w/ prolonged use.

Counseling: Advise on proper use to prevent bacterial contamination. Instruct to d/c medication and contact physician at the 1st sign of rash or an allergic reaction. Advise not to wear contact lenses if signs/symptoms of bacterial conjunctivitis are present.

MS CONTIN — morphine sulfate   CII

Class: Opioid analgesic

> Exposes users to the risks of opioid addiction, abuse, and misuse, leading to overdose and death; assess each patient's risk prior to prescribing therapy and monitor regularly for the development of these behaviors/conditions. Serious, life-threatening, or fatal respiratory depression may occur; monitor during initiation or following a dose increase. Crushing, chewing, or dissolving tab can cause rapid release and absorption of a potentially fatal dose; instruct to swallow tab whole. Accidental ingestion, especially in children, can result in fatal overdose. Prolonged use during pregnancy can result in neonatal opioid withdrawal syndrome; advise pregnant women of the risk and ensure availability of appropriate treatment.

ADULT DOSAGE	PEDIATRIC DOSAGE
Severe Pain (Daily, Around-the-Clock Management)	Pediatric use may not have been established
Use as 1st Opioid Analgesic:	
Initial: 15mg q8h or q12h	
Titrate: Dose adjustments may be done every 1-2 days	
Opioid Intolerant Patients:	
Initial: 15mg q12h	
Titrate: Dose adjustments may be done every 1-2 days	
Breakthrough Pain:	
May require a dose increase, or may need rescue medication w/ an immediate-release analgesic	
Conversions	
From Other Oral Morphine:	
Administer 1/2 of 24 hr requirement on an q12h schedule or administer 1/3 of the daily requirement on an q8h schedule	
From Other Opioids:	
D/C all other around-the-clock opioids when therapy is initiated and initiate dosing at 15mg q8-12h	
From Parenteral Morphine:	
Ratio: 2-6mg of oral morphine may be required to provide analgesia	

equivalent to 1mg of parenteral morphine; typically, a dose of morphine that is approximately 3X the previous daily parenteral morphine requirement is sufficient

From Other Non-Morphine Opioids (Parenteral or Oral):
Begin w/ 1/2 the estimated daily morphine requirement as initial dose, managing inadequate analgesia by supplementation w/ immediate-release morphine

---

DOSING CONSIDERATIONS
Discontinuation
Use a gradual downward titration of the dose; do not abruptly d/c

ADMINISTRATION
Oral route

Swallow tab whole; do not crush, dissolve, or chew

STORAGE
25°C (77°F); excursions permitted between 15-30°C (59-86°F).

HOW SUPPLIED
Tab, Extended-Release: 15mg, 30mg, 60mg, 100mg, 200mg

CONTRAINDICATIONS
Significant respiratory depression, acute or severe bronchial asthma in an unmonitored setting or in the absence of resuscitative equipment, known or suspected paralytic ileus, hypersensitivity (eg, anaphylaxis) to morphine.

WARNINGS/PRECAUTIONS
Reserve for use in patients for whom alternative treatment options are ineffective, not tolerated, or would be otherwise inadequate to provide sufficient management of pain. Should be prescribed only by healthcare professionals who are knowledgeable in the use of potent opioids for the management of chronic pain. Life-threatening respiratory depression is more likely to occur in elderly, cachectic, or debilitated patients. Consider alternative nonopioid analgesics in patients with significant COPD or cor pulmonale, and in patients having a substantially decreased respiratory reserve, hypoxia, hypercapnia, or preexisting respiratory depression. May cause severe hypotension, orthostatic hypotension, and syncope; increased risk in patients whose ability to maintain BP has already been compromised by a reduced blood volume or concurrent administration of certain CNS depressants. Avoid with circulatory shock, impaired consciousness, or coma. Monitor patients who may be susceptible to intracranial effects of carbon dioxide retention for signs of sedation and respiratory depression, particularly when initiating therapy. Therapy may obscure clinical course in patients with head injury. Avoid with GI obstruction. May cause spasm of sphincter of Oddi and increase in serum amylase; monitor for worsening symptoms with biliary tract disease (eg, acute pancreatitis). May aggravate convulsions in patients with convulsive disorders and may induce or aggravate seizures. May impair mental/physical abilities. Caution in elderly. Not recommended for use during or immediately prior to labor.

ADVERSE REACTIONS
Respiratory depression, constipation, dizziness, sedation, N/V, sweating, dysphoria, euphoric mood.

DRUG INTERACTIONS
Respiratory depression, hypotension, profound sedation, or coma may occur with CNS depressants (eg, sedatives, hypnotics, neuroleptics, alcohol); if coadministration is considered, reduce dose of one or both agents. Mixed agonist/antagonist (eg, pentazocine, nalbuphine, butorphanol) and partial agonist (buprenorphine) may reduce analgesic effect or precipitate withdrawal symptoms; avoid coadministration. May enhance neuromuscular-blocking action of skeletal muscle relaxants and produce increased respiratory depression. MAOIs have been reported to potentiate the effects of morphine anxiety, confusion, and significant depression of respiration or coma; avoid use or within 14 days of MAOI use. Cimetidine may potentiate morphine-induced respiratory depression. May reduce efficacy of diuretics. May lead to acute urine retention, particularly in men with enlarged prostates. Anticholinergics or other drugs with anticholinergic activity may increase risk of urinary retention and/or severe constipation, which may lead to paralytic ileus. Absorption/exposure may be increased with P-gp inhibitors (eg, quinidine) by about 2-fold; monitor for signs of respiratory and CNS depression.

PREGNANCY AND LACTATION
Category C, not for use in nursing.

MECHANISM OF ACTION
Opioid analgesic; acts as a full agonist, binding with and activating opioid receptors at sites in the periaqueductal and periventricular grey matter, the ventromedial medulla, and the spinal cord to produce analgesia.

PHARMACOKINETICS
Absorption: Oral bioavailability (20-40%). **Distribution:** V_d=3-4L/kg; plasma protein binding (30-35%); distributed to skeletal muscle, kidneys, liver, intestinal tract, lungs, spleen, and brain; crosses placental membranes; found in breast milk. **Metabolism:** Liver via glucuronidation and sulfation; (metabolites) morphine-3-glucuronide (M3G, about 50%), morphine-6-glucuronide (about 5-15%), morphine-3-ethereal sulfate. **Elimination:** Urine (primarily as M3G, 10% unchanged), bile (small amount of glucuronide conjugate); (IV) $T_{1/2}$=2-4 hrs.

PATIENT CONSIDERATIONS
Assessment: Assess for drug abuse/addiction risk, prior opioid therapy, opioid tolerance, respiratory depression, drug hypersensitivity, COPD or other respiratory

complications, GI obstruction, paralytic ileus, head injury, history of seizure, pregnancy/nursing status, possible drug interactions, and any other conditions where treatment is contraindicated or cautioned.

Monitoring: Monitor for signs/symptoms of respiratory depression (especially within first 24-72 hrs of initiation), hypotension, symptoms of worsening biliary tract disease, aggravation/induction of seizures, tolerance, physical dependence, mental/physical impairment, and other adverse reactions. Routinely monitor for signs of misuse, abuse, and addiction. Periodically reassess the continued need for therapy.

Counseling: Inform that use of drug can result in addiction, abuse, and misuse; instruct not to share drug with others and to take steps to protect from theft or misuse. Inform about risk of life-threatening respiratory depression; advise how to recognize respiratory depression and to seek medical attention if breathing difficulties develop. Advise to store drug securely; accidental exposure, especially in children, can result in serious harm/death. Instruct to dispose unused drug by flushing down the toilet. Inform females of reproductive potential that prolonged use during pregnancy may result in neonatal opioid withdrawal syndrome. Inform that potentially serious additive effects may occur when used with alcohol or other CNS depressants, and advise not to use such drugs unless supervised by physician. Instruct on how to take the medication properly. Inform that drug may cause orthostatic hypotension and syncope, and may impair the ability to perform potentially hazardous activities; advise to not perform such tasks until they know how they will react to medication. Advise of the potential for severe constipation (including management instructions), on how to recognize anaphylaxis, and when to seek medical attention. Inform females that drug can cause fetal harm; instruct to notify physician if pregnant/planning to become pregnant.

MULTAQ — dronedarone   Rx

Class: Class III antiarrhythmic

> Doubles the risk of death in patients with symptomatic heart failure (HF), with recent decompensation, requiring hospitalization or NYHA Class IV HF; contraindicated in these patients. Doubles the risk of death, stroke, and hospitalization for HF in patients with permanent A-fib; contraindicated in patients in A-fib who will not or cannot be cardioverted into normal sinus rhythm.

ADULT DOSAGE
Atrial Fibrillation

Reduce Risk of Hospitalization for Patients in Sinus Rhythm w/ History of Paroxysmal/Persistent A-Fib:
400mg bid (w/ am and pm meal)

PEDIATRIC DOSAGE
Pediatric use may not have been established

ADMINISTRATION
Oral route

Take once w/ am meal and again w/ pm meal

STORAGE
25°C (77°F); excursions permitted to 15-30°C (59-86°F).

HOW SUPPLIED
Tab: 400mg

CONTRAINDICATIONS
Permanent A-fib, symptomatic HF with recent decompensation requiring hospitalization or NYHA Class IV symptoms, 2nd- or 3rd-degree atrioventricular block or sick sinus syndrome (except when used with a functioning pacemaker), bradycardia <50 bpm, liver or lung toxicity related to previous use of amiodarone, QTc Bazett interval ≥500 msec or PR interval >280 msec, severe hepatic impairment, women who are or may become pregnant, nursing mothers. Concomitant use of strong CYP3A inhibitors (eg, ketoconazole, clarithromycin, nefazodone), drugs or herbal products that prolong QT interval and might increase risk of torsades de pointes (eg, phenothiazine antipsychotics, TCAs, certain oral macrolide antibiotics, Class I and III antiarrhythmics). Hypersensitivity to the active substance or to any of the excipients.

WARNINGS/PRECAUTIONS
Monitor cardiac rhythm no less than every 3 months. Cardiovert patients or d/c drug if patients are in A-fib. Only initiate in patients who are receiving appropriate antithrombotic therapy. New onset or worsening of HF reported; d/c if HF develops or worsens and requires hospitalization. Hepatocellular liver injury (including acute liver failure requiring transplant) reported; d/c if hepatic injury is suspected and test serum enzymes, AST, ALT, alkaline phosphatase, and serum bilirubin; do not restart therapy without another explanation for observed liver injury. Interstitial lung disease (including pneumonitis and pulmonary fibrosis) reported. Onset of dyspnea or nonproductive cough may be related to pulmonary toxicity; evaluate patients carefully. D/C if pulmonary toxicity is confirmed. K^+ levels should be within normal range prior to and during therapy. May induce moderate QTc (Bazett) prolongation. Increase in SrCr, prerenal azotemia, and acute renal failure often in the setting of HF or hypovolemia reported. Premenopausal women who have not undergone hysterectomy/oophorectomy must use effective contraception while on therapy.

ADVERSE REACTIONS
QT prolongation, SrCr increase, diarrhea, N/V, abdominal pain, asthenic conditions, bradycardia, rashes, pruritus, eczema, dermatitis, allergic dermatitis.

DRUG INTERACTIONS
See Contraindications. Hypokalemia/hypomagnesemia may occur with K^+-depleting diuretics. May increase exposure to digoxin. Digoxin may also potentiate electrophysiologic effects; consider discontinuing or 1/2 the dose of digoxin and closely monitor serum levels and for toxicity if digoxin treatment is continued.

Calcium channel blockers (CCBs) may potentiate effects on conduction and may increase exposure. Bradycardia more frequently observed with β-blockers. Give a low dose of CCBs or β-blockers initially and increase only after ECG verification of good tolerability. Avoid grapefruit juice, rifampin, or other CYP3A inducers (eg, phenobarbital, carbamazepine, St. John's wort). May increase exposure of simvastatin/simvastatin acid, CCBs, dabigatran, P-glycoprotein substrates, and CYP2D6 substrates (eg, β-blockers, TCAs, SSRIs). Avoid doses >10mg qd of simvastatin. May increase plasma levels of tacrolimus, sirolimus, and other CYP3A substrates with a narrow therapeutic range; monitor concentrations and adjust dosage appropriately. Clinically significant INR elevations with oral anticoagulants and increased S-warfarin exposure reported; monitor INR after initiating therapy in patients taking warfarin.

PREGNANCY AND LACTATION
Category X, not for use in nursing.

MECHANISM OF ACTION
Benzofuran derivative; has not been established. Has antiarrhythmic properties belonging to all 4 Vaughan-Williams classes.

PHARMACOKINETICS
Absorption: Absolute bioavailability (4% without food, 15% with high-fat meal); T_{max}=3-6 hrs (fed). **Distribution:** Plasma protein binding (>98%); (IV) V_d=1400L. **Metabolism:** Extensive via CYP3A; N-debutylation; N-debutyl metabolite (active). **Elimination:** Urine (6%, metabolites), feces (84%, metabolites); $T_{1/2}$=13-19 hrs.

PATIENT CONSIDERATIONS
Assessment: Assess for recent HF decompensation, permanent A-fib, hepatic impairment, any other conditions where treatment is contraindicated/cautioned, pregnancy/nursing status, and possible drug interactions. Assess serum K^+ levels.

Monitoring: Monitor for signs/symptoms of new/worsening HF, hepatic injury, pulmonary toxicity, and QT interval prolongation. Monitor cardiac rhythm no less than every 3 months, hepatic serum enzymes periodically, especially during first 6 months, and renal function periodically.

Counseling: Instruct to take with meals and not to take with grapefruit juice. If a dose is missed, advise to take next dose at the regularly scheduled time and not to double the dose. Counsel to consult physician if signs/symptoms of HF or potential liver injury occur and before stopping the treatment. Advise to inform physician of any history of HF, rhythm disturbance other than A-fib or atrial flutter, or predisposing conditions, such as uncorrected hypokalemia. Advise to report any use of other prescription, nonprescription medication, or herbal products, particularly St. John's wort. Counsel patients of childbearing potential about appropriate contraceptive choices while on therapy.

MUSE — alprostadil   Rx
Class: Prostaglandin E₁

ADULT DOSAGE	PEDIATRIC DOSAGE
Erectile Dysfunction **Initial:** 125 or 250mcg **Titrate:** Adjust in a stepwise manner to the lowest dose sufficient to achieve an erection for sexual intercourse; titration should be carried out under medical supervision **Max:** 2 administrations/24 hrs Administer prn to achieve an erection	Pediatric use may not have been established

ADMINISTRATION
Transurethral route

For single use only

STORAGE
2-8°C (36-46°F). May be stored at <30°C (86°F) for up to 14 days prior to use. Do not expose >30°C (86°F).

HOW SUPPLIED
Sup: 125mcg, 250mcg, 500mcg, 1000mcg

CONTRAINDICATIONS
Known hypersensitivity to alprostadil, abnormal penile anatomy (eg, urethral stricture, balanitis, severe hypospadias and curvature, acute/chronic urethritis), venous thrombosis predisposition or hyperviscosity syndrome (eg, sickle cell anemia/trait, thrombocythemia, polycythemia, multiple myeloma), men for whom sexual activity is inadvisable, sexual intercourse with pregnant woman unless condom barrier is used.

WARNINGS/PRECAUTIONS
Symptomatic hypotension and syncope reported; use lowest effective dose. May impair mental/physical abilities. Exclude reversible causes of erectile dysfunction prior to initiation and seek underlying disorders that might preclude therapy. May cause urethral abrasion resulting in minor bleeding or spotting when administered improperly, especially in patients with bleeding disorders. Examine cardiac fitness prior to treatment. Priapism (≥6 hrs erection) and prolonged erection (4-<6 hrs erection) reported; lower dose or consider d/c.

ADVERSE REACTIONS
Penile pain, urethral burning, minor urethral bleeding, testicular pain, flu symptoms, headache, body pain, respiratory infection.

DRUG INTERACTIONS
May increase risk of bleeding with anticoagulants; consider risk/benefit ratio before prescribing. May increase risk of hypotension with antihypertensives; use with caution. Drugs that attenuate erectile function may influence response.

PREGNANCY AND LACTATION
Category C, not for use in nursing.

MECHANISM OF ACTION
Prostaglandin E₁; acts as a vasodilator; vasodilatory effects in the cavernosal arteries and the trabecular smooth muscle of the corpora cavernosa result in rapid arterial inflow and expansion of the lacunar spaces within the corpora. As the expanded corporal sinusoids are compressed against the tunica albuginea, venous outflow through subtunical vessels is impeded and penile rigidity develops.

PHARMACOKINETICS
Absorption: Rapid. C_{max}= 11.4pg/mL; T_{max}=16 min. **Metabolism:** Via enzymatic oxidation. **Elimination:** (IV) Urine (90%), feces. (Transurethral) Lungs; $T_{1/2}$=30 sec-10 min.

PATIENT CONSIDERATIONS
Assessment: Assess for previous hypersensitivity to drug, abnormal penile anatomy, venous thrombosis predisposition or hyperviscosity syndrome, cardiac status, partner's pregnancy status, and possible drug interactions. Obtain a complete medical and physical examination.

Monitoring: Monitor for symptoms of hypotension, syncope, priapism, and prolonged erection.

Counseling: Inform that the drug offers no protection from the transmission of sexually transmitted diseases (STDs). Counsel about protective measures necessary to guard against spread of STDs, including HIV. Inform that drug may cause painful erection sustained for hours and unrelieved by sexual intercourse or masturbation; instruct to seek medical attention promptly if prolonged erection occurs. Advise on how to administer the drug. Instruct to use condoms during intercourse if partner is pregnant. Counsel couples to use adequate contraception while on therapy.

MYALEPT — metreleptin   Rx
Class: Leptin analogue

> Anti-metreleptin antibodies w/ neutralizing activity have been identified; consequences may include inhibition of endogenous leptin action and/or loss of drug efficacy. Severe infection and/or worsening metabolic control reported; test for anti-metreleptin antibodies w/ neutralizing activity if severe infections or signs suspicious for loss of drug efficacy during treatment develop. T-cell lymphoma reported in patients w/ acquired generalized lipodystrophy; carefully consider the benefits and risks of treatment in patients w/ significant hematologic abnormalities and/or acquired generalized lipodystrophy. Available only through a restricted program under a Risk Evaluation and Mitigation Strategy (REMS) called the Myalept REMS Program.

ADULT DOSAGE	PEDIATRIC DOSAGE
Leptin Deficiency Adjunct to diet as replacement therapy to treat the complications of leptin deficiency in patients w/ congenital or acquired generalized lipodystrophy **≤40kg:** **Initial:** **Males and Females:** 0.06mg/kg (0.012mL/kg) **Dose Adjustment:** 0.02mg/kg (0.004mL/kg) **Max Daily Dose:** 0.13mg/kg (0.026mL/kg) **>40kg:** **Initial:** **Male:** 2.5mg (0.5mL) **Female:** 5mg (1mL) **Dose Adjustment:** 1.25-2.5mg (0.25-0.5mL) **Max Daily Dose:** 10mg (2mL)	**Leptin Deficiency** Adjunct to diet as replacement therapy to treat the complications of leptin deficiency in patients w/ congenital or acquired generalized lipodystrophy **≤40kg:** **Initial:** **Males and Females:** 0.06mg/kg (0.012mL/kg) **Dose Adjustment:** 0.02mg/kg (0.004mL/kg) **Max Daily Dose:** 0.13mg/kg (0.026mL/kg) **>40kg:** **Initial:** **Male:** 2.5mg (0.5mL) **Female:** 5mg (1mL) **Dose Adjustment:** 1.25-2.5mg (0.25-0.5mL) **Max Daily Dose:** 10mg (2mL)

DOSING CONSIDERATIONS
Elderly
Start at lower end of dosing range

Discontinuation
Patients at Risk for Pancreatitis:
Taper dose over a 1-week period. During tapering, monitor TG levels and consider initiating or adjusting dose of lipid-lowering medications prn

Other Important Considerations
Dose adjustments, including possible large reductions, of insulin or insulin secretagogue (eg, sulfonylurea) may be necessary; monitor blood glucose in patients on concomitant insulin therapy, especially those on high doses, or insulin secretagogue

ADMINISTRATION
SQ route

Should be administered at the same time every day.
May administer at any time of the day, w/o regard to the timing of meals.

Administer into the SQ tissue of the abdomen, thigh or upper arm; use different inj site each day when injecting in the same region.

After choosing an inj site, pinch the skin and at a 45° angle, inject the sol.

Avoid IM inj, especially in patients w/ minimal SQ adipose tissue.

Doses exceeding 1mL can be administered as 2 inj (the total daily dose divided equally) to minimize potential inj-site discomfort due to volume; when dividing doses due to volume, doses can be administered one after the other.

Reconstitution
Reconstitute w/ 2.2mL of sterile bacteriostatic water for inj (0.9% benzyl alcohol), or w/ 2.2mL of sterile water for inj.

Use w/in 3 days when stored refrigerated between 2-8°C (36-46°F) and protected from light.

For neonates and infants, reconstitute w/ preservative-free sterile water for inj and administer immediately.

Compatibility
Do not mix w/, or transfer into, the contents of another vial of metreleptin.

Do not add other medications, including insulin; use a separate syringe for insulin inj.

STORAGE
2-8°C (36-46°F). Do not freeze. Protect from light. Do not shake or vigorously agitate reconstituted vial. Refer to PI for further storage and handling instructions.

HOW SUPPLIED
Inj: 5mg/mL [11.3mg]

CONTRAINDICATIONS
General obesity not associated w/ congenital leptin deficiency, prior severe hypersensitivity reactions to metreleptin or to any of the product components.

WARNINGS/PRECAUTIONS
Not indicated for use w/ HIV-related lipodystrophy, or in patients w/ metabolic disease, including diabetes mellitus and hypertriglyceridemia, w/o concurrent evidence of congenital or acquired generalized lipodystrophy. Case of anaplastic large cell lymphoma reported. Cases of progression of autoimmune hepatitis and membranoproliferative glomerulonephritis (associated w/ massive proteinuria and renal failure) reported in patients w/ acquired generalized lipodystrophy; carefully consider the potential benefits and risks of treatment in patients w/ autoimmune disease. Generalized hypersensitivity reported; consider discontinuing if a hypersensitivity reaction occurs.

Contains benzyl alcohol when reconstituted w/ Bacteriostatic Water for Inj; preservative-free Water for Inj is recommended for use in neonates and infants. Caution in elderly.

ADVERSE REACTIONS
Headache, hypoglycemia, decreased weight, abdominal pain, arthralgia, dizziness, ear infection, fatigue, nausea, ovarian cyst, URTI, anemia, back pain, diarrhea, paresthesia.

DRUG INTERACTIONS
See Dosing Considerations. Caution w/ drugs metabolized by CYP450 (eg, oral contraceptives, drugs w/ a narrow therapeutic index); effect of metreleptin on CYP450 enzymes may be clinically relevant for CYP450 substrates w/ a narrow therapeutic index, where dose is individually adjusted. Upon initiation or discontinuation of metreleptin, in patients being treated w/ CYP450 substrates w/ a narrow therapeutic index, perform therapeutic monitoring of effect (eg, warfarin) or drug concentration (eg, cyclosporine, theophylline) and adjust the individual dose of the agent PRN.

PREGNANCY AND LACTATION
Pregnancy: Category C.
Lactation: Not for use in nursing.

MECHANISM OF ACTION
Recombinant Human Leptin Analog; binds to and activates human leptin receptor, which belongs to the Class I cytokine family of receptors that signals through the JAK/STAT transduction pathway.

PHARMACOKINETICS
Absorption: (Single dose, 0.1-0.3mg/kg SQ) T_{max}=4-4.3 hrs. **Distribution:** (IV) V_d=370mL/kg (0.3mg/kg/day), 398mL/kg (1mg/kg/day), 463mL/kg (3mg/kg/day). **Elimination:** Renal (major route); (single dose, 0.01-0.3mg/mL SQ) $T_{1/2}$=3.8-4.7 hrs.

PATIENT CONSIDERATIONS
Assessment: Assess for hypersensitivity to the drug, general obesity not associated w/ congenital leptin deficiency, risk factors of pancreatitis, hematologic abnormalities, pregnancy/nursing status, and possible drug interactions.

Monitoring: Monitor for severe infections, worsening metabolic control, T-cell lymphoma in patients w/ acquired generalized lipodystrophy, hypersensitivity reactions, and other adverse events. Test for anti-metreleptin antibodies w/ neutralizing activity in patients who develop severe infections or show signs suspicious for loss of metreleptin efficacy during treatment. When discontinuing therapy in patients w/ risk factors for pancreatitis, monitor TG levels. Closely monitor blood glucose levels in patients on concomitant insulin or insulin secretagogue therapy.

Counseling: Inform about the risks/benefits of therapy. Instruct that if a dose is missed, administer dose as soon as noticed, and resume the normal dosing schedule the next day. Inform on the signs/symptoms that would warrant antibody testing. Inform on the signs/symptoms that indicate changes in hematologic status and the importance of routine lab assessment and physician monitoring. Advise that the risk of hypoglycemia is increased w/ insulin or an insulin secretagogue; instruct to closely monitor blood glucose levels. Advise

patients w/ history of autoimmune disease on signs/symptoms that indicate exacerbation of underlying autoimmune disease and the importance of routine lab assessments and physician monitoring. Instruct to seek medical advice if symptoms of hypersensitivity occur. Advise nursing mothers that breastfeeding is not recommended. Inform patients/caregivers about proper preparation and administration of drug; advise that 1st dose should be administered under the supervision of a qualified healthcare professional. Instruct patients w/ a history of pancreatitis and/or severe hypertriglyceridemia to taper dose over a 1-week period when discontinuing therapy; advise that additional monitoring of TG levels and possible initiation or dose adjustment of lipid-lowering medications may be considered.

MYFORTIC — mycophenolic acid   **Rx**
Class: Inosine monophosphate dehydrogenase (IMPDH) inhibitor

> Use during pregnancy is associated w/ increased risks of pregnancy loss and congenital malformations; counsel females of reproductive potential regarding pregnancy prevention and planning. Immunosuppression may lead to increased risk of development of lymphoma and other malignancies, particularly of the skin. Increased susceptibility to infections (bacterial, viral, fungal, protozoal, opportunistic). Only physicians experienced in immunosuppressive therapy and management of organ transplant patients should prescribe mycophenolic acid (MPA). Manage patients in facilities equipped and staffed w/ adequate lab and supportive medical resources. Physician responsible for maintenance therapy should have complete information requisite for patient follow-up.

ADULT DOSAGE
Organ Rejection Prophylaxis

Kidney Transplant:
720mg bid (1440mg/day)

Use in combination w/ cyclosporine and corticosteroids

PEDIATRIC DOSAGE
Organ Rejection Prophylaxis

≥5 Years:
At Least 6 Months Post Kidney Transplant:
400mg/m² bid
Max: 720mg bid

BSA 1.19-1.58m²: Dose either w/ three 180mg tabs, or one 180mg tab plus one 360mg tab bid (1080mg/day)
BSA >1.58m²: Dose either w/ four 180mg tabs, or two 360mg tabs bid (1440mg/day)

Use in combination w/ cyclosporine and corticosteroids

ADMINISTRATION
Oral route

Take on an empty stomach, 1 hr before or 2 hrs after food intake.

Swallow whole; do not crush, chew, or cut tabs.

STORAGE
25°C (77°F); excursions permitted to 15-30°C (59-86°F). Protect from moisture.

HOW SUPPLIED
Tab, Delayed-Release: 180mg, 360mg

CONTRAINDICATIONS
Hypersensitivity to mycophenolate sodium, mycophenolic acid, mycophenolate mofetil, or to any of its excipients.

WARNINGS/PRECAUTIONS
Should not be used interchangeably w/ mycophenolate mofetil (MMF) tabs and caps w/o medical supervision. Limit exposure to sunlight and UV light in patients at increased risk for skin cancer. Polyomavirus-associated nephropathy (PVAN), JC virus associated progressive multifocal leukoencephalopathy (PML), cytomegalovirus (CMV) infections, reactivation of hepatitis B (HBV) or hepatitis C (HCV) reported; consider reduction in immunosuppression for patients who develop evidence of new or reactivated viral infections. PVAN, especially due to BK virus infection, is associated w/ serious outcomes, including deteriorating renal function and renal graft loss. Consider PML in differential diagnosis in patients reporting neurological symptoms and consider consultation w/ a neurologist as clinically indicated. Cases of pure red cell aplasia (PRCA) reported when used w/ other immunosuppressive agents; monitor CBC weekly during the 1st month, twice monthly for the 2nd and 3rd month of therapy, and then monthly through 1st yr. Interrupt dosing or reduce dose, perform appropriate tests, and manage accordingly, if blood dyscrasias occur (neutropenia [ANC <1.3 x 10³/μL] or anemia). GI bleeding (requiring hospitalization), intestinal perforations, gastric ulcers, and duodenal ulcers reported; caution w/ active serious digestive system disease. Avoid w/ rare hereditary deficiency of hypoxanthine-guanine phosphoribosyl-transferase (HGPRT) (eg, Lesch-Nyhan and Kelley-Seegmiller syndromes). Caution in elderly.

ADVERSE REACTIONS
Anemia, leukopenia, constipation, N/V, diarrhea, dyspepsia, UTI, CMV infection, insomnia, postoperative pain.

DRUG INTERACTIONS
Caution w/ combination immunosuppressant therapy. Avoid live attenuated vaccines. Mg²⁺- and aluminum-containing antacids may decrease levels; do not administer simultaneously. Azathioprine and MMF inhibit purine metabolism; avoid concomitant use w/ azathioprine or MMF. Cholestyramine or other agents that may interfere w/ enterohepatic recirculation or drugs that may bind bile acids (eg, bile acid sequestrates or oral activated charcoal) may reduce efficacy; avoid concomitant use. Sevelamer may decrease levels; do not

administer simultaneously w/ sevelamer and other Ca^{2+}-free phosphate binders. Cyclosporine may decrease levels; there is a potential change of MPA levels after switching from cyclosporine to other immunosuppressive drugs or from other immunosuppressive drugs to cyclosporine. Concomitant norfloxacin and metronidazole may decrease levels; avoid w/ the combination of norfloxacin and metronidazole. Rifampin may decrease levels; avoid concomitant use unless the benefit outweighs the risk. May decrease levels and effects of hormonal contraceptives; coadminister w/ caution, and additional barrier contraceptive methods must be used. Drugs that undergo renal tubular secretion (eg, acyclovir/valacyclovir, ganciclovir/valganciclovir) may increase levels of both drugs; monitor blood cell counts. Drugs that alter the GI flora (eg, ciprofloxacin or amoxicillin plus clavulanic acid) may interact w/ MMF by disrupting enterohepatic recirculation.

PREGNANCY AND LACTATION
Pregnancy: Category D. For females using MPA during pregnancy and those becoming pregnant w/in 6 weeks of discontinuing therapy, report pregnancy to the Mycophenolate Pregnancy Registry. Strongly encourage patient to enroll in the registry. Associated w/ increased risk of 1st trimester pregnancy loss and an increased risk of congenital malformations. When appropriate, consider alternative immunosuppressants w/ less potential for embryofetal toxicity. In certain situations, the patient and her healthcare practitioner may decide that the maternal benefits outweigh the risks to the fetus.
Lactation: Not for use in nursing.
Reproductive Potential: Females of reproductive potential should have a serum or urine pregnancy test (sensitivity of at least 25 mIU/mL) immediately before starting therapy; repeat test after 8-10 days and during routine follow-up visits. In the event of a positive pregnancy test, counsel w/ regards to whether the maternal benefits may outweigh the risks to the fetus in certain situations. Females of reproductive potential should use acceptable contraception during therapy and for 6 weeks after discontinuation, unless patient chooses abstinence. Consider alternative immunosuppressants w/ less potential for embryofetal toxicity in patients considering pregnancy.

MECHANISM OF ACTION
IMPDH inhibitor; inhibits the de novo pathway of guanosine nucleotide synthesis w/o incorporation to DNA.

PHARMACOKINETICS
Absorption: Absolute bioavailability (72%); T_{max}=1.5-2.75 hrs (median).
Distribution: V_d=54L; plasma protein binding (>98% bound to albumin), (82% mycophenolic acid glucuronide [MPAG]). **Metabolism:** Glucuronyl transferase; MPAG (major metabolite). **Elimination:** Urine (>60% MPAG, 3% unchanged); bile; $T_{1/2}$=8-16 hrs, 13-17 hrs (MPAG).

PATIENT CONSIDERATIONS
Assessment: Assess for hypersensitivity to the drug, HBV or HCV infected patients, hereditary deficiency of HGPRT (eg, Lesch-Nyhan and Kelley-Seegmiller syndromes), active digestive disease, pregnancy/nursing status, and for possible drug interactions. Females of reproductive potential should have a serum or urine pregnancy test (sensitivity of at least 25 mIU/mL) immediately before starting therapy.

Monitoring: Monitor for signs/symptoms of lymphomas and other malignancies (eg, skin cancer), infections including reactivation of HBV or HCV, blood dyscrasias (eg, PRCA), GI complications, and other adverse reactions. Monitor CBC weekly during the 1st month, twice monthly for the 2nd and 3rd month of therapy, and then monthly through 1st yr. Monitor pregnancy status by doing a pregnancy test (sensitivity of at least 25 mIU/mL) 8-10 days after initiation of therapy and repeatedly during follow-up visits.

Counseling: Inform that use in pregnancy is associated w/ an increased risk of 1st trimester pregnancy loss and congenital malformation; discuss pregnancy testing, prevention (including acceptable contraception methods), and planning. Discuss appropriate alternative immunosuppressants w/ less potential for embryofetal toxicity in patients who are considering pregnancy. Advise not to breastfeed during therapy. Inform about increased risk of developing lymphomas and other malignancies; advise to limit exposure to sunlight and UV light by wearing protective clothing and using sunscreen w/ high protection factor. Inform about increased risk of developing a variety of infections, including opportunistic infections, due to immunosuppression. Inform about risk for developing blood dyscrasias. Instruct to report if experiencing any symptoms of infection, unexpected bruising, bleeding, or any other manifestation of bone marrow suppression. Inform that therapy may cause GI tract complications, including bleeding, intestinal perforations, and gastric or duodenal ulcers; advise to contact healthcare provider if symptoms of GI bleeding or sudden onset or persistent abdominal pain occurs. Inform that therapy may interfere w/ the usual response to immunizations and to avoid live vaccines. Advise to report to physician the use of any other medications while on therapy. Encourage to enroll in the pregnancy registry if patient becomes pregnant while on therapy.

MYLERAN — busulfan   Rx
Class: Alkylating agent

> **Do not use unless a diagnosis of chronic myelogenous leukemia (CML) is established and the responsible physician is knowledgeable in assessing response to chemotherapy. Can induce severe bone marrow hypoplasia; reduce or d/c dose immediately at the 1st sign of any unusual depression of bone marrow function. Perform bone marrow examination if the bone marrow status is uncertain.**

ADULT DOSAGE
Chronic Myelogenous Leukemia
Palliative Treatment of Chronic Myelogenous (Myeloid, Myelocytic, Granulocytic) Leukemia:
Remission Induction:
Weight Based: 60mcg/kg or 1.8mg/m^2, daily
Usual Range: 4-8mg daily; reserve doses >4mg/day for patients w/ the most compelling symptoms

Examine patient at monthly intervals and resume treatment w/ induction dosage when total leukocyte count reaches approx 50,000/mcL

Remission <3 Months:
Maint: 1-3mg daily

PEDIATRIC DOSAGE
Chronic Myelogenous Leukemia
Palliative Treatment of Chronic Myelogenous (Myeloid, Myelocytic, Granulocytic) Leukemia:
Remission Induction:
Weight Based: 60mcg/kg or 1.8mg/m^2, daily; reserve doses >4mg/day for patients w/ the most compelling symptoms

Examine patient at monthly intervals and resume treatment w/ induction dosage when total leukocyte count reaches approx 50,000/mcL

Remission <3 Months:
Maint: 1-3mg daily

DOSING CONSIDERATIONS
Elderly
Start at lower end of dosing range
Discontinuation
D/C prior to leukocyte count falling into normal range
Total Leukocyte Count Approx 15,000/mcL: Withhold therapy

ADMINISTRATION
Oral route

STORAGE
25°C (77°F); excursions permitted to 15-30°C (59-86°F).

HOW SUPPLIED
Tab: 2mg

CONTRAINDICATIONS
Lack of definitive diagnosis of CML, prior hypersensitivity to busulfan or any other component of the preparation.

WARNINGS/PRECAUTIONS
Induction of bone marrow failure resulting in severe pancytopenia reported; use w/ extreme caution and exceptional vigilance in patients whose bone marrow reserve may have been compromised by prior irradiation or chemotherapy, or whose marrow function is recovering from previous cytotoxic therapy. Bronchopulmonary dysplasia w/ pulmonary fibrosis reported to occur w/in 8 months to 10 yrs after initiation of therapy; d/c if this develops. Exclude more common conditions (eg, opportunistic infections or leukemic infiltration of the lungs) w/ appropriate diagnostic techniques. May cause cellular dysplasia in many organs. Chromosome aberrations reported. May be carcinogenic; malignant tumors and acute leukemias reported. Ovarian suppression and amenorrhea w/ menopausal symptoms may occur in premenopausal patients. Associated w/ ovarian failure including failure to achieve puberty in females. Sterility, azoospermia, and testicular atrophy reported in males. Hepatic veno-occlusive disease (HVOD), which may be life threatening, reported, usually w/ cyclophosphamide or other chemotherapeutic agents; possible risk factors include total busulfan dose >16mg/kg, and concurrent use of multiple alkylating agents. Cardiac tamponade reported in patients w/ thalassemia. May cause fetal harm. Seizures reported; caution w/ a history of seizure disorder or head trauma.

ADVERSE REACTIONS
Bone marrow hypoplasia, myelosuppression, hyperpigmentation, HVOD.

DRUG INTERACTIONS
Additive myelosuppression w/ other myelosuppressive drugs; may need to reduce busulfan dose. Caution w/ continuous therapy w/ thioguanine; portal hypertension and esophageal varices may occur. Additive pulmonary toxicity w/ other cytotoxic agents. Reduced clearance w/ systemic itraconazole; monitor for signs of busulfan toxicity. Caution w/ other potentially epileptogenic drugs.

PREGNANCY AND LACTATION
Category D, not for use in nursing.

MECHANISM OF ACTION
Bifunctional alkylating agent.

PHARMACOKINETICS
Absorption: Complete. Administration in multiple doses resulted in different parameters. **Distribution:** Plasma protein binding (32%). **Metabolism:** Liver (extensive) by enzymatic activity to at least 12 metabolites. **Elimination:** Urine (<2% unchanged); $T_{1/2}$=2.6 hrs.

PATIENT CONSIDERATIONS
Assessment: Confirm diagnosis of CML prior to therapy. Assess for hypersensitivity to the drug or any other component of the preparation, history of seizure disorder, head trauma, thalassemia, risk of developing HVOD, pregnancy/nursing status, and possible drug interactions. Assess hematological status and bone marrow function.

Monitoring: Monitor for signs of local infection, bleeding, secondary malignancy, bronchopulmonary/cellular dysplasia, HVOD, ovarian suppression, amenorrhea, sterility, azoospermia, testicular atrophy, seizures, and other adverse reactions. Obtain Hgb/Hct, total WBC and differential count, and quantitative platelet count weekly. Monitor serum transaminases, alkaline phosphatase, and bilirubin periodically. Monitor bone marrow status.

Counseling: Inform of the importance of having periodic blood counts. Instruct to immediately report any unusual bleeding, fever, difficulty breathing, persistent cough, congestion, abrupt weakness, unusual fatigue, anorexia, weight loss, N/V, or melanoderma. Inform about the risks and benefits of therapy. Instruct never to take medication w/o close medical supervision. Advise women of childbearing potential to avoid becoming pregnant. Explain the increased risk of a secondary malignancy.

MYRBETRIQ — mirabegron

Rx

Class: Beta-3 adrenergic agonist

ADULT DOSAGE	**PEDIATRIC DOSAGE**
Overactive Bladder	Pediatric use may not have been established
Initial: 25mg qd	
Titrate: May increase to 50mg qd based on individual efficacy and tolerability	

DOSING CONSIDERATIONS
Renal Impairment
Severe (CrCl 15-29mL/min or eGFR 15-29mL/min/1.73m^2):
Max: 25mg qd

ESRD: Not recommended

Hepatic Impairment
Moderate (Child-Pugh Class B):
Max: 25mg qd

Severe (Child-Pugh Class C): Not recommended

ADMINISTRATION
Oral route
Take w/ or w/o food.
Swallow whole w/ water; do not chew, divide, or crush.

STORAGE
25°C (77°F); excursions permitted from 15-30°C (59-86°F).

HOW SUPPLIED
Tab, Extended-Release: 25mg, 50mg

CONTRAINDICATIONS
Known hypersensitivity reactions to mirabegron or any component of the tab.

WARNINGS/PRECAUTIONS
May increase BP; not recommended in patients w/ severe uncontrolled HTN. Worsening of preexisting HTN reported infrequently. Urinary retention in patients w/ bladder outlet obstruction (BOO) reported. Angioedema of the face, lips, tongue, and/or larynx reported; if involvement of the tongue, hypopharynx, or larynx occurs, promptly d/c therapy and initiate appropriate therapy and/or measures necessary to ensure a patent airway.

ADVERSE REACTIONS
HTN, nasopharyngitis, UTI, headache.

DRUG INTERACTIONS
Increases systemic exposure of CYP2D6 substrates (eg, metoprolol, desipramine); monitoring and dose adjustment may be necessary, especially w/ narrow therapeutic index CYP2D6 substrates (eg, thioridazine, flecainide, propafenone). Increases digoxin levels; consider lowest dose for digoxin initially and monitor digoxin levels. May increase warfarin levels. Caution w/ antimuscarinic medications for overactive bladder (OAB); urinary retention reported w/ concomitant use.

PREGNANCY AND LACTATION
Pregnancy: Category C.
Lactation: Not for use in nursing.

MECHANISM OF ACTION
β-3 adrenergic agonist; relaxes the detrusor smooth muscle during the storage phase of the urinary bladder fill-void cycle by activation of β-3 adrenergic receptor, which increases bladder capacity.

PHARMACOKINETICS
Absorption: Absolute bioavailability (29% [25mg], 35% [50mg]); T_{max}=3.5 hrs. **Distribution:** V_d=1670L (IV); plasma protein binding (71%). **Metabolism:** Dealkylation, oxidation (via CYP2D6 and CYP3A4), direct glucuronidation, and amide hydrolysis. **Elimination:** Urine (6% unchanged) (25mg); $T_{1/2}$=50 hrs.

PATIENT CONSIDERATIONS
Assessment: Assess for HTN, BOO, renal/hepatic impairment, pregnancy/nursing status, and possible drug interactions.

Monitoring: Monitor for urinary retention in patients w/ BOO, angioedema, and other adverse reactions. Monitor BP periodically, especially in hypertensive patients.

Counseling: Inform that therapy may increase BP and has also been associated w/ infrequent UTI, rapid heartbeat, rash, and pruritus. Inform that urinary retention has been reported when therapy was taken w/ antimuscarinic drugs used in the treatment of OAB. Instruct to contact physician if these effects are experienced.

MYSOLINE — primidone

Rx

Class: Pyrimidinedione derivative

ADULT DOSAGE	**PEDIATRIC DOSAGE**
Seizures	**Seizures**
Grand Mal, Psychomotor, and Focal Epileptic Seizures (Alone or w/ Other Anticonvulsants):	**Grand Mal, Psychomotor, and Focal Epileptic Seizures (Alone or w/ Other Anticonvulsants):**
No Prior Antiepileptic Therapy:	**<8 Years:**
Initial:	**Days 1-3:** 50mg qhs
Days 1-3: 100-125mg qhs	**Days 4-6:** 50mg bid
Days 4-6: 100-125mg bid	**Days 7-9:** 100mg bid
Days 7-9: 100-125mg tid	**Days 10/Maint:** 125-250mg tid
Days 10/Maint: 250mg tid	**Usual Maint:** 125-250mg tid or 10-25mg/kg/day in divided doses
Usual Maint: 250mg tid or qid	**≥8 Years:**
Max: 500mg qid	**No Prior Antiepileptic Therapy:**
Already Receiving Other Anticonvulsants:	**Initial:**
Initial: 100-125mg qhs	**Days 1-3:** 100-125mg qhs
Titrate: Increase gradually to maint dose as other drug is gradually decreased. Continue until satisfactory dosage level achieved or other medication is completely withdrawn. When therapy w/ primidone alone is the objective, transition from concomitant therapy should not be completed in <2 weeks	**Days 4-6:** 100-125mg bid
	Days 7-9: 100-125mg tid
	Days 10/Maint: 250mg tid
	Usual Maint: 250mg tid or qid
	Max: 500mg qid
Max: 2g/day	**Already Receiving Other Anticonvulsants:**
May also control grand mal seizures refractory to other anticonvulsant therapy	**Initial:** 100-125mg qhs
	Titrate: Increase gradually to maint dose as other drug is gradually decreased. Continue until satisfactory dosage level achieved or other medication is completely withdrawn. When therapy w/ primidone alone is the objective, transition from concomitant therapy should not be completed in <2 weeks
	Max: 2g/day
	May also control grand mal seizures refractory to other anticonvulsant therapy

---

ADMINISTRATION
Oral route

STORAGE
20-25°C (68-77°F).

HOW SUPPLIED
Tab: 50mg*, 250mg* *scored

CONTRAINDICATIONS
Porphyria, phenobarbital hypersensitivity.

WARNINGS/PRECAUTIONS
Avoid abrupt withdrawal; may precipitate status epilepticus. Increased risk of suicidal thoughts or behavior; monitor for emergence or worsening of depression, suicidal thoughts/behavior, or any unusual changes in mood or behavior. Increased incidence of birth defects reported; encourage pregnant patients to enroll in the North American Antiepileptic Drug (NAAED) Pregnancy Registry. Neonatal hemorrhage reported in newborns; give pregnant women prophylactic vitamin K1 therapy for 1 month prior to, and during, delivery.

ADVERSE REACTIONS
Ataxia, vertigo, granulocytopenia, agranulocytosis, red-cell hypoplasia, aplasia.

PREGNANCY AND LACTATION
Safety not known in pregnancy, not for use in nursing.

MECHANISM OF ACTION
Pyrimidinedione derivative; not established. Raises electro- or chemoshock seizure thresholds or alters seizure patterns in experimental animals.

PHARMACOKINETICS
Distribution: Found in breast milk. **Metabolism:** Phenobarbital, phenylethylmalonamide (metabolites).

PATIENT CONSIDERATIONS
Assessment: Assess for porphyria, hypersensitivity to phenobarbital, prior anticonvulsant therapy, depression, and pregnancy/nursing status.

Monitoring: Monitor for status epilepticus, emergence or worsening of depression, suicidal thoughts/behavior, and any unusual changes in mood or behavior. Monitor CBC, drug serum blood level, and sequential multiple analysis-12 test every 6 months.

Counseling: Counsel patients, their caregivers, and families that the therapy may increase risk of suicidal thoughts and behavior and advise to be alert for the emergence or worsening of symptoms of depression, any unusual changes in mood or behavior, or the emergence of suicidal thoughts, behavior, or thoughts about self-harm. Instruct to immediately report behaviors of concern to healthcare providers. Encourage pregnant patients to enroll in the NAAED Pregnancy Registry (1-888-233-2334).

NABI-HB — hepatitis B immune globulin (human)　　Rx

Class: Immune globulin

ADULT DOSAGE
Postexposure Prophylaxis

Acute Exposure to Blood Containing HBsAg:
0.06mL/kg IM as soon as possible after exposure and w/in 24 hrs, if possible; give a 2nd dose 1 month after 1st dose for patients who refuse hepatitis B vaccine or are known non-responders to vaccine

Refer to PI for recommendations following percutaneous or permucosal exposure

Sexual Exposure to HBsAg-Positive Person:
0.06mL/kg IM single dose w/ hepatitis B vaccine series; give w/in 14 days of last sexual contact or if sexual contact w/ infected person will continue

Household Exposure to Persons w/ Acute Hepatitis B Virus Infection:
Prophylaxis not indicated unless there is an identifiable blood exposure to the index patient (eg, by sharing toothbrushes/razors); treat such exposures like sexual exposures

PEDIATRIC DOSAGE
Postexposure Prophylaxis

Safety/effectiveness not established

Perinatal Exposure of Infants Born to HBsAg Positive Mothers:
0.5mL IM after physiologic stabilization of infant and preferably w/in 12 hrs of birth; initiate hepatitis B vaccine series simultaneously

Household Exposure to Persons w/ Acute Hepatitis B Virus Infection: <12 Months of Age:
0.5mL IM along w/ hepatitis B vaccine Prophylaxis of other household contacts is not indicated unless there is an identifiable blood exposure to the index patient (eg, by sharing toothbrushes/razors); treat such exposures like sexual exposures

ADMINISTRATION
IM route

May be administered at the same time (but at a different site), or up to 1 month preceding hepatitis B vaccination
Preferred sites are anterolateral aspect of the upper thigh and deltoid muscle

STORAGE
2-8°C (36-46°F). Do not freeze. Use within 6 hrs once opened; do not reuse or save for future use, and partially used vials should be discarded.

HOW SUPPLIED
Inj: >312 IU [1mL]; >1560 IU [5mL]

CONTRAINDICATIONS
Anaphylactic or severe systemic reaction to human globulin or IgA-deficiency disorder.

WARNINGS/PRECAUTIONS
Caution in patients with severe thrombocytopenia or coagulation disorders that contraindicate IM administration; give only if expected benefits outweigh the potential risks. Products made from human plasma may contain infectious agents and cause disease. Must be administered IM.

ADVERSE REACTIONS
Headache, erythema, myalgia, malaise, nausea, injection-site pain, elevated alkaline phosphatase levels.

DRUG INTERACTIONS
May interfere with live virus vaccines; defer until 3 months following the last dose of vaccine.

PREGNANCY AND LACTATION
Category C, caution in nursing.

MECHANISM OF ACTION
Vaccine; passive immunization from HBV exposure resulting in reduction of HBV infection rate.

PHARMACOKINETICS
Absorption: T_{max}=6.5 days. Distribution: V_d=11.2L. Excretion: $T_{1/2}$=23.1 days.

PATIENT CONSIDERATIONS
Assessment: Assess HBsAg/HBeAg, thrombocytopenia, coagulation disorder, IgA-deficiency, previous history of severe anaphylactic or systemic reaction to human globulin, live virus vaccination, and pregnancy/nursing status. Assess for acute exposure to blood of HBsAg-positive mothers, sexual contact with HBsAg-positive persons, and household persons with acute HBV infection.

Monitoring: Monitor for erythema, headache, myalgia, malaise, nausea, and elevated alkaline phosphatase levels.

Counseling: Advise to avoid live virus vaccination for 3 months after hepatitis B immune globulin administration; revaccinate persons immediately after live virus administration.

NABUMETONE — nabumetone　　Rx

Class: NSAID

> NSAIDs cause an increased risk of serious cardiovascular (CV) thrombotic events (eg, MI, stroke), which can be fatal; risk may occur early in treatment and may increase w/ duration of use. Contraindicated in the setting of CABG surgery. NSAIDs cause an increased risk of serious GI adverse events (eg, bleeding, ulceration, perforation of the stomach/intestines), which can be fatal and can occur at any time during use and w/o warning symptoms; elderly patients are at greater risk.

ADULT DOSAGE
Osteoarthritis

Initial: 1000mg qd
Titrate: Adjust dose/frequency based on individual needs after observing response to initial therapy; some patients may obtain relief from 1500-2000mg/day
Max: 2000mg/day

May be given qd-bid; use lowest effective dose for chronic treatment

Rheumatoid Arthritis

Initial: 1000mg qd
Titrate: Adjust dose/frequency based on individual needs after observing response to initial therapy; some patients may obtain relief from 1500-2000mg/day
Max: 2000mg/day

May be given qd-bid; use lowest effective dose for chronic treatment

DOSING CONSIDERATIONS
Renal Impairment
Moderate (CrCl 30-49mL/min):
Initial: ≤750mg qd
Max: 1500mg/day
Severe (CrCl <30mL/min):
Initial: ≤500mg qd
Max: 1000mg/day

ADMINISTRATION
Oral route

Take w/ or w/o food.

STORAGE
20-25°C (68-77°F).

HOW SUPPLIED
Tab: 500mg, 750mg

CONTRAINDICATIONS
Known hypersensitivity to nabumetone or product excipients; history of asthma, urticaria, or allergic-type reactions after taking aspirin (ASA) or other NSAIDs; in the setting of CABG surgery.

WARNINGS/PRECAUTIONS
Use lowest effective dose for shortest duration possible. Increased CV thrombotic risk reported at higher doses. Avoid in patients w/ a recent MI unless benefits outweigh the risks; if used, monitor for signs of cardiac ischemia. May cause HTN or worsen preexisting HTN. Fluid retention and edema reported. Avoid in patients w/ severe heart failure (HF) unless benefits outweigh the risks; if used, monitor for signs of worsening HF. Use w/ extreme caution in patients w/ history of ulcer disease or GI bleeding, or risk factors for GI bleeding (eg, longer duration of NSAID therapy, older age, poor general health status). D/C if a serious GI adverse event is suspected, until event is ruled out; for high-risk patients, consider alternate therapies that do not involve NSAIDs. Renal papillary necrosis and other renal injury reported after long-term use. Renal toxicity also reported in patients in whom renal prostaglandins have a compensatory role in the maintenance of renal perfusion; increased risk w/ renal/hepatic impairment, HF, and in elderly. Not recommended w/ advanced renal disease; if therapy must be initiated, closely monitor renal function. D/C if renal disease develops. Anaphylactoid reactions may occur; avoid w/ ASA triad. May cause serious skin reactions (eg, exfoliative dermatitis, Stevens-Johnson syndrome, toxic epidermal necrolysis); d/c at 1st appearance of skin rash or any other sign of hypersensitivity. Avoid in late pregnancy; may cause premature closure of ductus arteriosus. Not a substitute for corticosteroids or for the treatment of corticosteroid insufficiency. May mask signs of inflammation and fever. May cause elevation of LFTs or severe hepatic reactions (eg, jaundice, fatal fulminant hepatitis, liver necrosis, hepatic failure); d/c if liver disease develops, systemic manifestations occur, or abnormal LFTs persist/ worsen. Anemia may occur; monitor Hgb/Hct if anemia develops. May inhibit platelet aggregation and prolong bleeding time; carefully monitor patients w/ coagulation disorders. Caution w/ preexisting asthma. May be associated w/ more reactions to sun exposure than might be expected based on skin tanning types.

ADVERSE REACTIONS
Diarrhea, dyspepsia, abdominal pain, constipation, flatulence, N/V, positive stool guaiac, dizziness, headache, pruritus, rash, tinnitus, edema.

DRUG INTERACTIONS
May diminish the antihypertensive effect of ACE inhibitors. Increased risk of renal toxicity w/ diuretics. Not recommended w/ ASA due to potential for increased adverse effects. May reduce the natriuretic effect of thiazide and loop diuretics. May increase lithium levels; monitor for lithium toxicity. May enhance methotrexate toxicity; caution w/ concomitant use. Synergistic effect on GI bleeding w/ warfarin. Monitor patients receiving anticoagulants. Increased risk of GI bleeding w/ oral corticosteroids, anticoagulants, smoking, and alcohol use. May blunt the CV effects of several therapeutic agents used to treat fluid retention and edema (eg, diuretics, ACE inhibitors, ARBs).

PREGNANCY AND LACTATION
Pregnancy: Category C.
Lactation: Not for use in nursing.

PEDIATRIC DOSAGE
Pediatric use may not have been established

MECHANISM OF ACTION

NSAID (naphthylalkanone derivative); mechanism not established. Suspected to inhibit prostaglandin synthesis and exerts anti-inflammatory, analgesic, and antipyretic actions.

PHARMACOKINETICS

Absorption: Well-absorbed. PO administration of variable doses resulted in different parameters. **Distribution:** Plasma protein binding (>99%, active metabolite). **Metabolism:** Liver (extensive biotransformation), 6-methoxy-2-naphthylacetic acid (active metabolite). **Elimination:** Urine (approximately 80%), feces (9%); $T_{1/2}$=24 hrs.

PATIENT CONSIDERATIONS

Assessment: Assess for history of asthma, urticaria, or allergic-type reactions w/ ASA or other NSAIDs, ASA triad, HTN, severe HF, history of ulcer disease or GI bleeding, coagulation disorders, renal/hepatic function, pregnancy/nursing status, any other conditions where treatment is contraindicated or cautioned, and possible drug interactions. Obtain baseline BP.

Monitoring: Monitor BP, CBC, bleeding time, LFTs, renal function, and chemistry profile periodically. Monitor for GI bleeding/ulceration/perforation, CV thrombotic events, MI, stroke, HTN, fluid retention, edema, skin/allergic reactions, photosensitivity, and other adverse reactions.

Counseling: Instruct to notify physician immediately if symptoms of CV thrombotic events, GI ulceration/bleeding, skin/hypersensitivity reactions, congestive HF, hepatotoxicity, or anaphylactoid reactions occur. Instruct to avoid in late pregnancy.

NALOXONE INJECTION — naloxone hydrochloride   Rx

Class: Opioid antagonist

ADULT DOSAGE

Opioid Depression

Complete or Partial Reversal of Opioid Depression Induced by Natural and Synthetic Opioids, and Certain Mixed Agonist-Antagonist Analgesics:

Initial: 0.1-0.2mg IV at 2- to 3- min intervals to the desired degree of reversal

Repeat doses may be required w/ in 1- to 2- hr intervals depending on the amount, type, and time interval since last administration of opioid; supplemental IM doses shown to produce longer lasting effect

Opioid Overdose

For the Diagnosis of Suspected or Known Acute Opioid Overdosage:

Initial: 0.4-2mg IV; may repeat at 2-3 min intervals if desired degree of counteraction and improvement in respiratory functions is not obtained

If no response is observed after 10mg, reassess diagnosis; may give IM or SQ if IV route is not available

Other Indications

May be useful as an adjunctive agent to increase BP in the management of septic shock

PEDIATRIC DOSAGE

Opioid Depression

Complete or Partial Reversal of Opioid Depression Induced by Natural and Synthetic Opioids, and Certain Mixed Agonist-Antagonist Analgesics:

Initial: 0.005mg-0.01mg IV at 2- to 3- min intervals to the desired degree of reversal
Follow recommendations and cautions as adults

Neonates:

When using in neonates, a product containing 0.02mg/mL should be used

Initial: 0.01mg/kg IV, IM, or SQ; may repeat this dose in accordance w/ adult administration guidelines

Opioid Overdose

For the Diagnosis of Suspected or Known Acute Opioid Overdosage:

Initial: 0.01mg/kg IV; may administer a subsequent dose of 0.1mg/kg if desired degree of clinical improvement is not obtained

May give IM or SQ in divided doses if IV route is not available

---

DOSING CONSIDERATIONS

Elderly

Start at lower end of dosing range

ADMINISTRATION

IV/IM/SQ routes

IV Infusion

May dilute drug for IV infusion in 0.9% NaCl inj or D5 inj; addition of 2mg of naloxone in 500mL of either sol provides a concentration of 0.004mg/mL. Mixtures should be used w/in 24 hrs.
Titrate rate of administration in accordance w/ patient's response.
Do not mix w/ preparations containing bisulfite, metabisulfite, long-chain or high molecular weight anions, or any sol having an alkaline pH.
No drug or chemical agent should be added to naloxone unless its effect on the chemical and physical stability of the sol has been established.

STORAGE

20-25°C (68-77°F). Protect from light.

HOW SUPPLIED

Inj: 0.4mg/mL [1mL, 10mL]

CONTRAINDICATIONS

Known hypersensitivity to naloxone HCl or to any of the other ingredients contained in the formulation.

WARNINGS/PRECAUTIONS

Caution with patients including newborns of mothers who are known or suspected to be physically dependent on opioids; abrupt and complete reversal of opioid

effects may precipitate acute withdrawal syndrome. Keep patients under continued surveillance and administer repeat doses PRN. Not effective against respiratory depression due to nonopioid drugs and in management of acute toxicity caused by levopropoxyphene. Reversal of respiratory depression by partial agonists or mixed agonist/antagonists may be incomplete or require higher doses of naloxone. Mechanically assist respirations as clinically indicated if incomplete response occurs. Other resuscitative measures (eg, artificial ventilation, cardiac massage) should be available and employed PRN. Abrupt postoperative reversal of opioid depression may result in N/V, sweating, tremulousness, tachycardia, increased BP, seizures, ventricular tachycardia and fibrillation, pulmonary edema, and cardiac arrest, which may result in death. Excessive dose in postoperative patients may result in significant reversal of analgesia and may cause agitation. Hypotension, HTN, ventricular tachycardia and fibrillation, pulmonary edema, and cardiac arrest reported in postoperative patients, which may lead to death, coma, and encephalopathy. May cause pulmonary edema. Caution with preexisting cardiac, renal, or hepatic disease, and in elderly.

ADVERSE REACTIONS

HTN, hypotension, ventricular tachycardia and fibrillation, dyspnea, pulmonary edema, cardiac arrest, N/V, sweating, seizures, body aches, fever, nervousness, weakness, diarrhea.

DRUG INTERACTIONS

Caution with drugs with potential adverse cardiovascular effects (eg, hypotension, ventricular tachycardia or fibrillation, pulmonary edema). Large doses may be required to antagonize buprenorphine. Barbiturate methohexital appears to block the acute onset of withdrawal symptoms induced by naloxone in opiate addicts.

PREGNANCY AND LACTATION

Category C, caution in nursing.

MECHANISM OF ACTION

Opioid antagonist; prevents or reverses effects of opioids, including respiratory depression, sedation, and hypotension, by competing for the mu, kappa, and sigma opiate receptor sites in the CNS, with the greatest affinity for the mu receptor.

PHARMACOKINETICS

Distribution: Rapid; crosses placenta. **Metabolism:** Liver via glucuronide conjugation; naloxone-3-glucuronide (major metabolite). **Elimination:** Urine (60-70% in 72 hrs); $T_{1/2}$=64 mins (adults), 3.1 hrs (neonates).

PATIENT CONSIDERATIONS

Assessment: Assess for known hypersensitivity to the drug, opioid dependency, cardiac/hepatic/renal disease, pregnancy/nursing status, and possible drug interactions.

Monitoring: Monitor for signs/symptoms of opioid withdrawal (eg, body aches, diarrhea, tachycardia, fever, runny nose, sneezing, piloerection, sweating, yawning, N/V, nervousness, restlessness, irritability, shivering or trembling, abdominal cramps, weakness, increase BP), postoperative effects, coma, and encephalopathy.

Counseling: Inform that withdrawal signs/symptoms (eg, body aches, diarrhea, tachycardia, fever) may occur. Inform that hypotension, HTN, ventricular tachycardia and fibrillation, dyspnea, pulmonary edema, and cardiac arrest have occurred in postoperative patients.

NAMENDA — memantine hydrochloride   Rx

Class: NMDA receptor antagonist

OTHER BRAND NAMES
Namenda XR

ADULT DOSAGE

Alzheimer's Disease

Moderate to Severe Dementia:

Sol, Tab:
Initial: 5mg qd
Titrate: Increase in 5mg increments to 10mg/day (5mg bid), 15mg/day (5mg and 10mg as separate doses), and 20mg/day (10mg bid) at ≥1-week intervals

Cap, ER:
Initial: 7mg qd
Titrate: Increase in 7mg increments to 28mg qd at ≥1-week intervals
Max/Target Dose: 28mg qd

Conversions

Switching from Tabs to Cap, ER:
Switch from 10mg bid tabs to 28mg qd caps the day following last dose of 10mg tab
Severe Renal Impairment: Switch from 5mg bid tabs to 14mg qd caps the day following last dose of 5mg tab

Missed Dose

Sol, Tab
If a single dose is missed, take next dose as scheduled and do not double dose; if missed for several days, resume dose at lower dose and retitrate

PEDIATRIC DOSAGE

Pediatric use may not have been established

DOSING CONSIDERATIONS
Renal Impairment
Severe (CrCl 5-29mL/min):
Target Dose:
Sol, Tab: 5mg bid
Cap, ER: 14mg/day

ADMINISTRATION
Oral route

May take w/ or w/o food

Sol
Do not mix w/ any other liquid
Administer w/ a dosing device (syringe, syringe adaptor cap, tubing, other supplies needed) that comes w/ the drug
Use syringe to withdraw correct volume of oral sol and squirt slowly into the corner of the mouth

Cap, ER
Swallow cap whole; do not divide, chew, or crush
May be opened, sprinkled on applesauce, and swallowed

STORAGE
25°C (77°F); excursions permitted to 15-30°C (59-86°F).

HOW SUPPLIED
Sol: 2mg/mL [360mL]; **Tab:** 5mg, 10mg; **Titration Pack:** 5mg [28^s], 10mg [21^s]. **Cap, ER:** 7mg, 14mg, 21mg, 28mg; **Titration Pack:** 7mg [7^s], 14mg [7^s], 21mg [7^s], 28mg [7^s].

CONTRAINDICATIONS
Known hypersensitivity to memantine HCl or to any excipients used in the formulation.

WARNINGS/PRECAUTIONS
Conditions that raise urine pH may decrease urinary elimination, resulting in increased plasma levels. Caution in patients w/ severe renal/hepatic impairment.

ADVERSE REACTIONS
Dizziness, headache, constipation, confusion, HTN, coughing, somnolence, hallucination, vomiting, back pain, (Sol, Tab) pain, (Cap, ER) diarrhea, influenza, weight gain, anxiety.

DRUG INTERACTIONS
Caution w/ other N-methyl-D-aspartate (NMDA) antagonists (eg, amantadine, ketamine, dextromethorphan) and drugs that alter urine pH towards the alkaline condition (eg, carbonic anhydrase inhibitors, sodium bicarbonate). (Cap, ER) Coadministration w/ drugs eliminated via renal (cationic system) mechanism (eg, HCTZ, triamterene, metformin, cimetidine, ranitidine) may result in altered plasma levels of both agents.

PREGNANCY AND LACTATION
Category B, caution in nursing.

MECHANISM OF ACTION
NMDA receptor antagonist; postulated to exert its therapeutic effect through its action as a low to moderate affinity uncompetitive (open-channel) NMDA receptor antagonist, which binds preferentially to the NMDA receptor-operated cation channels.

PHARMACOKINETICS
Absorption: (Sol, Tab) Well absorbed. T_{max}=3-7 hrs. (Cap, ER) Highly absorbed. T_{max}=9-12 hrs. **Distribution:** V_d=9-11L/kg. Plasma protein binding (45%). **Metabolism:** Liver (partial); N-glucuronide conjugate, 6-hydroxy memantine, 1-nitroso-deaminated memantine (metabolites). **Elimination:** Urine (48%, unchanged); $T_{1/2}$=60-80 hrs.

PATIENT CONSIDERATIONS
Assessment: Assess for hypersensitivity to drug, conditions that raise urine pH, renal/hepatic impairment, pregnancy/nursing status, and possible drug interactions.

Monitoring: Monitor for hypersensitivity reactions and other adverse reactions. Monitor renal/hepatic function.

Counseling: Instruct to take as prescribed. Inform about possible side effects and instruct to notify physician if any develop. (Sol, Tab) Instruct to follow dose titration schedule and not to resume dosing w/o consulting physician if there has been a failure to take the medication for several days. (Tab) Instruct not to use any damaged or tampered tabs. (Sol) Instruct on how to use the oral sol dosing device.

NAMZARIC — donepezil hydrochloride/memantine hydrochloride   Rx
Class: Acetylcholinesterase (AChE) inhibitor/NMDA receptor antagonist

ADULT DOSAGE
Alzheimer's Disease
Moderate to Severe Dementia of the Alzheimer's Type Stabilized on Donepezil 10mg:
28mg/10mg qd

Stabilized on Donepezil and Not Currently on Memantine:
Initial: 7mg/10mg qpm
Titrate: Increase in 7mg increments of memantine at a minimum interval of 1 week; increase only if previous dose is well tolerated
Maint: 28mg/10mg qd
Max: 28mg/10mg qd

PEDIATRIC DOSAGE
Pediatric use may not have been established

Stabilized on Both Donepezil 10mg qd and Memantine 10mg bid or 28mg Extended-Release (ER) qd:
Switch to Namzaric 28mg/10mg qpm; start the day following the last dose of memantine and donepezil administered separately

Missed Dose
If a dose is missed, the next dose should be taken as scheduled, w/o doubling up the dose

---

DOSING CONSIDERATIONS
Renal Impairment
Severe (CrCl 5-29mL/min):
Stabilized on Donepezil and Not Currently on Memantine:
Initial: 7mg/10mg qpm
Titrate: Increase after a minimum of 1 week to maint dose of 14mg/10mg qpm

Stabilized on Memantine 5mg bid or 14mg ER qd and Donepezil 10mg:
Switch to 14mg/10mg qd

ADMINISTRATION
Oral route
- May take w/ or w/o food.
- Swallow cap whole and intact; do not divide, chew, or crush.
- May be opened, sprinkled on applesauce, and swallowed w/o chewing.
- Consume entire contents of each cap; the dose should not be divided.

STORAGE
20-25°C (68-77°F); excursions permitted between 15-30°C (59-86°F).

HOW SUPPLIED
Cap, ER: (Memantine/Donepezil) 7mg/10mg, 14mg/10mg, 21mg/10mg, 28mg/10mg

CONTRAINDICATIONS
Known hypersensitivity to memantine HCl, donepezil HCl, piperidine derivatives, or to any excipients used in the formulation.

WARNINGS/PRECAUTIONS
Memantine: Conditions that raise urine pH may decrease urinary elimination, resulting in increased plasma levels. **Donepezil:** May exaggerate succinylcholine-type muscle relaxation during anesthesia. May have vagotonic effects on sinoatrial (SA) and atrioventricular (AV) nodes, manifesting as bradycardia or heart block. Syncopal episodes reported. May increase gastric acid secretion; monitor closely for symptoms of active or occult GI bleeding, especially in patients at increased risk for developing ulcers (eg, history of ulcer disease, concomitant use of NSAIDs). May produce diarrhea and N/V; observe closely at the initiation of treatment. May cause bladder outflow obstruction and generalized convulsions. Caution w/ history of asthma or obstructive pulmonary disease.

ADVERSE REACTIONS
Memantine: Headache, diarrhea, dizziness.
Donepezil: Diarrhea, anorexia, N/V, ecchymosis.

DRUG INTERACTIONS
Memantine: Caution w/ other N-methyl-D-aspartate (NMDA) antagonists (eg, amantadine, ketamine, dextromethorphan) and drugs that alter urine pH towards the alkaline condition (eg, carbonic anhydrase inhibitors, sodium bicarbonate). **Donepezil:** Inhibitors of CYP3A4 (eg, ketoconazole) and CYP2D6 (eg, quinidine) inhibit metabolism in vitro. CYP3A4 inducers (eg, phenytoin, carbamazepine, dexamethasone, rifampin, phenobarbital) may increase elimination rate. May interfere w/ the activity of anticholinergic medications. Synergistic effect w/ similar neuromuscular blocking agents (eg, succinylcholine) or cholinergic agonists (eg, bethanechol).

PREGNANCY AND LACTATION
Pregnancy: Adverse developmental effects observed in animal studies.
Lactation: There are no data on the presence of memantine or donepezil in human milk, the effects on the breastfed infant, or the effects of Namzaric or its metabolites on milk production; caution in nursing.

MECHANISM OF ACTION
Memantine: NMDA receptor antagonist; postulated to exert its therapeutic effect through its action as a low to moderate affinity uncompetitive (open-channel) NMDA receptor antagonist, which binds preferentially to the NMDA receptor-operated cation channels. **Donepezil:** Acetylcholinesterase inhibitor; postulated to exert its therapeutic effect by increasing acetylcholine concentration in the CNS through reversible inhibition of its hydrolysis by acetylcholinesterase.

PHARMACOKINETICS
Absorption: Memantine: Well-absorbed. (Multiple Dose) T_{max}=9-12 hrs. (Single Dose) T_{max}=18 hrs (fed), 25 hrs (fasted). Donepezil: T_{max}=3-4 hrs. **Distribution:** Memantine: V_d=9-11L/kg; plasma protein binding (45%). Donepezil: V_d=12-16L/kg; plasma protein binding (96%). **Metabolism:** Memantine: Hepatic (partial); N-glucuronide conjugate, 6-hydroxy memantine, 1-nitroso-deaminated memantine (active metabolites). Donepezil: Extensive; CYP2D6 and CYP3A4; glucuronidation; 6-O-desmethyl donepezil (active metabolite). **Elimination:** Memantine: Urine (48%, unchanged); $T_{1/2}$=60-80 hrs. Donepezil: Urine (57%, 17% unchanged), feces (15%); $T_{1/2}$=70 hrs.

PATIENT CONSIDERATIONS
Assessment: Assess for hypersensitivity to the drug or piperidine derivatives, underlying cardiac conduction abnormalities, risk for developing ulcers, conditions that raise urine pH, history of asthma or obstructive pulmonary disease, renal impairment, pregnancy/nursing status, and possible drug interactions.

Monitoring: Monitor for vagotonic effects on SA and AV nodes, syncopal episodes, active/occult GI bleeding, diarrhea, N/V, bladder outflow obstruction, generalized convulsions, and other adverse reactions.

Counseling: Instruct to take as prescribed. Inform that drug may cause headache, diarrhea, dizziness, anorexia, N/V, and ecchymosis.

NAPRELAN — naproxen sodium

Class: NSAID

Rx

> NSAIDs cause an increased risk of serious cardiovascular (CV) thrombotic events, including MI and stroke, which can be fatal. This risk may occur early in treatment and may increase w/ duration of use. Contraindicated in the setting of CABG surgery. NSAIDs cause an increased risk of serious GI adverse events (eg, bleeding, ulceration, stomach/intestinal perforation), which can be fatal and can occur anytime during use and w/o warning symptoms; elderly patients and patients w/ a prior history of peptic ulcer disease and/or GI bleeding are at a greater risk.

ADULT DOSAGE

Rheumatoid Arthritis

Initial: 750mg or 1000mg qd
Titrate:
Adjust dose/frequency depending on clinical response.
In patients who tolerate lower doses well, may increase to two 750mg tabs or three 500mg tabs once daily for limited periods, prn.

Osteoarthritis

Initial: 750mg or 1000mg qd
Titrate:
Adjust dose/frequency depending on clinical response.
In patients who tolerate lower doses well, may increase to two 750mg tabs or three 500mg tabs once daily for limited periods, prn.

Ankylosing Spondylitis

Initial: 750mg or 1000mg qd
Titrate:
Adjust dose/frequency depending on clinical response.
In patients who tolerate lower doses well, may increase to two 750mg tabs or three 500mg tabs once daily for limited periods, prn.

Mild to Moderate Pain

Initial: 1000mg qd; may give 1500mg qd for a limited period in patients requiring greater analgesia
Max: 1000mg/day after limited period of 1500mg qd

Primary Dysmenorrhea

Initial: 1000mg qd; may give 1500mg qd for a limited period in patients requiring greater analgesia
Max: 1000mg/day after limited period of 1500mg qd

Bursitis/Tendinitis

Acute:
Initial: 1000mg qd; may give 1500mg qd for a limited period in patients requiring greater analgesia
Max: 1000mg/day after limited period of 1500mg qd

Gout

Acute:
Day 1: 1000-1500mg qd
Succeeding Days: 1000mg qd until attack subsides

PEDIATRIC DOSAGE

Pediatric use may not have been established

DOSING CONSIDERATIONS

Renal Impairment
Consider lower dose

Hepatic Impairment
Consider lower dose

Elderly
If the anticipated benefit outweighs the potential risks, start at lower end of dosing range; monitor for adverse effects

Other Important Considerations
Rheumatoid Arthritis, Osteoarthritis, and Ankylosing Spondylitis:
Patients already taking naproxen 250mg, 375mg, or 500mg bid may have their total daily dose replaced w/ Naprelan as a qd dose

ADMINISTRATION
Oral route

STORAGE
20-25°C (68-77°F); excursions permitted to 15-30°C (59-86°F).

HOW SUPPLIED
Tab, Controlled-Release: 375mg, 500mg, 750mg

CONTRAINDICATIONS
Known hypersensitivity to naproxen or any components of the drug product; history of asthma, urticaria, or other allergic-type reactions after taking aspirin (ASA) or other NSAIDs; in the setting of CABG surgery.

WARNINGS/PRECAUTIONS
Use lowest effective dose for the shortest duration possible. Avoid in patients w/ a recent MI unless benefits outweigh the risks; if used, monitor for signs of cardiac ischemia. Increased risk for GI bleeding w/ longer duration of therapy, older age, poor general health status, and advanced liver disease and/or coagulopathy; avoid use in patients at higher risk unless benefits are expected to outweigh the increased risk and consider alternate therapies. Hepatotoxicity reported; d/c immediately and perform a clinical evaluation if clinical signs/symptoms consistent w/ liver disease develop, or if systemic manifestations occur. May cause new onset HTN or worsen preexisting HTN. Fluid retention and edema reported. Avoid use in patients w/ severe heart failure (HF) unless benefits outweigh risks; monitor for signs of worsening HF if used. Renal papillary necrosis and other renal injury reported w/ long-term use. Renal toxicity also reported in patients in whom renal prostaglandins have a compensatory role in the maintenance of renal perfusion; increased risk w/ renal/hepatic dysfunction, dehydration, hypovolemia, HF, and the elderly. Correct volume status in dehydrated or hypovolemic patients prior to initiating therapy. Avoid use in patients w/ advanced renal disease unless the benefits are expected to outweigh the risk; monitor for signs of worsening renal function if used in patients w/ advanced renal disease. Hyperkalemia reported. Associated w/ anaphylactic reactions. Monitor for changes in the signs/symptoms of asthma in patients w/ preexisting asthma (w/o known ASA sensitivity). May cause serious skin reactions (eg, exfoliative dermatitis, Stevens-Johnson syndrome, toxic epidermal necrolysis); d/c at 1st appearance of skin rash/hypersensitivity. Anemia reported. May increase the risk of bleeding events; coagulation disorders may increase this risk. May mask inflammation and fever. Lab test interactions may occur.

ADVERSE REACTIONS
Headache, dyspepsia, flu syndrome.

DRUG INTERACTIONS
Drugs that interfere w/ serotonin reuptake may potentiate the risk of bleeding. Synergistic effect on bleeding w/ anticoagulants (eg, warfarin); monitor for signs of bleeding w/ concomitant anticoagulants, antiplatelet agents, SSRIs, and SNRIs. May increase risk of GI bleeding w/ use of oral corticosteroids, anticoagulants, or SSRIs; smoking; and alcohol use. ASA may increase risk of bleeding and serious GI events; concomitant use w/ analgesic doses of ASA is not recommended. Monitor patients more closely for GI bleeding w/ concomitant use of low-dose ASA for cardiac prophylaxis. May diminish antihypertensive effect of ACE inhibitors, ARBs, and β-blockers (eg, propranolol); monitor BP. Coadministration w/ ACE inhibitors or ARBs may result in deterioration of renal function (including possible acute renal failure) in patients who are elderly, volume-depleted (including those on diuretic therapy), or have renal impairment; monitor for worsening renal function and adequately hydrate patient when these drugs are administered concomitantly. May reduce the natriuretic effect of loop diuretics (eg, furosemide) and thiazide diuretics; observe for signs of worsening renal function, in addition to assuring diuretic efficacy including antihypertensive effects. May increase digoxin serum concentrations and prolong the $T_{1/2}$ of digoxin; monitor digoxin levels. May elevate plasma lithium levels and reduce renal lithium clearance; monitor for signs of lithium toxicity. May increase the risk for methotrexate toxicity. May increase cyclosporine's nephrotoxicity; monitor for signs of worsening renal function. Use w/ other NSAIDs or salicylates (eg, diflunisal, salsalate) increases risk of GI toxicity; concomitant use not recommended. Concomitant use w/ pemetrexed may increase the risk of pemetrexed-associated myelosuppression, renal, and GI toxicity; refer to prescribing information for further information. Concomitant administration w/ some antacids (magnesium oxide or aluminum hydroxide), sucralfate, or cholestyramine is not recommended; may can delay absorption of naproxen. Probenecid increases naproxen anion plasma levels and extends its plasma $T_{1/2}$ significantly; observe for adjustment of dose if required. Theoretical potential for interaction w/ other albumin-bound drugs (eg, sulphonylureas, hydantoins); observe if dose adjustment is required in patients simultaneously receiving a hydantoin, sulphonamide, or sulphonylurea.

PREGNANCY AND LACTATION
Pregnancy: Use during the 3rd trimester of pregnancy increases the risk of premature closure of the fetal ductus arteriosus; avoid use in pregnant women starting at 30 weeks of gestation (3rd trimester).
Lactation: Found in breast milk; caution in nursing.
Reproductive Potential: May delay or prevent rupture of ovarian follicles, which has been associated w/ reversible infertility in some women. Small studies in women treated w/ NSAIDs have also shown a reversible delay in ovulation. Consider withdrawal of therapy in women who have difficulties conceiving or who are undergoing investigation of infertility.

MECHANISM OF ACTION
NSAID; mechanism not completely understood but involves inhibition of COX-1 and COX-2. Mode of action may be due to a decrease of prostaglandins in peripheral tissues; possesses anti-inflammatory, analgesic, and antipyretic activities.

PHARMACOKINETICS
Absorption: Rapid and complete. Bioavailability (95%); (1000mg qd multiple dose) C_{max}=94mcg/mL, T_{max}=5 hrs, AUC=1448mcg•hr/mL. **Distribution:** V_d=0.16L/kg; plasma protein binding (>99%); found in breast milk. **Metabolism:** Extensive; 6-O-desmethyl naproxen metabolite. **Elimination:** Urine (<1% unchanged, <1% 6-O-desmethyl naproxen, 66-92% conjugates), feces (<5%); $T_{1/2}$=15 hrs.

PATIENT CONSIDERATIONS

Assessment: Assess for hypersensitivity to naproxen or to any component of this product; history of asthma, urticaria, or other allergic-type reactions after taking ASA or other NSAIDs; asthma; CV disease (CVD) or risk factors for CVD; HTN; history of peptic ulcer disease or GI bleeding; coagulation disorders; renal/hepatic impairment; pregnancy/nursing status; or any other conditions where treatment is contraindicated or cautioned. Assess volume status. Assess for possible drug interactions. Obtain baseline BP, CBC, and chemistry profile.

Monitoring: Monitor for signs/symptoms of CV thrombotic events; cardiac ischemia in patients w/ a recent MI; GI bleeding/ulceration and perforation; hepatotoxicity; new or worsening HTN; HF; edema; renal papillary necrosis and other renal injury; hyperkalemia; anaphylactic reactions; serious skin reactions; anemia; and other adverse reactions. Monitor BP during initiation of therapy and throughout the course of therapy. Monitor for signs of bleeding in patients on concomitant therapy w/ anticoagulants, antiplatelet agents, SSRIs, or SNRIs. Monitor renal function in patients w/ renal/hepatic impairment, HF, dehydration, or hypovolemia. Periodically monitor CBC and chemistry profiles including LFTs in patients receiving long-term treatment.

Counseling: Advise to be alert for the symptoms of CV thrombotic events and to report symptoms immediately. Advise to report symptoms of ulcerations and bleeding. Inform of the increased risk for and the signs and symptoms of GI bleeding w/ ASA. Inform of the warning signs and symptoms of hepatotoxicity; instruct to d/c and seek immediate medical therapy. Advise to be alert for the symptoms of CHF and to contact healthcare provider if such symptoms occur. Inform of the signs of an anaphylactic reaction and instruct to seek immediate emergency help if these occur. Advise to d/c immediately if any type of rash develops, and to contact healthcare provider as soon as possible. Advise females of reproductive potential who desire pregnancy that NSAIDs may be associated w/ a reversible delay in ovulation. Inform pregnant women to avoid use of naproxen and other NSAIDs starting at 30 weeks' gestation. Inform patients that the concomitant use w/ other NSAIDs or salicylates is not recommended. Alert patients that NSAIDs may be present in OTC medications for treatment of colds, fever, or insomnia. Advise not to use low-dose ASA w/o consultation.

NAPROSYN — naproxen　　　　Rx

Class: NSAID

> NSAIDs may increase risk of serious cardiovascular thrombotic events, MI, and stroke; increased risk with duration of use and with cardiovascular disease (CVD) or risk factors for CVD. Increased risk of serious GI adverse events (eg, bleeding, ulceration, and stomach/intestinal perforation) that can be fatal and occur anytime during use without warning symptoms; elderly patients are at a greater risk. Contraindicated for treatment of perioperative pain in the setting of CABG surgery.

OTHER BRAND NAMES
Anaprox, Anaprox DS, EC-Naprosyn

ADULT DOSAGE
Gout
Acute Attack:

Naprosyn:
Initial: 750mg, then 250mg q8h until attack subsides

Anaprox:
Initial: 825mg, then 275mg q8h until attack subsides

Bursitis
Anaprox/Anaprox DS:
Initial: 550mg, then 550mg q12h or 275mg q6-8h as required
Max: 1375mg/day initially, 1100mg/day thereafter

Rheumatoid Arthritis
Naprosyn:
250mg, 375mg, or 500mg bid
EC-Naprosyn:
375mg or 500mg bid
Anaprox:
275mg bid
Anaprox DS:
550mg bid
Titrate: Adjust dose/frequency up or down depending on clinical response; may increase to 1500mg/day for ≤6 months if patient can tolerate lower doses well

Ankylosing Spondylitis
Naprosyn:
250mg, 375mg, or 500mg bid
EC-Naprosyn:
375mg or 500mg bid
Anaprox:
275mg bid
Anaprox DS:
550mg bid

PEDIATRIC DOSAGE
Juvenile Arthritis
≥2 Years:
Sus:
Usual: 5mg/kg bid

Titrate: Adjust dose/frequency up or down depending on clinical response; may increase to 1500mg/day for ≤6 months if patient can tolerate lower doses well

Pain
Anaprox/Anaprox DS:
Initial: 550mg, then 550mg q12h or 275mg q6-8h as required
Max: 1375mg/day initially, 1100mg/day thereafter

Primary Dysmenorrhea
Anaprox/Anaprox DS:
Initial: 550mg, then 550mg q12h or 275mg q6-8h as required
Max: 1375mg/day initially, 1100mg/day thereafter

Osteoarthritis
Naprosyn:
250mg, 375mg, or 500mg bid
EC-Naprosyn:
375mg or 500mg bid
Anaprox:
275mg bid
Anaprox DS:
550mg bid
Titrate: Adjust dose/frequency up or down depending on clinical response; may increase to 1500mg/day for ≤6 months if patient can tolerate lower doses well

---

DOSING CONSIDERATIONS
Renal Impairment
Start w/ lower end of dosing range
Moderate to Severe (CrCl <30mL/min): Not recommended

Hepatic Impairment
Start w/ lower end of dosing range

Elderly
Start w/ lower end of dosing range

ADMINISTRATION
Oral route
EC-Naprosyn
Do not chew, crush, or break

STORAGE
15-30°C (59-86°F). (Sus) Avoid excessive heat, >40°C (104°F). Shake gently before use.

HOW SUPPLIED
Sus: (Naprosyn) 125mg/5mL [473mL]; **Tab:** (Naprosyn) 250mg*, 375mg, 500mg*, (Anaprox [naproxen sodium]) 275mg, (Anaprox DS [naproxen sodium]) 550mg*; **Tab, Delayed-Release:** (EC-Naprosyn) 375mg, 500mg *scored

CONTRAINDICATIONS
Known hypersensitivity to naproxen and naproxen sodium; history of asthma, urticaria, or other allergic-type reactions w/ ASA or other NSAIDs; treatment of perioperative pain in the setting of CABG surgery.

WARNINGS/PRECAUTIONS
Use lowest effective dose for the shortest duration possible. May cause HTN or worsen preexisting HTN; monitor BP closely. Fluid retention and edema reported; caution with fluid retention, HTN, or HF. Caution with prior history of ulcer disease, GI bleeding, and risk factors for GI bleeding; monitor for GI ulceration/bleeding and d/c if serious GI event occurs. May exacerbate inflammatory bowel disease. Renal injury reported with long-term use; increased risk with renal/hepatic impairment, hypovolemia, HF, salt depletion, and in elderly. Not recommended with advanced renal disease or moderate to severe renal impairment (CrCl <30mL/min); monitor renal function closely and hydrate adequately. D/C if signs and symptoms consistent with renal disease develop. Anaphylactoid reactions may occur. Caution with asthma and avoid with ASA-sensitive asthma and the ASA triad. May cause serious skin adverse events (eg, exfoliative dermatitis, Stevens-Johnson syndrome, toxic epidermal necrolysis); d/c at 1st appearance of skin rash/hypersensitivity. Avoid in late pregnancy; may cause premature closure of ductus arteriosus. Not a substitute for corticosteroids or for the treatment of corticosteroid insufficiency. May mask signs of inflammation and fever. Periodically monitor Hgb if initial Hgb ≤10g and receiving long-term therapy. Perform ophthalmic studies if visual changes/disturbances occur. May cause elevations of LFTs or severe hepatic reactions; d/c if liver disease or systemic manifestations occur, or if abnormal LFTs persist/worsen. Caution with chronic alcoholic liver disease and other diseases with decreased/abnormal plasma proteins if high doses are administered; dosage adjustment may be required. Anemia reported; monitor Hgb/Hct if anemia develops. May inhibit platelet aggregation and prolong bleeding time; monitor patients with coagulation disorders. Monitor CBC and chemistry profile periodically with long-term treatment. (Sus, Anaprox/Anaprox DS) Contains Na⁺; caution with severely restricted Na⁺ intake. (EC-Naprosyn) Not recommended for initial treatment of acute pain.

ADVERSE REACTIONS

Cardiovascular (CV) thrombotic events, MI, stroke, GI adverse events, edema, drowsiness, dizziness, constipation, heartburn, abdominal pain, nausea, headache, tinnitus, dyspnea, pruritus.

DRUG INTERACTIONS

Avoid with other naproxen products. Not recommended with ASA. Risk of renal toxicity with diuretics, ACE inhibitors, and ARBs. May reduce natriuretic effect of loop (eg, furosemide) or thiazide diuretics; monitor for signs of renal failure and diuretic efficacy. May diminish antihypertensive effect of ACE inhibitors, ARBs, or β-blockers (eg, propranolol); monitor changes in BP. May result in deterioration of renal function, including possible acute renal failure with ACE inhibitors or ARBs; monitor closely for signs of worsening renal function. May enhance methotrexate toxicity; caution with concomitant use. May increase lithium levels and reduce renal lithium clearance; monitor for lithium toxicity. Increased risk of GI bleeding with SSRIs, oral corticosteroids, anticoagulants, alcohol, and smoking; monitor carefully. Synergistic effect on GI bleeding with warfarin. Potential for interaction with other albumin-bound drugs (eg, coumarin-type anticoagulants, sulfonylureas, hydantoins, other NSAIDs, ASA); dose adjustment with hydantoin, sulfonamide, or sulfonylurea may be required. Probenecid significantly increases plasma levels and extends $T_{1/2}$. Antacids, sucralfate, and cholestyramine can delay absorption. (EC-Naprosyn) Not recommended with H_2-blockers, sucralfate, or intensive antacid therapy.

PREGNANCY AND LACTATION

Category C, not for use in nursing.

MECHANISM OF ACTION

NSAID; not established. May be related to prostaglandin synthetase inhibition.

PHARMACOKINETICS

Absorption: Rapid and complete. Bioavailability (95%). Naprosyn: C_{max}=97.4mcg/mL, AUC=767mcg•hr/mL, T_{max}=2-4 hrs (tab), 1-4 hrs (sus). EC-Naprosyn: C_{max}=94.9mcg/mL, AUC=845mcg•hr/mL, T_{max}=4 hrs. Anaprox (naproxen sodium): T_{max}=1-2 hrs. **Distribution:** V_d=0.16L/kg; plasma protein binding (>99%); found in breast milk. **Metabolism:** Liver (extensive); 6-0-desmethyl naproxen (metabolite). **Elimination:** Urine (95%; <1% unchanged, <1% 6-0-desmethyl naproxen, 66-92% conjugates), feces (≤3%); $T_{1/2}$=12-17 hrs.

PATIENT CONSIDERATIONS

Assessment: Assess for history of asthma, urticaria, or allergic-type reactions with ASA or other NSAIDs, ASA triad, CVD, risk factors for CVD, HTN, fluid retention, HF, salt restriction, history of ulcer disease, history of/risk factors for GI bleeding, general health status, history of IBD, renal/hepatic impairment, hypovolemia, decreased/abnormal plasma proteins, coagulation disorders, pregnancy/nursing status, and for possible drug interactions. Obtain baseline CBC and BP.

Monitoring: Monitor for GI bleeding/ulceration/perforation, CV thrombotic events, MI, stroke, HTN, fluid retention, edema, and skin/allergic reactions. Monitor BP, CBC, LFTs, renal function, and chemistry profile periodically.

Counseling: Inform to seek medical advice if symptoms of CV events, GI ulceration/bleeding, skin/hypersensitivity reactions, unexplained weight gain or edema, hepatotoxicity, or anaphylactoid reactions occur. Instruct to avoid use in late pregnancy. Instruct to use caution when performing activities that require alertness if drowsiness, dizziness, vertigo, or depression occurs.

NASONEX — mometasone furoate monohydrate   Rx

Class: Corticosteroid

ADULT DOSAGE	PEDIATRIC DOSAGE
Seasonal/Perennial Allergic Rhinitis	**Seasonal/Perennial Allergic Rhinitis**
2 sprays/nostril qd	**2-11 Years:**
Prophylaxis:	1 spray/nostril qd
May start 2-4 weeks before pollen season	**≥12 Years:**
	2 sprays/nostril qd
Nasal Congestion:	**Prophylaxis:**
2 sprays/nostril qd	May start 2-4 weeks before pollen season (≥12 years)
Nasal Polyps	**Nasal Congestion:**
2 sprays/nostril qd-bid	**2-11 Years:**
	1 spray/nostril qd.
	≥12 Years:
	2 sprays/nostril qd

ADMINISTRATION

Intranasal route

STORAGE

25°C (77°F); excursions permitted to 15-30°C (59-86°F). Protect from light.

HOW SUPPLIED

Spray: 50mcg/spray [17g]

CONTRAINDICATIONS

Known hypersensitivity to mometasone furoate or any of its ingredients.

WARNINGS/PRECAUTIONS

Local nasal effects (eg, epistaxis, *Candida* infections of nose and pharynx, nasal septum perforation, impaired wound healing) may occur; d/c when infection occurs. Glaucoma and/or cataracts may develop; monitor closely in patients with change in vision, history of increased intraocular pressure (IOP), glaucoma, and/or cataracts. D/C if hypersensitivity reactions, including instances of wheezing, occur. May increase susceptibility to infections; caution with active/quiescent tuberculosis (TB), ocular herpes simplex, or untreated bacterial, fungal, and systemic viral infections. Hypercorticism and adrenal suppression may appear

when used at higher than recommended doses or in susceptible individuals at recommended doses; d/c slowly if such changes occur. May reduce growth velocity of pediatrics; monitor growth routinely.

ADVERSE REACTIONS

Headache, viral infection, pharyngitis, epistaxis/blood-tinged mucus, cough, upper respiratory tract infection, dysmenorrhea, musculoskeletal pain, sinusitis, N/V.

DRUG INTERACTIONS

May increase plasma concentrations with ketoconazole.

PREGNANCY AND LACTATION

Category C, caution with nursing.

MECHANISM OF ACTION

Corticosteroid; not established. Demonstrates anti-inflammatory properties and is shown to have wide range of effects on multiple cell types (eg, mast cells, eosinophils, neutrophils, macrophages, lymphocytes) and mediators (eg, histamine, eicosanoids, leukotrienes, cytokines) involved in inflammation.

PHARMACOKINETICS

Absorption: Bioavailability (<1%). **Distribution:** Plasma protein binding (98-99%). **Metabolism:** Liver (extensive) via CYP3A4. **Elimination:** Bile (as metabolites); urine (limited extent); (IV) $T_{1/2}$=5.8 hrs.

PATIENT CONSIDERATIONS

Assessment: Assess for previous hypersensitivity, active/quiescent TB, infections, ocular herpes simplex, change in vision, history of IOP, glaucoma or cataracts, recent nasal septum ulcers, nasal surgery/trauma, pregnancy/nursing status, and possible drug interactions.

Monitoring: Monitor for acute adrenal insufficiency, hypercorticism, nasal or pharyngeal *Candida* infections, suppression of growth velocity in children, hypersensitivity reactions, wheezing, nasal septum perforation, changes in vision, glaucoma, cataracts, increased IOP, epistaxis, wound healing, worsening of infections, and other adverse reactions.

Counseling: Advise to take ud at regular intervals and not to increase prescribed dosage. Inform patients that treatment may be associated with adverse reactions (eg, epistaxis, nasal septum perforation, *Candida* infection). Inform that glaucoma and/or cataracts may develop. Counsel to avoid exposure to chickenpox or measles and to immediately consult a physician if exposed. Contact physician if symptoms worsen or do not improve. Supervise young children during administration. Advise patient to take missed dose as soon as remembered. Counsel on proper priming and administration techniques.

NATAZIA — dienogest/estradiol valerate   Rx

Class: Estrogen/progestogen combination

> Cigarette smoking increases risk of serious cardiovascular (CV) events from combination oral contraceptive (COC) use. Risk increases w/ age (>35 yrs of age) and w/ the number of cigarettes smoked. Should not be used by women who are >35 yrs of age and smoke.

ADULT DOSAGE	PEDIATRIC DOSAGE
Contraception	**Contraception**
1 tab qd at the same time every day for 28 days, then repeat	Not indicated for use premenarche; refer to adult dosing
Start on Day 1 of menses	**Heavy Menstrual Bleeding**
Heavy Menstrual Bleeding	Not indicated for use premenarche; refer to adult dosing
In women w/o organic pathology who choose to use oral contraceptives as method of contraception	
1 tab qd at the same time every day for 28 days, then repeat	
Start on Day 1 of menses	
Conversions	
Switching from Combination Hormonal Method:	
Another Pill: Start on 1st day of withdrawal bleed. Do not continue taking pills from previous birth control pack. Rule out pregnancy before starting therapy if a withdrawal bleed does not occur	
Vaginal Ring/Transdermal Patch: Start on the day ring/patch is removed	
Switching from Progestin-Only Method (eg, Progestin-Only Pill, Implant, Intrauterine System, Inj): Start on the day the next progestin-only pill/inj would have been taken/administered, or on the day of removal of implant/intrauterine system	
Use a nonhormonal backup method (eg, condom, spermicide) for the first 9 days	

DOSING CONSIDERATIONS

Adverse Reactions

GI Disturbances:

In case of severe vomiting or diarrhea, absorption may not be complete and additional contraceptive measures should be taken. If vomiting or diarrhea occurs w/in 3-4 hrs after taking a colored tab, may regard as missed tab

Other Important Considerations

Postpartum Women Who Do Not Breastfeed/After Second Trimester Abortion: Start therapy no earlier than 4 weeks postpartum due to the increased risk of thromboembolism; if patient initiates therapy postpartum and has not yet had a period, use an additional method of contraception until patient has taken 9 consecutive days of therapy

ADMINISTRATION

Oral route

Take in the order directed on the blister pack.
Tabs should not be skipped or intake delayed by >12 hrs.
Use a nonhormonal contraceptive as backup during the first 9 days.

STORAGE

25°C (77°F); excursions permitted to 15-30°C (59-86°F).

HOW SUPPLIED

Tab: (Estradiol Valerate) 1mg, 3mg; **Tab:** (Estradiol Valerate/Dienogest) 2mg/2mg, 2mg/3mg

CONTRAINDICATIONS

High risk of arterial/venous thrombotic diseases (eg, smoking if >35 yrs of age, history/presence of deep vein thrombosis/pulmonary embolism, cerebrovascular disease, coronary artery disease, thrombogenic valvular or thrombogenic rhythm diseases of the heart [eg, subacute bacterial endocarditis w/ valvular disease, or A-fib], inherited/acquired hypercoagulopathies, uncontrolled HTN, diabetes mellitus [DM] w/ vascular disease, headaches w/ focal neurological symptoms or migraine w/ or w/o aura if >35 yrs of age), undiagnosed abnormal uterine bleeding, history/presence of breast cancer or other estrogen-/progestin-sensitive cancer, benign/malignant liver tumors, liver disease, pregnancy.

WARNINGS/PRECAUTIONS

Increased risk of venous thromboembolism (VTE) and arterial thrombosis (eg, stroke, MI); greatest risk of VTE is present after initially starting COC or restarting (after ≥4 weeks pill-free interval) the same or different COC. D/C if arterial/venous thrombotic event occurs. If feasible, d/c at least 4 weeks before and through 2 weeks after major surgery or other surgeries known to have an elevated risk of thromboembolism. D/C if there is unexplained loss of vision, proptosis, diplopia, papilledema, or retinal vascular lesions; evaluate for retinal vein thrombosis immediately. May increase risk of cervical cancer, intraepithelial neoplasia, or gallbladder disease. Hepatic adenomas are associated w/ COC use; increased risk of developing hepatocellular carcinoma in long-term COC users. D/C if jaundice develops. Cholestasis may occur in women w/ history of pregnancy-related cholestasis. Increased BP reported; d/c if BP rises significantly. May decrease glucose tolerance; monitor prediabetic and diabetic women. Consider alternative contraception w/ uncontrolled dyslipidemia. May increase risk of pancreatitis in women w/ hypertriglyceridemia or family history thereof. Evaluate the cause of new headaches that are recurrent, persistent, or severe, and d/c therapy if indicated; an increase in frequency/severity of migraine during use may be a reason for immediate discontinuation. May cause bleeding irregularities (eg, breakthrough bleeding, spotting, amenorrhea); rule out pregnancy or malignancies. Amenorrhea or oligomenorrhea after discontinuation may occur. Caution w/ history of depression; d/c if depression recurs to serious degree. May change results of some lab tests (eg, coagulation factors, lipids, glucose tolerance, binding proteins). Exogenous estrogens may induce/exacerbate angioedema in patients w/ hereditary angioedema. Chloasma may occur; women w/ a tendency to chloasma should avoid exposure to sun or UV radiation. Safety and efficacy not evaluated in women w/ BMI >30kg/m².

ADVERSE REACTIONS

N/V, headache (including migraines), menstrual disorders, breast pain/discomfort/tenderness, acne, increased weight, mood changes.

DRUG INTERACTIONS

Avoid w/ strong CYP3A4 inducers (eg, carbamazepine, phenytoin, rifampicin, St. John's wort) and for at least 28 days after discontinuation of these inducers. Drugs or herbal products that induce certain enzymes, including CYP3A4, may decrease the effectiveness or increase breakthrough bleeding; use an alternative or backup method of contraception when enzyme inducers are used and continue backup contraception for 28 days after discontinuing the enzyme inducer. Moderate or strong CYP3A4 inhibitors (eg, azole antifungals [eg, ketoconazole, itraconazole, voriconazole], verapamil, macrolides [eg, clarithromycin, erythromycin], grapefruit) increase levels of both estradiol and dienogest. Significant changes (increase/decrease) in estrogen and progestin levels reported w/ HIV/hepatitis C virus protease inhibitors or w/ non-nucleoside reverse transcriptase inhibitors. Pregnancy reported w/ antibiotics. May significantly decrease lamotrigine levels and may reduce seizure control; dosage adjustment of lamotrigine may be necessary. Increases thyroid-binding globulin levels; may need to increase dose of thyroid hormone in patients on thyroid hormone replacement therapy.

PREGNANCY AND LACTATION

Pregnancy: Contraindicated in pregnancy.
Lactation: Not for use in nursing.

MECHANISM OF ACTION

Estrogen/progestin oral contraceptive; acts primarily by suppressing ovulation. Other possible mechanisms may include cervical mucus changes that inhibit sperm penetration and endometrial changes that reduce the likelihood of implantation.

PHARMACOKINETICS

Absorption: Bioavailability (91%); C_{max}=91.7ng/mL, T_{max}=1 hr (median), $AUC_{(0-24\ hr)}$=964ng/mL; Estradiol: C_{max}=73.3pg/mL, T_{max}=6 hrs (median), $AUC_{(0-24\ hr)}$=1301pg•hr/mL. **Distribution:** Estradiol: V_d=1.2L/kg (IV); bound to sex hormone-binding globulin (38%) and albumin (60%); found in breast milk. Dienogest: V_d=46L (IV); bound to albumin (90%); found in breast milk. **Metabolism:** Estradiol: Extensive 1st pass effect; CYP3A; estrone and its sulfate or glucuronide conjugates (main metabolites); Dienogest: extensive (hydroxylation, conjugation), CYP3A4 (main). **Elimination:** Estradiol: Urine (main), feces (10%), $T_{1/2}$=14 hrs; Dienogest: Renal (main); $T_{1/2}$=11 hrs.

PATIENT CONSIDERATIONS

Assessment: Assess for abnormal uterine bleeding, risk of arterial or venous thrombotic diseases, pregnancy/nursing status, and for any other conditions where treatment is cautioned or contraindicated. Assess for possible drug interactions. Assess BP levels.

Monitoring: Monitor for bleeding irregularities, venous/arterial thrombotic events, cervical cancer or intraepithelial neoplasia, retinal vein thrombosis or any other ophthalmic changes, jaundice, new/worsening headaches or migraines, serious depression, cholestasis w/ history of pregnancy-related cholestasis, pancreatitis, and for other adverse reactions. Monitor thyroid function if receiving thyroid replacement therapy, glucose levels in diabetic and prediabetic women, depression in women w/ a history of depression, and lipids levels w/ dyslipidemia. Conduct yearly visit for a BP check and for other indicated healthcare.

Counseling: Inform that cigarette smoking increases the risk of serious CV events from COC use and that women who are >35 yrs of age and smoke should not use COCs. Inform about risk of VTE. Advise that drug does not protect against HIV infection and other sexually transmitted diseases. Instruct to d/c if pregnancy occurs during treatment. Instruct to take 1 tab daily at the same time every day in the exact order noted on the blister. Counsel on what to do if pills are missed. Instruct to use a backup or alternative method of contraception when weak or moderate enzyme inducers are used w/ therapy. Inform that COCs may reduce breast milk production. Instruct any patient who starts COCs postpartum, and who has not yet had a period, to use an additional method of contraception until they have taken 9 consecutive days of therapy. Inform that amenorrhea may occur.

NATESTO — testosterone   CIII

Class: Androgen

ADULT DOSAGE	PEDIATRIC DOSAGE
Testosterone Replacement Therapy	Pediatric use may not have been established
Congenital/Acquired Primary Hypogonadism or Hypogonadotropic Hypogonadism in Males:	
Usual: 11mg (2 pump actuations; 1 actuation/nostril) tid for a total dose of 33mg/day	
Consider alternative treatment if total testosterone concentration is consistently <300ng/dL; if total testosterone concentration is consistently >1050ng/dL, d/c therapy	

DOSING CONSIDERATIONS

Concomitant Medications
Use w/ other nasally administered drugs other than sympathomimetic decongestants (eg, oxymetazoline) is not recommended

Discontinuation
Severe Rhinitis: If patient experiences an episode of severe rhinitis, temporarily d/c therapy pending resolution of the severe rhinitis symptoms. If severe rhinitis symptoms persist, alternative testosterone replacement therapy is recommended

ADMINISTRATION

Intranasal route

Administer tid (in the am, afternoon, and pm) (6-8 hrs apart) preferably at the same time each day
Completely depress pump 1X in each nostril to receive total dose
Do not administer to other parts of the body
Replace dispenser when the top of the piston inside dispenser reaches the arrow at the top of the inside label

Preparing the Pump
Prime pump by inverting pump, and depressing pump 10X; discard any amount of product dispensed directly into a sink and thoroughly wash away the gel w/ warm water
Wipe tip w/ a clean, dry tissue
If gel gets on to the hands, wash hands w/ warm water and soap
Priming should be done only prior to the 1st use of each dispenser

Administering the Dose
1. Blow nose, then remove cap from dispenser
2. Place the right index finger on the pump of the actuator while in front of a mirror; slowly advance the tip of the actuator into the left nostril upwards until the finger on the pump reaches the base of the nose
3. Tilt actuator so that opening on the tip of the actuator is in contact w/ lateral wall of nostril to ensure application of gel to the nasal wall
4. Slowly depress pump until it stops
5. Remove actuator from nose while wiping the tip along the inside of the lateral nostril wall to fully transfer the gel
6. Using left index finger, repeat steps 2-5 for the right nostril
7. Use a clean, dry tissue to wipe tip of actuator and replace cap on dispenser
8. Press on nostrils at a point just below the bridge of the nose and lightly massage
9. Refrain from blowing nose or sniffing for 1 hr after administration

STORAGE

20-25°C (68-77°F); excursions permitted to 15-30°C (59-86°F). Discard used dispensers in household trash in a manner that prevents accidental exposure of children or pets.

HOW SUPPLIED

Gel: 5.5mg/actuation [60 actuations]

CONTRAINDICATIONS

Breast carcinoma or known/suspected prostate carcinoma in men; women who are or may become pregnant, or are breastfeeding.

WARNINGS/PRECAUTIONS

Nasal adverse reactions (eg, nasopharyngitis, rhinorrhea, epistaxis) reported; determine whether further evaluation or discontinuation of therapy is appropriate. Not recommended for use in patients w/ mucosal inflammatory disorders (eg, Sjogren's syndrome), sinus disease, and those w/ a history of nasal disorders, nasal/sinus surgery, or nasal fracture w/in the previous 6 months or nasal fracture that caused a deviated anterior nasal septum. Patients w/ BPH and geriatric patients may be at increased risk of worsening of signs/symptoms of BPH. May increase risk for prostate cancer. Increases in Hct, reflective of increases in RBC mass, may require discontinuation of therapy. If Hct becomes elevated, d/c until Hct decreases to an acceptable level. Increase in RBC mass may increase risk of thromboembolic events. Venous thromboembolic events (eg, deep vein thrombosis, pulmonary embolism) reported; d/c and initiate workup and management if a venous thromboembolic event is suspected. Increased risk of major adverse cardiovascular events (MACE) reported. Not indicated for use in women. Suppression of spermatogenesis may occur w/ large doses. Prolonged use of high doses of orally active 17-α-alkyl androgens has been associated w/ serious hepatic effects (eg, peliosis hepatis, hepatic neoplasms, cholestatic hepatitis); d/c promptly if any signs/symptoms of hepatic dysfunction occur. May promote retention of Na^+ and water. Risk of edema w/ or w/o CHF in patients w/ preexisting cardiac, renal, or hepatic disease; diuretic therapy, in addition to discontinuation of therapy, may be required. Gynecomastia may develop and persist. May potentiate sleep apnea, especially in those w/ risk factors (eg, obesity, chronic lung disease). Changes in serum lipid profile may occur and may require discontinuation of therapy. Caution in cancer patients at risk of hypercalcemia and associated hypercalciuria. May decrease levels of thyroxine-binding globulins, resulting in decreased total T4 serum levels and increased resin uptake of T3 and T4.

ADVERSE REACTIONS

Prostate-specific antigen increased, headache, rhinorrhea, epistaxis, nasal discomfort, nasopharyngitis, bronchitis, URTI, sinusitis, nasal scab, nasal dryness, nasal congestion, parosmia, pain in extremity.

DRUG INTERACTIONS

See Dosing Considerations. Changes in insulin sensitivity or glycemic control may occur; may decrease blood glucose and, therefore, may necessitate a dose reduction of anti-diabetic medication in diabetic patients. Changes in anticoagulant activity may occur; frequently monitor PT/INR in patients taking warfarin, especially at initiation and termination of androgen therapy. Concurrent use w/ corticosteroids may increase fluid retention; monitoring required, particularly in patients w/ cardiac, renal, or hepatic disease. Oxymetazoline given 30 min prior to therapy may decrease total testosterone levels.

PREGNANCY AND LACTATION

Category X, not for use in nursing.

MECHANISM OF ACTION

Androgen; responsible for normal growth and development of male sex organs and for maintenance of secondary sex characteristics.

PHARMACOKINETICS

Absorption: T_{max}=40 min. **Distribution:** Plasma protein binding (98%; 40% sex hormone-binding globulin). **Metabolism:** Estradiol and dihydrotestosterone (major active metabolites). **Elimination:** (IM) Urine (90% glucuronic and sulfuric acid conjugates), feces (6% unconjugated); $T_{1/2}$=10-100 min.

PATIENT CONSIDERATIONS

Assessment: Assess for mucosal inflammatory disorders; sinus disease, history of nasal disorders, nasal/sinus surgery, or nasal fracture w/in the previous 6 months or nasal fracture that caused a deviated anterior nasal septum; BPH; prostate cancer; cardiac/renal/hepatic disease; obesity; chronic lung disease, any other conditions where treatment is contraindicated or cautioned; and for possible drug interactions. Obtain baseline Hct and lipid levels. Confirm diagnosis of hypogonadism by measuring testosterone levels in am on at least 2 separate days prior to initiation.

Monitoring: Monitor for nasal adverse reactions, worsening of signs/symptoms of BPH, venous thromboembolic events, signs/symptoms of hepatic dysfunction, edema w/ or w/o CHF, gynecomastia, sleep apnea, MACE, and other adverse reactions. Monitor lipid profile periodically. Check serum testosterone levels periodically, starting as soon as 1 month after initiation of therapy. In cancer patients at risk for hypercalcemia, regularly monitor serum Ca^{2+} levels. Evaluate Hct level 3-6 months after starting therapy, then annually. Evaluate for prostate cancer 3-6 months after initiation of treatment, then in accordance w/ prostate cancer screening practices.

Counseling: Advise about possible adverse reactions, including risk of MACE. Inform that men w/ known/suspected prostate or breast cancer should not use therapy. Instruct to report to physician any nasal signs/symptoms or any signs/symptoms of hepatic dysfunction (eg, jaundice). Counsel to use ud, to report any changes in state of health to physician, and to never share medication w/ anyone.

NATPARA — parathyroid hormone

Rx

Class: Parathyroid hormone analogue

ADULT DOSAGE

Hypocalcemia with Hypoparathyroidism

Adjunct to Ca^{2+} and Vitamin D to Control Hypocalcemia:
Before Initiating and During Therapy:
Confirm 25-hydroxyvitamin D stores are sufficient; if insufficient, replace to sufficient levels
Confirm serum Ca^{2+} is >7.5mg/dL before initiating therapy

Initiating Therapy:
1. Initiate at 50mcg SQ qd
2. In patients using active forms of vitamin D, decrease dose of active vitamin D by 50%, if serum Ca^{2+} >7.5mg/dL
3. In patients using Ca^{2+} supplements, maintain Ca^{2+} supplement dose
4. Measure serum Ca^{2+} concentration w/in 3-7 days
5. Adjust dose of active vitamin D or Ca^{2+} supplement or both based on serum Ca^{2+} value and clinical assessment; refer to PI for suggested adjustments
6. Repeat steps 4 and 5 until target serum Ca^{2+} levels are w/in the lower 1/2 of the normal range (8-9mg/dL), active vitamin D has been discontinued, and Ca^{2+} supplementation is sufficient to meet daily requirements

Titration:
Dose Increase: May increase in increments of 25mcg every 4 weeks up to a max of 100mcg/day if serum Ca^{2+} cannot be maintained >8mg/dL w/o an active form of vitamin D and/or oral Ca^{2+} supplementation
Dose Decrease: May decrease to as low as 25mcg/day if total serum Ca^{2+} is repeatedly >9mg/dL after active form of vitamin D has been discontinued and Ca^{2+} supplement has been decreased to a dose sufficient to meet daily requirements After a dose change, monitor clinical response as well as serum Ca^{2+}; adjust active vitamin D and Ca^{2+} supplements per steps 4-6 above if indicated

Maint Dose:
Use lowest dose that achieves total serum Ca^{2+} (albumin-corrected) w/in the lower 1/2 of normal total serum Ca^{2+} range, w/o the need for active forms of vitamin D and w/ Ca^{2+} supplementation sufficient to meet daily requirements; monitor serum Ca^{2+} and 24 hr urinary calcium once maint dose is achieved

Missed Dose

Next dose should be administered as soon as reasonably feasible and additional exogenous Ca^{2+} should be taken in the event of hypocalcemia

----

DOSING CONSIDERATIONS
Elderly
Start at low end of dosing range

Dose Interruption or Discontinuation
Abrupt interruption or discontinuation can result in severe hypocalcemia; resume treatment w/, or increase the dose of, an active form of vitamin D and Ca^{2+} supplements if indicated in patients interrupting or discontinuing therapy

ADMINISTRATION
SQ route

Administer in thigh; alternate thigh every day
Refer to PI for the instructions to reconstitute using the mixing device for reconstitution and to administer using the pen delivery device (Q-Cliq pen)

STORAGE
(Cartridge) Prior to Reconstitution: 2-8°C (36-46°F). After Reconstitution: Store in the Q-Cliq pen at 2-8°C (36-46°F) and may be used for up to 14 days under these conditions; discard after 14 days. Store away from heat and light. Avoid exposure to elevated temperatures. Do not freeze or shake. (Mixing Device/Empty Q-Cliq Pen) Room temperature.

PEDIATRIC DOSAGE

Pediatric use may not have been established

HOW SUPPLIED
Inj: 25mcg/dose, 50mcg/dose, 75mcg/dose, 100mcg/dose

WARNINGS/PRECAUTIONS
Severe hypercalcemia reported; risk is highest when starting or increasing dose of parathyroid hormone but can occur at any time. Treat hypercalcemia per standard practice and consider holding and/or lowering parathyroid hormone dose if severe hypercalcemia occurs. Severe hypocalcemia reported; risk is highest when parathyroid hormone is withheld, missed, or abruptly discontinued. Resume treatment w/, or increase dose of, an active form of vitamin D or Ca^{2+} supplements or both if indicated in patients interrupting or discontinuing therapy. Caution in elderly.

ADVERSE REACTIONS
Paresthesia, hypo/hypercalcemia, headache, N/V, hypoaesthesia, diarrhea, arthralgia, hypercalciuria, pain in extremity, URTI, upper abdominal pain, sinusitis, HTN, neck pain.

DRUG INTERACTIONS
Not recommended w/ alendronate. Concomitant use w/ cardiac glycosides (eg, digoxin) may predispose patients to digitalis toxicity if hypercalcemia develops; carefully monitor serum Ca^{2+} and digoxin levels, and for signs/symptoms of digoxin toxicity. Adjustment of digoxin and/or parathyroid hormone may be needed.

PREGNANCY AND LACTATION
Pregnancy: Category C.
Lactation: Not for use in nursing.

MECHANISM OF ACTION
Parathyroid hormone; raises serum Ca^{2+} by increasing renal tubular Ca^{2+} reabsorption, increasing intestinal Ca^{2+} absorption, and by increasing bone turnover which releases Ca^{2+} into the circulation.

PHARMACOKINETICS
Absorption: Absolute bioavailability (53%); T_{max}=5-30 min (50mcg, 100mcg); 2nd small peak at 1-2 hrs. **Distribution:** V_d=5.35L. **Metabolism:** Liver, kidneys. **Elimination:** $T_{1/2}$=3.02 hrs (50mcg), 2.83 hrs (100mcg).

PATIENT CONSIDERATIONS
Assessment: Assess for increased baseline risk for osteosarcoma, pregnancy/nursing status, and for possible drug interactions. Assess serum Ca^{2+} levels, and 25-hydroxyvitamin D stores.

Monitoring: Monitor for signs and symptoms of osteosarcoma, hypo/hypercalcemia, and other adverse reactions. Monitor serum Ca^{2+} levels and 25-hydroxyvitamin D stores.

Counseling: Inform of the risks/benefits of therapy. Inform that the drug is available only through a restricted program called the Natpara REMS program. Advise of potential risk of osteosarcoma and to promptly report signs/symptoms of possible osteosarcoma (eg, persistent localized pain, occurrence of a new tissue mass that is tender to palpation). Advise that severe hypercalcemia may occur when initiating/adjusting dose and/or making changes to coadministered drugs known to raise serum Ca^{2+}; instruct to report symptoms promptly, report any changes to coadministered drugs known to influence Ca^{2+} levels, and follow recommended serum Ca^{2+} monitoring. Inform that severe hypocalcemia may occur when therapy is abruptly interrupted/discontinued; instruct to report symptoms of severe hypocalcemia promptly, report interruption in dosing, follow recommended serum Ca^{2+} monitoring, and to contact physician in the event of dose interruption as doses of active vitamin D and Ca^{2+} supplementation may need adjustment. Instruct to report use of digoxin-containing medication, and follow recommended serum Ca^{2+} monitoring. Counsel patient or caregiver on the proper technique for administering SQ inj using the mixing device and the Q-Cliq pen, including the use of aseptic technique.

NATROBA — spinosad   Rx

Class: Pediculicide

ADULT DOSAGE	PEDIATRIC DOSAGE
Head Lice	**Head Lice**
Depending on hair length, apply up to 120mL to adequately cover dry scalp and hair; leave on for 10 min, then thoroughly rinse off w/ warm water	**≥6 Months of Age:** Depending on hair length, apply up to 120mL to adequately cover dry scalp and hair; leave on for 10 min, then thoroughly rinse off w/ warm water
Apply 2nd treatment if live lice are seen 7 days after the 1st treatment	Apply 2nd treatment if live lice are seen 7 days after the 1st treatment

---

ADMINISTRATION
Topical route
Shake well before use
Avoid contact w/ eyes

STORAGE
25°C (77°F); excursions permitted between 15-30°C (59-86°F).

HOW SUPPLIED
Sus: 0.9% [120mL]

WARNINGS/PRECAUTIONS
Not for oral, ophthalmic, or intravaginal use. Contains benzyl alcohol; avoid in neonates and infants <6 months of age. Should be used in the context of an overall lice management program (eg, washing of recently worn clothing and personal care items).

ADVERSE REACTIONS
Application-site erythema/irritation, ocular erythema.

PREGNANCY AND LACTATION
Category B, caution in nursing.

MECHANISM OF ACTION
Pediculicide; causes neuronal excitation in insects; lice become paralyzed and die after periods of hyperexcitation.

PATIENT CONSIDERATIONS
Assessment: Assess pregnancy/nursing status.

Monitoring: Monitor for presence of live lice after 7 days of 1st treatment, and other adverse reactions.

Counseling: Advise to use only on dry scalp and hair. Instruct not to swallow. Instruct to repeat treatment only if live lice are seen 7 days after 1st treatment. Instruct to rinse thoroughly w/ water if medication gets in or near the eyes. Advise to wash hands after application. Inform to use on children only under direct supervision of an adult.

NATURE-THROID — thyroid   Rx

Class: Thyroid replacement hormone

ADULT DOSAGE	PEDIATRIC DOSAGE
Hypothyroidism	**Hypothyroidism**
Replacement/supplemental therapy in hypothyroidism of any etiology, except transient hypothyroidism during the recovery phase of subacute thyroiditis	**Congenital:**
	0-6 Months of Age: 4.8-6mg/kg/day (16.25-32.5mg/day)
Initial: 32.5mg/day; 16.25mg/day is recommended in patients w/ myxedema, particularly if cardiovascular impairment is suspected	**6-12 Months of Age:** 3.6-4.8mg/kg/day (32.5-48.75mg/day)
Titrate: Increase by 16.25mg every 2-3 weeks	**1-5 Years:** 3-3.6mg/kg/day (48.75-65mg/day)
Maint: 65-130mg/day	**6-12 Years:** 2.4-3mg/kg/day (65-97.5mg/day)
Myxedema Coma:	**>12 Years:** 1.2-1.8mg/kg/day (>97.5mg/day)
Initial: 400mcg (100mcg/mL) of levothyroxine sodium (T4) given rapidly; follow by daily supplements of 100-200mcg given IV	
Pituitary TSH Suppressant	
Used to treat/prevent various types of euthyroid goiters (eg, thyroid nodules, subacute or chronic lymphocytic thyroiditis [Hashimoto's], multinodular goiter) and to manage thyroid cancer	
1.56mg/kg/day of levothyroxine (T4) for 7-10 days	
Diagnostic Aid	
In Suppression Tests to Differentiate Suspected Mild Hyperthyroidism or Thyroid Gland Anatomy:	
1.56mg/kg/day of levothyroxine (T4) for 7-10 days	

DOSING CONSIDERATIONS
Adverse Reactions
Hypothyroidism:
Angina: Reduce dose if angina occurs

Elderly
Start at lower end of dosing range

ADMINISTRATION
Oral route

STORAGE
15-30°C (59-86°F).

HOW SUPPLIED
Tab: 16.25mg, 32.5mg, 48.75mg, 65mg, 81.25mg, 97.5mg, 113.75mg, 130mg, 146.25mg, 162.5mg, 195mg, 260mg, 325mg

CONTRAINDICATIONS
Uncorrected adrenal cortical insufficiency, untreated thyrotoxicosis, hypersensitivity to any of their active or extraneous constituents.

WARNINGS/PRECAUTIONS
Not for treatment of obesity; larger doses in euthyroid patients can cause serious or even life-threatening toxicity. Not for the treatment of male or female infertility unless accompanied by hypothyroidism. Caution with cardiovascular (CV) disorders (eg, angina pectoris) and elderly with risk of occult cardiac disease; initiate at low doses and reduce dose if aggravation of CV disease suspected. May aggravate diabetes mellitus (DM), diabetes insipidus (DI), or adrenal cortical insufficiency. Treatment of myxedema coma requires simultaneous administration of glucocorticoids. Excessive doses in infants may cause craniosynostosis. Caution with strong suspicion of thyroid gland autonomy. Androgens, corticosteroids, estrogens, iodine-containing preparations, and salicylates may interfere with lab tests.

DRUG INTERACTIONS

Large doses in euthyroid patients may cause serious or even life-threatening toxicity particularly with sympathomimetic amines. Closely monitor PT in patients on oral anticoagulants; dose reduction of anticoagulant may be required. May increase insulin or oral hypoglycemic requirements. Potentially impaired absorption with cholestyramine and colestipol; space dosing by 4-5 hrs. Estrogens may decrease free T4; increase in thyroid dose may be needed.

PREGNANCY AND LACTATION

Category A, caution in nursing.

MECHANISM OF ACTION

Thyroid replacement hormone; not established. Enhances oxygen consumption by most tissues of the body, increases the basal metabolic rate and the metabolism of carbohydrates, lipids, and proteins.

PHARMACOKINETICS

Distribution: Plasma protein binding (>99%); found in breast milk. **Metabolism:** (T4) Deiodination in liver, kidneys, other tissues.

PATIENT CONSIDERATIONS

Assessment: Assess for adrenal cortical insufficiency, thyrotoxicosis, apparent hypersensitivity to the drug, CV disorders (CAD, angina pectoris), DM/DI, myxedema coma, nursing status, and possible drug interactions.

Monitoring: Monitor response to treatment, urinary glucose levels in patients with DM, PT in patients receiving anticoagulants, and for aggravation of CV disease. Monitor thyroid function periodically.

Counseling: Inform that replacement therapy is taken essentially for life except in transient hypothyroidism. Instruct to immediately report to physician any signs/symptoms of thyroid hormone toxicity (eg, chest pain, increased pulse rate, palpitations, excessive sweating, heat intolerance, nervousness). Inform the importance of frequent/close monitoring of PT and urinary glucose and the need for dose adjustment of antidiabetic and/or oral anticoagulant medication. Inform that partial loss of hair may be seen in children in 1st few months of therapy.

NEBUPENT — pentamidine isethionate   Rx

Class: Antifungal agent

ADULT DOSAGE	PEDIATRIC DOSAGE
Pneumocystis Pneumonia	Pediatric use may not have been established
Prevention of *Pneumocystis jiroveci* pneumonia (PJP) in high-risk, HIV-infected patients that have history of ≥1 episode of PJP and/or have peripheral CD4+ (T4 helper/inducer) lymphocyte count ≤200/mm³	
Usual: 300mg once every 4 weeks via Respirgard II nebulizer	

ADMINISTRATION

Oral inhalational route

Deliver until nebulizer chamber is empty (approximately 30-45 min), w/ flow rate of 5-7L/min from 40-50 pounds per square inch (PSI) air or oxygen source; alternatively, use a 40-50 PSI air compressor w/ flowmeter at 5-7L/min or pressure at 22-25 PSI

Do not use Respirgard II nebulizer to administer a bronchodilator

Preparation

Dissolve contents of one 300mg vial in 6mL of sterile water for inj only; do not use saline sol for reconstitution

Do not mix w/ any other drugs

Place entire contents of vial into Respirgard II nebulizer reservoir for administration

STORAGE

Dry Product: 20-25°C (68-77°F). Reconstituted Sol: Room temperature; stable only for 48 hrs in original vial. Protect dry and reconstituted product from light.

HOW SUPPLIED

Sol (powder): 300mg/vial

WARNINGS/PRECAUTIONS

Potential for development of acute PJP still exists; monitor for symptoms of pulmonary infection (eg, dyspnea, fever, cough). May alter clinical and radiographic features of PJP and could result in atypical presentation (eg, mild disease, focal infection). Recommended dose is insufficient to treat acute PJP; evaluate for PJP prior to use. May induce bronchospasm or cough particularly with history of smoking or asthma; administration of inhaled bronchodilator prior to each dose may minimize recurrence of symptoms. Monitor for development of serious adverse reactions that have occurred with parenteral administration (eg, hypotension, hypoglycemia, hyperglycemia, hypocalcemia, anemia, thrombocytopenia, leukopenia, hepatic/renal dysfunction, ventricular tachycardia, pancreatitis, Stevens-Johnson syndrome [SJS], hyperkalemia, abnormal ST segment of ECG). Extrapulmonary infection with *P. jiroveci* reported infrequently. D/C if acute pancreatitis develops.

ADVERSE REACTIONS

Fatigue, cough, fever, decreased appetite, shortness of breath, dizziness/light-headedness, wheezing, nonspecific serious infection, bronchospasm, night sweats, diarrhea, nausea, anemia, pharyngitis.

DRUG INTERACTIONS

Avoid concomitant or sequential use with nephrotoxic drugs (eg, aminoglycosides, amphotericin B, cisplatin, foscarnet, vancomycin).

PREGNANCY AND LACTATION

Category C, not for use in nursing.

MECHANISM OF ACTION

Antifungal agent; mechanism not fully understood. Proposed to interfere with microbial nuclear metabolism by inhibition of DNA, RNA, phospholipid and protein synthesis.

PHARMACOKINETICS

Absorption: (Aerosolized) C_{max}=2.3ng/mL. (4mg/kg/day via Ultra Vent jet nebulizer) C_{max}=18.8ng/mL. (4mg/kg single 2-hr IV infusion) C_{max}=612ng/mL. **Elimination:** (4mg/kg single 2-hr IV infusion) $T_{1/2}$=6.4 hrs.

PATIENT CONSIDERATIONS

Assessment: Assess for PJP, history of smoking or asthma, history of anaphylactic reaction to the drug, pregnancy/nursing status, and possible drug interactions.

Monitoring: Monitor for acute PJP, opportunistic/nonopportunistic pathogens, symptoms of pulmonary infection, cough, bronchospasm, extrapulmonary pneumocystosis, acute pancreatitis, and other adverse reactions.

Counseling: Advise to seek medical evaluation and diagnostic tests if symptoms of pulmonary infection develop. Counsel to report if symptoms of acute pancreatitis occur. Instruct not to mix with any other drugs and not to use Respirgard II nebulizer to administer bronchodilator. Instruct to dissolve only in sterile water for injection, USP and not to use saline solution for reconstitution.

NEORAL — cyclosporine   Rx

Class: Calcineurin-inhibitor immunosuppressant

> Should only be prescribed by physicians experienced in management of systemic immunosuppressive therapy for indicated diseases. Manage patients in facilities equipped and staffed w/ adequate lab and supportive medical resources. Increased susceptibility to infection and development of neoplasia (eg, lymphoma) may result from immunosuppression. May be coadministered w/ other immunosuppressive agents in kidney, liver, and heart transplant patients. Not bioequivalent to Sandimmune and cannot be used interchangeably w/o physician supervision. Caution in switching from Sandimmune. Monitor cyclosporine blood concentrations in transplant and rheumatoid arthritis (RA) patients to avoid toxicity due to high concentrations. Dose adjustments should be made to minimize possible organ rejection due to low concentrations in transplant patients. Increased risk of developing skin malignancies in psoriasis patients previously treated w/ PUVA, methotrexate (MTX) or other immunosuppressive agents, UVB, coal tar, or radiation therapy. May cause systemic HTN and nephrotoxicity. Monitor for renal dysfunction, including structural kidney damage, during therapy.

ADULT DOSAGE	PEDIATRIC DOSAGE
Organ Transplant	**Organ Rejection Prophylaxis**
Organ Rejection Prophylaxis in Kidney, Liver, and Heart Allogeneic Transplants:	Transplant recipients as young as 1 year of age have received Neoral w/ no unusual adverse effects
Newly Transplanted Patients: Initial dose may be given 4-12 hrs prior to transplant or given postoperatively; dose varies depending on transplanted organ and other immunosuppressive agents included in protocol	
Suggested Initial Doses: **Renal Transplant:** 9mg/kg/day ± 3mg/kg/day **Liver Transplant:** 8mg/kg/day ± 4mg/kg/day **Heart Transplant:** 7mg/kg/day ± 3mg/kg/day	
Give bid	
Subsequently adjust dose to achieve a predefined blood concentration	
Adjunct therapy w/ adrenal corticosteroids is recommended initially	
Conversion from Sandimmune: Start w/ same daily dose as was previously used w/ Sandimmune (1:1 dose conversion); subsequently adjust dose to attain the pre-conversion blood trough concentration. After conversion, monitor blood trough concentration every 4-7 days while adjusting to trough levels until concentration attains pre-conversion value.	
Transplant Patients w/ Poor Sandimmune Absorption: Patients tend to have higher cyclosporine concentrations after conversion to therapy; caution when converting patients at doses >10mg/kg/day. Titrate dose individually based on trough concentrations, tolerability, and clinical response and measure blood trough concentration at least	

2X a week (daily if initial dose >10mg/kg/day) until stabilized w/in desired range.

Rheumatoid Arthritis

Severe, active rheumatoid arthritis where the disease has not adequately responded to methotrexate (MTX)

W/ or w/o MTX:
Initial: 2.5mg/kg/day, taken bid
Titrate: May increase by 0.5-0.75mg/kg/day after 8 weeks and again after 12 weeks
Max: 4mg/kg/day

Salicylates, NSAIDs, and oral corticosteroids may be continued

D/C if no benefit is seen by 16 weeks

Combination w/ MTX:
Most patients can be treated w/ doses of ≤3mg/kg/day when combined w/ MTX doses of up to 15mg/week

Plaque Psoriasis

In immunocompetent patients w/ severe, recalcitrant, plaque psoriasis who failed to respond to at least 1 systemic therapy (eg, PUVA, retinoids, methotrexate) or for whom other systemic therapies are contraindicated, or cannot be tolerated

Initial: 2.5mg/kg/day, taken bid, for at least 4 weeks
Titrate: If clinical improvement does not occur, increase dose at 2-week intervals by approx 0.5mg/kg/day
Max: 4mg/kg/day

D/C if satisfactory response cannot be achieved after 6 weeks at 4mg/kg/day or the patient's max tolerated dose

DOSING CONSIDERATIONS

Renal Impairment
In Kidney, Liver, and Heart Transplant:
Reduce dose if indicated
In Rheumatoid Arthritis/Plaque Psoriasis:
Not recommended for use

Hepatic Impairment
Severe: Dose reduction may be necessary

Elderly
Start at lower end of dosing range

Adverse Events
Rheumatoid Arthritis/Plaque Psoriasis:
Reduce dose by 25-50% to control adverse events; d/c therapy if dose reduction is not effective or if adverse event or abnormality is severe

Other Important Considerations
Avoid consumption of grapefruit or grapefruit juice during therapy

ADMINISTRATION
Oral route

Always administer daily dose in 2 divided doses (bid); administer on a consistent schedule w/ regard to time of day and relation to meals.

Sol
1. Dilute w/ room temperature orange or apple juice to make sol more palatable; avoid switching diluents frequently or diluting w/ grapefruit juice.
2. Take the prescribed amount of sol from the container using supplied dosing syringe, after removal of protective cover, and transfer sol to a glass of orange or apple juice (do not use a plastic container).
3. Stir well and drink at once; do not allow diluted oral sol to stand before drinking.
4. Rinse the glass w/ more diluent to ensure that the total dose is consumed.
5. After use, dry the outside of dosing syringe w/ a clean towel and replace protective cover.
6. Do not rinse dosing syringe w/ water or other cleaning agents; if syringe requires cleaning, it must be completely dry before resuming use.

STORAGE
20-25°C (68-77°F). (Sol) Use w/in 2 months upon opening. Do not refrigerate. At <20°C (68°F) may form gel; light flocculation, or formation of light sediment may occur; allow to warm to 25°C (77°F) to reverse changes.

HOW SUPPLIED
Cap: 25mg, 100mg; **Sol:** 100mg/mL [50mL]

CONTRAINDICATIONS
Hypersensitivity to cyclosporine or to any of the ingredients of the formulation. **RA/Psoriasis:** Abnormal renal function, uncontrolled HTN, malignancies. **Psoriasis:** Concomitant PUVA or UVB therapy, MTX, other immunosuppressants, coal tar, or radiation therapy.

WARNINGS/PRECAUTIONS
May cause hepatotoxicity and liver injury (eg, cholestasis, jaundice, hepatitis, liver failure). Elevations of SrCr and BUN may occur and reflect a reduction in GFR; closely monitor renal function and frequent dose adjustments may be indicated. Elevations in SrCr and BUN levels do not necessarily indicate rejection; evaluate patient before initiating dose adjustment. Thrombocytopenia and microangiopathic hemolytic anemia, resulting in graft failure, significant hyperkalemia (sometimes associated w/ hyperchloremic metabolic acidosis) and hyperuricemia reported. Avoid excessive ultraviolet light exposure. Oversuppression of the immune system may result in an increased risk of infection/malignancy; caution w/ a multiple immunosuppressant regimen. Increased risk of developing bacterial, viral, fungal, protozoal, and opportunistic infections (eg, polyomavirus infections). JC virus-associated progressive multifocal leukoencephalopathy and polyomavirus-/BK virus-associated nephropathy reported; consider reduction in immunosuppression if either develops. Convulsions, encephalopathy including posterior reversible encephalopathy syndrome, and rarely, optic disc edema reported. Evaluate before and during treatment for development of malignancies. In RA patients, monitor BP on at least 2 occasions and obtain 2 baseline SrCr levels before treatment, then monitor BP and SrCr every 2 weeks for the first 3 months of therapy, and then monthly if the patient is stable or more frequently during dose adjustments. In psoriasis patients, assess BP on at least 2 occasions and obtain baseline SrCr, BUN, CBC, Mg^{2+}, K^+, uric acid, and lipids before treatment, then monitor every 2 weeks for the first 3 months of therapy, and then monthly if the patient is stable or more frequently during dose adjustments. Monitor CBC and LFTs monthly w/ MTX. Monitor SrCr and BP after initiation or increases in NSAID dose for RA. Consider the alcohol content of the drug when given to patients in whom alcohol intake should be avoided or minimized (eg, pregnant or breastfeeding women, patients presenting w/ liver disease or epilepsy, alcoholic patients, or pediatric patients). HTN may occur and persist, and may require antihypertensive therapy.

ADVERSE REACTIONS
Increased susceptibility to infection, neoplasia, renal dysfunction, HTN, hirsutism/hypertrichosis, tremor, headache, gum hyperplasia, diarrhea, N/V, paresthesia, hypertriglyceridemia, hyperesthesia.

DRUG INTERACTIONS
See Boxed Warning, Dosing Considerations, and Contraindications. Avoid w/ K^+-sparing diuretics, aliskiren, orlistat, bosentan, or dabigatran. Vaccinations may be less effective; avoid live vaccines during therapy. Frequent gingival hyperplasia reported w/ nifedipine; avoid concomitant use w/ nifedipine in patients in whom gingival hyperplasia develops as a side effect of cyclosporine. Caution w/ rifabutin, nephrotoxic drugs, HIV protease inhibitors (eg, indinavir, nelfinavir, ritonavir, saquinavir), K^+-sparing drugs (eg, ACE inhibitors, ARBs), K^+-containing drugs, and K^+-rich diet. Ciprofloxacin, gentamicin, tobramycin, vancomycin, trimethoprim w/ sulfamethoxazole, melphalan, amphotericin B, ketoconazole, azapropazon, colchicine, diclofenac, naproxen, sulindac, cimetidine, ranitidine, tacrolimus, fibric acid derivatives (eg, bezafibrate, fenofibrate), MTX, and NSAIDs may potentiate renal dysfunction; closely monitor renal function and reduce dose of coadministered drug or consider alternative treatment if significant renal impairment occurs. Diltiazem, nicardipine, verapamil, fluconazole, itraconazole, ketoconazole, voriconazole, azithromycin, clarithromycin, erythromycin, quinupristin/dalfopristin, methylprednisolone, allopurinol, amiodarone, bromocriptine, colchicine, danazol, imatinib, metoclopramide, nefazodone, oral contraceptives, grapefruit, grapefruit juice, HIV protease inhibitors, boceprevir, and telaprevir may increase levels. Nafcillin, rifampin, carbamazepine, oxcarbazepine, phenobarbital, phenytoin, bosentan, octreotide, orlistat, sulfinpyrazone, terbinafine, ticlopidine, and St. John's wort may decrease levels. May increase levels of bosentan, dabigatran, and CYP3A4, P-gp, or organic anion transporter protein substrates. May increase levels of ambrisentan; do not titrate ambrisentan dose to the recommended max daily dose. CYP3A4 and/or P-gp inducers and inhibitors may alter levels; may require dose adjustments of cyclosporine if cyclosporine concentrations are significantly altered. May reduce clearance of digoxin, colchicine, prednisolone, HMG-CoA reductase inhibitors (statins), aliskiren, bosentan, dabigatran, repaglinide, NSAIDs, sirolimus, and etoposide. Digitalis toxicity reported when used w/ digoxin; monitor digoxin levels. May increase levels and enhance toxic effects (eg, myopathy, neuropathy) of colchicine; may reduce colchicine dose. Myotoxicity cases seen w/ lovastatin, simvastatin, atorvastatin, pravastatin, and, rarely fluvastatin; temporarily withhold or d/c statin therapy if signs of myopathy develop or w/ risk factors predisposing to severe renal injury, including renal failure, secondary to rhabdomyolysis. May increase levels of repaglinide, thereby increasing the risk of hypoglycemia; closely monitor blood glucose levels. High doses of cyclosporine may increase the exposure to anthracycline antibiotics (eg, doxorubicin, mitoxantrone, daunorubicin) in cancer patients. May double diclofenac blood levels; dose of diclofenac should be in the lower end of the therapeutic range. May increase MTX levels and decrease levels of active metabolite of MTX. May elevate SrCr and increase levels of sirolimus; give 4 hrs after cyclosporine administration. Convulsions reported w/ high-dose methylprednisolone. Calcium antagonists may interfere w/ cyclosporine metabolism. Avoid in psoriasis patients receiving other immunosuppressive agents or radiation therapy (including PUVA and UVB).

PREGNANCY AND LACTATION
Category C, not for use in nursing.

MECHANISM OF ACTION
Cyclic polypeptide immunosuppressant; results from specific and reversible inhibition of immunocompetent lymphocytes in the G_0- and G_1-phase of the cell cycle. T-lymphocytes are preferentially inhibited w/ T-helper cell as main target while also possibly suppressing T-suppressor cells. Also inhibits lymphokine production and release (eg, interleukin-2).

PHARMACOKINETICS
Absorption: Incomplete; T_{max}=1.5-2 hrs. Pharmacokinetic parameters varied w/ different indications (renal transplant, liver transplant, RA, and/or psoriasis).
Distribution: V_d=3-5L/kg (IV); plasma protein binding (90%); found in breast milk.
Metabolism: (Extensive) Liver via CYP3A, to a lesser extent GI tract and kidneys. M1, M9, and M4N (major metabolites); oxidation and demethylation pathways.
Elimination: Bile (primary), urine (6%, 0.1% unchanged); $T_{1/2}$=8.4 hrs.

PATIENT CONSIDERATIONS
Assessment: Assess for hypersensitivity to the drug, renal dysfunction, uncontrolled HTN, presence of malignancies, pregnancy/nursing status, and possible drug interactions. RA: Before initiating treatment, assess BP (on at least 2 occasions) and obtain 2 SrCr levels. Psoriasis: Prior to treatment, perform a dermatological and physical examination, including measuring BP. Assess for presence of occult infections and for the presence of tumors. Assess for atypical skin lesions and biopsy them. Obtain baseline SrCr (at least twice), BUN, LFTs, bilirubin, CBC, Mg^{2+}, K^+, uric acid, and lipid levels.

Monitoring: Monitor for signs/symptoms of hepatotoxicity, liver injury, nephrotoxicity, thrombocytopenia, microangiopathic hemolytic anemia, HTN, hyperkalemia, lymphomas and other malignancies, serious/polyoma virus infections, convulsions and other neurotoxicities, and other adverse reactions. Monitor cyclosporine blood concentrations routinely in transplant patients and periodically in RA patients. RA: Monitor BP and SrCr every 2 weeks during the initial 3 months of treatment, then monthly if patient is stable. Monitor SrCr and BP after an increase of the dose of NSAIDs and after initiation of new NSAID therapy. If coadministered w/ MTX, monitor CBC and LFTs monthly. Psoriasis: Monitor for occult infections and tumors. Monitor SrCr, BUN, BP, CBC, uric acid, K^+, lipids, and Mg^{2+} levels every 2 weeks during first 3 months of treatment, then monthly if stable.

Counseling: Instruct to contact physician before changing formulations of cyclosporine, which may require dose changes. Inform that repeated lab tests are required while on therapy. Advise of the potential risks if used during pregnancy and inform of the increased risk of neoplasia, HTN, and renal dysfunction. Inform that vaccinations may be less effective and to avoid live vaccines during therapy. Advise to take the medication on a consistent schedule w/ regard to time and meals, and to avoid grapefruit and grapefruit juice. Inform to avoid excessive sun exposure.

NESINA — alogliptin   Rx
Class: Dipeptidyl peptidase-4 (DPP-4) inhibitor

ADULT DOSAGE	PEDIATRIC DOSAGE
Type 2 Diabetes Mellitus	Pediatric use may not have been established
25mg qd	

DOSING CONSIDERATIONS
Renal Impairment
Mild (CrCl ≥60mL/min): No dosage adjustment needed
Moderate (CrCl ≥30 to <60mL/min): 12.5mg qd
Severe (CrCl ≥15 to <30mL/min): 6.25mg qd
ESRD (CrCl <15mL/min or Requiring Hemodialysis): 6.25mg qd

ADMINISTRATION
Oral route
May be taken w/ or w/o food.
May be administered w/o regard to timing of hemodialysis.

STORAGE
25°C (77°F); excursions permitted to 15-30°C (59-86°F).

HOW SUPPLIED
Tab: 6.25mg, 12.5mg, 25mg

CONTRAINDICATIONS
History of a serious hypersensitivity reaction (eg, anaphylaxis, angioedema, severe cutaneous adverse reactions) to alogliptin-containing products.

WARNINGS/PRECAUTIONS
Not for the treatment of type 1 diabetes mellitus (DM) or diabetic ketoacidosis. Acute pancreatitis reported; promptly d/c if suspected and initiate appropriate management. Hospitalization for CHF reported in patients w/ recent acute coronary syndrome; evaluate and manage accordingly and consider discontinuation if heart failure (HF) develops. Consider the risks and benefits of therapy prior to initiating treatment in patients at risk for HF. Serious hypersensitivity reactions reported; d/c if suspected, assess for other potential causes, and institute alternative treatment. Caution w/ history of angioedema w/ another DPP-4 inhibitor. Fatal/nonfatal hepatic failure and serum ALT >3X ULN reported; measure liver tests promptly in patients who report symptoms that may indicate liver injury. Interrupt treatment and assess for probable cause if clinically significant liver enzyme elevations exist and if abnormal LFTs persist/ worsen; do not restart w/o another explanation for abnormal LFTs. Severe and disabling arthralgia has been reported in patients taking DPP-4 inhibitors; d/c if appropriate. Caution in patients w/ liver disease.

ADVERSE REACTIONS
Nasopharyngitis, headache, URTI.

DRUG INTERACTIONS
Lower dose of insulin therapy or insulin secretagogue (eg, sulfonylurea) may be required to reduce risk of hypoglycemia.

PREGNANCY AND LACTATION
Pregnancy: Limited data w/ alogliptin in pregnant women are not sufficient to determine a drug-associated risk for major birth defects or miscarriage.

Lactation: There is no information regarding the presence of alogliptin in human milk, the effects on the breastfed infant, or the effects on milk production; caution in nursing.

MECHANISM OF ACTION
DPP-4 inhibitor; slows inactivation of incretin hormones, thereby increasing their bloodstream concentrations and reducing fasting and postprandial glucose concentrations in a glucose-dependent manner.

PHARMACOKINETICS
Absorption: Absolute bioavailability (100%); T_{max}=1-2 hrs. **Distribution:** V_d=417L; plasma protein binding (20%). **Metabolism:** Via CYP2D6 and CYP3A4; N-demethylated alogliptin, M-I (active metabolite) and N-acetylated alogliptin, M-II. **Elimination:** Feces (13%), urine (76%, 60-71% unchanged); $T_{1/2}$=21 hrs.

PATIENT CONSIDERATIONS
Assessment: Assess for previous hypersensitivity to the drug, renal/hepatic impairment, history of pancreatitis, type of DM, diabetic ketoacidosis, history of angioedema w/ another DPP-4 inhibitor, HF or risk factors for HF, pregnancy/ nursing status, and possible drug interactions. Obtain baseline FPG and HbA1c.

Monitoring: Monitor for pancreatitis, HF, arthralgia, hypersensitivity reactions, and other adverse reactions. Monitor FPG, HbA1c, and renal/hepatic function periodically.

Counseling: Inform of risks/benefits of therapy. Inform of signs/symptoms of pancreatitis; instruct to d/c promptly and contact physician if persistent severe abdominal pain occurs. Advise about the signs/symptoms of HF; instruct patients to contact their physician as soon as possible if they experience symptoms of HF (eg, increasing SOB, rapid increase in weight, swelling of the feet). Inform that allergic reactions and liver injury have been reported; instruct to d/c and seek medical advice promptly if these occur. Inform that hypoglycemia can occur, particularly when therapy is used in combination w/ an insulin secretagogue or insulin; explain risks/symptoms/appropriate management of hypoglycemia. Inform patients that severe and disabling joint pain may occur and the time to onset of symptoms can range from one day to years. Instruct patients to seek medical advice if severe joint pain occurs. Instruct to take only ud; if a dose is missed, advise not to double next dose. Instruct to inform physician if unusual symptom develops or if a symptom persists/worsens.

NEULASTA — pegfilgrastim   Rx
Class: Granulocyte colony-stimulating factor (G-CSF)

ADULT DOSAGE	PEDIATRIC DOSAGE
Chemotherapy-Associated Neutropenia	**Chemotherapy-Associated Neutropenia**

ADULT DOSAGE

Chemotherapy-Associated Neutropenia

To decrease the incidence of infection in patients w/ nonmyeloid malignancies receiving myelosuppressive anticancer drugs associated w/ febrile neutropenia

6mg SQ once per chemotherapy cycle; do not administer between 14 days before and 24 hrs after administration of cytotoxic chemotherapy

Hematopoietic Subsyndrome of Acute Radiation Syndrome

To increase survival in patients acutely exposed to myelosuppressive doses of radiation

2 doses of 6mg SQ, administered 1 week apart

Administer 1st dose as soon as possible after suspected or confirmed exposure to radiation levels >2 gray (Gy)

Obtain a baseline CBC; do not delay administration if a CBC is not readily available. Estimate a patient's absorbed radiation dose (eg, level of radiation exposure) based on information from public health authorities, biodosimetry if available, or clinical findings (eg, time to onset of vomiting, lymphocyte depletion kinetics)

PEDIATRIC DOSAGE

Chemotherapy-Associated Neutropenia

To decrease the incidence of infection in patients w/ nonmyeloid malignancies receiving myelosuppressive anticancer drugs associated w/ febrile neutropenia

<10kg: 0.1mg/kg (0.01mL/kg)
10-20kg: 1.5mg (0.15mL)
21-30kg: 2.5mg (0.25mL)
31-44kg: 4mg (0.40mL)
≥45kg: Refer to adult dosing

Administer once per chemotherapy cycle; do not administer between 14 days before and 24 hrs after administration of cytotoxic chemotherapy

Hematopoietic Subsyndrome of Acute Radiation Syndrome

To increase survival in patients acutely exposed to myelosuppressive doses of radiation

<10kg: 0.1mg/kg (0.01mL/kg)
10-20kg: 1.5mg (0.15mL)
21-30kg: 2.5mg (0.25mL)
31-44kg: 4mg (0.40mL)
≥45kg: Refer to adult dosing

Administer 1st dose as soon as possible after suspected or confirmed exposure to radiation levels >2 Gy

Administer 2nd dose 1 week after the 1st dose

Obtain a baseline CBC; do not delay administration if a CBC is not readily available. Estimate a patient's absorbed radiation dose (eg, level of radiation exposure) based on information from public health authorities, biodosimetry if available, or clinical findings (eg, time to onset of vomiting, lymphocyte depletion kinetics)

ADMINISTRATION
SQ route
Administer via a single-dose prefilled syringe for manual use or w/ the On-body Injector.
Use of the On-body Injector is not recommended for patients w/ hematopoietic subsydrome of acute radiation syndrome.
Use of On-body Injector has not been studied in pediatric patients.
Prefilled syringe is not designed to allow for direct administration of doses <0.6mL (6mg).
Prior to use, remove the carton from the refrigerator and allow the prefilled syringe to reach room temperature for a minimum of 30 min; discard any prefilled syringe left at room temperature for >48 hrs.
The needle cap on the prefilled syringes contain dry natural rubber (derived from latex); persons w/ latex allergies should not administer.

Instructions for On-body Injector
For Physicians:
- Fill the On-body Injector w/ pegfilgrastim using prefilled syringe and apply to patient's skin (abdomen or back of arm).
- Use back of the arm only if a caregiver is available to monitor the status of the On-body Injector.
- Approx 27 hrs after the application, pegfilgrastim will be delivered over approx 45 min.
- May initiate administration on the same day as the administration of cytotoxic chemotherapy, as long as On-body Injector delivers pegfilgrastim no less than 24 hrs after administration of cytotoxic chemotherapy.
- Do not use On-body Injector to deliver any other drug product except pegfilgrastim prefilled syringe co-packaged w/ On-body Injector.
- Apply to intact, non-irritated skin on the arm or abdomen.
- Missed dose may occur due to an On-body Injector failure/leakage; if a dose is missed, administer new dose by single-dose prefilled syringe for manual use, as soon as possible after detection.
- Refer to Healthcare Provider Instructions for Use for the On-body Injector for Neulasta for full administration information.

STORAGE
2-8°C (36-46°F). **Prefilled Syringe for Manual Use:** Protect from light. Do not shake. Discard syringes stored at room temperature for >48 hrs. Avoid freezing; if frozen, thaw in the refrigerator before administration. Discard syringe if frozen more than once. **Onpro Kit:** Do not hold Kit at room temperature >12 hrs prior to use; discard if stored at room temperature for >12 hrs.

HOW SUPPLIED
Inj: 6mg/0.6mL [prefilled syringe for manual use, Onpro Kit]

CONTRAINDICATIONS
History of serious allergic reactions to pegfilgrastim or filgrastim.

WARNINGS/PRECAUTIONS
Not indicated for the mobilization of peripheral blood progenitor cells for hematopoietic stem cell transplantation. Splenic rupture, including fatal cases, may occur; evaluate for an enlarged spleen or splenic rupture if left upper abdominal or shoulder pain occurs. Acute respiratory distress syndrome (ARDS) may occur; evaluate for ARDS if fever and lung infiltrates or respiratory distress develops, and d/c if ARDS develops. Serious allergic reactions (eg, anaphylaxis) may occur; permanently d/c if a serious allergic reaction occurs. Use of On-body Injector may result in a significant reaction in patients who have reactions to acrylic adhesives. Severe and sometimes fatal sickle cell crises may occur in patients w/ sickle cell disorders. Glomerulonephritis reported; evaluate for cause if glomerulonephritis is suspected and consider dose reduction or interruption of pegfilgrastim if causality is likely. WBC counts of ≥100 x 10^9/L reported; monitor CBC during therapy. May act as a growth factor for any tumor type. Capillary leak syndrome reported; closely monitor patients who develop symptoms and administer standard symptomatic treatment, which may include a need for intensive care. Increased hematopoietic activity of the bone marrow in response to therapy may result in transiently positive bone imaging changes; consider this when interpreting bone-imaging results.

ADVERSE REACTIONS
Bone pain, pain in extremity.

PREGNANCY AND LACTATION
Pregnancy: Category C.
Lactation: It is not known whether pegfilgrastim is secreted in human milk; caution in nursing.

MECHANISM OF ACTION
Granulocyte colony-stimulating factor; acts on hematopoietic cells by binding to specific cell surface receptors, thereby stimulating proliferation, differentiation, commitment, and end cell functional activation.

PHARMACOKINETICS
Elimination: $T_{1/2}$=15-80 hrs.

PATIENT CONSIDERATIONS
Assessment: Assess for history of hypersensitivity to pegfilgrastim or filgrastim, acrylic allergy, sickle cell disorders, and pregnancy/nursing status. In patients w/ hematopoietic subsyndrome of acute radiation syndrome, obtain CBC.

Monitoring: Monitor for enlarged spleen/splenic rupture, ARDS, serious allergic reactions, sickle cell crises (in patients w/ sickle cell disorders), glomerulonephritis, capillary leak syndrome, and other adverse reactions. Monitor CBC.

Counseling: Advise on the proper administration of pegfilgrastim and how to use the On-body Injector. Advise of the risks of therapy (eg, splenic rupture, ARDS, serious allergic reactions, sickle cell crisis, glomerulonephritis, capillary leak syndrome). Advise to avoid activities (eg, traveling, driving, operating heavy machinery) during 26-29 hrs following application of On-body Injector (this includes the 45-min delivery period plus 1 hr post-delivery). Advise female patients to notify physician if pregnant or nursing.

NEUMEGA — oprelvekin   Rx
Class: Thrombopoietic agent

Allergic or hypersensitivity reactions, including anaphylaxis, reported; permanently d/c if this develops.

ADULT DOSAGE	PEDIATRIC DOSAGE
Thrombocytopenia Prevention of severe thrombocytopenia and reduction of the need for platelet transfusions following myelosuppressive chemotherapy in adults w/ nonmyeloid malignancies who are at high risk of severe thrombocytopenia **Usual:** 50mcg/kg qd Initiate 6-24 hrs after chemotherapy completion. Continue therapy until post-nadir platelet count is ≥50,000/μL **Max:** 21 days/treatment course. D/C at least 2 days before starting the next chemotherapy cycle. May give for up to 6 cycles following chemotherapy	Pediatric use may not have been established

DOSING CONSIDERATIONS
Renal Impairment
Severe (CrCl <30mL/min): 25mcg/kg

ADMINISTRATION
SQ route
Administer in either the abdomen, thigh, or hip (upper arm if not self-injecting)

Preparation
1. Reconstitute using the 1mL of sterile water for inj (w/o preservative) contained in the prefilled syringe included in the kit
2. Administer oprelvekin w/in 3 hrs following reconstitution

STORAGE
2-8°C (36-46°F). Protect powder from light. Do not freeze. Reconstituted: 2-8°C (36-46°F) or up to 25°C (77°F). Do not freeze or shake.

HOW SUPPLIED
Inj: 5mg

CONTRAINDICATIONS
History of hypersensitivity to oprelvekin or any component of the product.

WARNINGS/PRECAUTIONS
Not indicated following myeloablative chemotherapy. May cause serious fluid retention; caution in congestive heart failure (CHF) patients, patients who may be susceptible to developing CHF, patients receiving aggressive hydration, patients with history of heart failure who are well-compensated and receiving appropriate medical therapy, and patients who may develop fluid retention as a result of associated medical conditions or whose medical condition may be exacerbated by fluid retention. Monitor preexisting fluid collections; consider drainage if medically indicated. Moderate decreases in Hgb, Hct, and RBCs reported. Cardiovascular events, including arrhythmias and pulmonary edema, reported. Caution with history of atrial arrhythmias. Papilledema reported; caution in patients with preexisting papilledema, or with tumors involving the CNS. Changes in visual acuity and/or visual field defects may occur in patients with papilledema. Obtain CBC before chemotherapy and at regular intervals during therapy. Monitor platelet counts during expected nadir time and until adequate recovery has occurred (post-nadir counts ≥50,000/μL).

ADVERSE REACTIONS
Edema, dyspnea, tachycardia, conjunctival injection, palpitations, atrial arrhythmias, pleural effusions, syncope, pneumonia, neutropenic fever, headache, N/V, mucositis, diarrhea.

DRUG INTERACTIONS
Perform close monitoring of fluid and electrolyte status in patients receiving chronic diuretic therapy.

PREGNANCY AND LACTATION
Category C, not for use in nursing.

MECHANISM OF ACTION
Thrombopoietic agent; stimulates megakaryocytopoiesis and thrombopoiesis.

PHARMACOKINETICS
Absorption: Absolute bioavailability (>80%); C_{max}=17.4ng/mL; T_{max}=3.2 hrs.
Elimination: Urine; $T_{1/2}$=6.9 hrs.

PATIENT CONSIDERATIONS
Assessment: Assess for conditions where treatment is contraindicated or cautioned, pregnancy/nursing status, and possible drug interactions. Obtain baseline CBC prior to chemotherapy.

Monitoring: Monitor for signs/symptoms of hypersensitivity reactions, papilledema, fluid retention, pleural/pericardial effusion, atrial arrhythmias, and other adverse reactions. Periodically monitor CBC (including platelet counts), fluid balance, fluid and electrolyte status (chronic diuretic therapy).

Counseling: Inform of pregnancy risks. Instruct on the proper dose, method for reconstituting and administering, and importance of proper disposal of the product when used outside of the hospital or office setting. Inform of the serious and most common adverse reactions associated with the product. Advise to immediately seek medical attention if any of the signs or symptoms of allergic or hypersensitivity reactions (edema, difficulty breathing, swallowing or talking, SOB, wheezing, chest pain, throat tightness, lightheadedness), worsening of dyspnea, or symptoms attributable to atrial arrhythmia occur.

NEUPOGEN — filgrastim   Rx

Class: Granulocyte colony-stimulating factor (G-CSF)

ADULT DOSAGE

Myelosuppressive Chemotherapy

Decrease the incidence of infection, as manifested by febrile neutropenia, in patients w/ nonmyeloid malignancies receiving myelosuppressive anti-cancer drugs associated w/ a significant incidence of severe neutropenia w/ fever

Initial: 5mcg/kg/day; administer as a single SQ inj, by short IV infusion (15-30 min), or by continuous IV infusion
Titrate: May increase in increments of 5mcg/kg for each chemotherapy cycle, according to duration and severity of ANC nadir

D/C if ANC increases beyond 10,000/mm^3

Administer at least 24 hrs after cytotoxic chemotherapy; do not administer w/in the 24-hr period prior to chemotherapy

Administer daily for up to 2 weeks or until the ANC has reached 10,000/mm^3 following the expected chemotherapy-induced neutrophil nadir

Induction or Consolidation Chemotherapy

To reduce the time to neutrophil recovery and the duration of fever, following induction or consolidation chemotherapy treatment of patients w/ acute myeloid leukemia (AML)
Initial: 5mcg/kg/day; administer as a single SQ inj, by short IV infusion (15-30 min), or by continuous IV infusion
Titrate: May increase in increments of 5mcg/kg for each chemotherapy cycle, according to duration and severity of ANC nadir

D/C if ANC increases beyond 10,000/mm^3

Administer at least 24 hrs after cytotoxic chemotherapy; do not administer w/in the 24-hr period prior to chemotherapy

Administer daily for up to 2 weeks or until the ANC has reached 10,000/mm^3 following the expected chemotherapy-induced neutrophil nadir

Bone Marrow Transplantation

To reduce the duration of neutropenia and neutropenia-related clinical sequelae (eg, febrile neutropenia) in patients w/ nonmyeloid malignancies undergoing myeloablative chemotherapy followed by bone marrow transplantation

10mcg/kg/day administered as an IV infusion no longer than 24 hrs; administer the first dose at least 24 hrs after cytotoxic chemotherapy and at least 24 hrs after bone marrow infusion

Dose Adjustments During Neutrophil Recovery:

When ANC >1000/mm^3 for 3 Consecutive Days: Reduce to 5mcg/kg/day*
If ANC Remains >1000/mm^3 for 3 More Consecutive Days: D/C therapy

PEDIATRIC DOSAGE

General Dosing

Studied in pediatric patients w/ chemotherapy-associated neutropenia and in pediatric patients w/ severe chronic neutropenia; refer to PI

If ANC Decreases to <1000/mm^3:
Resume at 5mcg/kg/day

*If ANC decreases to <1000/mm^3 at any time during the 5mcg/kg/day administration, increase dose to 10mcg/kg/day, and follow the above steps

Hematopoietic Progenitor Cell Mobilization

Mobilization of autologous hematopoietic progenitor cells into the peripheral blood for collection by leukapheresis

10mcg/kg/day SQ inj; administer for ≥4 days before the 1st leukapheresis procedure and continue until the last leukapheresis

Administration of therapy for 6-7 days w/ leukapheresis on Days 5, 6, and 7 was found to be safe and effective

Monitor neutrophil counts after 4 days of therapy, and d/c if WBC count rises to >100,000/mm^3

Severe Chronic Neutropenia

For chronic administration to reduce the incidence and duration of sequelae of neutropenia in symptomatic patients w/ congenital neutropenia, cyclic neutropenia, or idiopathic neutropenia

Initial:
Congenital Neutropenia: 6mcg/kg SQ bid
Idiopathic/Cyclic Neutropenia: 5mcg/kg SQ qd

Individualize dose based on the patient's clinical course as well as ANC; in rare instances, patients w/ congenital neutropenia have required doses ≥100mcg/kg/day

During the initial 4 weeks of therapy and during the 2 weeks following any dosage adjustment, monitor CBCs w/ differential and platelet counts. Once a patient is clinically stable, monitor CBCs w/ differential and platelet counts monthly during the first year of treatment. Thereafter, if the patient is clinically stable, less frequent routine monitoring is recommended

Hematopoietic Syndrome of Acute Radiation Syndrome

To increase survival in patients acutely exposed to myelosuppressive doses of radiation

10mcg/kg SQ qd; administer as soon as possible after suspected/confirmed exposure to radiation doses >2 gray

Obtain a baseline CBC and then serial CBCs approx every third day until the ANC remains >1000/mm^3 for 3 consecutive CBCs; do not delay administration if a CBC is not readily available

Continue administration of therapy until the ANC remains >1000/mm^3 for 3 consecutive CBCs or exceeds 10,000/mm^3 after a radiation-induced nadir

---

DOSING CONSIDERATIONS

Concomitant Medications

Cytotoxic Chemotherapy: Do not use Neupogen in the period 24 hrs before through 24 hrs after the administration of cytotoxic chemotherapy

ADMINISTRATION

SQ/IV route

- Prior to use, remove the vial or prefilled syringe from the refrigerator and allow Neupogen to reach room temperature for a minimum of 30 min and a max of 24 hrs; discard any vial or prefilled syringe left at room temperature for >24 hrs.
- Discard unused portion in vials or prefilled syringes; do not re-enter the vial or save unused drug for later administration.

SQ Inj

- Inject in the outer area of upper arms, abdomen, thighs, or upper outer areas of buttocks.

Instructions for Prefilled Syringe
- Persons w/ latex allergies should not administer the prefilled syringe, because the needle cap contains dry natural rubber (derived from latex).

Dilution Instructions (Vial Only)
- If required for IV administration, vials may be diluted in D5 inj from a concentration of 300mcg/mL to 5mcg/mL; do not dilute to a final concentration <5mcg/mL.
- Sol diluted to concentrations from 5mcg/mL to 15mcg/mL should be protected from adsorption to plastic materials by the addition of albumin (human) to a final concentration of 2mg/mL.
- When diluted in D5 inj or D5 plus albumin (human), Neupogen is compatible w/ glass bottles, polyvinylchloride and polyolefin IV bags, and polypropylene syringes.
- Do not dilute w/ saline; product may precipitate.
- Store diluted sol at room temperature for up to 24 hrs; this 24-hr time period includes the time during room temperature storage of the infusion sol and the duration of the infusion.

STORAGE
2-8°C (36-46°F). Protect from light. Avoid freezing; if frozen, thaw in the refrigerator before administration. Discard if frozen more than once. Avoid shaking.

HOW SUPPLIED
Inj: 300mcg/mL, 480mcg/1.6mL [vial]; 300mcg/0.5mL, 480mcg/0.8mL [prefilled syringe]

CONTRAINDICATIONS
History of serious allergic reactions to human granulocyte colony-stimulating factors (eg, filgrastim, pegfilgrastim).

WARNINGS/PRECAUTIONS
Splenic rupture, including fatal cases, reported. Acute respiratory distress syndrome (ARDS) reported; d/c in patients w/ ARDS. Serious allergic reactions, including anaphylaxis, reported; permanently d/c in patients w/ serious allergic reactions. Sickle cell crisis, in some cases fatal, reported in patients w/ sickle cell trait/disease. Glomerulonephritis has occurred, generally resolving after dose reduction or discontinuation. If glomerulonephritis is suspected, evaluate for cause; if causality is likely, consider dose-reduction or interruption of therapy. Not approved for peripheral blood progenitor cell mobilization in healthy donors. Capillary leak syndrome (CLS) reported. Myelodysplastic syndrome (MDS) and AML reported to occur in the natural history of congenital neutropenia w/o cytokine therapy. Cytogenetic abnormalities, transformation to MDS, and AML observed in patients treated for severe chronic neutropenia (SCN); carefully consider the risks and benefits of continuing therapy if a patient w/ SCN develops abnormal cytogenetics or myelodysplasia. Thrombocytopenia and leukocytosis reported. Cutaneous vasculitis reported. Hold therapy in patients w/ cutaneous vasculitis; treatment may be started at a reduced dose when the symptoms resolve and ANC has decreased. May act as a growth factor for any tumor type. Increased hematopoietic activity of the bone marrow in response to growth factor therapy has been associated w/ transient positive bone-imaging changes; consider this when interpreting bone-imaging results.

ADVERSE REACTIONS
W/ Nonmyeloid Malignancies Receiving Myelosuppressive Anti-Cancer Drugs: Pyrexia, pain, rash, cough, dyspnea.
W/ AML: Pain, epistaxis, rash.
W/ Nonmyeloid Malignancies Undergoing Myeloablative Chemotherapy followed by BMT: Rash.
Undergoing Peripheral Blood Progenitor Cell Mobilization and Collection: Bone pain, pyrexia, headache.
W/ Severe Chronic Neutropenia: Pain, anemia, epistaxis, diarrhea, hypoesthesia, alopecia.

DRUG INTERACTIONS
Avoid simultaneous use w/ chemotherapy and radiation therapy.

PREGNANCY AND LACTATION
Pregnancy: Category C.
Lactation: Caution in nursing.

MECHANISM OF ACTION
G-CSF; acts on hematopoietic cells by binding to specific cell surface receptors and stimulating proliferation, differentiation commitment, and some end-cell functional activation.

PHARMACOKINETICS
Absorption: (SQ) Absolute Bioavailability (60-70%); C_{max}=4ng/mL (3.45mcg/kg), 49ng/mL (11.5mcg/kg); T_{max}=2-8 hrs. **Distribution:** V_d=150mL/kg (IV); crosses placenta. **Elimination:** $T_{1/2}$=231 min (34.5mcg/kg IV), 210 min (3.45mcg/kg SQ).

PATIENT CONSIDERATIONS
Assessment: Assess for hypersensitivity to the drug, latex allergy, sickle cell disorder, pregnancy/nursing status, and possible drug interactions. Obtain baseline CBC and platelet count. Confirm diagnosis of SCN prior to therapy.
Monitoring: Monitor for splenic rupture, ARDS, serious allergic reactions, sickle cell crisis, glomerulonephritis, CLS, cutaneous vasculitis, thrombocytopenia, leukocytosis, and other adverse reactions. Monitor for cytogenetic abnormalities, transformation to MDS, and AML in patients w/ SCN. In patients receiving myelosuppressive chemotherapy or induction and/or consolidation chemotherapy for AML, monitor CBC and platelet count twice weekly. Monitor CBCs and platelet counts frequently following marrow transplantation. In patients w/ SCN, monitor CBCs w/ differential and platelet counts during the initial 4 weeks of therapy and during the 2 weeks following any dose adjustment. Once patient is clinically stable, monitor CBCs w/ differential and platelet counts monthly during the 1st yr of treatment; thereafter, if clinically stable, less frequent routine

monitoring is recommended. Monitor serial CBCs approx every 3rd day until the ANC remains >1000/mm^3 for 3 consecutive CBCs in patients acutely exposed to myelosuppressive doses of radiation.
Counseling: Train patients/caregivers on how to measure required dose and administer inj. Instruct to contact healthcare provider if a dose is missed. Inform that rupture or enlargement of the spleen may occur; advise to immediately report to physician if symptoms develop. Advise to seek immediate medical attention if signs/symptoms of hypersensitivity reaction occur. Advise to immediately report to physician if dyspnea develops. Discuss potential risks and benefits for patients w/ sickle cell disease prior to administration. Advise to immediately report signs/symptoms of glomerulonephritis to physician. Advise to immediately report to physician signs/symptoms of vasculitis. Advise females of reproductive potential that therapy should be used during pregnancy only if the potential benefit justifies the potential risk to the fetus. Advise patients acutely exposed to myelosuppressive doses of radiation that efficacy studies of therapy for this indication could not be conducted in humans for ethical and feasibility reasons; approval of this use was based on efficacy studies conducted in animals.

NEUPRO — rotigotine   Rx

Class: Dopamine receptor agonist

ADULT DOSAGE	PEDIATRIC DOSAGE
Parkinson's Disease	Pediatric use may not have been established
Early-Stage Parkinson's Disease (PD):	
Initial: 2mg/24 hrs	
Titrate: May increase weekly by 2mg/24 hrs based on response and tolerability, and if additional therapeutic effect is needed	
Lowest Effective Dose: 4mg/24 hrs	
Max: 6mg/24 hrs	
Advanced-Stage PD:	
Initial: 4mg/24 hrs	
Titrate: May increase weekly by 2mg/24 hrs based on response and tolerability, and if additional therapeutic effect is needed	
Max: 8mg/24 hrs	
Discontinuation of Therapy: Reduce daily dose by a max of 2mg/24 hrs preferably qod, until complete withdrawal is achieved	
Restless Legs Syndrome	
Moderate to Severe Primary Restless Leg Syndrome:	
Initial: 1mg/24 hrs	
Titrate: May increase weekly by 1mg/24 hrs based on response and tolerability, and if additional therapeutic effect is needed	
Lowest Effective Dose: 1mg/24 hrs	
Max: 3mg/24 hrs	
Discontinuation of Therapy: Reduce daily dose by 1mg/24 hrs preferably qod, until complete withdrawal is achieved	

ADMINISTRATION
Transdermal route

Apply 1 patch qd at approx the same time every day
Apply to clean, dry, intact healthy skin on the front of the abdomen, thigh, hip, flank, shoulder, or upper arm
Do not apply on oily, irritated, or damaged skin or where it will be rubbed by tight clothing
Rotate application site qd
Do not apply to same application site more than once every 14 days
Apply immediately upon removal from the pouch; press firmly in place for 30 sec
If applying to hairy area is necessary, shave area ≥3 days prior to application
Apply another patch if patient forgets to replace patch or if patch becomes dislodged

STORAGE
20-25°C (68-77°F); excursions permitted between 15-30°C (59-86°F).

HOW SUPPLIED
Patch, Extended-Release: 1mg/24 hrs, 2mg/24 hrs, 3mg/24 hrs, 4mg/24 hrs, 6mg/24 hrs, 8mg/24 hrs [30^s]

CONTRAINDICATIONS
Hypersensitivity to rotigotine or the components of the transdermal system.

WARNINGS/PRECAUTIONS
Contains sodium metabisulfite that may cause allergic-type reactions, including anaphylactic symptoms and life-threatening or less severe asthmatic episodes in certain susceptible people. Falling asleep during activities of daily living and somnolence reported. Should ordinarily d/c if daytime sleepiness or episodes of falling asleep during activities that require active participation occur. May impair mental/physical abilities. Hallucinations and new/worsening mental status and behavioral changes reported; avoid w/ major psychotic disorder. May cause

postural/orthostatic hypotension; monitor for signs/symptoms, especially during dose escalation. Syncope reported; patients w/ severe cardiovascular disease (CVD) should be monitored for symptoms of syncope and presyncope. May cause intense urges (eg, to gamble, have sex, to spend money, binge eating); consider dose reduction or discontinuation. BP and HR elevations reported. Weight gain and fluid retention reported; monitor patients w/ concomitant illnesses (eg, CHF, renal insufficiency). May cause or exacerbate preexisting dyskinesia. Application-site reactions reported; d/c if a generalized skin reaction is observed. Monitor for melanomas frequently and on a regular basis. Augmentation and rebound in RLS reported. Backing layer of patch contains aluminum; remove patch prior to MRI or cardioversion. Avoid exposing application site to external sources of direct heat. Symptom complex resembling neuroleptic malignant syndrome reported w/ rapid dose reduction, withdrawal of, or changes in antiparkinsonian therapy. Cases of retroperitoneal fibrosis, pulmonary infiltrates, pleural effusion, pleural thickening, pericarditis, and cardiac valvulopathy reported in some patients treated w/ ergot-derived dopaminergic agents.

ADVERSE REACTIONS
N/V, dizziness, somnolence, application-site reactions, hyperhidrosis, anorexia, headache, disturbances in initiating and maintaining sleep, visual disturbance, peripheral edema, dyskinesia, low Hgb/Hct, elevated serum BUN/CPK, low serum glucose.

DRUG INTERACTIONS
Sedating medications may increase risk of drowsiness. Dopamine antagonists (eg, antipsychotics, metoclopramide) may diminish effectiveness. May potentiate dopaminergic side effects of levodopa.

PREGNANCY AND LACTATION
Pregnancy: Category C.
Lactation: Caution in nursing.

MECHANISM OF ACTION
Non-ergoline dopamine agonist; mechanism of action not known. As a treatment for PD, suspected to be related to ability to stimulate dopamine receptors w/in the caudate-putamen in the brain. As a treatment for RLS, suspected to be related to ability to stimulate dopamine receptors.

PHARMACOKINETICS
Absorption: T_{max}=15-18 hrs. **Distribution:** V_d=84L/kg; plasma protein binding (92% in vitro, 89.5% in vivo). **Metabolism:** Extensive by conjugation and N-dealkylation via CYP isoenzymes, sulfotransferases, and UDP-glucuronosyltransferases. **Elimination:** Urine (<1%, unchanged), feces (23%); $T_{1/2}$=5-7 hrs.

PATIENT CONSIDERATIONS
Assessment: Assess for major psychotic disorder, sleep disorders, dyskinesia, CVD, CHF, renal insufficiency, hypersensitivity to drug or sulfites, pregnancy/nursing status, and possible drug interactions.

Monitoring: Monitor for drowsiness or sleepiness, hallucinations, new/worsening mental status and behavioral changes, symptomatic hypotension, syncope, impulse control/compulsive behaviors, BP and HR elevations, dyskinesia, application-site/generalized skin reactions, melanomas (frequently and regularly), and other adverse reactions.

Counseling: Advise about potential for sulfite sensitivity. Advise and alert about potential for sedating effects, including somnolence and possibility of falling asleep while engaged in activities of daily living; instruct not to drive a car or engage in potentially dangerous activities until effects have been determined. Advise to inform physician if taking alcohol, sedating medications, or other CNS depressants. Inform that hallucinations and other psychosis symptoms, symptomatic hypotension, syncope, BP and HR elevations, weight gain, fluid retention, dyskinesia, N/V, and general GI distress may occur. Instruct to notify physician if experiencing new/increased gambling urges, increased sexual urges, or other intense urges. Instruct not to apply patch to the same site more than once every 14 days and to report persistent application-site reaction (of more than a few days), increases in severity, or skin reactions that spread outside the application site. Advise to monitor for melanomas frequently and regularly. Inform that drug may cause RLS symptoms to have an earlier onset during the day or become worse. Instruct to avoid applying heating pads or other sources of heat to the area of the patch and to avoid direct sun exposure of the patch. Advise to d/c use only under the supervision of a physician to reduce risk for hyperpyrexia and confusion associated w/ sudden discontinuation or dose reduction.

Neurontin — gabapentin   Rx

Class: GABA analogue

ADULT DOSAGE
Postherpetic Neuralgia

Initial: 300mg single dose on Day 1, then 300mg bid (600mg/day) on Day 2, and 300mg tid (900mg/day) on Day 3
Titrate: May subsequently increase prn up to 600mg tid (1800mg/day)

Partial Seizures

Adjuvant Therapy for Partial Onset Seizures w/ Epilepsy, w/ and w/o Secondary Generalization:

Initial: 300mg tid
Maint: 300-600mg tid
Doses up to 2400mg/day (long-term)

PEDIATRIC DOSAGE
Partial Seizures

Adjuvant Therapy for Partial Onset Seizures w/ Epilepsy, w/ and w/o Secondary Generalization:

3-11 Years:
Initial: 10-15mg/kg/day in 3 divided doses
Titrate: Increase to recommended maint dose over a period of approx 3 days

3-4 Years:
Maint: 40mg/kg/day in 3 divided doses

and 3600mg/day (short-term) have been well tolerated
Administer tid using 300mg or 400mg caps, or 600mg or 800mg tabs
Dosing intervals should not exceed 12 hrs

5-11 Years:
Maint: 25-35mg/kg/day in 3 divided doses

Doses up to 50mg/kg/day have been well tolerated
Dosing intervals should not exceed 12 hrs

≥12 Years:
Initial: 300mg tid
Maint: 300-600mg tid
Doses up to 2400mg/day (long-term) and 3600mg/day (short-term) have been well tolerated
Administer tid using 300mg or 400mg caps, or 600mg or 800mg tabs
Dosing intervals should not exceed 12 hrs

DOSING CONSIDERATIONS
Renal Impairment
≥12 Years:
CrCl ≥60mL/min: 900-3600mg/day in 3 divided doses
CrCl >30-59mL/min: 400-1400mg/day in 2 divided doses
CrCl >15-29mL/min: 200-700mg single daily dose
CrCl 15mL/min: 100-300mg single daily dose
CrCl <15mL/min: Reduce daily dose in proportion to CrCl
Hemodialysis: Dose adjustment is necessary; see PI

Discontinuation
Dose Reduction/Substitution/Discontinuation: Should be done gradually over a minimum of 1 week

ADMINISTRATION
Oral route

Take w/ or w/o food.
Swallow caps whole w/ water.
If the scored tab is broken to administer a half-tab, take the unused half-tab as the next dose; discard half-tabs that are not used w/in 28 days of breaking the scored tab.

STORAGE
Cap/Tab: 25°C (77°F); excursions permitted to 15-30°C (59-86°F). **Sol:** 2-8°C (36-46°F).

HOW SUPPLIED
Cap: 100mg, 300mg, 400mg; **Sol:** 250mg/5mL [470mL]; **Tab:** 600mg*, 800mg* *scored

CONTRAINDICATIONS
Hypersensitivity to the drug or its ingredients.

WARNINGS/PRECAUTIONS
Drug reaction w/ eosinophilia and systemic symptoms (DRESS)/multiorgan hypersensitivity reported; evaluate immediately if signs/symptoms (eg, fever, lymphadenopathy) are present and d/c if an alternative etiology cannot be established. May cause anaphylaxis and angioedema; d/c and seek immediate medical care if experience signs/symptoms of anaphylaxis or angioedema. May cause significant driving impairment. Somnolence/sedation and dizziness reported. May impair mental/physical abilities. Do not abruptly d/c; may increase seizure frequency. Increases the risk of suicidal thoughts/behavior. Use in pediatric patients w/ epilepsy 3-12 yrs of age is associated w/ the occurrence of CNS-related adverse events. May have tumorigenic potential. Sudden and unexplained deaths reported in patients w/ epilepsy. Lab test interactions may occur. Caution in elderly.

ADVERSE REACTIONS
Dizziness, somnolence, fatigue, peripheral edema, hostility, diarrhea, asthenia, infection, dry mouth, nystagmus, constipation, N/V, ataxia, fever, amblyopia.

DRUG INTERACTIONS
Decreases hydrocodone exposure; consider the potential for alteration in hydrocodone exposure and effect when gabapentin is started or discontinued in a patient taking hydrocodone. Morphine may increase gabapentin concentrations; dose adjustment may be required. Observe for signs of CNS depression (eg, somnolence, sedation, respiratory depression) when used w/ other drugs w/ sedative properties (eg, morphine) because of potential synergy. Decreased bioavailability w/ Maalox; take gabapentin at least 2 hrs following Maalox administration.

PREGNANCY AND LACTATION
Pregnancy: Category C.
Lactation: Caution in nursing.

MECHANISM OF ACTION
GABA analogue; has not been established. Binds w/ high-affinity to the α2-delta subunit of voltage-activated Ca^{2+} channels.

PHARMACOKINETICS
Absorption: Administration of variable doses resulted in different parameters. **Distribution:** Plasma protein binding (<3%); found in breast milk; (150mg IV) V_d=58L. **Elimination:** Renal (unchanged); $T_{1/2}$=5-7 hrs.

PATIENT CONSIDERATIONS
Assessment: Assess for hypersensitivity to the drug, renal impairment, depression, pregnancy/nursing status, and possible drug interactions.

Monitoring: Monitor for DRESS, anaphylaxis, angioedema, somnolence/sedation, dizziness, emergence/worsening of depression, suicidal thoughts/behavior, unusual changes in mood/behavior, development/worsening of tumors, increased seizure frequency (upon abrupt discontinuation), and other adverse reactions.

Counseling: Instruct to immediately report to physician any rash or other signs/symptoms of hypersensitivity/anaphylaxis, angioedema, emergence/worsening of depression symptoms, any unusual changes in mood/behavior, emergence of suicidal thoughts/behavior, or thoughts of self-harm. Inform that therapy may cause a significant driving impairment, dizziness, somnolence, and other signs/symptoms of CNS depression; advise not to drive a car or operate other complex machinery until patient has gained sufficient experience on therapy. Instruct to notify physician if pregnant/breastfeeding or intending to become pregnant or to breastfeed during therapy; encourage enrollment in the North American Antiepileptic Drug Pregnancy Registry if patient becomes pregnant.

NEVANAC — nepafenac   Rx
Class: NSAID

ADULT DOSAGE	**PEDIATRIC DOSAGE**
Ocular Pain and Inflammation	**Ocular Pain and Inflammation**
1 drop to the affected eye tid, beginning 1 day prior to cataract surgery, continued on the day of surgery and through the first 2 weeks of the postoperative period	**≥10 Years:** 1 drop to the affected eye tid, beginning 1 day prior to cataract surgery, continued on the day of surgery and through the first 2 weeks of the postoperative period

---

DOSING CONSIDERATIONS
Concomitant Medications
If >1 topical ophthalmic medication is being used, administer at least 5 min apart

ADMINISTRATION
Ocular route

STORAGE
2-25°C (36-77°F).

HOW SUPPLIED
Ophthalmic Sus: 0.1% [3mL]

CONTRAINDICATIONS
Previously demonstrated hypersensitivity to any of the ingredients in the formula or to other NSAID.

WARNINGS/PRECAUTIONS
Potential for increased bleeding time due to interference w/ thrombocyte aggregation. Increased bleeding of ocular tissues (eg, hyphemas) reported in conjunction w/ ocular surgery; caution w/ known bleeding tendencies. May slow or delay healing, or result in keratitis. Continued use may result in epithelial breakdown and corneal thinning/erosion/ulceration/perforation, which may be sight threatening; immediately d/c if evidence of corneal epithelial breakdown occurs and closely monitor for corneal health. Caution w/ complicated ocular surgeries, corneal denervation, corneal epithelial defects, diabetes mellitus (DM), ocular surface diseases (eg, dry eye syndrome), rheumatoid arthritis (RA), or repeat ocular surgeries w/in a short period. Use >1 day prior to surgery or beyond 14 days postsurgery may increase risk and severity of corneal adverse events. Avoid use w/ contact lenses and during late pregnancy.

ADVERSE REACTIONS
Capsular opacity, decreased visual acuity, foreign body sensation, increased IOP, sticky sensation.

DRUG INTERACTIONS
May increase potential for healing problems w/ topical steroids. Caution w/ agents that may prolong bleeding time.

PREGNANCY AND LACTATION
Pregnancy: Category C.
Lactation: Caution in nursing.

MECHANISM OF ACTION
NSAID; thought to inhibit the action of prostaglandin H synthase (cyclooxygenase), an enzyme required for prostaglandin production.

PHARMACOKINETICS
Absorption: C_{max}=0.310ng/mL (nepafenac), 0.422ng/mL (amfenac). **Metabolism:** Hydrolysis via ocular tissue hydrolases to amfenac (metabolite).

PATIENT CONSIDERATIONS
Assessment: Assess for drug hypersensitivity, bleeding tendencies, complicated or repeated ocular surgeries, corneal denervation, corneal epithelial defects, DM, ocular surface diseases, RA, contact lens use, pregnancy/nursing status, and possible drug interactions.

Monitoring: Monitor for hypersensitivity reactions, wound healing problems, keratitis, increased bleeding time, bleeding of ocular tissues in conjunction w/ ocular surgery, epithelial corneal breakdown, corneal thinning/erosion/ulceration/perforation, and other adverse reactions.

Counseling: Inform of possibility that slow or delayed healing may occur. Instruct to avoid allowing the tip of the container to contact the eye or surrounding structures. Advise that use of the same bottle for both eyes is not recommended. Instruct not to use while wearing contact lens. Advise to notify physician if an intercurrent ocular condition (eg, trauma, infection) develops or if undergoing ocular surgery. If using >1 ophthalmic medication, instruct to separate administration by 5 min. Advise to shake bottle well.

NEXAVAR — sorafenib   Rx
Class: Kinase inhibitor

ADULT DOSAGE	**PEDIATRIC DOSAGE**
Hepatocellular Carcinoma	Pediatric use may not have been established
Unresectable: 400mg (two 200mg tabs) bid Continue until patient is no longer clinically benefiting from therapy or until unacceptable toxicity occurs	
Advanced Renal Cell Carcinoma 400mg (two 200mg tabs) bid Continue until patient is no longer clinically benefiting from therapy or until unacceptable toxicity occurs	
Differentiated Thyroid Carcinoma Locally recurrent or metastatic, progressive, differentiated thyroid carcinoma that is refractory to radioactive iodine treatment 400mg (two 200mg tabs) bid Continue until patient is no longer clinically benefiting from therapy or until unacceptable toxicity occurs	

DOSING CONSIDERATIONS
Adverse Reactions
Dermatologic Toxicities:
Hepatocellular/Renal Cell Carcinoma:
Grade 1 (Numbness/Dysesthesia/Paresthesia/Tingling/Painless Swelling/Erythema/Discomfort of Hands or Feet That Does Not Disrupt Normal Activities):
Any Occurrence: Continue treatment and consider topical therapy for symptomatic relief

Grade 2 (Painful Erythema and Swelling of Hands or Feet and/or Discomfort Affecting Normal Activities):
1st Occurrence: Continue treatment and consider topical therapy for symptomatic relief
No Improvement w/in 7 Days or 2nd/3rd Occurrence: Interrupt treatment until toxicity resolves to Grade 0-1; when resuming treatment, decrease dose by 1 dose level (400mg/day or 400mg qod)
4th Occurrence: D/C treatment

Grade 3 (Moist Desquamation/Ulceration/Blistering/Severe Pain of Hands or Feet, or Severe Discomfort That Causes Inability to Work or Perform Activities of Daily Living):
1st/2nd Occurrence: Interrupt treatment until toxicity resolves to Grade 0-1; when resuming treatment, decrease dose by 1 dose level (400mg/day or 400mg qod)
3rd Occurrence: D/C treatment

Differentiated Thyroid Carcinoma:
Grade 1:
Any Occurrence: Continue treatment

Grade 2:
1st Occurrence: Decrease dose to 600mg/day
No Improvement w/in 7 Days or 2nd/3rd Occurrence: Interrupt treatment until toxicity resolves or improves to Grade 1; if treatment is resumed, decrease dose as follows:
1st Dose Reduction: 600mg/day (400mg and 200mg 12 hrs apart)
2nd Dose Reduction: 400mg/day (200mg bid)
3rd Dose Reduction: 200mg qd
4th Occurrence: D/C treatment permanently

Grade 3:
1st Occurrence: Interrupt treatment until toxicity resolves or improves to Grade 1; if treatment is resumed, decrease dose to 600mg/day (400mg and 200mg 12 hrs apart)
2nd Occurrence: Interrupt treatment until toxicity resolves or improves to Grade 1; if treatment is resumed, decrease dose to 400mg/day (200mg bid)
3rd Occurrence: D/C treatment

Discontinuation
Temporary interruption or permanent discontinuation may be required for the following:
1. Cardiac ischemia or infarction
2. Hemorrhage requiring medical intervention
3. Severe or persistent HTN despite adequate anti-hypertensive therapy
4. GI perforation
5. QTc prolongation
6. Severe drug-induced liver injury

Other Important Considerations
Patients Undergoing Major Surgical Procedures: Temporarily interrupt therapy
Dose Reductions:
Hepatocellular Carcinoma/Renal Cell Carcinoma:
When dose reduction is necessary, reduce to 400mg qd; if additional dose reduction is required, reduce to a single 400mg dose qod

Differentiated Thyroid Carcinoma:
1st Dose Reduction: 600mg/day (400mg and 200mg 12 hrs apart)
2nd Dose Reduction: 400mg/day (200mg bid)
3rd Dose Reduction: 200mg qd

ADMINISTRATION
Oral route
Take w/o food (at least 1 hr ac or 2 hrs pc)

STORAGE
25°C (77°F); excursions permitted to 15-30°C (59-86°F). Store in a dry place.

HOW SUPPLIED
Tab: 200mg

CONTRAINDICATIONS
Known severe hypersensitivity to sorafenib or any other component of this medication, concomitant use w/ carboplatin and paclitaxel in patients w/ squamous cell lung cancer.

WARNINGS/PRECAUTIONS
HTN, cardiac ischemia, and/or infarction reported; consider temporary or permanent discontinuation. Increased risk of bleeding may occur; consider permanent discontinuation if bleeding necessitates medical intervention. Hand-foot skin reaction and rash reported; may require topical treatment, temporary interruption, and/or dose modification, or permanent discontinuation in severe or persistent cases. Severe dermatologic toxicities, including Stevens-Johnson syndrome (SJS) and toxic epidermal necrolysis (TEN) reported; d/c if SJS or TEN are suspected. D/C if GI perforation occurs. Temporarily interrupt therapy when undergoing major surgical procedures. May prolong the QT/QTc interval; avoid in patients w/ congenital long QT syndrome. Monitor electrolytes and ECG in patients w/ congestive heart failure (CHF), bradyarrhythmias, and in patients taking drugs known to prolong the QT interval (eg, Class Ia and III antiarrhythmics). Correct electrolyte abnormalities (Mg^{2+}, K^+, Ca^{2+}). Interrupt treatment if QTc interval is >500 msec or for an increase from baseline ≥60 msec. Drug-induced hepatitis, and increased bilirubin and INR may occur; d/c in case of significantly increased transaminases w/o alternative explanation (eg, viral hepatitis, progressing underlying malignancy). May impair exogenous thyroid suppression; monitor TSH levels monthly and adjust thyroid replacement medication as needed in patients w/ DTC. May cause fetal harm.

ADVERSE REACTIONS
HTN, fatigue, weight loss, rash, hand-foot skin reaction, alopecia, pruritus, diarrhea, N/V, abdominal pain, anorexia, constipation, hemorrhage, infection, decreased appetite.

DRUG INTERACTIONS
See Contraindications. Avoid w/ gemcitabine/cisplatin in squamous cell lung cancer patients. Avoid w/ strong CYP3A4 inducers (eg, carbamazepine, dexamethasone, St. John's wort); strong CYP3A4 inducers may decrease systemic exposure. Infrequent bleeding or increased INR w/ warfarin; monitor for changes in PT, INR, or bleeding episodes. Decreased exposure w/ oral neomycin.

PREGNANCY AND LACTATION
Category D, not for use in nursing.

MECHANISM OF ACTION
Kinase inhibitor; inhibits multiple intracellular (c-CRAF, BRAF and mutant BRAF) and cell surface kinases (KIT, FLT-3, RET, RET/PTC, VEGFR-1, VEGFR-2, VEGFR-3, and PDGFR-β) thought to be involved in tumor cell signaling, angiogenesis, and apoptosis.

PHARMACOKINETICS
Absorption: T_{max}=3 hrs. **Distribution:** Plasma protein binding (99.5%). **Metabolism:** Liver via oxidation and glucuronidation; CYP3A4, UGT1A9; pyridine N-oxide (metabolite). **Elimination:** (100mg Sol) Feces (77%, 51% unchanged), urine (19% glucuronidated metabolites). $T_{1/2}$=25-48 hrs.

PATIENT CONSIDERATIONS
Assessment: Assess for bleeding disorders, upcoming major surgical procedures, CHF, bradyarrhythmias, electrolyte abnormalities, congenital long QT syndrome, drug hypersensitivity, pregnancy/nursing status, and possible drug interactions.

Monitoring: Monitor for cardiac ischemia/infarction, hemorrhage, HTN, dermatologic toxicities, GI perforation, QT/QTc prolongation, and other adverse reactions. Monitor BP weekly during the first 6 weeks and periodically thereafter. Monitor electrolytes (eg, Mg^{2+}, Ca^{2+}, K^+) and ECG in patients w/ CHF, bradyarrhythmias, and in patients taking drugs known to prolong the QT interval. Monitor LFTs regularly, and TSH levels monthly. Monitor patients taking concomitant warfarin for changes in PT, INR, or clinical bleeding episodes.

Counseling: Inform about risks and benefits of therapy. Instruct to report to physician any episodes of bleeding or cardiac ischemia (eg, chest pain). Inform that HTN may develop, especially during the first 6 weeks; advise that BP should be monitored regularly during therapy. Inform of possible occurrence of hand-foot skin reaction and rash during therapy and appropriate countermeasures. Advise that GI perforation and drug-induced hepatitis may occur and to report signs/symptoms of hepatitis. Inform that temporary interruption of therapy is recommended in patients undergoing major surgical procedures. Counsel patients w/ a history of prolonged QT interval that drug can worsen the condition. Inform that the drug may cause birth defects or fetal loss during pregnancy; instruct both males and females to use effective birth control during treatment and for at least 2 weeks after stopping therapy. Instruct to notify physician if patient becomes pregnant while on therapy. Advise against breastfeeding while on therapy.

NEXIUM IV — esomeprazole sodium   Rx
Class: Proton pump inhibitor (PPI)

ADULT DOSAGE
Gastroesophageal Reflux Disease
W/ Erosive Esophagitis:
20mg or 40mg qd by IV inj (no less than 3 min) or IV infusion (10-30 min)
Safety and efficacy for >10 days have not been demonstrated.
Switch to oral therapy as soon as possible.

Gastric Ulcers
Risk Reduction of Rebleeding Following Therapeutic Endoscopy:
80mg as IV infusion over 30 min followed by 8mg/hr as a continuous infusion for a total treatment duration of 72 hrs (includes initial 30-min dose plus 71.5 hrs of continuous infusion)
Switch to oral therapy as soon as possible

Duodenal Ulcers
Risk Reduction of Rebleeding Following Therapeutic Endoscopy:
80mg as IV infusion over 30 min followed by 8mg/hr as a continuous infusion for a total treatment duration of 72 hrs (includes initial 30-min dose plus 71.5 hrs of continuous infusion)
Switch to oral therapy as soon as possible

PEDIATRIC DOSAGE
Gastroesophageal Reflux Disease
W/ Erosive Esophagitis:
1 Month to <1 Year:
0.5mg/kg qd
1-17 Years:
<55kg: 10mg qd
≥55kg: 20mg qd

Infuse IV over a period of 10-30 min. Switch to oral therapy as soon as possible.

DOSING CONSIDERATIONS
Hepatic Impairment
Adults:
GERD:
Mild to Moderate (Child Pugh Classes A and B):
No dosage adjustment required

Severe (Child Pugh Class C):
Max: 20mg qd

Risk Reduction of Rebleeding of Gastric/Duodenal Ulcers:
No dosage adjustment of the initial 80mg infusion is necessary

Mild to Moderate (Child-Pugh Classes A and B):
Max Continuous Infusion: 6mg/hr

Severe (Child Pugh Class C):
Max Continuous Infusion: 4mg/hr

ADMINISTRATION
IV route
Do not administer concomitantly w/ any other medications through same IV site and/or tubing.
Always flush IV line w/ 0.9% NaCl inj, lactated Ringer's inj, or D5 inj, both prior to and after administration.
Store admixture at room temperature up to 30°C (86°F).
Administer w/in 12 hrs after reconstitution w/ 0.9% NaCl inj or lactated Ringer's inj, or w/in 6 hrs if D5 inj is used.

GERD w/ Erosive Esophagitis
Adults:
- Reconstitute w/ 5mL of 0.9% NaCl.
- Withdraw 5mL of the reconstituted sol and administer as an IV inj over no less than 3 min.
Pediatrics:
- Reconstitute w/ 5mL of 0.9% NaCl, lactated Ringer's inj, or D5 inj, and further dilute the resulting sol to a final volume of 50mL. The resultant concentration after diluting is 0.8mg/mL (40mg vial) and 0.4mg/mL (20mg vial).
- Administer sol (admixture) as an IV infusion over 10-30 min.
- For patients 1 month to <1 yr of age, 1st calculate the dose (0.5mg/kg) to determine the vial size needed.

Risk Reduction of Rebleeding of Gastric/Duodenal Ulcers:
Preparation Instructions for LD and Continuous Infusion:
- Prepare by reconstituting two 40mg vials; reconstitute each vial w/ 5mL of 0.9% NaCl.
- Further dilute the contents of the 2 vials in 100mL 0.9% NaCl for IV use.
- Administer LD over 30 min; administer continuous infusion at a rate of 8mg/hr for 71.5 hrs.

STORAGE
25°C (77°F); excursions permitted to 15-30°C (59-86°F). Protect from light.

HOW SUPPLIED
Inj: 20mg, 40mg

CONTRAINDICATIONS
Known hypersensitivity to substituted benzimidazoles or to any component of the formulation.

WARNINGS/PRECAUTIONS

Symptomatic response does not preclude the presence of gastric malignancy in adults; consider additional follow-up and diagnostic testing in adults who have suboptimal response or an early symptomatic relapse after completing treatment w/ a PPI. Consider an endoscopy in older patients. Acute interstitial nephritis reported; d/c if this develops. May increase risk of *Clostridium difficile*-associated diarrhea (CDAD), especially in hospitalized patients. May increase risk of osteoporosis-related fractures of the hip, wrist, or spine, especially w/ high-dose and long-term therapy. Use lowest dose and shortest duration possible. Cutaneous lupus erythematosus (CLE) and systemic lupus erythematosus (SLE) reported; avoid administration of PPIs for longer than medically indicated, and d/c the drug if signs/symptoms consistent w/ CLE or SLE are noted. Hypomagnesemia reported (rarely) and may require Mg^{2+} replacement and discontinuation of therapy. Consider monitoring Mg^{2+} levels prior to initiation of treatment and periodically in patients expected to be on prolonged treatment.

ADVERSE REACTIONS

Headache, flatulence, nausea, abdominal pain, diarrhea, dry mouth, duodenal ulcer hemorrhage, inj-site reaction, pyrexia.

DRUG INTERACTIONS

Concomitant use of esomeprazole 40mg results in reduced plasma concentrations of the active metabolite of clopidogrel and a reduction in platelet inhibition; avoid concomitant administration w/ clopidogrel. Consider alternative antiplatelet therapy. Consider dose reduction of cilostazol from 100mg bid to 50mg bid; coadministration is expected to increase cilostazol concentrations. Concomitant administration w/ a combined inhibitor of CYP2C19 and CYP3A4 (eg, voriconazole) may result in more than doubling of the esomeprazole exposure; consider dose adjustment in patients who may require higher doses. Drugs known to induce CYP2C19 or CYP3A4 (eg, rifampin) may lead to decreased esomeprazole levels; avoid concomitant use w/ St. John's wort or rifampin. Concomitant use of atazanavir not recommended; coadministration is expected to substantially decrease atazanavir concentrations and thereby reduce its therapeutic effect. Caution w/ other antiretroviral drugs. May reduce the absorption of drugs where gastric pH is an important determinant of their bioavailability; absorption of ketoconazole, atazanavir, iron salts, erlotinib, and mycophenolate mofetil (MMF) may decrease, while the absorption of digoxin may increase. May increase digoxin exposure; monitor w/ concomitant use. Caution in transplant patients receiving MMF. Serum chromogranin A (CgA) levels increase secondary to PPI-induced decreases in gastric acidity and may cause false positive results in diagnostic investigations for neuroendocrine tumors; temporarily stop esomeprazole treatment at least 14 days before assessing CgA levels and consider repeating the test if initial CgA levels are high. Concomitant administration w/ tacrolimus may increase serum levels of tacrolimus. May elevate and prolong serum levels of methotrexate (MTX) and/or its metabolite, possibly leading to MTX toxicity; consider a temporary withdrawal of the PPI in high-dose MTX administration. May need to monitor for increases in INR and PT w/ concomitant warfarin. Caution w/ digoxin or other drugs that may cause hypomagnesemia (eg, diuretics).

PREGNANCY AND LACTATION

Pregnancy: Category C.
Lactation: Likely present in human milk. Caution in nursing.

MECHANISM OF ACTION

PPI; suppresses gastric acid secretion by specific inhibition of the H^+/K^+-ATPase in the gastric parietal cell. Blocks the final step of acid production, thus reducing gastric acidity.

PHARMACOKINETICS

Absorption: $C_{max}=3.86\mu mol/L$ (20mg), $7.51\mu mol/L$ (40mg); $AUC=5.11\mu mol\cdot hr/L$ (20mg), $16.21\mu mol\cdot hr/L$ (40mg). **Distribution:** $V_d=16L$; plasma protein binding (97%); likely present in breast milk. **Metabolism:** Liver (extensive) via CYP2C19 (major) into hydroxy and desmethyl metabolites, and via CYP3A4 into sulphone metabolite. **Elimination:** Urine (primary, <1% unchanged), feces; $T_{1/2}=1.05$ hrs (20mg), 1.41 hrs (40mg).

PATIENT CONSIDERATIONS

Assessment: Assess for hypersensitivity to substituted benzimidazoles or to any component of the formulation, hepatic dysfunction, risk for osteoporosis-related fractures, pregnancy/nursing status, and possible drug interactions. Obtain Mg^{2+} levels in patients expected to be on prolonged therapy.

Monitoring: Monitor for signs/symptoms of hypersensitivity reactions, acute interstitial nephritis, bone fractures, CLE/SLE, hypomagnesemia, CDAD, and other adverse reactions.

Counseling: Advise to report to physician if experiencing any signs/symptoms consistent w/ hypersensitivity reactions, acute interstitial nephritis, CDAD, bone fractures, CLE/SLE, or hypomagnesemia. Advise to notify physician if taking or beginning to take other medications. Inform that antacids may be used while on therapy. Advise to report and seek care for diarrhea that does not improve and for any cardiovascular/neurological symptoms.

NEXIUM ORAL — esomeprazole magnesium   Rx

Class: Proton pump inhibitor (PPI)

ADULT DOSAGE

Gastroesophageal Reflux Disease

Healing of Erosive Esophagitis:
20mg or 40mg qd for 4-8 weeks; may consider an additional 4-8 weeks of treatment if not healed

Maint of Healing of Erosive Esophagitis:
20mg qd; controlled studies did not extend beyond 6 months

Symptomatic GERD:
20mg qd for 4 weeks; may consider an additional 4 weeks of treatment if symptoms do not resolve completely

NSAID-Associated Gastric Ulcer

Risk Reduction of NSAID-Associated Gastric Ulcer:
20mg or 40mg qd for up to 6 months

Helicobacter pylori **Eradication**

Triple Therapy:
Esomeprazole 40mg qd + amoxicillin 1000mg bid + clarithromycin 500mg bid, all for 10 days

Pathological Hypersecretory Conditions

Eg, Zollinger-Ellison Syndrome:
40mg bid; adjust dose to individual patient needs

Doses up to 240mg/day have been administered

PEDIATRIC DOSAGE

Gastroesophageal Reflux Disease

Symptomatic GERD:
1-11 Years:
10mg qd for up to 8 weeks; doses >1mg/kg/day have not been studied

12-17 Years:
20mg qd for 4 weeks

Healing of Erosive Esophagitis:
1-11 Years:
<20kg: 10mg qd for 8 weeks
≥20kg: 10mg or 20mg qd for 8 weeks
Doses >1mg/kg/day have not been studied

12-17 Years:
20mg or 40mg qd for 4-8 weeks

Erosive Esophagitis Due to Acid-Mediated GERD:
1 Month to <1 Year:
3-5kg: 2.5mg qd for up to 6 weeks
>5-7.5kg: 5mg qd for up to 6 weeks
>7.5-12kg: 10mg qd for up to 6 weeks
Doses >1.33mg/kg/day have not been studied

DOSING CONSIDERATIONS

Hepatic Impairment
Mild to Moderate (Child Pugh Classes A and B):
No dosage adjustment necessary

Severe (Child-Pugh Class C):
Max Dose: 20mg/day

ADMINISTRATION

Oral route

Take at least 1 hr ac.

Cap
Swallow whole, or alternatively, open cap and add granules on 1 tbsp of applesauce, then swallow immediately; do not chew or crush the granules.

NG Tube:
1. Open and empty the intact granules into a 60mL catheter tipped syringe and mix w/ 50mL of water.
2. Replace the plunger and shake the syringe vigorously for 15 sec.
3. Attach the syringe to a NG tube and deliver the contents of the syringe into the stomach.
4. Flush the NG tube w/ additional water after use.

Sus
1. Empty the contents of a 2.5mg or 5mg pkt into 5mL of water. For the 10mg, 20mg, and 40mg pkts, empty into 15mL of water.
2. Stir and leave 2-3 min to thicken.
3. Stir and drink w/in 30 min. If any medicine remains after drinking, add more water, stir, and drink immediately.
4. In cases where 2 pkts need to be used, may mix in a similar way by adding twice the required amount of water or follow mixing instructions provided.

NG/Gastric Tube:
1. Add 5mL of water to a catheter tipped syringe, then add contents of a 2.5mg or 5mg pkt. For 10mg, 20mg, and 40mg pkts, volume of water in the syringe should be 15mL.
2. Immediately shake syringe and leave 2-3 min to thicken.
3. Shake syringe and inject through NG or gastric tube, French size ≥6, into the stomach w/in 30 min.
4. Refill the syringe w/ an equal amount of water (5mL or 15mL).
5. Shake and flush any remaining contents from NG or gastric tube into stomach.

STORAGE

25°C (77°F); excursions permitted to 15-30°C (59-86°F).

HOW SUPPLIED

Cap, Delayed-Release: 20mg, 40mg; **Oral Sus, Delayed-Release:** 2.5mg, 5mg, 10mg, 20mg, 40mg (granules/pkt)

CONTRAINDICATIONS

Known hypersensitivity to substituted benzimidazoles or to any component of the medication. When used w/ clarithromycin and amoxicillin, refer to the individual monographs.

WARNINGS/PRECAUTIONS

Symptomatic response does not preclude the presence of gastric malignancy in adults; consider additional follow-up and diagnostic testing in adults who have a suboptimal response or an early symptomatic relapse after completing treatment. In older patients, also consider an endoscopy. Acute interstitial nephritis reported; d/c if this develops. May increase risk of *Clostridium difficile* associated diarrhea (CDAD), especially in hospitalized patients. May increase risk for osteoporosis-related fractures of the hip, wrist, or spine, especially w/ high-dose and long-term therapy. Use lowest dose and shortest duration appropriate to the condition being treated. Cutaneous lupus erythematosus (CLE) and systemic lupus erythematosus (SLE) reported; avoid administration of PPIs for longer than medically indicated, and d/c therapy if signs/symptoms are consistent w/ CLE or SLE. Daily treatment w/ any acid-suppressing medications over a long period of time (eg, >3 years) may lead to malabsorption of cyanocobalamin (vitamin B12). Hypomagnesemia reported (rarely) and may require Mg^{2+} replacement and discontinuation of therapy.

ADVERSE REACTIONS

Adults: Headache, diarrhea, abdominal pain.
Pediatrics: (1-11 months) Irritability, vomiting. (1-11 years) Diarrhea, headache, somnolence. (12-17 years) Headache, abdominal pain, diarrhea, nausea.

DRUG INTERACTIONS

CYP2C19 or CYP3A4 inducers may decrease levels; avoid w/ St. John's wort or rifampin. Reduces pharmacological activity of clopidogrel; avoid concomitant use. May reduce atazanavir and nelfinavir levels; concomitant use not recommended. May change absorption or levels of antiretrovirals. May increase levels of saquinavir, cilostazol, and tacrolimus; consider saquinavir and cilostazol dose reduction. May reduce the absorption of drugs where gastric pH is an important determinant of bioavailability; ketoconazole, atazanavir, iron salts, erlotinib, and mycophenolate mofetil (MMF) absorption may decrease, while digoxin absorption may increase. Caution in transplant patients receiving MMF. Monitor for increases in INR and PT w/ warfarin. Decreases clearance of diazepam. Increased exposure w/ combined inhibitors of CYP2C19 and CYP3A4 (eg, voriconazole); consider dose adjustment w/ Zollinger-Ellison syndrome. Increased levels of esomeprazole and 14-hydroxyclarithromycin w/ amoxicillin and clarithromycin. Caution w/ digoxin or other drugs that may cause hypomagnesemia (eg, diuretics). May elevate and prolong levels of methotrexate (MTX) and/or its metabolite, possibly leading to toxicities; consider temporary withdrawal of therapy w/ high-dose MTX. Serum chromogranin A (CgA) levels increase secondary to PPI-induced decreases in gastric acidity and may cause false positive results in diagnostic investigations for neuroendocrine tumors; temporarily stop esomeprazole treatment at least 14 days before assessing CgA levels and consider repeating the test if initial CgA levels are high.

PREGNANCY AND LACTATION

Pregnancy: Category C.
Lactation: Likely present in human milk; caution in nursing.

MECHANISM OF ACTION

PPI; suppresses gastric acid secretion by specific inhibition of the H^+/K^+-ATPase in the gastric parietal cell. Blocks the final step of acid production, thus reducing gastric acidity.

PHARMACOKINETICS

Absorption: C_{max}=2.1μmol/L (20mg), 4.7μmol/L (40mg); T_{max}=1.6 hrs; AUC=4.2μmol•hr/L (20mg), 12.6μmol•hr/L (40mg). Refer to PI for pharmacokinetic parameters in pediatric patients. **Distribution:** V_d=16L; plasma protein binding (97%); likely found in breast milk. **Metabolism:** Liver (extensive) via CYP2C19 (major) into hydroxy and desmethyl metabolites, and via CYP3A4 into sulphone metabolites. **Elimination:** Urine (80% metabolites, <1% unchanged), feces; $T_{1/2}$=1.2 hrs (20mg), 1.5 hrs (40mg).

PATIENT CONSIDERATIONS

Assessment: Assess for hypersensitivity to substituted benzimidazoles or to any component of the formulation, hepatic dysfunction, risk for osteoporosis-related fractures, pregnancy/nursing status, and possible drug interactions. Obtain Mg^{2+} levels in patients expected to be on prolonged therapy.

Monitoring: Monitor for signs/symptoms of acute interstitial nephritis, CLE/SLE, cyanocobalamin deficiency, bone fractures, hypomagnesemia, CDAD, and other adverse reactions.

Counseling: Inform to take exactly ud. Advise to report to physician if experiencing any signs/symptoms consistent w/ hypersensitivity reactions, acute interstitial nephritis, CDAD, bone fracture, CLE/SLE, cyanocobalamin deficiency, or hypomagnesemia. Advise to report if taking or beginning to take any other medications.

NEXPLANON — etonogestrel   Rx

Class: Progestin contraceptive

ADULT DOSAGE	PEDIATRIC DOSAGE
Contraception	**Contraception**
No Preceding Hormonal Contraceptive Use in the Past Month: Insert subdermally in the upper arm between Day 1 (1st day of menstrual bleeding) and Day 5 of menstrual cycle, even if patient is still bleeding	Not indicated for use premenarche; refer to adult dosing
Following Abortion or Miscarriage: **1st Trimester:** Insert w/in 5 days following 1st trimester abortion or miscarriage **2nd Trimester:** Insert between 21-28 days following 2nd trimester abortion or miscarriage	
Postpartum: **Not Breastfeeding:** Insert between 21-28 days postpartum **Breastfeeding:** Insert after the 4th postpartum week	
Remove by the end of the 3rd year; if continued contraceptive protection is desired, may replace by a new implant at the time of removal using the same incision of the previous implant	

Conversions

Switching from Combination Hormonal Contraceptives:
Insert implant on the day after the last active tab of the previous combined oral contraceptive or on the day of the removal of the vaginal ring or transdermal patch. At the latest, insert implant on the day following the usual tab-free, ring-free, patch-free or placebo tab interval of the previous combined hormonal contraceptive

Switching from Progestin-Only Contraceptives:
Injectable Contraceptives: Insert implant on the day the next inj is due
Minipill: Insert implant on any day of the month, w/in 24 hrs after taking the last tab
Contraceptive Implant or Intrauterine System (IUS): Insert implant on the same day as the previous contraceptive implant or IUS is removed

---

ADMINISTRATION

Subdermal route

Insert implant at the inner side of the non-dominant upper arm about 8-10 cm (3-4 inches) above the medial epicondyle of the humerus, to reduce the risk of neural or vascular injury.
If inserted as recommended, backup contraception is not necessary.
If deviating from the recommended timing of insertion, advise to use a barrier method until 7 days after insertion; if intercourse has already occurred, pregnancy should be excluded.
In postpartum/breastfeeding women, advise to use a barrier method until 7 days after insertion; if intercourse has already occurred, pregnancy should be excluded.

Insertion Procedure

1. Anesthetize the insertion area (eg, w/ anesthetic spray or by injecting 2mL of 1% lidocaine).
2. Remove the transparent protection cap by sliding it horizontally in the direction of the arrow away from the needle.
3. Do not touch the purple slider until the needle is fully inserted subdermally.
4. Puncture the skin w/ the tip of the needle slightly angled <30°.
5. Lower the applicator to a horizontal position and insert needle to its full length.
6. Unlock the purple slider by pushing it slightly down and move the slider fully back until it stops.
7. Remove the applicator.
8. Verify the presence of the implant by palpation.

Refer to PI for further administration details and for removal procedure.

STORAGE

25°C (77°F); excursions permitted to 15-30°C (59-86°F). Avoid storing at temperatures >30°C (86°F).

HOW SUPPLIED

Implant: 68mg

CONTRAINDICATIONS

Known or suspected pregnancy, current/history of thrombosis or thromboembolic disorders, benign or malignant liver tumors, active liver disease, undiagnosed abnormal genital bleeding, known/suspected/personal history of breast cancer, current/history of other progestin-sensitive cancer, or allergic reaction to any of the components.

WARNINGS/PRECAUTIONS

Confirm by palpation immediately after insertion; failure to insert implant properly may lead to an unintended pregnancy. Complications related to insertion or removal procedures (eg, pain, paresthesias, bleeding, hematoma, scarring, infection) may occur. If infection develops at the insertion site, start suitable treatment; if infection persists, remove implant. Incomplete insertions or infections may lead to expulsion. Neural or vascular injury may occur if inserted too deeply. Implant removal may be difficult/impossible if inserted incorrectly, inserted too deeply, not palpable, if it is encased in fibrous tissue, or if it has migrated. Implant migration w/in the arm from the insertion site reported; may be related to a deep insertion. Reports of implants located w/in vessels of the arm and the pulmonary artery (rare); may be related to deep insertions or intravascular insertion. If at any time the implant cannot be palpated, it should be localized and removed. Failure to remove may result in continued effects of etonogestrel. May cause changes in menstrual bleeding patterns, ectopic pregnancy, thrombotic/vascular events, ovarian cysts, breast cancer, cervical cancer or intraepithelial neoplasia, hepatic adenomas, weight gain, gallbladder disease, and fluid retention. Perform appropriate measures to rule out malignancy if undiagnosed, persistent, or recurrent abnormal vaginal bleeding occurs. Carefully monitor women w/ a family history of breast cancer and those who develop breast nodules. Do not use prior to 21 days postpartum. Evaluate for retinal vein thrombosis immediately if there is unexplained loss of vision, proptosis, diplopia, papilledema, or retinal vascular lesions. Consider removal of implant if significant depression develops or in case of long-term immobilization due to surgery or illness. Remove implant in the event of thrombosis or if jaundice develops. Women w/ a history of HTN-related diseases or renal disease should be discouraged from using hormonal contraception. Remove implant if a significant increase in BP unresponsive to antihypertensive therapy or sustained HTN occurs. May induce mild insulin resistance and small changes in glucose levels; monitor prediabetic and diabetic women. May elevate LDL levels. Restart contraception immediately after removal for continued contraceptive protection. Contact lens wearers who develop visual changes or changes in lens tolerance should be assessed by an ophthalmologist. Broken or bent implants while in the patient's arm reported; broken or bent implant may slightly increase the release rate of etonogestrel. Remove implant in its entirety when it is removed. May decrease sex hormone-binding globulin (SHBG) and thyroxine levels initially, followed by gradual recovery. May be less effective in overweight women.

ADVERSE REACTIONS
Headache, vaginitis, weight increase, acne, breast pain, abdominal pain, pharyngitis, leukorrhea, influenza-like symptoms, dizziness, dysmenorrhea, back pain, emotional lability, nausea, pain.

DRUG INTERACTIONS
Drugs or herbal products that induce enzymes, including CYP3A4 that metabolize progestins (eg, barbiturates, bosentan, carbamazepine), may decrease levels of progestins and decrease the effectiveness therapy; recommended to remove implant if on long-term treatment w/ hepatic enzyme-inducing drugs. HIV protease inhibitors or non-nucleoside reverse transcriptase inhibitors have been reported in some cases to cause significant changes (increase or decrease) in plasma levels of progestins. CYP3A4 inhibitors (eg, itraconazole, ketoconazole) may increase levels of etonogestrel. May affect metabolism of other drugs and consequently may either increase (eg, cyclosporine) or decrease (eg, lamotrigine) plasma concentrations of coadministered drugs.

PREGNANCY AND LACTATION
Pregnancy: Contraindicated in pregnancy.
Lactation: May be used during breastfeeding after the 4th postpartum week. Small amounts of etonogestrel are excreted in breast milk.

MECHANISM OF ACTION
Progestin contraceptive; suppresses ovulation, increases viscosity of cervical mucus, and alters the endometrium.

PHARMACOKINETICS
Absorption: Bioavailability (100%); C_{max}=1200pg/mL; T_{max}=w/in the first 2 weeks after insertion. **Distribution:** V_d=201L; plasma protein binding [albumin (66%), SHBG (32%)]; found in breast milk. **Metabolism:** Liver via CYP3A4. **Elimination:** Urine (primary), feces; $T_{1/2}$=25 hrs.

PATIENT CONSIDERATIONS
Assessment: Assess for current or past history of thrombosis or thromboembolic disorders, benign or malignant liver tumors, active liver disease, undiagnosed abnormal genital bleeding, known/suspected/history of breast cancer or current or past history of other progestin-sensitive cancer, history of HTN-related diseases or renal disease, history of depressed mood, diabetes, hyperlipidemia, conditions that might be aggravated by fluid retention, pregnancy status, or for any other conditions where treatment is contraindicated or cautioned. Assess nursing status and for possible drug interactions.

Monitoring: Monitor for complications of insertion/removal of implant, changes in menstrual bleeding pattern, ectopic pregnancy, thrombotic/other vascular events, ovarian cysts, breast/cervical cancer, intraepithelial neoplasia, liver dysfunction, weight gain, gallbladder disease, fluid retention, and other adverse events. Monitor for visual changes or changes in lens tolerance in patients who wear contact lens and refer to an ophthalmologist if changes occur. Monitor glucose levels in diabetic and prediabetic patients, BP w/ history of HTN, lipid levels w/ a history of hyperlipidemia. Monitor for signs of depression w/ previous history. In cases of undiagnosed, persistent, or recurrent abnormal vaginal bleeding, perform appropriate measures to rule out malignancy. Perform BP check and other indicated healthcare annually.

Counseling: Inform of the risks and benefits of therapy. Counsel about insertion and removal procedure of the implant. Provide patient w/ a copy of the Patient Labeling and ensure information is understood before insertion and removal. Inform that consent form is included in the package and advise to complete consent form. Provide patient w/ the user card after insertion in order to have a record of the location of the implant in the upper arm and when it should be removed. Inform that the implant does not protect against HIV infection (AIDS) or other STDs. Advise that use may be associated w/ changes in normal menstrual bleeding patterns.

NIASPAN — niacin   Rx
Class: Nicotinic acid

ADULT DOSAGE
Hyperlipidemia

For use in patients w/ primary hyperlipidemia and mixed dyslipidemia. To reduce the risk of recurrent nonfatal MI in patients w/ a history of MI and hyperlipidemia. To slow progression or promote regression of atherosclerotic disease in patients w/ a history of coronary artery disease and hyperlipidemia in combination w/ a bile acid binding resin. To reduce elevated total cholesterol and LDL levels in patients w/ primary hyperlipidemia

PEDIATRIC DOSAGE
Pediatric use may not have been established

---

in combination w/ a bile acid binding resin. Adjunctive therapy in patients w/ severe hypertriglyceridemia who present a risk of pancreatitis and who do not respond adequately to a determined dietary effort to control them

>16 Years:
Initial: 500mg qhs after a low-fat snack
Titrate: Increase by 500mg every 4 weeks; after Week 8, titrate to patient response and tolerance; increase to 1500mg qd if response to 1000mg qd is inadequate and may subsequently increase to 2000mg qd
Do not increase daily dose by >500mg in any 4-week period
Maint: 1000-2000mg qhs
Max: 2000mg/day

Women may respond at lower doses than men

If therapy is discontinued for an extended period, reinstitution should include a titration phase

---

DOSING CONSIDERATIONS
Renal Impairment
Use caution

ADMINISTRATION
Oral route

Take at hs after a low-fat snack.
Swallow tab whole; do not break, crush, or chew.
Avoid administration on an empty stomach and slowly increase niacin dose to reduce flushing, pruritus, and GI distress.
May take aspirin (ASA) (up to 325mg) 30 min prior to treatment to reduce flushing.
Two of the 500mg tabs and one of the 1000mg tabs are interchangeable; do not interchange three 500mg tabs w/ two 750mg tabs.
Equivalent doses of niacin ER should not be substituted for sustained-release (modified-release, timed-release) niacin preparations or immediate-release (IR) (crystalline) niacin.

STORAGE
20-25°C (68-77°F).

HOW SUPPLIED
Tab, Extended-Release: 500mg, 750mg, 1000mg

CONTRAINDICATIONS
Active liver disease or unexplained persistent elevations in hepatic transaminases, active peptic ulcer disease (PUD), arterial bleeding. Hypersensitivity to niacin or any component of this medication.

WARNINGS/PRECAUTIONS
Do not substitute for equivalent doses of sustained-release (modified-release, timed-release) niacin or IR (crystalline) niacin; severe hepatic toxicity, including fulminant hepatic necrosis, have occurred in patients who have substituted sustained-release (modified-release, timed-release) niacin products for IR (crystalline) niacin at equivalent doses. If switching from IR niacin, initiate w/ low doses (eg, 500mg at hs) and titrate to desired therapeutic response. Caution in patients w/ unstable angina or in the acute phase of MI, particularly if also receiving vasoactive drugs (eg, nitrates, calcium channel blockers, adrenergic blocking agents). Caution in patients w/ renal impairment, or who consume substantial quantities of alcohol, and/or have history of liver disease. Closely observe patients w/ history of jaundice, hepatobiliary disease, or peptic ulcer. Has not been shown to reduce cardiovascular morbidity or mortality among patients already treated w/ a statin. Associated w/ abnormal LFTs; monitor LFTs (eg, AST, ALT) before treatment, every 6-12 weeks for the 1st yr, and periodically thereafter (eg, 6-month intervals). If elevated serum transaminase levels develop, measurements should be repeated promptly and then performed more frequently. D/C if transaminase levels progress, particularly if they rise to 3X ULN and are persistent, or if associated w/ nausea, fever, and/or malaise. May increase FPG; closely monitor diabetic/potentially diabetic patients (particularly during 1st few months of therapy or dose adjustment), and adjust diet and/or hypoglycemic therapy if necessary. Associated w/ dose-related reductions in platelet count and phosphorus (P) levels; periodically monitor P levels in patients at risk for hypophosphatemia. Associated w/ increases in PT; carefully evaluate patients undergoing surgery. Elevated uric acid levels reported; caution in patients predisposed to gout. Lab test interactions may occur.

ADVERSE REACTIONS
Flushing (warmth, redness, itching, and/or tingling), diarrhea, N/V, increased cough, pruritus, rash.

DRUG INTERACTIONS
Avoid ingestion of alcohol, hot drinks, or spicy foods around the time of administration; may increase flushing and pruritus. Use caution when prescribing niacin (≥1g/day) w/ statins; may increase risk of myopathy and rhabdomyolysis; consider performing periodic serum CPK and K+ determinations if used concomitantly w/ a statin. Separate dosing from bile acid-binding resins by at least 4-6 hrs. ASA may decrease the metabolic clearance of nicotinic acid.

May potentiate the effects of ganglionic blocking agents and vasoactive drugs, resulting in postural hypotension. Vitamins or other nutritional supplements containing large doses of niacin or related compounds (eg, nicotinamide) may potentiate adverse effects. Use caution w/ anticoagulants; monitor platelet counts and PT.

PREGNANCY AND LACTATION
Category C, not for use in nursing.

MECHANISM OF ACTION
Nicotinic acid; not established. May partially inhibit release of free fatty acids from adipose tissue, and increase lipoprotein lipase activity, which may increase the rate of chylomicron TG removal from plasma. Decreases the rate of hepatic synthesis of VLDL and LDL, and does not appear to affect fecal excretion of fats, sterols, or bile acids.

PHARMACOKINETICS
Absorption: T_{max}=5 hrs. **Distribution:** Found in breast milk. **Metabolism:** Liver (rapid; extensive and saturable 1st pass); nicotinuric acid (via conjugation), nicotinamide adenine dinucleotide (metabolites). **Elimination:** Urine (60-76%; up to 12% unchanged).

PATIENT CONSIDERATIONS
Assessment: Assess for history of/active liver disease or PUD, unexplained persistent hepatic transaminase elevations, predisposure to gout, arterial bleeding, history of jaundice or hepatobiliary disease, renal impairment, risk for hypophosphatemia, drug hypersensitivity, any other conditions where treatment is contraindicated or cautioned, pregnancy/nursing status, and possible drug interactions. Obtain baseline LFTs and lipid levels.

Monitoring: Monitor for signs/symptoms of liver dysfunction, decreases in platelet counts and P levels, increases in PT and uric acid levels, and other adverse reactions. Monitor LFTs every 6-12 weeks for the 1st yr, and periodically thereafter. Monitor lipid levels. Frequently monitor blood glucose levels. Periodically monitor P levels in patients at risk for hypophosphatemia. Monitor PT and platelet counts in patients on concomitant therapy w/ anticoagulants. Monitor patients on concomitant therapy w/ statins for any signs/symptoms of muscle pain, tenderness, or weakness, particularly during the initial months of therapy and during any periods of upward dosage titration; consider performing periodic serum CPK and K^+ determinations in such situations.

Counseling: Advise to adhere to the National Cholesterol Education Program-recommended diet, a regular exercise program, and periodic testing of a fasting lipid panel. Instruct to contact physician before restarting therapy if dosing is interrupted for any length of time. Instruct to notify physician of any unexplained muscle pain, tenderness or weakness, dizziness, changes in blood glucose if diabetic, and all medications being taken (eg, vitamins or other nutritional supplements containing niacin or nicotinamide). Inform that flushing may occur and may subside after several weeks of consistent use of therapy. Instruct that if awakened by flushing at night, to get up slowly, especially if feeling dizzy or faint, or taking BP medications. Advise of the symptoms of flushing and how they differ from the symptoms of MI. Instruct to avoid ingestion of alcohol, hot beverages, and spicy foods around the time of administration to minimize flushing. Advise to d/c use and contact physician if pregnant. Instruct not to use niacin if breastfeeding.

NICOTROL NASAL SPRAY — nicotine   Rx

Class: Nicotine

ADULT DOSAGE
Smoking Cessation Aid

For Relief of Nicotine Withdrawal Symptoms:
Stop smoking completely when beginning therapy
Individualize dose based on nicotine dependence and occurrence of symptoms of nicotine excess

Initial: 1 or 2 doses/hr (1 or 2 sprays in each nostril)
Titrate: May increase up to 40mg (80 sprays)/day; use at least the recommended minimum of 8 doses/day
Max Dose: 40 doses/day or 5 doses/hr
Max Duration: 3 months

D/C if unable to stop smoking by the 4th week of therapy
May taper or d/c abruptly

PEDIATRIC DOSAGE
Pediatric use may not have been established

DOSING CONSIDERATIONS
Elderly
Start at lower end of dosing range

ADMINISTRATION
Intranasal route

Do not sniff, swallow, or inhale through nose during administration
Administer spray w/ head slightly tilted back
1 dose is 1mg of nicotine (2 sprays, 1 in each nostril)

STORAGE
25°C (77°F); excursions permitted to 15-30°C (59-86°F).

HOW SUPPLIED
Spray: 10mg/mL (0.5mg/spray)

CONTRAINDICATIONS
Known hypersensitivity or allergy to nicotine or to any component of the product.

WARNINGS/PRECAUTIONS
Should be used as part of a comprehensive behavioral smoking cessation program. May be toxic and addictive. May cause fetal harm. Use beyond 6 months is not recommended. Exacerbation of bronchospasm with preexisting asthma reported; not recommended with severe reactive airway disease. May cause nasal irritation; risks and benefits should be considered. Not recommended with known chronic nasal disorders (eg, allergy, rhinitis, nasal polyps, sinusitis). Caution with coronary heart disease (eg, history of myocardial infarction [MI] and/or angina pectoris), serious cardiac arrhythmias, vasospastic diseases (eg, Buerger's disease, Prinzmetal's variant angina, and Raynaud's phenomena), hyperthyroidism, pheochromocytoma, insulin-dependent diabetes, active peptic ulcers, and in elderly. Tachycardia reported; d/c if cardiovascular (CV) events occur. Avoid in patients during the immediate post-MI period, with serious arrhythmias, or severe/worsening angina. Increased risk for malignant HTN in patients with accelerated HTN; use with caution. Not recommended for use during labor and delivery. Caution with hepatic/severe renal impairment.

ADVERSE REACTIONS
Dependence, nasal irritation, runny nose, throat irritation, watering eyes, sneezing, coughing, nasal congestion, sinus irritation, transient epistaxis, eye irritation, pharyngitis, paresthesias of the nose/mouth/head, earache, facial flushing.

DRUG INTERACTIONS
Nasal vasoconstrictor (eg, xylometazoline) may further prolong T_{max} in patients with rhinitis. May require dose reduction of acetaminophen, caffeine, imipramine, oxazepam, pentazocine, propranolol or other β-blockers, theophylline, insulin, adrenergic antagonists (eg, prazosin, labetalol) at smoking cessation. May require increase in dose of adrenergic agonists (eg, isoproterenol, phenylephrine) at smoking cessation.

PREGNANCY AND LACTATION
Category D, caution in nursing.

MECHANISM OF ACTION
Nicotine; binds stereo-selectively to nicotinic-cholinergic receptors at the autonomic ganglia, in the adrenal medulla, at neuromuscular junctions, and in the brain.

PHARMACOKINETICS
Absorption: C_{max}=2-12ng/mL, T_{max}=4-15 min. **Distribution:** V_d=2-3L/kg (IV); plasma protein binding (<5%); found in breast milk. **Metabolism:** Liver (major), kidneys and lungs; cotinine and trans-3-hydroxycotinine (primary urinary metabolites). **Elimination:** Urine (10%, unchanged); $T_{1/2}$=1-2 hrs, 15-20 hrs (cotinine).

PATIENT CONSIDERATIONS
Assessment: Assess for hypersensitivity or allergy to drug, preexisting asthma, severe reactive airway disease, chronic nasal disorders, coronary heart disease, arrhythmias, vasospastic diseases, hyperthyroidism, hepatic/severe renal impairment, pheochromocytoma, insulin-dependent diabetes, active peptic ulcers, accelerated HTN, pregnancy/nursing status, and possible drug interactions.

Monitoring: Monitor for exacerbation of bronchospasm, delay in healing with peptic ulcer disease, CV events, irritation of nasal mucosa, malignant HTN, withdrawal symptoms, and other adverse reactions.

Counseling: Instruct on the proper use of the drug. Instruct to stop smoking completely before beginning treatment. Inform that patients may experience adverse effects if they continue to smoke while on therapy. Counsel that patients are likely to experience nasal irritation, which may become less bothersome with continued use.

NINLARO — ixazomib   Rx

Class: Proteasome inhibitor

ADULT DOSAGE
Multiple Myeloma

Use in combination w/ lenalidomide and dexamethasone for the treatment of patients w/ multiple myeloma who have received at least one prior therapy; continue treatment until disease progression or unacceptable toxicity

Ixazomib:
Initial: 4mg once a week on Days 1, 8, and 15 of a 28-day treatment cycle

Lenalidomide:
Initial: 25mg qd on Days 1-21 of a 28-day treatment cycle

Dexamethasone:
Initial: 40mg on Days 1, 8, 15, and 22 of a 28-day treatment cycle

Prior to Initiation of a New Cycle of Therapy:
- ANC should be ≥1000/mm³
- Platelet count should be ≥75,000/mm³

PEDIATRIC DOSAGE
Pediatric use may not have been established

- Non-hematologic toxicities should, at the physician's discretion, generally be recovered to patient's baseline condition or ≤Grade 1

Missed Dose
If a dose is delayed or missed, take only if the next scheduled dose is ≥72 hrs away. A missed dose should not be taken w/in 72 hrs of the next scheduled dose. A double dose should not be taken to make up for the missed dose.

If vomiting occurs after taking a dose, do not repeat dose; resume dosing at the time of the next scheduled dose

---

DOSING CONSIDERATIONS
Renal Impairment
Severe Renal Impairment (CrCl <30mL/min)/ESRD Requiring Dialysis: Reduce starting dose to 3mg; administer w/o regard to the timing of dialysis

Hepatic Impairment
Moderate (Total Bilirubin >1.5-3X ULN) or Severe (Total Bilirubin >3X ULN): Reduce starting dose to 3mg

Adverse Reactions
Ixazomib Dose Reductions:
Recommended Starting Dose: 4mg
First Dose Reduction: 3mg
Second Dose Reduction: 2.3mg

Hematological Toxicities:
Thrombocytopenia (Platelet Count <30,000/mm³): Withhold ixazomib and lenalidomide until platelet count is ≥30,000/mm³; following recovery, resume lenalidomide at the next lower dose and resume ixazomib at its most recent dose. If platelet count falls to <30,000/mm³ again, withhold ixazomib and lenalidomide until platelet count is ≥30,000/mm³; following recovery, resume ixazomib at the next lower dose and resume lenalidomide at its most recent dose. For additional occurrences, alternate dose modification of lenalidomide and ixazomib

Neutropenia (ANC <500/mm³): Withhold ixazomib and lenalidomide until ANC is ≥500/mm³. Consider adding G-CSF as per guidelines. Following recovery, resume lenalidomide at the next lower dose and resume ixazomib at its most recent dose. If ANC falls to <500/mm³ again, withhold ixazomib and lenalidomide until ANC is at least 500/mm³; following recovery, resume ixazomib at the next lower dose and resume lenalidomide at its most recent dose. For additional occurrences, alternate dose modification of lenalidomide and ixazomib

Non-Hematological Toxicities:
Rash:
Grade 2 or 3: Withhold lenalidomide until rash recovers to ≤Grade 1; following recovery, resume lenalidomide at the next lower dose. If Grade 2 or 3 rash occurs again, withhold ixazomib and lenalidomide until rash recovers to ≤Grade 1; following recovery, resume ixazomib at the next lower dose and resume lenalidomide at its most recent dose. For additional occurrences, alternate dose modification of lenalidomide and ixazomib
Grade 4: D/C treatment regimen

Peripheral Neuropathy:
Grade 1 Peripheral Neuropathy w/ Pain or Grade 2 Peripheral Neuropathy: Withhold ixazomib until peripheral neuropathy recovers to ≤Grade 1 w/o pain or patient's baseline; following recovery, resume ixazomib at its most recent dose
Grade 2 Peripheral Neuropathy w/ Pain or Grade 3 Peripheral Neuropathy: Withhold ixazomib. Toxicities should generally recover to baseline condition or ≤Grade 1 prior to resuming; following recovery, resume ixazomib at the next lower dose
Grade 4 Peripheral Neuropathy: D/C treatment regimen

Other Non-Hematological Toxicities:
Other Grade 3 or 4 Non-Hematological Toxicities: Withhold ixazomib. Toxicities should generally recover to baseline condition or ≤Grade 1 prior to resuming; if attributable to ixazomib, resume at the next lower dose following recovery

Refer to the individual monographs for lenalidomide and dexamethasone for additional information

ADMINISTRATION
Oral route

Take once a week on the same day and at approx the same time for the first 3 weeks of a 4-week cycle.
Take at least 1 hr ac or at least 2 hrs pc.
Swallow whole w/ water; do not crush, chew, or open.

STORAGE
Room temperature. Do not store >30°C (86°F). Do not freeze. Store in original packaging until immediately prior to use.

HOW SUPPLIED
Cap: 2.3mg, 3mg, 4mg

WARNINGS/PRECAUTIONS
See Dosing Considerations. Thrombocytopenia reported; platelet nadirs typically occurring between Days 14-21 of each 28-day cycle and recovery to baseline by the start of the next cycle. Monitor platelet counts at least monthly during treatment; consider more frequent monitoring during the first three cycles. Rash, peripheral edema, diarrhea, constipation, and N/V reported. Peripheral neuropathy reported; monitor for symptoms of neuropathy. Drug-induced liver injury, hepatocellular injury, hepatic steatosis, hepatitis cholestatic, and hepatotoxicity

reported; monitor hepatic enzymes regularly and adjust dosing for Grade 3 or 4 symptoms. May cause fetal harm.

ADVERSE REACTIONS
Diarrhea, constipation, thrombocytopenia, peripheral neuropathy, N/V, peripheral edema, back pain.

DRUG INTERACTIONS
Avoid w/ strong CYP3A inducers (eg, rifampin, phenytoin, carbamazepine).

PREGNANCY AND LACTATION
Pregnancy: Avoid becoming pregnant while on therapy. May cause fetal harm.
Lactation: It is not known whether ixazomib or its metabolites are present in human milk; not for use in nursing.
Reproductive Potential: Males/females of childbearing potential must use effective contraception during and for 90 days following treatment.

MECHANISM OF ACTION
Reversible proteasome inhibitor; preferentially binds and inhibits the chymotrypsin-like activity of the beta 5 subunit of the 20S proteasome. Induces apoptosis of multiple myeloma cell lines and demonstrates in vitro cytotoxicity against myeloma cells from patients who had relapsed after multiple prior therapies. Combination of ixazomib/lenalidomide demonstrated synergistic cytotoxic effects in multiple myeloma cell lines.

PHARMACOKINETICS
Absorption: Absolute bioavailability (58%). T_{max}=1 hr (median). **Distribution:** V_d=543L; plasma protein binding (99%). **Metabolism:** Multiple CYP enzymes and non-CYP proteins (major). **Elimination:** $T_{1/2}$=9.5 days. Urine (62%, <3.5% unchanged), feces (22%).

PATIENT CONSIDERATIONS
Assessment: Assess for hypersensitivity to drug, preexisting renal or hepatic dysfunction, and pregnancy/nursing status. Obtain baseline platelet counts and ANC and assess non-hematologic toxicities.

Monitoring: Monitor platelet counts at least monthly during treatment; consider more frequent monitoring during the first three cycles. Monitor hepatic enzymes regularly. Monitor for signs/symptoms of neuropathy, edema, cutaneous reaction, and other adverse reactions. Monitor ANC, platelet counts, and non-hematologic toxicities before each new cycle of therapy. Monitor pregnancy status for females of reproductive potential.

Counseling: Instruct to take ud. Advise that ixazomib and dexamethasone should not be taken at the same time, because dexamethasone should be taken w/ food. Inform that direct contact w/ the cap contents should be avoided and instruct to avoid direct contact of cap contents w/ the skin or eyes, in case of cap breakage. If contact occurs w/ the skin, advise to wash thoroughly w/ soap and water; if contact occurs w/ the eyes, instruct to flush thoroughly w/ water. Advise to store caps in original packaging, and not to remove the cap from the packaging until just prior to administration. Advise patient that they may experience low platelet counts, diarrhea, constipation, N/V, new or worsening symptoms of peripheral neuropathy, unusual swelling of their extremities or weight gain due to swelling, new or worsening rash, jaundice, or right upper quadrant abdominal pain; advise to report any related symptoms to physician. Advise women of the potential risk to a fetus and to avoid becoming pregnant while on treatment and for 90 days following final dose; advise to contact physician immediately if patient becomes pregnant during treatment or w/in 90 days of the final dose. Advise to inform physician about other medications currently being taken and before starting any new medications.

NIPENT — pentostatin   Rx
Class: Adenosine deaminase (ADA) inhibitor

> Should be administered under the supervision of a physician qualified and experienced in the use of cancer chemotherapeutic agents. Higher doses than specified is not recommended; dose-limiting severe renal, liver, pulmonary, and CNS toxicities reported at higher doses (20-50mg/m² in divided doses over 5 days) than recommended. Use in combination with fludarabine phosphate is not recommended; severe or fatal pulmonary toxicity may occur.

ADULT DOSAGE
Untreated and α-Interferon-Refractory Hairy Cell Leukemia (HCL)
Hydrate with 500-1000mL of D5W in 0.5 normal saline or equivalent before drug administration and administer additional 500mL of D5W or equivalent after the drug is given

Usual: 4mg/m² every other week as IV bolus or infusion over 20-30 min

Give 2 additional doses after complete response is achieved
Assess for response in patients receiving treatment at 6 months; d/c if complete/partial response is not achieved
If partial response is achieved, continue treatment to achieve complete response; d/c if best response at the end of 12 months is a partial response
May need to withhold or d/c individual doses when severe adverse reactions occur

PEDIATRIC DOSAGE
Pediatric use may not have been established

ADMINISTRATION
IV route

Refer to PI for preparation of sol

STORAGE
2-8°C (36-46°F). Reconstituted/Further Diluted Vials: Room temperature and ambient light. Use within 8 hrs.

HOW SUPPLIED
Inj: 10mg

CONTRAINDICATIONS
Hypersensitivity to pentostatin.

WARNINGS/PRECAUTIONS
Myelosuppression may occur primarily during the 1st few courses of treatment. Worsening of infection leading to death reported; control the infection before treatment is initiated or resumed. Initial courses of treatment associated with worsening of neutropenia in patients with progressive HCL; frequently monitor CBC during this time. If severe neutropenia continues beyond initial cycles, evaluate disease status, including bone marrow examination. LFTs and SrCr elevations reported; withhold dose and determine CrCl in patients with elevated SrCr. Rashes, occasionally severe, reported and may worsen with continued treatment; withholding of treatment may be required. Withhold or d/c with evidence of nervous system toxicity. Temporarily withhold treatment if absolute neutrophil count falls to <200 cells/mm^3 in a patient who had an initial neutrophil count >500 cells/mm^3; may resume when the count returns to predose levels. May cause fetal harm. Treat patients with infection or renal impairment only when potential benefit of treatment justifies the potential risk.

ADVERSE REACTIONS
N/V, fever, rash, fatigue, leukopenia, pruritus, cough, myalgia, chills, headache, diarrhea, abdominal pain, anorexia, upper respiratory infection.

DRUG INTERACTIONS
See Boxed Warning. Acute pulmonary edema and hypotension, leading to death, reported when used in combination with carmustine, etoposide, and high dose cyclophosphamide as part of ablative regimen for bone marrow transplant. Hypersensitivity vasculitis that resulted in death reported with concomitant allopurinol. May enhance effects of vidarabine; combined use may increase adverse reactions associated with each drug.

PREGNANCY AND LACTATION
Category D, not for use in nursing.

MECHANISM OF ACTION
Adenosine deaminase inhibitor; has not been established. Elevates intracellular levels of dATP which can block DNA synthesis through inhibition of ribonucleotide reductase. Also, inhibits RNA synthesis and causes increased DNA damage.

PHARMACOKINETICS
Distribution: Plasma protein binding (4%). **Elimination:** Urine (90%); $T_{1/2}$=5.7 hrs.

PATIENT CONSIDERATIONS
Assessment: Assess for hypersensitivity to the drug, infection, pregnancy/nursing status, and possible drug interactions. Obtain CBC and SrCr before each dose and at other appropriate periods during therapy.

Monitoring: Monitor for myelosuppression, worsening of infection/neutropenia, LFTs/SrCr elevations, rashes, nervous system toxicity, and other adverse reactions. Monitor hematologic parameters and blood chemistry values. Perform periodic monitoring of the peripheral blood for hairy cells to assess response to treatment. Bone marrow aspirates and biopsies may be required at 2- to 3-month intervals to assess response to treatment.

Counseling: Inform of signs and symptoms of adverse events associated with therapy. Advise women of childbearing potential to avoid becoming pregnant during therapy.

NITRO-DUR — nitroglycerin   Rx
Class: Nitrate vasodilator

OTHER BRAND NAMES
Minitran

ADULT DOSAGE	PEDIATRIC DOSAGE
Angina Pectoris	Pediatric use may not have been established
Prevention:	
Initial: 0.2-0.4mg/hr patch for 12-14 hrs/day, remove patch for 10-12 hrs/day	

DOSING CONSIDERATIONS
Elderly

Start at lower end of dosing range

ADMINISTRATION
Transdermal route

STORAGE
25°C (77°F); excursions permitted to 15-30°C (59-86°F). Do not refrigerate.

HOW SUPPLIED
Patch: 0.1mg/hr, 0.2mg/hr, 0.3mg/hr, 0.4mg/hr, 0.6mg/hr, 0.8mg/hr [30^s]; (Minitran) 0.1mg/hr, 0.2mg/hr, 0.4mg/hr, 0.6mg/hr [30^s]

CONTRAINDICATIONS
Allergy to nitroglycerin or the adhesives used in the patches, concomitant use w/ phosphodiesterase inhibitors (eg, sildenafil, tadalafil, vardenafil) for erectile dysfunction or pulmonary arterial HTN, or the soluble guanylate cyclase stimulator riociguat.

WARNINGS/PRECAUTIONS
Use careful clinical or hemodynamic monitoring to avoid the hazards of hypotension and tachycardia if treating patients w/ acute MI or CHF. Do not discharge a cardioverter/defibrillator through a paddle electrode that overlies the patch; the arcing that may be seen in this situation is harmless in itself, but it may be associated w/ local current concentration that can cause damage to the paddles and burns to the patient. Severe hypotension, particularly w/ upright posture, may occur w/ even small doses, particularly in elderly; caution in elderly patients w/ volume depletion, hypotension, or on multiple medications. Nitroglycerin-induced hypotension may be accompanied by paradoxical bradycardia and increased angina pectoris. May aggravate the angina caused by hypertrophic cardiomyopathy, particularly in elderly. Tolerance and physical dependence may occur.

ADVERSE REACTIONS
Headache, lightheadedness, hypotension, syncope.

DRUG INTERACTIONS
See Contraindications. Vasodilating effects may be additive w/ those of other vasodilators (eg, alcohol).

PREGNANCY AND LACTATION
Category C, caution in nursing.

MECHANISM OF ACTION
Nitrate vasodilator; relaxes vascular smooth muscle and consequently dilates peripheral arteries and veins, especially the latter.

PHARMACOKINETICS
Distribution: V_d=3L/kg. **Metabolism:** Inorganic nitrate and 1,2- and 1,3-dinitroglycerols (metabolites). **Elimination:** $T_{1/2}$=3 min.

PATIENT CONSIDERATIONS
Assessment: Assess for hypersensitivity to drug, acute MI, CHF, volume depletion, hypotension, angina caused by hypertrophic cardiomyopathy, pregnancy/nursing status, and possible drug interactions.

Monitoring: Monitor for hypotension, paradoxical bradycardia, increased/aggravated angina pectoris, tolerance, physical dependence, and other adverse reactions. Perform careful clinical or hemodynamic monitoring in patients w/ acute MI or CHF.

Counseling: Inform that daily headaches sometimes accompany treatment and that the headaches may be a marker of the activity of the drug; advise to resist the temptation to avoid headaches by altering the schedule of treatment, since loss of headache may be associated w/ simultaneous loss of antianginal efficacy. Inform that therapy may be associated w/ lightheadedness on standing, especially just after rising from a recumbent or seated position; counsel that lightheadedness may be more frequent in patients who have consumed alcohol. Instruct to properly discard patches.

NITROMIST — nitroglycerin   Rx
Class: Nitrate vasodilator

ADULT DOSAGE	PEDIATRIC DOSAGE
Angina Pectoris	Pediatric use may not have been established
Acute Relief:	
1 or 2 sprays at the onset of attack onto or under the tongue; may repeat every 5 min prn.	
If 2 sprays are used initially, may only administer 1 more spray after 5 min.	
Max: 3 sprays/15 min.	
If chest pain persists after a total of 3 sprays, prompt medical attention is recommended.	
Prophylaxis:	
May be used 5-10 min before engaging in activities that might precipitate an acute attack.	

DOSING CONSIDERATIONS
Elderly

Start at lower end of dosing range

ADMINISTRATION
Sublingual route

Do not inhale.

Do not shake.

Do not expectorate medication or rinse mouth for 5-10 min after administration.

Priming Instructions
Spray 10X to prime initially; will remain adequately primed for 6 weeks.

Re-prime w/ 2 sprays if product is not used w/in 6 weeks.

Refer to PI for further administration instructions.

STORAGE
25°C (77°F); excursions permitted to 15-30°C (59-85°F).

HOW SUPPLIED
Spray: 400mcg/spray [90 metered sprays, 230 metered sprays]

CONTRAINDICATIONS
Concomitant use w/ selective inhibitor of cyclic guanosine monophosphate-specific PDE-5 inhibitors (eg, sildenafil, vardenafil, tadalafil) or to the soluble guanylate cyclase stimulator riociguat. Severe anemia, increased intracranial pressure (ICP), hypersensitivity to nitroglycerin or to other nitrates or nitrites.

WARNINGS/PRECAUTIONS
Excessive use may lead to tolerance; use only the smallest doses required for effective relief of the acute anginal attack. Severe hypotension may occur; caution w/ volume depleted patients or who are already hypotensive. Hypotension induced by nitroglycerin may be accompanied by paradoxical bradycardia and increased angina pectoris. Use careful clinical or hemodynamic monitoring in patients w/ acute MI or CHF. May aggravate angina caused by hypertrophic cardiomyopathy. Produces dose-related headaches, which may be severe; tolerance to headaches occurs. Caution in elderly.

ADVERSE REACTIONS
Headache, flushing, hypotension, syncope.

DRUG INTERACTIONS
See Contraindications. Possible additive hypotensive effects w/ antihypertensive and β-adrenergic blockers (eg, labetalol). Marked orthostatic hypotension reported w/ calcium channel blockers. Aspirin (ASA) may increase nitroglycerin maximum concentrations. Vasodilatory and hemodynamic effects of nitroglycerin may be enhanced w/ ASA. Caution during tissue-type plasminogen activator therapy. IV nitroglycerin reduces the anticoagulant effect of heparin; monitor activated PTT. Avoid concomitant use of ergotamine and related drugs; monitor for symptoms of ergotism when coadministered.

PREGNANCY AND LACTATION
Pregnancy: Category C.
Lactation: Caution in nursing.

MECHANISM OF ACTION
Nitrate vasodilator; relaxes vascular smooth muscle. Forms free radical nitric oxide, which activates guanylate cyclase, resulting in an increase of guanosine 3',5'-monophosphate in smooth muscle and other tissues, eventually leading to dephosphorylation of myosin light chains, which regulates the contractile state in smooth muscle and results in vasodilation.

PHARMACOKINETICS
Absorption: Rapid. (Healthy) C_{max}=0.8ng/mL (trinitroglycerin), 3.7ng/mL (1,2-dinitroglycerin), 1ng/mL (1,3-dinitroglycerin); T_{max}=8 min (trinitroglycerin), 34 min (1,2-dinitroglycerin), 41 min (1,3-dinitroglycerin). **Distribution:** (IV) V_d=3.3L/kg. **Metabolism:** Liver via reductase enzyme to glycerol di- and mononitrate metabolites and to glycerol and organic nitrates; 1,2- and 1,3-dinitroglycerin (major metabolites). **Elimination:** $T_{1/2}$=40 min (major metabolites).

PATIENT CONSIDERATIONS
Assessment: Assess for severe anemia, increased ICP, volume-depletion, hypotension, angina caused by hypertrophic cardiomyopathy, drug hypersensitivity, pregnancy/nursing status, and possible drug interactions.

Monitoring: Monitor for severe hypotension, paradoxical bradycardia, increased angina pectoris, tolerance, headache, and other adverse reactions. Perform clinical or hemodynamic monitoring in patients w/ acute MI or CHF.

Counseling: Inform about the risks and benefits of therapy. Instruct to use ud and not to use w/ certain medications for erectile dysfunction (PDE-5 inhibitors) because of the risk of hypotension. Instruct to familiarize w/ the position of the spray orifice to facilitate orientation for administration at night. Advise that headache, flushing, drug rash, and exfoliative dermatitis may occur. Inform that consuming alcohol may increase the risk of hypotension. Instruct not to forcefully open the bottle. Advise not to burn the container after use and not to spray directly towards flames.

NITROPRESS — sodium nitroprusside   Rx

Class: Vasodilator

> Not suitable for direct inj; dilute in sterile D5 inj before infusion. May cause precipitous decreases in BP; may lead to irreversible ischemic injuries or death if not monitored properly. Use only when available equipment and personnel allow BP to be continuously monitored. Except when used briefly or at low (<2mcg/kg/min) infusion rates, nitroprusside gives rise to important quantities of cyanide ion, which can reach toxic, potentially lethal levels. The usual dose rate is 0.5-10mcg/kg/min, but infusion at the max dose rate should never last >10 min; d/c immediately if BP has not been controlled by max rate after 10 min. Although acid-base balance and venous oxygen concentration should be monitored and may indicate cyanide toxicity, these tests provide imperfect guidance.

ADULT DOSAGE
Hypertensive Crisis

Initial: 0.3mcg/kg/min IV
Titrate: May increase every few min until the desired effect is achieved or the max infusion rate has been reached
Max: 10mcg/kg/min IV

Dosing varies by weight; refer to PI for infusion rates to achieve initial and maximal dosing of therapy

Surgical Bleeding

For producing controlled hypotension to reduce bleeding during surgery

PEDIATRIC DOSAGE
Hypertensive Crisis

Initial: 0.3mcg/kg/min IV
Titrate: May increase every few min until the desired effect is achieved or the max infusion rate has been reached
Max: 10mcg/kg/min IV

Dosing varies by weight; refer to PI for infusion rates to achieve initial and maximal dosing of therapy

Surgical Bleeding

For producing controlled hypotension to reduce bleeding during surgery

Initial: 0.3mcg/kg/min IV
Titrate: May increase every few min until the desired effect is achieved or the max infusion rate has been reached
Max: 10mcg/kg/min IV

Dosing varies by weight; refer to PI for infusion rates to achieve initial and maximal dosing of therapy

Acute Congestive Heart Failure
Titration of the infusion rate must be guided by the results of invasive hemodynamic monitoring w/ simultaneous monitoring of urine output

Initial: 0.3mcg/kg/min IV
Titrate: May increase every few min until the desired effect is achieved or the max infusion rate has been reached
Max: 10mcg/kg/min IV

Dosing varies by weight; refer to PI for infusion rates to achieve initial and maximal dosing of therapy

Initial: 0.3mcg/kg/min IV
Titrate: May increase every few min until the desired effect is achieved or the max infusion rate has been reached
Max: 10mcg/kg/min IV

Dosing varies by weight; refer to PI for infusion rates to achieve initial and maximal dosing of therapy

Acute Congestive Heart Failure
Titration of the infusion rate must be guided by the results of invasive hemodynamic monitoring w/ simultaneous monitoring of urine output

Initial: 0.3mcg/kg/min IV
Titrate: May increase every few min until the desired effect is achieved or the max infusion rate has been reached
Max: 10mcg/kg/min IV

Dosing varies by weight; refer to PI for infusion rates to achieve initial and maximal dosing of therapy

---

ADMINISTRATION
IV route

Dilute sol in 250-1000mL of sterile D5 inj, depending on the desired concentration
Do not administer other drugs in the same sol
Do not use flexible container in series connections
Do not infuse through ordinary IV apparatus, regulated only by gravity and mechanical clamps; use only an infusion pump, preferably a volumetric pump
Refer to PI for further administration instructions

STORAGE
20-25°C (68-77°F). Store in carton until used, to protect from light. Freshly diluted sol is stable for 24 hrs if properly protected from light.

HOW SUPPLIED
Inj: 25mg/mL [2mL]

CONTRAINDICATIONS
Compensatory HTN where the primary hemodynamic lesion is aortic coarctation or arteriovenous shunting, known inadequate cerebral circulation, moribund patients (A.S.A. Class 5E) coming to emergency surgery, congenital (Leber's) optic atrophy, tobacco amblyopia, acute CHF associated with reduced peripheral vascular resistance.

WARNINGS/PRECAUTIONS
Administer concomitant longer-acting antihypertensives to minimize duration of treatment. Drug-induced hypotension will be self-limited within 1-10 min after discontinuation; if hypotension persists more than a few min after discontinuation, therapy is not the cause, and the true cause must be sought. Hypertensive patients and patients concomitantly receiving other antihypertensives may be more sensitive to therapy. May increase intracranial pressure (ICP). May diminish patient's capacity to compensate for anemia and hypovolemia if used for controlled hypotension during anesthesia; correct preexisting anemia and hypovolemia prior to therapy. Hypotensive anesthetic techniques may cause abnormalities of pulmonary ventilation/perfusion ratio; may require higher fraction of inspired oxygen in patients intolerant of these abnormalities. Caution in patients who are especially poor surgical risks (A.S.A. Class 4 and 4E). Caution with hepatic insufficiency and in elderly.

ADVERSE REACTIONS
Excessive hypotension, cyanide toxicity, methemoglobinemia.

DRUG INTERACTIONS
May increase hypotensive effect with other hypotensive drugs (eg, ganglionic blocking agents, negative inotropic agents, inhaled anesthetics) and sodium thiosulfate.

PREGNANCY AND LACTATION
Category C, not for use in nursing.

MECHANISM OF ACTION
Vasodilator; relaxes vascular smooth muscle and dilates peripheral arteries, veins, and coronary arteries.

PHARMACOKINETICS
Metabolism: Converts to cyanmethemoglobin and cyanide ions. **Elimination:** Urine (as thiocyanate); $T_{1/2}$=2 min (nitroprusside); 3 days (thiocyanate).

PATIENT CONSIDERATIONS
Assessment: Assess for conditions where drug is contraindicated, hepatic insufficiency, pregnancy/nursing status, hypovolemia, anemia, and possible drug interactions.

Monitoring: Monitor for abnormalities of pulmonary ventilation/perfusion ratio, increased ICP, hepatic/renal dysfunction, and other adverse reactions. Monitor acid-base balance, venous oxygen concentration, BP, urine output, and cyanide/thiocyanate levels.

Counseling: Inform about risks/benefits of therapy. Instruct to notify physician if any signs of adverse reactions develop.

NITROSTAT — nitroglycerin   Rx

Class: Nitrate vasodilator

ADULT DOSAGE

Angina Pectoris

Acute Relief:
1 tab SL or in the buccal pouch at the 1st sign of an acute attack
May repeat approx every 5 min until relief is obtained
If pain persists after a total of 3 tabs in 15 min, or if pain is different than is typically experienced, prompt medical attention is recommended

Acute Prophylaxis:
May be used 5-10 min prior to engaging in activities that might precipitate an acute attack

PEDIATRIC DOSAGE
Pediatric use may not have been established

DOSING CONSIDERATIONS
Elderly
Start at lower end of dosing range

ADMINISTRATION
SL or buccal route

Dissolve under tongue or in buccal pouch; do not chew, crush, or swallow tabs
During administration the patient should rest, preferably in the sitting position

STORAGE
20-25°C (68-77°F).

HOW SUPPLIED
Tab, SL: 0.3mg, 0.4mg, 0.6mg

CONTRAINDICATIONS
Early MI, severe anemia, increased intracranial pressure (ICP), patients who are using a PDE-5 inhibitor (eg, sildenafil citrate, tadalafil, vardenafil hydrochloride), known hypersensitivity to nitroglycerin.

WARNINGS/PRECAUTIONS
Use careful clinical or hemodynamic monitoring in patients with acute MI (AMI) or CHF. Excessive use may lead to tolerance; use only the smallest dose required for effective relief of the acute anginal attack. Severe hypotension, particularly with upright posture, may occur with small doses; caution with volume depletion or hypotension. Nitroglycerin-induced hypotension may be accompanied by paradoxical bradycardia and increased angina pectoris. May aggravate angina caused by hypertrophic cardiomyopathy. As tolerance to other forms of nitroglycerin develops, effect on exercise tolerance is blunted. Physical dependence may occur. D/C if blurring of vision or drying of the mouth occurs. Excessive dosage may produce severe headaches. Lab test interactions may occur. Caution in elderly.

ADVERSE REACTIONS
Headache, vertigo, dizziness, weakness, palpitation, N/V, diaphoresis, pallor, collapse/syncope, flushing, drug rash, exfoliative dermatitis.

DRUG INTERACTIONS
See Contraindications. Hypotension may occur with alcohol. Enhanced vasodilatory and hemodynamic effects with ASA. Caution with alteplase therapy. IV nitroglycerin reduces the anticoagulant effect of heparin. TCAs (eg, amitriptyline, desipramine, doxepin) and anticholinergics may make SL tab dissolution difficult. Avoid ergotamine and related drugs or monitor for ergotism symptoms if unavoidable. Long-acting nitrates may decrease therapeutic effect.

PREGNANCY AND LACTATION
Category B, caution in nursing.

MECHANISM OF ACTION
Nitrate vasodilator; forms free radical nitric oxide, which activates guanylate cyclase, resulting in an increase of cGMP in smooth muscle and other tissues, leading to dephosphorylation of myosin light chains, which regulate the contractile state in smooth muscle and result in vasodilatation.

PHARMACOKINETICS
Absorption: Rapid. Absolute bioavailability (40%). (0.3mg x 2 doses) C_{max}=2.3ng/mL; T_{max}=6.4 min; AUC=14.9ng•mL/min. (0.6mg x 1 dose) C_{max}=2.1ng/mL; T_{max}=7.2 min; AUC=14.9ng•mL/min. **Distribution:** (IV) V_d=3.3L/kg; plasma protein binding (60%, 60% [1,2-dinitroglycerin], 30% [1,3-dinitroglycerin]). **Metabolism:** Liver via reductase enzyme to glycerol di- and mononitrate metabolites and to glycerol and organic nitrate; 1,2- and 1,3-dinitroglycerin (active metabolites). **Elimination:** $T_{1/2}$=2.8 min (0.3mg x 2 doses), 2.6 min (0.6mg x 1 dose).

PATIENT CONSIDERATIONS

Assessment: Assess for early MI, severe anemia, increased ICP, AMI, CHF, volume depletion, hypotension, angina caused by hypertrophic cardiomyopathy, drug hypersensitivity, pregnancy/nursing status, and possible drug interactions.

Monitoring: Monitor for hypotension, paradoxical bradycardia, increased/aggravated angina pectoris, tolerance, physical dependence, blurring of vision, drying of mouth, headache, and other adverse reactions. Perform careful clinical or hemodynamic monitoring in patients with AMI or CHF.

Counseling: Counsel on the proper dosage and administration of the drug. Advise to sit down when taking the drug and to use caution when returning to standing position. Inform about side effects of the drug (eg, burning or tingling sensation when administered SL, headaches, lightheadedness upon standing). Counsel that lightheadedness may be more frequent in patients who have consumed alcohol.

Instruct to keep in original glass container and to tightly cap after each use to prevent loss of potency.

NIZATIDINE — nizatidine   Rx

Class: H_2 blocker

OTHER BRAND NAMES
Axid

ADULT DOSAGE
Duodenal Ulcers

Treatment of Active Ulcer:
300mg qhs or 150mg bid up to 8 weeks

Maint of Healed Ulcer:
150mg qhs

Gastroesophageal Reflux Disease

Treatment of Endoscopically Diagnosed Esophagitis (Including Erosive and Ulcerative Esophagitis) and Associated Heartburn Due to GERD:
150mg bid up to 12 weeks

Gastric Ulcers

Treatment of Active Benign Ulcer:
300mg qhs or 150mg bid up to 8 weeks

PEDIATRIC DOSAGE
Gastroesophageal Reflux Disease

Treatment of Endoscopically Diagnosed Esophagitis (Including Erosive and Ulcerative Esophagitis) and Associated Heartburn Due to GERD:
≥12 Years:
Sol:
150mg (2 tsp) bid up to 8 weeks
Max: 300mg/day

DOSING CONSIDERATIONS
Renal Impairment
Active Duodenal Ulcer, GERD, and Benign Gastric Ulcer:
CrCl 20-50mL/min: 150mg/day
CrCl <20mL/min: 150mg qod

Maint Therapy:
CrCl 20-50mL/min: 150mg qod
CrCl <20mL/min: 150mg every 3 days

ADMINISTRATION
Oral route

In adults, sol may be substituted for any of the indications using equivalent doses of sol

STORAGE
Cap: 20-25°C (68-77°F). Sol: 25°C (77°F); excursions permitted to 15-30°C (59-86°F).

HOW SUPPLIED
Cap: 150mg, 300mg; **Sol:** (Axid) 15mg/mL [480mL]

CONTRAINDICATIONS
Known hypersensitivity to the drug, history of hypersensitivity to other H_2 receptor antagonists.

WARNINGS/PRECAUTIONS
Caution with moderate to severe renal insufficiency; reduce dose. Symptomatic response does not preclude the presence of gastric malignancy. False positive tests for urobilinogen with Multistix may occur. Caution in elderly.

ADVERSE REACTIONS
Headache, abdominal pain, pain, asthenia, diarrhea, N/V, flatulence, dyspepsia, rhinitis, pharyngitis, dizziness, cough, fever, irritability.

DRUG INTERACTIONS
May elevate serum salicylate levels with high dose (3900mg/day) aspirin. Inhibits gastric acid secretion stimulated by caffeine, betazole, and pentagastrin. May decrease absorption with antacids consisting of aluminum and magnesium hydroxides with simethicone. Fatal thrombocytopenia reported with concomitant use of another H_2-receptor antagonist.

PREGNANCY AND LACTATION
Category B, not for use in nursing.

MECHANISM OF ACTION
H_2-receptor antagonist; competitive, reversible inhibitor of histamine at the histamine H_2-receptors, particularly those in the gastric parietal cells.

PHARMACOKINETICS
Absorption: Absolute bioavailability (>70%); C_{max}=700-1800mcg/L (150mg dose), 1400-3600mcg/L (300mg dose); T_{max}=0.5-3 hrs. **Distribution:** V_d=0.8-1.5L/kg; plasma protein binding (35%); found in breast milk. **Metabolism:** N2-monodesmethylnizatidine (principal metabolite). **Elimination:** Urine (>90%, 60% unchanged); feces (<6%); $T_{1/2}$=1-2 hrs, 3.5-11 hrs.

PATIENT CONSIDERATIONS

Assessment: Assess for hypersensitivity to other H_2-receptor antagonists, renal dysfunction, presence of gastric malignancy, pregnancy/nursing status, and possible drug interactions.

Monitoring: Monitor for hypersensitivity, other adverse reactions, and signs of clinical improvement.

Counseling: Inform of the risks/benefits of therapy. Advise to take medication exactly as prescribed. Instruct to contact physician if signs/symptoms of hypersensitivity or other adverse reaction develops. Counsel pregnant/nursing females about risks of use.

NORCO — acetaminophen/hydrocodone bitartrate   CII

Class: Opioid analgesic

> Associated w/ cases of acute liver failure, at times resulting in liver transplant and death. Most cases of liver injury are associated w/ APAP use at doses >4000mg/day, and often involve >1 APAP-containing product.

ADULT DOSAGE
Moderate to Moderately Severe Pain
5mg/325mg:
Usual: 1 or 2 tabs q4-6h prn
Max: 8 tabs/day

7.5mg/325mg, 10mg/325mg:
Usual: 1 tab q4-6h prn
Max: 6 tabs/day

PEDIATRIC DOSAGE
Pediatric use may not have been established

DOSING CONSIDERATIONS
Elderly
Start at lower end of dosing range

ADMINISTRATION
Oral route

STORAGE
(5mg-325mg) 15-30°C (59-86°F). (7.5mg-325mg, 10mg-325mg) 20-25°C (68-77°F).

HOW SUPPLIED
Tab: (Hydrocodone/APAP) 5mg/325mg*, 7.5mg/325mg*, 10mg/325mg* *scored

CONTRAINDICATIONS
Hypersensitivity to hydrocodone or acetaminophen.

WARNINGS/PRECAUTIONS
Increased risk of acute liver failure in patients w/ underlying liver disease. May cause serious skin reactions (eg, acute generalized exanthematous pustulosis, Stevens-Johnson syndrome, toxic epidermal necrolysis); d/c at the 1st appearance of skin rash or any other sign of hypersensitivity. Hypersensitivity and anaphylaxis reported; d/c immediately if signs/symptoms occur. May produce dose-related respiratory depression and irregular/periodic breathing. Respiratory depressant effects and CSF pressure elevation capacity may be markedly exaggerated in the presence of head injury, other intracranial lesions, or a preexisting increase in intracranial pressure. May obscure clinical course of head injuries and acute abdominal conditions. Caution w/ hypothyroidism, Addison's disease, prostatic hypertrophy, urethral stricture, severe hepatic/renal impairment, or in elderly/debilitated. Suppresses cough reflex; caution w/ pulmonary disease and in postoperative use. Lab test interactions may occur. May be habit-forming.

ADVERSE REACTIONS
Acute liver failure, lightheadedness, dizziness, sedation, N/V.

DRUG INTERACTIONS
Increased risk of acute liver failure w/ alcohol. Additive CNS depression w/ other narcotics, antihistamines, antipsychotics, antianxiety agents, or other CNS depressants (eg, alcohol); reduce dose of one or both agents. Concomitant use w/ MAOIs or TCAs may increase the effect of either the antidepressant or hydrocodone.

PREGNANCY AND LACTATION
Category C, not for use in nursing.

MECHANISM OF ACTION
Hydrocodone: Opioid analgesic and antitussive; has not been established. Action believed to be related to the existence of opiate receptors in the CNS. APAP: Nonopiate, nonsalicylate analgesic, and antipyretic; has not been established. Antipyretic activity is mediated through hypothalamic heat-regulating centers; inhibits prostaglandin synthetase.

PHARMACOKINETICS
Absorption: Hydrocodone: (10mg) C_{max}=23.6ng/mL; T_{max}=1.3 hrs. APAP: Rapid. **Distribution:** APAP: Found in breast milk. **Metabolism:** Hydrocodone: O-demethylation, N-demethylation, and 6-keto reduction. APAP: Liver (conjugation). **Elimination:** Hydrocodone: (10mg) $T_{1/2}$=3.8 hrs. APAP: Urine (85%, mostly glucuronide conjugate); $T_{1/2}$=1.25-3 hrs.

PATIENT CONSIDERATIONS
Assessment: Assess for history of hypersensitivity to drug, level of pain intensity, type of pain, patient's general condition and medical status, renal/hepatic impairment, pregnancy/nursing status, any other conditions where treatment is cautioned, and possible drug interactions.

Monitoring: Monitor for signs/symptoms of hypersensitivity or anaphylaxis, serious skin reactions, acute liver failure, respiratory depression, elevations in CSF pressure, drug abuse/dependence/tolerance, and other adverse reactions. In patients w/ severe hepatic/renal disease, monitor effects w/ serial hepatic and/or renal function tests.

Counseling: Instruct to look for APAP on package labels and not to use >1 APAP-containing product. Instruct to seek medical attention immediately upon ingestion of >4000mg/day of APAP, even if feeling well. Advise to d/c use and contact physician immediately if signs of allergy develop. Inform about signs of serious skin reactions. Inform that drug may impair mental/physical abilities, and to use caution if performing potentially hazardous tasks (eg, driving, operating machinery). Instruct to avoid alcohol and other CNS depressants. Inform that drug may be habit-forming; instruct to take only ud.

NORDITROPIN — somatropin (rDNA origin)   Rx

Class: Recombinant human growth hormone (hGH)

ADULT DOSAGE
Growth Hormone Deficiency
Replacement of Endogenous Growth Hormone in Patients w/ Adult-Onset or Childhood-Onset Growth Hormone Deficiency:

Weight-Based:
Initial: ≤0.004mg/kg/day SQ
Titrate: May increase to ≤0.016mg/kg/day after 6 weeks according to individual requirements

Non-Weight Based:
Initial: 0.2mg/day SQ (range, 0.15-0.30mg/day)
Titrate: May increase gradually every 1-2 months by increments of 0.1-0.2mg/day based on response and serum insulin-like growth factor-I concentrations

PEDIATRIC DOSAGE
Growth Hormone Deficiency
Growth Failure Due to Inadequate Secretion of Endogenous Growth Hormone:
0.024-0.034mg/kg/day SQ 6-7X/week

Noonan Syndrome
Short Stature Associated w/ Noonan Syndrome:
Up to 0.066mg/kg/day SQ

Turner Syndrome
Short Stature Associated w/ Turner Syndrome:
Up to 0.067mg/kg/day SQ

Small for Gestational Age
Short Stature Born Small for Gestational Age w/ No Catch-Up Growth by Age 2-4 Years:
Up to 0.067mg/kg/day SQ

DOSING CONSIDERATIONS
Elderly
Consider lower starting dose and smaller dose increments

Other Important Considerations
Estrogen-replete women may need higher doses than men

ADMINISTRATION
SQ route

Rotate inj sites to avoid lipoatrophy

STORAGE
Unused: 2-8°C (36-46°F). Do not freeze. Avoid direct light. In-use: 2-8°C (36-46°F) and use w/in 4 weeks or store at room temperature ≤25°C (77°F) for up to 3 weeks.

HOW SUPPLIED
Inj: 5mg/1.5mL, 10mg/1.5mL, 15mg/1.5mL, 30mg/3mL

CONTRAINDICATIONS
Acute critical illness due to complications following open heart surgery, abdominal surgery, multiple accidental trauma, or w/ acute respiratory failure. Pediatric patients w/ Prader-Willi syndrome (PWS) who are severely obese, have a history of upper airway obstruction or sleep apnea, or have severe respiratory impairment. Pediatric patients who have growth failure due to genetically confirmed PWS. Active malignancy or evidence of progression or recurrence of underlying intracranial tumor. Active proliferative or severe nonproliferative diabetic retinopathy. Growth promotion in pediatric patients w/ closed epiphyses. Known hypersensitivity to somatropin or any of its excipients.

WARNINGS/PRECAUTIONS
Reevaluate adults who were treated w/ somatropin for growth hormone deficiency (GHD) in childhood and whose epiphyses are closed before continuation of somatropin therapy. Treatment for short stature should be discontinued when epiphyses are fused. Implement effective weight control in patients w/ PWS and treat respiratory infections aggressively; interrupt therapy if patient shows signs of upper airway obstruction and/or new onset sleep apnea. Increased risk of a 2nd neoplasm reported in childhood cancer survivors who were treated w/ radiation to the brain/head for 1st neoplasm and who developed subsequent GHD and were treated w/ somatropin. Increased risk of developing malignancies in children w/ certain rare genetic causes of short stature; monitor for development of neoplasms if treatment is initiated. Monitor for increased growth, or potential malignant changes, of preexisting nevi. Undiagnosed impaired glucose tolerance and overt diabetes mellitus (DM) may be unmasked and new-onset type 2 DM reported. Intracranial HTN w/ papilledema, visual changes, headache, or N/V reported; d/c if papilledema is observed. If drug-induced intracranial HTN is diagnosed, may restart therapy at a lower dose after signs/symptoms resolve. Fluid retention in adults may occur. Hypothyroidism may become evident or worsen, and undiagnosed/untreated hypothyroidism may prevent optimal response. Monitor standard hormonal replacement therapy in patients w/ hypopituitarism. Slipped capital femoral epiphysis (SCFE) and progression of scoliosis may occur in pediatric patients. Increased risk of ear/hearing disorders and cardiovascular (CV) disorders in TS patients; evaluate carefully for otitis media and other ear disorders, and monitor closely for CV disorders. Tissue atrophy may occur; rotate inj site. Allergic reactions (local or systemic) may occur. Serum levels of inorganic phosphorus, alkaline phosphatase, parathyroid hormone, and insulin-like growth factor may increase. Pancreatitis reported rarely. Caution in elderly.

ADVERSE REACTIONS
Gastroenteritis, ear infection, influenza, inj-site reaction, peripheral/leg edema, arthralgia, headache, increased sweating, myalgia, bronchitis, flu-like symptoms, HTN, paresthesia, skeletal pain, laryngitis.

DRUG INTERACTIONS
Glucocorticoid therapy may attenuate growth-promoting effects in children; carefully adjust glucocorticoid replacement dosing. May inhibit 11β-hydroxysteroid

dehydrogenase type 1, resulting in reduced serum cortisol concentrations; may need glucocorticoid replacement or dose adjustments of glucocorticoid therapy. May alter clearance of compounds metabolized by CYP450 liver enzymes (eg, corticosteroids, sex steroids, anticonvulsants, cyclosporine); monitor carefully. May increase clearance of antipyrine. May require greater dose w/ oral estrogen replacement. May need to adjust dose of insulin and/or oral/injectable hypoglycemic agents, and thyroid hormone replacement therapy.

PREGNANCY AND LACTATION
Category C, caution in nursing.

MECHANISM OF ACTION
Recombinant human growth hormone (GH); binds to dimeric GH receptor in cell membrane of target cells, resulting in intracellular signal transduction.

PHARMACOKINETICS
Absorption: T_{max}=4-5 hrs; C_{max}=13.8ng/mL (4mg), 17.1ng/mL (8mg). **Elimination:** $T_{1/2}$=7-10 hrs.

PATIENT CONSIDERATIONS

Assessment: Assess for PWS, preexisting DM or impaired glucose tolerance, history of scoliosis, hypothyroidism, hypopituitarism, hypersensitivity to drug, any other conditions where treatment is contraindicated or cautioned, pregnancy/nursing status, and possible drug interactions. Perform funduscopic exam.

Monitoring: Monitor growth and for clinical response, neoplasm, increased growth or malignant changes of preexisting nevi, fluid retention, intracranial HTN, allergic reactions, pancreatitis, and SCFE and progression of scoliosis in pediatric patients (eg, onset of limp, hip or knee pain). Perform periodic thyroid function tests, funduscopic exam, and monitoring of glucose levels. In patients w/ PWS, monitor weight as well as for signs of respiratory infection, sleep apnea, and upper airway obstruction. Monitor patients routinely w/ a history of GHD secondary to an intracranial neoplasm while on therapy for progression/recurrence of tumor. In patients w/ TS, monitor for ear/CV disorders.

Counseling: Inform about potential benefits and risks of therapy, proper administration, and usage/disposal. Caution against any reuse of needles. Counsel to never share pen w/ another person, even if the needle is changed.

NORINYL 1/50 — mestranol/norethindrone   Rx
Class: Estrogen/progestogen combination

> Cigarette smoking increases the risk of serious CV side effects. Risk increases with age (>35 yrs) and with heavy smoking (≥15 cigarettes/day). Women who use oral contraceptives should be strongly advised not to smoke.

OTHER BRAND NAMES
Necon 1/50

ADULT DOSAGE
Contraception

1 tab qd for 28 days, then repeat

Start 1st Sunday after menses begin or 1st day of menses

Missed Dose

Miss 1 Active Pill: Take as soon as dose is remembered; take next pill at regular time (may take 2 pills in 1 day). No backup birth control method is needed

Miss 2 Active Pills in a Row in Week 1 or 2: Take 2 pills on day it is remembered and 2 pills the next day, then take 1 pill qd until the pack is finished

Miss 2 Active Pills in a Row in Week 3 or Miss ≥3 Active Pills in a Row During the First 3 Weeks: (Day 1 starter) Throw out rest of the pack and start new pack the same day. (Sunday starter) Continue to take 1 pill qd until Sunday, then throw out the rest of the pack and start a new pack of pills that same day

Use a backup method of birth control for 7 days if ≥2 active pills are missed

PEDIATRIC DOSAGE
Contraception

Not indicated for use premenarche; refer to adult dosing

ADMINISTRATION
Oral route

Take tabs in the order directed on the package
Sunday Starter: Use a nonhormonal contraceptive as backup during the first 7 days of initiating therapy

STORAGE
15-25°C (59-77°F) (Norinyl 1/50); 20-25°C (68-77°F) (Necon 1/50).

HOW SUPPLIED
Tab: (Mestranol/Norethindrone) 0.05mg/1mg

CONTRAINDICATIONS
Thrombophlebitis, thromboembolic disorders, history of deep vein thrombophlebitis (DVT), cerebral vascular or coronary artery disease, carcinoma of the endometrium or other known or suspected estrogen-dependent neoplasia, undiagnosed abnormal genital bleeding, cholestatic jaundice of pregnancy or jaundice with prior pill use, hepatic adenomas or carcinomas, known or suspected carcinoma of the breast, and pregnancy. (Norinyl 1/50) Benign liver tumors.

WARNINGS/PRECAUTIONS
Increased risk of myocardial infarction, vascular disease, thromboembolism, stroke, gallbladder disease, and hepatic neoplasia. Increased risk of morbidity and mortality in patients with HTN, hyperlipidemias, obesity, and diabetes. May increase risk of breast cancer and cancer of the reproductive organs. Retinal thrombosis reported; d/c if unexplained partial or complete loss of vision occurs, onset of proptosis or diplopia, papilledema, or retinal vascular lesions develop. May cause glucose intolerance; monitor prediabetic and diabetic patients. May cause fluid retention and increase BP; monitor closely and d/c if significant elevation of BP occurs. Breakthrough bleeding and spotting reported; rule out malignancy or pregnancy. May cause onset or exacerbation of a migraine or development of a headache. May develop visual changes with contact lenses. May elevate LDL levels or cause other lipid effects. D/C if jaundice develops. Caution with history of depression; d/c if depression recurs to serious degree. Not indicated for use before menarche. Does not protect against HIV infection (AIDS) and other sexually transmitted diseases (STDs). May affect certain endocrine, LFTs, and blood components in laboratory tests. Ectopic and intrauterine pregnancies may occur with contraceptive failures. Should not be used to induce withdrawal bleeding as a test for pregnancy, or to treat threatened or habitual abortion during pregnancy.

ADVERSE REACTIONS
N/V, breakthrough bleeding, spotting, amenorrhea, migraine, mental depression, vaginal candidiasis, edema, weight changes, abdominal cramps/bloating, menstrual flow changes, melasma.

DRUG INTERACTIONS
Reduced effects, increased breakthrough bleeding, and menstrual irregularities with rifampin, barbiturates, phenylbutazone, phenytoin Na+, and possibly with griseofulvin, ampicillin, tetracyclines, and (Necon 1/50) carbamazepine.

PREGNANCY AND LACTATION
Category X, not for use in nursing.

MECHANISM OF ACTION
Estrogen/progestogen oral contraceptive; suppresses gonadotropins. Primarily inhibits ovulation. Also causes changes in cervical mucus (increases difficulty of sperm entry into uterus) and endometrium (reduces likelihood of implantation).

PHARMACOKINETICS
Distribution: Found in breast milk.

PATIENT CONSIDERATIONS

Assessment: Assess for thrombophlebitis, thromboembolic disorders, history of DVT or thromboembolic disorders, any other conditions where treatment is contraindicated or cautioned. Assess for pregnancy/nursing status, and for possible drug interactions. Assess use in patients with hyperlipidemia, HTN, obesity, diabetes, history of depression, and in patients >35 yrs of age who smoke ≥15 cigarettes/day. (Norinyl 1/50) Assess for benign liver tumors.

Monitoring: Monitor for MI, thromboembolism, stroke, and other adverse effects. Monitor glucose levels in diabetic or prediabetic patients, BP with history of HTN, and lipid levels with history of hyperlipidemia. Monitor for signs of liver dysfunction (eg, jaundice), and signs of worsening depression with previous history. Refer patients with contact lenses to ophthalmologist if ocular changes develop. Perform annual physical exam while on therapy.

Counseling: Inform that therapy does not protect against HIV infection and other STDs. Inform of potential risks/benefits of oral contraceptives. When initiating treatment, instruct to use additional form of contraception until after 7 days on therapy. Instruct to take 1 pill at same time daily at intervals not exceeding 24 hrs. Inform that if dose is missed, take as soon as possible; instruct to take next dose at regularly scheduled time. Instruct to continue medication if spotting or breakthrough bleeding occurs; instruct to notify physician if symptoms persist. Inform that missing a pill can cause spotting or light bleeding. Advise not to smoke while on therapy.

NORPACE — disopyramide phosphate   Rx
Class: Class I antiarrhythmic

> In a long-term clinical study in patients with asymptomatic non-life-threatening ventricular arrhythmias who had a myocardial infarction, an excessive mortality or non-fatal cardiac arrest rate was seen in patients treated with encainide or flecainide compared to placebo. Considering the known proarrhythmic properties of Norpace or Norpace CR and the lack of evidence of improved survival, its use should be reserved for patients with life-threatening ventricular arrhythmias.

OTHER BRAND NAMES
Norpace CR

ADULT DOSAGE
Ventricular Arrhythmias

Treatment of Documented Ventricular Arrhythmias (eg, Sustained Ventricular Tachycardia):
Individualize dose based on response and tolerance
Usual: 400-800mg/day in divided dose

PEDIATRIC DOSAGE
Ventricular Arrhythmias

Treatment of Documented Ventricular Arrhythmias (eg, Sustained Ventricular Tachycardia):
<1 Year: 10-30mg/kg/day
1-4 Years: 10-20mg/kg/day
4-12 Years: 10-15mg/kg/day
12-18 Years: 6-15mg/kg/day

Recommended:
<110 lbs: 100mg q6h immediate-release (IR) or 200mg q12h extended-release (CR)
≥110 lbs: 150mg q6h (600mg/day) IR or 300mg q12h CR
Rapid Control of Ventricular Arrhythmia:
LD: 300mg IR (200mg if <110 lbs) Follow w/ maint dose
Titrate:
If no response/evidence of toxicity w/in 6 hrs of LD, may give 200mg q6h IR
If no response to 200mg q6h of IR w/in 48 hrs; d/c disopyramide or consider hospitalizing patient for monitoring while subsequent 250mg or 300mg q6h IR is given
Patients w/ cardiomyopathy/cardiac decompensation, limit initial dose to 100mg q6-8h IR and adjust gradually; do not give LD
Switching from IR to CR:
Maint schedule of CR may be started 6 hrs after last dose of IR
Transferring to Norpace or Norpace CR from Quinidine Sulfate or Procainamide:
Norpace or Norpace CR should be started using the regular maint schedule w/o a LD 6-12 hrs after the last dose of quinidine sulfate or 3-6 hrs after the last dose of procainamide

Give in equally divided doses q6h
Hospitalize patient during initial therapy
Start dose titration at lower end of range

DOSING CONSIDERATIONS
Renal Impairment
CrCl >40mL/min: 100mg q6h IR or 200mg q12h CR
CrCl 30-40mL/min: 100mg q8h IR, w/ or w/o initial 150mg LD
CrCl 15-30mL/min: 100mg q12h IR, w/ or w/o initial 150mg LD
CrCl <15mL/min: 100mg q24h IR, w/ or w/o initial 150mg LD

Hepatic Impairment
Moderate: 100mg q6h IR or 200mg q12h CR

Elderly
Start at low end of dosing range

Adverse Reactions
Anticholinergic Side Effects:
Adjust dose based on side effects
Reduce recommended dose by 1/3 from 600mg/day to 400mg/day w/o changing the dosing interval

ADMINISTRATION
Oral route

Preparation of a 1mg/mL to 10mg/mL Liquid Sus
Add the entire contents of Norpace caps to cherry syrup (100mg caps contain 100mg of disopyramide base).
Prepare cherry syr as follows: cherry juice, 475mL; sucrose 800g; alcohol, 20mL; purified water, a sufficient quantity to make 1000mL.
The resulting sus, when refrigerated, is stable for 1 month and should be thoroughly shaken before the measurement of each dose.
The sus should be dispensed in an amber glass bottle with a child-resistant closure.
Norpace CR caps should not be used to prepare the above sus.

STORAGE
25°C (77°F); excursions permitted to 15-30°C (59-86°F).

HOW SUPPLIED
Cap: (Norpace) 100mg, 150mg; **Cap, Extended-Release:** (Norpace CR) 100mg, 150mg

CONTRAINDICATIONS
Known hypersensitivity to disopyramide, cardiogenic shock, 2nd- or 3rd-degree atrioventricular block (if no pacemaker present), congenital QT prolongation.

WARNINGS/PRECAUTIONS
May cause or worsen congestive heart failure (CHF) and produce hypotension due to negative inotropic properties. Reduce dose if 1st-degree heart block occurs. Avoid with urinary retention, glaucoma, and myasthenia gravis unless adequate overriding measures taken. Atrial flutter/fibrillation; digitalize 1st. Monitor closely or withdraw if QT prolongation >25% occurs and ectopy continues. D/C if QRS widening >25% occurs. Avoid LD with cardiomyopathy or cardiac decompensation. Correct K⁺ abnormalities before therapy. Reduce dose with renal/hepatic dysfunction; monitor ECG. Avoid CR formulation with CrCl ≤40mL/min. Caution with sick sinus syndrome, Wolff-Parkinson-White syndrome, bundle branch block, or elderly. May significantly lower blood glucose.

ADVERSE REACTIONS
Dry mouth, urinary retention/frequency/urgency, constipation, blurred vision, GI effects, dizziness, fatigue, headache.

DRUG INTERACTIONS
Avoid type IA and IC antiarrhythmics, and propranolol except in unresponsive, life-threatening arrhythmias. Hepatic enzyme inducers may lower levels. Avoid within 48 hrs before or 24 hrs after verapamil. Possible fatal interactions with CYP3A4 inhibitors. Monitor blood glucose with β-blockers, alcohol.

PREGNANCY AND LACTATION
Category C, not for use in nursing.

MECHANISM OF ACTION
Type I antiarrhythmic; decreases rate of diastolic depolarization in cells with augmented automaticity, decreases upstroke velocity, and increases action potential duration of normal cardiac cells. Decreases disparity in refractoriness between infracted and adjacent normally perfused myocardium and has no effect on α- or β-adrenergic receptors.

PHARMACOKINETICS
Absorption: Rapid and complete; C_{max}=2.22mcg/mL, T_{max}=4.5 hrs. **Distribution:** Plasma protein binding (50-65%). **Metabolism:** Liver. **Elimination:** Urine (50% unchanged), (20% mono-N-dealkylated metabolite), (10% other metabolite); $T_{1/2}$=11.65 hrs.

PATIENT CONSIDERATIONS
Assessment: Prior to therapy, patients with atrial flutter/fibrillation should be digitalized and K⁺ abnormalities should be corrected. Assess for cardiogenic shock, preexisting 2nd- or 3rd-degree heart block, presence of functioning pacemaker, sick sinus syndrome (bradycardia/tachycardia syndrome), Wolff-Parkinson-White syndrome, bundle branch block, congenital QT prolongation, myocardial infarction, life-threatening arrhythmia, CHF, cardiomyopathy or myocarditis, chronic malnutrition, hepatic/renal impairment, alcohol intake, glaucoma, myasthenia gravis, urinary retention or BPH, pregnancy/nursing status, and possible drug interactions.

Monitoring: Monitor for hypotension, HF, PR interval prolongation, widening of QRS, hypoglycemia, heart block, urinary retention, and myasthenia crisis.

Counseling: Inform about risks/benefits; report adverse reactions. Instruct to notify physician if pregnant/nursing.

NORTRIPTYLINE — nortriptyline hydrochloride   Rx
Class: Tricyclic antidepressant (TCA)

> Antidepressants increased the risk of suicidal thinking and behavior (suicidality) in short-term studies in children, adolescents, and young adults with major depressive disorder and other psychiatric disorders. Monitor and observe closely for clinical worsening, suicidality, or unusual changes in behavior in patients who are started on antidepressant therapy. Not approved for use in pediatric patients.

OTHER BRAND NAMES
Pamelor

ADULT DOSAGE
Depression
Usual: 25mg tid or qid; initiate at a low level and increase as required
Alternate Regimen: Total daily dose may be given qd
Max: 150mg/day

Monitor plasma levels w/ doses >100mg/day and maintain in the optimum range of 50-150ng/mL

Following remission, maintenance medication may be required for a longer period of time at the lowest dose that will maintain response

Dosing Considerations with MAOIs

Switching to/from an MAOI for Psychiatric Disorders:
Allow at least 14 days between discontinuation of an MAOI and initiation of treatment, and allow at least 14 days between discontinuation of treatment and initiation of an MAOI

Use w/ Other MAOIs (eg, Linezolid, IV Methylene Blue):
Do not start nortriptyline in a patient being treated w/ linezolid or IV methylene blue
In patients already receiving nortriptyline, if acceptable alternatives are not available and benefits outweigh risks, d/c nortriptyline and administer linezolid or IV methylene blue; monitor for serotonin syndrome for 2 weeks or until 24 hrs after the last dose of linezolid or IV methylene blue, whichever comes 1st. May resume nortriptyline therapy 24 hours after the last dose of linezolid or IV methylene blue

PEDIATRIC DOSAGE
Depression
Cap:
Adolescents:
30-50mg/day in single or divided doses

Following remission, maintenance medication may be required for a longer period of time at the lowest dose that will maintain remission

Dosing Considerations with MAOIs

Switching to/from an MAOI for Psychiatric Disorders:
Allow at least 14 days between discontinuation of an MAOI and initiation of treatment, and allow at least 14 days between discontinuation of treatment and initiation of an MAOI

Use w/ Other MAOIs (eg, Linezolid, IV Methylene Blue):
Do not start nortriptyline in a patient being treated w/ linezolid or IV methylene blue
In patients already receiving nortriptyline, if acceptable alternatives are not available and benefits outweigh risks, d/c nortriptyline and administer linezolid or IV methylene blue; monitor for serotonin syndrome for 2 weeks or until 24 hrs after the last dose of linezolid or IV methylene blue, whichever comes 1st. May resume nortriptyline therapy 24 hours after the last dose of linezolid or IV methylene blue

DOSING CONSIDERATIONS

Elderly
30-50mg/day in single or divided doses

Adverse Reactions
Reduce dose if a patient develops minor side effects and promptly d/c if adverse effects of a serious nature or allergic manifestations occur

ADMINISTRATION
Oral route

STORAGE
20-25°C (68-77°F).

HOW SUPPLIED
Cap: 10mg, 25mg, 50mg, 75mg; **Sol:** 10mg/5mL [16 fl oz]

CONTRAINDICATIONS
Use of an MAOI for psychiatric disorders either concomitantly or within 14 days of stopping treatment. Treatment within 14 days of stopping an MAOI for psychiatric disorders. Starting treatment in a patient being treated with other MAOIs (eg, linezolid, IV methylene blue). Hypersensitivity to nortriptyline HCl or other tricyclic antidepressants. During the acute recovery period following MI.

WARNINGS/PRECAUTIONS
Not approved for the treatment of bipolar depression. May precipitate mixed/manic episode in patients at risk for bipolar disorder. May produce sinus tachycardia and prolong conduction time; MI, arrhythmia, and strokes reported. Caution with cardiovascular disease (CVD), glaucoma, history of urinary retention, and hyperthyroidism. May lower seizure threshold, exacerbate psychosis or activate schizophrenia, or alter glucose levels. D/C several days prior to elective surgery. May impair mental/physical abilities. Serotonin syndrome reported; d/c immediately and initiate supportive symptomatic treatment. Pupillary dilation that occurs following use may trigger an angle-closure attack in a patient with anatomically narrow angles who does not have a patent iridectomy.

ADVERSE REACTIONS
Arrhythmias, hypotension, HTN, tachycardia, MI, heart block, stroke, confusion, hallucination, insomnia, tremors, ataxia, dry mouth, blurred vision, skin rash.

DRUG INTERACTIONS
See Contraindications. May cause serotonin syndrome with other serotonergic drugs (eg, triptans, TCAs, fentanyl) and with drugs that impair metabolism of serotonin; d/c immediately if this occurs. May block antihypertensive effect of guanethidine and similar agents. Caution in patients on thyroid medications. Alcohol may potentiate effects. May produce "stimulating" effect with reserpine. Monitor and adjust dose with anticholinergic and sympathomimetic drugs. Increased plasma levels with cimetidine. Hypoglycemia reported with chlorpropamide. Drugs that inhibit CYP2D6 (eg, quinidine, cimetidine, many CYP2D6 substrates [eg, other antidepressants, phenothiazines, propafenone, flecainide]) may increase plasma concentrations and may require lower doses for either TCA or the other drug and monitoring of TCA plasma levels. Caution with SSRI coadministration and when switching between TCAs and SSRIs; sufficient time must elapse before starting therapy when switching from fluoxetine (at least 5 weeks may be necessary). Longer $T_{1/2}$, higher exposure, and decreased clearance with quinidine.

PREGNANCY AND LACTATION
Safety not known in pregnancy/nursing.

MECHANISM OF ACTION
TCA; inhibits activity of histamine, 5-hydroxytryptamine, and acetylcholine. Increases pressor effect of norepinephrine, blocks pressor response of phenethylamine, and interferes with transport, release, and storage of catecholamines.

PATIENT CONSIDERATIONS
Assessment: Assess for recent MI, known hypersensitivity to drug, bipolar disorder risk, susceptibility to angle-closure glaucoma, CVD, hyperthyroidism, history of urinary retention/seizure disorder/mania/schizophrenia, any other conditions where treatment is cautioned or contraindicated, pregnancy/nursing status, and possible drug interactions.

Monitoring: Monitor for signs/symptoms of clinical worsening, suicidality, unusual changes in behavior, mixed manic episodes, arrhythmias, psychosis, serotonin syndrome, angle-closure glaucoma, changes in blood glucose levels, seizures, cognitive/motor impairment, and other adverse reactions.

Counseling: Advise to avoid alcohol. Instruct to seek medical attention for symptoms of activation of mania, seizures, clinical worsening, cardiovascular events, increasing psychosis, increasing anxiety/agitation, and hypo/hyperglycemia. Inform that physical/mental abilities may be impaired. Advise about the risk of angle-closure glaucoma in susceptible individuals.

NORVASC — amlodipine besylate   Rx
Class: Calcium channel blocker (CCB) (dihydropyridine)

ADULT DOSAGE
Hypertension
Alone or in combination w/ other antihypertensive agents

Initial: 5mg qd
Titrate: Adjust according to BP goals Wait 7-14 days between titration steps; if clinically warranted, titrate

PEDIATRIC DOSAGE
Hypertension
Alone or in combination w/ other antihypertensive agents

6-17 Years:
Usual: 2.5-5mg qd
Max: 5mg qd

more rapidly and assess patient frequently
Max: 10mg qd

Angina
Chronic stable angina or confirmed or suspected vasospastic (Prinzmetal's/variant) angina, alone or in combination w/ other antianginals

Usual: 5-10mg qd

Coronary Artery Disease
Reduces the risk of hospitalization due to angina and reduces risk of coronary revascularization procedures in patients w/ recently documented coronary artery disease by angiography and w/o heart failure or an ejection fraction <40%

Usual: 5-10mg qd

DOSING CONSIDERATIONS
Concomitant Medications
HTN:
Other Antihypertensives: 2.5mg qd

Hepatic Impairment
HTN:
Initial: 2.5mg qd

Angina: Give lower dose

Elderly
HTN:
Initial: 2.5mg qd

Angina: Give lower dose

Other Important Considerations
HTN:
Small/Fragile Patients:
Initial: 2.5mg qd

ADMINISTRATION
Oral route

STORAGE
15-30°C (59-86°F).

HOW SUPPLIED
Tab: 2.5mg, 5mg, 10mg

CONTRAINDICATIONS
Known sensitivity to amlodipine.

WARNINGS/PRECAUTIONS
May cause symptomatic hypotension, particularly in patients w/ severe aortic stenosis. Worsening angina and acute MI may develop after starting or increasing the dose, particularly w/ severe obstructive CAD. Titrate slowly in patients w/ severe hepatic impairment.

ADVERSE REACTIONS
Edema, palpitations, dizziness, fatigue, flushing.

DRUG INTERACTIONS
Increased systemic exposure w/ moderate and strong CYP3A inhibitors and may require dose reduction; monitor for symptoms of hypotension and edema to determine the need for dose adjustment. Closely monitor BP if coadministered w/ CYP3A inducers. Monitor for hypotension when coadministered w/ sildenafil. May increase simvastatin exposure; limit dose of simvastatin to 20mg daily. May increase systemic exposure of cyclosporine or tacrolimus; monitor trough blood levels of cyclosporine and tacrolimus frequently and adjust dose when appropriate.

PREGNANCY AND LACTATION
Category C, not for use in nursing.

MECHANISM OF ACTION
Calcium channel blocker (dihydropyridine); inhibits transmembrane influx of Ca^{2+} ions into vascular smooth muscle and cardiac muscle. Acts directly on vascular smooth muscle to cause a reduction in peripheral vascular resistance and reduction in BP.

PHARMACOKINETICS
Absorption: Absolute bioavailability (64-90%); T_{max}=6-12 hrs. **Distribution:** Plasma protein binding (approx 93%). **Metabolism:** Hepatic (extensive). **Elimination:** Urine (10% unchanged, 60% metabolites); $T_{1/2}$=30-50 hrs.

PATIENT CONSIDERATIONS
Assessment: Assess for hypersensitivity to the drug, severe aortic stenosis, severe obstructive CAD, hepatic impairment, pregnancy/nursing status, and possible drug interactions. Obtain baseline BP.

Monitoring: Monitor for worsening of angina, MI, and other adverse reactions. Monitor BP.

Counseling: Inform of the risks/benefits of therapy. Advise to seek medical attention if any adverse effects develop. Instruct to take as prescribed.

NORVIR — ritonavir

Rx

Class: Protease inhibitor

> Coadministration w/ several classes of drugs, including sedative hypnotics, antiarrhythmics, or ergot alkaloid preparations, may result in potentially serious and/or life-threatening adverse events due to possible effects of ritonavir (RTV) on the hepatic metabolism of certain drugs. Review medications taken by patients prior to prescribing RTV or when prescribing other medications to patients already taking RTV.

ADULT DOSAGE
HIV-1 Infection
In Combination w/ Other Antiretrovirals:
600mg bid; initiate at no less than 300mg bid and increase at 2- to 3-day intervals by 100mg bid
Max: 600mg bid

PEDIATRIC DOSAGE
HIV-1 Infection
In Combination w/ Other Antiretrovirals:
>1 Month of Age:
Initial: 250mg/m² bid
Titrate: Increase at 2- to 3-day intervals by 50mg/m² bid
Maint: 350-400mg/m² bid or highest tolerated dose
Max: 600mg bid

DOSING CONSIDERATIONS
Concomitant Medications
Reduce dose when used w/ other protease inhibitors

Hepatic Impairment
Severe (Child-Pugh Class C): Not recommended

Elderly
Start at lower end of dosing range

Other Important Considerations
Do not administer oral sol to neonates before a postmenstrual age (1st day of the mother's last menstrual period to birth plus the time elapsed after birth) of 44 weeks has been attained

ADMINISTRATION
Oral route

Take w/ meals.

Tab
Swallow tab whole; do not chew, break, or crush tab.

Sol
May improve the taste by mixing w/ chocolate milk, Ensure, or Advera w/in 1 hr of dosing.

STORAGE
Cap: 2-8°C (36-46°F). May not require refrigeration if used w/in 30 days and stored below 25°C (77°F). Protect from light. Avoid exposure to excessive heat. **Sol:** 20-25°C (68-77°F). Do not refrigerate. Avoid exposure to excessive heat. **Tab:** ≤30°C (86°F). Exposure up to 50°C (122°F) for 7 days permitted. Exposure to high humidity outside the original or USP equivalent tight container (≤60mL) for >2 weeks is not recommended.

HOW SUPPLIED
Cap: 100mg; **Sol:** 80mg/mL [240mL]; **Tab:** 100mg

CONTRAINDICATIONS
Known hypersensitivity (eg, toxic epidermal necrolysis or Stevens-Johnson syndrome) to RTV or any of its components. Coadministration w/ voriconazole or St. John's wort. Coadministration of RTV w/ several classes of drugs (including sedative hypnotics, antiarrhythmics, or ergot alkaloid preparations) is contraindicated and may result in potentially serious and/or life-threatening adverse events due to possible effects of RTV on the hepatic metabolism of these drugs (eg, alfuzosin HCl, amiodarone, flecainide, propafenone, quinidine, dihydroergotamine, ergotamine, methylergonovine, cisapride, lovastatin, simvastatin, pimozide, sildenafil when used for treatment of pulmonary arterial HTN, triazolam, oral midazolam).

WARNINGS/PRECAUTIONS
Hepatic transaminase elevations >5X ULN, clinical hepatitis, and jaundice reported; increased risk w/ underlying hepatitis B or C. Caution w/ preexisting liver diseases, liver enzyme abnormalities, or hepatitis; consider increased AST/ALT monitoring, especially during first 3 months of therapy. Pancreatitis observed; d/c if diagnosed. Allergic reactions, anaphylaxis, Stevens-Johnson syndrome, and toxic epidermal necrolysis reported; d/c if severe reactions develop. Prolonged PR interval and 2nd- or 3rd-degree atrioventricular (AV) block may occur; caution w/ underlying structural heart disease, preexisting conduction system abnormalities, ischemic heart disease, and cardiomyopathies. May elevate TG and total cholesterol levels. New onset or exacerbation of diabetes mellitus (DM), hyperglycemia, diabetic ketoacidosis, immune reconstitution syndrome, autoimmune disorders (eg, Graves' disease, polymyositis, Guillain-Barre syndrome) in the setting of immune reconstitution, and redistribution/accumulation of body fat reported. Increased bleeding in patients w/ hemophilia type A and B reported. Various degrees of cross-resistance observed. Lab test interactions may occur. **Sol:** Contains alcohol and propylene glycol. Avoid sol in preterm neonates in the immediate postnatal period; preterm neonates may be at increased risk of propylene glycol-associated adverse events and other toxicities. If benefit of treating infants immediately after birth outweighs potential risk, monitor closely for increases in serum osmolality and SrCr, and for drug-related toxicity.

ADVERSE REACTIONS
Diarrhea, N/V, abdominal pain, dizziness, dysgeusia, paresthesia, peripheral neuropathy, rash, fatigue/asthenia, arthralgia, back pain, coughing, oropharyngeal pain, pruritus, flushing.

DRUG INTERACTIONS
See Boxed Warning and Contraindications. Coadministration w/ CYP3A substrates for which elevated plasma concentrations are associated w/ serious and/or life-threatening reactions is contraindicated. May increase exposure of CYP2D6 substrates. Not recommended w/ fluticasone or other glucocorticoids that are metabolized by CYP3A, salmeterol, high doses of itraconazole or ketoconazole, and simeprevir. Avoid w/ colchicine in patients w/ renal/hepatic impairment, saquinavir/rifampin/RTV combination, avanafil, and rivaroxaban. Delavirdine may increase levels and rifampin may decrease levels. May increase levels of CYP3A substrates, atazanavir, darunavir, amprenavir, saquinavir, tipranavir, maraviroc, normeperidine, disopyramide, lidocaine, mexiletine, dasatinib, nilotinib, vincristine, vinblastine, rivaroxaban, carbamazepine, clonazepam, ethosuximide, nefazodone, SSRIs, TCAs, desipramine, trazodone, dronabinol, ketoconazole, itraconazole, colchicine, clarithromycin, bedaquiline, rifabutin and rifabutin metabolite, quinine, quetiapine, β-blockers, calcium channel blockers, digoxin, bosentan, simeprevir, atorvastatin, rosuvastatin, cyclosporine, tacrolimus, sirolimus, fluticasone, budesonide, salmeterol, fentanyl, perphenazine, risperidone, thioridazine, avanafil, sildenafil, tadalafil, vardenafil, buspirone, clorazepate, diazepam, estazolam, flurazepam, zolpidem, parenteral midazolam, dexamethasone, prednisone, and methamphetamine. May decrease levels of raltegravir, meperidine, divalproex, lamotrigine, phenytoin, bupropion, hydroxybupropion (active metabolite of bupropion), voriconazole, atovaquone, theophylline, methadone, and ethinyl estradiol. Caution w/ other drugs that prolong the PR interval, particularly w/ those drugs metabolized by CYP3A. May alter concentrations of warfarin (monitor INR) and indinavir. May need to decrease dose of tramadol and propoxyphene. RTV formulations contain alcohol; may produce disulfiram-like reactions w/ disulfiram or metronidazole. Refer to PI for dosing modifications when used w/ certain concomitant therapies.

PREGNANCY AND LACTATION
Pregnancy: Category B. Physicians are encouraged to register patients in the Antiretroviral Pregnancy Registry.
Lactation: Not for use in nursing.

MECHANISM OF ACTION
HIV-1 protease inhibitor; renders the enzyme incapable of processing the gag-pol polyprotein precursor, which leads to production of noninfectious immature HIV-1 particles.

PHARMACOKINETICS
Absorption: (Sol) T_{max}=2 hrs (fasting), 4 hrs (fed); (Cap) AUC=121.7mg•hr/mL (fed), (Sol) AUC=129mg•hr/mL (fed). **Distribution:** V_d=0.41L/kg; plasma protein binding (98-99%). **Metabolism:** CYP3A (major), CYP2D6 (oxidation); isopropylthiazole (major metabolite). **Elimination:** (Sol) Urine (11.3%, 3.5% unchanged), feces (86.4%, 33.8% unchanged); $T_{1/2}$=3-5 hrs.

PATIENT CONSIDERATIONS
Assessment: Assess for previous hypersensitivity to the drug, preexisting liver diseases, hepatitis, DM, hemophilia type A or B, underlying cardiac problems, lipid disorders, pregnancy/nursing status, and possible drug interactions. Obtain baseline ECG, LFTs, CPK, uric acid, TG, and cholesterol levels.

Monitoring: Monitor for signs/symptoms of anaphylaxis or allergic reactions, hepatitis, jaundice, hepatic dysfunction, new onset or exacerbation of DM, hyperglycemia, pancreatitis, AV block, cardiac conduction abnormalities, immune reconstitution syndrome, fat redistribution/accumulation, and for other adverse reactions. Monitor for increased bleeding in patients w/ hemophilia type A or B. Monitor ECG, LFTs, CPK, uric acid, TG, and cholesterol levels. Frequently monitor INR during coadministration w/ warfarin.

Counseling: Instruct to take prescribed dose ud. Instruct to inform physician if weight changes in children occur. Inform that therapy is not a cure for HIV-1 infection and illnesses associated w/ HIV-1 infection may still be experienced. Advise to practice safe sex; to use latex or polyurethane condoms; not to share personal items (eg, toothbrush, razor blades), needles, or other inj equipment; and not to breastfeed. Advise to notify physician of any use of prescription, OTC, or herbal products, particularly St. John's wort. Advise to use additional or alternative contraceptive measures if receiving estrogen-based hormonal contraceptives. Counsel about potential adverse effects; instruct to report signs/symptoms of worsening liver disease, pancreatitis, Stevens-Johnson syndrome, PR prolongation, and DM.

NOVOLIN 70/30 — NPH, human insulin isophane
(rDNA origin)/regular, human insulin (rDNA origin)

OTC

Class: Insulin (combination)

ADULT DOSAGE
Diabetes Mellitus
Individualize dose

PEDIATRIC DOSAGE
Diabetes Mellitus
Individualize dose

ADMINISTRATION
SQ route

To mix, roll gently and use right away.
Do not use if the liquid in the vial remains clear after the vial has been rolled gently.
Use only if cloudy or milky; there may be air bubbles.
Inject in stomach area, upper arms, buttocks, or upper legs.
Rotate inj site w/in the chosen area w/ each dose.
Do not mix w/ any insulins.

STORAGE

Unopened: 2-8°C (36-46°F) or if refrigeration is not possible, ≤25°C (77°F) for ≤6 weeks. Do not freeze. Protect from light. **Opened:** <25°C (77°F) for ≤6 weeks; discard unused portion after 6 weeks. Keep away from direct heat/light. Do not refrigerate an opened vial.

HOW SUPPLIED

Inj: (Isophane/Regular) (70 U/30 U)/mL [10mL]

WARNINGS/PRECAUTIONS

Avoid in patients w/ hypoglycemia. Any change of insulin should be made cautiously and only under medical supervision. Hyperglycemia may occur if dosage is not taken, which may lead to diabetic ketoacidosis if not treated. May need to change dosage w/ illness, stress, diet change, change in physical activity/ exercise, other medicines, or surgery. Hypoglycemia may occur; monitor for symptoms of hypoglycemia (eg, sweating, dizziness, blurred vision). May impair physical and mental abilities. Serious allergic reaction, inj-site reaction, hands/feet swelling, vision changes, and hypokalemia may occur. May cause lipodystrophy; rotate inj site. May cause or worsen heart failure (HF) w/ thiazolidinediones (TZDs); may need to adjust or d/c insulin and TZD if this occurs.

ADVERSE REACTIONS

Hypoglycemia, allergic reaction, inj-site reaction, lipodystrophy, hands/feet swelling, vision changes, hypokalemia.

DRUG INTERACTIONS

Avoid w/ alcohol (eg, beer, wine); may affect blood glucose.

PREGNANCY AND LACTATION

Has not been studied in pregnant or nursing women.

MECHANISM OF ACTION

Insulin; structurally identical to insulin produced by the human pancreas that is used to control high blood glucose in patients w/ diabetes mellitus.

PATIENT CONSIDERATIONS

Assessment: Assess for medical conditions, hypoglycemia, drug hypersensitivity, pregnancy/nursing status, and possible drug interactions. Obtain baseline blood glucose levels.

Monitoring: Monitor for signs and symptoms of hypoglycemia, lipodystrophy, allergic reactions, vision changes, hypokalemia, and other adverse effects. Monitor blood glucose levels. Monitor for HF if taking a TZD concomitantly.

Counseling: Inform about potential risks and benefits of taking insulin and possible adverse reactions. If taking a TZD concomitantly, advise to notify physician if any new or worsening symptoms of HF (eg, SOB, swelling of the ankles/feet, sudden weight gain) occur. Inform about proper administration techniques, lifestyle management, regular blood glucose monitoring, signs and symptoms of hypoglycemia/hyperglycemia, management of hypoglycemia/ hyperglycemia, and proper storage of insulin. Advise to consult physician if pregnant/nursing, stressed, ill, changing diet/physical activity, or having surgery, because changes in insulin dosage may be needed. Instruct to exercise caution when driving or operating machinery. Advise to always check carefully for correct type of insulin before administering. Instruct to notify physician of all medicines that are being taken.

NOVOLIN N — NPH, human insulin isophane (rDNA origin)   OTC

Class: Insulin (intermediate-acting)

ADULT DOSAGE	PEDIATRIC DOSAGE
Diabetes Mellitus	**Diabetes Mellitus**
Individualize dose	Individualize dose

ADMINISTRATION

SQ route

To mix, roll gently and use right away.
Do not use if the liquid in the vial remains clear after the vial has been rolled gently. Use only if cloudy or milky; there may be air bubbles.
Do not use if precipitate becomes lumpy, granular in appearance, or has formed deposit of solid particles on the wall of the vial.
Inject in stomach area, upper arms, buttocks, or upper legs; rotate inj site w/in chosen area w/ each dose.
Do not mix w/ any insulin other than regular human insulin in same syringe.

STORAGE

Unopened: 2-8°C (36-46°F) or if refrigeration is not possible, ≤25°C (77°F) for ≤6 weeks. Do not freeze; do not use if frozen. Protect from light. **Opened:** <25°C (77°F) for ≤6 weeks; discard unused portion after 6 weeks. Keep away from direct heat/light. Do not refrigerate an opened vial.

HOW SUPPLIED

Inj: 100 U/mL [10mL]

WARNINGS/PRECAUTIONS

Avoid in patients w/ hypoglycemia. Any change of insulin should be made cautiously and only under medical supervision. Hyperglycemia may occur if dosage is not taken. Hyperglycemia may lead to diabetic ketoacidosis if not treated; may cause loss of consciousness, coma, or death. May need to change dosage w/ illness, stress, change in diet, change in physical activity/exercise, other medicines, or surgery. May impair mental/physical abilities. Hypoglycemia may occur; monitor for symptoms of hypoglycemia (eg, sweating, dizziness, blurred vision). Serious allergic reaction, inj-site reactions, hands/feet swelling, vision changes, and hypokalemia may occur. May cause lipodystrophy; rotate inj site. May cause or worsen heart failure (HF) w/ thiazolidinediones (TZDs); may need to adjust or d/c insulin and TZD if this occurs.

ADVERSE REACTIONS

Hypoglycemia, allergic reaction, inj-site reaction, lipodystrophy, hands/feet swelling, vision changes, hypokalemia.

DRUG INTERACTIONS

Avoid w/ alcohol (eg, beer, wine); may affect blood glucose.

PREGNANCY AND LACTATION

Has not been studied in pregnant or nursing women.

MECHANISM OF ACTION

Insulin; structurally identical to insulin produced by the human pancreas that is used to control high blood glucose in patients w/ diabetes mellitus.

PATIENT CONSIDERATIONS

Assessment: Assess for medical conditions, hypoglycemia, drug hypersensitivity, pregnancy/nursing status, and possible drug interactions. Obtain baseline blood glucose levels.

Monitoring: Monitor for signs of hypoglycemia, hypokalemia, vision changes, lipodystrophy, allergic reactions, and other adverse reactions. Monitor blood glucose levels. Monitor for HF if taking a TZD concomitantly.

Counseling: Inform about potential risks and benefits of taking insulin and possible adverse reactions. If taking a TZD concomitantly, advise to notify physician if any new or worsening symptoms of HF (eg, SOB, swelling of the ankles/feet, sudden weight gain) occur. Counsel on proper administration techniques, lifestyle management, regular blood glucose monitoring, signs and symptoms of hypoglycemia/hyperglycemia, management of hypoglycemia/ hyperglycemia, and proper storage of insulin. Advise to consult physician if pregnant/nursing, stressed, ill, changing diet/physical activity, or having surgery, because changes in insulin dosage may be needed. Instruct to exercise caution when driving or operating machinery. Advise to always check carefully for correct type of insulin before administering. Instruct to notify physician of all medicines that are being taken.

NOVOLIN R — regular, human insulin (rDNA origin)   OTC

Class: Insulin (short-acting)

ADULT DOSAGE	PEDIATRIC DOSAGE
Diabetes Mellitus	**Type 1 Diabetes Mellitus**
Individualize dose and timing of administration	**≥2 Years:** Individualize dose and timing of administration
Total Daily Insulin Requirement: **Usual:** 0.5-1 U/kg/day	**Total Daily Insulin Requirement:** **Usual:** 0.5-1 U/kg/day

---

DOSING CONSIDERATIONS

Renal Impairment
Dose requirements may be reduced

Hepatic Impairment
Dose requirements may be reduced

ADMINISTRATION

SQ/IV route

Do not use in insulin pumps.
If Novolin R is mixed w/ NPH human insulin, Novolin R should be drawn into the syringe first and the mixture should be injected immediately after mixing.
Do not administer insulin mixtures IV.

SQ
Inject approx 30 min prior to the start of a meal.
Use w/ an intermediate or long-acting insulin.
Inject in abdominal region, buttocks, thigh, or upper arm; rotate inj sites w/in the same region.

IV
Use at concentrations from 0.05-1 U/mL in infusion systems using polypropylene infusion bags.
May be used w/ the following infusion fluids: 0.9% NaCl, D5, D10 w/ 40mmol/L potassium chloride.

STORAGE

Unopened: 2-8°C (36-46°F) or if carried as a spare or if refrigeration not possible, ≤25°C (77°F) for 42 days. Do not freeze. Protect from light. Do not expose to heat/light. **Opened:** <25°C (77°F) for 42 days, away from heat/light. Do not refrigerate after 1st use.

HOW SUPPLIED

Inj: 100 U/mL [10mL]

CONTRAINDICATIONS

During episodes of hypoglycemia or w/ hypersensitivity to Novolin R or one of its excipients.

WARNINGS/PRECAUTIONS

Any change of insulin dose should be made cautiously and only under medical supervision. Changing from one insulin product to another or changing the strength may result in the need for a change in dosage. May require dose adjustments in patients who change level of physical activity or meal plan. Stress, illness, or emotional disturbances may alter insulin requirements. Hypoglycemia may occur and may impair ability to concentrate and react; caution in patients w/ hypoglycemia unawareness and who may be predisposed to hypoglycemia (eg, patients who are fasting or have erratic food intake, pediatric patients, elderly). Hypokalemia may occur; caution in patients who may be at risk. Hyperglycemia, diabetic ketoacidosis, or hyperosmolar hyperglycemic non-ketotic syndrome may develop if taken less than needed. Redness, swelling, or itching at inj site may occur. Localized reactions and generalized myalgias reported w/ metacresol, an excipient in Novolin R. Severe, life-threatening, generalized allergy, including anaphylaxis, may occur. Increases in titers of anti-insulin antibodies reported. May be administered IV under medical supervision w/ close monitoring of blood glucose and K⁺ concentrations. Caution in elderly.

ADVERSE REACTIONS
Hypoglycemia, allergic reactions, lipodystrophy, weight gain, peripheral edema, transitory reversible ophthalmologic refraction disorder.

DRUG INTERACTIONS
May require dose adjustment and close monitoring w/ drugs that may increase blood glucose-lowering effect and susceptibility to hypoglycemia (eg, oral antidiabetic medications, ACE inhibitors, MAOIs), drugs that may reduce blood glucose-lowering effect leading to worsening of glycemic control (eg, corticosteroids, sympathomimetic agents, atypical antipsychotics), or drugs that may either potentiate or weaken blood glucose-lowering effect (eg, β-blockers, clonidine, lithium salts). Alcohol may increase susceptibility to hypoglycemia. Pentamidine may cause hypoglycemia, sometimes followed by hyperglycemia. Hypoglycemic signs may be reduced or absent w/ sympatholytics (eg, β-blockers, clonidine, guanethidine). Caution w/ K⁺-lowering medications or medications sensitive to serum K⁺ concentrations. Thiazolidinediones (TZDs) may cause dose-related fluid retention and heart failure (HF); observe for signs and symptoms of HF and consider dose reduction or discontinuation of TZDs if HF develops.

PREGNANCY AND LACTATION
Pregnancy: Category B.
Lactation: It is unknown whether Novolin R is excreted in breast milk. Use is compatible w/ breastfeeding, but insulin doses may need to be adjusted; lactation can reduce insulin requirements.

MECHANISM OF ACTION
Insulin; regulates glucose metabolism. Binds to insulin receptors on muscle and adipocytes and lowers blood glucose by facilitating the cellular uptake of glucose and simultaneously inhibiting the output of glucose from the liver.

PHARMACOKINETICS
Absorption: T_{max}=1.5-2.5 hrs (0.1 U/kg SQ).

PATIENT CONSIDERATIONS
Assessment: Assess for drug hypersensitivity, hypoglycemia unawareness, predisposal to hypoglycemia, risk of hypokalemia, renal/hepatic impairment, pregnancy/nursing status, and possible drug interactions. Obtain baseline blood glucose and HbA1c levels.

Monitoring: Monitor for signs and symptoms of hypoglycemia, lipodystrophy, hypersensitivity, allergic reactions, dose-related fluid retention, HF, and other adverse effects. Monitor blood glucose, HbA1c, and K⁺ concentrations (frequently during IV).

Counseling: Inform about potential risks and benefits of therapy, including possible adverse reactions. Offer continued education and advise on insulin therapies, inj technique, lifestyle management, regular glucose monitoring, periodic HbA1c testing, recognition and management of hypo/hyperglycemia, adherence to meal planning, complications of therapy, timing of dose, instruction in the use of inj devices, and proper storage. Inform that frequent, patient-performed blood glucose measurements are needed to achieve optimal glycemic control and to avoid both hyper/hypoglycemia. Advise to use caution when driving or operating machinery. Instruct to inform physician if patients intend to become pregnant, or if they become pregnant. Instruct to always carefully check that they are administering the correct insulin to avoid medication errors.

NOVOLOG — insulin aspart (rDNA origin)　　　　Rx
Class: Insulin (rapid-acting)

ADULT DOSAGE
Diabetes Mellitus

SQ/IV:
Total Daily Insulin Requirement:
Usual: 0.5-1 U/kg/day; generally used w/ an intermediate- or long-acting insulin

Meal-Related SQ Regimen:
50-70% of total requirement may be provided by insulin aspart; remainder provided by an intermediate- or long-acting insulin

PEDIATRIC DOSAGE
Type 1 Diabetes Mellitus

≥2 Years:
SQ:
Total Daily Insulin Requirement:
Usual: 0.5-1 U/kg/day; generally used w/ an intermediate- or long-acting insulin

Meal-Related SQ Regimen:
50-70% of total requirement may be provided by insulin aspart; remainder provided by an intermediate- or long-acting insulin

ADMINISTRATION
SQ/IV route
SQ
Administer in the abdominal region, buttocks, thigh, or upper arm; rotate inj sites w/in the same region
Administer immediately (w/in 5-10 min) ac
May be diluted w/ insulin diluting medium
If mixed w/ NPH insulin, draw insulin aspart into syringe first and inject immediately after mixing
Continuous SQ Insulin Infusion by External Pump
Infuse premeal boluses immediately (w/in 5-10 min) ac
Rotate infusion sites w/in the same region
Do not use diluted or mixed insulins w/ external pump

Initial Programming of External Insulin Infusion Pump:
Base on total daily insulin dose of previous regimen
Approx 50% of total dose given as meal-related boluses; remainder given as basal infusion
Change insulin in the reservoir at least every 6 days; change infusion sets and infusion set insertion site at least every 3 days
IV
Use at concentrations 0.05-1.0 U/mL in infusion systems using polypropylene infusion bags; stable in infusion fluids such as 0.9% NaCl
Do not administer insulin mixtures IV

STORAGE
Unused: 2-8°C (36-46°F) until expiration date. Do not freeze or store directly adjacent to the refrigerator cooling element; do not use if it has been frozen. Should not be drawn into a syringe and stored for later use. Opened: <30°C (86°F) for up to 28 days. (Vials) May refrigerate. (PenFill/FlexPen/FlexTouch) Do not refrigerate. Pump: Discard insulin in reservoir after exposure to >37°C (98.6°F). Diluted Sol: <30°C (86°F) for 28 days. Sol in Infusion Fluids: Stable at room temperature for 24 hrs. Protect from direct heat and light.

HOW SUPPLIED
Inj: 100 U/mL [3mL, PenFill cartridge, FlexPen, FlexTouch; 10mL, vial]

CONTRAINDICATIONS
During episodes of hypoglycemia, in patients with hypersensitivity to Novolog or one of its excipients.

WARNINGS/PRECAUTIONS
Insulin delivery devices should never be shared between patients, even if needle is changed; may carry a risk for transmission of blood-borne pathogens. Any change of insulin dose should be made cautiously and under medical supervision. Changing from 1 insulin product to another or changing the insulin strength may result in the need for a change in dosage. May require dosage adjustment w/ change in physical activity or meal plan. Illness, emotional disturbances, or other stresses may alter insulin requirements. Hypoglycemia may occur and may impair ability to concentrate and react; caution in patients w/ hypoglycemia unawareness and who may be predisposed to hypoglycemia. Hypokalemia, inj-site redness/swelling/itching, and severe, life-threatening, generalized allergy may occur. Contains metacresol as excipient; localized reactions and generalized myalgias reported. Increases in anti-insulin antibodies observed; may need to adjust insulin dose to correct a tendency towards hyper/hypoglycemia. Malfunction of the insulin pump or infusion set or insulin degradation can lead to a rapid onset of hyperglycemia and ketosis; prompt identification and correction of the cause is necessary. Train patients using continuous SQ infusion pump therapy to administer by inj and have alternate insulin therapy available in case of pump failure. IV administration should be under medical supervision w/ close monitoring of blood glucose and K⁺ levels. Caution w/ renal/hepatic impairment.

ADVERSE REACTIONS
Hypoglycemia, headache, hyporeflexia, onychomycosis, sensory disturbance, UTI, nausea, diarrhea, chest pain, abdominal pain, skin disorder, sinusitis.

DRUG INTERACTIONS
May require dose adjustment and increased frequency of glucose monitoring w/ drugs that may increase the risk of hypoglycemia (eg, ACE inhibitors, MAOIs, salicylates), drugs that may decrease the glucose-lowering effect (eg, atypical antipsychotics [eg, olanzapine, clozapine], corticosteroids, oral contraceptives), or drugs that may increase or decrease the glucose-lowering effect (eg, alcohol, β-blockers, clonidine, lithium salts). Pentamidine may cause hypoglycemia, sometimes followed by hyperglycemia. Signs and symptoms of hypoglycemia may be blunted w/ β-blockers, clonidine, guanethidine, and reserpine. Caution w/ K⁺-lowering drugs or drugs sensitive to serum K⁺ concentrations. Observe for signs/symptoms of heart failure (HF) if treated concomitantly w/ a peroxisome proliferator-activated receptor (PPAR)-gamma agonist (eg, thiazolidinedione); consider discontinuation or dose reduction of the PPAR-gamma agonist if HF develops.

PREGNANCY AND LACTATION
Category B, caution in nursing.

MECHANISM OF ACTION
Insulin aspart (rDNA origin); regulates glucose metabolism. Binds to the insulin receptors on muscle and fat cells and lowers blood glucose by facilitating the cellular uptake of glucose and simultaneously inhibiting the output of glucose from the liver.

PHARMACOKINETICS
Absorption: C_{max}=82 mU/L; T_{max}=40-50 min (median). **Distribution:** Plasma protein binding (<10%). **Elimination:** $T_{1/2}$=81 min.

PATIENT CONSIDERATIONS
Assessment: Assess for predisposition to hypoglycemia, risk of hypokalemia, hypersensitivity, renal/hepatic impairment, pregnancy/nursing status, and possible drug interactions. Obtain baseline blood glucose and HbA1c levels.

Monitoring: Monitor for signs/symptoms of hypoglycemia, hypokalemia, allergic reactions, and other adverse effects. Monitor blood glucose, HbA1c, K⁺ levels, and renal/hepatic function.

Counseling: Advise to never share insulin delivery device w/ another person, even if needle is changed. Inform about potential risks and benefits of therapy. Counsel on proper inj technique, lifestyle management, regular glucose monitoring, periodic HbA1c testing, recognition and management of hypo/hyperglycemia, adherence to meal planning, complications of insulin therapy, timing of dose, instruction in the use of inj or SQ insulin infusion pump, and proper storage of insulin. Inform that the ability to concentrate and react may be impaired as a result of hypoglycemia; advise to use caution when driving or operating machinery. Instruct to always carefully check that appropriate insulin is administered to avoid medication errors. Advise to inform physician if pregnant or intending to become pregnant.

NovoLog Mix 70/30 — insulin aspart protamine   Rx
(rDNA origin)/insulin aspart (rDNA origin)

Class: Insulin (combination)

ADULT DOSAGE	PEDIATRIC DOSAGE
Type 1 Diabetes Mellitus	Pediatric use may not have been established
Individualize dose; inject w/in 15 min ac	
Typically dosed bid (w/ each dose intended to cover 2 meals or a meal and snack)	
Type 2 Diabetes Mellitus	
Individualize dose; inject w/in 15 min ac or pc	
Typically dosed bid (w/ each dose intended to cover 2 meals or a meal and snack)	

DOSING CONSIDERATIONS
Elderly
Start at lower end of dosing range

ADMINISTRATION
SQ route

Administer in the abdominal region, buttocks, thigh, or upper arm; rotate inj sites w/in the same region
Do not use in insulin infusion pump; do not mix w/ any other insulin product
Always use a new needle for each inj and always remove needle after each inj to prevent contamination

Resuspension
Resuspension is easier when the insulin has reached room temperature
Vial:
1. Roll vial gently between hands in a horizontal position 10X to mix it
2. Repeat rolling procedure until the sus appears uniformly white and cloudy
3. Inject immediately
FlexPen:
1. Roll 10X gently between hands in a horizontal position
2. Turn FlexPen upside down so that the glass ball moves from 1 end of the reservoir to the other at least 10X
3. Repeat rolling and turning procedure until the sus appears uniformly white and cloudy
4. Inject immediately
5. Repeat turning procedure at least 10X before each subsequent inj

STORAGE
Unopened: 2-8°C (36-46°F) until expiration date, or room temperature (<30°C [86°F]) for 28 days (vial) or 14 days (FlexPen). Do not freeze; do not use if it has been frozen. Do not store directly adjacent to the refrigerator cooling element. Opened: <30°C (86°F) for 28 days (vial) or 14 days (FlexPen). Do not refrigerate FlexPen; store w/o a needle attached. Protect from excessive heat or sunlight.

HOW SUPPLIED
Inj: (Insulin Aspart Protamine/Insulin Aspart) (70 U/30 U)/mL [3mL, FlexPen; 10mL, vial]

CONTRAINDICATIONS
During episodes of hypoglycemia, hypersensitivity to Novolog Mix 70/30 or one of its excipients.

WARNINGS/PRECAUTIONS
FlexPens must never be shared between patients, even if needle is changed; may carry a risk for transmission of blood-borne pathogens. Any change of insulin dose should be made cautiously and under medical supervision. Changing from 1 insulin product to another or changing the insulin strength may result in the need for a change in dosage; changes may also be necessary during illness, emotional stress, and other physiologic stress in addition to changes in meals and exercise. Hypoglycemia may occur and may impair ability to concentrate and react. Hypokalemia, inj-site reactions (eg, erythema, edema, pruritus), and severe, life-threatening, generalized allergy may occur. Contains metacresol as excipient; localized reactions and generalized myalgias reported. Changes in cross-reactive anti-insulin antibodies reported; may need to adjust dose in order to correct a tendency towards hyper/hypoglycemia. Caution w/ renal/hepatic impairment.

ADVERSE REACTIONS
Hypoglycemia, headache, influenza-like symptoms, dyspepsia, back pain, diarrhea, pharyngitis, rhinitis, skeletal pain, URTI, neuropathy, abdominal pain.

DRUG INTERACTIONS
May require insulin dose adjustment and close monitoring w/ drugs that may increase blood glucose-lowering effect and susceptibility to hypoglycemia (eg, oral antidiabetic products, pramlintide, ACE inhibitors), drugs that may reduce blood glucose-lowering effect (eg, corticosteroids, niacin, danazol), or drugs that may potentiate or weaken blood glucose-lowering effect (β-blockers, clonidine, lithium salts, alcohol). Pentamidine may cause hypoglycemia, sometimes followed by hyperglycemia. Signs of hypoglycemia may be reduced or absent w/ sympatholytics (eg, β-blockers, clonidine, guanethidine). Caution w/ K+-lowering drugs or drugs sensitive to K+ concentrations. Observe for signs/symptoms of heart failure (HF) if treated concomitantly w/ a peroxisome proliferator-activated receptor (PPAR)-gamma agonist (eg, thiazolidinediones); consider discontinuation or dose reduction of the PPAR-gamma agonist if HF develops.

PREGNANCY AND LACTATION
Category B, caution in nursing.

MECHANISM OF ACTION
Insulin; regulates glucose metabolism. Binds to the insulin receptors on muscle, liver, and fat cells and lowers blood glucose by facilitating the cellular uptake of glucose and simultaneously inhibiting the output of glucose from the liver.

PHARMACOKINETICS
Absorption: Rapid. (0.2 U/kg) C_{max}=23.4 mU/L; T_{max}=60 min. (0.3 U/kg) C_{max}=61.3 mU/L; T_{max}=85 min. **Distribution:** Plasma protein binding (0-9%). **Elimination:** $T_{1/2}$=8-9 hrs.

PATIENT CONSIDERATIONS
Assessment: Assess for predisposition to hypoglycemia, risk of hypokalemia, renal/hepatic impairment, drug hypersensitivity, pregnancy/nursing status, and possible drug interactions. Obtain baseline blood glucose and HbA1c levels.

Monitoring: Monitor for signs/symptoms of hypoglycemia, hypokalemia, allergic reactions, and other adverse effects. Monitor blood glucose, HbA1c, K+ levels, and renal/hepatic function.

Counseling: Advise to never share FlexPen w/ another person, even if the needle is changed. Inform about potential risks and benefits of therapy. Counsel on proper inj technique, lifestyle management, regular glucose monitoring, periodic HbA1c testing, recognition and management of hypo/hyperglycemia, adherence to meal planning, complications of insulin therapy, timing of dose, instruction in the use of inj devices, and proper storage of insulin. Inform that the ability to concentrate and react may be impaired as a result of hypoglycemia; advise to use caution when driving or operating machinery. Instruct to always carefully check that appropriate insulin is administered to avoid medication errors. Advise to inform physician if pregnant/intending to become pregnant.

NovoSeven RT — coagulation factor VIIa (recombinant)   Rx
Class: Antihemophilic agent

> Serious arterial and venous thrombotic events reported. Monitor for signs/symptoms of activation of the coagulation system and for thrombosis.

ADULT DOSAGE	PEDIATRIC DOSAGE
Congenital Hemophilia	**Congenital Hemophilia**
Congenital Hemophilia A or B w/ Inhibitors:	**Congenital Hemophilia A or B w/ Inhibitors:**
Acute Bleeding Episodes:	**Acute Bleeding Episodes:**
Hemostatic: 90mcg/kg IV q2h until hemostasis is achieved, or until treatment has been judged to be inadequate; adjust dose based on severity of bleeding	**Hemostatic:** 90mcg/kg IV q2h until hemostasis is achieved, or until treatment has been judged to be inadequate; adjust dose based on severity of bleeding
Post-Hemostatic: 90mcg/kg IV q3-6h for severe bleeds until after homeostasis is achieved to maintain the hemostatic plug; monitor and minimize duration	**Post-Hemostatic:** 90mcg/kg IV q3-6h for severe bleeds until after homeostasis is achieved to maintain the hemostatic plug; monitor and minimize duration
Perioperative Management: **Minor Surgery:**	**Perioperative Management:** **Minor Surgery:**
Initial: 90mcg/kg IV immediately before surgery and repeat q2h for the duration of surgery	**Initial:** 90mcg/kg IV immediately before surgery and repeat q2h for the duration of surgery
Postsurgical: 90mcg/kg IV q2h for 48 hrs, then q2-6h until healing occurs	**Postsurgical:** 90mcg/kg IV q2h for 48 hrs, then q2-6h until healing occurs
Major Surgery:	**Major Surgery:**
Initial: 90mcg/kg IV immediately before surgery and repeat q2h for the duration of surgery	**Initial:** 90mcg/kg IV immediately before surgery and repeat q2h for the duration of surgery
Postsurgical: 90mcg/kg IV q2h for 5 days, then q4h until healing occurs Administer additional bolus doses if required	**Postsurgical:** 90mcg/kg IV q2h for 5 days, then q4h until healing occurs Administer additional bolus doses if required
Acquired Hemophilia	**Factor VII Deficiency**
Acute Bleeding Episodes: 70-90mcg/kg IV q2-3h until hemostasis is achieved	**Congenital:** **Acute Bleeding Episodes:** 15-30mcg/kg IV q4-6h until hemostasis is achieved
Perioperative Management: **Minor/Major Surgery:** 70-90mcg/kg IV immediately before surgery and repeat q2-3h for the duration of surgery, and until hemostasis is achieved	**Perioperative Management:** **Minor/Major Surgery:** 15-30mcg/kg IV immediately before surgery and repeat q4-6h for the duration of surgery and until hemostasis is achieved
Factor VII Deficiency	
Congenital: **Acute Bleeding Episodes:** 15-30mcg/kg IV q4-6h until hemostasis is achieved	Effective treatment has been achieved w/ doses as low as 10mcg/kg

Perioperative Management:
Minor/Major Surgery: 15-30mcg/kg IV immediately before surgery and repeat q4-6h for the duration of surgery and until hemostasis is achieved

Effective treatment has been achieved w/ doses as low as 10mcg/kg

Glanzmann's Thrombasthenia
Refractory to platelet transfusions, w/ or w/o antibodies to platelets

Acute Bleeding Episodes:
90mcg/kg IV q2-6h in severe bleeding episodes requiring systemic hemostatic therapy until hemostasis is achieved

Perioperative Management:
Minor/Major Surgery:
Initial: 90mcg/kg IV immediately before surgery and repeat q2h for the duration of the procedure
Postsurgical: 90mcg/kg IV q2-6h to prevent postoperative bleeding

Higher average infused doses (median dose of 100mcg/kg) were noted for surgical patients who had clinical refractoriness w/ or w/o platelet-specific antibodies compared to those w/ neither

Glanzmann's Thrombasthenia
Refractory to platelet transfusions, w/ or w/o antibodies to platelets

Acute Bleeding Episodes:
90mcg/kg IV q2-6h in severe bleeding episodes requiring systemic hemostatic therapy until hemostasis is achieved

Perioperative Management:
Minor/Major Surgery:
Initial: 90mcg/kg IV immediately before surgery and repeat q2h for the duration of the procedure
Postsurgical: 90mcg/kg IV q2-6h to prevent postoperative bleeding

Higher average infused doses (median dose of 100mcg/kg) were noted for surgical patients who had clinical refractoriness w/ or w/o platelet-specific antibodies compared to those w/ neither

ADMINISTRATION
IV route

For IV bolus only; administer as a slow bolus inj over 2-5 min, depending on the dose administered.
Do not mix w/ other infusion sol.
Use 0.9% NaCl inj if line needs to be flushed before/after administration.
Administer w/in 3 hrs after reconstitution and discard any unused sol.

Reconstitution
Bring the powder and diluent to room temperature but not >37°C (98.6°F).

Powder and Vial of Diluent:
Add 1.1mL, 2.1mL, 5.2mL, or 8.1mL of the histidine diluent to 1mg, 2mg, 5mg, or 8mg vial of the powder respectively.
Use syringe needles w/ 20-/26-gauge size.
Do not inject the diluent directly on the powder but aim the needle against the side so that the stream of liquid runs down the vial wall.
Gently swirl until all the material dissolves.

Powder and Prefilled Diluent Syringe:
Use the 1mL, 2mL, 5mL, or 8mL of the prefilled diluent syringe for the 1mg, 2mg, 5mg, or 8mg vial respectively.

Refer to PI for further administration instructions.

STORAGE
2-25°C (36-77°F). Do not freeze. Protect from light. **Reconstituted Sol:** Room temperature or refrigerated for up to 3 hrs. Do not freeze or store in syringes.

HOW SUPPLIED
Inj: 1mg, 2mg, 5mg, 8mg

WARNINGS/PRECAUTIONS
Coagulation parameters do not necessarily correlate w/ or predict effectiveness of therapy. Increased risk of developing thromboembolic events due to circulating tissue factor or predisposing coagulopathy in patients w/ disseminated intravascular coagulation (DIC), advanced atherosclerotic disease, crush injury, septicemia, and uncontrolled postpartum hemorrhage. Caution w/ administration to patients w/ an increased risk of thromboembolic complications (eg, history of coronary artery disease [CAD], liver disease, DIC, postoperative immobilization, elderly, neonates). Reduce dose or d/c treatment depending on patient's condition if there is lab confirmation of intravascular coagulation or presence of clinical thrombosis. Hypersensitivity reactions, including anaphylaxis, reported. Administer only if clearly needed in patients w/ known hypersensitivity to the drug or any of its components, or in patients w/ known hypersensitivity to mouse, hamster, or bovine proteins; if symptoms occur, d/c treatment, administer appropriate treatment, and weigh the benefit/risks prior to restarting treatment. Antibody formation may be suspected if FVIIa activity fails to reach expected level, PT is not corrected, or bleeding is not controlled after treatment w/ recommended doses; perform analysis for antibodies. Lab test interactions may occur.

ADVERSE REACTIONS
Arterial and venous thrombotic events, fever, pain, deep thrombophlebitis, pulmonary embolism, cerebrovascular disorder, angina pectoris, anaphylactic shock, abnormal hepatic function.

DRUG INTERACTIONS
Avoid simultaneous use w/ activated prothrombin complex concentrates or prothrombin complex concentrates. Thrombosis may occur if administered concomitantly w/ coagulation factor XIII.

PREGNANCY AND LACTATION
Pregnancy: There are no adequate and well-controlled studies in pregnant women to determine whether there is a drug-associated risk.

Lactation: There is no information regarding the presence of coagulation factor VIIa (recombinant) in human milk, the effect on the breastfed infant, and the effects on milk production.

MECHANISM OF ACTION
Antihemophilic agent: Recombinant FVIIa; when complexed w/ tissue factor, can activate coagulation factor X (FX) to FXa and coagulation factor IX (FIX) to FIXa. FXa, in complex w/ other factors, then converts prothrombin to thrombin, which leads to formation of a hemostatic plug by converting fibrinogen to fibrin and thereby inducing local hemostasis. This process may also occur on the surface of activated platelets.

PHARMACOKINETICS
Distribution: (Hemophilia A or B, Non-Bleeding State) V_d (median)=106.5mL/kg (15-63 yrs of age), 128mL/kg (30-45 yrs of age), 164mL/kg (2-12 yrs of age). (Congenital FVII Deficiency) V_d=(20-43 yrs of age) 280mL/kg (15mcg/kg dose), 290mL/kg (30mcg/kg dose). **Elimination:** (Hemophilia A or B) $T_{1/2}$=2.89 hrs (15-63 yrs of age), 3.1 hrs (30-45 yrs of age), 2.6 hrs (2-12 yrs of age). (Congenital FVII Deficiency) $T_{1/2}$=(20-43 yrs of age) 2.82 hrs (15mcg/kg dose), 3.11 hrs (30mcg/kg dose).

PATIENT CONSIDERATIONS

Assessment: Assess for risk of thromboembolic complications (eg, DIC, history of CAD, liver disease, postoperative immobilization), hypersensitivity to drug, mouse, hamster, or bovine proteins, pregnancy/nursing status, and for possible drug interactions. Obtain baseline PT and FVII coagulant activity in FVII-deficient patients.

Monitoring: Monitor for development of signs/symptoms of activation of the coagulation system or thrombosis. Monitor PT, FVII activity, and for antibody formation in FVII-deficient patients. Monitor for hypersensitivity reactions, including anaphylaxis, and other adverse reactions.

Counseling: Advise to immediately seek medical help if early signs of hypersensitivity reactions (eg, hives, urticaria, tightness of chest) and signs of thrombosis (eg, new onset swelling and pain in the limbs or abdomen, new onset chest pain, SOB) occur.

NOXAFIL — *posaconazole*   **Rx**
Class: Azole antifungal

ADULT DOSAGE	PEDIATRIC DOSAGE
Invasive *Aspergillus* and *Candida* Infections	**Invasive *Aspergillus* and *Candida* Infections**
Prophylaxis in patients who are at high risk of developing these infections due to being severely immunocompromised (eg, hematopoietic stem cell transplant recipients w/ graft-versus-host disease or those w/ hematologic malignancies w/ prolonged neutropenia from chemotherapy)	Prophylaxis in patients who are at high risk of developing these infections due to being severely immunocompromised (eg, hematopoietic stem cell transplant recipients w/ graft-versus-host disease or those w/ hematologic malignancies w/ prolonged neutropenia from chemotherapy)
Inj/Tab, Delayed-Release (DR): **LD:** 300mg bid on the 1st day **Maint:** 300mg qd, starting on the 2nd day	**≥13 Years:** **Tab, DR:** **LD:** 300mg bid on the 1st day **Maint:** 300mg qd, starting on the 2nd day
Oral Sus: 200mg (5mL) tid	**Oral Sus:** 200mg (5mL) tid
Duration of therapy is based on recovery from neutropenia or immunosuppression	Duration of therapy is based on recovery from neutropenia or immunosuppression
Oropharyngeal Candidiasis	**Oropharyngeal Candidiasis**
Oral Sus: **LD:** 100mg (2.5mL) bid on 1st day **Maint:** 100mg qd for 13 days	**≥13 Years:** **Oral Sus:** **LD:** 100mg (2.5mL) bid on 1st day **Maint:** 100mg qd for 13 days
Refractory to Itraconazole and/or Fluconazole: 400mg (10mL) bid; duration of therapy is based on severity of underlying disease and clinical response	**Refractory to Itraconazole and/or Fluconazole:** 400mg (10mL) bid; duration of therapy is based on severity of underlying disease and clinical response

DOSING CONSIDERATIONS
Concomitant Medications
Avoid coadministration w/ drugs that can decrease posaconazole levels; if such drugs are necessary, closely monitor for breakthrough fungal infections

Renal Impairment
Inj:
Moderate or Severe (eGFR <50mL/min): Avoid use; monitor SrCr levels closely and consider changing to oral posaconazole therapy if increases occur

ADMINISTRATION
IV/Oral route

Tab, DR and oral sus are not to be used interchangeably.

Inj
Administer via a central venous line, including a central venous catheter or peripherally inserted central catheter by slow IV infusion over approx 90 min.

If central venous catheter is not available, may administer through a peripheral venous catheter by slow IV infusion over 30 min only as a single dose in advance of central venous line placement or to bridge the period during which a central venous line is replaced or is in use for other IV treatment.

Infuse via a central venous line when multiple dosing is required.

Do not administer as an IV bolus inj.

Administer through a 0.22 micron polyethersulfone or polyvinylidene difluoride filter.

Preparation:
1. Equilibrate the refrigerated vial to room temperature.
2. Transfer contents of 1 vial (16.7mL) to an IV bag/bottle of a compatible admixture diluent, to achieve a final concentration of posaconazole that is between 1-2mg/mL.
3. Once admixed, use product immediately; if not used immediately, may store sol up to 24 hrs at 2-8°C (36-46°F).
4. Once admixed, the sol ranges from colorless to yellow; variations of color w/in this range do not affect the quality of the product.

Refer to PI for IV line compatibility and incompatible diluents.

Tab, DR
Administer w/ food.
Swallow tabs whole; do not divide, crush, or chew.

Oral Sus
Administer w/ a full meal or w/ a liquid nutritional supplement or an acidic carbonated beverage (eg, ginger ale) in patients who cannot eat a full meal; administer during or immediately (w/in 20 min) following a full meal.
Shake well before use.
Administer w/ measured dosing spoon provided.

STORAGE
Inj: 2-8°C (36-46°F). **Oral Sus:** 25°C (77°F); excursions permitted to 15-30°C (59-86°F). Do not freeze. **Tab, DR:** 20-25°C (68-77°F); excursions permitted to 15-30°C (59-86°F).

HOW SUPPLIED
Inj: 300mg/16.7mL; **Oral Sus:** 40mg/mL [105mL]; **Tab, DR:** 100mg

CONTRAINDICATIONS
Coadministration w/ sirolimus, CYP3A4 substrates that prolong the QT interval (eg, pimozide, quinidine), HMG-CoA reductase inhibitors that are primarily metabolized through CYP3A4 (eg, atorvastatin, lovastatin, simvastatin), and ergot alkaloids (ergotamine and dihydroergotamine).

WARNINGS/PRECAUTIONS
Tab, DR and oral sus are not interchangeable due to differences in the dosing of each formulation. Tab, DR provides higher plasma drug exposures than oral sus and is therefore the preferred oral formulation for the prophylaxis indication. Prolongation of the QT interval and cases of torsades de pointes reported; caution w/ potentially proarrhythmic conditions. Rigorous attempts to correct K⁺, Mg²⁺, and Ca²⁺ should be made before initiating treatment. Hepatic reactions (eg, mild-moderate elevations in ALT, AST, alkaline phosphatase, total bilirubin, and/or clinical hepatitis) reported. More severe hepatic reactions, including cholestasis or hepatic failure including deaths, reported in patients w/ serious underlying medical conditions (eg, hematologic malignancy). Evaluate LFTs at the start of and during the course of therapy; monitor for the development of more severe hepatic injury in patients who develop abnormal LFTs during therapy. Consider discontinuation if signs/symptoms of liver disease develop. Monitor closely for breakthrough fungal infections in patients weighing >120kg; may have lower plasma drug exposure. **Inj:** Avoid w/ moderate or severe renal impairment (estimated GFR <50mL/min), unless an assessment of the benefit/risk justifies the use of inj. Monitor SrCr levels closely in patients w/ moderate or severe renal impairment; consider changing to oral therapy if increases occur. **Oral Sus/Tab, DR:** Monitor closely for breakthrough fungal infections in patients w/ severe renal impairment and severe diarrhea or vomiting.

ADVERSE REACTIONS
Diarrhea, hypokalemia, pyrexia, N/V, headache, cough, neutropenia.

DRUG INTERACTIONS
See Contraindications and Dosing Considerations. May increase whole blood trough concentrations of cyclosporine and tacrolimus; frequently monitor tacrolimus or cyclosporine whole blood trough concentrations during and at discontinuation of posaconazole treatment, and adjust the dose of cyclosporine or tacrolimus accordingly. At initiation of posaconazole treatment, reduce tacrolimus dose to approx 1/3 of original dose and reduce cyclosporine dose to approx 3/4 of original dose. Inhibitors or inducers of UDP glucuronosyltransferase or P-gp may affect posaconazole levels. May increase levels of drugs predominantly metabolized by CYP3A4. Increases midazolam levels by approx 5-fold. Coadministration w/ other benzodiazepines metabolized by CYP3A4 (eg, alprazolam, triazolam) may increase levels of these benzodiazepines; closely monitor patients for adverse effects associated w/ high levels of benzodiazepines and ensure availability of benzodiazepine receptor antagonists. May increase levels of ritonavir and atazanavir; frequently monitor for adverse effects and toxicity. Fosamprenavir may decrease levels; if concomitant administration is required, closely monitor for breakthrough fungal infections. Avoid use w/ phenytoin, rifabutin, and efavirenz, unless benefit outweighs risk. If phenytoin is required, closely monitor for breakthrough fungal infections, frequently monitor phenytoin levels, and consider phenytoin dose reduction. If rifabutin is required, monitor for breakthrough fungal infections, and frequently monitor CBCs and adverse events due to increased rifabutin levels. May increase levels of vinca alkaloids (eg, vincristine, vinblastine); consider dose adjustment of vinca alkaloids. May increase levels of calcium channel blockers (CCBs) metabolized by CYP3A4 (eg, verapamil, diltiazem, nifedipine); monitor for adverse effects/toxicity and may need to reduce dose of CCBs. Increased digoxin levels reported;

monitor digoxin plasma levels during coadministration. Monitor glucose levels w/ glipizide. **Oral Sus:** Avoid use w/ cimetidine and esomeprazole, unless benefit outweighs risks; if concomitant administration is required, closely monitor for breakthrough fungal infections. Metoclopramide decreases levels; closely monitor for breakthrough fungal infections if coadministered.

PREGNANCY AND LACTATION
Pregnancy: There are no adequate and well-controlled studies in pregnant women. Should be used in pregnancy only if the potential benefit outweighs the potential risk to the fetus.
Lactation: Not for use in nursing.

MECHANISM OF ACTION
Azole antifungal agent; blocks the CYP450-dependent synthesis of ergosterol and weakens the structure and function of the fungal cell membrane.

PHARMACOKINETICS
Absorption: Administration of variable doses resulted in different pharmacokinetic parameters. **Distribution:** V_d=261L (IV); plasma protein binding (>98%, predominantly to albumin). **Metabolism:** Via UDP glucuronidation; glucuronide conjugates (metabolites). **Elimination:** (Oral sus) Feces (71%, 66% unchanged), urine (13%, <0.2% unchanged). $T_{1/2}$=27 hrs (inj), 26-31 hrs (tab, DR), 35 hrs (oral sus).

PATIENT CONSIDERATIONS
Assessment: Assess for hypersensitivity to any component of the drug or to other azole antifungals, proarrhythmic conditions, renal impairment, serious underlying medical conditions (eg, hematologic malignancy), pregnancy/nursing status, and for possible drug interactions. Obtain baseline LFTs.

Monitoring: Monitor for signs/symptoms of hypersensitivity reactions, hepatic reactions, QT prolongation, torsades de pointes, and other adverse reactions. Monitor LFTs during the course of therapy. Monitor closely for breakthrough fungal infections in patients weighing >120kg. **Oral Sus/Tab, DR:** Monitor closely for breakthrough fungal infections in patients w/ severe renal impairment and severe diarrhea or vomiting.

Counseling: Instruct to take oral sus and tab, DR ud. Advise patients to inform physician of all medications being taken and if they have a heart condition or circulatory disease; have liver disease; are pregnant, plan to become pregnant, or are breastfeeding; or if they have ever had an allergic reaction to other antifungal medications. Advise patients to inform physician if they develop severe diarrhea or vomiting, flu-like symptoms, itching, eyes/skin that turn yellow, swelling of a leg, or SOB. Instruct to notify physician if patients notice a change in HR/heart rhythm, or if they feel more tired than usual.

Nplate — romiplostim   Rx
Class: Thrombopoietin receptor agonist

ADULT DOSAGE	**PEDIATRIC DOSAGE**
Chronic Immune Thrombocytopenia	Pediatric use may not have been established
Use in patients who have had an insufficient response to corticosteroids, immunoglobulins, or splenectomy	
Initial: 1mcg/kg based on actual body weight	
Titrate: Adjust weekly dose by increments of 1mcg/kg until platelet count is ≥50 x 10⁹/L	
Platelet Count >200 x 10⁹/L for 2 Consecutive Weeks: Reduce dose by 1mcg/kg	
Platelet Count >400 x 10⁹/L: Do not dose; continue assessing platelet count weekly. After platelet count falls to <200 x 10⁹/L, resume therapy at a dose reduced by 1mcg/kg	
Max: 10mcg/kg/week	

DOSING CONSIDERATIONS
Concomitant Medications
Concomitant Medical Immune Thrombocytopenia (ITP) Therapies: May reduce or d/c medical ITP therapies (eg, corticosteroids, danazol, azathioprine, IV immunoglobulin, and anti-D immunoglobulin) if platelet count is ≥50 x 10⁹/L

Discontinuation
D/C if platelet count does not increase to a level sufficient to avoid clinically important bleeding after 4 weeks of therapy at the max weekly dose

ADMINISTRATION
SQ route

Administer as a weekly SQ inj.
Discard any unused portion; do not pool unused portions from vials and do not administer more than 1 dose from a single vial.

Preparation
Reconstitute 250mcg vial or 500mcg vial w/ 0.72mL or 1.2mL, respectively, of preservative-free sterile water for inj.
Gently swirl and invert vial to reconstitute; do not shake.
Use a syringe w/ 0.01mL graduations.
Withdraw appropriate volume of calculated dose from vial and administer SQ.
Reconstituted sol can be kept at 25°C (77°F) or 2-8°C (36-46°F) for up to 24 hrs prior to administration; protect reconstituted product from light.

STORAGE
2-8°C (36-46°F). Do not freeze. Protect from light.

HOW SUPPLIED
Inj: 250mcg, 500mcg [single-dose vial]

WARNINGS/PRECAUTIONS
Not for the treatment of thrombocytopenia due to myelodysplastic syndrome (MDS) or any cause of thrombocytopenia other than chronic ITP; progression from MDS to acute myelogenous leukemia has been observed. Use only in patients w/ ITP whose degree of thrombocytopenia and clinical condition increases the risk for bleeding. Do not use in an attempt to normalize platelet counts. Use lowest dose to achieve and maintain a platelet count ≥50 x 10⁹/L. Thrombotic/thromboembolic complications may occur. Portal vein thrombosis reported in patients w/ chronic liver disease. If hyporesponsiveness or failure to maintain a platelet response occurs, search for causative factors (eg, neutralizing antibodies). Caution in elderly.

ADVERSE REACTIONS
Headache, arthralgia, dizziness, insomnia, myalgia, pain in extremity, abdominal pain, shoulder pain, dyspepsia, paresthesia.

PREGNANCY AND LACTATION
Pregnancy: Category C. Women who become pregnant during treatment are encouraged to enroll in Amgen's Pregnancy Surveillance Program.
Lactation: Not for use in nursing.

MECHANISM OF ACTION
Thrombopoietin (TPO) receptor agonist; increases platelet production through binding and activation of the TPO receptor.

PHARMACOKINETICS
Absorption: T_{max}=14 hrs (median). **Elimination:** $T_{1/2}$=3.5 days (median).

PATIENT CONSIDERATIONS
Assessment: Assess for cause and degree of thrombocytopenia, hepatic impairment, and pregnancy/nursing status.

Monitoring: Obtain CBCs, including platelet counts, weekly during dose adjustment phase, then monthly after establishment of a stable dose, and then weekly for at least 2 weeks after discontinuation. Monitor for thrombotic/thromboembolic complications, hyporesponsiveness, and failure to maintain platelet response w/ therapy.

Counseling: Inform of risks and benefits of therapy. Advise that the risks associated w/ long-term administration are unknown. Advise to avoid situations or medications that may increase risk for bleeding. Inform pregnant women that they may enroll in the surveillance program.

NUCALA — mepolizumab   Rx
Class: Monoclonal antibody/interleukin-5 (IL-5) receptor antagonist

ADULT DOSAGE	PEDIATRIC DOSAGE
Asthma	**Asthma**
Add-on maint treatment of severe asthma in patients w/ an eosinophilic phenotype	Add-on maint treatment of severe asthma in patients w/ an eosinophilic phenotype
100mg SQ every 4 weeks into the upper arm, thigh, or abdomen	**≥12 Years:** 100mg SQ every 4 weeks into the upper arm, thigh, or abdomen

ADMINISTRATION
SQ route

Reconstitution Instructions
1. Reconstitute mepolizumab in the vial w/ 1.2mL sterile water for inj (SWFI), preferably using a 2 or 3mL syringe and a 21-gauge needle; the reconstituted sol will contain a concentration of 100mg/mL. Do not mix w/ other medications.
2. Direct the stream of SWFI vertically onto the center of the lyophilized cake. Gently swirl the vial for 10 sec w/ a circular motion at 15-sec intervals until the powder is dissolved. Do not shake the reconstituted sol.
3. If a mechanical reconstitution device (swirler) is used, swirl at 450 rpm for no longer than 10 min. Alternatively, swirling at 1000 rpm for no longer than 5 min is acceptable.
4. If the reconstituted sol is not used immediately, store at <30°C (86°F), do not freeze, and discard if not used w/in 8 hrs of reconstitution.

Administration
1. For SQ administration, preferably using a 1mL polypropylene syringe fitted w/ a disposable 21- to 27-gauge x 0.5-inch (13mm) needle.
2. Just before administration, remove 1mL of reconstituted mepolizumab. Do not shake the reconstituted sol.
3. Administer the 1mL inj (equivalent to 100mg mepolizumab) SQ into the upper arm, thigh, or abdomen.

STORAGE
<25°C (77°F). Do not freeze. Store in the original package to protect from light.

HOW SUPPLIED
Inj: 100mg

CONTRAINDICATIONS
History of hypersensitivity to mepolizumab or excipients in the formulation.

WARNINGS/PRECAUTIONS
Not indicated for treatment of other eosinophilic conditions or relief of acute bronchospasm or status asthmaticus. D/C in the event of a hypersensitivity reaction. Herpes zoster reported; consider varicella vaccination if medically appropriate prior to starting therapy. Do not d/c systemic or inhaled corticosteroids abruptly upon initiation of therapy; reductions in corticosteroid dose, if appropriate, should be gradual and performed under the direct supervision of a physician. Reduction in corticosteroid dose may be associated w/ systemic withdrawal symptoms and/or unmask conditions previously suppressed by systemic corticosteroid therapy. Treat patients w/ preexisting helminth infections before initiating therapy; if patients become infected while receiving treatment and do not respond to anti-helminth treatment, d/c mepolizumab until infection resolves.

ADVERSE REACTIONS
Headache, inj-site reactions, back pain, fatigue, influenza, UTI, upper abdominal pain, pruritus, eczema, muscle spasms.

PREGNANCY AND LACTATION
Pregnancy: There is a pregnancy exposure registry that monitors pregnancy outcomes in women exposed to mepolizumab during pregnancy. Monoclonal antibodies, such as mepolizumab, are transported across the placenta in a linear fashion as pregnancy progresses; therefore, potential effects on a fetus are likely to be greater during the 2nd and 3rd trimester of pregnancy.
Lactation: There is no information regarding the presence of mepolizumab in human milk, the effects on the breastfed infant, or the effects on milk production. However, mepolizumab is a humanized monoclonal antibody (IgG1 kappa), and IgG is present in human milk in small amounts. Caution in nursing.

MECHANISM OF ACTION
IL-5 antagonist monoclonal antibody; reduces the production and survival of eosinophils by inhibiting IL-5 signaling.

PHARMACOKINETICS
Absorption: Bioavailability (approx 80%). **Distribution:** V_d=3.6L (for a 70kg individual). **Metabolism:** Degraded by proteolytic enzymes. **Elimination:** $T_{1/2}$=16-22 days.

PATIENT CONSIDERATIONS
Assessment: Assess for other eosinophilic conditions, acute bronchospasm or status asthmaticus, preexisting helminth infections, hypersensitivity to drug or excipients in the formulation, and pregnancy/nursing status.

Monitoring: Monitor for hypersensitivity reactions, acute asthma symptoms or acute exacerbations, herpes zoster, parasitic infection, and other adverse reactions.

Counseling: Inform that hypersensitivity reactions have occurred after administration and instruct to contact physician if such reactions occur. Inform that mepolizumab does not treat acute asthma symptoms or acute exacerbations. Instruct to seek medical advice if asthma remains uncontrolled or worsens after initiation of treatment. Inform that herpes zoster infections have occurred and where medically appropriate, varicella vaccination should be considered before starting treatment. Instruct not to d/c systemic or inhaled corticosteroids except under the direct supervision of a physician. Inform women there is a pregnancy exposure registry that monitors pregnancy outcomes in women exposed to mepolizumab during pregnancy.

NUCYNTA — tapentadol   CII
Class: Centrally acting analgesic

ADULT DOSAGE	PEDIATRIC DOSAGE
Acute Pain	Pediatric use may not have been established
Moderate to Severe:	
Usual: 50mg, 75mg, or 100mg q4-6h depending upon pain intensity	
Day 1: May give 2nd dose 1 hr after 1st dose if pain relief is inadequate, then 50mg, 75mg, or 100mg q4-6h	
Adjust dose to maintain adequate analgesia w/ acceptable tolerability	
Max: 700mg on Day 1, then 600mg/day thereafter	
Periodically reassess continued need for use during chronic therapy, especially for noncancer-related pain	

DOSING CONSIDERATIONS
Hepatic Impairment
Moderate (Child-Pugh Score 7-9):
Initial: 50mg no more frequently than once q8h
Max: 3 doses/24 hrs

Elderly
Start at lower end of dosing range

Discontinuation
Taper dose gradually

ADMINISTRATION
Oral route

Take w/ or w/o food.

STORAGE
≤25°C (77°F); excursions permitted to 15-30°C (59-86°F). Protect from moisture.

HOW SUPPLIED
Tab: 50mg, 75mg, 100mg

CONTRAINDICATIONS

Significant respiratory depression, acute or severe bronchial asthma or hypercarbia in an unmonitored setting or in the absence of resuscitative equipment, known or suspected paralytic ileus, and patients receiving MAOIs or who have taken them within the last 14 days. Hypersensitivity (eg, anaphylaxis, angioedema) to tapentadol or to any other ingredients of the product.

WARNINGS/PRECAUTIONS

Abuse liability similar to other opioid agonists legal or illicit; assess each patient's risk for opioid abuse or addiction prior to prescribing. Routinely monitor all patients for signs of misuse, abuse, and addiction; misuse or abuse by crushing, chewing, snorting, or injecting will pose a significant risk that could result in overdose and death. Respiratory depression, if not immediately recognized and treated, may lead to respiratory arrest and death. Accidental ingestion, especially in children, can result in fatal overdose. Respiratory depression is more likely to occur in elderly, cachectic, or debilitated patients; monitor closely, particularly when given with drugs that depress respiration. Monitor for respiratory depression and consider use of alternative nonopioid analgesics in patients with significant COPD or cor pulmonale, and in patients with a substantially decreased respiratory reserve, hypoxia, hypercarbia, or preexisting respiratory depression. May cause severe hypotension. Monitor for signs of sedation and respiratory depression in patients susceptible to the intracranial effects of carbon dioxide retention (eg, those with evidence of increased intracranial pressure or brain tumors). May obscure clinical course in patients with a head injury. Avoid with circulatory shock, impaired consciousness, or coma. May aggravate convulsions in patients with convulsive disorders and may induce or aggravate seizures; monitor for worsened seizure control in patients with history of seizure disorders. May cause spasm of sphincter of Oddi; monitor for worsening symptoms in patients with biliary tract disease (eg, acute pancreatitis). Withdrawal symptoms may occur if discontinued abruptly. May impair mental/physical abilities. Monitor for respiratory/CNS depression with moderate hepatic impairment. Avoid use with severe renal/hepatic impairment. Not for use during and immediately prior to labor.

ADVERSE REACTIONS

N/V, dizziness, somnolence, constipation, pruritus, dry mouth, hyperhidrosis, fatigue.

DRUG INTERACTIONS

See Contraindications. Avoid use with alcoholic beverages or medications containing alcohol, other opioids, or drugs of abuse; may have additive effects. CNS depressants (eg, sedatives or hypnotics, general anesthetics, phenothiazines, tranquilizers, alcohol, anxiolytics, neuroleptics, muscle relaxants, other opioids, illicit drugs) may increase risk of respiratory depression, hypotension, profound sedation, or coma; start tapentadol at 1/3 to 1/2 of the usual dose and consider using a lower dose of concomitant CNS depressant. Serotonin syndrome may occur with serotonergic drugs (eg, SSRIs, SNRIs, TCAs, triptans, drugs that affect the serotonergic neurotransmitter system [eg, mirtazapine, trazodone, tramadol]), and drugs that may impair metabolism of serotonin (eg, MAOIs); use with caution. Avoid use with mixed agonist/antagonist analgesics (eg, butorphanol, nalbuphine, pentazocine), and partial agonists (eg, buprenorphine); may precipitate withdrawal symptoms. Anticholinergics may increase risk of urinary retention and/or severe constipation, which may lead to paralytic ileus.

PREGNANCY AND LACTATION

Pregnancy: Category C.
Lactation: Not for use in nursing.

MECHANISM OF ACTION

Centrally acting synthetic analgesic; not established. Suspected to be due to µ-opioid agonist activity and the inhibition of norepinephrine reuptake.

PHARMACOKINETICS

Absorption: T_{max}=1.25 hrs; absolute bioavailability (32%). **Distribution:** (IV) V_d=540L; plasma protein binding (20%); crosses placenta. **Metabolism:** Conjugation; N-desmethyl tapentadol by CYP2C9 and CYP2C19; hydroxy tapentadol by CYP2D6. **Elimination:** Kidneys (99%); urine (3% unchanged, 70% conjugated); $T_{1/2}$=4 hrs.

PATIENT CONSIDERATIONS

Assessment: Assess for personal/family history or risk factors for drug abuse or addiction, general condition and medical status, opioid experience/tolerance, pain type/severity, previous opioid daily dose, potency and type of prior analgesics used, respiratory depression, COPD or other respiratory complications, GI obstruction, paralytic ileus, renal/hepatic impairment, pregnancy/nursing status, possible drug interactions, and any other condition where treatment is contraindicated or cautioned.

Monitoring: Monitor for improvement of pain, signs/symptoms of respiratory depression, hypotension, symptoms of worsening biliary tract disease, aggravation/induction of seizure, tolerance, physical dependence, mental/physical impairment, serotonin syndrome, and other adverse reactions. Routinely monitor for signs of misuse, abuse, and addiction. Periodically reassess continued need for use during chronic therapy, especially for noncancer-related pain.

Counseling: Instruct to take only as prescribed and not to d/c without first discussing the need for a tapering regimen with prescriber. Inform that drug has potential for abuse; instruct not to share drug with others and to take steps to protect from theft or misuse. Discuss the risks of respiratory depression, orthostatic hypotension, syncope, severe constipation, and anaphylaxis; counsel on how to recognize symptoms and when to seek medical attention. Inform that accidental exposure may result in serious harm or death; advise to dispose unused tabs by flushing them down the toilet. Inform about risks of concomitant use of alcohol, other CNS depressants, MAOIs, and serotonergic drugs; instruct to notify physician if taking/planning to take additional medications. Instruct to not consume alcoholic beverages, or take prescription and OTC products that contain alcohol, during treatment. Counsel that drug may cause seizures if at risk for seizures or if patient has epilepsy; advise to d/c therapy and seek medical attention if seizures occur during therapy. Inform that drug may impair the ability to perform potentially hazardous activities (eg, driving a car or operating heavy machinery); advise not to perform such tasks until patients know how they will react to the medication. Advise females that drug can cause fetal harm; instruct to notify physician if pregnant/planning to become pregnant.

NUCYNTA ER — tapentadol   CII
Class: Centrally acting analgesic

> Exposes users to risks of addiction, abuse, and misuse, which can lead to overdose and death; assess each patient's risk prior to prescribing and monitor regularly for development of these behaviors/conditions. Serious, life-threatening, or fatal respiratory depression may occur; monitor during initiation or following a dose increase. Crushing, dissolving, or chewing tab can cause rapid release and absorption of potentially fatal dose; instruct patients to swallow tab whole. Accidental ingestion, especially by children, can result in a fatal overdose. Prolonged use during pregnancy can result in neonatal opioid withdrawal syndrome; advise pregnant women of the risk and ensure availability of appropriate treatment. Avoid use with alcoholic beverages or medications containing alcohol; may result in increased levels and potentially fatal overdose of tapentadol.

ADULT DOSAGE

Severe Pain (Daily, Around-the-Clock Management)

Pain severe enough to require daily, around-the-clock, long-term opioid treatment and for which alternative treatment options are inadequate

1st Opioid Analgesic/Opioid Intolerant Patients:
Initial: 50mg bid (q12h)
Titrate: Increase by 50mg no more than twice daily every 3 days

Diabetic Peripheral Neuropathy

Neuropathic pain severe enough to require daily, around-the-clock, long-term opioid treatment and for which alternative treatment options are inadequate

1st Opioid Analgesic/Opioid Intolerant Patients:
Initial: 50mg bid (q12h)
Titrate: Increase by 50mg no more than twice daily every 3 days

Conversions

From Immediate-Release (IR) to (Extended-Release) ER Tapentadol:
Use the equivalent total daily dose of IR tapentadol and divide it into 2 equal doses of ER tapentadol separated by approx 12-hr intervals

From Other Opioids:
D/C all other around-the-clock opioids when therapy is initiated; begin w/ 1/2 of the estimated daily tapentadol requirement as the initial dose, managing inadequate analgesia by supplementation w/ IR rescue medication

PEDIATRIC DOSAGE
Pediatric use may not have been established

DOSING CONSIDERATIONS

Renal Impairment
Severe: Not recommended

Hepatic Impairment
Moderate (Child-Pugh Score 7-9):
Initial: 50mg qd
Max: 100mg/day

Severe (Child-Pugh Score 10-15):
Not recommended

Elderly
Start at lower end of dosing range

Discontinuation
Use gradual downward titration

ADMINISTRATION
Oral route

Swallow tab whole; do not cut, crush, dissolve, or chew.
Take 1 tab at a time w/ enough water to ensure complete swallowing.

STORAGE
≤25°C (77°F); excursions permitted to 15-30°C (59-86°F). Protect from moisture.

HOW SUPPLIED
Tab, ER: 50mg, 100mg, 150mg, 200mg, 250mg

CONTRAINDICATIONS
Significant respiratory depression, acute or severe bronchial asthma or hypercarbia in an unmonitored setting or in the absence of resuscitative equipment, known or suspected paralytic ileus, patients receiving MAOIs or who have taken them within the last 14 days. Hypersensitivity (eg, anaphylaxis, angioedema) to tapentadol or to any other ingredients of the product.

WARNINGS/PRECAUTIONS

Reserve for use in patients for whom alternative treatment options are ineffective, not tolerated, or would be otherwise inadequate to provide sufficient management of pain. Should only be prescribed by healthcare professionals who are knowledgeable in the use of potent opioids for management of chronic pain. D/C all other tapentadol and tramadol products when initiating and during therapy. Life-threatening respiratory depression is more likely to occur in elderly, cachectic, or debilitated patients. Consider alternative nonopioid analgesics in patients with significant COPD or cor pulmonale, and in patients having a substantially decreased respiratory reserve, hypoxia, hypercarbia, or preexisting respiratory depression. May cause severe hypotension; increased risk in patients whose ability to maintain BP is compromised by a reduced blood volume or concurrent administration of certain CNS depressants. Avoid with circulatory shock, impaired consciousness, or coma. Monitor patients who may be susceptible to intracranial effects of carbon dioxide retention for signs of sedation and respiratory depression when initiating therapy. May obscure clinical course in patients with head injury. May aggravate convulsions and induce/aggravate seizures. May cause spasm of sphincter of Oddi; monitor patients with biliary tract disease (eg, acute pancreatitis). May impair mental/physical abilities. Monitor for respiratory/CNS depression with moderate hepatic impairment. Not recommended with severe renal/hepatic impairment.

ADVERSE REACTIONS

Respiratory depression, N/V, dizziness, constipation, headache, somnolence, fatigue, dry mouth, hyperhidrosis, pruritus, insomnia, dyspepsia, diarrhea, decreased appetite, anxiety.

DRUG INTERACTIONS

See Boxed Warning and Contraindications. Hypotension, profound sedation, coma, and respiratory depression may occur with CNS depressants (eg, sedatives, anxiolytics, hypnotics); if coadministration is required, consider dose reduction of one or both agents. Serotonin syndrome may occur with serotonergic drugs (eg, SSRIs, SNRIs, TCAs, triptans, drugs that affect serotonergic neurotransmitter system) and drugs that may impair metabolism of serotonin (eg, MAOIs). Avoid use of mixed agonist/antagonist (eg, nalbuphine, pentazocine, butorphanol) and partial agonists (eg, buprenorphine) analgesics; may reduce analgesic effects and/or precipitate withdrawal symptoms. Enhanced neuromuscular blocking action and increased degree of respiratory depression with skeletal muscle relaxants. Anticholinergics may increase risk of urinary retention and/or severe constipation, which may lead to paralytic ileus.

PREGNANCY AND LACTATION

Pregnancy: Category C.
Lactation: Not for use in nursing.

MECHANISM OF ACTION

Centrally acting synthetic analgesic; not established. Suspected to be due to μ-opioid receptor agonist activity and the inhibition of norepinephrine reuptake.

PHARMACOKINETICS

Absorption: T_{max}=3-6 hrs; absolute bioavailability (32%). **Distribution:** (IV) V_d=540L; plasma protein binding (20%); crosses placenta. **Metabolism:** Conjugation; N-desmethyl tapentadol by CYP2C9 and CYP2C19; hydroxy tapentadol by CYP2D6. **Elimination:** Kidneys (99%), urine (3% unchanged, 70% conjugated); $T_{1/2}$=5 hrs.

PATIENT CONSIDERATIONS

Assessment: Assess for abuse/addiction risk, opioid experience/tolerance, pain type/severity, pregnancy/nursing status, possible drug interactions, and any other condition where treatment is contraindicated or cautioned.

Monitoring: Monitor for signs/symptoms of respiratory depression, hypotension, symptoms of worsening biliary tract disease, aggravation/induction of seizure, mental/physical impairment, serotonin syndrome, and other adverse reactions. Routinely monitor for signs of misuse, abuse, and addiction.

Counseling: Inform that drug has potential for abuse and addiction; instruct not to share drug with others and to take steps to protect from theft or misuse. Inform about risk of accidental exposure and advise to store securely and to dispose unused tabs by flushing them down the toilet. Inform about the risks of life-threatening respiratory depression, orthostatic hypotension, and syncope. Inform about risks of concomitant use of alcohol, other CNS depressants, MAOIs, and serotonergic drugs; instruct to notify physician if taking/planning to take additional medications. Instruct to not consume alcoholic beverages or take prescription/OTC products that contain alcohol during treatment. Counsel on the risk for seizures and advise to d/c therapy and seek medical attention if seizures occur. Advise to use ud. Inform that drug may impair the ability to perform potentially hazardous activities; advise not to perform such tasks until patients know how they will react to medication. Advise of potential for severe constipation, including management instructions. Advise how to recognize anaphylaxis and when to seek medical attention. Advise females that drug can cause fetal harm; instruct to notify physician if pregnant/planning to become pregnant.

NUEDEXTA — dextromethorphan hydrobromide/quinidine sulfate   **Rx**

Class: CYP2D6 inhibitor/NMDA receptor antagonist

ADULT DOSAGE

Pseudobulbar Affect

Initial: 1 cap qd for 7 days
Maint: 1 cap q12h on Day 8 and thereafter

Periodically reassess need for continued treatment

PEDIATRIC DOSAGE

Pediatric use may not have been established

ADMINISTRATION

Oral route

May be taken w/o regard to meals

STORAGE

25°C (77°F); excursions permitted to 15-30°C (59-86°F).

HOW SUPPLIED

Cap: (Dextromethorphan-Quinidine) 20mg-10mg

CONTRAINDICATIONS

History of Nuedexta, quinine, mefloquine or quinidine-induced thrombocytopenia, hepatitis, bone marrow depression or lupus-like syndrome, known hypersensitivity to dextromethorphan (eg, rash, hives). Prolonged QT interval, congenital long QT syndrome or history suggestive of torsades de pointes, and heart failure. Complete AV block w/o implanted pacemakers, or high risk of complete AV block. During or w/in 14 days of MAOI therapy. Concomitant use w/ quinidine, quinine, mefloquine, and drugs that both prolong QT interval and are metabolized by CYP2D6 (eg, thioridazine and pimozide).

WARNINGS/PRECAUTIONS

May cause immune-mediated thrombocytopenia; d/c immediately if this occurs. Associated w/ lupus-like syndrome involving polyarthritis, rash, bronchospasm, lymphadenopathy, hemolytic anemia, vasculitis, uveitis, angioedema, agranulocytosis, sicca syndrome, myalgia, skeletal-muscle enzymes elevation, and pneumonitis. Hepatitis (eg, granulomatous hepatitis) reported. Fever and other signs of hypersensitivity may occur. QT prolongation reported; may cause torsades de pointes-type ventricular tachycardia. ECG evaluation should be conducted at baseline and 3-4 hrs after 1st dose in patients w/ left ventricular hypertrophy, left ventricular dysfunction, and those taking drugs that prolong the QT interval or that are strong or moderate CYP3A4 inhibitors. Reevaluate ECG if risk factors of arrhythmia change during therapy. Hypokalemia and hypomagnesemia should be corrected prior to therapy and monitored during treatment. D/C if cardiac arrhythmia (eg, syncope or palpitations) occurs. May cause dizziness; caution in patients w/ motor impairment affecting gait or w/ history of falls. Monitor for worsening clinical condition in myasthenia gravis and other conditions adversely affected by anticholinergic effects.

ADVERSE REACTIONS

Diarrhea, dizziness, cough, vomiting, asthenia, peripheral edema, UTI, influenza, increased gamma-glutamyltransferase, flatulence.

DRUG INTERACTIONS

See Contraindications. Recommend ECG in patients taking drugs that prolong QT interval and patients taking moderate or strong CYP3A4 inhibitors. Concomitant use w/ SSRIs or TCAs increases risk of serotonin syndrome. Adjust dose of desipramine or paroxetine if used concomitantly. May increase digoxin levels; monitor digoxin concentration and reduce dose if necessary. Caution w/ alcohol and other centrally acting drugs.

PREGNANCY AND LACTATION

Category C, caution in nursing.

MECHANISM OF ACTION

Dextromethorphan: Sigma-1 receptor and uncompetitive NMDA receptor antagonist; has not been established. Quinidine: CYP2D6 inhibitor; increases plasma levels of dextromethorphan by competitively inhibiting CYP2D6, which catalyzes a major biotransformation pathway for dextromethorphan.

PHARMACOKINETICS

Absorption: Dextromethorphan: Tmax=3-4 hrs. Quinidine: C_{max}=2-5mcg/mL; T_{max}=1-2 hrs. **Distribution:** Dextromethorphan: Plasma protein binding (60-70%). Quinidine: Plasma protein binding (80-89%). **Metabolism:** Liver. Dextromethorphan: CYP2D6. Quinidine: CYP3A4; 3-hydroxyquinidine (major metabolite). **Elimination:** Dextromethorphan: $T_{1/2}$=13 hrs. Quinidine: Urine (20%, unchanged); $T_{1/2}$=7 hrs.

PATIENT CONSIDERATIONS

Assessment: Assess for drug hypersensitivity, history of drug-induced thrombocytopenia, chronic HTN, known coronary artery disease, history of stroke, electrolyte abnormality (eg, hypokalemia, hypomagnesemia), bradycardia, family history of QT abnormality, or any other condition where treatment is contraindicated or cautioned. Assess renal/hepatic function, pregnancy/nursing status, and possible drug interactions. Obtain baseline ECG and genotyping.

Monitoring: Monitor for signs/symptoms of thrombocytopenia, lupus-like syndrome, hepatitis, fever, hypersensitivity, QTc prolongation, cardiac arrhythmias, dizziness, serotonin syndrome, hypokalemia, hypomagnesemia, and other adverse reactions. Monitor ECG 3-4 hrs after the 1st dose in patients at risk of QT prolongation and torsades de pointes. Reevaluate ECG if risk factors of arrhythmia change during therapy. Monitor for worsening clinical condition in myasthenia gravis and other conditions that may be adversely affected by anticholinergic effects. Periodically reassess need for continued treatment.

Counseling: Instruct to take medication as prescribed, not to take >2 caps in 24-hr period, and to make sure there is an approximate 12-hr interval between doses. Advise to inform physician if taking or planning to take other medications. Advise to seek immediate medical attention if hypersensitivity reactions, fainting, or loss of consciousness occurs. Instruct not to share or give medication to others even if w/ the same symptoms. Counsel to contact physician if PBA persists or worsens. Advise to use precautions to reduce risk of falls as dizziness may occur.

Nulojix — belatacept   Rx
Class: Selective costimulation modulator

> Increased risk for developing post-transplant lymphoproliferative disorder (PTLD), predominantly involving the CNS. Risk is increased in recipients without immunity to Epstein-Barr virus (EBV); use in EBV seropositive patients only. Do not use in transplant recipients who are EBV seronegative or with unknown serostatus. Should only be prescribed by physicians experienced in immunosuppressive therapy and management of kidney transplant patients. Manage patients in facilities equipped and staffed with adequate lab and supportive medical resources. Increased susceptibility to infection and the possible development of malignancies may result from immunosuppression. Use in liver transplant patients is not recommended due to an increased risk of graft loss and death.

ADULT DOSAGE
Organ Rejection Prophylaxis

Used in combination w/ basiliximab induction, mycophenolate mofetil, and corticosteroids in patients receiving a kidney transplant

The total infusion dose should be based on the actual body weight of the patient at the time of transplantation, and should not be modified during the course of therapy, unless there is a change in body weight of >10%

The prescribed dose must be evenly divisible by 12.5mg in order for the dose to be prepared accurately using the reconstituted sol and the silicone-free disposable syringe provided; evenly divisible increments are 0, 12.5, 25, 37.5, 50, 62.5, 75, 87.5, and 100

Initial Phase:
10mg/kg on Day 1 (day of transplantation, prior to implantation), Day 5 (approx 96 hrs after Day 1 dose), and end of Week 2, 4, 8, and 12 after transplantation

Maint Phase:
5mg/kg at the end of Week 16 after transplantation and every 4 weeks (± 3 days) thereafter

PEDIATRIC DOSAGE
Pediatric use may not have been established

ADMINISTRATION
IV route
Patients do not require premedication prior to administration

Preparation for Administration
1. Calculate the number of vials required to provide the total infusion dose; each vial contains 25mg of belatacept lyophilized powder
2. Reconstitute the contents of each vial w/ 10.5mL of a suitable diluent using the silicone-free disposable syringe provided w/ each vial and an 18- to 21-gauge needle; suitable diluents include: sterile water for inj (SWFI), 0.9% NaCl (NS), or D5W
Note: If the powder is accidentally reconstituted using a different syringe than the one provided, the sol may develop a few translucent particles; discard any sol prepared using siliconized syringes
3. To reconstitute the powder, insert the syringe needle into the vial through the center of the rubber stopper and direct the stream of diluent to the glass wall of the vial
4. To minimize foam formation, rotate the vial and invert w/ gentle swirling until the contents are completely dissolved; do not shake
5. The reconstituted sol contains a belatacept concentration of 25mg/mL and should be clear to slightly opalescent and colorless to pale yellow; do not use if opaque particles, discoloration, or other foreign particles are present
6. Calculate the total volume of the reconstituted 25mg/mL sol required to provide the total infusion dose
7. Prior to IV infusion, the required volume of the reconstituted sol must be further diluted w/ a suitable infusion fluid (NS or D5W). Nulojix reconstituted w/:
SWFI: Further dilute w/ either NS or D5W
NS: Further dilute w/ NS
D5W: Further dilute w/ D5W
8. From the appropriate size infusion bag or bottle, withdraw a volume of infusion fluid that is equal to the volume of the reconstituted sol required to provide the prescribed dose
9. W/ the same silicone-free disposable syringe used for reconstitution, withdraw the required amount of belatacept sol from the vial, inject it into the infusion bag or bottle, and gently rotate the infusion bag or bottle to ensure mixing
10. The final belatacept concentration in the infusion bag or bottle should range from 2-10mg/mL. Typically, an infusion volume of 100mL will be appropriate for most patients and doses, but total infusion volumes ranging from 50-250mL may be used; any unused sol remaining in the vials must be discarded
11. Administer entire infusion over a period of 30 min w/ an infusion set and a sterile, non-pyrogenic, low-protein-binding filter (w/ a pore size of 0.2-1.2μm)
12. Transfer the reconstituted sol from the vial to the infusion bag or bottle immediately; the infusion must be completed w/in 24 hrs of reconstitution of the lyophilized powder
13. Infuse in a separate line from other concomitantly infused agents; do not infuse concomitantly in the same IV line w/ other agents

STORAGE
Vial: 2-8°C (36-46°F). Protect from light by storing in the original package until time of use. Reconstituted Sol: 2-8°C (36-46°F) for up to 24 hrs. Protect from light. Max of 4 hrs of the total 24 hrs can be at room temperature (20-25°C) [68-77°F] and room light.

HOW SUPPLIED
Inj: 250mg

CONTRAINDICATIONS
Transplant recipients who are EBV seronegative or with unknown EBV serostatus.

WARNINGS/PRECAUTIONS
Administration of higher than recommended doses of drug or concomitant immunosuppressive agents or more frequent dosing is not recommended. Cytomegalovirus (CMV) infection and T-cell-depleting therapy are other known risk factors for PTLD; use T-cell depleting therapies cautiously. Patients who are EBV seropositive and CMV seronegative may also be at increased risk for PTLD. Limit exposure to sunlight and UV light. Progressive multifocal leukoencephalopathy (PML) reported at higher cumulative doses and more frequent regimens. Consider PTLD or PML if new or worsening neurological, cognitive, or behavioral signs/symptoms develop. If PML is diagnosed, consider reduction or withdrawal of immunosuppression taking into account the risk to the allograft. May increase risk of developing bacterial (tuberculosis [TB]), viral (CMV and herpes), fungal, and protozoal infections, including opportunistic infections; prophylaxis for CMV (for at least 3 months after transplantation) and *Pneumocystis jiroveci* are recommended after transplantation. Initiate treatment of latent TB infection prior to belatacept use. Polyoma virus-associated nephropathy (PVAN) reported; consider reductions in immunosuppression if evidence of PVAN develops. Increased rate and grade of acute rejection and graft loss reported with corticosteroid minimization to 5mg/day between Day 3 and Week 6 post-transplantation; corticosteroid utilization should be consistent with the belatacept clinical trial experience.

ADVERSE REACTIONS
PTLD, malignancies, anemia, diarrhea, urinary tract infection, peripheral edema, constipation, HTN, pyrexia, graft dysfunction, cough, N/V, headache, hypokalemia, hyperkalemia.

DRUG INTERACTIONS
Avoid use of live vaccines (eg, intranasal influenza, measles, mumps, rubella, oral polio, BCG, yellow fever, varicella, TY21a typhoid). Monitor for a need to adjust concomitant MMF dosage when therapy is switched between cyclosporine and belatacept, as cyclosporine decreases mycophenolic acid (MPA) exposure while belatacept does not. A higher MMF dosage may be needed after switching from belatacept to cyclosporine, since this may result in lower MPA concentrations and increase the risk of rejection. A lower MMF dosage may be needed after switching from cyclosporine to belatacept, since this may result in higher MPA concentrations and increase the risk for adverse reactions related to MPA.

PREGNANCY AND LACTATION
Category C, not for use in nursing.

MECHANISM OF ACTION
Selective T-cell costimulation blocker; binds to CD80 and CD86 on antigen-presenting cells, thereby blocking CD28 mediated costimulation of T lymphocytes.

PHARMACOKINETICS
Absorption: C_{max}=247mcg/mL (10mg/kg), 139mcg/mL (5mg/kg); AUC=22,252mcg•hr/mL (10mg/kg), 14,090mcg•hr/mL (5mg/kg). **Distribution:** V_d=0.11L/kg (10mg/kg), 0.12L/kg (5mg/kg). **Elimination:** $T_{1/2}$=9.8 days (10mg/kg), 8.2 days (5mg/kg).

PATIENT CONSIDERATIONS
Assessment: Assess for EBV serostatus, presence of infections, pregnancy/nursing status, possible drug interactions, and any other conditions where treatment is cautioned.

Monitoring: Monitor for PTLD, PML, infections, malignancies, TB, PVAN, and other adverse reactions.

Counseling: Instruct to immediately report any neurological, cognitive, or behavioral signs/symptoms during and after therapy (eg, changes in mood or usual behavior, confusion, problems thinking, memory loss, changes in walking or talking, decreased strength or weakness on one side of the body, changes in vision). Inform about increased risk of PTLD, malignancies (eg, skin cancer), PML, and infections. Advise to adhere to antimicrobial prophylaxis regimens as prescribed and to immediately report any signs/symptoms of infection during therapy. Instruct to limit exposure to sunlight and UV light by wearing protective clothing and using sunscreen with high protection factor. Instruct to look for any signs/symptoms of skin cancer (eg, suspicious moles or lesions). Advise to avoid live vaccines. Instruct to inform physician if pregnant/planning to become pregnant, or if breastfeeding.

NuLYTELY — polyethylene glycol 3350/potassium chloride/sodium bicarbonate/sodium chloride   Rx

Class: Bowel cleanser

OTHER BRAND NAMES
Trilyte

ADULT DOSAGE
Bowel Cleansing
Prior to Colonoscopy:
Oral:
240mL (8 oz) every 10 min until 4L consumed or rectal effluent is clear

NG Tube:
20-30mL/min (1.2-1.8L/hr)

PEDIATRIC DOSAGE
Bowel Cleansing
Prior to Colonoscopy:
≥6 Months of Age:
Oral/NG Tube:
25mL/kg/hr until rectal effluent is clear

ADMINISTRATION
Oral/NG Tube route

May be used w/ or w/o flavor pack.
Rapid drinking of each portion is preferred to drinking small amounts continuously.
First bowel movement should occur approx 1 hr after the start of administration.

Nulytely
Sol is more palatable if chilled prior to administration.
Patients may consume water or clear liquids during and after completion of the bowel preparation up until 2 hrs before the time of the colonoscopy.
Instructions Prior to Dosage:
On the day prior to colonoscopy, instruct patients to:
1. Take only clear liquids, but avoid red and purple liquids. Patients may consume a light breakfast.
2. If adding a flavor pack, pour the contents of the 2g flavor powder into the container prior to reconstitution. No additional flavorings should be added. Discard unused flavor packs. The flavor packs are for use only in combination w/ the contents of the accompanying 4L container.
3. Early in the pm prior to colonoscopy, fill the supplied container containing the powder (and if applicable, a flavor powder) w/ lukewarm water to the 4L fill line. The sol is clear and colorless when reconstituted to a final volume of 4L.
4. After capping the container, shake vigorously several times to ensure that the ingredients are dissolved.

Trilyte
Sol is more palatable if chilled prior to administration; chilled sol is not recommended for infants.
No solid food should be consumed during the 3- to 4-hr period before drinking the sol, but in no case should solid foods be eaten w/in 2 hr of taking Trilyte w/ flavor packs.
Preparation of Sol:
1. If adding a flavor pack, tear open 1 flavor pack at the indicated marking and pour contents into the bottle before reconstitution; discard unused flavor packs.
2. Shake well to incorporate flavoring into the powder.
3. Add tap water to fill line marked 4L.
4. Replace cap tightly and shake well until all ingredients have dissolved; no additional ingredients should be added to the sol.

STORAGE
25°C (77°F); excursions permitted between 15-30°C (59-86°F). Reconstituted Sol: Keep refrigerated. Use w/in 48 hrs.

HOW SUPPLIED
Sol (Powder): (Polyethylene Glycol (PEG) 3350/Potassium Chloride/Sodium Bicarbonate/Sodium Chloride) 420g/1.48g/5.72g/11.2g [4L]

CONTRAINDICATIONS
GI obstruction, ileus, or gastric retention; bowel perforation; toxic colitis or toxic megacolon; known allergy or hypersensitivity to any component of NuLYTELY.

WARNINGS/PRECAUTIONS
Slow administration or temporarily d/c if severe bloating, distention, or abdominal pain develops; caution w/ severe ulcerative colitis. Monitor for occurrence of possible hypoglycemia in children <2 years of age as the sol has no caloric substrate. Dehydration and hypokalemia reported in children. Caution in patients w/ impaired gag reflex, unconscious or semiconscious patients, and patients prone to regurgitation or aspiration; observe during administration especially if administered via NG tube. (Nulytely) Adequately hydrate before, during, and after use; caution w/ CHF when replacing fluids. Consider performing postcolonoscopy lab tests (electrolytes, SrCr, BUN) and treat accordingly if significant vomiting or signs of dehydration develop. Correct fluid and electrolyte abnormalities before treatment. Caution w/ conditions that increase risk for fluid and electrolyte disturbances or may increase risk of adverse events (eg, seizures, arrhythmias, and renal impairment). Serious arrhythmias reported rarely; caution in patients at increased risk of arrhythmias and consider predose and postcolonoscopy ECGs. Generalized tonic-clonic seizures and/or loss of consciousness reported; caution in patients w/ a history of or at increased risk of seizures (eg, w/ known/suspected hyponatremia). Caution w/ impaired renal function; consider performing baseline and postcolonoscopy lab tests. May produce colonic mucosal aphthous ulcerations; consider this when interpreting colonoscopy findings in patients w/ known/suspected inflammatory bowel disease. Serious cases of ischemic colitis reported. Not for direct ingestion; direct ingestion of undissolved powder may increase risk of N/V, dehydration, and electrolyte disturbances.

ADVERSE REACTIONS
Nausea, abdominal fullness, abdominal bloating.

DRUG INTERACTIONS
Oral medication administered w/in 1 hr of start of administration may be flushed from GI tract and may not be absorbed properly. (Nulytely) Caution w/ medications that increase risk for fluid and electrolyte disturbances or may increase risk of adverse events (eg, seizures, arrhythmias, prolonged QT, renal impairment). Caution w/ drugs that lower seizure threshold (eg, TCAs) and in patients withdrawing from alcohol or benzodiazepines. Caution w/ drugs that may affect renal function (eg, diuretics, ACE inhibitors, ARBs, NSAIDs). Avoid w/ stimulant laxatives (eg, bisacodyl, sodium picosulfate); may increase the risk of mucosal ulceration or ischemic colitis.

PREGNANCY AND LACTATION
Pregnancy: Category C.
Lactation: Caution in nursing.

MECHANISM OF ACTION
Osmotic laxative; primary mode of action is thought to be through the osmotic effect of PEG 3350 which causes water to be retained in the colon and produces a watery stool.

PHARMACOKINETICS
Absorption: Poor (Oral PEG 3350).

PATIENT CONSIDERATIONS
Assessment: Assess for drug hypersensitivity, GI obstruction, bowel perforation, gastric retention, ileus, toxic colitis, toxic megacolon, fluid and electrolyte abnormalities, renal impairment, any other conditions where treatment is cautioned, pregnancy/nursing status, and possible drug interactions. Consider predose ECG in patients at increased risk of serious cardiac arrhythmias.

Monitoring: Monitor arrhythmias, generalized tonic-clonic seizures, loss of consciousness, colonic mucosal aphthous ulceration, ischemic colitis, and other adverse reactions. Monitor patients w/ impaired gag reflex, unconscious or semiconscious patients, and patients prone to regurgitation/aspiration, especially if administered via NG tube. Monitor for hypoglycemia, dehydration, and hypokalemia in children. Consider performing postcolonoscopy lab tests (electrolytes, SrCr, BUN) in patients w/ dehydration or renal impairment.

Counseling: Inform that sol is more palatable if chilled. Instruct to inform physician if patient has trouble swallowing or is prone to regurgitation or aspiration. Instruct not to take other laxatives. Instruct to consume water or clear liquids during the bowel preparation and after completion of the bowel preparation up until 2 hrs before the time of the colonoscopy. If severe bloating, distention, or abdominal pain occurs, instruct to slow or temporarily d/c administration until symptoms abate; advise to report these events to physician. Instruct to d/c and contact physician if hives, rashes, or any allergic reaction develops. Instruct to notify physician if signs/symptoms of dehydration develop. Inform that oral medication administered w/in 1 hr of the start of administration may be flushed from the GI tract and the medication may not be absorbed completely. Counsel that rapid drinking of each portion is preferred rather than drinking small amounts continuously. Inform that 1st bowel movement should occur approximately 1 hr after start of administration and to continue drinking until the watery stool is clear and free of solid matter.

NUPLAZID — pimavanserin   Rx

Class: Atypical antipsychotic

> Elderly patients w/ dementia-related psychosis treated w/ antipsychotic drugs are at an increased risk of death. Not approved for the treatment of patients w/ dementia-related psychosis unrelated to the hallucinations and delusions associated w/ Parkinson's disease psychosis.

ADULT DOSAGE
Parkinson's Disease Psychosis
Treatment of hallucinations and delusions associated w/ Parkinson's disease psychosis

34mg qd, w/o titration

PEDIATRIC DOSAGE
Pediatric use may not have been established

DOSING CONSIDERATIONS
Concomitant Medications
Strong CYP3A4 Inhibitors:
17mg qd

Strong CYP3A4 Inducers:
Monitor for reduced efficacy; may need to increase pimavanserin dose

Renal Impairment
Severe (CrCl <30mL/min): Not recommended

Hepatic Impairment
Not recommended

ADMINISTRATION
Oral route

May take w/ or w/o food.

STORAGE
20-25°C (68-77°F); excursions permitted to 15-30°C (59-86°F).

HOW SUPPLIED
Tab: 17mg

WARNINGS/PRECAUTIONS

May prolong the QT interval; avoid in patients w/ known QT prolongation, a history of cardiac arrhythmias, and in circumstances that may increase the risk of the occurrence of torsades de pointes and/or sudden death (eg, symptomatic bradycardia, hypokalemia, hypomagnesemia, presence of congenital prolongation of the QT interval).

ADVERSE REACTIONS

Peripheral edema, confusional state.

DRUG INTERACTIONS

See Dosing Considerations. Avoid w/ other drugs known to prolong the QT interval (eg, quinidine, amiodarone, ziprasidone, chlorpromazine, thioridazine, moxifloxacin). Strong CYP3A4 inhibitors (eg, ketoconazole, clarithromycin, indinavir) may increase exposure. Strong CYP3A4 inducers (eg, carbamazepine, phenytoin, St. John's wort) may reduce exposure and result in a potential decrease in efficacy.

PREGNANCY AND LACTATION

Pregnancy: There are no data on pimavanserin use in pregnant women that would allow assessment of the drug-associated risk of major congenital malformations or miscarriage.
Lactation: There is no information regarding the presence of pimavanserin in human milk, the effects on the breastfed infant, or the effects on milk production.

MECHANISM OF ACTION

Atypical antipsychotic; mechanism not established. Effects could be mediated through a combination of inverse agonist and antagonist activity at serotonin 5-HT$_{2A}$ receptors and to a lesser extent at serotonin 5-HT$_{2C}$ receptors.

PHARMACOKINETICS

Absorption: T_{max}=6 hrs (median). **Distribution:** V_d=2173L; plasma protein binding (95%). **Metabolism:** Predominantly via CYP3A4 and CYP3A5, and lesser extent via CYP2J2, CYP2D6, and various other CYP and FMO enzymes; AC-279 (major active metabolite). **Elimination:** Urine (<1% of dose of pimavanserin and its active metabolite recovered, 0.55% unchanged), feces (1.53%); $T_{1/2}$=57 hrs (pimavanserin), 200 hrs (active metabolite).

PATIENT CONSIDERATIONS

Assessment: Assess for QT prolongation, history of cardiac arrhythmias, symptomatic bradycardia, hypokalemia, hypomagnesemia, renal/hepatic impairment, pregnancy/nursing status, and possible drug interactions.
Monitoring: Monitor for QT prolongation and any other adverse reaction.
Counseling: Advise to notify physician of all prescription and nonprescription medications currently taking.

NUTROPIN AQ — somatropin (rDNA origin)   Rx

Class: Recombinant human growth hormone (hGH)

ADULT DOSAGE

Growth Hormone Deficiency

Adult or Childhood-Onset Etiology:
Weight-Based:
Initial: ≤0.006mg/kg qd SQ
Titrate: May increase based on individual requirements
Maint: Individualize dose
Max:
≤35 Years: 0.025mg/kg qd
>35 Years: 0.0125mg/kg qd
Non-Weight-Based:
Initial: 0.2mg/day SQ (range, 0.15-0.30mg/day)
Titrate: May increase gradually every 1-2 months by increments of 0.1-0.2mg/day based on clinical response and serum insulin-like growth factor-I (IGF-I) concentrations
Maint: Individualize dose

PEDIATRIC DOSAGE

Growth Hormone Deficiency

Due to an inadequate secretion of endogenous growth hormone (GH)
Individualize dose
Recommended Dose: Up to 0.3mg/kg/week
Pubertal Patients: May use up to 0.7mg/kg/week
Divide weekly dose into daily SQ inj

Idiopathic Short Stature

Treatment of idiopathic short stature defined by height standard deviation score ≤-2.25, and associated w/ growth rates unlikely to permit attainment of adult height in the normal range, in pediatric patients whose epiphyses are not closed and for whom diagnostic evaluation excludes other causes associated w/ short stature that should be observed or treated by other means
Individualize dose
Recommended Dose: Up to 0.3mg/kg/week
Divide weekly dose into daily SQ inj

Growth Failure Secondary to Chronic Kidney Disease

Individualize dose
Recommended Dose: Up to 0.35mg/kg/week
Continue therapy up to the time of renal transplantation
Divide weekly dose into daily SQ inj
Hemodialysis: Give at hs or at least 3-4 hrs after dialysis
Chronic Cycling Peritoneal Dialysis: Give in am after completion of dialysis

Chronic Ambulatory Peritoneal Dialysis: Give in pm during overnight exchange

Turner Syndrome

Treatment of short stature associated w/ Turner syndrome (TS)
Individualize dose
Recommended Dose: Up to 0.375mg/kg/week divided into equal doses 3-7X/week SQ

DOSING CONSIDERATIONS

Concomitant Medications
Oral Estrogen: May increase the dose requirements in women
Elderly
Consider lower starting dose and smaller dose increments

ADMINISTRATION

SQ route
Rotate inj sites to avoid lipodystrophy.

Reconstitution

- The Nutropin AQ Pen 10 and 20mg cartridges are color-banded to help ensure appropriate use w/ the Nutropin AQ Pen delivery device. Each cartridge must be used w/ its corresponding color-coded Nutropin AQ Pen.
- Follow the directions provided in the Nutropin AQ Pen and Nutropin AQ NuSpin 5, 10, or 20 instructions for use.

STORAGE

2-8°C (36-46°F) for 28 days after initial use. Avoid freezing. Protect from light.

HOW SUPPLIED

Inj: 10mg/2mL, 20mg/2mL [pen cartridge], 5mg/2mL, 10mg/2mL, 20mg/2mL [NuSpin]

CONTRAINDICATIONS

Acute critical illness due to complications following open-heart surgery, abdominal surgery, multiple accidental trauma, or w/ acute respiratory failure. Pediatric patients w/ Prader-Willi syndrome (PWS) who are severely obese, have a history of upper airway obstruction or sleep apnea, or have severe respiratory impairment. Pediatric patients who have growth failure due to genetically confirmed PWS. Active malignancy, or evidence of progression or recurrence of an underlying intracranial tumor. Active proliferative or severe nonproliferative diabetic retinopathy. Growth promotion in pediatric patients w/ closed epiphysis. Known hypersensitivity to somatropin, excipients, or diluent.

WARNINGS/PRECAUTIONS

Reevaluate adults who were treated w/ somatropin for growth hormone deficiency (GHD) in childhood and whose epiphyses are closed. Treatment for short stature should be discontinued when epiphyses are fused. Implement effective weight control in patients w/ PWS and treat respiratory infections aggressively. Increased risk of developing malignancies in children w/ certain rare genetic causes of short stature; monitor for development of neoplasms if treatment is initiated. Monitor for increased growth, or potential malignant changes, of preexisting nevi. Undiagnosed impaired glucose tolerance and overt diabetes mellitus (DM) may be unmasked, and new-onset type 2 DM reported. Intracranial HTN w/ papilledema, visual changes, headache, and N/V reported; d/c therapy if papilledema occurs. Fluid retention in adults may occur. Monitor other hormonal replacement treatments in patients w/ hypopituitarism. Undiagnosed/untreated hypothyroidism may prevent optimal response. Hypothyroidism may become evident or worsen. Slipped capital femoral epiphysis (SCFE) and progression of scoliosis may occur in pediatric patients. Increased risk of ear/hearing disorders and cardiovascular (CV) disorders in TS patients. Periodically examine children w/ growth failure secondary to chronic kidney disease (CKD) for evidence of renal osteodystrophy progression. Tissue atrophy may occur; rotate inj site. Allergic reactions may occur. Serum levels of inorganic phosphorus, alkaline phosphatase, parathyroid hormone, and IGF-I may increase. Pancreatitis reported rarely. Obese individuals are more likely to manifest adverse effects when treated w/ a weight-based regimen. Estrogen replete women may need higher doses than men. Caution in elderly.

ADVERSE REACTIONS

Arthralgia, edema, joint disorders, otitis media, ear disorders, glucose intolerance, fluid retention.

DRUG INTERACTIONS

See Dosing Considerations. May inhibit 11β-hydroxysteroid dehydrogenase type 1, resulting in reduced serum cortisol concentrations; may need glucocorticoid replacement or dose adjustments of glucocorticoid therapy. Glucocorticoid therapy may attenuate growth-promoting effects in children; carefully adjust glucocorticoid replacement therapy. May increase clearance of antipyrine. May alter clearance of compounds metabolized by CYP450 liver enzymes (eg, corticosteroids, sex steroids, anticonvulsants, cyclosporine); monitor carefully. Oral estrogens may reduce IGF-1 response to treatment. May need to adjust dose of insulin, oral/injectable hypoglycemic agents, and/or thyroid hormone replacement therapy.

PREGNANCY AND LACTATION

Pregnancy: Category C.
Lactation: Caution in nursing.

MECHANISM OF ACTION

Recombinant human GH; binds to dimeric GH receptors in cell membranes of target tissue cells, resulting in intracellular signal transduction.

PHARMACOKINETICS

Absorption: Absolute bioavailability (81%); C_{max}=71.1mcg/L; T_{max}=3.9 hrs; AUC=677mcg•hr/L. **Distribution:** V_d=50mL/kg. **Metabolism:** Liver and kidneys. **Elimination:** $T_{1/2}$=2.1 hrs.

PATIENT CONSIDERATIONS

Assessment: Assess for PWS, preexisting DM or impaired glucose tolerance, hypothyroidism, hypopituitarism, history of scoliosis, hypersensitivity, any other conditions where treatment is contraindicated or cautioned, pregnancy/nursing status, and possible drug interactions. Perform funduscopic exam. Obtain x-rays of the hip in CKD patients.

Monitoring: Monitor for neoplasm, increased growth or malignant changes of preexisting nevi, fluid retention, intracranial HTN, allergic reactions, pancreatitis, and SCFE and progression of scoliosis in pediatric patients (eg, onset of limp, hip or knee pain), and for any other adverse reaction. Perform periodic thyroid function tests, funduscopic exam, and monitoring of glucose levels. In patients w/ PWS, monitor weight as well as for signs of respiratory infection, sleep apnea, and upper airway obstruction. Monitor patients w/ a history of GHD secondary to an intracranial neoplasm routinely for progression/recurrence of the tumor. In patients w/ TS, monitor for ear/CV disorders. In patients w/ CKD, periodically examine for evidence of progression of renal osteodystrophy. Monitor clinical response.

Counseling: Inform about potential benefits and risks of therapy, proper administration, and usage and disposal. Caution against any reuse of needles and syringes.

NUVARING — ethinyl estradiol/etonogestrel Rx

Class: Estrogen/progestogen combination

> Cigarette smoking increases the risk of serious cardiovascular (CV) events. Risk increases w/ age and w/ number of cigarettes smoked. Not for use by women who are >35 yrs of age and smoke.

ADULT DOSAGE

Contraception

1 ring, inserted in the vagina and left in place continuously for 3 weeks, then removed for 1 week. Insert new ring 1 week after the last ring was removed

No Hormonal Contraceptive Use in the Preceding Cycle:

May insert ring on Days 1-5 of menstrual bleeding; if inserted on Days 2-5 of cycle, use an additional barrier method of contraception (eg, male condom w/ spermicide) for the first 7 days

Changing from a Combination Hormonal Contraceptive:

May switch on any day, but at the latest on the day following the usual hormone-free interval

Changing from Progestin-Only Method (Progestin-Only Pill, Implant, Inj, or Progestin-Releasing Intrauterine System):

May switch on any day from the progestin-only pill; start using ring on the day after taking last progestin-only pill
May switch from an implant or intrauterine system on the day of its removal and from an injectable on the day when the next inj is due
In all cases, additional barrier method (eg, male condom w/ spermicide) should be used for the first 7 days

Use After Abortion/Miscarriage:

May start w/in the first 5 days following a complete 1st trimester abortion/miscarriage; no additional method of contraception needed
If not started w/in 5 days, follow instructions for "No Hormonal Contraceptive Use in the Preceding Cycle" and use a non-hormonal contraceptive method in the meantime

Following Childbirth or 2nd Trimester Abortion/Miscarriage:

Use may be initiated no earlier than 4 weeks postpartum in women who elect not to breastfeed, or 4 weeks after a 2nd trimester abortion/miscarriage
If use is begun postpartum, use an additional method of contraception (eg, male condom w/ spermicide) for the first 7 days

PEDIATRIC DOSAGE

Contraception

Not indicated for use premenarche; refer to adult dosing

DOSING CONSIDERATIONS

Other Important Considerations

Inadvertent Removal/Expulsion:

Ring is Left Outside of Vagina for <3 Hrs: Rinse and reinsert as soon as possible, but at the latest w/in 3 hrs. If ring is lost, insert new vaginal ring and continue regimen w/o alteration

Ring is Left Outside of Vagina for >3 Hrs During Weeks 1 and 2: Reinsert ring as soon as remembered and use barrier method (eg, condoms w/ spermicides) until ring has been used continuously for 7 days

Ring is Left Outside of Vagina for >3 Hrs During Week 3: Discard that ring and insert new ring immediately which will start the next 3-week use period. Alternatively, insert new ring no later than 7 days from the time the previous ring was removed/expelled if previous ring was used continuously for at least 7 days. In either case, use a barrier method (eg, condoms w/ spermicides) until new ring has been used continuously for 7 days

Prolonged Ring-Free Interval:
If ring-free interval has been extended beyond 1 week, must use additional method of contraception until ring has been used continuously for 7 days

Prolonged Use of Ring:
Left in Place for Up to 1 Extra Week (up to 4 Weeks Total): Remove ring and insert new ring after 1-week ring-free interval
Left in Place for >4 Weeks: Remove ring, and if pregnancy is ruled out, may restart ring w/ additional method of contraception until ring has been used continuously for 7 days

Ring Breakage:
Discard ring and replace w/ new ring

Use w/ Other Vaginal Products:
Use of diaphragm is not recommended as backup method w/ ring use; ring may interfere w/ correct placement/position of a diaphragm

ADMINISTRATION

Intravaginal route

Compress ring and insert into the vagina; exact position of ring inside the vagina is not critical for its function.
Ring must be inserted on the appropriate day and left in place for 3 consecutive weeks.
Remove ring 3 weeks later, on the same day of the week and at about the same time as it was inserted.

Removal/Reinsertion

Remove by hooking index finger under the forward rim or by grasping the rim between index and middle finger and pulling out.
Used ring should be placed in the sachet (foil pouch) and discarded in a waste receptacle; do not flush in toilet.
Reinsert new ring exactly 1 week after previous ring was removed, even if menstrual bleeding has not finished.

STORAGE

2-8°C (36-46°F). After dispensing, store up to 4 months at 25°C (77°F); excursions permitted to 15-30°C (59-86°F). Avoid direct sunlight or >30°C (86°F).

HOW SUPPLIED

Vaginal Ring: (Ethinyl Estradiol/Etonogestrel) (0.015mg/0.120mg)/day

CONTRAINDICATIONS

A high risk of arterial or venous thrombotic diseases (eg, women who are known to smoke [if >35 yrs of age]), current or history of deep vein thrombosis or pulmonary embolism, cerebrovascular disease, coronary artery disease, thrombogenic valvular or thrombogenic rhythm diseases of the heart (eg, subacute bacterial endocarditis w/ valvular disease, or atrial fibrillation), inherited or acquired hypercoagulopathies, uncontrolled HTN, diabetes mellitus w/ vascular disease, headaches w/ focal neurological symptoms or migraine headaches w/ aura, >35 yrs of age w/ any migraine headaches. Benign or malignant liver tumors or liver disease, undiagnosed abnormal uterine bleeding, pregnancy, current or history of breast cancer or other estrogen- or progestin-sensitive cancer. Hypersensitivity to any of the components of NuvaRing.

WARNINGS/PRECAUTIONS

Consider possibility of ovulation and conception prior to 1st use. Increased risk of a venous thromboembolic event (VTE) and arterial thromboses; d/c if these occur. D/C if unexplained loss of vision, proptosis, diplopia, papilledema, or retinal vascular lesions develop; evaluate for retinal vein thrombosis immediately. D/C at least 4 weeks prior to and 2 weeks after major surgery associated w/ an elevated risk of thromboembolism and during and following prolonged immobilization, if feasible. Caution in women w/ CV disease risk factors. If patient exhibits signs/symptoms of toxic shock syndrome (TSS), consider possibility of this diagnosis and initiate appropriate medical evaluation and treatment. Acute or chronic disturbances of liver function may necessitate discontinuation until LFTs return to normal and CHC causation has been excluded. D/C if jaundice develops. May increase risk of cervical cancer or intraepithelial neoplasia, hepatic adenoma, hepatocellular carcinoma, and gallbladder disease. Increase in BP reported; monitor BP and d/c if BP rises significantly. May not be suitable for women w/ conditions that make the vagina more susceptible to vaginal irritation or ulceration; vaginal/cervical erosion or ulceration reported. May increase risk of cholestasis w/ subsequent CHC use in patients w/ a history of CHC-related or pregnancy-related cholestasis. May decrease glucose tolerance; monitor prediabetic and diabetic women. Consider alternative contraception w/ uncontrolled dyslipidemia. May increase risk of pancreatitis w/ hypertriglyceridemia or a family history thereof. D/C if indicated and evaluate cause if new headaches that are recurrent, persistent, or severe develop. Consider discontinuation in case of increased frequency or severity of migraine during use. Unscheduled (breakthrough or intracyclic) bleeding and spotting reported; check for causes (eg, pregnancy, malignancy) if bleeding persists or occurs after previously regular cycles. Consider possibility of pregnancy if scheduled (withdrawal) bleeding does not occur and patient has not adhered to prescribed dosing schedule or has adhered to prescribed regimen and misses 2 consecutive periods; d/c if pregnancy confirmed. Caution w/ history of depression; d/c if it recurs to a serious degree. May induce or exacerbate angioedema in patients w/ hereditary angioedema. Chloasma may occur; avoid exposure to sun or UV radiation in women w/ a tendency to chloasma. Inadvertent insertion into urinary bladder reported; assess for ring insertion into urinary bladder w/ persistent urinary symptoms and if unable to locate ring. Cases of disconnection of the ring at the weld joint reported; discard the ring and replace it w/ a new ring if this occurs. May interfere w/ correct placement and position of a diaphragm. May influence results of certain lab tests.

ADVERSE REACTIONS
Vaginitis, headache, mood changes, device-related events, vaginal discharge, increased weight, N/V, vaginal discomfort, breast pain, dysmenorrhea, abdominal pain.

DRUG INTERACTIONS
May decrease plasma concentrations and potentially diminish effectiveness or increase breakthrough bleeding when used concomitantly w/ drugs or herbal products that induce CYP3A4 (eg, phenytoin, barbiturates, products containing St. John's wort); use an alternative method of contraception or a backup method when used concomitantly w/ enzyme inducers, and continue backup contraception for 28 days after discontinuing enzyme inducers. Atorvastatin, ascorbic acid, acetaminophen, CYP3A4 inhibitors (eg, itraconazole, grapefruit juice, ketoconazole), and vaginal miconazole nitrate may increase plasma hormone levels. HIV protease inhibitors (eg, nelfinavir, ritonavir, indinavir), hepatitis C virus protease inhibitors (eg, boceprevir, telaprevir), and non-nucleoside reverse transcriptase inhibitors (eg, nevirapine, etravirine) may cause significant changes in plasma levels. May inhibit the metabolism of other compounds (eg, cyclosporine, prednisolone, theophylline, tizanidine, voriconazole) and increase their plasma concentrations. May decrease levels of acetaminophen, clofibric acid, morphine, salicylic acid, and temazepam. May decrease levels of lamotrigine and reduce seizure control; dosage adjustments of lamotrigine may be necessary. May raise serum concentrations of thyroxine-binding globulin and cortisol-binding globulin; may need to increase dose of replacement thyroid hormone or cortisol therapy.

PREGNANCY AND LACTATION
Pregnancy: Contraindicated in pregnancy. **Lactation:** Not for use in nursing.

MECHANISM OF ACTION
Estrogen/progestogen combination; acts by suppression of gonadotropins. Primarily inhibits ovulation. Also produces other alterations, including changes in the cervical mucus (increasing difficulty of sperm entry into the uterus) and the endometrium (reducing likelihood of implantation).

PHARMACOKINETICS
Absorption: Etonogestrel: Rapid; bioavailability (100%); C_{max}=1716pg/mL; T_{max}=200.3 hrs. Ethinyl estradiol: Rapid; bioavailability (56%); C_{max}=34.7pg/mL; T_{max}=59.3 hrs. **Distribution:** Found in breast milk. Etonogestrel: Serum albumin binding (66%), sex hormone-binding globulin (32%). Ethinyl estradiol: Serum albumin binding (98.5%). **Metabolism:** Hepatic via CYP3A4. Ethinyl estradiol: aromatic hydroxylation. **Elimination:** Urine, bile, feces; Etonogestrel: $T_{1/2}$=29.3 hrs; Ethinyl estradiol: $T_{1/2}$=44.7 hrs.

PATIENT CONSIDERATIONS
Assessment: Assess for high risk of arterial or venous thrombotic diseases; benign or malignant liver tumors; liver disease; undiagnosed, abnormal uterine bleeding; presence or history of breast cancer or other estrogen- or progestin-sensitive cancer; pregnancy; and any other conditions where treatment is contraindicated/cautioned. Assess nursing status and for possible drug interactions.

Monitoring: Monitor for arterial thromboses or VTEs, TSS, hepatic adenomas, hepatocellular carcinoma, gallbladder disease, and other adverse effects. Monitor lipid levels w/ hyperlipidemia, BP, serum glucose levels in diabetic or prediabetic patients, and for signs of worsening depression w/ previous history. Have a yearly visit w/ patient for a BP check and for other indicated healthcare.

Counseling: Inform of risks and benefits of therapy. Inform that cigarette smoking increases risk of serious CV events. Inform of increased risk of VTE. Counsel that therapy does not protect against HIV infection (AIDS) or other STDs. Instruct not to use during pregnancy and to d/c if pregnancy is planned or occurs during use. Instruct to use a barrier method of contraception when ring is out for >3 continuous hrs until ring has been used continuously for at least 7 days. Counsel to use a backup or alternative method of contraception when enzyme inducers are concomitantly used. Inform that breast milk production may be reduced w/ use. Instruct postpartum women who have not yet had a normal period, to use an additional nonhormonal method of contraception for the first 7 days. Instruct on proper usage and what to do if not compliant w/ timing of insertion and removal. Inform that ring may be expelled while removing a tampon, during intercourse, or w/ straining during a bowel movement. Inform that amenorrhea may occur. Advise that pregnancy should be ruled out in the event of amenorrhea, if ring has been out of the vagina for >3 consecutive hrs, if ring-free interval was extended >1 week, if a period was missed for ≥2 consecutive cycles, or if ring has been retained for >4 weeks.

NUVESSA — metronidazole
Class: Nitroimidazole

Rx

ADULT DOSAGE
Bacterial Vaginosis

Non-Pregnant Women:
1 prefilled applicator (approx 5g of gel) administered once intravaginally at hs

PEDIATRIC DOSAGE
Pediatric use may not have been established

ADMINISTRATION
Intravaginal route

STORAGE
20-25°C (68-77°F); excursions permitted to 15-30°C (59-86°F). Protect from freezing. Do not refrigerate.

HOW SUPPLIED
Gel: 1.3% [5g]

CONTRAINDICATIONS
Hypersensitivity to metronidazole, parabens, other ingredients of the formulation, or other nitroimidazole derivatives; concurrent use w/ or w/in 2 weeks of disulfiram; consumption of ethanol or propylene glycol during treatment or for at least 24 hrs following treatment.

WARNINGS/PRECAUTIONS
Convulsive seizures and peripheral neuropathy reported w/ oral or IV metronidazole; caution w/ CNS diseases. Avoid unnecessary use; reserve for bacterial vaginosis treatment. May interfere w/ certain types of determinations of serum chemistry values (eg, AST, ALT, LDH, TGs, glucose hexokinase).

ADVERSE REACTIONS
Vulvovaginal candidiasis.

DRUG INTERACTIONS
See Contraindications. May potentiate anticoagulant effect of warfarin and other coumarin anticoagulants, resulting in a prolongation of PT. Elevated lithium levels and signs of lithium toxicity reported during short-term use of oral metronidazole w/ high doses of lithium. Cimetidine may prolong $T_{1/2}$ and decrease clearance; no dose adjustment of metronidazole is necessary.

PREGNANCY AND LACTATION
Category B, not for use in nursing.

MECHANISM OF ACTION
Nitroimidazole antimicrobial; acts primarily against anaerobic bacteria and selected protozoa. 5-nitro group on the metronidazole molecule is reduced by metabolically active anaerobes to its active state by the bacterial nitro-reductase enzyme after it diffuses into the bacterial cell. This results in the production of cytotoxic compounds that disrupt the helical structure of bacterial DNA thereby inhibiting bacterial nucleic acid synthesis, which leads to cell death.

PHARMACOKINETICS
Absorption: C_{max}=239ng/mL; T_{max}=7.3 hrs; AUC=5434ng•hr/mL. **Distribution:** Found in breast milk (PO); crosses placenta.

PATIENT CONSIDERATIONS
Assessment: Assess for hypersensitivity to the drug or other nitroimidazole derivatives, CNS diseases, pregnancy/nursing status, and possible drug interactions. Assess for clinical diagnosis of bacterial vaginosis.

Monitoring: Monitor for convulsive seizures, peripheral neuropathy, and other adverse reactions.

Counseling: Instruct not to consume alcoholic beverages and preparations containing ethanol or propylene glycol during and for at least 24 hrs after therapy. Instruct not to use the drug if disulfiram had been used w/in the last 2 weeks, and to inform physician if taking oral anticoagulants or lithium. Instruct not to engage in vaginal intercourse or use other vaginal products (eg, tampons, douches) following the single administration of the drug. Advise women who are breastfeeding, that they may consider discontinuing breastfeeding may or pump their breast milk and discard it during treatment and for 24 hrs after treatment. Instruct to d/c and consult physician if vaginal irritation occurs w/ the use of the drug. Inform that drug is supplied as a single dose in a prefilled applicator; instruct how to use the product and the vaginal applicator.

NUVIGIL — armodafinil
Class: Wakefulness-promoting agent

CIV

ADULT DOSAGE
Narcolepsy

Excessive Sleepiness Associated w/ Narcolepsy:
Usual: 150-250mg taken as a single dose qam

Shift Work Disorder

Excessive Sleepiness Associated w/ Shift Work Disorder:
Usual: 150mg qd taken as a single dose approx 1 hr prior to start of work shift

PEDIATRIC DOSAGE
Pediatric use may not have been established

Obstructive Sleep Apnea
Excessive Sleepiness Associated w/ Obstructive Sleep Apnea:
Usual: 150-250mg taken as a single dose qam

DOSING CONSIDERATIONS
Hepatic Impairment
Severe Impairment: Reduce dose

Elderly
Consider lower doses

ADMINISTRATION
Oral route

STORAGE
20-25°C (68-77°F).

HOW SUPPLIED
Tab: 50mg, 150mg, 200mg, 250mg

CONTRAINDICATIONS
Known hypersensitivity to modafinil or armodafinil or its inactive ingredients.

WARNINGS/PRECAUTIONS
Not indicated as treatment for underlying obstruction in OSA; if continuous positive airway pressure (CPAP) is the treatment of choice, treat w/ CPAP for an adequate period of time prior to initiation of therapy. Rare cases of serious or life-threatening rash, including Stevens-Johnson syndrome (SJS), toxic epidermal necrolysis (TEN), and drug rash w/ eosinophilia and systemic symptoms (DRESS) reported; d/c treatment at 1st sign of rash, unless rash is clearly not drug-related. Angioedema, anaphylaxis reactions, multiorgan hypersensitivity reactions, and psychiatric adverse reactions reported; d/c treatment if symptoms develop. Caution w/ cardiovascular disease (CVD) or history of psychosis, depression, or mania. Avoid in patients w/ history of left ventricular hypertrophy or w/ mitral valve prolapse who have experienced mitral valve prolapse syndrome (eg, ischemic ECG changes, chest pain, arrhythmia) w/ CNS stimulants. May impair mental/physical abilities. Level of wakefulness may not return to normal in patients w/ abnormal levels of sleepiness. Potential for abuse.

ADVERSE REACTIONS
Headache, nausea, dizziness, insomnia, diarrhea, dry mouth, anxiety, depression, rash.

DRUG INTERACTIONS
Reduced exposure of CYP3A4/5 substrates (eg, cyclosporine, midazolam, triazolam); consider dose adjustment of these drugs. Effectiveness of steroidal contraceptives may be reduced during and for 1 month after discontinuation of therapy; alternative or concomitant methods of contraception are recommended. Cyclosporine levels may be reduced; monitor levels and consider dosage adjustment. Increased exposure of CYP2C19 substrates (eg, omeprazole, diazepam, phenytoin); dosage reduction of these drugs may be required. Frequently monitor PT/INR w/ warfarin. Caution w/ MAOIs.

PREGNANCY AND LACTATION
Category C, caution in nursing.

MECHANISM OF ACTION
Wakefulness-promoting agent; not established. Binds to the dopamine transporter and inhibits dopamine reuptake.

PHARMACOKINETICS
Absorption: Readily absorbed. T_{max}=2 hrs (fasted). **Distribution:** V_d=42L. (Modafinil) Plasma protein binding (approx 60%). **Metabolism:** Liver via hydrolytic deamidation, S-oxidation, aromatic ring hydroxylation, and glucuronide conjugation; CYP3A4/5. **Elimination:** (Modafinil) Feces (1%), urine (80%, <10% parent compound). $T_{1/2}$=15 hrs.

PATIENT CONSIDERATIONS
Assessment: Assess for hypersensitivity to modafinil or to drug, hepatic impairment, psychosis, depression, mania, left ventricular hypertrophy, mitral valve prolapse, other CVDs, pregnancy/nursing status, and possible drug interactions.

Monitoring: Monitor for serious rash, SJS, TEN, DRESS, angioedema, anaphylaxis, hypersensitivity reactions, multiorgan hypersensitivity reactions, psychiatric adverse symptoms, and other adverse reactions. Monitor for signs of misuse or abuse. Monitor HR and BP. Frequently reassess degree of sleepiness. Consider close monitoring in elderly. Monitor PT/INR frequently w/ warfarin.

Counseling: Inform that drug is not a replacement for sleep. Inform that therapy may improve but not eliminate the abnormal tendency to fall asleep; instruct not to alter previous behavior w/ regard to potentially dangerous activities or other activities requiring appropriate levels of wakefulness, until and unless treatment has shown to produce levels of wakefulness that permit such activities. Inform of importance of continuing previously prescribed treatments. Advise to avoid alcohol during therapy. Advise to notify physician if pregnant, intending to become pregnant, or nursing. Caution about increased risk of pregnancy when using steroidal contraceptives and for 1 month after discontinuation of therapy. Instruct to inform physician if taking/planning to take any prescribed or OTC drugs. Instruct to d/c and notify physician if rash, hives, mouth sores, blisters, peeling skin, trouble swallowing or breathing or related allergic phenomenon, depression, anxiety, or signs of psychosis or mania develop.

NUWIQ — antihemophilic factor (recombinant)   Rx
Class: Antihemophilic factor (recombinant)

ADULT DOSAGE
Hemophilia A
Dosing Equations:
Required (IU) = Body Weight (kg) x Desired Factor VIII (FVIII) Rise (IU/dL or % of Normal) x 0.5 (IU/kg per IU/dL)

Expected FVIII Rise (% of Normal) = 2X Administered IU / Body Weight (kg)

Dose and duration of therapy depend on the severity of the FVIII deficiency, the location and extent of the bleeding, and clinical condition

Treatment/Control of Bleeding Episodes:

Minor Bleed:
20-40 (% of Normal or IU/dL)
Required FVIII Activity: Give q12-24h for at least 1 day, until bleeding episode is resolved

Moderate to Major Bleed:
30-60 (% of Normal or IU/dL)
Required FVIII Activity: Give q12-24h for 3-4 days or more, until bleeding episode is resolved

Life-Threatening Bleed:
60-100 (% of Normal or IU/dL)
Required FVIII Activity: Give q8-24h until bleeding risk is resolved

Perioperative Management:

Minor Surgery:
30-60 (% of Normal or IU/dL)
Required FVIII Activity (Pre-/Post-Operative): Give q24 hrs for at least 1 day, until healing is achieved

Major Surgery:
80-100 (% of Normal or IU/dL)
Required FVIII Activity (Pre-/Post-Operative): Give q8-24 hrs until adequate wound healing, then continue therapy for at least another 7 days to maintain a FVIII activity of 30-60 IU/dL

Routine Prophylaxis:
30-40 IU/kg IV qod

PEDIATRIC DOSAGE
Hemophilia A
Dosing Equations:
Required (IU) = Body Weight (kg) x Desired FVIII Rise (IU/dL or % of Normal) x 0.5 (IU/kg per IU/dL)

Expected FVIII Rise (% of Normal) = 2X Administered IU / Body Weight (kg)

Dose and duration of therapy depend on the severity of the FVIII deficiency, the location and extent of the bleeding, and clinical condition

Treatment/Control of Bleeding Episodes:

Minor Bleed:
20-40 (% of Normal or IU/dL)
Required FVIII Activity: Give q12-24h for at least 1 day, until bleeding episode is resolved

Moderate to Major Bleed:
30-60 (% of Normal or IU/dL)
Required FVIII Activity: Give q12-24h for 3-4 days or more, until bleeding episode is resolved

Life-Threatening Bleed:
60-100 (% of Normal or IU/dL)
Required FVIII Activity: Give q8-24h until bleeding risk is resolved

Perioperative Management:

Minor Surgery:
30-60 (% of Normal or IU/dL)
Required FVIII Activity (Pre-/Post-Operative): Give q24h for at least 1 day, until healing is achieved

Major Surgery:
80-100 (% of Normal or IU/dL)
Required FVIII Activity (Pre-/Post-Operative): Give q8-24h until adequate wound healing, then continue therapy for at least another 7 days to maintain a FVIII activity of 30-60 IU/dL

Routine Prophylaxis:
2-11 Years: 30-50 IU/kg qod or 3X/week
12-17 Years: 30-40 IU/kg IV qod

ADMINISTRATION
IV route

Do not administer in same tubing or container as other medications.
Perform IV bolus infusion; rate of administration should be determined by comfort level, at a max rate of 4mL/min.

Reconstitution
1. Allow vial and pre-filled syringe to come to room temperature.
2. Using supplied adapter and syringe, slowly inject all liquid from syringe into the concentrate vial.
3. Without removing syringe, dissolve concentrate powder in vial by gently moving or swirling; do not shake.
4. Turn the vial and syringe upside down (still attached).
5. Slowly withdraw sol into syringe. Make sure that all liquid is transferred to the syringe.
6. Detach syringe by turning counterclockwise.
7. Do not refrigerate reconstitution; use w/in 3 hrs after reconstitution. If not used w/in this time period, discard.

STORAGE
2-8°C (35-46°F) for up to 24 months. Do not freeze. Store in the original package to protect vials from light. During shelf life, may be kept at ≤25°C (77°F) for a single period ≤3 months. After storage at room temperature, do not return the product to the refrigerator. **Reconstituted Sol:** Keep at room temperature. Do not refrigerate. Use reconstituted sol immediately or w/in 3 hrs after reconstitution; discard any remaining sol.

HOW SUPPLIED
Inj: 250 IU, 500 IU, 1000 IU, 2000 IU

CONTRAINDICATIONS
Life-threatening hypersensitivity reactions to antihemophilic factor (recombinant) or its components.

WARNINGS/PRECAUTIONS
Not indicated for the treatment of von Willebrand disease. Hypersensitivity reactions, including anaphylaxis, may occur; d/c immediately and initiate appropriate treatment. Monitor plasma FVIII activity levels by the one-stage

clotting assay to confirm that adequate FVIII levels have been achieved and maintained. Formation of neutralizing antibodies may occur; monitor for development of FVIII inhibitors. If plasma FVIII level fails to increase as expected, or if bleeding is not controlled, suspect presence of an inhibitor; perform a Bethesda inhibitor assay.

ADVERSE REACTIONS
Paresthesia, headache, inj-site inflammation, inj-site pain, non-neutralizing anti-FVIII antibody formation, back pain, vertigo, dry mouth.

PREGNANCY AND LACTATION
Pregnancy: There are no data for use in pregnant women to inform of drug-associated risks; should be given to a pregnant woman only if clearly needed. **Lactation:** There is no information regarding the presence in human milk, the effect on the breastfed infant, or the effects on milk production; caution in nursing.

MECHANISM OF ACTION
Antihemophilic factor (recombinant); temporarily replaces the missing clotting FVIII that is needed for effective hemostasis.

PHARMACOKINETICS
Absorption: (50 IU/kg) AUC=18h·IU/mL. **Distribution:** (50 IU/kg) V_d=59.8mL/kg. **Elimination:** (50 IU/kg) $T_{1/2}$=17.1 hrs. Refer to PI for pediatric parameters.

PATIENT CONSIDERATIONS
Assessment: Assess for life-threatening hypersensitivity reactions (including anaphylaxis), location and extent of bleeding, patient's clinical condition, and pregnancy/nursing status. Assess FVIII activity levels.

Monitoring: Monitor for signs/symptoms of hypersensitivity reactions and other adverse reactions. Monitor plasma FVIII activity levels, clinical response, and development of FVIII inhibitors.

Counseling: Inform of the early signs of hypersensitivity reactions (eg, hives, generalized urticaria, tightness of the chest); advise to stop inj, contact physician, and seek prompt emergency treatment if any of these symptoms arise. Advise to contact physician or treatment center for further treatment and/or assessment if experiencing a lack of clinical response. Advise to consult w/ healthcare provider prior to traveling; while traveling, advise to bring an adequate supply.

NYMALIZE — nimodipine
Class: Calcium channel blocker (CCB) (dihydropyridine)

Rx

ADULT DOSAGE
Subarachnoid Hemorrhage

Improvement of neurological outcome by reducing the incidence and severity of ischemic deficits in adults w/ subarachnoid hemorrhage (SAH) from ruptured intracranial berry aneurysms regardless of their post-ictus neurological condition (eg, Hunt and Hess Grades I-V)

Usual: 20mL (60mg) q4h for 21 consecutive days, begin therapy w/in 96 hrs of onset of SAH

PEDIATRIC DOSAGE
Pediatric use may not have been established

DOSING CONSIDERATIONS
Hepatic Impairment
Cirrhosis:
Usual: 10mL (30mg) q4h

ADMINISTRATION
Enteral route only (eg, oral, NG/gastric tube route). Administer 1 hr ac or 2 hrs pc

Do not administer by IV or other parenteral routes

Administration Via NG/Gastric Tube
Use the supplied oral syringe
For each dose, refill the syringe w/ 20mL of 0.9% saline sol and then flush any remaining contents from NG/gastric tube into the stomach

STORAGE
25°C (77°F); excursions permitted to 15-30°C (59-86°F). Protect from light. Do not refrigerate.

HOW SUPPLIED
Sol: 60mg/20mL [473mL]

WARNINGS/PRECAUTIONS
Hypotension reported; carefully monitor BP during therapy. Increased risk of adverse reactions in patients with cirrhosis; closely monitor BP and pulse rate. Caution in elderly.

ADVERSE REACTIONS
Decreased BP, diarrhea.

DRUG INTERACTIONS
Risk of significant hypotension with strong CYP3A4 inhibitors (eg, some macrolide antibiotics [eg, clarithromycin, telithromycin], some HIV protease inhibitors [eg, indinavir, nelfinavir, ritonavir, saquinavir], some HCV protease inhibitors [eg, boceprevir, telaprevir], some azole antimycotics [eg, ketoconazole, itraconazole, posaconazole, voriconazole], conivaptan, delavirdine, nefazodone]; avoid concomitant use. Strong CYP3A4 inducers (eg, carbamazepine, phenobarbital, phenytoin, rifampin, St. John's wort) may significantly reduce levels and efficacy; avoid concomitant use. Moderate and weak CYP3A4 inhibitors (eg, cimetidine, erythromycin) may increase levels; monitor BP and reduce nimodipine dose if

necessary. Not recommended with grapefruit/grapefruit juice. Moderate and weak CYP3A4 inducers (eg, efavirenz, prednisone) may reduce efficacy; closely monitor for lack of effectiveness and increase nimodipine dose if needed. May increase the BP lowering effect of antihypertensives (eg, diuretics, β-blockers, ACE inhibitors, ARBs, other calcium channel blockers (CCB), α-adrenergic blockers, PDE-5 inhibitors, α-methyldopa); dose adjustment of the BP lowering drug may be necessary.

PREGNANCY AND LACTATION
Category C, not for use in nursing.

MECHANISM OF ACTION
CCB (dihydropyridine); not established. Inhibits Ca^{2+} ion transfer into smooth muscle cells and thus inhibits contractions of vascular smooth muscle.

PHARMACOKINETICS
Absorption: Rapid. Bioavailability (13%); T_{max}=1 hr. **Distribution:** Plasma protein binding (>95%). **Metabolism:** Via CYP3A4. **Elimination:** Urine (<1% unchanged); $T_{1/2}$=8-9 hrs.

PATIENT CONSIDERATIONS
Assessment: Assess for cirrhosis, pregnancy/nursing status, and possible drug interactions.

Monitoring: Carefully monitor pulse rate and BP.

Counseling: Inform that the most frequent adverse reaction associated with the drug is decreased BP. Instruct to avoid ingestion of grapefruit/grapefruit juice while on therapy. Advise to notify physician if pregnant or breastfeeding.

NYSTATIN ORAL — nystatin
Class: Polyene antifungal

Rx

ADULT DOSAGE
Oral Candidiasis

Oral Cavity Infections Caused by Candida albicans (Monilia):
Sus:
4-6mL qid (1/2 of dose in each side of mouth)
Continue treatment for at least 48 hrs after perioral symptoms disappear and cultures demonstrate eradication of C. albicans

Non-Esophageal GI Candidiasis
1-2 tab tid
Continue treatment for at least 48 hrs after clinical cure

Intestinal Candidiasis
Moniliasis:
Sus:
5-10mL tid
Continue treatment for at least 48 hrs after clinical cure

PEDIATRIC DOSAGE
Oral Candidiasis

Oral Cavity Infections Caused by Candida albicans (Monilia):
Sus:
Premature/Low Birth Weight Infants:
1mL qid
Infants: 2mL qid
Children: 4-6mL qid (1/2 of dose in each side of mouth)

Continue treatment for at least 48 hrs after perioral symptoms disappear and cultures demonstrate eradication of C. albicans

ADMINISTRATION
Oral route

Sus
Shake well before using
Retain in mouth as long as possible before swallowing
In infants and young children, use dropper to place 1/2 of dose in each side of mouth; avoid feeding for 5-10 min
Extemporaneous Preparation of Oral Sus: For adults and older children, add approx 500,000 U of powder to about 1/2 cup of water and stir well. Use immediately after mixing and do not store

STORAGE
20-25°C (68-77°F). (Sus) Avoid freezing.

HOW SUPPLIED
Sus: 100,000 U/mL [60mL, 473mL]; **Tab:** 500,000 U

CONTRAINDICATIONS
History of hypersensitivity to any of the components in this product.

WARNINGS/PRECAUTIONS
Not for use in treatment of systemic mycoses. D/C if sensitization/irritation occurs.

ADVERSE REACTIONS
Oral irritation/sensitization, diarrhea, N/V, GI upset/disturbances.

PREGNANCY AND LACTATION
Category C, caution in nursing.

MECHANISM OF ACTION
Polyene antifungal; binds to sterols in the cell membrane of susceptible Candida species with a resultant change in membrane permeability, allowing leakage of intracellular components.

PHARMACOKINETICS
Elimination: Feces (unchanged).

PATIENT CONSIDERATIONS
Assessment: Assess history of hypersensitivity to the drug or any of its components, and pregnancy/nursing status. Confirm diagnosis of candidiasis.

Monitoring: Monitor for oral irritation/sensitization, and other adverse reactions.

Counseling: Advise to notify physician if any adverse reactions (eg, sensitization, irritation) occur. Instruct to inform physician if pregnant, planning to become pregnant, or breastfeeding.

NYSTATIN TOPICAL — nystatin   Rx

Class: Polyene antifungal

OTHER BRAND NAMES
Nyamyc

ADULT DOSAGE	PEDIATRIC DOSAGE
Candida Infections	*Candida* Infections
Cutaneous or Mucocutaneous Mycotic Infections Caused by *Candida albicans* and Other Susceptible *Candida* Species:	**Cutaneous or Mucocutaneous Mycotic Infections Caused by *Candida albicans* and Other Susceptible *Candida* Species:**
Cre/Oint: Apply liberally to affected areas bid or as indicated until healing is complete	**Cre/Oint:** Apply liberally to affected areas bid or as indicated until healing is complete
Powder: Apply to lesions bid or tid until healing is complete	**Powder:** Apply to lesions bid or tid until healing is complete
***Candida* Infection of the Feet:** Dust the powder on the feet and in all footwear	***Candida* Infection of the Feet:** Dust the powder on the feet and in all footwear

ADMINISTRATION
Topical route

Cre is preferred to oint in candidiasis involving intertriginous areas, while very moist lesions are best treated with topical powder

STORAGE
(Cre/Oint) 20-25°C (68-77°F). (Cre) Avoid freezing. (Powder) 20-25°C (68-77°F); excursions permitted to 15-30°C (59-86°F). Avoid excessive heat (40°C [104°F]).

HOW SUPPLIED
Cre/Oint: 100,000 U/g [15g, 30g]; **Powder (Nyamyc):** 100,000 U/g [15g, 30g, 60g]

CONTRAINDICATIONS
History of hypersensitivity to any of its components.

WARNINGS/PRECAUTIONS
Not for systemic, oral, intravaginal, or ophthalmic use. D/C if irritation or sensitization develops and institute appropriate measures. Confirm diagnosis of *Candida* infection using potassium hydroxide smears, cultures, or other diagnostic methods; repeat tests if there is a lack of therapeutic response. Withdraw immediately if hypersensitivity reaction occurs, and take appropriate measures.

ADVERSE REACTIONS
(Cre/Powder) Allergic reactions, burning, itching, rash, eczema, pain on application site. (Oint) Irritation.

PREGNANCY AND LACTATION
(Cre/Powder) Category C, caution in nursing. (Oint) Safety not known in pregnancy/nursing.

MECHANISM OF ACTION
Polyene antifungal; binds to sterols in the cell membrane of susceptible species resulting in a change in membrane permeability and subsequent leakage of intracellular components.

PATIENT CONSIDERATIONS
Assessment: Assess for history of hypersensitivity to the drug or any of its components and for pregnancy/nursing status. Confirm diagnosis of *Candida* infection using appropriate diagnostic methods.

Monitoring: Monitor for hypersensitivity reaction, irritation, sensitization, other adverse reactions, and therapeutic response. Reassess diagnosis if there is a lack of therapeutic response.

Counseling: Instruct to use ud, including replacement of missed doses. Advise not to use for any disorder other than that for which it was prescribed. Instruct not to interrupt or d/c therapy until the prescribed course of treatment is completed, even if symptomatic relief occurs within the 1st few days of treatment. Advise to notify physician promptly if skin irritation develops.

NYSTATIN/TRIAMCINOLONE — nystatin/triamcinolone acetonide   Rx

Class: Corticosteroid/polyene antifungal

ADULT DOSAGE	PEDIATRIC DOSAGE
Cutaneous Candidiasis	**Cutaneous Candidiasis**
Apply gently bid (am and pm) D/C after 25 days if symptoms persist	Apply gently bid (am and pm) D/C after 25 days if symptoms persist

ADMINISTRATION
Topical route

Avoid use with occlusive dressings.

STORAGE
Room temperature; avoid freezing.

HOW SUPPLIED
Cre, Oint: (Nystatin-Triamcinolone) 100,000 U/g-0.1% [15g, 30g, 60g]

CONTRAINDICATIONS
History of hypersensitivity to any of the components.

WARNINGS/PRECAUTIONS
Avoid occlusive dressing. Monitor periodically for hypothalamic-pituitary-adrenal (HPA) axis suppression with prolonged use or when applied over a large area. D/C if hypersensitivity or irritation develops. Systemic absorption with topical corticosteroids reported; children are more prone to systemic toxicity. May cause Cushing's syndrome, hyperglycemia, and glucosuria.

ADVERSE REACTIONS
Acneiform eruption, burning, itching, irritation, secondary infection.

PREGNANCY AND LACTATION
Pregnancy: Category C.
Lactation: Caution in nursing.

MECHANISM OF ACTION
Nystatin: Polyene antifungal; binds to sterols in cell membrane, which renders cell membrane incapable of functioning as selective barrier. Triamcinolone: Synthetic corticosteroid; produces anti-inflammatory, antipruritic, and vasoconstrictive actions. Dermatological effects not established.

PHARMACOKINETICS
Absorption: Triamcinolone: Percutaneous; inflammation, other disease states, and the use of occlusive dressings may increase absorption. **Metabolism:** Triamcinolone: Liver. **Excretion:** Triamcinolone: Urine (primary); bile.

PATIENT CONSIDERATIONS
Assessment: Assess proper diagnosis (eg, KOH smears, cultures), pregnancy/status.

Monitoring: Monitor for signs/symptoms of reversible HPA axis suppression, impaired thermal homeostasis, Cushing's syndrome, hyperglycemia, glucosuria, irritation at treatment site, and hypersensitivity reactions. If applying large doses to large surface area, monitor for HPA-axis suppression by using urinary free cortisol and ACTH stimulation tests. In pediatric patients, monitor for signs/symptoms of systemic toxicity, HPA-axis suppression, Cushing's syndrome, and intracranial HTN. Monitor for response to therapy; if lack of response, repeat appropriate microbiological studies.

Counseling: Instruct to use exactly ud, topically. Avoid contact with eyes. Treatment area should not be bandaged or wrapped as to be occluded. Advise to contact physician if any adverse events develop. Inform that if applying to inguinal area, apply sparingly and wear loose clothing. Parents of pediatric patients should be instructed to avoid using tight fitting diapers or plastic pants when treating diaper area. Instruct to take preventative measures to avoid reinfection.

NYSTOP — nystatin   Rx

Class: Polyene antifungal

ADULT DOSAGE	PEDIATRIC DOSAGE
Candida Infections	*Candida* Infections
Cutaneous or Mucocutaneous Mycotic Infections Caused by *Candida albicans* and Other Susceptible *Candida* Species: Apply to lesions bid-tid until healing is complete	**Cutaneous or Mucocutaneous Mycotic Infections Caused by *Candida albicans* and Other Susceptible *Candida* Species:** Apply to lesions bid-tid until healing is complete
***Candida* Infection of the Feet:** Dust the powder on the feet and in all footwear	***Candida* Infection of the Feet:** Dust the powder on the feet and in all footwear

ADMINISTRATION
Topical route

STORAGE
15-30°C (59-86°F). Avoid excessive heat (40°C [104°F]).

HOW SUPPLIED
Powder: 100,000 U/g [15g, 30g, 60g]

CONTRAINDICATIONS
History of hypersensitivity to any of the components.

WARNINGS/PRECAUTIONS
Not for systemic, PO, intravaginal, or ophthalmic use. D/C if irritation or sensitization develops and institute appropriate measures. Confirm diagnosis of *Candida* infection using potassium hydroxide smears, cultures, or other diagnostic methods; repeat test if there is a lack of therapeutic response.

ADVERSE REACTIONS
Allergic reactions, burning, itching, rash, eczema, pain on application site.

PREGNANCY AND LACTATION
Pregnancy: Category C.
Lactation: Caution in nursing.

MECHANISM OF ACTION
Polyene antifungal; binds to sterols in the cell membrane of susceptible species resulting in a change in membrane permeability and subsequent leakage of intracellular components.

PATIENT CONSIDERATIONS
Assessment: Assess for history of hypersensitivity to the drug or any of its components and pregnancy/nursing status. Confirm diagnosis of *Candida* infection using appropriate diagnostic methods.

Monitoring: Monitor for irritation or sensitization, other adverse reactions, and therapeutic response. Reassess diagnosis if there is a lack of therapeutic response.

Counseling: Instruct to use exactly ud, including replacement of missed dose. Advise not to use the medication for any disorder other than prescribed. Instruct not to interrupt or d/c therapy until treatment is completed, even if symptomatic relief occurs within the first few days of treatment. Advise to notify physician promptly if skin irritation develops.

OBREDON — guaifenesin/hydrocodone bitartrate   CII
Class: Expectorant/opioid antitussive

ADULT DOSAGE
Cough

Symptomatic Relief of Cough and to Loosen Mucus Associated with the Common Cold:
>18 Years:
Usual: 10mL q4-6 hrs
Max: 6 doses (60mL)/24 hrs

PEDIATRIC DOSAGE
Pediatric use may not have been established

DOSING CONSIDERATIONS
Elderly
Start at lower end of dosing range
ADMINISTRATION
Oral route

Measure with an accurate mL measuring device
Do not use a household tsp to measure the dose
STORAGE
20-25°C (68-77°F).
HOW SUPPLIED
Sol: (Hydrocodone-Guaifenesin) 2.5mg-200mg/5mL [118mL, 473mL].
CONTRAINDICATIONS
Known hypersensitivity to hydrocodone bitartrate, guaifenesin, or any of the inactive ingredients of this medication; concomitant use w/ an MAOI or w/in 14 days of stopping such therapy.
WARNINGS/PRECAUTIONS
Do not use in patients with persistent or chronic cough such as occurs with smoking, asthma, chronic bronchitis, or emphysema, or where cough is accompanied by excessive phlegm. Caution with diabetes, thyroid disease, Addison's disease, prostatic hypertrophy/urethral stricture, asthma, severe renal/hepatic impairment, and in elderly. Hydrocodone: May produce dose-related respiratory depression. If respiratory depression occurs, it may be antagonized by use of naloxone HCl and other supportive measures when indicated. Potential for abuse. Psychic/physical dependence and tolerance may develop upon repeated administration of therapy. Respiratory depression effects of opioids and their capacity to elevate CSF pressure may be markedly exaggerated in the presence of head injury, other intracranial lesions, or a preexisting increase in intracranial pressure (ICP). May obscure clinical course of head injuries. Avoid in patients with head injury, intracranial lesions, or increased ICP. May obscure diagnosis or clinical course of patients with acute abdominal conditions. May impair mental/physical abilities.
ADVERSE REACTIONS
Headache, dizziness, sedation, nausea, diarrhea, decreased BP, hot flush.
DRUG INTERACTIONS
See Contraindications. Hydrocodone: Avoid with alcohol, opioids, antihistamines, antipsychotics, anti-anxiety agents, or other CNS depressants; may cause additive CNS depressant effect. Concomitant use with TCAs may increase effect of either the antidepressant or hydrocodone. May produce paralytic ileus and excessive anticholinergic effects with anticholinergics; exercise caution.
PREGNANCY AND LACTATION
Category C, not for use in nursing.
MECHANISM OF ACTION
Guaifenesin: Expectorant; mechanism unknown, but thought to act as an expectorant by increasing the volume and reducing the viscosity of secretions in the trachea and bronchi. Hydrocodone: Semisynthetic centrally acting opioid antitussive and analgesic; mechanism unknown, but believed to act directly on the cough center.
PHARMACOKINETICS
Absorption: Hydrocodone: C_{max}=12.6ng/mL; AUC_{0-inf}=80.9ng•hr/mL; T_{max}=1.25 hrs (median). Guaifenesin: C_{max}=3.7mcg/mL; AUC_{0-inf}=4.2mcg•hr/mL; T_{max}=20 min (median). **Distribution:** Hydrocodone: Found in breast milk. **Elimination:** Hydrocodone: $T_{1/2}$=5 hrs. Guaifenesin: $T_{1/2}$=1 hr.
PATIENT CONSIDERATIONS
Assessment: Assess for hypersensitivity to drug; respiratory depression; presence of head injury, other intracranial lesions, or a pre-existing increase in ICP conditions; acute abdominal conditions; persistent or chronic cough; diabetes; thyroid disease;

Addison's disease; prostatic hypertrophy or urethral stricture; asthma, hepatic/renal impairment; pregnancy/nursing status; or any other conditions where treatment is contraindicated or cautioned. Assess for possible drug interactions.

Monitoring: Monitor for respiratory depression, dependence/tolerance, elevations in CSF pressure, drowsiness, and other adverse reactions.

Counseling: Advise not to increase dose/dosing frequency, because serious adverse events (eg, respiratory depression) may occur with overdosage. Advise to measure sol with an accurate mL measuring device; inform that household tsp is not an accurate measuring device. Advise to avoid alcohol and other CNS depressants while on therapy, because additional reduction in mental alertness may occur. Advise to avoid engaging in hazardous tasks that require mental alertness and motor coordination (eg, operating machinery/driving). Inform that drug can produce drug dependence.

OCUFLOX — ofloxacin   Rx
Class: Fluoroquinolone

ADULT DOSAGE
Bacterial Conjunctivitis

Days 1-2:
1-2 drops in the affected eye(s) q2-4h
Days 3-7:
1-2 drops qid

Corneal Ulcers

Days 1-2:
1-2 drops into the affected eye every 30 min while awake; awaken at approx 4 and 6 hrs after retiring and instill 1-2 drops
Days 3 Through 7-9:
1-2 drops every hr while awake
Days 7-9 Through Treatment Completion:
1-2 drops qid

PEDIATRIC DOSAGE
Bacterial Conjunctivitis

≥1 Year:
Days 1-2:
1-2 drops in the affected eye(s) q2-4h
Days 3-7:
1-2 drops qid

Corneal Ulcers

≥1 Year:
Days 1-2:
1-2 drops into the affected eye every 30 min while awake; awaken at approx 4 and 6 hrs after retiring and instill 1-2 drops
Days 3 Through 7-9:
1-2 drops every hr while awake
Days 7-9 Through Treatment Completion:
1-2 drops qid

ADMINISTRATION
Ocular route
STORAGE
15-25°C (59-77°F).
HOW SUPPLIED
Sol: 0.3% [5mL]
CONTRAINDICATIONS
History of hypersensitivity to ofloxacin, to other quinolones, or to any of the components in this medication.
WARNINGS/PRECAUTIONS
Do not inject subconjunctivally or introduce directly into the eye's anterior chamber. Serious and occasionally fatal hypersensitivity (anaphylactic) reactions reported. Rare Stevens-Johnson syndrome (SJS), which progressed to toxic epidermal necrolysis (TEN) reported. May result in bacterial resistance with prolonged use or use in the absence of a proven/suspected bacterial infection or a prophylactic indication; take appropriate measures if superinfection develops. D/C at 1st appearance of skin rash or other signs of hypersensitivity reaction.
ADVERSE REACTIONS
Transient ocular burning/discomfort, stinging, redness, itching, chemical conjunctivitis/keratitis, ocular/periocular/facial edema, photophobia, blurred vision, tearing, dryness, eye pain, foreign body sensation.
DRUG INTERACTIONS
Systemic quinolone therapy may increase theophylline levels, interfere with caffeine metabolism, enhance effects of warfarin and its derivatives, and elevate SrCr with cyclosporine.
PREGNANCY AND LACTATION
Category C, not for use in nursing.
MECHANISM OF ACTION
Fluoroquinolone; exerts bactericidal effect on susceptible bacteria by inhibiting DNA gyrase, an essential bacterial enzyme that is a critical catalyst in duplication, transcription, and repair of bacterial DNA.
PHARMACOKINETICS
Absorption: C_{max}=1.1 ng/mL (Day 1, qid dosing), 1.9 ng/mL (Day 11, qid dosing). **Distribution:** (PO) Found in breast milk. **Excretion:** Urine (primarily unchanged).

PATIENT CONSIDERATIONS
Assessment: Assess for history of hypersensitivity to the drug, other quinolones, or any of its components, pregnancy/nursing status, and possible drug interactions.

Monitoring: Monitor for signs/symptoms of serious hypersensitivity/anaphylactic reactions, SJS, TEN, and other adverse reactions. Monitor for development of superinfection; examine with the aid of magnification (eg, slit lamp biomicroscopy) and fluorescein staining.

Counseling: Instruct to avoid contaminating applicator tip with material from eye, fingers, or other sources. Inform that systemic therapy has been associated with hypersensitivity reactions, even following a single dose; instruct to d/c immediately and contact physician at the 1st sign of a rash/allergic reaction.

ODEFSEY — emtricitabine/rilpivirine/tenofovir alafenamide   Rx

Class: Non-nucleoside reverse transcriptase inhibitor (NNRTI)/nucleoside reverse transcriptase inhibitor (NRTI) combination

> Lactic acidosis and severe hepatomegaly w/ steatosis, including fatal cases, reported w/ the use of nucleoside analogues in combination w/ other antiretrovirals. Not approved for the treatment of chronic hepatitis B virus (HBV) infection, and safety and efficacy has not been established in patients coinfected w/ HIV-1 and HBV. Severe acute exacerbations of hepatitis B reported in patients coinfected w/ HIV-1 and HBV and have discontinued products containing emtricitabine and/or tenofovir disoproxil fumarate, and may occur w/ discontinuation of Odefsey; closely monitor hepatic function w/ both clinical and laboratory follow-up for at least several months in patients who are coinfected w/ HIV-1 and HBV and d/c therapy. If appropriate, initiation of anti-hepatitis B therapy may be warranted.

ADULT DOSAGE
HIV-1 Infection

As a complete regimen for the treatment of HIV-1 infection as initial therapy in antiretroviral-naive patients w/ HIV-1 RNA ≤100,000 copies/mL; or to replace a stable antiretroviral regimen in those who are virologically suppressed (HIV-1 RNA <50 copies/mL) for at least 6 months w/ no history of treatment failure and no known substitutions associated w/ resistance to the individual drug components

Recommended Dose: 1 tab qd

In virologically suppressed patients, additional monitoring of HIV-1 RNA and regimen tolerability is recommended after replacing therapy to assess for potential virologic failure or rebound

PEDIATRIC DOSAGE
HIV-1 Infection

As a complete regimen for the treatment of HIV-1 infection as initial therapy in antiretroviral-naive patients w/ HIV-1 RNA ≤100,000 copies/mL; or to replace a stable antiretroviral regimen in those who are virologically suppressed (HIV-1 RNA <50 copies/mL) for at least 6 months w/ no history of treatment failure and no known substitutions associated w/ resistance to the individual drug components

≥12 Years:
≥35kg:
Recommended Dose: 1 tab qd

In virologically suppressed patients, additional monitoring of HIV-1 RNA and regimen tolerability is recommended after replacing therapy to assess for potential virologic failure or rebound

----

DOSING CONSIDERATIONS
Renal Impairment
Severe (CrCl <30mL/min): Not recommended

ADMINISTRATION
Oral route

Take w/ a meal.

STORAGE
<30°C (86°F).

HOW SUPPLIED
Tab: (Emtricitabine [FTC]/Rilpivirine [RPV]/Tenofovir Alafenamide [TAF]) 200mg/25mg/25mg

CONTRAINDICATIONS
Coadministration w/ carbamazepine, oxcarbazepine, phenobarbital, phenytoin, rifampin, rifapentine, proton pump inhibitors (eg, dexlansoprazole, esomeprazole, lansoprazole, omeprazole, pantoprazole, rabeprazole), systemic dexamethasone (more than a single dose), St. John's wort.

WARNINGS/PRECAUTIONS
Test for HBV before initiating therapy. Redistribution/accumulation of body fat reported. **FTC and TAF:** Lactic acidosis and severe hepatomegaly w/ steatosis reported; obesity and prolonged nucleoside exposure may be risk factors. Caution w/ known risk factors for liver disease. D/C if lactic acidosis or pronounced hepatotoxicity occur. **RPV:** Severe skin and hypersensitivity reactions including cases of drug reaction w/ eosinophilia and systemic symptoms reported; d/c immediately and initiate appropriate therapy if signs/symptoms develop. Higher than recommended doses of RPV reported to prolong the QTc interval; consider therapy alternatives when administered to patients at higher risk of torsades de pointes. Depressive disorders reported; promptly evaluate if severe depressive symptoms occur. Hepatic adverse events reported; patients w/ underlying hepatitis B or C, or marked liver-associated test elevations prior to treatment, may be at increased risk for worsening/development of liver-associated test elevations. **TAF:** Renal impairment (eg, acute renal failure, Fanconi syndrome) reported; d/c in patients who develop clinically significant decreases in renal function or evidence of Fanconi syndrome. Decreased bone mineral density (BMD), increased biochemical markers of bone metabolism, and osteomalacia reported. Consider assessment of BMD in patients w/ history of pathologic bone fracture or other risk factors for osteoporosis or bone loss. **FTC and RPV:** Immune reconstitution syndrome and autoimmune disorders (eg, Graves' disease, polymyositis, Guillain-Barre syndrome) in the setting of immune reconstitution reported.

ADVERSE REACTIONS
RPV: Depressive disorders, insomnia, headache.
FTC and TAF: Nausea.

DRUG INTERACTIONS
See Contraindications. May decrease ketoconazole levels. May decrease methadone levels; monitor levels. Methadone maint therapy may need to be adjusted. **RPV:** Coadministration w/ CYP3A inducers or drugs that increase gastric pH (eg, antacids, H$_2$-receptor antagonists [H$_2$-RAs]) may result in decreased levels, loss of virologic response, and possible resistance to rilpivirine or to the class of non-nucleoside reverse transcriptase inhibitors (NNRTIs). Administer antacids at least 2 hrs before or at least 4 hrs after dosing, and H$_2$-RAs at least 12 hrs before or at least 4 hrs after dosing. CYP3A inhibitors may increase levels.

Consider alternative medications in patients taking a drug w/ a known risk of torsade de pointes. Clarithromycin, erythromycin, or telithromycin may increase levels; consider alternatives (eg, azithromycin) where possible. **TAF:** P-gp inducers may decrease levels. P-gp inhibitors may increase levels. **FTC and TAF:** Drugs that reduce renal function or compete for active tubular secretion (eg, acyclovir, aminoglycosides [eg, gentamicin], high-dose or multiple NSAIDs) may increase levels of FTC, TAF, and other renally eliminated drugs. Patients taking nephrotoxic agents (eg, NSAIDs) are at increased risk of developing renal-related adverse reactions. **RPV and TAF:** Rifabutin may decrease levels; coadministration is not recommended. Azole antifungal agents may increase levels; clinically monitor for breakthrough fungal infections when azole antifungals are coadministered.

PREGNANCY AND LACTATION
Pregnancy: There are insufficient human data on the use of Odefsey during pregnancy to inform a drug-associated risk of birth defects and miscarriage. Healthcare providers are encouraged to register patients who are exposed to Odefsey during pregnancy in the Antiretroviral Pregnancy Registry.
Lactation: FTC has been shown to be present in human breast milk; it is unknown if RPV and TAF are present in human breast milk; not for use in nursing.

MECHANISM OF ACTION
FTC: Nucleoside analogue of cytidine; inhibits activity of HIV-1 reverse transcriptase (RT) by competing w/ natural substrate deoxycytidine 5'-triphosphate and by being incorporated into nascent viral DNA, resulting in chain termination. **RPV:** NNRTI; inhibits HIV-1 replication by noncompetitive inhibition of HIV-1 RT. **TAF:** Acyclic nucleoside phosphonate analogue of adenosine 5'-monophosphate; inhibits HIV-1 replication through incorporation into viral DNA by the HIV RT, which results in DNA chain termination.

PHARMACOKINETICS
Absorption: FTC: C_{max}=2.1µg/mL, AUC=11.7µg•hr/mL, T_{max}=3 hrs. RPV: AUC=2.2µg•hr/mL, T_{max}=4 hrs. TAF: C_{max}=0.16µg/mL, AUC=0.21µg•hr/mL, T_{max}=1 hr. **Distribution:** RPV: Plasma protein binding (approx 99%). FTC: Plasma protein binding (<4%); found in breast milk. TAF: Plasma protein binding (approx 80%). **Metabolism:** RPV: CYP3A. TAF: Via cathepsin A in peripheral blood mononuclear cells and macrophages and by carboxylesterase 1 in hepatocytes, CYP3A. **Excretion:** RPV: Feces (85%), urine (6%); $T_{1/2}$=50 hrs (median). FTC: Urine (70%), feces (13.7%); $T_{1/2}$=10 hrs (median). TAF: Feces (31.7%), urine (<1%); $T_{1/2}$=0.51 hrs (median).

PATIENT CONSIDERATIONS
Assessment: Assess for obesity, prolonged nucleoside exposure, HBV infection, risk of torsades de pointes, liver dysfunction or risk factors for liver disease, renal impairment, pregnancy/nursing status, and possible drug interactions. Assess BMD in patients w/ a history of pathological bone fracture or w/ other risk factors for osteoporosis/bone loss. Assess estimated CrCl, urine glucose, and urine protein.

Monitoring: Monitor for signs/symptoms of lactic acidosis, severe hepatomegaly w/ steatosis, severe skin and hypersensitivity reactions, depressive symptoms, hepatotoxicity, fat redistribution/accumulation, immune reconstitution syndrome, autoimmune disorders, renal impairment, decreased BMD, increased biochemical markers for bone metabolism, osteomalacia, and other adverse reactions. Monitor hepatic function closely in patients coinfected w/ HBV and HIV-1 w/ clinical and lab follow-up for at least several months upon discontinuation of therapy. Monitor estimated CrCl, urine glucose, and urine protein. Monitor serum phosphorus levels in patients w/ chronic kidney disease.

Counseling: Instruct to contact physician if symptoms of lactic acidosis or pronounced hepatotoxicity, depression, or infection occurs. Inform that hepatotoxicity has been reported during treatment. Inform that severe acute exacerbations of hepatitis B may occur in patients who are coinfected w/ HBV and HIV-1 and have discontinued therapy; advise not to d/c therapy w/o first informing physician. Instruct to immediately stop taking therapy and seek medical attention if patient develops a rash associated w/ any of the following symptoms: fever; blisters; mucosal involvement; eye inflammation (conjunctivitis); severe allergic reaction causing swelling of the face, eyes, lips, mouth, tongue, or throat; and any signs/symptoms of liver problems. Inform that laboratory tests will be performed and appropriate therapy will be initiated if severe rash occurs. Inform that fat redistribution/accumulation, renal impairment, and decreases in BMD may occur. Advise to inform physician if taking any other prescription/nonprescription medications or herbal products (eg, St. John's wort). Instruct to notify physician if pregnant or nursing.

ODOMZO — sonidegib   Rx

Class: Hedgehog pathway inhibitor

> May cause embryo-fetal death or severe birth defects when administered to a pregnant woman. Verify the pregnancy status of females of reproductive potential prior to initiating therapy. Advise females of reproductive potential to use effective contraception during treatment and for at least 20 months after the last dose. Advise males of the potential risk of exposure through semen and to use condoms w/ a pregnant partner or a female partner of reproductive potential during treatment and for at least 8 months after the last dose.

ADULT DOSAGE
Basal Cell Carcinoma

Locally advanced basal cell carcinoma that has recurred following surgery or radiation therapy, or for those who are not candidates for surgery or radiation therapy

200mg qd until disease progression or unacceptable toxicity

PEDIATRIC DOSAGE
Pediatric use may not have been established

DOSING CONSIDERATIONS
Adverse Reactions
Interrupt Therapy For:
- Severe or intolerable musculoskeletal adverse reactions
- First occurrence of serum creatine kinase (CK) elevation between 2.5 and 10X ULN
- Recurrent serum CK elevation between 2.5 and 5X ULN

Resume at 200mg/day upon resolution of clinical signs and symptoms

Permanently D/C Therapy For:
- Serum CK elevation >2.5X ULN w/ worsening renal function
- Serum CK elevation >10X ULN
- Recurrent serum CK elevation >5X ULN
- Recurrent severe or intolerable musculoskeletal adverse reactions

ADMINISTRATION
Oral route

Take on an empty stomach, at least 1 hr ac or 2 hrs pc.

STORAGE
25°C (77°F); excursions permitted to 15-30°C (59-86°F).

HOW SUPPLIED
Cap: 200mg

WARNINGS/PRECAUTIONS
Advise not to donate blood or blood products while taking sonidegib and for at least 20 months after the last dose. Musculoskeletal adverse reactions, which may be accompanied by serum CK elevations, reported; advise to report promptly any new unexplained muscle pain, tenderness, or weakness occurring during treatment or that persists after discontinuing therapy. Obtain baseline serum CK and creatinine levels prior to initiating therapy, periodically during treatment, and as clinically indicated (eg, if muscle symptoms are reported). Obtain SrCr and CK levels at least weekly in patients w/ musculoskeletal adverse reactions w/ concurrent serum CK elevation >2.5X ULN until resolution of clinical signs and symptoms.

ADVERSE REACTIONS
Muscle spasms, alopecia, dysgeusia, fatigue, abdominal pain, N/V, musculoskeletal pain, decreased weight, myalgia, diarrhea, decreased appetite, headache, pain, pruritus.

DRUG INTERACTIONS
Avoid w/ strong CYP3A inhibitors (eg, saquinavir, ketoconazole, nefazodone), and w/ moderate CYP3A inhibitors (eg, atazanavir, diltiazem, fluconazole). If a moderate CYP3A inhibitor must be used, administer the moderate CYP3A inhibitor for <14 days and monitor closely for adverse reactions, particularly musculoskeletal adverse reactions. Avoid w/ strong and moderate CYP3A inducers (eg, carbamazepine, efavirenz, modafinil).

PREGNANCY AND LACTATION
Pregnancy: May cause fetal harm.
Lactation: Not for use in nursing during treatment and for 20 months after the last dose.
Reproductive Potential: Advise females of reproductive potential to use effective contraception during treatment and for at least 20 months after the last dose. Advise males to use condoms, even after a vasectomy, during treatment and for at least 8 months after the last dose; advise not to donate semen during treatment and for at least 8 months after the last dose. May compromise female fertility.

MECHANISM OF ACTION
Hedgehog pathway inhibitor; binds to and inhibits smoothened, a transmembrane protein involved in hedgehog signal transduction.

PHARMACOKINETICS
Absorption: T_{max}=2-4 hrs (median); C_{max}=1030ng/mL; AUC=22mcg•h/mL.
Distribution: V_d=9166L; plasma protein binding (>97%). **Metabolism:** Liver via CYP3A. **Elimination:** Feces (70%), urine (30%); $T_{1/2}$=28 days.

PATIENT CONSIDERATIONS
Assessment: Assess for hypersensitivity to drug, pregnancy/nursing status, and for possible drug interactions. Obtain baseline CK levels and renal function tests.

Monitoring: Monitor for musculoskeletal adverse reactions (eg, rhabdomyolysis, muscle spasms, musculoskeletal pain) and for other adverse reactions. Monitor CK and SrCr levels periodically and as clinically indicated. Obtain SrCr and CK levels at least weekly in patients w/ musculoskeletal adverse reactions w/ concurrent serum CK elevations >2.5X ULN until clinical signs/symptoms are resolved.

Counseling: Advise females of reproductive potential that drug may cause fetal harm and to use effective contraception during treatment and for at least 20 months after the last dose. Advise males, even those w/ prior vasectomy, to use condoms, to avoid potential drug exposure in both pregnant partners and female partners of reproductive potential during treatment and for at least 8 months after the last dose. Instruct female patients and female partners of male patients to contact their healthcare provider if they become pregnant or suspect that they may be pregnant. Advise females who may have been exposed to sonidegib during pregnancy, either directly or through seminal fluid, to contact the Novartis Pharmaceuticals Corporation. Instruct not to donate blood or blood products while taking sonidegib and for 20 months after stopping treatment. Advise to contact healthcare provider immediately if new or worsening signs/symptoms of muscle toxicity, dark urine, decreased urine output, or the inability to urinate develops. Instruct to take on an empty stomach, at least 1 hr ac or 2 hrs pc. Advise women not to breastfeed during treatment and for up to 20 months after the last dose.

OFEV — nintedanib
Class: Kinase inhibitor

Rx

ADULT DOSAGE
Idiopathic Pulmonary Fibrosis
Recommended: 150mg bid approx 12 hrs apart
Max: 300mg/day

Missed Dose
If a dose is missed, the next dose should be taken at the next scheduled time; do not make up for a missed dose

PEDIATRIC DOSAGE
Pediatric use may not have been established

DOSING CONSIDERATIONS
Renal Impairment
Mild to Moderate: Adjustment of starting dose is not required
Severe (CrCl<30mL/min) and ESRD: Not studied

Hepatic Impairment
Mild (Child Pugh A):
100mg bid approx 12 hrs apart

Moderate (Child Pugh B) or Severe (Child Pugh C):
Not recommended

Adverse Reactions
In addition to symptomatic treatment, if applicable, dose reduction or temporary interruption may be required until the specific adverse reaction resolves to levels that allow continuation of therapy

Treatment may be resumed at the full dosage (150mg bid), or at the reduced dosage (100mg bid), which subsequently may be increased to the full dosage. If 100mg bid is not tolerated, d/c treatment

Liver Enzyme Elevations:
AST/ALT >3X to <5X ULN w/o Signs of Severe Liver Damage:
Interrupt treatment or reduce dose to 100mg bid; once LFTs return to baseline, may reintroduce at a reduced dosage (100mg bid), which subsequently may be increased to the full dosage (150mg bid)

AST/ALT Elevations >5X ULN or >3X ULN w/ Signs/Symptoms of Severe Liver Damage:
D/C treatment

Mild Hepatic Impairment (Child Pugh A):
Consider treatment interruption/discontinuation for management of adverse reactions

ADMINISTRATION
Oral route

Take w/ food.
Swallow whole w/ liquid; do not chew or crush caps.

STORAGE
25°C (77°F); excursions permitted to 15-30°C (59-86°F). Protect from exposure to high humidity and avoid excessive heat. If repackaged, use tight container.

HOW SUPPLIED
Cap: 100mg, 150mg

WARNINGS/PRECAUTIONS
See Dosing Considerations. Associated w/ elevations of liver enzymes and bilirubin; conduct LFTs prior to treatment, monthly for 3 months, and every 3 months thereafter, and as clinically indicated. Diarrhea reported; treat at 1st signs w/ adequate hydration and antidiarrheal medication (eg, loperamide) and consider treatment interruption if diarrhea continues. D/C treatment if severe diarrhea persists despite symptomatic treatment. N/V reported; may require dose reduction or treatment interruption if N/V persists despite appropriate supportive care including antiemetic therapy. D/C treatment if severe N/V does not resolve. Can cause fetal harm. Arterial thromboembolic events (eg, MI) reported; caution when treating patients at higher cardiovascular (CV) risk including known coronary artery disease. Consider treatment interruption in patients who develop signs or symptoms of acute myocardial ischemia. May increase the risk of bleeding and GI perforation. Caution in patients who have had recent abdominal surgery, and d/c therapy in patients who develop GI perforation.

ADVERSE REACTIONS
Diarrhea, N/V, abdominal pain, liver enzyme elevation, decreased appetite, weight decreased, headache, HTN.

DRUG INTERACTIONS
P-gp and CYP3A4 inhibitors (eg, erythromycin, ketoconazole) may increase exposure; monitor closely for tolerability. P-gp and CYP3A4 inducers (eg, carbamazepine, phenytoin, St. John's wort, rifampicin) may decrease exposure; avoid coadministration. Monitor closely for bleeding if on full anticoagulation therapy and adjust anticoagulation treatment as necessary. Smoking was associated w/ decreased exposure, which may alter the efficacy profile of nintedanib.

PREGNANCY AND LACTATION
Pregnancy: Can cause fetal harm based on findings from animal studies and mechanism of action.
Lactation: Not for use in nursing.
Reproductive Potential: May reduce fertility in females of reproductive potential based on animal data. Females of reproductive potential should use effective contraception during treatment and for at least 3 months after the last dose.

MECHANISM OF ACTION

Tyrosine kinase inhibitor; inhibits receptor tyrosine kinases implicated in IPF pathogenesis (eg, vascular endothelial growth factor receptor, fibroblast growth factor receptor, platelet-derived growth factor receptor). Binds competitively to the adenosine triphosphate binding pocket of these receptors and blocks the intracellular signaling that is crucial for the proliferation, migration, and transformation of fibroblasts representing essential mechanisms of the IPF pathology.

PHARMACOKINETICS

Absorption: Absolute bioavailability (4.7%); T_{max}=2-4 hrs (fed). **Distribution:** V_d=1050L (IV); plasma protein binding (97.8%). **Metabolism:** Hydrolytic cleavage by esterases resulting in the free acid moiety BIBF 1202 is the prevalent metabolic pathway. BIBF 1202 is subsequently glucuronidated by UGT enzymes, namely UGT1A1, UGT1A7, UGT1A8, and UGT1A10 to BIBF 1202 glucuronide. **Elimination:** Urine (0.05%, unchanged [oral]), (1.4%, unchanged [IV]); feces/biliary (93.4%); $T_{1/2}$=9.5 hrs.

PATIENT CONSIDERATIONS

Assessment: Assess for CV risk, hepatic impairment, risk of bleeding/GI perforation, recent abdominal surgery, nursing status, possible drug interactions, and if smoking. Conduct LFTs and a pregnancy test prior to treatment.

Monitoring: Monitor for GI disorders, arterial thromboembolic events, bleeding events, GI perforation, and other adverse reactions. Monitor for liver enzyme elevations; conduct LFTs (ALT, AST, bilirubin) monthly for 3 months, and every 3 months thereafter, and as clinically indicated.

Counseling: Advise that liver function testing will be needed periodically. Advise to immediately report any symptoms of a liver problem. Inform that GI disorders such as diarrhea or N/V were the most commonly reported GI events; advise that physician may recommend hydration, antidiarrheal medications (eg, loperamide), or antiemetic medications to treat these side effects. Instruct to contact physician at the 1st signs of diarrhea or for any severe or persistent diarrhea or N/V. Counsel on pregnancy planning and prevention. Advise females of childbearing potential of the potential hazard to a fetus, to avoid becoming pregnant while receiving treatment, and to use effective contraception during treatment and for at least 3 months after taking the last dose of the drug. Advise to notify physician if pregnancy occurs during therapy. Advise that breastfeeding is not recommended. Advise about the signs and symptoms of acute myocardial ischemia and other arterial thromboembolic events and the urgency to seek immediate medical care for these conditions. Advise to report unusual bleeding or any signs and symptoms of GI perforation. Encourage to stop smoking prior to treatment and to avoid smoking during treatment. If a dose is missed, instruct to take the next dose at the next scheduled time and to not make up for a missed dose.

OFIRMEV — acetaminophen   Rx

Class: Analgesic

> Caution when prescribing, preparing, and administering therapy to avoid dosing errors that could result in accidental overdose and death. Ensure that the dose in mg and mL is not confused, the dosing is based on weight for patients <50kg, infusion pumps are properly programmed, and the total daily dose of acetaminophen (APAP) from all sources does not exceed max daily limits. Associated w/ cases of acute liver failure, at times resulting in liver transplant and death. Most cases of liver injury are associated w/ APAP use at doses that exceed the max daily limits, and often involve >1 APAP-containing product.

ADULT DOSAGE

Moderate to Severe Pain

Adjunct to Opioid Analgesics:

<50kg:
Usual: 12.5mg/kg q4h or 15mg/kg q6h
Max: 15mg/kg (up to 750mg)/dose or 75mg/kg (up to 3750mg)/day

≥50kg:
Usual: 650mg q4h or 1000mg q6h
Max: 1000mg/dose or 4000mg/day

Mild to Moderate Pain

<50kg:
Usual: 12.5mg/kg q4h or 15mg/kg q6h
Max: 15mg/kg (up to 750mg)/dose or 75mg/kg (up to 3750mg)/day

≥50kg:
Usual: 650mg q4h or 1000mg q6h
Max: 1000mg/dose or 4000mg/day

Fever

<50kg:
Usual: 12.5mg/kg q4h or 15mg/kg q6h
Max: 15mg/kg (up to 750mg)/dose or 75mg/kg (up to 3750mg)/day

≥50kg:
Usual: 650mg q4h or 1000mg q6h
Max: 1000mg/dose or 4000mg/day

PEDIATRIC DOSAGE

Moderate to Severe Pain

Adjunct to Opioid Analgesics:

2-12 Years:
Usual: 12.5mg/kg q4h or 15mg/kg q6h
Max: 15mg/kg (up to 750mg)/dose or 75mg/kg (up to 3750mg)/day

≥13 Years:
<50kg:
Usual: 12.5mg/kg q4h or 15mg/kg q6h
Max: 15mg/kg (up to 750mg)/dose or 75mg/kg (up to 3750mg)/day

≥50kg:
Usual: 650mg q4h or 1000mg q6h
Max: 1000mg/dose or 4000mg/day

Mild to Moderate Pain

2-12 Years:
Usual: 12.5mg/kg q4h or 15mg/kg q6h
Max: 15mg/kg (up to 750mg)/dose or 75mg/kg (up to 3750mg)/day

≥13 Years:
<50kg:
Usual: 12.5mg/kg q4h or 15mg/kg q6h
Max: 15mg/kg (up to 750mg)/dose or 75mg/kg (up to 3750mg)/day

≥50kg:
Usual: 650mg q4h or 1000mg q6h
Max: 1000mg/dose or 4000mg/day

Fever

2-12 Years:
Usual: 12.5mg/kg q4h or 15mg/kg q6h
Max: 15mg/kg (up to 750mg)/dose or 75mg/kg (up to 3750mg)/day

≥13 Years:
<50kg:
Usual: 12.5mg/kg q4h or 15mg/kg q6h
Max: 15mg/kg (up to 750mg)/dose or 75mg/kg (up to 3750mg)/day

≥50kg:
Usual: 650mg q4h or 1000mg q6h
Max: 1000mg/dose or 4000mg/day

DOSING CONSIDERATIONS

Renal Impairment
Severe (CrCl ≤30mL/min): May need to give at longer dosing intervals and a reduced total daily dose

Hepatic Impairment
May need to reduce total daily dose

ADMINISTRATION
IV route

Minimum dosing interval should be 4 hrs.

Adults and Adolescents ≥50kg Requiring 1000mg Doses
Administer the dose by inserting a vented IV set through the septum of the 100mL vial.
May be administered w/o further dilution.
Administer contents of the vial IV over 15 min.

Doses <1000mg
Withdraw appropriate dose from vial and place into a separate empty, sterile container (eg, glass bottle, plastic IV container, syringe) for IV infusion.
The entire 100mL vial is not intended for use in patients weighing <50kg; discard the unused portion.
Place small volume pediatric doses up to 60mL in volume in a syringe and administer over 15 min using syringe pump.

Once vacuum seal of vial is penetrated, or contents transferred to another container, administer dose w/in 6 hrs.
Do not add other medications to sol; diazepam and chlorpromazine are physically incompatible.

STORAGE
20-25°C (68-77°F). Do not refrigerate or freeze.

HOW SUPPLIED
Inj: 10mg/mL [100mL]

CONTRAINDICATIONS
Known hypersensitivity to acetaminophen or to any of the excipients in the IV formulation, severe hepatic impairment or severe active liver disease.

WARNINGS/PRECAUTIONS
Caution w/ alcoholism, chronic malnutrition, or severe hypovolemia (eg, due to dehydration or blood loss). May cause hypersensitivity, anaphylaxis, and serious skin reactions (eg, acute generalized exanthematous pustulosis, Stevens-Johnson syndrome, toxic epidermal necrolysis); d/c at the 1st appearance of signs/symptoms.

ADVERSE REACTIONS
Liver failure, N/V, headache, insomnia, constipation, pruritus, agitation, atelectasis.

DRUG INTERACTIONS
Substances that induce or regulate CYP2E1 may alter the metabolism and increase hepatotoxic potential. Excessive alcohol use may induce hepatic cytochromes, but ethanol may also inhibit metabolism. Increased INR in some patients stabilized on sodium warfarin; more frequent assessment of INR may be appropriate.

PREGNANCY AND LACTATION
Pregnancy: Category C.
Lactation: Caution in nursing.

MECHANISM OF ACTION
Nonopiate, nonsalicylate analgesic and antipyretic; not established. Thought to primarily involve central actions.

PHARMACOKINETICS
Absorption: Administration of variable doses to different age groups resulted in different pharmacokinetic parameters. **Distribution:** Plasma protein binding (10-25%); widely distributed throughout most body tissues except fat. (Oral) Found in breast milk. **Metabolism:** Liver; glucuronide and sulfate conjugation, and oxidation via CYP2E1; N-acetyl-p-benzoquinone imine (intermediate metabolite). **Elimination:** Urine (>90% w/in 24 hrs, <5% unconjugated).

PATIENT CONSIDERATIONS

Assessment: Assess for previous hypersensitivity, alcoholism, chronic malnutrition, severe hypovolemia, hepatic/renal impairment, pregnancy/nursing status, and possible drug interactions.

Monitoring: Monitor for signs/symptoms of hypersensitivity and anaphylaxis, acute liver failure, serious skin reactions, and other adverse reactions. Monitor the end of infusion to prevent the possibility of air embolism, especially in cases where therapy is the primary infusion. Monitor INR frequently in patients stabilized on sodium warfarin.

Counseling: Inform about the risks and benefits of therapy. Instruct not to exceed the recommended dose. Instruct to notify physician if any adverse reactions occur or if pregnant/nursing or planning to become pregnant. Counsel about possible drug interactions.

OFLOXACIN — ofloxacin

Rx

Class: Fluoroquinolone

> Fluoroquinolones are associated with an increased risk of tendinitis and tendon rupture in all ages. Risk is further increased in patients >60 yrs of age, taking corticosteroids, and with kidney, heart, or lung transplants. May exacerbate muscle weakness with myasthenia gravis; avoid with known history of myasthenia gravis.

OTHER BRAND NAMES

Floxin (Discontinued)

ADULT DOSAGE

Acute Bacterial Exacerbation of Chronic Bronchitis
400mg q12h for 10 days

Community-Acquired Pneumonia
400mg q12h for 10 days

Skin and Skin Structure Infections
Uncomplicated:
400mg q12h for 10 days

Gonorrhea
Acute, Uncomplicated Urethral and Cervical:
400mg single dose

Nongonococcal Urethritis
300mg q12h for 7 days

Nongonococcal Cervicitis
300mg q12h for 7 days

Mixed Infection of the Urethra/Cervix
300mg q12h for 7 days

Acute Pelvic Inflammatory Disease
400mg q12h for 10-14 days

Uncomplicated Cystitis
Due to *Escherichia coli/Klebsiella pneumoniae*: 200mg q12h for 3 days
Due to Other Approved Pathogens:
200mg q12h for 7 days

Urinary Tract Infections
Complicated:
200mg q12h for 10 days

Prostatitis
300mg q12h for 6 weeks

PEDIATRIC DOSAGE
Pediatric use may not have been established

- -

DOSING CONSIDERATIONS
Renal Impairment
CrCl 20-50mL/min: Administer usual recommended unit dose q24h
CrCl <20mL/min: Administer 50% of the usual recommended unit dose q24h

Hepatic Impairment
Severe Liver Function Disorders (eg, Cirrhosis w/ or w/o Ascites):
Max: 400mg/day

ADMINISTRATION
Oral route
Administer w/o regard to meals

STORAGE
20-25°C (68-77°F).

HOW SUPPLIED
Tab: 200mg, 300mg, 400mg

CONTRAINDICATIONS
History of hypersensitivity associated w/ the use of ofloxacin or any member of the quinolone group of antimicrobial agents.

WARNINGS/PRECAUTIONS
D/C if pain, swelling, inflammation, or rupture of a tendon occurs. Convulsions, increased intracranial pressure (including pseudotumor cerebri), and toxic psychosis reported. CNS stimulation may occur; d/c and institute appropriate measures if reactions occur. Caution with CNS disorder or risk factors that may predispose to seizures or lower seizure threshold. Serious and occasionally fatal hypersensitivity and/or anaphylactic reactions reported; d/c immediately at the 1st appearance of skin rash, jaundice, or any other sign of hypersensitivity and institute supportive measures. Cases of sensory or sensorimotor axonal polyneuropathy resulting in paresthesias, hypoesthesias, dysesthesias, and weakness reported; d/c immediately if symptoms occur. *Clostridium difficile*-associated diarrhea (CDAD) reported; d/c if CDAD suspected or confirmed. May result in bacterial resistance when used in the absence of a proven/strongly suspected bacterial infection or a prophylactic indication. Not shown to be effective in the treatment of syphilis. Maintain adequate hydration to prevent formation of highly concentrated urine. D/C therapy if photosensitivity/phototoxicity occurs. Prolongation of the QT interval on ECG, arrhythmia, and torsades de pointes reported; avoid with known QT interval prolongation or uncorrected hypokalemia. Caution in the presence of renal or hepatic insufficiency/impairment and in elderly, especially those on corticosteroids. Lab test interactions may occur.

ADVERSE REACTIONS
Tendinitis, tendon rupture, N/V, insomnia, headache, dizziness, diarrhea, external genital pruritus in women, vaginitis, abdominal pain, chest pain, decreased appetite, dry mouth, dysgeusia, fatigue.

DRUG INTERACTIONS
See Boxed Warning. Caution with drugs that may lower the seizure threshold. May prolong QT interval; avoid with Class IA (eg, quinidine, procainamide) or Class III (eg, amiodarone, sotalol) antiarrhythmics. Administration with antacids containing Ca^{2+}, Mg^{2+}, or aluminum, with sucralfate, with divalent or trivalent cations (eg, iron), with multivitamins containing zinc or with didanosine, chewable/buffered tabs or pediatric powder for oral sol may result in lower systemic levels; do not take within the 2-hr period before or after ofloxacin administration. Cimetidine may interfere with elimination. May elevate cyclosporine levels. May prolong $T_{1/2}$ of drugs metabolized by CYP450 (eg, cyclosporine, methylxanthines). NSAIDs may increase risk of CNS stimulation and convulsive seizures. Probenecid may affect renal tubular secretion. May increase theophylline levels and increase risk of theophylline-related adverse reactions; monitor theophylline levels closely and adjust theophylline dose, if appropriate. May enhance effects of warfarin or its derivatives; monitor PT or other suitable coagulation test. Disturbances of blood glucose with antidiabetic agents reported; monitor blood glucose levels closely.

PREGNANCY AND LACTATION
Category C, not for use in nursing.

MECHANISM OF ACTION
Fluoroquinolone; inhibits bacterial topoisomerase IV and DNA gyrase, enzymes required for DNA replication, transcription, repair, and recombination.

PHARMACOKINETICS
Absorption: Bioavailability (98%); T_{max}=1-2 hrs. Oral administration of variable doses resulted in different parameters. **Distribution:** Plasma protein binding (32%); found in breast milk. **Elimination:** Urine (65-80% unchanged, <5% desmethyl and N-oxide metabolites), feces (4-8%); (Biphasic) $T_{1/2}$=4-5 hrs and 20-25 hrs (multiple doses).

PATIENT CONSIDERATIONS
Assessment: Assess for risk factors for developing tendinitis and tendon rupture, history of myasthenia gravis, drug hypersensitivity, epilepsy, CNS disorders, risk factors that may predispose to seizures or lower seizure threshold, QT interval prolongation, uncorrected hypokalemia, renal/hepatic dysfunction, pregnancy/nursing status, and possible drug interactions. Obtain baseline culture and susceptibility tests. Perform serologic test for syphilis in patients with gonorrhea.

Monitoring: Monitor for tendinitis or tendon rupture, CNS effects, signs/symptoms of hypersensitivity reactions, CDAD, peripheral neuropathy, photosensitivity/phototoxicity reactions, ECG changes, and other adverse reactions. Monitor renal/hepatic/hematopoietic function with prolonged use. Perform periodic culture and susceptibility testing. Perform follow-up serologic test for syphilis after 3 months in patients with gonorrhea. Monitor PT or other coagulation tests with warfarin or its derivatives.

Counseling: Advise to notify physician if pain, swelling, or inflammation of a tendon, or weakness or inability to move joints develops; instruct to d/c therapy and rest/refrain from exercise. Instruct to notify physician if experiencing worsening muscle weakness or breathing problems, sunburn-like reaction or skin eruption, and of all medications and supplements currently being taken. Inform that drug treats only bacterial, not viral, infections. Counsel to take exactly ud; inform that skipping doses or not completing full course of therapy may decrease effectiveness and increase bacterial resistance. Advise to drink fluids liberally. Instruct to d/c and notify physician if signs/symptoms of hypersensitivity reactions/allergic reactions or peripheral neuropathy develop. Inform that drug may cause dizziness and lightheadedness; advise to assess reaction to therapy before engaging in activities that require mental alertness or coordination. Counsel to minimize or avoid exposure to natural/artificial sunlight. Advise diabetic patients being treated with insulin or oral hypoglycemic drug to d/c therapy immediately if hypoglycemic reaction occurs and consult a physician. Instruct to notify physician of any history of convulsions. Advise to contact physician as soon as possible if watery and bloody stools (with or without stomach cramps and fever) develop. Instruct to notify physician if any symptoms of QT prolongation, including prolonged heart palpitations, or loss of consciousness occur. Advise not to take mineral supplements, vitamins with iron or minerals, antacids containing Ca^{2+}, Mg^{2+}, or aluminum, sucralfate, didanosine, chewable/buffered tabs, or pediatric powder for oral sol within the 2-hr period before or after taking ofloxacin.

OFLOXACIN OTIC — ofloxacin

Rx

Class: Fluoroquinolone

OTHER BRAND NAMES
Floxin Otic (Discontinued)

ADULT DOSAGE
Otitis Externa
Usual: 10 drops (0.5mL) into affected ear qd for 7 days

Otitis Media
Chronic Suppurative Otitis Media w/ Perforated Tympanic Membranes:
Usual: 10 drops (0.5mL) into affected ear bid for 14 days

PEDIATRIC DOSAGE
Otitis Externa
6 Months-13 Years:
Usual: 5 drops (0.25mL) into affected ear qd for 7 days
≥13 Years:
Usual: 10 drops (0.5mL) into affected ear qd for 7 days

Otitis Media

Chronic Suppurative Otitis Media w/ Perforated Tympanic Membranes:

≥12 Years:

Usual: 10 drops (0.5mL) into affected ear bid for 14 days

Acute Otitis Media w/ Tympanostomy Tubes:

1-12 Years:

Usual: 5 drops (0.25mL) into affected ear bid for 10 days

ADMINISTRATION

Otic route

Instillation

1. Warm sol by holding bottle in hand for 1-2 min.
2. Lie w/ affected ear upward then instill drops; maintain position for 5 min.
3. For acute otitis media w/ tympanostomy tubes and chronic suppurative otitis media w/ perforated tympanostomy tubes, pump tragus 4X by pushing inward to facilitate penetration into the middle ear.
4. Repeat for opposite ear if necessary.

STORAGE

20-25°C (68-77°F). Protect from light.

HOW SUPPLIED

Sol: 0.3% [5mL, 10mL]

CONTRAINDICATIONS

History of hypersensitivity to ofloxacin, to other quinolones, or to any of the components in the medication.

WARNINGS/PRECAUTIONS

D/C if hypersensitivity reaction occurs. Prolonged use may result in overgrowth of nonsusceptible organisms; reevaluate if no improvement after one week. If otorrhea persists after a full course, or if two or more episodes occur within 6 months, further evaluation is recommended. Not for injection or ophthalmic use.

ADVERSE REACTIONS

Pruritus, application-site reaction, taste perversion.

PREGNANCY AND LACTATION

Pregnancy: Category C.
Lactation: Not for use in nursing.

MECHANISM OF ACTION

Fluoroquinolone; exerts antibacterial activity by inhibiting DNA gyrase, an enzyme required for DNA replication, repair, deactivation, and transcription.

PHARMACOKINETICS

Absorption: (Perforated tympanic membrane) C_{max}=10ng/mL.

PATIENT CONSIDERATIONS

Assessment: Assess for drug hypersensitivity, preexisting cholesteatoma, foreign body or tumor, pregnancy/nursing status.

Monitoring: Monitor for anaphylactic reactions, cardiovascular collapse, loss of consciousness, angioedema, airway obstruction, dyspnea, urticaria and itching, overgrowth of nonsusceptible organisms, for improvement/persistence of otorrhea.

Counseling: Counsel to avoid touching applicator tip to fingers or other surfaces to avoid contamination. D/C and instruct to contact physician if signs of allergy occur. Instruct patients to warm bottle by holding for 1-2 min, to avoid dizziness that may result from instillation of a cold solution. Instruct to lie with affected ear upward, before instilling the drops; maintain position for 5 min. Instruct to repeat if necessary, for opposite ear.

OLEPTRO — trazodone hydrochloride   **Rx**

Class: Triazolopyridine derivative

> Antidepressants increased the risk of suicidal thinking and behavior (suicidality) in children, adolescents, and young adults in short-term studies of major depressive disorder (MDD) and other psychiatric disorders. Monitor and observe closely for clinical worsening, suicidality, or unusual changes in behavior. Not approved for use in pediatric patients.

ADULT DOSAGE

Major Depressive Disorder

Initial: 150mg qhs

Titrate: May increase by 75mg/day every 3 days (eg, start 225mg on Day 4 of therapy)

Max: 375mg/day

Maint: Generally recommended to continue treatment for several months after an initial response; maintain on the lowest effective dose

Once adequate response is achieved, may reduce dose gradually, w/ subsequent adjustment depending on therapeutic response

Dosing Considerations with MAOIs

Switching to/from an MAOI for Psychiatric Disorders:

Allow at least 14 days between discontinuation of an MAOI and initiation of treatment, and conversely allow at least 14 days between discontinuing treatment before starting an MAOI.

Use w/ Other MAOIs (eg, Linezolid, IV Methylene Blue):

Do not start trazodone in patients being treated w/ linezolid or IV methylene blue.

If acceptable alternatives are not available and benefits outweigh risks of serotonin syndrome, d/c trazodone promptly and administer linezolid or IV methylene blue; monitor for serotonin syndrome for 2 weeks or until 24 hrs after last dose of linezolid or IV methylene blue, whichever comes 1st. May resume trazodone therapy 24 hrs after last dose of linezolid or IV methylene blue.

PEDIATRIC DOSAGE

Pediatric use may not have been established

DOSING CONSIDERATIONS

Discontinuation

Gradually reduce dose whenever possible

ADMINISTRATION

Oral route

Take at the same time every day, in the late pm preferably hs, on an empty stomach.

May swallow whole or as a 1/2 tab by breaking the tab along the score line; do not chew or crush.

STORAGE

15-30°C (59-86°F).

HOW SUPPLIED

Tab, Extended Release: 150mg*, 300mg* *scored

CONTRAINDICATIONS

Use of an MAOI for psychiatric disorders either concomitantly or within 14 days of stopping treatment. Treatment within 14 days of stopping an MAOI for psychiatric disorders. Starting treatment in patients being treated with other MAOIs (eg, linezolid, IV methylene blue).

WARNINGS/PRECAUTIONS

Monitor for withdrawal symptoms when discontinuing treatment; reduce dose gradually. Serotonin syndrome reported; d/c immediately and initiate supportive symptomatic treatment. Pupillary dilation that occurs following use may trigger an angle-closure attack in a patient with anatomically narrow angles who does not have a patent iridectomy. May precipitate mixed/manic episode in patients at risk for bipolar disorder; screen for risk of bipolar disorder prior to initiating treatment. Not approved for treatment of bipolar depression. May cause QT/QTc interval prolongation, torsades de pointes, cardiac arrhythmias, and hypotension, including orthostatic hypotension and syncope. Not recommended for use during the initial recovery phase of myocardial infarction (MI). May increase risk of bleeding events. Priapism reported; caution in men with conditions that may predispose to priapism (eg, sickle cell anemia, multiple myeloma, leukemia) or with penile anatomical deformation; d/c with erection lasting >6 hrs (painful or not). Hyponatremia may occur; caution in elderly and volume-depleted patients. Consider discontinuation in patients with symptomatic hyponatremia and institute appropriate medical intervention. May cause somnolence or sedation and may impair mental/physical abilities. Caution with cardiac disease, hepatic/renal impairment, and in elderly.

ADVERSE REACTIONS

Somnolence, sedation, headache, dry mouth, dizziness, nausea, fatigue, diarrhea, constipation, back pain, blurred vision, sexual dysfunction.

DRUG INTERACTIONS

See Contraindications. May cause serotonin syndrome with other serotonergic drugs (eg, triptans, TCAs, fentanyl) and with drugs that impair serotonin metabolism; d/c immediately if this occurs. May enhance response to alcohol, barbiturates, and other CNS depressants. Increased risk of cardiac arrhythmia with drugs that prolong QT interval or CYP3A4 inhibitors. CYP3A4 inhibitors (eg, ritonavir, ketoconazole, indinavir) may increase levels with the potential for adverse effects. Potent CYP3A4 inhibitors may increase risk of cardiac arrhythmia; consider lower dose of trazodone. Carbamazepine (CYP3A4 inducer) may decrease levels; monitor to determine if a trazodone dose increase is required. Increased serum digoxin or phenytoin levels reported; monitor serum levels and adjust dosages PRN. Concomitant use with an antihypertensive may require a dose reduction of the antihypertensive drug. Monitor for potential risk of bleeding and use caution with NSAIDs, aspirin, and other drugs that affect coagulation or bleeding. Increased risk of hyponatremia with diuretics. Altered PT reported in patients on warfarin.

PREGNANCY AND LACTATION

Pregnancy: Category C.
Lactation: Caution in nursing.

MECHANISM OF ACTION

Triazolopyridine derivative; not established. Suspected to be related to its potentiation of serotonergic activity in the CNS. Preclinical studies show selective inhibition of neuronal reuptake of serotonin and activity as an antagonist at 5-HT-2A/2C serotonin receptors. Antagonizes α_1-adrenergic receptors.

PHARMACOKINETICS
Absorption: Well-absorbed; (300mg single dose) C_{max}=1188ng/mL, T_{max}=9 hrs.
Distribution: Plasma protein binding (89-95%). **Metabolism:** Liver (extensive); oxidative cleavage via CYP3A4; m-chlorophenylpiperazine (active metabolite). **Elimination:** Urine (70-75%, <1% unchanged); $T_{1/2}$=10 hrs.

PATIENT CONSIDERATIONS
Assessment: Assess for drug hypersensitivity, risk for bipolar disorder, cardiac disease (eg, recent MI), conditions that may predispose to priapism, penile anatomical deformation, susceptibility to angle-closure glaucoma, volume depletion, hepatic/renal impairment, pregnancy/nursing status, and possible drug interactions.

Monitoring: Monitor for clinical worsening, suicidality, unusual changes in behavior, mania/hypomania, serotonin syndrome, angle-closure glaucoma, QT/QTc interval prolongation, cardiac arrhythmias, hypotension, syncope, bleeding events, priapism, hyponatremia, withdrawal symptoms, and other adverse reactions. Periodically reassess to determine the continued need for maintenance treatment.

Counseling: Inform of the risks, benefits, and appropriate use of therapy. Instruct patients and caregivers to notify physician if signs of clinical worsening, changes in behavior, or suicidality occur. Instruct to report to physician the occurrence of anxiety, agitation, panic attacks, insomnia, irritability, hostility, aggressiveness, impulsivity, akathisia, hypomania, or mania. Instruct to inform physician if patient has history of bipolar disorder, cardiac disease, or MI. Caution about the risks of serotonin syndrome, angle-closure glaucoma, priapism, hypotension, syncope, bleeding, and withdrawal symptoms. Instruct men to immediately d/c use and contact physician if erection lasts >6 hrs, whether painful or not. Caution against performing potentially hazardous tasks (eg, operating machinery) until reasonably certain that treatment does not affect them. Inform that therapy may enhance response to alcohol. Instruct to notify physician if intending to become pregnant, or nursing.

OLUX-E — clobetasol propionate   Rx
Class: Corticosteroid

ADULT DOSAGE	PEDIATRIC DOSAGE
Inflammatory and Pruritic Manifestations of Corticosteroid-Responsive Dermatoses	**Inflammatory and Pruritic Manifestations of Corticosteroid-Responsive Dermatoses**
Apply a capful as a thin layer to affected area(s) bid (am and pm), for up to 2 consecutive weeks	**≥12 Years:** Apply a thin layer to affected area(s) bid (am and pm), for up to 2 consecutive weeks
Max: 50g/week or 21 capfuls/week	**Max:** 50g/week or 21 capfuls/week

ADMINISTRATION
Topical route

Shake can, hold upside down, and depress the actuator
Gently massage into the affected area(s) until foam is absorbed
STORAGE
20-25°C (68-77°F); excursions permitted between 15-30°C (59-86°F). Do not puncture or incinerate container. Do not expose to heat or store above 49°C (120°F).
HOW SUPPLIED
Foam: 0.05% [50g, 100g]
WARNINGS/PRECAUTIONS
May cause reversible hypothalamic-pituitary-adrenal (HPA) axis suppression with the potential for glucocorticosteroid insufficiency, Cushing's syndrome, hyperglycemia, and unmasking of latent diabetes mellitus; withdraw, reduce frequency, or substitute a less potent steroid if HPA axis suppression occurs. Manifestations of adrenal insufficiency may require systemic corticosteroids. Pediatric patients may be more susceptible to systemic toxicity. Local adverse reactions are more likely to occur with occlusive use, prolonged use, or use of higher potency corticosteroids. D/C if irritation occurs. Use appropriate antimicrobial agent with skin infections; d/c until infection is treated. Avoid application to eyes, face, groin, axillae, and area of skin atrophy. Flammable; avoid fire, flame, or smoking during and immediately following application. Do not apply on the chest if used during lactation. D/C if control is achieved.
ADVERSE REACTIONS
Application-site reaction, application-site atrophy, folliculitis, acneiform eruptions, hypopigmentation, perioral dermatitis, allergic contact dermatitis, secondary infection, irritation, striae, miliaria.
DRUG INTERACTIONS
Use of >1 corticosteroid-containing product may increase the total systemic corticosteroid exposure.
PREGNANCY AND LACTATION
Category C, caution in nursing.
MECHANISM OF ACTION
Corticosteroid; not established. Plays a role in cellular signaling, immune function, inflammation, and protein regulation.
PHARMACOKINETICS
Absorption: Percutaneous. C_{max}=59pg/mL, T_{max}=5 hrs (post-dose on Day 8). **Distribution:** Found in breast milk (systemically administered). **Metabolism:** Liver. **Elimination:** Kidneys, bile.

PATIENT CONSIDERATIONS
Assessment: Assess for presence of concomitant skin infections, severity of dermatoses, factors that predispose to HPA axis suppression, pregnancy/nursing status, and possible drug interactions.

Monitoring: Monitor for signs/symptoms of HPA axis suppression, Cushing's syndrome, hyperglycemia, irritation, allergic contact dermatitis (eg, failure to heal), and skin infections. Monitor for systemic toxicity, linear growth retardation, delayed weight gain, and intracranial HTN in pediatric patients. Monitor response to therapy.

Counseling: Counsel to use externally and exactly ud; avoid use on face, skin folds (eg, underarms, groin), eyes, or other mucous membranes. Advise to wash hands after use. Advise not to bandage or wrap treatment area, unless directed by physician. Counsel to contact physician if any local or systemic adverse reactions occur, if no improvement is seen after 2 weeks, or if surgery is contemplated. Advise that foam is flammable; avoid fire, flame, or smoking during application. Advise to d/c when control is achieved.

OLYSIO — simeprevir   Rx
Class: HCV NS3/4A protease inhibitor

ADULT DOSAGE	PEDIATRIC DOSAGE
Chronic Hepatitis C	Pediatric use may not have been established
Genotype 1 or 4 Infection: Recommended Dose: 150mg qd	
May be taken in combination w/ sofosbuvir or in combination w/ peginterferon alfa (Peg-IFN-alfa) and ribavirin (RBV); for specific dosing recommendations for the antiviral drugs used in combination w/ simeprevir, refer to their respective prescribing information	
Recommended Treatment Regimen and Duration:	
In Combination w/ Sofosbuvir in Patients w/ Genotype 1 Infection: Treatment-Naive and Treatment-Experienced w/o Cirrhosis: 12 weeks of simeprevir + sofosbuvir	
Treatment-Naive and Treatment-Experienced w/ Cirrhosis: 24 weeks of simeprevir + sofosbuvir	
In Combination w/ Peg-IFN-alfa and RBV in Patients w/ Genotype 1 or 4 Infection:	
Treatment-Naive and Prior Relapsers (w/ or w/o Cirrhosis, Not Coinfected w/ HIV or w/o Cirrhosis, Coinfected w/ HIV): Triple therapy (simeprevir/Peg-IFN-alfa/RBV) x 12 weeks; then dual therapy (Peg-IFN-alfa/RBV) x 12 weeks	
Treatment-Naive and Prior Relapsers (w/ Compensated Cirrhosis, Coinfected w/ HIV): Triple therapy x 12 weeks; then dual therapy x 36 weeks	
Prior Non-Responders, Including Partial and Null-Responders (w/ or w/o Cirrhosis, w/ or w/o HIV Coinfection): Triple therapy x 12 weeks; then dual therapy x 36 weeks	

DOSING CONSIDERATIONS
Hepatic Impairment
Moderate or Severe (Child-Pugh Class B or C): Use not recommended
Discontinuation
Use w/ Sofosbuvir:
No treatment stopping rules apply to the combination of simeprevir w/ sofosbuvir
Use w/ Peg-IFN-Alfa and RBV:
HCV RNA ≥25 IU/mL at Week 4: D/C triple therapy
HCV RNA ≥25 IU/mL at Week 12: D/C dual therapy (treatment w/ simeprevir is complete at Week 12)
HCV RNA ≥25 IU/mL at Week 24: D/C dual therapy (treatment w/ simeprevir is complete at Week 12)

Do not reinitiate if treatment is discontinued because of adverse reactions or inadequate on-treatment virologic response.

D/C therapy if any of the antiviral drugs used in combination w/ simeprevir for the treatment of chronic hepatitis C infection are permanently discontinued for any reason.

Other Important Considerations
Avoid reducing dose or interrupting treatment, to prevent treatment failure.

ADMINISTRATION
Oral route
Take w/ food.
Swallow whole.

STORAGE
Room temperature <30°C (86°F). Protect from light.

HOW SUPPLIED
Cap: 150mg

CONTRAINDICATIONS
When used in combination w/ other antiviral drugs (including Peg-IFN-alfa and RBV), refer to the respective prescribing information.

WARNINGS/PRECAUTIONS
Efficacy in combination w/ Peg-IFN-alfa and RBV is substantially reduced in patients infected w/ HCV genotype 1a w/ an NS3 Q80K polymorphism at baseline; consider alternative therapy for these patients. Not recommended in patients who previously failed therapy w/ a treatment regimen that included simeprevir or other HCV protease inhibitors. Not recommended as monotherapy. Caution in patients of East Asian ancestry; may exhibit higher simeprevir plasma exposures. Fatal cardiac arrest reported w/ sofosbuvir-containing regimen (ledipasvir/sofosbuvir). Hepatic decompensation and hepatic failure, including fatal cases, reported, mostly in patients w/ advanced and/or decompensated cirrhosis; d/c therapy if bilirubin elevation is accompanied by liver transaminase increases or clinical signs/symptoms of hepatic decompensation. Photosensitivity reactions and rash observed; consider discontinuation of treatment if a photosensitivity reaction or severe rash occurs and monitor patients until resolved. Contains a sulfonamide moiety; insufficient data to exclude association between sulfa allergy and frequency/severity of adverse reactions. Refer to the respective prescribing information when used w/ other antiviral drugs.

ADVERSE REACTIONS
When Used w/ Sofosbuvir: Fatigue, headache, nausea.
When Used in Combination w/ Peg-IFN-Alfa and RBV: Rash (including photosensitivity), pruritus, nausea.

DRUG INTERACTIONS
Coadministration of amiodarone w/ simeprevir in combination w/ sofosbuvir may result in serious symptomatic bradycardia; coadministration is not recommended. If coadministration is required, cardiac monitoring is recommended in an inpatient setting for the first 48 hrs, after which outpatient or self-monitoring of HR should occur on a daily basis for at least the first 2 weeks of treatment. Caution is warranted and therapeutic drug monitoring of amiodarone, if available, is recommended for concomitant use of amiodarone w/ a simeprevir-containing regimen that does not contain sofosbuvir. Use w/ moderate or strong inducers or inhibitors of CYP3A may lead to significantly lower or higher exposure, respectively, which may result in reduced therapeutic effect or adverse reactions; coadministration is not recommended. Increased levels of amiodarone, digoxin, oral antiarrhythmics (eg, disopyramide, flecainide, mexiletine, propafenone), oral calcium channel blockers (eg, amlodipine, diltiazem, felodipine), oral midazolam, oral triazolam, and PDE-5 inhibitors (eg, sildenafil, tadalafil, vardenafil). Use w/ caution w/ oral midazolam or triazolam. Concomitant use w/ systemic erythromycin may increase levels of both agents; coadministration is not recommended. May increase cisapride or cyclosporine levels; coadministration is not recommended. May increase levels of darunavir, rosuvastatin, atorvastatin, simvastatin, pitavastatin, pravastatin, and lovastatin. May increase or decrease sirolimus levels. Levels may be decreased w/ anticonvulsants (eg, carbamazepine, oxcarbazepine, phenobarbital), rifampin, rifabutin, rifapentine, systemic dexamethasone, St. John's wort, or efavirenz; coadministration is not recommended. Levels may be increased w/ systemic clarithromycin or telithromycin, systemic antifungals (eg, itraconazole, ketoconazole, posaconazole), milk thistle (*Silybum marianum*), cobicistat-containing products, darunavir/ritonavir, ritonavir, or cyclosporine; coadministration is not recommended. Levels may be increased or decreased w/ delavirdine, etravirine, nevirapine, or other ritonavir-boosted or unboosted HIV protease inhibitors (eg, atazanavir, fosamprenavir, lopinavir); coadministration is not recommended. May increase levels of CYP3A4, OATP1B1/3, and P-gp substrates. Refer to PI for dosing modifications and monitoring parameters when used w/ certain concomitant therapies.

PREGNANCY AND LACTATION
Pregnancy: Embryofetal developmental toxicity (including fetal loss) observed in mice; potential risk to fetus.
Lactation: Detected in plasma of nursing pups in animal studies; consider developmental and health benefits of breastfeeding along w/ mother's clinical need for treatment.

Refer to prescribing information of the drugs used in combination w/ simeprevir for information regarding use in pregnancy/nursing.

MECHANISM OF ACTION
HCV NS3/4A protease inhibitor; direct-acting antiviral agent against HCV.

PHARMACOKINETICS
Absorption: AUC_{24}=57,469ng•hr/mL; T_{max}=4-6 hrs. (150mg single dose) Absolute bioavailability (62%). **Distribution:** Plasma protein binding (>99.9%). **Metabolism:** Liver via CYP3A; oxidation. **Elimination:** (200mg single dose) Feces (91%, 31% unchanged), urine (<1%), bile; $T_{1/2}$=41 hrs (HCV-infected).

PATIENT CONSIDERATIONS
Assessment: Assess for presence of HCV genotype 1a w/ NS3 Q80K polymorphism, hepatic impairment, sulfa allergy, pregnancy/nursing status, and possible drug interactions. Obtain baseline HCV-RNA levels and liver chemistry tests.

Monitoring: Monitor for signs/symptoms of hepatic decompensation, photosensitivity reactions, rash, and other adverse reactions. Monitor HCV RNA levels and liver chemistry tests as clinically indicated.

Counseling: Instruct to take ud. Inform that drug must be used in combination w/ other antiviral drugs, and that therapy should be discontinued if any of the other antiviral drugs used in combination are permanently discontinued. Counsel about the risk of serious symptomatic bradycardia when coadministered w/ amiodarone in combination w/ sofosbuvir; advise to seek medical evaluation immediately if signs/symptoms of bradycardia (eg, near-fainting or fainting, dizziness or lightheadedness, malaise) develop. Inform of the potential risk to fetus. Instruct to watch for early warning signs of liver inflammation (eg, fatigue, weakness, lack of appetite, N/V) as well as later signs (eg, jaundice, discolored feces) and to contact physician if such symptoms occur. Inform of the risk of photosensitivity reactions/rash and that these reactions may become severe; instruct to contact physician if a photosensitivity reaction or rash develops and not to stop treatment unless instructed by physician. Advise to use effective sun protection measures to limit exposure to natural sunlight and to avoid artificial sunlight (tanning beds or phototherapy) during treatment. Advise that reducing or interrupting treatment may increase possibility of treatment failure.

OMECLAMOX-PAK — amoxicillin/clarithromycin/omeprazole   Rx
Class: H. pylori treatment combination

ADULT DOSAGE
Helicobacter pylori Eradication

Helicobacter Pylori Infection and Duodenal Ulcer Disease:
Usual: 20mg omeprazole + 500mg clarithromycin + 1000mg amoxicillin, each given bid (am and pm) ac for 10 days
Ulcer Present When Initiating Therapy:
Give an additional 18 days of omeprazole 20mg qd

PEDIATRIC DOSAGE
Pediatric use may not have been established

DOSING CONSIDERATIONS
Renal Impairment
Severe: Prolong clarithromycin dosing intervals

Hepatic Impairment
Avoid use

ADMINISTRATION
Oral route

Take each dose of 4 pills in the am and 4 pills in the pm ac.
Swallow whole; do not crush or chew.

STORAGE
20-25°C (68-77°F). Protect from light and moisture.

HOW SUPPLIED
Cap: (Amoxicillin) 500mg; **Cap, Delayed-Release:** (Omeprazole) 20mg; **Tab:** (Clarithromycin) 500mg

CONTRAINDICATIONS
Concomitant use with ergotamine or dihydroergotamine and pimozide, known hypersensitivity to omeprazole, any macrolide antibiotic, any penicillin, or any component of the formulations.

WARNINGS/PRECAUTIONS
Avoid use in Asian patients unless benefits outweigh risks. Lab test interactions may occur. Amoxicillin: Serious and occasionally fatal hypersensitivity (anaphylactic) reactions reported in patients on PCN therapy; caution with history of PCN hypersensitivity and/or a history of sensitivity to multiple allergens. Not recommended in patients with mononucleosis; may develop erythematosus skin rash. Caution in elderly. Clarithromycin: Use in pregnancy only when there is no appropriate alternative therapy. Exacerbation of symptoms of myasthenia gravis and new onset of myasthenic syndrome reported. Amoxicillin/Clarithromycin: *Clostridium difficile*-associated diarrhea (CDAD) reported; may need to d/c if CDAD is suspected or confirmed. May result in bacterial resistance with prolonged use in the absence of proven or suspected bacterial infection, or a prophylactic indication; d/c if superinfections occur and institute appropriate therapy. Omeprazole: Symptomatic response does not preclude the presence of gastric malignancy. Acute interstitial nephritis (AIN) reported; d/c if AIN develops.

ADVERSE REACTIONS
Diarrhea, taste perversion, headache.

DRUG INTERACTIONS
See Contraindications. Amoxicillin: May decrease renal tubular secretion when coadministered with probenecid. Clarithromycin: May lead to increased exposure to colchicine when coadministered; monitor for colchicine toxicity. May increase levels of drugs metabolized by CYP3A, digoxin, theophylline, carbamazepine, and statins (eg, lovastatin, simvastatin). May potentiate antiarrhythmic effects with concurrent use of antiarrhythmic drugs. Torsades de pointes may occur with quinidine or disopyramide. May increase systemic exposure of sildenafil; consider a reduction in sildenafil dose. May alter the effect of triazolobenziodiazepines/related benzodiazepines. CNS effects (eg, somnolence, confusion) reported with concomitant triazolam. Omeprazole: Monitor patients taking drugs metabolized by CYP450 (eg, cyclosporine, disulfiram, benzodiazepines). May reduce levels of atazanavir and nelfinavir; concomitant use not recommended. May increase levels of

saquinavir and tacrolimus; consider dose reduction of saquinavir. May increase systemic exposure of cilostazol; consider a reduction in cilostazol dose. May reduce absorption of drugs where gastric pH is an important determinant of bioavailability; absorption of ketoconazole, atazanavir, iron salts, erlotinib, and mycophenolate mofetil may decrease, while absorption of digoxin may increase. Monitor patients when digoxin is taken concomitantly. Caution with mycophenolate mofetil in transplant patients. Clarithromycin/Omeprazole: May alter the anticoagulant effects of warfarin and other anticoagulants; monitor PT and INR. May alter the antiretroviral effects of antiretrovirals.

PREGNANCY AND LACTATION
Pregnancy: Category C.
Lactation: Not for use in nursing.

MECHANISM OF ACTION
Omeprazole: Substituted benzimidazole; suppresses gastric acid secretion by specific inhibition of H^+/K^+ ATPase enzyme system at the secretory surface of the gastric parietal cells. Blocks the final step of acid production. Clarithromycin: Semi-synthetic macrolide antibiotic; exerts antibacterial action by binding to the 50S ribosomal subunit of susceptible microorganisms, resulting in inhibition of protein synthesis. Amoxicillin: Semi-synthetic antibiotic; acts through inhibition of biosynthesis of cell wall mucopeptide.

PHARMACOKINETICS
Absorption: Omeprazole: Rapid; absolute bioavailability (30-40% [20-40mg dose]); T_{max}=0.5-3.5 hrs. Clarithromycin: Rapid; absolute bioavailability (50% [250mg]). Administration of variable doses resulted in different parameters. Amoxicillin: Rapid. (500mg) T_{max}=1-2 hrs, C_{max}=5.5-7.5mcg/mL. Refer to PI for pharmacokinetic parameters of combination therapy of omeprazole with antimicrobials. **Distribution:** Found in breast milk. Omeprazole: Plasma protein binding (95%). Amoxicillin: Plasma protein binding (20%). **Metabolism:** Omeprazole: Extensive via CYP450; hydroxyomeprazole, carboxylic acid (metabolites). Clarithromycin: 14-OH clarithromycin (active metabolite). **Elimination:** Omeprazole: Urine (77%, metabolites), feces; $T_{1/2}$=0.5-1 hr. Clarithromycin: Urine (30%); $T_{1/2}$=5-7 hrs; 7-9 hrs (14-OH clarithromycin). Amoxicillin: Urine (60%, unchanged); $T_{1/2}$=61.3 min.

PATIENT CONSIDERATIONS
Assessment: Assess for hypersensitivity to the drug, macrolides, PCNs, cephalosporins, or other allergens. Assess for myasthenia gravis, mononucleosis, renal/hepatic impairment, gastric malignancy, pregnancy/nursing status, and possible drug interactions.

Monitoring: Monitor for hypersensitivity reactions, drug interactions, exacerbation of symptoms of myasthenia gravis and new onset of myasthenic syndrome, CDAD, superinfections, development of drug-resistant bacteria, erythematosus skin rash, AIN, and other adverse reactions. Monitor PT/INR with warfarin and other anticoagulants.

Counseling: Inform about risks/benefits of therapy. Advise that diarrhea may occur and will usually end when therapy is discontinued. Instruct to contact physician as soon as possible if watery/bloody stools (w/ or w/o stomach cramps and fever) develop even as late as 2 or more months after having taken the last dose of therapy. Counsel that therapy should only be used to treat bacterial, not viral, infections. Instruct to take exactly ud; inform that skipping doses or not completing full course may decrease effectiveness and increase antibiotic resistance.

OMIDRIA — ketorolac/phenylephrine   Rx

Class: Alpha₁ agonist/NSAID

ADULT DOSAGE
Ocular Surgery
Added to an ophthalmic irrigation sol used during cataract surgery or intraocular lens replacement to maintain pupil size by preventing intraoperative miosis and reducing postoperative ocular pain

Dilute 4mL in 500mL of ophthalmic irrigation sol; use irrigation sol prn for the surgical procedure

PEDIATRIC DOSAGE
Pediatric use may not have been established

ADMINISTRATION
Intraocular route
Dilute prior to use

STORAGE
20-25°C (68-77°F). Protect from light. Diluted Sol: ≤4 hrs at room temperature or 24 hrs under refrigerated conditions.

HOW SUPPLIED
Sol: (Phenylephrine/Ketorolac) 1%/0.3% [4mL]

CONTRAINDICATIONS
Known hypersensitivity to any of the ingredients in this product.

WARNINGS/PRECAUTIONS
Systemic exposure may cause elevations in BP. Potential for cross-sensitivity to acetylsalicylic acid (ASA), phenylacetic acid derivatives, and other NSAIDs; caution with previous sensitivities to these drugs. Bronchospasm or exacerbation of asthma reported in patients with known hypersensitivity to ASA/NSAIDs or past history of asthma. Avoid use during late pregnancy.

ADVERSE REACTIONS
Anterior chamber inflammation, posterior capsule opacification, increased intraocular pressure.

PREGNANCY AND LACTATION
Category C, caution in nursing.

MECHANISM OF ACTION
Ketorolac: NSAID; inhibits COX-1 and COX-2. Phenylephrine: α₁-adrenergic receptor agonist; mydriatic agent.

PHARMACOKINETICS
Absorption: Ketorolac: C_{max}=15ng/mL.

PATIENT CONSIDERATIONS
Assessment: Assess for previous hypersensitivity to the drug or cross-sensitivity to ASA, phenylacetic acid derivatives, and other NSAIDs, and pregnancy/nursing status.

Monitoring: Monitor for hypersensitivity reactions and other adverse reactions.

Counseling: Inform that sensitivity to light may be experienced.

OMNARIS — ciclesonide   Rx

Class: Non-halogenated glucocorticoid

ADULT DOSAGE
Seasonal/Perennial Allergic Rhinitis

2 sprays/nostril qd
Max: 2 sprays/nostril/day (200mcg/day)

PEDIATRIC DOSAGE
Perennial Allergic Rhinitis
≥12 Years:
2 sprays/nostril qd
Max: 2 sprays/nostril/day (200mcg/day)

Seasonal Allergic Rhinitis
≥6 Years:
2 sprays/nostril qd
Max: 2 sprays/nostril/day (200mcg/day)

DOSING CONSIDERATIONS
Elderly
Start at low end of dosing range

ADMINISTRATION
Intranasal route

Priming
Shake bottle gently and prime pump by actuating 8X before initial use. Reprime w/ 1 spray or until fine mist appears if not used for 4 consecutive days.

STORAGE
25°C (77°F); excursions permitted to 15-30°C (59-86°F). Do not freeze. Discard after 4 months after removal from pouch or after 120 actuations following initial priming, whichever comes 1st.

HOW SUPPLIED
Spray: 50mcg/spray [12.5g]

CONTRAINDICATIONS
Known hypersensitivity to ciclesonide or any of the ingredients of the nasal spray.

WARNINGS/PRECAUTIONS
Epistaxis reported. *Candida albicans* infections of the nose or pharynx may occur; examine periodically and treat accordingly. Nasal septal perforation may occur; avoid spraying directly onto nasal septum. May impair wound healing; avoid w/ recent nasal septal ulcers, nasal surgery, or nasal trauma until healing has occurred. Glaucoma and/or cataracts may develop. Risk for more severe/fatal course of infections (eg, chickenpox, measles); avoid exposure in patients who have not had these diseases or have not been properly immunized. May increase susceptibility to infections; caution w/ active or quiescent tuberculosis (TB), untreated local or systemic fungal/bacterial infections, systemic viral or parasitic infections, or ocular herpes simplex. D/C slowly if hypercorticism and adrenal suppression occur. Risk of adrenal insufficiency and withdrawal symptoms when replacing systemic corticosteroids w/ topical corticosteroids. May exacerbate symptoms of asthma and other conditions requiring long-term systemic corticosteroid use w/ rapid dose decrease. May reduce growth velocity in pediatric patients. Caution in elderly.

ADVERSE REACTIONS
Headache, epistaxis, nasopharyngitis, back pain, pharyngolaryngeal pain, sinusitis, influenza, nasal discomfort, bronchitis, UTI, cough.

DRUG INTERACTIONS
Ketoconazole may increase exposure of the active metabolite des-ciclesonide.

PREGNANCY AND LACTATION
Category C, caution in nursing.

MECHANISM OF ACTION
Non-halogenated glucocorticoid; not established. Shown to have a wide range of effects on multiple cell types and mediators involved in allergic inflammation.

PHARMACOKINETICS
Absorption: Des-ciclesonide: C_{max}=<30pg/mL. **Distribution:** (IV) V_d=2.9L/kg (Ciclesonide), 12.1L/kg (des-ciclesonide); plasma protein binding (≥99%). **Metabolism:** Hydrolysis by esterases to des-ciclesonide (active metabolite); further metabolism in liver, via CYP3A4, CYP2D6. **Elimination:** (IV) Feces (66%), urine (≤20%).

PATIENT CONSIDERATIONS

Assessment: Assess for drug hypersensitivity, TB, any infections, ocular herpes simplex, history of increased IOP, glaucoma, cataracts, recent nasal septal ulcers, nasal surgery/trauma, use of other inhaled or systemic corticosteroids, pregnancy/nursing status, and possible drug interactions. Assess if patients have not been immunized or exposed to infections, such as measles or chickenpox.

Monitoring: Monitor for hypercorticism, adrenal suppression, TB, infections, ocular herpes simplex, chickenpox, and measles. Monitor for epistaxis, nasal septal perforation, growth velocity in children, wound healing, visual changes, hypoadrenalism in infants born to mothers receiving corticosteroids during pregnancy, and hypersensitivity reactions. Monitor for adrenal insufficiency and withdrawal symptoms when replacing systemic w/ topical corticosteroids.

Counseling: Counsel on appropriate priming and administration of spray; avoid spraying in eyes or directly onto nasal septum. Instruct to take ud at regular intervals; not to exceed prescribed dosage. Instruct to contact physician if symptoms do not improve by a reasonable time (over 1-2 weeks in seasonal allergic rhinitis and 5 weeks in perennial allergic rhinitis) or if condition worsens. Counsel about risks of epistaxis, nasal ulceration, *Candida* infections, and other adverse reactions. Instruct to avoid exposure to chickenpox or measles and to consult physician if exposed to chickenpox or measles. Inform that worsening of existing TB infections, fungal/bacterial/viral/parasitic infections, or ocular herpes simplex may occur. Instruct to inform physician if change in vision occurs.

Omnipred — prednisolone acetate   Rx

Class: Corticosteroid

ADULT DOSAGE	PEDIATRIC DOSAGE
Steroid-Responsive Inflammatory Ocular Conditions	Pediatric use may not have been established
Treatment of palpebral and bulbar conjunctiva, cornea, and anterior segment of globe, such as allergic conjunctivitis, acne rosacea, superficial punctate keratitis, herpes zoster keratitis, iritis, cyclitis, or selected infective conjunctivitides	
Instill 2 drops in eye(s) qid	
Reevaluate if signs/symptoms do not improve after 2 days	
Corneal Injury	
Chemical, Radiation, or Thermal Burns, or Penetration of Foreign Bodies:	
Instill 2 drops in eye(s) qid	
Reevaluate if signs/symptoms do not improve after 2 days	

ADMINISTRATION
Ocular route
Shake well before use.
Use concomitantly with an anti-infective agent in cases of bacterial infections.

STORAGE
8-24°C (46-75°F); upright position.

HOW SUPPLIED
Sus: 1% [5mL, 10mL]

CONTRAINDICATIONS
Viral diseases of the cornea and conjunctiva (eg, epithelial herpes simplex keratitis, vaccinia, varicella); mycobacterial infection of the eye, and fungal diseases of ocular structures; known/suspected hypersensitivity to any of the ingredients of this preparation and to other corticosteroids.

WARNINGS/PRECAUTIONS
Prolonged use may result in glaucoma with damage to the optic nerve, defects in visual acuity and fields of vision, and in posterior subcapsular cataract formation. Prolonged use may suppress host immune response and increase hazard of secondary ocular infections. Use in the presence of thin corneal or scleral tissue, which may be caused by various ocular diseases or long-term use of topical corticosteroids, may lead to perforation. May enhance activity of or mask acute purulent infections of the eye. Routinely monitor intraocular pressure (IOP) if used for ≥10 days. Caution with glaucoma. Use after cataract surgery may delay healing and increase incidence of bleb formation. May prolong course and exacerbate severity of many viral infections of the eye; use with extreme caution with history of herpes simplex. Not effective in mustard gas keratitis and Sjogren's keratoconjunctivitis. Fungal infections of the cornea may develop coincidentally with long-term use; suspect fungal invasion in any persistent corneal ulceration. In chronic conditions, withdraw treatment by gradually decreasing frequency of application. Caution not to d/c therapy prematurely.

ADVERSE REACTIONS
Elevation of IOP, glaucoma, optic nerve damage, posterior subcapsular cataract formation, delayed wound healing, acute anterior uveitis, globe perforation.

PREGNANCY AND LACTATION
Pregnancy: Category C.
Lactation: Not for use in nursing.

MECHANISM OF ACTION

Corticosteroid; not established. Suspected to act by induction of phospholipase A_2 inhibitory proteins called lipocortins, which control the biosynthesis of potent inflammation mediators (eg, prostaglandins, leukotrienes) by inhibiting release of their precursor, arachidonic acid.

PHARMACOKINETICS

Distribution: Found in breast milk (systemic use).

PATIENT CONSIDERATIONS

Assessment: Assess for viral diseases of cornea and conjunctiva, mycobacterial infection of the eye, fungal diseases of ocular structures, hypersensitivity to drug or other corticosteroids, history of herpes simplex, thin corneal or scleral tissue, glaucoma, cataract surgery, and pregnancy/nursing status.

Monitoring: Monitor for glaucoma, optic nerve damage, visual acuity and fields of vision defects, posterior subcapsular cataracts, secondary ocular infections, perforation of the cornea/sclera, exacerbation of viral infections of eye, fungal invasion, and other adverse reactions. Routinely monitor IOP if used for ≥10 days. Monitor for improvement of signs/symptoms.

Counseling: Advise to d/c use and consult physician if inflammation or pain persists >48 hrs or becomes aggravated. Instruct to use caution to avoid touching the bottle tip to eyelids or to any other surfaces to prevent contamination. Instruct to keep bottle tightly closed when not in use and to keep it out of reach of children.

Omtryg — omega-3-acid ethyl esters A   Rx

Class: Lipid-regulating agent

ADULT DOSAGE	PEDIATRIC DOSAGE
Severe Hypertriglyceridemia (≥500mg/dL)	Pediatric use may not have been established
Usual: 4 caps qd or 2 caps bid	

ADMINISTRATION
Oral route
Take w/ meals
Swallow caps whole; do not break open, crush, dissolve, or chew

STORAGE
25°C (77°F); excursions permitted to 15-30°C (59-86°F). Do not freeze.

HOW SUPPLIED
Cap: 1.2g

CONTRAINDICATIONS
Known hypersensitivity (eg, anaphylactic reaction) to omega-3-acid ethyl esters or any component of this medication.

WARNINGS/PRECAUTIONS
Increases in ALT levels without a concurrent increase in AST levels reported. May increase LDL levels; monitor LDL levels periodically during therapy. Contains ethyl esters of omega-3 fatty acids (eicosapentaenoic acid [EPA] and docosahexaenoic acid [DHA]) obtained from oil of several fish sources; caution with known hypersensitivity to fish and/or shellfish. Recurrent symptomatic atrial fibrillation/flutter (A-fib/flutter) reported in patients with paroxysmal or persistent A-fib, particularly within the first 2-3 months of initiating therapy. Assess TG levels carefully before initiating therapy and monitor TG levels periodically during therapy.

ADVERSE REACTIONS
Eructation, taste perversion, dyspepsia.

DRUG INTERACTIONS
Periodically monitor patients receiving concomitant treatment with an anticoagulant or other drugs affecting coagulation (eg, antiplatelet agents). D/C or change medications known to exacerbate hypertriglyceridemia (eg, β-blockers, thiazides, estrogens), if possible, prior to consideration of therapy.

PREGNANCY AND LACTATION
Category C, caution in nursing.

MECHANISM OF ACTION
Lipid-regulating agent; not established. Potential mechanisms of action include inhibition of acyl-CoA: 1,2-diacylglycerol acyltransferase, increased mitochondrial and peroxisomal β-oxidation in the liver, decreased lipogenesis in the liver, and increased plasma lipoprotein lipase activity. May reduce the synthesis of TGs in the liver because EPA and DHA are poor substrates for the enzymes responsible for TG synthesis, and EPA and DHA inhibit esterification of other fatty acids.

PHARMACOKINETICS
Distribution: Found in breast milk.

PATIENT CONSIDERATIONS

Assessment: Assess for hypersensitivity to drug, fish, and/or shellfish; hepatic impairment; A-fib/flutter; pregnancy/nursing status; and possible drug interactions. Attempt to control serum lipids with appropriate diet, exercise, weight loss in obese patients, and control of any medical problems that are contributing to lipid abnormalities. Assess TG and LDL levels.

Monitoring: Monitor for recurrent symptomatic A-fib/flutter in patients with paroxysmal or persistent A-fib. Monitor for allergic reactions and other adverse reactions. Periodically monitor ALT and AST levels in patients with hepatic impairment. Periodically monitor LDL and TG levels.

Counseling: Instruct to notify physician if allergic to fish and/or shellfish. Advise that the use of lipid-regulating agents does not reduce the importance of adhering to diet. Instruct to take ud.

ONDANSETRON — ondansetron

Rx

Class: 5-HT₃ receptor antagonist

Class: 5-HT_3 receptor antagonist

OTHER BRAND NAMES
Zofran, Zofran ODT

ADULT DOSAGE

Chemotherapy-Induced Nausea/Vomiting

Inj:

Prevention of N/V Associated w/ Initial and Repeat Courses of Emetogenic Chemotherapy (Including High-Dose Cisplatin):
Three 0.15mg/kg IV doses (diluted) up to a max of 16mg/dose; infuse over 15 min. Give 1st dose 30 min before the start of chemotherapy, then give subsequent doses 4 and 8 hrs after the 1st dose

Oral:
Prevention of N/V Associated w/ Highly Emetogenic Chemotherapy (Including Cisplatin ≥50mg/m²):
24mg (given as three 8mg tabs) 30 min before start of single-day chemotherapy

Prevention of N/V Associated w/ Moderately Emetogenic Chemotherapy:
8mg bid; give 1st dose 30 min before chemotherapy, then give subsequent dose 8 hrs after 1st dose, then administer 8mg q12h for 1-2 days after completion of chemotherapy

Postoperative Nausea/Vomiting

Prevention:

Inj:
4mg IM/IV undiluted immediately before induction of anesthesia or postoperatively if prophylactic antiemetic was not received and N/V occurs w/in 2 hrs after surgery; infuse IV in not less than 30 sec, preferably over 2-5 min

Oral:
16mg given 1 hr before induction of anesthesia

Radiotherapy Associated Nausea/Vomiting

Oral:
Prevention in Patients Receiving Either Total Body Irradiation, Single High-Dose Fraction to the Abdomen, or Daily Fractions to the Abdomen:
Usual: 8mg tid

Total Body Irradiation:
8mg should be administered 1-2 hrs before each fraction of radiotherapy administered each day

Single High-Dose Fraction Radiotherapy to the Abdomen:
8mg should be administered 1-2 hrs before radiotherapy, w/ subsequent doses q8h after 1st dose for 1-2 days after completion of radiotherapy

Daily Fractionated Radiotherapy to the Abdomen:
8mg should be administered 1-2 hrs before radiotherapy, w/ subsequent doses q8h after 1st dose for each day radiotherapy is given

---

DOSING CONSIDERATIONS
Hepatic Impairment
Severe (Child-Pugh Score ≥10):
Oral:
Max: 8mg/day
Inj:
Max: 8mg/day infused over 15 min beginning 30 min prior to emetogenic chemotherapy

PEDIATRIC DOSAGE

Chemotherapy-Induced Nausea/Vomiting

Inj:

Prevention of N/V Associated w/ Initial and Repeat Courses of Emetogenic Chemotherapy (Including High-Dose Cisplatin):
6 Months-18 Years:
Three 0.15mg/kg IV doses (diluted) up to a max of 16mg/dose; infuse over 15 min. Give 1st dose 30 min before the start of chemotherapy, then give subsequent doses 4 and 8 hrs after the 1st dose

Oral:
Prevention of N/V Associated w/ Moderately Emetogenic Cancer Chemotherapy:
4-11 Years:
4mg tid; give 1st dose 30 min before chemotherapy, then give subsequent doses 4 and 8 hrs after 1st dose, then administer 4mg q8h for 1-2 days after completion of chemotherapy

≥12 Years:
8mg bid; give 1st dose 30 min before chemotherapy, then give subsequent dose 8 hrs after 1st dose, then administer 8mg q12h for 1-2 days after completion of chemotherapy

Postoperative Nausea/Vomiting

Prevention:
1 Month-12 Years:
Inj:
≤40kg: 0.1mg/kg IV single dose
>40kg: 4mg IV single dose

Infuse in not less than 30 sec, preferably over 2-5 min immediately before or after induction of anesthesia or postoperatively if prophylactic antiemetic was not received and N/V occurs shortly after surgery

ADMINISTRATION
IV/IM/Oral routes

ODT
Do not attempt to push tabs through the foil backing.
Peel back the foil backing of 1 blister and gently remove tab.
Immediately place tab on top of the tongue where it will dissolve in seconds, then swallow w/ saliva.

Inj
Should be diluted in 50mL of D5 or NaCl before administration.
Do not mix w/ alkaline sol as a precipitate may form.

STORAGE
20-25°C (68-77°F); excursions permitted to 15-30°C (59-86°F). Protect from light. Zofran: (Inj/ODT/Tab) 2-30°C (36-86°F). (Sol) 15-30°C (59-86°F); store bottles upright in cartons. (Inj/Sol/Tab) Protect from light. (Inj) Diluted Sol: Do not use beyond 24 hrs. Refer to PI for further information on stability and handling.

HOW SUPPLIED
Tab: 24mg; (Zofran) **Inj:** 2mg/mL [20mL], **Sol:** 4mg base/5mL [50mL], **Tab/Tab, Disintegrating (ODT):** 4mg, 8mg

CONTRAINDICATIONS
Concomitant use w/ apomorphine, known hypersensitivity to ondansetron or any of its components.

WARNINGS/PRECAUTIONS
Hypersensitivity reactions reported in patients hypersensitive to other selective 5-HT₃ receptor antagonists. ECG changes, including QT interval prolongation and torsades de pointes, reported; avoid in patients w/ congenital long QT syndrome. Monitor ECG in patients with electrolyte abnormalities (eg, hypokalemia, hypomagnesemia), CHF, bradyarrhythmias, and in patients taking other medications that lead to QT prolongation. Serotonin syndrome reported; d/c and initiate supportive treatment if symptoms occur. Use in patients following abdominal surgery or w/ chemotherapy-induced N/V may mask a progressive ileus and/or gastric distension. Does not stimulate gastric/intestinal peristalsis; do not use instead of NG suction. (ODT) Contains phenylalanine; caution in phenylketonuric patients.

ADVERSE REACTIONS
Headache, diarrhea, constipation, fever, pruritus, dizziness, bradycardia, drowsiness/sedation. (Inj) Inj-site reaction. (PO) Malaise/fatigue, anxiety/agitation, urinary retention.

DRUG INTERACTIONS
See Contraindications. Inducers or inhibitors of CYP3A4, CYP2D6, and CYP1A2 may change the clearance and $T_{1/2}$. Potent CYP3A4 inducers (eg, phenytoin, carbamazepine, rifampin) may significantly increase clearance and decrease blood levels. May reduce analgesic activity of tramadol. May cause serotonin syndrome w/ other serotonergic drugs (eg, SSRIs, SNRIs, MAOIs, mirtazapine, fentanyl, lithium, tramadol, IV methylene blue); d/c and initiate supportive treatment if symptoms occur.

PREGNANCY AND LACTATION
Pregnancy: Category B
Lactation: Caution in nursing.

MECHANISM OF ACTION
Selective 5-HT₃ receptor antagonist; has not been established.

PHARMACOKINETICS
Absorption: Administration in various age groups resulted in different parameters. (PO) Well absorbed from GI tract; mean bioavailability (56%). **Distribution:** Plasma protein binding (70-76%). **Metabolism:** Extensive; via CYP3A4, 1A2, 2D6; hydroxylation (primary), glucuronide/sulfate conjugation. **Elimination:** Urine (5% unchanged). Refer to PI for additional pharmacokinetic information.

PATIENT CONSIDERATIONS

Assessment: Assess for previous hypersensitivity to the drug, congenital long QT syndrome, electrolyte abnormalities, CHF, bradyarrhythmias, hepatic impairment, pregnancy/nursing status, and possible drug interactions. (ODT) Assess for phenylketonuria.

Monitoring: Monitor for QT interval prolongation, torsades de pointes, hypersensitivity reactions, serotonin syndrome, and other adverse reactions. Monitor ECG in patients w/ electrolyte abnormalities, CHF, bradyarrhythmias, and in patients taking other medications that lead to QT prolongation. In patients who recently underwent abdominal surgery or in patients w/ chemotherapy-induced N/V, monitor for masking of a progressive ileus and/or gastric distension.

Counseling: Inform about potential benefits/risks of therapy. Inform that drug may cause serious cardiac arrhythmias (eg, QT prolongation); instruct patients to contact physician if they perceive a change in their HR, if they feel lightheaded, or have a syncopal episode. Inform that chances of developing severe cardiac arrhythmias are higher in patients w/ a personal/family history of abnormal heart rhythms (eg, congenital long QT syndrome), patients taking medications (eg, diuretics) that may cause electrolyte abnormalities, and in patients w/ hypokalemia or hypomagnesemia. Advise of the possibility of serotonin syndrome; instruct to seek immediate medical attention if changes in mental status, autonomic instability, neuromuscular symptoms w/ or w/o GI symptoms occur. Inform that drug may cause hypersensitivity reactions, some as severe as anaphylaxis and bronchospasm; instruct to report any signs/symptoms of hypersensitivity reactions to physician. Advise to report the use of all medications to physician. Inform that drug may cause headache, drowsiness/sedation, constipation, fever, and diarrhea. Inform phenylketonuric patients that ODT contains phenylalanine.

ONEXTON — benzoyl peroxide/clindamycin phosphate   Rx

Class: Antibacterial/keratolytic

ADULT DOSAGE	PEDIATRIC DOSAGE
Acne Vulgaris	**Acne Vulgaris**
Apply a pea-sized amount to face qd	**>12 Years:**
	Apply a pea-sized amount to face qd

ADMINISTRATION

Topical route

Wash face gently with a mild soap, rinse with warm water, and pat skin dry before application

Avoid eyes, mouth, lips, mucous membranes, or areas of broken skin

STORAGE

Prior to Dispensing: 2-8°C (36-46°F). After Dispensing: ≤25°C (77°F). Do not freeze. Store pump upright.

HOW SUPPLIED

Gel: (Clindamycin-Benzoyl Peroxide) 1.2%-3.75% [50g]

CONTRAINDICATIONS

Hypersensitivity to clindamycin, benzoyl peroxide, any components of the formulation, or lincomycin; history of regional enteritis, ulcerative colitis, or antibiotic-associated colitis.

WARNINGS/PRECAUTIONS

Use of beyond 12 weeks has not been evaluated. Diarrhea, bloody diarrhea, and colitis (including pseudomembranous colitis) reported; d/c if significant diarrhea occurs. Minimize sun exposure (including use of tanning beds or sun lamps) following application.

ADVERSE REACTIONS

Local skin reactions (erythema, scaling, itching, burning, stinging).

DRUG INTERACTIONS

Avoid using in combination with topical or oral erythromycin-containing products. Caution with concomitant topical acne therapy; possible cumulative irritancy effect may occur, especially with use of peeling, desquamating, or abrasive agents; reduce frequency of application or temporarily interrupt treatment if irritancy or dermatitis occurs; resume once irritation subsides, and d/c if irritation persists. May enhance the action of other neuromuscular blocking agents; use with caution. Antiperistaltic agents (eg, opiates, diphenoxylate with atropine) may prolong and/or worsen severe colitis.

PREGNANCY AND LACTATION

Category C, caution in nursing.

MECHANISM OF ACTION

Clindamycin: Lincosamide antibacterial; binds to the 50S ribosomal subunits of susceptible bacteria and prevents elongation of peptide chains by interfering with peptidyl transfer, thereby suppressing bacterial protein synthesis. Benzoyl Peroxide: Not established; an oxidizing agent with bactericidal and keratolytic effects.

PHARMACOKINETICS

Absorption: Clindamycin: (Day 1) C_{max}=0.78ng/mL; AUC_{0-t}=5.29 hr•ng/mL. (Day 30) C_{max}=1.22ng/mL, AUC_{0-t}=8.42 hr•ng/mL. **Distribution:** Clindamycin: (PO/Parenteral) Found in breast milk. **Metabolism:** Benzoyl Peroxide: Converted to benzoic acid.

PATIENT CONSIDERATIONS

Assessment: Assess for history of hypersensitivity to drug/lincomycin, regional enteritis, ulcerative colitis, antibiotic-associated colitis, pregnancy/nursing status, and possible drug interactions.

Monitoring: Monitor for local skin reactions, diarrhea, colitis, and other adverse reactions.

Counseling: Instruct to d/c use and contact physician immediately if an allergic reaction (eg, severe swelling, SOB) develops. Inform that medication may cause irritation (eg, erythema, scaling, itching, burning), especially when used with other topical acne therapies. Instruct to limit excessive/prolonged exposure to sunlight by wearing a hat or other clothing and using sunscreen. Inform that medication may bleach hair or colored fabric.

ONFI — clobazam   CIV

Class: Benzodiazepine

ADULT DOSAGE	PEDIATRIC DOSAGE
Seizures	**Seizures**
Associated w/ Lennox-Gastaut Syndrome:	**Associated w/ Lennox-Gastaut Syndrome:**
≤30kg:	**≥2 Years:**
Initial: 5mg/day	**≤30kg:**
Starting Day 7: 10mg/day	**Initial:** 5mg/day
Starting Day 14: 20mg/day	**Starting Day 7:** 10mg/day
	Starting Day 14: 20mg/day
>30kg:	
Initial: 10mg/day	**>30kg:**
Starting Day 7: 20mg/day	**Initial:** 10mg/day
Starting Day 14: 40mg/day	**Starting Day 7:** 20mg/day
	Starting Day 14: 40mg/day
Do not proceed w/ dose escalation more rapidly than weekly	Do not proceed w/ dose escalation more rapidly than weekly
For doses >5mg/day, administer in divided doses bid	For doses >5mg/day, administer in divided doses bid

DOSING CONSIDERATIONS

Hepatic Impairment

Mild to Moderate (Child-Pugh Score 5-9):
Initial: 5mg/day
Titrate: Titrate according to weight, but to 1/2 the recommended dose, as tolerated; additional titration to the max dose (20mg/day or 40mg/day, depending on weight) may be started on day 21

Elderly

Initial: 5mg/day
Titrate: Titrate according to weight, but to 1/2 the recommended dose, as tolerated; additional titration to the max dose (20mg/day or 40mg/day, depending on weight) may be started on day 21

Discontinuation

Withdraw gradually; taper by decreasing total daily dose by 5-10mg/day on a weekly basis

Other Important Considerations

CYP2C19 Poor Metabolizers:
Initial: 5mg/day
Titrate: Titrate according to weight, but to 1/2 the recommended dose, as tolerated; additional titration to the max dose (20mg/day or 40mg/day, depending on weight) may be started on day 21

ADMINISTRATION

Oral route

Take w/ or w/o food

Tab

May administer whole, break in 1/2 along the score, or crush and mix in applesauce

Sus

Shake well before every administration

Administer using only the dosing syringe provided with the product

To Withdraw a Dose:
1. Insert the provided adapter firmly into the neck of the bottle before 1st use
2. Insert the dosing syringe into the adapter and invert bottle then slowly pull back plunger to prescribed dose
3. Remove the syringe from the bottle adapter and slowly squirt dose into the corner of the patient's mouth
4. Replace cap after each use (the cap fits over the adapter)

STORAGE

20-25°C (68-77°F). (Sus) Store in original bottle in an upright position. Use within 90 days of 1st opening the bottle; discard any remainder.

HOW SUPPLIED

Sus: 2.5mg/mL [120mL]; **Tab:** 10mg*, 20mg* *scored

CONTRAINDICATIONS

History of hypersensitivity to clobazam or its ingredients.

WARNINGS/PRECAUTIONS

Dose-related somnolence and sedation reported. May impair mental/physical abilities. Withdrawal symptoms reported to occur following abrupt discontinuation; withdraw gradually to minimize risk of precipitating seizures, seizure exacerbation, or status epilepticus. Serious skin reactions (eg, Stevens-Johnson syndrome [SJS], toxic epidermal necrolysis [TEN]) reported; d/c at the 1st sign of rash, unless the rash is clearly not drug-related. If signs/symptoms suggest SJS/TEN, do not resume therapy and consider alternative therapy. Monitor patients with history of substance abuse because of predisposition to habituation and dependence. May increase risk of suicidal thoughts or behavior; monitor for the emergence or worsening of depression, suicidal thoughts/behavior, and/or any unusual changes in mood/behavior.

ADVERSE REACTIONS

Somnolence, pyrexia, upper respiratory tract infection, lethargy, drooling, aggression, vomiting, irritability, constipation, fatigue, sedation, ataxia, insomnia, cough, pneumonia.

DRUG INTERACTIONS

May potentiate effects of other CNS depressants or alcohol; monitor for somnolence and sedation. May decrease effectiveness of hormonal contraceptives; additional nonhormonal forms of contraception are recommended. CYP2D6 substrates may require dose adjustment. Strong (eg, fluconazole, fluvoxamine, ticlopidine) and moderate (eg, omeprazole) inhibitors of CYP2C19 may increase exposure to N-desmethylclobazam; may require dose adjustment of clobazam. Alcohol may increase maximum plasma exposure.

PREGNANCY AND LACTATION

Category C, not for use in nursing.

MECHANISM OF ACTION

Benzodiazepine; not established. Thought to involve potentiation of gamma-aminobutyric acid (GABA)ergic neurotransmission resulting from binding at the benzodiazepine site of the $GABA_A$ receptor.

PHARMACOKINETICS

Absorption: Rapid and extensive. T_{max}=0.5-4 hrs (tab, single- or multiple-dose), 0.5-2 hrs (sus, single-dose). **Distribution:** Plasma protein binding (80-90%; 70% N-desmethylclobazam); V_d=100L; found in breast milk. **Metabolism:** Liver (extensive); via demethylation by CYP3A4 (primary), 2C19, 2B6; N-desmethylclobazam (major, active metabolite). **Elimination:** Urine (82%, 2% unchanged), feces (11%, 1% unchanged); $T_{1/2}$=36-42 hrs, 71-82 hrs (N-desmethylclobazam).

PATIENT CONSIDERATIONS

Assessment: Assess for hypersensitivity to drug, hepatic impairment, history of substance abuse, pregnancy/nursing status, and possible drug interactions. Assess if patient is a CYP2C19 poor metabolizer.

Monitoring: Monitor for somnolence, sedation, withdrawal symptoms, habituation, physical/psychological dependence, emergence or worsening of depression, suicidal thoughts/behavior, unusual changes in mood/behavior, and other adverse reactions. Closely monitor for signs/symptoms of SJS/TEN, especially during the first 8 weeks of treatment initiation or when reintroducing therapy.

Counseling: Caution about operating hazardous machinery, including automobiles, until the effect of the treatment is known. Inform to consult physician before increasing the dose or abruptly discontinuing the drug. Instruct to notify physician if a skin reaction occurs. Advise that abrupt withdrawal may increase risk of seizure. Counsel women to also use nonhormonal methods of contraception when clobazam is used with hormonal contraceptives and to continue these alternative methods for 28 days after discontinuation. Inform that clobazam may increase the risk of suicidal thoughts and behavior and counsel to be alert for the emergence or worsening of symptoms of depression, any unusual changes in mood/behavior, or the emergence of suicidal thoughts, behavior, or thoughts of self-harm; instruct to immediately report behaviors of concern to physician. Instruct to notify physician if pregnant/breastfeeding, or if intending to breastfeed or become pregnant during therapy. Encourage to enroll in the North American Antiepileptic Drug Pregnancy Registry if patient becomes pregnant.

ONGLYZA — saxagliptin   Rx

Class: Dipeptidyl peptidase-4 (DPP-4) inhibitor

ADULT DOSAGE	PEDIATRIC DOSAGE
Type 2 Diabetes Mellitus	Pediatric use may not have been established
2.5mg or 5mg qd	

DOSING CONSIDERATIONS
Concomitant Medications
Strong CYP3A4/5 Inhibitors: 2.5mg qd
Insulin Secretagogue (eg, Sulfonylurea)/Insulin: May require a lower dose of insulin secretagogue or insulin
Renal Impairment
Mild (CrCl>50mL/min): No dosage adjustment recommended
Moderate or Severe/ESRD Requiring Hemodialysis (CrCl ≤50mL/min): 2.5mg qd
Administer following hemodialysis

ADMINISTRATION
Oral route
Take regardless of meals.
Do not split or cut tab.

STORAGE
20-25°C (68-77°F); excursions permitted to 15-30°C (59-86°F).

HOW SUPPLIED
Tab: 2.5mg, 5mg

CONTRAINDICATIONS
History of a serious hypersensitivity reaction to saxagliptin (eg, anaphylaxis, angioedema, or exfoliative skin conditions).

WARNINGS/PRECAUTIONS
Not for treatment of type 1 diabetes mellitus (DM) or diabetic ketoacidosis. Acute pancreatitis reported; d/c if pancreatitis is suspected and initiate appropriate management. Increased incidence of hospitalization for heart failure (HF) reported in patients w/ established atherosclerotic cardiovascular disease (ASCVD) or multiple risk factors for ASCVD; consider the risks and benefits of therapy prior to initiating treatment in patients at a higher risk for HF. Evaluate and manage according to current standards of care and consider discontinuation of therapy if HF develops. Serious hypersensitivity reactions reported; if suspected, d/c therapy, assess for other potential causes, and institute alternative treatment. Caution in patients w/ history of angioedema to another DPP-4 inhibitor and in elderly. Severe and disabling arthralgia reported; d/c if appropriate.

ADVERSE REACTIONS
URTI, UTI, headache.

DRUG INTERACTIONS
See Dosing Considerations. Increased incidence of hypoglycemia reported w/ a sulfonylurea or insulin. Ketoconazole and other strong CYP3A4/5 inhibitors (eg, atazanavir, clarithromycin, itraconazole) may increase plasma levels.

PREGNANCY AND LACTATION
Pregnancy: Category B.
Lactation: Caution in nursing.

MECHANISM OF ACTION
DPP-4 inhibitor; slows the inactivation of the incretin hormones, thereby increasing their bloodstream concentrations and reducing fasting and postprandial glucose concentrations in a glucose-dependent manner.

PHARMACOKINETICS
Absorption: C_{max}=24ng/mL, 47ng/mL (5-hydroxy saxagliptin); AUC=78ng•hr/mL, 214ng•hr/mL (5-hydroxy saxagliptin); T_{max} (median)=2 hrs, 4 hrs (5-hydroxy saxagliptin). **Metabolism:** CYP3A4/5; 5-hydroxy saxagliptin (active metabolite). **Elimination:** Feces (22%), urine (24% unchanged, 36% 5-hydroxy saxagliptin); $T_{1/2}$=2.5 hrs, 3.1 hrs (5-hydroxy saxagliptin).

PATIENT CONSIDERATIONS

Assessment: Assess for previous hypersensitivity to the drug, history of pancreatitis, type of DM, diabetic ketoacidosis, HF or risk of HF, history of angioedema to another DPP-4 inhibitor, pregnancy/nursing status, and possible drug interactions. Obtain baseline renal function, and FPG and HbA1c levels.

Monitoring: Monitor for pancreatitis, HF, hypersensitivity reactions, severe and disabling arthralgia, and for other adverse reactions. Monitor FPG, HbA1c, and renal function periodically.

Counseling: Inform of the potential risks, benefits, and alternative modes of therapy. Advise on the importance of adherence to dietary instructions, regular physical activity, periodic blood glucose monitoring and HbA1c testing, recognition and management of hypo/hyperglycemia, and assessment of diabetic complications. Instruct to seek medical advice promptly during periods of stress as medication requirements may change. Instruct to d/c use and notify physician if signs and symptoms of pancreatitis or allergic reactions occur. Inform about the signs/symptoms of HF; instruct to contact physician as soon as possible if patient experiences symptoms of HF (eg, increasing SOB, rapid increase in weight or swelling of the feet). Counsel to inform physician if any unusual symptom develops, or if any existing symptom persists or worsens. Inform that severe and disabling joint pain may occur; instruct to seek medical advice if severe joint pain occurs. Inform that if a dose was missed, to take the next dose as prescribed, unless otherwise instructed by physician; instruct not to take an extra dose the next day.

ONIVYDE — irinotecan liposome   Rx

Class: Topoisomerase I inhibitor

> Fatal neutropenic sepsis reported. Severe or life-threatening neutropenic fever or sepsis and severe or life-threatening neutropenia reported in patients receiving irinotecan liposome in combination w/ fluorouracil (5-FU) and leucovorin (LV). Withhold therapy for ANC <1500/mm³ or neutropenic fever. Monitor blood cell counts periodically during treatment. Severe diarrhea reported in patients receiving irinotecan liposome in combination w/ 5-FU and LV; do not administer to patients w/ bowel obstruction. Withhold therapy for diarrhea of Grade 2-4 severity. Administer loperamide for late diarrhea of any severity and administer atropine, if not contraindicated, for early diarrhea of any severity.

ADULT DOSAGE	PEDIATRIC DOSAGE
Metastatic Pancreatic Adenocarcinoma	Pediatric use may not have been established
Treatment of metastatic adenocarcinoma of the pancreas, in combination w/ 5-FU and LV, after disease progression following gemcitabine-based therapy	
Recommended Dose: 70mg/m² IV over 90 min every 2 weeks Administer prior to LV and 5-FU	
Homozygous for the UGT1A1*28 Allele:	
Initial: 50mg/m² IV over 90 min	
Titrate: Increase to 70mg/m² as tolerated in subsequent cycles	
Premedication	
Administer a corticosteroid and an antiemetic 30 min prior to infusion	

DOSING CONSIDERATIONS
Adverse Reactions
NCI CTCAE Grade 3 or 4 Adverse Reactions:
Withhold drug. Initiate loperamide for late onset diarrhea of any severity. Administer IV or SQ atropine 0.25-1mg (unless contraindicated) for early onset diarrhea of any severity. Upon recovery to ≤Grade 1, resume therapy at:
1st Occurrence:
Patients Receiving 70mg/m²: 50mg/m²
Patients Homozygous for UGT1A1*28 w/o Previous Increase to 70mg/m²: 43mg/m²

2nd Occurrence:
Patients Receiving 70mg/m²: 43mg/m²
Patients Homozygous for UGT1A1*28 w/o Previous Increase to 70mg/m²: 35mg/m²

3rd Occurrence: D/C therapy

Interstitial Lung Disease (ILD): D/C therapy

Anaphylactic Reaction: D/C therapy

Refer to the full prescribing information, for recommended dose modifications for 5-FU or LV

ADMINISTRATION
IV route

Do not substitute irinotecan liposome for other drugs containing irinotecan HCl. Do not use in-line filters.

Preparation
1. Withdraw the calculated volume from vial.
2. Dilute in 500mL D5 or 0.9% NaCl inj and mix diluted sol by gentle inversion. Protect diluted sol from light.
3. Administer diluted sol w/in 4 hrs of preparation when stored at room temperature or w/in 24 hrs of preparation when stored under refrigerated conditions (2-8°C [36-46°F]). Do not freeze.
4. Allow diluted sol to come to room temperature prior to administration.

STORAGE
2-8°C (36-46°F). Do not freeze. Protect from light.

HOW SUPPLIED
Inj: (free base) 4.3mg/mL [10mL].

CONTRAINDICATIONS
Severe hypersensitivity reaction to this medication or irinotecan HCl.

WARNINGS/PRECAUTIONS
Not indicated as a single agent for the treatment of patients w/ metastatic adenocarcinoma of the pancreas. Monitor CBC on Days 1 and 8 of every cycle and more frequently if clinically indicated. Withhold therapy for ANC <1500/mm³ or if neutropenic fever occurs; resume when the ANC is ≥1500/mm³. Reduce dose for Grade 3-4 neutropenia or neutropenic fever following recovery in subsequent cycles. May cause severe and fatal ILD; withhold in patients w/ new or progressive dyspnea, cough, and fever, pending diagnostic evaluation. D/C therapy in patients w/ confirmed diagnosis of ILD. Severe hypersensitivity reactions, including anaphylactic reactions, may occur; permanently d/c in patients who experience a severe hypersensitivity reaction. May cause fetal harm when administered to a pregnant woman.

ADVERSE REACTIONS
Diarrhea, fatigue/asthenia, N/V, decreased appetite, stomatitis, pyrexia.

DRUG INTERACTIONS
Strong CYP3A4 inducers (eg, rifampin, St. John's wort, phenytoin) reported to reduce exposure of non-liposomal irinotecan or its active metabolite, SN-38; avoid concomitant use if possible. Substitute non-enzyme inducing therapies at least 2 weeks prior to initiation of irinotecan liposome therapy. CYP3A4 inhibitors (eg, clarithromycin, indinavir, itraconazole) or UGT1A1 inhibitors (eg, atazanavir, gemfibrozil, indinavir) may increase exposure to irinotecan liposome or SN-38; avoid the use of strong CYP3A4 or UGT1A1 inhibitors if possible. D/C strong CYP3A4 inhibitors at least 1 week prior to starting irinotecan liposome therapy.

PREGNANCY AND LACTATION
Pregnancy: May cause fetal harm. Embryotoxicity and teratogenicity were observed in animals following treatment w/ irinotecan HCl, at doses resulting in irinotecan exposures lower than those achieved w/ irinotecan liposome 70mg/m² in humans.
Lactation: There is no information regarding the presence of irinotecan liposome, irinotecan, or SN-38 in human milk, or the effects on the breastfed infant or on milk production. Not for use in nursing; nursing women should not breastfeed during treatment and for 1 month after the final dose.
Reproductive Potential: Females of reproductive potential should use effective contraception during treatment and for 1 month after the final dose. Males w/ female partners of reproductive potential should use condoms during treatment and for 4 months after the final dose.

MECHANISM OF ACTION
Topoisomerase I inhibitor; bind reversibly to the topoisomerase 1-DNA complex and prevents re-ligation of single strand DNA breaks, leading to exposure time-dependent double-strand DNA damage and cell death.

PHARMACOKINETICS
Absorption: Irinotecan: C_{max}=37.2mcg/mL; AUC=1364mcg•hr/mL. SN-38: C_{max}=5.4ng/mL; AUC=620ng•hr/mL. **Distribution:** Irinotecan: Plasma protein binding (<0.44%); V_d=4.1L **Metabolism:** Irinotecan: Liver (extensive) via esterases to SN-38 (active metabolite), and by CYP3A4 mediated oxidation. SN-38: UGT1A1 mediating glucuronidation to SN-38G. **Excretion:** Irinotecan HCl: Urine (11-20%); $T_{1/2}$=25.8 hrs. SN-38: Urine (<1%); $T_{1/2}$=67.8 hrs. SN-38G: Urine (3%).

PATIENT CONSIDERATIONS
Assessment: Assess for hypersensitivity to drug, bowel obstruction, pregnancy/nursing status, and for possible drug interactions. Assess for UGT1A1*28 allele status. Obtain baseline CBC.

Monitoring: Monitor for signs/symptoms of neutropenic sepsis, diarrhea, ILD (eg, new or progressive dyspnea, cough, fever), hypersensitivity reactions, and for any other adverse reactions. Monitor CBC on Days 1 and 8 of every cycle and more frequently if clinically indicated.

Counseling: Advise of the risk of neutropenia leading to severe and life-threatening infections and of the need for monitoring of blood counts. Instruct to contact physician if experiencing signs of infection. Inform of the risk of severe diarrhea; advise to contact physician if experiencing persistent vomiting or diarrhea, black or bloody stools, or symptoms of dehydration (eg, lightheadedness, dizziness, faintness). Inform of the risk of ILD; advise to contact physician as soon as possible for new onset cough or dyspnea. Instruct to seek immediate medical attention for signs of severe hypersensitivity reaction (eg, chest tightness; SOB; wheezing; dizziness or faintness; or swelling of the face, eyelids, or lips). Advise pregnant women of the potential risk to a fetus. Advise females of reproductive potential to use effective contraception during and for 1 month following the final dose of treatment and to inform physician of a known/suspected pregnancy. Advise males w/ female partners of reproductive potential to use condoms during and for 4 months after the final dose of treatment. Advise women not to breastfeed during treatment and for 1 month after the final dose.

ONZETRA XSAIL — sumatriptan   Rx

Class: 5-HT₁B/1D agonist (triptans)

ADULT DOSAGE	PEDIATRIC DOSAGE
Migraine	Pediatric use may not have been established
Acute Treatment of Migraine w/ or w/o Aura:	
22mg (2 nosepieces), using the Xsail breath-powered delivery device	

May administer a second 22mg dose if the migraine has not resolved by 2 hrs after taking the first dose, or returns after a transient improvement

Max Dose/24 hrs: 2 doses (44mg/4 nosepieces) or 1 dose of Onzetra Xsail and 1 dose of another sumatriptan product, separated by at least 2 hrs

Safety of treating an average of >4 headaches in a 30-day period has not been established

---

ADMINISTRATION
Nasal route
- Remove the clear device cap from the reusable delivery device.
- Remove a disposable nosepiece from its foil pouch and click the nosepiece into the device body.
- Fully press and promptly release the white piercing button on the device body to pierce the cap inside the nosepiece; the white piercing button should only be pressed once and released prior to administration to each nostril.
- Insert the nosepiece into the nostril so that it makes a tight seal; keeping the nosepiece in the nose, rotate the device to place the mouthpiece into the mouth.
- The patient blows forcefully through the mouthpiece to deliver the sumatriptan powder into the nasal cavity.
- Vibration (eg, a rattling noise) may occur, and indicates that the patient is blowing forcefully, as directed.
- Once the medication in the first nosepiece has been administered, remove and discard the nosepiece.
- The same process must then be repeated using a second 11mg nosepiece into the other nostril to administer the remainder of the total recommended 22mg dose.

STORAGE
20-25°C (68-77°F); excursions permitted between 15-30°C (59-86°F). Do not store in the refrigerator or freezer. Use nosepiece immediately after removing from foil pouch.

HOW SUPPLIED
Powder, Nasal: 11mg/nosepiece

CONTRAINDICATIONS
Ischemic coronary artery disease (CAD) (eg, angina pectoris, history of MI, silent ischemia), coronary artery vasospasm (eg, Prinzmetal's angina), or in patients w/ other significant underlying cardiovascular (CV) diseases. Wolff-Parkinson-White syndrome or arrhythmias associated w/ other cardiac accessory conduction pathway disorders, history of stroke or transient ischemic attack, history of hemiplegic/basilar migraine, peripheral vascular disease, ischemic bowel disease, uncontrolled HTN, hypersensitivity to sumatriptan, and severe hepatic impairment. Recent use (w/in 24 hrs) of another 5-HT₁ agonist, or of an ergotamine-containing or ergot-type medication (eg, dihydroergotamine, methysergide). Concurrent administration or recent use (w/in 2 weeks) of an MAO-A inhibitor.

WARNINGS/PRECAUTIONS
Use only if a clear diagnosis of migraine has been established. Reconsider diagnosis of migraine before treating any subsequent attacks if patient has no response to the first migraine attack treated w/ Onzetra Xsail. Not indicated for the prevention of migraine attacks. Serious cardiac adverse reactions (eg, acute MI) reported. May cause coronary artery vasospasm (Prinzmetal's angina). Perform CV evaluation in triptan-naive patients w/ multiple CV risk factors prior to therapy; if negative, consider administering 1st dose in a medically supervised setting and performing an ECG immediately following administration. Consider periodic CV evaluation in intermittent long-term users w/ multiple CV risk factors. Life-threatening disturbances of cardiac rhythm (eg, ventricular tachycardia, ventricular fibrillation leading to death) reported; d/c if these occur. Sensations of tightness, pain, pressure, and heaviness in the chest, throat, neck, and jaw, usually noncardiac in origin, reported; perform cardiac evaluation if at high cardiac risk. Cerebral/subarachnoid hemorrhage, stroke, and other cerebrovascular events may occur; d/c therapy if a cerebrovascular event occurs. May cause noncoronary vasospastic reactions (eg, peripheral vascular ischemia, GI vascular ischemia/infarction, splenic infarction, Raynaud's syndrome); rule out therapy-related vasospastic reactions before additional therapy is given. May cause transient/permanent blindness and significant partial vision loss. Overuse of acute migraine drugs may lead to exacerbation of headache; detoxification, including drug withdrawal, and treatment of withdrawal symptoms may be necessary. Serotonin syndrome may occur; d/c if suspected. Significant elevation in BP, including hypertensive crisis w/ acute impairment of organ systems, reported. Anaphylactic reactions may occur. Seizures reported; caution w/ history of epilepsy or conditions associated w/ a lowered seizure threshold.

ADVERSE REACTIONS
Abnormal taste, nasal discomfort, rhinorrhea, rhinitis.

DRUG INTERACTIONS
See Contraindications. Serotonin syndrome reported w/ SSRIs, SNRIs, TCAs, or MAOIs.

PREGNANCY AND LACTATION
Pregnancy: Category C.
Lactation: Excreted in human milk following SQ administration; infant exposure to sumatriptan can be minimized by avoiding breastfeeding for 12 hrs after treatment.

MECHANISM OF ACTION

Selective 5-HT$_{1B/1D}$ receptor agonist; presumably exerts its therapeutic effects through agonist effects at the 5-HT$_{1B/1D}$ receptors on intracranial blood vessels and sensory nerves of the trigeminal system, which result in cranial vessel constriction and inhibition of proinflammatory neuropeptide release.

PHARMACOKINETICS

Absorption: Bioavailability (approx 19%), C$_{max}$=21ng/mL, AUC=65ng•hr/mL, T$_{max}$=45 min. **Distribution:** V$_d$=2.7L/kg; plasma protein binding (14-21%). **Metabolism:** Via MAO-A; indole acetic acid (IAA) (major metabolite). **Elimination:** Urine (3% unchanged, 42% IAA); T$_{1/2}$=3 hrs.

PATIENT CONSIDERATIONS

Assessment: Confirm diagnosis of migraine and exclude other potentially serious neurologic conditions. Assess for CV disease, HTN, history of hemiplegic/basilar migraine, hypersensitivity to drug, and any other conditions where treatment is cautioned or contraindicated. Assess hepatic function, pregnancy/nursing status, and for possible drug interactions. Perform a CV evaluation in triptan-naive patients who have multiple CV risk factors.

Monitoring: Monitor for signs/symptoms of cardiac events, cerebrovascular events, noncoronary vasospastic reactions, serotonin syndrome, anaphylactic reactions, seizures, visual disorders, and other adverse reactions. Perform periodic CV evaluation in intermittent long-term users w/ multiple risk factors for CAD. Monitor BP.

Counseling: Inform that therapy may cause serious CV side effects and anaphylactic reactions. Instruct to seek medical attention if signs/symptoms of chest pain, SOB, irregular heartbeat, significant rise in BP, weakness, or slurring of speech occur. Caution about the risk of serotonin syndrome. Inform that use of acute migraine drugs for ≥10 days/month may lead to an exacerbation of headache; encourage to record headache frequency and drug use (eg, by keeping a headache diary). Inform that drug should not be used during pregnancy; instruct to notify physician if breastfeeding/planning to breastfeed. Inform that drug may cause somnolence and dizziness; instruct to evaluate ability to perform complex tasks during migraine attacks and after administration of drug. Inform that patient may experience local irritation of the nose and throat and that these symptoms will generally resolve in <2 hrs. Counsel on how to properly administer the medication.

OPANA — oxymorphone hydrochloride

CII

Class: Opioid analgesic

ADULT DOSAGE

Moderate to Severe Pain

Acute:
Opioid-Naive:
Initial: 10-20mg q4-6h depending on pain intensity; doses >20mg is not recommended
Titrate: Adjust dose to adequate pain relief (generally mild or no pain)

Maint:
Continually reevaluate; if level of pain increases, identify source of pain while adjusting the dose

Conversions

From Parenteral Oxymorphone:
Give 10X the total daily parenteral oxymorphone dose in 4-6 equally divided doses

From Other Oral Opioids:
Initial: 1/2 the calculated total daily dose in 4-6 equally divided doses, given q4-6h
Titrate: Gradually adjust until adequate pain relief and acceptable side effects achieved

PEDIATRIC DOSAGE

Pediatric use may not have been established

DOSING CONSIDERATIONS

Concomitant Medications
CNS Depressants (Sedatives/Hypnotics, General Anesthetics, Phenothiazines, Tranquilizers, and Alcohol):
Initial: 1/3 to 1/2 of the usual dose
MAOIs: Not recommended

Renal Impairment
<50mL/min:
Initial: 5mg; use caution
Titrate: Slowly adjust dose while monitoring side effects

Hepatic Impairment
Mild:
Initial: 5mg; use caution
Titrate: Slowly adjust to an acceptable level of analgesia based on response to initial dose

Elderly
Initial: Start at low end of dosing range (eg, 5mg)

Discontinuation
Taper doses gradually to prevent signs/symptoms of withdrawal

ADMINISTRATION

Oral route

STORAGE

25°C (77°F); excursions permitted to 15-30°C (59-86°F).

HOW SUPPLIED

Tab: 5mg, 10mg

CONTRAINDICATIONS

Known hypersensitivity to oxymorphone, morphine analogues (eg, codeine), or to any other ingredients in the product; respiratory depression (except in monitored settings with resuscitative equipment); acute/severe bronchial asthma or hypercarbia; paralytic ileus; moderate/severe hepatic impairment.

WARNINGS/PRECAUTIONS

Respiratory depression may occur; extreme caution in elderly or debilitated, or with conditions accompanied by hypoxia, hypercapnia, or decreased respiratory reserve (eg, asthma, chronic obstructive pulmonary disease or cor pulmonale, severe obesity, sleep apnea syndrome, myxedema, kyphoscoliosis, CNS depression, coma). May be abused in a manner similar to other opioid agonists. Respiratory depressant effects and potential to elevate CSF pressure may be markedly exaggerated in the presence of head injury, intracranial lesions, or preexisting increased intracranial pressure (ICP). May produce effects on papillary response and consciousness, which may obscure neurologic signs of further increases in ICP in patients with head injuries; extreme caution with increased ICP or impaired consciousness. May cause severe hypotension; caution with circulatory shock. Caution with adrenocortical insufficiency (eg, Addison's disease), prostatic hypertrophy or urethral stricture, severe pulmonary impairment, moderate/severe renal dysfunction, mild hepatic impairment, and toxic psychosis. May induce or aggravate convulsions/seizures. May diminish propulsive peristaltic waves in the GI tract; monitor for decreased bowel motility in postoperative patients. May obscure diagnosis or clinical course in patients with acute abdominal conditions. May cause spasm of the sphincter of Oddi; caution with biliary tract disease, including acute pancreatitis. May impair physical/mental abilities. Not recommended for use during and immediately prior to labor. Physical dependence and tolerance may occur. Avoid abrupt discontinuation.

ADVERSE REACTIONS

Constipation, N/V, pyrexia, somnolence, headache, dizziness, pruritus, confusion.

DRUG INTERACTIONS

Additive CNS depression with other CNS depressants (eg, sedatives, hypnotics, tranquilizers, general anesthetics, phenothiazines, other opioids, alcohol). Avoid with ethanol. Caution with MAOI; not recommended within 14 days of MAOI use. Anticholinergics may increase risk of urinary retention and/or severe constipation, which may lead to paralytic ileus. CNS side effects (eg, confusion, disorientation, respiratory depression, apnea, seizures) reported with cimetidine. Mixed agonist/antagonist analgesics (pentazocine, nalbuphine, butorphanol, buprenorphine) may reduce analgesic effect and/or precipitate withdrawal symptoms; use with caution. May cause severe hypotension with phenothiazines or other agents that compromise vasomotor tone.

PREGNANCY AND LACTATION

Pregnancy: Category C.
Lactation: Caution in nursing.

MECHANISM OF ACTION

Opioid analgesic; pure opioid agonist. Has not been established. Specific CNS opiate receptors and endogenous compounds with morphine-like activity have been identified throughout the brain and spinal cord and are likely to play a role in the expression and perception of analgesic effects.

PHARMACOKINETICS

Absorption: Absolute bioavailability (10%). Administration of variable doses resulted in different pharmacokinetic parameters. **Distribution:** Plasma protein binding (10-12%); crosses placenta. **Metabolism:** Liver (extensive) by reduction or conjugation with glucuronic acid; oxymorphone-3-glucuronide, 6-OH-oxymorphone (major metabolites). **Elimination:** Urine (<1% unchanged, 33-38% oxymorphone-3-glucuronide, 0.25-0.62% 6-OH-oxymorphone).

PATIENT CONSIDERATIONS

Assessment: Assess for level of pain intensity, type of pain, degree of opioid tolerance, patient's general condition and medical status, history of or risk factors for abuse and addiction, renal/hepatic impairment, pregnancy/nursing status, any other conditions where treatment is contraindicated or cautioned, and possible drug interactions.

Monitoring: Monitor for signs/symptoms of respiratory depression, hypotension, convulsions/seizures, decreased bowel motility in postoperative patients, spasm of sphincter of Oddi, physical dependence, tolerance, abuse/addiction, and other adverse reactions.

Counseling: Instruct to take drug ud. Inform that drug has potential for abuse and should be protected from theft. Instruct to dispose of any unused tabs by flushing down the toilet. Advise to contact physician if experiencing adverse events or inadequate pain control during therapy. Instruct not to adjust dose without consulting physician. Inform that drug may impair mental/physical abilities. Advise to avoid alcohol or other CNS depressants. Advise of the potential for severe constipation. Advise to consult physician if pregnant or planning to become pregnant. Inform that if taking medication for more than a few weeks, to avoid abrupt withdrawal; dosing will need to be tapered.

OPANA ER — oxymorphone hydrochloride   CII

Class: Opioid analgesic

> Exposes users to risks of addiction, abuse, and misuse, leading to overdose and death; assess each patient's risk prior to prescribing and monitor regularly for development of these behaviors/conditions. Serious, life-threatening, or fatal respiratory depression may occur; monitor upon initiation or following a dose increase. Crushing, chewing, or dissolving tab can cause rapid release and absorption of potentially fatal dose; instruct patients to swallow tab whole. Accidental ingestion of even 1 dose, especially by children, can result in a fatal overdose. Prolonged use during pregnancy can result in neonatal opioid withdrawal syndrome; advise pregnant women of the risk and ensure availability of appropriate treatment. Avoid use with alcoholic beverages or medications containing alcohol; co-ingestion may result in increased plasma levels and potentially fatal overdose.

ADULT DOSAGE

Severe Pain (Daily, Around-the-Clock Management)

1st Opioid Analgesic/Opioid Intolerant Patients:
Initial: 5mg q12h
Titrate: May adjust dose every 3-7 days in increments of 5-10mg q12h

Conversions
From Immediate-Release (IR) to Extended-Release (ER) Oxymorphone:
Administer 1/2 the total daily IR dose as ER, q12h
From Parenteral Oxymorphone:
Administer 10X the total daily parenteral oxymorphone dose as ER in 2 equally divided doses
From Other Oral Opioids:
D/C all other around-the-clock opioids when therapy is initiated; refer to PI for conversion factors and dose calculations

PEDIATRIC DOSAGE
Pediatric use may not have been established

DOSING CONSIDERATIONS
Renal Impairment
CrCl <50mL/min:
Opioid-Naive: Initiate treatment w/ 5mg dose
On Prior Opioid Therapy: Initiate at 50% lower than the starting dose for a patient w/ normal renal function on prior opioids and titrate slowly

Hepatic Impairment
Mild:
Opioid-Naive: Initiate treatment w/ 5mg dose
On Prior Opioid Therapy: Initiate at 50% lower than the starting dose for a patient w/ normal hepatic function on prior opioids and titrate slowly

Elderly
Opioid-Naive: Initiate treatment w/ 5mg dose
On Prior Opioid Therapy: Initiate at 50% lower than the starting dose for a younger patient on prior opioids and titrate slowly

Discontinuation
Use gradual downward dose titration every 2-4 days

ADMINISTRATION
Oral route
Do not presoak, lick, or otherwise wet tab prior to placing in mouth.
Swallow tab whole; do not crush, dissolve, or chew.
Take 1 tab at a time w/ enough water to ensure complete swallowing.
Take on an empty stomach, at least 1 hr ac or 2 hrs pc.

STORAGE
25°C (77°F); excursions permitted to 15-30°C (59-86°F).

HOW SUPPLIED
Tab, ER: 5mg, 7.5mg, 10mg, 15mg, 20mg, 30mg, 40mg

CONTRAINDICATIONS
Significant respiratory depression, acute/severe bronchial asthma or hypercarbia, known or suspected paralytic ileus and GI obstruction, moderate or severe hepatic impairment, hypersensitivity (eg, anaphylaxis) to oxymorphone, any other ingredients in the product, or to morphine analogs (eg, codeine).

WARNINGS/PRECAUTIONS
Reserve use in patients for whom alternative treatment options are ineffective, not tolerated, or would be otherwise inadequate to provide sufficient management of pain. Should only be prescribed by healthcare professionals who are knowledgeable in the use of potent opioids for management of chronic pain. Life-threatening respiratory depression is more likely to occur in elderly, cachectic, or debilitated patients. Consider alternative nonopioid analgesics in patients with significant COPD or cor pulmonale, and in patients having a substantially decreased respiratory reserve, hypoxia, hypercapnia, or preexisting respiratory depression. May cause severe hypotension, orthostatic hypotension, and syncope; increased risk in patients whose ability to maintain BP has already been compromised by a reduced blood volume or concurrent administration of certain CNS depressants. Avoid with circulatory shock. Monitor patients who may be susceptible to intracranial effects of carbon dioxide retention for signs of sedation and respiratory depression when initiating therapy. May obscure clinical course in a patient with head injury. Avoid with impaired consciousness or coma. Difficulty in swallowing tab, and intestinal obstruction reported; consider alternative analgesic in patients who have difficulty swallowing or have underlying GI disorders that may predispose them to obstruction. May cause spasm of sphincter of Oddi and increase in serum amylase; monitor patients for worsening symptoms with biliary tract disease. May aggravate convulsions and induce/aggravate seizures. May impair mental/physical abilities. Not for use during and immediately prior to labor.

ADVERSE REACTIONS
Respiratory depression, constipation, N/V, diarrhea, somnolence, headache, dizziness, pruritus, increased sweating, dry mouth, sedation, insomnia, fatigue, decreased appetite, abdominal pain.

DRUG INTERACTIONS
See Boxed Warning. Hypotension, profound sedation, coma, respiratory depression, and death may occur with CNS depressants (eg, sedatives, anxiolytics, neuroleptics); if coadministration is considered, reduce dose of 1 or both agents. Monitor use in elderly, cachectic, and debilitated patients when coadministered with other drugs that depress respiration. Mixed agonist/antagonist analgesics (pentazocine, nalbuphine, butorphanol) and partial agonists (buprenorphine) may reduce analgesic effect or precipitate withdrawal symptoms; avoid concomitant use. May enhance neuromuscular blocking action of skeletal muscle relaxants and increase degree of respiratory depression. Cimetidine may potentiate opioid-induced respiratory depression. Anticholinergics or other drugs with anticholinergic activity may increase risk of urinary retention and/or severe constipation, which may lead to paralytic ileus.

PREGNANCY AND LACTATION
Pregnancy: Category C.
Lactation: Caution in nursing.

MECHANISM OF ACTION
Opioid analgesic; opioid agonist. Has not been established. Specific CNS opiate receptors and endogenous compounds with morphine-like activity have been identified throughout the brain and spinal cord and are likely to play a role in the expression and perception of analgesic effects.

PHARMACOKINETICS
Absorption: Absolute bioavailability (10%). Administration of variable doses resulted in different pharmacokinetic parameters. **Distribution:** Plasma protein binding (10-12%); crosses placenta. **Metabolism:** Liver (extensive) by reduction or conjugation with glucuronic acid; oxymorphone-3-glucuronide, 6-OH-oxymorphone (major metabolites). **Elimination:** Urine (<1% unchanged), 33-38% oxymorphone-3 glucuronide, <1% 6-OH-oxymorphone.

PATIENT CONSIDERATIONS
Assessment: Assess for abuse/addiction risk, pain intensity, prior opioid therapy, opioid tolerance, respiratory depression, renal/hepatic impairment, GI obstruction, drug hypersensitivity, pregnancy/nursing status, possible drug interactions, or any other conditions where treatment is contraindicated or cautioned.

Monitoring: Monitor for sedation, respiratory depression (especially within first 24-72 hrs of initiation or following a dose increase), hypotension, seizures/convulsions, and other adverse reactions. Monitor BP and serum amylase levels. Routinely monitor for signs of misuse, abuse, and addiction. Periodically reassess the continued need for therapy.

Counseling: Inform that use of drug can result in addiction, abuse, and misuse; instruct not to share with others and to take steps to protect from theft or misuse. Inform about risk and signs/symptoms of respiratory depression. Advise to store securely and dispose of unused tabs by flushing down the toilet. Inform female patients of reproductive potential that prolonged use during pregnancy may result in neonatal opioid withdrawal syndrome. Advise that drug may cause fetal harm and instruct to inform physician if pregnant/planning to become pregnant. Instruct not to consume alcoholic beverages or prescription and OTC products that contain alcohol during treatment. Inform that potentially serious additive effects may occur when used with alcohol or other CNS depressants, and not to use such drugs unless supervised by physician. Instruct to take drug exactly as prescribed, and not to d/c without 1st discussing the need for a tapering regimen with the physician. Inform that occasionally, inactive ingredients may be eliminated as a soft mass in stool that may resemble the original tab; inform that the active medication has already been absorbed by the time they see the soft mass. Inform that drug may cause orthostatic hypotension and syncope. Inform that drug may impair the ability to perform potentially hazardous activities; advise not to perform such tasks until they know how they will react to medication. Advise of potential for severe constipation, including management instructions. Advise how to recognize anaphylaxis and when to seek medical attention.

OPDIVO — nivolumab   Rx

Class: Monoclonal antibody/programmed death receptor-1 (PD-1) blocker

ADULT DOSAGE
Unresectable or Metastatic Melanoma

As a Single Agent for the Treatment of BRAF V600 Wild-Type Unresectable/Metastatic Melanoma or BRAF V600 Mutation-Positive Unresectable/Metastatic Melanoma:
3mg/kg IV every 2 weeks until disease progression or unacceptable toxicity

Unresectable/Metastatic Melanoma, in Combination w/ Ipilimumab:
1mg/kg IV, followed by ipilimumab

PEDIATRIC DOSAGE
Pediatric use may not have been established

on the same day, every 3 weeks for 4 doses; the subsequent dose of nivolumab is 3mg/kg IV every 2 weeks until disease progression or unacceptable toxicity, as a single agent

Metastatic Non-Small Cell Lung Cancer

W/ Progression On or After Platinum-Based Chemotherapy: Patients w/ epidermal growth factor receptor or anaplastic lymphoma kinase genomic tumor aberrations should have disease progression on FDA-approved therapy for these aberrations prior to receiving nivolumab

3mg/kg IV every 2 weeks until disease progression or unacceptable toxicity

Advanced Renal Cell Carcinoma

In Patients Who Have Received Prior Anti-Angiogenic Therapy: 3mg/kg IV every 2 weeks until disease progression or unacceptable toxicity

Hodgkin Lymphoma

Treatment of patients w/ classical Hodgkin lymphoma that has relapsed or progressed after autologous hematopoietic stem cell transplantation (HSCT) and post-transplantation brentuximab vedotin

3mg/kg IV every 2 weeks until disease progression or unacceptable toxicity

---

DOSING CONSIDERATIONS
Adverse Reactions
Infusion Reactions:
Mild or Moderate: Interrupt or slow infusion rate
Severe or Life-Threatening: D/C
Colitis:
Grade 2 Diarrhea or Colitis: Withhold dose*
Grade 3 Diarrhea or Colitis: Withhold dose* (when administered as a single-agent) or permanently d/c (when administered w/ ipilimumab)
Grade 4 Diarrhea or Colitis: Permanently d/c
Pneumonitis:
Grade 2: Withhold dose*
Grade 3 or 4: Permanently d/c
Hepatitis:
AST or ALT >3 and up to 5X ULN or Total Bilirubin >1.5 and up to 3X ULN: Withhold dose*
AST or ALT >5X ULN or Total Bilirubin >3X ULN: Permanently d/c
Hypophysitis:
Grade 2 or 3: Withhold dose*
Grade 4: Permanently d/c
Adrenal Insufficiency:
Grade 2: Withhold dose*
Grade 3 or 4: Permanently d/c
Type 1 Diabetes Mellitus (DM):
Grade 3 Hyperglycemia: Withhold dose*
Grade 4 Hyperglycemia: Permanently d/c
Nephritis and Renal Dysfunction:
SrCr >1.5 and up to 6X ULN: Withhold dose*
SrCr >6X ULN: Permanently d/c
Rash:
Grade 3: Withhold dose*
Grade 4: Permanently d/c
Encephalitis:
New Onset Moderate or Severe Neurologic Signs or Symptoms: Withhold dose*
Immune-Mediated Encephalitis: Permanently d/c
Other:
Other Grade 3 Adverse Reaction:
1st Occurrence: Withhold dose*
Recurrence of Same Grade 3 Adverse Reactions: Permanently d/c
Life-Threatening or Grade 4 Adverse Reactions: Permanently d/c
Requirement for ≥10mg/day Prednisone or Equivalent for >12 Weeks: Permanently d/c
Persistent Grade 2 or 3 Adverse Reactions Lasting ≥12 Weeks: Permanently d/c
When administered w/ ipilimumab, if nivolumab is withheld, ipilimumab should also be withheld

*Resume treatment when adverse reaction returns to Grade 0 or 1

ADMINISTRATION
IV route
Preparation
1. Withdraw required volume of product and transfer into an IV container.

2. Dilute w/ either 0.9% NaCl inj or D5 inj to prepare an infusion w/ a final concentration ranging from 1-10mg/mL.
3. Mix diluted sol by gentle inversion; do not shake.
4. Discard partially used or empty vials.
5. After preparation, store infusion either at room temperature for ≤4 hrs from time of preparation (including room temperature storage of infusion in IV container and time for infusion administration) or at 2-8°C (36-46°F) for ≤24 hrs from time of infusion preparation; do not freeze.

Administration
Administer over 60 min through IV line containing a sterile, non-pyrogenic, low protein binding in-line filter (pore size 0.2-1.2μm).
Do not coadminister other drugs through the same IV line.
Flush IV line at end of infusion.
When administered w/ ipilimumab, infuse nivolumab 1st followed by ipilimumab on the same day. Use separate infusion bags and filters for each infusion.

STORAGE
2-8°C (36-46°F). Protect from light. Do not freeze or shake.

HOW SUPPLIED
Inj: 10mg/mL [4mL, 10mL]

WARNINGS/PRECAUTIONS
Refer to Dosing Considerations for recommendations to withhold or d/c therapy for the following adverse reactions. Refer to PI for corticosteroid dose in the management of the following adverse reactions. Immune-mediated pneumonitis, including fatal cases, reported; administer corticosteroids for ≥Grade 2 pneumonitis, followed by corticosteroid taper. Immune-mediated colitis may occur. Administer corticosteroids followed by corticosteroid taper for Grade 3 or 4 colitis. Administer corticosteroids followed by corticosteroid taper for Grade 2 colitis lasting >5 days; if worsening or no improvement occurs, increase corticosteroid dose. Permanently d/c therapy for recurrent colitis upon restarting therapy. Immune-mediated hepatitis may occur; administer corticosteroids for ≥Grade 2 transaminase elevations, w/ or w/o concomitant elevation in total bilirubin. Hypophysitis may occur; administer corticosteroids for ≥Grade 2 hypophysitis. Adrenal insufficiency may occur; administer corticosteroids for Grade 3 or 4 adrenal insufficiency. Thyroid disorders may occur; administer hormone replacement therapy for hypothyroidism and initiate medical management for control of hyperthyroidism. Type 1 DM may occur; administer insulin for type 1 diabetes. Immune-mediated nephritis and renal dysfunction may occur. For Grade 2 or 3 SrCr elevation, withhold therapy and administer corticosteroids followed by corticosteroid taper; if worsening or no improvement occurs, increase corticosteroid dose and permanently d/c therapy. Permanently d/c therapy and administer corticosteroids followed by corticosteroid taper for Grade 4 SrCr elevation. Immune-mediated rash may occur; administer corticosteroids for Grade 3 or 4 rash. Severe rash, including rare cases of fatal toxic epidermal necrolysis, reported. Immune-mediated encephalitis may occur; if other etiologies are ruled out, administer corticosteroids followed by corticosteroid taper. Other clinically significant immune-mediated adverse reactions (eg, uveitis, iritis, pancreatitis, facial and abducens nerve paresis, demyelination, polymyalgia rheumatica, autoimmune neuropathy) may occur during therapy and after discontinuation of therapy; exclude other causes. Based on severity of the adverse reaction, permanently d/c or withhold therapy, administer high-dose corticosteroids, and if appropriate, initiate hormone replacement therapy. Upon improvement to ≤Grade 1, initiate corticosteroid taper and continue to taper over at least 1 month. Consider restarting therapy after completion of corticosteroid taper based on the severity of the event. Severe infusion reactions reported. Complications, including fatal events, reported in patients who received allogeneic HSCT after nivolumab; follow patients closely for early evidence of transplant-related complications, such as hyperacute graft-versus-host-disease (GVHD), severe (Grade 3 to 4) acute GVHD, steroid-requiring febrile syndrome, hepatic veno-occlusive disease, and other immune-mediated adverse reactions, and intervene promptly. May cause fetal harm.

ADVERSE REACTIONS
Melanoma: (Single Agent) Fatigue, rash, musculoskeletal pain, pruritus, diarrhea, nausea. (W/ Ipilimumab) Fatigue, rash, diarrhea, N/V, pyrexia, dyspnea.
Metastatic Non-Small Cell Lung Cancer: Fatigue, musculoskeletal pain, cough, decreased appetite, constipation.
Advanced Renal Cell Carcinoma: Asthenic conditions, cough, nausea, rash, dyspnea, diarrhea, constipation, decreased appetite, back pain, arthralgia.
Classical Hodgkin Lymphoma: Fatigue, URTI, pyrexia, diarrhea, cough.

PREGNANCY AND LACTATION
Pregnancy: May cause fetal harm based on its mechanism of action and data from animal studies. Human IgG4 is known to cross the placenta and nivolumab is an IgG4; therefore, nivolumab has the potential to be transmitted from the mother to the developing fetus. Effects are likely to be greater during the 2nd and 3rd trimesters. Advise pregnant women of potential risk to fetus.
Lactation: Not for use in nursing.
Reproductive Potential: Females of reproductive potential should use effective contraception during treatment and for at least 5 months following the last dose.

MECHANISM OF ACTION
Human PD-1 blocking antibody; binds to PD-1 receptor and blocks its interaction w/ the PD-1 ligands, PD-L1 and PD-L2, releasing PD-1 pathway-mediated inhibition of the immune response, including the anti-tumor immune response. Combined nivolumab and ipilimumab (anti-CTLA-4) mediated inhibition results in enhanced T-cell function that is greater than the effects of either antibody alone, and results in improved anti-tumor responses in metastatic melanoma.

PHARMACOKINETICS
Distribution: V_d=8L, 7.92L (w/ ipilimumab); may cross placenta. **Elimination:** $T_{1/2}$=26.7 days, 24.8 days (w/ ipilimumab).

PATIENT CONSIDERATIONS

Assessment: Assess pregnancy/nursing status. Obtain baseline liver/renal (eg, SrCr)/thyroid function.

Monitoring: Monitor for signs w/ radiographic imaging and symptoms of pneumonitis. Monitor for signs/symptoms of immune-mediated colitis, hypophysitis, adrenal insufficiency, rash, encephalitis, hyperglycemia, transplant-related complications, and other adverse reactions. Monitor for abnormal liver tests, elevated SrCr, and thyroid function periodically.

Counseling: Inform of the risk of immune-mediated adverse reactions that may require corticosteroid treatment and withholding or discontinuation of therapy (eg, pneumonitis, colitis, hepatitis, endocrinopathies, nephritis and renal dysfunction, rash, encephalitis); instruct to immediately contact healthcare provider if signs/symptoms of an immune-mediated adverse reaction occur. Advise of the potential risk of infusion reaction. Advise of potential risk of posttransplant complications. Advise females of reproductive potential of the potential risk to a fetus and instruct to inform their healthcare provider of known/suspected pregnancy and to use effective contraception during treatment and for at least 5 months following the last dose of therapy. Advise women not to breastfeed while on therapy.

ORACEA — doxycycline

Rx

Class: Tetracyclines

ADULT DOSAGE	PEDIATRIC DOSAGE
Rosacea	Pediatric use may not have been established
Inflammatory Lesions (Papules/Pustules):	
Usual: 40mg qam	

DOSING CONSIDERATIONS
Elderly
Start at lower end of dosing range

ADMINISTRATION
Oral route

Take on an empty stomach, preferably at least 1 hr ac or 2 hrs pc. Administer w/ adequate amounts of fluid to reduce the risk of esophageal irritation and ulceration.

STORAGE
15-30°C (59-86°F).

HOW SUPPLIED
Cap: 40mg

CONTRAINDICATIONS
Hypersensitivity to doxycycline or any of the other tetracyclines.

WARNINGS/PRECAUTIONS
Do not use for treating bacterial infections, providing antibacterial prophylaxis, or reducing the numbers of (or eliminating) microorganisms associated w/ any bacterial disease. May cause fetal harm. May cause permanent discoloration of the teeth (yellow-gray-brown) if used during tooth development (last half of pregnancy, infancy, childhood up to 8 yrs of age). Enamel hypoplasia reported. Do not use during tooth development unless other drugs are not likely to be effective or are contraindicated. May decrease fibula growth rate in premature infants. *Clostridium difficile*-associated diarrhea (CDAD) reported; d/c if CDAD is suspected or confirmed. May result in overgrowth of non-susceptible microorganisms, including fungi; d/c and institute appropriate therapy if superinfection occurs. Caution in patients w/ a history of or predisposition to *Candida* overgrowth. Bacterial resistance may develop; use only as indicated and do not exceed recommended dosage. Photosensitivity manifested by an exaggerated sunburn reaction reported. Development of autoimmune syndromes reported; d/c immediately and perform LFTs, antinuclear antibody (ANA), CBC, and other appropriate tests in symptomatic patients. Tissue hyperpigmentation reported. May increase BUN. Caution in patients w/ renal impairment; may lead to excessive systemic accumulations and possible liver toxicity. Lower than usual total dosages are indicated and if therapy is prolonged, serum drug level determinations may be advisable. Associated w/ pseudotumor cerebri (benign intracranial HTN) in adults and bulging fontanels in infants. Lab test interactions may occur.

ADVERSE REACTIONS
Nasopharyngitis, sinusitis, diarrhea, HTN.

DRUG INTERACTIONS
Depresses plasma prothrombin activity; may require downward adjustment of anticoagulant dosage. May interfere w/ bactericidal action of penicillin; avoid concurrent use. Fatal renal toxicity reported w/ methoxyflurane. Bismuth subsalicylate, proton pump inhibitors, antacids containing aluminum, Ca^{2+}, or Mg^{2+}, and iron-containing preparations may impair absorption. May interfere w/ the effectiveness of low dose oral contraceptives. Avoid concurrent use w/ oral retinoids (eg, isotretinoin, acitretin); pseudotumor cerebri reported. Barbiturates, carbamazepine, and phenytoin decrease the $T_{1/2}$ of doxycycline.

PREGNANCY AND LACTATION
Pregnancy: Category D.
Lactation: Not for use in nursing.

MECHANISM OF ACTION
Tetracycline derivative; mechanism of action in the treatment of inflammatory lesions of rosacea has not been established.

PHARMACOKINETICS
Absorption: (Healthy) Single dose: C_{max}=510ng/mL; T_{max}=3 hrs; AUC=9227ng•hr/mL. Steady-state: C_{max}=600ng/mL; T_{max}=2 hrs; AUC=7543ng•hr/mL. **Distribution:** Plasma protein binding (>90%); crosses the placenta, found in breast milk. **Elimination:** Urine (unchanged), feces (unchanged); $T_{1/2}$=21.2 hrs (single dose), 23.2 hrs (steady-state).

PATIENT CONSIDERATIONS

Assessment: Assess for hypersensitivity to drug and other tetracyclines, renal impairment, history of or predisposition to *Candida* overgrowth, visual disturbances, pregnancy/nursing status, and possible drug interactions.

Monitoring: Monitor for signs/symptoms of CDAD, superinfection, photosensitivity, autoimmune syndromes, tissue hyperpigmentation, and other adverse reactions. Monitor serum drug levels in patients w/ renal impairment if therapy is prolonged. Routinely check for papilledema while on treatment. Perform periodic lab evaluations of organ systems, including hematopoietic, renal, and hepatic studies. If symptoms of autoimmune syndrome occur, perform LFTs, ANA, CBC, and other appropriate tests.

Counseling: Instruct to take exactly ud. Inform that drug should not be used by pregnant or breastfeeding women nor by individuals of either gender who are attempting to conceive a child. Inform that drug may render oral contraceptives less effective; advise females to use a 2nd form of contraception. Inform that pseudomembranous colitis and pseudotumor cerebri may occur; instruct to seek immediate medical attention if watery/bloody stools, or headache or blurred vision occur. Instruct to minimize/avoid exposure to natural or artificial sunlight and d/c at 1st evidence of sunburn, advise to wear loose-fitting clothes, and discuss other sun protection measures. Instruct to d/c and contact physician if arthralgia, fever, rash, or malaise develops. Inform that drug may cause discoloration of skin, scars, teeth, or gums.

ORAPRED ODT — prednisolone sodium phosphate

Rx

Class: Glucocorticoid

ADULT DOSAGE	PEDIATRIC DOSAGE
Steroid-Responsive Disorders	**Steroid-Responsive Disorders**
Initial: 10-60mg/day, depending on disease and response	**Initial:** 0.14-2mg/kg/day in 3 or 4 divided doses (4-60mg/m²/day)
Maint: Decrease initial dose in small decrements to lowest effective dose	**Nephrotic Syndrome**
Multiple Sclerosis	**>2 Years:**
Acute Exacerbations:	60mg/m²/day given in 3 divided doses for 4 weeks, followed by 4 weeks of single dose alternate-day therapy at 40mg/m²/day
200mg/day for a week, followed by 80mg qod for 1 month	**Asthma**
	Uncontrolled by Inhaled Corticosteroids and Long-Acting Bronchodilators:
	1-2mg/kg/day in single or divided doses; continue short course ("burst") therapy until peak expiratory flow rate of 80% of personal best is achieved or symptoms resolve (usually 3-10 days)

DOSING CONSIDERATIONS
Elderly
Start at lower end of dosing range

Discontinuation
Withdraw gradually after long-term therapy

ADMINISTRATION
Oral route

Take w/ food.
Place tab on tongue; may be swallowed whole or allowed to dissolve in mouth w/ or w/o water.
Do not break or use partial tabs.
Do not remove tab from blister until just prior to dosing.

STORAGE
20-25°C (68-77°F); excursions permitted to 15-30°C (59-86°F). Protect from moisture.

HOW SUPPLIED
Tab, Disintegrating: 10mg, 15mg, 30mg

CONTRAINDICATIONS
Hypersensitivity to corticosteroids (eg, prednisolone) or any components of this product.

WARNINGS/PRECAUTIONS
May produce reversible hypothalamic-pituitary-adrenal (HPA) axis suppression w/ the potential for glucocorticosteroid insufficiency after withdrawal; gradually reduce dose. May impair mineralocorticoid secretion; administer salt and/or mineralocorticoid concurrently. Metabolic clearance is decreased in hypothyroidism and increased in hyperthyroidism; changes in thyroid status may necessitate dose adjustment. May increase susceptibility to infections, mask signs of current infection, and increase risk of exacerbation, dissemination, or reactivation of latent infection. May exacerbate systemic fungal infections; avoid use in the presence of systemic fungal infections unless needed to control drug reactions. Rule out latent or active amebiasis before initiating therapy. May cause more serious/fatal course

of chickenpox or measles; avoid exposure, and if exposed, consider prophylaxis/treatment. Caution w/ *Strongyloides* infestation, active/latent tuberculosis (TB) or tuberculin reactivity, HTN, CHF, and renal insufficiency. May cause BP elevation, salt/water retention, and increased K⁺ and Ca²⁺ excretion; dietary salt restriction and K⁺ supplementation may be necessary. Caution w/ recent MI. Increased risk of GI perforation w/ certain GI disorders; signs of GI perforation (eg, peritoneal irritation) may be masked. Caution w/ probable impending perforation, abscess or other pyogenic infections; diverticulitis; fresh intestinal anastomoses; and active or latent peptic ulcers. Not for use in cerebral malaria and active ocular herpes simplex. May be associated w/ CNS effects (eg, euphoria, insomnia, psychotic manifestations); existing emotional instability or psychotic tendencies may be aggravated. May decrease bone formation and increase bone resorption, and may lead to inhibition of bone growth in pediatric patients and the development of osteoporosis at any age; caution w/ increased risk of osteoporosis. May produce posterior subcapsular cataracts, glaucoma w/ possible optic nerve damage, and may enhance the establishment of secondary ocular infections; not recommended in optic neuritis treatment. Acute myopathy w/ high doses reported, most often in patients w/ disorders of neuromuscular transmission (eg, myasthenia gravis). Elevation of CK or IOP may occur. Kaposi's sarcoma reported. Caution w/ ocular herpes simplex. May have negative effects on growth and development in children. May cause fetal harm. May suppress reactions to skin tests. Caution in elderly.

ADVERSE REACTIONS
Fluid retention, HTN, alteration of glucose tolerance, behavioral changes, increased appetite, weight gain.

DRUG INTERACTIONS
Live or live, attenuated vaccines are contraindicated w/ immunosuppressive doses. Killed or inactivated vaccines may be administered, although response is unpredictable. May exhibit a diminished response to toxoids and live or inactivated vaccines. May potentiate replication of some organisms contained in live, attenuated vaccines. Aminoglutethimide may lead to a loss of corticosteroid-induced adrenal suppression. Cardiac enlargement and CHF reported following concomitant use of amphotericin B and hydrocortisone. Concomitant use w/ anticholinesterase agents may produce severe weakness in patients w/ myasthenia gravis; d/c anticholinesterase agents at least 24 hrs before initiating therapy. May inhibit response to warfarin. May increase blood glucose levels; dosage adjustments of antidiabetic agents may be required. May decrease serum levels of isoniazid. CYP3A4 inducers (eg, barbiturates, phenytoin, carbamazepine, rifampin) may enhance metabolism and require corticosteroid dosage increase. Ketoconazole may decrease metabolism, leading to an increased risk of corticosteroid side effects. Cholestyramine may increase clearance. Increased activity of both drugs may occur w/ cyclosporine; convulsions reported w/ concurrent use. May increase risk of arrhythmias w/ digitalis glycosides. Estrogens, including oral contraceptives, may decrease hepatic metabolism and enhance effect. Aspirin (ASA) or other NSAIDs may increase risk of GI side effects; caution w/ ASA in hypoprothrombinemia patients. May increase clearance of salicylates. Closely monitor for hypokalemia w/ K⁺-depleting agents (eg, amphotericin B, diuretics). Acute myopathy reported w/ neuromuscular blocking drugs (eg, pancuronium).

PREGNANCY AND LACTATION
Pregnancy: Category D.
Lactation: Caution in nursing.

MECHANISM OF ACTION
Synthetic adrenocortical steroid; promotes gluconeogenesis, increases deposition of glycogen in the liver, inhibits glucose utilization, possesses anti-insulin activity, increases catabolism of protein and lipolysis, stimulates fat synthesis and storage, increases GFR that leads to increased urinary excretion of urate, and increases Ca²⁺ excretion.

PHARMACOKINETICS
Absorption: Rapid and well-absorbed. AUC=2408.1ng•hr/mL. **Distribution:** V_d=0.22-0.7L/kg; plasma protein binding (70-90%); found in breast milk. **Metabolism:** Liver. **Elimination:** Urine (as sulfate and glucuronide conjugates); T_{1/2}=2.6 hrs.

PATIENT CONSIDERATIONS
Assessment: Assess for hypersensitivity to drug or any of its components, unusual stress, current infections, systemic fungal infections, latent/active amebiasis, peptic ulcer and TB, cerebral malaria, ocular herpes simplex, CHF, HTN, recent MI, renal insufficiency, diverticulitis, intestinal anastomoses, psychotic tendencies, myasthenia gravis, thyroid disorders, any other conditions where treatment is contraindicated or cautioned, pregnancy/nursing status, and possible drug interactions.

Monitoring: Monitor for infections, changes in thyroid status, cataracts, glaucoma, Kaposi's sarcoma, growth/development (in pediatric patients), osteoporosis, acute myopathy, psychic derangements, emotional instability or psychotic tendencies aggravation, and other adverse reactions. Monitor BP, serum electrolytes, and CK. Monitor IOP if used for >6 weeks. Frequently monitor coagulation indices w/ warfarin. Monitor for HPA-axis suppression, Cushing's syndrome, and hyperglycemia w/ chronic use.

Counseling: Instruct not to d/c therapy abruptly or w/o medical supervision. Instruct to inform any physician of intake of corticosteroids and to seek medical advice at once if fever or other signs of infection develop. Instruct to avoid exposure to chickenpox or measles; instruct to seek medical advice w/o delay if exposed. Advise to take exactly as prescribed. Advise to report recent or ongoing infections, vaccination, and concurrent medicines. Counsel about common adverse reactions (eg, fluid retention, altered glucose tolerance, elevated BP, behavioral and mood changes, increased appetite, weight gain). Instruct to take missed dose as soon as remembered, but if it is almost time for next dose, skip missed dose and take at the next regularly scheduled time; advise not to take an extra dose to make up for missed dose.

ORAPRED ORAL SOLUTION — prednisolone sodium phosphate
Rx

Class: Glucocorticoid

ADULT DOSAGE	PEDIATRIC DOSAGE
Steroid-Responsive Disorders	**Steroid-Responsive Disorders**
Initial: 5-60mg/day (1.67-20mL), depending on disease and response	**Initial:** 0.14-2mg/kg/day in 3 or 4 divided doses (4-60mg/m²/day)
Maint: Decrease initial dose in small decrements to lowest effective dose	**Nephrotic Syndrome**
Multiple Sclerosis	**>2 Years:** 60mg/m²/day given in 3 divided doses for 4 weeks, followed by 4 weeks of single dose alternate-day therapy at 40mg/m²/day
Acute Exacerbations: 200mg/day for a week, followed by 80mg qod for 1 month	**Asthma**
	Uncontrolled by Inhaled Corticosteroids and Long-Acting Bronchodilators: 1-2mg/kg/day in single or divided doses; continue short course ("burst") therapy until peak expiratory flow rate of 80% of personal best is achieved or symptoms resolve (usually 3-10 days)

- -

DOSING CONSIDERATIONS
Elderly
Start at lower end of dosing range

Discontinuation
Withdraw gradually after long-term therapy

ADMINISTRATION
Oral route

STORAGE
2-8°C (36-46°F). Keep tightly closed.

HOW SUPPLIED
Sol: 15mg/5mL [237mL]

CONTRAINDICATIONS
Systemic fungal infections, hypersensitivity to the drug or any of its components.

WARNINGS/PRECAUTIONS
May need to increase dose before, during, and after stressful situations. May produce reversible hypothalamic-pituitary-adrenal (HPA) axis suppression with the potential for glucocorticoid insufficiency after withdrawal; gradually reduce dose. May impair mineralocorticoid secretion; administer salt and/or mineralocorticoid concurrently. Metabolic clearance is decreased in hypothyroidism and increased in hyperthyroidism; changes in thyroid status may necessitate dose adjustment. May increase susceptibility to infections, mask signs of current infection, activate latent disease, or exacerbate intercurrent infections. Rule out latent or active amebiasis before initiating therapy. May cause more serious/fatal course of chickenpox and measles; avoid exposure, and if exposed, consider prophylaxis/treatment. Caution w/ *Strongyloides* infestation, active/latent tuberculosis (TB) or tuberculin reactivity, HTN, CHF, and renal insufficiency. May cause BP elevation, salt/water retention, and increased K⁺ and Ca²⁺ excretion; dietary salt restriction and K⁺ supplementation may be necessary. Not for use in cerebral malaria and active ocular herpes simplex. Signs of GI perforation (eg, peritoneal irritation) may be masked, minimal, or absent. Caution with nonspecific ulcerative colitis; probable impending perforation, abscess, or other pyogenic infections; diverticulitis; fresh intestinal anastomoses; and active/latent peptic ulcers. Psychic derangements may appear and existing emotional instability or psychotic tendencies may be aggravated. May decrease bone formation and increase bone resorption, and may lead to inhibition of bone growth in children/adolescents and the development of osteoporosis at any age; caution with increased risk of osteoporosis. May produce posterior subcapsular cataracts, glaucoma with possible optic nerve damage, and may enhance the establishment of secondary ocular infections; not recommended in optic neuritis treatment. Acute myopathy with high doses reported, most often in patients with disorders of neuromuscular transmission (eg, myasthenia gravis). Elevation of CK or IOP may occur. May suppress reactions to skin tests. Kaposi's sarcoma reported. Enhanced effect in patients with cirrhosis and hypothyroidism. Caution in elderly.

ADVERSE REACTIONS
Fluid retention, HTN, decreased carbohydrate tolerance, abdominal distention, increased appetite, weight gain, glaucoma, osteoporosis, muscle weakness, development of cushingoid state, menstrual irregularities, convulsions, headache, impaired wound healing, increased sweating.

DRUG INTERACTIONS
Live or live, attenuated vaccines are contraindicated with immunosuppressive doses. Killed or inactivated vaccines may be administered, although response is unpredictable. May exhibit a diminished response to toxoids and live or inactivated vaccines. May potentiate replication of some organisms contained in live, attenuated vaccines. Hepatic enzyme inducers (eg, barbiturates, phenytoin, ephedrine) may enhance metabolism and require corticosteroid dosage increase. Increased activity of both drugs may occur with cyclosporine; convulsions reported with concurrent use. Estrogens may decrease hepatic metabolism and increase effect. Ketoconazole may decrease metabolism leading to an increased risk of corticosteroid side effects. May inhibit response to warfarin. ASA or other NSAIDs may increase risk of GI side effects; caution with

ASA in hypoprothrombinemia patients. May increase clearance of salicylates. Closely monitor for hypokalemia with K⁺-depleting agents (eg, amphotericin B, diuretics). May increase risk of arrhythmias with digitalis glycosides. Concomitant use with anticholinesterase agents may produce severe weakness in patients with myasthenia gravis; d/c anticholinesterase agents at least 24 hrs before initiating therapy. May increase blood glucose levels; dosage adjustments of antidiabetic agents may be required. Acute myopathy reported with neuromuscular blocking drugs (eg, pancuronium).

PREGNANCY AND LACTATION
Category C, caution in nursing.

MECHANISM OF ACTION
Synthetic adrenocortical steroid; promotes gluconeogenesis, increases deposition of glycogen in the liver, inhibits glucose utilization, possesses anti-insulin activity, increases catabolism of protein and lipolysis, stimulates fat synthesis and storage, increases GFR that leads to increased urinary excretion of urate, and increases Ca^{2+} excretion.

PHARMACOKINETICS
Absorption: Rapid and well-absorbed. **Distribution:** Plasma protein binding (70-90%); found in breast milk. **Metabolism:** Liver. **Elimination:** Urine (as sulfate and glucuronide conjugates); $T_{1/2}$=2-4 hrs.

PATIENT CONSIDERATIONS
Assessment: Assess for hypersensitivity to drug or any of its components, unusual stress, current infections, systemic fungal infections, latent/active amebiasis, peptic ulcer and TB, cerebral malaria, ocular herpes simplex, CHF, HTN, renal insufficiency, diverticulitis, intestinal anastomoses, ulcerative colitis, cirrhosis, psychotic tendencies, myasthenia gravis, thyroid disorders, any other conditions where treatment is contraindicated or cautioned, pregnancy/nursing status, and possible drug interactions.

Monitoring: Monitor for HPA axis suppression, infections, changes in thyroid status, cataracts, glaucoma, Kaposi's sarcoma, growth/development (in pediatric patients), osteoporosis, acute myopathy, psychic derangements, emotional instability or psychotic tendencies aggravation, and other adverse reactions. Monitor BP, serum electrolytes, and CK. Monitor IOP if used for >6 weeks. Frequently monitor coagulation indices with warfarin.

Counseling: Instruct not to d/c therapy abruptly or without medical supervision. Instruct to inform any physician of intake of corticosteroids and to seek medical advice at once if fever or other signs of infection develop. Instruct to avoid exposure to chickenpox or measles; instruct to seek medical advice without delay if exposed.

ORAQIX — lidocaine/prilocaine   Rx
Class: Local anesthetic

ADULT DOSAGE	PEDIATRIC DOSAGE
Localized Anesthesia in Periodontal Pockets **During Scaling and/or Root Planing:** **Usual:** 1 cartridge (1.7g) or less is sufficient for 1 quadrant of dentition **Max:** 5 cartridges (8.5g) per treatment session	Pediatric use may not have been established

DOSING CONSIDERATIONS
Elderly
Start at lower end of dosing range

ADMINISTRATION
Topical route

Do not inject

Instructions
1. Apply on the gingival margin around selected teeth using blunt-tipped applicator
2. Wait 30 sec, then fill the periodontal pockets until gel becomes visible at the gingival margin
3. Wait another 30 sec before starting treatment
4. Administer in liquid form; if gel forms, refrigerate until it becomes a liquid again (do not freeze)
5. May reapply if anesthesia starts to wear off; anesthetic effect has a duration of approx 20 min

STORAGE
25°C (77°F); excursions permitted to 15-30°C (59-86°F). May become opaque at <5°C; warm cartridge to room temperature for opacity to disappear. Do not freeze. Do not use dental cartridge warmers.

HOW SUPPLIED
Gel: (Lidocaine-Prilocaine) 2.5%-2.5% [1.7g]

CONTRAINDICATIONS
Known history of hypersensitivity to local anesthetics of the amide type or to any other component of the product.

WARNINGS/PRECAUTIONS
Dose-related methemoglobinemia reported; consider methemoglobinemia if central cyanosis unresponsive to oxygen therapy occurs. Patients with glucose-6-phosphate dehydrogenase (G6PD) deficiency are more susceptible to drug-induced methemoglobinemia. Avoid with congenital or idiopathic methemoglobinemia and in infants <12 months who are receiving

methemoglobin-inducing agents. Not for inj; do not use with standard dental syringes. Allergic and anaphylactic reactions may occur. Avoid contact with eyes; if this occurs, immediately rinse the eye with water or saline and protect it until normal sensation returns. Caution with renal impairment, severe hepatic disease, history of drug sensitivities, and in elderly.

ADVERSE REACTIONS
Application site reactions (eg, pain, soreness, irritation, numbness, vesicles, ulcerations, edema, abscess, redness).

DRUG INTERACTIONS
Greater risk of developing methemoglobinemia with drugs inducing methemoglobinemia (eg, sulfonamides, acetaminophen, acetanilide, aniline dyes, benzocaine, chloroquine, dapsone, naphthalene, nitrates and nitrites, nitrofurantoin, nitroglycerin, nitroprusside, pamaquine, para-aminosalicylic acid, phenacetin, phenobarbital, phenytoin, primaquine, quinine). Additive and potentially synergistic toxic effects in combination with dental inj anesthesia, other local anesthetics, or agents structurally related to local anesthetics (eg, Class 1 antiarrhythmics such as tocainide and mexiletine).

PREGNANCY AND LACTATION
Category B, caution in nursing.

MECHANISM OF ACTION
Amide local anesthetic; blocks Na⁺ ion channels required for the initiation and conduction of neuronal impulses, resulting in local anesthesia.

PHARMACOKINETICS
Absorption: (Single application) Lidocaine: C_{max}=182ng/mL, T_{max}=30 min (median); Prilocaine: C_{max}=77ng/mL, T_{max}=30 min (median). (Repeated applications) Lidocaine: C_{max}=284ng/mL, AUC=84,000ng·min/mL, T_{max}=200 min (median); Prilocaine: C_{max}=106ng/mL, AUC=26,000ng·min/mL, T_{max}=200 min (median). **Distribution:** Crosses placenta; found in breast milk. Lidocaine: Plasma protein binding (70%); (IV) V_d=90L. Prilocaine: Plasma protein binding (40%); (IV) V_d=156L. **Metabolism:** Lidocaine: Liver; N-dealkylation via CYP3A4, then hydrolysis to 2,6-xylidine, which is converted, via CYP2A6, to 4-hydroxy-2,6-xylidine (major urinary metabolite). Prilocaine: Liver; o-toluidine, which is converted further to 4- and 6-hydroxytoluidine (metabolites). **Elimination:** Kidney. Lidocaine: $T_{1/2}$=3.6 hrs. Prilocaine: $T_{1/2}$=2.8 hrs.

PATIENT CONSIDERATIONS
Assessment: Assess for G6PD deficiency, congenital or idiopathic methemoglobinemia, renal/hepatic impairment, history of hypersensitivity, pregnancy/nursing status, and possible drug interactions.

Monitoring: Monitor for allergic and anaphylactic reactions, and signs/symptoms of methemoglobinemia.

Counseling: Advise to avoid injury to the treated area, or exposure to extreme hot or cold temperatures, until complete sensation has returned.

ORAVIG — miconazole   Rx
Class: Azole antifungal

ADULT DOSAGE	PEDIATRIC DOSAGE
Oropharyngeal Candidiasis **≥16 Years:** Apply 1 tab qd for 14 consecutive days	Pediatric use may not have been established

ADMINISTRATION
Buccal route

Apply in the upper gum region qam w/ dry hands, after brushing the teeth
Either side of tab may be placed against the upper gum just above the incisor tooth (canine fossa), and held in place w/ slight pressure over the upper lip for 30 sec to ensure adhesion
For improved comfort, may apply rounded side surface of tab to gum
Subsequent applications should be made to alternate sides of the mouth; clear away any remaining tab material prior to next application
Do not crush, chew, or swallow
Food and drink can be taken normally when tab is in place

STORAGE
20-25°C (68-77°F); excursions between 15-30°C (59-86°F) permitted at room temperature. Protect from moisture.

HOW SUPPLIED
Tab, Buccal: 50mg

CONTRAINDICATIONS
Known hypersensitivity (eg, anaphylaxis) to miconazole, milk protein concentrate, or any other component of the product.

WARNINGS/PRECAUTIONS
Allergic reactions, including anaphylactic reactions and hypersensitivity, reported; d/c immediately at the 1st sign of hypersensitivity. Caution with hepatic impairment.

ADVERSE REACTIONS
Diarrhea, N/V, headache, dysgeusia.

DRUG INTERACTIONS
May enhance anticoagulant effects of warfarin; closely monitor PT, INR, or other suitable anticoagulation tests, and for evidence of bleeding. May interact with drugs metabolized through CYP2C9 and CYP3A4 (eg, oral hypoglycemics, phenytoin, ergot alkaloids).

PREGNANCY AND LACTATION
Category C, caution in nursing.

MECHANISM OF ACTION

Azole antifungal; inhibits the enzyme CYP450 14α-demethylase, leading to inhibition of ergosterol synthesis, an essential component of the fungal cell membrane. Affects the synthesis of TG and fatty acids and inhibits oxidative and peroxidative enzymes, increasing the amount of reactive oxygen species within the cell.

PHARMACOKINETICS

Absorption: Minimal systemic absorption (max salivary concentrations of 15mcg/mL at 7 hrs). **Metabolism:** Liver. **Elimination:** Urine (<1%, unchanged); $T_{1/2}$=24 hrs (healthy, systemic administration).

PATIENT CONSIDERATIONS

Assessment: Assess for hypersensitivity to drug, milk protein concentrate, or any other component of the product, hepatic impairment, pregnancy/nursing status, and possible drug interactions.

Monitoring: Monitor for signs/symptoms of hypersensitivity and other adverse reactions. Closely monitor PT, INR, or other suitable anticoagulation tests, and for evidence of bleeding with warfarin.

Counseling: Instruct on proper application of the tab. Inform that subsequent applications should be made to alternate sides of the gum. Advise that if tab does not stick or falls off within first 6 hrs, the same tab should be repositioned immediately; instruct to place a new tab if tab still does not adhere. Instruct to drink a glass of water and apply a new tab only once if tab is swallowed within first 6 hrs. Instruct to not apply a new tab until the next, regularly scheduled dose, if tab falls off or swallowed after it was in place for ≥6 hrs. Counsel to avoid situations that could interfere with the sticking of the tab (eg, touching/pressing tab after placement, wearing upper denture, chewing gum, hitting tab when brushing teeth, rinsing mouth too vigorously). Advise to d/c and contact physician if hives, skin rash, other symptoms of an allergic reaction, or application-site swelling/pain develops. Inform that patients may experience other adverse reactions, including diarrhea, headache, nausea, and change in taste.

ORBACTIV — oritavancin   Rx

Class: Lipoglycopeptide

ADULT DOSAGE	PEDIATRIC DOSAGE
Skin and Skin Structure Infections	Pediatric use may not have been established
Acute bacterial infections caused by *Staphylococcus aureus* (including methicillin-susceptible and methicillin-resistant isolates), *Streptococcus pyogenes, Streptococcus agalactiae, Streptococcus dysgalactiae, Streptococcus anginosus* group (includes *S. anginosus, S. intermedius,* and *S. constellatus*), and *Enterococcus faecalis* (vancomycin-susceptible isolates only)	
Single 1200mg dose by IV infusion over 3 hrs	

ADMINISTRATION

IV route

Preparation

Three 400mg vials need to be reconstituted and diluted to prepare a single 1200mg dose.

Reconstitution:

1. Add 40mL of sterile water for inj to reconstitute each vial to provide a 10mg/mL sol per vial.
2. Gently swirl each vial to avoid foaming and ensure that all powder is completely reconstituted in sol.

Dilution:

1. Use only D5W for dilution; do not use normal saline, as it is incompatible and may cause precipitation of the drug.
2. Withdraw and discard 120mL from a 1000mL IV bag of D5W.
3. Withdraw 40mL from each of the 3 reconstituted vials and add to D5W IV bag to bring the bag volume to 1000mL; this yields a concentration of 1.2mg/mL.

Diluted IV sol in an infusion bag should be used w/in 6 hrs when stored at room temperature, or w/in 12 hrs when refrigerated at 2-8°C (36-46°F). Combined storage time (reconstituted sol in the vial and diluted sol in the bag) and 3-hr infusion time should not exceed 6 hrs at room temperature or 12 hrs if refrigerated.

Incompatibilities

1. IV substances, additives, or other medications mixed in normal saline should not be added to oritavancin single-use vials or infused simultaneously through the same IV line or through a common IV port.
2. Drugs formulated at a basic or neutral pH may be incompatible.
3. Do not administer simultaneously w/ commonly used IV drugs through a common IV port; if the same IV line is used for sequential infusion of additional medications, the line should be flushed w/ D5W before and after infusion of oritavancin.

STORAGE

20-25°C (68-77°F); excursions permitted to 15-30°C (59-86°F). **Diluted Sol in Infusion Bag:** Use w/in 6 hrs when stored at room temperature or use w/in 12 hrs when refrigerated at 2-8°C (36-46°F). Combined storage time (reconstituted sol

in the vial and the diluted sol in the bag) and 3-hr infusion time should not exceed 6 hrs at room temperature or 12 hrs if refrigerated.

HOW SUPPLIED

Inj: 400mg

CONTRAINDICATIONS

Use of IV unfractionated heparin sodium for 120 hrs (5 days) after administration of therapy. Known hypersensitivity to oritavancin.

WARNINGS/PRECAUTIONS

May artificially prolong certain laboratory coagulation tests. Artificially prolongs activated PTT (aPTT) for 120 hrs, PT and INR for up to 12 hrs, and activated clotting time for up to 24 hrs by binding to and preventing action of the phospholipid reagents commonly used in lab coagulation tests. Has been shown to elevate D dimer concentrations up to 72 hrs after administration of therapy. For patients who require aPTT monitoring w/in 120 hrs of dosing, a non-phospholipid dependent coagulation test (eg, Factor Xa [chromogenic] assay) or an alternative anticoagulant not requiring aPTT monitoring may be considered. Serious hypersensitivity reactions reported; d/c immediately and institute appropriate supportive care if an acute hypersensitivity reaction occurs. Infusion-related reactions (eg, pruritus, urticaria, flushing) reported; consider slowing or interrupting drug infusion. *Clostridium difficile*-associated diarrhea (CDAD) reported; d/c if CDAD is suspected or confirmed. Osteomyelitis reported; institute appropriate alternate antibacterial therapy if suspected or diagnosed. May result in bacterial resistance if used in the absence of proven or suspected bacterial infection.

ADVERSE REACTIONS

Headache, N/V, limb and SQ abscesses, diarrhea.

DRUG INTERACTIONS

See Contraindications. Nonspecific, weak inhibitor (CYP2C9 and CYP2C19) or inducer (CYP3A4 and CYP2D6) of several CYP isoforms. Use caution when concomitantly administering w/ drugs w/ a narrow therapeutic window that are predominantly metabolized by 1 of the affected CYP450 enzymes (eg, warfarin); coadministration may increase (eg, CYP2C9 substrates) or decrease (eg, CYP2D6 substrates) concentrations of the narrow therapeutic range drug. Coadministration w/ warfarin may result in higher exposure of warfarin, which may increase the risk of bleeding. Use oritavancin in patients on chronic warfarin therapy only when the benefits can be expected to outweigh the risk of bleeding; frequently monitor for signs of bleeding.

PREGNANCY AND LACTATION

Pregnancy: Category C. **Lactation:** Caution in nursing.

MECHANISM OF ACTION

Semisynthetic lipoglycopeptide antibacterial agent; has 3 mechanisms of action: 1) inhibition of the transglycosylation (polymerization) step of cell-wall biosynthesis by binding to the stem peptide of peptidoglycan precursors; 2) inhibition of the transpeptidation (crosslinking) step of cell-wall biosynthesis by binding to the peptide bridging segments of the cell wall; and 3) disruption of bacterial membrane integrity, leading to depolarization, permeabilization, and cell death.

PHARMACOKINETICS

Absorption: C_{max}=138mcg/mL; AUC_{0-24}=1110mcg•hr/mL, $AUC_{0-infinity}$=2800mcg•hr/mL. **Distribution:** Plasma protein binding (85%); V_d=87.6L. **Elimination:** Urine (<5% unchanged), feces (<1% unchanged); $T_{1/2}$=245 hrs.

PATIENT CONSIDERATIONS

Assessment: Assess for hypersensitivity to drug or other glycopeptides, pregnancy/nursing status, and for possible drug interactions. Perform culture and susceptibility testing.

Monitoring: Monitor for hypersensitivity reactions, infusion-related reactions, CDAD, osteomyelitis, development of drug-resistant bacteria, and other adverse reactions. Frequently monitor for signs of bleeding w/ warfarin.

Counseling: Advise that allergic reactions may occur and that serious allergic reactions require immediate treatment. Advise to inform the physician about any previous hypersensitivity reactions to the drug, other glycopeptides, or other allergens. Inform that diarrhea is a common problem caused by therapy and usually resolves when therapy is discontinued; instruct to contact physician if severe watery or bloody diarrhea develops.

ORENCIA — abatacept   Rx

Class: Selective costimulation modulator

ADULT DOSAGE	PEDIATRIC DOSAGE
Rheumatoid Arthritis	**Juvenile Idiopathic Arthritis**
To reduce signs and symptoms, induce major clinical response, inhibit progression of structural damage, and improve physical function in adults w/ moderate to severe active rheumatoid arthritis; may be used as monotherapy or concomitantly w/ disease-modifying antirheumatic drugs other than TNF antagonists	To reduce signs and symptoms of moderately to severely active polyarticular juvenile idiopathic arthritis; may be used as monotherapy or concomitantly w/ methotrexate
IV Regimen:	**6-17 Years:**
Initial:	**IV Regimen:**
<60kg: 500mg	**Initial:**
60-100kg: 750mg	**<75kg:** 10mg/kg
>100kg: 1000mg	**≥75kg:** Follow adult IV dosing regimen; not to exceed 1000mg
Maint: Give succeeding infusions at 2	**Maint:** Give succeeding infusions at 2 and 4 weeks after the 1st infusion and every 4 weeks thereafter

and 4 weeks after the 1st infusion and every 4 weeks thereafter

SQ Regimen:
125mg SQ inj once weekly w/ or w/o an IV LD
If initiating w/ an IV LD, initiate w/ a single IV infusion (as per body weight categories listed in the IV regimen), followed by the first 125mg SQ inj w/in a day of the IV infusion

Switching from IV to SQ Regimen:
Give the 1st SQ dose instead of the next scheduled IV dose

ADMINISTRATION
IV/SQ route

IV
Give as an IV infusion over 30 min.
Do not infuse in the same IV line w/ other agents.

IV Infusion Preparation
Reconstitute w/ 10mL of sterile water for inj; only use silicone-free disposable syringe provided w/ each vial and an 18- to 21-gauge needle.
Rotate vial w/ gentle swirling until contents are completely dissolved; do not shake, and avoid prolonged/vigorous agitation.
Vent vial w/ needle to dissipate any foam after complete dissolution of powder.
Further dilute reconstituted sol w/ 0.9% NaCl inj using the same silicone-free disposable syringe to a total volume of 100mL.
Final concentration of abatacept in the bag or bottle will depend upon the amount of drug added, but will be ≤10mg/mL.
Do not shake bag or bottle.
May store fully diluted sol at room temperature or at 2-8°C (36-46°F) before use.
Infusion of fully diluted sol must be completed w/in 24 hrs of reconstitution; discard if not administered w/in 24 hrs.

SQ
Administer inj to front thigh or abdomen (except for the 2-inch area around navel) for self-inj, or outer area of the upper arm if a caregiver is administering dose.
Rotate inj site (at least 1 inch away from last inj site).
Do not inject into areas where the skin is tender, bruised, red, or hard.

STORAGE
2-8°C (36-46°F). Protect from light; store in original package until time of use.
Do not allow prefilled syringe to freeze. Fully Diluted Sol: May store at room temperature or at 2-8°C (36-46°F); discard if not administered w/in 24 hrs.

HOW SUPPLIED
Inj: 125mg/mL [prefilled syringe], 250mg [vial]

WARNINGS/PRECAUTIONS
Anaphylaxis or anaphylactoid reactions reported w/ IV use; permanently d/c and institute appropriate therapy if an anaphylactic or other serious allergic reaction occurs. Serious infections, including sepsis and pneumonia, reported; caution in patients w/ history of recurrent infections, underlying conditions that may predispose to infections, or chronic, latent, or localized infections. D/C if a serious infection develops. Screen for latent tuberculosis (TB) infection and viral hepatitis prior to initiation of therapy; treat patients testing (+) for TB prior to therapy. Hepatitis B reactivation may occur. JIA patients should be brought up-to-date w/ all immunizations prior to initiation of therapy. Caution in patients w/ COPD; monitor for worsening of respiratory status. May affect host defenses against infections and malignancies. Caution in elderly. (IV) Contains maltose that may react w/ glucose dehydrogenase pyrroloquinoline quinone-based glucose monitoring and may result in falsely elevated blood glucose readings on the day of infusion; consider methods that do not react w/ maltose in patients requiring blood glucose monitoring.

ADVERSE REACTIONS
Headache, URTI, nasopharyngitis, nausea, sinusitis, UTI, influenza, bronchitis, dizziness, cough, back pain, HTN, dyspepsia, rash, pain in extremities.

DRUG INTERACTIONS
May experience more infections and serious infections w/ TNF antagonists; concurrent use is not recommended. Monitor for signs of infection while transitioning from TNF antagonist to abatacept. Concomitant use w/ other biologic RA therapy (eg, anakinra) is not recommended. Do not give live vaccines concurrently w/ therapy or w/in 3 months of its discontinuation.

PREGNANCY AND LACTATION
Pregnancy: Category C.
Lactation: Not for use in nursing.

MECHANISM OF ACTION
Selective costimulation modulator; inhibits T-cell activation by binding to CD80 and CD86, thereby blocking interaction w/ CD28.

PHARMACOKINETICS
Absorption: (SQ) Bioavailability (78.6%). C_{max}=295mcg/mL (RA patients, IV), 48.1mcg/mL (RA patients, SQ), 217mcg/mL (JIA patients). **Distribution:** V_d=0.07L/kg (RA patients, IV), 0.11L/kg (RA patients, SQ). **Elimination:** $T_{1/2}$=13.1 days (RA patients, IV), 14.3 days (RA patients, SQ).

PATIENT CONSIDERATIONS
Assessment: Assess for previous hypersensitivity to drug, history of recurrent infections, chronic/latent/localized infections, underlying conditions that may predispose to infection, COPD, pregnancy/nursing status, and possible drug interactions. Assess immunization history in pediatric patients. Screen for latent TB infection w/ a tuberculin skin test and for viral hepatitis.

Monitoring: Monitor for signs/symptoms of hypersensitivity, infection, hepatitis B reactivation, worsening of respiratory status in COPD patients, immunosuppression, malignancies, and other adverse reactions.

Counseling: Instruct to immediately contact physician if an allergic reaction or infection occurs. Inform that may be tested for TB prior to therapy. Counsel not to receive live vaccines during therapy or w/in 3 months of its discontinuation. Inform caregivers that patients w/ JIA should be brought up-to-date w/ all immunizations prior to therapy and discuss how to best handle future immunizations once therapy has been initiated. Instruct to inform physician if pregnant/nursing or planning to become pregnant. Inform that the formulation for IV administration contains maltose, which can give falsely elevated blood glucose readings on the day of administration w/ certain blood glucose monitors; advise to discuss methods that do not react w/ maltose.

ORKAMBI — ivacaftor/lumacaftor   Rx
Class: CFTR potentiator

ADULT DOSAGE	PEDIATRIC DOSAGE
Cystic Fibrosis	**Cystic Fibrosis**
Treatment of cystic fibrosis in patients who are homozygous for the *F508del* mutation in the *CFTR* gene	Treatment of cystic fibrosis in patients who are homozygous for the *F508del* mutation in the *CFTR* gene
2 tabs q12h w/ fat-containing food	**≥12 Years:** 2 tabs q12h w/ fat-containing food
Missed Dose	**Missed Dose**
Take missed dose w/in 6 hrs, w/ fat-containing food. If >6 hrs have passed, skip missed dose and resume at normal schedule	Take missed dose w/in 6 hrs, w/ fat-containing food. If >6 hrs have passed, skip missed dose and resume at normal schedule

DOSING CONSIDERATIONS
Concomitant Medications
Initiating a CYP3A Inhibitor in Patients Already Taking Orkambi: No dose adjustment is necessary.
Initiating Orkambi in Patients Currently Taking Strong CYP3A Inhibitors: Reduce Orkambi dose to 1 tab daily for the 1st week of treatment; following this period, continue w/ the recommended daily dose

If Orkambi is interrupted for more than 1 week and then reinitiated while taking strong CYP3A inhibitors, reduce Orkambi dose to 1 tab daily for the 1st week of treatment reinitiation; following this period, continue w/ the recommended dose

Renal Impairment
Severe (CrCl ≤30mL/min) or ESRD: Use w/ caution

Hepatic Impairment
Moderate (Child-Pugh Class B): 2 tabs in the am and 1 tab in the pm
Severe (Child-Pugh Class C): Max dose of 1 tab in the am and 1 tab in the pm, or less

ADMINISTRATION
Oral route

Appropriate fat-containing foods include eggs, avocados, nuts, butter, peanut butter, cheese pizza, and whole-milk dairy products.

STORAGE
20-25°C (68-77°F); excursions permitted to 15-30°C (59-86°F).

HOW SUPPLIED
Tab: (Lumacaftor/Ivacaftor) 200mg/125mg

WARNINGS/PRECAUTIONS
Worsening of liver function (eg, hepatic encephalopathy) in patients w/ advanced liver disease reported; use w/ caution, and monitor closely. Elevated transaminases/serum bilirubin levels reported. Monitor closely if increased transaminases/bilirubin levels develop, until abnormalities resolve, and interrupt dosing w/ ALT or AST >5X ULN or w/ ALT or AST >3X ULN and bilirubin >2X ULN; consider benefits and risks of resuming dosing. Respiratory events observed more commonly during initiation of therapy; perform additional monitoring during initiation of therapy in patients w/ percent predicted FEV_1 (ppFEV$_1$) <40. Increased BP reported; monitor BP periodically in all patients. Non-congenital lens opacities reported in pediatric patients; baseline and follow-up ophthalmological exams are recommended in pediatric patients. Use FDA-cleared cystic fibrosis mutation test to detect the presence of *F508del* mutation on both alleles of the *CFTR* gene if patient's genotype is unknown. Use in transplanted patients is not recommended due to potential drug-drug interactions.

ADVERSE REACTIONS
Dyspnea, nasopharyngitis, nausea, diarrhea, URTI, fatigue, abnormal respiration, blood creatine phosphokinase increased, rash, flatulence, rhinorrhea, influenza.

DRUG INTERACTIONS
See Dosing Considerations. Increased ivacaftor exposure w/ concomitant itraconazole, a strong CYP3A inhibitor. May decrease systemic exposure of CYP3A substrates, which may decrease the therapeutic effect; co-administration is not recommended w/ sensitive CYP3A substrates or CYP3A substrates w/ a narrow therapeutic index. Consider an alternative to using midazolam or triazolam. Avoid use if taking cyclosporine, everolimus, sirolimus, or tacrolimus. May alter exposure of CYP2B6, CYP2C8, CYP2C9, CYP2C19, and P-gp substrates. Strong CYP3A inducers (eg, rifampin, St. John's wort) may significantly reduce ivacaftor exposure, which may reduce therapeutic effectiveness; co-administration w/ strong CYP3A inducers is not recommended. Monitor serum concentration of digoxin and titrate digoxin dose as needed. May decrease the

exposure of montelukast. May reduce the exposure/effectiveness of prednisone, methylprednisolone, ibuprofen, citalopram, escitalopram, and sertraline; may require higher doses. May decrease the exposure of clarithromycin, erythromycin, and telithromycin, which may reduce the effectiveness of these antibiotics; consider an alternative to these antibiotics (eg, ciprofloxacin, azithromycin, levofloxacin). May reduce exposure/effectiveness of itraconazole, ketoconazole, posaconazole, and voriconazole; concomitant use not recommended. Monitor patients closely for breakthrough fungal infections if use is necessary; consider an alternative (eg, fluconazole). May decrease hormonal contraceptive exposure/effectiveness and increase menstrual abnormality events; avoid concomitant use. Hormonal contraceptives should not be relied upon as an effective method of contraception when co-administered. May reduce exposure/effectiveness of repaglinide and alter the exposure of a sulfonylurea; a dose adjustment may be required. May reduce exposure/effectiveness of proton pump inhibitors (eg, omeprazole, esomeprazole, lansoprazole), and may alter the exposure of ranitidine; a dose adjustment may be required. May alter the exposure of warfarin; monitor INR.

PREGNANCY AND LACTATION
Pregnancy: There are limited and incomplete human data from clinical trials and postmarketing reports on use of Orkambi or its individual components, lumacaftor or ivacaftor, in pregnant women to inform a drug-associated risk.
Lactation: There is no information regarding the presence of lumacaftor or ivacaftor in human milk, the effects on the breastfed infant, or the effects on milk production; caution in nursing.

MECHANISM OF ACTION
Lumacaftor: Improves conformational stability of F508del-CFTR; increases processing/trafficking of mature protein to the cell surface.
Ivacaftor: CFTR potentiator; facilitates increased Cl⁻ transport by potentiating the channel-open probability (or gating) of the CFTR protein at the cell surface.

PHARMACOKINETICS
Absorption: Lumacaftor: C_{max}=25mcg/mL, AUC=198mcg•hr/mL, T_{max}=approx 4 hrs (median). Ivacaftor: C_{max}=0.602mcg/mL, AUC=3.66mcg•hr/mL, T_{max}=approx 4 hrs (median). **Distribution:** Lumacaftor: V_d=86L; plasma protein binding (approx 99%). Ivacaftor: plasma protein binding (approx 99%). **Metabolism:** Lumacaftor: via oxidation and glucuronidation. Ivacaftor: Extensive via CYP3A; M1 and M6 (major metabolites). **Elimination:** Lumacaftor: Feces (51%, unchanged), urine (8.6%, 0.18% as unchanged); $T_{1/2}$=25.2 hrs. Ivacaftor: Feces (87.8%), urine (6.6%); $T_{1/2}$=9.34 hrs.

PATIENT CONSIDERATIONS

Assessment: Assess for history of transaminase elevations, renal/hepatic impairment, pregnancy/nursing status, and possible drug interactions. Assess baseline ALT, AST, bilirubin, and BP levels. Obtain baseline ophthalmological examinations in pediatric patients. Use an FDA-cleared CF mutation test to detect the presence of *F508del* mutation on both alleles of the *CFTR* gene if patient's genotype is unknown.

Monitoring: Monitor for respiratory events, cataracts in pediatric patients, and other adverse reactions. Monitor ALT/AST/bilirubin levels every 3 months during the 1st yr of therapy and annually thereafter. Perform follow-up ophthalmological examinations in pediatric patients. Monitor patients w/ ppFEV₁ <40 during treatment initiation. Periodically monitor BP.

Counseling: Inform that treatment may worsen liver function in patients w/ advanced liver disease. Advise that abnormalities in liver function have occurred and that blood tests will be performed prior to initiating therapy, every 3 months during the 1st yr, and annually thereafter. Explain that chest discomfort, dyspnea, and abnormal respiration may occur. Instruct to notify physician of all medications currently being taking, including herbal supplements or vitamins; instruct how to properly take concomitant drugs. Instruct patients on alternative methods of birth control. Inform that drug is best absorbed by the body when taken w/ fat-containing food. Inform about missed dosing instructions. Advise that abnormality of the eye lens has been noted in some children and adolescents receiving therapy and that baseline and follow-up ophthalmological exam and follow-up exams are recommended in pediatric patients initiating therapy.

ORTHO TRI-CYCLEN — ethinyl estradiol/norgestimate   Rx
Class: Estrogen/progestogen combination

Cigarette smoking increases risk of serious cardiovascular (CV) events. Risk increases w/ age (>35 yrs of age) and w/ the number of cigarettes smoked. Contraindicated in women who are >35 yrs of age and smoke.

ADULT DOSAGE
Contraception
1 tab qd at the same time each day, for 28 days, then repeat

Start 1st Sunday after menses begin or 1st day of menses

Acne Vulgaris
Moderate Acne in Females Who Desire Oral Contraception:
1 tab qd at the same time each day, for 28 days, then repeat

Start 1st Sunday after menses begin or 1st day of menses

PEDIATRIC DOSAGE
Contraception
Not indicated for use premenarche; refer to adult dosing

Acne Vulgaris
Moderate Acne in Postpubertal Females ≥15 Years of Age Who Desire Oral Contraception:
1 tab qd at the same time each day, for 28 days, then repeat

Start 1st Sunday after menses begin or 1st day of menses

Missed Dose
Miss 1 Active Tab in Weeks 1, 2, or 3:
Take as soon as possible. Continue taking 1 tab qd until the pack is finished

Miss 2 Active Tabs in Weeks 1 or 2:
Take 2 missed tabs as soon as possible and the next 2 active tabs the next day. Continue taking 1 tab qd until pack is finished. Use additional nonhormonal contraception (eg, condom, spermicide) as backup if the patient has intercourse w/in 7 days after missing tabs

Miss 2 Active Tabs in Week 3 or Miss ≥3 Active Tabs in a Row in Weeks 1, 2, or 3:
(Day 1 Start) Throw out the rest of the pack and start a new pack that same day. (Sunday Start) Continue to take 1 tab qd until Sunday, then throw out the rest of the pack and start a new pack that same day. (Day 1 Start/Sunday Start) Use additional nonhormonal contraception as backup if the patient has intercourse w/in 7 days after missing tabs

Conversions
Switching from Another Oral Contraceptive:
Start on the same day that a new pack of the previous oral contraceptive would have started

Switching from Another Contraceptive Method:
Transdermal Patch/Vaginal Ring/Inj:
Start therapy on the day when next application would have been scheduled

Intrauterine Contraceptive:
Start on the day of removal; if the intrauterine device is not removed on the 1st day of menstrual cycle, additional nonhormonal contraceptive is needed for the first 7 days of the 1st cycle pack

Implant:
Start therapy on the day of removal

DOSING CONSIDERATIONS
Adverse Reactions
GI Disturbances: If vomiting/diarrhea occurs w/in 3-4 hrs after taking an active tab, handle this as a missed tab

Other Important Considerations
Starting Therapy after Abortion or Miscarriage:
1st Trimester: May start immediately; if starting therapy immediately, additional contraception is not needed. If therapy is not started w/in 5 days after termination of the pregnancy, use additional nonhormonal contraception for the first 7 days of 1st cycle pack
2nd Trimester: Do not start until 4 weeks after a 2nd trimester abortion or miscarriage

Starting Therapy after Childbirth:
Do not start until 4 weeks after delivery
ADMINISTRATION
Oral route

Take w/o regard to meals.
Sunday Start Regimen
Use additional nonhormonal contraception for the first 7 days of 1st cycle pack.
STORAGE
20-25°C (68-77°F); excursions permitted to 15-30°C (59-86°F). Protect from light.
HOW SUPPLIED
Tab: (Ethinyl Estradiol [EE]/Norgestimate) 0.035mg/0.18mg, 0.035mg/0.215mg, 0.035mg/0.25mg
CONTRAINDICATIONS
High risk of arterial/venous thrombotic diseases (eg, smoking [if >35 yrs of age], presence/history of deep vein thrombosis [DVT]/pulmonary embolism [PE], inherited or acquired hypercoagulopathies, cerebrovascular disease, coronary artery disease [CAD], thrombogenic valvular/ thrombogenic rhythm diseases of the heart [eg, subacute bacterial endocarditis w/ valvular disease or A-fib], uncontrolled HTN, diabetes mellitus [DM] w/ vascular disease, headaches w/ focal neurological symptoms or migraine headaches w/ aura [women >35 yrs of age w/ any migraine headaches]), benign/malignant liver tumors, liver disease, undiagnosed abnormal uterine bleeding, pregnancy, presence/history of breast cancer or other estrogen- or progestin-sensitive cancer.

WARNINGS/PRECAUTIONS

D/C if an arterial thrombotic event or venous thromboembolic event (VTE) occurs. D/C if there is unexplained loss of vision, proptosis, diplopia, papilledema, or retinal vascular lesions; evaluate for retinal vein thrombosis immediately. If feasible, d/c at least 4 weeks before and through 2 weeks after major surgery or other surgeries known to have an elevated risk of VTE as well as during and following prolonged immobilization. In women who are not breastfeeding, initiate therapy no earlier than 4 weeks after delivery; risk of postpartum VTE decreases after the 3rd postpartum week, whereas the risk of ovulation increases after the 3rd postpartum week. Increased risk of VTE and arterial thromboses (eg, strokes, MI). Caution w/ CV disease risk factors. D/C if jaundice develops. May increase risk of developing hepatocellular carcinoma. Increased BP reported; d/c if BP rises significantly. May worsen existing gallbladder disease. May increase risk of cholestasis in women w/ history of pregnancy-related cholestasis. May increase risk of cervical cancer or intraepithelial neoplasia, and gallbladder disease. May decrease glucose tolerance. Consider alternative contraception w/ uncontrolled dyslipidemia. Increased risk of pancreatitis w/ hypertriglyceridemia or family history of hypertriglyceridemia. Evaluate the cause of new headaches that are recurrent, persistent, or severe, and d/c if indicated; consider discontinuation in the case of increased frequency or severity of migraine during use. Unscheduled bleeding and spotting may occur; rule out pregnancy or malignancy. May cause amenorrhea; if scheduled bleeding does not occur, consider possibility of pregnancy. Administration of therapy to induce withdrawal bleeding should not be used as a test for pregnancy. Caution w/ history of depression; d/c if depression recurs to a serious degree. May interfere w/ lab tests (eg, coagulation factors, lipids, glucose tolerance, binding proteins). Chloasma may occur, especially w/ history of chloasma gravidarum; avoid exposure to the sun or UV radiation. EE: In women w/ hereditary angioedema, may induce/exacerbate angioedema.

ADVERSE REACTIONS

Irregular uterine bleeding, nausea, headache/migraine, abdominal/GI pain, vaginal infection, genital discharge, breast issues (eg, breast pain, discharge, and enlargement), mood disorders.

DRUG INTERACTIONS

Drugs or herbal products that induce certain enzymes, including CYP3A4 (eg, phenytoin, barbiturates, carbamazepine) may decrease levels and potentially diminish effectiveness of therapy or increase breakthrough bleeding; use an alternative or back-up method of contraception and continue back-up contraception for 28 days after discontinuing the enzyme inducer. CYP3A4 inhibitors (eg, itraconazole, voriconazole, grapefruit juice) may increase levels. Significant changes in levels when coadministered w/ HIV protease inhibitors; decreased levels w/ nelfinavir, ritonavir, darunavir/ritonavir, (fos)amprenavir/ritonavir, lopinavir/ritonavir, and tipranavir/ritonavir, and increased levels w/ indinavir and atazanavir/ritonavir. Decreased levels w/ boceprevir, telaprevir, and nevirapine, and increased levels w/ etravirine. May decrease levels of acetaminophen (APAP), clofibric acid, morphine, salicylic acid, and temazepam. May significantly decrease levels of lamotrigine and may reduce seizure control; dosage adjustment of lamotrigine may be needed. May need to increase dose of thyroid hormone in patients on thyroid hormone replacement therapy due to increased thyroid-binding globulin. EE: Colesevelam reported to significantly decrease EE exposure; decreased drug interaction reported when the 2 drug products are given 4 hrs apart. Atorvastatin or rosuvastatin may increase EE exposure; ascorbic acid and APAP may increase EE levels. May inhibit metabolism and increase levels of other compounds (eg, cyclosporine, prednisolone, theophylline, tizanidine, voriconazole).

PREGNANCY AND LACTATION

Pregnancy: Contraindicated in pregnancy.
Lactation: Not for use in nursing.

MECHANISM OF ACTION

Estrogen/progestogen oral contraceptive; acts by primarily suppressing ovulation. Also causes cervical mucus changes that inhibit sperm penetration and endometrial changes that reduce the likelihood of implantation. Acne: has not been established; increases sex hormone-binding globulin (SHBG) and decreases free testosterone.

PHARMACOKINETICS

Absorption: Rapid. Administration on various days of dosing cycle led to different parameters; refer to PI. **Distribution:** Found in breast milk. Norelgestromin and Norgestrel: Serum protein binding (>97%; norelgestromin bound to albumin; norgestrel bound primarily to SHBG). EE: Serum protein binding (>97% to albumin). **Metabolism:** Norgestimate: GI tract and/or liver (1st-pass). Norelgestromin (primary, active metabolite): Liver; norgestrel (active metabolite), hydroxylated and conjugated metabolites. EE: Hydroxylated metabolites and their glucuronide and sulfate conjugates. **Elimination:** Urine and feces (EE and norgestimate metabolites) (Norgestimate metabolites: 47% urine and 37% feces).

PATIENT CONSIDERATIONS

Assessment: Assess for DVT, PE, cerebrovascular disease, CAD, DM w/ vascular disease, headaches w/ focal neurological symptoms or migraine headaches w/ aura, pregnancy/nursing status, any other conditions where treatment is contraindicated or cautioned, and possible drug interactions.

Monitoring: Monitor for bleeding irregularities, venous/arterial thrombotic events, cervical cancer or intraepithelial neoplasia, retinal vein thrombosis or any other ophthalmic changes, jaundice, new/worsening headaches or migraines, depression, cholestasis w/ history of pregnancy-related cholestasis, pancreatitis, and other adverse reactions. Monitor BP in patients w/ HTN, glucose levels in diabetic or prediabetic patients, and lipid levels w/ dyslipidemia. Conduct a yearly visit in all patients for a BP check and for other indicated healthcare.

Counseling: Inform of risk/benefits of therapy. Advise to take ud. Counsel that cigarette smoking increases the risk of serious CV events and women who are >35 yrs of age and smoke should not use combination oral contraceptives (COCs). Inform of the risk of VTE. Inform that the drug does not protect against HIV infection (AIDS) and other sexually transmitted infections. Advise not to use during pregnancy; if pregnancy occurs during use, instruct to stop further use. Instruct on what to do in the event tabs are missed. Counsel to use a back-up or alternative method of contraception when enzyme inducers are used w/ therapy. Inform that COCs may reduce breast milk production. Counsel women who start COCs postpartum and have not yet had a period, to use an additional method of contraception until an active pill has been taken for 7 consecutive days. Inform that amenorrhea may occur; consider pregnancy in the event of amenorrhea at the time of 1st missed period, and rule out pregnancy in the event of amenorrhea in 2 or more consecutive cycles.

ORTHO TRI-CYCLEN LO — ethinyl estradiol/norgestimate **Rx**

Class: Estrogen/progestogen combination

> Cigarette smoking increases risk of serious cardiovascular (CV) events. Risk increases w/ age (>35 yrs of age) and w/ the number of cigarettes smoked. Contraindicated in women who are >35 yrs of age and smoke.

ADULT DOSAGE

Contraception

1 tab qd at the same time each day, for 28 days, then repeat

Start either on 1st day of menses or on 1st Sunday after onset of menses

Conversions

Switching from Another Oral Contraceptive:
Start on the same day that a new pack of the previous oral contraceptive would have been started

Switching from Another Contraceptive Method: Transdermal Patch/Vaginal Ring/Inj:
Start therapy on the day when the next application/insertion/inj would have been scheduled

Intrauterine Contraceptive:
Start on the day of removal; if the intrauterine device is not removed on the 1st day of menstrual cycle, additional nonhormonal contraceptive (eg, condom, spermicide) is needed for the first 7 days of the 1st cycle pack

Implant:
Start therapy on the day of removal

Missed Dose

Miss 1 Active Tab in Weeks 1, 2, or 3: Take tab as soon as possible. Continue taking 1 tab qd until the pack is finished

Miss 2 Active Tabs in Weeks 1 or 2: Take the 2 missed tabs as soon as possible and the next 2 active tabs the next day. Continue taking 1 tab qd until pack is finished. Use additional nonhormonal contraception as backup if the patient has intercourse w/in 7 days after missing tabs

Miss 2 Active Tabs in Week 3 or Miss ≥3 Active Tabs in a Row in Weeks 1, 2, or 3: (Day 1 Start) Throw out the rest of the pack and start a new pack that same day. (Sunday Start) Continue taking 1 tab qd until Sunday, then throw out the rest of the pack and start a new pack that same day. (Day 1 Start/Sunday Start) Use additional nonhormonal contraception as backup if the patient has intercourse w/in 7 days after missing tabs

PEDIATRIC DOSAGE

Contraception

Not indicated for use premenarche; refer to adult dosing

DOSING CONSIDERATIONS

Adverse Reactions

GI Disturbances: In case of severe vomiting/diarrhea, absorption may not be complete and additional contraceptive measures should be taken; if vomiting/diarrhea occurs w/in 3-4 hrs after taking an active tab, handle this as a missed tab

Other Important Considerations

Starting Therapy after Abortion or Miscarriage:

1st Trimester: May start immediately; if therapy is started immediately, additional method of contraception is not needed. If therapy is not started w/in 5 days after termination of the pregnancy, use additional nonhormonal contraception for the first 7 days of 1st cycle pack

2nd Trimester: Do not start until 4 weeks after a 2nd trimester abortion or miscarriage

Starting Therapy after Childbirth:

Do not start until 4 weeks after delivery; consider possibility of ovulation and conception in women who have not yet had a period postpartum

ADMINISTRATION

Oral route

Take w/o regard to meals.

Take tabs in the order directed on the blister pack.

Sunday Start Regimen

For the 1st cycle, use additional nonhormonal method of contraception for the first 7 consecutive days of administration.

STORAGE

20-25°C (68-77°F); excursions permitted to 15-30°C (59-86°F). Protect from light.

HOW SUPPLIED

Tab: (Ethinyl Estradiol [EE]/Norgestimate) 0.025mg/0.18mg, 0.025mg/0.215mg, 0.025mg/0.25mg

CONTRAINDICATIONS

High risk of arterial/venous thrombotic diseases (eg, smoking [if >35 yrs of age], presence/history of deep vein thrombosis [DVT]/pulmonary embolism [PE], inherited or acquired hypercagulopathies, cerebrovascular disease, coronary artery disease [CAD], thrombogenic valvular/thrombogenic rhythm diseases of the heart [eg, subacute bacterial endocarditis w/ valvular disease or A-fib], uncontrolled HTN, diabetes mellitus [DM] w/ vascular disease, headaches w/ focal neurological symptoms or migraine headaches w/ aura [women >35 yrs of age w/ any migraine headaches]), benign/malignant liver tumors, liver disease, undiagnosed abnormal uterine bleeding, pregnancy, presence/history of breast cancer or other estrogen- or progestin-sensitive cancer.

WARNINGS/PRECAUTIONS

D/C if an arterial thrombotic event or venous thromboembolic event (VTE) occurs. D/C if there is unexplained loss of vision, proptosis, diplopia, papilledema, or retinal vascular lesions; evaluate for retinal vein thrombosis immediately. If feasible, d/c at least 4 weeks before and through 2 weeks after major surgery or other surgeries known to have an elevated risk of VTE as well as during and following prolonged immobilization. In women who are not breastfeeding, initiate therapy no earlier than 4 weeks after delivery; risk of postpartum VTE decreases after the 3rd postpartum week, whereas the risk of ovulation increases after the 3rd postpartum week. Increased risk of VTE and arterial thromboses (eg, strokes, MI). D/C if jaundice develops. Hepatic adenomas may occur; increased risk of hepatocellular carcinoma reported in long-term users. Increased BP reported; d/c if BP rises significantly. May increase risk of gallbladder disease or worsen existing gallbladder disease. May increase risk of cholestasis in women w/ history of pregnancy-related cholestasis. May decrease glucose tolerance. Consider alternative contraception w/ uncontrolled dyslipidemia. May increase risk of pancreatitis in women w/ hypertriglyceridemia or family history thereof. Evaluate the cause of new headaches that are recurrent, persistent, or severe, and d/c therapy if indicated; consider discontinuation in the case of increased frequency or severity of migraine during use. Unscheduled bleeding and spotting may occur; rule out pregnancy or malignancy. May cause amenorrhea; amenorrhea or oligomenorrhea after discontinuation may occur. Caution w/ history of depression; d/c if depression recurs to a serious degree. May increase risk of cervical cancer or intraepithelial neoplasia. Chloasma may occur, especially w/ history of chloasma gravidarum; women w/ a tendency to chloasma should avoid exposure to the sun or UV radiation while on therapy. May interfere w/ lab tests (eg, coagulation factors, lipids, glucose tolerance, binding proteins). **EE:** In women w/ hereditary angioedema, may induce/exacerbate angioedema.

ADVERSE REACTIONS

Headache/migraine, N/V, breast issues (including tenderness, pain, enlargement, discharge), abdominal pain, menstrual disorders (including dysmenorrhea, menstrual discomfort, menstrual disorder), mood disorders (including mood alteration and depression), acne, vulvovaginal infection.

DRUG INTERACTIONS

Drugs or herbal products that induce certain enzymes, including CYP3A4 (eg, phenytoin, barbiturates, carbamazepine) may decrease levels and potentially diminish effectiveness of therapy or increase breakthrough bleeding; use an alternative or back-up method of contraception when using enzyme inducers and continue back-up contraception for 28 days after discontinuing the enzyme inducer. CYP3A4 inhibitors (eg, itraconazole, voriconazole, grapefruit juice) may increase levels. Significant changes (increase/decrease) in estrogen and/ or progestin levels reported w/ HIV/hepatitis C virus protease inhibitors or non-nucleoside reverse transcriptase inhibitors. May decrease levels of acetaminophen (APAP), clofibric acid, morphine, salicylic acid, and temazepam. May significantly decrease levels of lamotrigine and may reduce seizure control; dosage adjustment of lamotrigine may be necessary. Women on thyroid hormone replacement therapy may need to increase dose of thyroid hormone due to increased levels of thyroid-binding globulin. **EE:** Colesevelam reported to significantly decrease EE exposure; decreased drug interaction when the 2 drug products are given 4 hrs apart. Atorvastatin or rosuvastatin may increase EE exposure; ascorbic acid and APAP may increase EE levels. May inhibit metabolism and increase levels of other compounds (eg, cyclosporine, prednisolone, theophylline, tizanidine, voriconazole).

PREGNANCY AND LACTATION

Pregnancy: Contraindicated in pregnancy.

Lactation: Not for use in nursing.

MECHANISM OF ACTION

Estrogen/progestogen oral contraceptive; acts by primarily suppressing ovulation. Other possible mechanisms may include cervical mucus changes that inhibit sperm penetration and endometrial changes that reduce the likelihood of implantation.

PHARMACOKINETICS

Absorption: Rapid. Administration on various days of dosing cycle led to different parameters; refer to PI. **Distribution:** Found in breast milk. Norelgestromin (NGMN) and Norgestrel (NG): Serum protein binding (>97%; NGMN bound to albumin; NG bound primarily to sex hormone-binding globulin). EE: Serum protein binding (>97% to albumin). **Metabolism:** EE: Metabolized to various hydroxylated products and their glucuronide and sulfate conjugates. Norgestimate: Extensive by 1st pass mechanisms in GI tract and/or liver; NGMN and NG (major active metabolites). **Elimination:** Urine, feces; $T_{1/2}$=28.1 hrs (NGMN), 36.4 hrs (NG), 17.7 hrs (EE).

PATIENT CONSIDERATIONS

Assessment: Assess for DVT, PE, cerebrovascular disease, CAD, DM w/ vascular disease, headaches w/ focal neurological symptoms or migraine headaches w/ aura, pregnancy/nursing status, any other conditions where treatment is contraindicated or cautioned, and possible drug interactions.

Monitoring: Monitor for venous/arterial thrombotic events, cervical cancer or intraepithelial neoplasia, bleeding irregularities, retinal vein thrombosis or any other ophthalmic changes, jaundice, new/worsening headaches or migraines, depression, cholestasis w/ history of pregnancy-related cholestasis, pancreatitis, and other adverse reactions. Monitor BP in women w/ HTN, glucose levels in diabetic or prediabetic women, and lipid levels w/ dyslipidemia. Conduct a yearly visit in all patients for a BP check and for other indicated healthcare.

Counseling: Inform of risks/benefits of therapy. Advise to take ud. Explain that cigarette smoking increases the risk of serious CV events and women who are >35 yrs of age and smoke should not use combination oral contraceptives (COCs). Inform of the risk of VTE. Inform that the drug does not protect against HIV infection (AIDS) and other sexually transmitted infections. Advise not to use during pregnancy; if pregnancy occurs during use, instruct to stop further use. Instruct on what to do in the event tabs are missed. Instruct to use a back-up or alternative method of contraception when enzyme inducers are used w/ therapy. Inform that COCs may reduce breast milk production. Instruct women who start COCs postpartum and have not yet had a period to use an additional method of contraception until an active pill has been taken for 7 consecutive days. Inform that amenorrhea may occur; explain that patient and healthcare providers should consider pregnancy in the event of amenorrhea at the time of 1st missed period, and rule out pregnancy in the event of amenorrhea in ≥2 consecutive cycles.

ORTHO-CYCLEN — ethinyl estradiol/norgestimate   Rx

Class: Estrogen/progestogen combination

> Cigarette smoking increases risk of serious cardiovascular (CV) events. Risk increases w/ age (>35 yrs of age) and w/ the number of cigarettes smoked. Contraindicated in women who are >35 yrs of age and smoke.

ADULT DOSAGE

Contraception

1 tab qd at the same time each day, for 28 days, then repeat

Start 1st Sunday after menses begin or 1st day of menses

Missed Dose

Miss 1 Active Tab in Weeks 1, 2, or 3:
Take as soon as possible. Continue taking 1 tab qd until the pack is finished

Miss 2 Active Tabs in Weeks 1 or 2:
Take 2 missed tabs as soon as possible and the next 2 active tabs the next day. Continue taking 1 tab qd until pack is finished. Use additional nonhormonal contraception (eg, condom, spermicide) as backup if the patient has intercourse w/in 7 days after missing tabs

Miss 2 Active Tabs in Week 3 or Miss ≥3 Active Tabs in a Row in Weeks 1, 2, or 3:
(Day 1 Start) Throw out the rest of the pack and start a new pack that same day. (Sunday Start) Continue to take 1 tab qd until Sunday, then throw out the rest of the pack and start a new pack that same day. (Day 1 Start/Sunday Start) Use additional nonhormonal contraception as backup if the patient has intercourse w/in 7 days after missing tabs

PEDIATRIC DOSAGE

Contraception

Not indicated for use premenarche; refer to adult dosing

Conversions

Switching from Another Oral Contraceptive:
Start on the same day that a new pack of the previous oral contraceptive would have started

Switching from Another Contraceptive Method:
Transdermal Patch/Vaginal Ring/Injection:
Start therapy on the day when next application would have been scheduled

Intrauterine Contraceptive:
Start therapy on the day of removal; if the intrauterine device is not removed on the 1st day of menstrual cycle, additional nonhormonal contraceptive is needed for the first 7 days of the 1st cycle pack

Implant:
Start therapy on the day of removal

DOSING CONSIDERATIONS

Adverse Reactions
GI Disturbances: If vomiting/diarrhea occurs w/in 3-4 hrs after taking an active tab, handle this as a missed tab

Other Important Considerations

Starting Therapy after Abortion or Miscarriage:
1st Trimester: May start immediately; if starting therapy immediately, additional contraception is not needed. If therapy is not started w/in 5 days after termination of the pregnancy, use additional nonhormonal contraception for the first 7 days of 1st cycle pack
2nd Trimester: Do not start until 4 weeks after a 2nd trimester abortion or miscarriage

Starting Therapy after Childbirth:
Do not start until 4 weeks after delivery

ADMINISTRATION
Oral route

Take w/o regard to meals.

Sunday Start Regimen
Use additional nonhormonal contraception for the first 7 days of 1st cycle pack.

STORAGE
20-25°C (68-77°F); excursions permitted to 15-30°C (59-86°F). Protect from light.

HOW SUPPLIED
Tab: (Ethinyl Estradiol [EE]/Norgestimate) 0.035mg/0.25mg

CONTRAINDICATIONS
High risk of arterial/venous thrombotic diseases (eg, smoking [if >35 yrs of age], presence/history of deep vein thrombosis [DVT]/pulmonary embolism [PE], inherited or acquired hypercoagulopathies, cerebrovascular disease, coronary artery disease [CAD], thrombogenic valvular/ thrombogenic rhythm diseases of the heart [eg, subacute bacterial endocarditis w/ valvular disease or A-fib], uncontrolled HTN, diabetes mellitus [DM] w/ vascular disease, headaches w/ focal neurological symptoms or migraine headaches w/ aura [women >35 yrs of age w/ any migraine headaches]), benign/malignant liver tumors, liver disease, undiagnosed abnormal uterine bleeding, pregnancy, presence/history of breast cancer or other estrogen- or progestin-sensitive cancer.

WARNINGS/PRECAUTIONS
D/C if an arterial thrombotic event or venous thromboembolic event (VTE) occurs. D/C if there is unexplained loss of vision, proptosis, diplopia, papilledema, or retinal vascular lesions; evaluate for retinal vein thrombosis immediately. If feasible, d/c at least 4 weeks before and through 2 weeks after major surgery or other surgeries known to have an elevated risk of VTE as well as during and following prolonged immobilization. In women who are not breastfeeding, initiate therapy no earlier than 4 weeks after delivery; risk of postpartum VTE decreases after the 3rd postpartum week, whereas the risk of ovulation increases after the 3rd postpartum week. Increased risk of VTE and arterial thromboses (eg, strokes, MI). Caution w/ CV disease risk factors. D/C if jaundice develops. May increase risk of developing hepatocellular carcinoma. Increased BP reported; d/c if BP rises significantly. May worsen existing gallbladder disease. May increase risk of cholestasis in women w/ history of pregnancy-related cholestasis. May increase risk of cervical cancer or intraepithelial neoplasia, and gallbladder disease. May decrease glucose tolerance. Consider alternative contraception w/ uncontrolled dyslipidemia. Increased risk of pancreatitis w/ hypertriglyceridemia or family history of hypertriglyceridemia. Evaluate the cause of new headaches that are recurrent, persistent, or severe, and d/c if indicated; consider discontinuation in the case of increased frequency or severity of migraine during use. Unscheduled bleeding and spotting may occur; rule out pregnancy or malignancy. May cause amenorrhea; if scheduled bleeding does not occur, consider possibility of pregnancy. Administration of therapy to induce withdrawal bleeding should not be used as a test for pregnancy. Caution w/ history of depression; d/c if depression recurs to a serious degree. May interfere w/ lab tests (eg, coagulation factors, lipids, glucose tolerance, binding proteins). Chloasma may occur, especially w/ history of chloasma gravidarum; avoid exposure to the sun or UV radiation. **EE:** In women w/ hereditary angioedema, may induce/exacerbate angioedema.

ADVERSE REACTIONS
Irregular uterine bleeding, nausea, headache/migraine, abdominal/GI pain, vaginal infection, genital discharge, breast issues (eg, breast pain, discharge, and enlargement), mood disorders, flatulence.

DRUG INTERACTIONS
Drugs or herbal products that induce certain enzymes, including CYP3A4 (eg, phenytoin, barbiturates, carbamazepine) may decrease levels and potentially diminish effectiveness of therapy or increase breakthrough bleeding; use an alternative or back-up method of contraception and continue back-up contraception for 28 days after discontinuing the enzyme inducer. CYP3A4 inhibitors (eg, itraconazole, voriconazole, grapefruit juice) may increase levels. Significant changes in levels when coadministered w/ HIV protease inhibitors; decreased levels w/ nelfinavir, ritonavir, darunavir/ritonavir, (fos)amprenavir/ritonavir, lopinavir/ritonavir, and tipranavir/ritonavir, and increased levels w/ indinavir and atazanavir/ritonavir. Decreased levels w/ boceprevir, telaprevir, and nevirapine, and increased levels w/ etravirine. May decrease levels of acetaminophen (APAP), clofibric acid, morphine, salicylic acid, and temazepam. May significantly decrease levels of lamotrigine and may reduce seizure control; dosage adjustment of lamotrigine may be needed. May need to increase dose of thyroid hormone in patients on thyroid hormone replacement therapy due to increased thyroid-binding globulin. **EE:** Colesevelam reported to significantly decrease EE exposure; decreased drug interaction reported when the 2 drug products are given 4 hrs apart. Atorvastatin or rosuvastatin may increase EE exposure; ascorbic acid and APAP may increase EE levels. May inhibit metabolism and increase levels of other compounds (eg, cyclosporine, prednisolone, theophylline, tizanidine, voriconazole).

PREGNANCY AND LACTATION
Pregnancy: Contraindicated in pregnancy.
Lactation: Not for use in nursing.

MECHANISM OF ACTION
Estrogen/progestogen oral contraceptive; acts by primarily suppressing ovulation. Also causes cervical mucus changes that inhibit sperm penetration and endometrial changes that reduce the likelihood of implantation.

PHARMACOKINETICS
Absorption: Rapid. Administration on various days of dosing cycle led to different parameters; refer to PI. **Distribution:** Found in breast milk. Norelgestromin and Norgestrel: Serum protein binding (>97%; norelgestromin bound to albumin; norgestrel bound primarily to sex hormone-binding globulin). EE: Serum protein binding (>97% to albumin). **Metabolism:** Norgestimate: GI tract and/or liver (1st-pass). Norelgestromin (primary, active metabolite): Liver; norgestrel (active metabolite), hydroxylated and conjugated metabolites. EE: Hydroxylated metabolites and their glucuronide and sulfate conjugates. **Elimination:** Urine and feces (EE and norgestimate metabolites) (Norgestimate metabolites: 47% urine and 37% feces).

PATIENT CONSIDERATIONS

Assessment: Assess for DVT, PE, cerebrovascular disease, CAD, DM w/ vascular disease, headaches w/ focal neurological symptoms or migraine headaches w/ aura, pregnancy/nursing status, any other conditions where treatment is contraindicated or cautioned, and possible drug interactions.

Monitoring: Monitor for bleeding irregularities, venous/arterial thrombotic events, cervical cancer or intraepithelial neoplasia, retinal vein thrombosis or any other ophthalmic changes, jaundice, new/worsening headaches or migraines, depression, cholestasis w/ history of pregnancy-related cholestasis, pancreatitis, and other adverse reactions. Monitor BP in patients w/ HTN, glucose levels in diabetic or prediabetic patients, and lipid levels w/ dyslipidemia. Conduct a yearly visit in all patients for a BP check and for other indicated healthcare.

Counseling: Inform of risk/benefits of therapy. Advise to take ud. Counsel that cigarette smoking increases the risk of serious CV events and women who are >35 yrs of age and smoke should not use combination oral contraceptives (COCs). Inform of the risk of VTE. Inform that the drug does not protect against HIV infection (AIDS) and other sexually transmitted infections. Advise not to use during pregnancy; if pregnancy occurs during use, instruct to stop further use. Instruct on what to do in the event tabs are missed. Counsel to use a back-up or alternative method of contraception when enzyme inducers are used w/ therapy. Inform that COCs may reduce breast milk production. Counsel women who start COCs postpartum and have not yet had a period, to use an additional method of contraception until an active pill has been taken for 7 consecutive days. Inform that amenorrhea may occur; consider pregnancy in the event of amenorrhea at the time of 1st missed period, and rule out pregnancy in the event of amenorrhea in 2 or more consecutive cycles.

ORTHO-NOVUM 7/7/7 — ethinyl estradiol/norethindrone   Rx

Class: Estrogen/progestogen combination

> Cigarette smoking increases risk of serious cardiovascular events. Risk increases w/ age (>35 yrs of age) and w/ the number of cigarettes smoked. Should not be used by women who are >35 yrs of age and smoke.

OTHER BRAND NAMES
Necon 7/7/7, Cyclafem 7/7/7, Nortrel 7/7/7

ADULT DOSAGE	PEDIATRIC DOSAGE
Contraception	**Contraception**
1 tab qd at the same time each day for 28 days, then repeat	Not indicated for use premenarche; refer to adult dosing

Start 1st Sunday after menses begin or 1st day of menses

<u>Missed Dose</u>

Miss 1 Active Tab in Weeks 1, 2, or 3:
Take as soon as dose is remembered

Miss 2 Active Tabs in Week 1 or 2:
Take 2 tabs on day it is remembered and 2 tabs the next day, then take 1 tab qd until the pack is finished. Use backup method of contraception (eg, condom, spermicide) if having intercourse w/in 7 days after missing tabs

Miss 2 Active Tabs in Week 3 or Miss ≥3 Active Tabs in a Row: (Day 1 Start) Throw out rest of the pack and start new pack the same day. (Sunday Start) Continue to take 1 tab qd until Sunday, then throw out the rest of the pack and start a new pack that same day. (Day 1 Start/Sunday Start) Use backup method of birth control if having intercourse in the 7 days after missing pills

----

DOSING CONSIDERATIONS

<u>Other Important Considerations</u>

Postpartum Women Who Elect Not to Breastfeed:
May initiate therapy 4 weeks postpartum; consider the possibility of ovulation and conception prior to initiation

ADMINISTRATION
Oral route

Take exactly ud and at intervals not exceeding 24 hrs.

<u>Sunday Start Regimen</u>
Use another method of contraception until after the first 7 days of the 1st cycle pack.

STORAGE
25°C (77°F); excursions permitted to 15-30°C (59-86°F).

HOW SUPPLIED
Tab: (Ethinyl Estradiol [EE]/Norethindrone) 0.035mg/0.5mg, 0.035mg/0.75mg, 0.035mg/1mg

CONTRAINDICATIONS
Thrombophlebitis or thromboembolic disorders; history of deep vein thrombophlebitis or thromboembolic disorders; known thrombophilic conditions; cerebral vascular or coronary artery disease (current or history); valvular heart disease w/ complications; persistent BP values of ≥160mmHg systolic or ≥100mmHg diastolic; diabetes w/ vascular involvement; headaches w/ focal neurological symptoms; major surgery w/ prolonged immobilization; known or suspected breast carcinoma; carcinoma of the endometrium or other known or suspected estrogen-dependent neoplasia; undiagnosed abnormal genital bleeding; cholestatic jaundice of pregnancy or jaundice w/ prior pill use; acute or chronic hepatocellular disease w/ abnormal liver function; hepatic adenomas or carcinomas; known/suspected pregnancy; hypersensitivity to any component of the medication.

WARNINGS/PRECAUTIONS
Increased risk of morbidity and mortality w/ HTN, hyperlipidemias, obesity, and diabetes. Increased risk of MI; risk increases w/ other underlying risk factors for coronary artery disease (eg, HTN, hypercholesterolemia, morbid obesity). Increased risk of thromboembolic and thrombotic disease; venous thromboembolism (VTE) risk is highest in the 1st year of use and when restarting therapy after a break of ≥4 weeks. If feasible, d/c at least 4 weeks prior to and for 2 weeks after elective surgery of a type associated w/ an increased risk of thromboembolism, and during and following prolonged immobilization. Increased risk of cerebrovascular events (thrombotic and hemorrhagic strokes) and vascular disease. May increase risk of breast cancer and cervical intraepithelial neoplasia. Hepatic adenomas and increased risk of hepatocellular carcinoma (rare) reported. Retinal thrombosis reported; d/c if unexplained partial or complete loss of vision, onset of proptosis or diplopia, papilledema, or retinal vascular lesions develop. Should not be used to induce withdrawal bleeding as a test for pregnancy, or to treat threatened or habitual abortion during pregnancy. Rule out pregnancy if 2 consecutive periods are missed; d/c if pregnancy is confirmed. May increase risk of gallbladder disease. May decrease glucose tolerance; monitor prediabetic and diabetic patients. Changes in serum TGs and lipoprotein levels reported; may elevate LDL levels and render the control of hyperlipidemias more difficult. Increases in BP reported; monitor closely and d/c use if significant BP elevation occurs and cannot be adequately controlled. New onset/exacerbation of migraine or recurrent, persistent, severe headache may develop; d/c if this occurs. Breakthrough bleeding and spotting reported; rule out malignancy or pregnancy. Post-pill amenorrhea or oligomenorrhea may occur. Ectopic and intrauterine pregnancy may occur in contraceptive failures. D/C if jaundice develops. May cause fluid retention. Caution w/ history of depression; d/c if depression recurs to serious degree. Contact lens wearers who develop visual changes or changes in lens tolerance should be assessed by an ophthalmologist. Lab test interactions may occur.

ADVERSE REACTIONS
N/V, breakthrough bleeding, spotting, amenorrhea, migraine, vaginal candidiasis, edema, weight changes, melasma, breast changes, changes in cervical erosion and secretion, allergic reaction, mental depression, cholestatic jaundice, GI symptoms (eg, abdominal cramps, bloating).

DRUG INTERACTIONS
Drugs or herbal products that induce certain enzymes, including CYP3A4 (eg, bosentan, rifabutin, St. John's wort), may decrease levels and potentially diminish effectiveness or increase breakthrough bleeding; use an alternative or backup method of contraception and continue backup contraception for 28 days after discontinuing the enzyme inducer. Atorvastatin may increase EE exposure; ascorbic acid and acetaminophen (APAP) may increase EE levels. CYP3A4 inhibitors (eg, itraconazole, voriconazole, ketoconazole) may increase levels. Significant changes (increase/decrease) in estrogen and/or progestin levels sometimes noted when coadministered w/ HIV protease inhibitors (decreased [eg, nelfinavir, darunavir/ritonavir, (fos)amprenavir/ritonavir] or increased [eg, indinavir, atazanavir/ritonavir]), hepatitis C virus protease inhibitors (decreased [eg, boceprevir, telaprevir]), or non-nucleoside reverse transcriptase inhibitors (decreased [eg, nevirapine] or increased [eg, etravirine]). Colesevelam reported to significantly decrease EE exposure; decreased drug interaction reported when the 2 drug products are given 4 hrs apart. May inhibit metabolism and increase levels of other compounds (eg, cyclosporine, prednisolone, voriconazole). May decrease levels of APAP, clofibric acid, morphine, salicylic acid, and temazepam. May significantly decrease levels of lamotrigine; dosage adjustment of lamotrigine may be needed. May need to increase dose of thyroid hormone in patients on thyroid hormone replacement therapy due to increased thyroid-binding globulin.

PREGNANCY AND LACTATION
Pregnancy: Category X.
Lactation: Small amounts of drug identified in the milk of nursing mothers and a few adverse effects on the child reported; may decrease quantity and quality of breast milk. Not for use in nursing.

MECHANISM OF ACTION
Estrogen/progestogen oral contraceptive; acts by suppressing gonadotropins. Primarily inhibits ovulation and causes other alterations, including changes in the cervical mucus (increases difficulty of sperm entry into the uterus) and the endometrium (reduces likelihood of implantation).

PHARMACOKINETICS
Distribution: Found in breast milk.

PATIENT CONSIDERATIONS

Assessment: Assess for hypersensitivity to drug, thrombophlebitis or thromboembolic disorders, HTN, hyperlipidemia, diabetes, breast cancer, endometrial cancer or other estrogen-dependent neoplasia, undiagnosed abnormal genital bleeding, cholestatic jaundice of pregnancy or jaundice w/ prior pill use, pregnancy/nursing status, and for any other conditions where treatment is contraindicated/cautioned. Assess for possible drug interactions.

Monitoring: Monitor for MI, thromboembolism, VTE, stroke, hepatic neoplasia, and other adverse effects. Monitor BP w/ history of HTN, serum glucose levels in diabetic or prediabetic patients, lipid levels w/ hyperlipidemia, and for signs of worsening depression w/ previous history. Monitor liver function. Refer contact lens wearer to an ophthalmologist if ocular changes or changes in lens tolerance develop. Perform annual history and physical exam. Monitor women w/ a strong family history of breast cancer or who have breast nodules.

Counseling: Inform of the benefits and risks of therapy. Inform that drug does not protect against HIV infection (AIDS) and other sexually transmitted diseases. Counsel that cigarette smoking increases the risk of serious adverse effects on the heart and blood vessels and that women who are >35 yrs of age and smoke should not use oral contraceptives. Instruct to take exactly ud. Instruct on what to do if pills are missed. Inform that spotting or breakthrough bleeding may occur; advise not to d/c medication and instruct to notify physician if symptoms persist. Instruct to d/c if pregnancy is confirmed/suspected during treatment. Instruct to notify physician if breastfeeding. If scheduled for any lab test, advise patient to inform physician of the use of birth control pills. Inform that certain drugs may make therapy less effective and may need to use additional contraception.

Oseni — alogliptin/pioglitazone   Rx

Class: Dipeptidyl peptidase-4 (DPP-4) inhibitor/thiazolidinedione (glitazone)

> Thiazolidinediones, including pioglitazone, cause or exacerbate CHF in some patients. After initiation and dose increases, monitor carefully for signs and symptoms of heart failure (HF); manage accordingly and consider discontinuation or dose reduction if HF develops. Not recommended w/ symptomatic HF. Contraindicated w/ established NYHA Class III or IV HF.

ADULT DOSAGE

<u>Type 2 Diabetes Mellitus</u>

Adjunct to diet and exercise to improve glycemic control when treatment w/ both alogliptin and pioglitazone is appropriate

Initial:
Inadequately Controlled on Diet and Exercise:
25mg/15mg qd or 25mg/30mg qd
Inadequately Controlled on Metformin Monotherapy:
25mg/15mg qd or 25mg/30mg qd
On Alogliptin and Requiring Additional Glycemic Control:
25mg/15mg qd or 25mg/30mg qd

PEDIATRIC DOSAGE
Pediatric use may not have been established

OSENI

On Pioglitazone and Requiring Additional Glycemic Control:
25mg/15mg qd, 25mg/30mg qd, or 25mg/45mg qd as appropriate based upon current therapy
Switching from Alogliptin Coadministered w/ Pioglitazone:
Initiate at the dose of alogliptin and pioglitazone based upon current therapy
Patients w/ CHF (NYHA Class I or II):
25mg/15mg qd
Max: 25mg/45mg qd

DOSING CONSIDERATIONS
Concomitant Medications
Strong CYP2C8 Inhibitors (eg, Gemfibrozil):
Max: 25mg/15mg qd

Renal Impairment
Moderate (CrCl ≥30 to <60mL/min): 12.5mg/15mg qd, 12.5mg/30mg qd, or 12.5mg/45mg qd
Severe or ESRD: Not recommended for use; coadministration of pioglitazone and alogliptin 6.25mg qd based on individual requirements may be considered

ADMINISTRATION
Oral route

May be taken w/ or w/o food.
Do not split tabs before swallowing.

STORAGE
25°C (77°F); excursions permitted to 15-30°C (59-86°F). Protect from moisture and humidity.

HOW SUPPLIED
Tab: (Alogliptin/Pioglitazone) 12.5mg/15mg, 12.5mg/30mg, 12.5mg/45mg, 25mg/15mg, 25mg/30mg, 25mg/45mg

CONTRAINDICATIONS
History of a serious hypersensitivity reaction (eg, anaphylaxis, angioedema, severe cutaneous adverse reactions) to alogliptin or pioglitazone. NYHA Class III or IV HF.

WARNINGS/PRECAUTIONS
Not for the treatment of type 1 diabetes mellitus (DM) or for the treatment of diabetic ketoacidosis. Manage according to current standards of care and consider discontinuation of Oseni if CHF develops. Fatal and nonfatal hepatic failure and serum ALT >3X ULN reported; obtain baseline LFTs, and initiate w/ caution in patients w/ abnormal LFTs. Measure LFTs promptly in patients who report symptoms that may indicate liver injury; if results are abnormal (ALT >3X ULN), interrupt treatment and investigate for the probable cause, and do not restart therapy w/o another explanation for the LFT abnormalities. **Alogliptin:** Hospitalization for CHF reported in patients w/ recent acute coronary syndrome. Acute pancreatitis reported; promptly d/c if suspected and initiate appropriate management. Serious hypersensitivity reactions reported; d/c if suspected, assess for other potential causes, and institute alternative treatment for diabetes. Caution w/ history of angioedema to another DPP-4 inhibitor. Severe and disabling arthralgia reported in patients taking DPP-4 inhibitors; d/c if appropriate. **Pioglitazone:** May cause dose-related fluid retention when used alone or in combination w/ other antidiabetic medications; most common when used w/ insulin. Dose-related edema reported. Increased incidence of bone fractures reported in females. Not for use in patients w/ active bladder cancer; consider benefits versus risks in patients w/ a prior history of bladder cancer. Macular edema reported; promptly refer to an ophthalmologist if visual symptoms occur. May result in ovulation in some premenopausal anovulatory women, which may increase risk for pregnancy; adequate contraception is recommended in all premenopausal women.

ADVERSE REACTIONS
Nasopharyngitis, back pain, URTI.

DRUG INTERACTIONS
See Dosing Considerations. May require a lower dose of insulin or insulin secretagogue (eg, sulfonylurea) to minimize risk of hypoglycemia. **Pioglitazone:** Significantly increased exposure and $T_{1/2}$ w/ strong CYP2C8 inhibitors (eg, gemfibrozil). CYP2C8 inducers (eg, rifampin) may significantly decrease exposure; if a CYP2C8 inducer is started or stopped during treatment, changes in diabetes treatment dose may be needed based on clinical response w/o exceeding the maximum recommended daily dose of 45mg for pioglitazone.

PREGNANCY AND LACTATION
Pregnancy: Category C.
Lactation: Not for use in nursing.

MECHANISM OF ACTION
Alogliptin: DPP-4 inhibitor; slows inactivation of incretin hormones, thereby increasing their bloodstream concentrations and reducing fasting and postprandial glucose concentrations in a glucose-dependent manner.
Pioglitazone: Thiazolidinedione; improves insulin sensitivity in muscle and adipose tissue while inhibiting hepatic gluconeogenesis.

PHARMACOKINETICS
Absorption: Alogliptin: Absolute bioavailability (approx 100%). Pioglitazone: T_{max}=w/in 2 hrs, 3-4 hrs (w/ food). **Distribution:** Alogliptin: V_d=417L (IV); plasma protein binding (20%). Pioglitazone: V_d=0.63L/kg; plasma protein binding (>99%). **Metabolism:** Alogliptin: Via CYP2D6 and CYP3A4; N-demethylated alogliptin, M-I (minor, active metabolite). Pioglitazone: Via hydroxylation and oxidation (extensive), CYP2C8, and CYP3A4; M-III [keto derivative] and M-IV [hydroxyl derivative] (major, active metabolites). **Elimination:** Alogliptin: Urine (76%, 60-71% unchanged), feces (13%). Pioglitazone: Urine (15-30%), feces; $T_{1/2}$=3-7 hrs (pioglitazone), 16-24 hrs (metabolites).

PATIENT CONSIDERATIONS
Assessment: Assess for history of a serious hypersensitivity reaction to alogliptin or pioglitazone, type of DM, HF or risk of HF, edema, renal/hepatic impairment, bone health, history of pancreatitis, diabetic ketoacidosis, active/history of bladder cancer, history of angioedema to another DPP-4 inhibitor, pregnancy/nursing status, and possible drug interactions. Obtain FPG and HbA1c.

Monitoring: Monitor for signs/symptoms of CHF, pancreatitis, hypersensitivity reactions, edema, fractures, visual symptoms, severe and disabling arthralgia, and other adverse reactions. Monitor LFTs, FPG, and HbA1c. Monitor renal function periodically.

Counseling: Inform of the potential risks and benefits of therapy. Instruct to immediately report to physician any symptoms that may indicate HF. Inform that pancreatitis may occur; instruct to promptly d/c use and contact physician if persistent severe abdominal pain occurs. Instruct to d/c use and seek medical advice promptly if signs/symptoms of an allergic reaction, liver injury, or bladder cancer occur. Inform that hypoglycemia can occur; explain the risks, symptoms, and appropriate management. Counsel premenopausal women to use adequate contraception during treatment. Instruct to seek medical advice if severe joint pain occurs. Advise not to double the next dose if a dose is missed. Instruct to inform physician if an unusual symptom develops or if a symptom persists or worsens.

OSMOPREP — sodium phosphate dibasic anhydrous/sodium phosphate monobasic monohydrate   Rx
Class: Bowel cleanser

> Rare, but serious, acute phosphate nephropathy reported; some cases resulted in permanent renal impairment and some patients required long-term dialysis. Patients at increased risk may include those w/ increased age, hypovolemia, increased bowel transit time (eg, bowel obstruction), active colitis, or baseline kidney disease, and those using medicines that affect renal perfusion or function (eg, diuretics, ACE inhibitors, ARBs, and possibly NSAIDs). Use the dose and dosing regimen as recommended (pm/am split dose).

ADULT DOSAGE
Bowel Cleansing
Prior to Colonoscopy:
Evening Before Colonoscopy:
Take 4 tabs w/ 8 oz of clear liquids every 15 min for a total of 20 tabs

Day of Colonoscopy:
Starting 3-5 hrs before procedure, take 4 tabs w/ 8 oz of clear liquids every 15 min for a total of 12 tabs

PEDIATRIC DOSAGE
Pediatric use may not have been established

ADMINISTRATION
Oral route
- Do not drink any liquids colored purple or red.
- Adequately hydrate before, during, and after administration.

STORAGE
25°C (77°F); excursions permitted to 15-30°C (59-86°F).

HOW SUPPLIED
Tab: (Sodium Phosphate Monobasic Monohydrate/Sodium Phosphate Dibasic Anhydrous) 1.102g/0.398g

CONTRAINDICATIONS
Biopsy-proven acute phosphate nephropathy, GI obstruction, gastric bypass or stapling surgery, bowel perforation, toxic colitis, toxic megacolon, known allergy or hypersensitivity to sodium phosphate salts or any component of OsmoPrep.

WARNINGS/PRECAUTIONS
Do not use w/in 7 days of previous administration. Rare, but serious, renal failure and nephrocalcinosis reported. Caution w/ renal impairment (CrCl <30mL/min), history of acute phosphate nephropathy, known or suspected electrolyte disturbances (eg, dehydration), or w/ conditions that increase the risk for fluid and electrolyte disturbances or increase the risk of seizure (eg, hyponatremia). Adequately hydrate before, during, and after use. If significant vomiting or signs of dehydration develop, consider performing postcolonoscopy lab tests (electrolytes, SrCr, and BUN). Correct electrolyte abnormalities before treatment. Do not administer additional laxative or purgative agents, particularly additional sodium phosphate-based purgative or enema products. Serious arrhythmias rarely reported; consider predose and postcolonoscopy ECGs in patients at increased risk of serious cardiac arrhythmias. Generalized tonic-clonic seizures and/or loss of consciousness rarely reported; caution w/ history of seizures. May induce colonic mucosal aphthous ulcerations; consider this in patients w/ known or suspected inflammatory bowel disease (IBD). Caution w/ acute exacerbation of chronic IBD, impaired gag reflex, in patients prone to regurgitation or aspiration, and in elderly.

ADVERSE REACTIONS
Abdominal bloating, abdominal pain, N/V.

DRUG INTERACTIONS
See Boxed Warning. PO medication administered w/in 1 hr of the start of each dose may be flushed from GI tract and may not be absorbed properly. Caution

w/ drugs that may affect electrolyte levels (eg, diuretics), increase the risk of arrhythmias, prolong QT interval, and lower the seizure threshold (eg, TCAs). Caution in patients withdrawing from alcohol or benzodiazepines.

PREGNANCY AND LACTATION
Pregnancy: Category C.
Lactation: Caution in nursing.

MECHANISM OF ACTION
Osmotic laxative; thought to be through the osmotic effect of Na^+, causing large amounts of water to be drawn into the colon, promoting evacuation.

PATIENT CONSIDERATIONS
Assessment: Assess for biopsy-proven acute phosphate nephropathy, GI obstruction, gastric bypass or stapling surgery, bowel perforation, toxic colitis, toxic megacolon, risk of acute phosphate nephropathy, electrolyte abnormalities, or any other conditions where treatment is cautioned. Assess for hypersensitivity, pregnancy/nursing status, and possible drug interactions. Consider performing baseline lab tests (electrolytes, SrCr, and BUN). Consider predose ECGs in patients at increased risk of serious cardiac arrhythmias.

Monitoring: Monitor for acute phosphate nephropathy, arrhythmias, generalized tonic-clonic seizures, loss of consciousness, colonic mucosal aphthous ulcerations, and other adverse reactions. Consider performing postcolonoscopy lab tests. Consider postcolonoscopy ECGs in patients at increased risk of serious cardiac arrhythmias.

Counseling: Instruct to notify physician if patient has a history of renal disease or takes medication for BP, or cardiac/renal disease. Explain the importance of taking the recommended fluid regimen and advise to hydrate adequately before, during, and after use. Instruct to contact physician if experiencing symptoms of dehydration, or worsening of bloating, abdominal pain, N/V, or headache. Counsel not to take w/ other laxatives or enemas made w/ sodium phosphate.

OSPHENA — ospemifene   Rx
Class: Estrogen agonist/antagonist

> Has estrogen agonistic effects in the endometrium. Increased risk of endometrial cancer in a woman w/ a uterus who uses unopposed estrogens. Adding a progestin to estrogen therapy reduces the risk of endometrial hyperplasia. Perform adequate diagnostic measures to rule out malignancy in postmenopausal women w/ undiagnosed persistent/recurring abnormal genital bleeding. Increased risk of stroke and deep vein thrombosis (DVT) reported in postmenopausal women (50-79 yrs of age) who received daily oral conjugated estrogens-alone. Should be prescribed for the shortest duration consistent w/ treatment goals and risks.

ADULT DOSAGE
Dyspareunia

Moderate to Severe Dyspareunia, a Symptom of Vulvar and Vaginal Atrophy, Due to Menopause:
Usual: 60mg qd

Reevaluate periodically as clinically appropriate to determine if treatment is still necessary

PEDIATRIC DOSAGE
Pediatric use may not have been established

DOSING CONSIDERATIONS
Hepatic Impairment
Severe (Child-Pugh Class C): Should not be used

ADMINISTRATION
Oral route

Take w/ food.

STORAGE
20-25°C (68-77°F); excursions permitted to 15-30°C (59-86°F).

HOW SUPPLIED
Tab: 60mg

CONTRAINDICATIONS
Undiagnosed abnormal genital bleeding; known or suspected estrogen-dependent neoplasia; active DVT, pulmonary embolism (PE) or a history of these conditions; active arterial thromboembolic disease (eg, stroke, MI) or history of these conditions; hypersensitivity (eg, angioedema, urticaria, rash, pruritus) to ospemifene or any of the ingredients of the product; women who are or may become pregnant.

WARNINGS/PRECAUTIONS
Manage risk factors for cardiovascular disorders, arterial vascular disease (eg, HTN, diabetes mellitus, tobacco use, hypercholesterolemia, obesity), and/or venous thromboembolism (VTE) (eg, personal/family history of VTE, obesity, systemic lupus erythematosus) appropriately. MI reported. D/C immediately if thromboembolic/hemorrhagic stroke or VTE occurs or is suspected. If feasible, d/c therapy at least 4-6 weeks before surgery of the type associated w/ an increased risk of thromboembolism, or during periods of prolonged immobilization. Avoid w/ known/suspected breast cancer or w/ a history of breast cancer. Avoid w/ severe hepatic impairment.

ADVERSE REACTIONS
Hot flush, vaginal discharge, muscle spasms.

DRUG INTERACTIONS
Avoid w/ estrogens and estrogen agonists/antagonists. Fluconazole increases systemic exposure and may increase ospemifene-related adverse reactions; avoid concomitant use. Rifampin, a strong CYP3A4/moderate CYP2C9/moderate

CYP2C19 inducer, decreases systemic exposure; coadministration w/ CYP3A4, CYP2C9, and/or CYP2C19 inducers would be expected to decrease systemic exposure, which may decrease clinical effect. Ketoconazole increases systemic exposure; chronic ketoconazole administration may increase risk of ospemifene-related adverse reactions. Use w/ other drug products that are highly protein bound may increase exposure of either that drug or ospemifene. May increase risk of ospemifene-related adverse reactions w/ CYP3A4 and CYP2C9 inhibitors.

PREGNANCY AND LACTATION
Pregnancy: Category X.
Lactation: Safety not known in nursing.

MECHANISM OF ACTION
Estrogen agonist/antagonist; biological actions are mediated through binding to estrogen receptors, resulting in activation of estrogenic pathways in some tissues (agonism) and blockade of estrogenic pathway in others (antagonism).

PHARMACOKINETICS
Absorption: (Fasted) T_{max}=approx 2 hrs (median), C_{max}=533ng/mL, AUC_{0-inf}=4165ng•hr/mL. (Fed) T_{max}=approx 2.5 hrs, C_{max}=1198ng/mL, AUC_{0-inf}=7521ng•hr/mL. **Distribution:** V_d=448L; plasma protein binding (>99%). **Metabolism:** Via CYP3A4, 2C9, 2C19; 4-hydroxyospemifene (major metabolite). **Elimination:** Feces (approx 75%), urine (approx 7%, <0.2% unchanged); $T_{1/2}$=approx 26 hrs.

PATIENT CONSIDERATIONS
Assessment: Assess for drug hypersensitivity, undiagnosed abnormal genital bleeding, known/suspected estrogen-dependent neoplasia, active/history of DVT, active/history of PE, active/history of arterial thromboembolic disease, known/suspected or history of breast cancer, hepatic impairment, pregnancy/nursing status, possible drug interactions, or any other condition where treatment is cautioned or contraindicated.

Monitoring: Monitor for endometrial cancer, thromboembolic/hemorrhagic stroke, DVT, and other adverse reactions. Reevaluate periodically as clinically appropriate to determine if treatment is still necessary. Perform adequate diagnostic measures, including directed and random endometrial sampling when indicated, to rule out malignancy in postmenopausal women w/ undiagnosed persistent/recurring abnormal genital bleeding.

Counseling: Advise of risks and benefits of therapy. Inform that therapy may initiate/increase occurrence of hot flashes in some women. Inform postmenopausal women who have had hypersensitivity reactions to therapy not to take the drug. Inform postmenopausal women of the importance of reporting unusual vaginal bleeding to healthcare provider as soon as possible.

OTEZLA — apremilast   Rx
Class: Phosphodiesterase-4 (PDE-4) inhibitor

ADULT DOSAGE
Psoriatic Arthritis

Initial Dosage Titration:
Day 1: 10mg (am)
Day 2: 10mg bid (am and pm)
Day 3: 10mg (am) and 20mg (pm)
Day 4: 20mg bid (am and pm)
Day 5: 20mg (am) and 30mg (pm)

Maint:
Day 6 and Thereafter: 30mg bid (am and pm)

Plaque Psoriasis

Patients w/ Moderate to Severe Plaque Psoriasis Who Are Candidates for Phototherapy or Systemic Therapy:

Initial Dosage Titration:
Day 1: 10mg (am)
Day 2: 10mg bid (am and pm)
Day 3: 10mg (am) and 20mg (pm)
Day 4: 20mg bid (am and pm)
Day 5: 20mg (am) and 30mg (pm)

Maint:
Day 6 and Thereafter: 30mg bid (am and pm)

PEDIATRIC DOSAGE
Pediatric use may not have been established

DOSING CONSIDERATIONS
Renal Impairment
Severe (CrCl <30mL/min):
Initial Dosage Titration:
Days 1-3: 10mg qam
Days 4 and 5: 20mg qam
Maint:
Day 6 and Thereafter: 30mg qam

ADMINISTRATION
Oral route

May be administered w/o regard to meals.
Do not crush, split, or chew.

STORAGE
<30°C (86°F).

HOW SUPPLIED
Tab: 10mg, 20mg, 30mg

CONTRAINDICATIONS
Known hypersensitivity to apremilast or to any excipients in the formulation.

WARNINGS/PRECAUTIONS
Depression or depressed mood, and suicidal ideation and behavior reported; carefully evaluate the risks and benefits of continuing treatment if such events occur. Weight decrease reported; consider discontinuation if unexplained or clinically significant weight loss occurs.

ADVERSE REACTIONS
Diarrhea, headache/tension headache, N/V, URTI.

DRUG INTERACTIONS
Decreased exposure w/ strong CYP450 inducers (eg, rifampin), which may result in loss of efficacy; not recommended w/ CYP450 inducers (eg, rifampin, phenobarbital, carbamazepine).

PREGNANCY AND LACTATION
Pregnancy: Category C.
Nursing: Caution in nursing.

MECHANISM OF ACTION
PDE-4 inhibitor; not established. PDE-4 inhibition results in increased intracellular cAMP levels.

PHARMACOKINETICS
Absorption: Absolute bioavailability (73%); T_{max}=2.5 hrs (median). **Distribution:** V_d=87L; plasma protein binding (68%). **Metabolism:** Extensive. CYP oxidative metabolism (CYP3A4 [primary], CYP1A2, and CYP2A6 [minor]) w/ subsequent glucuronidation and non-CYP mediated hydrolysis. **Elimination:** Urine (58%, 3% unchanged), feces (39%, 7% unchanged); $T_{1/2}$=6-9 hrs.

PATIENT CONSIDERATIONS
Assessment: Assess for history of depression and/or suicidal thoughts or behavior, drug hypersensitivity, renal impairment, pregnancy/nursing status, and possible drug interactions.

Monitoring: Monitor for emergence or worsening of depression, suicidal thoughts, or other mood changes, and for other adverse reactions. Monitor weight regularly and monitor renal function.

Counseling: Inform of the risks and benefits of therapy. Advise patients, their caregivers, and families to be alert for emergence or worsening of depression, suicidal thoughts, or other mood changes, and to contact physician if such changes occur. Counsel to monitor weight regularly and to notify physician if unexplained or clinically significant weight loss occurs. Instruct to take only as prescribed.

OTIPRIO — ciprofloxacin　　　Rx
Class: Fluoroquinolone

PEDIATRIC DOSAGE
Otitis Media

Treatment of patients w/ bilateral otitis media w/ effusion undergoing tympanostomy tube placement

≥6 Months:
0.1mL (6mg) into each affected ear, following suctioning of middle ear effusion

Administer as a single intratympanic administration

ADMINISTRATION
Intratympanic route

Preparation
1. Keep product cold during preparation; if drug thickens during preparation, place the vial back in refrigeration.
2. To keep vial cold during shaking, hold vial by the aluminium seal to prevent gelation; shake for 5-8 sec until a visually homogenous sus is obtained.
3. Using an 18-21G needle, withdraw 0.3mL of the sus into the 1mL syringe.
4. Replace the needle w/ a 20-24G, 2-3 inch blunt, flexible needle to be used for administration.
5. Prime the needle leaving a dose of 0.1mL.
6. Using the same vial, prepare a second syringe for the other ear by repeating the steps above. Use a different syringe for each ear.
7. After preparation, syringes can be kept at room temperature or in the refrigerator prior to administration.
8. Keep syringes on their side; discard syringes if not administered in 3 hrs.

STORAGE
2-8°C (36-46°F). Protect from light.

HOW SUPPLIED
Otic Sus: 6% [1mL]

CONTRAINDICATIONS
History of hypersensitivity to ciprofloxacin, other quinolones, or any components in this medication.

WARNINGS/PRECAUTIONS
May result in overgrowth of nonsusceptible bacteria and fungi; institute alternative therapy if such infections occur.

ADVERSE REACTIONS
Nasopharyngitis, irritability, rhinorrhea.

PREGNANCY AND LACTATION
Pregnancy: No adequate and well-controlled studies have been performed in pregnant women. Due to negligible systemic exposure associated w/ clinical administration, the product is expected to be of minimal risk for maternal and fetal toxicity.
Lactation: Ciprofloxacin is excreted in human milk w/ systemic administration. Due to negligible systemic exposure after otic application, nursing infants of mothers receiving therapy should not be affected.

MECHANISM OF ACTION
Fluoroquinolone antibacterial; bactericidal action results from interference w/ the enzyme DNA gyrase, which is needed for the synthesis of bacterial DNA.

PATIENT CONSIDERATIONS
Assessment: Assess for hypersensitivity to drug or to other quinolones.

Monitoring: Monitor for overgrowth of nonsusceptible bacteria and fungi, and for other adverse reactions.

Counseling: Advise patients and their caregiver(s) that there may be drainage from the ear during the first few days following ear tube surgery; instruct to consult physician if the ear becomes painful, a continuous ear discharge is noted, or if a fever develops.

OTOVEL — ciprofloxacin/fluocinolone acetonide　　　Rx
Class: Antibacterial/corticosteroid combination

PEDIATRIC DOSAGE
Acute Otitis Media

Treatment of acute otitis media w/ tympanostomy tubes due to *Staphylococcus aureus, Streptococcus pneumoniae, Haemophilus influenzae, Moraxella catarrhalis*, and *Pseudomonas aeruginosa*

≥6 months:
0.25mL (one vial) into the affected ear canal bid for 7 days

ADMINISTRATION
Otic route
1. Warm vial in hand for 1-2 min.
2. Lie w/ affected ear upward, and then instill drops.
3. Pump the tragus 4 times by pushing inward to facilitate penetration of the medication into the middle ear.
4. Maintain this position for 1 min; repeat, if necessary, for the opposite ear.

STORAGE
20-25°C (68-77°F); excursions permitted to 15-30°C (59-86°F). Protect from light; store unused vials in pouch and discard 7 days after opening the pouch. Do not open until ready to use. Discard vial after use.

HOW SUPPLIED
Otic Sol: (Ciprofloxacin/Fluocinolone) 0.3%/0.025% [0.25mL]

CONTRAINDICATIONS
Known hypersensitivity to fluocinolone acetonide or other corticosteroids, ciprofloxacin or other quinolones, or to any other components of this product. Viral infections of the external ear canal (eg, varicella and herpes simplex infections) and fungal otic infections.

WARNINGS/PRECAUTIONS
D/C at 1st appearance of skin rash or any other sign of hypersensitivity. Serious and occasionally fatal hypersensitivity (anaphylactic) reactions reported; may require immediate emergency treatment. Prolonged use may result in overgrowth of nonsusceptible bacteria and fungi; perform culture testing if infection has not improved after 1 week and d/c and institute alternative therapy if such infections occur. If otorrhea persists after full course of therapy, or if ≥2 episodes of otorrhea occur w/in 6 months, evaluate further to exclude an underlying condition (eg, cholesteatoma, foreign body, tumor).

ADVERSE REACTIONS
Otorrhea, excessive granulation tissue, ear infection, ear pruritus, tympanic membrane disorder, auricular swelling, balance disorder.

PREGNANCY AND LACTATION
Pregnancy: Negligibly absorbed following otic administration; maternal use is not expected to result in fetal exposure to ciprofloxacin and fluocinolone.
Lactation: Breastfeeding is not expected to result in exposure of the infant to ciprofloxacin and fluocinolone.

MECHANISM OF ACTION
Ciprofloxacin: Fluoroquinolone antibacterial; bactericidal action results from interference w/ the enzyme, DNA gyrase, which is needed for the synthesis of bacterial DNA.
Fluocinolone: Corticosteroid; induces lipocortins. Lipocortins antagonize phospholipase A2, an enzyme which causes the breakdown of leukocyte lysosomal membranes to release arachidonic acid. This decreases the subsequent formation and release of endogenous inflammatory mediators including prostaglandins, kinins, histamine, liposomal enzymes, and the complement system.

PATIENT CONSIDERATIONS

Assessment: Assess for hypersensitivity to fluocinolone acetonide or other corticosteroids, ciprofloxacin or other quinolones, or to any other components of this product; viral infections of external ear canal (eg, varicella and herpes simplex infections); fungal ear infections; and pregnancy/nursing status.

Monitoring: Monitor for hypersensitivity reactions, overgrowth of non-susceptible bacteria and fungi, persistent otorrhea, and other adverse reactions.

Counseling: Inform that product is only for otic use. Advise not to use in the eyes. Instruct to warm the otic sol by holding the vial in the hand for 1-2 minutes before instilling it in the ear, to avoid dizziness. Instruct to d/c immediately at the first appearance of a skin rash or any other sign of hypersensitivity.

OTREXUP — methotrexate   Rx

Class: Dihydrofolic acid reductase inhibitor

Should be used only by physicians w/ knowledge and experience in the use of antimetabolite therapy. Use only in patients w/ psoriasis or rheumatoid arthritis (RA) w/ severe, recalcitrant, disabling disease not adequately responsive to other forms of therapy. Deaths reported in the treatment of malignancy, psoriasis, and RA. Closely monitor for bone marrow, liver, lung, skin, and kidney toxicities. Patients should be informed of the risks involved and be under physician's care throughout therapy. Fetal death and/or congenital anomalies reported; not recommended for females of childbearing potential unless benefits outweigh risks. Contraindicated in pregnant women. Reduced elimination w/ impaired renal function, ascites, or pleural effusions; monitor for toxicity and reduce dose or d/c in some cases. Unexpectedly severe (sometimes fatal) bone marrow suppression, aplastic anemia, and GI toxicity reported w/ coadministration of therapy (usually high dosage) w/ some NSAIDs. Causes hepatotoxicity, fibrosis, and cirrhosis (generally only after prolonged use); perform periodic liver biopsies in psoriatic patients on long-term therapy. Acutely, liver enzyme elevations frequently seen. Drug-induced lung disease may occur acutely at any time during therapy and reported at low doses. May need to interrupt therapy and carefully investigate if pulmonary symptoms (especially a dry, nonproductive cough) develop. Diarrhea and ulcerative stomatitis requires discontinuation of therapy. Malignant lymphomas, which may regress following withdrawal of treatment, may occur w/ low-dose therapy and, thus, may not require cytotoxic treatment; d/c therapy 1st and, if lymphoma does not regress, institute appropriate treatment. May induce tumor lysis syndrome in patients w/ rapidly growing tumors. Severe, occasionally fatal, skin reactions reported. Potentially fatal opportunistic infections, especially *Pneumocystis jiroveci* pneumonia, may occur. Concomitant use w/ radiotherapy may increase risk of soft tissue necrosis and osteonecrosis.

ADULT DOSAGE

Rheumatoid Arthritis

Severe, active RA (American College of Rheumatology criteria) in patients who have had an insufficient therapeutic response to, or are intolerant of, an adequate trial of 1st-line therapy including full-dose NSAIDs

Initial: 7.5mg once weekly
Titrate: Adjust dose gradually to achieve optimal response; significant increase in incidence and severity of serious toxic reactions, especially bone marrow suppression, reported at doses >20mg/week

Psoriasis

For symptomatic control of severe, recalcitrant, disabling psoriasis that is not adequately responsive to other forms of therapy, but only when the diagnosis has been established, as by biopsy and/or after dermatologic consultation

Initial: 10-25mg as a single weekly dose
Titrate: Adjust dose gradually to achieve optimal response; 30mg/week should not ordinarily be exceeded

Once optimal response is achieved, reduce dose to the lowest possible amount of drug and to the longest possible rest period

PEDIATRIC DOSAGE

Juvenile Idiopathic Arthritis

Active polyarticular juvenile idiopathic arthritis in patients who have had an insufficient therapeutic response to, or are intolerant of, an adequate trial of 1st-line therapy including full-dose NSAIDs

2-16 Years:
Initial: $10mg/m^2$ once weekly
Titrate: Adjust dose gradually to achieve optimal response; there is experience w/ doses up to $30mg/m^2$/week, however there are too few published data to assess how doses $>20mg/m^2$/week might affect the risk of serious toxicity

---

DOSING CONSIDERATIONS

Elderly

Consider relatively low doses and closely monitor for early signs of toxicity

ADMINISTRATION

SQ route

Patients may self-inject if determined that it is appropriate, if they have received proper training in how to prepare and administer the correct dose, and if they receive medical follow-up, as necessary; a trainer device is available for training purposes.

STORAGE

25°C (77°F); excursions permitted to 15-30°C (59-86°F). Protect from light.

HOW SUPPLIED

Inj: 7.5mg, 10mg, 12.5mg, 15mg, 17.5mg, 20mg, 22.5mg, 25mg [0.4mL]

CONTRAINDICATIONS

Pregnancy, nursing mothers, alcoholism, alcoholic liver disease, chronic liver disease, immunodeficiency syndromes, preexisting blood dyscrasias (eg, bone marrow hypoplasia, leukopenia, thrombocytopenia, significant anemia), known hypersensitivity to methotrexate (MTX).

WARNINGS/PRECAUTIONS

Use another formulation for alternative dosing in patients who require oral, IM, IV, intra-arterial, or intrathecal dosing, doses <7.5mg/week, doses >25mg/week, high-dose regimens, or dose adjustments between the available doses. Toxic effects may be related to dose/frequency of administration; if toxicity occurs, reduce dose or d/c therapy and take appropriate corrective measures, which may include use of leucovorin calcium and/or acute, intermittent hemodialysis w/ a high-flux dialyzer, if necessary. If therapy is reinstituted, carry it out w/ caution, w/ adequate consideration of further need for the drug and increased alertness as to possible recurrence of toxicity. Can suppress hematopoiesis and cause anemia, aplastic anemia, pancytopenia, leukopenia, neutropenia, and/or thrombocytopenia. Immediately d/c if there is a significant drop in blood counts; patients w/ profound granulocytopenia and fever should be evaluated immediately and usually require parenteral broad-spectrum antibiotic therapy. Neurologic toxicities may occur. May cause renal damage that may lead to acute renal failure; close attention to renal function including adequate hydration, urine alkalinization, and measurement of serum MTX and creatinine levels are essential for safe administration. Administered weekly; mistaken daily use has led to fatal toxicity. Caution in elderly/debilitated, patients w/ preexisting hematopoietic impairment, in the presence of preexisting liver damage or impaired hepatic function, and in the presence of active infection. May impair mental/physical abilities.

ADVERSE REACTIONS

Ulcerative stomatitis, leukopenia, nausea, abdominal distress, malaise, undue fatigue, chills, fever, dizziness, decreased resistance to infection.

DRUG INTERACTIONS

See Boxed Warning. NSAIDs may elevate and prolong levels; do not administer NSAIDs prior to or concomitantly w/ high doses of MTX, and use caution when NSAIDs and salicylates are administered concomitantly w/ lower doses of MTX. Proton pump inhibitors (PPIs) (eg, omeprazole, esomeprazole, pantoprazole) may elevate and prolong levels, possibly leading to toxicities; use caution if administering high-dose MTX w/ PPIs. Oral antibiotics (eg, tetracycline, chloramphenicol, nonabsorbable broad spectrum antibiotics) may decrease intestinal absorption or interfere w/ enterohepatic circulation. Penicillins may reduce renal clearance; increased serum concentrations of MTX w/ concomitant hematologic and GI toxicity reported w/ concomitant use w/ penicillins; carefully monitor. Trimethoprim/sulfamethoxazole reported rarely to increase bone marrow suppression. Closely monitor for increased risk of hepatotoxicity w/ hepatotoxins (eg, azathioprine, retinoids, sulfasalazine). May decrease theophylline clearance; monitor theophylline levels. Vitamin preparations containing folic acid or its derivatives may decrease response to systemically administered MTX; high doses of leucovorin may reduce efficacy of intrathecally administered MTX. Increases levels of mercaptopurine; may require dose adjustment. Toxicity may be increased due to displacement by salicylates, phenylbutazone, phenytoin, and sulfonamides. Renal tubular transport diminished by probenecid; carefully monitor w/ concomitant use. Combined use w/ gold, penicillamine, hydroxychloroquine, sulfasalazine, or cytotoxic agents may increase incidence of adverse effects. Immunization may be ineffective when given during therapy; immunization w/ live virus vaccines is generally not recommended. Disseminated vaccinia infections after smallpox immunizations reported. Lesions of psoriasis may be aggravated by concomitant exposure to UV radiation.

PREGNANCY AND LACTATION

Pregnancy: Category X.
Lactation: MTX has been detected in human breast milk; not for use in nursing.
Reproductive Potential: Avoid pregnancy if either partner is receiving MTX; during and for a minimum of three months after therapy for male patients, and during and for at least one ovulatory cycle after therapy for female patients. MTX has been reported to cause impairment of fertility, oligospermia, and menstrual dysfunction during and for a short period after cessation of therapy.

MECHANISM OF ACTION

Dihydrofolic acid reductase inhibitor; interferes w/ DNA synthesis, repair, and cellular replication. Mechanism in RA not established; may affect immune function.

PHARMACOKINETICS

Absorption: (PO) Well-absorbed. Bioavailability (60%) (adults). Administration of various doses and in different disease states resulted in different parameters.
Distribution: Plasma protein binding (50%); found in breast milk. (IV) V_d=0.18L/kg (initial), 0.4-0.8L/kg (steady-state). **Metabolism:** Hepatic and intracellular to polyglutamated forms (active); 7-hydroxymethotrexate (metabolite). (PO) Partially metabolized by intestinal flora. **Elimination:** $T_{1/2}$=3-10 hrs (psoriasis/RA/low-dose antineoplastic therapy), 8-15 hrs (high doses). (IV) Urine (80-90%, unchanged), bile (≤10%). Refer to PI for additional pharmacokinetic information.

PATIENT CONSIDERATIONS

Assessment: Assess for alcoholism, alcoholic/chronic liver disease, immunodeficiency, blood dyscrasias, ascites, pleural effusions, tumors, hypersensitivity to drug, pregnancy/nursing status, any other condition where treatment is cautioned or contraindicated, and possible drug interactions. Obtain baseline CBC w/ differential and platelet counts, hepatic enzymes, renal function tests, liver biopsy, and chest x-ray. Obtain baseline liver biopsy in psoriatic patients.

Monitoring: Monitor for toxicities of bone marrow, liver, lung, kidney, and GI tract, diarrhea, ulcerative stomatitis, malignant lymphomas, tumor lysis syndrome, skin reactions, opportunistic infections, and other adverse reactions. Monitor hematology at least monthly and renal/hepatic function every 1-2 months during therapy and more frequently during initial/changing doses, or during periods of increased risk of elevated drug levels (eg, dehydration). If drug-induced lung disease is suspected, perform pulmonary function tests. Perform periodic liver biopsies in psoriatic patients who are under long-term treatment.

Counseling: Inform of the risks of organ toxicity, the possible signs/symptoms for which the physician should be contacted, and the need for close follow-up, including periodic lab tests to monitor for organ toxicity. Emphasize that the recommended dose is taken weekly, and that mistaken daily use of recommended dose has led to fatal toxicity. Instruct not to self-administer until trained by physician. Advise that therapy can cause fetal harm; advise that pregnancy should be avoided if either partner is receiving MTX; during and for a minimum of 3 months after therapy for male patients, and during and for at least 1 ovulatory cycle after therapy for female patients. Instruct to contact physician if pregnancy is suspected. Inform that therapy is contraindicated in nursing mothers. Discuss the risk of effects on reproduction. Inform that adverse reactions such as dizziness and fatigue may affect ability to drive or operate machinery. Inform of the need for proper disposal after use, including the use of a sharps disposal container.

OVACE WASH — sodium sulfacetamide   Rx

Class: Sulfonamide

OTHER BRAND NAMES
Ovace Plus Wash

ADULT DOSAGE	**PEDIATRIC DOSAGE**
Scaling Dermatoses	**Scaling Dermatoses**
Seborrheic Dermatitis and Seborrhea Sicca (Dandruff):	**Seborrheic Dermatitis and Seborrhea Sicca (Dandruff):**
Wash affected area bid (am and pm) or ud; repeat application for 8-10 days or ud	**≥12 Years:** Wash affected area bid (am and pm) or ud; repeat application for 8-10 days or ud
May rinse cleanser off sooner or use less frequently if skin dryness occurs	May rinse cleanser off sooner or use less frequently if skin dryness occurs
May lengthen interval between applications as condition subsides; may apply once or twice weekly, or every other week to prevent recurrence	May lengthen interval between applications as condition subsides; may apply once or twice weekly, or every other week to prevent recurrence
If condition recurs after discontinuing therapy, reinitiate application as at the beginning of treatment	If condition recurs after discontinuing therapy, reinitiate application as at the beginning of treatment
Secondary Infections	**Secondary Infections**
Secondary Bacterial Infections of Skin Due to Organisms Susceptible to Sulfonamides:	**≥12 Years:** **Secondary Bacterial Infections of Skin Due to Organisms Susceptible to Sulfonamides:**
Wash affected area bid (am and pm) or ud	Wash affected area bid (am and pm) or ud
Repeat application for 8-10 days or ud	Repeat application for 8-10 days or ud
May rinse cleanser off sooner or use less frequently if skin dryness occurs	May rinse cleanser off sooner or use less frequently if skin dryness occurs

ADMINISTRATION
Topical route

Seborrheic Dermatitis/Dandruff:
Wet skin and liberally apply to areas to be cleansed, massage gently into skin working into a full lather, rinse thoroughly, pat dry, and repeat after 10-20 sec. Rinse w/ plain water to remove excess medication.
Shampoo hair at least once a week.

Secondary Infections:
Wet skin and liberally apply to areas to be cleansed, massage gently into skin for 10-20 sec working into a full lather, rinse thoroughly, and pat dry.
Rinse w/ plain water to remove excess medication.

STORAGE
20-25°C (68-77°F); excursions permitted between 15-30°C (59-86°F). Brief exposure up to 40°C (104°F) may be tolerated provided the mean kinetic temperature does not exceed 25°C (77°F); minimize such exposure. Protect from freezing and excessive heat. Product may tend to darken slightly on storage; slight discoloration does not impair efficacy or safety of product. Keep tightly closed.

HOW SUPPLIED
Wash: 10% [180mL, 355mL, 480mL], (Plus) 10% [473mL]

CONTRAINDICATIONS
Known or suspected hypersensitivity to any ingredients of the product, kidney disease.

WARNINGS/PRECAUTIONS
Stevens-Johnson syndrome (SJS) and drug-induced systemic lupus erythematosus (SLE) reported. May cause proliferation of nonsusceptible organisms, including fungi. Caution in patients who may be prone to hypersensitivity to topical sulfonamides; d/c if signs of hypersensitivity or other untoward reaction occurs. Local irritation or sensitization may occur during long-term therapy. Systemic toxic reactions (eg, agranulocytosis, acute hemolytic anemia, purpura hemorrhagica) indicate hypersensitivity to sulfonamides. Employ particular caution if areas of denuded or abraded skin are involved; systemic absorption is greater following application to large, infected, abraded, denuded, or severely burned areas.

ADVERSE REACTIONS
Irritation, hypersensitivity.

DRUG INTERACTIONS
Incompatible w/ silver preparations.

PREGNANCY AND LACTATION
Category C, caution in nursing.

MECHANISM OF ACTION
Sulfonamide; exerts a bacteriostatic effect against sulfonamide sensitive gram-positive and gram-negative microorganisms. Restricts the synthesis of folic acid required by bacteria for growth, by its competition w/ para-aminobenzoic acid.

PATIENT CONSIDERATIONS
Assessment: Assess for hypersensitivity to any of the ingredients of the product, kidney disease, pregnancy/nursing status, and possible drug interactions. Assess if treatment area contains denuded or abraded skin.

Monitoring: Monitor for signs/symptoms of hypersensitivity reactions, SJS, drug-induced SLE, systemic toxic reactions, and other adverse reactions. Monitor for local irritation or sensitization if used for long-term therapy. When applying to large, infected, abraded, denuded, or severely burned areas, monitor for occurrence of adverse events produced by systemic administration of sulfonamides and perform appropriate lab testing.

Counseling: Counsel to d/c therapy if condition worsens or if rash develops in the area being treated or elsewhere. Instruct to d/c promptly and notify physician if any signs of arthritis, fever, or mouth sores develop. Instruct to avoid contact w/ eyes, lips, and mucous membranes. Inform that a slight discoloration may occasionally occur when an excessive amount of the product is used and comes in contact w/ white fabrics; inform that this discoloration is readily removed by ordinary laundering w/o bleaches.

OVCON-35 — ethinyl estradiol/norethindrone   Rx

Class: Estrogen/progestogen combination

> Cigarette smoking increases the risk of serious cardiovascular side effects. Risk increases w/ age and w/ heavy smoking (≥15 cigarettes/day) and is quite marked in women >35 yrs of age. Women who use oral contraceptives should be strongly advised not to smoke.

OTHER BRAND NAMES
Balziva

ADULT DOSAGE	**PEDIATRIC DOSAGE**
Contraception	**Contraception**
1 tab qd for 28 days, then repeat regimen on the next day after the last tab	Not indicated for use premenarche; refer to adult dosing
Start on the 1st day of menses or 1st Sunday after menses begin	

DOSING CONSIDERATIONS
Adverse Reactions
GI Disturbances: Use a back-up method of contraception for the remainder of that cycle if significant GI disturbance occurs

ADMINISTRATION
Oral route

Take at the same time every day.
Use a nonhormonal contraceptive as backup during the 1st 7 days of therapy of initiating therapy (Sunday starter) or restarting after ≥2 missed doses.

STORAGE
20-25°C (68-77°F).

HOW SUPPLIED
Tab: (Ethinyl Estradiol/Norethindrone) 0.035mg/0.4mg

CONTRAINDICATIONS
Thrombophlebitis, current or history of thromboembolic disorders, past history of deep vein thrombophlebitis, cerebrovascular or coronary artery disease, known or suspected carcinoma of the breast, endometrial carcinoma or other known or suspected estrogen-dependent neoplasia, undiagnosed abnormal genital bleeding, cholestatic jaundice of pregnancy or jaundice w/ prior pill use, hepatic adenomas or carcinomas, known or suspected pregnancy.

WARNINGS/PRECAUTIONS
Increased risk of MI, thromboembolism, cerebrovascular events, gallbladder disease, and hepatic neoplasia. May increase risk of vascular disease. If feasible, d/c at least 4 weeks prior to and for 2 weeks after elective surgery of a type associated with an increase in risk of thromboembolism and during and following prolonged immobilization. Start therapy no earlier than 4-6 weeks after delivery in women who elect not to breastfeed. May increase risk of breast cancer and cervical intraepithelial neoplasia. Retinal thrombosis reported; d/c if unexplained partial or complete loss of vision, onset of proptosis or diplopia, papilledema, or retinal vascular lesions develop. Increased risk of gallbladder surgery reported. May cause glucose intolerance. Changes in serum TG and lipoprotein levels reported. May cause fluid retention and increase BP; d/c if significant elevation of BP occurs. D/C and evaluate the cause if onset/exacerbation of migraine or

headache w/ a new pattern that is recurrent, persistent, or severe develops. Breakthrough bleeding and spotting reported; rule out malignancy or pregnancy. D/C if jaundice develops. Monitor closely w/ depression and d/c if depression recurs to serious degree. Contact lens wearers who develop visual changes or changes in lens tolerance should be assessed by an ophthalmologist. May affect certain endocrine function tests, LFTs, and blood components in lab tests.

ADVERSE REACTIONS
N/V, breakthrough bleeding, GI symptoms, spotting, menstrual flow changes, amenorrhea, migraine, mental depression, vaginal candidiasis, edema, weight changes, cervical ectropion and secretion changes, melasma, breast changed (tenderness, enlargement, secretion), rash.

DRUG INTERACTIONS
Reduced effects, increased breakthrough bleeding, and menstrual irregularities w/ rifampin, barbiturates, phenylbutazone, phenytoin sodium, and possibly w/ griseofulvin, ampicillin, and tetracyclines.

PREGNANCY AND LACTATION
Pregnancy: Category X.
Lactation: Not for use in nursing.

MECHANISM OF ACTION
Estrogen/progestogen combination oral contraceptive; acts by suppressing gonadotropins. Primarily inhibits ovulation, but also causes other alterations including changes in the cervical mucus (which increase the difficulty of sperm entry into the uterus) and the endometrium (which reduce the likelihood of implantation).

PHARMACOKINETICS
Distribution: Found in breast milk.

PATIENT CONSIDERATIONS
Assessment: Assess for thrombophlebitis or thromboembolic disorders, HTN, hyperlipidemia, diabetes, breast cancer, undiagnosed abnormal genital bleeding, pregnancy/nursing status, possible drug interactions, and any other conditions where treatment is contraindicated or cautioned.

Monitoring: Monitor for signs/symptoms of thromboembolism, stroke, MI, and other adverse reactions. Monitor BP in patients w/ a history of HTN, HTN-related disease, or renal disease; for signs of depression in patients w/ a history of depression; serum glucose levels in prediabetic and diabetic patients; and lipid levels in patients w/ a history of hyperlipidemia. Perform annual history and physical exam including special reference to BP, breasts, abdomen and pelvic organs, including cervical cytology, and relevant laboratory tests. Monitor women w/ a strong family history of breast cancer or who have breast nodules.

Counseling: Inform that medication does not protect against HIV infection (AIDS) and other STDs. Counsel about possible serious side effects. Advise to avoid smoking while on therapy. Inform that if spotting, light bleeding, or nausea occurs during first 1-3 packs of pills, to not d/c medication, and if symptoms persist, to notify physician. Inform that if vomiting or diarrhea occurs, efficacy may decrease; instruct to use backup method of contraception and to contact physician. Advise to notify physician of all prescription/nonprescription medications currently taking. Instruct patients w/ contact lenses to notify physician if changes in vision or lens tolerance develop. Instruct to use additional method of protection until after patient has taken seven pills if using the Sunday-start method. Inform on what to do if pills are missed.

OVIDREL — choriogonadotropin alfa   Rx
Class: Recombinant human chorionic gonadotropin (hCG)

ADULT DOSAGE
Assisted Reproductive Technology
For induction of final follicular maturation and early luteinization in infertile women who have undergone pituitary desensitization and have been pretreated w/ follicle stimulating hormones as part of an assisted reproductive technology program

Usual: 250mcg administered 1 day following the last dose of the follicle stimulating agent
Do not administer until there is adequate follicular development
Withhold in cases of excessive ovarian response

Ovulation Induction
In anovulatory infertile women in whom the cause of infertility is functional and not due to primary ovarian failure

Usual: 250mcg administered 1 day following the last dose of the follicle stimulating agent
Do not administer until there is adequate follicular development
Withhold in cases of excessive ovarian response

PEDIATRIC DOSAGE
Pediatric use may not have been established

ADMINISTRATION
SQ route

STORAGE
Before Dispensing: 2-8°C (36-46°F). Following Dispensing: Refrigerate until expiry date or for no more than 30 days at room temperature up to 25°C (77°F) but must use within 30 days. Protect from light. Discard unused material.

HOW SUPPLIED
Inj: 250mcg/0.5mL

CONTRAINDICATIONS
Prior hypersensitivity to hCG preparations or one of their excipients, primary ovarian failure, uncontrolled thyroid or adrenal dysfunction, uncontrolled organic intracranial lesion (eg, pituitary tumor), abnormal uterine bleeding of undetermined origin, ovarian cyst or enlargement of undetermined origin, sex hormone dependent tumors of reproductive tract and accessory organs, pregnancy.

WARNINGS/PRECAUTIONS
Should only be used by physicians thoroughly familiar with infertility problems and their management. May cause ovarian hyperstimulation syndrome (OHSS) in women with or without pulmonary or vascular complications; risk of treatment should be considered for women with risk factors of thromboembolic events (eg, prior medical or family history). Withhold therapy if evidence of developing OHSS prior to administration. If severe OHSS occurs, d/c therapy and the patient should be hospitalized. Mild to moderate uncomplicated ovarian enlargement which may be accompanied by abdominal distention and/or abdominal pain may occur; withhold treatment if ovaries are abnormally enlarged on the last day of FSH therapy. May cause arterial thromboembolism. Multiple births and elevated ALT levels reported. Monitor ovarian response with serum estradiol and transvaginal ultrasound on a regular basis.

ADVERSE REACTIONS
Inj-site reactions (eg, pain, bruising), ovarian cyst, abdominal pain, nausea, OHSS.

PREGNANCY AND LACTATION
Category X, caution in nursing.

MECHANISM OF ACTION
Recombinant human chorionic gonadotropin; stimulates late follicular maturation and resumption of oocyte meiosis, and initiates rupture of preovulatory ovarian follicle.

PHARMACOKINETICS
Absorption: Absolute bioavailability (40%); C_{max}=121 IU/L, T_{max}=24 hrs, AUC=7701 h•IU/L. **Distribution:** (IV) V_d=5.9L. **Elimination:** Urine; $T_{1/2}$=29 hrs.

PATIENT CONSIDERATIONS
Assessment: Assess for primary ovarian failure, uncontrolled thyroid or adrenal dysfunction, uncontrolled organic intracranial lesion (eg, pituitary tumor), abnormal uterine bleeding of undetermined origin, ovarian cyst or enlargement of undetermined origin, sex hormone dependent tumors of reproductive tract and accessory organs, thromboembolic events risk factors, and pregnancy/nursing status.

Monitoring: Monitor for ovarian enlargement, OHSS, arterial thromboembolism, signs of multiple births, and other adverse reactions. Monitor ovarian response with serum estradiol and transvaginal ultrasound regularly.

Counseling: Inform about duration of therapy and the required monitoring procedures prior to therapy. Inform of the risks of OHSS, multiple pregnancies, and other possible adverse reactions.

OXACILLIN — oxacillin   Rx
Class: Penicillin (PCN) (penicillinase-resistant)

ADULT DOSAGE
General Dosing
Infections caused by penicillinase-producing staphylococci or for initial therapy in suspected cases of resistant staphylococcal infections prior to availability of susceptibility test results

Mild to Moderate Infections:
250-500mg IM/IV q4-6h
Severe Infections:
1g IM/IV q4-6h; continue for at least 14 days

Continue for at least 48 hrs after patient has become afebrile, asymptomatic, and cultures are negative; endocarditis/osteomyelitis may require longer duration of therapy

PEDIATRIC DOSAGE
General Dosing
Premature/Neonates:
25mg/kg/day IM/IV

Infants/Children <40kg (88 lbs):
Mild to Moderate Infections:
50mg/kg/day IM/IV in equally divided doses q6h
Severe Infections:
100mg/kg/day IM/IV in equally divided doses q4-6h; continue for at least 14 days

Continue for at least 48 hrs after patient has become afebrile, asymptomatic, and cultures are negative; endocarditis/osteomyelitis may require longer duration of therapy

DOSING CONSIDERATIONS
Elderly
Start at lower end of dosing range

ADMINISTRATION
IM/IV route
If another agent is used in conjunction, administer separately; do not physically mix w/ therapy.
Do not add supplementary medication to inj.

IM
Add 5.4mL of sterile water for inj (SWFI) to the 1g vial, and 10.6mL of SWFI to the 2g vial for reconstitution; shake well.
Reconstituted sol is stable for 3 days at 21°C (70°F) or for 1 week under refrigeration 4°C (40°F).

Direct IV Use
Use SWFI or NaCl inj and add 10mL to the 1g vial, and 20mL to the 2g vial for reconstitution.
Withdraw entire contents and administer slowly over a period of approx 10 min.

IV Drip
Reconstitute as directed above for Direct IV Use prior to diluting w/ compatible IV sol.
Adjust the rate and volume of the infusion so that the total dose is administered before the drug loses its stability in the sol in use.

Compatible IV Sol:
D5 in normal saline, 10% D-fructose in water, 10% D-fructose in normal saline, lactated potassic saline inj, 10% invert sugar in normal saline, 10% invert sugar plus 0.3% potassium chloride in water, Travert 10% electrolyte #1, Travert 10% electrolyte #2, Travert 10% electrolyte #3.

Refer to PI for further stability period information.

STORAGE
Dry Powder: 20-25°C (68-77°F).

HOW SUPPLIED
Inj: 1g, 2g

CONTRAINDICATIONS
History of a hypersensitivity (anaphylactic) reaction to any penicillin.

WARNINGS/PRECAUTIONS
Serious and occasionally fatal hypersensitivity (anaphylactic shock w/ collapse) reactions reported; initiate only after a comprehensive drug and allergy history has been obtained. D/C and institute supportive treatment if allergic reaction occurs. Avoid w/ history of sensitivity to any penicillin (PCN). *Clostridium difficile*-associated diarrhea (CDAD) reported; may need to d/c if CDAD is suspected/confirmed. Caution w/ histories of significant allergies and/or asthma. May result in overgrowth of nonsusceptible organisms; d/c and take appropriate measures if new infection due to bacteria or fungi occurs. May result in bacterial resistance w/ use in the absence of a proven or suspected bacterial infection or a prophylactic indication. Change to another active agent if culture tests fail to demonstrate the presence of staphylococci. Perform periodic urinalysis, BUN, and creatinine determinations; consider dosage alterations if these values become elevated. Consider dose reduction and monitor blood levels to avoid neurotoxic reactions if any impairment of renal function is suspected or known to exist.

ADVERSE REACTIONS
Allergic reactions, N/V, diarrhea, neurotoxic reactions, renal tubular damage, interstitial nephritis, agranulocytosis, neutropenia, bone marrow depression, hepatotoxicity.

DRUG INTERACTIONS
Tetracycline may antagonize bactericidal effect; avoid concomitant use. Probenecid may increase and prolong plasma concentrations; limit concomitant use to infections where high serum levels of oxacillin are necessary.

PREGNANCY AND LACTATION
Pregnancy: Category B.
Lactation: Caution in nursing.

MECHANISM OF ACTION
PCN (penicillinase-resistant); exerts bactericidal action against PCN-susceptible microorganisms during the state of active multiplication. Inhibits biosynthesis of bacterial cell wall.

PHARMACOKINETICS
Absorption: (IM) C_{max}=5.3mcg/mL (250mg), 10.9mcg/mL (500mg); T_{max}=30 min. (IV, 500mg) C_{max}=43mcg/mL; T_{max}=5 min. **Distribution:** Plasma protein binding (94.2%); found in breast milk. **Elimination:** Urine (primarily unchanged); $T_{1/2}$=20-30 min (IV, 500mg).

PATIENT CONSIDERATIONS

Assessment: Assess for previous hypersensitivity to PCN, history of significant allergies and/or asthma, renal dysfunction, pregnancy/nursing status, and possible drug interactions. Perform culture and susceptibility tests to determine causative organism and its susceptibility to the drug. Obtain baseline blood cultures, WBC counts, and differential counts.

Monitoring: Monitor for hypersensitivity/anaphylactic reactions, CDAD, neurotoxic reactions, and other adverse reactions. Monitor organ system function (eg, renal, hepatic, hematopoietic) periodically during prolonged therapy. Obtain blood cultures, WBC counts, and differential counts at least weekly during therapy. Perform urinalysis, BUN, LFTs including ALT/AST, and creatinine determinations periodically.

Counseling: Advise that therapy only treats bacterial, not viral, infections. Inform that skipping doses or not completing full course of therapy may decrease the effectiveness of treatment and increase resistance. Inform that diarrhea is a common problem that usually ends upon discontinuation; however, if watery and bloody stools occur (w/ or w/o stomach cramps and fever) even as late as ≥2 months after last dose, instruct to contact physician as soon as possible.

OXAYDO — oxycodone hydrochloride   CII
Class: Opioid analgesic

ADULT DOSAGE
Moderate to Severe Pain
Acute:
Patients Not Currently Receiving Opioid Analgesics:
Initial: 5-15mg q4-6h prn
Titrate: Adjust based on response to initial dose

Chronic:
Dose at lowest level that will achieve acceptable analgesia and tolerable adverse reactions, on an around-the-clock basis

Conversions
From Fixed-Ratio Oral Opioid/ Nonopioid Combinations:
Determine whether or not to continue nonopioid analgesic. Titrate dose in response to the level of analgesia and adverse reactions afforded by dosing regimen regardless of whether nonopioid is continued

From Other Oral Opioid Therapy:
Closely observe and adjust dose based on patient's response to therapy

PEDIATRIC DOSAGE
Pediatric use may not have been established

DOSING CONSIDERATIONS
Renal Impairment
Initial: Follow conservative approach and adjust according to clinical situation

Hepatic Impairment
Initial: Follow conservative approach and adjust according to clinical situation

Elderly
Start at low end of the dosing range

Discontinuation
Gradually taper over time to prevent development of withdrawal; generally can decrease therapy by 25% to 50% per day w/ careful monitoring

ADMINISTRATION
Oral route

Swallow tab whole.
Take each tab w/ enough water to ensure complete swallowing immediately after placing in the mouth.
Not for crushing and dissolution.
Do not administer via NG, gastric, or other feeding tubes.

STORAGE
25°C (77°F); excursions permitted to 15-30°C (59-86°F). Protect from moisture.

HOW SUPPLIED
Tab: 5mg, 7.5mg

CONTRAINDICATIONS
Respiratory depression in unmonitored settings and in the absence of resuscitative equipment; known or suspected paralytic ileus; acute or severe bronchial asthma or hypercarbia; known hypersensitivity to oxycodone, oxycodone salts, or any components of the product.

WARNINGS/PRECAUTIONS
Respiratory depression may occur; increased risk in elderly/debilitated patients, in those suffering from conditions accompanied by hypoxia, hypercapnia, or upper airway obstruction, or w/ large initial doses given to nontolerant patients. Extreme caution w/ COPD or cor pulmonale, in patients having substantially decreased respiratory reserve (eg, severe kyphoscoliosis), hypoxia, hypercapnia, or preexisting respiratory depression; consider alternative nonopioid analgesics. Potential for misuse and abuse. Respiratory depressant effects and its potential to elevate CSF pressure may be exaggerated in the presence of head injury, intracranial lesions, or preexisting increased intracranial pressure (ICP). May produce effects on pupillary response and consciousness. May cause severe hypotension in patients whose ability to maintain blood pressure has been compromised by a depleted intravascular volume. Orthostatic hypotension in ambulatory patients may occur. Caution w/ circulatory shock. Do not administer to patients w/ GI obstruction; may result in prolonged obstruction. May obscure diagnosis or clinical course of acute abdominal conditions. Caution w/ biliary tract disease; may cause spasm of sphincter of Oddi and diminish biliary/pancreatic secretions. Caution and reduce dose w/ severe renal/hepatic impairment, Addison's disease, hypothyroidism, prostatic hypertrophy, urethral stricture, and in elderly/debilitated patients. May induce/aggravate seizures. Caution in CNS depression, toxic psychosis, acute alcoholism, and delirium tremens. May impair mental/physical abilities.

ADVERSE REACTIONS
N/V, constipation, headache, pruritus, insomnia, dizziness, asthenia, somnolence.

DRUG INTERACTIONS
Caution and reduce dose w/ other CNS depressants (eg, sedatives, hypnotics, general anesthetics, antiemetics, phenothiazines, tranquilizers, alcohol); may increase risk of respiratory depression, hypotension, profound sedation, or

coma. Avoid alcoholic beverages/alcohol-containing medications. Risk of severe hypotension w/ phenothiazines, general anesthetics, or other agents that compromise vasomotor tone. May enhance neuromuscular blocking action of skeletal muscle relaxants and may increase respiratory depression. Mixed agonist/antagonist analgesics (eg, pentazocine, nalbuphine, butorphanol, buprenorphine) may reduce effect and/or precipitate withdrawal; do not administer mixed agonist/antagonist analgesics to patients who have received or are receiving a course of therapy w/ a pure opioid agonist. Not recommended in patients taking MAOIs or w/in 14 days of stopping treatment; may intensify effects causing anxiety, confusion, and significant respiratory depression or coma. Increased levels w/ voriconazole. Caution w/ CYP3A4 inhibitors (eg, macrolide antibiotics, azole-antifungal agents, protease inhibitors); may prolong opioid effects. May decrease levels/efficacy or result in development of abstinence syndrome w/ rifampin and other CYP3A4 inducers (eg, carbamazepine, phenytoin); use w/ caution. Urinary retention/severe constipation potentially leading to paralytic ileus may occur w/ anticholinergics. Caution w/ CYP2D6 inhibitors.

PREGNANCY AND LACTATION
Pregnancy: Category B.
Lactation: Not for use in nursing.

MECHANISM OF ACTION
Opioid analgesic; pure opioid agonist relatively selective for μ-receptor. Principal therapeutic action is analgesia.

PHARMACOKINETICS
Absorption: T_{max}=1.2-1.4 hrs. Oral bioavailability (60-87%). **Distribution:** V_d=2.6L/kg; plasma protein binding (approx 45%); crosses the placenta; found in the breast milk. **Metabolism:** Extensive via CYP3A4 and CYP2D6 to noroxycodone (major metabolite), oxymorphone, and noroxymorphone. **Elimination:** Urine; $T_{1/2}$=3.5-4 hrs.

PATIENT CONSIDERATIONS
Assessment: Assess for level of pain intensity, type of pain, respiratory depression, COPD, hypoxia, hypercarbia, asthma, GI obstruction, renal/hepatic impairment, or any other conditions where treatment is contraindicated or cautioned. Assess for pregnancy/nursing status and possible drug interactions.

Monitoring: Monitor for signs/symptoms of respiratory depression, CNS depression, seizures/convulsions, CSF pressure elevation, hypotension, and other adverse reactions. Monitor BP. Monitor for tolerance, physical dependence, and signs of misuse, abuse, and addiction.

Counseling: Advise to take ud and to take each tab w/ enough water to ensure complete swallowing. Instruct to swallow whole and not to crush/dissolve tab or pre-soak, lick, or otherwise wet the tablet prior to placing in the mouth. Advise to not adjust the dose w/o consulting healthcare provider. Advise that drowsiness, dizziness, or lightheadedness may occur. Inform that therapy may impair mental/physical abilities; instruct to refrain from potentially dangerous activities. Instruct to not combine w/ alcohol or other CNS depressants. Instruct to inform physician if pregnant or planning to become pregnant. Inform that dosing will need to be tapered if taking medication for more than a few weeks. Advise that medication has potential for abuse; protect from theft. Advise to not share or permit use by other individuals. Instruct to dispose of any unused medication by flushing down the toilet. Advise of possible occurrence of severe constipation and other adverse reactions.

OXTELLAR XR — oxcarbazepine   Rx
Class: Dibenzazepine

ADULT DOSAGE
Partial Seizures
Adjunctive Therapy:

Initial: 600mg qd for 1 week
Titrate: May increase at weekly intervals in 600mg/day increments
Recommended: 1200-2400mg qd

Conversions
Conversion from Immediate-Release (IR) Oxcarbazepine:
Higher doses may be necessary

PEDIATRIC DOSAGE
Partial Seizures
Adjunctive Therapy:

6-17 Years:
Initial: 8-10mg/kg (up to 600mg) qd for 1 week
Titrate: May increase at weekly intervals in 8-10mg/kg increments (up to 600mg) qd

Target Maint Dose (Achieved Over 2-3 Weeks):
20-29kg: 900mg qd
29.1-39kg: 1200mg qd
>39kg: 1800mg qd

Conversions
Conversion from IR Oxcarbazepine:
Higher doses may be necessary

DOSING CONSIDERATIONS
Concomitant Medications
Enzyme-Inducing Antiepileptic Drugs (AEDs):
Dose increases may be necessary; consider initiating therapy at 900mg qd

Renal Impairment
Severe (CrCl <30mL/min):
Initial: 1/2 the usual initial dose (300mg qd)
Titrate: May increase at weekly intervals in 300-450mg/day increments to achieve desired clinical response

ESRD on Dialysis:
Use IR oxcarbazepine

Hepatic Impairment
Severe: Not recommended
Elderly
Initial: Consider starting at 300-450mg qd
Titrate: May increase at weekly intervals in 300-450mg/day increments to achieve desired clinical effect

Discontinuation
Withdraw gradually to minimize potential of increased seizure frequency

ADMINISTRATION
Oral route

Take on an empty stomach (at least 1 hr ac or at least 2 hrs pc).
Swallow tabs whole w/ water or other liquid; do not cut, crush, or chew.
For ease of swallowing in pediatric patients or patients w/ difficulty swallowing, achieve daily dosages w/ multiples of appropriate lower strength tablets (eg, 150mg tabs).

STORAGE
25°C (77°F); excursions permitted to 15-30°C (59-86°F). Protect from light and moisture.

HOW SUPPLIED
Tab, Extended-Release: 150mg, 300mg, 600mg

CONTRAINDICATIONS
Known hypersensitivity to oxcarbazepine or to any of its components.

WARNINGS/PRECAUTIONS
Clinically significant hyponatremia may develop; measure serum Na^+ levels during treatment if symptoms occur, and particularly if receiving concomitant medications known to decrease serum Na^+ levels (eg, drugs associated w/ inappropriate antidiuretic hormone secretion). Anaphylaxis and angioedema involving the larynx, glottis, lips, and eyelids reported w/ IR oxcarbazepine (rare); d/c if any of these reactions develop, initiate alternative treatment, and do not rechallenge. Treat patients w/ history of hypersensitivity reactions to carbamazepine only if potential benefit justifies potential risk; d/c immediately if signs/symptoms of hypersensitivity develop. Serious dermatological reactions (eg, Stevens-Johnson syndrome [SJS], toxic epidermal necrolysis [TEN]) reported w/ IR oxcarbazepine; consider discontinuing and prescribing another AED if a skin reaction develops. Increased risk for SJS/TEN w/ HLA-B*1502 allele; avoid use in patients positive for HLA-B*1502 unless benefit clearly outweighs the risk. Increased risk of suicidal thoughts/behavior; monitor for emergence or worsening of depression, suicidal thoughts/behavior, and/or any unusual changes in mood/behavior. Multiorgan hypersensitivity reactions reported w/ IR oxcarbazepine; d/c and initiate an alternative treatment if suspected. Pancytopenia, agranulocytosis, and leukopenia reported w/ IR oxcarbazepine; consider discontinuing if any evidence of these hematologic events develops. Levels may decrease during pregnancy; monitor during pregnancy and through the postpartum period. IR oxcarbazepine associated w/ decreases in T4, w/o changes in T3 or TSH.

ADVERSE REACTIONS
Dizziness, somnolence, headache, balance disorder, tremor, vomiting, diplopia, asthenia.

DRUG INTERACTIONS
See Dosing Considerations. AEDs that are CYP450 inducers (eg, carbamazepine, phenobarbital, phenytoin), valproic acid, and verapamil may decrease 10-monohydroxy derivative (MHD) levels. May inhibit CYP2C19 and induce CYP3A4/5 w/ potentially important effects on levels of other drugs. May decrease levels of felodipine, oral contraceptives (eg, ethinyl estradiol, levonorgestrel), and cyclosporine. Consider avoiding the use of other drugs associated w/ SJS/TEN in HLA-B*1502 positive patients, when alternative therapies are otherwise equally acceptable.

PREGNANCY AND LACTATION
Pregnancy: Category C. Given that Oxtellar XR is closely related structurally to carbamazepine, and the results of animal studies, it is likely that Oxtellar XR is a human teratogen. Physicians are advised to recommend that pregnant patients enroll in the North American Antiepileptic Drug (NAAED) Pregnancy Registry.
Lactation: Found in breast milk; not for use in nursing.

MECHANISM OF ACTION
Dibenzazepine; mechanism not established. Oxcarbazepine and MHD suspected to exert antiseizure effects through blockade of voltage-sensitive Na^+ channels, resulting in stabilization of hyperexcited neural membranes, inhibition of repetitive neuronal firing, and diminution of propagation of synaptic impulses. Also, increased K^+ conductance and modulation of high-voltage activated Ca^{2+} channels may contribute to the anticonvulsant effects.

PHARMACOKINETICS
Absorption: (1200mg qd) T_{max}=7 hrs (MHD). **Distribution:** Found in breast milk. (MHD) V_d=49L; plasma protein binding (approx 40%). **Metabolism:** Liver; reduction by cytosolic enzymes to MHD (active metabolite). (MHD) Conjugation w/ glucuronic acid. **Elimination:** (IR Formulation) Urine (>95%, <1% unchanged), feces (<4%). $T_{1/2}$=7-11 hrs (oxcarbazepine), 9-11 hrs (MHD).

PATIENT CONSIDERATIONS
Assessment: Assess for hypersensitivity to drug, history of hypersensitivity to carbamazepine, depression, renal/hepatic impairment, pregnancy/nursing status, and for possible drug interactions. Consider testing for the presence of the HLA-B*1502 allele in patients w/ ancestry in genetically at-risk populations prior to initiating treatment.

Monitoring: Monitor for signs/symptoms of hyponatremia, anaphylaxis, angioedema, dermatological/hematologic reactions, emergence/worsening of depression, suicidal thoughts/behavior and/or any unusual changes in mood/

behavior, multiorgan hypersensitivity reactions, and other adverse reactions. Monitor patients during pregnancy and through the postpartum period.

Counseling: Advise to report symptoms of low Na+ and to report a fever associated w/ other organ system involvement (eg, rash, lymphadenopathy). Instruct to immediately report signs/symptoms suggesting angioedema and to d/c therapy until consulting w/ physician. Instruct to contact physician immediately if a hypersensitivity reaction, symptoms suggestive of blood disorders, or a skin reaction occurs. Inform female patients of childbearing age that concurrent use w/ hormonal contraceptives may render this method of contraception less effective; advise to use additional nonhormonal forms of contraception. Counsel that therapy may increase risk of suicidal thoughts or behavior and to be alert for emergence/worsening of symptoms of depression, any unusual changes in mood/behavior, or emergence of suicidal thoughts/behavior or thoughts about self-harm; instruct to immediately report behaviors of concern to healthcare providers. Advise to use caution if taking alcohol while on therapy, due to possible additive sedative effect. Inform that therapy may cause dizziness and somnolence; advise not to drive/operate machinery until effects have been determined. Encourage to enroll in the NAAED Pregnancy Registry if pregnancy occurs.

OXYBUTYNIN — oxybutynin chloride   Rx

Class: Anticholinergic

OTHER BRAND NAMES
Ditropan (Discontinued)

ADULT DOSAGE
Uninhibited Neurogenic or Reflex Neurogenic Bladder

Relief of Symptoms of Bladder Instability Associated with Voiding:
Usual: 5mg bid-tid
Max: 5mg qid

PEDIATRIC DOSAGE
Uninhibited Neurogenic or Reflex Neurogenic Bladder

Relief of Symptoms of Bladder Instability Associated with Voiding:
≥5 Years:
Usual: 5mg bid
Max: 5mg tid

DOSING CONSIDERATIONS
Elderly
Start at lower end of doing range

Frail Elderly:
Initial: 2.5mg bid-tid

ADMINISTRATION
Oral route

STORAGE
(Tab) 20-25°C (68-77°F). (Syrup) 15-30°C (59-86°F).

HOW SUPPLIED
Syrup: 5mg/5mL [118mL, 473mL]; **Tab:** 5mg* *scored

CONTRAINDICATIONS
Urinary retention, gastric retention and other severe decreased GI motility conditions, uncontrolled narrow-angle glaucoma, and in patients at risk for these conditions. Hypersensitivity to the drug substance or other components of the product.

WARNINGS/PRECAUTIONS
Angioedema of the face, lips, tongue, and/or larynx reported; d/c if involvement of the tongue, hypopharynx, or larynx occurs. Variety of CNS anticholinergic effects reported; consider dose reduction or discontinuation. May aggravate symptoms of hyperthyroidism, coronary heart disease (CHD), congestive heart failure (CHF), cardiac arrhythmias, hiatal hernia, tachycardia, HTN, myasthenia gravis, and prostatic hypertrophy. Caution with preexisting dementia treated with cholinesterase inhibitors, hepatic/renal impairment, myasthenia gravis, clinically significant bladder outflow obstruction, GI obstructive disorders, ulcerative colitis, intestinal atony, gastroesophageal reflux disorder, and in frail elderly.

ADVERSE REACTIONS
Dry mouth, dizziness, constipation, somnolence, nausea, blurred vision, urinary hesitation, headache, urinary tract infection, nervousness, dyspepsia, urinary retention, insomnia.

DRUG INTERACTIONS
May increase frequency and/or severity of adverse effects with other anticholinergics or with other agents that produce dry mouth, constipation, somnolence, and/or other anticholinergic effects. May alter GI absorption of other drugs due to GI motility effects; caution with drugs with narrow therapeutic index. Increased levels with ketoconazole. CYP3A4 inhibitors (eg, antimycotics, macrolides) may alter mean pharmacokinetic parameters; caution when coadministered. Caution with drugs that can cause or exacerbate esophagitis (eg, bisphosphonates).

PREGNANCY AND LACTATION
Category B, caution in nursing.

MECHANISM OF ACTION
Antispasmodic/anticholinergic agent; inhibits muscarinic action of acetylcholine on smooth muscle, exerting direct antispasmodic effect; relaxes smooth muscle of bladder.

PHARMACOKINETICS
Absorption: Rapid. Absolute bioavailability (6%); T_{max}=1 hr. Refer to PI for pediatric, isomer, and metabolite parameters. **Distribution:** (IV) V_d=193L; plasma protein binding (>99%, >97% desethyloxybutynin). **Metabolism:** Liver via CYP3A4; desethyloxybutynin (active metabolite). **Elimination:** Urine (<0.1%, unchanged; <0.1%, desethyloxybutynin); $T_{1/2}$=2-3 hrs.

PATIENT CONSIDERATIONS
Assessment: Assess for urinary and gastric retention, other severe decreased GI motility conditions, uncontrolled narrow-angle glaucoma, preexisting dementia, hepatic/renal impairment, myasthenia gravis, hyperthyroidism, CHD, CHF, hypersensitivity to the drug, other conditions where treatment is contraindicated or cautioned, pregnancy/nursing status, and possible drug interactions.

Monitoring: Monitor for aggravation of myasthenia gravis, hyperthyroidism, CHD, CHF, cardiac arrhythmias, hiatal hernia, tachycardia, HTN, and prostatic hypertrophy symptoms. Monitor for signs of anticholinergic CNS effects, hypersensitivity reactions, and other adverse reactions.

Counseling: Inform that angioedema may occur and could result in life-threatening airway obstruction; advise to promptly d/c therapy and seek medical attention if tongue/laryngopharynx edema or difficulty breathing occurs. Inform that heat prostration may occur when administered in high environmental temperature. Inform that drug may produce drowsiness or blurred vision; advise to exercise caution. Inform that alcohol may enhance drowsiness.

OXYCODONE CAPSULES — oxycodone hydrochloride   CII

Class: Opioid analgesic

ADULT DOSAGE
Moderate to Severe Pain

Acute and Chronic:
Opioid-Naive:
Initial: 5-15mg q4-6h prn
Titrate: Adjust dose based upon initial dose response
Maint: Periodically reassess the continued need for chronic therapy, especially for noncancer-related pain

PEDIATRIC DOSAGE
Pediatric use may not have been established

DOSING CONSIDERATIONS
Renal Impairment
Initiate dose conservatively and monitor closely

Hepatic Impairment
Initiate dose conservatively and monitor closely

Elderly
≥65 Years:
Start at lower end of dosing range

Discontinuation
Gradually taper dose

ADMINISTRATION
Oral route

STORAGE
25°C (77°F); excursions permitted to 15-30°C (59-86°F). Protect from moisture and light.

HOW SUPPLIED
Cap: 5mg

CONTRAINDICATIONS
Respiratory depression (in the absence of resuscitative equipment), paralytic ileus, acute or severe bronchial asthma or hypercarbia, known hypersensitivity to oxycodone, oxycodone salts, or any components of the product.

WARNINGS/PRECAUTIONS
Respiratory depression may occur; extreme caution with chronic obstructive pulmonary disease or cor pulmonale, substantially decreased respiratory reserve (eg, severe kyphoscoliosis), hypoxia, hypercapnia, preexisting respiratory depression, and in elderly/debilitated. Contains oxycodone, an opioid agonist and a Schedule II controlled substance, with an abuse liability similar to other opioids; assess patient's risk for opioid abuse or addiction prior to prescribing. Respiratory depressant effects and potential to elevate CSF pressure may be markedly exaggerated in the presence of head injury, intracranial lesions, or preexisting increased intracranial pressure (ICP). May produce effects on pupillary response and consciousness, which may obscure neurologic signs of further increases in ICP in patients with head injuries. May cause severe hypotension; caution with circulatory shock. May produce orthostatic hypotension and syncope in ambulatory patients. Avoid with GI obstruction as therapy diminishes propulsive peristaltic waves in the GI tract and may prolong the obstruction. May obscure diagnosis or clinical course in patients with acute abdominal conditions. May cause spasm of the sphincter of Oddi and diminish biliary and pancreatic secretions; caution with biliary tract disease, including acute pancreatitis. Caution with severe renal/hepatic impairment, Addison's disease, hypothyroidism, prostatic hypertrophy or urethral stricture, CNS depression, toxic psychosis, acute alcoholism, and delirium tremens. May aggravate convulsions with convulsive disorders and may induce or aggravate seizures in some clinical settings. Keep out of reach of children; seek emergency medical help immediately in cases of accidental ingestion. May impair mental/physical abilities. Not recommended for use during and immediately prior to labor.

ADVERSE REACTIONS

Respiratory depression/arrest, circulatory depression, cardiac arrest, hypotension, shock, N/V, constipation, headache, pruritus, insomnia, dizziness, asthenia, somnolence.

DRUG INTERACTIONS

Respiratory depression, hypotension, profound sedation, or coma may occur with other CNS depressants (eg, sedatives, hypnotics, general anesthetics, antiemetics, phenothiazines, tranquilizers, alcohol, other opioids); use with caution and in reduced dosages. May enhance neuromuscular blocking action of skeletal muscle relaxants and increase respiratory depression. Mixed agonist/antagonist analgesics (pentazocine, nalbuphine, butorphanol, buprenorphine) may reduce the analgesic effect and/or precipitate withdrawal symptoms; do not coadminister. CYP3A4 inhibitors, such as macrolide antibiotics (eg, erythromycin), azole-antifungal agents (eg, ketoconazole), and protease inhibitors (eg, ritonavir), may increase levels, prolonging opioid effects, while CYP3A4 inducers (eg, rifampin, carbamazepine, phenytoin) may decrease levels, leading to lack of efficacy or development of abstinence syndrome; if coadministration is necessary, use with caution, monitor patients, and consider dose adjustments. CYP2D6 inhibitors may block the partial metabolism to oxymorphone. Caution with MAOIs. Anticholinergics may increase risk of urinary retention and/or severe constipation, which may lead to paralytic ileus.

PREGNANCY AND LACTATION

Category B, not for use in nursing.

MECHANISM OF ACTION

Opioid analgesic; pure opioid agonist. Has not been established. Specific CNS opioid receptors for endogenous compounds with oxycodone-like activity have been identified throughout the brain and spinal cord and play a role in analgesic effects.

PHARMACOKINETICS

Absorption: Bioavailability (60-87%). **Distribution:** V_d=2.6L/kg (IV); plasma protein binding (45%); found in breast milk. **Metabolism:** Liver (extensive); N-demethylation via CYP3A4 to noroxycodone (major metabolite); O-demethylation via CYP2D6 to oxymorphone. **Elimination:** Urine; $T_{1/2}$=4 hrs.

PATIENT CONSIDERATIONS

Assessment: Assess for level of pain intensity, type of pain, patient's general condition and medical status, or any other conditions where treatment is contraindicated or cautioned. Assess for history of hypersensitivity, pregnancy/nursing status, renal/hepatic function, and possible drug interactions.

Monitoring: Monitor for signs/symptoms of respiratory depression, hypotension, convulsions/seizures, spasm of sphincter of Oddi, tolerance, physical dependence, and other adverse reactions.

Counseling: Instruct to take drug ud. Advise not to adjust dose without consulting physician. Inform that drug may impair mental/physical abilities. Counsel to avoid alcohol or other CNS depressants. Advise to consult physician if pregnant or planning to become pregnant. Inform that if taking medication for more than a few weeks, to avoid abrupt withdrawal; dosing will need to be tapered. Inform that drug has potential for abuse and should be protected from theft. Instruct to destroy unused cap by flushing down the toilet. Advise of the potential for severe constipation. Counsel on what to do if a dose is missed.

OXYCODONE ORAL SOLUTION — oxycodone

hydrochloride   **CII**

Class: Opioid analgesic

> The 100mg/5mL (20mg/mL) concentration is indicated for use in opioid-tolerant patients only. Use caution when prescribing and administering to avoid dosing errors due to confusion between mg and mL, and other oxycodone solutions with different concentrations, which could result in accidental overdose and death. Use caution to ensure the proper dose is communicated and dispensed. Keep out of reach of children; seek emergency medical help immediately in case of accidental ingestion.

ADULT DOSAGE

Moderate to Severe Pain

Opioid-Naive:

5mg/5mL:

Initial: 5-15mg q4-6h prn

Titrate: Adjust dose based upon initial dose response

Maint: Periodically reassess continued need for chronic therapy, especially for noncancer-related pain (or pain associated w/ other terminal illnesses)

Opioid Tolerant:

100mg/5mL:

Only use this strength for patients that have already been titrated to a stable analgesic regimen using lower strengths of oxycodone and can benefit from use of a smaller volume of oral sol

PEDIATRIC DOSAGE

Pediatric use may not have been established

DOSING CONSIDERATIONS

Renal Impairment

Initiate dose conservatively and monitor closely

Hepatic Impairment

Initiate dose conservatively and monitor closely

Elderly

≥65 Years:

Start at lower end of dosing range

Discontinuation

Gradually taper dose

ADMINISTRATION

Oral route

Always use the enclosed calibrated oral syringe to administer dose

STORAGE

25°C (77°F); excursions permitted to 15-30°C (59-86°F). Protect from moisture and light.

HOW SUPPLIED

Sol: 5mg/5mL [5mL, 100mL, 500mL], 100mg/5mL [30mL]

CONTRAINDICATIONS

Respiratory depression (in the absence of resuscitative equipment), paralytic ileus, acute or severe bronchial asthma or hypercarbia, known hypersensitivity to oxycodone, oxycodone salts, or any components of the product.

WARNINGS/PRECAUTIONS

Respiratory depression may occur; extreme caution with chronic obstructive pulmonary disease or cor pulmonale, substantially decreased respiratory reserve (eg, severe kyphoscoliosis), hypoxia, hypercapnia, preexisting respiratory depression, and in elderly/debilitated. Contains oxycodone, an opioid agonist and a Schedule II controlled substance, with an abuse liability similar to other opioids. Respiratory depressant effects and potential to elevate CSF pressure may be markedly exaggerated in the presence of head injury, intracranial lesions, or preexisting increased intracranial pressure (ICP). May produce effects on pupillary response and consciousness, which may obscure neurologic signs of further increases in ICP in patients with head injuries. May cause severe hypotension; caution with circulatory shock. May produce orthostatic hypotension and syncope in ambulatory patients. Avoid with GI obstruction as therapy diminishes propulsive peristaltic waves in the GI tract and may prolong the obstruction. May obscure diagnosis or clinical course in patients with acute abdominal condition. May cause spasm of the sphincter of Oddi and diminish biliary and pancreatic secretions; caution with biliary tract disease, including acute pancreatitis. Caution with renal/hepatic impairment, Addison's disease, hypothyroidism, prostatic hypertrophy or urethral stricture, CNS depression, toxic psychosis, acute alcoholism, and delirium tremens. May aggravate convulsions with convulsive disorders and may induce or aggravate seizures in some clinical settings. May impair mental/physical abilities. Not recommended for use during and immediately prior to labor.

ADVERSE REACTIONS

Respiratory depression/arrest, circulatory depression, cardiac arrest, hypotension, shock, N/V, constipation, headache, pruritus, insomnia, dizziness, asthenia, somnolence.

DRUG INTERACTIONS

Respiratory depression, hypotension, profound sedation, or coma may occur with other CNS depressants (eg, sedatives, hypnotics, general anesthetics, antiemetics, phenothiazines, tranquilizers, alcohol, other opioids); use with caution and in reduced dosages. May enhance neuromuscular blocking action of skeletal muscle relaxants and increase respiratory depression. Mixed agonist/antagonist analgesics (pentazocine, nalbuphine, butorphanol, buprenorphine) may reduce the analgesic effect and/or precipitate withdrawal symptoms; do not administer mixed agonist/antagonist analgesics to patients who have received or are receiving therapy. CYP3A4 inhibitors, such as macrolide antibiotics (eg, erythromycin), azole-antifungal agents (eg, ketoconazole), and protease inhibitors (eg, ritonavir), may increase levels, prolonging opioid effects, while CYP3A4 inducers (eg, rifampin, carbamazepine, phenytoin) may decrease levels, leading to lack of efficacy or development of abstinence syndrome; if coadministration is necessary, use with caution, monitor patients, and consider dose adjustments. CYP2D6 inhibitors may block the partial metabolism to oxymorphone. Caution with MAOIs. Anticholinergics may increase risk of urinary retention and/or severe constipation, which may lead to paralytic ileus.

PREGNANCY AND LACTATION

Category B, not for use in nursing.

MECHANISM OF ACTION

Opioid analgesic; pure opioid agonist. Has not been established. Specific CNS opioid receptors for endogenous compounds with opioid-like activity have been identified throughout the brain and spinal cord and play a role in analgesic effects.

PHARMACOKINETICS

Absorption: Absolute bioavailability (60-87%). **Distribution:** V_d=2.6L/kg (IV); plasma protein binding (45%); found in breast milk; crosses placenta. **Metabolism:** Extensive; N-demethylation via CYP3A4 to noroxycodone (major metabolite); O-demethylation via CYP2D6 to oxymorphone. **Elimination:** Urine; $T_{1/2}$=4 hrs.

PATIENT CONSIDERATIONS

Assessment: Assess for level of pain intensity, type of pain, patient's general condition and medical status, or any other conditions where treatment is contraindicated or cautioned. Assess for drug hypersensitivity, renal/hepatic impairment, pregnancy/nursing status, and possible drug interactions.

Monitoring: Monitor for signs/symptoms of respiratory depression, hypotension, convulsions/seizures, spasm of sphincter of Oddi, tolerance, physical dependence, and other adverse reactions. Periodically reassess the continued need for therapy.

Counseling: Instruct to take drug ud and how to measure and take the correct dose. Advise not to adjust dose without consulting physician. Inform that drug may impair mental/physical abilities required for the performance of potentially hazardous tasks (eg, operating machinery/driving). Counsel to avoid alcohol or other CNS depressants. Advise to consult physician if pregnant or planning to become pregnant. Inform that if taking medication for more than a few weeks and need to d/c therapy, to avoid abrupt withdrawal as dosing will need to be tapered. Inform that drug has potential for abuse and must be protected from theft. Instruct to destroy unused solution by flushing down the toilet. Advise of the potential for severe constipation.

OXYCODONE TABLETS — oxycodone hydrochloride   CII

Class: Opioid analgesic

OTHER BRAND NAMES
Roxicodone

ADULT DOSAGE	PEDIATRIC DOSAGE
Moderate to Severe Pain	Pediatric use may not have been
Opioid-Naive:	established
Initial: 5-15mg q4-6h prn	
Titrate: Adjust dose based upon response	
For chronic pain, give on an around-the-clock basis	
For severe chronic pain, give q4-6h at the lowest effective dose	
Conversions	
From Fixed-Ratio Opioid/ Acetaminophen, Opioid/Aspirin, or Opioid/Nonsteroidal Combination Drugs:	
Decision should be made whether or not to continue the nonopioid analgesic	
Discontinuing Nonopioid Analgesic:	
May be necessary to titrate to the minimum effective dose	
Continuing Nonopioid Regimen as a Separate Single Entity Agent:	
Starting dose of oxycodone should be based upon the most recent dose of opioid as a baseline for further titration of oxycodone Incremental increases should be gauged according to side effects to an acceptable level of analgesia	
From Other Opioids:	
Factor the potency of the prior opioid relative to oxycodone to select the total daily dose Closely observe and adjust dose based on response	

DOSING CONSIDERATIONS
Renal Impairment
Initial: Dose conservatively
Titrate: Adjust according to clinical situation

Hepatic Impairment
Initial: Dose conservatively
Titrate: Adjust according to clinical situation

Discontinuation
D/C gradually; decrease by 25-50% per day
Raise dose to previous level and titrate down more slowly if withdrawal symptoms occur

ADMINISTRATION
Oral route

STORAGE
25°C (77°F); excursions permitted to 15-30°C (59-86°F). Protect from moisture.

HOW SUPPLIED
Tab: 10mg*, 20mg*; (Roxicodone) 5mg*, 15mg*, 30mg* *scored

CONTRAINDICATIONS
Known hypersensitivity to oxycodone, significant respiratory depression (in unmonitored settings or the absence of resuscitative equipment), paralytic ileus, acute or severe bronchial asthma or hypercarbia.

WARNINGS/PRECAUTIONS
Respiratory depression may occur; extreme caution with significant chronic obstructive pulmonary disease or cor pulmonale, substantially decreased respiratory reserve, hypoxia, hypercapnia, preexisting respiratory depression, and in the elderly/debilitated. May cause severe hypotension; caution with circulatory shock. May produce orthostatic hypotension in ambulatory patients. Respiratory depressant effects and capacity to elevate CSF pressure may be markedly exaggerated in the presence of head injury, other intracranial lesions, or preexisting increased intracranial pressure. May obscure the clinical course of patients with head injuries. Caution with acute alcoholism, adrenocortical insufficiency (eg, Addison's disease), convulsive disorders, CNS depression or coma, delirium tremens, kyphoscoliosis associated with respiratory depression, myxedema or hypothyroidism, prostatic hypertrophy or urethral stricture, severe hepatic/renal/pulmonary impairment, and toxic psychosis. May obscure diagnosis or clinical course in patients with acute abdominal conditions. May aggravate convulsions with convulsive disorders and may induce or aggravate seizures in some clinical settings. Potential for tolerance and physical dependence. May cause spasm of the sphincter of Oddi; caution with biliary tract disease, including acute pancreatitis. May cause increases in serum amylase level. Not recommended for use during or immediately prior to labor. May impair mental/physical abilities.

ADVERSE REACTIONS
Respiratory depression/arrest, circulatory depression, cardiac arrest, hypotension, shock, N/V, constipation, headache, pruritus, insomnia, dizziness, asthenia, somnolence.

DRUG INTERACTIONS
CYP2D6 inhibitors may block the partial metabolism to oxymorphone. May enhance neuromuscular blocking action of skeletal muscle relaxants and increase respiratory depression. Additive CNS depression with other CNS depressants (eg, narcotics, general anesthetics, tranquilizers, alcohol); when combination is contemplated, reduce dose of one or both agents. Mixed agonist/antagonist analgesics (eg, pentazocine, nalbuphine, buprenorphine) may reduce analgesic effect and/or precipitate withdrawal symptoms. Not recommended with MAOIs or within 14 days of stopping such treatment. May cause severe hypotension with phenothiazines or other agents that compromise vasomotor tone. Muscle relaxants (eg, cyclobenzaprine), MAOIs (eg, phenelzine), and antidepressants (eg, TCAs, SSRIs, SNRIs) may enhance serotonergic activity, resulting in the development of serotonin syndrome.

PREGNANCY AND LACTATION
Category B, not for use in nursing.

MECHANISM OF ACTION
Opioid analgesic; pure opioid agonist. Has not been established. Specific CNS opioid receptors for endogenous compounds with opioid-like activity have been identified throughout the brain and spinal cord and play a role in analgesic effects.

PHARMACOKINETICS
Absorption: Absolute bioavailability (60-87%). Administration of multiple doses resulted in different parameters. **Distribution:** V_d=2.6L/kg (IV); plasma protein binding (45%); found in breast milk. **Metabolism:** Extensively metabolized to noroxycodone (major metabolite), oxymorphone (via CYP2D6), and their glucuronides. **Elimination:** Urine; $T_{1/2}$=3.5-4 hrs.

PATIENT CONSIDERATIONS
Assessment: Assess for level of pain intensity, type of pain, patient's general condition and medical status, or any other conditions where treatment is contraindicated or cautioned. Assess for drug hypersensitivity, renal/hepatic/pulmonary impairment, pregnancy/nursing status, and possible drug interactions.

Monitoring: Monitor for signs/symptoms of respiratory depression, hypotension, convulsions/seizures, spasm of the sphincter of Oddi, increases in serum amylase levels, tolerance, physical dependence, and other adverse reactions. Reassess the continued need for therapy.

Counseling: Advise to report episodes of breakthrough pain and adverse experiences occurring during therapy. Instruct to not adjust the dose without consulting physician. Inform that drug may impair mental/physical abilities required for the performance of potentially hazardous tasks. Counsel to avoid alcohol or other CNS depressants, except by the order of physician. Advise to consult physician regarding effects when used during pregnancy. Inform that drug has potential for abuse and should be protected from theft and never be given to anyone other than for whom it was prescribed. Counsel that if taking medication for more than a few weeks and need to d/c therapy, to avoid abrupt withdrawal, as dosing will need to be tapered.

OXYCONTIN — oxycodone hydrochloride   CII

Class: Opioid analgesic

> Exposes users to risks of addiction, abuse, and misuse, leading to overdose and death; assess each patient's risk prior to prescribing and monitor regularly for development of these behaviors/conditions. Serious, life-threatening, or fatal respiratory depression may occur; monitor during initiation or following a dose increase. Crushing, dissolving, or chewing tab can cause rapid release and absorption of potentially fatal dose; instruct patients to swallow tab whole. Accidental ingestion, especially by children, can result in a fatal overdose. Prolonged use during pregnancy can result in neonatal opioid withdrawal syndrome; advise pregnant women of the risk and ensure availability of appropriate treatment. Concomitant use of CYP3A4 inhibitors or discontinuation of CYP3A4 inducers can result in oxycodone overdose; monitor patients receiving concomitant CYP3A4 inhibitors/inducers.

ADULT DOSAGE	PEDIATRIC DOSAGE
Severe Pain (Daily, Around-the-Clock Management)	**Severe Pain (Daily, Around-the-Clock Management)**
1st Opioid Analgesic/Opioid-Intolerant Patients:	Use in patients ≥11 yrs already receiving and tolerating opioids for
Initial: 10mg q12h	at least 5 consecutive days; for the 2

Titrate: Increase total daily dose by 25-50% every 1-2 days when clinically indicated

Conversions

From Other Oral Oxycodone Formulations:
Administer 1/2 of total daily dose q12h

From Other Opioids:
D/C all other around-the-clock opioids when therapy is initiated and initiate dosing using 10mg q12h

From Transdermal Fentanyl:
Initiate treatment 18 hrs following removal of patch; 10mg q12h should be initially substituted for each 25mcg/hr fentanyl transdermal patch

days immediately preceding dosing w/ Oxycontin, patients must be taking a minimum of 20mg/day of oxycodone or its equivalent

Do not use if opioid requirement is <20mg/day; d/c all other opioids when initiating therapy

Conversion Formula:
Mg/Day of Prior Opioid x Conversion Factor = Mg/Day of Oxycontin

Divide the calculated total daily dose by 2 to get the q12h dose

Conversion Factors:
Oxycodone: 1
Hydrocodone: 0.9
Hydromorphone: 4 (oral), 20 (parenteral)
Morphine: 0.5 (oral), 3 (parenteral)
Tramadol: 0.17 (oral), 0.2 (parenteral)

For patients receiving high-dose parenteral opioids, a more conservative conversion is warranted; for high-dose parenteral morphine, use 1.5 instead of 3 as a multiplication factor

For patients taking ≥1 opioid, calculate the approx oxycodone dose for each opioid and sum the totals to obtain the approx Oxycontin daily dosage

For patients on a regimen of fixed-ratio opioid/nonopioid analgesic products, use only the opioid component of these products in the conversion

If using asymmetric dosing, give higher dose in the am and the lower dose in the pm

Conversion from Transdermal Fentanyl:
Initiate treatment 18 hrs following removal of patch; 10mg q12h should be initially substituted for each 25mcg/hr fentanyl transdermal patch

Initial: Round down to the nearest Oxycontin dose; if the rounded calculated dose is <20mg, do not initiate

Titrate: Increase total daily dose by 25% every 1-2 days when clinically indicated

----

DOSING CONSIDERATIONS
Concomitant Medications
If patient is currently on a CNS depressant, initiate Oxycontin at 1/3 to 1/2 the recommended starting dose and monitor

Hepatic Impairment
Initiate at 1/3 to 1/2 the recommended starting dose, followed by careful dose titration

Elderly
Reduce starting dose to 1/3 to 1/2 the recommended dose in debilitated, opioid-intolerant patients

Discontinuation
Use gradual downward titration

ADMINISTRATION
Oral route

Do not presoak, lick, or otherwise wet tab prior to placing in mouth. Swallow tab whole; do not crush, dissolve, or chew. Take 1 tab at a time w/ enough water to ensure complete swallowing.

STORAGE
25°C (77°F); excursions permitted to 15-30°C (59-86°F).

HOW SUPPLIED
Tab, Extended-Release: 10mg, 15mg, 20mg, 30mg, 40mg, 60mg, 80mg

CONTRAINDICATIONS
Significant respiratory depression, acute or severe bronchial asthma in unmonitored settings or in the absence of resuscitative equipment, known or suspected paralytic ileus and GI obstruction, hypersensitivity (eg, anaphylaxis) to oxycodone.

WARNINGS/PRECAUTIONS
Reserve use in patients for whom alternative treatment options are ineffective, not tolerated, or would be otherwise inadequate to provide sufficient management of pain. Should only be prescribed by healthcare professionals who are knowledgeable in the use of potent opioids for management of chronic pain. 60mg and 80mg tabs, a single dose >40mg, or a total daily dose >80mg are only for use in opioid-tolerant patients. Life-threatening respiratory depression is more likely to occur in elderly, cachectic, or debilitated patients. Consider alternative nonopioid analgesics in patients w/ significant COPD or cor pulmonale, and in patients having a substantially decreased respiratory reserve, hypoxia, hypercapnia, or preexisting respiratory depression. May cause severe hypotension, orthostatic hypotension, and syncope; increased risk in patients whose ability to maintain BP has already been compromised by a reduced blood volume or concurrent administration of certain CNS depressants. Avoid w/ circulatory shock. Monitor patients who may be susceptible to intracranial effects of carbon dioxide retention for signs of sedation and respiratory depression when initiating therapy. Therapy may obscure clinical course in patient w/ head injury. Avoid w/ impaired consciousness or coma. Difficulty in swallowing tab, intestinal obstruction, and exacerbation of diverticulitis reported; consider alternative analgesic in patients who have difficulty swallowing or have underlying GI disorders that may predispose them to obstruction. May cause spasm of sphincter of Oddi and increase in serum amylase; monitor patients w/ biliary tract disease. May aggravate convulsions and induce/aggravate seizures. May impair mental or physical abilities. Urine drug test may not detect oxycodone reliably. Not recommended for use immediately prior to labor.

ADVERSE REACTIONS
Respiratory depression, constipation, N/V, somnolence, dizziness, pruritus, headache, dry mouth, asthenia, sweating, apnea, respiratory arrest, circulatory depression, hypotension.

DRUG INTERACTIONS
See Boxed Warning. Respiratory depression, hypotension, and profound sedation or coma may occur w/ CNS depressants (eg, sedatives, anxiolytics, neuroleptics); if coadministration is required, consider dose reduction of one or both agents. Monitor use in elderly, cachectic, and debilitated patients when coadministered w/ other drugs that depress respiration. May enhance neuromuscular blocking action of true skeletal muscle relaxants and increase respiratory depression. CYP3A4 inhibitors (eg, erythromycin, ketoconazole, ritonavir) may increase levels of oxycodone and prolong opioid effects; these effects could be more pronounced w/ concomitant use of CYP2D6 and 3A4 inhibitors. CYP3A4 inducers (eg, rifampin, carbamazepine, phenytoin) may decrease levels and cause lack of efficacy, or development of abstinence syndrome. If coadministration is necessary, use w/ caution when initiating oxycodone treatment in patients currently taking or discontinuing CYP3A4 inhibitors/inducers. Mixed agonist/antagonists (eg, pentazocine, nalbuphine, butorphanol) or partial agonists (buprenorphine) may reduce analgesic effect or precipitate withdrawal symptoms; avoid coadministration. May reduce efficacy of diuretics and lead to acute urinary retention. Anticholinergics or other medications w/ anticholinergic activity may increase risk of urinary retention and/or severe constipation and lead to paralytic ileus.

PREGNANCY AND LACTATION
Pregnancy: Category C.
Lactation: Not for use in nursing.

MECHANISM OF ACTION
Full opioid agonist; not established. Specific CNS opioid receptors have been identified throughout the brain and spinal cord and are thought to play a role in analgesic effect.

PHARMACOKINETICS
Absorption: Oral bioavailability (60-87%). Administration of variable doses resulted in different parameters. **Distribution:** V_d=2.6L/kg (IV); plasma protein binding (45%); crosses placenta; found in breast milk. **Metabolism:** Extensive; via CYP3A mediated N-demethylation to noroxycodone and CYP2D6 mediated O-demethylation to oxymorphone; noroxycodone and noroxymorphone (major metabolites). **Elimination:** Urine; $T_{1/2}$=4.5 hrs.

PATIENT CONSIDERATIONS
Assessment: Assess for abuse/addiction risk, pain intensity, prior opioid therapy, opioid tolerance, respiratory depression, drug hypersensitivity, pregnancy/nursing status, possible drug interactions, or any other conditions where treatment is contraindicated or cautioned.

Monitoring: Monitor for respiratory depression (especially w/in first 24-72 hrs of initiation), hypotension, seizures/convulsions, and other adverse reactions. Monitor BP and serum amylase levels. Routinely monitor for signs of misuse, abuse, and addiction. Periodically reassess the continued need for therapy.

Counseling: Inform that use of drug can result in addiction, abuse, and misuse; instruct not to share w/ others and to take steps to protect from theft or misuse. Inform patients about risk of respiratory depression. Advise to store securely and dispose unused tabs by flushing down the toilet. Inform female patients of reproductive potential that prolonged use during pregnancy may result in neonatal opioid withdrawal syndrome and instruct to inform physician if pregnant or planning to become pregnant. Inform that potentially serious additive effects may occur when used w/ CNS depressants, and not to use such drugs unless supervised by healthcare provider. Instruct about proper administration instructions. Inform that drug may cause orthostatic hypotension, syncope, or may impair the ability to perform potentially hazardous activities; advise to not perform such tasks until they know how they will react to medication. Advise of potential for severe constipation, including management instructions. Advise how to recognize anaphylaxis and when to seek medical attention. Advise caregivers to strictly adhere to dosing when giving to pediatric patients.

PAMIDRONATE — pamidronate disodium

Rx

Class: Bisphosphonate

OTHER BRAND NAMES
Aredia (Discontinued)

ADULT DOSAGE

Hypercalcemia of Malignancy

In conjunction w/ adequate hydration for moderate or severe hypercalcemia associated w/ malignancy, w/ or w/o bone metastases

Moderate Hypercalcemia (Corrected Serum Ca²⁺ 12-13.5mg/dL):
Usual: 60-90mg single dose IV infusion over 2-24 hrs
Max: 90mg/single dose

Severe Hypercalcemia (Corrected Serum Ca²⁺ >13.5mg/dL):
Usual: 90mg single dose IV infusion over 2-24 hrs
Max: 90mg/single dose

Longer infusions (eg, >2 hours) may reduce the risk for renal toxicity, particularly in patients w/ preexisting renal insufficiency

Retreatment:
May be carried out in patients who show complete or partial response initially, if serum Ca²⁺ does not return to normal or remain normal after initial treatment; a minimum of 7 days should elapse before retreatment, to allow for full response to initial dose. The dose and manner of retreatment is identical to that of the initial therapy

Paget's Disease

Moderate to Severe:
Usual: 30mg/day as a 4-hr infusion on 3 consecutive days for a total dose of 90mg
Max: 90mg/single dose

Retreatment:
When indicated, retreat at the dose of initial therapy

Osteolytic Bone Metastases of Breast Cancer

In Conjunction w/ Standard Antineoplastic Therapy:
Usual: 90mg over a 2-hr infusion every 3-4 weeks
Max: 90mg/single dose

Pamidronate disodium has been frequently used w/ doxorubicin, fluorouracil, cyclophosphamide, methotrexate, mitoxantrone, vinblastine, dexamethasone, prednisone, melphalan, vincristine, megestrol, and tamoxifen

Osteolytic Bone Lesions of Multiple Myeloma

In Conjunction w/ Standard Antineoplastic Therapy:
Usual: 90mg as a 4-hr infusion given on a monthly basis
Max: 90mg/single dose

Patients with marked Bence-Jones proteinuria and dehydration should receive adequate hydration prior to pamidronate disodium infusion

PEDIATRIC DOSAGE

Pediatric use may not have been established

- -

DOSING CONSIDERATIONS

Renal Impairment
Osteolytic Bone Lesions of Multiple Myeloma/Osteolytic Bone Metastases of Breast Cancer:
Withhold treatment for renal deterioration and resume only when the creatinine returns to w/in 10% of baseline value

Renal deterioration is defined as follows:
For Patients w/ Normal Baseline Creatinine: Increase of 0.5mg/dL
For Patients w/ Abnormal Baseline Creatinine: Increase of 1mg/dL

Elderly
Start at lower end of dosing range

ADMINISTRATION
IV route
Do not mix w/ Ca²⁺-containing infusion sol (eg, Ringer's sol)
Administer in a single IV sol and line separate from all other drugs

Hypercalcemia of Malignancy
Avoid overhydration in patients w/ potential for cardiac failure
Administer daily dose as an IV infusion over at least 2-24 hrs for 60mg and 90mg doses
Dilute recommended dose in 1000mL of sterile 0.45% or 0.9% NaCl or D5 inj
Infusion sol is stable for up to 24 hrs at room temperature

Paget's Disease
Dilute recommended daily dose of 30mg in 500mL of sterile 0.45% or 0.9% NaCl or D5 inj

Osteolytic Bone Metastases of Breast Cancer
Dilute recommended dose of 90mg in 250mL of sterile 0.45% or 0.9% NaCl or D5 inj

Osteolytic Bone Lesions of Multiple Myeloma
Dilute recommended dose of 90mg in 500mL of sterile 0.45% or 0.9% NaCl or D5 inj

STORAGE
20-25°C (68-77°F).

HOW SUPPLIED
Inj: 3mg/mL, 6mg/mL, 9mg/mL [10mL]

CONTRAINDICATIONS
Clinically significant hypersensitivity to pamidronate disodium or other bisphosphonates.

WARNINGS/PRECAUTIONS
Patients with marked Bence-Jones proteinuria and dehydration should receive adequate hydration prior to infusion. Avoid overhydration in patients with hypercalcemia of malignancy who have potential for cardiac failure. Renal deterioration, progression to renal failure, and dialysis reported in patients after the initial or a single dose administration. Focal segmental glomerulosclerosis (including the collapsing variant) with or without nephrotic syndrome, which may lead to renal failure, has been reported, particularly in the setting of multiple myeloma and breast cancer. Avoid use during pregnancy; may cause fetal harm. Cases of asymptomatic hypophosphatemia, hypokalemia, hypomagnesemia, and hypocalcemia reported; rare cases of symptomatic hypocalcemia (including tetany) reported. Short-term Ca²⁺ therapy may be necessary if hypocalcemia occurs. Patients with a history of thyroid surgery may have relative hypoparathyroidism that may predispose to hypocalcemia. Not recommended in patients with bone metastases with severe renal impairment. Osteonecrosis of the jaw (ONJ) reported, predominantly in cancer patients; maintain good oral hygiene and perform dental exam with preventive dentistry prior to treatment and if possible, avoid invasive dental procedures while on treatment. Severe and occasionally incapacitating bone, joint, and/or muscle pain reported. Atypical subtrochanteric and diaphyseal femoral fractures reported; examine contralateral femur in patients who have sustained femoral shaft fracture. Any patient with a history of bisphosphonate exposure who presents with thigh/groin pain in the absence of trauma should be suspected of having an atypical fracture and should be evaluated; consider discontinuation in patients suspected to have an atypical femur fracture. Carefully monitor patients with preexisting anemia, leukopenia, or thrombocytopenia in the first 2 weeks post-treatment. Caution in elderly.

ADVERSE REACTIONS
Infusion-site reaction (eg, redness, swelling, induration, pain on palpation), fever, N/V, anorexia, constipation, dizziness, headache, paresthesia, increased sweating, somnolence, anemia.

DRUG INTERACTIONS
Caution when used with other potentially nephrotoxic drugs. Concomitant use with thalidomide may increase the risk of renal dysfunction in multiple myeloma.

PREGNANCY AND LACTATION
Category D, caution in nursing.

MECHANISM OF ACTION
Bisphosphonate; has not been established. Adsorbs to calcium phosphate crystals in bone and may directly block dissolution of this mineral component of bone. Inhibits osteoclast activity that contributes to inhibition of bone resorption.

PHARMACOKINETICS
Elimination: Urine (46%, unchanged); $T_{1/2}$=28 hrs.

PATIENT CONSIDERATIONS

Assessment: Assess for dehydration, hypersensitivity to the drug or other bisphosphonates, cardiac failure, renal impairment, history of thyroid surgery, anemia, leukopenia, thrombocytopenia, pregnancy/nursing status, and for possible drug interactions. Assess SrCr prior to each treatment. Obtain dental exam with preventive dentistry prior to treatment in cancer patients.

Monitoring: Monitor for renal toxicity, ONJ, musculoskeletal pain, atypical femur fracture, and other adverse reactions. Monitor standard hypercalcemia-related metabolic parameters (eg, serum Ca²⁺, phosphate, Mg²⁺, K⁺), electrolyte levels, CBC, differential, and Hct/Hgb. Monitor patients with preexisting anemia, leukopenia, or thrombocytopenia in the first 2 weeks post-treatment.

Counseling: Inform of the risks/benefits of therapy.

PARAGARD — copper Rx

Class: Intrauterine copper contraceptive

ADULT DOSAGE	PEDIATRIC DOSAGE
Contraception	**Contraception**
Place 1 sterile unit at the fundus of the uterine cavity at any time during cycle. Remove on or before 10 yrs from date of insertion	**>16 Years (Post-Menarche):** Place 1 sterile unit at the fundus of the uterine cavity at any time during cycle. Remove on or before 10 yrs from date of insertion

ADMINISTRATION

Intrauterine route

Before Placement

Establish the size and position of the uterus by pelvic examination
The uterus should sound to a depth of 6-9cm except when inserting immediately post-abortion or post-partum
Insertion into a uterine cavity <6cm may increase incidence of expulsion, bleeding, pain, and perforation

Placement

1. Fold the 2 horizontal arms of ParaGard against the stem and push the tips of the arms securely into the inserter tube; do not bend the arms earlier than 5 min before it is to be placed in the uterus
2. Introduce the solid white rod into the insertion tube from the bottom, alongside the threads
3. Pass the loaded insertion tube through the cervical canal until it just touches the fundus of the uterus
4. Hold the solid white rod steady and withdraw the insertion tube no more than 1cm to release the arms
5. Gently and carefully move the insertion tube upward toward the top of the uterus until slight resistance is felt
6. Hold the insertion tube steady and withdraw the solid white rod from the cervical canal; only the threads should be visible
7. Trim the threads so that 3-4cm protrude into the vagina

STORAGE

15-30°C (59-86°F).

HOW SUPPLIED

Intrauterine Insert: 313.4mg

CONTRAINDICATIONS

Pregnancy or suspicion of pregnancy, uterine abnormalities resulting in distortion of the uterine cavity, acute pelvic inflammatory disease (PID) or current behavior suggesting a high risk for PID, postpartum or postabortal endometritis in the past 3 months, known or suspected uterine or cervical malignancy, genital bleeding of unknown etiology, mucopurulent cervicitis, Wilson's disease, previously placed IUD that has not been removed.

WARNINGS/PRECAUTIONS

Should be placed and removed only by healthcare professionals who are experienced with product procedures. Evaluate for ectopic pregnancy and remove device (if string is visible) if pregnancy occurs. Increased risk of spontaneous abortion, premature delivery/labor, sepsis, septic shock, and (rare) death if pregnancy occurs and device is left in place. May increase risk of PID and actinomycosis; promptly assess and treat if signs/symptoms of PID develop. Not recommended for women at high risk for sexual infection. Avoid in women with AIDS unless clinically stable on antiretroviral therapy. Partial penetration or embedment of IUD in the myometrium may make removal difficult. Remove promptly if uterine wall or cervix perforation occurs; may lead to intraperitoneal adhesions. Intestinal penetration/obstruction and/or damage to adjacent organs may result if IUD is left in the peritoneal cavity. Expulsion may occur, usually during menses and in 1st few months after insertion, especially in nulliparous patients; unintended pregnancy may occur if unnoticed. May exacerbate Wilson's disease. Evaluate, treat, and consider discontinuation in women complaining of heavy vaginal bleeding. Vasovagal reactions, including fainting, may occur immediately after insertion. Increased risk of expulsion following placement immediately after delivery or abortion. Increased risk of perforation when inserted during 1st postpartum month (except for immediately after delivery); delay insertion to the 2nd postpartum month, unless done immediately postpartum. Medical diathermy may cause heat injury to surrounding tissue. May increase risk of perforation and expulsion if lactating.

ADVERSE REACTIONS

Intrauterine/ectopic pregnancy, septic abortion, pelvic infection, perforation, embedment, anemia, backache, dysmenorrhea, dyspareunia, leukorrhea, prolonged menstrual flow, menstrual spotting, cramping, vaginitis.

PREGNANCY AND LACTATION

Contraindicated in pregnancy, safe in nursing.

MECHANISM OF ACTION

Intrauterine copper contraceptive; copper enhances contraceptive efficacy by interfering with sperm transport and fertilization of an egg, and possibly preventing implantation.

PATIENT CONSIDERATIONS

Assessment: Assess for uterine abnormalities, acute PID or current behavior suggesting a high risk for PID, postpartum/postabortal endometritis, uterine/cervical malignancy, genital bleeding of unknown etiology, Wilson's disease, mucopurulent cervicitis, allergy to any component of IUD, presence of IUD, AIDS, and pregnancy/nursing status.

Monitoring: Monitor for intrauterine/ectopic pregnancy, septic abortion, PID, actinomycosis, embedment, perforation, expulsion, heavy vaginal bleeding, vasovagal reactions, allergic reactions, infection, and other adverse reactions. Check that IUD is in place following the 1st post-insertion menstrual period.

Counseling: Counsel that product does not protect against HIV infection (AIDS) and other sexually transmitted diseases (STDs). Inform about risks/benefits of using the device and other methods of contraception. Instruct to promptly report symptoms of infection, pregnancy, or missing strings.

PARCOPA — carbidopa/levodopa Rx

Class: Dopa-decarboxylase inhibitor/dopamine precursor

ADULT DOSAGE	PEDIATRIC DOSAGE
Parkinsonism	Pediatric use may not have been established

Treatment of Symptoms of Idiopathic Parkinson's Disease (Paralysis Agitans), Postencephalitic Parkinsonism, and Symptomatic Parkinsonism That May Follow Injury to the Nervous System by Carbon Monoxide Intoxication/Manganese Intoxication:

Initial: One 25mg/100mg tab tid or one 10mg/100mg tab tid-qid
Titrate: May increase by 1 tab (25mg/100mg or 10mg/100mg) qd or qod, as necessary, until a dose of 8 tabs/day is reached

Transfer from Levodopa:
D/C levodopa at least 12 hrs before starting therapy; choose a daily dose that will provide approx 25% of previous levodopa dose
Previously Taking <1500mg/day of Levodopa:
Initial: One 25mg/100mg tab tid or qid
Previously Taking >1500mg/day of Levodopa:
Initial: One 25mg/250mg tab tid or qid

Maint:
At least 70-100mg/day of carbidopa should be provided; may substitute one 25mg/100mg tab for each 10mg/100mg tab when greater proportion of carbidopa is required
When more levodopa is required, substitute 25mg/250mg tab for 25mg/100mg or 10mg/100mg; may increase dose of 25mg/250mg by 1/2 or 1 tab qd or qod to a max of 8 tabs/day if necessary

Max: 200mg/day of carbidopa

DOSING CONSIDERATIONS

Concomitant Medications

Addition of Other Antiparkinsonian Medications:
Standard drugs for Parkinson's disease, other than levodopa w/o a decarboxylase inhibitor, may be used concomitantly w/ therapy, although dosage adjustments may be required

Interruption of Therapy:

If general anesthesia is required, may continue therapy as long as patient is permitted to take fluids and medication by mouth. If therapy is interrupted temporarily, observe for symptoms resembling neuroleptic malignant syndrome, and administer usual daily dose as soon as patient is able to take oral medication

Adverse Reactions

Involuntary movements may require dosage reduction

ADMINISTRATION

Oral route

Just prior to administration, gently remove tab from bottle w/ dry hands and immediately place on top of tongue, then swallow w/ saliva; administration w/ liquid is not necessary

Available in a 1:4 ratio of carbidopa to levodopa (25/100) as well as a 1:10 ratio (25/250 and 10/100); tabs of the 2 ratios may be given separately or combined as needed to provide the optimum dosage

STORAGE

20-25°C (68-77°F); excursions permitted to 15-30°C (59-86°F). Protect from moisture and light.

HOW SUPPLIED

Tab, Disintegrating: (Carbidopa/Levodopa) 10mg/100mg*, 25mg/100mg*, 25mg/250mg* *scored

CONTRAINDICATIONS

During or w/in 2 weeks of using nonselective MAOIs; known hypersensitivity to any component of this drug; narrow-angle glaucoma; suspicious, undiagnosed skin lesions, or history of melanoma.

WARNINGS/PRECAUTIONS

Dyskinesias may occur; may require dose reduction. May cause mental disturbances; monitor for depression with concomitant suicidal tendencies. Caution with past or current psychoses, severe cardiovascular (CV) or pulmonary disease, bronchial asthma, renal/hepatic/endocrine disease, or chronic wide-angle glaucoma. Caution with history of myocardial infarction (MI) with residual atrial, nodal, or ventricular arrhythmias; monitor cardiac function with particular care during the period of initial dosage adjustment, in a facility with provisions for intensive cardiac care. May increase possibility of upper GI hemorrhage in patients with a history of peptic ulcer. Sporadic cases of a symptom complex resembling neuroleptic malignant syndrome (NMS) reported during dose reduction or withdrawal. Periodically evaluate hepatic, hematopoietic, CV, and renal function if on extended therapy. May be associated with somnolence and very rarely episodes of sudden onset of sleep; may impair physical/mental abilities. Monitor for melanomas frequently and on a regular basis. Abnormalities in lab tests may include elevations of LFTs (eg, alkaline phosphatase, AST, ALT, lactic dehydrogenase, bilirubin) and abnormalities in BUN and positive Coombs test, reported. May cause lab test interactions. Cases of falsely diagnosed pheochromocytoma reported very rarely; caution when interpreting the plasma and urine levels of catecholamines and their metabolites.

ADVERSE REACTIONS

Dyskinesias (eg, choreiform, dystonic, other involuntary movements), nausea.

DRUG INTERACTIONS

See Contraindications. Symptomatic postural hypotension reported with concomitant use of antihypertensives drugs; dosage adjustment of the antihypertensive drug may be required. Use with selegiline may cause severe orthostatic hypotension. HTN and dyskinesia may occur with TCAs. May reduce effects of levodopa when use concomitantly with dopamine D_2 receptor antagonists (eg, phenothiazines, butyrophenones, risperidone), and isoniazid. Beneficial effects of levodopa in Parkinson's disease reported to be reversed by phenytoin and papaverine; monitor for loss of therapeutic response. Iron salts may reduce the bioavailability of levodopa and carbidopa. Metoclopramide may increase the bioavailability of levodopa and may also adversely affect disease control.

PREGNANCY AND LACTATION

Category C, caution in nursing.

MECHANISM OF ACTION

Dopa-decarboxylase inhibitor/dopamine precursor. Carbidopa: Inhibits decarboxylation of peripheral levodopa. Levodopa: Crosses blood-brain barrier and presumably converted to dopamine in the brain.

PHARMACOKINETICS

Absorption: Carbidopa: Bioavailability (99%). **Elimination:** Urine.

PATIENT CONSIDERATIONS

Assessment: Assess for narrow-angle/chronic wide-angle glaucoma; suspicious/undiagnosed skin lesions or history of melanoma; presence of or history of psychoses; history of peptic ulcer; severe CV or pulmonary disease; bronchial asthma; hepatic, renal, or endocrine disease; history of MI with residual atrial, nodal, or ventricular arrhythmias; pregnancy/nursing status; and possible drug interactions.

Monitoring: Monitor for dyskinesias, mental disturbances, depression with suicidal tendencies, somnolence, NMS, upper GI hemorrhage in patients with a history of peptic ulcer, and other adverse reactions. Monitor cardiac function in patients with a history of MI who have residual atrial, nodal, or ventricular arrhythmias. Monitor for LFT elevations and BUN abnormalities. For patients on extended therapy, perform periodic evaluation of hepatic, hematopoietic, CV, and renal function. Monitor for melanomas frequently and on a regular basis. Monitor for changes in intraocular pressure in patients with chronic wide-angle glaucoma. Monitor closely during the dose adjustment period.

Counseling: Inform phenylketonuric patients that drug contains phenylalanine. Instruct not to remove tabs from the bottle until just prior to dosing. Instruct to gently remove the tab from the bottle with dry hands and to immediately place the tab on top of the tongue to dissolve and be swallowed with saliva. Inform that therapy is an immediate-release formulation designed to begin release of ingredients within 30 min. Advise to take at regular intervals according to the schedule outlined by the physician. Instruct to cautioned not to change the prescribed dosage regimen and not to add any additional antiparkinson medications, including other carbidopa and levodopa preparations, without consulting the physician. Advise that sometimes a "wearing-off" effect may occur at the end of the dosing interval; notify physician if such response poses a problem to lifestyle. Advise that occasionally, dark color (red, brown, or black) may appear in saliva, urine, or sweat after ingestion of therapy. Inform that high protein diet, excessive acidity, and iron salts may reduce clinical effectiveness. Advise to exercise caution while driving or operating machinery; instruct to refrain from these activities if have experienced somnolence and/or sudden sleep onset. Instruct to inform physician if new or increase gambling urges, or sexual or other intense urges develop.

PARLODEL — bromocriptine mesylate

Class: Dopamine receptor agonist

Rx

ADULT DOSAGE
Hyperprolactinemia-Associated Dysfunctions

Including Amenorrhea w/ or w/o Galactorrhea, Infertility, or Hypogonadism, in Patients w/ Prolactin-Secreting Adenomas:

Initial: 1/2-1 tab qd

Titrate: May add 1 tab (2.5mg) every 2-7 days, as tolerated until optimal response is achieved

Range: 2.5-15mg/day

In cases where adenectomy is elected, a course of therapy may be used to reduce tumor mass prior to surgery

Acromegaly
Alone or as Adjunctive Therapy w/ Pituitary Irradiation or Surgery:

Initial: 1/2-1 tab qhs w/ food for 3 days

Titrate: May add 1/2-1 tab every 3-7 days, as tolerated until optimal response is achieved; reevaluate monthly and adjust dose based on reductions of growth hormone or clinical response

Range: 20-30mg/day

Max: 100mg/day

Withdraw therapy for 4-8 weeks on a yearly basis if treated w/ pituitary irradiation to assess both the clinical effects of radiation on the disease process and effects of therapy

Parkinson's Disease
Signs/Symptoms of Idiopathic or Postencephalitic Parkinson's Disease:

Initial: 1/2 tab bid w/ meals

Titrate: May increase every 14-28 days by 2.5mg/day

Max: 100mg/day

Maintain levodopa dose during introductory period, if possible

PEDIATRIC DOSAGE
Hyperprolactinemia-Associated Dysfunctions

Including Amenorrhea w/ or w/o Galactorrhea, Infertility, or Hypogonadism, in Patients w/ Prolactin-Secreting Adenomas:

11-15 Years:

Initial: 1/2-1 tab qd

Titrate: May increase as tolerated until optimal response is achieved

Range: 2.5-10mg/day

In cases where adenectomy is elected, a course of therapy may be used to reduce tumor mass prior to surgery

---

DOSING CONSIDERATIONS

Elderly
Start at lower end of dosing range

Discontinuation
Acromegaly:
After a brief trial w/ therapy, if no significant reduction in growth hormone levels has taken place, carefully assess clinical features of disease; consider dose adjustment or discontinuation if no change has occurred

ADMINISTRATION
Oral route
Take w/ food

STORAGE
<25°C (77°F).

HOW SUPPLIED
Cap: 5mg; **Tab:** 2.5mg* *scored

CONTRAINDICATIONS
Hypersensitivity to bromocriptine or to any of the excipients of bromocriptine mesylate, uncontrolled HTN, postpartum period in women w/ history of coronary artery disease (CAD) and other severe cardiovascular (CV) conditions unless withdrawal is medically contraindicated, pregnancy if treating hyperprolactinemia. Hypertensive disorders of pregnancy (eg, eclampsia, preeclampsia, or pregnancy-induced HTN) if used to treat acromegaly, prolactinoma, or Parkinson's disease, unless withdrawal is medically contraindicated.

WARNINGS/PRECAUTIONS
Perform complete evaluation of the pituitary before treatment. Safety during pregnancy not established; use contraceptive measures, other than oral contraceptives, during treatment. D/C treatment if patient becomes pregnant. Somnolence and episodes of sudden sleep onset may occur, particularly to patients with Parkinson's disease; consider dose reduction or termination of therapy. May impair physical/mental abilities. Symptomatic hypotension may occur. HTN, myocardial infarction (MI), seizures, and stroke reported (rare) in postpartum women; not recommended for prevention of physiological lactation. D/C and evaluate promptly if HTN, severe, progressive or unremitting headache (with or without visual disturbance), or evidence of CNS toxicity develops. Pleural and pericardial effusions, pleural and pulmonary fibrosis, constrictive pericarditis, and retroperitoneal fibrosis reported, particularly on long-term and high-dose treatment; consider discontinuation of therapy. Caution with history of psychosis or CV disease. Avoid with hereditary problems of galactose intolerance, severe lactase deficiency, or glucose-galactose malabsorption. Visual field deterioration may develop; consider dose reduction in patients with macroprolactinoma. CSF rhinorrhea reported in patients with prolactin-secreting adenomas. Cold-sensitive digital vasospasm and possible tumor expansion reported in acromegalic patients; d/c therapy and consider alternative procedures if tumor expansion develops. Severe GI bleeding in patients with peptic ulcers reported. Safety during long-term use (>2 yrs) for Parkinson's disease not established. May cause confusion and mental disturbances with high doses; caution with mild degrees of dementia. May cause hallucinations (visual or auditory) with or without concomitant levodopa; dosage reduction or discontinuation of therapy may be required. May cause intense urges to gamble, increased sexual urges, intense urges to spend money uncontrollably, and other intense urges; consider dose reduction or d/c therapy.

Caution with history of MI with residual atrial, nodal, or ventricular arrhythmia. Regularly monitor for melanomas. Symptom complex resembling the neuroleptic malignant syndrome (NMS) reported with rapid dose reduction, withdrawal of, or changes in antiparkinsonian therapy. Caution with renal/liver impairment and in elderly.

ADVERSE REACTIONS
Confusion, hallucinations, headache, drowsiness, visual disturbance, hypotension, nasal congestion, N/V, dizziness, constipation, anorexia, dry mouth, indigestion/ dyspepsia, fatigue, lightheadedness.

DRUG INTERACTIONS
Not recommended with other ergot alkaloids. May potentiate side effects with alcohol. May interact with dopamine antagonists, butyrophenones, and certain other agents. May decrease efficacy with phenothiazines, haloperidol, metoclopramide, and pimozide. Caution with strong CYP3A4 inhibitors (eg, azole antimycotics, HIV protease inhibitors). Increased plasma levels with macrolide antibiotics (eg, erythromycin) and octreotide. Caution in patients recently treated or on concomitant therapy with drugs that can alter BP; concomitant use in puerperium is not recommended.

PREGNANCY AND LACTATION
Category B, not for use in nursing.

MECHANISM OF ACTION
Dopamine receptor agonist; activates postsynaptic dopamine receptors and modulates the secretion of prolactin from the anterior pituitary by secreting a prolactin inhibitory factor.

PHARMACOKINETICS
Absorption: (Healthy) C_{max} =465pg/mL (fasted, 2 x 2.5mg), 628pg/mL (5mg bid); AUC=2377pg•hr/mL; T_{max}=2.5 hrs. **Distribution:** Plasma protein binding (90-96%). **Metabolism:** Liver (extensive); via CYP3A and hydroxylation. **Elimination:** Feces (82%), urine (5.6%); $T_{1/2}$=4.85 hrs.

PATIENT CONSIDERATIONS
Assessment: Assess for previous hypersensitivity to ergot alkaloids, uncontrolled HTN, history of CAD or other severe CV conditions, pituitary tumors, dementia, history of psychosis, unexplained pleuropulmonary disorders, history of peptic ulcer or GI bleeding, hereditary problems of galactose intolerance, severe lactase deficiency or glucose-galactose malabsorption, macroadenomas, renal/hepatic disease, pregnancy/nursing status, and possible drug interactions. Perform complete pituitary evaluation.

Monitoring: Monitor for GI bleeding, somnolence, episodes of sudden sleep onset, seizures, stroke, MI; pleural and pericardial effusions, pleural and pulmonary fibrosis, constrictive pericarditis, retroperitoneal fibrosis, cold sensitive digital vasospasm, peptic ulcers, enlargement of a previously undetected or existing prolactin-secreting tumor, symptom complex resembling NMS, confusion and mental disturbances, and other adverse reactions. Monitor prolactin levels. Monitor visual fields in patients with macroprolactinoma; rapidly progressive visual field loss should be evaluated by a neurosurgeon. Periodically evaluate hepatic, hematopoietic, CV, and renal function. Periodic monitoring of BP, particularly during 1st weeks of therapy is prudent. Perform pregnancy test at least every 4 weeks during amenorrhea, and for every missed menstrual period once menses are reinitiated. Periodic skin exam should be performed by qualified individuals (eg, dermatologist).

Counseling: Inform that dizziness, drowsiness, faintness, fainting, and syncope may occur during treatment. Advise that somnolence and episodes of sudden sleep onset may occur and instruct not to engage in activities requiring rapid and precise responses. Instruct patients with hyperprolactinemic states associated with macroadenoma or those who have had previous transsphenoidal surgery to report any persistent watery nasal discharge. Inform patients with macroadenoma that discontinuation of therapy may be associated with rapid regrowth of tumor and recurrence of their original symptoms. Advise of the possibility that patients may experience intense urges to spend money uncontrollably, intense urges to gamble, increased sexual urges, and the inability to control these urges while on therapy. Inform that hypotensive reactions may occasionally occur and result in reduced alertness.

PAROMOMYCIN — paromomycin sulfate   Rx
Class: Aminoglycoside

ADULT DOSAGE
Amebiasis
Intestinal:
Usual: 25-35mg/kg/day, administered in 3 doses w/ meals, for 5-10 days

Hepatic Coma
Usual: 4g/day in divided doses, given at regular intervals for 5-6 days, as adjunctive therapy

PEDIATRIC DOSAGE
Amebiasis
Intestinal:
Usual: 25-35mg/kg/day, administered in 3 doses w/ meals, for 5-10 days

---

ADMINISTRATION
Oral route
Take w/ meals for intestinal amebiasis

STORAGE
20-25°C (68-77°F). Protect from moisture.

HOW SUPPLIED
Cap: 250mg

CONTRAINDICATIONS
Prior hypersensitivity to paromomycin, intestinal obstruction.

WARNINGS/PRECAUTIONS
May result in bacterial resistance if used in the absence of proven or suspected bacterial infection, or a prophylactic indication; take appropriate measures if superinfection develops. Caution with ulcerative lesions of the bowel to avoid renal toxicity through inadvertent absorption.

ADVERSE REACTIONS
Nausea, abdominal cramps, diarrhea.

PREGNANCY AND LACTATION
Safety not known in pregnancy/nursing.

MECHANISM OF ACTION
Aminoglycoside; closely parallels that of neomycin.

PHARMACOKINETICS
Absorption: Poor. **Elimination:** Feces (almost 100%).

PATIENT CONSIDERATIONS
Assessment: Assess for history of hypersensitivity to drug, intestinal obstruction, and ulcerative lesions of the bowel.

Monitoring: Monitor for superinfection and other adverse reactions.

Counseling: Counsel that therapy should only be used to treat bacterial, not viral (eg, common cold), infections. Instruct to take exactly ud. Inform that skipping doses or not completing the full course of therapy may decrease effectiveness of treatment and increase bacterial resistance.

PASER — aminosalicylic acid   Rx
Class: Hydroxybenzoic acid derivative

ADULT DOSAGE
Tuberculosis
Treatment of tuberculosis (TB) in combination w/ other active agents for patients w/ multidrug resistant TB or in situations when therapy w/ isoniazid and rifampin is not possible due to a combination of resistance and/or intolerance

4g tid

PEDIATRIC DOSAGE
Tuberculosis
Treatment of tuberculosis (TB) in combination w/ other active agents for patients w/ multidrug resistant TB or in situations when therapy w/ isoniazid and rifampin is not possible due to a combination of resistance and/or intolerance

Use smaller doses corresponding to the adult dose (4g tid)

ADMINISTRATION
Oral route
Sprinkle on applesauce or yogurt or by swirling contents in the glass to suspend the granules in an acidic drink (eg, tomato or orange juice)

STORAGE
Store below 15°C (59°F), refrigerate or freeze. Packets may be stored at room temperature for short periods of time. Avoid excessive heat.

HOW SUPPLIED
Granules, Delayed-Release: 4g/pkt

CONTRAINDICATIONS
Severe renal disease.

WARNINGS/PRECAUTIONS
Monitor for rash, or signs of intolerance during first 3 months. D/C if hypersensitivity (rash), fever, or other premonitory signs of intolerance occur. Can desensitize by administering small, gradually increasing doses.

ADVERSE REACTIONS
Diarrhea, N/V, abdominal pain, fever, dermatitis, lymphoma-like syndrome, leukocytosis, eosinophilia, agranulocytosis, thrombocytopenia, Coombs-positive hemolytic anemia, jaundice, hypoglycemia.

DRUG INTERACTIONS
Reduces acetylation of isoniazid, especially in rapid acetylators. Decreases vitamin B12 absorption; consider vitamin B12 maintenance treatment. Decreases digoxin levels.

PREGNANCY AND LACTATION
Category C, safety in nursing not known.

MECHANISM OF ACTION
Bacteriostatic agent; believed to inhibit folic acid synthesis and/or inhibition of synthesis of the cell-wall component, mycobactin, thus reducing iron uptake by *Mycobacterium tuberculosis.*

PHARMACOKINETICS
Absorption: C_{max}=20mcg/mL; T_{max}=6 hrs. **Distribution:** Plasma protein binding (50-60%), CSF penetration occurs only if the meninges is inflamed. **Metabolism:** Via acetylation. **Excretion:** Urine (80%); $T_{1/2}$=26.4 min.

PATIENT CONSIDERATIONS
Assessment: Assess for hepatic/renal impairment, hypersensitivity reactions, pregnancy/nursing status, and possible drug interactions. Obtain baseline CBC and platelet count, FPG, urinalysis, hepatic/renal function.

Monitoring: Monitor for N/V, diarrhea, abdominal pain, hepatomegaly, lymphadenopathy, leucocytosis, eosinophilia. Monitor for rash or signs of intolerance during first 3 months. Monitor CBC and platelet count, FPG, urinalysis, hepatic/renal function.

Counseling: Inform about risks and benefits of therapy. Instruct to d/c if hypersensitivity (eg, rash, fever, diarrhea) occurs. Inform that poor compliance in taking anti-TB drugs leads to treatment failure and resistance against organisms. Skeleton of the granules may be seen in stool. Sprinkle granules on acidic foods such as applesauce or yogurt or stir into a fruit drink and swirl to protect the coating from sinking. Store in refrigerator or freezer. Instruct not to use and inform pharmacist or physician if packets are swollen or the granules have lost their tan color and are dark brown or purple.

PAXIL — paroxetine hydrochloride   Rx

Class: Selective serotonin reuptake inhibitor (SSRI)

> Antidepressants increased the risk of suicidal thinking and behavior (suicidality) in children, adolescents, and young adults in short-term studies of major depressive disorder and other psychiatric disorders. Monitor and observe closely for clinical worsening, suicidality, or unusual changes in behavior in patients who are started on antidepressants. Not approved for use in pediatric patients.

ADULT DOSAGE

Major Depressive Disorder

Initial: 20mg/day
Titrate: May increase in 10mg/day increments at intervals of at least 1 week
Maint: Efficacy is maintained for periods of up to 1 yr w/ doses that averaged about 30mg
Max: 50mg/day

Obsessive Compulsive Disorder

Initial: 20mg/day
Titrate: May increase in 10mg/day increments at intervals of at least 1 week
Recommended: 40mg/day
Max: 60mg/day

Panic Disorder

W/ or w/o Agoraphobia:
Initial: 10mg/day
Titrate: May increase in 10mg/day increments at intervals of at least 1 week
Target Dose: 40mg/day
Max: 60mg/day

Anxiety Disorders

Social Anxiety Disorder:
Initial/Usual: 20mg/day
Titrate: May increase in 10mg/day increments at intervals of at least 1 week
Range: 20-60mg/day; no additional benefit for doses >20mg/day

Generalized Anxiety Disorder:
Initial/Usual: 20mg/day
Titrate: May increase in 10mg/day increments at intervals of at least 1 week
Range: 20-50mg/day

Post-traumatic Stress Disorder

Initial: 20mg/day
Titrate: May increase in 10mg/day increments at intervals of at least 1 week
Range: 20-50mg/day

Dosing Considerations with MAOIs

Switching to/from an MAOI for Psychiatric Disorders:
Allow at least 14 days between discontinuation of an MAOI and initiation of treatment, and conversely allow at least 14 days between discontinuing treatment before starting an MAOI

Use w/ Other MAOIs (eg, Linezolid, IV Methylene Blue):
If acceptable alternatives are not available and benefits outweigh risks of serotonin syndrome, d/c paroxetine promptly and administer linezolid or IV methylene blue; monitor for serotonin syndrome for 2 weeks or until 24 hrs after last dose of linezolid or IV methylene blue, whichever comes 1st. May resume paroxetine therapy 24 hrs after last dose of linezolid or IV methylene blue

PEDIATRIC DOSAGE

Pediatric use may not have been established

DOSING CONSIDERATIONS

Renal Impairment
Severe:
Initial: 10mg/day
Max: 40mg/day

Hepatic Impairment
Severe:
Initial: 10mg/day
Max: 40mg/day

Elderly
Elderly/Debilitated:
Initial: 10mg/day
Max: 40mg/day

Discontinuation
Reduce gradually; consider resuming previously prescribed dose if intolerable symptoms occur following a decrease in dose or upon discontinuation. Subsequently, may continue to decrease the dose, but at a more gradual rate

ADMINISTRATION
Oral route

Take w/ or w/o food.
Give qd, usually in the am.

Tab
Swallow whole; do not chew or crush.

Sus
Shake well before use.

STORAGE
Tab: 15-30°C (59-86°F). Sus: ≤25°C (77°F).

HOW SUPPLIED
Sus: 10mg/5mL [250mL]; **Tab:** 10mg*, 20mg*, 30mg, 40mg *scored

CONTRAINDICATIONS
Use of an MAOI for psychiatric disorders either concomitantly or within 14 days of stopping treatment. Treatment within 14 days of stopping an MAOI for psychiatric disorders. Starting treatment in a patient being treated with other MAOIs (eg, linezolid, IV methylene blue). Concomitant use with thioridazine or pimozide. Hypersensitivity to paroxetine or any of the inactive ingredients in this medication.

WARNINGS/PRECAUTIONS
May precipitate mixed/manic episode in patients at risk for bipolar disorder. Not approved for treatment of bipolar depression. Serotonin syndrome reported; d/c immediately and initiate supportive symptomatic treatment. Pupillary dilation that occurs following use may trigger an angle-closure attack in a patient with anatomically narrow angles who does not have a patent iridectomy. Increased risk of congenital malformations reported in 1st trimester of pregnancy; neonates exposed to therapy late in the 3rd trimester have developed complications. Activation of mania/hypomania reported; caution with history of mania. Seizures reported; d/c if seizures develop. Adverse reactions reported upon discontinuation; avoid abrupt withdrawal. Akathisia may develop. Hyponatremia may occur; caution in elderly and volume-depleted patients. Consider discontinuation in patients with symptomatic hyponatremia and institute appropriate medical intervention. May increase risk of bleeding events. Bone fracture risk following exposure to some antidepressants reported. Caution with diseases/conditions affecting hemodynamic responses or metabolism, severe hepatic/renal impairment, and in elderly/debilitated patients. Mydriasis reported; caution with narrow-angle glaucoma.

ADVERSE REACTIONS
Asthenia, nausea, somnolence, headache, insomnia, abnormal ejaculation, dry mouth, constipation, dizziness, diarrhea, decreased libido, sweating, decreased appetite, tremor, impotence.

DRUG INTERACTIONS
See Contraindications. Not recommended with SSRIs, SNRIs, tryptophan, and alcohol. May cause serotonin syndrome with other serotonergic drugs (eg, triptans, TCAs, fentanyl) and with drugs that impair metabolism of serotonin; d/c immediately if this occurs. Metabolism and pharmacokinetics may be affected by the induction or inhibition of drug-metabolizing enzymes. Increased risk of bleeding with aspirin, NSAIDs, warfarin, and other anticoagulants. Increased risk of hyponatremia with diuretics. Increased levels with cimetidine. Decreased levels with phenobarbital, phenytoin, and fosamprenavir/ritonavir. Caution with drugs that are metabolized by CYP2D6 (eg, phenothiazines, risperidone, type 1C antiarrhythmics) and with drugs that inhibit CYP2D6 (eg, quinidine). May increase levels of desipramine, risperidone, procyclidine and theophylline. May increase levels of atomoxetine; may require dose adjustments of atomoxetine. May inhibit metabolism of TCAs. May displace or be displaced by other highly protein-bound drugs. May reduce efficacy of tamoxifen. Caution with warfarin, TCAs, lithium, and digoxin. Severe hypotension reported when added to chronic metoprolol treatment.

PREGNANCY AND LACTATION
Pregnancy: Category D.
Lactation: Caution in nursing.

MECHANISM OF ACTION
SSRI; inhibits CNS neuronal reuptake of serotonin.

PHARMACOKINETICS
Absorption: Complete; C_{max}=61.7ng/mL, T_{max}=5.2 hrs (tab 30mg). **Distribution:** Plasma protein binding (95% [100ng/mL], 93% [400ng/mL]); found in breast milk. **Metabolism:** Extensive; oxidation and methylation via CYP2D6. **Elimination:** Urine (62% metabolites; 2% parent compound); feces (36%, <1% parent compound) (30mg oral sol); $T_{1/2}$=21 hrs (tab 30mg).

PATIENT CONSIDERATIONS

Assessment: Assess for drug hypersensitivity, risk of bipolar disorder, history of seizures or mania, volume depletion, diseases/conditions that affect metabolism or hemodynamic responses, hepatic/renal impairment, susceptibility to angle-closure glaucoma or narrow-angle glaucoma, pregnancy/nursing status, and for possible drug interactions.

Monitoring: Monitor for signs/symptoms of clinical worsening, suicidality, unusual changes in behavior, serotonin syndrome, angle-closure glaucoma, seizures, activation of mania/hypomania, akathisia, bone fracture, hyponatremia especially in the elderly, abnormal bleeding, and other adverse reactions. Periodically reevaluate long-term usefulness of therapy.

Counseling: Inform about benefits, risks, and appropriate use of therapy. Caution about risk of serotonin syndrome, angle-closure glaucoma, and bleeding. Counsel to be alert for emergence of unusual changes in behavior, worsening of depression, and suicidal ideation, especially during drug initiation or dose adjustment. Caution against operating hazardous machinery (including automobiles) until reasonably certain that therapy does not adversely affect ability to engage in such activities. Inform that improvement may be noticed in 1-4 weeks; instruct to continue therapy ud. Inform physician if taking, or planning to take, any prescription or OTC drugs. Instruct to notify physician if pregnant/intending to become pregnant, or if breastfeeding. Advise to avoid alcohol.

PAXIL CR — paroxetine hydrochloride   Rx

Class: Selective serotonin reuptake inhibitor (SSRI)

> Antidepressants increased the risk of suicidal thinking and behavior (suicidality) in short-term studies in children, adolescents, and young adults with major depressive disorder and other psychiatric disorders. Monitor and observe closely for clinical worsening, suicidality, or unusual changes in behavior in patients who are started on antidepressants. Not approved for use in pediatric patients.

ADULT DOSAGE

Major Depressive Disorder
Initial: 25mg/day
Titrate: May increase by 12.5mg/day increments at intervals of at least 1 week
Max: 62.5mg/day

Panic Disorder
W/ or w/o Agoraphobia:
Initial: 12.5mg/day
Titrate: May increase by 12.5mg/day increments at intervals of at least 1 week
Max: 75mg/day

Social Anxiety Disorder
Initial: 12.5mg/day
Titrate: May increase by 12.5mg/day increments at intervals of at least 1 week
Max: 37.5mg/day

Premenstrual Dysphoric Disorder
Initial: 12.5mg/day; give either qd throughout menstrual cycle or limit to luteal phase of menstrual cycle
Titrate: May increase to 25mg/day at intervals of at least 1 week

Dosing Considerations with MAOIs

Switching to/from an MAOI for Psychiatric Disorders:
Allow at least 14 days between discontinuation of an MAOI and initiation of treatment, and allow at least 14 days between discontinuation of treatment and initiation of an MAOI

Use w/ Other MAOIs (eg, Linezolid, IV Methylene Blue):
Do not start paroxetine in a patient being treated w/ linezolid or IV methylene blue.
In patients already receiving paroxetine, if acceptable alternatives are not available and benefits outweigh risks, d/c paroxetine and administer linezolid or IV methylene blue; monitor for serotonin syndrome for 2 weeks or until 24 hrs after the last dose of linezolid or IV methylene blue, whichever comes 1st. May resume paroxetine therapy 24 hrs after the last dose of linezolid or IV methylene blue.

PEDIATRIC DOSAGE

Pediatric use may not have been established

DOSING CONSIDERATIONS
Renal Impairment
Severe (CrCl <30mL/min):
Initial: 12.5mg/day
Max: 50mg/day

Hepatic Impairment
Severe:
Initial: 12.5mg/day
Max: 50mg/day

Elderly
Elderly/Debilitated:
Initial: 12.5mg/day
Max: 50mg/day

Discontinuation
Gradually reduce dose whenever possible; consider resuming previously prescribed dose if intolerable symptoms occur following a decrease in dose or upon discontinuation. Subsequently, may continue to decrease the dose, but at a more gradual rate

ADMINISTRATION
Oral route

Administer as a single daily dose, usually in the am.
Take w/ or w/o food.
Swallow whole; do not chew or crush.

STORAGE
≤25°C (77°F).

HOW SUPPLIED
Tab, Controlled-Release: 12.5mg, 25mg, 37.5mg

CONTRAINDICATIONS
Use of MAOIs intended to treat psychiatric disorders either concomitantly or within 14 days of stopping treatment. Treatment within 14 days of stopping an MAOI intended to treat psychiatric disorders. Starting treatment in patients being treated with MAOIs (eg, linezolid, IV methylene blue). Concomitant use with thioridazine or pimozide. Hypersensitivity to paroxetine or any of the inactive ingredients in this medication.

WARNINGS/PRECAUTIONS
May precipitate mixed/manic episode in patients at risk for bipolar disorder. Not approved for treatment of bipolar depression. Serotonin syndrome reported; d/c immediately and initiate supportive symptomatic treatment. Pupillary dilation that occurs following use may trigger an angle-closure attack in a patient with anatomically narrow angles who does not have a patent iridectomy. Increased risk of congenital malformations reported in 1st trimester of pregnancy; neonates exposed to therapy late in the 3rd trimester have developed complications. Activation of mania/hypomania reported; caution with history of mania. Seizures reported; d/c if seizures occur. Adverse reactions upon discontinuation (eg, dysphoric mood, irritability) reported; avoid abrupt withdrawal. Akathisia may develop. Hyponatremia reported; caution in elderly and volume-depleted patients. Consider discontinuation in patients with symptomatic hyponatremia and institute appropriate medical intervention. May increase risk of bleeding events. Bone fracture risk following exposure to some antidepressants reported. Caution with disease/conditions that could affect metabolism or hemodynamic responses, severe renal/hepatic impairment, pregnancy (3rd trimester), and in elderly/debilitated patients. May impair mental/physical abilities. Mydriasis reported; caution with narrow-angle glaucoma.

ADVERSE REACTIONS
Suicidality, somnolence, insomnia, nausea, asthenia, abnormal ejaculation, dry mouth, constipation, dizziness, diarrhea, decreased libido, sweating, abnormal vision, headache, tremor.

DRUG INTERACTIONS
See Contraindications. Serotonin syndrome reported with other serotonergic drugs (eg, triptans, TCAs, fentanyl, lithium, tramadol, tryptophan, buspirone, St. John's wort) and with drugs that impair serotonin metabolism. Use with other SSRIs, SNRIs, or tryptophan is not recommended. Avoid alcohol. Concomitant use with aspirin (ASA), NSAIDs, warfarin, and other anticoagulants may increase risk of bleeding events. Use with diuretics may increase risk of developing hyponatremia. Increased levels with cimetidine. Reduced levels with phenobarbital, phenytoin, and fosamprenavir/ritonavir. Caution with drugs that are metabolized by CYP2D6 (eg, nortriptyline, phenothiazines, risperidone, type 1C antiarrhythmics) and with drugs that inhibit CYP2D6 (eg, quinidine). May increase levels of desipramine, risperidone, atomoxetine, and theophylline. May reduce efficacy of tamoxifen. May displace or be displaced by other highly protein-bound drugs. May increase procyclidine levels; reduce dose if anticholinergic effects are seen. May inhibit metabolism of TCAs. Caution with digoxin, TCAs, and lithium.

PREGNANCY AND LACTATION
Pregnancy: Category D.
Lactation: Caution in nursing.

MECHANISM OF ACTION
SSRI; inhibits CNS neuronal reuptake of serotonin.

PHARMACOKINETICS
Absorption: Complete; administration of variable doses resulted in different parameters; T_{max}=6-10 hrs. **Distribution:** Plasma protein binding (95% [100ng/mL], 93% [400ng/mL]); found in breast milk. **Metabolism:** Extensive; oxidation and methylation via CYP2D6. **Elimination:** Sol: Urine (62% metabolites; 2% parent); feces (36% mostly metabolites; <1% parent). $T_{1/2}$=15-20 hrs.

PATIENT CONSIDERATIONS

Assessment: Assess for drug hypersensitivity, risk of bipolar disorder, history of seizures or mania, volume depletion, diseases/conditions that affect metabolism or hemodynamic response, hepatic/renal impairment, narrow-angle glaucoma, susceptibility to angle-closure glaucoma, pregnancy/nursing status, and for possible drug interactions.

Monitoring: Monitor for signs/symptoms of clinical worsening, suicidality, unusual changes in behavior, serotonin syndrome, seizures, activation of mania/hypomania, akathisia, bone fracture, hyponatremia especially in the elderly, abnormal bleeding, angle-closure glaucoma, and other adverse reactions. Upon discontinuation, monitor for symptoms. Periodically reassess need for continued therapy.

Counseling: Inform about the risks, benefits, and appropriate use of therapy. Advise to avoid alcohol use. Instruct to notify physician of all prescription or OTC drugs currently taking or planning to take. Caution about risk of serotonin syndrome, angle-closure glaucoma, and bleeding. Instruct patient, families, and caregivers to report emergence of anxiety, agitation, panic attacks, insomnia, irritability, hostility, aggressiveness, impulsivity, akathisia, hypomania, mania, unusual changes in behavior, worsening of depression, and suicidal ideation, especially during drug initiation or dose adjustment. Caution operating hazardous machinery (including automobiles) until reasonably certain that therapy does not adversely affect ability to engage in such activities. Inform that improvement may be noticed in 1-4 weeks; instruct to continue therapy ud. Instruct to notify physician if pregnant/intending to become pregnant, or if breastfeeding.

PAZEO — olopatadine hydrochloride   Rx

Class: H_1 antagonist and mast cell stabilizer

ADULT DOSAGE	PEDIATRIC DOSAGE
Allergic Conjunctivitis	**Allergic Conjunctivitis**
Itching:	**Itching:**
1 drop in each affected eye qd	**>2 Years:**
	1 drop in each affected eye qd

ADMINISTRATION
Ocular route

STORAGE
2-25°C (36-77°F). Keep bottle tightly closed when not in use.

HOW SUPPLIED
Sol: 0.7% [2.5mL]

WARNINGS/PRECAUTIONS
In order to prevent contaminating dropper tip of the bottle and sol, caution not to touch the eyelids or surrounding areas w/ the dropper tip. Contains benzalkonium chloride, which may be absorbed by soft contact lenses; patients who wear soft contact lenses and whose eyes are not red should wait at least 5 min after instilling sol before inserting contact lenses. Patient should not wear contact lens if eye is red.

ADVERSE REACTIONS
Blurred vision, dry eye, superficial punctate keratitis, dysgeusia, abnormal sensation in eye.

PREGNANCY AND LACTATION
Safety is not known in pregnancy, caution in nursing.

MECHANISM OF ACTION
H_1-antagonist and mast cell stabilizer. Also demonstrates decreased chemotaxis and inhibition of eosinophil activation.

PHARMACOKINETICS
Absorption: C_{max}=1.6ng/mL; AUC_{0-12}=9.7ng*hr/mL; T_{max}=2 hrs (median).
Elimination: $T_{1/2}$=3.4 hrs.

PATIENT CONSIDERATIONS

Assessment: Assess for contact lens use and pregnancy/nursing status.

Monitoring: Monitor for reddening of the eyes and other adverse reactions.

Counseling: Advise not to touch dropper tip to eyelids or any or surrounding area, in order to prevent contamination. Advise not to wear contact lenses if eyes are red. Advise not to use medication to treat contact lens-related irritation. Instruct to remove contact lenses prior to instillation of medication; inform that lenses may be reinserted 5 min following administration.

PEDIAPRED — prednisolone sodium phosphate   Rx

Class: Glucocorticoid

ADULT DOSAGE	PEDIATRIC DOSAGE
Steroid-Responsive Disorders	**Steroid-Responsive Disorders**
Initial: 5-60mg/day depending on disease and response	**Initial:** 0.14-2mg/kg/day in 3 or 4 divided doses (4-60mg/m²/day)
Maint: Decrease dose by small amounts to lowest effective dose	**Nephrotic Syndrome**
Multiple Sclerosis	**>2 Years:**
Acute Exacerbations:	**Usual:** 60mg/m²/day given in 3 divided doses for 4 weeks, followed by 4 weeks of single dose alternate-day therapy at 40mg/m²/day
Usual: 200mg/day for a week, followed by 80mg qod for 1 month	

Asthma
Uncontrolled by Inhaled Corticosteroids and Long-Acting Bronchodilators:
Usual: 1-2mg/kg/day in single or divided doses; continue short course ("burst") therapy until peak expiratory flow rate of 80% of personal best is achieved or symptoms resolve (usually 3-10 days)

DOSING CONSIDERATIONS
Elderly
Start at lower end of dosing range
Discontinuation
Withdraw gradually after long-term therapy

ADMINISTRATION
Oral route

STORAGE
4-25°C (39-77°F).

HOW SUPPLIED
Sol: 5mg/5mL [120mL]

CONTRAINDICATIONS
Systemic fungal infections, hypersensitivity to the drug or any of its components.

WARNINGS/PRECAUTIONS
May produce reversible hypothalamic-pituitary-adrenal axis suppression. Adjust dose during stress or change in thyroid status. May mask signs of infection or cause new infections. May activate latent amebiasis. Avoid with cerebral malaria. Avoid exposure to chickenpox or measles. Not for treatment of optic neuritis or active ocular herpes simplex. May cause elevation of BP or intraocular pressure (IOP), cataracts, glaucoma, optic nerve damage, Kaposi's sarcoma, psychic derangements, salt/water retention, increased excretion of K^+ and/or Ca^{2+}, osteoporosis, growth suppression in children, or secondary ocular infections. Caution with strongyloides, chronic heart failure, diverticulitis, HTN, renal insufficiency, fresh intestinal anastomoses, active or latent peptic ulcer, and ulcerative colitis. Enhanced effect in hypothyroidism or cirrhosis. Avoid abrupt withdrawal. Caution in elderly due to increased risk of corticosteroid-induced side effects; start at low end of dosing range and monitor bone mineral density.

ADVERSE REACTIONS
Edema, fluid/electrolyte disturbances, osteoporosis, muscle weakness, pancreatitis, peptic ulcer, impaired wound healing, increased intracranial pressure, cushingoid state, hirsutism, menstrual irregularities, growth suppression in children, glaucoma, nausea, weight gain.

DRUG INTERACTIONS
Enhanced metabolism with barbiturates, phenytoin, ephedrine, and rifampin. Use with cyclosporine may increase activity of both drugs; convulsions reported with concomitant use. Decreased metabolism with estrogens or ketoconazole. May inhibit response to warfarin. Increased risk of GI side effects with aspirin or other NSAIDs. May increase clearance of salicylates. High doses or concurrent neuromuscular drugs may cause acute myopathy. Enhanced possibility of hypokalemia when given with K^+-depleting agents. May produce severe weakness in myasthenia gravis patients on anticholinesterase agents. Avoid live vaccines with immunosuppressive doses. Possible diminished response with killed or inactivated vaccines. May increase blood glucose; adjust antidiabetic agents. May suppress reactions to skin tests.

PREGNANCY AND LACTATION
Category C, caution in nursing.

MECHANISM OF ACTION
Synthetic adrenocorticoid steroid; promotes gluconeogenesis, increases deposition of glycogen in the liver, inhibits glucose utilization, and increases catabolism of protein, lipolysis, and glomerular filtration that leads to increased urinary excretion of urate and Ca^{2+}.

PHARMACOKINETICS
Absorption: Rapidly absorbed from GI tract. **Distribution:** Plasma protein binding (70-90%); found in breast milk. **Metabolism:** Liver. **Elimination:** Urine (as sulfate and glucuronide conjugates); $T_{1/2}$=2-4 hrs.

PATIENT CONSIDERATIONS

Assessment: Assess for systemic fungal/other infections, active tuberculosis, vaccination history, HTN, congestive heart failure, renal insufficiency, ophthalmic disease, osteoporosis, thyroid status, hepatic impairment, nonspecific ulcerative colitis, ulcers, pregnancy/nursing status, and possible drug interactions.

Monitoring: Monitor for adrenocortical insufficiency, occurrence of infections, psychic derangement, cataracts, acute myopathy, Kaposi's sarcoma, fluid retention, and measurement of serum electrolytes, TSH, LFTs, glucose, IOP, and BP.

Counseling: Advise not to d/c therapy abruptly or without medical supervision. Instruct to avoid exposure to chickenpox or measles; report immediately if exposed. Advise to implement dietary salt restriction and K^+ supplementation.

PEDIARIX — diphtheria and tetanus toxoids and acellular pertussis adsorbed, hepatitis B (recombinant) and inactivated poliovirus vaccine Rx

Class: Toxoid/vaccine combination

PEDIATRIC DOSAGE

Active Immunization Against Diphtheria, Tetanus, Pertussis, Hepatitis B Virus, and Poliomyelitis

For Use in Infants Born of Hepatitis B Surface Antigen (HBsAg)-Negative Mothers:

6 Weeks to 6 Years (Prior to 7th Birthday):
0.5mL IM dose as a 3-dose series at 2, 4, and 6 months (at intervals of 6-8 weeks, preferably 8 weeks); 1st dose may be given as early as 6 weeks of age

Modified Schedules in Previously Vaccinated Children:

Children Previously Vaccinated w/ Diphtheria and Tetanus Toxoids and Acellular Pertussis Vaccine Adsorbed (DTaP):
May use to complete the first 3 doses of the DTaP series in children who have received 1 or 2 doses of Infanrix and are also scheduled to receive the other vaccine components of Pediarix

Children Previously Vaccinated w/ Hepatitis B Vaccine:
May be used to complete the hepatitis B vaccination series following 1 or 2 doses of another hepatitis B vaccine (monovalent or as part of a combination vaccine), including vaccines from other manufacturers, in children born of HBsAg-negative mothers who are also scheduled to receive the other vaccine components of Pediarix

A 3-dose series may be administered to infants born of HBsAg-negative mothers and who received a dose of hepatitis B vaccine at or shortly after birth

Children Previously Vaccinated w/ Inactivated Poliovirus Vaccine (IPV):
May be used to complete the first 3 doses of the IPV series in children who have received 1 or 2 doses of IPV from a different manufacturer and are also scheduled to receive the other vaccine components of Pediarix

Booster Immunization Following Pediarix:
Children who have received a 3-dose series w/ Pediarix should complete the DTaP and IPV series according to the recommended schedule; children should receive Infanrix as their 4th dose of DTaP and either Infanrix or Kinrix as their 5th dose of DTaP. Kinrix or another manufacturer's IPV may be used to complete the 4-dose IPV series

ADMINISTRATION
IM route

Administer in the anterolateral aspect of the thigh (children <1 yr) and in the deltoid muscle (older children); do not inject in the gluteal area or areas where there may be a major nerve trunk.
Shake vigorously; do not use if resuspension does not occur w/ vigorous shaking.
Do not mix w/ any other vaccine in the same syringe or vial.
Administer other vaccines separately, at different inj sites.

STORAGE
2-8°C (36-46°F). Do not freeze. Discard if frozen.

HOW SUPPLIED
Inj: 0.5mL [prefilled syringe]

CONTRAINDICATIONS
Severe allergic reaction (eg, anaphylaxis) after a previous dose of diphtheria toxoid-, tetanus toxoid-, pertussis antigen-, hepatitis B-, or poliovirus-containing vaccine or any component of this vaccine (eg, yeast, neomycin, polymyxin B). Encephalopathy (eg, coma, decreased level of consciousness, prolonged seizures) w/in 7 days of administration of a previous dose of pertussis-containing

vaccine that is not attributable to another identifiable cause. Progressive neurologic disorder (eg, infantile spasms, uncontrolled epilepsy, progressive encephalopathy).

WARNINGS/PRECAUTIONS
Use in infants is associated w/ higher risk of fever relative to separately administered vaccines. Evaluate potential benefits and risks of vaccine administration if Guillain-Barre syndrome occurs w/in 6 weeks of receipt of a prior tetanus toxoid-containing vaccine. Tip caps of prefilled syringes contain natural rubber latex; may cause allergic reactions. Syncope may occur and can be accompanied by transient neurological signs. Evaluate the potential benefits and risks of vaccine administration if any of the following events occur in temporal relation to receipt of a pertussis-containing vaccine: temperature ≥40.5°C (105°F) w/in 48 hrs not due to another identifiable cause; collapse or shock-like state occurring w/in 48 hrs; persistent, inconsolable crying lasting ≥3 hrs, occurring w/in 48 hrs; or seizures w/ or w/o fever occurring w/in 3 days. May administer an antipyretic at the time of vaccination and for the ensuing 24 hrs in children at higher risk for seizures. Apnea following IM administration observed in some premature infants; consider infant's medical status, and the potential benefits and possible risks of vaccination. Review immunization history for possible vaccine sensitivity; appropriate treatment should be available for possible allergic reactions.

ADVERSE REACTIONS
Local inj-site reactions (pain, redness, swelling), fever, irritability/fussiness, drowsiness, loss of appetite.

DRUG INTERACTIONS
Immunosuppressive therapies, including irradiation, antimetabolites, alkylating agents, cytotoxic drugs, and corticosteroids (used in greater than physiologic doses), may reduce immune response to vaccine.

PREGNANCY AND LACTATION
Pregnancy: Category C.

MECHANISM OF ACTION
Toxoid/vaccine combination; provides active immunization by producing antibodies against diphtheria toxin, tetanus toxin, pertussis, hepatitis B, and poliovirus infections.

PATIENT CONSIDERATIONS

Assessment: Assess for history of encephalopathy, development of Guillain-Barre syndrome following a prior tetanus toxoid-containing vaccine, progressive neurologic disorder, immunosuppression, risk for seizures, possible drug interactions, and hypersensitivity to latex, yeast, neomycin, or polymyxin B. Review immunization history for possible vaccine sensitivity and previous vaccination-related adverse reactions. Assess use in premature infants.

Monitoring: Monitor for signs/symptoms of Guillain-Barre syndrome, allergic reactions, syncope, neurological signs, apnea in premature infants, and other adverse reactions.

Counseling: Inform parents/guardians about potential benefits/risks of immunization, and of the importance of completing the immunization series. Counsel parents/guardians about potential adverse reactions; instruct to report any adverse events to physician.

PEGANONE — ethotoin Rx

Class: Hydantoin

ADULT DOSAGE	PEDIATRIC DOSAGE
Epilepsy	**Epilepsy**
Tonic-Clonic (Grand Mal) and Complex Partial (Psychomotor) Seizures:	**Tonic-Clonic (Grand Mal) and Complex Partial (Psychomotor) Seizures:**
Initial: ≤1g/day in 4-6 divided doses	**≥1 Year:**
Titrate: Increase gradually over several days based on individual response	Dose depends on age and weight
Maint: 2-3g/day	**Initial:** ≤750mg/day in 4-6 divided doses
	Maint: 500mg-1g/day, although occasionally 2g/day or (rarely) 3g/day may be necessary

DOSING CONSIDERATIONS
Concomitant Medications
Another Antiepileptic Drug:
Do not d/c other antiepileptic drug when therapy is begun; reduce dose of other antiepileptic drug gradually as dose of ethotoin is increased until therapy eventually replaces the other drug or optimal dose of both antiepileptics is established

Elderly
Start at lower end of dosing range

ADMINISTRATION
Oral route

Take after food
Space dose as evenly as possible

STORAGE
20-25°C (68-77°F).

HOW SUPPLIED
Tab: 250mg

CONTRAINDICATIONS
Hepatic abnormalities, hematologic disorders.

WARNINGS/PRECAUTIONS
May increase risk of suicidal thoughts/behavior; monitor for emergence or worsening of depression, suicidal thoughts/behavior, any unusual changes in mood/behavior, or thoughts about self-harm. May cause fetal harm; administer to women of childbearing potential only if found essential in seizure management. Do not d/c in pregnant women if being used for prevention of major seizures; status epilepticus may occur. Neonatal coagulation defect that may cause bleeding during the early (usually within 24 hrs of birth) neonatal period may possibly occur with maternal ingestion; give vitamin K prophylactically to mother 1 month prior to and during delivery, and to the infant, IV, immediately after birth. Blood dyscrasias reported; monitor for general malaise, sore throat, and other symptoms indicative of blood dyscrasias. May interfere with folic acid metabolism precipitating megaloblastic anemia; consider folic acid therapy if occurs during gestation. D/C if signs of liver damage or marked depression of blood count occurs. Caution in elderly.

ADVERSE REACTIONS
Lymphadenopathy, systemic lupus erythematosus, ataxia, gum hypertrophy, N/V, chest pain, nystagmus, diplopia, fever, dizziness, diarrhea, headache, insomnia, fatigue.

DRUG INTERACTIONS
Avoid with drugs known to adversely affect the hematopoietic system. Caution with coumarin anticoagulants.

PREGNANCY AND LACTATION
Category D, not for use in nursing.

MECHANISM OF ACTION
Hydantoin; likely similar to phenytoin, which appears to stabilize the normal seizure threshold and prevent the spread of seizure activity.

PHARMACOKINETICS
Absorption: Rapid. **Metabolism:** Liver; N-deethyl and p-hydroxyl-ethotoin (major metabolites). **Distribution:** Found in breast milk. **Elimination:** $T_{1/2}$=3-9 hrs.

PATIENT CONSIDERATIONS
Assessment: Assess for hepatic abnormalities, hematologic disorders, risk of suicidal thoughts/behavior, pregnancy/nursing status, and for possible drug interactions. Obtain baseline CBC and urinalyses.

Monitoring: Monitor for emergence or worsening of depression, suicidal thoughts/behavior, unusual changes in mood/behavior, symptoms of blood dyscrasias, signs of liver damage, and marked depression of blood count. Perform LFTs if clinical evidence suggests hepatic dysfunction. Monitor CBC and urinalyses at monthly intervals for several months after therapy is started.

Counseling: Advise to report immediately signs/symptoms such as sore throat, fever, malaise, easy bruising, petechiae, epistaxis, skin rash or others that may be indicative of an infection or bleeding tendency. Inform about increased risk of suicidal thoughts and behavior. Instruct to notify physician if there is emergence or worsening of symptoms of depression, any unusual changes in mood/behavior, or the emergence of suicidal thoughts, behavior, or thoughts of self-harm. If become pregnant, advise to enroll in the North American Antiepileptic Drug Pregnancy Registry. Inform of the benefits and risks associated with treatment and counsel about appropriate use.

PEGASYS — peginterferon alfa-2a   Rx
Class: Biological response modifier

> May cause or aggravate fatal or life-threatening neuropsychiatric, autoimmune, ischemic, and infectious disorders. Monitor closely w/ periodic clinical and lab evaluations. D/C w/ persistently severe or worsening signs/symptoms of these conditions.

ADULT DOSAGE
Chronic Hepatitis C with Compensated Liver Disease
W/O HIV Coinfection:
Monotherapy:
180mcg once weekly for 48 weeks

Combination Treatment:
Genotypes 1, 4:
180mcg once weekly for 48 weeks (if used w/ ribavirin only)

Genotypes 2, 3:
180mcg once weekly for 24 weeks (if used w/ ribavirin only)

W/ HIV Coinfection:
180mcg once weekly for 48 weeks (if used w/ ribavirin only)

Chronic Hepatitis B with Compensated Liver Disease
HBeAg-Positive and HBeAg-Negative:
180mcg once weekly for 48 weeks

PEDIATRIC DOSAGE
Chronic Hepatitis C with Compensated Liver Disease
≥5 Years:
Combination w/ Ribavirin:
180mcg/1.73m² x BSA once weekly
Max Dose: 180mcg

Treatment Duration:
Genotypes 2, 3: 24 weeks
Other Genotypes: 48 weeks

Treatment Initiation Prior to 18 Years:
Maintain pediatric dosing through the completion of therapy

DOSING CONSIDERATIONS
Renal Impairment
Adults:
CrCl <30mL/min and/or Hemodialysis: 135mcg once weekly
If severe adverse reactions or lab abnormalities develop, dose can be reduced to 90mcg once weekly until reactions abate; d/c if intolerance persists after dosage adjustment

Hepatic Impairment
Child Pugh-Score >6 (Class B and C): D/C Pegasys

Adverse Reactions
Neutropenia:
Adults:
ANC <750 cells/mm³: Reduce dose to 135mcg once weekly
ANC <500 cells/mm³: D/C until ANC values return to >1000 cells/mm³; restart at 90mcg once weekly
Pediatrics:
ANC 750-999 cells/mm³:
Weeks 1-2: Reduce dose to 135mcg/1.73m² x BSA
Weeks 3-48: No dose modification
ANC 500-749 cells/mm³:
Weeks 1-2: Hold dose until >750 cells/mm³ then resume at 135mcg/1.73m² x BSA
Weeks 3-48: Reduce dose to 135mcg/1.73m² x BSA
ANC 250-499 cells/mm³:
Weeks 1-2: Hold dose until >750 cells/mm³ then resume at 90mcg/1.73m² x BSA
Weeks 3-48: Hold dose until >750 cells/mm³ then resume at 135mcg/1.73m² x BSA
ANC <250 cells/mm³ (or Febrile Neutropenia): D/C treatment

Thrombocytopenia:
Adults:
Platelets <50,000 cells/mm³: Reduce dose to 90mcg once weekly
Platelets <25,000 cells/mm³: D/C treatment
Pediatrics:
Platelets <50,000 cells/mm³: 90mcg/1.73m² x BSA

Transaminase Elevations:
Adults:
Progressive ALT Increases After Dose Reduction: D/C therapy
ALT Increases w/ Increased Bilirubin/Evidence of Hepatic Decompensation: D/C therapy
Chronic Hepatitis C Patients:
Progressive ALT Increases Above Baseline: Reduce dose to 135mcg; resume therapy after flares subside
Chronic Hepatitis B Patients:
ALT Elevations >5X ULN: Reduce dose to 135mcg or temporarily d/c; resume therapy after flares subside
Persistent, Severe Flares (ALT >10X Above ULN): Consider discontinuation
Pediatrics:
Persistent/Increasing ALT Elevations ≥5 but <10X ULN: Modify dose to 135mcg/1.73m² x BSA; reduce dose further if necessary
Persistent ALT Elevations ≥10X ULN: D/C treatment

Depression:
Initial Management (4-8 Weeks):
Adults:
Moderate: Decrease dose to 135mcg or 90mcg once weekly
Severe: Permanently d/c treatment
Pediatrics:
Moderate: Decrease dose to 135mcg/1.73m² x BSA or 90mcg/1.73m² x BSA once weekly
Severe: Permanently d/c treatment
Worsening of Depression Severity After 8 Weeks:
Adults:
Mild: Decrease dose to 135mcg or 90mcg once weekly or d/c
Moderate: Permanently d/c treatment
Pediatrics:
Mild: Decrease dose to 135mcg/1.73m² x BSA or 90mcg/1.73m² x BSA once weekly
Moderate: Permanently d/c treatment
Refer to PI for psychiatric visit schedule

Discontinuation
Chronic Hepatic C Genotype 1 in Combination w/ Ribavirin or Alone:
D/C if at least a 2 log₁₀ HCV RNA reduction from baseline is not achieved by Week 12
D/C if undetectable HCV RNA is not achieved after 24 weeks

ADMINISTRATION
SQ route

Administer in abdomen or thigh.
Discard unused portion in single-use vials or prefilled syringes in excess of the labeled volume.

Recommended Volume to be Administered for Different Dosages
180mcg/mL in a Vial:
90mcg Dose: Use 0.5mL
135mcg Dose: Use 0.75mL
180mcg Dose: Use entire 1mL
180mcg/0.5mL in a Prefilled Syringe:
90mcg: Use 0.25mL
135mcg: Use 0.375mL
180mcg: Use entire 0.5mL
180mcg/0.5mL in an Autoinjector:
90mcg: Do not use
135mcg: Do not use
180mcg: May use

135mcg/0.5mL in an Autoinjector:
90mcg: Do not use
135mcg: May use
180mcg: Do not use

STORAGE
2-8°C (36-46°F). Do not leave out of the refrigerator for >24 hrs. Do not freeze or shake. Protect from light.

HOW SUPPLIED
Inj: 180mcg/0.5mL [prefilled syringe]; 180mcg/0.5mL, 135mcg/0.5mL [ProClick autoinjector]; 180mcg/mL [vial]

CONTRAINDICATIONS
Known hypersensitivity reactions (eg, urticaria, angioedema, bronchoconstriction, anaphylaxis, Stevens-Johnson syndrome) to alpha interferons or any component of this medication. autoimmune hepatitis, hepatic decompensation (Child-Pugh score >6 [Class B and C]) in cirrhotic patients before treatment, hepatic decompensation w/ Child-Pugh score ≥6 in cirrhotic CHC patients coinfected w/ HIV before treatment, neonates and infants (contains benzyl alcohol). When used with other HCV antiviral drugs, including ribavirin, refer to the individual monograph(s).

WARNINGS/PRECAUTIONS
Not recommended, alone or in combination w/ ribavirin w/o additional HCV antiviral drugs, in CHC patients who previously failed therapy w/ an interferon-alfa, and in CHC patients who have had a solid organ transplantation. Avoid in combination w/ ribavirin in pregnant women or men whose female partners are pregnant. Extreme caution w/ history of depression; d/c immediately in severe cases and institute psychiatric intervention. HTN, supraventricular arrhythmias, chest pain, and MI reported; caution w/ preexisting cardiac disease. May cause bone marrow suppression and severe cytopenias; d/c, at least temporarily, if severe decrease in neutrophil or platelet count develops. May cause or aggravate hypo/hyperthyroidism, ophthalmologic disorders, and pulmonary disorders. Hypo/hyperglycemia, diabetes mellitus, and ischemic and hemorrhagic cerebrovascular events reported. CHC patients w/ cirrhosis may be at risk for hepatic decompensation and death; d/c immediately w/ hepatic decompensation. Exacerbation of hepatitis B reported; d/c immediately if hepatic decompensation, progressive ALT increases, or increased bilirubin occurs. Ulcerative or hemorrhagic/ischemic colitis, pancreatitis, and severe acute hypersensitivity reactions reported; d/c if any of these develop. Consider discontinuation of treatment and immediately start appropriate anti-infective therapy if serious and severe infections occur. D/C w/ new or worsening ophthalmologic disorders, pulmonary infiltrates or pulmonary function impairment. Peripheral neuropathy reported in combination w/ telbivudine. May inhibit growth in pediatric patients. May impair fertility in women. Caution in renal impairment and in the elderly.

ADVERSE REACTIONS
Neuropsychiatric/autoimmune/ischemic/infectious disorders, inj-site reactions, fatigue/asthenia, diarrhea, pyrexia, rigors, N/V, anorexia, myalgia, headache, irritability/anxiety/nervousness.

DRUG INTERACTIONS
May inhibit CYP1A2 and increase exposure of theophylline; monitor theophylline serum levels and consider dose adjustments. May increase levels of methadone; monitor for toxicity. Hepatic decompensation can occur w/ peginterferon alfa-2a/ribavirin in combination w/ other HCV antiviral drugs and nucleoside reverse transcriptase inhibitors (NRTIs); refer to PI for other HCV antiviral drugs and the respective NRTIs for guidance regarding toxicity management. Concomitant use of peginterferon alfa-2a/ribavirin w/ zidovudine may cause severe neutropenia and severe anemia; consider discontinuation of zidovudine as medically appropriate and also consider dose reduction or discontinuation of peginterferon alfa-2a, ribavirin or both if worsening clinical toxicities are observed, including hepatic decompensation (eg, Child-Pugh >6). Pancytopenia and bone marrow suppression reported to occur w/in 3-7 weeks after the concomitant administration of pegylated interferon/ribavirin and azathioprine; d/c peginterferon alfa-2a, ribavirin, and azathioprine for pancytopenia, and do not re-introduce pegylated interferon/ribavirin w/ concomitant azathioprine.

PREGNANCY AND LACTATION
Pregnancy: Category C, Category X (w/ ribavirin).
Lactation: Not for use in nursing.

MECHANISM OF ACTION
Pegylated virus proliferation inhibitor; binds to human type 1 interferon receptor leading to receptor dimerization, which activates multiple intracellular signal transduction pathways initially mediated by the JAK/STAT pathway. Expected to have pleiotropic biological effects in the body.

PHARMACOKINETICS
Absorption: T_{max}=72-96 hrs. **Elimination:** $T_{1/2}$=160 hrs (CHC).

PATIENT CONSIDERATIONS
Assessment: Assess for neuropsychiatric, autoimmune, ischemic or infectious disorders, hepatic/renal impairment, known hypersensitivity reactions, history of treatment failure w/ interferon alfa in CHC patients, history of solid organ transplantation in CHC patients, nursing status, possible drug interactions, or any other conditions where treatment is contraindicated or cautioned. Obtain baseline CBC, TSH, CD4⁺ (HIV), and eye exam. Perform ECG for preexisting cardiac diseases. Obtain pregnancy test in women of childbearing potential.

Monitoring: Monitor for signs/symptoms of neuropsychiatric, autoimmune, ischemic, infectious, cardiovascular, cerebrovascular, endocrine, and pulmonary disorders; bone marrow toxicities; colitis; pancreatitis; delayed growth in pediatric patients; and other adverse reactions. Monitor hematological (Weeks 2, 4, and periodically thereafter) and biochemical tests (Week 4 and periodically thereafter), and TSH (every 12 weeks). Perform periodic eye exams in patients w/ preexisting ophthalmologic disorders. Perform monthly pregnancy tests if on combination therapy w/ ribavirin and for 6 months after discontinuation. Monitor clinical status and hepatic/renal function.

Counseling: Counsel on benefits and risks of therapy. Advise not to use drug in combination w/ ribavirin for pregnant women or men whose female partners are pregnant. Inform of the teratogenic/embryocidal risks w/ ribavirin; instruct to use 2 forms of effective contraception during ribavirin therapy and for 6 months post-therapy. Inform that drug is not known if drug will prevent transmission of HCV/HBV infection to others. Advise that it is not known if therapy will prevent cirrhosis, liver failure or liver cancer in HBV patients. Advise that laboratory evaluations are required prior to therapy, and periodically thereafter. Counsel to avoid alcohol, and avoid driving or operating machinery if dizziness, confusion, somnolence, or fatigue occurs. Instruct to remain well hydrated, and not to switch to another brand of interferon w/o consulting physician. Instruct on the proper preparation and administration, and disposal techniques for therapy.

PEGINTRON — peginterferon alfa-2b   **Rx**
Class: Biological response modifier

> May cause or aggravate fatal or life-threatening neuropsychiatric, autoimmune, ischemic, and infectious disorders. Closely monitor patients w/ periodic clinical and lab evaluations. D/C w/ persistently severe or worsening signs/symptoms of these conditions. When used w/ Rebetol, refer to the individual monograph.

ADULT DOSAGE
Chronic Hepatitis C with Compensated Liver Disease

Combination Therapy w/ Rebetol w/ or w/o Hepatitis C Virus (HCV) NS3/4A Protease Inhibitor:
Use w/ HCV NS3/4A protease inhibitor w/ HCV genotype 1 infection. Use w/o HCV NS3/4A protease inhibitor in genotypes other than 1, or w/ genotype 1 infection where use of an HCV NS3/4A protease inhibitor is not warranted based on tolerability, contraindications, or other clinical factors

1.5mcg/kg/week + 800-1400mg Rebetol (based on body weight)

Refer to the PI of the specific HCV NS3/4A protease inhibitor for dosing information

Treatment Duration:
Interferon-Alfa-Naive Patients:
Genotype 1: 48 weeks
Genotypes 2 and 3: 24 weeks
Retreatment of Prior Treatment Failure:
48 weeks (regardless of genotype)

Monotherapy:
Monotherapy should be used only if there are contraindications to or significant intolerance of Rebetol in previously untreated patients

1mcg/kg/week (same day of the week) for 1 yr

PEDIATRIC DOSAGE
Chronic Hepatitis C with Compensated Liver Disease

3-17 Years:
Combination Therapy w/ Rebetol:
60mcg/m²/week + 15mg/kg/day Rebetol in 2 divided doses

Remain on pediatric dosing regimen if 18th birthday was reached during therapy

Treatment Duration:
Genotype 1: 48 weeks
Genotype 2 and 3: 24 weeks

DOSING CONSIDERATIONS
Renal Impairment
Moderate (CrCl 30-50mL/min): Reduce dose by 25%
Severe (CrCl 10-29mL/min), Including Hemodialysis: Reduce dose by 50%
Decline in Renal Function During Treatment: D/C therapy

Adverse Reactions
Dose Reduction:
Adults:
Combination Therapy w/ Rebetol: Reduce to 1mcg/kg/week, then to 0.5mcg/kg/week, if needed
Monotherapy: Reduce to 0.5mcg/kg/week
Pediatrics:
Reduce to 40mcg/m²/week, then to 20mcg/m²/week, if needed

Depression:
Initial Management (4-8 Weeks):
Moderate: Reduce dose; see dose reduction above
Severe: Permanently d/c PegIntron/Rebetol

Refer to PI for psychiatric visit schedule and for recommendations based on depression status after initial management

Lab Parameters:
Reduce PegIntron Dose If (See Dose Reduction Above):
WBCs 1 to <1.5 x 10⁹/L, neutrophils 0.5 to <0.75 x 10⁹/L, platelets 25 to <50 x 10⁹/L (adults) or 50 to <70 x 10⁹/L (pediatrics)

Reduce PegIntron Dose by Half If:
≥2g/dL decrease in Hgb during any 4-week period during treatment in patients w/ history of stable cardiac disease; pediatric patients should have weekly evaluations and hematology testing

D/C Therapy If:
WBCs <1 x 10⁹/L, neutrophils <0.5 x 10⁹/L, platelets <25 x 10⁹/L (adults) or <50 x 10⁹/L (pediatrics), creatinine >2mg/dL (pediatrics), Hgb in patients w/o history of cardiac disease <8.5g/dL, Hgb in patients w/ history of stable cardiac disease <8.5g/dL or <12g/dL after 4 weeks of dose reduction
Refer to PI for Rebetol dose reductions

Discontinuation
Adults:
Genotype 1:
Interferon-Alfa-Naive Receiving PegIntron, Alone or in Combination w/ Rebetol:
D/C if there is not at least a 2 log₁₀ drop or loss of HCV-RNA at 12 weeks of therapy.
D/C if HCV-RNA levels remain detectable after 24 weeks of therapy.

All Genotypes:
Previously Treated Patients:
D/C if HCV-RNA levels remain detectable at Week 12 or 24

Pediatrics
3-17 Years and Excluding Genotype 2 and 3:
D/C therapy at 12 weeks if treatment Week 12 HCV-RNA drops <2 log₁₀ compared to pretreatment.
D/C therapy at 24 weeks if HCV-RNA is detectable at treatment Week 24.

ADMINISTRATION
SQ route
Do not reuse the vial/prefilled pen; discard unused portion.
Refer to Rebetol and specific HCV NS3/4A protease inhibitor labeling for dosing and administration.

STORAGE
Redipen: 2-8°C (36-46°F). **Vial:** 25°C (77°F); excursions permitted to 15-30°C (59-86°F). **Redipen/Vial:** (Reconstituted Sol) Should be used immediately, but may store for up to 24 hrs at 2-8°C (36-46°F). Do not freeze. Keep away from heat.

HOW SUPPLIED
Inj: 50mcg/0.5mL, 80mcg/0.5mL, 120mcg/0.5mL, 150mcg/0.5mL [vial, Redipen]

CONTRAINDICATIONS
Known hypersensitivity reactions (eg, urticaria, angioedema, bronchoconstriction, anaphylaxis, Stevens-Johnson syndrome, toxic epidermal necrolysis) to interferon alpha or any other component of the product. Autoimmune hepatitis, hepatic decompensation (Child-Pugh score >6 [Class B and C]) in cirrhotic chronic hepatitis C (CHC) patients before or during treatment. When used w/ Rebetol, refer to the individual monograph.

WARNINGS/PRECAUTIONS
Caution w/ history of psychiatric disorders. Monitor during treatment and in the 6-month follow-up period if psychiatric problems develop; d/c if symptoms persist or worsen, or if suicidal or homicidal ideation or aggressive behavior towards others is identified. Cases of encephalopathy reported in some w/ higher doses. Cardiovascular (CV) events reported; caution w/ CV disease (CVD) (eg, MI, arrhythmia). Hyperglycemia, diabetes mellitus, and new/worsening hypo/hyperthyroidism reported; do not begin/continue therapy in patients w/ these conditions who cannot be controlled w/ medication. Ophthalmologic disorders may be induced or aggravated; d/c if new or worsening ophthalmologic disorders develop. Ischemic and hemorrhagic cerebrovascular events reported. Suppresses bone marrow function; d/c if severe decreases in neutrophil or platelet counts develop. May rarely be associated w/ aplastic anemia. New/worsening of autoimmune disorders reported. Pancreatitis reported; suspend therapy w/ signs and symptoms suggestive of pancreatitis and d/c if diagnosed w/ pancreatitis. Ulcerative or hemorrhagic/ischemic colitis reported; d/c if signs/symptoms develop. Pulmonary disorders may be induced or aggravated; suspend combination treatment if pulmonary infiltrates or pulmonary function impairment develops. Caution w/ debilitating medical conditions (eg, history of pulmonary disease). CHC patients w/ cirrhosis may be at risk for hepatic decompensation and death. Cirrhotic CHC patients coinfected w/ HIV receiving highly active antiretroviral therapy (HAART) and alpha interferons w/ or w/o ribavirin may be at increased risk for hepatic decompensation compared to patients not receiving HAART. Increases SrCr levels in patients w/ renal insufficiency; monitor closely for signs and symptoms of interferon toxicity and adjust dose or d/c therapy. Use monotherapy w/ caution w/ CrCl <50mL/min. Serious, acute hypersensitivity reactions and cutaneous eruptions rarely reported; d/c treatment if such a reaction develops. Transient ALT increases and elevated TG levels reported; consider discontinuation in patients w/ persistently elevated TG levels (eg, TG >1000mg/dL). Dental/periodontal disorders reported w/ combination therapy w/ Rebetol. Weight loss and growth inhibition (including long-term growth inhibition) reported in pediatric patients during combination therapy w/ Rebetol.

ADVERSE REACTIONS
Adults: (Monotherapy or Combination Therapy w/ Rebetol) Inj-site inflammation/reaction, fatigue/asthenia, headache, rigors, fevers, N/V, myalgia, emotional lability/irritability. **Pediatric Patients:** Pyrexia, headache, vomiting, neutropenia, fatigue, anorexia, inj-site erythema, abdominal pain.

DRUG INTERACTIONS
Use caution when drugs w/ a narrow therapeutic range metabolized by CYP1A2 (eg, caffeine) or CYP2D6 (eg, thioridazine) are coadministered. Monitor blood cell count and suppressive effect on bone marrow function w/ zidovudine. Therapeutic monitoring of concomitant immunosuppressive agents recommended. May increase methadone, thioridazine, and theophylline levels; may need to reduce methadone dose, and monitor for thioridazine and theophylline adverse events. Closely monitor for toxicities, especially hepatic decompensation and anemia, when patient is receiving interferon w/ Rebetol and nucleoside reverse transcriptase inhibitors (NRTIs); consider dose reduction or discontinuation of interferon, Rebetol, or both if worsening clinical toxicities

occur, or discontinuation of NRTI if medically appropriate. Concomitant use of peginterferon alpha and Rebetol w/ zidovudine may cause severe neutropenia and severe anemia. Peripheral neuropathy reported when used in combination w/ telbivudine.

PREGNANCY AND LACTATION
Pregnancy: Category C; recommended for use in fertile women only when they are using effective contraception. Category X (w/ Rebetol).
Lactation: Not for use in nursing.

MECHANISM OF ACTION
Pegylated virus proliferation inhibitor; binds to and activates the human type 1 interferon receptor. Upon binding, the receptor subunits dimerize and activate multiple intracellular signal transduction pathways.

PHARMACOKINETICS
Absorption: T$_{max}$=15-44 hrs. **Elimination:** T$_{1/2}$=40 hrs.

PATIENT CONSIDERATIONS
Assessment: Assess for history of MI, arrhythmia, and psychiatric disorders; presence of CVD, endocrine, autoimmune, and ophthalmologic disorders; debilitating medical conditions; hepatic/renal impairment; drug hypersensitivity; any other conditions where treatment is contraindicated or cautioned; pregnancy/nursing status; and possible drug interactions. Obtain baseline CBC, blood chemistry, and eye exam. Perform ECG in patients w/ preexisting cardiac abnormalities.

Monitoring: Monitor CBC, blood chemistry, TG levels, and HCV-RNA periodically. Monitor hepatic/renal function. Perform periodic ophthalmologic exams w/ preexisting ophthalmologic disorders. Patients should have regular dental exams. Monitor growth in pediatric patients. Monitor for signs/symptoms of autoimmune, cerebrovascular, infectious, endocrine, and pulmonary disorders; CV and neuropsychiatric events; bone marrow toxicity; hepatic decompensation; colitis; pancreatitis; hypersensitivity reactions; and other adverse reactions.

Counseling: Inform of benefits/risks of therapy and about proper instructions for use. Advise to report immediately to physician any symptoms of depression or suicidal ideation. Instruct females and female partners of male patients to avoid pregnancy during combination treatment w/ Rebetol and for 6 months post-therapy; instruct to use at least 2 forms of effective contraception and to have monthly pregnancy tests during and for 6 months post-therapy. Instruct to brush teeth thoroughly bid and to have regular dental examinations when used in combination w/ Rebetol; if vomiting occurs, advise to rinse out mouth afterwards. Inform that there are no data regarding whether therapy will prevent HCV infection transmission to others. Advise that lab evaluations are required prior to starting therapy and periodically thereafter. Advise to remain well hydrated. Counsel that flu-like symptoms associated w/ treatment may be minimized by hs administration of the drug or by using antipyretics. Inform that chest x-ray or other tests may be needed if fever, cough, SOB, or other symptoms of a lung problem develop. Instruct self-administering patients on the importance of site selection, rotating inj sites, and proper disposal of needles, syringes, and Redipen.

PENICILLIN G SODIUM — penicillin G sodium   Rx

Class: Penicillin (PCN)

ADULT DOSAGE
Serious Infections

Septicemia, empyema, pneumonia, pericarditis, endocarditis, and meningitis due to susceptible strains of streptococci (including *Streptococcus pneumoniae*) and staphylococci

5-24 million U/day in divided equal doses q4-6h

Anthrax

Minimum of 8 million U/day in divided doses q6h; may require higher doses depending on susceptibility of organisms

Actinomycosis

Cervicofacial Disease:
1-6 million U/day in divided doses q4-6h

Thoracic and Abdominal Disease:
10-20 million U/day in divided doses q4-6h

Clostridial Infections

Botulism (adjunct to antitoxin), gas gangrene (debridement and/or surgery as indicated), tetanus (adjunct to human tetanus immune globulin)

20 million U/day q4-6h in divided doses

Diphtheria

Adjunctive to Antitoxin/For the Prevention of the Carrier State:
2-3 million U/day in divided doses q4-6h for 10-12 days

PEDIATRIC DOSAGE
Serious Infections

Serious infections (eg, pneumonia, endocarditis) due to susceptible strains of streptococci (including *Streptococci pneumoniae*) and meningococcus

150,000 U/kg/day in equally divided doses q4-6h

Meningitis

Susceptible Strains of Pneumococcus and Meningococcus:
250,000 U/kg/day in equally divided doses q4h for 7-14 days
Max: 12-20 million U/day

Gonococcal Infections

Disseminated Infections Caused by Susceptible Strains:

<45kg:
Arthritis: 100,000 U/kg/day in 4 equally divided doses for 7-10 days
Meningitis: 250,000 U/kg/day in equal doses q4h for 10-14 days
Endocarditis: 250,000 U/kg/day in equal doses q4h for 4 weeks

≥45kg:
Arthritis/Meningitis/Endocarditis:
10 million U/day in 4 equally divided doses

Syphilis

Congenital and Neurosyphilis After the Newborn Period:
200,000-300,000 U/kg/day (administered as 50,000 U/kg q4-6h) for 10-14 days

Erysipelothrix Endocarditis
12-20 million U/day in divided doses q4-6h for 4-6 weeks

Fusospirochetosis
Severe Infections of the Oropharynx (Vincent's), Lower Respiratory Tract, and Genital Area:
5-10 million U/day in divided doses q4-6h

Listeria Infections
Meningitis:
15-20 million U/day in divided doses q4-6h for 2 weeks

Endocarditis:
15-20 million U/day in divided doses q4-6h for 4 weeks

Pasteurella Infections
Including Bacteremia and Meningitis:
4-6 million U/day in divided doses q4-6h for 2 weeks

Haverhill Fever/Rat-bite Fever
12-20 million U/day in divided doses q4-6h for 3-4 weeks

Gonococcal Infections
Disseminated Infections Caused by Susceptible Organisms (eg, Meningitis, Endocarditis, Arthritis):
10 million U/day in divided doses q4-6h

Syphilis
Neurosyphilis:
12-24 million U/day, as 2-4 million U q4h for 10-14 days; may recommend additional therapy w/ IM benzathine penicillin G 2.4 million U/weekly for 3 doses after completion of IV therapy

Meningococcal Infections
Meningitis and/or Septicemia:
24 million U/day, as 2 million U q2h

Treatment Duration
Most Acute Infections:
Continue for at least 48-72 hrs after patient becomes asymptomatic

Group A β-Hemolytic Streptococcal Infections:
Maintain for at least 10 days

Diphtheria
Adjunctive to Antitoxin/For the Prevention of the Carrier State:
150,000-250,000 U/kg/day in equal doses q6h for 7-10 days

Haverhill Fever/Rat-bite Fever
W/ Endocarditis Caused by Streptobacillus moniliformis:
150,000-250,000 U/kg/day in equal doses q4h for 4 weeks

Treatment Duration
Most Acute Infections:
Continue for at least 48-72 hrs after patient becomes asymptomatic

Group A β-Hemolytic Streptococcal Infections:
Maintain for at least 10 days

- -

DOSING CONSIDERATIONS
Renal Impairment
Uremic Patients w/ CrCl >10mL/min: Administer a full LD followed by 1/2 of the LD q4-5h

CrCl <10mL/min: Administer a full LD followed by 1/2 of the LD q8-10h

ADMINISTRATION
IM/IV route

Pediatrics
Do not administer to patients requiring <1 million U/dose.

Preparation
Add 8mL for a final concentration of 500,000 U/mL or 3mL for a final concentration of 1 million U/mL.
Loosen powder; hold vial horizontally and rotate it while slowly directing stream of diluent against the wall of the vial.
Shake vial vigorously after all the diluent is added.
Depending on route of administration, use SWFI, 0.9% NaCl inj, dextrose inj.

STORAGE
(Dry Powder) 20-25°C (68-77°F). (Reconstituted Sol) May store at 2-8°C (36-46°F) for 3 days w/o significant loss of potency.

HOW SUPPLIED
Inj: 5,000,000 U

CONTRAINDICATIONS
History of hypersensitivity (anaphylactic) reaction to any penicillin.

WARNINGS/PRECAUTIONS
Not recommended as drug of choice in the treatment of gram-negative bacillary infections. Serious and occasionally fatal hypersensitivity reactions reported; d/c if an allergic reaction occurs and institute appropriate therapy. Carefully assess previous hypersensitivity to therapy, cephalosporins, and other allergens. Caution w/ a history of significant allergies and/or asthma. Clostridium difficile-associated diarrhea (CDAD) reported; may need to d/c if CDAD is suspected or confirmed. May result in bacterial resistance when used in the absence of a proven/suspected bacterial infection or a prophylactic indication; take appropriate measures if superinfection develops. Use by IV route in high doses (>10 million U) should be administered slowly because of potential electrolyte imbalance. Lab test interactions may occur.

ADVERSE REACTIONS
Jarisch-Herxheimer reaction, allergic reactions, pseudomembranous colitis, N/V, neutropenia, electrolyte disturbances, CHF (high dosage), neurotoxic reactions, renal tubular damage, interstitial nephritis, phlebitis, thrombophlebitis.

DRUG INTERACTIONS
Bacteriostatic antibacterials (eg, chloramphenicol, erythromycins, sulfonamides, tetracyclines) may antagonize the bactericidal effect; avoid concurrent use. Probenecid may prolong blood levels. Other drugs including ASA, phenylbutazone, sulfonamides, indomethacin, thiazide diuretics, furosemide, and ethacrynic acid may compete for renal tubular secretion and thus prolong the serum $T_{1/2}$ of penicillin (PCN).

PREGNANCY AND LACTATION
Category B, caution in nursing.

MECHANISM OF ACTION
PCN; bactericidal against PCN-susceptible microorganisms during the stage of active multiplication. Acts by inhibiting biosynthesis of cell-wall mucopeptide.

PHARMACOKINETICS
Absorption: Administration of variable doses resulted in different pharmacokinetic parameters. **Distribution:** Crosses the placenta; found in breast milk. **Metabolism:** Hepatic. **Elimination:** Urine (58-85%), bile; $T_{1/2}$=42 min (adults), 3.2 hrs (infants 0-6 days of age), 1.4 hrs (infants ≥14 days of age).

PATIENT CONSIDERATIONS
Assessment: Assess for previous hypersensitivity reactions to PCN, cephalosporins, or other allergens, history of asthma, renal impairment, pregnancy/nursing status, and possible drug interactions. Perform proper lab studies (eg, susceptibility tests) in suspected staphylococcal infection. Perform serologic test for syphilis prior to initiation of therapy in patients being treated for gonococcal infection.

Monitoring: Monitor for signs/symptoms of hypersensitivity reactions, CDAD, superinfection, and other adverse reactions. Perform adequate follow-up (eg, clinical and serological examinations) in all cases of PCN-treated syphilis. Perform periodic evaluation of organ system function (eg, electrolyte balance/hepatic/ renal/hematopoietic/cardiac/vascular status) if on prolonged therapy w/ high doses.

Counseling: Inform that drug treats only bacterial, not viral, infections. Instruct to take ud; inform that skipping doses or not completing the full course of therapy may decrease the effectiveness and increase the risk of bacterial resistance. Inform that diarrhea may occur, which usually ends when therapy is discontinued. Instruct to seek medical attention if watery and bloody stools (w/ or w/o stomach cramps and fever) occur even after ≥2 months of discontinuing therapy.

PENICILLIN VK — penicillin V potassium   Rx

Class: Penicillin (PCN)

ADULT DOSAGE

Fusospirochetosis
Mild to Moderately Severe Infections of the Oropharynx:
Usual: 250-500mg q6-8h

Streptococcal Infections
Mild to Moderately Severe URTIs, Scarlet Fever, and Mild Erysipelas:
Usual: 125-250mg q6-8h for 10 days

Respiratory Tract Infections
Mild to Moderately Severe Pneumococcal Infections:
Usual: 250-500mg q6h until patient has been afebrile for at least 2 days

Otitis Media
Mild to Moderately Severe Pneumococcal Infections:
Usual: 250-500mg q6h until patient has been afebrile for at least 2 days

Skin and Skin Structure Infections
Mild Staphylococcal Infections of the Skin and Soft Tissues:
Usual: 250-500mg q6-8h

Culture and sensitivity tests should be performed

Endocarditis
Prophylaxis against bacterial endocarditis in patients w/ congenital heart disease/rheumatic/other acquired valvular heart disease when undergoing dental procedures or surgical procedures of the upper respiratory tract

Usual: 2g 1 hr before the procedure, then 1g 6 hrs later

PEDIATRIC DOSAGE

Otitis Media
Mild to Moderately Severe Pneumococcal Infections:
≥12 Years:
Usual: 250-500mg q6h until patient has been afebrile for at least 2 days

Skin and Skin Structure Infections
Mild Staphylococcal Infections of the Skin and Soft Tissues:
≥12 Years:
Usual: 250-500mg q6-8h

Culture and sensitivity tests should be performed

Fusospirochetosis
Mild to Moderately Severe Infections of the Oropharynx:
≥12 Years:
Usual: 250-500mg q6-8h

Streptococcal Infections
Mild to Moderately Severe URTIs, Scarlet Fever, and Mild Erysipelas:
≥12 Years:
Usual: 125-250mg q6-8h for 10 days

Respiratory Tract Infections
Mild to Moderately Severe Pneumococcal Infections:
≥12 Years:
Usual: 250-500mg q6h until patient has been afebrile for at least 2 days

Other Indications
≥12 Years:

Prevention of Recurrence Following Rheumatic Fever and/or Chorea:
Usual: 125-500mg bid on a continuing basis

Other Indications
Prevention of Recurrence Following Rheumatic Fever and/or Chorea:
Usual: 125-500mg bid on a continuing basis

Prophylaxis Against Bacterial Endocarditis:
In patients w/ congenital heart disease/rheumatic/other acquired valvular heart disease when undergoing dental procedures or surgical procedures of the upper respiratory tract
<60 lbs:
Usual: 1g 1 hr before the procedure, then 500mg 6 hrs later

ADMINISTRATION
Oral route

Directions for Mixing Sol
125mg/mL Sol: Reconstitute 100mL or 200mL bottle size w/ 75mL or 150mL of water, respectively
250mg/5mL Sol: Reconstitute 100mL or 200mL bottle size w/ 75mL or 150mL of water, respectively
Add water in 2 portions, shaking vigorously between each aliquot

STORAGE
20-25°C (68-77°F). (Reconstituted Sol) Store in a refrigerator. Discard any unused portion after 14 days.

HOW SUPPLIED
Sol: 125mg/5mL [100mL, 200mL], 250mg/5mL [100mL, 200mL]; **Tab:** 250mg, 500mg

CONTRAINDICATIONS
Previous hypersensitivity reaction to any penicillin.

WARNINGS/PRECAUTIONS
Not for treatment of severe pneumonia, empyema, bacteremia, pericarditis, meningitis, and arthritis during the acute stage. Necessary dental care should be accomplished in infections involving the gum tissue. Oral penicillin should not be used in patients at particularly high risk for endocarditis (eg, those w/ prosthetic heart valves or surgically constructed systemic pulmonary shunts). Should not be used as adjunctive prophylaxis for genitourinary instrumentation/surgery, lower intestinal tract surgery, sigmoidoscopy, and childbirth. Serious and fatal anaphylactic reactions reported; caution w/ a history of hypersensitivity to PCN, cephalosporins, and/or multiple allergens. Caution w/ history of significant allergies and/or asthma. D/C if an allergic reaction occurs and institute appropriate therapy. *Clostridium difficile*-associated diarrhea (CDAD) reported; d/c therapy if CDAD is suspected/confirmed. Use in the absence of a proven/strongly suspected bacterial infection or a prophylactic indication is unlikely to provide benefit and increases the risk of drug-resistant bacteria. Prolonged use may promote overgrowth of nonsusceptible organisms; take appropriate measures if superinfection develops. Oral route of administration should not be relied upon w/ severe illness, N/V, gastric dilatation, cardiospasm, or intestinal hypermotility. Obtain cultures following completion of treatment for streptococcal infections.

ADVERSE REACTIONS
Epigastric distress, N/V, diarrhea, black hairy tongue, hypersensitivity reactions (skin eruptions, urticaria, other serum-sickness like reactions, laryngeal edema, anaphylaxis), fever, eosinophilia.

PREGNANCY AND LACTATION
Safety in pregnancy/nursing not known.

MECHANISM OF ACTION
PCN; exerts a bactericidal action against PCN-sensitive microorganisms during the stage of active multiplication. Acts through inhibition of biosynthesis of cell-wall mucopeptide.

PHARMACOKINETICS
Distribution: Plasma protein binding (80%). **Elimination:** Urine.

PATIENT CONSIDERATIONS
Assessment: Assess for previous hypersensitivity reactions to PCNs/cephalosporins or other allergens, history of asthma, N/V, gastric dilatation, severe illness, cardiospasm, intestinal hypermotility, and pregnancy/nursing status. Obtain cultures and sensitivity tests, especially in suspected staphylococcal infections.

Monitoring: Monitor for signs/symptoms of hypersensitivity reactions, CDAD, superinfections, and other adverse reactions. Obtain cultures following completion of treatment of streptococcal infections.

Counseling: Counsel that therapy only treats bacterial, not viral, infections. Instruct to take ud; inform that skipping doses or not completing the full course of therapy may decrease effectiveness and increase resistance. Inform that diarrhea may occur. Instruct to seek medical attention if watery and bloody stools (w/ or w/o stomach cramps and fever) occur even after ≥2 months of discontinuing therapy.

PENLAC — ciclopirox   Rx

Class: Broad-spectrum antifungal

ADULT DOSAGE	PEDIATRIC DOSAGE
Onychomycosis	**Onychomycosis**
Mild to Moderate Onychomycosis w/o Lunula Involvement Due to *Trichophyton rubrum*:	**Mild to Moderate Onychomycosis w/o Lunula Involvement Due to** *Trichophyton rubrum*:
Apply evenly over the entire plate qd (preferably at hs or 8 hrs before	**≥12 Years:** Apply evenly over the entire plate qd (preferably at hs or 8 hrs before

---

washing); when nail plate is free of nail bed (eg, onychomycosis), apply to the nail bed, hyponychium, and under the surface of the nail plate
Repeat regimen for up to 48 weeks

washing); when nail plate is free of nail bed (eg, onychomycosis), apply to the nail bed, hyponychium, and under the surface of the nail plate
Repeat regimen for up to 48 weeks

ADMINISTRATION
Topical route

Sol should not be removed on a daily basis; apply daily over previous coat and remove w/ alcohol every 7 days.
Removal of the unattached, infected nail, as frequently as monthly, by a healthcare professional, weekly trimming by the patient, and daily application of the medication are all integral parts of this therapy.

STORAGE
15-30°C (59-86°F). Flammable; keep away from heat and flame. Protect from light.

HOW SUPPLIED
Sol: 8% [6.6mL]

CONTRAINDICATIONS
Hypersensitivity to any of the components.

WARNINGS/PRECAUTIONS
Not for ophthalmic, oral, or intravaginal use; for use on nails and immediately adjacent skin only. Should be used as a component of a comprehensive management program for onychomycosis and should be used only under medical supervision by a healthcare professional who has special competence in the diagnosis and treatment of nail disorders, including minor nail procedures. D/C and treat appropriately if sensitivity reaction or chemical irritation occurs. Caution with removal of infected nail in patients with a history of insulin-dependent diabetes mellitus (DM) or diabetic neuropathy.

ADVERSE REACTIONS
Periungual erythema, erythema of the proximal nail fold, nail shape change, nail irritation, ingrown toenail, nail discoloration.

DRUG INTERACTIONS
Avoid with systemic antifungal agents for onychomycosis.

PREGNANCY AND LACTATION
Pregnancy: Category B.
Lactation: Caution in nursing.

MECHANISM OF ACTION
Broad spectrum antifungal; not established. Suggested to act by chelation of polyvalent cations, resulting in the inhibition of the metal-dependent enzymes responsible for degradation of peroxides within fungal cell.

PHARMACOKINETICS
Absorption: (PO) Rapid. **Metabolism:** Glucuronidation. **Elimination:** Urine (<5% of applied topical dose).

PATIENT CONSIDERATIONS
Assessment: Assess for insulin-dependent DM, diabetic neuropathy, drug hypersensitivity, pregnancy/nursing status, and possible drug interactions.

Monitoring: Monitor for sensitivity reactions, chemical irritation, and other adverse reactions. Perform frequent (eg, monthly) removal of unattached infected nails, trimming of onycholytic nail, and filing of any excess horny material.

Counseling: Advise to avoid contact with the eyes and mucous membranes. Instruct to apply medication evenly over entire nail plate and 5mm of surrounding skin. Advise that if possible, the medication should be applied to the nail bed, hyponychium, and the under surface of the nail plate when it is free of the nail bed (eg, onycholysis). Instruct to notify physician if signs of increased irritation at the application site develop. Instruct to inform physician if patient has diabetes or problems with numbness in toes or fingers for consideration of appropriate nail management program. Instruct to file away (with emery board) loose nail material and trim nails as required or ud. Advise to not use nail polish or other nail cosmetic products on the treated nails. Instruct not to use medication near open flame. Inform that it may take up to 48 weeks of daily application of the medication (including monthly professional removal of unattached infected nails) to achieve a clear or almost clear nail.

PENNSAID — diclofenac sodium   Rx

Class: NSAID

> NSAIDs cause an increased risk of serious cardiovascular (CV) thrombotic events, including MI and stroke, which can be fatal. This risk may occur early in treatment and may increase w/ duration of use. Contraindicated in the setting of CABG surgery. NSAIDs cause an increased risk of serious GI adverse events (eg, bleeding, ulceration, stomach/intestinal perforation), which can be fatal and can occur anytime during use and w/o warning symptoms; elderly patients and patients w/ a prior history of peptic ulcer disease and/or GI bleeding are at a greater risk.

ADULT DOSAGE	PEDIATRIC DOSAGE
Osteoarthritis	Pediatric use may not have been established
Knee:	
1.5%: 40 drops/knee qid	
2%: 40mg (2 pump actuations) on each painful knee bid	

DOSING CONSIDERATIONS
Elderly
If the anticipated benefit outweighs the potential risks, start at lower end of dosing range; monitor for adverse effects

ADMINISTRATION
Topical route
- Apply to clean, dry skin.
- Avoid showering/bathing ≥30 min after application.
- Do not apply to open wounds.
- Avoid contact w/ eyes and mucous membranes.
- Avoid wearing clothing over the treated knee(s) until dry.
- Do not apply external heat and/or occlusive dressings to treated knees; protect treated knees from sunlight.
- Wait until the treated area is dry before applying any topical product or medication to treated knee.
- Avoid skin-to-skin contact between others and the treated knee until knee is completely dry.

1.5%
- Dispense 10 drops at a time directly onto to knee or 1st into hand and then spread onto knee.
- Spread evenly around front, back, and sides of knee; repeat until 40 drops have been applied, completely covering knee w/ sol.

2%
- Prime pump before 1st use.
- Fully depress the pump mechanism (actuation) 4X while holding the bottle in an upright position and discard the dispensed portion.
- No further priming of the bottle should be required.
- Pump directly into palms and spread evenly around front, back, and sides of knees.

STORAGE
1.5%: 20-25°C (68-77°F); excursions permitted to 15-30°C (59-86°F). **2%:** 25°C (77°F); excursions permitted to 15-30°C (59-86°F).

HOW SUPPLIED
Sol: 1.5% [150mL], 2% [112g]

CONTRAINDICATIONS
Known hypersensitivity to diclofenac or any other component of this product, history of asthma, urticaria, or allergic-type reactions after taking aspirin (ASA) or other NSAIDs. In the setting of CABG surgery.

WARNINGS/PRECAUTIONS
Use the lowest effective dose for the shortest duration possible. Avoid in patients w/ a recent MI unless benefits outweigh the risks; if used, monitor for signs of cardiac ischemia. Increased risk for GI bleeding w/ longer duration of therapy, older age, poor general health status, and advanced liver disease and/or coagulopathy; avoid use in patients at higher risk unless benefits are expected to outweigh the increased risk, and consider alternate therapies. Promptly initiate evaluation and treatment if a serious GI adverse event is suspected; d/c until a serious GI adverse event is ruled out. Increases in LFTs reported; measure transaminases at baseline and periodically (w/in 4-8 weeks) if receiving long-term therapy. If abnormal liver tests persist or worsen, if clinical signs and/or symptoms consistent w/ liver disease develop, or if systemic manifestations occur, d/c immediately. May cause new onset HTN or worsen preexisting HTN; monitor BP during initiation and throughout course of therapy. Fluid retention and edema reported. Avoid use in patients w/ severe heart failure (HF) unless benefits outweigh risks; monitor for signs of worsening HF if used. Renal papillary necrosis and other renal injury reported w/ long-term use. Renal toxicity also reported in patients in whom renal prostaglandins have a compensatory role in the maintenance of renal perfusion; increased risk w/ renal/hepatic dysfunction, dehydration, hypovolemia, and HF, and in the elderly. Correct volume status in dehydrated or hypovolemic patients prior to initiating therapy. Avoid use in patients w/ advanced renal disease unless the benefits are expected to outweigh the risk; monitor for signs of worsening renal function if used in patients w/ advanced renal disease. Hyperkalemia reported. Associated w/ anaphylactic reactions. Monitor for changes in the signs/symptoms of asthma in patients w/ preexisting asthma (w/o known ASA sensitivity). May cause serious skin reactions (eg, exfoliative dermatitis, Stevens-Johnson syndrome, toxic epidermal necrolysis); d/c at 1st appearance of skin rash/hypersensitivity. Do not apply to open skin wounds, infections, inflammations, or exfoliative dermatitis. Anemia reported. May increase the risk of bleeding events; coagulation disorders may increase this risk. Monitor for signs of bleeding. May mask inflammation and fever.

ADVERSE REACTIONS
Application-site skin reactions.

DRUG INTERACTIONS
Drugs that interfere w/ serotonin reuptake may potentiate the risk of bleeding. Synergistic effect on bleeding w/ anticoagulants (eg, warfarin); monitor for signs of bleeding w/ concomitant anticoagulants, antiplatelet agents, SSRIs, and SNRIs. May increase risk of GI bleeding w/ use of oral corticosteroids, anticoagulants, and SSRIs; smoking; and alcohol use. ASA may increase risk of bleeding and serious GI events; concomitant use w/ analgesic doses of ASA is not recommended. Not a substitute for ASA for CV prophylaxis. May diminish antihypertensive effect of ACE inhibitors, ARBs, and β-blockers (eg, propranolol); monitor BP. Coadministration w/ ACE inhibitors or ARBs may result in deterioration of renal function (including possible acute renal failure) in patients who are elderly or volume-depleted (including those on diuretic therapy), or who have renal impairment; monitor for worsening renal function and adequately hydrate patient when these drugs are administered concomitantly. May reduce the natriuretic effect of loop diuretics (eg, furosemide) and thiazide diuretics; observe for signs of worsening renal function, in addition to assuring diuretic efficacy including antihypertensive effects. May increase digoxin serum concentrations and prolong the $T_{1/2}$ of digoxin; monitor digoxin levels. May elevate plasma lithium levels and reduce renal lithium clearance; monitor for signs of lithium toxicity. May increase the risk for methotrexate (MTX) toxicity; monitor for MTX toxicity. May increase cyclosporine's nephrotoxicity; monitor for signs of worsening renal function. Concomitant use w/ other NSAIDs or salicylates (eg, diflunisal, salsalate) increases the risk of GI toxicity; not recommended w/ other NSAIDs or salicylates. Avoid w/ oral NSAIDs unless benefit outweighs risk; conduct periodic lab evaluations. Concomitant use w/ pemetrexed may increase the risk of pemetrexed-associated myelosuppression, renal, and GI toxicity; refer to prescribing information for further information.

PREGNANCY AND LACTATION
Pregnancy: Category C, prior to 30 weeks' gestation; Category D, starting at 30 weeks' gestation. Use during the 3rd trimester of pregnancy increases the risk of premature closure of the fetal ductus arteriosus; avoid use in pregnant women starting at 30 weeks of gestation (3rd trimester).
Lactation: Maybe be present in human milk; caution in nursing.
Reproductive Potential: May delay or prevent rupture of ovarian follicles, which has been associated w/ reversible infertility in some women. Small studies in women treated w/ NSAIDs have also shown a reversible delay in ovulation. Consider withdrawal of therapy in women who have difficulties conceiving or who are undergoing investigation of infertility.

MECHANISM OF ACTION
NSAID; involves inhibition of COX-1 and COX-2. Has anti-inflammatory, analgesic, and antipyretic activities.

PHARMACOKINETICS
Absorption: Administration of multiple doses resulted in different parameters.
Distribution: Plasma protein binding (>99%). **Metabolism:** 4'-hydroxy-diclofenac (major metabolite) via CYP2C9; glucuronidation or sulfation, and acylglucuronidation (via UGT2B7) and oxidation (via CPY2C8). **Elimination:** Bile and urine. (1.5%) $T_{1/2}$=36.7 hrs (single dose), 79 hrs (multiple dose).

PATIENT CONSIDERATIONS
Assessment: Assess for history of hypersensitivity to diclofenac or to any component of this product; history of asthma, urticaria, pr other allergic-type reactions w/ ASA or other NSAIDs; asthma; CV disease (CVD) or risk factors for CVD; HTN; history of peptic ulcer disease or GI bleeding; coagulation disorders; renal/hepatic impairment; pregnancy/nursing status; or any other conditions where treatment is contraindicated or cautioned. Assess volume status. Assess for possible drug interactions. Obtain baseline LFTs, BP, CBC, and chemistry profile.

Monitoring: Monitor for signs/symptoms of CV thrombotic events; cardiac ischemia in patients w/ a recent MI; GI bleeding/ulceration and perforation; hepatotoxicity; new or worsening HTN; HF; edema; renal papillary necrosis and other renal injury; hyperkalemia; anaphylactic reactions; serious skin reactions; anemia; and other adverse reactions. Monitor BP during initiation of therapy and throughout the course of therapy. Monitor for signs of bleeding in patients on concomitant therapy w/ anticoagulants, antiplatelet agents, SSRIs, or SNRIs. Monitor renal function in patients w/ renal/hepatic impairment, HF, dehydration, or hypovolemia. Monitor LFTs, CBC, and chemistry profiles periodically during long-term treatment.

Counseling: Instruct on proper use. Inform of potential for CV thrombotic events, GI adverse events, hepatotoxicity, and worsening CHF/edema, and advise of symptoms; instruct to report symptoms to healthcare provider if any occur. Instruct to seek immediate emergency help if signs of an anaphylactic reaction occur. Advise to d/c immediately if rash develops and to contact healthcare provider as soon as possible. Advise females of reproductive potential who desire pregnancy that therapy may be associated w/ a reversible delay in ovulation. Instruct pregnant women to avoid use starting at 30 weeks of gestation. Instruct patient not to use other NSAIDs or salicylates concomitantly; notify of the presence of NSAIDs in OTC medications for colds, fever, or insomnia. Instruct patient to not use low-dose ASA concomitantly w/o talking to healthcare provider. Instruct to avoid contact w/ the eyes and mucosa and that if contact occurs, to immediately wash eye w/ water or saline and consult physician if irritation persists for >1 hr. Instruct to avoid skin-to-skin contact between other people and treated knee(s) until completely dry. Instruct not to apply drug to open skin wounds, infections, inflammations, or exfoliative dermatitis, as it may affect absorption and reduce tolerability of the drug. Instruct to wait until the area treated is completely dry before applying sunscreen, insect repellant, lotion, moisturizer, cosmetics, or other topical medication.

PENTASA — mesalamine   Rx
Class: 5-aminosalicylic acid derivative

ADULT DOSAGE	PEDIATRIC DOSAGE
Ulcerative Colitis	Pediatric use may not have been established
Mildly to Moderately Active:	
Induction of Remission/Treatment:	
1g (4 caps of 250mg or 2 caps of 500mg) qid. May be given up to 8 weeks	

- -

ADMINISTRATION
Oral route

May swallow cap whole or may open cap and sprinkle the entire contents of cap onto applesauce or yogurt.
Entire contents of cap should be consumed immediately.
Caps and contents of caps must not be crushed or chewed.

STORAGE
25°C (77°F); excursions permitted to 15-30°C (59-86°F).

HOW SUPPLIED
Cap, Controlled-Release: 250mg, 500mg

CONTRAINDICATIONS
Hypersensitivity to mesalamine, any other components of this medication, or salicylates.

WARNINGS/PRECAUTIONS
Caution w/ impaired hepatic or impaired renal function. Has been associated w/ an acute intolerance syndrome (eg, acute abdominal pain, cramping, bloody diarrhea) that may be difficult to distinguish from a flare of inflammatory bowel disease; d/c if acute intolerance syndrome is suspected. If a rechallenge is performed later in order to validate the hypersensitivity, it should be carried out under close medical supervision at reduced dose and only if clearly needed. Nephrotic syndrome and interstitial nephritis reported; monitor patients w/ preexisting renal disease, increased BUN or SrCr, or proteinuria, especially during the initial phase of therapy. Nephrotoxicity should be suspected in patients developing renal dysfunction during treatment. May interfere w/ lab tests.

ADVERSE REACTIONS
Diarrhea, headache, N/V, abdominal pain, dyspepsia, rash.

PREGNANCY AND LACTATION
Pregnancy: Category B.
Lactation: Caution in nursing.

MECHANISM OF ACTION
5-aminosalicylic acid derivative; not established. Suspected to diminish inflammation by blocking cyclooxygenase and inhibiting prostaglandin production in the colon.

PHARMACOKINETICS
Absorption: (1g dose) C_{max}=1mcg/mL, T_{max}=3 hrs. (N-acetylmesalamine) C_{max}=1.8mcg/mL, T_{max}=3 hrs. Distribution: Crosses the placenta; found in breast milk. Metabolism: N-acetylmesalamine (major metabolite). Elimination: Feces, urine (19-30%, N-acetylmesalamine); (IV) $T_{1/2}$=42 min.

PATIENT CONSIDERATIONS
Assessment: Assess for hypersensitivity to the drug or salicylates, hepatic/renal impairment, and pregnancy/nursing status.

Monitoring: Monitor for acute intolerance syndrome, interstitial nephritis, nephrotic syndrome, and other adverse reactions. Monitor renal function. Closely monitor patients w/ preexisting renal disease, increased BUN or SrCr, or proteinuria, especially during the initial phase of therapy.

Counseling: Inform of the risks/benefits of therapy. Advise to take ud. Advise to seek medical attention if symptoms of an acute intolerance syndrome, interstitial nephritis, or any adverse reaction develops.

PERCOCET — acetaminophen/oxycodone   CII

Class: Opioid analgesic

> Associated with cases of acute liver failure, at times resulting in liver transplant and death. Most cases of liver injury are associated with APAP use at doses >4000mg/day, and often involve >1 APAP-containing product.

OTHER BRAND NAMES
Endocet

ADULT DOSAGE
Moderate to Moderately Severe Pain

2.5mg/325mg Strength:
Usual: 1 or 2 tabs q6h prn
Max: 12 tabs/day

5mg/325mg Strength:
Usual: 1 tab q6h prn
Max: 12 tabs/day

7.5mg/325mg Strength:
Usual: 1 tab q6h prn
Max: 8 tabs/day

10mg/325mg Strength:
Usual: 1 tab q6h prn
Max: 6 tabs/day

If pain is constant, administer at regular intervals on an around-the-clock schedule
Max APAP Dose: 4g/day

PEDIATRIC DOSAGE
Pediatric use may not have been established

DOSING CONSIDERATIONS
Discontinuation
Taper dose gradually in patients treated for more than a few weeks

ADMINISTRATION
Oral route

STORAGE
20-25°C (68-77°F).

HOW SUPPLIED
Tab: (Oxycodone/APAP) 2.5mg/325mg, 5mg/325mg*, 7.5mg/325mg, 10mg/325mg *scored

CONTRAINDICATIONS
Known hypersensitivity to oxycodone, acetaminophen, or any other component of the product. Oxycodone: Significant respiratory depression (in unmonitored settings or absence of resuscitative equipment), acute or severe bronchial asthma or hypercarbia, suspected/known paralytic ileus.

WARNINGS/PRECAUTIONS
May be abused in a manner similar to other opioid agonists. Respiratory depression may occur; use extreme caution and consider alternative nonopioid analgesics in patients with acute asthma, chronic obstructive pulmonary disorder, cor pulmonale, preexisting respiratory impairment, or in the elderly or debilitated. Respiratory depressant effects may be markedly exaggerated in the presence of head injury, other intracranial lesions or preexisting increase in intracranial pressure. Produces effects on pupillary response and consciousness that may obscure neurologic signs of worsening in patients with head injuries. May cause severe hypotension; caution with circulatory shock. May produce orthostatic hypotension in ambulatory patients. Increased risk of acute liver failure in patients with underlying liver disease. May cause serious skin reactions (eg, acute generalized exanthematous pustulosis, Stevens-Johnson syndrome, toxic epidermal necrolysis), which can be fatal; d/c at the 1st appearance of skin rash or any other sign of hypersensitivity. Hypersensitivity and anaphylaxis reported; d/c immediately if signs/symptoms occur. May obscure diagnosis or clinical course in patients with acute abdominal conditions. Caution with CNS depression, hypothyroidism, Addison's disease, prostatic hypertrophy, urethral stricture, acute alcoholism, delirium tremens, kyphoscoliosis with respiratory depression, myxedema, toxic psychosis, hepatic/renal/pulmonary impairment, and in elderly/debilitated. May aggravate convulsions with convulsive disorders and may induce or aggravate seizures in some clinical settings. Monitor for decreased bowel motility in postoperative patients. May cause spasm of the sphincter of Oddi; caution with biliary tract disease, including acute pancreatitis. May cause increases in serum amylase level. Physical dependence and tolerance may occur. Do not abruptly d/c. Lab test interactions may occur. Not recommended for use during and immediately prior to labor and delivery.

ADVERSE REACTIONS
Lightheadedness, dizziness, drowsiness/sedation, N/V, respiratory depression, apnea, respiratory arrest, circulatory depression, hypotension, shock.

DRUG INTERACTIONS
Oxycodone: May cause severe hypotension after coadministration with drugs that compromise vasomotor tone (eg, phenothiazines). May enhance neuromuscular-blocking action of skeletal muscle relaxants and increase respiratory depression. Additive CNS depression with CNS depressants (eg, general anesthetics, phenothiazines, tranquilizers, alcohol); use in reduced dosages. Coadministration with anticholinergics may produce paralytic ileus. Agonist/antagonist analgesics (eg, pentazocine, nalbuphine, naltrexone, butorphanol) may reduce the analgesic effect or precipitate withdrawal symptoms; use with caution. APAP: Increased risk of acute liver failure with alcohol; hepatotoxicity reported in chronic alcoholics. Increase in glucuronidation, resulting in increased plasma clearance and decreased $T_{1/2}$ with oral contraceptives. Propranolol and probenecid may increase pharmacologic/therapeutic effects. May decrease effects of loop diuretics, lamotrigine, and zidovudine.

PREGNANCY AND LACTATION
Pregnancy: Category C.
Lactation: Not for use in nursing.

MECHANISM OF ACTION
Oxycodone: Opioid analgesic; semisynthetic pure opioid agonist whose principal therapeutic action is analgesia. Effects are mediated by receptors (eg, μ and kappa) in the CNS for endogenous opioid-like compounds (eg, endorphins, enkephalins). APAP: Nonopiate, nonsalicylate analgesic, and antipyretic; site and mechanism for the analgesic effect not established. Antipyretic effect is accomplished through inhibition of endogenous pyrogen action on the hypothalamic heat-regulating centers.

PHARMACOKINETICS
Absorption: Oxycodone: Absolute bioavailability (87%). APAP: Rapid and almost complete from GI tract. Distribution: Found in breast milk. Oxycodone: Plasma protein binding (45%); V_d=211.9L (IV); crosses the placenta. Metabolism: Oxycodone: N-dealkylation to noroxycodone (1st-pass); O-demethylation via CYP2D6 to oxymorphone. APAP: Liver via CYP450; conjugation with glucuronic acid and (lesser extent) sulfuric acid and cysteine; N acetyl-p-benzoquinoneimine (toxic metabolite). Elimination: Oxycodone: Urine (8-14% unchanged); $T_{1/2}$=3.51 hrs. APAP: Urine (90-100%).

PATIENT CONSIDERATIONS
Assessment: Assess for level of pain intensity, type of pain, patient's general condition and medical status, or any other conditions where treatment is contraindicated or cautioned. Assess for drug hypersensitivity, renal/hepatic/pulmonary impairment, pregnancy/nursing status, and possible drug interactions.

Monitoring: Monitor for acute liver failure, respiratory depression, hypotension, skin/hypersensitivity/anaphylactic reactions, convulsions/seizures, decreased bowel motility in postoperative patients, spasm of sphincter of Oddi, increases in serum amylase levels, physical dependence, tolerance, and other adverse reactions.

Counseling: Advise to d/c use and contact physician immediately if signs of allergy develop. Instruct to look for APAP on package labels and not to use >1 APAP-containing product. Instruct to seek medical attention immediately upon ingestion of >4000mg/day of APAP, even if patient is feeling well.

Inform about the signs of serious skin reactions. Advise to destroy unused tabs by flushing down the toilet. Inform that drug may impair mental/physical abilities required to perform hazardous tasks. Instruct to avoid alcohol or other CNS depressants. Advise not to adjust dose without consulting physician and not to abruptly d/c if on treatment for more than a few weeks. Inform that drug has potential for abuse and should be protected from theft. Instruct to consult physician if pregnant, planning to become pregnant, or breastfeeding.

PERFOROMIST — formoterol fumarate   Rx

Class: Long-acting beta₂ agonist (LABA)

> Long-acting β_2-adrenergic agonists (LABAs) increase the risk of asthma-related death. Contraindicated in asthma without use of a long-term asthma control medication.

ADULT DOSAGE	PEDIATRIC DOSAGE
Chronic Obstructive Pulmonary Disease	Pediatric use may not have been established
Long-Term Maint Treatment of Bronchoconstriction: 20mcg bid (am and pm) by nebulization **Max:** 40mcg/day	

ADMINISTRATION
Oral inh route
Administer via a standard jet nebulizer connected to an air compressor
Store in the foil pouch and only remove immediately before use

STORAGE
Prior to Dispensing: 2-8°C (36-46°F). After Dispensing: 2-25°C (36-77°F) for up to 3 months. Protect pouch from heat. Vial should always be stored in the foil pouch, and only removed immediately before use.

HOW SUPPLIED
Sol, Inhalation: 20mcg/2mL [30^s 60^s]

CONTRAINDICATIONS
Asthma without use of a long-term asthma control medication.

WARNINGS/PRECAUTIONS
Not indicated to treat asthma, acute deteriorations of COPD, or for the relief of acute symptoms (eg, as rescue therapy for acute bronchospasm episodes). D/C regular use of inhaled short-acting β_2-agonists (SABAs) when beginning treatment; use only for symptomatic relief of acute respiratory symptoms. Do not use more often or at higher doses than recommended; clinically significant cardiovascular (CV) effects and fatalities reported with excessive use. May produce paradoxical bronchospasm; d/c therapy immediately and institute alternative therapy. CV effects may occur; d/c if such effects occur. Caution with CV disorders, convulsive disorders, thyrotoxicosis, diabetes mellitus (DM), ketoacidosis, and in patients unusually responsive to sympathomimetic amines. May produce significant hypokalemia and transient hyperglycemia. Immediate hypersensitivity reactions may occur.

ADVERSE REACTIONS
Diarrhea, nausea, nasopharyngitis, dry mouth.

DRUG INTERACTIONS
Do not use with other medications containing LABAs. Adrenergic drugs may potentiate sympathetic effects; use with caution. Xanthine derivatives, steroids, or diuretics may potentiate hypokalemic effect. Caution is advised when coadministered with non-K$^+$-sparing diuretics (eg, loop, thiazide). Extreme caution with MAOIs, TCAs, or drugs known to prolong the QTc interval; effect on CV system may be potentiated. Drugs known to prolong the QTc interval have an increased risk of ventricular arrhythmias. β-blockers and formoterol may inhibit the effect of each other when administered concurrently. β-blockers may block therapeutic effects and produce severe bronchospasm in COPD patients; if such therapy is needed, consider cardioselective β-blockers and use with caution.

PREGNANCY AND LACTATION
Category C, caution in nursing.

MECHANISM OF ACTION
LABA; attributable to stimulation of intracellular adenyl cyclase, the enzyme that catalyzes the conversion of ATP to cAMP. Increased cAMP levels cause relaxation of bronchial smooth muscle and inhibition of release of mediators of immediate hypersensitivity from cells, especially from mast cells.

PHARMACOKINETICS
Distribution: Plasma protein binding (61-64%). **Metabolism:** Direct glucuronidation via UGT1A1, 1A8, 1A9, 2B7, 2B15; O-demethylation via CYP2D6, 2C19, 2C9, 2A6. **Elimination:** Urine (1.1-1.7%, unchanged).

PATIENT CONSIDERATIONS
Assessment: Assess for asthma, acute COPD deteriorations, CV disorders, convulsive disorders, thyrotoxicosis, DM, ketoacidosis, pregnancy/nursing status, and possible drug interactions. Assess use in patients unusually responsive to sympathomimetic amines.

Monitoring: Monitor for deteriorating disease, paradoxical bronchospasm, CV effects, hypokalemia, hyperglycemia, immediate hypersensitivity reactions, and other adverse reactions.

Counseling: Counsel about the risks and benefits of therapy. Inform that drug is not for treatment of asthma. Advise not to use to relieve acute symptoms; inform that acute symptoms should be treated with an inhaled SABA. Instruct to seek medical attention if symptoms worsen despite recommended doses, if treatment becomes less effective, or if experiencing a need for more inhalations of a SABA than usual. Advise not to stop therapy unless directed by physician, not to inhale more than the prescribed number of vials at any 1 time, and not to exceed recommended daily dosage. Instruct to d/c the regular use of inhaled SABAs (eg, albuterol) when beginning treatment. Counsel not to use with other inhaled medications containing LABAs, and not to stop or change the dose of other concomitant COPD therapy without medical advice, even if symptoms improve after initiating treatment. Inform of the common adverse reactions associated with therapy. Instruct on how to properly use the medication.

PERIDEX — chlorhexidine gluconate   Rx

Class: Antimicrobial

ADULT DOSAGE	PEDIATRIC DOSAGE
Gingivitis	Pediatric use may not have been established
For Use Between Dental Visits: Rinse w/ 15mL (undiluted) for 30 sec bid (am and pm) after toothbrushing; initiate directly following a dental prophylaxis	
Reevaluate and give a thorough prophylaxis at intervals no longer than 6 months	

ADMINISTRATION
Oral route
Not intended for ingestion; should be expectorated after rinsing.
Instruct to not rinse w/ water or other mouthwashes, brush teeth, or eat immediately after using.

STORAGE
20-25°C (68-77°F); excursions permitted to 15-30°C (59-86°F).

HOW SUPPLIED
Sol: 0.12% [15mL, 118mL, 473mL, 1893mL]

CONTRAINDICATIONS
Hypersensitivity to chlorhexidine gluconate or other formula ingredients.

WARNINGS/PRECAUTIONS
Has not been tested among patients with acute necrotizing ulcerative gingivitis (ANUG). Effect on periodontitis has not been determined. Presence or absence of gingival inflammation following treatment should not be used as a major indicator of underlying periodontitis in patients having coexisting gingivitis and periodontitis. Increase in supragingival calculus reported. Calculus deposits should be removed by a dental prophylaxis at intervals not greater than six months. Anaphylaxis, as well as serious allergic reactions, reported. May stain oral surfaces (eg, tooth surfaces, restorations, dorsum of tongue), and alter taste perception. Caution in patients with anterior facial restorations with rough surfaces or margins.

ADVERSE REACTIONS
Increase in staining of teeth and other oral surfaces, increase in calculus formation, alteration in taste perception, oral irritation, local allergy-type symptoms.

PREGNANCY AND LACTATION
Pregnancy: Category B.
Lactation: Caution in nursing.

MECHANISM OF ACTION
Antimicrobial agent; suspected to reduce bacterial assay count, both aerobic and anaerobic.

PHARMACOKINETICS
Absorption: Poorly absorbed. (300mg, PO dose) C_{max}=0.206µg/g, T_{max}=30 min. **Elimination:** (300mg, PO dose) Feces (90%), urine (<1%).

PATIENT CONSIDERATIONS
Assessment: Assess for drug hypersensitivity, ANUG, coexisting periodontitis and gingivitis, anterior facial restorations with rough surfaces or margins, and pregnancy/nursing status.

Monitoring: Monitor for staining of oral surfaces, alteration of taste, anaphylaxis and serious allergic reactions, and other adverse reactions.

Counseling: Advise to use the oral rinse bid (am and pm) for 30 sec after brushing. Instruct to not rinse with water or other mouthwashes, brush teeth, or eat immediately afterward. Instruct to expectorate after rinsing and not to ingest.

PERJETA — pertuzumab   Rx

Class: Monoclonal antibody/HER2 blocker

> May result in subclinical and clinical cardiac failure manifesting as decreased left ventricular ejection fraction (LVEF) and CHF; evaluate cardiac function prior to and during treatment. D/C treatment for a confirmed clinically significant decrease in left ventricular function. Exposure during pregnancy may result in embryo-fetal death and birth defects; advise patients of these risks and the need for effective contraception.

ADULT DOSAGE

Breast Cancer

Metastatic:
Combination w/ trastuzumab and docetaxel for HER2-positive metastatic breast cancer in patients who have not received prior anti-HER2 therapy or chemotherapy for metastatic disease

Initial: 840mg IV infusion over 60 min, followed every 3 weeks by 420mg IV infusion over 30-60 min

Trastuzumab:
Initial: 8mg/kg IV infusion over 90 min, followed every 3 weeks by a dose of 6mg/kg IV infusion over 30-90 min

Docetaxel:
Initial: 75mg/m^2 IV infusion
Titrate: May increase to 100mg/m^2 administered every 3 weeks if initial dose is well tolerated

Neoadjuvant Treatment:
Combination w/ trastuzumab and docetaxel for the neoadjuvant treatment of patients w/ HER2-positive, locally advanced, inflammatory, or early stage breast cancer (either >2cm in diameter or node positive) as part of a complete treatment regimen for early breast cancer

Initial: 840mg IV infusion over 60 min, followed every 3 weeks by a dose of 420mg IV infusion over 30-60 min

Trastuzumab:
Initial: 8mg/kg IV infusion over 90 min, followed every 3 weeks by a dose of 6mg/kg IV infusion over 30-90 min

Administer every 3 weeks for 3-6 cycles as part of 1 of the following treatment regimens for early breast cancer:
4 preoperative cycles of pertuzumab in combination w/ trastuzumab and docetaxel, followed by 3 postoperative cycles of fluorouracil, epirubicin, and cyclophosphamide (FEC)
OR
3 preoperative cycles of FEC alone, followed by 3 preoperative cycles of pertuzumab in combination w/ docetaxel and trastuzumab
OR
6 preoperative cycles of pertuzumab in combination w/ docetaxel, carboplatin, and trastuzumab (escalation of docetaxel >75mg/m^2 is not recommended)

Following surgery, patients should continue to receive trastuzumab to complete 1 yr of treatment

Missed Dose

Time Between 2 Sequential Infusions is <6 Weeks:
Administer the 420mg pertuzumab dose; do not wait until the next planned dose

Time Between 2 Sequential Infusions is ≥6 Weeks:
Readminister initial dose of 840mg pertuzumab as a 60-min IV infusion, followed every 3 weeks thereafter by a dose of 420mg administered as an IV infusion over 30-60 min

- -

DOSING CONSIDERATIONS

Concomitant Medications
D/C pertuzumab if trastuzumab treatment is discontinued

Adverse Reactions
LVEF:
<45% or 45-49% w/ a ≥10% Absolute Decrease Below Pretreatment Value:

PEDIATRIC DOSAGE

Pediatric use may not have been established

Withhold pertuzumab and trastuzumab dosing for ≥3 weeks. May resume if LVEF recovers to >49% or to 45-49% associated w/ <10% absolute decrease below pretreatment values. If after a repeat assessment w/in approx 3 weeks, LVEF has not improved or has declined further, d/c pertuzumab and trastuzumab, unless the benefits outweigh the risks

Infusion-Related Reactions:
May slow or interrupt the infusion

Hypersensitivity Reactions/Anaphylaxis:
D/C infusion immediately if serious hypersensitivity reaction occurs

ADMINISTRATION
IV route

Do not administer as IV push or bolus.
Do not mix w/ other drugs.
Administer pertuzumab, trastuzumab, and docetaxel sequentially.
Pertuzumab and trastuzumab can be given in any order; administer docetaxel after pertuzumab and trastuzumab.

Preparation
1. Withdraw the appropriate volume of pertuzumab sol from the vial(s).
2. Dilute into a 250mL 0.9% NaCl polyvinyl chloride (PVC) or non-PVC polyolefin infusion bag.
3. Mix diluted sol by gentle inversion; do not shake.
4. Administer immediately once prepared; if not used immediately, store at 2-8°C for up to 24 hrs.
5. Dilute w/ 0.9% NaCl inj only; do not use D5 sol.

STORAGE
2-8°C (36-46°F) until time of use. Protect from light. Do not freeze or shake.

HOW SUPPLIED
Inj: 30mg/mL [14mL]

CONTRAINDICATIONS
Known hypersensitivity to pertuzumab or to any of its excipients.

WARNINGS/PRECAUTIONS
Patients who have received prior anthracyclines or prior radiotherapy to the chest area may be at higher risk of decreased LVEF. Can cause fetal harm. Infusion-related reactions reported; observe closely for 60 min after the 1st infusion and for 30 min after subsequent infusions. Consider permanent discontinuation in patients w/ severe infusion reactions. Hypersensitivity/anaphylaxis reactions reported; medications/emergency equipment should be available for immediate use. Detection of HER2 protein overexpression is necessary for appropriate patient selection.

ADVERSE REACTIONS
Metastatic Breast Cancer in Combination w/ Trastuzumab and Docetaxel:
Diarrhea, alopecia, neutropenia, nausea, fatigue, rash, peripheral neuropathy.
Neoadjuvant Treatment in Combination w/ Trastuzumab and Docetaxel:
Alopecia, neutropenia, diarrhea, nausea.

PREGNANCY AND LACTATION
Pregnancy: Based on its mechanism of action and findings in animal studies, pertuzumab can cause fetal harm when administered to a pregnant woman. Monitor women who received pertuzumab in combination w/ trastuzumab during pregnancy or w/in 7 months prior to conception for oligohydramnios; if oligohydramnios occurs, perform fetal testing that is appropriate for gestational age and consistent w/ community standards of care. There is a pregnancy exposure registry that monitors pregnancy outcomes in women exposed to the drug during pregnancy. In addition, there is a pregnancy pharmacovigilance program.
Lactation: There is no information regarding the presence of pertuzumab in human milk, the effects on the breastfed infant, or the effects on milk production. Caution in nursing.
Reproductive Potential: Females of reproductive potential should use effective contraception during treatment and for 7 months following the last dose of pertuzumab in combination w/ trastuzumab. Verify the pregnancy status of females of reproductive potential prior to the initiation of therapy.

MECHANISM OF ACTION
Monoclonal antibody/HER2 blocker; inhibits ligand-initiated intracellular signaling pathways, which can result in cell growth arrest and apoptosis. Also mediates antibody-dependent cell-mediated cytotoxicity.

PHARMACOKINETICS
Elimination: $T_{1/2}$=18 days (median).

PATIENT CONSIDERATIONS

Assessment: Assess for hypersensitivity to drug and pregnancy/nursing status. Assess LVEF prior to initiation of therapy. Assess HER2 status; should be performed by laboratories w/ demonstrated proficiency in the specific technology being utilized.

Monitoring: Monitor for infusion-related reactions, hypersensitivity/anaphylaxis reactions, and other adverse reactions. Monitor LVEF at regular intervals (eg, every 3 months in the metastatic setting and every 6 weeks in the neoadjuvant setting).

Counseling: Advise to contact a healthcare professional immediately for new onset or worsening SOB, cough, swelling of the ankles/legs/face, palpitations, weight gain of >5 lbs in 24 hrs, dizziness, or loss of consciousness. Advise pregnant women and females of reproductive potential that exposure to pertuzumab in combination w/ trastuzumab during pregnancy or w/in 7 months prior to conception can result in fetal harm; advise to contact healthcare provider w/ a known or suspected pregnancy. Advise women who are exposed to pertuzumab in combination w/ trastuzumab during pregnancy or w/in 7 months prior to conception that there is a pregnancy exposure registry and a pregnancy pharmacovigilance program that monitors pregnancy outcomes. Advise females of reproductive potential to use effective contraception during treatment and for 7 months following the last dose of pertuzumab in combination w/ trastuzumab.

PERPHENAZINE — perphenazine   Rx

Class: Piperazine phenothiazine

> Increased mortality in elderly patients with dementia-related psychosis reported; most deaths appeared to be either cardiovascular (eg, heart failure, sudden death) or infectious (eg, pneumonia) in nature. Not approved for the treatment of dementia-related psychosis.

ADULT DOSAGE	PEDIATRIC DOSAGE
Schizophrenia	**Schizophrenia**
Moderately Disturbed Non-Hospitalized Patients:	**≥12 Years:**
Initial: 4-8mg tid	**Moderately Disturbed Non-Hospitalized Patients:**
Maint: Reduce to minimum effective dose, as soon as possible	**Initial:** 4-8mg tid
Hospitalized Patients:	**Maint:** Reduce to minimum effective dose, as soon as possible
Usual: 8-16mg bid-qid	**Hospitalized Patients:**
Max: 64mg/day	**Usual:** 8-16mg bid-qid
Nausea/Vomiting	**Max:** 64mg/day
Severe:	
Usual: 8-16mg/day in divided doses; may need 24mg/day	

DOSING CONSIDERATIONS
Elderly
Start at lower end of dosing range

ADMINISTRATION
Oral route

STORAGE
20-25°C (68-77°F); tight, light-resistant container.

HOW SUPPLIED
Tab: 2mg, 4mg, 8mg, 16mg

CONTRAINDICATIONS
Comatose or greatly obtunded patients; coadministration w/ large doses of CNS depressants (eg, barbiturates, alcohol, narcotics, analgesics, antihistamines); blood dyscrasias, bone marrow depression, or liver damage; hypersensitivity to perphenazine products, their components, or related compounds; subcortical brain damage w/ or w/o hypothalamic damage.

WARNINGS/PRECAUTIONS
Not effective for the management of behavioral complications in patients with mental retardation. Tardive dyskinesia reported; d/c if signs/symptoms appear. Neuroleptic Malignant Syndrome (NMS) reported; d/c therapy and carefully monitor for recurrences if therapy is reintroduced. Hypotension may occur; caution in patients with mitral insufficiency or pheochromocytoma. Rebound HTN may occur with pheochromocytoma. May lower convulsive threshold; caution with alcohol withdrawal and convulsive disorders. Caution with psychic depression. May impair mental/physical abilities. Increased risk of extrapyramidal and/or withdrawal symptoms in neonates if administered during the 3rd trimester. Leukopenia/neutropenia and agranulocytosis have been reported. Caution with preexisting low WBC or history of drug induced leukopenia/neutropenia; monitor CBC frequently and d/c at 1st sign of decline in WBC. Monitor for fever or infection with neutropenia; d/c if severe neutropenia (absolute neutrophil count <1000/mm^3) develops. Increased risk of suicide in depressed patients; avoid access to large quantities of the drug. May elevate prolactin levels; caution with previously detected breast cancer. Antiemetic effect may mask signs of overdosage of other drugs and obscure diagnosis of intestinal obstruction or brain tumor. D/C if significant rise in body temperature occurs; suggestive of intolerance. Monitor renal/hepatic function periodically; d/c therapy if abnormal LFTs/BUN. Caution with renal impairment, respiratory impairment due to acute pulmonary infections, or chronic respiratory disorders (eg, severe asthma, emphysema). Avoid abrupt cessation of high-dose therapy. Possibility of liver damage, corneal and lenticular deposits, and irreversible dyskinesias with long-term use. Avoid sun exposure; photosensitivity reported. Caution in elderly. Not recommended for pediatrics <12 yrs of age.

ADVERSE REACTIONS
Extrapyramidal reactions, cerebral edema, seizures, drowsiness, dry mouth, salivation, N/V, diarrhea, anorexia, constipation, urticaria, skin reactions, eczema, postural hypotension, tachycardia.

DRUG INTERACTIONS
See Contraindications. Additive effects with CNS depressants (eg, opiates, analgesics, antihistamines, barbiturates); use with caution and in reduced dosage. Avoid coadministration with alcohol; additive effects, hypotension and increased risk of suicide/overdose may occur. Additive anticholinergic effects with atropine/atropine-like drugs and phosphorous insecticide exposure; use with caution. Cytochrome P450 2D6 inhibitors (TCAs, SSRIs) may increase levels; monitor closely; lower doses may be required. May lower convulsive threshold; increased dosage of anticonvulsants may be required. May reverse effects of epinephrine; do not administer if hypotension develops. Hypotensive phenomena may occur in

patients undergoing surgery receiving large doses of the drug; reduce dosage of anesthetics and CNS depressants.

PREGNANCY AND LACTATION
Safety in pregnancy and nursing not known.

MECHANISM OF ACTION
Piperazinyl phenothiazine; unknown, has actions at all levels of the CNS, particularly the hypothalamus.

PHARMACOKINETICS
Absorption: C_{max}=984pg/mL; T_{max}=1-3 hrs. **Metabolism:** Liver (extensive) via CYP2D6; sulfoxidation, hydroxylation, dealkylation, and glucuronidation. **Elimination:** $T_{1/2}$=9-12 hrs.

PATIENT CONSIDERATIONS
Assessment: Assess for dementia-related psychosis, mental retardation with behavioral complications, state of consciousness, blood dyscrasia, bone marrow depression, respiratory/hepatic/renal impairment, subcortical brain damage with/without hypothalamic damage, mitral insufficiency, pheochromocytoma, alcohol withdrawal, convulsive disorder, psychic depression, low WBC count, history of drug-induced leukopenia/neutropenia, suicidal ideation, breast cancer, heat/sun exposure, alcohol use, hypersensitivity to drug, pregnancy/nursing status, and possible drug interactions.

Monitoring: Monitor for hypersensitivity reactions, tardive dyskinesia, NMS, hypotension, leukopenia/neutropenia/agranulocytosis, fever, infection, renal function, corneal and lenticular deposits, dyskinesias, and photosensitivity reactions. Monitor for hypotensive phenomena in patients undergoing surgery. Monitor temperature, CBC, LFTs, BUN, and prolactin levels periodically.

Counseling: Inform about benefits and risks of the drug. Advise to avoid hazardous tasks (operating machinery/driving) and sun exposure. Caution about additive effects with alcohol.

PERTZYE — pancrelipase   Rx

Class: Pancreatic enzyme supplement

ADULT DOSAGE	PEDIATRIC DOSAGE
Exocrine Pancreatic Insufficiency	**Exocrine Pancreatic Insufficiency**
Due to Cystic Fibrosis or Other Conditions:	**Due to Cystic Fibrosis or Other Conditions:**
Individualize dose based on clinical symptoms, degree of steatorrhea present, and fat content of diet; start at the lowest recommended dose and increase gradually	Individualize dose based on clinical symptoms, degree of steatorrhea present, and fat content of diet; start at the lowest recommended dose and increase gradually
Initial: 500 lipase U/kg/meal	**>12 Months to <4 Years:**
Max: 2500 lipase U/kg/meal (or ≤10,000 lipase U/kg/day) or <4000 lipase U/g fat ingested/day	**≥8kg:**
	Initial: 1000 lipase U/kg/meal
Refer to PI for dosing limitations	**Max:** 2500 lipase U/kg/meal (or ≤10,000 lipase U/kg/day) or <4000 lipase U/g fat ingested/day
	≥4 Years:
	≥16kg:
	Initial: 500 lipase U/kg/meal
	Max: 2500 lipase U/kg/meal (or ≤10,000 lipase U/kg/day) or <4000 lipase U/g fat ingested/day
	Refer to PI for dosing limitations

DOSING CONSIDERATIONS
Elderly
Reduce dose

ADMINISTRATION
Oral route

Take during meals or snacks, w/ sufficient fluid.
Swallow whole; do not crush or chew caps and cap contents.
1/2 of the dose used for an individualized full meal should be given w/ each snack. Patients unable to swallow intact caps may carefully open caps and mix contents w/ small amounts of acidic soft food w/ a pH of ≤4.5 (eg, applesauce); swallow soft food mixture immediately w/o crushing or chewing, and follow w/ water or juice.
Do not retain in mouth.

STORAGE
20-25°C (68-77°F); brief excursions permitted to 15-40°C (59-104°F). Protect from moisture.

HOW SUPPLIED
Cap, Delayed-Release: (Lipase/Protease/Amylase) 8000 U/28,750 U/30,250 U; 16,000 U/57,500 U/60,500 U

WARNINGS/PRECAUTIONS
Not interchangeable w/ other pancrelipase products. Fibrosing colonopathy reported; monitor closely for progression to stricture formation. Caution w/ doses >2500 lipase U/kg/meal (or >10,000 lipase U/kg/day); use only if these doses are documented to be effective by 3-day fecal fat measures indicating significant improvement. Examine patients receiving >6000 lipase U/kg/meal; immediately decrease dose or titrate dose downward to a lower range. Ensure that no drug

is retained in the mouth. Should not be mixed in foods w/ pH >4.5; may disrupt enteric coating of cap, resulting in early release of enzymes, irritation of oral mucosa, and/or loss of enzyme activity. May increase blood uric acid levels; consider monitoring serum uric acid levels in patients w/ hyperuricemia, gout, or renal impairment. Theoretical risk for transmission of viral diseases. Caution w/ known allergy to proteins of porcine origin; severe allergic reactions (eg, anaphylaxis, asthma, hives) reported.

ADVERSE REACTIONS
Diarrhea, dyspepsia, cough.

PREGNANCY AND LACTATION
Pregnancy: Category C.
Lactation: Caution in nursing.

MECHANISM OF ACTION
Pancreatic enzyme supplement; catalyzes the hydrolysis of fats to monoglyceride, glycerol and free fatty acids, proteins into peptides and amino acids, and starches into dextrins and short-chain sugars (eg, maltose, maltotriose) in the duodenum and proximal small intestine, thereby acting like digestive enzymes physiologically secreted by the pancreas.

PATIENT CONSIDERATIONS
Assessment: Assess for allergy to porcine protein, hyperuricemia, gout, renal impairment, and pregnancy/nursing status.

Monitoring: Monitor for fibrosing colonopathy, stricture formation, oral mucosal irritation, viral diseases, allergic reactions, and other adverse reactions. Monitor serum uric acid levels.

Counseling: Instruct to take ud, w/ food and sufficient fluids. Inform that if a dose is missed, take the next dose w/ the next meal/snack ud; instruct not to double doses. Inform that cap contents can be mixed w/ soft acidic foods (eg, applesauce), if necessary; instruct to discard unused portion of cap contents, and not to use for subsequent dosing. Inform that doses >6000 lipase U/kg/meal have been associated w/ colonic strictures in children <12 yrs of age. Advise to contact physician immediately if allergic reactions develop. Instruct to notify physician if pregnant/breastfeeding or if planning to become pregnant or breastfeed during therapy.

PEXEVA — paroxetine mesylate   Rx
Class: Selective serotonin reuptake inhibitor (SSRI)

> Antidepressants increased the risk of suicidal thinking and behavior (suicidality) in children, adolescents, and young adults in short-term studies of major depressive disorder (MDD) and other psychiatric disorders. Monitor and observe closely for clinical worsening, suicidality, or unusual changes in behavior. Not approved for use in pediatric patients.

ADULT DOSAGE
Major Depressive Disorder

Initial: 20mg/day
Titrate: If not responding to a 20mg dose, may increase in 10mg/day increments and at intervals of at least 1 week
Range: 20-50mg/day
Max: 50mg/day
Periodically reevaluate long-term usefulness of the drug

Obsessive Compulsive Disorder

Initial: 20mg/day
Titrate: May increase in 10mg/day increments and at intervals of at least 1 week
Usual: 40mg/day
Max: 60mg/day
Periodically reevaluate long-term usefulness of the drug

Panic Disorder

W/ or w/o Agoraphobia:

Initial: 10mg/day
Titrate: May increase in 10mg/day increments and at intervals of at least 1 week
Target Dose: 40mg/day
Max: 60mg/day
Periodically reevaluate long-term usefulness of the drug

Generalized Anxiety Disorder

Initial/Usual: 20mg/day; no sufficient evidence to suggest a greater benefit to doses >20mg/day
Titrate: May increase in 10mg/day increments and at intervals of at least 1 week
Range: 20-50mg/day
Periodically reevaluate long-term usefulness of the drug

PEDIATRIC DOSAGE
Pediatric use may not have been established

Dosing Considerations with MAOIs
Switching to/from an MAOI for Psychiatric Disorders:
Allow at least 14 days between discontinuation of an MAOI and initiation of treatment, and conversely allow at least 14 days between discontinuation of treatment and initiation of an MAOI

W/ Other MAOIs (eg, Linezolid, IV Methylene Blue):
Do not start paroxetine in patients being treated w/ linezolid or IV methylene blue.
In patients already receiving paroxetine, if acceptable alternatives are not available and benefits outweigh risks, d/c paroxetine and administer linezolid or IV methylene blue; monitor for serotonin syndrome for 2 weeks or until 24 hrs after the last dose of linezolid or IV methylene blue, whichever comes 1st. May resume paroxetine therapy 24 hrs after the last dose of linezolid or IV methylene blue

---

DOSING CONSIDERATIONS
Renal Impairment
Severe (CrCl <30mL/min):
Initial: 10mg/day; may increase if indicated
Max: 40mg/day

Hepatic Impairment
Severe:
Initial: 10mg/day; may increase if indicated
Max: 40mg/day

Elderly
Elderly/Debilitated:
Initial: 10mg/day; may increase if indicated
Max: 40mg/day

Discontinuation
Gradually reduce dose whenever possible
If intolerable symptoms occur following a decrease in dose or upon discontinuation of treatment, may resume the previously prescribed dose; subsequently, may continue decreasing dose but at a more gradual rate

ADMINISTRATION
Oral route

Administer as a single daily dose, usually in the am.
Take w/ or w/o food.
Swallow tab whole; do not chew or crush.

STORAGE
25°C (77°F); excursions permitted to 15-30°C (59-86°F). Protect from humidity.

HOW SUPPLIED
Tab: 10mg, 20mg*, 30mg, 40mg *scored

CONTRAINDICATIONS
Use of an MAOI for psychiatric disorders either concomitantly or w/in 14 days of stopping treatment. Treatment w/in 14 days of stopping an MAOI for psychiatric disorders. Starting treatment in a patient being treated w/ MAOIs (eg, linezolid, IV methylene blue). Concomitant use w/ thioridazine or pimozide. Hypersensitivity to paroxetine or any of the inactive ingredients in paroxetine mesylate.

WARNINGS/PRECAUTIONS
Not approved for the treatment of bipolar depression. Serotonin syndrome reported; d/c immediately and initiate supportive symptomatic treatment. Pupillary dilation that occurs following use may trigger an angle closure attack in a patient with anatomically narrow angles who does not have a patent iridectomy. Increased risk of congenital malformations reported in 1st trimester of pregnancy. Increased risk in 3rd trimester of pregnancy due to neonatal complications. Activation of mania/hypomania reported. Seizures reported; d/c if seizures occur. Avoid abrupt withdrawal; gradually reduce dose and monitor for discontinuation symptoms. Akathisia may develop. Hyponatremia may occur; caution in elderly and volume-depleted patients. Consider discontinuation in patients with symptomatic hyponatremia and institute appropriate medical intervention. May increase risk of bleeding events. Bone fracture risk following exposure to some antidepressants reported. Caution with conditions affecting hemodynamic responses or metabolism, severe hepatic/renal impairment, and in elderly.

ADVERSE REACTIONS
Asthenia, sweating, nausea, decreased appetite, somnolence, dizziness, insomnia, tremor, nervousness, abnormal ejaculation, dry mouth, constipation, decreased libido, impotence, headache.

DRUG INTERACTIONS
See Contraindications. Not recommended with SSRIs, SNRIs, tryptophan, and alcohol. May cause serotonin syndrome with other serotonergic drugs (eg, triptans, TCAs, fentanyl) and with drugs that impair metabolism of serotonin; d/c immediately if this occurs. Caution with warfarin, TCAs, lithium, and digoxin. Increased risk of bleeding with aspirin (ASA), NSAIDs, warfarin, and other anticoagulants. Increased risk of hyponatremia with diuretics. Increased levels with cimetidine. Decreased levels with phenobarbital, phenytoin, and fosamprenavir/

ritonavir. Caution with drugs that are metabolized by CYP2D6 (eg, antidepressants [eg, nortriptyline, amitriptyline, imipramine], phenothiazines, risperidone, Type 1C antiarrhythmics [eg, propafenone, flecainide, encainide]) and with drugs that inhibit CYP2D6 (eg, quinidine). May increase levels of desipramine, risperidone, procyclidine, and theophylline. May increase levels of atomoxetine; may require dose adjustments. May increase free concentrations of highly protein-bound drugs potentially resulting in adverse events. Severe hypotension reported when added to chronic metoprolol treatment. May decrease levels of active metabolite (endoxifen) and reduce efficacy of tamoxifen. May decrease phenytoin levels.

PREGNANCY AND LACTATION
Category D, caution in nursing.

MECHANISM OF ACTION
SSRI; inhibits CNS neuronal reuptake of serotonin.

PHARMACOKINETICS
Absorption: Complete; C_{max}=81.3ng/mL; T_{max}=8.1 hrs. **Distribution:** Plasma protein binding (95% [100ng/mL], 93% [400ng/mL]); found in breast milk. **Metabolism:** Extensive; oxidation and methylation via CYP2D6. **Elimination:** Urine (62% metabolites; 2% parent compound); feces (36% metabolites; <1% parent compound) (30mg oral sol); $T_{1/2}$=33.2 hrs.

PATIENT CONSIDERATIONS

Assessment: Assess for drug hypersensitivity, risk of bipolar disorder, history of seizures, history of mania, volume depletion, diseases/conditions that alter metabolism or hemodynamic responses, hepatic/renal impairment, susceptibility to angle closure glaucoma, history of drug abuse, pregnancy/nursing status, and possible drug interactions.

Monitoring: Monitor for signs/symptoms of clinical worsening, suicidality, unusual behavior changes, serotonin syndrome, angle closure glaucoma, seizures, hyponatremia, akathisia, bleeding events, and other adverse reactions. If abruptly discontinued, monitor for discontinuation symptoms. Periodically reevaluate long-term usefulness of therapy.

Counseling: Inform about the benefits and risks of therapy. Caution about the risk of serotonin syndrome, particularly with concomitant use of triptans, tramadol, or other serotonergic agents. Inform that drug may cause mild pupillary dilation, which in susceptible individuals, may lead to an episode of angle closure glaucoma. Advise to look for the emergence of unusual changes in behavior, worsening of depression, and suicidality, especially early during treatment and when the dose is adjusted up or down. Inform that concomitant use with ASA, NSAIDs, or other drugs that affect coagulation may increase the risk of bleeding. Caution against operating hazardous machinery (including automobiles) until reasonably certain that therapy does not adversely affect ability to engage in such activities. Inform that the patient may notice improvement in 1-4 weeks; instruct to continue therapy ud. Instruct to inform physician if taking, or plan to take, any prescription or OTC drugs. Advise to avoid alcohol. Instruct to notify physician if pregnant, intending to become pregnant, or breastfeeding.

PHENOBARBITAL — phenobarbital   CIV

Class: Barbiturate

ADULT DOSAGE
Sedation
Sedative:
Tab (15mg, 30mg, 60mg, 100mg):
30-120mg in 2-3 divided doses
Tab (16.2mg, 32.4mg, 64.8mg, 97.2mg):
30-120mg in 2-3 divided doses; individualize frequency by patient response
Doses >400mg/24 hrs not recommended
Elixir:
30-120mg in 2-3 divided doses; individualize dose based on patient response
Doses >400mg/24 hrs not recommended

Hypnotic:
Tab (15mg, 30mg, 60mg, 100mg):
100-320mg
Tab (16.2mg, 32.4mg, 64.8mg, 97.2mg):
100-200mg
Elixir:
100-200mg

Seizures
Generalized/Partial Seizures:
Tab (16.2mg, 32.4mg, 64.8mg, 97.2mg):
60-200mg/day
Elixir:
60-200mg/day
Anticonvulsant:
Tab (15mg, 30mg, 60mg, 100mg):
50-100mg bid or tid

PEDIATRIC DOSAGE
Sedation
Tab (15mg, 30mg, 60mg, 100mg):
6mg/kg/day in 3 divided doses

Seizures
Generalized/Partial Seizures:
Tab (16.2mg, 32.4mg, 64.8mg, 97.2mg):
3-6mg/kg/day
Elixir:
3-6mg/kg/day

Also used in the treatment/prophylaxis of febrile seizures

Anticonvulsant:
Tab (15mg, 30mg, 60mg, 100mg):
15-50mg bid or tid

DOSING CONSIDERATIONS
Renal Impairment
Reduce dose
Hepatic Impairment
Reduce dose
Elderly
Elderly/Debilitated: Reduce dose

ADMINISTRATION
Oral route

STORAGE
20-25°C (68-77°F). (15mg, 30mg, 60mg, 100mg Tab) Protect from light and moisture.

HOW SUPPLIED
Elixir: 20mg/5mL [473mL]; **Tab:** 15mg, 16.2mg*, 30mg*, 32.4mg*, 60mg, 64.8mg*, 97.2mg*, 100mg* *scored

CONTRAINDICATIONS
Hypersensitivity to barbiturates, marked impairment of liver function or respiratory disease in which dyspnea or obstruction is evident. (Elixir/16.2mg, 32.4mg, 64.8mg, 97.2mg Tab) History of manifest/latent porphyria. (15mg, 30mg, 60mg, 100mg Tab) Personal or familial history of acute intermittent porphyria, known previous addiction to sedative/hypnotic group.

WARNINGS/PRECAUTIONS
Caution w/ borderline hypoadrenal function and history of drug abuse or dependence. Caution in patients who are mentally depressed or w/ suicidal tendencies. Caution when prescribing large amounts to patients w/ a history of emotional disturbances. Elderly or debilitated patients may react w/ marked excitement, depression, or confusion. (15mg, 30mg, 60mg, 100mg Tab) May increase reaction to painful stimuli in small doses; cannot be relied upon to relieve pain or even produce sedation or sleep in the presence of severe pain if taken alone. Caution w/ decreased liver function. (Elixir/16.2mg, 32.4mg, 64.8mg, 97.2mg Tab) Caution w/ acute or chronic pain; may induce paradoxical excitement or mask important symptoms. Some persons, especially children, may repeatedly produce excitement rather than depression. Avoid in patients showing premonitory signs of hepatic coma. May cause fetal damage. Use during labor may result in respiratory depression in the newborn. Cognitive deficits reported in children taking drug for complicated febrile seizures. May be habit-forming; limit prescription and dispensing to amount required for the interval until the next appointment. Withdraw gradually in patients taking excessive doses over long periods of time.

ADVERSE REACTIONS
Respiratory/CNS depression, apnea, circulatory collapse, hypersensitivity reactions, N/V, headache, somnolence.

DRUG INTERACTIONS
May produce additive depressant effects w/ other CNS depressants (eg, other sedatives/hypnotics, antihistamines, tranquilizers, alcohol). May diminish systemic effects of exogenous corticosteroids (eg, hydrocortisone). Decreased anticoagulant response of oral anticoagulants (eg, warfarin, acenocoumarol, dicumarol, phenprocoumon); determine PT frequently. Dose adjustments of anticoagulants may be required if barbiturates are added to or withdrawn from the dosage regimen. (Elixir/16.2mg, 32.4mg, 64.8mg, 97.2mg Tab) Dose adjustments of corticosteroids may be required if barbiturates are added to or withdrawn from the dosage regimen. May decrease griseofulvin levels; avoid concomitant use. May shorten $T_{1/2}$ of doxycycline for as long as 2 weeks after barbiturate therapy is discontinued; monitor response to doxycycline closely if given concurrently. Monitor phenytoin and barbiturate blood levels frequently when given concurrently. Increased levels w/ sodium valproate and valproic acid; closely monitor barbiturate blood levels and adjust dose as indicated. MAOIs may prolong effects. May decrease effect of estradiol w/ pretreatment or w/ concurrent use. Pregnancy reported w/ oral contraceptives; may suggest use of alternative contraceptive method.

PREGNANCY AND LACTATION
Pregnancy: Category B (15mg, 30mg, 60mg, 100mg Tab) and D (Elixir/16.2mg, 32.4mg, 64.8mg, 97.2mg Tab).
Lactation: Caution in nursing.

MECHANISM OF ACTION
Barbiturate; CNS depressant. Depresses sensory cortex, decreases motor activity, alters cerebellar function, and produces drowsiness, sedation, and hypnosis.

PHARMACOKINETICS
Distribution: Crosses the placenta; found in breast milk. **Metabolism:** Hepatic. **Elimination:** Urine (25-50% unchanged), feces; $T_{1/2}$=53-118 hrs (adults), 60-180 hrs (children and newborns <48 hrs old).

PATIENT CONSIDERATIONS

Assessment: Assess for known barbiturate hypersensitivity, history of porphyria, respiratory disease w/ evident dyspnea or obstruction, hypoadrenal function, suicidal tendencies, history of drug abuse or dependence, mental depression, hepatic impairment, debilitation, pain, pregnancy/nursing status, and possible drug interactions. (Elixir/16.2mg, 32.4mg, 64.8mg, 97.2mg Tab) Assess for renal impairment.

Monitoring: Monitor for marked excitement, depression, and confusion in elderly and debilitated patients. Monitor for tolerance, psychological and physical dependence, and withdrawal symptoms. Monitor PT frequently if used w/ coumarin anticoagulants. (Elixir/16.2mg, 32.4mg, 64.8mg, 97.2mg Tab) Monitor for paradoxical excitement and for masking of symptoms in patients w/ acute/chronic pain. Monitor for cognitive deficits in children w/ complicated febrile seizures. Perform periodic lab evaluation of hematopoietic, renal, and hepatic systems during prolonged therapy.

Counseling: Inform that medication may impair mental/physical abilities required for the performance of potentially hazardous tasks (eg, driving/operating machinery); advise to use caution. (Elixir/16.2mg, 32.4mg, 64.8mg, 97.2mg Tab) Inform of the risk of psychological and/or physical dependence; instruct not to increase dose w/o consulting physician. Instruct to avoid alcohol while on therapy; inform that use of other CNS depressants (eg, alcohol, narcotics, tranquilizers, antihistamines) may result in additional CNS depressant effects.

PHENYTEK — phenytoin sodium   Rx

Class: Hydantoin

ADULT DOSAGE

Seizures

Generalized Tonic-Clonic (Grand Mal) and Psychomotor (Temporal Lobe) Seizures and Prevention/Treatment of Neurosurgery-Associated Seizures:

Divided Daily Dosing:
No Previous Treatment:
Initial: 100mg tid
Maint: 100mg tid-qid
Titrate: May increase up to 200mg tid, if necessary

QD Dosing:
May consider 300mg qd if seizure is controlled on divided doses of three 100mg caps daily

LD (Clinic/Hospital):
Initial: 1g in 3 divided doses (400mg, 300mg, 300mg) at 2-hr intervals
Maint: Start maint dose 24 hrs after LD
Do not give oral loading regimen in patients w/ history of renal/liver disease

Clinically effective serum level usually 10-20mcg/mL; do not change dose at intervals <7-10 days

PEDIATRIC DOSAGE

Seizures

Generalized Tonic-Clonic (Grand Mal) and Psychomotor (Temporal Lobe) Seizures and Prevention/Treatment of Neurosurgery-Associated Seizures:

Initial: 5mg/kg/day in 2 or 3 equally divided doses
Maint: 4-8mg/kg/day
Max: 300mg/day

>6 Years: May require the minimum adult dose (300mg/day)

Clinically effective serum level usually 10-20mcg/mL; do not change dose at intervals <7-10 days

---

DOSING CONSIDERATIONS

Renal Impairment
Caution when interpreting total phenytoin plasma concentrations; unbound phenytoin concentrations may be more useful

Hepatic Impairment
Caution when interpreting total phenytoin plasma concentrations; unbound phenytoin concentrations may be more useful

Elderly
May require lower or less frequent dosing

Other Important Considerations
Dosage adjustments and serum level monitoring may be necessary when switching from a product formulated w/ free acid to a product formulated w/ Na+ salt and vice versa

Hypoalbuminemia:
Caution when interpreting total phenytoin plasma concentrations; unbound phenytoin concentrations may be more useful

ADMINISTRATION
Oral route

STORAGE
20-25°C (68-77°F). Protect from light and moisture.

HOW SUPPLIED
Cap, Extended-Release: 200mg, 300mg

CONTRAINDICATIONS
History of hypersensitivity to phenytoin, its inactive ingredients, or other hydantoins; coadministration w/ delavirdine.

WARNINGS/PRECAUTIONS
Avoid abrupt withdrawal; may precipitate status epilepticus. May increase risk of suicidal thoughts/behavior. Serious and sometimes fatal dermatologic reactions, including toxic epidermal necrolysis (TEN) and Stevens-Johnson syndrome (SJS), reported; d/c at 1st sign of rash, unless the rash is clearly not drug-related. Do not resume therapy, and consider alternative therapy if signs/symptoms suggest SJS/TEN. Consider avoiding use as an alternative for carbamazepine in patients positive for HLA-B*1502. Drug reaction w/ eosinophilia and systemic symptoms (DRESS)/multiorgan hypersensitivity reported; evaluate immediately if signs/symptoms are present and d/c if an alternative etiology cannot be established. Caution w/ history/immediate family history of hypersensitivity to structurally similar drugs (eg, carboxamides, barbiturates, succinimides, oxazolidinediones); consider alternatives to therapy. Acute hepatotoxicity reported; d/c immediately and do not readminister. Hematopoietic complications and lymphadenopathy reported; follow-up observation for an extended period is indicated and every effort should be made to achieve seizure control using alternative antiepileptic drugs in all cases of lymphadenopathy. Decreased bone mineral density and bone fractures reported during chronic use; consider screening and initiating treatment as appropriate. Caution w/ porphyria, hepatic impairment, and in elderly or gravely ill patients. Increase in seizure frequency may occur during pregnancy. Potentially life-threatening bleeding disorder in newborns may occur; administer vitamin K to mother before delivery and to neonate after birth. Check plasma levels immediately if early signs of dose-related CNS toxicity develop. Hyperglycemia reported; may increase serum glucose levels in diabetics. Not indicated for seizures due to hypoglycemia or other metabolic causes. Not effective for absence (petit mal) seizures; if tonic-clonic (grand mal) and absence (petit mal) seizures are present, combined drug therapy is needed. May produce confusional states at levels sustained above optimal range; reduce dose if plasma levels are excessive, or d/c if symptoms persist. Lab test interactions may occur. May cause fetal harm.

ADVERSE REACTIONS
Rash, nystagmus, ataxia, slurred speech, decreased coordination, somnolence, mental confusion, dizziness, insomnia, transient nervousness, motor twitching, N/V, headache, altered taste sensation, Peyronie's disease.

DRUG INTERACTIONS
See Contraindications. Acute alcohol intake, amiodarone, antiepileptic agents (eg, ethosuximide, felbamate, oxcarbazepine), azoles (eg, fluconazole, ketoconazole, itraconazole), capecitabine, chloramphenicol, chlordiazepoxide, diazepam, disulfiram, estrogens, fluorouracil, fluoxetine, fluvastatin, fluvoxamine, H2-antagonists (eg, cimetidine), halothane, isoniazid, methylphenidate, phenothiazines, omeprazole, salicylates, sertraline, succinimides, sulfonamides (eg, sulfaphenazole, sulfadiazine, sulfamethoxazole-trimethoprim), ticlopidine, tolbutamide, trazodone, and warfarin may increase levels. Anticancer drugs usually in combination (eg, bleomycin, carboplatin, cisplatin), carbamazepine, chronic alcohol abuse, diazepam, diazoxide, folic acid, fosamprenavir, nelfinavir, reserpine, rifampin, ritonavir (RTV), St. John's wort, sucralfate, theophylline, and vigabatrin may decrease levels. Administration w/ preparations that increase gastric pH (eg, supplements or antacids containing calcium carbonate, aluminum hydroxide, and magnesium hydroxide) may affect absorption; do not take phenytoin and these drugs at the same time of day. Phenobarbital, sodium valproate, and valproic acid may increase/decrease levels. May impair efficacy of azoles, corticosteroids, doxycycline, estrogens, furosemide, irinotecan, oral contraceptives, paclitaxel, paroxetine, quinidine, rifampin, sertraline, teniposide, theophylline, and vitamin D. Increased and decreased PT/INR responses reported w/ warfarin. May decrease levels of active metabolites of albendazole, certain HIV antivirals (eg, efavirenz, lopinavir/RTV, indinavir), anti-epileptic agents (eg, carbamazepine, felbamate, lamotrigine), atorvastatin, chlorpropamide, clozapine, cyclosporine, digoxin, fluvastatin, folic acid, methadone, mexiletine, nifedipine, nimodipine, nisoldipine, praziquantel, simvastatin, and verapamil. May decrease levels of amprenavir (active metabolite) when given w/ fosamprenavir alone. May increase amprenavir levels when given w/ the combination of fosamprenavir and RTV. Resistance to the neuromuscular blocking action of pancuronium, vecuronium, rocuronium, and cisatracurium reported in patients chronically administered phenytoin; monitor closely for more rapid recovery from neuromuscular blockade than expected and for higher infusion rate requirements. Lower levels w/ enteral feeding preparations and/or related nutritional supplements; avoid w/ enteral feeding preparations.

PREGNANCY AND LACTATION
Pregnancy: Category D.
Lactation: Not for use in nursing.

MECHANISM OF ACTION
Hydantoin; inhibits seizure activity by promoting Na+ efflux from neurons and stabilizing the threshold against hyperexcitability caused by excessive stimulation or environmental changes capable of reducing membrane Na+ gradient. Reduces the maximal activity of the brain stem centers responsible for the tonic phase of tonic-clonic (grand mal) seizures.

PHARMACOKINETICS
Absorption: T_{max}=4-12 hrs. **Distribution:** Plasma protein binding (high); found in breast milk. **Metabolism:** Liver (hydroxylation). **Elimination:** Bile (mostly inactive metabolites), urine; $T_{1/2}$=22 hrs.

PATIENT CONSIDERATIONS

Assessment: Assess for history of hypersensitivity to the drug, its inactive ingredients, or other hydantoins, alcohol use, hepatic/renal impairment, hypoalbuminemia, grave illness, porphyria, seizures due to hypoglycemic or other metabolic causes, absence seizures, any other conditions where treatment is cautioned, pregnancy/nursing status, and possible drug interactions.

Monitoring: Monitor for allergic/hypersensitivity reactions, dermatologic reactions, DRESS/multiorgan hypersensitivity, hepatotoxicity, hematopoietic complications, lymphadenopathy, decreased bone mineral density, bone fractures, exacerbation of porphyria, hyperglycemia, and other adverse reactions. Monitor for emergence/worsening of depression, suicidal thoughts/behavior, and/or any unusual changes in mood/behavior. Monitor serum levels.

Counseling: Instruct to take only as prescribed. Advise of the importance of adhering strictly to the prescribed dosage regimen, and of informing physician of any clinical condition in which it is not possible to take the drug orally as prescribed (eg, surgery). Counsel about the early toxic signs/symptoms of potential hematologic, dermatologic, hypersensitivity, or hepatic reactions; instruct to immediately report any occurrence to physician even if mild or occurring after extended use. Caution on the use of other drugs or alcoholic beverages w/o first seeking physician's advice. Stress the importance of good dental hygiene to minimize development of gingival hyperplasia and its complications. Advise to notify physician immediately if depression, suicidal thoughts/behavior, or thoughts about self-harm emerge. Encourage patients to enroll in the North American Antiepileptic Drug Pregnancy Registry.

PHOSLYRA — calcium acetate   Rx

Class: Phosphate binder

ADULT DOSAGE
Hyperphosphatemia

In Patients w/ ESRD:
Initial: 10mL w/ each meal
Titrate: Increase dose gradually to
lower serum phosphorus (P) levels to
the target range, every 2-3 weeks until
acceptable serum P level is reached, as
long as hypercalcemia does not develop
Usual: 15-20mL w/ each meal

PEDIATRIC DOSAGE
Pediatric use may not have been
established

DOSING CONSIDERATIONS
Elderly
Start at lower end of dosing range

ADMINISTRATION
Oral route

STORAGE
25°C (77°F); excursions permitted to 15-30°C (59-86°F).

HOW SUPPLIED
Sol: 667mg (169mg Ca^{2+} base)/5mL [473mL]

CONTRAINDICATIONS
Hypercalcemia.

WARNINGS/PRECAUTIONS
May develop hypercalcemia. If hypercalcemia develops, reduce dose or d/c
immediately depending on severity. Chronic hypercalcemia may lead to vascular
calcification and other soft-tissue calcification; radiographic evaluation of
suspected anatomical regions may be helpful in early detection of soft-tissue
calcification. Maintain serum calcium-phosphorus (Ca x P) product <55mg^2/dL^2.

ADVERSE REACTIONS
Hypercalcemia, diarrhea, dizziness, edema, weakness.

DRUG INTERACTIONS
Avoid w/ other Ca^{2+} supplements, including Ca^{2+}-based nonprescription antacids.
Hypercalcemia may aggravate digitalis toxicity. May induce a laxative effect w/
other products containing maltitol. Fluoroquinolones must be taken at least 2
hrs before or 6 hrs after therapy. Tetracyclines must be taken at least 1 hr before
therapy. Levothyroxine must be taken at least 4 hrs before or 4 hrs after therapy.
Consider separating the timing of the administration of oral medications where a
reduction in the bioavailability of a medication would have a clinically significant
effect on its safety/efficacy. Consider monitoring clinical responses or blood levels
of concomitant medications that have a narrow therapeutic range.

PREGNANCY AND LACTATION
Pregnancy: Category C.
Lactation: Caution in nursing.

MECHANISM OF ACTION
Phosphate binder; combines w/ dietary phosphate to form insoluble calcium-
phosphate complex, resulting in decreased serum P concentrations.

PHARMACOKINETICS
Distribution: Found in breast milk.

PATIENT CONSIDERATIONS
Assessment: Assess for hypercalcemia, pregnancy/nursing status, and for possible
drug interactions.

Monitoring: Monitor for hypercalcemia, confusion, delirium, stupor, coma,
anorexia, N/V, vascular/other soft-tissue calcification, and other adverse reactions.
Monitor serum Ca^{2+} twice weekly early in treatment, during dose adjustment, and
periodically thereafter. Monitor for serum P levels periodically.

Counseling: Instruct to take w/ meals, adhere to prescribed diets, and to avoid
use of Ca^{2+} supplements including nonprescription antacids. Inform about
symptoms of hypercalcemia. Advise patients who are taking an oral medication to
take the drug 1 hr before or 3 hrs after calcium acetate.

PINDOLOL — pindolol   Rx

Class: Nonselective beta blocker

OTHER BRAND NAMES
Visken (Discontinued)

ADULT DOSAGE
Hypertension

Initial: 5mg bid
Titrate: May adjust dose in increments
of 10mg/day at 3- to 4-week intervals
if a satisfactory reduction in BP does
not occur
Max: 60mg/day

PEDIATRIC DOSAGE
Pediatric use may not have been
established

ADMINISTRATION
Oral route

STORAGE
20-25°C (68-77°F). Protect from light.

HOW SUPPLIED
Tab: 5mg*, 10mg* *scored

CONTRAINDICATIONS
Bronchial asthma, overt cardiac failure, cardiogenic shock, 2nd- and 3rd-degree
heart block, severe bradycardia.

WARNINGS/PRECAUTIONS
May precipitate more severe failure in patients with congestive heart failure
(CHF); if necessary, may be used with caution in patients with history of overt
CHF who are well-compensated, usually with digitalis and diuretics. May cause
cardiac failure in patients with latent cardiac insufficiency; fully digitalize
and/or give a diuretic, and closely observe the response at the 1st sign/
symptom of impending cardiac failure. If cardiac failure continues, despite
adequate digitalization and diuretic, withdraw therapy (gradually, if possible).
Hypersensitivity to catecholamines observed in patients withdrawn from therapy;
exacerbation of angina and, in some cases, myocardial infarction reported after
abrupt discontinuation. When discontinuing chronically administered therapy,
particularly with ischemic heart disease, gradually reduce dosage over 1-2 weeks
and carefully monitor the patient. If angina markedly worsens or acute coronary
insufficiency develops, reinstitute therapy promptly, at least temporarily, and
take other measures appropriate for the management of unstable angina.
Do not d/c therapy abruptly even in patients treated only for HTN. Avoid in
patients with bronchospastic diseases; if necessary, may use with caution.
Impairs the ability of the heart to respond to reflex stimuli and may increase
the risks of general anesthesia and surgical procedures, resulting in protracted
hypotension or low cardiac output; gradually withdraw therapy several days
prior to surgery. In the event of emergency surgery, inform the anesthesiologist
that patient is on β-blocker therapy. Difficulty in restarting and maintaining the
heart beat reported. May prevent the appearance of premonitory signs and
symptoms (eg, tachycardia, BP changes) of acute hypoglycemia, and reduces
the release of insulin in response to hyperglycemia. May mask certain clinical
signs (eg, tachycardia) of hyperthyroidism; carefully manage patients suspected
of developing thyrotoxicosis to avoid abrupt withdrawal of therapy that might
precipitate a thyroid crisis. Caution with hepatic/renal impairment. Patients
with a history of severe anaphylactic reaction to a variety of allergens may be
more reactive to repeated challenge and may be unresponsive to usual doses of
epinephrine.

ADVERSE REACTIONS
Insomnia, dizziness, fatigue, nervousness, joint pain, edema, dyspnea, bizarre/
many dreams, nausea, weakness, abdominal discomfort, muscle cramps/pain,
paresthesia.

DRUG INTERACTIONS
Increased risk of bradycardia with digitalis glycosides. May need to adjust the
dose of antidiabetic drugs. Additive effect with catecholamine-depleting drugs
(eg, reserpine); closely observe for evidence of hypotension and/or marked
bradycardia that may produce vertigo, syncope, or postural hypotension. Both
thioridazine and pindolol levels may increase when used concomitantly.

PREGNANCY AND LACTATION
Category B, not for use in nursing.

MECHANISM OF ACTION
Nonselective β-blocker; not established. Suspected to reduce sympathetic outflow
to the periphery, decrease cardiac output, and inhibit renin release. Possesses
intrinsic sympathomimetic activity.

PHARMACOKINETICS
Absorption: Rapidly absorbed. C_{max}=45-167ng/mL (20mg single dose); T_{max}=1 hr.
Distribution: (Healthy) V_d=2L/kg; plasma protein binding (40%); found in breast
milk. **Metabolism:** Extensive; hydroxy-metabolites. **Elimination:** Urine (35-40%,
unchanged), (IV) feces (6-9%); $T_{1/2}$=3-4 hrs, 8 hrs (polar metabolites).

PATIENT CONSIDERATIONS
Assessment: Assess for bronchial asthma, overt cardiac failure, cardiogenic shock,
2nd- and 3rd-degree heart block, severe bradycardia, history of well-compensated
CHF, latent cardiac insufficiency, ischemic heart disease, bronchospastic disease,
diabetes, thyrotoxicosis, hepatic/renal impairment, history of severe anaphylactic
reaction, any upcoming surgery, pregnancy/nursing status, and possible drug
interactions.

Monitoring: Monitor for signs/symptoms of cardiac failure, masking of
hypoglycemia/hyperthyroidism, and other adverse reactions.

Counseling: Instruct, especially those with evidence of coronary artery
insufficiency, not to interrupt or d/c therapy without consulting physician. Advise
to consult physician at the 1st sign/symptom of impending cardiac failure.

PLAQUENIL — hydroxychloroquine sulfate   Rx

Class: Aminoquinoline

> Before prescribing, physicians should be completely familiar w/ the complete PI.

ADULT DOSAGE
Rheumatoid Arthritis

Initial: 400-600mg (310-465mg
base)/day
Some patients may require temporary
reduction of initial dose due to
troublesome side effects; later
(usually from 5-10 days), dose may
be gradually increased to optimum
response level

PEDIATRIC DOSAGE
Malaria

**Due to *P. vivax*, *P. malariae*, *P.
ovale*, and susceptible strains of *P.
falciparum*:**

Infants and Children:

Suppression:
2 Weeks Prior to Exposure:
5mg base/kg weekly

Maint: When a good response is obtained (usually in 4-12 weeks), reduce dose by 50% and continue at 200-400mg (155-310mg base)/day

May resume therapy or continue on an intermittent schedule if relapse occurs after drug withdrawal if there are no ocular contraindications

Corticosteroids and salicylates may be used in conjunction and can generally be decreased gradually in dose or eliminated after drug has been used for several weeks

D/C if objective improvement (eg, reduced joint swelling, increased mobility) does not occur w/in 6 months

Malaria

Due to *Plasmodium vivax, P. malariae, P. ovale,* and susceptible strains of *P. falciparum:*

Suppression:
2 Weeks Prior to Exposure: 400mg (310mg base) on exactly the same day of each week
If Unable to Begin 2 Weeks Prior to Exposure: 800mg (620mg base) in 2 divided doses, 6 hrs apart

Continue suppressive therapy for 8 weeks after leaving endemic area

Treatment of Acute Attack:
800mg (620mg base), followed by 400mg (310mg base) 6-8 hrs later, then 400mg (310mg base) on each of 2 consecutive days
Alternative Dosing: 800mg (620mg base) single dose, or calculate on the basis of body weight (total of 25mg base/kg administered in 3 days; see Pediatric Dosage)

Lupus Erythematosus

Chronic Discoid and Systemic:
Initial: 400mg (310mg base) qd-bid for several weeks or months
Prolonged Maint: 200-400mg (155-310mg base)/day

ADMINISTRATION
Oral route

Rheumatoid Arthritis (RA)
Take w/ a meal or glass of milk.

STORAGE
Room temperature up to 30°C (86°F).

HOW SUPPLIED
Tab: 200mg (=155mg base)

CONTRAINDICATIONS
In the presence of retinal/visual field changes attributable to any 4-aminoquinoline compound; known hypersensitivity to 4-aminoquinoline compounds; for long-term therapy in children.

WARNINGS/PRECAUTIONS
Not effective against chloroquine-resistant strains of *P. falciparum*. Carefully examine for visual acuity, central visual field, and color vision (exam should include fundoscopy), prior to long-term therapy; repeat exam at least annually. Increased risk of retinal toxicity if recommended daily dose is exceeded sharply. Exam should be more frequent and adapted to patient in the following situations: daily dose >6.5mg/kg ideal body weight; renal insufficiency; cumulative dose >200g; elderly; impaired visual acuity. D/C immediately if any visual disturbance occurs and closely observe for possible progression of the abnormality. Retinal and visual disturbances may progress even after discontinuation of therapy. Suicidal behavior rarely reported. Children are especially sensitive to 4-aminoquinoline compounds. May precipitate a severe attack of psoriasis and may exacerbate porphyria; avoid use in these conditions unless benefit outweighs possible hazard. Avoid in pregnancy except in the suppression/treatment of malaria if benefit outweighs possible hazard. Caution w/ hepatic disease, alcoholism, and G6PD deficiency. Perform periodic blood cell counts w/ prolonged therapy; consider discontinuation of therapy if any severe blood disorder appears that is not attributable to the disease under treatment. **Lupus Erythematosus/RA:** Irreversible retinal damage reported w/ long-term or high dosage of 4-aminoquinoline therapy. Perform baseline and periodic (every 3 months) ophthalmologic exams w/ prolonged therapy. Examine all patients on long-term therapy periodically, including testing of knee and ankle reflexes; d/c treatment if muscular weakness occurs. Dermatologic reactions may occur.

ADVERSE REACTIONS
Malaria: Headache, dizziness, GI complaints, convulsions, nervousness, emotional lability, psychosis, suicidal behavior, retinopathy w/ changes in pigmentation, visual field defects, maculopathies, macular degeneration, bullous eruptions.
Lupus Erythematosus/RA: Irritability, nervousness, emotional changes, headache, dizziness, skeletal muscle palsies/skeletal muscle myopathy/neuromyopathy,

Max: 400mg (310mg base)/dose
If Unable to Begin 2 Weeks Prior to Exposure:
10mg base/kg in 2 divided doses, 6 hrs apart

Continue suppressive therapy for 8 weeks after leaving endemic area

Treatment of Acute Attack:
25mg base/kg administered in 3 days, as follows:
1st Dose: 10mg base/kg, not exceeding a single dose of 620mg base
2nd Dose: 5mg base/kg 6 hrs after 1st dose, not exceeding a single dose of 310mg base
3rd Dose: 5mg base/kg 18 hrs after 2nd dose
4th Dose: 5mg base/kg 24 hrs after 3rd dose

ocular reactions (eg, corneal changes), bleaching of hair, blood dyscrasias, anorexia, N/V, urticaria, weight loss.

DRUG INTERACTIONS
Caution w/ hepatotoxic drugs. **Lupus Erythematosus/RA:** Caution w/ drugs w/ a significant tendency to produce dermatitis.

PREGNANCY AND LACTATION
Pregnancy: Avoid except in the suppression or treatment of malaria when the benefit outweighs the possible hazard.

MECHANISM OF ACTION
Aminoquinoline; has not been established.

PATIENT CONSIDERATIONS
Assessment: Assess for retinal or visual field defects, psoriasis, porphyria, hepatic/renal disease, alcoholism, G6PD deficiency, chloroquine-resistant strains of *P. falciparum*, any other conditions where treatment is contraindicated or cautioned, pregnancy/nursing status, and possible drug interactions. Perform baseline ophthalmologic exams (eg, visual acuity, central visual field, color vision, fundoscopy) w/ prolonged therapy.

Monitoring: Monitor for retinal/visual disturbances, suicidal behavior, severe psoriasis attack, exacerbation of porphyria, dermatologic reactions, and other adverse reactions. Perform periodic (every 3 months) ophthalmologic exams, periodic blood cell counts, and periodic tests for knee and ankle reflexes w/ prolonged therapy.

Counseling: Inform about adverse effects and instruct to seek medical attention if any signs/symptoms develop. Advise about need for periodic follow-up.

PLAVIX — clopidogrel bisulfate   Rx

Class: Antiplatelet agent

> Effectiveness is dependent on activation to an active metabolite via CYP2C19. Poor metabolizers of CYP2C19 w/ acute coronary syndrome (ACS) or undergoing percutaneous coronary intervention treated w/ clopidogrel at recommended doses exhibit higher cardiovascular (CV) event rates than patients w/ normal CYP2C19 function. Tests are available to identify a patient's CYP2C19 genotype; these tests can be used as an aid in determining therapeutic strategy. Consider alternative treatment or treatment strategies in patients identified as CYP2C19 poor metabolizers.

ADULT DOSAGE	PEDIATRIC DOSAGE
Acute Coronary Syndrome **Unstable Angina/Non-ST-Elevation MI:** **LD:** 300mg **Maint:** 75mg qd. Initiate aspirin (ASA) (75-325mg qd) and continue in combination w/ clopidogrel **ST-Elevation MI:** 75mg qd w/ ASA (75-325mg qd), w/ or w/o thrombolytics May initiate w/ or w/o a LD **Recent Myocardial Infarction/Recent Stroke/Peripheral Arterial Disease** 75mg qd	Pediatric use may not have been established

----

ADMINISTRATION
Oral route
May be administered w/ or w/o food.

STORAGE
25°C (77°F); excursions permitted to 15-30°C (59-86°F).

HOW SUPPLIED
Tab: 75mg, 300mg

CONTRAINDICATIONS
Active pathological bleeding (eg, peptic ulcer, intracranial hemorrhage), hypersensitivity (eg, anaphylaxis) to clopidogrel or any component of the product.

WARNINGS/PRECAUTIONS
Increases the risk of bleeding; d/c 5 days prior to surgery if an antiplatelet effect is not desired. Avoid lapses in therapy; if therapy must be temporarily discontinued, restart as soon as possible. Premature discontinuation may increase risk of CV events. Thrombotic thrombocytopenic purpura (TTP) reported. Hypersensitivity (eg, rash, angioedema, hematologic reaction) reported, including in patients w/ a history of hypersensitivity or hematologic reaction to other thienopyridines.

ADVERSE REACTIONS
Bleeding.

DRUG INTERACTIONS
Reduced antiplatelet activity w/ omeprazole or esomeprazole; avoid concomitant use, or consider using another acid-reducing agent w/ minimal or no CYP2C19 inhibitory effect on the formation of clopidogrel active metabolite. Certain CYP2C19 inhibitors may reduce platelet inhibition. NSAIDs, warfarin, SSRIs, SNRIs, and ASA may increase risk of bleeding.

PREGNANCY AND LACTATION
Category B, not for use in nursing.

MECHANISM OF ACTION
Platelet activation and aggregation inhibitor; irreversibly and selectively inhibits the binding of adenosine diphosphate (ADP) to its platelet P2Y$_{12}$ receptor and the subsequent ADP-mediated activation of the glycoprotein GPIIb/IIIa complex.

PHARMACOKINETICS

Absorption: Rapid. T_{max}=30-60 min (active thiol metabolite). **Metabolism:** Extensive via esterases (leading to hydrolysis) and via multiple CYP450 enzymes; active thiol metabolite (principally by CYP2C19). **Elimination:** Urine (50%), feces (46%); $T_{1/2}$=6 hrs, 30 min (active thiol metabolite).

PATIENT CONSIDERATIONS

Assessment: Assess for active pathological bleeding, hypersensitivity to drug or another thienopyridine, CYP2C19 genotype, pregnancy/nursing status, and possible drug interactions. Assess use in patients at risk for increased bleeding (eg, undergoing surgery).

Monitoring: Monitor for bleeding, TTP, hypersensitivity, and other adverse reactions.

Counseling: Inform about the benefits and risks of treatment. Instruct to take exactly as prescribed and not to d/c w/o consulting the prescribing physician. Inform that they will bruise and bleed more easily and that bleeding will take longer than usual to stop. Advise to report any unanticipated, prolonged, or excessive bleeding, or blood in stool or urine. Instruct to seek prompt medical attention if unexplained fever, weakness, extreme skin paleness, purple skin patches, yellowing of the skin or eyes, or neurological changes occur. Instruct to notify physician or dentist about therapy before scheduling any invasive procedure. Advise to inform physician of all medications, including OTC medications and dietary supplements, they are taking or planning to take.

PLEGRIDY — peginterferon beta-1a   Rx

Class: Biological response modifier

ADULT DOSAGE	PEDIATRIC DOSAGE
Multiple Sclerosis	Pediatric use may not have been established
Treatment of Relapsing Forms:	
Day 1: 63mcg SQ	
Day 15: 94mcg SQ	
On Day 29 and Thereafter: 125mcg SQ every 14 days	
Premedication	
Prophylactic and concurrent use of analgesics and/or antipyretics may prevent or ameliorate flu-like symptoms sometimes experienced during treatment	

ADMINISTRATION

SQ route

Rotate inj sites; usual sites are abdomen, back of the upper arm, and thigh. Prefilled pens and syringes are for a single dose only; discard after use.

STORAGE

2-8°C (36-46°F). Protect from light. Do not freeze; discard if frozen. Once removed from the refrigerator, allow to warm to room temperature (about 30 min) prior to inj; do not use external heat sources (eg, hot water) to warm the product. If refrigeration is unavailable, may store at 2-25°C (36-77°F) for up to 30 days; protect from light. May be removed from, and returned to, a refrigerator if necessary. The total combined time out of refrigeration, w/in a temperature range of 2-25°C (36-77°F), should not exceed 30 days.

HOW SUPPLIED

Inj: 125mcg/0.5mL [prefilled pen, prefilled syringe]; (Starter Pack) 63mcg/0.5mL, 94mcg/0.5mL [prefilled pen, prefilled syringe]

CONTRAINDICATIONS

History of hypersensitivity to natural or recombinant interferon beta or peginterferon, or any other component of the formulation.

WARNINGS/PRECAUTIONS

Elevations in hepatic enzymes and hepatic injury reported. Depression and suicidal ideation reported; consider discontinuation if depression or other severe psychiatric symptoms develop. Seizures reported. Anaphylaxis and other serious allergic reactions (eg, angioedema, urticaria) reported; d/c if a serious allergic reaction occurs. Inj-site reactions reported; decision to d/c therapy following necrosis at a single inj site should be based on the extent of the necrosis. If therapy is continued after inj-site necrosis has occurred, avoid administration near the affected area until it is fully healed; if multiple lesions occur, d/c until healing occurs. Cardiovascular (CV) events reported; monitor patients w/ significant cardiac disease for worsening of their cardiac condition during initiation and continuation of treatment. Decreased peripheral blood counts reported; monitor for infections, bleeding, and symptoms of anemia. Cases of thrombotic microangiopathy (TMA) (eg, thrombotic thrombocytopenia purpura, hemolytic uremic syndrome), some fatal, reported w/ interferon β products; d/c and manage if TMA occurs. Autoimmune disorders reported; consider discontinuation if a new autoimmune disorder develops. Monitor for adverse reactions due to increased drug exposure in patients w/ severe renal impairment.

ADVERSE REACTIONS

Inj-site erythema, influenza-like illness, pyrexia, headache, myalgia, chills, inj-site pain, asthenia, inj-site pruritus, arthralgia.

PREGNANCY AND LACTATION

Pregnancy: Category C. There is a pregnancy exposure registry that monitors fetal outcomes in women exposed to therapy during pregnancy.
Lactation: Caution in nursing.

MECHANISM OF ACTION

Biological response modifier; has not been established.

PHARMACOKINETICS

Absorption: T_{max}=1-1.5 days; C_{max}=280pg/mL; AUC=34.8ng•hr/mL. **Distribution:** V_d=481L. **Elimination:** Renal; $T_{1/2}$=78 hrs.

PATIENT CONSIDERATIONS

Assessment: Assess for seizure disorder, cardiac disease, myelosuppression, renal/hepatic impairment, history of hypersensitivity to drug, and pregnancy/nursing status.

Monitoring: Monitor for signs/symptoms of hepatic injury; depression, suicidal ideation, or other severe psychiatric symptoms; seizures; serious allergic reactions; inj-site reactions/necrosis; CV events or worsening of cardiac condition; TMA, autoimmune disorders; and other adverse reactions. Monitor for infections, bleeding, and symptoms of anemia. Monitor CBCs, differential WBC count, and platelet counts; patients w/ myelosuppression may require more intensive monitoring. Monitor for adverse reactions due to increased drug exposure in patients w/ severe renal impairment.

Counseling: Advise not to change the dose or schedule of administration w/o medical consultation. Instruct on how to self-inject therapy and inform of the proper procedures to follow. Advise to rotate areas of inj w/ each dose, and not to inject into an area of the body where the skin is irritated, reddened, bruised, infected, or scarred in any way. Instruct to check the inj site after 2 hrs for redness, swelling, and tenderness, and to contact physician if a skin reaction occurs and does not clear up in a few days. Advise to inform physician if pregnant/breastfeeding. Encourage patients to enroll in the pregnancy registry if they become pregnant while taking therapy. Inform of the symptoms of hepatic dysfunction, depression, suicidal ideation, seizures, and worsening cardiac condition, and instruct to immediately report any of these symptoms to physician. Instruct to seek immediate medical attention if symptoms of allergic reactions and anaphylaxis occur. Advise that inj-site reactions may occur and to promptly report any signs of necrosis at inj site. Inform that flu-like symptoms are common following initiation of therapy.

PLETAL — cilostazol   Rx

Class: Phosphodiesterase-3 (PDE-3) inhibitor

> **Contraindicated in patients w/ heart failure (HF) of any severity. Cilostazol and several of its metabolites are PDE3 inhibitors; several drugs w/ this pharmacologic effect have caused decreased survival compared to placebo in patients w/ class III-IV HF.**

ADULT DOSAGE	PEDIATRIC DOSAGE
Intermittent Claudication	Pediatric use may not have been established
Reduction of Symptoms: 100mg bid	
D/C if symptoms have not improved after 3 months	

DOSING CONSIDERATIONS

Concomitant Medications
Strong or Moderate CYP3A4 or CYP2C19 Inhibitors: Reduce dose to 50mg bid

ADMINISTRATION

Oral route

Take at least 1/2 hr before or 2 hrs after breakfast and dinner.

STORAGE

25°C (77°F); excursions permitted to 15-30°C (59-86°F).

HOW SUPPLIED

Tab: 50mg, 100mg

CONTRAINDICATIONS

HF of any severity, hypersensitivity (eg, anaphylaxis, angioedema) to cilostazol or any components of the product.

WARNINGS/PRECAUTIONS

May induce tachycardia, palpitation, tachyarrhythmia, or hypotension; patients w/ a history of ischemic heart disease may be at risk for exacerbations of angina pectoris or MI. Cases of thrombocytopenia or leukopenia progressing to agranulocytosis reported. Avoid in patients w/ hemostatic disorders or active pathologic bleeding.

ADVERSE REACTIONS

Headache, diarrhea, abnormal stools, palpitation, dizziness, pharyngitis, infection, peripheral edema, rhinitis, dyspepsia, abdominal pain, tachycardia.

DRUG INTERACTIONS

See Dosing Considerations. Coadministration of strong (eg, ketoconazole) and moderate (eg, erythromycin, diltiazem, grapefruit juice) CYP3A4 inhibitors may increase exposure. Coadministration w/ CYP2C19 inhibitors (eg, ticlopidine, fluconazole, omeprazole) may increase exposure of active metabolites.

PREGNANCY AND LACTATION

Pregnancy: Category C.
Lactation: Not for use in nursing.

MECHANISM OF ACTION

PDE3 inhibitor; cilostazol and several of its metabolites inhibit PDE3 activity and suppress cAMP degradation w/ a resultant increase in cAMP in platelets and blood vessels, leading to inhibition of platelet aggregation and vasodilation, respectively.

PHARMACOKINETICS

Distribution: Plasma protein binding (95-98%). **Metabolism:** Liver (extensive) via CYP450 enzymes, mainly 3A4, and, to a lesser extent, 2C19; 3,4-dehydro-cilostazol, 4'-trans-hydroxy-cilostazol (major active metabolites). **Elimination:** Urine (74%), feces (20%); $T_{1/2}$=11-13 hrs.

PATIENT CONSIDERATIONS

Assessment: Assess for hypersensitivity to drug, HF of any severity, hemostatic disorders, active pathologic bleeding, history of ischemic heart disease, renal/hepatic impairment, pregnancy/nursing status, and possible drug interactions.

Monitoring: Monitor for tachycardia, palpitation, tachyarrhythmia, hypotension, and other adverse reactions. Periodically monitor platelets and WBC counts.

Counseling: Advise to take at least 1/2 hr ac or 2 hrs pc. Instruct to discuss w/ physician before taking any other medication. Inform that the beneficial effects of therapy may not be immediate; although benefit may be experienced in 2-4 weeks after initiation of therapy, advise that treatment for up to 12 weeks may be required before a beneficial effect is experienced. Instruct to d/c if symptoms do not improve after 3 months.

PLIAGLIS — lidocaine/tetracaine   Rx

Class: Local anesthetic

ADULT DOSAGE	PEDIATRIC DOSAGE
Topical Anesthetic	Pediatric use may not have been established
Dermal Filler Inj, Non-Ablative Laser Facial Resurfacing, Pulsed-Dye Laser Therapy: Apply 20-30 min prior to procedure	
Laser-Assisted Tattoo Removal: Apply for 60 min prior to procedure	

Amount of Cre According to Treatment Site Surface Area:
$10cm^2$: 3cm (1g) of cre
$20cm^2$: 6cm (3g) of cre
$40cm^2$: 12cm (5g) of cre
$80cm^2$: 24cm (11g) of cre
$100cm^2$: 30cm (13g) of cre
$150cm^2$: 46cm (20g) of cre
$200cm^2$: 61cm (26g) of cre
$250cm^2$: 76cm (33g) of cre
$300cm^2$: 91cm (40g) of cre
$350cm^2$: 106cm (46g) of cre
$400cm^2$: 121cm (53g) of cre

Do not exceed the recommended amount of drug to apply or the duration of application

ADMINISTRATION
Topical route

Application
1. Use a ruler supplied to squeeze out and measure the amount of cre that approximates the amount required
2. Spread cre evenly and thinly (approx 1mm or the thickness of a dime) across the treatment area using a flat-surfaced tool such as a metal spatula or tongue depressor
3. After waiting the required application time, remove cre by grasping a free-edge w/ your fingers and pulling it away from the skin

Important Administration Instructions
Remove cre if skin irritation or burning sensation occurs during application
Avoid eye contact w/ cre
Wash hands after application

STORAGE
2-8°C (36-46°F). Do not freeze. May be stored at room temperature for up to 3 months. Discard after storing at room temperature for 3 months.

HOW SUPPLIED
Cre: (Lidocaine/Tetracaine) 7%/7% [30g, 60g, 100g]

CONTRAINDICATIONS
Known history of sensitivity to lidocaine or tetracaine, local amide- or ester- type anesthetics, or to any other component of the product; para-aminobenzoic acid (PABA) hypersensitivity.

WARNINGS/PRECAUTIONS
Not recommended for use on mucous membranes or on areas with a compromised skin barrier. Application to broken or inflamed skin may result in toxic blood concentrations from increased absorption. Caution in patients who may be more sensitive to the systemic effects of lidocaine and tetracaine (eg, acutely ill, debilitated). May cause methemoglobinemia; increased risk in patients with congenital or idiopathic methemoglobinemia, and in patients with G6PD deficiencies. Carefully apply cream to ensure that the doses, areas of application, and duration of application are consistent with those recommended for the intended population. Allergic/anaphylactoid reactions (eg, urticaria, angioedema, bronchospasm, shock) may occur; manage by conventional means if an allergic reaction occurs. Avoid contact with the eyes; immediately wash out the eye with water or saline and protect the eye until sensation returns, if contact occurs. Increased risk of toxicity in patients with severe hepatic disease or pseudocholinesterase deficiency.

ADVERSE REACTIONS
Local erythema/skin discoloration/edema.

DRUG INTERACTIONS
Additive and potentially synergistic systemic toxic effects with Class I antiarrhythmics (eg, tocainide, mexiletine); use with caution. When used concomitantly with other products containing local anesthetic agents, consider the amount absorbed from all formulations, due to additive and potentially synergistic systemic toxic effects. Increased risk of methemoglobinemia if concomitantly taking drugs associated with drug-induced methemoglobinemia (eg, sulfonamides, acetaminophen, acetanilide, aniline dyes, benzocaine, chloroquine, dapsone, naphthalene, nitrates and nitrites, nitrofurantoin, nitroglycerin, nitroprusside, pamaquine, para-aminosalicylic acid, phenacetin, phenobarbital, phenytoin, primaquine, quinine).

PREGNANCY AND LACTATION
Category B, caution in nursing.

MECHANISM OF ACTION
Lidocaine: Amide-type local anesthetic. Tetracaine: Ester-type local anesthetic. Both drugs block Na^+ channels required for the initiation and conduction of neuronal impulses, resulting in local anesthesia.

PHARMACOKINETICS
Absorption: Lidocaine: Administration of multiple doses resulted in different parameters. Tetracaine: C_{max}=<0.9ng/mL. **Distribution:** Lidocaine: V_d=0.8-1.3L/kg (IV); plasma protein binding (75%); found in breast milk; crosses placenta. **Metabolism:** Lidocaine: Liver (rapid) by N-deethylation via CYP1A2 (primary) and CYP3A4 (minor); monoethylglycinexylidide, glycinexylidide (active metabolites). Tetracaine: Rapid hydrolysis by plasma esterases; PABA and diethylaminoethanol (primary metabolites). **Elimination:** Lidocaine: Urine (>98%; <10% unchanged); $T_{1/2}$=1.8 hrs (IV).

PATIENT CONSIDERATIONS
Assessment: Assess for hypersensitivity to drug, PABA, or local anesthetics of the amide- or ester-type. Assess for conditions that may increase sensitivity to the systemic effects of lidocaine and tetracaine (eg, acute illness, debilitation), risk of methemoglobinemia, hepatic disease, pseudocholinesterase deficiency, pregnancy/nursing status, and possible drug interactions.

Monitoring: Monitor for methemoglobinemia, allergic/anaphylactoid reactions, skin irritation, burning sensation, and other adverse reactions.

Counseling: Instruct to avoid contact with the eyes, and to immediately wash out the eye with water or saline and protect the eye until sensation returns, if contact occurs. Advise to remove the product if skin irritation or a burning sensation occurs during application. Instruct to seek immediate emergency help if signs of an allergic or anaphylactoid reaction (urticaria, angioedema, bronchospasm, and shock) occur. Inform that use may lead to diminished or blocked sensation in the treated skin; instruct to avoid inadvertent trauma (rubbing, scratching, or exposure to heat or cold) before complete sensation returns.

PNEUMOVAX 23 — pneumococcal vaccine polyvalent   Rx

Class: Vaccine

ADULT DOSAGE	PEDIATRIC DOSAGE
Prevention of Pneumococcal Disease	**Prevention of Pneumococcal Disease**
Active immunization against serotypes 1, 2, 3, 4, 5, 6B, 7F, 8, 9N, 9V, 10A, 11A, 12F, 14, 15B, 17F, 18C, 19F, 19A, 20, 22F, 23F, and 33F	Active immunization against serotypes 1, 2, 3, 4, 5, 6B, 7F, 8, 9N, 9V, 10A, 11A, 12F, 14, 15B, 17F, 18C, 19F, 19A, 20, 22F, 23F, and 33F
≥50 Years: Single 0.5mL dose	**≥2 Years and at Increased Risk for Pneumococcal Disease:** Single 0.5mL dose

ADMINISTRATION
IM/SQ route

Administer into the deltoid muscle or lateral mid-thigh.
Do not mix w/ other vaccines in the same syringe or vial.

Single-Dose and Multidose Vials
Withdraw 0.5mL from the vial using a sterile needle and syringe.

Single-Dose, Prefilled Syringe
Package does not contain a needle; attach a sterile needle to prefilled syringe by twisting in a clockwise direction until the needle fits securely on the syringe.

Revaccination
Advisory Committee on Immunization Practices has recommendations for revaccination against pneumococcal disease for persons at high risk who were previously vaccinated w/ Pneumovax 23; routine revaccination of immunocompetent persons previously vaccinated w/ a 23-valent vaccine is not recommended.

STORAGE
2-8°C (36-46°F).

HOW SUPPLIED
Inj: 0.5mL [prefilled syringe, single-dose vial, multidose vial]

CONTRAINDICATIONS
History of anaphylactic/anaphylactoid or severe allergic reaction to any component of the vaccine.

WARNINGS/PRECAUTIONS
Do not inject intravascularly or intradermally. Defer vaccination in patients with moderate or severe acute illness. Caution with severely compromised

cardiovascular (CV) and/or pulmonary function in whom a systemic reaction would pose a significant risk. Does not replace the need for antibiotic prophylaxis (eg, PCN) against pneumococcal infection; antibiotic prophylaxis should not be discontinued after vaccination in patients who require antibiotic prophylaxis. Response to vaccine may be diminished in immunocompromised individuals. May not be effective in preventing pneumococcal meningitis in patients with chronic CSF leakage resulting from congenital lesions, skull fractures, or neurosurgical procedures. Will not prevent disease caused by capsular types of pneumococcus other than those contained in the vaccine. Caution in elderly.

ADVERSE REACTIONS
Local inj-site reactions (eg, pain, soreness, tenderness, swelling, induration, erythema), asthenia, fatigue, myalgia, headache.

DRUG INTERACTIONS
Persons receiving immunosuppressive therapies may have a diminished immune response to the vaccine. Reduced immune response to zoster vaccine live reported; consider separation of vaccinations by at least 4 weeks.

PREGNANCY AND LACTATION
Pregnancy: Category C.
Lactation: Caution in nursing.

MECHANISM OF ACTION
Vaccine; induces antibodies that enhance opsonization, phagocytosis, and killing of pneumococci by leukocytes and other phagocytic cells.

PATIENT CONSIDERATIONS
Assessment: Assess for moderate/severe acute illness, severely compromised CV and/or pulmonary function, chronic CSF leakage, vaccination history, history of anaphylactic/anaphylactoid or severe allergic reaction to any component of the vaccine, immunocompromised conditions, pregnancy/nursing status, and for possible drug interactions.

Monitoring: Monitor for hypersensitivity reactions and other adverse reactions.

Counseling: Inform of potential benefits/risks of vaccination. Inform that the vaccine may not offer 100% protection from pneumococcal infection. Instruct to report any serious adverse reactions to physician.

POLYTRIM — polymyxin B sulfate/trimethoprim   Rx
Class: Antibiotic/dihydrofolate reductase inhibitor

ADULT DOSAGE	PEDIATRIC DOSAGE
Ocular Infections	**Ocular Infections**
Mild-Moderate Surface Bacterial Infections:	**Mild-Moderate Surface Bacterial Infections:**
(eg, blepharoconjunctivitis, acute bacterial conjunctivitis)	(eg, blepharoconjunctivitis, acute bacterial conjunctivitis)
Instill 1 drop in affected eye(s) q3h for 7-10 days	**≥2 Months of Age:**
Max: 6 doses/day	Instill 1 drop in affected eye(s) q3h for 7-10 days
	Max: 6 doses/day

ADMINISTRATION
Ocular route

STORAGE
15-25°C (59-77°F). Protect from light.

HOW SUPPLIED
Sol: (Trimethoprim/Polymyxin B) (1mg/10,000 U)/mL [10mL]

CONTRAINDICATIONS
Known hypersensitivity to any of the components.

WARNINGS/PRECAUTIONS
Do not inject into eye. Not indicated for the prophylaxis or treatment of ophthalmia neonatorum.

ADVERSE REACTIONS
Local irritation, lid edema, itching, increased redness, tearing, burning, stinging, circumocular rash, superinfection (prolonged use).

PREGNANCY AND LACTATION
Pregnancy: Category C.
Lactation: Caution in nursing.

MECHANISM OF ACTION
Dihydrofolate reductase inhibitor/antibiotic. Polymyxin B: Increases permeability of bacterial cell membrane by interacting with phospholipid components of membrane. Trimethoprim: Blocks production of tetrahydrofolic acid from dihydrofolic acid by binding to and reversibly inhibiting the enzyme dihydrofolate reductase. Binding is stronger for bacterial enzyme than for corresponding mammalian enzyme, therefore selectively interferes with bacterial biosynthesis of nucleic acids and proteins.

PHARMACOKINETICS
Absorption: C_{max}=0.03mcg/mL (trimethoprim), 1 unit/mL (polymyxin B) (following two-time dosing of 2 drops of ophthalmic solution containing 1mg of trimethoprim and 10,000 units of polymyxin B).

PATIENT CONSIDERATIONS
Assessment: Assess proper diagnosis of causative organisms, that medication is not being used as treatment for patients with ophthalmia neonatorum, and use in pregnant/nursing females.

Monitoring: Monitor for signs/symptoms of hypersensitivity reactions (eg, lid edema, itching, increased redness, tearing, and circumocular rash). For patients on prolonged therapy, monitor for overgrowth of nonsusceptible organisms (eg, fungi) and for the development of a superinfection.

Counseling: Advise to avoid contaminating applicator tip with material from eye, fingers, or other sources. Instruct to d/c therapy if redness, irritation, swelling, or pain persists or worsens. Advise not to wear contact lenses if there are signs/symptoms of ocular bacterial infections.

POMALYST — pomalidomide   Rx
Class: Thalidomide analogue

> Contraindicated in pregnancy; may cause severe birth defects or embryo-fetal death. Females of reproductive potential should have 2 negative pregnancy tests before starting treatment and must use 2 forms of contraception or continuously abstain from heterosexual sex during and for 4 weeks after stopping treatment. Available only through a restricted distribution program called Pomalyst Risk Evaluation and Mitigation Strategy. Deep vein thrombosis, pulmonary embolism, MI, and stroke reported; thromboprophylaxis is recommended, and the choice of regimen should be based on assessment of the patient's underlying risk factors.

ADULT DOSAGE	PEDIATRIC DOSAGE
Multiple Myeloma	Pediatric use may not have been established
In combination w/ dexamethasone, for patients who have received ≥2 prior therapies including lenalidomide and a proteasome inhibitor and have demonstrated disease progression on or w/in 60 days of completion of the last therapy	
Initial: 4mg qd on Days 1-21 of repeated 28-day cycles until disease progression	

DOSING CONSIDERATIONS
Concomitant Medications
Strong CYP1A2 Inhibitors: Avoid concomitant use; consider alternative treatments. If a strong CYP1A2 inhibitor must be used, reduce pomalidomide dose by 50%

Renal Impairment
Severe Renal Impairment Requiring Dialysis:
Initial: 3mg qd (25% dose reduction); take pomalidomide after completion of dialysis procedure on hemodialysis days

Hepatic Impairment
Mild or Moderate (Child-Pugh Classes A or B):
Initial: 3mg qd (25% dose reduction)

Severe (Child-Pugh Class C):
Initial: 2mg qd (50% dose reduction)

Adverse Reactions
Neutropenia:
ANC <500/μL or Febrile Neutropenia (Fever ≥38.5°C and ANC <1000/μL): Interrupt treatment; follow CBC weekly
ANC Return to ≥500/μL: Resume treatment at 3mg/day
For Each Subsequent Drop <500/μL: Interrupt treatment
Return to ≥500/μL: Resume treatment at 1mg less than previous dose

Thrombocytopenia:
Platelets <25,000/μL: Interrupt treatment; follow CBC weekly
Platelets Return to >50,000/μL: Resume treatment at 3mg daily
For Each Subsequent Drop <25,000/μL: Interrupt treatment
Return to ≥50,000/μL: Resume treatment at 1mg less than previous dose

To initiate a new cycle, neutrophil count must be at least 500/μL and platelet count must be at least 50,000/μL; if toxicities occur after dose reductions to 1mg, then d/c treatment

Angioedema, Skin Exfoliation, Bullae, or Any Other Severe Dermatologic Reaction: Permanently d/c

Other Grade 3 or 4 Toxicities: Hold treatment and restart at 1mg less than previous dose when toxicity has resolved to ≤Grade 2

ADMINISTRATION
Oral route

May take w/ water.
May be taken w/ or w/o food.
Do not break, chew, or open caps.

STORAGE
20-25°C (68-77°F); excursions permitted to 15-30°C (59-86°F).

HOW SUPPLIED
Cap: 1mg, 2mg, 3mg, 4mg

CONTRAINDICATIONS
Pregnancy.

WARNINGS/PRECAUTIONS
See Dosing Considerations. Avoid blood donation during treatment and for 1 month following discontinuation. Greater risk of arterial thromboembolism and venous thromboembolism (VTE) may exist in patients w/ known risk factors (eg, prior thrombosis); try to minimize all modifiable factors (eg, hyperlipidemia, HTN, smoking). Neutropenia, anemia, and thrombocytopenia reported; may require

dose interruption and/or modification. Monitor CBC weekly for the first 8 weeks of therapy and monthly thereafter. Hepatic failure, including fatal cases, and elevated levels of ALT and bilirubin reported; monitor LFTs monthly. D/C therapy upon elevation of liver enzymes and evaluate; after return to baseline values, consider treatment at a lower dose. Angioedema and severe dermatologic reactions reported. Dizziness, confusional state, and neuropathy reported. Cases of acute myelogenous leukemia reported in patients receiving pomalidomide as an investigational therapy outside of multiple myeloma. Tumor lysis syndrome (TLS) may occur; caution in patients w/ high tumor burden prior to treatment.

ADVERSE REACTIONS
Fatigue/asthenia, neutropenia, anemia, constipation, diarrhea, nausea, URTI, back pain, dyspnea, pyrexia.

DRUG INTERACTIONS
See Dosing Considerations. Coadministration of fluvoxamine, a strong CYP1A2 inhibitor, increased levels, which increases the risk of exposure-related toxicities. Cigarette smoking may reduce exposure due to CYP1A2 induction and may reduce efficacy.

PREGNANCY AND LACTATION
Pregnancy: Based on the mechanism of action and findings from animal studies, Pomalyst can cause embryo-fetal harm when administered to a pregnant female and is contraindicated during pregnancy. There is a pregnancy exposure registry that monitors pregnancy outcomes in females exposed to Pomalyst during pregnancy as well as female partners of male patients who are exposed to Pomalyst.
Lactation: Not for use in nursing.
Reproductive Potential:
Pregnancy Testing: Verify the pregnancy status of females of reproductive potential prior to initiating therapy and for at least 4 weeks after completing therapy; avoid pregnancy while on therapy. Females of reproductive potential must have 2 negative pregnancy tests before initiating therapy; the 1st test should be performed w/in 10-14 days, and the 2nd test w/in 24 hrs prior to prescribing Pomalyst. Once treatment has started and during dose interruptions, pregnancy testing for females of reproductive potential should occur weekly during the first 4 weeks of use, then be repeated every 4 weeks (females w/ regular menstrual cycles), or every 2 weeks (irregular menstrual cycles).
Contraception: (Females) Females of reproductive potential must commit either to abstain continuously from heterosexual sexual intercourse or to use 2 methods of reliable birth control simultaneously (1 highly effective form of contraception and 1 additional effective contraceptive method). Contraception must begin 4 weeks prior to initiating treatment and must continue during therapy, during dose interruptions, and for 4 weeks following discontinuation of therapy. (Males) Pomalidomide is present in the semen of males; must always use a latex or synthetic condom during any sexual contact w/ females of reproductive potential while on therapy and for up to 4 weeks after discontinuing therapy, even if they have undergone a successful vasectomy. Must not donate sperm.
Infertility: Based on findings in animals, female fertility may be compromised by treatment.
Refer to PI for further details on pregnancy testing/contraception.

MECHANISM OF ACTION
Thalidomide analogue; immunomodulatory agent w/ antineoplastic activity. Enhances T cell- and natural killer cell-mediated immunity and inhibits production of pro-inflammatory cytokines (eg, TNF-α and IL-6) by monocytes.

PHARMACOKINETICS
Absorption: T_{max}=2-3 hrs; AUC=860ng•hr/mL; C_{max}=75ng/mL. **Distribution:** V_d=62-138L; plasma protein binding (12-44%). **Metabolism:** Liver via CYP1A2 and CYP3A4 (major), CYP2C19 and CYP2D6 (minor). **Elimination:** Urine (73%, 2% unchanged), feces (15%, 8% unchanged); $T_{1/2}$=approx 7.5 hrs (median).

PATIENT CONSIDERATIONS
Assessment: Assess nursing status, renal/hepatic function, and for risk factors for arterial thromboembolism or VTE, high tumor burden, and possible drug interactions. Obtain pregnancy test 10-14 days before and 24 hrs prior to therapy.
Monitoring: Perform pregnancy test weekly during 1st month, then monthly thereafter (regular menstrual cycle) or every 2 weeks (irregular menstrual cycle). Monitor CBC weekly for the first 8 weeks of therapy and monthly thereafter. Monitor LFTs monthly. Monitor for signs/symptoms of arterial thromboembolism, VTE, hematologic toxicities (especially neutropenia), hypersensitivity reactions, dizziness, confusional state, neuropathy, second primary malignancies, TLS, and for other adverse reactions.
Counseling: Instruct females of reproductive potential to avoid pregnancy while on therapy and for at least 4 weeks after completing therapy, to have monthly pregnancy tests, and to use 2 different forms of contraception, including at least 1 highly effective form simultaneously during therapy, during dose interruption, and for 4 weeks after completing therapy. Instruct to immediately d/c and contact physician if patient becomes pregnant, misses her menstrual period, experiences unusual menstrual bleeding, or she stops taking birth control. Instruct males (including those w/ vasectomy) to always use latex/synthetic condoms during any sexual contact w/ females of reproductive potential during therapy and for up to 4 weeks after discontinuation. Advise males not to donate sperm. Instruct all patients not to donate blood during therapy and for 1 month following discontinuation. Inform females that there is a pregnancy exposure registry that monitors pregnancy outcomes in females exposed to pomalidomide during pregnancy. Inform of the other risks associated w/ therapy. Instruct to avoid situations where dizziness or confusional state may be a problem and not to take other medications that may cause dizziness or confusional state w/o adequate medical advice. Instruct to take ud. Advise patients that smoking tobacco may reduce the efficacy of the drug.

PORTRAZZA — necitumumab   Rx
Class: Monoclonal antibody/EGFR blocker

> Cardiopulmonary arrest and/or sudden death reported. Closely monitor serum electrolytes, including serum Mg^+, K^+, and Ca^+ w/ aggressive replacement when warranted during and after administration. Hypomagnesemia reported; monitor patients for hypomagnesemia, hypocalcemia, and hypokalemia prior to each dose during treatment and for at least 8 weeks following completion. Withhold for Grade 3 or 4 electrolyte abnormalities. Replete electrolytes as medically appropriate.

ADULT DOSAGE	PEDIATRIC DOSAGE
Metastatic Squamous Non-Small Cell Lung Cancer	Pediatric use may not have been established
1st-Line Treatment in Combination w/ Gemcitabine and Cisplatin: 800mg IV over 60 min on Days 1 and 8 of each 3-week cycle prior to gemcitabine and cisplatin infusion	
Continue until disease progression or unacceptable toxicity	
Premedication	
Previous Grade 1 or 2 Infusion-Related Reaction (IRR): Premedicate w/ diphenhydramine hydrochloride (or equivalent) prior to all subsequent infusions	
2nd Grade 1 or 2 Occurrence of IRR: Premedicate for all subsequent infusions, w/ diphenhydramine hydrochloride (or equivalent), acetaminophen (or equivalent), and dexamethasone (or equivalent) prior to each infusion	

DOSING CONSIDERATIONS
Adverse Reactions
IRR:
Grade 1: Reduce the infusion rate by 50%
Grade 2: Stop the infusion until signs and symptoms have resolved to Grade 0 or 1; resume at 50% reduced rate for all subsequent infusions
Grade 3 or 4: Permanently d/c
Dermatologic Toxicity:
Grade 3 Rash or Acneiform Rash: Withhold until symptoms resolve to Grade ≤2, then resume at reduced dose of 400mg for at least 1 treatment cycle. If symptoms do not worsen, may increase dose to 600mg and 800mg in subsequent cycles
Permanently D/C If:
- Grade 3 rash or acneiform rash does not resolve to Grade ≤2 w/in 6 weeks
- Reactions worsen or become intolerable at a dose of 400mg
- Patient experiences Grade 3 skin induration/fibrosis
- Patient experiences Grade 4 dermatologic toxicity

ADMINISTRATION
IV route
Administer via infusion pump over 60 min through a separate infusion line; flush the line w/ 0.9% NaCl inj at the end of infusion.

Preparation for Administration
1. Dilute the required volume of necitumumab w/ 0.9% NaCl inj, in an IV infusion container to a final volume of 250mL; do not use sol containing dextrose.
2. Gently invert the container to ensure adequate mixing.
3. Do not freeze or shake the infusion sol. Do not dilute w/ other sol or co-infuse w/ other electrolytes or medication.
4. Store diluted infusion sol for no >24 hrs at 2-8°C (36-46°F), or no >4 hrs at room temperature (up to 25°C [77°F]).
5. Discard vial w/ any unused portion.

STORAGE
2-8°C (36-46°F). Protect from light. Do not freeze or shake the vial.

HOW SUPPLIED
Inj: 800mg/50mL

WARNINGS/PRECAUTIONS
See Dosing Considerations. Once electrolyte abnormalities and hypomagnesemia improve to Grade ≤2, subsequent cycles may be administered. Venous thromboembolic events (VTEs) and arterial thromboembolic events (ATEs) reported w/ combination treatment; d/c in patients w/ serious/life-threatening VTE or ATE. The most common ATEs were cerebral stroke, ischemia, and MI. Dermatologic toxicities, including rash, dermatitis acneiform, acne, dry skin, pruritus, generalized rash, skin fissures, maculopapular rash, and erythema reported; limit sun exposure. IRR reported; d/c for serious or life-threatening IRR. Not indicated for the treatment of patients w/ non-squamous non-small cell lung cancer. May cause fetal harm.

ADVERSE REACTIONS
Rash, vomiting, diarrhea, dermatitis acneiform.

PREGNANCY AND LACTATION
Pregnancy: Can cause fetal harm.
Lactation: Do not breastfeed during treatment and for 3 months following the final dose.
Reproductive Potential: Females of reproductive potential should use effective contraception during treatment and for 3 months following the final dose.

MECHANISM OF ACTION

Recombinant human IgG1 monoclonal antibody; binds to EGFR and blocks the binding of EGFR to its ligands. Binding of necitumumab induces EGFR internalization and degradation in vitro. In vitro, binding of necitumumab also led to antibody-dependent cellular cytotoxicity in EGFR-expressing cells.

PHARMACOKINETICS

Distribution: V_d=7.0L. **Elimination:** $T_{1/2}$=14 days.

PATIENT CONSIDERATIONS

Assessment: Assess for presence or history of cardiopulmonary and dermatologic disease, pregnancy/nursing status, and for possible drug interactions. Obtain serum electrolyte levels (Mg^{2+}, K^+, Ca^{2+}).

Monitoring: Monitor for signs/symptoms of cardiopulmonary arrest, dermatologic toxicities, IRR, VTEs/ATEs, and other adverse reactions. Monitor electrolytes (eg, hypomagnesemia, hypokalemia, hypocalcemia) periodically during and for up to 8 weeks after completion of therapy.

Counseling: Advise patients of risk of decreased blood levels of Mg^{2+}, K^+, and Ca^{2+} and instruct to take medicines to replace the electrolytes exactly as advised. Inform of the increased risk of VTEs/ATEs. Instruct to minimize sun exposure w/ protective clothing and use of sunscreen. Advise to report if signs/symptoms of an infusion reaction develop. Instruct to notify physician if pregnant or nursing; inform of the potential risk to a fetus and instruct to not breastfeed during treatment and for 3 months following final dose. Advise of the need for adequate contraception in females during therapy and for 3 months after the last dose.

POTABA — aminobenzoate potassium   Rx

Class: Vitamin B complex

ADULT DOSAGE
Dietary/Nutritional Supplement

Possibly effective in the treatment of scleroderma, dermatomyositis, morphea, linear scleroderma, pemphigus, and Peyronie's disease

Usual: 12g/day, given in 4-6 divided doses

PEDIATRIC DOSAGE
Dietary/Nutritional Supplement

Possibly effective in the treatment of scleroderma, dermatomyositis, morphea, linear scleroderma, pemphigus, and Peyronie's disease

Usual: 1g/day, given in divided doses for each 10 lbs of body weight

---

ADMINISTRATION

Oral route

Take w/ meals and at hs w/ a snack

HOW SUPPLIED

Cap: 0.5g

CONTRAINDICATIONS

Concomitant use with sulfonamides.

WARNINGS/PRECAUTIONS

If anorexia or nausea occurs, interrupt therapy until the patient is eating normally again. Caution with renal disease. D/C if hypersensitivity reaction occurs.

ADVERSE REACTIONS

Anorexia, nausea, fever, rash.

DRUG INTERACTIONS

See Contraindications.

PREGNANCY AND LACTATION

Safety not known in pregnancy/nursing.

MECHANISM OF ACTION

Vitamin B complex; it is suggested that the antifibrosis action is due to its mediation of increased oxygen uptake at the tissue level, which enhances MAO activity and prevents or brings about regression of fibrosis.

PATIENT CONSIDERATIONS

Assessment: Assess for renal disease, pregnancy/nursing status, and possible drug interactions.

Monitoring: Monitor for anorexia, nausea, hypersensitivity reactions, and other adverse reactions.

Counseling: Inform of the possible adverse reactions (eg, anorexia, nausea, fever, rash). Advise to d/c if hypersensitivity reaction should occur.

POTIGA — ezogabine   CV

Class: Potassium channel opener

> May cause retinal abnormalities w/ funduscopic features similar to those seen in retinal pigment dystrophies, which are known to result in damage to the photoreceptors and vision loss. Macular abnormalities characterized as vitelliform lesions have also been observed. Some patients w/ retinal abnormalities have been found to have abnormal visual acuity; it is not possible to determine whether therapy caused this decreased visual acuity. Reversibility of retinal pigmentary abnormalities and partial resolution of vitelliform lesions has been reported after discontinuation of therapy in some patients. Should only be used in patients who have responded inadequately to several alternative treatments and for whom the benefits outweigh the potential risk of vision loss. D/C in patients who fail to show substantial clinical benefit after adequate titration. All patients should have baseline and periodic (every 6 months) systematic visual monitoring by an ophthalmic professional. Testing should include visual acuity, dilated fundus photography, and optical coherence tomography. Additional testing may include fluorescein angiograms, perimetry, and electroretinograms. D/C if retinal pigmentary abnormalities or vision changes are detected unless no other suitable treatment options are available and the benefits outweigh the potential risk of vision loss.

ADULT DOSAGE
Partial Onset Seizures

Adjunctive treatment in patients who have responded inadequately to several alternative treatments and for whom the benefits outweigh the risk of retinal abnormalities and potential decline in visual acuity

Initial: 100mg tid
Titrate: Increase gradually at weekly intervals by no more than 50mg tid based on response and tolerability
Maint: 200-400mg tid
Max: 400mg tid

PEDIATRIC DOSAGE

Pediatric use may not have been established

DOSING CONSIDERATIONS
Renal Impairment
CrCl <50mL/min or ESRD on Dialysis:
Initial: 50mg tid
Titrate: Increase by no more than 50mg tid, at weekly intervals
Max: 200mg tid
Hemodialysis: A single supplemental dose is recommended immediately following hemodialysis. An additional supplemental dose may be considered at the start of subsequent dialysis sessions if breakthrough seizures occur toward the end of hemodialysis

Hepatic Impairment
Moderate (Child-Pugh 7-9):
Initial: 50mg tid
Titrate: Increase by no more than 50mg tid, at weekly intervals
Max: 250mg tid

Severe (Child-Pugh >9):
Initial: 50mg tid
Titrate: Increase by no more than 50mg tid, at weekly intervals
Max: 200mg tid

Elderly
≥65 Years:
Initial: 50mg tid
Titrate: Increase by no more than 50mg tid, at weekly intervals
Max: 250mg tid

Adverse Reactions
Retinal Pigmentary Abnormalities or Vision Changes: D/C unless no other suitable treatment options are available and the benefits of treatment outweigh the potential risk of vision loss

Discontinuation
If discontinued, gradually reduce dose over a period of at least 3 weeks, unless safety concerns require abrupt withdrawal

ADMINISTRATION

Oral route

Take w/ or w/o food.
Swallow tab whole.

STORAGE

25°C (77°F); excursions permitted to 15-30°C (59-86°F).

HOW SUPPLIED

Tab: 50mg, 200mg, 300mg, 400mg

WARNINGS/PRECAUTIONS

See Dosing Considerations. Patients whose visual function cannot be monitored should usually not be treated. Urinary retention, urinary hesitation, dysuria, and hydronephrosis reported. Perform closer monitoring for patients who have other risk factors for urinary retention (eg, benign prostatic hyperplasia), patients who are unable to communicate clinical symptoms (eg, cognitively impaired patients), or patients who use concomitant medications that may affect voiding (eg, anticholinergics). May cause skin discoloration; consider changing to an alternative medication if skin discoloration develops. Neuropsychiatric symptoms (eg, confusional state, psychotic symptoms, hallucinations) reported. May cause dose-related increases in dizziness and somnolence. Prolonged QT interval reported; monitor the QT interval when used concomitantly w/ medicines known to increase the QT interval, and in patients w/ known prolonged QT interval, CHF, ventricular hypertrophy, hypokalemia, or hypomagnesemia. May increase risk of suicidal thoughts or behavior. Withdraw gradually to minimize the potential of increased seizure frequency when therapy is discontinued. May interfere w/ clinical laboratory assays of both serum and urine bilirubin, which can result in falsely elevated readings.

ADVERSE REACTIONS

Dizziness, somnolence, fatigue, confusional state, vertigo, tremor, abnormal coordination, diplopia, disturbance in attention, memory impairment, asthenia, blurred vision, gait disturbance, aphasia, dysarthria.

DRUG INTERACTIONS

Decreased levels w/ carbamazepine and phenytoin; consider an increase in dose of ezogabine when adding carbamazepine or phenytoin and a decrease in dose of ezogabine when discontinuing carbamazepine or phenytoin. Increased exposure and worsening of dose-related adverse reactions reported w/ alcohol.

PREGNANCY AND LACTATION

Pregnancy: Category C. Physicians are advised to recommend that pregnant patients enroll in the North American Antiepileptic Drug (NAAED) Pregnancy Registry.
Lactation: Not for use in nursing.

MECHANISM OF ACTION

Potassium channel opener; not established. Enhances transmembrane K^+ currents mediated by the KCNQ (Kv7.2 to 7.5) family of ion channels; by activating KCNQ channels, it is thought to stabilize the resting membrane potential and reduce brain excitability. May exert therapeutic effects through augmentation of GABA-mediated currents.

PHARMACOKINETICS

Absorption: Rapid. T_{max}=0.5-2 hrs (median). Absolute bioavailability (60%). **Distribution:** Plasma protein binding (80%, 45% metabolite); V_d=2-3L/kg (IV). **Metabolism:** Extensive via glucuronidation and acetylation; N-acetyl metabolite of ezogabine (active metabolite). **Elimination:** Urine (85%, 36% unchanged, 18% metabolite), feces (14%, 3% unchanged); $T_{1/2}$=7-11 hrs.

PATIENT CONSIDERATIONS

Assessment: Assess for risk factors for urinary retention, known prolonged QT interval, CHF, ventricular hypertrophy, hypokalemia, hypomagnesemia, renal/hepatic impairment, pregnancy/nursing status, and possible drug interactions. Obtain baseline visual function. Perform a baseline comprehensive evaluation of urologic symptoms in patients w/ risk factors for urinary retention.

Monitoring: Monitor for urinary retention/hesitation, dysuria, hydronephrosis, neuropsychiatric symptoms, dizziness, somnolence, emergence or worsening of depression, suicidal thoughts/behavior, unusual changes in mood/behavior, increased seizure frequency, retinal abnormalities or vision changes, skin discoloration, and other adverse reactions. Periodically perform a comprehensive evaluation of urologic symptoms in patients w/ risk factors for urinary retention. Monitor visual function every 6 months. Monitor QT interval when drug is prescribed w/ medicines known to increase QT interval and in patients w/ known prolonged QT interval, CHF, ventricular hypertrophy, hypokalemia, or hypomagnesemia.

Counseling: Inform of the risk of retinal abnormalities and possible risk of vision loss; instruct to notify physician immediately if any changes in vision are suspected. Instruct to seek immediate medical assistance if experiencing any symptoms of urinary retention, inability to urinate, and/or pain with urination. Inform that therapy may cause discoloration of nails, lips, skin, palate, and parts of the eye; instruct to notify physician if skin discoloration develops. Inform that psychiatric symptoms may occur; instruct to notify physician if experiencing psychotic symptoms. Inform that drug may cause dizziness, somnolence, memory impairment, abnormal coordination/balance, disturbance in attention, and ophthalmological effects; advise to avoid operating hazardous machinery or driving a car until effects of drug are known. Inform patients, caregivers, and families that therapy may increase the risk of suicidal thoughts and behavior; advise of the need to be alert for the emergence or worsening of symptoms of depression, any unusual changes in mood or behavior, or the emergence of suicidal thoughts, behavior, or thoughts about self-harm, and instruct to notify physician immediately. Advise to notify physician if pregnant or intending to become pregnant or if breastfeeding or intending to breastfeed. Encourage patients to enroll in the NAAED Pregnancy Registry if they become pregnant.

Pradaxa — dabigatran etexilate mesylate   Rx

Class: Direct thrombin inhibitor (DTI)

> Premature discontinuation of therapy increases the risk of thrombotic events. If therapy is discontinued for a reason other than pathological bleeding or completion of a course of therapy, consider coverage w/ another anticoagulant. Epidural or spinal hematomas may occur in patients treated w/ dabigatran who are receiving neuraxial anesthesia or undergoing spinal puncture; may result in long-term or permanent paralysis. Consider these risks when scheduling for spinal procedures. Increased risk of developing epidural or spinal hematomas w/ the use of indwelling epidural catheters, concomitant use of other drugs that affect hemostasis (eg, NSAIDs, platelet inhibitors, other anticoagulants), history of traumatic or repeated epidural or spinal punctures, history of spinal deformity or spinal surgery, or unknown optimal timing between the administration of therapy and neuraxial procedures. Monitor frequently for signs/symptoms of neurological impairment; if noted, urgent treatment is necessary. Consider benefits and risks before neuraxial intervention in patients anticoagulated or to be anticoagulated.

ADULT DOSAGE

Reduce Risk of Stroke and Systemic Embolism in Nonvalvular Atrial Fibrillation

150mg bid

Deep Vein Thrombosis/Pulmonary Embolism

Treatment in Patients Treated w/ a Parenteral Anticoagulant for 5-10 Days:
150mg bid

Reduce Risk of Recurrent Deep Vein Thrombosis (DVT)/Pulmonary Embolism (PE) in Previously Treated Patients:
150mg bid

Prophylaxis of DVT and PE Following Hip Replacement Surgery:
110mg taken 1-4 hrs after surgery and after hemostasis has been achieved, then 220mg taken qd for 28-35 days; if therapy is not started on the day of surgery, after hemostasis has been achieved, initiate treatment w/ 220mg qd

PEDIATRIC DOSAGE

Pediatric use may not have been established

Conversions

Conversion from Warfarin:
D/C warfarin and start therapy when INR <2.0

Conversion to Warfarin:
CrCl ≥50mL/min: Start warfarin 3 days before discontinuing therapy
CrCl 30-50mL/min: Start warfarin 2 days before discontinuing therapy
CrCl 15-30mL/min: Start warfarin 1 day before discontinuing therapy
CrCl <15mL/min: No recommendations can be made

Conversion from Parenteral Anticoagulants:
Start 0-2 hrs before the time that the next dose of the parenteral drug was to have been administered, or at time of discontinuation of a continuously administered parenteral drug (eg, IV unfractionated heparin)

Conversion to Parenteral Anticoagulant:
CrCl ≥30mL/min: Wait 12 hrs after last dose before initiating treatment w/ a parenteral anticoagulant
CrCl <30mL/min: Wait 24 hrs after last dose before initiating treatment w/ a parenteral anticoagulant

Missed Dose

Take missed dose as soon as possible on the same day; skip the missed dose if it cannot be taken at least 6 hrs before the next scheduled dose

---

DOSING CONSIDERATIONS

Concomitant Medications

Reduction in Risk of Stroke and Systemic Embolism in Nonvalvular A-Fib:
CrCl 30-50mL/min w/ Concomitant P-gp Inhibitors: Reduce dose to 75mg bid if given w/ P-gp inhibitors dronedarone or systemic ketoconazole
CrCl <30mL/min w/ Concomitant P-gp Inhibitors: Avoid coadministration

Treatment and Reduction in Risk of Recurrent DVT/PE:
CrCl <50mL/min w/ Concomitant P-gp Inhibitors: Avoid coadministration

Prophylaxis of DVT and PE Following Hip Replacement Surgery:
CrCl <50mL/min w/ Concomitant P-gp Inhibitors: Avoid coadministration

Renal Impairment

Reduction in Risk of Stroke and Systemic Embolism in Nonvalvular A-Fib:
CrCl 15-30mL/min: 75mg bid
CrCl <15mL/min or on Dialysis: Dosing recommendations cannot be provided

Treatment and Reduction in the Risk of Recurrent DVT/PE:
CrCl ≤30mL/min or on Dialysis: Dosing recommendations cannot be provided

Prophylaxis of DVT and PE Following Hip Replacement Surgery:
CrCl ≤30mL/min or on Dialysis: Dosing recommendations cannot be provided

Other Important Considerations

Surgery/Other Interventions:
CrCl ≥50mL/min: D/C 1-2 days before invasive or surgical procedures, if possible
CrCl <50mL/min: D/C 3-5 days before invasive or surgical procedures, if possible
Consider longer times for patients undergoing major surgery, spinal puncture, or placement of spinal/epidural catheter or port.
Use a specific reversal agent (idarucizumab) in case of emergency surgery or urgent procedures when reversal of dabigatran is needed; refer to idarucizumab PI for additional information. Restart dabigatran as soon as medically appropriate.

ADMINISTRATION

Oral route

Take w/ or w/o food w/ a full glass of water.
Swallow cap whole.

STORAGE

25°C (77°F); excursions permitted to 15-30°C (59-86°F). Store in original package to protect from moisture. Once bottle is opened, use w/in 4 months; keep tightly closed.

HOW SUPPLIED

Cap: 75mg, 110mg, 150mg

CONTRAINDICATIONS

Active pathological bleeding, mechanical prosthetic heart valve, serious hypersensitivity reaction to dabigatran (eg, anaphylaxis reaction or anaphylactic shock).

WARNINGS/PRECAUTIONS

Renal impairment may increase anticoagulant activity and $T_{1/2}$. D/C therapy in patients who develop acute renal failure and consider alternative anticoagulant therapy. Increases risk of bleeding and may cause significant and, sometimes, fatal bleeding; promptly evaluate for any signs/symptoms of blood loss. D/C therapy in patients w/ active pathological bleeding. Consider administration of platelet concentrates in cases where thrombocytopenia is present or long-acting antiplatelet drugs have been used. Use for the prophylaxis of thromboembolic events in patients w/ A-fib in the setting of other forms of valvular heart disease (including the presence of a bioprosthetic heart valve) is not recommended.

ADVERSE REACTIONS
GI reactions (eg, dyspepsia, gastritis-like symptoms), bleeding events.

DRUG INTERACTIONS
See Boxed Warning and Dosing Considerations. **Reduction of Risk of Stroke and Systemic Embolism in Non-valvular A-Fib:** P-gp inducers (eg, rifampin) may reduce exposure to dabigatran; should generally avoid concomitant use. Concomitant use w/ P-gp inhibitors in patients w/ renal impairment may produce increased exposure of dabigatran compared to that seen with either factor alone. **Prophylaxis of DVT and PE Following Hip Replacement Surgery:** May be helpful to separate timing of administration of dabigatran and the P-gp inhibitor by several hours, in patients w/ CrCl ≥50mL/min who have concomitant administration of P-gp inhibitors (eg, dronedarone, systemic ketoconazole).

PREGNANCY AND LACTATION
Pregnancy: Category C.
Lactation: Not for use in nursing.

MECHANISM OF ACTION
Direct thrombin inhibitor; prevents the development of a thrombus. Both free and clot-bound thrombin and thrombin-induced platelet aggregation are inhibited by the active moieties.

PHARMACOKINETICS
Absorption: Absolute bioavailability (approx 3-7%); T_{max}=1 hr (fasted).
Distribution: Plasma protein binding (approx 35%); V_d=50-70L. **Metabolism:** Esterase-catalyzed hydrolysis. **Elimination:** Urine (7%), feces (86%); $T_{1/2}$=12-17 hrs. Refer to PI for pharmacokinetic parameters in renally impaired patients.

PATIENT CONSIDERATIONS
Assessment: Assess for history of serious hypersensitivity reaction to drug, active pathological bleeding, mechanical prosthetic heart valve, A-fib in the setting of other forms of valvular heart disease, risk factors for bleeding and epidural or spinal hematomas, renal impairment, pregnancy/nursing status, and possible drug interactions.

Monitoring: Monitor for bleeding, GI adverse reactions, hypersensitivity reactions, and other adverse events. Periodically monitor renal function as clinically indicated. When necessary, monitor anticoagulant activity by using activated PTT or ecarin clotting time, and not INR. Monitor for signs/symptoms of neurological impairment (eg, midline back pain, sensory/motor deficits [numbness, tingling, weakness in lower limbs], bowel/bladder dysfunction) frequently in patients receiving neuraxial anesthesia or undergoing spinal puncture.

Counseling: Instruct to take exactly as prescribed and not to d/c w/o talking to physician. Instruct to keep drug in original bottle to protect from moisture and not to put it in pill boxes/organizers. When >1 bottle is dispensed, instruct to open only 1 bottle at a time. Instruct to remove only 1 cap from the opened bottle at the time of use and to immediately and tightly close bottle. Inform that bleeding may be longer and occur more easily. Instruct to call physician if any signs/symptoms of bleeding, dyspepsia, or gastritis occur. Advise patients who have had neuraxial anesthesia or spinal puncture to watch for signs and symptoms of spinal/epidural hematoma, particularly if concomitantly taking NSAIDs or platelet inhibitors; instruct to contact physician immediately if symptoms occur. Instruct to inform physician of intake of dabigatran before any invasive procedure (including dental procedures) is scheduled. Advise patients to list all prescription/OTC medications or dietary supplements they may be taking or planning to take. Instruct to inform healthcare provider if planning to undergo surgery or already had surgery to place a prosthetic heart valve.

PRALUENT — alirocumab   Rx
Class: Proprotein Convertase Subtilisin Kexin Type 9 (PCSK9) Inhibitor

ADULT DOSAGE	PEDIATRIC DOSAGE
Primary Hyperlipidemia	Pediatric use may not have been established
Adjunct to diet and maximally tolerated statin therapy for the treatment of patients w/ heterozygous familial hypercholesterolemia or clinical atherosclerotic cardiovascular disease, who require additional lowering of LDL-C	
Initial: 75mg SQ once every 2 weeks **Titrate:** May increase to max dose if LDL-C response is inadequate **Max:** 150mg every 2 weeks	
Missed Dose	
If a dose is missed, administer the inj w/in 7 days from the missed dose and then resume the original schedule. If the missed dose is not administered w/in 7 days, wait until the next dose on the original schedule	

ADMINISTRATION
SQ route

Allow alirocumab to warm to room temperature for 30-40 min prior to use; use as soon as possible after it has warmed up. Do not use if it has been at room temperature for ≥24 hrs.

Administer in the thigh, abdomen, or upper arm; rotate inj site w/ each inj. Do not inject into areas of active skin disease or injury (eg, sunburns, skin rashes, inflammation, skin infections).
Do not coadminister w/ other injectable drugs at the same inj site.

STORAGE
2-8°C (36-46°F). Store in the outer carton in order to protect from light. Do not freeze. Do not expose to extreme heat. Do not shake.

HOW SUPPLIED
Inj: 75mg/mL, 150mg/mL [prefilled pen, prefilled syringe]

CONTRAINDICATIONS
History of a serious hypersensitivity reaction to alirocumab.

WARNINGS/PRECAUTIONS
Hypersensitivity reactions, including some serious events (eg, hypersensitivity vasculitis and hypersensitivity reactions requiring hospitalization), reported; if signs/symptoms of serious allergic reactions occur, d/c treatment, treat according to the standard of care, and monitor until signs/symptoms resolve.

ADVERSE REACTIONS
Nasopharyngitis, inj-site reactions, influenza, UTI, diarrhea, bronchitis, myalgia, muscle spasms, sinusitis.

PREGNANCY AND LACTATION
Pregnancy: FDA's experience w/ monoclonal antibodies in humans indicates that they are unlikely to cross the placenta in the 1st trimester; however, they are likely to cross the placenta in increasing amounts in the 2nd and 3rd trimester. Consider the benefits and risks of alirocumab and possible risks to the fetus before prescribing to pregnant women.
Lactation: There is no information regarding the presence of alirocumab in human milk, the effects on the breastfed infant, or the effects on milk production; caution in nursing.

MECHANISM OF ACTION
Human monoclonal antibody (IgG1 isotype) that targets PCSK9; PCSK9 binds to the low-density lipoprotein receptors (LDLRs) on the surface of hepatocytes to promote LDLR degradation w/in the liver. By inhibiting the binding of PCSK9 to LDLR, alirocumab increases the number of LDLRs available to clear LDL, thereby lowering LDL-C levels.

PHARMACOKINETICS
Absorption: Absolute bioavailability (85%); T_{max}=3-7 days (median). **Distribution:** (IV) V_d=0.04-0.05L/kg. **Metabolism:** Expected to degrade to small peptides and individual amino acids. Does not affect CYP450 enzymes, P-gp, and OATP. **Elimination:** $T_{1/2}$=17-20 days (median).

PATIENT CONSIDERATIONS
Assessment: Assess for drug hypersensitivity and pregnancy/nursing status. Obtain baseline lipid levels.

Monitoring: Monitor for hypersensitivity reactions. Measure LDL-C levels w/in 4-8 weeks of initiating or titrating therapy.

Counseling: Instruct on proper inj technique, including aseptic technique, and how to use the prefilled pen/syringe correctly; inform that it may take up to 20 sec to inject alirocumab. Caution that the prefilled pen/syringe must not be reused and inform about the proper technique of disposal in a puncture-resistant container. Advise to d/c therapy and seek prompt medical attention if any signs/symptoms of serious allergic reactions occur.

PRANDIMET — metformin hydrochloride/repaglinide   Rx
Class: Biguanide/meglitinide

> Lactic acidosis may occur due to metformin accumulation; risk increases with conditions such as sepsis, dehydration, excess alcohol intake, hepatic impairment, renal impairment, and acute CHF. If acidosis is suspected, d/c and hospitalize patient immediately.

ADULT DOSAGE	PEDIATRIC DOSAGE
Type 2 Diabetes Mellitus	Pediatric use may not have been established
In patients who are already treated w/ a meglitinide and metformin or who have inadequate glycemic control on a meglitinide alone or metformin alone	
May administer bid-tid	
Inadequately Controlled w/ Metformin Monotherapy: **Initial:** 1mg/500mg bid w/ meals **Titrate:** Gradually escalate dose based on glycemic response	
Inadequately Controlled w/ Meglitinide Monotherapy: **Initial:** 500mg of metformin component bid **Titrate:** Gradually escalate dose based on glycemic response	
Currently Using Repaglinide and Metformin Concomitantly: **Initial:** Initiate at a dose similar to, but not exceeding, doses of current repaglinide and metformin therapy	

Titrate: Increase as necessary to achieve targeted glycemic control

Max: (10mg/2500mg)/day or (4mg/1000mg)/meal

ADMINISTRATION
Oral route

Take dose w/in 15 min ac; timing may vary from immediately preceding meal up to 30 min before meal.

If meal is skipped, skip dose for that meal.

STORAGE
≤25°C (77°F). Protect from moisture.

HOW SUPPLIED
Tab: (Repaglinide/Metformin) 1mg/500mg, 2mg/500mg

CONTRAINDICATIONS
Renal impairment (eg, SrCr ≥1.5mg/dL [males], ≥1.4mg/dL [females], or abnormal CrCl), acute or chronic metabolic acidosis, including diabetic ketoacidosis, concomitant gemfibrozil, known hypersensitivity to PrandiMet or any inactive ingredients in the product.

WARNINGS/PRECAUTIONS
Do not initiate in patients ≥80 yrs of age unless renal function is normal. Temporarily d/c at the time of or prior to intravascular contrast studies with iodinated materials, and withhold for 48 hrs subsequent to the procedure and reinstitute only if renal function is normal. Avoid with hepatic impairment. May cause hypoglycemia; risk increased in elderly, debilitated, or malnourished patients, or with adrenal or pituitary insufficiency. May decrease vitamin B12 levels; measure hematologic parameters annually. Suspend temporarily for any surgical procedure (except minor procedures not associated with restricted food and fluid intake); restart when oral intake is resumed and renal function is normal. Temporary loss of glycemic control may occur when exposed to stress; may need to withhold therapy and temporarily administer insulin. D/C promptly in hypoxic states (eg, acute CHF, shock, acute myocardial infarction). Evaluate promptly for evidence of ketoacidosis or lactic acidosis if laboratory abnormalities or clinical illness develops; d/c immediately if acidosis occurs.

ADVERSE REACTIONS
Lactic acidosis, GI system disorder, symptomatic hypoglycemia, headache, diarrhea, nausea, upper respiratory tract infection.

DRUG INTERACTIONS
See Contraindications. May increase C_{max} of fenofibrate. Metformin: Alcohol potentiates effect of metformin on lactate metabolism. Caution with drugs that may affect renal function or result in significant hemodynamic change or may interfere with the disposition of metformin, such as cationic drugs eliminated by renal tubular secretion (eg, amiloride, digoxin, morphine). Cimetidine, furosemide, nifedipine, and ibuprofen may increase levels. Propranolol may decrease levels. May decrease levels of furosemide. Repaglinide: Not for use in combination with NPH-insulin. Risk of hypoglycemia increased with alcohol. Hypoglycemia may be difficult to recognize with β-adrenergic blocking drugs. CYP2C8 inhibitors, CYP3A4 inhibitors, or CYP2C8/3A4 inducers may alter pharmacokinetics and pharmacodynamics. Clarithromycin, deferasirox, fenofibrate, gemfibrozil, itraconazole, ketoconazole, simvastatin, trimethoprim, and OATP1B1 inhibitors (eg, cyclosporine) may increase levels. Levonorgestrel/ethinyl estradiol combination may decrease area under the curve and increase C_{max}. Nifedipine and rifampin may decrease levels. May increase levels of ethinyl estradiol.

PREGNANCY AND LACTATION
Pregnancy: Category C.
Lactation: Not for use in nursing.

MECHANISM OF ACTION
Metformin: Biguanide; decreases hepatic glucose production, decreases intestinal absorption of glucose, and improves insulin sensitivity by increasing peripheral glucose uptake and utilization. Repaglinide: Meglitinide; lowers blood glucose levels by stimulating the release of insulin from the pancreas.

PHARMACOKINETICS
Absorption: Administration of variable doses resulted in different pharmacokinetic parameters. Metformin: Absolute bioavailability (50-60%) (fasted). Repaglinide: Absolute bioavailability (56%); T_{max}=1 hr. **Distribution:** Metformin: V_d=654L. Repaglinide: (IV) V_d=31L; plasma protein binding (>98%). **Metabolism:** Repaglinide: Complete. CYP2C8, 3A4; oxidation, and direct conjugation with glucuronic acid; oxidized dicarboxylic acid (M2), aromatic amine (M1), acyl glucuronide (M7) (major metabolites). **Elimination:** Metformin: Urine (90%); $T_{1/2}$=6.2 hrs (plasma), 17.6 hrs (blood). Repaglinide: Feces (90%, <2% unchanged), urine (8%, 0.1% unchanged); $T_{1/2}$=1 hr.

PATIENT CONSIDERATIONS
Assessment: Assess for metabolic acidosis, diabetic ketoacidosis, type of DM, renal/hepatic function, risk factors for lactic acidosis, susceptibility to hypoglycemia, drug hypersensitivity, pregnancy/nursing status, and possible drug interactions. Assess if patient is planning to undergo any surgical procedure or is under any form of stress. Obtain baseline FPG and HbA1c.

Monitoring: Monitor for lactic acidosis, clinical illness, hypoxic states, and other adverse reactions. Monitor renal function, especially in elderly patients, at least annually. Monitor vitamin B12 levels in patients predisposed to develop subnormal vitamin B12 levels. Monitor FPG, HbA1c, and hematologic parameters periodically.

Counseling: Inform of potential risks/advantages of therapy, alternative modes of therapy, the importance of adherence to dietary instructions, regular exercise program, and regular testing of blood glucose, HbA1c, renal function, and hematologic parameters. Inform about risks of hypoglycemia and lactic acidosis,

---

their symptoms and treatment, and predisposing conditions. Instruct to seek medical advice during periods of stress as medication needs may change. Advise to d/c drug immediately and notify physician if unexplained hyperventilation, myalgia, malaise, unusual somnolence, or other nonspecific symptoms occur. Instruct to take drug with meals; if a meal is skipped, instruct to skip the dose for that meal. Counsel against excessive alcohol intake.

PRANDIN — repaglinide   Rx
Class: Meglitinide

ADULT DOSAGE
Type 2 Diabetes Mellitus
Administer dose w/in 15-30 min ac, bid-qid in response to changes in meal pattern

Initial:
Not Previously Treated or HbA1c <8%: 0.5mg w/ each meal preprandially
Previously Treated and HbA1c ≥8%: 1mg or 2mg w/ each meal preprandially
Titrate: May double preprandial dose up to 4mg until satisfactory blood glucose response; at least 1 week should elapse to assess response after each dose adjustment
Range: 0.5-4mg w/ meals preprandially
Max: 16mg/day

Replacing Other Oral Hypoglycemics:
Repaglinide may be started on the day after the final dose is given; observe carefully for hypoglycemia due to potential overlapping drug effects. Close monitoring for up to 1 week or longer may be indicated when transferred from longer half-life sulfonylurea agents (eg, chlorpropamide)

Combination Therapy:
May add metformin or a thiazolidinedione if repaglinide monotherapy does not result in adequate glycemic control; may add repaglinide if metformin or thiazolidinedione monotherapy does not provide adequate control
Starting dose and dose adjustments for repaglinide combination therapy is the same as for repaglinide monotherapy

PEDIATRIC DOSAGE
Pediatric use may not have been established

DOSING CONSIDERATIONS
Concomitant Medications
W/ Thiazolidinedione or w/ Metformin:
If hypoglycemia occurs in patients taking a combination of repaglinide and a thiazolidinedione or repaglinide and metformin, reduce dose of repaglinide

Renal Impairment
Severe (CrCl 20-40mL/min):
Initial: 0.5mg ac; titrate carefully

Hepatic Impairment
Utilize longer intervals between dose adjustments to fully assess response

ADMINISTRATION
Oral route
Take w/in 15-30 min ac.

STORAGE
≤25°C (77°F). Protect from moisture.

HOW SUPPLIED
Tab: 0.5mg, 1mg, 2mg

CONTRAINDICATIONS
Diabetic ketoacidosis w/ or w/o coma, type 1 DM, concomitant gemfibrozil, known hypersensitivity to the drug or its inactive ingredients.

WARNINGS/PRECAUTIONS
May cause hypoglycemia; risk increased in elderly, debilitated or malnourished patients, or with adrenal, pituitary, hepatic, or severe renal insufficiency. Loss of glycemic control may occur when exposed to stress; may need to d/c therapy and administer insulin. Secondary failure may occur; assess adequate dose adjustment and adherence to diet before classifying a patient as a secondary failure. Caution with hepatic impairment.

ADVERSE REACTIONS
Hypoglycemia, upper respiratory infection, headache, rhinitis, sinusitis, bronchitis, arthralgia, back pain, N/V, diarrhea, dyspepsia, constipation, paresthesia, chest pain.

DRUG INTERACTIONS

See Contraindications. Not for use in combination with NPH-insulin. CYP3A4 and/or CYP2C8 inducers (eg, barbiturates, carbamazepine), CYP3A4 inhibitors (eg, erythromycin), and CYP2C8 inhibitors (eg, montelukast) may alter metabolism; use with caution. OATP1B1 inhibitors (eg, cyclosporine), itraconazole, ketoconazole, clarithromycin, trimethoprim, and deferasirox may increase levels. Rifampin may decrease levels. NSAIDs, highly protein-bound drugs, salicylates, sulfonamides, cyclosporine, chloramphenicol, coumarins, probenecid, MAOIs, β-blockers, alcohol, and >1 glucose-lowering drug may potentiate hypoglycemic action. Thiazides and other diuretics, corticosteroids, phenothiazines, thyroid products, estrogens, oral contraceptives, phenytoin, nicotinic acid, sympathomimetics, calcium channel blockers, and isoniazid tend to produce hyperglycemia and may lead to loss of glycemic control. β-blockers may mask hypoglycemia. May increase ethinyl estradiol levels and levonorgestrel C_{max}. Levonorgestrel/ethinyl estradiol combination and simvastatin may increase C_{max}.

PREGNANCY AND LACTATION

Pregnancy: Category C.
Lactation: Not for use in nursing.

MECHANISM OF ACTION

Meglitinide; lowers blood glucose levels by stimulating the release of insulin from the pancreas.

PHARMACOKINETICS

Absorption: Rapid and complete. Absolute bioavailability (56%); T_{max}=1 hr. See PI for parameters of different doses. **Distribution:** (IV) V_d=31L; plasma protein binding (>98%). **Metabolism:** CYP2C8, 3A4; oxidation, and direct conjugation with glucuronic acid; oxidized dicarboxylic acid (M2), aromatic amine (M1), acyl glucuronide (M7) (major metabolites). **Elimination:** Feces (90%, <2% unchanged), urine (8%, 0.1% unchanged); $T_{1/2}$=1-1.4 hrs.

PATIENT CONSIDERATIONS

Assessment: Assess for diabetic ketoacidosis, type 1 DM, adrenal/pituitary/hepatic/severe renal insufficiency, drug hypersensitivity, pregnancy/nursing status, and possible drug interactions. Assess FPG, postprandial glucose (PPG), and HbA1c.

Monitoring: Monitor for hypo/hyperglycemia, secondary failure, and other adverse events. Monitor FPG, PPG, HbA1c, and renal/hepatic function.

Counseling: Inform of potential risks/benefits of therapy, alternative modes of therapy, the importance of adherence to dietary instructions, regular exercise program, and regular blood glucose and HbA1c testing. Inform about risks of hypoglycemia, its symptoms and treatment, and predisposing conditions. Instruct to take drug ac (bid-qid preprandially); if a meal is skipped (or an extra meal is added), instruct to skip (or add) a dose for that meal.

PRAVASTATIN — pravastatin sodium   Rx

Class: HMG-CoA reductase inhibitor (statin)

OTHER BRAND NAMES

Pravachol

ADULT DOSAGE

Hyperlipidemia

Primary Hypercholesterolemia/ Mixed Dyslipidemia/Primary Dysbetalipoproteinemia:
Initial: 40mg qd
Titrate: Increase to 80mg qd if 40mg qd does not achieve desired cholesterol levels

Maximal effect of a given dose is seen w/in 4 weeks; perform periodic lipid determinations at this time and adjust dose accordingly

Prevention of Cardiovascular Disease

Dose based on current clinical practice

PEDIATRIC DOSAGE

Heterozygous Familial Hypercholesterolemia

8-13 Years:
20mg qd
Doses >20mg have not been studied in this patient population

14-18 Years:
Initial: 40mg qd
Doses >40mg have not been studied in this patient population

DOSING CONSIDERATIONS

Concomitant Medications

Bile Acid Resins:
Administer pravastatin either 1 hr or more before or at least 4 hrs following the resin

Clarithromycin:
Limit pravastatin dose to 40mg qd

Immunosuppressive Drugs (eg, Cyclosporine):
Initial: 10mg qhs
Titrate: Increase dose cautiously
Max: 20mg/day

Renal Impairment

Severe:
Initial: 10mg qd

ADMINISTRATION

Oral route

Administer as a single dose at any time of the day, w/ or w/o food.

STORAGE

20-25°C (68-77°F); excursions permitted to 15-30°C (59-86°F). Protect from light and moisture. **Pravachol:** 25°C (77°F); excursions permitted to 15-30°C (59-86°F). Protect from light and moisture.

HOW SUPPLIED

Tab: 10mg; (Pravachol) 20mg, 40mg, 80mg

CONTRAINDICATIONS

Hypersensitivity to any component of the medication; active liver disease or unexplained, persistent elevations of serum transaminases; pregnancy; nursing mothers.

WARNINGS/PRECAUTIONS

Rare cases of rhabdomyolysis w/ acute renal failure secondary to myoglobinuria reported. Increased risk of rhabdomyolysis w/ history of renal impairment; closely monitor for skeletal muscle effects. Uncomplicated myalgia and myopathy (including immune-mediated necrotizing myopathy [IMNM]) reported; d/c if markedly elevated CPK levels occur or myopathy is diagnosed/suspected. Temporarily withhold in any patient experiencing an acute or serious condition predisposing to development of renal failure secondary to rhabdomyolysis. May cause biochemical liver function abnormalities; perform LFTs prior to initiation of therapy and when clinically indicated. Caution in patients who have recent (<6 months) history of liver disease, have signs that may suggest liver disease, are heavy alcohol users, or are elderly. Fatal and nonfatal hepatic failure reported (rare); promptly interrupt therapy if serious liver injury w/ clinical symptoms and/or hyperbilirubinemia or jaundice occurs and do not restart if no alternate etiology found. May blunt adrenal or gonadal steroid hormone production. Evaluate patients who display clinical evidence of endocrine dysfunction. Not studied in conditions where the major lipoprotein abnormality is elevation of chylomicrons (Fredrickson Types I and V). Not evaluated in patients w/ rare homozygous familial hypercholesterolemia; statins reported to be less effective because patients lack functional LDL receptors.

ADVERSE REACTIONS

Musculoskeletal pain, N/V, URTI, diarrhea, headache.

DRUG INTERACTIONS

See Dosing Considerations. Increased risk of myopathy/rhabdomyolysis w/ cyclosporine, colchicine, gemfibrozil, and other fibrates; avoid w/ gemfibrozil and use caution w/ colchicine and other fibrates. Niacin (nicotinic acid) may enhance risk of skeletal muscle effects; consider dose reduction of pravastatin. Increased risk of myopathy/rhabdomyolysis w/ clarithromycin. Other macrolides (eg, erythromycin, azithromycin) may increase pravastatin exposure and increase risk of myopathies; use w/ caution. Caution w/ drugs that may diminish levels or activity of steroid hormones (eg, ketoconazole, spironolactone, cimetidine).

PREGNANCY AND LACTATION

Pregnancy: May cause fetal harm; contraindicated.
Lactation: Present in human milk; contraindicated.
Reproductive Potential: Females should use effective contraception during treatment.

MECHANISM OF ACTION

HMG-CoA reductase inhibitor; inhibits the enzyme that catalyzes the conversion of HMG-CoA to mevalonate, an early and rate-limiting step in the biosynthetic pathway for cholesterol. Reduces VLDL and TGs and increases HDL.

PHARMACOKINETICS

Absorption: Absolute bioavailability (17%); T_{max}=1-1.5 hrs; (fasted) C_{max}=26.5ng/mL, AUC=59.8ng•hr/mL. **Distribution:** Plasma protein binding (50%); found in breast milk. **Metabolism:** Liver (extensive 1st pass), by isomerization and enzymatic ring hydroxylation; 3α-hydroxyisomeric metabolite (active). **Elimination:** Feces (70%), urine (20%); $T_{1/2}$=1.8 hrs.

PATIENT CONSIDERATIONS

Assessment: Assess for history of or active liver disease, unexplained persistent serum transaminase elevations, predisposing factors for myopathy, alcohol consumption, renal impairment, hypersensitivity to the drug, pregnancy/nursing status, and possible drug interactions. Obtain baseline lipid profile and LFTs.

Monitoring: Monitor for signs/symptoms of rhabdomyolysis, myopathy (including IMNM), liver/endocrine dysfunction, and other adverse reactions. Monitor lipid profile, LFTs when clinically indicated, and CPK levels.

Counseling: Advise to report promptly any unexplained muscle pain, tenderness, or weakness, particularly if accompanied by malaise or fever or if muscle signs/symptoms persist after discontinuing therapy. Advise females of reproductive potential of the risk to a fetus, to use effective contraception during treatment, and to inform their healthcare provider of a known or suspected pregnancy. Instruct women not to breastfeed during treatment. Advise to promptly report any symptoms that may indicate liver injury (eg, fatigue, anorexia, right upper abdominal discomfort, dark urine, jaundice).

PRAXBIND — idarucizumab   Rx

Class: Antidote

ADULT DOSAGE

Dabigatran Reversal

For use in emergency surgery/urgent procedures, or in the event of life-threatening or uncontrolled bleeding, to reverse the anticoagulant effects of dabigatran

5g IV, provided as 2 separate vials each containing 2.5g/50mL; limited data to support administration of an additional 5g

If reappearance of bleeding w/ elevated coagulation parameters

PEDIATRIC DOSAGE

Pediatric use may not have been established

occurs after 1 dose of 5g, may give another 5g dose.
Similarly, patients who require a 2nd emergency surgery/urgent procedure and have elevated coagulation parameters may receive an additional 5g dose.

Dabigatran treatment can be initiated 24 hrs after administration

ADMINISTRATION
IV route

Do not mix w/ other products.
Administer w/in 1 hr after withdrawing from vial.
Administer dose as 2 consecutive infusions or a bolus inj by injecting both vials consecutively.
A preexisting IV line may be used for administration; the line must be flushed w/ 0.9% NaCl prior to infusion.

STORAGE
2-8°C (36-46°F). Do not freeze. Do not shake. Unopened vial may be kept at 25°C (77°F) for ≤48 hrs if stored in the original package to protect from light, or ≤6 hrs when exposed to light.

HOW SUPPLIED
Inj: 2.5g/50mL

WARNINGS/PRECAUTIONS
Reversing dabigatran therapy exposes patients to the thrombotic risk of their underlying disease; consider resuming anticoagulant therapy as soon as medically appropriate. Elevated coagulation parameters (eg, aPTT, ECT) have been observed. If an anaphylactic reaction or other serious allergic reaction occurs, immediately d/c. Serious adverse reactions reported in patients w/ hereditary fructose intolerance due to sorbitol excipient. Recommended dose of idarucizumab contains 4g of sorbitol; consider the combined daily metabolic load of sorbitol/fructose from all sources, including idarucizumab and other drugs containing sorbitol when prescribing.

ADVERSE REACTIONS
Headache, hypokalemia, delirium, constipation, pyrexia, pneumonia.

PREGNANCY AND LACTATION
Pregnancy: There are no adequate/well-controlled studies in pregnant women to inform on associated risks. Use in pregnant women only if clearly needed.
Lactation: There are no data on the effects on the breastfed child or on milk production.

MECHANISM OF ACTION
Dabigatran reversal agent; monoclonal antibody fragment binds to dabigatran and its acylglucuronide metabolites, neutralizing their anticoagulant effect.

PHARMACOKINETICS
Distribution: V_d = 8.9L. **Metabolism:** Biodegradation to smaller molecules.
Elimination: Urine (32.1%); $T_{1/2}$ = 10.3 hrs.

PATIENT CONSIDERATIONS
Assessment: Assess for thromboembolic risk, hereditary fructose intolerance, and pregnancy/nursing status.

Monitoring: Monitor for allergic/anaphylactic reaction, signs/symptoms of thromboembolism, coagulation parameters (aPTT, ECT), bleeding, and other adverse reactions.

Counseling: Inform patients that reversing dabigatran therapy exposes them to the thromboembolic risk of their underlying disease. Instruct to get immediate medical attention for any signs/symptoms of bleeding. Inform of signs/symptoms of allergic hypersensitivity reactions. Inform patients w/ hereditary fructose intolerance that drug contains sorbitol.

PRECEDEX — dexmedetomidine hydrochloride   Rx

Class: Alpha₂ agonist

ADULT DOSAGE
Sedation

Intensive Care Unit Sedation:
Initiation:
LD: 1mcg/kg over 10 min
Conversion from Alternate Sedative Therapy:
LD may not be required

Maint:
0.2-0.7mcg/kg/hr; adjust rate of infusion to achieve desired level of sedation

Procedural Sedation:
Initiation:
LD: 1mcg/kg over 10 min
Less Invasive Procedures (eg, Ophthalmic Surgery):
LD: 0.5mcg/kg over 10 min
Awake Fiberoptic Intubation:
LD: 1mcg/kg over 10 min

PEDIATRIC DOSAGE
Pediatric use may not have been established

Maint:
Initiate at 0.6mcg/kg/hr; titrate to achieve desired clinical effect
Range: 0.2-1mcg/kg/hr; adjust rate of infusion to achieve the targeted level of sedation
Awake Fiberoptic Intubation:
Maint infusion of 0.7mcg/kg/hr until the endotracheal tube is secured

DOSING CONSIDERATIONS
Concomitant Medications
A dose reduction in Precedex or other concomitant anesthetics, sedatives, hypnotics, or opioids may be required when coadministered

Hepatic Impairment
Consider dose reduction

Elderly
>65 Years:
Intensive Care Unit Sedation:
Initiation/Maint: Consider a dose reduction
Procedural Sedation:
Initiation: LD: 0.5mcg/kg over 10 min
Maint: Consider a dose reduction

ADMINISTRATION
IV route

Administer using a controlled infusion device; not indicated for infusions lasting >24 hrs.

Preparation of Sol
Precedex Inj, 200mcg/2mL (100mcg/mL):
Dilute w/ 0.9% NaCl inj to achieve required concentration (4mcg/mL) prior to administration.
Preparation is the same, whether for the LD or maint infusion.
1. Withdraw 2mL of Precedex inj and add to 48mL of 0.9% NaCl inj to a total of 50mL.
2. Shake gently to mix well.

Precedex in 0.9% NaCl Inj, 80mcg/20mL (4mcg/mL), 200mcg/50mL (4mcg/mL), and 400mcg/100mL (4mcg/mL):
Precedex in 0.9% NaCl inj is supplied in glass containers containing a premixed, ready to use dexmedetomidine HCl sol in 0.9% NaCl in water; no further dilution necessary.

Administration w/ Other Fluids
Do not coadminister through the same IV catheter w/ blood or plasma.
Incompatible when administered w/ the following drugs:
- amphotericin B
- diazepam
Compatible when administered w/ the following IV fluids:
- 0.9% NaCl in water
- 5% dextrose in water
- 20% mannitol
- lactated Ringer's sol
- 100mg/mL magnesium sulfate sol
- 0.3% potassium chloride sol

Compatibility w/ Natural Rubber
Advisable to use administration components made w/ synthetic or coated natural rubber gaskets.

STORAGE
25°C (77°F); excursions allowed from 15-30°C (59-86°F).

HOW SUPPLIED
Inj: 100mcg/mL [2mL, vial]; (0.9% NaCl) 4mcg/mL [50mL, 100mL, bottle; 20mL, vial]

WARNINGS/PRECAUTIONS
Should be administered only by persons skilled in the management of patients in the intensive care or operating room setting. Continuously monitor patients during administration. Hypotension, bradycardia, and sinus arrest reported; treat appropriately. Hypotension and/or bradycardia may be more pronounced in patients w/ hypovolemia, diabetes mellitus (DM), chronic HTN, or who are elderly. Caution w/ advanced heart block and/or severe ventricular dysfunction. Transient HTN observed primarily during the LD; reduction of loading infusion rate may be desirable. Arousability and alertness reported in some patients upon stimulation; this alone should not be considered as lack of efficacy in the absence of other clinical signs and symptoms. Withdrawal events reported w/ intensive care unit sedation; if tachycardia and/or HTN occurs after discontinuation, supportive therapy is indicated. Use beyond 24 hrs has been associated w/ tolerance, tachyphylaxis, and a dose-related increase in adverse reactions.

ADVERSE REACTIONS
Hypotension, bradycardia, dry mouth.

DRUG INTERACTIONS
See Dosing Considerations. Coadministration w/ anesthetics, sedatives, hypnotics, and opioids (eg, sevoflurane, isoflurane, propofol, alfentanil, midazolam) may lead to enhancement of effects. Caution w/ vasodilators or negative chronotropic agents.

PREGNANCY AND LACTATION
Pregnancy: Category C.
Lactation: Caution in nursing.

MECHANISM OF ACTION
Selective α_2-adrenergic agonist; possesses sedative properties.

PHARMACOKINETICS
Distribution: V_d=118L; plasma protein binding (94%). **Metabolism:** Direct N-glucuronidation, aliphatic hydroxylation (via CYP2A6), and N-methylation. **Elimination:** Urine (95%), feces (4%); $T_{1/2}$=2 hrs.

PATIENT CONSIDERATIONS
Assessment: Assess for advanced heart block, severe ventricular dysfunction, hepatic impairment, hypovolemia, DM, chronic HTN, pregnancy/nursing status, and possible drug interactions.

Monitoring: Monitor for hypotension, bradycardia, sinus arrest, transient HTN, withdrawal events, and other adverse reactions.

Counseling: When infused for >6 hrs, instruct to report nervousness, agitation, and headaches that may occur for up to 48 hrs. Instruct to report symptoms that may occur w/in 48 hrs after administration (eg, weakness, confusion, excessive sweating, weight loss, abdominal pain, salt cravings, diarrhea, constipation, dizziness, lightheadedness).

PREDNISOLONE — prednisolone   Rx

Class: Glucocorticoid

ADULT DOSAGE	PEDIATRIC DOSAGE
Steroid-Responsive Disorders	**Steroid-Responsive Disorders**
Syr/Tab:	**Syr/Tab:**
Initial: 5-60mg/day depending on disease and response	**Initial:** 5-60mg/day depending on disease and response
Maint: Decrease initial dose in small decrements to lowest effective dose	**Maint:** Decrease dose by small amounts to lowest effective dose
Tab:	**Tab:**
Alternate-Day Therapy: Administer twice the usual daily dose every other am; refer to PI for more detailed information	**Alternate-Day Therapy:** Administer twice the usual daily dose every other am; refer to PI for more detailed information

---

DOSING CONSIDERATIONS
Discontinuation
Withdraw gradually after long-term therapy

ADMINISTRATION
Oral route

STORAGE
20-25°C (68-77°F). (Syrup) Do not refrigerate.

HOW SUPPLIED
Syrup: 5mg/5mL [120mL], 15mg/5mL [240mL, 480mL]; **Tab:** 5mg* *scored

CONTRAINDICATIONS
Systemic fungal infections.

WARNINGS/PRECAUTIONS
May need to increase dose before, during, and after stressful situation. May mask signs of infection or cause new infections. May decrease resistance and inability to localize infection. Possible benefits should be weighed against potential hazards if used during pregnancy/nursing. Prolonged use may produce posterior subcapsular cataracts, glaucoma, optic nerve damage, and secondary ocular infections. May cause BP elevation, increased K^+/Ca^{2+} excretion, and salt/water retention. Dietary salt restriction and K^+ supplementation may be necessary when used in large doses. More serious/fatal course of infections reported with chickenpox and measles; avoid exposure. Reactivation of disease may occur with latent TB or tuberculin reactivity. Caution with hypothyroidism, cirrhosis, ocular herpes simplex, HTN, diverticulitis, fresh intestinal anastomoses, nonspecific ulcerative colitis, osteoporosis, myasthenia gravis, renal insufficiency, and active or latent peptic ulcer. Growth and development of children on prolonged therapy should be monitored. May cause psychic derangements or aggravate existing emotional instability or psychotic tendencies. Avoid abrupt withdrawal. (Syrup) D/C treatment if a period of spontaneous remission occurs in a chronic condition.

ADVERSE REACTIONS
Fluid and electrolyte disturbances, osteoporosis, muscle weakness, cushingoid state, menstrual irregularities, facial erythema, convulsions, impaired wound healing, increased sweating, decreased carbohydrate tolerance, glaucoma, posterior subcapsular cataracts, vertigo, headache, abdominal distention.

DRUG INTERACTIONS
Caution with ASA in hypoprothrombinemia. Avoid smallpox vaccination and other immunization procedures, especially if on high doses of corticosteroids. Increased insulin and PO hypoglycemic requirements in diabetics.

PREGNANCY AND LACTATION
Safety not known in pregnancy/nursing.

MECHANISM OF ACTION
Anti-inflammatory glucocorticoid; causes profound and varied metabolic effects and modifies the body's immune response to diverse stimuli.

PHARMACOKINETICS
Absorption: Readily absorbed from GI tract.

PATIENT CONSIDERATIONS
Assessment: Assess for systemic fungal infections/other current infections, active TB, vaccination history, hypothyroidism, cirrhosis, renal insufficiency, HTN, ocular

herpes simplex, ulcerative colitis, diverticulitis, fresh intestinal anastomoses, active or latent peptic ulcer, osteoporosis, myasthenia gravis, psychotic tendencies, pregnancy/nursing status, and for possible drug interactions.

Monitoring: Monitor for adrenocortical insufficiency, salt/water retention, new infections, psychic derangements, posterior subcapsular cataracts, glaucoma, optic nerve damage, and secondary ocular infections. Monitor BP, serum K^+ and Ca^{2+} levels. Monitor growth and development of infants/children on prolonged therapy (including bone growth) and for hypoadrenalism in infants born to mothers who received substantial doses. (Syrup) Obtain BP, weight, routine lab studies (including 2-hr postprandial blood glucose and serum K^+), chest x-ray, and upper GI x-rays (with known/suspected peptic ulcer disease) at regular intervals during prolonged therapy.

Counseling: Advise not to d/c abruptly. Counsel to avoid exposure to chickenpox or measles if on an immunosuppressant dose of corticosteroids; instruct to report immediately if exposed.

PREDNISONE — prednisone   Rx

Class: Glucocorticoid

OTHER BRAND NAMES
Prednisone Intensol

ADULT DOSAGE	PEDIATRIC DOSAGE
Steroid-Responsive Disorders	**Steroid-Responsive Disorders**
Initial: 5-60mg/day, depending on disease and response	**Initial:** 5-60mg/day, depending on disease and response
Maint: Decrease initial dose in small decrements at appropriate time intervals until lowest effective dose	**Maint:** Decrease initial dose in small decrements at appropriate time intervals until lowest effective dose
Alternate-Day Therapy: Administer twice the usual daily dose every other am; refer to PI for more detailed information	**Alternate-Day Therapy:** Administer twice the usual daily dose every other am; refer to PI for more detailed information
Multiple Sclerosis	**Multiple Sclerosis**
Acute Exacerbations: 200mg/day for 1 week, followed by 80mg qod for 1 month	**Acute Exacerbations:** 200mg/day for 1 week, followed by 80mg qod for 1 month

---

DOSING CONSIDERATIONS
Elderly
Start at lower end of dosing range

Discontinuation
Withdraw gradually after long-term therapy

ADMINISTRATION
Oral route

Take before, during, or immediately pc or w/ food or milk to reduce gastric irritation.
Administer in the am prior to 9 am; when large doses are given, administer antacids between meals to prevent peptic ulcers.
Multiple dose therapy should be evenly distributed in evenly spaced intervals throughout the day.

STORAGE
20-25°C (68-77°F). **Tab:** Protect from moisture. **Prednisone Intensol:** Discard opened bottle after 90 days.

HOW SUPPLIED
Oral Sol: 5mg/5mL [120mL, 500mL]; (Prednisone Intensol) 5mg/mL [30mL]; **Tab:** 1mg*, 2.5mg*, 5mg*, 10mg*, 20mg*, 50mg* *scored

CONTRAINDICATIONS
Systemic fungal infections, known hypersensitivity to the components of the medication.

WARNINGS/PRECAUTIONS
Monitor for situations that may make dosage adjustments necessary (eg, change in clinical status secondary to remissions/exacerbations in the disease process, individual drug responsiveness, effect of patient exposure to stress). Anaphylactoid reactions may occur. May need to increase dose before, during, and after stressful situations. May cause BP elevation, salt/water retention, and increased K^+ and Ca^{2+} excretion; dietary salt restriction and K^+ supplementation may be necessary. Caution in patients w/ a recent MI; may be associated w/ left ventricular free wall rupture after a recent MI. May produce reversible hypothalamic-pituitary-adrenal (HPA) axis suppression w/ the potential for corticosteroid insufficiency after withdrawal of treatment. Metabolic clearance is decreased in hypothyroid patients and increased in hyperthyroid patients; changes in thyroid status may necessitate dose adjustment. May increase susceptibility to infections, mask signs of current infection, activate latent disease, or exacerbate intercurrent infections. Avoid use in the presence of systemic fungal infections unless needed to control life-threatening drug reactions. Rule out latent or active amebiasis before initiating therapy. Caution w/ known/suspected *Strongyloides* infestation, active/latent TB or tuberculin reactivity, HTN, CHF, and renal insufficiency. Caution w/ active or latent peptic ulcers, diverticulitis, fresh intestinal anastomoses, and nonspecific ulcerative colitis; may increase risk of perforation. Signs of peritoneal irritation following GI perforation may be minimal/absent. Not for use in cerebral malaria and active ocular herpes simplex. May cause more serious/fatal course of chickenpox and measles; avoid exposure, and if exposed, consider prophylaxis/treatment. May

produce posterior subcapsular cataracts, glaucoma w/ possible optic nerve damage, and may enhance the establishment of secondary ocular infections due to bacteria, fungi, or viruses. Kaposi's sarcoma reported. Not recommended in optic neuritis treatment. Drug-induced secondary adrenocortical insufficiency may be minimized by gradual dose reduction. Enhanced effect in patients w/ hypothyroidism and cirrhosis. May decrease bone formation and increase bone resorption, and may lead to inhibition of bone growth in pediatric patients and development of osteoporosis at any age; caution w/ increased risk of osteoporosis. Acute myopathy w/ high doses reported, most often in patients w/ neuromuscular transmission disorders (eg, myasthenia gravis). Psychiatric derangements may appear and existing emotional instability or psychotic tendencies may be aggravated. Elevation of creatine kinase (CK) may occur. May elevate IOP; monitor IOP if used for >6 weeks. May suppress reactions to skin tests.

ADVERSE REACTIONS
Anaphylactoid reactions, HTN, osteoporosis, muscle weakness, menstrual irregularities, insomnia, impaired wound healing, ulcerative esophagitis, increased sweating, decreased carbohydrate tolerance, glaucoma, weight gain, nausea, malaise, anemia.

DRUG INTERACTIONS
Live or live, attenuated vaccines are contraindicated w/ immunosuppressive doses. Killed or inactivated vaccines may be administered; however, response to such vaccines may be diminished and cannot be predicted. May diminish response to toxoids and live or inactivated vaccines. Defer routine administration of vaccines or toxoids until corticosteroid therapy is discontinued, if possible. Closely monitor for hypokalemia when administered w/ K⁺-depleting agents (eg, amphotericin B, diuretics). Reports of cardiac enlargement and CHF following concomitant use of amphotericin B and hydrocortisone. Macrolide antibiotics may decrease clearance. Concomitant use w/ anticholinesterase agents (eg, neostigmine, pyridostigmine) may produce severe weakness in myasthenia gravis patients; d/c anticholinesterase agents at least 24 hrs before start of therapy. May inhibit response to warfarin; frequently monitor coagulation indices. May increase blood glucose levels; dose adjustment of antidiabetic agents may be required. May decrease serum concentration of isoniazid. Extreme caution w/ bupropion; employ low initial dosing and small gradual increases. Cholestyramine may increase clearance. Increased activity of both drugs may occur w/ cyclosporine; convulsions reported w/ concurrent use. May increase risk of arrhythmias due to hypokalemia w/ digitalis glycosides. Estrogens, including oral contraceptives, may decrease hepatic metabolism and increase effect. Increased risk of tendon rupture, especially in elderly, w/ concomitant fluoroquinolones. CYP3A4 inducers (eg, barbiturates, phenytoin, carbamazepine, rifampin) may enhance metabolism and may require increase in corticosteroid dose. CYP3A4 inhibitors (eg, ketoconazole, ritonavir, macrolide antibiotics such as erythromycin) may increase plasma levels. May increase clearance of other drugs that are metabolized by CYP3A4 (eg, indinavir, erythromycin), resulting in decreased plasma levels. Increased risk of corticosteroid side effects w/ ketoconazole. Aspirin (ASA) or other NSAIDs may increase risk of GI side effects. Caution w/ ASA in hypoprothrombinemia patients. May increase clearance of salicylates. Decreased therapeutic effect w/ phenytoin. Increased doses of quetiapine may be required to maintain control of schizophrenia symptoms. Caution w/ thalidomide; toxic epidermal necrolysis reported w/ concomitant use. Acute myopathy reported w/ neuromuscular blocking drugs (eg, pancuronium).

PREGNANCY AND LACTATION
Pregnancy: Category C. Infants born to mothers who have received substantial doses of corticosteroids during pregnancy should be carefully observed for signs of hypoadrenalism.
Lactation: Systemically administered corticosteroids appear in human milk and could suppress growth, interfere with endogenous corticosteroid production, or cause other untoward effects. Not for use in nursing.

MECHANISM OF ACTION
Glucocorticoid; causes profound and varied metabolic effects and modifies the body's immune responses to diverse stimuli.

PHARMACOKINETICS
Absorption: Readily absorbed (GI tract). **Distribution:** Found in breast milk (systemically administered).

PATIENT CONSIDERATIONS
Assessment: Assess for hypersensitivity to drug, CHF, HTN, renal impairment, systemic fungal infections, other current infections, active TB, latent/active amebiasis, cerebral malaria, active ocular herpes simplex, emotional instability or psychotic tendencies, recent MI, vaccination history, thyroid status, any other conditions where treatment is cautioned, pregnancy/nursing status, and for possible drug interactions.

Monitoring: Monitor for anaphylactoid reactions, HPA axis suppression, adrenocortical insufficiency, salt/water retention, infections, change in thyroid status, cataracts, glaucoma, Kaposi's sarcoma, emotional instability or psychotic tendencies aggravation, and other adverse reactions. Monitor IOP, BP, CK, and serum electrolytes. Monitor growth and development of infants/children on prolonged therapy. Frequently monitor coagulation indices w/ warfarin.

Counseling: Instruct not to d/c therapy abruptly or w/o medical supervision. Instruct to inform any medical attendants of intake of corticosteroids and to seek medical advice at once if fever or other signs of infection develop. Advise to avoid exposure to chickenpox or measles; instruct to seek medical advice w/o delay if exposed.

PREMARIN TABLETS — conjugated estrogens   Rx
Class: Estrogen

> Estrogens increase the risk of endometrial cancer. Perform adequate diagnostic measures, including endometrial sampling, to rule out malignancy in postmenopausal women w/ undiagnosed persistent or recurring abnormal genital bleeding. Should not be used for the prevention of cardiovascular (CV) disease or dementia. Increased risks of MI, stroke, invasive breast cancer, pulmonary embolism (PE), and deep vein thrombosis (DVT) in postmenopausal women (50-79 yrs of age) reported. Increased risk of developing probable dementia in postmenopausal women ≥65 yrs of age reported. Should be prescribed at the lowest effective dose and for the shortest duration consistent w/ treatment goals and risks.

ADULT DOSAGE
Postmenopausal Osteoporosis
Prevention:
Initial: 0.3mg qd continuously or cyclically (eg, 25 days on, 5 days off)
Titrate: Adjust subsequent dose based on clinical and bone mineral density responses

Use lowest effective dose and for the shortest duration consistent w/ treatment goals and risk

Menopausal Vasomotor Symptoms
Moderate to Severe:
Initial: 0.3mg/day continuously or cyclically (eg, 25 days on followed by 5 days off)
Titrate: Subsequent dose adjustment may be made based on response

Use lowest effective dose for the shortest duration; reevaluate periodically

Menopausal Vulvar/Vaginal Atrophy
Moderate to Severe:
Initial: 0.3mg/day continuously or cyclically (eg, 25 days on followed by 5 days off)
Titrate: Subsequent dose adjustment may be made based on response

Use lowest effective dose for the shortest duration; reevaluate periodically

Hypoestrogenism
Female Hypogonadism:
0.3 or 0.625mg qd cyclically (eg, 3 weeks on and 1 week off)
Titrate: Adjust dose based on severity of symptoms and response of the endometrium

Female Castration/Primary Ovarian Failure:
Usual: 1.25mg qd cyclically
Titrate: Adjust dose based on severity of symptoms and response

Use lowest effective dose and for the shortest duration consistent w/ treatment goals and risk

Metastatic Breast Cancer
Palliative Treatment in Appropriately Selected Women and Men:
10mg tid for a minimum of 3 months

Use lowest effective dose and for the shortest duration consistent w/ treatment goals and risk

Prostate Carcinoma
Palliative Treatment of Advanced Androgen-Dependent Carcinoma:
1.25-2.5mg (two 1.25mg tabs) tid

Use lowest effective dose and for the shortest duration consistent w/ treatment goals and risk

PEDIATRIC DOSAGE
Pediatric use may not have been established

ADMINISTRATION
Oral route
May take w/o regard to meals.

STORAGE
20-25°C (68-77°F); excursions permitted to 15-30°C (59-86°F).

HOW SUPPLIED
Tab: 0.3mg, 0.45mg, 0.625mg, 0.9mg, 1.25mg

CONTRAINDICATIONS
Undiagnosed abnormal genital bleeding; known/suspected/history of breast cancer except in appropriately selected patients being treated for metastatic disease; known/suspected estrogen-dependent neoplasia; active/history of DVT/PE/arterial thromboembolic disease (eg, stroke, MI); known anaphylactic reaction/

angioedema w/ conjugated estrogens; liver impairment/disease; known protein C, protein S, antithrombin deficiency, or other known thrombophilic disorders; known/suspected pregnancy.

WARNINGS/PRECAUTIONS

D/C immediately if stroke, DVT, PE, and MI occurs or is suspected. Caution in patients w/ risk factors for arterial vascular disease and/or venous thromboembolism. If feasible, d/c at least 4-6 weeks before surgery of the type associated w/ an increased risk of thromboembolism, or during periods of prolonged immobilization. May increase risk of ovarian cancer and gallbladder disease requiring surgery. May lead to severe hypercalcemia in patients w/ breast cancer and bone metastases; d/c and take appropriate measures if hypercalcemia occurs. Retinal vascular thrombosis reported; if visual abnormalities or migraine occurs, d/c therapy pending examination. If examination reveals papilledema or retinal vascular lesions, d/c permanently. Anaphylaxis and angioedema involving tongue, larynx, face, hands, and feet requiring medical intervention reported; d/c if anaphylactic reaction w/ or w/o angioedema occurs. Cases of malignant transformation of residual endometrial implants reported in women treated post-hysterectomy w/ estrogen-alone therapy; consider addition of progestin for women known to have residual endometriosis post-hysterectomy. May elevate BP and thyroid-binding globulin levels. May elevate plasma TGs leading to pancreatitis in patients w/ preexisting hypertriglyceridemia; consider discontinuation if pancreatitis occurs. Caution w/ history of cholestatic jaundice associated w/ past estrogen use or w/ pregnancy; d/c in case of recurrence. May cause fluid retention; caution w/ cardiac/renal dysfunction. Caution w/ hypoparathyroidism; estrogen-induced hypocalcemia may occur. May exacerbate symptoms of angioedema in women w/ hereditary angioedema. May exacerbate asthma, diabetes mellitus, epilepsy, migraine, porphyria, systemic lupus erythematosus, and hepatic hemangiomas; use w/ caution. May affect certain endocrine and blood components in lab tests.

ADVERSE REACTIONS

Abdominal pain, asthenia, back pain, headache, pain, depression, insomnia, dizziness, leukorrhea, breast pain, vaginal hemorrhage, vaginitis, flatulence, nausea, weight gain.

DRUG INTERACTIONS

CYP3A4 inducers (eg, St. John's wort, phenobarbital, carbamazepine, rifampin) may decrease levels, which may decrease therapeutic effects and/or change uterine bleeding profile. CYP3A4 inhibitors (eg, erythromycin, clarithromycin, ketoconazole) may increase levels, which may result in side effects. Women concomitantly receiving thyroid hormone replacement therapy may require increased doses of their thyroid replacement therapy; monitor thyroid function.

PREGNANCY AND LACTATION

Pregnancy: Contraindicated in pregnancy.
Lactation: Not for use in nursing.

MECHANISM OF ACTION

Estrogen; binds to nuclear receptors in estrogen-responsive tissues. Circulating estrogens modulate pituitary secretion of gonadotropins, luteinizing hormone, and follicle-stimulating hormone, through a negative feedback mechanism. Reduces elevated levels of these hormones in postmenopausal women.

PHARMACOKINETICS

Absorption: Administration of variable doses resulted in different parameters. **Distribution:** Largely bound to sex hormone-binding globulin and albumin; found in breast milk. **Metabolism:** Liver to estrone; estriol (major urinary metabolite); sulfate and glucuronide conjugation (liver); biliary secretion of conjugates into the intestine; hydrolysis; reabsorption. **Elimination:** Urine (parent compound and metabolites).

PATIENT CONSIDERATIONS

Assessment: Assess for undiagnosed abnormal genital bleeding, estrogen-dependent neoplasia, presence or history of breast cancer, active/history of DVT/PE/arterial thromboembolic disease, thrombophilic disorders, pregnancy/nursing status, any other conditions where treatment is contraindicated or cautioned, need for progestin therapy, and possible drug interactions.

Monitoring: Monitor for signs/symptoms of CV events, malignant neoplasms, dementia, gallbladder disease, hypercalcemia, visual abnormalities, anaphylaxis, angioedema, BP and serum TG elevations, fluid retention, exacerbation of endometriosis and other conditions, and other adverse reactions. Perform annual breast exam; schedule mammography based on age, risk factors, and prior mammogram results. Monitor thyroid function in women on thyroid replacement therapy. In cases of undiagnosed persistent or recurring genital bleeding, perform adequate diagnostic measures (eg, endometrial sampling) to rule out malignancies. Periodically reevaluate to determine the need of therapy.

Counseling: Inform of the risks/benefits of therapy. Inform of the importance of reporting vaginal bleeding to physician as soon as possible. Inform of possible serious adverse reactions and of possible less serious but common adverse reactions of estrogen therapy.

PREMARIN VAGINAL — conjugated estrogens   Rx

Class: Estrogen

Increased risk of endometrial cancer in a woman w/ a uterus who uses unopposed estrogens. Adding a progestin to estrogen therapy reduces the risk of endometrial hyperplasia. Adequate diagnostic measures (eg, directed or random endometrial sampling) should be undertaken to rule out malignancy in postmenopausal women w/ undiagnosed, persistent or recurring abnormal genital bleeding. Should not be used for the prevention of cardiovascular disease (CVD) or dementia. Increased risk of stroke and deep vein thrombosis (DVT) reported in postmenopausal women (50-79 yrs of age) treated w/ daily oral conjugated estrogens (CEs) alone and when combined w/ medroxyprogesterone acetate (MPA). Increased risk of developing probable dementia reported in postmenopausal women ≥65 yrs of age treated w/ daily CEs alone and when combined w/ MPA. Increased risks of pulmonary embolism (PE), MI, and invasive breast cancer reported in postmenopausal women (50-79 yrs of age) treated w/ daily oral CEs combined w/ MPA. Should be prescribed at the lowest effective dose and for the shortest duration consistent w/ treatment goals and risks.

ADULT DOSAGE

Atrophic Vaginitis and Kraurosis Vulvae

Initial: 0.5g intravaginally in a cyclic regimen (daily for 21 days, and then off for 7 days)
Titrate: Dose adjustments (0.5-2g) may be made based on individual response

Dyspareunia

Moderate to Severe Dyspareunia Due to Menopause:
0.5g intravaginally 2X/week (eg, Monday and Thursday) continuously or in a cyclic regimen (21 days of therapy followed by 7 days off of therapy)

PEDIATRIC DOSAGE

Pediatric use may not have been established

ADMINISTRATION

Intravaginal route

STORAGE

20-25°C (68-77°F); excursions permitted to 15-30°C (59-86°F).

HOW SUPPLIED

Vaginal Cre: 0.625mg/g [30g]

CONTRAINDICATIONS

Undiagnosed abnormal genital bleeding; known/suspected/history of breast cancer; known/suspected estrogen-dependent neoplasia; active or history of DVT/PE; active or history of arterial thromboembolic disease (eg, stroke, MI); known anaphylactic reaction or angioedema to CEs vaginal cream; known liver dysfunction/disease; known protein C, protein S, or antithrombin deficiency or other known thrombophilic disorders; known/suspected pregnancy.

WARNINGS/PRECAUTIONS

Systemic absorption reported. D/C therapy immediately if stroke, DVT, PE, or MI occurs or is suspected. Caution in patients w/ risk factors for arterial vascular disease and/or venous thromboembolism. If feasible, d/c at least 4-6 weeks before surgery of the type associated w/ an increased risk of thromboembolism, or during periods of prolonged immobilization. May increase risk of gallbladder disease requiring surgery and risk of ovarian cancer. May lead to severe hypercalcemia in patients w/ breast cancer and bone metastases; d/c and take appropriate measures if hypercalcemia occurs. Retinal vascular thrombosis reported; d/c therapy pending examination if sudden partial/complete loss of vision or sudden onset of proptosis, diplopia, or migraine occurs. If examination reveals papilledema or retinal vascular lesions, d/c therapy permanently. May elevate BP and thyroid-binding globulin levels. May be associated w/ elevations of plasma TGs, leading to pancreatitis in patients w/ preexisting hypertriglyceridemia; consider discontinuation if pancreatitis occurs. Caution w/ history of cholestatic jaundice associated w/ past estrogen use or pregnancy; d/c in case of recurrence. May cause fluid retention. Caution in patients w/ hypoparathyroidism; estrogen-induced hypocalcemia may occur. Cases of malignant transformation of residual endometrial implants reported in women treated posthysterectomy w/ estrogen-alone therapy; consider addition of progestin for these patients. Anaphylaxis and angioedema reported w/ orally administered Premarin. May exacerbate symptoms of angioedema in women w/ hereditary angioedema. May exacerbate asthma, diabetes mellitus (DM), epilepsy, migraine, porphyria, systemic lupus erythematosus, and hepatic hemangiomas; use w/ caution. May weaken latex condoms; consider potential for CEs vaginal cream to weaken and contribute to the failure of condoms, diaphragms, or cervical caps made of latex or rubber. May affect certain endocrine function tests, HDL, LDL, TG levels, and blood components in lab tests. Consider addition of progestin for postmenopausal women w/ a uterus to reduce the risk of endometrial cancer.

ADVERSE REACTIONS

Headache, pelvic pain, vasodilation, breast pain, leukorrhea, vaginitis, vulvovaginal disorder.

DRUG INTERACTIONS

CYP3A4 inducers (eg, St. John's wort preparations, phenobarbital, carbamazepine) may decrease levels, which may result in a decrease in therapeutic effects and/or changes in the uterine bleeding profile. CYP3A4 inhibitors (eg, erythromycin, ketoconazole, grapefruit juice) may increase levels and may result in side effects. Patients dependent on thyroid hormone replacement therapy who are also receiving estrogens may require increased doses of thyroid replacement therapy; monitor thyroid function.

PREGNANCY AND LACTATION

Pregnancy: Contraindicated in pregnancy.
Lactation: Not for use in nursing. Estrogen administration to nursing women has been shown to decrease the quantity and quality of breast milk. Found in breast milk.

MECHANISM OF ACTION

Estrogen; binds to nuclear receptors in estrogen-responsive tissues. Circulating estrogens modulate pituitary secretion of the gonadotropins, luteinizing hormone, and follicle-stimulating hormone, through a (-) feedback mechanism. Reduces elevated levels of these hormones in postmenopausal women.

PHARMACOKINETICS

Absorption: Refer to PI for conjugated and unconjugated estrogen parameters.
Distribution: Largely bound to sex hormone-binding globulin and albumin; found in breast milk. **Metabolism:** Liver to estrone (metabolite); estriol (major urinary metabolite); enterohepatic recirculation via sulfate and glucuronide conjugation

in the liver, biliary secretion of conjugates into the intestine; hydrolysis in the intestine; reabsorption; CYP3A4 (partial metabolism). **Elimination:** Urine (parent compound and metabolites).

PATIENT CONSIDERATIONS

Assessment: Assess for abnormal genital bleeding, estrogen-dependent neoplasia, presence/history of breast cancer, arterial thromboembolic disease, DVT/PE, hereditary angioedema, previous hypersensitivity, thrombophilic disorders, or any other conditions where treatment is contraindicated or cautioned. Assess use in women ≥65 yrs of age and in those w/ DM, asthma, epilepsy, migraines or porphyria, SLE, or hepatic hemangiomas. Assess for cardiac or renal dysfunction, pregnancy/nursing status, need for progestin therapy, and possible drug interactions.

Monitoring: Monitor for signs/symptoms of cardiovascular events, malignant neoplasms, dementia, gallbladder disease, hypercalcemia, visual abnormalities, pancreatitis, hypertriglyceridemia, cholestatic jaundice, hypothyroidism, fluid retention, exacerbation of endometriosis and other conditions. Perform annual breast exam; schedule mammography based on age, risk factors, and prior mammogram results. Regularly monitor BP, thyroid function in women on thyroid replacement therapy, and periodically evaluate to determine need for treatment. Perform adequate diagnostic measures (eg, endometrial sampling) to rule out malignancies if undiagnosed persistent or recurring genital bleeding occurs.

Counseling: Advise to notify physician if signs/symptoms of unusual vaginal bleeding occur. Inform about possible serious adverse reactions (eg, CVD, malignant neoplasms, and probable dementia) and possible less serious but common adverse reactions (eg, headache, breast pain/tenderness, N/V). Instruct to perform monthly breast self-examination. Inform that medication may weaken barrier contraceptives (eg, latex or rubber condoms, diaphragms, cervical caps).

PREMPHASE — conjugated estrogens/medroxyprogesterone acetate

Rx

Class: Estrogen/progestogen combination

> Estrogens increase the risk of endometrial cancer. Perform adequate diagnostic measures, including endometrial sampling, to rule out malignancy in postmenopausal women w/ undiagnosed persistent or recurring abnormal genital bleeding. Should not be used for the prevention of cardiovascular disease (CVD) or dementia. Increased risk of MI, stroke, invasive breast cancer, PE, and DVT in postmenopausal women (50-79 yrs of age) reported. Increased risk of developing probable dementia in postmenopausal women ≥65 yrs of age reported. Should be prescribed at the lowest effective dose and for the shortest duration consistent w/ treatment goals and risks.

OTHER BRAND NAMES
Prempro

ADULT DOSAGE

Menopausal Vasomotor Symptoms

Moderate to Severe:
Prempro:
1 tab qd

Premphase:
Days 1-14: One maroon 0.625mg conjugated estrogens (CE) tab qd
Days 15-28: One light-blue tab containing 0.625mg CE and 5mg medroxyprogesterone acetate qd

Use lowest effective dose for the shortest duration; reevaluate periodically

Menopausal Vulvar/Vaginal Atrophy

Moderate to Severe:
Prempro:
1 tab qd

Premphase:
Days 1-14: One maroon 0.625mg conjugated estrogens (CE) tab qd
Days 15-28: One light-blue tab containing 0.625mg CE and 5mg medroxyprogesterone acetate qd

Use lowest effective dose for the shortest duration; reevaluate periodically

Postmenopausal Osteoporosis

Prevention:
Prempro:
1 tab qd

Premphase:
Days 1-14: One maroon 0.625mg conjugated estrogens (CE) tab qd
Days 15-28: One light-blue tab containing 0.625mg CE and 5mg medroxyprogesterone acetate qd

Use lowest effective dose for the shortest duration; reevaluate periodically

PEDIATRIC DOSAGE
Pediatric use may not have been established

ADMINISTRATION
Oral route

STORAGE
20-25°C (68-77°F); excursions permitted to 15-30°C (59-86°F).

HOW SUPPLIED
Tab: (Premphase) (Conjugated Estrogens [CE]) 0.625mg, (CE/Medroxyprogesterone) 0.625mg/5mg; (Prempro) (CE/Medroxyprogesterone) 0.3mg/1.5mg, 0.45mg/1.5mg, 0.625mg/2.5mg, 0.625mg/5mg

CONTRAINDICATIONS
Undiagnosed abnormal genital bleeding; known/suspected/history of breast cancer; known/suspected estrogen-dependent neoplasia; active or history of DVT/PE/arterial thromboembolic disease (eg, stroke, MI); known anaphylactic reaction/angioedema to Prempro/Premphase; known liver dysfunction/disease; known protein C, protein S, antithrombin deficiency, or other known thrombophilic disorders; known/suspected pregnancy.

WARNINGS/PRECAUTIONS
D/C immediately if PE, DVT, stroke, or MI occurs or is suspected. If feasible, d/c at least 4-6 weeks before surgery of the type associated w/ an increased risk of thromboembolism, or during periods of prolonged immobilization. May increase risk of ovarian cancer. May increase risk of gallbladder disease requiring surgery. May lead to severe hypercalcemia in patients w/ breast cancer and bone metastases; d/c and take appropriate measures if hypercalcemia occurs. Retinal vascular thrombosis reported; d/c therapy pending examination if sudden partial/complete loss of vision or sudden onset of proptosis, diplopia, or migraine occurs. D/C permanently if examination reveals papilledema or retinal vascular lesions. May increase BP and thyroid-binding globulin levels. May be associated w/ elevations of plasma TGs; consider discontinuation if pancreatitis occurs. Caution w/ history of cholestatic jaundice associated w/ past estrogen use or w/ pregnancy; d/c in case of recurrence. May cause fluid retention. Caution w/ hypoparathyroidism; hypocalcemia may occur. Anaphylaxis and angioedema reported. May exacerbate symptoms of angioedema in women w/ hereditary angioedema. May exacerbate endometriosis, asthma, diabetes mellitus, epilepsy, migraine, porphyria, systemic lupus erythematosus, and hepatic hemangiomas. May affect certain endocrine and blood components in lab tests.

ADVERSE REACTIONS
Headache, breast pain, abdominal pain, back pain, depression, nausea, flatulence, peripheral edema, weight gain, pruritus, breast enlargement, dysmenorrhea, leukorrhea, vaginitis, asthenia.

DRUG INTERACTIONS
CYP3A4 inducers (eg, St. John's wort, phenobarbital, carbamazepine) may decrease levels, which may decrease therapeutic effects and/or cause changes in the uterine bleeding profile. CYP3A4 inhibitors (eg, erythromycin, ketoconazole, grapefruit juice) may increase levels and may result in side effects. Aminoglutethimide may significantly depress bioavailability of medroxyprogesterone acetate (MPA). Patients concomitantly receiving thyroid hormone replacement therapy and estrogens may require increased doses of their thyroid replacement therapy; monitor thyroid function.

PREGNANCY AND LACTATION
Contraindicated in pregnancy, not for use in nursing.

MECHANISM OF ACTION
CE: Estrogen; binds to nuclear receptors in estrogen-responsive tissues. Reduces elevated levels of gonadotropins, luteinizing hormone and follicle-stimulating hormone, in postmenopausal women. MPA: Progesterone derivative; parenterally administered MPA inhibits gonadotropin production, which prevents follicular maturation and ovulation.

PHARMACOKINETICS
Absorption: Well-absorbed. Administration of variable doses resulted in different parameters. **Distribution:** Found in breast milk. CE: Largely bound to sex hormone-binding globulin and albumin. MPA: Plasma protein binding (approx 90%). **Metabolism:** CE: Liver to estrone (metabolite) and estriol (major urinary metabolite); enterohepatic recirculation via sulfate and glucuronide conjugation in the liver; biliary secretion of conjugates into the intestine; hydrolysis in the intestine; reabsorption. MPA: Liver via hydroxylation, w/ subsequent conjugation. **Elimination:** CE: Urine (parent compound and metabolites). MPA: Urine (metabolites).

PATIENT CONSIDERATIONS

Assessment: Assess for abnormal genital bleeding, presence/history of breast cancer, estrogen-dependent neoplasia, active or history of DVT/PE/arterial thromboembolic disease, liver dysfunction/disease, thrombophilic disorders, known anaphylactic reaction or angioedema to the drug, cardiac or renal dysfunction, other conditions where treatment is contraindicated or cautioned, pregnancy/nursing status, and possible drug interactions.

Monitoring: Monitor for signs/symptoms of CVD, malignant neoplasms, dementia, gallbladder disease, hypercalcemia, visual abnormalities, BP and plasma TG elevations, pancreatitis, cholestatic jaundice, hypothyroidism, fluid retention, anaphylaxis, angioedema, exacerbation of endometriosis, and for other adverse reactions. Perform annual breast examinations; schedule mammography based on patient age, risk factors, and prior mammogram results. Perform adequate diagnostic measures (eg, endometrial sampling) in patients w/ undiagnosed persistent or recurring genital bleeding. Perform periodic evaluation to determine treatment need.

Counseling: Inform of the importance of reporting abnormal vaginal bleeding to physician as soon as possible. Advise of possible serious adverse reactions of therapy (eg, CVD, malignant neoplasms, probable dementia) and of possible less serious but common adverse reactions (eg, headache, breast pain and tenderness, N/V). Instruct to have yearly breast examinations by a healthcare provider and to perform monthly breast self-examinations.

PRENATE AM — calcium carbonate/folic acid/ginger extract/lingonberry/vitamin B6 (pyridoxine hydrochloride)/vitamin B12 (cyanocobalamin)

Rx

Class: Prenatal vitamin

> Concomitant use of ginger in patients with bleeding disorders, or who are on anticoagulant or antiplatelet therapy, may increase the risk of bleeding. Folic acid alone is improper therapy in the treatment of pernicious anemia and other megaloblastic anemias where vitamin B12 is deficient. Folic acid >0.1mg/day may obscure pernicious anemia; hematologic remission may occur while neurological manifestations progress. Consider medical condition and any drugs, herbs and/or supplements consumption when prescribing.

ADULT DOSAGE	PEDIATRIC DOSAGE
Dietary/Nutritional Supplement	Pediatric use may not have been established
1 tab qd or ud	

ADMINISTRATION
Oral route

STORAGE
20-25°C (68-77°F); excursions permitted to 15-30°C (59-86°F).

HOW SUPPLIED
Tab: Pyridoxine HCl 75mg-Cyanocobalamin 12mcg-Calcium carbonate 200mg-Folic acid 1mg-Ginger extract 500mg-Lingonberry 25mg

DRUG INTERACTIONS
See Boxed Warning.

MECHANISM OF ACTION
Prenatal vitamins/minerals.

PATIENT CONSIDERATIONS
Assessment: Assess for bleeding disorders, pernicious anemia, other megaloblastic anemias, and possible drug interactions.

Monitoring: Monitor for masking of pernicious anemia and other adverse reactions.

Counseling: Instruct to take ud.

PREPOPIK — anhydrous citric acid/magnesium oxide/sodium picosulfate

Rx

Class: Bowel cleanser

ADULT DOSAGE
Bowel Cleansing

Prior to Colonoscopy:
Split-Dose Regimen (Preferred Method):
1st Dose: Take during the pm before colonoscopy (eg, 5-9 pm), followed by five 8-oz drinks (upper line on dosing cup) of clear liquids hs. Consume clear liquids w/in 5 hrs
2nd Dose: Take the next day, approx 5 hrs before colonoscopy, followed by at least three 8-oz drinks of clear liquids before the colonoscopy. Consume clear liquids w/in 5 hrs up until 2 hrs before time of the colonoscopy

Day-Before Regimen (Alternative Method):
1st Dose: Take in afternoon or early pm (eg, 4-6 pm) before colonoscopy, followed by five 8-oz drinks of clear liquids before next dose. Consume clear liquids w/in 5 hrs
2nd Dose: Take approx 6 hrs later in the late pm (eg, 10 pm-12 am) the night before colonoscopy, followed by three 8-oz drinks of clear liquids hs. Consume clear liquids w/in 5 hrs

PEDIATRIC DOSAGE
Pediatric use may not have been established

DOSING CONSIDERATIONS
Adverse Reactions
Severe Bloating/Distention/Abdominal Pain Following 1st Dose: Delay 2nd dose until symptoms resolve

ADMINISTRATION
Oral route

Only clear liquids (no solid food or milk) should be consumed on the day before the colonoscopy up until 2 hrs before the time of the colonoscopy.

Reconstitution
1. Reconstitute the powder right before each administration; do not prepare sol in advance.

2. Fill the supplied dosing cup w/ cold water up to the lower (5 oz) line on the cup and pour in the contents of 1 pkt of powder.
3. Stir for 2-3 min; reconstituted sol may become slightly warm as the powder dissolves.

STORAGE
25°C (77°F); excursions permitted to 15-30°C (59-86°F).

HOW SUPPLIED
Sol (Powder): (Sodium Picosulfate/Magnesium Oxide/Anhydrous Citric Acid) 10mg/3.5g/12g [16.1g, 16.2g]

CONTRAINDICATIONS
Severely reduced renal function (CrCl <30mL/min); GI obstruction or ileus, bowel perforation; toxic colitis or toxic megacolon; gastric retention; allergy to any of the ingredients in the product.

WARNINGS/PRECAUTIONS
May cause fluid/electrolyte disturbances, arrhythmias, and generalized tonic-clonic seizures; correct fluid and electrolyte abnormalities prior to treatment. Caution with CHF when replacing fluids. If vomiting or signs of dehydration (including signs of orthostatic hypotension) develop after treatment, perform postcolonoscopy lab tests (eg, electrolytes, SrCr, BUN) and treat accordingly. Caution with patients at risk of seizure (eg, known/suspected hyponatremia). Caution with impaired renal function and severe active ulcerative colitis. May produce colonic mucosal aphthous ulceration. Serious cases of ischemic colitis reported. Caution in patients prone to regurgitation/aspiration or with impaired gag reflex. Direct ingestion of undissolved powder may increase risk of N/V, dehydration, and electrolyte disturbance. Rule out GI obstruction/perforation before administration.

ADVERSE REACTIONS
Headache, N/V.

DRUG INTERACTIONS
Increased risk of colonic mucosal aphthous ulceration with stimulant laxatives. Caution with drugs that increase the risk of fluid and electrolyte abnormalities, drugs that affect renal function (eg, diuretics, ACE inhibitors, ARBs, NSAIDs), drugs associated with hypokalemia (eg, corticosteroid, cardiac glycosides) or hyponatremia, drugs that lower seizure threshold (eg, TCAs), drugs known to induce antidiuretic hormone secretion (eg, SSRIs, antipsychotics, carbamazepine), and in patients withdrawing from alcohol or benzodiazepines. Caution with drugs that increase the risk for arrhythmias and prolonged QT in the setting of fluid and electrolyte abnormalities. Oral medications given within 1 hr of administration may be flushed from GI tract and may not be absorbed. Take tetracycline and fluoroquinolone antibiotics, iron, digoxin, chlorpromazine, and penicillamine at least 2 hrs before and not <6 hrs after administration. Reduced efficacy with antibiotics.

PREGNANCY AND LACTATION
Pregnancy: Category B.
Lactation: Caution in nursing.

MECHANISM OF ACTION
Bowel cleanser: Stimulant and osmotic laxative; produces a purgative effect that produces watery diarrhea.

PHARMACOKINETICS
Absorption: Sodium Picosulfate: C_{max}=3.2ng/mL, T_{max}=7 hrs. Mg^{2+}: (Post-initial pkt) C_{max}=1.9mEq/L, T_{max}=10 hrs. **Metabolism:** Sodium Picosulfate: intestinal bacteria to bis-(p-hydroxy-phenyl)-pyridyl-2-methane (active metabolite). **Elimination:** Sodium Picosulfate; Urine (0.19% unchanged), $T_{1/2}$=7.4 hrs.

PATIENT CONSIDERATIONS
Assessment: Assess for previous hypersensitivity to any of the components, electrolyte abnormalities, risk for arrhythmias, CHF, risk/history of seizures, renal impairment, ileus, GI obstruction/perforation, gastric retention, toxic colitis/megacolon, ulcerative colitis, impaired gag reflex, regurgitation or aspiration tendencies, pregnancy/nursing status, and possible drug interactions. Perform predose lab tests (eg, electrolytes, SrCr, BUN) and ECG.

Monitoring: Monitor for fluid/electrolyte disturbances, arrhythmias, seizures, GI ulceration, colitis, bloating, abdominal distention/pain, and other adverse reactions. Perform postcolonoscopy lab tests and ECG.

Counseling: Advise to adequately hydrate before, during, and after use. Instruct not to take other laxatives during therapy. Inform patients that if they experience severe bloating, distention or abdominal pain following the 1st pkt, delay the 2nd administration until the symptoms resolve. Instruct patients to contact their healthcare provider if they develop signs/symptoms of dehydration, have trouble swallowing, or are prone to regurgitation or aspiration. Inform that product is not for direct ingestion.

PRESTALIA — amlodipine/perindopril arginine

Rx

Class: ACE inhibitor/calcium channel blocker (CCB) (dihydropyridine)

> D/C as soon as possible when pregnancy is detected. Drugs that act directly on the renin-angiotensin system (RAS) can cause injury/death to the developing fetus.

ADULT DOSAGE	PEDIATRIC DOSAGE
Hypertension	Pediatric use may not have been established
In Patients Inadequately Controlled w/ Monotherapy or as Initial Therapy in Patients Who Require Multiple Drugs to Achieve BP Goals:	
Initial: 3.5mg/2.5mg qd	
Titrate: Adjust based on BP goals; wait 7-14 days between titration steps	
Max: 14mg/10mg qd	

DOSING CONSIDERATIONS
Renal Impairment
CrCl <60mL/min: Not recommended
Hepatic Impairment
Not recommended
Elderly
Not recommended in patients >65 yrs
ADMINISTRATION
Oral route

Take w/ or w/o food.
STORAGE
25°C (77°F); excursions permitted to 15-30°C (59-86°F). Protect from moisture.
HOW SUPPLIED
Tab: (Perindopril/Amlodipine) 3.5mg/2.5mg, 7mg/5mg, 14mg/10mg
CONTRAINDICATIONS
Hereditary or idiopathic angioedema, w/ or w/o previous ACE inhibitor treatment; hypersensitivity to perindopril, to any other ACE inhibitor, or to amlodipine. Coadministration w/ aliskiren in patients w/ diabetes.
WARNINGS/PRECAUTIONS
Not recommended w/ heart failure (HF). Worsening angina and acute MI may develop after starting or increasing the dose, particularly w/ severe obstructive coronary artery disease (CAD). Symptomatic hypotension may occur and is most likely to occur in patients w/ volume/salt depletion as a result of prolonged diuretic therapy, dietary salt restriction, dialysis, diarrhea, or vomiting. Closely monitor patients at risk for excessive hypotension; follow patients closely during the first 2 weeks of treatment and whenever dose is increased or a diuretic is added or its dose is increased. Patients w/ severe aortic stenosis may be more likely to experience symptomatic hypotension. Hypotension may occur w/ major surgery or during anesthesia; correct by volume expansion. May cause changes in renal function; consider withholding or discontinuing therapy in patients who develop a clinically significant decrease in renal function. **Perindopril:** Angioedema of the face, extremities, lips, tongue, glottis, or larynx reported; d/c and administer appropriate therapy. Intestinal angioedema reported. Higher incidence of angioedema in blacks than nonblacks. May cause hyperkalemia; risk factors include renal insufficiency and diabetes mellitus (DM). Persistent nonproductive cough reported; consider ACE inhibitor-induced cough in the differential diagnosis of cough.
ADVERSE REACTIONS
Peripheral edema, cough.
DRUG INTERACTIONS
See Contraindications. Patients taking concomitant mTOR inhibitor (eg, temsirolimus) therapy may be at increased risk for angioedema. **Perindopril:** May occasionally experience an excessive reduction of BP w/ diuretics after initiation of perindopril; closely monitor w/ the 1st dose of perindopril, for at least 2 hrs and until BP has stabilized for another hr. May attenuate K^+ loss caused by thiazide diuretics. Increased risk of hyperkalemia w/ K^+-sparing diuretics (eg, spironolactone, amiloride, triamterene), K^+ supplements, K^+-containing salt substitutes, or other drugs capable of increasing serum K^+ (eg, indomethacin, heparin, cyclosporine); frequently monitor serum K^+. Increased serum lithium levels and symptoms of lithium toxicity reported; frequently monitor serum lithium levels. Nitritoid reactions reported w/ injectable gold (sodium aurothiomalate). Coadministration w/ NSAIDs, including selective COX-2 inhibitors, may attenuate antihypertensive effect of perindopril, and in patients who are elderly, volume-depleted (including those on diuretic therapy), or w/ compromised renal function, coadministration may result in deterioration of renal function, including possible acute renal failure. Dual blockade of the RAS w/ ARBs, ACE inhibitors, or aliskiren is associated w/ increased risks of hypotension, hyperkalemia, and changes in renal function (including acute renal failure); avoid combined use of RAS inhibitors, or closely monitor BP, renal function, and electrolytes w/ concomitant agents that affect the RAS. Avoid w/ aliskiren in patients w/ renal impairment (GFR <60mL/min). **Amlodipine:** May increase simvastatin exposure; limit simvastatin dose to 20mg/day. May increase trough cyclosporine levels in renal transplant patients; frequently monitor trough blood levels of cyclosporine. Moderate CYP3A inhibitor diltiazem increases exposure. Strong CYP3A inhibitors (eg, itraconazole) may increase plasma concentrations; monitor for symptoms of hypotension and edema w/ moderate or strong CYP3A inhibitors to determine the need for dose adjustment.
PREGNANCY AND LACTATION
Pregnancy: Category D.
Lactation: Not for use in nursing.
MECHANISM OF ACTION
Perindopril: ACE inhibitor; inhibits ACE activity, resulting in decreased plasma angiotensin II, leading to decreased vasoconstriction, increased plasma renin activity, and decreased aldosterone secretion. **Amlodipine:** Dihydropyridine CCB; inhibits transmembrane influx of Ca^{2+} ions into vascular smooth muscle and cardiac muscle. Acts directly on vascular smooth muscle to cause a reduction in peripheral vascular resistance and reduction in BP.
PHARMACOKINETICS
Absorption: T_{max}=1 hr (perindopril), 4 hrs (perindoprilat), 6-12 hrs (amlodipine). Amlodipine: Absolute bioavailability (64-90%). **Distribution:** Amlodipine: Plasma protein binding (approx 93%). **Metabolism:** Perindopril: Hepatic (extensive); hydrolysis, glucuronidation, cyclization via dehydration; perindoprilat (active metabolite). Amlodipine: Liver (extensive). **Elimination:** $T_{1/2}$=1.3 hrs (perindopril), 100 hrs (perindoprilat), 30-50 hrs (amlodipine). Amlodipine: Urine (10% unchanged, 60% metabolites).

PATIENT CONSIDERATIONS
Assessment: Assess for hypersensitivity to the drug, hereditary or idiopathic angioedema, volume/salt depletion, HF, severe obstructive CAD, severe aortic stenosis, hepatic/renal impairment, DM, pregnancy/nursing status, and possible drug interactions.

Monitoring: Monitor for signs/symptoms of worsening angina, acute MI, anaphylactoid reactions, head/neck/intestinal angioedema, persistent nonproductive cough, and other adverse reactions. Monitor renal function, BP, and K^+ levels periodically.

Counseling: Advise of risks and benefits of therapy. Inform of pregnancy risks and discuss treatment options w/ women planning to become pregnant; advise to report pregnancy to physician as soon as possible. Instruct to resume the usual dose at the next scheduled time in case of a missed dose. Instruct to notify physician if any adverse reactions develop.

PREVACID — lansoprazole   Rx
Class: Proton pump inhibitor (PPI)
OTHER BRAND NAMES
Prevacid SoluTab

ADULT DOSAGE
Pathological Hypersecretory Conditions
Treatment Including Zollinger-Ellison Syndrome:

Initial: 60mg qd
Titrate: Individualize dose

Doses up to 90mg bid have been administered
Divide dose if >120mg/day
Active Duodenal Ulcer
Treatment:
15mg qd for 4 weeks
Maint of Healing of Duodenal Ulcer:
15mg qd
NSAID-Associated Gastric Ulcer
Healing:
30mg qd for 8 weeks
Risk Reduction:
15mg qd for up to 12 weeks
Helicobacter pylori Eradication
W/ Duodenal Ulcer Disease to Reduce the Risk of Duodenal Ulcer Recurrence:

Triple Therapy:
30mg cap + clarithromycin 500mg + amoxicillin 1000mg, all bid for 10 or 14 days
Dual Therapy:
Allergic/Intolerant/Resistant to Clarithromycin:
30mg cap + amoxicillin 1000mg, all tid w/ for 14 days
Gastroesophageal Reflux Disease
Symptomatic GERD:
15mg qd for up to 8 weeks
Treatment of Erosive Esophagitis:
30mg qd for up to 8 weeks; may give for 8 more weeks if healing does not occur
May consider an additional 8-week course if there is a recurrence of erosive esophagitis
Maint of Healing of Erosive Esophagitis:
15mg qd
Gastric Ulcers
Benign:
30mg qd for up to 8 weeks

PEDIATRIC DOSAGE
Gastroesophageal Reflux Disease
Symptomatic GERD:
1-11 Years:
≤30kg: 15mg qd for up to 12 weeks; may increase up to 30mg bid after ≥2 weeks if still symptomatic
>30kg: 30mg qd for up to 12 weeks; may increase up to 30mg bid after ≥2 weeks if still symptomatic
Symptomatic Nonerosive GERD:
12-17 Years:
15mg qd for up to 8 weeks
Treatment of Erosive Esophagitis:
1-11 Years:
≤30kg: 15mg qd for up to 12 weeks; may increase up to 30mg bid after ≥2 weeks if still symptomatic
>30kg: 30mg qd for up to 12 weeks; may increase up to 30mg bid after ≥2 weeks if still symptomatic
12-17 Years:
30mg qd for up to 8 weeks

DOSING CONSIDERATIONS
Hepatic Impairment
Severe: Consider dose adjustment
ADMINISTRATION
Oral route

Take ac.
Cap
Swallow whole; do not crush or chew.
If trouble swallowing, may sprinkle intact granules on 1 tbsp of either applesauce,

Ensure pudding, cottage cheese, yogurt or strained pears, or into 60mL of either apple juice, orange juice, or tomato juice and swallow immediately.

NG Tube (≥16 French):
Mix intact granules into 40mL of apple juice; do not use other liquids.
Inject through the NG tube into the stomach.
Flush w/ additional apple juice to clear the tube.

Disintegrating SoluTab
Do not break, crush, chew, or cut.
Allow tab to disintegrate on tongue, w/ or w/o water, until particles can be swallowed.
Oral Syringe:
Place a 15mg tab in oral syringe and draw up 4mL of water, or place a 30mg tab w/ 10mL of water.
Shake gently to allow for a quick dispersal.
After the tab has dispersed, administer w/in 15 min.
Refill the syringe w/ approx 2mL (5mL for the 30mg tab) of water, shake gently, and administer any remaining contents.
NG Tube (≥8 French):
Place a 15mg tab in a syringe and draw up 4mL of water, or place a 30mg tab w/ 10mL of water.
Shake gently to allow for a quick dispersal.
After the tab has dispersed, inject through the NG tube into the stomach w/in 15 min.
Refill the syringe w/ approx 5mL of water, shake gently, and flush the NG tube.

STORAGE
25°C (77°F); excursions permitted to 15-30°C (59-86°F).

HOW SUPPLIED
Cap, Delayed-Release: 15mg, 30mg; **Tab, Disintegrating (SoluTab):** 15mg, 30mg

CONTRAINDICATIONS
Known severe hypersensitivity to any component of the formulation. When used w/ clarithromycin and/or amoxicillin, refer to the individual PIs.

WARNINGS/PRECAUTIONS
Symptomatic response does not preclude the presence of gastric malignancy. Acute interstitial nephritis reported; d/c if this develops. Cyanocobalamin (vitamin B12) deficiency may occur due to malabsorption with daily long-term treatment (eg, >3 yrs) with any acid-suppressing medications. May increase risk for *Clostridium difficile*-associated diarrhea (CDAD), especially in hospitalized patients. May increase risk for osteoporosis-related fractures of the hip, wrist, or spine, especially with high-dose and long-term therapy. Use lowest dose and shortest duration appropriate to the condition being treated. Hypomagnesemia reported; Mg^{2+} replacement and discontinuation of therapy may be required. (Tab, Disintegrating) Contains phenylalanine.

ADVERSE REACTIONS
Abdominal pain, constipation, diarrhea, nausea, dizziness, headache.

DRUG INTERACTIONS
May reduce the absorption of drugs where gastric pH is an important determinant of bioavailability; ampicillin esters, ketoconazole, atazanavir, nelfinavir, iron salts, erlotinib and mycophenolate mofetil (MMF) absorption may decrease, while digoxin absorption may increase. May substantially decrease concentrations of HIV protease inhibitors (eg, atazanavir, nelfinavir); avoid coadministration. Caution in transplant patients receiving MMF. May increase theophylline clearance; may require theophylline dose titration when lansoprazole is started or stopped. Monitor for increases in INR and PT with warfarin. May increase tacrolimus levels. May elevate and prolong levels of MTX leading to toxicities; consider temporary withdrawal of therapy with high-dose MTX. Caution with digoxin or other drugs that may cause hypomagnesemia (eg, diuretics).

PREGNANCY AND LACTATION
Pregnancy: Category B.
Lactation: Not for use in nursing.

MECHANISM OF ACTION
Proton pump inhibitor; suppresses gastric acid secretion by specific inhibition of the (H^+/K^+)-ATPase enzyme system at the secretory surface of the gastric parietal cell. Blocks the final step of acid production.

PHARMACOKINETICS
Absorption: Rapid; absolute bioavailability (>80%); T_{max}=1.7 hrs. **Distribution:** Plasma protein binding (97%). **Metabolism:** Liver (extensive). **Elimination:** Urine (1/3), feces (2/3); $T_{1/2}$<2 hrs.

PATIENT CONSIDERATIONS
Assessment: Assess for hepatic insufficiency, risk for osteoporosis, phenylketonuria, previous hypersensitivity to the drug, pregnancy/nursing status, and possible drug interactions. Obtain baseline Mg^{2+} levels in patients expected to be on prolonged treatment.

Monitoring: Monitor for signs/symptoms of acute interstitial nephritis, cyanocobalamin deficiency, bone fractures, CDAD, hypersensitivity reactions, and other adverse reactions. Monitor Mg^{2+} levels periodically in patients expected to be on prolonged treatment.

Counseling: Advise to seek immediate medical attention if diarrhea does not improve or cardiovascular/neurological symptoms (eg, palpitations, dizziness, seizures, tetany) develop. Instruct to take exactly ud. Inform of alternative methods of administration if patient has swallowing difficulties.

PREVALITE — cholestyramine   **Rx**
Class: Bile acid sequestrant

ADULT DOSAGE
Hyperlipidemia
Initial: 1 pkt or 1 level scoopful (4g) qd or bid
Maint: 2-4 pkts or scoopfuls (8-16g) daily in 2 divided doses
Titrate: Increase gradually w/ periodic assessment of lipid/lipoprotein levels at intervals of ≥4 weeks
Max: 6 pkts or scoopfuls (24g) daily
May also give in 1-6 doses/day

Partial Biliary Obstruction
Relief of pruritus associated w/ partial biliary obstruction
Initial: 1 pkt or 1 level scoopful (4g) qd or bid
Maint: 2-4 pkts or scoopfuls (8-16g) daily in 2 divided doses
Titrate: Increase gradually w/ periodic assessment of lipid/lipoprotein levels at intervals of ≥4 weeks
Max: 6 pkts or scoopfuls (24g) daily
May also give in 1-6 doses/day

PEDIATRIC DOSAGE
Hyperlipidemia
Usual: 240mg/kg/day in 2-3 divided doses
Titrate: Based on response and tolerance
Max: 8g/day

Partial Biliary Obstruction
Relief of pruritus associated w/ partial biliary obstruction
Usual: 240mg/kg/day in 2-3 divided doses
Titrate: Based on response and tolerance
Max: 8g/day

ADMINISTRATION
Oral route

Do not take in its dry form; mix w/ water or other fluids.
May also mix w/ highly fluid soups or pulpy fruits w/ high moisture content (eg, applesauce, crushed pineapple).
Suggested time of administration is mealtime but may be modified to avoid interference w/ absorption of other medications.

Preparation
1. Place 1 single-dose pkt or 1 level scoopful in a glass or cup.
2. Add at least 2-3 oz of water or beverage of choice.
3. Stir to a uniform consistency.

STORAGE
20-25°C (68-77°F); excursions permitted to 15-30°C (59-86°F).

HOW SUPPLIED
Powder: 4g/pkt or 1 level scoopful [42s, 60s, 231g]

CONTRAINDICATIONS
Complete biliary obstruction, hypersensitivity to any of the components of the medication.

WARNINGS/PRECAUTIONS
Contains phenylalanine; caution w/ phenylketonurics. Chronic use may increase bleeding tendency due to hypoprothrombinemia associated w/ vitamin K deficiency; may be managed/prevented by vitamin K1 administration. Reduction of serum or red cell folate reported w/ long-term use; consider folic acid supplementation. May produce hyperchloremic acidosis w/ prolonged use, especially in younger or smaller patients. Caution w/ renal insufficiency or volume depletion. May produce or worsen preexisting constipation, which may aggravate hemorrhoids. Avoid constipation w/ symptomatic coronary artery disease (CAD).

ADVERSE REACTIONS
Constipation, abdominal discomfort/pain, flatulence, N/V, diarrhea, dyspepsia, eructation, anorexia, steatorrhea, bleeding tendencies, osteoporosis.

DRUG INTERACTIONS
May prevent absorption of fat-soluble vitamins (eg, A, D, E, K); consider concomitant supplementation w/ water-miscible (or parenteral) forms of fat-soluble vitamins when given cholestyramine resin for long periods of time. May interfere w/ the pharmacokinetics of drugs that undergo enterohepatic circulation. Enhanced lipid-lowering effect w/ HMG-CoA reductase inhibitors (eg, pravastatin, lovastatin, simvastatin, fluvastatin). Additive effect on LDL-cholesterol w/ nicotinic acid. Caution w/ spironolactone. May reduce or delay absorption of oral medications, such as phenylbutazone, warfarin, thiazide diuretics (acidic), propranolol (basic), tetracycline, penicillin G, phenobarbital, thyroid and thyroxine preparations, estrogens and progestins, and digitalis. Discontinuance of cholestyramine resin could pose a health hazard if potentially toxic drug (eg, digitalis) has been titrated to maint level while patient was taking cholestyramine resin. May bind other drugs given concurrently; take other drugs ≥1 hr before or 4-6 hrs after cholestyramine resin. Interference w/ the absorption of oral phosphate supplements has been observed w/ another positively-charged bile acid sequestrant.

PREGNANCY AND LACTATION
Pregnancy: Category C.
Lactation: Caution in nursing.

MECHANISM OF ACTION
Bile acid sequestrant; adsorbs and combines w/ bile acids in the intestine to form an insoluble complex excreted in the feces, resulting in partial removal of bile acids from enterohepatic circulation by preventing their absorption. This leads to increased oxidation of cholesterol to bile acids, a decrease in β-lipoprotein or LDL plasma levels, and a decrease in serum cholesterol levels.

PHARMACOKINETICS
Elimination: Feces.

PATIENT CONSIDERATIONS

Assessment: Assess weight and need for caloric restriction for weight normalization in overweight patients. Assess for phenylketonuria, renal insufficiency, volume depletion, presence of biliary obstruction, CAD, pregnancy/nursing status, and possible drug interactions. Exclude secondary causes of hypercholesterolemia (eg, poorly controlled diabetes mellitus, hypothyroidism, nephrotic syndrome, dysproteinemias, obstructive liver disease, alcoholism). Obtain baseline lipid profile (total-C, HDL-C, TG).

Monitoring: Monitor for signs/symptoms of increased bleeding tendencies (vitamin K deficiency), hyperchloremic acidosis, worsening of preexisting constipation, and hemorrhoids. Monitor serum cholesterol frequently during the first few months and periodically thereafter. Monitor serum TGs periodically. Monitor for reduction in serum or red cell folate.

Counseling: Advise to inform physician if pregnant, planning to become pregnant, or breastfeeding. Instruct to drink plenty of fluids and to mix each single-dose pkt or scoopful in at least 2-3 oz of fluid before taking. Inform that sipping or holding the resin sus in the mouth for prolonged periods may lead to changes in the surface of the teeth (eg, discoloration, erosion of enamel, or decay). Advise to maintain good oral hygiene.

PREVIDENT — sodium fluoride   Rx

Class: Fluoride preparation

OTHER BRAND NAMES
PreviDent 5000 Plus, Denta 5000 Plus

ADULT DOSAGE	**PEDIATRIC DOSAGE**
Dental Caries Prevention	**Prevention and Control of Dental Caries**
Apply a thin ribbon to toothbrush and brush thoroughly qd for 2 min, preferably at hs; expectorate after use	**6-16 Years:** Apply a thin ribbon to toothbrush and brush thoroughly qd for 2 min, preferably at hs; expectorate and rinse mouth thoroughly after use

---

ADMINISTRATION
Topical route (teeth)

For best results, do not eat, drink, or rinse for 30 min.

STORAGE
20-25°C (68-77°F).

HOW SUPPLIED
Gel: (PreviDent) 1.1% [2 oz (56g)]; Cre: (PreviDent 5000 Plus/Denta 5000 Plus) 1.1% [1.8 oz (51g)]

CONTRAINDICATIONS
Not for pediatrics <6 yrs unless recommended by dentist or physician.

WARNINGS/PRECAUTIONS
Prolonged ingestion may lead to dental fluorosis in pediatrics <6 yrs. Not for systemic treatment. Do not swallow.

ADVERSE REACTIONS
Allergic reactions.

PREGNANCY AND LACTATION
Pregnancy: Category B.
Lactation: Caution in nursing.

MECHANISM OF ACTION
Fluoride preparation; increases tooth resistance to acid dissolution and enhances penetration of fluoride ion into tooth enamel.

PATIENT CONSIDERATIONS
Assessment: Assess for dental caries, dental fluorosis, patient age, and pregnancy/nursing status.

Monitoring: Monitor for allergic reactions and other idiosyncrasies.

Counseling: Instruct patient not to swallow after use. Adults should not eat, drink, or rinse for 30 min after use; however, pediatrics 6-16 yrs should rinse mouth thoroughly after use. Keep out of reach of children.

PREVNAR 13 — pneumococcal 13-valent conjugate vaccine (diphtheria CRM197 protein)   Rx

Class: Vaccine

ADULT DOSAGE	**PEDIATRIC DOSAGE**
***Streptococcus pneumoniae* Immunization**	***Streptococcus pneumoniae* Immunization**
Active immunization for the prevention of pneumonia and invasive disease caused by *S. pneumoniae* serotypes 1, 3, 4, 5, 6A, 6B, 7F, 9V, 14, 18C, 19A, 19F, and 23F	**6 Weeks-5 Years (Prior to 6th Birthday):** Active immunization for the prevention of invasive disease caused by *S. pneumoniae* serotypes 1, 3, 4, 5, 6A, 6B, 7F, 9V, 14, 18C, 19A, 19F, and 23F. Also indicated for active immunization for the prevention of otitis media caused by *S. pneumoniae*
≥18 Years: 0.5mL IM as a single dose	

serotypes 4, 6B, 9V, 14, 18C, 19F, and 23F

Vaccination Schedule for Infants and Toddlers:
0.5mL IM as a 4-dose series at 2, 4, and 6 months of age (at intervals of 4-8 weeks), and then at 12-15 months of age (at least 2 months after 3rd dose); 1st dose may be given as early as 6 weeks of age

Vaccination Schedule for Unvaccinated Children 7 Months-5 Years:

7-11 Months: Three 0.5mL IM doses; administer first 2 doses at least 4 weeks apart, and 3rd dose after 1st birthday, at least 2 months after 2nd dose
12-23 Months: Two 0.5mL IM doses at least 2 months apart
24 Months-5 Years (Prior to 6th Birthday): One 0.5mL IM dose

Vaccination Schedule for Children 15 Months-5 Years Previously Vaccinated w/ Prevnar Pneumococcal 7-Valent Conjugate Vaccine:
May give 1 dose of Prevnar 13 to elicit immune response to the 6 additional serotypes; this catch-up dose should be administered at least 8 weeks after the final dose of Prevnar

6-17 Years (Prior to 18th Birthday):
Active immunization for the prevention of invasive disease caused by *S. pneumoniae* serotypes 1, 3, 4, 5, 6A, 6B, 7F, 9V, 14, 18C, 19A, 19F, and 23F

Vaccination Schedule:
0.5mL IM as a single dose; if Prevnar was previously administered, at least 8 weeks should elapse before receiving Prevnar 13

ADMINISTRATION
IM route

Shake vigorously immediately prior to use; do not use if the vaccine cannot be resuspended.
Do not mix w/ other vaccines/products in the same syringe.
When administered at the same time as another injectable vaccine(s), administer w/ different syringes and at different inj sites.

Preferred Sites for Inj:
Infants: Anterolateral aspect of the thigh.
Toddlers/Children/Adults: Deltoid muscle of the upper arm.

Do not inject in the gluteal area or areas where there may be a major nerve trunk and/or blood vessel.

STORAGE
After Shipping: May arrive at 2-25°C (36-77°F). **Upon Receipt:** 2-8°C (36-46°F). Do not freeze; discard if frozen.

HOW SUPPLIED
Inj: 0.5mL

CONTRAINDICATIONS
Severe allergic reaction (eg, anaphylaxis) to any component of Prevnar 13 or any diphtheria toxoid-containing vaccine.

WARNINGS/PRECAUTIONS
Epinephrine and other appropriate agents must be immediately available should an acute anaphylactic reaction occur following administration. Individuals w/ altered immunocompetence, including those at higher risk for invasive pneumococcal disease (eg, individuals w/ congenital or acquired splenic dysfunction, HIV infection, malignancy, hematopoietic stem cell transplant, nephrotic syndrome), may have reduced antibody responses to immunization. Apnea following IM vaccination observed in some premature infants; consider infant's medical status, and the potential benefits and possible risks of vaccination.

ADVERSE REACTIONS
Pediatrics 12-15 Months of Age: Irritability, inj-site tenderness, decreased appetite, decreased sleep, increased sleep, fever, inj-site redness, inj-site swelling.
Pediatrics 5-17 Years: Inj-site tenderness, inj-site redness, inj-site swelling, irritability, decreased appetite, increased sleep, fever, decreased sleep.
Adults ≥18 Years: Pain at the inj site, fatigue, headache, muscle pain, vomiting, joint pain, decreased appetite, inj-site redness, inj-site swelling, arm movement limitation, chills, rash.

DRUG INTERACTIONS
Patients receiving immunosuppressive therapy (eg, irradiation, corticosteroids, antimetabolites, alkylating agents, cytotoxic agents) may not respond optimally to

active immunization. Prior receipt of Pneumovax 23 w/in 1 yr results in diminished immune response to Prevnar 13.

PREGNANCY AND LACTATION
Pregnancy: Available data on Prevnar 13 administered to pregnant women are insufficient to inform vaccine-associated risks in pregnancy.
Lactation: Data are not available to assess the effects of Prevnar 13 on the breastfed infant or on milk production/excretion. Caution in nursing.

MECHANISM OF ACTION
Vaccine; elicits a T-cell dependent immune response. Protein carrier-specific T-cells provide the signals needed for maturation of the B-cell response.

PATIENT CONSIDERATIONS
Assessment: Assess for altered immunocompetence, hypersensitivity/vaccination history, pregnancy/nursing status, and possible drug interactions.

Monitoring: Monitor for allergic/anaphylactic reactions, inj-site reactions, and other possible adverse reactions.

Counseling: Inform of the potential benefits/risks of vaccination, and of the importance of completing the immunization series unless contraindicated. Instruct to report any suspected adverse reactions to physician.

PREVPAC — amoxicillin/clarithromycin/lansoprazole   Rx

Class: *H. pylori* treatment combination

ADULT DOSAGE	PEDIATRIC DOSAGE
Helicobacter pylori Eradication **H. pylori Infection and Duodenal Ulcer Disease (Active or 1-Year History):** Usual: 30mg lansoprazole, 1g amoxicillin, and 500mg clarithromycin administered together bid (am and pm) for 10 or 14 days	Pediatric use may not have been established

DOSING CONSIDERATIONS
Renal Impairment
Severe (w/ or w/o Coexisting Hepatic Impairment): May need to decrease dosage or prolong dosing intervals of clarithromycin
CrCl <30mL/min: Not recommended

Hepatic Impairment
Severe: Consider reduction of lansoprazole dosage

ADMINISTRATION
Oral route
Take each dose ac.
Swallow each pill whole.

STORAGE
20-25°C (68-77°F). Protect from light and moisture.

HOW SUPPLIED
Cap: (Amoxicillin) 500mg; **Cap, Delayed-Release:** (Lansoprazole) 30mg; **Tab:** (Clarithromycin) 500mg

CONTRAINDICATIONS
Lansoprazole: Known severe hypersensitivity to any component of the formulation. **Amoxicillin:** History of severe hypersensitivity reactions (eg, anaphylaxis, Stevens-Johnson syndrome) to amoxicillin or other beta-lactam antibiotics (eg, penicillins, cephalosporins). **Clarithromycin:** Known hypersensitivity to clarithromycin, erythromycin, or any of the macrolide antibiotics. History of cholestatic jaundice/hepatic dysfunction associated w/ prior use of clarithromycin. History of QT prolongation or ventricular cardiac arrhythmia, including torsades de pointes. Concomitant administration w/ cisapride, pimozide, astemizole, terfenadine, ergotamine, dihydroergotamine, or HMG-CoA reductase inhibitors (statins) that are extensively metabolized by CYP3A4 (lovastatin or simvastatin). Concomitant administration w/ colchicine in patients w/ renal/hepatic impairment.

WARNINGS/PRECAUTIONS
Not recommended with CrCl <30mL/min. Lab test interactions may occur. Caution in elderly. **Amoxicillin:** Serious and occasionally fatal hypersensitivity (anaphylactic) reactions reported in patients on penicillin (PCN) therapy; caution with history of PCN hypersensitivity and/or a history of sensitivity to multiple allergens. Immediately d/c therapy and initiate appropriate treatment if severe acute hypersensitivity reactions occur. **Clarithromycin:** Use in pregnancy only when there is no appropriate alternative therapy. Exacerbation of symptoms of myasthenia gravis and new onset of myasthenic syndrome reported. Hepatic dysfunction reported; d/c immediately if signs/symptoms of hepatitis occur. May cause QT interval prolongation, arrhythmia, and torsades de pointes; avoid with ongoing proarrhythmic conditions (eg, uncorrected hypokalemia or hypomagnesemia), and clinically significant bradycardia. **Lansoprazole:** Symptomatic response does not preclude the presence of gastric malignancy. Acute interstitial nephritis (AIN) reported; d/c if AIN develops. Amoxicillin/Clarithromycin: *Clostridium difficile*-associated diarrhea (CDAD) reported; d/c if CDAD is suspected or confirmed. May result in bacterial resistance with prolonged use in the absence of proven or suspected bacterial infection, or a prophylactic indication; d/c if superinfections occur and institute appropriate therapy.

ADVERSE REACTIONS
Diarrhea, taste perversion, headache.

DRUG INTERACTIONS
See Contraindications. **Amoxicillin:** Probenecid decreases renal tubular secretion. Chloramphenicol, macrolides, sulfonamides, and tetracyclines may interfere with bactericidal effects of PCN. May affect the gut flora, leading to lower estrogen reabsorption and reduced efficacy of combined oral estrogen/progesterone contraceptives. **Clarithromycin:** Avoid with class IA (quinidine, procainamide) or class III (dofetilide, amiodarone, sotalol) antiarrhythmic agents. Hypotension may occur with calcium channel blockers metabolized by CYP3A4 (eg, verapamil, amlodipine, diltiazem). Concomitant use with oral hypoglycemic agents and/or insulin may result in significant hypoglycemia; monitor glucose levels. May increase theophylline, carbamazepine, digoxin, colchicine, tolterodine, itraconazole, and saquinavir levels. Tolterodine 1mg bid is recommended in patients deficient in CYP2D6 activity (poor metabolizers). Bradyarrhythmias and lactic acidosis observed with verapamil. May decrease zidovudine levels; separate administration by at least 2 hrs. Fluconazole, itraconazole, and saquinavir may increase levels. Ritonavir and atazanavir may increase clarithromycin exposure and significantly decrease 14-OH clarithromycin exposure; consider alternative antibacterial therapy for indications other than infections due to *Mycobacterium avium* complex. Do not coadminister doses >1000mg/day with protease inhibitors. Decrease dose by 50% when coadministered with atazanavir. May increase concentrations of CYP3A substrates, which may lead to increased/prolonged therapeutic and adverse effects; caution with CYP3A substrates, especially those with narrow safety margin (eg, carbamazepine) and/or extensively metabolized by CYP3A enzyme. CYP3A inducers (eg, efavirenz, nevirapine, rifampicin, rifabutin, rifapentine) may decrease clarithromycin levels and increase 14-OH clarithromycin levels; consider alternative antibacterial treatment. May increase exposure of sildenafil, tadalafil, and vardenafil; coadministration is not recommended. May increase midazolam exposure; dose adjustments may be necessary when oral midazolam is coadministered. Caution and consider appropriate dose adjustments with triazolam or alprazolam. CNS effects reported with triazolam. Torsades de pointes reported with quinidine or disopyramide; monitor ECG. Interactions with drugs not thought to be metabolized by CYP3A (eg, hexobarbital, phenytoin, valproate) reported. **Lansoprazole:** May elevate and prolong levels of methotrexate (MTX) and/or its metabolite, possibly leading to toxicities; consider temporary withdrawal of therapy with high-dose MTX. May reduce absorption of drugs where gastric pH is an important determinant of bioavailability (eg, absorption of ampicillin esters, ketoconazole, atazanavir, iron salts, erlotinib, and mycophenolate mofetil may decrease, while absorption of digoxin may increase). Caution with mycophenolate mofetil in transplant patients. May interact with drugs metabolized by CYP450 enzymes (CYP1A2, CYP2C9, CYP2C19, CYP2D6, CYP3A). May increase theophylline clearance; may require additional titration of theophylline dosage when lansoprazole is started or stopped. May increase tacrolimus levels, especially in transplant patients who are intermediate or poor metabolizers of CYP2C19. Delayed absorption and reduced bioavailability with sucralfate; give at least 30 min prior to sucralfate. **Clarithromycin/Lansoprazole:** May alter the anticoagulant effects of warfarin and other anticoagulants; monitor PT and INR. Refer to PI for additional drug interaction information.

PREGNANCY AND LACTATION
Pregnancy: Category C.
Lactation: Not for use in nursing.

MECHANISM OF ACTION
Lansoprazole: Substituted benzimidazole; inhibits gastric acid secretion.
Amoxicillin: Semisynthetic antibiotic; has broad spectrum of bactericidal activity against many gram-positive and gram-negative microorganisms. **Clarithromycin:** Semisynthetic macrolide antibiotic.

PHARMACOKINETICS
Absorption: Lansoprazole: Rapid; absolute bioavailability (>80%); T_{max}=1.7 hrs. Amoxicillin: Rapid; T_{max}=1-2 hrs; C_{max}=5.5-7.5mcg/mL. Clarithromycin: Rapid; absolute bioavailability (50% [250mg]); T_{max}=2-2.5 hrs (500mg). Administration of variable doses resulted in different parameters. **Distribution:** Lansoprazole: Plasma protein binding (97%). Amoxicillin: Plasma protein binding (20%); found in breast milk. **Metabolism:** Lansoprazole: Liver (extensive). Clarithromycin: 14-OH clarithromycin (active metabolite). **Elimination:** Lansoprazole: Urine (1/3), feces (2/3). Amoxicillin: Urine (60%, unchanged); $T_{1/2}$=61.3 min. Clarithromycin: Urine (30%); $T_{1/2}$=5-7 hrs, 7-9 hrs (14-OH clarithromycin).

PATIENT CONSIDERATIONS
Assessment: Assess for history of hypersensitivity to drug, macrolides, β-lactam antibiotics (PCNs, cephalosporins), or other allergens. Assess for ongoing proarrhythmic conditions, bradycardia, myasthenia gravis, renal/hepatic impairment, any other conditions where treatment is contraindicated or cautioned, pregnancy/nursing status, and possible drug interactions.

Monitoring: Monitor for hypersensitivity reactions, hepatic dysfunction, QT prolongation, CDAD, superinfections, exacerbation of myasthenia gravis symptoms, new onset of symptoms of myasthenic syndrome, AIN, and other adverse reactions. Periodically monitor renal/hepatic/hematopoietic function during prolonged therapy. Monitor PT/INR with warfarin and other anticoagulants.

Counseling: Inform about risks/benefits of therapy. Advise to report the use of any other medications. Advise that diarrhea may occur and will usually end if therapy is discontinued. Instruct to contact physician as soon as possible if watery/bloody stools (with/without stomach cramps and fever) develop even as late as 2 or more months after having taken the last dose of therapy. Counsel that therapy should only be used to treat bacterial, not viral, infections. Instruct to take exactly ud; inform that skipping doses or not completing full course may decrease effectiveness and increase antibiotic resistance. Instruct to immediately report and seek care for any cardiovascular/neurological symptoms.

PREZCOBIX — cobicistat/darunavir   Rx

Class: CYP3A inhibitor/protease inhibitor

ADULT DOSAGE

HIV-1 Infection

In treatment-naive and treatment-experienced patients w/ no darunavir resistance-associated substitutions

1 tab qd; administer in conjunction w/ other antiretroviral agents

HIV Genotypic Testing Prior to Initiation of Therapy:
Recommended for antiretroviral treatment-experienced patients; when genotypic testing is not feasible, therapy may be used in protease inhibitor-naive patients, but is not recommended in protease inhibitor-experienced patients

PEDIATRIC DOSAGE

Pediatric use may not have been established

DOSING CONSIDERATIONS

Renal Impairment
CrCl <70mL/min: Do not coadminister w/ tenofovir disoproxil fumarate (TDF)

Hepatic Impairment
Severe: Not recommended

ADMINISTRATION

Oral route

Take w/ food.

STORAGE

20-25°C (68-77°F); excursions permitted to 15-30°C (59-86°F).

HOW SUPPLIED

Tab: (Darunavir/Cobicistat) 800mg/150mg

CONTRAINDICATIONS

Concomitant use w/ alfuzosin, ranolazine, dronedarone, colchicine (in patients w/ renal and/or hepatic impairment), rifampin, lurasidone, pimozide, dihydroergotamine, ergotamine, methylergonovine, cisapride, St. John's wort, lovastatin, simvastatin, sildenafil (when used to treat pulmonary arterial HTN), oral midazolam, or triazolam due to the potential for serious and/or life-threatening events or loss of therapeutic effect.

WARNINGS/PRECAUTIONS

Redistribution/accumulation of body fat, immune reconstitution syndrome, and autoimmune disorders (eg, Graves' disease, polymyositis, Guillain-Barre syndrome) in the setting of immune reconstitution reported. Caution in elderly. **Darunavir:** Drug-induced hepatitis and liver injury, including some fatalities, reported. Consider performing increased AST/ALT monitoring in patients w/ underlying chronic hepatitis, cirrhosis, or those w/ pretreatment transaminase elevations, especially during the 1st several months of treatment. Consider interruption or discontinuation of therapy if evidence of new/worsening liver dysfunction occurs. Severe skin reactions (eg, Stevens-Johnson syndrome, toxic epidermal necrolysis, drug rash w/ eosinophilia and systemic symptoms), accompanied by fever and/or transaminase elevations in some cases, reported; d/c immediately if signs/symptoms of severe skin reactions develop. Contains a sulfonamide moiety; monitor patients w/ a known sulfonamide allergy. May develop new onset diabetes mellitus (DM), exacerbation of preexisting DM, hyperglycemia, and diabetic ketoacidosis; may require either initiation or dose adjustments of insulin or oral hypoglycemic agents. Increased bleeding including spontaneous skin hematomas and hemarthrosis reported in patients w/ hemophilia type A and B. **Cobicistat:** Decreases estimated CrCl; consider effect when interpreting changes in CrCl in patients initiating therapy particularly in patients w/ medical conditions or receiving drugs needing monitoring w/ estimated CrCl. Closely monitor patients w/ confirmed increase in SrCr >0.4mg/dL from baseline for renal safety.

ADVERSE REACTIONS

Darunavir: Diarrhea, N/V, rash, headache, abdominal pain.
Cobicistat: Refer to cobicistat PI for adverse reactions reported w/ cobicistat.

DRUG INTERACTIONS

See Dosing Considerations and Contraindications. Coadministration w/ TDF in combination w/ concomitant or recent use of a nephrotoxic agent is not recommended. Coadministration w/ drugs that are primarily metabolized by CYP3A and/or CYP2D6 or are substrates of P-gp, BCRP, OATP1B1, or OATP1B3 may increase plasma concentrations of such drugs, which could increase or prolong their therapeutic effect and can be associated w/ adverse events. CYP3A inducers may decrease levels, which may lead to loss of therapeutic effect and development of resistance. CYP3A inhibitors may increase levels. Give didanosine 1 hr before or 2 hrs after administration w/ therapy. Not recommended w/ products containing the individual components of Prezcobix, ritonavir (RTV), other antiretroviral drugs that require pharmacokinetic boosting (eg, another protease inhibitor, elvitegravir), efavirenz, etravirine, nevirapine, apixaban, dabigatran etexilate (in specific renal impairment groups), rivaroxaban, rifapentine, boceprevir, simeprevir, telaprevir, everolimus, avanafil, salmeterol, or voriconazole. Caution w/ SSRIs and w/ narcotics used for treatment of opioid dependence (buprenorphine, buprenorphine/naloxone, methadone). May increase levels of maraviroc, antiarrhythmics, digoxin, dasatinib, nilotinib, vinblastine, vincristine, anticonvulsants metabolized by CYP3A (eg, carbamazepine, clonazepam), TCAs, itraconazole, ketoconazole, trazodone, colchicine, rifabutin, antipsychotics (eg, perphenazine, risperidone, thioridazine), quetiapine, β-blockers, calcium channel blockers, corticosteroids, bosentan, atorvastatin, fluvastatin, pravastatin, rosuvastatin, immunosuppressants (cyclosporine, sirolimus, tacrolimus), narcotic analgesics metabolized by CYP3A (eg, fentanyl, oxycodone), tramadol, PDE-5 inhibitors, sedatives/hypnotics metabolized by CYP3A (eg, buspirone, diazepam, estazolam), clarithromycin, erythromycin, and telithromycin. Itraconazole, ketoconazole, posaconazole, clarithromycin, erythromycin, and telithromycin may increase levels. Monitor INR w/ warfarin. Monitor phenobarbital or phenytoin levels. Monitor for a potential decrease of antimalarial efficacy or potential QT prolongation if coadministered w/ artemether/lumefantrine. Coadministration w/ inhaled/nasal fluticasone or other corticosteroids that are metabolized by CYP3A may result in reduced serum cortisol concentrations. Coadministration w/ corticosteroids that are metabolized by CYP3A, particularly long-term use, may increase the risk of development of systemic corticosteroid effects. Coadministration w/ dexamethasone or other corticosteroids that induce CYP3A may result in loss therapeutic effect and development of resistance to darunavir. Consider additional or alternative (nonhormonal) forms of contraception if taking hormonal contraceptives. Coadministration w/ parenteral midazolam should be done in a setting that ensures close clinical monitoring and appropriate medical management in case of respiratory depression and/or prolonged sedation. Bosentan may decrease levels. **Cobicistat:** Renal impairment, including cases of acute renal failure and Fanconi syndrome, reported when used in an antiretroviral regimen w/ TDF. Anticonvulsants that induce CYP3A (eg, carbamazepine, oxcarbazepine, phenobarbital) may decrease levels; consider alternative anticonvulsant or antiretroviral therapy, and if coadministration is necessary, monitor for lack or loss of virologic response. Refer to PI for further detailed information on drug interactions, including dosing modifications required when used w/ certain concomitant therapies.

PREGNANCY AND LACTATION

Pregnancy: Category C. Physicians are encouraged to register patients in the Antiretroviral Pregnancy Registry.
Lactation: Not for use in nursing.

MECHANISM OF ACTION

Darunavir: Protease inhibitor; selectively inhibits the cleavage of HIV-1 encoded Gag-Pol polyproteins in infected cells, thereby preventing the formation of mature virus particles. **Cobicistat:** CYP3A inhibitor; inhibits CYP3A-mediated metabolism by cobicistat that enhances the systemic exposure of CYP3A substrates.

PHARMACOKINETICS

Absorption: (Fed) Darunavir: T_{max}=4-4.5 hrs. (Fed) Cobicistat: T_{max}=4-5 hrs. **Distribution:** Darunavir: Plasma protein binding (95%). Cobicistat: Plasma protein binding (97-98%). **Metabolism:** Darunavir: Liver (extensive); oxidation via CYP3A. Cobicistat: CYP3A, CYP2D6 (minor). **Elimination:** Darunavir/RTV: Feces (79.5%, 41.2% unchanged), urine (13.9%, 7.7% unchanged); Darunavir: $T_{1/2}$=7 hrs (fed state). Cobicistat: Feces (86.2%), urine (8.2%); $T_{1/2}$=4 hrs (fed state).

PATIENT CONSIDERATIONS

Assessment: Assess for hypersensitivity to drug, sulfonamide allergy, liver dysfunction, autoimmune disorders, hemophilia, preexisting DM, pregnancy/nursing status, and possible drug interactions. Assess estimated CrCl. When coadministering w/ TDF, assess estimated CrCl, urine glucose, and urine protein at baseline. If feasible, perform HIV genotypic testing in antiretroviral treatment-experienced patients.

Monitoring: Monitor for signs/symptoms of hepatotoxicity, severe skin reactions, new onset/ worsening renal impairment when coadministered w/ TDF, new onset/ exacerbation of DM, hyperglycemia, diabetic ketoacidosis, fat redistribution/ accumulation, immune reconstitution syndrome, autoimmune disorders, and other adverse reactions. In patients w/ hemophilia, monitor for bleeding events. Consider performing increased AST/ALT monitoring in patients w/ underlying chronic hepatitis, cirrhosis, or those w/ pretreatment transaminase elevations, especially during the 1st several months of treatment. Monitor INR during coadministration w/ warfarin. Perform routine monitoring of estimated CrCl, urine glucose, and urine protein when used w/ TDF. Measure serum phosphorus in patients w/ or at risk for renal impairment when used w/ TDF.

Counseling: Inform that therapy is not a cure for HIV and that patient may continue to experience illnesses associated w/ HIV-1 infection. Advise to avoid doing things that can spread HIV infection to others. Instruct to take w/ food qd as prescribed. Instruct not to alter dose or d/c w/o consulting physician. Counsel to take drug immediately for missed dose <12 hrs and to take the next dose at regular scheduled time. Instruct that if a dose is missed by >12 hrs, to take the next dose as scheduled; instruct not to double the dose. Advise about the signs/symptoms of liver problems. Inform that mild to severe skin reactions may develop; advise to immediately contact physician if signs/symptoms of severe skin reactions develop. Inform that renal impairment, including cases of acute renal failure and Fanconi syndrome, has been reported when used in combination w/ TDF-containing regimen. Instruct to notify physician of the use of any other prescription, OTC, or herbal medication. Instruct patients receiving hormonal contraceptives to use additional or alternative contraceptive (non-hormonal) measures during therapy. Inform that redistribution and accumulation of body fat may occur.

PREZISTA — darunavir   Rx

Class: Protease inhibitor

ADULT DOSAGE

HIV-1 Infection

Coadministered w/ Ritonavir (RTV) and in Combination w/ Other Antiretrovirals:

Treatment-Naive:
800mg (8mL) + RTV 100mg (1.25mL) qd

PEDIATRIC DOSAGE

HIV-1 Infection

Coadministered w/ RTV and in Combination w/ Other Antiretrovirals:

3 to <18 Years:
Treatment-Naive Patients or Treatment-Experienced Patients w/

Treatment-Experienced:
No Darunavir Resistance Associated Substitutions:
800mg (8mL) + RTV 100mg (1.25mL) qd

≥1 Darunavir Resistance Associated Substitutions or w/ No Baseline Resistance Information:
600mg (6mL) + RTV 100mg (1.25mL) bid

No Darunavir Resistance Associated Substitutions:
Weight-Based Dose: 35mg/kg + RTV 7mg/kg qd using the following recommendations
≥10 to <11kg: 350mg (3.6mL) + RTV 64mg (0.8mL) qd
≥11 to <12kg: 385mg (4mL) + RTV 64mg (0.8mL) qd
≥12 to <13kg: 420mg (4.2mL) + RTV 80mg (1mL) qd
≥13 to <14kg: 455mg (4.6mL) + RTV 80mg (1mL) qd
≥14 to <15kg: 490mg (5mL) + RTV 96mg (1.2mL) qd
≥15 to <30kg: 600mg (6mL) + RTV 100mg (1.25mL) qd
≥30 to <40kg: 675mg (6.8mL) + RTV 100mg (1.25mL) qd
≥40kg: 800mg (8mL) + RTV 100mg (1.25mL) qd

Treatment-Experienced Patients w/ ≥1 Darunavir Resistance Associated Substitution:
Weight-Based Dose: 20mg/kg + RTV 3mg/kg bid using the following recommendations
≥10 to <11kg: 200mg (2mL) + RTV 32mg (0.4mL) bid
≥11 to <12kg: 220mg (2.2mL) + RTV 32mg (0.4mL) bid
≥12 to <13kg: 240mg (2.4mL) + RTV 40mg (0.5mL) bid
≥13 to <14kg: 260mg (2.6mL) + RTV 40mg (0.5mL) bid
≥14 to <15kg: 280mg (2.8mL) + RTV 48mg (0.6mL) bid
≥15 to <30kg: 375mg (3.8mL) + RTV 48mg (0.6mL) bid
≥30 to <40kg: 450mg (4.6mL) + RTV 60mg (0.75mL) bid
≥40kg: 600mg (6mL) + RTV 100mg (1.25mL) bid

Dose should not exceed the recommended dose for adults

DOSING CONSIDERATIONS
Hepatic Impairment
Mild-Moderate: No dose adjustment required
Severe: Not recommended

Pregnancy
Recommended Dose: 600mg + RTV 100mg bid
Only consider 800mg + RTV 100mg qd in certain pregnant patients who are already on a stable 800mg + RTV 100mg qd regimen prior to pregnancy, are virologically suppressed (HIV-1 RNA <50 copies/mL), and in whom a change to 600mg + RTV 100mg bid may compromise tolerability or compliance

ADMINISTRATION
Oral route

Take w/ food.

Oral Sus
- Shake well before each use.
- An 8mL darunavir dose should be taken as two 4mL administrations w/ the included oral dosing syringe.
- Patients who have difficulty swallowing tabs can use the oral sus.
- Before prescribing therapy, assess children weighing ≥15kg for the ability to swallow tabs; if a child is unable to reliably swallow tab, consider the use of oral sus.
- Use oral sus for pediatric patients weighing ≤10kg.

STORAGE
25°C (77°F); excursions permitted to 15-30°C (59-86°F). **Oral Sus:** Do not refrigerate or freeze. Avoid exposure to excessive heat. Store in the original container.

HOW SUPPLIED
Oral Sus: 100mg/mL [200mL]; **Tab:** 75mg, 150mg, 600mg, 800mg

CONTRAINDICATIONS
Coadministration w/ drugs that are highly dependent on CYP3A for clearance and for which elevated plasma concentrations are associated w/ serious and/or life-threatening events (narrow therapeutic index), and w/ certain other drugs that may lead to reduced efficacy of darunavir (eg, alfuzosin, dronedarone, colchicine [in patients w/ renal and/or hepatic impairment], ranolazine, pimozide, dihydroergotamine, ergotamine, methylergonovine, cisapride, oral midazolam, triazolam, St. John's wort, lovastatin, simvastatin, rifampin, sildenafil [when used to treat pulmonary arterial HTN]). Refer to RTV PI for a description of RTV contraindications.

WARNINGS/PRECAUTIONS
Must be coadministered w/ RTV and food to achieve desired antiviral effect; refer to RTV PI for additional information on precautory measures. Drug-induced hepatitis reported; increased risk for liver function abnormalities, including severe hepatic adverse events, in patients w/ preexisting liver dysfunction, including chronic active hepatitis B or C. Cases of liver injury reported; consider performing increased AST/ALT monitoring in patients w/ underlying chronic hepatitis, cirrhosis, or those w/ pretreatment transaminase elevations, especially during the first several months of treatment. Consider interruption or discontinuation of therapy if evidence of new/worsening liver dysfunction occurs. Severe skin reactions sometimes accompanied by fever and/or transaminase elevations, Stevens-Johnson syndrome (rare), toxic epidermal necrolysis, drug rash w/ eosinophilia and systemic symptoms, and acute generalized exanthematous pustulosis reported; d/c immediately if severe skin reactions develop. Caution in patients w/ a known sulfonamide allergy. New onset diabetes mellitus (DM), exacerbation of preexisting DM, hyperglycemia, and diabetic ketoacidosis reported. Immune reconstitution syndrome, autoimmune disorders (eg, Graves' disease, polymyositis, Guillain-Barre syndrome) in the setting of immune reconstitution, redistribution/accumulation of body fat, and increased bleeding in hemophilia type A and B reported. Caution in elderly.

ADVERSE REACTIONS
Diarrhea, N/V, headache, abdominal pain, rash.

DRUG INTERACTIONS
See Contraindications. Not recommended w/ lopinavir/RTV, saquinavir, other HIV protease inhibitors (except atazanavir), apixaban, dabigatran etexilate (in specific renal impairment groups), rivaroxaban, rifapentine, boceprevir, simeprevir, everolimus, salmeterol, and avanafil. Avoid use of tadalafil during initiation therapy; d/c tadalafil at least 24 hrs prior to starting darunavir/RTV. Not recommended w/ voriconazole unless an assessment comparing predicted benefit to risk ratio justifies use of voriconazole. May increase levels of indinavir, maraviroc, antiarrhythmics, digoxin, clarithromycin, anticoagulant, carbamazepine, amitriptyline, desipramine, imipramine, nortriptyline, trazodone, itraconazole, ketoconazole, colchicine, rifabutin, antineoplastics, quetiapine, antipsychotics, β-blockers, calcium channel blockers, systemic corticosteroids (metabolized by CYP3A), inhaled/nasal corticosteroid, bosentan, simeprevir, HMG-CoA reductase inhibitors, immunosuppressants, salmeterol, norbuprenorphine, PDE-5 inhibitors (eg, avanafil, sildenafil, vardenafil, tadalafil), sedatives/hypnotics (metabolized by CYP3A), and CYP3A, CYP2D6, and P-gp substrates. May decrease levels of warfarin, phenytoin, phenobarbital, paroxetine, sertraline, voriconazole, boceprevir, methadone, ethinyl estradiol, norethindrone, and omeprazole. CYP3A inhibitors, P-gp inhibitors, indinavir, itraconazole, ketoconazole, posaconazole, rifabutin, and simeprevir may increase levels. CYP3A inducers, lopinavir/RTV, saquinavir, rifapentine, systemic dexamethasone, and boceprevir may decrease levels. Give didanosine 1 hr before or 2 hrs after administration. Increased lumefantrine exposure may increase the risk of QT prolongation; caution w/ artemether/lumefantrine. May increase risk for development of systemic corticosteroid effects including Cushing's syndrome and adrenal suppression w/ corticosteroids metabolized by CYP3A. May require initiation or dose adjustments of insulin or oral hypoglycemics for treatment of DM. Refer to PI for dosing modifications when used w/ certain concomitant therapies.

PREGNANCY AND LACTATION
Pregnancy: There is a pregnancy exposure registry that monitors pregnancy outcomes in women exposed to Prezista during pregnancy.
Lactation: Not for use in nursing.
Reproductive Potential: May reduce efficacy of combined hormonal contraceptives and the progestin only pill; use an effective alternative contraceptive method or add a barrier method of contraception.

MECHANISM OF ACTION
Protease inhibitor; selectively inhibits the cleavage of HIV-1 encoded Gag-Pol polyproteins in infected cells, thereby preventing the formation of mature virus particles.

PHARMACOKINETICS
Absorption: Absolute oral bioavailability (37% darunavir), (82% darunavir/RTV); T_{max}=approx 2.5-4 hrs. **Distribution:** Plasma protein binding (approx 95%). **Metabolism:** Hepatic (extensive); oxidation via CYP3A. **Elimination:** Darunavir/RTV: Feces (approx 79.5%, approx 41.2% unchanged darunavir), urine (approx 13.9%, approx 7.7% unchanged darunavir); $T_{1/2}$=approx 15 hrs.

PATIENT CONSIDERATIONS
Assessment: Assess for sulfonamide allergy, liver dysfunction, hemophilia, preexisting DM, pregnancy/nursing status, and possible drug interactions. Assess ability to swallow tab in children ≥15kg. In treatment-experienced patients, assess treatment history and perform genotypic and/or phenotypic testing. Conduct appropriate lab testing such as serum liver biochemistries.

Monitoring: Monitor for signs/symptoms of hepatotoxicity, severe skin reactions, new onset/exacerbation of DM, diabetic ketoacidosis, fat redistribution/accumulation, immune reconstitution syndrome, autoimmune disorders, and other adverse reactions. In patients w/ hemophilia, monitor for bleeding events. Consider performing increased AST/ALT monitoring in patients w/ underlying chronic hepatitis, cirrhosis, or those w/ pretreatment transaminase elevations, especially during the first several months of treatment. Monitor INR during coadministration w/ warfarin.

Counseling: Advise to take darunavir and RTV w/ food every day on a regular dosing schedule and instruct not to alter dose, d/c RTV, or d/c therapy w/ darunavir w/o consulting physician. Advise about the signs and symptoms of liver problems. Instruct to d/c immediately if signs or symptoms of severe skin reactions develop. Advise to report to physician the use of any other prescription or nonprescription medication or herbal products, including St. John's wort. Instruct patients receiving combined hormonal contraception or the progestin only pill to use an effective alternative contraceptive method or add a barrier method during therapy because hormonal levels may decrease. Inform that redistribution/accumulation of body fat may occur. Advise to inform physician immediately of any symptoms of infection. Inform that there is an antiretroviral pregnancy registry to monitor fetal outcomes of pregnant women exposed to therapy. Instruct women w/ HIV-1 infection not to breastfeed because HIV-1 can be passed to the baby in breast milk.

PRIFTIN — rifapentine   Rx
Class: Rifamycin derivative

ADULT DOSAGE
Tuberculosis
Active Pulmonary Tuberculosis (TB) Caused by *Mycobacterium tuberculosis*:
Initial Phase:
600mg twice weekly for 2 months by direct observation of therapy w/ an interval of not <3 consecutive days (72 hrs) between doses in combination w/ other anti-TB drugs (eg, isoniazid [INH], ethambutol, pyrazinamide)
Continuation Phase:
Following initial phase, 600mg once weekly for 4 months in combination w/ INH or an appropriate anti-TB agent by direct observation therapy

Latent TB Infection Caused by *M. tuberculosis* in Patients at High Risk of Progression to TB Disease:
Administer once-weekly in combination w/ INH for 12 weeks as directly observed therapy
Usual:
10-14kg: 300mg once weekly
14.1-25kg: 450mg once weekly
25.1-32kg: 600mg once weekly
32.1-50kg: 750mg once weekly
>50kg: 900mg once weekly
Max: 900mg/week
INH Dosing:
Usual: 15mg/kg (rounded to the nearest 50mg or 100mg)
Max: 900mg once weekly

PEDIATRIC DOSAGE
Tuberculosis
Active Pulmonary Tuberculosis (TB) Caused by *Mycobacterium tuberculosis*:
≥12 Years:
Initial Phase:
600mg twice weekly for 2 months by direct observation of therapy w/ an interval of not <3 consecutive days (72 hrs) between doses in combination w/ other anti-TB drugs (eg, isoniazid [INH], ethambutol, pyrazinamide)
Continuation Phase:
Following initial phase, 600mg once weekly for 4 months in combination w/ INH or an appropriate anti-TB agent by direct observation therapy

Latent TB Infection Caused by *M. tuberculosis* in Patients at High Risk of Progression to TB Disease:
Administer once-weekly in combination w/ INH for 12 weeks as directly observed therapy
Usual:
10-14kg: 300mg once weekly
14.1-25kg: 450mg once weekly
25.1-32kg: 600mg once weekly
32.1-50kg: 750mg once weekly
>50kg: 900mg once weekly
Max: 900mg/week
INH Dosing:
2-11 Years: 25mg/kg (rounded to the nearest 50mg or 100mg)
≥12 Years: 15mg/kg (rounded to the nearest 50mg or 100mg)
Max: 900mg once weekly

ADMINISTRATION
Oral route
Take w/ meals
May crush tab and add to a small amount of semi-solid food for patients who cannot swallow tabs
STORAGE
25°C (77°F); excursions permitted to 15-30°C (59-86°F). Protect from excessive heat and humidity.
HOW SUPPLIED
Tab: 150mg
CONTRAINDICATIONS
History of hypersensitivity to rifamycins.
WARNINGS/PRECAUTIONS
Do not use in the treatment of active pulmonary TB caused by rifampin-resistant strains. Elevations of liver transaminases may occur; d/c therapy if evidence of liver injury occurs. Should only give therapy in cases of necessity and under strict medical supervision in patients with abnormal liver tests and/or liver disease or patients initiating treatment for active pulmonary TB. Hypersensitivity reactions and anaphylaxis reported; administer supportive measures and d/c therapy if symptoms occur. Higher rate of failure and/or relapse with rifampin-resistant organisms in patients with active pulmonary TB that are HIV-infected; do not use as a once-weekly continuation phase regimen. Higher relapse rates may occur with cavitary pulmonary lesions and/or positive sputum cultures after initial phase of active TB treatment and in patients with evidence of bilateral pulmonary disease. Poor adherence to therapy is associated with high relapse rate; emphasize the importance of compliance with therapy. May produce a red-orange discoloration of body tissues and/or fluids. May stain/discolor contact lenses or dentures. *Clostridium difficile*-associated diarrhea (CDAD) reported; if suspected/confirmed, d/c and institute appropriate therapy. Avoid with porphyria. Administration with a meal increases oral bioavailability and may reduce the incidence of GI upset, nausea and/or vomiting. Lab interactions may occur; consider alternative assay methods.
ADVERSE REACTIONS
Anemia, neutropenia, lymphopenia, hemoptysis, coughing, thrombocytosis, back pain, anorexia, increased ALT/AST, increased sweating, arthralgia, headache, rash.
DRUG INTERACTIONS
Decrease activity of drugs metabolized by CYP3A4, CYP2C8, and CYP2C9 due to enzyme induction; dose adjustments of these drugs may be necessary. May

decrease concentration and loss of therapeutic effect of protease inhibitors and certain reverse transcriptase inhibitors. May reduce effectiveness of hormonal contraceptives; may need to change to nonhormonal methods of birth control.
PREGNANCY AND LACTATION
Category C, not for use in nursing.
MECHANISM OF ACTION
Cyclopentyl rifamycin; inhibits DNA-dependent RNA polymerase in susceptible strains of *M. tuberculosis* but does not affect mammalian cells at concentrations that are active against these bacteria. It also inhibits RNA transcription by preventing the initiation of RNA chain formation.
PHARMACOKINETICS
Absorption: C_{max}=15.05mcg/mL; AUC=319.54mcg/mL•hr/mL; T_{max}=4.83 hrs. **Distribution:** V_d=70.2L; plasma protein binding (97.7%), (93.2%, metabolite). **Metabolism:** 25-desacetyl rifapentine (active metabolite). **Elimination:** Urine (17%), feces (70%); $T_{1/2}$=13.19 hrs.

PATIENT CONSIDERATIONS
Assessment: Assess for history of hypersensitivity to drug, porphyria, pregnancy/nursing status, and possible drug interactions. Rule out active TB before initiating treatment for latent TB infection. Obtain baseline serum transaminase levels in patients with abnormal liver tests and/or liver disease or patients initiating treatment for active pulmonary TB.

Monitoring: Monitor for signs/symptoms of liver injury, hypersensitivity reactions, TB relapse, CDAD, red-orange discoloration of body tissues/fluids, and other adverse reactions. Monitor serum transaminases every 2-4 weeks during therapy in patients with abnormal liver tests and/or liver disease or in patients initiating treatment for active pulmonary TB.

Counseling: Emphasize the importance of compliance with the full course of therapy and the importance of not missing any doses of therapy or companion medications in the treatment of active pulmonary TB or latent TB infection. Inform of the signs and symptoms of hypersensitivity reactions and advise to d/c use and contact physician if any of these symptoms are experienced. Instruct to stop medication and promptly notify physician if symptoms of hepatitis are experienced. Inform of the possible drug interactions. Inform that drug produces a reddish coloration of urine, sweat, sputum, tears, and breast milk and that contact lenses or dentures may be permanently stained. Advise nursing mothers that breastfeeding is not recommended with therapy use.

PRILOSEC — omeprazole   Rx
Class: Proton pump inhibitor (PPI)

ADULT DOSAGE
Helicobacter pylori Eradication
To Reduce the Risk of Duodenal Ulcer Recurrence:
Triple Therapy:
Omeprazole 20mg + clarithromycin 500mg + amoxicillin 1000mg, each given bid x 10 days. Give additional 18 days of omeprazole 20mg qd if ulcer is present at the time of initiation of therapy
Dual Therapy:
Omeprazole 40mg qd + clarithromycin 500mg tid x 14 days. Give additional 14 days of omeprazole 20mg qd if ulcer is present at the time of initiation of therapy

Active Duodenal Ulcer
20mg qd for 4 weeks; some patients may require an additional 4 weeks

Gastroesophageal Reflux Disease
Symptomatic Treatment:
20mg qd for up to 4 weeks
Erosive Esophagitis
Treatment Due to Acid-Mediated GERD:
20mg qd for 4-8 weeks. Efficacy used for >8 weeks has not been established. If a patient does not respond to 8 weeks of treatment, an additional 4 weeks may be given; if there is recurrence of erosive esophagitis or GERD symptoms, additional 4- to 8-week courses may be considered
Maint of Healing Due to Acid-Mediated GERD:
20mg qd. Controlled studies do not extend beyond 12 months

Gastric Ulcers
Active Benign:
40mg qd for 4-8 weeks

PEDIATRIC DOSAGE
Erosive Esophagitis
Treatment Due to Acid-Mediated GERD:
1 Month to <1 Year of Age:
3 to <5kg: 2.5mg qd for up to 6 weeks
5 to <10kg: 5mg qd for up to 6 weeks
≥10kg: 10mg qd for up to 6 weeks

1-16 Years:
5 to <10kg: 5mg qd for 4-8 weeks
10 to <20kg: 10mg qd for 4-8 weeks
≥20kg: 20mg qd for 4-8 weeks
Efficacy used for >8 weeks has not been established. If a patient does not respond to 8 weeks of treatment, an additional 4 weeks may be given; if there is recurrence of erosive esophagitis or GERD symptoms, additional 4- to 8-week courses may be considered

Maint of Healing Due to Acid-Mediated GERD:
1-16 Years:
5 to <10kg: 5mg qd
10 to <20kg: 10mg qd
≥20kg: 20mg qd
Controlled studies do not extend beyond 12 months

Gastroesophageal Reflux Disease
Symptomatic Treatment:
1-16 Years:
5 to <10kg: 5mg qd for up to 4 weeks
10 to <20kg: 10mg qd for up to 4 weeks
≥20kg: 20mg qd for up to 4 weeks

Pathological Hypersecretory Conditions

Long-Term Treatment:
Initial: 60mg qd
Titrate: Individualize and continue for as long as clinically indicated. Doses up to 120mg tid have been administered

Doses >80mg/day should be administered in divided doses

- -

DOSING CONSIDERATIONS
Hepatic Impairment
Child-Pugh Class A, B, or C:
Reduce dose to 10mg qd when used for the maint of healing of erosive esophagitis

Other Important Considerations
Asian Population:
Reduce dose to 10mg qd when used for the maint of healing of erosive esophagitis

ADMINISTRATION
Oral route

Take ac.
May be used concomitantly w/ antacids.

Cap, Delayed-Release
Swallow whole; do not chew.
May also be opened and administered as follows if unable to swallow intact capsule:
1. Place 1 tbsp of applesauce in a clean container; the applesauce used should not be hot and should be soft enough to be swallowed w/o chewing.
2. Open the cap and carefully empty all of the pellets inside the cap on the applesauce.
3. Mix the pellets w/ the applesauce and swallow applesauce and pellets immediately w/ a glass of cool water to ensure complete swallowing of the pellets. Do not chew/crush the pellets, and do not save for future use.

Oral Sus, Delayed-Release
Oral Administration in Water:
1. Empty the contents of a 2.5mg pkt into 5mL of water or 10mg pkt into 15mL of water.
2. Stir and leave 2-3 min to thicken.
3. Stir and drink w/in 30 min.
4. If any material remains after drinking, add more water, stir, and drink immediately.

Administration w/ Water via NG or Gastric Tube (Size 6 or Larger):
1. Add 5mL of water to a catheter-tipped syringe and then add the contents of a 2.5mg pkt (or 15mL of water for the 10mg pkt).
2. Immediately shake the syringe and leave 2-3 min to thicken.
3. Shake the syringe and inject through the NG or gastric tube into the stomach w/in 30 min.
4. Refill the syringe w/ an equal amount of water; shake and flush any remaining contents into the stomach.

STORAGE
Cap: 15-30°C (59-86°F). Protect from light and moisture. **Oral Sus:** 25°C (77°F); excursions permitted to 15-30°C (59-86°F).

HOW SUPPLIED
Cap, Delayed-Release: 10mg, 20mg, 40mg; **Oral Sus, Delayed-Release:** 2.5mg, 10mg (granules/pkt)

CONTRAINDICATIONS
Known hypersensitivity to substituted benzimidazoles or to any component of the formulation. Concomitant use w/ rilpivirine-containing products. When used w/ clarithromycin and amoxicillin, refer to the individual monographs.

WARNINGS/PRECAUTIONS
Symptomatic response to therapy does not preclude the presence of gastric malignancy in adults; consider additional follow-up and diagnostic testing in adults who have a suboptimal response or an early symptomatic relapse after completing treatment. In older patients, also consider an endoscopy. Acute interstitial nephritis reported; d/c if this develops. May increase risk of *Clostridium difficile*-associated diarrhea (CDAD), especially in hospitalized patients. May increase risk for osteoporosis-related fractures of the hip, wrist, or spine, especially w/ high-dose and long-term therapy. Use lowest dose and shortest duration appropriate to the condition being treated. Cutaneous lupus erythematosus (CLE) and systemic lupus erythematosus (SLE) reported; avoid administration of PPIs for longer than medically indicated, and d/c if signs/symptoms are consistent w/ CLE or SLE. Daily treatment w/ any acid-suppressing medications over a long period of time (eg, >3 years) may lead to malabsorption of cyanocobalamin (vitamin B12). Hypomagnesemia reported (rarely) and may require Mg^{2+} replacement and discontinuation of therapy.

ADVERSE REACTIONS
Headache, abdominal pain, N/V, diarrhea, flatulence.

DRUG INTERACTIONS
See Contraindications. Decreased exposure of some antiretroviral drugs (eg, rilpivirine, atazanavir, nelfinavir) when used concomitantly w/ omeprazole may reduce antiviral effect and promote development of drug resistance. Increased exposure of other antiretroviral drugs (eg, saquinavir) may increase toxicity. Avoid concomitant use w/ atazanavir and nelfinavir. Increased INR and PT w/ concomitant warfarin; monitor INR and PT and adjust dose of warfarin, if needed.

Concomitant use w/ methotrexate (MTX) may elevate and prolong serum levels of MTX and/or its metabolite, possibly leading to MTX toxicities; may consider temporary withdrawal of omeprazole in patients receiving high-dose MTX. Concomitant use of omeprazole 80mg reduced levels of active metabolite of clopidogrel and reduced platelet inhibition; avoid concomitant use and consider alternative antiplatelet therapy. Increased exposure of citalopram leading to increased risk of QT prolongation. Increased exposure of one of the active metabolites of cilostazol. Potential for increased exposure of phenytoin; monitor phenytoin levels and adjust dose as needed. Increased exposure of diazepam; monitor for increased sedation and reduce diazepam dose as needed. Potential for increased exposure of digoxin; monitor digoxin levels and adjust dose as needed. May reduce absorption of other drugs dependent on gastric pH for absorption (eg, iron salts, erlotinib, mycophenolate mofetil, ketoconazole) due to its effect on reducing intragastric acidity. Use w/ caution in transplant patients receiving mycophenolate mofetil. Potential for increased exposure of tacrolimus, especially in transplant patients who are intermediate or poor metabolizers of CYP2C19; monitor tacrolimus whole blood concentration and adjust dose as needed. Serum chromogranin A (CgA) levels increase secondary to PPI-induced decreases in gastric acidity and may cause false positive results in diagnostic investigations for neuroendocrine tumors; temporarily stop omeprazole treatment at least 14 days before assessing CgA levels and consider repeating the test if initial CgA levels are high. May cause hyper-response in gastrin secretion in response to secretin stimulation test, falsely suggesting gastrinoma; temporarily stop omeprazole treatment at least 14 days before assessing. False positive urine screening tests for tetrahydrocannabinol reported; consider alternative confirmatory method to verify positive results. Interactions w/ other drugs metabolized via CYP450 (eg, cyclosporine, disulfiram) reported; monitor and determine if necessary to adjust dose of these other drugs. Decreased exposure of omeprazole when used concomitantly w/ strong CYP2C19 or CYP3A4 inducers; avoid concomitant use w/ St. John's wort and rifampin. Increased exposure of omeprazole w/ CYP2C19 or CYP3A4 inhibitors; consider dose adjustment of omeprazole in patients w/ Zollinger-Ellison syndrome who may require higher doses and are taking voriconazole. Monitor Mg^{2+} levels prior to initiation and periodically during treatment in patients who take PPIs w/ medications such as digoxin or drugs that may cause hypomagnesemia (eg, diuretics). Refer to PI for further information on drug interactions.

PREGNANCY AND LACTATION
Pregnancy: There are no adequate and well-controlled studies in pregnant women.
Lactation: Limited data suggest omeprazole may be present in human milk; there is no information on the effects on the breastfed infant or on milk production. Caution in nursing.

MECHANISM OF ACTION
PPI; substituted benzimidazole that suppresses gastric acid secretion by specific inhibition of the H$^+$/K$^+$ ATPase enzyme system at the secretory surface of the gastric parietal cell. Blocks the final step of acid production.

PHARMACOKINETICS
Absorption: Rapid. Absolute bioavailability (30-40%); T$_{max}$=0.5-3.5 hrs.
Distribution: Plasma protein binding (95%); may be present in breast milk.
Metabolism: Extensive via CYP450. Formation of hydroxyomeprazole (major metabolite) via CYP2C19 (major). Formation of omeprazole sulphone via CYP3A4.
Elimination: Urine (77%, metabolites), feces; T$_{1/2}$=0.5-1 hr.

PATIENT CONSIDERATIONS
Assessment: Assess for hypersensitivity to the drug or to substituted benzimidazoles, risk for osteoporosis-related fractures, hepatic impairment, pregnancy/nursing status, and possible drug interactions. Obtain baseline Mg^{2+} levels in patients expected to be on prolonged therapy.

Monitoring: Monitor for signs/symptoms of acute interstitial nephritis, CLE/SLE, cyanocobalamin deficiency, bone fractures, hypersensitivity reactions, CDAD, and other adverse reactions. Monitor Mg^{2+} levels periodically in patients expected to be on prolonged therapy. Monitor INR and PT when given w/ warfarin.

Counseling: Inform to take exactly ud. Advise to report to physician if experiencing any signs/symptoms consistent w/ hypersensitivity reactions, acute interstitial nephritis, cyanocobalamin deficiency, CDAD, bone fracture, CLE/SLE, or hypomagnesemia. Advise to report to physician if starting treatment w/ clopidogrel, St. John's wort, or rifampin. Advise to notify physician if taking high-dose MTX.

PRINIVIL — lisinopril
Class: ACE inhibitor

Rx

D/C when pregnancy is detected. Drugs that act directly on the renin-angiotensin system (RAS) can cause injury and death to the developing fetus.

ADULT DOSAGE	PEDIATRIC DOSAGE
Hypertension	**Hypertension**
Initial: 10mg qd or 5mg qd in patients taking diuretics	**≥6 Years:**
Usual Range: 20-40mg qd. Doses up to 80mg have been used but do not appear to give a greater effect	**GFR >30mL/min/1.73m^2:**
	Initial: 0.07mg/kg qd (up to 5mg total)
May add a low-dose diuretic (eg, hydrochlorothiazide 12.5mg) if BP is not controlled	**Titrate:** Adjust dose according to BP response
	Max: 0.61mg/kg (up to 40mg) qd

Heart Failure

Reduce Signs/Symptoms in Patients Not Responding Adequately to Diuretics and Digitalis:

Adjunct w/ Diuretics and (Usually) Digitalis:

Initial: 5mg qd; 2.5mg qd w/ hyponatremia (serum Na$^+$ <130mEq/L)

Max: 40mg qd

Diuretic dose may need to be adjusted to help minimize hypovolemia

Acute Myocardial Infarction

Reduction of Mortality in Treatment of Hemodynamically Stable Patients w/in 24 Hrs of Acute MI (AMI):

5mg w/in 24 hrs of onset of symptoms, followed by 5mg after 24 hrs, 10mg after 48 hrs, and then 10mg qd for at least 6 weeks

In patients w/ low systolic BP (SBP) (100-120mmHg) during the first 3 days after infarct, initiate therapy w/ 2.5mg. If hypotension occurs (SBP ≤100mmHg) consider doses of 2.5mg or 5mg. D/C therapy if prolonged hypotension occurs (SBP <90mmHg for >1 hr)

DOSING CONSIDERATIONS

Renal Impairment

CrCl 10-30mL/min:
Reduce initial dose to 1/2 of the usual recommended dose (eg, HTN, 5mg; heart failure or AMI, 2.5mg)

Hemodialysis or CrCl <10mL/min:
Initial: 2.5mg qd

Pediatric Patients:
GFR <30mL/min/1.73m^2: Not recommended

ADMINISTRATION
Oral route

STORAGE
15-30°C (59-86°F). Protect from moisture.

HOW SUPPLIED
Tab: 5mg*, 10mg*, 20mg* *scored

CONTRAINDICATIONS
History of ACE inhibitor-associated angioedema or hypersensitivity, hereditary or idiopathic angioedema. Coadministration w/ aliskiren in patients w/ diabetes.

WARNINGS/PRECAUTIONS
Head/neck angioedema reported; d/c and administer appropriate therapy. Patients w/ a history of angioedema unrelated to ACE inhibitor therapy may be at increased risk of angioedema during therapy. Higher rate of angioedema in blacks than nonblacks. Intestinal angioedema reported; monitor for abdominal pain. Anaphylactoid reactions reported during desensitization w/ hymenoptera venom, dialysis w/ high-flux membranes, and LDL apheresis w/ dextran sulfate absorption. May cause changes in renal function, including acute renal failure, especially in patients whose renal function may depend in part on the activity of the RAS; consider withholding or discontinuing therapy if a clinically significant decrease in renal function develops. May cause symptomatic hypotension, sometimes complicated by oliguria, progressive azotemia, acute renal failure, or death; closely monitor patients at risk of excessive hypotension for the first 2 weeks of treatment and whenever therapy and/or diuretic dose is increased. Avoid in patients who are hemodynamically unstable after an AMI. Symptomatic hypotension may occur in patients w/ severe aortic stenosis or hypertrophic cardiomyopathy. Hypotension may occur w/ major surgery or during anesthesia. May cause hyperkalemia; periodically monitor serum K$^+$ during therapy. Associated w/ a syndrome that starts w/ cholestatic jaundice or hepatitis and progresses to fulminant hepatic necrosis and sometimes death; d/c therapy if jaundice or marked hepatic enzyme elevations develop.

ADVERSE REACTIONS
Headache, dizziness, cough, hypotension, chest pain, increased creatinine, hyperkalemia, syncope.

DRUG INTERACTIONS
See Contraindications. Initiation of therapy in patients on diuretics may result in excessive reduction of BP. Decrease or d/c diuretic or increase the salt intake prior to initiation of therapy; if this is not possible, reduce the starting dose of lisinopril. Attenuates K$^+$ loss caused by thiazide-type diuretics. K$^+$-sparing diuretics (eg, spironolactone, amiloride, triamterene) may increase hyperkalemia risk; frequently monitor serum K$^+$ if concomitant use of such agents is indicated. Increased risk of hyperkalemia w/ K$^+$ supplements or K$^+$-containing salt substitutes. May cause an increased blood-glucose-lowering effect w/ risk of hypoglycemia w/ antidiabetic medicines (insulins, oral hypoglycemic agents). NSAIDs, including selective COX-2 inhibitors, may result in deterioration of renal function, including possible acute renal failure in elderly, volume depleted or patients w/ compromised renal function. Antihypertensive effect may be attenuated by NSAIDs. Dual blockade of the RAS is associated w/ increased risks of hypotension, syncope, hyperkalemia, and changes in renal function (including acute renal failure); avoid combined use of RAS inhibitors, and monitor BP, renal function, and electrolytes w/ other agents that affect the RAS. Avoid w/ aliskiren in patients w/ renal impairment (GFR <60mL/min). Lithium toxicity reported; monitor serum lithium levels during concurrent use. Nitritoid reactions reported w/ injectable gold. Increased BUN and SrCr w/ diuretics. Coadministration w/ mTOR inhibitors (eg, temsirolimus, sirolimus, everolimus) may increase risk for angioedema.

PREGNANCY AND LACTATION
Pregnancy: Category D.
Lactation: Not for use in nursing.

MECHANISM OF ACTION
ACE inhibitor; decreases plasma angiotensin II, which leads to decreased vasopressor activity and decreased aldosterone secretion.

PHARMACOKINETICS
Absorption: T_{max}=7 hrs (adults), 6 hrs (pediatric patients). **Elimination:** Urine (unchanged); $T_{1/2}$=12 hrs.

PATIENT CONSIDERATIONS

Assessment: Assess for hypersensitivity to the drug, hereditary or idiopathic angioedema, history of ACE inhibitor-associated angioedema, risk factors for hyperkalemia, risk of excessive hypotension, renal artery stenosis, severe aortic stenosis or hypertrophic cardiomyopathy, renal impairment, pregnancy/nursing status, and possible drug interactions.

Monitoring: Monitor for angioedema, anaphylactoid reactions, hyperkalemia, and other adverse reactions. Monitor BP, LFTs, serum K$^+$, and renal function.

Counseling: Inform of pregnancy risks and discuss treatment options for women planning to become pregnant; instruct to report pregnancy to physician as soon as possible. Instruct to immediately report signs/symptoms of angioedema and to avoid drug until they have consulted w/ prescribing physician. Instruct to report lightheadedness, especially during 1st few days of therapy; if syncope occurs, advise to d/c therapy until physician is consulted. Advise that excessive perspiration, dehydration, and other causes of volume depletion (eg, vomiting, diarrhea) may lead to excessive fall in BP; instruct to consult w/ a physician. Advise not to use salt substitutes containing K$^+$ w/o consulting physician. Advise diabetic patients treated w/ oral antidiabetic agents or insulin to closely monitor for hypoglycemia, especially during the 1st month of combined use. Instruct to report promptly any indication of infection, which may be a sign of leukopenia/neutropenia.

PRISTIQ — desvenlafaxine   **Rx**

Class: Serotonin and norepinephrine reuptake inhibitor (SNRI)

> Antidepressants increased the risk of suicidal thoughts and behavior in children, adolescents, and young adults in short-term studies. In patients of all ages who are started on antidepressant therapy, monitor closely for worsening, and emergence of suicidal thoughts and behaviors. Not approved for use in pediatric patients.

ADULT DOSAGE

Major Depressive Disorder

50mg qd

In clinical studies, doses of 50-400mg/day were effective; no additional benefit was demonstrated at doses >50mg/day and adverse reactions/discontinuations were more frequent at higher doses

Switching from Other Antidepressants:
May need to taper initial antidepressant to minimize discontinuation symptoms

Dosing Considerations with MAOIs

Switching to/from an MAOI for Psychiatric Disorders:
Allow at least 14 days between discontinuation of an MAOI and initiation of desvenlafaxine, and allow at least 7 days between discontinuation of desvenlafaxine and initiation of an MAOI

W/ Other MAOIs (eg, Linezolid, IV Methylene Blue):
Do not start desvenlafaxine in a patient being treated w/ linezolid or IV methylene blue.
In patients already receiving desvenlafaxine, if acceptable alternatives are not available and benefits outweigh risks, d/c desvenlafaxine promptly and administer linezolid or IV methylene blue; monitor for serotonin syndrome for 7 days or until 24 hrs after the last dose of linezolid or IV methylene blue, whichever comes 1st. May resume desvenlafaxine therapy 24 hrs after the last dose of linezolid or IV methylene blue.

PEDIATRIC DOSAGE

Pediatric use may not have been established

DOSING CONSIDERATIONS
Renal Impairment
Mild:
No dose adjustment
Moderate (CrCl 30-50mL/min):
Max: 50mg/day
Severe (CrCl <30mL/min)/ESRD:
Max: 25mg qd or 50mg qod; do not give supplemental doses after dialysis
Hepatic Impairment
Mild:
No dose adjustment
Moderate to Severe:
50mg/day
Max: Dose escalation >100mg/day not recommended
Discontinuation
Gradually reduce dose; if intolerable symptoms occur following a decrease in dose or upon discontinuation, consider resuming the previously prescribed dose and continue decreasing the dose at a more gradual rate. The 25mg dose is available for discontinuing therapy

ADMINISTRATION
Oral route
Take at approx the same time each day, w/ or w/o food.
Swallow tab whole w/ fluid; do not divide, crush, chew, or dissolve.

STORAGE
20-25°C (68-77°F); excursions permitted to 15-30°C (59-86°F).

HOW SUPPLIED
Tab, Extended-Release: 25mg, 50mg, 100mg

CONTRAINDICATIONS
Hypersensitivity to desvenlafaxine succinate, venlafaxine HCl, or to any excipients in the formulation. Use of an MAOI intended to treat psychiatric disorders either concomitantly or w/in 7 days of stopping treatment. Treatment w/in 14 days of stopping an MAOI intended to treat psychiatric disorders. Starting treatment in patients being treated w/ MAOIs (eg, linezolid, IV methylene blue).

WARNINGS/PRECAUTIONS
Not approved for the treatment of bipolar depression; screen patients to determine risk for bipolar disorder prior to initiating therapy. Serotonin syndrome reported; d/c immediately if symptoms occur and initiate supportive symptomatic treatment. May increase BP; caution w/ preexisting HTN or cardiovascular (CV)/cerebrovascular conditions that might be compromised by increases in BP. Consider dose reduction or discontinuation of therapy if sustained increases in BP occur. May increase risk of bleeding events. Pupillary dilation that occurs following use may trigger an angle-closure attack in a patient w/ anatomically narrow angles who does not have a patent iridectomy. Activation of mania/hypomania reported. Discontinuation symptoms reported. Avoid abrupt discontinuation. Seizures reported. Hyponatremia may occur; caution in elderly and volume-depleted patients. Consider discontinuation in patients w/ symptomatic hyponatremia. Interstitial lung disease and eosinophilic pneumonia may occur; consider diagnosis for either in patients w/ progressive dyspnea, cough, or chest discomfort, and consider discontinuing therapy. False (+) urine immunoassay screening tests for phencyclidine and amphetamines reported.

ADVERSE REACTIONS
Nausea, dizziness, insomnia, hyperhidrosis, constipation, somnolence, decreased appetite, anxiety, specific male sexual function disorders.

DRUG INTERACTIONS
See Contraindications. Avoid w/ other desvenlafaxine-containing products or venlafaxine products; may increase desvenlafaxine levels and increase dose-related adverse reactions. Avoid alcohol consumption. May cause serotonin syndrome w/ other serotonergic drugs (eg, triptans, TCAs, fentanyl) and w/ drugs that impair metabolism of serotonin; d/c desvenlafaxine and any concomitant serotonergic agent immediately if serotonin syndrome occurs. Caution w/ NSAIDs, aspirin (ASA), warfarin, and other drugs that affect coagulation or bleeding, due to increased risk of bleeding. May increase risk of hyponatremia w/ diuretics. Potent CYP3A4 inhibitors (eg, ketoconazole) may increase levels. CYP2D6 substrates (eg, desipramine, atomoxetine, dextromethorphan) should be dosed at the original level when coadministered w/ 100mg desvenlafaxine or lower, or when desvenlafaxine is discontinued; reduce the dose of these substrates by up to 1/2 if coadministered w/ 400mg desvenlafaxine.

PREGNANCY AND LACTATION
Pregnancy: Category C.
Lactation: Found in breast milk; not for use in nursing.

MECHANISM OF ACTION
SNRI; has not been established. Thought to be related to the potentiation of serotonin and norepinephrine in the CNS through inhibition of their reuptake.

PHARMACOKINETICS
Absorption: Absolute bioavailability (80%). **Distribution:** Plasma protein binding (30%); V_d=3.4L/kg (IV); found in breast milk. **Metabolism:** Conjugation via UGT isoforms (primary) and N-demethylation via CYP3A4 (minor). **Elimination:** Urine (45% unchanged, 19% glucuronide metabolite, <5% oxidative metabolite). $T_{1/2}$=10-11.1 hrs.

PATIENT CONSIDERATIONS
Assessment: Assess for risk for bipolar disorder, history of mania/hypomania, seizure disorders, HTN, CV/cerebrovascular conditions, susceptibility to angle-closure glaucoma, volume depletion, hypersensitivity to the drug, hepatic/renal impairment, pregnancy/nursing status, and possible drug interactions.

Monitoring: Monitor for signs/symptoms of clinical worsening (eg, suicidality, unusual changes in behavior), serotonin syndrome, abnormal bleeding, angle-closure glaucoma, activation of mania/hypomania, seizures, hyponatremia, interstitial lung disease, eosinophilic pneumonia, and other adverse reactions. Monitor BP, LFTs, and renal function. Monitor for discontinuation symptoms (eg, dysphoric mood, irritability, agitation) when discontinuing therapy, Carefully monitor patients receiving concomitant warfarin therapy when treatment w/ desvenlafaxine is initiated or discontinued. Periodically reassess to determine the need for continued treatment.

Counseling: Advise patients, families, and caregivers about the benefits and risks of treatment and counsel on its appropriate use. Counsel patients, families, and caregivers to look for the emergence of suicidality, especially early during treatment and when the dose is adjusted up or down. Caution about the risk of serotonin syndrome, particularly w/ the concomitant use w/ other serotonergic agents. Inform that concomitant use w/ ASA, NSAIDs, warfarin, or other drugs that affect coagulation may increase the risk of bleeding. Advise to monitor BP regularly, to observe for signs/symptoms of activation of mania/hypomania, to avoid alcohol, and not to d/c therapy w/o notifying physician. Inform that discontinuation effects may occur when stopping treatment and a dose of 25mg/day is available for discontinuing therapy. Caution about risk of angle-closure glaucoma. Caution against operating hazardous machinery (including automobiles) until reasonably certain that therapy does not adversely affect ability to engage in such activities. Advise to notify physician if allergic phenomena develop, if pregnant, intending to become pregnant, or if breastfeeding. Inform that an inert matrix tab may pass in the stool or via colostomy.

PRIVIGEN — immune globulin intravenous (human)   Rx
Class: Immune globulin

> Thrombosis may occur. Renal dysfunction, acute renal failure, osmotic nephrosis, and death may occur w/ immune globulin intravenous (IGIV) products in predisposed patients. Renal dysfunction and acute renal failure occur more commonly w/ IGIV products containing sucrose; this product does not contain sucrose. For patients at risk of thrombosis (eg, using estrogens), renal dysfunction (eg, receiving known nephrotoxic drugs), or renal failure, administer at the minimum dose and infusion rate practicable. Ensure adequate hydration before administration. Monitor for signs/symptoms of thrombosis and assess blood viscosity if at risk for hyperviscosity.

ADULT DOSAGE
Primary Humoral Immunodeficiency
Replacement Therapy:
Usual: 200-800mg/kg (2-8mL/kg) every 3-4 weeks
Titrate: Adjust to achieve desired serum trough levels and clinical response
Initial Infusion Rate:
0.5mg/kg/min (0.005mL/kg/min)
Maint Infusion Rate:
Increase to 8mg/kg/min (0.08mL/kg/min) as tolerated

If a dose is missed, administer the missed dose as soon as possible, and then resume scheduled treatments every 3 or 4 weeks, as applicable

Chronic Immune Thrombocytopenic Purpura
Usual: 1g/kg (10mL/kg) daily for 2 consecutive days (total dosage of 2g/kg)
Initial Infusion Rate:
0.5mg/kg/min (0.005mL/kg/min)
Maint Infusion Rate:
Increase to 4mg/kg/min (0.04mL/kg/min) as tolerated

PEDIATRIC DOSAGE
Primary Humoral Immunodeficiency
Replacement Therapy:
≥3 Years:
Usual: 200-800mg/kg (2-8mL/kg) every 3-4 weeks
Titrate: Adjust to achieve desired serum trough levels and clinical response
Initial Infusion Rate:
0.5mg/kg/min (0.005mL/kg/min)
Maint Infusion Rate:
Increase to 8mg/kg/min (0.08mL/kg/min) as tolerated

If a dose is missed, administer the missed dose as soon as possible, and then resume scheduled treatments every 3 or 4 weeks, as applicable

Chronic Immune Thrombocytopenic Purpura
≥15 Years:
Usual: 1g/kg (10mL/kg) daily for 2 consecutive days (total dosage of 2g/kg)
Initial Infusion Rate:
0.5mg/kg/min (0.005mL/kg/min)
Maint Infusion Rate:
Increase to 4mg/kg/min (0.04mL/kg/min) as tolerated

DOSING CONSIDERATIONS
Elderly
Do not exceed recommended doses, and administer at the minimum dose and infusion rate practicable

Adverse Reactions
Slow or stop infusion if adverse reactions occur; may resume at a lower rate if symptoms subside promptly

ADMINISTRATION
IV route

Preparation and Administration
Do not shake.
Do not freeze; do not use if product has been frozen.
Should be at room temperature at the time of administration.
Infuse using a separate infusion line; prior to use, infusion line may be flushed w/ D5W or 0.9% NaCl for inj.
Do not mix w/ other IGIV products or other IV medications; may be diluted w/ D5W.

May use an infusion pump to control rate of administration.
If large doses are to be administered, several vials may be pooled using aseptic technique; begin infusion w/in 8 hrs of pooling.

STORAGE
Room temperature up to 25°C (77°F) for up to 36 months. Do not freeze; do not use if it has been frozen. Protect from light.

HOW SUPPLIED
Inj: 10% [50mL, 100mL, 200mL, 400mL]

CONTRAINDICATIONS
History of anaphylactic or severe systemic reaction to human immune globulin, hyperprolinemia, IgA-deficient patients w/ antibodies to IgA, and a history of hypersensitivity.

WARNINGS/PRECAUTIONS
Contains trace amounts of IgA; severe hypersensitivity reactions may occur. D/C infusion immediately and institute appropriate treatment if hypersensitivity develops. Ensure that patients w/ preexisting renal insufficiency are not volume depleted; consider discontinuation if renal function deteriorates. Hyperproteinemia, increased serum viscosity, and hyponatremia may occur. Distinguish true hyponatremia from pseudohyponatremia (as demonstrated by a decreased calculated serum osmolality or elevated osmolar gap); treatment aimed at decreasing serum free water in patients w/ pseudohyponatremia may lead to volume depletion, a further increase in serum viscosity, and a possible predisposition to thromboembolic events. Aseptic meningitis syndrome (AMS) reported and may occur more frequently w/ high doses (2g/kg) and/or rapid infusion; rule out other causes of meningitis. Delayed hemolytic anemia may develop; acute hemolysis reported. Severe hemolysis-related renal dysfunction/ failure or disseminated intravascular coagulation reported. Noncardiogenic pulmonary edema may occur; if transfusion-related acute lung injury (TRALI) is suspected, perform tests for presence of antineutrophil antibodies and anti-human leukocyte antigen (HLA) antibodies in both the product and patient's serum. Caution w/ high-dose regimen (for chronic ITP) in patients at increased risk of thrombosis, hemolysis, acute kidney injury, or volume overload. May carry a risk of transmitting infectious agents (eg, viruses, and, theoretically, the Creutzfeldt-Jakob disease agent). May interfere w/ some serological tests. Caution in elderly.

ADVERSE REACTIONS
Thrombosis, renal dysfunction, acute renal failure, osmotic nephrosis, headache, fatigue, N/V, chills, back pain, pain, elevated body temperature, anemia, epistaxis, blood bilirubin increased, Hct decreased.

DRUG INTERACTIONS
See Boxed Warning. May interfere w/ the response to live virus vaccines (eg, measles, mumps, rubella, varicella).

PREGNANCY AND LACTATION
Category C, safety not known in nursing.

MECHANISM OF ACTION
Immune globulin; not established. Replacement therapy for PI; supplies a broad spectrum of opsonic and neutralizing IgG antibodies against bacterial, viral, parasitic, and mycoplasma agents and their toxins.

PHARMACOKINETICS
Absorption: (3-Week Dosing Interval) C_{max}=2550mg/dL; $AUC_{0-t,0-inf}$=32,820 day•mg/dL, 79,315 day•mg/dL. (4-Week Dosing Interval) C_{max}=2260mg/dL; $AUC_{0-t,0-inf}$=36,390 day•mg/dL, 104,627 day•mg/dL. **Distribution:** Crosses placenta. (3-Week Dosing Interval) V_d=50mL/kg. (4-Week Dosing Interval) V_d=84mL/kg. **Elimination:** (3-Week Dosing Interval) $T_{1/2}$=27.6 days. (4-Week Dosing Interval) $T_{1/2}$=45.4 days.

PATIENT CONSIDERATIONS
Assessment: Assess for history of anaphylactic or severe systemic reactions to human immune globulin, hyperprolinemia, IgA deficiency, risk of thrombosis/ renal dysfunction/renal failure/hemolysis/volume overload, pregnancy/nursing status, and possible drug interactions. Assess renal function. Consider baseline assessment of blood viscosity in patients at risk for hyperviscosity, including those w/ cryoglobulins, fasting chylomicronemia/markedly high TGs, or monoclonal gammopathies. Consider appropriate lab testing in patients at higher risk for hemolysis, including measurement of Hgb/Hct prior to infusion.

Monitoring: Monitor for thrombosis, hypersensitivity reactions, hyperproteinemia, hyperviscosity, hyponatremia, hemolytic anemia, pulmonary adverse reactions, infection, and other adverse reactions. Monitor renal function and urine output periodically. Perform neurological exam, including CSF studies, if AMS is suspected. Consider testing in patients at higher risk for hemolysis, including measurement of Hgb/Hct w/in 36-96 hrs post infusion. Perform confirmatory lab testing if signs/symptoms of hemolysis or a significant drop in Hgb/Hct have been observed. Perform tests for presence of antineutrophil antibodies and anti-HLA antibodies in both the product and patient's serum if TRALI is suspected. Monitor vital signs throughout the infusion.

Counseling: Instruct to immediately report to physician any signs/symptoms of hypersensitivity reactions, kidney problems, thrombosis, AMS, hemolysis, TRALI, and infection. Inform that drug is made from human blood and may contain infectious agents that can cause disease. Inform that product may interfere w/ the response to live virus vaccines; instruct to notify immunizing physician of recent therapy w/ this product.

ProAir HFA — albuterol sulfate   Rx
Class: Short-acting beta₂ agonist (SABA)

ADULT DOSAGE	PEDIATRIC DOSAGE
Bronchospasm	**Bronchospasm**
Treatment/Prevention of Bronchospasm w/ Reversible Obstructive Airway Disease: 2 inh q4-6h; 1 inh q4h may be sufficient in some patients	**Treatment/Prevention of Bronchospasm w/ Reversible Obstructive Airway Disease:** **≥4 Years:** 2 inh q4-6h; 1 inh q4h may be sufficient in some patients
Exercise-Induced Bronchospasm	**Exercise-Induced Bronchospasm**
Prevention: 2 inh 15-30 min prior to exercise	**Prevention:** **≥4 Years:** 2 inh 15-30 min prior to exercise

DOSING CONSIDERATIONS
Elderly
Start at lower end of dosing range

ADMINISTRATION
Oral inh route
Shake well before each spray.

Priming
Prime inhaler before using for the 1st time and when inhaler has not been used for >2 weeks by releasing 3 sprays into the air, away from the face.

STORAGE
15-25°C (59-77°F). Protect from freezing and direct sunlight. Contents under pressure; do not puncture or incinerate. Exposure to temperatures >49°C (120°F) may cause bursting.

HOW SUPPLIED
MDI: 90mcg of albuterol base/inh [200 actuations]

CONTRAINDICATIONS
History of hypersensitivity to albuterol or any components of the medication.

WARNINGS/PRECAUTIONS
May produce paradoxical bronchospasm; d/c immediately and institute alternative therapy if this occurs. More doses than usual may be a marker of destabilization of asthma and may require reevaluation of the patient and treatment regimen; anti-inflammatory treatment (eg, corticosteroids) may be needed. May produce clinically significant cardiovascular (CV) effects; may need to d/c. ECG changes and immediate hypersensitivity reactions may occur. Fatalities reported w/ excessive use. Caution w/ CV disorders (eg, coronary insufficiency, arrhythmias, HTN), convulsive disorders, hyperthyroidism, diabetes mellitus (DM), and in patients unusually responsive to sympathomimetic amines. May produce significant hypokalemia and BP changes. Aggravation of preexisting DM and ketoacidosis reported w/ large doses of IV albuterol. Caution w/ renal impairment.

ADVERSE REACTIONS
Pharyngitis, headache, rhinitis, dizziness, musculoskeletal pain, tachycardia.

DRUG INTERACTIONS
Avoid w/ other short-acting sympathomimetic aerosol bronchodilators; caution w/ additional adrenergic drugs administered by any route. Use w/ β-blockers may block pulmonary effect and produce severe bronchospasm in asthmatic patients; avoid concomitant use. If needed, consider cardioselective β-blockers and use w/ caution. ECG changes and/or hypokalemia caused by non-K⁺-sparing diuretics (eg, loop, thiazide) may be acutely worsened; use caution and consider monitoring K⁺ levels. May decrease digoxin levels; monitor serum digoxin levels. Use extreme caution w/ MAOIs and TCAs, or w/in 2 weeks of discontinuation of such agents; consider alternative therapy in patients taking MAOIs or TCAs.

PREGNANCY AND LACTATION
Pregnancy: Category C.
Lactation: Not for use in nursing.

MECHANISM OF ACTION
β₂-agonist; activates β₂-adrenergic receptors on airway smooth muscle, leading to activation of adenylcyclase and to an increase in cAMP. Increased cAMP leads to activation of protein kinase A, which inhibits the phosphorylation of myosin and lowers intracellular ionic calcium concentrations, resulting in relaxation of smooth muscle of all airways, from the trachea to the terminal bronchioles.

PHARMACOKINETICS
Absorption: C_{max}=4100pg/mL; AUC=28,426pg/mL•hr. **Metabolism:** GI tract via SULTIA3 (sulfotransferase). **Elimination:** Urine (80-100%), feces (<20%); $T_{1/2}$=6 hrs.

PATIENT CONSIDERATIONS
Assessment: Assess for history of hypersensitivity to drug, CV disorders, convulsive disorders, hyperthyroidism, DM, renal impairment, pregnancy/nursing status, and possible drug interactions. Assess use in patients unusually responsive to sympathomimetic amines.

Monitoring: Monitor for paradoxical bronchospasm, deterioration of asthma, CV effects, ECG changes, hypokalemia, immediate hypersensitivity reactions, and other adverse reactions. Monitor BP, HR, and ECG changes. Monitor renal function in elderly.

Counseling: Inform not to increase dose/frequency of doses w/o consulting physician. Advise to seek immediate medical attention if treatment becomes less effective for symptomatic relief, symptoms become worse, and/or there is a need to use product more frequently than usual. Instruct to keep plastic mouthpiece clean to prevent medication build-up and blockage; advise to wash, shake to remove excess water, and air dry mouthpiece thoroughly at least once a week. Inform that inhaler may cease to deliver medication if not cleaned properly. Inform that drug may cause paradoxical bronchospasm; instruct to d/c if this occurs. Instruct to take concurrent inhaled drugs and other asthma medications only ud. Inform of the common adverse effects of treatment (eg, palpitations, chest pain, rapid HR, tremor, nervousness). Instruct to notify physician if pregnant/nursing. Instruct to use only w/ supplied actuator and not to use actuator w/ other aerosol medications.

PROAIR RESPICLICK — albuterol sulfate   Rx

Class: Short-acting beta$_2$ agonist (SABA)

ADULT DOSAGE	PEDIATRIC DOSAGE
Bronchospasm	**Bronchospasm**
Treatment/Prevention w/ Reversible Obstructive Airway Disease: 2 inh q4-6h; 1 inh q4h may be sufficient in some patients	**≥4 Years:** **Treatment/Prevention w/ Reversible Obstructive Airway Disease:** 2 inh q4-6h; 1 inh q4h may be sufficient in some patients
Exercise-Induced Bronchospasm	**Exercise-Induced Bronchospasm**
Prevention: 2 inh 15-30 min prior to exercise	**≥4 Years:** **Prevention:** 2 inh 15-30 min prior to exercise

---

DOSING CONSIDERATIONS
Elderly
Start at lower end of dosing range

ADMINISTRATION
Oral inh route

Priming
Does not require priming.
Do not use w/ a spacer or volume holding chamber.

STORAGE
15-25°C (59-77°F). Avoid exposure to extreme heat, cold, or humidity.

HOW SUPPLIED
MDI: 90mcg of albuterol base/inh [200 actuations]

CONTRAINDICATIONS
History of hypersensitivity to albuterol and/or severe milk protein hypersensitivity.

WARNINGS/PRECAUTIONS
May produce paradoxical bronchospasm; d/c immediately and institute alternative therapy if this occurs. More doses than usual may be a marker of destabilization of asthma and may require reevaluation of the patient and treatment regimen; give special consideration to the possible need for anti-inflammatory treatment (eg, corticosteroids). May produce cardiovascular (CV) effects; may need to d/c if CV effects occur. ECG changes reported. Immediate hypersensitivity reactions may occur. Fatalities reported w/ excessive use; do not exceed recommended dose. Caution w/ CV disorders (eg, coronary insufficiency, arrhythmias, HTN), convulsive disorders, hyperthyroidism, diabetes mellitus (DM), and in patients unusually responsive to sympathomimetic amines. May produce significant hypokalemia and BP changes. Aggravation of preexisting DM and ketoacidosis reported w/ large doses of IV albuterol. Caution when administering high doses in patients w/ renal impairment.

ADVERSE REACTIONS
Back pain, pain, gastroenteritis viral, sinus headache, UTI.

DRUG INTERACTIONS
Avoid w/ other short-acting sympathomimetic bronchodilators; caution w/ additional adrenergic drugs administered by any route. Use w/ β-blockers may block pulmonary effect and produce severe bronchospasm in asthmatic patients; avoid concomitant use. If needed, consider cardioselective β-blockers and administer w/ caution. ECG changes and/or hypokalemia caused by non-K$^+$-sparing diuretics (eg, loop, thiazide) may be worsened; consider monitoring K$^+$ levels. May decrease digoxin levels; monitor serum digoxin levels. Use extreme caution w/ MAOIs and TCAs, or w/in 2 weeks of discontinuation of such agents; consider alternative therapy in patients taking MAOIs or TCAs.

PREGNANCY AND LACTATION
Pregnancy: There are no randomized clinical studies of use of albuterol during pregnancy. Available data from published epidemiological studies and postmarketing case reports of pregnancy outcomes following inhaled albuterol use do not consistently demonstrate a risk of major birth defects or miscarriage. Closely monitor pregnant women and adjust medication as necessary to maintain optimal control.
Lactation: There are no available data on the presence of albuterol in human milk, the effects on the breastfed child, or the effects on milk production; plasma levels of albuterol after inhaled therapeutic doses are low in humans, and if present in breast milk, albuterol has a low oral bioavailability.

MECHANISM OF ACTION
β$_2$-agonist; activates β$_2$-adrenergic receptors on airway smooth muscle, leading to activation of adenylcyclase and to an increase in cAMP.

PHARMACOKINETICS
Absorption: Rapid. T$_{max}$=30 min. **Distribution:** Plasma protein binding (10%). **Metabolism:** GI tract via SULT1A3 (sulfotransferase). **Elimination:** Urine (80-100%), feces (<20%); T$_{1/2}$=approx 5 hrs.

PATIENT CONSIDERATIONS

Assessment: Assess for history of hypersensitivity to drug, milk protein hypersensitivity, CV disorders, convulsive disorders, hyperthyroidism, DM, renal impairment, pregnancy/nursing status, and possible drug interactions. Assess use in patients unusually responsive to sympathomimetic amines.

Monitoring: Monitor for paradoxical bronchospasm, deterioration of asthma, CV effects, ECG changes, hypokalemia, immediate hypersensitivity reactions, and other adverse reactions. Monitor BP and HR. Monitor renal function in elderly.

Counseling: Counsel not to increase dose/frequency of doses w/o consulting physician. Advise to seek immediate medical attention if treatment becomes less effective for symptomatic relief, symptoms become worse, and/or there is a need to use product more frequently than usual. Instruct not to open the inhaler unless taking a dose. Advise to keep the inhaler clean and dry at all times. Instruct not to wash or put any part of the inhaler in water. If the mouthpiece needs cleaning, instruct to gently wipe the mouthpiece w/ a dry cloth or tissue prn. Instruct to never take the inhaler apart. Inform that drug may cause paradoxical bronchospasm; instruct to d/c if this occurs. Instruct to take concurrent inhaled drugs and other asthma medications only ud. Inform of the common adverse effects of treatment (eg, palpitations, chest pain, rapid HR). Instruct to notify physician if pregnant/nursing. Advise that the inhaler has a dose counter attached to the actuator. Inform that when the patient receives the inhaler, the number 200 will be displayed. Advise that the dose counter will count down each time the inhaler is actuated and that when the dose counter reaches 20, the color of the numbers will change to red to remind the patient to contact their pharmacist for a refill of medication or consult their physician for a prescription refill. Inform that when the dose counter reaches 0, the background will change to solid red; instruct to discard inhaler 13 months after opening the foil pouch, when the dose counter displays 0, or after the expiration date on the product, whichever comes first.

PROBENECID/COLCHICINE — colchicine/probenecid   Rx

Class: Uricosuric

ADULT DOSAGE	PEDIATRIC DOSAGE
Gouty Arthritis	Pediatric use may not have been established
Treatment of chronic gouty arthritis when complicated by frequent, recurrent acute attacks of gout	
Usual: 1 tab qd for 1 week, then 1 tab bid thereafter **Titrate:** Daily dose may be increased by 1 tab every 4 weeks w/in tolerance (and usually not >4 tabs/day) if symptoms are not controlled or the 24-hr uric acid excretion is <700mg	
When acute attacks have been absent for ≥6 months and serum urate levels remain w/in normal limits, the daily dose may be decreased by 1 tab every 6 months	

DOSING CONSIDERATIONS
Renal Impairment
2 tabs/day may be adequate
Chronic Renal Insufficiency (GFR ≤30mL/min): Probenecid may not be effective

Adverse Reactions
Gastric Intolerance: May be indicative of overdose; correct by decreasing the dose

ADMINISTRATION
Oral route

Do not initiate therapy until an acute gouty attack has subsided; however, if an acute attack is precipitated during therapy, probenecid and colchicine may be continued w/o changing the dose, and additional colchicine or other appropriate therapy should be given to control the acute attack.

A liberal fluid intake is recommended, as well as sufficient sodium bicarbonate (3-7.5g/day) or potassium citrate (7.5g/day) to maintain an alkaline urine.

STORAGE
20-25°C (68-77°F). Protect from light.

HOW SUPPLIED
Tab: (Probenecid/Colchicine) 500mg/0.5mg

CONTRAINDICATIONS
Hypersensitivity to this product or to probenecid or colchicine. Blood dyscrasias, uric acid kidney stones, children <2 yrs of age, pregnancy, initiating therapy before acute gout attack subsides, coadministration with salicylates.

WARNINGS/PRECAUTIONS
Exacerbation of gout may occur. Severe allergic reactions and anaphylaxis reported rarely; d/c if hypersensitivity occurs. Caution with history of peptic ulcer. Hematuria, renal colic, costovertebral pain, and formation of uric acid stones reported; maintain liberal fluid intake and alkalization of urine. May not be effective in chronic renal insufficiency (GFR ≤30mL/min). Reversible azoospermia reported. Colchicine is an established mutagen; may be carcinogenic.

ADVERSE REACTIONS
Headache, dizziness, fever, pruritus, acute gouty arthritis, purpura, leukopenia, peripheral neuritis, muscular weakness, N/V, urticaria, anemia, dermatitis, alopecia.

DRUG INTERACTIONS

See Contraindications. Salicylates and pyrazinamide antagonize uricosuric effects; use acetaminophen (APAP) if mild analgesic is needed. Probenecid increases plasma levels of penicillin and other β-lactams; psychic disturbances reported. Methotrexate levels increased with coadministration; reduce dose and monitor levels. May prolong/enhance effects of sulfonylureas; increased risk of hypoglycemia. Increased $T_{1/2}$ levels of indomethacin, naproxen, ketoprofen, meclofenamate, lorazepam, APAP, and rifampin. Increased levels of sulindac and sulfonamides; monitor sulfonamide levels with prolonged use. Inhibits renal transport of amino hippuric acid, aminosalicylic acid, indomethacin, sodium iodomethamate and related iodinated organic acids, 17-ketosteroids, pantothenic acid, phenolsulfonphthalein, sulfonamides, and sulfonylureas. Possible falsely high plasma levels of theophylline. Decreases hepatic/renal excretion of sulfobromophthalein. May require significantly less thiopental for induction of anesthesia.

PREGNANCY AND LACTATION

Pregnancy: Contraindicated in pregnancy.
Lactation: Safety not known in nursing.

MECHANISM OF ACTION

Probenecid: Uricosuric/renal tubular blocking agent; increases urinary excretion of uric acid and decreases serum urate levels. Colchicine: Colchicum alkaloid; not established. Has prophylactic, suppressive effect helping to reduce incidence of acute attacks and to relieve residual pain and mild discomfort.

PATIENT CONSIDERATIONS

Assessment: Assess for known blood dyscrasias, uric acid kidney stones, acute/chronic gout attack, history of peptic ulcer, renal function, hypersensitivity to drug, pregnancy/nursing status, and possible drug interactions.

Monitoring: Monitor for signs/symptoms of gout exacerbation, allergic reactions, hematuria, renal colic, costovertebral pain, and uric acid stone formation. Monitor serum uric acid levels.

Counseling: Inform about the risks and benefits of therapy and importance of liberal fluid intake. Advise to seek medical attention if symptoms of allergic reaction, hematuria, renal colic, or costovertebral pain occur.

PROCARDIA XL — nifedipine   Rx

Class: Calcium channel blocker (CCB) (dihydropyridine)

OTHER BRAND NAMES

Nifedical XL

ADULT DOSAGE

Angina

Vasospastic Angina/Chronic Stable Angina (Effort-Associated Angina):
Initial: 30 or 60mg qd
Titrate: Adjust dose over a 7- to 14-day period, but may proceed more rapidly if symptoms warrant
Max: 120mg/day; caution w/ doses >90mg

Use nearest equivalent total daily dose when switching to extended-release tab from nifedipine caps alone or in combination w/ other antianginal medications; titrate as clinically warranted

Hypertension

Initial: 30 or 60mg qd
Titrate: Adjust dose over a 7- to 14-day period, but may proceed more rapidly if symptoms warrant
Max: 120mg/day

May use alone or in combination w/ other antihypertensive agents

PEDIATRIC DOSAGE

Pediatric use may not have been established

DOSING CONSIDERATIONS

Discontinuation

Gradually decrease w/ close supervision

Other Important Considerations

Avoid w/ grapefruit juice

ADMINISTRATION

Oral route

Swallow tab whole; do not crush, divide, or chew.

STORAGE

Protect from moisture and humidity. **Procardia XL:** <30°C (86°F). **Nifedical XL:** 25°C (77°F); excursions permitted to 15-30°C (59-86°F).

HOW SUPPLIED

Tab, Extended-Release: 30mg, 60mg, 90mg; (Nifedical XL) 30mg, 60mg

CONTRAINDICATIONS

Known hypersensitivity reaction to nifedipine.

WARNINGS/PRECAUTIONS

May cause excessive hypotension; monitor BP initially and w/ titration. May increase frequency, duration, and/or severity of angina or acute MI (AMI), particularly w/ severe obstructive coronary artery disease (CAD). May develop heart failure (HF) after beginning therapy, w/ a higher risk in patients w/ tight aortic stenosis. GI obstruction and bezoars reported rarely; caution w/ altered GI anatomy (eg, severe GI narrowing, colon cancer, small bowel obstruction), hypomotility disorders, and concomitant medications (eg, H_2-histamine blockers, NSAIDs, laxatives). Tab adherence to GI wall w/ ulceration reported. Mild to moderate peripheral edema, typically associated w/ arterial vasodilation, may occur; differentiate peripheral edema from the effects of increasing left ventricular dysfunction in patients w/ angina or HTN complicated by CHF. Transient elevations of enzymes (eg, alkaline phosphatase, creatine phosphokinase, lactate dehydrogenase, AST, ALT), cholestasis w/ or w/o jaundice, and allergic hepatitis reported (rare). May decrease platelet aggregation and increase bleeding time. Positive direct Coombs test w/ or w/o hemolytic anemia reported. Reversible elevation in BUN and SrCr reported rarely in patients w/ chronic renal insufficiency. Decreased clearance resulting in higher exposure reported in the elderly.

ADVERSE REACTIONS

Edema, headache.

DRUG INTERACTIONS

β-blockers may increase the likelihood of CHF, severe hypotension, or angina exacerbation; avoid abrupt β-blocker withdrawal. Severe hypotension and/or increased fluid volume reported together w/ β-blockers and fentanyl or other narcotic analgesics; if condition permits, allow sufficient time (at least 36 hrs) for nifedipine to be washed out prior to surgery w/ fentanyl. May increase digoxin levels; monitor digoxin when initiating, adjusting, and discontinuing nifedipine to avoid possible over- or under-digitalization. May increase PT w/ coumarin anticoagulants. Cimetidine may increase levels; caution during titration. Monitor w/ other medications known to lower BP. Phenytoin may lower systemic exposure to nifedipine; avoid w/ phenytoin or any known CYP3A4 inducer. CYP3A inhibitors (eg, fluconazole, itraconazole, clarithromycin) may result in increased exposure to nifedipine when coadministered; monitor carefully and consider initiating nifedipine at the lowest dose available. Grapefruit juice increases levels; avoid ingestion of grapefruit/grapefruit juice while on therapy.

PREGNANCY AND LACTATION

Pregnancy: Category C.
Lactation: Therapy is transferred through breast milk; caution in nursing.

MECHANISM OF ACTION

Calcium channel blocker (dihydropyridine); selectively inhibits Ca^{2+} influx into cardiac muscle and smooth muscle: **Angina:** has not been established; believed to act by relaxation and prevention of coronary artery spasm and reduction of oxygen utilization. **HTN:** Peripheral arterial vasodilation, resulting in reduction in peripheral vascular resistance.

PHARMACOKINETICS

Absorption: Complete. Bioavailability (86%). **Distribution:** Plasma protein binding (92-98%); found in breast milk. **Metabolism:** Liver, extensive. **Elimination:** Urine (<0.1%, unchanged), feces (metabolites); $T_{1/2}$=2 hrs.

PATIENT CONSIDERATIONS

Assessment: Assess for acute coronary syndrome, severe obstructive CAD, aortic stenosis, recent β-blocker withdrawal, renal impairment, altered GI anatomy, hypomotility disorders, hypersensitivity to the drug, pregnancy/nursing status, and possible drug interactions.

Monitoring: Monitor for excessive hypotension, increased frequency, duration, and/or severity of angina and/or AMI, HF, signs/symptoms of GI obstruction, bezoars, peripheral edema, cholestasis w/ or w/o jaundice, allergic hepatitis, and other adverse reactions. Monitor BP, BUN, SrCr, and for decreased platelet aggregation and increased bleeding time.

Counseling: Inform about potential risks/benefits of drug. Instruct to notify physician if pregnant/nursing or if any adverse reactions occur. Inform that it is normal to occasionally observe a tab-like material in the stool.

PROCENTRA — dextroamphetamine sulfate   CII

Class: CNS stimulant

> **High potential for abuse. Prolonged use may lead to drug dependence and must be avoided. Misuse may cause sudden death and serious cardiovascular (CV) adverse events.**

ADULT DOSAGE

Narcolepsy

Initial: 10mg/day
Titrate: May increase in increments of 10mg at weekly intervals until optimal response is obtained
Usual: 5-60mg/day in divided doses

Give 1st dose on awakening; additional doses (1 or 2) at intervals of 4-6 hrs

PEDIATRIC DOSAGE

Narcolepsy

Usual: 5-60mg/day in divided doses

Give 1st dose on awakening; additional doses (1 or 2) at intervals of 4-6 hrs

6-12 Years:
Initial: 5mg/day
Titrate: May increase in increments of 5mg at weekly intervals until optimal response is obtained

≥12 Years:
Initial: 10mg/day
Titrate: May increase in increments of 10mg at weekly intervals until optimal response is obtained

Attention-Deficit Hyperactivity Disorder

3-5 Years:
Initial: 2.5mg/day
Titrate: May increase in increments of 2.5mg at weekly intervals until optimal response is obtained

≥6 Years:
Initial: 5mg qd or bid
Titrate: May increase in increments of 5mg at weekly intervals until optimal response is obtained. Only in rare cases will it be necessary to exceed a total of 40mg/day

Give 1st dose on awakening; additional doses (1 or 2) at intervals of 4-6 hrs

DOSING CONSIDERATIONS
Adverse Reactions
Narcolepsy:
Reduce dose if bothersome adverse reactions appear (eg, insomnia, anorexia)

ADMINISTRATION
Oral route
Avoid late pm doses.

STORAGE
20-25°C (68-77°F).

HOW SUPPLIED
Oral Sol: 5mg/5mL (473mL)

CONTRAINDICATIONS
Advanced arteriosclerosis, symptomatic CV disease (CVD), moderate to severe HTN, hyperthyroidism, known hypersensitivity or idiosyncrasy to the sympathomimetic amines, glaucoma, agitated states, and history of drug abuse. During or w/in 14 days following MAOI use.

WARNINGS/PRECAUTIONS
Sudden death reported in children and adolescents w/ structural cardiac abnormalities or other serious heart problems. Sudden death, stroke, and MI reported in adults. Avoid w/ known serious structural cardiac abnormalities, cardiomyopathy, serious heart rhythm abnormalities, coronary artery disease, or other serious cardiac problems. May cause a modest increase in average BP and HR. Prior to treatment, obtain medical history and perform physical exam to assess for presence of cardiac disease. Promptly perform cardiac evaluation if symptoms of cardiac disease develop during treatment. May exacerbate symptoms of behavior disturbance and thought disorder in patients w/ preexisting psychotic disorder. May induce mixed/manic episodes in patients w/ comorbid bipolar disorder. May cause treatment-emergent psychotic or manic symptoms in children and adolescents w/o a prior history of psychotic illness or mania; consider discontinuation if such symptoms occur. Aggressive behavior or hostility reported in children and adolescents w/ ADHD. May cause long-term suppression of growth in children; monitor growth, and may need to interrupt treatment in patients not growing or gaining height or weight as expected. May lower convulsive threshold; d/c if seizures occur. Associated w/ peripheral vasculopathy, including Raynaud's phenomenon. Difficulties w/ accommodation and blurring of vision reported. May exacerbate motor and phonic tics and Tourette's syndrome. May elevate plasma corticosteroid levels and interfere w/ urinary steroid determinations.

ADVERSE REACTIONS
Palpitations, tachycardia, BP elevation, dizziness, insomnia, euphoria, tremor, headache, dryness of mouth, diarrhea, constipation, urticaria, impotence, changes in libido, rhabdomyolysis.

DRUG INTERACTIONS
See Contraindications. GI acidifying agents (eg, guanethidine, reserpine, glutamic acid) and urinary acidifying agents (eg, ammonium chloride, sodium acid phosphate) lower blood levels and efficacy. Inhibits adrenergic blockers. GI alkalinizing agents (eg, sodium bicarbonate) and urinary alkalinizing agents (eg, acetazolamide, some thiazides) increase blood levels and therefore potentiate actions. May enhance activity of TCAs or sympathomimetic agents. Desipramine or protriptyline and possibly other TCAs cause striking and sustained increases in the concentration of *d*-amphetamine in the brain; CV effects can be potentiated. May counteract sedative effects of antihistamines. May antagonize effect of antihypertensives. Chlorpromazine and haloperidol block dopamine and norepinephrine reuptake, thus inhibiting central stimulant effects. May delay intestinal absorption of ethosuximide, phenobarbital, and phenytoin; coadministration w/ phenobarbital or phenytoin may produce a synergistic anticonvulsant action. Lithium carbonate may inhibit stimulatory effects. Potentiates analgesic effect of meperidine. Acidifying agents used in methenamine therapy increase urinary excretion and reduce efficacy. Enhances adrenergic effect of norepinephrine. In cases of propoxyphene overdosage, CNS stimulation is potentiated and fatal convulsions can occur. Inhibits hypotensive effect of veratrum alkaloids.

PREGNANCY AND LACTATION
Pregnancy: Category C. Infants born to mothers dependent on amphetamines have an increased risk of premature delivery and low birth weight, and may experience withdrawal symptoms.
Lactation: Found in breast milk; mothers should be advised to refrain from nursing.

MECHANISM OF ACTION
Sympathomimetic amine w/ CNS stimulant activity; not established.

PHARMACOKINETICS
Absorption: C_{max}=33.2ng/mL. **Distribution:** Found in breast milk. **Elimination:** Urine (38%); $T_{1/2}$=11.75 hrs.

PATIENT CONSIDERATIONS
Assessment: Assess for hypersensitivity/idiosyncrasy to sympathomimetic amines, advanced arteriosclerosis, symptomatic CVD, moderate to severe HTN, hyperthyroidism, glaucoma, agitated states, history of drug abuse, tics, Tourette's syndrome, preexisting psychotic disorder, risk for/comorbid bipolar disorder, cardiac disease, medical conditions that might be compromised by increases in BP or HR, any other conditions where treatment is cautioned, pregnancy/nursing status, and possible drug interactions.
Monitoring: Monitor for changes in HR and BP, signs/symptoms of cardiac disease, exacerbation of behavioral disturbance and thought disorder, psychosis, mania, appearance or worsening of aggressive behavior or hostility, seizures, visual disturbances, exacerbation of motor and phonic tics or Tourette's syndrome, and other adverse reactions. Monitor growth and weight in pediatric patients. Observe carefully for signs and symptoms of peripheral vasculopathy; further clinical evaluation (eg, rheumatology referral) may be appropriate for certain patients.
Counseling: Inform about benefits and risks of treatment. Inform that drug has high potential for abuse. Caution against engaging in potentially hazardous activities. Instruct patients beginning treatment about the risk of peripheral vasculopathy and associated signs/symptoms. Instruct to report any new numbness, pain, skin color change, or sensitivity to temperature in fingers/toes, and to call physician immediately w/ any signs of unexplained wounds appearing on fingers/toes.

PROCHLORPERAZINE — prochlorperazine edisylate; prochlorperazine maleate   Rx
Class: Phenothiazine derivative

> Elderly patients with dementia-related psychosis treated with antipsychotic drugs are at an increased risk of death; most deaths appeared to be cardiovascular (CV) (eg, heart failure, sudden death) or infectious (eg, pneumonia) in nature. Treatment with conventional antipsychotic drugs may similarly increase mortality. Not approved for the treatment of patients with dementia-related psychosis.

OTHER BRAND NAMES
Compazine (Discontinued)

ADULT DOSAGE
Nausea/Vomiting
Tab:
Usual: 5mg or 10mg tid-qid
Daily dose >40mg should only be used in resistant cases
IM:
Initial: 5-10mg q3-4h prn
Max: 40mg/day
IV:
2.5-10mg slow inj or infusion at rate ≤5mg/min
Max: 10mg single dose and 40mg/day
N/V w/ Surgery:
IM:
5-10mg 1-2 hrs before induction of anesthesia (repeat once in 30 min if necessary)
IV:
5-10mg as slow inj or infusion 15-30 min before induction of anesthesia. To control acute symptoms during or after surgery, repeat once if necessary
Max: 40mg/day

Psychotic Disorders
Tab:
Nonpsychotic Anxiety
Usual: 5mg tid-qid
Max: 20mg/day, not longer than 12 weeks
Mild Conditions Including Schizophrenia:
Usual: 5 or 10mg tid-qid
Moderate-Severe Conditions (Hospitalized/Supervised):
Initial: 10mg tid-qid
Titrate: Increase gradually until controlled or bothersome side effects
More Severe Disturbances:
Usual: 100-150mg/day
IM:
Start w/ lowest recommended dose and adjust based on severity

PEDIATRIC DOSAGE
Nausea/Vomiting
≥2 Years:
Tab:
20-29 lbs:
Usual: 2.5mg qd-bid
Max: 7.5mg/day
30-39 lbs:
Usual: 2.5mg bid-tid
Max: 10mg/day
40-85 lbs:
Usual: 2.5mg tid or 5mg bid
Max: 15mg/day
Severe N/V:
IM:
Usual: 0.06mg/lb; control is usually obtained w/ 1 dose

Schizophrenia
Tab:
2-12 Years:
Initial: 2.5mg bid-tid; do not give >10mg on the 1st day
Titrate: Increase according to response
Max:
2-5 Years: 20mg/day
6-12 Years: 25mg/day
IM:
<12 Years:
Usual: 0.06mg/lb. Control is usually obtained with 1 dose. Switch to PO after obtaining control at the same dosage level or higher

Schizophrenia w/ Severe Symptomatology:
Initial: 10-20mg, may repeat q2-4h if necessary (or, in resistant cases, every hr)
Switch to PO after obtaining control at the same dosage level or higher
Prolonged Parenteral Therapy:
10-20mg IM q4-6h

DOSING CONSIDERATIONS
Elderly
Start at lower end of dosing range and increase more gradually

Other Important Considerations
Debilitated or Emaciated Adults:
Increase more gradually

ADMINISTRATION
IV, IM, Oral route

Inj
Inject deeply into upper, outer quadrant of the buttock.
SQ is not advisable because of local irritation.
May be administered either undiluted or diluted in isotonic sol.
When given IV, do not use bolus inj.
Do not mix w/ other agents in the syringe.
Avoid getting injection sol on hands or clothing because of potential contact dermatitis.

STORAGE
Tab, Inj: 20-25°C (68-77°F). Protect from light. (Inj) Do not freeze.

HOW SUPPLIED
Inj: (Edisylate) 5mg/mL [2mL, 10mL]; **Tab:** (Maleate) 5mg, 10mg

CONTRAINDICATIONS
Known hypersensitivity to phenothiazines, comatose states, concomitant large doses of CNS depressants (eg, alcohol, barbiturates, narcotics), pediatric surgery, pediatrics <2 yrs of age or <20 lbs.

WARNINGS/PRECAUTIONS
Secondary extrapyramidal symptoms can occur. Tardive dyskinesia (TD) may develop, especially in elderly and during long-term use. Neuroleptic malignant syndrome (NMS) reported; d/c if it occurs and institute appropriate treatment. Caution during reintroduction of therapy as NMS recurrence reported. Avoid in patients with bone marrow depression, previous hypersensitivity reaction, and in pregnant women. May impair mental and/or physical abilities, especially during the 1st few days of therapy. May mask symptoms of overdose of other drugs, and obscure diagnosis of intestinal obstruction, brain tumor, and Reye's syndrome; avoid in children/adolescents whose signs and symptoms suggest Reye's syndrome. May cause hypotension; caution with large doses and parenteral administration in patients with impaired CV system. May interfere with thermoregulation; caution in patients exposed to extreme heat. Evaluate therapy periodically with prolonged use. Leukopenia/neutropenia/agranulocytosis reported; monitor during 1st few months of therapy, and d/c at 1st sign of leukopenia or if severe neutropenia (absolute neutrophil count <1000/mm^3) occurs. Caution with glaucoma, in children with dehydration or acute illness, and in elderly. May produce α-adrenergic blockade, lower seizure threshold, or elevate prolactin levels. D/C 48 hrs before myelography; may resume after 24 hrs postprocedure.

ADVERSE REACTIONS
NMS, cholestatic jaundice, leukopenia, agranulocytosis, drowsiness, dizziness, amenorrhea, blurred vision, skin reactions, hypotension, motor restlessness, extrapyramidal symptoms, TD, dystonia, pseudoparkinsonism.

DRUG INTERACTIONS
See Contraindications. May intensify and prolong action of CNS depressants (eg, alcohol, anesthetics, narcotics), atropine, and organophosphorus insecticides. May decrease oral anticoagulant effects. Thiazide diuretics accentuate orthostatic hypotension. Increased levels of both drugs with propranolol. Anticonvulsants may need dosage adjustment; may lower convulsive threshold. May interfere with metabolism of phenytoin and precipitate toxicity. Risk of encephalopathic syndrome occurs with lithium. May antagonize antihypertensive effects of guanethidine and related compounds. Avoid use prior to myelography with metrizamide; vomiting as a sign of toxicity of cancer chemotherapeutic drugs may be obscured by the antiemetic effect. May reverse effect of epinephrine. May cause paradoxical further lowering of BP with epinephrine and other pressor agents (excluding norepinephrine bitartrate and phenylephrine HCl).

PREGNANCY AND LACTATION
Pregnancy: Safety is not known in pregnancy.
Lactation: Caution in nursing.

MECHANISM OF ACTION
Phenothiazine derivative; antiemetic and antipsychotic.

PHARMACOKINETICS
Distribution: Excreted in breast milk.

PATIENT CONSIDERATIONS
Assessment: Assess for Reye's syndrome, TD, pregnancy/nursing status, possible drug interactions, impaired CV system, breast cancer, glaucoma, bone marrow depression, preexisting low WBC count, history of drug-induced leukopenia/neutropenia, history of psychosis, and seizure disorder. Assess use in children with acute illness or dehydration, elderly, debilitated, or emaciated patients.

Monitoring: Monitor for extrapyramidal symptoms, signs/symptoms of TD, NMS, hypotension, fever, sore throat, infection, jaundice, motor restlessness, dystonia,

pseudoparkinsonism, and hypersensitivity reactions. Monitor CBC, WBC, and prolactin levels. Conduct liver studies if fever with grippe-like symptoms occur.

Counseling: Inform about the risks and benefits of therapy. Instruct to avoid engaging in hazardous activities and exposure to extreme heat. Counsel to seek medical attention if symptoms of TD, NMS, hypotension, mydriasis, encephalopathic syndrome, sore throat, infection, deep sleep, or hypersensitivity reactions occur.

PROCRIT — epoetin alfa   Rx
Class: Erythropoiesis-stimulating agent (ESA)

> Increased risk of death, MI, stroke, venous thromboembolism (VTE), thrombosis of vascular access, and tumor progression or recurrence. Use the lowest dose sufficient to reduce/avoid the need for RBC transfusions. Chronic Kidney Disease (CKD): Greater risks for death, serious adverse cardiovascular (CV) reactions, and stroke when administered to target Hgb level >11g/dL. Cancer: Shortened overall survival and/or increased risk of tumor progression or recurrence in patients w/ breast, non-small cell lung, head and neck, lymphoid, and cervical cancers. Must enroll in and comply w/ the ESA APPRISE Oncology Program to prescribe and/or dispense drug to patients. Use only for anemia from myelosuppressive chemotherapy. Not indicated for patients receiving myelosuppressive chemotherapy when anticipated outcome is cure. D/C following completion of chemotherapy course. Perisurgery: Due to increased risk of deep venous thrombosis (DVT), DVT prophylaxis is recommended.

ADULT DOSAGE
Anemia

Chronic Kidney Disease Associated Anemia:
Patients on Dialysis:
Initiate treatment when Hgb is <10g/dL
If Hgb approaches/exceeds 11g/dL, reduce or interrupt dose
Initial: 50-100 U/kg IV/SQ 3X weekly; IV recommended for hemodialysis patients
Patients Not on Dialysis:
Consider initiating treatment when Hgb is <10g/dL AND the following considerations apply:
1. Rate of Hgb decline indicates likelihood of requiring a RBC transfusion AND,
2. Reducing the risk of alloimmunization and/or other RBC transfusion-related risks is a goal
If Hgb exceeds 10g/dL, reduce or interrupt dose and use lowest dose sufficient to reduce the need for RBC transfusion
Initial: 50-100 U/kg IV/SQ 3X weekly
All Patients:
Do not increase dose more frequently than once every 4 weeks; decreases in dose may occur more frequently
If Hgb Rises Rapidly (eg, >1g/dL in any 2-Week Period): Reduce dose by ≥25% prn to reduce rapid responses
If Hgb Has Not Increased by >1g/dL After 4 Weeks: Increase dose by 25% If adequate response is not achieved over a 12-week escalation period, use lowest dose that will maintain a Hgb level sufficient to reduce need for RBC transfusions and evaluate other causes of anemia; d/c if responsiveness does not improve

Zidovudine Associated Anemia in HIV-Infected Patients:
Initial: 100 U/kg IV/SQ 3X weekly
Titrate:
No Hgb Increase After 8 Weeks:
Increase dose by approx 50-100 U/kg at 4- to 8-week intervals until Hgb reaches level needed to avoid RBC transfusions or 300 U/kg
Hgb >12g/dL: Withhold therapy until Hgb <11g/dL; then resume at a dose 25% below previous dose
D/C therapy if an increase in Hgb is not achieved at 300 U/kg for 8 weeks

Chemotherapy Associated Anemia:
Initiate if Hgb <10g/dL and if there is a minimum of 2 additional months of planned chemotherapy
Initial: 150 U/kg SQ 3X weekly or 40,000 U SQ weekly until completion of a chemotherapy course
Dose Reduction: Reduce by 25% if:
1. Hgb increases >1g/dL in any 2-week period

PEDIATRIC DOSAGE
Anemia

Chronic Kidney Disease Associated Anemia:
1 Month-16 Years on Dialysis:
Initiate treatment when Hgb is <10g/dL
If Hgb approaches/exceeds 11g/dL, reduce or interrupt dose
Initial: 50 U/kg IV/SQ 3X weekly; IV recommended for hemodialysis patients
Do not increase dose more frequently than once every 4 weeks; decreases in dose may occur more frequently
If Hgb Rises Rapidly (eg, >1g/dL in any 2-Week Period): Reduce dose by ≥25% prn to reduce rapid responses
If Hgb Has Not Increased by >1g/dL After 4 Weeks: Increase dose by 25% If adequate response is not achieved over a 12-week escalation period, use lowest dose that will maintain a Hgb level sufficient to reduce need for RBC transfusions and evaluate other causes of anemia; d/c if responsiveness does not improve

Chemotherapy Associated Anemia: 5-18 Years:
Initiate if Hgb <10g/dL and if there is a minimum of 2 additional months of planned chemotherapy
Initial: 600 U/kg IV weekly until completion of a chemotherapy course
Dose Reduction: Reduce by 25% if
1. Hgb increases >1g/dL in any 2-week period
2. Hgb reaches a level needed to avoid a RBC transfusion
Withhold dose if Hgb exceeds level needed to avoid RBC transfusion; reinitiate at a dose 25% below previous dose when Hgb approaches a level where RBC transfusions may be required
Dose Increase: After initial 4 weeks of therapy, if Hgb increases by <1g/dL and remains below 10g/dL increase dose to 900 U/kg (max 60,000 U) weekly
D/C therapy if there is no response in Hgb levels or if RBC transfusions are still required after 8 weeks

2. Hgb reaches a level needed to avoid a RBC transfusion
Withhold dose if Hgb exceeds level needed to avoid RBC transfusion; reinitiate at a dose 25% below previous dose when Hgb approaches a level where RBC transfusions may be required

Dose Increase: After initial 4 weeks of therapy, if Hgb increases by <1g/dL and remains below 10g/dL increase dose to 300 U/kg 3X weekly or 60,000 U weekly
D/C therapy if there is no response in Hgb levels or if RBC transfusions are still required after 8 weeks

Surgery Patients:
300 U/kg/day SQ for 10 days before, on the day of, and for 4 days after surgery; or 600 U/kg SQ in 4 doses administered 21, 14, and 7 days before surgery and on the day of surgery
DVT prophylaxis is recommended

ADMINISTRATION
IV/SQ route

Do not shake; do not use if shaken or frozen.
Discard unused portions in preservative-free vials; do not re-enter preservative-free vials.
Do not dilute.
Preservative-free vials may be admixed in a syringe w/ bacteriostatic 0.9% NaCl inj, w/ benzyl alcohol 0.9% in a 1:1 ratio.

STORAGE
2-8°C (36-46°F). Do not freeze; do not use if it has been frozen. Protect from light. Discard unused portions of multidose vials 21 days after initial entry.

HOW SUPPLIED
Inj: 2000 U/mL, 3000 U/mL, 4000 U/mL, 10,000 U/mL, 40,000 U/mL [single-dose vial]; 10,000 U/mL [2mL], 20,000 U/mL [1mL] [multidose vial]

CONTRAINDICATIONS
Uncontrolled HTN, pure red cell aplasia (PRCA) that begins after treatment w/ epoetin alfa or other erythropoietin protein drugs, serious allergic reactions to epoetin alfa. (Multidose Vials) Neonates, infants, pregnant women, and nursing mothers.

WARNINGS/PRECAUTIONS
Not indicated for use in patients w/ cancer receiving hormonal agents, biologic products, or radiotherapy, unless also receiving concomitant myelosuppressive chemotherapy; in patients scheduled for surgery who are willing to donate autologous blood; in patients undergoing cardiac/vascular surgery, or as a substitute for RBC transfusions in patients requiring immediate correction of anemia. Evaluate transferrin saturation and serum ferritin prior to and during treatment; administer supplemental iron when serum ferritin is <100mcg/L or serum transferrin saturation is <20%. Correct/exclude other causes of anemia (eg, vitamin deficiency, metabolic/chronic inflammatory conditions, bleeding) before initiating therapy. Hypertensive encephalopathy and seizures reported in patients w/ CKD. Appropriately control HTN prior to initiation of and during treatment; reduce/withhold therapy if BP becomes difficult to control. PRCA and severe anemia, w/ or w/o other cytopenias that arise following development of neutralizing antibodies to erythropoietin reported. Withhold and evaluate for neutralizing antibodies to erythropoietin if severe anemia and low reticulocyte count develop; d/c permanently if PRCA develops, and do not switch to other erythropoiesis-stimulating agents. Serious allergic reactions may occur; immediately and permanently d/c therapy. Contains albumin; may carry an extremely remote risk for transmission of viral diseases or Creutzfeldt-Jakob disease. Patients may require adjustments in their dialysis prescriptions after initiation of therapy, or require increased anticoagulation w/ heparin to prevent clotting of extracorporeal circuit during hemodialysis. Multidose vial contains benzyl alcohol; benzyl alcohol is associated w/ serious adverse events and death, particularly in pediatric patients.

ADVERSE REACTIONS
MI, stroke, VTE, thrombosis of vascular access, tumor progression/recurrence, pyrexia, N/V, HTN, cough, arthralgia, pruritus, rash, headache, dizziness.

PREGNANCY AND LACTATION
Pregnancy: Category C (single-dose vials only).
Lactation: Caution in nursing (single-dose vials only).

MECHANISM OF ACTION
Erythropoiesis-stimulating glycoprotein; stimulates erythropoiesis by the same mechanism as endogenous erythropoietin.

PHARMACOKINETICS
Absorption: Adults and Pediatrics w/ CKD: (SQ) T_{max}=5-24 hrs. Anemic Cancer Patients: (SQ) T_{max}=13.3 hrs (150 U/kg), 38 hrs (40,000 U). **Elimination:** Adults and Pediatrics w/ CKD: (IV) $T_{1/2}$=4-13 hrs. Anemic Cancer Patients: (SQ) $T_{1/2}$=16-67 hrs.

PATIENT CONSIDERATIONS
Assessment: Assess for uncontrolled HTN, previous hypersensitivity to the drug, causes of anemia, pregnancy/nursing status, and other conditions where treatment is contraindicated or cautioned. Obtain baseline Hgb levels, transferrin saturation, and serum ferritin.

Monitoring: Monitor for signs/symptoms of an allergic reaction, CV/thromboembolic events, stroke, premonitory neurologic symptoms, PRCA, severe anemia, progression/recurrence of tumor, and other adverse reactions. Monitor BP, transferrin saturation, and serum ferritin. Following initiation of therapy and after each dose adjustment, monitor Hgb weekly until Hgb is stable and sufficient to minimize need for RBC transfusion.

Counseling: Inform of the risks/benefits of therapy and of the increased risks of mortality, serious CV reactions, thromboembolic reactions, stroke, and tumor progression. Advise of the need to have regular lab tests for Hgb. Inform cancer patients that they must sign the patient-physician acknowledgment form prior to therapy. Instruct to undergo regular BP monitoring, adhere to prescribed antihypertensive regimen, and follow recommended dietary restrictions. Advise to contact physician for new-onset neurologic symptoms or change in seizure frequency. Instruct regarding proper disposal of used syringes and caution against the reuse of needles, syringes, or unused portions of single-dose vials.

PROCTOCORT SUPPOSITORY — hydrocortisone acetate   Rx
Class: Corticosteroid

ADULT DOSAGE	PEDIATRIC DOSAGE
Colorectal Disorders	Pediatric use may not have been established
For use in inflamed hemorrhoids, postirradiation (factitial) proctitis, as an adjunct in the treatment of chronic ulcerative colitis, cryptitis, and other inflammatory conditions of anorectum and pruritus ani	
Usual: 1 sup rectally bid (am and pm) for 2 weeks, in nonspecific proctitis. In more severe cases, 1 sup rectally tid or 2 sup rectally bid. In factitial proctitis, recommended duration is 6-8 weeks or less, according to response	

ADMINISTRATION
Rectal route

Detach 1 sup from strip; remove foil wrapper
Avoid excessive handling of sup
Insert sup into rectum w/ gentle pressure, pointed end 1st

STORAGE
20-25°C (68-77°F). Store away from heat. Protect from freezing.

HOW SUPPLIED
Sup: 30mg

CONTRAINDICATIONS
History of hypersensitivity to hydrocortisone acetate or any of the components.

WARNINGS/PRECAUTIONS
Use only after adequate proctologic exam. D/C if irritation develops and institute appropriate therapy. In presence of infection, if favorable response does not occur promptly, d/c until infection has been adequately controlled.

ADVERSE REACTIONS
Burning, itching, irritation, dryness, folliculitis, hypopigmentation, allergic contact dermatitis, secondary infection.

PREGNANCY AND LACTATION
Category C, not for use in nursing.

MECHANISM OF ACTION
Corticosteroid; anti-inflammatory, antipruritic, and vasoconstrictive action.

PATIENT CONSIDERATIONS
Assessment: Assess for drug hypersensitivity, presence of infection, and pregnancy/nursing status. Perform adequate proctologic examination prior to treatment.

Monitoring: Monitor for signs/symptoms of irritation, hypersensitivity, infection, and local adverse reactions.

Counseling: Advise to d/c therapy if irritation occurs. Advise to inform physician if adverse reactions occur. Inform patient of proper handling/administration of the suppositories. Advise to avoid excessive handling of the sup.

PROCTOFOAM-HC — hydrocortisone acetate/pramoxine hydrochloride   Rx
Class: Anesthetic/corticosteroid

ADULT DOSAGE	PEDIATRIC DOSAGE
Inflammatory and Pruritic Manifestations of Corticosteroid-Responsive Dermatoses	**Inflammatory and Pruritic Manifestations of Corticosteroid-Responsive Dermatoses**
Anal Region:	**Anal Region:**
Apply to affected area tid-qid	Apply to affected area tid-qid; use least amount effective for condition
D/C if no evidence of improvement w/in 2 or 3 weeks after starting therapy, or if condition worsens	D/C if no evidence of improvement w/in 2 or 3 weeks after starting therapy, or if condition worsens

---

ADMINISTRATION
Topical route

For anal administration, use the applicator supplied.
For perianal use, transfer a small quantity to a tissue and rub in gently.

Directions for Use
1. Shake foam container vigorously for 5-10 sec before each use; do not remove container cap during use of the product.
2. Hold container upright on a level surface and gently place the tip of the applicator onto the nose of the container cap; pull plunger past the fill line on the applicator barrel.
3. To fill applicator barrel, press down firmly on cap flanges, hold for 1-2 sec, and release.
4. Wait 5-10 sec to allow foam to expand in applicator barrel; repeat until foam reaches fill line. It usually requires 3-4 pumps for foam to reach fill line.
5. Remove applicator from container cap; if foam goes beyond fill line, it will continue to expand and flow backwards, resulting in foam build-up under cap.
6. Gently insert tip into anus; once in place, push plunger to expel foam, then withdraw applicator.
7. After each use, applicator parts should be pulled apart for thorough cleaning w/ warm water. Since some foam will appear under the cap, the cap and underlying tip should be pulled apart and rinsed to help prevent build-up of foam and possible blockage.

Priming
Prime the container by pressing down firmly on flanges and then release. W/ initial priming, a burst of air may come out of the container; it usually requires 1-2 pumps for foam to appear.

STORAGE
20-25°C (68-77°F). Do not store at temperatures >49°C (120°F). Do not refrigerate.

HOW SUPPLIED
Foam: (Hydrocortisone/Pramoxine) 1%/1% [10g]

CONTRAINDICATIONS
History of hypersensitivity to any components of the preparation.

WARNINGS/PRECAUTIONS
Do not insert any part of the aerosol container directly into the anus. Avoid contact with eyes. Contents of the container are under pressure; do not burn or puncture. Systemic absorption may produce reversible hypothalamic-pituitary-adrenal (HPA) axis suppression, manifestations of Cushing's syndrome, hyperglycemia, and glucosuria. Application of more potent steroids, use over large surface areas, prolonged use, and the addition of occlusive dressings may augment systemic absorption. Periodically evaluate for evidence of HPA axis suppression when a large dose is applied to a large surface area or under an occlusive dressing; if noted, withdraw the drug, reduce frequency of application, or substitute with a less potent steroid. Infrequently, signs and symptoms of steroid withdrawal may occur, requiring supplemental systemic corticosteroids. D/C and institute appropriate therapy if irritation develops. Use appropriate antifungal or antibacterial agent in the presence of dermatological infections; if a favorable response does not occur promptly, d/c until infection has been adequately controlled. Pediatric patients may be more susceptible to systemic toxicity. Chronic therapy may interfere with growth and development of pediatric patients. Caution in elderly.

ADVERSE REACTIONS
Burning, itching, irritation, dryness, folliculitis, hypertrichosis, acneiform eruptions, hypopigmentation, perioral dermatitis, allergic contact dermatitis, skin maceration, secondary infection, skin atrophy, striae, miliaria.

PREGNANCY AND LACTATION
Pregnancy: Category C.
Lactation: Caution in nursing.

MECHANISM OF ACTION
Hydrocortisone: Corticosteroid; possesses anti-inflammatory, antipruritic, and vasoconstrictive properties. Mechanism of anti-inflammatory activity not established. Pramoxine: Local anesthetic.

PHARMACOKINETICS
Absorption: (Corticosteroids) Percutaneous; extent of absorption is determined by many factors (eg, vehicle, integrity of the epidermal barrier, use of occlusive dressings). **Distribution:** (Corticosteroids) Bound to plasma proteins in varying degrees; found in breast milk (systemically administered). **Metabolism:** (Corticosteroids) Liver. **Elimination:** (Corticosteroids) Kidneys, bile.

PATIENT CONSIDERATIONS
Assessment: Assess for drug hypersensitivity, conditions that augment systemic absorption, dermatological infections, and pregnancy/nursing status.

Monitoring: Monitor for signs/symptoms of HPA axis suppression, Cushing's syndrome, hyperglycemia, glucosuria, steroid withdrawal, irritation, dermatological infections, systemic toxicity in pediatric patients, and other adverse reactions. When a large dose is applied to a large surface area or under an occlusive dressing, monitor for HPA axis suppression by using urinary free cortisol and adrenocorticotropic hormone stimulation tests. Monitor for improvement or worsening of condition.

Counseling: Instruct to use ud (anal or perianal use only) and to avoid contact with eyes. Advise not to use for any disorder other than for which it was prescribed. Instruct to report any signs of adverse reactions.

PROCYSBI — cysteamine bitartrate   Rx
Class: Cystine-depleting agent

ADULT DOSAGE
Nephropathic Cystinosis

Cysteamine-Naive Patients:
Start treatment immediately after diagnosis
Initial: 0.2-0.3g/m^2/day (1/6 to 1/4 of the maint dose) divided q12h
Titrate: Increase gradually over 4-6 weeks until maint dose is achieved
Maint: 1.3g/m^2/day divided q12h
Max: 1.95g/m^2/day

Refer to PI for weight-based starting and maint doses

Switching from Immediate-Release (IR) Cysteamine Bitartrate Caps:
Initial: Total daily dose should be equal to previous total daily dose of IR cysteamine bitartrate
Max: 1.95g/m^2/day

Dose Titration:
Target WBC cystine concentration is <1nmol 1/2 cystine/mg protein; adjust dose as needed to achieve target WBC cystine concentration. If a dose adjustment is required, increase by 10%. If adverse reactions occur, decrease dose; for patients who have initial intolerance, temporarily d/c therapy and then restart at a lower dose and gradually increase to the target dose

Lab Monitoring:
Cysteamine-Naive Patients: Measure WBC cystine concentration after reaching maint dose, then monthly for 3 months, quarterly for 1 yr, and then twice yearly, at a minimum
Patients Switching from IR Cysteamine: Measure WBC cystine concentration after 2 weeks of treatment while titrating the dose, then quarterly for 6 months, then twice yearly, at a minimum

Obtain blood samples for WBC cystine concentration measurement 12 hrs after dosing; accurately record time of the last dose, actual dose, and time the blood sample was taken

Missed Dose

If a dose is missed, take as soon as possible up to 8 hrs after the scheduled time. However, if a dose is missed and the next scheduled dose is due in <4 hrs, do not take missed dose and take the next dose at the usual scheduled time. Do not take 2 doses at one time to make up for a missed dose

PEDIATRIC DOSAGE
Nephropathic Cystinosis

≥2 Years:
Cysteamine-Naive Patients:
Start treatment immediately after diagnosis
Initial: 0.2-0.3g/m^2/day (1/6 to 1/4 of the maint dose) divided q12h
Titrate: Increase gradually over 4-6 weeks until maint dose is achieved
Maint: 1.3g/m^2/day divided q12h
Max: 1.95g/m^2/day

Refer to PI for weight-based starting and maint doses

Switching from IR Cysteamine Bitartrate Caps:
Initial: Total daily dose should be equal to previous total daily dose of IR cysteamine bitartrate
Max: 1.95g/m^2/day

Dose Titration:
Target WBC cystine concentration is <1nmol 1/2 cystine/mg protein; adjust dose as needed to achieve target WBC cystine concentration. If a dose adjustment is required, increase by 10%. If adverse reactions occur, decrease dose; for patients who have initial intolerance, temporarily d/c therapy and then re-start at a lower dose and gradually increase to the target dose

Laboratory Monitoring:
Cysteamine-Naive Patients: Measure WBC cystine concentration after reaching maint dose, then monthly for 3 months, quarterly for 1 yr, and then twice yearly, at a minimum
Patients Switching from IR Cysteamine: Measure WBC cystine concentration after 2 weeks of treatment while titrating the dose, then quarterly for 6 months, then twice yearly, at a minimum

Obtain blood samples for WBC cystine concentration measurement 12 hrs after dosing; accurately record time of the last dose, actual dose, and time the blood sample was taken

Missed Dose

If a dose is missed, take as soon as possible up to 8 hrs after the scheduled time. However, if a dose is missed and the next scheduled dose is due in <4 hrs, do not take missed dose and take the next dose at the usual scheduled time. Do not take 2 doses at one time to make up for a missed dose

---

DOSING CONSIDERATIONS
Concomitant Medications
Medications Containing Bicarbonate or Carbonate: Administer Procysbi at least 1 hr before or 1 hr after these agents
Alcohol: Avoid alcohol while on therapy

ADMINISTRATION
Oral route

Swallow whole; do not crush/chew caps or cap contents.
Take w/ fruit juice (except grapefruit juice).
Do not eat for at least 2 hrs before and for at least 30 min after. If unable to take w/o eating, take w/ food and limit amount of food to approx 4 oz (1/2 cup) w/in 1 hr before dose through 1 hr after.
Take in a consistent manner in regard to food; avoid high-fat food close to dosing.

Difficulty Swallowing Caps
Administration w/ Applesauce or Berry Jelly:
1. Open caps and sprinkle intact granules on 4 oz applesauce or berry jelly; mix granules.
2. Consume entire contents w/in 30 min of mixing; do not chew granules. Do not save applesauce or berry jelly and granules for later use.

Administration w/ Fruit Juice (Except Grapefruit Juice):
1. Open caps and sprinkle intact granules into 4 oz of juice; gently stir until mixed.
2. Drink entire contents w/in 30 min of mixing; do not chew granules. Do not save fruit juice and granules for later use.

Administration w/ Applesauce via a Gastrostomy Tube (14 French or larger)

A bolus (straight) feeding tube is recommended.
1. Flush the gastrostomy tube button 1st w/ 5mL of water to clear the button.
2. Open cap and empty granules into a clean container w/ approx 4 oz of applesauce (use only strained applesauce w/ no chunks). A minimum of 1 oz (1/8 cup) of applesauce may be used for children ≤25kg starting at a dose of 1 or 2 caps. Mix intact granules into applesauce.
3. Draw up the mixture into a syringe. Keep the feeding tube horizontal during administration and apply rapid and steady pressure (10mL/10 sec) to dispense the syringe contents into the tube w/in 30 min of preparation.
4. Do not save applesauce and granule mixture for later use.
5. Draw up a minimum of 10mL of fruit juice into another syringe, swirl gently, and flush the tube.

STORAGE

20-25°C (68-77°F). Prior to dispensing, store at 2-8°C (36-46°F). Protect from light and moisture.

HOW SUPPLIED

Cap, Delayed-Release: 25mg, 75mg

CONTRAINDICATIONS

Serious hypersensitivity reaction, including anaphylaxis, to penicillamine or cysteamine bitartrate.

WARNINGS/PRECAUTIONS

Skin and bone lesions that resemble Ehlers-Danlos-like syndrome may occur. Monitor for development of skin or bone lesions and interrupt dosing if these lesions develop; may restart at a lower dose under close supervision, then slowly increase to the appropriate therapeutic dose. Severe skin rashes (eg, erythema multiforme bullosa, toxic epidermal necrolysis) may occur; permanently d/c use if severe skin rashes develop. GI ulceration/bleeding and GI tract symptoms (eg, N/V, anorexia, abdominal pain) may occur; consider decreasing the dose if severe GI tract symptoms develop. CNS symptoms may occur; carefully evaluate/monitor patients who develop CNS symptoms and interrupt or adjust dose as necessary for patients w/ severe symptoms or w/ symptoms that persist or progress. May impair mental/physical abilities. Associated w/ reversible leukopenia and elevated alkaline phosphatase levels; monitor WBC counts and alkaline phosphatase levels and consider decreasing dose or discontinuing drug if tests values remain elevated, until values revert to normal. Benign intracranial HTN (pseudotumor cerebri) and/or papilledema may occur. Monitor for signs/symptoms of pseudotumor cerebri; interrupt or decrease dose and refer patient to an ophthalmologist if signs/symptoms persist and permanently d/c use if diagnosis is confirmed.

ADVERSE REACTIONS

N/V, abdominal pain/discomfort, headache, diarrhea, anorexia/decreased appetite, breath odor, fatigue, dizziness, skin odor, rash.

DRUG INTERACTIONS

See Dosing Considerations. Drugs that increase gastric pH (eg, proton pump inhibitors, medications containing bicarbonate or carbonate) may alter the pharmacokinetics of cysteamine and increase WBC cystine concentration; monitor WBC cystine concentration w/ concomitant use. Alcohol may increase the rate of cysteamine release and/or adversely alter the pharmacokinetic properties, as well as the effectiveness/safety of therapy; do not consume alcoholic beverages during treatment.

PREGNANCY AND LACTATION

Pregnancy: No available data on use in pregnant women to inform any drug-associated risks for birth defects or miscarriage.
Lactation: Not for use in nursing.

MECHANISM OF ACTION

Cystine-depleting agent; participates w/in lysosomes in a thiol-disulfide interchange reaction converting cystine into cysteine and cysteine-cysteamine mixed disulfide, both of which can exit the lysosome in patients w/ cystinosis.

PHARMACOKINETICS

Absorption: C_{max}=3.6mg/L; T_{max}=188 min; AUC=785mg•min/L. **Distribution:** V_d=382L. Plasma protein binding (52%, predominantly to albumin). **Elimination:** $T_{1/2}$=253 min.

PATIENT CONSIDERATIONS

Assessment: Assess for hypersensitivity to the drug or to penicillamine, pregnancy/nursing status, and possible drug interactions.

Monitoring: Monitor for skin/bone lesions, severe skin rashes, GI ulceration/bleeding, GI tract symptoms, CNS symptoms, pseudotumor cerebri, and other adverse reactions. Monitor WBC counts and alkaline phosphatase levels. For cysteamine-naive patients, measure WBC cystine levels after reaching maint dose, then monthly for 3 months, quarterly for 1 yr, and then twice yearly, at a minimum. For patients switching from IR cysteamine, measure WBC cystine levels after 2 weeks of treatment while titrating dose, then quarterly for 6 months, then twice yearly, at a minimum.

Counseling: Advise that drug may cause abnormalities of the skin, bones, and joints; instruct to report any skin changes or problems w/ bones/joints to physician. Instruct to contact physician immediately if a skin rash is experienced. Inform that drug may cause ulcers/bleeding; advise to contact physician immediately if stomach pain, N/V, loss of appetite, or vomiting blood occurs. Inform that ability to perform tasks (eg, driving/operating machinery) may be impaired; instruct to contact physician immediately if seizures, lethargy, somnolence, depression, and encephalopathy are experienced. Advise that drug may cause benign intracranial HTN; advise to contact physician immediately if headache, tinnitus, dizziness, nausea, double vision, blurry vision, loss of vision, or eye pain occurs. Instruct to contact physician immediately if pregnancy is suspected. Discuss the risks/benefits of continuing

therapy during pregnancy. Advise that breastfeeding is not recommended during therapy. Inform to take ud and discuss the importance of required lab testing.

PROGLYCEM — diazoxide   Rx

Class: Nondiuretic benzothiadiazine

ADULT DOSAGE

Hypoglycemia

Due to hyperinsulinism associated w/ inoperable islet cell adenoma/carcinoma, or extrapancreatic malignancy

Initial: 3mg/kg/day, divided into 3 equal doses q8h
Usual: 3-8mg/kg/day, divided into 2 or 3 equal doses q8h or q12h
Refractory Hypoglycemia: May require higher doses

PEDIATRIC DOSAGE

Hypoglycemia

Due to hyperinsulinism associated w/ leucine sensitivity, islet cell hyperplasia, nesidioblastosis, extrapancreatic malignancy, islet cell adenoma, or adenomatosis; may be used preoperatively as a temporary measure, and postoperatively, if hypoglycemia persists

Infants and Newborns:
Initial: 10mg/kg/day, divided into 3 equal doses q8h
Usual: 8-15mg/kg/day, divided into 2 or 3 equal doses q8-12h

Children:
Initial: 3mg/kg/day, divided into 3 equal doses q8h
Usual: 3-8mg/kg/day, divided into 2 or 3 equal doses q8h or q12h

Refractory Hypoglycemia: May require higher doses

ADMINISTRATION

Oral route

Shake well before each use.

STORAGE

25°C (77°F); excursions permitted to 15-30°C (59-86°F). Protect from light.

HOW SUPPLIED

Sus: 50mg/mL [30mL]

CONTRAINDICATIONS

Functional hypoglycemia, hypersensitivity to diazoxide or to other thiazides.

WARNINGS/PRECAUTIONS

May lead to significant fluid retention, which may precipitate CHF in patients w/ compromised cardiac reserve. Ketoacidosis and nonketotic hyperosmolar coma reported. Transient cataracts in association w/ hyperosmolar coma reported in an infant. Development of abnormal facial features in children treated chronically (>4 yrs) reported. Pulmonary HTN reported in infants and neonates; monitor for respiratory distress and d/c if pulmonary HTN is suspected. Initiate under close clinical supervision. Monitor blood glucose and clinical response until condition has stabilized; d/c if not effective after 2-3 weeks. Regularly monitor urine for sugar and ketones during prolonged treatment, especially under stress conditions. Caution w/ hyperuricemia or history of gout. Consider reduced dose and evaluate serum electrolyte levels in patients w/ renal impairment. May displace bilirubin from albumin; caution in newborns w/ increased bilirubinemia. Increased renin secretion and immunoglobulin G concentrations, and decreased cortisol secretions reported. May cause false-negative insulin response to glucagon.

ADVERSE REACTIONS

Na^+ and fluid retention, hirsutism of the lanugo type, hyperglycemia, glycosuria, GI intolerance, tachycardia, palpitations, increased serum uric acid levels, thrombocytopenia, transient neutropenia, skin rash, headache, weakness, malaise.

DRUG INTERACTIONS

May displace protein-bound substances (eg, bilirubin or coumarin and its derivatives), resulting in higher blood levels of these substances; may require dose reduction of the anticoagulant. May enhance antihypertensive effect of other drugs; caution w/ antihypertensive agents. Concomitant use w/ diphenylhydantoin may result in loss of seizure control. Thiazides or other commonly used diuretics may potentiate the hyperglycemic and hyperuricemic effects.

PREGNANCY AND LACTATION

Pregnancy: Category C.
Lactation: Not for use in nursing.

MECHANISM OF ACTION

Nondiuretic benzothiadiazine; produces a prompt dose-related increase in blood glucose level, due primarily to an inhibition of insulin release from the pancreas, and also to an extrapancreatic effect.

PHARMACOKINETICS

Distribution: Plasma protein binding (>90%); crosses the placenta. **Elimination:** Kidney; $T_{1/2}$=24-36 hrs (adults), 9.5-24 hrs (children 4 months-6 yrs).

PATIENT CONSIDERATIONS

Assessment: Assess for functional hypoglycemia, compromised cardiac reserve, hyperuricemia, history of gout, renal impairment, increased bilirubinemia in newborns, risk factors for pulmonary HTN, drug hypersensitivity, pregnancy/nursing status, and possible drug interactions.

Monitoring: Monitor for fluid retention, ketoacidosis, nonketotic hyperosmolar coma, respiratory distress, and other adverse reactions. Monitor clinical response and blood glucose (until condition has stabilized), BUN, CrCl, CBC, serum AST and uric acid levels, and urine for glucose and ketones. Monitor electrolyte levels in patients w/ renal impairment.

Counseling: Advise to consult regularly with the physician and to cooperate in the periodic monitoring of their condition by laboratory tests. Advise to take drug on a regular schedule as prescribed, not to skip doses, and not to take extra doses. Instruct not to use drug with other medications unless done with physician's advice, not to allow anyone else to take the medication, and to follow dietary instructions. Counsel to report promptly any adverse effects (increased urinary frequency, increased thirst, fruity breath odor), and to report pregnancy or discuss plans for pregnancy.

PROGRAF — tacrolimus   Rx

Class: Calcineurin-inhibitor immunosuppressant

> Immunosuppression may lead to increased risk of lymphoma and other malignancies, particularly of the skin. Increased susceptibility to infections (bacterial, viral, fungal, protozoal, opportunistic). Should only be prescribed by physicians experienced in immunosuppressive therapy and management of organ transplant patients. Manage patients in facilities equipped and staffed w/ adequate lab and supportive medical resources. Physician responsible for maintenance therapy should have complete information requisite for patient follow-up.

ADULT DOSAGE

Hepatic Transplant
Prophylaxis of organ rejection in patients receiving allogeneic liver transplant; recommended to be used concomitantly w/ adrenal corticosteroids early post-transplant

Cap:
Initial: 0.1-0.15mg/kg/day as 2 divided doses, q12h; administer no sooner than 6 hrs after liver transplant
Titrate: Based on clinical assessments of rejection and tolerability
Maint: Lower dosages than the initial dosage may be sufficient

Observed Tacrolimus Whole Blood Trough Concentrations w/ Liver Transplant:
Months 1-12: 5-20ng/mL
IV:
Initial: 0.03-0.05mg/kg/day
If receiving tacrolimus IV infusion, give 1st oral dose 8-12 hrs after discontinuing the IV infusion

Renal Transplant
Prophylaxis of organ rejection in patients receiving allogeneic kidney transplant; recommended to be used concomitantly w/ azathioprine or mycophenolate mofetil (MMF) and adrenal corticosteroids (early post-transplant)

Cap:
Initial: 0.2mg/kg/day in combination w/ azathioprine or 0.1mg/kg/day in combination w/ MMF/Interleukin (IL)-2 receptor antagonist; give as 2 divided doses, q12h. May administer w/in 24 hrs of kidney transplant, but should be delayed until renal function has recovered
Titrate: Based on clinical assessments of rejection and tolerability
Maint: Lower dosages than the initial dosage may be sufficient

Observed Tacrolimus Whole Blood Trough Concentrations w/ Kidney Transplant:
W/ Azathioprine:
Months 1-3: 7-20ng/mL
Months 4-12: 5-15ng/mL
W/ MMF/IL-2 Receptor Antagonist:
Months 1-12: 4-11ng/mL
IV:
Initial: 0.03-0.05mg/kg/day
If receiving tacrolimus IV infusion, give 1st oral dose 8-12 hrs after discontinuing the IV infusion

Cardiac Transplant
Prophylaxis of organ rejection in patients receiving allogeneic heart transplant; recommended to be used concomitantly w/ azathioprine or

PEDIATRIC DOSAGE

Hepatic Transplant
Prophylaxis of organ rejection in patients receiving allogeneic liver transplant; recommended to be used concomitantly w/ adrenal corticosteroids early post-transplant

Cap:
Initial: 0.15-0.2mg/kg/day as 2 divided doses, q12h; administer no sooner than 6 hrs after liver transplant

Observed Tacrolimus Whole Blood Trough Concentrations w/ Liver Transplant:
Months 1-12: 5-20ng/mL
IV:
Initial: 0.03-0.05mg/kg/day

mycophenolate mofetil (MMF) and adrenal corticosteroids (early post-transplant)

Cap:
Initial: 0.075mg/kg/day as 2 divided doses, q12h; administer no sooner than 6 hrs after heart transplant
Titrate: Based on clinical assessments of rejection and tolerability
Maint: Lower dosages than the initial dosage may be sufficient

Observed Tacrolimus Whole Blood Trough Concentrations w/ Heart Transplant:
Months 1-3: 10-20ng/mL
Months ≥4: 5-15ng/mL
IV:
Initial: 0.01mg/kg/day
If receiving tacrolimus IV infusion, give 1st oral dose 8-12 hrs after discontinuing the IV infusion

---

DOSING CONSIDERATIONS
Concomitant Medications
Cyclosporine: Do not use simultaneously; d/c tacrolimus or cyclosporine at least 24 hrs before initiating the other

Renal Impairment
Liver/Heart Transplant:
Preexisting Renal Impairment: Start at lower end of dosing range
Kidney Transplant:
Postoperative Oliguria: Initial dose should be administered no sooner than 6 hrs and w/in 24 hrs of transplantation, but may be delayed until renal function shows evidence of recovery

Hepatic Impairment
Severe (Child-Pugh ≥10): May require lower doses

Elderly
Start at lower end of dosing range

Other Important Considerations
Black patients may require higher doses
Do not eat grapefruit or drink grapefruit juice

ADMINISTRATION
Oral/IV route

Inj should be used only as a continuous IV infusion and when the patient cannot tolerate oral administration of cap.

Cap
Take consistently, either w/ or w/o food.

IV
Dilute product w/ 0.9% NaCl inj or D5 inj to concentration between 0.004mg/mL and 0.02mg/mL prior to use.
Diluted infusion sol should be stored in glass or polyethylene containers and should be discarded after 24 hrs; do not store in PVC container due to decreased stability and potential for extraction of phthalates; in situations where more dilute sol are utilized (eg, pediatric dosing), PVC-free tubing should likewise be used to minimize the potential for significant drug adsorption onto tubing.
Should not be mixed or co-infused w/ sol of pH ≥9 (eg, ganciclovir, acyclovir).

STORAGE
(Cap) 25°C (77°F); excursions permitted to 15-30°C (59-86°F). (Inj) 5-25°C (41-77°F).

HOW SUPPLIED
Cap: 0.5mg, 1mg, 5mg; **Inj:** 5mg/mL [1mL]

CONTRAINDICATIONS
Hypersensitivity to tacrolimus. **Inj:** Hypersensitivity to polyoxyl 60 hydrogenated castor oil (HCO-60).

WARNINGS/PRECAUTIONS
Limit exposure to sunlight and UV light in patients at increased risk for skin cancer. Increased risk for polyoma virus infections, CMV viremia, and CMV disease. Polyoma virus-associated nephropathy (PVAN) reported; may lead to renal function deterioration and kidney graft loss. Progressive multifocal leukoencephalopathy (PML) reported; consider PML in differential diagnosis in patients reporting neurological symptoms and consider consultation w/ a neurologist. Consider reductions in immunosuppression if CMV viremia, CMV disease, or if evidence of PVAN or PML develops. May cause new onset diabetes mellitus; closely monitor blood glucose concentrations. May cause acute/chronic nephrotoxicity; closely monitor patients w/ renal dysfunction. Consider changing to another immunosuppressive therapy in patients w/ persistent SrCr elevations unresponsive to dose adjustments. May cause neurotoxicity (eg, posterior reversible encephalopathy syndrome [PRES], delirium, coma); if PRES is suspected or diagnosed, maintain BP control and immediately reduce immunosuppression. Hyperkalemia and HTN reported. May prolong the QT/QTc interval and may cause torsades de pointes; avoid in patients w/ congenital long QT syndrome and consider obtaining ECGs and monitoring electrolytes (Mg^{2+}, K^+, Ca^{2+}) periodically in patients w/ CHF, bradyarrhythmias, those taking certain antiarrhythmic medications or other medicinal products that lead to QT prolongation, and those w/ electrolyte disturbances. Myocardial hypertrophy reported; consider dose reduction or discontinuation if diagnosed and consider

echocardiographic evaluation in patients who develop renal failure or clinical manifestations of ventricular dysfunction. Pure red cell aplasia (PRCA) reported; consider discontinuation if diagnosed. GI perforation reported; institute appropriate medical/surgical management promptly. (Inj) Anaphylactic reactions may occur; should be reserved for patients unable to take cap orally. Patients should be under continuous observation for at least the first 30 min following the start of infusion and at frequent intervals thereafter; d/c infusion if signs/symptoms of anaphylaxis occur.

ADVERSE REACTIONS
Lymphoma, malignancies, infections, tremor, HTN, abnormal renal function, headache, insomnia, hyperglycemia, hyperkalemia, hypomagnesemia, diarrhea, N/V, paresthesia.

DRUG INTERACTIONS
See Dosing Considerations. Not recommended w/ sirolimus in liver or heart transplants; safety and efficacy not established in kidney transplant. Due to potential for additive/synergistic renal impairment, caution w/ drugs that may be associated w/ renal dysfunction (eg, aminoglycosides, ganciclovir, amphotericin B). Increased whole blood concentrations w/ CYP3A inhibitors (eg, antifungals, calcium channel blockers [CCBs], macrolide antibiotics), and magnesium and aluminum hydroxide antacids. Decreased whole blood concentrations w/ CYP3A inducers. May increase mycophenolic acid (MPA) exposure after crossover from cyclosporine to tacrolimus in patients concomitantly receiving MPA-containing products. Avoid w/ nelfinavir unless the benefits outweigh the risks. Monitor whole blood concentrations and adjust tacrolimus dose if used concomitantly w/ protease inhibitors (eg, ritonavir, telaprevir, boceprevir), CCBs (eg, verapamil, diltiazem, nifedipine), erythromycin, clarithromycin, troleandomycin, chloramphenicol, rifampin, rifabutin, phenytoin, carbamazepine, phenobarbital, St. John's wort, magnesium and aluminum hydroxide antacids, bromocriptine, nefazodone, metoclopramide, danazol, ethinyl estradiol, amiodarone, methylprednisolone, herbal products containing *Schisandra sphenanthera* extracts, or CYP3A inhibitors/inducers. Monitor whole blood concentrations and adjust tacrolimus dose when concomitant use of antifungal drugs (eg, azoles, caspofungin) w/ tacrolimus is initiated or discontinued; initially reduce tacrolimus dose to 1/3 of the original dose when initiating therapy w/ voriconazole or posaconazole. May increase levels of phenytoin; monitor phenytoin levels and adjust phenytoin dose as needed. Caution w/ antihypertensive agents (eg, K⁺-sparing diuretics, ACE inhibitors, ARBs) or other agents associated w/ hyperkalemia. Reduce tacrolimus dose, closely monitor tacrolimus whole blood concentrations, and monitor for QT prolongation when coadministered w/ CYP3A4 substrates and/or inhibitors that also have the potential to prolong the QT interval. Amiodarone may increase whole blood concentrations w/ or w/o concurrent QT prolongation. Avoid live vaccines during therapy. Caution w/ concomitant immunosuppressants.

PREGNANCY AND LACTATION
Pregnancy: Category C.
Lactation: Not for use in nursing.

MECHANISM OF ACTION
Macrolide immunosuppressant; not established. Inhibits T-lymphocyte activation. Binds to an intracellular protein, FKBP-12, forming a complex of tacrolimus-FKBP-12, Ca²⁺, calmodulin, and calcineurin, and inhibiting phosphatase activity of calcineurin. This effect may prevent dephosphorylation and translocation of nuclear factor of activated T-cells, a nuclear component thought to initiate gene transcription for the formation of lymphokines.

PHARMACOKINETICS
Absorption: (Oral) Incomplete and variable. Administration of variable doses in different populations resulted in different pharmacokinetic parameters.
Distribution: Plasma protein binding (approx 99%); crosses placenta; found in breast milk. **Metabolism:** Liver, via CYP3A (demethylation and hydroxylation); 13-demethyl tacrolimus (major metabolite); 31-demethyl (active metabolite).
Elimination: (Oral) Feces (92.6%), urine (2.3%). (IV) Feces (92.4%); urine (<1% unchanged). Refer to PI for $T_{1/2}$ values in different populations.

PATIENT CONSIDERATIONS
Assessment: Assess for drug hypersensitivity, congenital long QT syndrome, CHF, bradyarrhythmias, electrolyte disturbances, renal/hepatic impairment, pregnancy/nursing status, and possible drug interactions. (Inj) Assess for hypersensitivity to HCO-60.

Monitoring: Monitor tacrolimus blood concentrations in conjunction w/ other laboratory and clinical parameters. Monitor for lymphomas and other malignancies, infections, neurotoxicity, HTN, QT prolongation, PRCA, GI perforation, and other adverse reactions. Monitor serum K⁺ and glucose concentrations. (Inj) Monitor for anaphylactic reactions.

Counseling: Inform of the risks and benefits of therapy. Advise to take medicine at the same 12-hr interval every day and not to eat grapefruit or drink grapefruit juice in combination w/ the drug. Advise to limit exposure to sunlight and UV light by wearing protective clothing and to use a sunscreen w/ a high protection factor. Instruct to contact physician if frequent urination, increased thirst or hunger, vision changes, deliriums, tremors, or any symptoms of infection develop. Advise to attend all visits and complete all blood tests ordered by medical team. Inform that therapy may cause high BP, which may require treatment w/ antihypertensive therapy. Instruct to inform physician if planning to become pregnant or breastfeed or when starting or stopping any medication (prescription and nonprescription medicines, natural/herbal remedies, nutritional supplements, vitamins). Inform that therapy may interfere w/ the usual response to immunizations and that live vaccines should be avoided.

PROLENSA — bromfenac sodium
Class: NSAID   Rx

ADULT DOSAGE	PEDIATRIC DOSAGE
Ocular Pain and Inflammation 1 drop to the affected eye qd beginning 1 day prior to cataract surgery, continued on the day of surgery, and through the first 14 days of the postoperative period	Pediatric use may not have been established

- -

DOSING CONSIDERATIONS
Concomitant Medications
Administer at least 5 min apart if using other topical ophthalmic medications

ADMINISTRATION
Ocular route

STORAGE
15-25°C (59-77°F).

HOW SUPPLIED
Sol: 0.07% [1.6mL, 3mL]

WARNINGS/PRECAUTIONS
Contains sodium sulfite; may cause allergic-type reactions, including anaphylactic symptoms and life-threatening or less severe asthmatic episodes in certain susceptible people. May slow or delay healing. Potential for cross-sensitivity to acetylsalicylic acid (ASA), phenylacetic acid derivatives, and other NSAIDs; caution with previous sensitivities to these drugs. May cause increased bleeding of ocular tissues (eg, hyphemas) in conjunction with ocular surgery; caution with known bleeding tendencies. May result in keratitis. Continued use may result in sight-threatening epithelial breakdown or corneal thinning/erosion/ulceration/perforation; d/c use and monitor for corneal health if corneal epithelial breakdown occurs. Caution in patients with complicated ocular surgeries, corneal denervation, corneal epithelial defects, diabetes mellitus (DM), ocular surface diseases (eg, dry eye syndrome), rheumatoid arthritis (RA), or repeat ocular surgeries within a short period. Use >24 hrs prior to surgery or use beyond 14 days postsurgery may increase risk for occurrence and severity of corneal adverse events. Do not instill while wearing contact lenses; remove contact lenses prior to instillation, and may reinsert after 10 min following administration. Avoid use during late pregnancy because of the known effects on the fetal cardiovascular system (closure of ductus arteriosus).

ADVERSE REACTIONS
Anterior chamber inflammation, foreign body sensation, eye pain, photophobia, vision blurred.

DRUG INTERACTIONS
Caution with medications that may prolong bleeding time. Increased potential for healing problems with topical steroids.

PREGNANCY AND LACTATION
Safety not known in pregnancy, caution in nursing.

MECHANISM OF ACTION
NSAID; blocks prostaglandin synthesis by inhibiting COX-1 and -2.

PATIENT CONSIDERATIONS
Assessment: Assess for hypersensitivity (eg, to sodium sulfite) or cross-sensitivity (eg, to ASA) reactions, history of complicated or repeated ocular surgeries, corneal denervation, corneal epithelial defects, DM, ocular surface diseases (eg, dry eye syndrome), RA, bleeding tendencies, pregnancy/nursing status, and possible drug interactions.

Monitoring: Monitor for anaphylactic symptoms, severe asthma attacks, wound-healing problems, keratitis, corneal epithelial breakdown, corneal thinning/erosion/ulceration/perforation, bleeding of ocular tissues, and other adverse reactions.

Counseling: Inform of the possibility that slow or delayed healing may occur. Advise to replace bottle cap after using, to not touch dropper tip to any surface, and to use a single bottle to treat only 1 eye. Advise to remove contact lenses prior to instillation, and that lenses may be reinserted after 10 min following administration. Advise to administer at least 5 min apart if >1 topical ophthalmic medication is being used.

PROLIA — denosumab
Class: IgG₂ monoclonal antibody   Rx

ADULT DOSAGE	PEDIATRIC DOSAGE
Osteoporosis **Postmenopausal Osteoporosis:** Postmenopausal women at high risk for fracture, or patients who have failed or are intolerant to other available osteoporosis therapy 60mg as a single SQ inj once every 6 months **To Increase Bone Mass in Men w/ Osteoporosis:** Men at high risk for fracture, or patients who have failed or	Pediatric use may not have been established

are intolerant to other available osteoporosis therapy

60mg as a single SQ inj once every 6 months

Calcium and Vitamin D Supplementation:
All patients should receive Ca^{2+} 1000mg/day and $\geq$400 IU vitamin D daily

Bone Loss
In Men Receiving Androgen Deprivation Therapy for Nonmetastatic Prostate Cancer:
60mg as a single SQ inj once every 6 months

In Women Receiving Adjuvant Aromatase Inhibitor Therapy for Breast Cancer:
60mg as a single SQ inj once every 6 months

Calcium and Vitamin D Supplementation:
All patients should receive Ca^{2+} 1000mg/day and $\geq$400 IU vitamin D daily

Missed Dose
If a dose is missed, administer as soon as patient is available, then schedule inj every 6 months from date of last inj

----

ADMINISTRATION
SQ route

Administer in the upper arm/thigh or abdomen.
People sensitive to latex should not handle the grey needle cap on the single-use prefilled syringe, which contains dry natural rubber (a derivative of latex).
Prior to administration, remove from the refrigerator and bring to room temperature up to 25°C (77°F), by standing in the original container for 15-30 min.

Instructions for Prefilled Syringe w/ Needle Safety Guard:
Do not slide the green safety guard forward over the needle before administering the inj; it will lock in place and prevent inj.
Insert needle and inject all the liquid SQ.

Instructions for Single-Use Vial:
Use a 27-gauge needle to withdraw and inject the 1mL dose.
Do not re-enter the vial; discard vial and any liquid remaining in the vial.

STORAGE
2-8°C (36-46°F). Do not freeze. Use w/in 14 days once removed from the refrigerator and do not expose to temperatures >25°C (77°F). Protect from direct light and heat. Avoid vigorous shaking.

HOW SUPPLIED
Inj: 60mg/mL [prefilled syringe, vial]

CONTRAINDICATIONS
Hypocalcemia, pregnancy, history of systemic hypersensitivity to any component of the product.

WARNINGS/PRECAUTIONS
Should be administered by a healthcare professional. Do not give w/ other drugs that contain the same active ingredient (eg, Xgeva). Hypersensitivity, including anaphylaxis, reported; d/c further use and initiate appropriate therapy if an anaphylactic or other clinically significant allergic reaction occurs. Hypocalcemia may be exacerbated; correct preexisting hypocalcemia prior to initiating therapy. Monitor Ca^{2+} and mineral levels (phosphorus [P] and Mg^{2+}) w/in 14 days of inj in patients predisposed to hypocalcemia and disturbances of mineral metabolism (eg, history of hypoparathyroidism, malabsorption syndromes, excision of the small intestine). Significant risk of hypocalcemia following administration w/ severe renal impairment (CrCl <30mL/min) or receiving dialysis; marked elevations of serum parathyroid hormone (PTH) may develop. Osteonecrosis of the jaw (ONJ) may occur; increased risk w/ duration of exposure to therapy. A dental examination is recommended w/ appropriate preventive dentistry prior to treatment in patients w/ risk factors for ONJ (eg, invasive dental procedures, diagnosis of cancer, concomitant therapies [eg, chemotherapy, corticosteroids, angiogenesis inhibitors]). Atypical low-energy or low-trauma fractures of the femoral shaft reported; evaluate patients w/ thigh/groin pain to rule out an incomplete femur fracture and consider interruption of therapy. Endocarditis and serious skin, abdomen, urinary tract, and ear infections leading to hospitalization reported; assess need for continued therapy if serious infections develop. Increased risk for serious infections in patients w/ an impaired immune system. Epidermal and dermal adverse events may occur; consider discontinuing therapy if severe symptoms develop. Severe and occasionally incapacitating bone, joint, and/or muscle pain reported; consider discontinuing use if severe symptoms develop. Significant suppression of bone remodeling as evidenced by markers of bone turnover and bone histomorphometry reported.

ADVERSE REACTIONS
Postmenopausal Osteoporosis: Back pain, pain in extremity, musculoskeletal pain, hypercholesterolemia, cystitis.
Men w/ Osteoporosis: Back pain, arthralgia, nasopharyngitis.
Patients Receiving Androgen Deprivation Therapy/Adjuvant Aromatase Inhibitor: Arthralgia, back pain.

DRUG INTERACTIONS
Immunosuppressant agents may increase the risk of serious infections. Concomitant administration of drugs associated w/ ONJ may increase risk of developing ONJ.

PREGNANCY AND LACTATION
Pregnancy: Category X. May cause fetal harm. Physicians are advised to recommend that pregnant patients enroll in Amgen's Pregnancy Surveillance Program.
Lactation: Not for use in nursing.

MECHANISM OF ACTION
IgG_2 monoclonal antibody; binds to receptor activator of nuclear factor kappa-B ligand (RANKL) and prevents RANKL from activating its receptor, RANK, on the surface of osteoclasts and their precursors, thereby decreasing bone resorption and increasing bone mass and strength in both cortical and trabecular bone.

PHARMACOKINETICS
Absorption: Fasting: C_{max}=6.75mcg/mL, T_{max}=10 days (median), $AUC_{0-16\ weeks}$ =316mcg•day/mL. **Distribution:** Crosses placenta. **Elimination:** $T_{1/2}$=25.4 days.

PATIENT CONSIDERATIONS
Assessment: Assess for drug hypersensitivity, preexisting hypocalcemia, history of hypoparathyroidism, thyroid/parathyroid surgery, malabsorption syndromes, excision of the small intestine, renal impairment, impairment of the immune system, risk factors for ONJ, pregnancy/nursing status, and possible drug interactions. Perform routine oral exam, and dental examination w/ appropriate preventive dentistry in patients w/ risk factors for ONJ.

Monitoring: Monitor for signs/symptoms of hypocalcemia, infections, hypersensitivity, dermatological reactions, serum PTH elevation, ONJ, atypical femoral fractures, delayed fracture healing, musculoskeletal pain, and other adverse reactions. Monitor Ca^{2+} and mineral levels (P and Mg^{2+}) w/in 14 days of inj in patients predisposed to hypocalcemia and disturbances of mineral metabolism.

Counseling: Advise not to take w/ other drugs w/ the same active ingredient. Inform about the importance of maintaining Ca^{2+} levels w/ adequate Ca^{2+} and vitamin D supplementation. Advise to seek prompt medical attention if signs/symptoms of hypocalcemia, infections, dermatological reactions, or hypersensitivity reactions develop. Advise to maintain good oral hygiene during treatment and to inform dentist prior to dental procedures of current treatment. Instruct to inform physician or dentist if patient experiences persistent pain and/ or slow healing of the mouth or jaw after dental surgery. Advise to report new or unusual thigh, hip, or groin pain. Inform that severe bone, joint, and/or muscle pain reported during therapy; instruct to report development of severe symptoms. Inform that therapy should not be used if pregnant or nursing. Advise to adhere to proper schedule of administration.

PROMACTA — eltrombopag   Rx

Class: Thrombopoietin receptor agonist

> May increase risk of hepatic decompensation in patients w/ chronic hepatitis C when given in combination w/ interferon and ribavirin.

ADULT DOSAGE	PEDIATRIC DOSAGE
Chronic Immune Thrombocytopenia	**Chronic Immune Thrombocytopenia**
W/ Insufficient Response to Corticosteroids, Immunoglobulins, or Splenectomy:	**W/ Insufficient Response to Corticosteroids, Immunoglobulins, or Splenectomy:**
Initial: 50mg qd	**Initial:**
Titrate: Adjust the dose to achieve and maintain a platelet count $\geq$50 x 10^9/L	**1-5 Years:** 25mg qd
Max: 75mg/day	**$\geq$6 Years:** 50mg qd
	Titrate: Adjust the dose to achieve and maintain a platelet count $\geq$50 x 10^9/L
Dose Adjustment Based on Platelet Counts:	**Max:** 75mg/day
<50 x 10^9/L Following at Least 2 Weeks of Therapy:	**Dose Adjustment Based on Platelet Counts:**
Increase daily dose by 25mg to a max of 75mg/day; patients taking 12.5mg qd, increase to 25mg qd before increasing dose amount by 25mg	**<50 x 10^9/L Following at Least 2 Weeks of Therapy:**
$\geq$200 to $\leq$400 x 10^9/L at Any Time:	Increase daily dose by 25mg to a max of 75mg/day; patients taking 12.5mg qd, increase to 25mg qd before increasing dose amount by 25mg
Decrease daily dose by 25mg; wait 2 weeks to assess the effects and any subsequent dose adjustments Patients taking 25mg qd, decrease to 12.5mg qd	**$\geq$200 to $\leq$400 x 10^9/L at Any Time:**
>400 x 10^9/L:	Decrease daily dose by 25mg; wait 2 weeks to assess the effects and any subsequent dose adjustments Patients taking 25mg qd, decrease to 12.5mg qd
Stop therapy and increase frequency of platelet monitoring to twice weekly; once platelet count is <150 x 10^9/L, reinitiate at a daily dose reduced by 25mg or reinitiate at a daily dose of 12.5mg for patients taking 25mg qd	**>400 x 10^9/L:**
>400 x 10^9/L After 2 Weeks of Therapy at Lowest Dose:	Stop therapy and increase frequency of platelet monitoring to twice weekly; once platelet count is <150 x 10^9/L, reinitiate at a daily dose reduced by 25mg or reinitiate at a daily dose of 12.5mg for patients taking 25mg qd
D/C therapy	**>400 x 10^9/L After 2 Weeks of Therapy at Lowest Dose:**
Chronic Hepatitis C-Associated Thrombocytopenia	D/C therapy
To allow the initiation and maint of interferon-based therapy	

Initial: 25mg qd
Titrate: Adjust dose in 25mg increments every 2 weeks as necessary to achieve target platelet count required to initiate antiviral therapy. During antiviral therapy, adjust dose to avoid dose reductions of peginterferon
Max: 100mg/day
Dose Adjustment Based on Platelet Counts:
<50 x 10^9/L Following at Least 2 Weeks of Therapy:
Increase daily dose by 25mg to a max of 100mg/day
≥200 to ≤400 x 10^9/L at Any Time:
Decrease daily dose by 25mg; wait 2 weeks to assess the effects and any subsequent dose adjustments
>400 x 10^9/L:
Stop therapy and increase frequency of platelet monitoring to twice weekly; once platelet count is <150 x 10^9/L, reinitiate at a daily dose reduced by 25mg or reinitiate at a daily dose of 12.5mg for patients taking 25mg qd
>400 x 10^9/L After 2 Weeks of Therapy at Lowest Dose:
D/C therapy

Severe Aplastic Anemia

W/ Insufficient Response to Immunosuppressive Therapy:
Initial: 50mg qd
Titrate: Adjust dose in 50mg increments every 2 weeks as necessary to achieve the target platelet count ≥50 x 10^9/L
Max: 150mg/day
Dose Adjustment Based on Platelet Counts:
<50 x 10^9/L Following at Least 2 Weeks of Therapy:
Increase daily dose by 50mg to a max of 150mg/day; patients taking 25mg qd, increase to 50mg qd before increasing dose amount by 50mg
≥200 to ≤400 x 10^9/L at Any Time:
Decrease daily dose by 50mg; wait 2 weeks to assess the effects and any subsequent dose adjustments
>400 x 10^9/L:
Stop therapy for 1 week; once platelet count is <150 x 10^9/L, reinitiate therapy at a dose reduced by 50mg
>400 x 10^9/L After 2 Weeks of Therapy at Lowest Dose:
D/C therapy

DOSING CONSIDERATIONS
Concomitant Medications
Chronic Immune Thrombocytopenia:
Modify dosage regimen of concomitant medications for therapy to avoid excessive increases in platelet counts; do not administer >1 dose of eltrombopag w/in any 24-hr period
Hepatic Impairment
≥6 Years:
Mild to Severe (Child-Pugh Class A, B, C):
Chronic Immune Thrombocytopenia:
Initial: 25mg qd; after initiating therapy or after any subsequent dosing increase, wait 3 weeks before increasing the dose
Severe Aplastic Anemia:
Initial: 25mg qd
East Asian Ancestry w/ Hepatic Impairment (Child-Pugh Class A, B, C):
Chronic Immune Thrombocytopenia:
Initial: 12.5mg qd
Discontinuation
Chronic Immune Thrombocytopenia: D/C if platelet count does not increase to a sufficient level after 4 weeks of therapy at max daily dose of 75mg
Chronic Hepatitis C-Associated Thrombocytopenia: D/C therapy when antiviral therapy is discontinued; important liver test abnormalities may necessitate discontinuation
Severe Aplastic Anemia: D/C therapy if no hematologic response occurs after 16 weeks of therapy. Consider discontinuation if new cytogenetic abnormalities or important liver test abnormalities are observed
Other Important Considerations
≥6 Years:
Chronic Immune Thrombocytopenia/Severe Aplastic Anemia:

Assess platelet counts weekly for 2 weeks, and then monitor monthly when switching between oral sus and tab

East Asian Ancestry:
Initial: 25mg qd
ADMINISTRATION
Oral route
- Take on empty stomach (1 hr ac or 2 hrs pc).
- Take sus/tab at least 2 hrs before or 4 hrs after other medications (eg, antacids), Ca^{2+}-rich foods (eg, dairy products, Ca^{2+}-fortified juices), or supplements containing polyvalent cations (eg, iron, Ca^{2+}, aluminum, Mg^{2+}, selenium, zinc).
- Do not crush tabs and mix w/ food or liquids.
Sus
- Administer immediately after preparation.
- Discard any sus not administered w/in 30 min after preparation.
- Prepare w/ water only; do not use hot water.
- For details on preparation and administration of sus, see Instructions for Use.
STORAGE
20-25°C (68-77°F); excursions permitted to 15-30°C (59-86°F). **Reconstituted Sus:** 20-25°C (68-77°F) for 30 min; discard if not used w/in 30 min.
HOW SUPPLIED
Sus: 25mg/pkt; **Tab:** 12.5mg, 25mg, 50mg, 75mg, 100mg
WARNINGS/PRECAUTIONS
Should not be used to normalize platelet counts. Should only be used in patients w/ immune thrombocytopenia whose degree of thrombocytopenia and clinical condition increase the risk for bleeding. Liver enzyme elevations and indirect hyperbilirubinemia may occur; if bilirubin is elevated, perform fractionation. D/C if ALT levels increase to ≥3X ULN in patients w/ normal liver function or ≥3X baseline in patients w/ pretreatment elevations in transaminases, and are progressively increasing or persistent for ≥4 weeks, or are accompanied by increased direct bilirubin or by clinical symptoms of liver injury or evidence for hepatic decompensation. Hepatotoxicity may reoccur w/ reinitiation; caution w/ reintroduction of therapy and measure LFTs weekly during the dose adjustment phase. If liver test abnormalities persist, worsen, or reoccur, then permanently d/c therapy. Thrombotic/thromboembolic complications may result from increases in platelet counts; caution in patients w/ known risk factors for thromboembolism (eg, factor V Leiden, antithrombin III deficiency, antiphospholipid syndrome, chronic liver disease). Development or worsening of cataracts reported.
ADVERSE REACTIONS
Chronic Immune Thrombocytopenia:
Adults: N/V, diarrhea, URTI, increased ALT, myalgia, UTI.
Peds >1 Year: URTI, nasopharyngitis.
Chronic Hepatitis C-Associated Thrombocytopenia: Anemia, pyrexia, fatigue, headache, nausea, diarrhea, decreased appetite, influenza-like illness, asthenia, insomnia, cough, pruritus, chills, myalgia, alopecia, peripheral edema.
Severe Aplastic Anemia: Nausea, fatigue, cough, diarrhea, headache.
DRUG INTERACTIONS
See Boxed Warning. Take at least 2 hrs before or 4 hrs after any medications or products containing polyvalent cations (eg, antacids, dairy products, mineral supplements). Increases rosuvastatin levels; recommended to reduce rosuvastatin by 50%. Caution w/ substrates of organic anion transporting polypeptide 1B1 (eg, atorvastatin, bosentan, glyburide) or breast cancer resistance protein (eg, imatinib, irinotecan, methotrexate); monitor for signs/symptoms of excessive exposure and consider dose reduction of these drugs. Lopinavir/ritonavir may decrease plasma exposure.
PREGNANCY AND LACTATION
Pregnancy: Category C.
Lactation: Not for use in nursing.
MECHANISM OF ACTION
Thrombopoietin (TPO)-receptor agonist; interacts w/ the transmembrane domain of the human TPO receptor and initiates signaling cascades that induce proliferation and differentiation from bone marrow progenitor cells.
PHARMACOKINETICS
Absorption: T_{max}=2-6 hrs; (50mg dose qd) C_{max}=7.03mcg/mL (adults), 6.8mcg/mL (12-17 yrs of age), 10.3mcg/mL (6-11 yrs of age), 11.6mcg/mL (1-5 yrs of age); AUC=101mcg•hr/mL (adults), 103mcg•hr/mL (12-17 yrs of age), 153mcg•hr/mL (6-11 yrs of age), 162mcg•hr/mL (1-5 yrs of age). **Distribution:** Plasma protein binding (>99%). **Metabolism:** Extensive; cleavage, oxidation (via CYP1A2, CYP2C8), and conjugation w/ glucuronic acid (via UGT1A1, UGT1A3), glutathione, or cysteine. **Elimination:** Urine (31%), feces (59%, 20% unchanged); $T_{1/2}$=26-35 hrs (immune thrombocytopenia), 21-32 hrs (healthy subjects).

PATIENT CONSIDERATIONS

Assessment: Assess for degree of thrombocytopenia, risk factors for thromboembolism, renal/hepatic impairment, pregnancy/nursing status, and for possible drug interactions. Obtain baseline CBCs w/ differential, including platelet count, and LFTs. Perform a baseline ocular exam.

Monitoring: Monitor for thrombotic/thromboembolic complications, hepatotoxicity, hepatic decompensation in patients w/ chronic hepatitis C, cataracts, and other adverse reactions. Closely monitor patients w/ renal impairment. Monitor LFTs every 2 weeks during dose adjustment phase, then monthly following establishment of a stable dose. If abnormal LFT levels are detected, repeat tests w/in 3-5 days. If the abnormalities are confirmed, monitor serum LFT tests weekly until resolved or stabilized. Perform a regular ocular exam. Monitor platelet counts every week prior to starting antiviral therapy in patients w/ chronic hepatitis C. Monitor CBCs w/ differentials, including platelets counts, weekly during therapy until a stable platelet count is achieved. Obtain CBCs w/ differentials, including platelet counts, monthly thereafter and then weekly for at least 4 weeks after discontinuation.

Counseling: Ensure patients or caregivers receive training on proper dosing, preparation, and administration of sus. Inform about the risks and benefits of therapy. Inform that therapy may be associated w/ hepatobiliary lab abnormalities. Advise patients w/ chronic hepatitis C and cirrhosis that hepatic decompensation may occur when receiving alfa interferon therapy. Advise to avoid situations or medications that may increase risk for bleeding and to report to physician any signs/symptoms of liver problems immediately. Inform that thrombocytopenia and risk of bleeding may reoccur upon discontinuation, particularly if therapy is discontinued while on anticoagulants/antiplatelet agents. Inform that excessive dose may result in excessive platelet counts and risk for thrombotic/thromboembolic complications. Advise to have a baseline ocular exam prior to administration of therapy and be monitored for signs/symptoms of cataracts during therapy. Advise to take sus/tab at least 2 hrs before or 4 hrs after foods, mineral supplements, and antacids which contain polyvalent cations.

PROMETHAZINE — promethazine hydrochloride   Rx

Class: Phenothiazine derivative

> Do not be use in pediatric patients <2 yrs of age; potential for fatal respiratory depression. Caution when administering to patients ≥2 yrs of age; use lowest effective dose and avoid concomitant administration of other drugs w/ respiratory depressant effects.

OTHER BRAND NAMES
Promethegan, Phenadoz

ADULT DOSAGE

Nausea/Vomiting

Active Therapy:
12.5-25mg q4-6h, prn

Prophylaxis During Surgery and Postoperative Period:
25mg q4-6h, prn

Sedation

Nighttime, Presurgical, or Obstetrical Sedation:
25-50mg

Pre- and Postoperative Use

Preoperative Medication:
50mg in combination w/ reduced dose of narcotic or barbiturate and the required amount of a belladonna alkaloid

Postoperative Sedation/Adjunctive Use w/ Analgesics:
25-50mg

Allergies
25mg qhs or 12.5mg ac and hs; may give 6.25-12.5mg tid

Adjust to lowest effective dose

Motion Sickness
Initial: 25mg 30-60 min before travel and repeat after 8-12 hrs, if necessary
Maint: 25mg bid (on arising and before pm meal)

Other Indications
Perennial and seasonal allergic rhinitis, vasomotor rhinitis, allergic conjunctivitis due to inhalant allergens and foods, mild uncomplicated allergic skin manifestations of urticaria and angioedema, amelioration of allergic reactions to blood or plasma, and dermographism. Adjunct therapy in anaphylactic reactions. Pre/postoperative or obstetric sedation. Prevention and control of N/V associated w/ certain types of anesthesia and surgery. Adjunct therapy w/ meperidine or other analgesics for control of postoperative pain. Sedation, relief of apprehension, and production of light sleep. Active and prophylactic treatment of motion sickness. Antiemetic in postoperative patients.

PEDIATRIC DOSAGE

Allergies

≥2 Years:
25mg qhs or 12.5mg ac and hs; may give 6.25-12.5mg tid

Adjust to lowest effective dose

Nausea/Vomiting

≥2 Years:

Active Therapy:
Usual: 0.5mg/lb; adjust dose based on patient age/weight and severity of condition

Prophylaxis During Surgery and the Postoperative Period:
25mg q4-6h, prn

Sedation

≥2 Years:
12.5-25mg qhs

Pre- and Postoperative Use

≥2 Years:

Preoperative Medication:
0.5mg/lb in combination w/ reduced dose of narcotic or barbiturate and the appropriate dose of an atropine-like drug

Postoperative Sedation/Adjunctive Use w/ Analgesics:
12.5-25mg

Motion Sickness

≥2 Years:
12.5-25mg bid

Other Indications
Perennial and seasonal allergic rhinitis, vasomotor rhinitis, allergic conjunctivitis due to inhalant allergens and foods, mild uncomplicated allergic skin manifestations of urticaria and angioedema, amelioration of allergic reactions to blood or plasma, and dermographism. Adjunct therapy in anaphylactic reactions. Pre/postoperative or obstetric sedation. Prevention and control of N/V associated w/ certain types of anesthesia and surgery. Adjunct therapy w/ meperidine or other analgesics for control of postoperative pain. Sedation, relief of apprehension, and production of light sleep. Active and prophylactic treatment of motion sickness. Antiemetic in postoperative patients.

DOSING CONSIDERATIONS
Elderly
Start at lower end of dosing range

ADMINISTRATION
Oral/rectal route

STORAGE
Keep tightly closed. (Syrup/Tab) 20-25°C (68-77°F). (Sup) 2-8°C (36-46°F). (Syrup/Tab) Protect from light.

HOW SUPPLIED
Sup: (Phenadoz) 12.5mg, 25mg, (Promethegan) 50mg; **Syrup:** 6.25mg/5mL [118mL, 237mL, 473mL] **Tab:** 12.5mg*, 25mg*, 50mg *scored

CONTRAINDICATIONS
Pediatric patients <2 yrs of age; comatose states; known hypersensitivity or idiosyncratic reaction to promethazine or to other phenothiazines; treatment of lower respiratory tract symptoms, including asthma.

WARNINGS/PRECAUTIONS
Not recommended for uncomplicated vomiting in pediatric patients; should be limited to prolonged vomiting of known etiology. Avoid in pediatric patients whose signs and symptoms may suggest Reye's syndrome or other hepatic diseases. May impair mental/physical abilities. May lead to potentially fatal respiratory depression; avoid w/ compromised respiratory function. May lower seizure threshold. Caution w/ bone marrow depression; leukopenia and agranulocytosis reported. Neuroleptic malignant syndrome (NMS) reported alone or w/ antipsychotics; d/c immediately and monitor. Hallucinations and convulsions may occur in pediatric patients. Acutely ill pediatric patients associated w/ dehydration may have an increased susceptibility to dystonias. Cholestatic jaundice reported. Caution w/ narrow-angle glaucoma, prostatic hypertrophy, stenosing peptic ulcer, bladder-neck or pyloroduodenal obstruction, cardiovascular disease, and liver function impairment. Lab test interactions may occur. Caution in elderly patients.

ADVERSE REACTIONS
Drowsiness, sedation, blurred vision, dizziness, increased or decreased BP, urticaria, dry mouth, N/V, hallucination, leukopenia, asthma, apnea, photosensitivity, angioneurotic edema.

DRUG INTERACTIONS
See Boxed Warning. May increase incidence of extrapyramidal effects w/ MAOIs. May increase, prolong, or intensify the sedative action of other CNS depressants, (eg, alcohol, sedatives/hypnotics, narcotics, TCAs); avoid such agents or reduce dosage. Reduce dose of barbiturates by at least 50% if given concomitantly. Reduce dose of narcotics by 25-50% if given concomitantly. May reverse vasopressor effect of epinephrine; do not use to treat hypotension associated w/ promethazine overdose. Caution w/ anticholinergics. Caution w/ medications that may affect seizure threshold (eg, narcotics, local anesthetics). Leukopenia and agranulocytosis reported when used w/ other known marrow-toxic agents.

PREGNANCY AND LACTATION
Pregnancy: Category C.
Lactation: Not for use in nursing.

MECHANISM OF ACTION
Phenothiazine derivative; H_1 receptor-blocking agent w/ antihistaminic action. Provides sedative and antiemetic effects.

PHARMACOKINETICS
Absorption: Well-absorbed from GI tract. **Metabolism:** Liver; sulfoxides, N-demethylpromethazine (metabolites). **Elimination:** Urine.

PATIENT CONSIDERATIONS
Assessment: Assess for drug hypersensitivity or past idiosyncratic reaction to phenothiazines, bone marrow depression, narrow-angle glaucoma, pregnancy/nursing status, possible drug interactions, or any other conditions where treatment is contraindicated or cautioned. Assess for signs/symptoms of hepatic diseases, and for Reye's syndrome in pediatric patients.

Monitoring: Monitor for signs/symptoms of CNS/respiratory depression, NMS, seizures, cholestatic jaundice, leukopenia, agranulocytosis, and other adverse reactions. Monitor for hallucinations, convulsions, extrapyramidal symptoms, and respiratory depression, and for dystonias in pediatric patients.

Counseling: Inform that therapy may cause drowsiness and impairment of mental and/or physical abilities. Counsel to report any involuntary muscle movements. Instruct to avoid alcohol use, prolonged sun exposure, and concomitant use of other CNS depressants.

PROMETHAZINE DM — dextromethorphan hydrobromide/ promethazine hydrochloride   Rx

Class: Antitussive/phenothiazine derivative

> Promethazine HCl should not be used in patients <2 yrs; potential for fatal respiratory depression. Caution when administering to patients ≥2 yrs; use lowest effective dose and avoid concomitant administration of respiratory depressants.

ADULT DOSAGE
Antihistamine/Cough Suppressant

Temporary relief of coughs and upper respiratory symptoms associated with allergy or the common cold

5mL q4-6h
Max: 30mL/24 hrs

PEDIATRIC DOSAGE
Antihistamine/Cough Suppressant

Temporary relief of coughs and upper respiratory symptoms associated with allergy or the common cold

2 to <6 Years:
1.25-2.5mL q4-6h
Max: 10mL/24 hrs

6 to <12 Years:
2.5-5mL q4-6h
Max: 20mL/24 hrs

≥12 Years:
5mL q4-6h
Max: 30mL/24 hrs

DOSING CONSIDERATIONS
Elderly
Start at lower end of dosing range

ADMINISTRATION
Oral route

STORAGE
20-25°C (68-77°F). Protect from light. Keep bottle tightly closed. Dispense in a tight, light-resistant container with a child-resistant closure.

HOW SUPPLIED
Syrup: (Dextromethorphan/Promethazine) (15mg/6.25mg)/5mL

CONTRAINDICATIONS
Dextromethorphan: Concomitant MAOIs. **Promethazine:** Comatose states; known hypersensitivity or idiosyncratic reaction to promethazine or to other phenothiazines; treatment of lower respiratory tract symptoms, including asthma.

WARNINGS/PRECAUTIONS
Should be given to a pregnant woman only if clearly needed. Avoid prolonged exposure to sunlight. Promethazine: Caution in pediatrics ≥2 yrs. Respiratory depression and apnea, sometimes associated with death, are strongly associated with promethazine products and are not directly related to individualized weight-based dosing. Avoid in pediatric patients whose signs and symptoms may suggest Reye's syndrome or hepatic diseases. May impair mental/physical abilities. May lower seizure threshold; caution with seizure disorders. May lead to potentially fatal respiratory depression; avoid with compromised respiratory function (eg, COPD, sleep apnea). Caution with bone marrow depression; leukopenia and agranulocytosis reported. Neuroleptic malignant syndrome (NMS) reported; d/c immediately. Hallucinations and convulsions may occur in pediatrics with therapeutic doses or overdoses. Acutely ill, dehydrated pediatric patients may have increased susceptibility to dystonias. Caution with narrow-angle glaucoma, prostatic hypertrophy, stenosing peptic ulcer, bladder neck or pyloroduodenal obstruction, CV disease, hepatic impairment. Cholestatic jaundice reported. May increase blood glucose. Dextromethorphan: Caution in atopic children, sedated, or debilitated patients, and patients confined to supine position.

ADVERSE REACTIONS
Drowsiness, dizziness, sedation, blurred vision, dry mouth, increased or decreased BP, rash, N/V, respiratory depression, apnea, leukopenia, agranulocytosis, NMS.

DRUG INTERACTIONS
See Boxed Warning and Contraindications. Promethazine: May increase, prolong, or intensify the sedative action of other CNS depressants, such as alcohol, sedatives/hypnotics (including barbiturates), narcotics, narcotic analgesics, general anesthetics, TCAs, and tranquilizers; avoid such agents or administer in reduced dosages. Reduce barbiturate dose by at least 1/2 and narcotic analgesics by 1/4 to 1/2. May reverse vasopressor effect of epinephrine. Caution with concomitant medications that may also affect seizure threshold (eg, narcotics, local anesthetics). Caution with concomitant use of other agents with anticholinergic properties. Leukopenia and agranulocytosis reported, usually when used in association with other marrow-toxic agents. NMS reported alone or in combination with antipsychotic drugs. Dextromethorphan: Hyperpyrexia, hypotension, and death have been reported coincident with the coadministration of MAOIs and products containing dextromethorphan.

PREGNANCY AND LACTATION
Pregnancy: Category C.
Lactation: Caution in nursing.

MECHANISM OF ACTION
Dextromethorphan: Antitussive agent; acts centrally and elevates the threshold for coughing. Promethazine: Phenothiazine derivative; blocks H_1 receptor (antihistaminic action) and provides clinically useful sedative and antiemetic effects.

PHARMACOKINETICS
Absorption: Dextromethorphan: Rapid. Promethazine: Well-absorbed. **Metabolism:** Dextromethorphan: Liver via O-demethylation, N-demethylation, and partial conjugation with glucuronic acid and sulfate. Promethazine: Liver, sulfoxides and N-demethylpromethazine (metabolites). **Elimination:** Dextromethorphan: Urine [(+)-3-hydroxy-N-methylmorphinan, (+)-3-hydroxymorphinan, traces of unmetabolized drug]. Promethazine: Urine (sulfoxides and N-demethylpromethazine).

PATIENT CONSIDERATIONS
Assessment: Assess for drug hypersensitivity or idiosyncrasy, or any other conditions where treatment is contraindicated or cautioned. Assess for pregnancy/nursing status and possible drug interactions. Assess use in atopic children, elderly, debilitated, and for signs/symptoms of Reye's syndrome, hepatic diseases, or encephalopathy in pediatrics.

Monitoring: Monitor for signs/symptoms of CNS/respiratory depression, NMS, seizures, cholestatic jaundice, leukopenia, and agranulocytosis. Monitor children for hallucinations, convulsions, extrapyramidal symptoms, and dystonias. Monitor for false positive and false negative pregnancy tests, blood glucose levels, and BP.

Counseling: Inform that therapy may cause marked drowsiness or may impair mental and/or physical abilities required for performing hazardous tasks (eg, operating machinery, driving). Instruct to report involuntary muscle movements. Counsel to avoid the use of alcohol and other CNS depressants while on therapy. Instruct to avoid prolonged exposure to the sun.

PROMETHAZINE INJECTION — promethazine hydrochloride **Rx**
Class: Phenothiazine derivative

> Do not use in pediatric patients <2 yrs of age; potential for fatal respiratory depression. Caution when administering to pediatric patients ≥2 yrs of age. May cause severe chemical irritation and damage to tissue regardless of the route of administration. Irritation and damage may result from perivascular extravasation, unintentional intra-arterial inj, and intraneuronal/perineuronal infiltration; surgical intervention may be required. Preferred route of administration is deep IM inj. SQ inj is contraindicated.

OTHER BRAND NAMES
Phenergan (Discontinued)

ADULT DOSAGE
Allergic Reactions
25mg; may repeat w/in 2 hrs if necessary; adjust to smallest amount adequate to relieve symptoms

Continued therapy, if indicated, should be via oral route as soon as existing circumstances permit

Sedation
Nighttime Sedation in Hospitalized Patients:
25-50mg

Nausea/Vomiting
Usual: 12.5-25mg, not to be repeated more frequently than q4h

Pre- and Postoperative Use
25-50mg; may be combined w/ appropriately reduced doses of analgesics and atropine-like drugs as desired

Obstetrics
Early Stages of Labor:
50mg

Established Labor:
25-75mg; may be given w/ an appropriately reduced dose of any desired narcotic. If necessary, may repeat once or twice at 4-hr intervals in the course of a normal labor
Max: 100mg/24 hrs

Other Indications
Amelioration of allergic reactions to blood/plasma

Adjunct to epinephrine and other standard measures in anaphylaxis after acute symptoms have been controlled

For other uncomplicated allergic conditions of the immediate type when oral therapy is impossible or contraindicated

For sedation and relief of apprehension and to produce light sleep

Active treatment of motion sickness

Prevention and control of N/V associated w/ certain types of anesthesia and surgery

Adjunct to analgesics for the control of postop pain

Preop, postop, and obstetric sedation

IV in special surgical situations (eg, repeated bronchoscopy, ophthalmic surgery, poor-risk patients) w/ reduced amounts of meperidine or other narcotic analgesic as an adjunct to anesthesia and analgesia

PEDIATRIC DOSAGE
General Dosing
≥2 Years:
Dose should not exceed 1/2 of suggested adult dose; use lowest effective dose

Premedication Adjunct:
Usual: 1.1mg/kg in combination w/ an appropriately reduced dose of narcotic or barbiturate and appropriate dose of an atropine-like drug

- -

DOSING CONSIDERATIONS
Elderly
≥60 Years:
Reduce dose

ADMINISTRATION
Deep IM/IV route

The preferred parenteral route of administration is by deep IM inj

When administered IV, give in a concentration no greater than 25mg/mL and at a rate not to exceed 25mg/min; preferable to inject through the tubing of IV infusion set that is known to be functioning satisfactorily

STORAGE
20-25°C (68-77°F). Protect from light.

HOW SUPPLIED
Inj: 25mg/mL, 50mg/mL

CONTRAINDICATIONS

Children <2 yrs of age, comatose states, intra-arterial or SQ inj, idiosyncratic reaction or hypersensitivity to promethazine or other phenothiazines.

WARNINGS/PRECAUTIONS

If pain occurs during IV inj, d/c immediately to evaluate for possible arterial inj or perivascular extravasation. Not recommended for uncomplicated vomiting in pediatric patients; should be limited to prolonged vomiting of known etiology. May lead to potentially fatal respiratory depression; avoid with compromised respiratory function or in patients at risk of respiratory failure (eg, chronic obstructive pulmonary disease, sleep apnea). May impair physical/mental abilities and lower seizure threshold. Caution with bone marrow depression; leukopenia and agranulocytosis reported. Neuroleptic malignant syndrome (NMS) reported alone and in combination with antipsychotics; d/c immediately and monitor. Contains sodium metabisulfite, which may cause allergic-type reactions. Cholestatic jaundice reported. Caution with narrow-angle glaucoma, prostatic hypertrophy, stenosing peptic ulcer, bladder-neck or pyloroduodenal obstruction, cardiovascular disease, and hepatic dysfunction. Avoid in pediatric patients whose signs/symptoms may suggest Reye's syndrome or other hepatic diseases. Hallucinations and convulsions may occur in pediatric patients. Increased susceptibility to dystonias in acutely ill pediatric patients. Lab test interactions may occur. Caution in elderly.

ADVERSE REACTIONS

Respiratory depression, severe tissue injury, drowsiness, dizziness, tinnitus, blurred vision, dry mouth, increased/decreased BP, urticaria, N/V, tachycardia, photosensitivity, gangrene.

DRUG INTERACTIONS

Avoid concomitant use of other drugs with respiratory depressant effects in pediatric patients. May increase, prolong, or intensify sedative action of CNS depressants (eg, alcohol, sedative/hypnotics, narcotics, TCAs); avoid concomitant use or reduce dose of such agents. Reduce dose of barbiturates by at least 50% if given concomitantly. Reduce dose of narcotics by 25-50% if given concomitantly. Caution with drugs that alter seizure threshold (eg, narcotics, local anesthetics). Leukopenia and agranulocytosis reported when used with other known marrow-toxic agents. May reverse vasopressor effect of epinephrine; do not use to treat promethazine overdose. Caution with anticholinergics. May increase incidence of extrapyramidal effects with MAOIs.

PREGNANCY AND LACTATION

Category C, not for use in nursing.

MECHANISM OF ACTION

Phenothiazine derivative; H_1 receptor antagonist (does not block release of histamine). Possesses antihistaminic, sedative, antimotion-sickness, antiemetic, and anticholinergic effects.

PHARMACOKINETICS

Metabolism: Liver; sulfoxides, N-desmethylpromethazine (metabolites).
Elimination: Urine; $T_{1/2}$=9-16 hrs (IV), 9.8 hrs (IM).

PATIENT CONSIDERATIONS

Assessment: Assess for drug hypersensitivity or idiosyncratic reaction to phenothiazines, bone marrow depression, sulfite sensitivity, seizure disorders, pregnancy/nursing status, possible drug interactions, or any other conditions where treatment is contraindicated or cautioned. Assess for signs/symptoms of Reye's syndrome or hepatic diseases in pediatric patients.

Monitoring: Monitor for signs/symptoms of CNS/respiratory depression, seizures, leukopenia, NMS, cholestatic jaundice, and other adverse reactions. Monitor for hallucinations, convulsions, extrapyramidal symptoms, respiratory depression, and dystonias in pediatric patients.

Counseling: Advise of the risk of respiratory depression and severe tissue injury. Instruct to immediately report persistent/worsening pain or burning at the inj site. Inform that drowsiness or impairment of mental/physical abilities may occur. Counsel to report any involuntary muscle movements. Instruct to avoid alcohol use, prolonged sun exposure, and concomitant use of other CNS depressants.

PROMETHAZINE VC WITH CODEINE — codeine phosphate/phenylephrine hydrochloride/promethazine hydrochloride CV

Class: Antitussive/phenothiazine derivative/sympathomimetic

> Contraindicated in pediatric patients <6 yrs of age. Concomitant administration of promethazine products with other respiratory depressants is associated with respiratory depression, and sometimes death, in pediatric patients. Respiratory depression, including fatalities, have been reported with use of promethazine in patients <2 yrs of age. Respiratory depression and death reported in children who received codeine following tonsillectomy and/or adenoidectomy and had evidence of being ultra-rapid metabolizers of codeine due to a CYP2D6 polymorphism.

ADULT DOSAGE
Antihistamine/Cough Suppressant/Nasal Decongestant

Temporary relief of coughs and upper respiratory symptoms (eg, nasal congestion) associated with allergy or the common cold

5mL q4-6h
Max: 30mL/24 hrs

PEDIATRIC DOSAGE
Antihistamine/Cough Suppressant/Nasal Decongestant

Temporary relief of coughs and upper respiratory symptoms (eg, nasal congestion) associated with allergy or the common cold

6 to <12 Years:
2.5-5mL q4-6h
Max: 30mL/24 hrs

≥12 Years:
5mL q4-6h
Max: 30mL/24 hrs

DOSING CONSIDERATIONS

Elderly
Start at lower end of dosing range

ADMINISTRATION

Oral route

Measure w/ an accurate measuring device.

STORAGE

20-25°C (68-77°F).

HOW SUPPLIED

Syrup: (Codeine/Promethazine/Phenylephrine) (10mg/6.25mg/5mg)/5mL [118mL, 237mL, 473mL]

CONTRAINDICATIONS

Pediatric patients <6 yrs of age. **Codeine:** Postoperative pain management in children who have undergone tonsillectomy and/or adenoidectomy, known hypersensitivity to the drug, treatment of lower respiratory tract symptoms (eg, asthma). **Promethazine:** Comatose states, known hypersensitivity or idiosyncratic reaction to promethazine or to other phenothiazines, treatment of lower respiratory tract symptoms (eg, asthma). **Phenylephrine:** HTN, peripheral vascular insufficiency, known hypersensitivity to the drug, concomitant use w/ MAOIs.

WARNINGS/PRECAUTIONS

Should only be given to a pregnant woman if clearly needed. Caution in elderly. Lab test interactions may occur. Codeine: Do not increase dose if cough fails to respond to treatment. May cause/aggravate constipation. May release histamine; caution in atopic children. Capacity to elevate CSF pressure and respiratory depressant effects may be markedly exaggerated in head injury, intracranial lesions, or with preexisting increase in intracranial pressure. May obscure clinical course in patients with head injuries. Avoid with acute febrile illness with productive cough or in chronic respiratory disease. May produce orthostatic hypotension in ambulatory patients. Give with caution and reduce initial dose with acute abdominal conditions, convulsive disorders, significant hepatic/renal impairment, fever, hypothyroidism, Addison's disease, ulcerative colitis, prostatic hypertrophy, recent GI or urinary tract surgery, and in very young, elderly, or debilitated patients. Use lowest effective dose for the shortest period of time. Potential for abuse and dependence. Promethazine: May impair mental/physical abilities. May lead to potentially fatal respiratory depression; avoid with compromised respiratory function (eg, COPD, sleep apnea). May lower seizure threshold; caution with seizure disorders. Leukopenia and agranulocytosis reported, especially when given with other marrow-toxic agents; caution with bone-marrow depression. Neuroleptic malignant syndrome (NMS) reported; d/c immediately if NMS occurs. Hallucinations and convulsions reported in pediatric patients. Acutely ill pediatric patients who are dehydrated may have increased susceptibility to dystonias. Cholestatic jaundice reported. Caution with narrow-angle glaucoma, prostatic hypertrophy, stenosing peptic ulcer, pyloroduodenal/bladder-neck obstruction, cardiovascular disease, or impaired liver function. Increased blood glucose reported. Phenylephrine: Caution with diabetes mellitus and thyroid/heart diseases. May cause urinary retention in men with symptomatic BPH. May decrease cardiac output; use extreme caution with arteriosclerosis, in elderly, and/or patients with initially poor cerebral or coronary circulation.

ADVERSE REACTIONS

Respiratory depression, drowsiness, dizziness, somnolence, anxiety, sedation, tremor, blurred vision, dry mouth, increased or decreased BP, N/V, urinary retention, NMS, constipation.

DRUG INTERACTIONS

See Boxed Warning and Contraindications. Promethazine: May increase, prolong, or intensify the sedative action of other CNS depressants (eg, alcohol, narcotics, general anesthetics, tranquilizers); avoid such agents or administer in reduced doses. Reduce dose of barbiturate by at least 1/2 and narcotic analgesics by 1/4 to 1/2; individualize dose. Do not use epinephrine to treat hypotension associated with promethazine overdose; may reverse vasopressor effect of epinephrine. Caution with other agents with anticholinergic properties and drugs that also affect seizure threshold (eg, narcotics, local anesthetics). Phenylephrine: Pressor response increased with TCAs and decreased with prior administration of phentolamine or other α-adrenergic blockers. Ergot alkaloids may cause excessive rise in BP. Tachycardia or other arrhythmias may occur with bronchodilator sympathomimetics, epinephrine, or other sympathomimetics. Reflex bradycardia blocked and pressor response enhanced with atropine sulfate. Cardiostimulating effects blocked with prior administration of propranolol or other β-adrenergic blockers. Synergistic adrenergic response with diet preparations (eg, amphetamines, phenylpropanolamine).

PREGNANCY AND LACTATION

Pregnancy: Category C.
Lactation: Caution in nursing.

MECHANISM OF ACTION

Codeine: Narcotic analgesic/antitussive; primary effects are on CNS and GI tract. Promethazine: Phenothiazine derivative; blocks H_1 receptor and provides sedative and antiemetic effects. Phenylephrine: Sympathomimetic amine; potent postsynaptic-α-receptor agonist with little effect on β-receptors of heart. Causes vasoconstriction and has a mild central stimulant effect.

PHARMACOKINETICS

Absorption: Codeine/Promethazine: Well-absorbed. Phenylephrine: Irregularly absorbed. **Distribution:** Codeine: Crosses placenta; found in breast milk. **Metabolism:** Codeine: Liver via O-demethylation, N-demethylation, and partial conjugation with glucuronic acid. Promethazine: Liver; sulfoxides and N-demethylpromethazine (metabolites). Phenylephrine: Liver and intestine via monoamine oxidase. **Elimination:** Codeine: Urine (small amounts of free and conjugated morphine). Promethazine: Urine (metabolites).

PATIENT CONSIDERATIONS

Assessment: Assess for drug hypersensitivity or idiosyncrasy, history of drug abuse/dependence, head injury, compromised respiratory function, poor cerebral/

coronary circulation, or any other conditions where treatment is contraindicated or cautioned, pregnancy/nursing status, and for possible drug interactions.

Monitoring: Monitor for signs/symptoms of CNS and respiratory depression, constipation, leukopenia, agranulocytosis, cholestatic jaundice, seizures, NMS, orthostatic hypotension, abuse/dependence, increased blood glucose levels, and other adverse reactions. Monitor for urinary retention in men with BPH. Monitor pediatric patients for hallucinations, convulsions, and dystonias. Reevaluate 5 days or sooner if cough is unresponsive to treatment.

Counseling: Inform that therapy may cause marked drowsiness and may impair mental and/or physical abilities required for performing hazardous tasks; advise to avoid such activities until it is known that they do not become drowsy or dizzy with therapy. Instruct to avoid the use or reduce dose of alcohol and other CNS depressants while on therapy. Advise to report any involuntary muscle movements, and to avoid prolonged sun exposure. Inform that therapy may produce orthostatic hypotension. Advise patients that some people have a genetic variation that results in codeine changing into morphine more rapidly and completely than other people; instruct caregivers of children receiving codeine for other reasons to monitor for signs of respiratory depression. Inform about risks and the signs of morphine overdose. Instruct nursing mothers to notify pediatrician immediately, or get emergency medical attention, if signs of morphine toxicity (eg, increased sleepiness, difficulty breastfeeding, breathing difficulties, limpness) are noticed in their infants.

PROMETHAZINE WITH CODEINE — codeine phosphate/ promethazine hydrochloride

CV

Class: Antitussive/phenothiazine derivative

> Contraindicated in pediatric patients <6 yrs of age. Concomitant administration of promethazine products with other respiratory depressants is associated with respiratory depression, and sometimes death, in pediatric patients. Respiratory depression, including fatalities, have been reported with use of promethazine in pediatric patients <2 yrs of age. Respiratory depression and death reported in children who received codeine following tonsillectomy and/or adenoidectomy and had evidence of being ultra-rapid metabolizers of codeine due to a CYP2D6 polymorphism.

ADULT DOSAGE	**PEDIATRIC DOSAGE**
Antihistamine/Cough Suppressant	**Antihistamine/Cough Suppressant**
Temporary relief of coughs and upper respiratory symptoms associated with allergy or the common cold	Temporary relief of coughs and upper respiratory symptoms associated with allergy or the common cold
5mL q4-6h	
Max: 30mL/24 hrs	**6 to <12 Years:**
	2.5-5mL q4-6h
	Max: 30mL/24 hrs
	≥12 Years:
	5mL q4-6h
	Max: 30mL/24 hrs

DOSING CONSIDERATIONS
Elderly
Start at lower end of dosing range

ADMINISTRATION
Oral route
Measure w/ an accurate measuring device

STORAGE
20-25°C (68-77°F).

HOW SUPPLIED
Syrup: (Codeine/Promethazine) 10mg/6.25mg/5mL [473mL]

CONTRAINDICATIONS
Pediatric patients <6 yrs of age. **Codeine:** Postoperative pain management in children who have undergone tonsillectomy and/or adenoidectomy, known hypersensitivity to the drug, treatment of lower respiratory tract symptoms (eg, asthma). **Promethazine:** Comatose states, known hypersensitivity or idiosyncratic reaction to promethazine or to other phenothiazines, treatment of lower respiratory tract symptoms (eg, asthma).

WARNINGS/PRECAUTIONS
Should only be given to a pregnant woman if clearly needed. Caution in elderly. Lab test interactions may occur. Codeine: Do not increase dose if cough fails to respond to treatment. May cause/aggravate constipation. May release histamine; caution in atopic children. Capacity to elevate CSF pressure and respiratory depressant effects may be markedly exaggerated in head injury, intracranial lesions, or with preexisting increase in intracranial pressure. May obscure clinical course in patients with head injuries. Avoid with acute febrile illness with productive cough or in chronic respiratory disease. May produce orthostatic hypotension in ambulatory patients. Give with caution and reduce initial dose with acute abdominal conditions, convulsive disorders, significant hepatic/renal impairment, fever, hypothyroidism, Addison's disease, ulcerative colitis, prostatic hypertrophy, recent GI or urinary tract surgery, and in the very young, elderly, or debilitated patients. Use lowest effective dose for the shortest period of time. Potential for abuse and dependence. Promethazine: May impair mental/physical abilities. May lead to potentially fatal respiratory depression; avoid with compromised respiratory function (eg, COPD, sleep apnea). May lower seizure threshold; caution with seizure disorders. Leukopenia and agranulocytosis reported, especially when given with other marrow-toxic agents; caution with bone-marrow depression. Neuroleptic malignant syndrome (NMS) reported; d/c immediately if NMS occurs. Hallucinations and convulsions reported in pediatric

patients. Acutely ill pediatric patients who are dehydrated may have increased susceptibility to dystonias. Cholestatic jaundice reported. Caution with narrow-angle glaucoma, prostatic hypertrophy, stenosing peptic ulcer, pyloroduodenal/bladder-neck obstruction, cardiovascular disease, or impaired liver function. Increased blood glucose reported.

ADVERSE REACTIONS
Drowsiness, dizziness, sedation, blurred vision, dry mouth, increased or decreased BP, N/V, constipation, urinary retention, leukopenia, agranulocytosis, respiratory depression, apnea, NMS.

DRUG INTERACTIONS
See Boxed Warning. Possible interaction with MAOIs (eg, increased incidence of extrapyramidal effects); consider initial small test dose. Promethazine: May increase, prolong, or intensify the sedative action of other CNS depressants (eg, alcohol, narcotics, general anesthetics, tranquilizers); avoid such agents or administer in reduced doses. Reduce dose of barbiturate by at least 1/2 and narcotics by 1/4 to 1/2; individualize dose. Do not use epinephrine to treat hypotension associated with promethazine overdose; may reverse vasopressor effect of epinephrine. Caution with other agents with anticholinergic properties and drugs that also affect seizure threshold (eg, narcotics, local anesthetics).

PREGNANCY AND LACTATION
Category C, caution in nursing.

MECHANISM OF ACTION
Codeine: Narcotic analgesic/antitussive; primary effects are on CNS and GI tract. Promethazine: Phenothiazine derivative; blocks H_1 receptor and provides sedative and antiemetic effects.

PHARMACOKINETICS
Absorption: Well absorbed. **Distribution:** Codeine: Crosses placenta; found in breast milk. **Metabolism:** Codeine: Liver via O-demethylation, N-demethylation, and partial conjugation with glucuronic acid. Promethazine: Liver; sulfoxides and N-demethylpromethazine (metabolites). **Elimination:** Codeine: Urine (small amounts of free and conjugated morphine). Promethazine: Urine (metabolites).

PATIENT CONSIDERATIONS
Assessment: Assess for drug hypersensitivity or idiosyncrasy, history of drug abuse/dependence, head injury, or any other conditions where treatment is contraindicated or cautioned, pregnancy/nursing status, and for possible drug interactions.

Monitoring: Monitor for signs/symptoms of CNS and respiratory depression, constipation, leukopenia, agranulocytosis, cholestatic jaundice, seizures, NMS, orthostatic hypotension, abuse/dependence, increased blood glucose levels, and other adverse reactions. Monitor pediatric patients for hallucinations, convulsions, and dystonias. Reevaluate 5 days or sooner if cough is unresponsive to treatment.

Counseling: Inform that therapy may cause drowsiness and may impair mental and/or physical abilities required for performing potentially hazardous tasks (eg, driving or operating machinery); advise to avoid such activities until it is known that they do not become drowsy or dizzy with therapy. Instruct to avoid the use or reduce dose of alcohol and other CNS depressants while on therapy. Instruct to report any involuntary muscle movements. Instruct to avoid prolonged sun exposure. Inform that therapy may produce orthostatic hypotension. Advise patients that some people have a genetic variation that results in codeine changing into morphine more rapidly and completely than other people; instruct caregivers of children receiving codeine for other reasons to monitor for signs of respiratory depression. Inform about risks and the signs of morphine overdose. Instruct nursing mothers to notify pediatrician immediately, or get emergency medical attention, if signs of morphine toxicity (eg, increased sleepiness, difficulty breastfeeding, breathing difficulties, limpness) are noticed in their infants.

PROMETRIUM — progesterone

Rx

Class: Progestogen

> Estrogens plus progestin therapy should not be used for the prevention of cardiovascular disease or dementia. Increased risks of DVT, PE, stroke, MI, and invasive breast cancer reported in postmenopausal women (50-79 yrs of age) on estrogen plus progestin therapy. Increased risk of probable dementia reported in postmenopausal women ≥65 yrs of age on estrogen plus progestin therapy. Progestins with estrogens should be prescribed at the lowest effective dose and for the shortest duration consistent with treatment goals and risks.

ADULT DOSAGE	**PEDIATRIC DOSAGE**
Endometrial Hyperplasia	Pediatric use may not have been established
Prevention in Nonhysterectomized Postmenopausal Women Receiving Conjugated Estrogens Tabs:	
200mg qhs for 12 days sequentially per 28-day cycle	
Secondary Amenorrhea	
400mg qhs for 10 days	

ADMINISTRATION
Oral route

In patients w/ difficulty swallowing caps, take w/ a glass of water while in standing position

STORAGE
25°C (77°F); excursions permitted to 15-30°C (59-86°F). Protect from excessive moisture.

HOW SUPPLIED
Cap: 100mg, 200mg

CONTRAINDICATIONS
Known hypersensitivity to progesterone or any components (eg, peanuts) of the medication. Undiagnosed abnormal genital bleeding, known/suspected/history of breast cancer, active or history of DVT/PE, active or history of arterial thromboembolic disease (eg, stroke, MI), known liver dysfunction or disease, known or suspected pregnancy.

WARNINGS/PRECAUTIONS
Caution in patients with risk factors for arterial vascular disease and/or VTE. If feasible, d/c at least 4 to 6 weeks before surgery of the type associated with an increased risk of thromboembolism, or during periods of prolonged immobilization. Increased risk of endometrial cancer reported with the use of unopposed estrogen therapy in women with a uterus. Rule out malignancy in all cases of undiagnosed persistent or recurring abnormal genital bleeding. Adding a progestin to estrogen therapy in women with a uterus reported to reduce risk of endometrial hyperplasia. May increase risk of ovarian cancer. Retinal vascular thrombosis reported; d/c therapy pending examination if there is sudden partial or complete loss of vision, or if there is sudden onset of proptosis, diplopia, or migraine. If examination reveals papilledema or retinal vascular lesions, d/c permanently. May cause fluid retention; caution with cardiac/renal dysfunction. May impair physical/mental abilities. May affect certain endocrine, hepatic, and blood components in lab tests.

ADVERSE REACTIONS
Headache, breast tenderness, joint pain, depression, dizziness, abdominal bloating, hot flashes, urinary problems, abdominal pain, vaginal discharge, N/V, worry, chest pain, diarrhea, breast pain.

PREGNANCY AND LACTATION
Category B, caution in nursing.

MECHANISM OF ACTION
Progestogen; chemically identical to progesterone of ovarian origin.

PHARMACOKINETICS
Absorption: Administration of different doses resulted in different pharmacokinetic parameters. **Distribution:** Plasma protein binding (96-99%); found in breast milk. **Metabolism:** Liver to pregnanediols and pregnanolones, and sulfate/glucuronide conjugation; intestine via reduction, dehydroxylation, and epimerization. **Elimination:** Bile, urine, feces.

PATIENT CONSIDERATIONS
Assessment: Assess for drug hypersensitivity, peanut allergy, undiagnosed abnormal genital bleeding, known/suspected/history of breast cancer, active/history of DVT/PE, active/history of arterial thromboembolic disease, and any other conditions where treatment is contraindicated or cautioned.

Monitoring: Monitor for signs/symptoms of cardiovascular disorders, breast cancer, endometrial cancer, ovarian cancer, dementia, visual abnormalities, fluid retention, and other adverse reactions. Perform annual breast exam; schedule mammography based on age, risk factors, and prior mammogram results. In cases of undiagnosed, persistent, or recurrent vaginal bleeding in women with uterus, perform adequate diagnostic measures (eg, endometrial sampling) to rule out malignancies.

Counseling: Inform that the drug contains peanut oil and should not be used if allergic to peanuts. Inform that medication may increase chances for heart attack, stroke, visual loss/blindness, and blood clots. Advise to contact physician if breast lumps, unusual vaginal bleeding, dizziness or faintness, changes in speech, severe headaches, chest pain, SOB, leg pain, visual changes, or vomiting occurs. Advise to have yearly breast examinations by a physician and to perform monthly breast self-examinations.

PROPAFENONE — propafenone hydrochloride Rx
Class: Class IC antiarrhythmic

> Increased rate of death or reversed cardiac arrest rate reported in patients treated w/ encainide or flecainide (Class 1C antiarrhythmics) in a study of patients w/ asymptomatic non-life-threatening ventricular arrhythmias who had a MI >6 days but <2 yrs previously. Consider any 1C antiarrhythmic to have a significant proarrhythmic risk in patients w/ structural heart disease. Avoid in patients w/ non-life-threatening ventricular arrhythmias, even if experiencing unpleasant, but not life-threatening signs/symptoms.

OTHER BRAND NAMES
Rythmol

ADULT DOSAGE
Paroxysmal Atrial Fibrillation/Flutter
Associated w/ Disabling Symptoms in Patients w/o Structural Heart Disease:

Initial: 150mg q8h (450mg/day)
Titrate: May increase at a minimum of 3- to 4-day intervals to 225mg q8h (675mg/day). May increase to 300mg q8h (900mg/day) if additional therapeutic effect is needed
Max: 900mg/day

Paroxysmal Supraventricular Tachycardia
Associated w/ Disabling Symptoms in Patients w/o Structural Heart

PEDIATRIC DOSAGE
Pediatric use may not have been established

Disease:
Initial: 150mg q8h (450mg/day)
Titrate: May increase at a minimum of 3- to 4-day intervals to 225mg q8h (675mg/day). May increase to 300mg q8h (900mg/day) if additional therapeutic effect is needed
Max: 900mg/day

Ventricular Arrhythmias
Initial: 150mg q8h (450mg/day)
Titrate: May increase at a minimum of 3- to 4-day intervals to 225mg q8h (675mg/day). May increase to 300mg q8h (900mg/day) if additional therapeutic effect is needed
Max: 900mg/day
Initiate therapy in the hospital

DOSING CONSIDERATIONS
Concomitant Medications
CYP2D6 and CYP3A4 Inhibitors:
Avoid simultaneous use of propafenone w/ both a CYP2D6 inhibitor and a CYP3A4 inhibitor

Hepatic Impairment
Consider reducing dose

Elderly
Start at lower end of dosing range. Increase dose more gradually during initial phase of treatment

Other Important Considerations
Significant QRS Widening/2nd- or 3rd-Degree Atrioventricular (AV) Block:
Consider reducing dose

Ventricular Arrhythmia w/ Marked Previous Myocardial Damage: Increase dose more gradually during initial phase of treatment

ADMINISTRATION
Oral route

STORAGE
20-25°C (68-77°F). (Rythmol) 25°C (77°F); excursions permitted to 15-30°C (59-86°F).

HOW SUPPLIED
Tab: 300mg*; (Rythmol) 150mg*, 225mg* *scored

CONTRAINDICATIONS
Heart failure (HF), cardiogenic shock, known Brugada syndrome, bradycardia, marked hypotension, bronchospastic disorders or severe obstructive pulmonary disease, marked electrolyte imbalance, and sinoatrial, AV, and intraventricular disorders of impulse generation or conduction (eg, sick sinus node syndrome, AV block) in the absence of an artificial pacemaker.

WARNINGS/PRECAUTIONS
Do not use to control ventricular rate during A-fib. Concomitant treatment w/ drugs that increase the functional AV nodal refractory period is recommended. May cause new or worsened arrhythmias; evaluate ECG prior to and during therapy to determine if response supports continued treatment. Brugada syndrome may be unmasked after exposure to therapy; perform ECG after initiation of treatment and d/c if changes are suggestive of Brugada syndrome. May provoke overt HF. Conduction disturbances (eg, 1st to 3rd-degree AV block, bundle branch block, intraventricular conduction delay, bradycardia), agranulocytosis, positive antinuclear antibody (ANA) titers, and exacerbation of myasthenia gravis reported. D/C if persistent or worsening elevation of ANA titers detected. May alter pacing and sensing thresholds of implanted pacemakers and defibrillators; monitor and reprogram devices accordingly during and after therapy. Carefully evaluate patients who develop an abnormal ANA test and consider discontinuing therapy, if persistent or worsening elevation of ANA titers is detected. Reversible, short-term drop (w/in normal range) in sperm count may occur. Caution in patients w/ hepatic dysfunction and in the elderly. Monitor for signs of overdosage in patients w/ impaired renal function.

ADVERSE REACTIONS
Unusual taste, N/V, dizziness, constipation, headache, fatigue, blurred vision, weakness.

DRUG INTERACTIONS
See Dosing Considerations. Avoid w/ Class IA and III antiarrhythmics (eg, quinidine, amiodarone) and withhold these agents for at least 5 half-lives prior to therapy. Inhibitors of CYP2D6 (eg, desipramine, paroxetine, ritonavir) and CYP3A4 (eg, ketoconazole, saquinavir, erythromycin) may increase levels. Amiodarone can affect conduction and repolarization; coadministration is not recommended. Fluoxetine may increase levels in extensive metabolizers. Rifampin may decrease propafenone and 5-OH-propafenone (active metabolite) levels and may increase norpropafenone (active metabolite) levels. May increase levels of digoxin, propranolol, metoprolol, and warfarin; monitor digoxin levels and INR. Orlistat may limit the fraction of propafenone available for absorption; abrupt cessation of orlistat in patients stabilized on propafenone may result in severe adverse events (eg, convulsions, AV block, acute circulatory failure). May increase risk of CNS side effects of lidocaine. CYP1A2 inhibitors (eg, amiodarone, tobacco smoke) and cimetidine may increase levels.

PREGNANCY AND LACTATION
Pregnancy: Category C.
Lactation: Excreted in human milk; not for use in nursing.

MECHANISM OF ACTION
Class 1C antiarrhythmic; has local anesthetic effects and direct stabilizing action on myocardial membranes. Reduces upstroke velocity (phase 0) of the monophasic action potential. Reduces the fast inward current carried by Na$^+$ ions in Purkinje fibers and myocardial fibers. Diastolic excitability threshold is increased and effective refractory period prolonged. Reduces spontaneous automaticity and depresses triggered activity.

PHARMACOKINETICS
Absorption: Complete; absolute bioavailability (3.4%, 150mg dose), (10.6%, 300mg dose); T$_{max}$=3.5 hrs. **Distribution:** (IV) V$_d$=252L; plasma protein binding (>95%); found in breast milk. **Metabolism:** Liver (rapid, extensive) via CYP3A4, 1A2, and 2D6; 5-hydroxypropafenone and N-depropylpropafenone (active metabolites). **Elimination:** T$_{1/2}$=2-10 hrs (>90% of patients), 10-32 hrs (<10% of patients).

PATIENT CONSIDERATIONS
Assessment: Assess for HF, cardiogenic shock, sinoatrial/AV/intraventricular disorders, implanted pacemaker/defibrillator, bradycardia, marked hypotension, bronchospastic disorders or severe obstructive pulmonary disease, marked electrolyte imbalance, MI, renal/hepatic dysfunction, known Brugada syndrome, pregnancy/nursing status, and possible drug interactions. Evaluate ECG prior to therapy.

Monitoring: Monitor for proarrhythmic effects, signs/symptoms of conduction disturbances, agranulocytosis, HF, unmasking of Brugada syndrome, exacerbation of myasthenia gravis, and other adverse reactions. Monitor implanted pacemakers and defibrillators during and after therapy and reprogram accordingly. Evaluate ECG during therapy. Monitor ANA titers and renal/hepatic function. Monitor INR when given w/ warfarin.

Counseling: Inform about risks/benefits of therapy. Advise to report symptoms that may be associated w/ electrolyte imbalance to physician. Instruct to notify physician of all prescriptions, herbal/natural preparations, and OTC medications currently being taken or of any changes w/ these products. Instruct not to double the next dose if a dose is missed but to take next dose at the usual time.

PROPECIA — finasteride   Rx
Class: Type II 5 alpha-reductase inhibitor (5-ARI)

ADULT DOSAGE	PEDIATRIC DOSAGE
Male Pattern Hair Loss	Pediatric use may not have been established
Androgenetic Alopecia:	
1 tab (1mg) qd for ≥3 months	
Continued use is recommended to sustain benefit; reevaluate periodically	

ADMINISTRATION
Oral route

Take w/ or w/o meals

STORAGE
15-30°C (59-86°F). Protect from moisture.

HOW SUPPLIED
Tab: 1mg

CONTRAINDICATIONS
Pregnancy, women of childbearing potential, hypersensitivity to any component of this medication.

WARNINGS/PRECAUTIONS
Withdrawal of treatment may lead to reversal of effect within 12 months. Potential risk to male fetus; broken or crushed tabs should not be handled by pregnant women or women who may potentially be pregnant. May decrease serum prostate specific antigen (PSA) levels during therapy or in the presence of prostate cancer; any confirmed increase from lowest PSA value during treatment may signal presence of prostate cancer and should be evaluated. May increase risk of high-grade prostate cancer. Caution with liver dysfunction.

ADVERSE REACTIONS
Decreased libido, erectile dysfunction, ejaculation disorder.

PREGNANCY AND LACTATION
Category X, not for use in nursing.

MECHANISM OF ACTION
Type II 5α-reductase inhibitor; blocks peripheral conversion of testosterone to 5α-dihydrotestosterone (DHT), resulting in significant decreases in serum and tissue DHT concentrations.

PHARMACOKINETICS
Absorption: Absolute bioavailability (65%); C$_{max}$=9.2ng/mL; T$_{max}$=1-2 hrs; AUC$_{(0-24\,hr)}$=53ng•hr/mL. **Distribution:** V$_d$=76L; plasma protein binding (90%). **Metabolism:** Liver (extensive) via CYP3A4; t-butyl side chain monohydroxylated and monocarboxylic acid (metabolites). **Elimination:** Urine (39%, metabolites), feces (57%); T$_{1/2}$=5-6 hrs (18-60 yrs of age), 8 hrs (>70 yrs of age).

PATIENT CONSIDERATIONS
Assessment: Assess for liver dysfunction and previous hypersensitivity to the drug and its components. Obtain baseline PSA levels.

Monitoring: Monitor for hypersensitivity reactions or other adverse reactions. Monitor PSA levels.

Counseling: Instruct pregnant or potentially pregnant women not to handle crushed or broken tabs due to possible absorption and potential risk to male fetus; advise to immediately wash contact area with soap and water if contact occurs. Inform that there was an increase in high-grade prostate cancer in men treated with 5α-reductase inhibitors indicated for BPH treatment. Instruct to promptly report any changes in breasts (eg, lumps, pain, nipple discharge) to physician.

PROPRANOLOL — propranolol hydrochloride   Rx
Class: Nonselective beta blocker

OTHER BRAND NAMES
Inderal (Discontinued)

ADULT DOSAGE

Hypertension
Sol/Tab:
Initial: 40mg bid
Titrate: May increase gradually until adequate BP control is achieved
Maint: 120-240mg/day

In some instances, 640mg/day may be required

If control is not adequate w/ bid dosing, a larger dose, or tid therapy may achieve better control

Angina Pectoris
Due to coronary atherosclerosis to decrease angina frequency and increase exercise tolerance

Sol/Tab:
80-320mg/day given bid, tid or qid

Reduce dose gradually over a period of a few weeks if therapy is to be discontinued

Atrial Fibrillation
Sol/Tab:
10-30mg tid or qid ac and hs

Myocardial Infarction
To reduce cardiovascular mortality in patients who have survived the acute phase of MI and are clinically stable
Sol/Tab:
Initial: 40mg tid
Titrate: Increase to 60-80mg tid after 1 month as tolerated
Maint: 180-240mg/day in divided doses (either bid or tid)
Max: 240mg/day

Migraine
Prophylaxis:
Sol/Tab:
Initial: 80mg/day in divided doses
Usual: 160-240mg/day
Titrate: May increase gradually for optimum prophylaxis

D/C gradually if a satisfactory response is not obtained w/in 4-6 weeks after reaching max dose

Essential Tremor
Familial or Hereditary:
Sol/Tab:
Initial: 40mg bid
Usual: 120mg/day
May be necessary to give 240-320mg/day

Hypertrophic Subaortic Stenosis
Sol/Tab:
Usual: 20-40mg tid or qid ac and hs

Pheochromocytoma
Sol/Tab:
Usual: 60mg/day in divided doses for 3 days before surgery w/ α-adrenergic blocker

Inoperable Tumor:
Usual: 30mg/day in divided doses w/ α-adrenergic blocker

Arrhythmias
Life-threatening or those occurring under anesthesia (supraventricular/ventricular tachycardia, tachyarrhythmia of digitalis intoxication, resistant tachyarrhythmia due to excessive catecholamine action during anesthesia)

PEDIATRIC DOSAGE
Pediatric use may not have been established

Inj:
Usual: 1-3mg IV at ≤1mg/min

May give a 2nd dose if necessary after 2 min then do not give additional drug in <4 hrs

Do not give additional dose when desired alteration in rate/rhythm is achieved

Transfer to oral therapy as soon as possible

DOSING CONSIDERATIONS

Hepatic Impairment
Hepatic Insufficiency:
Inj:
Consider lower dose

Elderly
Start at lower end of dosing range

ADMINISTRATION
Oral/IV route

STORAGE
20-25°C (68-77°F); (Sol) excursions permitted to 15-30°C (59-86°F). (Inj) Protect from freezing and excessive heat. (Tab) Protect from light.

HOW SUPPLIED
Inj: 1mg/mL; **Sol:** 20mg/5mL, 40mg/5mL [500mL]; **Tab:** 10mg*, 20mg*, 40mg*, 60mg*, 80mg* *scored

CONTRAINDICATIONS
Cardiogenic shock, sinus bradycardia and >1st-degree block, bronchial asthma, known hypersensitivity to propranolol HCl.

WARNINGS/PRECAUTIONS
Exacerbation of angina and MI following abrupt discontinuation reported; when discontinuation is planned, reduce dose gradually over at least a few weeks. Reinstitute therapy if exacerbation of angina occurs upon interruption and take other measures for management of angina pectoris; follow same procedure in patients at risk of occult atherosclerotic heart disease who are given propranolol for other indication since coronary artery disease may be unrecognized. May precipitate more severe failure in patients w/ CHF; avoid w/ overt CHF and caution in patients w/ history of heart failure (HF) who are well-compensated and are receiving additional therapies. Caution w/ bronchospastic lung disease, hepatic/renal impairment, Wolff-Parkinson-White (WPW) syndrome, and tachycardia. Chronically administered therapy should not be routinely withdrawn prior to major surgery; however, may augment risks of general anesthesia and surgical procedures. May mask acute hypoglycemia and hyperthyroidism signs/symptoms. May be more difficult to adjust insulin dose in labile insulin-dependent diabetics. Abrupt withdrawal may be followed by an exacerbation of symptoms of hyperthyroidism, including thyroid storm. May reduce IOP. Hypersensitivity/anaphylactic/cutaneous reactions reported. Patients w/ history of severe anaphylactic reaction to a variety of allergens may be more reactive to repeated accidental/diagnostic/therapeutic challenge; may be unresponsive to usual doses of epinephrine. Elevated serum K+, transaminases, and alkaline phosphatase levels reported. Increases in BUN reported in patients w/ severe HF. Not for treatment of hypertensive emergencies. (Oral) Not indicated for migraine attack that has started and tremor associated w/ parkinsonism. Continued use in patients w/o history of HF may lead to cardiac failure.

ADVERSE REACTIONS
Bradycardia, CHF, hypotension, lightheadedness, mental depression, N/V, agranulocytosis, respiratory distress.

DRUG INTERACTIONS
Administration w/ CYP450 (2D6, 1A2, 2C19) substrates, inducers, and inhibitors may lead to clinically relevant drug interactions. Increased levels and/or toxicity w/ substrates/inhibitors of CYP2D6 (eg, amiodarone, cimetidine, fluoxetine, ritonavir), CYP1A2 (eg, imipramine, ciprofloxacin, isoniazid, theophylline), and CYP2C19 (eg, fluconazole, teniposide, tolbutamide). Decreased blood levels w/ hepatic enzyme inducers (eg, rifampin, ethanol, phenytoin, phenobarbital). May increase levels of propafenone, lidocaine, nifedipine, zolmitriptan, rizatriptan, diazepam and its metabolites. Increased levels w/ nisoldipine, nicardipine, and chlorpromazine. May decrease theophylline clearance. Increased thioridazine plasma and metabolite (mesoridazine) concentrations w/ doses ≥160mg/day. Decreased levels w/ aluminum hydroxide gel, cholestyramine, and colestipol. May decrease levels of lovastatin and pravastatin. Increased warfarin levels and PT; monitor PT. Additive effect w/ propafenone and amiodarone. Caution w/ drugs that slow atrioventricular (AV) nodal conduction (eg, digitalis, lidocaine, calcium channel blockers); increased risk of bradycardia w/ digitalis. Significant bradycardia, HF, and CV collapse reported w/ concomitant verapamil. Bradycardia, hypotension, high-degree heart block, and HF reported w/ concomitant diltiazem. Concomitant ACE inhibitors may cause hypotension. May antagonize effects of clonidine; administer cautiously to patients withdrawing from clonidine. Prolongation of 1st dose hypotension may occur w/ concomitant prazosin. Postural hypotension reported w/ concomitant terazosin or doxazosin. Monitor for excessive reduction of resting sympathetic nervous activity w/ catecholamine-depleting drugs (eg, reserpine). Patients on long-term therapy may experience uncontrolled HTN w/ concomitant epinephrine. β-receptor agonists (eg, dobutamine, isoproterenol) may reverse effects. NSAIDs (eg, indomethacin) may blunt the antihypertensive effect. Coadministration w/ methoxyflurane and trichloroethylene may depress myocardial contractility. Hypotension and cardiac arrest reported w/ concomitant haloperidol. Thyroxine may result in a lower than expected T3 concentration when coadministered w/ propranolol. May exacerbate hypotensive effects of MAOIs or TCAs. (Inj) Severe bradycardia, asystole, and HF reported w/ concomitant disopyramide. Increased bronchial hyperreactivity w/ ACE inhibitors. (Oral) Increased levels w/ alcohol.

PREGNANCY AND LACTATION
Category C, caution in nursing.

MECHANISM OF ACTION
Nonselective β-adrenergic receptor blocker. (Oral) HTN: Not established; proposed to decrease cardiac output, inhibit renin release, and lessen tonic sympathetic nerve outflow from vasomotor centers in the brain. Angina: Reduces the oxygen requirement of the heart at any given level of effort by blocking the catecholamine-induced increases in the HR, systolic BP, and the velocity and extent of myocardial contraction. Migraine: Not established; β-adrenergic receptors have been demonstrated in the pial vessels of the brain. Tremor: Not established; β_2 receptors may be involved and a central effect is also possible. (Inj) Arrhythmia: Decreases the activity of both normal and ectopic pacemaker cells and AV nodal conduction velocity.

PHARMACOKINETICS
Absorption: (Oral) Almost complete. Bioavailability (25%); T_{max}=1-4 hrs. **Distribution:** V_d=4-5L/kg; plasma protein binding (90%); found in breast milk, (Oral) crosses placenta. **Metabolism:** Liver (extensive); hydroxylation (CYP2D6), N-dealkylation, oxidation (CYP1A2, 2D6), and glucuronidation. Propranolol glucuronide, naphthyloxylactic acid, glucuronic acid, and sulfate conjugates of 4-hydroxy propranolol (major metabolites). **Elimination:** Urine; $T_{1/2}$=3-6 hrs (Oral), 2-5.5 hrs (Inj).

PATIENT CONSIDERATIONS

Assessment: Assess for cardiogenic shock, sinus bradycardia, AV heart block, bronchial asthma, CHF, bronchospastic lung disease, hyperthyroidism, diabetes, WPW syndrome, tachycardia, hepatic/renal impairment, history/presence of HF, risk for occult atherosclerotic heart disease, hypersensitivity to drug, pregnancy/nursing status, and possible drug interactions.

Monitoring: Monitor for signs/symptoms of cardiac failure, hypoglycemia, decreased IOP, hyperthyroidism, withdrawal symptoms, hypersensitivity reactions, and other adverse reactions. (Inj) Monitor ECG and central venous pressure. (Oral) For HTN (bid dosing), measure BP near the end of dosing interval to determine satisfactory BP control.

Counseling: Inform of the risk/benefits of therapy. Instruct not to interrupt or d/c therapy w/o physician's advice. Inform that therapy may interfere w/ glaucoma screening test.

PROPYLTHIOURACIL — propylthiouracil   Rx

Class: Thiourea-derivative antithyroid agent

> Severe liver injury and acute liver failure reported; some cases have been fatal or required liver transplantation. Reserve use only for those who cannot tolerate methimazole and in whom radioactive iodine therapy or surgery are not appropriate treatments for the management of hyperthyroidism. Treatment of choice during or just prior to the 1st trimester of pregnancy.

ADULT DOSAGE
Hyperthyroidism

Symptomatic hyperthyroidism in preparation for thyroidectomy or radioactive iodine therapy in patients who are intolerant of methimazole

Initial: 300mg/day
Severe Hyperthyroidism/Very Large Goiters: 400mg/day; occasionally may require 600-900mg/day
Maint: 100-150mg/day

Graves' Disease

In patients w/ Graves' disease w/ hyperthyroidism or toxic multinodular goiter who are intolerant of methimazole and for whom surgery or radioactive iodine therapy is not an appropriate treatment option

Initial: 300mg/day
Severe Hyperthyroidism/Very Large Goiters: 400mg/day; occasionally may require 600-900mg/day
Maint: 100-150mg/day

PEDIATRIC DOSAGE
Hyperthyroidism

Symptomatic hyperthyroidism in preparation for thyroidectomy or radioactive iodine therapy in patients who are intolerant of methimazole

≥6 Years:
Initial: 50mg/day
Titrate: Carefully increase based on clinical response and evaluation of TSH and free T4 levels

Studies evaluating appropriate dosing regimen have not been conducted in the pediatric population

Graves' Disease

In patients w/ Graves' disease w/ hyperthyroidism or toxic multinodular goiter who are intolerant of methimazole and for whom surgery or radioactive iodine therapy is not an appropriate treatment option

≥6 Years:
Initial: 50mg/day
Titrate: Carefully increase based on clinical response and evaluation of TSH and free T4 levels

Studies evaluating appropriate dosing regimen have not been conducted in the pediatric population

---

ADMINISTRATION
Oral route

Give total daily dose in 3 equal doses at approx 8-hr intervals.

STORAGE
15-30°C (59-86°F).

HOW SUPPLIED
Tab: 50mg* *scored

CONTRAINDICATIONS
Hypersensitivity to the drug or any of the other product components.

WARNINGS/PRECAUTIONS
Not recommended for pediatric patients except when methimazole is not well-tolerated and surgery or radioactive iodine therapy are not appropriate treatments. D/C if hepatic dysfunction occurs and obtain LFTs and ALT and AST levels. Cases of liver injury, including liver failure and death, reported during pregnancy; may cause fetal harm. Crosses the placenta and fetal goiter and cretinism may occur when given during pregnancy. Use alternative antithyroid medication after the 1st trimester of pregnancy. Agranulocytosis reported; d/c if agranulocytosis, aplastic anemia (pancytopenia), anti-neutrophilic cytoplasmic antibodies (ANCA)-positive vasculitis, hepatitis, interstitial pneumonitis, fever, or exfoliative dermatitis develops or is suspected. May cause hypothyroidism; adjust dose to maintain euthyroid state. May cause hypoprothrombinemia and bleeding. Caution in elderly.

ADVERSE REACTIONS
Skin rash, N/V, epigastric distress, arthralgia, paresthesias, taste perversion, abnormal loss of hair, myalgia, headache, drowsiness, neuritis, edema, vertigo, skin pigmentation, lymphadenopathy.

DRUG INTERACTIONS
May increase activity of oral anticoagulants (eg, warfarin); consider additional monitoring of PT/INR, especially before surgical procedures. Hyperthyroidism may increase clearance of β-blockers; may need reduced β-blocker dose when patient becomes euthyroid. Digitalis glycoside levels may be increased when patient becomes euthyroid; may need to reduce digitalis glycoside dose. Theophylline clearance may decrease when patient becomes euthyroid; may need reduced theophylline dose. Caution w/ other drugs that cause agranulocytosis.

PREGNANCY AND LACTATION
Pregnancy: Category D. Crosses placental membranes and can induce goiter and cretinism in the developing fetus.
Lactation: Present in breast milk to a small extent and likely results in clinically insignificant doses to the nursing infant.

MECHANISM OF ACTION
Thiourea-derivate antithyroid agent; inhibits the synthesis of thyroid hormones and the conversion of thyroxine to triiodothyronine in peripheral tissues.

PHARMACOKINETICS
Absorption: Readily absorbed. **Distribution:** Found in breast milk, crosses placenta. **Metabolism:** Extensive. **Elimination:** Urine (approx 35%).

PATIENT CONSIDERATIONS
Assessment: Assess for previous hypersensitivity to the drug, hepatic impairment, pregnancy/nursing status, and possible drug interactions. Obtain baseline WBC and differential counts and thyroid function tests.

Monitoring: Monitor for signs/symptoms of hepatic dysfunction, agranulocytosis, leukopenia, thrombocytopenia, aplastic anemia/pancytopenia, ANCA-positive vasculitis, interstitial pneumonitis, fever, exfoliative dermatitis, hypothyroidism, and other adverse reactions. Monitor WBC and differential counts, AST, ALT, bilirubin, and alkaline phosphatase. Monitor PT, especially before surgical procedures. Monitor thyroid function tests (eg, TSH, free T4 levels) periodically.

Counseling: Instruct to inform physician if pregnant/nursing or planning to become pregnant. Inform the patient of the rare potential hazard to the mother and fetus of liver damage. Inform about the risk of liver failure. Advise to report signs/symptoms of illness (eg, fever, sore throat, skin eruptions) and hepatic dysfunction.

PROSCAR — finasteride   Rx

Class: Type II 5 alpha-reductase inhibitor (5-ARI)

ADULT DOSAGE	PEDIATRIC DOSAGE
Benign Prostatic Hyperplasia	Pediatric use may not have been established
Monotherapy or in Combination w/ Doxazosin:	
1 tab (5mg) qd	

ADMINISTRATION
Oral route
Take w/ or w/o meals.

STORAGE
Room temperature <30°C (86°F). Protect from light.

HOW SUPPLIED
Tab: 5mg

CONTRAINDICATIONS
Hypersensitivity to any component of this medication. Women who are or may potentially be pregnant.

WARNINGS/PRECAUTIONS
Not approved for the prevention of prostate cancer. May decrease serum prostate specific antigen (PSA) concentration during therapy or in the presence of prostate cancer; establish a new baseline PSA at least 6 months after starting treatment and monitor PSA periodically thereafter. Any confirmed increase from lowest PSA value during treatment may signal presence of prostate cancer. May increase risk of high-grade prostate cancer. Potential risk to male fetus; broken or crushed tabs should not be handled by pregnant women or women who may potentially be pregnant. May decrease ejaculate volume and total sperm per ejaculate. Prior to treatment initiation, consider other urological conditions that may cause similar symptoms; BPH and prostate cancer may coexist. Monitor for obstructive uropathy in patients with large residual urinary volume and/or severely diminished urinary flow; such patients may not be candidates for therapy. Caution with liver dysfunction.

ADVERSE REACTIONS
Impotence, decreased libido, decreased ejaculate volume, asthenia, postural hypotension, dizziness, abnormal ejaculation.

PREGNANCY AND LACTATION
Pregnancy: Category X.
Lactation: Not for use in nursing.

MECHANISM OF ACTION
Type II 5α-reductase inhibitor; competitively and specifically inhibits type II 5α-reductase with which it forms a stable enzyme complex, inhibiting metabolism of testosterone to 5α-dihydrotestosterone.

PHARMACOKINETICS
Absorption: Absolute bioavailability (63%); C_{max}=37ng/mL; T_{max}=1-2 hrs. Refer to PI for different pharmacokinetic parameters of different age groups. **Distribution:** V_d=76L; plasma protein binding (90%). **Metabolism:** Liver (extensive) via CYP3A4; t-butyl side chain monohydroxylated and monocarboxylic acid (metabolites). **Elimination:** Urine (39% as metabolites), feces (57%); $T_{1/2}$=6 hrs (45-60 yrs of age), 8 hrs (≥70 yrs of age).

PATIENT CONSIDERATIONS
Assessment: Assess for liver dysfunction, previous hypersensitivity to the drug, other urological conditions that may cause similar symptoms, residual urinary volume, and diminished urinary flow.

Monitoring: Monitor for obstructive uropathy in patients with large residual urinary volume and/or severely diminished urinary flow. Monitor for signs/symptoms of prostate cancer, hypersensitivity reactions, and other adverse reactions. Obtain baseline PSA levels at least 6 months after starting treatment and monitor PSA periodically thereafter.

Counseling: Inform that therapy may increase risk of high-grade prostate cancer. Instruct pregnant or potentially pregnant females not to handle crushed or broken tabs due to possible absorption and potential risk to male fetus; advise to immediately wash contact area with soap and water if contact occurs. Advise that the volume of ejaculate may be decreased and impotence/decreased libido may occur. Instruct to promptly report to physician any changes in breasts (eg, lumps, pain, nipple discharge).

PROTONIX — pantoprazole sodium   Rx

Class: Proton pump inhibitor (PPI)

OTHER BRAND NAMES
Protonix IV

ADULT DOSAGE	PEDIATRIC DOSAGE
Gastroesophageal Reflux Disease	**Gastroesophageal Reflux Disease**
Short-Term Treatment of Erosive Esophagitis Associated w/ GERD: 40mg qd for up to 8 weeks; may consider additional 8-week course if not healed after 8 weeks of treatment	**Short-Term Treatment of Erosive Esophagitis Associated w/ GERD:** **Tab/Sus:** **≥5 Years:** **≥15kg to <40kg:** 20mg qd for up to 8 weeks **≥40kg:** 40mg qd for up to 8 weeks
Maint of Healing of Erosive Esophagitis: 40mg qd; no controlled studies beyond 12 months	
GERD Associated w/ History of Erosive Esophagitis: 40mg qd by IV infusion for 7-10 days; d/c as soon as patient is able to receive oral formulation	
Pathological Hypersecretory Conditions	
Long-term treatment of pathological hypersecretory conditions, including Zollinger-Ellison syndrome	
Tab/Sus: 40mg bid **Titrate:** Adjust to individual needs and continue for as long as clinically indicated; doses up to 240mg have been administered	
IV: 80mg q12h **Titrate:** Adjust based on acid output measurements; 80mg IV q8h is expected to maintain acid output <10mEq/h. Doses >240mg/day or >6 days of use have not been studied	
Ensure continuity of suppression of acid secretion during transition from oral to IV and from IV to oral formulations	

ADMINISTRATION
Oral/IV route

Tab/Sus
- Do not split, chew, or crush.

Tab
- Swallow whole, w/ or w/o food.
- If patients are unable to swallow a 40mg tab, two 20mg tabs may be taken.

Sus
- Administer approx 30 min ac via oral administration in apple juice or applesauce or NG tube in apple juice only; do not administer in other liquids/foods.
- Do not divide the 40mg pkt to create a 20mg dosage.

Oral Administration in Applesauce:
- Sprinkle granules on 1 tsp of applesauce and take w/in 10 min of preparation.
- Take sips of water to ensure granules are washed down.

Oral Administration in Apple Juice:
- Empty granules into a small cup or tsp containing 1 tsp of apple juice.
- Stir for 5 sec and swallow immediately.
- Rinse container once or twice w/ apple juice and swallow immediately to ensure entire dose is taken.

NG Tube/Gastrostomy Tube Administration:
- Remove plunger from barrel of 60mL catheter-tip syringe and connect catheter tip to a 16 French (or larger) tube.
- Empty the contents of the pkt into the barrel of the syringe.
- Add 10mL (2 tsp) of apple juice and gently tap and/or shake the barrel of the syringe to help rinse the syringe and tube.
- Repeat at least twice more using the same amount of apple juice each time; no granules should remain in the syringe.

IV
- May be administered through a dedicated line or through a Y-site.
- Flush w/ D5 inj, 0.9% NaCl, or lactated Ringer's inj before and after administration.
- Compatible w/ D5 inj, 0.9% NaCl, or lactated Ringer's inj when administered through a Y-site.
- Incompatible w/ midazolam (at Y-site) and may not be compatible w/ products containing zinc.
- D/C immediately if precipitation/discoloration occurs during Y-site administration.

GERD Associated w/ History of Erosive Esophagitis:
15-Min Infusion:
- Reconstitute w/ 10mL of 0.9% NaCl and further dilute w/ 100mL of D5 inj, 0.9% NaCl, or lactated Ringer's inj to a final concentration of approx 0.4mg/mL.
- May store reconstituted sol for up to 6 hrs at room temperature prior to further dilution.
- Admixed sol must be used w/in 24 hrs from the time of initial reconstitution.
- Administer over approx 15 min at a rate of approx 7mL/min.

2-Min Infusion:
- Reconstitute w/ 10mL of 0.9% NaCl to a final concentration of approx 4mg/mL.
- The reconstituted sol may be stored for up to 24 hrs at room temperature prior to IV infusion.
- Administer over at least 2 min.

Pathological Hypersecretion Including Zollinger-Ellison Syndrome:
15-Min Infusion:
- Reconstitute each vial w/ 10mL of 0.9% NaCl.
- Combine contents of 2 vials and further dilute w/ 80mL of D5 in, 0.9% NaCl, or lactated Ringer's inj, to a total volume of 100mL w/ a final concentration of approx 0.8mg/mL.
- May store reconstituted sol for up to 6 hrs at room temperature prior to further dilution.
- Admixed sol must be used w/in 24 hrs from the time of initial reconstitution.
- Administer over approx 15 min at a rate of approx 7mL/min.

2-Min Infusion:
- Reconstitute w/ 10mL of 0.9% NaCl per vial to a final concentration of approx 4mg/mL.
- The reconstituted sol may be stored for up to 24 hrs at room temperature prior to IV infusion.
- Administer total volume from both vials over at least 2 min.

STORAGE
20-25°C (68-77°F); excursions permitted to 15-30°C (59-86°F). (IV) Protect from light.

HOW SUPPLIED
Inj: 40mg; **Sus, Delayed-Release:** 40mg (granules/pkt); **Tab, Delayed-Release:** 20mg, 40mg

CONTRAINDICATIONS
Known hypersensitivity reactions (eg, anaphylaxis) to any component of the formulation or any substituted benzimidazole.

WARNINGS/PRECAUTIONS
Symptomatic response does not preclude the presence of gastric malignancy. Acute interstitial nephritis reported; d/c if this develops. May increase risk of *Clostridium difficile*-associated diarrhea (CDAD), especially in hospitalized patients. May increase risk for osteoporosis-related fractures of the hip, wrist, or spine, especially w/ high-dose and long-term therapy. Use lowest dose and shortest duration appropriate to the condition being treated. Hypomagnesemia reported and may require Mg^{2+} replacement and discontinuation of therapy; consider monitoring Mg^{2+} levels prior to and periodically during therapy w/ prolonged treatment. Anaphylaxis and other serious reactions (eg, erythema multiforme, Stevens-Johnson syndrome, toxic epidermal necrolysis) reported; may require emergency medical treatment. Lab test interactions may occur.

(Oral) Atrophic gastritis noted w/ long-term therapy, particularly in patients who were *Helicobacter pylori* positive. Vitamin B12 deficiency caused by hypo- or achlorhydria may occur w/ long-term use (eg, >3 yrs). (IV) Thrombophlebitis reported. Contains EDTA, a chelator of metal ions including zinc; consider zinc supplementation in patients prone to zinc deficiency. Mild, transient transaminase elevations observed in clinical studies.

ADVERSE REACTIONS
Adults: Headache, diarrhea, N/V, abdominal pain, flatulence, dizziness, rash, fever, URI, arthralgia.
Pediatrics: URI, headache, fever, diarrhea, vomiting, rash, abdominal pain.

DRUG INTERACTIONS
Concomitant use w/ atazanavir or nelfinavir is not recommended; may substantially decrease atazanavir or nelfinavir concentrations. Monitor for increases in INR and PT w/ warfarin. May reduce the absorption of drugs where gastric pH is an important determinant of bioavailability; ketoconazole, ampicillin esters, atazanavir, iron salts, erlotinib, and mycophenolate mofetil (MMF) absorption may decrease. Caution in transplant patients receiving MMF. Caution w/ digoxin or other drugs that may cause hypomagnesemia (eg, diuretics). May elevate and prolong levels of methotrexate (MTX) and/or its metabolite, possibly leading to toxicities; consider temporary withdrawal of therapy w/ high-dose MTX. (IV) Use caution when other EDTA-containing products are also coadministered IV.

PREGNANCY AND LACTATION
Pregnancy: Category B.
Lactation: Not for use in nursing.

MECHANISM OF ACTION
Proton pump inhibitor; suppresses the final step in gastric acid production by covalently binding to the (H^+/K^+)-ATPase enzyme system at the secretory surface of the gastric parietal cell.

PHARMACOKINETICS
Absorption: Tab: Absolute bioavailability (77%). (40mg) C_{max}=2.5mcg/mL; T_{max}=2.5 hrs; AUC=4.8mcg•hr/mL. IV: (40mg) C_{max}=5.52mcg/mL; AUC=5.4mcg•hr/mL. Sus: Refer to PI. **Distribution:** V_d=11-23.6L; plasma protein binding (98%); (Oral) found in breast milk. **Metabolism:** Liver (extensive) via demethylation, by CYP2C19, w/ subsequent sulfation; oxidation by CYP3A4. **Elimination:** Urine (71%), feces (18%); $T_{1/2}$=1 hr.

PATIENT CONSIDERATIONS
Assessment: Assess for hypersensitivity to the drug, risk for osteoporosis-related fractures, pregnancy/nursing status, and possible drug interactions. Obtain baseline Mg^{2+} levels. (IV) Assess if prone to zinc deficiency.

Monitoring: Monitor for signs/symptoms of acute interstitial nephritis, CDAD, bone fractures, hypersensitivity reactions, and other adverse reactions. Monitor Mg^{2+} levels periodically. Monitor INR and PT when given w/ warfarin. (Oral) Monitor for signs/symptoms of atrophic gastritis and vitamin B12 deficiency. (IV) Monitor for thrombophlebitis, zinc deficiency, and transaminase elevations.

Counseling: Instruct to take ud. Inform of the most frequently occurring adverse reactions. Instruct to inform physician if any unusual symptom develops, or if any known symptom persists or worsens; advise to immediately report and seek care for any cardiovascular or neurological symptoms (eg, palpitation, dizziness, seizures, tetany) and for diarrhea that does not improve. Instruct to inform physician of all medications currently being taken, including OTC medications, as well as allergies to any medications. Inform that concomitant administration of antacids does not affect the absorption of the tabs. Advise that oral sus pkt is a fixed dose and cannot be divided to make smaller dose.

PROTOPIC — tacrolimus   **Rx**
Class: Calcineurin-inhibitor immunosuppressant

> Rare cases of malignancy (eg, skin and lymphoma) reported with topical calcineurin inhibitors, including tacrolimus oint, although causal relationship has not been established. Avoid long-term use, and application should be limited to areas of involvement with atopic dermatitis. Not indicated for children <2 yrs of age; only 0.03% oint is indicated for children 2-15 yrs of age.

ADULT DOSAGE
Atopic Dermatitis
2nd-line therapy for short-term and non-continuous chronic treatment of moderate to severe atopic dermatitis

0.03%/0.1%:
Apply a thin layer to the affected skin bid until signs and symptoms resolve

Reexamine patient if signs and symptoms do not improve w/in 6 weeks

PEDIATRIC DOSAGE
Atopic Dermatitis
2nd-line therapy for short-term and non-continuous chronic treatment of moderate to severe atopic dermatitis

2-15 Years:
0.03%:
Apply a thin layer to the affected skin bid until signs and symptoms resolve

Reexamine patient if signs and symptoms do not improve w/in 6 weeks

ADMINISTRATION
Topical route

Rub minimum amount in gently and completely
Moisturizers can be used w/ oint

STORAGE
25°C (77°F); excursions permitted to 15-30°C (59-86°F).

HOW SUPPLIED
Oint: 0.03%, 0.1% [30g, 60g, 100g]

CONTRAINDICATIONS

History of hypersensitivity to tacrolimus or any other component of this product.

WARNINGS/PRECAUTIONS

Long-term safety, beyond 1 yr of noncontinuous use, has not been established. Avoid with premalignant and malignant skin conditions. Not recommended for oral application, or in patients having skin conditions with a skin barrier defect where there is potential for increased systemic absorption (eg, Netherton's syndrome, lamellar ichthyosis, generalized erythroderma, cutaneous graft-versus-host disease). May cause local symptoms, such as skin burning or pruritus and may improve as the lesions of atopic dermatitis resolve. Resolve bacterial or viral infections at treatment sites before starting treatment. Increased risk of varicella zoster and herpes simplex virus (HSV) infection, or eczema herpeticum. Lymphadenopathy reported; d/c if etiology of lymphadenopathy is unknown, or in the presence of acute infectious mononucleosis. Minimize or avoid natural or artificial sunlight exposure during treatment. Rare cases of acute renal failure reported. Not for ophthalmic use. Do not use with occlusive dressings.

ADVERSE REACTIONS

Skin burning, pruritus, flu-like symptoms, allergic reaction, skin erythema, headache, skin infection, fever, herpes simplex, rhinitis, increased cough, asthma, pharyngitis, pustular rash, folliculitis.

DRUG INTERACTIONS

Caution with CYP3A4 inhibitors (eg, erythromycin, ketoconazole, calcium channel blockers, cimetidine) in patients with widespread and/or erythrodermic disease.

PREGNANCY AND LACTATION

Category C, not for use in nursing.

MECHANISM OF ACTION

Macrolide immunosuppressant; not established in atopic dermatitis. Inhibits T-lymphocyte activation by 1st binding to an intracellular protein, FKBP-12. A complex of tacrolimus-FKBP-12, Ca^{2+}, calmodulin, and calcineurin is then formed and the phosphatase activity of calcineurin is inhibited. This has been shown to prevent the dephosphorylation and translocation of nuclear factor of activated T-cells, a nuclear component thought to initiate gene transcription for the formation of lymphokines.

PHARMACOKINETICS

Absorption: Absolute bioavailability (0.5%), C_{max}=<2ng/mL. **Distribution:** Plasma protein binding (99%); crosses placenta; found in breast milk. **Metabolism:** Extensive via CYP3A; demethylation and hydroxylation; 13-demethyl tacrolimus (major metabolite).

PATIENT CONSIDERATIONS

Assessment: Assess for history of hypersensitivity to drug, premalignant/malignant skin conditions, conditions where there is potential for increased systemic absorption, bacterial or viral infections at treatment sites, renal impairment, pregnancy/nursing status, and possible drug interactions.

Monitoring: Monitor for skin malignancy, lymphoma, infections, local symptoms, lymphadenopathy, and acute renal failure. Monitor improvement of signs/symptoms of atopic dermatitis within 6 weeks.

Counseling: Instruct to use drug exactly as prescribed, only on areas of skin that have eczema, and not to use continuously for a prolonged period. Advise to d/c medication when signs/symptoms of eczema subside. Instruct to consult physician if symptoms get worse, if skin infection develops, or if symptoms do not improve after 6 weeks. Advise caregivers applying the oint, or patients not treating their hands, to wash hands with soap and water after application. Counsel to not bathe, shower, or swim right after application. Advise to avoid getting oint in the eyes or mouth. Instruct to avoid artificial sunlight exposure during treatment, limit sun exposure, wear loose-fitting clothing that protects treated area from the sun, and not cover treated skin with bandages, dressings, or wraps.

PROVENGE — sipuleucel-T   Rx

Class: Immunomodulatory agent

ADULT DOSAGE	PEDIATRIC DOSAGE
Metastatic Castration-Resistant Prostate Cancer	Pediatric use may not have been established
Asymptomatic or Minimally Symptomatic, Hormone Refractory Prostate Cancer: 3 complete doses (250mL each) given at approx 2-week intervals via IV infusion over 60 min	
If unable to give scheduled infusion, additional leukapheresis is needed	
Premedication	
Oral acetaminophen and antihistamine (eg, diphenhydramine) 30 min prior to administration	

ADMINISTRATION

IV route

Begin infusion prior to expiration date and time; do not infuse expired product

Administration Instructions

1. Gently mix and resuspend contents of infusion bag; do not administer if clumps remain in the bag
2. Do not use a cell filter during infusion

3. Observe patient for at least 30 min after each infusion
4. Keep infusion bag at room temperature if infusion is interrupted
5. If infusion bag has been at room temperature >3 hrs, do not resume infusion

STORAGE

Infusion bag must remain w/in the insulated polyurethane container inside the outer cardboard shipping box until the time of administration; stable for ≤3 hrs at room temperature once removed. Do not remove from the outer cardboard shipping box. Refer to PI for complete handling instructions.

HOW SUPPLIED

Sus: 250mL

WARNINGS/PRECAUTIONS

For autologous use only. Acute infusion reactions may occur; if reactions occur, decrease the rate or stop the infusion depending on severity of reaction and administer appropriate medical therapy prn. Closely monitor patients w/ cardiac or pulmonary conditions. Thromboembolic events (eg, deep vein thrombosis [DVT], pulmonary embolism) may occur. Vascular disorders (eg, cerebrovascular disease, cardiovascular disorders) reported. Not tested for transmissible infectious diseases and may carry the risk of transmitting infectious diseases to healthcare professionals handling the product; employ universal precautions. Do not use until confirmation of product release is received.

ADVERSE REACTIONS

Chills, fatigue, fever, back pain, N/V, joint ache, headache, citrate toxicity, paresthesia, anemia, constipation, pain, dizziness, muscle ache, asthenia.

DRUG INTERACTIONS

Immunosuppressive agents may alter efficacy and/or safety; evaluate whether it is appropriate to reduce or d/c immunosuppressive agents prior to treatment.

PREGNANCY AND LACTATION

Safety in pregnancy and nursing not known.

MECHANISM OF ACTION

Immunomodulatory agent (autologous cellular immunotherapy); not established. Induces an immune response targeted against prostatic acid phosphatase, an antigen expressed in most prostate cancer.

PATIENT CONSIDERATIONS

Assessment: Assess for history of cardiac or pulmonary conditions, risk factors for thromboembolic events, and possible drug interactions.

Monitoring: Monitor for signs and symptoms of infusion reactions, especially w/ cardiac or pulmonary conditions, thromboembolic events, vascular disorders, and other adverse reactions. Monitor for infectious sequelae in patients w/ central venous catheters.

Counseling: Counsel on the importance of adhering to preparation instructions for leukapheresis procedure, possible side effects, and postprocedure care. Advise to report signs and symptoms of acute infusion reactions and symptoms suggestive of cardiac arrhythmia, cerebral ischemia, DVT, and pulmonary embolism. Instruct to notify physician if taking immunosuppressive agents. Inform of the need for a central venous catheter placement if peripheral venous access is not adequate, and counsel on the importance of catheter care; advise to inform physician if fever or any swelling or redness around the catheter site occurs. Inform of the need to undergo an additional leukapheresis if a scheduled dose is missed.

PROVENTIL HFA — albuterol sulfate   Rx

Class: Short-acting beta₂ agonist (SABA)

ADULT DOSAGE	PEDIATRIC DOSAGE
Bronchospasm	**Bronchospasm**
Treatment/Prevention: Usual: 2 inh q4-6h; 1 inh q4h may be sufficient in some patients	**≥4 Years: Treatment/Prevention:** Usual: 2 inh q4-6h; 1 inh q4h may be sufficient in some patients
Exercise-Induced Bronchospasm	**Exercise-Induced Bronchospasm**
Prevention: Usual: 2 inh 15-30 min before exercise	**≥4 Years: Prevention:** Usual: 2 inh 15-30 min before exercise

---

ADMINISTRATION

Oral inh route

Shake well before use.
Discard canister after 200 sprays have been used.

Priming

Prime inhaler before using for 1st time or if inhaler has not been used for >2 weeks by releasing 4 test sprays into air, away from the face.

STORAGE

15-25°C (59-77°F). Store inhaler w/ the mouthpiece down. Contents under pressure; do not puncture or incinerate. Exposure to temperatures >49°C (120°F) may cause bursting.

HOW SUPPLIED

MDI: 90mcg of albuterol base/inh [200 inh]

CONTRAINDICATIONS

History of hypersensitivity to albuterol or any other components in this medication.

WARNINGS/PRECAUTIONS

May produce paradoxical bronchospasm that may be life threatening; d/c immediately and institute alternative therapy if this occurs. More doses than usual may be a marker of destabilization of asthma and may require reevaluation of the patient and treatment regimen; give special consideration to the possible need for anti-inflammatory treatment (eg, corticosteroids). May produce clinically significant cardiovascular (CV) effects; may need to d/c. ECG changes reported. Immediate hypersensitivity reactions may occur. Fatalities reported w/ excessive use. Caution w/ CV disorders (eg, coronary insufficiency, arrhythmias, HTN), convulsive disorders, hyperthyroidism, diabetes mellitus (DM), and in patients unusually responsive to sympathomimetic amines. May cause significant BP changes and hypokalemia. Aggravation of preexisting DM and ketoacidosis reported w/ large doses of IV albuterol. Caution in elderly.

ADVERSE REACTIONS
Tachycardia, tremor, rhinitis, URTI, fever, inhalation-site sensation, inhalation-taste sensation, nervousness, allergic reaction, respiratory disorder, N/V.

DRUG INTERACTIONS
Use w/ β-blockers may block pulmonary effects and produce severe bronchospasm in asthmatic patients; avoid concomitant use. If needed, consider cardioselective β-blockers and use w/ caution. ECG changes and/or hypokalemia caused by non-K+-sparing diuretics (eg, loop or thiazide diuretics) may be acutely worsened; use caution during coadministration. May decrease serum digoxin levels. Use extreme caution w/ MAOIs and TCAs, or w/in 2 weeks of discontinuation of such agents.

PREGNANCY AND LACTATION
Pregnancy: Category C.
Lactation: Not for use in nursing.

MECHANISM OF ACTION
β_2-agonist; activates β_2-adrenergic receptors on airway smooth muscle leading to activation of adenylcyclase and to an increase in intracellular cyclic-3',5'-adenosine monophosphate (cAMP). Increased cAMP leads to activation of protein kinase A, which inhibits the phosphorylation of myosin and lowers intracellular ionic calcium concentrations, resulting in relaxation of smooth muscle of all airways, from the trachea to the terminal bronchioles.

PATIENT CONSIDERATIONS
Assessment: Assess for history of hypersensitivity to the drug, CV disorders, convulsive disorders, hyperthyroidism, DM, pregnancy/nursing status, and possible drug interactions. Assess use in patients unusually responsive to sympathomimetic amines.

Monitoring: Monitor for paradoxical bronchospasm, deterioration of asthma, CV effects, ECG changes, hypokalemia, immediate hypersensitivity reactions, and other adverse effects. Monitor BP and HR.

Counseling: Instruct not to increase dose/frequency of doses w/o consulting physician. Advise to seek immediate medical attention if treatment becomes less effective for symptomatic relief, symptoms become worse, and/or there is a need to use the product more frequently than usual. Instruct to keep plastic mouthpiece clean to prevent medication build-up and blockage; advise to wash, shake to remove excess water, and air dry mouthpiece thoroughly at least once a week. Inform that inhaler may cease to deliver medication if not cleaned properly. Instruct to take concurrent inhaled drugs/asthma medications only as directed. Inform of the common side effects of treatment, such as chest pain, palpitations, rapid HR, tremor, or nervousness. Advise to notify physician if pregnant/nursing. Advise to avoid spraying in eyes. Instruct to use only w/ supplied actuator and not to use actuator w/ other aerosol medications.

PROVERA — medroxyprogesterone acetate   Rx
Class: Progestogen

> Estrogen plus progestin therapy should not be used for the prevention of cardiovascular disease (CVD) or dementia. Increased risk of deep vein thrombosis (DVT), pulmonary embolism (PE), stroke, and MI reported in postmenopausal women (50-79 yrs of age) treated w/ daily oral conjugated estrogens (CEs) combined w/ medroxyprogesterone acetate (MPA). Increased risk of developing probable dementia reported in postmenopausal women ≥65 yrs of age treated w/ daily CEs combined w/ MPA. Increased risk of invasive breast cancer reported w/ estrogen plus progestin. Should be prescribed at the lowest effective dose and for the shortest duration consistent w/ treatment goals and risks.

ADULT DOSAGE
Abnormal Uterine Bleeding
Due to Hormonal Imbalance in the Absence of Organic Pathology (eg, Fibroids, Uterine Cancer):
5 or 10mg/day for 5-10 days beginning on Day 16 or 21 of cycle; 10mg/day for 10 days, beginning on Day 16 of the cycle is recommended to produce an optimum secretory transformation of an endometrium that has been adequately primed w/ either endogenous or exogenous estrogen

Endometrial Hyperplasia
Reduce Incidence in Non-Hysterectomized Postmenopausal Women Receiving Daily Oral CEs 0.625mg Tabs:
5 or 10mg/day for 12-14 consecutive days/month, beginning on Day 1 or 16 of cycle

PEDIATRIC DOSAGE
Pediatric use may not have been established

Secondary Amenorrhea
5 or 10mg/day for 5-10 days. 10mg/day for 10 days is a dose for inducing an optimum secretory transformation of an endometrium that has been adequately primed w/ either endogenous or exogenous estrogen. May start therapy at any time

---

ADMINISTRATION
Oral route

STORAGE
20-25°C (68-77°F).

HOW SUPPLIED
Tab: 2.5mg*, 5mg*, 10mg* *scored

CONTRAINDICATIONS
Undiagnosed abnormal genital bleeding, known/suspected/history of breast cancer, known/suspected estrogen- or progesterone-dependent neoplasia, active/history of DVT/PE or arterial thromboembolic disease (eg, stroke, MI), known anaphylactic reaction or angioedema to medroxyprogesterone acetate, known liver impairment or disease, known/suspected pregnancy.

WARNINGS/PRECAUTIONS
D/C estrogen plus progestin therapy immediately if PE, DVT, stroke, or MI occurs or is suspected. If feasible, d/c estrogen plus progestin therapy at least 4-6 weeks before surgery of the type associated w/ an increased risk of thromboembolism, or during periods of prolonged immobilization. Increased risk of endometrial cancer reported w/ use of unopposed estrogen therapy in women w/ a uterus; adding a progestin to estrogen therapy has been shown to reduce risk of endometrial hyperplasia, which may be a precursor to endometrial cancer. Estrogen plus progestin therapy may increase risk of ovarian cancer. D/C estrogen plus progestin therapy pending exam if there is sudden partial or complete loss of vision, or a sudden onset of proptosis, diplopia or migraine; d/c permanently if exam reveals papilledema or retinal vascular lesions. In cases of unexpected abnormal vaginal bleeding, perform adequate diagnostic measures. Monitor BP at regular intervals w/ estrogen plus progestin therapy. Estrogen plus progestin therapy may increase plasma TGs, leading to pancreatitis in women w/ preexisting hypertriglyceridemia; consider discontinuation of treatment if pancreatitis occurs. Caution w/ history of cholestatic jaundice associated w/ past estrogen use or w/ pregnancy; d/c in case of recurrence. May cause fluid retention; caution in cardiac or renal impairment. Caution in women w/ hypoparathyroidism as estrogen-induced hypocalcemia may occur. Estrogen plus progestin therapy may exacerbate asthma, diabetes mellitus, epilepsy, migraine, porphyria, systemic lupus erythematosus, and hepatic hemangiomas. Withdrawal bleeding may occur w/in 3-7 days after discontinuing therapy. May affect LFTs and certain endocrine and blood components in lab tests.

ADVERSE REACTIONS
Abnormal uterine bleeding, breast tenderness, galactorrhea, urticaria, pruritus, edema, rash, menstrual changes, change in weight, mental depression, insomnia, somnolence, dizziness, headache, nausea.

DRUG INTERACTIONS
Women on thyroid replacement therapy may require higher doses of thyroid hormone.

PREGNANCY AND LACTATION
Category X, not for use in nursing.

MECHANISM OF ACTION
Progestogen; transforms proliferative endometrium into secretory endometrium.

PHARMACOKINETICS
Absorption: Rapid. Administration of different doses resulted in different pharmacokinetic parameters; refer to PI. **Distribution:** Plasma protein binding (approx 90%); found in breast milk. **Metabolism:** Extensive (hepatic) via hydroxylation w/ subsequent conjugation. **Elimination:** Urine.

PATIENT CONSIDERATIONS
Assessment: Assess for abnormal genital bleeding, cardiac or renal impairment, presence or history of breast cancer, estrogen- or progesterone-dependent neoplasias, active/history of DVT/PE or arterial thromboembolic disease, any other conditions where treatment is contraindicated or cautioned, and for possible drug interactions.

Monitoring: Monitor for signs/symptoms of CVD, malignant neoplasms, visual abnormalities, hypertriglyceridemia, fluid retention, exacerbation of asthma, and other adverse reactions. Perform annual breast exam; schedule mammography based on age, risk factors, and prior mammogram results. Regularly monitor BP in patients on estrogen plus progestin therapy. Monitor thyroid function in patients on thyroid replacement therapy. Periodically reevaluate (every 3-6 months) need for therapy. In cases of undiagnosed, persistent, or recurrent genital bleeding in women w/ a uterus, perform adequate diagnostic measures (eg, endometrial sampling) to rule out malignancy.

Counseling: Advise of risks and benefits of therapy. Instruct to have annual breast exams and perform monthly breast self-exams. Advise to schedule mammography exams based on age, risk factors, and prior mammogram results. Inform of possible increased risk of minor birth defects in children whose mothers are exposed to progestins during the 1st trimester of pregnancy; inform of the importance of reporting exposure of therapy in early pregnancy.

PROVIGIL — modafinil   CIV
Class: Wakefulness-promoting agent

ADULT DOSAGE
Excessive Sleepiness
Associated w/ Narcolepsy/ Obstructive Sleep Apnea/Shift Work Disorder:
200mg qd
Max: 400mg/day as a single dose

PEDIATRIC DOSAGE
Pediatric use may not have been established

DOSING CONSIDERATIONS
Hepatic Impairment
Severe: 100mg qd

Elderly
Consider using lower doses

ADMINISTRATION
Oral route

Narcolepsy/Obstructive Sleep Apnea
Take as single dose in am

Shift Work Disorder
Take 1 hr prior to start of work shift

STORAGE
20-25°C (68-77°F).

HOW SUPPLIED
Tab: 100mg, 200mg* *scored

CONTRAINDICATIONS
Known hypersensitivity to modafinil or armodafinil or its inactive ingredients.

WARNINGS/PRECAUTIONS
Not indicated as treatment for underlying obstruction in OSA; if continuous positive airway pressure (CPAP) is the treatment of choice, treat w/ CPAP for an adequate period of time prior to initiating and during treatment. Rare cases of serious or life-threatening rash, including Stevens-Johnson syndrome (SJS), toxic epidermal necrolysis (TEN), and drug rash w/ eosinophilia and systemic symptoms (DRESS), reported; d/c at the 1st sign of rash, unless the rash is clearly not drug-related. Angioedema reported; d/c if angioedema or anaphylaxis occurs. Multiorgan hypersensitivity reactions reported; d/c if suspected. Level of wakefulness may not return to normal in patients w/ abnormal levels of sleepiness. Psychiatric adverse reactions reported; caution w/ history of psychosis, depression, or mania. Consider discontinuation if psychiatric symptoms develop in association w/ drug administration. May impair mental and/or physical abilities. Cardiovascular (CV) adverse reactions reported; not recommended in patients w/ a history of left ventricular hypertrophy (LVH) or in patients w/ mitral valve prolapse who have experienced mitral valve prolapse syndrome (eg, ischemic ECG changes, chest pain, arrhythmia) when previously receiving CNS stimulants. Caution w/ known CV disease (CVD). Caution in elderly. Potential for abuse.

ADVERSE REACTIONS
Headache, nausea, nervousness, anxiety, insomnia, rhinitis, diarrhea, back pain, dizziness, dyspepsia, anorexia, dry mouth, pharyngitis, chest pain, HTN.

DRUG INTERACTIONS
May reduce exposure of CYP3A4/5 substrates (eg, midazolam, triazolam); consider dose adjustment of these drugs. Effectiveness of steroidal contraceptives (eg, ethinyl estradiol) may be reduced when used w/ therapy and for 1 month after discontinuation of therapy; alternative or concomitant methods of contraception are recommended. May reduce levels of cyclosporine; consider dose adjustment for cyclosporine. May increase exposure of CYP2C19 substrates (eg, phenytoin, diazepam, propranolol). In individuals deficient in the CYP2D6 enzyme, levels of CYP2D6 substrates, which have ancillary routes of elimination through CYP2C19 (eg, TCAs, SSRIs) may be increased; dose adjustments of these drugs and other drugs that are substrates for CYP2C19 may be necessary. Consider more frequent monitoring of PT/INR w/ warfarin. Caution w/ MAOIs.

PREGNANCY AND LACTATION
Category C, caution in nursing.

MECHANISM OF ACTION
Wakefulness-promoting agent; has not been established. Binds to the dopamine transporter and inhibits dopamine reuptake.

PHARMACOKINETICS
Absorption: Readily absorbed. T_{max}=2-4 hrs, delayed by 1 hr (fed). **Distribution:** V_d=0.9L/kg; plasma protein binding (60%). **Metabolism:** Liver via hydrolytic deamidation, S-oxidation, aromatic ring hydroxylation, and glucuronide conjugation; CYP3A4. **Elimination:** Urine (80%) and feces (1%), <10% unchanged; $T_{1/2}$=15 hrs.

PATIENT CONSIDERATIONS
Assessment: Assess for hypersensitivity to the drug, history of psychosis, depression, mania, or LVH, mitral valve prolapse, other CVD, hepatic impairment, pregnancy/nursing status, and possible drug interactions.

Monitoring: Monitor for rash, SJS, TEN, DRESS, angioedema, anaphylaxis, multiorgan hypersensitivity reactions, psychiatric symptoms, CV events (especially in patients w/ a history of MI or unstable angina), and other adverse reactions. Monitor for signs of misuse or abuse. Monitor HR and BP. Frequently reassess degree of sleepiness. Monitor PT/INR frequently w/ warfarin.

Counseling: Instruct to d/c use and notify physician immediately if allergic reactions and other adverse reactions (eg, chest pain, rash, depression, anxiety, signs of psychosis/mania) develop. Advise not to alter previous behavior w/ regard to potentially dangerous activities (eg, driving, operating machinery) or other activities requiring appropriate levels of wakefulness, until and unless treatment has been shown to produce levels of wakefulness that permit such activities. Inform that drug is not a replacement for sleep. Counsel patients that it may be critical that they continue to take their previously prescribed treatments (eg, patients w/ OSA receiving CPAP). Advise to notify physician if pregnancy occurs, if intending to become pregnant, or if breastfeeding. Caution regarding the potential increased risk of pregnancy when using steroidal contraceptives w/ therapy and for 1 month after discontinuation of therapy. Instruct to inform physician if taking/planning to take any prescription/OTC drugs, and to avoid alcohol.

PROZAC — fluoxetine hydrochloride   Rx
Class: Selective serotonin reuptake inhibitor (SSRI)

> Antidepressants increased the risk of suicidal thoughts and behavior in children, adolescents, and young adults in short-term studies. Monitor closely for worsening and for emergence of suicidal thoughts and behaviors in patients who are started on antidepressant therapy. Not approved for use in children <7 yrs of age.

OTHER BRAND NAMES
Prozac Weekly

ADULT DOSAGE
Major Depressive Disorder
Initial: 20mg/day qam
Titrate: Consider a dose increase after several weeks if improvement is insufficient; administer doses >20mg/day qam or bid (am and noon)
Max: 80mg/day

Prozac Weekly:
Initiate 7 days after the last daily dose of 20mg cap
Consider reestablishing a daily dosing regimen if satisfactory response is not maintained

Switching to a TCA:
May need to reduce TCA dose and monitor plasma concentrations temporarily w/ coadministration or when fluoxetine has been recently discontinued

Obsessive Compulsive Disorder
Initial: 20mg/day qam
Titrate: Consider a dose increase after several weeks if improvement is insufficient; administer doses >20mg/day qam or bid (am and noon)
Range: 20-60mg/day
Max: 80mg/day

Bulimia Nervosa
Initial: 60mg/day qam; may titrate up to this target dose over several days
Max: 60mg/day

Panic Disorder
W/ or w/o Agoraphobia:
Initial: 10mg/day
Titrate: Increase to 20mg/day after 1 week; consider a dose increase after several weeks if no improvement
Max: 60mg/day

Bipolar I Disorder
Depressive Episodes:
In Combination w/ Olanzapine:
Initial: 20mg fluoxetine + 5mg olanzapine qpm
Range: 20-50mg fluoxetine + 5-12.5mg olanzapine
Max: 75mg fluoxetine + 18mg olanzapine

Major Depressive Disorder
Use in patients who do not respond to 2 separate trials of different antidepressants of adequate dose and duration in the current episode

In Combination w/ Olanzapine:
Initial: 20mg fluoxetine + 5mg olanzapine qpm
Range: 20-50mg fluoxetine + 5-20mg olanzapine
Max: 75mg fluoxetine + 18mg olanzapine

Dosing Considerations with MAOIs
Switching to/from an MAOI for Psychiatric Disorders:

PEDIATRIC DOSAGE
Major Depressive Disorder
≥8 Years:
Initial: 10 or 20mg/day
Titrate: After 1 week at 10mg/day, increase to 20mg/day

Lower Weight Children:
Initial/Target: 10mg/day
Titrate: Consider a dose increase to 20mg/day after several weeks if improvement is insufficient

Switching to a TCA:
May need to reduce TCA dose and monitor plasma concentrations temporarily w/ coadministration or when fluoxetine has been recently discontinued

Obsessive Compulsive Disorder
≥7 Years:
Initial: 10mg/day
Titrate: Increase to 20mg/day after 2 weeks; consider additional dose increases after several more weeks if improvement is insufficient
Range: 20-60mg/day

Lower Weight Children:
Initial: 10mg/day
Titrate: Consider additional dose increases after several weeks if improvement is insufficient
Range: 20-30mg/day
Max: 60mg/day

Bipolar I Disorder
Depressive Episodes:
In Combination w/ Olanzapine:
10-17 Years:
Initial: 20mg fluoxetine + 2.5mg olanzapine qpm
Max: 50mg fluoxetine + 12mg olanzapine

Dosing Considerations with MAOIs
Switching to/from an MAOI for Psychiatric Disorders:
Allow at least 14 days between discontinuation of an MAOI and initiation of treatment, and allow at least 5 weeks between discontinuation of treatment and initiation of an MAOI

W/ Other MAOIs (eg, Linezolid, IV Methylene Blue):
Do not start fluoxetine in patients being treated w/ linezolid or IV methylene blue.
In patients already receiving fluoxetine, if acceptable alternatives are not available and benefits outweigh risks, d/c fluoxetine and administer linezolid or IV methylene blue; monitor for serotonin syndrome for 5 weeks or until 24 hrs after the last dose of linezolid or IV methylene blue, whichever comes 1st. May

Allow at least 14 days between discontinuation of an MAOI and initiation of treatment, and allow at least 5 weeks between discontinuation of treatment and initiation of an MAOI

W/ Other MAOIs (eg, Linezolid, IV Methylene Blue):
Do not start fluoxetine in patients being treated w/ linezolid or IV methylene blue.
In patients already receiving fluoxetine, if acceptable alternatives are not available and benefits outweigh risks, d/c fluoxetine and administer linezolid or IV methylene blue; monitor for serotonin syndrome for 5 weeks or until 24 hrs after the last dose of linezolid or IV methylene blue, whichever comes 1st. May resume fluoxetine therapy 24 hrs after the last dose of linezolid or IV methylene blue.

resume fluoxetine therapy 24 hrs after the last dose of linezolid or IV methylene blue.

DOSING CONSIDERATIONS
Concomitant Medications
Combination w/ Olanzapine:
Patients Predisposed to Hypotensive Reactions w/ Hepatic Impairment, Slow Metabolizers, Pharmacodynamic Olanzapine Sensitivity:
Initial: 20mg fluoxetine + 2.5-5mg olanzapine
Titrate slowly and adjust dosage prn

Hepatic Impairment
Use lower or less frequent dosage

Elderly
Consider lower or less frequent dosage

Other Important Considerations
Concomitant Illness: May require dose adjustments

ADMINISTRATION
Oral route
Take w/ or w/o food.

STORAGE
15-30°C (59-86°F). (Cap) Protect from light.

HOW SUPPLIED
Cap: 10mg, 20mg, 40mg; **Cap, Delayed-Release:** (Prozac Weekly) 90mg

CONTRAINDICATIONS
Use of an MAOI for psychiatric disorders either concomitantly or within 5 weeks of stopping treatment. Treatment within 14 days of stopping an MAOI for psychiatric disorders. Starting treatment in patients being treated with other MAOIs (eg, linezolid, IV methylene blue). Concomitant use with pimozide or thioridazine.

WARNINGS/PRECAUTIONS
Serotonin syndrome reported; d/c immediately and initiate supportive symptomatic treatment. Anaphylactoid and pulmonary reactions reported; d/c if unexplained allergic reaction or rash occurs. May precipitate mixed/manic episode in patients at risk for bipolar disorder. Weight loss and anorexia reported. May increase risk of bleeding reactions. Pupillary dilation that occurs following use may trigger an angle-closure attack in a patient with anatomically narrow angles who does not have a patent iridectomy. Hyponatremia may occur; caution in elderly and volume-depleted patients. Consider discontinuation in patients with symptomatic hyponatremia and institute appropriate medical intervention. Convulsions, mania/hypomania, anxiety, insomnia, and nervousness reported. QT interval prolongation and ventricular arrhythmia (eg, torsades de pointes) reported. Caution in patients with congenital long QT syndrome, previous history of QT prolongation, family history of long QT syndrome or sudden cardiac death, and other conditions that predispose to QT prolongation and ventricular arrhythmia. Consider discontinuing treatment and obtaining cardiac evaluation if signs or symptoms of ventricular arrhythmia develop. Caution in patients with diseases/conditions that could affect hemodynamic responses or metabolism. May alter glycemic control in patients with diabetes. May impair mental/physical abilities. Long elimination $T_{1/2}$; changes in dose may not be fully reflected in plasma for several weeks. Adverse reactions reported upon discontinuation; avoid abrupt withdrawal.

ADVERSE REACTIONS
Somnolence, anorexia, anxiety, asthenia, diarrhea, dry mouth, dyspepsia, headache, insomnia, tremor, pharyngitis, flu syndrome, dizziness, nausea, nervousness.

DRUG INTERACTIONS
See Contraindications. Do not use thioridazine within 5 weeks of discontinuing therapy. Caution with CNS-active drugs. Avoid with other drugs that cause QT prolongation (eg, ziprasidone, erythromycin, quinidine). May cause serotonin syndrome with other serotonergic drugs (eg, triptans, TCAs, fentanyl) and with drugs that impair metabolism of serotonin; d/c immediately if this occurs. Increased risk of bleeding with aspirin, NSAIDs, warfarin, and other anticoagulants. Rare reports of prolonged seizures with electroconvulsive therapy. Drugs that are tightly bound to plasma proteins (eg, warfarin, digitoxin) may cause a shift in plasma concentrations, resulting in an adverse effect. Caution with CYP2D6 substrates, including antidepressants (eg, TCAs), antipsychotics (eg, phenothiazines and most atypicals), and antiarrhythmics (eg, propafenone,

flecainide). Consider decreasing dose of drugs metabolized by CYP2D6, especially drugs with a narrow therapeutic index (eg, flecainide, propafenone, vinblastine). May prolong $T_{1/2}$ of diazepam. May increase levels of phenytoin, carbamazepine, haloperidol, clozapine, imipramine, and desipramine. Coadministration with alprazolam resulted in increased alprazolam levels and further psychomotor performance decrement. Anticonvulsant toxicity reported with phenytoin and carbamazepine. Antidiabetic drugs (eg, insulin, oral hypoglycemics) may require dose adjustment. May cause lithium toxicity; monitor lithium levels. Increased risk of hyponatremia with diuretics. Increased levels with CYP2D6 inhibitors.

PREGNANCY AND LACTATION
Pregnancy: Category C.
Lactation: Not for use in nursing.

MECHANISM OF ACTION
SSRI; has not been established. Presumed to be linked to its inhibition of CNS neuronal uptake of serotonin.

PHARMACOKINETICS
Absorption: (Single 40mg dose) C_{max}=15-55ng/mL, T_{max}=6-8 hrs. **Distribution:** Plasma protein binding (94.5%); crosses the placenta; found in breast milk. **Metabolism:** Liver (extensive) via CYP2D6; demethylation into norfluoxetine (active metabolite). **Elimination:** Kidney; $T_{1/2}$=1-3 days (acute administration), 4-6 days (chronic administration), 4-16 days (norfluoxetine, acute and chronic administration).

PATIENT CONSIDERATIONS
Assessment: Assess for volume depletion, history of seizures, risk for/presence of bipolar disorder, diseases/conditions that affect metabolism or hemodynamic responses, diabetes, susceptibility to angle-closure glaucoma, congenital long QT syndrome, previous history of QT prolongation, family history of long QT syndrome or sudden cardiac death, other conditions that predispose to QT prolongation and ventricular arrhythmia, pregnancy/nursing status, and possible drug interactions. Consider ECG assessment if initiating treatment in patients with risk factors for QT prolongation and ventricular arrhythmia.

Monitoring: Monitor for clinical worsening, suicidality, unusual changes in behavior, allergic reactions, serotonin syndrome, bleeding reactions, angle-closure glaucoma, altered appetite and weight, hyponatremia, seizures, activation of mania/hypomania, hypoglycemia/hyperglycemia, QT interval prolongation, ventricular arrhythmia, and other adverse reactions. Monitor height and weight in children periodically. Consider periodic ECG monitoring if initiating treatment in patients with risk factors for QT prolongation and ventricular arrhythmia. Periodically reassess need for continued/maintenance treatment.

Counseling: Inform of risks, benefits, and appropriate use of therapy. Counsel to be alert for the emergence of suicidality, unusual changes in behavior, or worsening of depression, especially early during treatment and when the dose is adjusted up or down. Inform about risk of serotonin syndrome with concomitant use with other serotonergic agents. Counsel to seek medical care immediately if rash/hives or unusual bruising/bleeding develops, or if experiencing signs/symptoms associated with serotonin syndrome or hyponatremia. Inform that drug may cause mild pupillary dilation, which in susceptible individuals, may lead to an episode of angle-closure glaucoma. Inform that QT interval prolongation and ventricular arrhythmia (eg, torsades de pointes) have been reported. Advise to avoid operating hazardous machinery or driving a car until effects of drug are known. Advise to inform physician if taking or planning to take any prescription or OTC drugs, if pregnant/intending to become pregnant, or if breastfeeding. Instruct to take ud, not to stop taking medication without consulting physician, and to consult physician if symptoms do not improve.

PULMICORT — budesonide   Rx
Class: Corticosteroid

OTHER BRAND NAMES
Pulmicort Flexhaler, Pulmicort Respules

ADULT DOSAGE
Asthma

Flexhaler:
Maint:
Initial: 180-360mcg bid
Max: 720mcg bid

PEDIATRIC DOSAGE
Asthma

1-8 Years:
Respules:
Maint/Prophylaxis:
Previously on Bronchodilators Alone:
Initial: 0.5mg qd or 0.25mg bid
Max: 0.5mg/day

Previously on Inhaled Corticosteroids:
Initial: 0.5mg qd or 0.25mg bid
Max: 1mg/day

Previously on Oral Corticosteroids:
Initial: 1mg qd or 0.5mg bid
Max: 1mg/day

Symptomatic Children Not Responding to Nonsteroidal Therapy:
Initial: 0.25mg qd

≥6 Years:
Flexhaler:
Prophylaxis:
Initial: 180-360mcg bid
Max: 360mcg bid

DOSING CONSIDERATIONS
Elderly
Flexhaler:
Start at lower end of dosing range

ADMINISTRATION
Oral inhalation route

Patients should rinse mouth w/ water w/o swallowing after inh.

Flexhaler
Priming is required prior to initial use.

Respules
Administer via jet nebulizer connected to air compressor w/ adequate air flow (eg, Pari-LC-Jet Plus Nebulizer [w/ face mask or mouthpiece] connected to a Pari Master compressor).
Administer separately from other nebulizable medications in the nebulizer.

STORAGE
(Flexhaler): 20-25°C (68-77°F). Cover tightly. Store in a dry place. (Respules): 20-25°C (68-77°F). Protect from light. Do not freeze. After aluminum foil opened, unused ampules stable for 2 weeks. Once opened, use promptly.

HOW SUPPLIED
Powder, Inhalation: (Flexhaler) 90mcg/dose, 180mcg/dose. **Sus, Inhalation:** (Respules) 0.25mg/2mL, 0.5mg/2mL, 1mg/2mL [2mL]

CONTRAINDICATIONS
Primary treatment of status asthmaticus or other acute episodes of asthma where intensive measures are required. Hypersensitivity to budesonide or any components of the medication. (Flexhaler) Severe hypersensitivity to milk proteins.

WARNINGS/PRECAUTIONS
Candida albicans infections of mouth and pharynx reported; treat and/or d/c if needed. Not indicated for the rapid relief of bronchospasm or other acute episodes of asthma; may require oral corticosteroids. Increased susceptibility to infections (eg, chickenpox, measles), may lead to serious/fatal course; if exposed, consider prophylaxis/treatment. Caution w/ tuberculosis, untreated systemic fungal, bacterial, viral or parasitic infections, and ocular herpes simplex. Deaths due to adrenal insufficiency reported w/ transfer from systemic to inhaled corticosteroids (ICS); if oral corticosteroids are required, wean slowly from systemic steroid use after transferring to ICS. Transfer from systemic to inhalation therapy may unmask allergic conditions (eg, rhinitis, conjunctivitis). Observe for systemic corticosteroid withdrawal effects. Hypercorticism and adrenal suppression may appear; reduce dose slowly. Decreases in bone mineral density (BMD) reported; caution w/ chronic use of drugs that can reduce bone mass (eg, anticonvulsants, corticosteroids). May cause reduction in growth velocity in pediatrics. Glaucoma, increased IOP, and cataracts reported. Bronchospasm, w/ immediate increase in wheezing, may occur; d/c immediately. Rare cases of systemic eosinophilic conditions and vasculitis consistent w/ Churg-Strauss syndrome reported. Hypersensitivity reactions reported; d/c if signs and symptoms occur. (Flexhaler) Caution in elderly.

ADVERSE REACTIONS
Respiratory infection. (Flexhaler) Nasopharyngitis, headache, fever, sinusitis, pain, N/V, insomnia, dry mouth, weight gain. (Respules) Rhinitis, otitis media, coughing, viral infection, ear infection, gastroenteritis.

DRUG INTERACTIONS
Oral ketoconazole increases plasma levels of oral budesonide. Inhibition of metabolism and increased exposure w/ CYP3A4 inhibitors. Caution w/ ketoconazole and other known strong CYP3A4 inhibitors (eg, ritonavir, clarithromycin, itraconazole, nefazodone).

PREGNANCY AND LACTATION
Pregnancy: Category B.
Lactation: Caution in nursing.

MECHANISM OF ACTION
Corticosteroid; not established. Shown to have inhibitory activities against multiple cell types and mediators involved in inflammatory and asthmatic response.

PHARMACOKINETICS
Absorption: Flexhaler: (Adults) T_{max}=10 min; C_{max}=0.6nmol/L (180mcg qd), 1.6nmol/L (360mcg bid). (Peds) T_{max}=15-30 min; C_{max}=0.4nmol/L (180mcg qd), 1.5nmol/L (360mcg bid). Respules: (4-6 yrs of age) Absolute bioavailability (6%); C_{max}=2.6nmol/L; T_{max}=20 min. **Distribution:** V_d=3L/kg; plasma protein binding (85-90%); found in breast milk. **Metabolism:** Liver (extensive) via CYP450 and CYP3A4; 16α-hydroxyprednisolone and 6β-hydroxybudesonide (major metabolites). **Elimination:** Urine and feces (metabolites); (IV) Urine (60%). Flexhaler: $T_{1/2}$=2-3 hrs. Respules: $T_{1/2}$=2.3 hrs.

PATIENT CONSIDERATIONS
Assessment: Assess for concomitant diseases (eg, status asthmaticus, acute bronchospasm, other acute episodes of asthma), infections, major risk factors for decreased bone mineral content, history of eye disorders, hypersensitivity, pregnancy/nursing status, and possible drug interactions. Obtain baseline cortisol production levels. Assess lung function in oral corticosteroids withdrawal. (Flexhaler) Assess for severe milk protein hypersensitivity and hepatic disease.

Monitoring: Monitor for localized oral infections w/ *C. albicans*, worsening or acutely deteriorating asthma, systemic corticosteroid effects, decreased BMD, height in children, vision change, bronchospasm, and hypersensitivity reactions. (Flexhaler) Monitor for hepatic disease.

Counseling: Advise to use at regular intervals and rinse mouth after inhalation; effectiveness depends on regular use. Instruct to d/c if oral candidiasis or hypersensitivity reactions occur. Inform that medication is not meant to relieve acute asthma symptoms and extra doses should not be used for that purpose. Instruct not to d/c w/o physician's guidance; symptoms may recur after discontinuation.

Warn to avoid exposure to chickenpox or measles; if exposed, consult physician. Counsel that max benefit may not be achieved for ≥1-2 weeks (Flexhaler) or ≥4-6 weeks (Respules); instruct to notify physician if symptoms worsen or do not improve in that time frame. (Flexhaler) Instruct not to repeat inhalation even if the patient did not feel medication when inhaling; discard whole device after labeled number of inhalations have been used. Advise to carry a warning card indicating need for supplemental systemic corticosteroid during periods of stress or severe asthma attack if chronic systemic corticosteroids have been reduced or withdrawn. Instruct to consult physician if pregnant/breastfeeding or intend to become pregnant.

PULMOZYME — dornase alfa   Rx

Class: Enzyme

ADULT DOSAGE	PEDIATRIC DOSAGE
Cystic Fibrosis	**Cystic Fibrosis**
Improves pulmonary function in conjunction with standard therapies	Improves pulmonary function in conjunction with standard therapies
2.5mg qd via nebulizer/compressor system (may benefit with bid dosing)	**≥5 Years:** 2.5mg qd via nebulizer/compressor system (may benefit with bid dosing)

ADMINISTRATION
Inhalation route

Should not be diluted or mixed with other drugs in the nebulizer.
Squeeze each ampule prior to use to check for leaks.
Once opened, entire contents of the ampule must be used or discarded.
Refer to PI for the recommended nebulizer/compressor systems.

STORAGE
Store in the protective foil pouch at 2-8°C (36-46°F). Protect from light. Refrigerate during transport and do not expose to room temperatures for a total time of 24 hrs.

HOW SUPPLIED
Sol: 2.5mg/2.5mL

CONTRAINDICATIONS
Known hypersensitivity to dornase alfa, Chinese Hamster ovary cell products, or any component of the product.

WARNINGS/PRECAUTIONS
May consider use for pediatric patients younger than 5 years of age who may experience potential benefit in pulmonary function or who may be at risk of RTI.

ADVERSE REACTIONS
Voice alteration, pharyngitis, rash, laryngitis, chest pain, conjunctivitis, rhinitis, fever, dyspnea, dyspepsia, antibodies development.

PREGNANCY AND LACTATION
Safety not known in pregnancy/nursing.

MECHANISM OF ACTION
Enzyme; hydrolyzes the deoxyribonucleic acid in sputum of CF patients and reduces sputum viscoelasticity.

PATIENT CONSIDERATIONS
Assessment: Assess for hypersensitivity to the drug, Chinese hamster ovary cell products, or any component of the drug, and nursing status.

Monitoring: Monitor for worsening of the condition and other adverse reactions.

Counseling: Instruct on the proper techniques to store and handle therapy. Advise to squeeze each ampule prior to use in order to check for leaks. Instruct to discard sol if cloudy or discolored. Inform that entire contents of ampule must be used or discarded once opened. Instruct on the proper use and maintenance of the nebulizer and compressor system. Instruct to not dilute or mix with other drugs in the nebulizer.

PURIXAN — mercaptopurine   Rx

Class: Purine analogue

ADULT DOSAGE	PEDIATRIC DOSAGE
Acute Lymphoblastic Leukemia	**Acute Lymphoblastic Leukemia**
Component of a Multi-agent Combination Chemotherapy Maint Regimen:	**Component of a Multi-agent Combination Chemotherapy Maint Regimen:**
Initial: 1.5-2.5mg/kg (50-75mg/m²) as a single daily dose	**Initial:** 1.5-2.5mg/kg (50-75mg/m²) as a single daily dose
Continuation of appropriate dosing requires periodic monitoring of absolute neutrophil count and platelet count to assure sufficient drug exposure and to adjust for excessive hematological toxicity	Continuation of appropriate dosing requires periodic monitoring of absolute neutrophil count and platelet count to assure sufficient drug exposure and to adjust for excessive hematological toxicity

DOSING CONSIDERATIONS
Renal Impairment
Consider starting at lower end of dosing range or increasing the dosing interval to 36-48 hrs

Hepatic Impairment
Consider starting at lower end of dosing range

Elderly
Consider starting at lower end of dosing range

Other Important Considerations

Thiopurine S-Methyltransferase (TPMT) Deficiency:

Homozygous TPMT Deficiency: May require up to a 90% dosage reduction

Heterozygous TPMT Deficiency: May require dose reduction based on toxicities

ADMINISTRATION

Oral route

Shake vigorously for at least 30 sec.
Once opened, use within 6 weeks.

STORAGE

15-25°C (59-77°F) in a dry place. Do not store >25°C.

HOW SUPPLIED

Sus: 20mg/mL [100mL]

WARNINGS/PRECAUTIONS

Increased risk for severe mercaptopurine toxicity in patients with inherited little or no TPMT activity; evaluate TPMT status in patients with evidence of severe bone marrow toxicity or with repeated episodes of myelosuppression. Dose-related bone marrow suppression may occur; adjust dose for severe neutropenia and thrombocytopenia. Hepatotoxicity reported; interrupt therapy in patients with evidence of hepatotoxicity. Monitor LFTs more frequently in patients who are receiving mercaptopurine with other hepatotoxic drugs or with known pre-existing liver disease. Therapy is immunosuppressive and may impair the immune response to infectious agents. May cause fetal harm. May increase risk of secondary malignancies. Caution with renal/hepatic impairment and in elderly.

ADVERSE REACTIONS

Myelosuppression, anorexia, N/V, diarrhea, malaise, rash.

DRUG INTERACTIONS

Allopurinol inhibits 1st-pass oxidative metabolism, leading to mercaptopurine toxicity (bone marrow suppression, N/V); avoid concomitant use. May decrease anticoagulant effectiveness of warfarin; monitor PT/INR and adjust warfarin dose if necessary. Drugs that inhibit TPMT (eg, aminosalicylate derivatives [eg, olsalazine, mesalamine, sulfasalazine]), drugs whose primary or secondary toxicity is myelosuppression, and trimethoprim-sulfamethoxazole may exacerbate myelosuppression; if coadministration with aminosalicylate derivatives is necessary, use the lowest possible doses of each drug and closely monitor for bone marrow suppression. May impair the immune response to vaccines; response to all vaccines may be diminished and there is a risk of infection with live virus vaccines.

PREGNANCY AND LACTATION

Pregnancy: Category D.

Lactation: Not for use in nursing.

MECHANISM OF ACTION

Purine analogue; activation occurs via hypoxanthine-guanine phosphoribosyl transferase and several enzymes to form 6-thioguanine nucleotides (6-TGNs). Incorporation of 6-TGN into nucleic acids (instead of purine bases) results in cell-cycle arrest and cell death.

PHARMACOKINETICS

Absorption: Incomplete and variable. (Single 50mg dose, fasting conditions) AUC=136ng•hr/mL (median); C_{max}=95ng/mL (median). **Metabolism:** Thiol methylation via TPMT and oxidation via xanthine oxidase. **Elimination:** Urine; $T_{1/2}$=2 hrs.

PATIENT CONSIDERATIONS

Assessment: Assess for TPMT deficiency, renal/hepatic impairment, pregnancy/nursing status, and possible drug interactions.

Monitoring: Monitor for myelosuppression, hepatotoxicity, immunosuppression, secondary malignancies, and other adverse reactions. Monitor serum transaminase levels, alkaline phosphatase, and bilirubin levels at weekly intervals when first beginning therapy and at monthly intervals thereafter. Monitor CBC. Evaluate bone marrow in patients with prolonged or repeated marrow suppression to assess leukemia status and marrow cellularity. Evaluate TPMT status in patients with clinical or lab evidence of severe bone marrow toxicity, or with repeated episodes of myelosuppression.

Counseling: Instruct on proper handling, storage, administration, disposal and clean-up of accidental spillage of the medication; counsel regarding which syringe to use and how to administer a specified dose. Inform that the major toxicities of therapy are related to myelosuppression, hepatotoxicity, and GI toxicity; instruct to contact physician if patient experiences fever, sore throat, jaundice, N/V, signs of local infection, bleeding from any site, or symptoms suggestive of anemia. Advise women of childbearing potential to avoid becoming pregnant. Inform that the oral dispensing syringe is intended for multiple use; instruct on how to clean the syringe.

PYLERA — bismuth subcitrate potassium/metronidazole/tetracycline hydrochloride

Rx

Class: *H. pylori* treatment combination

ADULT DOSAGE

Helicobacter pylori Eradication

H. pylori Infection and Duodenal Ulcer Disease (Active or History of w/in the Past 5 Years):

Usual: 3 caps qid (pc and hs) for 10 days; take w/ omeprazole 20mg bid for 10 days (after am and pm meals)

PEDIATRIC DOSAGE

Pediatric use may not have been established

ADMINISTRATION

Oral route

Swallow cap whole w/ a full glass of water (8 oz.)

STORAGE

20-25°C (68-77°F).

HOW SUPPLIED

Cap: (Bismuth/Metronidazole/Tetracycline) 140mg/125mg/125mg

CONTRAINDICATIONS

Use of methoxyflurane concomitantly; disulfiram w/in the last 2 weeks; alcoholic beverages or other products containing propylene glycol during therapy and for at least 3 days after therapy; severe renal impairment; known hypersensitivity (eg; urticaria, erythematous rash, flushing, and fever) to bismuth subcitrate potassium, metronidazole or other nitroimidazole derivatives, or tetracycline.

WARNINGS/PRECAUTIONS

May result in bacterial resistance if used in the absence of a proven or strongly suspected bacterial infection or a prophylactic indication. Caution with hepatic impairment and in the elderly. Bismuth: Neurotoxicity associated with excessive doses reported. May cause temporary and harmless darkening of the tongue and/or black stool. May interfere with x-ray diagnostic procedures of the GI tract. Metronidazole: Encephalopathy, optic and peripheral neuropathy, convulsive seizures, and aseptic meningitis reported. Known or previously unrecognized candidiasis may present more prominent symptoms; treat with an antifungal agent. Caution with evidence of or history of blood dyscrasia. Mild leukopenia reported; obtain total and differential leukocyte counts prior to and after therapy. May interfere with certain types of determinations of serum chemistry values (eg, AST, ALT, LDH, TG, and hexokinase glucose). Tetracycline: May cause fetal harm. May cause permanent teeth discoloration during tooth development (last half of pregnancy, infancy, and childhood to the age of 8 yrs) and enamel hypoplasia; avoid use in this age group. Maternal hepatotoxicity may occur if given during pregnancy at high doses (>2g IV). Pseudotumor cerebri reported. May result in overgrowth of nonsusceptible organisms (eg, fungi); d/c if superinfection occurs. Photosensitivity reported; avoid exposure to the sun or sun lamps and d/c treatment at the 1st evidence of skin erythema. May increase BUN.

ADVERSE REACTIONS

Abnormal feces, nausea, diarrhea, abdominal pain, asthenia, headache, dysgeusia.

DRUG INTERACTIONS

See Contraindications. May alter anticoagulant effects of warfarin and other oral coumarin anticoagulants; monitor PT, INR, or other suitable anticoagulation tests and for evidence of bleeding. Metronidazole: Short-term use may cause elevation of serum lithium concentrations and signs of lithium toxicity with high doses of lithium. Drugs that inhibit microsomal liver enzymes (eg, cimetidine) may decrease plasma clearance and prolong $T_{1/2}$. Drugs that induce microsomal liver enzymes (eg, phenytoin, phenobarbital) may accelerate elimination and reduce plasma concentrations. Impaired clearance of phenytoin reported; monitor phenytoin concentrations. Tetracycline: Oral contraceptives may become less effective and may cause breakthrough bleeding if given concomitantly. Antacids containing aluminum, Ca^{2+}, or Mg^{2+}; preparations containing iron, zinc, or sodium bicarbonate; or milk and dairy products may reduce absorption; do not consume concomitantly. May interfere with bactericidal action of penicillin; avoid coadministration.

PREGNANCY AND LACTATION

Category D, not for use in nursing.

MECHANISM OF ACTION

H. pylori treatment combination; antimicrobial agent. Bismuth: Antibacterial action not well understood. Metronidazole: Metabolized through reductive pathways into reactive intermediates that have cytotoxic action. Tetracycline: Interacts with 30S subunit of the bacterial ribosome and inhibits protein synthesis.

PHARMACOKINETICS

Absorption: Metronidazole: Well-absorbed. Tetracycline: 60-90% (stomach and upper small intestine). Administration of the individual drugs as separate cap formulations or as Pylera resulted in variable pharmacokinetic parameters. **Distribution:** Bismuth: Plasma protein binding (>90%). Metronidazole: Plasma protein binding (<20%); found in breast milk. Tetracycline: Plasma protein binding (varying degrees); crosses placenta, found in breast milk. **Metabolism:** Metronidazole: Side-chain oxidation and glucuronide conjugation. **Elimination:** Bismuth: Urinary, biliary; $T_{1/2}$=5 days (blood and urine). Metronidazole: Urine (60-80%, 20% unchanged), feces (6-15%); $T_{1/2}$=8 hrs (normal patients). Tetracycline: Urine, feces.

PATIENT CONSIDERATIONS

Assessment: Assess for drug hypersensitivity, history of blood dyscrasia, known or previously unrecognized candidiasis, hepatic/renal impairment, pregnancy/nursing status, and possible drug interactions. Obtain total and differential leukocyte counts prior to therapy.

Monitoring: Monitor for encephalopathy, peripheral neuropathy, convulsive seizures, aseptic meningitis, leukopenia, enamel hypoplasia, pseudotumor cerebri, superinfections, photosensitivity reactions, skin erythema, and other adverse reactions. Monitor total and differential leukocyte counts and BUN levels. Monitor PT, INR, or other suitable anticoagulation tests and for evidence of bleeding with warfarin and other oral coumarin anticoagulants.

Counseling: Advise pregnant women that therapy may cause fetal harm. Advise to avoid breastfeeding while on therapy; instruct to d/c feeding or pump and discard breast milk during treatment and for 24 hrs after the last dose. Inform that therapy may cause allergic reactions; instruct to d/c therapy at 1st sign of urticaria, erythematous rash, flushing, fever or other symptoms of an allergic reaction. Inform of the risk of central and peripheral nervous system effects; inform to d/c and notify physician immediately if any neurologic symptoms occur. Instruct to avoid exposure to sun or sun lamps. Advise patients to notify physician of the use of any other medications while on therapy. Inform that temporary and harmless darkening of tongue, and/or black stool may occur. Inform of proper dosing information and instruct to take exactly ud; inform that skipping doses or not completing the full course of therapy may decrease effectiveness and increase likelihood of bacterial resistance. Advise not to take double doses; if a dose is missed, advise to continue normal dosing schedule until medication is gone. Instruct to inform physician if >4 doses are missed. Counsel that therapy should only be used to treat bacterial, not viral (eg, common cold), infections.

PYRAZINAMIDE — pyrazinamide   Rx

Class: Nicotinamide analogue

ADULT DOSAGE	PEDIATRIC DOSAGE
Tuberculosis	**Tuberculosis**
Initial treatment of active tuberculosis (TB) when combined w/ other anti-TB agents and for the use after treatment failure w/ other primary drugs in any form of active TB	Initial treatment of active tuberculosis (TB) when combined w/ other anti-TB agents and for the use after treatment failure w/ other primary drugs in any form of active TB
Usual: 15-30mg/kg qd **Max:** 3g/day	**Usual:** 15-30mg/kg qd **Max:** 3g/day
Alternate Regimen: 50-70mg/kg twice weekly based on lean body weight	**Alternate Regimen:** 50-70mg/kg twice weekly based on lean body weight
Always administer w/ other effective anti-TB drugs; administer for the initial 2 months of a 6-month or longer treatment regimen	Always administer w/ other effective anti-TB drugs; administer for the initial 2 months of a 6-month or longer treatment regimen
Patients w/ HIV infection may require longer courses of therapy	Patients w/ HIV infection may require longer courses of therapy

DOSING CONSIDERATIONS
Renal Impairment
May start at lower end of dosing range

Elderly
Start at lower end of dosing range

ADMINISTRATION
Oral route

STORAGE
20-25°C (68-77°F).

HOW SUPPLIED
Tab: 500mg* *scored

CONTRAINDICATIONS
Severe hepatic damage, hypersensitivity to pyrazinamide, acute gout.

WARNINGS/PRECAUTIONS
Should only be used in conjunction with other effective anti-TB agents. Closely monitor patients with preexisting liver disease or those at increased risk for drug-related hepatitis (eg, alcohol abusers). D/C and do not resume therapy if signs of hepatocellular damage or hyperuricemia with acute gouty arthritis appear. Perform in vitro susceptibility tests with recent cultures of *Mycobacterium tuberculosis* against pyrazinamide and the usual primary drugs in cases with known or suspected drug resistance. Interference with Acetest and Ketostix urine tests to produce a pink-brown color reported. Caution with history of diabetes mellitus (DM) and in elderly.

ADVERSE REACTIONS
Gout, hepatotoxicity, N/V, anorexia, arthralgia, myalgia, rash, urticaria, pruritus.

PREGNANCY AND LACTATION
Category C, caution in nursing.

MECHANISM OF ACTION
Nicotinamide analogue; not established. Suspected to act as bacteriostatic or bactericidal against *M. tuberculosis* depending on the concentration of the drug attained at the site of infection.

PHARMACOKINETICS
Absorption: Well-absorbed from GI tract. T_{max}=2 hrs. **Distribution:** Plasma protein binding (10%); found in breast milk. **Metabolism:** Liver via hydrolysis; pyrazinoic acid (major active metabolite). **Elimination:** Urine (70%); $T_{1/2}$=9-10 hrs.

PATIENT CONSIDERATIONS
Assessment: Assess for risk for drug-related hepatitis, history of DM, drug hypersensitivity, and pregnancy/nursing status. Obtain baseline serum uric acid levels, LFTs, and renal function.

Monitoring: Monitor for drug resistance, signs of hepatocellular damage, hyperuricemia with acute gouty arthritis, and other adverse reactions. Perform appropriate lab testing periodically and if any clinical signs/symptoms occur.

Counseling: Instruct to notify physician if fever, loss of appetite, malaise, N/V, darkened urine, yellowish discoloration of skin and eyes, or joint pain/swelling occurs. Emphasize compliance with full course of therapy and importance of not missing any doses.

PYRIDIUM — phenazopyridine hydrochloride   Rx

Class: Urinary tract analgesic

ADULT DOSAGE	PEDIATRIC DOSAGE
Irritation of Lower Urinary Tract Mucosa	Pediatric use may not have been established
Symptomatic Relief of Pain, Burning, Urgency, Frequency, and Other Discomforts Caused by Infection, Trauma, Surgery, Endoscopic Procedures, or Passage of Sounds/ Catheters:	
Usual: 200mg tid	
Max Duration: 2 days, when used concomitantly w/ an antibacterial agent for treatment of UTI	

ADMINISTRATION
Oral route
Take pc.

STORAGE
20-25°C (68-77°F); excursions permitted to 15-30°C (59-86°F).

HOW SUPPLIED
Tab: 100mg, 200mg

CONTRAINDICATIONS
Hypersensitivity to phenazopyridine HCl, renal insufficiency.

WARNINGS/PRECAUTIONS
D/C when symptoms are controlled. A yellowish tinge of the skin/sclera may indicate accumulation due to impaired renal excretion and the need to d/c therapy. Produces a reddish-orange discoloration of the urine and may stain fabric; staining of contact lenses reported. May interfere with urinalysis based on spectrometry or color reactions.

ADVERSE REACTIONS
Headache, rash, pruritus, GI disturbance, anaphylactoid-like reaction.

PREGNANCY AND LACTATION
Pregnancy: Category B.
Lactation: Safety not known in nursing.

MECHANISM OF ACTION
Urinary tract analgesic; has not been established. Excreted in urine where it exerts a topical analgesic effect on urinary tract mucosa.

PHARMACOKINETICS
Elimination: Urine (as much as 66% unchanged).

PATIENT CONSIDERATIONS
Assessment: Assess for previous hypersensitivity to the drug, renal insufficiency, cause of urinary pain, and pregnancy/nursing status.

Monitoring: Monitor for control of symptoms, development of yellowish tinge of the skin/sclera, and other adverse reactions.

Counseling: Inform that drug produces a reddish-orange discoloration of urine and may stain fabric and contact lenses.

QNASL — beclomethasone dipropionate   Rx

Class: Corticosteroid

ADULT DOSAGE	PEDIATRIC DOSAGE
Seasonal/Perennial Allergic Rhinitis	**Seasonal/Perennial Allergic Rhinitis**
Nasal Symptoms:	**Nasal Symptoms:**
Usual: 2 actuations/nostril qd	**4-11 Years:**
Max: 4 actuations/day	**Usual:** 1 actuation/nostril qd **Max:** 2 actuations/day
	≥12 Years:
	Usual: 2 actuations/nostril qd **Max:** 4 actuations/day

ADMINISTRATION
Intranasal route

Priming
Spray 4X into the air, away from eyes and face.
The dose counter should read 120 after initial priming.
If not used for 7 consecutive days it should be primed by spraying 2X.

STORAGE
25°C (77°F); excursions permitted between 15-30°C (59-86°F). Do not puncture. Do not store near heat or open flame.

HOW SUPPLIED
Aerosol: 40mcg/actuation, 80mcg/actuation [8.7g]

CONTRAINDICATIONS
History of hypersensitivity to beclomethasone dipropionate and/or any other ingredients of the product.

WARNINGS/PRECAUTIONS
Epistaxis, nasal erosions, nasal ulcerations reported; d/c if these occur. *Candida albicans* infections of the nose and pharynx may occur; treat and, if needed, d/c therapy. Monitor for evidence of *Candida* infection or possible changes in the nasal

mucosa periodically during prolonged use. Nasal septal perforation may occur. May impair wound healing; avoid with recent nasal septal ulcers, nasal surgery, or nasal trauma until healed. Glaucoma and/or cataracts may develop; monitor patients with a change in vision or with a history of increased intraocular pressure (IOP), glaucoma, and/or cataracts. Hypersensitivity reactions (eg, anaphylaxis, angioedema, urticaria, rash) may occur; d/c if such reactions develop. May lead to serious/fatal course of chickenpox or measles; avoid exposure and if exposed, consider prophylaxis/treatment. Caution with active or quiescent tuberculous infections, untreated local or systemic fungal or bacterial infections, systemic viral or parasitic infections, or ocular herpes simplex. Risk of adrenal insufficiency and withdrawal symptoms when replacing systemic corticosteroid with topical corticosteroid; monitor closely. D/C slowly if symptoms of hypercorticism and adrenal suppression occur. May reduce growth velocity in pediatric patients. Caution in elderly.

ADVERSE REACTIONS
Nasal discomfort, epistaxis, headache.

PREGNANCY AND LACTATION
Pregnancy: Category C.
Lactation: Caution in nursing.

MECHANISM OF ACTION
Corticosteroid; has not been established. Shown to have multiple anti-inflammatory effects, inhibiting both inflammatory cells (eg, mast cells, eosinophils, basophils, lymphocytes, macrophages, neutrophils) and the release of inflammatory mediators (eg, histamine, eicosanoids, leukotrienes, cytokines).

PHARMACOKINETICS
Absorption: C_{max}=262.7pg/mL (beclomethasone-17-monopropionate [17-BMP]). **Distribution:** Plasma protein binding (94-96%) (17-BMP); V_d=20L, 424L (17-BMP). **Metabolism:** Extensive 1st-pass metabolism via CYP3A4; 17-BMP (major/most active metabolite). **Elimination:** Urine (<10%), feces; $T_{1/2}$=0.3 hr, 4.5 hrs (17-BMP).

PATIENT CONSIDERATIONS
Assessment: Assess for drug hypersensitivity, active or quiescent tuberculous infections, local/systemic infections, ocular herpes simplex, recent nasal ulcers/surgery/trauma, history of increased IOP, glaucoma, cataracts, immunization status, and pregnancy/nursing status.

Monitoring: Monitor for systemic corticosteroid effects (eg, hypercorticism, adrenal suppression), epistaxis, nasal discomfort/ulceration, nasal septal perforation, infections, nasal or pharyngeal *C. albicans* infections, hypersensitivity reactions, growth velocity in children, hypoadrenalism (in infants born to mothers receiving corticosteroids during pregnancy), and other adverse reactions. Monitor for adrenal insufficiency and withdrawal symptoms in the event of replacing systemic corticosteroid with topical corticosteroid.

Counseling: Counsel on appropriate priming and administration. Counsel about risks of epistaxis, nasal ulceration, nasal discomfort, *Candida* infections, and other adverse reactions. Inform that glaucoma and cataracts may develop; instruct to inform physician if visual changes occur. Advise to d/c therapy if hypersensitivity reactions occur. Advise to avoid exposure to chickenpox or measles and to consult physician if exposed. Inform of potential worsening of existing tuberculosis, fungal/bacterial/viral/parasitic infections, or ocular herpes simplex. Instruct to contact physician immediately if symptoms do not improve, or if the condition worsens. Advise to avoid spraying in the eyes or mouth.

QSYMIA — phentermine/topiramate   CIV

Class: Anorectic sympathomimetic amine/sulfamate-substituted monosaccharide

ADULT DOSAGE
Weight Loss

Adjunct to a reduced-calorie diet and increased physical activity for chronic weight management in patients w/ initial BMI ≥30kg/m^2, or ≥27kg/m^2 in the presence of ≥1 weight-related comorbidity

Initial: 3.75mg/23mg qd for 14 days
Titrate: After 14 days, increase to 7.5mg/46mg qd; d/c or escalate dose if patient has not lost at least 3% of baseline weight after 12 weeks
Dose Escalation: Increase to 11.25mg/69mg qd for 14 days, followed by 15mg/92mg qd; d/c if patient has not lost at least 5% of baseline weight after 12 weeks on 15mg/92mg

Use 3.75mg/23mg and 11.25mg/69mg strengths for titration purposes only

Discontinuation: D/C 15mg/92mg gradually by taking a dose qod for at least 1 week prior to stopping treatment

PEDIATRIC DOSAGE
Pediatric use may not have been established

DOSING CONSIDERATIONS
Renal Impairment
Moderate (CrCl ≥30-<50mL/min) to Severe (CrCl <30mL/min):
Max: 7.5mg/46mg qd

ESRD on Dialysis:
Avoid use

Hepatic Impairment
Moderate (Child-Pugh Score 7-9):
Max: 7.5mg/46mg qd

Severe (Child-Pugh Score 10-15):
Avoid use

Elderly
Start at lower end of dosing range

ADMINISTRATION
Oral route

Take w/ or w/o food.
Take qam; avoid pm dosing due to the possibility of insomnia.

STORAGE
15-25°C (59-77°F). Protect from moisture.

HOW SUPPLIED
Cap, Extended-Release: (Phentermine/Topiramate) 3.75mg/23mg, 7.5mg/46mg, 11.25mg/69mg, 15mg/92mg

CONTRAINDICATIONS
Pregnancy, glaucoma, hyperthyroidism, during or w/in 14 days of administration of MAOIs, known hypersensitivity or idiosyncrasy to the sympathomimetic amines.

WARNINGS/PRECAUTIONS
May cause fetal harm; use effective contraception to prevent pregnancy. Available through a limited program under the Risk Evaluation and Mitigation Strategy. May increase resting HR; monitor resting HR regularly in all patients, especially those with cardiac or cerebrovascular disease or when initiating or increasing dose. Reduce dose or d/c if sustained increase in resting HR or persistent SrCr elevations occur. Increased risk of suicidal thoughts/behavior; monitor for emergence/worsening of depression, suicidal thoughts/behavior, and/or any unusual changes in mood or behavior, and d/c if these occur. Avoid with history of suicidal attempts or active suicidal ideation. Acute myopia associated with secondary angle-closure glaucoma reported; d/c immediately to reverse symptoms. Mood/sleep disorders, including anxiety and insomnia, may occur; consider dose reduction or withdrawal for clinically significant or persistent symptoms. May impair physical/mental abilities; consider dose reduction or withdrawal if cognitive dysfunction persists. Hyperchloremic, non-anion gap, metabolic acidosis reported. Conditions that predispose to acidosis (eg, renal disease, severe respiratory disorders, status epilepticus, diarrhea, surgery, ketogenic diet) may be additive to the bicarbonate lowering effects of topiramate. Weight loss may increase risk of hypoglycemia in patients with type 2 DM treated with insulin and/or insulin secretagogues (eg, sulfonylureas), and risk of hypotension in those treated with antihypertensives; appropriate changes should be made to antidiabetic or antihypertensive therapy if hypoglycemia or hypotension develops. Seizures associated with abrupt withdrawal in individuals without history of seizures or epilepsy; taper dose gradually if using 15mg/92mg and monitor for seizures in situations where immediate termination of therapy is required. Avoid with ESRD on dialysis or severe hepatic impairment (Child-Pugh 10-15). Associated with kidney stone formation; increase fluid intake to increase urine output. Oligohidrosis reported; monitor for decreased sweating and increased body temperature during physical activity, especially in hot weather. May increase risk of hypokalemia. Potential for abuse. Lab test interactions may occur. Caution in elderly.

ADVERSE REACTIONS
Paresthesia, dry mouth, constipation, URTI, headache, dysgeusia, insomnia, nasopharyngitis, dizziness, sinusitis, bronchitis, nausea, back pain, diarrhea, blurred vision.

DRUG INTERACTIONS
See Contraindications. May decrease exposure of ethinyl estradiol and increase exposure of norethindrone with single dose of oral contraceptive. Alcohol or CNS depressants (eg, barbiturates, benzodiazepines, sleep medications) may potentiate CNS depression. May potentiate the K$^+$ wasting action of non-K$^+$-sparing diuretics; monitor for hypokalemia. Avoid with other drugs that inhibit carbonic anhydrase (eg, zonisamide, acetazolamide, methazolamide, dichlorphenamide); may increase severity of metabolic acidosis and kidney stone formation. Caution with other drugs that predispose patients to heat-related disorders (eg, other carbonic anhydrase inhibitors, drugs with anticholinergic activity). Phenytoin or carbamazepine may decrease plasma levels. Concurrent administration of valproic acid has been associated with hyperammonemia with or without encephalopathy, and hypothermia.

PREGNANCY AND LACTATION
Pregnancy: Category X.
Lactation: Not for use in nursing.

MECHANISM OF ACTION
Phentermine: Anorectic sympathomimetic amine; has not been established. Releases catecholamines in the hypothalamus, resulting in reduced appetite and decreased food consumption. Topiramate: Sulfamate-substituted monosaccharide; has not been established. Effect may be due to its effects on both appetite suppression and satiety enhancement, induced by combination of pharmacologic effects including augmenting the activity of the neurotransmitter gamma-aminobutyrate, modulation of voltage-gated ion channels, inhibition of AMPA/kainite excitatory glutamate receptors, or inhibition of carbonic anhydrase.

PHARMACOKINETICS
Absorption: (15mg-92mg Single Dose) Phentermine: C_{max}=49.1ng/mL, T_{max}=6 hrs, AUC_{0-t}=1990ng•hr/mL, AUC_{0-inf}=2000ng•hr/mL. Topiramate: C_{max}=1020ng/mL, T_{max}=9 hrs, AUC_{0-t}=61,600ng•hr/mL, AUC_{0-inf}=68,000ng•hr/mL. **Distribution:** Found in breast milk; Phentermine: V_d=348L; plasma protein binding (17.5%). Topiramate: Plasma protein binding (15-41%). **Metabolism:** Phentermine: CYP3A4 by p-hydroxylation and N-oxidation. Topiramate: Hydroxylation, hydrolysis,

glucuronidation. **Elimination:** Phentermine: Urine (70-80% unchanged); $T_{1/2}$=20 hrs. Topiramate: Urine (70% unchanged); $T_{1/2}$=65 hrs.

PATIENT CONSIDERATIONS

Assessment: Assess for known hypersensitivity or idiosyncrasy to sympathomimetic amines, glaucoma, hyperthyroidism, cardiac and cerebrovascular disease, history of behavioral/mood disorders, history of seizures, renal/hepatic dysfunction, any other conditions where treatment is contraindicated or cautioned, pregnancy/nursing status, and possible drug interactions. Obtain baseline HR and blood chemistry profile (eg, bicarbonate, creatinine, K^+, glucose).

Monitoring: Monitor for acute myopia, secondary angle-closure glaucoma, emergence/worsening of depression, suicidal thoughts or behavior, mood/sleep disorders, cognitive dysfunction, hyperchloremic metabolic acidosis, seizures, kidney stone formation, oligohidrosis, and hyperthermia. Monitor HR regularly and blood chemistry profile (eg, bicarbonate, creatinine, K^+, glucose) periodically. Assess pregnancy status monthly during therapy.

Counseling: Inform that therapy is for chronic weight management in conjunction with a reduced-calorie diet and increased physical activity. Inform that drug is only available through certified pharmacies. Instruct to inform physician about all medications, nutritional supplements, and vitamins (including any weight loss products) taken while on therapy. Instruct on how to properly take the medication. Instruct to avoid pregnancy/breastfeeding while on therapy and to notify physician immediately if patient becomes pregnant during treatment. Advise to report symptoms of sustained periods of heart pounding or racing while at rest, suicidal behavior/ideation, mood changes, depression, severe/persistent eye pain or significant visual changes, any changes in attention/concentration/memory, and/or difficulty finding words. Advise not to drive/operate machinery until reaction to the medication is known. Instruct to notify physician about any factors that can increase the risk of acidosis (eg, prolonged diarrhea, surgery, high protein/low carbohydrate diet, and/or concomitant medications such as other carbonic anhydrase inhibitors) and to avoid alcohol while on therapy. Instruct diabetic patients to monitor blood glucose levels and to report symptoms of hypoglycemia to physician. Advise not to abruptly d/c therapy without notifying physician. Advise to increase fluid intake and report symptoms of severe side or back pain, and/or blood in urine to physician. Advise to monitor for decreased sweating and increased body temperature during physical activity, especially in hot weather.

QUALAQUIN — *quinine sulfate*   Rx

Class: Cinchona alkaloid

> Use for treatment/prevention of nocturnal leg cramps may result in serious and life-threatening hematological reactions (eg, thrombocytopenia and hemolytic uremic syndrome/thrombotic thrombocytopenic purpura [HUS/TTP]). Chronic renal impairment associated with the development of TTP reported. Risks associated with therapy for treatment/prevention of nocturnal leg cramps outweighs any potential benefits.

ADULT DOSAGE	PEDIATRIC DOSAGE
Malaria	**Malaria**
Treatment of Uncomplicated *Plasmodium falciparum* Malaria: 648mg (2 caps) q8h for 7 days	**Treatment of Uncomplicated *Plasmodium falciparum* Malaria:** **≥16 Years:** 648mg (2 caps) q8h for 7 days

DOSING CONSIDERATIONS
Renal Impairment
Severe Chronic:
LD: 648mg
Maint: 324mg q12h, starting 12 hrs after LD

Hepatic Impairment
Severe (Child-Pugh C): Avoid use

ADMINISTRATION
Oral route
Take w/ food

STORAGE
20-25°C (68-77°F).

HOW SUPPLIED
Cap: 324mg

CONTRAINDICATIONS
Prolonged QT interval, G6PD deficiency, known hypersensitivity reactions to quinine, known hypersensitivity to mefloquine or quinidine, myasthenia gravis, optic neuritis.

WARNINGS/PRECAUTIONS
Not for severe or complicated *P. falciparum* malaria or prevention of malaria. May cause immune-mediated thrombocytopenia that is more severe and more rapid in onset on subsequent reexposure. QT prolongation, ventricular arrhythmias, and concentration-dependent PR and QRS intervals prolongation reported; caution with risk factors and conditions causing PR or QRS intervals prolongation. Serious hypersensitivity reactions reported; d/c if any signs/symptoms of hypersensitivity occur. Caution with atrial fibrillation, atrial flutter, and chronic renal/hepatic impairment. May cause hypoglycemia, especially in pregnancy. Do not administer in patients with severe (Child-Pugh C) hepatic impairment.

ADVERSE REACTIONS
Headache, vasodilation/sweating, N/V, tinnitus, hearing impairment, vertigo/dizziness, blurred vision, disturbance in color perception, diarrhea, abdominal pain, deafness, blindness, disturbance in cardiac rhythm or conduction.

DRUG INTERACTIONS
Not recommended with drugs known to prolong QT interval (eg, Class IA and Class III antiarrhythmic agents). Fatal torsades de pointes with concomitant quinine, erythromycin, and dopamine. Avoid with CYP3A4 substrates with QT prolongation potential (eg, astemizole, cisapride, terfenadine, halofantrine, pimozide, quinidine), rifampin, antacids containing aluminum and/or Mg^{2+}, macrolide antibiotics (eg, erythromycin, troleandomycin), and ritonavir. May enhance the neuromuscular blocking effects of neuromuscular blocking agents; avoid concomitant use. Decreased levels with carbamazepine, phenobarbital, and phenytoin. Monitor for quinine-associated adverse events when used with tetracycline, ranitidine, cimetidine, ketoconazole, theophylline, or aminophylline. Monitor for adverse reactions of CYP2D6 substrates, carbamazepine, phenytoin, and phenobarbital. Urinary alkalinizing agents may increase levels. May increase levels of atorvastatin and other statins that are CYP3A4 substrates (eg, simvastatin, lovastatin), thereby increasing the risk of myopathy and rhabdomyolysis; d/c statin if marked CPK elevation occurs or myopathy is diagnosed/suspected. May increase levels of halofantrine and mefloquine, which may result in ECG abnormalities. May increase risk of seizure with mefloquine. May reduce biliary clearance of digoxin; monitor digoxin levels and adjust digoxin dose as necessary. May interfere with anticoagulant effects of heparin and enhance action of warfarin and other oral anticoagulants; monitor PT, PTT, and INR.

PREGNANCY AND LACTATION
Category C, caution in nursing.

MECHANISM OF ACTION
Cinchona alkaloid; inhibits nucleic acid synthesis, protein synthesis, and glycolysis in *P. falciparum* and can bind with hemazoin in parasitized erythrocytes.

PHARMACOKINETICS
Absorption: Bioavailability (76-88%). C_{max}=8.4mcg/mL, T_{max}=5.9 hrs, AUC_{0-12}=73mcg•hr/mL. **Distribution:** V_d=2.5-7.1L/kg (600mg single oral dose); plasma protein binding (78-95%); crosses placenta, found in breast milk. **Metabolism:** Liver oxidation via CYP3A4; 3-hydroxyquinine (major metabolite). **Elimination:** Urine (20% unchanged); $T_{1/2}$=9.7-12.5 hrs.

PATIENT CONSIDERATIONS
Assessment: Assess the severity of *P. falciparum* malaria and cardiac function, Assess for prolonged QT interval, G6PD deficiency, myasthenia gravis, optic neuritis, hypersensitivity, renal/hepatic impairment, pregnancy/nursing status, and possible drug interactions.

Monitoring: Monitor platelet function, renal/hepatic/cardiac function, glucose levels. Monitor for hypersensitivity, QT prolongation, and other adverse reactions.

Counseling: Discuss risks and benefits of therapy. Instruct to take ud. Counsel not to double the next dose if a dose is missed; if >4 hrs has elapsed since the missed dose, instruct to wait and take the next dose as previously scheduled. Advise to seek medical attention if any signs/symptoms of adverse effects develop.

QUDEXY XR — *topiramate*   Rx

Class: Sulfamate-substituted monosaccharide antiepileptic

ADULT DOSAGE
Epilepsy
Monotherapy:
Partial Onset Seizures or Primary Generalized Tonic-Clonic Seizures:

Usual: 400mg qd
Titration Schedule:
Week 1: 50mg qd
Week 2: 100mg qd
Week 3: 150mg qd
Week 4: 200mg qd
Week 5: 300mg qd
Week 6: 400mg qd

Adjunctive Therapy:
Partial Onset Seizures, Primary Generalized Tonic-Clonic Seizures, or Lennox-Gastaut Syndrome:

≥17 Years:
Initial: 25-50mg qd
Titrate: Increase in increments of 25-50mg every week to achieve effective dose
Usual:
Partial Onset Seizures or Lennox-Gastaut Syndrome: 200-400mg qd
Primary Generalized Tonic-Clonic Seizures: 400mg qd

Titrate: May increase to 50mg qd in the 2nd week, then by 25-50mg qd each subsequent week. Titration to the minimum maint dose should be attempted over 5-7 weeks; additional titration to a higher dose (up to the max maint dose) can be attempted in weekly increments by 25-50mg qd, up to the max recommended maint dose for each range of body weight

Up to 11kg:
Minimum Maint Dose: 150mg/day
Max Maint Dose: 250mg/day
12-22kg:
Minimum Maint Dose: 200mg/day
Max Maint Dose: 300mg/day
23-31kg:
Minimum Maint Dose: 200mg/day
Max Maint Dose: 350mg/day
32-38kg:
Minimum Maint Dose: 250mg/day
Max Maint Dose: 350mg/day
>38kg:
Minimum Maint Dose: 250mg/day
Max Maint Dose: 400mg/day

≥10 Years:
Usual: 400mg qd
Titration Schedule:
Week 1: 50mg qd
Week 2: 100mg qd
Week 3: 150mg qd
Week 4: 200mg qd
Week 5: 300mg qd
Week 6: 400mg qd

Adjunctive Therapy:
Partial Onset Seizures, Primary Generalized Tonic-Clonic Seizures, or

PEDIATRIC DOSAGE

Epilepsy

Monotherapy:
Partial Onset Seizures or Primary Generalized Tonic-Clonic Seizures:
2-<10 Years:
Initial: 25mg qpm for the 1st week

Lennox-Gastaut Syndrome:
2-16 Years:
Usual: 5-9mg/kg qd
Titrate: Begin titration at 25mg qpm (based on a range of 1-3mg/kg/day) for 1st week. Subsequently, increase at 1- or 2-week intervals by increments of 1-3mg/kg to achieve optimal clinical response; longer intervals between dose adjustments may be used if required

---

DOSING CONSIDERATIONS
Concomitant Medications
Phenytoin and/or Carbamazepine
May require an adjustment of the dose of phenytoin to achieve optimal clinical outcome.
Addition or withdrawal of phenytoin and/or carbamazepine during adjunctive therapy may require dose adjustment of topiramate.

Renal Impairment
CrCl <70mL/min: Use 1/2 the usual starting and maint dose
Hemodialysis: Supplemental dose may be required

ADMINISTRATION
Oral route
May take w/o regard to meals.
May swallow whole or carefully open and sprinkle entire contents on a small amount (tsp) of soft food; swallow drug/food mixture immediately and do not chew/crush.

STORAGE
20-25°C (68-77°F); excursions permitted to 15-30°C (59-86°F). Protect from moisture.

HOW SUPPLIED
Cap, Extended-Release: 25mg, 50mg, 100mg, 150mg, 200mg

CONTRAINDICATIONS
Patients w/ metabolic acidosis taking concomitant metformin.

WARNINGS/PRECAUTIONS
Acute myopia associated w/ secondary angle-closure glaucoma reported; d/c as rapidly as possible to reverse symptoms. Visual field defects reported in patients independent of elevated IOP; consider discontinuing therapy if visual problems occur. Oligohydrosis and hyperthermia reported, mostly in pediatric patients; monitor for decreased sweating and increased body temperature. Hyperchloremic, non-anion gap, metabolic acidosis reported; conditions or therapies that predispose to acidosis may be additive to the bicarbonate lowering effects. Consider discontinuing or reducing dose if metabolic acidosis develops/persists. If decision is to continue therapy, consider alkali treatment. Increased risk of suicidal thoughts/behavior; monitor for the emergence/worsening of depression, suicidal thoughts/behavior, and/or any unusual changes in mood or behavior. Cognitive-related dysfunction, psychiatric/behavioral disturbances, and somnolence or fatigue reported. May cause fetal harm; increased risk for cleft lip and/or palate in infants if used during pregnancy. Gradually withdraw therapy to minimize the potential for seizures or increased seizure frequency; appropriate monitoring is recommended when rapid withdrawal is required. Patients w/ inborn errors of metabolism or reduced hepatic mitochondrial activity may be at an increased risk for hyperammonemia w/ or w/o encephalopathy; consider hyperammonemic encephalopathy and measure ammonia levels in patients who develop unexplained lethargy, vomiting, or changes in mental status associated w/ therapy. Kidney stone formation reported; hydration is recommended to reduce new stone formation. Paresthesia may occur.

ADVERSE REACTIONS
Anorexia, anxiety, dizziness, fatigue, fever, infection, weight decrease, cognitive problems, paresthesia, somnolence, psychomotor slowing, mood problems, difficulty w/ memory, nervousness, confusion.

DRUG INTERACTIONS
See Dosing Considerations and Contraindications. May decrease contraceptive efficacy and increase breakthrough bleeding w/ combination oral contraceptives. Phenytoin or carbamazepine may decrease levels. Concomitant administration of valproic acid has been associated w/ hyperammonemia w/ or w/o encephalopathy and hypothermia. Concomitant administration w/ other CNS depressants or alcohol can result in significant CNS depression; use w/ extreme caution and avoid w/ alcohol. Concomitant use w/ other carbonic anhydrase inhibitors (eg, zonisamide, acetazolamide, dichlorphenamide) may increase the severity of metabolic acidosis and may also increase the risk of kidney stone formation; monitor for appearance or worsening of metabolic acidosis. Increase in systemic exposure of lithium observed following topiramate doses of ≤600mg/day; monitor lithium levels. Caution w/ agents that predispose patients to heat-related disorders (eg, carbonic anhydrase inhibitors, anticholinergics).

PREGNANCY AND LACTATION
Pregnancy: Category D.
Lactation: Caution in nursing.

MECHANISM OF ACTION
Sulfamate-substituted monosaccharide antiepileptic; has not been established. Suspected to block voltage-dependent Na⁺ channels, augment activity of the neurotransmitter gamma-aminobutyrate at some subtypes of the GABA-A receptor, antagonize the AMPA/kainate subtype of the glutamate receptor, and inhibit the carbonic anhydrase enzyme, particularly isoenzymes II and IV.

PHARMACOKINETICS
Absorption: T_{max}=approx 20 hrs (200mg). **Distribution:** Plasma protein binding (15-41%). Found in breast milk. **Metabolism:** Hydroxylation, hydrolysis, glucuronidation. **Elimination:** Urine (approx 70% unchanged); $T_{1/2}$=approx 56 hrs.

PATIENT CONSIDERATIONS
Assessment: Assess for metabolic acidosis in patients taking concomitant metformin, predisposing factors for metabolic acidosis, renal dysfunction, inborn errors of metabolism, reduced hepatic mitochondrial activity, pregnancy/nursing status, and possible drug interactions. Obtain baseline serum bicarbonate, CrCl, and blood ammonia levels.

Monitoring: Monitor for signs/symptoms of acute myopia, secondary angle-closure glaucoma, visual field defects, oligohydrosis, hyperthermia, depression or suicidal thoughts/behavior, cognitive or neuropsychiatric adverse reactions, kidney stones, renal dysfunction, metabolic acidosis, paresthesia, hyperammonemia, and other adverse reactions. Monitor serum bicarbonate and blood ammonia levels.

Counseling: Instruct to take only as prescribed. Instruct to seek immediate medical attention if blurred vision, visual disturbances, periorbital pain, high or persistent fever, or decreased sweating occurs. Inform about the risk for metabolic acidosis that may be asymptomatic and may be associated w/ adverse effects on kidneys, bones, and growth in pediatric patients, and on the fetus. Instruct to immediately report to the physician if emergence or worsening of depression, unusual changes in mood/behavior, emergence of suicidal thoughts, or behavior/thoughts about self-harm occur. Advise to use caution when engaging in activities where loss of consciousness may result in serious danger. Inform of pregnancy risks; encourage pregnant women to enroll in the North American Antiepileptic Drug Pregnancy Registry. Warn about possible development of hyperammonemia w/ or w/o encephalopathy; instruct to contact physician if unexplained lethargy, vomiting, or mental status changes develop. Instruct to maintain adequate fluid intake to minimize risk of kidney stones. Inform that therapy may cause reduction in body temperature that can lead to alterations in mental status; if changes are noted, instruct to measure body temperature and contact physician. Instruct to consult physician if tingling in the arms and legs occurs.

QUILLICHEW ER — methylphenidate hydrochloride   CII
Class: CNS stimulant

> **High potential for abuse and dependence; assess risk of abuse prior to prescribing, and monitor for signs of abuse/dependence while on therapy.**

ADULT DOSAGE
Attention-Deficit Hyperactivity Disorder

Initial: 20mg qam
Titrate: May increase or decrease weekly in increments of 10mg, 15mg, or 20mg
Max: 60mg/day

D/C if improvement is not observed after appropriate dose adjustment over a 1-month period

Conversions

Switching from Other Methylphenidate Products:
D/C other treatment, and titrate w/ QuilliChew ER using above titration schedule

Do not substitute for other methylphenidate products on a mg-per-mg basis

PEDIATRIC DOSAGE
Attention-Deficit Hyperactivity Disorder

≥6 Years:
Initial: 20mg qam
Titrate: May increase or decrease weekly in increments of 10mg, 15mg, or 20mg
Max: 60mg/day

Periodically d/c to assess the child's condition.

D/C if improvement is not observed after appropriate dose adjustment over a 1-month period.

Conversions

Switching from Other Methylphenidate Products:
D/C other treatment, and titrate w/ QuilliChew ER using above titration schedule

Do not substitute for other methylphenidate products on a mg-per-mg basis

---

DOSING CONSIDERATIONS
Adverse Reactions
If paradoxical aggravation of symptoms or other adverse effects occur, reduce dose or, if necessary, d/c therapy

ADMINISTRATION
Oral route
Take w/ or w/o food.

STORAGE
20-25°C (68-77°F); excursions permitted from 15-30°C (59-86°F).

HOW SUPPLIED
Chewable Tab, Extended-Release: 20mg*, 30mg*, 40mg *scored

CONTRAINDICATIONS
Hypersensitivity to methylphenidate or other components of QuilliChew ER. Concomitant treatment w/ MAOIs and w/in 14 days following discontinuation of treatment w/ an MAOI.

WARNINGS/PRECAUTIONS
Sudden death, stroke, and MI reported in adults. Sudden death reported in pediatric patients w/ structural cardiac abnormalities and other serious cardiac problems. Avoid use w/ known structural cardiac abnormalities, cardiomyopathy, serious cardiac arrhythmias, coronary artery disease, or other serious cardiac problems. Evaluate patients who develop exertional chest pain, unexplained

syncope, or arrhythmias during treatment. May cause an increase in BP/HR; monitor for HTN and tachycardia. May exacerbate symptoms of behavior disturbance and thought disorder in patients w/ a preexisting psychotic disorder. May induce a manic or mixed episode in patients w/ bipolar disorder; screen patients for risk factors for developing a manic episode prior to initiation of treatment. May cause psychotic or manic symptoms in patients w/o prior history of psychotic illness or mania; consider discontinuing treatment if symptoms occur. Priapism reported. Associated w/ peripheral vasculopathy (eg, Raynaud's phenomenon); carefully monitor digital changes. Associated w/ weight loss and slowing of growth rate in pediatric patients; closely monitor growth and may need to interrupt treatment in patients who are not growing or gaining height or weight as expected. Contains phenylalanine; caution w/ phenylketonuria.

ADVERSE REACTIONS
Decreased appetite, aggression, emotional poverty, nausea, headache, decreased weight.

DRUG INTERACTIONS
See Contraindications.

PREGNANCY AND LACTATION
Pregnancy: Can cause vasoconstriction and thereby decrease placental perfusion. Premature delivery and low birth weight infants have been reported in amphetamine-dependent mothers.
Lactation: Present in human milk; caution in nursing. Monitor breastfeeding infants for adverse reactions (eg, agitation, insomnia, anorexia, reduced weight gain).

MECHANISM OF ACTION
CNS stimulant; thought to block the reuptake of norepinephrine and dopamine into the presynaptic neuron and increase release of these monoamines into extraneuronal space.

PHARMACOKINETICS
Absorption: T_{max}=5 hrs (median, 40mg single dose). **Distribution:** Found in breast milk. **Metabolism:** Via deesterification to α-phenyl-piperidine acetic acid [PPAA] (metabolite). **Elimination:** Urine (90%, 80% PPAA), $T_{1/2}$=approx 5.2 hrs (40mg single dose).

PATIENT CONSIDERATIONS

Assessment: Assess for drug hypersensitivity, cardiac problems, psychotic disorders, bipolar disorder, phenylketonuria, pregnancy/nursing status, and for possible drug interactions. Obtain baseline height/weight in children. Screen patients for risk factors for developing a manic episode and the risk of abuse before starting therapy.

Monitoring: Monitor for stroke, MI, HTN, tachycardia, exacerbations of behavior disturbances and thought disorders, psychotic or manic symptoms, digital changes, priapism, and other adverse reactions. Monitor growth in children. Monitor for signs of abuse and dependence. Periodically reevaluate long-term usefulness.

Counseling: Inform patients/families/caregivers about risks, benefits, and appropriate use of treatment. Advise that there is a potential for serious cardiovascular risks; instruct to contact healthcare provider immediately if symptoms such as exertional chest pain, unexplained syncope, or other symptoms suggestive of cardiac disease develop. Advise that treatment may elevate BP/HR. Inform that treatment can cause psychotic/manic symptoms. Instruct to seek immediate medical attention in the event of priapism. Inform of the risk of peripheral vasculopathy, including Raynaud's phenomenon and instruct to report to physician if symptoms occur (eg, new numbness, pain, skin color change, sensitivity to temperature in fingers or toes, unexplained wounds on fingers or toes). Advise that treatment can cause slowing of growth and weight loss. Advise patients to avoid alcohol during treatment. Inform that drug contains phenylalanine.

QUILLIVANT XR — methylphenidate hydrochloride   CII

Class: CNS stimulant

> High potential for abuse and dependence. Assess the risk of abuse prior to prescribing, and monitor for signs of abuse and dependence while on therapy.

ADULT DOSAGE	PEDIATRIC DOSAGE
Attention-Deficit Hyperactivity Disorder	**Attention-Deficit Hyperactivity Disorder**
Initial: 20mg qam	**≥6 Years:**
Titrate: May be titrated weekly in increments of 10mg to 20mg	**Initial:** 20mg qam
	Titrate: May be titrated weekly in increments of 10mg to 20mg
Daily doses >60mg have not been studied and are not recommended.	Daily doses >60mg have not been studied and are not recommended.
D/C if improvement is not observed after appropriate dose adjustment over a 1-month period.	Periodically d/c to assess the child's condition.
	D/C if improvement is not observed after appropriate dose adjustment over a 1-month period.

DOSING CONSIDERATIONS
Adverse Reactions
If paradoxical aggravation of symptoms or other adverse effects occur, reduce dose or, if necessary, d/c therapy

ADMINISTRATION
Oral route

Take w/ or w/o food.
Vigorously shake bottle for at least 10 sec before each dose to ensure that the proper dose is administered.
Use only w/ the oral dosing dispenser provided.

Reconstitution Instructions for Pharmacist
- Supplied as a powder for oral sus; must be reconstituted w/ water prior to dispensing.
- Tap bottle until powder flows freely. Remove bottle cap, and add specified amount of water to the bottle (see below). Insert bottle adapter into neck of bottle, replace bottle cap, and shake vigorously for at least 10 sec to prepare sus.
300mg Bottle: Add 53mL of water; final reconstituted volume is 60mL
600mg Bottle: Add 105mL of water; final reconstituted volume is 120mL
750mg Bottle: Add 131mL of water; final reconstituted volume is 150mL
900mg Bottle: Add 158mL of water; final reconstituted volume is 180mL
Store reconstituted sus at 25°C (77°F); excursions permitted from 15-30°C (59-86°F); stable for up to 4 months after reconstitution.

STORAGE
25°C (77°F); excursions permitted from 15-30°C (59-86°F). Dispense in original container.

HOW SUPPLIED
Oral Sus, Extended-Release: 5mg/mL [60mL, 120mL, 150mL, 180mL]

CONTRAINDICATIONS
Known hypersensitivity to methylphenidate, or other components of the product. Concomitant treatment w/ MAOIs and w/in 14 days following discontinuation of treatment w/ an MAOI.

WARNINGS/PRECAUTIONS
Sudden death reported in children and adolescents w/ structural cardiac abnormalities and other serious cardiac problems. Sudden death, stroke, and MI reported in adults. Avoid use w/ known structural cardiac abnormalities, cardiomyopathy, serious cardiac arrhythmias, coronary artery disease, or other serious cardiac problems. Evaluate patients who develop exertional chest pain, unexplained syncope, or arrhythmias during treatment. May cause an increase in BP/HR. May exacerbate symptoms of behavior disturbance and thought disorder in patients w/ a preexisting psychotic disorder. May induce a manic or mixed episode in patients w/ bipolar disorder; screen patients for risk factors for developing a manic episode prior to initiation of treatment. May cause psychotic or manic symptoms in patients w/o prior history of psychotic illness or mania; consider discontinuing treatment if symptoms occur. Priapism reported. Associated w/ peripheral vasculopathy, including Raynaud's phenomenon; carefully monitor for digital changes. Associated w/ weight loss and slowing of growth rate in pediatric patients; closely monitor growth and may need to interrupt treatment in patients who are not growing or gaining height or weight as expected.

ADVERSE REACTIONS
Affect lability, excoriation, initial insomnia, tic, decreased appetite, vomiting, motion sickness, eye pain, rash.

DRUG INTERACTIONS
See Contraindications.

PREGNANCY AND LACTATION
Pregnancy: CNS stimulant medications, such as Quillivant XR, can cause vasoconstriction and thereby decrease placental perfusion. Premature delivery and low birth weight infants have been reported in amphetamine-dependent mothers.
Lactation: Limited published literature reports that methylphenidate is present in human milk. Caution in nursing. Monitor breastfeeding infants for adverse reactions, such as agitation, insomnia, anorexia, and reduced weight gain.

MECHANISM OF ACTION
CNS stimulant; thought to block the reuptake of norepinephrine and dopamine into the presynaptic neuron and increase the release of these monoamines into the extraneuronal space.

PHARMACOKINETICS
Absorption: d-methylphenidate: C_{max}=34.4ng/mL (children), 21.1ng/mL (adolescents), 17ng/mL (healthy adults); T_{max}=4.05 hrs (median, children), 2 hrs (median, adolescents), 4 hrs (median, healthy adults); AUC_{inf}=378hr•ng/mL (children), 178hr•ng/mL (adolescents), 163.2hr•ng/mL (healthy adults). **Distribution:** Found in breast milk. **Metabolism:** Via deesterification to α-phenyl-piperidine acetic acid [PPAA] (metabolite). **Elimination:** Urine (90%, 80% PPAA); (d-methylphenidate) $T_{1/2}$=5.2 hrs (children/healthy adults), 5 hrs (adolescents).

PATIENT CONSIDERATIONS

Assessment: Assess for drug hypersensitivity, cardiac problems, psychotic disorders, bipolar disorder, pregnancy/nursing status, and for possible drug interactions. Obtain baseline height/weight in children. Screen patients for risk factors for developing a manic episode and the risk of abuse before starting therapy.

Monitoring: Monitor for stroke, MI, HTN, tachycardia, exacerbations of behavior disturbances and thought disorders, psychotic or manic symptoms, digital changes, priapism, and other adverse reactions. Monitor growth in children. Monitor for signs of abuse and dependence. Periodically reevaluate long-term usefulness.

Counseling: Inform about risks, benefits, and appropriate use of treatment. Counsel that drug has potential for abuse and dependence; instruct to keep medication in a safe place to prevent abuse. Advise of the potential for serious cardiovascular risks, including sudden death, MI, and stroke; instruct to contact physician immediately if symptoms, such as exertional chest pain, unexplained syncope, or other symptoms suggestive of cardiac disease develop. Advise that the drug can elevate BP and HR. Inform that treatment can cause psychotic or manic symptoms even in patients w/o a prior history of psychotic symptoms or mania. Advise that therapy can cause slowing of growth and weight loss. Advise of the possibility of priapism; instruct to seek immediate medical attention in the event of priapism. Inform about the risk of peripheral vasculopathy, including Raynaud's phenomenon; instruct to report to the physician any numbness, pain, skin color change, sensitivity to temperature in fingers or toes, and any signs of unexplained wounds appearing on fingers or toes. Instruct to inform physician if pregnant/intending to become pregnant during therapy. Advise of the potential fetal effects from use during pregnancy.

QUINIDINE SULFATE — quinidine sulfate　　　　Rx

Class: Class IA antiarrhythmic/schizonticide antimalarial

> Increased mortality reported w/ non-life-threatening arrhythmias; risk is greatest w/ structural heart disease. Meta-analysis described that mortality was >3X as great as placebo when used to prevent or defer recurrence of A-flutter/A-fib. Another meta-analysis showed that mortality was greater than that associated w/ alternative antiarrhythmics in patients w/ non-life-threatening ventricular arrhythmias.

ADULT DOSAGE

Atrial Fibrillation/Flutter

Conversion to Sinus Rhythm:
Extended-Release (ER) Tab:
Initial: 300mg q8-12h
Dose may be cautiously raised if regimen is well tolerated, serum level is w/in therapeutic range, and regimen has not resulted in conversion

Tab:
Initial: 400mg q6h
Cautiously increase dose if conversion not achieved after 4 or 5 doses of this regimen

D/C therapy and consider other means of conversion (eg, direct-current cardioversion) if QRS complex widens to 130% of its pretreatment duration, QTc interval widens to 130% of its pretreatment duration and is longer than 500 msec; P waves disappear, or patient if develops significant tachycardia, symptomatic bradycardia, or hypotension

Reduction of Frequency of Relapse into A-Fib/A-Flutter:
ER Tab:
Initial: 300mg q8-12h
Tab:
Initial: 200mg q6h

Dose may be cautiously raised if regimen is well tolerated, serum level is w/in therapeutic range, and average time between arrhythmic episodes have not been satisfactorily increased

Reduce total daily dose if QRS complex widens to 130% of its pretreatment duration, QTc interval widens to 130% of its pretreatment duration and is longer than 500 msec; P waves disappear, or patient if develops significant tachycardia, symptomatic bradycardia, or hypotension

Malaria

Tab:
Refer to quinidine gluconate inj

Ventricular Arrhythmias

Dosing regimens for suppressing life-threatening ventricular arrhythmias have not been adequately studied

Regimens have generally been similar to regimen for prophylaxis of symptomatic A-fib/A-flutter
Therapy should be guided by results of programmed electrical stimulation/ Holter monitoring w/ exercise

DOSING CONSIDERATIONS
Elderly
Consider dose reduction

Other Important Considerations
Congestive Heart Failure: Reduce dose

PEDIATRIC DOSAGE

Malaria

Tab:
Refer to quinidine gluconate inj

ADMINISTRATION
Oral route

STORAGE
20-25°C (68-77°F). (Tab) Protect from light and moisture.

HOW SUPPLIED
Tab: 200mg*, 300mg*; **Tab, Extended-Release (ER):** 300mg *scored

CONTRAINDICATIONS
Thrombocytopenic purpura w/ previous quinidine or quinine treatment, cardiac rhythm that is dependent upon a junctional or idioventricular pacemaker (including complete atrioventricular [AV] block) in the absence of a functioning artificial pacemaker, patients who might be adversely affected by anticholinergics (eg, myasthenia gravis).

WARNINGS/PRECAUTIONS
May prolong QTc interval leading to torsades de pointes (TdP) and other ventricular arrhythmias; use w/ extreme care in patients w/ preexisting long QT syndromes, histories of TdP, or who have previously responded to drug (or other drugs that prolong ventricular repolarization) w/ marked lengthening of QTc interval. May cause paradoxical increase in ventricular rate in A-fib/A-flutter. May exacerbate bradycardia in sick sinus syndrome. Physical/pharmacologic vagal maneuvers to terminate paroxysmal supraventricular tachycardia may be ineffective. Hypersensitivity/anaphylactoid reactions may occur especially during 1st weeks of therapy. Renal/hepatic dysfunction and CHF may cause toxicity. Caution in patients w/o implanted pacemakers who are at high risk of complete AV block (eg, digitalis intoxication, 2nd-degree AV block, severe intraventricular conduction defects). Perform initiation or dose adjustment in a setting where facilities and personnel for monitoring and resuscitation are available, especially in patients w/ structural heart disease or other risk factors for toxicity. Treat symptomatic A-fib/A-flutter only after ventricular rate control (eg, w/ digitalis or β-blockers) has failed to provide satisfactory control of symptoms. (Tab, ER) D/C if blood dyscrasias or evidence of hepatic/renal dysfunction occurs.

ADVERSE REACTIONS
Diarrhea, upper GI distress, lightheadedness, headache, fatigue, palpitations, angina-like pain, weakness, rash, visual problems, change in sleep habits, N/V, heartburn, esophagitis.

DRUG INTERACTIONS
Urine alkalinizers (eg, carbonic anhydrase inhibitors, sodium bicarbonate, thiazide diuretics) reduce renal elimination. Amiodarone, cimetidine, and ketoconazole may increase levels. Nifedipine may decrease levels. CYP3A4 inducers (eg, phenobarbital, phenytoin, rifampin) may accelerate hepatic elimination. Verapamil and propranolol decrease clearance. Caution w/ drugs metabolized by CYP2D6 (eg, mexiletine, phenothiazines, polycyclic antidepressants, codeine, hydrocodone). May cause slowing of metabolism of drugs metabolized by CYP3A4 (eg, nifedipine, felodipine, nicardipine, nimodipine). May increase levels of digoxin, digitoxin, procainamide, and haloperidol; may need to reduce digoxin dose. Potentiates action of warfarin, and depolarizing (eg, succinylcholine, decamethonium) and nondepolarizing (eg, d-tubocurarine, pancuronium) neuromuscular blockers; may need to reduce anticoagulant dose. Additive effects w/ anticholinergics, vasodilators and negative inotropics. Antagonistic effects w/ cholinergics, vasoconstrictors, and positive inotropes. (Tab, ER) Diltiazem decreases clearance. Avoid grapefruit juice. Decrease in dietary salt intake may increase levels.

PREGNANCY AND LACTATION
Category C, not for use in nursing.

MECHANISM OF ACTION
Class IA antiarrhythmic/schizonticide antimalarial. Arrhythmia: Slows phase-0 depolarization by depressing the inward depolarizing Na^+ current, which slows conduction, prolongs effective refractory period, and reduces automaticity in the heart. Malaria: Acts as intra-erythrocytic schizonticide w/ little effect upon sporozites or upon pre-erythrocytic parasites.

PHARMACOKINETICS
Absorption: Absolute bioavailability (70%); T_{max}=2 hrs (tab), 6 hrs (tab, ER).
Distribution: V_d=2-3L/kg; plasma protein binding (80-88%, adults and older children; 50-70%, pregnant, infants and neonates). Found in breast milk.
Metabolism: Liver via CYP3A4. 3-hydroxy-quinidine (3HQ) (active major metabolite). **Elimination:** Urine (5-20% unchanged); $T_{1/2}$=6-8 hrs (adults), 3-4 hrs (pediatrics), 12 hrs (3HQ).

PATIENT CONSIDERATIONS
Assessment: Assess for previous allergy/thrombocytopenic purpura to the drug or quinine, myasthenia gravis, structural heart disease, preexisting long-QT syndrome, history of TdP, marked lengthening of QTc interval w/ previous drug use, implanted pacemaker, sick sinus syndrome, CHF, renal/hepatic dysfunction, pregnancy/nursing status, and possible drug/diet interactions.

Monitoring: Monitor for exacerbated bradycardia in sick sinus syndrome, paradoxical increase in ventricular rate in A-fib/A-flutter, ventricular arrhythmias (eg, TdP), hypotension, hypersensitivity, renal/hepatic dysfunction, and other adverse reactions. Perform ECG monitoring. Continue monitoring for toxicity for 2 or 3 days after initiation of regimen on which patient will be discharged. (Tab, ER) Monitor blood counts periodically during long-term therapy.

Counseling: Inform about risks/benefits of the drug, including the goal of therapy and the increased risk of death. (Tab, ER) Counsel to avoid consuming grapefruit juice.

QUIXIN — levofloxacin   Rx
Class: Fluoroquinolone

ADULT DOSAGE	PEDIATRIC DOSAGE
Bacterial Conjunctivitis	**Bacterial Conjunctivitis**
Days 1-2:	**≥1 Year:**
1-2 drops in the affected eye(s) q2h while awake, up to 8X/day	**Days 1-2:**
Days 3-7:	1-2 drops in the affected eye(s) q2h while awake, up to 8X/day
1-2 drops in the affected eye(s) q4h while awake, up to qid	**Days 3-7:**
	1-2 drops in the affected eye(s) q4h while awake, up to qid

ADMINISTRATION
Ocular route
STORAGE
15-25°C (59-77°F).
HOW SUPPLIED
Sol: 0.5% [5mL]
CONTRAINDICATIONS
History of hypersensitivity to levofloxacin, to other quinolones, or to any of the components in this medication.
WARNINGS/PRECAUTIONS
Should not be injected subconjunctivally nor introduced directly to anterior chamber of the eye. D/C if allergic reaction or superinfection occurs; prolonged use may cause overgrowth of nonsusceptible organisms. Avoid wearing contact lenses if signs/symptoms of conjunctivitis present.
ADVERSE REACTIONS
Transient ocular burning, transient decreased vision, fever, foreign body sensation, headache, ocular pain/discomfort, pharyngitis, photophobia.
DRUG INTERACTIONS
Systemic quinolone therapy may increase theophylline levels, interfere with caffeine metabolism, enhance warfarin effects, and elevate SrCr with cyclosporine.
PREGNANCY AND LACTATION
Category C, caution in nursing.
MECHANISM OF ACTION
Fluoroquinolone; inhibits bacterial topoisomerase IV and DNA gyrase, which are enzymes required for DNA replication, transcription, repair, and recombination.
PHARMACOKINETICS
Absorption: C_{max}=0.94ng/mL (single dose), 2.15ng/mL (multiple doses).
Distribution: Presumed to be excreted in breast milk.

PATIENT CONSIDERATIONS

Assessment: Assess for hypersensitivity to the drug or to other quinolones, use of contact lenses, pregnancy/nursing status, possible drug interactions, or any other conditions where treatment is contraindicated or cautioned.

Monitoring: Monitor for signs/symptoms of hypersensitivity or anaphylactic reaction, and overgrowth of nonsusceptible organisms. Perform eye exam using magnification (eg, slit-lamp biomicroscopy, fluorescein staining) if necessary.

Counseling: Instruct to avoid contaminating applicator tip with material from eye, fingers, or other sources. Advise to not wear contact lenses if there are signs/symptoms of bacterial conjunctivitis. Instruct to d/c medication and contact physician if signs of hypersensitivity reaction (eg, rash) develop.

QVAR — beclomethasone dipropionate   Rx
Class: Corticosteroid

ADULT DOSAGE	PEDIATRIC DOSAGE
Asthma	**Asthma**
Previously on Bronchodilators Alone:	**5-11 Years:**
Initial: 40-80mcg bid	**Previously on Bronchodilators Alone or Inhaled Corticosteroids:**
Max: 320mcg bid	**Initial:** 40mcg bid
Previously on Inhaled Corticosteroids:	**Max:** 80mcg bid
Initial: 40-160mcg bid	**≥12 Years:**
Max: 320mcg bid	**Previously on Bronchodilators Alone:**
	Initial: 40-80mcg bid
	Max: 320mcg bid
	Previously on Inhaled Corticosteroids:
	Initial: 40-160mcg bid
	Max: 320mcg bid

DOSING CONSIDERATIONS
Concomitant Medications
Systemic Corticosteroids (eg, Prednisone):
Slowly wean patient beginning after at least 1 week of therapy

Elderly
Start at lower end of dosing range
ADMINISTRATION
Oral inh route
Advise patient to rinse mouth after inh.
Priming
Actuate into the air twice before using for the 1st time or if not used for >10 days.
STORAGE
25°C (77°F); excursions permitted to 15-30°C (59-86°F). For optimal results, canister should be at room temperature when used. Do not puncture, use/store near heat or open flame, or throw container into fire/incinerator. Exposure to temperatures >49°C (120°F) may cause bursting.
HOW SUPPLIED
MDI: 40mcg/inh, 80mcg/inh [120 actuations]
CONTRAINDICATIONS
Primary treatment of status asthmaticus or other acute episodes of asthma where intensive measures are required. Known hypersensitivity to beclomethasone dipropionate or any of the ingredients in the product.
WARNINGS/PRECAUTIONS
Candida albicans infections of mouth and pharynx may occur; treat and/or interrupt therapy if needed. Not indicated for relief of acute bronchospasm. Deaths due to adrenal insufficiency have occurred during and after transfer from systemic to inhaled corticosteroids; wean slowly from systemic corticosteroid use after transferring to therapy. Resume oral corticosteroids (in large doses) immediately during periods of stress or a severe asthmatic attack in patients previously withdrawn from systemic corticosteroids. Transfer from systemic to inhaled corticosteroids may unmask allergic conditions previously suppressed by systemic therapy (eg, rhinitis, conjunctivitis, eczema). Increased susceptibility to infections. May lead to more serious/fatal course of chickenpox or measles; avoid exposure, and if exposed, consider prophylaxis/treatment. Caution w/ active or quiescent tuberculosis (TB), untreated systemic fungal/bacterial/parasitic/viral infections, or ocular herpes simplex. Paradoxical bronchospasm, w/ immediate increase in wheezing, may occur after dosing; treat immediately w/ a short-acting inhaled bronchodilator; d/c and institute alternative therapy. Hypersensitivity reactions (eg, urticaria, angioedema, rash) may occur; d/c if these occur. Monitor for systemic corticosteroid effects; reduce dose slowly if hypercorticism and adrenal suppression occur. Caution should be taken in observing patients postoperatively or during periods of stress for evidence of inadequate adrenal response. May cause reduction in growth velocity in pediatric patients; monitor growth. Decreases in bone mineral density (BMD) reported w/ long-term use; monitor in patients w/ major risk factors (eg, prolonged immobilization, family history of osteoporosis, chronic use of drugs that can reduce bone mass). Glaucoma, increased intraocular pressure (IOP), and cataracts reported w/ long-term use. Caution in elderly.
ADVERSE REACTIONS
Headache, pharyngitis, URTI, rhinitis, increased asthma symptoms, oral symptoms (inhalation route), sinusitis, dysphonia, dysmenorrhea, coughing.
PREGNANCY AND LACTATION
Pregnancy: Category C.
Lactation: Caution in nursing.
MECHANISM OF ACTION
Corticosteroid; has multiple anti-inflammatory effects, inhibiting both inflammatory cells (eg, mast cells, eosinophils, basophils, lymphocytes, macrophages, neutrophils) and release of inflammatory mediators (eg, histamine, eicosanoids, leukotrienes, cytokines).
PHARMACOKINETICS
Absorption: C_{max}=88pg/mL, T_{max}=0.5 hr. (Beclomethasone-17-monopropionate [17-BMP] C_{max}=1419pg/mL, T_{max}=0.7 hr. **Distribution:** Plasma protein binding (94-96%, 17-BMP); found in breast milk. **Metabolism:** Liver (biotransformation) via CYP3A; 17-BMP, beclomethasone-21-monopropionate, and beclomethasone (major metabolites). **Elimination:** Feces, urine (<10%); $T_{1/2}$= 2.8 hrs (17-BMP).

PATIENT CONSIDERATIONS

Assessment: Assess for status asthmaticus, acute asthma episodes, acute bronchospasm, active/quiescent TB, untreated systemic infections, ocular herpes simplex, known hypersensitivity to drug or to any of the ingredients, risk factors for BMD, history of increased IOP/glaucoma/cataracts, and pregnancy/nursing status.

Monitoring: Monitor for paradoxical bronchospasm, hypercorticism, adrenal suppression/insufficiency, BMD, changes in vision, glaucoma, increased IOP, cataracts, infections, hypersensitivity reactions, asthma instability, and other adverse reactions. Monitor growth in pediatric patients.

Counseling: Advise to contact physician if oropharyngeal candidiasis develops. Instruct to avoid exposure to chickenpox or measles, and, if exposed, to consult physician w/o delay. Inform about risks of immunosuppression, hypercorticism, adrenal suppression, reduction in bone mineral density, reduced growth velocity in pediatric patients, glaucoma, and cataracts. Advise that drug is not intended for use in the treatment of acute asthma; instruct to immediately contact physician if asthma deteriorates. Advise to use medication at regular intervals since its effectiveness depends on regular use. Instruct to contact physician if symptoms do not improve after 2 weeks of therapy or if condition worsens. Counsel about the proper priming/use of inhaler. Instruct not to stop abruptly and to immediately contact physician if drug is discontinued.

RANEXA — ranolazine   Rx

Class: Miscellaneous antianginal

ADULT DOSAGE

Chronic Angina

Initial: 500mg bid
Titrate: Increase to 1000mg bid prn
Max: 1000mg bid

May be used w/ β-blockers, nitrates, calcium channel blockers, antiplatelet therapy, lipid-lowering therapy, ACE inhibitors, and ARBs

Missed Dose

If a dose is missed, take the prescribed dose at the next scheduled time; do not double the next dose

PEDIATRIC DOSAGE

Pediatric use may not have been established

DOSING CONSIDERATIONS

Concomitant Medications

Moderate CYP3A Inhibitors (eg, Diltiazem, Verapamil, Erythromycin):
Max Dose: 500mg bid

P-gp Inhibitors (eg, Cyclosporine):
Titrate ranolazine based on clinical response

Elderly

Start at lower end of dosing range

ADMINISTRATION

Oral route

Take w/ or w/o meals.
Swallow tab whole; do not crush, break, or chew.

STORAGE

25°C (77°F); excursions permitted to 15-30°C (59-86°F).

HOW SUPPLIED

Tab, Extended-Release: 500mg, 1000mg

CONTRAINDICATIONS

Liver cirrhosis, concomitant use w/ CYP3A inducers (eg, rifampin, phenobarbital, phenytoin) or strong CYP3A inhibitors (eg, ketoconazole, itraconazole, clarithromycin).

WARNINGS/PRECAUTIONS

May prolong QTc interval in a dose-related manner. Acute renal failure reported in patients w/ severe renal impairment (CrCl <30mL/min); d/c and treat appropriately if acute renal failure develops. Monitor renal function after initiation and periodically in patients w/ moderate to severe renal impairment (CrCl <60mL/min) for increases in SrCr accompanied by an increase in BUN.

ADVERSE REACTIONS

Dizziness, headache, constipation, nausea.

DRUG INTERACTIONS

See Contraindications and Dosing Considerations. P-gp inhibitors (eg, cyclosporine) may increase concentrations. May increase levels of simvastatin; limit simvastatin dose to 20mg qd. May increase concentrations of other sensitive CYP3A substrates (eg, lovastatin) and CYP3A substrates w/ a narrow therapeutic range (eg, cyclosporine, tacrolimus, sirolimus); may require dose adjustment of these drugs. May increase exposure to digoxin and CYP2D6 substrates (eg, TCAs, antipsychotics); may require digoxin dose adjustment and lower doses of CYP2D6 substrates. May increase levels of metformin; do not exceed 1700mg/day of metformin if coadministered w/ ranolazine 1000mg bid and monitor blood glucose levels and risks associated w/ high metformin exposure.

PREGNANCY AND LACTATION

Pregnancy: There are no available data on use in pregnant women to inform any drug-associated risks.
Lactation: There are no data on the presence in human milk, the effects on the breastfed infant, or the effects on milk production. However, ranolazine is present in rat milk. Caution in nursing.

MECHANISM OF ACTION

Antianginal; has not been established. Can inhibit the cardiac late Na^+ current.

PHARMACOKINETICS

Absorption: Highly variable. C_{max}=2600ng/mL (1000mg bid), T_{max}=2-5 hrs.
Distribution: Plasma protein binding (62%). **Metabolism:** Intestine and liver (rapid and extensive) by CYP3A (major) and CYP2D6 (minor). **Elimination:** (Sol) Urine (75%), feces (25%); urine and feces (<5% unchanged); $T_{1/2}$=7 hrs, 6-22 hrs (metabolites).

PATIENT CONSIDERATIONS

Assessment: Assess for liver cirrhosis, QT interval prolongation, renal impairment, pregnancy/nursing status, and possible drug interactions.

Monitoring: Monitor for ECG changes (eg, QT interval prolongation) and other adverse reactions. Monitor renal function (eg, SrCr, BUN) after initiation and periodically in patients w/ moderate to severe renal impairment.

Counseling: Inform that drug will not abate an acute angina episode. Inform that drug should not be used w/ drugs that are strong CYP3A inhibitors or CYP3A inducers. Inform that drug should not be used in patients w/ liver cirrhosis. Advise to inform physician if receiving drugs that are moderate CYP3A inhibitors or P-gp inhibitors. Advise to limit grapefruit juice or grapefruit products. Inform that drug may produce QTc interval prolongation, and

to inform physician of any personal or family history of QTc prolongation, congenital long QT syndrome, or if receiving drugs that prolong QTc interval. Advise to inform physician of any renal function impairment before or while taking drug. Inform that drug may cause dizziness and lightheadedness, and instruct to contact physician if experiencing fainting spells; instruct patients to know how they react to the drug before engaging in activities requiring mental alertness or coordination (eg, operating machinery, driving). Instruct to take exactly ud.

RANITIDINE — ranitidine hydrochloride   Rx

Class: H₂ blocker

OTHER BRAND NAMES

Zantac Oral, Zantac Injection

ADULT DOSAGE

General Dosing

Inj:
For hospitalized patients w/ pathological hypersecretory conditions or intractable duodenal ulcers, or as an alternative to the oral dosage form for short-term use in patients who are unable to take oral medication
IM:
50mg q6-8h
IV:
50mg q6-8h as intermittent bolus/ infusion or 6.25mg/hr continuous IV infusion
Max: 400mg/day

Gastric Ulcers

Short-Term Treatment of Active, Benign Ulcers:
PO:
150mg bid
Maint: 150mg hs

Gastroesophageal Reflux Disease

PO:
150mg bid

Erosive Esophagitis

Endoscopically Diagnosed:
PO:
150mg qid
Maint: 150mg bid

Duodenal Ulcers

Short-Term Treatment of Active Ulcers:
PO:
150mg bid or 300mg qd after pm meal or hs
Maint: 150mg hs

Pathological Hypersecretory Conditions

Treatment of pathological hypersecretory conditions (eg, Zollinger-Ellison syndrome, systemic mastocytosis)

PO:
150mg bid; adjust dose according to patient needs and continue as long as clinically indicated. Doses up to 6g/ day have been employed w/ severe disease

Continuous IV Infusion:
Zollinger-Ellison Syndrome:
Initial: 1mg/kg/hr
Titrate: May increase after 4 hrs by 0.5mg/kg/hr increments if gastric acid output is >10mEq/hr or patient becomes symptomatic.
Doses up to 2.5mg/kg/hr and infusion rates as high as 220mg/hr have been used.

PEDIATRIC DOSAGE

Erosive Esophagitis

Endoscopically Diagnosed:
1 Month-16 Years:
PO:
5-10mg/kg/day given as 2 divided doses

Duodenal Ulcers

Short-Term Treatment of Active Ulcers:
1 Month-16 Years:
PO:
2-4mg/kg bid
Maint: 2-4mg/kg qd
Max: 300mg/day (treatment), 150mg/ day (maint)

Inj:
2-4mg/kg/day IV given q6-8h
Max: 50mg IV q6-8h

Gastric Ulcers

Short-Term Treatment of Active, Benign Ulcers:
1 Month-16 Years:
PO:
2-4mg/kg bid
Maint: 2-4mg/kg qd
Max: 300mg/day (treatment), 150mg/ day (maint)

Gastroesophageal Reflux Disease

1 Month-16 Years:
PO:
5-10mg/kg/day given as 2 divided doses

Other Indications

Inj:
<1 Month of Age:
Limited data in neonatal patients receiving extracorporeal membrane oxygenation suggest that ranitidine may be useful and safe for increasing gastric pH for patients at risk of GI hemorrhage

2mg/kg given q12-24h or as a continuous infusion should be considered

----

DOSING CONSIDERATIONS

Renal Impairment

CrCl <50mL/min: 150mg PO q24h or 50mg IV/IM q18-24h; may increase dosing frequency to q12h or even further, w/ caution
Hemodialysis: Give dose at the end of treatment

ADMINISTRATION

Oral/IM/IV routes

PO
Administer concomitant antacids prn for pain relief to patients w/ active duodenal ulcer; active, benign gastric ulcer; hypersecretory states; GERD; or erosive esophagitis.

Inj
IV:
Intermittent Bolus:
Dilute ranitidine 50mg inj in 0.9% NaCl inj or other compatible IV sol to a concentration ≤2.5mg/mL (20mL).
Inject at a rate ≤4mL/min (5 min).
Intermittent Infusion:
Dilute ranitidine 50mg inj in D5 inj or other compatible IV sol to a concentration ≤0.5mg/mL (100mL).
Infuse at a rate ≤5-7mL/min (15-20 min).
Continuous Infusion:
Add ranitidine inj to D5 inj or other compatible IV sol; deliver at a rate of 6.25mg/hr (eg, 150mg of ranitidine inj in 250mL of D5 inj at 10.7mL/hr).
For Zollinger-Ellison patients, dilute ranitidine inj in D5 inj or other compatible IV sol to a concentration ≤2.5mg/mL.

IM:
No dilution necessary.

Stability:
Stable for 48 hrs at room temperature when added to or diluted w/ most commonly used IV sol (eg, 0.9% NaCl inj, D5 inj, 10% dextrose inj, lactated Ringer's inj, 5% sodium bicarbonate inj).

STORAGE
Cap: 20-25°C (68-77°F) in a dry place. Protect from light. Tab: 15-30°C (59-86°F) in a dry place. Protect from light. Syrup: 4-25°C (39-77°F). Do not freeze. Inj: 4-25°C (39-77°F); excursions permitted to 30°C (86°F). Protect from light. Avoid excessive heat; brief exposure up to 40°C (104°F) does not adversely affect the product. Protect from freezing.

HOW SUPPLIED
Cap: 150mg, 300mg; **Syrup:** 15mg/mL [16 fl oz]; (Zantac) **Inj:** 25mg/mL [2mL, 6mL], **Tab:** 150mg, 300mg

CONTRAINDICATIONS
Hypersensitivity to ranitidine or any of the ingredients.

WARNINGS/PRECAUTIONS
Symptomatic response does not preclude the presence of gastric malignancy. Caution w/ hepatic/renal dysfunction. May precipitate acute porphyric attacks in patients w/ acute porphyria; avoid w/ history of acute porphyria. False (+) tests for urine protein w/ Multistix may occur. Caution in elderly. D/C immediately if hepatocellular, cholestatic, or mixed hepatitis occurs. (Inj) Do not exceed recommended administration rates; bradycardia reported w/ rapid infusion. ALT elevations may occur; monitor if on IV therapy for ≥5 days at doses ≥100mg qid.

ADVERSE REACTIONS
Headache, constipation, diarrhea, N/V, abdominal discomfort/pain, rash.

DRUG INTERACTIONS
Affects bioavailability of other drugs through several mechanisms (eg, competition for renal tubular secretion, alteration of gastric pH, CYP450 inhibition). Increased plasma levels of procainamide w/ high doses of ranitidine; monitor for procainamide toxicity when administered w/ oral ranitidine at a dose >300mg/day. Altered PT w/ warfarin; closely monitor PT. May alter absorption of drugs in which gastric pH is an important determinant of bioavailability; may increase absorption of triazolam, midazolam, and glipizide and decrease absorption of ketoconazole, atazanavir, delavirdine, and gefitinib. Monitor for excessive/prolonged sedation w/ oral midazolam and triazolam. Chronic use w/ delavirdine is not recommended.

PREGNANCY AND LACTATION
Pregnancy: Category B.
Lactation: Caution in nursing.

MECHANISM OF ACTION
H_2-blocker; competitive, reversible inhibitor of histamine at histamine H_2-receptors, including receptors found on gastric cells.

PHARMACOKINETICS
Absorption: (Oral, 150mg) Absolute bioavailability (50%); C_{max}=440-545ng/mL, T_{max}=2-3 hrs. (IM, 50mg) Rapid. Absolute bioavailability (90-100%); C_{max}=576ng/mL, T_{max}=≤15 min. Refer to PI for pediatric parameters. **Distribution:** V_d=1.4L/kg; serum protein binding (15%); found in breast milk. **Metabolism:** Liver, N-oxide (principal metabolite). **Elimination:** Feces, urine (30% unchanged [oral], 70% unchanged [IV]); $T_{1/2}$=2.5-3 hrs (oral), 2-2.5 hrs (IV).

PATIENT CONSIDERATIONS
Assessment: Assess for hypersensitivity to the drug, renal/hepatic impairment, history of acute porphyria, pregnancy/nursing status, and possible drug interactions.

Monitoring: Monitor for signs/symptoms of hepatic effects (eg, hepatitis, elevations in ALT values), hypersensitivity reactions, and other adverse reactions. Monitor PT in patients receiving warfarin.

Counseling: Inform that antacids may be taken prn for relief of pain. Instruct to notify physician if any adverse events develop.

RAPAFLO — silodosin   Rx
Class: Alpha₁ antagonist

ADULT DOSAGE	**PEDIATRIC DOSAGE**
Benign Prostatic Hyperplasia	Pediatric use may not have been established
8mg qd w/ a meal	

DOSING CONSIDERATIONS
Renal Impairment
CrCl 30-50mL/min: 4mg qd w/ a meal

ADMINISTRATION
Oral route

Take w/ a meal.
Patients who have difficulty swallowing caps may sprinkle the cap powder on a tbsp of applesauce (should not be hot).
Swallow immediately (w/in 5 min) w/o chewing and follow with 8 oz of cool water.
Do not subdivide the contents of cap or store any powder/applesauce mixture for future use.

STORAGE
25°C (77°F); excursions permitted to 15-30°C (59-86°F). Protect from light and moisture.

HOW SUPPLIED
Cap: 4mg, 8mg

CONTRAINDICATIONS
Severe renal impairment (CrCl <30mL/min), severe hepatic impairment (Child-Pugh score ≥10), concomitant administration w/ strong CYP3A4 inhibitors (eg, ketoconazole, clarithromycin, itraconazole, ritonavir), history of hypersensitivity to silodosin or any of the ingredients of the product.

WARNINGS/PRECAUTIONS
Not for treatment of HTN. Postural hypotension and syncope may occur; may impair mental/physical abilities. Caution in patients with moderate renal impairment. Examine patients prior to therapy to rule out prostate cancer. Intraoperative floppy iris syndrome (IFIS) observed during cataract surgery in some patients on α₁-blockers or previously treated with α₁-blockers.

ADVERSE REACTIONS
Retrograde ejaculation, dizziness, diarrhea, orthostatic hypotension, headache, nasopharyngitis, nasal congestion.

DRUG INTERACTIONS
See Contraindications. Avoid with other α-blockers and strong P-glycoprotein (P-gp) inhibitors (eg, cyclosporine). Caution with antihypertensives. Coadministration with PDE-5 inhibitors may cause symptomatic hypotension; caution with use. Increased concentrations with P-gp inhibitors and moderate CYP3A4 inhibitors (eg, diltiazem, erythromycin, verapamil). UGT2B7 inhibitors (eg, probenecid, valproic acid, fluconazole) may potentially increase exposure.

PREGNANCY AND LACTATION
Pregnancy: Category B.
Lactation: Safety not known in nursing.

MECHANISM OF ACTION
α₁-antagonist; blocks α₁-adrenoreceptors, causing smooth muscle relaxation in the bladder neck/base and prostate, resulting in improved urine flow and reduction in BPH symptoms.

PHARMACOKINETICS
Absorption: Absolute bioavailability (32%), C_{max}=61.6ng/mL, T_{max}=2.6 hrs, AUC_{ss}=373.4ng•hr/mL. **Distribution:** V_d=49.5L; plasma protein binding (97%). **Metabolism:** Glucuronidation, alcohol and aldehyde dehydrogenase, CYP3A4; KMD-3213G (main metabolite), KMD-3293 (2nd major metabolite). **Elimination:** Urine (33.5%), feces (54.9%); $T_{1/2}$=13.3 hrs.

PATIENT CONSIDERATIONS
Assessment: Assess for drug hypersensitivity, renal/hepatic impairment, prostate cancer, and possible drug interactions.

Monitoring: Monitor for signs/symptoms of postural hypotension, syncope, IFIS during cataract surgery, and other adverse reactions.

Counseling: Counsel about possible occurrence of symptoms related to postural hypotension (eg, dizziness); advise to use caution when driving, operating machinery, or performing hazardous tasks, particularly in patients with low BP or taking antihypertensives. Inform that most common side effect seen is an orgasm with reduced or no semen; inform that this side effect does not pose a safety concern and is reversible when drug is discontinued. Advise to notify ophthalmologist about the use of the drug before cataract surgery or other eye procedures, even if no longer taking silodosin.

RAPAMUNE — sirolimus   Rx
Class: Immunosuppressant

Increased susceptibility to infection and the possible development of lymphoma and other malignancies may result from immunosuppression. Only physicians experienced in immunosuppressive therapy and management of renal transplant patients should use sirolimus for prophylaxis of organ rejection in patients receiving renal transplants. Use not recommended in liver or lung transplant patients. Use in combination w/ tacrolimus was associated w/ excess mortality and graft loss in de novo liver transplant patients. Use in combination w/ cyclosporine or tacrolimus was associated w/ increased hepatic artery thrombosis in de novo liver transplant patients. Cases of bronchial anastomotic dehiscence, most fatal, reported in de novo lung transplant patients when sirolimus was used as part of an immunosuppressive regimen.

ADULT DOSAGE

Renal Transplant

Prophylaxis of Organ Rejection in Renal Transplantation:

General:

Give initial dose as soon as possible after transplantation, and 4 hrs after cyclosporine (MODIFIED)

Once maint dose is adjusted, continue on the new maint dose for ≥7-14 days before further dose adjustment

Dosage adjustment may be based on simple proportion:
New Rapamune Dose = Current Dose x (Target Concentration/Current Concentration)

LD should be considered in addition to new maint dose when it is necessary to increase sirolimus trough concentrations:
Rapamune LD = 3 x (New Maint Dose - Current Maint Dose)

Max: 40mg/day

If estimated dose is >40mg/day due to addition of LD, administer LD over 2 days; monitor trough concentrations at least 3-4 days after LD(s)

2mg of sol are clinically equivalent to 2mg tab and are interchangeable on a mg-to-mg basis; unknown if higher doses of sol are clinically equivalent to higher doses of tabs on a mg-to-mg basis

Low- to Moderate-Immunologic Risk:
LD: Give LD equivalent to 3X the maint dose

Give w/ cyclosporine and corticosteroids in de novo renal transplant patients; progressively d/c cyclosporine over 4-8 weeks at 2-4 months following transplantation

Adjust dose to maintain blood trough concentration w/in target-range

Target Sirolimus Whole Blood Trough Concentrations Following Cyclosporine Withdrawal:
1st Year: 16-24ng/mL
Thereafter: 12-20ng/mL

High-Immunologic Risk:

Give w/ cyclosporine and corticosteroids for the first 12 months following transplantation. Safety and efficacy of this combination not studied beyond first 12 months; after 12 months, consider adjustments to immunosuppressive regimen based on patient's clinical status
LD: Up to 15mg on Day 1 post-transplantation
Maint: 5mg/day beginning on Day 2; obtain trough level between Days 5 and 7 and adjust daily dose thereafter

Cyclosporine Dosing:
Initial: Up to 7mg/kg/day in divided doses; subsequently adjust to achieve target whole blood trough concentrations

Prednisone Dosing:
Minimum of 5mg/day

Antibody induction therapy may be used

Lymphangioleiomyomatosis

Initial: 2mg/day

Measure sirolimus whole blood trough concentrations in 10-20 days, w/ a dosage adjustment to maintain concentrations between 5-15ng/mL

Dosage adjustment may be based on simple proportion:
New Rapamune Dose = Current Dose x (Target Concentration/Current Concentration)

Once maint dose is adjusted, continue on the new maint dose for at least 7-14 days before further dose adjustment

PEDIATRIC DOSAGE

Renal Transplant

Prophylaxis of Organ Rejection in Renal Transplantation:

≥13 Years:
General:

Give initial dose as soon as possible after transplantation, and 4 hrs after cyclosporine (MODIFIED)

Once maint dose is adjusted, continue on the new maint dose for ≥7-14 days before further dose adjustment

Dosage adjustment can be based on simple proportion:
New Rapamune Dose = Current Dose x (Target Concentration/Current Concentration)

LD should be considered in addition to new maint dose when it is necessary to increase sirolimus trough concentrations:
Rapamune LD = 3 x (New Maint Dose - Current Maint Dose)

Max: 40mg/day

If estimated dose is >40mg/day due to addition of LD, administer LD over 2 days; monitor trough concentrations at least 3-4 days after LD(s)

2mg of sol are clinically equivalent to 2mg tab and are interchangeable on a mg-to-mg basis; unknown if higher doses of sol are clinically equivalent to higher doses of tabs on a mg-to-mg basis

Low- to Moderate-Immunologic Risk:
LD: Give LD equivalent to 3X the maint dose

Give w/ cyclosporine and corticosteroids in de novo renal transplant patients; progressively d/c cyclosporine over 4-8 weeks at 2-4 months following transplantation

Adjust dose to maintain blood trough concentration w/in target range

Target Sirolimus Whole Blood Trough Concentrations Following Cyclosporine Withdrawal:
1st Year: 16-24ng/mL
Thereafter: 12-20ng/mL

Once a stable dose is achieved, perform therapeutic drug monitoring at least every 3 months

---

DOSING CONSIDERATIONS

Hepatic Impairment
Mild or Moderate: Reduce maint dose by approx 1/3
Severe: Reduce maint dose by approx 1/2

Elderly
Start at lower end of dosing range

Other Important Considerations
Low Body Weight (<40kg): Adjust initial dose based on BSA to 1mg/m²/day w/ a LD of 3mg/m²

ADMINISTRATION
Oral route

Administer qd.
Give consistently w/ or w/o food.

Tab
Do not crush, chew, or split.

Sol
Once the bottle is opened, use w/in 1 month.
Contains polysorbate 80, which is known to increase the rate of di-(2-ethylhexyl) phthalate extraction from polyvinyl chloride.
Instructions for Dilution:
1. Use amber oral dose syringe to withdraw the prescribed amount of sol from bottle.
2. Empty the correct amount of sirolimus from syringe into only a glass or plastic container holding at least 2 oz (1/4 cup, 60mL) of water or orange juice; no other liquids, including grapefruit juice, should be used for dilution.
3. Stir vigorously and drink at once.
4. Refill the container w/ an additional volume (minimum of 4 oz [1/2 cup, 120mL]) of water or orange juice, stir vigorously, and drink at once.

STORAGE
Sol: (Bottle) 2-8°C (36-46°F). Protect from light. May store at room temperatures up to 25°C (77°F) for a short period (eg, not >15 days). (Syringe) May be kept in syringe for max of 24 hrs at room temperatures up to 25°C (77°F) or at 2-8°C (36-46°F). **Tab:** 20-25°C (68-77°F). Protect from light.

HOW SUPPLIED
Sol: 1mg/mL [60mL]; **Tab:** 0.5mg, 1mg, 2mg

CONTRAINDICATIONS
Hypersensitivity to sirolimus.

WARNINGS/PRECAUTIONS
Hypersensitivity reactions reported. Associated w/ the development of angioedema. Impaired/delayed wound healing, including lymphocele and wound dehiscence, and fluid accumulation (eg, peripheral edema, lymphedema, pleural effusion, ascites, pericardial effusions) reported. May increase serum cholesterol and TGs. Long-term administration w/ cyclosporine associated w/ renal function deterioration; consider appropriate adjustment of immunosuppressive regimen w/ elevated or increasing SrCr levels. May delay recovery of renal function in patients w/ delayed graft function. Proteinuria observed in maint renal transplant patients when converting from calcineurin inhibitors (CNIs) to sirolimus; safety and efficacy of conversion in maint renal transplant patients not established. Increased risk for opportunistic infections, including activation of latent viral infections. BK virus-associated nephropathy reported. Progressive multifocal leukoencephalopathy (PML) reported. Consider reduction in immunosuppression if BK virus-associated nephropathy is suspected or if PML develops. Interstitial lung disease (ILD) (eg, pneumonitis, bronchiolitis obliterans organizing pneumonia, pulmonary fibrosis) reported. In some cases, ILD was associated w/ pulmonary HTN. Safety and efficacy of de novo use w/o cyclosporine is not established in renal transplant patients. Provide 1 yr prophylaxis for *Pneumocystis carinii* pneumonia and 3 months for CMV after transplant. Patient sample concentration values from different assays may not be interchangeable. Increased risk of skin cancer; limit exposure to sunlight and UV light.

ADVERSE REACTIONS
Peripheral edema, hypertriglyceridemia, HTN, constipation, hypercholesterolemia, increased creatinine, abdominal pain, nausea, diarrhea, headache, fever, acne, chest pain, stomatitis, nasopharyngitis.

DRUG INTERACTIONS
See Boxed Warning and Dosage. CYP3A4 and P-gp inducers may decrease concentrations. CYP3A4 and P-gp inhibitors may increase concentrations. Avoid w/ strong inhibitors (eg, ketoconazole, erythromycin, clarithromycin) and strong inducers (eg, rifampin, rifabutin) of CYP3A4 and P-gp. Cyclosporine, bromocriptine, cimetidine, cisapride, clotrimazole, danazol, diltiazem, fluconazole, protease inhibitors, metoclopramide, nicardipine, troleandomycin, and verapamil may increase levels. Carbamazepine, phenobarbital, phenytoin, rifapentine, and St. John's wort may decrease levels. May increase verapamil concentration. Vaccines may be less effective; avoid live vaccines. May increase risk of angioedema w/ drugs known to cause angioedema (eg, ACE inhibitors). Increased risk of CNIs-induced hemolytic uremic syndrome/thrombotic thrombocytopenic purpura/thrombotic microangiography w/ concomitant CNIs. Do not administer w/ grapefruit juice or use grapefruit juice for dilution. Caution w/ other nephrotoxic drugs (eg, aminoglycosides, amphotericin B). Monitor for possible development of rhabdomyolysis and other adverse effects w/ HMG-CoA inhibitors and/or fibrates.

PREGNANCY AND LACTATION

Pregnancy: Category C; effective contraception must be initiated before, during, and for 12 weeks after therapy.
Lactation: Not for use in nursing.

MECHANISM OF ACTION

Immunosuppressive agent; inhibits T-lymphocyte activation and proliferation that occurs in response to antigenic and cytokine (interleukin [IL]-2, IL-4, and IL-15) stimulation by a mechanism distinct from that of other immunosuppressants. Also inhibits antibody production. Inhibits activated mTOR pathway and proliferation of lymphangioleiomyomatosis cells.

PHARMACOKINETICS

Absorption: (Sol) Bioavailability (14%); AUC=194ng•hr/mL, C_{max}=14.4ng/mL, T_{max}=2.1 hrs. (Tab) AUC=230ng•hr/mL, C_{max}=15ng/mL, T_{max}=3.5 hrs. Different pharmacokinetic data resulted from concentration-controlled trials of pediatric renal transplants. **Distribution:** V_d=12L/kg; plasma protein binding (approx 92%). **Metabolism:** CYP3A4, P-gp; extensively in intestinal wall and liver via O-demethylation and/or hydroxylation; 7 major metabolites including hydroxy, demethyl, and hydroxydemethyl. **Elimination:** Feces (91%), urine (2.2%); $T_{1/2}$=62 hrs.

PATIENT CONSIDERATIONS

Assessment: Assess for drug hypersensitivity, immunologic risk, hepatic impairment, body weight/BMI, hyperlipidemia, infections, pregnancy/nursing status, and possible drug interactions.

Monitoring: Monitor for infections including opportunistic infections and activation of latent infections, development of PML, lymphoma, other malignancies (particularly of the skin), hypersensitivity reactions, ILD, hyperlipidemia, and other adverse reactions. Monitor trough concentrations, especially in patients w/ altered drug metabolism, in patients who weigh <40kg, in patients w/ hepatic impairment, when a change is made to sirolimus dosage form, and during concurrent administration of strong CYP3A4 inducers or inhibitors. Monitor urinary protein excretion, renal function w/ concomitant cyclosporine, hepatic function, cholesterol, TGs, and BP.

Counseling: Instruct to limit sunlight and UV light exposure by wearing protective clothing and using a sunscreen w/ a high protection. Inform about the potential risks during pregnancy and instruct to use effective contraception prior to, during, and 12 weeks after therapy has been stopped.

RAPIVAB — peramivir   Rx

Class: Neuraminidase inhibitor

ADULT DOSAGE	PEDIATRIC DOSAGE
Influenza	Pediatric use may not have been established
Treatment of Acute Uncomplicated Influenza:	
Single 600mg dose, via IV infusion for 15-30 min	

- -

DOSING CONSIDERATIONS

Renal Impairment
CrCl 30-49mL/min: 200mg
CrCl 10-29mL/min: 100mg

ADMINISTRATION

IV route

Administer w/in 2 days of onset of symptoms of influenza.
In patients w/ chronic renal impairment maintained on hemodialysis, administer after dialysis.

Dilute an appropriate dose of peramivir 10mg/mL sol in 0.9% or 0.45% NaCl, D5, or lactated Ringer's to a max volume of 100mL.
Administer diluted sol via IV infusion for 15-30 min.

Compatible w/ 0.9% or 0.45% NaCl, D5, or lactated Ringer's.
Do not mix or coinfuse w/ other IV medications.
If diluted sol refrigerated, allow to reach room temperature then administer immediately.
Refer to PI for further administration instructions.

STORAGE

20-25°C (68-77°F); excursions permitted to 15-30°C (59-86°F). Diluted Sol: 2-8°C (36-46°F) for up to 24 hrs.

HOW SUPPLIED

Inj: 10mg/mL [20mL]

WARNINGS/PRECAUTIONS

Emergence of resistance substitutions can decrease drug effectiveness; consider available information on influenza drug susceptibility patterns and treatment effects when deciding whether to use peramivir. Rare cases of serious skin reactions (eg, erythema multiforme, Stevens-Johnson syndrome) reported; institute appropriate treatment if a serious skin reaction occurs or is suspected. Neuropsychiatric events (eg, hallucinations, delirium, abnormal behavior), in some cases resulting in fatal outcomes, reported; monitor for signs of abnormal behavior. Serious bacterial infections may begin with influenza-like symptoms or may coexist with or occur during the course of influenza; peramivir does not prevent these complications.

ADVERSE REACTIONS

Diarrhea, increased alanine aminotransferase/serum glucose/CPK, decreased neutrophils.

DRUG INTERACTIONS

Avoid use of live attenuated influenza vaccine within 2 weeks before or 48 hrs after administration of peramivir, unless medically indicated.

PREGNANCY AND LACTATION

Pregnancy: Category C.
Lactation: Caution in nursing.

MECHANISM OF ACTION

Neuraminidase inhibitor; inhibits influenza virus neuraminidase, an enzyme that releases viral particles from the plasma membrane of infected cells.

PHARMACOKINETICS

Absorption: C_{max}=46,800ng/mL; AUC$_{0-inf}$=102,700ng•hr/mL. **Distribution:** Plasma protein binding (<30%); V_d=12.56L. **Elimination:** Kidney (90% as unchanged); $T_{1/2}$=20 hrs.

PATIENT CONSIDERATIONS

Assessment: Assess for renal impairment, pregnancy/nursing status, and possible drug interactions.

Monitoring: Monitor for signs/symptoms of serious skin/hypersensitivity reactions, neuropsychiatric events, and other adverse reactions.

Counseling: Advise of the risk of serious skin reactions and to seek immediate medical attention if a skin reaction occurs. Advise of the risk of neuropsychiatric events in patients with influenza and to contact physician if experiencing signs of abnormal behavior after receiving treatment.

RASUVO — methotrexate   Rx

Class: Dihydrofolic acid reductase inhibitor

> Should be used only by physicians w/ knowledge and experience in the use of antimetabolite therapy. Use only in patients w/ psoriasis or rheumatoid arthritis (RA) w/ severe, recalcitrant, disabling disease not adequately responsive to other forms of therapy. Deaths reported in the treatment of malignancy, psoriasis, and RA. Closely monitor for bone marrow, liver, lung, skin, and kidney toxicities. Patients should be informed of the risks involved and be under physician's care throughout therapy. Fetal death and/or congenital anomalies reported; not recommended for females of childbearing potential unless benefits outweigh risks. Contraindicated in pregnant women. Reduced elimination w/ impaired renal function, ascites, or pleural effusions; monitor for toxicity and reduce dose or d/c in some cases. Unexpectedly severe (sometimes fatal) bone marrow suppression, aplastic anemia, and GI toxicity reported w/ coadministration of therapy (usually high dosage) w/ some NSAIDs. Causes hepatotoxicity, fibrosis, and cirrhosis (generally only after prolonged use); perform periodic liver biopsies in psoriatic patients on long-term therapy. Acutely, liver enzyme elevations frequently seen. Drug-induced lung disease may occur acutely at any time during therapy and reported at low doses. Pulmonary symptoms (especially a dry, nonproductive cough) may require an interruption of therapy. Diarrhea and ulcerative stomatitis require interruption of therapy. Malignant lymphomas, which may regress following withdrawal of treatment, may occur w/ low-dose therapy and, thus, may not require cytotoxic treatment; d/c therapy 1st and, if lymphoma does not regress, institute appropriate treatment. May induce tumor lysis syndrome in patients w/ rapidly growing tumors. Severe, occasionally fatal, skin reactions reported. Potentially fatal opportunistic infections, especially *Pneumocystis jiroveci* pneumonia, may occur. Concomitant use w/ radiotherapy may increase risk of soft tissue necrosis and osteonecrosis.

ADULT DOSAGE	PEDIATRIC DOSAGE
Rheumatoid Arthritis	**Juvenile Idiopathic Arthritis**
Management of selected adults w/ severe, active RA (American College of Rheumatology criteria) who have had insufficient therapeutic response to, or are intolerant of, an adequate trial of 1st-line therapy including full-dose NSAIDs	Management of children w/ active polyarticular juvenile idiopathic arthritis, who have had insufficient therapeutic response to, or are intolerant of, an adequate trial of 1st-line therapy including full-dose NSAIDs
Initial: 7.5mg as single dose once weekly **Titrate:** May adjust gradually to achieve optimal response	**2-16 Years:** **Initial:** 10mg/m^2 once weekly **Titrate:** May adjust gradually to achieve optimal response
Significant increase in incidence and severity of serious toxic reactions, especially bone marrow suppression, reported at doses >20mg/week	Limited data to assess how doses >20mg/m^2/week might affect the risk of serious toxicity; refer to PI for further information
Psoriasis	**Conversions**
Symptomatic control of severe, recalcitrant, disabling psoriasis not adequately responsive to other forms of therapy, but only when the diagnosis has been established, as by a biopsy and/or after dermatologic consultation	**Switching from Oral to SQ Therapy:** Consider any differences in bioavailability between oral and SQ therapy
Initial: 10-25mg as single dose once weekly **Titrate:** May adjust gradually to achieve optimal response **Max:** 30mg/week **Maint:** Once optimal response is achieved, reduce dosage to lowest possible amount of drug and to longest possible rest period	
Conversions	
Switching from Oral to SQ Therapy: Consider any differences in bioavailability between oral and SQ therapy	

DOSING CONSIDERATIONS
Renal Impairment
Reduce dose and monitor carefully for toxicity

Elderly
Consider relatively low doses and closely monitor for early signs of toxicity

Other Important Considerations
Ascites or Pleural Effusions: Reduce dose and monitor carefully for toxicity

ADMINISTRATION
SQ route

Administer in the abdomen or the thigh

Administration and Handling
Patients may self-inject if physician determines that it is appropriate, if they received proper training in how to prepare and administer the correct dose, and if they receive medical follow-up, as necessary
The patient must be explicitly informed about the once weekly dosing schedule
It is advisable to determine an appropriate fixed day of the week for the inj
Visually inspect for particulate matter and discoloration prior to administration
Do not use if the seal is broken
Handle and dispose inj consistent w/ recommendations for handling and disposal of cytotoxic drugs

Important Dosing Information
Only available in doses between 7.5-30mg in 2.5mg increments
Use another formulation of methotrexate for alternative dosing in patients who require oral, IM, IV, intra-arterial, or intrathecal dosing, doses <7.5mg/week, doses >30mg/week, high-dose regimens, or dose adjustments in increments <2.5mg

STORAGE
25°C (77°F); excursions permitted to 15-30°C (59-86°F). Protect from light.

HOW SUPPLIED
Inj: 7.5mg/0.15mL, 10mg/0.20mL, 12.5mg/0.25mL, 15mg/0.30mL, 17.5mg/0.35mL, 20mg/0.40mL, 22.5mg/0.45mL, 25mg/0.50mL, 27.5mg/0.55mL, 30mg/0.60mL

CONTRAINDICATIONS
Pregnancy, nursing mothers, alcoholism, alcoholic liver disease, chronic liver disease, immunodeficiency syndromes, preexisting blood dyscrasias (eg, bone marrow hypoplasia, leukopenia, thrombocytopenia, significant anemia), known hypersensitivity to methotrexate.

WARNINGS/PRECAUTIONS
Not indicated for the treatment of neoplastic diseases. Toxic effects may be related to dose/frequency of administration; if toxicity occurs, reduce dose or d/c therapy and take appropriate corrective measures, which may include use of leucovorin calcium and/or acute, intermittent hemodialysis w/ high-flux dialyzer, if necessary. If therapy is reinstituted, carry it out w/ caution, w/ adequate consideration of further need for the drug and increased alertness as to possible recurrence of toxicity. May cause multiple organ system toxicities (eg, GI, hematologic). Caution in debilitated patients. Avoid pregnancy if either partner is receiving therapy (during and for a minimum of 3 months after therapy for male patients, and during and for at least 1 ovulatory cycle after therapy for female patients). May cause impairment of fertility, oligospermia, and menstrual dysfunction, during and for a short period after cessation of therapy. May impair mental/physical abilities.

ADVERSE REACTIONS
Bone marrow/liver/lung/skin/kidney toxicities, diarrhea, ulcerative stomatitis, hemorrhagic enteritis, opportunistic infections, malignant lymphomas, tumor lysis syndrome, N/V, abdominal distress, malaise, undue fatigue, chills, fever, dizziness.

DRUG INTERACTIONS
See Boxed Warning. Elevated and prolonged levels w/ NSAIDs; do not administer NSAIDs prior to or concomitantly w/ high doses of therapy, and use caution when NSAIDs and salicylates are administered concomitantly w/ lower doses of therapy. Proton pump inhibitors (PPIs) (eg, omeprazole, esomeprazole, pantoprazole) may elevate and prolong levels, possibly leading to toxicities; use caution if administering high-dose therapy w/ PPIs. Oral antibiotics (eg, tetracycline, chloramphenicol, nonabsorbable broad-spectrum antibiotics) may decrease intestinal absorption or interfere w/ enterohepatic circulation. Penicillins may reduce renal clearance; hematologic and GI toxicity observed. Trimethoprim/sulfamethoxazole may increase bone marrow suppression by decreasing tubular secretion and/or an additive antifolate effect. Closely monitor for increased risk of hepatotoxicity w/ potential hepatotoxins (eg, azathioprine, retinoids, sulfasalazine). May decrease theophylline clearance; monitor theophylline levels. Vitamin preparations containing folic acid or its derivatives may decrease responses to methotrexate; high doses of leucovorin may reduce efficacy of intrathecally administered drug. Increases levels of mercaptopurine; may require dose adjustment. Toxicity may be increased due to displacement by certain drugs (eg, salicylates, phenylbutazone, phenytoin, sulfonamides). Renal tubular transport diminished by probenecid. Combined use w/ gold, penicillamine, hydroxychloroquine, sulfasalazine, or cytotoxic agents may increase incidence of adverse effects. Immunization may be ineffective when given during therapy; immunization w/ live virus vaccines is generally not recommended. Disseminated vaccinia infections after smallpox immunizations reported.

PREGNANCY AND LACTATION
Category X, not for use in nursing.

MECHANISM OF ACTION
Dihydrofolic acid reductase inhibitor; interferes w/ DNA synthesis, repair, and cellular replication. Mechanism in RA not established; may affect immune function.

PHARMACOKINETICS
Absorption: (Oral) Well-absorbed. Bioavailability (60%) (adults). Administration of various doses and in different disease states resulted in different parameters.
Distribution: Plasma protein binding (50%); found in breast milk. (IV) V_d=0.18L/ kg (initial), 0.4-0.8L/kg (steady-state). **Metabolism:** Hepatic and intracellular to polyglutamated forms (active); 7-hydroxymethotrexate (metabolite). (Oral) Partially metabolized by intestinal flora. **Elimination:** $T_{1/2}$=3-10 hrs (psoriasis/RA/low-dose antineoplastic therapy), 8-15 hrs (high doses). (IV) Urine (80-90%, unchanged), bile (≤10%). Refer to PI for additional pharmacokinetic information.

PATIENT CONSIDERATIONS
Assessment: Assess for alcoholism, alcoholic/chronic liver disease, immunodeficiency syndromes, blood dyscrasias, ascites, pleural effusions, tumors, hypersensitivity to drug, pregnancy/nursing status, any other conditions where treatment is cautioned or contraindicated, and possible drug interactions. Obtain baseline CBC w/ differential and platelet counts, hepatic enzymes, renal function tests, liver biopsy, and chest x-ray.

Monitoring: Monitor for toxicities of bone marrow, liver, lung, kidney, and GI tract; diarrhea; ulcerative stomatitis; malignant lymphoma; tumor lysis syndrome; skin reactions; opportunistic infections; and other adverse reactions. Monitor hematology at least monthly and renal/hepatic function every 1-2 months during therapy and more frequently during initial/changing doses, or during periods of increased risk of elevated drug levels (eg, dehydration). If drug-induced lung disease is suspected, perform pulmonary function tests.

Counseling: Inform of the risks of organ toxicity, the possible signs/symptoms for which physician should be contacted, and the need for close follow-up, including periodic lab tests to monitor toxicity. Emphasize that the recommended dose is taken once weekly, and that mistaken daily use of recommended dose has led to fatal toxicity. Instruct not to self-administer until trained by physician. Advise women of childbearing potential that drug should not be started until pregnancy is excluded; counsel on the serious risk to the fetus should pregnancy occur while undergoing treatment. Instruct to contact physician if pregnancy is suspected. Advise to avoid pregnancy if either partner is receiving therapy (during and for a minimum of 3 months after therapy for male patients, and during and for at least 1 ovulatory cycle after therapy for female patients). Discuss the risk of effects on reproduction. Inform that adverse reactions such as dizziness and fatigue may affect ability to drive or operate machinery. Inform of the need for proper disposal after use, including the use of a sharps disposal container.

RAVICTI — glycerol phenylbutyrate Rx
Class: Urea cycle disorder agent

ADULT DOSAGE
Urea Cycle Disorders

In patients who cannot be managed by dietary protein restriction and/or amino acid supplementation alone

Switching from Sodium Phenylbutyrate:
Should receive the dose of glycerol phenylbutyrate that contains the same amount of phenylbutyric acid; refer to PI for conversion

Phenylbutyrate-Naive Patients:
Initial: $4.5-11.2mL/m^2/day$ (5-12.4g/m^2/day); $4.5mL/m^2$/day for patients w/ some residual enzyme activity who are not adequately controlled w/ protein restrictions

Consider patient's residual urea synthetic capacity, dietary protein requirements, and diet adherence in determining the initial dose in treatment-naive patients

For Both Subpopulations:
Administer in 3 equally divided doses, each rounded up to the nearest 0.5mL
Max: 17.5mL/day (19g/day)

PEDIATRIC DOSAGE
Urea Cycle Disorders

In patients who cannot be managed by dietary protein restriction and/or amino acid supplementation alone

≥2 Years:
Switching from Sodium Phenylbutyrate:
Should receive the dose of glycerol phenylbutyrate that contains the same amount of phenylbutyric acid; refer to PI for conversion

Phenylbutyrate-Naive Patients:
Initial: $4.5-11.2mL/m^2/day$ (5-12.4g/m^2/day); $4.5mL/m^2$/day for patients w/ some residual enzyme activity who are not adequately controlled w/ protein restrictions

Consider patient's residual urea synthetic capacity, dietary protein requirements, and diet adherence in determining the initial dose in treatment-naive patients

For Both Subpopulations:
Administer in 3 equally divided doses, each rounded up to the nearest 0.5mL
Max: 17.5mL/day (19g/day)

DOSING CONSIDERATIONS
Hepatic Impairment
Moderate to Severe: Recommended starting dosage is at the lower end of the range

Elderly
Start at lower end of dosing range

Other Important Considerations
Adjustment Based on Plasma Ammonia: Adjust dose to produce a fasting plasma ammonia level that is <1/2 the ULN according to age

Adjustment Based on Urinary Phenylacetylglutamine (U-PAGN): Adjust dose upward if U-PAGN excretion is insufficient to cover daily dietary protein intake and the fasting ammonia is >1/2 the ULN; the amount of dose adjustment should factor in the amount of dietary protein that has not been covered, as indicated by the 24-hr U-PAGN level and the estimated Ravicti dose needed per gram of dietary protein ingested and the max total daily dose

Consider use of concomitant medications (eg, probenecid) when making dosage adjustment decisions based on U-PAGN; probenecid may result in a decrease of the U-PAGN excretion

Refer to PI for adjustment based on plasma phenylacetate

ADMINISTRATION

Oral route, NG or gastrostomy tube

Take w/ food.

Administer directly into the mouth via oral syringe or dosing cup.

Use w/ dietary protein restriction and, in some cases, dietary supplements (eg, essential amino acids, arginine, citrulline, protein-free calorie supplements).

Preparation for NG or Gastrostomy Tube Administration

1. Utilize an oral syringe to withdraw the prescribed dosage of Ravicti from the bottle.
2. Place the tip of the syringe into to the tip of the gastrostomy/NG tube.
3. Utilizing the plunger of the syringe, administer Ravicti into the tube.
4. Flush once w/ 30mL of water and allow the flush to drain.
5. Flush a 2nd time w/ an additional 30mL of water to clear the tube.

STORAGE

20-25°C (68-77°F); excursions permitted to 15-30°C (59-86°F).

HOW SUPPLIED

Liquid: 1.1g/mL [25mL]

CONTRAINDICATIONS

Pediatric patients <2 months of age.

WARNINGS/PRECAUTIONS

Not indicated for the treatment of acute hyperammonemia in patients w/ UCDs. Should be prescribed by a physician experienced in the management of UCDs. The major metabolite, phenylacetate (PAA), is associated w/ neurotoxicity; reduce dose if symptoms of N/V, headache, somnolence, confusion, or sleepiness are present in the absence of high ammonia or other intercurrent illnesses. Low or absent pancreatic enzymes or intestinal disease resulting in fat malabsorption may result in reduced or absent digestion of glycerol phenylbutyrate and/or absorption of phenylbutyrate and reduced control of plasma ammonia; monitor ammonia levels closely in patients w/ pancreatic insufficiency or intestinal malabsorption and when starting therapy in patients w/ renal impairment.

ADVERSE REACTIONS

Diarrhea, flatulence, headache.

DRUG INTERACTIONS

Use of corticosteroids may cause breakdown of body protein and increase plasma ammonia levels; monitor ammonia levels closely. Hyperammonemia may be induced by haloperidol and by valproic acid; monitor ammonia levels closely when concurrent use is necessary. Probenecid may inhibit the renal excretion of metabolites.

PREGNANCY AND LACTATION

Pregnancy: Category C. A voluntary patient registry will include evaluation of pregnancy outcomes in patients w/ UCDs.

Lactation: It is not known whether glycerol phenylbutyrate or its metabolites are present in breast milk; not for use in nursing.

MECHANISM OF ACTION

Prodrug of PBA; provides an alternate vehicle for waste nitrogen excretion.

PHARMACOKINETICS

Absorption: T_{max}=8 hrs (PBA), 12 hrs (PAA), 10 hrs (PAGN). Refer to PI for parameters in different populations. **Distribution:** Plasma protein binding (80.6-98% PBA, 37.1-65.6% PAA, 7-12% PAGN). **Metabolism:** Hydrolysis via pancreatic lipases; PBA via β-oxidation to PAA; conjugation (hepatic) and via L-glutamine-N-acetyltransferase (renal) to PAGN. **Elimination:** Urine=68.9% (PAGN [adults]); 66.4% (PAGN [pediatric patients]); <1% (PAA); <1% (PBA).

PATIENT CONSIDERATIONS

Assessment: Assess for drug hypersensitivity, acute hyperammonemia, N-acetylglutamate synthase deficiency, pancreatic insufficiency, intestinal malabsorption, renal/hepatic impairment, pregnancy/nursing status, and possible drug interactions.

Monitoring: Monitor for neurotoxicity, symptoms of N/V, headache, somnolence, confusion, or sleepiness in the absence of high ammonia or other intercurrent illnesses, and other adverse reactions. Monitor ammonia levels.

Counseling: Inform of the possible benefits/risks of therapy. Advise of the common/possible adverse reactions and instruct to call the doctor immediately if symptoms are experienced or if neurological toxicity (eg, somnolence, fatigue, lightheadedness, headache, dysgeusia, hypoacusis, disorientation, impaired memory) occurs. Encourage patients and caregivers to participate in the registry for UCD patients and advise that their participation is voluntary. Instruct to take drug exactly as prescribed and inform that treatment must be used w/ dietary protein restriction, and in some cases, dietary supplements (eg, essential amino acids, arginine, citrulline, protein-free calorie supplements).

RAXIBACUMAB — raxibacumab   Rx

Class: Monoclonal antibody

ADULT DOSAGE	PEDIATRIC DOSAGE
Inhalational Anthrax	**Inhalational Anthrax**
Treatment of inhalational anthrax due to *Bacillus anthracis* in combination w/ appropriate antibacterial drugs and for prophylaxis of inhalational anthrax when alternative therapies are not available/not appropriate	Treatment of inhalational anthrax due to *B. anthracis* in combination w/ appropriate antibacterial drugs and for prophylaxis of inhalational anthrax when alternative therapies are not available/not appropriate
40mg/kg IV as a single dose over 2 hrs and 15 min	**≤15kg:** 80mg/kg IV as a single dose over 2 hrs and 15 min

Premedication

Administer 25-50mg diphenhydramine w/in 1 hr prior to infusion to reduce the risk of infusion reactions; diphenhydramine route of administration (oral or IV) should be based on the temporal proximity to the start of raxibacumab infusion

>15-50kg:

60mg/kg IV as a single dose over 2 hrs and 15 min

>50kg:

40mg/kg IV as a single dose over 2 hrs and 15 min

Premedication

Premedicate w/ diphenhydramine w/in 1 hr prior to infusion; diphenhydramine route of administration (oral or IV) should be based on the temporal proximity to the start of raxibacumab infusion

---

DOSING CONSIDERATIONS

Adverse Reactions

May slow or interrupt infusion if patient develops any signs of adverse reactions (eg, infusion-associated symptoms)

ADMINISTRATION

IV route

Give as an IV infusion after dilution in a compatible sol to a final volume of 250mL (adults and children ≥50kg) or to a volume indicated based on the child's weight (refer to PI).

Compatible Sol

- NaCl 0.9% inj
- NaCl 0.45% inj

The prepared sol is stable for 8 hrs stored at room temperature.

Refer to PI for further information on preparation and administration instructions, including diluents, infusion volumes, and rates based on weight.

STORAGE

2-8°C (36-46°F). Do not freeze. Protect from exposure to light, prior to use; brief exposure to light, as w/ normal use, is acceptable.

HOW SUPPLIED

Inj: 50mg/mL [34mL]

WARNINGS/PRECAUTIONS

Does not prevent or treat meningitis. Infusion-related reactions (eg, rash, urticaria, pruritus) reported; slow or interrupt infusion and administer appropriate treatment if these reactions occur.

ADVERSE REACTIONS

Rash, pain in extremity, pruritus, somnolence.

PREGNANCY AND LACTATION

Pregnancy: Category B.

Lactation: Safety not known in nursing.

MECHANISM OF ACTION

Monoclonal antibody; binds free protective antigen (PA) of *B. anthracis*. Inhibits the binding of PA to its cellular receptors, preventing the intracellular entry of the anthrax lethal factor and edema factor, the enzymatic toxin components responsible for the pathogenic effects of anthrax toxin.

PHARMACOKINETICS

Absorption: AUC=15,845.8mcg•day/mL; C_{max}=1020.3mcg/mL.

PATIENT CONSIDERATIONS

Assessment: Assess for drug hypersensitivity and pregnancy/nursing status.

Monitoring: Monitor for infusion reactions and other adverse reactions.

Counseling: Instruct to inform physician if patients are pregnant, become pregnant, or are thinking about becoming pregnant, or are planning to breastfeed. Instruct to notify physician if any adverse reactions develop.

RAYOS — prednisone   Rx

Class: Glucocorticoid

ADULT DOSAGE	PEDIATRIC DOSAGE
Steroid-Responsive Disorders	**Steroid-Responsive Disorders**
Initial: 5-60mg/day depending on disease being treated	**Initial:** 5-60mg/day depending on disease being treated
If currently on immediate-release prednisone, prednisolone, or methylprednisolone, switch to an equivalent dose based on relative potency	If currently on immediate-release prednisone, prednisolone, or methylprednisolone, switch to an equivalent dose based on relative potency
Maintain/adjust initial dose until response is satisfactory	Maintain/adjust initial dose until response is satisfactory
If no satisfactory clinical response after a reasonable period, D/C and transfer to other appropriate therapy	If no satisfactory clinical response after a reasonable period, D/C and transfer to other appropriate therapy
Maint: Decrease initial dosage in small decrements at appropriate time intervals to lowest effective dose	**Maint:** Decrease initial dosage in small decrements at appropriate time intervals to lowest effective dose
D/C if a period of spontaneous remission occurs in a chronic condition	D/C if a period of spontaneous remission occurs in a chronic condition

DOSING CONSIDERATIONS

Elderly
Start at lower end of dosing range

Discontinuation
Withdraw gradually after long-term therapy

ADMINISTRATION
Oral route

Take PO w/ food
Do not break, divide, or chew tab

STORAGE
25°C (77°F); excursions permitted to 15-30°C (59-86°F). Protect from light and moisture.

HOW SUPPLIED
Tab, Delayed-Release: 1mg, 2mg, 5mg

CONTRAINDICATIONS
Known hypersensitivity to prednisone or to any of the excipients.

WARNINGS/PRECAUTIONS
Monitor for situations which may make dosage adjustments necessary (eg, change in clinical status secondary to remissions/exacerbations in the disease process, individual drug responsiveness, effect of patient exposure to stress). May need to increase dose for a period of time consistent with patient's condition during stressful situations. May produce reversible hypothalamic-pituitary adrenal (HPA) axis suppression with potential for corticosteroid insufficiency after withdrawal. Drug-induced secondary adrenocortical insufficiency may be minimized by gradual dose reduction. Changes in thyroid status may necessitate dose adjustment. May mask signs of infection, and increase risk of dissemination, reactivation, or exacerbation of latent infection. May reduce resistance to new infections. More serious or fatal course of chickenpox and measles in non-immune patients reported; avoid exposure. May exacerbate systemic fungal infections; avoid use unless needed to control drug reactions. May activate latent amebiasis; rule out latent or active amebiasis before initiating therapy. Not for use in cerebral malaria and active ocular herpes simplex. Increased risk of GI perforation in patients with certain GI disorders; Signs of GI perforation may be masked. Caution with known or suspected *Strongyloides* (threadworm) infestation, active/latent tuberculosis (TB) or tuberculin reactivity, diverticulitis, fresh intestinal anastomoses, active or latent peptic ulcer, left ventricular free wall rupture after a recent myocardial infarction, probable impending perforation, abscess or other pyogenic infections. May cause BP elevation, salt/water retention, increased K+ and Ca2+ excretion; caution with congestive heart failure (CHF), HTN, or renal insufficiency. May be associated with CNS effects and may aggravate existing emotional instability or psychotic tendencies. May decrease bone formation and increase bone resorption, and may lead to inhibition of bone growth in pediatric patients and development of osteoporosis at any age; caution with increased risk of osteoporosis (eg, postmenopausal women). May produce posterior subcapsular cataracts, glaucoma with possible optic nerve damage, and enhance establishment of secondary ocular infections. Not recommended in optic neuritis treatment. May elevate intraocular pressure (IOP); monitor IOP if used for >6 weeks. Caution with ocular herpes simplex. Monitor growth and development of pediatric patients on prolonged therapy. May cause fetal harm. Acute myopathy reported with use of high doses, most often occurring in patients with neuromuscular transmission disorders (eg, myasthenia gravis). Creatine kinase elevation and Kaposi's sarcoma may occur. May suppress reactions to skin tests. Caution in elderly.

ADVERSE REACTIONS
Fluid retention, glucose tolerance alteration, BP elevation, behavioral/mood changes, increased appetite, weight gain.

DRUG INTERACTIONS
Live or live, attenuated vaccines are contraindicated with immunosuppressive doses. May diminish response to toxoids and live or inactivated vaccines. Aminoglutethimide may lead to loss of corticosteroid-induced adrenal suppression. Cardiac enlargement and CHF may occur with concomitant use of amphotericin B. May produce severe weakness in myasthenia gravis patients with anticholinesterase agents; d/c anticholinesterase agents at least 24 hrs before initiating therapy. Monitor coagulation indices frequently with warfarin. Dose adjustment of antidiabetic agents may be required. May decrease serum concentrations of isoniazid. CYP3A4 inducers (eg, barbiturates, phenytoin, carbamazepine, ephedrine, rifampin) may enhance metabolism and may require increase in corticosteroid dose. CYP3A4 inhibitors (eg, ketoconazole, macrolide antibiotics) may decrease metabolism leading to increased risk of corticosteroid side effects. Cholestyramine may increase clearance. Increased activity of both drugs may occur with cyclosporine; convulsions reported with concurrent use. May increase risk of arrhythmias due to hypokalemia with digitalis glycosides. Estrogens may decrease hepatic metabolism, thereby increasing the effect. Aspirin (ASA) or other NSAIDs may increase risk of GI side effects. Caution with ASA in hypoprothrombinemia patients. May increase clearance of salicylates. Closely monitor for hypokalemia when administered with K+-depleting agents (eg, amphotericin B, diuretics). Acute myopathy reported with neuromuscular blocking drugs (eg, pancuronium).

PREGNANCY AND LACTATION
Category D, caution in nursing.

MECHANISM OF ACTION
Glucocorticoid; causes profound and varied metabolic effects and modifies the body's immune responses to diverse stimuli.

PHARMACOKINETICS
Absorption: T_{max}=6-6.5 hrs (median). **Distribution:** Found in breast milk. **Metabolism:** Liver; prednisolone (active metabolite). **Elimination:** Urine; $T_{1/2}$=2-3 hrs.

PATIENT CONSIDERATIONS

Assessment: Assess for systemic fungal/other current infections, active TB, latent/active amebiasis, cerebral malaria, active ocular herpes simplex, emotional instability or psychotic tendencies, hypersensitivity to drug, and for any other condition where treatment is contraindicated or cautioned. Assess pregnancy/nursing status, vaccination history, thyroid status, and for possible drug interactions.

Monitoring: Monitor for HPA axis suppression, adrenocortical insufficiency, salt/water retention, infections/secondary ocular infections, change in thyroid status, posterior subcapsular cataracts, glaucoma with optic nerve damage, Kaposi's sarcoma, emotional instability or psychotic tendencies aggravation, and other adverse reactions. Monitor BP, body weight, routine laboratory studies (eg, 2-hr postprandial blood glucose and serum K+ levels), and chest X-ray at regular intervals during prolonged therapy. Monitor growth and development of pediatric patients on prolonged therapy. Monitor for hypoadrenalism in infants born to mothers who received substantial doses during pregnancy. Monitor bone density in patients on long term therapy.

Counseling: Instruct to take exactly as prescribed, not to d/c therapy abruptly or without medical supervision, to advise any medical attendants that taking the drug, and to seek medical advice if fever or other signs of infection develop. Instruct to discuss with physician if had recent or ongoing infections or if have recently received a vaccine. Advise if on immunosuppressant doses, to avoid exposure to chickenpox or measles; instruct to seek medical advice if exposed. Instruct to inform physician of all the medicines being taken, including OTC and prescription drugs, dietary supplements, and herbal products. Inform that for missed doses, take the missed dose as soon as remember; counsel that if it is almost time for the next dose, instruct to skip the missed dose and take medicine at the next regularly schedule time. Advise about common adverse reactions that could occur with therapy.

RAZADYNE ER — galantamine hydrobromide   Rx

Class: Acetylcholinesterase (AChE) inhibitor

OTHER BRAND NAMES
Razadyne

ADULT DOSAGE	PEDIATRIC DOSAGE
Alzheimer's Disease	Pediatric use may not have been established
Mild to Moderate Dementia of the Alzheimer's Type:	
Sol/Tab: **Initial:** 4mg bid (8mg/day) **Titrate:** Increase to initial maint dose of 8mg bid (16mg/day) after ≥4 weeks, then may increase to 12mg bid (24mg/day) after ≥4 weeks **Range:** 16-24mg/day	
If therapy is interrupted for >3 days, restart at the lowest dose and escalate to current dose	
Cap, Extended-Release (ER): **Initial:** 8mg/day **Titrate:** Increase to initial maint dose of 16mg/day after ≥4 weeks, then increase to 24mg/day after ≥4 weeks **Range:** 16-24mg/day	
Converting from Immediate-Release (IR) Tab/Sol: Use same total daily dose of IR; take last dose of IR tab/sol in pm and start ER cap the next am	

DOSING CONSIDERATIONS

Renal Impairment
CrCl 9-59mL/min: Do not exceed 16mg/day
<9mL/min: Not recommended

Hepatic Impairment
Child-Pugh 7-9: Do not exceed 16mg/day
Child-Pugh 10-15: Not recommended

ADMINISTRATION
Oral route

Take w/ food.
Cap, ER: Administer once daily in the am.
Tab/Sol: Administer twice a day, w/ am and pm meals.
Ensure adequate fluid intake during treatment.

STORAGE
25°C (77°F); excursions permitted to 15-30°C (59-86°F). (Sol) Do not freeze.

HOW SUPPLIED
Cap, ER: 8mg, 16mg, 24mg; **Sol:** 4mg/mL [100mL]; **Tab:** 4mg, 8mg, 12mg

CONTRAINDICATIONS
Known hypersensitivity to galantamine hydrobromide or to any excipients used in the formulation.

WARNINGS/PRECAUTIONS

Serious skin reactions (Stevens-Johnson syndrome and acute generalized exanthematous pustulosis) reported; d/c at the 1st appearance of skin rash, unless the rash is clearly not drug-related. Do not resume, and consider alternative therapy if signs/symptoms suggest a serious skin reaction. Bradycardia and all types of heart block reported in patients w/ and w/o known underlying cardiac conduction abnormalities; all patients should be considered at risk. May increase gastric acid secretion. May produce N/V, diarrhea, anorexia, or weight loss. May cause bladder outflow obstruction. Potential to cause generalized convulsions. Caution in patients w/ history of severe asthma or obstructive pulmonary disease. Deaths reported w/ mild cognitive impairment.

ADVERSE REACTIONS

N/V, dizziness, decreased appetite, diarrhea, headache.

DRUG INTERACTIONS

Potential to interfere w/ anticholinergics. Expected synergistic effect w/ succinylcholine, other cholinesterase inhibitors, similar neuromuscular blockers, or cholinergic agonists (eg, bethanechol). Monitor closely for symptoms of active/ occult GI bleeding w/ concurrent NSAIDs.

PREGNANCY AND LACTATION

Pregnancy: Category C.
Lactation: Caution in nursing.

MECHANISM OF ACTION

Acetylcholinesterase inhibitor; not established. Increases concentration of acetylcholine through reversible inhibition of its hydrolysis by cholinesterase.

PHARMACOKINETICS

Absorption: Absolute bioavailability (90%), T_{max}=1 hr. **Distribution:** V_d=175L; plasma protein binding (18%). **Metabolism:** Glucuronidation via CYP2D6 and CYP3A4. **Elimination:** (IV/PO) Urine (20% unchanged); $T_{1/2}$=7 hrs.

PATIENT CONSIDERATIONS

Assessment: Assess for known hypersensitivity to drug, cardiovascular conditions, history of ulcer disease, severe asthma or obstructive pulmonary disease, renal/ hepatic impairment, pregnancy/nursing status, and possible drug interactions.

Monitoring: Monitor closely for symptoms of active/occult GI bleeding, serious skin reactions, bradycardia, heart block, bladder outflow obstruction, seizures, and other adverse reactions. Closely monitor respiratory function. Monitor weight during therapy.

Counseling: Advise patients and caregivers to d/c therapy and seek immediate medical attention at the 1st appearance of skin rash. Instruct to take ud in order to minimize adverse reactions. Inform that dose escalation should follow a minimum of 4 weeks at prior dose. Inform that if therapy has been interrupted for >3 days, patient should be restarted w/ the lowest dose and then retitrated to an appropriate dosage. Advise to ensure adequate fluid intake during treatment. (Sol) Inform that there is an Instruction Sheet describing how sol should be given; urge to read prior to administration.

REBETOL — ribavirin   Rx

Class: Nucleoside analogue

> Not for monotherapy treatment of chronic hepatitis C virus infection. Primary toxicity is hemolytic anemia. Anemia associated w/ therapy may result in worsening of cardiac disease and lead to fatal and nonfatal MIs. Avoid w/ history of significant/unstable cardiac disease. Contraindicated in women who are pregnant and in male partners of pregnant women. Extreme care must be taken to avoid pregnancy during therapy and for 6 months after completion of therapy in both female patients and in female partners of male patients who are taking therapy. Use at least 2 reliable forms of effective contraception during treatment and for 6 months after discontinuation.

ADULT DOSAGE

Chronic Hepatitis C with Compensated Liver Disease

Combination Therapy w/ PegIntron:
Treat w/ PegIntron 1.5mcg/kg/ week SQ

<66kg: 400mg qam and 400mg qpm
66-80kg: 400mg qam and 600mg qpm
81-105kg: 600mg qam and 600mg qpm
>105kg: 600mg qam and 800mg qpm

Interferon Alfa-Naive:
Genotype 1: Treat for 48 weeks
Genotype 2 and 3: Treat for 24 weeks

Retreatment:
Treat for 48 weeks, regardless of hepatitis C virus genotype

Combination Therapy w/ Intron A:
Treat w/ Intron A 3 million IU 3X weekly SQ

≤75kg: 400mg qam and 600mg qpm
>75kg: 600mg qam and 600mg qpm

Interferon Alfa-Naive:
Treat for 24-48 weeks

Retreatment:
Treat for 24 weeks

PEDIATRIC DOSAGE

Chronic Hepatitis C with Compensated Liver Disease

Combination Therapy w/ PegIntron/ Intron A:
≥3 Years:
Sol:
<47kg: 15mg/kg/day divided into two doses; may use sol regardless of body weight

Cap:
47-59kg: 400mg qam and 400mg qpm
60-73kg: 400mg qam and 600mg qpm
>73kg: 600mg qam and 600mg qpm

Treat w/ Intron A 3 million IU/m² 3X weekly SQ for 25-61kg (refer to adult dosing for >61kg) or PegIntron 60mcg/m²/week SQ

Genotype 1: Treat for 48 weeks
Genotype 2 or 3: Treat for 24 weeks

Remain on pediatric dosing while receiving therapy in combination w/ PegIntron when 18th birthday is reached

DOSING CONSIDERATIONS
Renal Impairment
CrCl <50mL/min: Not recommended
Elderly
Start at lower end of dosing range
Adverse Reactions
Refer to PI for dose modification/discontinuation based on lab parameters in adults and pediatric patients

Discontinuation
Adults:
Genotype 1:
Interferon-Alfa Naive:
D/C therapy if at least a 2 log_{10} drop or loss of hepatitis C virus (HCV)-RNA at 12 weeks of therapy is not achieved
D/C therapy if HCV-RNA levels remain detectable after 24 weeks of therapy

All Genotypes:
Previously Treated Patients:
Consider discontinuation if fail to achieve undetectable HCV-RNA at Week 12 of therapy, or if HCV-RNA remains detectable after 24 weeks of therapy

Pediatric Patients (3-17 Years):
All Genotypes (Excluding Genotype 2 and 3):
D/C therapy at 12 weeks if treatment Week 12 HCV-RNA drops <2 log_{10} compared to pretreatment
D/C therapy at 24 weeks if HCV-RNA is detectable at treatment Week 24

ADMINISTRATION

Oral route

Take w/ food.

Refer to PegIntron or Intron A PIs for further information on dosing, dosing modifications, and administration for these drugs.

Cap
Do not open, crush, or break.

STORAGE
(Cap) 25°C (77°F); excursions permitted to 15-30°C (59-86°F). (Sol) 2-8°C (36-46°F) or at 25°C (77°F); excursions permitted to 15-30°C (59-86°F).

HOW SUPPLIED
Cap: 200mg; **Sol:** 40mg/mL [100mL]

CONTRAINDICATIONS
Women who are or may become pregnant, men whose female partners are pregnant, autoimmune hepatitis, hemoglobinopathies (eg, thalassemia major, sickle cell anemia), CrCl <50mL/min, coadministration w/ didanosine. Known hypersensitivity reactions (eg, Stevens-Johnson syndrome, toxic, epidermal necrolysis, erythema multiforme) to ribavirin or any component of the product.

WARNINGS/PRECAUTIONS
Do not start therapy unless a negative pregnancy test has been obtained immediately prior to therapy. Suspend therapy in patients w/ signs and symptoms of pancreatitis; d/c therapy w/ confirmed pancreatitis. Pulmonary symptoms (eg, dyspnea, pulmonary infiltrates, pneumonitis) reported; closely monitor if pulmonary infiltrates or pulmonary function impairment develops and if appropriate, d/c therapy. Alfa interferons may induce or aggravate ophthalmologic disorders (eg, decrease or loss of vision, retinopathy); perform eye exam in all patients prior to therapy, periodically w/ preexisting ophthalmologic disorders (eg, diabetic or hypertensive retinopathy), and if ocular symptoms develop during therapy. D/C if new or worsening ophthalmologic disorders develop. Severe decreases in neutrophil and platelet counts, and hematologic, endocrine (eg, TSH), and hepatic abnormalities may occur in combination w/ PegIntron; perform hematology and blood chemistry testing prior to therapy and periodically thereafter. Dental/periodontal disorders reported in patients receiving ribavirin and interferon or peginterferon combination therapy. Weight changes and growth inhibition (including long-term growth inhibition) reported in pediatric patients during combination therapy w/ PegIntron or Intron A. Use w/ PegIntron or Intron A is associated w/ significant adverse reactions (eg, severe depression and suicidal or homicidal ideation, suppression of bone marrow function, autoimmune and infectious disorders). Caution w/ preexisting cardiac disease; d/c if cardiovascular (CV) status deteriorates.

ADVERSE REACTIONS
Hemolytic anemia, inj-site reactions, headache, fatigue, rigors, fever, N/V, anorexia, myalgia, arthralgia, insomnia, irritability, depression, neutropenia, alopecia.

DRUG INTERACTIONS
See Contraindications. Closely monitor for toxicities, especially hepatic decompensation and anemia when receiving interferon w/ribavirin and nucleoside reverse transcriptase inhibitors (NRTIs); consider dose reduction or discontinuation of interferon, ribavirin, or both, or discontinuation of NRTI if medically appropriate. May antagonize the cell culture antiviral activity of stavudine and zidovudine against HIV; caution w/ concomitant use of ribavirin with either of these drugs. Severe pancytopenia and bone marrow suppression reported w/ concomitant administration of pegylated interferon/ribavirin and azathioprine; d/c pegylated interferon/ribavirin and azathioprine if pancytopenia develops and do not reintroduce pegylated interferon/ribavirin w/ concomitant azathioprine.

PREGNANCY AND LACTATION
Category X, not for use in nursing.

MECHANISM OF ACTION
Nucleoside analogue; has not been established. Has direct antiviral activity in tissue culture against many RNA viruses; increases mutation frequency in the genomes of several viruses and ribavirin triphosphate inhibits HCV polymerase in a biochemical reaction.

PHARMACOKINETICS

Absorption: Rapid and extensive. Absolute bioavailability (64%). Multiple Dose: (Cap) (Adults) C_{max}=3680ng/mL, T_{max}=3 hrs, AUC=228,000ng•hr/mL. (Pediatrics) C_{max}=3275ng/mL, T_{max}=1.9 hrs, AUC=29,774ng•hr/mL. **Distribution:** (Adults) (Cap) Single Dose: V_d=2825L. **Metabolism:** Nucleated cells (phosphorylation); deribosylation and amide hydrolysis. **Elimination:** Urine (61%), feces (12%). (Adults) (Cap) Multiple Dose: $T_{1/2}$=298 hrs.

PATIENT CONSIDERATIONS

Assessment: Assess for autoimmune hepatitis, hemoglobinopathies, depression, preexisting ophthalmologic disorders, history of or preexisting cardiac disease, hypersensitivity, and possible drug interactions. Assess nursing status and hepatic/renal/pulmonary function. Conduct pregnancy test (including female partners of male patients), standard hematologic tests, blood chemistries, ECG in patients w/ preexisting cardiac disease, and eye examination.

Monitoring: Monitor for anemia, worsening of cardiac disease, pancreatitis, renal/hepatic dysfunction, CV deterioration, pulmonary function impairment, new/worsening ophthalmologic disorders, and other adverse reactions. Monitor height and weight in pediatric patients. Perform standard hematologic tests, blood chemistries (eg, TSH), ECG, and HCV-RNA periodically. Obtain Hct and Hgb (Week 2 and 4 of therapy, and as clinically appropriate). Perform pregnancy test monthly during therapy and for 6 months after discontinuation of therapy (including female partners of male patients). Schedule regular dental exams.

Counseling: Counsel on risk/benefits associated w/ treatment. Inform that anemia may develop. Advise that lab evaluations are required prior to starting therapy and periodically thereafter. Advise to be well-hydrated, especially during the initial stages of treatment. Inform of pregnancy risks. Instruct to use at least 2 forms of contraception and perform a monthly pregnancy test during therapy and for 6 months post-therapy (including female partners of male patients); advise to notify physician in the event of a pregnancy. Inform that appropriate precautions to prevent HCV transmission should be taken. Instruct to brush teeth bid and have regular dental exams; if vomiting occurs, advise to rinse out mouth afterwards.

REBIF — interferoh beta-1a   Rx

Class: Biological response modifier

ADULT DOSAGE	PEDIATRIC DOSAGE
Multiple Sclerosis	Pediatric use may not have been established
Treatment of Relapsing Forms: 22mcg or 44mcg 3X/week	
Titration Schedule for 22mcg Prescribed Dose:	
Week 1: 4.4mcg (half of 8.8mcg syringe)	
Week 2: 4.4mcg (half of 8.8mcg syringe)	
Week 3: 11mcg (half of 22mcg syringe)	
Week 4: 11mcg (half of 22mcg syringe)	
Week 5 and After: 22mcg Use only prefilled syringes to titrate to the 22mcg prescribed dose	
Titration Schedule for 44mcg Prescribed Dose:	
Week 1: 8.8mcg	
Week 2: 8.8mcg	
Week 3: 22mcg	
Week 4: 22mcg	
Week 5 and After: 44mcg Prefilled syringes or autoinjectors can be used to titrate to the 44mcg prescribed dose	
Premedication	
Concurrent use of analgesics and/or antipyretics may help ameliorate flu-like symptoms on treatment days	

- -

DOSING CONSIDERATIONS

Elderly
Start at lower end of dosing range

Adverse Reactions
Decreased Peripheral Blood Counts: May necessitate dose reduction or discontinuation until toxicity is resolved
Elevated LFTs: May necessitate dose reduction or discontinuation until toxicity is resolved

ADMINISTRATION

SQ route

Administer at the same time (preferably late afternoon or pm) on the same 3 days at least 48 hrs apart each week.
Rotate site of inj w/ each dose.
Refer to PI for additional instructions.

STORAGE

2-8°C (36-46°F). Do not freeze. If needed, may store at 2-25°C (36-77°F) for up to 30 days and away from heat and light, but refrigeration is preferred.

HOW SUPPLIED

Inj: 22mcg/0.5mL, 44mcg/0.5mL [prefilled syringe, Rebidose autoinjector]; (Titration Pack) 8.8mcg/0.2mL, 22mcg/0.5mL [prefilled syringe, Rebidose autoinjector]

CONTRAINDICATIONS

History of hypersensitivity to natural or recombinant interferon beta, human albumin, or any other component of the formulation.

WARNINGS/PRECAUTIONS

Depression, suicidal ideation, and suicide attempts reported; consider cessation of treatment if depression develops. Severe liver injury reported rarely; d/c immediately if jaundice or other symptoms of liver dysfunction appear. Asymptomatic elevation of hepatic transaminases (particularly ALT) may occur; caution w/ active liver disease, alcohol abuse, increased serum ALT (>2.5X ULN), or history of significant liver disease. Consider dose reduction if ALT rises >5X ULN; may gradually re-escalate dose when enzyme levels have normalized. Anaphylaxis (rare) and other allergic reactions (eg, skin rash, urticaria) reported; d/c if anaphylaxis occurs. Inj-site reactions (eg, necrosis), decreased peripheral blood counts in all cell lines (including pancytopenia), thrombotic microangiopathy (including thrombotic thrombocytopenic purpura and hemolytic uremic syndrome), seizures, and new or worsening thyroid abnormalities reported. D/C if clinical symptoms and lab findings consistent w/ thrombotic microangiopathy occur. Caution in patients w/ preexisting seizure disorders.

ADVERSE REACTIONS

Inj-site disorders, headache, fatigue, fever, rigors, chest pain, back pain, myalgia, abdominal pain, depression, elevation of liver enzymes, hematologic abnormalities.

DRUG INTERACTIONS

Consider the potential for hepatic injury when used in combination w/ known hepatotoxic products, or when new agents are added to the regimen.

PREGNANCY AND LACTATION

Pregnancy: Category C.
Lactation: Caution in nursing.

MECHANISM OF ACTION

Biological response modifier; mechanism not established.

PHARMACOKINETICS

Absorption: (Single 60mcg SQ inj) C_{max}=5.1 IU/mL, T_{max}=16 hrs (median), AUC_{0-96h}=294 IU•hr/mL. **Elimination:** $T_{1/2}$=69 hrs.

PATIENT CONSIDERATIONS

Assessment: Assess for depression, history of or active liver disease, alcohol abuse, preexisting seizure disorder, thyroid dysfunction, myelosuppression, history of hypersensitivity to drug or to human albumin, pregnancy/nursing status, and possible drug interactions.

Monitoring: Monitor for depression, suicidal ideation, jaundice, anaphylaxis, allergic reactions, inj-site reactions, seizures, thrombotic microangiopathy, and other adverse reactions. Perform CBC and LFTs at regular intervals (1, 3, and 6 months) following initiation of therapy and then periodically thereafter in the absence of clinical symptoms; patients w/ myelosuppression may require more intensive monitoring of CBC, w/ differential and platelet counts. Perform thyroid function tests every 6 months in patients w/ a history of thyroid dysfunction, or as clinically indicated.

Counseling: Inform of the symptoms of depression, suicidal ideation, hepatic injury, decreased peripheral blood counts, and seizures, and instruct to immediately report any of these symptoms to physician. Instruct to seek immediate medical attention if symptoms of allergic reactions and anaphylaxis occur. Advise patients that inj-site reactions may occur and to promptly report any signs of necrosis at inj site. Inform that flu-like symptoms are common following initiation of therapy; advise on concurrent use of analgesics and/or antipyretics to help reduce flu-like symptoms on treatment days. Instruct on the use of aseptic technique when self-administering the drug and on the importance of rotating inj sites. Explain the importance of proper disposal of prefilled syringes and autoinjectors, and caution against reuse of these items. Inform about the risks/benefits of treatment during pregnancy.

RECLAST — zoledronic acid   Rx

Class: Bisphosphonate

ADULT DOSAGE	PEDIATRIC DOSAGE
Osteoporosis	Pediatric use may not have been established
Treatment in Men and Postmenopausal Women: 5mg IV once a yr	
Prevention in Postmenopausal Women: 5mg IV once every 2 yrs	
Glucocorticoid-Induced Osteoporosis: In men and women who are either initiating or continuing systemic glucocorticoids in a daily dosage ≥7.5mg of prednisone and who are expected to remain on glucocorticoids for ≥12 months **Treatment/Prevention:** 5mg IV once a yr	

Paget's Disease

5mg IV

May consider retreatment in patients who have relapsed (based on increases in serum alkaline phosphatase), failed to achieve normalization of serum alkaline phosphatase, or those w/ symptoms

---

DOSING CONSIDERATIONS

Other Important Considerations

Recommended Intake of Ca²⁺ and Vitamin D:

In Osteoporosis: At least 1200mg of Ca^{2+} daily and 800-1000 IU of vitamin D daily

In Paget's Disease of Bone: 1500mg of Ca^{2+} daily in divided doses (750mg bid or 500mg tid) and 800 IU of vitamin D daily, particularly in the 2 weeks following administration

ADMINISTRATION

IV route

Infuse IV over ≥15 min at a constant rate.

Hydrate patients appropriately prior to administration.

IV infusion should be followed by a 10mL normal saline flush of the IV line.

Do not allow sol to come in contact w/ any Ca^{2+} or other divalent cation-containing sol.

Administer as a single IV sol through a separate vented infusion line.

May give acetaminophen following administration to reduce incidence of acute-phase reaction symptoms.

If refrigerated, allow refrigerated sol to reach room temperature before administration.

After opening, sol is stable for 24 hrs at 2-8°C (36-46°F).

STORAGE

25°C (77°F); excursions permitted to 15-30°C (59-86°F).

HOW SUPPLIED

Inj: 5mg/100mL

CONTRAINDICATIONS

Hypocalcemia, CrCl <35mL/min, acute renal impairment, known hypersensitivity to zoledronic acid or any components of this medication.

WARNINGS/PRECAUTIONS

Consider discontinuation after 3-5 yrs of use in patients at low-risk for fracture; periodically reevaluate risk for fracture in patients who d/c therapy. Contains same active ingredient as Zometa; do not treat w/ Reclast if on concomitant therapy w/ Zometa. Treat preexisting hypocalcemia and disturbances of mineral metabolism prior to treatment. Risk of hypocalcemia in Paget's disease. Withhold therapy until normovolemic status has been achieved if history or physical signs suggest dehydration. Caution w/ chronic renal impairment. Acute renal impairment, including renal failure, reported, especially in patients w/ preexisting renal compromise, advanced age, concomitant nephrotoxic medications or diuretic therapy, or severe dehydration. Transient increase in SrCr may be greater w/ impaired renal function; interim monitoring of CrCl should be performed in at-risk patients. Assess fluid status in patients at increased risk of acute renal failure (ARF) (eg, elderly, concomitant diuretic therapy). Osteonecrosis of the jaw (ONJ) reported; risk may increase w/ duration of exposure to drug or w/ concomitant administration of drugs associated w/ ONJ. Consider a dental examination w/ appropriate preventive dentistry prior to treatment in patients w/ a history of concomitant risk factors (eg, cancer, chemotherapy, angiogenesis inhibitors, radiotherapy, corticosteroids, poor oral hygiene, preexisting dental disease or infection, anemia, coagulopathy) and if possible, avoid invasive dental procedures while on treatment. Atypical, low-energy, or low-trauma fractures of the femoral shaft reported; evaluate any patient w/ a history of bisphosphonate exposure who presents w/ thigh/groin pain to rule out an incomplete femur fracture, and consider interruption of therapy. Avoid use in pregnancy; may cause fetal harm. Severe and occasionally incapacitating bone, joint, and/or muscle pain reported; consider withholding future treatment if severe symptoms develop. Caution w/ aspirin (ASA) sensitivity; bronchoconstriction reported.

ADVERSE REACTIONS

Treatment of Osteoporosis in Postmenopausal Women: Arthralgia, pyrexia, HTN, headache, myalgia, pain in extremity, osteoarthritis, influenza-like illness, dizziness, shoulder pain, diarrhea, bone pain, fatigue, chills, asthenia.

Prevention of Osteoporosis in Postmenopausal Women: Arthralgia, pain, pyrexia, myalgia, back pain, chills, N/V, headache, fatigue, pain in extremity, abdominal pain, diarrhea, musculoskeletal pain, dizziness, dyspepsia.

Osteoporosis in Men: Myalgia, fatigue, headache, musculoskeletal pain/stiffness, pain, chills, influenza-like illness, abdominal pain, malaise, dyspnea, increased C-reactive protein, acute phase reaction, lethargy, A-fib.

Glucocorticoid-Induced Osteoporosis: Abdominal pain, musculoskeletal pain, nausea, dyspepsia.

Paget's Disease of Bone: Influenza-like illness, pyrexia, bone pain, dizziness, nausea, fatigue, rigors, myalgia, influenza, constipation, lethargy, dyspnea, dyspepsia, pain, hypocalcemia.

DRUG INTERACTIONS

Caution w/ aminoglycosides; may have an additive effect to lower serum Ca^{2+} levels for prolonged periods. Caution w/ loop diuretics; may increase risk of hypocalcemia. Caution w/ other potentially nephrotoxic drugs (eg, NSAIDs). In patients w/ renal impairment, exposure to concomitant medications that are primarily renally excreted (eg, digoxin) may increase.

PREGNANCY AND LACTATION

Pregnancy: Category D.

Lactation: Not for use in nursing.

MECHANISM OF ACTION

Bisphosphonate; acts primarily on bone. Inhibits osteoclast-mediated bone resorption.

PHARMACOKINETICS

Distribution: Plasma protein binding (28% at 200ng/mL, 53% at 50ng/mL).

Elimination: Urine (39%), feces (<3%); $T_{1/2}$=146 hrs.

PATIENT CONSIDERATIONS

Assessment: Assess for hypocalcemia, disturbances of mineral metabolism, risk factors for developing renal impairment and ONJ, ASA sensitivity, previous hypersensitivity to the drug, pregnancy/nursing status, and possible drug interactions. Obtain SrCr and calculate CrCl based on actual body weight before each dose. Assess fluid status in patients at increased risk of ARF. Perform routine oral exam, and consider appropriate preventive dentistry in patients w/ a history of risk factors for ONJ.

Monitoring: Monitor for ONJ, atypical femur fracture, musculoskeletal pain, bronchoconstriction, and other adverse events. Monitor renal function and serum Ca^{2+}/mineral levels. Reevaluate the need for continued therapy on a periodic basis.

Counseling: Inform about benefits/risks of therapy, the symptoms of hypocalcemia, and the importance of Ca^{2+} and vitamin D supplementation. Instruct to notify physician if patient had surgery to remove some or all of parathyroid glands, had sections of intestine removed, takes any other medications, or is unable to take Ca^{2+} supplements. Advise to avoid becoming pregnant during treatment. Advise to eat and drink normally (at least 2 glasses of fluid, such as water, w/in a few hrs prior to infusion) on the day of treatment, w/in a few hrs prior to infusion. Inform of the most commonly associated side effects of therapy and instruct to consult physician if these symptoms persist. Instruct to maintain good oral hygiene and to undergo routine dental check-ups. Advise to report physician or dentist if experiencing persistent pain and/or nonhealing sore of the mouth or jaw.

RECOMBIVAX HB — *hepatitis B vaccine (recombinant)*   Rx

Class: Vaccine

ADULT DOSAGE	PEDIATRIC DOSAGE
Hepatitis B Vaccine	**Hepatitis B Vaccine**
Prevention of Infection Caused by All Known Subtypes:	**Prevention of Infection Caused by All Known Subtypes:**
≥20 Years (Adult Formulation): 10mcg at 0, 1, 6 months; if suggested dose (10mcg) is not available, the appropriate dosage can be achieved w/ two 5mcg doses	**0-19 Years (Pediatric/Adolescent Formulation):** **3-Dose Regimen:** 5mcg at 0, 1, 6 months
Predialysis/Dialysis (Dialysis Formulation):	**11-15 Years (Adult Formulation):** **2-Dose Regimen:** 10mcg at 0 and 4-6 months; if suggested dose (10mcg) is not available, the appropriate dosage can be achieved w/ two 5mcg doses
≥18 Years: 40mcg at 0, 1, 6 months; consider booster/revaccination if anti-hepatitis B surface (anti-HBs) level is <10 mIU/mL at 1-2 months after 3rd dose Assess the need for a booster dose annually by antibody testing, and give a booster dose when the anti-HBs level declines to <10 mIU/mL	Adolescents may receive either regimen of 3 x 5mcg (pediatric formulation) or 2 x 10mcg (adult formulation)
Known or Presumed Exposure to Hepatitis B Surface Antigen: Refer to recommendations of the Advisory Committee on Immunization Practices (ACIP) and to the package insert for hepatitis B immune globulin (HBIG) When recommended, administer the vaccine w/ HBIG IM at separate sites as soon as possible after exposure; administer additional doses of the vaccine in accordance w/ ACIP recommendations	**Known or Presumed Exposure to Hepatitis B Surface Antigen:** Refer to recommendations of the Advisory Committee on Immunization Practices (ACIP) and to the package insert for hepatitis B immune globulin (HBIG) When recommended, administer the vaccine w/ HBIG IM at separate sites as soon as possible after exposure; administer additional doses of the vaccine in accordance w/ ACIP recommendations

---

ADMINISTRATION

IM route

Administer into the deltoid muscle or the anterolateral thigh for infants <1 yr of age; do not administer in the gluteal region

May be given SQ if at risk of hemorrhage (eg, hemophiliacs)

Do not mix w/ any other vaccine; 1st dose of vaccine may be given at the same time as HBIG, but administer at different sites

Shake well before use

For single-dose vials, withdraw and administer entire dose using a sterile needle and syringe

For single-dose prefilled syringes, securely attach a needle by twisting in a clockwise direction and administer dose

STORAGE

2-8°C (36-46°F). Do not freeze.

HOW SUPPLIED
Inj: (Pediatric/Adolescent) 5mcg/0.5mL [vial, prefilled syringe]; (Adult) 10mcg/mL [vial, prefilled syringe]; (Dialysis) 40mcg/mL [vial]

CONTRAINDICATIONS
History of severe allergic or hypersensitivity reactions (eg, anaphylaxis) after a previous dose of any hepatitis B-containing vaccine or to any component of this product, including yeast

WARNINGS/PRECAUTIONS
Vial stopper, syringe plunger stopper, and tip cap contain dry natural latex rubber; allergic reactions may occur in latex-sensitive individuals. Apnea in premature infants following IM administration observed; decisions about when to administer vaccine should be based on consideration of medical status, and the potential benefits and possible risks of vaccination. Delay vaccine until 1 month of age or hospital discharge in infants weighing <2000g if the mother is documented to be HBsAg negative at the time of infant's birth. Infants weighing <2000g born to HBsAg positive or HBsAg unknown mothers should receive vaccine and HBIG in accordance with ACIP recommendations if HBsAg status cannot be determined. Appropriate medical treatment and supervision must be available for possible anaphylactic reactions following administration. May not prevent hepatitis B infection in patients with an unrecognized hepatitis B infection at time of vaccination. Vaccination may not protect all individuals.

ADVERSE REACTIONS
Irritability, fever, diarrhea, fatigue/weakness, diminished appetite, rhinitis, inj-site reactions.

PREGNANCY AND LACTATION
Category C, caution in nursing.

MECHANISM OF ACTION
Vaccine; has been shown to elicit antibodies to HBV.

PATIENT CONSIDERATIONS
Assessment: Assess current health status, hypersensitivity to yeast or any component of the vaccine, latex hypersensitivity, and pregnancy/nursing status. Review vaccination history for previous vaccination-related adverse reactions.

Monitoring: Monitor for signs/symptoms of hypersensitivity reactions, inj-site reactions, immune response, and for systemic reactions. Perform annual antibody testing in predialysis/dialysis patients to assess the need for booster doses.

Counseling: Inform of potential benefits/risks of vaccination and the importance of completing the immunization series. Instruct to report inj-site reactions or any serious adverse reactions to physician.

RECTIV — nitroglycerin   Rx

Class: Nitrate vasodilator

ADULT DOSAGE	PEDIATRIC DOSAGE
Moderate to Severe Pain	Pediatric use may not have been established
Associated w/ Chronic Anal Fissure: Apply 1 inch of oint (375mg) intra-anally q12h for up to 3 weeks	

ADMINISTRATION
Intra-anal route

1. Gently squeeze tube until a line of oint the length of the measuring line is expressed onto a covered finger.
2. Insert the oint into the anal canal using a covered finger no further than to the 1st finger joint.
3. Apply oint around the side of the anal canal; if unable to reach the anal canal due to pain, apply the oint directly to the outside of the anus.

STORAGE
20-25°C (68-77°F); excursions permitted to 15-30°C (59-85°F). Keep tube tightly closed; use within 8 weeks of 1st opening.

HOW SUPPLIED
Oint: 0.4% (4mg/g) [30g tube]

CONTRAINDICATIONS
Concomitant use w/ PDE-5 (eg, sildenafil, vardenafil, and tadalafil); severe anemia; increased intracranial pressure (ICP); known hypersensitivity to nitroglycerin, other nitrates and nitrites, or any components of the oint.

WARNINGS/PRECAUTIONS
Not for oral, ophthalmic, or intravaginal use. Venous and arterial dilatation reported; may decrease venous blood return and reduce arterial vascular resistance and systolic pressure. Caution with blood volume depletion, existing hypotension, cardiomyopathies, congestive heart failure (CHF), acute MI, or poor cardiac function for other reasons; monitor cardiovascular (CV) status and clinical condition. May produce dose-related headaches, which may be severe.

ADVERSE REACTIONS
Headache, dizziness, hypotension, flushing, allergic reactions, application-site reactions, methemoglobinemia.

DRUG INTERACTIONS
See Contraindications. Marked orthostatic hypotension reported with calcium channel blockers. Additive hypotensive effects with antihypertensive drugs, β-adrenergic blockers, and other nitrates. May increase levels with aspirin. Monitor anticoagulation status when administered with IV heparin. Decreased 1st-pass metabolism of dihydroergotamine. Consider the possibility of ergotism with ergotamine. Caution with tissue-type plasminogen activator; may decrease thrombolytic effect. May potentiate additive effects with alcohol.

PREGNANCY AND LACTATION
Pregnancy: Category C.
Lactation: Caution in nursing.

MECHANISM OF ACTION
Nitrate vasodilator; forms free radical nitric oxide, which activates guanylate cyclase, resulting in an increase of cyclic GMP in smooth muscle and other tissues leading to dephosphorylation of myosin light chains, which regulates the contractile state in smooth muscle and results in vasodilation.

PHARMACOKINETICS
Absorption: Absolute bioavailability (50%, 0.75mg dose of 0.2% oint).
Metabolism: Liver via reductase enzyme to glycerol nitrate metabolites and organic nitrate. **Elimination:** $T_{1/2}$=2-3 min.

PATIENT CONSIDERATIONS
Assessment: Assess for known hypersensitivity, anemia, ICP, blood volume depletion, existing hypotension, cardiomyopathies, CHF, acute MI, cardiac function, pregnancy/nursing status, and possible drug interactions.

Monitoring: Monitor for CV status, clinical conditions, headaches, and other adverse reactions.

Counseling: Advise patients that treatment may be associated with lightheadedness on standing, especially just after rising from lying or seated position. Inform patient that headaches and dizziness has been reported. Tolerance to headaches occurs. Instruct to avoid driving or operating machinery immediately after applying the ointment. Advise not to use medications for erectile dysfunction (eg, sildenafil, vardenafil, tadalafil); may increase hypotensive effects of nitroglycerin.

REFISSA — tretinoin   Rx

Class: Retinoid

ADULT DOSAGE	PEDIATRIC DOSAGE
Fine Facial Wrinkles	Pediatric use may not have been established
Adjunct to comprehensive skin care and sunlight avoidance programs for mitigation (palliation) of fine wrinkles of facial skin	
18-50 Years: **Usual:** Apply to face qd before retiring, using only enough (pea-sized amount) to cover the entire affected area lightly **Max:** 48 weeks of therapy	
Pigmentation Disorders	
Adjunct to comprehensive skin care and sunlight avoidance programs for mitigation (palliation) of mottled hyperpigmentation of facial skin	
18-50 Years: **Usual:** Apply to face qd before retiring, using only enough (pea-sized amount) to cover the entire affected area lightly **Max:** 48 weeks of therapy	
Tactile Roughness of Facial Skin	
Adjunct to comprehensive skin care and sunlight avoidance programs for mitigation (palliation) of tactile roughness of facial skin	
18-50 Years: **Usual:** Apply to face qd before retiring, using only enough (pea-sized amount) to cover the entire affected area lightly **Max:** 48 weeks of therapy	

ADMINISTRATION
Topical route

Gently wash face w/ a mild soap, pat skin dry, and wait 20-30 min before application. Avoid applying to eyes, ears, nostrils, and mouth.
May use cosmetics; thoroughly cleanse areas to be treated before medication is applied.

STORAGE
20-25°C (68-77°F). Do not freeze.

HOW SUPPLIED
Cre: 0.05% [40g]

CONTRAINDICATIONS
History of sensitivity reactions to any component of this medication.

WARNINGS/PRECAUTIONS
Should be used under medical supervision. Avoid or minimize exposure to sunlight (including sunlamps); may heighten sunburn susceptibility. During use, wear protective clothing and use sunscreens (minimum SPF of 15). Avoid use in patients

with sunburn until fully recovered. Caution in patients who may have considerable sun exposure, (eg, due to occupation or with inherent sensitivity to sunlight). Keep away from eyes, mouth, angles of the nose, and mucous membranes. May cause severe local erythema, pruritus, burning, stinging, and peeling at application site. If the degree of local irritation warrants, use less medication, reduce frequency of application, d/c temporarily, or d/c use altogether. Caution in patients with eczematous skin; may cause severe irritation. Application of larger amounts than recommended may not lead to more rapid or better results, and marked redness, peeling, or discomfort may occur. D/C if drug sensitivity, chemical irritation, or systemic adverse reaction develops. Weather extremes (eg, wind, cold) may cause irritation. Application may cause a transitory feeling of warmth or slight stinging. Majority of patients may lose the mitigating effects on fine wrinkles, mottled hyperpigmentation, and tactile roughness of facial skin with discontinuation of therapy. Do not use if patient is pregnant or attempting to become pregnant or is at high risk of pregnancy, is inherently sensitive to sunlight and if patient has eczema or other chronic skin conditions.

ADVERSE REACTIONS
Peeling, dry skin, burning, stinging, erythema, pruritus.

DRUG INTERACTIONS
Avoid with photosensitizers (eg, thiazides, tetracyclines, fluoroquinolones, phenothiazines, sulfonamides); may cause augmented phototoxicity. Caution with topical medications, medicated or abrasive soaps, shampoos, cleansers, cosmetics with strong drying effects, products with high concentrations of alcohol, astringents, spices or lime, permanent wave solutions, electrolysis, hair depilatories or waxes, and products that may irritate the skin.

PREGNANCY AND LACTATION
Category C, caution in nursing.

MECHANISM OF ACTION
Retinoid; exact mechanism unknown. Believed to exert an effect on the growth and differentiation of various epithelial cells.

PATIENT CONSIDERATIONS
Assessment: Assess for drug hypersensitivity, sunburned skin, eczema or other chronic skin conditions, sun exposure, inherent sensitivity to sunlight, pregnancy/nursing status, and for possible drug interactions.

Monitoring: Monitor for irritation, erythema, pruritus, burning, stinging or peeling at application site, and other adverse reactions.

Counseling: Instruct to use ud, and to keep away from eyes, ears, nostrils, angles of the nose, mouth, and mucous membranes. Instruct to wear protective clothing and sunscreens with minimum SPF of 15 when using the medication. Instruct not to use medication if pregnant or planning to become pregnant and to notify physician immediately if the patient becomes pregnant. Instruct to avoid sunlight and other medicines that may increase sensitivity to sunlight. Inform that therapy does not remove wrinkles, repair sun-damaged skin, reverse photoaging, or restore a more youthful or younger dermal histologic pattern.

RELISTOR — methylnaltrexone bromide   Rx
Class: Opioid antagonist

ADULT DOSAGE
Opioid-Induced Constipation

In Patients w/ Chronic Non-Cancer Pain:
Inj:
12mg SQ qd
Tab:
450mg qd in the am

In Patients w/ Advanced Illness Receiving Palliative Care w/ Insufficient Response to Laxative Therapy:
Inj:
Recommended Dose/Inj Volume Based on Weight:
38 to <62kg: 8mg SQ (0.4mL) qod prn
62-114kg: 12mg SQ (0.6mL) qod prn
<38kg or >114kg: 0.15mg/kg SQ qod prn; calculate inj volume by multiplying weight in kg by 0.0075 and rounding up the volume to the nearest 0.1mL
Max: 1 dose/24 hrs

DOSING CONSIDERATIONS
Renal Impairment
Moderate and Severe (CrCl <60mL/min):
Chronic Non-Cancer Pain:
Tab:
150mg qd in the am
Inj:
6mg SQ qd

Advanced Illness:
Inj:
Recommended Dose/Inj Volume Based on Weight:

PEDIATRIC DOSAGE
Pediatric use may not have been established

38 to <62kg: 4mg SQ (0.2mL) qod prn
62-114kg: 6mg SQ (0.3mL) qod prn
<38kg or >114kg: 0.075mg/kg SQ qod prn; calculate inj volume by multiplying weight in kg by 0.0075 and rounding up the volume to the nearest 0.1mL

Hepatic Impairment
Chronic Non-Cancer Pain:
Tab:
Moderate or Severe (Child-Pugh Class B or C): 150mg qd in the am
Inj:
Severe: Not studied; if considering dose adjustment, follow the recommendations below:
Recommended Dose/Inj Volume Based on Weight:
38 to <62kg: 4mg SQ (0.2mL)
62-114kg: 6mg SQ (0.3mL)
<38kg or >114kg: 0.075mg/kg SQ; calculate inj volume by multiplying weight in kg by 0.0075 and rounding up the volume to the nearest 0.1mL

Discontinuation
D/C if treatment w/ opioid pain medication is also discontinued

Other Important Considerations
Chronic Non-Cancer Pain:
Shown to be efficacious in patients who have taken opioids for at least 4 weeks; sustained exposure to opioids prior to starting therapy may increase patient's sensitivity to the effects of methylnaltrexone.
D/C all maint laxative therapy prior to initiation of therapy; laxative(s) can be used prn, if suboptimal response to therapy after 3 days.
Reevaluate the continued need for therapy when the opioid regimen is changed to avoid adverse reactions.

ADMINISTRATION
Oral/SQ route

Patient should be w/in close proximity to toilet facilities once administered.
In patients w/ chronic non-cancer pain, take tabs w/ water on an empty stomach at least 30 min before the first meal of the day.

Inj
Inject in the upper arm, abdomen, or thigh; rotate inj sites.

Single-Use Vials
Once drawn into the syringe, if immediate administration is not possible, store at ambient room temperature and administer w/in 24 hrs.

Single-Use Prefilled Syringes
Use only for patients requiring an 8mg or 12mg dose; use the vial if other doses are required.
Do not remove prefilled syringe from the tray until ready to administer.

STORAGE
Inj: 20-25°C (68-77°F); excursions permitted to 15-30°C (59-86°F). Do not freeze. Protect from light. **Tab:** 25°C (77°F); excursions permitted to 15-30°C (59-86°F).

HOW SUPPLIED
Inj: 12mg/0.6mL [vial, prefilled syringe], 8mg/0.4mL [prefilled syringe]; **Tab:** 150mg

CONTRAINDICATIONS
Known/suspected GI obstruction and at increased risk of recurrent obstruction.

WARNINGS/PRECAUTIONS
Use of inj beyond 4 months has not been studied in the advanced illness population. Cases of GI perforation reported in patients w/ conditions that may be associated w/ localized or diffuse reduction of structural integrity in the wall of GI tract (eg, peptic ulcer disease, Ogilvie's syndrome, diverticular disease); consider overall risk-benefit w/ these conditions or w/ other conditions which might result in impaired integrity of the GI tract wall (eg, Crohn's disease). D/C if severe, persistent, or worsening abdominal pain develops. D/C if severe/persistent diarrhea occurs. Symptoms consistent w/ opioid withdrawal (eg, hyperhidrosis, chills, diarrhea) may occur. May be at increased risk for opioid withdrawal and/or reduced analgesia in patients who have disruptions to the blood-brain barrier; consider overall risk-benefit profile.

ADVERSE REACTIONS
Chronic Non-Cancer Pain: (Inj) Abdominal pain, nausea, diarrhea, hyperhidrosis, hot flush, tremor, chills. (Tab) Abdominal pain, diarrhea, headache, abdominal distention, vomiting, hyperhidrosis, anxiety, muscle spasms, rhinorrhea, chills.
Advanced Illness: (Inj) Abdominal pain, flatulence, nausea, dizziness, diarrhea.

DRUG INTERACTIONS
Potential for additive effects of opioid receptor antagonism and increased risk of opioid withdrawal if used concomitantly w/ other opioid antagonists; avoid use.

PREGNANCY AND LACTATION
Pregnancy: The limited available data w/ methylnaltrexone in pregnant women are not sufficient to inform a drug-associated risk for major birth defects and miscarriages. Use of methylnaltrexone during pregnancy may precipitate opioid withdrawal in a fetus due to the immature fetal blood-brain barrier.
Lactation: Not for use in nursing.

MECHANISM OF ACTION
Opioid antagonist; peripherally acting μ-opioid receptor antagonist in tissues such as the GI tract. Decreases constipating effects of opioids w/o impacting opioid-mediated analgesic effects on the CNS.

PHARMACOKINETICS
Absorption: (Inj) (0.15mg/kg single dose) C_{max}=117ng/mL, AUC=175ng•hr/mL, T_{max}=0.5 hrs; (Tab) T_{max}=1.5 hrs, C_{max}=48.1ng/mL (healthy), AUC=382ng•hr/mL (healthy). **Distribution:** V_d=1.1L/kg; plasma protein binding (11-15%). **Metabolism:** Conjugated by sulfotransferase SULT1E1 and SULT2A1 isoforms to methylnaltrexone sulfate (weak metabolite); aldo-keto reductase 1C enzymes to

methyl-6-naltrexol isomers (active metabolites). **Elimination:** (IV) Urine (54%, primarily unchanged), feces (17%, primarily unchanged); (Tab) $T_{1/2}$=15 hrs. Refer to prescribing information for further details.

PATIENT CONSIDERATIONS

Assessment: Assess for GI obstruction, increased risk of recurrent GI obstruction, conditions which might result in impaired integrity of GI tract wall, disruptions to the blood-brain barrier, renal/hepatic impairment, pregnancy/nursing status, and other possible drug interactions.

Monitoring: Monitor for signs/symptoms of GI perforation, severe/persistent/worsening abdominal pain, severe/persistent diarrhea, adequacy of analgesia, opioid withdrawal symptoms, and other adverse reactions.

Counseling: Advise of risks/benefits of therapy. Instruct to d/c therapy and promptly notify physician if unusually severe, persistent, or worsening abdominal pain develops. Advise to d/c treatment if patient experiences severe/persistent diarrhea. Inform that symptoms consistent w/ opioid withdrawal may occur (eg, sweating, chills, diarrhea) while taking therapy. Advise to be w/in close proximity to toilet facilities once medication is administered. Advise females of reproductive potential who become pregnant or are planning to become pregnant that the use of drug during pregnancy may precipitate opioid withdrawal in a fetus due to the undeveloped blood-brain barrier. Advise patients that breastfeeding is not recommended during treatment. **Inj:** Inform of proper SQ technique. **Tab:** For patients w/ chronic non-cancer pain, instruct to take tabs w/ water on an empty stomach at least 30 min before the first meal of the day.

RELPAX — eletriptan hydrobromide   Rx

Class: 5-HT$_{1B/1D}$ agonist (triptans)

ADULT DOSAGE	PEDIATRIC DOSAGE
Migraine	Pediatric use may not have been established
W/ or w/o Aura:	
Single Dose: 20mg or 40mg	
Max Single Dose: 40mg	
May give a 2nd dose at least 2 hrs after 1st dose if migraine has not resolved by 2 hrs or returns after transient improvement	
Max Daily Dose: 80mg	
Safety of treating >3 migraine attacks/30 days not known	

ADMINISTRATION
Oral route
Take w/ or w/o food.

STORAGE
20-25°C (68-77°F); excursions permitted to 15-30°C (59-86°F).

HOW SUPPLIED
Tab: 20mg, 40mg

CONTRAINDICATIONS
Ischemic coronary artery disease (CAD) (eg, angina pectoris, history of MI, documented silent ischemia); coronary artery vasospasm (eg, Prinzmetal's angina); Wolff-Parkinson-White syndrome or arrhythmias associated w/ other cardiac accessory conduction pathway disorders; history of stroke, transient ischemic attack, or hemiplegic/basilar migraine; peripheral vascular disease; ischemic bowel disease; uncontrolled HTN; hypersensitivity to eletriptan hydrobromide. Recent use (w/in 24 hrs) of another 5-HT$_1$ agonist, ergotamine-containing, or ergot-type medication (eg, dihydroergotamine, methysergide). Recent use (w/in 72 hrs) of the following potent CYP3A4 inhibitors: ketoconazole, itraconazole, nefazodone, troleandomycin, clarithromycin, ritonavir, or nelfinavir.

WARNINGS/PRECAUTIONS
If no treatment response for the 1st migraine attack, reconsider diagnosis before treating any subsequent attacks. Not intended for prevention of migraine attacks. Serious cardiac adverse reactions (eg, acute MI) reported. May cause coronary artery vasospasm (Prinzmetal's angina). Perform cardiovascular (CV) evaluation in triptan-naive patients who have multiple CV risk factors (eg, increased age, diabetes, HTN, smoking, obesity, strong family history of CAD) prior to therapy; if CV evaluation is negative, consider administering 1st dose in a medically-supervised setting and performing an ECG immediately following administration. Consider periodic CV evaluation in long-term intermittent users with risk factors for CAD. Life-threatening cardiac rhythm disturbances, including ventricular tachycardia and ventricular fibrillation leading to death, reported; d/c if these occur. Sensations of tightness, pain, and pressure in the chest, throat, neck, and jaw commonly occur, usually noncardiac in origin. Cerebral/subarachnoid hemorrhage and stroke reported; exclude other potentially serious neurological conditions prior to therapy in patients not previously diagnosed as migraineurs, and in migraineurs who present with atypical symptoms. May cause noncoronary vasospastic reactions (eg, peripheral vascular ischemia, GI vascular ischemia/infarction, Raynaud's syndrome). Overuse of acute migraine drugs may lead to exacerbation of headache; detoxification, including drug withdrawal and treatment of withdrawal symptoms may be necessary. Serotonin syndrome may occur; d/c if suspected. Significant elevation in BP, including hypertensive crisis with acute impairment of organ systems, reported. Anaphylaxis, anaphylactoid, and hypersensitivity reactions reported. Not recommended with severe hepatic impairment.

ADVERSE REACTIONS
Asthenia, dizziness, somnolence, nausea, headache, paresthesia, dry mouth, chest tightness/pain/pressure.

DRUG INTERACTIONS
See Contraindications. Serotonin syndrome reported with SSRIs, SNRIs, TCAs, or MAOIs.

PREGNANCY AND LACTATION
Category C, caution in nursing.

MECHANISM OF ACTION
Selective 5-HT$_{1B/1D}$ receptor agonist; thought to be due to the agonist effects at the 5-HT$_{1B/1D}$ receptors located on intracranial blood vessels (including arteriovenous anastomoses) and sensory nerves of the trigeminal system that result in cranial vessel constriction and inhibition of proinflammatory neuropeptide release.

PHARMACOKINETICS
Absorption: Well-absorbed. Absolute bioavailability (50%); T_{max}=2 hrs (median). **Distribution:** V_d=138L (IV); plasma protein binding (85%), found in breast milk. **Metabolism:** via CYP3A4; N-demethylated metabolite (active). **Elimination:** $T_{1/2}$=4 hrs (eletriptan), 13 hrs (metabolite).

PATIENT CONSIDERATIONS
Assessment: Confirm diagnosis of migraine and exclude other potentially serious neurological conditions prior to therapy. Assess for ischemic CAD, HTN, hemiplegic/basilar migraine, hypersensitivity to drug, or any other conditions where treatment is contraindicated or cautioned. Assess for hepatic dysfunction, pregnancy/nursing status, and possible drug interactions. Perform a CV evaluation for patients who have multiple CV risk factors.

Monitoring: Monitor for signs/symptoms of cardiac events, cerebrovascular events, noncoronary vasospastic reactions, serotonin syndrome, hypersensitivity reactions, HTN, and other adverse reactions. Perform periodic CV evaluation in intermittent long-term users with risk factors for CAD.

Counseling: Inform that therapy may cause serious CV side effects and anaphylactic/anaphylactoid reactions. Instruct to seek medical attention if signs/symptoms of chest pain, SOB, weakness, slurring of speech, or other vasospastic reactions occur. Inform that use of acute migraine drugs for ≥10 days/month may lead to an exacerbation of headache; encourage to record headache frequency and drug use (eg, by keeping a headache diary). Inform about the risk of serotonin syndrome. Inform that medication should not be used during pregnancy and instruct to notify physician if breastfeeding or planning to breastfeed.

REMICADE — infliximab   Rx

Class: Monoclonal antibody/TNF blocker

> Increased risk for developing serious infections (eg, active tuberculosis [TB], latent TB reactivation, invasive fungal infections, bacterial/viral infections, opportunistic infections) leading to hospitalization or death, mostly w/ concomitant use w/ immunosuppressants (eg, methotrexate [MTX], corticosteroids). D/C if serious infection or sepsis develops. Active/latent reactivation TB may present w/ disseminated or extrapulmonary disease; test for latent TB before and during therapy and initiate treatment for latent TB prior to infliximab use. Invasive fungal infections reported; consider empiric antifungal therapy in patients at risk who develop severe systemic illness. Consider risks and benefits prior to therapy in patients w/ chronic or recurrent infection. Monitor patients for development of infection during and after treatment, including development of TB in patients who tested (-) for latent TB infection prior to therapy. Lymphoma and other malignancies, some fatal, reported in children and adolescents. Postmarketing cases of aggressive and fatal hepatosplenic T-cell lymphoma (HSTCL) reported, and the majority of cases were in patients w/ Crohn's disease (CD) or ulcerative colitis (UC) and mostly in adolescent and young adult males; almost all of these patients were treated concomitantly w/ azathioprine or 6-mercaptopurine.

ADULT DOSAGE	PEDIATRIC DOSAGE
Rheumatoid Arthritis	**Crohn's Disease**
Moderately to Severely Active: For reducing signs/symptoms, inhibiting progression of structural damage, and improving physical function	**Moderately to Severely Active w/ Inadequate Response to Conventional Therapy:** For reducing signs/symptoms and inducing/maintaining clinical remission
In Combination w/ MTX:	**≥6 Years:**
Induction: 3mg/kg at 0, 2, and 6 weeks	**Induction:** 5mg/kg at 0, 2, and 6 weeks
Maint: 3mg/kg every 8 weeks	**Maint:** 5mg/kg every 8 weeks
Incomplete Response: May give up to 10mg/kg or treat every 4 weeks	**Ulcerative Colitis**
Ankylosing Spondylitis	**Moderately to Severely Active w/ Inadequate Response to Conventional Therapy:** For reducing signs/symptoms and inducing/maintaining clinical remission
Active:	
Induction: 5mg/kg at 0, 2, and 6 weeks	**≥6 Years:**
Maint: 5mg/kg every 6 weeks	**Induction:** 5mg/kg at 0, 2, and 6 weeks
Psoriatic Arthritis	**Maint:** 5mg/kg every 8 weeks
For reducing signs/symptoms of active arthritis, inhibiting progression of structural damage, and improving physical function	
W/ or w/o MTX:	
Induction: 5mg/kg at 0, 2, and 6 weeks	
Maint: 5mg/kg every 8 weeks	
Plaque Psoriasis	
Chronic Severe (eg, Extensive and/or Disabling):	
Induction: 5mg/kg at 0, 2, and 6 weeks	

Maint: 5mg/kg every 8 weeks

Crohn's Disease

Moderately to Severely Active w/ Inadequate Response to Conventional Therapy:
For reducing signs/symptoms and inducing/maintaining clinical remission

Induction: 5mg/kg at 0, 2, and 6 weeks

Maint: 5mg/kg every 8 weeks

May give 10mg/kg to patients who respond and then lose their response Consider discontinuation if no response by Week 14

Also indicated for reducing number of draining enterocutaneous and rectovaginal fistulas and maintaining fistula closure in patients w/ fistulizing Crohn's disease

Ulcerative Colitis

Moderately to Severely Active w/ Inadequate Response to Conventional Therapy:
For reducing signs/symptoms, inducing/maintaining clinical remission and mucosal healing, and eliminating corticosteroid use

Induction: 5mg/kg at 0, 2, and 6 weeks

Maint: 5mg/kg every 8 weeks

ADMINISTRATION

IV route

Do not dilute reconstituted sol w/ any other diluent.
Begin infusion w/in 3 hrs of reconstitution and dilution.
Administer infusion over a period of not less than 2 hrs.
Do not infuse concomitantly in the same IV line w/ other agents.
Refer to PI for further instructions.

STORAGE

2-8°C (36-46°F). May also be stored up to 30°C (86°F) for a single period of up to 6 months, but not exceeding the original expiration date. Do not return to refrigerated storage after removing from refrigerated storage.

HOW SUPPLIED

Inj: 100mg

CONTRAINDICATIONS

Moderate to severe heart failure (HF) (NYHA Class III/IV) w/ doses >5mg/kg, re-administration to patients who have experienced a severe hypersensitivity reaction to infliximab, known hypersensitivity to inactive components of the product or to any murine proteins.

WARNINGS/PRECAUTIONS

Do not initiate w/ an active infection. Increased risk of infection in patients >65 yrs of age and in patients w/ comorbid conditions; consider risks and benefits prior to therapy for those who have resided or traveled in areas of endemic TB or mycoses, and w/ any underlying conditions predisposing to infection. Cases of acute/chronic leukemia, melanoma, and Merkel cell carcinoma reported. Caution in patients w/ moderate to severe COPD, history of malignancy, or in continuing treatment in patients who develop malignancy during therapy. Hepatitis B virus (HBV) reactivation reported; if reactivation occurs, d/c and initiate antiviral therapy w/ appropriate supportive treatment. Severe hepatic reactions (eg, acute liver failure, jaundice, hepatitis, cholestasis) reported; d/c if jaundice or marked elevations of liver enzymes (eg, ≥5X ULN) develop. New onset (rare) HF and worsening of HF reported; d/c if new or worsening symptoms of HF occur. Leukopenia, neutropenia, thrombocytopenia, and pancytopenia reported; consider discontinuation of therapy if significant hematologic abnormalities occur. Caution in patients who have ongoing or history of significant hematologic abnormalities. Hypersensitivity reactions reported; d/c for severe hypersensitivity reactions. CNS manifestation of systemic vasculitis, seizures, and new onset/exacerbation of CNS demyelinating disorders reported (rare); caution in patients w/ these neurologic disorders and consider discontinuation if these disorders develop. Caution when switching from one biologic disease-modifying antirheumatic drug to another; overlapping biological activity may further increase risk of infection. May cause autoantibody formation and, rarely, may develop lupus-like syndrome; d/c if lupus-like syndrome develops. Live vaccines may lead to clinical infections; concurrent administration is not recommended. All pediatric patients should be up to date w/ all vaccinations prior to therapy. Fatal outcome due to disseminated BCG infection reported in infants who received BCG vaccine after in utero exposure to infliximab; wait at least 6 months following birth before administering any live vaccine to infants exposed in utero. Caution in elderly.

ADVERSE REACTIONS

Infusion reactions, nausea, abdominal pain, diarrhea, dyspepsia, URTI, sinusitis, pharyngitis, coughing, bronchitis, rash, headache.

DRUG INTERACTIONS

See Boxed Warning. Avoid w/ live vaccines or therapeutic infectious agents. Avoid use w/ tocilizumab; possible increased immunosuppression and increased risk of infection. Not recommended w/ anakinra or abatacept; may increase risk of serious infections. Not recommended w/ other biological therapeutics used to treat the same conditions. MTX may decrease the incidence of anti-infliximab antibody production and increase infliximab concentrations. Upon initiation or discontinuation of infliximab in patients being treated w/ CYP450 substrates w/ a narrow therapeutic index, monitor therapeutic effect (eg, warfarin) or drug concentration (eg, cyclosporine, theophylline) and adjust individual dose of the drug product as needed.

PREGNANCY AND LACTATION

Pregnancy: Category B.
Lactation: Not for use in nursing.

MECHANISM OF ACTION

Monoclonal antibody/TNF-α receptor blocker; neutralizes biological activity of TNF-α by binding w/ high affinity to the soluble and transmembrane forms of TNF-α and inhibits binding of TNF-α w/ its receptors.

PHARMACOKINETICS

Distribution: Crosses placenta. **Elimination:** $T_{1/2}$=7.7-9.5 days (median).

PATIENT CONSIDERATIONS

Assessment: Assess for active/chronic/recurrent infection (eg, TB, HBV), history of an opportunistic infection, recent travel to areas of endemic TB or endemic mycoses, underlying conditions that may predispose to infection, HF, history of malignancy, moderate to severe COPD, presence or history of significant hematologic abnormalities, neurologic disorders, previous hypersensitivity to drug or to murine proteins, risk factors for skin cancer, pregnancy/nursing status, and for possible drug interactions. Assess vaccination history in pediatric patients. Perform test for latent TB infection.

Monitoring: Monitor for sepsis, TB (active, reactivation, or latent), invasive fungal infections, or bacterial, viral, and other infections caused by opportunistic pathogens during and after therapy. Monitor for development of lymphoma, HSTCL, or other malignancies. Monitor for nonmelanoma skin cancers in psoriasis patients, melanoma and Merkel cell carcinoma, new or worsening symptoms of HF, HBV infection reactivation, hepatotoxicity, hematological events, hypersensitivity reactions, CNS demyelinating disorders, lupus-like syndrome, and other adverse reactions. Monitor LFTs. Perform periodic skin examination, particularly in patients w/ risk factors for skin cancer.

Counseling: Advise of potential risks and benefits of therapy. Inform that therapy may lower the ability of immune system to fight infections; instruct to immediately contact physician if any signs/symptoms of an infection develop, including TB and HBV reactivation. Inform about the risks of lymphoma and other malignancies while on therapy. Advise to report to physician signs of new or worsening medical conditions (eg, heart disease, neurological disease, autoimmune disorders) and symptoms of cytopenia.

RENAGEL — sevelamer hydrochloride   Rx

Class: Phosphate binder

ADULT DOSAGE	PEDIATRIC DOSAGE
Hyperphosphatemia	Pediatric use may not have been established
Chronic Kidney Disease on Dialysis:	
Not Taking a Phosphate Binder:	
Initial:	
800mg Tab:	
Serum Phosphorus:	
>5.5 and <7.5mg/dL: 1 tab tid	
≥7.5 and <9.0mg/dL: 2 tabs tid	
≥9.0mg/dL: 2 tabs tid	
400mg Tab:	
Serum Phosphorus:	
>5.5 and <7.5mg/dL: 2 tabs tid	
≥7.5 and <9.0mg/dL: 3 tabs tid	
≥9.0mg/dL: 4 tabs tid	
Switching from Calcium Acetate:	
Initial:	
800mg Tab:	
Calcium Acetate 667mg (Tabs per Meal):	
1 Tab: 1 tab/meal	
2 Tabs: 2 tabs/meal	
3 Tabs: 3 tabs/meal	
400mg Tab:	
Calcium Acetate 667mg (Tabs per Meal):	
1 Tab: 2 tabs/meal	
2 Tabs: 3 tabs/meal	
3 Tabs: 5 tabs/meal	
Dose Titration (All Patients):	
Serum Phosphorus:	
<3.5mg/dL: Decrease 1 tab per meal	
3.5-5.5mg/dL: Maintain current dose	
>5.5mg/dL: Increase 1 tab per meal at 2-week intervals	

DOSING CONSIDERATIONS
Elderly
Start at the lower end of dosing range

ADMINISTRATION
Oral route

Take w/ meals.

STORAGE
25°C (77°F); excursions permitted to 15-30°C (59-86°F). Protect from moisture.

HOW SUPPLIED
Tab: 400mg, 800mg

CONTRAINDICATIONS
Bowel obstruction, known hypersensitivity to sevelamer hydrochloride or to any of the excipients.

WARNINGS/PRECAUTIONS
Dysphagia and esophageal tab retention reported w/ use of tab formulation; consider use of sus formulation in patients w/ a history of swallowing disorders. Bowel obstruction and perforation reported.

ADVERSE REACTIONS
N/V, diarrhea, dyspepsia, abdominal pain, flatulence, constipation.

DRUG INTERACTIONS
Consider separating timing of administration of therapy and an oral medication where a reduction in bioavailability of that medication would have a clinically significant effect on its safety or efficacy (eg, cyclosporine, tacrolimus, levothyroxine). Take oral ciprofloxacin at least 2 hrs before or 6 hrs after therapy. Take oral mycophenolate mofetil at least 2 hrs before therapy. Where possible, consider monitoring clinical response and/or blood levels of concomitant drugs that have a narrow therapeutic range. Cases of increased phosphate levels reported w/ coadministration of proton pump inhibitors.

PREGNANCY AND LACTATION
Pregnancy: Category C.
Lactation: Safety not known in nursing.

MECHANISM OF ACTION
Phosphate binder; contains multiple amines that exist in a protonated form in the intestine and interact w/ phosphate molecules through ionic and hydrogen bonding, decreasing absorption, and lowering phosphate concentration in the serum.

PATIENT CONSIDERATIONS
Assessment: Assess for hypersensitivity to the drug, presence of bowel obstruction and other GI disorders (eg, dysphagia, swallowing disorders), pregnancy/nursing status, and possible drug interactions.

Monitoring: Monitor for bowel obstruction and perforation, dysphagia, esophageal tab retention, and other adverse reactions. Monitor bicarbonate and Cl⁻ levels, and for reduced vitamin D, E, K (clotting factors), and folic acid levels.

Counseling: Advise to take w/ meals and adhere to prescribed diet. Instruct on concomitant oral medications that should be dosed apart from therapy. Inform that drug may cause constipation and if left untreated, may lead to severe complications; caution to report new onset or worsening of existing constipation promptly to physician.

RENVELA — sevelamer carbonate   Rx
Class: Phosphate binder

ADULT DOSAGE	PEDIATRIC DOSAGE
Hyperphosphatemia	Pediatric use may not have been established
Chronic Kidney Disease on Dialysis:	
Not Taking a Phosphate Binder:	
Initial:	
800mg Tab:	
Serum Phosphorus:	
>5.5 and <7.5mg/dL: 1 tab tid	
≥7.5mg/dL: 2 tabs tid	
Powder:	
Serum Phosphorus:	
>5.5 and <7.5mg/dL: 0.8g tid	
≥7.5mg/dL: 1.6g tid	
Dose Titration (All Patients):	
Titrate by 0.8g tid w/ meals at 2-week intervals as necessary	
Conversions	
Switching from Sevelamer HCl Tabs/ Switching Between Sevelamer Carbonate Tabs and Powder:	
Use the same dose in grams; further titration may be necessary to achieve desired phosphorus levels	
Switching from Calcium Acetate:	
Initial:	
1 Calcium Acetate 667mg Tab/Meal:	
1 sevelamer carbonate 800mg tab/meal	
2 Calcium Acetate 667mg Tabs/Meal: 2 sevelamer carbonate 800mg tabs/meal	

3 Calcium Acetate 667mg Tabs/Meal:
3 sevelamer carbonate 800mg tabs/meal

1 Calcium Acetate 667mg Tab/Meal:
0.8g sevelamer carbonate powder
2 Calcium Acetate 667mg Tabs/Meal:
1.6g sevelamer carbonate powder
3 Calcium Acetate 667mg Tabs/Meal:
2.4g sevelamer carbonate powder

DOSING CONSIDERATIONS
Elderly
Start at low end of dosing range

ADMINISTRATION
Oral route

Take w/ meals.

Powder Preparation Instructions
The entire contents of each pkt should be placed in a cup and mixed thoroughly w/ the appropriate amount of water.
Multiple pkts may be mixed together w/ the appropriate amount of water.
Stir the mixture vigorously (it does not dissolve) and drink the entire preparation w/in 30 min and resuspend the preparation right before drinking.

Minimum Amount of Water for Dose Preparation:
0.8g Powder Pkt: Use 30mL water
2.4g Powder Pkt: Use 60mL water

STORAGE
25°C (77°F); excursions permitted to 15-30°C (59-86°F). Protect from moisture.

HOW SUPPLIED
Tab: 800mg; **Powder:** 0.8g/pkt, 2.4g/pkt

CONTRAINDICATIONS
Bowel obstruction, known hypersensitivity to sevelamer carbonate or to any of the excipients.

WARNINGS/PRECAUTIONS
Dysphagia and esophageal tab retention reported w/ use of tab formulation; consider use of sus formulation in patients w/ a history of swallowing disorders. Bowel obstruction and perforation reported.

ADVERSE REACTIONS
N/V, diarrhea, dyspepsia, abdominal pain, flatulence, constipation.

DRUG INTERACTIONS
Consider separating administration of therapy and an oral medication where a reduction in bioavailability of that medication would have a clinically significant effect on its safety or efficacy (eg, cyclosporine, tacrolimus, levothyroxine). Take oral ciprofloxacin at least 2 hrs before or 6 hrs after therapy. Take oral mycophenolate mofetil at least 2 hrs before therapy. Where possible, consider monitoring clinical response and/or blood levels of concomitant drugs that have a narrow therapeutic range. Cases of increased phosphate levels reported w/ coadministration of proton pump inhibitors.

PREGNANCY AND LACTATION
Pregnancy: Category C.
Lactation: Safety not known in nursing.

MECHANISM OF ACTION
Phosphate binder; contains multiple amines that exist in a protonated form in the intestine and interact w/ phosphate molecules through ionic and hydrogen bonding, decreasing absorption, and lowering phosphate concentration in the serum.

PATIENT CONSIDERATIONS
Assessment: Assess for hypersensitivity to the drug, presence of bowel obstruction and other GI disorders (eg, dysphagia, swallowing disorders), pregnancy/nursing status, and possible drug interactions.

Monitoring: Monitor for bowel obstruction and perforation, dysphagia, esophageal tab retention, and other adverse reactions. Monitor bicarbonate and Cl⁻ levels, and for reduced vitamin D, E, K (clotting factors), and folic acid levels.

Counseling: Advise to take w/ meals and adhere to prescribed diet. If taking an oral medication where reduced bioavailability would produce a clinically significant effect on safety or efficacy, advise to take medication ≥1 hr before or 3 hrs after dosing. Inform that drug may cause constipation that if left untreated may lead to severe complications; caution to report new onset or worsening of existing constipation promptly to physician.

REOPRO — abciximab   Rx
Class: Glycoprotein IIb/IIIa inhibitor

ADULT DOSAGE	PEDIATRIC DOSAGE
Percutaneous Coronary Intervention	Pediatric use may not have been established
Adjunct to percutaneous coronary intervention (PCI) for the prevention of cardiac ischemic complications	
Usual: 0.25mg/kg IV bolus administered 10-60 min before start of PCI, followed by continuous IV infusion of 0.125µg/kg/min (to a max of 10µg/min) for 12 hrs	

PATIENT CONSIDERATIONS

Assessment: Assess for presence of sleep disorders (other than RLS), known hypersensitivity/allergic reaction to drug or to any of the excipients, CVD, dyskinesia, major psychotic disorder, renal impairment, pregnancy/nursing status, and possible drug interactions.

Monitoring: Monitor for hypersensitivity reactions, psychotic-like behavior, impulse control/compulsive behaviors, syncope, bradycardia, hallucinations, dyskinesia, fibrotic complications, symptom complex resembling NMS, melanomas, and other adverse reactions. Monitor for signs/symptoms of hypotension, especially during dose escalation. Continually reassess for drowsiness or sleepiness. Perform periodic skin examinations. (Tab) Monitor for augmentation or early-am rebound in RLS patients. (Tab, XL) Monitor for BP elevation and HR changes.

Counseling: Instruct to take only as prescribed. Advise not to double next dose if a dose is missed. Advise about the potential for developing a hypersensitivity/allergic reaction; instruct patients to immediately contact physician if they experience these or similar reactions. Advise and alert about potential sedating effects; instruct patients not to drive a car, operate machinery, or engage in other dangerous activities until they have gained sufficient experience with therapy. Advise of possible additive effects when taking other sedating medications, alcohol, or other CNS depressants concomitantly, or when taking a concomitant medication (eg, ciprofloxacin) that increases ropinirole plasma levels. Advise patients that they may experience syncope and that hypotension/orthostatic hypotension may develop with/without symptoms; caution against standing rapidly after sitting or lying down, especially at treatment initiation. Inform that hallucinations or other psychotic-like behavior may occur; advise patients to promptly report these to physician should they develop. Inform that medication may cause and/or exacerbate preexisting dyskinesia. Advise to inform physician if new or increased gambling urges, sexual urges, uncontrolled spending, binge or compulsive eating, or other urges develop while on therapy. Advise patients to contact physician if they wish to d/c drug or decrease its dose. Advise of the higher risk of developing melanoma; instruct to have skin examined on a regular basis by a qualified healthcare provider when using medication. Instruct to notify physician if pregnant/intending to become pregnant during therapy. Advise that drug may inhibit lactation. (Tab) Inform RLS patients that augmentation and/or rebound may occur after starting treatment. (Tab, XL) Alert to the possibility of increases in BP and that significant increases/decreases in HR may be experienced during treatment.

RESCRIPTOR — delavirdine mesylate

Rx

Class: Non-nucleoside reverse transcriptase inhibitor (NNRTI)

ADULT DOSAGE	**PEDIATRIC DOSAGE**
HIV-1 Infection	**HIV-1 Infection**
Combination w/ at Least 2 Other Antiretrovirals:	**Combination with at Least 2 Other Antiretrovirals:**
400mg (four 100mg or two 200mg tabs) tid	**≥16 Years:** 400mg (four 100mg or two 200mg tabs) tid

DOSING CONSIDERATIONS
Concomitant Medications
Antacids: Take at least 1 hr apart

ADMINISTRATION
Oral route

Take w/ or w/o food
Take w/ acidic beverage if achlorhydric
Take 200mg tabs intact; not dispersible in water

Dispersion of 100mg Tab
1. Add four 100mg tabs to at least 3 oz of water
2. Allow to stand for a few minutes
3. Stir until a uniform dispersion occurs
4. Consume dispersion promptly
5. Rinse glass with water and swallow the rinse

STORAGE
20-25°C (68-77°F). Protect from high humidity.

HOW SUPPLIED
Tab: 100mg, 200mg

CONTRAINDICATIONS
Known hypersensitivity to delavirdine mesylate or any components of the medication. Coadministration w/ CYP3A substrates that are associated w/ serious and/or life-threatening events at elevated plasma concentrations (eg, astemizole, terfenadine, dihydroergotamine, ergonovine, ergotamine, methylergonovine, cisapride, pimozide, alprazolam, midazolam, triazolam).

WARNINGS/PRECAUTIONS
Immune reconstitution syndrome reported. Autoimmune disorders (eg, Graves' disease, polymyositis, Guillain-Barre syndrome) have been reported to occur in the setting of immune reconstitution. Redistribution/accumulation of body fat reported. May confer cross-resistance to the other non-nucleoside reverse transcriptase inhibitors (NNRTIs). Severe rash (eg, erythema multiforme, Stevens-Johnson syndrome) reported; d/c use if this occurs. Caution with hepatic impairment and in elderly.

ADVERSE REACTIONS
Headache, fatigue, N/V, diarrhea, increased ALT/AST, rash, maculopapular rash, pruritus, erythema, insomnia, upper respiratory infection, depressive symptoms, generalized abdominal pain.

DRUG INTERACTIONS
See Contraindications. Avoid with another NNRTI. Not recommended with lovastatin, simvastatin, St. John's wort, phenytoin, phenobarbital, carbamazepine, rifabutin, rifampin, or chronic use of H_2-receptor antagonists or PPIs. Increased risk of myopathy with HMG-CoA reductase inhibitors metabolized by CYP3A4 (eg, atorvastatin, cerivastatin). May increase levels of nelfinavir, lopinavir, ritonavir, amphetamines, trazodone, antiarrhythmics, warfarin (monitor INR), calcium channel blockers, atorvastatin, cerivastatin, fluvastatin, immunosuppressants, CYP3A substrates, fluticasone, methadone, and ethinyl estradiol. May increase levels of maraviroc; maraviroc dose should be reduced. May increase levels of indinavir; consider dose reduction of indinavir. May increase levels of saquinavir; consider dose reduction of saquinavir (soft gelatin cap). May decrease levels of didanosine. Ketoconazole, fluoxetine, and CYP3A inhibitors may increase levels. Nelfinavir, didanosine, antacids, CYP3A inducers, H_2-receptor antagonists, PPIs, and dexamethasone may decrease levels. May increase levels of clarithromycin; adjust clarithromycin dose in patients with impaired renal function. May increase levels of sildenafil; do not exceed a max single sildenafil dose of 25mg in a 48-hr period. Doses of an antacid and didanosine (buffered tabs) should be separated by at least 1 hr.

PREGNANCY AND LACTATION
Category C, not for use in nursing.

MECHANISM OF ACTION
NNRTI; binds directly to reverse transcriptase and blocks RNA-dependent and DNA-dependent DNA polymerase activities.

PHARMACOKINETICS
Absorption: Rapid. (400mg tid) C_{max}=35µM, AUC=180µM•hr; T_{max}=1 hr.
Distribution: Plasma protein binding (98%). **Metabolism:** Hepatic (N-desalkylation, pyridine hydroxylation) via CYP3A (major), 2D6. **Elimination:** (300mg tid multiple dose) Urine (51%, <5% unchanged), feces (44%); (400mg tid) $T_{1/2}$=5.8 hrs.

PATIENT CONSIDERATIONS
Assessment: Assess for hypersensitivity, achlorhydria, hepatic impairment, pregnancy/nursing status, and possible drug interactions.

Monitoring: Monitor for severe rash or rash accompanied by symptoms (eg, fever, blistering, oral lesions, conjunctivitis, swelling, muscle joint aches), immune reconstitution syndrome, cross-resistance to other NNRTIs, fat redistribution, and other adverse reactions.

Counseling: Inform patient that drug is not a cure for HIV-1 infection and that they may continue to experience illnesses associated with HIV-1 infection. Advise to avoid doing things that can spread HIV-1 infection to others. Inform to take as prescribed and to not alter the dose without consulting the physician. Advise patients with achlorhydria to take with acidic beverage (eg, orange or cranberry juice). Inform to take at least 1 hr apart if taking antacids. Advise to d/c and seek medical attention if severe rash or rash with symptoms such as fever, blistering, oral lesions, conjunctivitis, swelling, muscle or joint aches occur. Counsel that fat redistribution may occur. Advise to report use of any prescription or nonprescription medication or herbal products, particularly St. John's wort. Inform patients receiving sildenafil about increased risk of sildenafil-associated adverse events (eg, hypotension, visual changes, prolonged penile erection), and instruct to promptly report any symptoms to the physician. Counsel to notify physician if pregnant or breastfeeding.

RESTASIS — cyclosporine

Rx

Class: Topical immunomodulator

ADULT DOSAGE	**PEDIATRIC DOSAGE**
Keratoconjunctivitis Sicca	**Keratoconjunctivitis Sicca**
Instill 1 drop in ou q12h	**≥16 Years:** Instill 1 drop in ou q12h

ADMINISTRATION
Ocular route

Invert unit dose vial a few times to obtain uniform, white, opaque emulsion before using.
Can be used concomitantly with artificial tears, allowing 15-min interval between products.

STORAGE
15-25°C (59-77°F).

HOW SUPPLIED
Emulsion: 0.05% [0.4mL]

CONTRAINDICATIONS
Known or suspected hypersensitivity to any of the ingredients in the formulation.

WARNINGS/PRECAUTIONS
Increased tear production not seen in patients currently taking topical anti-inflammatory drugs or using punctal plugs. Do not touch vial tip to the eye or other surfaces to avoid the potential for eye injury and contamination. Do not administer in patients wearing contact lenses. Remove contact lenses prior to administration; may reinsert 15 min after administration.

ADVERSE REACTIONS
Ocular burning, conjunctival hyperemia, discharge, epiphora, eye pain, foreign body sensation, pruritus, stinging, visual disturbance (eg, blurring).

PREGNANCY AND LACTATION
Pregnancy: Category C.
Lactation: Caution in nursing.

MECHANISM OF ACTION
Topical immunomodulator; not established. Thought to act as a partial immunomodulator.

PHARMACOKINETICS
Distribution: Found in breast milk (systemic administration).

PATIENT CONSIDERATIONS
Assessment: Assess for hypersensitivity, contact lens use, and pregnancy/nursing status.

Monitoring: Monitor for signs/symptoms of ocular burning and other adverse reactions.

Counseling: Instruct not to allow the vial tip to touch the eye or any surface. Advise to remove contact lenses before administration; inform that lenses may be reinserted 15 min following administration. Advise to use single-use vial immediately after opening and to discard the remaining contents immediately after administration.

RESTORIL — temazepam CIV

Class: Benzodiazepine

ADULT DOSAGE
Insomnia
Short-Term Treatment (Generally 7 to 10 Days):
Usual: 15mg before retiring
7.5mg may be sufficient for some patients and others may need 30mg
Transient Insomnia:
7.5mg before retiring

PEDIATRIC DOSAGE
Pediatric use may not have been established

DOSING CONSIDERATIONS
Elderly
Elderly/Debilitated Patients:
Initial: 7.5mg before retiring

ADMINISTRATION
Oral route

STORAGE
20-25°C (68-77°F).

HOW SUPPLIED
Cap: 7.5mg, 15mg, 22.5mg, 30mg

CONTRAINDICATIONS
Women who are or may become pregnant.

WARNINGS/PRECAUTIONS
Initiate only after careful evaluation; failure of insomnia to remit after 7-10 days of treatment may indicate primary psychiatric and/or medical illness. Worsening of insomnia and emergence of thinking or behavior abnormalities may occur, especially in elderly; use lowest possible effective dose. Behavioral changes (eg, decreased inhibition, bizarre behavior, agitation, hallucinations, depersonalization) and complex behavior (eg, sleep-driving) reported; strongly consider discontinuation if sleep-driving episode occurs. Amnesia and other neuropsychiatric symptoms may occur unpredictably. Worsening of depression, including suicidal thinking, reported. Withdrawal symptoms may occur after abrupt discontinuation. Rare cases of angioedema and anaphylaxis reported; do not rechallenge. Oversedation, confusion, and/or ataxia may develop w/ large doses in elderly and debilitated patients. Caution w/ hepatic/renal impairment, chronic pulmonary insufficiency, debilitated, severe or latent depression, and in elderly. Abnormal LFTs, renal function tests, and blood dyscrasias reported.

ADVERSE REACTIONS
Drowsiness, headache, fatigue, nervousness, lethargy, dizziness, nausea.

DRUG INTERACTIONS
Increased risk of complex behaviors w/ alcohol and CNS depressants. Potential additive effects w/ hypnotics and CNS depressants. Possible synergistic effect w/ diphenhydramine.

PREGNANCY AND LACTATION
Pregnancy: Category X.
Lactation: Caution in nursing.

MECHANISM OF ACTION
Benzodiazepine hypnotic agent.

PHARMACOKINETICS
Absorption: Well-absorbed; C_{max}=865ng/mL; T_{max}=1.5 hrs. Distribution: Plasma protein binding (96% unchanged); crosses placenta. Metabolism: Complete; conjugation. Elimination: Urine (80-90%); $T_{1/2}$=3.5-18.4 hrs.

PATIENT CONSIDERATIONS
Assessment: Assess for physical and/or psychiatric disorder, medical illness, severe or latent depression, renal/hepatic dysfunction, chronic pulmonary

insufficiency, pregnancy/nursing status, alcohol use, and possible drug interactions.

Monitoring: Monitor for signs/symptoms of withdrawal, tolerance, abuse, dependence, abnormal thinking, behavioral changes, agitation, depersonalization, hallucinations, complex behaviors, amnesia, anxiety, neuropsychiatric symptoms, worsening of depression, suicidal thoughts and actions, angioedema, driving/psychomotor impairment, worsening of insomnia, thinking or behavioral abnormalities, and possible abuse/dependence.

Counseling: Inform about the benefits and risks of treatment. Instruct patient to take as prescribed. Inform about the risks and possibility of physical/psychological dependence; memory problems, and complex behaviors (eg, sleep-driving). Caution against hazardous tasks (eg, operating machinery/driving). Advise not to drink alcohol. Instruct to notify physician if pregnant/planning to become pregnant.

RETAVASE — reteplase Rx

Class: Thrombolytic agent

ADULT DOSAGE
Acute Myocardial Infarction
Management of acute MI (AMI) for the improvement of ventricular function following AMI, reduction of the incidence of CHF, and the reduction of mortality associated w/ AMI

Treatment should be initiated as soon as possible after onset of AMI symptoms

Two 10 U bolus inj; administer each bolus as IV inj over 2 min
Give 2nd bolus 30 min after initiation of 1st bolus inj

PEDIATRIC DOSAGE
Pediatric use may not have been established

ADMINISTRATION
IV route

Reconstitution
Reconstitute using the provided diluent and dispensing pin. Reconstitute w/ 10mL of sterile water for inj
Swirl vial gently to dissolve. Do not shake
Slight foaming upon reconstitution is not unusual; allow vial to stand undisturbed for several min to allow dissipation of large bubbles

Administration
Reconstitute immediately before use; reconstituted preparation contains 1 U/mL
Use w/in 4 hrs of reconstitution when stored at 2-30°C (36-86°F)
Do not administer other medications simultaneously via the same IV line
Heparin and reteplase are incompatible when combined in sol; if reteplase is to be injected through an IV line containing heparin, normal saline or D5W sol should be flushed through the line prior to and following reteplase inj

STORAGE
Unused vial: 2-25°C (36-77°F). Box should remain sealed until use to protect the lyophilisate from exposure to light. Reconstituted: 2-30°C (36-86°F); use within 4 hrs.

HOW SUPPLIED
Inj: 10.4 U (18.1mg)

CONTRAINDICATIONS
Active internal bleeding; history of cerebrovascular accident (CVA); recent intracranial or intraspinal surgery or trauma; intracranial neoplasm; arteriovenous malformation or aneurysm; known bleeding diathesis; severe uncontrolled HTN.

WARNINGS/PRECAUTIONS
Bleeding is the most common complication during therapy; careful attention to all potential bleeding sites is required. If arterial puncture is necessary during administration, use an upper extremity vessel that is accessible to manual compression. Avoid IM inj and nonessential handling of patients. Perform venipuncture carefully and only if required. Weigh benefits/risks of therapy with recent major surgery, previous puncture of noncompressible vessels, cerebrovascular disease, recent GI or genitourinary (GU) bleeding, recent trauma, HTN, high likelihood of left heart thrombus, acute pericarditis, subacute bacterial endocarditis, hemostatic defects, severe hepatic or renal dysfunction, pregnancy, diabetic hemorrhagic retinopathy or other hemorrhagic ophthalmic conditions, septic thrombophlebitis or occluded AV cannula at a seriously infected site, advanced age, or any other condition in which bleeding would constitute a significant hazard or be difficult to manage. Cholesterol embolism reported. Coronary thrombolysis may result in arrhythmias associated with reperfusion. Do not administer 2nd bolus if an anaphylactoid reaction occurs. May affect results of coagulation tests and/or measurements of fibrinolytic activity.

ADVERSE REACTIONS
Bleeding, allergic reactions.

DRUG INTERACTIONS
Increased risk of bleeding with heparin, vitamin K antagonists, and drugs that alter platelet function (eg, ASA, dipyridamole, abciximab) if administered before, during, or after therapy. Concomitant use of anticoagulant therapy should be terminated if serious bleeding occurs.

PREGNANCY AND LACTATION
Category C, caution in nursing.

MECHANISM OF ACTION

Thrombolytic agent; recombinant plasminogen activator that catalyzes the cleavage of endogenous plasminogen to generate plasmin. Plasmin in turn degrades the fibrin matrix of the thrombus, thereby exerting its thrombolytic action.

PHARMACOKINETICS

Metabolism: Hepatic. **Elimination:** Renal; $T_{1/2}$=13-16 min.

PATIENT CONSIDERATIONS

Assessment: Assess for active internal bleeding, history of CVA, or any other conditions where treatment is contraindicated or cautioned. Assess for age, renal/hepatic function, pregnancy/nursing status, and possible drug interactions.

Monitoring: Monitor for signs/symptoms of bleeding, internal and superficial bleeding sites, bleeding at recent puncture sites, cholesterol embolism (eg, livedo reticularis, "purple toe" syndrome, MI, cerebral infarction, HTN, gangrenous digits), and arrhythmias. Monitor renal/hepatic function.

Counseling: Inform the patient about the risks and benefits of the therapy. Instruct to contact physician if any unusual bleeding occurs or if any other adverse reaction develops. Advise to avoid IM injections while on therapy.

RETIN-A — tretinoin

Rx

Class: Retinoid

OTHER BRAND NAMES

Retin-A Micro

ADULT DOSAGE

Acne Vulgaris

Apply qpm/qhs to the skin where acne lesions appear, using enough to cover the entire affected area in a thin layer

PEDIATRIC DOSAGE

Acne Vulgaris

≥12 Years:
Retin-A Micro:
Apply qpm to the skin where acne lesions appear, using enough to cover the entire affected area in a thin layer

ADMINISTRATION

Topical route

Thoroughly cleanse the areas to be treated before applying the medication. To help limit skin irritation, wash treated skin gently, using a mild, non-medicated soap, and pat it dry; avoid washing treated skin too often or scrubbing hard when washing.

Keep away from eyes, mouth, paranasal creases of the nose, and mucous membranes.

Patients treated w/ therapy may use cosmetics.

STORAGE

(Retin-A) Cre: <27°C (80°F). **Gel:** <30°C (86°F). **(Retin-A Micro) Gel:** 20-25°C (68-77°F); excursions permitted from 15-30°C (59-86°F). Store pump upright.

HOW SUPPLIED

(Retin-A) Cre: 0.025%, 0.05%, 0.1% [20g, 45g]; **Gel:** 0.01%, 0.025% [15g, 45g]; **(Retin-A Micro) Gel:** 0.04%, 0.1% [20g, 45g, 50g], 0.08% [50g]

CONTRAINDICATIONS

Hypersensitivity to any of the ingredients.

WARNINGS/PRECAUTIONS

Severe irritation on eczematous skin reported; use caution in patients w/ this condition. If the degree of local irritation warrants, temporarily reduce the amount/frequency of application, d/c use temporarily, or d/c use all together. D/C therapy if a reaction suggesting sensitivity or chemical irritation occurs. Avoid or minimize unprotected exposure to sunlight, including sunlamps (UV light); avoid use w/ sunburn until fully recovered. Caution in patients who may be required to have considerable sun exposure and those w/ inherent sensitivity to the sun. Use of sunscreen products and protective clothing over treated areas is recommended when exposure cannot be avoided. Weather extremes (eg, cold, wind) may irritate skin. An apparent exacerbation of inflammatory lesions may occur during early weeks of therapy. A transitory feeling of warmth or slight stinging may be noted on application. **Retin-A:** May induce severe local erythema and peeling at application site. Gels are flammable. **Retin-A Micro:** Skin may become excessively dry, red, swollen, or blistered; apply topical moisturizer if dryness is bothersome.

ADVERSE REACTIONS

Skin irritation/burning, erythema, dermatitis, hyper/hypopigmentation.

DRUG INTERACTIONS

Caution w/ topical medications, medicated/abrasive soaps and cleansers, products w/ strong drying effect, and products w/ high concentrations of alcohol, astringents, limes, or spices. Caution w/ medications that cause photosensitivity. Caution w/ preparations containing sulfur, resorcinol, or salicylic acid; allow effects of these agents to subside before initiation of treatment. **Retin-A Micro:** Caution w/ OTC acne preparations containing benzoyl peroxide.

PREGNANCY AND LACTATION

Pregnancy: Category C (Retin-A). There are no well-controlled studies in pregnant women; should be used during pregnancy only if the potential benefit justifies the potential risk to the fetus.

Lactation: It is not known whether the drug is excreted in human milk; caution in nursing.

MECHANISM OF ACTION

Retinoid; exact mode of action not established. Current evidence suggests that topical tretinoin decreases cohesiveness of follicular epithelial cells w/ decreased microcomedo formation. Additionally, stimulates mitotic activity and increased turnover of follicular epithelial cells causing extrusion of the comedones.

PHARMACOKINETICS

Absorption: Bioavailability (Retin-A Micro Gel 0.1%) 0.82% (single applications), 1.41% (multiple daily applications for 28 days).

PATIENT CONSIDERATIONS

Assessment: Assess for drug hypersensitivity, sun exposure, sensitivity to sun, sunburn, eczematous skin, pregnancy/nursing status, and possible drug interactions.

Monitoring: Monitor for sensitivity reactions, irritation, local erythema or peeling at application site, and other adverse reactions. Closely monitor alterations of vehicle, drug concentration, or dose frequency by carefully observing therapeutic response and skin tolerance.

Counseling: Instruct to d/c use and consult physician if irritation occurs. Instruct not to use more than the recommended amount and not to apply more than qd. Advise to minimize exposure to sunlight, including sunlamps, and to use sunscreen products and protective clothing over treated areas when exposure to sun cannot be avoided. Inform that weather extremes may be irritating to treated skin. Instruct to use ud, and to keep away from eyes, mouth, angles of the nose, and mucous membranes. Advise to inform physician of other acne preparations being used and if pregnant or breastfeeding. Inform that during the early weeks of therapy, an apparent exacerbation of inflammatory lesions may occur, which should not be considered a reason for discontinuation. **Retin-A Micro:** Advise to apply moisturizer if dryness is bothersome.

REVATIO — sildenafil

Rx

Class: Phosphodiesterase-5 (PDE-5) inhibitor

ADULT DOSAGE

Pulmonary Arterial Hypertension

Treatment of pulmonary arterial HTN (WHO Group I) to improve exercise ability and delay clinical worsening

PO:
5mg or 20mg tid, 4-6 hrs apart
Max: 20mg tid

IV:
For continued treatment in patients currently taking tabs/sus and who are temporarily unable to take oral medications

2.5mg or 10mg IV bolus tid

PEDIATRIC DOSAGE

Pediatric use may not have been established

ADMINISTRATION

Oral/IV route

Refer to PI for reconstitution of the powder for oral sus.

Incompatibilities

Do not mix w/ any other medication or additional flavoring agent.

STORAGE

(Tab/Inj) 20-25°C (68-77°F); excursions permitted to 15-30°C (59-86°F). (Sus) <30°C (86°F). Protect from moisture. Constituted: <30°C (86°F) or 2-8°C (36-46°F). Do not freeze. Shelf-life: 60 days.

HOW SUPPLIED

Inj: 10mg [12.5mL]; **Sus:** 10mg/mL [112mL]; **Tab:** 20mg

CONTRAINDICATIONS

Concomitant use of organic nitrates in any form, either regularly/intermittently, or riociguat, a guanylate cyclase stimulator. Known hypersensitivity to sildenafil or any component of the tablet, injection, or oral suspension.

WARNINGS/PRECAUTIONS

Adding sildenafil to bosentan therapy does not result in any beneficial effect on exercise capacity. Not recommended in children. Vasodilatory effects may adversely affect patients w/ resting hypotension (BP <90/50), fluid depletion, severe left ventricular outflow obstruction, or autonomic dysfunction. Not recommended w/ pulmonary veno-occlusive disease (PVOD); consider possibility of associated PVOD if signs of pulmonary edema occur. Epistaxis reported in patients w/ pulmonary HTN secondary to connective tissue disorder. When used to treat erectile dysfunction, non-arteritic anterior ischemic optic neuropathy (NAION) was reported. Caution w/ previous NAION in 1 eye and w/ retinitis pigmentosa. Cases of sudden decrease or loss of hearing, possibly accompanied by tinnitus and dizziness, reported. Caution in patients w/ anatomical penile deformation (eg, angulation, cavernosal fibrosis, Peyronie's disease) or w/ predisposition to priapism (eg, sickle-cell anemia, multiple myeloma, leukemia). Penile tissue damage and permanent loss of potency may result if priapism is not immediately treated. Vaso-occlusive crises requiring hospitalization reported in patients w/ pulmonary HTN secondary to sickle-cell disease. Caution in elderly.

ADVERSE REACTIONS

Headache, dyspepsia, gastritis, epistaxis, paresthesia, flushing, diarrhea, insomnia, dyspnea exacerbation, myalgia, nausea, sinusitis, erythema, pyrexia, rhinitis.

DRUG INTERACTIONS

See Contraindications. Vasodilatory effects may adversely affect patients on antihypertensive therapy; monitor BP when given w/ antihypertensives. Reports of epistaxis w/ oral vitamin K antagonists. Avoid w/ other PDE-5 inhibitors. Not recommended w/ ritonavir and other potent CYP3A inhibitors. Symptomatic postural hypotension w/ doxazosin reported. Additional reduction of supine BP w/ oral amlodipine reported.

PREGNANCY AND LACTATION
Pregnancy: Category B.
Lactation: Caution in nursing.

MECHANISM OF ACTION
PDE-5 inhibitor; increases cGMP w/in pulmonary vascular smooth muscle cells, resulting in relaxation and vasodilation of pulmonary vascular bed and (to a lesser degree) systemic circulation.

PHARMACOKINETICS
Absorption: (Oral) Rapid; absolute bioavailability (41%); T_{max}=60 min (median) (fasted). **Distribution:** V_d=105L; plasma protein binding (96%). **Metabolism:** CYP3A (major route) and CYP2C9 (minor route); N-desmethyl metabolite (active metabolite). **Elimination:** Feces (80% metabolites), urine (13% metabolites); $T_{1/2}$=4 hrs.

PATIENT CONSIDERATIONS

Assessment: Assess for hypotension, fluid depletion, left ventricular outflow obstruction, autonomic dysfunction, PVOD, risk factors for developing NAION, previous NAION in 1 eye, retinitis pigmentosa, anatomical deformities of the penis, conditions predisposing to priapism, pulmonary HTN secondary to sickle-cell disease, hypersensitivity to drug, pregnancy/nursing status, and possible drug interactions. Obtain baseline BP.

Monitoring: Monitor for signs of pulmonary edema, decreased/sudden loss of vision or hearing, tinnitus, dizziness, epistaxis, priapism, vaso-occlusive crises, hypersensitivity reactions, and other adverse reactions. Monitor BP.

Counseling: Counsel about risks and benefits of the drug. Inform that drug is also marketed as Viagra for male erectile dysfunction. Advise not to take Viagra or other PDE-5 inhibitors and organic nitrates during therapy. Advise to notify physician if sudden decrease/loss of vision or hearing occurs. Instruct to seek immediate medical attention if an erection persists >4 hrs.

REVIA — naltrexone hydrochloride   Rx

Class: Opioid antagonist

ADULT DOSAGE	PEDIATRIC DOSAGE
Alcohol Dependence	Pediatric use may not have been established
Usual: 50mg qd up to 12 weeks	
Prior to initiating therapy, an opioid-free interval of a minimum of 7-10 days is recommended for patients previously dependent on short-acting opioids	
Alternative Dosing Schedules: May receive 50mg every weekday w/ a 100mg dose on Saturday, 100mg qod, or 150mg every 3rd day; may reduce the degree of blockade produced by therapy by these extended dosing intervals	
Opioid Dependence	
For Blockade of Effects of Exogenously Administered Opioids:	
Initial: 25mg; if no withdrawal signs occur, may start on 50mg qd thereafter	
Prior to initiating therapy, an opioid-free interval of a minimum of 7-10 days is recommended for patients previously dependent on short-acting opioids	
Alternative Dosing Schedules: May receive 50mg every weekday w/ a 100mg dose on Saturday, 100mg qod, or 150mg every 3rd day; may reduce the degree of blockade produced by therapy by these extended dosing intervals	
Conversions	
Switching from Buprenorphine, Buprenorphine/Naloxone, or Methadone: Be prepared to manage withdrawal symptomatically w/ nonopioid medications	

ADMINISTRATION
Oral route

STORAGE
20-25°C (68-77°F). Protect from light.

HOW SUPPLIED
Tab: 50mg* *scored

CONTRAINDICATIONS
Patient receiving opioid analgesics; patients currently dependent on opioids, including those currently maintained on opiate agonists (eg, methadone) or partial agonists (eg, buprenorphine); patients in acute opioid withdrawal; any individual who failed the naloxone challenge test or who has a positive urine screen for opioids; history of sensitivity to this medication or any other components of this product.

WARNINGS/PRECAUTIONS
Patients may have reduced tolerance to opioids after opioid detoxification; may result in potentially life-threatening opioid intoxication with use of previously tolerated opioid doses. Potential risk of patients attempting to overcome antagonism by taking opioids; may lead to life-threatening opioid intoxication or fatal overdose. Withdrawal syndrome, severe enough to require hospitalization, may occur when withdrawal is precipitated abruptly by the administration of an opioid antagonist to an opioid-dependent patient. Opioid-dependent patients, including those being treated for alcohol dependence, should be opioid-free before starting treatment to reduce risk of either precipitated withdrawal in patients dependent on opioids or exacerbation of a preexisting subclinical withdrawal syndrome; an opioid-free interval of a minimum of 7-10 days is recommended for patients previously dependent on short-acting opioids. May experience severe manifestations of precipitated withdrawal when being switched from opioid agonist to opioid antagonist therapy; patients transitioning from buprenorphine or methadone may be vulnerable to precipitation of withdrawal symptoms for as long as 2 weeks. A naloxone challenge test may be helpful to determine if patient is opioid-free; however, precipitated withdrawal may occur despite having negative urine toxicology screen or tolerating a naloxone challenge test. Cases of hepatitis, clinically significant liver dysfunction, and transient, asymptomatic liver transaminase elevations reported; d/c in the event of symptoms and/or signs of acute hepatitis. Depression, suicide, attempted suicide, and suicidal ideation reported. In emergency situations, suggested plan for pain management is regional analgesia, conscious sedation with benzodiazepine, use of nonopioid analgesics, or general anesthesia. In a situation requiring opioid analgesia, amount of opioid required may be greater than usual, and the resulting respiratory depression may be deeper and more prolonged. Rapidly acting opioid analgesic is preferred. Caution with renal or hepatic impairment. Appropriate compliance-enhancing techniques should be implemented for all components of the treatment program.

ADVERSE REACTIONS
N/V, headache, dizziness, nervousness, fatigue, low energy, insomnia, anxiety, difficulty sleeping, abdominal pain/cramps, joint/muscle pain.

DRUG INTERACTIONS
See Contraindications. Concomitant use with other hepatotoxic medications (eg, disulfiram) is not ordinarily recommended unless the probable benefits outweigh the known risks. Lethargy and somnolence reported with thioridazine. Patients may not benefit from opioid-containing medications (eg, cough and cold preparations, antidiarrheal preparations, opioid analgesics).

PREGNANCY AND LACTATION
Category C, caution in nursing.

MECHANISM OF ACTION
Opioid antagonist; markedly attenuates or completely blocks, reversibly, the subjective effects of intravenously administered opioids.

PHARMACOKINETICS
Absorption: Rapid and nearly complete. Bioavailability (5-40%); T_{max}=1 hr (naltrexone and 6-β-naltrexol). **Distribution:** (IV) V_d=1350L; plasma protein binding (21%). **Metabolism:** Liver; 6-β-naltrexol (major metabolite). **Elimination:** Urine (53-79%; <2% unchanged, 43% unchanged/conjugated 6-β-naltrexol), feces; $T_{1/2}$=4 hrs, 13 hrs (6-β-naltrexol).

PATIENT CONSIDERATIONS

Assessment: Assess for renal/hepatic impairment, any other conditions where treatment is contraindicated or cautioned, pregnancy/nursing status, and possible drug interactions. Assess patients, including patients treated for alcohol dependence, for underlying opioid dependence and for any recent use of opioids.

Monitoring: Monitor for opioid intoxication/overdose, withdrawal syndrome, liver impairment, depression, suicidality, and other adverse reactions.

Counseling: Instruct to take ud. Advise patient that if they previously used opioids, they may be more sensitive to lower doses of opioids and at risk of accidental overdose if they use opioids after treatment is discontinued or temporarily interrupted. Advise that patients will not perceive any effect if they attempt to self-administer heroin or any other opioid drug in small doses while on therapy. Inform that administration of large doses of heroin or any other opioid to try to bypass the blockade may lead to serious injury, coma, or death. Inform that patient may not experience the expected effects from opioid-containing analgesic, antidiarrheal, or antitussive medications. Instruct to be off all opioids for a minimum of 7-10 days before starting therapy in order to avoid precipitation of opioid withdrawal. Advise not to take therapy if they have any symptoms of opioid withdrawal. Advise all patients, including those with alcohol dependence, to notify physician of any recent use of opioids or any history of opioid dependence before starting therapy. Inform that drug may cause liver injury; instruct to immediately notify physician if symptoms and/or signs of liver disease develop. Inform that depression may be experienced while taking therapy; instruct to contact physician if they become depressed or symptoms of depression are experienced. Advise that therapy has been shown to be effective only when used as part of a treatment program that includes counseling and support. Advise that dizziness may occur; instruct to avoid driving or operating heavy machinery. Advise to notify physician if pregnant or intending to become pregnant during treatment, breastfeeding, or experiencing other unusual or significant side effects while on therapy.

REVLIMID — lenalidomide

Class: Thalidomide analogue

Rx

Do not use during pregnancy; may cause birth defects or embryo-fetal death. Females of reproductive potential should have 2 negative pregnancy tests prior to treatment and must use 2 forms of contraception or continuously abstain from heterosexual sex during and for 4 weeks after treatment. Available only through a restricted distribution program, the Revlimid REMS program. May cause significant neutropenia and thrombocytopenia. Patients on therapy for del 5q myelodysplastic syndrome (MDS) should have their CBC monitored weekly for the first 8 weeks of therapy and at least monthly thereafter; may require dose interruption and/or reduction and use of blood product support and/or growth factors. Increased risk of deep vein thrombosis (DVT) and pulmonary embolism (PE), as well as risk of MI and stroke, reported in patients w/ multiple myeloma (MM) treated w/ lenalidomide and dexamethasone; monitor for and advise patients about signs/symptoms of thromboembolism. Advise patients to seek immediate medical care if symptoms such as SOB, chest pain, or arm or leg swelling develop. Thromboprophylaxis is recommended and the choice of regimen should be based on assessment of individual's underlying risks.

ADULT DOSAGE

Multiple Myeloma

Initial: 25mg qd on Days 1-21 of repeated 28-day cycles in combination w/ dexamethasone; may reduce initial dose of dexamethasone for patients >75 yrs

Continue until disease progression or unacceptable toxicity

In Patients who are not eligible for autologous stem cell transplantation (ASCT), continue treatment until disease progression or unacceptable toxicity. For patients who are ASCT-eligible, hematopoietic stem cell mobilization should occur w/in 4 cycles of a lenalidomide-containing therapy

Myelodysplastic Syndromes

Patients w/ transfusion-dependent anemia due to low- or intermediate-1-risk myelodysplastic syndromes associated w/ a deletion 5q cytogenetic abnormality w/ or w/o additional cytogenetic abnormalities

Initial: 10mg/day

Continue or modify treatment based upon clinical and lab findings

Mantle Cell Lymphoma

Patients whose disease has relapsed or progressed after 2 prior therapies, 1 of which included bortezomib

Initial: 25mg/day on Days 1-21 of repeated 28-day cycles for relapsed or refractory disease

Continue until disease progression or unacceptable toxicity

PEDIATRIC DOSAGE

Pediatric use may not have been established

DOSING CONSIDERATIONS

Renal Impairment

Multiple Myeloma (MM):
Moderate (CrCl 30-50mL/min): Initial: 10mg q24h
Severe (CrCl <30mL/min Not Requiring Dialysis): Initial: 15mg q48h
ESRD (CrCl <30mL/min Requiring Dialysis): Initial: 5mg qd. On dialysis days, administer dose following dialysis

Myelodysplastic Syndromes (MDS):
Moderate (CrCl 30-60mL/min): Initial: 5mg q24h
Severe (CrCl <30mL/min Not Requiring Dialysis): Initial: 2.5mg q24h
ESRD (CrCl <30mL/min Requiring Dialysis): Initial: 2.5mg qd. On dialysis days, administer dose following dialysis

Mantle Cell Lymphoma (MCL):
Moderate (CrCl 30-60mL/min): Initial: 10mg q24h
Severe (CrCl <30mL/min Not Requiring Dialysis): Initial: 15mg q48h
ESRD (CrCl <30mL/min Requiring Dialysis): Initial: 5mg qd. On dialysis days, administer dose following dialysis

Adverse Reactions

MM:
Thrombocytopenia:
Platelets:
Fall to <30,000/µL: Interrupt treatment and follow CBC weekly
Return to ≥30,000/µL: Resume at next lower dose. Do not dose <2.5mg/day
For Each Subsequent Drop <30,000/µL: Interrupt treatment
Return to ≥30,000/µL: Resume at next lower dose; do not dose <2.5mg/day
Neutropenia:
Neutrophils:
Fall to <1000/µL: Interrupt treatment, follow CBC weekly
Return to ≥1000/µL and Neutropenia is Only Toxicity: Resume at 25mg/day or initial starting dose

Return to ≥1000/µL and if Other Toxicity: Resume at next lower dose. Do not dose <2.5mg/day
For Each Subsequent Drop <1000/µL: Interrupt treatment
Return to ≥1000/µL: Resume at next lower dose. Do not dose <2.5mg/day
Other Toxicities in MM:
For other Grade 3/4 toxicities judged to be related to treatment, hold treatment and restart at physician's discretion at next lower dose level when toxicity has resolved to ≤Grade 2

MDS:
Thrombocytopenia w/in 4 Weeks at Starting Dose 10mg/day (Baseline ≥100,000/µL):
Platelets:
Fall to <50,000/µL: Interrupt treatment
Return to ≥50,000/µL: Resume at 5mg/day
Thrombocytopenia w/in 4 Weeks at Starting Dose 10mg/day (Baseline <100,000/µL):
Platelets:
Falls to 50% of Baseline: Interrupt treatment
If Baseline ≥60,000/µL and Return to ≥50,000/µL: Resume at 5mg/day
If Baseline <60,000/µL and Return to ≥30,000/µL: Resume at 5mg/day
Thrombocytopenia after 4 Weeks at Starting Dose 10mg/day:
Platelets:
<30,000/µL or <50,000/µL w/ Platelet Transfusions: Interrupt treatment
Return to ≥30,000/µL (w/o Hemostatic Failure): Resume at 5mg/day
Thrombocytopenia During Treatment at 5mg/day:
Platelets:
<30,000/µL or <50,000/µL w/ Platelet Transfusions: Interrupt treatment
Return to ≥30,000/µL (w/o Hemostatic Failure): Resume at 2.5mg/day
Neutropenia w/in 4 Weeks of Starting Treatment at 10mg/day (Baseline ANC ≥1000/µL):
Neutrophils:
Fall to <750/µL: Interrupt treatment
Return to ≥1000/µL: Resume at 5mg/day
Neutropenia w/in 4 Weeks of Starting Treatment at 10mg/day (Baseline ANC <1000/µL):
Neutrophils:
Fall to <500/µL: Interrupt treatment
Return to ≥500/µL: Resume at 5mg/day
Neutropenia After 4 Weeks of Starting Treatment at 10mg/day:
Neutrophils:
<500/µL for ≥7 days or <500/µL Associated w/ Fever (≥38.5°C): Interrupt treatment
Return to ≥500/µL: Resume at 5mg/day
Neutropenia During Treatment at 5mg/day:
Neutrophils:
<500/µL for ≥7 Days or <500/µL Associated w/ Fever (≥38.5°C): Interrupt treatment
Return to ≥500/µL: Resume at 2.5mg/day
Other Toxicities in MDS:
For other Grade 3/4 toxicities judged to be related to treatment, hold treatment and restart at the physician's discretion at next lower dose level when toxicity has resolved to ≤Grade 2

MCL:
Thrombocytopenia During Treatment:
Platelets:
Fall to <50,000/µL: Interrupt treatment and follow CBC weekly
Return to ≥50,000/µL: Resume at 5mg less than the previous dose. Do not dose <5mg daily
Neutropenia During Treatment:
Neutrophils:
Fall to <1000/µL for at Least 7 Days or Falls to <1000/µL w/ an Associated Temperature ≥38.5°C or Fall to <500/µL: Interrupt treatment and follow CBC weekly
Return to ≥1000/µL: Resume at 5mg less than previous dose. Do not dose <5mg/day
Other Toxicities in MCL:
For other Grade 3/4 toxicities judged to be related to treatment, hold treatment and restart at next lower dose level when toxicity has resolved to ≤Grade 2

ADMINISTRATION

Oral route

Take at about the same time each day, w/ or w/o food. Swallow cap whole w/ water; do not open, crush, break, or chew.

Handling Precautions

Wash skin immediately and thoroughly w/ soap and water if powder from cap contacts the skin. If drug contacts the mucous membranes, flush thoroughly w/ water.

STORAGE

20-25°C (68-77°F); excursions permitted to 15-30°C (59-86°F).

HOW SUPPLIED

Cap: 2.5mg, 5mg, 10mg, 15mg, 20mg, 25mg

CONTRAINDICATIONS

Pregnancy, hypersensitivity (eg, angioedema, Stevens-Johnson syndrome, toxic epidermal necrolysis) to lenalidomide.

WARNINGS/PRECAUTIONS

Not indicated and not recommended for the treatment of patients w/ chronic lymphocytic leukemia outside of controlled clinical trials; increased risk of death and serious adverse cardiovascular (CV) reactions reported. Avoid pregnancy for at least 4 weeks before beginning therapy, during therapy, during dose interruptions, and for at least 4 weeks after completing therapy. Male patients (including those who had a vasectomy) must always use a latex/synthetic condom during any sexual contact w/ females of reproductive potential during therapy and for up to 28 days after discontinuing therapy. Avoid sperm donation during therapy. Avoid blood donation during treatment and for 1 month following discontinuation. Greater risk of MI or stroke in patients w/ known risk factors, including prior thrombosis; minimize all modifiable factors (eg, hyperlipidemia, HTN, smoking). Increase of invasive 2nd primary malignancies notably acute myelogenous leukemia and MDS reported in patients w/ MM, predominantly in those receiving therapy in combination w/ oral melphalan or immediately following high dose IV melphalan and ASCT. Hepatic failure, including fatal cases, reported in combination w/ dexamethasone. D/C treatment upon elevation of liver enzymes and consider treatment at a lower dose after values return to baseline. Angioedema and serious dermatologic reactions reported; d/c if angioedema, Stevens-Johnson syndrome (SJS), toxic epidermal necrolysis (TEN), Grade 4 rash, or exfoliative or bullous rash is suspected and do not resume following discontinuation for these reactions. Consider treatment interruption or discontinuation for Grade 2-3 skin rash. Avoid w/ a prior history of Grade 4 rash associated w/ thalidomide treatment. Contains lactose. Fatal instances of tumor lysis syndrome reported; caution in patients w/ high tumor burden prior to treatment. Tumor flare reaction (TFR) reported in patients w/ MCL; withhold treatment in patients w/ Grade 3 or 4 TFR until TFR resolves to ≤Grade 1. A decrease in the number of CD34+ cells collected after treatment (>4 cycles) reported; in patients who are ASCT candidates, referral to a transplant center should occur early in treatment to optimize the timing of the stem cell collection. Consider granulocyte-colony stimulating factor (G-CSF) w/ cyclophosphamide or the combination of G-CSF w/ a CXCR4 inhibitor in patients who received >4 cycles of a lenalidomide-containing treatment or for whom inadequate numbers of CD34+ cells have been collected w/ G-CSF alone.

ADVERSE REACTIONS

Thrombocytopenia, neutropenia, PE, pruritus, rash, diarrhea, constipation, nausea, anemia, fatigue, cough, back pain, pyrexia, muscle cramp, asthenia.

DRUG INTERACTIONS

May increase levels of digoxin; monitor digoxin levels periodically. Closely monitor PT and INR w/ warfarin in MM patients. Caution w/ erythropoietic agents or other agents that may increase the risk of thrombosis (eg, estrogen-containing therapies).

PREGNANCY AND LACTATION

Pregnancy: Category X.
Lactation: Not for use in nursing.

MECHANISM OF ACTION

Thalidomide analogue; w/ immunomodulatory, antiangiogenic, and antineoplastic properties. Inhibits proliferation and induces apoptosis of certain hematopoietic tumor cells. Immunomodulatory properties include activation of T cells and natural killer T (NKT) cells, increased numbers of NKT cells, and inhibition of proinflammatory cytokines (eg, TNF-α and IL-6) by monocytes.

PHARMACOKINETICS

Absorption: Rapid. (Single/Multiple Doses) T_{max}=0.5-6 hrs. **Distribution:** Plasma protein binding (approx 30%). **Metabolism:** 5-hydroxy-lenalidomide and N-acetyl-lenalidomide (metabolites). **Elimination:** Urine (approx 90%, approx 82% unchanged), feces (approx 4%); $T_{1/2}$=3-5 hrs.

PATIENT CONSIDERATIONS

Assessment: Assess for renal/hepatic impairment, history of Grade 4 rash, risk factors for MI and stroke, prior thrombosis, high tumor burden, lactose intolerance, hypersensitivity to the drug, pregnancy/nursing status, and possible drug interactions. Perform pregnancy test 10-14 days before and 24 hrs prior to therapy. Obtain baseline CBC.

Monitoring: Monitor for signs/symptoms of thromboembolism, neutropenia, thrombocytopenia, angioedema, SJS, TEN, tumor lysis syndrome, TFR, 2nd primary malignancies, serious adverse CV reactions, and other adverse reactions. Perform pregnancy test weekly during 1st month, then repeat monthly (regular menstrual cycle) or every 2 weeks (irregular menstrual cycle) and perform pregnancy test if period is missed or if there is any abnormal menstrual bleeding. Monitor CBC periodically; every 7 days (weekly) for the first 2 cycles, on Days 1 and 15 of cycle 3, and every 28 days (4 weeks) thereafter (MM patients taking concomitant dexamethasone); weekly for the first 8 weeks of therapy and at least monthly thereafter (MDS); and weekly for the 1st cycle (28 days), every 2 weeks during cycles 2-4, and monthly thereafter (MCL). Monitor patients w/ neutropenia for signs of infection. Monitor renal/hepatic function. Closely monitor patients w/ high tumor burden. Closely monitor PT and INR w/ warfarin in MM patients.

Counseling: Instruct females of reproductive potential to avoid pregnancy, have monthly pregnancy tests, and to use 2 different forms of contraception, including at least 1 highly effective form, simultaneously during therapy, during dose interruption, and for 4 weeks after completing therapy. Instruct to immediately d/c and contact physician if patient becomes pregnant, misses her menstrual period, experiences unusual menstrual bleeding, stops taking birth control, or believes for any reason that she is pregnant. Instruct males (including those who had a vasectomy) to always use a latex/synthetic condom during any sexual contact w/ females of reproductive potential during therapy and for up to 28 days after discontinuing therapy. Advise males not to donate sperm. Instruct not to

donate blood during therapy, during dose interruptions, and for 1 month following discontinuation. Inform of the other risks associated w/ therapy. Instruct that if a dose is missed, may still take dose up to 12 hrs after the time dose is normally taken. Advise that if >12 hrs have elapsed, the dose for that day should be skipped, and the dose for the next day should be taken at the usual time. Advise to observe for bleeding/bruising, especially w/ use of concomitant medication that may increase risk of bleeding.

REXULTI — brexpiprazole   Rx

Class: Atypical antipsychotic

> Elderly patients w/ dementia-related psychosis treated w/ antipsychotic drugs are at an increased risk of death. Not approved for treatment of patients w/ dementia-related psychosis. Antidepressants increased the risk of suicidal thoughts and behaviors in patients aged 24 years and younger in short-term studies. Monitor closely for clinical worsening and for emergence of suicidal thoughts and behaviors. Safety and efficacy of brexpiprazole have not been established in pediatric patients.

ADULT DOSAGE	PEDIATRIC DOSAGE
Major Depressive Disorder	Pediatric use may not have been established
Adjunctive Treatment:	
Initial: 0.5mg or 1mg qd	
Titrate: Titrate to 1mg qd, then up to target dose of 2mg qd; increase dose at weekly intervals based on clinical response and tolerability	
Max: 3mg/day	
Schizophrenia	
Initial: 1mg qd on Days 1-4	
Titrate: Titrate to 2mg qd on Days 5-7, then to 4mg on Day 8 based on clinical response and tolerability	
Target Dose: 2-4mg qd	
Max: 4mg/day	

DOSING CONSIDERATIONS

Concomitant Medications
Strong CYP2D6 Inhibitors:
Administer 1/2 of brexpiprazole usual dose; adjust to original level if coadministered drug is discontinued. Dose adjustment not needed in patients who are being treated for major depressive disorder (MDD)

Strong CYP3A4 Inhibitors:
Administer 1/2 of brexpiprazole usual dose; adjust to original level if coadministered drug is discontinued

Strong/Moderate CYP2D6 Inhibitors w/ Strong/Moderate CYP3A4 Inhibitors:
Administer 1/4 of brexpiprazole usual dose; adjust to original level if coadministered drug is discontinued

Strong CYP3A4 Inducers:
Double brexpiprazole usual dose over 1-2 weeks; reduce to original level over 1-2 weeks if the coadministered CYP3A4 inducer is discontinued

Renal Impairment
Moderate, Severe, or ESRD (CrCl <60mL/min):
Max Dose:
MDD: 2mg qd
Schizophrenia: 3mg qd

Hepatic Impairment
Moderate to Severe (Child-Pugh Score ≥7):
Max Dose:
MDD: 2mg qd
Schizophrenia: 3mg qd

Elderly
Start at lower end of dosing range

Other Important Considerations
CYP2D6 Poor Metabolizers:
Administer 1/2 of usual dose

Known CYP2D6 Poor Metabolizers Taking Strong/Moderate CYP3A4 Inhibitors:
Administer 1/4 of usual dose

ADMINISTRATION

Oral route
Take w/ or w/o food.

STORAGE

20-25°C (68-77°F); excursions permitted to 15-30°C (59-86°F).

HOW SUPPLIED

Tab: 0.25mg, 0.5mg, 1mg, 2mg, 3mg, 4mg

CONTRAINDICATIONS

Known hypersensitivity to Rexulti or any of its components.

WARNINGS/PRECAUTIONS

Neuroleptic malignant syndrome (NMS) may occur; d/c immediately, institute symptomatic treatment, and monitor. May cause tardive dyskinesia (TD), especially in the elderly; consider discontinuation if signs/symptoms appear. Hyperglycemia, in some cases extreme and associated w/ ketoacidosis or hyperosmolar coma or death, reported w/ atypical antipsychotics. Undesirable alterations in lipids and weight gain have been observed in patients treated w/ atypical antipsychotics. Leukopenia, neutropenia, and agranulocytosis reported w/ atypical antipsychotics. Consider discontinuation at the 1st sign of a clinically significant decline in WBC count in the absence of other causative factors in patients w/ a history of a clinically significant low WBC count/ANC or drug-induced leukopenia/neutropenia. Monitor patients w/ clinically significant neutropenia for fever or other signs/symptoms of infection and treat promptly if such signs/symptoms occur. D/C in patients w/ severe neutropenia (ANC<1000/mm³) and follow their WBC count until recovery. May cause orthostatic hypotension and syncope; consider using a lower starting dosage and slower titration, and monitor orthostatic vital signs in patients at increased risk of these adverse reactions or at increased risk of developing complications from hypotension. Caution w/ history of seizures or w/ conditions that potentially lower seizure threshold. May disrupt the body's ability to reduce core body temperature; caution w/ conditions that may contribute to an elevation in core body temperature (eg, exercising strenuously, receiving concomitant medication w/ anticholinergic activity, being subject to dehydration). May cause esophageal dysmotility and aspiration; caution in patients at risk for aspiration pneumonia. May impair physical/mental abilities.

ADVERSE REACTIONS
MDD: Akathisia, headache, somnolence, tremor, dizziness, fatigue, nasopharyngitis, weight increased, increased appetite, anxiety, restlessness.
Schizophrenia: Akathisia, dyspepsia, diarrhea, weight increased, tremor.

DRUG INTERACTIONS
See Dosing Considerations. Strong CYP3A4 inhibitors (eg, itraconazole, clarithromycin, ketoconazole) and strong CYP2D6 inhibitors (eg, paroxetine, fluoxetine, quinidine) may increase exposure. Concomitant use w/ a strong CYP3A4 inhibitor and a strong CYP2D6 inhibitor; or a moderate CYP3A4 inhibitor and a strong CYP2D6 inhibitor; or a strong CYP3A4 inhibitor and a moderate CYP2D6 inhibitor; or a moderate CYP3A4 inhibitor and a moderate CYP2D6 inhibitor, may increase exposure. Strong CYP3A4 inducers (eg, rifampin, St. John's wort) may decrease exposure.

PREGNANCY AND LACTATION
Pregnancy: There is a pregnancy exposure registry that monitors pregnancy outcomes in women exposed to brexpiprazole during pregnancy. Adequate and well-controlled studies have not been conducted w/ brexpiprazole in pregnant women to inform drug-associated risks. However, neonates whose mothers are exposed to antipsychotic drugs, like brexpiprazole, during the 3rd trimester are at risk for extrapyramidal and/or withdrawal symptoms.
Lactation: Lactation studies have not been conducted to assess the presence of brexpiprazole in human milk, the effects of brexpiprazole on the breastfed infant, or the effects of brexpiprazole on milk production. Caution in nursing.

MECHANISM OF ACTION
Atypical antipsychotic; mechanism not established. Efficacy may be mediated through a combination of partial agonist activity at serotonin 5-HT$_{1A}$ and dopamine D$_2$ receptors, and antagonist activity at serotonin 5-HT$_{2A}$ receptors.

PHARMACOKINETICS
Absorption: Absolute oral bioavailability (95%); T$_{max}$=w/in 4 hrs. **Distribution:** V$_d$=1.56L/kg (IV); plasma protein binding (>99%, albumin and α1-acid glycoprotein). **Metabolism:** Mainly via CYP3A4 and CYP2D6; DM-3411 (major metabolite). **Excretion:** Urine (25%, <1% unchanged), feces (46%, 14% unchanged); T$_{1/2}$= 91 hrs (brexpiprazole), 86 hrs (DM-3411).

PATIENT CONSIDERATIONS
Assessment: Assess for dementia-related psychosis, drug hypersensitivity, renal/hepatic impairment, history of seizures or conditions that potentially lower the seizure threshold, any other conditions where treatment is cautioned, pregnancy/nursing status, and possible drug interactions. Obtain baseline FPG in patients w/ diabetes mellitus (DM) or at risk for DM. Obtain baseline CBC in patients w/ a history of a clinically significant low WBC count/ANC or drug-induced leukopenia/neutropenia.

Monitoring: Monitor for clinical worsening of depression, emergence of suicidal thoughts and behaviors, NMS, TD, hyperglycemia, dyslipidemia, weight gain, orthostatic hypotension, seizures, esophageal dysmotility, aspiration, and other adverse reactions. Monitor CBC frequently during the 1st few months of therapy in patients w/ a history of a clinically significant low WBC count/ANC or drug-induced leukopenia/neutropenia. Monitor for fever or other signs/symptoms of infection in patients w/ neutropenia. Monitor for worsening of glucose control in patients w/ DM. Monitor FPG periodically during therapy in patients at risk for DM. Periodically reassess to determine the continued need for maintenance treatment.

Counseling: Advise patients and caregivers to look for the emergence of suicidality and instruct them to report such symptoms to the healthcare provider. Advise to contact healthcare provider or report to the emergency room if signs/symptoms of NMS are experienced. Counsel on the signs/symptoms of TD and to contact healthcare provider if these abnormal movements occur. Educate about the risk of metabolic changes, how to recognize symptoms of hyperglycemia and DM, and the need for specific monitoring, including blood glucose, lipids, and weight. Advise patients w/ a preexisting low WBC count or a history of drug induced leukopenia/neutropenia that they should have their CBCs monitored during therapy. Educate about the risk of orthostatic hypotension and syncope. Counsel regarding appropriate care in avoiding overheating and dehydration. Caution about performing activities requiring mental alertness (eg, operating hazardous machinery) until reasonably certain that therapy does not adversely affect ability to engage in such activities. Advise to notify healthcare provider of any changes to prescription/OTC medications currently taking and if pregnant/nursing.

REYATAZ — atazanavir
Class: Protease inhibitor

Rx

ADULT DOSAGE
HIV-1 Infection
Treatment-Naive Patients:
300mg + Ritonavir (RTV) 100mg qd, or
400mg qd (w/o RTV) if intolerant to RTV

In Combination w/ Efavirenz for Treatment-Naive Patients:
400mg + RTV 100mg qd

Treatment-Experienced Patients:
300mg + RTV 100mg qd

In Combination w/ H$_2$-Receptor Antagonist and Tenofovir for Treatment-Experienced Patients:
400mg + RTV 100mg qd

PEDIATRIC DOSAGE
HIV-1 Infection
Powder:
≥3 Months of Age:
Treatment-Naive/Treatment-Experienced Patients:
5 to <15kg: 200mg + RTV 80mg qd
15 to <25kg: 250mg + RTV 80mg qd
≥25kg: 300mg + RTV 100mg qd

Treatment-Naive and Intolerant to 200mg Atazanavir Powder:
5 to <10kg: 150mg + RTV 80mg qd w/ close HIV viral load monitoring

Caps:
6 to <18 Years:
Treatment-Naive/Treatment-Experienced Patients:
15 to <20kg: 150mg + RTV 100mg qd
20 to <40kg: 200mg + RTV 100mg qd
≥40kg: 300mg + RTV 100mg qd

≥13 Years:
Treatment-Naive and Intolerant to RTV:
≥40kg: 400mg qd (w/o RTV)

DOSING CONSIDERATIONS
Concomitant Medications
H$_2$-Receptor Antagonists/Proton-Pump Inhibitors:
Dose separation may be required

Renal Impairment
ESRD w/ Hemodialysis:
Treatment-Naive: 300mg + RTV 100mg qd
Treatment-Experienced: Not recommended for use

Hepatic Impairment
Coadministration w/RTV is not recommended w/ any degree of hepatic impairment

Treatment-Naive:
Mild (Child-Pugh Class A): 400mg qd (w/o RTV)
Moderate (Child-Pugh Class B): 300mg qd (w/o RTV)
Severe (Child-Pugh Class C): Not recommended for use

Pregnancy
Treatment-Naive and Treatment-Experienced:
300mg + RTV 100mg qd
Treatment-Experienced During 2nd/3rd Trimester w/ Either H$_2$-Receptor Antagonist or Tenofovir:
400mg + RTV 100mg qd

ADMINISTRATION
Oral route

Take w/ food.

Cap
Do not open.
Use w/o RTV is not recommended for treatment-experienced adults/pediatric patients w/ prior virologic failure.

Powder
Must be taken w/ RTV.

Instructions for Mixing Oral Powder
Preferred Method:
1. Mix the recommended number of pkts w/ a minimum of 1 tbsp of food (eg, applesauce or yogurt).
2. Feed the mixture to the infant or young child.
3. Add an additional 1 tbsp of food to the container, mix, and feed the child the residual mixture.

For Infants Who Can Drink from a Cup:
1. Mix the recommended number of pkts w/ a minimum of 30mL of a beverage (eg, milk or water).
2. Have the child drink the mixture.
3. Add an additional 15mL of beverage to the cup, mix, and have the child drink the residual mixture. If water is used, food should also be taken at the same time.

For Infants <6 Months Who Cannot Eat Solid Food or Drink from a Cup:
1. Mix the recommended number of pkts w/ 10mL of prepared liquid infant formula.
2. Draw up the full amount of the mixture into an oral syringe and administer into either right or left inner cheek of infant.
3. Pour another 10mL of formula into the medicine cup to rinse off remaining oral powder in cup.
4. Draw up residual mixture into the syringe and administer into either inner cheek again.

Administer RTV immediately after powder administration.

Administer the entire dose of oral powder (mixed in the food or beverage) w/in 1 hr (may leave the mixture at room temperature during this 1-hr period).

Ensure that the patient eats or drinks all the food or beverage that contains the powder.
Additional food may be given after consumption of the entire mixture.

STORAGE
Cap: 25°C (77°F); excursions permitted to 15-30°C (59-86°F). **Powder:** <30°C (86°F); may be kept at room temperature 20-30°C (68-86°F) for up to 1 hr prior to administration once powder is mixed w/ food/beverages. Store in original pkt and do not open until ready to use.

HOW SUPPLIED
Cap: 150mg, 200mg, 300mg; **Powder:** 50mg/pkt [30ˢ]

CONTRAINDICATIONS
Coadministration w/ drugs that are highly dependent on CYP3A or UGT1A1 for clearance, and for which elevated plasma concentrations are associated w/ serious and/or life-threatening events, and w/ strong CYP3A inducers (eg, alfuzosin, rifampin, irinotecan, triazolam, oral midazolam, dihydroergotamine, ergotamine, ergonovine, methylergonovine, cisapride, St. John's wort, lovastatin, simvastatin, pimozide, sildenafil when used for pulmonary arterial HTN, indinavir, nevirapine). Previously demonstrated clinically significant hypersensitivity (eg, Stevens-Johnson syndrome, erythema multiforme, or toxic skin eruptions) to any of the components of this medication.

WARNINGS/PRECAUTIONS
May prolong PR interval; consider ECG monitoring w/ preexisting conduction system disease. Rash and cases of Stevens-Johnson syndrome, erythema multiforme, and toxic skin eruptions, including drug rash w/ eosinophilia and systemic symptoms (DRESS) syndrome, reported; d/c if severe rash develops. May cause hyperbilirubinemia; dose reduction is not recommended. Powder contains phenylalanine; caution w/ phenylketonuria. Increased risk for further transaminase elevations or hepatic decompensation in patients w/ underlying hepatitis B or C infections or marked transaminase elevations before treatment; obtain LFTs prior to and during treatment. Nephrolithiasis and/or cholelithiasis reported; consider temporary interruption or discontinuation of therapy if signs/symptoms occur. New onset or exacerbation of diabetes mellitus (DM), hyperglycemia, diabetic ketoacidosis, immune reconstitution syndrome, autoimmune disorders (eg, Graves' disease, polymyositis, Guillain-Barre syndrome) in the setting of immune reconstitution, redistribution/accumulation of body fat, and increased bleeding in patients w/ hemophilia A and B reported. Various degrees of cross-resistance observed. Caution in elderly.

ADVERSE REACTIONS
N/V, jaundice/scleral icterus, rash, myalgia, headache, abdominal pain, insomnia, peripheral neurologic symptoms, diarrhea, cough, fever, AST/ALT elevations, neutropenia, hypoglycemia, extremity pain.

DRUG INTERACTIONS
See Contraindications and Dosing Considerations. Not recommended w/ salmeterol. Use w/o RTV not recommended w/ drugs highly dependent on CYP2C8 w/ narrow therapeutic indices (eg, paclitaxel, repaglinide), carbamazepine, phenytoin, phenobarbital, bosentan, and buprenorphine. ATV/RTV is not recommended w/ other protease inhibitors, voriconazole, fluticasone propionate, and boceprevir. Not recommended w/ efavirenz or proton pump inhibitors (PPIs) in treatment-experienced patients. Avoid w/ colchicine in patients w/ renal/hepatic impairment. Caution w/ oral contraceptives. CYP3A4 inducers, tenofovir, carbamazepine, boceprevir, phenytoin, phenobarbital, bosentan, efavirenz, PPIs, antacids, buffered medications, and H$_2$-receptor antagonists may decrease levels. RTV and clarithromycin may increase levels. Administer 2 hrs before or 1 hr after buffered formulations (eg, didanosine buffered or enteric-coated formulations)/antacids, ≥10 hrs after H$_2$-receptor antagonists, and 12 hrs after PPIs. May increase levels of CYP3A or UGT1A1 substrates, tenofovir, saquinavir, amiodarone, bepridil, lidocaine (systemic), quinidine, TCAs, trazodone, itraconazole, ketoconazole, colchicine, rifabutin, quetiapine, parenteral midazolam, warfarin (monitor INR), diltiazem and other calcium channel blockers, bosentan, atorvastatin, rosuvastatin, norgestimate, norethindrone, fluticasone propionate, clarithromycin, buprenorphine, norbuprenorphine, immunosuppressants, and PDE-5 inhibitors. ATV/RTV may increase levels of carbamazepine. Rosuvastatin dose should not exceed 10mg/day. May decrease levels of didanosine, and 14-OH clarithromycin (clarithromycin active metabolite). ATV/RTV may decrease levels of phenytoin, phenobarbital, and lamotrigine. Voriconazole may alter levels. May alter levels of ethinyl estradiol. Initiation of medications that inhibit or induce CYP3A may increase or decrease concentrations of ATV/RTV, respectively. Refer to PI for dosing modifications when used w/ certain concomitant therapies.

PREGNANCY AND LACTATION
Pregnancy: Physicians are encouraged to register patients in the Antiretroviral Pregnancy Registry. Lactic acidosis syndrome, symptomatic hyperlactatemia, and hyperbilirubinemia reported in pregnant women.
Lactation: Mothers should be instructed not to breastfeed due to potential for HIV-1 transmission and the potential for serious adverse reactions in breastfed infants.

MECHANISM OF ACTION
HIV-1 protease inhibitor; selectively inhibits virus-specific processing of viral Gag and Gag-Pol polyproteins in HIV-1 infected cells, preventing formation of mature virions.

PHARMACOKINETICS
Absorption: Rapid. C_{max}=3152ng/mL, T_{max}=approx 2.5 hrs, AUC=22262ng•hr/mL.
Distribution: Plasma protein binding (86%). **Metabolism:** Liver (extensive); mono- and dioxygenation via CYP3A. **Elimination:** Urine (13%, approx 7% unchanged), feces (79%, approx 20% unchanged); $T_{1/2}$=approx 7 hrs.

PATIENT CONSIDERATIONS
Assessment: Assess for treatment history, known hypersensitivity, DM, hemophilia, conduction system disease, phenylketonuria, renal/hepatic impairment, pregnancy/nursing status, and possible drug interactions. Obtain baseline LFTs

in patients w/ underlying hepatitis B or C infections or marked transaminase elevations.
Monitoring: Monitor for cardiac conduction abnormalities, PR interval prolongation, rash, DRESS, hyperbilirubinemia, nephrolithiasis, cholelithiasis, new onset or exacerbation of DM, hyperglycemia, diabetic ketoacidosis, autoimmune disorders, immune reconstitution syndrome, fat redistribution/accumulation, cross-resistance among protease inhibitors, and other adverse reactions. Monitor LFTs in patients w/ underlying hepatitis B or C infections or marked transaminase elevations. Monitor for bleeding in patients w/ hemophilia. Closely monitor for adverse events during the first 2 months postpartum.
Counseling: Inform that therapy is not a cure for HIV infection, and patients may continue to experience illnesses associated w/ HIV infections. Advise to avoid doing things that can spread HIV infection to others. Advise to take ud and to take w/ food. Instruct not to alter the dose or d/c therapy w/o consulting physician. Advise caregiver on how to mix oral powder w/ a food or beverage, and to carefully follow the instructions for use and storage of powder formulation. Inform caregivers of patients w/ phenylketonuria that oral powder contains phenylalanine, and advise to call healthcare providers if they have any questions. Instruct to report use of any other medications or herbal products. Advise to consult physician if dizziness or lightheadedness occurs. Inform that mild rashes w/o other symptoms, redistribution or accumulation of body fat, or yellowing of the skin or whites of the eyes may occur. Inform that kidney stones and/or gallstones have been reported. Advise to d/c and seek medical evaluation immediately if signs or symptoms of severe skin reactions or hypersensitivity reactions develop.

REZIRA — hydrocodone bitartrate/pseudoephedrine hydrochloride CII
Class: Antitussive/decongestant

ADULT DOSAGE	PEDIATRIC DOSAGE
Cough Suppressant/Nasal Decongestant	Pediatric use may not have been established
Relief of cough and nasal congestion associated w/ common cold	
5mL q4-6h PRN	
Max: 20mL/24 hrs	

DOSING CONSIDERATIONS
Elderly
Start at lower end of dosing range

ADMINISTRATION
Oral route

STORAGE
20-25°C (68-77°F).

HOW SUPPLIED
Sol: (Hydrocodone-Pseudoephedrine) 5mg-60mg/5mL [480mL]

CONTRAINDICATIONS
Known hypersensitivity to hydrocodone bitartrate, pseudoephedrine hydrochloride, or any of the inactive ingredients of this medication; narrow-angle glaucoma; urinary retention; severe HTN/coronary artery disease; MAOI therapy or w/in 14 days of stopping such therapy.

WARNINGS/PRECAUTIONS
Caution with diabetes, thyroid disease, Addison's disease, prostatic hypertrophy/urethral stricture, asthma, severe renal/hepatic impairment, and in elderly. Hydrocodone: May produce dose-related respiratory depression; d/c and treat appropriately if it occurs. Risk of psychic/physical dependence, tolerance, and abuse. May elevate CSF pressure in presence of head injury, other intracranial lesions, or a preexisting increase in intracranial pressure; avoid use. May obscure clinical course of head injuries and acute abdominal conditions. May impair mental/physical abilities. Pseudoephedrine: May produce cardiovascular (CV) and CNS effects (eg, insomnia, dizziness, weakness, tremors, arrhythmias). CNS stimulation with convulsions or CV collapse with accompanying hypotension reported. Caution with CV disorders and do not use in patients with severe hypotension or coronary artery disease.

ADVERSE REACTIONS
Sedation, drowsiness, mental clouding, lethargy, impairment of mental and physical performance, anxiety, fear, dysphoria, dizziness, psychic dependence, mood changes, nervousness, sleeplessness, tremor, arrhythmia.

DRUG INTERACTIONS
See Contraindications. Avoid with alcohol, opioids, antihistamines, antipsychotics, anti-anxiety agents, or other CNS depressants; may cause additive CNS depressant effect. May produce paralytic ileus and excessive anticholinergic effects with anticholinergics; exercise caution. May increase effects of/with TCAs.

PREGNANCY AND LACTATION
Category C, not for use in nursing.

MECHANISM OF ACTION
Antitussive/decongestant. Hydrocodone: semisynthetic centrally acting opioid antitussive; mechanism unknown, but believed to act directly on the cough center. Pseudoephedrine: sympathomimetic amine; exerts a decongestant action on the nasal mucosa.

PHARMACOKINETICS
Absorption: Hydrocodone: C_{max}=10.6ng/mL, T_{max}=1.4 hrs. Pseudoephedrine: C_{max}=212ng/mL, T_{max}=1.8 hrs. **Distribution:** Found in breast milk. **Metabolism:**

Pseudoephedrine: Liver. **Elimination:** Hydrocodone: $T_{1/2}$=4.9 hrs. Pseudoephedrine: Urine (unchanged); $T_{1/2}$=5.6 hrs.

PATIENT CONSIDERATIONS

Assessment: Assess for conditions where treatment is contraindicated or cautioned, renal/hepatic function, hypersensitivity to drug, pregnancy/nursing status, and possible drug interactions.

Monitoring: Monitor for respiratory depression, dependence/tolerance, increased intracranial pressure, CV/CNS effects, hepatic/renal function, and other adverse reactions.

Counseling: Advise not to increase dose/dosing frequency, because respiratory depression may occur. Advise to measure sol with an accurate mL measuring device; inform that household tsp is not an accurate measuring device. Advise to avoid alcohol and other CNS depressants while on therapy. Advise to avoid engaging in hazardous tasks (eg, operating machinery/driving). Inform that drug can produce drug dependence. Advise not to use with an MAOI or within 14 days of stopping an MAOI.

RHEUMATREX — methotrexate

Rx

Class: Dihydrofolic acid reductase inhibitor

> Should be used only by physicians w/ knowledge and experience in the use of antimetabolite therapy. Use only in life-threatening neoplastic diseases, or in patients w/ psoriasis or rheumatoid arthritis (RA) w/ severe, recalcitrant, disabling disease not adequately responsive to other forms of therapy. Deaths reported in the treatment of malignancy, psoriasis, and RA. Closely monitor for bone marrow, liver, lung, and kidney toxicities. Patients should be informed of the risks involved and be under a physician's care throughout therapy. Fetal death and/or congenital anomalies reported; not recommended for women of childbearing potential unless benefits outweigh risks. Contraindicated in pregnant women w/ psoriasis or RA. Reduced elimination w/ impaired renal function, ascites, or pleural effusions; monitor for toxicity and reduce dose or d/c in some cases. Unexpectedly severe (sometimes fatal) bone marrow suppression, aplastic anemia, and GI toxicity reported w/ coadministration of therapy (usually high dosage) w/ some NSAIDs. Causes hepatotoxicity, fibrosis, and cirrhosis (generally only after prolonged use); perform periodic liver biopsies in psoriatic patients on long-term therapy. Acutely, liver enzyme elevations frequently seen. Drug-induced lung disease may occur acutely at any time during therapy and reported at low doses. Interrupt therapy if pulmonary symptoms (especially a dry, nonproductive cough), diarrhea, or ulcerative stomatitis occurs. Malignant lymphomas, which may regress following withdrawal of treatment, may occur w/ low-dose therapy and, thus, may not require cytotoxic treatment; d/c therapy 1st and, if lymphoma does not regress, institute appropriate treatment. May induce tumor lysis syndrome in patients w/ rapidly growing tumors; may be prevented/alleviated w/ appropriate supportive and pharmacologic measures. Severe, occasionally fatal, skin reactions reported. Potentially fatal opportunistic infections, especially *Pneumocystis carinii* pneumonia, may occur. Concomitant use w/ radiotherapy may increase risk of soft tissue necrosis and osteonecrosis.

OTHER BRAND NAMES
Methotrexate Tablets

ADULT DOSAGE

Choriocarcinoma/Trophoblastic Diseases
Gestational choriocarcinoma, chorio-adenoma destruens, and hydatidiform mole

15-30mg/day for a 5-day course

Courses are usually repeated 3-5X as required, w/ rest periods of 1 or more weeks interposed between courses, until any manifesting toxic symptoms subside

Acute Lymphoblastic Leukemia
Induction: 3.3mg/m²/day + prednisone 60mg/m²/day
Maint of Remission: 30mg/m²/week, administered 2X weekly

If and when relapse occurs, repeat the initial induction regimen to obtain reinduction of remission

Lymphomas
Burkitt's Tumor:
Stages I-II:
Recommended: 10-25mg/day for 4-8 days
Stage III:
Methotrexate is commonly given concomitantly w/ other anti-tumor agents

Treatment in all stages usually consists of several courses of the drug interposed w/ 7- to 10-day rest periods

Lymphosarcoma:
Stage III: May respond to combined drug therapy w/ methotrexate given in doses of 0.625-2.5mg/kg/day

Mycosis Fungoides (Cutaneous T-Cell Lymphoma)
Early Stages:
Usual: 5-50mg once weekly

PEDIATRIC DOSAGE

Acute Lymphoblastic Leukemia
Induction: 3.3mg/m²/day + prednisone 60mg/m²/day
Maint of Remission: 30mg/m²/week, administered 2X weekly

If relapse occurs, repeat the initial induction regimen to obtain reinduction of remission

Juvenile Rheumatoid Arthritis
Active polyarticular-course juvenile RA (JRA) in patients who have had an insufficient therapeutic response to, or are intolerant of, an adequate trial of 1st-line therapy including full dose NSAIDs

2-16 Years:
Initial: 10mg/m² once weekly
Titrate: Adjust dose gradually to achieve optimal response; there is experience w/ doses up to 30mg/m²/week, however there are too few published data to assess how doses >20mg/m²/week might affect the risk of serious toxicity

---

Methotrexate has also been administered twice weekly in doses ranging from 15-37.5mg in patients who have responded poorly to weekly therapy

Rheumatoid Arthritis
Severe, active RA (ACR criteria) in patients who have had an insufficient therapeutic response to, or are intolerant of, an adequate trial of 1st-line therapy including full-dose NSAIDs

Initial:
Single-Dose Schedule: 7.5mg once weekly
Divided-Dose Schedule: 2.5mg at 12-hr intervals for 3 doses given as a course once weekly
Titrate: Adjust dose gradually to achieve optimal response; significant increase in incidence and severity of serious toxic reactions, especially bone marrow suppression, reported at doses >20mg/week

Psoriasis
Symptomatic control of severe, recalcitrant, disabling psoriasis not adequately responsive to other forms of therapy, but only when the diagnosis has been established, as by a biopsy and/or after dermatologic consultation

Initial:
Single-Dose Schedule: 10-25mg/week until adequate response is achieved
Divided-Dose Schedule: 2.5mg at 12-hr intervals for 3 doses
Titrate: Adjust dose gradually to achieve optimal response; 30mg/week should not ordinarily be exceeded

Once optimal response is achieved, each dosage schedule should be reduced to the lowest possible amount of drug and to the longest possible rest period

Other Indications
Alone or in combination w/ other anticancer agents in the treatment of breast cancer, epidermoid cancers of the head and neck, and lung cancer, particularly squamous cell and small cell types. Methotrexate is also used in combination w/ other chemotherapeutic agents in the treatment of advanced-stage non-Hodgkin's lymphomas

---

DOSING CONSIDERATIONS
Elderly
Consider relatively low doses and closely monitor for early signs of toxicity

ADMINISTRATION
Oral route

RA and JRA
Weekly therapy may be instituted w/ the Rheumatrex Dose Packs which are designed to provide doses over a range of 5-20mg administered as a single weekly dose; the dose packs are not recommended for administration of methotrexate in weekly doses >20mg.

STORAGE
20-25°C (68-77°F). Protect from light.

HOW SUPPLIED
Tab: 2.5mg* *scored

CONTRAINDICATIONS
Pregnant women w/ psoriasis or RA (should be used in treatment of pregnant women w/ neoplastic diseases only when potential benefit outweighs risk to the fetus), nursing mothers. Psoriasis or RA patients w/ alcoholism, alcoholic liver disease, chronic liver disease, immunodeficiency syndromes, or preexisting blood dyscrasias (eg, bone marrow hypoplasia, leukopenia, thrombocytopenia, significant anemia). Known hypersensitivity to methotrexate.

WARNINGS/PRECAUTIONS
Toxic effects may be related to dose/frequency of administration; if toxicity occurs, reduce dose or d/c therapy and take appropriate corrective measures, which may include use of leucovorin calcium and/or acute, intermittent

hemodialysis w/ high-flux dialyzer, if necessary. If therapy is reinstituted, carry it out w/ caution, w/ adequate consideration of further need for the drug and increased alertness as to possible recurrence of toxicity. Caution in elderly/debilitated. Avoid pregnancy if either partner is receiving therapy (during and for a minimum of 3 months after therapy for male patients, and during and for at least 1 ovulatory cycle after therapy for female patients). May cause multiple organ system toxicities (eg, GI, hematologic). May cause impairment of fertility, oligospermia, and menstrual dysfunction during and for a short period after cessation of therapy.

ADVERSE REACTIONS

Ulcerative stomatitis, leukopenia, nausea, abdominal distress.

DRUG INTERACTIONS

See Boxed Warning. Elevated and prolonged levels w/ coadministration of high-dose therapy w/ NSAIDs; caution w/ NSAIDs or salicylates when used w/ lower doses of therapy. Toxicity may be increased due to displacement by salicylates, phenylbutazone, phenytoin, and sulfonamides. Renal tubular transport diminished by probenecid. Oral antibiotics (eg, tetracycline, chloramphenicol, nonabsorbable broad spectrum) may decrease intestinal absorption or interfere w/ enterohepatic circulation. Penicillins may reduce renal clearance; hematologic and GI toxicity observed. Closely monitor for increased risk of hepatotoxicity w/ hepatotoxins (eg, azathioprine, retinoids, sulfasalazine). May decrease theophylline clearance; monitor theophylline levels. Trimethoprim/sulfamethoxazole may increase bone marrow suppression by an additive antifolate effect. Immunization may be ineffective when given during therapy; immunization w/ live virus vaccines is generally not recommended. Disseminated vaccinia infections after smallpox immunizations reported. Combined use w/ gold, penicillamine, hydroxychloroquine, sulfasalazine, or cytotoxic agents may increase incidence of adverse effects.

PREGNANCY AND LACTATION

Pregnancy: Category X (psoriasis, RA).
Lactation: Contraindicated.

MECHANISM OF ACTION

Dihydrofolic acid reductase inhibitor; interferes w/ DNA synthesis, repair, and cellular replication. Mechanism in RA not established; may affect immune function.

PHARMACOKINETICS

Absorption: Well-absorbed. Bioavailability (60%) (adults). Administration of various doses and in different disease states resulted in different parameters.
Distribution: Plasma protein binding (50%); found in breast milk. (IV) V_d=0.18L/kg (initial), 0.4-0.8L/kg (steady-state). **Metabolism:** Hepatic and intracellular to polyglutamated forms (active); 7-hydroxymethotrexate (metabolite). Partially metabolized by intestinal flora. **Elimination:** $T_{1/2}$=3-10 hrs (psoriasis/RA/low-dose antineoplastic therapy), 8-15 hrs (high dose). (IV) Urine (80-90%, unchanged), bile (≤10%). Refer to PI for additional pharmacokinetic information.

PATIENT CONSIDERATIONS

Assessment: Assess for alcoholism, alcoholic/chronic liver disease, immunodeficiency, blood dyscrasias, ascites, pleural effusions, tumors, hypersensitivity to drug, pregnancy/nursing status, any other condition where treatment is cautioned or contraindicated, and possible drug interactions. Obtain baseline CBC w/ differential and platelet counts, hepatic enzymes, renal function tests, liver biopsy, and chest x-ray.

Monitoring: Monitor for toxicities of bone marrow, liver, lung, and kidney; GI toxicities; diarrhea; ulcerative stomatitis; malignant lymphoma; tumor lysis syndrome; skin reactions; opportunistic infections; and other adverse reactions. Monitor hematology at least monthly and renal/hepatic function every 1-2 months during therapy of RA/psoriasis and more frequently during antineoplastic therapy, during initial/changing doses, or during periods of increased risk of elevated drug levels (eg, dehydration). If drug-induced lung disease is suspected, perform pulmonary function tests.

Counseling: Inform of the early signs/symptoms of toxicity, the need to see physician promptly if toxicity occurs, and the need for close follow-up, including periodic lab tests to monitor toxicity. Emphasize that the recommended dose is taken weekly in RA and psoriasis, and that mistaken daily use of recommended dose has led to fatal toxicity. Counsel about risks/benefits of therapy, and effects on reproduction.

RIFADIN — rifampin   Rx

Class: Rifamycin derivative

ADULT DOSAGE

Tuberculosis

Treatment of All Forms of Tuberculosis:
10mg/kg qd
Max: 600mg/day

Initial phase of short course therapy consists of rifampin + isoniazid (INH) + pyrazinamide for 2 months; add streptomycin or ethambutol unless the likelihood of INH resistance is very low. Following initial phase, continue treatment w/ rifampin + INH for at least 4 months; treat longer if the patient is still sputum or culture positive, if resistant organisms are present, or if the patient is HIV positive

PEDIATRIC DOSAGE

Tuberculosis

Treatment of All Forms of Tuberculosis:
10-20mg/kg qd
Max: 600mg/day

Initial phase of short course therapy consists of rifampin + isoniazid (INH) + pyrazinamide for 2 months; add streptomycin or ethambutol unless the likelihood of INH resistance is very low. Following initial phase, continue treatment w/ rifampin + INH for at least 4 months; treat longer if the patient is still sputum or culture positive, if resistant organisms are present, or if the patient is HIV positive

Meningococcal Carrier State

Treatment of symptomatic carriers of *Neisseria meningitidis* to eliminate meningococci from the nasopharynx
Usual: 600mg bid for 2 days

Meningococcal Carrier State

Treatment of symptomatic carriers of *Neisseria meningitidis* to eliminate meningococci from the nasopharynx
<1 Month of Age:
5mg/kg q12h for 2 days
≥1 Month of Age:
10mg/kg q12h for 2 days
Max: 600mg/dose

ADMINISTRATION

Oral/IV route

PO

Administer 1 hr ac or 2 hrs pc w/ a full glass of water.

IV

Preparation:

Reconstitute lyophilized powder by transferring 10mL of sterile water for inj to a vial containing 600mg of rifampin for inj; swirl vial gently to completely dissolve antibiotic.

Prior to administration, withdraw from reconstituted sol a volume equivalent to amount of rifampin calculated to be administered and add to 500mL of infusion medium.

Mix well and infuse at a rate allowing for complete infusion w/in 3 hrs.

Alternatively, add amount of rifampin calculated to be administered to 100mL of infusion medium and infuse in 30 min.

May dilute w/ D5 for inj and normal saline (NS).

Incompatibilities:

Undiluted (5mg/mL) and diluted (1mg/mL in NS) diltiazem hydrochloride and rifampin (6mg/mL in NS) during simulated Y-site administration

Oral Sus

Compound using simple syrup (Syrup NF), simple syrup (Humco Laboratories), Syrpalta syrup (Emerson Laboratories), or raspberry syrup (Humco Laboratories) Compounding procedure results in a 1% w/v sus containing 10mg/mL of rifampin

Preparation:

Empty contents of four 300mg caps or eight 150mg caps onto a piece of weighing paper and gently crush the contents w/ a spatula to produce a fine powder.

Transfer powder blend to a 4 oz amber glass or plastic bottle.

Rinse paper and spatula w/ 20mL of 1 of above-mentioned syrups, and add rinse to bottle.

Add 100mL of syrup to the bottle and shake vigorously.

STORAGE

25°C (77°F); excursions permitted to 15-30°C (59-86°F). (Cap) Store in dry place. Avoid excessive heat. (IV) Avoid excessive heat (>40°C [104°F]). Protect from light. Reconstituted Sol: Room temperature for 24 hrs. Dilutions in D5W: Room temperature for up to 4 hrs. Dilutions in Normal Saline: Room temperature for up to 24 hrs. Prepare and use within this time.

HOW SUPPLIED

Cap: 150mg, 300mg; **Inj:** 600mg

CONTRAINDICATIONS

History of hypersensitivity to rifampin or any of the components, or to any of the rifamycins. Patients who are taking ritonavir-boosted saquinavir due to an increased risk of severe hepatocellular toxicity. Patients who are receiving atazanavir, darunavir, fosamprenavir, saquinavir, or tipranavir.

WARNINGS/PRECAUTIONS

May produce liver dysfunction; caution with impaired liver function. Monitor LFTs prior to therapy and every 2-4 weeks during therapy; d/c if signs of hepatocellular damage occur. Hyperbilirubinemia and porphyria exacerbation reported. Not for treatment of meningococcal disease. Caution with history of diabetes mellitus (DM); diabetes management may be more difficult. Higher doses than recommended may result in higher incidence of adverse reactions including flu syndrome (fever, chills, and malaise), hematopoietic reactions (leukopenia, thrombocytopenia, or acute hemolytic anemia), cutaneous, GI, and hepatic reactions, SOB, shock, anaphylaxis, and renal failure. Not recommended for intermittent therapy; caution against intentional or accidental interruption of the daily dosage regimen since rare renal hypersensitivity reactions reported when therapy was resumed. IV doses are the same as those for oral. Caution in elderly. (IV) For IV infusion only; do not administer IM or SQ. Avoid extravasation; d/c infusion if local irritation and inflammation occur and restart at another site.

ADVERSE REACTIONS

Heartburn, N/V, headache, fever, drowsiness, dizziness, muscle weakness, visual disturbances, menstrual disturbances, BUN elevation, serum uric acid elevation, flushing, urticaria, rash, edema.

DRUG INTERACTIONS

See Contraindications. Induces certain CYP450 enzymes; dosages of drugs metabolized by these enzymes may require adjustment when starting/stopping therapy. May accelerate the metabolism of anticonvulsants, digitoxin, antiarrhythmics, oral anticoagulants, antifungals, barbiturates, β-blockers, calcium channel blockers, chloramphenicol, clarithromycin, corticosteroids, cyclosporine, cardiac glycoside preparations, clofibrate, oral or other systemic hormonal contraceptives, dapsone, diazepam, doxycycline, fluoroquinolones, haloperidol, oral hypoglycemic agents, levothyroxine, methadone, narcotic analgesics, progestins, quinine, tacrolimus, theophylline, TCAs, and zidovudine; dose adjustments of these drugs may be necessary. May increase requirements for coumarin-type anticoagulants; perform PT daily or as frequently as necessary. Decreased levels of enalaprilat and atovaquone. Increased levels with atovaquone. Concomitant ketoconazole decreases serum levels of both drugs. Antacids may reduce absorption; give daily doses of rifampin at least 1 hr before ingestion of antacids. Increased blood level with probenecid and cotrimoxazole. Increased risk of hepatotoxicity with halothane or isoniazid; avoid concomitant use with halothane and monitor closely for hepatotoxicity when given with isoniazid. Caution with other hepatotoxic agents. Coadministration with sulfasalazine may reduce plasma concentrations of sulfapyridine.

PREGNANCY AND LACTATION
Pregnancy: Category C.
Lactation: Not for use in nursing.

MECHANISM OF ACTION
Rifamycin derivative; inhibits DNA-dependent RNA polymerase activity in susceptible *Mycobacterium tuberculosis* organisms. Interacts with bacterial RNA polymerase; does not inhibit the mammalian enzyme.

PHARMACOKINETICS
Absorption: PO/IV administration resulted in different parameters; refer to PI for further information. **Distribution:** Distributed in body fluids and CSF; crosses the placenta; plasma protein binding (80%); (IV; 300mg, 600mg) V_d=0.66L/kg, 0.64L/kg. **Metabolism:** Via deacetylation; 25-desacetyl-rifampin (primary metabolite). **Elimination:** Bile, urine (≤30%; 50% unchanged [PO]), (<30% unchanged or metabolites [IV]); $T_{1/2}$ varies based on age and dosing; refer to PI for further information.

PATIENT CONSIDERATIONS
Assessment: Assess for drug hypersensitivity, history of DM, meningococcal disease, hepatic/renal impairment, pregnancy/nursing status, and possible drug interactions. Obtain baseline CBC. Obtain bacteriologic cultures to confirm susceptibility of organism prior to therapy.

Monitoring: Monitor for liver dysfunction, hyperbilirubinemia, porphyria exacerbation, and other adverse reactions. Monitor for LFTs every 2-4 weeks, SrCr, CBC, and platelet count. Monitor treatment response by performing serotyping and susceptibility tests. (IV) Monitor for local irritation and inflammation at infusion site.

Counseling: Counsel that drug treats bacterial and not viral infections. Instruct to take exactly as prescribed. Inform that skipping doses or not completing full course of therapy may decrease effectiveness and increase bacterial resistance. Inform that the drug may produce reddish urine, sweat, sputum, and tears, and that soft contact lenses may be permanently stained. Advise that the reliability of oral or systemic hormonal contraceptives may be affected; instruct to use alternative contraceptive measures. Instruct to notify physician if fever, loss of appetite, malaise, N/V, darkened urine, yellowish discoloration of skin and eyes, and joint pain/swelling occur. Emphasize the compliance with full course of therapy and the importance of not missing any doses.

RIFAMATE — isoniazid/rifampin   Rx

Class: Isonicotinic acid hydrazide/rifamycin derivative

> Severe and sometimes fatal hepatitis associated with isoniazid (INH) therapy may occur and may develop even after many months of treatment. The risk of developing hepatitis is age-related and increased with daily alcohol consumption. Monitor LFTs monthly. D/C promptly if signs of hepatic damage are detected. Give appropriate alternative treatment in patients with tuberculosis (TB). If INH must be reinstituted, do so only after symptoms and lab abnormalities have cleared. Restart in very small and gradually increasing doses and withdraw immediately if there is any indication of recurrent liver involvement. Defer treatment in persons with acute hepatic diseases.

ADULT DOSAGE
Tuberculosis

Treatment of pulmonary tuberculosis when the patient has been titrated on the individual components and has been established to be therapeutically effective

Usual: 2 caps qd

Initial phase of short course therapy consists of rifampin + isoniazid (INH) + pyrazinamide for 2 months; add streptomycin or ethambutol unless likelihood of INH or rifampin resistance is very low. Following initial phase, continue treatment w/ rifampin + INH for at least 4 months; treat longer if the patient is still sputum or culture positive, if resistant organisms are present, or if the patient is HIV positive

Concomitant Administration of Pyridoxine (B6):
Recommended in malnourished patients and in those predisposed to neuropathy (eg, alcoholics and diabetics)

PEDIATRIC DOSAGE
Tuberculosis

Treatment of pulmonary tuberculosis when the patient has been titrated on the individual components and has been established to be therapeutically effective

≥15 Years:
Usual: 2 caps qd

Initial phase of short course therapy consists of rifampin + isoniazid (INH) + pyrazinamide for 2 months; add streptomycin or ethambutol unless likelihood of INH or rifampin resistance is very low. Following initial phase, continue treatment w/ rifampin + INH for at least 4 months; treat longer if the patient is still sputum or culture positive, if resistant organisms are present, or if the patient is HIV positive

Concomitant Administration of Pyridoxine (B6):
Recommended in malnourished patients and in those predisposed to neuropathy (eg, alcoholics and diabetics)

ADMINISTRATION
Oral route
Take 1 hr ac or 2 hrs pc w/ a full glass of water

STORAGE
25°C (77°F); excursions permitted to 15-30°C (59-86°F). Protect from excessive humidity.

HOW SUPPLIED
Cap: (INH/Rifampin) 150mg/300mg

CONTRAINDICATIONS
History of hypersensitivity to rifampin or isoniazid, or any of the components, or to any of the rifamycins. **INH:** Severe hepatic damage, severe adverse reactions to INH (eg, drug fever, chills, arthritis), acute liver disease, acute gout. **Rifampin:** Concomitant administration of atazanavir, darunavir, fosamprenavir, saquinavir, tipranavir, and ritonavir-boosted saquinavir.

WARNINGS/PRECAUTIONS
Not recommended for initial therapy of TB or preventive therapy. Not indicated for the treatment of meningococcal infections or asymptomatic carriers of *Neisseria meningitidis* to eliminate meningococci from the nasopharynx. Associated with liver dysfunction. Caution with impaired liver function; d/c if signs of hepatocellular damage occur. Caution with history of diabetes mellitus (DM) and in elderly. Concomitant administration of pyridoxine is recommended in the malnourished, in those predisposed to neuropathy (eg, alcoholics, diabetics), and in adolescents. Lab test interactions may occur. Rifampin: Hyperbilirubinemia may occur in the early days of treatment; assess need for treatment interruption. Porphyria exacerbation reported (isolated). Doses of >600mg qd or 2X weekly resulted in higher incidence of adverse reactions (flu syndrome, hematopoietic/cutaneous/GI/hepatic reactions, SOB, shock, anaphylaxis, renal failure). Not recommended for intermittent therapy; caution against intentional or accidental interruption of treatment since renal hypersensitivity reactions (rare) reported when therapy is resumed. May enhance metabolism of endogenous substrates (eg, adrenal/thyroid hormones, vitamin D). INH: D/C all drugs and evaluate patient at 1st sign of a hypersensitivity reaction. Carefully monitor patients with current chronic liver disease or severe renal dysfunction.

ADVERSE REACTIONS
Hepatitis, thrombocytopenia, hemolytic anemia, abnormal LFTs, fever, vasculitis, epigastric distress, anaphylactic reactions, peripheral neuropathy, N/V, BUN/serum uric acid elevations, eosinophilia, jaundice, pyridoxine deficiency, pellagra.

DRUG INTERACTIONS
See Contraindications. Avoid with halothane. Caution with other hepatotoxic drugs. Rifampin: Induces certain CYP450 enzymes; dosages of drugs metabolized by these enzymes may require adjustment when starting/stopping concomitant rifampin. May accelerate metabolism of anticonvulsants, digitoxin, antiarrhythmics, oral anticoagulants, antifungals, barbiturates, β-blockers, calcium channel blockers, chloramphenicol, clarithromycin, fluoroquinolones, corticosteroids, cyclosporine, cardiac glycosides, clofibrate, oral/systemic hormonal contraceptives, dapsone, diazepam, doxycycline, haloperidol, oral hypoglycemics, levothyroxine, methadone, narcotic analgesics, TCAs, progestins, quinine, tacrolimus, theophylline, and zidovudine; dosage adjustment of these drugs may be necessary. Decreased concentration of atovaquone, ketoconazole, enalaprilat, or sulfapyridine; adjust ketoconazole or enalapril dose if indicated. Decreased concentration with ketoconazole. Increased blood levels with atovaquone, probenecid, or cotrimoxazole. Antacids may reduce absorption; give daily doses at least 1 hr before antacids. Increases requirements for anticoagulant drugs of the coumarin type; perform PT daily or as frequently as necessary to establish and maintain required anticoagulant dose. Monitor for hepatotoxicity with INH. INH: Higher incidence of hepatitis with daily alcohol ingestion. Monitor renal function with enflurane. Inhibits certain CYP450 enzymes; dosages of drugs metabolized by these enzymes may require adjustment when starting/stopping therapy. Inhibits metabolism of anticonvulsants (eg, carbamazepine, phenytoin), benzodiazepines, haloperidol, ketoconazole, theophylline, and warfarin; dose adjustments of these drugs may be necessary. Decreased levels with corticosteroids (eg, prednisolone). Para-aminosalicylic acid may increase levels and $T_{1/2}$. Monitor for hepatotoxicity with rifampin. Exaggerates CNS effects of meperidine, cycloserine, and disulfiram. Levodopa may produce symptoms of excess catecholamine stimulation or lack of levodopa effect. May produce hyperglycemia and lead to loss of glucose control with oral hypoglycemics. Avoid foods containing tyramine (eg, cheese, red wine) or histamine (eg, skipjack, tuna, other tropical fish).

PREGNANCY AND LACTATION
Category C, not for use in nursing.

MECHANISM OF ACTION
INH: Isonicotinic acid hydrazide; Inhibits the biosynthesis of mycolic acids, which are major components of the cell wall of *Mycobacterium tuberculosis*. Rifampin: Rifamycin derivative; inhibits DNA-dependent RNA polymerase activity in susceptible *M. tuberculosis* cells; interacts with bacterial RNA polymerase but does not inhibit the mammalian enzyme.

PHARMACOKINETICS
Absorption: Readily absorbed from GI tract. (INH) T_{max}=1-2 hrs. (Rifampin) C_{max}=10mcg/mL, T_{max}=1.5-3 hrs. **Distribution:** Crosses placenta; found in breast milk. (Rifampin) Plasma protein binding (80%). **Metabolism:** (INH) Liver via acetylation and dehydrazination. (Rifampin) Via deacetylation. **Elimination:** (INH) Urine (50-70% metabolites); $T_{1/2}$=1-4 hrs. (Rifampin) Bile, urine (≤30%, 50% unchanged); refer to PI for $T_{1/2}$.

PATIENT CONSIDERATIONS
Assessment: Assess for history of hypersensitivity to any components of the drug, severe adverse reactions to INH, severe hepatic damage, acute liver disease, acute

gout, DM, pregnancy/nursing status, and possible drug interactions. Perform bacteriologic smears or cultures and susceptibility tests to confirm diagnosis. Obtain baseline LFTs, bilirubin, SrCr, CBC, platelet count, and blood uric acid. Perform ophthalmologic exam.

Monitoring: Monitor for liver dysfunction, hyperbilirubinemia, hypersensitivity reactions, porphyria exacerbation, and other adverse reactions. Monitor LFTs every 2-4 weeks with impaired liver function. Perform periodic ophthalmologic exams, even without occurrence of visual symptoms. Repeat bacteriologic smears or cultures and susceptibility tests throughout therapy to monitor response to treatment. Monitor patients at least monthly.

Counseling: Instruct to avoid foods containing tyramine (eg, cheese, red wine) and histamine (eg, skipjack, tuna, other tropical fish). Inform that drug may produce reddish discoloration of urine, sweat, sputum, and tears, and may permanently stain soft contact lenses. Inform that reliability of oral or other systemic contraceptives may be affected; advise to change to nonhormonal methods of birth control during therapy. Instruct to notify physician if fever, loss of appetite, malaise, N/V, darkened urine, yellowish discoloration of the skin and eyes, or pain/swelling of joints occurs. Advise to comply with the full course of therapy; inform of the importance of not missing any doses.

RIFATER — isoniazid/pyrazinamide/rifampin   Rx

Class: Isonicotinic acid hydrazide/nicotinamide analogue/rifamycin derivative

> Severe and sometimes fatal hepatitis associated with isoniazid (INH) therapy may occur even after many months of treatment. The risk of developing hepatitis is age-related and increased with daily alcohol consumption. Monitor LFTs at monthly intervals. D/C promptly if symptoms appear or signs of hepatic damage occur and give appropriate alternative treatment. If INH must be reinstituted, do so only after symptoms and lab abnormalities have cleared. Restart in very small and gradually increasing doses and withdraw immediately if there is any indication of recurrent liver involvement. Defer treatment in patients with acute hepatic diseases.

ADULT DOSAGE
Tuberculosis

Initial Phase of the Short-Course Treatment of Pulmonary Tuberculosis:
≤44kg: 4 tabs qd for 2 months
45-54kg: 5 tabs qd for 2 months
≥55kg: 6 tabs qd for 2 months

Add streptomycin or ethambutol unless the likelihood of isoniazid (INH) or rifampin resistance is very low. Following the initial phase, continue treatment w/ rifampin + INH for at least 4 months; treat longer if the patient is still sputum or culture positive, if resistant organisms are present, or if the patient is HIV positive

Concomitant Administration of Pyridoxine (B6):
Recommended in malnourished patients, in those predisposed to neuropathy (eg, alcoholics and diabetics), and in adolescents

PEDIATRIC DOSAGE
Tuberculosis

Initial Phase of the Short-Course Treatment of Pulmonary Tuberculosis:
≥15 Years:
≤44kg: 4 tabs qd for 2 months
45-54kg: 5 tabs qd for 2 months
≥55kg: 6 tabs qd for 2 months

Add streptomycin or ethambutol unless the likelihood of isoniazid (INH) or rifampin resistance is very low. Following the initial phase, continue treatment w/ rifampin + INH for at least 4 months; treat longer if the patient is still sputum or culture positive, if resistant organisms are present, or if the patient is HIV positive

Concomitant Administration of Pyridoxine (B6):
Recommended in malnourished patients, in those predisposed to neuropathy (eg, alcoholics and diabetics), and in adolescents

---

ADMINISTRATION
Oral route

Take 1 hr ac or 2 hrs pc w/ a full glass of water

STORAGE
25°C (77°F); excursions permitted to 15-30°C (59-86°F). Protect from excessive humidity.

HOW SUPPLIED
Tab: (INH/Pyrazinamide/Rifampin) 50mg/300mg/120mg

CONTRAINDICATIONS
History of hypersensitivity to rifampin, isoniazid, pyrazinamide or any of the components, or to any of the rifamycins. **INH:** Severe hepatic damage, adverse reactions to INH (eg, drug fever, chills, arthritis), acute liver disease, and acute gout. **Rifampin:** Concomitant administration of atazanavir, darunavir, fosamprenavir, saquinavir, tipranavir, and ritonavir-boosted saquinavir.

WARNINGS/PRECAUTIONS
Associated with liver dysfunction. Caution in patients with impaired liver function; d/c if signs of hepatocellular damage occur. Caution with history of diabetes mellitus (DM) and in elderly. Concomitant administration of pyridoxine is recommended in the malnourished, in those predisposed to neuropathy (eg, alcoholics, diabetics), and in adolescents. Lab test interactions may occur. Rifampin: Hyperbilirubinemia may occur in the early days of treatment. A decision to interrupt treatment should be made after repeating tests, noting trends in levels, and considering clinical condition. Porphyria exacerbation reported (isolated). Doses of >600mg qd or 2X weekly resulted in higher incidence of adverse reactions (eg, flu syndrome, hematopoietic/cutaneous/GI/hepatic reactions, SOB, shock, anaphylaxis, renal failure). Not recommended for intermittent therapy; caution against intentional or accidental interruption of treatment since renal hypersensitivity reactions (rare) reported when therapy

is resumed. May enhance metabolism of endogenous substrates (eg, adrenal/thyroid hormones, vitamin D). INH: Perform periodic ophthalmologic exams before and periodically thereafter. D/C all drugs and evaluate patient at the 1st sign of a hypersensitivity reaction. Carefully monitor patients with current chronic liver disease or severe renal dysfunction. Pyrazinamide: D/C and do not resume treatment if signs of hepatocellular damage or hyperuricemia accompanied by acute gouty arthritis appear; transfer to a regimen not containing pyrazinamide if acute gouty arthritis occurs without liver dysfunction.

ADVERSE REACTIONS
Hepatitis, N/V, digestive pain, diarrhea, sweating, headache, insomnia, rash, arthralgia, tightness in chest, coughing, angina, palpitation, hemoptysis, total pneumothorax, phlebitis.

DRUG INTERACTIONS
See Contraindications. Rifampin: Induces certain CYP450 enzymes; dosages of drugs metabolized by these enzymes may require adjustment when starting/stopping concomitant rifampin. May accelerate metabolism of anticonvulsants, digitoxin, antiarrhythmics (eg, disopyramide, mexiletine, quinidine, tocainide), oral anticoagulants, antifungals (eg, fluconazole, itraconazole, ketoconazole), barbiturates, β-blockers, calcium channel blockers (eg, diltiazem, nifedipine, verapamil), chloramphenicol, clarithromycin, fluoroquinolones (eg, ciprofloxacin), corticosteroids, cyclosporine, cardiac glycosides, clofibrate, oral or systemic hormonal contraceptives, dapsone, diazepam, doxycycline, haloperidol, oral hypoglycemics (eg, sulfonylureas), levothyroxine, methadone, narcotic analgesics, TCAs (eg, amitriptyline, nortriptyline), progestins, quinine, tacrolimus, theophylline, and zidovudine; dosage adjustment of these drugs may be necessary. Decreased concentration of atovaquone, ketoconazole, enalaprilat (active metabolite of enalapril) or sulfapyridine; adjust ketoconazole or enalapril dose if indicated. Decreased concentration with ketoconazole. Increased concentration with atovaquone, probenecid, or cotrimoxazole. Antacids may reduce absorption; give daily doses at least 1 hr before antacids. Increased requirements for anticoagulant drugs of the coumarin type; perform PT daily or as frequently as necessary to establish and maintain required anticoagulant dose. Avoid with halothane. Monitor for hepatotoxicity with INH. INH: Higher incidence of hepatitis with daily alcohol ingestion. Monitor renal function with enflurane. Inhibits certain CYP450 enzymes; dosages of drugs metabolized by these enzymes may require adjustment when starting/stopping therapy. Inhibits metabolism of anticonvulsants (eg, carbamazepine, phenytoin, primidone, valproic acid), benzodiazepines (eg, diazepam), haloperidol, ketoconazole, theophylline, and warfarin; dose adjustments of these drugs may be necessary. Antacids and food may reduce absorption; take therapy on an empty stomach at least 1 hr before antacids/food. Decreased levels with corticosteroids (eg, prednisolone). Para-aminosalicylic acid may increase levels and $T_{1/2}$. Monitor for hepatotoxicity with rifampin. Exaggerates CNS effects of meperidine, cycloserine, and disulfiram. Levodopa may produce symptoms of excess catecholamine stimulation or lack of levodopa effect. May produce hyperglycemia and lead to loss of glucose control with oral hypoglycemics. Avoid foods containing tyramine (eg, cheese, red wine) or histamine (eg, skipjack, tuna, other tropical fish).

PREGNANCY AND LACTATION
Category C, not for use in nursing.

MECHANISM OF ACTION
INH: Isonicotinic acid hydrazide; inhibits the biosynthesis of mycolic acids, which are major components of the cell wall of *Mycobacterium tuberculosis*. Pyrazinamide: Nicotinamide analogue; has not been established. Rifampin: Rifamycin derivative; inhibits DNA-dependent RNA polymerase activity in susceptible *M. tuberculosis* organisms. Interacts with bacterial RNA polymerase, but does not inhibit the mammalian enzyme.

PHARMACOKINETICS
Absorption: (5 tabs single dose) INH: Readily absorbed. Bioavailability (100.6%), C_{max}=3.09mcg/mL, T_{max}=1-2 hrs. Pyrazinamide: Well-absorbed. Bioavailability (96.8%), C_{max}=28.02mcg/mL, T_{max}=2 hrs. Rifampin: Readily absorbed. Bioavailability (88.8%), C_{max}=11.04mcg/mL. **Distribution:** Found in breast milk. INH: Crosses placenta. Pyrazinamide: Plasma protein binding (10%). Rifampin: Protein binding (80%). **Metabolism:** INH: Acetylation and dehydrazination. Pyrazinamide: Liver, via hydroxylation; pyrazinoic acid (major active metabolite). Rifampin: Via deacetylation. **Elimination:** INH: Urine (50-70% mostly metabolites); $T_{1/2}$=1-4 hrs. Pyrazinamide: Urine (70%, 4-14% unchanged); $T_{1/2}$=9-10 hrs. Rifampin: Urine (≤30%, 50% unchanged), bile. Refer to PI for $T_{1/2}$.

PATIENT CONSIDERATIONS
Assessment: Assess for history of hypersensitivity to any components of the drug, severe adverse reactions to INH, severe hepatic damage, renal/hepatic impairment, acute gout, DM, pregnancy/nursing status, and possible drug interactions. Perform bacteriologic smears or cultures and susceptibility tests to confirm diagnosis. Obtain baseline LFTs, bilirubin, SrCr, CBC and platelet count, and blood uric acid. Perform ophthalmologic exam.

Monitoring: Monitor for liver dysfunction, hyperbilirubinemia, hyperuricemia, hypersensitivity reactions, acute gouty arthritis, porphyria exacerbation, and other adverse reactions. Monitor LFTs every 2-4 weeks with impaired liver function. Perform ophthalmologic exam periodically, even without occurrence of visual symptoms. Repeat bacteriologic smears or cultures and susceptibility tests throughout therapy to monitor response to treatment. Monitor PT daily or as frequently as necessary if used with anticoagulants. Monitor patients at least monthly; those with lab abnormalities should have follow-up lab testing if necessary.

Counseling: Instruct to avoid foods containing tyramine and histamine. Inform that medication may produce reddish coloration of urine, sweat, sputum, and tears, and may permanently stain soft contact lenses. Inform that reliability of oral or other systemic contraceptives may be affected; advise to change to nonhormonal methods of birth control during therapy. Instruct to notify physician if fever, loss of appetite, malaise, N/V, darkened urine, yellowish discoloration of the skin and eyes, pain or swelling of joints occur. Advise to comply with the full course of therapy; inform of the importance of not missing any doses.

RILUTEK — riluzole

Rx

Class: Benzothiazole

ADULT DOSAGE	PEDIATRIC DOSAGE
Amyotrophic Lateral Sclerosis	Pediatric use may not have been established
50mg bid	

ADMINISTRATION
Oral route

Take at least 1 hr ac or 2 hrs pc.

STORAGE
20-25°C (68-77°F); protect from bright light.

HOW SUPPLIED
Tab: 50mg

CONTRAINDICATIONS
History of severe hypersensitivity reactions to riluzole or to any of its components.

WARNINGS/PRECAUTIONS
Cases of drug-induced liver injury, some fatal, and asymptomatic elevations of hepatic transaminases reported; monitor for hepatic injury every month for the first 3 months of therapy, and periodically thereafter. Not recommended in patients who develop hepatic transaminase levels >5X ULN. D/C if there is evidence of liver dysfunction. Severe neutropenia (ANC <500/mm³) w/in the first 2 months of therapy reported. Interstitial lung disease, including hypersensitivity pneumonitis, reported; d/c if this develops. Caution in elderly. Japanese patients are more likely to have higher drug levels; risk of adverse reactions may be greater.

ADVERSE REACTIONS
Asthenia, nausea, dizziness, decreased lung function, abdominal pain.

DRUG INTERACTIONS
CYP1A2 inhibitors (eg, ciprofloxacin, enoxacin, fluvoxamine) may increase levels and the risk of riluzole-associated adverse reactions. CYP1A2 inducers may decrease levels and efficacy. Concomitant use w/ other potentially hepatotoxic drugs (eg, allopurinol, methyldopa, sulfasalazine) may increase the risk for hepatotoxicity.

PREGNANCY AND LACTATION
Pregnancy: There are no studies in pregnant women, and case reports have been inadequate to inform the drug-associated risk.
Lactation: Caution in nursing.

MECHANISM OF ACTION
Benzothiazole; mechanism not established.

PHARMACOKINETICS
Absorption: Oral bioavailability (approx 60%). **Distribution:** Plasma protein binding (96%). **Metabolism:** Oxidation via CYP1A2; direct and sequential glucoronidation via UGT-HP4. **Elimination:** Urine (90%, 2% unchanged), feces (5%); $T_{1/2}$=12 hrs.

PATIENT CONSIDERATIONS
Assessment: Assess for history of severe hypersensitivity reactions to riluzole or to any of its components, pregnancy/nursing status, and possible drug interactions. Obtain baseline LFTs.

Monitoring: Monitor for hepatic injury every month during first 3 months, then periodically thereafter. Monitor for signs/symptoms of febrile illness, neutropenia, interstitial lung disease, and for other adverse reactions.

Counseling: Instruct to notify healthcare provider if patient experiences yellowing of the whites of the eyes, fever, or respiratory symptoms (eg, dry cough, difficult or labored breathing). Advise to notify healthcare provider if pregnant, nursing, or if taking any concomitant medications.

RISPERDAL CONSTA — risperidone

Rx

Class: Atypical antipsychotic

> Elderly patients w/ dementia-related psychosis treated w/ antipsychotic drugs are at an increased risk of death; most deaths appeared to be cardiovascular (CV) (eg, heart failure, sudden death) or infectious (eg, pneumonia) in nature. Not approved for the treatment of patients w/ dementia-related psychosis.

ADULT DOSAGE	PEDIATRIC DOSAGE
Schizophrenia	Pediatric use may not have been established
Recommended Dose: 25mg IM every 2 weeks	
Titrate: May increase to 37.5mg or 50mg if unresponsive to 25mg; upward dose adjustment should not be made more frequently than every 4 weeks	
Max: 50mg every 2 weeks	
May give a lower initial dose of 12.5mg if clinically warranted (eg, history	

of poor tolerability to psychotropic medications).
Oral risperidone (or another antipsychotic) should be given w/ the 1st inj of Risperdal Consta, continued for 3 weeks, and then discontinued. For patients who have never taken oral risperidone, establish tolerability w/ oral risperidone prior to initiating treatment w/ Risperdal Consta.

Bipolar I Disorder

Monotherapy or Adjunctive Therapy to Lithium or Valproate for Maint Treatment:
Recommended Dose: 25mg IM every 2 weeks
Titrate: May increase to 37.5mg or 50mg; upward dose adjustment should not be made more frequently than every 4 weeks
Max: 50mg every 2 weeks
May give a lower initial dose of 12.5mg if clinically warranted (eg, history of poor tolerability to psychotropic medications).
Oral risperidone (or another antipsychotic) should be given w/ the 1st inj of Risperdal Consta, continued for 3 weeks, and then discontinued. For patients who have never taken oral risperidone, establish tolerability w/ oral risperidone prior to initiating treatment w/ Risperdal Consta.

Conversions

Switching from Other Antipsychotics:
Continue previous antipsychotic for 3 weeks after 1st inj of Risperdal Consta

For patients who have never taken oral risperidone, establish tolerability w/ oral risperidone prior to initiating treatment w/ Risperdal Consta.

DOSING CONSIDERATIONS
Concomitant Medications
Carbamazepine or Other CYP3A4 Inducers (eg, Phenytoin, Rifampin, Phenobarbital):
Initiation of Carbamazepine or Other CYP3A4 Inducers: Closely monitor patients during the first 4-8 weeks; consider dose increase or administration of additional oral risperidone.
Discontinuation of Carbamazepine or Other CYP3A4 Inducers: Reevaluate Risperdal Consta dose and decrease, if necessary. May place patients on lower dose of Risperdal Consta 2-4 weeks before the planned discontinuation of carbamazepine or other CYP3A4 inducers. Patients treated w/ the recommended 25mg dose of Risperdal Consta and discontinuing from carbamazepine or other CYP3A4 inducers should continue 25mg dose unless clinical judgment necessitates a lower dose of 12.5mg or treatment interruption.

CYP2D6 Inhibitors (eg, Fluoxetine, Paroxetine):
Initiation of Risperdal Consta in Patients Receiving Fluoxetine or Paroxetine: Consider a starting dose of 12.5mg.
Initiation of Fluoxetine/Paroxetine: May place patients on a lower dose of Risperdal Consta 2-4 weeks before the planned start of concomitant therapy. When fluoxetine or paroxetine is initiated in patients receiving the recommended 25mg dose of Risperdal Consta, it is recommended to continue treatment w/ 25mg dose unless clinical judgment necessitates a lower dose of 12.5mg or treatment interruption.

Renal Impairment
Titrate w/ oral risperidone prior to initiating treatment w/ Risperdal Consta
Initial: 0.5mg oral risperidone bid during 1st week
Titrate: May increase to 1mg bid or 2mg qd PO during 2nd week. If total daily oral dose of ≥2mg is well tolerated, may administer 25mg IM of Risperdal Consta every 2 weeks (or alternatively, an initial dose of 12.5mg may be appropriate)

Continue oral supplementation for 3 weeks after 1st inj

Hepatic Impairment
Titrate w/ oral risperidone prior to initiating treatment w/ Risperdal Consta
Initial: 0.5mg oral risperidone bid during 1st week
Titrate: May increase to 1mg bid or 2mg qd PO during 2nd week. If total daily oral dose of ≥2mg is well tolerated, may administer 25mg IM of Risperdal Consta every 2 weeks (or alternatively, an initial dose of 12.5mg may be appropriate)
Continue oral supplementation for 3 weeks after 1st inj

Elderly
Recommended Dose: 25mg IM every 2 weeks
Oral risperidone (or another antipsychotic) should be given w/ the 1st inj and continued for 3 weeks

Other Important Considerations

Reinitiation of Treatment After Previous Discontinuation:
Administer supplementation w/ oral risperidone (or another antipsychotic) when restarting patients who have had an interval off treatment w/ Risperdal Consta

ADMINISTRATION

IM route
Administer by deep IM deltoid or gluteal inj only.
Deltoid Administration: Use the 1-inch needle alternating inj between the 2 arms.
Gluteal Administration: Use the 2-inch needle alternating inj between the 2 buttocks.
Do not combine 2 different dose strengths in a single administration.

Instructions for Use
1. Use components provided in dose pack; must reconstitute only in diluent supplied in dose pack.
2. Do not substitute any components of dose pack.
3. Do not store sus after reconstitution; administer dose as soon as possible after reconstitution to avoid settling.
4. Entire contents of vial must be administered to ensure intended dose is delivered.

Refer to PI for further administration instructions.

STORAGE

2-8°C (36-46°F). Protect from light. If refrigeration is unavailable, may store at ≤25°C (77°F) for no more than 7 days prior to administration.

HOW SUPPLIED

Inj: 12.5mg, 25mg, 37.5mg, 50mg

CONTRAINDICATIONS

Known hypersensitivity to either risperidone or paliperidone, or to any of the excipients in the product.

WARNINGS/PRECAUTIONS

Each inj should be administered by a healthcare professional. Neuroleptic malignant syndrome (NMS) reported; immediately d/c and institute symptomatic treatment and medical monitoring. May cause tardive dyskinesia (TD), especially in the elderly; consider discontinuation if signs/symptoms appear. Associated w/ metabolic changes (eg, hyperglycemia, dyslipidemia, weight gain) that may increase CV/cerebrovascular risk. Hyperglycemia and diabetes mellitus (DM), in some cases extreme and associated w/ ketoacidosis or hyperosmolar coma or death, reported; monitor for worsening of glucose control in patients w/ DM and FPG in patients at risk for DM. Somnolence, seizures, and hyperprolactinemia reported. May induce orthostatic hypotension; consider dose reduction if hypotension occurs. Caution w/ known CV disease, cerebrovascular disease, and conditions that predispose to hypotension. Elderly patients and those w/ a predisposition to hypotensive reactions should avoid Na^+ depletion or dehydration, and circumstances that accentuate hypotension (alcohol intake, high ambient temperature). Leukopenia, neutropenia, and agranulocytosis reported; consider discontinuation at the 1st sign of a clinically significant decline in WBC count in the absence of other causative factors in patients w/ a history of a clinically significant low WBC count or a drug-induced leukopenia/neutropenia. D/C therapy and follow WBC counts until recovery in patients w/ severe neutropenia (ANC <1000/mm³). May impair mental/physical abilities. Associated w/ esophageal dysmotility and aspiration; caution in patients at risk for aspiration pneumonia. Priapism and thrombotic thrombocytopenic purpura (TTP) reported. May cause disruption of body temperature regulation; caution when exposed to temperature extremes. May be associated w/ an antiemetic effect and may mask signs/symptoms of overdosage w/ certain drugs or of conditions (eg, intestinal obstruction, Reye's syndrome, brain tumor). Closely supervise patients at high-risk of suicide. Increased sensitivity to antipsychotic medications reported in patients w/ Parkinson's disease or dementia w/ Lewy bodies. Caution w/ diseases/conditions affecting metabolism or hemodynamic responses. Avoid inadvertent inj into a blood vessel.

ADVERSE REACTIONS

Schizophrenia: Headache, parkinsonism, dizziness, akathisia, fatigue, constipation, dyspepsia, sedation, weight increased, pain in extremity, dry mouth.
Bipolar Disorder: (Monotherapy) Weight increased. (Adjunctive Treatment) Tremor, parkinsonism.

DRUG INTERACTIONS

See Dosing Considerations. Caution w/ other centrally-acting drugs or alcohol. May enhance hypotensive effects of other therapeutic agents w/ this potential. May antagonize effects of levodopa and dopamine agonists. Cimetidine or ranitidine may increase bioavailability. Ranitidine may increase exposure. Chronic administration of clozapine may decrease clearance. May increase valproate C_{max}. Fluoxetine, paroxetine, and other CYP2D6 inhibitors may increase levels. Carbamazepine and other CYP3A4 inducers may decrease levels and lead to decreased efficacy.

PREGNANCY AND LACTATION

Pregnancy: Category C. Neonates exposed to antipsychotic drugs during the 3rd trimester of pregnancy are at risk for extrapyramidal and/or withdrawal symptoms following delivery.
Lactation: Excreted in human breast milk. Not for use in nursing during treatment and for at least 12 weeks after last inj.

MECHANISM OF ACTION

Atypical antipsychotic. Benzisoxazole derivative; has not been established. In schizophrenia, the therapeutic activity is proposed to be mediated through a combination of dopamine type 2 and serotonin type 2 receptor antagonism.

PHARMACOKINETICS

Distribution: Rapid; V_d=1-2L/kg; plasma protein binding (90% [risperidone]), (77% [9-hydroxyrisperidone]); found in breast milk. **Metabolism:** Liver (extensive).

Hydroxylation (main pathway) via CYP2D6; N-dealkylation (minor pathway); 9-hydroxyrisperidone (major active metabolite). **Elimination:** (Oral) Urine (70%), feces (14%); $T_{1/2}$=3-6 days.

PATIENT CONSIDERATIONS

Assessment: Assess for known hypersensitivity to drug or paliperidone, dementia-related psychosis, DM, risk for hypotension, history of seizures, hepatic/renal impairment, any other conditions where treatment is cautioned, pregnancy/nursing status, and for possible drug interactions. Obtain baseline FPG in patients at risk for DM.

Monitoring: Monitor for NMS, TD, hyperprolactinemia, orthostatic hypotension, cognitive and motor impairment, seizures, esophageal dysmotility, aspiration, priapism, TTP, metabolic changes, disruption of body temperature, and other adverse reactions. Monitor for glucose control; perform periodic FPG in patients at risk for DM. Monitor for signs/symptoms of leukopenia, neutropenia, and agranulocytosis; perform frequent monitoring of CBC during the 1st few months of therapy in patients w/ history of clinically significant low WBC count or drug-induced leukopenia/neutropenia. Periodically reevaluate long-term risks and benefits of the drug.

Counseling: Advise of risk of orthostatic hypotension and of nonpharmacologic interventions that help to reduce its occurrence. Inform that therapy has the potential to impair judgment, thinking, or motor skills; advise to use caution when operating hazardous machinery, including automobiles. Instruct to notify physician if pregnant/intending to become pregnant during therapy and for at least 12 weeks after last inj. Instruct not to breastfeed while on therapy and for at least 12 weeks after last inj. Advise to inform physician if taking/planning to take any prescription or OTC drugs, and to avoid alcohol during treatment.

RISPERIDONE — risperidone   Rx

Class: Atypical antipsychotic

> Elderly patients w/ dementia-related psychosis treated w/ antipsychotic drugs are at an increased risk of death. Not approved for the treatment of patients w/ dementia-related psychosis.

OTHER BRAND NAMES

Risperdal, Risperdal M-Tab

ADULT DOSAGE

Schizophrenia
May be administered qd or bid
Initial: 2mg/day
Titrate: May increase at intervals of ≥24 hrs, by 1-2mg/day
Target: 4-8mg/day; efficacy demonstrated in a range of 4-16mg/day
Maint: 2-8mg/day
Max: 16mg/day

Bipolar Mania
Acute Manic or Mixed Episodes Associated w/ Bipolar I Disorder:
Initial: 2-3mg/day
Titrate: May increase at intervals of ≥24 hrs, by 1mg/day
Target: 1-6mg/day
Max: 6mg/day

Also indicated as adjunctive therapy w/ lithium or valproate for the treatment of acute manic or mixed episodes associated w/ bipolar I disorder

PEDIATRIC DOSAGE

Schizophrenia
13-17 Years:
Initial: 0.5mg qd in am or pm
Titrate: May increase at intervals of ≥24 hrs, by 0.5 or 1mg/day
Target: 3mg/day; efficacy demonstrated in a range of 1-6mg/day
Max: 6mg/day
If experiencing persistent somnolence, may administer 1/2 daily dose bid

Bipolar Mania
Acute Manic or Mixed Episodes Associated w/ Bipolar I Disorder:
Monotherapy:
10-17 Years:
Initial: 0.5mg qd in am or pm
Titrate: May increase at intervals of ≥24 hrs, by 0.5 or 1mg/day
Target: 1-2.5mg/day; efficacy demonstrated in range of 0.5-6mg/day
Max: 6mg/day
If experiencing persistent somnolence, may administer 1/2 daily dose bid

Autistic Disorder
Irritability Associated w/ Autistic Disorder (eg, Symptoms of Aggression Towards Others, Deliberate Self-Injuriousness, Temper Tantrums, Quickly Changing Moods):
5-17 Years:
Total daily dose may be administered qd or divided bid
Initial:
<20kg: 0.25mg/day
≥20kg: 0.5mg/day
Titrate: May increase after a minimum of 4 days
Target:
<20kg: 0.5mg/day
≥20kg: 1mg/day
Maintain target dose for a minimum of 14 days. If not achieving sufficient response, may increase at intervals of ≥2 weeks, by 0.25mg/day (<20kg) or 0.5mg/day (≥20kg)

Range: 0.5-3mg/day

Once sufficient response is achieved and maintained, consider gradually lowering the dose.

If experiencing persistent somnolence, may give qd dose hs, divide daily dose bid, or reduce dose.

DOSING CONSIDERATIONS
Concomitant Medications
Enzyme Inducers (eg, Carbamazepine, Phenytoin, Rifampin): Increase risperidone dose up to double usual dose when coadministered; may need to decrease dose when enzyme inducers are discontinued

Enzyme Inhibitors (eg, Fluoxetine, Paroxetine): Reduce risperidone dose during coadministration and titrate slowly when initiating therapy; may need to increase dose when enzyme inhibitors are discontinued

Max: 8mg/day of risperidone in adults during coadministration

Renal Impairment
Adults:
Severe (CrCl <30mL/min):
Initial: 0.5mg bid
Titrate: May increase by ≤0.5mg, administered bid. For doses >1.5mg bid, increase in intervals of ≥1 week

Hepatic Impairment
Adults:
10-15 Points on Child-Pugh System:
Initial: 0.5mg bid
Titrate: May increase by ≤0.5mg, administered bid. For doses >1.5mg bid, increase in intervals of ≥1 week

Elderly
Start at lower end of dosing range; limiting initial dose to 0.5mg bid w/ careful titration may minimize risk of orthostatic hypotension

Other Important Considerations
Schizophrenia:
Reinitiation of Treatment in Patients Previously Discontinued:
After an interval off risperidone, follow initial titration schedule

ADMINISTRATION
Oral route

May be given w/ or w/o meals.

Oral Sol
May be administered directly from calibrated pipette, or may be mixed w/ a beverage (eg, water, coffee, orange juice, low-fat milk) prior to administration (not compatible w/ cola or tea).

Tab, Disintegrating
Do not push tab through the foil; peel back foil to expose the tab.
Immediately place the entire tab on the tongue after removing from blister.
Swallow w/ or w/o liquid.
Do not split or chew the tab.

STORAGE
20-25°C (68-77°F). **Risperdal/Risperdal M-Tab:** 15-25°C (59-77°F). **Oral Sol:** Protect from light and freezing. **Tab:** Protect from light and moisture.

HOW SUPPLIED
Tab, Disintegrating: 0.25mg, (Risperdal M-Tab) 0.5mg, 1mg, 2mg, 3mg, 4mg; (Risperdal) **Oral Sol:** 1mg/mL [30mL]; **Tab:** 0.25mg, 0.5mg, 1mg, 2mg, 3mg, 4mg

CONTRAINDICATIONS
Known hypersensitivity to either risperidone or paliperidone, or to any of the excipients in the formulation.

WARNINGS/PRECAUTIONS
May cause neuroleptic malignant syndrome (NMS); d/c immediately and institute symptomatic treatment and medical monitoring. Tardive dyskinesia (TD) may develop; consider discontinuation if signs/symptoms appear. Hyperglycemia and diabetes mellitus (DM), in some cases extreme and associated w/ ketoacidosis or hyperosmolar coma or death, reported; monitor for worsening of glucose control in patients w/ DM, and perform FPG testing in patients at risk for DM. Undesirable alterations in lipids and weight gain reported. Somnolence, seizures, and elevation of prolactin levels reported. May induce orthostatic hypotension and syncope; consider dose reduction if hypotension occurs. Caution w/ known cardiovascular (CV) disease, cerebrovascular disease, and conditions that predispose to hypotension. Leukopenia, neutropenia, and agranulocytosis reported; monitor CBC in patients w/ history of clinically significant low WBC counts or drug-induced leukopenia/neutropenia, and consider discontinuation at 1st sign of clinically significant decline in WBC counts w/o other causative factors. D/C and follow WBC counts until recovery in patients w/ severe neutropenia (ANC <1000/mm³). May impair mental/physical abilities. Esophageal dysmotility and aspiration reported; caution in patients at risk for aspiration pneumonia. Priapism reported. May disrupt body temperature regulation; caution when prescribing for patients who will be exposed to temperature extremes. Patients w/ Parkinson's disease or dementia w/ Lewy bodies may experience increased sensitivity. Caution in elderly.
Tab, Disintegrating: Contains phenylalanine.

ADVERSE REACTIONS
Parkinsonism, akathisia, dystonia, tremor, sedation, dizziness, anxiety, blurred vision, N/V, upper abdominal pain, stomach discomfort, dyspepsia, diarrhea, salivary hypersecretion, constipation, dry mouth, increased appetite, increased weight, fatigue, rash, nasal congestion, URTI, nasopharyngitis, pharyngolaryngeal pain.

DRUG INTERACTIONS
See Dosing Considerations. Adjust dose when used w/ CYP2D6 inhibitors (eg, fluoxetine, paroxetine) and enzyme inducers (eg, carbamazepine). May increase valproate peak plasma concentrations. Caution w/ other centrally acting drugs and alcohol. May enhance hypotensive effects of other therapeutic agents w/ this potential. May antagonize effects of levodopa and dopamine agonists. Chronic administration of clozapine may decrease clearance.

PREGNANCY AND LACTATION
Pregnancy: Category C. Neonates exposed to antipsychotic drugs during the 3rd trimester of pregnancy are at risk for extrapyramidal and/or withdrawal symptoms following delivery.
Lactation: Risperidone and 9-hydroxyrisperidone are present in human breast milk; not for use in nursing.

MECHANISM OF ACTION
Benzisoxazole derivative; has not been established. In schizophrenia, proposed to be mediated through a combination of dopamine type 2 and serotonin type 2 receptor antagonism.

PHARMACOKINETICS
Absorption: Well-absorbed. Absolute bioavailability (70%); T_{max}=1 hr, 3 hrs (9-hydroxyrisperidone, extensive metabolizers), 17 hrs (9-hydroxyrisperidone, poor metabolizers). **Distribution:** V_d=1-2L/kg; plasma protein binding (90% [risperidone]), (77% [9-hydroxyrisperidone]); found in breast milk. **Metabolism:** Liver (extensive) via CYP2D6; hydroxylation (major pathway), N-dealkylation (minor pathway); 9-hydroxyrisperidone (major active metabolite). **Elimination:** Urine (70%), feces (14%); $T_{1/2}$=3 hrs (extensive metabolizers), 20 hrs (poor metabolizers), 21 hrs (9-hydroxyrisperidone, extensive metabolizers), 30 hrs (9-hydroxyrisperidone, poor metabolizers).

PATIENT CONSIDERATIONS
Assessment: Assess for dementia-related psychosis, DM, CV disease, cerebrovascular disease, conditions which would predispose to hypotension, hepatic/renal impairment, history of seizures, drug hypersensitivity, any other conditions where treatment is cautioned, pregnancy/nursing status, and possible drug interactions. Obtain FPG in patients at risk for DM.

Monitoring: Monitor for NMS, TD, hyperglycemia, weight gain, dyslipidemia, hyperprolactinemia, orthostatic hypotension, leukopenia, neutropenia, agranulocytosis, cognitive/motor impairment, seizures, esophageal dysmotility, aspiration, priapism, disruption of body temperature, and other adverse reactions. Monitor for worsening of glucose control in patients w/ DM and monitor FPG in patients at risk for DM. Monitor CBC frequently during the 1st few months of therapy in patients w/ history of clinically significant low WBC count or drug-induced leukopenia/neutropenia. In patients w/ clinically significant neutropenia, monitor for fever or other symptoms or signs of infection. Periodically reevaluate long-term risks and benefits of the drug.

Counseling: Advise about the risk of orthostatic hypotension, especially during the period of initial dose titration. Inform that therapy has the potential to impair judgment, thinking, or motor skills; advise to use caution when operating hazardous machinery. Instruct to notify physician if pregnant/planning to become pregnant, nursing, and if taking/planning to take any prescription or OTC drugs. Advise to avoid alcohol during treatment. Inform that orally disintegrating tab contains phenylalanine. Inform that treatment can be associated w/ hyperglycemia, DM, dyslipidemia, and weight gain. Inform about risk of TD.

RITALIN — methylphenidate hydrochloride
Class: CNS stimulant

CII

> Caution w/ history of drug dependence or alcoholism. Chronic abuse may lead to marked tolerance and psychological dependence w/ varying degrees of abnormal behavior. Frank psychotic episodes may occur, especially w/ parenteral abuse. Careful supervision is required during withdrawal from abusive use, since severe depression may occur. Withdrawal following chronic use may unmask symptoms of underlying disorder that may require follow-up.

OTHER BRAND NAMES
Ritalin-SR

ADULT DOSAGE
Attention Deficit Disorders
Tab:
20-30mg/day given in divided doses bid-tid, preferably 30-45 min ac; some patients may require 40-60mg/day and others, 10-15mg/day may be adequate
Last dose should be taken before 6 pm if patient is unable to sleep as a result of taking medication late in the day

Tab, Sustained-Release (SR):
May be used in place of methylphenidate immediate-release (IR) tabs when the 8-hr dosage of SR tab corresponds to the titrated 8-hr dosage of methylphenidate IR tabs

Narcolepsy
Tab:
20-30mg/day given in divided doses bid-tid, preferably 30-45 min ac;

PEDIATRIC DOSAGE
Attention Deficit Disorders
≥6 Years:
Tab:
Initial: 5mg bid before breakfast and lunch
Titrate: Increase gradually by 5-10mg weekly
Max: 60mg/day

Tab, Sustained-Release (SR):
May be used in place of methylphenidate immediate release (IR) tabs when the 8-hr dosage of SR tab corresponds to the titrated 8-hr dosage of methylphenidate IR tabs

D/C if no improvement seen after appropriate dosage adjustment over 1 month

D/C periodically to assess the child's condition; therapy should not be indefinite some patients may require 40-60mg/day and others, 10-15mg/day may be adequate

Last dose should be taken before 6 pm if patient is unable to sleep as a result of taking medication late in the day

Tab, SR:
May be used in place of methylphenidate IR tabs when the 8-hr dosage of SR tab corresponds to the titrated 8-hr dosage of methylphenidate IR tabs

Narcolepsy
≥6 Years:
Tab:
Initial: 5mg bid before breakfast and lunch
Titrate: Increase gradually by 5-10mg weekly
Max: 60mg/day

Tab, SR:
May be used in place of methylphenidate IR tabs when the 8-hr dosage of SR tab corresponds to the titrated 8-hr dosage of methylphenidate IR tabs

D/C if no improvement seen after appropriate dosage adjustment over 1 month

D/C periodically to assess the child's condition; therapy should not be indefinite

---

DOSING CONSIDERATIONS
Adverse Reactions
Children ≥6 Years:
Reduce dose or, if necessary, d/c if paradoxical aggravation of symptoms or other adverse effects occur

ADMINISTRATION
Oral route

Tab, SR
Swallow tabs whole; do not crush or chew.

STORAGE
Ritalin/Ritalin-SR: 25°C (77°F); excursions permitted to 15-30°C (59-86°F).
Generic: 20-25°C (68-77°F). **Tab:** Protect from light. **Tab, SR:** Protect from moisture.

HOW SUPPLIED
Tab: (Ritalin) 5mg, 10mg*, 20mg*; **Tab, SR:** (Generic) 10mg, (Ritalin-SR) 20mg
*scored

CONTRAINDICATIONS
Marked anxiety, tension, agitation, known hypersensitivity to the drug, glaucoma, motor tics or family history or diagnosis of Tourette's syndrome. Treatment w/ MAOIs or w/in a minimum of 14 days following discontinuation of an MAOI.

WARNINGS/PRECAUTIONS
Avoid w/ known serious structural cardiac abnormalities, cardiomyopathy, serious heart rhythm abnormalities, coronary artery disease, or other serious cardiac problems. Sudden death reported in children and adolescents w/ structural cardiac abnormalities or other serious heart problems. Sudden death, stroke, and MI reported in adults. May increase BP and HR; caution w/ conditions that may be compromised by increases in BP/HR (eg, preexisting HTN, heart failure, recent MI). Prior to treatment, obtain medical history (including assessment for family history of sudden death or ventricular arrhythmia) and perform a physical exam to assess for the presence of cardiac disease. Promptly perform cardiac evaluation if symptoms of cardiac disease develop. May exacerbate symptoms of behavior disturbance and thought disorder in patients w/ preexisting psychotic disorder. Caution in patients w/ comorbid bipolar disorder; may induce mixed/manic episode. May cause treatment-emergent psychotic or manic symptoms (eg, hallucinations, delusional thinking, mania) in children and adolescents w/o prior history of psychotic illness or mania; consider discontinuation if such symptoms occur. Aggressive behavior or hostility reported in children and adolescents. May cause long-term suppression of growth in children; monitor growth, and may need to interrupt treatment in patients not growing or gaining height or weight as expected. May lower convulsive threshold; d/c if seizures occur. Priapism, sometimes requiring surgical intervention, reported. Associated w/ peripheral vasculopathy, including Raynaud's phenomenon. Difficulties w/ accommodation and blurring of vision reported. Patients w/ an element of agitation may react adversely; d/c if necessary.

ADVERSE REACTIONS
Nervousness, insomnia, hypersensitivity reactions, anorexia, nausea, dizziness, palpitations, headache, dyskinesia, drowsiness, BP and pulse changes, tachycardia, angina, cardiac arrhythmia, abdominal pain.

DRUG INTERACTIONS
See Contraindications. Caution w/ pressor agents. May decrease effectiveness of drugs used to treat HTN. May inhibit metabolism of coumarin anticoagulants, anticonvulsants (eg, phenobarbital, phenytoin, primidone), and TCAs (eg, imipramine, clomipramine, desipramine); downward dose adjustment and monitoring of plasma drug concentration (or coagulation times for coumarin) of these drugs may be necessary when initiating or discontinuing methylphenidate.

PREGNANCY AND LACTATION
Pregnancy: Category C.
Lactation: Caution in nursing.

MECHANISM OF ACTION
Mild CNS stimulant; has not been established. Thought to activate the brain stem arousal system and cortex to produce its stimulant effect.

PHARMACOKINETICS
Absorption: (Children) T_{max}=4.7 hrs (Tab, SR), 1.9 hrs (Tab). **Metabolism:** Deesterification to α-phenyl-2-piperidine acetic acid (ritalinic acid) (major metabolite). **Elimination:** Urine (Tab, SR) (86%; 67% [Children]).

PATIENT CONSIDERATIONS
Assessment: Assess for hypersensitivity to the drug, marked anxiety, tension, agitation, glaucoma, motor tics or family history or diagnosis of Tourette's syndrome, cardiovascular conditions, history of drug dependence or alcoholism, psychotic disorder, comorbid bipolar disorder, any other conditions where treatment is contraindicated or cautioned, pregnancy/nursing status, and possible drug interactions.

Monitoring: Monitor for changes in HR and BP, signs/symptoms of cardiac disease, exacerbation of behavior disturbance and thought disorder, psychosis, mania, appearance of or worsening of aggressive behavior or hostility, seizures, priapism, digital changes, visual disturbances, and other adverse reactions. In pediatric patients, monitor growth. Perform periodic monitoring of CBC, differential, and platelet counts during prolonged therapy.

Counseling: Inform about the benefits and risks of therapy and counsel about appropriate use. Instruct to seek immediate medical attention in the event of priapism. Instruct to report to physician any new numbness, pain, skin color change, or sensitivity in fingers or toes, and to contact physician immediately if any signs of unexplained wounds appear on fingers or toes while taking the drug.

RITALIN LA — methylphenidate hydrochloride   CII
Class: CNS stimulant

> Caution w/ history of drug dependence or alcoholism. Chronic abuse may lead to marked tolerance and psychological dependence w/ varying degrees of abnormal behavior. Frank psychotic episodes may occur, especially w/ parenteral abuse. Careful supervision is required during withdrawal from abusive use since severe depression may occur. Withdrawal following chronic use may unmask symptoms of underlying disorder that may require follow-up.

ADULT DOSAGE	PEDIATRIC DOSAGE
Attention-Deficit Hyperactivity Disorder	**Attention-Deficit Hyperactivity Disorder**
Refer to pediatric dosing	**≥6 Years:**
	Initial: 20mg qam; may begin w/ 10mg when a lower initial dose is appropriate
	Titrate: May adjust in weekly 10mg increments
	Max: 60mg/day qam
	Maint/Extended Treatment: Periodically reevaluate long-term usefulness of drug for the individual patient w/ trials off medication
	D/C if no improvement seen after appropriate dosage adjustment over 1 month
	Conversions
	Patients Currently Receiving Methylphenidate:
	5mg Methylphenidate BID: 10mg Ritalin LA qd
	10mg Methylphenidate Bid or 20mg Methylphenidate-SR: 20mg Ritalin LA qd
	15mg Methylphenidate BID: 30mg Ritalin LA qd
	20mg Methylphenidate Bid or 40mg Methylphenidate-SR: 40mg Ritalin LA qd
	30mg Methylphenidate Bid or 60mg Methylphenidate-SR: 60mg Ritalin LA qd

---

DOSING CONSIDERATIONS
Adverse Reactions
Reduce dose or d/c if paradoxical aggravation of symptoms or other adverse events occur

ADMINISTRATION
Oral route

May be swallowed whole or cap may be opened and cap contents sprinkled over a spoonful of applesauce and consumed immediately, and not stored for future use. Do not crush, chew, or divide cap and/or cap contents.

STORAGE
25°C (77°F); excursions permitted to 15-30°C (59-86°F).

HOW SUPPLIED
Cap, Extended-Release: 10mg, 20mg, 30mg, 40mg, 60mg

CONTRAINDICATIONS
Marked anxiety, tension, agitation, known hypersensitivity to methylphenidate or other components of the product, glaucoma, motor tics, or family history or diagnosis of Tourette's syndrome. Treatment w/ MAOIs or w/in a minimum of 14 days following discontinuation of an MAOI.

WARNINGS/PRECAUTIONS
Sudden death reported in children and adolescents w/ structural cardiac abnormalities or other serious heart problems. Sudden death, stroke, and MI

reported in adults. Avoid w/ known serious structural cardiac abnormalities, cardiomyopathy, serious heart rhythm abnormalities, coronary artery disease, or other serious cardiac problems. May increase BP and HR; caution w/ conditions that might be compromised by increases in BP/HR (eg, preexisting HTN, HF, recent MI, ventricular arrhythmia). Promptly perform cardiac evaluation if symptoms of cardiac disease develop. May exacerbate symptoms of behavior disturbance and thought disorder in patients w/ preexisting psychotic disorder. Caution in patients w/ comorbid bipolar disorder; may induce mixed/manic episode. May cause treatment-emergent psychotic or manic symptoms (eg, hallucinations, delusional thinking, mania) in children and adolescents w/o prior history of psychotic illness or mania; consider discontinuation if such symptoms occur. Aggressive behavior or hostility reported in children and adolescents. May cause long-term suppression of growth in children; monitor growth, and may need to interrupt treatment in patients not growing or gaining height or weight as expected. May lower convulsive threshold; d/c if seizures occur. Priapism, sometimes requiring surgical intervention, reported. Associated w/ peripheral vasculopathy, including Raynaud's phenomenon; carefully observe for digital changes. Difficulties w/ accommodation and blurring of vision reported.

ADVERSE REACTIONS
Headache, insomnia, upper abdominal pain, appetite decreased, anorexia, nervousness.

DRUG INTERACTIONS
See Contraindications. Antacids or acid suppressants may alter release. May decrease effectiveness of drugs used to treat HTN. Caution w/ pressor agents. May be associated w/ pharmacodynamic interactions when coadministered w/ direct and indirect dopamine agonists (eg, dihydroxyphenylalanine, TCAs) as well as dopamine antagonists (antipsychotics [eg, haloperidol]). Potential interaction w/ coumarin anticoagulants, anticonvulsants (eg, phenobarbital, phenytoin, primidone), and TCAs (eg, imipramine, clomipramine, desipramine); downward dose adjustment of these drugs and monitoring of plasma drug concentrations (or coagulation times for coumarin) may be necessary when initiating/discontinuing methylphenidate. Avoid w/ alcohol.

PREGNANCY AND LACTATION
Pregnancy: Category C.
Lactation: Caution in nursing.

MECHANISM OF ACTION
Sympathomimetic amine; CNS stimulant. Has not been established; thought to block reuptake of norepinephrine and dopamine into presynaptic neuron and increase release of these monoamines into extraneuronal space.

PHARMACOKINETICS
Absorption: Children: Absolute bioavailability (22% [d-methylphenidate], 5% [l-methylphenidate]); T_{max1}=2 hrs; C_{max1}=10.3ng/mL; T_{max2}=6.6 hrs; C_{max2}=10.2ng/mL; AUC=86.6ng•hr/mL. Adults: T_{max1}=2 hrs; C_{max1}=5.3ng/mL; T_{max2}=5.5 hrs; C_{max2}=6.2ng/mL; AUC=45.8ng•hr/mL. **Distribution:** Plasma protein binding (10-33%); V_d=2.65L/kg (d-methylphenidate), 1.8L/kg (l-methylphenidate). **Metabolism:** Rapid and extensive by carboxylesterase CES1A1 to α-phenyl-2-piperidine acetic acid (ritalinic acid) (main deesterified metabolite). **Elimination:** (Immediate-Release) Urine (78-97% metabolites [60-86% ritalinic acid], <1% unchanged), feces (1-3% metabolites). $T_{1/2}$=3-4 hrs (ritalinic acid), 2.4 hrs (children), 3.3 hrs (adults).

PATIENT CONSIDERATIONS

Assessment: Assess for hypersensitivity to the drug, marked anxiety, tension, agitation, glaucoma, motor tics, family history or diagnosis of Tourette's syndrome, history of drug dependence or alcoholism, psychotic disorder, comorbid bipolar disorder, any other conditions where treatment is contraindicated or cautioned, pregnancy/nursing status, and possible drug interactions. Prior to treatment, obtain medical history (including assessment for family history of sudden death or ventricular arrhythmia) and perform physical exam to assess for presence of cardiac disease.

Monitoring: Monitor for changes in HR and BP, signs/symptoms of cardiac disease, exacerbation of behavior disturbance and thought disorder, psychosis, mania, appearance of or worsening of aggressive behavior or hostility, seizures, priapism, peripheral vasculopathy, visual disturbances, and other adverse reactions. In pediatric patients, monitor growth. Perform periodic monitoring of CBC, differential, and platelet counts during prolonged therapy. Periodically reevaluate long-term usefulness of drug.

Counseling: Advise to avoid alcohol while taking the drug. Inform about the benefits and risks of therapy and counsel about appropriate use. Instruct to seek immediate medical attention in the event of priapism. Instruct to report to physician any new numbness, pain, skin color change, or sensitivity to temperature in fingers or toes, and to contact physician immediately if any signs of unexplained wounds appear on fingers or toes while taking the drug.

RITUXAN — rituximab

Rx

Class: Monoclonal antibody/CD20 blocker

Serious infusion reactions and severe mucocutaneous reactions, some fatal (death has occurred within 24 hrs of infusion), may occur. Monitor patients closely. D/C infusion for severe reaction and treat for Grade 3/4 infusion reactions. Hepatitis B virus (HBV) reactivation can occur, in some cases resulting in fulminant hepatitis, hepatic failure, and death. Screen all patients for HBV infection before treatment initiation; monitor patients during and after treatment. D/C therapy and concomitant medications in the event of HBV reactivation. Fatal progressive multifocal leukoencephalopathy (PML) may occur.

ADULT DOSAGE
Non-Hodgkin's Lymphoma

$375mg/m^2$ as an IV infusion

Relapsed/Refractory, Low-Grade/Follicular, CD20-Positive, B-Cell Non-Hodgkin's Lymphoma (NHL) as a Single Agent:
Administer once weekly for 4 or 8 doses
Retreatment: Administer once weekly for 4 doses

Previously Untreated Follicular, CD20-Positive, B-Cell NHL:
In Combination w/ Chemotherapy:
Administer on Day 1 of each chemotherapy cycle for up to 8 doses
Maint in Complete/Partial Responders: Administer as a single agent every 8 weeks for 12 doses; initiate 8 weeks following completion of combination treatment w/ chemotherapy

Non-Progressing, Low-Grade, CD20-Positive, B-Cell NHL as a Single Agent After 1st Line Cyclophosphamide, Vincristine, and Prednisone (CVP) Chemotherapy:
Administer once weekly for 4 doses at 6-month intervals following completion of 6-8 CVP chemotherapy cycles
Max: 16 doses

Previously Untreated Diffuse Large B-Cell, CD20-Positive NHL in Combination w/ Cyclophosphamide, Doxorubicin, Vincristine, and Prednisone (CHOP) or Other Anthracycline-Based Chemotherapy:
Administer on Day 1 of each chemotherapy cycle for up to 8 infusions

As a Component of Zevalin:
Infuse $250mg/m^2$ w/in 4 hrs prior to the administration of Indium-111 (In-111) Zevalin and w/in 4 hrs prior to the administration of Yttrium-90 (Y-90) Zevalin; administer rituximab and In-111 Zevalin 7-9 days prior to rituximab and Y-90 Zevalin

Refer to the Zevalin PI for additional information

Chronic Lymphocytic Leukemia

In combination w/ fludarabine and cyclophosphamide, for previously untreated and previously treated CD20-positive chronic lymphocytic leukemia

$375mg/m^2$ the day prior to initiation of fludarabine and cyclophosphamide chemotherapy, then $500mg/m^2$ on Day 1 of cycles 2-6 (every 28 days)

Pneumocystis jiroveci pneumonia and anti-herpetic viral prophylaxis is recommended during treatment and for up to 12 months following treatment as appropriate

Rheumatoid Arthritis

In combination w/ methotrexate for moderately to severely active rheumatoid arthritis in patients who have had an inadequate response to ≥1 TNF antagonist therapy

Two 1000mg IV infusions separated by 2 weeks

Administer subsequent courses every 24 weeks or based on evaluation, but not sooner than every 16 weeks

Granulomatosis with Polyangiitis and Microscopic Polyangiitis

In Combination w/ Glucocorticoids:
$375mg/m^2$ IV infusion once weekly for 4 weeks

Glucocorticoid Administration:
Methylprednisolone 1000mg/day IV for 1-3 days, followed by oral prednisone 1mg/kg/day (not to exceed 80mg/day and tapered per clinical need); begin regimen w/in

PEDIATRIC DOSAGE
Pediatric use may not have been established

14 days prior to or w/ initiation of rituximab and continue during and after the 4-week course of treatment

Pneumocystis jiroveci pneumonia prophylaxis is recommended during treatment and for at least 6 months following the last infusion

Premedication

Premedicate before each infusion w/ acetaminophen and an antihistamine

For patients administered rituximab according to the 90-min infusion rate, the glucocorticoid component of their chemotherapy regimen should be administered prior to infusion

Rheumatoid Arthritis Patients:
Methylprednisolone 100mg IV (or its equivalent) 30 min prior to each infusion

- -

DOSING CONSIDERATIONS

Adverse Reactions

Infusion Reactions: Interrupt or slow the infusion; continue at 1/2 the previous rate upon improvement of symptoms

ADMINISTRATION

IV route

For IV infusion only; do not administer as IV push or bolus.
Do not mix or dilute w/ other drugs.
Single-use vial; discard any unused portion left in vial.

1st Infusion

Initiate at a rate of 50mg/hr; in the absence of infusion toxicity, increase rate by 50mg/hr increments every 30 min, to a max of 400mg/hr

Subsequent Infusions

Standard Infusion: Initiate at a rate of 100mg/hr; in the absence of infusion toxicity, increase by 100mg/hr increments every 30 min, to a max of 400mg/hr

Previously Untreated Follicular and Diffuse Large B-Cell Non-Hodgkin's Lymphoma Patients:

Grade 3 or 4 Infusion-Related Adverse Event Not Experienced During Cycle 1:
Administer a 90-min infusion in Cycle 2 w/ a glucocorticoid-containing chemotherapy regimen; initiate at a rate of 20% of the total dose given in the first 30 min and the remaining 80% of the total dose given over the next 60 min. If 90-min infusion is tolerated in cycle 2, use the same rate when administering the remainder of the treatment regimen (through Cycle 6 or 8)

Clinically Significant Cardiovascular Disease/Circulating Lymphocyte Count ≥5000/mm³ Before Cycle 2:
Do not administer the 90-min infusion

Preparation

1. Withdraw the necessary amount of rituximab and dilute to a final concentration of 1-4mg/mL in an infusion bag containing either 0.9% normal saline or D5W.
2. Gently invert bag to mix the sol.

STORAGE

2-8°C (36-46°F). Protect from direct sunlight. Do not freeze or shake. **Sol for Infusion:** 2-8°C (36-46°F) for 24 hrs. Stable for additional 24 hrs at room temperature; however, store diluted solutions at 2-8°C (36-46°F).

HOW SUPPLIED

Inj: 100mg/10mL, 500mg/50mL

WARNINGS/PRECAUTIONS

Should only be administered by a healthcare professional with appropriate medical support to manage severe infusion reactions that can be fatal if they occur. Not recommended for use with severe, active infections. *Pneumocystis jiroveci* pneumonia (PCP) and antiherpetic viral prophylaxis is recommended for patients with CLL during treatment and for up to 12 months following treatment as appropriate. PCP prophylaxis is recommended for patients with GPA and MPA during treatment and for at least 6 months following last infusion. Potential for immunogenicity. Acute renal failure, hyperkalemia, hypocalcemia, hyperuricemia, and/or hyperphosphatemia from tumor lysis may occur within 12-24 hrs after the 1st infusion. A high number of circulating malignant cells (≥25,000/mm³) or high tumor burden confers greater risk of tumor lysis syndrome (TLS); administer aggressive IV hydration and antihyperuricemic therapy in patients at high risk of TLS. Correct electrolyte abnormalities, monitor renal function and fluid balance, and administer supportive care, including dialysis as indicated. Serious, including fatal, bacterial, fungal, and new/reactivated viral infections may occur during and following the completion of therapy; d/c for serious infections and institute anti-infective therapy. Infections reported in some patients with prolonged hypogammaglobulinemia (>11 months after rituximab exposure). D/C if severe mucocutaneous reactions, PML, or serious/life-threatening cardiac arrhythmias occur. Perform cardiac monitoring during and after all infusions if arrhythmias develop or with history of arrhythmia/angina. Severe renal toxicity may occur in NHL patients; d/c if SrCr rises or oliguria occurs. Abdominal pain, bowel obstruction, and perforation may occur in combination with chemotherapy. Follow current immunization guidelines and administer non-live vaccines at least 4 weeks prior to therapy for RA patients. Obtain CBC and platelet count prior to each course in lymphoid malignancy patients, at weekly to monthly intervals (more frequently if cytopenia develops) during treatment with rituximab and chemotherapy, and at 2- to 4-month intervals during therapy in RA, GPA, or MPA patients. Not recommended in patients with RA who have not had prior inadequate response to one or more TNF antagonists.

ADVERSE REACTIONS

Infusion reactions, mucocutaneous reactions, hepatitis B reactivation, PML, infections, fever, lymphopenia, chills, asthenia, neutropenia, headache, leukopenia, diarrhea, muscle spasms.

DRUG INTERACTIONS

Renal toxicity reported with cisplatin. Vaccination with live viral vaccines not recommended. Observe closely for signs of infection if biologic agents and/or disease-modifying antirheumatic drugs are used concomitantly.

PREGNANCY AND LACTATION

Pregnancy: Category C.
Lactation: Caution in nursing.

MECHANISM OF ACTION

Chimeric murine/human monoclonal IgG_1 kappa antibody/CD20 antigen blocker; binds to CD20 antigen expressed on the surface of pre-B and mature B-lymphocytes, mediates B-cell lysis, possibly by complement-dependent cytotoxicity and antibody-dependent cell-mediated cytotoxicity.

PHARMACOKINETICS

Absorption: RA: C_{max}=157mcg/mL (1st infusion), 183mcg/mL (2nd infusion), 318mcg/mL (2 x 500mg dose), 381mcg/mL (2 x 1000mg dose). **Distribution:** RA: V_d=3.1L. GPA/MPA: V_d=4.5L. **Elimination:** NHL: $T_{1/2}$=22 days, RA: $T_{1/2}$=18 days, CLL: $T_{1/2}$=32 days. GPA/MPA: $T_{1/2}$=23 days.

PATIENT CONSIDERATIONS

Assessment: Assess for severe active infections, preexisting cardiac/pulmonary conditions, prior experience of cardiopulmonary adverse reactions, high number of circulating malignant cells (≥25,000/mm³), high tumor burden, electrolyte abnormalities, risk/preexisting HBV infection, hypogammaglobulinemia, any other conditions where treatment is cautioned, pregnancy/nursing status, and possible drug interactions. Perform HBsAg and anti-HBc measurement before initiating treatment. Obtain CBC and platelet count.

Monitoring: Monitor fluid and electrolyte balance, cardiac/renal function, CBC, and platelet counts periodically. Monitor for signs/symptoms of infusion reactions, mucocutaneous reactions, hepatitis B reactivation, PML, new-onset neurologic manifestations, TLS, infections, arrhythmias, bowel obstruction/perforation, cytopenias, and other adverse reactions. Closely monitor for infusion reactions in patients with preexisting cardiac/pulmonary conditions, those who experienced prior cardiopulmonary adverse reactions, and those with high numbers of circulating malignant cells. Monitor patients with evidence of current or prior HBV infection for clinical and lab signs of hepatitis or HBV reactivation during and for several months following therapy.

Counseling: Inform of risks of therapy and importance of assessing overall health status at each visit. Inform that drug is detectable in serum for up to 6 months following completion of therapy. Advise to use effective contraception during and for 12 months after therapy.

RIXUBIS — coagulation factor IX (recombinant)   Rx

Class: Antihemophilic factor (recombinant)

ADULT DOSAGE	PEDIATRIC DOSAGE
Hemophilia B	Pediatric use may not have been established
Control/Prevention of Bleeding Episodes:	
Minor Bleeding: Required Factor IX (FIX) Level 20-30 IU/dL: q12-24h for at least 1 day, until healing is achieved	
Moderate Bleeding: Required FIX Level 25-50 IU/dL: q12-24h for 2-7 days, until bleeding stops and healing is achieved	
Major Bleeding: Required FIX Level 50-100 IU/dL: q12-24h for 7-10 days, until bleeding stops and healing is achieved	
Perioperative Management:	
Minor Surgery: Required FIX Level 30-60 IU/dL: q24h for at least 1 day, until healing is achieved	
Major Surgery: Required FIX Level 80-100 IU/dL: q8-24h for 7-10 days, until bleeding stops and healing is achieved	
Routine Prophylaxis: 40-60 IU/kg IV twice weekly; adjust dose based on response	
Dosing Equation: Initial Dose = Body Weight (kg) x Desired FIX Increase (% of normal or IU/dL) x Reciprocal of Observed Recovery (IU/kg per IU/dL)	

- -

ADMINISTRATION
IV bolus infusion route

Use a plastic syringe

Use w/in 3 hrs of reconstitution

STORAGE
2-8°C (36-46°F) for up to 24 months; do not freeze. May store at room temperature ≤30°C (86°F) for up to 12 months within the 24-month period; do not return to refrigerator after storage at room temperature.

HOW SUPPLIED
Inj: 250 IU, 500 IU, 1000 IU, 2000 IU, 3000 IU

CONTRAINDICATIONS
Known hypersensitivity to this product or its excipients, including hamster protein; disseminated intravascular coagulation (DIC); signs of fibrinolysis.

WARNINGS/PRECAUTIONS
Not indicated for induction of immune tolerance in patients with hemophilia B. Initiate therapy under the supervision of a physician experienced in the treatment of hemophilia. Hypersensitivity reactions reported; immediately d/c and initiate appropriate treatment if an allergic/anaphylactic-type reaction occurs. Contains trace amounts of Chinese hamster ovary proteins; may develop hypersensitivity to these proteins. May develop FIX inhibitors; perform an assay that measures FIX inhibitor concentration if expected FIX activity plasma levels are not attained, or if bleeding is not controlled with expected dose. Association between occurrence of FIX inhibitor and allergic reactions reported; increased risk of severe hypersensitivity reactions or anaphylaxis if these patients are re-exposed to therapy. Nephrotic syndrome reported following attempted immune tolerance induction in hemophilia B patients with FIX inhibitors. Associated with the development of thromboembolic complications; monitor for early signs of thromboembolic and consumptive coagulopathy in patients with liver disease, with signs of fibrinolysis, peri/postoperatively, or at risk for thromboembolic events or DIC.

ADVERSE REACTIONS
Dysgeusia, pain in extremity, (+) furin antibody test, FIX/furin antibodies.

PREGNANCY AND LACTATION
Category C, caution in nursing.

MECHANISM OF ACTION
Recombinant antihemophilic factor; temporarily replaces the missing coagulation FIX that is required for effective hemostasis.

PHARMACOKINETICS
Absorption: (Non-bleeding subjects) (Dose range: 71.3-79.4 IU/kg) AUC_{0-inf}=1207 IU•hrs/dL (single dose), 1305 IU•hrs/dL (repeated dose); C_{max}=66.2 IU/dL (single dose), 72.7 IU/dL (repeated dose). **Distribution:** V_d=201.9mL/kg (single dose), 178.6mL/kg (repeated dose). **Elimination:** $T_{1/2}$=26.7 hrs (single dose), 25.4 hrs (repeated dose).

PATIENT CONSIDERATIONS
Assessment: Assess for known hypersensitivity to drug or to its excipients, including hamster protein; severity of bleeding; DIC or risk for DIC; liver disease; signs of fibrinolysis; risk for thromboembolic events; presence of FIX inhibitors; and pregnancy/nursing status.

Monitoring: Monitor for hypersensitivity reactions, DIC, thromboembolic complications, nephrotic syndrome, and other adverse reactions. Monitor FIX activity plasma levels. Monitor for the development of FIX inhibitors if expected FIX activity plasma levels are not attained or if bleeding is not controlled with an expected dose.

Counseling: Advise to report to physician any adverse reactions or problems following administration. Inform of the early signs of hypersensitivity reactions and anaphylaxis; instruct to d/c and contact physician if these symptoms occur. Advise to contact physician or treatment facility for further treatment and/or assessment if experiencing a lack of clinical response to FIX replacement therapy. Instruct to follow the specific preparation and administration procedures provided by physician.

ROBAXIN — methocarbamol

Rx

Class: Muscular analgesic (centrally acting)

OTHER BRAND NAMES
Robaxin-750

ADULT DOSAGE
Musculoskeletal Conditions
Adjunct for relief of discomfort associated w/ acute, painful musculoskeletal conditions

Oral:
≥16 Years:
Robaxin:
Initial: 3 tabs qid
Maint: 2 tabs qid

Robaxin-750:
Initial: 2 tabs qid
Maint: 1 tab q4h or 2 tabs tid

6g/day are recommended for the first 48-72 hrs; 8g/day may be administered for severe conditions. Thereafter, the dose can usually be reduced to approx 4g/day

PEDIATRIC DOSAGE
Tetanus
Inj:
Initial: 15mg/kg or 500mg/m²; repeat q6h prn
Max: 1.8g/m² for 3 consecutive days

Maint dose may be administered by inj into tubing or by IV infusion w/ an appropriate quantity of fluid

---

Inj:
Moderate Symptoms:
Single 1g (10mL) dose IV/IM; administration of oral form will usually sustain relief initiated by the inj
Max: 3g/day for no more than 3 consecutive days

Severe Cases/Postop Conditions:
Single 1g (10mL) dose IV/IM; may administer additional doses of 1g q8h
Max: 3g/day for no more than 3 consecutive days

Tetanus
Inj:
1 or 2 vials directly into the tubing of the previously inserted indwelling needle; additional 10mL or 20mL may be added to infusion bottle so that a total of up to 30mL (3 vials) is given as initial dose

Repeat q6h until conditions allow for insertion of NG tube; crushed methocarbamol tabs suspended in water or saline may then be given through this tube

Total oral doses up to 24g/day may be required

ADMINISTRATION
Oral/IV/IM route

Directions for IV Use
Inj may be administered undiluted at a max rate of 3mL/min or added to an IV drip of NaCl inj or D5 inj.
One vial given as a single dose should not be diluted to more than 250mL for IV infusion.
Do not refrigerate after mixing w/ IV infusion fluids.
Avoid vascular extravasation of this hypertonic sol, which may result in thrombophlebitis.
Patient should be in a recumbent position during and for at least 10-15 min following inj.

Directions for IM Use
Not more than 5mL (1/2 vial) should be injected into each gluteal region.
Inj may be repeated at 8-hr intervals, if necessary.
When satisfactory relief of symptoms is achieved, it can usually be maintained w/ tabs.
Not recommended for SQ administration.

STORAGE
20-25°C (68-77°F), in tight container; excursions permitted to 15-30°C (59-86°F).

HOW SUPPLIED
Inj: 100mg/mL [10mL]; **Tab:** 500mg, 750mg

CONTRAINDICATIONS
Hypersensitivity to methocarbamol or to any components in the formulation. **Inj:** Known/suspected renal pathology due to propylene glycol content.

WARNINGS/PRECAUTIONS
May impair mental/physical abilities. May cause color interference in certain screening tests for 5-hydroxy-indoleacetic acid (5-HIAA) and vanillylmandelic acid (VMA). Caution in epilepsy with the inj. Inj rate should not exceed 3mL/min. Avoid extravasation with inj. Avoid use in women who are or may become pregnant and particularly during early pregnancy.

ADVERSE REACTIONS
Lightheadedness, dizziness, drowsiness, nausea, urticaria, pruritus, rash, conjunctivitis, nasal congestion, blurred vision, headache, fever, seizures, syncope, flushing.

DRUG INTERACTIONS
Additive adverse effects with alcohol and other CNS depressants. May inhibit effect of pyridostigmine; caution in patients with myasthenia gravis receiving anticholinergics.

PREGNANCY AND LACTATION
Pregnancy: Category C.
Lactation: Caution in nursing.

MECHANISM OF ACTION
Carbamate derivative of guaifenesin; not established, suspected to have CNS depressant with sedative and musculoskeletal relaxant properties.

PHARMACOKINETICS
Distribution: Plasma protein binding (46-50%). Found in breast milk. **Metabolism:** Via dealkylation, hydroxylation, and conjugation pathways. **Elimination:** Urine; $T_{1/2}$=1-2 hrs.

PATIENT CONSIDERATIONS
Assessment: Assess for renal/hepatic impairment, myasthenia gravis, seizures, pregnancy/nursing status, alcohol intake, and drug interactions.

Monitoring: Monitor for congenital and fetal abnormalities if taken during pregnancy, for color interference in certain screening tests for 5-HIAA using nitrosonaphthol reagent, and in screening tests for urinary VMA using Gitlow method.

Counseling: Instruct to use caution while performing hazardous tasks. Warn to avoid alcohol or other CNS depressants. Instruct to notify physician if pregnant/ nursing or if planning to become pregnant.

ROCALTROL — calcitriol   Rx

Class: Vitamin D analogue

ADULT DOSAGE

Hypoparathyroidism
Initial: 0.25mcg/day qam
Titrate: May increase at 2- to 4-week intervals
Range: 0.5-2mcg/day

Secondary Hyperparathyroidism
Predialysis Patients:
Initial: 0.25mcg/day
Titrate: May increase to 0.5mcg/day

Hypocalcemia
Dialysis Patients:
Initial: 0.25mcg/day
Titrate: May increase by 0.25mcg/day at 4- to 8-week intervals

Patients w/ normal or only slightly reduced serum Ca^{2+} levels may respond to doses of 0.25mcg every other day; most patients respond to doses between 0.5 and 1 mcg/day

PEDIATRIC DOSAGE

Hypoparathyroidism
1-5 Years:
Usual: 0.25-0.75mcg/day qam
≥6 Years:
Range: 0.5-2mcg/day qam

Secondary Hyperparathyroidism
Predialysis Patients:
<3 Years:
Initial: 10-15ng/kg/day
≥3 Years:
Initial: 0.25mcg/day
Titrate: May increase to 0.5mcg/day

DOSING CONSIDERATIONS

Elderly
Start at lower end of dosing range

Adverse Reactions
Hypercalcemia: Immediately d/c until normocalcemia ensues; when normal levels return, continue treatment at a daily dose 0.25mcg lower than that previously used

ADMINISTRATION
Oral route

STORAGE
15-30°C (59-86°F). Protect from light.

HOW SUPPLIED
Cap: 0.25mcg, 0.5mcg; **Sol:** 1mcg/mL [15mL]

CONTRAINDICATIONS
Hypercalcemia or evidence of vitamin D toxicity, known hypersensitivity to calcitriol (or drugs of the same class) or any of the inactive ingredients is contraindicated.

WARNINGS/PRECAUTIONS
Administration in excess of daily requirements may cause hypercalcemia, hypercalciuria, and hyperphosphatemia. Chronic hypercalcemia may lead to generalized vascular calcification, nephrocalcinosis, and other soft tissue calcification. Serum Ca^{2+} times phosphate (Ca x P) product should not exceed $70mg^2/dL^2$. May increase serum inorganic phosphate levels, leading to ectopic calcification in patients with renal failure; use non-aluminum phosphate binders and low phosphate diet to control serum phosphate in dialysis patients. Caution in elderly and immobilized patients. If treatment switched from ergocalciferol, may take several months for ergocalciferol level in blood to return to baseline. In patients with normal renal function, chronic hypercalcemia may be associated with an increase in SrCr. Avoid dehydration in patients with normal renal function. When indicated, estimate daily dietary Ca^{2+} intake and adjust accordingly.

ADVERSE REACTIONS
Hypercalcemia, hypercalciuria, SrCr elevation, weakness, N/V, dry mouth, constipation, muscle and bone pain, metallic taste, polyuria, polydipsia, weight loss, hypersensitivity reactions.

DRUG INTERACTIONS
Avoid pharmacological doses of vitamin D products and derivatives during therapy. Avoid uncontrolled intake of additional Ca^{2+}-containing preparations. Avoid with Mg^{2+}-containing preparations (eg, antacids) in patients on chronic renal dialysis; use may lead to hypermagnesemia. May impair intestinal absorption with cholestyramine. Reduced blood levels with phenytoin or phenobarbital. Caution with thiazides; may cause hypercalcemia. Reduced serum endogenous concentrations with ketoconazole reported. Hypercalcemia may precipitate cardiac arrhythmias in patients on digitalis; use with caution. Functional antagonism with corticosteroids. Adjust dose of concomitant phosphate-binding agent.

PREGNANCY AND LACTATION
Category C, not for use in nursing.

MECHANISM OF ACTION
Synthetic vitamin D analogue; regulates absorption of Ca^{2+} from the GI tract and its utilization in the body.

PHARMACOKINETICS
Absorption: Rapid (intestine). T_{max}=3-6 hrs, 8-12 hrs (hemodialysis); C_{max}=116pmol/L (pediatrics). **Distribution:** Found in breast milk. **Metabolism:** Hydroxylation to 1α, 25R(OH)₂-26, 23S-lactone D₃ (major metabolite). **Elimination:**
Feces (primary), urine (10%, 1mcg dose); $T_{1/2}$=5-8 hrs (normal subjects), 16.2 hrs and 21.9 hrs (hemodialysis).

PATIENT CONSIDERATIONS
Assessment: Assess for hypercalcemia, evidence of vitamin D toxicity, renal function, presence of immobilization, pregnancy/nursing status, and possible drug interactions. Obtain baseline levels of serum Ca^{2+}, P, alkaline phosphatase, creatinine, and intact parathyroid hormone (iPTH).

Monitoring: Monitor for hypercalcemia, hypercalciuria, and hyperphosphatemia. For dialysis patients, perform periodic monitoring of serum Ca^{2+}, P, Mg^{2+}, and alkaline phosphatase. For hypoparathyroid patients, perform periodic monitoring of serum Ca^{2+}, P, and 24-hr urinary Ca^{2+}. For predialysis patients, perform monthly monitoring of serum Ca^{2+}, P, alkaline phosphatase, and creatinine for 6 months; then periodically, and periodic monitoring of iPTH every 3- to 4-months. Monitor serum Ca^{2+} levels ≥2X/week after all dosage changes and during titration periods.

Counseling: Inform about compliance with dosage instructions, adherence to instructions about diet and Ca^{2+} supplementation, and avoidance of the use of unapproved nonprescription drugs. Carefully inform about symptoms of hypercalcemia. Advise to maintain adequate Ca^{2+} intake at a minimum of 600mg/ day.

ROTARIX — rotavirus vaccine, live, oral   Rx

Class: Vaccine

PEDIATRIC DOSAGE
Rotavirus Gastroenteritis Prevention
Caused by G1 and non-G1 types (G3, G4, and G9):
6-24 Weeks of Age:
Vaccination series consists of two 1mL doses

Administer 1st dose beginning at 6 weeks of age and administer 2nd dose after an interval of at least 4 weeks; the 2-dose series should be completed by 24 weeks of age

If infant spits out or regurgitates most of vaccine dose, may consider a single replacement dose at same vaccination visit

---

ADMINISTRATION
Oral route

No restrictions on infant's liquid consumption (eg, breast milk), either before or after vaccination.
Administer w/in 24 hrs of reconstitution.

Reconstitution Instructions for Oral Administration
Reconstitute only w/ accompanying diluents; do not mix w/ other vaccines or sol.
1. Remove vial cap and push transfer adapter onto vial (lyophilized vaccine).
2. Shake diluent in oral applicator; connect oral applicator to transfer adapter.
3. Push plunger of oral applicator to transfer diluents into vial.
4. Withdraw vaccine into oral applicator.
5. Twist and remove oral applicator.
6. Do not use a needle; not for inj.

STORAGE
Vials: 2-8°C (36-46°F). Protect from light. **Diluent:** 2-8°C (36-46°F) or room temperature up to 25°C (77°F). Do not freeze; discard if it has been frozen.
Reconstituted Sus: 2-8°C (36-46°F) or room temperature up to 25°C (77°F). Discard if not used w/in 24 hrs. Do not freeze; discard if it has been frozen.

HOW SUPPLIED
Oral Sus: 1mL

CONTRAINDICATIONS
History of hypersensitivity to any component of the vaccine, severe combined immunodeficiency disease (SCID), history of uncorrected congenital malformation of the GI tract (eg, Meckel's diverticulum) that would predispose infant for intussusception, and history of intussusception.

WARNINGS/PRECAUTIONS
Tip caps of the prefilled oral applicators of diluent contain natural rubber latex, which may cause allergic reactions. Delay administration in infants suffering from acute diarrhea or vomiting. Safety and effectiveness have not been evaluated in infants w/ chronic GI disorders, w/ known primary or secondary immunodeficiencies (including HIV), on immunosuppressive therapy, or w/ malignant neoplasms affecting the bone marrow or lymphatic system, or when administered after exposure to rotavirus. Rotavirus shedding in stool occurs after vaccination w/ peak excretion around Day 7. Transmission of vaccine virus from vaccinees to healthy seronegative contacts reported; caution when considering whether to administer to individuals w/ immunodeficient close contacts. Intussusception reported.

ADVERSE REACTIONS
Fussiness, irritability, loss of appetite, vomiting, diarrhea.

DRUG INTERACTIONS
Immunosuppressive therapies, including irradiation, antimetabolites, alkylating agents, cytotoxic drugs, and corticosteroids (used in greater than physiologic doses), may reduce immune response to vaccine.

PREGNANCY AND LACTATION
Pregnancy: Category C.
MECHANISM OF ACTION
Vaccine; exact immunologic mechanism is unknown. Replicates in small intestine and induces immunity.

PATIENT CONSIDERATIONS
Assessment: Assess for previous hypersensitivity to the vaccine, history of uncorrected congenital malformation of the GI tract, history of intussusception, SCID, latex sensitivity, GI disorders, immunocompromised conditions, immunization history, and possible drug interactions.

Monitoring: Monitor for hypersensitivity reactions, intussusception, and other adverse events.

Counseling: Inform parents/guardians of the potential benefits and risks of immunization, and of the importance of completing the immunization series. Inform about the potential for adverse reactions that have been temporally associated w/ administration of the vaccine or other vaccines containing similar components. Instruct to immediately report any signs and/or symptoms of intussusception.

ROTATEQ — rotavirus vaccine, live, oral, pentavalent   Rx

Class: Vaccine

PEDIATRIC DOSAGE
Rotavirus Gastroenteritis Prevention
Caused by the Serotypes G1, G2, G3, and G4:
6-32 Weeks of Age:
Administer series of 3 (2mL) doses PO starting at 6-12 weeks of age, w/ subsequent doses administered at 4- to 10-week intervals; 3rd dose should not be given after 32 weeks of age

ADMINISTRATION
Oral route

Administer as soon as possible after being removed from refrigeration
No restrictions on food/liquid consumption (eg, breast milk) either before or after vaccination
Do not mix w/ any other vaccines or sol
Do not reconstitute or dilute
Gently squeeze liquid into infant's mouth toward inner cheek until dosing tube is empty
A replacement dose is not recommended if an incomplete dose is administered (eg, infant spits or regurgitates vaccine); infant should continue to receive any remaining doses in the recommended series

STORAGE
2-8°C (36-46°F). Protect from light.

HOW SUPPLIED
Sol: 2mL

CONTRAINDICATIONS
History of hypersensitivity to any component of the vaccine, severe combined immunodeficiency disease (SCID) and history of intussusception.

WARNINGS/PRECAUTIONS
For PO use only. Appropriate treatment and supervision must be available to manage possible anaphylactic reactions following administration. Safety and efficacy data not available for administration to infants who are potentially immunocompromised. Caution in infants with a history of GI disorders (eg, active acute GI illness, chronic diarrhea, failure to thrive, history of congenital abdominal disorders, abdominal surgery). Intussusception reported. Shedding of vaccine virus in stool reported. Transmission of vaccine virus from vaccinees to unvaccinated contacts reported; caution when administering to individuals with immunodeficient close contacts. Consider delaying use with febrile illness. May not protect all vaccine recipients against rotavirus. Clinical data not available for postexposure prophylaxis or for level of protection provided with administration of an incomplete regimen. If an incomplete dose is administered (eg, infant spits or regurgitates vaccine), do not give replacement dose; continue to give any remaining doses in the recommended series.

ADVERSE REACTIONS
Irritability, fever, diarrhea, vomiting, nasopharyngitis, otitis media.

DRUG INTERACTIONS
Immunosuppressive therapies, including irradiation, antimetabolites, alkylating agents, cytotoxic drugs, and corticosteroids (used in greater than physiologic doses) may reduce immune response to vaccine.

PREGNANCY AND LACTATION
Category C, safety not known in nursing.

MECHANISM OF ACTION
Vaccine; exact immunologic mechanism is unknown. Replicates in small intestine and induces immunity.

PATIENT CONSIDERATIONS
Assessment: Assess for previous hypersensitivity to the vaccine, SCID, history of intussusception, immunization history, immunocompromised conditions, history of GI disorders, febrile illness, and possible drug interactions.

Monitoring: Monitor for hypersensitivity/anaphylactic reactions, intussusception, and other adverse events.

Counseling: Inform parent/guardian of potential benefits/risks of vaccine. Instruct parent/guardian to inform physician of the current health status of patient and to report if patient has close contact with a family/household member who has a weak immune system. Advise to contact physician immediately if patient develops vomiting, diarrhea, severe stomach pain, or blood in the stool and advise to contact physician if any other adverse reactions develop.

ROXICET — acetaminophen/oxycodone   CII

Class: Opioid analgesic

> Associated w/ cases of acute liver failure, at times resulting in liver transplant and death. Most cases of liver injury are associated w/ acetaminophen (APAP) use at doses >4000mg/day, and often involve >1 APAP-containing product.

ADULT DOSAGE	PEDIATRIC DOSAGE
Moderate to Moderately Severe Pain	Pediatric use may not have been established
Usual: 1 tab or 5mL (1 tsp) q6h prn	
Max: 12 tabs/day or 60mL/day (12 tsp/day)	
If pain is constant, give at regular intervals on an around-the-clock schedule	
Max: 4g/day of APAP	

DOSING CONSIDERATIONS
Discontinuation
Taper dose gradually in patients treated for more than a few weeks
ADMINISTRATION
Oral route
STORAGE
20-25°C (68-77°F). (Tab) Protect from moisture.
HOW SUPPLIED
(Oxycodone/APAP) Sol: 5mg/325mg/5mL [500mL]; **Tab:** 5mg/325mg* *scored
CONTRAINDICATIONS
Known hypersensitivity to oxycodone, acetaminophen, or any other component of this product. **Oxycodone:** Significant respiratory depression (in unmonitored settings or absence of resuscitative equipment), acute or severe bronchial asthma or hypercarbia, suspected/known paralytic ileus.

WARNINGS/PRECAUTIONS
May be abused in a manner similar to other opioid agonists. Respiratory depression may occur; use extreme caution and consider alternative nonopioid analgesics in patients w/ acute asthma, chronic obstructive pulmonary disorder (COPD), cor pulmonale, preexisting respiratory impairment, or in the elderly or debilitated. Respiratory depressant effects may be markedly exaggerated in the presence of head injury, other intracranial lesions, or preexisting increase in intracranial pressure. Produces effects on pupillary response and consciousness, which may obscure neurologic signs of worsening in patients w/ head injuries. May cause severe hypotension; caution w/ circulatory shock. May produce orthostatic hypotension in ambulatory patients. Increased risk of acute liver failure in patients w/ underlying liver disease. May cause serious skin reactions (eg, acute generalized exanthematous pustulosis, Stevens-Johnson syndrome, toxic epidermal necrolysis), which can be fatal; d/c at the 1st appearance of skin rash or any other sign of hypersensitivity/anaphylaxis. Hypersensitivity and anaphylaxis reported. May obscure diagnosis or clinical course in patients w/ acute abdominal conditions. Caution w/ CNS depression, hypothyroidism, Addison's disease, prostatic hypertrophy, urethral stricture, acute alcoholism, delirium tremens, kyphoscoliosis w/ respiratory depression, myxedema, toxic psychosis, hepatic/renal/pulmonary impairment, and in elderly/debilitated. May aggravate convulsions w/ convulsive disorders and may induce or aggravate seizures in some clinical settings. Monitor for decreased bowel motility in postoperative patients. May cause spasm of the sphincter of Oddi; caution w/ biliary tract disease, including acute pancreatitis. May cause increases in serum amylase level. Physical dependence and tolerance may occur. Do not abruptly d/c. Lab test interactions may occur. Not recommended for use during and immediately prior to labor and delivery.

ADVERSE REACTIONS
Acute liver failure, respiratory depression, apnea, respiratory arrest, circulatory depression, hypotension, shock, lightheadedness, dizziness, drowsiness/sedation, N/V.

DRUG INTERACTIONS
Oxycodone: May cause severe hypotension w/ drugs that compromise vasomotor tone (eg, phenothiazines). May enhance neuromuscular-blocking action of skeletal muscle relaxants and increase respiratory depression. Additive CNS depression w/ CNS depressants (eg, general anesthetics, phenothiazines, tranquilizers, alcohol); reduce dose of one or both agents. Coadministration w/ anticholinergics may produce paralytic ileus. Agonist/antagonist analgesics (eg, pentazocine, nalbuphine, butorphanol) may reduce analgesic effect and/or precipitate withdrawal symptoms; use w/ caution. APAP: Increased risk of acute liver failure w/ alcohol; hepatotoxicity occurred in chronic alcoholics. Increase in glucuronidation and plasma clearance and decreased $T_{1/2}$ w/ oral contraceptives. Probenecid and propranolol may increase pharmacologic/therapeutic effects. May decrease effects of loop diuretics, lamotrigine, and zidovudine.

PREGNANCY AND LACTATION
Category C, not for use in nursing.

MECHANISM OF ACTION
Oxycodone: Opioid analgesic; semisynthetic pure opioid agonist whose principal therapeutic action is analgesia. Effects are mediated by receptors (notably μ and kappa) in the CNS for endogenous opioid-like compounds (eg, endorphins, enkephalins). APAP: Nonopiate, nonsalicylate analgesic and antipyretic; site and mechanism for the analgesic effect not established. Antipyretic effect is accomplished through inhibition of endogenous pyrogen action on the hypothalamic heat-regulating centers.

PHARMACOKINETICS
Absorption: Oxycodone: Absolute bioavailability (87%). APAP: Rapid and almost complete. **Distribution:** Found in breast milk. Oxycodone: Plasma protein binding (45%); (IV) V_d=211.9L; crosses placenta. APAP: Plasma protein binding during acute intoxication (20-50%). **Metabolism:** Oxycodone: N-dealkylated to noroxycodone (1st-pass); O-demethylation via CYP2D6 to oxymorphone; noroxycodone, oxymorphone (metabolites). APAP: Liver via CYP450 conjugation w/ glucuronic acid and (lesser extent) sulfuric acid and cysteine; N acetyl-p-benzoquinoneimine, N-acetylimidoquinone (toxic metabolite). **Elimination:** Oxycodone: Urine (8-14%, unchanged); $T_{1/2}$=3.51 hrs. APAP: Urine (90-100%).

PATIENT CONSIDERATIONS

Assessment: Assess for risks for opioid abuse, addiction, or misuse, patient's general condition and medical status, severity and type of pain, respiratory depression, bronchial asthma, COPD, cor pulmonale, hypercarbia, paralytic ileus, acute alcoholism, drug hypersensitivity, renal/hepatic impairment, pregnancy/nursing status, or any other conditions where treatment is contraindicated or cautioned, and possible drug interactions.

Monitoring: Monitor for development of addiction, abuse, or misuse, physical dependence, tolerance, acute liver failure, respiratory depression, altered consciousness, hypotension, convulsions, hypersensitivity/anaphylactic/serious skin reactions, decreased bowel motility in postoperative patients, spasm of the sphincter of Oddi, and other adverse reactions. Monitor serum amylase levels.

Counseling: Inform that drug contains oxycodone, which is a morphine-like substance. Instruct to keep in a secure place out of reach of children or from theft; advise to seek emergency medical care immediately in case of accidental ingestions. Advise to destroy the unused tabs/oral sol by flushing down the toilet. Advise not to adjust dosing w/o consulting physician. Inform that drug may impair mental/physical abilities required to perform potentially hazardous tasks (eg, driving, operating heavy machinery). Instruct not to combine w/ alcohol, opioid analgesics, tranquilizers, sedatives, or other CNS depressants unless under recommendation and guidance of a physician. Inform that drug may cause dangerous additive CNS or respiratory depression if coadministered w/ another CNS depressant. Instruct to consult physician if pregnant, planning to become pregnant, or if breastfeeding. Advise not to adjust dose w/o consulting physician and not to abruptly d/c if on treatment for more than a few weeks. Advise to d/c and contact physician immediately if signs of allergy develop. Inform about signs of serious skin reactions. Instruct to look for APAP on package labels and not to use >1 APAP-containing product. Instruct to seek medical attention immediately upon ingestion of >4000mg/day of APAP, even if patient is feeling well.

ROZEREM — ramelteon   Rx
Class: Melatonin receptor agonist

ADULT DOSAGE	**PEDIATRIC DOSAGE**
Insomnia	Pediatric use may not have been established
Difficulty w/ Sleep Onset: 8mg w/in 30 min of hs	
Max: 8mg/day	

ADMINISTRATION
Oral route

Do not take w/ or immediately after high-fat meal.

STORAGE
25°C (77°F); excursions permitted to 15-30°C (59-86°F). Protect from moisture and humidity.

HOW SUPPLIED
Tab: 8mg

CONTRAINDICATIONS
Rechallenge in patients who developed angioedema after treatment w/ ramelteon. Coadministration w/ fluvoxamine.

WARNINGS/PRECAUTIONS
Angioedema reported; do not rechallenge if angioedema develops. Sleep disturbances may manifest as a physical and/or psychiatric disorder; symptomatic treatment of insomnia should be initiated only after careful evaluation. Failure of insomnia to remit after 7-10 days of therapy may indicate presence of psychiatric and/or medical illness. Cognitive and behavior changes, hallucinations, amnesia, anxiety, other neuropsychiatric symptoms, and complex behaviors reported; d/c if complex sleep behavior occurs. Worsening of depression reported in primarily depressed patients. May impair physical/mental abilities. May affect reproductive hormones (eg, decreased testosterone levels, increased prolactin levels). Not recommended with severe sleep apnea. Do not use with severe hepatic impairment. Caution with moderate hepatic impairment.

ADVERSE REACTIONS
Dizziness, somnolence, fatigue, nausea, exacerbated insomnia.

DRUG INTERACTIONS
See Contraindications. Decreased efficacy with strong CYP inducers (eg, rifampin). Caution with less strong CYP1A2 inhibitors, strong CYP3A4 inhibitors (eg, ketoconazole), and strong CYP2C9 inhibitors (eg, fluconazole). Increased levels with donepezil and doxepin; monitor patients closely. Increased T_{max} of zolpidem; avoid use. Increased risk of complex behaviors with alcohol and other CNS depressants. Additive effect with alcohol; avoid alcohol use.

PREGNANCY AND LACTATION
Pregnancy: Category C.
Lactation: Caution in nursing.

MECHANISM OF ACTION
Melatonin receptor agonist; activity at MT_1 and MT_2 receptors believed to contribute to sleep-promoting properties. These receptors, acted upon by endogenous melatonin, are thought to be involved in the maintenance of the circadian rhythm underlying the normal sleep-wake cycle.

PHARMACOKINETICS
Absorption: Rapid. Absolute bioavailability (1.8%); T_{max}=0.75 hr (fasted). **Distribution:** Plasma protein binding (82%). **Metabolism:** Oxidation via CYP1A2 (major), CYP2C, CYP3A4 (minor). M-II, M-IV, M-I, M-III (principal metabolites). **Elimination:** Urine and feces (<0.1% parent compound); $T_{1/2}$=1-2.6 hrs, 2-5 hrs (M-II). Refer to PI for PK parameters in elderly patients.

PATIENT CONSIDERATIONS

Assessment: Assess for hepatic impairment, manifestations of physical and/or psychiatric disorder, depression, sleep apnea, other comorbid diagnoses, hypersensitivity, pregnancy/nursing status, and possible drug interactions.

Monitoring: Monitor for signs/symptoms of angioedema, exacerbations of insomnia, emergence of cognitive or behavioral abnormalities, worsening of depression, complex sleep behaviors, and anaphylactic/anaphylactoid reactions.

Counseling: Inform patients, families, and caregivers about benefits and risks associated with treatment. Counsel for appropriate use and instruct to read Medication Guide. Inform that severe anaphylactic and anaphylactoid reactions may occur; advise to seek immediate medical attention. Instruct to report sleep-driving to doctor immediately. Instruct to consult healthcare provider if cessation of menses, galactorrhea in females, decreased libido, or fertility problems occur. Instruct to take within 30 min prior to hs and confine activities to those necessary to prepare for bed. Instruct to swallow tab whole and to not break tab.

RYANODEX — dantrolene sodium   Rx
Class: Direct-acting skeletal muscle relaxant

ADULT DOSAGE	**PEDIATRIC DOSAGE**
Malignant Hyperthermia	**Malignant Hyperthermia**
Treatment:	**Treatment:**
Usual: Minimum of 1mg/kg IV push; administer additional IV boluses up to a max cumulative dose of 10mg/kg if physiologic and metabolic abnormalities continue	**Usual:** Minimum of 1mg/kg IV push; administer additional IV boluses up to a max cumulative dose of 10mg/kg if physiologic and metabolic abnormalities continue
May repeat IV push dosing starting w/ 1mg/kg if abnormalities reappear	May repeat IV push dosing starting w/ 1mg/kg if abnormalities reappear
Prevention in High-Risk Patients:	**Prevention in High Risk Patients:**
Usual: 2.5mg/kg IV over at least 1 min, starting approx 75 min prior to surgery; administer additional individualized doses during anesthesia and surgery if surgery is prolonged	**Usual:** 2.5mg/kg IV over at least 1 min, starting approx 75 min prior to surgery; administer additional individualized doses during anesthesia and surgery if surgery is prolonged

ADMINISTRATION
IV route

Do not dilute or transfer reconstituted sus to another container to infuse product Administer reconstituted sus into the IV catheter while an IV infusion of 0.9% NaCl inj or D5 inj is freely running or into the indwelling catheter w/o a freely running infusion; flush line to assure no residual product remaining in the catheter
Use w/in 6 hrs after reconstitution

Preparation
Reconstitute each vial by adding 5mL of sterile water for inj (w/o a bacteriostatic agent); do not reconstitute w/ any other sol
Shake vial to ensure an orange-colored sus

STORAGE
20-25°C (68-77°F). Excursions permitted to 15-30°C (59-86°F). Avoid prolonged exposure to light. Reconstituted Sol: 20-25°C (68-77°F). Use within 6 hrs after reconstitution. Protect from light.

HOW SUPPLIED
Inj: 250mg

WARNINGS/PRECAUTIONS
Institute the following supportive measures; d/c use of triggering anesthetic agents (eg, volatile anesthetic gases, succinylcholine), manage the metabolic acidosis, institute cooling when necessary, and administer diuretics to prevent late kidney injury due to myoglobinuria (amount of mannitol in drug is insufficient to maintain diuresis). Somnolence and dizziness may occur and may persist up to 48 hrs post-dose. Associated with skeletal muscle weakness, dyspnea, respiratory

muscle weakness, decreased inspiratory capacity, and dysphasia. Patients should not be permitted to ambulate without assistance until they have normal strength and balance. Care must be taken to prevent extravasation due to potential for tissue necrosis. Caution in elderly.

ADVERSE REACTIONS
Flushing, somnolence, dysphonia, dysphagia, N/V, feeling abnormal, headache, vision blurred, pain in extremity, muscular weakness/asthenia, atrioventricular block, tachycardia, infusion-site pain, dizziness.

DRUG INTERACTIONS
Concomitant use of sedative agents may increase risk of somnolence and dizziness. Coadministration with calcium channel blockers is not recommended; cardiovascular collapse in association with marked hyperkalemia reported. Concomitant administration with muscle relaxants may potentiate the neuromuscular block. Concomitant antipsychotic and antianxiety agents may potentiate their effects on the CNS.

PREGNANCY AND LACTATION
Category C, not for use in nursing.

MECHANISM OF ACTION
Direct-acting skeletal muscle relaxant; dissociates excitation-contraction coupling, probably by interfering with Ca^{2+} release from the sarcoplasmic reticulum.

PHARMACOKINETICS
Absorption: (2.5mg/kg single dose) C_{max}=9mcg/mL, AUC_{0-inf}=77.7mcg•hr/mL, T_{max}=1 min (median). **Distribution:** V_d=36.4L; found in breast milk; crosses the placenta; significant amounts are bound to plasma proteins, mostly albumin. **Metabolism:** Liver; hydrolysis and subsequent oxidation; 5-hydroxy dantrolene and acetylamino metabolite (major metabolites). **Elimination:** Urine; $T_{1/2}$=10.8 hrs.

PATIENT CONSIDERATIONS
Assessment: Assess for difficulty swallowing, choking, pregnancy/nursing status, and for possible drug interactions.

Monitoring: Monitor for extravasation, kidney injury, skeletal muscle weakness, somnolence, dizziness, dysphasia, and other adverse reactions. Monitor adequacy of ventilation.

Counseling: Inform patients, families, and caregivers that muscle weakness, dizziness, and somnolence may occur and that patients should be provided assistance with standing and walking until their strength has returned to normal. Inform that dysphagia has been reported; caution at meals on the day of administration. Inform that lightheadedness may occur and may persist for up to 48 hrs after treatment; caution against performing hazardous activities during this time.

RYTARY — carbidopa/levodopa

Rx

Class: Dopa-decarboxylase inhibitor/dopamine precursor

ADULT DOSAGE
Parkinson's Disease

Levodopa Naive:
Initial: 23.75mg/95mg tid for the first 3 days. On the 4th day of treatment, may increase to 36.25mg/145mg tid
Titrate: May increase up to 97.5mg/390mg tid to 5X/day based on clinical response and tolerability
Max: (612.5mg/2450mg)/day

Parkinsonism

Postencephalitic Parkinsonism and Parkinsonism Following Carbon Monoxide/Manganese Intoxication:
Levodopa Naive:
Initial: 23.75mg/95mg tid for the first 3 days. On the 4th day of treatment, may increase to 36.25mg/145mg tid
Titrate: May increase up to 97.5mg/390mg tid to 5X/day based on clinical response and tolerability
Max: (612.5mg/2450mg)/day

Conversions

From Immediate-Release (IR) Carbidopa-Levodopa:
Total Daily Dose of Levodopa in IR Combination:
400-549mg IR: Three 23.75mg/95mg cap tid
550-749mg IR: Four 23.75mg/95mg cap tid
750-949mg IR: Three 36.25mg/145mg cap tid
950-1249mg IR: Three 48.75mg/195mg cap tid
>1250mg IR: Four 48.7mg/195mg cap tid or three 61.25mg/245mg cap tid

PEDIATRIC DOSAGE
Pediatric use may not have been established

DOSING CONSIDERATIONS
Concomitant Medications
Currently Treated w/ Carbidopa and Levodopa Plus Catechol-O-Methyl Transferase Inhibitors:
Initial: May need to increase initial total daily dose of levodopa

Discontinuation
Avoid sudden discontinuation or rapid dose reduction; taper daily dose at time of treatment discontinuation

ADMINISTRATION
Oral route

Swallow whole w/ or w/o food.
Do not chew, divide or crush cap.
May administer by carefully opening cap and sprinkling entire contents on a small amount of applesauce (1-2 tbsp) and consuming immediately; do not store drug/food mixture for future use.

STORAGE
25°C (77°F); excursions permitted to 15-30°C (59-86°F). Protect from light and moisture.

HOW SUPPLIED
Cap, Extended-Release: (Carbidopa/Levodopa) 23.75mg/95mg, 36.25mg/145mg, 48.75mg/195mg, 61.25mg/245mg

CONTRAINDICATIONS
Patients who are currently taking a nonselective MAOI (eg, phenelzine, tranylcypromine) or have recently (within 2 weeks) taken a nonselective MAOI.

WARNINGS/PRECAUTIONS
A symptom complex resembling neuroleptic malignant syndrome (hyperpyrexia and confusion) reported in association with rapid dose reduction, withdrawal of, or changes in dopaminergic therapy; avoid sudden discontinuation/rapid dose reduction, or taper dose if discontinuing therapy. Cardiovascular ischemic events reported; monitor cardiac function in an intensive cardiac care facility during the period of initial dosage adjustment, in patients with a history of MI who have residual atrial, nodal, or ventricular arrhythmias. Increased risk for hallucinations and psychosis; do not use in patients with a major psychotic disorder. Intense urge to gamble, increased sexual urges, intense urges to spend money, binge eating, and/or other intense urges, and the inability to control these urges may occur; consider dose reduction or discontinuation if such urges develop. May cause dyskinesias; may require dose reduction of Rytary or other medications used for the treatment of Parkinson's disease. May increase the possibility of upper GI hemorrhage in patients with history of peptic ulcer. May cause increased intraocular pressure (IOP) in patients with glaucoma. Perform periodic skin examinations to monitor for melanoma. Levodopa: Falling asleep while engaged in activities of daily living and somnolence reported; consider discontinuation if significant daytime sleepiness or episodes of falling asleep during activities that require active participation occur. May impair mental/physical abilities.

ADVERSE REACTIONS
N/V, dizziness, headache, insomnia, abnormal dreams, dry mouth, dyskinesia, anxiety, constipation, orthostatic hypotension.

DRUG INTERACTIONS
See Contraindications. Selective MAO-B inhibitors (eg, rasagiline, selegiline) may be associated with orthostatic hypotension; monitor patients who are taking these drugs concurrently. Iron salts or multivitamins containing iron salts may form chelates and may cause a reduction in bioavailability; monitor patients for worsening Parkinson's symptoms. Levodopa: Caution with concomitant use of sedating medications; may increase the risk for somnolence. Dopamine D2 receptor antagonists (eg, phenothiazines, butyrophenones, risperidone, metoclopramide) and isoniazid may reduce the effectiveness of levodopa; monitor patients for worsening Parkinson's symptoms.

PREGNANCY AND LACTATION
Pregnancy: Category C.
Lactation: Caution in nursing.

MECHANISM OF ACTION
Dopa-decarboxylase inhibitor/dopamine precursor. Carbidopa: Inhibits decarboxylation of peripheral levodopa, making more levodopa available for delivery to the brain. Levodopa: Crosses blood-brain barrier and presumably is converted to dopamine in the brain.

PHARMACOKINETICS
Absorption: Carbidopa: T_{max}=3 hrs. **Distribution:** Carbidopa: Plasma protein binding (36%). Levodopa: Plasma protein binding (10-30%); crosses the placenta; found in breast milk. **Metabolism:** Carbidopa: α-methyl-3-methoxy-4-hydroxyphenylpropionic acid and α-methyl-3,4-dihydroxy-phenylpropionic acid (main metabolites). Levodopa: Decarboxylation and O-methylation. **Elimination:** Carbidopa: Urine (30% unchanged); $T_{1/2}$=2 hrs. Levodopa: $T_{1/2}$=2 hrs (in the presence of carbidopa).

PATIENT CONSIDERATIONS
Assessment: Assess for major psychotic disorder, glaucoma, risk factors that may increase risk for somnolence (eg, presence of sleep disorders), history of peptic ulcer, history of MI with residual atrial, nodal, or ventricular arrhythmias, pregnancy/nursing status, and possible drug interactions.

Monitoring: Monitor for hallucinations, psychosis, control/compulsive behaviors, dyskinesias, drowsiness/sleepiness, somnolence, upper GI hemorrhage in patients with a history of peptic ulcer, increased IOP in patients with glaucoma, and other adverse reactions. Monitor cardiac function in an intensive cardiac care facility during the initial dosage adjustment period in patients with a history of MI who have residual atrial, nodal, or ventricular arrhythmias. Monitor for hyperpyrexia and confusion if sudden discontinuation or rapid dose reduction occurs. Perform periodic skin examinations to monitor for melanoma.

Counseling: Instruct to take ud. Instruct to call physician before stopping therapy and to call physician if withdrawal symptoms (eg, fever, confusion, severe muscle stiffness) develop. Advise that certain side effects (eg, sleepiness and dizziness) that have been reported may affect some patients' ability to drive and operate machinery safely. Inform that hallucinations may occur with levodopa products. Inform of the potential for experiencing intense urges to gamble, increased sexual urges, and other intense urges, and the inability to control these urges while on therapy. Instruct to notify physician if abnormal involuntary movements appear or get worse during treatment. Advise that may develop orthostatic hypotension with or without symptoms (eg, dizziness, nausea, syncope, sweating); advise to rise slowly after sitting or lying down, especially if patient has been doing so for a prolonged period. Advise of the possible additive sedative effects when taking other CNS depressants in combination with therapy. Instruct to notify physician if pregnant/breastfeeding an infant, or intend to breastfeed/become pregnant.

RYTHMOL SR — propafenone hydrochloride   Rx

Class: Class IC antiarrhythmic

> Increased rate of death or reversed cardiac arrest rate reported in patients treated with encainide or flecainide (Class 1C antiarrhythmics) in a study of patients with asymptomatic non-life-threatening ventricular arrhythmias who had a MI >6 days but <2 yrs previously. Consider any 1C antiarrhythmics to have significant proarrhythmic risk in patients with structural heart disease. Avoid in patients with non-life-threatening ventricular arrhythmias, even if experiencing unpleasant, but not life-threatening signs/symptoms.

ADULT DOSAGE	PEDIATRIC DOSAGE
Atrial Fibrillation	Pediatric use may not have been established
In Patients w/ No Structural Heart Disease:	
Initial: 225mg q12h	
Titrate: May increase at a minimum of 5-day intervals to 325mg q12h. May increase to 425mg q12h if additional therapeutic effect is needed	

DOSING CONSIDERATIONS
Hepatic Impairment
Reduce dose

Other Important Considerations
Significant QRS Widening/2nd- or 3rd-degree Atrioventricular Block: Reduce dose

ADMINISTRATION
Oral route
Take w/ or w/o food.
Do not crush or further divide cap contents.

STORAGE
25°C (77°F); excursions permitted to 15-30°C (59-86°F).

HOW SUPPLIED
Cap, Extended-Release: 225mg, 325mg, 425mg

CONTRAINDICATIONS
Heart failure (HF), cardiogenic shock, known Brugada syndrome, bradycardia, marked hypotension, bronchospastic disorders or severe obstructive pulmonary disease, marked electrolyte imbalance, and sinoatrial, AV and intraventricular disorders of impulse generation or conduction (eg, sick sinus node syndrome, AV block) in the absence of an artificial pacemaker.

WARNINGS/PRECAUTIONS
Do not use to control ventricular rate during A-fib. Concomitant treatment with drugs that increase the functional AV nodal refractory period is recommended. May cause new or worsened arrhythmias; evaluate ECG prior to and during therapy. Brugada syndrome may be unmasked after exposure to therapy; perform ECG after initiation of treatment and d/c if changes are suggestive of Brugada syndrome. May provoke overt HF. Proarrhythmic effects more likely occur in patients with HF or severe MI. Conduction disturbances (eg, 1st-degree AV block), agranulocytosis, positive antinuclear antibody (ANA) titers, and exacerbation of myasthenia gravis reported. D/C if persistent or worsening elevation of ANA titers detected. May alter pacing and sensing thresholds of implanted pacemakers and defibrillators; monitor and reprogram devices accordingly during and after therapy. Reversible, short-term drop (within normal range) in sperm count may occur. Caution with renal/hepatic dysfunction.

ADVERSE REACTIONS
Dizziness, palpitations, chest pain, dyspnea, taste disturbance, nausea, fatigue, anxiety, constipation, URTI, edema, influenza.

DRUG INTERACTIONS
Avoid with Class Ia and III antiarrhythmics (eg, quinidine, amiodarone) and withhold these agents for at least 5 half-lives prior to therapy. Inhibitors of CYP2D6 (eg, desipramine, paroxetine, ritonavir) and CYP3A4 (eg, ketoconazole, ritonavir, erythromycin, grapefruit juice) may increase levels; avoid simultaneous use with both a CYP2D6 and a CYP3A4 inhibitor. Amiodarone can affect conduction and repolarization; coadministration is not recommended. Fluoxetine may increase levels in extensive metabolizers. Rifampin may decrease levels and may increase norpropafenone (active metabolite) levels. May increase levels of digoxin, propranolol, metoprolol, and warfarin; monitor digoxin levels and INR. May result in severe adverse events (eg, convulsions, AV block, acute circulatory

failure) with abrupt cessation of orlistat. May increase risk of CNS side effects of lidocaine. CYP1A2 inhibitors (eg, amiodarone, tobacco smoke) and cimetidine may increase levels.

PREGNANCY AND LACTATION
Pregnancy: Category C.
Lactation: Not for use in nursing.

MECHANISM OF ACTION
Class 1C antiarrhythmic; has local anesthetic effects and direct stabilizing action on myocardial membranes. Reduces upstroke velocity (Phase 0) of the monophasic action potential. Reduces the fast inward current carried by Na+ ions in Purkinje fibers and myocardial fibers. Diastolic excitability is increased and effective refractory period is prolonged. Reduces spontaneous automaticity and depresses triggered activity.

PHARMACOKINETICS
Absorption: T_{max}=3-8 hrs. **Distribution:** (IV) V_d=252L; plasma protein binding (>95%); found in breast milk. **Metabolism:** Liver (rapid, extensive) via CYP2D6, 3A4, and 1A2. 5-hydroxypropafenone and N-depropylpropafenone (active metabolites). **Elimination:** $T_{1/2}$=2-10 hrs (>90% of patients), $T_{1/2}$=10-32 hrs (<10% of patients).

PATIENT CONSIDERATIONS
Assessment: Assess for HF, cardiogenic shock, sinoatrial/AV/intraventricular disorders, implanted pacemaker/defibrillator, bradycardia, marked hypotension, bronchospastic disorders or severe obstructive pulmonary disease, marked electrolyte imbalance, MI, renal/hepatic dysfunction, known Brugada syndrome, pregnancy/nursing status, and possible drug interactions. Evaluate ECG prior to therapy.

Monitoring: Monitor for proarrhythmic effects, signs/symptoms of conduction disturbances, agranulocytosis, HF, unmasking of Brugada syndrome, exacerbation of myasthenia gravis, and other adverse reactions. Monitor implanted pacemakers and defibrillators during and after therapy and reprogram accordingly. Evaluate ECG during therapy. Monitor ANA titers, LFTs, and renal/hepatic function.

Counseling: Inform about risks/benefits of therapy. Advise to report symptoms that may be associated with electrolyte imbalance (eg, excessive/prolonged diarrhea, sweating, vomiting, loss of appetite, thirst). Inform to notify physician of all prescription, herbal/natural preparations, and OTC medications currently being taken or of any changes with these products. Instruct not to double the next dose if a dose is missed and to take next dose at the usual time.

SABRIL — vigabatrin   Rx

Class: GABA analogue

> Can cause permanent bilateral concentric visual field constriction including tunnel vision that can result in disability; in some cases, treatment may also damage the central retina and may decrease visual acuity. Onset of vision loss is unpredictable. Risk of vision loss increases w/ increasing dose and cumulative exposure, but there is no dose or exposure known to be free of risk of vision loss. Vision loss may not be recognized until it is severe. Vision should be assessed at baseline (no later than 4 weeks after starting therapy), at least every 3 months during therapy, and about 3-6 months after therapy is discontinued. Once detected, vision loss due to treatment is not reversible. Consider discontinuation, balancing benefit and risk, if visual loss is documented. Risk of new or worsening vision loss continues as long as therapy is used. Vision loss may worsen despite discontinuation of therapy. D/C in patients who fail to show clinical benefit w/in 2-4 weeks (infantile spasms) or 3 months (refractory complex partial seizures) of initiation, or sooner if treatment failure is obvious. Unless benefit clearly outweighs the risk, avoid use w/ other drugs associated w/ serious adverse ophthalmic effects (eg, retinopathy, glaucoma) and in patients w/, or at high risk of, other types of irreversible vision loss. Use lowest dose and shortest exposure to treatment. Available only through a restricted program under a Risk Evaluation and Mitigation Strategy (REMS) called the Sabril REMS Program.

ADULT DOSAGE	PEDIATRIC DOSAGE
Refractory Complex Partial Seizures	**Refractory Complex Partial Seizures**
Adjunctive Therapy:	**Adjunctive Therapy:**
≥17 Years:	**10-16 Years:**
Initial: 1000mg/day (500mg bid)	**25-60kg:**
Titrate: May increase total daily dose in 500mg increments at weekly intervals to a recommended dose of 3000mg/day (1500mg bid)	**Initial:** 500mg/day (250mg bid)
	Titrate: May increase weekly in 500mg/day increments to a total maint dose of 2000mg/day (1000mg bid)
Use lowest dose and shortest exposure to treatment	**>60kg:** Dose according to adult recommendations
	Use lowest dose and shortest exposure to treatment
	Infantile Spasms
	Monotherapy:
	1 Month-2 Years:
	Initial: 50mg/kg/day in 2 divided doses (25mg/kg bid)
	Titrate: Subsequent dosing can be titrated by 25-50mg/kg/day increments every 3 days
	Max: 150mg/kg/day in 2 divided doses (75mg/kg bid)
	Use lowest dose and shortest exposure to treatment

DOSING CONSIDERATIONS
Renal Impairment
Infants:
Information about how to adjust the dose is unavailable
Adults and Pediatric Patients ≥10 Years:
Mild (CrCl >50-80mL/min): Decrease dose by 25%
Moderate (CrCl >30-50mL/min): Decrease dose by 50%
Severe (CrCl >10-30mL/min): Decrease dose by 75%
Discontinuation
Reduce dose gradually to d/c

ADMINISTRATION
Oral route

Take w/ or w/o food.
Either tab or powder for oral sol can be used for complex partial seizures.
Use powder for oral sol for infantile spasms; do not use tabs.

Preparation/Administration of Oral Sol
Mix powder for oral sol w/ water prior to administration.
Empty entire contents of each pkt into a clean cup, and dissolve in 10mL of cold or room temperature water per pkt.
Administer the resulting sol using the 10mL oral syringe supplied w/ medication. The concentration of the final sol is 50mg/mL.
Each individual dose should be prepared and used immediately; discard any unused portion of sol.

STORAGE
20-25°C (68-77°F).

HOW SUPPLIED
Sol: 500mg/pkt [50ˢ]; **Tab:** 500mg* *scored

WARNINGS/PRECAUTIONS
Not indicated as a 1st line agent for complex partial seizures. Abnormal MRI signal changes involving the thalamus, basal ganglia, brain stem, and cerebellum observed in some infants. May increase risk of suicidal thoughts/behavior. Withdraw therapy gradually; rapid discontinuation can be considered if withdrawal is needed because of a serious adverse event. May cause anemia, somnolence, fatigue, peripheral neuropathy, weight gain, and edema. May impair physical/mental abilities. May decrease ALT and AST plasma activity and may preclude the use of these markers, especially ALT, to detect early hepatic injury. May increase amount of amino acids in the urine, possibly leading to false (+) test for certain rare genetic metabolic diseases (eg, alpha aminoadipic aciduria). Caution in elderly.

ADVERSE REACTIONS
Refractory Complex Partial Seizures:
Adults: Fatigue, somnolence, nystagmus, tremor, blurred vision, memory impairment, weight gain, arthralgia, abnormal coordination, confusional state.
Pediatrics (10-16 Years): Weight gain, URTI, tremor, fatigue, aggression, diplopia.
Infantile Spasms:
Somnolence, bronchitis, ear infection, acute otitis media.

DRUG INTERACTIONS
See Boxed Warning. May decrease phenytoin plasma levels; consider dose adjustment of phenytoin if clinically indicated. May increase C_{max} of clonazepam resulting in an increase of clonazepam-associated adverse reactions.

PREGNANCY AND LACTATION
Pregnancy: Category C. Physicians are advised to recommend that pregnant patients taking Sabril enroll in the North American Antiepileptic Drug (NAAED) Pregnancy Registry.
Lactation: Not for use in nursing.

MECHANISM OF ACTION
GABA analogue; has not been established. Believed to be the result of its action as an irreversible inhibitor of GABA transaminase, which results in increased levels of GABA in the CNS.

PHARMACOKINETICS
Absorption: Complete. T_{max}=1 hr (adults/children), 2.5 hrs (infants). **Distribution:** V_d=1.1L/kg; found in breast milk. **Elimination:** Urine (95%, 80% parent drug); $T_{1/2}$=10.5 hrs (adults), 9.5 hrs (children), 5.7 hrs (infants).

PATIENT CONSIDERATIONS
Assessment: Assess for renal impairment, underlying suicidal behavior/ideation, pregnancy/nursing status, and possible drug interactions. Perform baseline vision assessment (no later than 4 weeks after starting therapy).
Monitoring: Monitor for abnormal MRI signal changes, suicidal thoughts/behavior, emergence/worsening of depression, unusual changes in thoughts or behavior, anemia, somnolence, fatigue, peripheral neuropathy, weight gain, edema, and other adverse reactions. Perform vision assessment at least every 3 months during therapy and about 3-6 months after discontinuation of therapy. Periodically reassess response to and continued need for treatment.
Counseling: Inform of the risk of permanent vision loss, particularly loss of peripheral vision, and the need for vision monitoring. Instruct to notify physician if changes in vision are suspected. Inform caregiver(s) of the possibility that infants may develop an abnormal MRI signal of unknown clinical significance. Counsel that therapy may increase risk of suicidal thoughts and behavior; advise of the need to be alert for the emergence or worsening of symptoms of depression, any unusual changes in mood or behavior, or the emergence of suicidal thoughts, behavior, or thoughts of self-harm. Instruct to report immediately to physician behaviors of concern. Instruct to notify physician if pregnant, intending to become pregnant during therapy, or if breastfeeding or intending to breastfeed during therapy; encourage to enroll in the NAAED Pregnancy Registry if pregnant. Advise not to drive a car or operate other complex machinery until familiar w/ the effects of therapy on ability to perform such activities. Instruct not to abruptly d/c therapy.

SAFYRAL — drospirenone/ethinyl estradiol/levomefolate calcium   **Rx**
Class: Estrogen/progestogen combination

> Cigarette smoking increases the risk of serious cardiovascular (CV) events. Risk increases w/ age (>35 yrs of age) and w/ the number of cigarettes smoked. Should not be used by women who are >35 yrs of age and smoke.

ADULT DOSAGE
Contraception
1 tab qd at the same time every day for 28 days, then repeat
Start either on 1st day of menses or on 1st Sunday after onset of menses
Other Indications
May be used to raise folate levels for the purpose of reducing the risk of neural tube defect in a pregnancy conceived while taking the product or shortly after discontinuation
Conversions
Switching from Different Birth Control Pill:
Start on the same day that a new pack of the previous oral contraceptive would have been started
Switching from a Method Other Than a Birth Control Pill:
Transdermal Patch/Vaginal Ring/Inj:
Start when next application or dose would have been due
Intrauterine Contraceptive/Implant:
Start on day of removal

PEDIATRIC DOSAGE
Contraception
Not indicated for use premenarche; refer to adult dosing

DOSING CONSIDERATIONS
Adverse Reactions
GI Disturbances:
In case of severe vomiting or diarrhea, absorption may not be complete and additional contraceptive measures should be taken. If vomiting occurs w/in 3-4 hrs after taking tab, may regard as missed tab

Other Important Considerations
Postpartum Women Who Do Not Breastfeed/After Second Trimester Abortion:
Start therapy no earlier than 4 weeks postpartum; if patient initiates therapy postpartum and has not yet had a period, use an additional method of contraception until patient has taken 7 consecutive days of therapy

ADMINISTRATION
Oral route

Take tabs in the order directed on blister pack, preferably after pm meal or hs.
May be taken w/o regard to meals.
Take single missed pills as soon as remembered.
If 1st taken later than Day 1 of menstrual cycle, use a nonhormonal contraceptive as backup during the first 7 days of therapy.

STORAGE
25°C (77°F); excursions permitted to 15-30°C (59-86°F).

HOW SUPPLIED
Tab: (Drospirenone [DRSP]/Ethinyl Estradiol [EE]/Levomefolate calcium) 3mg/0.03mg/0.451mg; **Tab:** (Levomefolate calcium) 0.451mg

CONTRAINDICATIONS
Renal impairment, adrenal insufficiency, high risk of arterial/venous thrombotic disease (eg, smoking if >35 yrs of age, presence/history of deep vein thrombosis/pulmonary embolism, cerebrovascular disease, coronary artery disease (CAD), thrombogenic valvular or thrombogenic rhythm diseases of the heart [eg, subacute bacterial endocarditis w/ valvular disease, or A-fib], inherited/acquired hypercoagulopathies, uncontrolled HTN, diabetes mellitus [DM] w/ vascular disease, headaches w/ focal neurological symptoms or migraine w/ or w/o aura if >35 yrs of age), undiagnosed abnormal uterine bleeding, presence/history of breast cancer or other estrogen- or progestin-sensitive cancer, benign/malignant liver tumors, liver disease, pregnancy.

WARNINGS/PRECAUTIONS
Increased risk of venous thromboembolism (VTE) and arterial thrombosis (eg, stroke, MI); greatest risk of VTE during the first 6 months of combination oral contraceptive (COC) use and is present after initially starting COC or restarting the same or different COC. D/C if arterial/venous thrombotic event occurs. If feasible, d/c at least 4 weeks before and through 2 weeks after major surgery or other surgeries known to have an elevated risk of thromboembolism. D/C if there is unexplained loss of vision, proptosis, diplopia, papilledema, or retinal vascular lesions; evaluate for retinal vein thrombosis immediately. Potential for hyperkalemia in high-risk patients; contraindicated in patients predisposed to hyperkalemia. May increase risk of cervical cancer, intraepithelial neoplasia, and gallbladder disease. Hepatic adenoma and increased risk of hepatocellular carcinoma reported; d/c if jaundice develops. Cholestasis may occur w/ history of pregnancy-related cholestasis. Increased BP reported; d/c if BP rises significantly. May decrease glucose tolerance; monitor prediabetic and diabetic women. Consider alternative contraception w/ uncontrolled dyslipidemia. May increase risk of pancreatitis w/ hypertriglyceridemia or family history thereof. D/C if new headaches that are recurrent, persistent, or severe develop. Unscheduled bleeding

and spotting may occur; rule out pregnancy or malignancy. May encounter post-pill amenorrhea or oligomenorrhea. Caution w/ history of depression; d/c if depression recurs to serious degree. May change results of some lab tests (eg, coagulation factors, lipids, glucose tolerance, binding proteins). Folate may mask vitamin B12 deficiency. May induce/exacerbate angioedema in patients w/ hereditary angioedema. Chloasma may occur; women w/ a tendency to chloasma should avoid sun exposure or UV radiation.

ADVERSE REACTIONS
Premenstrual syndrome, headache/migraine, breast pain/tenderness/discomfort, N/V.

DRUG INTERACTIONS
Consider monitoring serum K^+ levels in high-risk patients who take a strong CYP3A4 inhibitor long-term and concomitantly. Potential for an increase in serum K^+ levels w/ use of other drugs that may increase serum K^+ (eg, ACE inhibitors, heparin, aldosterone antagonists, NSAIDs); monitor K^+ levels during 1st treatment cycle in women receiving daily, long-term treatment for chronic conditions/ diseases. Agents that induce certain enzymes, including CYP3A4 (eg, phenytoin, barbiturates, products containing St. John's wort), may decrease COC efficacy or increase breakthrough bleeding; use an alternative contraceptive or a backup method when using inducers and continue backup contraception for 28 days after discontinuation of the inducer. Significant changes (increase or decrease) in plasma estrogen and progestin concentrations reported w/ HIV/hepatitis C virus protease inhibitors or non-nucleoside reverse transcriptase inhibitors. Pregnancy reported w/ antibiotics. Atorvastatin may increase EE exposure. Ascorbic acid and acetaminophen may increase EE concentrations. Moderate or strong CYP3A4 inhibitors such as azole antifungals (eg, ketoconazole, itraconazole, voriconazole, fluconazole), verapamil, macrolides (eg, clarithromycin, erythromycin), diltiazem, and grapefruit juice may increase plasma concentrations of estrogen or progestin or both. May decrease concentrations of lamotrigine and reduce seizure control; dosage adjustments of lamotrigine may be necessary. May increase plasma concentrations of CYP3A4 substrates (eg, midazolam), CYP2C19 substrates (eg, omeprazole, voriconazole), and CYP1A2 substrates (eg, theophylline, tizanidine). Increases thyroid-binding globulin levels; may need to increase dose of thyroid hormone in patients on thyroid hormone replacement therapy. May decrease pharmacological effect of antifolate drugs (eg, antiepileptics, methotrexate [MTX], pyrimethamine). Reduced folate concentrations via inhibition of dihydrofolate reductase enzyme (eg, MTX, sulfasalazine), reduction of folate absorption (eg, cholestyramine), or via unknown mechanisms (eg, antiepileptics, such as carbamazepine, phenytoin, phenobarbital, primidone, valproic acid).

PREGNANCY AND LACTATION
Pregnancy: Contraindicated in pregnancy.
Lactation: Not for use in nursing.

MECHANISM OF ACTION
Estrogen/progestogen oral contraceptive; acts by primarily suppressing ovulation. Other possible mechanisms may include cervical mucus changes that inhibit sperm penetration and endometrial changes that reduce the likelihood of implantation.

PHARMACOKINETICS
Absorption: DRSP: Absolute bioavailability (76%); T_{max}=1-2 hrs. EE: Absolute bioavailability (40%); T_{max}=1-2 hrs. Levomefolate: T_{max}=0.5-1.5 hrs. Refer to PI for further information on absorption parameters. **Distribution:** Found in breast milk; DRSP: V_d=4L/kg; serum protein binding (97%). EE: V_d=4-5L/kg; serum albumin binding (98.5%). **Metabolism:** DRSP: Reduction, subsequent sulfation, oxidation catalyzed by CYP3A4. EE: Gut and liver (1st-pass), conjugation w/ glucuronide or sulfate, hydroxylation (via CYP3A4). **Elimination:** DRSP: Urine, feces; $T_{1/2}$=30 hrs. EE: Urine, feces; $T_{1/2}$=24 hrs. Levomefolate (L-5-methyl-THF): Urine, feces; $T_{1/2}$=4-5 hrs.

PATIENT CONSIDERATIONS
Assessment: Assess for renal impairment, abnormal uterine bleeding, adrenal insufficiency, CAD, thrombogenic valvular or thrombogenic rhythm diseases of the heart, pregnancy/nursing status, and for any other conditions where treatment is cautioned or contraindicated. Assess for possible drug interactions. Assess BP levels.

Monitoring: Monitor for bleeding irregularities, venous/arterial thrombotic events, cervical cancer or intraepithelial neoplasia, retinal vein thrombosis, jaundice, new/ worsening headaches or migraines, serious depression, cholestasis w/ history of pregnancy-related cholestasis, pancreatitis, and for other adverse reactions. Monitor K^+ levels, thyroid function if receiving thyroid replacement therapy, glucose levels in diabetic and prediabetic patients, depression in patients w/ a history of depression, lipids levels in patients w/ dyslipidemia, and BP in patients w/ HTN. Conduct yearly visit w/ all patients for a BP check and for other indicated healthcare.

Counseling: Inform of benefits and risks of therapy. Counsel that cigarette smoking increases the risk of serious CV events. Inform that drug does not protect against HIV infection and other STDs. Instruct to take at the same time every day preferably after pm meal or hs. Instruct on what to do if pills are missed or vomiting occurs w/in 3-4 hrs after taking tab. Inform that COCs may reduce breast milk production. Inform that amenorrhea may occur and pregnancy should be ruled out if amenorrhea occurs in ≥2 consecutive cycles. Counsel to report if taking folate supplements and advise to maintain folate supplementation upon discontinuation due to pregnancy. Advise to inform physician of preexisting medical conditions and/or drugs currently being taken. Counsel women who start COCs postpartum and have not yet had a period to use additional method of contraception until drug is taken for 7 consecutive days. Instruct to d/c if pregnancy occurs during treatment.

SAIZEN — somatropin (rDNA origin)   Rx
Class: Recombinant human growth hormone (hGH)

ADULT DOSAGE	PEDIATRIC DOSAGE
Growth Hormone Deficiency	**Growth Hormone Deficiency**
Adult or Childhood Onset Etiology:	**Due to Inadequate Secretion of**
Weight-Based:	**Endogenous Growth Hormone:**
Initial: ≤0.005mg/kg qd SQ	**Usual:** 0.18mg/kg/week SQ divided
Titrate: May increase to ≤0.01mg/kg/ day after 4 weeks based on individual requirements	into equal doses given either on 3 alternate days, 6X/week or daily
Non-Weight-Based:	
Initial: 0.2mg/day SQ (range, 0.15-0.30mg/day)	
Titrate: May increase gradually every 1-2 months by increments of 0.1-0.2mg/day based on clinical response and serum insulin-like growth factor-I (IGF-I) concentrations	
Maint: Individualize dose	

DOSING CONSIDERATIONS
Concomitant Medications
Oral Estrogen: Adult women may require a larger dose of somatropin

Elderly
Consider lower starting dose and smaller dose increments

ADMINISTRATION
SQ route

Reconstitution
1. Determine the appropriate patient dose 1st and then each vial should be reconstituted as follows: 5mg vial w/ 1-3mL of bacteriostatic water for inj (benzyl alcohol preserved); 8.8mg vial w/ 2-3mL of bacteriostatic water for inj (benzyl alcohol preserved)
2. If sensitivity to the diluent occurs, may reconstitute w/ sterile water for inj, the reconstituted sol should be used immediately and any unused sol should be discarded
3. Following reconstitution, swirl the vial w/ a gentle rotary motion until contents are completely dissolved; do not shake and use it only if it is clear and colorless

STORAGE
15-30°C (59-86°F). Reconstituted Sol: 2-8°C (36-46°F) for up to 14 days for vials and for up to 21 days for click.easy. Avoid freezing.

HOW SUPPLIED
Inj: 5mg [vial], 8.8mg [vial, click.easy]

CONTRAINDICATIONS
Acute critical illness due to complications following open heart surgery, abdominal surgery, multiple accidental trauma, or with acute respiratory failure. Pediatric patients with Prader-Willi syndrome (PWS) who are severely obese or have severe respiratory impairment. Long-term treatment of pediatric patients who have growth failure due to genetically confirmed PWS. Active malignancy, or evidence of progression or recurrence of an underlying intracranial tumor. Active proliferative or severe nonproliferative diabetic retinopathy. Growth promotion in pediatric patients with closed epiphysis. Known sensitivity to benzyl alcohol (bacteriostatic water for inj diluent), somatropin, or any components of the medication.

WARNINGS/PRECAUTIONS
Reevaluate adults who were treated with somatropin for GHD in childhood and whose epiphyses are closed. D/C when epiphyses are fused. Implement effective weight control in patients with PWS and treat respiratory infections aggressively. Increased risk of developing malignancies in children with certain rare genetic causes of short stature; monitor for development of neoplasms if treatment is initiated. Monitor for increased growth, or potential malignant changes of preexisting nevi. Undiagnosed impaired glucose tolerance and overt diabetes mellitus (DM) may be unmasked, and new-onset type 2 DM reported. Intracranial HTN with papilledema, visual changes, headache, N/V reported; d/c therapy if papilledema occurs. Fluid retention in adults may occur. Undiagnosed/untreated hypothyroidism may prevent optimal response. Hypothyroidism may become evident or worsen. Slipped capital femoral epiphysis (SCFE) and progression of scoliosis may occur in pediatric patients. Tissue atrophy may occur; rotate inj site. Allergic reactions may occur. Monitor other hormonal replacement treatments in patients with hypopituitarism. Serum levels of inorganic phosphorus, alkaline phosphatase, parathyroid hormone, and IGF-I may increase. Pancreatitis reported rarely. Bacteriostatic water for inj diluent contains benzyl alcohol, which has been associated with serious adverse events and death, particularly in pediatric patients. Caution in elderly.

ADVERSE REACTIONS
Arthralgia, headache, peripheral edema, myalgia, paresthesia, hypoaesthesia, skeletal pain, insomnia, carpal tunnel syndrome, generalized edema, depression, chest pain, hypothyroidism, dependent edema.

DRUG INTERACTIONS
May inhibit 11β-hydroxysteroid dehydrogenase type 1, resulting in reduced serum cortisol concentrations; may need glucocorticoid replacement or dose adjustments of glucocorticoid therapy. Glucocorticoid therapy may attenuate

growth-promoting effects in children; carefully adjust glucocorticoid replacement dosing. May increase clearance of antipyrine. May alter clearance of compounds metabolized by CYP450 liver enzymes (eg, corticosteroids, sex steroids, anticonvulsants, cyclosporine); monitor carefully. Oral estrogen replacement may increase dose requirements. May need to adjust dose of insulin and/or oral/injectable hypoglycemic agents, and thyroid hormone replacement therapy.

PREGNANCY AND LACTATION
Category B, caution in nursing.

MECHANISM OF ACTION
Recombinant human GH; binds to dimeric GH receptors in cell membranes of target tissue cells resulting in intracellular signal transduction.

PHARMACOKINETICS
Absorption: Absolute bioavailability (70-90%). **Distribution:** V_d=12L (IV). **Metabolism:** Liver and kidneys. **Elimination:** $T_{1/2}$=2 hrs.

PATIENT CONSIDERATIONS
Assessment: Assess for PWS, preexisting DM or impaired glucose tolerance, hypothyroidism, hypopituitarism, history of scoliosis, hypersensitivity to drug or to benzyl alcohol, any other conditions where treatment is contraindicated or cautioned, pregnancy/nursing status, and possible drug interactions. Perform funduscopic exam.

Monitoring: Monitor growth, for clinical response, compliance, neoplasm, increased growth or malignant changes of preexisting nevi, intracranial HTN, fluid retention, allergic reactions, pancreatitis, and SCFE and progression of scoliosis in pediatric patients. Perform periodic thyroid function tests, funduscopic exam, and monitor glucose levels. In patients with PWS, monitor weight as well as for signs of respiratory infection, sleep apnea, and upper airway obstruction. Monitor patients with a history of GHD secondary to an intracranial neoplasm routinely for progression/recurrence of the tumor.

Counseling: Inform about potential benefits and risks of therapy, proper administration, usage and disposal, and caution against any reuse of needles and syringes.

SAMSCA — tolvaptan
Rx

Class: Arginine vasopressin antagonist

> Initiate and reinitiate therapy in patients only in a hospital where serum Na+ can be monitored closely. Osmotic demyelination resulting in dysarthria, mutism, dysphagia, lethargy, affective changes, spastic quadriparesis, seizures, coma, and death may occur due to rapid correction of hyponatremia (eg, >12mEq/L/24 hrs). Slower rates of correction may be advisable in susceptible patients (eg, with severe malnutrition, alcoholism, advanced liver disease).

ADULT DOSAGE
Hyponatremia

Hypervolemic and Euvolemic Hyponatremia:
Including Patients w/ HF and SIADH:
Initial: 15mg qd
Titrate: Increase to 30mg qd, after at least 24 hrs
Max Dose: 60mg qd
Max Duration: 30 days

Patients should be in a hospital for initiation and reinitiation of therapy

Avoid fluid restriction during the first 24 hrs of therapy; patients can continue ingestion of fluid in response to thirst. Following discontinuation, patients should be advised to resume fluid restriction

PEDIATRIC DOSAGE
Pediatric use may not have been established

DOSING CONSIDERATIONS
Concomitant Medications
Moderate CYP3A Inhibitors: Avoid coadmistration
Potent CYP3A Inducers: Monitor response and adjust dose accordingly
P-gp Inhibitors: Coadmistration may necessitate a decrease in tolvaptan dose
Renal Impairment
CrCl <10mL/min: Not recommended for use
Hepatic Impairment
Underlying Liver Disease: Avoid use
ADMINISTRATION
Oral route

Take w/o regard to meals
STORAGE
25°C (77°F); excursions permitted between 15-30°C (59-86°F).
HOW SUPPLIED
Tab: 15mg, 30mg
CONTRAINDICATIONS
Urgent need to raise serum Na+ acutely, inability to autoregulate fluid balance, hypovolemic hyponatremia, anuria, and concomitant use of strong CYP3A inhibitors (eg, clarithromycin, ketoconazole, itraconazole, ritonavir, indinavir, nelfinavir, saquinavir, nefazodone, telithromycin). Hypersensitivity (eg, anaphylactic shock, rash generalized) to tolvaptan or any component of the product.

WARNINGS/PRECAUTIONS
Frequently monitor for changes in serum electrolytes and volume during initiation and titration. Allow to continue fluid ingestion in response to thirst. Resume fluid restriction and monitor for serum Na+ and volume status changes following discontinuation of therapy. D/C or interrupt therapy if patient develops elevation in serum Na+ too rapidly; consider hypotonic fluid administration. Serious and potentially fatal liver injury may occur; avoid use in patients with underlying liver disease, including cirrhosis, and d/c therapy in patients with symptoms that may indicate liver injury. May induce copious aquaresis. Dehydration and hypovolemia may occur, especially in potentially volume-depleted patients receiving diuretics or those who are fluid restricted; interrupt or d/c therapy and provide supportive care with careful management of vital signs, fluid balance, and electrolytes if signs/symptoms of hypovolemia develop. Concomitant use with hypertonic saline is not recommended. Increased serum K+ levels may occur; monitor serum K+ levels after initiation of therapy in patients with serum K+ >5mEq/L and those receiving drugs known to increase serum K+ levels. Not recommended for patients with CrCl <10mL/min.

ADVERSE REACTIONS
Osmotic demyelination, thirst, dry mouth, pollakiuria/polyuria, nausea, asthenia, constipation, hyperglycemia, pyrexia, anorexia.

DRUG INTERACTIONS
See Contraindications. Avoid with moderate CYP3A inhibitors (eg, erythromycin, fluconazole, aprepitant, diltiazem, verapamil). Avoid with CYP3A inducers (eg, rifampin, rifabutin, rifapentin, barbiturates, phenytoin, carbamazepine, St. John's wort); if coadministered, the dose of tolvaptan may need to be increased. Dose reduction of tolvaptan may be required when coadministered with P-gp inhibitors (eg, cyclosporine). Grapefruit juice may increase exposure. Increases exposure of digoxin. Higher incidence of hyperkalemia with ARBs, ACE inhibitors, and K+-sparing diuretics; monitor serum K+ levels. Not recommended with vasopressin V_2 agonist (eg, desmopressin).

PREGNANCY AND LACTATION
Category C, not for use in nursing.

MECHANISM OF ACTION
Arginine vasopressin antagonist; antagonizes the effect of vasopressin and causes an increase in urine water excretion, resulting in an increase in free water clearance (aquaresis), a decrease in urine osmolality, and an increase in serum Na+ concentrations.

PHARMACOKINETICS
Absorption: T_{max}=2-4 hrs. **Distribution:** V_d=3L/kg; plasma protein binding (99%). **Metabolism:** Via CYP3A. **Elimination:** $T_{1/2}$=12 hrs.

PATIENT CONSIDERATIONS
Assessment: Assess serum Na+ levels, neurologic status, ability to respond to thirst, renal/hepatic function, for hypersensitivity to drug, any other conditions where treatment is cautioned or contraindicated, pregnancy/nursing status, and possible drug interactions.

Monitoring: Monitor for osmotic demyelination, changes in serum Na+/electrolytes/volume, neurologic status, signs/symptoms of hypovolemia, liver injury, hypersensitivity reactions, and other adverse reactions. Monitor serum K+ levels in patients with serum K+ >5mEq/L and those receiving drugs known to increase serum K+ levels.

Counseling: Advise to continue ingestion of fluid in response to thirst. Advise to resume fluid restriction following discontinuation of therapy. Instruct to inform physician if taking or planning to take any prescription or OTC drugs. Advise not to breastfeed during therapy.

SANCUSO — granisetron
Rx

Class: 5-HT$_3$ receptor antagonist

ADULT DOSAGE
Chemotherapy-Induced Nausea/Vomiting

Prevention of N/V in Patients Receiving Moderately and/or Highly Emetogenic Chemotherapy Regimens of up to 5 Consecutive Days Duration:
Apply a single patch to the upper outer arm a minimum of 24 hrs before chemotherapy; may apply up to a max of 48 hrs before chemotherapy as appropriate. Remove patch a minimum of 24 hrs after completion of chemotherapy; may be worn for up to 7 days depending on duration of chemotherapy regimen

PEDIATRIC DOSAGE
Pediatric use may not have been established

ADMINISTRATION
Transdermal route

Apply to clean, dry, intact, healthy skin on the upper outer arm; do not place on skin that is red, irritated, or damaged.
Apply directly after the pouch has been opened.
Do not cut the patch into pieces.
STORAGE
20-25°C (68-77°F); excursions permitted between 15-30°C (59-86°F).

HOW SUPPLIED
Patch: 3.1mg/24 hrs

CONTRAINDICATIONS
Known hypersensitivity to granisetron or to any of the components of this medication.

WARNINGS/PRECAUTIONS
May mask a progressive ileus and/or gastric distention caused by the underlying condition. Serotonin syndrome may develop; d/c therapy and initiate supportive treatment if symptoms occur. Application-site reactions reported; remove patch if a severe reaction or a generalized skin reaction occurs. Avoid applying a heat pad over or in vicinity of patch and avoid prolonged exposure to heat; plasma concentration continues increasing during the period of heat exposure. May be affected by direct natural or artificial sunlight; cover the patch application site if there is a risk of exposure to sunlight throughout the period of wear and for 10 days following its removal because of a potential skin reaction. Caution in elderly.

ADVERSE REACTIONS
Constipation.

DRUG INTERACTIONS
CYP1A1 and CYP3A4 inducers or inhibitors may change clearance and hence, the $T_{1/2}$. Ketoconazole inhibited ring oxidation (in vitro). Phenobarbital may increase clearance. May cause serotonin syndrome w/ serotonergic drugs (eg, SSRIs, SNRIs, MAOIs, mirtazapine, fentanyl, lithium, tramadol, IV methylene blue); d/c therapy and initiate supportive treatment if symptoms occur.

PREGNANCY AND LACTATION
Pregnancy: Category B.
Lactation: It is not known whether granisetron is excreted in human milk; caution in nursing.

MECHANISM OF ACTION
5-HT$_3$ receptor antagonist; antinauseant and antiemetic. Blocks serotonin stimulation and subsequent vomiting after emetogenic stimuli.

PHARMACOKINETICS
Absorption: T_{max}=48 hrs; C_{max}=5ng/mL; $AUC_{0-168hr}$=527ng•hr/mL. Distribution: Plasma protein binding (65%). Metabolism: CYP3A; N-demethylation and aromatic ring oxidation followed by conjugation. Elimination: (IV) Urine (49% metabolites, 12% unchanged), feces (34% metabolites).

PATIENT CONSIDERATIONS
Assessment: Assess for drug hypersensitivity, pregnancy/nursing status, and possible drug interactions.

Monitoring: Monitor for masking of progressive ileus and/or gastric distention, application-site/skin reactions, serotonin syndrome, and other adverse reactions.

Counseling: Advise to inform physician if patient has abdominal pain/swelling. Instruct to remove patch if a severe or a generalized skin reaction occurs; advise to peel off gently when removing the patch. Advise to cover the patch application site (eg, w/ clothing) if there is a risk of exposure to sunlight or sunlamps throughout the period of wear and for 10 days following its removal. Inform of the possibility of serotonin syndrome and instruct to seek immediate medical attention if symptoms occur. Advise not to apply a heat pad over or near the patch and avoid prolonged exposure to heat.

SANDOSTATIN — octreotide acetate   Rx

Class: Somatostatin analogue

ADULT DOSAGE

Acromegaly
To reduce blood levels of growth hormone and insulin-like growth factor-1 (IGF-I) (somatomedin C) in acromegaly patients who have had inadequate response to or cannot be treated w/ surgical resection, pituitary irradiation, and bromocriptine mesylate at maximally tolerated doses

Initial: 50mcg tid
Usual: 100mcg tid; some patients require up to 500mcg tid

If an increase in dose fails to provide additional benefit, the dose should be reduced

Withdraw yearly for approx 4 weeks from patients who have received irradiation to assess disease activity; if growth hormone or IGF-I (somatomedin C) levels increase and signs and symptoms recur, therapy may be resumed

Carcinoid Tumors
Symptomatic treatment of patients w/ metastatic carcinoid tumors where it suppresses or inhibits the severe diarrhea and flushing episodes associated w/ the disease

Usual: 100-600mcg/day in 2-4 divided doses (mean dose is 300mcg/day) for the first 2 weeks of therapy

PEDIATRIC DOSAGE
Pediatric use may not have been established

In clinical studies, the median maint dose was approx 450mcg/day, but benefits were obtained in some patients w/ as little as 50mcg, while others required up to 1500mcg/day; experience w/ doses >750mcg/day is limited

Vasoactive Intestinal Peptide-Secreting Tumors
Treatment of the profuse watery diarrhea associated w/ vasoactive intestinal peptide-secreting tumors

Usual: 200-300mcg/day in 2-4 divided doses during the initial 2 weeks of therapy (range 150-750mcg)
Titrate: Adjust dose to achieve a therapeutic response; usually doses >450mcg/day are not required

---

DOSING CONSIDERATIONS
Elderly
Start at lower end of dosing range

ADMINISTRATION
IV/SQ routes
Avoid multiple SQ inj at the same site w/in short periods of time; rotate sites in a systematic manner.
Not compatible in TPN sol.
Stable in sterile isotonic saline sol or sterile sol of D5W for 24 hrs.

Preparation and Administration
Octreotide may be diluted in volumes of 50-200mL and infused IV over 15-30 min or administered by IV push over 3 min; in emergency situations (eg, carcinoid crisis) it may be given by rapid bolus.

STORAGE
2-8°C (36-46°F) for prolonged storage. Protect from light. Stable for 14 days at 20-30°C (70-86°F) if protected from light. Do not warm artificially; sol can be allowed to come to room temperature prior administration. After initial use, multidose vials should be discarded within 14 days. Open ampuls prior to administration and discard unused portion.

HOW SUPPLIED
Inj: 50mcg/mL, 100mcg/mL, 200mcg/mL, 500mcg/mL, 1000mcg/mL

CONTRAINDICATIONS
Sensitivity to this drug or any of its components.

WARNINGS/PRECAUTIONS
May inhibit gallbladder contractility and decrease bile secretion; increased risk of gallbladder abnormalities. May alter balance between the counter-regulatory hormones, insulin, glucagon, and GH and lead to hypo- or hyperglycemia; monitor glucose tolerance periodically. May cause hypothyroidism; monitor thyroid levels periodically. Cardiac conduction and other cardiovascular abnormalities (eg, bradycardia, arrhythmias) may occur; caution in patients at risk. Risk of pregnancy with normalization of IGF-1 and GH in acromegalic women. Pancreatitis, depressed vitamin B12 levels, alteration in fat absorption, and abnormal Schilling's test reported. Caution in elderly.

ADVERSE REACTIONS
Gallbladder abnormalities, cardiac abnormalities, abdominal discomfort, diarrhea, loose stool, N/V, abdominal distention, flatulence, constipation, headache, dizziness, hypoglycemia, hyperglycemia, hypothyroidism.

DRUG INTERACTIONS
May alter absorption of orally administered drugs. May decrease blood levels of cyclosporine and may result in transplant rejection. May require dose adjustments of insulin, oral hypoglycemics, β-blockers, calcium channel blockers, or agents that control fluid and electrolyte balance. Increased availability of bromocriptine. May decrease the metabolic clearance of compounds known to be metabolized by CYP450; caution with other drugs mainly metabolized by CYP3A4 and which have a low therapeutic index (eg, quinidine, terfenadine).

PREGNANCY AND LACTATION
Pregnancy: Category B.
Lactation: Caution in nursing.

MECHANISM OF ACTION
Somatostatin analog; exerts similar pharmacologic actions to natural hormone somatostatin, but is more potent in inhibiting GH, glucagon, and insulin. Like somatostatin, it also suppresses luteinizing hormone response to gonadotropin-releasing hormone, decreases splanchnic blood flow, and inhibits release of serotonin, gastrin, vasoactive intestinal peptide (VIP), secretin, motilin, and pancreatic polypeptide.

PHARMACOKINETICS
Absorption: (SQ) Rapid and complete; (100mcg) C_{max}=5.2ng/mL, T_{max}=0.4 hrs; (Acromegaly, 100mcg SQ) C_{max}=2.8ng/mL, T_{max}=0.7 hr. Distribution: V_d=13.6L, plasma protein binding (65%); (Acromegaly) V_d=21.6L, plasma protein binding (41.2%). Elimination: Urine (32% unchanged); $T_{1/2}$=1.7-1.9 hrs. $T_{1/2}$ varies based on the severity of renal and liver disease; refer to PI for further details.

PATIENT CONSIDERATIONS
Assessment: Assess for drug hypersensitivity, renal impairment, diabetes mellitus, cardiac dysfunction, pregnancy/nursing status, and possible drug interactions. Obtain baseline thyroid function tests (TSH, total and/or free T4).

Monitoring: Monitor for biliary tract abnormalities, hypo- and hyperglycemia, hypothyroidism, cardiac conduction abnormalities, and pancreatitis. Monitor GH levels at 1-4 hr intervals for 8-12 hrs post-dose or IGF-1 levels at 2 weeks after drug initiation or dose change with acromegaly. Monitor urinary 5-hydroxyindole acetic acid, plasma serotonin, and plasma Substance P levels with carcinoid tumors. Monitor VIP levels in patients with VIPomas. Monitor thyroid function (periodically) and vitamin B12 levels with chronic therapy.

Counseling: Advise of risks and benefits of treatment. Instruct patients and other persons who may administer the medication about sterile SQ inj technique. Advise female patients of childbearing potential to use contraception during therapy.

SANDOSTATIN LAR — octreotide acetate

Class: Somatostatin analogue

Rx

ADULT DOSAGE

Acromegaly

Long-Term Maint Therapy in Patients Who Have Had an Inadequate Response to Surgery and/or Radiotherapy, or if Surgery and/or Radiotherapy is Not an Option:

Not Currently Receiving Octreotide:
Begin therapy w/ Sandostatin SQ (initial dose of 50mcg tid; most patients require doses of 100-200mcg tid but some patients require up to 500mcg tid) and maintain for at least 2 weeks to determine tolerance

Patients considered to be responders to the drug and who tolerate it may be switched to Sandostatin LAR

Currently Receiving Sandostatin Inj:
Initial: 20mg at 4-week intervals for 3 months

Titrate:
After 3 Months:
Growth Hormone (GH) ≤2.5ng/mL, Normal Insulin-Like Growth Factor-1 (IGF-1), and Controlled Clinical Symptoms: Maintain at 20mg every 4 weeks
GH >2.5ng/mL, Elevated IGF-1, and/or Uncontrolled Clinical Symptoms: Increase to 30mg every 4 weeks
GH ≤1ng/mL, Normal IGF-1, and Controlled Clinical Symptoms: Reduce to 10mg every 4 weeks
GH, IGF-1, or Symptoms Are Not Adequately Controlled at 30mg: May increase to 40mg every 4 weeks

Max: 40mg every 4 weeks

In patients who have received pituitary irradiation, withdraw therapy yearly for 8 weeks to assess disease activity; may resume therapy if GH or IGF-1 levels increase and signs/symptoms recur

Carcinoid Tumors

Long-Term Treatment of Severe Diarrhea and Flushing Episodes Associated w/ Metastatic Carcinoid Tumors:

Not Currently Receiving Octreotide:
Begin therapy w/ Sandostatin SQ (100-600mcg/day in 2-4 divided doses; some patients may require doses up to 1500mcg/day) and maintain for at least 2 weeks to determine tolerance

Patients considered to be responders to the drug and who tolerate it may be switched to Sandostatin LAR

Currently Receiving Sandostatin Inj:
Initial: 20mg at 4-week intervals for 2 months; patients should continue to receive Sandostatin SQ for at least 2 weeks in the same dosage taken before the switch

Titrate:
If Symptoms Are Adequately Controlled After 2 Months:
Consider reducing to 10mg for a trial period; if symptoms recur, then increase to 20mg every 4 weeks

PEDIATRIC DOSAGE
Pediatric use may not have been established

If Symptoms Are Not Adequately Controlled After 2 Months:
Increase to 30mg every 4 weeks; lower to 10mg for a trial period if good control is achieved on 20mg dose and if symptoms recur, increase to 20mg every 4 weeks

Max: 30mg every 4 weeks

For exacerbation of symptoms, may give Sandostatin SQ for a few days at the dosage received prior to switching to Sandostatin LAR; d/c when symptoms are again controlled

Vasoactive Intestinal Peptide-Secreting Tumors

Long-Term Treatment of Profuse Watery Diarrhea Associated w/ Vasoactive Intestinal Peptide-Secreting Tumors (VIPomas):

Not Currently Receiving Octreotide:
Begin therapy w/ Sandostatin SQ (200-300mcg in 2-4 divided doses [range 150-750mcg]; doses >450mcg/day are usually not required) and maintain for at least 2 weeks to determine tolerance

Patients considered to be responders to the drug and who tolerate it may be switched to Sandostatin LAR

Currently Receiving Sandostatin Inj:
Initial: 20mg at 4-week intervals for 2 months; patients should continue to receive Sandostatin SQ for at least 2 weeks in the same dosage taken before the switch

Titrate:
If Symptoms Are Adequately Controlled After 2 Months:
Consider reducing to 10mg for a trial period; if symptoms recur, then increase to 20mg every 4 weeks
If Symptoms Are Not Adequately Controlled After 2 Months:
Increase to 30mg every 4 weeks; lower to 10mg for a trial period if good control is achieved on 20mg dose and if symptoms recur, increase to 20mg every 4 weeks

Max: 30mg every 4 weeks

For exacerbation of symptoms, may give Sandostatin SQ for a few days at the dosage received prior to switching to Sandostatin LAR; d/c when symptoms are again controlled

---

DOSING CONSIDERATIONS
Renal Impairment
Renal Failure Requiring Dialysis:
Initial: 10mg every 4 weeks

Hepatic Impairment
Cirrhotic Patients:
Initial: 10mg every 4 weeks

Elderly
Start at lower end of dosing range

ADMINISTRATION
IM route

Administer in the gluteal region; avoid deltoid inj.
Rotate inj sites to avoid irritation.
Administer immediately after reconstitution; do not directly inject diluent w/o preparing sus.
Refer to PI for further administration instructions.

STORAGE
2-8°C (36-46°F). Protect from light until time of use. Drug product kit should remain at room temperature for 30-60 min prior to preparation of drug sus.

HOW SUPPLIED
Inj, Depot: 10mg, 20mg, 30mg

WARNINGS/PRECAUTIONS
Should be administered by a trained healthcare provider. Rotate inj sites in a systematic manner to avoid irritation. May inhibit gallbladder contractility and decrease bile secretion, which may lead to gallbladder abnormalities or sludge. Alters balance between the counter-regulatory hormones, insulin, glucagon, and GH, which may result in hypo/hyperglycemia. Hypothyroidism may occur. Bradycardia, arrhythmias, and cardiac conduction abnormalities reported. May alter dietary fat absorption. Depressed vitamin B12 levels and abnormal Schilling

test reported. Serum zinc may rise excessively when fluid loss is reversed in patients on TPN. Caution in elderly.

ADVERSE REACTIONS

Acromegaly: Diarrhea, cholelithiasis, abdominal pain, flatulence.
Carcinoid Tumors and VIPomas: Back pain, fatigue, headache, abdominal pain, nausea, dizziness.

DRUG INTERACTIONS

Associated w/ nutrient absorption alterations; may alter absorption of orally administered drugs. May decrease cyclosporine levels and result in transplant rejection. May need dose adjustments of insulin, oral hypoglycemics, and drugs w/ bradycardic effects (eg, β-blockers). Increases availability of bromocriptine. May decrease metabolic clearance of drugs metabolized by CYP450; caution w/ other drugs mainly metabolized by CYP3A4 and which have a low therapeutic index (eg, quinidine, terfenadine).

PREGNANCY AND LACTATION

Pregnancy: Category B.
Lactation: Caution in nursing.

MECHANISM OF ACTION

Somatostatin analogue; long acting. Exerts similar actions to natural hormone somatostatin, but is more potent in inhibiting GH, glucagon, and insulin. Like somatostatin, it also suppresses luteinizing hormone response to gonadotropin-releasing hormone, decreases splanchnic blood flow, and inhibits release of serotonin, gastrin, vasoactive intestinal peptide, secretin, motilin, and pancreatic polypeptide.

PHARMACOKINETICS

Absorption: (Acromegaly; Day 1) C_{max}=0.3ng/mL (10mg), 0.8ng/mL (20mg), 1.3ng/mL (30mg).

PATIENT CONSIDERATIONS

Assessment: Assess for renal/hepatic impairment, cardiac dysfunction, pregnancy/nursing status, and possible drug interactions. Obtain baseline thyroid function tests (TSH, total and/or free T4) and glucose levels. Obtain baseline plasma vasoactive intestinal peptide levels in patients w/ VIPoma.

Monitoring: Monitor for signs/symptoms of gallbladder abnormalities or sludge, hypo/hyperglycemia, hypothyroidism, bradycardia, arrhythmia, cardiac conduction abnormalities, and other adverse reactions. Monitor zinc levels if receiving TPN. Monitor vitamin B12 levels. Monitor thyroid function periodically during chronic therapy. Monitor GH and IGF-1 levels in patients w/ acromegaly. Monitor urinary 5-hydroxyindole acetic acid, plasma serotonin, and plasma substance P levels in patients w/ carcinoids. Monitor glucose levels when the dose is altered.

Counseling: Inform of the risks and benefits of treatment. Advise patients w/ carcinoid tumors and VIPomas to adhere closely to scheduled return visits for reinjection to minimize exacerbation of symptoms. Instruct patients w/ acromegaly to adhere to a return visit schedule to help assure steady control of GH and IGF-1 levels.

SAPHRIS — asenapine   Rx

Class: Atypical antipsychotic

> Elderly patients w/ dementia-related psychosis treated w/ antipsychotic drugs are at an increased risk of death. Not approved for treatment of patients w/ dementia-related psychosis.

ADULT DOSAGE

Schizophrenia

5mg bid
Titrate: May increase to 10mg bid after 1 week
Max: 10mg bid

Bipolar I Disorder

Acute Treatment of Manic or Mixed Episodes:
Monotherapy:
Initial: 10mg bid
Titrate: May decrease to 5mg bid if warranted by adverse effects
Max: 10mg bid

Adjunctive Therapy (w/ Lithium or Valproate):
Initial: 5mg bid
Titrate: May increase to 10mg bid
Max: 10mg bid

PEDIATRIC DOSAGE

Bipolar I Disorder

Acute Treatment of Manic or Mixed Episodes:
10-17 Years:
Monotherapy:
Initial: 2.5mg bid
Titrate: May increase to 5mg bid after 3 days, and from 5mg to 10mg bid after 3 additional days
Max: 10mg bid

Pediatric patients appear to be more sensitive to dystonia w/ initial dosing when recommended escalation schedule is not followed

ADMINISTRATION

SL route
Place tab under the tongue and allow it to dissolve completely.
Do not split, crush, chew, or swallow tabs.
Do not eat/drink for 10 min after administration.

STORAGE

15-30°C (59-86°F).

HOW SUPPLIED

Tab, SL: 2.5mg, 5mg, 10mg

CONTRAINDICATIONS

Severe hepatic impairment (Child-Pugh C), history of hypersensitivity reactions to asenapine.

WARNINGS/PRECAUTIONS

Neuroleptic malignant syndrome (NMS) reported; d/c therapy and institute symptomatic treatment. May cause tardive dyskinesia (TD), especially in the elderly; consider discontinuation of therapy if this occurs. Associated w/ metabolic changes that may increase cardiovascular (CV) and cerebrovascular risk (eg, hyperglycemia sometimes associated w/ ketoacidosis or hyperosmolar coma, dyslipidemia, weight gain). Hypersensitivity reactions reported, usually after the 1st dose. May induce orthostatic hypotension and syncope; consider dose reduction if hypotension occurs. Caution w/ known CV disease, cerebrovascular disease, conditions that predispose to hypotension, and in elderly. Leukopenia, neutropenia, and agranulocytosis may occur; consider discontinuation at 1st sign of a clinically significant decline in WBC count w/o causative factors. D/C therapy and follow WBC count until recovery in patients w/ severe neutropenia (ANC <1000/mm³). May prolong QTc interval; avoid use w/ history of cardiac arrhythmias and in other circumstances that may increase the risk of torsades de pointes. May elevate prolactin levels. Seizures and somnolence reported. May impair mental/physical abilities. May disrupt body's ability to reduce core body temperature. Caution w/ those at risk for suicide. May cause esophageal dysmotility and aspiration; do not use in patients at risk for aspiration pneumonia.

ADVERSE REACTIONS

Somnolence, insomnia, headache, dizziness, extrapyramidal symptoms, akathisia, vomiting, oral hypoesthesia, constipation, weight increase, fatigue, increased appetite, anxiety, dysgeusia, dyspepsia.

DRUG INTERACTIONS

Avoid use w/ other drugs known to prolong QTc including Class 1A antiarrhythmics (eg, quinidine, procainamide), Class 3 antiarrhythmics (eg, amiodarone, sotalol), antipsychotics (eg, ziprasidone, chlorpromazine, thioridazine), and antibiotics (eg, gatifloxacin, moxifloxacin). Caution w/ other drugs that can induce hypotension/bradycardia/respiratory or CNS depression and drugs w/ anticholinergic activity. May enhance the effects of certain antihypertensive agents; monitor BP and adjust dosage of antihypertensive drug accordingly. May cause greater increase in asenapine exposure when used w/ fluvoxamine; dose reduction of asenapine based on clinical response may be necessary. May enhance the inhibitory effects of paroxetine on its own metabolism and increase exposure of paroxetine; reduce paroxetine dose by 1/2 when used in combination.

PREGNANCY AND LACTATION

Pregnancy: There is a pregnancy exposure registry that monitors pregnancy outcomes in women exposed to asenapine during pregnancy. Neonates exposed to antipsychotic drugs during the 3rd trimester of pregnancy are at risk for extrapyramidal and/or withdrawal symptoms; monitor and manage symptoms accordingly.
Lactation: Lactation studies have not been conducted to assess the presence of asenapine in human milk, the effects of asenapine on the breastfed infant, or the effects of asenapine on milk production. Asenapine is excreted in rat milk.

MECHANISM OF ACTION

Atypical antipsychotic; has not been established. Suggested that efficacy in schizophrenia could be mediated through a combination of antagonist activity at dopamine type 2 and serotonin type 2A receptors.

PHARMACOKINETICS

Absorption: Rapid. (5mg) Absolute bioavailability (35%); C_{max}=4ng/mL; T_{max}=1 hr. **Distribution:** V_d=20-25L/kg; plasma protein binding (95%). **Metabolism:** Direct glucuronidation via UGT1A4 and oxidation via CYP1A2, and to a lesser extent 3A4 and 2D6. **Elimination:** Urine (50%), feces (40%); $T_{1/2}$=24 hrs.

PATIENT CONSIDERATIONS

Assessment: Assess for dementia-related psychosis, history of cardiac arrhythmias, factors that may increase risk of torsades de pointes, risk for aspiration pneumonia, hepatic impairment, known hypersensitivity to the drug, history of seizures/conditions that lower seizure threshold, any other conditions where treatment is contraindicated or cautioned, pregnancy/nursing status, and possible drug interactions. Obtain baseline FPG in patients w/ diabetes mellitus (DM) or at risk for DM. Obtain baseline CBC if at risk for leukopenia/neutropenia.

Monitoring: Monitor for QT prolongation, NMS, TD, orthostatic hypotension, seizures, esophageal dysmotility, aspiration, suicidal ideation, hypersensitivity reactions, metabolic changes, and other adverse reactions. Monitor CBC frequently during 1st few months in patients w/ preexisting low WBC count/ANC or drug-induced leukopenia/neutropenia. Monitor for fever or other signs/symptoms of infection in patients w/ clinically significant neutropenia. Monitor worsening of glucose control in patients w/ DM or FPG in patients at risk for DM. Periodically reevaluate long-term risks/benefits if used for extended periods in bipolar patients.

Counseling: Inform of the risks/benefits and appropriate administration instructions of therapy. Inform of the signs/symptoms of serious allergic reaction; instruct to seek immediate medical attention if these develop. Inform that application-site reactions, primarily in the sublingual area, including oral ulcers, blisters, peeling/sloughing, and inflammation have been reported; instruct to monitor for these reactions. Inform that numbness or tingling of the mouth or throat may occur directly after administration and usually resolves w/in 1 hr. Counsel on the signs and symptoms of tardive dyskinesia and advise to contact their physician if these abnormal movements occur. Counsel about the risk of developing NMS and explain its signs and symptoms. Counsel about the risk of metabolic changes, how to recognize symptoms of hyperglycemia and DM, and the need for specific monitoring. Inform about risk of orthostatic hypotension especially early in the treatment, and also at times of reinitiating treatment or increases in dose. Advise patients w/ preexisting low WBC counts or history of drug-induced leukopenia/neutropenia to have their CBC monitored. Caution about performing activities requiring mental alertness. Counsel regarding appropriate care in avoiding overheating and dehydration. Advise to notify physician if taking/planning to take any prescription or OTC medications, or w/ known or suspected pregnancy during therapy. Advise that there is a pregnancy exposure registry that monitors pregnancy outcomes in women exposed during pregnancy.

SAVAYSA — edoxaban

Class: Selective factor Xa inhibitor

Rx

Reduced efficacy reported in nonvalvular A-fib (NVAF) patients w/ CrCl >95 mL/min; should not be used in NVAF patients w/ CrCl >95mL/min; use another anticoagulant. Increased risk of ischemic events w/ premature discontinuation of any oral anticoagulant in the absence of adequate alternative anticoagulation; consider coverage w/ another anticoagulant if therapy is discontinued for a reason other than pathological bleeding or completion of a course of therapy. Epidural or spinal hematomas may occur in patients treated w/ edoxaban who are receiving neuraxial anesthesia or undergoing spinal puncture; hematomas may result in long-term or permanent paralysis. Increased risk of developing epidural or spinal hematomas in patients using indwelling epidural catheters, concomitant use of other drugs that affect hemostasis (eg, NSAIDs, platelet inhibitors, other anticoagulants), history of traumatic or repeated epidural or spinal punctures, history of spinal deformity or spinal surgery, or unknown optimal timing between the administration of edoxaban and neuraxial procedures. Monitor frequently for signs/symptoms of neurologic impairment; if neurologic compromise noted, urgent treatment is necessary. Consider benefits and risks before neuraxial intervention in patients anticoagulated or to be anticoagulated.

ADULT DOSAGE

Nonvalvular Atrial Fibrillation

Reduce Risk of Stroke and Systemic Embolism:
60mg qd

Deep Vein Thrombosis/Pulmonary Embolism

Treatment:
60mg qd following 5-10 days of initial therapy w/ a parenteral anticoagulant

Conversions

Transition to Edoxaban:
From Warfarin/Other Vitamin K Antagonists: D/C warfarin and start edoxaban when INR ≤2.5
From Oral Anticoagulants Other Than Warfarin/Other Vitamin K Antagonists: D/C current oral anticoagulant and start edoxaban at the time of next scheduled dose of the other oral anticoagulant
From Low Molecular Weight Heparin (LMWH): D/C LMWH and start edoxaban at the time of next schedule administration of LMWH
From Unfractionated Heparin: D/C infusion and start edoxaban 4 hrs later

Transition from Edoxaban:
To Warfarin:
Oral Option: For patients taking 60mg, reduce dose to 30mg and begin warfarin concomitantly. For patients taking 30mg, reduce dose to 15mg and begin warfarin concomitantly. INR must be measured at least weekly and just prior to the daily dose of edoxaban to minimize the influence of edoxaban on INR measurements. D/C edoxaban and continue warfarin once a stable INR ≥2 is achieved
Parenteral Option: D/C and administer a parenteral anticoagulant and warfarin at the time of next scheduled edoxaban dose. Once a stable INR ≥2.0 is achieved, d/c parenteral anticoagulant and continue warfarin
To Non-Vitamin-K Dependent Oral Anticoagulants or Parenteral Anticoagulants:
D/C edoxaban and start other PO/parenteral anticoagulant at the time the next dose of edoxaban

---

PEDIATRIC DOSAGE

Pediatric use may not have been established

DOSING CONSIDERATIONS

Concomitant Medications

DVT and PE:
Certain P-gp Inhibitors: 30mg qd

Renal Impairment

Nonvalvular A-Fib:
CrCl >95mL/min: Do not use
CrCl 15-50mL/min: 30mg qd

DVT and PE:
CrCl 15-50mL/min: 30mg qd

Discontinuation

D/C at least 24 hrs before invasive/surgical procedure. May restart edoxaban after the procedure as soon as adequate hemostasis has been established noting that the time to onset of pharmacodynamic effect is 1-2 hrs. Administer a parenteral anticoagulant and then switch to edoxaban if oral medication cannot be taken during/after surgical intervention

Other Important Considerations

DVT and PE:
≤60kg: 30mg qd

ADMINISTRATION

Oral route

May take w/o regard to food.

STORAGE

20-25°C (68-77°F); excursions permitted to 15-30°C (59-86°F).

HOW SUPPLIED

Tab: 15mg, 30mg, 60mg

CONTRAINDICATIONS

Active pathological bleeding.

WARNINGS/PRECAUTIONS

Increases risk of bleeding and can cause serious and potentially fatal bleeding; promptly evaluate any signs or symptoms of blood loss. D/C in patients w/ active pathological bleeding. No established way to reverse anticoagulant effects of edoxaban; effects can be expected to persist for approx 24 hrs after last dose. Indwelling epidural or intrathecal catheters should not be removed earlier than 12 hrs after the last administration of edoxaban; next dose of edoxaban should not be administered earlier than 2 hrs after removal of the catheter. Not recommended w/ mechanical heart valves or moderate to severe mitral stenosis, CrCl <15mL/min, moderate/severe hepatic impairment (Child-Pugh B and C). Increased risk for ischemic stroke in patients w/ NVAF, as renal function improves and edoxaban blood levels decrease.

ADVERSE REACTIONS

Bleeding, rash, abnormal LFTs, anemia.

DRUG INTERACTIONS

See Boxed Warning and Dosing Considerations. May increase risk of bleeding w/ drugs affecting hemostasis (eg, ASA and other antiplatelet agents, anticoagulants, fibrinolytics, thrombolytics, chronic use of NSAIDs); promptly evaluate any signs or symptoms of blood loss if patients are treated concomitantly w/ anticoagulants, ASA, other platelet aggregation inhibitors, and/or NSAIDs. Long-term concomitant treatment w/ other anticoagulants is not recommended; short-term coadministration may be needed for patients transitioning to or from edoxaban. Avoid use w/ rifampin.

PREGNANCY AND LACTATION

Pregnancy: Category C.
Lactation: Not for use in nursing.

MECHANISM OF ACTION

Selective factor Xa (FXa) inhibitor; inhibits free FXa, and prothrombinase activity and inhibits thrombin-induced platelet aggregation. Inhibition of FXa in the coagulation cascade reduces thrombin generation and reduces thrombus formation.

PHARMACOKINETICS

Absorption: Absolute bioavailability (62%); T_{max}=1-2 hrs. **Distribution:** Plasma protein binding (55%); V_d=107L. **Metabolism:** Minimal metabolism via hydrolysis (mediated by carboxylesterase 1), conjugation, oxidation via CYP3A4; M-4 (predominant metabolite). **Elimination:** Urine (50% unchanged), biliary/intestinal; $T_{1/2}$=10-14 hrs.

PATIENT CONSIDERATIONS

Assessment: Assess for active pathological bleeding, risk factors of developing epidural/spinal hematomas, mechanical heart valves, moderate to severe mitral stenosis, renal/hepatic impairment, pregnancy/nursing status, and possible drug interactions. Assess if patient is receiving neuraxial anesthesia or scheduled to undergo spinal puncture.

Monitoring: Monitor for signs/symptoms of ischemic events w/ premature discontinuation of therapy, bleeding, and other adverse reactions.

Counseling: Inform of the risks and benefits of therapy. Advise that may bleed/bruise more easily or may bleed longer while on therapy. Instruct to report any unusual bleeding immediately to physician. Advise to take exactly as prescribed. Counsel not to d/c therapy w/o talking to physician. Advise to inform all healthcare providers and dentists that patient is taking edoxaban before any surgery, medical or dental procedure is scheduled. Instruct to inform all healthcare providers and dentists if patient is taking/planning to take any prescription medications, OTC drugs, or herbal products. Counsel to inform physician immediately if pregnant/breastfeeding or intending to become pregnant/breastfeed during treatment. Advise patients who are having neuraxial anesthesia or spinal puncture to watch for signs and symptoms of spinal/epidural hematoma; instruct to contact physician immediately if symptoms occur.

SAVELLA — milnacipran hydrochloride

Class: Serotonin and norepinephrine reuptake inhibitor (SNRI)

Rx

Savella is a selective SNRI, similar to some drugs used for the treatment of depression and other psychiatric disorders. Antidepressants increased the risk of suicidal thinking and behavior (suicidality) in children, adolescents, and young adults in short-term studies of major depressive disorder (MDD) and other psychiatric disorders. Monitor appropriately and observe closely for clinical worsening, suicidality, or unusual behavioral changes in patients who are started on milnacipran. Not approved for use in the treatment of MDD and in pediatric patients.

ADULT DOSAGE

Fibromyalgia

Recommended Dose: 50mg bid

Titration Schedule:
Day 1: 12.5mg once
Days 2-3: 12.5mg bid
Days 4-7: 25mg bid
After Day 7: 50mg bid

Based on individual response, may increase to 100mg bid

Max: 200mg/day

Dosing Considerations with MAOIs

Switching to/from an MAOI for Psychiatric Disorders:
Allow at least 14 days between discontinuation of an MAOI and initiation of treatment w/ milnacipran, and allow at least 5 days between discontinuation of milnacipran and initiation of an MAOI

W/ Other MAOIs (eg, Linezolid, IV Methylene Blue):
-Do not start milnacipran in patients being treated w/ linezolid or IV methylene blue. Consider other interventions (eg, hospitalization) in patients who require more urgent treatment of a psychiatric condition.
-In patients already receiving milnacipran, if acceptable alternatives are not available and benefits outweigh risks, d/c milnacipran promptly and administer linezolid or IV methylene blue; monitor for serotonin syndrome for 5 days or until 24 hrs after the last dose of linezolid or IV methylene blue, whichever comes 1st. May resume milnacipran therapy 24 hrs after the last dose of linezolid or IV methylene blue

- -

DOSING CONSIDERATIONS

Renal Impairment
Moderate: Use w/ caution
Severe (CrCl 5-29mL/min): Reduce maint dose by 50% to 25mg bid; may increase to 50mg bid based on individual response
ESRD: Not recommended

Discontinuation
Taper gradually and do not abruptly d/c after extended use

ADMINISTRATION
Oral route

Take w/ or w/o food.
Taking w/ food may improve tolerability.

STORAGE
25°C (77°F); excursions permitted to 15-30°C (59-86°F).

HOW SUPPLIED
Tab: 12.5mg, 25mg, 50mg, 100mg

CONTRAINDICATIONS
Use of an MAOI for psychiatric disorders either concomitantly or w/in 5 days of stopping treatment. Treatment w/in 14 days of stopping an MAOI for psychiatric disorders. Starting treatment in patients being treated w/ other MAOIs (eg, linezolid, IV methylene blue).

WARNINGS/PRECAUTIONS
Serotonin syndrome reported; d/c immediately and initiate supportive symptomatic treatment. Increases in BP and HR reported; treat preexisting HTN, preexisting tachyarrhythmias, and other cardiac diseases before starting therapy. Caution w/ significant HTN or cardiac disease. Consider dose reduction or discontinuation of therapy if sustained increase in BP or HR occurs. Increased liver enzymes and severe liver injury reported; d/c if jaundice or other evidence of liver dysfunction develops. Withdrawal symptoms and physical dependence reported upon discontinuation of therapy; therapy should be tapered and not abruptly discontinued after extended use. If intolerable symptoms occur following a decrease in the dose or upon discontinuation of treatment, consider resuming the previously prescribed dose; subsequently, may continue decreasing dose but at a more gradual rate. Hyponatremia may occur; elderly and volume-depleted patients may be at greater risk. Consider discontinuation in patients w/ symptomatic hyponatremia. May increase risk of bleeding events. Caution w/ history of a seizure disorder or mania. May affect urethral resistance and micturition; caution w/ history of dysuria, notably in male patients w/ prostatic hypertrophy, prostatitis, and other lower urinary tract obstructive disorders. Male patients may experience testicular pain or ejaculation disorders. Pupillary dilation that occurs following use may trigger an angle-closure attack in a patient w/ anatomically narrow angles who does not have a patent iridectomy. May aggravate preexisting liver disease; avoid in patients w/ substantial alcohol use or chronic liver disease. Caution in the elderly.

PEDIATRIC DOSAGE
Pediatric use may not have been established

ADVERSE REACTIONS
N/V, headache, constipation, dizziness, insomnia, hot flush, hyperhidrosis, palpitations, heart rate increased, dry mouth, HTN.

DRUG INTERACTIONS
See Contraindications. May cause serotonin syndrome w/ other serotonergic drugs (eg, triptans, TCAs, fentanyl) and w/ drugs that impair metabolism of serotonin; immediately d/c therapy and any concomitant serotonergic agent if this occurs and initiate supportive symptomatic treatment. If concomitant treatment w/ a triptan is clinically warranted, careful observe the patient, particularly during treatment initiation and dose increases. Paroxysmal HTN and possible arrhythmia may occur w/ epinephrine and norepinephrine. Increase in euphoria and postural hypotension observed in patients who switched from clomipramine; caution w/ other centrally acting drugs. Concomitant use w/ digoxin may potentiate adverse hemodynamic effects. Avoid w/ IV digoxin; postural hypotension and tachycardia reported. May inhibit antihypertensive effect of clonidine. Caution w/ NSAIDs, aspirin (ASA), warfarin, and other drugs that affect coagulation due to potential increased risk of bleeding. Caution w/ drugs that increase BP and HR. May increase risk of hyponatremia w/ diuretics.

PREGNANCY AND LACTATION
Pregnancy: Category C. Physicians are advised to recommend that pregnant patients enroll in the Savella Pregnancy Registry.
Lactation: Caution in nursing.

MECHANISM OF ACTION
Selective SNRI; not established. Potent inhibitor of neuronal norepinephrine and serotonin reuptake w/o directly affecting uptake of dopamine or other neurotransmitters.

PHARMACOKINETICS
Absorption: Well-absorbed. Absolute bioavailability (85-90%); T_{max}=2-4 hrs.
Distribution: Found in breast milk. (IV) V_d=400L; plasma protein binding (13%). **Metabolism:** l-milnacipran carbamoyl-O-glucuronide (major metabolite).
Elimination: Urine (55% unchanged, 17% major metabolite); $T_{1/2}$=6-8 hrs.

PATIENT CONSIDERATIONS
Assessment: Assess for HTN, tachyarrhythmias, cardiac disease, depression, history of seizure disorder/mania/dysuria, prostatic hypertrophy, prostatitis, lower urinary tract obstructive disorders, volume depletion, susceptibility to angle-closure glaucoma, renal/hepatic impairment, pregnancy/nursing status, and possible drug interactions. Assess alcohol use. Obtain baseline BP and HR.

Monitoring: Monitor for clinical worsening, suicidality, unusual changes in behavior, serotonin syndrome, hyponatremia, bleeding events, urethral resistance, micturition, withdrawal symptoms, hepatotoxicity, angle-closure glaucoma, and other adverse reactions. Monitor for mania/hypomania in patients w/ mood disorders. Monitor for testicular pain and ejaculation disorders in male patients. Monitor BP and HR.

Counseling: Inform about benefits, risks, and appropriate use of therapy. Advise patients, their families, and their caregivers to look for the emergence of suicidality, especially early during treatment and when the dose is adjusted up or down. Inform about the risk of serotonin syndrome, particularly w/ concomitant use w/ other serotonergic agents. Instruct to consult physician if symptoms of serotonin syndrome and emergence of suicidality occur. Advise to have BP and HR monitored regularly. Caution about the increased risk of abnormal bleeding w/ concomitant use of NSAIDs, ASA, and other drugs that affect coagulation. Caution about the risk of angle closure glaucoma. Inform that drug may impair mental/physical abilities; caution against operating machinery/driving motor vehicles until effects of drug are known. Instruct to discuss alcohol intake w/ physician prior to initiating therapy. Advise that withdrawal symptoms may occur, particularly w/ abrupt discontinuation. Advise that if a dose is missed, to skip the dose and take the next dose at the regular time. Instruct to notify physician if pregnant, intending to become pregnant, or if breastfeeding. Encourage patients to enroll in the Savella Pregnancy Registry if they become pregnant.

SAXENDA — liraglutide (rDNA origin)   Rx

Class: Glucagon-like peptide-1 (GLP-1) receptor agonist

> Causes dose-dependent and treatment-duration-dependent thyroid C-cell tumors at clinically relevant exposures in animal studies. It is unknown whether drug causes thyroid C-cell tumors (eg, medullary thyroid carcinoma [MTC]) in humans. Contraindicated in patients w/ a personal or family history of MTC and in patients w/ multiple endocrine neoplasia syndrome type 2 (MEN 2). Counsel patients on the risk of MTC and symptoms of thyroid tumors. Routine monitoring of serum calcitonin or using thyroid ultrasound is of uncertain value for early detection of MTC.

ADULT DOSAGE

Chronic Weight Management

Adjunct to a reduced-calorie diet and increased physical activity in patients w/ BMI ≥30kg/m² or ≥27kg/m² w/ at least 1 weight-related comorbid condition

Usual: 3mg daily; dose escalation should be used to reduce the likelihood of GI symptoms

Dose Escalation:
Week 1: 0.6mg/day
Week 2: 1.2mg/day
Week 3: 1.8mg/day
Week 4: 2.4mg/day

PEDIATRIC DOSAGE
Pediatric use may not have been established

Week 5 and Onward: 3mg/day

May delay dose escalation for 1 additional week if unable to tolerate increased dose

D/C if patient is unable to tolerate 3mg dose.

D/C if patient has not lost at least 4% of baseline body weight 16 weeks after initiating therapy.

Missed Dose

If a dose is missed, resume once-daily regimen w/ next scheduled dose; do not take an extra dose or increase dose to make up for missed dose

If >3 days have elapsed since last dose, reinitiate at 0.6mg/day and retitrate following dose escalation schedule

------

DOSING CONSIDERATIONS
Concomitant Medications
Insulin Secretagogues: Consider reducing dose of insulin secretagogue (eg, reduce by 1/2

ADMINISTRATION
SQ route

Administer qd at any time of day, w/o regard to timing of meals.
May inject in the abdomen, thigh, or upper arm; inj site/timing can be changed w/o dose adjustment.

STORAGE
2-8°C (36-46°F). Do not store in the freezer or directly adjacent to the refrigerator cooling element. Do not freeze and do not use if it has been frozen. After Initial Use: 15-30°C (59-86°F) or 2-8°C (36-46°F) for 30 days. Protect from excessive heat and sunlight. Remove and safely discard the needle after each inj; store the pen w/o an inj needle attached.

HOW SUPPLIED
Inj: 6mg/mL [3mL]

CONTRAINDICATIONS
MEN 2, personal or family history of MTC, prior serious hypersensitivity reaction to liraglutide or to any of the product components, pregnancy.

WARNINGS/PRECAUTIONS
Should not be used w/ other drugs containing the active ingredient or w/ any other glucagon-like peptide-1 (GLP-1) receptor agonist. Acute pancreatitis, including fatal and nonfatal hemorrhagic or necrotizing pancreatitis, reported; d/c if suspected, and do not restart if confirmed. Acute gallbladder disease reported; if cholelithiasis is suspected, gallbladder studies and appropriate clinical follow up are indicated. May lower blood glucose. Increases in HR reported; d/c if a sustained increase in resting HR develops. Acute renal failure and worsening of chronic renal failure, sometimes requiring hemodialysis, reported. Serious hypersensitivity reactions reported; d/c if a hypersensitivity reaction occurs. Caution w/ history of angioedema w/ another GLP-1 receptor agonist. Suicidal ideation reported; avoid w/ history of suicidal attempts or active suicidal ideation. Monitor for emergence or worsening of depression, suicidal thoughts or behavior, and/or any unusual changes in mood or behavior; d/c if suicidal thoughts/ behaviors develop. Slows gastric emptying. Caution w/ renal/hepatic impairment.

ADVERSE REACTIONS
N/V, diarrhea, constipation, hypoglycemia in type 2 DM, decreased appetite, headache, dyspepsia, fatigue, dizziness, abdominal pain, increased lipase, GERD, gastroenteritis, abdominal distention, eructation.

DRUG INTERACTIONS
See Dosage. Do not use w/ insulin. Increased risk for serious hypoglycemia w/ insulin secretagogues (eg, sulfonylureas) in patients w/ type 2 DM. Adjust coadministered antidiabetic drugs, if needed, based on glucose monitoring results and risk of hypoglycemia, in patients w/ type 2 DM. Causes a delay of gastric emptying, and therefore may affect the absorption of concomitantly administered oral medications; use w/ caution.

PREGNANCY AND LACTATION
Pregnancy: Category X.
Lactation: Not for use in nursing.

MECHANISM OF ACTION
GLP-1 receptor agonist; binds to and activates the GLP-1 receptor, a cell-surface receptor coupled to adenylyl cyclase activation through the stimulatory G-protein, Gs.

PHARMACOKINETICS
Absorption: Absolute bioavailability (55%); T_{max}=11 hrs; AUC=116ng/mL.
Distribution: Plasma protein binding (>98%); V_d=20-25L (3mg, 100kg person).
Elimination: Urine (6%, metabolites), feces (5%, metabolites); $T_{1/2}$=13 hrs.

PATIENT CONSIDERATIONS
Assessment: Assess for previous hypersensitivity to the drug, MEN 2, personal or family history of MTC, history of pancreatitis, type 2 DM, history of angioedema w/ another GLP-1 receptor agonist, history of suicidal attempts or active suicidal ideation, renal/hepatic impairment, pregnancy/nursing status, and possible drug interactions. Obtain blood glucose parameters in patients w/ type 2 DM.

Monitoring: Monitor for thyroid C-cell tumors, elevated serum calcitonin, pancreatitis, acute gallbladder disease, renal impairment, hypersensitivity

reactions, emergence or worsening of depression, suicidal thoughts or behavior, any unusual changes in mood or behavior, and other adverse reactions. Monitor blood glucose, especially in patients w/ type 2 DM. Monitor HR at regular intervals.

Counseling: Advise to take exactly as prescribed. Counsel to report symptoms of thyroid tumors (eg, a lump in the neck, hoarseness, dysphagia, dyspnea) to physician. Inform of risk of acute pancreatitis and instruct to d/c therapy and contact physician if persistent severe abdominal pain occurs. Inform that substantial or rapid weight loss can increase the risk of cholelithiasis; advise to contact physician if cholelithiasis is suspected. Advise patients w/ type 2 DM on antidiabetic therapy to monitor blood glucose levels and report symptoms of hypoglycemia to physician. Counsel to report symptoms of sustained periods of heart pounding or racing while at rest to physician, and to d/c therapy if a sustained increase in resting HR occurs. Inform of the potential risk of dehydration due to GI adverse reactions and to take precautions to avoid fluid depletion. Inform of the potential risk of worsening renal function. Instruct to d/c therapy and seek medical advice if symptoms of hypersensitivity reactions occur. Advise to report emergence or worsening of depression, suicidal thoughts or behavior, and/or any unusual changes in mood or behavior, and to d/c therapy if suicidal thoughts or behaviors develop. Instruct to contact physician if jaundice develops. Counsel to never share a pen w/ another person, even if the needle is changed.

SEASONIQUE — ethinyl estradiol/levonorgestrel   Rx
Class: Estrogen/progestogen combination

> Cigarette smoking increases risk of serious cardiovascular (CV) events. Risk increases with age (>35 yrs of age) and with the number of cigarettes smoked. Should not be used by women who are >35 yrs of age and smoke.

OTHER BRAND NAMES
Camrese

ADULT DOSAGE	PEDIATRIC DOSAGE
Contraception	**Contraception**
1 tab qd at the same time every day for 91 days, then repeat	Not indicated for use premenarche; refer to adult dosing
Start on the 1st Sunday after onset of menstruation	

DOSING CONSIDERATIONS
Other Important Considerations
Postpartum Women Who Do Not Breastfeed:
Initiate therapy no earlier than 4-6 weeks postpartum; if patient has not yet had a period, she should use additional method of contraception until she has taken tabs for 7 consecutive days

ADMINISTRATION
Oral route

Take at the same time every day at intervals not exceeding 24 hrs
For initial cycle, use a nonhormonal backup method of contraception until a light blue-green tab has been taken for 7 consecutive days

STORAGE
20-25°C (68-77°F).

HOW SUPPLIED
Tab: (Levonorgestrel/Ethinyl Estradiol [EE]) 0.15mg/0.03mg; **Tab:** (EE) 0.01mg

CONTRAINDICATIONS
High risk of arterial/venous thrombotic diseases (eg, smoking if >35 yrs of age, history/presence of deep vein thrombosis/pulmonary embolism, cerebrovascular disease, coronary artery disease, thrombogenic valvular or thrombogenic rhythm diseases of the heart [eg, subacute bacterial endocarditis with valvular disease, or atrial fibrillation], inherited/acquired hypercoagulopathies, uncontrolled HTN, diabetes with vascular disease, headaches with focal neurological symptoms or migraine with/without aura if >35 yrs of age), undiagnosed abnormal genital bleeding, history/presence of breast or other estrogen-/progestin-sensitive cancer, benign/malignant liver tumors, liver disease, pregnancy.

WARNINGS/PRECAUTIONS
Increased risk of venous thromboembolism and arterial thrombosis (eg, stroke, myocardial infarction); d/c if an arterial/deep venous thrombotic event occurs. D/C at least 4 weeks before and through 2 weeks after major surgery or other surgeries known to have an elevated risk of thromboembolism. Start therapy no earlier than 4-6 weeks postpartum in women who do not breastfeed. Caution with CV disease risk factors. D/C if there is unexplained loss of vision, proptosis, diplopia, papilledema, or retinal vascular lesions; evaluate for retinal vein thrombosis immediately. May increase risk of cervical cancer, intraepithelial neoplasia, and gallbladder disease. D/C if jaundice develops. Hepatic adenoma and increased risk of hepatocellular carcinoma reported. Cholestasis may occur in women with a history of pregnancy-related cholestasis. Increase in BP reported. Monitor BP in women with well-controlled HTN; d/c if BP rises significantly. May decrease glucose tolerance; monitor prediabetic and diabetic women. Consider alternative contraception with uncontrolled dyslipidemias. May increase risk of pancreatitis with hypertriglyceridemia or family history thereof. Evaluate the cause and d/c if indicated if new headaches that are recurrent, persistent, or severe develop. Unscheduled bleeding and spotting may occur; rule out pregnancy or malignancies. Amenorrhea or oligomenorrhea may occur after discontinuing therapy. Caution with history of depression; d/c if depression recurs to a serious degree. May change results of laboratory tests (eg, coagulation factors, lipids, glucose tolerance, binding proteins). May induce/exacerbate angioedema in

patients with hereditary angioedema. Chloasma may occur; women with chloasma should avoid sun exposure or UV radiation.

ADVERSE REACTIONS
Irregular and/or heavy uterine bleeding, weight gain, acne.

DRUG INTERACTIONS
Agents that induce certain enzymes, including CYP3A4 (eg, barbiturates, bosentan, carbamazepine, felbamate, griseofulvin, oxcarbazepine, phenytoin, rifampin, St. John's wort, topiramate), may decrease combination oral contraceptive (COC) efficacy or increase breakthrough bleeding; use additional or alternative contraceptive method. Significant changes (increase or decrease) in plasma estrogen and progestin levels reported with HIV protease inhibitors or non-nucleoside reverse transcriptase inhibitors. Pregnancy reported with antibiotics. Atorvastatin may increase ethinyl estradiol exposure; ascorbic acid and acetaminophen may increase ethinyl estradiol levels. CYP3A4 inhibitors (eg, itraconazole, ketoconazole) may increase plasma hormone levels. May decrease concentrations of lamotrigine and reduce seizure control; dosage adjustments of lamotrigine may be needed. Increases thyroid-binding globulin; may need to increase dose of thyroid hormone in patients on thyroid hormone replacement therapy.

PREGNANCY AND LACTATION
Contraindicated in pregnancy, not for use in nursing.

MECHANISM OF ACTION
Estrogen/progestogen COC; acts primarily by suppressing ovulation. Also causes cervical mucus changes that inhibit sperm penetration and endometrial changes that reduce the likelihood of implantation.

PHARMACOKINETICS
Absorption: T_{max}=2 hrs. Levonorgestrel: Complete. Bioavailability (nearly 100%). EE: Bioavailability (43%). Administration on different days resulted in variable parameters; refer to PI. **Distribution:** Found in breast milk. Levonorgestrel: V_d=1.8L/kg; plasma protein binding (97.5-99%). EE: V_d=4.3L/kg; plasma protein binding (95-97%, albumin). **Metabolism:** Levonorgestrel: Sulfate and glucuronide conjugation. EE: 1st-pass (gut wall); liver by hydroxylation via CYP3A4; methylation and/or conjugation. **Elimination:** Levonorgestrel: Urine (45%) (levonorgestrel and metabolites), feces (32%)(mostly metabolites); $T_{1/2}$=34 hrs. EE: Urine, feces (metabolites); $T_{1/2}$=18 hrs.

PATIENT CONSIDERATIONS
Assessment: Assess for high risk of arterial or venous thrombotic diseases; benign or malignant liver tumors; liver disease; undiagnosed abnormal genital bleeding; presence or history of breast cancer or other estrogen- or progestin-sensitive cancer; pregnancy; and any other conditions where treatment is contraindicated/cautioned. Assess nursing status and for possible drug interactions.

Monitoring: Monitor for arterial/deep venous thrombotic events, retinal vein thrombosis, cervical cancer or intraepithelial neoplasia, hepatic impairment, liver tumors, gallbladder disease, pancreatitis, new headaches or increased frequency or severity of migraines, bleeding irregularities, worsening depression with previous history, and other adverse reactions. Monitor BP with history of HTN, glucose levels in diabetic or prediabetic women, lipid levels with dyslipidemia, and thyroid function if receiving thyroid replacement therapy. Schedule a yearly visit with patient for a BP check and for other indicated health care.

Counseling: Inform of benefits and risks of therapy. Counsel that cigarette smoking increases the risk of serious CV events, and that women who are >35 yrs of age and smoke should not use COCs. Inform that drug does not protect against HIV infection and other sexually transmitted diseases. Instruct on what to do if pills are missed. Inform that COCs may reduce breast milk production. Advise to inform physician of preexisting medical conditions and/or drugs currently being taken. Counsel women who start COCs postpartum, and who have not yet had a period, to use an additional method of contraception until after the first 7 consecutive days of administration. Inform that amenorrhea may occur and pregnancy should be ruled out if amenorrhea is associated with symptoms of pregnancy. Instruct to d/c if pregnancy occurs during treatment.

SECTRAL — acebutolol hydrochloride   Rx

Class: Selective beta₁ blocker

ADULT DOSAGE	PEDIATRIC DOSAGE
Hypertension	Pediatric use may not have been established
Uncomplicated Mild to Moderate HTN:	
Initial: 400mg/day, given qd-bid	
Maint: 200-800mg/day	
Severe/Inadequate Control HTN:	
Maint: 1200mg/day, given bid or add second antihypertensive agent	
Ventricular Arrhythmias	
Initial: 200mg bid	
Maint: Increase gradually to 600-1200mg/day	
Gradually reduce dose over a period of about 2 weeks to d/c	

DOSING CONSIDERATIONS
Renal Impairment
CrCl <50mL/min: Reduce daily dose by 50%
CrCl <25mL/min: Reduce daily dose by 75%

Elderly
Start at lower end of dosing range
Max: 800mg/day

ADMINISTRATION
Oral route

STORAGE
20-25°C (68-77°F). Protect from light.

HOW SUPPLIED
Cap: 200mg, 400mg

CONTRAINDICATIONS
Persistently severe bradycardia, 2nd- and 3rd-degree heart block, overt cardiac failure, cardiogenic shock.

WARNINGS/PRECAUTIONS
Caution in patients with history of heart failure (HF) who are controlled with digitalis and/or diuretics. Cardiac failure may occur in patients with aortic or mitral valve disease or compromised left ventricular function; digitalize and/or give diuretic, and d/c acebutolol if cardiac failure continues. Exacerbation of ischemic heart disease and death reported with coronary artery disease (CAD); avoid abrupt withdrawal. Use low doses in patients with bronchospastic disease who do not respond to or cannot tolerate alternative treatment. Do not routinely withdraw prior to major surgery. Can precipitate/aggravate arterial insufficiency in patients with peripheral vascular disease (PVD). Caution with hepatic or renal dysfunction. May mask hypoglycemia in diabetics or hyperthyroidism symptoms (eg, tachycardia). Abrupt withdrawal may precipitate thyroid storm; thyrotoxicosis may occur. May be more reactive to repeated challenge with history of severe anaphylactic reaction to variety of allergens; may be unresponsive to usual doses of epinephrine. May develop antinuclear antibodies (ANAs).

ADVERSE REACTIONS
Fatigue, dizziness, headache, constipation, diarrhea, dyspepsia, nausea, dyspnea, flatulence, micturition, insomnia.

DRUG INTERACTIONS
Possible additive effects with catecholamine-depleting drugs (eg, reserpine); monitor closely for hypotension and bradycardia. NSAIDs may reduce antihypertensive effects. Exaggerated hypertensive responses with α-adrenergic stimulants reported. May potentiate insulin-induced hypoglycemia. Digitalis glycosides may increase risk of bradycardia. May augment the risks of general anesthesia.

PREGNANCY AND LACTATION
Category B, not for use in nursing.

MECHANISM OF ACTION
Cardioselective β-adrenoreceptor blocking agent; reduction in resting HR and decrease in exercise-induced tachycardia, reduction in cardiac output at rest and after exercise, reduction of systolic and diastolic BP at rest and post-exercise, and inhibition of isoproterenol-induced tachycardia.

PHARMACOKINETICS
Absorption: Well-absorbed; absolute bioavailability (40%); T_{max}=2.5 hrs; 3.5 hrs (diacetolol). **Distribution:** Plasma protein binding (26%); crosses placental barrier; found in breast milk. **Metabolism:** Diacetolol (major active metabolite). **Elimination:** Renal (30-40%), nonrenal (50-60%); $T_{1/2}$=3-4 hrs (acebutolol), 8-13 hrs (diacetolol).

PATIENT CONSIDERATIONS
Assessment: Assess for bradycardia, cardiogenic shock, 2nd- and 3rd-degree heart block, overt cardiac failure, thyroid problems, hepatic/renal function, history of severe anaphylactic reaction, HF, CAD, bronchospastic disease, PVD, diabetes mellitus, pregnancy/nursing status, and possible drug interactions.

Monitoring: Monitor for cardiac failure, renal dysfunction, exacerbation of angina pectoris, and MI following abrupt withdrawal, thyrotoxicosis, ANA, and other adverse reactions.

Counseling: Instruct to not interrupt or d/c therapy without consulting physician. Advise to consult physician if signs/symptoms of impending congestive heart failure or unexplained respiratory symptoms develop. Warn about possible hypertensive reactions from concomitant use of α-adrenergic stimulants, such as nasal decongestants used in OTC cold preparations.

SEEBRI NEOHALER — glycopyrrolate   Rx

Class: Anticholinergic

ADULT DOSAGE	PEDIATRIC DOSAGE
Chronic Obstructive Pulmonary Disease	Pediatric use may not have been established
Long-Term, Maint Treatment of Airflow Obstruction:	
Recommended: Orally inhale the contents of 1 cap bid using the Neohaler device	
Max: 1 cap bid	

ADMINISTRATION
Oral inh route
Caps should only be used w/ Neohaler device.
Do not swallow caps.
Administer at the same time every day.
Store caps in the blister; only remove immediately before use.

STORAGE

77°F (25°C); excursions permitted to 59-86°F (15-30°C). Do not use the Neohaler device w/ any other caps. Store caps in the blister protected from moisture; remove caps from the blister immediately before use. Always use the new Neohaler inhaler provided w/ each new prescription.

HOW SUPPLIED

Cap, Inh: 15.6mcg [60ˢ]

CONTRAINDICATIONS

Hypersensitivity to glycopyrrolate or to any of the ingredients.

WARNINGS/PRECAUTIONS

Do not initiate during acutely deteriorating or potentially life-threatening episodes of COPD. Do not use for the relief of acute symptoms (eg, rescue therapy). May produce paradoxical bronchospasm; treat immediately w/ an inhaled, short acting bronchodilator and d/c and institute alternative therapy. Immediate hypersensitivity reactions reported; d/c immediately and institute alternative therapy if signs suggesting an allergic reaction occur. Caution in patients w/ severe hypersensitivity to milk proteins, narrow-angle glaucoma, and urinary retention.

ADVERSE REACTIONS

URTI, nasopharyngitis.

DRUG INTERACTIONS

Avoid w/ other anticholinergic-containing drugs; may lead to an increase in anticholinergic effects.

PREGNANCY AND LACTATION

Pregnancy: Category C.
Lactation: Not for use in nursing.

MECHANISM OF ACTION

Anticholinergic; exhibits effects through inhibition of M3-receptors at the smooth muscle, leading to bronchodilation.

PHARMACOKINETICS

Absorption: Absolute bioavailability (40%); T_{max}=5 min. Distribution: (IV) V_d=83L (steady state); 376L (terminal phase); plasma protein binding (38-41%). Metabolism: Hydroxylation and direct hydrolysis, multiple CYP isoenzymes; M9 (carboxylic acid derivative). Elimination: Urine (60-70%); biliary; $T_{1/2}$=33-53 hrs.

PATIENT CONSIDERATIONS

Assessment: Assess for hypersensitivity to glycopyrrolate, milk proteins, or any component of the product. Assess for acutely deteriorating COPD, narrow-angle glaucoma, urinary retention, pregnancy/nursing status, and possible drug interactions.

Monitoring: Monitor for deteriorating disease, paradoxical bronchospasm, hypersensitivity reactions, narrow-angle glaucoma, urinary retention, and other adverse reactions.

Counseling: Inform that drug is not for relief of acute symptoms of COPD. Advise that acute symptoms should be treated w/ a rescue inhaler (eg, albuterol). Instruct to seek medical attention immediately if experiencing worsening of symptoms or a need for more inhalations than usual of the rescue inhaler. Advise not to d/c therapy w/o physician guidance. Instruct to d/c therapy if paradoxical bronchospasm occurs. Inform about risks of acute narrow-angle glaucoma and urinary retention associated w/ therapy; instruct to consult physician immediately if any signs/symptoms develop. Instruct on how to correctly administer caps using the Neohaler device. Inform that the contents of the caps are for oral inhalation only and must not be swallowed. Advise to contact physician if pregnancy occurs while on therapy.

SELENIUM SULFIDE — selenium sulfide

Class: Antifungal/antiseborrheic

Rx

ADULT DOSAGE

Tinea Versicolor

Apply to affected areas qd for 7 days or ud; lather w/ a small amount of water and rinse off after 10 min

Seborrheic Dermatitis

Scalp:
2 applications/week for 2 weeks; subsequently may use at less frequent intervals (eg, weekly, every 2 weeks, or every 3-4 weeks)

Dandruff

2 applications/week for 2 weeks; subsequently may use at less frequent intervals (eg, weekly, every 2 weeks, or every 3-4 weeks)

PEDIATRIC DOSAGE

Pediatric use may not have been established

ADMINISTRATION

Topical route

Shake well before use.

Lot

Seborrheic Dermatitis/Dandruff:
Massage 1-2 tsp into wet scalp; rinse off after 2-3 min
Repeat application and rinse thoroughly
Wash hands well after treatment

STORAGE

Lotion: 20-25°C (68-77°F). Shampoo: 20-25°C (68-77°F), excursions permitted to 15-30°C (59-86°F). May tolerate brief exposure up to 40°C (104°F) provided the mean temperature does not exceed 25°C (77°F); minimize such exposure. Protect from freezing.

HOW SUPPLIED

Lot: 2.5% [4 fl oz]; Shampoo: 2.25% [180mL]

CONTRAINDICATIONS

Known or suspected hypersensitivity to any of the components.

WARNINGS/PRECAUTIONS

For external use only; not for ophthalmic use. Avoid use on broken skin and areas where inflammation or exudation is present; increased absorption may occur. D/C if allergic/sensitivity reactions occur. Avoid contact w/ eyes. Lot: When used for tinea versicolor, application may produce skin irritation, especially in the genital area and skin folds; rinse these areas thoroughly after application. Shampoo: Avoid contact w/ genital areas and skin folds; may cause irritation and burning.

ADVERSE REACTIONS

Skin irritation, increased loss of hair, hair discoloration, oiliness/dryness of hair and scalp.

PREGNANCY AND LACTATION

Pregnancy: Category C. (Lot) Should not be used to treat for tinea versicolor in pregnant women. (Shampoo) Should not be used under ordinary circumstances by pregnant women.
Lactation: (Lot) Safety not known in nursing, (Shampoo) Caution in nursing.

MECHANISM OF ACTION

Antiseborrheic/antifungal; appears to have a cytostatic effect on cells of the epidermis and follicular epithelium, reducing corneocyte production.

PATIENT CONSIDERATIONS

Assessment: Assess for known/suspected hypersensitivity to the drug, broken skin, presence of inflammation/exudation, and pregnancy/nursing status.

Monitoring: Monitor for allergic reactions, irritation or burning, and other possible side effects.

Counseling: Advise patients that treatment is for external use only and not for ophthalmic use; instruct to avoid contact w/ eyes. Inform that application may produce irritation or sensitization; instruct to d/c if sensitivity reactions occur. Instruct to apply ud. Lot: For treatment of tinea versicolor, inform that skin irritation may occur, especially in genital area and where skin folds occur; instruct to thoroughly rinse these areas after application. Advise that product may damage jewelry; remove jewelry before use. Shampoo: Instruct to avoid contact w/ genital areas and skin folds because irritation and burning may result; if accidental contact occurs, advise to rinse thoroughly w/ water.

SELZENTRY — maraviroc

Class: CCR5 co-receptor antagonist

Rx

> Hepatotoxicity reported; may be preceded by severe rash or evidence of systemic allergic reaction (eg, fever, eosinophilia, elevated IgE). Immediately evaluate patients w/ signs/symptoms of hepatitis or allergic reaction.

ADULT DOSAGE

CCR5-Tropic HIV-1

Use in combination w/ other antiretroviral agents

Concomitant Potent CYP3A Inhibitors (w/ or w/o Potent CYP3A Inducer):
150mg bid

Concomitant Potent CYP3A Inducers (w/o Potent CYP3A Inhibitor):
600mg bid

Other Concomitant Medications (eg, Tipranavir/Ritonavir, Nevirapine, Raltegravir, All Nucleoside Reverse Transcriptase Inhibitors [NRTIs], Enfuvirtide):
300mg bid

PEDIATRIC DOSAGE

Pediatric use may not have been established

DOSING CONSIDERATIONS

Renal Impairment

Concomitant Potent CYP3A Inhibitors (w/ or w/o a CYP3A Inducer):
CrCl <30mL/min or ESRD on Regular Hemodialysis: Not recommended for use

Concomitant Potent CYP3A Inducers (w/o a Potent CYP3A Inhibitor):
CrCl <30mL/min or ESRD on Regular Hemodialysis: Not recommended for use

Other Concomitant Medications (eg, Tipranavir/Ritonavir, Nevirapine, Raltegravir, All NRTIs, Enfuvirtide):
CrCl <30mL/min or ESRD on Regular Hemodialysis: Reduce dose to 150mg bid if symptoms of postural hypotension develop

ADMINISTRATION

Oral route

Take w/ or w/o food.

STORAGE
25°C (77°F); excursions permitted between 15-30°C (59-86°F).

HOW SUPPLIED
Tab: 150mg, 300mg

CONTRAINDICATIONS
In patients w/ severe renal impairment or ESRD (CrCl <30mL/min) who are taking potent CYP3A inhibitors or inducers.

WARNINGS/PRECAUTIONS
Caution in patients w/ preexisting liver dysfunction or who are coinfected w/ hepatitis B and/or C virus. Consider discontinuation in patients w/ signs/ symptoms of hepatitis, or w/ increased liver transaminases combined w/ rash or other systemic symptoms. Severe, potentially life-threatening skin and hypersensitivity reactions reported (eg, Stevens-Johnson syndrome, toxic epidermal necrolysis, drug rash w/ eosinophilia and systemic symptoms); d/c therapy and other suspected agents immediately if signs/symptoms develop. Cardiovascular (CV) events (eg, myocardial ischemia/infarction) and postural hypotension reported; caution in patients at increased risk for CV events and w/ history of or risk factors for postural hypotension or CV comorbidities. Increased risk of postural hypotension in patients w/ severe renal insufficiency or ESRD. Immune reconstitution syndrome reported. Autoimmune disorders (eg, Graves' disease, polymyositis, Guillain-Barre syndrome) reported in the setting of immune reconstitution and can occur many months after initiation of treatment. May increase risk of developing infections. May affect immune surveillance and lead to increased risk of malignancy. In treatment-naive patients, more subjects treated w/ maraviroc experienced virologic failure and developed lamivudine resistance compared w/ efavirenz. Caution in elderly.

ADVERSE REACTIONS
Treatment-Experienced: URTIs, cough, pyrexia, rash, dizziness.

DRUG INTERACTIONS
See Dosing Considerations and Contraindications. Not recommended w/ St. John's wort or products containing St. John's wort; may substantially decrease levels and lead to loss of virologic response and possible resistance. Dose adjustment may be required w/ CYP3A inhibitors/inducers and P-gp inhibitors/ inducers. Caution w/ medication known to lower BP.

PREGNANCY AND LACTATION
Pregnancy: Category B. Physicians are encouraged to register patients in the Antiretroviral Pregnancy Registry.
Lactation: Not for use in nursing.

MECHANISM OF ACTION
CCR5 co-receptor antagonist; selectively binds to human chemokine receptor CCR5 present on the cell membrane, preventing interaction of HIV-1 gp120 and CCR5 necessary for CCR5-tropic HIV-1 to enter cells.

PHARMACOKINETICS
Absorption: T_{max}=0.5-4 hrs (1-1200mg in uninfected volunteers); absolute bioavailability (23% [100mg], 33% [300mg]). Refer to PI for other pharmacokinetic parameters. **Distribution:** V_d=194L; plasma protein binding (76%). **Metabolism:** CYP3A (major); secondary amine (metabolite) via N-dealkylation. **Elimination:** Urine (20%, 8% unchanged), feces (76%, 25% unchanged); $T_{1/2}$=14-18 hrs.

PATIENT CONSIDERATIONS
Assessment: Assess for renal and liver dysfunction, coinfection w/ hepatitis B and/or C, risk for CV events, history of or risk factors for postural hypotension and CV comorbidities, pregnancy/nursing status, and possible drug interactions. Conduct tropism testing to identify appropriate patients. Obtain baseline LFTs.

Monitoring: Monitor for signs/symptoms of hepatotoxicity, allergic/skin/ hypersensitivity reactions, immune reconstitution syndrome, CV events, postural hypotension, infections, malignancy, and other adverse reactions. Monitor LFTs as clinically indicated.

Counseling: Inform that liver problems have been reported and that they should d/c therapy and seek medical attention immediately if signs/symptoms of hepatitis or allergic reaction develop. Advise that lab tests may be ordered before therapy, during therapy, and if severe rash or signs/symptoms of hepatitis or an allergic reaction develop. Inform that therapy is not a cure for HIV-1 infection and patients may continue to experience illnesses associated w/ HIV-1 infection, including opportunistic infections. Advise to remain under the care of a physician. Advise to avoid doing things that can spread HIV-1 infection to others (eg, reusing/sharing of needles/inj equipment or personal items that can have blood/body fluids on them). Advise to always practice safer sex by using latex or polyurethane condoms. Advise females not to breastfeed. Inform that it is important to take all anti-HIV medicines as prescribed and at the same time(s) each day. Instruct not to change dose or d/c therapy w/o consulting physician. If a dose is missed, instruct to take missed dose as soon as possible and then to take next scheduled dose at the regular time; instruct to skip missed dose if it is <6 hrs before next scheduled dose and to take next dose at the regular time. Instruct to avoid driving/operating machinery if dizziness occurs.

SENSIPAR — cinacalcet

Rx

Class: Calcimimetic agent

ADULT DOSAGE
Secondary Hyperparathyroidism

In Patients w/ Chronic Kidney Disease on Dialysis:
Initial: 30mg qd

PEDIATRIC DOSAGE
Pediatric use may not have been established

Titrate: Increase no more frequently than every 2-4 weeks through sequential doses of 30mg, 60mg, 90mg, 120mg, and 180mg qd to target intact parathyroid (iPTH) hormone of 150-300pg/mL

Measure serum Ca^{2+} and phosphorus w/in 1 week and measure iPTH hormone 1-4 weeks after initiation/ dose adjustment; serum iPTH levels should be assessed no earlier than 12 hrs after dosing

Once maint dose is established, measure serum Ca^{2+} monthly

May be used alone or in combination w/ vitamin D sterols and/or phosphate binders

Hypercalcemia

In Patients w/ Primary Hyperparathyroidism who are Unable to Undergo Parathyroidectomy and Patients w/ Parathyroid Carcinoma:
Initial: 30mg bid
Titrate: Increase every 2-4 weeks through sequential doses of 30mg bid, 60mg bid, 90mg bid, and 90mg tid-qid as necessary to normalize serum Ca^{2+} levels

Measure serum Ca^{2+} w/in 1 week after initiation/dose adjustment; once maint dose is established, measure serum Ca^{2+} every 2 months

---

DOSING CONSIDERATIONS
Adverse Reactions
Secondary Hyperparathyroidism in Patients w/ Chronic Kidney Disease on Dialysis:
If serum Ca^{2+} falls <7.5mg/dL, or if hypocalcemia symptoms persist and vitamin D dose cannot be increased, withhold administration until Ca^{2+} levels reach 8.0mg/ dL and/or symptoms of hypocalcemia resolve. Treatment should be reinitiated using next lowest dose of cinacalcet

ADMINISTRATION
Oral route

Take whole; do not divide.
Take w/ food or shortly after a meal.

STORAGE
25°C (77°F); excursions permitted to 15-30°C (59-86°F).

HOW SUPPLIED
Tab: 30mg, 60mg, 90mg

CONTRAINDICATIONS
Hypocalcemia.

WARNINGS/PRECAUTIONS
Avoid use in patients with CKD not on dialysis. Lowers serum Ca^{2+}; monitor for occurrence of hypocalcemia during treatment. Life-threatening events and fatal outcomes associated with hypocalcemia reported in patients treated with the drug, including pediatric patients. QT prolongation and ventricular arrhythmia secondary to hypocalcemia reported. Seizures reported; monitor serum Ca^{2+}, particularly in patients with history of seizure disorder. Hypotension, worsening HF, and/or arrhythmia reported in patients with impaired cardiac function. Adynamic bone disease may develop with iPTH levels <100pg/mL; reduce dose or d/c therapy if iPTH levels <150pg/mL. Monitor patients with moderate and severe hepatic impairment throughout treatment.

ADVERSE REACTIONS
N/V, diarrhea, myalgia, dizziness, HTN, asthenia, anorexia, paresthesia, fatigue, fracture, hypercalcemia, dehydration, anemia, arthralgia, depression.

DRUG INTERACTIONS
May require dose adjustment with CYP2D6 substrates (eg, desipramine, metoprolol, carvedilol) and particularly those with narrow therapeutic index (eg, flecainide, most TCAs). May require dose adjustment if a patient initiates or discontinues therapy with strong CYP3A4 inhibitors (eg, ketoconazole, itraconazole); closely monitor iPTH and serum Ca^{2+} levels.

PREGNANCY AND LACTATION
Pregnancy: Category C.
Lactation: Not for use in nursing.

MECHANISM OF ACTION
Calcimimetic agent; lowers PTH levels by increasing the sensitivity of the Ca^{2+}- sensing receptor to extracellular Ca^{2+}.

PHARMACOKINETICS
Absorption: T_{max}=2-6 hrs. **Distribution:** V_d=1000L; plasma protein binding (93-97%). **Metabolism:** Via CYP3A4, 2D6, and 1A2; hydrocinnamic acid and glucuronidated dihydrodiols (major metabolites). **Elimination:** Urine (80%), feces (15%); $T_{1/2}$=30-40 hrs.

PATIENT CONSIDERATIONS

Assessment: Assess for hypocalcemia, history of seizure disorder, hepatic impairment, cardiac function, pregnancy/nursing status, and possible drug interactions. Assess serum Ca^{2+} levels prior to administration.

Monitoring: Monitor for signs/symptoms of hypocalcemia, adynamic bone disease, and other adverse reactions. In patients with impaired cardiac function, monitor for hypotension, worsening HF, and/or arrhythmias. Monitor iPTH/Ca^{2+}/phosphorus levels with moderate and severe hepatic impairment. Monitor serum Ca^{2+} carefully for the occurrence of hypocalcemia during treatment.

Counseling: Inform of the importance of regular blood tests. Advise to report to physician if N/V and potential symptoms of hypocalcemia occur. Advise to report to their physician if taking medication to prevent seizures, have had seizures in the past, and experience any seizure episodes while on therapy. Encourage patients who are nursing during treatment to enroll in Amgen's Lactation Surveillance Program.

SEREVENT DISKUS — salmeterol xinafoate

Class: Long-acting beta₂ agonist (LABA)   **Rx**

> **Long-acting β₂-adrenergic agonists (LABAs)** increase the risk of asthma-related death. Contraindicated in asthma without use of a concomitant long-term asthma control medication (eg, inhaled corticosteroid). Do not use if asthma is adequately controlled on low- or medium-dose inhaled corticosteroids. LABAs may increase the risk of asthma-related hospitalization in pediatric and adolescent patients.

ADULT DOSAGE

Asthma

Use only as concomitant therapy w/ a long-term asthma control medication (eg, inhaled corticosteroid) in patients w/ reversible obstructive airway disease, including patients w/ symptoms of nocturnal asthma

1 inh bid (12 hrs apart)

Chronic Obstructive Pulmonary Disease

Long-Term Maint Treatment of Bronchospasm:
1 inh bid (12 hrs apart)

Exercise-Induced Bronchospasm

Prevention:
1 inh ≥30 min before exercise (additional doses should not be used for 12 hrs after administration or if already on bid dose)

PEDIATRIC DOSAGE

Asthma

Use only as concomitant therapy w/ a long-term asthma control medication (eg, inhaled corticosteroid) in patients w/ reversible obstructive airway disease, including patients w/ symptoms of nocturnal asthma

≥4 Years:
1 inh bid (12 hrs apart)

Exercise-Induced Bronchospasm

Prevention:
≥4 Years:
1 inh ≥30 min before exercise (additional doses should not be used for 12 hrs after administration or if already on bid dose)

ADMINISTRATION
Oral inh route

STORAGE
20-25°C (68-77°F); excursions permitted from 15-30°C (59-86°F). Store in a dry place away from direct heat or sunlight. Store inside the unopened moisture-protective foil pouch and only remove from the pouch immediately before initial use. Discard 6 weeks after opening the foil pouch or when the counter reads "0," whichever comes 1st.

HOW SUPPLIED
Disk: 50mcg/inh [28, 60 blisters]

CONTRAINDICATIONS
Treatment of asthma without concomitant use of long-term asthma control medication (eg, inhaled corticosteroid). Primary treatment of status asthmaticus or other acute episodes of asthma/COPD where intensive measures are required. Severe hypersensitivity to milk proteins.

WARNINGS/PRECAUTIONS
Not indicated for acute bronchospasm relief. Do not initiate during rapidly deteriorating or potentially life-threatening episodes of asthma or COPD; serious acute respiratory events reported. D/C regular use of oral/inhaled short-acting β₂-agonist (SABA) when beginning treatment. Not a substitute for corticosteroids. Do not use more often or at higher doses than recommended; clinically significant cardiovascular (CV) effects and fatalities reported with excessive use. May produce paradoxical bronchospasm; treat immediately with an inhaled, short acting bronchodilator; d/c and institute alternative therapy. Upper airway symptoms reported. Immediate hypersensitivity reactions and CV/CNS effects may occur. Caution with CV disorders, convulsive disorders, thyrotoxicosis, hepatic disease, diabetes mellitus (DM), ketoacidosis, and in patients unusually responsive to sympathomimetic amines. Clinically significant and dose-related changes in blood glucose and/or serum K^+ reported.

ADVERSE REACTIONS
Nasal/sinus congestion, pharyngitis, cough, viral respiratory infection, musculoskeletal pain, rhinitis, headache, tracheitis/bronchitis, influenza, throat irritation.

DRUG INTERACTIONS
Do not use with other medicines containing a LABA. Not recommended with strong CYP3A4 inhibitors (eg, ketoconazole, ritonavir, clarithromycin); increased CV adverse effects may occur. Extreme caution with MAOIs or TCAs, or within

2 weeks of discontinuation of such agents; action on the vascular system may be potentiated. β-blockers may block pulmonary effects and produce severe bronchospasm; if such therapy is needed, consider cardioselective β-blockers and use with caution. Caution is advised when coadministered with non-K^+-sparing diuretics (eg, loop, thiazide).

PREGNANCY AND LACTATION
Category C, caution in nursing.

MECHANISM OF ACTION
LABA; attributable to stimulation of intracellular adenyl cyclase, the enzyme that catalyzes the conversion of ATP to cAMP. Increased cAMP levels cause relaxation of bronchial smooth muscle and inhibition of release of mediators of immediate hypersensitivity from cells, especially from mast cells.

PHARMACOKINETICS
Absorption: C_{max}=167pg/mL; T_{max}=20 min. **Distribution:** Plasma protein binding (96%). **Metabolism:** Liver (extensive) by hydroxylation; α-hydroxysalmeterol (aliphatic oxidation) via CYP3A4. **Elimination:** Urine (25%), feces (60%); $T_{1/2}$=5.5 hrs.

PATIENT CONSIDERATIONS
Assessment: Assess for hypersensitivity to milk proteins, status asthmaticus, asthma/COPD status, CV disorders, convulsive disorders, thyrotoxicosis, DM, ketoacidosis, hepatic disease, pregnancy/nursing status, and possible drug interactions.

Monitoring: Monitor for deteriorating disease, paradoxical bronchospasm, upper airway symptoms, immediate hypersensitivity reactions, CV and CNS effects, changes in blood glucose and/or serum K^+, and other adverse reactions.

Counseling: Counsel about the risks and benefits of therapy. Inform that the medication should only be used as additional therapy when long-term asthma control medications do not adequately control asthma symptoms. Inform that drug is not meant to relieve acute asthma or exacerbations of COPD symptoms and extra doses should not be used for that purpose; advise to treat acute symptoms with an inhaled SABA (eg, albuterol). Instruct to seek medical attention immediately if experiencing a decrease in effectiveness of inhaled SABA, a need for more inhalations than usual of inhaled SABA, or a significant decrease in lung function. Advise not to d/c therapy without physician guidance and not to use other LABA. Advise that therapy is not a substitute for oral or inhaled corticosteroids; instruct not to change dosage or stop therapy without consulting physician. Advise that immediate hypersensitivity reactions may occur; instruct to d/c if such reactions occur. Inform of adverse effects (eg, palpitations, chest pain, rapid HR, tremor, nervousness). Inform patients treated for EIB not to use additional doses for 12 hrs and not to use additional doses for prevention of EIB if receiving therapy bid. Inform that the inhaler is not reusable and advise not to take the inhaler apart.

SERNIVO — betamethasone dipropionate

Class: Corticosteroid   **Rx**

ADULT DOSAGE

Plaque Psoriasis

Mild to Moderate:
Apply to affected skin areas bid and rub in gently

D/C when control is achieved; use for up to 4 weeks

Do not use if atrophy is present at the treatment site

PEDIATRIC DOSAGE
Pediatric use may not have been established

ADMINISTRATION
Topical route

Do not bandage, cover, or wrap the treated skin area unless directed.
Avoid use on the face, scalp, axilla, groin, or other intertriginous areas.
Shake well before use.

STORAGE
20-25°C (68-77°F); excursions permitted to 15-30°C (59-86°F).

HOW SUPPLIED
Spray: 0.05% [60mL, 120mL]

WARNINGS/PRECAUTIONS
May produce reversible hypothalamic-pituitary-adrenal (HPA) axis suppression w/ the potential for glucocorticosteroid insufficiency during or after treatment. Factors predisposing to HPA axis suppression include the use of high-potency corticosteroids, use over large treatment surface areas, prolonged use, use of occlusive dressings, altered skin barrier, liver failure, and young age. Evaluation for HPA axis suppression may be done by using the ACTH stimulation test. Gradually withdraw the drug, reduce the frequency of application, or substitute w/ a less potent corticosteroid if HPA axis suppression is documented. Supplemental systemic corticosteroids may be required if signs/symptoms of steroid withdrawal occur. Systemic effects of therapy may manifest as Cushing's syndrome, hyperglycemia, and glucosuria. Allergic contact dermatitis is usually diagnosed by observing failure to heal rather than noting a clinical exacerbation; perform appropriate diagnostic patch testing if such an observation is seen. D/C and institute appropriate therapy if irritation develops.

ADVERSE REACTIONS
Application-site reactions (pruritus, burning and/or stinging, pain, atrophy).

PREGNANCY AND LACTATION
Pregnancy: Category C.
Lactation: Caution in nursing.

MECHANISM OF ACTION
Corticosteroid; has not been established. Plays a role in cellular signaling, immune function, inflammation, and protein regulation.

PHARMACOKINETICS
Absorption: Percutaneous; extent of absorption is determined by many factors (eg, vehicle, integrity of epidermal barrier, use of occlusive dressings); C_{max}=119pg/mL (betamethasone after 15 days), 57.6pg/mL (betamethasone after 29 days), 120pg/mL (betamethasone-17-propionate after 15 days), 63.9pg/mL (betamethasone-17-propionate after 29 days). **Distribution:** Found in breast milk (systemically administered).

PATIENT CONSIDERATIONS
Assessment: Assess for drug hypersensitivity, predisposing factors to HPA axis suppression, treatment-site atrophy, pregnancy/nursing status, and possible drug interactions.

Monitoring: Monitor for signs/symptoms of HPA axis suppression, glucocorticosteroid insufficiency, Cushing's syndrome, hyperglycemia, glucosuria, allergic contact dermatitis, and other adverse reactions.

Counseling: Advise to d/c therapy when control is achieved, unless otherwise directed. Instruct not use for >4 consecutive weeks. Instruct to avoid contact w/ the eyes and to avoid use of the drug on the face, scalp, underarms, groin, or other intertriginous areas, unless otherwise directed. Advise not to occlude the treatment area w/ bandage or other covering, unless otherwise directed. Inform that local reactions and skin atrophy are more likely to occur w/ occlusive use, prolonged use, or use of higher potency corticosteroids.

SEROQUEL — quetiapine fumarate   Rx

Class: Atypical antipsychotic

> Elderly patients w/ dementia-related psychosis treated w/ antipsychotic drugs are at an increased risk of death. Not approved for the treatment of patients w/ dementia-related psychosis. Antidepressants increased the risk of suicidal thoughts and behavior in children, adolescents, and young adults in short-term studies. Monitor closely for worsening, and for emergence of suicidal thoughts and behaviors in patients who are started on antidepressant therapy. Not approved for use in pediatric patients <10 yrs of age.

ADULT DOSAGE
Schizophrenia
Day 1: 25mg bid
Days 2-3: Increase by 25-50mg divided bid or tid to a range of 300-400mg by Day 4
Titrate: Further adjustments can be made in increments of 25-50mg bid, in intervals of ≥2 days
Recommended Dose: 150-750mg/day
Max: 750mg/day

Maint:
Recommended Dose: 400-800mg/day
Max: 800mg/day

Switching from Depot Antipsychotics:
Initiate quetiapine therapy in place of the next scheduled inj if medically appropriate

Bipolar I Disorder
Acute Treatment of Manic Episodes: Monotherapy/Adjunct to Lithium or Divalproex:
Day 1: 100mg/day given bid
Day 2: 200mg/day given bid
Day 3: 300mg/day given bid
Day 4: 400mg/day given bid
Titrate: Further adjustments up to 800mg/day by Day 6 should be in increments of ≤200mg/day
Recommended Dose: 400-800mg/day
Max: 800mg/day

Maint Treatment of Bipolar I Disorder as Adjunct to Lithium or Divalproex:
Recommended Dose: 400-800mg/day given bid
Max: 800mg/day

Bipolar Disorder
Acute Treatment of Depressive Episodes:
Monotherapy:
Day 1: 50mg qhs
Day 2: 100mg qhs
Day 3: 200mg qhs
Day 4: 300mg qhs
Recommended Dose: 300mg/day
Max: 300mg/day

PEDIATRIC DOSAGE
Schizophrenia
13-17 Years:
Day 1: 25mg bid
Day 2: 100mg/day given bid
Day 3: 200mg/day given bid
Day 4: 300mg/day given bid
Day 5: 400mg/day given bid
Titrate: Further adjustments should be in increments ≤100mg/day
Recommended Dose: 400-800mg/day
Max: 800mg/day

May administer tid based on response and tolerability

Switching from Depot Antipsychotics:
Initiate quetiapine therapy in place of the next scheduled inj if medically appropriate

Bipolar I Disorder
Acute Treatment of Manic Episodes:
10-17 Years:
Monotherapy:
Day 1: 25mg bid
Day 2: 100mg/day given bid
Day 3: 200mg/day given bid
Day 4: 300mg/day given bid
Day 5: 400mg/day given bid
Titrate: Further adjustments should be in increments ≤100mg/day
Recommended Dose: 400-600mg/day
Max: 600mg/day

May administer tid based on response and tolerability

DOSING CONSIDERATIONS
Concomitant Medications
CYP3A4 Inhibitors:
Reduce quetiapine dose to 1/6 of original dose when coadministered w/ a potent CYP3A4 inhibitor.
When the CYP3A4 inhibitor is discontinued, increase quetiapine dose by 6-fold.

CYP3A4 Inducers:
Increase quetiapine dose up to 5-fold of the original dose when used in combination w/ a chronic treatment (eg, >7-14 days) of a potent CYP3A4 inducer. When the CYP3A4 inducer is discontinued, reduce quetiapine dose to original level w/in 7-14 days.

Hepatic Impairment
Initial: 25mg/day
Titrate: May increase by 25-50mg/day

Elderly
Initial: 50mg/day
Titrate: May increase by 50mg/day

Other Important Considerations
Debilitated Patients/Predisposed to Hypotension:
Consider slower rate of titration and lower target dose

Reinitiation of Treatment in Patients Previously Discontinued:
Discontinued <1 Week: Gradual dose escalation may not be required; may reinitiate maint dose
Discontinued >1 Week: Follow initial dosing schedule

ADMINISTRATION
Oral route
Take w/ or w/o food.

STORAGE
25°C (77°F); excursions permitted to 15-30°C (59-86°F).

HOW SUPPLIED
Tab: 25mg, 50mg, 100mg, 200mg, 300mg, 400mg

CONTRAINDICATIONS
Hypersensitivity to quetiapine or to any excipients in the formulation.

WARNINGS/PRECAUTIONS
Initiate in pediatric patients only after a thorough diagnostic evaluation is conducted and careful consideration is given to the risks of therapy. Neuroleptic malignant syndrome (NMS) reported; d/c and institute symptomatic treatment. Associated w/ metabolic changes that include hyperglycemia/diabetes mellitus (DM), dyslipidemia, and body weight gain. May cause tardive dyskinesia (TD), especially in the elderly; consider discontinuation if this occurs. May induce orthostatic hypotension; caution w/ known cardiovascular/cerebrovascular disease or conditions that predispose patients to hypotension. May increase BP in children and adolescents. Leukopenia, neutropenia, and agranulocytosis reported; d/c at 1st sign of decline in WBC count w/o causative factors in patients w/ preexisting low WBC count or a history of drug induced leukopenia/neutropenia. D/C therapy and follow WBC count until recovery in patients w/ severe neutropenia (ANC <1000/mm³). Lens changes reported during long-term treatment. May prolong QT interval; avoid in circumstances that may increase the risk of torsades de pointes and/or sudden death. Seizures reported; caution w/ conditions that lower seizure threshold. Decrease in thyroid hormone levels reported; measure TSH and free T4 at baseline and at follow-up in addition to clinical assessment. May elevate prolactin levels. May impair physical/mental abilities. May disrupt body's ability to reduce core body temperature. May cause esophageal dysmotility and aspiration; caution in patients at risk for aspiration pneumonia. Acute withdrawal symptoms (eg, N/V, insomnia) may occur after abrupt cessation; d/c gradually.

ADVERSE REACTIONS
Adults: Somnolence, dizziness, dry mouth, constipation, ALT increased, weight gain, dyspepsia, asthenia, abdominal pain, postural hypotension, pharyngitis, lethargy.
Children and Adolescents: Somnolence, dizziness, dry mouth, tachycardia, fatigue, increased appetite, N/V, weight increased, diarrhea.

DRUG INTERACTIONS
See Dosing Considerations. Caution w/ other centrally acting drugs and alcohol. Increased exposure w/ CYP3A4 inhibitors (eg, ketoconazole, ritonavir, nefazodone) and decreased exposure w/ CYP3A4 inducers (eg, phenytoin, carbamazepine, rifampin). May enhance the effects of certain antihypertensives. May antagonize the effects of levodopa and dopamine agonists. QT prolongation reported w/ drugs known to cause electrolyte imbalance. Avoid w/ other drugs that are known to prolong QTc interval (eg, quinidine, amiodarone, ziprasidone). Caution w/ anticholinergic medications.

PREGNANCY AND LACTATION
Pregnancy: Category C.
Lactation: Excreted into human milk; not for use in nursing.

MECHANISM OF ACTION
Dibenzothiazepine derivative; not established. Suspected to be mediated through a combination of dopamine type 2 and serotonin type 2 antagonism.

PHARMACOKINETICS
Absorption: Rapid. T_{max}=1.5 hrs. **Distribution:** V_d=10L/kg; plasma protein binding (83%); found in breast milk. **Metabolism:** Liver (extensive) via sulfoxidation and oxidation (CYP3A4); N-desalkyl quetiapine (active metabolite). **Elimination:** Urine (approx 73%), feces (approx 20%); $T_{1/2}$=6 hrs.

PATIENT CONSIDERATIONS
Assessment: Assess for history of dementia-related psychosis, risk for hypotension, drug hypersensitivity, psychiatric disorders, hepatic impairment,

other conditions where treatment is cautioned, pregnancy/nursing status, and possible drug interactions. Obtain baseline FPG in patients w/ DM or at risk for DM. Obtain baseline CBC if at risk for leukopenia/neutropenia. Obtain baseline TSH and free T4. Obtain baseline BP in children and adolescents. Assess for cataracts by performing lens exam (eg, slit-lamp exam).

Monitoring: Monitor for clinical worsening, suicidality, unusual changes in behavior, NMS, TD, hyperglycemia, orthostatic hypotension, hypothyroidism, seizures, aspiration, and other adverse effects. Monitor CBC frequently during 1st few months in patients w/ preexisting low WBC count or history of drug-induced leukopenia/neutropenia. Monitor for fever or other signs/symptoms of infection in patients w/ neutropenia. Monitor weight regularly, and lipids, hepatic function, and FPG periodically. Monitor for cataract formation shortly after start of treatment, and at 6-month intervals during chronic treatment. Monitor BP periodically during treatment in children and adolescents. Periodically reassess for continued need for maintenance treatment.

Counseling: Inform of the risks and benefits of therapy. Instruct caregivers and patients to contact physician if signs of agitation, anxiety, panic attacks, insomnia, hostility, aggressiveness, impulsivity, akathisia, hypomania, mania, irritability, worsening of depression, changes in behavior, or suicidal ideation develop. Advise about signs/symptoms of NMS, hyperglycemia/DM, and weight gain, and of the risk of orthostatic hypotension and hyperlipidemia. Instruct to avoid overheating and dehydration. Caution about performing activities requiring mental alertness. Instruct to notify physician if patient becomes pregnant or intends to become pregnant during therapy, and if patient is taking or plans to take any prescription or OTC drugs.

SEROQUEL XR — quetiapine fumarate

Class: Atypical antipsychotic

Rx

Elderly patients w/ dementia-related psychosis treated w/ antipsychotic drugs are at an increased risk of death. Not approved for the treatment of patients w/ dementia-related psychosis. Antidepressants increased the risk of suicidal thoughts and behavior in children, adolescents, and young adults in short-term studies. Monitor closely for worsening, and for emergence of suicidal thoughts and behaviors in patients who are started on antidepressant therapy. Not approved for use in pediatric patients <10 yrs of age.

ADULT DOSAGE

Schizophrenia

Day 1: 300mg/day
Titrate: May increase at intervals as short as 1 day and in increments of up to 300mg/day
Recommended Dose: 400-800mg/day
Max: 800mg/day

Maint:
Monotherapy:
Recommended Dose: 400-800mg/day
Max: 800mg/day

Bipolar I Disorder

Manic/Mixed Episodes:
Monotherapy or Adjunct to Lithium/Divalproex:
Day 1: 300mg/day
Day 2: 600mg/day
Day 3 Onward: 400-800mg/day
Max: 800mg/day

Maint Treatment of Bipolar I Disorder as Adjunct to Lithium or Divalproex:
Recommended Dose: 400-800mg/day
Max: 800mg/day

Bipolar Disorder

Depressive Episodes:
Day 1: 50mg/day
Day 2: 100mg/day
Day 3: 200mg/day
Day 4 Onward: 300mg/day
Max: 300mg/day

Major Depressive Disorder

Adjunct to Antidepressants:
Days 1 & 2: 50mg/day
Day 3: 150mg/day
Recommended Dose: 150-300mg/day
Max: 300mg/day

Conversions

Switching from Seroquel Immediate-Release (IR) to Seroquel XR:
Switch at the equivalent total daily dose taken qd

Switching from Depot Antipsychotics:
Initiate quetiapine therapy in place of next scheduled inj if medically appropriate

PEDIATRIC DOSAGE

Schizophrenia

13-17 Years:
Day 1: 50mg/day
Day 2: 100mg/day
Day 3: 200mg/day
Day 4: 300mg/day
Day 5: 400mg/day
Recommended Dose: 400-800mg/day
Max: 800mg/day

Bipolar I Disorder

Mania:
10-17 Years:
Monotherapy:
Day 1: 50mg/day
Day 2: 100mg/day
Day 3: 200mg/day
Day 4: 300mg/day
Day 5: 400mg/day
Recommended Dose: 400-600mg/day
Max: 600mg/day

Conversions

Switching from Seroquel IR to Seroquel XR:
Switch at the equivalent total daily dose taken qd

Switching from Depot Antipsychotics:
Initiate quetiapine therapy in place of next scheduled inj if medically appropriate

DOSING CONSIDERATIONS

Concomitant Medications

CYP3A4 Inhibitors:
Reduce quetiapine dose to 1/6 of original dose when coadministered w/ a potent CYP3A4 inhibitor.
When the CYP3A4 inhibitor is discontinued, increase quetiapine dose by 6-fold.

CYP3A4 Inducers:
Increase quetiapine dose up to 5-fold of the original dose when used in combination w/ a chronic treatment (eg, >7-14 days) of a potent CYP3A4 inducer.
When the CYP3A4 inducer is discontinued, reduce quetiapine dose to original level w/in 7-14 days.

Hepatic Impairment

Initial: 50mg/day
Titrate: May increase in increments of 50mg/day

Elderly

Initial: 50mg/day
Titrate: May increase in increments of 50mg/day

Other Important Considerations

Debilitated Patients/Predisposed to Hypotension:
Consider slower rate of titration and lower target dose

Reinitiation of Treatment in Patients Previously Discontinued:
Discontinued <1 Week: Gradual dose escalation may not be required; may reinitiate maint dose
Discontinued >1 Week: Follow initial dosing schedule

ADMINISTRATION

Oral route

Swallow tab whole; do not split, crush, or chew.
Take w/o food or w/ a light meal (approx 300 calories).
Administer qd, preferably in the pm.

STORAGE

25°C (77°F); excursions permitted to 15-30°C (59-86°F).

HOW SUPPLIED

Tab, Extended-Release: 50mg, 150mg, 200mg, 300mg, 400mg

CONTRAINDICATIONS

Hypersensitivity to quetiapine or to any excipients in the formulation.

WARNINGS/PRECAUTIONS

Initiate in pediatric patients only after a thorough diagnostic evaluation is conducted and careful consideration is given to the risks of therapy. Neuroleptic malignant syndrome (NMS) reported; d/c and institute symptomatic treatment. Associated w/ metabolic changes that include hyperglycemia/diabetes mellitus (DM), dyslipidemia, and body weight gain. May cause tardive dyskinesia (TD), especially in the elderly; consider discontinuation if this occurs. May induce orthostatic hypotension; caution w/ known cardiovascular/cerebrovascular disease or conditions which predispose patients to hypotension. May increase BP in children and adolescents. Leukopenia, neutropenia, and agranulocytosis reported; d/c at 1st sign of decline in WBC count w/o causative factors in patients w/ preexisting low WBC count or a history of drug induced leukopenia/neutropenia. D/C therapy and follow WBC count until recovery in patients w/ severe neutropenia (ANC <1000/mm³). Lens changes reported during long-term treatment. May prolong QT interval; avoid in circumstances that may increase the risk of torsades de pointes and/or sudden death. Seizures reported; caution w/ conditions that lower seizure threshold. Decrease in thyroid hormone levels reported; measure TSH and free T4 at baseline and at follow-up in addition to clinical assessment. May elevate prolactin levels. May impair physical/mental abilities. May disrupt body's ability to reduce core body temperature. May cause esophageal dysmotility and aspiration; caution in patients at risk for aspiration pneumonia. Acute withdrawal symptoms (eg, N/V, insomnia) may occur after abrupt cessation; d/c gradually.

ADVERSE REACTIONS

Adults: Somnolence, dry mouth, dizziness, dyspepsia, constipation, weight gain, dysarthria, nasal congestion, increased appetite, fatigue.
Children and Adolescents: Somnolence, dizziness, fatigue, diarrhea, dry mouth, tachycardia, increased appetite, N/V, weight increased.

DRUG INTERACTIONS

See Dosing Considerations. Caution w/ other centrally acting drugs and alcohol. Increased exposure w/ CYP3A4 inhibitors (eg, ketoconazole, ritonavir, nefazodone) and decreased exposure w/ CYP3A4 inducers (eg, phenytoin, carbamazepine, rifampin). May enhance the effects of certain antihypertensives. May antagonize the effects of levodopa and dopamine agonists. QT prolongation reported w/ drugs known to cause electrolyte imbalance. Avoid w/ other drugs that are known to prolong QTc interval. Avoid w/ other drugs that are known to prolong QTc interval (eg, quinidine, amiodarone, ziprasidone). Caution w/ anticholinergic medications.

PREGNANCY AND LACTATION

Pregnancy: Category C.
Lactation: Excreted into human milk; not for use in nursing.

MECHANISM OF ACTION

Dibenzothiazepine derivative; not established. Suspected to be mediated through a combination of dopamine type 2 and serotonin type 2A antagonism.

PHARMACOKINETICS

Absorption: T_{max}=approx 6 hrs. **Distribution:** V_d=10L/kg; plasma protein binding (83%); found in breast milk. **Metabolism:** Liver (extensive) via sulfoxidation and oxidation (CYP3A4); norquetiapine (major active metabolite). **Elimination:** Urine (approx 73%), feces (approx 20%); $T_{1/2}$=approx 7 hrs (quetiapine), approx 12 hrs (norquetiapine).

PATIENT CONSIDERATIONS

Assessment: Assess for history of dementia-related psychosis, risk for hypotension, drug hypersensitivity, psychiatric disorders, hepatic impairment, other conditions where treatment is cautioned, pregnancy/nursing status, and possible drug interactions. Obtain baseline FPG in patients w/ DM or at risk for DM. Obtain baseline CBC if at risk for leukopenia/neutropenia. Obtain baseline TSH and free T4. Obtain baseline BP in children and adolescents. Assess for cataracts by performing lens exam (eg, slit-lamp exam).

Monitoring: Monitor for clinical worsening, suicidality, unusual changes in behavior, NMS, TD, hyperglycemia, orthostatic hypotension, hypothyroidism, seizures, aspiration, and other adverse effects. Monitor CBC frequently during 1st few months in patients w/ preexisting low WBC count or history of drug-induced leukopenia/neutropenia. Monitor for fever or other signs/symptoms of infection in patients w/ neutropenia. Monitor weight regularly, and lipids, hepatic function, and FPG periodically. Monitor for cataract formation shortly after start of treatment, and at 6-month intervals during chronic treatment. Monitor BP periodically during treatment in children and adolescents. Periodically reassess for continued need for maintenance treatment.

Counseling: Inform of the risks and benefits of therapy. Instruct caregivers and patients to contact physician if signs of agitation, anxiety, panic attacks, insomnia, hostility, aggressiveness, impulsivity, akathisia, hypomania, mania, irritability, worsening of depression, changes in behavior, or suicidal ideation develop. Advise about signs/symptoms of NMS, hyperglycemia/DM, and weight gain, and of the risk of orthostatic hypotension and hyperlipidemia. Instruct to avoid overheating and dehydration. Caution about performing activities requiring mental alertness. Instruct to notify physician if patient becomes pregnant or intends to become pregnant during therapy, and if patient is taking or plans to take any prescription or OTC drugs.

SEROSTIM — somatropin (rDNA origin)   Rx

Class: Recombinant human growth hormone (hGH)

ADULT DOSAGE	PEDIATRIC DOSAGE
HIV-associated Wasting or Cachexia	Pediatric use may not have been established
To increase lean body mass and weight, and improve physical endurance. Concomitant antiretroviral therapy is necessary.	
Initial: 0.1mg/kg (up to a total dose of 6mg) SQ qhs; consider 0.1mg/kg qod in patients at increased risk for adverse effects related to therapy (eg, glucose intolerance)	
Weight-Based Recommendations (SQ QD):	
<35kg: 0.1mg/kg	
35-45kg: 4mg	
45-55kg: 5mg	
>55kg: 6mg	
Most of the effect was apparent after 12 weeks of treatment and maintained during an additional 12 weeks of therapy; no safety or efficacy data available from controlled studies for treatment >48 weeks	

DOSING CONSIDERATIONS

Elderly
Consider a lower starting dose and smaller dose increments

Adverse Reactions
Consider dose reductions (eg, reducing total daily dose or number of doses/week) for side effects potentially related to therapy

ADMINISTRATION
SQ route
Therapy should be carried out under the regular guidance of a physician who is experienced in HIV infection diagnosis and management.
Rotate inj sites (thigh, upper arm, abdomen, buttock).

Reconstitution
Each vial of Serostim 5mg or 6mg is reconstituted w/ 0.5-1mL sterile water for inj (SWFI).
Each vial of Serostim 4mg is reconstituted in 0.5-1mL of bacteriostatic water for inj (0.9% benzyl alcohol preserved); for patients sensitive to benzyl alcohol, may reconstitute w/ SWFI.
When reconstituted w/ SWFI, the reconstituted sol should be used immediately and any unused portion should be discarded.
When reconstituted w/ bacteriostatic water for inj, the reconstituted sol may be refrigerated (2-8°C/36-46°F) for up to 14 days.
Approx 10% mechanical loss can be associated w/ reconstitution and administration from multidose vials.
Inject the diluent into the vial aiming the liquid against the glass vial wall. Swirl the vial w/ a gentle rotary motion until contents are dissolved completely.
Do not shake and use it only if it is clear and colorless.

Serostim can be administered using (1) a standard sterile, disposable syringe and needle, (2) a compatible Serostim needle-free inj device, or (3) a compatible Serostim needle inj device.
For proper use, refer to the instructions for use provided w/ the administration device.

STORAGE
Before Reconstitution: 15-30°C (59-86°F). **After Reconstitution w/ SWFI (Single-Use Vials):** Use immediately and discard any unused portion. **After Reconstitution w/ Bacteriostatic Water for Injection (Multi-Use Vials):** 2-8°C (36-46°F) for up to 14 days. **Reconstituted Sol:** Avoid freezing.

HOW SUPPLIED
Inj: 4mg [multi-use vial]; 5mg, 6mg [single-use vial]

CONTRAINDICATIONS
Active malignancy, active proliferative or severe nonproliferative diabetic retinopathy, and acute critical illness due to complications following open heart or abdominal surgery, multiple accidental trauma, or acute respiratory failure.

WARNINGS/PRECAUTIONS
Somatropin has been shown to potentiate HIV replication; maintain on antiretroviral therapy for the duration of treatment. New onset impaired glucose tolerance, new onset type 2 diabetes mellitus (DM), exacerbation of preexisting DM, diabetic ketoacidosis, and diabetic coma reported. Intracranial HTN w/ papilledema, visual changes, headache, and N/V reported; perform funduscopic exam before and during therapy. D/C if papilledema is observed by funduscopy; if somatropin-induced intracranial HTN is diagnosed, may restart at a lower dose after signs/symptoms have resolved. Increased tissue turgor and musculoskeletal discomfort may occur; may resolve spontaneously, w/ analgesic therapy, or after reducing frequency of dosing. Carpal tunnel syndrome may occur; d/c if symptoms do not resolve after decreasing the weekly number of doses. Tissue atrophy may result if administered SQ at the same site over a long period; rotate inj site. Local/systemic allergic reactions may occur. Monitor for the development of neoplasms in all patients and routinely monitor for progression or recurrence of a tumor in patients w/ a history of any neoplasm. Pancreatitis reported rarely. Caution in the elderly.

ADVERSE REACTIONS
Tissue turgor (swelling, particularly of hands or feet); musculoskeletal discomfort.

DRUG INTERACTIONS
Inhibits 11β-hydroxysteroid dehydrogenase type 1; patients treated w/ glucocorticoid replacement (eg, cortisone acetate, prednisone) for previously diagnosed hypoadrenalism may require an increase in maintenance or stress doses following initiation of somatropin therapy. May alter clearance of compounds metabolized by CYP450 liver enzymes (eg, corticosteroids, sex steroids, anticonvulsants, cyclosporine); careful monitoring is advised w/ concomitant use. Oral estrogens may reduce serum insulin-like growth factor-1 (IGF-1) response to somatropin; may require greater somatropin doses if taking oral estrogen replacement concomitantly. May require adjustment of doses of insulin and/or other hypoglycemic agents.

PREGNANCY AND LACTATION
Pregnancy: Category B.
Lactation: Caution in nursing.

MECHANISM OF ACTION
Recombinant hGH; anabolic and anticatabolic agent. Interacts w/ specific receptors on a variety of cell types, including myocytes, hepatocytes, adipocytes, lymphocytes, and hematopoietic cells. Some effects are mediated by IGF-1.

PHARMACOKINETICS
Absorption: Absolute bioavailability (70-90%). **Distribution:** (IV) V_d=12L. **Metabolism:** Liver, kidneys. **Elimination:** Urine; $T_{1/2}$=4.28 hrs (6mg SQ).

PATIENT CONSIDERATIONS

Assessment: Assess for hypersensitivity to drug or diluent; acute critical illness due to complications following open heart/abdominal surgery, multiple accidental trauma, or acute respiratory failure; active malignancy; active proliferative or severe nonproliferative diabetic retinopathy; risk factors for glucose intolerance; DM; history of any neoplasm; preexisting nevi; pregnancy/nursing status; and possible drug interactions. Obtain baseline glucose levels and perform funduscopic exam.

Monitoring: Monitor for signs/symptoms of intracranial HTN, increased tissue turgor, musculoskeletal discomfort, carpal tunnel syndrome, local/systemic reactions, glucose intolerance, pancreatitis, and other adverse reactions. Monitor glucose levels, and perform funduscopic exam periodically. Carefully monitor for development of neoplasms, progression/recurrence of tumor in patients w/ history of any neoplasm, and for increased growth, or potential malignant changes of preexisting nevi.

Counseling: Inform about benefits and risks of therapy. Instruct to contact physician if side effects or discomfort occurs. Inform about management of common side effects relating to tissue turgor, glucose intolerance, and musculoskeletal discomfort. Instruct to use sterile, disposable syringes/needles and caution against reuse; inform of the importance of proper disposal. Instruct to rotate inj sites to avoid localized tissue atrophy. Counsel to never share drug or inj devices w/ another person, even if needle/nozzle is changed; inform that sharing inj devices may pose a risk of transmission of infection. Inform that allergic reactions are possible and that prompt medical attention should be sought if these occur.

SF ROWASA — mesalamine

Class: 5-aminosalicylic acid derivative

Rx

OTHER BRAND NAMES
Rowasa

ADULT DOSAGE
Ulcerative Colitis

Active Mild-Moderate Distal Ulcerative Colitis, Proctosigmoiditis, or Proctitis:
Usual: One rectal instillation of 60mL (4g) qhs for 3-6 weeks; retain for 8 hrs

PEDIATRIC DOSAGE
Pediatric use may not have been established

ADMINISTRATION
Rectal route

- Shake bottle well.
- Remove the protective sheath from applicator tip; hold bottle at the neck.
- Position most often used is obtained by lying on the left side w/ the lower leg extended and the upper right leg flexed forward for balance; an alternative is the knee-chest position.
- Insert applicator tip gently in the rectum pointing toward the umbilicus; a steady squeezing of the bottle will discharge most of the preparation.

STORAGE
20-25°C (68-77°F). Excursions permitted. Discard unwrapped bottles after 14 days. Discard product if contents are dark brown.

HOW SUPPLIED
Sus: 4g/60mL

CONTRAINDICATIONS
Hypersensitivity to mesalamine or any component of the medication.

WARNINGS/PRECAUTIONS
Acute intolerance syndrome (eg, cramping, bloody diarrhea, abdominal pain, headache) may develop; d/c if signs and symptoms occur. Reevaluate history of sulfasalazine intolerance; if rechallenge is considered, perform under close supervision. Caution w/ sulfasalazine hypersensitivity; d/c if rash or fever occurs. Carefully monitor w/ preexisting renal disease; obtain baseline/periodic urinalysis, BUN, and creatinine. Worsening of colitis or symptoms of inflammatory bowel disease, including melena and hematochezia, may occur. Pancolitis and pericarditis (rare) reported.

ADVERSE REACTIONS
Abdominal pain/cramps/discomfort, headache, flatulence, flu, fever, nausea, malaise/fatigue.

PREGNANCY AND LACTATION
Pregnancy: Category B.
Lactation: Not for use in nursing.

MECHANISM OF ACTION
5-aminosalicylic acid; has not been established. Suspected to diminish inflammation by blocking cyclo-oxygenase and inhibiting prostaglandin production in the colon.

PHARMACOKINETICS
Absorption: Colon: Poor. Extent dependent on retention time. Metabolism: Acetylation, N-acetyl-5-aminosalicylic acid (metabolite). Elimination: Urine (10-30%), feces, $T_{1/2}$=0.5-1.5 hrs.

PATIENT CONSIDERATIONS

Assessment: Assess for history of sulfasalazine intolerance, preexisting renal disease, hypersensitivity, pregnancy/nursing status, and possible drug interactions. Obtain baseline urinalysis, BUN, and creatinine.

Monitoring: Monitor urinalysis, BUN, and creatinine periodically. Monitor for signs/symptoms of acute intolerance syndrome, hypersensitivity, or allergic reaction.

Counseling: Instruct on how to use. Advise that best results achieved if bowel emptied immediately before administration. Advise to seek medical attention if symptoms of acute intolerance syndrome, hypersensitivity, or allergic reactions occur. Instruct that if signs of rash or fever develop, patient should d/c therapy. Advise to choose a suitable location for administration, as sus will stain direct contact surfaces (eg, fabrics, flooring).

SILENOR — doxepin

Class: H_1 antagonist

Rx

ADULT DOSAGE
Insomnia

Difficulty w/ Sleep Maint:
Initial: 6mg qd w/in 30 min of hs; may use 3mg qd if clinically indicated
Max: 6mg/day

PEDIATRIC DOSAGE
Pediatric use may not have been established

DOSING CONSIDERATIONS
Concomitant Medications
Cimetidine:
Max: 3mg
Hepatic Impairment
Initial: 3mg

Elderly
≥65 Years:
Initial: 3mg qd; may increase to 6mg

ADMINISTRATION
Oral route
Do not take w/in 3 hrs of a meal.

STORAGE
20-25°C (68-77°F). Protect from light.

HOW SUPPLIED
Tab: 3mg, 6mg

CONTRAINDICATIONS
Hypersensitivity to doxepin HCl, any of its inactive ingredients, or other dibenzoxepines; untreated narrow angle glaucoma; severe urinary retention; administration w/ or w/in 2 weeks of MAOIs.

WARNINGS/PRECAUTIONS
Evaluate comorbid diagnoses prior to initiation of treatment. Failure of remission after 7-10 days may indicate the presence of primary psychiatric and/or medical illness that should be evaluated. Complex behaviors (eg, sleep-driving), amnesia, anxiety, and other neuropsychiatric symptoms reported; consider discontinuation if sleep-driving episode occurs. Worsening of depression reported. May impair physical/mental abilities. Caution in patients w/ compromised respiratory function. Avoid in patients w/ severe sleep apnea.

ADVERSE REACTIONS
Somnolence/sedation, URTI/nasopharyngitis, HTN.

DRUG INTERACTIONS
See Contraindications and Dosing Considerations. Sedative effects of alcohol, CNS depressants, and sedating antihistamines may be potentiated w/ concomitant use. Increased exposure w/ inhibitors of CYP2C19, CYP2D6, CYP1A2, and CYP2C9. Exposure doubled w/ cimetidine. Hypoglycemia reported when therapy added to tolazamide regimen.

PREGNANCY AND LACTATION
Pregnancy: Category C.
Lactation: Caution in nursing.

MECHANISM OF ACTION
H_1-antagonist; has not been established. Suspected to exert its sleep maintenance effect by antagonizing the H_1 receptor.

PHARMACOKINETICS
Absorption: T_{max}=3.5 hrs. Distribution: V_d=11,930L; plasma protein binding (80%); found in breast milk. Metabolism: Extensive by oxidation and demethylation via CYP2C19, CYP2D6, CYP1A2, CYP2C9; N-desmethyldoxepin (nordoxepin) (primary metabolite). Elimination: Urine (<3%); $T_{1/2}$=15.3 hrs, 31 hrs (nordoxepin).

PATIENT CONSIDERATIONS

Assessment: Assess for drug hypersensitivity, untreated narrow-angle glaucoma, urinary retention, presence of a primary psychiatric and/or medical illness that may cause insomnia, depression, hepatic impairment, sleep apnea, pregnancy/nursing status, and possible drug interactions.

Monitoring: Monitor for treatment response, complex behaviors/neuropsychiatric symptoms, worsening of depression, and other adverse reactions.

Counseling: Inform of benefits and risks associated w/ therapy. Counsel on appropriate use of medication. Instruct to contact physician if sleep-driving occurs or if patient performs other complex behaviors while not fully awake. Instruct to seek medical attention if symptoms of cognitive or behavioral abnormalities or if worsening of insomnia occurs. Inform that medication may cause sedation; caution against operating machinery (eg, automobiles) during therapy. Advise to avoid alcohol consumption during therapy.

SILVADENE — silver sulfadiazine

Class: Sulfonamide

Rx

OTHER BRAND NAMES
SSD

ADULT DOSAGE
Burns

Adjunct for the Prevention and Treatment of Wound Sepsis in Patients w/ 2nd- and 3rd-Degree Burns:
Apply qd-bid to a thickness of approx 1/16 inch

Whenever necessary, reapply to any areas from which it has been removed due to patient activity

Reapply immediately after hydrotherapy

Continue treatment until satisfactory healing has occurred or until the burn site is ready for grafting; do not withdraw from therapeutic regimen while there remains possibility of infection, except if a significant adverse reaction occurs

PEDIATRIC DOSAGE
Pediatric use may not have been established

ADMINISTRATION
Topical route

Cleanse and debride burn wounds prior to application, under sterile conditions.
Burn areas should be covered w/ cre at all times.
Dressings are not required, however if individual patient requirements make dressings necessary, they may be used.

STORAGE
20-25°C (68-77°F). **SSD:** 15-30°C (59-86°F).

HOW SUPPLIED
Cre: 1% [50g, 400g, 1000g (jar); 20g, 25g, 50g, 85g (tube)]; (SSD) 1% [50g, 400g (jar); 25g, 50g, 85g (tube)]

CONTRAINDICATIONS
Hypersensitivity to silver sulfadiazine or any of the other ingredients in the preparation. Pregnant women approaching or at term, premature infants, newborn infants during the first 2 months of life.

WARNINGS/PRECAUTIONS
Potential cross-sensitivity w/ other sulfonamides; if allergic reactions attributable to treatment occur, weigh continuation of therapy against potential hazards of the particular allergic reaction. Fungal proliferation in and below the eschar may occur. Caution w/ G6PD deficiency; hemolysis may occur. Drug accumulation may occur if hepatic and renal functions become impaired and elimination of drug decreases; weigh discontinuation of therapy against the therapeutic benefit being achieved. In the treatment of burn wounds involving extensive areas of the body, serum sulfa concentrations may approach adult therapeutic levels (8-12mg%); monitor serum sulfa concentrations in these patients. Monitor renal function and check urine for sulfa crystals. Lab test interactions may occur. Adverse reactions associated w/ sulfonamides (eg, blood dyscrasias, dermatologic and allergic reactions, GI reactions, hepatitis and hepatocellular necrosis, CNS reactions, toxic nephrosis) may occur.

ADVERSE REACTIONS
Transient leukopenia, skin necrosis, erythema multiforme, skin discoloration, burning sensation, rash, interstitial nephritis.

DRUG INTERACTIONS
May inactivate topical proteolytic enzymes.

PREGNANCY AND LACTATION
Pregnancy: Category B.
Lactation: It is not known whether silver sulfadiazine is excreted in human milk. However, sulfonamides are known to be excreted in human milk, and all sulfonamide derivatives are known to increase the possibility of kernicterus. Not for use in nursing.

MECHANISM OF ACTION
Sulfonamide; topical antibacterial. Bactericidal for many gram-negative and gram-positive bacteria as well as being effective against yeast; acts only on cell membrane and cell wall to produce bactericidal effect.

PATIENT CONSIDERATIONS
Assessment: Assess for hypersensitivity to drug, G6PD deficiency, renal/hepatic impairment, pregnancy/nursing status, and possible drug interactions.

Monitoring: Monitor for allergic reactions, fungal proliferation, renal/hepatic dysfunction, and other adverse reactions. Check urine for sulfa crystals. Monitor serum sulfa concentrations in patients w/ wounds involving extensive areas of the body.

Counseling: Inform of the risks and benefits of therapy. Instruct to use ud. Advise to notify physician if adverse reactions occur.

SIMBRINZA — brimonidine tartrate/brinzolamide   Rx

Class: Alpha₂ agonist/carbonic anhydrase inhibitor

ADULT DOSAGE	PEDIATRIC DOSAGE
Elevated Intraocular Pressure	**Elevated Intraocular Pressure**
Open-Angle Glaucoma/Ocular HTN: 1 drop in the affected eye(s) tid	**Open-Angle Glaucoma/Ocular HTN:** **≥2 Years:** 1 drop in the affected eye(s) tid

- - - - - - - - - -

DOSING CONSIDERATIONS
Concomitant Medications
If >1 topical ophthalmic drug is being used, administer drugs at least 5 min apart

ADMINISTRATION
Ocular route
Shake well before use.

STORAGE
2-25°C (36-77°F).

HOW SUPPLIED
Ophthalmic Sus: (Brinzolamide/Brimonidine) 1%/0.2% [8mL]

CONTRAINDICATIONS
Hypersensitivity to any component of this product, neonates and infants (<2 yrs of age).

WARNINGS/PRECAUTIONS
Caution w/ low endothelial cell counts; increased potential for corneal edema. Not recommended w/ severe renal impairment (CrCl <30mL/min). Contains benzalkonium chloride, which may be absorbed by soft contact lenses; contact lenses should be removed during instillation, but may be reinserted 15 min after instillation. Caution w/ severe cardiovascular disease (CVD) and hepatic impairment. Bacterial keratitis reported w/ multidose containers. **Brimonidine:** May potentiate syndromes associated w/ vascular insufficiency; caution w/ depression, cerebral or coronary insufficiency, Raynaud's phenomenon, orthostatic hypotension, or thromboangiitis

obliterans. **Brinzolamide:** Systemically absorbed. Fatalities occurred due to severe reactions to sulfonamides, including Stevens-Johnson syndrome, toxic epidermal necrolysis, fulminant hepatic necrosis, agranulocytosis, aplastic anemia, and other blood dyscrasias. Sensitization may recur when a sulfonamide is readministered irrespective of route. D/C if signs of serious reactions or hypersensitivity occur.

ADVERSE REACTIONS
Blurred vision, eye irritation, dysgeusia, dry mouth, eye allergy.

DRUG INTERACTIONS
Potential additive systemic effects w/ oral carbonic anhydrase inhibitors; coadministration is not recommended. Acid-base alterations reported w/ high-dose salicylate therapy in patients treated w/ oral carbonic anhydrase inhibitors. Possible additive or potentiating effect w/ CNS depressants (eg, alcohol, opiates, barbiturates, sedatives, anesthetics). Caution w/ antihypertensives and/or cardiac glycosides. Caution w/ TCAs and MAOIs, which can affect the metabolism and uptake of circulating amines.

PREGNANCY AND LACTATION
Pregnancy: Category C.
Lactation: Not for use in nursing.

MECHANISM OF ACTION
Brinzolamide: Carbonic anhydrase inhibitor; inhibits carbonic anhydrase in the ciliary processes of the eye to decrease aqueous humor secretion. Results in a reduction in elevated IOP. **Brimonidine:** α₂-adrenergic receptor agonist; reduces aqueous humor production and increases uveoscleral outflow. Results in a reduction in IOP.

PHARMACOKINETICS
Absorption: Brinzolamide: Systemic. Brimonidine: T_{max}=1-4 hrs. **Distribution:** Brinzolamide: Plasma protein binding (60%). **Metabolism:** Brinzolamide: N-desethyl brinzolamide (metabolite). Brimonidine: Liver (extensive). **Elimination:** Brinzolamide: Urine (unchanged, metabolites); $T_{1/2}$=111 days (whole blood). Brimonidine: (PO) Urine (74%, unchanged and metabolites). $T_{1/2}$=3 hrs.

PATIENT CONSIDERATIONS
Assessment: Assess for hypersensitivity to drug or to sulfonamides, low endothelial cell counts, renal/hepatic impairment, contact lens use, severe CVD, depression, cerebral or coronary insufficiency, Raynaud's phenomenon, orthostatic hypotension, thromboangiitis obliterans, pregnancy/nursing status, and possible drug interactions.

Monitoring: Monitor for sulfonamide hypersensitivity reactions, potentiation of syndromes associated w/ vascular insufficiency, bacterial keratitis, and other adverse reactions.

Counseling: Advise to d/c use and consult physician if serious or unusual ocular or systemic reactions or signs of hypersensitivity occur. Inform that vision may be temporarily blurred following dosing and fatigue and/or drowsiness may be experienced; instruct to use caution in operating machinery, driving a motor vehicle, and engaging in other hazardous activities. Instruct that ocular sol, if handled improperly or if the tip of dispensing container contacts the eye or surrounding structures, can become contaminated by common bacteria known to cause infections. Advise that using contaminated sol may result in serious eye damage and subsequent loss of vision. Instruct to always replace cap after using. Advise not to use if sol changes color or becomes cloudy. Instruct to consult physician about the continued use of the present multidose container if having ocular surgery or if an intercurrent ocular condition (eg, trauma, infection) develops. If using >1 topical ophthalmic drug, instruct to administer the drugs at least 5 min apart. Advise that contact lenses should be removed during instillation, but may be reinserted 15 min after instillation.

SIMCOR — niacin/simvastatin   Rx

Class: HMG-CoA reductase inhibitor (statin)/nicotinic acid

ADULT DOSAGE	PEDIATRIC DOSAGE
Hypertriglyceridemia	Pediatric use may not have been established
When treatment w/ simvastatin monotherapy or niacin extended-release (ER) monotherapy is considered inadequate	
Not Currently on Niacin ER or Switching from Non-ER Niacin: **Initial:** 500mg/20mg at hs	
Titrate (Niacin ER Component): Increase by no more than 500mg qd every 4 weeks; after Week 8, titrate to patient response and tolerance	
Maint: 1000mg/20mg to 2000mg/40mg qd depending on tolerability and lipid levels	
Max: 2000mg/40mg qd	
If discontinued for >7 days, retitrate as tolerated	
Additional Lipid Level Management Needed Despite Simvastatin 20-40mg Only: **Initial:** 500mg/40mg qd at hs	
Primary Hypercholesterolemia/Mixed Dyslipidemia	
When treatment w/ simvastatin monotherapy or niacin ER monotherapy is considered inadequate	

Not Currently on Niacin ER or Switching from Non-ER Niacin:
Initial: 500mg/20mg qd at hs
Titrate (Niacin ER Component):
Increase by no more than 500mg qd every 4 weeks; after Week 8, titrate to patient response and tolerance
Maint: 1000mg/20mg to 2000mg/40mg qd depending on tolerability and lipid levels
Max: 2000mg/40mg qd

If discontinued for >7 days, retitrate as tolerated

Additional Lipid Level Management Needed Despite Simvastatin 20-40mg Only:
Initial: 500mg/40mg qd at hs

DOSING CONSIDERATIONS
Concomitant Medications
Amiodarone, Amlodipine, or Ranolazine:
Max: 1000mg/20mg/day

Renal Impairment
Mild/Moderate: No studies have been conducted
Severe: Do not start unless already tolerated ≥10mg simvastatin; exercise caution and monitor closely

Other Important Considerations
Chinese Patients:
Caution w/ doses >(1000mg/20mg)/day

ADMINISTRATION
Oral route

Take at hs w/ a low-fat snack.
Swallow whole; do not break, crush, or chew.
Avoid administration on an empty stomach to reduce flushing, pruritus, and GI distress.
May take aspirin (ASA) (up to 325mg) 30 min prior to treatment to reduce flushing.

STORAGE
20-25°C (68-77°F).

HOW SUPPLIED
Tab: (Niacin ER/Simvastatin) 500mg/20mg, 500mg/40mg, 750mg/20mg, 1000mg/20mg, 1000mg/40mg

CONTRAINDICATIONS
Active liver disease or unexplained persistent elevations in hepatic transaminase levels, active peptic ulcer disease (PUD), arterial bleeding, women who are or may become pregnant, and nursing mothers. Concomitant administration w/ strong CYP3A4 inhibitors (eg, itraconazole, ketoconazole, posaconazole, HIV protease inhibitors, boceprevir, telaprevir, erythromycin, clarithromycin, telithromycin, nefazodone), gemfibrozil, cyclosporine, danazol, verapamil, or diltiazem. Known hypersensitivity to any component of this product.

WARNINGS/PRECAUTIONS
No incremental benefit of Simcor on cardiovascular (CV) morbidity and mortality over and above that demonstrated for simvastatin monotherapy and niacin monotherapy has been established. Niacin ER, at doses of 1500-2000mg/day, in combination w/ simvastatin, did not reduce the incidence of CV events more than simvastatin in patients w/ CV disease and mean baseline LDL levels of 74mg/dL. Should only be substituted for equivalent doses of niacin ER (Niaspan); do not substitute for equivalent doses of immediate-release (crystalline) niacin. Dose-related myopathy and/or rhabdomyolysis reported; predisposing factors include advanced age (≥65 yrs of age), female gender, uncontrolled hypothyroidism, and renal impairment. Immune-mediated necrotizing myopathy (IMNM) reported. D/C if markedly elevated CPK levels occur or myopathy is diagnosed/suspected, and temporarily withhold in any patient experiencing an acute or serious condition predisposing to development of renal failure secondary to rhabdomyolysis. Stop treatment for a few days before elective major surgery and when any major acute medical/surgical condition supervenes. Severe hepatic toxicity, including fulminant hepatic necrosis, reported when substituting sustained-release niacin for IR niacin at equivalent doses. Caution w/ substantial alcohol consumption and/or history of liver disease. May cause abnormal LFTs; obtain LFTs prior to initiation and repeat as clinically indicated. Fatal and nonfatal hepatic failure (rare) reported; promptly interrupt therapy if serious liver injury w/ clinical symptoms and/or hyperbilirubinemia or jaundice occurs and do not restart if an alternate etiology is not found. Increases in HbA1c and FPG levels reported; closely monitor diabetic/potentially diabetic patients (particularly during 1st few months of therapy), and adjust diet and/or hypoglycemic therapy or d/c Simcor if necessary. May reduce platelet count or phosphorus (P) levels, and increase PT or uric acid levels. Caution in patients predisposed to gout or w/ renal impairment, and in elderly.

ADVERSE REACTIONS
Flushing, headache, back pain, diarrhea, nausea, pruritus.

DRUG INTERACTIONS
See Contraindications. Avoid ingestion of alcohol, hot drinks, or spicy foods around the time of administration; may increase flushing and pruritus.
Simvastatin: Due to the risk of myopathy, avoid w/ large quantities of grapefruit juice (>1 quart/day) and drugs that cause myopathy/rhabdomyolysis when given alone (eg, fibrates). Caution w/ colchicine; do not exceed 1000mg/20mg/day w/ amiodarone, amlodipine, and ranolazine. Voriconazole may increase concentration; consider dose adjustment of Simcor to reduce risk of myopathy/rhabdomyolysis. Decreased C_{max} w/ propranolol. May increase digoxin concentrations; monitor patients taking digoxin when therapy is initiated. May potentiate effect of coumarin anticoagulants; determine PT before initiation and monitor frequently during early therapy and at usual recommended intervals once a stable PT has been documented. **Niacin:** ASA may decrease metabolic clearance. May potentiate effects of ganglionic blocking agents and vasoactive drugs, resulting in postural hypotension. Separate administration from bile acid-binding resins (eg, colestipol, cholestyramine) by at least 4-6 hrs. Nutritional supplements containing large doses of niacin or related compounds may potentiate adverse effects.

PREGNANCY AND LACTATION
Pregnancy: Category X.
Lactation: Not for use in nursing. It is not known whether simvastatin is excreted into human milk; however, a small amount of another drug in this class does pass into breast milk. Niacin is excreted into human milk but the actual infant dose or infant dose as a percent of the maternal dose is not known.

MECHANISM OF ACTION
Niacin: Nicotinic acid; has not been established. May partially inhibit release of free fatty acids from adipose tissue, and increase lipoprotein lipase activity (which may increase rate of chylomicron TG removal from plasma). Decreases rate of hepatic synthesis of VLDL-C and LDL-C. **Simvastatin:** HMG-CoA reductase inhibitor; inhibits conversion of HMG-CoA to mevalonate. Reduces VLDL and TGs, and increases HDL-C.

PHARMACOKINETICS
Absorption: Niacin: T_{max}=4.6-4.9 hrs. Simvastatin: T_{max}=1.9-2 hrs, 6.56 hrs (simvastatin acid); C_{max}=3.29ng/mL, $AUC_{(0-t)}$=30.81ng•hr/mL (simvastatin acid). **Distribution:** Niacin: Found in breast milk. **Metabolism:** Niacin: Liver (rapid and extensive 1st-pass); nicotinuric acid (via conjugation), nicotinamide adenine dinucleotide (metabolites). Simvastatin: Liver (rapid and extensive 1st-pass) via CYP3A4; β-hydroxyacid (simvastatin acid), 6'-hydroxy, 6'-hydroxymethyl, and 6'-exomethylene derivatives (major active metabolites). **Elimination:** Niacin: Urine (54%, 3.6% unchanged). Simvastatin: Feces (60%), urine (13%); $T_{1/2}$=4.2-4.9 hrs, 4.6-5 hrs (simvastatin acid).

PATIENT CONSIDERATIONS
Assessment: Assess for history of/active liver disease, unexplained persistent hepatic transaminase elevations, active PUD, arterial bleeding, predisposing factors for myopathy, renal impairment, diabetes, any other conditions where treatment is contraindicated or cautioned, drug hypersensitivity, pregnancy/nursing status, and possible drug interactions. Assess lipid profile and LFTs.

Monitoring: Monitor for signs/symptoms of myopathy (including IMNM), rhabdomyolysis, liver/renal dysfunction, decreases in platelet counts and P levels, increases in PT and uric acid levels, and other adverse reactions. Monitor lipid profile, LFTs, blood glucose, and CPK levels. Check PT w/ coumarin anticoagulants.

Counseling: Advise to adhere to their National Cholesterol Education Program-recommended diet, a regular exercise program, and periodic testing of a fasting lipid panel. Inform about substances that should be avoided during therapy, and advise to discuss all medications, both prescription and OTC, including vitamins or other nutritional supplements containing niacin or nicotinamide, w/ their physician. Instruct to report promptly any unexplained muscle pain, tenderness, or weakness, particularly if accompanied by malaise or fever or if these muscle signs or symptoms persist after discontinuation, any symptoms that may indicate liver injury, or if symptoms of dizziness occur. Advise to notify physician prior to restarting therapy if dosing is interrupted for any length of time, and of changes in blood glucose if diabetic. Inform that flushing may occur but may subside after several weeks of consistent use of therapy. If awakened by flushing at night, instruct to get up slowly, especially if feeling dizzy or faint, or taking BP medications. Instruct women to use an effective method of birth control to prevent pregnancy while on therapy, to d/c therapy and call physician if pregnant, and not to breastfeed while on therapy.

SIMPONI — golimumab

Class: Monoclonal antibody/TNF blocker

Rx

Increased risk for developing serious infections (eg, active tuberculosis [TB], latent TB reactivation, invasive fungal infections, bacterial/viral infections, opportunistic infections) leading to hospitalization or death, mostly w/ concomitant use of immunosuppressants (eg, methotrexate [MTX] or corticosteroids). D/C if serious infection develops. Active TB/latent TB reactivation may present w/ disseminated or extrapulmonary disease; test for latent TB before and during therapy and initiate treatment for latent TB prior to therapy. Invasive fungal infections reported; consider empiric antifungal therapy in patients at risk who develop severe systemic illness. Consider risks and benefits prior to therapy in patients w/ chronic or recurrent infection. Monitor patients for development of infection during and after treatment, including development of TB in patients who tested (-) for latent TB infection prior to therapy. Lymphoma and other malignancies, some fatal, reported in children and adolescents.

ADULT DOSAGE
Ulcerative Colitis

Moderately to severely active ulcerative colitis (UC) in patients w/ an inadequate response or intolerant to prior treatment or in patients who have demonstrated corticosteroid dependence

PEDIATRIC DOSAGE
Pediatric use may not have been established

Initial: 200mg SQ at Week 0, followed by 100mg SQ at Week 2
Maint: 100mg SQ every 4 weeks

Psoriatic Arthritis

Treatment of Active Psoriatic Arthritis w/ or w/o MTX or Other Nonbiologic Disease Modifying Antirheumatic Drugs (DMARDs):
50mg SQ once a month

May continue corticosteroids, nonbiologic DMARDs, and/or NSAIDs during treatment

Rheumatoid Arthritis

Moderately to Severely Active in Combination w/ MTX:
50mg SQ once a month

May continue corticosteroids, nonbiologic DMARDs, and/or NSAIDs during treatment

Ankylosing Spondylitis

Treatment of Active Ankylosing Spondylitis w/ or w/o MTX or Other Nonbiologic DMARDs:
50mg SQ once a month

May continue corticosteroids, nonbiologic DMARDs, and/or NSAIDs during treatment

---

ADMINISTRATION
SQ route

Allow the prefilled syringe or autoinjector to sit at room temperature outside the carton for 30 min prior to SQ inj. Do not warm in any other way.
If multiple inj are required, administer the inj at different sites on the body.
Rotate inj sites; avoid areas where skin is tender, bruised, red, or hard.
Refer to PI for further instructions.

STORAGE
2-8°C (36-46°F). Protect from light. Do not freeze or shake.

HOW SUPPLIED
Inj: 50mg/0.5mL, 100mg/mL [prefilled SmartJect autoinjector, prefilled syringe]

WARNINGS/PRECAUTIONS
Do not initiate in patients w/ an active infection. Increased risk of infection in patients >65 yrs of age and in patients w/ comorbid conditions; consider the risks and benefits prior to therapy in patients who have resided or traveled in areas of endemic TB or endemic mycoses, and w/ any underlying conditions predisposing to infection. D/C if an opportunistic infection or sepsis develops. Hepatitis B virus (HBV) reactivation reported in chronic carriers; closely monitor for signs of active HBV infection during and for several months after therapy. D/C if reactivation occurs and initiate antiviral therapy. Consider risks and benefits prior to initiating therapy in patients w/ a known malignancy other than a successfully treated nonmelanoma skin cancer or when considering continuing therapy in patients who develop a malignancy. Cases of acute/chronic leukemia, melanoma, and Merkel cell carcinoma reported. Rare postmarketing cases of hepatosplenic T-cell lymphoma reported, and nearly all of the cases occurred in patients w/ Crohn's disease or UC and mostly in adolescent and young adult males; almost all of these patients were treated concomitantly w/ azathioprine or 6-mercaptopurine. All patients w/ UC who are at increased risk for dysplasia or colon carcinoma, or who had a prior history of dysplasia or colon carcinoma should be screened for dysplasia at regular intervals before therapy and throughout their disease course. Worsening and new onset congestive heart failure (CHF) reported; caution w/ CHF and d/c if new/worsening symptoms appear. Associated w/ rare cases of new onset or exacerbation of CNS demyelinating disorders (eg, multiple sclerosis) and peripheral demyelinating disorders (eg, Guillain-Barre syndrome); consider discontinuation if these disorders develop. May result in the formation of antinuclear antibodies and, rarely, in the development of a lupus-like syndrome; d/c treatment if symptoms suggestive of a lupus-like syndrome develop. Caution when switching from one biologic DMARD to another; overlapping biological activity may further increase risk of infection. Hematologic cytopenias (eg, pancytopenia, leukopenia, neutropenia, thrombocytopenia) reported; caution in patients who have or have had significant cytopenias. Serious systemic hypersensitivity reactions reported; d/c immediately and institute appropriate therapy if these reactions occur. Caution in elderly.

ADVERSE REACTIONS
URTI, viral infections, inj-site reactions, HTN, increased ALT/AST.

DRUG INTERACTIONS
See Boxed Warning. Not recommended w/ anakinra, abatacept, or biologics approved to treat rheumatoid arthritis, psoriatic arthritis, or ankylosing spondylitis; may increase risk of serious infections. Avoid w/ live vaccines and therapeutic infectious agents (eg, live attenuated bacteria [eg, Bacille Calmette-Guerin bladder instillation for the treatment of cancer]). Avoid administration of live vaccines to infants for 6 months following the mother's last golimumab inj during pregnancy. Upon initiation or discontinuation of therapy in patients being treated w/ CYP450 substrates w/ a narrow therapeutic index, monitor effect (eg, warfarin) or drug concentration (eg, cyclosporine, theophylline) and may adjust individual dose of the drug product as needed.

PREGNANCY AND LACTATION
Pregnancy: Category B. IgG antibodies cross placenta during pregnancy and have been detected in the serum of infants born to patients treated w/ these antibodies; infants born to women treated w/ Simponi during their pregnancy may be at increased risk of infection for up to 6 months. Administration of live vaccines to infants exposed to Simponi in utero is not recommended for 6 months following the mother's last infusion during pregnancy.
Lactation: Not for use in nursing.

MECHANISM OF ACTION
Monoclonal antibody/TNF-α receptor blocker; prevents the binding of TNF-α to its receptors, thereby inhibiting the biological activity of TNF-α.

PHARMACOKINETICS
Absorption: Absolute bioavailability (53%); C_{max}=3.2mcg/mL; T_{max}=2-6 days (median). **Distribution:** V_d=58-126mL/kg (IV); crosses the placenta. **Elimination:** (IV) $T_{1/2}$=2 weeks (median).

PATIENT CONSIDERATIONS
Assessment: Assess for active/chronic/recurrent infection, history of an opportunistic infection, recent travel to areas of endemic TB or endemic mycoses, underlying conditions that may predispose to infection, malignancies, dysplasia (in UC patients), CHF, demyelinating disorders, significant cytopenias, latex sensitivity, risk factors for skin cancer, pregnancy/nursing status, and possible drug interactions. Test for latent TB infection and for HBV infection.

Monitoring: Monitor for development of infection during and after treatment. Monitor for HBV reactivation, malignancies, dysplasia, new or worsening CHF, demyelinating disorders, hematological events, hypersensitivity reactions, and other adverse reactions. Periodically evaluate for active TB and test for latent TB infection. Perform periodic skin examination, particularly in patients w/ risk factors for skin cancer.

Counseling: Advise of the potential risks and benefits of therapy. Inform that therapy may lower the ability of immune system to fight infections; instruct to contact physician if any symptoms of infection develop. Counsel about the risk of lymphoma and other malignancies. Instruct patients sensitive to latex to not handle the needle cover on the prefilled syringe as well as the needle cover of the prefilled syringe w/in the autoinjector cap because it contains dry natural rubber (a derivative of latex). Advise to report any signs of new/worsening medical conditions (eg, CHF, demyelinating disorders, autoimmune diseases, liver disease, cytopenias, psoriasis). Inform about proper administration instructions.

SIMPONI ARIA — golimumab   Rx
Class: Monoclonal antibody/TNF blocker

> Increased risk for developing serious infections (eg, active tuberculosis [TB], latent TB reactivation, invasive fungal infections, bacterial/viral infections, and opportunistic infections) leading to hospitalization or death, mostly w/ concomitant use w/ immunosuppressants (eg, methotrexate [MTX] or corticosteroids). D/C if serious infection develops. Active/latent reactivation TB may present w/ disseminated or extrapulmonary disease; test for latent TB before and during therapy and initiate treatment for latent TB prior to therapy. Invasive fungal infections reported; consider empiric antifungal therapy in patients at risk who develop severe systemic illness. Consider risks and benefits prior to therapy in patients w/ chronic or recurrent infection. Monitor patients for development of infection during and after treatment, including development of TB in patients who tested (-) for latent TB infection prior to therapy. Lymphoma and other malignancies, some fatal, reported in children and adolescents.

ADULT DOSAGE
Rheumatoid Arthritis

Moderately to Severely Active in Combination w/ MTX:
2mg/kg IV infusion over 30 min at Weeks 0 and 4, then every 8 weeks thereafter

May continue other non-biologic disease-modifying antirheumatic drugs (DMARDs), corticosteroids, NSAIDs, and/or analgesics during treatment

PEDIATRIC DOSAGE
Pediatric use may not have been established

ADMINISTRATION
IV route

Dilute w/ 0.9% w/v NaCl to a final volume of 100mL; gently mix.
Alternatively, may dilute w/ 0.45% w/v NaCl.
Use only an infusion set w/ an in-line, sterile, non-pyrogenic, low protein-binding filter (pore size 0.22µM or less).
Do not infuse concomitantly in the same IV line w/ other agents.
Infuse diluted sol over 30 min.
Once diluted, may store infusion sol for 4 hrs at room temperature.
Refer to PI for further administration instructions.

STORAGE
2-8°C (36-46°F). Protect from light. Do not freeze or shake.

HOW SUPPLIED
Inj: 50mg/4mL

WARNINGS/PRECAUTIONS
Do not initiate in patients w/ an active infection. Increased risk of infection in patients >65 yrs of age and in patients w/ comorbid conditions; consider the risks and benefits prior to therapy in patients who have resided or traveled in areas of endemic TB or endemic mycoses, and w/ any underlying conditions predisposing

to infection. D/C if an opportunistic infection or sepsis develops. Hepatitis B virus (HBV) reactivation reported in chronic carriers; closely monitor for signs of active HBV infection during and for several months after therapy. D/C if reactivation occurs and initiate antiviral therapy; caution when considering resuming TNF blockers. Consider risks and benefits prior to initiating therapy in patients w/ a known malignancy other than a successfully treated non-melanoma skin cancer or when considering continuing therapy in patients who develop a malignancy. Cases of acute/chronic leukemia, melanoma, and Merkel cell carcinoma reported. Rare postmarketing cases of hepatosplenic T-cell lymphoma reported, and nearly all of the cases occurred in patients w/ Crohn's disease or ulcerative colitis and mostly in adolescent and young adult males; almost all of these patients were treated concomitantly w/ azathioprine or 6-mercaptopurine. Worsening and new onset CHF reported; caution w/ CHF and d/c if new/worsening symptoms appear. Associated w/ rare cases of new onset or exacerbation of CNS demyelinating disorders (eg, multiple sclerosis) and peripheral demyelinating disorders (eg, Guillain-Barre syndrome); consider discontinuation if these disorders develop. May result in the formation of antinuclear antibodies and, rarely, in the development of a lupus-like syndrome; d/c treatment if symptoms suggestive of a lupus-like syndrome develop. Caution when switching from one biologic DMARD to another; overlapping biological activity may further increase risk of infection. Pancytopenia, leukopenia, neutropenia, and thrombocytopenia reported; caution in patients who have or have had significant cytopenias. Serious systemic hypersensitivity reactions may occur; d/c immediately and institute appropriate therapy if anaphylactic or other serious allergic reactions occur. Caution in elderly.

ADVERSE REACTIONS
URTI, viral infections, bronchitis, HTN, rash.

DRUG INTERACTIONS
See Boxed Warning. MTX decreases clearance. Not recommended w/ anakinra, abatacept, or biologics approved to treat rheumatoid arthritis; may increase risk of serious infections. Avoid w/ live vaccines and therapeutic infectious agents (eg, live attenuated bacteria [eg, bacille Calmette-Guerin bladder instillation for the treatment of cancer]). Avoid administration of live vaccines to infants for 6 months following the mother's last golimumab infusion during pregnancy. Upon initiation or discontinuation of therapy in patients being treated w/ CYP450 substrates w/ a narrow therapeutic index, monitor effect (eg, warfarin) or drug concentration (eg, cyclosporine, theophylline) and adjust individual dose of the drug product as needed.

PREGNANCY AND LACTATION
Pregnancy: Category B. IgG antibodies cross placenta during pregnancy and have been detected in the serum of infants born to patients treated w/ these antibodies; infants born to women treated w/ Simponi Aria during their pregnancy may be at increased risk of infection for up to 6 months. Administration of live vaccines to infants exposed to Simponi Aria in utero is not recommended for 6 months following the mother's last infusion during pregnancy.
Lactation: Not for use in nursing.

MECHANISM OF ACTION
Monoclonal antibody/TNF-α receptor blocker; binds to both soluble and transmembrane bioactive forms of human TNF-α. Prevents the binding of TNF-α to its receptors, thereby inhibiting the biological activity of TNF-α.

PHARMACOKINETICS
Absorption: C_{max}=44.4mcg/mL. **Distribution:** V_d=151mL/kg; crosses the placenta. **Elimination:** $T_{1/2}$=14 days.

PATIENT CONSIDERATIONS
Assessment: Assess for active/chronic/recurrent infection, history of an opportunistic infection, recent travel to areas of endemic TB or endemic mycoses, underlying conditions that may predispose to infection, malignancies, CHF, demyelinating disorders, significant cytopenias, risk factors for skin cancer, pregnancy/nursing status, and possible drug interactions. Test for latent TB infection and for HBV infection.

Monitoring: Monitor for development of infection during and after treatment. Monitor for HBV reactivation, malignancies, new or worsening CHF, demyelinating disorders, hematological events, hypersensitivity reactions, and other adverse reactions. Periodically evaluate for active TB and test for latent TB infection. Perform periodic skin examination, particularly in patients w/ risk factors for skin cancer.

Counseling: Advise of the potential risks and benefits of therapy. Inform that therapy may lower the ability of the immune system to fight infections; instruct to contact physician if any symptoms of infection develop. Inform of the risk of lymphoma and other malignancies. Advise to report any signs of new/worsening medical conditions (eg, CHF, demyelinating disorders, autoimmune diseases, liver disease, cytopenias, psoriasis).

SINEMET CR — carbidopa/levodopa
Class: Dopa-decarboxylase inhibitor/dopamine precursor   Rx

OTHER BRAND NAMES
Sinemet

ADULT DOSAGE
Parkinsonism

Treatment of Parkinson's Disease, Postencephalitic Parkinsonism, and Symptomatic Parkinsonism Following Carbon Monoxide/Manganese Intoxication:

PEDIATRIC DOSAGE
Pediatric use may not have been established

Tab:
Usual Dose:
Initial: One 25mg/100mg tab tid or one 10mg/100mg tab tid-qid
Titrate: May increase by 1 tab (25mg/100mg or 10mg/100mg) qd or qod, as necessary, until a dose of 8 tabs/day is reached

Transfer from Levodopa:
D/C levodopa at least 12 hrs before starting therapy; choose a daily dose of therapy that will provide approx 25% of the previous levodopa dose
Previously Taking <1500mg/day of Levodopa:
Initial: One 25mg/100mg tab tid or qid
Previously Taking >1500mg/day of Levodopa:
Initial: One 25mg/250mg tab tid or qid

Maint:
At least 70-100mg/day of carbidopa should be provided; may substitute one 25mg/100mg tab for each 10mg/100mg tab when greater proportion of carbidopa is required. When more levodopa is required, substitute 25mg/250mg tab for 25mg/100mg or 10mg/100mg; may increase dose of 25mg/250mg by 1/2 or 1 tab qd or qod to a max of 8 tabs/day if necessary

Max: 200mg/day of carbidopa

Tab, Sustained-Release (SR):
Initial Dosage:
Currently Treated w/ Conventional Carbidopa Levodopa Preparations:
Dosage w/ SR tabs should be substituted at an amount that provides approx 10% more levodopa per day. May need to increase to a dose that provides up to 30% more levodopa per day depending on clinical response; interval between doses should be 4-8 hrs during the waking day

Initial Conversion from IR to SR Tabs (Based on Levodopa Component):
300-400mg: 200mg bid
500-600mg: 300mg bid or 200mg tid
700-800mg: Total of 800mg in ≥3 divided doses (eg, 300mg am, 300mg early pm, and 200mg later pm)
900-1000mg: Total of 1000mg in ≥3 divided doses (eg, 400mg am, 400mg early pm, and 200mg later pm)

Currently Treated w/ Levodopa w/o a Decarboxylase Inhibitor:
D/C levodopa at least 12 hrs before starting therapy; substitute at a dose that will provide approx 25% of the previous levodopa dose
Mild to Moderate Disease:
Initial: One 50mg/200mg tab bid

Patients Not Receiving Levodopa:
Mild to Moderate Disease:
Initial: One 50mg/200mg tab bid at ≥6-hr intervals

Titration:
Following therapy initiation, may increase/decrease doses and dosing intervals depending on response. Most patients have been adequately treated w/ doses that provide 400-1600mg/day of levodopa given in divided doses at 4- to 8-hr intervals during the waking day.
When given at intervals of <4 hrs, and/or if the divided doses are not equal, give the smaller doses at the end of the day.
An interval of at least 3 days between dosage adjustments is recommended.

DOSING CONSIDERATIONS
Concomitant Medications
Addition of Other Antiparkinsonian Medications:
Tab/Tab, SR:
Standard drugs for Parkinson's disease, other than levodopa w/o a decarboxylase inhibitor, may be used concomitantly w/ therapy, although their dosage may have to be adjusted
Tab, SR:
Anticholinergic agents, dopamine agonists, and amantadine may be given w/ therapy; dosage adjustment of therapy may be necessary when these agents are added
A dose of 25mg/100mg IR or 10mg/100mg IR (1/2 tab or whole tab) may be added to the dosage regimen in selected patients w/ advanced disease who need additional IR levodopa for a brief time during daytime hrs

Interruption of Therapy:
Tab/Tab, SR:
If general anesthesia is required, may continue therapy as long as patient is permitted to take fluids and medication by mouth. If therapy is interrupted temporarily, observe for symptoms resembling neuroleptic malignant syndrome and administer usual daily dose as soon as patient is able to take oral medication

Adverse Reactions
Tab:
Involuntary movements may require dosage reduction

ADMINISTRATION
Oral route

Tab
Tabs w/ different ratios of carbidopa to levodopa may be given separately or combined as needed to provide the optimum dosage.

Tab, SR
Do not chew or crush.

STORAGE
25°C (77°F); excursions permitted to 15-30°C (59-86°F). Protect from light and moisture.

HOW SUPPLIED
(Carbidopa/Levodopa) **Tab, SR (CR):** 25mg/100mg, 50mg/200mg; (Sinemet)
Tab: 10mg/100mg, 25mg/100mg, 25mg/250mg

CONTRAINDICATIONS
During or within 2 weeks of using nonselective MAOIs. Narrow-angle glaucoma, known hypersensitivity to any component of this drug.

WARNINGS/PRECAUTIONS
May cause or increase dyskinesias; may require dose reduction. Monitor for depression with concomitant suicidal tendencies. Caution with severe cardiovascular (CV) or pulmonary disease, bronchial asthma, renal/hepatic/ endocrine disease, chronic wide-angle glaucoma, or history of MI with residual atrial, nodal, or ventricular arrhythmias. May increase the possibility of upper GI hemorrhage in patients with history of peptic ulcer. Falling asleep during activities of daily living and somnolence reported; consider discontinuation if significant daytime sleepiness or episodes of falling asleep during activities that require active participation occur. May impair mental/physical abilities. Sporadic cases of a symptom complex resembling neuroleptic malignant syndrome (hyperpyrexia and confusion) reported during dose reductions or withdrawal; observed carefully when the dosage of levodopa is reduced abruptly or discontinued, especially if the patient is receiving neuroleptics. Hallucinations and psychotic-like behavior reported; do not use in patients with a major psychotic disorder. Intense urge to gamble, increased sexual urges, intense urges to spend money, binge eating, and/or other intense urges, and the inability to control these urges may occur; consider dose reduction or discontinuation if such urges develop. Monitor for melanomas frequently and on a regular basis. Abnormalities in lab tests, including elevations of LFTs, and abnormalities in BUN and (+) Coombs test reported. Lab test interactions may occur. Cases of falsely diagnosed pheochromocytoma reported very rarely; caution when interpreting the plasma and urine levels of catecholamines and their metabolites. Caution in elderly.

ADVERSE REACTIONS
Dyskinesias (eg, choreiform, dystonic, other involuntary movements), nausea, hallucinations, confusion.

DRUG INTERACTIONS
See Contraindications. Caution with concomitant use of sedating medications; may increase the risk for somnolence. Certain medications used to treat psychosis may exacerbate the symptoms of Parkinson's disease and may decrease effectiveness of carbidopa-levodopa. Symptomatic postural hypotension reported with concomitant use of some antihypertensive drugs; dosage adjustment of the antihypertensive drug may be required. Use with selegiline may cause severe orthostatic hypotension. Adverse reactions, including HTN and dyskinesia, reported rarely with TCAs. Dopamine D$_2$ receptor antagonists (eg, phenothiazines, butyrophenones, risperidone) and isoniazid may reduce effects of levodopa. Beneficial effects of levodopa in Parkinson's disease reported to be reversed by phenytoin and papaverine; monitor for loss of therapeutic response. Not recommended with dopamine-depleting agents (eg, reserpine, tetrabenazine) or other drugs known to deplete monoamine stores. Iron salts may reduce bioavailability; caution with iron salts or multivitamins containing iron salts. Metoclopramide may increase bioavailability of levodopa and may also adversely affect disease control.

PREGNANCY AND LACTATION
Pregnancy: Category C.
Lactation: Caution in nursing.

MECHANISM OF ACTION
Dopa-decarboxylase inhibitor/dopamine precursor. Carbidopa: Inhibits decarboxylation of peripheral levodopa. Levodopa: Crosses blood-brain barrier and presumably is converted to dopamine in the brain.

PHARMACOKINETICS
Absorption: Administration of variable doses resulted in different parameters. **Distribution:** Levodopa: Crosses the placenta; found in breast milk. **Elimination:** Levodopa: $T_{1/2}$=50 min, 1.5 hrs (in the presence of carbidopa).

PATIENT CONSIDERATIONS
Assessment: Assess for hypersensitivity to drug; narrow-angle/chronic wide-angle glaucoma; major psychotic disorder; history of peptic ulcer; risk factors that may increase risk for somnolence (eg, presence of sleep disorders); severe CV or pulmonary disease; bronchial asthma; renal/hepatic/endocrine disease; history of MI with residual atrial, nodal, or ventricular arrhythmias; pregnancy/nursing status; and possible drug interactions.

Monitoring: Monitor for dyskinesias, depression with suicidal tendencies, drowsiness/sleepiness, somnolence, hyperpyrexia and confusion, hallucinations/ psychotic-like behavior, impulse control/compulsive behaviors, upper GI hemorrhage in patients with a history of peptic ulcer, and other adverse reactions. In patients with a history of MI who have residual atrial, nodal, or ventricular arrhythmias, monitor cardiac function with particular care during the period of initial dosage adjustment. Monitor for LFT elevations and BUN abnormalities. For patients on extended therapy, perform periodic evaluation of hepatic, hematopoietic, CV, and renal function. Monitor for melanomas frequently and on a regular basis. Monitor for changes in intraocular pressure in patients with chronic wide-angle glaucoma. Monitor closely during the dose adjustment period.

Counseling: Instruct to take ud and not to change the prescribed dosage regimen or add any additional antiparkinson medications, including other carbidopa-levodopa preparations, without 1st consulting the physician. Inform that, occasionally, dark color (red, brown, or black) may appear in saliva, urine, or sweat after ingestion of therapy. Inform that high protein diet, excessive acidity, and iron salts may reduce clinical effectiveness. Instruct to exercise caution while driving or operating machinery, and that if somnolence and/or sudden sleep onset is experienced, to refrain from these activities. Instruct to inform physician if new/increased gambling urges, increased sexual urges, or other intense urges develop. (Tab, IR) Advise that sometimes a "wearing-off" effect may occur at the end of the dosing interval; instruct to notify physician if such response poses a problem to lifestyle. (Tab, SR) Instruct to notify physician if abnormal involuntary movements appear or get worse during treatment. Advise that sometimes the onset of effect of the 1st am dose may be delayed for up to 1 hr compared with the response usually obtained from the 1st am dose of IR tab; instruct to notify physician if such delayed responses pose a problem in treatment.

SINGULAIR — montelukast sodium
Rx

Class: Leukotriene receptor antagonist

ADULT DOSAGE
Asthma
Prophylaxis/Chronic Treatment:
10mg tab qpm

Patients w/ both asthma and allergic rhinitis should take only 1 dose qpm

Perennial Allergic Rhinitis
10mg tab qd

Patients w/ both asthma and allergic rhinitis should take only 1 dose qpm

Seasonal Allergic Rhinitis
10mg tab qd

Patients w/ both asthma and allergic rhinitis should take only 1 dose qpm

Exercise-Induced Bronchoconstriction
Prevention:
10mg tab at least 2 hrs before exercise

Do not take an additional dose w/in 24 hrs of a previous dose.
Patients already taking montelukast daily for another indication (including chronic asthma) should not take an additional dose to prevent exercise-induced bronchoconstriction (EIB).

PEDIATRIC DOSAGE
Asthma
Prophylaxis/Chronic Treatment:
12-23 Months:
4mg oral granules qpm

2-5 Years:
4mg chewable tab or 4mg oral granules qpm

6-14 Years:
5mg chewable tab qpm

≥15 Years:
10mg tab qpm

Patients w/ both asthma and allergic rhinitis should take only 1 dose qpm

Perennial Allergic Rhinitis
6-23 Months:
4mg oral granules qd

2-5 Years:
4mg chewable tab or 4mg oral granules qd

6-14 Years:
5mg chewable tab qd

≥15 Years:
10mg tab qd

Patients w/ both asthma and allergic rhinitis should take only 1 dose qpm

Seasonal Allergic Rhinitis
2-5 Years:
4mg chewable tab or 4mg oral granules qd

6-14 Years:
5mg chewable tab qd

≥15 Years:
10mg tab qd

Patients w/ both asthma and allergic rhinitis should take only 1 dose qpm

Exercise-Induced Bronchoconstriction

Prevention:

6-14 Years:
5mg chewable tab at least 2 hrs before exercise

≥15 Years:
10mg tab at least 2 hrs before exercise

Do not take an additional dose w/in 24 hrs of a previous dose. Patients already taking montelukast daily for another indication (including chronic asthma) should not take an additional dose to prevent EIB.

ADMINISTRATION
Oral route

Take w/o regard to time of meals.

Instructions for Administration of Oral Granules
May be administered either directly in the mouth, dissolved in 1 tsp (5mL) of cold or room temperature baby formula or breast milk, or mixed w/ a spoonful of cold or room temperature soft foods; only applesauce, carrots, rice, or ice cream should be used.

Do not open packet until ready to use.

After opening the packet, the full dose (w/ or w/o mixing w/ baby formula, breast milk, or food) must be administered w/in 15 min.

If mixed w/ baby formula, breast milk, or food, oral granules must not be stored for future use.

Not intended to be dissolved in any liquid other than baby formula or breast milk for administration; however, liquids may be taken subsequent to administration.

STORAGE
25°C (77°F); excursions permitted to 15-30°C (59-86°F). Protect from light and moisture.

HOW SUPPLIED
Oral Granules: 4mg/pkt [30s]; **Tab, Chewable:** 4mg, 5mg; **Tab:** 10mg

CONTRAINDICATIONS
Hypersensitivity to any component of this product.

WARNINGS/PRECAUTIONS
Not for use in the reversal of bronchospasm in acute asthma attacks, including status asthmaticus; have appropriate rescue medication available. Therapy may be continued during acute exacerbations of asthma. Patients who have exacerbations of asthma after exercise should have short-acting inhaled β-agonist available for rescue. Should not be abruptly substituted for inhaled or oral corticosteroids. Avoid aspirin (ASA) and NSAIDs in patients w/ known ASA sensitivity while on therapy; although effective in improving airway function in asthmatics w/ documented ASA sensitivity, it has not been shown to truncate bronchoconstrictor response to ASA and other NSAIDs in ASA-sensitive asthmatic patients. Neuropsychiatric events reported; evaluate risks and benefits of continuing treatment if such events occur. Patients on therapy may present w/ systemic eosinophilia, sometimes presenting w/ clinical features of vasculitis consistent w/ Churg-Strauss syndrome; monitor for eosinophilia, vasculitic rash, worsening pulmonary symptoms, cardiac complications, and/or neuropathy. Chewable tabs contain phenylalanine; caution w/ phenylketonuria.

ADVERSE REACTIONS
URI, fever, headache, pharyngitis, cough, abdominal pain, diarrhea, otitis media, influenza, rhinorrhea, sinusitis, otitis.

PREGNANCY AND LACTATION
Pregnancy: Category B.
Lactation: Caution in nursing.

MECHANISM OF ACTION
Leukotriene receptor antagonist; binds to cysteinyl leukotriene (CysLT) receptors found in the airway (including airway smooth muscle cells and airway macrophages) and on other proinflammatory cells (including eosinophils and certain myeloid stem cells). Inhibits physiologic actions of leukotriene D4 at the CysLT type 1 receptor.

PHARMACOKINETICS
Absorption: Rapid. (10mg tab) T_{max}=3-4 hrs; oral bioavailability (64%). (5mg Chewable tab) T_{max}=2-2.5 hrs; oral bioavailability: fasted (73%), fed (63%). 2-5 Yrs: (4mg Chewable tab) T_{max}=2 hrs (fasted). (4mg Oral Granules) T_{max}=2.3 hrs (fasted), 6.4 hrs (fed). **Distribution:** V_d=8-11L; plasma protein binding (>99%). **Metabolism:** Liver (extensive); CYP3A4, 2C8, and 2C9. **Elimination:** Biliary (major), feces (86%), urine (<0.2%); $T_{1/2}$=2.7-5.5 hrs.

PATIENT CONSIDERATIONS
Assessment: Assess for hypersensitivity to drug, phenylketonuria, pregnancy/nursing status, and possible drug interactions.

Monitoring: Monitor for signs/symptoms of eosinophilia, vasculitic rash, worsening pulmonary symptoms, cardiac complications, neuropathy, neuropsychiatric events, hypersensitivity reactions, and other adverse reactions.

Counseling: Advise to take daily as prescribed, even when asymptomatic, as well as during periods of worsening asthma; instruct to contact physician if asthma is not well controlled. Inform that drug is not for treatment of acute asthma attacks; advise to have appropriate short-acting inhaled β-agonist medication available to treat asthma exacerbations. Advise to seek medical attention if short-acting inhaled bronchodilators are needed more often than usual while on therapy or if more than the max number of inhalations of short-acting bronchodilator treatment prescribed for a 24-hr period are needed. Instruct not to decrease dose or d/c other antiasthma medications unless instructed by physician. Instruct to notify physician if symptoms of neuropsychiatric events occur. Advise patients w/ ASA sensitivity to continue avoiding ASA and NSAIDs while on therapy. Inform phenylketonuric patients that the 4mg and 5mg chewable tabs contain phenylalanine.

SIRTURO — bedaquiline

Class: Diarylquinoline antimycobacterial agent

Rx

> Increased risk of death reported; only use when an effective treatment regimen cannot otherwise be provided. QT prolongation may occur. Use w/ drugs that prolong the QT interval may cause additive QT prolongation. Monitor ECGs. D/C therapy if significant ventricular arrhythmia or if QTcF interval prolongation of >500 msec develops.

ADULT DOSAGE
Tuberculosis

As part of a combination therapy for pulmonary multidrug resistant tuberculosis (MDR-TB), for use when an effective treatment regimen cannot otherwise be provided

Weeks 1-2: 400mg qd
Weeks 3-24: 200mg 3X/week (w/ at least 48 hrs between doses)

Use only in combination w/ at least 3 other drugs to which the patient's MDR-TB isolate is susceptible; if in vitro testing results are unavailable, may initiate treatment in combination w/ at least 4 other drugs to which patient's MDR-TB isolate is likely susceptible. Refer to PI of drugs used in combination.

Missed Dose

If a dose is missed during the first 2 weeks of treatment, do not administer missed dose (skip the dose and then continue the daily dosing regimen)

From Week 3 onwards, if 200mg dose is missed, administer the missed dose as soon as possible, and then resume the 3X/week dosing regimen

PEDIATRIC DOSAGE
Pediatric use may not have been established

ADMINISTRATION
Oral route

Swallow tab whole w/ water; take w/ food.
Administer by directly observed therapy.

STORAGE
25°C (77°F); excursions permitted to 15-30°C (59-86°F).

HOW SUPPLIED
Tab: 100mg

WARNINGS/PRECAUTIONS
Not for use for the treatment of latent infection due to *Mycobacterium tuberculosis* or infections caused by non-tuberculous mycobacteria. Increased risk of QT prolongation w/ history of torsades de pointes, congenital long QT syndrome, and uncompensated heart failure; history of or ongoing hypothyroidism or bradyarrhythmias; and serum Ca^{2+}, Mg^{2+}, or K^+ levels below the lower limits of normal. If necessary, consider treatment initiation after a favorable benefit risk assessment and w/ frequent ECG monitoring. If syncope occurs, obtain an ECG to detect QT prolongation. Hepatic-related adverse reactions reported. Test for viral hepatitis and d/c other hepatotoxic drugs if evidence of new/worsening liver dysfunction occurs. D/C therapy if aminotransferase elevations are accompanied by total bilirubin elevation >2X ULN, aminotransferase elevations are >8X ULN, or aminotransferase elevations are >5X ULN and persist >2 weeks. Caution in severe hepatic/renal impairment or in ESRD requiring hemodialysis/peritoneal dialysis.

ADVERSE REACTIONS
Nausea, arthralgia, headache, increased transaminases, hemoptysis, chest pain, anorexia, rash.

DRUG INTERACTIONS
See Boxed Warning. More hepatic-related adverse drug reactions reported w/ the addition of other drugs used to treat tuberculosis. Avoid w/ alcohol, other hepatotoxic drugs, strong CYP3A4 inducers (eg, rifamycins [eg, rifampin, rifapentine, rifabutin]), or moderate CYP3A4/CYP3A inducers (eg, efavirenz). Avoid use w/ strong CYP3A4 inhibitors (eg, ketoconazole, itraconazole) for >14 consecutive days, unless benefit outweighs the risk. Decreased exposure w/ CYP3A4 inducers and increased exposure w/ CYP3A4 inhibitors. Caution w/ lopinavir/ritonavir.

PREGNANCY AND LACTATION
Pregnancy: Category B.
Lactation: Not for use in nursing.

MECHANISM OF ACTION

Diarylquinoline antimycobacterial; inhibits mycobacterial adenosine 5'-triphosphate synthase, an enzyme that is essential for the generation of energy in *M. tuberculosis*.

PHARMACOKINETICS

Absorption: T_{max}=5 hrs (post-dose). **Distribution:** Plasma protein binding (>99.9%), V_d=164L. **Metabolism:** CYP3A4; N-monodesmethyl metabolite (M2) (active metabolite). **Elimination:** Urine (≤0.001% unchanged), feces; $T_{1/2}$=5.5 months.

PATIENT CONSIDERATIONS

Assessment: Assess for risk for QT prolongation, severe hepatic/renal impairment, pregnancy/nursing status, and possible drug reactions. Obtain baseline ECG, serum K^+, Ca^{2+}, and Mg^{2+} concentrations, and liver enzymes. Perform susceptibility tests for the background regimen against the *M. tuberculosis* isolate if possible.

Monitoring: Monitor for evidence of new/worsening liver dysfunction, syncope, QT interval prolongation, ventricular arrhythmia, and other adverse reactions. Obtain ECG at least 2, 12, and 24 weeks after starting treatment. Monitor serum electrolytes if QT prolongation is detected. Monitor lab tests (ALT, AST, alkaline phosphatase, bilirubin) monthly while on treatment, and prn.

Counseling: Advise to take in combination w/ other antimycobacterial drugs as prescribed; emphasize the need for compliance w/ the full course of therapy. Advise about serious adverse reactions (eg, death, heart rhythm abnormalities, hepatitis) and other potential side effects (eg, nausea, joint pain, headache). Advise about instructions for missed dose. Instruct to take w/ food and to abstain from alcohol, hepatotoxic drugs, or herbal products. Advise to discuss w/ physician the other drugs being taken and other medical conditions before starting treatment.

SITAVIG — acyclovir   Rx

Class: Nucleoside analogue

ADULT DOSAGE
Herpes Labialis (Cold Sores)

Recurrent Herpes Labialis in Immunocompetent Patients:

Usual: Apply one 50mg buccal tab as a single dose to the upper gum region (canine fossa)

Apply w/in 1 hr after the onset of prodromal symptoms and before the appearance of any signs of herpes labialis lesions

PEDIATRIC DOSAGE
Pediatric use may not have been established

ADMINISTRATION
Buccal route

Apply w/ a dry finger immediately after removing from blister.
Place tab to the upper gum just above the incisor tooth (canine fossa) and hold in place w/ slight pressure over upper lip for 30 sec.
Apply tab on the same side of the mouth as the herpes labialis symptoms.
Do not crush, chew, suck, or swallow tab.
Avoid any situation that may interfere w/ tab adhesion (eg, chewing gum, touching or pressing tab after placement, wearing upper denture, brushing teeth); rinse mouth gently if teeth need to be cleaned while tab is in place.
May take food/drink normally when tab is in place; drink plenty of liquids in case of dry mouth.

If Tab Does not Adhere or Falls Off w/in the First 6 Hrs
Reposition same tab immediately or place new tab if tab cannot be repositioned.

If Tab is Swallowed w/in the First 6 Hrs
Drink a glass of water and apply new tab.

Do not reapply if tab falls out or is swallowed after first 6 hrs.

STORAGE
20-25°C (68-77°F); excursions permitted between 15-30°C (59-86°F). Protect from moisture.

HOW SUPPLIED
Tab, Buccal: 50mg

CONTRAINDICATIONS
Known hypersensitivity (eg, anaphylaxis) to acyclovir, milk protein concentrate, or any other component of the product.

WARNINGS/PRECAUTIONS
Do not administer during labor and delivery.

ADVERSE REACTIONS
Headache.

PREGNANCY AND LACTATION
Category B, caution in nursing.

MECHANISM OF ACTION
Synthetic purine nucleoside analogue; inhibits replication of herpes viral DNA by competing with nucleotides for binding to the viral DNA polymerase and by incorporation into and termination of the growing viral DNA chain.

PHARMACOKINETICS
Absorption: Minimal systemic absorption (max salivary concentrations of 440mcg/mL at 8 hrs). **Distribution:** (PO) Found in breast milk. **Metabolism:** Oxidation and hydroxylation to 9-[(carboxymethoxy)methyl]guanine and 8-hydroxy-acyclovir. **Elimination:** Urine (unchanged).

PATIENT CONSIDERATIONS

Assessment: Assess for hypersensitivity to drug or to milk protein concentrate, immune status, and pregnancy/nursing status.

Monitoring: Monitor for hypersensitivity and other adverse reactions.

Counseling: Inform that drug is not a cure for cold sores. Instruct to reapply tab if it comes out before 6 hrs have gone by; advise that if this does not work, a new tab should be applied. Instruct to apply ud and not to apply to the inside of the lip or cheek. Instruct not to reapply if it falls out or if swallowed after it has been in place ≥6 hrs. Advise to drink a glass of water and place a new tab if swallowed within the first 6 hrs of applying it. Inform that adverse reactions, including headache and application-site pain, may occur.

SIVEXTRO — tedizolid phosphate   Rx

Class: Oxazolidinone class antibacterial

ADULT DOSAGE
Skin and Skin Structure Infections

Acute bacterial infections caused by *Staphylococcus aureus* (including methicillin-resistant and methicillin-susceptible isolates), *Streptococcus pyogenes, Streptococcus agalactiae, Streptococcus anginosus* Group (including *Streptococcus anginosus, Streptococcus intermedius,* and *Streptococcus constellatus*), and *Enterococcus faecalis*

IV:
200mg qd infused over 1 hr for 6 days

Oral:
200mg qd for 6 days

PEDIATRIC DOSAGE
Pediatric use may not have been established

ADMINISTRATION
Oral/IV route

No dose adjustment is necessary when changing from IV to oral route.
If patients miss a dose, they should take it as soon as possible anytime up to 8 hrs prior to their next scheduled dose; if <8 hrs remain before the next dose, wait until their next scheduled dose.

Preparation of IV Sol
1. Reconstitute the vial w/ 4mL of SWFI.
2. Gently swirl the contents and let the vial stand until the cake has completely dissolved and any foam disperses.
3. Inspect the vial to ensure the sol contains no particulate matter and no cake or powder remains attached to the sides of the vial; if necessary, invert the vial to dissolve any remaining powder and swirl gently to prevent foaming.
4. Tilt the upright vial and insert a syringe w/ appropriately sized needle into the bottom corner of the vial and remove 4mL of the reconstituted sol; do not invert the vial during extraction.
5. The reconstituted sol must be further diluted in 250mL of 0.9% NaCl inj. Slowly inject the 4mL of reconstituted sol into a 250mL bag of 0.9% NaCl inj and invert the bag gently to mix; do not shake the bag.

Administration of IV Sol
Administer as an IV infusion only.
Incompatibilities:
1. Any sol containing divalent cations (eg, Ca^{2+}, Mg^{2+}), including lactated Ringer's Inj and Hartmann's sol.
2. Do not add other IV substances, additives, or other medications to the single-use vials or infuse simultaneously; if the same IV line is used for sequential infusion of several different drugs, the line should be flushed before and after infusion of tedizolid phosphate w/ 0.9% NaCl inj.

STORAGE
20-25°C (68-77°F); excursions permitted to 15-30°C (59-86°F). (Inj) Reconstituted Sol: Do not exceed 24 hrs at room temperature or under 2-8°C (36-46°F).

HOW SUPPLIED
Inj/Tab: 200mg

WARNINGS/PRECAUTIONS
Consider alternative therapies when treating patients with neutropenia and acute bacterial skin and skin structure infections. *Clostridium difficile*-associated diarrhea (CDAD) reported; d/c if CDAD is suspected or confirmed. May result in bacterial resistance if used in the absence of proven or suspected bacterial infection or a prophylactic indication.

ADVERSE REACTIONS
N/V, headache, diarrhea.

PREGNANCY AND LACTATION
Pregnancy: Category C.
Lactation: Caution in nursing.

MECHANISM OF ACTION
Oxazolidinone antibacterial; inhibits bacterial protein synthesis by binding to the 50S subunit of the bacterial ribosome.

PHARMACOKINETICS
Absorption: Absolute bioavailability (91%); (IV) C_{max}=3mcg/mL, T_{max}=1.2 hr, AUC=29.2mcg•hr/mL; (PO) C_{max}=2.2mcg/mL, T_{max}=3.5 hrs, AUC=25.6mcg•hr/mL.

Distribution: V_d=67-80L (IV); plasma protein binding (70-90%). **Elimination:** Urine (18%, <3% unchanged), feces (82%, <3% unchanged); $T_{1/2}$=12 hrs.

PATIENT CONSIDERATIONS

Assessment: Assess for neutropenia, pregnancy/nursing status, and possible drug interactions.

Monitoring: Monitor for CDAD and other adverse reactions.

Counseling: Counsel that therapy should only be used to treat bacterial, not viral, infections. Instruct to take exactly ud even if the patient feels better early in the course of therapy. Inform that skipping doses or not completing full course of therapy may decrease effectiveness of immediate treatment and increase bacterial resistance. Inform that diarrhea is a common problem caused by therapy and usually resolves when therapy is discontinued. Instruct to contact physician if severe watery or bloody diarrhea develops.

SKYLA — levonorgestrel   Rx

Class: Progestin contraceptive

ADULT DOSAGE	PEDIATRIC DOSAGE
Contraception	**Contraception**

ADULT DOSAGE

Contraception

Timing of Insertion:
Insert into the uterine cavity during the first 7 days of the menstrual cycle

Following 1st Trimester Abortion:
Insert immediately after a 1st trimester abortion

Following 2nd Trimester Abortion/ Postpartum: Postpone insertion a minimum of 6 weeks or until the uterus is fully involuted; if involution is delayed, wait until involution is complete before insertion

Timing of Removal:
Should not remain in the uterus after 3 yrs.
If pregnancy is not desired, removal should be carried out during menstruation, provided the woman is still experiencing regular menses.
If removal will occur at other times during the cycle, consider starting a new contraceptive method a week prior to removal

Continuation of Contraception after Removal:
If pregnancy is not desired and if a woman wishes to continue using Skyla, a new system can be inserted immediately after removal any time during the cycle

Conversions

Switching to a Different Birth Control Method:

Patients w/ Regular Cycles:
Time removal and initiation of new method to ensure continuous contraception. Either remove Skyla during the first 7 days of the menstrual cycle and start the new method, or start the new method at least 7 days prior to removing Skyla if removal is to occur at other times during the cycle

Patients w/ Irregular Cycles or Amenorrhea:
Start the new method at least 7 days before removal

PEDIATRIC DOSAGE

Contraception

Not indicated for use premenarche; refer to adult dosing

ADMINISTRATION
Intrauterine route

Should be inserted by a trained healthcare provider.
Backup contraception is not needed when inserted as directed.
Consider administering analgesics prior to insertion.
Remove Skyla if it is not positioned completely w/in the uterus; do not reinsert once it is removed.
Must be removed by the end of the 3rd yr.
Refer to PI for additional insertion and removal instructions.

STORAGE
25°C (77°F); excursions permitted to 15-30°C (59-86°F).

HOW SUPPLIED
Intrauterine Insert: 13.5mg

CONTRAINDICATIONS
Pregnancy or suspicion of pregnancy (cannot be used for post-coital contraception), congenital or acquired uterine anomaly (including fibroids if they distort the uterine cavity), acute or history of pelvic inflammatory disease (PID) (unless there has been a subsequent intrauterine pregnancy), postpartum endometritis or infected abortion in the past 3 months, known/suspected uterine or cervical neoplasia, known/suspected or history of breast cancer or other progestin-sensitive cancer, uterine bleeding of unknown etiology, untreated acute cervicitis or vaginitis (including bacterial vaginosis or other lower genital tract infections until infection is controlled), acute liver disease or liver tumor (benign or malignant), conditions associated w/ increased susceptibility to pelvic infections, and previously inserted IUD that has not been removed, hypersensitivity to any component of this product.

WARNINGS/PRECAUTIONS
Evaluate for ectopic pregnancy and remove device if pregnancy occurs w/ device in place. Increased risk of septic abortion, miscarriage, sepsis, premature delivery/labor, and possible congenital anomalies if pregnancy occurs and device is left in place. Severe infection or sepsis, including Group A streptococcal sepsis, may occur; use aseptic technique during insertion of device. Associated w/ increased risk of PID and actinomycosis. Remove device in cases of recurrent endometritis or PID, or if an acute pelvic infection is severe or does not respond to treatment. May alter bleeding pattern and result in spotting, irregular bleeding, heavy bleeding, oligomenorrhea, and amenorrhea; perform appropriate diagnostic measures to rule out endometrial pathology if bleeding irregularities develop during prolonged use. Consider possibility of pregnancy if menstruation does not occur w/in 6 weeks of the onset of a previous menstruation. Perforation may occur and may reduce contraceptive effectiveness; risk increased if inserted in lactating women and may be increased if inserted when the uterus is fixed retroverted or not completely involuted during the postpartum period. Partial or complete expulsion may occur; may be replaced w/in 7 days of a menstrual period after ruling out pregnancy. Ovarian cysts reported. Breast cancer reported w/ a levonorgestrel-releasing intrauterine system. Caution in patients w/ coagulopathy or receiving anticoagulants, migraine, focal migraine w/ asymmetrical visual loss or other symptoms indicating transient cerebral ischemia, exceptionally severe headache, marked increase in BP, and in patients w/ severe arterial disease. Consider removing device if uterine/cervical malignancy or jaundice arises during use. Consider possibility that device may have been displaced (eg, expelled or perforated the uterus) if the threads are not visible or are significantly shortened; exclude pregnancy and verify location of device. If device is displaced, remove it. May be safely scanned on MRI only under specific conditions. MRI quality may be compromised if area of interest is in exact same area or relatively close to position of the device.

ADVERSE REACTIONS
Increased bleeding, vulvovaginitis, abdominal/pelvic pain, acne/seborrhea, ovarian cyst, headache, dysmenorrhea, breast pain/discomfort, nausea.

DRUG INTERACTIONS
Drugs or herbal products that induce enzymes, including CYP3A4 that metabolize progestins (eg, barbiturates, bosentan, carbamazepine), may decrease levels. HIV protease inhibitors or non-nucleoside reverse transcriptase inhibitors may significantly increase or decrease plasma levels. CYP3A4 inhibitors (eg, itraconazole, ketoconazole) may increase plasma hormone levels.

PREGNANCY AND LACTATION
Pregnancy: Contraindicated in pregnancy.
Lactation: Small amounts of progestins reported to pass into the breast milk, resulting in detectable steroid levels in infant serum; caution in nursing.

MECHANISM OF ACTION
Progestin contraceptive; local mechanism by which continuously released levonorgestrel enhances contraceptive effectiveness has not been conclusively demonstrated. Thickens cervical mucus (preventing passage of sperm into uterus), inhibits sperm capacitation or survival, and alters endometrium.

PHARMACOKINETICS
Absorption: C_{max}=192pg/mL; T_{max}=2 days (median). **Distribution:** Plasma protein binding (bound non-specifically to serum albumin and specifically to sex hormone binding globulin); V_d=1.8L/kg; found in breast milk. **Metabolism:** Conjugation; sulfate and glucuronide (lesser extent) conjugates (metabolites). **Elimination:** Urine (45%), feces (32%, glucuronide conjugates); $T_{1/2}$=20 hrs (parenteral).

PATIENT CONSIDERATIONS
Assessment: Assess for congenital or acquired uterine anomaly, acute or history of PID, known/suspected or history of breast cancer or other progestin-sensitive cancer, acute liver disease or liver tumor, pregnancy/nursing status, any other conditions where treatment is contraindicated or cautioned, and for possible drug interactions. Perform a complete medical and social history and if indicated, a physical examination, and appropriate tests for any forms of genital or other sexually transmitted infections (STIs).

Monitoring: Monitor for intrauterine/ectopic pregnancy, sepsis, PID, actinomycosis, bleeding pattern alterations, perforation, migraine/exceptionally severe headache, jaundice, marked BP increase, and other adverse reactions. Reexamine and evaluate 4-6 weeks after insertion and once a yr thereafter, or more frequently if clinically indicated. Monitor if thread is still visible and length of thread.

Counseling: Inform that product does not protect against HIV infection (AIDS) and other STDs. Inform of the risks/benefits/side effects of the device. Inform of the risk of ectopic pregnancy, including loss of fertility; instruct to promptly report symptoms of ectopic pregnancy to physician. Inform of the possibility of PID and of the symptoms of PID; instruct to promptly notify physician if any symptoms of PID develop. Inform that irregular/prolonged bleeding and spotting, and/or cramps may occur during the 1st few weeks after insertion; instruct to report to physician if symptoms continue or are severe. Instruct on how to check if the device's threads still protrude from the cervix and caution not to pull on the threads and displace device. Inform that no contraceptive protection exists if device is displaced or expelled. Instruct to contact physician if any adverse reactions develop, if pregnancy is suspected or occurs, if HIV positive seroconversion occurs in the patient or her partner, or if possible exposure to STIs occurs. Inform that device may be safely scanned w/ MRI only under specific conditions; instruct patients who will have an MRI to notify their physician that they have an IUD.

SOLARAZE — diclofenac sodium   Rx

Class: NSAID

> NSAIDs cause an increased risk of serious cardiovascular (CV) thrombotic events (eg, MI, stroke), which can be fatal; risk may occur early in treatment and may increase w/ duration of use. Contraindicated in the setting of CABG surgery.

ADULT DOSAGE

Actinic Keratosis

Apply to lesions bid for 60-90 days; complete healing or optimal effect may not be evident for up to 30 days following cessation

Reevaluate lesions that do not respond to therapy and reconsider management

Sun avoidance is indicated during therapy

PEDIATRIC DOSAGE

Pediatric use may not have been established

ADMINISTRATION
Topical route

Use 0.5g of gel on each 5cm x 5cm lesion site.

STORAGE
20-25°C (68-77°F); excursions permitted between 15-30°C (59-86°F). Protect from heat. Avoid freezing.

HOW SUPPLIED
Gel: 3% [100g]

CONTRAINDICATIONS
Known hypersensitivity to diclofenac, benzyl alcohol, polyethylene glycol monomethyl ether 350, and/or hyaluronate sodium; in the setting of CABG surgery.

WARNINGS/PRECAUTIONS
Use lowest effective dose for shortest duration possible. Anaphylactoid reactions may occur; caution w/ aspirin (ASA) triad. Monitor for CV events throughout entire treatment course, even in the absence of previous CV symptoms. Avoid use w/ recent MI unless benefits are expected to outweigh risk of recurrent CV thrombotic events; if used w/ recent MI, monitor for signs of cardiac ischemia. Heart failure (HF) and edema/fluid retention reported w/ NSAID use; avoid use w/ severe HF unless benefits are expected to outweigh risk of worsening HF. Monitor for signs of worsening HF in patients w/ severe HF. Caution w/ active GI ulceration or bleeding and severe renal or hepatic impairments. Do not apply to open skin wounds, infections, or exfoliative dermatitis; avoid contact w/ eyes.

ADVERSE REACTIONS
Flu syndrome, back pain, infection, application-site reaction, contact dermatitis, dry skin, edema, exfoliation, paresthesia, pruritus, rash.

DRUG INTERACTIONS
Use w/ ASA may increase risk of GI bleed. May blunt CV effects of therapeutic agents used to treat HF/edema/fluid retention (eg, diuretics, ACE inhibitors, ARBs). Use w/ oral NSAIDs or ASA may result in increased NSAID adverse effects.

PREGNANCY AND LACTATION
Pregnancy: Category B; avoid in late pregnancy.
Lactation: Not for use in nursing.

MECHANISM OF ACTION
NSAID; mechanism not established.

PHARMACOKINETICS
Absorption: C_{max}=4ng/mL, T_{max}=4.5 hrs, AUC_{0-t}=9ng•hr/mL. **Distribution:** (PO) V_d=550mL/kg. **Metabolism:** Conjugation, hydroxylation, and glucuronidation. **Elimination:** (PO) $T_{1/2}$=1-2 hours.

PATIENT CONSIDERATIONS
Assessment: Assess for drug hypersensitivity, ASA-triad, active GI ulceration or bleeding, renal/hepatic impairment, open wounds, infections or exfoliative dermatitis, pregnancy/nursing status, and for possible drug interactions.

Monitoring: Monitor for anaphylactoid reactions and other adverse reactions. Monitor response to treatment.

Counseling: Advise of the importance of monitoring and follow-up evaluation, signs/symptoms of dermal adverse reactions, and the possibility of irritant or allergic contact dermatitis. Instruct to d/c therapy until condition subsides if severe dermal reactions occur. Inform that exposure to sunlight and the use of sun lamps should be avoided. Advise to be alert for the symptoms of CV thrombotic events and CHF and to report any symptoms to their healthcare provider immediately.

SOLIRIS — eculizumab   Rx

Class: Monoclonal antibody/protein C5 blocker

> Life-threatening and fatal meningococcal infections reported; may become rapidly life-threatening or fatal if not recognized and treated early. Comply with the most current Advisory Committee on Immunization Practices (ACIP) recommendations for meningococcal vaccination. Immunize patients with meningococcal vaccine at least 2 weeks prior to administering the 1st dose, unless risks of delaying therapy outweigh risk of meningococcal infection development. Monitor for early signs of meningococcal infections and evaluate immediately if infection suspected. Available only through a restricted program under a Risk Evaluation and Mitigation Strategy.

ADULT DOSAGE

Paroxysmal Nocturnal Hemoglobinuria

Reduction of Hemolysis:
Initial: 600mg weekly for the first 4 weeks
Maint: 900mg for the 5th dose 1 week later, then 900mg every 2 weeks thereafter

Atypical Hemolytic Uremic Syndrome

Inhibition of Complement-Mediated Thrombotic Microangiopathy:
Initial: 900mg weekly for the first 4 weeks
Maint: 1200mg for the 5th dose 1 week later, then 1200mg every 2 weeks thereafter

Supplemental Dose After Plasmapheresis/Plasma Exchange:
If Most Recent Dose is 300mg:
300mg w/in 60 min after each plasmapheresis/plasma exchange
If Most Recent Dose is ≥600mg:
600mg w/in 60 min after each plasmapheresis/plasma exchange

Supplemental Dose After Fresh Frozen Plasma Infusion:
If Most Recent Dose is ≥300mg:
300mg w/in 60 min prior to each infusion of fresh frozen plasma

PEDIATRIC DOSAGE

Atypical Hemolytic Uremic Syndrome

Inhibition of Complement-Mediated Thrombotic Microangiopathy:
<18 Years:
5-<10kg:
Induction: 300mg weekly x 1 dose
Maint: 300mg at week 2, then 300mg every 3 weeks
10-<20kg:
Induction: 600mg weekly x 1 dose
Maint: 300mg at week 2, then 300mg every 2 weeks
20-<30kg:
Induction: 600mg weekly x 2 doses
Maint: 600mg at week 3, then 600mg every 2 weeks
30-<40kg:
Induction: 600mg weekly x 2 doses
Maint: 900mg at week 3, then 900mg every 2 weeks
≥40kg:
Induction: 900mg weekly x 4 doses
Maint: 1200mg at week 5, then 1200mg every 2 weeks

Supplemental Dose After Plasmapheresis/Plasma Exchange:
If Most Recent Dose is 300mg:
300mg w/in 60 min after each plasmapheresis/plasma exchange
If Most Recent Dose is ≥600mg:
600mg w/in 60 min after each plasmapheresis/plasma exchange

Supplemental Dose After Fresh Frozen Plasma Infusion:
If Most Recent Dose is ≥300mg:
300mg w/in 60 min prior to each infusion of fresh frozen plasma

ADMINISTRATION
IV route

Administer by IV infusion over 35 min in adults and 1-4 hrs in pediatric patients; do not administer as an IV push or bolus inj.

May slow or stop infusion if an adverse reaction occurs during administration; if infusion is slowed, total infusion time should not exceed 2 hrs in adults.

Monitor for at least 1 hr following completion of infusion for signs/symptoms of infusion reaction.

Preparation
Withdraw required amount from vial into sterile syringe and transfer recommended dose to an infusion bag.

Dilute to a final concentration of 5mg/mL by adding the appropriate amount (equal volume of diluent to drug volume) of 0.9% NaCl inj, 0.45% NaCl inj, D5W, or Ringer's inj to the infusion bag.

Final admixed infusion volume is 60mL (300mg), 120mL (600mg), 180mL (900mg), or 240mL (1200mg).

Gently invert infusion bag to ensure thorough mixing of product and diluent. Discard unused portion left in vial.

Prior to administration, allow admixture to adjust to room temperature; do not heat in microwave or w/ any heat source other than ambient air temperatures.

STORAGE
2-8°C (36-46°F). Protect from light. Do not freeze or shake. Admixed Sol: Stable for 24 hrs at 2-8°C (36-46°F) and at room temperature.

HOW SUPPLIED
Inj: 10mg/mL [30mL]

CONTRAINDICATIONS
Patients with unresolved serious *Neisseria meningitidis* infection and patients not currently vaccinated against it.

WARNINGS/PRECAUTIONS
Not indicated for treatment of Shiga toxin *Escherichia coli*-related hemolytic uremic syndrome. May increase susceptibility to infections, especially with encapsulated bacteria. Aspergillus infections reported in immunocompromised and neutropenic patients. Administer vaccinations for the prevention of *Streptococcus pneumoniae* and *Haemophilus influenza* type b (Hib) infections according to ACIP guidelines, and use caution with any systemic infection. Monitor PNH patients for at least 8 weeks after discontinuing therapy to detect

hemolysis. Monitor aHUS patients for signs/symptoms of TMA complications for at least 12 weeks after discontinuing therapy; consider reinstitution of therapy, plasma therapy, or appropriate organ-specific supportive measures if TMA complications occur after discontinuing therapy. May result in infusion reactions, including anaphylaxis or other hypersensitivity reactions; interrupt infusion and institute appropriate supportive measures if signs of cardiovascular instability or respiratory compromise occur.

ADVERSE REACTIONS
Meningococcal infections, headache, nasopharyngitis, N/V, urinary tract infection, HTN, upper respiratory tract infection, diarrhea, anemia, pyrexia, renal impairment, nasal congestion, tachycardia, abdominal pain, peripheral edema.

PREGNANCY AND LACTATION
Category C, caution in nursing.

MECHANISM OF ACTION
Monoclonal antibody/complement protein C5 blocker; specifically binds to complement protein C5 with high affinity, thereby inhibiting its cleavage to C5a and C5b and preventing the generation of the terminal complement complex C5b-9. Inhibits terminal complement-mediated intravascular hemolysis in PNH patients and complement-mediated TMA in patients with aHUS.

PHARMACOKINETICS
Absorption: C_{max}=194mcg/mL (PNH). **Distribution:** V_d=7.7L (PNH), 6.14L (aHUS); crosses the placenta; found in breast milk. **Elimination:** $T_{1/2}$=272 hrs (PNH), 291 hrs (aHUS).

PATIENT CONSIDERATIONS
Assessment: Assess for unresolved serious *N. meningitidis* infection, meningococcal vaccination status, presence of a systemic infection, and pregnancy/nursing status.

Monitoring: Monitor for signs/symptoms of meningococcal infections, other infections, infusion/hypersensitivity reactions, and other adverse reactions. Monitor PNH patients after discontinuing therapy for at least 8 weeks to detect hemolysis. Monitor aHUS patients for signs/symptoms of TMA complications for at least 12 weeks after discontinuing therapy.

Counseling: Counsel about risks/benefits of therapy, in particular, the risk of meningococcal infection, and the need to be monitored by a physician after discontinuing therapy. Inform that patients are required to receive meningococcal vaccination at least 2 weeks prior to receiving the 1st dose of treatment, if not previously vaccinated, and that they are required to be revaccinated while on therapy. Inform about the signs/symptoms of a meningococcal infection, and advise to seek immediate medical attention if these signs/symptoms occur. Instruct patients to carry the Soliris Patient Safety Information Card with them at all times, until 3 months after the last dose. Inform parents/caregivers that their child being treated for aHUS should be vaccinated against *S. pneumoniae* and Hib.

SOLU-CORTEF — hydrocortisone sodium succinate   Rx

Class: Glucocorticoid

ADULT DOSAGE
Steroid-Responsive Disorders

When oral therapy is not feasible

Initial: 100-500mg IV/IM, depending on disease being treated; administer IV over 30 sec (eg, 100mg) to 10 min (eg, ≥500mg).
May repeat dose at intervals of 2, 4, or 6 hrs.
High-dose therapy should be continued only until patient is stabilized, usually not beyond 48-72 hrs
Maint: After a favorable response is noted, decrease initial dose in small decrements at appropriate time intervals until lowest effective dose. Withdraw gradually after long-term therapy

Acute Exacerbations of Multiple Sclerosis:
800mg/day for 1 week followed by 320mg qod for 1 month

PEDIATRIC DOSAGE
Steroid-Responsive Disorders

When oral therapy is not feasible

Initial: 0.56-8mg/kg/day IV/IM in 3 or 4 divided doses (20-240mg/m²BSA/day), depending on disease being treated
Maint: After a favorable response is noted, decrease initial dose in small decrements at appropriate time intervals until lowest effective dose. Withdraw gradually after long-term therapy

DOSING CONSIDERATIONS
Elderly
Start at lower end of dosing range

ADMINISTRATION
IM/IV routes
IV inj preferred for initial emergency use; consider longer acting inj preparation or oral preparation after initial emergency period.
Avoid inj into deltoid muscle.
Should not be diluted or mixed w/ other sol.

Preparation
IV or IM Inj:
Add not more than 2mL of bacteriostatic water for inj or bacteriostatic NaCl inj to contents of one 100mg vial.

IV Infusion:
1. Add not more than 2mL of bacteriostatic water for inj to vial.
2. 100mg sol may then be added to 100-1000mL of D5W (or isotonic saline sol or D5 in isotonic saline sol if patient is not on Na⁺ restriction); 250mg sol may be added to 250-1000mL; 500mg sol may be added to 500-1000mL; and 1000mg sol may be added to 1000mL of same diluents.
3. If administration of small volume of fluid is desirable, 100mg-3000mg may be added to 50mL of above diluents.

Act-O-Vial System:
Refer to PI for directions.

STORAGE
20-25°C (68-77°F). Protect from light. Discard unused sol after 3 days.

HOW SUPPLIED
Inj: 100mg, 250mg, 500mg, 1000mg

CONTRAINDICATIONS
Systemic fungal infections, known hypersensitivity to the product and its constituents, intrathecal administration. **IM Preparations:** Idiopathic thrombocytopenic purpura.

WARNINGS/PRECAUTIONS
Serious neurologic events reported with epidural inj; not approved for epidural administration. May result in dermal and/or subdermal changes forming depressions in the skin at the inj site; avoid inj into the deltoid muscle. Anaphylactoid reactions may occur. May need to increase dose before, during, and after stressful situations. High doses should not be used for the treatment of traumatic brain injury. May cause elevation of BP, salt/water retention, and increased excretion of K⁺ and Ca²⁺; dietary salt restriction and K⁺ supplementation may be necessary. Caution in patients with recent MI. Hypothalamic-pituitary-adrenal (HPA) axis suppression, Cushing's syndrome, and hyperglycemia reported; monitor with chronic use. May produce reversible HPA axis suppression with the potential for glucocorticosteroid insufficiency after withdrawal of treatment; reduce dose gradually. May cause decreased resistance and inability to localize infection. May mask some signs of current infection or cause new infections; do not use intra-articularly, intrabursally, or for intratendinous administration for local effect in the presence of acute local infection. May exacerbate systemic fungal infections; avoid use in the presence of such infections unless needed to control drug reactions. Rule out latent or active amebiasis before initiating therapy. Caution with *Strongyloides* infestation, active or latent tuberculosis (TB), CHF, HTN, renal insufficiency, osteoporosis, and ocular herpes simplex. Not for use in cerebral malaria or active ocular herpes simplex. May cause more serious/fatal course of chickenpox and measles. Severe medical events associated with intrathecal route of administration reported. May produce posterior subcapsular cataracts, glaucoma with possible damage to the optic nerves, and may enhance the establishment of secondary ocular infections due to bacteria, fungi, or viruses. Sensitive to heat; should not be autoclaved when it is desirable to sterilize the exterior of the vial. Kaposi's sarcoma reported. Caution with active or latent peptic ulcers, diverticulitis, fresh intestinal anastomoses, and nonspecific ulcerative colitis; may increase risk of perforation. Signs of peritoneal irritation following GI perforation may be minimal or absent. Enhanced effect in patients with cirrhosis. May decrease bone formation and increase bone resorption, which may lead to inhibition of bone growth in pediatric patients and development of osteoporosis at any age. Local inj into a previously infected site is not recommended. Acute myopathy with high doses reported most often in patients with disorders of neuromuscular transmission (eg, myasthenia gravis). Elevation of creatine kinase (CK) may occur. Changes in thyroid status may necessitate dose adjustment. Psychic derangements may appear and existing emotional instability or psychotic tendencies may be aggravated. May elevate intraocular pressure (IOP); monitor IOP if steroid therapy is continued for >6 weeks. May suppress reactions to skin tests. Caution in elderly.

ADVERSE REACTIONS
Bradycardia, cardiac arrest, acne, allergic dermatitis, decreased carbohydrate and glucose tolerance, fluid retention, abdominal distention, bowel/bladder dysfunction, negative nitrogen balance, aseptic necrosis of femoral and humeral heads, convulsions, emotional instability, exophthalmoses, glaucoma, abnormal fat deposits.

DRUG INTERACTIONS
Aminoglutethimide may lead to a loss of corticosteroid-induced adrenal suppression. Closely monitor for the development of hypokalemia with K⁺-depleting agents (eg, amphotericin B, diuretics). Reports of cardiac enlargement and CHF with amphotericin B. Macrolide antibiotics may decrease clearance. Concomitant use with anticholinesterase agents may produce severe weakness in patients with myasthenia gravis; d/c anticholinesterase agents at least 24 hrs before initiating therapy. May inhibit response to warfarin; frequently monitor coagulation indices. May increase blood glucose levels; may require dose adjustments of antidiabetic agents. May decrease serum levels of isoniazid. Cholestyramine may increase clearance. Increased activity of both drugs may occur with cyclosporine; convulsions reported with concurrent use. May increase risk of arrhythmias with digitalis glycosides. Estrogens, including oral contraceptives, may decrease hepatic metabolism and increase effect. Drugs that induce CYP3A4 (eg, barbiturates, phenytoin, carbamazepine) may enhance metabolism and require corticosteroid dosage increase. Drugs that inhibit CYP3A4 (eg, ketoconazole, macrolide antibiotics) may increase plasma levels. Ketoconazole may increase risk of corticosteroid side effects. Aspirin (ASA) or other NSAIDs may increase risk of GI side effects; caution with ASA in hypoprothrombinemia. May increase clearance of salicylates. Administration of live or live, attenuated vaccines is contraindicated in patients receiving immunosuppressive doses. Killed or inactivated vaccines may be administered, although response is unpredictable. Acute myopathy reported with neuromuscular blocking drugs (eg, pancuronium).

PREGNANCY AND LACTATION
Pregnancy: Category C.
Lactation: Not for use in nursing.

MECHANISM OF ACTION
Glucocorticoid; causes profound and varied metabolic effects and modifies the body's immune responses to diverse stimuli.

PHARMACOKINETICS
Absorption: (IM) Rapid. **Distribution:** Found in breast milk.

PATIENT CONSIDERATIONS
Assessment: Assess for hypersensitivity to drug, traumatic brain injury, CHF, renal insufficiency, systemic fungal infections, active/latent TB, vaccination status, unusual stress, ulcerative colitis, diverticulitis, HTN, recent MI, intestinal anastomoses, active or latent peptic ulcer, myasthenia gravis, psychotic tendencies, cerebral malaria, active ocular herpes simplex, any other conditions where treatment is contraindicated or cautioned, pregnancy/nursing status, and possible drug interactions.

Monitoring: Monitor for anaphylactoid reactions, dermal and/or subdermal changes, growth/development (in pediatric patients), intestinal perforation, Kaposi's sarcoma, cataracts, glaucoma, osteoporosis, and other adverse reactions. Monitor for HPA axis suppression, Cushing's syndrome, and hyperglycemia with chronic use. Monitor BP, CK, serum electrolytes, and IOP. Frequently monitor coagulation indices with warfarin.

Counseling: Warn not to d/c abruptly or without medical supervision. Advise patients to inform any medical attendants that they are taking corticosteroids. Instruct to seek medical advice at once if fever or other signs of infection develop. Warn to avoid exposure to chickenpox or measles; advise to report immediately if exposed.

SOLU-MEDROL — methylprednisolone sodium succinate   Rx

Class: Glucocorticoid

ADULT DOSAGE
Steroid-Responsive Disorders

When Oral Therapy is Not Feasible:
Initial: 10-40mg IV/IM inj or IV infusion, depending on disease
Maint: Decrease initial dosage in small decrements at appropriate time intervals until lowest effective dose

High-Dose Therapy: 30mg/kg IV over at least 30 min; may be repeated q4-6h for 48 hrs.
High-dose therapy should continue only until patient is stabilized, usually not beyond 48-72 hrs.

Multiple Sclerosis
Acute Exacerbations:
Usual: 160mg qd for a week followed by 64mg qod for 1 month
D/C if a period of spontaneous remission occurs in a chronic condition

PEDIATRIC DOSAGE
Steroid-Responsive Disorders

When Oral Therapy is Not Feasible:
Initial: 0.11-1.6mg/kg/day in 3 or 4 divided doses (3.2-48mg/m²/day)

Asthma
Uncontrolled Asthma: 1-2mg/kg/day in single or divided doses.
Continue short-course ("burst") therapy until patient achieves a peak expiratory flow rate of 80% of personal best, or symptoms resolve (usually 3-10 days).
Dose may be reduced, but should be governed by severity of condition/response; should not be <0.5mg/kg/24 hrs.
D/C if a period of spontaneous remission occurs in a chronic condition

---

DOSING CONSIDERATIONS
Elderly
Start at lower end of dosing range

Discontinuation
If after long-term therapy the drug is to be stopped, withdraw gradually rather than abruptly

ADMINISTRATION
IM/IV route

Do not dilute or mix w/ other sol.
Avoid inj into deltoid muscle.

Refer to PI for preparation and administration instructions.

STORAGE
20-25°C (68-77°F). Protect from light. Use w/in 48 hrs after mixing.

HOW SUPPLIED
Inj: 40mg, 125mg, 500mg, 1g, 2g

CONTRAINDICATIONS
Systemic fungal infections, known hypersensitivity to the product and its constituents, intrathecal administration, premature infants (formulations preserved w/ benzyl alcohol). **IM Preparations:** Idiopathic thrombocytopenic purpura. **40mg:** Known hypersensitivity to cow's milk or its components or other dairy products.

WARNINGS/PRECAUTIONS
Serious neurologic events (some resulting in death) reported w/ epidural inj; not approved for epidural administration. Formulations w/ preservative contain benzyl alcohol, which is potentially toxic when administered locally to neural tissue. Exposure to excessive amounts of benzyl alcohol has been associated w/ toxicity, particularly in neonates. May result in dermal and/or subdermal changes forming depressions in the skin at the inj site. Anaphylactoid reactions may occur. May need to increase dose before, during, and after stressful situations. High systemic doses should not be used to treat traumatic brain injury. May cause elevation of BP, salt/water retention, and increased excretion of K⁺ and Ca²⁺; dietary salt restriction and K⁺ supplementation may be necessary. Monitor for hypothalamic-pituitary-adrenal (HPA) axis suppression, Cushing's syndrome, and hyperglycemia w/ chronic use. May produce reversible HPA axis suppression w/ the potential for glucocorticosteroid insufficiency after withdrawal of treatment; reduce dose gradually. May increase susceptibility to, mask signs of, or cause new infections; may exacerbate systemic fungal infections. Avoid use intra-articularly, intrabursally, or for intratendinous administration for local effect in the presence of acute local infection. Latent disease may be activated or intercurrent infections due to certain pathogens exacerbated. Rule out latent or active amebiasis before initiating therapy. Caution w/ recent myocardial infarction (MI), *Strongyloides* infestation, active or latent tuberculosis (TB), ocular herpes simplex, HTN, CHF, and renal insufficiency. May cause more serious/fatal course of chickenpox and measles. May produce posterior subcapsular cataracts, glaucoma w/ possible damage to the optic nerves, and may enhance the establishment of secondary ocular infections. Not for use in active ocular herpes simplex or in cerebral malaria. Sensitive to heat. Kaposi's sarcoma reported. Metabolic clearance is decreased in hypothyroidism and increased in hyperthyroidism; changes in thyroid status may necessitate dose adjustment. Caution w/ active or latent peptic ulcers, diverticulitis, fresh intestinal anastomoses, and nonspecific ulcerative colitis; may increase risk of perforation. Signs of peritoneal irritation following GI perforation may be minimal/absent. Enhanced effect in patients w/ cirrhosis. May decrease bone formation and increase bone resorption, and may lead to inhibition of bone growth in pediatric patients and development of osteoporosis at any age; caution w/ increased risk of osteoporosis. Acute myopathy w/ high doses reported, most often in patients w/ disorders of neuromuscular transmission (eg, myasthenia gravis). Elevation of creatine kinase (CK) or intraocular pressure (IOP) may occur; monitor IOP if used >6 weeks. Psychic derangements may appear, and existing emotional instability or psychotic tendencies may be aggravated. May suppress reactions to skin tests. Caution in elderly.

ADVERSE REACTIONS
Anaphylactoid reaction, HTN, osteoporosis, muscle weakness, menstrual irregularities, insomnia, impaired wound healing, manifestations of latent diabetes mellitus, ulcerative esophagitis, increased sweating, increased intracranial pressure, decreased carbohydrate/glucose tolerance, glaucoma, posterior subcapsular cataracts.

DRUG INTERACTIONS
Aminoglutethimide may lead to a loss of corticosteroid-induced adrenal suppression. Closely monitor for hypokalemia w/ K⁺-depleting agents (eg, amphotericin B, diuretics). Reports of cardiac enlargement and CHF following concomitant use of amphotericin B and hydrocortisone. Macrolide antibiotics may decrease clearance and cholestyramine may increase clearance. Concomitant use w/ anticholinesterase agents may produce severe weakness in patients w/ myasthenia gravis; d/c anticholinesterase agents at least 24 hrs before initiating therapy. May inhibit response to warfarin; frequently monitor coagulation indices. May increase blood glucose levels; dosage adjustments of antidiabetic agents may be required. May decrease serum levels of isoniazid. Increased activity of both drugs may occur w/ cyclosporine; convulsions reported w/ concurrent use. May increase risk of arrhythmias w/ digitalis glycosides. Estrogens, including oral contraceptives, may decrease hepatic metabolism and enhance effect. Drugs that induce CYP3A4 (eg, barbiturates, phenytoin, carbamazepine) may enhance metabolism and require corticosteroid dosage increase. Drugs that inhibit CYP3A4 (eg, ketoconazole, macrolide antibiotics such as erythromycin and troleandomycin) may increase plasma levels. Ketoconazole may increase risk of corticosteroid side effects. Aspirin (ASA) or other NSAIDs may increase risk of GI side effects; caution w/ ASA in hypoprothrombinemia patients. May increase clearance of salicylates. Administration of live or live, attenuated vaccines is contraindicated in patients receiving immunosuppressive doses. Killed or inactivated vaccines may be administered, although response is unpredictable. Acute myopathy reported w/ neuromuscular blocking drugs (eg, pancuronium).

PREGNANCY AND LACTATION
Pregnancy: Category C. Infants born to mothers who have received corticosteroids during pregnancy should be carefully observed for signs of hypoadrenalism.
Lactation: Systemically administered corticosteroids appear in human milk and could suppress growth, interfere w/ endogenous corticosteroid production, or cause other untoward effects. Not for use in nursing.

MECHANISM OF ACTION
Glucocorticoid; causes profound and varied metabolic effects and modifies the body's immune responses to diverse stimuli.

PHARMACOKINETICS
Absorption: (IM) Rapid. **Distribution:** Found in breast milk.

PATIENT CONSIDERATIONS
Assessment: Assess for hypersensitivity to drug, traumatic brain injury, CHF, renal insufficiency, cirrhosis, systemic fungal infections, active/latent TB, HTN, recent MI, active or latent peptic ulcer, ocular herpes simplex, any other conditions where treatment is contraindicated or cautioned, pregnancy/nursing status, and possible drug interactions.

Monitoring: Monitor for anaphylactoid reactions, dermal and/or subdermal changes, growth/development (in pediatric patients), intestinal perforation, infections, cataracts, glaucoma, osteoporosis, CK/IOP elevation, and other adverse reactions. Monitor for HPA-axis suppression, Cushing's syndrome, and hyperglycemia w/ chronic use. Frequently monitor coagulation indices w/ warfarin.

Counseling: Warn not to d/c abruptly or use w/o medical supervision. Instruct to seek medical advice at once if fever or other signs of infection develop. Warn to avoid exposure to chickenpox or measles; advise to report immediately if exposed.

SOMA — carisoprodol   CIV

Class: Skeletal muscle relaxant (centrally acting)

ADULT DOSAGE	PEDIATRIC DOSAGE
Musculoskeletal Conditions	Pediatric use may not have been established
Relief of Discomfort Associated w/ Acute Painful Conditions:	
16-65 Years:	
250-350mg tid and hs for up to 2-3 weeks	

ADMINISTRATION
Oral route

Take w/ or w/o food.

STORAGE
20-25°C (68-77°F).

HOW SUPPLIED
Tab: 250mg, 350mg

CONTRAINDICATIONS
History of acute intermittent porphyria, hypersensitivity reaction to a carbamate (eg, meprobamate).

WARNINGS/PRECAUTIONS
May impair mental/physical abilities. Abuse and dependence reported w/ prolonged use and a history of drug abuse. Withdrawal symptoms reported following abrupt cessation after prolonged use. Assess risk of abuse prior to prescribing; after prescribing, limit the length of treatment to 3 weeks for acute musculoskeletal discomfort, keep careful prescription records, and educate about abuse and on proper storage and disposal. Seizures reported. Caution w/ renal/hepatic impairment.

ADVERSE REACTIONS
Drowsiness, dizziness, headache.

DRUG INTERACTIONS
Additive sedative effects w/ other CNS depressants (eg, alcohol, benzodiazepines, opioids, TCAs); caution when coadministering. Concomitant use w/ meprobamate is not recommended. Increased exposure of carisoprodol and decreased exposure of meprobamate w/ CYP2C19 inhibitors (eg, omeprazole, fluvoxamine). Decreased exposure of carisoprodol and increased exposure of meprobamate w/ CYP2C19 inducers (eg, rifampin, St. John's wort). Induction effect on CYP2C19 seen w/ low-dose aspirin.

PREGNANCY AND LACTATION
Pregnancy: Category C.
Lactation: Limited data show drug is present in breast milk; based on animal studies, may lead to reduced or less effective infant feeding and/or decreased milk production. Caution in nursing.

MECHANISM OF ACTION
Centrally acting muscle relaxant; mechanism not established. Suspected to be associated w/ altered interneuronal activity in the spinal cord and the descending reticular formation of the brain. Meprobamate, a metabolite, has anxiolytic and sedative properties.

PHARMACOKINETICS
Absorption: Carisoprodol: (250mg) C_{max}=1.2mcg/mL, T_{max}=1.5 hrs, AUC=4.5mcg•hr/mL; (350mg) C_{max}=1.8mcg/mL, T_{max}=1.7 hrs, AUC=7.0mcg•hr/mL. Meprobamate: (250mg) C_{max}=1.8mcg/mL, T_{max}=3.6 hrs, AUC=32mcg•hr/mL; (350mg) C_{max}=2.5mcg/mL, T_{max}=4.5 hrs, AUC=46mcg•hr/mL. **Distribution:** Found in breast milk. **Metabolism:** Liver via CYP2C19. Meprobamate (metabolite). **Elimination:** Renal/Nonrenal route, Carisoprodol: $T_{1/2}$=1.7 hrs (250mg), 2.0 hrs (350mg). Meprobamate: $T_{1/2}$=9.7 hrs (250mg), 9.6 hrs (350mg).

PATIENT CONSIDERATIONS
Assessment: Assess for acute intermittent porphyria, renal/hepatic impairment, history of drug abuse, abuse potential, pregnancy/nursing status, and possible drug interactions.

Monitoring: Monitor for sedation, drug abuse/dependence, and seizures.

Counseling: Advise that drug may cause drowsiness and/or dizziness; instruct to avoid taking carisoprodol before engaging in hazardous tasks. Instruct to avoid alcohol, and to check w/ physician before taking other CNS depressants. Inform that drug is limited to acute use. Instruct to notify physician if musculoskeletal symptoms persist. Inform of drug dependence/abuse potential.

SONATA — zaleplon   CIV

Class: Pyrazolopyrimidine (non-benzodiazepine)

ADULT DOSAGE	PEDIATRIC DOSAGE
Insomnia	Pediatric use may not have been established
Short-Term Treatment:	
10mg qhs; for certain low weight individuals, 5mg may be a sufficient dose	
Max: 20mg	

DOSING CONSIDERATIONS
Concomitant Medications
Concomitant Use w/ Cimetidine:
Initial: 5mg

Hepatic Impairment
Mild to Moderate Impairment: 5mg
Severe Impairment: Not recommended

Elderly
Elderly/Debilitated:
Usual: 5mg
Max: 10mg

ADMINISTRATION
Oral route

Take immediately before hs or after patient has gone to bed and has experienced difficulty falling asleep

STORAGE
20-25°C (68-77°F).

HOW SUPPLIED
Cap: 5mg, 10mg

CONTRAINDICATIONS
Hypersensitivity to zaleplon or any excipients in the formulation.

WARNINGS/PRECAUTIONS
Initiate only after careful evaluation; failure of insomnia to remit after 7-10 days of treatment may indicate presence of a primary psychiatric and/or medical illness. Use lowest effective dose, especially in elderly. Abnormal thinking and behavior changes reported. Complex behaviors (eg, sleep-driving) reported; consider discontinuation if sleep-driving occurs. Amnesia and other neuropsychiatric symptoms may occur unpredictably. Worsening of depression, including suicidal thoughts and actions, reported in primarily depressed patients; caution with signs/symptoms of depression. Withdrawal signs/symptoms reported following rapid dose decrease or abrupt discontinuation. May impair mental/physical abilities. Severe anaphylactic and anaphylactoid reactions reported; do not rechallenge if angioedema develops. May result in short-term memory impairment, hallucinations, impaired coordination, dizziness, and lightheadedness when taken while still up and about. Caution with diseases or conditions affecting metabolism or hemodynamic responses, or with compromised respiratory function. Carefully monitor patients with compromised respiration due to preexisting illness. Not recommended for use in patients with severe hepatic impairment or in women during pregnancy. Contains tartrazine, which may cause allergic-type reactions (including bronchial asthma) in certain susceptible persons. Has an abuse potential. Monitor patients at risk of habituation and dependence (eg, history of addiction to, or abuse of, drugs or alcohol).

ADVERSE REACTIONS
Headache, dizziness, nausea, asthenia, abdominal pain, somnolence, amnesia, eye pain, dysmenorrhea, paresthesia.

DRUG INTERACTIONS
Additive CNS depression with other psychotropic medications, anticonvulsants, antihistamines, narcotic analgesics, anesthetics, ethanol, and other CNS depressants; dosage adjustment may be necessary. Do not take with alcohol. Increased risk of complex behaviors with alcohol and other CNS depressants. Decreased C_{max} with promethazine. Decreased levels with rifampin (a potent CYP3A4 inducer); coadministration of a potent CYP3A4 inducer can lead to ineffectiveness of zaleplon. May consider alternative non-CYP3A4 substrate hypnotic agent in patients taking CYP3A4 inducers (eg, phenytoin, carbamazepine, phenobarbital). Strong selective CYP3A4 inhibitors (eg, erythromycin, ketoconazole) may increase levels. Increased levels with cimetidine; give an initial dose of 5mg.

PREGNANCY AND LACTATION
Category C, not for use in nursing.

MECHANISM OF ACTION
Pyrazolopyrimidine (non-benzodiazepine) hypnotic agent; interacts with gamma-aminobutyric acid-benzodiazepine receptor complex.

PHARMACOKINETICS
Absorption: Rapid and almost complete. Absolute bioavailability (30%); T_{max}=1 hr. **Distribution:** Plasma protein binding (60%); found in breast milk. (IV) V_d=1.4L/kg. **Metabolism:** Liver (extensive) via aldehyde oxidation (primary), CYP3A4 (lesser extent). **Elimination:** Urine (<1% unchanged, 70% within 48 hrs, 71% within 6 days), feces (17% within 6 days); $T_{1/2}$=1 hr.

PATIENT CONSIDERATIONS
Assessment: Assess for physical and/or psychiatric disorders, medical illness, depression, diseases/conditions affecting metabolism or hemodynamic responses, compromised respiratory function, hepatic impairment, risk of habituation and dependence, hypersensitivity, pregnancy/nursing status, and possible drug interactions.

Monitoring: Monitor for complex behaviors, emergence of any new behavioral signs/symptoms, anaphylactic/anaphylactoid reactions, angioedema, abuse, habituation, dependence, withdrawal symptoms, and other adverse reactions. Monitor elderly and/or debilitated patients closely.

Counseling: Inform of the risks and benefits of therapy. Caution against engaging in hazardous occupations requiring complete mental alertness (eg, operating machinery, driving). Instruct to immediately report to physician if any adverse reactions (eg, sleep-driving or other complex behaviors) occur. Instruct to notify physician if pregnant/nursing or planning to become pregnant. Instruct not to take with alcohol. Inform that taking the drug with or immediately after a heavy, high-fat meal results in slower absorption and may reduce the effect of the drug on sleep latency.

SOOLANTRA — ivermectin   Rx

Class: Avermectin derivative

ADULT DOSAGE

Rosacea

Inflammatory Lesions:

Apply to the affected areas of the face qd

Use a pea-size amount for each area of the face (forehead, chin, nose, each cheek) that is affected

Spread as a thin layer, avoiding the eyes and lips

PEDIATRIC DOSAGE

Pediatric use may not have been established

ADMINISTRATION

Topical route

STORAGE

20-25°C (68-77°F); excursions permitted to 15-30°C (59-86°F).

HOW SUPPLIED

Cre: 1% [30g, 45g, 60g]

WARNINGS/PRECAUTIONS

Not for oral, ophthalmic, or intravaginal use.

ADVERSE REACTIONS

Skin burning sensation, skin irritation.

PREGNANCY AND LACTATION

Category C, not for use in nursing.

MECHANISM OF ACTION

Avermectin derivative; has not been established.

PHARMACOKINETICS

Absorption: C_{max}=2.10ng/mL, T_{max}=10 hrs, $AUC_{0-24 hr}$=36.14ng•hr/mL. **Distribution:** Plasma protein binding (>99%); found in breast milk (PO). **Metabolism:** CYP3A4 (primary). **Elimination:** $T_{1/2}$=6.5 days.

PATIENT CONSIDERATIONS

Assessment: Assess for history of drug hypersensitivity and pregnancy/nursing status.

Monitoring: Monitor for skin burning sensation, skin irritation, and other adverse reactions.

Counseling: Instruct to use ud. Advise to report any adverse reactions to physician. Instruct to notify physician if pregnant or nursing.

SORIATANE — acitretin   Rx

Class: Retinoid

Avoid in pregnancy and avoid becoming pregnant during therapy and for at least 3 yrs after discontinuation of therapy; use 2 effective forms of contraception simultaneously. Females of childbearing potential should avoid ethanol during and for 2 months after discontinuation of therapy because it may increase the duration of teratogenic potential. Only use in females of reproductive potential w/ severe psoriasis unresponsive to or contraindicated w/ other therapies. Patient must have 2 negative urine/serum pregnancy tests w/ a sensitivity of at least 25 mIU/mL before receiving initial prescription; if 2nd pregnancy test is negative, initiation of treatment should begin w/in 7 days of specimen collection. Therapy should be limited to a monthly supply. Contraception counseling should be done on a regular basis. It is not known whether residual acitretin in seminal fluid poses risk to a fetus while a male patient is taking the drug or after it is discontinued. Severe birth defects reported. Interferes w/ contraceptive effect of microdosed progestin "minipill" oral contraceptives. Caution not to self-medicate w/ herbal St. John's wort, because a possible interaction has been suggested w/ hormonal contraceptives, based on reports of breakthrough bleeding. Potential for hepatotoxicity; d/c if hepatotoxicity is suspected.

ADULT DOSAGE

Psoriasis

Severe:

Initial: 25-50mg/day as a single dose w/ main meal

Maint: 25-50mg/day

May treat relapses as outlined for initial therapy

PEDIATRIC DOSAGE

Pediatric use may not have been established

DOSING CONSIDERATIONS

Elderly

Start at lower end of dosing range

Other Important Considerations

When used w/ phototherapy, decrease phototherapy dose, dependent on patient's individual response

ADMINISTRATION

Oral route

STORAGE

15-25°C (59-77°F). Protect from light. Avoid exposure to high temperatures and humidity after the bottle is opened.

HOW SUPPLIED

Cap: 10mg, 17.5mg, 25mg

CONTRAINDICATIONS

Pregnancy, severely impaired liver or kidney function, chronic abnormally elevated blood lipid values. Coadministration w/ methotrexate or tetracyclines. Hypersensitivity (eg, angioedema, urticaria) to the preparation (acitretin or excipients) or to other retinoids.

WARNINGS/PRECAUTIONS

Risk of skeletal abnormalities, pancreatitis, and pseudotumor cerebri (benign intracranial HTN). D/C and refer for ophthalmologic evaluation if visual difficulties occur. Bone abnormalities of the vertebral column, knees, and ankles reported. Increased TG and cholesterol and decreased HDL levels reported; perform blood lipid determinations before therapy and again at 1- to 2-week intervals until lipid response to therapy is established, usually w/in 4-8 weeks. Caution in patients w/ an increased tendency to develop hypertriglyceridemia (eg, disturbances of lipid metabolism, diabetes mellitus [DM], obesity, increased alcohol intake, or familial history of these conditions). Capillary leak syndrome reported; d/c if this develops during therapy. Rhabdomyolysis and myalgias reported in association w/ capillary leak syndrome, and may reveal neutrophilia, hypoalbuminemia, and an elevated Hct in lab tests. Exfoliative dermatitis/erythroderma reported; d/c if this occurs during therapy. Blood sugar control problems and new cases of diabetes, including diabetic ketoacidosis, reported; monitor blood sugar levels very carefully in diabetics. Not indicated for treatment of acne.

ADVERSE REACTIONS

Hepatotoxicity, cheilitis, alopecia, skin peeling, rhinitis, dry skin, nail disorder, pruritus, rigors, xerophthalmia, dry mouth, epistaxis, arthralgia, spinal hyperostosis, erythematous rash.

DRUG INTERACTIONS

See Boxed Warning, Dosing Considerations, and Contraindications. Potentiates the blood glucose-lowering effect of glyburide; careful supervision of diabetic patients is recommended. Reduced protein binding of phenytoin. Avoid use w/ vitamin A and/or other oral retinoids; may increase risk of hypervitaminosis A.

PREGNANCY AND LACTATION

Category X, not for use in nursing.

MECHANISM OF ACTION

Retinoid; has not been established.

PHARMACOKINETICS

Absorption: (50mg) C_{max}=416ng/mL, T_{max}=2.7 hrs. **Distribution:** Plasma protein binding (>99.9%); found in breast milk. **Metabolism:** Extensive; via isomerization to cis-acitretin; both parent compound and isomer are further metabolized into chain-shortened breakdown products and conjugates. **Elimination:** Urine (16-53%, metabolites and conjugates); feces (34-54%, metabolites and conjugates); $T_{1/2}$=49 hrs (multiple dose), 63 hrs (cis-acitretin).

PATIENT CONSIDERATIONS

Assessment: Assess for DM, obesity, alcohol intake, or familial history of these conditions, cardiovascular status, preexisting abnormalities of the spine or extremities, renal/hepatic function, drug hypersensitivity, pregnancy/nursing status, and possible drug interactions. Perform blood lipid determinations before initiating therapy.

Monitoring: Monitor for hepatotoxicity, skeletal abnormalities, hypertriglyceridemia, MI or other thromboembolic events, pancreatitis, pseudotumor cerebri, visual difficulties, capillary leak syndrome, exfoliative dermatitis/erythroderma, and other adverse reactions. Perform appropriate examinations periodically in view of possible ossification abnormalities. Monitor blood sugar levels very carefully in diabetic patients. Repeat pregnancy test every month, during therapy, and every 3 months for at least 3 yrs after discontinuation of therapy. Monitor blood lipid determinations at 1- to 2-week intervals until lipid response to the drug is established during therapy.

Counseling: Inform about the Pregnancy Prevention Actively Required During and After Treatment (*Do Your P.A.R.T.*) program and the risks of therapy. Advise to notify physician if pregnant or nursing. Advise to use 2 effective forms of contraception simultaneously at least 1 month prior to initiation of therapy. Advise against donating blood during or for at least 3 yrs following completion of therapy. Counsel to d/c therapy and notify physician immediately if psychiatric symptoms develop. Instruct not to ingest beverages or products containing ethanol while taking therapy and for 2 months after discontinuation of therapy. Advise to be cautious when driving or operating a vehicle at night, and not to give the drug to any other person. Inform to use caution when taking vitamin A supplements to avoid additive toxic effects. Instruct to avoid use of sun lamps and excessive exposure to sunlight. Advise that a transient worsening of psoriasis may be seen during initial treatment period, and that patients may have to wait 2-3 months before they get the full benefit of therapy.

SORILUX — calcipotriene   Rx

Class: Vitamin D3 derivative

ADULT DOSAGE

Plaque Psoriasis

Scalp and Body:

Apply a thin layer bid to the affected areas and rub in gently and completely

PEDIATRIC DOSAGE

Pediatric use may not have been established

ADMINISTRATION

Topical route

Avoid contact w/ the face and eyes

STORAGE

20-25°C (68-77°F); excursions permitted to 15-30°C (59-86°F). Do not puncture or incinerate. Do not expose to heat or to temperatures >49°C (120°F).

HOW SUPPLIED

Foam: 0.005% [60g, 120g]

CONTRAINDICATIONS

Hypercalcemia.

WARNINGS/PRECAUTIONS

Propellant in drug is flammable; avoid fire, flame, and smoking during and immediately following application. Hypercalcemia may occur; d/c treatment until normal Ca^{2+} levels are restored if elevation outside normal range occurs. Avoid excessive exposure of treated areas to natural or artificial sunlight. Limit or avoid use of phototherapy. Use not evaluated with erythrodermic, exfoliative, or pustular psoriasis. Avoid contact with the face and eyes.

ADVERSE REACTIONS

Application-site erythema/pain.

PREGNANCY AND LACTATION

Category C, caution in nursing.

MECHANISM OF ACTION

Vitamin D3 analog; not established.

PATIENT CONSIDERATIONS

Assessment: Assess for hypercalcemia and pregnancy/nursing status.

Monitoring: Monitor serum Ca^{2+} levels and for development of application-site erythema and/or pain.

Counseling: Advise not to refrigerate or freeze the product. Instruct to avoid fire, flame, and smoking during and immediately following application and excessive exposure of the treated areas to natural or artificial sunlight (eg, tanning beds, sun lamps). If the foam gets on the face or in or near the eyes, advise to rinse thoroughly with water. Instruct to consult physician if there are no improvements after 8 weeks of treatment. Counsel to wash hands after application, unless treating the hands. Instruct to apply foam to the scalp when hair is dry.

SOTYLIZE — sotalol hydrochloride   Rx

Class: Beta blocker (group II/III antiarrhythmic)

> To minimize risk of induced arrhythmia, patients initiated or reinitiated on therapy and patients converted from IV sotalol to oral administration should be hospitalized in a facility that can provide cardiac resuscitation, continuous ECG monitoring, and calculations of CrCl. May cause life-threatening ventricular tachycardia associated w/ QT interval prolongation. Do not initiate therapy if the baseline QTc is >450 msec. If the QT interval prolongs to ≥500 msec, reduce dose, prolong interval between doses, or d/c drug. Adjust the dosing interval based on CrCl.

ADULT DOSAGE

Ventricular Arrhythmias

Documented Life-Threatening Ventricular Arrhythmias (eg, Sustained Ventricular Tachycardia):
Initial: 80mg qd or bid based on CrCl
Titrate: May increase in increments of 80mg/day every 3 days prn, provided QTc <500 msec
Usual: 80-160mg qd or bid

Refractory Life-Threatening Arrhythmia:
240-320mg qd or bid

Atrial Fibrillation/Flutter

Maint of Normal Sinus Rhythm in Patients w/ Symptomatic A-fib/A-Flutter Who Are Currently in Sinus Rhythm:
Initial: 80mg qd or bid based on CrCl
Titrate: If that dose level at steady-state does not acceptably reduce time to recurrence of arrhythmia and is tolerated w/ QTc <520 msec, increase dose to 160mg qd or bid every 3 days

PEDIATRIC DOSAGE

Ventricular Arrhythmias

Documented Life-Threatening Ventricular Arrhythmias (eg, Sustained Ventricular Tachycardia):
<2 Years:
Refer to PI for dosing chart

≥2 Years:
Initial: 30mg/m² tid (90mg/m² total daily dose)
Titrate: Allow at least 36 hrs between dose increments; monitor QTc and HR
Max: 60mg/m² (approx equivalent to 360mg total daily dose for adults)

DOSING CONSIDERATIONS

Renal Impairment

Adults:
CrCl >60mL/min: Administer bid
CrCl 40-60mL/min: Administer qd
CrCl <40mL/min: Not recommended

Pediatrics:
Lower doses or increase intervals between doses

ADMINISTRATION

Oral route

STORAGE

20-25°C (68-77°F); excursions permitted between 15-30°C (59-86°F).

HOW SUPPLIED

Sol: 5mg/mL [250mL, 480mL]

CONTRAINDICATIONS

Sinus bradycardia (<50bpm during waking hrs), sick sinus syndrome or 2nd and 3rd degree atrioventricular (AV) block unless a functioning pacemaker is present, congenital or acquired long QT syndromes, baseline QT interval >450 msec, cardiogenic shock, uncontrolled heart failure (HF), CrCl <40mL/min, serum K^+ <4mEq/L, bronchial asthma or related bronchospastic conditions, known hypersensitivity to sotalol.

WARNINGS/PRECAUTIONS

May not enhance survival in patients w/ ventricular arrhythmias. Reserve use for patients in whom A-fib/A-flutter is highly symptomatic. Should usually not be given to patients w/ paroxysmal A-fib whose A-fib/A-flutter is easily reversed (eg, by Valsalva maneuver). Avoid w/ asymptomatic ventricular premature contractions. May cause serious ventricular arrhythmias. Bradycardia/heart block reported. Not recommended w/ sick sinus syndrome associated w/ symptomatic arrhythmias. May cause hypotension, including decompensated HF; monitor hemodynamics in patients w/ marginal cardiac compensation. Careful dose titration is especially important in the first 2 weeks post-MI, particularly in patients w/ markedly impaired ventricular function. Exacerbation of angina pectoris, arrhythmias, and MI reported after abrupt discontinuation; if possible, reduce dose gradually over a period of 1-2 weeks. When discontinuing chronically administered sotalol, particularly in patients w/ ischemic heart disease, carefully monitor and consider temporary use of an alternate β-blocker if appropriate. Abrupt discontinuation in patients w/ arrhythmias may unmask latent coronary insufficiency. Do not use w/ hypokalemia or hypomagnesemia prior to correction of imbalance; caution w/ severe or prolonged diarrhea or w/ concomitant diuretic drugs. Avoid w/ bronchospastic diseases; if drug is to be administered, use smallest effective dose. May mask premonitory signs of acute hypoglycemia (eg, tachycardia) in patients w/ diabetes (especially labile diabetes) or w/ a history of episodes of spontaneous hypoglycemia. May mask certain clinical signs (eg, tachycardia) of hyperthyroidism; avoid abrupt withdrawal. Patients w/ a history of anaphylactic reaction to various allergens may have a more severe reaction on repeated challenge and may be unresponsive to usual doses of epinephrine. Impaired ability of the heart to respond to reflex adrenergic stimuli may augment the risks of general anesthesia and surgical procedures; chronically administered therapy should not be routinely withdrawn prior to major surgery.

ADVERSE REACTIONS

Ventricular tachycardia associated w/ QT interval prolongation, bradycardia, dyspnea, fatigue, N/V, diarrhea, hyperhidrosis, weakness, dizziness, ECG abnormality.

DRUG INTERACTIONS

Not recommended w/ other drugs that prolong the QT interval (eg, many antiarrhythmics, some phenothiazines, TCAs, certain oral macrolides and quinolone antibiotics). Class I or Class III antiarrhythmic agents should be withheld for at least 3 half-lives prior to dosing w/ sotalol. Avoid w/ Class Ia (eg, disopyramide, quinidine, procainamide) and other Class III (eg, amiodarone) antiarrhythmics. Proarrhythmic events reported more commonly w/ concomitant digoxin therapy. Additive effects on AV conduction, ventricular function, and BP w/ calcium-blocking drugs. May produce an excessive reduction of resting sympathetic nervous tone w/ catecholamine-depleting drugs (eg, reserpine, guanethidine). Hyperglycemia may occur; may require dose adjustment of insulin or antidiabetic agents. $β_2$-agonists (eg, albuterol, terbutaline, isoproterenol) may need a dose increase. May potentiate rebound HTN w/ clonidine withdrawal. Avoid administration of therapy w/in 2 hrs of antacids containing aluminum oxide and magnesium hydroxide; may reduce levels.

PREGNANCY AND LACTATION

Category B, not for use in nursing.

MECHANISM OF ACTION

β-blocker (group II/III antiarrhythmic); has both β-adrenoreceptor blocking and cardiac action potential duration prolongation antiarrhythmic properties.

PHARMACOKINETICS

Absorption: Oral bioavailability (90-100%); T_{max}=2.5-4 hrs. **Distribution:** Crosses placenta; found in breast milk. **Elimination:** Urine (unchanged); $T_{1/2}$=12 hrs.

PATIENT CONSIDERATIONS

Assessment: Assess for hypersensitivity to drug, sinus bradycardia, sick sinus syndrome, 2nd- and 3rd-degree AV block, cardiogenic shock, uncontrolled HF, bronchial asthma or related bronchospastic conditions, marginal cardiac compensation, recent MI, ischemic heart disease, diabetes, hypoglycemia, hyperthyroidism, upcoming major surgery, any other conditions where treatment is contraindicated or cautioned, pregnancy/nursing status, and possible drug interactions. Obtain baseline ECG, serum K^+ and Mg^{2+}, and renal function (eg, SrCr, CrCl).

Monitoring: Monitor for ECG changes, arrhythmias, hypotension, electrolyte imbalance, tachycardia, anaphylaxis, and other adverse reactions.

Counseling: Advise to contact physician if syncope, pre-syncopal symptoms, cardiac palpitations, conditions conducive to electrolyte changes (eg, severe diarrhea, unusual sweating, vomiting, less appetite than normal or excessive thirst), or bradycardia develops. Advise that doses for children and infants should be measured using an appropriate measuring device (eg, oral syringe). Advise to not interrupt or d/c therapy w/o physician's advice. Counsel not to start taking other medications w/o 1st discussing new medications w/ physician. Instruct to avoid taking drug w/in 2 hrs of taking antacids that contain aluminum oxide or magnesium hydroxide.

SOVALDI — sofosbuvir   Rx

Class: HCV nucleotide analogue NS5B polymerase inhibitor

ADULT DOSAGE	PEDIATRIC DOSAGE
Chronic Hepatitis C	Pediatric use may not have been established
HCV Mono-Infected and HCV/HIV-1 Coinfected:	
Genotype 1 or 4:	
400mg qd in combination w/ peginterferon alfa and ribavirin for 12 weeks	
Genotype 1 Ineligible for Interferon-Based Regimen:	
400mg qd in combination w/ ribavirin for 24 weeks	
Genotype 2:	
400mg qd in combination w/ ribavirin for 12 weeks	
Genotype 3:	
400mg qd in combination w/ ribavirin for 24 weeks	
Hepatocellular Carcinoma Awaiting Liver Transplantation:	
400mg qd in combination w/ ribavirin for up to 48 weeks or until time of transplant, whichever occurs 1st	

DOSING CONSIDERATIONS

Adverse Reactions

Serious Reaction Potentially Related to Peginterferon Alfa and/or Ribavirin: Reduce dose of or d/c peginterferon alfa and/or ribavirin; refer to each respective PI for instructions

ADMINISTRATION

Oral route

Take w/ or w/o food.
D/C sofosbuvir if concomitant agents are permanently discontinued.

STORAGE

Room temperature <30°C (86°F).

HOW SUPPLIED

Tab: 400mg

CONTRAINDICATIONS

Refer to the individual PIs for peginterferon alfa and ribavirin.

WARNINGS/PRECAUTIONS

Fatal cardiac arrest reported w/ sofosbuvir-containing regimen (ledipasvir/sofosbuvir).

ADVERSE REACTIONS

Fatigue, headache, nausea, insomnia, anemia, pruritus, asthenia, rash, decreased appetite, influenza-like illness, pyrexia, diarrhea, myalgia, irritability.

DRUG INTERACTIONS

Coadministration of amiodarone w/ sofosbuvir in combination w/ another direct-acting antiviral (DAA) may result in serious symptomatic bradycardia; coadministration is not recommended. If coadministration is required, cardiac monitoring is recommended in an inpatient setting for the first 48 hrs, after which outpatient or self-monitoring of HR should occur on a daily basis for at least the first 2 weeks. Intestine P-gp inducers (eg, rifampin, St. John's wort) may significantly decrease concentration and may lead to a reduced therapeutic effect; do not use w/ rifampin and St. John's wort. Carbamazepine, phenytoin, phenobarbital, oxcarbazepine, rifabutin, rifapentine, and tipranavir/ritonavir may decrease concentration, leading to reduced therapeutic effects; coadministration is not recommended w/ other products containing sofosbuvir.

PREGNANCY AND LACTATION

Pregnancy: Category B. If administered w/ ribavirin or peginterferon and ribavirin, combination regimen is contraindicated in pregnant women and in men whose female partners are pregnant.
Lactation: The developmental and health benefits of breastfeeding should be considered along with the mother's clinical need and any potential adverse effects on the breastfed child from the drug or from the underlying maternal condition. If sofosbuvir is administered in a regimen containing ribavirin, refer to the ribavirin PI for more information.

MECHANISM OF ACTION

HCV nucleotide analogue NS5B polymerase inhibitor; direct-acting antiviral agent against HCV.

PHARMACOKINETICS

Absorption: T_{max}=0.5-2 hrs, 2-4 hrs (GS-331007); (w/ ribavirin) AUC_{0-24}=969ng•hr/mL, 6790ng•hr/mL (GS-331007). **Distribution:** Plasma protein binding (approx 61-65%). **Metabolism:** Liver (extensive) to GS-461203 (active); dephosphorylation to GS-331007 (major). **Elimination:** Urine (80%; 78% GS-331007, 3.5% unchanged), feces (14%); $T_{1/2}$ (median)=0.4 hr, 27 hrs (GS-331007).

PATIENT CONSIDERATIONS

Assessment: Assess for pregnancy/nursing status and possible drug interactions.
Monitoring: Monitor for adverse reactions.

Counseling: Advise to seek medical evaluation immediately for symptoms of bradycardia. Advise patients to avoid pregnancy during combination treatment w/ sofosbuvir and ribavirin or sofosbuvir and peginterferon and ribavirin; instruct to notify physician immediately in the event of a pregnancy. Inform that the effect of treatment of hepatitis C on transmission is unknown and that appropriate precautions should be taken to prevent HCV transmission during treatment or in the event of treatment failure. Advise to take ud.

SPIRIVA — tiotropium bromide   Rx

Class: Anticholinergic

ADULT DOSAGE	PEDIATRIC DOSAGE
Chronic Obstructive Pulmonary Disease	Pediatric use may not have been established
Long-Term Maint Treatment of Bronchospasm/Reduction of COPD Exacerbations:	
2 inh of the powder contents of 1 cap qd via HandiHaler device	

ADMINISTRATION

Orally inhaled powder

Do not swallow caps.
Use w/ HandiHaler device only and inhale through the mouth.
Do not use HandiHaler device to take any other medicine.

Instructions
1. Place cap into the center chamber of the HandiHaler device.
2. Spiriva cap is pierced by pressing and releasing the green piercing button on the side of the device.
3. The formulation will be dispersed into the air stream when the patient inhales through the mouthpiece.

STORAGE

25°C (77°F); excursions permitted to 15-30°C (59-86°F). Do not expose to extreme temperatures or moisture. Do not store caps in the HandiHaler device.

HOW SUPPLIED

Cap, Inhalation: 18mcg

CONTRAINDICATIONS

Hypersensitivity to tiotropium, ipratropium, or any components of this medication.

WARNINGS/PRECAUTIONS

Not for relief of acute symptoms (eg, as rescue therapy for the treatment of acute episodes of bronchospasm). D/C and consider alternative treatments if immediate hypersensitivity reactions (eg, angioedema, itching, rash) or paradoxical bronchospasm occurs. Caution w/ hypersensitivity to milk proteins or to atropine. Caution w/ narrow-angle glaucoma; observe for signs/symptoms of acute narrow-angle glaucoma. Caution w/ urinary retention; observe for signs/symptoms of urinary retention especially in patients w/ prostatic hyperplasia or bladder-neck obstruction. Monitor for anticholinergic effects in patients w/ moderate to severe renal impairment (CrCl ≤60mL/min).

ADVERSE REACTIONS

Dry mouth, sinusitis, constipation, abdominal pain, UTI, URTI, chest pain, edema, vomiting, myalgia, moniliasis, rash, dyspepsia, pharyngitis, rhinitis.

DRUG INTERACTIONS

Avoid w/ other anticholinergic-containing drugs; may lead to an increase in anticholinergic adverse effects.

PREGNANCY AND LACTATION

Pregnancy: Category C
Lactation: It is not known whether tiotropium is excreted in human milk; caution in nursing.

MECHANISM OF ACTION

Anticholinergic bronchodilator; inhibits M_3-receptors on smooth muscle, leading to bronchodilation.

PHARMACOKINETICS

Absorption: Absolute bioavailability (19.5%); T_{max}=7 min. **Distribution:** V_d=32L/kg; plasma protein binding (72%). **Metabolism:** Liver (oxidation, conjugation) via CYP2D6, 3A4. **Elimination:** (IV) Urine (74%, unchanged). (5mcg qd, inhaled) $T_{1/2}$=25 hrs.

PATIENT CONSIDERATIONS

Assessment: Assess for hypersensitivity to atropine or its derivatives, hypersensitivity to milk proteins, narrow-angle glaucoma, urinary retention, prostatic hyperplasia or bladder-neck obstruction, renal impairment, pregnancy/nursing status, and possible drug interactions.

Monitoring: Monitor for signs/symptoms of hypersensitivity reactions, paradoxical bronchospasm, urinary retention, worsening narrow-angle glaucoma, and other adverse reactions.

Counseling: Inform that contents of cap are for oral inhalation only and must not be swallowed. Advise to administer only via the HandiHaler device and that the device should not be used for other medications. Advise not to use as a rescue medication for immediate relief of breathing problems. Advise to seek medical attention if signs/symptoms of narrow-angle glaucoma or urinary retention develop. Advise to use caution when engaging in activities such as driving a vehicle or operating appliances/machinery. Inform that paradoxical bronchospasm may occur; d/c if this develops. Instruct not to allow the powder to enter into the eyes.

SPIRIVA RESPIMAT — tiotropium bromide   Rx

Class: Anticholinergic

ADULT DOSAGE

Chronic Obstructive Pulmonary Disease

Long-Term Maint Treatment of Bronchospasm/Reduction of Exacerbations:
5mcg (2 inh; 2.5mcg/actuation) qd
Max: 1 dose (2 inh)/24 hrs

Asthma

Long-Term Maint Treatment:
2.5mcg (2 inh; 1.25mcg/actuation) qd
Max: 1 dose (2 inh)/24 hrs

Max benefits in lung function may take up to 4-8 weeks of dosing

PEDIATRIC DOSAGE

Asthma

Long-Term Maint Treatment:
>12 Years:
2.5mcg (2 inh; 1.25mcg/actuation) qd
Max: 1 dose (2 inh)/24 hrs

Max benefits in lung function may take up to 4-8 weeks of dosing

---

ADMINISTRATION
Oral inh route

Priming
First-Time Use:
Actuate the inhaler toward the ground until an aerosol cloud is visible and repeat the process 3 additional times.
If Not Used for >3 Days:
Actuate the inhaler once.
If Not Used for >21 Days:
Actuate the inhaler until an aerosol cloud is visible and repeat the process 3 additional times.

STORAGE
25°C (77°F); excursions permitted to 15-30°C (59-86°F). Avoid freezing. After assembly, discard the inhaler at the latest 3 months after 1st use or when the locking mechanism is engaged, whichever comes 1st.

HOW SUPPLIED
Spray, Inh: (Tiotropium) 1.25mcg/actuation [60 actuations], 2.5mcg/actuation [60 actuations]

CONTRAINDICATIONS
Hypersensitivity to tiotropium, ipratropium, or any component of this medication.

WARNINGS/PRECAUTIONS
Not for relief of acute symptoms (eg, acute episodes of bronchospasm). Immediate hypersensitivity reactions may occur; d/c and consider alternative treatments if such a reaction occurs. Closely monitor patients w/ a history of hypersensitivity reactions to atropine, or its derivatives. May cause paradoxical bronchospasm; d/c and consider other treatments, and treat immediately w/ an inhaled, short-acting β_2-agonist. Caution w/ narrow-angle glaucoma; monitor for signs and symptoms. Caution w/ urinary retention; monitor for signs and symptoms, especially in patients w/ prostatic hyperplasia or bladder neck obstruction. Closely monitor for anticholinergic effects in patients w/ moderate to severe renal impairment (CrCl <60mL/min).

ADVERSE REACTIONS
COPD: Pharyngitis, cough, dry mouth, sinusitis.
Asthma: Pharyngitis, sinusitis, bronchitis, headache.

DRUG INTERACTIONS
Possible increase in anticholinergic adverse effects w/ other anticholinergic-containing drugs; avoid coadministration.

PREGNANCY AND LACTATION
Pregnancy: Category C.
Lactation: It is not known whether tiotropium is excreted in human milk. Caution in nursing.

MECHANISM OF ACTION
Anticholinergic (long-acting) bronchodilator; exhibits effects through inhibition of M_3-receptors at the smooth muscle, leading to bronchodilation.

PHARMACOKINETICS
Absorption: Absolute bioavailability (2-3%, oral sol); T_{max}=5-7 min. **Distribution:** (IV) V_d=32L/kg; plasma protein binding (72%). **Metabolism:** Liver (oxidation, conjugation) via CYP2D6 and 3A4. **Elimination:** Urine (74%, unchanged, IV); $T_{1/2}$=25 hrs (COPD), 44 hrs (asthma).

PATIENT CONSIDERATIONS
Assessment: Assess for hypersensitivity to drug, atropine or its derivatives, narrow-angle glaucoma, urinary retention, prostatic hyperplasia, bladder neck obstruction, renal impairment, pregnancy/nursing status, and possible drug interactions.

Monitoring: Monitor for hypersensitivity reactions, paradoxical bronchospasm, narrow-angle glaucoma, and other adverse reactions. Monitor for urinary retention, especially in those w/ prostatic hyperplasia or bladder neck obstruction.

Counseling: Advise to d/c if paradoxical bronchospasm occurs. Instruct to consult physician immediately if any signs/symptoms of narrow-angle glaucoma and urinary retention develop. Advise not to allow the aerosol cloud to enter into the eyes. Caution when engaging in activities such as driving a vehicle or operating appliances/machinery. Instruct asthma patients that the max benefits of therapy may only be apparent after 4-8 weeks of therapy. Inform that drug is not for immediate relief of breathing problems. Instruct to administer ud.

SPORANOX CAPSULES — itraconazole   Rx

Class: Azole antifungal

> Should not be administered for the treatment of onychomycosis in patients w/ evidence of ventricular dysfunction (eg, CHF, history of CHF). D/C use if signs/symptoms of CHF occur. Contraindicated w/ methadone, disopyramide, dofetilide, dronedarone, quinidine, ergot alkaloids (eg, dihydroergotamine, ergometrine [ergonovine], ergotamine, methylergometrine [methylergonovine]), irinotecan, lurasidone, oral midazolam, pimozide, triazolam, felodipine, nisoldipine, ranolazine, eplerenone, cisapride, lovastatin, simvastatin, ticagrelor, and, in subjects w/ varying degrees of renal or hepatic impairment, colchicine, fesoterodine, telithromycin, and solifenacin; may cause elevated levels of these drugs and may increase or prolong both the pharmacologic effects and/or adverse reactions to these drugs.

ADULT DOSAGE

Aspergillosis

Pulmonary/extrapulmonary aspergillosis in patients intolerant or refractory to amphotericin B therapy who are immunocompromised/nonimmunocompromised

Usual: 200-400mg/day

Blastomycosis

Pulmonary/extrapulmonary blastomycosis in immunocompromised/nonimmunocompromised patients

Usual: 200mg qd
Titrate: May increase in 100mg increments if no improvement or if w/ evidence of progressive fungal disease
Max: 400mg/day

Administer in 2 divided doses for doses >200mg/day

Histoplasmosis

Pulmonary/extrapulmonary histoplasmosis in immunocompromised/nonimmunocompromised patients

Usual: 200mg qd
Titrate: May increase in 100mg increments if no improvement or if w/ evidence of progressive fungal disease
Max: 400mg/day

Administer in 2 divided doses for doses >200mg/day

Onychomycosis

Nonimmunocompromised Patients:
Toenails (w/ or w/o Fingernail Involvement):
Usual: 200mg qd for 12 consecutive weeks

Fingernails Only:
Usual: 2 treatment pulses, each consisting of 200mg bid for 1 week; separate pulses by a 3-week period w/o itraconazole

Life-Threatening Infections

LD: 200mg tid for the first 3 days

Continue treatment for a minimum of 3 months and until infection subsides

PEDIATRIC DOSAGE
Pediatric use may not have been established

ADMINISTRATION
Oral route

Swallow caps whole; take w/ a full meal

STORAGE
15-25°C (59-77°F). Protect from light and moisture.

HOW SUPPLIED
Cap: 100mg

CONTRAINDICATIONS
Coadministration of a number of CYP3A4 substrates (eg, methadone, disopyramide, dofetilide, dronedarone, quinidine, ergot alkaloids [eg, dihydroergotamine, ergometrine (ergonovine), ergotamine, methylergometrine (methylergonovine)], irinotecan, lurasidone, oral midazolam, pimozide, triazolam, felodipine, nisoldipine, ranolazine, eplerenone, cisapride, lovastatin, simvastatin, ticagrelor, and, in subjects w/ varying degrees of renal or hepatic impairment, colchicine, fesoterodine, telithromycin, and solifenacin). Treatment of onychomycosis in pregnant patients, women contemplating pregnancy, and in patients w/ evidence of ventricular dysfunction (eg, CHF, history of CHF), hypersensitivity to itraconazole.

WARNINGS/PRECAUTIONS
Sol and caps should not be used interchangeably. Rare cases of serious hepatotoxicity reported, including liver failure and death; d/c if clinical signs/

symptoms that are consistent w/ liver disease develop. Caution w/ cardiac disease (eg, ischemic/valvular disease); pulmonary disease (eg, COPD); and renal failure and other edematous disorders. Itraconazole reported to have a negative inotropic effect. CHF, peripheral edema, and pulmonary edema reported. D/C if neuropathy occurs. Consider switching to alternative therapy if a cystic fibrosis patient does not respond to therapy. Transient/permanent hearing loss reported. Absorption of itraconazole may be decreased in HIV-infected individuals who have hypochlorhydria. Caution in hepatic/renal impairment and in the elderly.

ADVERSE REACTIONS
N/V, edema, headache, rash, diarrhea, fatigue, fever, rhinitis, URTI, sinusitis, abdominal pain, dizziness, elevated liver enzymes, HTN, flatulence.

DRUG INTERACTIONS
See Boxed Warning and Contraindications. Not recommended w/ potent CYP3A4 inducers (eg, rifabutin, carbamazepine, efavirenz), tamsulosin, apixaban, rivaroxaban, axitinib, dabrafenib, dasatinib, ibrutinib, nilotinib, sunitinib, simeprevir, aliskiren, sildenafil (for the treatment of pulmonary HTN), everolimus, temsirolimus, salmeterol, darifenacin, vardenafil, conivaptan, and tolvaptan. Avoid CYP3A4 inducers from 2 weeks before and during treatment w/ itraconazole, unless the benefits outweigh the risk of potentially reduced itraconazole efficacy; monitor antifungal activity and increase itraconazole dose as necessary. Drugs that reduce the gastric acidity (eg, aluminum hydroxide, H_2-receptor antagonists, proton pump inhibitors) may impair absorption; use w/ caution. Potent CYP3A4 inhibitors (eg, ciprofloxacin, clarithromycin, telaprevir) may increase levels; use w/ caution, monitor closely for signs/symptoms of increased/prolonged itraconazole pharmacologic effects, and decrease itraconazole dose as necessary. Caution w/ alfentanil, buprenorphine (IV and SL), fentanyl, oxycodone, sufentanil, digoxin, coumarins, cilostazol, dabigatran, repaglinide, saxagliptin, praziquantel, eletriptan, bortezomib, busulphan, docetaxel, erlotinib, imatinib, ixabepilone, lapatinib, ponatinib, trimetrexate, vinca alkaloids, alprazolam, aripiprazole, buspirone, diazepam, haloperidol, midazolam IV, perospirone, quetiapine, ramelteon, risperidone, maraviroc, indinavir, ritonavir, saquinavir, nadolol, dihydropyridine calcium channel blockers [except felodipine and nisoldipine], verapamil, bosentan, riociguat, aprepitant, budesonide, ciclesonide, dexamethasone, cyclosporine, fluticasone, methylprednisolone, sirolimus, tacrolimus, atorvastatin, oxybutynin, sildenafil (for the treatment of erectile dysfunction), tadalafil, tolterodine, and cinacalcet. May decrease levels of meloxicam; use w/ caution and monitor effects/side effects; adjust meloxicam dose if necessary. May inhibit metabolism of drugs metabolized by CYP3A4 and can inhibit drug transport by P-gp, which may result in increased plasma concentrations of these drugs and/or their active metabolite(s). Refer to PI for more information on drug interactions.

PREGNANCY AND LACTATION
Category C, caution in nursing.

MECHANISM OF ACTION
Azole antifungal agent; inhibits the CYP450-dependent synthesis of ergosterol, which is a vital component of fungal cell membranes.

PHARMACOKINETICS
Absorption: Rapid. Absolute oral bioavailability (55%); T_{max}=2-5 hrs. **Distribution:** V_d>700L; plasma protein binding (99.8%, itraconazole), (99.6%, hydroxy-metabolite); found in breast milk. **Metabolism:** Liver (extensive via CYP3A4; hydroxyitraconazole (major metabolite). **Elimination:** (IV) Urine (<1% unchanged and hydroxyitraconazole); (PO) feces (3-18% unchanged).

PATIENT CONSIDERATIONS
Assessment: Assess for hypersensitivity to the drug or to other azole antifungal agents, ventricular dysfunction, ischemic/valvular disease, pulmonary disease, renal/hepatic impairment, edematous disorders, or any other conditions where treatment is cautioned or contraindicated. Assess pregnancy/nursing status and for possible drug interactions. Obtain specimens for fungal cultures and other relevant lab studies to isolate and identify causative organisms.

Monitoring: Monitor for signs/symptoms of CHF, peripheral/pulmonary edema, hepatotoxicity, neuropathy, transient/permanent hearing loss, and other adverse reactions. Monitor LFTs.

Counseling: Instruct not to interchange caps and oral sol. Instruct to take w/ a full meal. Instruct on signs/symptoms of CHF and liver dysfunction; advise to d/c use if these occur and contact physician immediately. Instruct to contact physician before taking any concomitant medications w/ the drug. Instruct to d/c therapy and inform physicians if hearing loss occurs. Instruct that dizziness or blurred/double vision may sometimes occur; advise not to drive or use machines if these events occur.

SPRITAM — levetiracetam Rx
Class: Pyrrolidine derivative

ADULT DOSAGE	PEDIATRIC DOSAGE
Partial Onset Seizures	**Partial Onset Seizures**
Adjunctive Therapy in Patients w/ Epilepsy:	**Adjunctive Therapy in Patients w/ Epilepsy:**
>40kg:	**≥4 Years:**
Initial: 500mg bid	**20-40kg:**
Titrate: May increase by 1000mg/day every 2 weeks	**Initial:** 250mg bid
Max: 3000mg/day	**Titrate:** May increase by 500mg/day every 2 weeks
Myoclonic Seizures	**Max:** 1500mg/day
Adjunctive Therapy in Patients w/ Juvenile Myoclonic Epilepsy:	**>40kg:**
Initial: 500mg bid	**Initial:** 500mg bid
	Titrate: May increase by 1000mg/day every 2 weeks

Titrate: Increase by 1000mg/day every 2 weeks to recommended dose of 3000mg/day

Tonic-Clonic Seizures
Adjunctive Therapy in the Treatment of Primary Generalized Tonic-Clonic Seizures w/ Idiopathic Generalized Epilepsy:
>40kg:
Initial: 500mg bid
Titrate: Increase by 1000mg/day every 2 weeks to recommended dose of 3000mg/day

Max: 3000mg/day
Myoclonic Seizures
Adjunctive Therapy in Patients w/ Juvenile Myoclonic Epilepsy:
≥12 Years:
Initial: 500mg bid
Titrate: Increase by 1000mg/day every 2 weeks to recommended dose of 3000mg/day

Tonic-Clonic Seizures
Adjunctive Therapy in the Treatment of Primary Generalized Tonic-Clonic Seizures w/ Idiopathic Generalized Epilepsy:
≥6 Years:
20-40kg:
Initial: 250mg bid
Titrate: Increase by 500mg/day every 2 weeks
Max: 750mg bid
>40kg:
Initial: 500mg bid
Titrate: Increase by 1000mg/day every 2 weeks to recommended dose of 3000mg/day

---

DOSING CONSIDERATIONS
Renal Impairment
Adults:
Mild (CrCl 50-80mL/min): 500-1000mg q12h
Moderate (CrCl 30-50mL/min): 250-750mg q12h
Severe (CrCl <30mL/min): 250-500mg q12h
ESRD Using Dialysis: 500-1000mg q24h; following dialysis, a supplemental dose of 250-500mg is recommended

ADMINISTRATION
Oral route

- Give w/ or w/o food.
- Foil should be peeled from blister by bending up and lifting the peel tab around the blister seal; do not push through foil.
- Place tab on the tongue w/ a dry hand, follow w/ a sip of liquid, and swallow only after tab disintegrates.
- May add whole tab to small volume of liquid in a cup (1 tbsp or enough to cover medicine); allow tab to disperse prior to consuming immediately. Resuspend any residue and swallow full amount.
- Partial tabs should not be administered; do not attempt to administer partial quantities of dispersed tabs.
- Do not swallow intact.

STORAGE
25°C (77°F); excursions permitted to 15-30°C (59-86°F).

HOW SUPPLIED
Tab, Disintegrating: 250mg, 500mg, 750mg, 1000mg

WARNINGS/PRECAUTIONS
May cause behavioral abnormalities, psychotic symptoms, somnolence, fatigue, and coordination difficulties. May impair mental/physical abilities. Serious dermatological reactions (eg, Stevens-Johnson syndrome [SJS], toxic epidermal necrolysis [TEN]), and recurrence of serious skin reactions following rechallenge reported; d/c at the 1st sign of rash, unless the rash is clearly not drug-related. Do not resume, and consider alternative therapy if signs/symptoms suggest SJS/TEN. Increased risk of suicidal thoughts or behavior. Withdraw gradually to minimize the potential of increased seizure frequency. Hematologic abnormalities and agranulocytosis reported. Physiological changes may decrease plasma levels throughout pregnancy; monitor patients during pregnancy and through the postpartum period, especially if the dose was changed during pregnancy. Caution in elderly. Increased diastolic BP reported.

ADVERSE REACTIONS
Adults: Somnolence, asthenia, infection, dizziness, neck pain, pharyngitis, nasopharyngitis.
Ped: Fatigue, aggression, nasal congestion, decreased appetite, irritability.

PREGNANCY AND LACTATION
Pregnancy: Category C.
Lactation: Not for use in nursing.

MECHANISM OF ACTION
Pyrrolidine derivative; has not been established. Inhibits burst firing w/o affecting normal neuronal excitability, suggesting that it may selectively prevent hypersynchronization of epileptiform burst firing and propagation of seizure activity.

PHARMACOKINETICS
Absorption: Oral bioavailability (100%); T_{max}=1 hr. **Distribution:** Plasma protein binding (<10%); found in breast milk. **Metabolism:** Enzymatic hydrolysis of acetamide group; ucb L057 (metabolite). **Elimination:** Renal (66%, unchanged); $T_{1/2}$=7 hrs.

PATIENT CONSIDERATIONS
Assessment: Assess for renal impairment, depression, suicidal thoughts/behavior, pregnancy/nursing status, and possible drug interactions.

Monitoring: Monitor for signs/symptoms of psychiatric reactions, behavior abnormalities, somnolence and fatigue, coordination difficulties, suicidal behavior/ideation, serious dermatological reactions, hematologic abnormalities, agranulocytosis, and other adverse reactions. Monitor patients during pregnancy and continue close monitoring through the postpartum period, especially if the dose was changed during pregnancy. Monitor for increase in diastolic BP in patients 1 month to <4 yrs of age.

Counseling: Advise to take ud. Advise patients and their caregivers that the drug may cause behavioral changes and psychotic symptoms. Inform that the drug may increase the risk of suicidal thoughts and behavior; advise to be alert for the emergence or worsening of symptoms of depression, unusual changes in mood/behavior, or the emergence of suicidal thoughts, behavior, or thoughts about self-harm. Instruct to immediately report behaviors of concern to physician. Inform that dizziness and somnolence may occur; advise not to drive, operate heavy machinery, or engage in other hazardous activities until the patient has gained sufficient experience to gauge whether it adversely affects his or her performance of these activities. Inform that serious dermatological adverse reactions have been reported; advise to notify physician immediately if a rash develops. Advise to notify physician if patient becomes pregnant or intends to become pregnant; encourage to enroll in the North American Antiepileptic Drug Pregnancy Registry if the patient becomes pregnant during therapy.

SPRIX — ketorolac tromethamine
Class: NSAID

Rx

> May cause an increased risk of serious cardiovascular (CV) thrombotic events (eg, MI, stroke), which can be fatal; risk may occur early in treatment and may increase w/ duration of use. Contraindicated in the setting of CABG surgery. May cause an increased risk of serious GI adverse events (eg, bleeding, ulceration, perforation of the stomach/intestines), which can be fatal; events may occur at any time during use and w/o warning symptoms. Elderly patients and patients w/ prior history of peptic ulcer disease (PUD) and/or GI bleeding are at greater risk for serious GI events.

ADULT DOSAGE

Moderate to Moderately Severe Pain

<65 Years:
31.5mg (one 15.75mg spray in each nostril) q6-8h for up to 5 days
Max: 126mg/day (4 doses)

PEDIATRIC DOSAGE
Pediatric use may not have been established

DOSING CONSIDERATIONS
Concomitant Medications
Do not use w/ other formulations of ketorolac or other NSAIDs
Total duration of use of Sprix alone or sequentially w/ other formulations of ketorolac (IM/IV or oral) must not exceed 5 days

Renal Impairment
15.75mg (1 spray in 1 nostril) q6-8h
Max: 63mg/day (4 doses)

Elderly
≥65 Years:
15.75mg (1 spray in 1 nostril) q6-8h
Max: 63mg/day (4 doses)

Other Important Considerations
<50kg (110 lbs):
15.75mg (1 spray in 1 nostril) q6-8h
Max: 63mg/day (4 doses)

ADMINISTRATION
Intranasal route
Do not inhale when administering.

Instructions
1. Activate the pump before using the bottle for the 1st time by holding the bottle at arm's length away from the body and pressing down evenly and releasing the pump 5X.
2. Blow nose gently to clear nostrils then sit straight or stand w/ head slightly tilted forward.
3. Insert tip of the container into the right nostril and point the container away from the center of the nose.
4. Hold breath and spray once into the right nostril, pressing down evenly on both sides.
5. Resume breathing through mouth immediately after administration; may pinch nose to help retain spray.
6. If a 2nd spray is needed, repeat directions for left nostril.
7. Discard bottle no more than 24 hrs after the 1st dose.

STORAGE
Protect from light and freezing. (Unopened) 2-8°C (36-46°F). (During Use) 15-30°C (59-86°F), out of direct sunlight. Discard w/in 24 hrs of priming.

HOW SUPPLIED
Spray: 15.75mg/spray [1.7g]

CONTRAINDICATIONS
Known hypersensitivity to ketorolac or any components of the drug product; history of asthma, urticaria, or other allergic-type reactions after taking aspirin (ASA) or other NSAIDs; setting of CABG surgery; active PUD; recent GI bleeding or perforation; use as a prophylactic analgesic before any major surgery; advanced renal disease or risk for renal failure due to volume depletion; use in labor and delivery; suspected or confirmed cerebrovascular bleeding, hemorrhagic

diathesis, incomplete hemostasis, or those for whom hemostasis is critical; use w/ probenecid or pentoxifylline.

WARNINGS/PRECAUTIONS
Total duration of use of Sprix alone or sequentially w/ other forms of ketorolac is not to exceed 5 days. Use lowest effective dose for shortest duration possible. Remain alert for the development of CV events, throughout entire treatment course, even in absence of previous CV symptoms. Avoid the use of patients w/ a recent MI unless the benefits are expected to outweigh the risks; if used, monitor for signs of cardiac ischemia. Increased risk of GI bleeding w/ longer duration of therapy; smoking; use of alcohol; older age; and poor general health status. Avoid use in patients at higher risk unless benefits are expected to outweigh the increased risk of bleeding; consider alternate therapies other than NSAIDs. Do not use w/ active GI bleed. If serious GI adverse event is suspected, promptly evaluate, initiate treatment, and d/c until serious GI adverse event is ruled out. Use w/ great care w/ history of inflammatory bowel disease. ALT/AST elevations reported; d/c immediately if systemic manifestations of hepatotoxicity occur. May lead to new onset of HTN or worsening of preexisting HTN; monitor BP during initiation and throughout course of therapy. Fluid retention and edema reported. Avoid use w/ severe heart failure (HF) unless benefits outweigh risks of worsening HF; monitor for signs of worsening HF. Renal papillary necrosis and other renal injury reported w/ long-term use. Renal toxicity also reported in patients in whom renal prostaglandins have a compensatory role in the maintenance of renal perfusion; increased risk w/ renal/hepatic dysfunction, dehydration, hypovolemia, HF, and in the elderly. Correct volume status if dehydrated or hypovolemic prior to initiating therapy. Monitor renal function w/ renal or hepatic impairment, HF, dehydration, or hypovolemia during use. Increases in K⁺, including hyperkalemia, reported. Associated w/ anaphylactic reactions w/ and w/o known hypersensitivity to ketorolac and w/ ASA-sensitive asthma. Monitor for changes in the signs/symptoms of asthma in patients w/ preexisting asthma (w/o known ASA sensitivity). May cause serious skin adverse reactions (eg, exfoliative dermatitis, Stevens-Johnson syndrome, toxic epidermal necrolysis); d/c at the 1st appearance of skin rash or any other sign of hypersensitivity. May cause premature closure of the fetal ductus arteriosus; avoid use in pregnant women starting at 30 weeks of gestation (3rd trimester). Anemia reported; monitor Hgb or Hct if signs/symptoms of anemia develop. May increase the risk of bleeding events; coagulation disorders may increase this risk. May diminish the utility of diagnostic signs in detecting infections. Avoid contact w/ eyes; if contact occurs, wash out eye w/ water or saline.

ADVERSE REACTIONS
Nasal discomfort, rhinalgia, increased lacrimation, throat irritation, oliguria, rash, bradycardia, decreased urine output, increased ALT and/or AST, HTN, rhinitis.

DRUG INTERACTIONS
See Dosing Considerations/Contraindications. Drugs that interfere w/ serotonin reuptake may potentiate the risk of bleeding. Concurrent use w/ therapy that affects hemostasis (eg, prophylactic low dose heparin [2500-5000 U q12h], anticoagulants [eg, warfarin], dextrans, and oral corticosteroids) may be associated w/ an increased risk of bleeding; use w/ extreme caution. Monitor patients for signs of bleeding w/ concomitant use of anticoagulants, antiplatelet agents (eg, ASA), SSRIs, and SNRIs. Increased incidence of GI adverse reactions w/ analgesic doses of ASA; concomitant use not recommended. May diminish antihypertensive effect of ACE inhibitors, ARBs, or β-blockers (eg, propranolol); monitor BP. Coadministration w/ ACE inhibitors or ARBs may result in deterioration of renal function (including possible acute renal failure) in patients who are elderly, volume-depleted (including those on diuretic therapy), or have renal impairment; monitor for worsening renal function. Adequately hydrate and assess renal function at the beginning of the concomitant treatment and periodically thereafter. May reduce natriuretic effect of loop diuretics (eg, furosemide) and thiazide diuretics; observe for signs of worsening renal function, in addition to assuring diuretic efficacy including antihypertensive effects. May increase serum concentration and prolong $T_{1/2}$ of digoxin; monitor serum digoxin levels. May cause elevations in plasma lithium levels and reductions in renal lithium clearance; monitor for signs of lithium toxicity. May increase risk for methotrexate toxicity. May increase cyclosporine's nephrotoxicity; monitor for signs of worsening renal function. Use w/ other NSAIDs or salicylates (eg, diflunisal, salsalate) increases risk of GI toxicity; concomitant use not recommended. May increase the risk of pemetrexed-associated myelosuppression, renal, and GI toxicity; refer to prescribing information for further information. Possible increase in $T_{1/2}$ and systemic exposure of probenecid. Sporadic cases of seizures reported w/ antiepileptic drugs (eg, phenytoin, carbamazepine). Hallucinations reported w/ psychoactive drugs (eg, fluoxetine, thiothixene, alprazolam). Possible apnea w/ nondepolarizing muscle relaxants.

PREGNANCY AND LACTATION
Pregnancy: Category C (prior to 30 weeks gestation) and D (starting at 30 weeks gestation).
Lactation: Excreted in human milk; caution in nursing.
Females and Males of Reproductive Potential: May delay or prevent rupture of ovarian follicles. Consider withdrawal in women who have difficulties conceiving or who are undergoing investigation of infertility.

MECHANISM OF ACTION
NSAID; inhibits cyclooxygenase (COX-1 and COX-2), resulting in reduced synthesis of prostaglandins, thromboxanes, and prostacyclin. Exerts anti-inflammatory, analgesic, and antipyretic actions.

PHARMACOKINETICS
Absorption: C_{max}=1805.8ng/mL, T_{max}=0.75 hr, AUC=7477.3ng•hr/mL. **Distribution:** V_d=13L; plasma protein binding (99.2%); found in breast milk. **Metabolism:** Liver via hydroxylation and conjugation. **Elimination:** Urine (92%; 40% metabolites, 60%, unchanged), feces (6%); $T_{1/2}$= 5.24 hrs (31.5mg), 2.5 hrs (S-enantiomer), 5 hrs (R-enantiomer).

PATIENT CONSIDERATIONS

Assessment: Assess for hypersensitivity to ketorolac or to any component of this product; history of asthma, urticaria, or other allergic-type reactions after taking ASA or other NSAIDs; CABG surgery; active PUD/GI bleed or history of PUD/GI bleeding or perforation; advanced renal disease or risk for renal failure due to volume depletion; suspected or confirmed cerebrovascular bleeding, hemorrhagic diathesis, incomplete hemostasis, or when hemostasis is critical; inflammatory bowel disease; HTN; HF; pregnancy/nursing status; and other conditions where use is cautioned/contraindicated. Assess renal function and other NSAID use. Assess for possible drug interactions.

Monitoring: Monitor signs/symptoms of CV thrombotic events; cardiac ischemia in patients w/ a recent MI; GI bleeding/ulceration and perforation; hepatotoxicity; fluid retention; edema; renal papillary necrosis and other renal injury; hyperkalemia; anaphylactoid/skin/hypersensitivity reactions; hematological effects; and other adverse reactions. Monitor BP during initiation of therapy and throughout the course of therapy. Monitor renal function in patients w/ renal/hepatic impairment, HF, dehydration, or hypovolemia. Monitor for signs of bleeding in patients w/ on concomitant therapy w/ anticoagulants, antiplatelet agents, SSRIs, or SNRIs. Monitor CBC and chemistry profiles periodically during long-term treatment.

Counseling: Instruct patients not to use for >5 days. Instruct not to use any single bottle for >1 day. Advise to be alert for the symptoms of CV thrombotic events. Advise to report symptoms of ulcerations/bleeding. In the setting of concomitant use of low-dose ASA for cardiac prophylaxis, inform of the increased risk for and the signs/symptoms of GI bleeding. Inform of the warning signs/symptoms of hepatotoxicity and advise to d/c use and seek immediate medical therapy if signs/symptoms occur. Advise to be alert for the symptoms of CHF and to contact healthcare provider if such symptoms occur. Inform of the signs of an anaphylactic reaction and to seek immediate emergency help if signs/symptoms occur. Advise to d/c and contact healthcare provider if immediately any type of rash develops. Advise females of reproductive potential who desire pregnancy that therapy may be associated w/ a reversible delay in ovulation. Inform pregnant women to avoid use starting at 30 weeks gestation. Inform that concomitant use w/ other NSAIDs or salicylates is not recommended. Advise that NSAIDs may be present in OTC medications for treatment of colds, fever, or insomnia. Inform not to use low-dose ASA w/o the patient talking his or her physician. Advise to maintain adequate fluid intake and request medical advice if urine output decreases significantly. Advise that transient, mild to moderate nasal irritation or discomfort may occur upon dosing.

SPRYCEL — dasatinib   Rx

Class: Kinase inhibitor

ADULT DOSAGE	PEDIATRIC DOSAGE
Ph+ Chronic Phase CML	Pediatric use may not have been established

Newly Diagnosed Ph+ CML in Chronic Phase:
Initial: 100mg qd
Titrate: If no hematologic or cytogenetic response, increase to 140mg qd

Chronic Phase Ph+ CML w/ Resistance or Intolerance to Prior Therapy (Including Imatinib):
Initial: 100mg qd
Titrate: If no hematologic or cytogenetic response, increase to 140mg qd

Accelerated Phase CML/Myeloid or Lymphoid Blast Phase CML/Ph+ ALL

Accelerated or myeloid/lymphoid blast phase Ph+ CML w/ resistance or intolerance to prior therapy (including imatinib) and Ph+ ALL w/ resistance or intolerance to prior therapy

Initial: 140mg qd
Titrate: If no hematologic or cytogenetic response, increase to 180mg qd

- -

DOSING CONSIDERATIONS
Concomitant Medications
Strong CYP3A4 Inducers:
Avoid use; if necessary, consider dose increase of dasatinib w/ careful monitoring for toxicity

Strong CYP3A4 Inhibitors:
Avoid use; if necessary, consider dose decrease of dasatinib to 20mg if taking 100mg qd, and to 40mg if taking 140mg qd
If therapy is not tolerated after dose reduction, either d/c concomitant inhibitor and allow a washout period of approx 1 week before increasing dasatinib dose, or d/c dasatinib until end of treatment w/ inhibitor

Grapefruit Juice:
Avoid grapefruit juice

Adverse Reactions
Neutropenia and Thrombocytopenia:
Chronic Phase CML:
ANC <0.5 x 10^9/L or Platelets <50 x 10^9/L:
1. Stop therapy until ANC ≥1.0 x 10^9/L and platelets ≥50 x 10^9/L
2. Resume therapy at the original starting dose if recovery occurs in ≤7 days
3. If platelets <25 x 10^9/L or recurrence of ANC <0.5 x 10^9/L for >7 days, repeat Step 1 and resume at a reduced dose of 80mg qd for 2nd episode. For 3rd episode, further reduce dose to 50mg qd (for newly diagnosed patients) or d/c (for patients resistant or intolerant to prior therapy, including imatinib)

Accelerated Phase CML, Blast Phase CML, and Ph+ ALL (Starting Dose 140mg QD):
ANC <0.5 x 10^9/L or Platelets <10 x 10^9/L:
1. If cytopenia is unrelated to leukemia, stop until ANC ≥1.0 x 10^9/L and platelets ≥20 x 10^9/L and resume at the original starting dose
2. If recurrence of cytopenia, repeat Step 1 and resume at a reduced dose of 100mg qd (2nd episode) or 80mg qd (3rd episode)
3. If cytopenia is related to leukemia, consider dose escalation to 180mg qd

Nonhematological Adverse Reactions:
If a severe nonhematological adverse reaction develops, withhold until the event has resolved or improved
May resume at a reduced dose depending on the severity and recurrence of the event

ADMINISTRATION
Oral route

Take w/ or w/o meal, either in am or pm.
Swallow whole; do not crush or cut.

STORAGE
20-25°C (68-77°F); excursions permitted between 15-30°C (59-86°F).

HOW SUPPLIED
Tab: 20mg, 50mg, 70mg, 80mg, 100mg, 140mg

WARNINGS/PRECAUTIONS
Severe thrombocytopenia, neutropenia, and anemia reported earlier and more frequently in patients w/ advanced phase CML than in patients w/ chronic phase CML. In patients w/ chronic phase CML, perform CBCs every 2 weeks for 12 weeks, then every 3 months thereafter, or as clinically indicated. In patients w/ advanced phase CML or Ph+ ALL, perform CBCs weekly for the first 2 months and then monthly thereafter, or as clinically indicated. ≥Grade 3 CNS and GI hemorrhages, including fatalities and other cases of ≥Grade 3 hemorrhage, reported. Fluid retention may occur; perform chest x-ray if symptoms suggestive of pleural effusion or other fluid retention develop (eg, dyspnea, pleuritic chest pain, dry cough). Cardiac adverse reactions reported; monitor for signs/symptoms consistent w/ cardiac dysfunction and treat appropriately. May increase risk of developing pulmonary arterial HTN (PAH); d/c permanently if PAH is confirmed. QT prolongation reported; correct hypokalemia or hypomagnesemia prior to and during dasatinib administration. Cases of severe mucocutaneous dermatologic reactions (eg, Stevens-Johnson syndrome) reported; d/c permanently in patients who experience a severe mucocutaneous reaction during treatment if no other etiology can be identified. Tumor lysis syndrome reported; maintain adequate hydration and correct uric acid levels prior to initiating therapy w/ dasatinib, and monitor electrolyte levels. Caution w/ hepatic impairment.

ADVERSE REACTIONS
Fluid retention, diarrhea, N/V, headache, musculoskeletal pain, abdominal pain, hemorrhage, pneumonia, pyrexia, dyspnea, rash, fatigue, arthralgia, infection, muscle spasms.

DRUG INTERACTIONS
See Dosing Considerations. CYP3A4 inhibitors (eg, ketoconazole, clarithromycin, ritonavir) and grapefruit juice may increase levels. CYP3A4 inducers (eg, dexamethasone, phenytoin, carbamazepine) and St. John's wort may decrease levels. Avoid w/ antacids (eg, aluminum hydroxide/magnesium hydroxide); if use is necessary, administer antacid dose at least 2 hrs prior to or 2 hrs after dasatinib dose. H_2 antagonists (eg, famotidine) or proton pump inhibitors (eg, omeprazole) may reduce exposure; concomitant use is not recommended. May increase levels of simvastatin (a CYP3A4 substrate); caution w/ CYP3A4 substrates w/ narrow therapeutic index (eg, alfentanil, astemizole, ergotamine). Medications that inhibit platelet function or anticoagulants may increase the risk of hemorrhage. Antiarrhythmics or other QT-prolonging agents and cumulative high-dose anthracycline therapy may increase risk of QT prolongation.

PREGNANCY AND LACTATION
Pregnancy: Can cause fetal harm; adverse pharmacologic effects (eg, hydrops fetalis, fetal leukopenia, fetal thrombocytopenia) reported w/ maternal exposure to dasatinib.
Lactation: No data are available regarding the presence of dasatinib in human milk, the effects of the drug on the breastfed infant or the effects of the drug on milk production; breastfeeding is not recommended during treatment w/ dasatinib and for 2 weeks after the final dose.
Females and Males Reproductive Potential: Females of reproductive potential should avoid pregnancy, which may include the use of effective contraceptive methods during treatment and for 30 days after the final dose. Dasatinib may result in damage to female and male reproductive tissues.

MECHANISM OF ACTION
Kinase inhibitor; inhibits BCR-ABL, SRC family, c-KIT, EPHA2, and PDGFRβ kinases.

PHARMACOKINETICS
Absorption: T_{max}=0.5-6 hrs. **Distribution:** V_d=2505L; plasma protein binding (96% [parent], 93% [active metabolite]); crosses placenta. **Metabolism:** Extensive, primarily via CYP3A4. **Elimination:** Feces (85%, 19% unchanged), urine (4%, 0.1% unchanged); $T_{1/2}$=3-5 hrs.

PATIENT CONSIDERATIONS

Assessment: Assess for signs/symptoms of underlying cardiopulmonary disease, hepatic impairment, presence or risk of QT prolongation, hypokalemia, hypomagnesemia, pregnancy/nursing status, and possible drug interactions.

Monitoring: Monitor for bleeding events, fluid retention, cardiac dysfunction, myelosuppression, QT prolongation, PAH, tumor lysis syndrome, severe mucocutaneous dermatologic reactions, and other adverse reactions. Perform chest x-ray if symptoms of pleural effusion develop. In patients w/ chronic phase CML, perform CBCs every 2 weeks for 12 weeks, then every 3 months thereafter, or as clinically indicated. In patients w/ advanced phase CML or Ph+ ALL, perform CBCs weekly for the first 2 months and then monthly thereafter, or as clinically indicated.

Counseling: Inform of pregnancy risks; instruct females of reproductive potential to avoid becoming pregnant during therapy and for 30 days after the final dose of therapy. Advise females of reproductive potential to contact physician if patient becomes pregnant, or if pregnancy is suspected, while on therapy. Instruct to seek medical attention if symptoms of hemorrhage, myelosuppression, fluid retention, significant N/V, diarrhea, headache, musculoskeletal pain, fatigue, or rash develop. Inform that product contains lactose.

STALEVO — carbidopa/entacapone/levodopa   Rx

Class: COMT inhibitor/dopa-decarboxylase inhibitor/dopamine precursor

ADULT DOSAGE

Parkinson's Disease

May be used:
1. To substitute (w/ equivalent strengths of each of the 3 components) carbidopa/levodopa and entacapone previously administered as individual products
2. To replace carbidopa/levodopa therapy (w/o entacapone) for patients experiencing signs/symptoms of end-of-dose "wearing-off" and who have been taking a total daily dose of levodopa of ≤600mg and have not been experiencing dyskinesias

Converting from Carbidopa, Levodopa, and Entacapone:

In patients currently treated w/ entacapone 200mg w/ each dose of non-extended release carbidopa/levodopa tab may switch to corresponding strength of Stalevo w/ same amounts of carbidopa and levodopa

Converting from Carbidopa and Levodopa Products:

Titrate patients initially to a dose that is tolerated and that meets individual therapeutic need using a separate carbidopa/levodopa tab (1:4 ratio) plus an entacapone tab; switch to the corresponding single tab of Stalevo once the individual dose of carbidopa/levodopa plus entacapone has been established

When less levodopa is required, reduce the total daily dose of carbidopa/levodopa either by decreasing the strength of Stalevo at each administration or by decreasing the frequency of administration by extending time between doses

Max: 8 tabs/day (Stalevo 50, 75, 100, 125, 150); 6 tabs/day (Stalevo 200)

Determine optimum daily dose by careful titration in each patient

Administer only 1 tab at each dosing interval

PEDIATRIC DOSAGE

Pediatric use may not have been established

DOSING CONSIDERATIONS

Concomitant Medications

Other Anti-Parkinson's Disease Drugs: May need to adjust concomitant medication or Stalevo

Other Important Considerations

Decrease or Interruption of Dosing: Avoid interruption of Stalevo dosing; hyperpyrexia reported when levodopa is suddenly discontinued or reduced

ADMINISTRATION

Oral route

Do not split, crush, or chew tabs.

Take w/ or w/o food; a high-fat, high-calorie meal may delay absorption of levodopa by about 2 hrs.

STORAGE

25°C (77°F); excursions permitted to 15-30°C (59-86°F).

HOW SUPPLIED

Tab: (Carbidopa/Levodopa/Entacapone): **Stalevo 50:** 12.5mg/50mg/200mg; **Stalevo 75:** 18.75mg/75mg/200mg; **Stalevo 100:** 25mg/100mg/200mg; **Stalevo 125:** 31.25mg/125mg/200mg; **Stalevo 150:** 37.5mg/150mg/200mg; **Stalevo 200:** 50mg/200mg/200mg

CONTRAINDICATIONS

Narrow-angle glaucoma. Nonselective MAOIs (eg, phenelzine, tranylcypromine); d/c nonselective MAOIs at least 2 weeks prior to therapy.

WARNINGS/PRECAUTIONS

Falling asleep suddenly w/o prior warning of sleepiness while engaged in activities of daily living and somnolence reported; reassess for drowsiness or sleepiness, and should ordinarily be discontinued if significant daytime sleepiness or episodes of falling asleep during activities that require active participation occur. May impair mental/physical abilities. Dyskinesia may occur or be exacerbated at lower dosages and sooner than w/ carbidopa/levodopa; may require dose reductions. Monitor for depression w/ concomitant suicidal tendencies. Caution w/ past or current psychoses. May cause intense urges to gamble/spend money uncontrollably, increased sexual urges, and other intense urges; consider dose reduction or discontinuation if such urges develop. Caution w/ biliary obstruction or hepatic disease/impairment. Cases of hyperpyrexia and confusion resembling neuroleptic malignant syndrome (NMS) reported in association w/ dose reduction or withdrawal; decrease dose slowly if a patient needs to d/c or reduce daily dose. Syncope, orthostatic hypotension, hypotension, hallucinations and/or psychotic-like behavior, and rhabdomyolysis reported. Cases of retroperitoneal fibrosis, pulmonary infiltrates, pleural effusion, and pleural thickening reported in patients treated w/ ergot derived dopaminergic agents. Pulmonary fibrosis reported w/ entacapone treatment. Diarrhea and colitis reported w/ entacapone use; d/c and consider appropriate medical therapy if prolonged diarrhea is suspected to be related to therapy. Monitor for melanomas frequently and regularly; perform periodic skin examination. May increase the possibility of upper GI hemorrhage in patients w/ history of peptic ulcer. Lab test abnormalities, including elevations of LFTs, BUN abnormalities, and (+) Coombs test reported. May cause a false-positive reaction for urinary ketone bodies when a test tape is used for determination of ketonuria and may cause false-negative tests w/ the use of glucose-oxidase methods of testing for glucosuria. Cases of falsely diagnosed pheochromocytoma in patients on carbidopa/levodopa rarely reported; caution when interpreting the plasma and urine levels of catecholamines and their metabolites. Levodopa is known to depress prolactin secretion and increase growth hormone levels.

ADVERSE REACTIONS

Dyskinesia, N/V, hyperkinesia, diarrhea, urine discoloration, hypokinesia, dizziness, abdominal pain, constipation, fatigue, back pain, dry mouth, dyspnea.

DRUG INTERACTIONS

See Contraindications. Caution w/ concomitant use of alcohol, sedating medications, and other CNS depressants (eg, benzodiazepines, antipsychotics, antidepressants); may produce additive effects. Iron salts may reduce bioavailability; caution w/ iron salts or multivitamins containing iron salts. Adjust dose of Stalevo as clinically needed in patients using other drugs metabolized via CYP2C9. **Entacapone:** Caution w/ drugs metabolized by catechol-O-methyltransferase (COMT) (eg, epinephrine, dopamine, α-methyldopa, isoetherine); increased HR, possibly arrhythmias, and excessive changes in BP may occur. Caution w/ drugs known to interfere w/ biliary excretion, glucuronidation, and intestinal β-glucuronidase (eg, probenecid, cholestyramine, erythromycin, ampicillin). Increased R-warfarin exposure and INR values reported w/ warfarin; monitor INR when initiating therapy in patents receiving warfarin. **Levodopa:** Beneficial effects of levodopa in Parkinson's disease reported to be reversed by phenytoin and papaverine; monitor for loss of therapeutic response and increase dosage of Stalevo as clinically needed. Isoniazid and dopamine D₂ receptor antagonists (eg, phenothiazines, butyrophenones, risperidone, metoclopramide) may reduce therapeutic effects. **Carbidopa/Levodopa:** Symptomatic postural hypotension reported when added w/ antihypertensives; dosage adjustment of the antihypertensive drug may be required when starting therapy. Adverse reactions, including HTN and dyskinesia, reported w/ TCAs.

PREGNANCY AND LACTATION

Pregnancy: Category C.
Lactation: Caution in nursing.

MECHANISM OF ACTION

Carbidopa: Dopa-decarboxylase inhibitor; inhibits the decarboxylation of peripheral levodopa, making more levodopa available for delivery to the brain. **Levodopa:** Dopamine precursor; crosses blood-brain barrier and presumably converts to dopamine in brain. **Entacapone:** COMT inhibitor; selective and reversible inhibitor of COMT.

PHARMACOKINETICS

Absorption: Levodopa: Rapid. (PO) Administration of variable doses resulted in different parameters. Entacapone: Rapid. C_{max}=1200-1500ng/mL; T_{max}=0.8-1.2 hrs; AUC=1250-1750ng•hr/mL. Carbidopa: Slower; C_{max}=40-225ng/mL; T_{max}=2.5-3.4 hrs; AUC=170-1200ng•hr/mL. **Distribution:** Plasma protein binding: Levodopa: (10-30%); Entacapone: (98%); Carbidopa: (36%). Levodopa: Crosses the placenta. **Metabolism:** Levodopa: Extensive decarboxylation by dopa decarboxylase and O-methylation by COMT. Entacapone: Isomerization; *cis*-isomer (active metabolite). Carbidopa: α-methyl-3-methoxy-4-hydroxyphenylpropionic acid, α-methyl-3,4-dihydroxyphenylpropionic acid (metabolites). **Elimination:** Levodopa: $T_{1/2}$=1.7 hrs. Entacapone: Feces (90%), urine (10%, 0.2% unchanged); $T_{1/2}$=0.8-1 hr. Carbidopa: Urine (30%, unchanged); $T_{1/2}$=1.6-2 hrs.

PATIENT CONSIDERATIONS

Assessment: Assess for narrow-angle glaucoma, sleep disorder, past/current psychoses, history of peptic ulcer, hypotension, biliary obstruction, hepatic impairment, pregnancy/nursing status, any other conditions where treatment is contraindicated or cautioned, and possible drug interactions.

Monitoring: Monitor for signs/symptoms of falling asleep during activities of daily living, hypotension/orthostatic hypotension, syncope, dyskinesia, depression, suicidal tendencies, hallucinations/psychotic-like behavior, impulse control/compulsive behaviors, withdrawal-emergent hyperpyrexia and confusion, diarrhea, colitis, melanoma, rhabdomyolysis, and other adverse reactions. Perform skin examination periodically. Monitor INR w/ warfarin.

Counseling: Inform of the risks and benefits of therapy. Advise about the potential for sedating effects including somnolence and the possibility of falling asleep while engaged in activities of daily living; instruct not to drive or participate in potentially dangerous activities until aware of how medication affects mental and/or motor performance. Advise to speak w/ physician before taking alcohol, sedating medications, or other CNS depressants because of the possible additive effects in combination w/ therapy. Inform that symptomatic (or asymptomatic) postural (orthostatic) hypotension or non-orthostatic hypotension may develop; advise not to rise rapidly after sitting or lying down, especially if doing so for prolonged periods and especially at the initiation of treatment. Inform about the possibility of syncope. Inform that therapy may cause and/or exacerbate preexisting dyskinesias. Inform that hallucinations and other psychotic-like behavior may occur. Instruct to inform physician of new or increased gambling urges, sexual urges, or other intense urges while on therapy. Advise that fever and confusion may develop as part of a syndrome resembling NMS, possibly w/ other clinical features; instruct to contact physician if wishing to d/c or decrease dose, or if fever and confusion develop. Inform that diarrhea, colitis, rhabdomyolysis, myalgia, and N/V may occur. Inform of higher risk of developing melanoma; instruct to have skin examined on a regular basis by a qualified healthcare provider (eg, dermatologist) and to monitor for melanomas frequently and on a regular basis when using therapy.

STARLIX — nateglinide   Rx

Class: Meglitinide

ADULT DOSAGE	PEDIATRIC DOSAGE
Type 2 Diabetes Mellitus	Pediatric use may not have been established
Monotherapy and Combination w/ Metformin or a Thiazolidinedione: **Initial/Maint:** 120mg tid ac; may use 60mg dose in patients near goal HbA1c when treatment is initiated	

DOSING CONSIDERATIONS
Hepatic Impairment
Moderate to Severe: Use caution

ADMINISTRATION
Oral route
Take 1-30 min ac.
Patients who skip meals should also skip their scheduled dose of nateglinide to reduce risk of hypoglycemia.

STORAGE
25°C (77°F); excursions permitted to 15-30°C (59-86°F).

HOW SUPPLIED
Tab: 60mg, 120mg

CONTRAINDICATIONS
Known hypersensitivity to the drug or its inactive ingredients, type 1 diabetes mellitus (DM), diabetic ketoacidosis.

WARNINGS/PRECAUTIONS
Risk of hypoglycemia increased with strenuous exercise, adrenal/pituitary insufficiency, severe renal impairment, and in elderly/malnourished patients. Autonomic neuropathy may mask hypoglycemia. Caution in moderate to severe hepatic impairment. Transient loss of glucose control may occur with fever, infection, trauma, or surgery; may need insulin therapy instead of nateglinide. Secondary failure (reduced effectiveness over a period of time) may occur.

ADVERSE REACTIONS
Upper respiratory infection (URI), flu symptoms, dizziness, arthropathy, diarrhea, hypoglycemia, back pain, jaundice, cholestatic hepatitis, elevated liver enzymes.

DRUG INTERACTIONS
Alcohol, NSAIDs, salicylates, MAOIs, nonselective β-blockers, guanethidine, and CYP2C9 inhibitors (eg, fluconazole, amiodarone, miconazole, oxandrolone) may potentiate hypoglycemia. Thiazides, corticosteroids, thyroid products, sympathomimetics, somatropin, rifampin, phenytoin, and dietary supplements (St. John's wort) may reduce hypoglycemic action of drug. Somatostatin analogues may potentiate/attenuate hypoglycemia. Reduced levels reported with liquid meals. β-blockers may mask hypoglycemic effects. Caution with highly protein-bound drugs.

PREGNANCY AND LACTATION
Category C, not for use in nursing.

MECHANISM OF ACTION
Meglitinide; lowers blood glucose levels by stimulating insulin secretion from the pancreas.

PHARMACOKINETICS
Absorption: Rapidly absorbed. Absolute bioavailability (73%); T_{max}=1 hr.
Distribution: V_d=10L (IV); plasma protein binding (98%). **Metabolism:** CYP2C9, 3A4; hydroxylation, glucuronide conjugation. **Elimination:** Urine (75%), feces; $T_{1/2}$=1.5 hrs.

PATIENT CONSIDERATIONS
Assessment: Assess for diabetic ketoacidosis, type 1 DM, renal/hepatic impairment, adrenal/pituitary insufficiency, pregnancy/nursing status, other conditions where treatment is cautioned, and possible drug interactions. Assess FPG and HbA1c.

Monitoring: Monitor for hypo/hyperglycemia, diabetic ketoacidosis, secondary failure, URI, and other adverse reactions. Monitor FPG, HbA1c, renal function, and LFTs.

Counseling: Inform of potential risks, benefits, alternate modes of therapy, and drug interactions. Instruct to take 1-30 min ac, but to skip scheduled dose if meal is skipped. Inform about importance of adherence to meal planning, regular physical activity, regular blood glucose monitoring, periodic HbA1c testing, recognition and management of hypo/hyperglycemia, and periodic assessment for diabetes complications. Advise to notify physician if any adverse events occur.

STAXYN — vardenafil hydrochloride   Rx

Class: Phosphodiesterase-5 (PDE-5) inhibitor

ADULT DOSAGE	PEDIATRIC DOSAGE
Erectile Dysfunction	Pediatric use may not have been established
10mg prn, approx 60 min before sexual activity	
Max: 1 tab/day	

DOSING CONSIDERATIONS
Concomitant Medications
α-blocker:
In patients taking α-blockers, do not initiate vardenafil therapy w/ Staxyn; use lower doses of vardenafil film-coated tab as initial therapy. Patients taking α-blockers who have previously used vardenafil film-coated tablets may change to Staxyn at the advice of their healthcare provider; consider a time interval between dosing when Staxyn is prescribed concomitantly w/ an α-blocker

Potent or Moderate CYP3A4 Inhibitors: Avoid use

Renal Impairment
Dialysis: Avoid use

Hepatic Impairment
Moderate or Severe (Child-Pugh B or C): Avoid use

ADMINISTRATION
Oral route

Place on tongue to disintegrate.
Take w/o liquid and immediately upon removal from blister.
Take w/ or w/o food.

STORAGE
25°C (77°F); excursions permitted to 15-30°C (59-86°F).

HOW SUPPLIED
Tab, Disintegrating: 10mg

CONTRAINDICATIONS
Concomitant use w/ nitrates (regularly and/or intermittently), nitric oxide donors, or guanylate cyclase (GC) stimulators (eg, riociguat).

WARNINGS/PRECAUTIONS
Not interchangeable w/ vardenafil 10mg film-coated tab (Levitra); prescribe film-coated tab if requiring a lower/higher dose. Do not use in men for whom sexual activity is not recommended due to underlying cardiovascular (CV) status; not recommended w/ unstable angina; hypotension (resting SBP <90mmHg); uncontrolled HTN (>170/110mmHg); recent history of stroke, life-threatening arrhythmia, or MI (w/in last 6 months); or severe cardiac failure. Patients w/ left ventricular outflow obstruction (eg, aortic stenosis, idiopathic hypertrophic subaortic stenosis) may be sensitive to the action of vasodilators. Has systemic vasodilatory properties that resulted in transient decreases in supine BP. Rare reports of prolonged erections >4 hrs and priapism (painful erections >6 hrs in duration); caution w/ anatomical deformation of the penis (eg, angulation, cavernosal fibrosis, Peyronie's disease) or predispositions to priapism (eg, sickle cell anemia, multiple myeloma, leukemia). D/C if sudden loss of vision in 1 or both eyes occurs as this may be a sign of nonarteritic anterior ischemic optic neuropathy (NAION). Caution in patients w/ underlying NAION risk factors; increased risk in patients w/ previous history of NAION or "crowded" optic disc. Not recommended w/ hereditary degenerative retinal disorders (including retinitis pigmentosa). D/C if sudden decrease or loss of hearing occurs. May prolong QT interval; avoid w/ congenital QT prolongation. Caution w/ bleeding disorders or significant active peptic ulceration. Contains aspartame, which may be harmful in phenylketonurics. Contains sorbitol; do not use in patients w/ hereditary problems of fructose intolerance. Does not protect against STDs.

ADVERSE REACTIONS
Headache, flushing, nasal congestion.

DRUG INTERACTIONS
See Dosing Considerations and Contraindications. Potent CYP3A4 inhibitors (eg, ritonavir, indinavir, ketoconazole) or moderate CYP3A4 inhibitors (eg,

erythromycin) increase vardenafil levels. Vardenafil may reduce levels of ritonavir or indinavir. Step-wise increases in α-blocker dose may be associated w/ further lowering of BP. Caution w/ medications known to prolong the QT interval; avoid w/ Class IA (eg, quinidine, procainamide) or Class III (eg, amiodarone, sotalol) antiarrhythmics. Not recommended for use w/ other treatments for erectile dysfunction (ED). Additive hypotensive effect w/ antihypertensive agents.

PREGNANCY AND LACTATION
Pregnancy: Category B; not for use in women.
Lactation: Not for use in women.

MECHANISM OF ACTION
PDE5 inhibitor; increases the amount of cGMP, triggering smooth muscle relaxation and allowing increased blood flow into the penis.

PHARMACOKINETICS
Absorption: T_{max}=1.5 hrs (median). **Distribution:** V_{ss}=208L; plasma protein binding (95%). **Metabolism:** Predominantly via CYP3A4, w/ contributions from CYP3A5 and CYP2C; M1 (major metabolite). **Excretion:** Feces (91-95%), urine (2-6%); $T_{1/2}$=4-6 hrs (vardenafil), 3-5 hrs (M1).

PATIENT CONSIDERATIONS
Assessment: Assess for hypersensitivity to drug, potential underlying causes of ED, CV disease, left ventricular outflow obstruction, anatomical deformation of the penis, predisposition to priapism, NAION risk factors, hereditary degenerative retinal disorders, congenital QT prolongation, renal/hepatic impairment, bleeding disorders, active peptic ulceration, phenylketonuria, fructose intolerance, any other conditions where treatment is contraindicated or cautioned, and for possible drug interactions. Obtain baseline BP.

Monitoring: Monitor for priapism, changes in vision/hearing, QT prolongation, and other adverse reactions.

Counseling: Inform that drug is not interchangeable w/ vardenafil film-coated tab (Levitra). Inform that therapy is contraindicated w/ regular and/or intermittent use of organic nitrates and GC stimulators. Inform that use w/ nitrates may cause BP to suddenly drop to an unsafe level, resulting in dizziness, syncope, or even heart attack or stroke. Inform patients w/ preexisting CV risk factors of the potential cardiac risk of sexual activity. Inform that concomitant use w/ α-blockers may lower BP significantly, leading to symptomatic hypotension; advise of the possible occurrence of symptoms related to postural hypotension and appropriate countermeasures. Discuss the appropriate use and anticipated benefits of therapy. Explain that sexual stimulation is required for an erection to occur after taking the drug. Instruct to contact physician if not satisfied w/ the quality of sexual performance or in the case of an unwanted effect. Instruct to seek immediate medical assistance if an erection persists >4 hrs. Instruct to d/c treatment and seek medical attention in the event of sudden loss of vision in 1 or both eyes; inform of the increased risk of NAION w/ history of NAION in 1 eye or w/ a "crowded" optic disc. Instruct to d/c treatment and seek prompt medical attention in the event of sudden decrease or loss of hearing. Inform that drug does not protect against STDs; advise to consider protective measures necessary to guard against STDs, including HIV. Advise to examine blister pack before use and not to use if blisters are torn, broken, or missing.

STELARA — ustekinumab   Rx
Class: Monoclonal antibody/interleukin-12 (IL-12) and IL-23 antagonist

ADULT DOSAGE	PEDIATRIC DOSAGE
Psoriasis	Pediatric use may not have been established

ADULT DOSAGE

Psoriasis

Patients w/ Moderate to Severe Plaque Psoriasis who are Candidates for Phototherapy or Systemic Therapy:
≤100kg (≤220 lbs): 45mg initially and 4 weeks later, followed by 45mg every 12 weeks
>100kg (>220 lbs): 90mg initially and 4 weeks later, followed by 90mg every 12 weeks

Psoriatic Arthritis

Active:
45mg initially and 4 weeks later, followed by 45mg every 12 weeks

Coexistent Moderate to Severe Plaque Psoriasis:
>100kg (>220 lbs): 90mg initially and 4 weeks later, followed by 90mg every 12 weeks

Can be used alone or in combination w/ methotrexate

PEDIATRIC DOSAGE
Pediatric use may not have been established

ADMINISTRATION
SQ route

Administer each inj at a different anatomic location (eg, upper arms, gluteal regions, thighs, any quadrant of abdomen) than the previous inj; do not administer into areas where the skin is tender, bruised, erythematous, or indurated. When using the single-use vial, a 27-gauge, 1/2-inch needle is recommended.

Administration Instructions
1. To prevent premature activation of the needle safety guard, do not touch the needle guard activation clips at any time during use.
2. Hold body and remove needle cover; do not hold plunger or plunger head while removing needle cover and do not use prefilled syringe if it is dropped w/o needle cover in place.
3. Inject SQ as recommended; inject all of the medication by pushing in plunger until plunger head is completely between needle guard wings; inj of entire prefilled syringe contents is necessary to activate needle guard.
4. After injection, maintain pressure on plunger head and remove needle from skin.
5. Slowly take your thumb off plunger head to allow empty syringe to move up until entire needle is covered by needle guard; discard used syringes in puncture-resistant container.

STORAGE
2-8°C (36-46°F). Store vials upright. Protect from light. Do not freeze or shake.

HOW SUPPLIED
Inj: 45mg/0.5mL, 90mg/mL [prefilled syringe, vial]

CONTRAINDICATIONS
Clinically significant hypersensitivity to ustekinumab or to any of the excipients.

WARNINGS/PRECAUTIONS
Serious bacterial, fungal, and viral infections, and infections requiring hospitalization reported. Do not give to patients with any clinically important active infection or until infection resolves or is adequately treated. Caution with chronic infection or a history of recurrent infection. Individuals genetically deficient in interleukin (IL)-12/IL-23 are particularly vulnerable to disseminated infections from mycobacteria (eg, nontuberculous, environmental mycobacteria), salmonella (eg, nontyphi strains), and Bacillus Calmette-Guerin (BCG) vaccinations; consider appropriate diagnostic testing. Evaluate for tuberculosis (TB) infection prior to, during, and after treatment; do not administer to patients with active TB. Consider anti-TB therapy prior to initiation in patients with history of latent or active TB when an adequate course of treatment cannot be confirmed. Rapid appearance of multiple cutaneous squamous cell carcinomas reported in patients who had preexisting risk factors for developing non-melanoma skin cancer; closely monitor patients with history of prolonged immunosuppressant therapy, history of PUVA treatment, and patients >60 yrs of age. Hypersensitivity reactions (eg, anaphylaxis, angioedema) reported; institute appropriate therapy and d/c. Reversible posterior leukoencephalopathy syndrome (RPLS) reported; administer appropriate treatment and d/c if suspected. Prior to initiating therapy, patients should receive all immunizations appropriate for age as recommended by current immunization guidelines. Needle cover on prefilled syringe contains dry natural rubber and should not be handled by latex-sensitive individuals. Should only be given to patients who will be closely monitored and have regular follow-up visits with a physician.

ADVERSE REACTIONS
Infection, nasopharyngitis, upper respiratory tract infection, headache, fatigue, arthralgia, nausea.

DRUG INTERACTIONS
Do not give with live vaccines; caution when administering live vaccines to household contacts of patients receiving ustekinumab. BCG vaccines should not be given during, for 1 yr prior to initiating, or 1 yr following discontinuation of treatment. Non-live vaccinations received during course of therapy may not elicit an immune response sufficient to prevent disease. Consider monitoring for therapeutic effect (eg, for warfarin) or drug concentration (eg, for cyclosporine) with concomitant CYP450 substrates, particularly those with a narrow therapeutic index; adjust individual dose prn. May decrease protective effect of allergen immunotherapy (decrease tolerance), which may increase the risk of an allergic reaction to a dose of allergen immunotherapy; caution in patients receiving or who have received allergen immunotherapy.

PREGNANCY AND LACTATION
Pregnancy: Category B.
Lactation: Caution in nursing.

MECHANISM OF ACTION
Monoclonal antibody; binds with specificity to the shared p40 protein subunit used by both the IL-12 and IL-23 cytokines.

PHARMACOKINETICS
Absorption: (Psoriasis) T_{max}=13.5 days (median, 45mg), 7 days (median, 90mg). **Distribution:** (Psoriasis) V_d=161mL/kg (45mg), 179mL/kg (90mg); found in breast milk. **Elimination:** (Psoriasis) $T_{1/2}$=14.9-45.6 days.

PATIENT CONSIDERATIONS
Assessment: Assess for drug hypersensitivity, active/chronic/serious infections, history of recurrent infection, IL-12/IL-23 genetic deficiency, TB, immunization history, pregnancy/nursing status, and possible drug interactions.

Monitoring: Monitor for signs/symptoms of infection, appearance of non-melanoma skin cancer, TB during and after treatment, malignancies, hypersensitivity reactions, RPLS, and other adverse reactions.

Counseling: Advise that therapy may lower the ability of the immune system to fight infections. Inform of the importance of communicating any history of infections to physician and instruct to contact physician if any signs/symptoms of infection develop. Counsel about the risk of malignancies while on therapy. Advise to seek immediate medical attention if experiencing any symptoms of a serious allergic reaction. Inform of inj techniques and procedures. Advise not to reuse needles/syringes and instruct on proper disposal procedures.

STENDRA — avanafil   Rx

Class: Phosphodiesterase-5 (PDE-5) inhibitor

ADULT DOSAGE

Erectile Dysfunction

Initial: 100mg prn, as early as 15 min before sexual activity

Titrate: May increase to 200mg as early as 15 min before, or decrease to 50mg 30 min before sexual activity, based on individual efficacy and tolerability

Max Dosing Frequency: qd

Use lowest effective dose. Sexual stimulation is required for response to treatment

PEDIATRIC DOSAGE

Pediatric use may not have been established

DOSING CONSIDERATIONS

Concomitant Medications

α-Blocker:
Initial: 50mg

Moderate CYP3A4 Inhibitors (eg, Erythromycin, Amprenavir, Diltiazem):
Max: 50mg/24 hrs

Strong CYP3A4 Inhibitors (eg, Ketoconazole, Ritonavir, Atazanavir):
Do not use

ADMINISTRATION

Oral route

Take w/ or w/o food.

STORAGE

20-25°C (68-77°F); excursions permitted to 30°C (86°F). Protect from light.

HOW SUPPLIED

Tab: 50mg, 100mg, 200mg

CONTRAINDICATIONS

Concomitant use (regularly and/or intermittently) w/ organic nitrates. Known hypersensitivity to any component of the tablet. Do not use in patients who are using a guanylate cyclase stimulator (eg, riociguat).

WARNINGS/PRECAUTIONS

In a patient who has taken avanafil, where nitrate administration is necessary, allow at least 12 hrs to elapse after the last dose of therapy before considering nitrate administration; only administer under close medical supervision w/ appropriate hemodynamic monitoring. Potential for cardiac risk during sexual activity in patients w/ preexisting cardiovascular (CV) disease; avoid if sexual activity is inadvisable due to underlying CV status. Patients w/ left ventricular outflow obstruction (eg, aortic stenosis, idiopathic hypertrophic subaortic stenosis) and those w/ severely impaired autonomic control of BP may be sensitive to therapy. Not recommended in patients w/ MI, stroke, life-threatening arrhythmia, or coronary revascularization w/in the last 6 months; resting hypotension (BP <90/50mmHg) or HTN (BP >170/100mmHg), or unstable angina, angina w/ sexual intercourse, or NYHA Class 2 or greater CHF. Has vasodilatory properties resulting in transient decreases in sitting BP. Prolonged erection >4 hrs and priapism may occur; caution w/ anatomical deformation of the penis (eg, angulation, cavernosal fibrosis, Peyronie's disease), or conditions that may predispose to priapism (eg, sickle cell anemia, multiple myeloma, leukemia). Nonarteritic anterior ischemic optic neuropathy (NAION) reported (rare); d/c if sudden loss of vision in 1 or both eyes occurs. Caution w/ underlying NAION risk factors; increased risk w/ previous history of NAION and in individuals w/ "crowded" optic disc. Sudden decrease or loss of hearing that may be accompanied by tinnitus or dizziness reported; d/c if this occurs. Avoid in patients w/ severe renal disease, on renal dialysis, or w/ severe hepatic disease.

ADVERSE REACTIONS

Headache, flushing, nasopharyngitis, nasal congestion, back pain, URI, ECG abnormal.

DRUG INTERACTIONS

See Contraindications and Dosage. Not recommended w/ other PDE-5 inhibitors or ED therapy combinations. Not recommended w/ CYP inducers. Caution w/ α-blockers; may augment BP-lowering effect of α-blockers and other antihypertensives. May increase BP-lowering effect of each compound w/ concomitant alcohol use and the risk of orthostatic signs/symptoms w/ substantial alcohol consumption. Do not use w/ strong CYP3A4 inhibitors (eg, ketoconazole, ritonavir, clarithromycin, nefazodone). Increased levels w/ strong, moderate, and likely w/ other CYP3A4 inhibitors (eg, grapefruit juice). May increase levels of desipramine or omeprazole. May affect rosiglitazone levels. Amlodipine may increase levels and prolong $T_{1/2}$. May decrease amlodipine levels. May potentiate the antiaggregatory effect of sodium nitroprusside.

PREGNANCY AND LACTATION

Pregnancy: Category C.
Lactation: Safety not known in nursing.

MECHANISM OF ACTION

PDE-5 inhibitor; enhances effect of nitric oxide, which activates the enzyme guanylate cyclase resulting in increased levels of cGMP, producing smooth muscle relaxation in the corpus cavernosum and allowing inflow of blood.

PHARMACOKINETICS

Absorption: Rapid; (fasted) T_{max}=30-45 min (median). **Distribution:** Plasma protein binding (99%). **Metabolism:** Liver (extensive); CYP3A4 (major), CYP2C (minor); M4 and M16 (major circulating metabolites). **Elimination:** Feces (62% metabolites), urine (21% metabolites); $T_{1/2}$=5 hrs.

PATIENT CONSIDERATIONS

Assessment: Assess for hypersensitivity to the drug, CV disease, left ventricular outflow obstruction, anatomical deformation of the penis, conditions that predispose to priapism, potential underlying causes of ED, risk for NAION, renal/hepatic impairment, any other conditions where treatment is contraindicated/cautioned, and possible drug interactions. Obtain baseline BP.

Monitoring: Monitor for hypersensitivity reactions, CV risk, priapism, changes in vision/hearing, and other adverse reactions.

Counseling: Instruct to take ud and explain that sexual stimulation is required for an erection to occur. Inform about the contraindication of avanafil w/ regular and/or intermittent use of organic nitrates; instruct patients who experience anginal chest pain after taking medication to seek immediate medical attention. Inform patients w/ preexisting CV risk factors of the potential cardiac risk of sexual activity; advise patients who experience symptoms upon initiation of sexual activity to refrain from further sexual activity and seek immediate medical attention. Advise to contact prescribing physician if new medications that may interact w/ therapy are prescribed by another healthcare provider. Instruct to seek emergency medical attention if erection persists >4 hrs; inform that priapism, if not treated promptly, may result in irreversible erectile tissue damage. Inform of the increased risk of NAION w/ history of NAION in 1 eye and in patients w/ a "crowded" optic disc. Instruct to d/c and seek medical attention in the event of sudden loss of vision in 1 or both eyes, or if a sudden decrease or loss of hearing that may be accompanied by tinnitus and dizziness occurs. Inform that substantial alcohol consumption (eg, >3 units) in combination w/ medication may increase the potential for orthostatic signs/symptoms. Inform that drug does not protect against STDs; counsel about protective measures necessary to guard against STDs, including HIV. Inform about the contraindication of avanafil w/ the use of guanylate cyclase stimulators.

STIOLTO RESPIMAT — olodaterol/tiotropium bromide   Rx

Class: Anticholinergic/long-acting beta₂ agonist (LABA)

> **Long-acting β₂-adrenergic agonists (LABAs)** increase the risk of asthma-related death. Not indicated for the treatment of asthma.

ADULT DOSAGE

Chronic Obstructive Pulmonary Disease

Long-Term Maint Treatment of Airflow Obstruction:
Recommended: 2 inh qd at the same time of day
Max: 2 inh/24 hrs

PEDIATRIC DOSAGE

Pediatric use may not have been established

ADMINISTRATION

Oral inh route

Insert cartridge into inhaler and prime the unit prior to 1st use.

Priming Instructions
1. Actuate the inhaler toward the ground until the aerosol cloud is visible.
2. Repeat 3 more times.

If not used for >3 days, actuate inhaler once to prepare for use.
If not used for >21 days, repeat priming instructions.

STORAGE

25°C (77°F); excursions permitted to 15-30°C (59-86°F). Avoid freezing.

HOW SUPPLIED

Spray, Inh: (Tiotropium/Olodaterol) (2.5mcg/2.5mcg)/actuation [60 actuations]

CONTRAINDICATIONS

Hypersensitivity to tiotropium, ipratropium, olodaterol, or any component of this product. **Olodaterol:** Asthma w/o use of a long-term asthma control medication.

WARNINGS/PRECAUTIONS

Do not initiate in acutely deteriorating COPD patients or use for the relief of acute symptoms. D/C regular use of inhaled short-acting β₂-agonists (SABAs) when beginning treatment; use only for symptomatic relief of acute respiratory symptoms. Immediate hypersensitivity reactions (eg, angioedema, anaphylaxis) may occur; d/c therapy immediately and consider alternative treatment. May produce paradoxical bronchospasm; d/c therapy immediately and institute alternative therapy. Should be used w/ caution in patients w/ narrow-angle glaucoma and urinary retention. **Tiotropium:** Patients w/ moderate to severe renal impairment (CrCl <60mL/min) should be monitored closely for anticholinergic side effects. **Olodaterol:** Do not use more often or at higher doses than recommended; clinically significant cardiovascular (CV) effects and fatalities reported w/ excessive use. CV effects may occur; may need to d/c if such effects occur. Caution w/ CV disorders, convulsive disorders, thyrotoxicosis, and in patients unusually responsive to sympathomimetic amines. Doses of the related β₂-agonist albuterol, administered intravenously, have been reported to aggravate preexisting diabetes mellitus (DM) and ketoacidosis. May produce significant hypokalemia and increases in plasma glucose.

ADVERSE REACTIONS

COPD exacerbation, pneumonia, nasopharyngitis, cough, back pain.

DRUG INTERACTIONS

Tiotropium: Avoid w/ other anticholinergic-containing drugs. **Olodaterol:** Do not use w/ other medications containing LABAs. Adrenergic drugs may potentiate sympathetic effects; use w/ caution. Xanthine derivatives, steroids, or diuretics may potentiate any hypokalemic effect. Caution w/ non-K⁺-sparing diuretics (eg, loop or thiazide diuretics). Extreme caution w/ MAOIs, TCAs, or other drugs known to prolong the QTc interval; action on CV system may be potentiated. Drugs known to prolong the QTc interval may be associated w/ an increased risk of ventricular arrhythmias. β-blockers and olodaterol may interfere w/ the effect of each other when administered concurrently. β-blockers may block therapeutic effects and produce severe bronchospasm in COPD patients; if such therapy is needed, consider cardioselective β-blockers and use w/ caution. Ketoconazole (a strong dual CYP and P-gp inhibitor) may increase levels.

PREGNANCY AND LACTATION
Pregnancy: Category C.
Lactation: It is not known whether tiotropium and olodaterol are excreted in human milk. Caution in nursing.

MECHANISM OF ACTION
Tiotropium: Anticholinergic; exhibits effects through inhibition of M_3-receptors at the smooth muscle, leading to bronchodilation. **Olodaterol:** LABA; binds and activates β_2-adrenoceptors. Activation of these receptors in the airways results in a stimulation of intracellular adenyl cyclase, an enzyme that mediates the synthesis of cAMP. Elevated levels of cAMP induce bronchodilation by relaxation of airway smooth muscle cells.

PHARMACOKINETICS
Absorption: Tiotropium: (Oral Sol) Absolute bioavailability (2-3%). T_{max}=5-7 min. Olodaterol: Absolute bioavailability (approx 30%); T_{max}=10-20 min. **Distribution:** Tiotropium: V_d=32L/kg; plasma protein binding (72%). Olodaterol: V_d=1110L; plasma protein binding (approx 60%). **Metabolism:** Tiotropium: Liver (oxidation, conjugation) via CYP2D6 and 3A4. Olodaterol: Direct glucuronidation via UGT2B7, UGT1A1, 1A7, and 1A9; O-demethylation via CYP2C9, CYP2C8, and CYP3A4 (negligible). **Elimination:** Tiotropium: Urine (18.6%); $T_{1/2}$=approx 25 hrs. Olodaterol: Urine (5-7%, unchanged); $T_{1/2}$=7.5 hrs (effective), 45 hrs (terminal).

PATIENT CONSIDERATIONS

Assessment: Assess for hypersensitivity to tiotropium, ipratropium, olodaterol, or any component of the product. Assess for asthma, acutely deteriorating COPD, CV disorders, convulsive disorders, thyrotoxicosis, DM, ketoacidosis, narrow-angle glaucoma, urinary retention, renal impairment, pregnancy/nursing status, and possible drug interactions. Evaluate use in patients unusually responsive to sympathomimetic amines.

Monitoring: Monitor for deteriorating COPD, paradoxical bronchospasm, CV effects, hypokalemia, hyperglycemia, immediate hypersensitivity reactions, and other adverse reactions.

Counseling: Counsel about the risks and benefits of therapy. Inform that drug is not for treatment of asthma. Advise not to use to relieve acute symptoms; inform that acute symptoms should be treated w/ an inhaled SABA. Instruct to notify physician immediately if experiencing worsening of symptoms, decreasing effectiveness of inhaled SABA, a need for more inhalations than usual of inhaled SABA, or a significant decrease in lung function. Advise not to stop therapy w/o physician guidance since symptoms may recur after discontinuation. Advise not to use additional medications containing LABAs. Inform of adverse effects associated w/ therapy. Advise to d/c therapy if paradoxical bronchospasm occurs. Instruct to consult physician immediately if signs/symptoms of new/worsening prostatic hyperplasia, bladder outlet obstruction, or acute narrow-angle glaucoma develops. Inform that care must be taken not to allow the aerosol cloud enter into the eyes as this may cause blurring of vision and pupil dilation. Caution patients about engaging in activities such as driving a vehicle or operating machinery, since dizziness and blurred vision may occur w/ use of therapy.

STIVARGA — regorafenib   Rx
Class: Kinase inhibitor

> Severe and sometimes fatal hepatotoxicity reported. Monitor hepatic function prior to and during treatment. Interrupt and then reduce or d/c treatment for hepatotoxicity as manifested by elevated LFTs or hepatocellular necrosis, depending upon severity and persistence.

ADULT DOSAGE
Metastatic Colorectal Cancer

Previously treated w/ fluoropyrimidine-, oxaliplatin-, and irinotecan-based chemotherapy, an antivascular endothelial growth factor therapy, and, if RAS wild-type, an anti-epidermal growth factor receptor therapy.

160mg qd for the first 21 days of each 28-day cycle until disease progression or unacceptable toxicity

Locally Advanced, Unresectable or Metastatic Gastrointestinal Stromal Tumor

Previously treated w/ imatinib mesylate and sunitinib malate.

160mg qd for the first 21 days of each 28-day cycle until disease progression or unacceptable toxicity

PEDIATRIC DOSAGE
Pediatric use may not have been established

DOSING CONSIDERATIONS
Renal Impairment
Mild (CrCl 60-89mL/min): No dose adjustment recommended
Moderate (CrCl 30-59mL/min): Limited pharmacokinetic data available
Severe or ESRD: Has not been studied
Hepatic Impairment
Severe (Child-Pugh Class C): Not recommended
Adverse Reactions
Interrupt For:
- Grade 2 hand-foot skin reaction (HFSR) that is recurrent or does not improve w/ in 7 days despite dose reduction; interrupt therapy for a minimum of 7 days for Grade 3 HFSR
- Symptomatic Grade 2 HTN
- Any Grade 3 or 4 adverse reaction
Reduce to 120mg:
- For the 1st occurrence of Grade 2 HFSR of any duration
- After recovery of any Grade 3 or 4 adverse reaction
- For Grade 3 AST/ALT elevation; only resume if the potential benefit outweighs the risk of hepatotoxicity
Reduce to 80mg:
- For reoccurrence of Grade 2 HFSR at the 120mg dose
- After recovery of any Grade 3 or 4 adverse reaction at the 120mg dose (except hepatotoxicity)
Discontinue For:
- Failure to tolerate 80mg dose
- Any occurrence of AST or ALT >20X ULN
- Any occurrence of AST or ALT >3X ULN w/ concurrent bilirubin >2X ULN
- Reoccurrence of AST or ALT >5X ULN despite dose reduction to 120mg
- For any Grade 4 adverse reaction; only resume if the potential benefit outweighs the risks
Other Important Considerations
A higher incidence of HFSR and LFT abnormalities occurred in Asian patients as compared w/ White patients

ADMINISTRATION
Oral route
Take at the same time each day.
Swallow tab whole w/ water after a low-fat meal that contains <600 calories and <30% fat.
Do not take 2 doses of therapy on the same day to make up for a missed dose from the previous day.

STORAGE
25°C (77°F); excursions permitted to 15-30°C (59-86°F). Store tabs in original bottle and do not remove the desiccant. Keep the bottle tightly closed after 1st opening. Discard any unused tabs 7 weeks after opening the bottle.

HOW SUPPLIED
Tab: 40mg

WARNINGS/PRECAUTIONS
See Dosing Considerations. Increased incidence of hemorrhage reported. Increased incidence of adverse reactions involving the skin and SQ tissues (eg, HFSR, toxic epidermal necrolysis, severe rash). Increased incidence of HTN reported. Avoid initiation unless BP is adequately controlled. Increased incidence of myocardial ischemia and infarction; withhold if new or acute onset cardiac ischemia or infarction develops. Resume treatment only after resolution of acute cardiac ischemic events, if benefits outweigh risks of further cardiac ischemia. Reversible posterior leukoencephalopathy syndrome (RPLS) reported; perform evaluation for RPLS in any patient presenting w/ seizures, headache, visual disturbances, confusion, or altered mental function. D/C if RPLS develops. GI perforation or fistula reported; permanently d/c if GI perforation or fistula develops. May impair wound healing; d/c at least 2 weeks prior to scheduled surgery. D/C in patients w/ wound dehiscence. May cause fetal harm.

ADVERSE REACTIONS
Asthenia/fatigue, HFSR, diarrhea, decreased appetite/food intake, HTN, mucositis, dysphonia, infection, pain, decreased weight, GI and abdominal pain, rash, fever, nausea.

DRUG INTERACTIONS
Decreased mean exposure of regorafenib and increased mean exposure of active metabolite M-5 w/ coadministration of rifampin. Increased mean exposure of regorafenib and decreased mean exposure of active metabolites M-2 and M-5 w/ coadministration of ketoconazole. Avoid w/ strong CYP3A4 inducers (eg, rifampin, phenytoin, carbamazepine) and strong CYP3A4 inhibitors (eg, clarithromycin, grapefruit juice, itraconazole). Monitor INR levels more frequently in patients receiving warfarin.

PREGNANCY AND LACTATION
Pregnancy: Based on animal studies and mechanism of action, can cause fetal harm.
Lactation: Do not breastfeed during treatment and for 2 weeks after the final dose.
Reproductive Potential: Females and male patients w/ female partners of reproductive potential should use effective contraception during treatment and for 2 months after the final dose.

MECHANISM OF ACTION
Multikinase inhibitor; inhibits multiple membrane-bound and intracellular kinases involved in normal cellular functions and in pathologic processes, such as oncogenesis, tumor angiogenesis, and maintenance of the tumor microenvironment.

PHARMACOKINETICS

Absorption: (Single 160mg dose) C_{max}=2.5mcg/mL, T_{max}=4 hrs (median), AUC=70.4mcg•hr/mL. (Steady state) C_{max}=3.9mcg/mL, AUC=58.3mcg•hr/mL. **Distribution:** Plasma protein binding (99.5%). **Metabolism:** CYP3A4, UGT1A9; M-2 (N-oxide) and M-5 (N-oxide and N-desmethyl) (active metabolites). **Elimination:** Urine (19%; 17% glucuronides), feces (approx 71%; 47% parent compound, 24% metabolites); $T_{1/2}$=28 hrs (regorafenib), 25 hrs (M-2), 51 hrs (M-5).

PATIENT CONSIDERATIONS

Assessment: Assess for scheduled/recent surgical procedures, hepatic impairment, HTN, pregnancy/nursing status, and possible drug interactions. Obtain baseline LFTs (ALT, AST, and bilirubin).

Monitoring: Monitor for hepatotoxicity, hemorrhage, dermatologic toxicity, HTN, myocardial ischemia or infarction, RPLS, wound dehiscence, GI perforation or fistula, and other adverse reactions. Monitor BP weekly for the first 6 weeks of treatment and then every cycle, or more frequently, as clinically indicated. Monitor LFTs at least every 2 weeks during the first 2 months of treatment, then monthly or more frequently as clinically indicated; monitor weekly in patients experiencing elevated LFTs until improvement to <3X ULN or baseline. Monitor INR levels more frequently in patients receiving warfarin.

Counseling: Advise to take ud. Advise of the need to undergo monitoring for liver damage and to report immediately any signs/symptoms of severe liver damage. Advise to contact physician for unusual bleeding, bruising, or symptoms of bleeding (such as lightheadedness). Advise to contact physician if experiencing skin changes associated w/ redness, pain, blisters, bleeding or swelling. Advise of the need to undergo BP monitoring and to contact physician if BP is elevated or if symptoms from HTN occur (including severe headache, lightheadedness, or neurologic symptoms). Advise to seek immediate emergency help if experiencing chest pain, SOB, feeling dizzy, or feel like passing out. Advise to contact physician if experiencing signs/symptoms of RPLS. Advise to contact physician immediately if experiencing severe pains in abdomen, persistent swelling of abdomen, high fever, chills, N/V, or dehydration. Advise to contact physician if planning to undergo surgical procedure or had recent surgery. Advise that drug can cause fetal harm and to use effective contraception during treatment and for 2 months after completion of treatment. Instruct women of reproductive potential to immediately contact physician if pregnancy is suspected or confirmed during or w/in 2 months of completing treatment. Advise nursing mothers that it is not known whether drug is present in breast milk.

STRATTERA — atomoxetine   Rx

Class: Selective norepinephrine reuptake inhibitor

> Increased risk of suicidal ideation in short-term studies in children or adolescents with attention-deficit hyperactivity disorder (ADHD); balance this risk with the clinical need. Closely monitor for suicidality (suicidal thinking and behavior), clinical worsening, or unusual changes in behavior. Not approved for major depressive disorder.

ADULT DOSAGE
Attention-Deficit Hyperactivity Disorder

Initial: 40mg/day
Titrate: Increase after a minimum of 3 days to target dose of approx 80mg/day; may increase after 2-4 additional weeks if optimal response is not achieved
Max: 100mg/day

Periodically reevaluate long-term usefulness

May d/c w/o tapering

PEDIATRIC DOSAGE
Attention-Deficit Hyperactivity Disorder

≤70kg:
Initial: 0.5mg/kg/day
Titrate: Increase after a minimum of 3 days to target dose of approx 1.2mg/kg/day
Max: 1.4mg/kg/day or 100mg/day, whichever is less

>70kg:
Initial: 40mg/day
Titrate: Increase after a minimum of 3 days to target dose of approx 80mg/day; may increase after 2-4 additional weeks if optimal response is not achieved
Max: 100mg/day

Periodically reevaluate long-term usefulness

May d/c w/o tapering

DOSING CONSIDERATIONS
Concomitant Medications
Strong CYP2D6 Inhibitors:
<70kg:
Initial: 0.5mg/kg/day
Titrate: Only increase to target dose of 1.2mg/kg/day if symptoms fail to improve after 4 weeks and initial dose is well tolerated

>70kg or Adults:
Initial: 40mg/day
Titrate: Only increase to target dose of 80mg/day if symptoms fail to improve after 4 weeks and initial dose is well tolerated

Hepatic Impairment
Moderate Impairment (Child-Pugh Class B):
Initial/Target: Reduce to 50% of normal dose

Severe Impairment (Child-Pugh Class C):
Initial/Target: Reduce to 25% of normal dose

Other Important Considerations
CYP2D6 Poor Metabolizers:
Initial: 0.5mg/kg/day
Titrate: Only increase to target dose of 1.2mg/kg/day if symptoms fail to improve after 4 weeks and initial dose is well tolerated

ADMINISTRATION
Oral route

Take whole, w/ or w/o food; do not open cap.
Take as a single dose in the am or as evenly divided doses in the am and late afternoon/early pm.

STORAGE
25°C (77°F); excursions permitted to 15-30°C (59-86°F).

HOW SUPPLIED
Cap: 10mg, 18mg, 25mg, 40mg, 60mg, 80mg, 100mg

CONTRAINDICATIONS
Narrow-angle glaucoma, presence/history of pheochromocytoma, and severe cardiac/vascular disorders that would deteriorate w/ increases in BP/HR that would be clinically important (eg, 15-20mmHg in BP or 20 bpm in HR). Use of an MAOI either concomitantly or w/in 2 weeks of stopping treatment. Treatment w/ in 2 weeks of stopping an MAOI. Known hypersensitivity to atomoxetine or other constituents of the product.

WARNINGS/PRECAUTIONS
May cause severe liver injury; d/c in patients with jaundice or lab evidence of liver injury, and do not restart therapy. Perform LFTs upon the 1st sign/symptom of liver dysfunction. Sudden death reported in children and adolescents with structural cardiac abnormalities or other serious heart problems. Sudden death, stroke, and MI reported in adults. Avoid in patients with known serious structural cardiac abnormalities, cardiomyopathy, serious heart rhythm abnormalities, coronary artery disease, or other serious cardiac problems. Promptly perform cardiac evaluation if symptoms suggestive of cardiac disease develop. May increase BP/HR; caution in patients whose underlying medical conditions could be worsened by increases in BP or HR. Orthostatic hypotension and syncope reported; caution with conditions predisposing to hypotension, or conditions associated with abrupt HR/BP changes. Caution in patients with comorbid bipolar disorder; may induce mixed/manic episode. May cause treatment-emergent psychotic or manic symptoms in children/adolescents without prior history of psychotic illness or mania; consider discontinuation if such symptoms occur. Monitor for appearance/worsening of aggressive behavior or hostility. Allergic reactions and priapism reported. May cause urinary retention/hesitation. Monitor growth in children.

ADVERSE REACTIONS
Abdominal pain, N/V, fatigue, decreased appetite, somnolence, headache, dry mouth, dizziness, insomnia, constipation, urinary hesitation, erectile dysfunction, irritability, weight decreased, hyperhidrosis.

DRUG INTERACTIONS
See Contraindications. Caution with systemically administered albuterol or other β_2 agonists; may potentiate cardiovascular (CV) effects of albuterol. Caution with antihypertensive drugs and pressor agents (eg, dopamine, dobutamine) or other drugs that increase BP. CYP2D6 inhibitors (eg, paroxetine, fluoxetine, quinidine) increase levels in extensive metabolizers (EMs).

PREGNANCY AND LACTATION
Pregnancy: Category C.
Lactation: Caution in nursing.

MECHANISM OF ACTION
Selective norepinephrine reuptake inhibitor; not established. May selectively inhibit the presynaptic norepinephrine transporter.

PHARMACOKINETICS
Absorption: Rapid; well-absorbed; absolute bioavailability (63% [EMs], 94% [PMs]); T_{max}=1-2 hrs. **Distribution:** V_d=0.85L/kg (IV); plasma protein binding (98%). **Metabolism:** Via CYP2D6; 4-hydroxyatomoxetine (major active metabolite), N-desmethylatomoxetine. **Elimination:** $T_{1/2}$=5 hrs. 4-hydroxyatomoxetine-O-glucuronide: Urine (>80%), feces (<17%).

PATIENT CONSIDERATIONS

Assessment: Assess for hypersensitivity to drug, narrow-angle glaucoma, presence/history of pheochromocytoma, comorbid bipolar disorder, CV disorders, hepatic impairment, any other conditions where treatment is contraindicated or cautioned, pregnancy/nursing status, and possible drug interactions. Obtain baseline pulse and BP.

Monitoring: Monitor for signs/symptoms of CV events, liver injury, allergic reactions, emergence of psychosis/mania, suicidality, clinical worsening, aggressive or unusual changes in behavior, hostility, urinary retention/hesitation, priapism, and other adverse reactions. Monitor growth in children. Monitor pulse and BP following dose increases and periodically during therapy. Periodically reevaluate long-term usefulness.

Counseling: Inform about risks, benefits, and appropriate use of therapy. Encourage patients, families, and caregivers to be alert for the emergence of agitation, irritability, and unusual changes in behavior, as well as the emergence of suicidality, especially early during treatment and when dose is adjusted; advise to report such symptoms to physician, especially if severe, abrupt in onset, or not part of presenting symptoms. Advise to contact physician if symptoms of liver injury develop. Inform that priapism requires prompt medical attention. Inform that drug is an ocular irritant; if content of cap comes in contact with eye, instruct to immediately flush affected eye with water and obtain medical advice. Tell to notify physician if taking or planning to take any prescription or OTC medicines, dietary supplements, or herbal remedies. Instruct to notify physician if nursing, pregnant, or thinking of becoming pregnant. Advise to use caution when driving a car/operating hazardous machinery until reasonably certain that performance is not affected by therapy.

STRIANT — testosterone   CIII

Class: Androgen

ADULT DOSAGE

Testosterone Replacement Therapy

Congenital/Acquired Primary Hypogonadism or Hypogonadotropic Hypogonadism in Males:

Usual: Apply 1 buccal system (30mg) to the gum region bid; am and pm (about 12 hrs apart)

Measure am, predose serum testosterone concentrations at 4-12 weeks after initiation of therapy to ensure proper concentrations are achieved

PEDIATRIC DOSAGE

Pediatric use may not have been established

DOSING CONSIDERATIONS
Discontinuation
D/C therapy if serum testosterone concentrations are consistently outside of the normal range (300-1050ng/dL) despite the use of 1 buccal system applied bid

ADMINISTRATION
Buccal Route

Do not chew or swallow buccal system.
Place in a comfortable position just above the incisor tooth (on either side of the mouth); rotate to alternate sides of the mouth w/ each application.
Place the rounded side surface of the buccal system against the gum and hold firmly in place w/ a finger over the lip and against the product for 30 sec to ensure adhesion; if the system fails to properly adhere to the gum or should fall off during the 12-hr dosing interval, remove the old system and apply a new one. Check to see if tab is in place following consumption of food or beverages.

If Buccal System Falls Out of Position
W/in the First 8 Hrs of Dosing: Replace w/ a new system and continue for a total of 12 hrs from the placement of the 1st system
After 8 Hrs of Dosing: Apply a new buccal system; it may remain in place for 12 hrs, then continue w/ the next regularly scheduled dosing

Removal of Buccal System
Gently slide it downwards from the gum toward the tooth to avoid scratching the gum; remove before routine am and pm oral care is performed, followed by application of a new buccal system

STORAGE
20-25°C (68-77°F). Protect from heat and moisture.

HOW SUPPLIED
Tab, Buccal: 30mg [6 blister packs, 10 buccal systems/blister pack]

CONTRAINDICATIONS
Breast carcinoma or known/suspected prostate carcinoma in men, women who are or may become pregnant or who are breastfeeding.

WARNINGS/PRECAUTIONS
Gum-related adverse reactions reported. Patients w/ BPH may be at increased risk for worsening of signs/symptoms of BPH. May increase risk for prostate cancer. Increases in Hct/RBC mass may increase risk for thromboembolic events; lower dose or d/c therapy until Hct decreases to acceptable level. Venous thromboembolic events reported; d/c treatment and initiate appropriate workup and management if suspected. Increased risk of major adverse cardiovascular events (MACE) reported. Suppression of spermatogenesis may occur w/ large doses. Prolonged use of high doses of orally active 17-α-alkyl androgens has been associated w/ serious hepatic effects; promptly d/c while cause is evaluated if signs/symptoms of hepatic dysfunction develop. May promote retention of Na+ and water. Edema w/ or w/o CHF in patients w/ preexisting cardiac, renal, or hepatic disease may occur; may require diuretic therapy in addition to discontinuation of therapy. Gynecomastia may develop and persist. May potentiate sleep apnea. Changes in serum lipid profile may occur. Caution in cancer patients at risk of hypercalcemia and associated hypercalciuria. May decrease concentrations of thyroxine-binding globulins, resulting in decreased total T4 concentrations and increased resin uptake of T3 and T4.

ADVERSE REACTIONS
Gum/mouth irritation, bitter taste, gum pain/tenderness, headache.

DRUG INTERACTIONS
Changes in insulin sensitivity or glycemic control may occur; may decrease blood glucose and therefore may necessitate a decrease in the dose of antidiabetic medications. Changes in anticoagulant activity may occur; monitor more frequently the INR and PT in patients taking warfarin, especially at initiation and termination of androgen therapy. Corticosteroids may increase fluid retention; carefully monitor, especially in patients w/ cardiac, renal, or hepatic disease.

PREGNANCY AND LACTATION
Category X, not for use in nursing.

MECHANISM OF ACTION
Androgen; responsible for normal growth and development of male sex organs and maintenance of secondary sex characteristics.

PHARMACOKINETICS
Absorption: T_{max}=10-12 hrs. **Distribution:** Plasma protein binding (approx 40% sex hormone-binding globulin). **Metabolism:** Estradiol and dihydrotestosterone (major active metabolites). **Elimination:** (IM) Urine (90%), feces (6%); $T_{1/2}$=10-100 min.

PATIENT CONSIDERATIONS
Assessment: Assess for BPH, breast carcinoma, prostate cancer, cardiac/renal/hepatic disease, risk factors for sleep apnea, any other conditions where treatment is contraindicated or cautioned, and possible drug interactions. Obtain baseline Hct level, lipid levels, and serum testosterone level. Confirm diagnosis of hypogonadism by measuring testosterone levels in the am on at least 2 separate days prior to initiation.

Monitoring: Monitor for gum-related adverse reactions, prostate cancer, edema w/ or w/o CHF, gynecomastia, sleep apnea, venous thromboembolic events, worsening of BPH, and other adverse reactions. Monitor serum lipid profile, testosterone serum levels, and LFTs periodically. In cancer patients at risk for hypercalcemia, regularly monitor serum Ca^{2+} levels. Obtain Hct level 3-6 months after start of therapy, then annually.

Counseling: Inform that men w/ known or suspected prostate/breast cancer should not use this therapy. Advise patients to regularly inspect the gum region of the application site and to report any abnormality to physician. Inform about potential adverse reactions. Instruct on proper application of the buccal system. Inform of the possible risk of MACE when deciding to use or continue use of therapy.

STRIBILD — cobicistat/elvitegravir/emtricitabine/tenofovir disoproxil fumarate   Rx

Class: CYP3A inhibitor/HIV integrase strand transfer inhibitor/nucleoside reverse transcriptase inhibitor (NRTI) combination

> Lactic acidosis and severe hepatomegaly w/ steatosis, including fatal cases, reported w/ the use of nucleoside analogues in combination w/ other antiretrovirals. Not approved for the treatment of chronic hepatitis B virus (HBV) infection. Severe acute exacerbations of hepatitis B reported in patients coinfected w/ HBV and HIV-1 upon discontinuation of therapy; closely monitor hepatic function w/ both clinical and lab follow-up for at least several months. If appropriate, initiation of anti-hepatitis B therapy may be warranted.

ADULT DOSAGE
HIV-1 Infection

For use as a complete regimen for the treatment of HIV-1 infection in adults who have no antiretroviral treatment history or to replace the current antiretroviral regimen in those who are virologically-suppressed (HIV-1 RNA <50 copies/mL) on a stable antiretroviral regimen for at least 6 months w/ no history of treatment failure and no known substitutions associated w/ resistance to the individual components of the drug

1 tab qd

PEDIATRIC DOSAGE
Pediatric use may not have been established

DOSING CONSIDERATIONS
Renal Impairment
CrCl <70mL/min: Initiation of treatment not recommended
CrCl Declines <50mL/min During Treatment: D/C therapy

Hepatic Impairment
Severe (Child-Pugh Class C): Not recommended

ADMINISTRATION
Oral route

Take w/ food.

STORAGE
25°C (77°F); excursions permitted to 15-30°C (59-86°F).

HOW SUPPLIED
Tab: (Cobicistat/Elvitegravir/Emtricitabine/Tenofovir Disoproxil Fumarate [TDF]) 150mg/150mg/200mg/300mg

CONTRAINDICATIONS
Concomitant use w/ drugs that are highly dependent on CYP3A for clearance and for which elevated plasma concentrations are associated w/ serious and/or life-threatening events and w/ other drugs that may lead to reduced efficacy and possible resistance (e.g, alfuzosin, carbamazepine, phenobarbital, phenytoin, rifampin, dihydroergotamine, ergotamine, methylergonovine, cisapride, St. John's wort, lovastatin, simvastatin, pimozide, sildenafil [when dosed as Revatio for the treatment of pulmonary arterial HTN], triazolam, oral midazolam).

WARNINGS/PRECAUTIONS
Test for HBV infection and document estimated CrCl, urine glucose, and urine protein prior to initiation of therapy. Not recommended for use in patients w/ severe hepatic impairment. Renal impairment, including cases of acute renal failure and Fanconi syndrome, reported; d/c if estimated CrCl <50mL/min. Do not initiate therapy in patients w/ estimated CrCl <70mL/min. Immune reconstitution syndrome, autoimmune disorders (eg, Graves' disease, polymyositis, Guillain-Barre syndrome) in the setting of immune reconstitution, and redistribution/

accumulation of body fat reported. Caution in elderly. **Cobicistat:** May cause modest increases in SrCr and modest declines in estimated CrCl w/o affecting renal glomerular function; closely monitor patients w/ confirmed increase in SrCr >0.4mg/dL from baseline for renal safety. **TDF:** Obesity and prolonged nucleoside exposure may be risk factors for lactic acidosis and severe hepatomegaly. Caution w/ known risk factors for liver disease. D/C if lactic acidosis or pronounced hepatotoxicity occurs. Decreased bone mineral density (BMD), increased biochemical markers of bone metabolism, and osteomalacia reported. Consider hypophosphatemia and osteomalacia secondary to proximal renal tubulopathy in patients at risk of renal dysfunction who present w/ persistent/worsening bone or muscle symptoms.

ADVERSE REACTIONS
Diarrhea, nausea, fatigue, headache, dizziness, insomnia, abnormal dreams, rash, creatine kinase/amylase elevation, hematuria, AST elevation.

DRUG INTERACTIONS
See Contraindications. Avoid w/ cobicistat, elvitegravir, adefovir dipivoxil, rifabutin, rifapentine, salmeterol, ledipasvir/sofosbuvir, nephrotoxic agents (eg, high-dose or multiple NSAIDs), other antiretrovirals, or w/ products containing emtricitabine, TDF, lamivudine, or ritonavir. Avoid w/ colchicine in patients w/ renal or hepatic impairment. Antacids (eg, aluminum and magnesium hydroxide) may decrease elvitegravir levels; separate administration by at least 2 hrs. May increase levels of antiarrhythmics (eg, digoxin), clonazepam, ethosuximide, ketoconazole, itraconazole, voriconazole, colchicine, β-blockers, calcium channel blockers, inhaled or nasal fluticasone, bosentan, atorvastatin, immunosuppressants, salmeterol, neuroleptics, PDE-5 inhibitors, and sedative/hypnotics (eg, benzodiazepines). May increase levels of quetiapine; consider alternative antiretroviral therapy. Concomitant use w/ inhaled or nasal fluticasone may reduce serum cortisol concentrations. May increase norgestimate and decrease ethinyl estradiol levels; caution w/ contraceptives containing norgestimate/ethinyl estradiol. Consider alternative (nonhormonal) methods of contraception. May increase levels of buprenorphine and norbuprenorphine and may decrease levels of naloxone; monitor for sedation and cognitive effects upon coadministration w/ buprenorphine/naloxone. Monitor INR upon coadministration w/ warfarin. May increase levels of antidepressants (eg, SSRIs, TCAs, trazodone); carefully titrate antidepressant dose and monitor response. May increase levels of clarithromycin; reduce clarithromycin dose by 50% in patients w/ CrCl 50-60mL/min. Anticonvulsants (eg, oxcarbazepine, clonazepam, ethosuximide) may decrease elvitegravir and cobicistat levels; consider alternative anticonvulsants. Rifabutin, rifapentine, and dexamethasone may decrease elvitegravir and cobicistat levels. Ketoconazole, itraconazole, or voriconazole may increase levels of elvitegravir and cobicistat. May increase levels of drugs that are primarily metabolized by CYP3A/2D6, or are substrates of P-gp, breast cancer resistance protein, or organic anion transporting polypeptides 1B1/1B3. Elvitegravir may decrease levels of CYP2C9 substrates. CYP3A inducers may decrease elvitegravir and cobicistat levels and may result in loss of therapeutic effect and development of resistance. Drugs that reduce renal function or compete for active tubular secretion (eg, acyclovir, cidofovir, gentamicin) may increase levels of emtricitabine, TDF, and other renally eliminated drugs and may increase risk of adverse reactions. CYP3A inhibitors and clarithromycin may increase plasma levels of cobicistat. Cases of acute renal failure after initiation of high-dose or multiple NSAIDs reported in patients w/ risk factors for renal dysfunction who appeared stable on TDF; consider alternatives to NSAIDs, if needed, in patients at risk for renal dysfunction. Ledipasvir/sofosbuvir may increase tenofovir levels. Refer to PI for dosing modifications when used w/ certain concomitant therapies.

PREGNANCY AND LACTATION
Pregnancy: Category B. An antiretroviral pregnancy registry has been established to monitor fetal outcomes of pregnant women.
Lactation: Not for use in nursing.

MECHANISM OF ACTION
Elvitegravir: HIV-1 integrase strand inhibitor; inhibits the strand transfer activity of HIV-1 integrase, preventing the integration of HIV-1 DNA into host genomic DNA, blocking the formation of HIV-1 provirus and propagation of the viral infection.
Cobicistat: CYP3A inhibitor; enhances the systemic exposure of CYP3A substrates (eg, elvitegravir). **Emtricitabine:** Nucleoside analogue of cytidine; inhibits the activity of HIV-1 reverse transcriptase (RT) by competing w/ the natural substrate deoxycytidine 5'-triphosphate and by being incorporated into nascent viral DNA, resulting in chain termination. **TDF:** Acyclic nucleoside phosphonate diester analogue of adenosine monophosphate; inhibits the activity of HIV-1 RT by competing w/ the natural substrate deoxyadenosine 5'-triphosphate and, after incorporation into DNA, by DNA chain termination.

PHARMACOKINETICS
Absorption: Elvitegravir: C_{max}=1.7 ± 0.4mcg/mL, AUC=23 ± 7.5mcg•hr/mL, T_{max}=4 hrs. Cobicistat: C_{max}=1.1 ± 0.4mcg/mL, AUC=8.3 ± 3.8mcg•hr/mL, T_{max}=3 hrs. Emtricitabine: C_{max}=1.9 ± 0.5mcg/mL, AUC=12.7 ± 4.5mcg•hr/mL, T_{max}=3 hrs. TDF: C_{max}=0.45 ± 0.2mcg/mL, AUC=4.4 ± 2.2mcg•hr/mL, T_{max}=2 hrs. **Distribution:** Elvitegravir: Plasma protein binding (approx 99%). Cobicistat: Plasma protein binding (approx 98%). Emtricitabine: Plasma protein binding (<4%); found in breast milk. TDF: Plasma protein binding (<0.7%); found in breast milk. **Metabolism:** Elvitegravir: CYP3A (major), UGT1A1/3 (minor). Cobicistat: CYP3A (major), CYP2D6 (minor). **Elimination:** Elvitegravir: Feces (94.8%), urine (6.7%); $T_{1/2}$=12.9 hrs (median). Cobicistat: Feces (86.2%), urine (8.2%); $T_{1/2}$=3.5 hrs (median). Emtricitabine: Feces (13.7%), urine (70%); $T_{1/2}$=10 hrs (median). TDF: Urine (70-80%); $T_{1/2}$=12-18 hrs (median).

PATIENT CONSIDERATIONS
Assessment: Assess for obesity, prolonged nucleoside exposure, risk factors for liver disease, renal/hepatic impairment, pregnancy/nursing status, and possible drug interactions. Assess BMD in patients who have a history of pathological bone

fracture or w/ other risk factors for osteoporosis or bone loss. Obtain baseline estimated CrCl, urine glucose, and urine protein. Perform test for HBV infection prior to therapy.

Monitoring: Monitor for signs/symptoms of lactic acidosis, severe hepatomegaly w/ steatosis, new onset/worsening renal impairment, immune reconstitution syndrome, autoimmune disorders, fat redistribution/accumulation, increased biochemical markers for bone metabolism, osteomalacia, and other adverse reactions. Monitor for exacerbations of hepatitis B in patients w/ coinfection for at least several months upon discontinuation of therapy. Monitor BMD, estimated CrCl, urine glucose, and urine protein. Monitor serum phosphorus levels in patients at risk for renal impairment. Monitor INR upon coadministration w/ warfarin.

Counseling: Advise to remain under care of a physician during therapy. Inform that therapy does not cure HIV-1 infection and continuous therapy is necessary to control HIV-1 infection and decrease HIV-related illnesses. Advise to practice safe sex, to use latex or polyurethane condoms, not to share personal items (eg, toothbrush, razor blades), needles, or other inj equipment, and not to breastfeed. Instruct to take on a regular dosing schedule w/ food and to avoid missing doses. Instruct to contact physician if symptoms of lactic acidosis/pronounced hepatotoxicity, or any symptoms of infection occur. Advise that fat redistribution/accumulation, renal impairment, and decreases in BMD may occur. Inform that hepatitis B testing is recommended prior to initiating therapy. Advise to report use of any prescription or nonprescription medication or herbal products, including St. John's wort.

STRIVERDI RESPIMAT — olodaterol   **Rx**
Class: Long-acting beta₂ agonist (LABA)

> **Long-acting β₂-adrenergic agonists (LABAs) increase the risk of asthma-related death. Not indicated for the treatment of asthma.**

ADULT DOSAGE	PEDIATRIC DOSAGE
Chronic Obstructive Pulmonary Disease **Long-Term Maint Treatment of Airflow Obstruction:** **Maint:** 2 inh qd at the same time of day **Max:** 2 inh/24 hrs	Pediatric use may not have been established

DOSING CONSIDERATIONS
Hepatic Impairment
Mild and Moderate: No dosage adjustment is required
Severe: No data available

ADMINISTRATION
Oral inh route

Insert cartridge into inhaler and prime the unit prior to 1st use.

Priming Instructions
1. Actuate the inhaler toward the ground until an aerosol cloud is visible.
2. Repeat 3 more times.

If Not Used >3 Days: Actuate inhaler once to prepare for use.
If Not Used >21 Days: Repeat priming instructions.

STORAGE
25°C (77°F); excursions permitted to 15-30°C (59-86°F). Avoid freezing.

HOW SUPPLIED
Spray, Inh: 2.5mcg/actuation [60 actuations]

CONTRAINDICATIONS
Asthma w/o use of a long-term asthma control medication.

WARNINGS/PRECAUTIONS
Do not initiate in acutely deteriorating COPD patients or use for the relief of acute symptoms. D/C regular use of inhaled short-acting β₂-agonists (SABAs) when beginning treatment; use them only for symptomatic relief of acute respiratory symptoms. Do not use more often or at higher doses than recommended; clinically significant cardiovascular (CV) effects and fatalities reported w/ excessive use. May produce paradoxical bronchospasm; d/c therapy immediately and institute alternative therapy. CV effects may occur; therapy may need to be discontinued if such effects occur. Caution w/ CV disorders, convulsive disorders, thyrotoxicosis, diabetes mellitus (DM), ketoacidosis, and in patients unusually responsive to sympathomimetic amines. May produce significant hypokalemia and increases in plasma glucose. Immediate hypersensitivity reactions may occur; d/c therapy immediately and consider alternative treatment.

ADVERSE REACTIONS
Nasopharyngitis, URTI, bronchitis, cough, back pain.

DRUG INTERACTIONS
Do not use w/ other medications containing LABAs. Adrenergic drugs may potentiate sympathetic effects; use w/ caution. Xanthine derivatives, steroids, or diuretics may potentiate any hypokalemic effect. Caution is advised when coadministered w/ non-K⁺-sparing diuretics (eg, loop, thiazide). Extreme caution w/ MAOIs, TCAs, or other drugs known to prolong the QTc interval; action on CV system may be potentiated. Drugs known to prolong the QTc interval may be associated w/ an increased risk of ventricular arrhythmias. β-blockers and olodaterol may interfere w/ the effect of each other when administered concurrently. β-blockers may block therapeutic effects and produce severe bronchospasm in COPD patients; if such therapy is needed, consider cardioselective β-blockers and use w/ caution. Ketoconazole (a strong dual CYP and P-gp inhibitor) may increase levels.

PREGNANCY AND LACTATION
Pregnancy: Category C.
Lactation: Excretion into human milk is probable; caution in nursing.

MECHANISM OF ACTION
LABA; binds and activates β_2-adrenoceptors. Activation of these receptors in the airways results in a stimulation of intracellular adenyl cyclase, an enzyme that mediates the synthesis of cAMP. Elevated levels of cAMP induce bronchodilation by relaxation of airway smooth muscle cells.

PHARMACOKINETICS
Absorption: Absolute bioavailability (30%); T_{max}=10-20 min. **Distribution:** V_d=1110L; plasma protein binding (60%). **Metabolism:** Direct glucuronidation via UGT2B7, UGT1A1, 1A7, and 1A9; O-demethylation via CYP2C9, CYP2C8, and CYP3A4 (negligible). **Elimination:** Urine (5-7%, unchanged); $T_{1/2}$=7.5 hrs.

PATIENT CONSIDERATIONS
Assessment: Assess for asthma, acute COPD deteriorations, CV disorders, convulsive disorders, thyrotoxicosis, DM, ketoacidosis, pregnancy/nursing status, and possible drug interactions. Assess use in patients unusually responsive to sympathomimetic amines.

Monitoring: Monitor for deteriorating disease, paradoxical bronchospasm, CV effects, hypokalemia, hyperglycemia, immediate hypersensitivity reactions, and other adverse reactions.

Counseling: Counsel about the risks and benefits of therapy. Inform that drug is not for treatment of asthma. Advise not to use olodaterol to relieve acute symptoms; inform that acute symptoms should be treated w/ an inhaled SABA. Instruct to notify physician immediately if experiencing worsening of symptoms, decreasing effectiveness of inhaled SABA, a need for more inhalations than usual of inhaled SABA, or a significant decrease in lung function. Advise not to stop therapy w/o physician guidance, not to use additional LABA, and not to use more than the recommended once-daily dose. Instruct to d/c the regular use of inhaled SABAs when beginning treatment. Inform of adverse effects associated w/ therapy.

SUBOXONE — buprenorphine/naloxone   CIII

Class: Partial opioid agonist/opioid antagonist

ADULT DOSAGE

Opioid Dependence
Use as part of a complete treatment plan to include counseling and psychosocial support

Prior to Induction:
Consider type of opioid dependence (eg, long- or short-acting opioid products), the time since last opioid use, and degree or level of opioid dependence. The 1st dose of therapy should be started only when objective signs of moderate withdrawal appear

Induction:
Day 1:
Initial: 2mg/0.5mg or 4mg/1mg
Titrate: May titrate upwards in 2mg or 4mg increments of buprenorphine, at approx 2-hr intervals to 8mg/2mg based on the control of acute withdrawal symptoms. Induction dosage of up to 8mg/2mg is recommended

Day 2:
Up to 16mg/4mg as single daily dose

Naloxone exposure is somewhat higher after buccal than after SL administration; the SL site of administration is recommended to be used during induction to minimize naloxone exposure, to reduce risk of precipitated withdrawal

On Methadone/Long-Acting Opioids:
May be more susceptible to precipitated and prolonged withdrawal during induction therapy; buprenorphine monotherapy is recommended when used according to approved administration instructions. Following induction, may then be transitioned to qd SL film dose

On Heroin/Other Short-Acting Opioids:
May be inducted w/ SL film or w/ SL buprenorphine monotherapy. Administer 1st dose when objective signs of moderate opioid withdrawal appear, and not <6 hrs after last

PEDIATRIC DOSAGE
Pediatric use may not have been established

opioid use. Achieve adequate maint dose, titrated to clinical effectiveness as soon as possible

Maint:
For maint, SL film may be administered buccally or sublingually
Day 3 Onwards:
Progressively adjust dose in increments/decrements of 2mg/0.5mg or 4mg/1mg to a level that maintains treatment and suppresses opioid withdrawal signs/symptoms. After treatment induction and stabilization, the maint dose is generally in the range of 4mg/1mg to 24mg/6mg per day depending on the patient/response
Target Dose: (16mg/4mg)/day as single daily dose

Dosages higher than (24mg/6mg)/day have not been demonstrated to provide clinical advantage

Conversions
Switching Between Buprenorphine or Buprenorphine/Naloxone SL Tabs and Buprenorphine/Naloxone SL Film:
Start on the corresponding dosage of the previously administered product; adjust dose prn. Refer to PI for switching between SL film strengths

---

DOSING CONSIDERATIONS
Hepatic Impairment
Mild: No clinically significant changes have been observed
Moderate: Use may not be appropriate
Severe: Avoid use

Elderly
Start at lower end of dosing range

Discontinuation
Decision to d/c therapy should be made as part of a comprehensive treatment plan; taper patients to avoid opioid withdrawal signs/symptoms

Other Important Considerations
Unstable Patients:
Patients who continue to misuse, abuse, or divert buprenorphine products or other opioids should be provided w/, or referred to, more intensive and structured treatment

ADMINISTRATION
Buccal/SL route

Administer SL film whole; do not cut, chew, or swallow film.
Do not move film after placement.

SL Administration
Place 1 film under the tongue, close to the base on the left or right side.
If an additional film is necessary, place film SL on the opposite side from the 1st film; place film in a manner to minimize overlapping as much as possible. Keep under the tongue until completely dissolved.
If a 3rd film is necessary, place it under the tongue on either side after the first 2 films have dissolved.

Buccal Administration
Place 1 film on the inside of the right or left cheek.
If an additional film is necessary, place on the inside of the opposite cheek. Keep on the inside of the cheek until completely dissolved.
If a 3rd film is necessary, place it on the inside of the right or left cheek after the first 2 films have dissolved.

Switching Between SL and Buccal Sites of Administration
Buprenorphine exposure between buccal and SL administration is similar; therefore, once induction is complete, may switch between buccal and SL administration w/o significant risk of under- or over-dosing.

STORAGE
25°C (77°F); excursions permitted to 15-30°C (59-86°F).

HOW SUPPLIED
Film, SL: (Buprenorphine/Naloxone) 2mg/0.5mg, 4mg/1mg, 8mg/2mg, 12mg/3mg

CONTRAINDICATIONS
Hypersensitivity to buprenorphine or naloxone

WARNINGS/PRECAUTIONS
Not appropriate as an analgesic. Hypersensitivity reactions, bronchospasm, angioneurotic edema, and anaphylactic shock reported. May precipitate opioid withdrawal signs and symptoms if administered before the agonist effects of the opioid have subsided. Not recommended for initiation of treatment in patients w/ moderate hepatic impairment; may be used w/ caution for maintenance treatment in patients w/ moderate hepatic impairment who have initiated treatment on a buprenorphine product w/o naloxone. May impair mental/physical abilities. May produce orthostatic hypotension in ambulatory patients. Caution w/ myxedema, hypothyroidism, adrenal cortical insufficiency (eg, Addison's

disease), CNS depression/coma, toxic psychoses, prostatic hypertrophy, urethral stricture, acute alcoholism, delirium tremens, kyphoscoliosis, and in debilitated patients. **Buprenorphine:** Potential for abuse. Significant respiratory depression and death reported; caution w/ compromised respiratory function. Reestablish adequate ventilation in case of overdose; higher than normal doses and repeated administration of naloxone may be necessary. Accidental pediatric exposure can cause severe, possibly fatal, respiratory depression. Neonatal opioid withdrawal syndrome (NOWS) is an expected and treatable outcome of prolonged use of opioids during pregnancy; observe newborns for signs of NOWS and manage accordingly. Chronic use produces physical dependence. Cytolytic hepatitis and hepatitis w/ jaundice reported; obtain LFTs prior to initiation and periodically during treatment. If a hepatic event is suspected, biological and etiological evaluation is recommended; careful discontinuation may be needed depending on the case. Caution w/ preexisting liver enzyme abnormalities, hepatitis B or C infection, use w/ other potentially hepatotoxic drugs, and ongoing injecting drug use. May elevate CSF pressure; caution w/ head injury, intracranial lesions, and other circumstances when CSF pressure may be increased. May produce miosis and changes in the level of consciousness that may interfere w/ patient evaluation. May increase intracholedochal pressure; caution w/ biliary tract dysfunction. May obscure the diagnosis or clinical course of patients w/ acute abdominal conditions.

ADVERSE REACTIONS
Oral hypoesthesia, constipation, glossodynia, oral mucosal erythema, vomiting, intoxication, disturbance in attention, palpitations, insomnia, withdrawal syndrome, hyperhidrosis, blurred vision, restlessness.

DRUG INTERACTIONS
May cause respiratory depression, coma, and death w/ benzodiazepines or other CNS depressants (eg, alcohol); use w/ caution. Opioid analgesics, general anesthetics, benzodiazepines, phenothiazines, other tranquilizers, sedative/hypnotics, or other CNS depressants (eg, alcohol) may increase CNS depression; consider dose reduction of 1 or both agents. Concomitant use w/ CYP3A4 inhibitors (eg, azole antifungals, macrolides, HIV protease inhibitors) should be monitored and may require dose reduction of 1 or both agents. Monitor for signs and symptoms of opioid withdrawal w/ CYP3A4 inducers (eg, efavirenz, phenobarbital, carbamazepine, phenytoin, rifampicin). Monitor dose of patients who are on chronic buprenorphine treatment if non-nucleoside reverse transcriptase inhibitors are added to treatment regimen. Atazanavir and atazanavir/ritonavir may increase levels and sedation; monitor and consider dose reduction of buprenorphine.

PREGNANCY AND LACTATION
Pregnancy: There are no adequate and well-controlled studies in pregnant women. Use of buprenorphine prior to delivery may result in respiratory depression in the newborn; closely monitor neonates for signs of respiratory depression. Should be used during pregnancy only if the potential benefit justifies the potential risk to the fetus.
Lactation: Buprenorphine and the metabolite norbuprenorphine are present at low levels in human milk and infant urine. Monitor the infant for increased drowsiness and breathing difficulties. Caution in nursing.

MECHANISM OF ACTION
Buprenorphine: Partial agonist at the mu-opioid receptor and an antagonist at the kappa-opioid receptor. **Naloxone:** Potent antagonist at the mu-opioid receptor.

PHARMACOKINETICS
Distribution: Plasma protein binding (96% buprenorphine; 45% naloxone); found in breast milk (buprenorphine and norbuprenorphine). **Metabolism:** Buprenorphine: N-dealkylation via CYP3A4 and glucuronidation; norbuprenorphine (major metabolite). Naloxone: Glucuronidation, N-dealkylation, and reduction; naloxone-3-glucuronide (metabolite). **Elimination:** Buprenorphine: Urine (30%), feces (69%); $T_{1/2}$=24-42 hrs. Naloxone: $T_{1/2}$=2-12 hrs.

PATIENT CONSIDERATIONS
Assessment: Assess for history of hypersensitivity to drug, myxedema, hypothyroidism, adrenal cortical insufficiency, CNS depression or coma, toxic psychoses, prostatic hypertrophy, urethral stricture, acute alcoholism, delirium tremens, kyphoscoliosis, debilitation, compromised respiratory function, hepatic impairment, hepatitis B or C infection, head injury, intracranial lesions and other circumstances in which CSF pressure may be increased, biliary tract dysfunction, acute abdominal conditions, pregnancy/nursing status, and possible drug interactions. Obtain baseline LFTs prior to therapy.
Monitoring: Monitor for hypersensitivity reactions, signs/symptoms of precipitated opioid withdrawal, impaired mental/physical ability, orthostatic hypotension, respiratory depression, drug abuse/dependence, cytolytic hepatitis, hepatitis w/ jaundice, elevation of CSF pressure and intracholedochal pressure, miosis, changes in consciousness levels, and other adverse reactions. Monitor LFTs periodically. Monitor for symptoms related to over-dosing or under-dosing when switching between buprenorphine or other buprenorphine/naloxone products.
Counseling: Warn about danger of self-administration of benzodiazepines and other CNS depressants, including alcohol, while on therapy. Advise that drug contains opioid that can be a target for abuse; instruct to keep film in a safe place protected from theft and children. Instruct to seek medical attention immediately if a child is exposed to the drug. Caution that drug may impair mental/physical abilities and cause orthostatic hypotension. Advise to take film qd and to not change dose w/o consulting physician. Inform that treatment can cause dependence and that withdrawal syndrome may occur upon discontinuation. Advise patients seeking to d/c treatment w/ buprenorphine for opioid dependence to work closely w/ physician on a tapering schedule, and apprise of the potential to relapse to illicit drug use associated w/ discontinuation of treatment. Advise to report to physician all medications prescribed or currently being used. Advise women that if they are pregnant while on therapy, that the

baby may have signs of withdrawal at birth and that withdrawal is treatable. Instruct women who are breastfeeding to monitor the infant for drowsiness and difficulty breathing. Advise to instruct family members that, in event of emergency, the treating physician or staff should be informed that patient is physically dependent on an opioid and that the patient is being treated w/ SL film. Advise to dispose of unused drugs as soon as they are no longer needed by flushing films down the toilet.

SUBSYS — fentanyl   CII
Class: Opioid analgesic

> Fatal respiratory depression may occur. Contraindicated in the management of acute or postoperative pain (eg, headache/migraine) and in opioid-nontolerant patients. Death reported upon accidental ingestion in children; keep out of reach of children. Concomitant use w/ CYP3A4 inhibitors may increase plasma levels, and may cause fatal respiratory depression. Do not convert patients on a mcg-per-mcg basis from any other fentanyl product to Subsys. Do not substitute for any other fentanyl products; may result in fatal overdose. Contains fentanyl w/ an abuse liability similar to other opioid analgesics. Available only through a restricted program called the Transmucosal Immediate-Release Fentanyl Risk Evaluation and Mitigation Strategy (TIRF REMS) Access program due to risk for misuse, abuse, addiction, and overdose. Outpatients, healthcare professionals who prescribe to outpatients, pharmacies, and distributors must enroll in the program.

ADULT DOSAGE	PEDIATRIC DOSAGE
Cancer Pain	Pediatric use may not have been established
Breakthrough Pain in Patients Already Receiving and Tolerant to Around-the-Clock Opioid Therapy:	
Initial: 100mcg	
Titrate: May take only 1 additional dose of the same strength for each breakthrough pain episode if pain is not relieved after 30 min	
100mcg: 1 x 100mcg unit	
200mcg: 1 x 200mcg unit	
400mcg: 1 x 400mcg unit	
600mcg: 1 x 600mcg unit	
800mcg: 1 x 800mcg unit	
1200mcg: 2 x 600mcg unit	
1600mcg: 2 x 800mcg unit	
Maint: Once titrated to an effective dose, use only 1 dose of the appropriate strength per breakthrough pain episode; only increase dose when single administration of current dose fails to adequately treat the breakthrough pain episode for several consecutive episodes	
Max: 2 doses for any breakthrough pain episode; limit consumption to ≤4 doses/day	
Wait at least 4 hrs before treating another episode of breakthrough pain. If >4 breakthrough pain episodes/day are experienced, reevaluate maint dose (around-the-clock) used for persistent pain	
Conversions	
Switching from Actiq to Subsys:	
Initial:	
200 or 400mcg Actiq: 100mcg Subsys	
600 or 800mcg Actiq: 200mcg Subsys	
1200 or 1600mcg Actiq: 400mcg Subsys	
Titrate:	
≤400mcg Actiq: Proceed using multiples of 100mcg Subsys	
600 and 800mcg Actiq: Proceed using multiples of 200mcg Subsys	
1200 and 1600mcg Actiq: Proceed using multiples of 400mcg Subsys	

DOSING CONSIDERATIONS
Adverse Reactions
Oral Mucositis:
Grade 1: Monitor closely for respiratory depression and CNS depression particularly during initiation of therapy
Grade ≥2: Avoid use unless benefits outweigh potential risk
Excessive Opioid Effects: Decrease subsequent doses

ADMINISTRATION
SL route

Open blister package w/ scissors immediately prior to use
Carefully spray contents into mouth underneath the tongue

Disposal
Use the charcoal-lined disposal pouch to dispose of the contents of any unneeded unit dose systems

STORAGE
20-25°C (68-77°F); excursions permitted between 15-30°C (59-86°F) until ready to use.

HOW SUPPLIED
Spray: 100mcg/spray, 200mcg/spray, 400mcg/spray, 600mcg/spray, 800mcg/spray

CONTRAINDICATIONS
Opioid-nontolerant patients, management of acute or postoperative pain (eg, headache/migraine).

WARNINGS/PRECAUTIONS
Increased risk of respiratory depression in patients w/ underlying respiratory disorders and in elderly/debilitated. May impair mental and/or physical abilities. Caution w/ COPD or preexisting medical conditions predisposing to respiratory depression; may further decrease respiratory drive to the point of respiratory failure. Extreme caution in patients who may be susceptible to intracranial effects of carbon dioxide retention (eg, those w/ evidence of increased intracranial pressure or impaired consciousness). May obscure clinical course of head injuries; use only if clinically warranted. Caution w/ bradyarrhythmias. Avoid use during labor and delivery. Caution w/ renal/hepatic impairment.

ADVERSE REACTIONS
Respiratory depression, circulatory depression, hypotension, shock, N/V, constipation, somnolence, dizziness, asthenia, dyspnea, anxiety, known intolerance or hypersensitivity to fentanyl or any of the components of this medication.

DRUG INTERACTIONS
See Boxed Warning. Monitor for an extended period of time w/ concomitant use w/ moderate or strong CYP3A4 inhibitors. Not recommended w/ an MAOI or w/ in 14 days of MAOI discontinuation. Increased depressant effects w/ other CNS depressants (eg, other opioids, sedatives/hypnotics, general anesthetics); adjust dose of Subsys if warranted and monitor for a change in opioid effects. CYP3A4 inducers (eg, barbiturates, carbamazepine, efavirenz) may decrease levels; monitor and adjust dose of Subsys accordingly. Respiratory depression may be more likely to occur when given in conjunction w/ other drugs that depress respiration.

PREGNANCY AND LACTATION
Category C, not for use in nursing.

MECHANISM OF ACTION
Opioid analgesic; has not been established. Known to be μ-opioid receptor agonist; specific CNS opioid receptors for endogenous compounds w/ opioid-like activity have been identified throughout the brain and spinal cord and play a role in analgesic effects.

PHARMACOKINETICS
Absorption: Absolute bioavailability (76%). Administration of variable doses resulted in different parameters. **Distribution:** V_d=4L/kg; plasma protein binding (80-85%); crosses placenta; found in breast milk. **Metabolism:** Liver and intestinal mucosa via CYP3A4; norfentanyl (metabolite). **Elimination:** Urine (<7%, unchanged), feces (1%, unchanged); $T_{1/2}$=5-12 hrs.

PATIENT CONSIDERATIONS
Assessment: Assess for degree of opioid tolerance, previous opioid dose, level of pain intensity, type of pain, patient's general condition and medical status, underlying respiratory disorders, or any other conditions where treatment is contraindicated or cautioned. Assess for intolerance or previous hypersensitivity, renal/hepatic function, pregnancy/nursing status, and possible drug interactions.

Monitoring: Monitor for signs/symptoms of respiratory depression, impairment of mental/physical abilities, drug abuse/addiction, and other adverse reactions. Closely monitor patients w/ Grade 1 mucositis or hepatic/renal impairment, and monitor elderly for respiratory depression and CNS effects.

Counseling: Inform outpatients to enroll in the TIRF REMS Access program; instruct to sign a patient-prescriber agreement form to confirm understanding. Instruct to properly dispose of consumed units. Instruct not to take medication for acute or postoperative pain, pain from injuries, headache, migraine, or any other short-term pain. Advise to take drug as prescribed and avoid sharing it w/ anyone else. Inform of the high risk of fatal respiratory depression in children if exposed to therapy. Instruct to notify physician if breakthrough pain is not alleviated or worsens after taking the medication. Inform that medication use may impair mental/physical abilities; caution against performing activities that require a high level of attention. Advise not to combine w/ alcohol, sleep aids, or tranquilizers, except if ordered by physician. Instruct to inform physician if pregnant or planning to become pregnant.

SUCLEAR — magnesium sulfate/potassium sulfate/sodium sulfate, polyethylene glycol 3350/potassium chloride/sodium bicarbonate/sodium chloride   Rx

Class: Bowel cleanser

ADULT DOSAGE
Bowel Cleansing

Prior to Colonoscopy:
Split-Dose (2-Day) Regimen (Preferred Method):
Take Dose 1 the pm before the colonoscopy (10-12 hrs prior to Dose 2), then Dose 2 the next am on the

PEDIATRIC DOSAGE
Pediatric use may not have been established

day of the colonoscopy, starting at least 3.5 hrs prior to colonoscopy

Day-Before (1-Day) Regimen (Alternative Method):
On the pm before the colonoscopy, take Dose 1 beginning at least 3.5 hrs prior to hs, then Dose 2 approx 2 hrs after starting Dose 1

ADMINISTRATION
Oral route

Additional fluids must be consumed in both dosing regimens.
Consume only clear liquids (no solid food or milk) and avoid alcohol on the day before colonoscopy until after completion of the colonoscopy.

Split-Dose (2-Day) Regimen (Preferred Method)
Dose 1 (PM Before Colonoscopy):
1. Dilute the 6-oz oral sol prior to use by pouring entire contents of the bottle into the 16-oz mixing container and then filling the container w/ cool water to the fill line and mix.
2. Drink entire sol in container; best to complete drinking the sol w/in 20 min.
3. Refill container w/ 16 oz of water to the fill line and drink it over the next 2 hrs.
4. Refill container w/ 16 oz of water to the fill line and finish drinking it before going to bed.

Dose 2 (Next Morning on the Day of Colonoscopy):
1. Dissolve powder of Dose 2 by adding water to the fill line on the jug.
2. Shake jug until all powder is dissolved; sol can be used w/ or w/o the addition of a flavor pack.
3. Sol may be refrigerated after adding water and should be used w/in 48 hrs of reconstitution.
4. Using the 16-oz container provided w/ the kit, drink all the sol in the jug at a rate of one 16-oz container every 20 min (eg, four 16-oz containers over a period of 1.5 hrs).
5. Complete drinking sol at least 2 hrs before colonoscopy.
6. Consume only clear liquids until 2 hrs prior to colonoscopy; thereafter, nothing should be consumed until the completion of colonoscopy.

Day-Before (1-Day) Regimen (Alternative Method)
PM Before Colonoscopy:
Dose 1:
1. Dilute the 6-oz oral sol prior to use by pouring entire contents of the bottle into the 16-oz mixing container and then filling the container w/ cool water to the fill line and mix.
2. Drink entire sol in container; best to complete drinking the sol w/in 20 min.
3. Refill container w/ 16 oz of water to the fill line and drink it over the next 2 hrs.
Dose 2:
1. Dissolve powder of Dose 2 by adding water to the fill line on the jug.
2. Shake jug until all the powder is dissolved; sol can be used w/ or w/o the addition of a flavor pack.
3. Sol may be refrigerated after adding water and should be used w/in 48 hrs of reconstitution.
4. Using the 16-oz container provided w/ the kit, drink all the sol in the jug at a rate of one 16-oz container every 20 min (eg, four 16-oz containers over a period of 1.5 hrs).
5. Refill container w/ 16 oz of water to the fill line and finish drinking it before going to bed.
6. Consume only clear liquids until 2 hrs prior to colonoscopy; thereafter, nothing should be consumed until the completion of colonoscopy.

STORAGE
20-25°C (68-77°F); excursions permitted between 15-30°C (59-86°F). Reconstituted Sol: May be refrigerated. Use within 48 hrs.

HOW SUPPLIED
Sol: (Liquid) Dose 1 (Sodium Sulfate/Potassium Sulfate/Magnesium Sulfate) 17.5g/3.13g/1.6g [6 oz]; (Powder) Dose 2 (Polyethylene Glycol [PEG] 3350/Sodium Chloride/Sodium Bicarbonate/Potassium Chloride) 210g/5.6g/2.86g/0.74g/2L

CONTRAINDICATIONS
GI obstruction or ileus, bowel perforation, gastric retention, toxic colitis or toxic megacolon, known allergies to any components of Suclear.

WARNINGS/PRECAUTIONS
Consume only clear liquids (no solid food or milk) and avoid alcohol on the day before colonoscopy until after completion of the colonoscopy. Adequately hydrate before, during, and after use. If significant vomiting or signs of dehydration develop, perform postcolonoscopy lab tests (electrolytes, SrCr, BUN). Correct electrolyte abnormalities before treatment. Caution with conditions that increase risk of fluid and electrolyte disturbances or may increase risk of seizure, arrhythmias, prolonged QT, and renal impairment. Serious arrhythmias reported rarely; use with caution and consider predose and postcolonoscopy ECGs in patients at increased risk of serious cardiac arrhythmias. Generalized tonic-clonic seizures reported; caution in patients with a history of or at increased risk of seizures (eg, with known/suspected hyponatremia). Caution with impaired renal function; consider performing baseline and postcolonoscopy lab tests. May produce colonic mucosal aphthous ulcerations; consider this when interpreting colonoscopy findings in patients with known/suspected inflammatory bowel disease. Serious cases of ischemic colitis reported. Patients with severe active ulcerative colitis may be at increased risk of exacerbation of their disease with therapy. Monitor patients with impaired gag reflex and patients prone to

regurgitation/aspiration. Not for direct ingestion; direct ingestion of undiluted solution may increase the risk of N/V, dehydration, or other serious adverse reactions.

ADVERSE REACTIONS
Discomfort, abdominal distension, abdominal pain, N/V.

DRUG INTERACTIONS
Caution with medications that increase risk for fluid and electrolyte disturbances or may increase risk of seizure, arrhythmias, prolonged QT, and renal impairment. Caution with drugs associated with hypokalemia (eg, diuretics, corticosteroids, drugs where hypokalemia is a particular risk [eg, cardiac glycosides]) or hyponatremia, NSAIDs, and drugs known to induce antidiuretic hormone secretion (eg, TCAs, SSRIs, antipsychotics, carbamazepine). Alcohol may increase the risk of dehydration. Caution with drugs that lower seizure threshold (eg, TCAs) and in patients withdrawing from alcohol or benzodiazepines. Caution with drugs that may affect renal function (eg, diuretics, ACE inhibitors, ARBs, NSAIDs). Increased risk of mucosal ulceration or ischemic colitis with stimulant laxatives (eg, bisacodyl, sodium picosulfate); avoid concurrent use. Oral medication administered within 1 hr of the start of each dose may be flushed from GI tract and may not be absorbed properly.

PREGNANCY AND LACTATION
Pregnancy: Category C.
Lactation: Caution in nursing.

MECHANISM OF ACTION
Bowel cleanser; primary mode of action is the osmotic effect of the unabsorbed PEG and sulfate salts, which causes water to be retained within the GI tract.

PHARMACOKINETICS
Absorption: (Sulfate salts) T_{max}=5.5 hrs (healthy). (PEG 3350) Poor. **Elimination:** (Sulfate salts/PEG 3350) Urine, feces. (Sulfate salts) $T_{1/2}$=8.5 hrs (healthy).

PATIENT CONSIDERATIONS
Assessment: Assess for drug hypersensitivity, GI obstruction or ileus, bowel perforation, gastric retention, toxic colitis, toxic megacolon, fluid and electrolyte abnormalities, renal impairment, any other conditions where treatment is cautioned, pregnancy/nursing status, and possible drug interactions. Consider predose ECGs in patients at increased risk of serious cardiac arrhythmias.

Monitoring: Monitor for arrhythmias, generalized tonic-clonic seizures, colonic mucosal aphthous ulcerations, ischemic colitis, and other adverse reactions. Monitor patients with impaired gag reflex and patients prone to regurgitation/aspiration. Consider postcolonoscopy ECGs in patients at increased risk of serious cardiac arrhythmias.

Counseling: Instruct to inform physician if patient has trouble swallowing or is prone to regurgitation/aspiration. Inform that each bottle needs to be diluted in water before ingestion and instruct to drink additional water according to the instructions. Inform that oral medications may not be absorbed properly if taken within 1 hr of starting each dose of drug. Instruct not to take other laxatives during therapy. Advise to hydrate adequately before, during, and after use. Instruct to consume only clear liquids (no solid food or milk) and to avoid alcohol on the day before colonoscopy until after completion of the colonoscopy.

SUFENTA — sufentanil citrate   CII

Class: Opioid analgesic

ADULT DOSAGE
Analgesia (Surgical)
Adjunct in the maint of balanced general anesthesia in patients who are intubated and ventilated

Expected Duration of Anesthesia 1-2 Hrs:
Incremental or Infusion:
Usual: 1-2mcg/kg w/ nitrous oxide/oxygen.
Approx ≥75% of total sufentanil dose may be administered prior to intubation by either slow inj or infusion titrated to patient response
Maint:
Incremental: 10-25mcg (0.2-0.5mL) may be administered in increments prn.
Supplemental doses should be individualized and adjusted to remaining operative time anticipated
Infusion: Administer as an intermittent or continuous infusion prn.
Adjust based upon the induction dose so that total dose does not exceed 1mcg/kg/hr of expected surgical time

Expected Duration of Anesthesia 2-8 Hrs:
Incremental or Infusion:
Usual: 2-8mcg/kg w/ nitrous oxide/oxygen.
Approx ≤75% of the total calculated sufentanil dose may be administered

PEDIATRIC DOSAGE
General Anesthesia
Induction/Maint of Anesthesia:
<12 Years:
Undergoing Cardiovascular Surgery:
Usual: 10-25mcg/kg w/ 100% oxygen
Maint: Supplemental doses of up to 25-50mcg may be given based on response to initial dose

by slow inj or infusion prior to intubation, titrated to individual patient response
Maint:
Incremental: 10-50mcg (0.2-1mL) may be administered in increments prn.
Supplemental doses should be individualized and adjusted to the remaining operative time anticipated
Infusion: May administer as an intermittent or continuous infusion prn.
Adjust based upon the induction dose so that total dose does not exceed 1mcg/kg/hr of expected surgical time

Anesthesia (Surgical)
As a primary anesthetic agent for the induction and maint of anesthesia w/ 100% oxygen in patients undergoing major surgical procedures who are intubated and ventilated

Incremental or Infusion:
Total Dose: 8-30mcg/kg (anesthetic doses) administered as slow inj, infusion, or inj followed by infusion. Produces sleep and maintains deep level of anesthesia w/o use of additional anesthetics at doses ≥8mcg/kg when administered w/ 100% oxygen and a muscle relaxant
Maint:
Incremental: Depending on initial dose, 0.5-10mcg/kg may be administered by slow inj
Infusion: May be administered by continuous or intermittent infusion as needed.
Maint infusion rate should be based upon the induction dose so that the total dose for the procedure does not exceed 30mcg/kg

Labor Pain
Analgesic During Labor and Vaginal Delivery:
Usual: 10-15mcg administered w/ 10mL bupivacaine 0.125% w/ or w/o epinephrine.
Doses can be repeated twice (for a total of 3 doses) at ≥1-hr intervals until delivery

---

DOSING CONSIDERATIONS
Concomitant Medications
Benzodiazepines, Barbiturates, Inhalation Agents, Other Opioids/CNS Depressants: Reduce sufentanil dose or dose of concomitant drug
Elderly/Debilitated
Reduce dose
Other Important Considerations
Neonates: Reduce dose accordingly, especially in those w/ cardiovascular disease
ADMINISTRATION
IV route

For purposes of administering small volumes accurately, use of tuberculin syringe or equivalent is recommended

Epidural Use in Labor and Delivery:
Administer by slow inj
Should be mixed together w/ bupivacaine before administration

STORAGE
20-25°C (68-77°F). Protect from light.
HOW SUPPLIED
Inj: 50mcg/mL
CONTRAINDICATIONS
Known hypersensitivity to this product or known intolerance to other opioid agonists.

WARNINGS/PRECAUTIONS
Should only be administered by persons specifically trained in the use of IV and epidural anesthetics and management of the respiratory effects of potent opioids. An opioid antagonist, resuscitative and intubation equipment and oxygen should be readily available. Prior to catheter insertion, the physician should be familiar with patient conditions (such as infection at the injection site, bleeding diathesis, anticoagulation therapy) which call for special evaluation of the benefit versus risk potential. May cause muscle rigidity of the neck and extremities. Adequate facilities should be available for postoperative monitoring and ventilation. Monitor vital signs routinely. Reduce dose for elderly and debilitated patients. Caution with pulmonary disease, decreased respiratory reserve, liver and kidney dysfunction, cardiac bradyarrhythmias. Reports of bradycardia responsive to atropine. May obscure clinical course of patients with head injuries.

ADVERSE REACTIONS
Respiratory depression, skeletal muscle rigidity, bradycardia, HTN, hypotension, chest wall rigidity, somnolence, pruritus, N/V.

DRUG INTERACTIONS
Reports of cardiovascular depression with nitrous oxide. High doses of pancuronium may produce increase in HR. Reports of bradycardia and hypotension with other muscle relaxants. Greater incidence and degree of bradycardia and hypotension with chronic CCB and β-blocker therapy. Additive or potentiating effects with other CNS depressants (eg, barbiturates, tranquilizers, narcotics, general anesthetics). Reduce dose of either agent. Decrease in mean arterial pressure and systemic vascular resistance with benzodiazepines.

PREGNANCY AND LACTATION
Category C, caution in nursing.

MECHANISM OF ACTION
An opioid analgesic.

PHARMACOKINETICS
Distribution: Plasma protein binding (healthy males: 93%, mothers: 91%, neonates: 79%). **Elimination:** $T_{1/2}$=164 min (adults), 97 min (neonates).

PATIENT CONSIDERATIONS
Assessment: Assess for pulmonary disease, decreased respiratory reserve, hepatic/renal dysfunction, cardiac bradyarrhythmias, head injury, pregnancy/nursing status, and possible drug interactions.

Monitoring: Monitor for cardiovascular depression (eg, bradycardia and hypotension), respiratory depression, muscle rigidity of the neck and extremities, N/V, chills, arrhythmias, chest wall rigidity. Monitor vital signs routinely. Appropriate postoperative monitoring should ensure that adequate spontaneous breathing is established and maintained prior to discharging patient.

Counseling: Counsel about side effects of drug and abuse potential.

SULAR — nisoldipine   Rx
Class: Calcium channel blocker (CCB) (dihydropyridine)

ADULT DOSAGE	PEDIATRIC DOSAGE
Hypertension	Pediatric use may not have been established
Initial: 17mg qd	
Titrate: Increase by 8.5mg/week or longer intervals	
Maint: 17-34mg qd	
Max: 34mg qd	

DOSING CONSIDERATIONS
Hepatic Impairment
Initial: ≤8.5mg qd
Elderly
Initial: ≤8.5mg qd

ADMINISTRATION
Oral route

Take on an empty stomach (1 hr ac or 2 hrs pc)
Swallow whole; do not bite, divide, or crush

STORAGE
20-25°C (68-77°F); excursions permitted to 15-30°C (59-86°F). Protect from light and moisture.

HOW SUPPLIED
Tab, Extended-Release: 8.5mg, 17mg, 34mg

CONTRAINDICATIONS
Known hypersensitivity to dihydropyridine calcium channel blockers.

WARNINGS/PRECAUTIONS
Increased angina and/or acute myocardial infarction (MI) may occur in patients with severe obstructive coronary artery disease (CAD). May cause hypotension. Caution with heart failure (HF) or compromised ventricular function, particularly with concomitant β-blockers. Caution with severe hepatic dysfunction and in the elderly.

ADVERSE REACTIONS
Peripheral edema, headache, dizziness, pharyngitis, vasodilation, sinusitis, palpitation.

DRUG INTERACTIONS
Increased levels with cimetidine. Avoid with CYP3A4 inducers or inhibitors. Phenytoin decreased concentrations; avoid concomitant use. Quinidine decreased bioavailability. Avoid grapefruit products before and after dosing.

PREGNANCY AND LACTATION
Category C, not for use in nursing.

MECHANISM OF ACTION
Calcium channel blocker (dihydropyridine); inhibits transmembrane influx of Ca^{2+} into vascular smooth muscle and cardiac muscle, resulting in dilation of arterioles and decreased peripheral vascular resistance.

PHARMACOKINETICS
Absorption: Relatively well-absorbed. Absolute bioavailability (5%); T_{max}=9.2 hrs. **Distribution:** Plasma protein binding (<1% unbound). **Metabolism:** Hydroxylation by CYP450; hydroxylated derivative of the side chain (active metabolite). **Elimination:** Urine (60-80%; trace amounts, unchanged), feces; $T_{1/2}$=13.7 hrs.

PATIENT CONSIDERATIONS
Assessment: Assess for hypersensitivity to drug, CAD, HF, compromised ventricular function, hepatic impairment, pregnancy/nursing status, and possible drug interactions. Obtain baseline BP.

Monitoring: Monitor for increased angina or MI, and other adverse effects. Monitor BP.

Counseling: Instruct to avoid grapefruit products. Inform that drug contains tartrazine, which may cause allergic-type reactions in certain susceptible persons.

SULFAMETHOXAZOLE/TRIMETHOPRIM —
sulfamethoxazole/trimethoprim   Rx
Class: Sulfonamide/tetrahydrofolic acid inhibitor

OTHER BRAND NAMES
Bactrim, Bactrim DS, Sulfatrim

ADULT DOSAGE
Traveler's Diarrhea
Sus/Tab:
Usual: One 800mg/160mg tab or two 400mg/80mg tabs or 4 tsp (20mL) sus q12h for 5 days

Urinary Tract Infections
Inj:
Severe Infections: 8-10mg/kg/day (based on the trimethoprim component) given in 2 or 4 equally divided doses q6h, q8h, or q12h for up to 14 days
Max: 60mL/day
Sus/Tab:
Usual: One 800mg/160mg tab or two 400mg/80mg tabs or 4 tsp (20mL) sus q12h for 10-14 days

Acute Bacterial Exacerbation of Chronic Bronchitis
Sus/Tab:
Usual: One 800mg/160mg tab or two 400mg/80mg tabs or 4 tsp sus (20mL) q12h for 14 days

Shigellosis
Inj:
8-10mg/kg/day (based on the trimethoprim component) given in 2 or 4 equally divided doses q6h, q8h, or q12h for up to 5 days
Max: 60mL/day
Sus/Tab:
Usual: One 800mg/160mg tab or two 400mg/80mg tabs or 4 tsp (20mL) sus q12h for 5 days

Pneumonia
Pneumocystis jiroveci Pneumonia Treatment:
Inj:
15-20mg/kg/day (based on the trimethoprim component) given in 3 or 4 equally divided doses q6-8h for up to 14 days
Sus/Tab:
75-100mg/kg sulfamethoxazole and 15-20mg/kg trimethoprim per 24 hrs given in equally divided doses q6h for 14-21 days

P. jiroveci Pneumonia Prophylaxis in Immunosuppressed Patients:
Sus/Tab:
One 800mg/160mg tab or 4 tsp (20mL) sus daily

PEDIATRIC DOSAGE
Pneumonia
≥2 Months of Age:
P. jiroveci Pneumonia Treatment:
Inj:
15-20mg/kg/day (based on the trimethoprim component) given in 3 or 4 equally divided doses q6-8h for up to 14 days
Sus/Tab:
75-100mg/kg sulfamethoxazole and 15-20mg/kg trimethoprim per 24 hrs given in equally divided doses q6h for 14-21 days

P. jiroveci Pneumonia Prophylaxis in Immunosuppressed Patients:
Sus/Tab:
750mg/m²/day sulfamethoxazole w/ 150mg/m²/day trimethoprim given in equally divided doses bid, on 3 consecutive days/week
Max: 1600mg/day sulfamethoxazole and 320mg/day trimethoprim

Acute Otitis Media
Use only when sulfamethoxazole/ trimethoprim offers some advantage over the use of other antimicrobial agents
≥2 Months of Age:
Sus/Tab:
40mg/kg sulfamethoxazole and 8mg/kg trimethoprim per 24 hrs, given in 2 divided doses q12h for 10 days

Shigellosis
≥2 Months of Age:
Inj:
8-10mg/kg/day (based on the trimethoprim component) given in 2 or 4 equally divided doses q6h, q8h, or q12h for up to 5 days
Max: 60mL/day
Sus/Tab:
40mg/kg sulfamethoxazole and 8mg/kg trimethoprim per 24 hrs, given in 2 divided doses q12h for 5 days

Urinary Tract Infections
≥2 Months of Age:
Inj:
Severe Infections: 8-10mg/kg/day (based on the trimethoprim component) given in 2 or 4 equally divided doses q6h, q8h, or q12h for up to 14 days
Max: 60mL/day
Sus/Tab:
40mg/kg sulfamethoxazole and 8mg/kg trimethoprim per 24 hrs, given in 2 divided doses q12h for 10 days

---

DOSING CONSIDERATIONS
Renal Impairment
CrCl 15-30mL/min: 1/2 the usual regimen
CrCl <15mL/min: Use not recommended

ADMINISTRATION
IV/Oral route

IV
Must be diluted prior to administration.

Administer by IV infusion over 60-90 min; avoid rapid infusion or bolus inj. Do not mix w/ other drugs or sol.

IV Preparation/Dilution:
Each 5mL of the drug should be added to 125mL D5W; use w/in 6 hrs after dilution and do not refrigerate.
If 5mL/100mL D5W dilution is desired, use w/in 4 hrs.
If fluid restriction is desired, each 5mL of the drug may be added to 75mL D5W; administer w/in 2 hrs.
Multidose vials must be used w/in 48 hrs after initial entry into vial.

Compatible Infusion Systems:
Unit-dose glass containers, unit-dose polyvinyl chloride and polyolefin containers.

Sus
Shake well before using.
Refer to PI for specific weight-dose recommendations for sus/tab use in pediatrics.

STORAGE
20-25°C (68-77°F). **Inj:** Do not refrigerate. **Sus:** Protect from light.

HOW SUPPLIED
Sulfamethoxazole/Trimethoprim (SMX/TMP) **Inj:** (80mg/16mg)/mL [5mL, 10mL, 30mL]; **Sus:** (Sulfatrim) (200mg/40mg)/5mL [473mL]; **Tab:** (Bactrim) 400mg/80mg*, (Bactrim DS) 800mg/160mg* *scored

CONTRAINDICATIONS
Known hypersensitivity to TMP or sulfonamides, documented megaloblastic anemia due to folate deficiency, history of drug-induced immune thrombocytopenia w/ use of TMP and/or sulfonamides, and pediatric patients <2 months of age. **Inj/Sus:** Pregnant and nursing women. **Sus/Tab:** Marked hepatic damage or severe renal insufficiency when renal function status cannot be monitored.

WARNINGS/PRECAUTIONS
Fatalities, although rare, have occurred due to severe reactions, including Stevens-Johnson syndrome, toxic epidermal necrolysis, fulminant hepatic necrosis, agranulocytosis, aplastic anemia, thrombocytopenia, and other blood dyscrasias; d/c at the 1st appearance of skin rash or any sign of adverse reaction. Cough, SOB, and pulmonary infiltrates reported. Do not use for treatment of group A β-hemolytic streptococcal infections. *Clostridium difficile*-associated diarrhea (CDAD) reported; may need to d/c if CDAD is suspected or confirmed. May result in bacterial resistance if used in the absence of proven or suspected bacterial infection or a prophylactic indication. Caution w/ hepatic/renal impairment, possible folate deficiency (eg, the elderly, chronic alcoholics, those receiving anticonvulsant therapy, malabsorption syndrome, malnutrition states), severe allergies or bronchial asthma, porphyria, and thyroid dysfunction. Hematological changes indicative of folic acid deficiency may occur in the elderly, or w/ preexisting folic acid deficiency or kidney failure; effects are reversible by folinic acid therapy. Hemolysis may occur in patients w/ G6PD deficiency. Cases of hypoglycemia in nondiabetic patients reported rarely; increased risk w/ renal dysfunction, liver disease, malnutrition, and high doses. TMP may impair phenylalanine metabolism. AIDS patients may not tolerate or respond to therapy in the same manner as non-AIDS patients; increased incidence of side effects, particularly rash, fever, leukopenia, and elevated transaminase values in AIDS patients being treated for *P. jiroveci* pneumonia; reevaluate therapy if skin rash or any sign of adverse reaction develops. May cause hyperkalemia in patients receiving high dosage of TMP, w/ underlying disorders of K⁺ metabolism, w/ renal insufficiency, or when used concomitantly w/ drugs known to induce hyperkalemia; closely monitor serum K⁺. Ensure adequate fluid intake and urinary output during treatment to prevent crystalluria. Slow acetylators may be more prone to idiosyncratic reactions to sulfonamides. D/C if a significant reduction in the count of any formed blood element is noted. Lab test interactions may occur. **Inj:** Contains sodium metabisulfite, which may cause allergic-type reactions, including anaphylactic symptoms and life-threatening or less severe asthmatic episodes in certain susceptible people. Contains benzyl alcohol, which has been associated w/ an increased incidence of neurological and other complications (sometimes fatal) in newborns. Local irritation and inflammation due to extravascular infiltration of the infusion reported; d/c infusion and restart at another site if these occur. **Tab:** Severe and symptomatic hyponatremia may occur, particularly in patients treated for *P. jiroveci* pneumonia; evaluation for hyponatremia and appropriate correction is necessary in symptomatic patients to prevent life-threatening complications. Use during pregnancy may be associated w/ an increased risk of congenital malformations.

ADVERSE REACTIONS
GI disturbances (N/V, anorexia), allergic skin reactions (eg, rash, urticaria).

DRUG INTERACTIONS
Increased incidence of thrombocytopenia w/ purpura reported in elderly concurrently receiving certain diuretics, primarily thiazides. May prolong PT w/ warfarin; caution w/ anticoagulants. May inhibit the hepatic metabolism of phenytoin; monitor for possible excessive phenytoin effect. May increase free methotrexate concentrations. Marked but reversible nephrotoxicity reported w/ cyclosporine in renal transplant recipients. May increase digoxin levels, especially in the elderly; monitor digoxin levels. Increased SMX levels w/ indomethacin. Megaloblastic anemia may develop if used in patients receiving pyrimethamine as malaria prophylaxis in doses >25mg/week. May decrease efficacy of TCAs. Potentiates the effect of oral hypoglycemics. Toxic delirium reported w/ amantadine. Hyperkalemia in elderly patients reported after concomitant use w/ an ACE inhibitor. **Inj/Tab:** Treatment failure and excess mortality reported when used concomitantly w/ leucovorin for the treatment of HIV positive patients w/ *P. jiroveci* pneumonia; avoid coadministration during treatment of *P.*

jiroveci pneumonia. **Tab:** Caution w/ drugs that are substrates of CYP2C8 (eg, pioglitazone, repaglinide, rosiglitazone), CYP2C9 (eg, glipizide, glyburide), or OCT2 (eg, memantine, metformin).

PREGNANCY AND LACTATION
Pregnancy: (Inj/Sus) Category C; contraindicated. (Tab) Category D.
Lactation: (Inj/Sus) Contraindicated. (Tab) Levels of drug in breast milk are approx 2-5% of the recommended daily dose for infants >2 months of age; caution in nursing due to potential risk of bilirubin displacement and kernicterus.

MECHANISM OF ACTION
SMX: Sulfonamide; inhibits bacterial synthesis of dihydrofolic acid by competing w/ para-aminobenzoic acid. **TMP:** Tetrahydrofolic acid inhibitor; blocks the production of tetrahydrofolic acid from dihydrofolic acid by binding to and reversibly inhibiting the required enzyme, dihydrofolate reductase. Thus, this combination blocks 2 consecutive steps in biosynthesis of nucleic acids and proteins essential to many bacteria.

PHARMACOKINETICS
Absorption: (PO) Rapid. T_{max}=1-4 hrs. (Inj) SMX: C_{max}=46.3mcg/mL. TMP: C_{max}=3.4mcg/mL. **Distribution:** Crosses placenta; found in breast milk. Plasma protein binding (70% [SMX], 44% [TMP]). **Metabolism:** SMX: N_4-acetylation. TMP: 1- and 3-oxides, 3'- and 4'-hydroxy derivatives (major metabolites). **Elimination:** (PO) Urine (84.5% total sulfonamide [30% as free SMX and remaining as N_4-acetylated metabolite], 66.8% free TMP). SMX: $T_{1/2}$=10 hrs. TMP: $T_{1/2}$=8-10 hrs. (Inj) Urine (7-12.7% free SMX, 17-42.4% free TMP, 36.7-56% total SMX). SMX: $T_{1/2}$=12.8 hrs. TMP: Refer to PI for $T_{1/2}$.

PATIENT CONSIDERATIONS
Assessment: Assess for hypersensitivity to the drug, megaloblastic anemia, history of drug-induced immune thrombocytopenia, hepatic/renal impairment, folate deficiency, severe allergies, bronchial asthma, G6PD deficiency, porphyria, thyroid dysfunction, underlying disorders of K⁺ metabolism, pregnancy/nursing status, and possible drug interactions.

Monitoring: Monitor for hypersensitivity and other fatal reactions, CDAD, folate deficiency, hypoglycemia, hyperkalemia, and other adverse reactions. Monitor hydration status. Perform CBC frequently, and urinalysis w/ careful microscopic exam and renal function tests. **Inj:** Monitor for infusion reactions. **Tab:** Monitor for hyponatremia.

Counseling: Advise that therapy should only be used to treat bacterial, not viral, infections. Instruct to take exactly ud even if patient feels better early in the course of therapy. Inform that skipping doses or not completing the full course of therapy may decrease effectiveness of treatment and increase bacterial resistance. Instruct to maintain an adequate fluid intake. Inform that diarrhea is a common problem caused by therapy, which usually ends when therapy is discontinued. Instruct to immediately contact physician if watery and bloody stools (w/ or w/o stomach cramps and fever) occur, even as late as ≥2 months after having taken the last dose.

SUMAVEL DOSEPRO — sumatriptan   Rx
Class: 5-HT₁ᵦ/₁ᴅ agonist (triptans)

ADULT DOSAGE	PEDIATRIC DOSAGE
Migraine	Pediatric use may not have been established
Acute Treatment of Migraine w/ or w/o Aura:	
Max Single Dose: 6mg; if side effects are dose limiting, 4mg may be used	
Max Cumulative Dose: 12mg/24 hrs; separate doses by at least 1 hr	
Only consider a 2nd dose if some response to a 1st dose was observed. May be given at least 1 hr following a dose of another sumatriptan product.	
Cluster Headache	
Acute Treatment:	
Max Single Dose: 6mg	
Max Cumulative Dose: 12mg/24 hrs; separate doses by at least 1 hr	
Only consider a 2nd dose if some response to a 1st dose was observed. May be given at least 1 hr following a dose of another sumatriptan product.	

DOSING CONSIDERATIONS
Hepatic Impairment
Severe: Not recommended

Elderly
Use caution; start at lower end of dosing range

ADMINISTRATION
SQ route

Administer to the abdomen or thigh w/ an adequate SQ thickness to accommodate penetration of sumatriptan inj into the SQ space; do not administer to other areas of the body, including the arm.
Do not administer w/in 2 inches of the naval.

STORAGE
20-25°C (68-77°F); excursions permitted between 15-30°C (59-86°F). Do not freeze. Protect from light.

HOW SUPPLIED
Inj: 4mg/0.5mL, 6mg/0.5mL

CONTRAINDICATIONS
Ischemic coronary artery disease (CAD) (eg, angina pectoris, history of MI, documented silent ischemia), coronary artery vasospasm (eg, Prinzmetal's angina), Wolff-Parkinson-White syndrome or arrhythmias associated w/ other cardiac accessory conduction pathway disorders, history of stroke or transient ischemic attack (TIA), history of hemiplegic/basilar migraine, peripheral vascular disease, ischemic bowel disease, uncontrolled HTN. Recent use (w/in 24 hrs) of ergotamine-containing medication, ergot-type medication (eg, dihydroergotamine, methysergide), or another 5-HT₁ agonist. Concurrent administration or recent use (w/in 2 weeks) of an MAO-A inhibitor. Hypersensitivity to Sumavel DosePro.

WARNINGS/PRECAUTIONS
Use only if a clear diagnosis of migraine or cluster headache has been established. Reconsider diagnosis of migraine before treating any subsequent attacks if patient has no response to the first migraine attack treated w/ Sumavel DosePro. Not indicated for the prevention of migraine attacks. Serious cardiac adverse reactions (eg, acute MI) reported. May cause coronary artery vasospasm (Prinzmetal's angina). Perform a cardiovascular (CV) evaluation in triptan-naive patients w/ multiple CV risk factors (eg, diabetes, HTN, smoking) prior to therapy; if negative, consider administering 1st dose in a medically supervised setting and performing an ECG immediately following administration. Consider periodic CV evaluation in intermittent long-term users w/ multiple CV risk factors. Life-threatening cardiac rhythm disturbances (eg, ventricular tachycardia, ventricular fibrillation leading to death) reported; d/c if these occur. Sensations of tightness, pain, pressure, and heaviness in the precordium, throat, neck, and jaw, usually noncardiac in origin, reported; perform cardiac evaluation if at high cardiac risk. Cerebral/subarachnoid hemorrhage, stroke, and other cerebrovascular events may occur; d/c therapy if a cerebrovascular event occurs. May cause noncoronary vasospastic reactions (eg, peripheral vascular ischemia, GI vascular ischemia/infarction, splenic infarction, Raynaud's syndrome); rule out therapy-related vasospastic reactions before additional therapy is given in patients who experience signs/symptoms of noncoronary vasospasm reaction. May cause transient/permanent blindness and significant partial vision loss. Overuse of acute migraine drugs may lead to exacerbation of headache; detoxification, including withdrawal of the overused drugs, and treatment of withdrawal symptoms may be necessary. Serotonin syndrome may occur; d/c if suspected. Significant elevation in BP, including hypertensive crisis w/ acute impairment of organ systems, reported. Anaphylactic, anaphylactoid, and hypersensitivity reactions may occur; caution w/ history of sensitivity to multiple allergens. Seizures reported; caution w/ history of epilepsy or conditions associated w/ a lowered seizure threshold. Caution in elderly.

ADVERSE REACTIONS
Inj-site reaction, tingling, warm sensation, burning sensation, feeling of heaviness, pressure sensation, feeling of tightness, numbness, flushing, chest discomfort, weakness, dizziness, neck pain, paresthesia, N/V.

DRUG INTERACTIONS
See Contraindications. Serotonin syndrome reported w/ SSRIs, SNRIs, TCAs, or MAOIs.

PREGNANCY AND LACTATION
Pregnancy: Category C.
Lactation: Not for use in nursing.

MECHANISM OF ACTION
5-HT₁B/₁D agonist; presumably exerts its therapeutic effects through agonist effects at the 5-HT₁B/₁D receptors on intracranial blood vessels and sensory nerves of the trigeminal system, which result in cranial vessel constriction and inhibition of proinflammatory neuropeptide release.

PHARMACOKINETICS
Absorption: Bioavailability (97%); C_{max}=71.9ng/mL (thigh), 78.6ng/mL (abdomen); T_{max}=12 min. **Distribution:** (Healthy) Plasma protein binding (14-21%). **Metabolism:** Via MAO-A; indole acetic acid (major metabolite). **Elimination:** $T_{1/2}$=103 min (thigh), 102 min (abdomen).

PATIENT CONSIDERATIONS
Assessment: Assess for CV disease, HTN, hemiplegic or basilar migraine, hypersensitivity to drug, hepatic impairment, any other conditions where treatment is contraindicated or cautioned, pregnancy/nursing status, and possible drug interactions. Confirm diagnosis of migraine or cluster headache and exclude other potentially serious neurological conditions. Perform a CV evaluation in triptan-naive patients who have multiple CV risk factors.

Monitoring: Monitor for signs/symptoms of cardiac events (eg, coronary vasospasm, acute MI, arrhythmia, ECG changes), cerebrovascular events (eg, hemorrhage, stroke, TIA), noncoronary vasospastic reactions, visual disorders, serotonin syndrome, anaphylactic/anaphylactoid/hypersensitivity reactions, HTN, seizures, and other adverse reactions. Perform periodic CV evaluation in patients on long-term intermittent use w/ risk factors for CAD. Reassess diagnosis if clinical response does not occur following 1st dose of therapy.

Counseling: Inform that therapy may cause serious CV side effects and anaphylactic/anaphylactoid reactions. Instruct to seek medical attention

if signs/symptoms of chest pain, SOB, irregular heartbeat, significant rise in BP, weakness, or slurring of speech occur. Inform that use of acute migraine drugs for ≥10 days/month may lead to an exacerbation of headache; encourage to record headache frequency and drug use (eg, by keeping a headache diary). Inform about the risk of serotonin syndrome, particularly during combined use w/ SSRIs, SNRIs, TCAs, and MAOIs. Inform that drug may cause somnolence and dizziness; instruct to evaluate ability to perform complex tasks during migraine attacks and after administration of drug. Inform that medication should not be used during pregnancy unless the potential benefit justifies the potential risk to the fetus. Instruct to notify physician if breastfeeding or planning to breastfeed. Instruct on proper use of product and to avoid IM or IV use. Instruct to use inj sites on the abdomen (but not w/in 2 inches of the navel) or thigh w/ adequate SQ thickness to accommodate penetration of drug into the SQ space, and not on the arms or other areas of the body. Instruct patients not to use a device if the tip of the device is tilted or broken off upon removal from packaging.

SUPRAX — cefixime   Rx

Class: Cephalosporin (3rd generation)

ADULT DOSAGE	PEDIATRIC DOSAGE
General Dosing	**General Dosing**
400mg tab/cap qd or 1/2 tab q12h	**≥6 Months of Age:**
	Sus:
***Streptococcus pyogenes* Infection:**	8mg/kg qd or 4mg/kg q12h
Administer for at least 10 days	
	>12 Years or >45kg:
Gonorrhea	Use adult dose
Uncomplicated Cervical/Urethral Infections:	***Streptococcus pyogenes* Infection:**
400mg single dose	Administer for at least 10 days
Other Indications	**Otitis Media:**
- Uncomplicated UTIs	Treat w/ chewable tab or sus; do not
- Otitis media	substitute tab or cap for chewable
- Pharyngitis	tab or sus
- Tonsillitis	
- Acute exacerbation of chronic	Refer to PI for Pediatric Dosage Chart
bronchitis	

DOSING CONSIDERATIONS
Renal Impairment
Adults:
CrCl 21-59mL/min or on Hemodialysis: 13mL/day of 100mg/5mL sus; 6.5mL/day of 200mg/5mL sus; 2.6mL/day of 500mg/5mL sus
CrCl ≤20mL/min or on Continuous Peritoneal Dialysis: 8.6mL of 100mg/5mL sus; 4.4mL/day of 200mg/5mL sus; 1.8mL/day of 500mg/5mL sus; 200mg/day of tab; or 200mg of tab, chewable

ADMINISTRATION
Oral route

Cap/Tab
Take w/ or w/o food.

Tab, Chewable
Chew or crush before swallowing.

Sus
Refer to PI for reconstitution directions.
After reconstitution, may keep sus for 14 days either at room temperature or under refrigeration.
Keep tightly closed; shake well before using.
Discard unused portion after 14 days.

STORAGE
20-25°C (68-77°F).

HOW SUPPLIED
Cap: 400mg; **Sus:** 100mg/5mL [50mL, 75mL, 100mL], 200mg/5mL [25mL, 37.5mL, 50mL, 75mL, 100mL], 500mg/5mL [10mL, 20mL]; **Tab, Chewable:** 100mg, 150mg, 200mg; **Tab:** 400mg* *scored

CONTRAINDICATIONS
Known allergy to cefixime or other cephalosporins.

WARNINGS/PRECAUTIONS
Anaphylactic/anaphylactoid reactions reported. Cross hypersensitivity among β-lactam antibiotics reported; caution in patients w/ penicillin (PCN) sensitivity. D/C if an allergic reaction occurs. *Clostridium difficile*-associated diarrhea (CDAD) reported; may need to d/c if CDAD is suspected or confirmed. Carefully monitor patients on dialysis. May be associated w/ fall in prothrombin activity; caution in patients w/ renal/hepatic impairment, poor nutritional state, protracted course of antimicrobial therapy, and those previously stabilized on anticoagulant therapy. May result in bacterial resistance if used in the absence of proven/suspected bacterial infection. Lab test interactions may occur.

ADVERSE REACTIONS
Diarrhea, loose or frequent stools, abdominal pain, nausea, dyspepsia, flatulence.

DRUG INTERACTIONS
May increase levels of carbamazepine. Increased PT, w/ or w/o bleeding, w/ anticoagulants (eg, warfarin).

PREGNANCY AND LACTATION
Pregnancy: Category B.
Lactation: Not for use in nursing.

MECHANISM OF ACTION
Cephalosporin (3rd generation); bactericidal action results from inhibition of cell-wall synthesis.

PHARMACOKINETICS
Absorption: (Tab/Sus) 40-50%. C_{max}=2mcg/mL (200mg tab), 3.7mcg/mL (400mg tab), 3mcg/mL (200mg tab), 4.6mcg/mL (400mg sus); T_{max}=2-6 hrs (200mg tab, 400mg tab/sus), 2-5 hrs (200mg sus), 3-8 hrs (400mg cap). **Distribution:** Serum protein binding (65%). **Elimination:** Urine (50% unchanged); $T_{1/2}$=3-4 hrs but may range up to 9 hrs.

PATIENT CONSIDERATIONS
Assessment: Assess for previous hypersensitivity to cephalosporins, PCNs, or other drugs. Assess renal/hepatic function, nutritional status, history of antimicrobial or anticoagulants use, pregnancy/nursing status, and for possible drug interactions.

Monitoring: Monitor for signs/symptoms of anaphylactic/anaphylactoid reactions and CDAD. Monitor PT and renal function.

Counseling: Inform that therapy only treats bacterial, not viral, infections. Instruct to take exactly ud; inform that skipping doses or not completing full course of therapy may decrease effectiveness and increase risk of bacterial resistance. Inform that diarrhea may be experienced as late as 2 or more months after last dose; instruct to contact physician if watery/bloody stools (w/ or w/o stomach cramps and fever) occur. Inform that chewable tabs contain phenylalanine.

SUPREP — magnesium sulfate/potassium sulfate/sodium sulfate   Rx

Class: Bowel cleanser

ADULT DOSAGE
Bowel Cleansing
Prior to Colonoscopy:
Split-Dose (2-Day) Regimen:
Day Prior to Colonoscopy:
1. A light breakfast may be consumed, or have only clear liquids; avoid red and purple liquids, milk, and alcoholic beverages
2. Early in the pm, pour the contents of 1 bottle into the mixing container provided, fill the container w/ water to the 16 oz fill line, and drink the entire amount
3. Drink 2 additional containers filled to the 16 oz line w/ water over the next hr

Day of Colonoscopy:
1. Have only clear liquids until after the colonoscopy; avoid red and purple liquids, milk, and alcoholic beverages
2. The morning of colonoscopy (10-12 hrs after the evening dose), pour the contents of the 2nd bottle into the mixing container provided, fill the container w/ water to the 16 oz fill line, and drink the entire amount
3. Drink 2 additional containers filled to the 16 oz line w/ water over the next hr
4. Complete all Suprep Bowel Prep Kit and required water at least 1 hr prior to colonoscopy

PEDIATRIC DOSAGE
Pediatric use may not have been established

ADMINISTRATION
Oral route

STORAGE
20-25°C (68-77°F); excursions permitted between 15-30°C (59-86°F).

HOW SUPPLIED
Sol: (Sodium Sulfate/Potassium Sulfate/Magnesium Sulfate) 17.5g/3.13g/1.6g

CONTRAINDICATIONS
GI obstruction, bowel perforation, gastric retention, ileus, toxic colitis or toxic megacolon, known allergies to components of the kit.

WARNINGS/PRECAUTIONS
Hydrate adequately before, during, and after use. If significant vomiting or signs of dehydration occur, consider performing postcolonoscopy tests (eg, electrolytes, creatinine, BUN). Correct electrolyte abnormalities prior to use. Caution w/ conditions that may increase the risk of fluid/electrolyte disturbances and renal impairment. May increase uric acid levels. Serious arrhythmias reported rarely; caution in patients at increased risk of arrhythmias. Generalized tonic-clonic seizures and/or loss of consciousness reported; caution in patients at increased risk of seizures (eg, hyponatremia, alcohol or benzodiazepine withdrawal). May produce colonic mucosal aphthous ulcerations and ischemic colitis. If suspected, rule out GI obstruction or perforation prior to administration. Caution in patients w/ impaired gag reflex and patients prone to regurgitation/aspiration; observe during administration. Not for direct ingestion.

ADVERSE REACTIONS
Overall discomfort, abdominal distention, abdominal pain, N/V.

DRUG INTERACTIONS
Caution w/ concomitant use of medications that increase the risk for fluid and electrolyte disturbances or increase the risk of seizures (eg, TCAs), arrhythmias and prolonged QT. Caution w/ medications that may affect renal function (eg, diuretics, ACE inhibitors, ARBs, NSAIDs). Concurrent use w/ stimulant laxatives may increase risk of colonic mucosal ulcerations and ischemic colitis. Absorption of oral medications may not occur if administered w/in an hr of the start of a Suprep dose.

PREGNANCY AND LACTATION
Category C, caution in nursing.

MECHANISM OF ACTION
Bowel cleanser: sulfate salts provide sulfate anions that are poorly absorbed. The osmotic effect of the unabsorbed sulfate anions and the associated cations causes water to be retained w/in the GI tract.

PHARMACOKINETICS
Absorption: T_{max}=17 hrs (1st dose), 5 hrs (2nd dose). **Elimination:** Feces (primary), $T_{1/2}$=8.5 hrs.

PATIENT CONSIDERATIONS
Assessment: Assess for GI obstruction, bowel perforation, or any other conditions where treatment is contraindicated or cautioned. Assess for pregnancy/nursing status, and for possible drug interactions. Obtain baseline electrolytes, creatinine, and BUN in patients w/ renal impairment. Perform baseline ECGs in patients at risk for arrhythmias.

Monitoring: Monitor for electrolyte abnormalities, cardiac arrhythmias, seizures, loss of consciousness, colonic mucosal ulcerations, ischemic colitis, and aspiration. Perform ECG in patients at increased risk of serious cardiac arrhythmias. Monitor electrolytes, creatinine, and BUN in patients w/ renal impairment.

Counseling: Instruct to notify physician if patient has difficulty swallowing or is prone to regurgitation/aspiration. Instruct to dilute each bottle w/ water prior to ingestion and drink additional water ud by instructions. Advise that ingestion of undiluted solution may increase risk of N/V and dehydration. Inform that oral medications may not be absorbed properly if they are taken w/in 1 hr of starting each dose of Suprep Bowel Kit. Instruct not to take additional laxatives.

SURFAXIN — lucinactant   Rx

Class: Lung surfactant

PEDIATRIC DOSAGE
Respiratory Distress Syndrome
Prevention in Premature Infants at High Risk:
Reduces incidence at 24 hrs and mortality due to respiratory distress syndrome

Usual: 5.8mL/kg birth weight. Up to 4 doses can be administered in the first 48 hrs of life; give doses no more frequently than q6h

---

ADMINISTRATION
Intratracheal route

Preparation
Before use, warm vial for 15 min in a preheated dry block heater set at 44°C (111°F). After warming, shake vial vigorously until product is a uniform and free-flowing sus.
If not used immediately after warming, may be stored, protected from light, at room temperature for up to 2 hrs; do not return to refrigerator after warming and discard if not used w/in 2 hrs of warming.

Administration
1. Draw up appropriate amount into a single, appropriately sized syringe, depending on total dose volume, using a 16- or 18-gauge needle
2. Before administering, assure proper placement and patency of the endotracheal tube; at the discretion of the clinician, endotracheal tube may be suctioned before administering; allow infant to stabilize before proceeding w/ dosing
3. Position infant in the right lateral decubitus position w/ head and thorax inclined upward 30°
4. Attach syringe containing sus to a 5 French end-hole catheter; thread catheter through a Bodai valve or equivalent device that allows maintenance of positive end-expiratory pressure and then advance the tip of the catheter into the endotracheal tube. Position the catheter such that its tip is slightly distal to the end of the endotracheal tube
5. Each dose should be delivered in 4 aliquots
6. Instill 1st aliquot of the dose (1/4 of total volume) as a bolus while continuing positive pressure mechanical ventilation and maintaining positive end-expiratory pressure of 4-5cm H_2O

7. Ventilator settings may be adjusted at the discretion of the clinician to maintain appropriate oxygenation and ventilation. Ventilate until infant is stable, (ie, has an oxygen saturation of at least 90% and a HR>120bpm)

8. Repeat procedure w/ infant in the left decubitus position while maintaining adequate positive pressure ventilation

9. Repeat procedure w/ infant in the right, then left decubitus position to deliver a total of 4 aliquots; a pause should separate administration of the aliquots to allow for an evaluation of the infant's respiratory status

10. After instillation of last aliquot, remove catheter and resume usual ventilator management and critical care while keeping the head of the infant's bed elevated at least 10° for at least 1-2 hrs. Do not suction the infant during the 1st hr after dosing unless signs of significant airway obstruction occur

STORAGE
2-8°C (36-46°F). Protect from light. Do not freeze. Warmed Vial: Room temperature, protected from light (in the carton), for up to 2 hrs. Do not return to the refrigerator after warming. Discard if not used within 2 hours of warming.

HOW SUPPLIED
Sus: 8.5mL

WARNINGS/PRECAUTIONS
For intratracheal administration only. Can rapidly affect lung compliance and oxygenation; should be administered only by clinicians trained and experienced in the resuscitation, intubation, stabilization, and ventilatory management of premature infants in a clinical setting with the capacity to care for critically ill neonates. Perform frequent clinical assessments so that oxygen and ventilatory support can be modified to respond to changes in respiratory status. Administration-related adverse reactions (eg, bradycardia, oxygen desaturation, reflux of drug into the endotracheal tube [ETT], airway/ETT obstruction) frequently reported; if any of these occur, interrupt dosing, and assess/stabilize infant's clinical condition. Suctioning of the ETT or reintubation may be required if airway obstruction persists or is severe. Dosing may proceed with appropriate monitoring once patient is stable.

ADVERSE REACTIONS
Oxygen desaturation, bradycardia, ETT reflux/obstruction, pallor, apnea, intraventricular hemorrhage, periventricular leukomalacia, acquired sepsis, patent ductus arteriosus, retinopathy of prematurity, necrotizing enterocolitis, pulmonary interstitial emphysema, pneumothorax, pulmonary hemorrhage.

PREGNANCY AND LACTATION
Safety in pregnancy and nursing not known.

MECHANISM OF ACTION
Lung surfactant; lowers surface tension at the air-liquid interface of the alveolar surfaces during respiration and stabilizes the alveoli against collapse at resting transpulmonary pressures. Compensates for the deficiency of surfactant and restores surface activity to the lungs of infants.

PATIENT CONSIDERATIONS
Assessment: Assess respiratory status.

Monitoring: Monitor for acute changes in lung compliance, administration-related adverse reactions (eg, bradycardia, oxygen desaturation, ETT reflux, airway/ETT obstruction), and other adverse effects.

Counseling: Inform parent/caregiver about the risks/benefits of therapy.

SURVANTA INTRATRACHEAL SUSPENSION –
beractant   **Rx**

Class: Lung surfactant

PEDIATRIC DOSAGE
Respiratory Distress Syndrome

Reduces incidence and mortality due to respiratory distress syndrome and air leak complications

100mg of phospholipids/kg birth weight (4mL/kg) per dose. May administer 4 doses in the first 48 hrs of life; administer no more frequently than q6h

Prevention:
Administer as soon as possible, preferably w/in 15 min of birth in premature infants <1250g birth weight or w/ evidence of surfactant deficiency

Rescue Treatment:
Administer as soon as possible, preferably by 8 hrs of age for treatment of premature infants w/ respiratory distress syndrome confirmed by x-ray and requiring mechanical ventilation

---

ADMINISTRATION
Intratracheal route

Directions for Use
Gently swirl vial to redisperse if settling occurs during storage; do not shake. Before administration, product should be warmed by standing at room temperature for at least 20 min or warmed in the hand for at least 8 min; do not use artificial warming methods.
If a prevention dose is to be given, begin preparation before the infant's birth. Unopened, unused vials that have been warmed to room temperature may be returned to the refrigerator w/in 24 hrs of warming, and stored for future use; should not be warmed and returned to the refrigerator more than once.
Does not require reconstitution or sonication before use.

Dosing Procedures
Administer intratracheally by instillation through a 5 French end-hole catheter; catheter may be inserted into the infant's endotracheal tube w/o interrupting ventilation by passing the catheter through a neonatal suction valve attached to the endotracheal tube.
Alternatively, may be instilled through the catheter by briefly disconnecting the endotracheal tube from the ventilator.
Do not instill into a mainstem bronchus.
Divide each dose into 4 quarter-doses to ensure homogenous distribution throughout lungs; each quarter-dose is administered w/ the infant in a different position.
Refer to PI for further administration instructions.

STORAGE
Unopened Vial: 2-8°C. Protect from light.

HOW SUPPLIED
Sus: 25mg/mL [4mL, 8mL]

WARNINGS/PRECAUTIONS
For intratracheal use only. May rapidly affect oxygenation and lung compliance; restrict use for within a highly supervised clinical setting. Perform frequent monitoring with arterial or transcutaneous measurement of systemic oxygen and carbon dioxide. Transient episodes of bradycardia and decreased oxygen saturation reported; d/c if occurs and initiate appropriate measures. Use not studied in infants <600g birth weight or >1750g birth weight. Increased probability of post-treatment nosocomial sepsis reported. Rales and moist breath sounds may occur transiently following administration.

ADVERSE REACTIONS
Transient bradycardia, oxygen desaturation, intracranial hemorrhage, necrotizing enterocolitis, apnea, post-treatment sepsis, post-treatment infection, pulmonary hemorrhage.

MECHANISM OF ACTION
Lung surfactant; replenishes surfactant and restores surface activity to the lungs.

PATIENT CONSIDERATIONS
Assessment: Assess for RDS, blood oxygenation, and lung compliance.

Monitoring: Monitor for bradycardia, decreased oxygen saturation, rales, moist breath sounds, and for sepsis. Perform frequent monitoring with arterial or transcutaneous measurement of systemic oxygen and carbon dioxide.

Counseling: Inform parent/caregiver about risks/benefits of therapy.

SUTENT — sunitinib malate   **Rx**

Class: Kinase inhibitor

Hepatotoxicity has been observed; may be severe, and deaths have been reported.

ADULT DOSAGE
Gastrointestinal Stromal Tumor

After Disease Progression or Intolerance to Imatinib Mesylate:
50mg qd, on a schedule of 4 weeks on, followed by 2 weeks off

Advanced Renal Cell Carcinoma
50mg qd, on a schedule of 4 weeks on, followed by 2 weeks off

Advanced Pancreatic Neuroendocrine Tumors

Progressive, Well-Differentiated Tumors w/ Unresectable Locally Advanced or Metastatic Disease:
37.5mg qd continuously w/o a scheduled off-treatment period

PEDIATRIC DOSAGE
Pediatric use may not have been established

DOSING CONSIDERATIONS
Concomitant Medications
Selection of an alternate concomitant medication w/ no or minimal enzyme inhibition/induction potential is recommended

Strong CYP3A4 Inhibitors:
GI Stromal Tumors/Advanced Renal Cell Carcinoma: Consider dose reduction to a minimum of 37.5mg qd

Advanced Pancreatic Neuroendocrine Tumors: Consider dose reduction to a minimum of 25mg qd

CYP3A4 Inducers:
GI Stromal Tumors/Advanced Renal Cell Carcinoma: Consider dose increase to a max of 87.5mg qd
Advanced Pancreatic Neuroendocrine Tumors: Consider dose increase to a max of 62.5mg qd

Renal Impairment
ESRD on Hemodialysis: May increase gradually up to 2-fold based on safety and tolerability for subsequent doses

Other Important Considerations
Interruption and/or modification in 12.5mg increments or decrements is recommended based on individual safety and tolerability

ADMINISTRATION
Oral route

Take w/ or w/o food.

STORAGE
25°C (77°F); excursions permitted to 15-30°C (59-86°F).

HOW SUPPLIED
Cap: 12.5mg, 25mg, 37.5mg, 50mg

WARNINGS/PRECAUTIONS
Interrupt therapy for Grade 3 or 4 hepatic adverse events; d/c if no resolution. Do not restart treatment if subsequent severe changes in LFTs or other signs/symptoms of liver failure occur. May cause fetal harm; avoid pregnancy. D/C in the presence of clinical manifestations of CHF, and interrupt and/or reduce dose in patients w/o clinical evidence of CHF but w/ ejection fraction <50% and >20% below baseline. Cardiovascular (CV) events, including heart failure, cardiomyopathy, myocardial ischemia, and MI reported; use w/ caution in patients who are at risk for, or have a history of, these events. Decline in left ventricular ejection fraction (LVEF) reported. Dose-dependent QT interval prolongation and torsades de pointes reported; caution w/ history of QT interval prolongation or preexisting cardiac disease, bradycardia, or electrolyte disturbances. Monitor for HTN and treat prn; temporarily suspend in cases of severe HTN until controlled. Hemorrhagic events, including tumor-related hemorrhage and pulmonary hemorrhage, reported. Serious, sometimes fatal GI complications (eg, GI perforation) reported w/ intra-abdominal malignancies. Tumor lysis syndrome (TLS) reported; closely monitor patients presenting w/ a high tumor burden prior to treatment and treat as clinically indicated. Thrombotic microangiopathy (TMA), including thrombotic thrombocytopenic purpura and hemolytic syndrome, reported; d/c if TMA develops. Proteinuria and nephrotic syndrome reported; interrupt and reduce dose for 24-hr urine protein ≥3g. D/C therapy for patients w/ nephrotic syndrome or repeat episodes of urine protein ≥3g despite dose reductions. Severe cutaneous reactions (eg, erythema multiforme, Stevens Johnson syndrome [SJS], toxic epidermal necrolysis [TEN]) reported; d/c therapy if signs/symptoms are present and do not restart treatment if a diagnosis of SJS or TEN is suspected. Necrotizing fasciitis reported; d/c therapy in patients who develop necrotizing fasciitis. Hyperthyroidism, some followed by hypothyroidism, reported; observe closely for signs/symptoms of thyroid dysfunction (eg, hypo/hyperthyroidism, thyroiditis). Associated w/ symptomatic hypoglycemia, resulting in loss of consciousness, or requiring hospitalization; reductions in blood glucose may be worse in diabetic patients. Osteonecrosis of the jaw (ONJ) reported; exposure to risk factors (eg, dental disease) may increase the risk of ONJ. Impaired wound healing reported; interrupt temporarily in patients undergoing major surgical procedures. Monitor for adrenal insufficiency in patients w/ stress, trauma, or severe infection.

ADVERSE REACTIONS
Fatigue, asthenia, fever, diarrhea, N/V, mucositis/stomatitis, dyspepsia, abdominal pain, constipation, HTN, peripheral edema, rash, hand-foot syndrome, skin discoloration.

DRUG INTERACTIONS
See Dosing Considerations. Caution w/ antiarrhythmics for QT interval prolongation/torsades de pointes. Strong CYP3A4 inhibitors (eg, ketoconazole, nefazodone, ritonavir) and grapefruit may increase levels. CYP3A4 inducers (eg, dexamethasone, phenytoin, rifampin) may decrease levels. Avoid w/ St. John's wort. TMA reported w/ bevacizumab. Concomitant use w/ bisphosphonates may increase the risk of ONJ.

PREGNANCY AND LACTATION
Pregnancy: Category D. May cause fetal harm; avoid pregnancy.
Lactation: Not for use in nursing.

MECHANISM OF ACTION
Multikinase inhibitor; inhibits multiple receptor tyrosine kinases, some of which are implicated in tumor growth, pathologic angiogenesis, and metastatic cancer progression.

PHARMACOKINETICS
Absorption: T_{max}=6-12 hrs. **Distribution:** V_d=2230L; plasma protein binding (95%, 90%[primary active metabolite]). **Metabolism:** Liver via CYP3A4. **Elimination:** Feces (61%), urine (16%); $T_{1/2}$=40-60 hrs, 80-110 hrs (primary active metabolite).

PATIENT CONSIDERATIONS
Assessment: Assess for risk/history of cardiac events, cardiac disease, bradycardia, electrolyte disturbances, dental disease, high tumor burden, diabetes, pregnancy/nursing status, and possible drug interactions. Obtain baseline LFTs, LVEF, thyroid function, CBC w/ platelet count, serum chemistries (eg, phosphate), and urinalysis.

Monitoring: Monitor for signs/symptoms of CV events, HTN, hemorrhagic events, ONJ, TLS, TMA, adrenal insufficiency, hepatotoxicity, nephrotic syndrome, severe cutaneous reactions, necrotizing fasciitis, and other adverse reactions. Monitor LFTs, LVEF (in patients w/ cardiac risk factors), ECG, electrolytes (Mg^{2+}, K^+), thyroid function, CBC w/ platelet count, and serum chemistries (eg, phosphate). Monitor blood glucose levels regularly during and after discontinuation of treatment. Perform periodic urinalysis w/ follow-up measurement of 24-hr urine protein as clinically indicated.

Counseling: Inform about the most commonly reported GI disorders and other adverse reactions that may occur. Advise that depigmentation of the hair or skin and other possible dermatologic effects may occur during treatment. Inform that severe dermatologic toxicities (eg, SJS, TEN) have been reported; advise to immediately inform physician if severe dermatologic reactions occur. Advise to consider a dental examination and appropriate preventive dentistry prior to treatment. Instruct to avoid invasive dental procedures if previously or concomitantly taking bisphosphonates. Advise of the signs, symptoms, and risks associated w/ hypoglycemia that may occur while on therapy; instruct to immediately inform physician if severe signs/symptoms of hypoglycemia occur. Inform of the signs/symptoms of TMA; instruct to inform physician if TMA occurs. Advise that urinalysis will be performed prior to and during treatment. Advise to inform physician of all concomitant medications, including OTC medications and dietary supplements. Inform of pregnancy risks; advise women of childbearing potential to avoid becoming pregnant.

SYLATRON — peginterferon alfa-2b   **Rx**
Class: Biological response modifier

> Increased risk of serious depression, w/ suicidal ideation and completed suicides, and other serious neuropsychiatric disorders. Permanently d/c in patients w/ persistently severe or worsening signs or symptoms of depression, psychosis, or encephalopathy; may not resolve after stopping therapy.

ADULT DOSAGE	**PEDIATRIC DOSAGE**
Melanoma	Pediatric use may not have been established
Adjuvant treatment of melanoma w/ microscopic or gross nodal involvement w/in 84 days of definitive surgical resection including complete lymphadenectomy	
Initial: 6mcg/kg/week SQ for 8 doses **Follow-Up:** 3mcg/kg/week SQ for up to 5 yrs	
Premedication	
Acetaminophen 500-1000mg PO 30 min prior to 1st dose and prn for subsequent doses	

- -

DOSING CONSIDERATIONS
Renal Impairment
Moderate (CrCl 30-50mL/min/1.73m²):
Initial: 4.5mcg/kg/week for 8 weeks
Follow-Up: 2.25mcg/kg/week for 5 yrs
Severe (CrCl <30mL/min/1.73m²)/ESRD on Dialysis:
Initial: 3mcg/kg/week for 8 weeks
Follow-Up: 1.5mcg/kg/week for 5 yrs

Adverse Reactions
Permanently D/C Therapy for:
- Persistent or worsening severe neuropsychiatric disorders
- Grade 4 non-hematologic toxicity
- Inability to tolerate a dose of 1mcg/kg/week
- New or worsening retinopathy

Withhold Dose for Any of the Following:
- ANC <0.5 x 10⁹/L
- Platelet count (PLT) <50 x 10⁹/L
- ECOG PS ≥2
- Non-hematologic toxicity ≥Grade 3

Resume Dosing at Reduced Dose When All of the Following Are Present:
- ANC ≥0.5 x 10⁹/L
- PLT ≥50 x 10⁹/L
- ECOG PS 0-1
- Non-hematologic toxicity has completely resolved or improved to Grade 1

Sylatron Dose Modifications:
Patients Using 6mcg/kg/week for Doses 1-8:
1st Dose Modification: 3mcg/kg/week
2nd Dose Modification: 2mcg/kg/week
3rd Dose Modification: 1mcg/kg/week
Permanently d/c if unable to tolerate 1mcg/kg/week

Patients Using 3mcg/kg/week for Doses 9-260:
1st Dose Modification: 2mcg/kg/week
2nd Dose Modification: 1mcg/kg/week
Permanently d/c if unable to tolerate 1mcg/kg/week

ADMINISTRATION
SQ route

Rotate inj sites.
If reconstituted sol is not used immediately, store at 2-8°C (36-46°F) for no more than 24 hrs; discard after 24 hrs. Do not freeze.

Preparation and Administration

1. Reconstitute w/ 0.7mL of sterile water for inj.
2. Swirl gently to dissolve the lyophilized powder; do not shake.
3. Do not withdraw >0.5mL of reconstituted sol from each vial.

STORAGE
25°C (77°F); excursions permitted to 15-30°C (59-86°F). Do not freeze.

HOW SUPPLIED
Inj: 200mcg, 300mcg, 600mcg

CONTRAINDICATIONS
History of anaphylaxis to peginterferon alfa-2b or interferon alfa-2b, autoimmune hepatitis, hepatic decompensation (Child-Pugh score >6 [class B and C]).

WARNINGS/PRECAUTIONS
Monitor and evaluate for depression and other psychiatric symptoms every 3 weeks during the first 8 weeks of therapy, every 6 months thereafter, and for at least 6 months after the last dose. Cardiac adverse reactions reported; permanently d/c for new onset of ventricular arrhythmia or cardiovascular decompensation. May cause decrease in visual acuity or blindness due to retinopathy; retinal and ocular changes may be induced or aggravated by treatment. Perform an eye exam at baseline in patients w/ preexisting retinopathy and during therapy if visual changes occur; permanently d/c if new/worsening retinopathy develops. Increases risk of hepatic decompensation and death in patients w/ cirrhosis; permanently d/c for evidence of severe (Grade 3) hepatic injury/decompensation (Child-Pugh score >6 [class B and C]). Monitor hepatic function w/ serum bilirubin, ALT, AST, alkaline phosphatase, and LDH at 2 and 8 weeks, and 2 and 3 months following initiation, then every 6 months thereafter. May cause new onset/worsening of hypo/hyperthyroidism, and diabetes mellitus (DM); permanently d/c if any of these conditions develop and cannot be effectively managed. Obtain TSH levels w/in 4 weeks prior to initiation of therapy, at 3 and 6 months following initiation, then every 6 months thereafter while on therapy.

ADVERSE REACTIONS
Fatigue, increased AST/ALT, pyrexia, headache, anorexia, myalgia, nausea, chills, inj-site reaction.

DRUG INTERACTIONS
Increased exposure to caffeine (CYP1A2 substrate) or desipramine (CYP2D6 substrate) during coadministration; monitor for potential toxicities of drugs w/ a narrow therapeutic range metabolized by CYP1A2 or CYP2D6.

PREGNANCY AND LACTATION
Pregnancy: Category C.
Lactation: It is not known whether the components of Sylatron are excreted in human milk; not for use in nursing.

MECHANISM OF ACTION
Pleiotropic cytokine; mechanism not established.

PHARMACOKINETICS
Absorption: (6mcg/kg/week) C_{max}=4.4ng/mL, AUC=430ng•hr/mL; (3mcg/kg/week) C_{max}=2.5ng/mL, AUC=228ng•hr/mL. **Elimination:** $T_{1/2}$=(6mcg/kg/week) 51 hrs; (3mcg/kg/week) 43 hrs.

PATIENT CONSIDERATIONS
Assessment: Assess for history of autoimmune hepatitis, hepatic decompensation, cirrhosis, neuropsychiatric disorders, history of anaphylaxis to peginterferon alfa-2b or interferon alfa-2b, hypo/hyperthyroidism, DM, renal impairment, pregnancy/nursing status, and possible drug interactions. Perform baseline eye exam in patients w/ preexisting retinopathy. Obtain TSH levels w/in 4 weeks prior to therapy.

Monitoring: Monitor for cardiac adverse events, new/worsening retinopathy, and other adverse reactions. Obtain TSH levels at 3 and 6 months following initiation, then every 6 months thereafter while on therapy. Monitor and evaluate for depression and other psychiatric symptoms every 3 weeks during the first 8 weeks of therapy, every 6 months thereafter, and for at least 6 months after the last dose. Monitor CBC and platelet counts periodically. Monitor hepatic function w/ serum bilirubin, ALT, AST, alkaline phosphatase, and LDH at 2 and 8 weeks, and 2 and 3 months following initiation, then every 6 months thereafter. Perform eye exam if visual changes develop.

Counseling: Advise that drug may be administered w/ antipyretics at hs to minimize common flu-like symptoms, and advise to maintain hydration if symptoms occur. Instruct to report immediately any symptoms of depression or suicidal ideation to physician during treatment and up to 6 months after the last dose. Advise to notify physician in the event of pregnancy. Instruct not to reuse or share syringes and needles. Instruct on proper disposal of vials, syringes, and needles.

SYLVANT — siltuximab   Rx

Class: Monoclonal antibody/interleukin-6 (IL-6) receptor antagonist

ADULT DOSAGE
Multicentric Castleman's Disease

Treatment of patients who are HIV negative and human herpesvirus-8 negative

11mg/kg given over 1 hr as an IV infusion administered every 3 weeks until treatment failure

Perform hematology lab tests prior to

PEDIATRIC DOSAGE
Pediatric use may not have been established

each dose for the first 12 months and every 3 dosing cycles thereafter. If treatment criteria outlined below are not met, consider delaying treatment; do not reduce dose

Treatment Criteria
Requirements Prior to 1st Dose:
ANC: ≥1.0 x 10^9/L
Platelet Count: ≥75 x 10^9/L
Hgb: <17 g/dL
Retreatment Criteria:
ANC: ≥1.0 x 10^9/L
Platelet Count: ≥50 x 10^9/L
Hgb: <17 g/dL

DOSING CONSIDERATIONS
Adverse Reactions
D/C in patients w/ severe infusion related reactions, anaphylaxis, severe allergic reactions, or cytokine release syndromes; do not reinstitute treatment

Other Important Considerations
Do not administer to patients w/ severe infections until the infection resolves

ADMINISTRATION
IV route

Preparation
1. Calculate the dose (mg), total volume (mL) of reconstituted sol required, and the number of vials needed. A 21-gauge 1-1/2 inch needle is recommended for preparation. Infusion bags (250mL) must contain D5W and must be made of polyvinyl chloride, polyolefin, polypropylene, or polyethylene. Alternatively, polyethylene bottles may be used.
2. Allow the vial(s) to come to room temperature over approx 30 min. Sylvant should remain at room temperature for the duration of the preparation.
3. Reconstitute each vial as follows:
100mg Vial: Reconstitute w/ 5.2mL of sterile water for inj (SWFI)
400mg Vial: Reconstitute w/ 20mL of SWFI
4. Gently swirl reconstituted vials; do not shake or swirl vigorously. The lyophilized powder should dissolve in <60 min. Reconstituted product should be kept for no more than 2 hrs prior to addition into the infusion bag.
5. Dilute the reconstituted sol dose to 250mL w/ sterile D5W by withdrawing a volume equal to the total calculated volume of reconstituted sol from the D5W, 250 mL bag.
6. Slowly add the total calculated volume (mL) of reconstituted sol to the D5W infusion bag. Gently invert the bag to mix the sol.

Administration
Administer the diluted sol by IV infusion over a period of 1 hr using administration sets lined w/ polyvinyl chloride, polyurethane, or polyethylene, containing a 0.2µm inline polyethersulfone filter. The infusion should be completed w/in 4 hrs of the dilution of the reconstituted sol to the infusion bag.
Do not infuse concomitantly in the same IV line w/ other agents.
Do not store any unused portion of the reconstituted product or of the infusion sol.

STORAGE
2-8°C (36-46°F). Protect from light.

HOW SUPPLIED
Inj: 100mg, 400mg

CONTRAINDICATIONS
Severe hypersensitivity reaction to siltuximab or any of the excipients in the product.

WARNINGS/PRECAUTIONS
May increase Hgb levels. Do not administer to patients w/ severe infections until the infection resolves. May mask signs and symptoms of acute inflammation including suppression of fever and of acute phase reactants (eg, C-reactive protein). D/C if signs of anaphylaxis or mild to moderate infusion reaction develops. If the infusion reaction resolves, may restart infusion at a lower infusion rate and consider medication w/ antihistamines, acetaminophen, and corticosteroids; d/c if the patient does not tolerate the infusion following these interventions. Administer in a setting that provides resuscitation equipment, medication, and personnel trained to provide resuscitation. GI perforation reported. Women of childbearing potential should use contraception during and for 3 months after treatment.

ADVERSE REACTIONS
Pruritus, increased weight, rash, hyperuricemia, URTI.

DRUG INTERACTIONS
Do not administer live vaccines. May increase metabolism of CYP450 substrates; upon initiation or discontinuation of siltuximab, in patients being treated w/ CYP450 substrates w/ a narrow therapeutic index, perform therapeutic monitoring of effect (eg, warfarin) or drug concentration (eg, cyclosporine, theophylline) prn and adjust dose. Caution w/ CYP3A4 substrates where a decrease in effectiveness would be undesirable (eg, oral contraceptives, lovastatin, atorvastatin).

PREGNANCY AND LACTATION
Pregnancy: Category C. Infants born to pregnant women treated w/ siltuximab may be at increased risk of infection. Women of childbearing potential should use contraception during and for 3 months after treatment.
Lactation: Not for use in nursing.

MECHANISM OF ACTION

Monoclonal antibody/IL-6 receptor antagonist; binds human IL-6 and prevents the binding of IL-6 to both soluble and membrane-bound IL-6 receptors.

PHARMACOKINETICS

Absorption: C_{max}=332mcg/mL. **Distribution:** V_d=4.5L (70kg male). **Elimination:** $T_{1/2}$=20.6 days.

PATIENT CONSIDERATIONS

Assessment: Assess for infection, risk for GI perforation, drug hypersensitivity, pregnancy/nursing status, and possible drug interactions. Perform hematology lab tests prior to each dose of therapy for the first 12 months and every 3 dosing cycles thereafter.

Monitoring: Monitor for signs/symptoms of infection, infusion-related reactions, hypersensitivity, GI perforation, and other adverse reactions.

Counseling: Inform of benefits and risks of treatment. Instruct to immediately contact physician when symptoms suggesting infection or any signs of new/worsening medical conditions appear. Advise to seek immediate medical attention if any symptoms of a serious allergic reaction occur during the infusion. Advise patients of childbearing potential to avoid pregnancy; instruct to use contraception during and for 3 months after treatment.

SYMBICORT — budesonide/formoterol fumarate dihydrate   Rx

Class: Corticosteroid/long-acting beta₂ agonist (LABA)

> Long-acting β₂-adrenergic agonists (LABAs), such as formoterol, increase the risk of asthma-related death. LABAs may increase the risk of asthma-related hospitalization in pediatric patients and adolescents. Use only for patients not adequately controlled on a long-term asthma-control medication or whose disease severity clearly warrants initiation of treatment with both inhaled corticosteroids and LABA. Do not use if asthma is adequately controlled on low- or medium-dose inhaled corticosteroids.

ADULT DOSAGE

Asthma

2 inh bid (am and pm, approx q12h)
Initial: Based on severity
Max: (160mcg/4.5mcg)/inh bid

Not Responding After 1-2 Weeks of Therapy w/ (80mcg/4.5mcg)/inh: Replace w/ (160mcg/4.5mcg)/inh for better asthma control

Chronic Obstructive Pulmonary Disease

Maint Treatment of Airflow Obstruction:
2 inh ([160mcg/4.5mcg]/inh) bid

PEDIATRIC DOSAGE

Asthma

≥12 Years:
2 inh bid (am and pm, approx q12h)
Initial: Based on severity
Max: (160mcg/4.5mcg)/inh bid

Not Responding After 1-2 Weeks of Therapy w/ (80mcg/4.5mcg)/inh: Replace w/ (160mcg/4.5mcg)/inh for better asthma control

ADMINISTRATION

Oral inh route

After inh, rinse mouth w/ water w/o swallowing.
Shake well for 5 sec before use.

Priming

1. Shake the inhaler well for 5 sec.
2. Hold the inhaler pointing away from the face and then release a test spray.
3. Shake it again for 5 sec and release a 2nd test spray.
4. Depending on which size was provided, the counter will read either 120 or 60 after it has been primed.

If inhaler is not used for more than 7 days or if it is dropped, prime again.

STORAGE

20-25°C (68-77°F). Store with mouthpiece down. Contents under pressure; do not puncture, incinerate, or store near heat or open flame. Discard when labeled number of inhalations have been used or within 3 months after removal from pouch.

HOW SUPPLIED

MDI: (Budesonide/Formoterol) (80mcg/4.5mcg)/inh, (160mcg/4.5mcg)/inh [60 inhalations, 120 inhalations]

CONTRAINDICATIONS

Primary treatment of status asthmaticus or other acute episodes of asthma or COPD where intensive measures are required. Hypersensitivity to any of the ingredients in Symbicort.

WARNINGS/PRECAUTIONS

Not indicated for the relief of acute bronchospasm; take inhaled short-acting β₂-agonists (SABAs) for immediate relief. Do not initiate during rapidly deteriorating/potentially life-threatening asthma or COPD. D/C regular use of oral/inhaled SABAs when beginning treatment. Cardiovascular (CV) effects and fatalities reported with excessive use; do not use more often or at higher doses than recommended. *Candida albicans* infections of the mouth and pharynx reported; treat with appropriate local or systemic (eg, antifungal) therapy or, interrupt therapy if needed. Lower respiratory tract infections (eg, pneumonia) reported in patients with COPD. Increased susceptibility to infections. May lead to serious/fatal course of chickenpox or measles; avoid exposure and, if exposed, consider prophylaxis/treatment. Caution with active/quiescent tuberculosis (TB); untreated systemic fungal, bacterial, viral, or parasitic infections; or ocular herpes simplex. Deaths due to adrenal insufficiency reported with transfer from systemic to inhaled corticosteroids; if systemic corticosteroids are required, wean slowly from systemic steroid after transferring to therapy. Resume oral corticosteroids during periods of stress or a severe asthma attack if patient was previously withdrawn from systemic corticosteroid. Carefully monitor during withdrawal of oral corticosteroid. Transferring from systemic to inhalation therapy may unmask previously suppressed allergic conditions (eg, rhinitis, conjunctivitis, eczema, arthritis, eosinophilic conditions); monitor for systemic corticosteroid withdrawal effects. Observe carefully for any evidence of systemic corticosteroid effects; caution should be taken in observing patients postoperatively or during periods of stress for evidence of inadequate adrenal response. Reduce dose slowly if hypercorticism or adrenal suppression (including adrenal crisis) appears. May produce paradoxical bronchospasm; d/c immediately and institute alternative therapy. Immediate hypersensitivity reactions (eg, urticaria, angioedema, rash, bronchospasm) may occur. Caution with CV disorders (eg, coronary insufficiency, cardiac arrhythmias, HTN). Decreases in bone mineral density (BMD) reported; caution with major risk factors for decreased bone mineral content (eg, prolonged immobilization, family history of osteoporosis, postmenopausal status, tobacco use, advanced age, poor nutrition). May reduce growth velocity in pediatrics; use lowest effective dose. Glaucoma, increased IOP, cataracts, rare cases of systemic eosinophilic conditions, and vasculitis consistent with Churg-Strauss syndrome reported. Caution with convulsive disorders, thyrotoxicosis, diabetes mellitus (DM), ketoacidosis, hepatic impairment, and in patients unusually responsive to sympathomimetic amines. Clinically significant changes in blood glucose and/or serum K⁺ reported. Caution in elderly.

ADVERSE REACTIONS

Nasopharyngitis, headache, URTI, pharyngolaryngeal pain, sinusitis, influenza, back pain, nasal congestion, stomach discomfort, oral candidiasis, bronchitis, vomiting.

DRUG INTERACTIONS

Do not use with other medications containing LABAs (eg, salmeterol, formoterol fumarate, arformoterol tartrate); increased risk of CV effects. Caution with ketoconazole, other known strong CYP3A4 inhibitors (eg, ritonavir, nefazodone, telithromycin, itraconazole), and non-K⁺-sparing diuretics (eg, loop, thiazide). Caution with MAOIs or TCAs, or within 2 weeks of discontinuation of such agents. Concomitant use with β-blockers may produce severe bronchospasm in patients with asthma; consider cardioselective β-blockers and administer with caution. Caution with chronic use of drugs that can reduce bone mass (eg, anticonvulsants, oral corticosteroids).

PREGNANCY AND LACTATION

Pregnancy: Category C.
Lactation: Not for use in nursing.

MECHANISM OF ACTION

Budesonide: Corticosteroid; shown to have inhibitory activities on multiple cell types and mediators involved in allergic and nonallergic mediated inflammation. Formoterol: LABA; attributable to stimulation of intracellular adenyl cyclase, that catalyzes the conversion of ATP to cAMP. Increased cAMP levels cause relaxation of bronchial smooth muscle and inhibition of release of mediators of immediate hypersensitivity from cells, especially mast cells.

PHARMACOKINETICS

Absorption: Rapid. Administration of various doses resulted in different pharmacokinetic parameters. **Distribution:** Budesonide: V_d=3L/kg; plasma protein binding (85-90%). Formoterol: Plasma protein binding (RR enantiomer, 46%), (SS enantiomer, 58%). **Metabolism:** Budesonide: Liver (rapid and extensive) via CYP3A4. Formoterol: Liver (direct glucuronidation and O-demethylation) via CYP2D6, CYP2C. **Elimination:** Budesonide: Urine (60%); feces. $T_{1/2}$=2-3 hrs. Formoterol: (Healthy) Urine (62%); feces (24%).

PATIENT CONSIDERATIONS

Assessment: Assess use of long-term asthma control medication (eg, inhaled corticosteroids), status asthmaticus, acute asthma episodes, rapidly deteriorating asthma, bronchospasm, known hypersensitivity to any component of drug, risk factors for decreased bone mineral content, CV or convulsive disorders, other conditions where treatment is contraindicated or cautioned, pregnancy/nursing status, and possible drug interactions. Assess use in patients unusually responsive to sympathomimetic amines. Obtain baseline BMD, eye exam, and lung function.

Monitoring: Monitor for localized oral *C. albicans* infections, worsening or acutely deteriorating asthma, development of glaucoma, increased IOP, cataracts, CV/CNS effects, inhalation induced paradoxical bronchospasm, pneumonia, lower respiratory tract in patients with COPD, hypercorticism, adrenal suppression, hypersensitivity reactions, signs of increased drug exposure with hepatic impairment, and other adverse reactions. Monitor lung function, pulse rate, BP, ECG changes, blood glucose, and serum K⁺ levels. Monitor BMD periodically. Monitor growth in children.

Counseling: Inform about increased risk of asthma-related death/hospitalization in pediatrics and adolescents. Instruct not to use to relieve acute asthma symptoms; treat acute symptoms with an inhaled SABA for immediate relief. Instruct to notify physician immediately if experiencing decreased effectiveness of inhaled SABA, need for more inhalations of inhaled SABA than usual, or significant decrease in lung function. Instruct not to d/c without physician's guidance. Instruct not to use with other LABA for asthma and COPD. Advise that localized infections with *C. albicans* may occur in the mouth and pharynx. Instruct to contact physician if symptoms of pneumonia develop. Instruct to avoid exposure to chickenpox or measles and to consult physician without delay, if exposed. Inform of potential worsening of existing TB, fungal, bacterial, viral, or parasitic infections, or ocular herpes simplex.

Inform about risks of hypercorticism and adrenal suppression, decreased BMD, cataracts or glaucoma, and reduced growth velocity in pediatric patients. Instruct to taper slowly from systemic corticosteroids if transferring to budesonide-formoterol. Inform of adverse effects associated with β₂-agonists (eg, palpitations, chest pain, rapid HR, tremor, nervousness).

SYMBYAX — fluoxetine/olanzapine   Rx

Class: Atypical antipsychotic/selective serotonin reuptake inhibitor (SSRI)

> Antidepressants increased the risk of suicidal thoughts and behavior in children, adolescents, and young adults in short-term studies. Monitor closely for worsening and emergence of suicidal thoughts and behaviors in patients who are started on antidepressant therapy. Elderly patients with dementia-related psychosis treated with antipsychotic drugs are at an increased risk of death. Not approved for use in children <10 yrs of age or for the treatment of dementia-related psychosis.

ADULT DOSAGE
Bipolar I Disorder
Acute Depressive Episodes:
Initial: 6mg/25mg qpm
Titrate: Adjust dosage, if indicated, according to efficacy and tolerability
Effective Range: 6-12mg (olanzapine) and 25-50mg (fluoxetine)
Max: 18mg/75mg
Periodically reexamine need for continued pharmacotherapy

Depression
Treatment Resistant:
Initial: 6mg/25mg qpm
Titrate: Adjust dosage, if indicated, according to efficacy and tolerability
Effective Range: 6-18mg (olanzapine) and 25-50mg (fluoxetine)
Max: 18mg/75mg
Periodically reexamine need for continued pharmacotherapy

Dosing Considerations with MAOIs
Switching to/from an MAOI for Psychiatric Disorders:
Allow at least 14 days between discontinuation of an MAOI and initiation of treatment, and allow at least 5 weeks between discontinuation of treatment and initiation of an MAOI

With Other MAOIs (eg, Linezolid, IV Methylene Blue):
Do not start in a patient being treated with linezolid or IV methylene blue. If acceptable alternatives are not available, d/c and administer linezolid or IV methylene blue; monitor for serotonin syndrome for 5 weeks or until 24 hrs after the last dose of linezolid or IV methylene blue, whichever comes first. May resume therapy 24 hrs after the last dose of linezolid or IV methylene blue

PEDIATRIC DOSAGE
Bipolar I Disorder
Acute Depressive Episodes:
10-17 Years:
Initial: 3mg/25mg qpm
Usual/Target Dosing Range:
6mg/25mg to 12mg/50mg
Max: 12mg/50mg

DOSING CONSIDERATIONS
Hepatic Impairment
Initial: 3mg/25mg or 6mg/25mg qpm
Elderly
Use w/ caution and start at lower end of dosing range
Discontinuation
Gradually reduce dose
Other Important Considerations
Predisposition to Hypotension Risk/Slow Metabolizers (Female, Geriatric Age, Nonsmoker)/Olanzapine-Sensitive:
Initial: 3mg-25mg or 6mg-25mg qpm
Titrate: Increase slowly and adjust dose prn in slow metabolizers

ADMINISTRATION
Oral route

STORAGE
25°C (77°F); excursions permitted to 15-30°C (59-86°F). Protect from moisture.

HOW SUPPLIED
Cap: (Olanzapine/Fluoxetine) 3mg/25mg, 6mg/25mg, 6mg/50mg, 12mg/25mg, 12mg/50mg

CONTRAINDICATIONS
Use of an MAOI intended to treat psychiatric disorders either concomitantly or within 5 weeks of stopping treatment. Treatment within 14 days of stopping an MAOI intended to treat psychiatric disorders. Starting treatment in patients being treated with other MAOIs (eg, linezolid or IV methylene blue). Concomitant use with pimozide or thioridazine.

WARNINGS/PRECAUTIONS
Associated with metabolic changes (eg, hyperglycemia, dyslipidemia, weight gain [dose-related]) that may increase cardiovascular/cerebrovascular risk. Hyperglycemia, in some cases extreme and associated with ketoacidosis/hyperosmolar coma/death reported; caution in patients with diabetes mellitus (DM) or borderline increased blood glucose level. Dose-related hyperprolactinemia reported. Pupillary dilation that occurs following use may trigger an angle-closure attack in a patient with anatomically narrow angles who does not have a patent iridectomy. Anaphylactoid and pulmonary reactions reported; d/c if unexplained allergic reaction occurs. May increase precipitation of a manic episode in patients at risk for bipolar disorder. Tardive dyskinesia (TD) may develop; consider discontinuation if signs and symptoms appear. May induce orthostatic hypotension; caution with cardiovascular disease (CVD), cerebrovascular disease, or conditions that would predispose to hypotension. Leukopenia, neutropenia, and agranulocytosis reported; consider discontinuing at 1st sign of clinically significant decline in WBC count without causative factors, or discontinuing if severe neutropenia (ANC <1000/mm³) develops. May cause esophageal dysmotility and aspiration. Not approved for treatment of patients with Alzheimer's disease. Seizures reported; caution with history of seizures or with conditions that potentially lower the seizure threshold. May impair physical/mental abilities. May disrupt body's ability to reduce core body temperature; caution with conditions that may elevate core temperature (eg, strenuous exercise, extreme heat exposure, dehydration). Caution with conditions affecting hemodynamic responses, hepatic impairment, in cardiac patients, and in the elderly. Fluoxetine: Serotonin syndrome reported; d/c immediately and initiate supportive symptomatic treatment. May increase risk of bleeding reactions. Hyponatremia reported; consider discontinuation in patients with symptomatic hyponatremia. QT interval prolongation and ventricular arrhythmia, including torsades de pointes, reported; caution in patients with congenital long QT syndrome, a previous history of QT prolongation, a family history of long QT syndrome or sudden cardiac death, and other conditions that predispose to QT prolongation and ventricular arrhythmia. Consider discontinuing treatment and obtaining a cardiac evaluation if signs/symptoms of ventricular arrhythmia develop. Because of long elimination $T_{1/2}$, changes in dose will not be fully reflected for several weeks. Adverse reactions reported upon discontinuation; avoid abrupt withdrawal. Olanzapine: Neuroleptic malignant syndrome (NMS) reported; d/c and instill intensive symptomatic treatment and monitoring. Caution with clinically significant prostatic hypertrophy, angle-closure glaucoma, history of paralytic ileus or related conditions.

ADVERSE REACTIONS
Asthenia, somnolence, weight gain, increased appetite, disturbance in attention, peripheral edema, tremor, dry mouth, arthralgia, blurred vision, sedation, fatigue, flatulence, restlessness, hypersomnia.

DRUG INTERACTIONS
See Contraindications. Caution with CNS-active drugs and anticholinergic drugs. May potentiate sedation and orthostatic hypotension with alcohol. Fluoxetine: May cause serotonin syndrome with other serotonergic drugs (eg, triptans, tramadol, St. John's wort) and with drugs that impair metabolism of serotonin; d/c immediately if this occurs. Increased risk of bleeding with ASA, NSAIDs, warfarin, and other anticoagulants. Rare reports of prolonged seizures with combined use of electroconvulsive therapy. Caution with drugs that cause QT prolongation (eg, specific antipsychotics [eg, ziprasidone, iloperidone, chlorpromazine], specific antibiotics [eg, erythromycin, moxifloxacin, sparfloxacin], class 1A antiarrhythmics [eg, quinidine, procainamide], class III antiarrhythmics [eg, amiodarone, sotalol], and others [eg, pentamidine, methadone, tacrolimus]). May increase levels of TCAs (eg, imipramine, desipramine). May prolong $T_{1/2}$ of diazepam. May increase levels of carbamazepine, alprazolam, clozapine, phenytoin, and haloperidol. Caution with CYP2D6 substrates, including antidepressants (eg, TCAs), antipsychotics (eg, phenothiazines, most atypicals), vinblastine, and antiarrhythmics (eg, propafenone, flecainide). May cause lithium toxicity; monitor lithium levels. May cause a shift in plasma concentration with drugs that are tightly bound to protein (eg, warfarin, digitoxin), resulting in an adverse effect. CYP2D6 inhibitors or other highly protein-bound drugs may increase levels. Olanzapine: May potentiate orthostatic hypotension with diazepam. Inducers of CYP1A2 or glucuronyl transferase (eg, carbamazepine, omeprazole, rifampin) may increase clearance. Fluvoxamine may increase levels; consider lower doses of the olanzapine component when used concomitantly. May enhance effects of certain antihypertensive agents. May antagonize effects of levodopa and dopamine agonists.

PREGNANCY AND LACTATION
Category C, not for use in nursing.

MECHANISM OF ACTION
SSRI/Thienobenzodiazepine; unknown. Proposed that activation of 3 monoaminergic neural systems (serotonin, norepinephrine, and dopamine) is responsible for its enhanced antidepressant effect. Fluoxetine: SSRI; inhibits serotonin transport; weak inhibitor of norepinephrine and dopamine transporters. Olanzapine: Thienobenzodiazepine; psychotropic agent with high affinity binding to 5HT$_{2A/2C}$, 5HT$_6$, D$_{1-4}$, H$_1$, and adrenergic (α)$_1$-receptors.

PHARMACOKINETICS
Absorption: Fluoxetine (single PO 40mg): C$_{max}$=15-55ng/mL, T$_{max}$=6-8 hrs. Olanzapine: Well-absorbed; T$_{max}$=6 hrs. **Distribution:** Found in breast milk. Fluoxetine: Crosses placenta; plasma protein binding (94.5%). Olanzapine:

V_d=1000L; plasma protein binding (93%). **Metabolism:** Fluoxetine: Liver (extensive) via CYP2D6; norfluoxetine (active metabolite). Olanzapine: Via direct glucuronidation and CYP450-mediated oxidation; 10-N-glucuronide and 4'-N-desmethyl olanzapine (major metabolites). **Elimination:** Fluoxetine: Kidneys; $T_{1/2}$=1-3 days (acute administration), 4-6 days (chronic administration), 4-16 days (norfluoxetine, acute and chronic administration). Olanzapine: Urine (57%, 7% unchanged), feces (30%); $T_{1/2}$=21-54 hrs.

PATIENT CONSIDERATIONS

Assessment: Assess for DM, susceptibility to angle-closure glaucoma, CVD, cerebrovascular disease, history of seizures, or any other conditions where treatment is contraindicated or cautioned. Assess for bipolar disorder, dementia-related psychosis, Alzheimer's disease, pregnancy/nursing status, and possible drug interactions. Assess for predisposition to hypotension, hepatic impairment, slow metabolism, and pharmacodynamic sensitivity to olanzapine. Obtain baseline FPG, CBC, and lipid levels. Consider ECG assessment if initiating treatment in patients with risk factors for QT prolongation and ventricular arrhythmia. Consider potential consequences of weight gain.

Monitoring: Monitor for signs/symptoms of NMS, serotonin syndrome, TD, clinical worsening, suicidality, unusual changes in behavior, hyperglycemia, hyperlipidemia, rash or other possible allergic phenomena, orthostatic hypotension, mania/hypomania, QT prolongation, angle-closure glaucoma, and other adverse reactions. Frequently monitor CBC in patients with a history of clinically significant low WBC counts or drug-induced leukopenia/neutropenia. Monitor FPG, lipid levels, and weight of patient. In patients with clinically significant neutropenia, monitor for fever or other signs/symptoms of infection. Consider periodic ECG monitoring in patients with risk factors for QT prolongation and ventricular arrhythmia. Periodically reassess need for continued treatment.

Counseling: Inform about risks and benefits of therapy. Advise patient, family, and caregivers to be alert for signs of behavioral changes, worsening of depression, suicidal ideation, and signs/symptoms of NMS. Inform patient of the potential risk of hyperglycemia, dyslipidemia, weight gain, and hyponatremia. Caution about risk of serotonin syndrome with other serotonergic agents (eg, triptans, buspirone, St. John's wort); instruct to seek medical care immediately if experiencing symptoms of serotonin syndrome. Inform about risk of bleeding with ASA, warfarin, or other drugs that affect coagulation; advise to seek medical care immediately if experiencing any increased or unusual bruising or bleeding. Caution about risk of angle-closure glaucoma. Counsel to seek medical care immediately if a rash or hives, or signs/symptoms associated with orthostatic hypotension occur. Explain that drug may impair physical/mental abilities and instruct to use caution when operating hazardous machinery, including automobiles. Advise about appropriate care in avoiding overheating and dehydration and instruct to notify physician if sever illness or symptoms of dehydration develop. Instruct to notify physician if taking other drugs or if pregnant/planning to become pregnant. Instruct to avoid breastfeeding and alcohol. Instruct to take exactly as prescribed and to continue even if symptoms improve.

SYMLIN — pramlintide acetate   Rx

Class: Synthetic amylin analogue

> Use w/ insulin increases risk of severe hypoglycemia, particularly in patients w/ type 1 diabetes. Severe hypoglycemia occurs w/in 3 hrs following inj. Serious injuries may occur if severe hypoglycemia occurs while operating a motor vehicle, heavy machinery, or while engaging in other high-risk activities. Appropriate patient selection, careful patient instruction, and insulin dose reduction are critical elements for reducing this risk.

ADULT DOSAGE
Type 1 Diabetes Mellitus

Adjunctive treatment in patients w/ type 1 diabetes who use mealtime insulin therapy and who have failed to achieve desired glucose control despite optimal insulin therapy

Reduce mealtime insulin doses (including premixed insulins) by 50% when initiating pramlintide acetate

Initial: 15mcg SQ immediately prior to each major meal
Titrate: Increase to the next increment (30mcg, 45mcg, 60mcg) when no clinically significant nausea has occurred for ≥3 days

If significant nausea persists at the 45 or 60mcg dose, decrease to 30mcg
If 30mcg dose is not tolerated, consider discontinuation of therapy

If pramlintide acetate is discontinued for any reason, the same initiation protocol should be followed when therapy is reinstituted

PEDIATRIC DOSAGE
Pediatric use may not have been established

Type 2 Diabetes Mellitus

Adjunctive treatment in patients w/ type 2 diabetes who use mealtime insulin therapy and who have failed to achieve desired glucose control despite optimal insulin therapy

Reduce mealtime insulin doses (including premixed insulins) by 50% when initiating pramlintide acetate

Initial: 60mcg SQ immediately prior to each major meal
Titrate: Increase to 120mcg when no clinically significant nausea has occurred for ≥3 days

If significant nausea persists at the 120mcg dose, decrease to 60mcg

If pramlintide acetate is discontinued for any reason, the same initiation protocol should be followed when therapy is reinstituted

Missed Dose

Wait until the next scheduled dose and administer the usual amount if dose is missed

---

DOSING CONSIDERATIONS
Discontinuation
Criteria:
Recurrent unexplained hypoglycemia requiring medical assistance
Persistent clinically significant nausea
Noncompliance w/ self-monitoring of blood glucose, insulin dose adjustments, or scheduled healthcare provider contacts or recommended clinic visits

ADMINISTRATION
SQ route

Administer immediately prior to each major meal (≥250 kcal or ≥30g of carbohydrate).
Inj should be at room temperature before administration.
Inject in the abdominal wall or thigh; rotate inj sites w/in the same region.
Inj site for any concomitant insulin inj should be distinct from therapy inj site.
Should not be mixed w/ any type of insulin; administer as separate inj.

STORAGE
Not in Use: 2-8°C (36-46°F). Protect from light. Do not freeze; do not use if sol has been frozen. In Use: After 1st use, refrigerate or keep at ≤30°C (86°F) for 30 days. Use w/in 30 days, whether or not refrigerated.

HOW SUPPLIED
Inj: 1000mcg/mL [1.5mL, 2.7mL]

CONTRAINDICATIONS
Serious hypersensitivity reaction to Symlin or to any of its product components, hypoglycemia unawareness, confirmed gastroparesis.

WARNINGS/PRECAUTIONS
Should be used only in patients who can fully understand and adhere to proper insulin adjustments and glucose monitoring. Caution w/ visual or dexterity impairment. Pen must never be shared between patients, even if the needle is changed; poses a risk for transmission of blood-borne pathogens. Erythema, edema, or pruritus at the inj site may occur.

ADVERSE REACTIONS
N/V, headache, anorexia, abdominal pain, fatigue, dizziness, cough, pharyngitis, arthralgia, allergic reaction.

DRUG INTERACTIONS
See Boxed Warning. Not recommended w/ other medications that alter GI motility (eg, anticholinergic agents [atropine]) or medications that slow intestinal absorption of nutrients (eg, α-glucosidase inhibitors). May delay the absorption of concomitantly administered oral medications; when the rapid onset or threshold concentration of a concomitant orally administered medication is a critical determinant of effectiveness (eg, analgesics, antibiotics, oral contraceptives), the medication should be administered at least 1 hr prior to or 2 hrs after pramlintide inj. Caution w/ other medications that may increase the susceptibility to hypoglycemia (eg, ACE inhibitors, fibrates, MAOIs).

PREGNANCY AND LACTATION
Category C, caution in nursing.

MECHANISM OF ACTION
Synthetic amylin analogue; slows gastric emptying, reduces the postprandial rise in plasma glucagon, and modulates satiety leading to decreased caloric intake.

PHARMACOKINETICS
Absorption: Absolute bioavailability (approx 30-40%). Administration of variable doses resulted in different parameters. **Distribution:** Not extensively bound to RBCs or albumin (approx 40% unbound). **Metabolism:** Des-lys pramlintide (primary metabolite). **Elimination:** $T_{1/2}$=approx 48 min.

PATIENT CONSIDERATIONS

Assessment: Assess for drug hypersensitivity, gastroparesis, hypoglycemia unawareness, visual or dexterity impairment, pregnancy/nursing status, and possible drug interactions. Review HbA1c, recent blood glucose monitoring data, history of insulin-induced hypoglycemia, current insulin regimen, and body weight.

Monitoring: Monitor for signs/symptoms of hypoglycemia, erythema, edema, or pruritus at the inj site, and other adverse reactions. Monitor blood glucose frequently.

Counseling: Inform about the risks and benefits of therapy. Inform about the importance of self-management practices, including glucose monitoring and timing of dosing. Reinforce the importance of adherence to meal planning, physical activity, recognition and management of hypo/hyperglycemia, and assessment of diabetic complications. Advise not to share pen w/ another person, even if the needle is changed. Advise women w/ diabetes to inform physician if pregnant or contemplating pregnancy. Instruct on the proper inj technique, proper storage, and on handling special situations (eg, intercurrent conditions [illness, stress], inadequate or omitted insulin dose, inadvertent administration of increased insulin or pramlintide dose, inadequate food intake, missed meals).

SYNAGIS — palivizumab
Rx

Class: Monoclonal antibody/RSV F-protein blocker

PEDIATRIC DOSAGE
Respiratory Syncytial Virus
Prevention of serious lower respiratory tract disease in children at high risk of RSV disease

≤24 Months of Age:
15mg/kg monthly throughout RSV season; administer first dose prior to start of RSV season

Undergoing Cardiopulmonary Bypass:
Administer an additional dose as soon as possible after the procedure (even if <1 month from previous dose) then monthly thereafter, as scheduled

---

ADMINISTRATION
IM route
If RSV infection develops, continue monthly doses throughout RSV season.
Give inj volumes >1mL as a divided dose.
Do not dilute, shake, or vigorously agitate vial.
Administer immediately after withdrawal from vial.
Administer preferably into the anterolateral aspect of the thigh.
Refer to PI for further instructions.

STORAGE
2-8°C (36-46°F). Do not freeze.

HOW SUPPLIED
Inj: 50mg/0.5mL, 100mg/mL

CONTRAINDICATIONS
Previous significant hypersensitivity reaction to palivizumab.

WARNINGS/PRECAUTIONS
Anaphylaxis, anaphylactic shock, and other acute hypersensitivity reactions reported; permanently d/c if a significant hypersensitivity reaction occurs, and use caution during readministration if a mild hypersensitivity reaction occurs. Caution with thrombocytopenia or any coagulation disorder. May interfere with immunological-based RSV diagnostic tests and viral culture assays; diagnostic test results should be used in conjunction with clinical findings.

ADVERSE REACTIONS
Fever, rash, anaphylaxis.

PREGNANCY AND LACTATION
Pregnancy: Category C.
Lactation: Safety not known in nursing.

MECHANISM OF ACTION
Monoclonal antibody/RSV F-protein blocker; provides passive immunity against RSV. Acts by blocking the RSV envelope fusion protein on the surface of the virus and blocking a critical step in the membrane fusion process. Also prevents cell-to-cell fusion of RSV-infected cells.

PHARMACOKINETICS
Absorption: Bioavailability (70%). **Elimination:** $T_{1/2}$=20 days.

PATIENT CONSIDERATIONS
Assessment: Assess for previous hypersensitivity to the drug, thrombocytopenia, and coagulation disorders. Assess if patient is undergoing cardiopulmonary bypass.

Monitoring: Monitor for anaphylaxis, hypersensitivity reactions, and other adverse reactions.

Counseling: Counsel parents/guardians about the potential risks and benefits of therapy. Inform parents/guardians of the possible side effects and of the signs/symptoms of potential allergic reactions; advise of the appropriate actions. Advise parents/guardians of the dosing schedule and the importance of compliance with the full course of therapy.

SYNERCID — dalfopristin/quinupristin
Rx

Class: Streptogramin

ADULT DOSAGE
Skin and Skin Structure Infections

Complicated *Staphylococcus aureus* (methicillin-susceptible) or *Streptococcus pyogenes* Infections:
7.5mg/kg q12h for at least 7 days

PEDIATRIC DOSAGE
Skin and Skin Structure Infections

Complicated *Staphylococcus aureus* (methicillin-susceptible) or *Streptococcus pyogenes* Infections:
≥12 Years:
7.5mg/kg q12h for at least 7 days

DOSING CONSIDERATIONS
Hepatic Impairment
Hepatic Cirrhosis (Child-Pugh A or B): May need dose reduction

ADMINISTRATION
IV route
Administer by IV infusion in D5W sol over a 60-min period.
Flush only w/ D5W to minimize venous irritation.
May use an infusion pump or device to control the rate of infusion.
May use central venous access (eg, peripherally inserted central catheter) to decrease incidence of venous irritation.

Preparation
Reconstitute 500mg single dose vial by slowly adding 5mL of D5W or sterile water for inj.
Gently swirl the vial while limiting foam formation; allow the sol to sit for a few min until all the foam disappears.
Further dilution is required before infusion; dilute w/in 30 min of reconstitution.
Based on patient's weight, add the reconstituted sol to 250mL of D5W; may use 100mL infusion volume for central line infusions.
Consider increasing the infusion volume to 500mL or 750mL or changing the infusion site if moderate to severe venous irritation occurs.

Compatibility and Stability
Saline solutions are not compatible w/ treatment.
Compatible by Y-site inj in D5W w/ aztreonam 20mg/mL, ciprofloxacin 1mg/mL, haloperidol 0.2mg/mL, metoclopramide. 5mg/mL, potassium chloride 40mEq/L, and fluconazole 2mg/mL used as the undiluted sol.
Flush w/ D5W before and after administration of other drugs through a common IV line.

STORAGE
2-8°C (36-46°F). Dilute reconstituted solution w/in 30 min. Diluted Sol: Stable for 5 hrs at room temperature or for 54 hrs at 2-8°C (36-46°F). Do not freeze.

HOW SUPPLIED
Inj: (Dalfopristin/Quinupristin) 350mg/150mg

CONTRAINDICATIONS
Known hypersensitivity to Synercid, or w/ prior hypersensitivity to other streptogramins.

WARNINGS/PRECAUTIONS
Clostridium difficile-associated diarrhea (CDAD) reported; d/c if CDAD is suspected or confirmed. May result in bacterial resistance if used in the absence of a proven/strongly suspected bacterial infection or a prophylactic indication; take appropriate measures if superinfection develops. Flush vein w/ D5W following completion of a peripheral infusion to minimize venous irritation; do not flush w/ saline or heparin. If moderate to severe venous irritation occurs after peripheral infusion of the drug diluted in 250mL of D5W, consider increasing infusion volume to 500 or 750mL, changing infusion site, or infusing by a peripherally inserted central catheter or central venous catheter. Arthralgia and myalgia, sometimes severe, reported. Total bilirubin elevation >5X ULN observed.

ADVERSE REACTIONS
Inflammation at infusion site, pain at infusion site, edema at infusion site, infusion site reaction, nausea.

DRUG INTERACTIONS
May increase plasma concentrations of drugs metabolized by CYP3A4 (eg, astemizole, terfenadine, delavirdine, nevirapine, indinavir, ritonavir, vinca alkaloids [eg, vinblastine], docetaxel, paclitaxel, midazolam, diazepam, dihydropyridines [eg, nifedipine], verapamil, diltiazem, HMG-CoA reductase inhibitors [eg, lovastatin], cisapride, cyclosporine, tacrolimus, methylprednisolone, carbamazepine, quinidine, lidocaine, disopyramide). Coadministration w/ CYP3A4 substrates that possess a narrow therapeutic window requires caution and monitoring of these drugs (eg, cyclosporine). Avoid w/ drugs metabolized by CYP3A4 that may prolong QTc interval. May inhibit gut metabolism of digoxin.

PREGNANCY AND LACTATION
Pregnancy: Category B.
Lactation: Caution in nursing.

MECHANISM OF ACTION
Streptogramin antibiotic; components act synergistically on bacterial ribosome. Quinupristin: Inhibits the late phase of protein synthesis. Dalfopristin: Inhibits the early phase of protein synthesis.

PHARMACOKINETICS
Absorption: Quinupristin: C_{max}=3.2mcg/mL, AUC=7.2mcg•hr/mL; Dalfopristin: C_{max}=7.96mcg/mL, AUC=10.57mcg•hr/mL. **Distribution:** V_d=0.45L/kg (quinupristin); 0.24L/kg (dalfopristin). **Metabolism:** Quinupristin: 2 conjugated active metabolites (1 w/ glutathione; 1 w/ cysteine); Dalfopristin: 1 nonconjugated

active metabolite, via hydrolysis. **Elimination:** Urine: 15% (quinupristin), 19% (dalfopristin), feces (75-77%); $T_{1/2}$=0.85 hrs (quinupristin), 0.70 hrs (dalfopristin).

PATIENT CONSIDERATIONS

Assessment: Assess for known hypersensitivity to the drug or prior hypersensitivity to other streptogramins (eg, pristinamycin, virginiamycin), hepatic impairment, pregnancy/nursing status, and possible drug interactions. Perform culture and susceptibility testing.

Monitoring: Monitor for CDAD, venous irritation, arthralgia, myalgia, superinfection, and other adverse reactions. Monitor total bilirubin levels.

Counseling: Inform about risks/benefits of therapy. Inform that diarrhea is a common problem caused by therapy that usually ends when therapy is discontinued; advise to contact physician immediately if watery and bloody stools (w/ or w/o stomach cramps and fever) develop, even as late as ≥2 months after the last dose. Counsel that drug only treats bacterial, not viral (eg, common cold), infections. Instruct to take ud; inform that skipping doses or not completing the full course of therapy may decrease effectiveness of the drug and increase resistance of bacteria.

SYNJARDY — empagliflozin/metformin hydrochloride   Rx

Class: Biguanide/sodium-glucose cotransporter 2 (SGLT2) inhibitor

> Cases of metformin-associated lactic acidosis resulting in death, hypothermia, hypotension, and resistant bradyarrhythmias reported. Risk factors include renal impairment; concomitant use of certain drugs (eg, carbonic anhydrase inhibitors such as topiramate); age ≥65 years; having a radiological study w/ contrast, surgery, and other procedures; hypoxic states (eg, acute CHF); excessive alcohol intake; and hepatic impairment. D/C therapy immediately and institute general supportive measures in a hospital setting if metformin-associated lactic acidosis is suspected. Prompt hemodialysis is recommended.

ADULT DOSAGE

Type 2 Diabetes Mellitus

When treatment w/ both empagliflozin and metformin is appropriate

Patients on Metformin:
Switch to Synjardy containing empagliflozin 5mg w/ a similar total daily dose of metformin

Patients on Empagliflozin:
Switch to Synjardy containing metformin 500mg w/ a similar total daily dose of empagliflozin

Patients Already Treated w/ Empagliflozin and Metformin:
Switch to Synjardy containing the same total daily doses of each component

Max Daily Dose: Metformin 2000mg and empagliflozin 25mg

Take bid w/ meals, w/ gradual dose escalation to reduce GI side effects

PEDIATRIC DOSAGE

Pediatric use may not have been established

DOSING CONSIDERATIONS

Renal Impairment
eGFR <45mL/min/1.73m²:
Contraindicated

Hepatic Impairment
Avoid use in patients w/ clinical or laboratory evidence of hepatic disease

Other Important Considerations
Patients w/ Volume-Depletion Not Previously Treated w/ Empagliflozin:
Correct this condition before initiating treatment

Iodinated Contrast Imaging Procedures:
D/C therapy at the time of, or prior to, an iodinated contrast imaging procedure in patients w/ an eGFR 45-60mL/min/1.73m²; in patients w/ a history of liver disease, alcoholism, or heart failure; or in patients who will be administered intra-arterial iodinated contrast. Reevaluate eGFR 48 hrs after the imaging procedure and restart therapy if renal function is stable

ADMINISTRATION
Oral route

STORAGE
25°C (77°F); excursions permitted to 15-30°C (59-86°F).

HOW SUPPLIED
Tab: (Empagliflozin/Metformin) 5mg/500mg, 5mg/1000mg, 12.5mg/500mg, 12.5mg/1000mg

CONTRAINDICATIONS
Moderate to severe renal impairment (eGFR <45mL/min/1.73m²), ESRD, or dialysis; acute or chronic metabolic acidosis, including diabetic ketoacidosis; history of a serious hypersensitivity reaction to empagliflozin or metformin.

WARNINGS/PRECAUTIONS
See Dosing Considerations. Not recommended in patients w/ type 1 diabetes mellitus (DM) or for treatment of diabetic ketoacidosis. **Empagliflozin:** Causes intravascular volume contraction. Symptomatic hypotension may occur,

particularly in patients w/ renal impairment, the elderly, patients w/ low systolic BP, and patients on diuretics. Ketoacidosis reported; if suspected, d/c and institute prompt treatment. Assess for ketoacidosis in patients presenting w/ signs/symptoms consistent w/ severe metabolic acidosis regardless of presenting blood glucose levels. Consider temporarily discontinuing therapy in clinical situations known to predispose to ketoacidosis (eg, prolonged fasting due to acute illness or surgery). Increases SrCr and decreases eGFR; risk of impaired renal function is increased in elderly patients and patients w/ renal impairment. Serious UTIs (eg, urosepsis, pyelonephritis), requiring hospitalization, reported; evaluate for signs/symptoms of UTIs and treat promptly, if indicated. Increases the risk for genital mycotic infections and UTIs; monitor and treat as appropriate. Increases LDL levels; monitor and treat as appropriate. Monitoring glycemic control w/ urine glucose tests or w/ 1,5-anhydroglucitol assay is not recommended; use alternative methods. **Metformin:** Withholding of food and fluids during surgical or other procedures may increase the risk for volume depletion, hypotension, and renal impairment; temporarily d/c while patient has restricted food and fluid intake. D/C if a condition associated w/ hypoxemia occurs (eg, cardiovascular collapse, acute MI, sepsis). Elderly, debilitated, or malnourished patients, and those w/ adrenal or pituitary insufficiency or alcohol intoxication, may be particularly susceptible to hypoglycemic effects; monitor a need to lower the dose of Synjardy to minimize risk of hypoglycemia in these patients. Hypoglycemia may be difficult to recognize in the elderly. May decrease vitamin B12 levels; monitor hematologic parameters annually.

ADVERSE REACTIONS
Empagliflozin: UTI, female genital mycotic infections, URTI, dyslipidemia.
Metformin: Diarrhea, N/V, flatulence, abdominal discomfort, indigestion, asthenia, headache.

DRUG INTERACTIONS
See Boxed Warning and Dosing Considerations. **Empagliflozin:** Risk of hypoglycemia is increased when used in combination w/ insulin secretagogues (eg, sulfonylurea) or insulin; a lower dose of the insulin secretagogue or insulin may be required. Coadministration w/ diuretics resulted in increased urine volume and frequency of voids, which might enhance potential for volume depletion. **Metformin:** Hypoglycemia may be difficult to recognize in people who are taking β-adrenergic blocking drugs; monitor for a need to lower the dose of Synjardy to minimize the risk of hypoglycemia in these patients. Hypoglycemia may occur during concomitant use w/ other glucose-lowering agents (eg, sulfonylureas, insulin) or ethanol. Drugs that impair renal function, result in significant hemodynamic change, interfere w/ acid-base balance, or increase metformin accumulation (eg, cationic drugs) may increase the risk of lactic acidosis; consider more frequent monitoring of these patients. Drugs that are eliminated by renal tubular secretion (eg, cimetidine) may increase the accumulation of metformin and the risk for lactic acidosis; consider more frequent monitoring of these patients. Topiramate or other carbonic anhydrase inhibitors (eg, zonisamide, acetazolamide, dichlorphenamide) frequently cause a decrease in serum bicarbonate and induce non-anion gap, hyperchloremic metabolic acidosis; consider more frequent monitoring of these patients. Thiazides and other diuretics, corticosteroids, phenothiazines, thyroid products, estrogens, oral contraceptives, phenytoin, nicotinic acid, sympathomimetics, calcium channel blockers, and isoniazid may produce hyperglycemia and lead to loss of glycemic control; monitor for loss of blood glucose control when such drugs are administered and monitor for hypoglycemia when such drugs are withdrawn.

PREGNANCY AND LACTATION
Pregnancy: Based on animal data showing adverse renal effects, not recommended during the 2nd and 3rd trimesters of pregnancy.
Lactation: Not for use in nursing.
Reproductive Potential: Discuss the potential for unintended pregnancy w/ premenopausal women as therapy w/ metformin may result in ovulation in some anovulatory women.

MECHANISM OF ACTION
Empagliflozin: SGLT2 inhibitor; reduces renal reabsorption of filtered glucose and lowers the renal threshold for glucose, and thereby increases urinary glucose excretion. **Metformin:** Biguanide; decreases hepatic glucose production, decreases intestinal absorption of glucose, and improves insulin sensitivity by increasing peripheral glucose uptake and utilization.

PHARMACOKINETICS
Absorption: Empagliflozin: T_{max}=1.5 hrs; (10mg qd) C_{max}=259nmol/L, AUC=1870nmol•h/L; (25mg qd) C_{max}=687nmol/L, AUC=4740nmol•h/L. Metformin: (500mg, fasted) Absolute bioavailability (50-60%). **Distribution:** Empagliflozin: Plasma protein binding (86.2%); V_d=73.8L. Metformin: (850mg) V_d=654L. **Metabolism:** Empagliflozin: Glucuronidation via UGT2B7, UGT1A3, UGT1A8, and UGT1A9. **Elimination:** Empagliflozin: Feces (41.2%), urine (54.4%); $T_{1/2}$=12.4 hrs. Metformin: Urine (90%); $T_{1/2}$=6.2 hrs (plasma), 17.6 hrs (blood).

PATIENT CONSIDERATIONS
Assessment: Assess for metabolic acidosis (including diabetic ketoacidosis), risk factors for lactic acidosis, type of DM, alcoholism, hypoxemia, presence of malnourishment or debilitation, adrenal/pituitary insufficiency, risk for genital mycotic infections, inadequate vitamin B12 or Ca^{2+} intake/absorption, drug hypersensitivity, any other conditions where treatment is cautioned, pregnancy/nursing status, and possible drug interactions. Assess if patient is planning to undergo any surgical procedure or any radiologic studies involving the use of intravascular iodinated contrast materials. Assess volume status.

Obtain baseline FPG and HbA1c levels, renal/hepatic function, and hematologic parameters.

Monitoring: Monitor for signs/symptoms of lactic acidosis, hypotension, ketoacidosis, UTIs, genital mycotic infections, hypersensitivity reactions, hypoxic states, and other adverse reactions. Monitor renal function at least annually. Monitor hematologic parameters annually. Perform routine serum vitamin B12 measurements at 2- to 3-yr intervals in patients predisposed to developing subnormal vitamin B12 levels. Monitor FPG and HbA1c and LDL levels.

Counseling: Inform of the potential risks and benefits of therapy and of alternative modes of therapy. Advise about the importance of adherence to dietary instructions, regular physical activity, periodic blood glucose monitoring and HbA1c testing, recognition and management of hypo/ hyperglycemia, and assessment for diabetes complications. Instruct to seek medical advice promptly during periods of stress (eg, fever, trauma, infection, surgery), as medication requirements may change. Inform of the risks of lactic acidosis; advise to d/c therapy immediately and to notify physician promptly if unexplained hyperventilation, malaise, myalgia, unusual somnolence, slow or irregular heartbeat, sensation of feeling cold (especially in the extremities), or other nonspecific symptoms occur. Instruct to report to physician if pregnant, nursing, or experiencing symptoms of hypotension. Instruct to have adequate fluid intake. Instruct to d/c and seek medical advice immediately if symptoms of ketoacidosis occur. Counsel on the signs/symptoms of ketoacidosis, UTI, vaginal yeast infection, balanitis, and balanoposthitis; inform of treatment options and when to seek medical advice.

SYNRIBO — omacetaxine mepesuccinate   Rx

Class: Protein synthesis inhibitor

ADULT DOSAGE	PEDIATRIC DOSAGE
Chronic Myeloid Leukemia	Pediatric use may not have been established
Chronic or accelerated phase w/ resistance and/or intolerance to ≥2 tyrosine kinase inhibitors	
Induction: 1.25mg/m^2 bid (approx 12-hr intervals) for 14 consecutive days every 28 days, over a 28-day cycle; repeat cycle every 28 days until hematologic response is achieved	
Maint: 1.25mg/m^2 bid (approx 12-hr intervals) for 7 consecutive days every 28 days, over a 28-day cycle	

DOSING CONSIDERATIONS
Adverse Reactions
Hematologic Toxicity:
Grade 4 Neutropenia (ANC <0.5 x 10^9/L) or Grade 3 Thrombocytopenia (Platelet Counts <50 x 10^9/L) During a Cycle:
Delay starting next cycle until ANC ≥1.0 x 10^9/L and platelet count ≥50 x 10^9/L; reduce number of dosing days by 2 days for next cycle

Non-Hematologic Toxicity:
Manage symptomatically; interrupt and/or delay therapy until toxicity is resolved

ADMINISTRATION
SQ route
Reconstitution Instructions
1. Reconstitute w/ 1mL of 0.9% NaCl inj prior to SQ inj.
2. After addition of diluent, gently swirl until a clear sol is obtained; lyophilized powder should be completely dissolved in <1 min.
3. The resulting sol contains 3.5mg/mL.

Handling Precautions
If contact w/ skin occurs, immediately and thoroughly wash affected area w/ soap and water.
If contact w/ the eyes occurs, thoroughly flush the eyes w/ water.

STORAGE
20-25°C (68-77°F); excursions permitted from 15-30°C (59-86°F). Protect from light. **Reconstituted Sol:** Use w/in 12 hrs if stored at 20-25°C (68-77°F) or use w/ in 6 days if stored at 2-8°C (36-46°F).

HOW SUPPLIED
Inj: 3.5mg

WARNINGS/PRECAUTIONS
Severe and fatal myelosuppression (eg, thrombocytopenia, neutropenia, anemia) reported; delay next cycle and/or reduce the number of days of treatment. Increased risk of infection in neutropenic patients; monitor frequently. Monitor CBC weekly during induction and initial maintenance cycles, and every 2 weeks during later maintenance cycles, as clinically indicated. Cerebral hemorrhage and severe, nonfatal GI hemorrhages observed; monitor platelet counts. Glucose intolerance and hyperglycemia, including hyperosmolar non-ketotic hyperglycemia reported; monitor blood glucose levels frequently, especially in patients w/ diabetes mellitus (DM) or risk factors for DM. Avoid w/ poorly controlled DM until

glycemic control is established. May cause fetal harm if administered during pregnancy.

ADVERSE REACTIONS
Thrombocytopenia, anemia, neutropenia, lymphopenia, bone marrow failure, infections/infestations, diarrhea, N/V, inj-site related reactions, fatigue, pyrexia, asthenia, arthralgia.

DRUG INTERACTIONS
Increased risk of bleeding w/ anticoagulants, aspirin, and NSAIDs; avoid when platelet count is <50,000/μL.

PREGNANCY AND LACTATION
Pregnancy: Category D.
Lactation: Not for use in nursing.

MECHANISM OF ACTION
Protein synthesis inhibitor; not fully elucidated. Binds to the A-site cleft in the peptidyl-transferase center of the large ribosomal subunit from a strain of archaeabacteria. In vitro, reduces protein levels of the Bcr-Abl oncoprotein and Mcl-1, an antiapoptotic Bcl-2 family member.

PHARMACOKINETICS
Absorption: T$_{max}$=30 min. **Distribution:** V$_d$=141L; plasma protein binding (≤50%). **Metabolism:** Hydrolyzed via plasma esterases; 4'-DMHHT (metabolite). **Elimination:** Urine (<15%, unchanged); T$_{1/2}$=6 hrs.

PATIENT CONSIDERATIONS
Assessment: Assess for thrombocytopenia, neutropenia, anemia, hemorrhage, DM, risk factors for DM, pregnancy/nursing status, and possible drug interactions.

Monitoring: Monitor for signs and symptoms of myelosuppression, hemorrhage, infection, and other adverse reactions. Monitor CBC and blood glucose levels.

Counseling: Advise patient to read medication guide and provide instructions for appropriate use. Advise of the possibility of serious bleeding due to low platelet counts; instruct to report immediately any signs/symptoms suggestive of hemorrhage. Instruct to report in advance if patients plan to have any dental or surgical procedures. Inform that hematological parameters (eg, WBCs, platelets, RBCs) will need to be monitored. Instruct to report if fever or any signs/symptoms of infection (eg, SOB, significant fatigue, bleeding) develop. Advise diabetic patients of the possibility of hyperglycemia and the need to monitor blood glucose levels carefully. Advise females of reproductive potential to avoid pregnancy/nursing while on treatment. Inform that N/V, diarrhea, abdominal pain, and constipation may develop; instruct to seek medical attention if symptoms persist. Instruct to avoid driving/operating any dangerous tools or machinery if tiredness is experienced. Inform that skin rash may occur and to immediately report severe/worsening rash or itching. Inform that hair loss may be experienced.

SYNTHROID — levothyroxine sodium   Rx

Class: Thyroid replacement hormone

> Do not use for the treatment of obesity or weight loss; doses within range of daily hormonal requirements are ineffective for weight reduction in euthyroid patients. Serious or life-threatening manifestations of toxicity may occur when given in larger doses, particularly when given in association with sympathomimetic amines.

ADULT DOSAGE	PEDIATRIC DOSAGE
Hypothyroidism	**Hypothyroidism**
Replacement/supplemental therapy in hypothyroidism of any etiology, except transient hypothyroidism during the recovery phase of subacute thyroiditis	**Usual:** **0-3 Months of Age:** 10-15mcg/kg/day **3-6 Months of Age:** 8-10mcg/kg/day **6-12 Months of Age:** 6-8mcg/kg/day **1-5 Years:** 5-6mcg/kg/day **6-12 Years:** 4-5mcg/kg/day **>12 Years:**
Usual: 1.7mcg/kg/day; >200mcg/day seldom required	**Growth/Puberty Incomplete:** 2-3mcg/kg/day
Severe: **Initial:** 12.5-25mcg/day **Titrate:** Increase by 25mcg/day every 2-4 weeks until TSH level normalized	**Growth/Puberty Complete:** 1.7mcg/kg/day
Secondary (Pituitary) or Tertiary (Hypothalamic) Hypothyroidism: **Titrate:** Increase until clinically euthyroid and serum free-T4 level is restored to the upper half of the normal range	**Infants w/ Very Low (<5mcg/dL) or Undetectable Serum T4:** **Initial:** 50mcg/day
Subclinical Hypothyroidism: Lower doses (eg, 1mcg/kg/day) may be adequate to normalize serum TSH level	**Chronic/Severe Hypothyroidism:** **Initial:** 25mcg/day **Titrate:** Increase by 25mcg every 2-4 weeks
Pituitary TSH Suppressant Used to treat/prevent various types of euthyroid goiters (eg, thyroid nodules, subacute or chronic lymphocytic thyroiditis, multinodular goiter) and to manage thyroid cancer	

Well-Differentiated (Papillary and Follicular) Thyroid Cancer: Adjunct to Surgery and Radioiodine Therapy:
Usual: >2mcg/kg/day, w/ target TSH level <0.1 mU/L
High-Risk Tumors: Target TSH level <0.01 mU/L

Benign Nodules and Nontoxic Multinodular Goiter:
TSH is suppressed to a higher target (eg, 0.1 to 0.5 or 1.0 mU/L)

DOSING CONSIDERATIONS
Pregnancy
May increase levothyroxine requirements
Elderly
Hypothyroidism:
>50 Years:
Initial: 25-50mcg/day
Titrate: Increase by 12.5-25mcg increments every 6-8 weeks prn

W/ Underlying Cardiac Disease:
Initial: 12.5-25mcg/day
Titrate: Increase by 12.5-25mg increments every 4-6 weeks

Adverse Reactions
Minimize Hyperactivity in Older Children:
Initial: Give 1/4 of full replacement dose
Titrate: Increase on a weekly basis by 1/4 the full recommended replacement dose until the full recommended replacement dose is reached

Other Important Considerations
Underlying Cardiac Disease:
Hypothyroidism:
Infants (Risk for Cardiac Failure):
Initial: Consider lower dose (eg, 25mcg/day)
Titrate: Increase dose in 4-6 weeks prn
<50 Years:
Initial: 25-50mcg/day
Titrate: Increase by 12.5-25mcg increments every 6-8 weeks prn

ADMINISTRATION
Oral route

Administer as a single daily dose, preferably 30-60 min before breakfast. Take at least 4 hrs apart from drugs that are known to interfere w/ its absorption.
Pediatrics
Unable to Swallow Intact Tab:
1. Crush tab and suspend in small amount (5-10mL or 1-2 tsp) of water.
2. Administer using a spoon or dropper.
3. Do not store sus for later use.
4. Do not use foods that decrease absorption of levothyroxine (eg, soybean infant formula) to administer.
STORAGE
25°C (77°F); excursions permitted to 15-30°C (59-86°F). Protect from light and moisture.

HOW SUPPLIED
Tab: 25mcg*, 50mcg*, 75mcg*, 88mcg*, 100mcg*, 112mcg*, 125mcg*, 137mcg*, 150mcg*, 175mcg*, 200mcg*, 300mcg* *scored

CONTRAINDICATIONS
Untreated subclinical (suppressed serum TSH level with normal T3 level and T4 levels) or overt thyrotoxicosis of any etiology, acute MI, and uncorrected adrenal insufficiency. Hypersensitivity to any of the inactive components in this medication.

WARNINGS/PRECAUTIONS
Should not be used in the treatment of male or female infertility unless associated with hypothyroidism. Contraindicated in patients with nontoxic diffuse goiter or nodular thyroid disease, particularly in the elderly or with underlying cardiovascular (CV) disease if serum TSH level is already suppressed; use with caution if TSH level is not suppressed and carefully monitor thyroid function. Has narrow therapeutic index; carefully titrate dose to avoid over- or under-treatment. May decrease bone mineral density (BMD) with long-term use; give minimum dose necessary to achieve desired clinical and biochemical response. Caution with CV disorders and the elderly. If cardiac symptoms develop or worsen, reduce or withhold dose for 1 week and then restart at lower dose. Overtreatment may produce CV effects (eg, increase in HR, increase in cardiac wall thickness, increase in cardiac contractility, precipitation of angina or arrhythmias). Monitor patients with CAD closely during surgical procedures; may precipitate cardiac arrhythmias. Caution in patients with diabetes mellitus (DM). Patients with concomitant adrenal insufficiency should be treated with replacement glucocorticoids prior to therapy.

ADVERSE REACTIONS
Fatigue, increased appetite, weight loss, heat intolerance, headache, hyperactivity, irritability, insomnia, palpitations, arrhythmias, dyspnea, hair loss, menstrual irregularities, pseudotumor cerebri (children), slipped capital femoral epiphysis (children).

DRUG INTERACTIONS
Concurrent sympathomimetics may increase effects of sympathomimetics or thyroid hormone; may increase risk of coronary insufficiency with CAD. Upward dose adjustments may be needed for insulin and oral hypoglycemic agents. May decrease absorption with soybean flour, cottonseed meal, walnuts, and dietary fiber. May increase oral anticoagulant activity; adjust dose of anticoagulant and monitor PT. May decrease levels and effects of digitalis glycosides. Transient reduction in TSH secretion with dopamine/dopamine agonists, glucocorticoids, octreotide. Decreased thyroid hormone secretion with aminoglutethimide, amiodarone, iodide (including iodine-containing radiographic contrast agents), lithium, methimazole, propylthiouracil (PTU), sulfonamides, and tolbutamide. May increase thyroid hormone secretion with amiodarone and iodide. May decrease T4 absorption with antacids (aluminum and magnesium hydroxides), simethicone, bile acid sequestrants (cholestyramine, colestipol), calcium carbonate, cation exchange resins (kayexalate), ferrous sulfate, orlistat, and sucralfate; administer at least 4 hrs apart. May increase serum thyroxine-binding globulin (TBG) concentrations with clofibrate, estrogen-containing oral contraceptives, oral estrogens, heroin/methadone, 5-fluorouracil, mitotane, and tamoxifen. May decrease serum TBG concentrations with androgens/anabolic steroids, asparaginase, glucocorticoids, and slow-release nicotinic acid. May cause protein-binding site displacement with furosemide (>80mg IV), heparin, hydantoins, NSAIDs (fenamates, phenylbutazone), and salicylates (>2g/day). May alter T4 and T3 metabolism with carbamazepine, hydantoins, phenobarbital, and rifampin. May decrease T4 5'-deiodinase activity with amiodarone, β-adrenergic antagonists (eg, propranolol >160mg/day), glucocorticoids (eg, dexamethasone >4mg/day), and PTU. Concurrent use with tricyclic (eg, amitriptyline) and tetracyclic (eg, maprotiline) antidepressants may increase the therapeutic and toxic effects of both drugs. Coadministration with sertraline in patients stabilized on levothyroxine may result in increased levothyroxine requirements. Interferon-α may cause development of antithyroid microsomal antibodies and transient hypothyroidism, hyperthyroidism, or both. Interleukin-2 has been associated with transient painless thyroiditis. Excessive use with growth hormones (eg, somatropin, somatrem) may accelerate epiphyseal closure. Ketamine may produce marked HTN and tachycardia. May reduce uptake of radiographic agents. Decreased theophylline clearance may occur in hypothyroid patients. Altered levels of thyroid hormone and/or TSH levels with choral hydrate, diazepam, ethionamide, lovastatin, metoclopramide, 6-mercaptopurine, nitroprusside, para-aminosalicylate sodium, perphenazine, resorcinol (excessive topical use), and thiazide diuretics.

PREGNANCY AND LACTATION
Pregnancy: Category A.
Lactation: Caution in nursing.

MECHANISM OF ACTION
Thyroid replacement hormone; mechanism not established. Suspected that principal effects are exerted through control of DNA transcription and protein synthesis.

PHARMACOKINETICS
Absorption: Majority absorbed from jejunum and upper ileum. **Distribution:** Plasma protein binding (>99%); found in breast milk. **Metabolism:** Sequential deiodination and conjugation in the liver (mainly), kidneys, and other tissues. **Elimination:** Urine; feces (approximately 20% unchanged). $T_{1/2}$=6-7 days (T4),≤2 days (T3).

PATIENT CONSIDERATIONS
Assessment: Assess for untreated subclinical or overt thyrotoxicosis, acute MI, uncorrected adrenal insufficiency, CAD, CV disorders, nontoxic diffuse goiter, nodular thyroid disease, DM, hypersensitivity, pregnancy/nursing status, and for possible drug interactions. In patients with secondary or tertiary hypothyroidism, assess for additional hypothalamic/pituitary hormone deficiencies. Assess TSH levels. In infants with congenital hypothyroidism, assess for other congenital anomalies.

Monitoring: Monitor for CV effects. In patients on long-term therapy, monitor for signs/symptoms of decreased BMD. In patients with nontoxic diffuse goiter or nodular thyroid disease, monitor for precipitation of thyrotoxicosis. In adults with primary hypothyroidism, perform periodic monitoring of serum TSH levels. In pediatric patients with congenital hypothyroidism, perform periodic monitoring of serum TSH levels and total or free T4 levels. In patients with secondary and tertiary hypothyroidism, perform periodic monitoring of serum free-T4 levels. Refer to PI for TSH and T4 monitoring parameters. Closely monitor PT if coadministered with an oral anticoagulant.

Counseling: Instruct to notify physician if allergic to any foods or medicines, pregnant/planning to become pregnant, breastfeeding, or taking any other drugs, including prescriptions and OTC preparations. Instruct to notify physician of any other medical conditions, particularly heart disease, diabetes, clotting disorders, and adrenal or pituitary gland problems. Instruct not to stop or change dose unless directed by physician. Instruct to take on empty stomach, at least 30-60 min before eating breakfast. Advise that partial hair loss may occur during the 1st few months of therapy, but is usually temporary. Instruct to notify physician or dentist prior to surgery about levothyroxine therapy. Inform that drug should not be used for weight control. Instruct to notify physician if rapid or irregular heartbeat, chest pain, SOB, leg cramps, headache, or any other unusual medical event occurs. Inform that dose may be increased during pregnancy. Inform that drug should not be administered within 4 hrs of agents such as iron/calcium supplements and antacids.

TABLOID — thioguanine   Rx

Class: Purine analogue

ADULT DOSAGE

Acute Non-Lymphocytic Leukemia

Remission Induction and Remission Consolidation:

Single Agent Chemotherapy:

Initial: 2mg/kg/day

Titrate: May cautiously increase to 3mg/kg/day if no improvement and no leukocyte/platelet depression after 4 weeks

Total daily dose may be given at one time

Other Neoplasms

Not effective in chronic lymphocytic leukemia, Hodgkin's lymphoma, multiple myeloma, or solid tumors. Although thioguanine is one of several agents w/ activity in the treatment of the chronic phase of chronic myelogenous leukemia, more objective responses are observed w/ busulfan, and therefore busulfan is usually regarded as the preferred drug

PEDIATRIC DOSAGE

Acute Non-Lymphocytic Leukemia

Remission Induction and Remission Consolidation:

Single Agent Chemotherapy:

Initial: 2mg/kg/day

Titrate: May cautiously increase to 3mg/kg/day if no improvement and no leukocyte/platelet depression after 4 weeks

Total daily dose may be given at one time

Other Neoplasms

Not effective in chronic lymphocytic leukemia, Hodgkin's lymphoma, multiple myeloma, or solid tumors. Although thioguanine is one of several agents w/ activity in the treatment of the chronic phase of chronic myelogenous leukemia, more objective responses are observed w/ busulfan, and therefore busulfan is usually regarded as the preferred drug

DOSING CONSIDERATIONS

Elderly

Start at lower end of dosing range

Other Important Considerations

Thiopurine Methyltransferase (TPMT) Deficiency: May require substantial dose reductions

ADMINISTRATION

Oral route

STORAGE

15-25°C (59-77°F). Store in a dry place.

HOW SUPPLIED

Tab: 40mg* *scored

CONTRAINDICATIONS

Prior resistance to thioguanine, cross-resistance with mercaptopurine.

WARNINGS/PRECAUTIONS

Potentially hazardous; should only be administered by physicians experienced in the risks of therapy and knowledgeable in acute nonlymphocytic leukemias. Not for use in maint therapy/similar long-term continuous treatments due to high risk of liver toxicity associated with vascular endothelial damage; prevalent in males and usually presents with clinical syndrome of hepatic veno-occlusive disease or signs of portal HTN. D/C if evidence of liver toxicity; reversal of signs and symptoms of liver toxicity reported upon withdrawal. Dose-related bone-marrow suppression (eg, anemia, leukopenia, thrombocytopenia) may occur; d/c temporarily at 1st sign of abnormal large fall in any formed blood elements. Caution in patients with inherited TPMT enzyme deficiency; may be sensitive to myelosuppressive effects and develop rapid bone marrow suppression; closely monitor clinical and hematologic parameters. May cause myelosuppression; modify or d/c dose based on underlying disease response and carefully consider available supportive facilities (eg, granulocyte and platelet transfusion). Life-threatening infections and bleeding reported. May cause fetal harm. D/C therapy with evidence of toxic hepatitis/biliary stasis/clinical jaundice. Caution in elderly.

ADVERSE REACTIONS

Myelosuppression, hyperuricemia, liver toxicity (hepatic veno-occlusive disease, portal HTN), N/V, anorexia, stomatitis, intestinal necrosis/perforation.

DRUG INTERACTIONS

Avoid live vaccines in immunocompromised patients. Caution with TPMT inhibitors, such as aminosalicylate derivatives (eg, olsalazine, mesalazine, sulphasalazine); may exacerbate bone marrow suppression. May need dose reduction when used with other drugs whose primary toxicity is myelosuppression (eg, other chemotherapeutic agents).

PREGNANCY AND LACTATION

Category D, not for use in nursing.

MECHANISM OF ACTION

Purine analog; competes with hypoxanthine and guanine for hypoxanthine-guanine phosphoribosyltransferase (HGPRTase) and is converted to 6-thioguanylic acid (TGMP), resulting in sequential blockade of the synthesis and utilization of purine nucleotides.

PHARMACOKINETICS

Absorption: Incomplete and variable; T_{max}=8 hrs. **Metabolism:** Via HGPRTase converted to TGMP (metabolite); via methylation to 2-amino-6-methylthiopurine (MTG) (metabolite). **Elimination:** Urine (Parent compound in trace amounts; MTG; thiouric acid in small amounts; inorganic sulfates).

PATIENT CONSIDERATIONS

Assessment: Assess for prior resistance to the drug, cross-resistance with mercaptopurine, TPMT deficiency, hepatic impairment, pregnancy/nursing status, and possible drug interactions. Assess LFTs (serum transaminases, alkaline phosphatase, bilirubin) and hematological parameters including Hgb, Hct, WBC and differential count, and quantitative platelet count.

Monitoring: Monitor for signs and symptoms of liver toxicity (eg, hepatic veno-occlusive disease, portal HTN), bone-marrow suppression, infection, bleeding, and other adverse reactions. Perform frequent monitoring of Hgb, Hct, total WBC and differential count, and quantitative platelet count. Perform bone marrow evaluation. Monitor LFTs (serum transaminases, alkaline phosphatase, bilirubin) at weekly intervals when 1st beginning therapy and at monthly intervals thereafter; more frequently in patients with preexisting liver disease or concomitantly taking other hepatotoxic drugs.

Counseling: Inform about major toxicities associated with therapy (eg, myelosuppression, hepatotoxicity, GI toxicity). Advise to never take medication without medical supervision. Instruct to consult physician if experience fever, sore throat, jaundice, N/V, signs of local infection, bleeding from any site, or symptoms suggestive of anemia. Advise women of childbearing potential to avoid becoming pregnant.

TACHOSIL — fibrin sealant   Rx

Class: Fibrinogen/topical thrombin

ADULT DOSAGE

Hemostasis

For use w/ manual compression as an adjunct to hemostasis in cardiovascular and hepatic surgery when control of bleeding by standard surgical techniques is ineffective/impractical

Determine the number of patches to be applied by the size of the bleeding area

Max Number of Patches to be Applied:

Patch Size 9.5cm x 4.8cm: 10

Patch Size 4.8cm x 4.8cm: 14

Patch Size 3.0cm x 2.5cm: 42

Repeat application (w/o removing already applied patch) if not satisfied w/ placement of patch, or if bleeding still occurs during or after specified duration of compression

PEDIATRIC DOSAGE

Hemostasis

For use w/ manual compression as an adjunct to hemostasis in cardiovascular and hepatic surgery when control of bleeding by standard surgical techniques is ineffective/impractical

≥1 Month of Age:

Determine the number of patches to be applied by the size of the bleeding area

Max Number of Patches to be Applied:

Patch Size 9.5cm x 4.8cm: 10

Patch Size 4.8cm x 4.8cm: 14

Patch Size 3.0cm x 2.5cm: 42

Repeat application (w/o removing already applied patch) if not satisfied w/ placement of patch, or if bleeding still occurs during or after specified duration of compression

ADMINISTRATION

Topical route

For topical use on cardiovascular or hepatic tissue only.

Preparation of Application

1. When in the operating room, the outer aluminum foil pouch may be opened in a nonsterile environment; the inner sterile blister must be opened in a sterile environment.
2. Remove patch from blister.
3. Determine the size of patch(es) to be applied. Select the appropriate patch so that it extends 1-2cm beyond the margins of the wound. May cut patch to the correct size and shape if desired. If >1 patch used, overlap patches by at least 1cm.
4. Before application, cleanse area to be treated. Alcohol, iodine, or heavy metal ions can denature fibrinogen and thrombin proteins; if any of these substances are used to clean, thoroughly irrigate area before application.
5. Apply directly to bleeding area either wet or dry. If applied wet, premoisten in 0.9% saline sol for no more than 1 min and then apply immediately. If wet tissue surface, may apply w/o premoistening.

Method of Application

1. Cleanse surgical instruments and gloves w/ saline sol to reduce the adherence.
2. Apply yellow, active side of the patch to the bleeding area and hold in place w/ gentle pressure applied through moistened gloves or a moist pad for at least 3 min.
3. To avoid pulling the patch loose, place a premoistened surgical instrument at one end of the patch before relieving the pressure; gentle irrigation may also aid in removal of premoistened pad or gloved hand w/o removing patch from bleeding area.
4. Leave in place once it adheres to organ tissue. Removed unattached patches (or part of) and replace w/ new patches.

STORAGE

2-25°C (36-77°F). Does not require refrigeration. Do not freeze. Do not use if package is opened/damaged.

HOW SUPPLIED

Patch: (Human fibrinogen/Human thrombin) 5.5mg/2.0 U/cm² [9.5cm x 4.8cm, 1s; 4.8cm x 4.8cm, 2s; 3.0cm x 2.5cm, 1s, 5s]

CONTRAINDICATIONS

Intravascular application, known anaphylactic or severe systemic reaction to human blood products or horse proteins.

WARNINGS/PRECAUTIONS

Not for use in place of sutures or other form of mechanical ligation for the treatment of major arterial/venous bleeding. Thrombosis may occur if applied intravascularly; ensure that patch is applied to the surface of cardiac, vascular, or hepatic tissue only. Hypersensitivity or allergic/anaphylactoid reactions may occur. Avoid application to contaminated or infected areas of the body, or in the presence of active infection. Contains collagen, which may adhere to bleeding surfaces. Avoid over-packing when placing into cavities or closed spaces; may cause compression of underlying tissue. Use only the minimum amount of patches necessary to achieve hemostasis; do not pack. Excess patch material can become dislodged and migrate to other areas of the body. Remove unattached pieces of patch. Made from human blood; may carry risk of transmitting infectious agents (eg, viruses, variant Creutzfeldt-Jakob disease [CJD] agent, CJD agent).

ADVERSE REACTIONS
A-fib, pleural effusion, pyrexia, nausea, anemia, diarrhea, HTN, transaminases increased.

PREGNANCY AND LACTATION
Category C, caution in nursing.

MECHANISM OF ACTION
Fibrinogen/topical thrombin; fibrinogen-thrombin reaction initiates the last step in the cascade of biochemical reactions-conversion of fibrinogen into fibrin monomers that further polymerize to form the fibrin clot. Hemostasis is achieved when the formed fibrin clot adheres the collagen patch to the wound surface, thus providing a physical barrier to bleeding.

PATIENT CONSIDERATIONS
Assessment: Assess for hypersensitivity reactions to human blood products or horse proteins, size of the bleeding area, presence of contamination or infection at application site, and pregnancy/nursing status.

Monitoring: Monitor for signs/symptoms of thrombosis, hypersensitivity reactions, transmission of infectious agents (eg, viruses, CJD agent), and other adverse reactions.

Counseling: Advise that drug is made from human blood, and may carry a risk of transmitting infectious agents (eg, viruses, CJD agent). Inform that patch may cause clot formation in blood vessels if exposed intravascularly; advise to consult physician if chest pain, SOB, difficulty speaking/swallowing, or leg tenderness/swelling develops. Instruct to consult physician if symptoms of B19 virus infection appear (fever, drowsiness, chills) followed about 2 weeks later by a rash and joint pain; inform that pregnant women (fetal infection), immunocompromised individuals, or those w/ increased erythropoiesis (eg, hemolytic anemia) are most seriously affected.

TACLONEX OINTMENT — betamethasone dipropionate/calcipotriene
RX

Class: Corticosteroid/vitamin D3 analogue

ADULT DOSAGE	**PEDIATRIC DOSAGE**
Plaque Psoriasis	**Plaque Psoriasis**
≥18 Years:	**12-17 Years:**
Apply an adequate layer to affected area(s) qd for up to 4 weeks.	Apply an adequate layer to affected area(s) qd for up to 4 weeks.
D/C therapy when control is achieved.	D/C therapy when control is achieved.
Max: 100g/week	**Max:** 60g/week
Treatment of >30% BSA is not recommended	Treatment of >30% BSA is not recommended

ADMINISTRATION
Topical route

Rub in gently and completely.
Wash hands after application.
Avoid use on the face, groin, axillae, or if skin atrophy is present at the treatment site.
Avoid use w/ occlusive dressings unless directed by a physician.

STORAGE
20-25°C (68-77°F); excursions permitted to 15-30°C (59-86°F).

HOW SUPPLIED
Oint: (Calcipotriene/Betamethasone) 0.005%/0.064% [60g, 100g]

WARNINGS/PRECAUTIONS
Not for oral, ophthalmic, or intravaginal use. Hypercalcemia and hypercalciuria observed; d/c until parameters of Ca²⁺ metabolism have normalized. May cause reversible hypothalamic-pituitary-adrenal (HPA) axis suppression w/ the potential for glucocorticosteroid insufficiency during and after withdrawal of treatment. Factors predisposing to HPA axis suppression include the use of high-potency corticosteroids, large treatment surface areas, prolonged use, concomitant use of >1 corticosteroids-containing product, use of occlusive dressings, altered skin barrier, liver failure, and young age. Gradually withdraw drug, reduce frequency of application, or substitute to a less potent steroid if HPA axis suppression is documented. Cushing's syndrome, and hyperglycemia may occur. Pediatric patients may be more susceptible to systemic toxicity. Allergic contact dermatitis may occur; may be confirmed by patch testing. D/C and institute appropriate therapy if irritation develops. Avoid excessive exposure of treated areas to natural or artificial sunlight; limit or avoid use of phototherapy.

ADVERSE REACTIONS
Pruritus.

DRUG INTERACTIONS
Use w/ other corticosteroid-containing products may increase total systemic exposure.

PREGNANCY AND LACTATION
Pregnancy: Category C.
Lactation: Caution in nursing.

MECHANISM OF ACTION
Calcipotriene: Synthetic vitamin D3 analogue; has not been established.
Betamethasone: Synthetic corticosteroid; has not been established.

PHARMACOKINETICS
Distribution: Betamethasone: Found in breast milk (systemically administered).
Metabolism: Betamethasone: Betamethasone 17-propionate (major metabolite). Calcipotriene: Liver (rapid); MC1080 (major metabolite).

PATIENT CONSIDERATIONS
Assessment: Assess for predisposing factors to HPA axis suppression, treatment-site atrophy, use of phototherapy, pregnancy/nursing status, and possible drug interactions.

Monitoring: Monitor for hypercalcemia, hypercalciuria, HPA axis suppression, Cushing's syndrome, hyperglycemia, allergic contact dermatitis, irritation, and other adverse reactions.

Counseling: Instruct adult patients not to use >100g/week and pediatric patients not to use >60g/week. Instruct to d/c therapy when control is achieved unless directed otherwise by the physician. Advise to avoid use on the face, underarms, groin, or eyes; instruct to wash area right away if medicine gets on face or in eyes. Instruct not to occlude the treatment area w/ a bandage or other covering unless directed by physician. Inform that local reactions and skin atrophy are more likely to occur w/ occlusive use, prolonged use or use of higher potency corticosteroids. Instruct to wash hands after application. Counsel not to use other products containing calcipotriene or a corticosteroid w/o first consulting the physician. Instruct to avoid excessive exposure to either natural or artificial sunlight (eg, tanning booths, sun lamps).

TAFINLAR — dabrafenib
Rx

Class: Kinase inhibitor

ADULT DOSAGE	**PEDIATRIC DOSAGE**
Unresectable or Metastatic Melanoma with BRAF V600E Mutation	Pediatric use may not have been established
150mg bid, approx 12 hrs apart, as a single agent until disease progression or unacceptable toxicity occurs	
Unresectable or Metastatic Melanoma with BRAF V600E or V600K Mutations	
150mg bid, approx 12 hrs apart, in combination w/ trametinib until disease progression or unacceptable toxicity occurs	
Missed Dose	
Do not take a missed dose w/in 6 hrs of the next dose	

DOSING CONSIDERATIONS
Adverse Reactions
Dose Reductions for Dabrafenib:
First Dose Reduction: 100mg bid
Second Dose Reduction: 75mg bid
Third Dose Reduction: 50mg bid
Subsequent Modification: Permanently d/c if unable to tolerate 50mg bid

New Primary Noncutaneous Malignancies:
Permanently d/c if RAS mutation-positive noncutaneous malignancies develop

Febrile Drug Reaction:
Fever of 101.3-104°F: Withhold until fever resolves, then resume at same or lower dose level
Fever >104°F or Fever Complicated by Rigors, Hypotension, Dehydration, or Renal Failure: Withhold until fever resolves, then resume at a lower dose level or permanently d/c

Cutaneous:
Grade 3 or 4 Skin Toxicity or Intolerable Grade 2 Skin Toxicity: Withhold for up to 3 weeks; resume at a lower dose level if improved or permanently d/c if not improved

Cardiac:
Symptomatic CHF: Withhold; if improved, then resume at the same dose
Absolute Decrease in Left Ventricular Ejection Fraction (LVEF) >20% from Baseline That is Below Lower Limit of Normal: Withhold; if improved, then resume at the same dose

Uveitis Including Iritis and Iridocyclitis:
If mild or moderate uveitis does not respond to ocular therapy, or for severe uveitis, withhold for up to 6 weeks; resume at the same or at a lower dose level if improved to Grade 0-1, or permanently d/c if not improved

Other:

Any Grade 3 Adverse Reaction or Intolerable Grade 2 Adverse Reactions:
Withhold; resume at a lower dose level if improved to Grade 0-1, or permanently
d/c if not improved

First Occurrence of Any Grade 4 Adverse Reaction: Withhold until adverse
reaction improves to Grade 0-1, then resume at a lower dose level; or permanently
d/c

Recurrent Grade 4 Adverse Reaction: Permanently d/c

Refer to trametinib PI for trametinib modifications

ADMINISTRATION

Oral route

Take at least 1 hr ac or 2 hrs pc.

Do not open, crush, or break caps.

STORAGE

25°C (77°F); excursions permitted to 15-30°C (59-86°F).

HOW SUPPLIED

Cap: 50mg, 75mg

WARNINGS/PRECAUTIONS

See Dosing Considerations. Not indicated for treatment of patients w/ wild-type
BRAF melanoma. New primary cutaneous and noncutaneous malignancies may
occur when dabrafenib is administered alone or in combination w/ trametinib;
perform dermatologic evaluations prior to initiation, every 2 months while
on therapy, and for up to 6 months following discontinuation. Increased cell
proliferation may occur in BRAF wild-type cells exposed to BRAF inhibitors;
confirm evidence of BRAF V600E or V600K mutation status prior to treatment
initiation. Hemorrhages (eg, major hemorrhages) may occur when administered
w/ trametinib; permanently d/c for all Grade 4 hemorrhagic events and for any
persistent Grade 3 hemorrhagic events. Cardiomyopathy may occur; assess
LVEF by echocardiogram or multigated acquisition (MUGA) scan before
initiation of dabrafenib w/ trametinib, 1 month after initiation, and then at 2- to
3-month intervals while on treatment. Uveitis may occur; monitor for visual
signs/symptoms (eg, change in vision, photophobia, eye pain). Permanently d/c
for persistent Grade 2 or greater uveitis of >6 weeks duration. Serious febrile
reactions and fever of any severity complicated by hypotension, rigors/chills,
dehydration, or renal failure may occur; incidence and severity of pyrexia are
increased w/ trametinib. Monitor SrCr and other evidence of renal function during
and following severe pyrexia. Serious skin toxicity may occur. Hyperglycemia may
occur; monitor serum glucose levels upon initiation and as clinically appropriate
in patients w/ preexisting diabetes or hyperglycemia. Potential risk of hemolytic
anemia in patients w/ G6PD deficiency; closely monitor such patients for signs of
hemolytic anemia. May cause fetal harm.

ADVERSE REACTIONS

Single Agent Dabrafenib: Hyperkeratosis, headache, pyrexia, arthralgia, papilloma,
alopecia, palmar-plantar erythrodysesthesia syndrome.

W/ Trametinib: Pyrexia, rash, chills, headache, arthralgia, cough.

DRUG INTERACTIONS

Strong inhibitors of CYP3A4 or CYP2C8 may increase concentrations and strong
inducers of CYP3A4 or CYP2C8 may decrease concentrations; substitution of
these medications is recommended during treatment. If concomitant use of
strong inhibitors (eg, ketoconazole, nefazodone, clarithromycin, gemfibrozil)
or strong inducers (eg, rifampin, phenytoin, carbamazepine, phenobarbital, St.
John's wort) of CYP3A4 or CYP2C8 is unavoidable, monitor closely for adverse
reactions when taking strong inhibitors or loss of efficacy when taking strong
inducers. May decrease systemic exposures of midazolam (CYP3A4 substrate),
S-warfarin (CYP2C9 substrate), and R-warfarin (CYP3A4/CYP1A2 substrate).
Monitor INR levels more frequently in patients receiving warfarin during initiation
or discontinuation of dabrafenib. Coadministration w/ CYP3A4 and CYP2C9
substrates (eg, dexamethasone, hormonal contraceptives) may result in decreased
concentrations and loss of efficacy; substitute for these medications or monitor
for loss of efficacy if use of these medications is unavoidable.

PREGNANCY AND LACTATION

Pregnancy: May cause fetal harm.

Lactation: Advise women not to breastfeed during treatment and for 2 weeks
following the last dose.

Reproductive Potential: Females of reproductive potential should use effective
nonhormonal contraception during treatment and for 2 weeks after the last dose.
May impair fertility in females of reproductive potential. Potential risk for impaired
spermatogenesis that may be irreversible in males.

MECHANISM OF ACTION

Kinase inhibitor; inhibits BRAF V600 mutation-positive melanoma cell growth. Use
of dabrafenib and trametinib in combination resulted in greater growth inhibition
of BRAF V600 mutation-positive melanoma cell lines in vitro and prolonged
inhibition of tumor growth in BRAF V600 mutation-positive melanoma xenografts
compared w/ either drug alone.

PHARMACOKINETICS

Absorption: Absolute bioavailability (95%); T_{max}=2 hrs (median). **Distribution:**
Plasma protein binding (99.7%); V_d=70.3L. **Metabolism:** Via CYP2C8 and CYP3A4
to hydroxy-dabrafenib (active), hydroxy-dabrafenib is oxidized via CYP3A4
to carboxy-dabrafenib, carboxy-dabrafenib is decarboxylated to desmethyl-
dabrafenib (active), desmethyl-dabrafenib via CYP3A4 to oxidative metabolites.
Elimination: Feces (71%), urine (23%, metabolites); $T_{1/2}$=8 hrs, 10 hrs (hydroxy-
dabrafenib), 21-22 hrs (carboxy- and desmethyl-dabrafenib).

PATIENT CONSIDERATIONS

Assessment: Assess for diabetes, hyperglycemia, G6PD deficiency, pregnancy/
nursing status, and possible drug interactions. Assess for presence of BRAF
V600E or V600K mutation in tumor specimens. Perform dermatologic

---

evaluations. Assess LVEF by echocardiogram or MUGA scan before initiation of
dabrafenib w/ trametinib.

Monitoring: Monitor for new primary malignancies, hemorrhagic events,
cardiomyopathy, uveitis, febrile reactions, fever, skin toxicity, hyperglycemia,
and other adverse reactions. Perform dermatologic evaluations every 2 months
during therapy and for up to 6 months following discontinuation. Monitor LVEF by
echocardiogram and MUGA scan 1 month after initiation and then at 2- to 3-month
intervals during therapy. Monitor SrCr and other evidence of renal function during
and following severe pyrexia. Monitor serum glucose levels upon initiation and
as clinically appropriate in patients w/ preexisting diabetes or hyperglycemia.
Closely monitor patients w/ G6PD deficiency for signs of hemolytic anemia.
Monitor INR levels more frequently in patients receiving warfarin during initiation
or discontinuation.

Counseling: Inform that evidence of BRAF V600E or V600K mutation in
the tumor specimen is necessary to identify patients for whom treatment is
indicated. Inform of increased risk of developing new primary cutaneous and
noncutaneous malignancies; instruct to contact healthcare provider immediately
for any new lesions, changes to existing lesions on the skin, or signs/symptoms
of other malignancies. Inform that combined use w/ trametinib may increase
risk of intracranial and GI hemorrhage; advise to contact healthcare provider or
seek immediate medical attention for unusual bleeding or hemorrhage. Advise
that therapy may cause cardiomyopathy and to report signs/symptoms of
heart failure. Advise that therapy may cause uveitis and to contact healthcare
provider if changes in vision occur. Inform that therapy may cause pyrexia,
including serious febrile reactions, and that incidence and severity are increased
w/ trametinib; advise to contact healthcare provider if fever develops. Advise of
risk of serious skin reactions and to contact healthcare provider for progressive
or intolerable rash. Advise diabetic patients that therapy may impair glucose
control and to report severe hyperglycemia symptoms to healthcare provider.
Advise patients w/ known G6PD deficiency to contact healthcare provider to
report signs/symptoms of anemia or hemolysis. Instruct female patients to use
effective nonhormonal contraception during treatment and for 2 weeks after
discontinuation of dabrafenib; advise to contact healthcare provider if pregnancy
occurs, or is suspected, while on therapy. Advise breastfeeding mothers to d/c
nursing while on therapy and for 2 weeks after the last dose. Inform males and
females of reproductive potential that treatment may impair fertility.

TAGRISSO — osimertinib　　　　　　　　　　　　　Rx

Class: Kinase inhibitor

ADULT DOSAGE	PEDIATRIC DOSAGE
Metastatic Non-Small Cell Lung Cancer	Pediatric use may not have been established
Treatment of patients w/ metastatic epidermal growth factor receptor (EGFR) T790M mutation-positive non-small cell lung cancer (NSCLC), as detected by an FDA-approved test, who have progressed on or after EGFR tyrosine kinase inhibitor therapy	
80mg qd until disease progression or unacceptable toxicity	
Missed Dose	
If a dose is missed, do not make up the missed dose and take the next dose as scheduled	

DOSING CONSIDERATIONS

Adverse Reactions

Pulmonary:

Interstitial Lung Disease (ILD)/Pneumonitis: Permanently d/c

Cardiac:

QTc Interval >500 msec on at Least 2 Separate ECGs: Withhold until QTc interval
is <481 msec or recovery to baseline if baseline QTc is ≥481 msec, then resume at
40mg dose

QTc Interval Prolongation w/ Signs/Symptoms of Life-Threatening Arrhythmia:
Permanently d/c

**Asymptomatic, Absolute Decrease in Left Ventricular Ejection Fraction (LVEF)
of 10% from Baseline and <50%:** Withhold for up to 4 weeks. Resume if LVEF
improves to baseline, or permanently d/c if LVEF does not improve to baseline

Symptomatic CHF: Permanently d/c

Other:

Grade ≥3 Adverse Reaction: Withhold for up to 3 weeks

If Improvement to Grade 0-2 w/in 3 Weeks: Resume at 80mg or 40mg qd

If No Improvement w/in 3 Weeks: Permanently d/c

ADMINISTRATION

Oral route

Take w/ or w/o food.

Administration to Patients Who Have Difficulty Swallowing Solids

1. Disperse tab in 4 tbsp (approx 50mL) of non-carbonated water only; stir until
tab is completely dispersed.

2. Swallow or administer through NG tube immediately.

3. Do not crush, heat, or ultrasonicate during preparation.

4. Rinse container w/ 4-8 oz of water and immediately drink or administer through
the NG tube.

STORAGE
25°C (77°F); excursions permitted to 15-30°C (59-86°F).

HOW SUPPLIED
Tab: 40mg, 80mg

WARNINGS/PRECAUTIONS
See Dosing Considerations. ILD/pneumonitis reported; withhold therapy and promptly investigate for ILD in any patient who presents w/ worsening of respiratory symptoms. QTc interval prolongation reported; periodically monitor ECGs and electrolytes in patients w/ congenital long QTc syndrome, CHF, or electrolyte abnormalities. Cardiomyopathy reported; assess LVEF before initiation and then at 3-month intervals while on treatment. May cause fetal harm.

ADVERSE REACTIONS
Diarrhea, rash, dry skin, nail toxicity.

DRUG INTERACTIONS
Avoid w/ strong CYP3A inhibitors (eg, telithromycin, itraconazole, ritonavir). Concomitant use of strong CYP3A inhibitors may increase osimertinib levels; if no other alternative exists, monitor patients more closely for adverse reactions. Avoid w/ strong CYP3A inducers (eg, phenytoin, carbamazepine, St. John's wort); may decrease osimertinib levels. Avoid w/ drugs that are sensitive substrates of CYP3A, breast cancer resistance protein, or CYP1A2 w/ narrow therapeutic indices (eg, fentanyl, cyclosporine, quinidine); osimertinib may increase or decrease levels of these drugs. Periodically monitor ECGs and electrolytes in patients taking medications known to prolong the QTc interval.

PREGNANCY AND LACTATION
Pregnancy: May cause fetal harm.
Lactation: Lactating women should not breastfeed during treatment and for 2 weeks after final dose.
Reproductive Potential: Advise females of reproductive potential to use effective contraception during treatment and for 6 weeks after the final dose. Advise male patients w/ female partners of reproductive potential to use effective contraception during and for 4 months following the final dose. May impair fertility in females and males of reproductive potential.

MECHANISM OF ACTION
Kinase inhibitor; binds irreversibly to certain mutant forms of EGFR. Exhibits anti-tumor activity against NSCLC lines harboring EGFR-mutations (T790M/L858R, L858R, T790M/exon 19 deletion, and exon 19 deletion) and, to a lesser extent, wild-type EGFR amplifications.

PHARMACOKINETICS
Absorption: T_{max}=6 hrs (median). **Distribution:** V_d=986L. Plasma protein binding is likely high. **Metabolism:** Oxidation (predominantly CYP3A) and dealkylation. AZ7550 and AZ5104 (active metabolites). **Elimination:** Feces (68%), urine (14%), unchanged (2%). $T_{1/2}$=48 hrs.

PATIENT CONSIDERATIONS
Assessment: Assess for congenital long QTc syndrome, CHF, and electrolyte abnormalities. Assess LVEF, pregnancy/nursing status, and for possible drug interactions.

Monitoring: Monitor for ILD, pneumonitis, QTc interval prolongation, and cardiomyopathy. Periodically monitor ECGs and electrolytes in patients w/ congenital long QTc syndrome, CHF, electrolyte abnormalities, or those who are taking medications known to prolong the QTc interval. Assess LVEF at 3-month intervals.

Counseling: Inform of the risks of severe or fatal ILD, including pneumonitis; advise to contact physician immediately to report new or worsening respiratory symptoms. Inform patients of symptoms that may be indicative of significant QTc prolongation (eg, dizziness, lightheadedness, syncope) and advise to report these symptoms. Advise to inform physician about the use of any heart or blood pressure medications. Advise to immediately report any signs or symptoms of heart failure. Inform that drug can cause fetal harm if taken during pregnancy. Advise pregnant women of the potential risk to a fetus. Advise females to inform physician if they become pregnant or if pregnancy is suspected while on therapy. Instruct females of reproductive potential to use effective contraception during treatment and for 6 weeks after the final dose. Instruct males w/ female partners of reproductive potential to use effective contraception during treatment and for 4 months after the final dose. Advise women not to breastfeed during treatment and for 2 weeks after the final dose.

TALTZ — ixekizumab   Rx

Class: Monoclonal antibody/IL-17A antagonist

ADULT DOSAGE
Plaque Psoriasis

In Patients Who Are Candidates for Systemic/Phototherapy:
Moderate to Severe:
160mg (two 80mg inj) at Week 0, followed by 80mg at Weeks 2, 4, 6, 8, 10, and 12, then 80mg every 4 weeks

PEDIATRIC DOSAGE
Pediatric use may not have been established

ADMINISTRATION
SQ route

Administer each inj at a different anatomic location (eg, upper arms, thighs, any quadrant of abdomen) than previous inj.
Do not inject into areas where the skin is tender, bruised, erythematous, indurated, or affected by psoriasis.

Before inj, remove from refrigerator and allow to reach room temperature (30 min) w/o removing needle cap.
Product does not contain preservatives; discard any unused product remaining in the autoinjector or prefilled syringe.
Refer to prescribing information for further instructions for administration.

STORAGE
2-8°C (36-46°F). Protect from light. Do not freeze; do not use if product has been frozen. Do not shake.

HOW SUPPLIED
Inj: 80mg/mL [autoinjector, prefilled syringe]

CONTRAINDICATIONS
Previous serious hypersensitivity reaction to ixekizumab or to any of the excipients in the product.

WARNINGS/PRECAUTIONS
Intended for use under the guidance and supervision of a physician. May increase risk of infection. If a serious infection develops or if not responding to standard therapy, monitor the patient closely and d/c therapy until the infection resolves. Evaluate for tuberculosis (TB) infection prior to initiating treatment; do not administer to patients w/ active TB infection. Initiate treatment of latent TB prior to administering therapy; consider anti-TB therapy prior to initiation in patients w/ a past history of latent or active TB in whom an adequate course of treatment cannot be confirmed. Serious hypersensitivity reactions (eg, angioedema, urticaria) reported; d/c immediately and initiate appropriate therapy if a serious hypersensitivity reaction occurs. Crohn's disease and ulcerative colitis, including exacerbations, reported. Prior to initiating therapy, consider completion of all age-appropriate immunizations according to current immunization guidelines.

ADVERSE REACTIONS
Inj-site reactions, URTIs, nausea, tinea infections.

DRUG INTERACTIONS
Avoid w/ live vaccines. May normalize formation of CYP450 enzymes; upon initiation or discontinuation of therapy in patients who are receiving concomitant CYP450 substrates, particularly those w/ a narrow therapeutic index, consider monitoring for therapeutic effect (eg, warfarin) or drug concentration (eg, cyclosporine) and consider dosage modification of the CYP450 substrate.

PREGNANCY AND LACTATION
Pregnancy: There are no available data on ixekizumab use in pregnant women to inform any drug-associated risks. Human IgG is known to cross the placental barrier; therefore, ixekizumab may be transmitted from the mother to the developing fetus.
Lactation: There are no data on the presence of ixekizumab in human milk, the effects on the breastfed infant, or the effects on milk production; caution in nursing.

MECHANISM OF ACTION
Monoclonal antibody/interleukin-17A (IL-17A) antagonist; selectively binds to the IL-17A cytokine and inhibits its interaction w/ the IL-17 receptor. Inhibits the release of proinflammatory cytokines and chemokines.

PHARMACOKINETICS
Absorption: Bioavailability (60-81%); C_{max}=16.2mcg/mL (160mg); T_{max}=4 days.
Distribution: V_d=7.11L. **Elimination:** $T_{1/2}$=13 days.

PATIENT CONSIDERATIONS
Assessment: Assess for previous hypersensitivity to the drug or to any of the excipients of the product, infection including TB infection, inflammatory bowel disease, immunization status, pregnancy/nursing status, and possible drug interactions.

Monitoring: Monitor for signs/symptoms of infection, inflammatory bowel disease, hypersensitivity reactions, and other adverse reactions. Monitor for signs/symptoms of active TB during and after treatment.

Counseling: Advise of the potential benefits and risks of therapy. Instruct on proper SQ inj technique, including aseptic technique, and how to use the autoinjector or prefilled syringe correctly. Inform that drug may lower the ability of immune system to fight infections; instruct to contact physician if any symptoms of infection develop. Advise to seek immediate medical attention if any symptoms of a serious hypersensitivity reaction occur.

TAMIFLU — oseltamivir phosphate   Rx

Class: Neuraminidase inhibitor

ADULT DOSAGE
Influenza

Treatment of Acute/Uncomplicated Illness Due to Influenza A and B Infection W/In 48 Hrs of Symptoms:
75mg bid for 5 days

Prophylaxis of Influenza A and B:
Initiate post-exposure prophylaxis w/in 48 hrs following close contact w/ an infected individual or during a community outbreak for seasonal prophylaxis
Post-Exposure Prophylaxis:
75mg qd for at least 10 days
Community Outbreak (Seasonal/Pre-Exposure Prophylaxis):
75mg qd for up to 6 weeks, or up to 12 weeks in immunocompromised patients

PEDIATRIC DOSAGE
Influenza

Treatment of Acute/Uncomplicated Illness Due to Influenza A and B Infection W/In 48 Hrs of Symptoms:
2 Weeks to <1 Year:
3mg/kg bid for 5 days

1-12 Years:
≤15kg: 30mg bid for 5 days
15.1-23kg: 45mg bid for 5 days
23.1-40kg: 60mg bid for 5 days
≥40.1kg: 75mg bid for 5 days

≥13 Years:
75mg bid for 5 days

Prophylaxis of Influenza A and B:
Initiate post-exposure prophylaxis w/in 48 hrs following close contact

w/ an infected individual or during a community outbreak for seasonal prophylaxis

Post-Exposure Prophylaxis:
1-12 Years:
≤15kg: 30mg qd for 10 days
15.1-23kg: 45mg qd for 10 days
23.1-40kg: 60mg qd for 10 days
≥40.1kg: 75mg qd for 10 days

≥13 Years:
75mg qd for at least 10 days

Community Outbreak (Seasonal/Pre-Exposure Prophylaxis):
Prophylaxis dose for up to 6 weeks, or up to 12 weeks in immunocompromised patients

---

DOSING CONSIDERATIONS
Renal Impairment
Adults:
Mild (CrCl >60-90mL/min): No dosage adjustment needed

Moderate (CrCl >30-60mL/min):
Treatment: 30mg bid for 5 days
Prophylaxis: 30mg qd
Prophylaxis Duration: At least 10 days for post-exposure prophylaxis and for up to 6 weeks (or up to 12 weeks in immunocompromised patients) for community outbreak prophylaxis

Severe (CrCl >10-30mL/min):
Treatment: 30mg qd for 5 days
Prophylaxis: 30mg qod
Prophylaxis Duration: At least 10 days for post-exposure prophylaxis and for up to 6 weeks (or up to 12 weeks in immunocompromised patients) for community outbreak prophylaxis

ESRD on Hemodialysis (CrCl ≤10mL/min):
Treatment: 30mg immediately and then 30mg after every hemodialysis cycle; treatment duration not to exceed 5 days
Prophylaxis: 30mg immediately and then 30mg after alternate hemodialysis cycles
Prophylaxis Duration: At least 10 days for post-exposure prophylaxis and for up to 6 weeks (or up to 12 weeks in immunocompromised patients) for community outbreak prophylaxis

ESRD on Continuous Ambulatory Peritoneal Dialysis (CrCl ≤10mL/min):
Treatment: A single 30mg dose administered immediately
Prophylaxis: 30mg immediately and then 30mg once weekly
Prophylaxis Duration: At least 10 days for post-exposure prophylaxis and for up to 6 weeks (or up to 12 weeks in immunocompromised patients) for community outbreak prophylaxis

ESRD Not on Dialysis:
Not recommended

Hepatic Impairment
Mild to Moderate: No dosage adjustment needed
Severe: Not evaluated

ADMINISTRATION
Oral route

Take w/ or w/o food; enhanced tolerability w/ food.
Oral sus is the preferred formulation for patients who cannot swallow caps. When oral sus is not available, caps may be opened and mixed w/ sweetened liquids such as regular or sugar-free chocolate syrup, corn syrup, caramel topping, or light brown sugar (dissolved in water).
Shake oral sus well before use.
Use an oral dosing dispensing device that measures the appropriate volume in mL w/ the oral sus.

Preparation of Oral Sus
1. Tap the closed bottle containing the supplied white powder several times to loosen the powder.
2. Add 55mL of water to the bottle.
3. Close the bottle and shake well for 15 sec.
Storage:
Refrigerated (2-8°C [36-46°F]): Use constituted oral sus w/in 17 days of preparation
Room Temperature (25°C [77°F]): Use w/in 10 days

Emergency Preparation of Oral Sus from 75mg Caps
Refer to PI for number of caps and amount of water and vehicle needed.
1. Place the specified amount of water into a polyethyleneterephthalate (PET) or glass bottle.
2. Open the required number of caps and pour the contents of caps into the PET or glass bottle.
3. Gently swirl the sus for at least 2 min.
4. Slowly add the specified amount of vehicle to the bottle.
5. Close the bottle and shake well for 30 sec.
Storage:
Refrigerated (2-8°C [36-46°F]): Stable for 5 weeks
Room Temperature (25°C [77°F]): Stable for 5 days

STORAGE
Cap/Dry Powder: 25°C (77°F); excursions permitted to 15-30°C (59-86°F).
Constituted Sus: 2-8°C (36-46°F) for up to 17 days, or at 25°C (77°F) for up to 10 days w/ excursions permitted to 15-30°C (59-86°F). Do not freeze.

HOW SUPPLIED
Cap: 30mg, 45mg, 75mg; **Sus:** 6mg/mL [60mL]

CONTRAINDICATIONS
Known serious hypersensitivity to oseltamivir or any component of the product.

WARNINGS/PRECAUTIONS
Not a substitute for early influenza vaccination on an annual basis. Emergence of resistance substitutions can decrease drug effectiveness; consider available information on influenza drug susceptibility patterns and treatment effects when deciding whether to use treatment. Anaphylaxis and serious skin reactions (eg, toxic epidermal necrolysis, Stevens-Johnson syndrome, erythema multiforme) reported; d/c and institute appropriate treatment if an allergic-like reaction occurs or is suspected. Neuropsychiatric events (eg, delirium, abnormal behavior leading to injury), in some cases resulting in fatal outcomes, reported; monitor for abnormal behavior and evaluate risks and benefits of continuing treatment if neuropsychiatric symptoms occur. Serious bacterial infections may begin w/ influenza-like symptoms or may coexist w/ or occur during the course of influenza; treatment does not prevent these complications. One dose of 75mg oseltamivir for oral sus delivers 2g of sorbitol, which is above the daily max limit of sorbitol for patients w/ hereditary fructose intolerance and may cause dyspepsia and diarrhea.

ADVERSE REACTIONS
Treatment: N/V, headache.
Prophylaxis: N/V, headache, pain.

DRUG INTERACTIONS
Avoid administration of live attenuated influenza vaccine w/in 2 weeks before or 48 hrs after oseltamivir, unless medically indicated.

PREGNANCY AND LACTATION
Pregnancy: Category C. There are no adequate and well-controlled studies in pregnant women. Use only if the potential benefit justifies the potential risk to the fetus.
Lactation: Based on limited published data, oseltamivir and oseltamivir carboxylate are present in human milk at low levels considered unlikely to lead to toxicity in the breastfed infant; caution in nursing.

MECHANISM OF ACTION
Neuraminidase inhibitor; inhibits influenza virus neuraminidase affecting release of viral particles.

PHARMACOKINETICS
Absorption: Absorbed from GI tract. Oseltamivir: C_{max}=65ng/mL; AUC_{0-12h}=112ng•hr/mL. Oseltamivir Carboxylate: C_{max}=348ng/mL; AUC_{0-12h}=2719ng•hr/mL. **Distribution:** Oseltamivir: Plasma protein binding (42%). Oseltamivir Carboxylate: Plasma protein binding (3%); (IV) V_d=23-26L. **Metabolism:** Extensive via hepatic esterases; oseltamivir carboxylate (active metabolite). **Elimination:** Oseltamivir: Feces (<20%); $T_{1/2}$=1-3 hrs. Oseltamivir Carboxylate: Urine (>99%); $T_{1/2}$=6-10 hrs.

PATIENT CONSIDERATIONS
Assessment: Assess for drug hypersensitivity, renal impairment, pregnancy/nursing status, and possible drug interactions.

Monitoring: Monitor for signs/symptoms of neuropsychiatric events, anaphylaxis/serious skin reactions, and other adverse reactions.

Counseling: Advise of the risk of severe allergic reactions or serious skin reactions and to d/c and seek immediate medical attention if an allergic-like reaction occurs or is suspected. Advise of the risk of neuropsychiatric events and to contact physician if experiencing signs of abnormal behavior during treatment. Instruct to begin treatment as soon as possible from the 1st appearance of flu symptoms (w/in 48 hrs of onset), and as soon as possible after exposure (for prevention). Instruct to take missed doses as soon as remembered, unless next scheduled dose is w/in 2 hrs, and then to continue at the usual times. Inform that the medication is not a substitute for flu vaccination. Inform that oral sus delivers 2g sorbitol/75mg dose; inform that this is above the daily max limit of sorbitol for patients w/ hereditary fructose intolerance and may cause dyspepsia and diarrhea.

TAMOXIFEN — tamoxifen citrate   Rx

Class: Antiestrogen

> Serious and life-threatening uterine malignancies (endometrial adenocarcinoma and uterine sarcoma), stroke, and pulmonary embolism (PE) reported in the risk-reduction setting; some of these events were fatal. Discuss the potential benefits versus the potential risks of these serious events w/ women at high-risk for breast cancer and women w/ ductal carcinoma in situ (DCIS) considering therapy for breast cancer risk reduction.

OTHER BRAND NAMES
Soltamox

ADULT DOSAGE
Breast Cancer

Treatment of metastatic breast cancer in women and men. Treatment of node-positive breast cancer in postmenopausal women or axillary node-negative breast cancer in women following total or segmental mastectomy, axillary dissection, and breast irradiation. To reduce risk of invasive breast cancer in women w/ DCIS following breast surgery and

PEDIATRIC DOSAGE
Pediatric use may not have been established

radiation. To reduce incidence of breast cancer in high-risk women (those at least 35 yrs of age w/ a 5-yr predicted risk of breast cancer ≥1.67%, as calculated by the Gail Model)

Treatment:
20-40mg/day
Give dosages >20mg/day in divided doses (am and pm)

Incidence Reduction in High-Risk Women/DCIS:
20mg qd for 5 yrs

ADMINISTRATION
Oral route

STORAGE
Protect from light. **Oral Sol:** Up to 25°C (77°F). Do not freeze or refrigerate. Use w/in 3 months of opening. **Tab:** 20-25°C (68-77°F).

HOW SUPPLIED
Tab: (Base) 10mg, 20mg; **Oral Sol (Soltamox):** (Base) 10mg/5mL [150mL]

CONTRAINDICATIONS
Known hypersensitivity to the drug or any of its ingredients. **Breast Cancer Incidence Reduction in High-Risk Women/Women w/ DCIS:** Women who require coumarin-type anticoagulant therapy or w/ history of deep vein thrombosis (DVT) or PE.

WARNINGS/PRECAUTIONS
Hypercalcemia reported in patients w/ bone metastases; take appropriate measures if hypercalcemia occurs, and, if severe, d/c therapy. Increased incidence of uterine malignancies reported; promptly evaluate any patient receiving or who has previously received therapy who reports abnormal vaginal bleeding. Perform annual gynecological examinations in patients receiving or who have previously received therapy. Increased incidence of endometrial changes, including hyperplasia and polyps, reported. Endometriosis, uterine fibroids, ovarian cysts (in premenopausal patients w/ advanced breast cancer), and menstrual irregularity or amenorrhea reported. Increased incidence of thromboembolic events (eg, DVT, PE) reported; for treatment of breast cancer, carefully consider the risks and benefits of therapy in women w/ history of thromboembolic events. Liver cancer and nonmalignant (eg, changes in liver enzyme levels) effects on the liver, secondary primary tumors (non-uterine), ocular disturbances, increased incidence of cataracts and risk of having cataract surgery, thrombocytopenia, leukopenia, neutropenia, and pancytopenia reported. May cause fetal harm. Hyperlipidemias reported; may consider periodic monitoring of plasma TGs and cholesterol in patients w/ preexisting hyperlipidemias. T4 elevations, not accompanied by clinical hyperthyroidism, reported in a few postmenopausal patients.

ADVERSE REACTIONS
Hot flashes, vaginal discharge, irregular menses, fatigue/asthenia, weight loss, skin changes, N/V, fluid retention, pain, cough, vasodilatation, flu syndrome.

DRUG INTERACTIONS
See Contraindications. A significant increase in anticoagulant effect when used in combination w/ coumarin-type anticoagulants may occur; where such coadministration exists, carefully monitor patient's PT. Increased risk of thromboembolic events w/ cytotoxic agents. May reduce letrozole concentrations. Reduced concentrations w/ rifampin, aminoglutethimide, and phenobarbital. Medroxyprogesterone reduces concentrations of N-desmethyl tamoxifen (active metabolite). Aminoglutethimide may reduce tamoxifen and N-desmethyl tamoxifen plasma concentrations. Bromocriptine may increase tamoxifen and N-desmethyl tamoxifen plasma concentrations. May reduce anastrozole concentrations; avoid w/ anastrozole.

PREGNANCY AND LACTATION
Pregnancy: Category D. May cause fetal harm when administered to a pregnant woman. Avoid pregnancy while on therapy or w/in 2 months of discontinuing therapy; use barrier or nonhormonal contraceptive measures if sexually active. Initiate therapy during menstruation for sexually active women of childbearing potential; a negative β-HCG immediately prior to the initiation of therapy is sufficient in women w/ menstrual irregularity.
Lactation: Reported to inhibit lactation. It is not known if tamoxifen is excreted in human milk; not for use in nursing.

MECHANISM OF ACTION
Nonsteroidal antiestrogen; competes w/ estrogen for binding sites in target tissues such as breast.

PHARMACOKINETICS
Absorption: C_{max}=40ng/mL, 15ng/mL (N-desmethyl tamoxifen); T_{max}=5 hrs.
Metabolism: Extensive; N-desmethyl tamoxifen (active metabolite). **Elimination:** Feces; $T_{1/2}$=5-7 days.

PATIENT CONSIDERATIONS
Assessment: Assess for history of thromboembolic events, preexisting hyperlipidemias, known hypersensitivity, pregnancy/nursing status, and possible drug interactions.

Monitoring: Monitor for signs/symptoms of uterine malignancies, thromboembolic events, hypercalcemia, endometrial changes, uterine fibroids, menstrual irregularity, ocular disturbances, and other adverse reactions. Periodically monitor plasma TG and cholesterol levels in patients w/ preexisting hyperlipidemias.

Periodically monitor CBCs, including platelet counts and LFTs. Perform annual gynecological examinations.

Counseling: Inform about potential risks and benefits of treatment. Advise premenopausal women not to become pregnant and to use nonhormonal contraception during therapy and for 2 months after discontinuation if sexually active. Instruct women to seek prompt medical attention if new breast lumps, vaginal bleeding, gynecologic symptoms (eg, menstrual irregularities), changes in vaginal discharge, pelvic pain/pressure), symptoms of leg swelling/tenderness, unexplained SOB, or changes in vision occur. Inform women taking tamoxifen for the purpose of reducing the incidence of breast cancer and in women taking tamoxifen as adjuvant breast cancer therapy, that they should have a breast examination, a mammogram, and a gynecologic examination prior to the initiation of therapy and at regular intervals while on therapy.

TANDEM DHA — docosahexaenoic acid (DHA)/ eicosapentaenoic acid (EPA)/ferrous fumarate/polysaccharide iron complex/vitamin B6 (pyridoxine hydrochloride)/vitamin B9 (folic acid)/ vitamin C (sodium ascorbate)   RX

Class: Prenatal vitamin

> Accidental overdose of iron-containing products is the leading cause of fatal poisoning in children <6 yrs. Keep out of reach of children. In case of accidental overdose, call a doctor or poison control center immediately.

ADULT DOSAGE
Dietary/Nutritional Supplement
For use prior to conception, throughout pregnancy, and during postnatal period (lactating and nonlactating mothers)

>12 Years:
1 cap qd or ud

PEDIATRIC DOSAGE
Pediatric use may not have been established

ADMINISTRATION
Oral route
Administer between meals

STORAGE
15-30°C (59-86°F). Keep in a cool, dry place.

HOW SUPPLIED
Cap: Ferrous fumarate 15mg-Polysaccharide Iron Complex 15mg-Vitamin C 20mg-Folic acid 1mg-Vitamin B_6 25mg-Omega-3 fatty acids 310.1mg

CONTRAINDICATIONS
Hemosiderosis, hemochromatosis, hemolytic anemias, pernicious anemia, hypersensitivity to this product or its ingredients, including fish or fish oil.

WARNINGS/PRECAUTIONS
Ingestion of >3g/day of omega-3 fatty acids from fish oils may have potential antithrombotic effects, including increased bleeding time and INR; avoid docosahexaenoic acid with inherited or acquired bleeding diatheses. Folic acid alone is improper therapy in the treatment for pernicious anemia and other megaloblastic anemias where vitamin B_{12} is deficient. Folic acid doses >0.1-0.4mg/ day may obscure pernicious anemia in that hematological remission can occur, while neurological manifestations remain progressive. Caution in elderly. Do not exceed recommended dosage.

ADVERSE REACTIONS
Allergic sensitizations, GI disturbances (eg, anorexia, nausea, diarrhea, constipation).

DRUG INTERACTIONS
Calcium may inhibit iron absorption; prescribe calcium salts separately for women at high nutritional risk. Omega-3 fatty acids may have potential antithrombotic effects; avoid with anticoagulants.

MECHANISM OF ACTION
Prenatal vitamin.

PATIENT CONSIDERATIONS
Assessment: Assess for hypersensitivity to the drug and its ingredients including fish and fish oil, pernicious/hemolytic anemia, hemosiderosis, hemochromatosis, and possible drug interactions.

Monitoring: Monitor for hypersensitivity/adverse reactions, increased bleeding time, increased INR and obscuring of pernicious anemia.

Counseling: Inform to immediately call a doctor or poison control center in case of accidental overdose. Advise to keep out of reach of children. Advise to take medication as prescribed. Counsel about possible adverse reactions.

TANZEUM — albiglutide   Rx

Class: Glucagon-like peptide-1 (GLP-1) receptor agonist

> Carcinogenicity of albiglutide could not be assessed in rodents, but other glucagon-like peptide-1 (GLP-1) receptor agonists have caused thyroid C-cell tumors in rodents at clinically relevant exposures; human relevance of GLP-1 receptor agonist induced C-cell tumors has not been determined. It is unknown whether albiglutide causes thyroid C-cell tumors (eg, medullary thyroid carcinoma [MTC]) in humans. Contraindicated in patients w/ a personal or family history of MTC or in patients w/ multiple endocrine neoplasia syndrome type 2 (MEN 2). Routine monitoring of serum calcitonin or using thyroid ultrasound monitoring is of uncertain value for early detection of MTC in patients treated w/ albiglutide.

ADULT DOSAGE
Type 2 Diabetes Mellitus
Usual: 30mg once weekly on the same day each week

Titrate: May increase to 50mg once weekly if glycemic response is inadequate

Day of weekly administration may be changed if necessary as long as the last dose was administered ≥4 days before

Missed Dose
If a dose is missed, administer as soon as possible w/in 3 days after the missed dose; if >3 days after the missed dose, wait until the next regularly scheduled weekly dose

PEDIATRIC DOSAGE
Pediatric use may not have been established

DOSING CONSIDERATIONS
Concomitant Medications
Insulin Secretagogue (eg, Sulfonylurea)/Insulin: Consider reducing dose of insulin secretagogues or insulin

Renal Impairment
Caution when initiating/escalating doses

ADMINISTRATION
SQ route

Administer at any time of the day w/o regard to meals
Inject in the abdomen, thigh, or upper arm region
When used w/ insulin, administer separately and never mix products
May inj insulin in the same body region but inj should not be adjacent to each other; if injecting in the same body region, use different inj site each week

Reconstitution of Lyophilized Powder
Pen Reconstitution/Preparation for Inj:
1. Hold the pen body w/ the clear cartridge pointing up to see the [1] in the number window
2. To reconstitute the lyophilized powder w/ the diluent in the pen, twist the clear cartridge on the pen in the direction of the arrow until the pen is felt/heard to "click" into place and the [2] is seen in the number window
3. Slowly and gently rock the pen side-to-side 5X to mix the reconstituted sol; do not shake the pen hard to avoid foaming
4. Wait 15 min for the 30mg pen and 30 min for the 50mg pen to ensure that the reconstituted sol is mixed
5. Slowly and gently rock the pen side-to-side 5 additional times to mix the reconstituted sol
6. The reconstituted sol will be yellow in color; after reconstitution, use w/in 8 hrs
7. Holding the pen upright, attach the needle to the pen
8. Gently tap the clear cartridge to bring large bubbles to the top

Alternate Method of Reconstitution (Healthcare Professional Use Only):
1. Inspect the pen for [1] in the number window and expiration date
2. Twist the clear cartridge until [2] appears in the number window and a "click" is heard; this combines the medicine powder and liquid in the clear cartridge
3. Hold the pen w/ the clear cartridge pointing up and maintain this orientation throughout the reconstitution
4. Gently swirl the pen in small circular motions for at least 1 min; avoid shaking as this can result in foaming
5. Inspect the sol, and if needed, continue to gently swirl the pen until all the powder is dissolved and you see a clear yellow sol that is free of particles (a small amount of foam on top of the sol at the end of reconstitution is normal)
For 30mg Pen: Complete dissolution usually occurs w/in 2 min but may take up to 5 min
For 50mg Pen: Complete dissolution usually occurs w/in 7 min but may take up to 10 min

Important Administration Instructions
1. Use pen w/in 8 hrs of reconstitution prior to attaching the needle
2. After attaching the supplied needle, remove air bubbles by slowly twisting the pen until you see the [3] in the number window; at the same time, the inj button will be automatically released from the bottom of the pen
3. Use immediately after the needle is attached and primed
4. After SQ inserting the needle into the skin, press the inj button; hold button until you hear a "click" and then hold the button for 5 additional sec to deliver the full dose

STORAGE
2-8°C (36-46°F). May store at room temperature not exceeding 30°C (86°F) for up to 4 weeks prior to use. Do not freeze.

HOW SUPPLIED
Inj: 30mg, 50mg

CONTRAINDICATIONS
Prior serious hypersensitivity reaction to albiglutide or to any of the product components, personal or family history of MTC, MEN 2.

WARNINGS/PRECAUTIONS
Not recommended as 1st-line therapy for patients inadequately controlled on diet and exercise; weigh potential benefits/risks. Not a substitute for insulin; do not use in type 1 DM or for treatment of diabetic ketoacidosis. Not recommended w/ preexisting severe GI disease. Acute pancreatitis reported; d/c promptly if suspected, and do not restart therapy if confirmed. Consider other antidiabetic therapies in patients w/ a history of pancreatitis. Serious hypersensitivity reactions reported; d/c and treat promptly. Acute renal failure and worsening of chronic renal failure reported.

ADVERSE REACTIONS
URTI, diarrhea, N/V, inj-site reaction, cough, back pain, arthralgia, sinusitis, influenza, GERD, dyspepsia.

DRUG INTERACTIONS
See Dosing Considerations. Increased risk of hypoglycemia w/ insulin secretagogues (eg, sulfonylureas) or insulin. May affect the absorption of oral medications; use w/ caution.

PREGNANCY AND LACTATION
Category C, not for use in nursing.

MECHANISM OF ACTION
GLP-1 receptor agonist; augments glucose-dependent insulin secretion. Slows gastric emptying.

PHARMACOKINETICS
Absorption: C_{max}=1.74mcg/mL; AUC=465mcg•hr/mL; T_{max}=3-5 days. **Distribution:** V_d=11L. **Metabolism:** Degradation by proteolytic enzymes. **Elimination:** $T_{1/2}$=approx 5 days.

PATIENT CONSIDERATIONS

Assessment: Assess for previous hypersensitivity reactions, MEN 2, personal or family history of MTC, history of pancreatitis, renal impairment, severe GI disease, pregnancy/nursing status, and possible drug interactions. Further evaluate patients w/ thyroid nodules and/or elevated calcitonin levels.

Monitoring: Monitor for signs/symptoms of thyroid tumor, pancreatitis, elevated serum calcitonin levels, hypoglycemia, hypersensitivity reactions, renal impairment, and other adverse reactions. Monitor renal function in patients w/ renal impairment reporting severe adverse GI reactions.

Counseling: Counsel regarding the potential risk of MTC and instruct to report symptoms of thyroid tumors (eg, lump in the neck, dysphagia) to physician. Inform about self-management practices, including importance of proper storage, inj technique, timing of dosage and concomitant oral drugs, and recognition and management of hypoglycemia. Instruct to d/c therapy promptly and contact physician if persistent severe abdominal pain and/or symptoms of hypersensitivity reactions occur. Advise on the proper use, storage, and disposal of pen. Advise to seek medical advice if any unusual symptom develops, or if any known symptom persists or worsens. Instruct to administer once a week on the same day each week. Instruct not to take an extra dose to make up for a missed dose.

TAPAZOLE — methimazole   Rx

Class: Thyroid hormone synthesis inhibitor

ADULT DOSAGE
Hyperthyroidism

Treatment in patients w/ Graves' disease w/ hyperthyroidism or toxic multinodular goiter for whom surgery or radioactive iodine therapy is not an appropriate treatment option. To ameliorate symptoms of hyperthyroidism in preparation for thyroidectomy or radioactive iodine therapy.

Initial:
Mild Hyperthyroidism: 15mg/day
Moderately Severe Hyperthyroidism: 30-40mg/day
Severe Hyperthyroidism: 60mg/day

Maint: 5-15mg/day

Give total daily dose in 3 divided doses at approx 8-hr intervals

PEDIATRIC DOSAGE
Hyperthyroidism

Treatment in patients w/ Graves' disease w/ hyperthyroidism or toxic multinodular goiter for whom surgery or radioactive iodine therapy is not an appropriate treatment option. To ameliorate symptoms of hyperthyroidism in preparation for thyroidectomy or radioactive iodine therapy.

Initial: 0.4mg/kg/day given in 3 divided doses at 8-hr intervals
Maint: Approx 1/2 of initial dose

ADMINISTRATION
Oral route

STORAGE
15-30°C (59-86°F).

HOW SUPPLIED
Tab: 5mg*, 10mg* *scored

CONTRAINDICATIONS
Hypersensitivity to the drug or any of the other product components.

WARNINGS/PRECAUTIONS

May cause fetal harm when administered in the 1st trimester of pregnancy; rare instances of congenital defects occurred in infants born to mothers who received methimazole in the 1st trimester of pregnancy. Agranulocytosis, leukopenia, thrombocytopenia, and aplastic anemia (pancytopenia) may occur. D/C therapy in the presence of agranulocytosis, aplastic anemia, ANCA-positive vasculitis, hepatitis, or exfoliative dermatitis, and monitor bone marrow indices. Hepatotoxicity (including acute liver failure) reported; promptly evaluate liver function (bilirubin, alkaline phosphatase) and hepatocellular integrity (ALT, AST) if symptoms suggestive of hepatic dysfunction occur. D/C treatment promptly w/ evidence of liver abnormality including hepatic transaminases >3X ULN. May cause hypothyroidism; routinely monitor TSH and free T4 levels and adjust dose to maintain a euthyroid state. May cause fetal goiter and cretinism; lowest possible dose should be given during pregnancy. May cause hypoprothrombinemia and bleeding; monitor PT during therapy, especially before surgical procedures. Monitor thyroid function tests periodically during therapy; use lower maintenance dose once clinical evidence of hyperthyroidism has resolved.

ADVERSE REACTIONS

Agranulocytosis, granulocytopenia, thrombocytopenia, aplastic anemia, drug fever, lupus-like syndrome, insulin autoimmune syndrome, hepatitis, periarteritis, hypoprothrombinemia, skin rash, urticaria, N/V, arthralgia, paresthesia.

DRUG INTERACTIONS

May increase oral anticoagulant (eg, warfarin) activity; consider additional PT/INR monitoring, especially before surgical procedures. β-blockers, digitalis glycosides, and theophylline may need dose reduction when patient becomes euthyroid. Caution w/ other drugs that cause agranulocytosis.

PREGNANCY AND LACTATION

Pregnancy: Category D. Methimazole crosses placental membranes and can induce goiter and cretinism in the developing fetus. Due to the rare occurrence of congenital malformations associated w/ methimazole use, it may be appropriate to use an alternative anti-thyroid medication in pregnant women requiring treatment for hyperthyroidism particularly in the 1st trimester of pregnancy during organogenesis.

Lactation: Methimazole is present in breast milk. However, several studies found no effect on clinical status in nursing infants of mothers taking methimazole. Monitor thyroid function at frequent (weekly or biweekly) intervals.

MECHANISM OF ACTION

Thyroid hormone synthesis inhibitor.

PHARMACOKINETICS

Absorption: Readily absorbed in the GI tract. **Distribution:** Crosses placenta; found in breast milk. **Metabolism:** Liver. **Elimination:** Urine.

PATIENT CONSIDERATIONS

Assessment: Assess for hypersensitivity to drug, pregnancy/nursing status, and possible drug interactions.

Monitoring: Monitor for agranulocytosis, leukopenia, thrombocytopenia, aplastic anemia, hepatotoxicity, hypothyroidism, and other adverse reactions. Monitor PT, especially before surgical procedures. Monitor TSH and free T4 levels periodically.

Counseling: Inform of the benefits/risks of therapy. Instruct to inform physician if pregnant/nursing or planning to become pregnant. Inform of the potential hazard to the fetus if used during pregnancy or if patient becomes pregnant while taking this drug. Instruct to immediately report any evidence of illness, particularly sore throat, skin eruptions, fever, headache, or general malaise.

TARCEVA — erlotinib   Rx

Class: Kinase inhibitor

ADULT DOSAGE

Non-Small Cell Lung Cancer

1st-line treatment of patients w/ metastatic non-small cell lung cancer (NSCLC) whose tumors have epidermal growth factor receptor (EGFR) exon 19 deletions or exon 21 (L858R) substitution mutations; treatment of locally advanced or metastatic NSCLC after failure of at least 1 prior chemotherapy regimen; maint treatment of locally advanced or metastatic NSCLC that has not progressed after 4 cycles of platinum-based 1st-line chemotherapy

Recommended Dose: 150mg qd; continue until disease progression or unacceptable toxicity occurs

Pancreatic Cancer

1st-line treatment of locally advanced, unresectable, or metastatic pancreatic cancer

Recommended Dose: 100mg qd in combination w/ gemcitabine; continue until disease progression or unacceptable toxicity occurs

PEDIATRIC DOSAGE

Pediatric use may not have been established

DOSING CONSIDERATIONS

Concomitant Medications

Reduce by 50mg Decrements If:

If severe reactions occur w/ concomitant use of strong CYP3A4 inhibitors or when using concomitantly w/ an inhibitor of both a CYP3A4 and CYP1A2 (eg, ciprofloxacin); avoid concomitant use if possible

Increase by 50mg Increments As Tolerated For:

- Concomitant use w/ CYP3A4 inducers; increase by 50mg increments at 2-week intervals to a max of 450mg; avoid concomitant use if possible
- Concurrent cigarette smoking; increase by 50mg increments at 2-week intervals to a max of 300mg; immediately reduce the dose to the recommended dose (150mg or 100mg qd) upon cessation of smoking

Drugs Affecting Gastric pH:

- Avoid concomitant use w/ proton pump inhibitors if possible
- If treatment w/ an H2-receptor antagonist is required, dose must be taken 10 hrs after the H2-receptor antagonist dosing and at least 2 hrs before the next dose of the H2-receptor antagonist
- If an antacid is necessary, antacid dose and erlotinib dose should be separated by several hrs

Renal Impairment

No clinical studies have been conducted in patients w/ compromised renal function

Hepatic Impairment

Total Bilirubin >ULN or Child-Pugh A, B, and C: Closely monitor; use w/ extra caution in patients w/ total bilirubin >3X ULN

Adverse Reactions:

D/C For:

- Interstitial Lung Disease (ILD)
- Severe hepatic toxicity that does not improve significantly or resolve w/in 3 weeks
- GI perforation
- Severe bullous, blistering, or exfoliating skin conditions
- Corneal perforation or severe ulceration

Withhold For:

- During diagnostic evaluation for possible ILD
- For severe (CTCAE Grade 3-4) renal toxicity, and consider discontinuation
- In patients w/o preexisting hepatic impairment for total bilirubin levels >3X ULN or transaminases >5X ULN, and consider discontinuation
- In patients w/ preexisting hepatic impairment or biliary obstruction for doubling of bilirubin or tripling of transaminases values over baseline and consider discontinuation
- For persistent severe diarrhea not responsive to medical management (eg, loperamide)
- For severe rash not responsive to medical management
- For keratitis of (NCI-CTC version 4.0) Grade 3-4 or for Grade 2 lasting more than 2 weeks
- For acute/worsening ocular disorders such as eye pain, and consider discontinuation

Reduce by 50mg Decrements:

When restarting therapy following withholding treatment for a dose-limiting toxicity that has resolved to baseline or Grade ≤1

ADMINISTRATION

Oral route

Take on an empty stomach (at least 1 hr ac or 2 hrs pc).

STORAGE

25°C (77°F); excursions permitted to 15-30°C (59-86°F).

HOW SUPPLIED

Tab: 25mg, 100mg, 150mg

WARNINGS/PRECAUTIONS

See Dosing Considerations. Not recommended for use in combination w/ platinum-based chemotherapy. Cases of serious ILD may occur; withhold for acute onset of new/progressive unexplained pulmonary symptoms and permanently d/c therapy if ILD is confirmed. Hepatorenal syndrome; severe acute renal failure; renal insufficiency; hepatotoxicity w/ or w/o hepatic impairment; bullous, blistering, and exfoliative skin conditions (eg, Stevens-Johnson syndrome/ toxic epidermal necrolysis); MI/ischemia; cerebrovascular accidents (CVAs); microangiopathic hemolytic anemia w/ thrombocytopenia; and fetal harm may occur. Decreased tear production, abnormal eyelash growth, keratoconjunctivitis sicca, or keratitis may occur and can lead to corneal perforation/ulceration. GI perforation may occur; increased risk in patients w/ prior history of peptic ulceration or diverticular disease.

ADVERSE REACTIONS

Rash, diarrhea, anorexia, asthenia, dyspnea, cough, N/V.

DRUG INTERACTIONS

See Dosing Considerations. Concomitant use w/ antiangiogenic agents, corticosteroids, NSAIDs, and/or taxane-based chemotherapy may increase risk of GI perforation. Increased levels w/ potent CYP3A4 inhibitors (eg, ketoconazole), and w/ inhibitors of both CYP3A4 and CYP1A2 (eg, ciprofloxacin). Decreased levels w/ CYP3A4 inducers (eg, rifampicin). Cigarette smoking and drugs affecting gastric pH (eg, omeprazole, ranitidine) may decrease levels. INR elevations and bleeding events reported w/ coumarin-derived anticoagulants (eg, warfarin); monitor PT/INR regularly.

PREGNANCY AND LACTATION

Pregnancy: Category D; based on its mechanism of action, erlotinib can cause fetal harm when administered to a pregnant woman.

Lactation: Not for use in nursing.

Reproductive Potential: Females of reproductive potential should use effective contraception during treatment and for at least 2 weeks after the last dose.

MECHANISM OF ACTION

EGFR tyrosine kinase inhibitor; reversibly inhibits the kinase activity of EGFR, preventing autophosphorylation of tyrosine residues associated w/ the receptor and thereby inhibiting further downstream signaling.

PHARMACOKINETICS

Absorption: Bioavailability (60% w/o food, 100% w/ food); T_{max}=4 hrs.
Distribution: V_d=232L; plasma protein binding (93%). **Metabolism:** CYP3A4 (major); 1A2, 1A1 (minor). **Elimination:** Feces (83%; 1% parent drug), urine (8%; 0.3% parent drug); $T_{1/2}$=36.2 hrs (median).

PATIENT CONSIDERATIONS

Assessment: Assess for hepatic/renal impairment, dehydration, history of peptic ulceration or diverticular disease, pregnancy/nursing status, and possible drug interactions.

Monitoring: Monitor for signs and symptoms of ILD, hepatotoxicity, GI perforation, MI/ischemia, renal failure/insufficiency, CVAs, microangiopathic hemolytic anemia w/ thrombocytopenia, ocular disorders, bullous and exfoliative skin disorders, and other adverse reactions. Monitor LFTs, renal function, and serum electrolytes periodically.

Counseling: Inform of risks/benefits of therapy. Instruct to notify physician if onset or worsening of skin rash or development of bullous lesions or desquamation; severe/persistent diarrhea, N/V, or anorexia; unexplained SOB or cough; or eye irritation occurs. Instruct to stop smoking and advise to contact physician for any changes in smoking status. Advise on the presentation of skin, hair, and nail disorders. Instruct on initial management of rash or diarrhea. Counsel on pregnancy planning and prevention; advise females of reproductive potential to use highly effective contraception during treatment and for at least 2 weeks after the last dose. Advise to contact physician if pregnant or if pregnancy is suspected and to d/c nursing during treatment.

TARGRETIN CAPSULES – bexarotene   **Rx**

Class: Retinoid

> Associated w/ birth defects. Do not administer to a pregnant woman.

ADULT DOSAGE

Cutaneous T-Cell Lymphoma

Treatment of cutaneous manifestations of cutaneous T-cell lymphoma in patients who are refractory to at least 1 prior systemic therapy

Initial: 300mg/m^2/day
Titrate: If no tumor response after 8 weeks of treatment and if initial dose of 300mg/m^2/day is well-tolerated, may increase to 400mg/m^2/day w/ careful monitoring

Continue as long as the patient is deriving benefit (administered for up to 97 weeks in clinical trials)

PEDIATRIC DOSAGE

Pediatric use may not have been established

DOSING CONSIDERATIONS

Adverse Reactions

May adjust the 300mg/m^2/day dose level to 200mg/m^2/day then to 100mg/m^2/day, or temporarily suspend, if necessitated by toxicity. When toxicity is controlled, may carefully readjust upward

ADMINISTRATION

Oral route

Take as a single daily dose.
Take w/ a meal.

STORAGE

2-25°C (36-77°F). Avoid exposing to high temperatures and humidity after bottle is opened. Protect from light.

HOW SUPPLIED

Cap: 75mg

CONTRAINDICATIONS

Females who are pregnant, known serious hypersensitivity to bexarotene or other components of the product.

WARNINGS/PRECAUTIONS

May induce substantial elevations in lipids; if fasting TGs are elevated or become elevated during treatment, institute antilipemic therapy, and if necessary, reduce or interrupt dose of bexarotene. Fasting TGs should be normal or normalized w/ appropriate intervention prior to initiating therapy; maintain TG levels <400mg/dL to reduce risk of clinical sequelae. Acute pancreatitis (including a fatal case) reported; interrupt therapy and evaluate if pancreatitis is suspected. May be at greater risk for pancreatitis if risk factors exist (eg, prior pancreatitis, uncontrolled hyperlipidemia, excessive alcohol consumption, uncontrolled diabetes mellitus, biliary tract disease, medications known to increase TG levels or to be associated w/ pancreatic toxicity). Elevations in LFTs, cholestasis, and liver failure reported; obtain baseline LFTs and monitor LFTs after 1, 2 and 4 weeks of treatment initiation, and if stable, at least every 8 weeks thereafter during treatment.

Interrupt or d/c therapy if test results exceed >3X ULN values for AST, ALT, or bilirubin. Hypothyroidism reported; consider treatment w/ thyroid hormone supplementation. Leukopenia and neutropenia reported. New cataracts or worsening of previous cataracts reported; perform ophthalmologic evaluation if visual difficulties occur. May cause photosensitivity; minimize exposure to sunlight and artificial UV light. Lab test interactions may occur.

ADVERSE REACTIONS

Hyperlipemia, hypercholesterolemia, headache, hypothyroidism, asthenia, leukopenia, rash, diarrhea, anemia, N/V, peripheral edema, infection, abdominal pain, exfoliative dermatitis, dry skin.

DRUG INTERACTIONS

Limit vitamin A supplements to avoid potential additive toxic effects. May enhance action of insulin, agents enhancing insulin secretion (eg, sulfonylureas), or insulin-sensitizers (eg, thiazolidinedione class), resulting in hypoglycemia. Gemfibrozil increased bexarotene concentrations; coadministration is not recommended. May reduce concentrations of CYP3A4 substrates (eg, oral/systemic hormonal contraceptives); strongly consider using a non-hormonal contraception if treatment w/ bexarotene is intended for a female w/ reproductive potential.

PREGNANCY AND LACTATION

Pregnancy: May cause fetal harm. Must not be given to a pregnant female or a female who intends to become pregnant. If pregnancy does occur during treatment, immediately d/c the drug and advise the pregnant female of the potential risk to a fetus.
Lactation: There is no information regarding the presence of bexarotene in human milk, the effects on the breast fed infant, or the effects on milk production; not for use in nursing.
Reproductive Potential: Obtain a negative pregnancy test w/ a sensitivity of at least 50 mIU/L w/in 1 week prior to therapy; obtain another pregnancy test at monthly intervals while the patient remains on therapy. Females must use effective contraception for 1 month prior to the initiation of therapy, during therapy, and for ≥1 month following discontinuation of therapy; use 2 reliable forms of contraception simultaneously (1 of which should be nonhormonal) unless abstinence is the chosen method. Initiate therapy on the 2nd or 3rd day of a normal menstrual period. No more than a 1 month supply of therapy should be given to female patients to allow assessment of pregnancy test and reinforcement of counseling regarding avoidance of pregnancy and birth defects. Male patients w/ sexual partners who are pregnant, possibly pregnant, or who could become pregnant must use condoms during sexual intercourse while on therapy and for ≥1 month after the last dose.

MECHANISM OF ACTION

Retinoid; has not been established. Selectively binds and activates retinoid X receptor subtypes. Once activated, these receptors function as transcription factors that regulate the expression of genes that control cellular differentiation and proliferation. Inhibits the growth in vitro of some tumor cell lines of hematopoietic and squamous cell origin.

PHARMACOKINETICS

Absorption: T_{max}=2 hrs. **Distribution:** Plasma protein binding (>99%). **Metabolism:** Oxidation by CYP3A4; 6- and 7-hydroxy-bexarotene and 6- and 7-oxo-bexarotene (metabolites). **Elimination:** Urine (<1% unchanged); $T_{1/2}$=7 hrs.

PATIENT CONSIDERATIONS

Assessment: Assess for risk factors for pancreatitis, hepatic insufficiency, hypersensitivity to bexarotene or other components of the product, nursing status, and possible drug interactions. Obtain a negative pregnancy test w/ a sensitivity of at least 50 mIU/L w/in 1 week prior to therapy. Perform fasting blood lipid determinations before therapy. Obtain baseline LFTs, thyroid function tests, and CBC (including WBC count w/ differential).

Monitoring: Monitor for pancreatitis, visual difficulties, photosensitivity, and other adverse reactions. Perform pregnancy test at monthly intervals. Perform fasting blood lipid determinations weekly until lipid response is established (usually occurs w/in the initial 2-4 weeks), and monitor at 8-week intervals thereafter. Monitor LFTs after 1, 2, and 4 weeks of treatment initiation, and if stable, at least every 8 weeks thereafter during treatment. Monitor thyroid function tests as indicated, and CBC (including WBC count w/ differential) periodically during treatment.

Counseling: Inform of the risks/benefits of therapy. Inform that drug may cause fetal harm; instruct to d/c use immediately and notify physician if pregnancy occurs. Instruct females of reproductive potential on the importance of monthly pregnancy testing while taking therapy. Instruct females of reproductive potential to use effective contraception for 1 month prior to initiation of therapy, during therapy, and for at least 1 month following discontinuation of therapy; advise to use 2 reliable forms of contraception simultaneously, one of which should be non-hormonal. Instruct male patients w/ sexual partners who are pregnant, possibly pregnant, or who could become pregnant to use condoms during sexual intercourse while on therapy and for at least 1 month after the last dose. Instruct to notify physician if signs/symptoms of pancreatitis, hepatotoxicity, or neutropenia develop. Instruct to inform physician about any changes in vision during treatment. Advise patients to limit vitamin A intake to ≤15,000 IU/day to avoid potential additive toxic effects. Advise to minimize exposure to sunlight and artificial UV light. Inform of the possibility of developing hypoglycemia when using insulin, agents enhancing insulin secretion, or insulin-sensitizers while on therapy; instruct patients on these medications to check their blood sugar frequently and to notify physician of any changes in blood sugar level. Instruct to take w/ a meal. Advise patients of laboratory testing that will occur during therapy.

TARKA — trandolapril/verapamil hydrochloride   Rx

Class: ACE inhibitor/calcium channel blocker (CCB) (nondihydropyridine)

> **D/C when pregnancy is detected. Drugs that act directly on the renin-angiotensin system (RAS) can cause injury/death to the developing fetus.**

ADULT DOSAGE

Hypertension

Begin therapy only after patient has either failed to achieve desired antihypertensive effect w/ monotherapy at max recommended dose and shortest dosing interval, or monotherapy dose cannot be increased further because of dose-limiting side effects

Usual: Trandolapril 1-4mg/day; verapamil extended-release (ER) 120-480mg/day

Replacement Therapy: For patients receiving trandolapril (up to 8mg) and verapamil ER (up to 240mg) in separate tabs, administered qd, combination may be substituted for same component doses

Not for initial therapy of HTN

PEDIATRIC DOSAGE

Pediatric use may not have been established

DOSING CONSIDERATIONS

Renal Impairment

Tarka has not been evaluated.
Dose adjustment of trandolapril is recommended.
Use verapamil w/ caution.

Hepatic Impairment

Tarka has not been evaluated.
Consider lower doses of trandolapril.
Use verapamil w/ caution; give approx 30% of the normal verapamil dose in severe hepatic dysfunction.

ADMINISTRATION

Oral route

Take qd w/ food.

STORAGE

15-25°C (59-77°F).

HOW SUPPLIED

Tab, ER: (Trandolapril/Verapamil ER) 2mg/180mg, 1mg/240mg, 2mg/240mg, 4mg/240mg

CONTRAINDICATIONS

Hypersensitivity to any ACE inhibitor or verapamil. **Verapamil:** Severe left ventricular dysfunction, hypotension (systolic BP <90mmHg) or cardiogenic shock, sick sinus syndrome (except w/ functioning artificial ventricular pacemaker), 2nd- or 3rd-degree atrioventricular (AV) block (except w/ functioning artificial ventricular pacemaker), A-fib/A-flutter and an accessory bypass tract (eg, Wolff-Parkinson-White, Lown-Ganong-Levine syndromes). **Trandolapril:** History of ACE inhibitor-associated angioedema, coadministration w/ aliskiren in patients w/ diabetes.

WARNINGS/PRECAUTIONS

Trandolapril: Symptomatic hypotension may occur and is most likely in patients who are salt- or volume-depleted; correct the depletion prior to therapy. May cause excessive hypotension, which may be associated w/ oliguria or azotemia and, rarely, w/ acute renal failure and death in patients w/ CHF, w/ or w/o associated renal insufficiency. Associated w/ a syndrome of cholestatic jaundice, fulminant hepatic necrosis, and death rarely; d/c if jaundice develops. Angioedema reported; d/c if laryngeal stridor or angioedema of the face, tongue, or glottis occurs and administer appropriate therapy. Anaphylactoid reactions reported during desensitization w/ hymenoptera venom, dialysis w/ high-flux membranes, and LDL apheresis w/ dextran sulfate absorption. Potential for agranulocytosis and neutropenia; monitor WBCs in patients w/ collagen vascular disease and/or renal disease. Changes in renal function may occur. May increase BUN and SrCr w/ renal artery stenosis and w/o preexisting renal vascular disease; consider dose reduction and/or discontinuation. Hyperkalemia and persistent, nonproductive cough reported. Hypotension may occur w/ major surgery or during anesthesia; can be corrected by volume expansion. **Verapamil:** Caution w/ impaired renal function. Has a negative inotropic effect; avoid w/ severe left ventricular dysfunction and w/ any degree of ventricular dysfunction if receiving a β-adrenergic blocker. May decrease BP, which may result in dizziness or symptomatic hypotension. Elevated transaminases w/ or w/o alkaline phosphatase/bilirubin elevation and hepatocellular injury reported. May lead to asymptomatic 1st-degree AV block and transient bradycardia. Reduce dose or d/c in marked 1st-degree block or progression to 2nd- or 3rd-degree AV block. Sinus bradycardia, 2nd-degree AV block, sinus arrest, and pulmonary edema/severe hypotension reported in patients w/ hypertrophic cardiomyopathy. May decrease neuromuscular transmission in patients w/ Duchenne muscular dystrophy; may need to reduce dose w/ attenuated neuromuscular transmission.

ADVERSE REACTIONS

1st-degree AV block, constipation, cough, dizziness.

DRUG INTERACTIONS

See Contraindications. May cause additive hypotensive effects w/ diuretics, vasodilators, β-adrenergic blockers, and α-antagonists. **Trandolapril:** Avoid w/ aliskiren in patients w/ renal impairment (GFR <60mL/min). May increase lithium levels and symptoms of lithium toxicity. Dual blockade of the RAS is associated w/ increased risk of hypotension, hyperkalemia, and changes in renal function (including acute renal failure); avoid combined use of RAS inhibitors, or closely monitor BP, renal function, and electrolytes w/ concomitant agents that also affect the RAS. Excessive BP reduction reported w/ diuretics; d/c diuretic or cautiously increase salt intake prior to Tarka initiation, and if it is not possible to d/c diuretic, reduce starting dose of Tarka. May attenuate K+ loss caused by diuretics. May increase risk of hyperkalemia w/ K+-sparing diuretics, K+ supplements, or K+-containing salt substitutes. May result in deterioration of renal function w/ NSAIDs, including selective COX-2 inhibitors, in the elderly or volume-depleted or those w/ compromised renal function. NSAIDs may also attenuate antihypertensive effect. Nitritoid reactions reported rarely w/ injectable gold. Concomitant use w/ mTOR inhibitors (eg, temsirolimus, sirolimus, everolimus) may increase risk for angioedema. May increase blood glucose-lowering effect w/ antidiabetic medications. **Verapamil:** CYP3A4 inhibitors (eg, erythromycin, telithromycin, ritonavir) may increase levels. CYP3A4 inducers (eg, rifampin, phenobarbital, sulfinpyrazone, St. John's wort) may decrease levels. Avoid w/ ivabradine; may increase exposure to ivabradine and may exacerbate bradycardia and conduction disturbances. May increase levels of digoxin, prazosin, terazosin, simvastatin, lovastatin, atorvastatin, carbamazepine, cyclosporine, sirolimus, tacrolimus, theophylline, buspirone, midazolam, almotriptan, imipramine, doxorubicin, quinidine, metoprolol, propranolol, colchicine, and glyburide; reduce maintenance doses of digoxin. Increased sensitivity to the effects of lithium. Hypotension, bradyarrhythmias, and lactic acidosis were seen w/ clarithromycin and erythromycin ethylsuccinate. Clearance may be reduced w/ cimetidine. Avoid disopyramide w/in 48 hrs before or 24 hrs after administration. Additive negative inotropic effect and prolongation of AV conduction w/ flecainide. Avoid concomitant quinidine use w/ hypertrophic cardiomyopathy; significant hypotension reported. Additive negative effects on HR, AV conduction, and/or cardiac contractility w/ β-adrenergic blockers. Asymptomatic bradycardia w/ a wandering atrial pacemaker has been observed w/ concomitant use of timolol eye drops. Myopathy/rhabdomyolysis reported w/ HMG-CoA reductase inhibitors that are CYP3A4 substrates; limit simvastatin dose to 10mg/day, lovastatin dose to 40mg/day, and consider lower starting and maintenance doses for others. Not recommended w/ colchicine. Inhalational anesthetics may depress cardiovascular activity; inhalation anesthetics and verapamil should be titrated carefully to avoid excessive cardiovascular depression. May increase exposure to dabigatran. May potentiate activity of neuromuscular blocking agents (curare-like and depolarizing); may need to reduce dose of either or both drugs. Refer to prescribing information for further details.

PREGNANCY AND LACTATION

Pregnancy: Category D.
Lactation: Verapamil is found in breast milk; not for use in nursing.

MECHANISM OF ACTION

Verapamil: Calcium channel blocker; modulates influx of ionic Ca^{2+} across the cell membrane of the arterial smooth muscle as well as in conductile and contractile myocardial cells. Decreases systemic vascular resistance, usually w/o orthostatic decreases in BP or reflex tachycardia. **Trandolapril:** ACE inhibitor; inhibition results in decreased plasma angiotensin II, which leads to decreased vasopressor activity and decreased aldosterone secretion.

PHARMACOKINETICS

Absorption: Verapamil: Absolute bioavailability (20-35%), T_{max}=4-15 hrs, 5-15 hrs (norverapamil). Trandolapril: Absolute bioavailability (10%, 70% trandolaprilat), T_{max}=0.5-2 hrs, 2-12 hrs (trandolaprilat). **Distribution:** Verapamil: Plasma protein binding (90%); found in breast milk. Trandolapril: Plasma protein binding (80%). **Metabolism:** Verapamil: Liver (extensive); norverapamil (active metabolite). Trandolapril: Trandolaprilat (active metabolite). **Elimination:** Verapamil: Urine (70% metabolite, 3-4% unchanged), feces (≥16% metabolite); $T_{1/2}$=6-11 hrs. Trandolapril: Urine (33%, <1% unchanged), feces (66%); $T_{1/2}$=6 hrs.

PATIENT CONSIDERATIONS

Assessment: Assess for drug hypersensitivity, ventricular dysfunction, cardiogenic shock, sick sinus syndrome, AV block, A-fib/A-flutter and an accessory bypass tract, history of angioedema, diabetes, hepatic/renal impairment, CHF, hypertrophic cardiomyopathy, Duchenne muscular dystrophy, volume/salt depletion, collagen vascular disease, pregnancy/nursing status, and possible drug interactions.

Monitoring: Monitor for angioedema, cough, anaphylactoid reactions, hypotension, hepatic/renal impairment, cholestatic jaundice, fulminant hepatic necrosis, heart block, bradycardia, agranulocytosis, and other adverse reactions. Monitor for abnormal prolongation of PR interval or other signs of excessive pharmacologic effects w/ impaired hepatic/renal function. Monitor BP. Monitor WBC counts in patients w/ collagen vascular disease and/or renal disease.

Counseling: Counsel regarding adverse effects (eg, angioedema, neutropenia, jaundice) and instruct to report any signs/symptoms. Inform of risks when taken during pregnancy; instruct to notify physician if patient is pregnant or becomes pregnant. Educate about need for periodic follow-ups and blood tests to rule out adverse effects and to monitor therapeutic effects.

TASIGNA — nilotinib   Rx

Class: Kinase inhibitor

Prolongs QT interval. Monitor for hypokalemia or hypomagnesemia and correct deficiencies prior to administration and periodically. Obtain ECGs to monitor QTc at baseline, 7 days after initiation, and periodically thereafter, and following any dose adjustments. Sudden deaths reported. Do not administer to patients w/ hypokalemia, hypomagnesemia, or long QT syndrome. Avoid w/ drugs known to prolong the QT interval and strong CYP3A4 inhibitors. Avoid food 2 hrs before and 1 hr after taking the dose.

ADULT DOSAGE

Ph+ Chronic Myeloid Leukemia

Newly Diagnosed Philadelphia Chromosome-Positive Chronic Myeloid Leukemia (Ph+ CML)- Chronic Phase (CP):
300mg bid

Resistant or Intolerant Ph+ CML-CP and CML-Accelerated Phase (AP):
In patients resistant/intolerant to prior therapy that included imatinib
400mg bid

May be given in combination w/ hematopoietic growth factors (eg, erythropoietin, granulocyte colony-stimulating factor), hydroxyurea, or anagrelide if clinically indicated

PEDIATRIC DOSAGE

Pediatric use may not have been established

DOSING CONSIDERATIONS

Concomitant Medications

Strong CYP3A4 Inhibitors (eg, Ketoconazole, Clarithromycin, Atazanavir):
- Avoid concomitant use
- If treatment w/ any of these agents is required, interrupt nilotinib treatment
- If coadministration is a must, consider dose reduction to 300mg qd w/ resistant or intolerant Ph+ CML or to 200mg qd w/ newly diagnosed Ph+ CML; closely monitor for QT interval prolongation in patients who cannot avoid use of strong inhibitor
- If the strong inhibitor is discontinued, allow a washout period before nilotinib dose is adjusted upward to the indicated dose
- Avoid grapefruit products

Strong CYP3A4 Inducers (eg, Dexamethasone, Phenytoin, Carbamazepine):
- Avoid concomitant use
- Avoid St. John's wort

Hepatic Impairment

Newly Diagnosed Ph+ CML:
Mild, Moderate, or Severe (Child-Pugh Class A, B, or C): 200mg bid initially, followed by dose escalation to 300mg bid based on tolerability

Resistant or Intolerant Ph+ CML:
Mild or Moderate (Child-Pugh Score A or B): 300mg bid initially, followed by dose escalation to 400mg bid based on tolerability
Severe (Child-Pugh Score C): 200mg bid initially, followed by sequential dose escalation to 300mg bid and then to 400mg bid based on tolerability

Adverse Reactions

ECGs w/ a QTc >480 msec:
1. Withhold nilotinib, and perform an analysis of serum K^+ and Mg^{2+}, and if below lower limit of normal, correct w/ supplements to w/in normal limits. Concomitant medication usage must be reviewed
2. Resume w/in 2 weeks at prior dose if QTcF returns to <450 msec and to w/in 20 msec of baseline
3. If QTcF is between 450 msec and 480 msec after 2 weeks, reduce dose to 400mg qd
4. If, following dose reduction to 400mg qd, QTcF returns to >480 msec, d/c therapy
5. An ECG should be repeated approx 7 days after any dose adjustment

Neutropenia and Thrombocytopenia (Not Related to Underlying Leukemia): ANC <1.0 x 10^9/L and/or Platelet Counts <50 x 10^9/L:
1. Stop nilotinib, and monitor blood counts
2. Resume w/in 2 weeks at prior dose if ANC >1.0 x 10^9/L and platelets >50 x 10^9/L
3. If blood counts remain low for >2 weeks, reduce dose to 400mg qd

Selected Nonhematologic Lab Abnormalities:
Elevated Serum Lipase or Amylase ≥Grade 3:
1. Withhold nilotinib, and monitor serum lipase or amylase
2. Resume at 400mg qd if serum lipase or amylase returns to ≤Grade 1

Elevated Bilirubin ≥Grade 3:
1. Withhold nilotinib, and monitor bilirubin
2. Resume at 400mg qd if bilirubin returns to ≤Grade 1

Elevated Hepatic Transaminases ≥Grade 3:
1. Withhold nilotinib, and monitor hepatic transaminases
2. Resume at 400mg qd if hepatic transaminases returns to ≤Grade 1

Other Nonhematologic Toxicities:
Grade 3 to 4 Lipase Elevations, Grade 3 to 4 Bilirubin, or Hepatic Transaminase Elevations:
Withhold dose and may resume at 400mg qd

Other Significant Moderate or Severe Toxicities:
Withhold dose and resume at 400mg qd when the toxicity has resolved. If clinically appropriate, consider escalating dose back to 300mg bid (newly diagnosed Ph+ CML) or 400mg bid (resistant or intolerant Ph+ CML).

ADMINISTRATION

Oral route
Take on an empty stomach.
Avoid food for at least 2 hrs before and 1 hr after taking the dose.
Take at approx 12-hr intervals.
Swallow whole w/ water.
May disperse contents of each cap in 1 tsp of applesauce if unable to swallow; take immediately (w/in 15 min) and do not store for future use.

STORAGE

25°C (77°F); excursions permitted between 15-30°C (59-86°F).

HOW SUPPLIED

Cap: 150mg, 200mg

CONTRAINDICATIONS

Hypokalemia, hypomagnesemia, long QT syndrome.

WARNINGS/PRECAUTIONS

May cause myelosuppression (eg, Grade 3/4 thrombocytopenia, neutropenia, and anemia); perform CBCs every 2 weeks for the first 2 months, then monthly thereafter, or as clinically indicated. Cardiovascular (CV) events, including arterial vascular occlusive events, reported; evaluate CV status and monitor and actively manage CV risk factors during therapy. May increase serum lipase; increased risk in patients w/ history of pancreatitis. Interrupt dosing and consider appropriate diagnostics to exclude pancreatitis if lipase elevations are accompanied by abdominal symptoms. May result in hepatotoxicity as measured by elevations in bilirubin, AST/ALT, and alkaline phosphatase. May cause hypophosphatemia, hypo/hyperkalemia, hypocalcemia, and hyponatremia; correct electrolyte abnormalities prior to initiation and during therapy. Exposure is increased in patients w/ impaired hepatic function; monitor QT interval frequently. Tumor lysis syndrome cases reported in patients w/ resistant or intolerant CML; maintain adequate hydration and correct uric acid levels prior to initiation. Hemorrhage reported in patients w/ newly diagnosed Ph+ CML. Reduced exposure in patients w/ total gastrectomy; perform more frequent monitoring and consider dose increase or alternative therapy. Contains lactose; not recommended for patients w/ rare hereditary problems of galactose intolerance, severe lactase deficiency w/ a severe degree of intolerance to lactose-containing products, or of glucose-galactose malabsorption. May cause fetal harm. Severe (Grade 3 or 4) fluid retention, effusions (eg, pleural effusion, pericardial effusion, ascites) or pulmonary edema reported w/ newly diagnosed Ph+ CML-CP. Monitor patients for signs of severe fluid retention and for symptoms of respiratory/cardiac compromise during treatment; evaluate etiology and treat patients accordingly. Caution w/ relevant cardiac disorders.

ADVERSE REACTIONS

Non-Hematologic: Rash, pruritus, headache, N/V, fatigue, alopecia, myalgia, upper abdominal pain, constipation, diarrhea.
Hematologic: Myelosuppression (thrombocytopenia, neutropenia, anemia).

DRUG INTERACTIONS

See Boxed Warning and Dosing Considerations. May increase concentrations of drugs eliminated by CYP3A4 (eg, midazolam, certain HMG-CoA reductase inhibitors), CYP2C8, CYP2C9, CYP2D6, and UGT1A1 enzymes; dose adjustment may be necessary for CYP3A4 substrates, especially those that have narrow therapeutic indices (eg, alfentanil, cyclosporine, dihydroergotamine). May decrease concentrations of drugs eliminated by CYP2B6, CYP2C8, and CYP2C9 enzymes; monitor patients closely when nilotinib is coadministered w/ drugs that have a narrow therapeutic index and are substrates for these enzymes. May increase concentrations of P-gp substrates; use w/ caution. Concomitant administration of strong CYP3A4 inhibitors or inducers may increase or decrease nilotinib concentrations significantly. Decreased solubility and reduced bioavailability w/ drugs that inhibit gastric acid secretion to elevate the gastric pH; concomitant use w/ proton pump inhibitors is not recommended. When the concurrent use of a H_2 blocker is necessary, administer approx 10 hrs before and 2 hrs after the dose of nilotinib. If antacid administration is necessary, administer approx 2 hrs before or 2 hrs after the dose of nilotinib. P-gp inhibitors may increase concentrations; use w/ caution. Avoid w/ drugs that may prolong the QT interval (eg, antiarrhythmic drugs), and grapefruit products and other foods that inhibit CYP3A4.

PREGNANCY AND LACTATION

Pregnancy: Category D. May cause fetal harm when administered to a pregnant woman. Women of childbearing potential should avoid becoming pregnant while on therapy.
Lactation: Not for use in nursing.

MECHANISM OF ACTION

Kinase inhibitor; inhibits BCR-ABL kinase. Binds to and stabilizes the inactive conformation of the kinase domain of ABL protein.

PHARMACOKINETICS

Absorption: T_{max}=3 hrs. **Distribution:** Plasma protein binding (98%). **Metabolism:** Via oxidation and hydroxylation. **Elimination:** Feces (93%, 69% unchanged); $T_{1/2}$=17 hrs.

PATIENT CONSIDERATIONS

Assessment: Assess for electrolyte abnormalities, history of pancreatitis, long QT syndrome, cardiac disorders, total gastrectomy, hepatic impairment, galactose intolerance, lactase deficiency, glucose-galactose malabsorption, pregnancy/nursing status, and possible drug interactions. Obtain baseline ECG, uric acid levels, and chemistry panels, including lipid profile and glucose.

Monitoring: Monitor for myelosuppression; perform CBCs every 2 weeks for the first 2 months of therapy, then monthly thereafter or as clinically indicated. Perform chemistry panels, including electrolytes and liver enzymes periodically. Monitor lipid profiles and glucose periodically during 1st yr of therapy and at least yearly during chronic therapy. Monitor for signs/symptoms of QT prolongation; obtain ECG 7 days after initiation, periodically thereafter, and after any dose adjustments. Maintain adequate hydration, evaluate CV status, and monitor CV risk factors. Monitor serum lipase levels and LFTs monthly or as clinically indicated. Monitor for signs of severe fluid retention, symptoms of respiratory/cardiac compromise, tumor lysis syndrome, hemorrhage, and other adverse reactions.

Counseling: Instruct to take ud. Advise to seek immediate medical attention w/ any symptoms suggestive of a CV event. Instruct not to consume grapefruit products at any time during treatment. Instruct to inform physician of other medicines being taken, including OTC drugs or herbal supplements (eg, St. John's wort). Advise that use of drug during pregnancy may cause harm to the fetus and that nilotinib should not be taken during pregnancy unless necessary. Instruct women of childbearing potential to use highly effective contraceptives while on therapy. Instruct not to d/c or change dose w/o consulting physician.

TASMAR — tolcapone

Rx

Class: COMT inhibitor

> Because of the risk of potentially fatal, acute fulminant liver failure, tolcapone should be used in patients w/ Parkinson's disease (PD) on levodopa/carbidopa who are experiencing symptom fluctuations and are not responding satisfactorily to or are not appropriate candidates for other adjunctive therapies. Withdraw treatment if patient fails to show substantial clinical benefit w/in 3 weeks of initiation. Do not initiate therapy if liver disease is clinically evident or if 2 ALT/AST values are >ULN. Caution w/ severe dyskinesia or dystonia. Patients who develop evidence of hepatocellular injury while on therapy and are withdrawn from the drug for any reason may be at increased risk for liver injury if tolcapone is reintroduced; do not consider such patients for retreatment. Monitor for evidence of emergent liver injury if used in face of the increased risk of liver injury. Determine ALT/AST at baseline/before increasing dose to 200mg tid and periodically (eg, every 2-4 weeks) for the first 6 months of therapy, then periodically thereafter at intervals deemed clinically relevant. D/C therapy if ALT/AST exceed 2X ULN or if clinical signs/symptoms suggest the onset of hepatic dysfunction (eg, persistent nausea, fatigue, lethargy, anorexia, jaundice, dark urine, pruritus, right upper quadrant tenderness).

ADULT DOSAGE	PEDIATRIC DOSAGE
Parkinson's Disease	Pediatric use may not have been established
Adjunct to Levodopa and Carbidopa for the Treatment of Signs/Symptoms of Idiopathic PD:	
Initial/Usual: 100mg tid; use 200mg tid only if anticipated clinical benefit is justified	
D/C if patient fails to show substantial clinical benefit w/in 3 weeks of initiation of treatment	
Take 1st dose of the day together w/ 1st dose of the day of levodopa/carbidopa; take subsequent doses 6 and 12 hrs later	
May need to reduce daily levodopa dose to optimize response if daily levodopa dose is >600mg or if patient has moderate/severe dyskinesias prior to therapy	
May be combined w/ both the immediate and sustained-release formulations of levodopa/carbidopa	

DOSING CONSIDERATIONS
Discontinuation
If a decision is made to d/c treatment, closely monitor patient and adjust other dopaminergic treatments prn

ADMINISTRATION
Oral route
Take w/ or w/o food.

STORAGE
20-25°C (68-77°F).

HOW SUPPLIED
Tab: 100mg

CONTRAINDICATIONS
Liver disease, patients withdrawn from therapy due to drug-induced hepatocellular injury, hypersensitivity to tolcapone or the ingredients in this medication, history of nontraumatic rhabdomyolysis or hyperpyrexia and confusion possibly related to medication.

WARNINGS/PRECAUTIONS
Falling asleep during activities of daily living and somnolence reported; continually reassess for drowsiness or sleepiness, and consider discontinuing therapy in patients who report significant daytime sleepiness or episodes of falling asleep during activities that require active participation (eg, conversations, eating). May impair mental/physical abilities. Orthostatic hypotension, syncope, and hallucinations reported. Incidence of hallucination may be increased in elderly patients >75 yrs of age. Diarrhea reported; appropriate work-up (including occult blood samples) is recommended in all cases of persistent diarrhea. May experience new or worsening mental status and behavioral changes, which may be severe, including psychotic-like behavior during treatment or after starting or increasing the dose. Avoid in patients w/ major psychotic disorder. May cause

and/or exacerbate preexisting dyskinesia. May cause intense urges (eg, intense urges to gamble, increased sexual urges, intense urges to spend money, binge eating); consider dose reduction or discontinuation. Severe rhabdomyolysis and hematuria reported. A symptom complex resembling neuroleptic malignant syndrome (NMS) (hyperpyrexia and confusion) reported in association w/ the abrupt withdrawal or lowering of the dose of tolcapone. Caution w/ severe renal impairment. Retroperitoneal fibrosis, pulmonary infiltrates, pleural effusion, and pleural thickening reported w/ ergot derived dopaminergic agents; unknown if nonergot derived dopaminergic drugs cause these complications. PD patients have a higher risk of developing melanoma; frequently monitor for melanomas. Withdrawal or abrupt dose reduction may lead to emergence of signs and symptoms of PD, or hyperpyrexia and confusion.

ADVERSE REACTIONS
Dyskinesia, dystonia, anorexia, muscle cramps, diarrhea, orthostatic complaints, hallucination, N/V, sleep disorder, somnolence, increased sweating, confusion, urine discoloration, dizziness.

DRUG INTERACTIONS
Consider dose reduction of drugs metabolized by COMT (eg, α-methyldopa, dobutamine, apomorphine) if coadministered. Avoid w/ nonselective MAOIs (eg, phenelzine, tranylcypromine). Caution w/ desipramine. Monitor coagulation parameters if coadministered w/ warfarin.

PREGNANCY AND LACTATION
Pregnancy: Category C.
Lactation: Caution in nursing.

MECHANISM OF ACTION
COMT inhibitor; has not been established. Suspected to alter the plasma pharmacokinetics of levodopa, leading to more sustained plasma levels of levodopa when given in conjunction w/ levodopa/carbidopa. These sustained plasma levels of levodopa believed to result in more constant dopaminergic stimulation in the brain.

PHARMACOKINETICS
Absorption: Rapid; absolute bioavailability (65%); C_{max}=3mcg/mL (100mg), 6mcg/mL (200mg); T_{max}=2 hrs. **Distribution:** V_d=9L; plasma protein binding (>99.9%). **Metabolism:** Liver; glucuronidation (main metabolic pathway), methylation via COMT, oxidation via CYP3A4 and CYP2A6. **Elimination:** Urine (60%, 0.5% unchanged), feces (40%); $T_{1/2}$=2-3 hrs.

PATIENT CONSIDERATIONS
Assessment: Assess for hypersensitivity to the drug, liver disease, drug-induced hepatocellular injury, history of nontraumatic rhabdomyolysis or hyperpyrexia and confusion, renal impairment, dyskinesia, dystonia, major psychotic disorder, pregnancy/nursing status, other conditions where treatment is contraindicated or cautioned, and possible drug interactions. Obtain baseline LFTs.

Monitoring: Monitor for hypotension/syncope, diarrhea, dyskinesia, rhabdomyolysis, hematuria, fibrotic complications, melanomas, hallucinations, hyperpyrexia and confusion, mental/behavioral changes, impulse control/compulsive behaviors, drowsiness or sleepiness, and other adverse reactions. Perform skin exams periodically. Monitor liver enzymes periodically (eg, every 2-4 weeks) for the first 6 months of therapy, then periodically thereafter at intervals deemed clinically relevant.

Counseling: Inform of the benefits/risks of therapy and instruct to take ud. Inform about signs/symptoms that suggest onset of hepatic injury; advise to contact physician immediately if symptoms of hepatic failure occur. Inform of the need to have regular blood tests to monitor liver enzymes. Advise that sleepiness or drowsiness may occur; instruct to avoid driving a car or operating other complex machinery until sufficient experience is gained on therapy. Inform that nausea (especially at the initiation of treatment), hallucinations, other psychotic-like behavior, and hypotension may occur. Advise about the possibility of developing or worsening of existing dyskinesia and/or dystonia. Advise that postural (orthostatic) hypotension w/ or w/o symptoms (eg, dizziness, nausea, syncope, sweating) may develop; advise to rise slowly, especially after long periods of sitting or lying down. Instruct patients/caregivers to report intense urges to gamble, increased sexual urges, increase in spending money, binge eating, and other intense urges to physician. Advise to notify physician if pregnant/intending to become pregnant, or if breastfeeding/intending to breastfeed during therapy.

TAZICEF — ceftazidime

Rx

Class: Cephalosporin (3rd generation)

ADULT DOSAGE	PEDIATRIC DOSAGE
General Dosing	**General Dosing**
Usual: 1g IM/IV q8-12h	**Neonates (0-4 Weeks of Age):** 30mg/kg IV q12h
Severe Life-threatening Infections, Especially in Immunocompromised Patients: 2g IV q8h	**Infants and Children (1 Month-12 Years):** 30-50mg/kg IV q8h
Urinary Tract Infections	**Max:** 6g/day
Uncomplicated: 250mg IM/IV q12h	Reserve higher doses for immunocompromised, cystic fibrosis, or meningitis
Complicated: 500mg IM/IV q8-12h	Continue for 2 days after signs/symptoms of infection disappear; may require longer therapy w/ complicated infections
Bone/Joint Infections 2g IV q12h	

Pneumonia
Uncomplicated:
500mg-1g IM/IV q8h

Skin and Skin Structure Infections
Mild:
500mg-1g IM/IV q8h

Gynecologic Infections
Serious Infections:
2g IV q8h

Intra-Abdominal Infections
Serious Infections:
2g IV q8h

Meningitis
2g IV q8h

Lung Infection
Caused by *Pseudomonas* species in Patients w/ Cystic Fibrosis w/ Normal Renal Function:
30-50mg/kg IV q8h
Max: 6g/day

Treatment Duration
Continue for 2 days after signs/symptoms of infection disappear; may require longer therapy w/ complicated infections

Other Indications
Treatment of the Following Infections Caused by Susceptible Strains of Microorganisms:
Lower respiratory tract
CNS infections
Bacterial septicemia
Sepsis

DOSING CONSIDERATIONS
Renal Impairment
Adults:
LD: May give 1g
Maint:
CrCl 31-50mL/min: 1g q12h
CrCl 16-30mL/min: 1g q24h
CrCl 6-15mL/min: 500mg q24h
CrCl <5mL/min: 500mg q48h
If usual dose is lower than recommended dose for renal impairment, the lower dose should be used
Renal Impairment and Severe Infection: May increase dose by 50% or the dosing frequency may be increased appropriately
Hemodialysis: Give 1g LD, followed by 1g after each hemodialysis period
Intraperitoneal Dialysis/Continuous Ambulatory Peritoneal Dialysis: Give 1g LD, followed by 500mg q24h, or add to dialysis fluid at 250mg/2L

Pediatrics:
Adjust CrCl for BSA or lean body mass; reduce dosing frequency in renal insufficiency

ADMINISTRATION
IV/IM routes

Avoid intra-arterial administration
Do not add to sol of aminoglycoside; administer separately
May administer as intermittent IV infusion w/ a Y-type administration set w/ compatible sol; during infusion of ceftazidime, desirable to d/c other sol

ADD-Vantage
Not intended for direct IV/IM inj
Intended for single dose administration w/ ADD-Vantage flexible diluent container
Constitute ADD-Vantage vials w/ 50mL or 100mL of D5 inj, 0.9% NaCl inj, or 50mL of 0.45% NaCl inj in ADD-Vantage diluent; constitute only when it is certain patient is ready to receive drug

Refer to PI for further administration procedures, direction for use of inj in ADD-Vantage vials, compatibility, and stability

STORAGE
(Dry state) 20-25°C (68-77°F). Protect from light.

HOW SUPPLIED
Inj: 1g, 2g. Also available as a Pharmacy Bulk Package. Refer to individual package insert for more information.

CONTRAINDICATIONS
Hypersensitivity to ceftazidime or the cephalosporin group of antibiotics.

WARNINGS/PRECAUTIONS
Caution in penicillin (PCN)-sensitive patients; determine whether patient has had previous hypersensitivity reactions to cephalosporins, PCN, or other drugs. D/C if an allergic reaction occurs. *Clostridium difficile*-associated diarrhea (CDAD) reported; d/c if CDAD is suspected or confirmed. May result in overgrowth of nonsusceptible organisms with prolonged use or use in the absence of a proven or strongly suspected bacterial infection or prophylactic indication; take appropriate measures if superinfection develops. High and prolonged serum concentrations may occur in patients with transient or persistent reduction of urinary output.

Elevated levels with renal insufficiency can lead to seizures, encephalopathy, coma, asterixis, neuromuscular excitability, and myoclonia. Risk of decreased prothrombin activity in patients with renal/hepatic impairment, poor nutritional state, and patients receiving a protracted course of therapy; monitor PT. Distal necrosis may occur after inadvertent intra-arterial administration. Lab test interactions may occur. Caution with impaired renal function, history of GI disease, particularly colitis, and in elderly.

ADVERSE REACTIONS
Phlebitis and inflammation at inj site, pruritus, rash, fever, diarrhea, N/V, abdominal pain, increased ALT/AST/GGT/LDH, eosinophilia.

DRUG INTERACTIONS
Nephrotoxicity reported with concomitant aminoglycosides or potent diuretics (eg, furosemide). Avoid with chloramphenicol; may antagonize effect of β-lactam antibiotics. May affect the gut flora, leading to lower estrogen reabsorption and reduced efficacy of combined estrogen/progesterone oral contraceptives.

PREGNANCY AND LACTATION
Category B, caution in nursing.

MECHANISM OF ACTION
Cephalosporin (3rd generation); bactericidal, exerting effect by inhibition of enzymes responsible for cell-wall synthesis.

PHARMACOKINETICS
Absorption: (IV/IM) Administration of variable doses resulted in different parameters. **Distribution:** Plasma protein binding (<10%); found in breast milk. **Elimination:** Urine (80-90% unchanged); $T_{1/2}$=1.9 hrs (IV), 2 hrs (IM).

PATIENT CONSIDERATIONS
Assessment: Assess for previous hypersensitivity reaction to cephalosporins, PCNs or other drugs, renal/hepatic impairment, poor nutritional status, patients receiving protracted course of antibiotics, history of GI disease (eg, colitis), pregnancy/nursing status, and possible drug interactions.

Monitoring: Monitor for signs/symptoms of allergic reactions, CDAD, superinfection, and other adverse reactions. Monitor for seizures, encephalopathy, coma, asterixis, neuromuscular excitability, and myoclonia with renal impairment. Monitor renal function and PT. Perform periodic susceptibility testing.

Counseling: Inform that drug only treats bacterial, not viral, infections. Instruct to take exactly ud; skipping doses or not completing full course of therapy may decrease effectiveness and increase the likelihood of bacterial resistance. Inform that diarrhea may occur and will usually end when therapy is discontinued. Instruct to contact physician as soon as possible if watery/bloody stools (with/without stomach cramps, fever) develop even as late as 2 months or more after having taken the last dose of therapy.

TAZORAC — tazarotene   Rx
Class: Retinoid

ADULT DOSAGE	PEDIATRIC DOSAGE
Plaque Psoriasis	**Plaque Psoriasis**
Gel 0.5%: **Stable Psoriasis Up to 20% BSA:** **Initial:** Apply thin film (2mg/cm²) to cover only affected area qpm **Max:** 0.1% if tolerated and medically indicated	**≥12 Years:** **Gel 0.5%:** **Stable Psoriasis Up to 20% BSA:** **Initial:** Apply thin film (2mg/cm²) to cover only affected area qpm **Max:** 0.1% if tolerated and medically indicated
Cre 0.5%: **Initial:** Apply thin film to cover only affected area qpm **Max:** 0.1% if tolerated and medically indicated	**Cre 0.5%:** **Initial:** Apply thin film (2mg/cm²) to cover only affected area qpm **Max:** 0.1% if tolerated and medically indicated
Acne Vulgaris Apply thin film (2mg/cm²) of 0.1% gel/cre to cover the entire affected area qpm Gel indicated for mild to moderate facial acne	**Acne Vulgaris** **≥12 Years:** Apply thin film (2mg/cm²) of 0.1% gel/cre to cover the entire affected area qpm Gel indicated for mild to moderate facial acne

----

ADMINISTRATION
Topical route
Wash hands after application
Avoid application to unaffected skin

Psoriasis
If a bath or shower is taken prior to application, the skin should be dry prior to application
If emollients are used, they should be applied at least an hr before application

Acne
Cleanse face gently and dry prior to application

STORAGE
(Cre) 20-25°C (68-77°F); excursions permitted from -5 to 30°C (23-86°F). (Gel) 25°C (77°F); excursions permitted to 15-30°C (59-86°F).

HOW SUPPLIED
Cre: 0.05%, 0.1% [30g, 60g]; **Gel:** 0.05%, 0.1% [30g, 100g]

CONTRAINDICATIONS

Women who are or may become pregnant. Hypersensitivity to any of components of the product.

WARNINGS/PRECAUTIONS

Avoid contact with eyes, eyelids, and mouth; rinse thoroughly with water if contact with eyes occurs. Females of childbearing potential should use adequate birth-control measures during treatment. Initiate therapy during normal menstrual period. May cause excessive skin irritation; do not use on eczematous skin. May cause excessive pruritus, burning, skin redness, or peeling; d/c therapy until integrity of skin is restored or reduce dosing interval if these occur. Patients with psoriasis being treated with 0.1% concentration can be switched to lower concentration. Weather extremes (eg, wind, cold) may be more irritating. Avoid exposure to sunlight (including sunlamps); if exposure is medically necessary, minimize exposure during therapy. Avoid use in patients with sunburn until fully recovered.

ADVERSE REACTIONS

Pruritus, burning/stinging, erythema, worsening of psoriasis, irritation, skin pain, desquamation, dry skin, rash, contact dermatitis, skin inflammation.

DRUG INTERACTIONS

Avoid concomitant topical medications and cosmetics that have a strong drying effect. Possibility of augmented photosensitivity increased with photosensitizers (eg, thiazides, tetracyclines, fluoroquinolones, phenothiazines, sulfonamides); use with caution. If emollients are used, they should be applied at least 1 hr before gel/cre application.

PREGNANCY AND LACTATION

Category X; caution in nursing (gel), not for use in nursing (cre).

MECHANISM OF ACTION

Retinoid; not established. Binds to all 3 members of the retinoic acid receptor (RAR) family: RAR α, RAR β, and RAR gamma, but shows relative selectivity for RAR β and RAR gamma, and may modify gene expression.

PHARMACOKINETICS

Absorption: Administration of gel/cre resulted in different pharmacokinetic parameters. **Distribution:** Tazarotenic Acid: Plasma protein binding (>99%). **Metabolism:** Esterase hydrolysis to form tazarotenic acid (active metabolite). **Elimination:** Urine, feces. Tazarotenic Acid: $T_{1/2}$=18 hrs.

PATIENT CONSIDERATIONS

Assessment: Assess for eczematous skin, sunburn, considerable sun exposure due to occupation, sunlight sensitivity, hypersensitivity, pregnancy/nursing status, and possible drug interactions. Obtain negative result for pregnancy test within 2 weeks prior to therapy.

Monitoring: Monitor for local irritation (excessive pruritus, burning, skin redness, peeling) and other adverse reactions. Monitor application frequency by careful observation of the clinical therapeutic response and skin tolerance.

Counseling: Advise females of childbearing potential to use an effective method of contraception during treatment to avoid pregnancy, and to stop medication and notify physician if pregnancy occurs. Instruct to reduce frequency of application or temporarily interrupt treatment if undue irritation (redness, peeling, discomfort) occurs; inform that treatment may be resumed once irritation subsides. Inform that moisturizers may be used as frequently as desired. Advise patients with psoriasis that a cre or lot may be used to soften or moisten skin at least 1 hr before application. Instruct to avoid exposure of treated areas to either natural/artificial sunlight (eg, tanning beds, sunlamps); advise to use sunscreen and wear protective clothing if exposure to sunlight is unavoidable during use. Instruct to avoid contact with eyes and to rinse thoroughly with water if contact with eyes occurs.

TECENTRIQ — atezolizumab   Rx

Class: Monoclonal antibody/programmed death ligand-1 (PD-L1) blocker

ADULT DOSAGE	**PEDIATRIC DOSAGE**
Locally Advanced or Metastatic Urothelial Carcinoma	Pediatric use may not have been established
Use in patients w/ disease progression during or following platinum-containing chemotherapy or disease progression w/in 12 months of neoadjuvant or adjuvant treatment w/ platinum-containing chemotherapy	
1200mg q3wks until disease progression or unacceptable toxicity	

DOSING CONSIDERATIONS

Adverse Reactions
Withhold for Any of the Following:
- Grade 2 pneumonitis
- AST or ALT >3-5X ULN or total bilirubin >1.5-3X ULN
- Grade 2 or 3 diarrhea or colitis
- Symptomatic hypophysitis, adrenal insufficiency, hypothyroidism, hyperthyroidism, or Grade 3 or 4 hyperglycemia
- Grade 2 ocular inflammatory toxicity
- Grade 2 or 3 pancreatitis, or Grade 3 or 4 increases in amylase or lipase levels (>2X ULN)
- Grade 3 or 4 infection
- Grade 2 infusion-related reactions
- Grade 3 rash

Permanently D/C for Any of the Following:
- Grade 3 or 4 pneumonitis
- AST or ALT >5X ULN or total bilirubin >3X ULN
- Grade 4 diarrhea or colitis
- Grade 4 hypophysitis
- Myasthenic syndrome/myasthenia gravis, Guillain-Barre syndrome, or meningoencephalitis (all grades)
- Grade 3 or 4 ocular inflammatory toxicity
- Grade 4 or any grade of recurrent pancreatitis
- Grade 3 or 4 infusion-related reactions
- Grade 4 rash

ADMINISTRATION

IV route

- Administer initial infusion over 60 min through an IV line w/ or w/o a sterile, non-pyrogenic, low-protein binding in-line filter (pore size of 0.2-0.22 micron).
- If first infusion is tolerated, all subsequent infusions may be delivered over 30 min.
- Do not coadminister other drugs through the same IV line.
- Do not administer as an IV push or bolus.

Preparation
1. Withdraw 20mL from vial.
2. Dilute into a 250 mL polyvinyl chloride, polyethylene, or polyolefin infusion bag containing 0.9% NaCl inj.
3. Dilute w/ 0.9% NaCl inj only.
4. Mix diluted sol by gentle inversion; do not shake.
5. Discard partially used or empty vials.
6. Administer immediately once prepared.

If diluted infusion sol is not used immediately, it can be stored either:
- At room temperature for ≤6 hrs from the time of preparation (including time for administration).
- Under refrigeration at 2-8°C (36-46°F) for ≤24 hrs.
Do not shake or freeze.

STORAGE

2-8°C (36-46°F) in original carton to protect from light. Do not freeze. Do not shake.

HOW SUPPLIED

Inj: 1200mg/20mL

WARNINGS/PRECAUTIONS

See Dosing Considerations. Refer to PI for corticosteroid dose in the management of the following adverse reactions. Immune-mediated pneumonitis or interstitial lung disease reported; monitor for signs w/ radiographic imaging and symptoms of pneumonitis. Immune-mediated hepatitis reported; monitor AST, ALT, and bilirubin prior to and periodically during treatment. Withhold for Grade 2 and permanently d/c for Grade 3 or 4 immune-mediated hepatitis. Immune-mediated colitis or diarrhea reported. Immune-related thyroid disorders, adrenal insufficiency, hypophysitis, and type 1 diabetes mellitus (DM), including diabetic ketoacidosis, reported. Initiate treatment w/ insulin for type 1 DM. Other immune-related adverse reactions (eg, meningoencephalitis, myasthenic syndrome/myasthenia gravis, Guillain-Barre, ocular inflammatory toxicity, pancreatitis) reported. Monitor for clinical signs/symptoms of meningitis or encephalitis, symptoms of motor and sensory neuropathy, hepatitis, diarrhea or colitis, endocrinopathies, and acute pancreatitis. Severe infections, (eg, sepsis, herpes encephalitis, mycobacterial infection leading to retroperitoneal hemorrhage) reported; monitor for signs/symptoms of infection and treat w/ antibiotics for suspected or confirmed bacterial infections. Severe infusion reactions reported; interrupt or slow rate of infusion w/ mild or moderate infusion reactions. May cause fetal harm.

ADVERSE REACTIONS

Fatigue, decreased appetite, nausea, UTI, pyrexia, constipation.

PREGNANCY AND LACTATION

Pregnancy: May cause fetal harm.
Lactation: Not for use in nursing and for at least 5 months after last dose.
Reproductive Potential: Females of reproductive potential should use effective contraception during treatment and for at least 5 months following the last dose. May impair fertility in females while receiving treatment.

MECHANISM OF ACTION

Monoclonal antibody/programmed death ligand-1 (PD-L1) blocker; binds to PD-L1 and blocks its interactions w/ both PD-1 and B7.1 receptors, releasing the PD-L1/PD-1 mediated inhibition of the immune response, including activation of the anti-tumor immune response w/o inducing antibody-dependent cellular cytotoxicity.

PHARMACOKINETICS

Distribution: V_d=6.9L. **Elimination:** $T_{1/2}$=27 days.

PATIENT CONSIDERATIONS

Assessment: Assess pregnancy/nursing status. Obtain baseline thyroid function and AST, ALT, and bilirubin levels.

Monitoring: Monitor for signs of immune-mediated pneumonitis w/ radiographic imaging and monitor for symptoms of pneumonitis. Monitor for signs/symptoms of immune-mediated hepatitis, diarrhea/colitis, hypophysitis, thyroid disorders, adrenal insufficiency, meningitis/encephalitis, hyperglycemia, motor and sensory neuropathy, pancreatitis, severe infections, infusion-related reactions, and other adverse reactions. Periodically monitor thyroid function and AST, ALT, and bilirubin levels.

Counseling: Inform of the risk of immune-related adverse reactions that may require corticosteroid treatment and interruption or discontinuation of atezolizumab. Advise to contact healthcare provider immediately for any new or worsening cough, chest pain, SOB, jaundice, severe N/V, pain on the right side of abdomen, lethargy, easy bruising or bleeding, diarrhea, severe abdominal pain, and signs/symptoms of hypophysitis, hyperthyroidism, hypothyroidism, adrenal insufficiency, type 1 DM, meningitis, myasthenic syndrome/myasthenia gravis, Guillain-Barre syndrome, ocular inflammatory toxicity, pancreatitis, infection, infusion-related reactions, and rash. Advise that treatment may cause fetal harm. Instruct females of reproductive potential to use effective contraception during treatment and for at least 5 months after the last dose. Advise not to breastfeed while on therapy and for at least 5 months after the last dose.

Tecfidera — dimethyl fumarate   Rx

Class: Immunomodulatory agent

ADULT DOSAGE
Multiple Sclerosis
Relapsing Forms:
Initial: 120mg bid
Titrate: Increase to 240mg bid after 7 days
Maint: 240mg bid. Consider temporary dose reductions to 120mg bid for individuals who do not tolerate the maint dose; resume the recommended dose of 240mg bid w/ in 4 weeks. Consider discontinuation for patients unable to tolerate return to maint dose

PEDIATRIC DOSAGE
Pediatric use may not have been established

ADMINISTRATION
Oral route

Take w/ or w/o food.
Swallow whole and intact; do not crush or chew.
Do not sprinkle cap contents on food.
To reduce flushing, take w/ food or take up to 325mg of non-enteric coated aspirin 30 min prior to therapy.

STORAGE
15-30°C (59-86°F). Protect from light.

HOW SUPPLIED
Cap, Delayed-Release: 120mg, 240mg

CONTRAINDICATIONS
Known hypersensitivity to dimethyl fumarate (DMF) or to any of the excipients of this medication.

WARNINGS/PRECAUTIONS
May cause anaphylaxis and angioedema; d/c if signs/symptoms occur. Progressive multifocal leukoencephalopathy (PML) reported; withhold treatment and perform appropriate diagnostic evaluation at the 1st sign/symptom suggestive of PML. May decrease lymphocyte counts; obtain CBC, including lymphocyte count, before initiating treatment, after 6 months of starting treatment, and then every 6-12 months thereafter, and as clinically indicated. Consider interruption of therapy w/ lymphocyte counts <0.5 x 10^9/L persisting for >6 months; continue to obtain lymphocyte counts until their recovery if therapy is discontinued or interrupted due to lymphopenia. Consider withholding treatment in patients w/ serious infections until resolution; decisions about whether or not to restart therapy should be individualized based on clinical circumstances. May cause flushing; administration w/ food may reduce the incidence of flushing. Alternatively, administration of non-enteric coated aspirin (up to a dose of 325mg) 30 min prior to dosing may reduce the incidence or severity of flushing.

ADVERSE REACTIONS
Flushing, abdominal pain, diarrhea, nausea.

PREGNANCY AND LACTATION
Pregnancy: Category C. Encourage pregnant patients to enroll in the Tecfidera Pregnancy Registry.
Lactation: Caution in nursing.

MECHANISM OF ACTION
Immunomodulatory agent; not established. DMF and the metabolite (monomethyl fumarate [MMF]) have been shown to activate the nuclear factor (erythroid-derived 2)-like 2 (Nrf2) pathway. Nrf2 pathway is involved in the cellular response to oxidative stress.

PHARMACOKINETICS
Absorption: MMF: C_{max}=1.87mg/L (w/ food), AUC=8.21mg•hr/L (w/ food), T_{max}=2-2.5 hrs (median). **Distribution:** MMF: V_d=53-73L; plasma protein binding (27-45%). **Metabolism:** Extensive via rapid presystemic hydrolysis by esterases to MMF (active metabolite). **Elimination:** Primary Route: Exhalation of CO_2 (60%). Minor Route: Urine (16%), feces (1%); $T_{1/2}$=1 hr (MMF).

PATIENT CONSIDERATIONS
Assessment: Assess for known hypersensitivity to drug or any of the excipients, and pregnancy/nursing status. Obtain baseline CBC including lymphocyte count.

Monitoring: Monitor for anaphylaxis, angioedema, PML, lymphopenia, flushing, and other adverse reactions. Monitor CBC including lymphocyte count after 6 months of treatment, every 6-12 months thereafter, and as clinically indicated.

Counseling: Instruct to take ud. Advise to d/c therapy and seek medical care if signs/symptoms of anaphylaxis or angioedema develop. Inform that PML has occurred in patients who received therapy and is characterized by progression

of deficits and usually leads to death or severe disability; instruct to contact physician if any symptoms suggestive of PML develop. Inform that therapy may decrease lymphocyte counts. Advise to contact physician if patient experiences persistent and/or severe flushing or GI reactions. Inform patients experiencing flushing that taking w/ food or taking a non-enteric coated aspirin prior to taking therapy may help. Instruct to inform physician if patient is pregnant or plans to become pregnant while on therapy; encourage enrollment in the Tecfidera pregnancy registry if patient becomes pregnant while on therapy.

Technivie — ombitasvir/paritaprevir/ritonavir   Rx

Class: CYP3A inhibitor/HCV NS5A inhibitor/HCV NS3/4A protease inhibitor

ADULT DOSAGE
Chronic Hepatitis C (Genotype 4)
Combination w/ Ribavirin (RBV) in Patients w/o Cirrhosis:
2 tabs qd (am) w/ RBV at 1000mg/day (<75kg) and 1200mg/day (≥75kg) in 2 divided doses for 12 weeks

May be given w/o RBV for 12 weeks for treatment-naive patients who cannot take or tolerate RBV

PEDIATRIC DOSAGE
Pediatric use may not have been established

DOSING CONSIDERATIONS
Hepatic Impairment
Moderate to Severe (Child-Pugh B and C): Contraindicated

ADMINISTRATION
Oral route
Take in the am w/ a meal w/o regard to fat or calorie content.

STORAGE
≤30°C (86°F).

HOW SUPPLIED
Tab: (Ombitasvir/Paritaprevir/Ritonavir [RTV]) 12.5mg/75mg/50mg

CONTRAINDICATIONS
Moderate to severe hepatic impairment (Child-Pugh Class B and C). Drugs that are highly dependent on CYP3A for clearance and for which elevated plasma concentrations are associated w/ serious and/or life-threatening events, and drugs that are moderate or strong inducers of CYP3A and may lead to reduced efficacy (alfuzosin HCl, colchicine, ranolazine, dronedarone, carbamazepine, phenytoin, phenobarbital, rifampin, lurasidone, pimozide, ergotamine, dihydroergotamine, methylergonovine, ethinyl estradiol-containing medications such as combined oral contraceptives, cisapride, St. John's wort, lovastatin, simvastatin, efavirenz, sildenafil [when dosed as Revatio for the treatment of pulmonary arterial hypertension], triazolam, oral midazolam). Known hypersensitivity to RTV (eg, toxic epidermal necrolysis, Stevens-Johnson syndrome). Refer to the RBV prescribing information for a list of contraindications for RBV.

WARNINGS/PRECAUTIONS
Hepatic decompensation and hepatic failure, including liver transplantation or fatal outcomes, reported; d/c treatment in patients who develop evidence of hepatic decompensation. ALT elevations to >5X ULN reported; occurred during first 4 weeks of treatment and declined w/in 2-8 weeks w/ continued dosing. Perform hepatic lab testing during first 4 weeks of treatment and as clinically indicated thereafter. Monitor closely if ALT is elevated above baseline. Consider discontinuing if ALT levels remain persistently >10X ULN. D/C if ALT elevation is accompanied by signs/symptoms of liver inflammation or increasing direct bilirubin, alkaline phosphatase, or INR. Any hepatitis C virus (HCV)/HIV-1 coinfected patients should also be on a suppressive antiretroviral drug regimen to reduce the risk of HIV-1 protease inhibitor drug resistance. Refer to the RBV prescribing information for a full list of the warnings and precautions for RBV.

ADVERSE REACTIONS
Asthenia, fatigue, nausea, insomnia, pruritus, skin reactions, serum bilirubin elevations.

DRUG INTERACTIONS
See Contraindications. ALT elevation reported more frequently w/ ethinyl estradiol-containing medications (eg, combined oral contraceptives, contraceptive patches, contraceptive vaginal rings); d/c ethinyl estradiol-containing medications prior to starting therapy. Alternative methods of contraception (eg, progestin only contraception, nonhormonal methods) are recommended during therapy; ethinyl estradiol-containing medications can be restarted approx 2 weeks following completion of treatment. Caution w/ estrogens other than ethinyl estradiol (eg, estradiol and conjugated estrogens) used in hormone replacement therapy. Coadministration w/ drugs that are substrates of CYP3A, P-gp, BCRP, OATP1B1, or OATP1B3 may result in increased plasma concentrations of such drugs. Coadministration w/ strong inhibitors of CYP3A may increase paritaprevir and RTV concentrations. Inhibition of P-gp, BCRP, OATP1B1, or OATP1B3 may increase the plasma concentrations of the various components of Technivie. May increase levels of angiotensin receptor blockers, digoxin, antiarrhythmics, ketoconazole, quetiapine, calcium channel blockers, inhaled/nasal fluticasone, furosemide (C_{max}), rilpivirine, pravastatin, cyclosporine, tacrolimus, salmeterol, buprenorphine, norbuprenorphine, hydrocodone, or alprazolam. Concomitant use w/ inhaled or nasal fluticasone may reduce serum cortisol concentrations. May decrease levels of carisoprodol, cyclobenzaprine, norcyclobenzaprine, diazepam, nordiazepam, omeprazole, darunavir (C_{trough}), or voriconazole. Atazanavir, atazanavir/RTV, or lopinavir/RTV may increase paritaprevir levels. Not recommended w/

voriconazole, atazanavir, atazanavir/RTV, lopinavir/RTV, rilpivirine once daily, or salmeterol. Refer to PI for further information on drug interactions, including dosing modifications when used w/ certain concomitant therapies.

PREGNANCY AND LACTATION

Pregnancy: Category B. When therapy is administered w/ RBV, the combination regimen is contraindicated in pregnant women and in men whose female partners are pregnant.

Lactation: It is not known whether any of the components of the drug or their metabolites are present in human milk. Caution in nursing.

MECHANISM OF ACTION

Ombitasvir: Inhibitor of HCV NS5A, which is essential for viral RNA replication and virion assembly. **Paritaprevir:** Inhibitor of HCV NS3/4A protease which is necessary for the proteolytic cleavage of the HCV encoded polyprotein (into mature forms of the NS3, NS4A, NS4B, NS5A, and NS5B proteins) and is essential for viral replication. **RTV:** Not active against HCV but it is a potent CYP3A inhibitor that increases peak and trough plasma drug concentrations of paritaprevir and overall drug exposure.

PHARMACOKINETICS

Absorption: Absolute bioavailability (48% [ombitasvir], 53% [paritaprevir]). AUC_{0-24}=1239 (ombitasvir), 2276 (paritaprevir), 6072 (RTV) ng•hr/mL (median); C_{max}=82 (ombitasvir), 194 (paritaprevir), 543 (RTV) ng/mL (median); T_{max}=4-5 hrs. **Distribution:** Plasma protein binding (99.9%, ombitasvir), (97-98.6%, paritaprevir), (>99%, RTV); V_d=173L (ombitasvir), 103L (paritaprevir). **Metabolism:** Ombitasvir: Amide hydrolysis followed by oxidative metabolism. Paritaprevir: Via CYP3A4 (major), CYP3A5. RTV: Via CYP3A (major), CYP2D6. **Elimination:** Ombitasvir: Feces (90.2%, 87.8% unchanged), Urine (1.91%, 0.03% unchanged); $T_{1/2}$=21-25 hrs. Paritaprevir: Feces (88%, 1.1% unchanged), Urine (8.8%, 0.05% unchanged); $T_{1/2}$=5.5 hrs. RTV: Feces (86.4%, 33.8% unchanged), Urine (11.3%, 3.5% unchanged); $T_{1/2}$=4 hrs.

PATIENT CONSIDERATIONS

Assessment: Assess for cirrhosis, hepatic impairment, pregnancy/nursing status, hypersensitivity to any component in drug, and possible drug interactions. Assess baseline hepatic laboratory and clinical parameters. Assess HCV genotype.

Monitoring: Monitor for signs/symptoms of hepatic decompensation, hepatic failure, liver inflammation, ALT elevations, and other adverse reactions. Perform hepatic lab testing during first 4 weeks of treatment and as clinically indicated thereafter.

Counseling: Advise to take ud. Inform patients to watch for signs of liver inflammation or failure (eg, fatigue, weakness, lack of appetite); instruct to notify physician w/o delay if such symptoms develop. Advise to avoid pregnancy during treatment and w/in 6 months of stopping treatment w/ Technivie w/ RBV; instruct to notify physician immediately in the event of a pregnancy. Inform of drug interactions that may occur; instruct to report to physician use of any prescription, nonprescription medication, or herbal products. Inform that contraceptives containing ethinyl estradiol should not be used.

TEFLARO — ceftaroline fosamil   Rx

Class: Cephalosporin

ADULT DOSAGE

Skin and Skin Structure Infections

Acute Infections:
600mg q12h IV over 5-60 min for 5-14 days

Community-Acquired Pneumonia
600mg q12h IV over 5-60 min for 5-7 days

PEDIATRIC DOSAGE

Skin and Skin Structure Infections

Acute Infections:
≥2 Months to <2 Years: 8mg/kg q8h
≥2 Years to <18 Years (≤33kg): 12mg/kg q8h
≥2 Years to <18 Years (>33kg): 400mg q8h or 600mg q12h

Administer IV over 5-60 min for 5-14 days

Community-Acquired Pneumonia
≥2 Months to <2 Years: 8mg/kg q8h
≥2 Years to <18 Years (≤33kg): 12mg/kg q8h
≥2 Years to <18 Years (>33kg): 400mg q8h or 600mg q12h

Administer IV over 5-60 min for 5-14 days

DOSING CONSIDERATIONS

Renal Impairment

Adults:
CrCl >50mL/min: No dosage adjustment necessary
CrCl >30 to ≤50mL/min: 400mg IV over 5-60 min q12h
CrCl ≥15 to ≤30mL/min: 300mg IV over 5-60 min q12h
ESRD (CrCl <15mL/min), Including Hemodialysis: 200mg IV over 5-60 min q12h; administer after hemodialysis on hemodialysis days

Pediatric Patients:
CrCl >50mL/min/1.73m²: No dosage adjustment is required
CrCl <50mL/min/1.73m²: There is insufficient information to recommend a dosage regimen

ADMINISTRATION

IV route

Preparation for Administration

Constitution of Powder for Inj:
1. Constitute contents of vial w/ 20mL of sterile water for inj (SWFI), 0.9% NaCl inj, D5 inj, or lactated Ringer's inj. Constitution time is <2 min.
2. Mix gently to constitute and check to see that the contents have dissolved completely.
3. Refer to PI for volume to be withdrawn.

Dilution of Constituted Sol:
1. Further dilute the constituted sol in a range between 50-250mL before IV infusion.
2. Use the same diluent used for constitution of the powder for this dilution, unless SWFI was used earlier. If SWFI was used earlier, then appropriate infusion sol include 0.9% NaCl inj, D5 inj, 2.5% dextrose inj, 0.45% NaCl inj, or lactated Ringer's inj.

Refer to PI for dilution of the constituted sol in the 50mL infusion bag.

Storage of Constituted Sol

Stability in Baxter Mini-Bag Plus:
Sol in concentrations ranging from 4-12mg/mL in containers w/ 0.9% NaCl inj may be stored for up to 6 hrs at room temperature or for up to 24 hrs at 2-8°C (36-46°F).

Stability in Infusion Bag:
Use constituted sol w/in 6 hrs when stored at room temperature or w/in 24 hrs when stored at 2-8°C (36-46°F).

Drug Compatibilities
Compatibility w/ other drugs has not been established; do not mix w/ or physically add to sol containing other drugs.

STORAGE

Unreconstituted Vials: 25°C (77°F); excursions permitted to 15-30°C (59-86°F).

HOW SUPPLIED

Inj: 400mg, 600mg

CONTRAINDICATIONS

Known serious hypersensitivity to ceftaroline or other members of the cephalosporin class.

WARNINGS/PRECAUTIONS

Serious and occasionally fatal hypersensitivity (anaphylactic) reactions and serious skin reactions reported; d/c and institute appropriate treatment and supportive measures if an allergic reaction occurs. Caution w/ penicillin (PCN) or other β-lactam allergy; cross-sensitivity may occur. *Clostridium difficile*-associated diarrhea (CDAD) reported; may need to d/c if CDAD is suspected or confirmed and institute appropriate fluid and electrolyte management, protein supplementation, antibiotic treatment of *C. difficile*, and surgical evaluation as clinically indicated. Seroconversion from a negative to a positive direct Coombs' test reported. If anemia develops during and after treatment, drug-induced hemolytic anemia should be considered. If drug-induced hemolytic anemia is suspected, consider discontinuation of therapy and administer supportive care if clinically indicated. Increased risk of bacterial resistance if used in the absence of a proven or strongly suspected bacterial infection. Caution in elderly.

ADVERSE REACTIONS

Adults: Diarrhea, nausea, rash.
Pediatric Patients: Diarrhea, N/V, pyrexia, rash.

PREGNANCY AND LACTATION

Pregnancy: There are no adequate studies in pregnant women that informed any drug-associated risks.

Lactation: No data is available regarding the presence of ceftaroline in human milk, the effects of ceftaroline on breastfed infants, or the effects on milk production. Caution in nursing.

MECHANISM OF ACTION

Cephalosporin; bactericidal action is mediated through binding to essential PCN-binding proteins.

PHARMACOKINETICS

Absorption: C_{max}=19mcg/mL (single 600mg dose), 21.3mcg/mL (multiple 600mg doses); T_{max}=1 hr (single 600mg dose), 0.92 hrs (multiple 600mg doses); AUC=56.8mcg•hr/mL (single 600mg dose), 56.3mcg•hr/mL (multiple 600mg doses). **Distribution:** V_d=20.3L (median) (single 600mg dose); plasma protein binding (20%). **Metabolism:** Ceftaroline fosamil (prodrug) converted into ceftaroline via a phosphatase enzyme. **Elimination:** (single 600mg dose) Urine (88%, 64% as ceftaroline and 2% as metabolite), feces (6%); $T_{1/2}$=1.6 hrs (single 600mg dose), 2.66 hrs (multiple 600mg doses).

PATIENT CONSIDERATIONS

Assessment: Assess for cephalosporin or other β-lactam allergy, drug hypersensitivity, renal impairment, pregnancy/nursing status, and possible drug interactions. Obtain appropriate specimens for microbiological examination to identify pathogen and determine susceptibility.

Monitoring: Monitor for signs/symptoms of hypersensitivity reactions, skin reactions, CDAD, drug-induced hemolytic anemia, and other adverse reactions. Monitor renal function, especially in elderly.

Counseling: Advise that allergic reactions could occur and that serious reactions require immediate treatment. Advise to inform the physician about any previous hypersensitivity reactions to the drug, other β-lactams (including cephalosporins), or other allergens. Advise that antibacterial drugs should be used to treat only bacterial, not viral, infections. Instruct to take ud; inform that skipping doses or not completing the full course may decrease effectiveness of treatment and increase risk of bacterial resistance. Advise that diarrhea may occur; instruct to notify physician if severe watery or bloody diarrhea develops.

TEKAMLO — aliskiren/amlodipine   Rx

Class: Calcium channel blocker (CCB) (dihydropyridine)/renin inhibitor

> D/C when pregnancy is detected. Drugs that act directly on the renin-angiotensin system (RAS) can cause injury/death to the developing fetus.

ADULT DOSAGE	PEDIATRIC DOSAGE
Hypertension	Pediatric use may not have been established
Initial: 150mg/5mg qd	
Titrate: If BP remains uncontrolled after 2-4 weeks of therapy, titrate dose prn	
Max: 300mg/10mg qd	
Add-On Therapy:	
Use for patients not adequately controlled w/ aliskiren alone or amlodipine (or another dihydropyridine CCB) alone; if dose-limiting adverse reactions occur on either component alone, switch to Tekamlo containing a lower dose of that component in combination w/ the other to achieve similar BP reductions	
Replacement Therapy:	
Switch patients receiving aliskiren and amlodipine from separate tabs to Tekamlo containing the same component doses; if BP is uncontrolled when substituting for individual components, increase the dose of one or both of the components	
May be used alone or w/ other antihypertensive agents	

DOSING CONSIDERATIONS

Hepatic Impairment
Consider lower doses

Elderly
Consider starting w/ the lowest available dose of amlodipine

ADMINISTRATION

Oral route

Establish a routine pattern for taking the drug either w/ or w/o a meal; high-fat meals decrease absorption substantially.

STORAGE

25°C (77°F); excursions permitted to 15-30°C (59-86°F). Protect from heat and moisture.

HOW SUPPLIED

Tab: (Aliskiren/Amlodipine) 150mg/5mg, 150mg/10mg, 300mg/5mg, 300mg/10mg

CONTRAINDICATIONS

Concomitant use w/ ARBs or ACE inhibitors in patients w/ diabetes. Known hypersensitivity to any of the components of the product.

WARNINGS/PRECAUTIONS

Symptomatic hypotension may occur in patients w/ marked volume/salt depletion, w/ severe aortic stenosis; correct volume/salt depletion prior to administration, or start treatment under close supervision. May cause changes in renal function, including acute renal failure; consider withholding or discontinuing therapy if significant decrease in renal function develops. Patients whose renal function may depend in part on the activity of the renin-angiotensin-aldosterone system (RAAS) (eg, renal artery stenosis, severe heart failure [HF], post-MI, volume depletion) may be at particular risk for developing acute renal failure. **Aliskiren:** Hypersensitivity reactions and head/neck angioedema reported; d/c therapy immediately if anaphylactic reactions or edema occurs and do not readminister. May cause hyperkalemia; periodically monitor serum K^+. **Amlodipine:** Worsening angina and acute MI may develop after starting or increasing dose, particularly w/ severe obstructive coronary artery disease (CAD).

ADVERSE REACTIONS

Peripheral edema.

DRUG INTERACTIONS

See Contraindications. **Aliskiren:** Cyclosporine or itraconazole may increase levels; avoid concomitant use. NSAIDs (including selective COX-2 inhibitors) may result in deterioration of renal function, including possible acute renal failure, in elderly, volume depleted, or those w/ compromised renal function. Antihypertensive effect may be attenuated by NSAIDs. Dual blockade of the RAAS is associated w/ increased risks of hypotension, hyperkalemia, and changes in renal function (including acute renal failure); avoid combined use w/ ACE inhibitors or ARBs, particularly in patients w/ CrCl <60mL/min. Oral coadministration w/ furosemide reduced exposure to furosemide; monitor diuretic effects. Risk of developing hyperkalemia w/ NSAIDs (eg, selective COX-2 inhibitors), K^+ supplements, or K^+-sparing diuretics. **Amlodipine:** May increase simvastatin exposure; limit simvastatin dose to 20mg/day. CYP3A inhibitors (moderate and strong) result in increased systemic exposure to amlodipine warranting dose reduction; monitor for symptoms of hypotension and edema to determine need for dose adjustment. Monitor BP when coadministered w/ CYP3A4 inducers.

PREGNANCY AND LACTATION

Pregnancy: Category D. Use of drugs that act on the RAS during the 2nd and 3rd trimesters of pregnancy reduces fetal renal function and increases fetal and neonatal morbidity and death. Resulting oligohydramnios can be associated w/ fetal lung hypoplasia and skeletal deformations. When pregnancy is detected, d/c Tekamlo as soon as possible.
Lactation: Not for use in nursing.

MECHANISM OF ACTION

Aliskiren: Direct renin inhibitor; decreases plasma renin activity and inhibits the conversion of angiotensinogen to angiotensin I. **Amlodipine:** Dihydropyridine CCB; inhibits the transmembrane influx of Ca^{2+} ions into vascular smooth muscle and cardiac muscle. Acts directly on vascular smooth muscle to cause a reduction in peripheral vascular resistance and reduction in BP.

PHARMACOKINETICS

Absorption: Aliskiren: Poor. Bioavailability (2.5%); T_{max}=1-3 hrs. Amlodipine: Absolute bioavailability (64-90%); T_{max}=6-12 hrs. **Distribution:** Amlodipine: Plasma protein binding (approx 93%); V_d=21L/kg. **Metabolism:** Aliskiren: Via CYP3A4. Amlodipine: Hepatic (extensive). **Elimination:** Aliskiren: Urine (25%, unchanged); $T_{1/2}$=24 hrs. Amlodipine: Urine (10%, unchanged; 60% metabolites); $T_{1/2}$=30-50 hrs.

PATIENT CONSIDERATIONS

Assessment: Assess for drug hypersensitivity, volume/salt depletion, renal artery stenosis, HF, post-MI status, severe aortic stenosis, CAD, hyperkalemia risk factors, renal/hepatic impairment, pregnancy/nursing status, and possible drug interactions.

Monitoring: Monitor for signs/symptoms of hypotension, worsening of angina, acute MI, hyperkalemia, hypersensitivity reactions, airway obstruction, angioedema, and other adverse reactions. Monitor BP, renal function, and serum K^+ periodically.

Counseling: Inform female patients of childbearing age of the consequences of exposure to therapy during pregnancy and of the treatment options for women planning to become pregnant. Advise to report pregnancies as soon as possible. Caution that lightheadedness may occur, especially during the 1st days of therapy; advise to contact physician if lightheadedness occurs. Advise to d/c until physician has been consulted if syncope occurs. Caution that inadequate fluid intake, excessive perspiration, diarrhea, or vomiting can lead to an excessive fall in BP. Advise to d/c and immediately report any signs/symptoms of a severe allergic reaction or angioedema. Inform that angioedema (eg, laryngeal edema) may occur anytime during treatment. Instruct not to use K^+ supplements or salt substitutes containing K^+ w/o consulting physician.

TEKTURNA — aliskiren   Rx

Class: Renin inhibitor

> D/C when pregnancy is detected. Drugs that act directly on the renin-angiotensin system can cause injury/death to the developing fetus.

ADULT DOSAGE	PEDIATRIC DOSAGE
Hypertension	Pediatric use may not have been established
Initial: 150mg qd	
Titrate: May increase to 300mg qd if BP is not adequately controlled	
Max: 300mg/day	

ADMINISTRATION

Oral route

Establish a routine pattern for taking drug w/ regard to meals; high-fat meals decrease absorption substantially.

STORAGE

25°C (77°F); excursions permitted to 15-30°C (59-86°F). Protect from moisture.

HOW SUPPLIED

Tab: 150mg, 300mg

CONTRAINDICATIONS

Coadministration w/ ARBs or ACE inhibitors in patients w/ diabetes. Known hypersensitivity to any of the components of the product.

WARNINGS/PRECAUTIONS

Hypersensitivity reactions and head/neck angioedema reported; d/c therapy immediately and do not readminister if anaphylactic reactions or angioedema develop. Symptomatic hypotension may occur in patients w/ marked volume depletion or w/ salt depletion; correct volume/salt depletion prior to administration, or start treatment under close medical supervision. May cause changes in renal function, including acute renal failure; caution in patients whose renal function may depend in part on the activity of the renin-angiotensin-aldosterone system (RAAS) (eg, renal artery stenosis, severe heart failure [HF], post-MI, volume depletion). Consider withholding or discontinuing therapy if clinically significant decrease in renal function develops. May cause hyperkalemia.

ADVERSE REACTIONS

Edema, diarrhea, cough, seizures, rash, elevated uric acid, gout, renal stones, increased BUN/SrCr/creatine kinase.

DRUG INTERACTIONS

See Contraindications. Cyclosporine or itraconazole may increase levels; avoid concomitant use. NSAIDs, including selective COX-2 inhibitors, may deteriorate renal function and may attenuate antihypertensive effect. Dual blockade of the RAAS is associated w/ increased risk of hypotension, hyperkalemia, and changes in renal function (including acute renal failure); avoid combined use w/ ACE inhibitors or ARBs, particularly in patients w/ CrCl <60mL/min. Reduced furosemide exposure w/ concomitant use. May develop hyperkalemia w/ NSAIDs, K+ supplements, or K+-sparing diuretics.

PREGNANCY AND LACTATION
Pregnancy: Category D. Use of drugs that act on the renin-angiotensin system during the 2nd and 3rd trimesters of pregnancy reduces fetal renal function and increases fetal and neonatal morbidity and death. When pregnancy is detected, d/c aliskiren as soon as possible.
Lactation: Not for use in nursing.

MECHANISM OF ACTION
Direct renin inhibitor; decreases plasma renin activity and inhibits conversion of angiotensinogen to angiotensin I.

PHARMACOKINETICS
Absorption: Poor. Bioavailability (2.5%); T_{max}=1-3 hrs. **Metabolism:** Via CYP3A4. **Elimination:** Urine (25%, unchanged); $T_{1/2}$=24 hrs.

PATIENT CONSIDERATIONS
Assessment: Assess for hypersensitivity to the drug, diabetes, volume/salt depletion, renal artery stenosis, HF, post-MI status, pregnancy/nursing status, and possible drug interactions.

Monitoring: Monitor for hypersensitivity reactions, angioedema, airway obstruction, and other adverse reactions. Monitor BP, renal function, and serum K+ periodically.

Counseling: Inform female patients of childbearing age of the consequences of exposure during pregnancy and of the treatment options for women planning to become pregnant. Advise to report pregnancies to physicians as soon as possible. Advise to d/c therapy and to report immediately any signs/symptoms of a severe allergic reaction or angioedema. Advise that lightheadedness may occur, especially during the 1st days of therapy; instruct to contact physician if lightheadedness occurs. Advise to d/c treatment until physician has been consulted if syncope occurs. Caution that inadequate fluid intake, excessive perspiration, diarrhea, or vomiting can lead to an excessive fall in BP. Advise not to use K+ supplements or salt substitutes containing K+ w/o consulting physician. Instruct patients to establish a routine pattern for taking aliskiren w/ regard to meals.

TEKTURNA HCT — aliskiren/hydrochlorothiazide   Rx

Class: Renin inhibitor/thiazide diuretic

> D/C when pregnancy is detected. Drugs that act directly on the renin-angiotensin system can cause injury and death to the developing fetus.

ADULT DOSAGE	PEDIATRIC DOSAGE
Hypertension	Pediatric use may not have been established
Add-On/Initial Therapy: Patients whose BP is not adequately controlled w/ aliskiren alone or hydrochlorothiazide (HCTZ) alone may be switched to Tekturna HCT, patients whose BP is controlled w/ HCTZ alone but who experience hypokalemia may be switched to Tekturna HCT, or patients who experience dose-limiting adverse reactions on either component alone may be switched to Tekturna HCT containing a lower dose of that component in combination w/ the other. May be used as initial therapy in patients likely to need multiple drugs to achieve BP goals	
Initial: 150mg/12.5mg qd prn to control BP **Titrate:** May increase if BP remains uncontrolled after 2-4 weeks **Max:** 300mg/25mg qd	
Replacement Therapy: May substitute for individually titrated components	

ADMINISTRATION
Oral route

Establish a routine pattern for taking drug w/ regard to meals; high-fat meals decrease absorption substantially.

STORAGE
25°C (77°F); excursions permitted to 15-30°C (59-86°F). Protect from moisture.

HOW SUPPLIED
Tab: (Aliskiren/HCTZ) 150mg/12.5mg, 150mg/25mg, 300mg/12.5mg, 300mg/25mg

CONTRAINDICATIONS
Coadministration w/ ARBs or ACE inhibitors in patients w/ diabetes, known anuria, hypersensitivity to sulfonamide-derived drugs (eg, HCTZ) or to any of the components.

WARNINGS/PRECAUTIONS
Not for initial therapy w/ intravascular volume depletion. Symptomatic hypotension may occur in patients w/ marked volume depletion or w/ salt depletion; correct volume/salt depletion prior to administration or begin therapy under close medical supervision. Renal function changes may occur, including acute renal failure; caution in patients whose renal function may depend in part on the activity of the renin-angiotensin-aldosterone system (RAAS) (eg, renal artery stenosis, severe heart failure [HF], post-MI, or volume depletion). Consider withholding or discontinuing therapy if clinically significant decrease in renal function develops. May cause hypo/hyperkalemia; d/c if hypokalemia is accompanied by clinical signs (eg, muscular weakness, paresis, ECG alterations). **Aliskiren:** Hypersensitivity reactions (eg, anaphylactic reactions) and head/neck angioedema reported; d/c therapy immediately and do not readminister if anaphylactic reactions or angioedema develops. May cause hyperkalemia. **HCTZ:** May cause hypersensitivity reactions, w/ or w/o bronchial asthma, and exacerbation or activation of systemic lupus erythematosus (SLE). May cause hypokalemia and hyponatremia; hypomagnesemia may result in hypokalemia. Correct hypokalemia and any coexisting hypomagnesemia prior to initiation of thiazides. May cause idiosyncratic reaction, resulting in acute transient myopia and acute angle-closure glaucoma; d/c as rapidly as possible. May alter glucose tolerance and increase serum cholesterol and TG levels. May cause or exacerbate hyperuricemia and precipitate gout in susceptible patients. May cause hypercalcemia. Minor alterations of fluid and electrolyte balance may precipitate hepatic coma in patients w/ hepatic impairment or progressive liver disease.

ADVERSE REACTIONS
Dizziness, influenza, diarrhea, cough, vertigo, asthenia, arthralgia.

DRUG INTERACTIONS
See Contraindications. **Aliskiren:** Cyclosporine or itraconazole may increase levels; avoid concomitant use. NSAIDs (eg, selective COX-2 inhibitors) may deteriorate renal function, including possible acute renal failure, and may attenuate antihypertensive effect. Dual blockade of the RAAS is associated w/ increased risk of hypotension, hyperkalemia, and changes in renal function (including acute renal failure); in general, avoid combined use w/ ACE inhibitors or ARBs, particularly in patients w/ CrCl <60mL/min. Reduced furosemide exposure w/ concomitant use. May develop hyperkalemia w/ NSAIDs (eg, selective COX-2 inhibitors), K+ supplements, or K+-sparing diuretics. **HCTZ:** Dosage adjustment of antidiabetic drugs (oral agents and insulin) may be required. May increase risk of lithium toxicity; monitor serum lithium levels. Observe patients closely to determine if the desired effect of the diuretic is obtained when used concomitantly w/ NSAIDs and COX-2 selective agents. Administer ≥4 hrs before or 4-6 hrs after the administration of ion exchange resins (eg, cholestyramine, colestipol).

PREGNANCY AND LACTATION
Pregnancy: Category D. Use of drugs that act on the renin-angiotensin system during the 2nd and 3rd trimesters of pregnancy reduces fetal renal function and increases fetal and neonatal morbidity and death. When pregnancy is detected, d/c therapy as soon as possible. Thiazides cross the placenta and their use is associated w/ risk of fetal or neonatal jaundice, thrombocytopenia, and possible other adverse reactions.
Lactation: Not for use in nursing. Thiazides appear in human milk.

MECHANISM OF ACTION
Aliskiren: Direct renin inhibitor; decreases plasma renin activity and inhibits conversion of angiotensinogen to angiotensin I. **HCTZ:** Thiazide diuretic; has not been established. Affects renal tubular mechanisms of electrolyte reabsorption, directly increasing excretion of Na+ and Cl-, and indirectly reduces plasma volume.

PHARMACOKINETICS
Absorption: Aliskiren: Poor. Bioavailability (2.5%); T_{max}=1 hr (median). HCTZ: Absolute bioavailability (70%); T_{max}=2.5 hrs (median). **Distribution:** HCTZ: Plasma protein binding (40-70%, albumin); crosses placenta; found in breast milk. **Metabolism:** Aliskiren: Via CYP3A4. **Elimination:** Aliskiren: Urine (25%, unchanged); $T_{1/2}$=24 hrs. HCTZ: Urine (70%, unchanged); $T_{1/2}$=10 hrs.

PATIENT CONSIDERATIONS
Assessment: Assess for diabetes, anuria, sulfonamide-derived drug hypersensitivity, history of penicillin allergy, volume/salt depletion, renal artery stenosis, HF, post-MI status, SLE, hepatic/renal impairment, pregnancy/nursing status, and possible drug interactions. Correct electrolyte abnormalities (eg, hypokalemia, hypomagnesemia) prior to initiating therapy.

Monitoring: Monitor for signs/symptoms of idiosyncratic reactions, hypersensitivity reactions, angioedema, airway obstruction, exacerbation/activation of SLE, hyperuricemia, precipitation of gout, and other adverse reactions. Monitor BP, renal function, serum electrolytes, cholesterol, and TG levels.

Counseling: Inform female patients of childbearing age of the consequences of exposure during pregnancy and of the treatment options for women planning to become pregnant. Advise to report pregnancies to physicians as soon as possible. Inform that lightheadedness may occur, especially during the 1st days of therapy; instruct to contact physician if lightheadedness occurs. Advise to d/c treatment until physician has been consulted if syncope occurs. Caution that inadequate fluid intake, excessive perspiration, diarrhea, or vomiting can lead to an excessive fall in BP. Advise to d/c therapy and immediately report any signs/symptoms of a severe allergic reaction or angioedema. Advise not to use K+ supplements or salt substitutes containing K+ w/o consulting physician. Instruct to establish a routine pattern for taking the medication w/ regard to meals.

Temodar – temozolomide

Rx

Class: Alkylating agent

ADULT DOSAGE

Newly Diagnosed High Grade Glioblastoma Multiforme

Concomitant Phase:

$75mg/m^2$/day for 42 days concomitant w/ focal radiotherapy

Dose should be continued throughout the 42-day concomitant period up to 49 days if all of the following conditions are met:
- ANC $\geq$1.5 x 10^9/L
- Platelet count $\geq$100 x 10^9/L
- Common toxicity criteria (CTC) nonhematological toxicity $\leq$Grade 1 (except for alopecia, N/V)

Maint Phase:

Four weeks after completing the concomitant phase, temozolomide is administered for an additional 6 cycles of maint treatment

Cycle 1: $150mg/m^2$ qd for 5 days followed by 23 days w/o treatment

Cycles 2-6: May increase to $200mg/m^2$ at start of Cycle 2 if nonhematologic toxicity for Cycle 1 is $\leq$Grade 2 (except alopecia, N/V), ANC $\geq$1.5 x 10^9/L, and platelet count $\geq$100 x 10^9/L. The dose remains at $200mg/m^2$/day for the first 5 days of each subsequent cycle unless toxicity occurs; if the dose was not escalated at Cycle 2, do not escalate in subsequent cycles.

Refractory Anaplastic Astrocytoma

Patients Who Have Experienced Disease Progression on a Drug Regimen Containing Nitrosourea and Procarbazine:

Initial: $150mg/m^2$ qd for 5 consecutive days per 28-day cycle

Titrate: May increase to $200mg/m^2$/day for 5 consecutive days per 28-day treatment cycle if both the nadir and day of dosing (Day 29, Day 1 of next cycle) ANC are $\geq$1.5 x 10^9/L (1500/μL) and both the nadir and Day 29, Day 1 of next cycle platelet counts are $\geq$100 x 10^9/L (100,000/μL)

Therapy may be continued until disease progression

PEDIATRIC DOSAGE

Pediatric use may not have been established

DOSING CONSIDERATIONS

Adverse Reactions

Glioblastoma Multiforme (GBM) During Concomitant Radiotherapy:

Interrupt Dose If:
1. ANC $\geq$0.5 and <1.5 x 10^9/L
2. Platelet count $\geq$10 and <100 x 10^9/L
3. Nonhematologic toxicity (except alopecia, N/V) CTC Grade 2

D/C Therapy If:
1. ANC <0.5 x 10^9/L
2. Platelet count <10 x 10^9/L
3. Nonhematologic toxicity (except alopecia, N/V) CTC Grade 3 or 4

GBM During Maint Treatment:

Dose Levels for Maint Treatment:

Dose Level -1 (Reduction for Prior Toxicity): $100mg/m^2$/day

Dose Level 0 (Dose During Cycle 1): $150mg/m^2$/day

Dose Level 1 (Dose During Cycles 2-6 in Absence of Toxicity): $200mg/m^2$/day

Reduce by 1 Dose Level If:
1. ANC <1.0 x 10^9/L
2. Platelet count <50 x 10^9/L
3. Nonhematologic toxicity (except alopecia, N/V) CTC Grade 3

D/C Therapy If:
1. Dose reduction to <$100mg/m^2$ is required
2. The same Grade 3 nonhematological toxicity (except for alopecia, N/V) recurs after dose reduction
3. Nonhematologic toxicity (except alopecia, N/V) CTC Grade 4

Refractory Anaplastic Astrocytoma:

Refer to PI for dose modification

Other Important Considerations

Dose must be adjusted according to nadir neutrophil and platelet counts in the previous cycle and the neutrophil and platelet counts at the time of initiating the next cycle

ADMINISTRATION

Oral/IV route

Cap

Take on an empty stomach; bedtime administration may be advised.

Swallow whole w/ a glass of water; do not open or chew.

Antiemetic therapy may be administered prior to and/or following administration.

Inj

Infuse IV over 90 min.

When reconstituted w/ 41mL sterile water for inj, the resulting sol will contain 2.5mg/mL temozolomide.

Bring vial to room temperature prior to reconstitution.

Gently swirl the vials; do not shake.

Do not further dilute the reconstituted sol.

After reconstitution, store at room temperature (25°C [77°F]) and use w/in 14 hrs, including infusion time.

Withdraw up to 40mL from each vial to make up the total dose and transfer into an empty 250mL infusion bag.

Infuse IV using a pump over 90 min; flush the lines before and after each infusion.

May be administered in the same IV line w/ 0.9% NaCl inj only.

Do not infuse other medications simultaneously through the same IV line.

STORAGE

Cap: 25°C (77°F); excursions permitted to 15-30°C (59-86°F). **Inj:** 2-8°C (36-46°F). After reconstitution, store reconstituted product at 25°C (77°F); must be used w/in 14 hrs, including infusion time.

HOW SUPPLIED

Cap: 5mg, 20mg, 100mg, 140mg, 180mg, 250mg; **Inj:** 100mg

CONTRAINDICATIONS

History of hypersensitivity reaction (eg, urticaria, allergic reaction including anaphylaxis, toxic epidermal necrolysis, and Stevens-Johnson syndrome) to any components of the product. History of hypersensitivity to dacarbazine (DTIC).

WARNINGS/PRECAUTIONS

See Dosing Considerations. Myelosuppression, including prolonged pancytopenia, which may result in aplastic anemia, may occur. Prior to dosing, patients must have an ANC$\geq$1.5 x 10^9/L and a platelet count $\geq$100 x 10^9/L. For the concomitant treatment phase w/ radiotherapy, obtain a CBC prior to initiation of treatment and weekly during treatment. For the 28-day treatment cycles, obtain a CBC prior to treatment on Day 1 and on Day 22 (21 days after the first dose) of each cycle or w/in 48 hrs of that day, and weekly until the ANC is >1.5 x 10^9/L and platelet count exceeds 100 x 10^9/L. Greater risk of myelosuppression in women and elderly patients. Cases of myelodysplastic syndrome and secondary malignancies, including myeloid leukemia, observed. *Pneumocystis carinii* pneumonia (PCP) prophylaxis is required in all patients w/ newly diagnosed GBM who are receiving concomitant radiotherapy for 42-day regimen, and should be continued in patients who develop lymphocytopenia until recovery from lymphocytopenia (CTC $\leq$Grade 1); higher occurrence of PCP when temozolomide is administered during a longer dosing regimen. Fatal and severe hepatotoxicity reported; perform LFTs at baseline, midway through 1st cycle, prior to each subsequent cycle, and approx 2-4 weeks after last dose. May cause fetal harm. Caution w/ severe renal/hepatic impairment and in elderly. **Inj:** Bioequivalence established only when inj is given over 90 min; infusion over a shorter or longer period may result in suboptimal dosing and may increase possibility of infusion related adverse reactions.

ADVERSE REACTIONS

Alopecia, N/V, anorexia, headache, constipation, fatigue, convulsions, thrombocytopenia.

DRUG INTERACTIONS

Valproic acid may decrease oral clearance.

PREGNANCY AND LACTATION

Pregnancy: Category D. May cause fetal harm.

Lactation: Not for use in nursing.

MECHANISM OF ACTION

Alkylating agent (imidazotetrazine derivative); not directly active but undergoes rapid nonenzymatic conversion at physiologic pH to the reactive compound 5-(3-methyltriazen-1-yl)-imidazole-4-carboxamide (MTIC). Cytotoxicity of MTIC is thought to be primarily due to alkylation of DNA. Alkylation (methylation) occurs mainly at the O^6 and N^7 positions of guanine.

PHARMACOKINETICS

Absorption: (PO) Rapid and complete, T_{max}=1 hr (median); C_{max}=7.5mcg/mL, 282ng/mL (MTIC); AUC=23.4mcg•hr/mL, 864ng•hr/mL (MTIC). (IV) C_{max}=7.3mcg/mL, 276ng/mL (MTIC); AUC=24.6mcg•hr/mL, 891ng•hr/mL (MTIC). **Distribution:** V_d=0.4L/kg; plasma protein binding (15%). **Metabolism:** Spontaneous hydrolysis to the active species, MTIC, and to temozolomide acid metabolite. MTIC is further hydrolyzed to 5-amino-imidazole-4-carboxamide and methylhydrazine. **Elimination:** Urine (37.7%, 5.6% unchanged), feces (0.8%); $T_{1/2}$=1.8 hrs.

PATIENT CONSIDERATIONS

Assessment: Assess for previous hypersensitivity to drug or DTIC, myelosuppression, hepatic/renal impairment, pregnancy/nursing status, and possible drug interactions. Obtain baseline LFTs, CBC, and ANC.

Monitoring: Monitor for myelosuppression, PCP, myelodysplastic syndrome, secondary malignancies, and other adverse reactions. For the concomitant treatment phase w/ radiotherapy, obtain a CBC weekly during treatment. For the 28-day treatment cycles, obtain a CBC on Day 22 (21 days after the first dose) of each cycle or w/in 48 hrs of that day. If ANC falls <1.5 x 10^9/L and the platelet count falls <100 x 10^9/L, obtain blood counts weekly until recovery. Perform LFTs midway through the 1st cycle, prior to each subsequent cycle, and approx 2-4 weeks after the last dose. **Inj:** Monitor for infusion-related reactions.

Counseling: Instruct to take exactly as prescribed. Instruct to take rigorous precautions to avoid inhalation or contact w/ skin or mucous membranes if caps or vials are accidentally opened or damaged. Inform about the most frequently occurring adverse effects (eg, N/V).

TENEX — guanfacine hydrochloride   Rx

Class: Alpha₂ agonist

ADULT DOSAGE	PEDIATRIC DOSAGE
Hypertension	**Hypertension**
Initial: 1mg at hs	**≥12 Years:**
Titrate: If result is not satisfactory after 3-4 weeks, may increase dose to 2mg	**Initial:** 1mg at hs
	Titrate: If result is not satisfactory after 3-4 weeks, may increase dose to 2mg
Higher daily doses have been used, but adverse reactions increase significantly w/ doses >3mg/day	Higher daily doses have been used, but adverse reactions increase significantly w/ doses >3mg/day

DOSING CONSIDERATIONS
Elderly
Start at lower end of dosing range

ADMINISTRATION
Oral route

STORAGE
20-25°C (68-77°F).

HOW SUPPLIED
Tab: 1mg, 2mg

CONTRAINDICATIONS
Known hypersensitivity to guanfacine HCl.

WARNINGS/PRECAUTIONS
Caution with severe coronary insufficiency, recent MI, cerebrovascular disease, or chronic renal or hepatic failure. May cause sedation or drowsiness, especially when beginning therapy. Abrupt cessation of therapy may be associated with increases in plasma and urinary catecholamines, symptoms of "nervousness/anxiety," and increases in BP to levels significantly greater than those prior to therapy. Caution in elderly.

ADVERSE REACTIONS
Dry mouth, somnolence, asthenia, dizziness, headache, impotence, constipation, fatigue, insomnia.

DRUG INTERACTIONS
Additive sedative effects with other centrally active depressants (eg, phenothiazines, barbiturates, benzodiazepines). Concomitant use with known microsomal enzyme inducers (eg, phenobarbital, phenytoin) in patients with renal impairment may decrease levels; more frequent dosing may be required to achieve/maintain hypotensive response; taper guanfacine dose upon discontinuation to avoid rebound phenomena.

PREGNANCY AND LACTATION
Category B, caution in nursing.

MECHANISM OF ACTION
α₂-adrenoceptor agonist; reduces sympathetic nerve impulses from the vasomotor center to the heart and blood vessels, resulting in decreased peripheral vascular resistance and reduction in HR.

PHARMACOKINETICS
Absorption: Absolute bioavailability (80%); T_{max}=2.6 hrs. **Distribution:** V_d=6.3L/kg; plasma protein binding (70%). **Metabolism:** Oxidation of the aromatic ring. **Elimination:** Urine (50% unchanged); $T_{1/2}$=17 hrs.

PATIENT CONSIDERATIONS
Assessment: Assess for previous hypersensitivity to the drug, recent MI, severe coronary insufficiency, cerebrovascular disease, chronic renal/hepatic failure, pregnancy/nursing status, and possible drug interactions.

Monitoring: Monitor for drowsiness, sedation, and other adverse reactions. Monitor BP, LFTs, and renal function.

Counseling: Advise to exercise caution when operating dangerous machinery or driving motor vehicles. Inform that tolerance for alcohol and other CNS depressants may be diminished. Instruct not to d/c therapy abruptly.

TENORETIC — atenolol/chlorthalidone   Rx

Class: Monosulfamyl diuretic/selective beta₁ blocker

ADULT DOSAGE	PEDIATRIC DOSAGE
Hypertension	Pediatric use may not have been established
Initial: 50mg/25mg tab qd	
Titrate: May increase to 100mg/25mg tab qd, if optimal response not achieved	

DOSING CONSIDERATIONS
Renal Impairment
CrCl 15-35mL/min:
Max: 50mg atenolol/day
CrCl <15mL/min:
Max: 50mg atenolol qod
Elderly
Start at lower end of dosing range

ADMINISTRATION
Oral route

STORAGE
20-25°C (68-77°F).

HOW SUPPLIED
Tab: (Atenolol/Chlorthalidone) 50mg/25mg*, 100mg/25mg *scored

CONTRAINDICATIONS
Sinus bradycardia, >1st-degree heart block, cardiogenic shock, overt cardiac failure, anuria, hypersensitivity to this product or to sulfonamide-derived drugs.

WARNINGS/PRECAUTIONS
Not for initial therapy. Avoid w/ untreated pheochromocytoma. May aggravate peripheral arterial circulatory disorders. Caution in elderly. **Atenolol:** May cause/precipitate HF; d/c if cardiac failure continues despite adequate treatment. Caution in patients w/ impaired renal function. Avoid abrupt discontinuation; exacerbation of angina and MI reported. Avoid w/ bronchospastic disease, but may use w/ caution if unresponsive/intolerant of other antihypertensive treatment. Chronically administered therapy should not be routinely withdrawn prior to major surgery; however, may augment risks of general anesthesia and surgical procedures. Caution in diabetic patients; may mask tachycardia occurring w/ hypoglycemia. May mask clinical signs of hyperthyroidism and precipitate thyroid storm w/ abrupt discontinuation. May cause fetal harm. **Chlorthalidone:** May precipitate azotemia w/ renal disease. If progressive renal impairment becomes evident, d/c therapy. Caution w/ impaired hepatic function or progressive liver disease; may precipitate hepatic coma. D/C prior to parathyroid function test. Decreased Ca²⁺ excretion observed. Altered parathyroid glands, w/ hypercalcemia and hypophosphatemia, seen w/ prolonged therapy. Hyperuricemia may occur, or acute gout may be precipitated. Fluid/electrolyte imbalance may develop. Sensitivity reactions may occur. Exacerbation/activation of systemic lupus erythematous (SLE) reported. May enhance effects in postsympathectomy patients.

ADVERSE REACTIONS
Bradycardia, dizziness, fatigue, nausea.

DRUG INTERACTIONS
May potentiate other antihypertensive agents. Observe for hypotension and/or marked bradycardia w/ catecholamine-depleting drugs (eg, reserpine). Additive effects w/ calcium channel blockers. **Atenolol:** Bradycardia, heart block, and rise of left ventricular end diastolic pressure may occur w/ verapamil or diltiazem. May cause severe bradycardia, asystole, and HF w/ disopyramide. Additive effects w/ amiodarone. Prostaglandin synthase inhibitors (eg, indomethacin) may decrease hypotensive effects. Exacerbates rebound HTN w/ clonidine withdrawal. May be unresponsive to usual doses of epinephrine. Digitalis glycosides may slow AV conduction and increase risk of bradycardia. **Chlorthalidone:** May alter insulin requirements in diabetic patients; latent diabetes mellitus (DM) may manifest. May develop hypokalemia w/ concomitant corticosteroids or adrenocorticotropic hormone. May decrease arterial response to norepinephrine. May increase responsiveness to tubocurarine. Avoid w/ lithium; risk of lithium toxicity.

PREGNANCY AND LACTATION
Pregnancy: Category D.
Lactation: Caution in nursing.

MECHANISM OF ACTION
Atenolol: Cardioselective β-adrenoreceptor blocking agent; has not been established. Suspected to competitively antagonize catecholamines at peripheral adrenergic neuron sites, leading to decreased cardiac output; a central effect leading to reduced sympathetic outflow to the periphery and suppression of renin activity. **Chlorthalidone:** Monosulfamyl diuretic; acts on cortical diluting segment of ascending limb of Henle's loop and produces diuresis w/ increased excretion of Na⁺ and Cl⁻.

PHARMACOKINETICS
Absorption: Atenolol: Rapid, incomplete; T_{max}=2-4 hrs. **Distribution:** Crosses placenta. Atenolol: Plasma protein binding (6-16%); found in breast milk. **Elimination:** Atenolol: Renal excretion; feces (unchanged); $T_{1/2}$=6-7 hrs.

PATIENT CONSIDERATIONS
Assessment: Assess for bradycardia, cardiogenic shock, >1st-degree heart block, overt cardiac failure, impaired renal/hepatic function, bronchospastic disease, peripheral vascular disease, DM, hyperthyroidism, pheochromocytoma, anuria, hypersensitivity to sulfonamide-derived drugs, serum electrolytes, parathyroid disease, pregnancy/nursing status, SLE, CAD, and possible drug interactions.

Monitoring: Monitor for cardiac failure, hepatic/renal function, withdrawal symptoms, hypersensitivity reactions, hyperuricemia or acute gout, and signs/symptoms of electrolyte imbalance. Monitor serum glucose, serum electrolytes, and BP.

Counseling: Instruct not to interrupt or d/c therapy w/o consulting physician. Instruct to notify physician if signs/symptoms of impending CHF or unexplained respiratory symptoms develop. Counsel about signs/symptoms of electrolyte imbalance, and advise to seek prompt medical attention. Inform that drug may cause potential harm to fetus; instruct to inform physician if pregnant/planning to become pregnant.

TENORMIN — atenolol   Rx

Class: Selective beta₁ blocker

> Avoid abrupt discontinuation of therapy in patients w/ coronary artery disease (CAD). Severe exacerbation of angina and occurrence of MI and ventricular arrhythmias reported in angina patients following abrupt discontinuation w/ β-blockers. If planning to d/c therapy, carefully observe and advise to limit physical activity. Promptly reinstitute therapy, at least temporarily, if angina worsens or acute coronary insufficiency develops. CAD may be unrecognized; may be prudent to avoid abrupt discontinuation in patients only treated for HTN.

ADULT DOSAGE

Hypertension
Initial: 50mg qd, either alone or w/ diuretic therapy
Titrate: May increase to 100mg qd after 1-2 weeks
Max: 100mg qd

Angina Pectoris
Long-term Management:
Initial: 50mg qd
Titrate: May increase to 100mg qd after 1 week
Max: 200mg qd

Acute Myocardial Infarction
Management of hemodynamically stable patients w/ definite/suspected acute MI to reduce cardiovascular mortality

Usual: Following IV dose, 50mg 10 min after IV dose followed by 50mg 12 hrs later, then 100mg qd or 50mg bid for 6-9 days or until discharge from the hospital

Atenolol is an additional treatment to standard coronary unit therapy

PEDIATRIC DOSAGE
Pediatric use may not have been established

DOSING CONSIDERATIONS
Renal Impairment
Max Dose for CrCl 15-35mL/min: 50mg/day
Max Dose for CrCl <15mL/min: 25mg/day

Hemodialysis:
25mg or 50mg after each dialysis

HTN:
Initial: May require a lower dose of 25mg qd

Elderly
HTN:
Initial: May require a lower dose of 25mg qd

ADMINISTRATION
Oral route

STORAGE
20-25°C (68-77°F).

HOW SUPPLIED
Tab: 25mg, 50mg*, 100mg *scored

CONTRAINDICATIONS
Sinus bradycardia, >1st-degree heart block, cardiogenic shock, overt cardiac failure, history of hypersensitivity to atenolol or any of the drug product's components.

WARNINGS/PRECAUTIONS
May cause/precipitate heart failure (HF); d/c if cardiac failure continues despite adequate treatment. Avoid w/ bronchospastic disease; may use w/ caution if unresponsive to/intolerant of other antihypertensive treatment. Chronically administered therapy should not be routinely withdrawn prior to major surgery; however, may augment risks of general anesthesia and surgical procedures. Caution in diabetic patients; may mask tachycardia occurring w/ hypoglycemia. May mask clinical signs of hyperthyroidism and may precipitate thyroid storm w/ abrupt discontinuation. Avoid w/ untreated pheochromocytoma. May cause fetal harm. May aggravate peripheral arterial circulatory disorders.

ADVERSE REACTIONS
Tiredness, dizziness, cold extremities, depression, fatigue, dyspnea, postural hypotension, bradycardia, leg pain, lightheadedness, lethargy, diarrhea, nausea, wheeziness.

DRUG INTERACTIONS
Additive effects w/ catecholamine-depleting drugs (eg, reserpine), calcium channel blockers, and amiodarone. May cause severe bradycardia, asystole, and HF w/ disopyramide. Bradycardia and heart block can occur and left ventricular end diastolic pressure can rise w/ verapamil or diltiazem. Exacerbates rebound HTN w/ clonidine withdrawal; withdraw β-blocker therapy several days before gradual withdrawal of clonidine or delay introduction of β-blockers for several days after stopping clonidine. Prostaglandin synthase inhibitors (eg, indomethacin) may decrease hypotensive effects. May be unresponsive to usual doses of epinephrine. Concomitant use w/ digitalis glycosides may increase risk of bradycardia.

PREGNANCY AND LACTATION
Category D, caution in nursing.

MECHANISM OF ACTION
Cardioselective β-adrenoreceptor-blocking agent; not established. Suspected to competitively antagonize catecholamines at peripheral (especially cardiac) adrenergic neuron sites, leading to decreased cardiac output; a central effect leading to reduced sympathetic outflow to the periphery and suppression of renin activity.

PHARMACOKINETICS
Absorption: Rapid, incomplete; T_max=2-4 hrs. **Distribution:** Plasma protein binding (6-16%); found in breast milk; crosses the placenta. **Elimination:** Urine (approx 50%), feces (unchanged); T_1/2=approx 6-7 hrs.

PATIENT CONSIDERATIONS
Assessment: Assess for history of hypersensitivity, bradycardia, cardiogenic shock, >1st-degree heart block, overt cardiac failure, acute MI, renal dysfunction, bronchospastic disease, conduction abnormalities, left ventricular dysfunction, peripheral arterial circulatory disorders, diabetes mellitus, hyperthyroidism, pheochromocytoma, pregnancy/nursing status, and for possible drug interactions.

Monitoring: Monitor for signs/symptoms of cardiac failure, for masking of hyperthyroidism/hypoglycemia, and for other adverse reactions. Monitor renal function, pulse, and BP. Following abrupt discontinuation, monitor for thyroid storm and in patients w/ angina, monitor for severe exacerbation of angina, MI, and ventricular arrhythmias.

Counseling: Instruct to take as prescribed. Advise not to interrupt or d/c therapy w/o first consulting physician. Inform that drug may cause fetal harm; instruct to notify physician if pregnant or if considering becoming pregnant.

TERAZOL 3 — terconazole   Rx

Class: Azole antifungal

OTHER BRAND NAMES
Terazol 7

ADULT DOSAGE

Vaginal Candidiasis
Local Treatment:
Terazol 7:
1 full applicator (5g) intravaginally qhs for 7 consecutive days

Terazol 3 Cream:
1 full applicator (5g) intravaginally qhs for 3 consecutive days

Terazol 3 Suppositories:
1 suppository intravaginally qhs for 3 consecutive days

PEDIATRIC DOSAGE
Pediatric use may not have been established

ADMINISTRATION
Intravaginal route

STORAGE
15-30°C (59-86°F).

HOW SUPPLIED
Cre: (Terazol 7) 0.4% [45g], (Terazol 3) 0.8% [20g]; **Sup:** (Terazol 3) 80mg [3ˢ]

CONTRAINDICATIONS
Hypersensitivity to terconazole or to any of the components.

WARNINGS/PRECAUTIONS
Effective only for vulvovaginitis caused by the genus Candida; confirm diagnosis by potassium hydroxide (KOH) smears and/or cultures. Therapeutic effect is not affected by menstruation. Anaphylaxis and toxic epidermal necrolysis (TEN) reported; d/c if these reactions develop. D/C use and do not retreat if sensitization, irritation, fever, chills, or flu-like symptoms occur. Repeat microbiologic studies to confirm diagnosis and rule out other pathogens if there is lack of response. Base contained in suppository formulation may interact with certain rubber or latex products (eg, vaginal contraceptive diaphragms, latex condoms); concurrent use is not recommended. Do not use in the 1st trimester of pregnancy unless considered essential to the welfare of the patient; may be used during the 2nd and 3rd trimester if potential benefit outweighs the possible risks to the fetus.

ADVERSE REACTIONS
Headache. (0.8%, Cre) Dysmenorrhea, abdominal pain. (Sup) Genital burning, female genital pain, body pain.

PREGNANCY AND LACTATION
Category C, not for use in nursing.

MECHANISM OF ACTION
Azole antifungal; inhibits fungal CYP450-mediated 14 α-lanosterol demethylase enzyme which functions to convert lanosterol to ergosterol resulting in subsequent loss of ergosterol in the fungal cell wall and may be responsible for its antifungal activity.

PHARMACOKINETICS
Absorption: T_max=5-10 hrs. **Distribution:** Plasma protein binding (94.9%). **Metabolism:** Extensive. **Elimination:** (Sup) Urine (3-10%), feces (2-6%); T_1/2=6.4-8.5 hrs.

PATIENT CONSIDERATIONS
Assessment: Assess for hypersensitivity to drug or to any of its components, use of certain rubber or latex products, and pregnancy/nursing status. Confirm diagnosis by KOH smears and/or cultures.

Monitoring: Monitor for signs/symptoms of hypersensitivity reactions, anaphylaxis, TEN, sensitization, irritation, fever, chills, flu-like symptoms, and other adverse reactions. Monitor response to treatment; if there is lack of response, repeat standard KOH smear and/or cultures to confirm diagnosis and rule out other pathogens.

Counseling: Inform that therapeutic effect is not affected by menstruation. Instruct to use as prescribed, even if symptoms improve quickly. Advise to consult physician if anaphylaxis, TEN, sensitization, irritation, fever, chills, or flu-like symptoms occur. Advise to consult physician if partner has any penile itching, redness, or discomfort. Instruct to avoid scratching as more irritation and the spread of infection may occur. Advise to avoid douching unless instructed by physician. Instruct on how to use applicator. (Sup) Instruct not to use concurrently with rubber or latex products (eg, diaphragms, latex condoms).

TERAZOSIN — terazosin hydrochloride　　　Rx

Class: Alpha₁ blocker (quinazoline)

OTHER BRAND NAMES
Hytrin (Discontinued)

ADULT DOSAGE

Hypertension

Initial: 1mg hs
Usual: 1-5mg qd
If response is substantially diminished at 24 hrs, may slowly increase dose or use bid regimen
Max: 40mg/day

If discontinued for several days or longer, restart using the initial dosing regimen

Benign Prostatic Hyperplasia

Initial: 1mg hs
Titrate: Increase stepwise to 2mg, 5mg, or 10mg qd
Max: 20mg/day

If discontinued for several days or longer, restart using the initial dosing regimen

PEDIATRIC DOSAGE
Pediatric use may not have been established

ADMINISTRATION
Oral route

STORAGE
20-25°C (68-77°F).

HOW SUPPLIED
Cap: 1mg, 2mg, 5mg, 10mg

CONTRAINDICATIONS
Hypersensitivity to terazosin HCl.

WARNINGS/PRECAUTIONS
May cause marked lowering of BP, especially postural hypotension, and syncope with the 1st dose or 1st few days of therapy; similar effect may be anticipated if therapy is interrupted for several days and then restarted. May impair physical/mental abilities. Examine patients with BPH to rule out prostate cancer prior to initiation of therapy. Priapism reported. Intraoperative floppy iris syndrome observed during cataract surgery. Decreases in Hct, Hgb, WBCs, total protein, and albumin reported.

ADVERSE REACTIONS
Asthenia, postural hypotension, headache, dizziness, dyspnea, nasal congestion, somnolence, palpitations, nausea, peripheral edema, pain in extremities.

DRUG INTERACTIONS
Caution with other antihypertensive agents, especially verapamil; may need dose reduction or retitration of either agent. Increased levels with captopril. Hypotension reported with PDE-5 inhibitors.

PREGNANCY AND LACTATION
Category C, caution in nursing.

MECHANISM OF ACTION
Alpha₁-blocker; (BPH) relaxes smooth muscle in bladder neck and prostate; (HTN) decreases total peripheral vascular resistance, causing decreased BP.

PHARMACOKINETICS
Absorption: Complete; T_{max}=1 hr. **Distribution:** Plasma protein binding (90-94%). **Elimination:** Feces (60%), urine (40%); $T_{1/2}$=12 hrs, 14 hrs (≥70 yrs), 11.4 hrs (20-39 yrs).

PATIENT CONSIDERATIONS
Assessment: Assess BP, pregnancy/nursing status, and possible drug interactions. Rule out prostate cancer with BPH.

Monitoring: Monitor for signs/symptoms of hypotension, priapism, and other adverse reactions. Monitor Hct, Hgb, WBCs, total protein/albumin, and BP periodically.

Counseling: Inform of possibility of syncope and orthostatic symptoms, especially at initiation of therapy. Caution against driving or hazardous tasks for 12 hrs after 1st dose, dosage increase, or when resuming therapy after interruption. Avoid situations where injury could result, should syncope occur. Advise to sit or lie down when symptoms of low BP occur. Inform of possibility of priapism; advise to seek medical attention if this occurs and inform that priapism can lead to permanent erectile dysfunction if not brought to immediate medical attention.

TESTIM — testosterone　　　CIII

Class: Androgen

> Virilization reported in children secondarily exposed to testosterone gel. Children should avoid contact w/ unwashed or unclothed application sites in men using testosterone gel. Advise patients to strictly adhere to recommended instructions for use.

ADULT DOSAGE

Testosterone Replacement Therapy

Congenital/Acquired Primary Hypogonadism or Hypogonadotropic Hypogonadism in Males:

Initial: Apply 50mg (1 tube) qd
Measure am, predose serum testosterone levels approx 14 days after initiation of therapy
Titrate: May increase to 100mg (2 tubes) qd if serum testosterone levels are below normal range
Max: 100mg (2 tubes) qd

PEDIATRIC DOSAGE
Pediatric use may not have been established

ADMINISTRATION
Topical route

Apply qd at approx the same time (preferably in am) each day to clean, dry skin of the shoulders and/or upper arms; do not apply to scrotum, penis, or abdomen. Wash hands thoroughly w/ soap and water after application.
Avoid swimming, showering, or washing the administration site for a minimum of 2 hrs after application.
Refer to PI for further administration instructions.

STORAGE
20-25°C (68-77°F); excursions permitted to 15-30°C (59-86°F).

HOW SUPPLIED
Gel: 1% [5g, 30ˢ]

CONTRAINDICATIONS
Breast carcinoma or known/suspected prostate carcinoma in men; women who are or may become pregnant, and women who are breastfeeding.

WARNINGS/PRECAUTIONS
Topical testosterone products may have different doses, strengths, or application instructions that may result in different systemic exposure. Application site and dose are not interchangeable w/ other topical testosterone products. Patients w/ BPH are at an increased risk for worsening of signs/symptoms of BPH. May increase risk for prostate cancer. Increases in Hct/RBC mass may increase risk for thromboembolic events; may require lowering of dose or discontinuation of therapy. Venous thromboembolic events (VTE) reported; d/c treatment and initiate appropriate workup and management if VTE is suspected. Increased risk of major adverse cardiovascular events (MACE) reported. Suppression of spermatogenesis may occur w/ large doses. Prolonged use of high doses of orally active 17-α-alkyl androgens has been associated w/ serious hepatic effects; promptly d/c while cause is evaluated if signs/symptoms of hepatic dysfunction develop. Edema, w/ or w/o CHF may be a serious complication in patients w/ preexisting cardiac, renal, or hepatic disease; may require diuretic therapy in addition to discontinuation of therapy. Gynecomastia may develop and persist. May potentiate sleep apnea. Changes in serum lipid profile may occur. Caution in cancer patients at risk of hypercalcemia and associated hypercalciuria. May decrease concentrations of thyroxine-binding globulins, resulting in decreased total T4 concentrations and increased resin uptake of T3 and T4. Flammable; avoid fire, flame, or smoking until the gel has dried.

ADVERSE REACTIONS
Application-site reactions.

DRUG INTERACTIONS
Changes in insulin sensitivity or glycemic control may occur; may decrease blood glucose and therefore, may necessitate a decrease in the dose of antidiabetic medications. Changes in anticoagulant activity may occur; frequently monitor INR and PT in patients taking warfarin, especially at initiation and termination of androgen therapy. Corticosteroids may increase fluid retention; carefully monitor, especially in patients w/ cardiac, renal, or hepatic disease.

PREGNANCY AND LACTATION
Category X, not for use in nursing.

MECHANISM OF ACTION
Androgen; responsible for normal growth and development of male sex organs and maintenance of secondary sex characteristics.

PHARMACOKINETICS
Absorption: 10% absorbed systemically. **Distribution:** Plasma protein binding (98% [40% sex hormone-binding globulin]). **Metabolism:** Estradiol and dihydrotestosterone (major active metabolites). **Elimination:** (IM) Urine (90% glucuronic and sulfuric acid conjugates), feces (6% unconjugated); $T_{1/2}$=10-100 min

PATIENT CONSIDERATIONS
Assessment: Assess for breast carcinoma, prostate cancer, BPH, cardiac/renal/hepatic disease, risk factors for sleep apnea, and any other conditions where treatment is contraindicated or cautioned, and possible drug interactions. Obtain baseline Hct and lipid levels. Confirm diagnosis of hypogonadism by measuring testosterone levels in the am on at least 2 separate days prior to initiation.

Monitoring: Monitor for worsening of BPH, prostate cancer, edema w/ or w/o CHF, sleep apnea, VTE, MACE, gynecomastia, and other adverse reactions.

Monitor prostate specific antigen, serum lipid profile, and LFTs periodically. Monitor serum Ca^{2+} levels regularly in cancer patients at risk of hypercalcemia. Obtain Hct 3-6 months after starting therapy, then annually. Measure am, predose serum testosterone levels approx 14 days after initiation of therapy and periodically thereafter.

Counseling: Inform that men w/ known or suspected prostate/breast cancer should not use this therapy. Advise to report signs and symptoms of hepatic dysfunction and secondary exposure in children and women to physician. Inform about possible adverse reactions. Inform that children and women should avoid contact w/ unwashed or unclothed application sites of men. Instruct to apply ud and to wash hands w/ soap and water immediately after application, cover application site w/ clothing after gel dries, and wash application site thoroughly w/ soap and water prior to direct skin-to-skin contact w/ others. Inform that drug is flammable; instruct to avoid fire, flame, or smoking until the gel has dried. Advise not to share the medication w/ anyone. Advise about the importance of adhering to all the recommended monitoring, to report changes in state of health, and to wait 2 hrs before swimming or washing. Inform of the possible risk of MACE when deciding whether to use or continue to use drug.

TESTOPEL — testosterone   CIII

Class: Androgen

ADULT DOSAGE

Testosterone Replacement Therapy

Congenital/Acquired Primary Hypogonadism or Hypogonadotropic Hypogonadism in Males:
Usual: 150-450mg SQ every 3-6 months; implant two 75mg pellets for each 25mg testosterone propionate required weekly

Prior to initiating, confirm diagnosis by ensuring that serum testosterone concentrations have been measured in the morning on at least 2 separate days and that these concentrations are below the normal range.
Consider chronological and skeletal age in determining the initial dose and in adjusting the dose.

PEDIATRIC DOSAGE

Testosterone Replacement Therapy

Congenital/Acquired Primary Hypogonadism or Hypogonadotropic Hypogonadism in Males:
Usual: 150-450mg SQ every 3-6 months; implant two 75mg pellets for each 25mg testosterone propionate required weekly

Prior to initiating, confirm diagnosis by ensuring that serum testosterone concentrations have been measured in the morning on at least 2 separate days and that these concentrations are below the normal range.
Consider chronological and skeletal age in determining the initial dose and in adjusting the dose.

Delayed Puberty in Males

Usual: Lower range of 150-450mg for a limited duration (eg, 4-6 months)

Consider chronological and skeletal age in determining the initial dose and in adjusting the dose

---

ADMINISTRATION
SQ route

STORAGE
25°C (77°F); excursions permitted to 15-30°C (59-86°F).

HOW SUPPLIED
Pellet: 75mg

CONTRAINDICATIONS
Breast carcinoma or known/suspected prostate carcinoma in men, women who are or may become pregnant.

WARNINGS/PRECAUTIONS
May cause hypercalcemia by stimulating osteolysis in patients w/ breast cancer; d/c if this occurs. Prolonged use of high doses has been associated w/ the development of peliosis hepatitis and hepatic neoplasms (eg, hepatocellular carcinoma). May increase risk for the development of prostatic hypertrophy and prostatic carcinoma. Venous thromboembolic events (VTEs) (eg, deep vein thrombosis, pulmonary embolism) reported; d/c if a VTE is suspected. Increased risk of major adverse cardiovascular events (MACEs) reported w/ testosterone replacement therapy in men. Edema w/ or w/o CHF may be a serious complication in patients w/ preexisting cardiac, renal, or hepatic disease; may require diuretic therapy in addition to discontinuation of therapy. Gynecomastia may develop and persist. Caution in healthy males w/ delayed puberty; monitor bone maturation by assessing bone age of the wrist and hand every 6 months. May accelerate bone maturation w/o producing compensatory gain in linear growth in children; compromised adult stature may result. Implant site infection (cellulitis and abscess) and/or pellet extrusion at or near the implantation site may occur; infection and extrusion may occur concurrently or separately. Should not be used for enhancement of athletic performance. Caution when estimating amount of testosterone needed. In the face of complications where the effects of therapy should be discontinued, pellets should be removed. May decrease levels of thyroxine-binding globulins, resulting in decreased total T_4 serum levels and increased resin uptake of T_3 and T_4.

ADVERSE REACTIONS
Implantation site infection, pellet extrusion, gynecomastia, excessive frequency and duration of penile erections, hirsutism, male pattern of baldness, acne, myocardial infarction, stroke, nausea, cholestatic jaundice, increased or decreased libido, headache, anxiety, depression.

DRUG INTERACTIONS
May decrease oral anticoagulant requirements; close monitoring is required, especially when androgens are started or stopped. May increase oxyphenbutazone levels. May decrease blood glucose and insulin requirements in diabetic patients.

PREGNANCY AND LACTATION
Pregnancy: Category X.
Lactation: Not for use in nursing.

MECHANISM OF ACTION
Androgen; responsible for the normal growth and development of the male sex organs and for the maintenance of secondary sex characteristics.

PHARMACOKINETICS
Distribution: Plasma protein binding (98% bound to a specific testosterone-estradiol binding globulin). **Metabolism:** Liver. **Elimination:** Urine (90%, glucuronic and sulfuric acid conjugates), feces (6%, mostly unconjugated); $T_{1/2}$=10-100 min.

PATIENT CONSIDERATIONS

Assessment: Assess for breast carcinoma, prostate carcinoma, preexisting cardiac/renal/hepatic disease, or any other conditions where treatment is contraindicated or cautioned, and possible drug interactions. Confirm diagnosis of hypogonadism by measuring testosterone levels in am on at least 2 separate days prior to initiation.

Monitoring: Monitor for signs/symptoms of edema w/ or w/o CHF, prostatic hypertrophy, prostatic carcinoma, gynecomastia, implant site infection and/or pellet extrusion, VTEs, MACEs, and other adverse reactions. Monitor LFTs periodically. Perform periodic (every 6 months) x-ray exam of bone age during treatment of prepubertal males. Monitor Hgb and Hct periodically for polycythemia in patients receiving high doses of therapy.

Counseling: Instruct to report to physician any of the following side effects: too frequent or persistent erections of the penis, any N/V, changes in skin color, or ankle swelling. Inform that implantation site infection and/or pellet extrusion can occur and may be associated w/ implant site induration, inflammation, fibrosis, bleeding, bruising, wound drainage, pain, itching, and pellet extrusion. Inform that any male adolescent receiving therapy for delayed puberty should have bone development checked every 6 months.

TEVETEN — eprosartan mesylate   Rx

Class: Angiotensin II receptor blocker (ARB)

> **D/C when pregnancy is detected. Drugs that act directly on the renin-angiotensin system (RAS) can cause injury/death to the developing fetus.**

ADULT DOSAGE

Hypertension

Initial: 600mg qd
Usual: 400-800mg/day, given qd or bid
Max: 800mg/day
Twice-a-day regimen at the same total daily dose or an increase in dose may give a more satisfactory response

PEDIATRIC DOSAGE
Pediatric use may not have been established

DOSING CONSIDERATIONS
Renal Impairment
Moderate and Severe:
Max: 600mg/day

ADMINISTRATION
Oral route
Take w/ or w/o food.

STORAGE
20-25°C (68-77°F).

HOW SUPPLIED
Tab: 400mg, 600mg

CONTRAINDICATIONS
Hypersensitivity to this product or any of its components. Coadministration w/ aliskiren in patients w/ diabetes.

WARNINGS/PRECAUTIONS
Symptomatic hypotension may occur in patients w/ an activated RAS (eg, volume- and/or salt-depleted patients [eg, those being treated w/ diuretics]); correct volume or salt depletion prior to therapy or monitor closely. Changes in renal function reported. Oliguria and/or progressive azotemia and (rarely) acute renal failure and/or death may occur in patients whose renal function may depend on the renin-angiotensin-aldosterone system activity (eg, severe CHF). Increases in SrCr or BUN reported in patients w/ renal artery stenosis.

ADVERSE REACTIONS
Upper respiratory tract infection, rhinitis, pharyngitis, cough.

DRUG INTERACTIONS
See Contraindications. Dual blockade of the RAS is associated w/ increased risks of hypotension, hyperkalemia, and changes in renal function (including acute renal failure); avoid combined use of RAS inhibitors, or closely monitor BP, renal function, and electrolytes w/ concomitant agents that also affect the RAS. Avoid w/ aliskiren in patients w/ renal impairment (GFR <60mL/min). NSAIDs, including selective COX-2 inhibitors, may attenuate antihypertensive effect and may

deteriorate renal function. Increases in serum lithium concentrations and lithium toxicity may occur; monitor lithium levels.

PREGNANCY AND LACTATION
Pregnancy: Category D.
Lactation: Not for use in nursing.

MECHANISM OF ACTION
Angiotensin II receptor antagonist; blocks the vasoconstrictor and aldosterone-secreting effects of angiotensin II by selectively blocking the binding of angiotensin II to AT_1 receptor found in many tissues.

PHARMACOKINETICS
Absorption: Absolute bioavailability (13%) (single 300mg dose); T_{max}=1-2 hrs (fasted). **Distribution:** V_d=308L; plasma protein binding (98%). **Elimination:** Feces (90%), urine (7%; 80%, unchanged); (multiple doses of 600mg) $T_{1/2}$=20 hrs.

PATIENT CONSIDERATIONS
Assessment: Assess for hypersensitivity to the drug, volume/salt depletion, renal impairment, CHF, renal artery stenosis, diabetes, pregnancy/nursing status, and possible drug interactions.

Monitoring: Monitor for signs/symptoms of hypotension, renal dysfunction, and other adverse reactions.

Counseling: Inform about the consequences of exposure during pregnancy in females of childbearing age. Discuss treatment options w/ women planning to become pregnant. Instruct to report pregnancies to physician as soon as possible.

TEVETEN HCT — eprosartan mesylate/hydrochlorothiazide   Rx
Class: Angiotensin II receptor blocker (ARB)/thiazide diuretic

> D/C when pregnancy is detected. Drugs that act directly on the renin-angiotensin system (RAS) can cause injury/death to the developing fetus.

ADULT DOSAGE	PEDIATRIC DOSAGE
Hypertension	Pediatric use may not have been established
Replacement Therapy: May be substituted for individual components	
Usual (Not Volume-Depleted): 600mg/12.5mg qd	
Titrate: May increase to 600mg/25mg qd	
Max: 600mg/25mg qd	
If additional BP control required, or to maintain a bid dosing schedule of monotherapy, 300mg eprosartan may be added as pm dose	

DOSING CONSIDERATIONS
Renal Impairment
Moderate and Severe:
Max Eprosartan: 600mg/day

ADMINISTRATION
Oral route
Take w/ or w/o food

STORAGE
20-25°C (68-77°F).

HOW SUPPLIED
Tab: (Eprosartan-HCTZ) 600mg/12.5mg, 600mg/25mg

CONTRAINDICATIONS
Hypersensitivity to Teveten HCT, any of its components, or to other sulfonamide-derived drugs; patients w/ anuria. Coadministration w/ aliskiren in patients w/ diabetes.

WARNINGS/PRECAUTIONS
Not indicated for initial therapy. Symptomatic hypotension may occur in patients with an activated RAS (eg, volume- and/or salt-depleted patients [eg, those being treated with diuretics]); correct volume or salt depletion prior to therapy or monitor closely. Changes in renal function reported. Oliguria and/or progressive azotemia and (rare) acute renal failure and/or death may occur in patients whose renal function may depend on the renin-angiotensin-aldosterone system activity (eg, severe CHF). Increases in SrCr or BUN reported in patients with renal artery stenosis. Consider withholding or discontinuing therapy if progressive renal impairment becomes evident. HCTZ: Caution with severe renal disease; may precipitate azotemia. Caution with hepatic impairment or progressive liver disease; may precipitate hepatic coma. May cause hypersensitivity reactions (with or without a history of allergy or bronchial asthma), exacerbation or activation of systemic lupus erythematosus (SLE), hyperuricemia or precipitation of frank gout, hypomagnesemia, hypercalcemia, hyperglycemia, and manifestations of latent diabetes mellitus (DM). May cause idiosyncratic reaction, resulting in acute transient myopia and acute angle-closure glaucoma; d/c as rapidly as possible. D/C before testing for parathyroid function. Enhanced effects in postsympathectomy patients. Observe for signs of fluid/electrolyte imbalance (eg, hyponatremia, hypochloremic alkalosis, hypokalemia). Hypokalemia may sensitize/exaggerate the response of the heart to toxic effects of digitalis.

ADVERSE REACTIONS
Dizziness, headache.

DRUG INTERACTIONS
See Contraindications. Dual blockade of the RAS is associated with increased risks of hypotension, hyperkalemia, and changes in renal function (including acute renal failure); avoid combined use of RAS inhibitors, or closely monitor BP, renal function, and electrolytes with concomitant agents that also affect the RAS. Avoid with aliskiren in patients with renal impairment (GFR <60mL/min). NSAIDs, including selective COX-2 inhibitors, may decrease effects of diuretics and angiotensin II receptor antagonists and may deteriorate renal function. Increases in serum lithium concentrations and lithium toxicity reported; monitor lithium levels. Eprosartan: K⁺-sparing diuretics (eg, spironolactone, triamterene, amiloride), K⁺ supplements, or K⁺-containing salt substitutes may increase serum K⁺. HCTZ: Potentiation of orthostatic hypotension may occur with alcohol, barbiturates, or narcotics. Dose adjustment of antidiabetic drugs (oral agents and insulin) may be required. Additive effect or potentiation with other antihypertensives. Anionic exchange resins (eg, cholestyramine, colestipol) may impair absorption. Corticosteroids and adrenocorticotropic hormone may intensify electrolyte depletion, particularly hypokalemia. May decrease response to pressor amines (eg, norepinephrine). May increase responsiveness to nondepolarizing skeletal muscle relaxants (eg, tubocurarine).

PREGNANCY AND LACTATION
Category D, not for use in nursing.

MECHANISM OF ACTION
Eprosartan: Angiotensin II receptor antagonist; blocks the vasoconstrictor and aldosterone-secreting effects of angiotensin II by selectively blocking the binding of angiotensin II to AT_1 receptor found in many tissues. HCTZ: Thiazide diuretic; has not been established. Affects the renal tubular mechanisms of electrolyte reabsorption, directly increasing excretion of Na⁺ and Cl⁻ in approximately equivalent amounts.

PHARMACOKINETICS
Absorption: Eprosartan: Absolute bioavailability (13%) (single 300mg dose); T_{max}=1-2 hrs (fasted). **Distribution:** Eprosartan: V_d=308L; plasma protein binding (98%). HCTZ: Crosses placenta; found in breast milk. **Elimination:** Eprosartan: Feces (90%), urine (7%; 80%, unchanged); (multiple doses of 600mg) $T_{1/2}$=20 hrs. HCTZ: Kidney (≥61% unchanged); $T_{1/2}$=5.6-14.8 hrs.

PATIENT CONSIDERATIONS
Assessment: Assess for hypersensitivity to the drug or sulfonamide-derived drugs, anuria, volume/salt depletion, CHF, renal artery stenosis, SLE, DM, postsympathectomy status, renal/hepatic impairment, pregnancy/nursing status, and possible drug interactions.

Monitoring: Monitor for signs/symptoms of hypotension, renal/hepatic impairment, hypersensitivity reactions, exacerbation/activation of SLE, hyperuricemia, precipitation of gout, fluid/electrolyte imbalance, latent DM, idiosyncratic reaction, and other adverse reactions. Monitor BP and serum electrolytes periodically.

Counseling: Inform about the consequences of exposure during pregnancy in females of childbearing age. Discuss treatment options with women planning to become pregnant. Instruct to report pregnancies to physician as soon as possible. Caution that lightheadedness may occur, especially during the 1st days of therapy; instruct to report to physician. Instruct to d/c therapy and consult physician if syncope occurs. Caution that inadequate fluid intake, excessive perspiration, diarrhea, or vomiting may lead to an excessive fall in BP, with the same consequences of lightheadedness and possible syncope. Instruct not to use K⁺ supplements or salt substitutes containing K⁺ without consulting physician.

THEO-24 — theophylline anhydrous   Rx
Class: Xanthine bronchodilator

ADULT DOSAGE	PEDIATRIC DOSAGE
Chronic Lung Disease	**Chronic Lung Disease**
Symptoms and Reversible Airflow Obstruction Associated w/ Chronic Asthma and Other Chronic Lung Diseases:	**Symptoms and Reversible Airflow Obstruction Associated w/ Chronic Asthma and Other Chronic Lung Diseases:**
Individualize dose based on peak serum levels	Individualize dose based on peak serum levels and ideal body weight
16-60 Years:	**12-15 Years:**
Initial: 300-400mg/day divided q24h	**<45kg:**
Titrate: After 3 days, increase to 400-600mg/day if tolerated; consider giving a lower dose and titrating more slowly if caffeine-like adverse effects occur.	**Initial:** 12-14mg/kg/day up to a max of 300mg/day divided q24h
After 3 more days, if needed and tolerated, may increase to >600mg/day.	**Titrate:** After 3 days, increase to 16mg/kg/day up to a max of 400mg/day divided q24h.
	After 3 more days, if tolerated and needed, may increase to 20mg/kg/day up to a max of 600mg/day.
	>45kg:
	Initial: 300-400mg/day divided q24h
	Titrate: After 3 days, increase to 400-600mg/day if tolerated; consider giving a lower dose and titrating more slowly if caffeine-like adverse effects occur.
	After 3 more days, if needed and tolerated, may increase to >600mg/day.

DOSING CONSIDERATIONS

Elderly
>60 Years:
Max: 400mg/day

Other Important Considerations
Rapid Metabolizers:
Give smaller dose more frequently to prevent breakthrough symptoms

Risk Factors for Impaired Clearance/If Not Feasible to Monitor Serum Theophylline Concentrations:
12-15 Years:
Max: 16mg/kg/day up to a max of 400 mg/day
≥16 Years:
Max: 400mg/day

Dose Adjustments Based on Peak Serum Concentration:
<9.9mcg/mL: If symptoms are not controlled and current dosage is tolerated, increase dose about 25%; recheck serum concentration after 3 days for further dosage adjustment
10-14.9mcg/mL: If symptoms are controlled and current dosage is tolerated, maintain dose and recheck serum concentration at 6- to 12-month intervals. If symptoms are not controlled and current dosage is tolerated, consider adding additional medication(s) to treatment regimen.
15-19.9mcg/mL: Consider 10% decrease in dose to provide greater margin of safety even if current dosage is tolerated
20-24.9mcg/mL: Decrease dose by 25% even if no adverse effects are present; recheck serum concentration after 3 days to guide further dosage adjustment
25-30mcg/mL: Skip next dose and decrease subsequent doses at least 25% even if no adverse effects present; recheck serum concentration after 3 days to guide further dosage adjustment.
If symptomatic, consider whether overdose treatment is indicated (see PI).
>30mcg/mL: Treat overdose as indicated (see PI); if therapy is subsequently resumed, decrease dose by at least 50% and recheck serum concentration after 3 days to guide further dosage adjustment

ADMINISTRATION
Oral route

Take dose at approx the same time each am.
For twice daily dosing, 2nd dose should be taken 10-12 hours after the morning dose and before the pm meal.

STORAGE
Below 25°C (77°F).

HOW SUPPLIED
Cap, Extended-Release: 100mg, 200mg, 300mg, 400mg

CONTRAINDICATIONS
History of hypersensitivity to theophylline or other components in the product.

WARNINGS/PRECAUTIONS
Extreme caution w/ active peptic ulcer disease (PUD), seizure disorders, and cardiac arrhythmias (not including bradyarrhythmias); increased risk of exacerbation of the concurrent condition. Caution w/ risk factors for reduced clearance (eg, neonates [term/premature], children <1 yr of age, elderly [>60 yrs of age], acute pulmonary edema, CHF, cor pulmonale, fever [≥102°F for 24 hrs or more, lesser temperature elevations for longer periods], hypothyroidism, liver disease [eg, cirrhosis, acute hepatitis], reduced renal function in infants <3 months of age, sepsis w/ multiorgan failure, shock, cessation of smoking); severe and potentially fatal toxicity can occur if total daily dose is not appropriately reduced. Carefully consider benefits and risks of therapy and the need for more intensive monitoring of serum drug levels. Whenever N/V (particularly repetitive N/V) or other signs/symptoms of toxicity develop (even if another cause may be suspected), withhold additional doses and measure serum levels immediately. Avoid dose increases in response to acute exacerbation of symptoms of chronic lung disease. Measure peak steady-state serum theophylline concentration before increasing the dose and limit dose increases to about 25% of the previous total daily dose to reduce risk of unintended excessive increases in serum levels. Lab test interactions may occur. Caution in elderly and with selection of maintenance dose in pediatric patients.

ADVERSE REACTIONS
N/V, headache, insomnia, diarrhea, irritability, restlessness, fine skeletal muscle tremors, transient diuresis.

DRUG INTERACTIONS
Adding a drug that inhibits metabolism (eg, cimetidine, erythromycin, tacrine) or stopping a concurrently administered drug that enhances metabolism (eg, carbamazepine, rifampin) may reduce clearance. Blocks adenosine receptors; higher dose of adenosine may be required to achieve desired effect. Benzodiazepines increase CNS concentrations of adenosine; larger doses of benzodiazepines may be required to produce desired level of sedation. Alcohol, allopurinol, cimetidine, ciprofloxacin, clarithromycin, disulfiram, enoxacin, erythromycin, estrogen, fluvoxamine, human recombinant interferon α-A, methotrexate, mexiletine, pentoxifylline, propafenone, propranolol, tacrine, thiabendazole, ticlopidine, troleandomycin, and verapamil may decrease clearance and increase effect. Aminoglutethimide, carbamazepine, IV isoproterenol, moricizine, phenobarbital (after 2 weeks of concurrent phenobarbital use), phenytoin, rifampin, and sulfinpyrazone may increase clearance and decrease effect. May decrease phenytoin concentration. Increased risk of ventricular arrhythmias w/ halothane. Ketamine may lower theophylline seizure threshold. May increase renal lithium clearance. May antagonize nondepolarizing neuromuscular blocking effects of pancuronium; larger doses of pancuronium may be required. Synergistic CNS effects w/ ephedrine; increased frequency of nausea, nervousness and insomnia. St. John's wort may decrease plasma levels; higher doses of theophylline may be required. Discontinuing St. John's wort may result in theophylline toxicity.

PREGNANCY AND LACTATION
Pregnancy: Category C.
Lactation: Caution in nursing.

MECHANISM OF ACTION
Methylxanthine; not established. Acts via smooth muscle relaxation and suppression of airway response to stimuli. Bronchodilatation suggested to be mediated by inhibition of 2 isozymes of PDE while non-bronchodilator prophylactic actions are probably mediated through one or more different molecular mechanisms that do not involve inhibition of PDE-3 or antagonism of adenosine receptors. Also increases the force of contraction of diaphragmatic muscles due to enhancement of Ca^{2+} uptake through an adenosine-mediated channel.

PHARMACOKINETICS
Absorption: Rapid, complete (oral sol, immediate-release); C_{max}=18.1mcg/mL. **Distribution:** V_d=0.45L/kg; plasma protein binding (40%); crosses placenta; found in breast milk. **Metabolism:** Liver (extensive); demethylation via CYP1A2, and hydroxylation via CYP2E1, 3A3; caffeine and 3-methylxanthine (active metabolites). **Elimination:** Urine (10% unchanged, >3 months of age), (50% unchanged, neonates), (35-40% 1,3-dimethyluric acid, 20-25% 1-methyluric acid, 15-20% 3-methylxanthine). Refer to PI for $T_{1/2}$.

PATIENT CONSIDERATIONS
Assessment: Assess for hypersensitivity to drug, active PUD, seizure disorders, cardiac arrhythmias, conditions that alter theophylline clearance, any condition where treatment is contraindicated or cautioned, pregnancy/nursing status, and possible drug interactions. Obtain baseline serum levels when initiating therapy to guide final dosage adjustment after titration.

Monitoring: Measure serum levels before a dose increase in patients who continue to be symptomatic, whenever signs/symptoms of toxicity are present, and whenever there is a new illness, worsening of a chronic illness, or a change in treatment regimen that may alter clearance. Monitor serum levels at 6-month intervals for rapidly growing children and at yearly intervals for all others; acutely ill patients should be monitored at frequent intervals (eg, q24h). Monitor for signs/symptoms of toxicity, exacerbation of active PUD, seizure disorders or cardiac arrhythmias, and other adverse reactions.

Counseling: Instruct to seek medical attention if N/V, persistent headache, insomnia, or rapid heartbeat occurs. Instruct to contact physician if new illness (especially if accompanied by a persistent fever) develops, if a chronic illness worsens, if patient starts/stops smoking cigarettes or marijuana, or if another physician adds a new medication or discontinues a previously prescribed medication. Inform that theophylline interacts w/ a wide variety of drugs. Instruct to inform all physicians of theophylline use, especially if a medication is being added or removed from treatment. Instruct not to alter dose, timing of dose, or frequency of administration w/o 1st consulting physician; if a dose is missed, instruct to take next dose at the usually scheduled time and to not attempt to make up for the missed dose. Instruct to take medication each am at approximately the same time and not to exceed the prescribed dose. Instruct to d/c any dosage that causes adverse effects, to withhold subsequent doses until symptoms have resolved, and to then resume therapy at a lower, previously tolerated dose.

THIOTHIXENE — thiothixene   Rx
Class: Thioxanthene

> Elderly patients w/ dementia-related psychosis treated w/ antipsychotic drugs are at an increased risk of death; most deaths appeared to be cardiovascular (CV) (eg, heart failure, sudden death) or infectious (eg, pneumonia) in nature. Not approved for the treatment of patients w/ dementia-related psychosis.

OTHER BRAND NAMES
Navane (Discontinued)

ADULT DOSAGE	PEDIATRIC DOSAGE
Schizophrenia	**Schizophrenia**
Mild Condition:	**>12 Years:**
Initial: 2mg tid	**Mild Condition:**
Titrate: May increase to 15mg/day	**Initial:** 2mg tid
	Titrate: May increase to 15mg/day
Severe Condition:	
Initial: 5mg bid	**Severe Condition:**
Usual: 20-30mg/day	**Initial:** 5mg bid
Max: 60mg/day	**Usual:** 20-30mg/day
	Max: 60mg/day

ADMINISTRATION
Oral route

STORAGE
20-25°C (68-77°F). Protect from light.

HOW SUPPLIED
Cap: 1mg, 2mg, 5mg, 10mg

CONTRAINDICATIONS
Circulatory collapse, comatose states, CNS depression, blood dyscrasias, hypersensitivity to thiothixene.

WARNINGS/PRECAUTIONS
Tardive dyskinesia (TD) may develop, especially in the elderly; consider discontinuation if signs/symptoms develop. Neuroleptic malignant syndrome (NMS) reported; d/c and instill intensive symptomatic treatment and monitoring.

May impair mental/physical abilities. May mask signs of overdosage of toxic drugs and obscure conditions, such as intestinal obstruction and brain tumor. Extreme caution w/ history of convulsive disorders or in a state of alcohol withdrawal; may lower convulsive threshold. Caution w/ CV disease and in patients who might be exposed to extreme heat. Liver damage reported w/ related drugs. Pigmentary retinopathy and lenticular pigmentation noted w/ prolonged therapy. May elevate prolactin levels; galactorrhea, amenorrhea, gynecomastia, and impotence reported. Leukopenia, neutropenia, and agranulocytosis reported. In patients w/ a history of a clinically significant low WBC or drug induced leukopenia/neutropenia, frequently monitor CBC during the 1st few months of therapy and consider discontinuation at 1st sign of a clinically significant decline in WBC counts in the absence of other causative factors. D/C if severe neutropenia (ANC <1000/mm³) develops.

ADVERSE REACTIONS
Tachycardia, hypotension, lightheadedness, syncope, drowsiness, restlessness, agitation, insomnia, extrapyramidal symptoms, dystonia, cerebral edema, CSF abnormalities, allergic reactions, hematologic effects, dry mouth.

DRUG INTERACTIONS
Possible additive effects w/ hypotensive agents and alcohol. Possible additive effects w/ other CNS depressants; caution and careful adjustment of the dosages is indicated. Increased clearance w/ hepatic microsomal enzyme inducers (eg, carbamazepine); observe closely for signs of reduced thiothixene effectiveness. Potentiates the actions of barbiturates; do not reduce anticonvulsant dose when administered concurrently. Caution w/ atropine or related drugs. If hypotension occurs, do not use epinephrine as a pressor agent, since a paradoxical further lowering of BP may result.

PREGNANCY AND LACTATION
Safety is not known in pregnancy and nursing.

MECHANISM OF ACTION
Thioxanthene derivative; antipsychotic agent.

PATIENT CONSIDERATIONS
Assessment: Assess for history of convulsive disorders, state of alcohol withdrawal, circulatory collapse, comatose state, CNS depression, CV disease, previous hypersensitivity to the drug, any other conditions where treatment is contraindicated or cautioned, pregnancy/nursing status, and possible drug interactions. Obtain baseline CBC.

Monitoring: Monitor for signs/symptoms of TD, NMS, hyperprolactinemia, pigmentary retinopathy, lenticular pigmentation, and other adverse reactions. Monitor CBC.

Counseling: Inform about the risks of treatment, particularly about the possibility of developing TD. Instruct to use caution when performing hazardous tasks (operating machinery/driving). Advise about possible additive effects (eg, hypotension) when drug is combined w/ hypotensive agents, CNS depressants, and/or alcohol.

Tiazac — diltiazem hydrochloride   Rx

Class: Calcium channel blocker (CCB) (nondihydropyridine)

OTHER BRAND NAMES
Taztia XT

ADULT DOSAGE

Hypertension

Initial (Monotherapy): 120-240mg qd
Titrate: Max effect usually observed by 14 days of therapy; schedule dose adjustments accordingly
Usual Range: 120-540mg qd
Max: 540mg qd

Angina

Chronic Stable:
Initial: 120-180mg qd
Titration should be carried out over 7-14 days, when necessary
Max: 540mg qd

Conversions

Hypertensive/Anginal Patients Treated w/ Other Diltiazem Formulations:
May be switched to therapy at the nearest equivalent total daily dose

PEDIATRIC DOSAGE
Pediatric use may not have been established

DOSING CONSIDERATIONS
Elderly
Start at lower end of dosing range

ADMINISTRATION
Oral route
May sprinkle cap contents on a spoonful of applesauce.
Swallow applesauce immediately w/o chewing and follow w/ a glass of cool water; do not store for future use.
Subdividing contents of cap is not recommended.

STORAGE
25°C (77°F); excursions permitted to 15-30°C (59-86°F). Avoid excessive humidity. (Taztia XT) 20-25°C (68-77°F). Avoid excessive humidity.

HOW SUPPLIED
Cap, Extended-Release: 120mg, 180mg, 240mg, 300mg, 360mg, 420mg; (Taztia XT) 120mg, 180mg, 240mg, 300mg, 360mg

CONTRAINDICATIONS
Sick sinus syndrome and 2nd- or 3rd-degree atrioventricular (AV) block (except w/ a functioning ventricular pacemaker), severe hypotension (<90mmHg systolic), hypersensitivity to the drug, acute myocardial infarction (AMI) and pulmonary congestion documented by x-ray on admission.

WARNINGS/PRECAUTIONS
Prolongs AV node refractory periods without significantly prolonging sinus node recovery time, except in patients with sick sinus syndrome. Periods of asystole reported in a patient with Prinzmetal's angina. Worsening of CHF reported in patients with preexisting ventricular dysfunction. Symptomatic hypotension may occur. Mild elevations of transaminases with and without concomitant alkaline phosphatase and bilirubin elevation reported. Significant elevations in enzymes (eg, alkaline phosphatase, LDH, AST, ALT) and other phenomena consistent with acute hepatic injury reported in rare instances. Monitor LFTs and renal function at regular intervals; caution with renal/hepatic dysfunction. Transient dermatological reactions and skin eruptions progressing to erythema multiforme and/or exfoliative dermatitis have been reported; d/c if a dermatologic reaction persists. Caution in elderly.

ADVERSE REACTIONS
Peripheral edema, dizziness, headache, infection, pain, pharyngitis, dyspepsia, dyspnea, bronchitis, AV block, asthenia, vasodilation.

DRUG INTERACTIONS
Potential additive effects with other agents known to affect cardiac contractility and/or conduction; caution and careful titration are warranted. Additive effects in prolonging cardiac conduction with β-blockers or digitalis. CYP3A4 substrates, inhibitors, or inducers may have a significant impact on the efficacy and side effect profile of diltiazem; patients taking CYP3A4 substrates, especially patients with renal and/or hepatic impairment, may require dosage adjustment when starting or stopping concomitantly administered diltiazem. May potentiate depression of cardiac contractility, conductivity and automaticity, and vascular dilation associated with anesthetics; carefully titrate anesthetics and calcium channel blockers (CCBs) when used concomitantly. May increase levels of midazolam, triazolam, carbamazepine, quinidine, and lovastatin. May increase levels of propranolol; adjustment of the propranolol dose may be warranted. May increase levels of buspirone; dose adjustments may be necessary. Increased levels with cimetidine; adjustment of diltiazem dose may be warranted. Sinus bradycardia resulting in hospitalization and pacemaker insertion reported with clonidine; monitor HR. Monitor cyclosporine/digoxin concentrations, especially when diltiazem therapy is initiated, adjusted, or discontinued. Rifampin may decrease concentrations; avoid rifampin or any CYP3A4 inducer when possible, and consider alternative therapy. May increase simvastatin exposure; limit daily doses of simvastatin to 10mg and diltiazem to 240mg if coadministration is required. Risk of myopathy and rhabdomyolysis with statins metabolized by CYP3A4 may be increased. When possible, use a non-CYP3A4-metabolized statin; otherwise, consider dose adjustments for both agents and closely monitor for signs and symptoms of any statin-related adverse events. Additive antihypertensive effect when used with other antihypertensive agents; dosage of diltiazem or the concomitant antihypertensive may need to be adjusted.

PREGNANCY AND LACTATION
Pregnancy: Category C.
Lactation: Not for use in nursing.

MECHANISM OF ACTION
CCB; inhibits cellular influx of Ca^{2+} during membrane depolarization of cardiac and vascular smooth muscle. HTN: Relaxes vascular smooth muscle, resulting in decreased peripheral vascular resistance. Angina: Produces increases in exercise tolerance, probably due to its ability to reduce myocardial oxygen demand; accomplished via reductions in HR and systemic BP at submaximal and maximal workloads.

PHARMACOKINETICS
Absorption: Well-absorbed from GI tract. (Immediate-Release) Absolute bioavailability (40%). **Distribution:** Plasma protein binding (70-80%); found in breast milk. **Metabolism:** Liver (extensive; substantial 1st-pass effect); desacetyldiltiazem (active), desmethyldiltiazem (primary metabolites). **Elimination:** Urine (2-4%, unchanged), bile; $T_{1/2}$=6.5 hrs.

PATIENT CONSIDERATIONS
Assessment: Assess for sick sinus syndrome, 2nd- or 3rd-degree AV block, hypotension, AMI, pulmonary congestion, ventricular/renal/hepatic dysfunction, drug hypersensitivity, pregnancy/nursing status, and possible drug interactions.

Monitoring: Monitor for bradycardia, AV block, worsening of CHF, symptomatic hypotension, dermatological reactions, and other adverse reactions. Monitor LFTs and renal function at regular intervals. Monitor HR with clonidine.

Counseling: Inform of risks and benefits of therapy. Instruct to take ud. Counsel to report any adverse reactions to physician. Inform that when administering with applesauce, it should not be hot and it should be soft enough to be swallowed without chewing.

TIGAN — trimethobenzamide hydrochloride Rx

Class: Emetic response modifier

ADULT DOSAGE

Nausea/Vomiting

Postoperative N/V and Nausea Associated w/ Gastroenteritis:
Adjust according to indication, severity of symptoms, and response of patient
Usual:
Cap:
300mg tid-qid
Inj:
200mg IM tid-qid

PEDIATRIC DOSAGE
Pediatric use may not have been established

DOSING CONSIDERATIONS

Renal Impairment
CrCl ≤70mL/min: Consider reducing total dose administered at each dosing or increasing dosing interval

Elderly
Start at lower end of dosing range

ADMINISTRATION
Oral/IM route

IM administration can be a deep inj into the upper quadrant of the gluteal region. Avoid the escape of sol along the route to prevent inj-related adverse effects.

STORAGE
25°C (77°F); excursions permitted to 15-30°C (59-86°F).

HOW SUPPLIED
Cap: 300mg; **Inj:** 100mg/mL

CONTRAINDICATIONS
Known hypersensitivity to trimethobenzamide. **(Inj)** Pediatric patients.

WARNINGS/PRECAUTIONS
May impair physical/mental abilities. Caution with acute febrile illness, encephalitides, gastroenteritis, dehydration, electrolyte imbalance, especially in children/elderly/debilitated; CNS reactions reported. Caution in the elderly and patients with renal impairment. May obscure diagnosis of appendicitis and signs of toxicity due to overdosage of other drugs. **(Cap)** Caution in children; may cause extrapyramidal symptoms (EPS), which may be confused with CNS signs of undiagnosed primary disease (eg, Reye's syndrome, other encephalopathy) and may unfavorably alter the course of Reye's syndrome due to hepatotoxic potential. Not recommended for uncomplicated vomiting in children.

ADVERSE REACTIONS
Parkinsonian-like symptoms, blood dyscrasias, blurred vision, coma, convulsions, mood depression, diarrhea, disorientation, dizziness, drowsiness, headache, jaundice, muscle cramps, opisthotonos.

DRUG INTERACTIONS
Caution w/ CNS-acting agents (phenothiazines, barbiturates, belladonna derivatives) in acute febrile illness, encephalitides, gastroenteritis, dehydration, and electrolyte imbalance due to potential CNS reactions. Adverse drug interaction reported w/ alcohol.

PREGNANCY AND LACTATION
Pregnancy: Safety in pregnancy not known.
Lactation: Safety in nursing not known.

MECHANISM OF ACTION
Not established; thought to involve chemoreceptor trigger zone, through which emetic impulses are conveyed to vomiting center (direct impulses to vomiting center apparently not similarly inhibited).

PHARMACOKINETICS
Absorption: T_{max}=30 min (IM 200mg), 45 min (cap 300mg). **Metabolism:** (Cap) Oxidation, trimethobenzamide N-oxide (major metabolite). **Elimination:** Urine (30-50%, unchanged); $T_{1/2}$=7-9 hrs.

PATIENT CONSIDERATIONS
Assessment: Assess for renal/hepatic impairment, Reye's syndrome in children, alcohol intake, acute febrile illness, encephalitides, gastroenteritis, dehydration, electrolyte imbalance, appendicitis, previous hypersensitivity to the drug, possible drug interactions, and any other conditions where treatment is contraindicated or cautioned.

Monitoring: Monitor renal function and for signs of hepatotoxicity, CNS reactions (eg, opisthotonos, convulsions, coma), EPS, hydration status, and electrolytes.

Counseling: Advise that may cause drowsiness; caution against performing hazardous tasks (operating machinery/driving). Advise patients to not consume alcohol due to a potential drug interaction.

TIKOSYN — dofetilide Rx

Class: Class III antiarrhythmic

> To minimize risk of induced arrhythmia, for a minimum of 3 days, place patients initiated or reinitiated on therapy in a facility that can provide calculations of CrCl, continuous ECG monitoring, and cardiac resuscitation.

ADULT DOSAGE

Atrial Fibrillation

Conversion of A-Fib/A-Flutter to Normal Sinus Rhythm and Maint of Normal Sinus Rhythm in Patients w/ Highly Symptomatic A-Fib/A-Flutter of >1 Week Duration Who Were Converted to Normal Sinus Rhythm:
Reserve for patients in whom A-fib/A-flutter is highly symptomatic. Hypokalemia should be corrected before initiation; maintain serum K⁺ levels >3.6-4.0mEq/L.

Initial:
Individualize dose based on CrCl and QTc (use QT interval if HR <60bpm); QTc must be ≤440 msec to proceed
CrCl >60mL/min: 500mcg bid
CrCl 40-60mL/min: 250mcg bid
CrCl 20 to <40mL/min: 125mcg bid
CrCl <20mL/min: Contraindicated

Post Dose Adjustment:
After 2-3 hrs if the QTc has increased ≤15%, continue current dose; if QTc has increased >15% compared to the baseline or if the QTc is >500 msec (550 msec w/ ventricular conduction abnormalities), adjust subsequent doses as such:
Initial Dose of 500mcg bid: Reduce dose to 250mcg bid
Initial Dose of 250mcg bid: Reduce dose to 125mcg bid
Initial Dose of 125mcg bid: Reduce dose to 125mcg qd

Maint:
If at any time after the 2nd dose the QTc increases >500 msec (550 msec in patients w/ ventricular conduction abnormalities), d/c dofetilide

If renal function deteriorates, adjust dose based on CrCl as seen above

Max:
CrCl >60mL/min: 500mcg bid

Cardioversion:
If patients do not convert to normal sinus rhythm w/in 24 hrs of initiation, electrical conversion should be considered. Patients continuing on dofetilide after successful electrical cardioversion should continue to be monitored by ECG for 12 hrs post cardioversion, or a minimum of 3 days after initiation of dofetilide therapy, whichever is greater

Conversions

Switching from Class I or Other Class III Antiarrhythmics:
Withdraw previous antiarrhythmic therapy under careful monitoring for a minimum of 3 plasma half-lives before initiating therapy; do not initiate dofetilide following amiodarone therapy until amiodarone plasma levels are <0.3mcg/mL or until withdrawn for at least 3 months

DOSING CONSIDERATIONS

Discontinuation
If dofetilide needs to be discontinued to allow dosing of other potentially interacting drugs, a washout period of ≥2 days should be followed before starting the other drug

ADMINISTRATION
Oral route

Take PO w/ or w/o food.
Initiate/titrate in presence of continuous ECG monitoring and personnel trained in management of serious ventricular arrhythmias.

STORAGE
15-30°C (59-86°F). Protect from humidity and moisture.

HOW SUPPLIED
Cap: 125mcg, 250mcg, 500mcg

CONTRAINDICATIONS
Congenital or acquired long QT syndromes, baseline QT interval or QTc >440 msec (500 msec w/ ventricular conduction abnormalities), severe renal impairment (CrCl <20mL/min), known hypersensitivity to the drug. Concomitant

PEDIATRIC DOSAGE
Pediatric use may not have been established

verapamil, HCTZ (alone/in combinations [eg, triamterene]), and inhibitors of renal cation transport system (eg, cimetidine, trimethoprim [alone/combination w/ sulfamethoxazole], ketoconazole, prochlorperazine, dolutegravir, megestrol).

WARNINGS/PRECAUTIONS

May cause serious ventricular arrhythmias, primarily torsades de pointes (TdP); risk of TdP can be reduced by controlling the plasma concentration through adjustment of the initial dofetilide dose according to CrCl and by monitoring the ECG. Calculate CrCl before 1st dose. Caution in patients w/ severe hepatic impairment. Do not discharge patients w/in 12 hrs of conversion to normal sinus rhythm. Maintain normal K^+ levels prior to and during administration. Patients w/ A-fib should be anticoagulated prior to cardioversion and may continue to use after cardioversion. Rehospitalize patient for 3 days anytime dose is increased. Consider electrical cardioversion if patient does not convert to normal sinus rhythm w/in 24 hrs of initiation of therapy. If dofetilide needs to be discontinued to allow dosing of other potentially interacting drug(s), a washout period of at least 2 days should be followed before starting the other drug(s). Caution in elderly.

ADVERSE REACTIONS

Headache, chest pain, dizziness, ventricular arrhythmia, ventricular tachycardia, TdP, respiratory tract infection, dyspnea, nausea, flu syndrome, insomnia, back pain, diarrhea, rash, abdominal pain.

DRUG INTERACTIONS

See Contraindications. Hypokalemia or hypomagnesemia may occur w/ K^+-depleting diuretics, increasing the potential for TdP. CYP3A4 inhibitors (eg, macrolides, protease inhibitors, serotonin reuptake inhibitors) and drugs actively secreted by cationic secretion (eg, triamterene, metformin, amiloride) may increase levels; caution when coadministered. Not recommended w/ drugs that prolong the QT interval (eg, phenothiazines, TCAs, certain oral macrolides). Withhold Class I and III antiarrhythmics for at least 3 half-lives prior to dosing w/ dofetilide. Do not initiate therapy until amiodarone levels are <0.3mcg/mL or until amiodarone has been withdrawn for at least 3 months. Higher occurrence of TdP w/ digoxin.

PREGNANCY AND LACTATION

Pregnancy: Category C.
Lactation: Not for use in nursing.

MECHANISM OF ACTION

Class III antiarrhythmic; blocks cardiac ion channel carrying rapid component of delayed rectifier K^+ current, I_{Kr}.

PHARMACOKINETICS

Absorption: T_{max}=2-3 hrs (fasted). **Distribution:** V_d=3L/kg; plasma protein binding (60-70%). **Metabolism:** Liver via CYP3A4 through N-dealkylation and N-oxidation pathways. **Elimination:** Urine (80% unchanged, 20% metabolites); $T_{1/2}$=10 hrs.

PATIENT CONSIDERATIONS

Assessment: Assess for previous hypersensitivity to drug, congenital or acquired long QT syndrome, renal/hepatic impairment, pregnancy/nursing status, and possible drug interactions. Correct K^+ levels prior to therapy. Obtain baseline ECG and CrCl prior to therapy.

Monitoring: Monitor serum K^+ levels and for development of ventricular arrhythmias (eg, TdP). After initiation or cardioversion, continuously monitor by ECG for a minimum of 3 days, or for a minimum of 12 hrs after electrical/pharmacological conversion to normal sinus rhythm, whichever is greater. Reevaluate renal function and QTc every 3 months, as medically warranted.

Counseling: Inform about risks/benefits, need for compliance w/ prescribed dosing, potential drug interactions, and the need for periodic monitoring of QTc and renal function. Instruct to notify physician of any changes in medications and supplements or if hospitalized or prescribed a new medication for any condition. Counsel to report immediately any symptoms associated w/ electrolyte imbalance (eg, excessive/prolonged diarrhea, sweating, vomiting, loss of appetite, thirst). Instruct not to double the next dose if a dose is missed and to take the next dose at the usual time.

TIMOLOL — timolol maleate   Rx

Class: Nonselective beta blocker

> Hypersensitivity to catecholamines observed in patients withdrawn from β-blocker therapy; exacerbation of angina and myocardial infarction (MI) reported after abrupt discontinuation. When discontinuing chronic therapy, particularly with ischemic heart disease, taper over 1-2 weeks with careful monitoring. If angina markedly worsens or acute coronary insufficiency develops, promptly reinstitute therapy, at least temporarily, and take other measures appropriate for management of unstable angina. Warn against interruption or discontinuation of therapy without physician's advice. Coronary artery disease may be unrecognized; avoid abrupt discontinuation of therapy even in patients treated only for HTN.

ADULT DOSAGE

Hypertension

Initial: 10mg bid
Titrate: May increase or decrease dose depending on HR and BP response; wait for an interval of at least 7 days between dose increases
Maint: 20-40mg/day
Max: 60mg/day in 2 divided doses

May be used with a thiazide diuretic or other antihypertensive agents

PEDIATRIC DOSAGE

Pediatric use may not have been established

Myocardial Infarction

Long-Term Prophylactic Use:
Usual: 10mg bid

Migraine

Initial: 10mg bid
Titrate: May increase total daily dosage to max dose of 30mg or decrease to 10mg qd, depending on clinical response and tolerability
Maint: 20mg/day; may be administered as a single dose
Max: 30mg/day in divided doses

D/C if satisfactory response is not obtained after 6-8 weeks with max dose

- -

DOSING CONSIDERATIONS

Elderly
Start at lower end of dosing range

ADMINISTRATION

Oral route

STORAGE

20-25°C (68-77°F). Protect from light.

HOW SUPPLIED

Tab: 5mg, 10mg*, 20mg* *scored

CONTRAINDICATIONS

Presence/history of bronchial asthma, severe chronic obstructive pulmonary disease (COPD), sinus bradycardia, 2nd- and 3rd-degree atrioventricular (AV) block, overt cardiac failure, cardiogenic shock, hypersensitivity to timolol maleate.

WARNINGS/PRECAUTIONS

May precipitate more severe failure in patients with diminished myocardial contractility; if necessary, may be used with caution in patients with history of failure who are well-compensated. May lead to cardiac failure in patients without a history of cardiac failure; digitalize and/or give a diuretic at the 1st sign/symptom of cardiac failure and closely observe response; d/c if cardiac failure persists despite adequate treatment. Avoid with mild or moderate COPD, and history/known bronchospastic disease; if therapy is necessary, use with caution. May augment risks of general anesthesia in surgical procedures; difficulty in restarting and maintaining HR reported; gradual withdrawal of therapy is recommended in patients undergoing elective surgery. May mask signs/symptoms of acute hypoglycemia; caution in patients subject to spontaneous hypoglycemia or in diabetic patients receiving insulin or oral hypoglycemics. May mask certain clinical signs of hyperthyroidism (eg, tachycardia) and may precipitate a thyroid storm with abrupt withdrawal. May increase muscle weakness with myasthenia gravis or myasthenic symptoms. Dosage reductions may be necessary with hepatic and/or renal insufficiency. Caution with marked renal impairment undergoing dialysis after 20mg doses. Caution with cerebrovascular insufficiency; consider discontinuing therapy if signs/symptoms suggesting reduced cerebral blood flow are observed. Patients with a history of atopy or a history of severe anaphylactic reaction to a variety of allergens may be more reactive to repeated challenge and may be unresponsive to usual doses of epinephrine. Caution in elderly.

ADVERSE REACTIONS

Fatigue, nausea, dizziness, asthenia, bradycardia, nonfatal cardiac failure, cold hands/feet, claudication, hypotension.

DRUG INTERACTIONS

Caution with catecholamine-depleting drugs (eg, reserpine); possible additive effects. NSAIDs may blunt antihypertensive effects. Potentiated systemic β-blockade reported with concomitant CYP2D6 inhibitors (eg, quinidine). Concomitant use with digitalis and either diltiazem or verapamil may have additive effects in prolonging AV conduction time. Hypotension, AV conduction disturbances, and left ventricular failure reported with oral calcium antagonists; caution with IV calcium antagonists. Avoid calcium antagonists with cardiac dysfunction. May exacerbate rebound HTN following clonidine withdrawal; withdraw therapy several days before the gradual clonidine withdrawal. If replacing clonidine, delay initiation of therapy for several days after clonidine has been discontinued.

PREGNANCY AND LACTATION

Category C, not for use in nursing.

MECHANISM OF ACTION

Nonselective β-blocker; antihypertensive mechanism not established. Thought to reduce cardiac output and plasma renin activity, and to have a CNS sympatholytic action.

PHARMACOKINETICS

Absorption: Rapid and nearly complete; T_{max}=1-2 hrs. **Distribution:** Plasma protein binding (<10% by equilibrium dialysis, 60% by ultrafiltration); found in breast milk. **Metabolism:** Liver (partial). **Elimination:** Kidneys; $T_{1/2}$=4 hrs.

PATIENT CONSIDERATIONS

Assessment: Assess for hypersensitivity to drug, sinus bradycardia, cardiogenic shock, 2nd- and 3rd-degree AV block, overt cardiac failure, impaired hepatic/renal function, bronchial asthma or history thereof, COPD, thyrotoxicosis, myasthenia gravis, any other conditions where treatment is contraindicated or cautioned, pregnancy/nursing status, and possible drug interactions.

Monitoring: Monitor for cardiac failure, exacerbation of ischemia following abrupt withdrawal, hypersensitivity reactions, hypoglycemia, and other adverse reactions. Carefully monitor patients when discontinuing chronically administered therapy, especially those with ischemic heart disease.

Counseling: Inform of the benefits and risks of therapy. Warn against interruption or discontinuation of therapy without a physician's advice.

TIMOPTIC — timolol maleate   Rx

Class: Nonselective beta blocker

OTHER BRAND NAMES
Timoptic-XE, Timoptic in Ocudose

ADULT DOSAGE

Elevated Intraocular Pressure

In Patients w/ Ocular HTN or Open-Angle Glaucoma:

Timoptic/Timoptic in Ocudose:
1 drop of 0.25% sol in the affected eye(s) bid; may change to 1 drop of 0.5% sol bid if response is inadequate. Dosage schedule may be changed to 1 drop qd in the affected eye(s) if IOP maintained at satisfactory levels

Doses >1 drop of 0.5% bid generally have not been shown to produce further reduction in IOP

Timoptic-XE:
1 drop of either 0.25% or 0.5% sol in the affected eye(s) qd

Doses >1 drop of 0.5% qd have not been studied

PEDIATRIC DOSAGE
Pediatric use may not have been established

DOSING CONSIDERATIONS
Concomitant Medications
Administer other topically applied ophthalmic medications at least 10 min before Timoptic-XE

ADMINISTRATION
Ocular route

Timoptic in Ocudose
May be used when a patient is sensitive to the preservative in Timoptic, benzalkonium chloride, or when use of a preservative-free topical medication is advisable.

Timoptic-XE
Invert closed container and shake once before each use.

STORAGE
Timoptic/Timoptic in Ocudose: 15-30°C (59-86°F). Protect from freezing. Protect from light. **Timoptic in Ocudose:** Keep unit dose container in protective foil overwrap and use w/in 1 month after opening the foil package. **Timoptic-XE:** 15-25°C (59-77°F). Avoid freezing. Protect from light.

HOW SUPPLIED
Ophthalmic Sol: (Timoptic) 0.25% [5mL], 0.5% [5mL, 10mL]; (Timoptic in Ocudose) 0.25%, 0.5% [0.3mL, 60^s]; **Ophthalmic Sol, Gel-Forming:** (Timoptic-XE) 0.25%, 0.5% [5mL]

CONTRAINDICATIONS
Bronchial asthma, history of bronchial asthma, severe COPD, sinus bradycardia, 2nd- or 3rd-degree atrioventricular (AV) block, overt cardiac failure, cardiogenic shock, hypersensitivity to any component of the product.

WARNINGS/PRECAUTIONS
Absorbed systemically. Severe respiratory and cardiac reactions, including death due to bronchospasm in patients w/ asthma and, rarely, death associated w/ cardiac failure, reported. May precipitate more severe failure in individuals w/ diminished myocardial contractility. In patients w/o a history of cardiac failure, continued depression of the myocardium w/ β-blocking agents over a period of time can, in some cases, lead to cardiac failure; d/c at the 1st sign/symptom of cardiac failure. Avoid w/ COPD (eg, chronic bronchitis, emphysema) of mild or moderate severity, bronchospastic disease, or a history of bronchospastic disease. Impairs the ability of the heart to respond to β-adrenergically mediated reflex stimuli and may augment the risk of general anesthesia in surgical procedures; consider gradual withdrawal of therapy in patients undergoing elective surgery. May mask signs/symptoms of acute hypoglycemia; caution in patients subject to spontaneous hypoglycemia and in diabetic patients (especially those w/ labile diabetes) receiving insulin or hypoglycemic agents. May mask certain clinical signs of hyperthyroidism (eg, tachycardia); carefully manage patients suspected of developing thyrotoxicosis to avoid abrupt withdrawal that may precipitate a thyroid storm. Caution w/ cerebrovascular insufficiency; consider alternative therapy if signs/symptoms suggesting reduced cerebral blood flow develop. Choroidal detachment after filtration procedures reported. Should not be used alone in the treatment of angle-closure glaucoma. Patients w/ a history of atopy or a history of severe anaphylactic reactions to a variety of allergens may be more reactive to repeated challenge w/ such allergens; may be unresponsive to usual doses of epinephrine. May potentiate muscle weakness consistent w/ certain myasthenic symptoms (eg, diplopia, ptosis, generalized weakness); increased muscle weakness in some patients w/ myasthenia gravis or myasthenic symptoms reported rarely w/ timolol.

Timoptic/Timoptic-XE: Bacterial keratitis reported w/ the use of multiple-dose containers.

ADVERSE REACTIONS
Timoptic: Burning/stinging upon instillation.
Timoptic in Ocudose: Burning/stinging upon instillation.
Timoptic-XE: (Ocular) Burning/stinging upon instillation, transient blurred vision, pain, conjunctivitis, discharge, foreign body sensation, itching, tearing. (Systemic) Headache, dizziness, URIs.

DRUG INTERACTIONS
Monitor for potentially additive effects, both systemic and on IOP, w/ concomitant oral β-blockers; concomitant use of 2 topical β-blocking agents is not recommended. Possible AV conduction disturbances, left ventricular failure, and hypotension may occur w/ oral or IV calcium antagonists; use w/ caution and avoid coadministration in patients w/ impaired cardiac function. Closely observe patients receiving catecholamine-depleting drugs (eg, reserpine) because of possible additive effects and the production of hypotension and/or marked bradycardia. Concomitant use w/ digitalis or calcium antagonists may have additive effects in prolonging AV conduction time. Potentiated systemic β-blockade (eg, decreased HR, depression) reported w/ concomitant CYP2D6 inhibitors (eg, quinidine, SSRIs). **Timoptic/Timoptic in Ocudose:** Mydriasis occasionally reported w/ concomitant use w/ epinephrine.

PREGNANCY AND LACTATION
Pregnancy: There are no adequate and well-controlled studies in pregnant women; should be used during pregnancy only if the potential benefit justifies the potential risk to the fetus.
Lactation: Timolol has been detected in human milk following oral and ophthalmic drug administration. Not for use in nursing.

MECHANISM OF ACTION
Nonselective β-blocker; reduces elevated and normal IOP, whether or not accompanied by glaucoma. Ocular hypotensive action not clearly established; may be related to reduced aqueous formation and a slight increase in outflow capacity.

PHARMACOKINETICS
Absorption: (Timoptic/Timoptic in Ocudose) C_{max}=0.46ng/mL (am dose), 0.35ng/mL (afternoon dose); (Timoptic-XE) C_{max}=0.28ng/mL (am dose). (Timoptic) T_{max}=1-2 hrs. **Distribution:** Found in breast milk.

PATIENT CONSIDERATIONS

Assessment: Assess for presence or history of bronchial asthma, COPD (eg, bronchitis, emphysema), or any other conditions where treatment is contraindicated or cautioned. Assess pregnancy/nursing status and for possible drug interactions.

Monitoring: Monitor for signs/symptoms of cardiac failure, masking of signs/symptoms of hypoglycemia or hyperthyroidism, reduced cerebral blood flow, choroidal detachment, muscle weakness, and other adverse reactions. Evaluate IOP after 4 weeks of treatment.

Counseling: Advise not to use product if patient has a presence or history of bronchial asthma, severe COPD, sinus bradycardia, 2nd- or 3rd-degree AV block, or cardiac failure. **Timoptic/Timoptic-XE:** Instruct to avoid touching tip of container to eye or surrounding structures. Advise to seek physician's advice on continued use of product if patient had prior ocular surgery or develops intercurrent ocular condition (eg, trauma or infection). Instruct to handle ocular sol properly to avoid contamination; inform that using contaminated sol may result in serious eye damage. **Timoptic:** Inform that drug contains benzalkonium chloride, which may be absorbed by soft contact lenses. Instruct to remove contact lenses prior to administration and explain that lenses may be reinserted 15 min following administration. **Timoptic in Ocudose:** Instruct about proper administration. Advise to use immediately after opening, and discard the individual unit and any remaining contents immediately after use. **Timoptic-XE:** Instruct to invert the closed container and shake once before each use. Patients requiring concomitant topical ophthalmic medications should be instructed to administer these at least 10 min before instilling Timoptic-XE. Inform that ability to perform hazardous tasks (eg, operating machinery, driving motor vehicle) may be impaired.

TINDAMAX — tinidazole   Rx

Class: Antiprotozoal agent

> Carcinogenicity has been seen in mice and rats treated chronically with metronidazole. Although not reported for tinidazole, the two drugs are structurally related and have similar biologic effects. Use only for approved indications.

ADULT DOSAGE
Trichomoniasis
Usual: 2g single dose

Sexual partners should be treated w/ the same dose at the same time

Giardiasis
Usual: 2g single dose taken w/ food

Amebiasis
Intestinal:
Usual: 2g/day for 3 days taken w/ food

PEDIATRIC DOSAGE
Giardiasis
>3 Years:
Usual: 50mg/kg single dose taken w/ food
Max: 2g/day

Amebiasis
>3 Years:

Intestinal:
Usual: 50mg/kg/day for 3 days taken w/ food
Max: 2g/day

Amebic Liver Abscess:
Usual: 2g/day for 3-5 days taken w/ food

Bacterial Vaginosis
In Nonpregnant Woman:
Usual: 2g qd for 2 days taken w/ food or 1g qd for 5 days taken w/ food

Amebic Liver Abscess:
Usual: 50mg/kg/day for 3-5 days taken w/ food; closely monitor when treatment duration is >3 days
Max: 2g/day

DOSING CONSIDERATIONS
Renal Impairment
Hemodialysis: If given on same day and prior to hemodialysis, give additional dose equivalent to 1/2 of recommended dose at the end of dialysis

ADMINISTRATION
Oral route

Take w/ food

Avoid alcoholic beverages when taking tinidazole and for 3 days afterwards

May crush tabs in artificial cherry syrup to be taken w/ food if unable to swallow whole tab; shake well before use

Pharmacy Compounding
Pulverize four 500mg tabs w/ a mortar and pestle

Add approx 10mL of cherry syrup to the powder and mix until smooth; transfer sus to a graduated amber container

Use small rinses of cherry syrup to transfer remaining drug to final sus for a final volume of 30mL

STORAGE
20-25°C (68-77°F); excursions permitted to 15-30°C (59-86°F). Protect contents from light.

HOW SUPPLIED
Tab: 250mg*, 500mg* *scored

CONTRAINDICATIONS
Treatment during 1st trimester of pregnancy, nursing mothers during therapy and 3 days following last dose.

WARNINGS/PRECAUTIONS
Seizures, peripheral neuropathy reported. D/C if abnormal neurologic signs occur. Caution with hepatic impairment or blood dyscrasias. May develop vaginal candidiasis. May develop drug resistance if prescribed in absence of proven or strongly suspected bacterial infection. Caution in elderly.

ADVERSE REACTIONS
Metallic/bitter taste, N/V, vaginal fungal infection, anorexia, headache, dizziness, constipation, dyspepsia, cramps/epigastric discomfort, weakness, fatigue, malaise, convulsions, peripheral neuropathy.

DRUG INTERACTIONS
Avoid alcohol during therapy and for 3 days after use. Do not give if patient has taken disulfiram within the last 2 weeks. May potentiate oral anticoagulants. May prolong $T_{1/2}$ and reduce clearance of phenytoin (IV). May decrease clearance of fluorouracil, causing increased side effects; if concomitant use needed, monitor for toxicities. May increase levels of lithium, cyclosporine, and tacrolimus. Separate dosing with cholestyramine. Phenobarbital, rifampin, phenytoin, fosphenytoin, and other CYP3A4 inducers may decrease levels. Cimetidine, ketoconazole, and other CYP3A4 inhibitors may increase levels. Therapeutic effect antagonized by oxytetracycline.

PREGNANCY AND LACTATION
Category C, not for use in nursing.

MECHANISM OF ACTION
Antiprotozoal, antibacterial agent; nitro group of tinidazole is reduced by cell extracts of *Trichomonas*. Free nitro radical generated as a result of this reduction may be responsible for antiprotozoal activity.

PHARMACOKINETICS
Absorption: Rapid, complete. (Fasted) C_{max}=47.7mcg/mL, T_{max}=1.6 hrs, AUC=901.6mcg.hr/mL at 72 hrs. **Distribution:** V_d=50L; plasma protein binding (12%); crosses blood-brain and placental barrier; found in breast milk. **Metabolism:** Mainly via oxidation, hydroxylation, conjugation; CYP3A4 mainly involved. **Elimination:** Urine (20-25% unchanged), feces (12%); $T_{1/2}$=12-14 hrs.

PATIENT CONSIDERATIONS
Assessment: Assess for blood dyscrasias, seizures, pregnancy/nursing status, hypersensitivity and possible drug interactions. Assess for proven or strongly suspected bacterial infection to avoid drug resistance.

Monitoring: Monitor for convulsive seizures, peripheral neuropathy, vaginal candidiasis, drug resistance, hypersensitivity reactions (urticaria, pruritus, angioedema, erythema multiforme, Stevens-Johnson syndrome).

Counseling: Advise to take with food to minimize epigastric discomfort and other GI side effects. Instruct to avoid alcohol and preparations containing ethanol and propylene glycol during therapy and for 3 days afterward to prevent abdominal cramps, N/V, headache, and flushing. Inform that therapy only treats bacterial, not viral (eg, common cold), infections. Instruct to take ud; skipping doses or not completing full course may decrease effectiveness and increase resistance.

TIVICAY — dolutegravir   Rx
Class: HIV-integrase strand transfer inhibitor

ADULT DOSAGE
HIV-1 Infection

Used in combination w/ other antiretrovirals

Treatment-Naive/Treatment-Experienced Integrase Strand Transfer Inhibitor (INSTI)-Naive:
50mg qd

INSTI-Experienced w/ Certain INSTI-Associated Resistance Substitutions or Clinically Suspected INSTI Resistance:
50mg bid

PEDIATRIC DOSAGE
HIV-1 Infection

Used in combination w/ other antiretrovirals

Treatment-Naive/Treatment-Experienced Integrase Strand Transfer Inhibitor (INSTI)-Naive:
30 to <40kg:
35mg qd
≥40kg:
50mg qd

DOSING CONSIDERATIONS
Concomitant Medications
Treatment-Naive/Treatment-Experienced INSTI-Naive in Combination w/ Certain UGT1A/CYP3A Inducers (eg, Efavirenz, Fosamprenavir/Ritonavir [RTV], Tipranavir/RTV, Carbamazepine, Rifampin):
Adults:
50mg bid
Pediatric Patients:
30 to <40kg:
35mg bid
≥40kg:
50mg bid

Hepatic Impairment
Severe (Child-Pugh Score C): Not recommended
Mild to Moderate (Child-Pugh Score A or B): No dose adjustment needed

ADMINISTRATION
Oral route

Take w/ or w/o food.

STORAGE
25°C (77°F); excursions permitted to 15-30°C (59-86°F).

HOW SUPPLIED
Tab: 10mg, 25mg, 50mg

CONTRAINDICATIONS
Previous hypersensitivity reaction to dolutegravir, coadministration w/ dofetilide.

WARNINGS/PRECAUTIONS
Hypersensitivity reactions reported; d/c therapy and other suspect agents immediately if signs/symptoms develop, monitor clinical status (eg, liver aminotransferases), and initiate appropriate therapy. Patients w/ underlying hepatitis B or C may be at increased risk for worsening or development of transaminase elevations. Redistribution/accumulation of body fat observed. Immune reconstitution syndrome reported. Autoimmune disorders (eg, Graves' disease, polymyositis, Guillain-Barre syndrome) reported in the setting of immune reconstitution and can occur many months after initiation of treatment. Caution in elderly. Caution in INSTI-experienced patients (w/ certain INSTI-associated resistance substitutions or clinically suspected INSTI resistance) w/ severe renal impairment.

ADVERSE REACTIONS
Insomnia, fatigue, headache.

DRUG INTERACTIONS
See Dosing Considerations and Contraindications. Drugs that induce/inhibit UGT1A1, CYP3A, UGT1A3, UGT1A9, breast cancer resistance protein, and P-gp may decrease/increase levels, respectively. Decreased levels w/ etravirine; etravirine use w/o coadministration of atazanavir/RTV, darunavir/RTV, or lopinavir/RTV is not recommended. Decreased levels w/ carbamazepine, efavirenz, fosamprenavir/RTV, and tipranavir/RTV; use alternative combinations that do not include metabolic inducers where possible for INSTI-experienced patients w/ certain INSTI-associated resistance substitutions or clinically suspected INSTI resistance. Decreased levels w/ nevirapine, oxcarbazepine, phenytoin, phenobarbital, and St. John's wort; avoid coadministration. Administer 2 hrs before or 6 hrs after taking medications containing polyvalent cations (eg, cation-containing antacids/laxatives, sucralfate, buffered medications) and oral Ca^{2+} or iron supplements (eg, multivitamins); alternatively, dolutegravir and supplements containing Ca^{2+} or iron can be taken together w/ food. May increase levels of drugs eliminated via renal organic cation transporters, OCT2, or multidrug and toxin extrusion transporter 1 (eg, metformin); limit the total daily dose of metformin to 1000mg when starting metformin or dolutegravir. When stopping dolutegravir, the metformin dose may require an adjustment; monitor blood glucose when initiating concomitant use and after withdrawal of dolutegravir. Decreased levels w/ rifampin; use alternatives to rifampin where possible for INSTI-experienced patients w/ certain INSTI-associated resistance substitutions or clinically suspected INSTI resistance.

PREGNANCY AND LACTATION
Pregnancy: There are insufficient human data on the use of dolutegravir during pregnancy. Physicians are encouraged to register patients in the Antiretroviral Pregnancy Registry.
Lactation: Not for use in nursing.

MECHANISM OF ACTION
HIV-1 INSTI; inhibits HIV integrase by binding to integrase active site and blocking the strand transfer step of retroviral DNA integration, which is essential for the HIV replication cycle.

PHARMACOKINETICS

Absorption: Adults: AUC_{0-24}=53.6mcg•hr/mL (50mg qd), 75.1mcg•hr/mL (50mg bid); C_{max}=3.67mcg/mL (50mg qd), 4.15mcg/mL (50mg bid); T_{max}=2-3 hrs. Pediatrics: 30 to <40kg (35mg qd): C_{max}=4.4mcg/mL, AUC_{0-24}=64.6mcg•hr/mL. ≥40kg (50mg qd): C_{max}=3.89mcg/mL, AUC_{0-24}=50.1mcg•hr/mL. **Metabolism:** Via UGT1A1, CYP3A. **Elimination:** Urine (31%, <1% unchanged), feces (53% unchanged); $T_{1/2}$=approx 14 hrs.

PATIENT CONSIDERATIONS

Assessment: Assess for previous hypersensitivity to the drug, hepatitis B or C infection, renal/hepatic impairment, pregnancy/nursing status, and possible drug interactions.

Monitoring: Monitor for signs/symptoms of hypersensitivity reactions, redistribution/accumulation of body fat, immune reconstitution syndrome, autoimmune disorders, and other adverse reactions. If a hypersensitivity reaction develops, monitor clinical status, including liver aminotransferases. In patients w/ underlying hepatic disease, monitor for hepatotoxicity.

Counseling: Instruct to d/c immediately and seek medical attention if rash develops and is associated w/ other symptoms of hypersensitivity. Advise patients w/ underlying hepatitis B or C to have lab testing before and during therapy. Inform that fat redistribution/accumulation may occur. Advise to inform physician immediately of any symptoms of infection. Advise that therapy is not a cure for HIV-1 infection and that patients may continue to experience illnesses associated w/ HIV-1 infection, including opportunistic infections. Advise to take all HIV medications exactly as prescribed. Advise to avoid doing things that can spread HIV to others. Instruct to inform physician if any unusual symptom develops, or if any known symptom persists or worsens. Counsel patients on missed dose instructions. Advise not to breastfeed.

TIZANIDINE — tizanidine   Rx

Class: Alpha₂ agonist

OTHER BRAND NAMES
Zanaflex

ADULT DOSAGE	PEDIATRIC DOSAGE
Spasticity	Pediatric use may not have been established
Management:	
Initial: 4mg, (Zanaflex) 2mg May repeat at 6- to 8-hr intervals, prn, up to a max of 3 doses in 24 hrs **Titrate:** May gradually increase by 2-4mg/dose, w/ 1-4 days between increases, until a satisfactory reduction in muscle tone is achieved **Max:** 36mg/day	

DOSING CONSIDERATIONS

Renal Impairment
CrCl <25mL/min:
Reduce individual doses during titration
If higher doses are required, increase individual doses

Hepatic Impairment
Reduce individual doses during titration
If higher doses are required, increase individual doses

Discontinuation
Decrease dose slowly, particularly in patients who have been receiving high doses for long periods or who may be on concomitant treatment w/ narcotics

ADMINISTRATION
Oral route

Take w/ or w/o food
Do not alter regimen once formulation has been selected and the decision to take w/ or w/o food has been made

STORAGE
20-25°C (68-77°F). (Zanaflex) 25°C (77°F); excursions permitted to 15-30°C (59-86°F).

HOW SUPPLIED
Tab: 2mg* **(Zanaflex) Cap:** 2mg, 4mg, 6mg; **Tab:** 4mg* *scored

CONTRAINDICATIONS
Concomitant use with potent CYP1A2 inhibitors (eg, fluvoxamine, ciprofloxacin), hypersensitivity to tizanidine or its ingredients.

WARNINGS/PRECAUTIONS
May cause hypotension; may be minimized by dose titration and by focusing attention on signs/symptoms of hypotension prior to dose advancement. May cause hepatocellular liver injury; avoid or caution with hepatic impairment. May cause sedation. Associated with hallucinations/psychosis; consider discontinuation if hallucinations develop. Caution with renal insufficiency (CrCl <25mL/min); monitor closely for the onset or increase in severity of the common adverse events (dry mouth, somnolence, asthenia, dizziness). Withdrawal adverse reactions (eg, rebound HTN, tachycardia, hypertonia) may occur; decrease dose slowly. Caution in elderly. (Zanaflex) May cause anaphylaxis; d/c if signs/ symptoms of anaphylaxis occur.

ADVERSE REACTIONS
Dry mouth, somnolence, asthenia, dizziness, UTI, infection, constipation, LFT abnormality, vomiting, speech disorder, amblyopia (blurred vision), urinary frequency, dyskinesia, nervousness, pharyngitis.

DRUG INTERACTIONS
See Contraindications and Dosage. Avoid with other CYP1A2 inhibitors (eg, zileuton, amiodarone, mexiletine, cimetidine); if use is clinically necessary, use with caution. Avoid with oral contraceptives; if use is clinically necessary, the starting dose and subsequent titration rate of tizanidine should be reduced. May have additive sedative effects with alcohol and other CNS depressants (eg, benzodiazepines, opioids, TCAs); monitor for symptoms of excess sedation. Monitor for hypotension in patients receiving concurrent antihypertensive therapy. Not recommended with other α₂-adrenergic agonists. Withdrawal symptoms are more likely to occur with concomitant use of narcotics. May delay T_{max} of acetaminophen.

PREGNANCY AND LACTATION
Category C, caution in nursing.

MECHANISM OF ACTION
Centrally acting α₂-agonist: presumably reduces spasticity by increasing presynaptic inhibition of motor neurons.

PHARMACOKINETICS
Absorption: Complete; absolute oral bioavailability (40%). (Single Dose) T_{max}=1 hr (two 4mg caps/tabs, fasted); T_{max}=85 min (two 4mg tabs, fed); T_{max}=2-3 hrs (median)(two 4mg caps, fed). **Distribution:** (IV, Healthy) V_d=2.4L/kg; plasma protein binding (30%). **Metabolism:** Liver (extensive) via CYP1A2. **Elimination:** Urine (60%), feces (20%); $T_{1/2}$=2.5 hrs.

PATIENT CONSIDERATIONS
Assessment: Assess for hypersensitivity to drug, hypotension, hepatic/renal impairment, pregnancy/nursing status, and possible drug interactions. Obtain baseline aminotransferase levels.

Monitoring: Monitor for hypotension, hepatocellular liver injury, anaphylaxis, sedation, hallucinations/psychosis, syncope, and other adverse reactions. Monitor aminotransferase levels at 1 month after max dose is achieved, or if hepatic injury is suspected. Monitor renal function with renal impairment and in elderly.

Counseling: Instruct to inform physician of all medications being taken, including if starting/stopping any medication. Instruct to take exactly ud, and not to switch between tab and cap. Advise not to suddenly d/c therapy, because rebound HTN and tachycardia may occur. Inform that hypotension may occur; advise to be careful when changing from lying/sitting to standing position. Inform that medication may cause somnolence or sedation; instruct to be careful when performing activities that require alertness (eg, driving/ operating machinery). Inform that sedation may be additive when taken with drugs (baclofen, benzodiazepines) or substances (eg, alcohol) that act as CNS depressants. Inform that medication decreases spasticity; advise to use caution if dependent on spasticity to sustain posture and balance in locomotion, or whenever spasticity is utilized to obtain increased function. Inform of the signs/ symptoms of severe allergic reactions; instruct to d/c and seek immediate medical care if these occur.

TOBI — tobramycin   Rx

Class: Aminoglycoside

OTHER BRAND NAMES
TOBI Podhaler

ADULT DOSAGE	PEDIATRIC DOSAGE
Cystic Fibrosis	**Cystic Fibrosis**
Management of Cystic Fibrosis w/ *Pseudomonas aeruginosa*:	**Management of Cystic Fibrosis w/ *Pseudomonas aeruginosa*:**
Sol:	**≥6 Years:**
300mg bid (as close to 12 hrs apart as possible; not <6 hrs apart) for 28 days by inh over approx 15 min, using a nebulizer	**Sol:** 300mg bid (as close to 12 hrs apart as possible; not <6 hrs apart) for 28 days by inh over approx 15 min, using a nebulizer
Cap:	**Cap:**
Inh of four 28mg caps bid (as close to 12 hrs apart as possible; not <6 hrs apart) for 28 days using the Podhaler device	Inh of four 28mg caps bid (as close to 12 hrs apart as possible; not <6 hrs apart) for 28 days using the Podhaler device
After 28 days of therapy, stop for the next 28 days, then resume for the next 28 day on and 28 day off cycle	After 28 days of therapy, stop for the next 28 days, then resume for the next 28 day on and 28 day off cycle

---

ADMINISTRATION
Oral inh route

Sol
Do not dilute or mix w/ dornase alfa or other medications in the nebulizer
Use w/ handheld PARI LC PLUS reusable nebulizer w/ a DeVilbiss Pulmo-Aide compressor

Cap
Do not swallow cap
Use w/ Podhaler device only; always use the new Podhaler device provided w/ each weekly pack
Only remove cap from blister immediately before use

Refer to PI for preparation and administration instructions

STORAGE
(Sol) 2-8°C (36-46°F). Upon removal from the refrigerator, or if refrigeration is unavailable, may be stored at room temperature (up to 25°C [77°F]) for up to 28 days. Do not expose to intense light. (Cap) 25°C (77°F); excursions permitted to 15-30°C (59-86°F). Protect from moisture.

HOW SUPPLIED
Sol, Inhalation: 300mg/5mL; **Cap, Inhalation (Podhaler):** 28mg [8, 56, 224 caps]

CONTRAINDICATIONS
Known hypersensitivity to any aminoglycoside.

WARNINGS/PRECAUTIONS
Ototoxicity (eg, tinnitus), nephrotoxicity, or bronchospasm may occur. May aggravate muscle weakness. If ototoxicity or nephrotoxicity occurs, d/c therapy until serum concentrations fall <2mcg/mL. May cause fetal harm.

ADVERSE REACTIONS
Cough, lung disorder, dyspnea, hemoptysis, N/V, pulmonary function test decreased, headache, fever, chest pain, diarrhea, dysgeusia, dysphonia.

DRUG INTERACTIONS
Avoid concurrent and/or sequential use w/ other drugs w/ neurotoxic, nephrotoxic, or ototoxic potential. Some diuretics may enhance toxicity by altering concentrations in serum and tissue; do not administer w/ ethacrynic acid, furosemide, urea, or IV mannitol.

PREGNANCY AND LACTATION
Category D, not for use in nursing.

MECHANISM OF ACTION
Aminoglycoside; acts primarily by disrupting protein synthesis, leading to altered cell membrane permeability, progressive disruption of the cell envelope, and eventual cell death.

PHARMACOKINETICS
Absorption: (Sol) C_{max}=1.04mcg/mL; T_{max}=1 hr (median); AUC=4.8mcg•hr/mL. (Cap) C_{max}=1.02mcg/mL (single dose), 1.48-1.99mcg/mL (multiple dose); T_{max}=1 hr (median); AUC=4.6mcg•hr/mL. **Distribution:** Crosses placenta. (Cap) V_d=85.1L. **Elimination:** Urine (unchanged). (Sol) Expectorated sputum (unabsorbed). (Cap) $T_{1/2}$=3 hrs.

PATIENT CONSIDERATIONS
Assessment: Assess for auditory, vestibular, renal, or neuromuscular dysfunction, drug hypersensitivity, pregnancy/nursing status, and possible drug interactions. Consider an audiogram at baseline, particularly for patients at increased risk of auditory dysfunction.

Monitoring: Monitor for ototoxicity, nephrotoxicity, neuromuscular effects, bronchospasm, and other adverse reactions. Consider an audiogram for patients who show any evidence of auditory dysfunction.

Counseling: Instruct to take drug ud, and to complete a full 28-day course of therapy even if feeling better. Inform of adverse reactions associated w/ therapy, such as ototoxicity, bronchospasm, nephrotoxicity, and neuromuscular disorders; instruct to inform physician if new or worsening symptoms develop, or if ringing in the ears, dizziness, or any changes in hearing occur. Inform of the need to monitor hearing, serum concentrations, or renal function during treatment. Advise to inform physician if patient has any history of kidney problems, is pregnant/nursing, or plans to become pregnant. (Cap) Advise that tobramycin inhalation sol or alternative therapeutic options may be considered if coughing that may be experienced w/ therapy becomes bothersome or cannot be tolerated. Advise to count each day of use towards the 28 day on-treatment part of the cycle if prescribed a 1-day or 7-day pack either immediately before or during a 28-day treatment w/ therapy; instruct to take only a total of 28 consecutive days of treatment during a cycle.

TobraDex — dexamethasone/tobramycin   Rx
Class: Aminoglycoside/corticosteroid

OTHER BRAND NAMES
TobraDex ST

ADULT DOSAGE	PEDIATRIC DOSAGE
Steroid-Responsive Inflammatory Ocular Conditions	**Steroid-Responsive Inflammatory Ocular Conditions**
Use for conditions for which a corticosteroid is indicated and where superficial bacterial ocular infection or a risk of bacterial ocular infection exists	Use for conditions for which a corticosteroid is indicated and where superficial bacterial ocular infection or a risk of bacterial ocular infection exists
	≥2 Years:
Sus:	**Sus:**
1-2 drops into the conjunctival sac(s) q4-6h	1-2 drops into the conjunctival sac(s) q4-6h
Titrate: May increase to 1-2 drops q2h during the initial 24-48 hrs; decrease frequency gradually as condition improves	**Titrate:** May increase to 1-2 drops q2h during the initial 24-48 hrs; decrease frequency gradually as condition improves
ST:	**ST:**
1 drop into the conjunctival sac(s) q4-6h	1 drop into the conjunctival sac(s) q4-6h
Titrate: May increase to 1 drop q2h during the initial 24-48 hrs; decrease frequency gradually as condition improves	**Titrate:** May increase to 1 drop q2h during the initial 24-48 hrs; decrease frequency gradually as condition improves
Sus/ST:	**Sus/ST:**
Do not prescribe more than 20mL initially	Do not prescribe more than 20mL initially
Care should be taken not to d/c therapy prematurely	Care should be taken not to d/c therapy prematurely
Oint:	**Oint:**
Apply a small amount (1/2 inch ribbon) into the conjunctival sac(s) up to tid-qid	Apply a small amount (1/2 inch ribbon) into the conjunctival sac(s) up to tid-qid
Do not prescribe more than 8g initially	Do not prescribe more than 8g initially

---

ADMINISTRATION
Ocular route
Sus/ST
Shake well before use.
Oint
1. Tilt head back.
2. Place finger on cheek just under the eye and gently pull down until a "V" pocket is formed between eyeball and lower lid.
3. Apply recommended dose, making sure to avoid touching tip of tube to eye.
4. Look downward before closing the eye.

STORAGE
(Sus) 8-27°C (46-80°F); store upright. (Oint/ST): 2-25°C (36-77°F); protect ST from light.

HOW SUPPLIED
Oint: (Tobramycin/Dexamethasone) 0.3%/0.1% [3.5g]; **Sus:** 0.3%/0.1% [2.5mL, 5mL, 10mL]; **Sus (ST):** 0.3%/0.05% [2.5mL, 5mL, 10mL]

CONTRAINDICATIONS
Most viral diseases of the cornea and conjunctiva, including epithelial herpes simplex keratitis (dendritic keratitis), vaccinia, and varicella; mycobacterial infection of the eye; fungal diseases of ocular structures; hypersensitivity to a component of the medication.

WARNINGS/PRECAUTIONS
Prolonged use may result in glaucoma with optic nerve damage, visual acuity and field of vision defects, posterior subcapsular cataract formation, and may suppress host response and increase risk of secondary ocular infections. Perforations may occur with diseases causing thinning of the cornea or sclera. May mask/enhance existing infection in acute purulent conditions. Fungal infections of the cornea may occur; consider fungal invasion in any persistent corneal ulceration. (Oint/Sus) Not for injection into the eye. Routinely monitor intraocular pressure (IOP). D/C if sensitivity occurs. Cross-sensitivity to other aminoglycoside antibiotics may occur; d/c and institute appropriate therapy if hypersensitivity develops. May result in overgrowth of nonsusceptible organisms, including fungi; initiate appropriate therapy if superinfection occurs. (ST) Monitor IOP if to be used for ≥10 days. Reevaluate after 2 days if patient fails to improve. Use may prolong the course and may exacerbate the severity of many viral infections of the eye (including herpes simplex). May delay healing and increase the incidence of bleb formation after cataract surgery. (Oint) May retard corneal wound healing.

ADVERSE REACTIONS
Hypersensitivity, localized ocular toxicity, secondary infection, increased IOP, posterior subcapsular cataract formation, impaired wound healing.

DRUG INTERACTIONS
Monitor total serum concentrations if used concomitantly with systemic aminoglycoside antibiotics.

PREGNANCY AND LACTATION
Pregnancy: Category C.
Lactation: Caution in nursing.

MECHANISM OF ACTION
Tobramycin: Aminoglycoside antibiotic; provides action against susceptible organisms. **Dexamethasone:** Corticoid; suppresses inflammatory response and probably delays or slows healing.

PATIENT CONSIDERATIONS
Assessment: Assess for epithelial herpes simplex keratitis (dendritic keratitis), vaccinia, varicella, other viral diseases of cornea or conjunctiva, mycobacterial infection and fungal diseases of eye, diseases that may cause thinning of cornea or sclera, other existing infections, pregnancy/nursing status, and for drug interactions. (ST) Assess for history of herpes simplex.

Monitoring: Monitor for signs/symptoms of hypersensitivity reactions, glaucoma, defects in visual acuity and fields of vision, posterior subcapsular cataracts, perforations, secondary infections, delayed wound healing. (ST) Monitor for IOP if used for ≥10 days, exacerbation of ocular viral infections, and bleb formation. (Oint/Sus) Routinely monitor IOP, and for development of superinfections.

Counseling: Instruct not to touch dropper tip to any surface to avoid contaminating contents and not to wear contact lenses during therapy.

Tofranil — imipramine hydrochloride   Rx
Class: Tricyclic antidepressant (TCA)

> Antidepressants increased the risk of suicidal thinking and behavior (suicidality) in children, adolescents, and young adults in short-term studies of major depressive disorder and other psychiatric disorders. Monitor and observe closely for clinical worsening, suicidality, or unusual changes in behavior in patients who are started on antidepressant therapy. Not approved for use in pediatric patients.

ADULT DOSAGE

Depression

Hospitalized Patients:
Initial: 100mg/day in divided doses
Titrate: Increase gradually to 200mg/day as required; increase to 250-300mg/day if no response after 2 weeks

Outpatients:
Initial: 75mg/day
Titrate: Increase to 150mg/day
Maint: 50-150mg/day
Max: 200mg/day

Following remission, may require maint for a longer period of time at the lowest effective dose

PEDIATRIC DOSAGE

Depression

Adolescents:
Initial: 30-40mg/day
Max: 100mg/day

Following remission, may require maint for a longer period of time at the lowest effective dose

Enuresis

Temporary Adjunctive Therapy in Reducing Enuresis After Possible Organic Causes Have Been Excluded by Appropriate Tests:

≥6 Years:
Initial: 25mg/day 1 hr before hs
Titrate: If no satisfactory response w/in 1 week, increase to 50mg nightly in children <12 yrs; may give up to 75mg nightly in children >12 yrs
Max: 2.5mg/kg/day

In early night bedwetters, drug is more effective given earlier and in divided doses (eg, 25mg in midafternoon, repeated hs)

Consider a drug-free period following an adequate trial w/ favorable response

Dosage should be tapered off gradually rather than abruptly discontinued; may reduce tendency to relapse

DOSING CONSIDERATIONS

Elderly
Initial: 30-40mg/day
Max: 100mg/day

ADMINISTRATION
Oral route

STORAGE
20-25°C (68-77°F).

HOW SUPPLIED
Tab: 10mg, 25mg, 50mg

CONTRAINDICATIONS
Use of an MAOI concomitantly. Treatment w/in 14 days of stopping an MAOI. During the acute recovery period following myocardial infarction (MI). Known hypersensitivity to this product.

WARNINGS/PRECAUTIONS
Not approved for the treatment of bipolar depression. May precipitate mixed/manic episode in patients at risk for bipolar disorder; screen for risk for bipolar disorder prior to initiating treatment. Pupillary dilation that occurs following therapy may trigger an angle-closure attack in a patient with anatomically narrow angles who does not have a patent iridectomy. Use extreme caution in patients with cardiovascular disease (CVD); cardiac surveillance required. Caution in patients with history of urinary retention, narrow-angle glaucoma, or seizure disorder. Caution in patients with hyperthyroidism, serious depression, significant renal/hepatic impairment, and in elderly. May impair mental/physical abilities. Hypomanic or manic episodes may occur, particularly in patients with cyclic disorders; may require discontinuation and, if needed, may resume at lower dosage when episodes are relieved. May activate psychosis in schizophrenic patients; may require dose reduction and addition of a phenothiazine. Hazards may be increased with electroshock therapy. Photosensitization reported; avoid excessive exposure to sunlight. May alter blood glucose levels. Perform leukocyte and differential blood counts if fever and sore throat develop; d/c if there is evidence of pathological neutrophil depression. Prior to elective surgery, d/c treatment for as long as the clinical situation will allow.

ADVERSE REACTIONS
Nervousness, sleep disorders, tiredness, mild GI disturbances, orthostatic hypotension, HTN, confusion, hallucinations, numbness, tremors, dry mouth, skin rash, bone marrow depression, anorexia, jaundice.

DRUG INTERACTIONS
See Contraindications. Caution in patients on thyroid medication. May block pharmacological effects of guanethidine, clonidine, or similar agents; use with caution. Methylphenidate HCl may inhibit metabolism; may require downward dose adjustment of imipramine. May enhance CNS depressant effects of alcohol. Drugs that inhibit CYP2D6 (eg, quinidine, cimetidine, many CYP2D6 substrates [other antidepressants, phenothiazines, propafenone, flecainide]) may increase plasma concentrations; may require lower doses for either TCA or the other drug, and monitoring of TCA plasma levels. Caution with SSRI coadministration and when switching between TCAs and SSRIs (eg, fluoxetine, sertraline, paroxetine); sufficient time must elapse before starting therapy when switching from fluoxetine (at least 5 weeks may be necessary). Hepatic enzyme inhibitors (eg, cimetidine, fluoxetine) may increase plasma concentration and hepatic enzyme inducers (eg, barbiturates, phenytoin) may decrease plasma concentration; may require dosage adjustment of imipramine. Atropine-like effects may become more pronounced (eg, paralytic ileus) with anticholinergics (including antiparkinsonism agents); close supervision and careful dose adjustment is required when coadministered with anticholinergic drugs. May potentiate effects of catecholamines; avoid use of preparations (eg, decongestants, local anesthetics) that contain any sympathomimetic amine (eg, epinephrine, norepinephrine). Caution with agents that lower BP. May potentiate effects of CNS depressants.

PREGNANCY AND LACTATION
Safety not known in pregnancy; not for use in nursing.

MECHANISM OF ACTION
TCA; has not been established. Suspected to potentiate adrenergic synapses by blocking uptake of norepinephrine at nerve endings. Mechanism in controlling childhood enuresis is thought to be apart from its antidepressant effect.

PATIENT CONSIDERATIONS
Assessment: Assess for acute recovery period following MI, known hypersensitivity to drug, history of urinary retention or seizure disorder, history of/susceptibility to narrow-angle glaucoma, risk for bipolar disorder, CVD, hyperthyroidism, schizophrenia, serious depression, renal/hepatic impairment, pregnancy/nursing status, and possible drug interactions. Obtain ECG recording prior to initiation of larger-than-usual doses of therapy.

Monitoring: Monitor for signs/symptoms of clinical worsening, suicidality, unusual changes in behavior, hypomanic/manic episodes, psychosis activation, angle-closure glaucoma, changes in blood glucose levels, and other adverse reactions. Take ECG recording at appropriate intervals until steady state is achieved; perform cardiac surveillance in patients with CVD. Perform leukocyte and differential blood counts if fever and sore throat develop.

Counseling: Inform about benefits, risks, and appropriate use of therapy. Advise to monitor for unusual changes in behavior, worsening of depression, and suicidal ideation on a day-to-day basis, and to report such symptoms to physician. Inform that drug can cause mild pupillary dilation, which in susceptible individuals, can lead to an episode of angle-closure glaucoma. Advise to use caution when performing potentially hazardous tasks (eg, driving, operating machinery). Instruct to avoid excessive exposure to sunlight.

TOPAMAX — topiramate   **Rx**

Class: Sulfamate-substituted monosaccharide antiepileptic

OTHER BRAND NAMES
Topamax Sprinkle

ADULT DOSAGE

Epilepsy

Monotherapy:
Partial Onset/Primary Generalized Tonic-Clonic Seizures:
Week 1: 25mg bid (am and pm)
Week 2: 50mg bid (am and pm)
Week 3: 75mg bid (am and pm)
Week 4: 100mg bid (am and pm)
Week 5: 150mg bid (am and pm)
Week 6 & Onward: 200mg bid (am and pm).

Adjunctive Therapy:
Partial Onset Seizure/Primary Generalized Tonic-Clonic Seizures/Lennox-Gastaut Syndrome:
≥17 Years:
Initial: 25-50mg/day
Titrate: Increase in increments of 25-50mg/day every week

Partial Onset Seizures:
Usual: 200-400mg/day in 2 divided doses

Primary Generalized Tonic-Clonic:
Usual: 400mg/day in 2 divided doses

Migraine

Prophylaxis:
Week 1: 25mg qpm
Week 2: 25mg bid
Week 3: 25mg qam and 50mg qpm
Week 4 & Onward: 50mg bid

PEDIATRIC DOSAGE

Epilepsy

Monotherapy:
Partial Onset/Primary Generalized Tonic-Clonic Seizures:

2-<10 Years:
Initial: 25mg qpm for the 1st week
Titrate: May increase to 50mg qd in the 2nd week, then by 25-50mg qd each subsequent week. Titration to the minimum maint dose should be attempted over 5-7 weeks; additional titration to a higher dose (up to the max maint dose) can be attempted in weekly increments by 25-50mg qd, up to the max maint dose for each range of body weight

Up to 11kg:
Minimum Maint Dose: 150mg/day
Max Maint Dose: 250mg/day
12-22kg:
Minimum Maint Dose: 200mg/day
Max Maint Dose: 300mg/day
23-31kg:
Minimum Maint Dose: 200mg/day
Max Maint Dose: 350mg/day
32-38kg:
Minimum Maint Dose: 250mg/day
Max Maint Dose: 350mg/day
>38kg:
Minimum Maint Dose: 250mg/day
Max Maint Dose: 400mg/day

Administer in 2 equally divided doses; refer to PI for titration instructions

≥10 Years:
Week 1: 25mg bid (am and pm)
Week 2: 50mg bid (am and pm)
Week 3: 75mg bid (am and pm)
Week 4: 100mg bid (am and pm)
Week 5: 150mg bid (am and pm)
Week 6 & Onward: 200mg bid (am and pm)

Adjunctive Therapy:
Partial Onset Seizure/Primary Generalized Tonic-Clonic Seizures/Lennox-Gastaut Syndrome:
2-16 Years:
Week 1: 1-3mg/kg/day (≤25mg/day) qpm

Titrate: Increase dose at 1- or 2-week intervals by increments of 1-3mg/kg/day (administered in 2 divided doses)
Usual: 5-9mg/kg/day in 2 divided doses

Migraine
Prophylaxis:
≥12 Years:
Week 1: 25mg qpm
Week 2: 25mg bid
Week 3: 25mg qam and 50mg qpm
Week 4 & Onward: 50mg bid

DOSING CONSIDERATIONS
Renal Impairment
CrCl <70mL/min: Administer 50% of usual adult dose
Patients Undergoing Hemodialysis: May require a supplemental dose

ADMINISTRATION
Oral route

Take w/o regard to meals.

Sprinkle Caps
May be swallowed whole or administered by carefully opening the cap and sprinkling entire contents on a small amount (tsp) of soft food; swallow drug/food mixture immediately and do not chew or store mixture for later use.

STORAGE
Protect from moisture. (Tab) 15-30°C (59-86°F). (Cap) ≤25°C (77°F).

HOW SUPPLIED
Cap: (Sprinkle) 15mg, 25mg; **Tab:** 25mg, 50mg, 100mg, 200mg

WARNINGS/PRECAUTIONS
Acute myopia associated with secondary angle-closure glaucoma reported; d/c immediately to reverse symptoms. Elevated IOP of any etiology may lead to serious adverse events (eg, permanent loss of vision) if left untreated. Visual field defects (independent of elevated IOP) reported; consider discontinuing therapy if visual problems occur. Oligohidrosis and hyperthermia reported, mostly in pediatric patients. Hyperchloremic, non-anion gap, metabolic acidosis reported; d/c or reduce dose if metabolic acidosis develops/persists. If decision is to continue therapy, consider alkali treatment. Conditions or therapies that predispose to acidosis (eg, renal disease, severe respiratory disorders, status epilepticus, diarrhea, ketogenic diet, specific drugs) may be additive to the bicarbonate lowering effects. Increased risk of suicidal thoughts/behavior. Cognitive-related dysfunction, psychiatric/behavioral disturbances, and somnolence or fatigue reported. May cause cleft lip and/or palate in infants if used during pregnancy. D/C gradually to minimize the potential for seizure or increased seizure frequency; appropriate monitoring is recommended when rapid withdrawal is required. Sudden unexplained deaths in epilepsy reported. Patients with inborn errors of metabolism or reduced hepatic mitochondrial activity may be at an increased risk for hyperammonemia with or without encephalopathy; consider hyperammonemic encephalopathy and measure ammonia levels in patients who develop unexplained lethargy, vomiting, or changes in mental status associated with therapy. Kidney stone formation reported; hydration is recommended to reduce new stone formation. Paresthesia may occur. Lab abnormalities may occur. Caution with renal/hepatic impairment and in elderly.

ADVERSE REACTIONS
Anorexia, anxiety, diarrhea, fatigue, fever, infection, weight decrease, cognitive problems, paresthesia, somnolence, taste perversion, mood problems, nausea, nervousness, confusion.

DRUG INTERACTIONS
Phenytoin or carbamazepine may decrease levels. Increase in systemic exposure of lithium observed following topiramate doses of ≤600mg/day; monitor lithium levels. May cause CNS depression and cognitive/neuropsychiatric adverse events with alcohol and other CNS depressants; use with extreme caution. May decrease contraceptive efficacy and increase breakthrough bleeding with combination oral contraceptives. Concurrent administration of valproic acid has been associated with hyperammonemia with or without encephalopathy, and hypothermia. Other carbonic anhydrase inhibitors (eg, zonisamide, acetazolamide, dichlorphenamide) may increase the severity of metabolic acidosis and may also increase the risk of kidney stone formation. Caution with agents that predispose patients to heat-related disorders (eg, carbonic anhydrase inhibitors, anticholinergics).

PREGNANCY AND LACTATION
Pregnancy: Category D.
Lactation: Caution in nursing.

MECHANISM OF ACTION
Sulfamate-substituted monosaccharide; not established. Suspected to block voltage-dependent Na⁺ channels, augment activity of the neurotransmitter gamma-aminobutyrate at some subtypes of the GABA-A receptor, antagonize the AMPA/kainate subtype of the glutamate receptor, and inhibit the carbonic anhydrase enzyme, particularly isoenzymes II and IV.

PHARMACOKINETICS
Absorption: Rapid. T_{max}=2 hrs (400mg). **Distribution:** Plasma protein binding (15-41%). **Metabolism:** Hydroxylation, hydrolysis, glucuronidation. **Elimination:** Urine (70% unchanged); $T_{1/2}$=21 hrs.

PATIENT CONSIDERATIONS
Assessment: Assess for renal/hepatic dysfunction, predisposing factors for metabolic acidosis, inborn errors of metabolism, reduced hepatic mitochondrial activity, pregnancy/nursing status, and possible drug interactions. Obtain baseline serum bicarbonate and blood ammonia levels.

Monitoring: Monitor for signs/symptoms of acute myopia, secondary angle-closure glaucoma, visual field defects, oligohidrosis, hyperthermia, cognitive or neuropsychiatric adverse reactions, kidney stones, renal dysfunction, metabolic acidosis, paresthesia, hyperammonemia, and other adverse reactions. Monitor serum bicarbonate and blood ammonia levels.

Counseling: Instruct to seek immediate medical attention if blurred vision, visual disturbances, periorbital pain, changes in mood/behavior, or suicidal thoughts/behavior occur and to closely monitor for decreased sweating or high/persistent fever. Warn about risk for metabolic acidosis. Advise to use caution when engaging in activities where loss of consciousness may result in serious danger. Inform about risk for hyperammonemia with or without encephalopathy; instruct to contact physician if unexplained lethargy, vomiting, or mental status changes develop. Instruct to maintain adequate fluid intake to minimize risk of kidney stones. Inform of pregnancy risks. Encourage to enroll in the North American Antiepileptic Drug Pregnancy Registry if patient becomes pregnant. Instruct that if a single dose is missed, to take that dose as soon as possible, skip it if cannot be taken at least 6 hrs before the next scheduled dose, and not to double the dose. Advise to contact physician if >1 dose is missed.

TOPICORT — desoximetasone   Rx
Class: Corticosteroid

ADULT DOSAGE	PEDIATRIC DOSAGE
Inflammatory and Pruritic Manifestations of Corticosteroid-Responsive Dermatoses	**Inflammatory and Pruritic Manifestations of Corticosteroid-Responsive Dermatoses**
Apply a thin film to affected area(s) bid and rub in gently	**Cre/Gel/0.05% Oint:** Apply a thin film to affected area(s) bid and rub in gently
	0.25% Oint: **≥10 Years:** Apply a thin film to affected area(s) bid and rub in gently

---

ADMINISTRATION
Topical route

STORAGE
Cre/Gel/0.05% Oint: 20-25°C (68-77°F); excursions permitted to 15-30°C (59-86°F). **0.25% Oint:** 15-30°C (59-86°F).

HOW SUPPLIED
Cre: 0.05%, 0.25% [15g, 30g, 60g, 100g]; **Gel:** 0.05% [15g, 30g, 60g]; **Oint:** 0.05% [15g, 30g, 60g, 100g], 0.25% [15g, 60g, 100g]

CONTRAINDICATIONS
History of hypersensitivity to any of the components of the medication.

WARNINGS/PRECAUTIONS
Not for oral, ophthalmic, or intravaginal use. May produce reversible hypothalamic-pituitary-adrenal (HPA) axis suppression w/ potential for clinical glucocorticosteroid insufficiency; periodically evaluate patient and when noted, gradually withdraw the drug, reduce the frequency of application, or substitute a less potent steroid. Caution w/ factors predisposing to HPA axis suppression (eg, use of more potent steroids, large surface areas, prolonged use, use under occlusion, altered skin barrier, liver failure). May produce Cushing's syndrome, hyperglycemia, and unmasking of latent diabetes mellitus (DM). Local adverse reactions (eg, atrophy, striae, irritation) may occur. Allergic contact dermatitis may occur; confirm by patch testing. Use appropriate antimicrobial agent w/ skin infections; d/c until infection has been adequately treated. Pediatric patients may be more susceptible to systemic toxicity. Limit administration to the least amount compatible w/ an effective therapeutic regimen in pediatric patients; chronic use may interfere w/ growth and development.

ADVERSE REACTIONS
Burning, itching, irritation, dryness, folliculitis, hypertrichosis, acneiform eruptions, hypopigmentation, perioral dermatitis, allergic contact dermatitis, skin maceration, secondary infection, skin atrophy, striae, miliaria.

DRUG INTERACTIONS
Use w/ other corticosteroid-containing products may increase exposure.

PREGNANCY AND LACTATION
Pregnancy: Category C; drugs of this class should not be used extensively on pregnant patients.
Lactation: It is not known whether topical administration could result in sufficient systemic absorption to produce detectable quantities in breast milk. Caution in nursing.

MECHANISM OF ACTION
Corticosteroid; not established. Has anti-inflammatory, antipruritic, and vasoconstrictive actions.

PHARMACOKINETICS
Distribution: Found in breast milk (systemically administered). **Metabolism:** Liver. **Elimination:** (Oint) Urine, feces. (Cre [0.25%, under occlusion]) Urine (4.1%), feces (1.1%); $T_{1/2}$=15 hrs (urine), 17 hrs (feces).

PATIENT CONSIDERATIONS
Assessment: Assess for predisposing factors to HPA axis suppression, skin infections, hypersensitivity to drug, pregnancy/nursing status, and possible drug interactions.

Monitoring: Monitor for HPA axis suppression, Cushing's syndrome, hyperglycemia, glucosuria, unmasking of latent DM, local adverse reactions, allergic contact dermatitis, development of infections, and other adverse reactions. Perform periodic monitoring of HPA axis suppression using adrenocorticotropic hormone stimulation test or urinary free cortisol test. Monitor for systemic toxicity (eg, adrenal suppression, intracranial HTN) in pediatric patients.

Counseling: Instruct to use externally ud, to avoid contact w/ the eyes, and not to use for any disorder other than prescribed. Advise not to bandage or occlude the treated skin area unless directed by physician. Instruct to report any signs of local adverse reactions to physician. Instruct not to use w/ other corticosteroid-containing products w/o first consulting w/ physician, to d/c therapy when control is achieved, and to contact physician if no improvement is seen w/in 4 weeks. Advise parents of pediatric patients not to use tight-fitting diapers or plastic pants on a child being treated in the diaper area.

TOPROL-XL — metoprolol succinate   Rx

Class: Selective beta₁ blocker

> Exacerbations of angina and MI reported following abrupt discontinuation. When discontinuing chronic therapy, particularly w/ ischemic heart disease, taper over 1-2 weeks w/ careful monitoring. If worsening of angina or acute coronary insufficiency develops, reinstate therapy promptly, at least temporarily, and take other appropriate measures. Caution patients against interruption or discontinuation of therapy w/o physician's advice.

ADULT DOSAGE	PEDIATRIC DOSAGE
Hypertension	**Hypertension**
Initial: 25-100mg qd	**≥6 Years:**
Titrate: May increase at weekly (or longer) intervals	**Initial:** 1mg/kg qd up to 50mg qd
Max: 400mg/day	**Titrate:** Adjust dose according to BP response
Angina Pectoris	**Max:** 2mg/kg (or up to 200mg) qd
Initial: 100mg qd	
Titrate: May gradually increase weekly	
Max: 400mg/day	
Reduce dose gradually over a period of 1-2 weeks if to be discontinued	
Heart Failure	
Initial:	
NYHA Class II HF: 25mg qd for 2 weeks	
Severe Heart Failure: 12.5mg qd for 2 weeks	
Titrate: Double dose every 2 weeks to the highest dose level tolerated	
Max: 200mg	
Dose should not be increased until symptoms of worsening HF have been stabilized.	
Reduce dose if experiencing symptomatic bradycardia.	

DOSING CONSIDERATIONS
Hepatic Impairment
May require lower initial dose; gradually increase dose to optimize therapy

Elderly
Start at low initial dose

ADMINISTRATION
Oral route

Tab may be divided; do not crush or chew whole or half tab.

STORAGE
25°C (77°F); excursions permitted to 15-30°C (59-86°F).

HOW SUPPLIED
Tab, Extended-Release: 25mg*, 50mg*, 100mg*, 200mg* *scored

CONTRAINDICATIONS
Severe bradycardia, 2nd- or 3rd-degree heart block, cardiogenic shock, decompensated cardiac failure, sick sinus syndrome (unless w/ a permanent pacemaker), hypersensitivity to any component of this product.

WARNINGS/PRECAUTIONS
Worsening cardiac failure may occur during up-titration; lower dose or temporarily d/c therapy. Avoid w/ bronchospastic disease; may be used only w/ those who do not respond to or cannot tolerate other antihypertensive treatment. If used in the setting of pheochromocytoma, should be given in combination w/ α-blockers, and only after α-blocker has been initiated; may cause a paradoxical increase in BP if administered alone. Avoid initiation of a high-dose regimen in patients undergoing noncardiac surgery. Chronically administered therapy should not be routinely withdrawn prior to major surgery; however, the impaired ability of the heart to respond to reflex adrenergic stimuli may augment the risks of general anesthesia and surgical procedures. May mask tachycardia occurring w/ hypoglycemia. May mask signs of hyperthyroidism (eg, tachycardia); abrupt withdrawal may precipitate thyroid storm. Patients w/ a history of severe anaphylactic reactions to variety of allergens may be more reactive to repeated challenge and may be unresponsive to usual doses of epinephrine. May precipitate or aggravate symptoms of arterial insufficiency w/ peripheral vascular disease (PVD). Caution w/ hepatic impairment and in elderly.

ADVERSE REACTIONS
Tiredness, dizziness, depression, diarrhea, SOB, bradycardia, rash.

DRUG INTERACTIONS
Additive effects w/ catecholamine-depleting drugs (eg, reserpine, MAOIs). CYP2D6 inhibitors (eg, quinidine, fluoxetine, propafenone) may increase levels. Caution when used w/ verapamil and diltiazem. May increase the risk of bradycardia w/ digitalis glycosides, clonidine, diltiazem, and verapamil. When given concomitantly w/ clonidine, d/c several days before clonidine is gradually withdrawn; may exacerbate rebound HTN.

PREGNANCY AND LACTATION
Pregnancy: Category C.
Lactation: Caution in nursing.

MECHANISM OF ACTION
β₁-selective adrenergic receptor blocker; not established. Proposed to decrease cardiac output, reduce sympathetic outflow to the periphery, and suppress renin activity.

PHARMACOKINETICS
Absorption: Rapid, complete. **Distribution:** Found in breast milk. **Metabolism:** Liver via CYP2D6. **Elimination:** Urine (<5% unchanged); $T_{1/2}$=3-7 hrs.

PATIENT CONSIDERATIONS
Assessment: Assess for severe bradycardia, 2nd- or 3rd-degree heart block, cardiogenic shock, decompensated cardiac failure, sick sinus syndrome, presence of pacemaker, ischemic heart disease, bronchospastic disease, diabetes, hyperthyroidism, PVD, hepatic impairment, pheochromocytoma, history of anaphylactic reactions, pregnancy/nursing status, and possible drug interactions.

Monitoring: Monitor for signs/symptoms of worsening cardiac failure during up-titration, hypoglycemia, precipitation of thyroid storm, precipitation/aggravation of arterial insufficiency in patients w/ PVD, anaphylactic reactions, and other adverse reactions. Monitor patients w/ ischemic heart disease.

Counseling: Advise to take drug regularly and continuously, ud, preferably w/ or immediately following meals. Counsel that if dose is missed, take only the next scheduled dose (w/o doubling). Instruct not to interrupt or d/c therapy w/o consulting physician. Advise to avoid operating automobiles and machinery or engaging in other tasks requiring alertness. Instruct to contact physician if any difficulty in breathing occurs. Instruct to inform physician or dentist of medication use before any type of surgery. Advise HF patients to consult physician if experience signs/symptoms of worsening HF.

TORSEMIDE — torsemide   Rx

Class: Loop diuretic

OTHER BRAND NAMES
Demadex

ADULT DOSAGE	PEDIATRIC DOSAGE
Edema	Pediatric use may not have been established
IV/PO:	
CHF:	
Initial: 10 or 20mg qd	
Titrate: Double dose until desired response is obtained	
Max Single Dose: 200mg	
Chronic Renal Failure:	
Initial: 20mg qd	
Titrate: Double dose until desired response is obtained	
Max Single Dose: 200mg	
Hepatic Cirrhosis:	
Initial: 5 or 10mg qd w/ an aldosterone antagonist or K⁺-sparing diuretic	
Titrate: Double dose until desired response is obtained	
Max Single Dose: 40mg	
Hypertension	
IV/PO:	
Initial: 5mg qd	
Titrate: May increase to 10mg qd after 4-6 weeks if BP reduction is inadequate	
An additional antihypertensive agent should be added to the treatment regimen if response to 10mg is insufficient	

DOSING CONSIDERATIONS
IV to PO Conversion
May switch to/from IV form w/ no change in dose

ADMINISTRATION
IV/Oral route

Inj
Administer either slowly as a bolus over 2 min or as continuous infusion.
Flush IV line w/ normal saline before and after administration.
Refer to PI for further administration instructions.

Compatibility
D5W
0.9% NaCl
0.45% NaCl

Tab
May be given at any time in relation to a meal.

STORAGE
(Inj) 20-25°C (68-77°F). Do not freeze. Continuous Infusion Sol: Stable for 24 hrs at room temperature in plastic containers. Refer to PI for IV fluids and concentrations. (Tab) 15-30°C (59-86°F).

HOW SUPPLIED
Inj: 10mg/mL [2mL, 5mL]; **Tab:** (Demadex) 5mg*, 10mg*, 20mg*, 100mg* *scored

CONTRAINDICATIONS
Known hypersensitivity to torsemide or to sulfonylureas, anuria.

WARNINGS/PRECAUTIONS
Caution in patients with hepatic disease with cirrhosis and ascites as sudden alterations of fluid/electrolyte balance may precipitate hepatic coma; diuresis is best initiated in a hospital. Tinnitus and hearing loss (usually reversible) reported. Excessive diuresis may cause dehydration, blood-volume reduction, and possible thrombosis and embolism, especially in elderly. Monitor for electrolyte imbalance, hypovolemia, or prerenal azotemia; d/c until situation is corrected and may restart at a lower dose, if signs/symptoms occur. Increased risk of hypokalemia with liver cirrhosis, brisk diuresis, and inadequate oral intake of electrolytes. Diuretic-induced hypokalemia may be a risk factor for the development of arrhythmias in patients with cardiovascular disease (CVD), especially with concomitant digitalis glycosides. Hyperglycemia, hypomagnesemia, hypercalcemia, and symptomatic gout reported. May increase BUN, SrCr, serum uric acid, total cholesterol, and TGs. Associated with small decreases in Hgb, Hct, erythrocyte count, and small increases in WBC count, platelet count, and alkaline phosphatase.

ADVERSE REACTIONS
Headache, excessive urination, dizziness, hypotension, chest pain, A-fib, diarrhea, GI hemorrhage, rectal bleeding, rash, shunt thrombosis, syncope, ventricular tachycardia, hyperglycemia, hyperuricemia.

DRUG INTERACTIONS
Reduced renal clearance and increased levels of spironolactone. Salicylate toxicity may occur with concomitant high-dose salicylates. Possible renal dysfunction with NSAIDs (including aspirin). Indomethacin partially inhibits natriuretic effect. Digoxin may increase exposure by 50%. Simultaneous administration with cholestyramine is not recommended. Probenecid may decrease diuretic activity. Caution with lithium; high risk of lithium toxicity. Increased ototoxic potential of aminoglycoside antibiotics and ethacrynic acid reported, especially in the presence of renal impairment. Increased risk of hypokalemia with adrenocorticotropic hormone or corticosteroids.

PREGNANCY AND LACTATION
Pregnancy: Category B.
Lactation: Caution in nursing.

MECHANISM OF ACTION
Loop diuretic; acts from within the lumen of the thick ascending limb of loop of Henle, inhibiting $Na^+/K^+/2Cl^-$-carrier system.

PHARMACOKINETICS
Absorption: (Tab) Bioavailability (80%); T_{max}=1 hr. **Distribution:** V_d=12-15L; plasma protein binding (>99%). **Metabolism:** Liver; carboxylic acid derivative (major metabolite). **Elimination:** Urine (20%); $T_{1/2}$=3.5 hrs.

PATIENT CONSIDERATIONS
Assessment: Assess for history of hypersensitivity to the drug or to sulfonylureas, anuria, CVD, renal/hepatic impairment, pregnancy/nursing status, and possible drug interactions.

Monitoring: Monitor for hypovolemia, prerenal azotemia, tinnitus, hearing loss, hypersensitivity reactions, renal/hepatic impairment, arrhythmias in patients with CVD, and other adverse reactions. Monitor serum electrolytes periodically.

Counseling: Inform of risks and benefits of therapy. Advise to seek medical attention if symptoms of hypokalemia, fluid/electrolyte imbalance, hypersensitivity reactions, hearing loss, or tinnitus occur.

TOUJEO — insulin glargine   Rx

Class: Insulin (long-acting)

ADULT DOSAGE

Type 1 Diabetes Mellitus
Initial:

Insulin-Naive Patients:
Approx 1/3 to 1/2 of the total daily insulin dose; 0.2-0.4 U/kg can be used to calculate the initial total daily insulin dose
Give the remainder of the total daily insulin dose as a short-acting insulin and divide between each daily meal

Changing from QD Long-Acting or Intermediate-Acting Insulin:
Can be the same as the qd long-acting dose

PEDIATRIC DOSAGE
Pediatric use may not have been established

For patients controlled on Lantus (insulin glargine, 100 U/mL), expect that a higher daily dose of Toujeo will be needed to maintain the same level of glycemic control

Changing from BID NPH Insulin:
80% of the total daily NPH dosage

Titrate: Based on individual's metabolic needs, blood glucose monitoring results, and glycemic control goal; titrate dose no more frequently than every 3-4 days
Range: 1-80 U/inj

Type 2 Diabetes Mellitus
Initial:

Insulin-Naive Patients:
0.2 U/kg qd

Changing from QD Long-Acting or Intermediate-Acting Insulin:
Can be the same as the qd long-acting dose
For patients controlled on Lantus (insulin glargine, 100 U/mL), expect that a higher daily dose of Toujeo will be needed to maintain the same level of glycemic control

Changing from BID NPH Insulin:
80% of the total daily NPH dosage

Titrate: Based on individual's metabolic needs, blood glucose monitoring results, and glycemic control goal; titrate dose no more frequently than every 3-4 days
Range: 1-80 U/inj

DOSING CONSIDERATIONS
Concomitant Medications
Dosage of other antidiabetic drugs may need to be adjusted when starting Toujeo in patients w/ type 2 diabetes

Elderly
Dose conservatively

Other Important Considerations
Dosage adjustments may be needed w/ changes in physical activity, changes in meal patterns (eg, macronutrient content, timing of food intake), changes in renal/hepatic function, or during acute illness

ADMINISTRATION
SQ route

Do not administer IV, IM, or in an insulin pump.
Inject qd into the abdominal area, thigh, or deltoid at the same time each day.
Rotate inj sites w/in the same region from 1 inj to the next.
Do not dilute or mix w/ any other insulin products or sol.
Patients should follow the directions provided in the "Instructions for Use" to correctly use the pen device and administer the drug.

STORAGE
Do not freeze; discard if prefilled pen has been frozen. **Unopened:** 2-8°C (36-46°F) until expiration date. **Opened:** <30°C (86°F). Do not refrigerate. Protect from direct heat and light. Discard after 42 days.

HOW SUPPLIED
Inj: 300 U/mL [1.5mL]

CONTRAINDICATIONS
During episodes of hypoglycemia, hypersensitivity to insulin glargine or one of its excipients.

WARNINGS/PRECAUTIONS
Not recommended for the treatment of diabetic ketoacidosis. Never share pen between patients, even if the needle is changed; poses risk for transmission of blood-borne pathogens. Changes in insulin strength, manufacturer, type, or method of administration may affect glycemic control and predispose to hypo/hyperglycemia; these changes should be made cautiously and only under close medical supervision, and the frequency of blood glucose monitoring should be increased. In type 1 diabetes patients treated w/ IV insulin, consider the longer onset of action of insulin glargine before stopping IV insulin. The full glucose lowering effect may not be apparent for at least 5 days. Hypoglycemia may occur and may impair concentration ability and reaction time. Symptomatic awareness of hypoglycemia may be less pronounced in patients w/ longstanding diabetes, diabetic nerve disease, on medications that block the sympathetic nervous system, or in patients who experience recurrent hypoglycemia. Accidental mix-ups between basal insulin products and other insulins, particularly rapid-acting insulins, reported. Severe, life-threatening, generalized allergy, including anaphylaxis, may occur. If hypersensitivity reactions occur, d/c therapy; treat per standard of care and monitor until signs/symptoms resolve. May cause hypokalemia; caution in patients at risk for hypokalemia (eg, patients using K^+-lowering medications or medications sensitive to serum K^+ concentrations). Caution in elderly and in patients w/ renal or hepatic impairment.

ADVERSE REACTIONS
Nasopharyngitis, URTI, hypoglycemia.

DRUG INTERACTIONS

See Dosing Considerations. Dose adjustment and increased frequency of glucose monitoring may be required w/ drugs that may increase the risk of hypoglycemia (eg, ACE inhibitors, ARBs, disopyramide, fibrates, fluoxetine, MAOIs, pentoxifylline, pramlintide, propoxyphene, salicylates, somatostatin analogues [eg, octreotide], sulfonamide antibiotics), drugs that may decrease blood glucose-lowering effect (eg, atypical antipsychotics [eg, olanzapine, clozapine], corticosteroids, danazol, diuretics, estrogens, glucagon, isoniazid, niacin, oral contraceptives, phenothiazines, progestogens [eg, in oral contraceptives], protease inhibitors, somatropin, sympathomimetic agents [eg, albuterol, epinephrine, terbutaline], thyroid hormones), or drugs that may increase/decrease blood glucose-lowering effect (eg, alcohol, β-blockers, clonidine, lithium salts, pentamidine). Signs/symptoms of hypoglycemia may be blunted w/ β-blockers, clonidine, guanethidine, or reserpine. Observe for signs/symptoms of heart failure (HF) if treated concomitantly w/ a peroxisome proliferator-activated receptor (PPAR)-gamma agonist (eg, thiazolidinedione); consider discontinuation or dose reduction of the PPAR-gamma agonist if HF develops.

PREGNANCY AND LACTATION

Pregnancy: Use has not been studied in pregnant women; use during pregnancy only if potential benefit justifies potential risk to the fetus.
Lactation: It is not known if insulin glargine is excreted in human milk; caution in nursing. Use is compatible w/ breastfeeding, but women may require adjustments of insulin doses.

MECHANISM OF ACTION

Insulin glargine; regulates glucose metabolism. Lowers blood glucose by stimulating peripheral glucose uptake and by inhibiting hepatic glucose production. Inhibits lipolysis and proteolysis, and enhances protein synthesis.

PHARMACOKINETICS

Absorption: T_{max} (median)=12 hrs (0.4 U/kg dose, 0.6 U/kg dose), 16 hrs (0.9 U/kg dose). **Metabolism:** M1 (21A-Gly-insulin) and M2 (21A-Gly-des-30B-Thr-insulin) (active metabolites).

PATIENT CONSIDERATIONS

Assessment: Assess for hypoglycemia, diabetic ketoacidosis, predisposition to hypo/hyperglycemia, risk factors for hypokalemia, hypersensitivity, renal/hepatic impairment, pregnancy/nursing status, and possible drug interactions. Obtain baseline blood glucose and HbA1c levels.

Monitoring: Monitor for signs/symptoms of hypoglycemia, hypersensitivity/allergic reactions, and other adverse reactions. Monitor for changes in physical activity, changes in meal patterns, changes in renal/hepatic function, or acute illness. Monitor blood glucose and HbA1c levels; increase frequency of blood glucose monitoring in patients at higher risk for hypoglycemia and in those w/ reduced symptomatic awareness of hypoglycemia. Monitor K⁺ levels in patients at risk for hypokalemia if indicated.

Counseling: Inform of the risks/benefits of therapy. Advise to never share SoloStar pen w/ another person, even if needle is changed. Inform of the symptoms of hypoglycemia, including impairment of the ability to concentrate and react; advise to use caution when driving/operating machinery. Inform that if change from other basal insulins to insulin glargine, may experience higher average FPG levels in the 1st weeks of therapy; advise to monitor glucose daily when initiating therapy. Instruct to always check the label before each inj to avoid medication errors. Inform that the dose counter of SoloStar pen shows the number of units of therapy to be injected and that no dose recalculation is required. Instruct not to reuse needles and to never use a syringe to remove drug from SoloStar pen if it malfunctions. Instruct on self-management procedures, including glucose monitoring, proper inj technique, management of hypo/hyperglycemia, and on handling of special situations (eg, intercurrent conditions, inadequate or skipped dose, inadvertent administration of increased insulin dose, inadequate food intake, skipped meals). Advise to inform physician if pregnant or contemplating pregnancy.

TOVIAZ — fesoterodine fumarate   Rx

Class: Muscarinic antagonist

ADULT DOSAGE	**PEDIATRIC DOSAGE**
Overactive Bladder	Pediatric use may not have been established
Initial: 4mg qd	
Titrate: May increase to 8mg qd based on individual response and tolerability	

- -

DOSING CONSIDERATIONS

Concomitant Medications
Strong CYP3A4 Inhibitors:
Max: 4mg/day

Renal Impairment
CrCl <30mL/min:
Max: 4mg/day

ADMINISTRATION

Oral route

Take w/ or w/o food.
Take tab w/ liquid and swallow whole; do not crush, chew, or divide.

STORAGE

20-25°C (68-77°F); excursions permitted between 15-30°C (59-86°F). Protect from moisture.

HOW SUPPLIED

Tab, Extended-Release (ER): 4mg, 8mg

CONTRAINDICATIONS

Urinary/gastric retention; uncontrolled narrow-angle glaucoma; known hypersensitivity to the drug or its ingredients, or to tolterodine tartrate tabs or ER caps.

WARNINGS/PRECAUTIONS

Not recommended with severe hepatic impairment (Child-Pugh C). Angioedema of the face, lips, tongue, and/or larynx reported; d/c and promptly provide appropriate therapy if angioedema occurs. Risk of urinary retention; caution with clinically significant bladder outlet obstruction. Caution with decreased GI motility (eg, severe constipation), controlled narrow-angle glaucoma, and myasthenia gravis. CNS anticholinergic effects (eg, headache, dizziness, somnolence) reported; monitor for signs, particularly after beginning treatment or increasing the dose, and consider dose reduction or discontinuation if such effects occur.

ADVERSE REACTIONS

Dry mouth, constipation, urinary tract infection, dry eyes.

DRUG INTERACTIONS

May increase the frequency and/or severity of dry mouth, constipation, urinary retention, and other anticholinergic pharmacologic effects with other antimuscarinic agents that produce such effects. May potentially alter the absorption of some concomitantly administered drugs due to anticholinergic effects on GI motility. CYP3A4 inhibitors may increase levels; doses >4mg are not recommended in patients taking potent CYP3A4 inhibitors (eg, ketoconazole, itraconazole, clarithromycin). CYP2D6 inhibitors may increase levels. Rifampin or rifampicin may decrease levels.

PREGNANCY AND LACTATION

Pregnancy: Category C.
Lactation: Caution in nursing.

MECHANISM OF ACTION

Muscarinic receptor antagonist; inhibits muscarinic receptors, which mediate contractions of urinary bladder smooth muscle and stimulation of salivary secretion.

PHARMACOKINETICS

Absorption: Well-absorbed. Bioavailability (52%, 5-hydroxymethyl tolterodine [5-HMT]); T_{max}=5 hrs (5-HMT). Variable doses resulted in different pharmacokinetic parameters in extensive and poor CYP2D6 metabolizers. **Distribution:** Plasma protein binding (50%, 5-HMT); V_d=169L (IV, 5-HMT). **Metabolism:** Rapid and extensive via hydrolysis; 5-HMT (active metabolite). 5-HMT further metabolized in liver via CYP2D6 and CYP3A4. **Elimination:** Urine (70%; 16%, 5-HMT), feces (7%); $T_{1/2}$=7 hrs (5-HMT).

PATIENT CONSIDERATIONS

Assessment: Assess for hypersensitivity to the drug or tolterodine tartrate, urinary/gastric retention, narrow-angle glaucoma, bladder outlet obstruction, decreased GI motility, severe constipation, myasthenia gravis, severe hepatic/renal impairment, pregnancy/nursing status, and possible drug interactions.

Monitoring: Monitor for angioedema, upper airway swelling, urinary retention, CNS anticholinergic effects, and other adverse reactions.

Counseling: Inform that therapy may produce angioedema; instruct to promptly d/c therapy and seek immediate medical attention if edema of the tongue/laryngopharynx or difficulty in breathing occurs. Counsel that therapy may produce clinically significant adverse effects (eg, constipation, urinary retention). Inform that blurred vision may occur; advise to exercise caution in decisions to engage in potentially dangerous activities until effects have been determined. Inform that heat prostration (due to decreased sweating) may occur when used in a hot environment. Inform that alcohol may enhance drowsiness caused by therapy.

TRACLEER — bosentan   Rx

Class: Endothelin receptor antagonist

> Available only through a restricted program called the Tracleer REMS Program, a component of the Tracleer Risk Evaluation and Mitigation Strategy (REMS); prescribers, patients, and pharmacies must enroll in the program. Elevation of liver aminotransferases (ALT and AST) and bilirubin reported; measure serum aminotransferase levels prior to initiation of treatment and then monthly. Hepatic cirrhosis (after prolonged therapy in patients w/ multiple comorbidities and drug therapies) and liver failure reported. Avoid w/ elevated aminotransferases (>3X ULN) at baseline; d/c if liver aminotransferase elevations are accompanied by clinical symptoms of hepatotoxicity (eg, N/V, fever, jaundice) or increases in bilirubin ≥2X ULN. Likely to cause major birth defects if used during pregnancy; exclude pregnancy before start of treatment. Throughout treatment, and for 1 month after discontinuing, females of reproductive potential must use 2 reliable methods of contraception unless the patient has an IUD or tubal sterilization, in which case, no other contraception is needed. Hormonal contraceptives, including oral, injectable, transdermal, and implantable contraceptives, may not be effective in patients receiving bosentan; do not use as the sole means of contraception. Obtain monthly pregnancy tests.

ADULT DOSAGE	**PEDIATRIC DOSAGE**
Pulmonary Arterial Hypertension	Pediatric use may not have been established
Treatment of pulmonary arterial HTN (WHO Group 1) to improve exercise ability and to decrease clinical worsening	
Initial: 62.5mg bid (in am and pm) for 4 weeks	
Maint/Max: 125mg bid	

Low Body Weight:
<40kg and >12 Years:
Initial/Maint: 62.5mg bid
There is limited information about the safety and efficacy of therapy in children between 12-18 yrs of age

DOSING CONSIDERATIONS
Concomitant Medications
Patients on Ritonavir for at Least 10 Days:
Initial: 62.5mg qd or qod based on individual tolerability

Adding Ritonavir:
D/C bosentan at least 36 hrs prior to initiation of ritonavir.
After at least 10 days following initiation of ritonavir, resume therapy at 62.5mg qd or qod based on individual tolerability.

Hepatic Impairment
Preexisting Impairment:
Moderate/Severe: Not recommended
Aminotransferases >3X ULN: Not recommended

Development of Aminotransferase Elevations:
D/C treatment if aminotransferase elevations are accompanied by clinical symptoms of hepatotoxicity (eg, N/V, abdominal pain, jaundice) or increases in bilirubin ≥2X ULN

ALT/AST >3 and ≤5X ULN:
Confirm by another aminotransferase test; if confirmed, reduce daily dose to 62.5mg bid or interrupt treatment. Monitor aminotransferase levels at least every 2 weeks thereafter.
If the aminotransferase levels return to pretreatment values, continue/reintroduce the treatment as appropriate. Reintroduce at the starting dose and check aminotransferase levels w/in 3 days and every 2 weeks thereafter.

ALT/AST >5 and ≤8X ULN:
Confirm by another aminotransferase test; if confirmed, stop treatment and monitor aminotransferase levels at least every 2 weeks thereafter.
Once aminotransferase levels return to pretreatment values, consider reintroduction of treatment. Reintroduce at the starting dose and check aminotransferase levels w/in 3 days and every 2 weeks thereafter.

ALT/AST >8X ULN:
D/C treatment; reintroduction of treatment should not be considered

Discontinuation
Consider gradual dose reduction (62.5mg bid for 3-7 days)

ADMINISTRATION
Oral route

Take w/ or w/o food.

STORAGE
20-25°C (68-77°F); excursions permitted to 15-30°C (59-86°F).

HOW SUPPLIED
Tab: 62.5mg, 125mg

CONTRAINDICATIONS
Females who are or may become pregnant. Coadministration w/ cyclosporine A or w/ glyburide. Hypersensitivity to bosentan or any component of product.

WARNINGS/PRECAUTIONS
Not recommended w/ moderate or severe liver impairment. Fluid retention and peripheral edema reported. If clinically significant fluid retention develops, evaluate further to determine cause and possible need for treatment or discontinuation of therapy. If signs of pulmonary edema occur, consider possibility of associated pulmonary veno-occlusive disease (PVOD) and consider discontinuing therapy. Decreased sperm counts reported. May cause a dose-related decrease in Hgb and Hct; check Hgb concentrations after 1 and 3 months, and every 3 months thereafter.

ADVERSE REACTIONS
Respiratory tract infection, headache, edema, chest pain, syncope, flushing, hypotension, sinusitis, arthralgia, abnormal serum aminotransferases, palpitations, anemia.

DRUG INTERACTIONS
See Boxed Warning, Contraindications, and Dosing Considerations.
Coadministration w/ both a CYP2C9 inhibitor (eg, fluconazole, amiodarone) and a strong CYP3A inhibitor (eg, ketoconazole, itraconazole) or a moderate CYP3A inhibitor (eg, amprenavir, erythromycin, fluconazole) may largely increase levels; coadministration of such combinations is not recommended. Increased levels w/ ketoconazole; increased effects of bosentan should be considered. May decrease levels of CYP3A/CYP2C9 substrates; estrogens and progestins in hormonal contraceptives; oral hypoglycemic agents predominantly metabolized by CYP2C9/CYP3A; simvastatin and other statins significantly metabolized by CYP3A (eg, lovastatin, atorvastatin); S-warfarin (a CYP2C9 substrate) and R-warfarin (a CYP3A substrate); and sildenafil. Monitor cholesterol levels after bosentan is initiated in patients using CYP3A-metabolized statins to see whether the statin dose needs adjustment. Increased trough levels w/ lopinavir/ritonavir; adjust dose of bosentan when initiating lopinavir/ritonavir. Rifampin may increase trough levels after 1st concomitant dose, but decrease levels at steady-state; measure serum aminotransferases weekly for first 4 weeks before reverting to normal monitoring. Caution w/ tacrolimus. Increased levels w/ sildenafil.

PREGNANCY AND LACTATION
Pregnancy: Category X. Females of reproductive potential should have a negative pregnancy test before treatment initiation; a urine or serum pregnancy test should be performed during the first 5 days of a normal menstrual period and at least 11 days after the last unprotected act of sexual intercourse. Obtain follow-up urine or serum pregnancy tests monthly in females of reproductive potential. Females of reproductive potential must use acceptable methods of contraception during treatment and for 1 month after treatment; patient must choose 1 highly effective form of contraception (IUD or tubal sterilization) or a combination of methods (hormone method w/ a barrier method or 2 barrier methods). If partner's vasectomy is chosen, a hormone or barrier method must be used along w/ this method.
Lactation: Not for use in nursing.

MECHANISM OF ACTION
Endothelin receptor antagonist; specific and competitive antagonist at endothelin receptor types ET_A and ET_B w/ slightly higher affinity for ET_A receptors than ET_B receptors.

PHARMACOKINETICS
Absorption: Absolute bioavailability (50%); T_{max}=3-5 hrs. **Distribution:** V_d=18L; plasma protein binding (>98%). **Metabolism:** Liver via CYP2C9 and CYP3A. **Elimination:** Biliary, urine (<3%); $T_{1/2}$=5 hrs.

PATIENT CONSIDERATIONS
Assessment: Assess for liver impairment, hypersensitivity, pregnancy/nursing status, and possible drug interactions. Obtain baseline serum aminotransferase levels.
Monitoring: Monitor for clinical symptoms of hepatotoxicity, increases in bilirubin ≥2X ULN, fluid retention, signs of pulmonary edema, PVOD, and other adverse reactions. Monitor serum aminotransferase levels monthly. Obtain monthly pregnancy tests. Check Hgb concentrations after 1 and 3 months of therapy and then every 3 months thereafter.
Counseling: Advise that drug is only available through a restricted access program called the Tracleer REMS Program and from specialty pharmacies enrolled in the Tracleer REMS Program. Inform of hepatotoxicity risk; discuss the requirement for monthly monitoring of serum aminotransferases. Inform that drug may cause serious birth defects if used by pregnant women. Inform females of reproductive potential to have monthly pregnancy tests and to use 2 reliable methods of contraception during and for 1 month after treatment discontinuation. Inform females who have an IUD or tubal sterilization that they can use these forms of contraception alone. Instruct to immediately contact physician if pregnancy is suspected. Educate regarding use of emergency contraception in the event of unprotected sex or contraceptive failure. Advise prepubertal females to report changes in reproductive status to prescriber. Inform that patient must sign the Tracleer Patient Enrollment and Consent Form to confirm the patient's understanding of the risks. Inform of other risks associated w/ therapy (eg, decreases in Hgb, Hct, and sperm count; fluid retention). Advise of the importance of Hgb testing.

TRADJENTA — linagliptin   Rx

Class: Dipeptidyl peptidase-4 (DPP-4) inhibitor

ADULT DOSAGE	PEDIATRIC DOSAGE
Type 2 Diabetes Mellitus	Pediatric use may not have been established
5mg qd	

DOSING CONSIDERATIONS
Concomitant Medications
W/ Insulin Secretagogue (eg, Sulfonylurea)/Insulin:
May require lower dose of insulin secretagogue or insulin

ADMINISTRATION
Oral route

Take w/ or w/o food.

STORAGE
25°C (77°F); excursions permitted to 15-30°C (59-86°F).

HOW SUPPLIED
Tab: 5mg

CONTRAINDICATIONS
History of a hypersensitivity reaction to linagliptin (eg, anaphylaxis, angioedema, exfoliative skin conditions, urticaria, or bronchial hyperreactivity).

WARNINGS/PRECAUTIONS
Not for use in patients w/ type 1 diabetes mellitus (DM) or for the treatment of diabetic ketoacidosis. Acute pancreatitis reported; d/c if pancreatitis is suspected. Serious hypersensitivity reactions reported; if suspected, d/c therapy, assess for other potential causes for the event, and institute alternative treatment for diabetes. Caution in patients w/ a history of angioedema w/ another DPP-4 inhibitor. Severe and disabling arthralgia reported in patients taking DPP-4 inhibitors. Consider as a possible cause for severe joint pain and d/c therapy if appropriate.

ADVERSE REACTIONS
Hypoglycemia, nasopharyngitis, diarrhea.

DRUG INTERACTIONS
See Dosing Considerations. Strong inducers of P-gp or CYP3A4 (eg, rifampin) may reduce efficacy; use of alternative treatments is strongly recommended.

PREGNANCY AND LACTATION
Pregnancy: Category B.
Lactation: Caution in nursing.

MECHANISM OF ACTION
DPP-4 inhibitor; increases the concentrations of active incretin hormones, stimulating the release of insulin in a glucose-dependent manner, and decreasing glucagon levels in the circulation.

PHARMACOKINETICS

Absorption: Absolute bioavailability (approx 30%); C_{max}=8.9nmol/L, T_{max}=1.5 hrs, AUC=139nmol•hr/L. **Distribution:** (IV) V_d=approx 1110L; plasma protein binding (concentration-dependent). **Elimination:** Enterohepatic (80%), urine (5%); $T_{1/2}$=12 hrs (effective), >100 hrs (terminal).

PATIENT CONSIDERATIONS

Assessment: Assess for history of hypersensitivity, type of DM, diabetic ketoacidosis, history of pancreatitis, history of angioedema w/ another DPP-4 inhibitor, pregnancy/nursing status, and possible drug interactions. Obtain baseline FPG and HbA1c levels.

Monitoring: Monitor for pancreatitis, arthralgia, hypersensitivity reactions, and other adverse reactions. Monitor FPG and HbA1c levels periodically.

Counseling: Inform of the potential risks/benefits and alternative modes of therapy. Advise on the importance of adherence to dietary instructions, regular physical activity, periodic blood glucose monitoring and HbA1c testing, recognition/management of hypo/hyperglycemia, and assessment for diabetes complications. Instruct to seek medical advice promptly during periods of stress as medication requirements may change. Inform that acute pancreatitis and serious allergic reactions reported; instruct to d/c use and notify physician if signs and symptoms of pancreatitis or allergic reactions occur. Inform that severe and disabling joint pain may occur w/ this class of drugs; instruct to seek medical advice if severe joint pain occurs. Instruct to take as prescribed. Instruct to inform physician or pharmacist if any unusual symptom develops, or if any known symptom persists or worsens.

TRANSDERM SCOP — scopolamine   Rx

Class: Anticholinergic

ADULT DOSAGE	PEDIATRIC DOSAGE
Motion Sickness	Pediatric use may not have been established
Prevention of N/V:	
1 patch at least 4 hrs before the antiemetic effect is required. Replace patch after 3 days if therapy is required for >3 days.	
Postoperative Nausea/Vomiting	
Prevention of N/V Associated w/ Recovery from Anesthesia and/or Opiate Analgesia and Surgery:	
1 patch on the pm before surgery or 1 hr prior to cesarean section. Remove patch 24 hrs following surgery.	

ADMINISTRATION

Transdermal route

Apply only to skin in the postauricular area.
After application, wash hands thoroughly w/ soap and water and dry.
Wear only 1 patch at any time.
Do not cut patch.
Discard patch if displaced and replace w/ a fresh patch.

STORAGE

20-25°C (68-77°F).

HOW SUPPLIED

Patch: 1.5mg [4^s]

CONTRAINDICATIONS

Angle-closure glaucoma, hypersensitivity to scopolamine or other belladonna alkaloids or to any ingredient/component in the formulation or delivery system.

WARNINGS/PRECAUTIONS

May increase IOP with open-angle glaucoma; monitor therapy and adjust during use. May cause temporary dilation of pupils and blurred vision if contact with eyes occurs. Caution with pyloric obstruction, urinary bladder neck obstruction, and intestinal obstruction. May aggravate seizures or psychosis. Idiosyncratic reactions may occur with ordinary therapeutic doses. Increased CNS effects may occur in elderly and with hepatic/renal impairment. May impair physical/mental abilities. Remove patch before undergoing a MRI scan; skin burns at the patch site reported. May interfere with gastric secretion test.

ADVERSE REACTIONS

Dry mouth, dizziness, somnolence, urinary retention, agitation, visual impairment, confusion, mydriasis, pharyngitis.

DRUG INTERACTIONS

May decrease absorption of oral medications due to decreased gastric motility and delayed gastric emptying. Caution with other drugs with CNS effects (eg, sedatives, tranquilizers, alcohol) and anticholinergic properties (eg, meclizine, TCAs, muscle relaxants).

PREGNANCY AND LACTATION

Pregnancy: Category C.
Lactation: Caution in nursing.

MECHANISM OF ACTION

Anticholinergic agent; acts as competitive inhibitor at postganglionic muscarinic receptor sites of parasympathetic nervous system and on smooth muscles that respond to acetylcholine but lack cholinergic innervation. Acts in the CNS by blocking cholinergic transmission from vestibular nuclei to higher centers in the CNS and from reticular formation to the vomiting center.

PHARMACOKINETICS

Absorption: Well-absorbed. T_{max}=24 hrs. **Distribution:** Crosses placenta; found in breast milk. **Metabolism:** Extensive; conjugation. **Elimination:** Urine (<10%, <5% unchanged); $T_{1/2}$=9.5 hrs.

PATIENT CONSIDERATIONS

Assessment: Assess for known hypersensitivity to the drug, glaucoma, pyloric obstruction, urinary bladder neck obstruction, intestinal obstruction, history of seizures or psychosis, hepatic/renal impairment, pregnancy/nursing status, and for possible drug interactions.

Monitoring: Monitor for aggravation of seizures or psychosis, idiosyncratic reactions (eg, agitation, hallucinations, paranoid behaviors, delusions), CNS effects, drowsiness, disorientation, confusion, withdrawal symptoms, and other adverse reactions. Monitor IOP in patients with open-angle glaucoma.

Counseling: Inform elderly that patch may cause a greater likelihood of CNS effects and to seek medical care if patient becomes confused, disoriented, or dizzy while wearing the patch or after removing. Inform that patch may cause drowsiness, disorientation, and confusion; advise to use caution when engaging in activities that require mental alertness. Instruct to avoid alcohol. Instruct to seek medical care if withdrawal symptoms occur following abrupt discontinuation. Inform that patch may cause temporary dilation of pupils and blurred vision. Instruct to wash hands thoroughly with soap and water immediately after handling patch. Instruct to dispose the patch properly to avoid contact with children or pets. Advise to remove patch before undergoing an MRI to avoid skin burns. Instruct to use ud. Advise to remove the patch immediately and promptly contact physician if symptoms of acute angle-closure glaucoma or difficulty in urinating is experienced.

TRANXENE — clorazepate dipotassium   CIV

Class: Benzodiazepine

ADULT DOSAGE	PEDIATRIC DOSAGE
Anxiety Disorders	**Partial Seizures**
Management or Short-Term Relief:	**Adjunctive Therapy:**
Usual: 30mg/day in divided doses	**9-12 Years:**
Titrate: May adjust gradually w/in the range of 15-60mg/day	**Max Initial:** 7.5mg bid
	Titrate: Increase by no more than 7.5mg/week
When administered as a single daily dose hs, initial dose is 15mg; may require dosage adjustment	**Max:** 60mg/day
Alcohol Withdrawal	**>12 Years:**
Symptomatic Relief of Acute Withdrawal:	**Max Initial:** 7.5mg tid
Day 1: 30mg initially, then 30-60mg in divided doses	**Titrate:** Increase by no more than 7.5mg/week
Day 2: 45-90mg in divided doses	**Max:** 90mg/day
Day 3: 22.5-45mg in divided doses	
Day 4: 15-30mg in divided doses	
Titrate: Gradually reduce dose to 7.5-15mg/day; d/c when stable	
Max: 90mg/day	
Partial Seizures	
Adjunctive Therapy:	
Max Initial: 7.5mg tid	
Titrate: Increase by no more than 7.5mg/week	
Max: 90mg/day	

DOSING CONSIDERATIONS

Elderly
Elderly/Debilitated:
Anxiety:
Initial: 7.5-15mg/day

ADMINISTRATION

Oral route

STORAGE

20-25°C (68-77°F). Protect from moisture.

HOW SUPPLIED

Tab: 3.75mg*, 7.5mg*, 15mg* *scored

CONTRAINDICATIONS

Known hypersensitivity to the drug, acute narrow-angle glaucoma.

WARNINGS/PRECAUTIONS

Avoid w/ depressive neuroses or psychotic reactions. May impair mental/physical abilities. Withdrawal symptoms (eg, delirium, tremors, abdominal and muscle cramps, insomnia, irritability, memory impairment) may occur following abrupt discontinuation; taper gradually following extended therapy. Caution w/ known drug dependency or renal/hepatic impairment. May increase the risk of suicidal thoughts and behavior; monitor for emergence or worsening of depression, suicidal thoughts or behavior, and/or any unusual changes in mood or behavior. Suicidal tendencies may be present in patients who have depression along w/ anxiety; least amount of drug that is feasible should be available to such patients.

Caution in elderly/debilitated; dose adjustments should be made slowly to preclude ataxia or excessive sedation.

ADVERSE REACTIONS
Drowsiness, dizziness, GI complaints, nervousness, blurred vision, dry mouth, headache, mental confusion.

DRUG INTERACTIONS
Additive CNS depression w/ CNS depressants, and alcohol. Barbiturates, narcotics, phenothiazines, MAOIs, and other antidepressants may potentiate the actions of the benzodiazepines. Increased sedation w/ hypnotics.

PREGNANCY AND LACTATION
Pregnancy: An increased risk of congenital malformation associated w/ the use of minor tranquilizers (eg, chlordiazepoxide, diazepam, meprobamate) during the 1st trimester of pregnancy has been suggested in several studies. Clorazepate has not been studied adequately to determine the risk of fetal abnormality; its use during pregnancy should almost always be avoided. **Lactation:** Not for use in nursing.

MECHANISM OF ACTION
Benzodiazepine; antianxiety/hypnotic agent that has CNS depressant effects.

PHARMACOKINETICS
Distribution: (Nordiazepam) Found in breast milk; plasma protein binding (97-98%). **Metabolism:** Liver; rapidly decarboxylated to nordiazepam (primary metabolite); hydroxylation. **Elimination:** Urine (62-67%), feces (15-19%); (Nordiazepam) $T_{1/2}$=40-50 hrs.

PATIENT CONSIDERATIONS
Assessment: Assess for acute narrow-angle glaucoma, renal/hepatic impairment, depressive neurosis, psychotic reactions, depression, hypersensitivity to drug, pregnancy/nursing status, and for possible drug interactions. Assess psychological potential for drug dependence.

Monitoring: Monitor for signs/symptoms of depression, suicidal thoughts or behavior, unusual changes in mood or behavior, drug dependence, withdrawal symptoms, and other adverse reactions. Monitor blood counts and LFTs periodically w/ prolonged therapy.

Counseling: Inform about benefits/risks and appropriate use of therapy. Counsel patients, caregivers, and family members that therapy may increase the risk of suicidal thoughts and behavior and advise of the need to be alert for the emergence or worsening of signs and symptoms of depression, any unusual changes in mood/behavior, suicidal thoughts/behavior, or thoughts about self-harm; instruct to immediately report behaviors of concern. Caution against engaging in hazardous tasks requiring mental alertness (eg, operating machinery/driving). Inform that therapy may produce psychological and physical dependence; instruct to contact physician before either increasing the dose or discontinuing therapy. Encourage patients to enroll in the North American Antiepileptic Drug Pregnancy Registry if they become pregnant.

TRAVATAN Z — travoprost   Rx
Class: Prostaglandin analogue

ADULT DOSAGE	PEDIATRIC DOSAGE
Elevated Intraocular Pressure	**Elevated Intraocular Pressure**
Open-Angle Glaucoma/Ocular HTN: 1 drop in affected eye(s) qd in pm	**Open-Angle Glaucoma/Ocular HTN:** **≥16 Years:** 1 drop in affected eye(s) qd in pm

---

DOSING CONSIDERATIONS
Concomitant Medications
Space by at least 5 min if using >1 topical ophthalmic drug

ADMINISTRATION
Ocular route

STORAGE
2-25°C (36-77°F).

HOW SUPPLIED
Sol: 0.004% [2.5mL, 5mL]

WARNINGS/PRECAUTIONS
Changes to pigmented tissues, including increased pigmentation of iris (may be permanent), eyelid and eyelashes (may be reversible) reported. Regularly examine patients w/ noticeably increased iris pigmentation. May cause changes to eyelashes and vellus hair in the treated eye. May exacerbate active intraocular inflammation (eg, uveitis). Macular edema, including cystoid macular edema, reported; caution w/ aphakic patients, pseudophakic patients w/ torn posterior lens capsule, or patients at risk of macular edema. Treatment of angle-closure, inflammatory, or neovascular glaucoma has not been evaluated. Bacterial keratitis reported w/ multidose containers. Remove contact lenses prior to instillation; may reinsert 15 min after administration.

ADVERSE REACTIONS
Ocular hyperemia, foreign body sensation, decreased visual acuity, eye discomfort/pruritus/pain.

PREGNANCY AND LACTATION
Pregnancy: Category C. **Lactation:** Caution in nursing.

MECHANISM OF ACTION
Prostaglandin analogue; not established. Selective FP prostanoid receptor agonist believed to reduce IOP by increasing uveoscleral outflow.

PHARMACOKINETICS
Absorption: C_{max}=0.018ng/mL; T_{max}=30 min. **Metabolism:** Cornea, via esterases to active free acid and systemically to inactive metabolites via β-oxidation and reduction. **Elimination:** Urine (<2%); $T_{1/2}$=45 min.

PATIENT CONSIDERATIONS
Assessment: Assess for active intraocular inflammation (uveitis), risk factors for macular edema, aphakic/pseudophakic patients w/ torn posterior lens capsule, angle-closure, inflammatory, or neovascular glaucoma, and pregnancy/nursing status.

Monitoring: Monitor for increased pigmentation of the iris and eyelid, changes in eyelashes, macular edema, and bacterial keratitis.

Counseling: Inform about risk of brown pigmentation of iris and darkening of eyelid skin. Inform about the possibility of eyelash and vellus hair changes. Advise to avoid touching tip of dispensing container to eye, surrounding structures, fingers, or any other surface, in order to avoid contamination of the sol. Advise to consult physician if having ocular surgery or if intercurrent ocular conditions (eg, trauma or infection) or ocular reactions develop. Instruct to remove contact lenses prior to instillation; reinsert 15 min after administration. Instruct to administer at least 5 min apart if using >1 topical ophthalmic drugs.

TREANDA — bendamustine hydrochloride   Rx
Class: Alkylating agent

ADULT DOSAGE	PEDIATRIC DOSAGE
Chronic Lymphocytic Leukemia	Pediatric use may not have been established
100mg/m² IV over 30 min on Days 1 and 2 of a 28-day cycle, up to 6 cycles	
B-Cell Non-Hodgkin Lymphoma	
Indolent B-Cell Non-Hodgkin Lymphoma That Has Progressed During or w/in 6 Months of Treatment w/ Rituximab or a Rituximab-Containing Regimen: 120mg/m² IV over 60 min on Days 1 and 2 of a 21-day cycle, up to 8 cycles	

DOSING CONSIDERATIONS
Renal Impairment
CrCl <40mL/min: Not recommended for use

Hepatic Impairment
Moderate (AST or ALT 2.5-10X ULN and Total Bilirubin 1.5-3X ULN): Not recommended for use
Severe (Total Bilirubin >3X ULN): Not recommended for use

Adverse Reactions
Chronic Lymphocytic Leukemia:
Grade 4 Hematologic Toxicity: Delay
Clinically Significant ≥Grade 2 Nonhematologic Toxicity: Delay
Nonhematologic Toxicity Has Recovered to ≤Grade 1 and/or the Blood Counts Have Improved (ANC ≥1 x 10⁹/L, Platelets ≥75 x 10⁹/L): Reinitiate; dose reduction may be warranted
≥Grade 3 Hematologic Toxicity: Reduce to 50mg/m² on Days 1 and 2 of each cycle
≥Grade 3 Hematologic Toxicity Recurs: Reduce to 25mg/m² on Days 1 and 2 of each cycle
≥Grade 3 Nonhematologic Toxicity: Reduce to 50mg/m² on Days 1 and 2 of each cycle

May consider dose re-escalation in subsequent cycles

B-Cell Non-Hodgkin Lymphoma:
Grade 4 Hematologic Toxicity: Delay
Clinically Significant ≥Grade 2 Nonhematologic Toxicity: Delay
Nonhematologic Toxicity Has Recovered to ≤Grade 1 and/or the Blood Counts Have Improved (ANC ≥1 x 10⁹/L, Platelets ≥75 x 10⁹/L): Reinitiate; dose reduction may be warranted
Grade 4 Hematologic Toxicity: Reduce to 90mg/m² on Days 1 and 2 of each cycle
Grade 4 Hematologic Toxicity Recurs: Reduce to 60mg/m² on Days 1 and 2 of each cycle
≥Grade 3 Nonhematologic Toxicity: Reduce to 90mg/m² on Days 1 and 2 of each cycle
≥Grade 3 Nonhematologic Toxicity Recurs: Reduce to 60mg/m² on Days 1 and 2 of each cycle

ADMINISTRATION
IV route

Selection/Preparation
Do not mix or combine the 2 formulations.
Admixture should be prepared as close as possible to the time of patient administration.

Sol:
Withdraw and transfer for dilution in a biosafety cabinet or containment isolator using only a polypropylene syringe w/ a metal needle and a polypropylene hub. Do not use w/ devices containing polycarbonate or acrylonitrile-butadiene-styrene (ABS) (eg, closed system transfer devices [CSTDs], adapters, syringes) prior to dilution in the infusion bag.
After dilution of into the infusion bag, devices that contain polycarbonate or ABS, including infusion sets, may be used.

1. Withdraw the volume needed for the required dose (from the 90mg/mL sol).
2. Immediately transfer to a 500mL infusion bag of 0.9% NaCl. As an alternative, a 500mL infusion bag of 2.5% dextrose/0.45% NaCl may be considered. The resulting final concentration should be w/in 0.2-0.7mg/mL.
3. Administer diluted sol w/in 24 hrs when stored at 2-8°C (36-46°F) or w/in 2 hrs when stored at 15-30°C (59-86°F).

Powder:
Only use powder for inj if a CSTD or adapter that contains polycarbonate or ABS is used as supplemental protection during preparation.

1. Reconstitute 25mg vial w/ 5mL of sterile water for inj (SWFI) and 100mg vial w/ 20mL of SWFI.
2. Shake well to yield a clear, colorless to a pale yellow sol w/ a concentration of 5mg/mL; should completely dissolve in 5 min and transfer reconstituted sol to infusion bag w/in 30 min of reconstitution.
3. Withdraw the volume needed for the required dose and immediately transfer to 500mL infusion bag of 0.9% NaCl; as an alternative, a 500mL infusion bag of 2.5% dextrose/0.45% NaCl may be considered.
4. The resulting final concentration should be w/in 0.2-0.6mg/mL; thoroughly mix the contents of the infusion bag after transferring.
5. Administer w/in 24 hrs when stored at 2-8°C (36-46°F) or w/in 3 hrs when stored at 15-30°C (59-86°F).

STORAGE
Sol: 2-8°C (36-47°F). Protect from light. **Powder:** Up to 25°C (77°F); excursions permitted up to 30°C (86°F). Protect from light.

HOW SUPPLIED
Inj: (Powder) 25mg, 100mg; (Sol) 45mg/0.5mL, 180mg/2mL

CONTRAINDICATIONS
Known hypersensitivity to bendamustine.

WARNINGS/PRECAUTIONS
Severe myelosuppression reported; may require dose delays and/or subsequent dose reductions if recovery to the recommended values has not occurred by the 1st day of the next scheduled cycle. Monitor leukocytes, platelets, Hgb, and neutrophils frequently if treatment-related myelosuppression occurs. Infection (eg, pneumonia, sepsis, hepatitis) and death reported. Increased risk for reactivation of infections (eg, hepatitis B, cytomegalovirus, herpes zoster); patients should undergo appropriate measures for infection and infection reactivation prior to administration. Infusion reactions and severe anaphylactic/anaphylactoid reactions reported; monitor clinically and d/c for severe reactions. Consider measures to prevent severe reactions (eg, antihistamines, antipyretics, corticosteroids) in subsequent cycles in patients who have experienced Grade 1 or 2 infusion reactions. Consider discontinuation for Grade 3 infusion reactions as clinically appropriate; d/c for Grade 4 infusion reactions. Do not rechallenge in patients who experience ≥Grade 3 allergic-type reactions. Tumor lysis syndrome reported; preventive measures include vigorous hydration and close monitoring of blood chemistry, particularly K+ and uric acid levels. Skin reactions (eg, rash, toxic skin reactions, bullous exanthema) reported; monitor closely and withhold or d/c if skin reactions are severe or progressive. Premalignant and malignant diseases (eg, myelodysplastic syndrome, myeloproliferative disorders, acute myeloid leukemia, bronchial carcinoma) reported. Extravasations reported; assure good venous access prior to starting infusion and monitor for infusion-site redness, swelling, pain, infection, and necrosis during and after administration. May cause fetal harm. Caution w/ mild/moderate renal impairment and w/ mild hepatic impairment.

ADVERSE REACTIONS
Chronic Lymphocytic Leukemia: Pyrexia, N/V.
Non-Hodgkin Lymphoma: N/V, fatigue, diarrhea, pyrexia.

DRUG INTERACTIONS
CYP1A2 inhibitors (eg, fluvoxamine, ciprofloxacin) may increase plasma concentrations of bendamustine and may decrease plasma concentrations of active metabolites. CYP1A2 inducers (eg, omeprazole, smoking) may decrease plasma concentrations of bendamustine and may increase plasma concentrations of active metabolites. Use caution or consider alternative treatments if treatment w/ CYP1A2 inhibitors/inducers is needed. May increase risk of severe skin toxicity w/ allopurinol.

PREGNANCY AND LACTATION
Pregnancy: Category D.
Lactation: Not for use in nursing.

MECHANISM OF ACTION
Alkylating agent; has not been established. Bifunctional mechlorethamine derivative containing a purine-like benzimidazole ring; forms electrophilic alkyl groups that form covalent bonds w/ electron-rich nucleophilic moieties, resulting in interstrand DNA crosslinks. Bifunctional covalent linkage can lead to cell death via several pathways. Active against both quiescent and dividing cells.

PHARMACOKINETICS
Distribution: Plasma protein binding (94-96%); V_d=20-25L. **Metabolism:** Extensive via hydrolytic (primary), oxidative, and conjugative pathways; gamma-hydroxy-bendamustine (M3), N-desmethyl-bendamustine (M4) (active minor metabolites) via CYP1A2. **Elimination:** Urine (50%, 3.3% unchanged, <1% as M3 and M4), feces (25%); $T_{1/2}$=40 min, 3 hrs (M3), 30 min (M4).

PATIENT CONSIDERATIONS
Assessment: Assess for renal/hepatic impairment, hypersensitivity to drug, pregnancy/nursing status, and possible drug interactions.
Monitoring: Monitor for signs/symptoms of myelosuppression, infections, anaphylaxis/infusion reactions, tumor lysis syndrome, skin reactions, premalignant/malignant diseases, extravasation, lab abnormalities, and other adverse reactions. Monitor CBCs and blood chemistry, particularly K+ and uric acid levels.

Counseling: Inform of the possibility of mild/serious allergic reactions and instruct to immediately report rash, facial swelling, or difficulty breathing during or soon after infusion. Inform that therapy may cause a decrease in WBC counts, platelets, and RBC counts, and of the need for frequent monitoring of blood counts; instruct to report SOB, significant fatigue, bleeding, fever, or other signs of infection. Advise that therapy may cause tiredness; instruct to avoid driving or operating dangerous tools or machinery if tiredness occurs. Inform that therapy may cause N/V, diarrhea, and mild rash or itching; instruct to report any adverse reactions immediately to physician. Advise women to avoid becoming pregnant and men to use reliable contraception throughout treatment and for 3 months after discontinuation of therapy; instruct to immediately report pregnancy and to avoid nursing while on therapy.

TRESIBA — insulin degludec Rx

Class: Insulin (long-acting)

ADULT DOSAGE	PEDIATRIC DOSAGE
Type 1 Diabetes Mellitus	Pediatric use may not have been established
Initial:	
Insulin Naive:	
Approx 1/3 to 1/2 of total daily insulin dose; as a general rule, 0.2-0.4 U/kg can be used to calculate initial total daily insulin dose. Give the remainder of the total daily insulin dose as a short-acting insulin and divided between each daily meal.	
Patients Already on Insulin Therapy: Start at the same unit dose as the total daily long- or intermediate-acting insulin unit dose	
Titrate: Adjust dose based on the patient's metabolic needs, blood glucose monitoring results, and glycemic control goal; recommended days between dose increases is 3 to 4 days	
Type 2 Diabetes Mellitus	
Initial: **Insulin Naive:** 10 U qd	
Patients Already on Insulin Therapy: Start at the same unit dose as the total daily long- or intermediate-acting insulin unit dose	
Titrate: Adjust dose based on the patient's metabolic needs, blood glucose monitoring results, and glycemic control goal; recommended days between dose increases is 3 to 4 days	
Missed Dose Inject daily dose during waking hrs upon discovering the missed dose; ensure that at least 8 hrs have elapsed between consecutive inj	

- -

DOSING CONSIDERATIONS
Renal Impairment
Intensify glucose monitoring and adjust dose prn

Hepatic Impairment
Intensify glucose monitoring and adjust dose prn

Elderly
Dose conservatively

Other Important Considerations
Dosage adjustments may be needed w/ changes in physical activity, changes in meal patterns (eg, macronutrient content, timing of food intake), changes in renal/hepatic function, or during acute illness

ADMINISTRATION
SQ route

Inject into the thigh, upper arm, or abdomen, and rotate inj sites w/in the same region from 1 inj to the next.
Inject qd at any time of day.
Do not administer IV, IM, or in an insulin infusion pump.
Do not dilute or mix w/ any other insulin products or sol.
Do not transfer from the pen into a syringe for administration.
Do not perform dose conversion when using the U-100 or U-200 FlexTouch pens; dose window for both the U-100 and U-200 FlexTouch pens shows the number of insulin units to be delivered and no conversion is needed.

STORAGE
Unopened: 2-8°C (36-46°F) until expiration date. Do not store in freezer or directly adjacent to the refrigerator cooling element. Do not freeze and do not use

if frozen. May also store at room temperature <30°C (86°F) for 56 days. **Open (In-Use):** 2-8°C (36-46°F) or room temperature <30°C (86°F) for up to 56 days. Keep away from direct heat and light.

HOW SUPPLIED
Inj: 100 U/mL, 200 U/mL [3mL]

CONTRAINDICATIONS
During episodes of hypoglycemia. Hypersensitivity to Tresiba or one of its excipients.

WARNINGS/PRECAUTIONS
Not recommended for the treatment of diabetic ketoacidosis. Never share prefilled pen between patients, even if the needle is changed; sharing poses a risk for transmission of blood-borne pathogens. Changes in insulin, manufacturer, type, or method of administration may affect glycemic control and predispose to hypo/hyperglycemia; these changes should be made cautiously and only under medical supervision and the frequency of blood glucose monitoring should be increased. Hypoglycemia may occur and may impair concentration ability and reaction time. Symptomatic awareness of hypoglycemia may be less pronounced in patients w/ longstanding diabetes, diabetic nerve disease, w/ medications that block the sympathetic nervous system (eg, β-blockers), or in patients who experience recurrent hypoglycemia. Accidental mix-ups between basal insulin products and other insulins, particularly rapid-acting insulins, reported. Do not transfer from the pen to a syringe; markings on the insulin syringe will not measure the dose correctly and can result in overdosage and severe hypoglycemia. Severe, life-threatening, generalized allergy, including anaphylaxis, may occur. D/C if a hypersensitivity reaction occurs; treat per standard of care and monitor until signs/symptoms resolve. May cause hypokalemia; monitor K⁺ levels in patients at risk for hypokalemia (eg, patients using K⁺-lowering medications or medications sensitive to serum K⁺ concentrations) if indicated.

ADVERSE REACTIONS
Hypoglycemia, nasopharyngitis, URTI, headache, sinusitis, gastroenteritis, diarrhea.

DRUG INTERACTIONS
Observe for signs/symptoms of CHF if treated concomitantly w/ a peroxisome proliferator-activated receptor (PPAR)-gamma agonist (eg, thiazolidinedione); consider discontinuation or dose reduction of the PPAR-gamma agonist if CHF develops. Antidiabetic agents, ACE inhibitors, ARBs, disopyramide, fibrates, fluoxetine, MAOIs, pentoxifylline, pramlintide, propoxyphene, salicylates, somatostatin analogues (eg, octreotide), sulfonamide antibiotics, GLP-1 receptor agonists, DPP-4 inhibitors, and SGLT-2 inhibitors may increase the risk of hypoglycemia; dose reductions and increased frequency of glucose monitoring may be required when coadministered w/ these drugs. Atypical antipsychotics (eg, olanzapine, clozapine), corticosteroids, danazol, diuretics, estrogens, glucagon, isoniazid, niacin, oral contraceptives, phenothiazines, progestogens (eg, in oral contraceptives), protease inhibitors, somatropin, sympathomimetic agents (eg, albuterol, epinephrine, terbutaline), and thyroid hormones may decrease the blood glucose lowering effect; dose increases and increased frequency of glucose monitoring may be required when coadministered w/ these drugs. Alcohol, β-blockers, clonidine, and lithium salts may increase or decrease the blood glucose lowering effect; dose adjustment and increased frequency of glucose monitoring may be required when coadministered w/ these drugs. Pentamidine may cause hypoglycemia, which may sometimes be followed by hyperglycemia; dose adjustment and increased frequency of glucose monitoring may be required when coadministered w/ this drug. β-blockers, clonidine, guanethidine, and reserpine may blunt signs/symptoms of hypoglycemia; increased frequency of glucose monitoring may be required when coadministered w/ these drugs. May need adjustments in concomitant oral antidiabetic treatment in patients w/ type 2 diabetes.

PREGNANCY AND LACTATION
Pregnancy: Category C.
Lactation: It is unknown whether insulin degludec is excreted in human milk. Caution in nursing.

MECHANISM OF ACTION
Insulin degludec; regulates glucose metabolism. Lowers blood glucose by stimulating peripheral glucose uptake and by inhibiting hepatic glucose production. Also inhibits lipolysis and proteolysis, and enhances protein synthesis.

PHARMACOKINETICS
Absorption: C_{max}=4472 pmol/L; T_{max}=9 hrs (median). **Distribution:** Plasma protein binding (>99%). **Elimination:** $T_{1/2}$=25 hrs.

PATIENT CONSIDERATIONS
Assessment: Assess for diabetic ketoacidosis, predisposition to hypoglycemia, hypersensitivity, renal/hepatic impairment, pregnancy/nursing status, and possible drug interactions. Obtain baseline blood glucose, HbA1c, and K⁺ levels.

Monitoring: Monitor for signs/symptoms of hypoglycemia, allergic reactions, hypokalemia, and other adverse reactions. Monitor blood glucose and HbA1c levels, and renal/hepatic function. Perform increased frequency of blood glucose monitoring in patients at higher risk for hypoglycemia and in patients who have reduced symptomatic awareness of hypoglycemia. Monitor K⁺ levels in patients at risk for hypokalemia.

Counseling: Advise to never share pen device w/ another person, even if the needle is changed. Inform of hypoglycemia symptoms, including impairment of the ability to concentrate and react; advise to use caution when driving/operating machinery. Advise that changes in insulin regimen can predispose to hypo/hyperglycemia and that changes should be made under close medical supervision. Instruct to always check the label before each inj to avoid medication errors and to not dilute or mix w/ any other insulin or sol. Instruct on self-management procedures, including glucose monitoring, proper inj technique, management

of hypo/hyperglycemia, and on handling of special situations (eg, intercurrent conditions, inadequate or skipped dose, inadvertent administration of increased insulin dose, inadequate food intake, skipped meals). Advise to inform physician if pregnant or contemplating pregnancy.

TRETIN-X — tretinoin   Rx
Class: Retinoid

ADULT DOSAGE	PEDIATRIC DOSAGE
Acne Vulgaris	**Acne Vulgaris**
Lightly cover affected area qd, before retiring; may apply less frequently or use other dosage forms once acne lesions have responded satisfactorily	**≥12 Yrs:** Lightly cover affected area qd, before retiring; may apply less frequently or use other dosage forms once acne lesions have responded satisfactorily

ADMINISTRATION
Topical route

If using cosmetics, thoroughly clean the areas to be treated before applying the medication

STORAGE
<27°C (80°F). Do not expose to heat or store at temperatures >49°C (120°F).

HOW SUPPLIED
Cre: 0.1%, 0.075%, 0.05%, 0.0375%, 0.025% [35g]

CONTRAINDICATIONS
Hypersensitivity to any of the ingredients in this product.

WARNINGS/PRECAUTIONS
D/C if a reaction suggesting sensitivity or chemical irritation occurs. Minimize exposure to sunlight, including sunlamps. Heightened susceptibility to sunlight; do not use in patients with sunburn until fully recovered. Caution in patients who may have considerable sun exposure due to occupation or those with inherent sensitivity to the sun. Use sunscreen products and protective clothing over treated areas when exposure to sun cannot be avoided. Weather extremes (eg, wind, cold) may cause irritation. Keep away from eyes, mouth, angles of the nose, and mucous membranes. May induce severe local erythema and peeling at application site. If the degree of irritation warrants, use less frequently, d/c use temporarily, or d/c use altogether. May cause severe irritation on eczematous skin; caution in patients with this condition. Application may cause a transitory feeling of warmth or slight stinging; in cases where it has been necessary to temporarily d/c therapy or to reduce frequency of application, therapy may be resumed or frequency of application increased when the patient becomes able to tolerate treatment. Closely monitor alterations of vehicle, drug concentration, or dose frequency by carefully observing therapeutic response and skin tolerance. An apparent exacerbation of deep, previously unseen inflammatory lesions may occur; should not be considered a reason to d/c therapy.

ADVERSE REACTIONS
Red/edematous/blistered/crusted skin, hyper-/hypopigmentation.

DRUG INTERACTIONS
Caution with topical medication, medicated or abrasive soaps and cleansers, soaps and cosmetics with strong drying effects, and products with high concentrations of alcohol, astringents, spices, or lime. Caution with preparations containing sulfur, resorcinol, or salicylic acid. Allow effects of such preparations to subside before initiation of treatment.

PREGNANCY AND LACTATION
Category C, caution in nursing.

MECHANISM OF ACTION
Retinoid; not established. Suspected to decrease cohesiveness of follicular epithelial cells with decreased microcomedo formation. Stimulates mitotic activity and increased turnover of follicular epithelial cells, causing extrusion of the comedones.

PATIENT CONSIDERATIONS
Assessment: Assess for drug hypersensitivity, sunburn, sun exposure, sensitivity to sun, eczematous skin, pregnancy/nursing status, and possible drug interactions.

Monitoring: Monitor for hypersensitivity reactions, irritation, local erythema or peeling at application site, and other adverse reactions. Closely monitor alterations of vehicle, drug concentration, or dose frequency by carefully observing therapeutic response and skin tolerance.

Counseling: Instruct to d/c use and consult physician if hypersensitivity or irritation occurs. Advise to minimize exposure to sunlight, including sunlamps, or use sunscreen products and protective clothing over treated areas when exposure to sun cannot be avoided. Inform that weather extremes (eg, wind, cold) may be irritating to treated skin. Instruct to use ud, and to keep away from eyes, mouth, angles of the nose, and mucous membranes. Advise to inform physician of other topical medication or preparations being used, and if pregnant or breastfeeding. Inform that during the early weeks of therapy, an apparent exacerbation of inflammatory lesions may occur, which should not be considered a reason for discontinuation.

TREXALL — methotrexate   Rx

Class: Dihydrofolic acid reductase inhibitor

> Should be used only by physicians with knowledge and experience in the use of antimetabolite therapy. Use only in life-threatening neoplastic diseases, or in patients with psoriasis or rheumatoid arthritis (RA) with severe, recalcitrant, disabling disease not adequately responsive to other forms of therapy. Deaths reported in the treatment of malignancy, psoriasis, and RA. Closely monitor for bone marrow, liver, lung, and kidney toxicities. Patients should be informed of the risks involved and be under physician's care throughout therapy. Fetal death and/or congenital anomalies reported; not recommended for women of childbearing potential unless benefits outweigh risks. Contraindicated in pregnant women with psoriasis or RA. Reduced elimination with impaired renal function, ascites, or pleural effusions; monitor for toxicity and reduce dose or d/c in some cases. Unexpectedly severe (sometimes fatal) bone marrow suppression, aplastic anemia, and GI toxicity reported with coadministration of therapy (usually high dosage) with some NSAIDs. Causes hepatotoxicity, fibrosis, and cirrhosis (generally only after prolonged use); perform periodic liver biopsies in psoriatic patients on long-term therapy. Acutely, liver enzyme elevations frequently seen. Drug-induced lung disease may occur acutely at any time during therapy and reported at low doses. Interrupt therapy if pulmonary symptoms (especially a dry, nonproductive cough), diarrhea, or ulcerative stomatitis occurs. Malignant lymphomas, which may regress following withdrawal of treatment, may occur with low-dose therapy and, thus, may not require cytotoxic treatment; d/c therapy 1st and, if lymphoma does not regress, institute appropriate treatment. May induce tumor lysis syndrome in patients with rapidly growing tumors; may be prevented/alleviated by appropriate supportive and pharmacologic measures. Severe, occasionally fatal, skin reactions reported. Potentially fatal opportunistic infections, especially *Pneumocystis carinii* pneumonia, may occur. Concomitant use with radiotherapy may increase risk of soft tissue necrosis and osteonecrosis.

ADULT DOSAGE

Choriocarcinoma/Trophoblastic Diseases

Gestational choriocarcinoma, chorioadenoma destruens, and hydatidiform mole

15-30mg/day for a 5-day course

Courses are usually repeated 3-5X as required, w/ rest periods of one or more weeks interposed between courses, until any manifesting toxic symptoms subside

Acute Lymphoblastic Leukemia

Induction: $3.3mg/m^2/day$ + prednisone $60mg/m^2/day$
Maint of Remission: $30mg/m^2/week$, administered 2X weekly

If and when relapse occurs, repeat the initial induction regimen to obtain reinduction of remission

Lymphomas

Burkitt's Tumor:
Stages I-II:
Usual: 10-25mg/day for 4-8 days
Stage III:
Methotrexate is commonly given concomitantly w/ other anti-tumor agents

Treatment in all stages usually consists of several courses of the drug interposed w/ 7- to 10-day rest periods

Lymphosarcoma:
Stage III: May respond to combined drug therapy w/ methotrexate given in doses of 0.625-2.5mg/kg/day

Mycosis Fungoides (Cutaneous T-Cell Lymphoma)

Early Stages:
Usual: 5-50mg once weekly

Methotrexate has also been administered twice weekly in doses ranging from 15-37.5mg in patients who have responded poorly to weekly therapy

Rheumatoid Arthritis

Severe, active rheumatoid arthritis (ACR criteria) in patients who have had an insufficient therapeutic response to, or are intolerant of, an adequate trial of 1st-line therapy including full-dose NSAIDs

Initial:
Single-Dose Schedule: 7.5mg once weekly
Divided-Dose Schedule: 2.5mg at 12-hr intervals for 3 doses given as a course once weekly
Titrate: Adjust dose gradually to achieve optimal response; significant increase in incidence and severity

PEDIATRIC DOSAGE

Acute Lymphoblastic Leukemia

Induction: $3.3mg/m^2/day$ + prednisone $60mg/m^2/day$
Maint of Remission: $30mg/m^2/week$, administered 2X weekly

If and when relapse occurs, repeat the initial induction regimen to obtain reinduction of remission

Juvenile Rheumatoid Arthritis

Active polyarticular-course juvenile rheumatoid arthritis in patients who have had an insufficient therapeutic response to, or are intolerant of, an adequate trial of 1st-line therapy including full dose NSAIDs

2-16 Years:
Initial: $10mg/m^2$ once weekly
Titrate: Adjust dose gradually to achieve optimal response; there is experience w/ doses up to $30mg/m^2/week$, however there are too few published data to assess how doses $>20mg/m^2/week$ might affect the risk of serious toxicity

---

of serious toxic reactions, especially bone marrow suppression, reported at doses >20mg/week

Psoriasis

Symptomatic control of severe, recalcitrant, disabling psoriasis not adequately responsive to other forms of therapy, but only when the diagnosis has been established, as by a biopsy and/or after dermatologic consultation

Initial:
Single-Dose Schedule: 10-25mg/week until adequate response is achieved
Divided-Dose Schedule: 2.5mg at 12-hr intervals for 3 doses
Titrate: Adjust dose gradually to achieve optimal response; 30mg/week should not ordinarily be exceeded

Once optimal response is achieved, each dosage schedule should be reduced to the lowest possible amount of drug and to the longest possible rest period

Other Indications

Alone or in combination w/ other anticancer agents in the treatment of breast cancer, epidermoid cancers of the head and neck, and lung cancer, particularly squamous cell and small cell types. Methotrexate is also used in combination w/ other chemotherapeutic agents in the treatment of advanced stage non-Hodgkin's lymphomas

---

DOSING CONSIDERATIONS

Elderly
Consider relatively low doses and closely monitor for early signs of toxicity

ADMINISTRATION
Oral route

STORAGE
20-25°C (68-77°F). Protect from light.

HOW SUPPLIED
Tab: 5mg*, 7.5mg*, 10mg*, 15mg* *scored

CONTRAINDICATIONS
Pregnant women with psoriasis or RA (should be used in treatment of pregnant women with neoplastic diseases only when potential benefit outweighs risk to the fetus), nursing mothers. Psoriasis or RA patients with alcoholism, alcoholic liver disease, chronic liver disease, immunodeficiency syndromes, or preexisting blood dyscrasias (eg, bone marrow hypoplasia, leukopenia, thrombocytopenia, significant anemia). Known hypersensitivity to methotrexate.

WARNINGS/PRECAUTIONS
Toxic effects may be related to dose/frequency of administration; if toxicity occurs, reduce dose or d/c therapy and take appropriate corrective measures, which may include use of leucovorin calcium and/or acute, intermittent hemodialysis with high-flux dialyzer, if necessary. If therapy is reinstituted, carry it out with caution, with adequate consideration of further need for the drug and increased alertness as to possible recurrence of toxicity. Caution in elderly/debilitated. Avoid pregnancy if either partner is receiving therapy (during and for a minimum of 3 months after therapy for male patients, and during and for at least 1 ovulatory cycle after therapy for female patients). May cause multiple organ system toxicities (eg, GI, hematologic). May cause impairment of fertility, oligospermia, and menstrual dysfunction during and for a short period after cessation of therapy.

ADVERSE REACTIONS
Bone marrow/liver/lung/kidney toxicities, diarrhea, ulcerative stomatitis, malignant lymphomas, tumor lysis syndrome, skin reactions, opportunistic infections, nausea, abdominal distress, malaise, undue fatigue, chills.

DRUG INTERACTIONS
See Boxed Warning. Elevated and prolonged levels with coadministration of high-dose therapy with NSAIDs; caution when NSAIDs or salicylates are administered concomitantly with lower doses of therapy. Toxicity may be increased due to displacement by salicylates, phenylbutazone, phenytoin, and sulfonamides. Renal tubular transport diminished by probenecid. Oral antibiotics (eg, tetracycline, chloramphenicol, nonabsorbable broad spectrum antibiotics) may decrease intestinal absorption or interfere with enterohepatic circulation. Penicillins may reduce renal clearance; hematologic and GI toxicity observed. Closely monitor for increased risk of hepatotoxicity with hepatotoxins (eg, azathioprine, retinoids, sulfasalazine). May decrease theophylline clearance; monitor theophylline levels. Vitamin preparations containing folic acid or its derivatives may decrease responses; high doses of leucovorin may reduce efficacy of intrathecally administered drug. Trimethoprim/sulfamethoxazole may increase bone marrow suppression by an additive antifolate effect. Immunization may be ineffective when given during therapy; immunization with live virus vaccines is generally not

recommended. Disseminated vaccinia infections after smallpox immunizations reported. Combined use with gold, penicillamine, hydroxychloroquine, sulfasalazine, or cytotoxic agents may increase incidence of adverse effects.

PREGNANCY AND LACTATION
Category X (psoriasis, RA), not for use in nursing.

MECHANISM OF ACTION
Dihydrofolic acid reductase inhibitor; interferes with DNA synthesis, repair, and cellular replication. Mechanism in RA not established; may affect immune function.

PHARMACOKINETICS
Absorption: Rapid and well-absorbed. Bioavailability (60%) (adults). Administration of various doses and in different disease states resulted in different parameters. **Distribution:** Plasma protein binding (50%); found in breast milk. (IV) V_d=0.18L/kg (initial), 0.4-0.8L/kg (steady-state). **Metabolism:** Hepatic and intracellular to polyglutamated forms (active); 7-hydroxymethotrexate (metabolite). Partially metabolized by intestinal flora. **Elimination:** $T_{1/2}$=3-10 hrs (psoriasis/RA/low-dose antineoplastic therapy), 8-15 hrs (high doses). (IV) Urine (80-90%, unchanged), bile (≤10%). Refer to PI for additional pharmacokinetic information.

PATIENT CONSIDERATIONS

Assessment: Assess for alcoholism, alcoholic/chronic liver disease, immunodeficiency, blood dyscrasias, ascites, pleural effusions, tumors, hypersensitivity to drug, pregnancy/nursing status, any other condition where treatment is cautioned or contraindicated, and possible drug interactions. Obtain baseline CBC with differential and platelet counts, hepatic enzymes, renal function tests, liver biopsy, and chest x-ray.

Monitoring: Monitor for toxicities of bone marrow, liver, lung, kidney and GI, diarrhea, ulcerative stomatitis, malignant lymphoma, tumor lysis syndrome, skin reactions, opportunistic infections, and other adverse reactions. Monitor hematology at least monthly and renal/hepatic function every 1-2 months during therapy of RA/psoriasis and more frequently during antineoplastic therapy, during initial/changing doses, or during periods of increased risk of elevated drug levels (eg, dehydration). If drug-induced lung disease is suspected, perform pulmonary function tests.

Counseling: Inform of the early signs/symptoms of toxicity, the need to see physician promptly if toxicity occurs, and the need for close follow-up, including periodic lab tests to monitor toxicity. Emphasize that the recommended dose is taken weekly in RA and psoriasis, and that mistaken daily use of recommended dose has led to fatal toxicity. Counsel about risks/benefits of therapy, and effects on reproduction.

TREXIMET — naproxen sodium/sumatriptan   Rx
Class: 5-HT$_1$ agonist/NSAID

> NSAIDs cause an increased risk of serious cardiovascular (CV) thrombotic events (eg, MI, stroke), which can be fatal. This risk may occur early in treatment and may increase w/ duration of use. Contraindicated in the setting of CABG surgery. NSAIDs cause an increased risk of serious GI adverse events (eg, bleeding, ulceration, stomach/intestinal perforation), which can be fatal and can occur at any time during use and w/o warning symptoms; elderly patients and patients w/ a prior history of peptic ulcer disease and/or GI bleeding are at a greater risk.

ADULT DOSAGE
Migraine

Acute Treatment of Migraine w/ or w/o Aura:
1 tab of 85mg/500mg
Max: 2 tabs of 85mg/500mg in a 24-hr period, taken at least 2 hrs apart

PEDIATRIC DOSAGE
Migraine

Acute Treatment of Migraine w/ or w/o Aura:
12-17 Years:
1 tab of 10mg/60mg
Max: 1 tab of 85mg/500mg in a 24-hr period

DOSING CONSIDERATIONS
Renal Impairment
Severe (CrCl <30mL/min): Not recommended

Hepatic Impairment
Mild to Moderate: 1 tab of 10mg/60mg in a 24-hr period
Severe: Contraindicated

Elderly
Not recommended in elderly patients who have decreased renal function, higher risk for unrecognized coronary artery disease (CAD), and increases in BP

ADMINISTRATION
Oral route

Take w/ or w/o food.
Do not split, crush, or chew.

STORAGE
25°C (77°F); excursions permitted to 15-30°C (59-86°F).

HOW SUPPLIED
Tab: (Sumatriptan/Naproxen) 10mg/60mg, 85mg/500mg

CONTRAINDICATIONS
Ischemic CAD (angina pectoris, history of MI, documented silent ischemia); coronary artery vasospasm, including Prinzmetal's angina; in the setting of CABG surgery; Wolff-Parkinson-White syndrome or arrhythmias associated w/ other cardiac accessory conduction pathway disorders; history of stroke or transient ischemic attack (TIA) or history of hemiplegic/basilar migraine; peripheral vascular disease; ischemic bowel disease; uncontrolled HTN; recent use (w/in 24 hrs) of ergotamine-containing medication, ergot-type medication (eg, dihydroergotamine, methysergide), or another 5-HT$_1$-agonist; concurrent administration or recent use (w/in 2 weeks) of an MAO-A inhibitor; history of asthma, urticaria, or allergic-type reactions after taking aspirin (ASA) or other NSAIDs; known hypersensitivity (eg, anaphylactic reactions, angioedema, serious skin reactions) to sumatriptan, naproxen, or any components of Treximet; 3rd trimester of pregnancy; severe hepatic impairment.

WARNINGS/PRECAUTIONS
Use lowest effective dose for the shortest duration possible. Use only if a clear diagnosis of migraine headache has been established; reconsider diagnosis before treating any subsequent attacks if patient has no response to the 1st migraine attack treated w/ therapy. Safety of treating >5 migraine headaches (adults) or >2 migraine headaches (pediatric patients) in a 30-day period not established. Serotonin syndrome may occur; d/c if suspected. Monitor renal function in patients w/ mild (CrCl=60-89mL/min) or moderate (CrCl=30-59mL/min) renal impairment, preexisting kidney disease, or dehydration. Renal effects associated w/ therapy may hasten the progression of renal dysfunction in patients w/ preexisting renal disease. Correct volume status in dehydrated or hypovolemic patients prior to initiating therapy. Avoid use in patients w/ advanced renal disease unless the benefits are expected to outweigh the risk; monitor for signs of worsening renal function if used in patients w/ advanced renal disease. Anaphylactic reactions may occur; avoid w/ ASA triad. May cause premature closure of the ductus arteriosus; avoid use in pregnant women starting at 30 weeks of gestation (3rd trimester). Caution in patients w/ preexisting asthma; monitor for changes in the signs/symptoms of asthma in these patients. May mask inflammation and fever. **Naproxen:** Increased CV thrombotic risk reported at higher doses. Patients treated w/ NSAIDs in the post-MI period may be at increased risk of reinfarction, CV-related death, and all-cause mortality. Increased risk for GI bleeding w/ longer duration of therapy, older age, poor general health status, and advanced liver disease and/or coagulopathy; avoid use in patients at higher risk unless benefits are expected to outweigh the increased risk and consider alternate therapies. Promptly initiate evaluation and treatment if a serious GI adverse event is suspected; d/c until a serious GI adverse event is ruled out. Hepatotoxicity reported; d/c immediately and perform a clinical evaluation if clinical signs/symptoms consistent w/ liver disease develop, if systemic manifestations occur, or if abnormal liver tests persist/worsen. May cause HTN or worsen preexisting HTN. Fluid retention and edema reported. Avoid use in patients w/ severe heart failure (HF) unless benefits outweigh risks; monitor for signs of worsening HF if used. Caution in patients whose overall Na+ intake must be severely restricted. Renal papillary necrosis and other renal injury reported w/ long-term use. Renal toxicity also reported in patients in whom renal prostaglandins have a compensatory role in the maintenance of renal perfusion; increased risk w/ renal/hepatic dysfunction, dehydration, hypovolemia, HF, salt depletion, and in the elderly. D/C if clinical signs/symptoms consistent w/ renal disease develop or if systemic manifestations occur. Hyperkalemia reported. May cause serious skin adverse events (eg, exfoliative dermatitis, Stevens-Johnson syndrome, toxic epidermal necrolysis); d/c at 1st appearance of skin rash or any sign of hypersensitivity. Anemia reported; monitor Hgb/Hct if signs/symptoms of anemia develop. May increase the risk of bleeding events; coagulation disorders may increase this risk. Monitor patients on long-term therapy w/ a CBC and a chemistry profile periodically. May decrease platelet aggregation and prolong bleeding time. Lab test interactions may occur. Not recommended in labor and delivery. **Sumatriptan:** Serious cardiac adverse reactions (eg, acute MI) reported; some reactions occurred in patients w/o known CAD. May cause coronary artery vasospasm, even in patients w/o a history of CAD. Life-threatening cardiac rhythm disturbances (eg, ventricular tachycardia, ventricular fibrillation) leading to death reported; d/c if these disturbances occur. Sensations of tightness, pain, pressure, and heaviness in the precordium, throat, neck, and jaw reported after treatment and are usually noncardiac in origin; perform a cardiac evaluation if these patients are at high cardiac risk. Cerebral/subarachnoid hemorrhage and stroke reported; d/c therapy if a cerebrovascular event occurs. Exclude other potentially serious neurological conditions prior to treating headaches in patients not previously diagnosed as migraineurs, and in migraineurs who present w/ atypical symptoms. May cause noncoronary vasospastic reactions (eg, peripheral vascular ischemia, GI vascular ischemia/infarction, splenic infarction, Raynaud's syndrome); rule out a vasospastic reaction before giving additional doses in patients who experience signs/symptoms. May cause transient/permanent blindness and significant partial vision loss. Significant elevation in BP, including hypertensive crisis w/ acute impairment of organ systems, reported. Overuse of acute migraine drugs may lead to exacerbation of headache; detoxification of patients, including withdrawal of the overused drugs, and treatment of withdrawal symptoms may be necessary. Seizures reported; caution w/ history of epilepsy or conditions associated w/ a lowered seizure threshold.

ADVERSE REACTIONS
Adults: Dizziness, somnolence, nausea, chest discomfort/pain, neck/throat/jaw pain/tightness/pressure.
Pediatric Patients: Hot flush, muscle tightness.

DRUG INTERACTIONS
See Contraindications. Serotonin syndrome reported during coadministration of triptans and SSRIs, SNRIs, TCAs, and MAOIs; d/c if suspected. **Naproxen:** Synergistic effect on bleeding w/ anticoagulants (eg, warfarin); monitor for signs of bleeding w/ concomitant anticoagulants, antiplatelet agents (eg, ASA), SSRIs, and SNRIs. Concomitant use w/ drugs that interfere w/ serotonin reuptake may potentiate the risk of bleeding. May increase risk of GI bleeding w/ use of oral corticosteroids, anticoagulants, SSRIs, smoking, and alcohol use. ASA may increase risk of bleeding and serious GI events; concomitant use w/ analgesic doses of ASA is not recommended. Monitor patients more closely for GI bleeding w/ concomitant use of low-dose ASA for cardiac prophylaxis. May diminish antihypertensive effect of ACE inhibitors, ARBs, and β-blockers (eg,

propranolol); monitor BP. Coadministration w/ ACE inhibitors or ARBs may result in deterioration of renal function (including possible acute renal failure) in patients who are elderly, volume-depleted (including those on diuretic therapy), or have renal impairment; monitor for worsening renal function. May reduce the natriuretic effect of loop diuretics (eg, furosemide) and thiazide diuretics; observe for signs of worsening renal function, in addition to assuring diuretic efficacy including antihypertensive effects. May increase digoxin serum concentrations and prolong the $T_{1/2}$ of digoxin; monitor digoxin levels. May elevate plasma lithium levels and reduce renal lithium clearance; monitor for signs of lithium toxicity. May increase the risk for methotrexate (MTX) toxicity; monitor for MTX toxicity. May increase cyclosporine's nephrotoxicity; monitor for signs of worsening renal function. Concomitant use w/ other NSAIDs or salicylates (eg, diflunisal, salsalate) increases the risk of GI toxicity; not recommended w/ other NSAIDs or salicylates. Concomitant use w/ pemetrexed may increase the risk of pemetrexed-associated myelosuppression, renal, and GI toxicity; refer to prescribing information for further information. Probenecid increases naproxen anion plasma levels and extends its plasma $T_{1/2}$ significantly; reduce frequency of administration of Treximet when given concurrently w/ probenecid.

PREGNANCY AND LACTATION
Pregnancy: First 2 trimesters (Category C). Third trimester (Category X); inhibitors of prostaglandin synthesis (including naproxen) are known to cause premature closure of the ductus arteriosus in humans.
Lactation: Found in breast milk; not for use in nursing.

MECHANISM OF ACTION
Naproxen: NSAID; mechanism not completely understood but involves inhibition of COX-1 and COX-2. Mode of action may be due to a decrease of prostaglandins in peripheral tissues; possesses analgesic, anti-inflammatory, and antipyretic activities. **Sumatriptan:** 5-HT₁-receptor agonist; presumably exerts its therapeutic effects through agonist effects at the 5-HT$_{1B/1D}$-receptors on intracranial blood vessels and sensory nerves of the trigeminal system, which result in cranial vessel constriction and inhibition of neuropeptide release.

PHARMACOKINETICS
Absorption: Naproxen: Bioavailability (95%); T_{max}=5 hrs (median). Sumatriptan: Bioavailability (approx 15%), T_{max}=1 hr. **Distribution:** Naproxen: V_d=0.16L/kg; plasma protein binding (>99%); found in breast milk. Sumatriptan: V_d=2.7L/kg; plasma protein binding (14-21%); found in breast milk. **Metabolism:** Naproxen: Extensively metabolized to 6-0-desmethyl naproxen. Sumatriptan: Via MAO-A; indole acetic acid (IAA) (major metabolite). **Elimination:** Naproxen: Urine (95%; <1% unchanged, <1% 6-0-desmethyl naproxen, 66-92% conjugates), $T_{1/2}$=approx 19 hrs. Sumatriptan: Urine (60%, mostly IAA or the IAA glucuronide, 3% unchanged), feces (40%); $T_{1/2}$=approx 2 hrs.

PATIENT CONSIDERATIONS
Assessment: Assess for history of asthma, urticaria, or allergic-type reactions after taking ASA or other NSAIDs; asthma; CV disease; HTN; history of hemiplegic or basilar migraine; history of stroke or TIA; peripheral vascular disease; ischemic bowel disease; Na⁺ restriction; fluid retention; HF; renal/hepatic impairment; drug hypersensitivity; other conditions where treatment is contraindicated or cautioned; pregnancy/nursing status; and possible drug interactions. Assess volume status. Perform a CV evaluation in patients who have multiple CV risk factors prior to therapy.

Monitoring: Monitor for signs/symptoms of CV thrombotic events; GI bleeding/ulceration and perforation; hepatotoxicity; noncoronary vasospastic reactions; new or worsening HTN; HF; edema; renal papillary necrosis and other renal injury; hyperkalemia; medication overuse headache; serotonin syndrome; anaphylactic reactions; seizures; serious skin reactions; anemia; and other adverse reactions. Perform ECG immediately after administration of therapy in patients w/ multiple CV risk factors who have a negative CV evaluation; consider periodic CV evaluation in intermittent long-term users. Monitor CBC and chemistry profile periodically during long-term treatment. Monitor renal function in patients w/ renal/hepatic impairment, HF, dehydration, or hypovolemia. Monitor for signs of bleeding in patients on concomitant therapy w/ anticoagulants, antiplatelet agents, SSRIs, or SNRIs.

Counseling: Inform about risks/benefits of therapy. Advise of potential for CV thrombotic events, GI adverse events, and worsening CHF/edema, and inform of symptoms; instruct to report symptoms to healthcare provider immediately if any occur. Inform of the potential for hepatotoxicity, and advise of signs/symptoms; if signs/symptoms occur, instruct to d/c and seek immediate medical therapy. Instruct to seek immediate emergency help if signs of an anaphylactic reaction occur. Advise to d/c immediately if rash develops and to contact healthcare provider as soon as possible. Inform that drug should be used during the 1st and 2nd trimester of pregnancy only if the potential benefit justifies the potential risk to the fetus; inform that drug should not be used during the 3rd trimester of pregnancy. Advise to notify physician if breastfeeding or planning to breastfeed. Instruct to report to physician all medications being used. Caution about the risk of serotonin syndrome. Inform that use of acute migraine drugs for ≥10 days/month may lead to an exacerbation of headache; encourage to record headache frequency and drug use (eg, by keeping a headache diary). Inform that treatment may cause somnolence and dizziness; instruct to evaluate ability to perform complex tasks after drug administration. Advise patients w/ preexisting asthma to seek immediate medical attention if their asthma worsens after taking Treximet. Advise patient to not use other NSAIDs or salicylates concomitantly; notify of the presence of NSAIDs in OTC medications for colds, fever, or insomnia. Instruct patient to not use low-dose ASA concomitantly w/o talking to healthcare provider.

TREZIX — acetaminophen/caffeine/dihydrocodeine bitartrate   CIII
Class: Opioid analgesic

> Respiratory depression and death have occurred in children who received codeine following tonsillectomy and/or adenoidectomy and had evidence of being ultra-rapid metabolizers of codeine due to a CYP2D6 polymorphism. Acetaminophen (APAP) has been associated with cases of acute liver failure, at times resulting in liver transplant and death. Most cases of liver injury are associated with APAP use at doses >4000mg/day, and often involve >1 APAP-containing product.

ADULT DOSAGE	**PEDIATRIC DOSAGE**
Moderate to Moderately Severe Pain	Pediatric use may not have been established
Usual: 2 caps q4h prn	
Max: 2 caps/4 hr; 5 doses (10 caps)/24 hrs	

DOSING CONSIDERATIONS
Renal Impairment
Reduce dose

ADMINISTRATION
Oral route

STORAGE
20-25°C (68-77°F). Dispense in a tight, light-resistant container with a child-resistant closure. Protect from moisture.

HOW SUPPLIED
Cap: (APAP/Caffeine/Dihydrocodeine) 320.5mg/30mg/16mg

CONTRAINDICATIONS
Postoperative pain management in children who have undergone tonsillectomy and/or adenoidectomy; hypersensitivity to dihydrocodeine, codeine, acetaminophen, caffeine, or any of the inactive components; significant respiratory depression (in unmonitored settings or in the absence of resuscitative equipment); acute or severe bronchial asthma or hypercapnia; paralytic ileus.

WARNINGS/PRECAUTIONS
May produce orthostatic hypotension in ambulatory patients; caution in patients in circulatory shock. May aggravate convulsions in patients with convulsive disorders. Caution in elderly or debilitated patients or those with acute alcoholism, adrenocortical insufficiency (eg, Addison's disease), asthma, CNS depression or coma, chronic obstructive pulmonary disease, decreased respiratory reserve (eg, emphysema, severe obesity, cor pulmonale, kyphoscoliosis), delirium tremens, head injury, hypotension, increased intracranial pressure (ICP), myxedema or hypothyroidism, prostatic hypertrophy or urethral stricture, toxic psychosis, and hepatic/renal impairment. May obscure diagnosis or clinical course of acute abdominal conditions. Not recommended for use by women during and immediately before labor and delivery; may cause respiratory depression in the newborn. APAP: Increased risk of acute liver failure in patients with underlying liver disease. Rarely, may cause serious skin reactions (eg, acute generalized exanthematous pustulosis, Stevens-Johnson syndrome, toxic epidermal necrolysis), which can be fatal; d/c at the 1st appearance of skin rash or any other sign of hypersensitivity. Hypersensitivity and anaphylaxis reported; avoid in patients with APAP allergy. Caution when using large doses in malnourished patients or those with history of chronic alcohol abuse; may be more susceptible to hepatic damage. Dihydrocodeine: Deaths reported in nursing infants exposed to high levels of morphine because their mothers were ultra-rapid metabolizers of codeine. Ultra-rapid metabolizers, due to specific CYP2D6 genotype (gene duplications denoted as *1/*1xN or *1/*2xN), may have life-threatening or fatal respiratory depression or experience signs of overdose (eg, extreme sleepiness, confusion, shallow breathing). Use lowest effective dose for the shortest period. May impair mental and/or physical abilities. May cause respiratory depression, most frequently in elderly or debilitated patients, usually after large initial doses in nontolerant patients; caution in patients with cor pulmonale, hypoxia, hypercapnia, or respiratory depression; consider alternative nonopioid analgesics and administer opioids only under careful medical supervision. May obscure neurologic signs of increases in ICP in patients with head injuries. Respiratory depressant effects and secondary elevation of CSF pressure may be markedly exaggerated in the presence of head injury, intracranial lesions, or other causes of increased ICP. May cause hypotension in patients whose ability to maintain BP has been compromised by a depleted blood volume. May produce drug dependence and has potential for abuse. May cause spasms of the sphincter of Oddi; caution with biliary tract disease, including pancreatitis. Caffeine: May produce CNS and cardiovascular (CV) stimulation and GI irritation.

ADVERSE REACTIONS
Respiratory depression, acute liver failure, light-headedness, dizziness, drowsiness, headache, fatigue, sedation, sweating, N/V, constipation, pruritus, skin reactions, anxiety, excitement.

DRUG INTERACTIONS
Agonist/antagonist analgesics (eg, pentazocine, nalbuphine, butorphanol, buprenorphine) may reduce analgesic effect. Dihydrocodeine: Concomitant administration with other opioid analgesics, sedatives or hypnotics, muscle relaxants, general anesthetics, centrally acting antiemetics, phenothiazines or other tranquilizers, or alcohol may cause additive CNS depressant effects; when combination is contemplated, reduce dose of one or both agents. May cause respiratory depression with other agents that depress respiration. Concurrent use with phenothiazines or other agents that compromise vasomotor tone may cause hypotension. Caution with MAOIs; may cause CNS excitation and HTN. APAP: Chronic/excessive alcohol consumption may increase hepatotoxic risk. Risk may also be increased in patients receiving anticonvulsants that induce hepatic microsomal enzymes (eg, phenytoin, barbiturates, carbamazepine) or

isoniazid. Chronic ingestion of large doses may slightly potentiate the effects of warfarin- and indandione-derivative anticoagulants. Severe hypothermia is possible with phenothiazines. Caffeine: May enhance the cardiac inotropic effects of β-adrenergic stimulating agents. Coadministration with disulfiram may decrease clearance. May increase the metabolism of phenobarbital and aspirin. Caffeine accumulation may occur when products or foods containing caffeine are consumed concomitantly with quinolones (eg, ciprofloxacin).

PREGNANCY AND LACTATION
Category C, not for use in nursing.

MECHANISM OF ACTION
Dihydrocodeine: Semisynthetic narcotic analgesic; multiple actions, qualitatively similar to those of codeine. Principal action of therapeutic value is analgesia. APAP: Nonopiate, nonsalicylate analgesic and antipyretic. Caffeine: Analgesic adjuvant. Also a CNS and CV stimulant.

PHARMACOKINETICS
Distribution: Found in breast milk. **Metabolism:** Dihydrocodeine: Liver via CYP2D6; dihydromorphine (active metabolite).

PATIENT CONSIDERATIONS
Assessment: Assess for severity of pain, hypersensitivity to drug, significant respiratory depression, bronchial asthma, hypercapnia, paralytic ileus, hepatic/renal impairment, head injury, intracranial lesions, acute abdominal conditions, history of drug abuse or seizures, any other conditions where treatment is cautioned, pregnancy/nursing status, and possible drug interactions.

Monitoring: Monitor for signs/symptoms of hepatotoxicity, respiratory depression, hypotension, skin reactions, hypersensitivity, anaphylaxis, elevation in CSF pressure, drug abuse, tolerance, dependence, GI irritation, and other adverse reactions.

Counseling: Instruct to d/c therapy and contact physician immediately if signs of allergy develop. Instruct to look for APAP on package labels and not to use >1 APAP-containing product. Instruct to seek medical attention immediately upon ingestion of >4000mg/day APAP, even if feeling well. Advise that drug may impair mental/physical abilities. Advise to report adverse experiences occurring during therapy. Advise not to adjust dose without consulting prescribing physician. Instruct not to combine medication with alcohol or other CNS depressants (sleep aids, tranquilizers) except by the orders of the prescribing physician, because additive effects may occur. Advise women of childbearing potential who become or are planning to become pregnant to consult their physician regarding the effects of analgesics and other drug use during pregnancy on themselves and their unborn child. Advise of the potential for abuse; instruct to protect drug from theft and never to give to anyone other than the individual for whom it was prescribed.

TRI-LUMA — fluocinolone acetonide/hydroquinone/tretinoin   Rx
Class: Corticosteroid/depigmenting agent/retinoid

ADULT DOSAGE	PEDIATRIC DOSAGE
Melasma of the Face	Pediatric use may not have been established
Moderate to Severe:	
Apply a thin film to affected area qd, at least 30 min before hs. Apply to hyperpigmented areas of melasma, including about 1/2 inch of normal appearing skin surrounding each lesion; rub lightly and uniformly into the skin	
D/C when control is achieved	

DOSING CONSIDERATIONS
Elderly
Start at lower end of dosing range

ADMINISTRATION
Topical route

Gently wash the face and neck w/ a mild cleanser.
Rinse and pat the skin dry.
Wash hands after each application.
Avoid sunlight exposure; use a sunscreen of SPF 30, and wear protective clothing during the day.
May use moisturizers and/or cosmetics during the day.

STORAGE
2-8°C (36-46°F). Protect from freezing. Keep tightly closed.

HOW SUPPLIED
Cre: (Fluocinolone-Hydroquinone-Tretinoin) 0.01%-4%-0.05% [30g]

CONTRAINDICATIONS
History of hypersensitivity to Tri-Luma or any of its components.

WARNINGS/PRECAUTIONS
Melasma usually recurs upon discontinuation of treatment. Excessive bleaching may occur in patients w/ darker skin. Contains sodium metabisulfite, which may cause allergic-type reactions (eg, anaphylactic symptoms, life-threatening asthmatic episodes) in susceptible individuals; d/c and institute appropriate therapy if anaphylaxis, asthma, or other clinically significant hypersensitivity reactions occur. Allergic contact dermatitis may occur. Cutaneous hypersensitivity reported. May cause mild to moderate irritation; d/c use if reaction suggests hypersensitivity or chemical irritation. Caution in elderly. **Hydroquinone:** Promptly

d/c if exogenous ochronosis occurs. **Fluocinolone:** Systemic absorption of topical corticosteroids may produce reversible hypothalamic pituitary adrenal (HPA)-axis suppression w/ the potential for glucocorticosteroid insufficiency after withdrawal of treatment; d/c if HPA-axis suppression is noted. May also produce manifestations of Cushing's syndrome, hyperglycemia, and glucosuria.

ADVERSE REACTIONS
Erythema, desquamation, burning, dryness, pruritus at application site.

DRUG INTERACTIONS
Avoid medicated/abrasive soaps and cleansers, soaps and cosmetics w/ drying effects, products w/ high concentrations of alcohol and astringents, and other irritants or keratolytic drugs while on treatment. Caution w/ medications that are known to be photosensitizing.

PREGNANCY AND LACTATION
Pregnancy: Category C.
Lactation: Caution in nursing.

MECHANISM OF ACTION
Fluocinolone: Corticosteroid. **Hydroquinone:** Melanin synthesis inhibitor. **Tretinoin:** Retinoid.

PHARMACOKINETICS
Absorption: Hydroquinone: C_{max}=25.55-86.52ng/mL. Tretinoin: (1g dose) C_{max}=2.01-5.34ng/mL, (6g dose) C_{max}=2-4.99ng/mL. **Distribution:** Fluocinolone: Found in breast milk (systemically administered).

PATIENT CONSIDERATIONS
Assessment: Assess for drug hypersensitivity, pregnancy/nursing status, and possible drug interactions.

Monitoring: Monitor for allergic-type reactions, local irritation, exogenous ochronosis, Cushing's syndrome, hyperglycemia, glucosuria, and other adverse reactions. Monitor for HPA-axis suppression by using adrenocorticotropic hormone or cosyntropin stimulation tests.

Counseling: Advise patients to change to nonhormonal forms of birth control, if hormonal methods are used. Instruct to use ud and not to use for any disorder other than that for which it was prescribed. Instruct to avoid exposure to sunlight, sunlamp, or UV light. Instruct to exercise caution when consistently exposed to sunlight or skin irritants. Advise to use sunscreen and protective covering over the treated areas. Due to the drying effect of this medication, inform that moisturizer may be applied to the face the am after washing. Instruct to keep away from eyes, nose, angles of mouth, or open wounds. Advise to d/c medication and consult physician if local irritation persists or becomes severe. Instruct to seek medical attention if allergic contact dermatitis, blistering, crusting, and severe burning or swelling of the skin, and irritation of the mucous membranes of eyes, nose, and mouth are experienced. Inform that marked redness, peeling, or discomfort may occur if medication is applied excessively.

TRI-SPRINTEC — ethinyl estradiol/norgestimate   Rx
Class: Estrogen/progestogen combination

> Cigarette smoking increases risk of serious cardiovascular (CV) events. Risk increases w/ age (>35 yrs of age) and w/ the number of cigarettes smoked. Contraindicated in women who are >35 yrs of age and smoke.

ADULT DOSAGE	PEDIATRIC DOSAGE
Contraception	**Contraception**
1 tab qd at the same time each day, for 28 days, then repeat	Not indicated for use premenarche; refer to adult dosing
Start either on 1st day of menses or on 1st Sunday after onset of menses	**Acne Vulgaris**
Acne Vulgaris	**Moderate Acne in Postpubertal Females ≥15 Years Who Desire Oral Contraception:**
Moderate Acne in Females Who Desire Oral Contraception:	1 tab qd at the same time each day, for 28 days, then repeat
1 tab qd at the same time each day, for 28 days, then repeat	Start either on 1st day of menses or on 1st Sunday after onset of menses
Start either on 1st day of menses or on 1st Sunday after onset of menses	
Missed Dose	
Miss 1 Active Tab in Weeks 1, 2, or 3: Take as soon as possible. Continue taking 1 tab qd until the pack is finished	
Miss 2 Active Tabs in Weeks 1 or 2: Take the 2 missed tabs as soon as possible and the next 2 active tabs the next day. Continue taking 1 tab qd until pack is finished. Use additional nonhormonal contraception (eg, condom, spermicide) as backup if the patient has intercourse w/in 7 days after missing tabs	
Miss 2 Active Tabs in Week 3 or Miss ≥3 Active Tabs in a Row in Weeks 1, 2, or 3: (Day 1 Start) Throw out the rest of the pack and start a new pack that same day. (Sunday Start) Continue taking 1 tab qd until Sunday, then throw out the rest	

of the pack and start a new pack that same day. (Day 1 Start/Sunday Start) Use additional nonhormonal contraception as backup if the patient has intercourse w/in 7 days after missing tabs

Conversions

Switching from Another Oral Contraceptive:
Start on the same day that a new pack of the previous oral contraceptive would have started

Switching from Another Contraceptive Method:
Transdermal Patch/Vaginal Ring/Inj: Start therapy on the day when next application/insertion/inj would have been scheduled

Intrauterine Contraceptive:
Start on the day of removal; if the intrauterine device is not removed on the 1st day of menstrual cycle, additional nonhormonal contraceptive is needed for the first 7 days of the 1st cycle pack

Implant:
Start therapy on the day of removal

- -

DOSING CONSIDERATIONS
Adverse Reactions
GI Disturbances: In case of severe vomiting/diarrhea, absorption may not be complete and additional contraceptive measures should be taken; if vomiting/diarrhea occurs w/in 3-4 hrs after taking an active tab, handle this as a missed tab

Other Important Considerations
Starting Therapy after Abortion or Miscarriage:
1st Trimester: May start immediately; if starting therapy immediately, additional method of contraception is not needed. If therapy is not started w/in 5 days after termination of the pregnancy, use additional nonhormonal contraception for the first 7 days of 1st cycle pack
2nd Trimester: Do not start until 4 weeks after a 2nd trimester abortion or miscarriage

Starting Therapy after Childbirth:
Do not start until 4 weeks after delivery; consider possibility of ovulation and conception in women who have not yet had a period postpartum

ADMINISTRATION
Oral route

Take tabs in the order directed on the blister pack.
Take w/o regard to meals.

Sunday Start Regimen
Use additional nonhormonal method of contraception for the first 7 days of 1st cycle pack.

STORAGE
20-25°C (68-77°F). Protect from light.

HOW SUPPLIED
Tab: (Ethinyl Estradiol [EE]/Norgestimate) 0.035mg/0.18mg, 0.035mg/0.215mg, 0.035mg/0.25mg

CONTRAINDICATIONS
High risk of arterial/venous thrombotic diseases (eg, smoking [if >35 yrs of age], presence/history of deep vein thrombosis [DVT]/pulmonary embolism [PE], inherited or acquired hypercoagulopathies, cerebrovascular disease, coronary artery disease [CAD], thrombogenic valvular/ thrombogenic rhythm diseases of the heart [eg, subacute bacterial endocarditis w/ valvular disease or A-fib], uncontrolled HTN, diabetes mellitus [DM] w/ vascular disease, headaches w/ focal neurological symptoms or migraine headaches w/ aura [women >35 yrs of age w/ any migraine headaches]), benign/malignant liver tumors, liver disease, undiagnosed abnormal uterine bleeding, pregnancy, presence/history of breast cancer or other estrogen- or progestin-sensitive cancer.

WARNINGS/PRECAUTIONS
D/C if an arterial thrombotic event or venous thromboembolic event (VTE) occurs. D/C if there is unexplained loss of vision, proptosis, diplopia, papilledema, or retinal vascular lesions; evaluate for retinal vein thrombosis immediately. If feasible, d/c at least 4 weeks before and through 2 weeks after major surgery or other surgeries known to have an elevated risk of VTE as well as during and following prolonged immobilization. In women who are not breastfeeding, initiate therapy no earlier than 4 weeks after delivery; risk of postpartum VTE decreases after the 3rd postpartum week, whereas the risk of ovulation increases after the 3rd postpartum week. Increased risk of VTE and arterial thromboses (eg, strokes, MI). D/C if jaundice develops. Hepatic adenomas and increased risk of hepatocellular carcinoma reported. Increased BP reported; d/c if BP rises significantly. May increase risk of gallbladder disease or worsen existing gallbladder disease. May increase risk of cholestasis in women w/ history of pregnancy-related cholestasis. May decrease glucose tolerance. Consider alternative contraception w/ uncontrolled dyslipidemia. May increase risk of pancreatitis w/ hypertriglyceridemia or family history thereof. Evaluate the cause of new headaches that are recurrent, persistent, or

severe, and d/c if indicated; consider discontinuation in the case of increased frequency or severity of migraine during use. Unscheduled bleeding and spotting may occur; rule out pregnancy or malignancy. May cause amenorrhea; amenorrhea or oligomenorrhea after discontinuation may occur. Caution w/ history of depression; d/c if depression recurs to a serious degree. May increase risk of cervical cancer or intraepithelial neoplasia. Chloasma may occur, especially w/ history of chloasma gravidarum; women w/ a tendency to chloasma should avoid exposure to the sun or UV radiation while on therapy. May interfere w/ lab tests (eg, coagulation factors, lipids, glucose tolerance, binding proteins). **EE:** In women w/ hereditary angioedema, may induce/exacerbate angioedema.

ADVERSE REACTIONS
Headache/migraine, breast issues (including breast pain, enlargement, discharge), vaginal infection, abdominal/GI pain, mood disorders (including mood alteration and depression), genital discharge, and changes in weight.

DRUG INTERACTIONS
Drugs or herbal products that induce certain enzymes, including CYP3A4 (eg, phenytoin, barbiturates, carbamazepine) may decrease levels and potentially diminish effectiveness of therapy or increase breakthrough bleeding; use an alternative or back-up method of contraception when using enzyme inducers and continue back-up contraception for 28 days after discontinuing the enzyme inducer. CYP3A4 inhibitors (eg, itraconazole, voriconazole, grapefruit juice) may increase levels. Significant changes (increase/decrease) in estrogen and/or progestin levels reported w/ HIV/hepatitis C virus protease inhibitors or non-nucleoside reverse transcriptase inhibitors. May decrease levels of acetaminophen (APAP), clofibric acid, morphine, salicylic acid, and temazepam. May significantly decrease levels of lamotrigine and may reduce seizure control; dosage adjustment of lamotrigine may be necessary. Women on thyroid hormone replacement therapy may need to increase dose of thyroid hormone due to increased levels of thyroid-binding globulin. **EE:** Colesevelam reported to significantly decrease EE exposure; decreased drug interaction when the 2 drug products are given 4 hrs apart. Atorvastatin or rosuvastatin may increase EE exposure; ascorbic acid and APAP may increase EE levels. May inhibit metabolism and increase levels of other compounds (eg, cyclosporine, prednisolone, theophylline, tizanidine, voriconazole).

PREGNANCY AND LACTATION
Pregnancy: Contraindicated in pregnancy.
Lactation: Not for use in nursing.

MECHANISM OF ACTION
Estrogen/progestogen oral contraceptive; acts by primarily suppressing ovulation. Other possible mechanisms may include cervical mucus changes that inhibit sperm penetration and endometrial changes that reduce the likelihood of implantation. Acne: has not been established; increases sex hormone-binding globulin (SHBG) and decreases free testosterone.

PHARMACOKINETICS
Absorption: Rapid. Administration on various days of dosing cycle led to different parameters; refer to PI. **Distribution:** Found in breast milk. Norelgestromin (NGMN) and Norgestrel (NG): Serum protein binding (>97%; NGMN bound to albumin; NG bound primarily to SHBG. EE: Serum protein binding (>97% to albumin). **Metabolism:** EE: Metabolized to various hydroxylated products and their glucuronide and sulfate conjugates. Norgestimate: Extensive by 1st pass mechanisms in GI tract and/or liver; NGMN and NG (major active metabolites). **Elimination:** EE: Urine and feces (metabolites). Norgestimate: Urine (47%) and feces (37%) as metabolites.

PATIENT CONSIDERATIONS
Assessment: Assess for DVT, PE, cerebrovascular disease, CAD, DM w/ vascular disease, headaches w/ focal neurological symptoms or migraine headaches w/ aura, pregnancy/nursing status, any other conditions where treatment is contraindicated or cautioned, and possible drug interactions.

Monitoring: Monitor for bleeding irregularities, venous/arterial thrombotic events, cervical cancer or intraepithelial neoplasia, retinal vein thrombosis or any other ophthalmic changes, jaundice, new/worsening headaches or migraines, depression, cholestasis w/ history of pregnancy-related cholestasis, pancreatitis, and other adverse reactions. Monitor BP in women w/ HTN, glucose levels in diabetic or prediabetic women, and lipid levels w/ dyslipidemia. Conduct a yearly visit in all patients for a BP check and for other indicated healthcare.

Counseling: Inform of risks/benefits of therapy. Advise to take ud. Counsel that cigarette smoking increases the risk of serious CV events and women who are >35 yrs of age and smoke should not use combination oral contraceptives (COCs). Inform of the risk of VTE. Inform that the drug does not protect against HIV infection (AIDS) and other sexually transmitted infections. Advise not to use during pregnancy; if pregnancy occurs during use, instruct to stop further use. Instruct on what to do in the event tabs are missed. Counsel to use a back-up or alternative method of contraception when enzyme inducers are used w/ therapy. Inform that COCs may reduce breast milk production. Counsel women who start COCs postpartum and have not yet had a period, to use an additional method of contraception until an active pill has been taken for 7 consecutive days. Inform that amenorrhea may occur; consider pregnancy in the event of amenorrhea at the time of 1st missed period, and rule out pregnancy in the event of amenorrhea in ≥2 consecutive cycles.

TRIBENZOR — amlodipine/hydrochlorothiazide/olmesartan medoxomil

RX

Class: Angiotensin II receptor blocker (ARB)/calcium channel blocker (CCB) (dihydropyridine)/ thiazide diuretic

> D/C as soon as possible when pregnancy is detected. Drugs that act directly on the renin-angiotensin system (RAS) can cause injury/death to the developing fetus.

ADULT DOSAGE

Hypertension
Usual: Dose qd
Titrate: May increase dose after 2 weeks
Max: 40mg/10mg/25mg qd

Replacement Therapy:
May substitute for individually titrated components

Add-On/Switch Therapy:
May use for patients not adequately controlled on any 2 of the following classes: ARBs, CCBs, and diuretics. Patients w/ dose-limiting adverse reactions to an individual component while on any dual combination of the components of therapy may be switched to therapy containing a lower dose of that component.

Not indicated for initial therapy of HTN.
May be administered w/ other antihypertensive agents.

PEDIATRIC DOSAGE
Pediatric use may not have been established

DOSING CONSIDERATIONS

Renal Impairment
Severe (CrCl <30mL/min): Avoid use

Hepatic Impairment
Severe:
Initial: 2.5mg amlodipine (not available w/ Tribenzor)

Elderly
≥75 Years:
Initial: 2.5mg amlodipine (not available w/ Tribenzor)

ADMINISTRATION
Oral route
Take w/ or w/o food.

STORAGE
25°C (77°F); excursions permitted to 15-30°C (59-86°F).

HOW SUPPLIED
Tab: (Olmesartan/Amlodipine/Hydrochlorothiazide [HCTZ]) 20mg/5mg/12.5mg, 40mg/5mg/12.5mg, 40mg/5mg/25mg, 40mg/10mg/12.5mg, 40mg/10mg/25mg

CONTRAINDICATIONS
Anuria, sulfonamide-derived drug hypersensitivity. Coadministration w/ aliskiren in patients w/ diabetes.

WARNINGS/PRECAUTIONS
Renal impairment reported; consider withholding or discontinuing either diuretic or ARB therapies if progressive renal impairment becomes evident. **Olmesartan:** Symptomatic hypotension may occur in patients w/ an activated RAS (eg, volume- and/or salt-depleted patients [eg, those being treated w/ high doses of diuretics]). Oliguria or progressive azotemia and (rarely) acute renal failure and/or death may occur in patients whose renal function may be compromised upon the activity of the renin-angiotensin-aldosterone system (eg, w/ severe CHF). May increase SrCr and BUN levels in patients w/ renal artery stenosis. Increased blood creatinine levels and hyperkalemia reported. Sprue-like enteropathy w/ symptoms of severe, chronic diarrhea w/ substantial weight loss reported; exclude other etiologies if these symptoms develop and consider discontinuation in cases where no other etiology is identified. **Amlodipine:** May develop increased frequency, duration, or severity of angina or acute MI, particularly w/ severe obstructive coronary artery disease (CAD). Rare reports of acute hypotension; caution w/ severe aortic stenosis. Hepatic enzyme elevations reported. **HCTZ:** May precipitate azotemia w/ renal disease and hepatic coma due to fluid and electrolyte imbalance. Observe for clinical signs of fluid or electrolyte imbalance (eg, hyponatremia, hypochloremic alkalosis, hypokalemia). Hypokalemia may sensitize/exaggerate the response of the heart to toxic effects of digitalis. May cause metabolic acidosis, hyperuricemia or precipitation of frank gout, hyperglycemia, manifestation of latent diabetes mellitus (DM), hypomagnesemia, hypersensitivity reactions (w/ or w/o a history of allergy or bronchial asthma), exacerbation/activation of systemic lupus erythematosus (SLE), and increased cholesterol and TG levels. Enhanced effects in postsympathectomy patients. D/C before carrying out tests for parathyroid function. May cause idiosyncratic reaction, resulting in acute transient myopia and acute angle-closure glaucoma; d/c as rapidly as possible.

ADVERSE REACTIONS
Dizziness, peripheral edema, headache, fatigue, nasopharyngitis, muscle spasms, nausea, URTI, diarrhea, UTI, joint swelling.

DRUG INTERACTIONS
See Contraindications. **Olmesartan:** NSAIDs, including selective COX-2 inhibitors, may attenuate antihypertensive effect and result in deterioration of renal function, including possible acute renal failure. Dual blockade of the RAS is associated w/ increased risk of hypotension, hyperkalemia, and changes in renal function (including acute renal failure); avoid combined use of RAS inhibitors or closely monitor BP, renal function, and electrolytes w/ concomitant agents that affect the RAS. Avoid w/ aliskiren in patients w/ renal impairment (GFR <60mL/min). Reduced systemic exposure and levels w/ colesevelam; administer at least 4 hrs before colesevelam dose. **Amlodipine:** May increase simvastatin exposure; limit simvastatin dose to 20mg daily. **HCTZ:** Alcohol, barbiturates, or narcotics may potentiate orthostatic hypotension. Dose adjustment of antidiabetic drugs (eg, oral agents, insulin) may be required. Additive effect or potentiation w/ other antihypertensives. Anionic exchange resins (eg, cholestyramine, colestipol) may impair absorption. Corticosteroids and adrenocorticotropic hormone may intensify electrolyte depletion, particularly hypokalemia. May decrease response to pressor amines (eg, norepinephrine). May increase response to nondepolarizing skeletal muscle relaxants (eg, tubocurarine). NSAIDs may reduce diuretic, natriuretic, and antihypertensive effects. **Olmesartan/HCTZ:** Increases in serum lithium concentrations and lithium toxicity reported.

PREGNANCY AND LACTATION
Pregnancy: Category D.
Lactation: Not for use in nursing.

MECHANISM OF ACTION
Olmesartan: ARB; blocks vasoconstrictor effects of angiotensin II by selectively blocking the binding of angiotensin II to the AT_1 receptor in vascular smooth muscle. **Amlodipine:** Dihydropyridine CCB; inhibits transmembrane influx of Ca^{2+} ions into vascular smooth muscle and cardiac muscle. **HCTZ:** Thiazide diuretic; has not been established. Affects renal tubular mechanisms of electrolyte reabsorption, directly increasing excretion of Na^+ and Cl^- and indirectly reducing plasma volume.

PHARMACOKINETICS
Absorption: Olmesartan: Absolute bioavailability (26%); T_{max}=1-2 hrs. Amlodipine: Absolute bioavailability (64-90%); T_{max}=6-12 hrs. HCTZ: T_{max}=1.5-2 hrs. **Distribution:** Olmesartan: V_d=17L; plasma protein binding (99%). Amlodipine: Plasma protein binding (93%). HCTZ: Crosses placenta; found in breast milk. **Metabolism:** Olmesartan: Ester hydrolysis to olmesartan. Amlodipine: Hepatic (extensive). **Elimination:** Olmesartan: Urine (35-50%), feces; $T_{1/2}$=13 hrs. Amlodipine: Urine (60% metabolites, 10% parent), $T_{1/2}$=30-50 hrs. HCTZ: Kidney (≥61% unchanged); $T_{1/2}$=5.6-14.8 hrs.

PATIENT CONSIDERATIONS

Assessment: Assess for anuria, sulfonamide-derived drug hypersensitivity, aortic stenosis, renal artery stenosis, SLE, CHF, volume/salt depletion, electrolyte imbalances, postsympathectomy status, DM, CAD, renal/hepatic impairment, pregnancy/nursing status, any other conditions where treatment is cautioned, and possible drug interactions.

Monitoring: Monitor for signs/symptoms of hypotension, angina, MI, fluid/ electrolyte imbalance, latent DM, sprue-like enteropathy, exacerbation/activation of SLE, hypersensitivity/idiosyncratic reactions, metabolic disturbances, myopia and angle-closure glaucoma, and other adverse reactions. Monitor BP, serum electrolytes, cholesterol and TG levels, and renal/hepatic function.

Counseling: Inform females of childbearing potential of the consequences of exposure during pregnancy and of the treatment options for women planning to become pregnant; instruct to report pregnancy to physician as soon as possible. Counsel that lightheadedness may occur, especially during the 1st days of therapy; instruct to report to physician. Instruct to d/c therapy and consult physician if syncope occurs. Advise that inadequate fluid intake, excessive perspiration, diarrhea, or vomiting may lead to an excessive fall in BP, which may result in lightheadedness and possible syncope.

TRICOR — fenofibrate

Rx

Class: Fibric acid derivative

ADULT DOSAGE

Primary Hypercholesterolemia/Mixed Dyslipidemia
Initial/Max: 145mg qd
Titrate: May consider reducing dose if lipid levels fall significantly below the targeted range

D/C if no adequate response after 2 months of treatment w/ max dose

Severe Hypertriglyceridemia
Initial: 48-145mg/day
Titrate: Adjust dose if necessary following repeat lipid determinations at 4- to 8-week intervals; may consider reducing dose if lipid levels fall significantly below the targeted range
Max: 145mg qd

D/C if no adequate response after 2 months of treatment w/ max dose

PEDIATRIC DOSAGE
Pediatric use may not have been established

DOSING CONSIDERATIONS
Renal Impairment
Mild to Moderate:
Initial: 48mg/day
Titrate: Increase only after evaluation of effects on renal function and lipid levels

Severe: Avoid use

ADMINISTRATION
Oral route

May be taken w/o regard to meals.
Swallow tab whole.

STORAGE
25°C (77°F); excursions permitted to 15-30°C (59-86°F). Protect from moisture.

HOW SUPPLIED
Tab: 48mg, 145mg

CONTRAINDICATIONS
Severe renal impairment (including dialysis), active liver disease (including primary biliary cirrhosis and unexplained persistent liver function abnormalities), preexisting gallbladder disease, nursing mothers, known hypersensitivity to fenofibrate or fenofibric acid.

WARNINGS/PRECAUTIONS
Not shown to reduce coronary heart disease morbidity and mortality in patients w/ type 2 diabetes mellitus (DM). Increases risk of myopathy and associated w/ rhabdomyolysis; risk for serious muscle toxicity increased w/ DM, renal insufficiency, and hypothyroidism, and in elderly. Consider myopathy in any patient w/ diffuse myalgias, muscle tenderness or weakness, and/or marked elevations of creatine phosphokinase (CPK) levels; d/c therapy if marked CPK elevation occurs or myopathy/myositis is suspected or diagnosed. Increases in serum transaminases; hepatocellular, chronic active, and cholestatic hepatitis; and cirrhosis (extremely rare) reported. Perform baseline and regular periodic monitoring of liver function, including serum ALT during duration of therapy; d/c if enzyme levels persist >3X the normal limit. Elevations in SrCr reported; monitor renal function in patients w/ renal impairment or at risk for renal insufficiency (eg, elderly, patients w/ diabetes). May cause cholelithiasis; d/c if gallstones are found. Pancreatitis and acute hypersensitivity reactions (eg, Stevens-Johnson syndrome, toxic epidermal necrolysis) reported. Mild to moderate Hgb, Hct, and WBC decreases; thrombocytopenia; and agranulocytosis reported. Periodically monitor RBC and WBC counts during the first 12 months of therapy. May cause venothromboembolic disease. Severe decreases in HDL levels reported; check HDL levels w/in the 1st few months after initiation of therapy. If a severely depressed HDL level is detected, withdraw therapy, monitor HDL level until it has returned to baseline, and do not reinitiate therapy. Estrogen therapy, thiazide diuretics, and β-blockers may be associated w/ massive rises in plasma TGs; discontinuation of these agents may obviate the need for specific drug therapy of hypertriglyceridemia.

ADVERSE REACTIONS
Abnormal LFTs, respiratory disorder, abdominal pain, back pain, headache, increased AST/ALT/CPK.

DRUG INTERACTIONS
Increased risk of rhabdomyolysis w/ HMG-CoA reductase inhibitors (statins); avoid combination unless benefit outweighs risk. Cases of myopathy, including rhabdomyolysis, reported when coadministered w/ colchicine; caution when prescribing w/ colchicine. May potentiate anticoagulant effects of coumarin anticoagulants; use w/ caution, reduce anticoagulant dosage, and monitor PT/INR frequently. Immunosuppressants (eg, cyclosporine, tacrolimus) may produce nephrotoxicity; consider benefits and risks, use lowest effective dose, and monitor renal function w/ immunosuppressants and other potentially nephrotoxic agents. Bile acid-binding resins may bind other drugs given concurrently; take at least 1 hr before or 4-6 hrs after the bile acid-binding resin to avoid impeding its absorption.

PREGNANCY AND LACTATION
Pregnancy: Category C.
Lactation: Not for use in nursing.

MECHANISM OF ACTION
Fibric acid derivative; activates peroxisome proliferator-activated receptor α. Increases lipolysis and elimination of TG-rich particles from plasma by activating lipoprotein lipase and reducing production of apoprotein C-III (lipoprotein lipase activity inhibitor). Also, induces an increase in the synthesis of apolipoproteins A-I, A-II, and HDL.

PHARMACOKINETICS
Absorption: Well-absorbed. T_{max}=6-8 hrs. **Distribution:** Plasma protein binding (99%). **Metabolism:** Rapid by ester hydrolysis to fenofibric acid (active metabolite); fenofibric acid is primarily conjugated w/ glucuronic acid. **Elimination:** Urine (60%, fenofibric acid and glucuronate conjugate), feces (25%); $T_{1/2}$=20 hrs.

PATIENT CONSIDERATIONS
Assessment: Assess for renal impairment, active liver disease, preexisting gallbladder disease, other medical conditions (eg, DM, hypothyroidism), hypersensitivity to drug, pregnancy/nursing status, and possible drug interactions. Obtain baseline LFTs.

Monitoring: Monitor for signs/symptoms of myositis, myopathy, or rhabdomyolysis; measure CPK levels in patients reporting such symptoms. Monitor for cholelithiasis, pancreatitis, hypersensitivity reactions, pulmonary embolism, and deep vein thrombosis. Monitor renal function, LFTs, CBC, and lipid levels. Monitor PT/INR frequently w/ coumarin anticoagulants.

Counseling: Advise of potential benefits and risks of therapy, and of medications to avoid during treatment. Instruct to continue to follow an appropriate lipid-modifying diet during therapy and to take drug qd, at the prescribed dose. Instruct to inform physician of all medications, supplements, and herbal preparations being taken, and any changes in medical condition. Instruct to notify physician of any muscle pain, tenderness, or weakness; onset of abdominal pain; or any other new symptoms. Advise to return for routine monitoring.

TRILEPTAL — oxcarbazepine   Rx

Class: Dibenzazepine

ADULT DOSAGE
Partial Seizures
Adjunctive Therapy:
Initial: 300mg bid
Titrate: Increase by a max of 600mg/day at weekly intervals
Usual: 1200mg/day

Conversion to Monotherapy:
Initial: 300mg bid
Titrate: Increase by a max of 600mg/day at weekly intervals
Usual: 2400mg/day

Reduce dose and withdraw concomitant antiepileptic drugs over 3-6 weeks, while reaching max oxcarbazepine dose in about 2-4 weeks

Initiation of Monotherapy:
Initial: 300mg bid
Titrate: Increase by 300mg/day every third day
Usual: 1200mg/day

PEDIATRIC DOSAGE
Partial Seizures
Adjunctive Therapy:
2-<4 Years:
Initial: 8-10mg/kg/day, not to exceed 600mg/day; may consider 16-20mg/kg for patients <20kg
Titrate: Increase to max maint dose over 2-4 weeks
Max: 60mg/kg/day

4-16 Years:
Initial: 8-10mg/kg/day, not to exceed 600mg/day
Maint: Increase to target dose over 2 weeks
20-29kg: 450mg bid
29.1-39kg: 600mg bid
>39kg: 900mg bid

W/ Epilepsy:
Conversion to Monotherapy:
4-16 Years:
Initial: 8-10mg/kg/day
Titrate: Increase by a max of 10mg/kg/day at weekly intervals

Reduce dose and withdraw concomitant antiepileptic drugs over 3-6 weeks

Initiation of Monotherapy:
4-16 Years:
Initial: 8-10mg/kg/day
Titrate: Increase by 5mg/kg/day every third day

Conversion to/Initiation of Monotherapy:
Maint:
20kg: 600-900mg/day
25-30kg: 900-1200mg/day
35-40kg: 900-1500mg/day
45kg: 1200-1500mg/day
50-55kg: 1200-1800mg/day
60-65kg: 1200-2100mg/day
70kg: 1500-2100mg/day

DOSING CONSIDERATIONS
Renal Impairment
CrCl <30mL/min:
Initial: 1/2 the usual starting dose (300mg/day)
Titrate: Increase slowly

ADMINISTRATION
Oral route

All dosing should be given in a bid regimen.
Sus and tabs may be interchanged at equal doses.
Take w/ or w/o food.

Sus
1. Before use, shake well and prepare dose immediately afterwards.
2. Use the supplied oral dosing syringe to withdraw the prescribed amount from the bottle.
3. Sus may be mixed in a small glass of water just prior to administration or may be swallowed directly from the syringe.
4. Close the bottle and rinse the syringe w/ warm water and allow it to dry thoroughly after each use.

STORAGE
25°C (77°F); excursions permitted to 15-30°C (59-86°F). (Sus) Use w/in 7 weeks of 1st opening the bottle.

HOW SUPPLIED
Sus: 300mg/5mL [250mL]; **Tab:** 150mg*, 300mg*, 600mg* *scored

CONTRAINDICATIONS
Known hypersensitivity to oxcarbazepine or to any of its components.

WARNINGS/PRECAUTIONS
Clinically significant hyponatremia may develop; consider measurement of serum Na+ levels during maintenance treatment, particularly if patient is receiving other medications known to decrease serum Na+ levels (eg, drugs associated w/ inappropriate antidiuretic hormone secretion) or if symptoms indicating hyponatremia develop. Anaphylaxis and angioedema involving the larynx, glottis, lips, and eyelids reported; d/c therapy if any of these reactions develop, start

alternative treatment, and do not rechallenge. Caution in patients w/ history of hypersensitivity reactions to carbamazepine; d/c immediately if signs/symptoms of hypersensitivity develop. Serious dermatological reactions (eg, Stevens-Johnson syndrome [SJS], toxic epidermal necrolysis [TEN]) reported; consider discontinuing use and prescribing another antiepileptic drug (AED) if a skin reaction develops. Patients carrying the human leukocyte antigen (HLA)-B*1502 allele may be at increased risk for SJS/TEN; consider testing for presence of HLA-B*1502 allele in patients w/ ancestry in genetically at-risk populations, and avoid use in patients positive for HLA-B*1502 unless benefits clearly outweigh risks. Increased risk of suicidal thoughts or behavior. Withdraw gradually to minimize the potential of increased seizure frequency. Associated w/ CNS-related adverse events (cognitive symptoms, somnolence or fatigue, coordination abnormalities). Drug reaction w/ eosinophilia and systemic symptoms (DRESS)/ multiorgan hypersensitivity reported; evaluate immediately if signs/symptoms (eg, rash, fever, lymphadenopathy) are present, and d/c if an alternative etiology cannot be established. Pancytopenia, agranulocytosis, and leukopenia reported; consider discontinuation if any evidence of hematologic events develop. Levels may decrease during pregnancy; monitor patients during pregnancy and through the postpartum period. Associated w/ decreases in T4, without changes in T3 or TSH. Caution w/ severe hepatic impairment.

ADVERSE REACTIONS
Dizziness, somnolence, diplopia, fatigue, N/V, ataxia, abnormal vision, tremor, abnormal gait, dyspepsia, abdominal pain.

DRUG INTERACTIONS
Verapamil, valproic acid, and strong CYP450 inducers (eg, carbamazepine, phenytoin, phenobarbital) may decrease levels. May decrease levels of dihydropyridine calcium antagonists, oral contraceptives (eg, ethinyl estradiol, levonorgestrel), cyclosporine, and felodipine. May increase levels of phenytoin, phenobarbital, and CYP2C19 substrates; may require dose reduction of phenytoin when using oxcarbazepine doses >1200mg/day. Decreased levels w/ AEDs that are CYP450 inducers.

PREGNANCY AND LACTATION
Pregnancy: Category C.
Lactation: Not for use in nursing.

MECHANISM OF ACTION
Dibenzazepine; has not been established. Suspected to exert antiseizure effects through blockade of voltage-sensitive Na^+ channels, resulting in stabilization of hyperexcited neural membranes, inhibition of repetitive neuronal firing, and diminution of propagation of synaptic impulses. Also, increased K^+ conductance and modulation of high-voltage activated Ca^{2+} channels may contribute to the anticonvulsant effects.

PHARMACOKINETICS
Absorption: (Tab) Complete. T_{max}=4.5 hrs (median). (Sus) T_{max}=6 hrs (median).
Distribution: Found in breast milk. 10-monohydroxy derivative (MHD): V_d=49L; plasma protein binding (40%). **Metabolism:** Liver (extensive); reduction by cytosolic enzymes to MHD (active metabolite). MHD: Conjugation w/ glucuronic acid.
Elimination: Urine (>95%, <1% unchanged), feces (<4%); $T_{1/2}$=2 hrs. MHD: $T_{1/2}$=9 hrs.

PATIENT CONSIDERATIONS
Assessment: Assess for history of hypersensitivity to drug or to carbamazepine, presence of HLA-B*1502 allele, depression, renal/hepatic impairment, pregnancy/ nursing status, and possible drug interactions.

Monitoring: Monitor for signs/symptoms of hyponatremia, angioedema, anaphylactic/hypersensitivity/dermatological reactions, emergence/worsening of depression, suicidal thoughts/behavior, unusual changes in mood/behavior, cognitive/neuropsychiatric events, DRESS, hematologic events, and other adverse reactions. Monitor patients during pregnancy and through the postpartum period.

Counseling: Advise to report symptoms of low Na^+, and fever to physician. Instruct to d/c and contact physician immediately if signs/symptoms suggesting angioedema develop. Advise to consult physician immediately if experiencing a hypersensitivity reaction, skin reaction, or symptoms suggestive of blood disorders. Warn female patients of childbearing age that concurrent use w/ hormonal contraceptives may render this method of contraception less effective; advise to use additional nonhormonal forms of contraception. Advise of the need to be alert for the emergence/worsening of symptoms of depression, any unusual changes in mood/behavior, or the emergence of suicidal thoughts, behavior, or thoughts about self-harm; instruct to immediately report behaviors of concern to physician. Instruct to use caution if taking alcohol while on therapy. Advise that drug may cause dizziness and somnolence, and not to drive or operate machinery until effects have been determined. Encourage to enroll in the North American Antiepileptic Drug Pregnancy Registry if patient becomes pregnant.

TRILIPIX — fenofibric acid   Rx
Class: Fibric acid derivative

ADULT DOSAGE
Severe Hypertriglyceridemia
Initial: 45-135mg qd
Titrate: Adjust dose if necessary following repeat lipid determinations at 4- to 8-week intervals
Max: 135mg qd

Primary Hypercholesterolemia/Mixed Dyslipidemia
135mg qd

PEDIATRIC DOSAGE
Pediatric use may not have been established

DOSING CONSIDERATIONS
Renal Impairment
Mild to Moderate:
Initial: 45mg qd
Titrate: Increase only after evaluation of effects on renal function and lipid levels

Other Important Considerations
D/C or change medications known to exacerbate hypertriglyceridemia (eg, β-blockers, thiazides, estrogens) if possible before considering therapy. Address excessive alcohol intake before therapy is considered.

ADMINISTRATION
Oral route

May be taken w/o regard to meals.
Swallow cap whole; do not open, crush, dissolve, or chew.

STORAGE
25°C (77°F); excursions permitted to 15-30°C (59-86°F). Protect from moisture.

HOW SUPPLIED
Cap, Delayed-Release: 45mg, 135mg

CONTRAINDICATIONS
Severe renal impairment (including dialysis), active liver disease (including primary biliary cirrhosis and unexplained persistent liver function abnormalities), preexisting gallbladder disease, and nursing mothers. Known hypersensitivity to fenofibrate or fenofibric acid.

WARNINGS/PRECAUTIONS
Not shown to reduce coronary heart disease morbidity and mortality in patients w/ type 2 diabetes mellitus (DM). Not indicated for patients who have elevations of chylomicrons and plasma TGs, but have normal VLDL levels. Increased risk of myositis/myopathy and rhabdomyolysis; risk increased w/ DM, renal failure, hypothyroidism, and in elderly. D/C therapy if markedly elevated CPK levels occur or myopathy/myositis is suspected or diagnosed. Increases in serum transaminases; hepatocellular, chronic active, and cholestatic hepatitis; and cirrhosis (rare) reported. Perform baseline and regular monitoring of LFTs, and d/c therapy if enzyme levels persist >3X ULN. Reversible elevations in SrCr reported. May cause cholelithiasis; d/c if gallstones are found. Acute hypersensitivity reactions (eg, Stevens-Johnson syndrome, toxic necrolysis) and pancreatitis reported. Mild to moderate decreases in Hgb, Hct, and WBCs reported. Thrombocytopenia and agranulocytosis reported; periodically monitor RBC and WBC counts during the first 12 months of therapy. May cause venothromboembolic disease. Severe decreases in HDL levels reported; check HDL levels w/in the 1st few months after initiation of therapy. If a severely depressed HDL level is detected, withdraw therapy, monitor HDL level until it has returned to baseline, and do not reinitiate therapy.

ADVERSE REACTIONS
Headache, back pain, abdominal pain, respiratory disorder, diarrhea, dyspepsia, pain, nasopharyngitis, sinusitis, URTI, arthralgia, myalgia, pain in extremity, dizziness.

DRUG INTERACTIONS
Increased risk of rhabdomyolysis w/ HMG-CoA reductase inhibitors (statins). May potentiate anticoagulant effects of coumarin anticoagulants prolonging PT/INR; use w/ caution, reduce anticoagulant dosage, and monitor PT/INR frequently. Bile acid-binding resins may bind other drugs given concurrently; take at least 1 hr before or 4-6 hrs after the bile acid resin to avoid impeding its absorption. Immunosuppressants (eg, cyclosporine, tacrolimus) may produce nephrotoxicity; consider benefits and risks, and use lowest effective dose w/ immunosuppressants and other potentially nephrotoxic agents. Cases of myopathy, including rhabdomyolysis, reported when coadministered w/ colchicine; caution when prescribing w/ colchicine.

PREGNANCY AND LACTATION
Pregnancy: Category C.
Lactation: Not for use in nursing.

MECHANISM OF ACTION
Fibric acid derivative; activates peroxisome proliferator-activated receptor α. Increases lipolysis and elimination of TG-rich particles from plasma by activating lipoprotein lipase and reducing production of Apo CIII (lipoprotein lipase activity inhibitor). Also induces an increase in the synthesis of HDL and Apo AI and AII.

PHARMACOKINETICS
Absorption: Well-absorbed. Absolute bioavailability (81%); T_{max}=4-5 hrs.
Distribution: Plasma protein binding (99%). **Metabolism:** Conjugation w/ glucuronic acid. **Elimination:** Urine; $T_{1/2}$=20 hrs.

PATIENT CONSIDERATIONS
Assessment: Assess for renal impairment, active liver disease, preexisting gallbladder disease, other medical conditions (eg, DM, hypothyroidism), hypersensitivity to drug, pregnancy/nursing status, and possible drug interactions. Obtain baseline LFTs.

Monitoring: Monitor for signs/symptoms of myositis, myopathy, or rhabdomyolysis; measure CPK levels in patients reporting such symptoms. Monitor for cholelithiasis, pancreatitis, hypersensitivity reactions, pulmonary embolism, and deep vein thrombosis. Monitor renal function, LFTs, CBC, and lipid levels. Monitor PT/INR frequently w/ coumarin anticoagulants.

Counseling: Advise of the potential benefits and risks of therapy, and of medications to avoid during treatment. Advise to read the Medication Guide before therapy and reread each time prescription is renewed. Instruct to follow appropriate lipid-modifying diet during therapy, and to take drug ud. Advise to return for routine monitoring. Instruct to inform physician of all medications, supplements, and herbal preparations being taken, any changes in medical condition, development of muscle pain, tenderness, or weakness, and onset of abdominal pain or any other new symptoms.

TRINTELLIX — vortioxetine   Rx

Class: Miscellaneous antidepressant

> Antidepressants increased the risk of suicidal thoughts and behavior in children, adolescents, and young adults in short-term studies. Monitor closely for worsening and for emergence of suicidal thoughts and behaviors in patients who are started on antidepressant therapy. Not evaluated for use in pediatric patients.

OTHER BRAND NAMES
Brintellix

ADULT DOSAGE

Major Depressive Disorder

Initial: 10mg qd
Titrate: Increase to 20mg/day, as tolerated. May consider decreasing dose to 5mg/day for patients who do not tolerate higher doses
Max: 20mg/day
Maint: Acute episodes of major depression should be followed by several months or longer of sustained therapy to decrease risk of recurrence

Dosing Considerations with MAOIs

Switching to/from an MAOI for Psychiatric Disorders:
Allow at least 14 days between discontinuation of an MAOI and initiation of treatment, and allow at least 21 days between discontinuation of treatment and initiation of an MAOI

Use w/ Other MAOIs (eg, Linezolid, IV Methylene Blue):
Do not start vortioxetine in a patient being treated w/ linezolid or IV methylene blue
In patients already receiving vortioxetine, if acceptable alternatives are not available and benefits outweigh risks, d/c vortioxetine and administer linezolid or IV methylene blue; monitor for serotonin syndrome for 21 days or until 24 hrs after the last dose of linezolid or IV methylene blue, whichever comes 1st. May resume vortioxetine therapy 24 hrs after the last dose of linezolid or IV methylene blue

PEDIATRIC DOSAGE
Pediatric use may not have been established

DOSING CONSIDERATIONS

Concomitant Medications

Use w/ Strong CYP2D6 Inhibitors:
Reduce vortioxetine dose by 1/2; increase dose to original level when CYP2D6 inhibitor is discontinued

Use w/ Strong CYP Inducers:
Consider increasing vortioxetine dose when a strong CYP inducer is coadministered for >14 days; max recommended dose should not exceed 3X original dose
Reduce dose to original level w/in 14 days, when the inducer is discontinued

Hepatic Impairment
Severe: Not recommended

Discontinuation
Decrease dose to 10mg/day for 1 week before full discontinuation of 15mg/day or 20mg/day

Other Important Considerations
CYP2D6 Poor Metabolizers:
Max: 10mg/day

ADMINISTRATION
Oral route
Take w/o regard to meals.

STORAGE
25°C (77°F); excursions permitted to 15-30°C (59-86°F).

HOW SUPPLIED
Tab: 5mg, 10mg, 15mg, 20mg

CONTRAINDICATIONS
Hypersensitivity to vortioxetine or any components of the formulation, use of an MAOI for psychiatric disorders either concomitantly or w/in 21 days of stopping treatment, treatment w/in 14 days of stopping an MAOI for psychiatric disorders, starting treatment in patients being treated w/ other MAOIs (eg, linezolid, IV methylene blue).

WARNINGS/PRECAUTIONS
May increase likelihood of precipitation of a mixed/manic episode in patients at risk for bipolar disorder. Screen patient to determine if at risk for bipolar disorder; not approved for treatment of bipolar depression. Serotonin syndrome reported; d/c immediately and initiate supportive symptomatic treatment. May increase risk of bleeding events. Activation of mania/hypomania reported; caution in patients w/ a history or family history of bipolar disorder, mania, or hypomania. Pupillary dilation that occurs following use may trigger an angle-closure attack in a patient w/ anatomically narrow angles who does not have a patent iridectomy. Transient adverse reactions (eg, headache, muscle tension) reported following abrupt discontinuation of doses of 15mg/day or 20mg/day. Hyponatremia reported; caution in the elderly and in volume-depleted patients. D/C in patients w/ symptomatic hyponatremia and institute appropriate medical intervention.

ADVERSE REACTIONS
N/V, constipation.

DRUG INTERACTIONS
See Dosage, Dosing Considerations, and Contraindications. May cause serotonin syndrome when coadministered w/ other serotonergic drugs (eg, SSRIs, triptans, TCAs, fentanyl, lithium) and w/ drugs that impair metabolism of serotonin; d/c immediately if this occurs and initiate supportive symptomatic treatment. May increase risk of bleeding w/ aspirin (ASA), NSAIDs, warfarin, and other anticoagulants; monitor patients receiving other drugs that interfere w/ hemostasis when vortioxetine is initiated or discontinued. Increased risk of hyponatremia w/ diuretics. Coadministration w/ another drug that is highly protein bound may increase free concentrations of the other drug.

PREGNANCY AND LACTATION
Pregnancy: Category C. Neonates exposed to SSRIs or SNRIs late in the 3rd trimester have developed complications requiring prolonged hospitalization, respiratory support, and tube feeding. Neonates exposed to SSRIs in pregnancy may have an increased risk for persistent pulmonary HTN of the newborn.
Lactation: Not for use in nursing.

MECHANISM OF ACTION
Antidepressant; has not been established. Thought to be related to its enhancement of serotonergic activity in the CNS through inhibition of the reuptake of 5-HT. Also has several other activities, including 5-HT$_3$ receptor antagonism and 5-HT$_{1A}$ receptor agonism.

PHARMACOKINETICS
Absorption: Absolute bioavailability (75%); C_{max}=9, 18, and 33ng/mL following doses of 5, 10, 20mg/day, T_{max}=7-11 hrs. **Distribution:** V_d: 2600L. Plasma protein binding (98%). **Metabolism:** Extensive. Oxidation via CYP2D6 (primary), CYP3A4/5, CYP2C19, CYP2C9, CYP2A6, CYP2C8, and CYP2B6, and glucuronic acid conjugation. **Elimination:** Urine (59%), feces (26%); $T_{1/2}$=66 hrs.

PATIENT CONSIDERATIONS

Assessment: Assess for hypersensitivity to drug or any of its components, volume depletion, susceptibility to angle-closure glaucoma, hepatic dysfunction, pregnancy/nursing status, and for possible drug interactions. Screen for risk for bipolar disorder; perform a detailed psychiatric history, including a family history of suicide, bipolar disorder, and depression.

Monitoring: Monitor for clinical worsening, suicidality, unusual changes in behavior, serotonin syndrome, abnormal bleeding, activation of mania/hypomania, angle-closure glaucoma, hyponatremia, hypersensitivity reactions, and other adverse reactions. If discontinuing therapy (particularly if abrupt), monitor for discontinuation symptoms.

Counseling: Inform of risks, benefits, and appropriate use of therapy. Advise patients and caregivers to look for the emergence of suicidality, especially early during treatment and when the dose is adjusted up or down. Inform that if patient is taking 15mg/day or 20mg/day, that he or she may experience headache, muscle tension, mood swings, sudden outburst of anger, dizziness, and runny nose if therapy is abruptly discontinued; advise not to d/c w/o notifying physician. Advise to inform physician if taking or planning to take any prescription or OTC drugs. Caution about risk of bleeding w/ NSAIDs, ASA, warfarin, or other drugs that affect hemostasis. Advise to look for signs of activation of mania/hypomania. Inform that drug may cause mild pupillary dilation, which in susceptible individuals may lead to an episode of angle-closure glaucoma. Inform of the greater risk of hyponatremia if treated w/ diuretics, if volume depleted, or if elderly. Inform that nausea is the most common adverse reaction, and is dose related. Instruct to notify physician if an allergic reaction occurs, if pregnant/planning to become pregnant, or if breastfeeding/planning to breastfeed.

TRIOSTAT — liothyronine sodium   Rx

Class: Thyroid replacement hormone

> Drugs with thyroid hormone activity, alone or together with other therapeutic agents, have been used for the treatment of obesity. Doses within the range of daily hormonal requirements are ineffective for weight reduction in euthyroid patients. Larger doses may produce serious or life-threatening manifestations of toxicity, particularly when given in association with sympathomimetic amines, such as those used for their anorectic effects.

ADULT DOSAGE

Myxedema Coma/Precoma

Initial: 25-50mcg IV (emergency treatment) or 10-20mcg IV (w/ known/suspected cardiovascular disease)

Initial and subsequent doses should be based on continuous monitoring of clinical status and response to therapy

At least 4 hrs and no more than 12 hrs should elapse between doses

PEDIATRIC DOSAGE
Pediatric use may not have been established

Conversions
Switching to Oral Therapy:
Resume as soon as clinical situation has been stabilized and patient is able to take oral medication

Switching to Liothyronine Sodium:
D/C therapy, initiate oral therapy at a low dose, and increase gradually according to response

Switching to L-thyroxine:
D/C gradually if L-thyroxine rather than liothyronine sodium is used in initiating oral therapy due to the delay of several days in the onset of L-thyroxine activity

DOSING CONSIDERATIONS
Elderly
Start at lower end of dosing range

ADMINISTRATION
IV route

IV administration only; should not be given IM or SQ. Administer at least 4 hrs and not more than 12 hrs apart.

STORAGE
2-8°C (36-46°F).

HOW SUPPLIED
Inj: 10mcg/mL [1mL]

CONTRAINDICATIONS
Uncorrected adrenal cortical insufficiency, untreated thyrotoxicosis, artificial rewarming. Hypersensitivity to any of the active or extraneous constituents of Triostat.

WARNINGS/PRECAUTIONS
Not for IM or SQ route. Use is unjustified for the treatment of male or female infertility unless accompanied by hypothyroidism. Caution with CVD (eg, angina pectoris) or in elderly; monitor cardiac function. Caution in myxedematous patients; start at a low dose level and increase gradually. Supplemental adrenocortical steroids may be necessary in patients with severe and prolonged hypothyroidism. May precipitate a hyperthyroid state or aggravate hyperthyroidism. May aggravate symptoms of diabetes mellitus (DM), diabetes insipidus (DI), or adrenal cortical insufficiency. Monitor and treat infection appropriately in myxedema coma patients. Therapy of myxedema coma requires simultaneous administration of glucocorticoids. Concurrent use with androgens, corticosteroids, estrogens, oral contraceptives containing estrogens, iodine-containing preparations, and salicylates may interfere with thyroid laboratory tests.

ADVERSE REACTIONS
Arrhythmia, tachycardia.

DRUG INTERACTIONS
See Boxed Warning. Hypothyroidism decreases and hyperthyroidism increases sensitivity to anticoagulants; monitor PT closely and adjust anticoagulants based on frequent PT determinations. May cause increases in insulin or oral hypoglycemic requirements during thyroid replacement initiation. Estrogens increase thyroxine-binding globulin; increase in thyroid dose may be needed in patients without a functioning thyroid gland. Increased effects of both agents with TCAs (eg, imipramine). May cause HTN and tachycardia with ketamine; use with caution and treat HTN if necessary. May potentiate toxic effects of digitalis. Increased adrenergic effect of catecholamines (eg, epinephrine, norepinephrine). May increase risk of precipitating coronary insufficiency, especially with coronary artery disease (CAD) with vasopressors; use with caution. Caution when administering fluid therapy.

PREGNANCY AND LACTATION
Pregnancy: Category A.
Lactation: Caution in nursing.

MECHANISM OF ACTION
Synthetic thyroid hormone; enhances oxygen consumption by most tissues of the body and increases the basal metabolic rate and metabolism of carbohydrates, lipids, and proteins.

PATIENT CONSIDERATIONS
Assessment: Assess thyroid status, CVD (eg, CAD, angina pectoris), DM/DI, adrenal cortical insufficiency, nursing status, and for possible drug interactions.

Monitoring: Monitor for signs/symptoms of precipitation of adrenocortical insufficiency, aggravation of DM/DI, infection, hypersensitivity reactions, and other adverse reactions. Monitor thyroid function periodically. Monitor patient's clinical status and response to therapy. Monitor PT closely in thyroid-treated patients on anticoagulants and adjust anticoagulants based on frequent PT determinations.

Counseling: Inform of the risks/benefits of therapy. Instruct to seek medical attention if symptoms of toxicity, aggravation of DM/DI, or hypersensitivity reactions occur.

TRIUMEQ — abacavir/dolutegravir/lamivudine   Rx
Class: Integrase strand transfer inhibitor/nucleoside reverse transcriptase inhibitor (NRTI) combination

> Lactic acidosis and severe hepatomegaly w/ steatosis, including fatal cases, reported w/ nucleoside analogues; d/c if clinical or lab findings suggestive of lactic acidosis or pronounced hepatotoxicity occur. **Abacavir:** Serious and sometimes fatal hypersensitivity reactions, w/ multiple organ involvement, reported; d/c immediately if a hypersensitivity reaction is suspected and never restart therapy or any other abacavir-containing product. Patients who carry the HLA-B*5701 allele are at a higher risk of a hypersensitivity reaction; screen all patients for HLA-B*5701 allele prior to initiating or reinitiating therapy, unless patient has a previously documented HLA-B*5701 allele assessment. **Lamivudine:** Severe acute exacerbations of hepatitis B reported in patients coinfected w/ hepatitis B virus (HBV) and HIV-1 and have discontinued therapy; closely monitor hepatic function for at least several months. If appropriate, initiation of antihepatitis B therapy may be warranted.

ADULT DOSAGE	PEDIATRIC DOSAGE
HIV-1 Infection	Pediatric use may not have been established
1 tab qd	

DOSING CONSIDERATIONS
Concomitant Medications
Efavirenz, Fosamprenavir/Ritonavir (RTV), Tipranavir/RTV, Carbamazepine, or Rifampin: Take an additional dolutegravir 50mg tab, separated by 12 hrs from therapy

Renal Impairment
CrCl <50mL/min: Not recommended

Hepatic Impairment
Mild (Child-Pugh Score A): Not recommended
Moderate (Child-Pugh Class B) or Severe (Child-Pugh Class C): Contraindicated

ADMINISTRATION
Oral route

Take w/ or w/o food.
Screen for the HLA-B*5701 allele prior to initiating therapy.

STORAGE
25°C (77°F); excursions permitted to 15-30°C (59-86°F). Protect from moisture.

HOW SUPPLIED
Tab: (Abacavir/Dolutegravir/Lamivudine) 600mg/50mg/300mg

CONTRAINDICATIONS
Patients w/ HLA-B*5701 allele; prior hypersensitivity reaction to abacavir, dolutegravir, or lamivudine; coadministration w/ dofetilide; moderate or severe hepatic impairment.

WARNINGS/PRECAUTIONS
Not recommended for use w/ current or past history of resistance to any components of therapy. Therapy alone is not recommended w/ resistance-associated integrase substitutions or clinically suspected integrase strand transfer inhibitor resistance. Immune reconstitution syndrome reported. Autoimmune disorders (eg, Graves' disease, polymyositis, Guillain-Barre syndrome) reported to occur in the setting of immune reconstitution and may occur many months after initiation of treatment. Redistribution/accumulation of body fat may occur. Caution in elderly. **Abacavir:** May increase risk of MI. Consider underlying risk of coronary heart disease (CHD) when prescribing therapy; minimize all modifiable risk factors. **Dolutegravir:** Hypersensitivity reactions reported; d/c therapy and other suspect agents immediately if signs/symptoms develop. May be at increased risk for worsening or development of transaminase elevations in patients w/ underlying hepatitis B or C. **Lamivudine:** Emergence of lamivudine-resistant HBV reported.

ADVERSE REACTIONS
Insomnia, headache, fatigue.

DRUG INTERACTIONS
See Dosing Considerations and Contraindications. Closely monitor for treatment-associated toxicities, especially hepatic decompensation in patients receiving interferon alfa w/ or w/o ribavirin; consider dose reduction or discontinuation of interferon alfa, ribavirin, or both if worsening clinical toxicities are observed, including hepatic decompensation (eg, Child-Pugh >6); consider discontinuation of Triumeq as medically appropriate. Not recommended w/ other abacavir- or lamivudine-containing products. **Abacavir:** May increase oral methadone clearance; an increased methadone dose may be required in a small number of patients. **Dolutegravir:** Drugs that induce/inhibit UGT1A1, CYP3A, UGT1A3, UGT1A9, breast cancer resistance protein, and P-gp may decrease/increase levels, respectively. Decreased levels w/ etravirine; use of Triumeq w/ etravirine w/o coadministration of atazanavir/RTV, darunavir/RTV, or lopinavir/RTV is not recommended. Decreased levels w/ efavirenz, fosamprenavir/RTV, tipranavir/RTV, rifampin, and carbamazepine. Decreased levels w/ nevirapine, oxcarbazepine, phenytoin, phenobarbital, and St. John's wort; avoid coadministration w/ Triumeq. Administer 2 hrs before or 6 hrs after taking medications containing polyvalent cations (eg, cation-containing antacids/laxatives, sucralfate, buffered medications) or taking oral Ca²⁺ or iron supplements (eg, multivitamins); alternatively, therapy and supplements containing Ca²⁺ or iron can be taken together w/ food. May increase levels of drugs eliminated via organic cation transporter 2 or multidrug and toxin extrusion transporter 1 (eg, metformin); limit the total daily dose of metformin to 1000mg when starting either metformin or Triumeq; monitoring of blood glucose when initiating concomitant use and after withdrawal of Triumeq is recommended. When stopping Triumeq, metformin dose may require adjustment.

PREGNANCY AND LACTATION
Pregnancy: Category C.
Lactation: Not for use in nursing.

MECHANISM OF ACTION

Abacavir: Carbocyclic synthetic nucleoside analogue; inhibits HIV-1 reverse transcriptase (RT) activity by competing w/ natural substrate deoxyguanosine-5'-triphosphate and by incorporating into viral DNA. **Dolutegravir:** HIV-1 integrase strand transfer inhibitor; inhibits HIV integrase by binding to integrase active site and blocking the strand transfer step of retroviral DNA integration, which is essential for the HIV replication cycle. **Lamivudine:** Synthetic nucleoside analogue; inhibits RT via DNA chain termination after incorporation of the nucleotide analogue.

PHARMACOKINETICS

Absorption: Abacavir: Rapid. C_{max}=4.26mcg/mL; AUC=11.95mcg•hr/mL. Dolutegravir: AUC_{0-24}=53.6mcg•hr/mL; C_{max}=3.67mcg/mL; T_{max}=2-3 hrs. Lamivudine: Rapid. C_{max}=2.04mcg/mL; AUC=8.87mcg•hr/mL. **Distribution:** Abacavir: Plasma protein binding (50%). Dolutegravir: V_d=17.4L; plasma protein binding (≥98.9%). Lamivudine: Found in breast milk. **Metabolism:** Abacavir: Via alcohol dehydrogenase and glucuronyl transferase; 5'-carboxylic acid, 5'-glucuronide (metabolites). Dolutegravir: Via UGT1A1, CYP3A. Lamivudine: Trans-sulfoxide (metabolite). **Elimination:** Abacavir: $T_{1/2}$=1.54 hrs. Dolutegravir: Urine (31%, <1% unchanged), feces (53% unchanged); $T_{1/2}$=14 hrs. Lamivudine: Urine (70%, unchanged) (IV); $T_{1/2}$=5-7 hrs.

PATIENT CONSIDERATIONS

Assessment: Assess for previous hypersensitivity to the drug, hepatic/renal impairment, hepatitis B or C infection, risk factors for CHD, pregnancy/nursing status, and possible drug interactions. Screen for HLA-B*5701 allele prior to initiation/reinitiation of therapy. Assess medical history for prior exposure to any abacavir-containing product.

Monitoring: Monitor for signs/symptoms of hypersensitivity reactions, lactic acidosis, hepatomegaly w/ steatosis, immune reconstitution syndrome, autoimmune disorders, fat redistribution/accumulation, MI, and other adverse reactions. Monitor hepatic function. Monitor for exacerbations of hepatitis B in patients who are coinfected w/ HBV; closely monitor hepatic function for at least several months after stopping therapy in patients coinfected w/ HBV.

Counseling: Inform about the risks and benefits of therapy. Advise to report the use of any prescription or nonprescription medication or herbal products. Advise about hypersensitivity reactions; instruct to contact physician immediately if symptoms develop and not to restart or replace w/ any drug containing abacavir w/o medical consultation. Inform that the drug may cause lactic acidosis and severe hepatomegaly w/steatosis. Inform patients w/ underlying hepatitis B or C that they may be at increased risk of worsening or development of transaminase elevations. Inform that hepatic decompensation has occurred in HIV-1/HCV-coinfected patients receiving combination antiretroviral therapy and interferon alfa w/ or w/o ribavirin. Inform that fat redistribution/accumulation may occur. Advise that drug is not a cure for HIV-1 infection and that illness associated w/ HIV-1 infection may continue, including opportunistic infections. Instruct to take all HIV medications exactly as prescribed. Advise to avoid doing things that can spread HIV-1 infection to others. Advise to inform physician immediately of any symptoms of infection or if any unusual symptom develops, or if any known symptom persists or worsens. Explain missed dose instructions.

TRIZIVIR — abacavir/lamivudine/zidovudine　　　　　Rx
Class: Nucleoside reverse transcriptase inhibitor (NRTI) combination

> Lactic acidosis and severe hepatomegaly w/ steatosis, including fatal cases, reported w/ nucleoside analogues and other antiretrovirals. D/C if clinical or lab findings suggestive of lactic acidosis or pronounced hepatotoxicity occur. **Abacavir:** Serious and sometimes fatal hypersensitivity reactions w/ multiple organ involvement reported; d/c immediately if a hypersensitivity reaction is suspected and never restart therapy or any other abacavir-containing product. Patients who carry the HLA-B*5701 allele are at a higher risk of a hypersensitivity reaction; screen all patients for HLA-B*5701 allele prior to initiating or reinitiating therapy, unless patient has a previously documented HLA-B*5701 allele assessment. **Zidovudine:** Associated w/ hematologic toxicity (eg, neutropenia, severe anemia), particularly w/ advanced HIV-1 disease. Symptomatic myopathy associated w/ prolonged use. **Lamivudine:** Severe acute exacerbations of hepatitis B reported in patients coinfected w/ hepatitis B virus (HBV) and HIV-1 and have discontinued therapy; closely monitor hepatic function w/ both clinical and lab follow-up for at least several months. If appropriate, initiation of antihepatitis B therapy may be warranted.

ADULT DOSAGE
HIV-1 Infection
1 tab bid

PEDIATRIC DOSAGE
HIV-1 Infection
>40kg:
1 tab bid

DOSING CONSIDERATIONS
Renal Impairment
CrCl <50mL/min: Not recommended for use

Hepatic Impairment
Mild: Not recommended for use
Moderate/Severe: Contraindicated

ADMINISTRATION
Oral route

Take w/ or w/o food.
Screen for the HLA-B*5701 allele prior to initiating therapy.

STORAGE
25°C (77°F); excursions permitted to 15-30°C (59-86°F).

HOW SUPPLIED
Tab: (Abacavir Sulfate/Lamivudine/Zidovudine) 300mg/150mg/300mg

CONTRAINDICATIONS
Prior hypersensitivity reaction to Trizivir, moderate or severe hepatic impairment, patients w/ HLA-B*5701 allele.

WARNINGS/PRECAUTIONS
Obesity and prolonged nucleoside exposure may be risk factors for lactic acidosis and severe hepatomegaly w/ steatosis; suspend therapy if clinical or lab findings suggestive of lactic acidosis or pronounced hepatotoxicity develop. Immune reconstitution syndrome reported. Autoimmune disorders (eg, Graves' disease, polymyositis, Guillain-Barre syndrome) reported to occur in the setting of immune reconstitution and can occur many months after initiation of treatment. Redistribution/accumulation of body fat may occur. Cross-resistance potential w/ nucleoside reverse transcriptase inhibitors reported. Caution w/ any known risk factors for liver disease and in elderly. Avoid use in adolescents weighing <40kg and in patients requiring dose adjustments (eg, renal impairment [CrCl <50mL/min]). **Abacavir:** Consider underlying risk of coronary heart disease (CHD) when prescribing therapy. **Lamivudine:** Emergence of lamivudine-resistant HBV reported. **Zidovudine:** Caution w/ compromised bone marrow evidenced by granulocyte count <1000 cells/mm^3 or Hgb <9.5g/dL; monitor blood counts frequently w/ advanced HIV-1 disease and periodically in other HIV-1 infected patients. Interrupt therapy if anemia or neutropenia develops.

ADVERSE REACTIONS
N/V, headache, malaise, fatigue, hypersensitivity reaction, diarrhea, fever, chills, depressive disorders, musculoskeletal pain, skin rashes, anxiety, ear/nose/throat infections.

DRUG INTERACTIONS
Avoid w/ other abacavir-, lamivudine-, zidovudine-, and/or emtricitabine-containing products. Closely monitor for treatment associated toxicities, especially hepatic decompensation, neutropenia, and anemia, in patients receiving interferon alfa w/ or w/o ribavirin and Trizivir; consider discontinuation of Trizivir as medically appropriate and consider dose reduction or discontinuation of interferon alfa, ribavirin, or both if worsening clinical toxicities are observed. **Abacavir:** Ethanol may decrease elimination, causing an increase in overall exposure. May increase oral methadone clearance; an increased methadone dose may be required in a small number of patients. **Zidovudine:** Avoid w/ stavudine, doxorubicin, and nucleoside analogues (eg, ribavirin). May increase hematologic toxicity w/ ganciclovir, interferon alfa, ribavirin, and other bone marrow suppressive or cytotoxic agents.

PREGNANCY AND LACTATION
Pregnancy: Category C.
Lactation: Not for use in nursing.

MECHANISM OF ACTION
Abacavir: Carbocyclic synthetic nucleoside analogue; inhibits HIV-1 reverse transcriptase (RT) by competing w/ natural substrate deoxyguanosine-5'-triphosphate and by incorporating into viral DNA. **Lamivudine/Zidovudine:** Synthetic nucleoside analogue; inhibits RT via DNA chain termination after incorporation of the nucleotide analogue.

PHARMACOKINETICS
Absorption: Rapid. Abacavir: Oral Bioavailability: (86%); C_{max}=3 mcg/mL; AUC=6.02mcg•hr/mL. Lamivudine: Oral Bioavailability: (86%). Zidovudine: Oral Bioavailability: (64%). **Distribution:** Abacavir: V_d=0.86L/kg; plasma protein binding (50%). Lamivudine: V_d=1.3L/kg; plasma protein binding (low). Zidovudine: V_d=1.6L/kg; plasma protein binding (low); crosses the placenta. **Metabolism:** Abacavir: Via alcohol dehydrogenase and glucuronyl transferase; 5'-carboxylic acid, 5'-glucuronide (metabolites). Lamivudine: Trans-sulfoxide (metabolite). Zidovudine: Hepatic via glucuronyl transferase; 3'-azido-3'-deoxy-5'-O-β-D-glucopyranuronosylthymidine (GZDV) (major metabolite). **Elimination:** Abacavir: $T_{1/2}$=1.45 hrs. Lamivudine: (IV) Urine (70%, unchanged); $T_{1/2}$=5-7 hrs. Zidovudine: Urine (14% unchanged, 74% GZDV); $T_{1/2}$=0.5-3 hrs.

PATIENT CONSIDERATIONS
Assessment: Assess for history of hypersensitivity reactions, advanced HIV disease, hepatic/renal impairment, risk factors for lactic acidosis, risk factors for CHD, bone marrow compromise, HBV infection, pregnancy/nursing status, and possible drug interactions. Screen for HLA-B*5701 allele prior to initiation of therapy. Assess medical history for prior exposure to any abacavir-containing product.

Monitoring: Monitor for signs/symptoms of hypersensitivity reactions, hematologic toxicity, lactic acidosis, hepatomegaly w/ steatosis, myopathy, immune reconstitution syndrome, autoimmune disorders, fat redistribution/accumulation, MI, and other adverse reactions. Monitor hepatic/renal function. Monitor hepatic function closely for at least several months in patients who d/c therapy and are coinfected w/ HIV-1 and HBV. Perform frequent blood counts in patients w/ advanced HIV-1 disease and perform periodic blood counts for other HIV-1-infected patients.

Counseling: Inform about hypersensitivity reactions; instruct to contact physician immediately if symptoms develop and not to restart or replace w/ any drug containing abacavir w/o medical consultation. Inform about risk for hematologic toxicities and advise on importance of close blood count monitoring while on therapy. Counsel about the possible occurrence of myopathy and myositis w/ pathological changes during prolonged use and that therapy may cause a rare but serious condition called lactic acidosis w/ hepatomegaly. Inform patients coinfected w/ HBV that deterioration of liver disease has occurred in some cases when treatment was discontinued; instruct to discuss any changes in regimen w/ physician. Inform that hepatic decompensation has occurred in HIV-1/hepatitis C virus coinfected patients receiving combination antiretroviral therapy and interferon alfa w/ or w/o ribavirin. Inform that redistribution/accumulation of body fat may occur. Advise that drug is not a cure for HIV-1 infection and that illness associated w/ HIV-1 may still be experienced. Advise to avoid doing things that can spread HIV-1 infection to others. Inform patients to take all HIV medications exactly as prescribed.

TROKENDI XR — topiramate

Class: Sulfamate-substituted monosaccharide antiepileptic

Rx

ADULT DOSAGE

Epilepsy

Partial Onset Seizures or Primary Generalized Tonic-Clonic Seizures:
Monotherapy:
Titration Schedule:
Week 1: 50mg qd
Week 2: 100mg qd
Week 3: 150mg qd
Week 4: 200mg qd
Week 5: 300mg qd
Week 6: 400mg qd
Recommended Dose: 400mg qd

Adjunctive Therapy:
≥17 Years:
Initial: 25-50mg qd
Titrate: Increase in increments of 25-50mg every week to achieve effective dose
Recommended Dose:
Partial Onset Seizures: 200-400mg qd
Primary Generalized Tonic-Clonic Seizures: 400mg qd

Daily doses >1600mg have not been studied

Lennox-Gastaut Syndrome:
Adjunctive Therapy:
≥17 Years:
Initial: 25-50mg qd
Titrate: Increase in increments of 25-50mg every week to achieve effective dose
Recommended Dose: 200-400mg qd

Daily doses >1600mg have not been studied

PEDIATRIC DOSAGE

Epilepsy

Partial Onset Seizures or Primary Generalized Tonic-Clonic Seizures:
Monotherapy:
6 to <10 Years:
Initial: 25mg qpm for the 1st week
Titrate: May increase to 50mg/day in the 2nd week, then may increase by 25-50mg/day each subsequent week. Titration to the minimum maint dose should be attempted over 5-7 weeks of the total titration period; additional titration to a higher dose (up to the max maint dose) can be attempted in weekly increments at 25-50mg/day weekly increments up to the max recommended maint dose for each range of body weight

Up to 11kg:
Minimum Maint Dose: 150mg/day
Max Maint Dose: 250mg/day

12-22kg:
Minimum Maint Dose: 200mg/day
Max Maint Dose: 300mg/day

23-31kg:
Minimum Maint Dose: 200mg/day
Max Maint Dose: 350mg/day

32-38kg:
Minimum Maint Dose: 250mg/day
Max Maint Dose: 350mg/day

>38kg:
Minimum Maint Dose: 250mg/day
Max Maint Dose: 400mg/day

≥10 Years:
Titration Schedule:
Week 1: 50mg qd
Week 2: 100mg qd
Week 3: 150mg qd
Week 4: 200mg qd
Week 5: 300mg qd
Week 6: 400mg qd
Recommended Dose: 400mg qd

Partial Onset Seizures, Primary Generalized Tonic-Clonic Seizures, or Lennox-Gastaut Syndrome:
Adjunctive Therapy:
6-16 Years:
Initial: 25mg qpm (based on a range of 1-3mg/kg/day) for 1st week
Titrate: Increase at 1- or 2-week intervals by increments of 1-3mg/kg to achieve optimal clinical response; longer intervals between dose adjustments may be used if required
Recommended Dose: 5-9mg/kg qd

- -

DOSING CONSIDERATIONS
Concomitant Medications
Phenytoin and/or Carbamazepine:
May require an adjustment of the dose of phenytoin to achieve optimal clinical outcome.
Addition or withdrawal of phenytoin and/or carbamazepine during adjunctive therapy may require dose adjustment of topiramate.

Renal Impairment
CrCl <70mL/min: Use 1/2 the usual starting and maint dose
Hemodialysis: Supplemental dose may be required

ADMINISTRATION
Oral route

May be taken w/o regard to meals.
Swallow cap whole and intact; do not sprinkle on food, chew, or crush.
Completely avoid alcohol use w/in 6 hrs prior to and 6 hrs after administration.

STORAGE
25°C (77°F); excursions permitted to 15-30°C (59-86°F). Protect from moisture and light.

HOW SUPPLIED
Cap, Extended-Release: 25mg, 50mg, 100mg, 200mg

CONTRAINDICATIONS
Patients w/ recent alcohol use (eg, w/in 6 hrs prior to and 6 hrs after use), patients w/ metabolic acidosis taking concomitant metformin.

WARNINGS/PRECAUTIONS
Acute myopia associated w/ secondary angle-closure glaucoma reported; d/c as rapidly as possible to reverse symptoms. Oligohydrosis and hyperthermia reported, mostly in pediatric patients; monitor closely for decreased sweating and increased body temperature. Hyperchloremic, non-anion gap, metabolic acidosis reported; conditions or therapies that predispose to acidosis may be additive to the bicarbonate lowering effects. Consider discontinuing or reducing dose if metabolic acidosis develops and persists. If decision is made to continue therapy, consider alkali treatment. Increased risk of suicidal thoughts/behavior; monitor for the emergence/worsening of depression, suicidal thoughts/behavior, and/or any unusual changes in mood or behavior. May cause cognitive-related dysfunction, psychiatric/behavioral disturbances, somnolence, or fatigue. May cause fetal harm. D/C gradually to minimize the potential for seizures or increased seizure frequency; appropriate monitoring is recommended when rapid withdrawal is required. Patients w/ inborn errors of metabolism or reduced hepatic mitochondrial activity may be at an increased risk for hyperammonemia w/ or w/o encephalopathy; consider hyperammonemic encephalopathy and measure ammonia levels in patients who develop unexplained lethargy, vomiting, or changes in mental status associated w/ therapy. Kidney stone formation reported; hydration recommended to reduce new stone formation. Ketogenic diet may increase the risk of kidney stone formation; avoid use. Paresthesia may occur. Visual field defects (independent of elevated IOP) reported; consider discontinuation if visual problems occur at any time during treatment. Lab abnormalities may occur.

ADVERSE REACTIONS
Paresthesia, anorexia, weight decrease, speech disorders/related speech problems, fatigue, dizziness, somnolence, nervousness, psychomotor slowing, abnormal vision, difficulty w/ memory, difficulty w/ concentration/attention, fever.

DRUG INTERACTIONS
See Dosing Considerations and Contraindications. May decrease contraceptive efficacy and increase breakthrough bleeding w/ combination oral contraceptives. Avoid use w/ other drugs producing metabolic acidosis. Phenytoin or carbamazepine may decrease levels. Concurrent administration of valproic acid has been associated w/ hyperammonemia w/ or w/o encephalopathy and hypothermia; consider stopping topiramate or valproate in patients who develop hypothermia. Concomitant administration w/ other CNS depressant drugs or alcohol can result in significant CNS depression. Other carbonic anhydrase inhibitors (eg, zonisamide, acetazolamide, dichlorphenamide) may increase the severity of metabolic acidosis and may also increase the risk of kidney stone formation; monitor for appearance or worsening of metabolic acidosis. Increase in systemic exposure of lithium observed following topiramate doses of ≤600mg/day; monitor lithium levels. Caution w/ agents that predispose patients to heat-related disorders (eg, carbonic anhydrase inhibitors, anticholinergics).

PREGNANCY AND LACTATION
Pregnancy: Can cause fetal harm. Data from pregnancy registries indicate that infants exposed to topiramate in utero have increased risk for cleft lip and/or cleft palate and for being small for gestational age. Physicians are advised to recommend that pregnant patients enroll in the North American Antiepileptic Drug (NAAED) Pregnancy Registry.
Lactation: Topiramate is excreted in human milk; caution in nursing.
Reproductive Potential: Women of childbearing potential who are not planning a pregnancy should use effective contraception because of the risks to the fetus.

MECHANISM OF ACTION
Sulfamate-substituted monosaccharide antiepileptic; has not been established. Suspected to block voltage-dependent Na^+ channels, augment activity of the neurotransmitter gamma-aminobutyrate at some subtypes of the GABA-A receptor, antagonize the AMPA/kainate subtype of the glutamate receptor, and inhibit the carbonic anhydrase enzyme, particularly isoenzymes II and IV.

PHARMACOKINETICS
Absorption: T_{max}=24 hrs (200mg). **Distribution:** Plasma protein binding (15-41%). Found in breast milk. **Metabolism:** Hydroxylation, hydrolysis, glucuronidation. **Elimination:** Urine (approx 70% unchanged); $T_{1/2}$=approx 31 hrs.

PATIENT CONSIDERATIONS
Assessment: Assess for recent alcohol use, metabolic acidosis in patients taking concomitant metformin, predisposing factors for metabolic acidosis, renal dysfunction, inborn errors of metabolism, reduced hepatic mitochondrial activity, pregnancy/nursing status, and possible drug interactions. Obtain baseline serum bicarbonate levels. Obtain baseline estimated GFR measurement in patients at high risk for renal insufficiency.

Monitoring: Monitor for signs/symptoms of acute myopia, secondary-angle glaucoma, oligohydrosis, hyperthermia, suicidal behavior and ideation, cognitive or neuropsychiatric adverse reactions, kidney stones, metabolic acidosis, paresthesias, hyperammonemia, visual field defects, and other adverse reactions. Periodically measure serum bicarbonate levels.

Counseling: Instruct to take ud. Advise to completely avoid consumption of alcohol at least 6 hrs prior to and 6 hrs after taking the drug. Instruct to seek immediate medical attention if blurred vision, visual disturbances, periorbital pain, decreased sweating, or increased body temperature occurs. Inform about the potentially significant risk for metabolic acidosis that may be asymptomatic and may be associated w/ adverse effects on kidneys, bones, and growth in pediatric patients, and on the fetus. Instruct to immediately report to the physician if emergence or worsening of depression, unusual changes in mood/behavior, emergence of suicidal thoughts, or behavior/thoughts about self-harm occur. Instruct to use caution when engaging in any activities where loss of consciousness may result in serious danger. Inform of pregnancy risks; encourage pregnant women to enroll in the NAAED Pregnancy Registry. Warn about the possible development of hyperammonemia w/ or w/o encephalopathy; instruct to contact physician if unexplained lethargy, vomiting, or mental status changes develop. Instruct to maintain an adequate fluid intake to minimize risk of kidney stones. Inform that therapy may cause a reduction in body temperature that can lead to alterations in mental status; if changes are noted, instruct patients to measure their body temperature and to contact physician. Instruct to consult physician if tingling in the arms and legs occurs.

TRULICITY — dulaglutide   Rx

Class: Glucagon-like peptide-1 (GLP-1) receptor agonist

> Causes dose-related and treatment-duration-dependent increase in the incidence of thyroid C-cell tumors (adenomas, carcinomas) after lifetime exposure in animal studies. It is unknown whether drug causes thyroid C-cell tumors (eg, medullary thyroid carcinoma [MTC]) in humans; human relevance of dulaglutide-induced thyroid C-cell tumors in rodents has not been determined. Contraindicated in patients w/ a personal or family history of MTC and in patients w/ multiple endocrine neoplasia syndrome type 2 (MEN 2). Routine monitoring of serum calcitonin or using thyroid ultrasound is of uncertain value for early detection of MTC in patients treated w/ therapy.

ADULT DOSAGE

Type 2 Diabetes Mellitus

Initial: 0.75mg once weekly; may increase to 1.5mg once weekly
Max: 1.5mg once weekly

Day of weekly administration may be changed if necessary as long as the last dose was administered ≥3 days before

Missed Dose

If a dose is missed, administer as soon as possible if there are ≥3 days (72 hrs) until the next scheduled dose; if <3 days remain before the next scheduled dose, skip the missed dose and administer the next dose on the regularly scheduled day

Patients may then resume regular once weekly dosing schedule in each case

PEDIATRIC DOSAGE

Pediatric use may not have been established

DOSING CONSIDERATIONS

Concomitant Medications

Insulin Secretagogue (eg, Sulfonylurea)/Insulin: Consider reducing dose of insulin secretagogues or insulin when initiating therapy

ADMINISTRATION

SQ route

Administer once weekly, any time of day, w/ or w/o food
Inject in the abdomen, thigh, or upper arm

Use w/ Insulin

Administer as separate inj; never mix products
May inject in the same body region; inj should not be adjacent to each other
If injecting in the same body region, use a different inj site each week

STORAGE

2-8°C (36-46°F). If needed, keep at room temperature, not to exceed 30°C (86°F) for a total of 14 days. Do not freeze. Do not use if it has been frozen. Protect from light. Discard after use in a puncture-resistant container.

HOW SUPPLIED

Inj: 0.75mg/0.5mL, 1.5mg/0.5mL [pen, prefilled syringe]

CONTRAINDICATIONS

Prior serious hypersensitivity reaction to dulaglutide or to any of the product components, personal or family history of MTC, MEN 2.

WARNINGS/PRECAUTIONS

Not recommended as 1st-line therapy for patients who have inadequate glycemic control on diet and exercise; weigh potential benefits/risks. Not recommended w/ preexisting severe GI disease (eg, gastroparesis). Not a substitute for insulin; do not use in type 1 DM or for treatment of diabetic ketoacidosis. Pancreatitis related adverse reactions reported; d/c promptly if suspected, and do not restart therapy if confirmed. Consider other antidiabetic therapies in patients w/ a history of pancreatitis. Systemic hypersensitivity reactions reported; d/c and promptly seek medical advice if reaction occurs. Acute renal failure and worsening of chronic renal failure reported; caution when initiating/escalating doses in patients w/ renal impairment. Caution w/ hepatic impairment.

ADVERSE REACTIONS

N/V, diarrhea, abdominal pain, decreased appetite, dyspepsia, fatigue.

DRUG INTERACTIONS

See Dosing Considerations. May slow gastric emptying and thus has the potential to reduce the rate of absorption of concomitant oral medications; use w/ caution. Adequately monitor drug levels of oral medications w/ a narrow therapeutic index.

PREGNANCY AND LACTATION

Category C, not for use in nursing.

MECHANISM OF ACTION

Glucagon-like peptide-1 receptor agonist; increases intracellular cAMP in β cells, leading to glucose-dependent insulin release. Also decreases glucagon secretion and slows gastric emptying.

PHARMACOKINETICS

Absorption: Absolute bioavailability (65% [0.75mg], 47% [1.5mg]); T_{max}=24-72 hrs. (Multiple-dose of 1.5mg) C_{max}=114ng/mL, AUC=14,000ng•hr/mL. **Distribution:** V_d=approx 19.2L (0.75mg), approx 17.4L (1.5mg). **Metabolism:** Degradation to amino acids by general protein catabolism pathways. **Elimination:** $T_{1/2}$=approx 5 days.

PATIENT CONSIDERATIONS

Assessment: Assess for previous hypersensitivity reactions, MEN 2, personal or family history of MTC, history of pancreatitis, renal/hepatic impairment, GI disease, pregnancy/nursing status, and possible drug interactions. Further evaluate patients w/ thyroid nodules and/or elevated calcitonin levels.

Monitoring: Monitor for signs/symptoms of thyroid tumor, pancreatitis, elevated serum calcitonin levels, hypoglycemia, systemic hypersensitivity reactions, renal impairment, and other adverse reactions. Monitor renal function in patients w/ renal impairment reporting severe adverse GI reactions.

Counseling: Counsel regarding the potential risk of MTC and inform patient of symptoms of thyroid tumors (eg, mass in the neck, dysphagia, persistent hoarseness). Inform of the potential risks/benefits of therapy and of alternative modes of therapy. Instruct to report symptoms of thyroid tumors to physician. Instruct to d/c therapy promptly, and contact physician if persistent severe abdominal pain and/or symptoms of hypersensitivity reactions occur. Advise of the potential risk of dehydration due to GI adverse reactions and instruct to take precautions to avoid fluid depletion. Inform patients treated w/ therapy of the potential risk of worsening renal function and explain the associated signs and symptoms of renal impairment, as well as the possibility of dialysis as a medical intervention if renal failure occurs. Instruct to inform physician if pregnant/ intending to become pregnant. Inform about the importance of adherence to dietary instructions, regular physical activity, periodic blood glucose monitoring and HbA1c testing, proper inj technique, recognition and management of hypo/hyperglycemia, and assessment for diabetes complications. Inform that medication requirements may change during periods of stress; advise to seek medical advice promptly. Advise that if a dose is missed, administer as soon as noticed, provided the next regularly scheduled dose is due at least 3 days later. Instruct to then resume the usual dosing schedule thereafter. Instruct that if a dose is missed and the next regularly scheduled dose is due in 1 or 2 days, not to administer the missed dose and instead resume w/ the next regularly scheduled dose. Advise of the potential risk of GI side effects. Advise to inform physician if any unusual symptom develops, or if any known symptom persists or worsens.

TRUMENBA — meningococcal group B vaccine   Rx

Class: Vaccine

ADULT DOSAGE

Meningococcal Vaccine

Active Immunization to Prevent Invasive Disease Caused by *Neisseria meningitidis* Serogroup B:
≤25 Years:
Three Dose Schedule: Administer 0.5mL at 0, 1-2, and 6 months.
Two Dose Schedule: Administer 0.5mL at 0 and 6 months.

PEDIATRIC DOSAGE

Meningococcal Vaccine

Active Immunization to Prevent Invasive Disease Caused by *Neisseria meningitidis* Serogroup B:
≥10 Years:
Three Dose Schedule: Administer 0.5mL at 0, 1-2, and 6 months.
Two Dose Schedule: Administer 0.5mL at 0 and 6 months.

ADMINISTRATION

IM route

Shake syringe vigorously; do not use if vaccine cannot be re-suspended.
Preferred site for inj is the deltoid muscle of the upper arm.
Do not mix w/ any other vaccine in the same syringe.

STORAGE

2-8°C (36-46°F). Store syringes in the refrigerator horizontally (laying flat on the shelf) to minimize the re-dispersion time. Do not freeze; discard if the vaccine has been frozen.

HOW SUPPLIED

Inj: 0.5mL

CONTRAINDICATIONS

Severe allergic reaction after a previous dose of Trumenba.

WARNINGS/PRECAUTIONS

Epinephrine and other appropriate agents used to manage immediate allergic reactions must be immediately available should an acute anaphylactic reaction occur. Individuals w/ altered immunocompetence may have reduced immune responses to therapy.

ADVERSE REACTIONS

Pain at inj site, fatigue, headache, muscle pain, chills.

PREGNANCY AND LACTATION

Pregnancy: Category B.
Lactation: It is not known whether Trumenba is excreted in human milk. Caution in nursing.

MECHANISM OF ACTION

Vaccine; protection against invasive meningococcal disease is conferred mainly by complement-mediated antibody-dependent killing of *N. meningitidis*.

PATIENT CONSIDERATIONS

Assessment: Assess for hypersensitivity/vaccination history, altered immunocompetence, and pregnancy/nursing status.

Monitoring: Monitor for allergic/anaphylactic reactions, and other adverse reactions.

Counseling: Inform of the importance of completing the immunization series. Instruct to report any suspected adverse reactions to physician.

TRUSOPT — dorzolamide hydrochloride   Rx

Class: Carbonic anhydrase inhibitor

ADULT DOSAGE	PEDIATRIC DOSAGE
Elevated Intraocular Pressure	**Elevated Intraocular Pressure**
Ocular HTN/Open-Angle Glaucoma: 1 drop in the affected eye(s) tid	**Ocular HTN/Open-Angle Glaucoma:** 1 drop in the affected eye(s) tid

---

DOSING CONSIDERATIONS
Concomitant Medications
Administer at least 5 min apart if >1 topical ophthalmic drug is being used

ADMINISTRATION
Ocular route

STORAGE
15-30°C (59-86°F). Protect from light.

HOW SUPPLIED
Sol: 2% [10mL]

CONTRAINDICATIONS
Hypersensitivity to any component of Trusopt.

WARNINGS/PRECAUTIONS
Systemically absorbed. Rare fatalities have occurred due to severe sulfonamide reactions (eg, Stevens-Johnson syndrome, toxic epidermal necrolysis, fulminant hepatic necrosis, agranulocytosis, aplastic anemia, other blood dyscrasias); d/c if signs of hypersensitivity or other serious reactions occur. Sensitization may recur when readministered irrespective of the route of administration. Bacterial keratitis reported with use of multiple-dose containers of topical ophthalmic products that had been inadvertently contaminated by patients with a concurrent corneal disease or a disruption of the ocular epithelial surface. Caution in patients with low endothelial cell counts; increased potential for corneal edema. Local ocular adverse effects (eg, conjunctivitis, lid reactions) reported with chronic use; d/c use and evaluate patient before considering restarting therapy. The management of acute angle-closure glaucoma requires therapeutic interventions in addition to ocular hypotensive agents. Not recommended with severe renal impairment (CrCl <30mL/min). Caution with hepatic impairment.

ADVERSE REACTIONS
Ocular burning/stinging/discomfort, bitter taste, superficial punctate keratitis, ocular allergic reactions, conjunctivitis, lid reactions, blurred vision, eye redness, tearing, dryness, photophobia.

DRUG INTERACTIONS
Concomitant administration of oral carbonic anhydrase inhibitor is not recommended due to potential for additive effects. Acid-base and electrolyte disturbances reported with oral carbonic anhydrase inhibitors; drug interactions (eg, toxicity associated with high-dose salicylate therapy) may occur.

PREGNANCY AND LACTATION
Category C, not for use in nursing.

MECHANISM OF ACTION
Carbonic anhydrase inhibitor; decreases aqueous humor secretion, presumably by slowing the formation of bicarbonate ions with subsequent reduction in Na^+ and fluid transport, resulting in a reduction in IOP.

PHARMACOKINETICS
Absorption: Systemic. **Distribution:** Plasma protein binding (33%). **Metabolism:** N-desethyl (metabolite). **Elimination:** Urine (unchanged, metabolite); $T_{1/2}$=4 months.

PATIENT CONSIDERATIONS

Assessment: Assess for hypersensitivity to drug, acute angle-closure glaucoma, low endothelial cell counts, renal/hepatic impairment, pregnancy/nursing status, and possible drug interactions.

Monitoring: Monitor for sulfonamide hypersensitivity reactions, ocular reactions, bacterial keratitis, and other adverse reactions. Monitor for improvement in IOP.

Counseling: Advise to d/c use if serious or unusual reactions (eg, severe skin reactions, signs of hypersensitivity) occur. Instruct to immediately seek physician's advice concerning the continued use of present multidose container if patients have ocular surgery or develop an intercurrent ocular condition (eg, trauma, infection). Advise to d/c use and seek physician's advice if patient develops any ocular reactions (eg, conjunctivitis, lid reactions). Instruct to avoid allowing tip of dispensing container to contact eye or surrounding structures. Inform that ocular sol can become contaminated by common bacteria known to cause ocular infections if handled improperly or if the tip of the dispensing container contacts the eye or surrounding structures, and may result in serious damage to the eye and subsequent loss of vision. Instruct to administer at least 5 min apart if >1 topical ophthalmic drug is being used. Instruct to remove contact lenses prior to administration and inform that they may be reinserted 15 min after administration.

TRUVADA — emtricitabine/tenofovir disoproxil fumarate   Rx

Class: Nucleoside reverse transcriptase inhibitor (NRTI) combination

> Lactic acidosis and severe hepatomegaly w/ steatosis, including fatal cases, reported w/ the use of nucleoside analogues in combination w/ other antiretrovirals. Not approved for treatment of chronic hepatitis B virus (HBV) infection. Severe acute exacerbations of hepatitis B reported in patients coinfected w/ HBV and HIV-1 and who have discontinued therapy; closely monitor hepatic function w/ both clinical and lab follow-up for at least several months. If appropriate, initiation of anti-hepatitis B therapy may be warranted. Drug-resistant HIV-1 variants have been identified w/ use for preexposure prophylaxis (PrEP) indication following undetected acute HIV-1 infection. PrEP use must only be prescribed to individuals confirmed to be HIV-negative immediately prior to initiating and periodically (at least every 3 months) during use; do not initiate if signs/symptoms of acute HIV-1 infection are present unless negative infection status is confirmed.

ADULT DOSAGE	PEDIATRIC DOSAGE
HIV-1 Infection	**HIV-1 Infection**
Combination w/ Other Antiretrovirals: 1 tab (200mg/300mg) qd	**Combination w/ Other Antiretrovirals:** **17 to <22kg:** 1 tab (100mg/150mg) qd
HIV-1 Pre-Exposure Prophylaxis	**22 to <28kg:** 1 tab (133mg/200mg) qd
Combination w/ Safer Sex Practices for High-Risk Patients: 1 tab (200mg/300mg) qd	**28 to <35kg:** 1 tab (167mg/250mg) qd
	≥35kg: 1 tab (200mg/300mg) qd
	Monitor weight periodically and adjust dose accordingly

DOSING CONSIDERATIONS
Renal Impairment
HIV-1 Infection:
CrCl 30-49mL/min: 1 tab q48h
CrCl <30mL/min (Including Hemodialysis): Not recommended for use

HIV-1 PrEP:
CrCl <60mL/min: Not recommended for use

ADMINISTRATION
Oral route

Take w/ or w/o food.
Swallow tab whole.

STORAGE
25°C (77°F); excursions permitted to 15-30°C (59-86°F).

HOW SUPPLIED
Tab: (Emtricitabine/Tenofovir Disoproxil Fumarate [TDF]) 100mg/150mg, 133mg/200mg, 167mg/250mg, 200mg/300mg

CONTRAINDICATIONS
Individuals w/ unknown or positive HIV-1 status when used for PrEP. Use in HIV-infected patients w/o other concomitant antiretroviral agents.

WARNINGS/PRECAUTIONS
Obesity and prolonged nucleoside exposure may be risk factors for lactic acidosis and severe hepatomegaly w/ steatosis. Caution w/ known risk factors for liver disease. D/C if findings suggestive of lactic acidosis or pronounced hepatotoxicity develop. Test for the presence of chronic HBV before initiating therapy; offer vaccination to HBV-uninfected individuals. Redistribution/accumulation of body fat and immune reconstitution syndrome reported. Autoimmune disorders (eg, Graves' disease, polymyositis, Guillain-Barre syndrome) reported in the setting of immune reconstitution and can occur many months after initiation of treatment. Early virological failure and high rates of resistance substitutions reported w/ certain regimens that only contain 3 nucleoside reverse transcriptase inhibitors; consider treatment modification in these patients. Use for PrEP only as part of a comprehensive prevention strategy that includes other prevention measures (eg, safer sex practices). Delay starting PrEP therapy for at least 1 month and reconfirm HIV-1 status or use an FDA-approved test to diagnose acute or primary HIV-1 infection if symptoms of acute viral infection are present and recent (<1 month) exposures are suspected. D/C PrEP therapy if symptoms of acute HIV-1 infection develop following potential exposure event until negative status is confirmed using an FDA-approved test. Caution in elderly. **TDF:** Renal impairment (eg, acute renal failure, Fanconi syndrome) reported; caution in patients at risk of renal dysfunction, including patients who have previously experienced renal events while receiving adefovir dipivoxil. Promptly evaluate renal function in at-risk patients w/ persistent/worsening bone pain, pain in extremities, fractures, and/or muscular pain/weakness. Decreased bone mineral density (BMD) and increased biochemical markers of bone metabolism reported. Osteomalacia associated w/ proximal renal tubulopathy reported; consider hypophosphatemia and osteomalacia secondary to proximal renal tubulopathy in patients at risk of renal dysfunction who present w/ persistent or worsening bone/muscle symptoms.

ADVERSE REACTIONS
HIV-1 Infected Patients: Diarrhea, nausea, fatigue, headache, dizziness, depression, insomnia, abnormal dreams, rash.
HIV-1 Uninfected Patients: Headache, abdominal pain, decreased weight.

DRUG INTERACTIONS
Avoid w/ concurrent or recent use of nephrotoxic agents (eg, high-dose or multiple NSAIDs). Do not coadminister w/ emtricitabine-, TDF-, or tenofovir alafenamide-containing products, drugs containing lamivudine, or w/ adefovir dipivoxil. Coadministration w/ drugs eliminated by active tubular secretion (eg, acyclovir, cidofovir, ganciclovir, valacyclovir, aminoglycosides [eg, gentamicin], high-dose or multiple NSAIDs) may increase levels of emtricitabine, TDF, and/ or the coadministered drug. Drugs that decrease renal function may increase levels of emtricitabine and/or TDF. Refer to PI for dosing modifications when used w/ concomitant therapies. **TDF:** May increase levels of didanosine; d/c

w/ pulmonary disease or SOB, or whenever ventilator function is depressed. May produce drug dependence and has potential for abuse. Psychological dependence, physical dependence, and tolerance may develop upon repeated administration; use w/ caution. Respiratory depression effects and capacity to elevate CSF pressure may be markedly exaggerated in the presence of head injury, other intracranial lesions, or a preexisting increase in intracranial pressure. May obscure clinical course of patients w/ head injuries; avoid use in these patients. Chronic use may result in constipation or obstructive bowel disease, especially in patients w/ underlying intestinal motility disorders. May obscure diagnosis or clinical course of patients w/ acute abdominal conditions.

ADVERSE REACTIONS
Allergic laryngospasm, nasal stuffiness, asthenia, HTN, skin rash, glycosuria, hypoglycemia, N/V, constipation, ureteral spasm, blurred vision, urinary retention, diplopia, tinnitus, confusion.

DRUG INTERACTIONS
May cause additive CNS depressant effect w/ opioids, antihistamines, antipsychotics, antianxiety agents, or other CNS depressants (eg, alcohol); avoid use. Concomitant use w/ MAOIs or TCAs may increase the effect of either the antidepressant or codeine; do not prescribe if patient is taking an MAOI or for 2 weeks after stopping an MAOI drug. May produce paralytic ileus and excessive anticholinergic effects w/ anticholinergics; use w/ caution. **Codeine:** Drugs that inhibit codeine O-demethylation (via CYP2D6) may decrease levels of codeine's active metabolites, morphine and morphine-6-glucuronide. **Chlorpheniramine:** May inhibit hepatic metabolism of phenytoin; monitor for evidence of phenytoin toxicity.

PREGNANCY AND LACTATION
Pregnancy: Category C. Babies born to mothers who have been taking opioids regularly prior to delivery will be physically dependent; intensity of the syndrome does not always correlate w/ the duration of maternal opioid use or dose. **Lactation:** Excreted in human milk; caution in nursing.

MECHANISM OF ACTION
Codeine: Semisynthetic narcotic antitussive/analgesic; has not been established, but believed to act centrally on the cough center. **Chlorpheniramine:** Antihistamine (H_1-receptor antagonist); possesses anticholinergic and sedative activity. Prevents released histamine from dilating capillaries and causing edema of the respiratory mucosa.

PHARMACOKINETICS
Absorption: Codeine: (Single dose) C_{max}=51.4ng/mL; T_{max}=2.19 hrs; AUC=348.5ng•hr/mL; (Multiple dose) C_{max}=64.6ng/mL; T_{max}=1.86 hrs; AUC=348.8ng•hr/mL. Chlorpheniramine: (Single dose) C_{max}=7.84ng/mL; T_{max}=6.52 hrs; AUC=304.3ng•hr/mL; (Multiple dose) C_{max}=38.7ng/mL; T_{max}=5.77 hrs; AUC=392.4ng•hr/mL. **Distribution:** Found in breast milk and crosses placenta. Codeine: V_d=approx 3-6L/kg; plasma protein binding (7-25%). Chlorpheniramine: V_d=approx 3.2L/kg; plasma protein binding (70%). **Metabolism:** Codeine: Glucuronidation to codeine-6-glucuronide via UDP-glucuronosyltransferase 2B7 and 2B4; O-demethylation to morphine (active metabolite) via CYP2D6; N-demethylation to norcodeine via CYP3A4. Chlorpheniramine: Liver (rapid, extensive) via demethylation forming mono- and didesmethyl derivatives; oxidative metabolism catalyzed by CYP2D6. **Elimination:** Codeine: Kidneys (approx 90%, 10% unchanged); (Single dose) $T_{1/2}$=5 hrs. Chlorpheniramine: Kidneys; (Single dose) $T_{1/2}$=21.45 hrs.

PATIENT CONSIDERATIONS
Assessment: Assess for drug hypersensitivity, asthma, persistent or chronic cough, intestinal motility disorder, acute abdominal conditions, hypothyroidism, Addison's disease, prostatic hypertrophy or urethral stricture, hepatic/renal impairment, any other conditions where treatment is cautioned or contraindicated, pregnancy/nursing status, and possible drug interactions.

Monitoring: Monitor for respiratory depression, drug abuse/dependence, constipation, and other adverse reactions.

Counseling: Advise not to increase the dose or dosing frequency because serious adverse events may occur w/ overdosage. Counsel on how to utilize an oral dosing dispenser that measures the appropriate volume in mL. Instruct to avoid the use of alcohol and other CNS depressants while on therapy. Counsel that drug may produce marked drowsiness and impair mental and/or physical abilities required for the performance of potentially hazardous tasks such as driving a car or operating machinery. Advise that drug contains codeine and can produce drug dependence.

TWYNSTA — amlodipine/telmisartan   Rx
Class: Angiotensin II receptor blocker (ARB)/calcium channel blocker (CCB) (dihydropyridine)

> D/C as soon as possible when pregnancy is detected. Drugs that act directly on the renin-angiotensin system (RAS) can cause injury/death to the developing fetus.

ADULT DOSAGE
Hypertension
Initial Therapy:
Initial: 40mg/5mg qd or, if requiring larger BP reductions, 80mg/5mg qd
Titrate: May be increased after at least 2 weeks
Max: 80mg/10mg qd

Initial therapy is not recommended in patients ≥75 yrs old or w/ hepatic impairment

PEDIATRIC DOSAGE
Pediatric use may not have been established

Replacement Therapy:
May substitute for individual components; increase dose if BP control is unsatisfactory

Add-On Therapy:
May be used if BP not adequately controlled w/ amlodipine (or another dihydropyridine calcium channel blocker [CCB]) alone or w/ telmisartan (or another ARB) alone. Patients w/ dose-limiting adverse reactions to amlodipine 10mg may be switched to telmisartan/amlodipine 40mg/5mg qd.

DOSING CONSIDERATIONS
Renal Impairment
Severe: Titrate slowly
Hepatic Impairment
Initial: 2.5mg amlodipine; titrate slowly
Elderly
≥75 Years:
Initial: 2.5mg amlodipine; titrate slowly

ADMINISTRATION
Oral route
Take w/ or w/o food.

STORAGE
25°C (77°F); excursions permitted to 15-30°C (59-86°F). Do not remove from blisters until immediately before administration. Protect from light and moisture.

HOW SUPPLIED
Tab: (Telmisartan/Amlodipine) 40mg/5mg, 40mg/10mg, 80mg/5mg, 80mg/10mg

CONTRAINDICATIONS
Known hypersensitivity to Twynsta or any component of the medication, coadministration w/ aliskiren in patients w/ diabetes.

WARNINGS/PRECAUTIONS
Symptomatic hypotension may occur in patients w/ an activated RAS (eg, volume- or salt-depleted patients) and in patients w/ severe aortic stenosis. Correct volume/salt depletion prior to therapy or start therapy under close medical supervision w/ a reduced dose. **Amlodipine:** Worsening angina and acute MI may develop after starting or increasing the dose, particularly in patients w/ severe obstructive coronary artery disease (CAD). Closely monitor patients w/ heart failure (HF); pulmonary edema reported. Caution in elderly. **Telmisartan:** Hyperkalemia may occur, particularly in patients w/ advanced renal impairment, renal replacement therapy, or HF; periodically monitor serum electrolytes. Clearance is reduced in patients w/ biliary obstructive disorders or hepatic insufficiency. Changes in renal function may occur; oliguria and/or progressive azotemia and (rare) acute renal failure and/or death reported in patients whose renal function may depend on the RAS (eg, severe congestive HF or renal dysfunction). May increase SrCr/BUN w/ renal artery stenosis.

ADVERSE REACTIONS
Peripheral edema, dizziness, back pain.

DRUG INTERACTIONS
See Contraindications. **Amlodipine:** Increased exposure to simvastatin reported; limit dose of simvastatin to 20mg daily. May increase exposure of cyclosporine or tacrolimus; monitor cyclosporine/tacrolimus trough levels and adjust dose when appropriate. Diltiazem may increase systemic exposure. Strong CYP3A4 inhibitors (eg, ketoconazole, itraconazole, ritonavir) may increase concentrations to a greater extent; monitor for symptoms of hypotension and edema. Monitor for adequate clinical effect when coadministered w/ CYP3A4 inducers. **Telmisartan:** Dual blockade of the RAS is associated w/ increased risks of hypotension, hyperkalemia, and changes in renal function (eg, acute renal failure); avoid combined use of RAS inhibitors and closely monitor BP, renal function, and electrolytes w/ concomitant agents that affect the RAS. Avoid w/ aliskiren in patients w/ renal impairment (GFR <60mL/min). May increase digoxin concentrations; monitor digoxin levels upon initiation, adjustment, and discontinuation of therapy. Increases in lithium concentrations/toxicity reported; monitor lithium levels during concurrent use. NSAIDs, including selective COX-2 inhibitors, may attenuate antihypertensive effect and may deteriorate renal function in patients who are elderly, volume-depleted, or w/ compromised renal function. Coadministration w/ ramipril may increase ramipril/ramiprilat levels and decrease telmisartan levels; not recommended w/ ramipril. Increased risk of hyperkalemia w/ K⁺-sparing diuretics, K⁺ supplements, K⁺-containing salt substitutes, or other drugs that increase K⁺ levels. May possibly inhibit metabolism of drugs metabolized by CYP2C19.

PREGNANCY AND LACTATION
Pregnancy: Category D.
Lactation: Not for use in nursing.

MECHANISM OF ACTION
Amlodipine: Dihydropyridine CCB; inhibits transmembrane influx of Ca^{2+} ions into vascular smooth muscle and cardiac muscle. **Telmisartan:** ARB; blocks vasoconstrictor and aldosterone-secreting effects of angiotensin II by selectively blocking the binding of angiotensin II to the AT_1 receptor in many tissues.

PHARMACOKINETICS
Absorption: Amlodipine: Absolute bioavailability (64-90%); T_{max}=6-12 hrs. Telmisartan: Absolute bioavailability (42%, 40mg), (58%, 160mg); T_{max}=0.5-1 hr.
Distribution: Amlodipine: V_d=21L/kg; plasma protein binding (93%).

Telmisartan: V_d=500L; plasma protein binding (>99.5%). **Metabolism:** Amlodipine: Liver (extensive). Telmisartan: Conjugation. **Elimination:** Amlodipine: Urine (10% unchanged, 60% metabolites); $T_{1/2}$=30-50 hrs. Telmisartan: Feces (>97%, unchanged), urine (0.49%); $T_{1/2}$=24 hrs.

PATIENT CONSIDERATIONS

Assessment: Assess for severe obstructive CAD, severe aortic stenosis, HF, volume/salt depletion, biliary obstructive disorders, renal artery stenosis, diabetes, hepatic/renal dysfunction, hypersensitivity to drug, pregnancy/nursing status, and possible drug interactions.

Monitoring: Monitor for worsening angina and acute MI, particularly in patients w/ severe obstructive CAD, and for other adverse reactions. Monitor BP, renal function, and serum electrolytes (especially K^+ levels).

Counseling: Inform of consequences if exposure occurs during pregnancy, and of treatment options in women planning to become pregnant. Instruct to report pregnancies to physician as soon as possible.

TYBOST — cobicistat   Rx

Class: CYP3A inhibitor

ADULT DOSAGE

HIV-1 Infection

To increase systemic exposure of atazanavir or darunavir (once daily dosing regimen) in combination w/ other antiretroviral agents

Treatment-Naive/Experienced:
150mg qd + atazanavir 300mg qd

Treatment-Naive; Treatment-Experienced w/ No Darunavir Resistance-Associated Substitutions:
150mg qd + darunavir 800mg qd

PEDIATRIC DOSAGE

Pediatric use may not have been established

DOSING CONSIDERATIONS

Renal Impairment
CrCl <70mL/min: Do not coadminister w/ tenofovir disoproxil fumarate (TDF)

ADMINISTRATION

Oral route

Take w/ food.
Must be coadministered at the same time as atazanavir or darunavir.

STORAGE

25°C (77°F); excursions permitted to 15-30°C (59-86°F). Keep tightly closed.

HOW SUPPLIED

Tab: 150mg

CONTRAINDICATIONS

Concomitant use w/ alfuzosin, ranolazine, dronedarone, carbamazepine, phenobarbital, phenytoin, colchicine (in patients w/ renal and/or hepatic impairment), rifampin, irinotecan (when coadministered w/ atazanavir only), lurasidone, pimozide, dihydroergotamine, ergotamine, methylergonovine, cisapride, St. John's wort, lovastatin, simvastatin, nevirapine (when coadministered w/ atazanavir only), sildenafil (when used to treat pulmonary arterial HTN), indinavir (when coadministered w/ atazanavir only), triazolam, and oral midazolam.

WARNINGS/PRECAUTIONS

Not interchangeable w/ ritonavir to increase systemic exposure of darunavir 600mg bid, fosamprenavir, saquinavir, or tipranavir, Decreases estimated CrCl due to inhibition of tubular secretion of creatinine w/o affecting actual renal glomerular function; consider this effect when interpreting changes in estimated CrCl in patients initiating therapy, particularly in patients w/ medical conditions or receiving drugs needing monitoring w/ estimated CrCl. Consider alternative medications that do not require dosage adjustments in patients w/ renal impairment. Closely monitor patients who experience a confirmed increase in SrCr of >0.4mg/dL from baseline for renal safety.

ADVERSE REACTIONS

Jaundice, rash.

DRUG INTERACTIONS

See Contraindications. Renal impairment, including cases of acute renal failure and Fanconi syndrome, reported w/ TDF; coadministration is not recommended in patients w/ estimated CrCl <70mL/min. Coadministration w/ TDF in combination w/ concomitant or recent use of a nephrotoxic agent is not recommended. Not recommended w/ >1 antiretroviral that requires pharmacokinetic enhancement (eg, 2 protease inhibitors or a protease inhibitor in combination w/ elvitegravir); darunavir in combination w/ efavirenz, nevirapine, or etravirine; atazanavir in combination w/ etravirine; atazanavir in combination w/ efavirenz in treatment-experienced patients; darunavir 600mg bid; other HIV-1 protease inhibitors (eg, fosamprenavir, saquinavir, tipranavir); fixed-dose combination tablets that contain cobicistat; and lopinavir/ritonavir or regimens containing ritonavir. Not recommended w/ boceprevir, simeprevir, salmeterol, avanafil, or voriconazole. May increase concentration of drugs that are primarily metabolized by CYP3A (eg, maraviroc, clonazepam, corticosteroids [eg, dexamethasone, inhaled/nasal fluticasone or budesonide], cyclosporine, everolimus, sirolimus, tacrolimus) or CYP2D6, or are substrates of P-gp, BCRP, OATP1B1, or OATP1B3. Coadministration w/ inhaled or nasal fluticasone or other corticosteroids that are metabolized by CYP3A may result in reduced serum cortisol concentrations. Coadministration w/ dexamethasone or other corticosteroids that induce CYP3A may result in decreased concentrations of cobicistat, atazanavir, and darunavir, which may lead to loss of therapeutic effect and possible development of resistance. CYP3A inhibitors may increase concentrations, which may lead to clinically significant adverse reactions. Coadministration w/ atazanavir in combination w/ antacids (eg, aluminum and magnesium hydroxide) may decrease atazanavir levels; administer a minimum of 2 hrs apart. May increase levels of antiarrhythmics (eg, amiodarone, quinidine, digoxin), dasatinib, nilotinib, vinblastine, vincristine, itraconazole, ketoconazole, colchicine, rifabutin, β-blockers, calcium channel blockers, bosentan, HMG-CoA reductase inhibitors (eg, atorvastatin, rosuvastatin), fentanyl, tramadol, antipsychotic (eg, perphenazine, risperidone, thioridazine, quetiapine), PDE-5 inhibitors (eg, sildenafil, tadalafil), and sedatives/hypnotics (eg, buspirone, diazepam, parenteral midazolam). When coadministering w/ digoxin, titrate digoxin dose and monitor digoxin concentrations. Coadministration w/ macrolide/ketolide antibiotics (clarithromycin, erythromycin, telithromycin) may increase levels of the antibiotic and of cobicistat, atazanavir, and darunavir; consider alternative antibiotics. Monitor for hematologic or GI side effects w/ vincristine and vinblastine. Monitor INR w/ warfarin. Avoid w/ rivaroxaban. Clinical monitoring of anticonvulsants that are metabolized by CYP3A (eg, clonazepam) is recommended. Coadministration w/ anticonvulsants w/ CYP3A induction effects that are not contraindicated (eg, eslicarbazepine, oxcarbazepine) may decrease cobicistat and atazanavir level; consider alternative anticonvulsant or antiretroviral therapy to avoid potential changes in exposures and monitor for lack or loss of virologic response if coadministration is necessary. Caution w/ SSRIs (eg, paroxetine), TCAs (eg, amitriptyline, desipramine), and trazodone; may increase levels of TCAs and trazodone. Bosentan may decrease levels. Coadministration w/ atazanavir in combination w/ H_2-receptor antagonists (eg, famotidine) may decrease atazanavir levels; administer atazanavir/cobicistat coadministration at either the same time or a minimum of 10 hrs after administering H_2-receptor antagonists. Consider additional or alternative (nonhormonal) forms of contraception if to be used w/ hormonal contraceptives. Caution w/ buprenorphine, buprenorphine/naloxone, and methadone. Coadministration w/ atazanavir in combination w/ proton pump inhibitors (eg, omeprazole), may decrease atazanavir levels; administer cobicistat w/ atazanavir a minimum of 12 hrs after administering proton pump inhibitors (PPIs) in treatment-naive patients; coadministration w/ PPIs, w/ or w/o tenofovir, is not recommended in treatment-experienced patients. Refer to PI for further information including dosing modifications when used w/ certain concomitant therapies.

PREGNANCY AND LACTATION

Pregnancy: There are no data w/ cobicistat in pregnant women to inform a drug-associated risk. There is a pregnancy exposure registry that monitors fetal outcomes in women exposed to therapy during pregnancy.
Lactation: Not for use in nursing.

MECHANISM OF ACTION

CYP3A inhibitor; increases the systemic exposure of CYP3A substrates atazanavir and darunavir.

PHARMACOKINETICS

Absorption: (W/ Darunavir) T_{max}=3.5 hrs (median); C_{max}=0.99mcg/mL; AUC=7.6mcg•hr/mL. **Distribution:** Plasma protein binding (97-98%). **Metabolism:** CYP3A, CYP2D6 (minor). **Elimination:** Feces (86.2%), urine (8.2%); $T_{1/2}$=3-4 hrs.

PATIENT CONSIDERATIONS

Assessment: Assess pregnancy/nursing status and for possible drug interactions. Assess estimated CrCl. When used w/ TDF, assess estimated CrCl, urine glucose, and urine protein.

Monitoring: Monitor for adverse reactions. Monitor CrCl. When used w/ TDF, perform routine monitoring of estimated CrCl, urine glucose, and urine protein and measure serum phosphorus in patients w/ or at risk for renal impairment.

Counseling: Inform of the risks and benefits of therapy. Inform patients that they should remain under the care of a physician when using therapy. Counsel about the risks of developing resistance to HIV-1 medications. Instruct that if a dose of the drug and atazanavir or darunavir is missed by <12 hrs, to take the missed dose of the drug w/ atazanavir or darunavir together right away, and the next dose together as usual; if a dose of the drug w/ atazanavir or darunavir is missed by >12 hrs, instruct to wait and take the next dose at the usual time. If a dose of the drug w/ atazanavir or darunavir is skipped, instruct not to double the next dose. Inform that therapy may interact w/ many drugs w/ potential serious implications and that some drugs should not be taken w/ therapy; advise to report to physician the use of any other prescription or nonprescription medication or herbal products, including St. John's wort. Inform patients that there is a pregnancy exposure registry that monitors pregnancy outcomes in women exposed to cobicistat during pregnancy. Instruct mothers not to breastfeed while on therapy.

TYKERB — lapatinib   Rx

Class: Kinase inhibitor

> Hepatotoxicity observed; may be severe and deaths have been reported.

ADULT DOSAGE

HER2-Positive Metastatic Breast Cancer

In combination w/ capecitabine in patients who have received prior therapy, including an anthracycline, a taxane, and trastuzumab

PEDIATRIC DOSAGE

Pediatric use may not have been established

1250mg qd on Days 1-21 continuously w/ capecitabine 2000mg/m²/day (administered PO in 2 doses approx 12 hrs apart) on Days 1-14 in a repeating 21-day cycle; take capecitabine w/ food or w/in 30 min after food

Continue until disease progression or unacceptable toxicity occurs

Hormone Receptor-Positive, HER2-Positive Metastatic Breast Cancer

In combination w/ letrozole for the treatment of postmenopausal women for whom hormonal therapy is indicated

1500mg qd continuously w/ letrozole 2.5mg qd

DOSING CONSIDERATIONS

Concomitant Medications

Strong CYP3A4 Inhibitors:
Avoid use; if coadministration is required, reduce lapatinib dose to 500mg/day
If strong inhibitor is discontinued, a washout period of approx 1 week should be allowed before the lapatinib dose is adjusted upward to the indicated dose
Avoid w/ grapefruit

Strong CYP3A4 Inducers:
Avoid use; if coadministration is required, titrate dose gradually as follows:
HER2-Positive Metastatic Breast Cancer: Titrate up to 4500mg/day
Hormone Receptor-Positive, HER2-Positive Metastatic Breast Cancer: Titrate up to 5500mg/day
If strong inducer is discontinued, reduce lapatinib dose to the indicated dose

Hepatic Impairment

Severe (Child-Pugh Class C):
HER2-Positive Metastatic Breast Cancer: Reduce dose to 750mg/day
Hormone Receptor-Positive, HER2-Positive Metastatic Breast Cancer: Reduce dose to 1000mg/day

Adverse Reactions

Cardiac Events:
D/C Therapy in Patients w/:
1. Decreased left ventricular ejection fraction (LVEF) ≥Grade 2 by National Cancer Institute Common Terminology Criteria for Adverse Events (NCI CTCAE v3)
2. LVEF that drops below the lower limit of normal
If LVEF Recovers to Normal and Patient is Asymptomatic for ≥2 Weeks:
In Combination w/ Capecitabine: Restart dose at 1000mg/day
In Combination w/ Letrozole: Restart dose at 1250mg/day

Diarrhea:
NCI CTCAE Grade 3 or Grade 1 or 2 w/ Complicating Features: Interrupt therapy
When Diarrhea Resolves to ≤Grade 1:
HER2-Positive Metastatic Breast Cancer: Reduce dose to 1000mg/day
Hormone Receptor-Positive, HER2-Positive Metastatic Breast Cancer: Reduce dose to 1250mg/day
NCI CTCAE Grade 4: Permanently d/c therapy

Other Toxicities:
≥Grade 2 NCI CTCAE Toxicity: Consider discontinuation/dose interruption
When Toxicity Improves to ≤Grade 1: Restart at standard dose
If Toxicity Recurs:
In Combination w/ Capecitabine: Restart at 1000mg/day
In Combination w/ Letrozole: Restart at 1250mg/day

ADMINISTRATION
Oral route

Take at least 1 hr ac or 1 hr pc
Do not divide the daily dose

STORAGE
25°C (77°F); excursions permitted to 15-30°C (59-86°F).

HOW SUPPLIED
Tab: 250mg

CONTRAINDICATIONS
Known severe hypersensitivity (eg, anaphylaxis) to lapatinib or any components of the medication.

WARNINGS/PRECAUTIONS
Patients should have disease progression on trastuzumab prior to initiation of treatment w/ lapatinib in combination w/ capecitabine. Decreased LVEF reported; confirm normal LVEF prior to therapy. D/C if severe liver function changes occur, and do not retreat. Diarrhea, including severe cases and deaths, reported; early identification and intervention is critical. Prompt treatment of diarrhea w/ antidiarrheals (eg, loperamide) after the 1st unformed stool is recommended. Severe diarrhea may require administration of oral or IV electrolytes/fluids, use of antibiotics such as fluoroquinolones (especially if diarrhea persists >24 hrs, there is fever, or Grade 3 or 4 neutropenia), and interruption or discontinuation of therapy. Associated w/ interstitial lung disease and pneumonitis; d/c if pulmonary symptoms indicative of interstitial lung disease/pneumonitis (≥Grade 3) occur. QT prolongation observed; caution in patients who have or may develop prolongation of QTc (eg, taking antiarrhythmics or other drugs that prolong the QT interval, cumulative high-dose anthracycline therapy). Correct hypokalemia and hypomagnesemia before administration. Severe cutaneous reactions reported; d/c treatment if life-threatening reactions (eg, erythema multiforme, Stevens-Johnson syndrome, toxic epidermal necrolysis) are suspected. May cause fetal harm.

ADVERSE REACTIONS
Hepatotoxicity, diarrhea, N/V, stomatitis, dyspepsia, palmar-plantar erythrodysesthesia, rash, dry skin, mucosal inflammation, pain in extremity, back pain, dyspnea, fatigue, headache, alopecia.

DRUG INTERACTIONS
See Dosing Considerations. Caution w/ substrates of CYP3A4, CYP2C8, and P-gp; consider dose reduction of the concomitant substrate drug when dosing lapatinib concurrently w/ concomitant substrate drugs w/ narrow therapeutic windows. Increased levels w/ P-gp inhibitors; use w/ caution. Increased levels w/ grapefruit. May increase exposure of paclitaxel and midazolam. May increase exposure of digoxin; monitor serum digoxin concentrations prior to initiation of lapatinib and throughout coadministration. If digoxin level is >1.2ng/mL, reduce digoxin dose by 1/2.

PREGNANCY AND LACTATION
Category D, not for use in nursing.

MECHANISM OF ACTION
Kinase inhibitor; inhibits both epidermal growth factor receptor (ErbB1) and HER2 (ErbB2), resulting in tumor cell growth inhibition.

PHARMACOKINETICS
Absorption: Incomplete and variable. C_{max}=2.43mcg/mL (1250mg daily); T_{max}=approx 4 hrs; AUC=36.2mcg•hr/mL (1250mg daily). **Distribution:** Plasma protein binding (>99%). **Metabolism:** Liver (extensive); (major) CYP3A4, CYP3A5; (minor) CYP2C19, CYP2C8. **Elimination:** Feces (27% [median] parent), urine (<2%); $T_{1/2}$=14.2 hrs (single dose).

PATIENT CONSIDERATIONS

Assessment: Assess for severe hepatic impairment, decreased LVEF or conditions that may impair left ventricular function, QT prolongation, hypokalemia, hypomagnesemia, pregnancy/nursing status, drug hypersensitivity, and possible drug interactions. Obtain baseline ECG, LFTs, serum K⁺, and Mg²⁺ levels.

Monitoring: Monitor for hepatotoxicity, diarrhea, bowel changes, pulmonary symptoms indicative of interstitial lung disease or pneumonitis, decreased LVEF, QT prolongation, severe cutaneous reactions, and other adverse reactions. Consider ECG and electrolyte monitoring. Monitor LFTs every 4-6 weeks during therapy and as clinically indicated.

Counseling: Instruct to notify physician if SOB, palpitations, or fatigue occurs. Advise that diarrhea is a common side effect and instruct on how it should be managed/prevented; instruct to contact physician immediately if any change in bowel patterns or severe diarrhea occurs. Counsel to report use of any prescription/nonprescription drugs or herbal products. Instruct not to take w/ grapefruit products. Advise women not to become pregnant while on therapy.

TYSABRI — natalizumab   **Rx**

Class: Monoclonal antibody/integrin receptor antagonist

> Increases risk of progressive multifocal leukoencephalopathy (PML). Risk factors for development of PML include duration of therapy, prior use of immunosuppressants, and presence of anti-JC virus (JCV) antibodies. Monitor for any new signs/symptoms of PML; withhold dosing immediately at the 1st sign/symptom suggestive of PML. For diagnosis, an evaluation that includes a gadolinium-enhanced MRI scan of the brain and, when indicated, CSF analysis for JC viral DNA are recommended. Due to the risk of PML, available only through a restricted program under a Risk Evaluation and Mitigation Strategy (REMS) called the TOUCH Prescribing Program.

ADULT DOSAGE

Multiple Sclerosis

Monotherapy for the Treatment of Relapsing Forms of Multiple Sclerosis (MS):
300mg IV infusion over 1 hr every 4 weeks

Crohn's Disease

To induce and maintain clinical response and remission in patients w/ moderately to severely active Crohn's disease (CD) w/ evidence of inflammation who have had an inadequate response to, or are unable to tolerate, conventional CD therapies and TNF-α inhibitors

300mg IV infusion over 1 hr every 4 weeks

- Aminosalicylates may be continued during treatment
- D/C therapy if therapeutic benefit is not experienced by 12 weeks of induction therapy
- For patients starting therapy while on chronic oral corticosteroids, commence steroid tapering as soon as a therapeutic benefit has occurred; if patient cannot be tapered off oral corticosteroids w/in 6 months of starting therapy, d/c natalizumab
- Consider discontinuation for patients who require additional steroid use that exceeds 3 months in a calendar year to control their CD

PEDIATRIC DOSAGE
Pediatric use may not have been established

ADMINISTRATION
IV route

Dilution
1. To prepare sol, withdraw 15mL from the vial and inject the concentrate into 100mL of 0.9% NaCl inj; no other IV diluents may be used to prepare the sol.
2. Gently invert sol to mix completely; do not shake.
3. The final dosage sol has a concentration of 2.6mg/mL.
4. Following dilution, infuse sol immediately, or refrigerate at 2-8°C (36-46°F), and use w/in 8 hrs; if refrigerated, allow sol to warm to room temperature prior to infusion. Do not freeze.

Administration
1. Infuse 300mg in 100mL 0.9% NaCl inj, over approx 1 hr (infusion rate approx 5mg/min).
2. Do not administer as an IV push or bolus inj.
3. Observe patients during infusion and for 1 hr after completion of infusion.
4. After the infusion is complete, flush w/ 0.9% NaCl inj.
5. Do not inject other medications into infusion set side ports or mix w/ therapy. Use of filtration devices during administration has not been evaluated.

STORAGE
2-8°C (36-46°F). Do not shake or freeze. Protect from light.

HOW SUPPLIED
Inj: 300mg/15mL

CONTRAINDICATIONS
PML or history of PML. Hypersensitivity reaction to natalizumab.

WARNINGS/PRECAUTIONS
Anti-JCV antibody testing should not be used to diagnose PML. Avoid anti-JCV antibody testing during and for at least 2 weeks following plasma exchange due to the removal of antibodies from the serum. Retest patients w/ negative anti-JCV antibody test result periodically. PML reported following discontinuation in patients who did not have findings suggestive of PML at the time of discontinuation; monitor for any new signs or symptoms that may be suggestive of PML for at least 6 months following discontinuation. Immune reconstitution inflammatory syndrome (IRIS) reported in patients who developed PML and subsequently discontinued therapy; monitor for development of IRIS and treat appropriately. Increases the risk of developing encephalitis and meningitis caused by herpes simplex and varicella zoster viruses; d/c and treat appropriately if herpes encephalitis or meningitis occurs. Liver injury, including acute liver failure requiring transplant, reported; d/c in patients w/ jaundice or other evidence of significant liver injury (eg, lab evidence). Hypersensitivity reactions, including serious systemic reactions (eg, anaphylaxis) reported; d/c administration, initiate appropriate therapy, and do not retreat. Patients who receive natalizumab for a short exposure (1 to 2 infusions) followed by an extended period w/o treatment are at higher risk of developing anti-natalizumab antibodies and/or hypersensitivity reactions on re-exposure; consider testing for the presence of antibodies in patients who wish to recommence therapy following a dose interruption. May increase risk for infections. Avoid in patients w/ systemic medical conditions resulting in significantly compromised immune system function. Induces increases in circulating lymphocytes, monocytes, eosinophils, basophils, and nucleated RBCs or transient decreases in Hgb levels.

ADVERSE REACTIONS
MS: Headache, fatigue, arthralgia, UTI, lower respiratory tract infection, gastroenteritis, vaginitis, depression, pain in extremity, abdominal discomfort, diarrhea, rash.
CD: Headache, fatigue, URTI, nausea.

DRUG INTERACTIONS
Avoid w/ immunomodulatory therapy, immunosuppressants (eg, 6-mercaptopurine, azathioprine, cyclosporine, methotrexate) or TNF-α inhibitors. Concurrent use of antineoplastic, immunosuppressant, or immunomodulating agents may further increase risk of infections, including PML and other opportunistic infections.

PREGNANCY AND LACTATION
Pregnancy: Category C.
Lactation: Detected in human milk. The effects of this exposure on infants are unknown.

MECHANISM OF ACTION
Monoclonal antibody/integrin receptor antagonist; specific mechanisms by which natalizumab exerts its effects in MS and CD have not been fully defined. Binds to the α4-subunit of α4β1 and α4β7 integrins expressed on the surface of all leukocytes except neutrophils, and inhibits the α4-mediated adhesion of leukocytes to their counter-receptor(s).

PHARMACOKINETICS
Absorption: (MS) C_{max}=110mcg/mL; (CD) C_{max}=101mcg/mL. Distribution: Found in breast milk; (MS) V_d=5.7L; (CD) V_d=5.2L. Elimination: (MS) $T_{1/2}$=11 days; (CD) $T_{1/2}$=10 days.

PATIENT CONSIDERATIONS
Assessment: Assess for risk of PML, immunosuppression, drug hypersensitivity, pregnancy/nursing status, and possible drug interactions. Obtain MRI prior to initiating therapy. Test for anti-JCV antibody status; retest periodically in patients w/ negative result.

Monitoring: Monitor for PML, IRIS, encephalitis, meningitis, hepatotoxicity, hypersensitivity/antibody formation, infections, and other adverse reactions. Evaluate patients 3 and 6 months after the 1st infusion, every 6 months thereafter, and for at least 6 months after discontinuing treatment. Consider periodic monitoring for radiographic signs consistent w/ PML to allow for an early diagnosis of PML.

Counseling: Educate on risks/benefits of therapy. Instruct to promptly report any new or continuously worsening symptoms that persist over several days to physician. Advise patients to inform all of their physicians that they are receiving natalizumab. Counsel about the follow-up schedule (3 and 6 months after 1st infusion, every 6 months thereafter, and for at least 6 months after discontinuation). Instruct to seek medical attention if symptoms suggestive of PML develop, including progressive weakness on one side of the body or clumsiness of the limbs, disturbance of vision, and changes in thinking, memory, and orientation leading to confusion and personality changes. Instruct patients to continue to look for new signs and symptoms suggestive of PML for approx 6 months following treatment discontinuation. Advise that therapy is only available through a restricted program called the TOUCH Prescribing Program and inform about requirements. Instruct to report symptoms of infections, hypersensitivity reactions, hepatotoxicity, and herpes encephalitis/meningitis.

TYZEKA — telbivudine   Rx

Class: Nucleoside reverse transcriptase inhibitor (NRTI)

> Lactic acidosis and severe hepatomegaly with steatosis, including fatal cases, reported with nucleoside analogues alone or in combination with other antiretrovirals. Severe acute exacerbations of hepatitis B reported in patients who discontinued therapy; monitor hepatic function closely for at least several months. If appropriate, resumption of anti-hepatitis B therapy may be warranted.

ADULT DOSAGE	PEDIATRIC DOSAGE
Chronic Hepatitis B	**Chronic Hepatitis B**
Tab: 600mg qd	**≥16 Years:** **Tab:** 600mg qd
Sol: 30mL qd	**Sol:** 30mL qd

DOSING CONSIDERATIONS
Renal Impairment
CrCl 30-49mL/min:
Tab: 600mg q48h
Sol: 20mL qd
CrCl <30mL/min (Not Requiring Dialysis):
Tab: 600mg q72h
Sol: 10mL qd
ESRD:
Tab: 600mg q96h; administer after hemodialysis, when administered on hemodialysis days
Sol: 6mL qd; administer after hemodialysis, when administered on hemodialysis days

Other Important Considerations
HBV DNA ≥300 copies/mL After 24 Weeks of Treatment:
Institute alternate therapy

ADMINISTRATION
Oral route
Take with or without food

STORAGE
25°C (77°F); excursions permitted to 15-30°C (59-86°F). (Sol) Use within 2 months after opening. Do not freeze.

HOW SUPPLIED
Sol: 100mg/5mL [300mL]; Tab: 600mg

CONTRAINDICATIONS
Combination with pegylated interferon alfa-2a.

WARNINGS/PRECAUTIONS
Initiate only if pretreatment HBV DNA and ALT levels are known. HBV DNA should be <9 $\log_{10}$ copies/mL and ALT should be ≥2X ULN in HBeAg-positive patients prior to therapy. HBV DNA should be <7 $\log_{10}$ copies/mL in HBeAg-negative patients prior to therapy. Institute alternate therapy in patients with incomplete viral suppression (HBV DNA ≥300 copies/mL) after 24 weeks of treatment or if patients test positive for HBV DNA at any time after initial response. Female gender, obesity, and prolonged nucleoside exposure may be risk factors for developing lactic acidosis and hepatomegaly with steatosis; d/c therapy if lactic acidosis or hepatotoxicity develops. Caution with known risk factors for liver disease. Myopathy/myositis and peripheral neuropathy reported; interrupt therapy if suspected and d/c if confirmed. Rhabdomyolysis and uncomplicated myalgia reported. Caution in elderly.

ADVERSE REACTIONS
Fatigue, creatinine kinase increase, headache, cough, diarrhea, abdominal pain, nausea, pharyngolaryngeal pain, arthralgia, pyrexia, rash, lactic acidosis, severe hepatomegaly with steatosis, back pain, dizziness.

DRUG INTERACTIONS
See Contraindications. Drugs that alter renal function may alter plasma concentrations. Combination with interferons may be associated with risk of peripheral neuropathy.

PREGNANCY AND LACTATION
Category B, not for use in nursing.

MECHANISM OF ACTION
Thymidine nucleoside analogue; inhibits HBV DNA polymerase (reverse transcriptase) by competing with the natural substrate thymidine 5'-triphosphate and causing DNA chain termination after incorporation into viral DNA.

PHARMACOKINETICS

Absorption: (600mg qd) C_{max}=3.69mcg/mL, T_{max}=2 hrs, AUC=26.1mcg•h/mL. Administration with varying degrees of renal function resulted in different pharmacokinetic parameters. **Distribution:** Plasma protein binding (3.3%). **Elimination:** (600mg single dose) Urine (42%), $T_{1/2}$=40-49 hrs.

PATIENT CONSIDERATIONS

Assessment: Assess for renal/hepatic impairment, use in women, obesity, nucleoside exposure duration, risk factors for liver disease, pregnancy/nursing status, and possible drug interactions. Obtain HBV DNA and ALT levels prior to therapy.

Monitoring: Monitor hepatic function periodically and for several months after discontinuation. Monitor for exacerbation of HBV after discontinuation, lactic acidosis, hepatomegaly, hepatotoxicity, myopathy, and peripheral neuropathy. Monitor HBV DNA levels at 24 weeks of therapy and every 6 months thereafter. Monitor renal function in elderly patients. Closely monitor for any signs/symptoms of unexplained muscle pain, tenderness, or weakness when initiating with any drug associated with myopathy.

Counseling: Advise patients to remain under care of a physician during therapy and to discuss any new symptoms or concurrent medications. Advise to report promptly unexplained muscle weakness, tenderness or pain, numbness, tingling, and/or burning sensations in the arms and/or legs with or without difficulty walking. Inform that medication is not a cure for hepatitis B and long-term treatment benefits are unknown. Inform that deterioration of liver disease may occur in some cases if treatment is discontinued; advise to discuss any changes in regimen with physician. Inform that therapy has not shown to reduce risk of transmission of HBV to others through sexual contact or blood contamination and counsel on HBV prevention strategies. Advise patients on low-sodium diet that sol contains 47mg sodium/600mg. Advise to dispose of unused/expired drug properly, and to remove all identifying information from the original container prior to disposal.

UCERIS EXTENDED-RELEASE TABLETS — budesonide Rx

Class: Corticosteroid

ADULT DOSAGE	**PEDIATRIC DOSAGE**
Ulcerative Colitis	Pediatric use may not have been established
Induction of Remission in Active, Mild to Moderate Ulcerative Colitis: 9mg qam for up to 8 weeks	

ADMINISTRATION

Oral route

Take w/ or w/o food
Swallow whole w/ water; do not chew, crush, or break

STORAGE

25°C (77°F); excursions permitted to 15-30°C (59-86°F). Protect from light and moisture.

HOW SUPPLIED

Tab, ER: 9mg

CONTRAINDICATIONS

Hypersensitivity to budesonide or any of the ingredients in this product.

WARNINGS/PRECAUTIONS

Systemic effects (eg, hypercorticism, adrenal suppression) may occur when used chronically. May reduce response of hypothalamus-pituitary-adrenal axis to stress; supplement with a systemic glucocorticosteroid during surgery or other stress situations. Caution in patients who are transferred from glucocorticosteroid treatment with higher systemic effects to glucocorticosteroids with lower systemic effects; withdrawal symptoms (eg, acute adrenal suppression, benign intracranial HTN) may develop. Cautiously reduce dose of glucocorticosteroid treatment with high systemic effects. Increased susceptibility to infection. Chickenpox and measles may lead to serious/fatal course; avoid exposure in patients who have not had these diseases and consider prophylaxis/treatment if exposed. Caution with active/quiescent TB, untreated fungal, bacterial, systemic viral or parasitic infections, HTN, diabetes mellitus (DM), osteoporosis, peptic ulcer, glaucoma, cataracts, family history of DM or glaucoma, and in elderly. Replacement of systemic glucocorticosteroids with the drug may unmask allergies (eg, rhinitis, eczema). Increased systemic availability reported in patients with liver cirrhosis; consider discontinuation in patients with moderate to severe liver disease.

ADVERSE REACTIONS

Headache, nausea, decreased blood cortisol, upper abdominal pain, fatigue, flatulence, abdominal distension, acne, UTI, arthralgia, constipation, mood changes, sleep changes.

DRUG INTERACTIONS

CYP3A4 inhibitors (eg, ketoconazole, ritonavir, erythromycin) may increase levels; consider discontinuation of the drug or the CYP3A4 inhibitor. If coadministration is indicated, closely monitor for increased signs and/or symptoms of hypercorticism. Avoid grapefruit or grapefruit juice. Release properties and uptake may be altered when used after treatment with gastric acid reducing agents (eg, proton pump inhibitors, H_2-blockers, antacids).

PREGNANCY AND LACTATION

Category C, not for use in nursing.

MECHANISM OF ACTION

Glucocorticosteroid.

PHARMACOKINETICS

Absorption: C_{max}=1.35ng/mL; T_{max}=13.3 hrs; AUC=16.43ng•hr/mL. **Distribution:** V_d=2.2-3.9L/kg; plasma protein binding (85-90%); found in breast milk. **Metabolism:** Liver (rapid and extensive) via CYP3A4; 6β-hydroxy budesonide and 16α-hydroxy prednisolone (major metabolites). **Elimination:** Urine (60%), feces; (IV) $T_{1/2}$=2-3.6 hrs.

PATIENT CONSIDERATIONS

Assessment: Assess for liver disease, active/quiescent TB, untreated infections, history of chickenpox or measles, HTN, DM, osteoporosis, peptic ulcer, glaucoma, cataracts, family history of DM or glaucoma, hypersensitivity to drug, pregnancy/nursing status, and possible drug interactions.

Monitoring: Monitor for hypercorticism, adrenal suppression, infection, and other adverse reactions. Monitor adrenocortical function in patients who are transferred from glucocorticosteroid treatment with higher systemic effects.

Counseling: Advise that the drug may cause systemic glucocorticosteroid effects of hypercorticism and adrenal suppression; instruct to taper slowly from systemic corticosteroids if transferring to the drug. Advise to avoid exposure to chickenpox or measles and, if exposed, to consult physician immediately. Inform of potential worsening of existing TB; fungal, bacterial, viral or parasitic infections; or ocular herpes simplex. Instruct to avoid consumption of grapefruit or grapefruit juice during therapy.

UCERIS RECTAL FOAM — budesonide Rx

Class: Corticosteroid

ADULT DOSAGE	**PEDIATRIC DOSAGE**
Ulcerative Colitis	Pediatric use may not have been established
1 metered dose rectally bid (am and hs) for 2 weeks, followed by 1 metered dose rectally hs for 4 weeks	

DOSING CONSIDERATIONS

Concomitant Medications

CYP3A4 Inhibitors (eg, Ketoconazole, Grapefruit Juice):
Avoid concomitant use

Elderly
Start at lower end of dosing range

ADMINISTRATION

Rectal route

STORAGE

20-25°C (68-77°F); excursions permitted to 15-30°C (59-86°F). Do not burn the canister after use and do not spray contents directly towards flames. Do not expose to heat or store at >49°C (120°F). Contents under pressure; do not puncture or incinerate. Do not refrigerate.

HOW SUPPLIED

Foam: 2mg/metered dose [14 metered doses]

CONTRAINDICATIONS

Known hypersensitivity to budesonide or any of the ingredients in Uceris rectal foam.

WARNINGS/PRECAUTIONS

Systemic effects (eg, hypercorticism, adrenal suppression) may occur when used chronically. May reduce response of hypothalamus-pituitary-adrenal axis to stress; supplement with a systemic glucocorticosteroid during surgery or other stress situations. Increased systemic availability of oral budesonide reported in patients with liver cirrhosis; consider discontinuation in patients with moderate to severe hepatic impairment (Child-Pugh class B or C) if signs of hypercorticism are observed. Monitor patients who are transferred from glucocorticosteroid treatment with higher systemic effects to glucocorticosteroids with lower systemic effects; withdrawal symptoms (eg, acute adrenal suppression, benign intracranial HTN) may develop. Cautiously reduce dose of glucocorticosteroid treatment with high systemic effects. Replacement of systemic glucocorticosteroids with the drug may unmask allergies (eg, rhinitis, eczema). Increased susceptibility to infection. Chickenpox and measles may have a more serious/fatal course; avoid exposure in patients who have not had these diseases and consider prophylaxis/treatment if exposed. Caution with active/quiescent tuberculosis (TB), untreated fungal, bacterial, systemic viral or parasitic infections, or ocular herpes simplex, and in elderly. Monitor patients with HTN, diabetes mellitus (DM), osteoporosis, peptic ulcer, glaucoma, cataracts, family history of DM or glaucoma, or with any other condition where glucocorticosteroids may have unwanted effects. Contains n-butane, isobutane and propane as propellants which are flammable; temporarily d/c use before initiation of bowel preparation for colonoscopy.

ADVERSE REACTIONS

Decreased blood cortisol, adrenal insufficiency, nausea.

DRUG INTERACTIONS

See Dosing Considerations. CYP3A4 inhibitors (eg, ritonavir, erythromycin, cyclosporine) may increase levels.

PREGNANCY AND LACTATION

Category C, caution in nursing.

MECHANISM OF ACTION

Glucocorticosteroid.

PHARMACOKINETICS

Absorption: AUC_{0-12}=4.31ng•hr/mL. **Distribution:** V_d=2.2-3.9L/kg; plasma protein binding (85-90%); found in breast milk. **Metabolism:** Liver (rapid and extensive) via CYP3A4; 6β-hydroxy budesonide and 16α-hydroxy prednisolone (major metabolites). **Elimination:** Urine (60%) (Oral/IV), feces.

PATIENT CONSIDERATIONS

Assessment: Assess for hepatic impairment, active/quiescent TB, untreated infections, ocular herpes simplex, HTN, DM, osteoporosis, peptic ulcer, glaucoma, cataracts, family history of DM or glaucoma, hypersensitivity to drug, pregnancy/nursing status, and possible drug interactions.

Monitoring: Monitor for hypercorticism, adrenal suppression, infection, and other adverse reactions. Monitor adrenocortical function in patients who are transferred from glucocorticosteroid treatment with higher systemic effects. Monitor patients with HTN, DM, osteoporosis, peptic ulcer, glaucoma, cataracts, family history of DM or glaucoma, or with any other condition where glucocorticosteroids may have unwanted effects.

Counseling: Advise that drug is only to be applied rectally; it is not for oral use. Instruct to use the bathroom to empty bowels before use and to try not to empty bowels again until the next morning. Advise that each applicator is coated with a lubricant; petrolatum or petroleum jelly can also be used if additional lubrication is needed. Advise to warm the canister in hands while shaking vigorously for 10-15 sec prior to use. Instruct that drug may be used in a standing, lying, or sitting position (eg, while using the toilet). Instruct to avoid consumption of grapefruit or grapefruit juice during therapy. Advise to avoid fire, flame, and smoking during and immediately following administration. Advise that the drug may cause hypercorticism and adrenal suppression; instruct to taper slowly from systemic corticosteroids if transferring to the drug. Advise that replacement of systemic glucocorticosteroids with drug may unmask allergies. Advise to avoid exposure to chickenpox or measles and, if exposed, to consult physician. Inform that patients are at increased risk of developing a variety of infections, including worsening of existing TB, fungal, bacterial, viral, or parasitic infections, or ocular herpes simplex; instruct to contact physician if any symptoms of infection develop. Instruct to consult physician before resuming therapy if temporarily discontinued prior to colonoscopy.

ULORIC — febuxostat   Rx

Class: Xanthine oxidase inhibitor

ADULT DOSAGE	**PEDIATRIC DOSAGE**
Hyperuricemia	Pediatric use may not have been established
Chronic Management in Patients w/ Gout:	
Initial: 40mg qd	
Titrate: If serum uric acid is not <6mg/dL after 2 weeks, increase dose to 80mg qd	

ADMINISTRATION
Oral route
May be taken w/o regard to food or antacid use.

STORAGE
25°C (77°F); excursions permitted to 15-30°C (59-86°F). Protect from light.

HOW SUPPLIED
Tab: 40mg, 80mg

CONTRAINDICATIONS
Patients being treated with azathioprine or mercaptopurine.

WARNINGS/PRECAUTIONS
Not recommended for treatment of asymptomatic hyperuricemia. Increase in gout flares observed after initiation; concurrent prophylactic treatment with NSAIDs or colchicine is recommended. Cardiovascular (CV) thromboembolic events (eg, CV deaths, MIs, strokes) reported; monitor for signs and symptoms of MI and stroke. Fatal and nonfatal hepatic failure reported; obtain baseline LFTs before initiation. Measure LFTs promptly in patients who report symptoms that may indicate liver injury; d/c if LFTs are abnormal (ALT >3X ULN) and do not restart if no alternative etiology is found. D/C permanently in patients with ALT >3X ULN with serum total bilirubin >2X ULN without alternative etiologies; use with caution in patients with lesser ALT or bilirubin elevations and with an alternate probable cause. Caution with severe hepatic impairment (Child-Pugh Class C) and severe renal impairment (CrCl <30mL/min). Avoid use in patients whom the rate of urate formation is greatly increased (eg, malignant disease and its treatment, Lesch-Nyhan syndrome).

ADVERSE REACTIONS
Liver function abnormalities, nausea, arthralgia, rash.

DRUG INTERACTIONS
See Contraindications. Caution with theophylline.

PREGNANCY AND LACTATION
Pregnancy: Category C.
Lactation: Caution in nursing.

MECHANISM OF ACTION
Xanthine oxidase inhibitor; achieves its therapeutic effect by decreasing sUA.

PHARMACOKINETICS
Absorption: C_{max}=1.6mcg/mL (40mg), 2.6mcg/mL (80mg); T_{max}=1-1.5 hrs.
Distribution: V_d=50L; plasma protein binding (99.2%). **Metabolism:** Conjugation via uridine diphosphate glucuronosyltransferase enzymes and oxidation via CYP450 enzymes. **Elimination:** Urine (49%, 3% unchanged); feces (45%, 12% unchanged); $T_{1/2}$=5-8 hrs.

PATIENT CONSIDERATIONS

Assessment: Assess for asymptomatic hyperuricemia, hepatic/renal impairment, malignant disease, Lesch-Nyhan syndrome, pregnancy/nursing status, and possible drug interactions. Obtain baseline serum uric acid (sUA) and LFTs.

Monitoring: Monitor sUA levels as early as 2 weeks after initiation of therapy. Monitor for signs/symptoms of liver injury, MI, and stroke.

Counseling: Advise of the potential benefits and risks of therapy. Inform that gout flares, elevated liver enzymes, and adverse CV events may occur. Instruct to notify physician if rash, chest pain, SOB, or neurologic symptoms suggesting a stroke occur. Instruct to inform physician of any other medications, including OTC drugs, currently being taken.

ULTRACET — acetaminophen/tramadol hydrochloride   CIV

Class: Centrally acting analgesic

> Associated with cases of acute liver failure, at times resulting in liver transplant and death. Most cases of liver injury are associated with acetaminophen (APAP) use at doses >4000mg/day and often involve >1 APAP-containing product.

ADULT DOSAGE	**PEDIATRIC DOSAGE**
Acute Pain	Pediatric use may not have been established
Short-Term (≤5 Days) Management:	
2 tabs q4-6h prn for ≤5 days	
Max: 8 tabs/day	

DOSING CONSIDERATIONS
Renal Impairment
CrCl <30mL/min:
Max: 2 tabs q12h

ADMINISTRATION
Oral route

STORAGE
25°C (77°F); excursions permitted to 15-30°C (59-86°F).

HOW SUPPLIED
Tab: (Tramadol/APAP) 37.5mg/325mg

CONTRAINDICATIONS
Previously demonstrated hypersensitivity to tramadol, acetaminophen, any other component of Ultracet, or opioids. Any situation where opioids are contraindicated, including acute intoxication with alcohol, hypnotics, narcotics, centrally acting analgesics, opioids, or psychotropic drugs.

WARNINGS/PRECAUTIONS
Do not exceed recommended dose. May complicate clinical assessment of acute abdominal conditions. Not recommended in patients with hepatic impairment; increased risk of acute liver failure in patients with underlying liver disease. Not for use in pregnant women prior to or during labor unless benefits outweigh risks. Not recommended for obstetrical preoperative medication or for postdelivery analgesia in nursing mothers. Caution in elderly. Serious and fatal anaphylactic reactions reported; avoid use in patients with a history of anaphylactoid reactions to codeine or other opioids. D/C use if anaphylaxis develops. APAP: Avoid in patients with APAP allergy. May cause serious skin reactions (eg, acute generalized exanthematous pustulosis, Stevens-Johnson syndrome, toxic epidermal necrolysis), which can be fatal; d/c at the 1st appearance of skin rash or any other sign of hypersensitivity. Tramadol: Seizures reported; risk increases in patients with epilepsy, history/risk of seizures, and with naloxone coadministration. Avoid in patients who are suicidal or addiction-prone; caution with emotional disturbances or depression. Reports of tramadol-related deaths with previous history of emotional disturbances, suicidal ideation/attempts, and misuse of tranquilizers/alcohol/CNS-active drugs. Potentially life-threatening serotonin syndrome, including mental status changes, autonomic instability, neuromuscular aberrations, and GI symptoms, may occur. Caution if at risk for respiratory depression; consider alternative nonopioid analgesic. Caution with CNS depression, head injury, and increased intracranial pressure (ICP). May impair mental/physical abilities. May cause withdrawal symptoms; do not d/c abruptly.

ADVERSE REACTIONS
Acute liver failure, constipation, somnolence, increased sweating, diarrhea, nausea, anorexia, dizziness.

DRUG INTERACTIONS
See Contraindications. Do not use concomitantly with alcohol, other APAP- or tramadol-containing products; increased risk of acute liver failure with alcohol ingestion. May alter effects of warfarin; periodically monitor PT with warfarin-like compounds. Tramadol: Increased seizure risk with SSRIs, TCAs, other tricyclic compounds (eg, cyclobenzaprine, promethazine), MAOIs, other opioids, neuroleptics, and drugs that reduce seizure threshold. Serotonin syndrome may occur when coadministered with SSRIs, SNRIs, TCAs, MAOIs, triptans, α_2-adrenergic blockers, linezolid, lithium, St. John's wort, or drugs that impair tramadol metabolism; observe carefully, especially during initiation and dose increases. Caution and reduce dose with CNS depressants (eg, alcohol, opioids, anesthetics); increased risk of CNS/respiratory depression. Caution with antidepressants and muscle relaxants; additive CNS depressant effects. CYP2D6 inhibitors (eg, quinidine, fluoxetine, paroxetine, amitriptyline) and/or CYP3A4 inhibitors (eg, ketoconazole, erythromycin) may reduce metabolic clearance; increased risk of serious adverse effects. CYP3A4 inhibitors or inducers (eg, rifampin, St. John's wort) may alter drug exposure. Digoxin toxicity may occur with concomitant use. Carbamazepine may reduce analgesic effect; avoid coadministration.

PREGNANCY AND LACTATION
Category C, not for use in nursing.

MECHANISM OF ACTION
Tramadol: Centrally acting synthetic opioid analgesic; has not been established. Suspected to be due to the binding of parent and M1 metabolite to μ-opioid

receptors and weak inhibition of reuptake of norepinephrine and serotonin. APAP: Nonopiate, nonsalicylate analgesic, and antipyretic.

PHARMACOKINETICS

Absorption: Tramadol: Absolute bioavailability (75%); T_{max}=2 hrs. APAP: T_{max}=1 hr.
Distribution: Tramadol: (100mg IV) V_d=2.6L/kg (male), 2.9L/kg (female); plasma protein binding (20%); found in breast milk; crosses the placenta. APAP: V_d=0.9L/kg; plasma protein binding (20%). **Metabolism:** Tramadol: Liver (extensive) via CYP2D6, 3A4; M1 (active metabolite). APAP: Liver via CYP2E1, 1A2, 3A4.
Elimination: Tramadol: Urine (30% unchanged, 60% metabolites); $T_{1/2}$=5-6 hrs. APAP: Urine (<9% unchanged); $T_{1/2}$= 2-3 hrs.

PATIENT CONSIDERATIONS

Assessment: Assess for known hypersensitivity to the drug and other opioids, acute intoxication with alcohol, hypnotics, narcotics, centrally acting analgesics, opioids, or psychotropic drugs, epilepsy, seizure and respiratory depression risks, suicidal ideation, emotional disturbance or depression, increased ICP, head injury, drug abuse potential, suicidal or addiction proneness, renal/hepatic impairment, pregnancy/nursing status, and possible drug interactions.

Monitoring: Monitor for acute liver failure, skin hypersensitivity/anaphylactic reactions, respiratory/CNS depression, physical dependence/abuse, misuse, tolerance, seizures, development of serotonin syndrome, withdrawal symptoms with abrupt discontinuation, and other adverse reactions. Periodically monitor PT with warfarin-like compounds.

Counseling: Instruct to d/c therapy and notify physician if signs of allergy occur. Advise patients of dose limits. Instruct to seek medical attention immediately upon ingestion of >4000mg/day APAP, even if feeling well. Counsel not to use with other tramadol or APAP-containing products, including OTC preparations. Inform that seizures and serotonin syndrome may occur when used with serotonergic agents or drugs that reduce the clearance of tramadol. Inform that therapy may impair physical/mental abilities. Instruct to notify physician if pregnant or planning to become pregnant. Instruct to avoid alcohol-containing beverages while on therapy. Inform about the signs of serious skin reactions and of possible drug interactions.

ULTRAM — tramadol hydrochloride   CIV

Class: Centrally acting analgesic

ADULT DOSAGE	PEDIATRIC DOSAGE
Moderate to Moderately Severe Pain	Pediatric use may not have been established
≥17 Years:	
Initial: 25mg/day qam	
Titrate: Increase in 25mg increments every 3 days to reach 100mg/day (25mg qid), then may increase total daily dose by 50mg as tolerated every 3 days to reach 200mg/day (50mg qid)	
After Titration/Rapid Onset Required: 50-100mg q4-6h prn	
Max: 400mg/day	

DOSING CONSIDERATIONS
Renal Impairment
CrCl <30mL/min:
Increase dosing interval to 12 hrs
Dialysis patients may receive regular dose on the day of dialysis
Max: 200mg/day

Hepatic Impairment
Cirrhosis: 50mg q12h

Elderly
Start at lower end of dosing range
>75 Years:
Max: 300mg/day

ADMINISTRATION
Oral route
Administer w/o regard to food.

STORAGE
25°C (77°F); excursions permitted to 15-30°C (59-86°F).

HOW SUPPLIED
Tab: 50mg* *scored

CONTRAINDICATIONS
Previously demonstrated hypersensitivity to tramadol, any other component of Ultram, or opioids. Any situation where opioids are contraindicated, including acute intoxication with alcohol, hypnotics, narcotics, centrally acting analgesics, opioids, or psychotropic drugs.

WARNINGS/PRECAUTIONS
Do not exceed recommended dose. Seizures reported; risk increases in patients with epilepsy, history of seizures, recognized risk for seizures, and with naloxone coadministration. Anaphylactoid reactions and potentially life-threatening serotonin syndrome may occur. Avoid in patients who are suicidal or addiction-prone, and with history of anaphylactoid reactions to codeine and other opioids. Caution with emotional disturbances or depression, and in elderly. Tramadol-related deaths reported with previous histories of emotional disturbances, suicidal ideation/attempts, and misuse of tranquilizers, alcohol, and other CNS active drugs. Caution in patients at risk for respiratory depression; consider alternative

nonopioid analgesics. Caution with increased intracranial pressure (ICP) or head injury. May impair mental/physical abilities. Withdrawal symptoms may occur if discontinued abruptly. May complicate clinical assessment of acute abdominal conditions. Not for use in pregnant women prior to or during labor unless benefits outweigh risks. Not recommended for obstetrical preoperative medication or for postdelivery analgesia in nursing mothers.

ADVERSE REACTIONS
Dizziness/vertigo, N/V, constipation, headache, somnolence, sweating, asthenia, dyspepsia, dry mouth, diarrhea, pruritus.

DRUG INTERACTIONS
See Contraindications. Caution and reduce dose with CNS depressants (eg, alcohol, opioids, anesthetics); increased risk of CNS/respiratory depression. CYP2D6 inhibitors (eg, quinidine, fluoxetine, paroxetine, amitriptyline) and CYP3A4 inhibitors (eg, ketoconazole, erythromycin) may reduce metabolic clearance and increase risk for serious adverse events including seizures and serotonin syndrome. Altered exposure with CYP3A4 inducers (eg, rifampin, St. John's wort). Increased seizure risk with SSRIs, TCAs, other tricyclic compounds (eg, cyclobenzaprine, promethazine), MAOIs, other opioids, neuroleptics, and drugs that reduce seizure threshold. Caution with SSRIs, SNRIs, TCAs, MAOIs, α2-adrenergic blockers, triptans, linezolid, lithium, St. John's wort, and drugs that impair tramadol metabolism, due to potential serotonin syndrome. Not recommended with carbamazepine; may significantly reduce analgesic effect. Digoxin toxicity and alteration of warfarin effect, including elevation of PT, reported rarely.

PREGNANCY AND LACTATION
Category C, not for use in nursing.

MECHANISM OF ACTION
Centrally acting synthetic opioid analgesic; has not been established. Suspected to be due to binding of parent and (O-desmethyltramadol) M1 metabolite to μ-opioid receptors and weak inhibition of norepinephrine and serotonin reuptake.

PHARMACOKINETICS
Absorption: Absolute bioavailability (75%, 100mg). Administration of multiple doses resulted in different parameters. **Distribution:** (100mg IV) V_d=2.6L/kg (male), 2.9L/kg (female); plasma protein binding (20%); found in breast milk (IV); crosses placenta. **Metabolism:** Extensive via CYP2D6, 3A4 and 2B6; N- and O-demethylation and glucuronidation or sulfation (major pathway); M1 (active metabolite). **Elimination:** Urine (30% unchanged, 60% as metabolites); $T_{1/2}$=6.3 hrs, 7.4 hrs (M1).

PATIENT CONSIDERATIONS

Assessment: Assess for previous hypersensitivity to the drug and other opioids, acute intoxication with alcohol/hypnotics/narcotics/centrally acting analgesics/opioids/psychotropic drugs, epilepsy, seizure and respiratory depression risks, suicidal ideation, emotional disturbance or depression, increased ICP, head injury, drug abuse potential, suicidal/addiction proneness, pain severity, renal/hepatic impairment, pregnancy/nursing status, any other conditions where treatment is contraindicated or cautioned, and possible drug interactions.

Monitoring: Monitor for signs/symptoms of anaphylactoid reactions, respiratory/CNS depression, tolerance, physical dependence, seizures, serotonin syndrome, withdrawal symptoms, and other adverse reactions.

Counseling: Inform of the risks and benefits of therapy. Inform that drug may cause seizures and/or serotonin syndrome with concomitant use of serotonergic agents or drugs that significantly reduce the metabolic clearance of therapy. Inform that drug may impair physical/mental abilities required for the performance of hazardous tasks (eg, driving a car, operating machinery). Instruct not to take drug with alcohol containing beverages. Inform to use drug with caution when taking tranquilizers, hypnotics, other opiate containing analgesics). Instruct to inform physician if pregnant, think or trying to become pregnant. Educate about single-dose and 24-hr dose limits and time interval between doses; advise not to exceed the recommended dose.

ULTRAM ER — tramadol hydrochloride   CIV

Class: Centrally acting analgesic

ADULT DOSAGE	PEDIATRIC DOSAGE
Moderate to Moderately Severe Pain	Pediatric use may not have been established
Chronic Pain Requiring Around-the-Clock Treatment for an Extended Period:	
Not Currently on Tramadol Immediate-Release (IR):	
Initial: 100mg qd	
Titrate: Increase as necessary by 100mg increments every 5 days	
Max: 300mg/day	
Currently on Tramadol IR:	
Initial: Calculate 24-hr tramadol IR dose and initiate total daily dose rounded down to next lowest 100mg increment	
Titrate: Individualize according to patients need	
Max: 300mg/day	

DOSING CONSIDERATIONS
Renal Impairment
CrCl <30mg/mL: Do not use

Hepatic Impairment
Severe (Child-Pugh Class C): Do not use

Elderly
Start at low end of dosing range

ADMINISTRATION
Oral route

Swallow whole; do not chew, crush, or split.

STORAGE
25°C (77°F); excursions permitted to 15-30°C (59-86°F).

HOW SUPPLIED
Tab, Extended-Release: 100mg, 200mg, 300mg

CONTRAINDICATIONS
Previously demonstrated hypersensitivity to tramadol, any other component of Ultram ER, or opioids. Any situation where opioids are contraindicated, including acute intoxication w/ alcohol, hypnotics, narcotics, centrally acting analgesics, opioids, or psychotropic drugs.

WARNINGS/PRECAUTIONS
Do not exceed recommended dose. Seizures reported; risk increases in patients w/ epilepsy, history of seizures, recognized risk for seizures, and w/ naloxone coadministration. Anaphylactoid reactions and potentially life-threatening serotonin syndrome may occur. Avoid in patients who are suicidal or addiction-prone, and w/ history of anaphylactoid reactions to codeine and other opioids. Tramadol-related deaths reported w/ previous histories of emotional disturbances, suicidal ideation/attempts, and misuse of tranquilizers, alcohol, and other CNS-active drugs. Caution in patients at risk for respiratory depression; consider alternative nonopioid analgesics. Caution w/ increased intracranial pressure (ICP) or head injury. May impair mental/physical abilities. Withdrawal symptoms may occur if discontinued abruptly. May complicate clinical assessment of acute abdominal conditions. Not for use in pregnant women prior to or during labor unless benefits outweigh risks. Not recommended for obstetrical preoperative medication or for postdelivery analgesia in nursing mothers.

ADVERSE REACTIONS
Dizziness, N/V, constipation, headache, somnolence, flushing, insomnia, increased sweating, asthenia, dry mouth, diarrhea, pruritus, postural hypotension.

DRUG INTERACTIONS
See Contraindications. Caution and reduce dose w/ CNS depressants (eg, alcohol, opioids, anesthetics); increased risk of CNS/respiratory depression. CYP2D6 inhibitors (eg, quinidine, fluoxetine, paroxetine, amitriptyline) and CYP3A4 inhibitors (eg, ketoconazole, erythromycin) may reduce metabolic clearance and increase risk for serious adverse events, including seizures and serotonin syndrome. Altered exposure w/ CYP3A4 inducers (eg, rifampin, St. John's wort) and inhibitors (ketoconazole, erythromycin). Increased seizure risk w/ SSRIs, TCAs, other tricyclic compounds (eg, cyclobenzaprine, promethazine), MAOIs, other opioids, neuroleptics, and drugs that reduce seizure threshold. Caution w/ SSRIs, SNRIs, TCAs, MAOIs, α_2-adrenergic blockers, triptans, linezolid, lithium, St. John's wort, and drugs that impair tramadol metabolism, due to potential serotonin syndrome. Not recommended w/ carbamazepine; may significantly reduce analgesic effect. Digoxin toxicity and alterations of warfarin effect, including elevation of PT, reported rarely. Use w/ other tramadol products is not recommended.

PREGNANCY AND LACTATION
Pregnancy: Category C.
Lactation: Not for use in nursing.

MECHANISM OF ACTION
Centrally acting synthetic opioid analgesic; has not been established. Suspected to be due to binding of parent and (O-desmethyltramadol) M1 metabolite to µ-opioid receptors and weak inhibition of norepinephrine and serotonin reuptake.

PHARMACOKINETICS
Absorption: Administration of multiple doses resulted in different parameters. **Distribution:** (100mg IV) V_d=2.6L/kg (male), 2.9L/kg (female); plasma protein binding (20%); found in breast milk (IV); crosses placenta. **Metabolism:** Extensive via CYP2D6, CYP3A4, and CYP2B6; N- and O-demethylation and glucuronidation or sulfation (major pathway); M1 (active metabolite). **Elimination:** Urine (30% unchanged, 60% metabolites); $T_{1/2}$=7.9 hrs, 8.8 hrs (M1).

PATIENT CONSIDERATIONS
Assessment: Assess for previous hypersensitivity to the drug and other opioids, acute intoxication w/ alcohol/hypnotics/narcotics/centrally acting analgesics/opioids/psychotropic drugs, epilepsy, seizure and respiratory depression risks, suicidal ideation, emotional disturbance or depression, increased ICP, head injury, drug abuse potential, suicidal/addiction proneness, pain severity, renal/hepatic impairment, pregnancy/nursing status, any other conditions where treatment is contraindicated or cautioned, and possible drug interactions.

Monitoring: Monitor for signs/symptoms of anaphylactoid reactions, respiratory/CNS depression, tolerance, physical dependence, seizures, serotonin syndrome, withdrawal symptoms, and other adverse reactions.

Counseling: Inform of the risks/benefits of therapy. Inform that drug may cause seizures and/or serotonin syndrome w/ concomitant use of serotonergic agents or drugs that significantly reduce the metabolic clearance of therapy. Inform that drug may impair physical/mental abilities required for the performance of hazardous tasks (eg, driving a car, operating machinery). Instruct not to take drug w/ alcohol containing beverages. Inform to use drug w/ caution when taking tranquilizers, hypnotics, and other opiate containing analgesics. Instruct to inform physician if pregnant, thinking/trying to become pregnant. Educate regarding the single-dose and 24-hr dosing regimen; advise not to exceed the recommended dose.

ULTRAVATE — halobetasol propionate   Rx
Class: Corticosteroid

ADULT DOSAGE	PEDIATRIC DOSAGE
Inflammatory and Pruritic Manifestations of Corticosteroid-Responsive Dermatoses	**Inflammatory and Pruritic Manifestations of Corticosteroid-Responsive Dermatoses**
Apply a thin layer to affected skin qd or bid ud and rub in gently and completely	**≥12 Years:** Apply a thin layer to affected skin qd or bid ud and rub in gently and completely
Max Dose: 50g/week	**Max Dose:** 50g/week
Max Duration: 2 weeks; reassess diagnosis if no improvement w/in 2 weeks	**Max Duration:** 2 weeks; reassess diagnosis if no improvement w/in 2 weeks
D/C when control is achieved	D/C when control is achieved

ADMINISTRATION
Topical route
Avoid w/ occlusive dressings.

STORAGE
15-30°C (59-86°F).

HOW SUPPLIED
Cre, Oint: 0.05% [50g]

CONTRAINDICATIONS
History of hypersensitivity to any of the components of Ultravate.

WARNINGS/PRECAUTIONS
For dermatologic use only; not for ophthalmic use. May produce reversible hypothalamic-pituitary-adrenal (HPA) axis suppression, manifestations of Cushing's syndrome, hyperglycemia or glucosuria; evaluate periodically for evidence of HPA axis suppression when applying to a large surface area or to areas under occlusion. Attempts should be made to withdraw treatment, reduce frequency of application, or substitute to a less potent corticosteroid if HPA axis suppression is noted. Signs and symptoms of glucocorticosteroid insufficiency may occur (infrequent), requiring supplemental systemic corticosteroids. Pediatric patients may be more susceptible to systemic toxicity. D/C and treat appropriately if irritation develops. Allergic contact dermatitis reported. Use appropriate antibacterial or antifungal agent if skin infections are present or develop; if no favorable prompt response, may need to d/c until infection is controlled. Not for use in rosacea or perioral dermatitis. Do not use on the face, groin, or in the axillae.

ADVERSE REACTIONS
Stinging, burning, itching, dry skin, erythema, skin atrophy, leukoderma, rash.

PREGNANCY AND LACTATION
Pregnancy: Category C.
Lactation: Caution in nursing.

MECHANISM OF ACTION
Corticosteroid; has anti-inflammatory, antipruritic, and vasoconstrictive properties. Mechanism of anti-inflammatory action not established; thought to act by the induction of phospholipase A_2 inhibitory proteins called lipocortins, which control the biosynthesis of potent mediators of inflammation by inhibiting release of arachidonic acid.

PHARMACOKINETICS
Absorption: Percutaneous; extent is determined by many factors, including vehicle, integrity of epidermal barrier, use of occlusive dressings, inflammation and/or other disease processes. **Distribution:** Found in breast milk (systemically administered).

PATIENT CONSIDERATIONS
Assessment: Assess for previous hypersensitivity to any components of the drug, dermatological conditions, pregnancy/nursing status, and conditions that increase systemic absorption of the medication.

Monitoring: Monitor for HPA axis suppression, manifestations of Cushing's syndrome, hyperglycemia, glucosuria, skin irritation, allergic contact dermatitis (eg, failure to heal), skin infections (eg, bacterial, fungal), and other adverse reactions. Monitor for glucocorticosteroid insufficiency following withdrawal from therapy.

Counseling: Instruct to use externally and ud. Instruct to avoid contact with eyes. Advise not to use for any disorder other than for which it was prescribed. Instruct not to bandage, cover, or wrap treated skin, unless directed by physician. Instruct to report any signs of local adverse reactions to physician.

UNASYN — ampicillin sodium/sulbactam sodium   Rx
Class: Beta-lactamase inhibitor/semisynthetic penicillin (PCN)

ADULT DOSAGE	PEDIATRIC DOSAGE
General Dosing	**Skin and Skin Structure Infections**
Skin and skin structure infections, intra-abdominal infections, and gynecological infections caused by susceptible strains of microorganisms	**≥1 Year:** 300mg/kg/day (200mg ampicillin + 100mg sulbactam) IV in equally divided doses q6h
1.5g (1g ampicillin + 0.5g sulbactam)-3g (2g ampicillin + 1g sulbactam) IM/IV q6h	**≥40kg:** 1.5g (1g ampicillin + 0.5g sulbactam)-3g (2g ampicillin + 1g sulbactam) IV q6h
Max: 4g sulbactam/day	**Max:** 4g sulbactam/day
	Therapy should not routinely exceed 14 days

DOSING CONSIDERATIONS
Renal Impairment
CrCl ≥30mL/min: 1.5-3g q6-8h
CrCl 15-29mL/min: 1.5-3g q12h
CrCl 5-14mL/min: 1.5-3g q24h

ADMINISTRATION
IV/IM route

Do not reconstitute/administer w/ aminoglycosides.

IM
Administer by deep IM inj.

IV
Administer slowly over at least 10-15 min or 15-30 min in greater dilutions.
Refer to PI for directions for use, preparation, compatibility, and stability.

STORAGE
Prior to Reconstitution: ≤30°C (86°F). **Reconstituted:** Refer to PI for storage requirements.

HOW SUPPLIED
Inj: (Ampicillin/Sulbactam) 1g/0.5g, 2g/1g. Also available as a Pharmacy Bulk Package. Refer to individual package insert for more information.

CONTRAINDICATIONS
History of serious hypersensitivity reactions to ampicillin, sulbactam or to other beta-lactam antibacterial drugs (eg, penicillins, cephalosporins). Previous history of cholestatic jaundice/hepatic dysfunction associated with therapy.

WARNINGS/PRECAUTIONS
Serious and occasionally fatal hypersensitivity reactions reported; d/c and institute appropriate therapy if allergic reaction occurs. Hepatic dysfunction (eg, hepatitis, cholestatic jaundice) reported. *Clostridium difficile*-associated diarrhea (CDAD) reported and may range in severity from mild diarrhea to fatal colitis; may need to d/c if CDAD is suspected or confirmed. Ampicillin class antibacterial should not be administered to patients with mononucleosis. May result in bacterial resistance in the absence of proven or suspected bacterial infection or a prophylactic indication; d/c and/or take appropriate measures if superinfection develops. Decrease in total conjugated estriol, estriol-glucuronide, conjugated estrone, and estradiol reported in pregnant women. Lab test interactions may occur. Caution with renal impairment.

ADVERSE REACTIONS
Inj-site pain, thrombophlebitis, diarrhea.

DRUG INTERACTIONS
Probenecid decreases renal tubular secretion and may increase and prolong blood levels. **Ampicillin:** Increased incidence of rash with allopurinol.

PREGNANCY AND LACTATION
Pregnancy: Category B.
Lactation: Caution in nursing.

MECHANISM OF ACTION
Ampicillin: Semi-synthetic PCN; acts through inhibition of cell wall mucopeptide biosynthesis. Has a broad spectrum of bactericidal activity against many gram-positive and gram-negative aerobic and anaerobic bacteria. **Sulbactam:** β-lactamase inhibitor; provides good inhibitory activity against clinically important plasmid mediated β-lactamases most frequently responsible for transferred drug resistance.

PHARMACOKINETICS
Absorption: IV/IM administration of variable doses resulted in different parameters. **Distribution:** Plasma protein binding (28% ampicillin, 38% sulbactam); found in breast milk. **Elimination:** Urine (75-85% unchanged); $T_{1/2}$=1 hr.

PATIENT CONSIDERATIONS
Assessment: Assess for history of hypersensitivity to drug, PCNs, cephalosporins, or other allergens, history of cholestatic jaundice/hepatic dysfunction, mononucleosis, renal impairment, pregnancy/nursing status, and for possible drug interactions. Perform culture and susceptibility testing.

Monitoring: Monitor for signs/symptoms of hypersensitivity reactions, CDAD, superinfection, and other adverse reactions. Monitor for changes in estrogen levels in pregnant women. Monitor hepatic function at regular intervals in patients with hepatic impairment.

Counseling: Inform that therapy should only be used to treat bacterial, not viral, infections. Advise to take exactly ud even if patient feels better early in the course of therapy. Inform that skipping doses or not completing full course may decrease effectiveness and increase resistance. Inform that diarrhea is a common problem caused by therapy and will usually end upon discontinuation of therapy. Inform that diarrhea may occur as late as ≥2 months after last dose of therapy; instruct to notify physician as soon as possible if watery/bloody stools (with or without stomach cramps and fever) occur.

UNIRETIC — hydrochlorothiazide/moexipril hydrochloride   Rx
Class: ACE inhibitor/thiazide diuretic

> D/C when pregnancy is detected. Drugs that act directly on the renin-angiotensin system (RAS) can cause death/injury to developing fetus.

ADULT DOSAGE
Hypertension

Uncontrolled BP on Moexipril/HCTZ Monotherapy:
Initial: 7.5mg-12.5mg, 15mg-12.5mg, or 15mg-25mg qd

Titrate: Based on clinical response. May increase HCTZ dose after 2-3 weeks
Max: 30mg-50mg qd

Controlled BP on HCTZ 25mg qd with Hypokalemia: Switch to 3.75mg-6.25mg (1/2 of 7.5mg-12.5mg tab)
Excessive BP Reduction with 7.5mg-12.5mg: Switch to 3.75mg-6.25mg
Replacement Therapy: May substitute for titrated components

PEDIATRIC DOSAGE
Pediatric use may not have been established

ADMINISTRATION
Oral route
Take 1 hr ac

STORAGE
20-25°C (68-77°F). Protect from excessive moisture.

HOW SUPPLIED
Tab: (Moexipril-HCTZ) 7.5mg-12.5mg*, 15mg-12.5mg*, 15mg-25mg* *scored

CONTRAINDICATIONS
Hypersensitivity to any component of this product, history of ACE inhibitor-associated angioedema, anuria, hypersensitivity to sulfonamide-derived drugs. Coadministration with aliskiren in patients with diabetes.

WARNINGS/PRECAUTIONS
Not for initial therapy. Not recommended with severe renal impairment (CrCl ≤40mL/min/1.73m²). Symptomatic hypotension may occur, most likely in patients with salt and/or volume depletion; correct such conditions before therapy. May precipitate hepatic coma with hepatic impairment or progressive liver disease. Caution in elderly. HCTZ: Enhanced antihypertensive effects in postsympathectomy patients. May precipitate azotemia with severe renal disease. May cause idiosyncratic reaction, resulting in acute transient myopia and acute angle-closure glaucoma; d/c as rapidly as possible. May cause exacerbation or activation of systemic lupus erythematosus (SLE), hyperuricemia, precipitation of frank gout or overt diabetes, hypercalcemia, hypophosphatemia, hypomagnesemia, reduced glucose tolerance, and increased cholesterol and TG levels. Observe for signs of fluid and electrolyte imbalance; monitor serum electrolytes periodically. Hypokalemia may sensitize or exaggerate the response of the heart to toxic effects of digitalis. Moexipril: Angioedema of the face, extremities, lips, tongue, glottis, and/or larynx reported; d/c and administer appropriate therapy if symptoms develop. Intestinal angioedema reported; monitor for abdominal pain. More reports of angioedema in blacks than nonblacks. Anaphylactoid reactions reported during desensitization with hymenoptera venom, dialysis with high-flux membranes, and LDL apheresis with dextran sulfate absorption. Excessive hypotension, which may be associated with oliguria or progressive azotemia, and rarely, with acute renal failure and/or death, may occur in congestive heart failure (CHF) patients; monitor closely upon initiation and during first 2 weeks of therapy and whenever dose is increased. May cause changes in renal function. May increase BUN/SrCr in patients with no preexisting renal vascular disease or with renal artery stenosis; monitor renal function during the 1st few weeks of therapy in patients with renal artery stenosis. May cause agranulocytosis and bone marrow depression; monitor WBCs with collagen vascular disease. Rarely, associated with syndrome of cholestatic jaundice, hepatic necrosis, and death; d/c if jaundice or marked hepatic enzyme elevation occurs. Hyperkalemia and persistent nonproductive cough reported. Hypotension may occur with major surgery or during anesthesia.

ADVERSE REACTIONS
Cough, dizziness, angioedema, hypotension, fatigue.

DRUG INTERACTIONS
See Contraindications. Dual blockade of the RAS is associated with increased risks of hypotension, hyperkalemia, and changes in renal function (including acute renal failure); closely monitor BP, renal function, and electrolytes with concomitant agents that affect the RAS. Avoid with aliskiren in patients with renal impairment (GFR <60mL/min). NSAIDs, including selective COX-2 inhibitors, may attenuate diuretic, natriuretic, and antihypertensive effects. HCTZ: Potentiation of orthostatic hypotension may occur with alcohol, barbiturates, or narcotics. Dosage adjustment of antidiabetic drugs (oral agents and insulin) may be required. Cholestyramine and colestipol resins may reduce absorption. Corticosteroids and adrenocorticotropic hormone may intensify electrolyte depletion, particularly hypokalemia. May decrease response to pressor amines (eg, norepinephrine). May increase responsiveness to nondepolarizing skeletal muscle relaxants (eg, tubocurarine). Increased absorption with guanabenz or propantheline. May potentiate action of other antihypertensives, especially ganglionic or peripheral adrenergic-blocking drugs. Moexipril: NSAIDs may deteriorate renal function. Increased lithium levels and symptoms of toxicity reported; use with caution and monitor lithium levels. Increased risk of hyperkalemia with K⁺-sparing diuretics (spironolactone, amiloride, triamterene), K⁺ supplements, or K⁺-containing salt substitutes; use with caution and monitor serum K⁺. Nitritoid reactions reported with injectable gold (sodium aurothiomalate).

PREGNANCY AND LACTATION
Category D, not for use in nursing.

MECHANISM OF ACTION
Moexipril: ACE inhibitor; decreases angiotensin II formation, leading to decreased vasoconstriction, increased plasma renin activity, and decreased aldosterone secretion. HCTZ: Thiazide diuretic; not established. Affects distal renal tubular mechanisms of electrolyte reabsorption, directly increasing excretion of Na⁺ and Cl⁻ in approximately equivalent amounts.

PHARMACOKINETICS

Absorption: Moexipril: Incomplete. Bioavailability (13%, moexiprilat); T_{max}=0.8 hr, 1.5-1.6 hrs (moexiprilat); C_{max} and AUC reduced by 70% and 40%, respectively, with low-fat breakfast, or 80% and 50%, respectively, with high-fat breakfast. **Distribution:** Moexipril: V_d=2.8L/kg (moexiprilat); plasma protein binding (50%, moexiprilat). HCTZ: V_d=1.5-4.2L/kg; plasma protein binding (21-24%); crosses placenta; found in breast milk. **Metabolism:** Rapid via de-esterification; moexiprilat (active metabolite). **Elimination:** Moexipril: Urine (1% unchanged, 7% moexiprilat, 5% other metabolites), feces (1% unchanged, 52% moexiprilat); $T_{1/2}$=1.3 hrs, 2-9 hrs (moexiprilat). HCTZ: Kidney (>60% unchanged); $T_{1/2}$=5.6-14.8 hrs.

PATIENT CONSIDERATIONS

Assessment: Assess for history of ACE inhibitor-associated angioedema, anuria, hypersensitivity to drug or sulfonamide-derived drugs, history of allergy or bronchial asthma, volume/salt depletion, CHF, collagen vascular disease, renal artery stenosis, SLE, risk factors for hyperkalemia, hepatic/renal function, pregnancy/nursing status, and possible drug interactions. Obtain baseline serum electrolytes.

Monitoring: Monitor for signs of angioedema, hypotension, exacerbation/ activation of SLE, idiosyncratic reaction, and other adverse reactions. Monitor hepatic/renal function, BP, WBC counts (collagen vascular disease), serum electrolytes, blood glucose, cholesterol, TG, and uric acid.

Counseling: Advise to take therapy 1 hr ac. Instruct to d/c use and report immediately to physician if signs/symptoms of angioedema occur. Inform that lightheadedness may occur, especially during the 1st few days of therapy; instruct to d/c use and consult physician if fainting occurs. Inform that excessive perspiration, dehydration, and other causes of volume depletion may lead to excessive fall in BP; advise to consult physician if these conditions develop. Instruct not to use K⁺ supplements or salt substitutes containing K⁺ without consulting physician, and to report promptly any indication of infection. Inform of the consequences of exposure during pregnancy and discuss treatment options in women planning to become pregnant. Instruct to report pregnancies to physician as soon as possible.

UNITHROID — levothyroxine sodium   Rx

Class: Thyroid replacement hormone

> **Do not use for the treatment of obesity or weight loss; doses within range of daily hormonal requirements are ineffective for weight reduction in euthyroid patients. Serious or life-threatening manifestations of toxicity may occur when given in larger doses, particularly when given in association with sympathomimetic amines.**

ADULT DOSAGE

Hypothyroidism

Replacement/supplemental therapy in hypothyroidism of any etiology, except transient hypothyroidism during the recovery phase of subacute thyroiditis

The average full replacement dose is approx. 1.7mcg/kg/day; >200mcg/day seldom required

Severe:
Initial: 12.5-25mcg/day
Titrate: Increase by 25mcg/day every 2-4 weeks until TSH level normalized

Secondary (Pituitary)/Tertiary (Hypothalamic) Hypothyroidism:
Titrate: Increase until euthyroid and serum free-T4 level is restored to the upper 1/2 of the normal range

Subclinical Hypothyroidism:
Lower doses (eg, 1mcg/kg/day) may be adequate to normalize the serum TSH level

Pituitary TSH Suppressant

Used to treat/prevent various types of euthyroid goiters (eg, thyroid nodules, subacute or chronic lymphocytic thyroiditis, multinodular goiter) and to manage thyroid cancer

Well-Differentiated (Papillary and Follicular) Thyroid Cancer:
Adjunct to Surgery and Radioiodine Therapy:
>2 mcg/kg/day, w/ target TSH level <0.1 mU/L
High-Risk Tumors: Target TSH level <0.01 mU/L

Benign Nodules and Nontoxic Multinodular Goiter:
TSH is suppressed to a higher target (eg, 0.1 to 0.5 for nodules and 1.0 mU/L for multinodular goiter)

PEDIATRIC DOSAGE

Hypothyroidism

0-3 Months of Age: 10-15mcg/kg/day
3-6 Months of Age: 8-10mcg/kg/day
6-12 Months of Age: 6-8mcg/kg/day
1-5 Years: 5-6mcg/kg/day
6-12 Years: 4-5mcg/kg/day
>12 Years (Growth/Puberty Incomplete): 2-3mcg/kg/day
Growth/Puberty Complete: 1.7mcg/kg/day

Infants w/ Very Low (<5mcg/dL) or Undetectable Serum T4:
Initial: 50mcg/day

Chronic/Severe Hypothyroidism:
Initial: 25mcg/day
Titrate: Increase by 25mcg increments every 2-4 weeks

DOSING CONSIDERATIONS

Pregnancy
May increase levothyroxine requirements

Elderly
Hypothyroidism:
>50 Years:
Initial: 25-50mcg/day
Titrate: Increase by 12.5-25mcg increments every 6-8 weeks prn
W/ Underlying Cardiac Disease:
Initial: 12.5-25mcg/day
Titrate: Increase by 12.5-25mg increments every 4-6 weeks

Adverse Reactions
Minimize Hyperactivity in Older Children:
Initial: Give 1/4 of full replacement dose
Titrate: Increase on a weekly basis by 1/4 the full recommended replacement dose until the full recommended replacement dose is reached

Other Important Considerations
Hypothyroidism:
W/ Underlying Cardiac Disease:
Infants (Risk for Cardiac Failure):
Initial: Consider lower dose (eg, 25mcg/day)
Titrate: Increase dose in 4-6 weeks prn
<50 Years:
Initial: 25-50mcg/day
Titrate: Increase by 12.5-25mcg increments every 6-8 weeks prn

ADMINISTRATION
Oral route
Take in the am on an empty stomach at least 1/2-1 hr before food
Take at least 4 hrs apart from drugs that are known to interfere w/ its absorption

Pediatrics
Unable to Swallow Intact Tab:
1. Crush tab and suspend in small amount (5-10mL or 1-2 tsp) of water
2. Administer using a spoon or dropper
3. Do not store sus for later use
4. Do not use foods that decrease absorption of levothyroxine (eg, soybean infant formula) to administer

STORAGE
20-25°C (68-77°F); excursions permitted to 15-30°C (59-86°F). Store away from heat, moisture, and light.

HOW SUPPLIED
Tab: 25mcg*, 50mcg*, 75mcg*, 88mcg*, 100mcg*, 112mcg*, 125mcg*, 137mcg*, 150mcg*, 175mcg*, 200mcg*, 300mcg* *scored

CONTRAINDICATIONS
Untreated subclinical (suppressed serum TSH level with normal T3 and T4levels) or overt thyrotoxicosis, acute MI, uncorrected adrenal insufficiency, hypersensitivity to any of the inactive ingredients in this medication.

WARNINGS/PRECAUTIONS
Should not be used in the treatment of male or female infertility unless associated with hypothyroidism. Contraindicated in patients with nontoxic diffuse goiter or nodular thyroid disease, particularly in the elderly or with underlying cardiovascular (CV) disease if serum TSH level is already suppressed; use with caution if TSH level is not suppressed and carefully monitor thyroid function. Has narrow therapeutic index; carefully titrate dose to avoid over- or under-treatment. May decrease bone mineral density (BMD) with long-term use; give minimum dose necessary to achieve desired clinical and biochemical response. Caution with CV disorders and the elderly. If cardiac symptoms develop or worsen, reduce or withhold dose for 1 week and then restart at lower dose. Overtreatment may produce CV effects (eg, increase in HR, increase in cardiac wall thickness, increase in cardiac contractility, precipitation of angina or arrhythmias). Monitor patients with coronary artery disease (CAD) closely during surgical procedures; may precipitate cardiac arrhythmias. Caution in patients with diabetes mellitus (DM). Patients with concomitant adrenal insufficiency should be treated with replacement glucocorticoids prior to therapy.

ADVERSE REACTIONS
Fatigue, increased appetite, weight loss, heat intolerance, headache, hyperactivity, irritability, insomnia, palpitations, arrhythmias, dyspnea, hair loss, menstrual irregularities, pseudotumor cerebri (children), slipped capital femoral epiphysis (children).

DRUG INTERACTIONS
Concurrent sympathomimetics may increase effects of sympathomimetics or thyroid hormone; may increase risk of coronary insufficiency with CAD. Upward dose adjustments may be needed for insulin and oral hypoglycemic agents. May decrease absorption with soybean flour, cottonseed meal, walnuts, and dietary fiber. May increase oral anticoagulant activity; adjust dose of anticoagulant and monitor PT. May decrease levels and effects of digitalis glycosides. Transient reduction in TSH secretion with dopamine/dopamine agonists, glucocorticoids, octreotide. Decreased thyroid hormone secretion with aminoglutethimide, amiodarone, iodide (including iodine-containing radiographic contrast agents), lithium, methimazole, propylthiouracil (PTU), sulfonamides, and tolbutamide. May increase thyroid hormone secretion with amiodarone and iodide. May decrease T4 absorption with antacids (aluminum and magnesium hydroxides), simethicone, bile acid sequestrants (cholestyramine, colestipol), calcium carbonate, cation exchange resins (kayexalate), ferrous sulfate, orlistat, and sucralfate; administer at least 4 hrs apart. May increase serum thyroxine-binding globulin (TBG) concentrations with clofibrate, estrogen-containing oral contraceptives, oral estrogens, heroin/methadone, 5-fluorouracil, mitotane, and tamoxifen. May decrease serum TBG concentrations with androgens/anabolic steroids,

asparaginase, glucocorticoids, and slow-release nicotinic acid. May cause protein-binding site displacement with furosemide (>80mg IV), heparin, hydantoins, NSAIDs (fenamates, phenylbutazone), and salicylates (>2g/day). May alter T4 and T3 metabolism with carbamazepine, hydantoins, phenobarbital, and rifampin. May decrease T4 5'-deiodinase activity with amiodarone, β-adrenergic antagonists (eg, propranolol >160mg/day), glucocorticoids (eg, dexamethasone >4mg/day), and PTU. Concurrent use with tricyclic (eg, amitriptyline) and tetracyclic (eg, maprotiline) antidepressants may increase the therapeutic and toxic effects of both drugs. Coadministration with sertraline in patients stabilized on levothyroxine may result in increased levothyroxine requirements. Interferon-α may cause development of antithyroid microsomal antibodies and transient hypothyroidism, hyperthyroidism, or both. Interleukin-2 has been associated with transient painless thyroiditis. Excessive use with growth hormones (eg, somatropin, somatrem) may accelerate epiphyseal closure. Ketamine may produce marked HTN and tachycardia. May reduce uptake of radiographic agents. Decreased theophylline clearance may occur in hypothyroid patients. Altered levels of thyroid hormone and/or TSH levels with choral hydrate, diazepam, ethionamide, lovastatin, metoclopramide, 6-mercaptopurine, nitroprusside, para-aminosalicylate sodium, perphenazine, resorcinol (excessive topical use), and thiazide diuretics.

PREGNANCY AND LACTATION
Category A, caution in nursing.

MECHANISM OF ACTION
Thyroid replacement hormone; mechanism not established. Suspected that principal effects are exerted through control of DNA transcription and protein synthesis.

PHARMACOKINETICS
Administration: Majority absorbed from jejunum and upper ileum. **Distribution:** Plasma protein binding (>99%), found in breast milk. **Metabolism:** Sequential deiodination and conjugation in liver (mainly), kidneys, other tissues. **Elimination:** Urine; feces (20% unchanged); $T_{1/2}$=6-7 days (T4), ≤2 days (T3).

PATIENT CONSIDERATIONS

Assessment: Assess for untreated subclinical or overt thyrotoxicosis, acute MI, uncorrected adrenal insufficiency, CAD, CV disorders, nontoxic diffuse goiter, nodular thyroid disease, DM, hypersensitivity, pregnancy/nursing status, and possible drug interactions. In patients with secondary or tertiary hypothyroidism, assess for additional hypothalamic/pituitary hormone deficiencies. Assess TSH levels. In infants with congenital hypothyroidism, assess for other congenital anomalies.

Monitoring: Monitor for CV effects. In patients on long-term therapy, monitor for signs/symptoms of decreased BMD. In patients with nontoxic diffuse goiter or nodular thyroid disease, monitor for precipitation of thyrotoxicosis. In adults with primary hypothyroidism, perform periodic monitoring of serum TSH levels. In pediatric patients with congenital hypothyroidism, perform periodic monitoring of serum TSH levels and total or free T4 levels. In patients with secondary and tertiary hypothyroidism, perform periodic monitoring of serum free-T4 levels. Refer to PI for TSH and T4 monitoring parameters. Closely monitor PT if coadministered with an oral anticoagulant.

Counseling: Instruct to notify physician if allergic to any foods or medicines, pregnant or planning to become pregnant, breastfeeding or taking any other drugs, including prescriptions and OTC preparations. Instruct to notify physician of any other medical conditions, particularly heart disease, diabetes, clotting disorders, and adrenal or pituitary gland problems. Instruct not to stop or change dose unless directed by physician. Instruct to take on empty stomach, at least 1/2 to 1 hr before eating breakfast. Instruct to notify physician if rapid or irregular heartbeat, chest pain, SOB, leg cramps, headache, or any other unusual medical event occurs. Inform that dose may be increased during pregnancy. Instruct to notify physician or dentist prior to surgery about levothyroxine therapy. Advise that partial hair loss may occur during the 1st few months of therapy, but is usually temporary. Inform that drug should not be used as a primary or adjunctive therapy in a weight control program. Inform that drug should not be administered within 4 hrs of agents such as iron/Ca^{2+} supplements and antacids.

UNITUXIN — dinutuximab

Rx

Class: GD2-binding monoclonal antibody

> Serious and potentially life-threatening infusion reactions reported; administer required prehydration and premedication including antihistamines prior to each infusion. Monitor closely for signs/symptoms of an infusion reaction during and for at least 4 hrs following completion of each infusion. Immediately interrupt therapy for severe infusion reactions and permanently d/c for anaphylaxis. May cause severe neuropathic pain; administer IV opioid prior to, during, and for 2 hrs following completion of infusion. Grade 3 peripheral sensory neuropathy reported. Severe motor neuropathy reported in adults. D/C therapy for severe unresponsive pain, severe sensory neuropathy, or moderate to severe peripheral motor neuropathy.

PEDIATRIC DOSAGE
Neuroblastoma

In combination w/ granulocyte-macrophage colony-stimulating factor, interleukin-2 and 13-cis-retinoic acid, for the treatment of patients w/ high-risk neuroblastoma who achieve at least a partial response to prior 1st-line multiagent, multimodality therapy

Usual: 17.5mg/m^2/day as IV infusion over 10-20 hrs for 4 consecutive days for a max of 5 cycles

Initiate at an infusion rate of 0.875mg/m^2/hr for 30 min; may gradually increase as tolerated to a max rate of 1.75mg/m^2/hr

Schedule of Administration:
Cycles 1, 3, and 5:
Take on Days 4, 5, 6, and 7
Cycles 1, 3, and 5 are 24 days in duration

Cycles 2 and 4:
Take on Days 8, 9, 10, and 11
Cycles 2 and 4 are 32 days in duration

Required Pretreatment and Guidelines for Pain Management:
IV Hydration: Administer 10mL/kg IV infusion of 0.9% NaCl inj over 1 hr just prior to initiating each dinutuximab infusion

Analgesics: Administer 50mcg/kg morphine sulfate IV immediately prior to initiation of dinutuximab, then continue as a morphine sulfate drip at an infusion rate of 20-50mcg/kg/hr during and for 2 hrs following completion of dinutuximab. Administer additional 25-50mcg/kg IV doses of morphine sulfate prn for pain for up to once q2h followed by an increase in morphine sulfate infusion rate in clinically stable patients. Consider using fentanyl or hydromorphone if morphine sulfate is not tolerated.
If pain is inadequately managed w/ opioids, consider use of gabapentin or lidocaine in conjunction w/ IV morphine.

Antihistamines/Antipyretics:
Administer 0.5-1mg/kg (max dose of 50mg) of antihistamine (eg, diphenhydramine) IV over 10-15 min starting 20 min prior to initiation of dinutuximab and as tolerated q4-6h during dinutuximab infusion. Administer 10-15mg/kg (max dose of 650mg) of acetaminophen 20 min prior to each dinutuximab infusion and q4-6h prn for fever or pain. Administer 5-10mg/kg of ibuprofen q6h prn for control of persistent fever or pain.

DOSING CONSIDERATIONS
Adverse Reactions
Infusion-Related Reactions:
Mild to moderate adverse reactions (eg, transient rash, fever, rigors, localized urticaria) that respond promptly to symptomatic treatment
Onset of Reaction: Reduce infusion rate to 50% of the previous rate and monitor closely
After Resolution: Gradually increase infusion rate up to a max rate of 1.75mg/m^2/hr
Prolonged or Severe Adverse Reactions (eg, Mild Bronchospasm w/o Other Symptoms, Angioedema That Does Not Affect the Airway):
Onset of Reaction: Interrupt immediately
After Resolution: Resume at 50% of the previous rate and observe closely, if signs and symptoms resolve rapidly
1st Recurrence: D/C until the following day. If symptoms resolve and continued treatment is warranted, premedicate w/ 1mg/kg (max dose of 50mg) hydrocortisone IV and administer dinutuximab at a rate of 0.875mg/m^2/hr in an intensive care unit
2nd Recurrence: D/C permanently

Capillary Leak Syndrome:
Moderate to Severe but Not Life-Threatening:
Onset of Reaction: Interrupt immediately
After Resolution: Resume at 50% of the previous rate
Life-Threatening:
Onset of Reaction: D/C for the current cycle
After Resolution: Administer at 50% of the previous rate in subsequent cycles
1st Recurrence: D/C permanently

Hypotension Requiring Medical Intervention:
Symptomatic Hypotension, Systolic BP (SBP) < Lower Limit of Normal for Age, or SBP Decreased by >15% Compared to Baseline:
Onset of Reaction: Interrupt infusion
After Resolution: Resume infusion at 50% of the previous rate. Increase infusion rate as tolerated up to a max rate of 1.75mg/m^2/hr if BP remains stable for at least 2 hrs

Severe Systemic Infection or Sepsis:
Onset of Reaction: D/C until resolution of infection, and then proceed w/ subsequent cycles of therapy

Neurological Disorders of the Eye:
Onset of Reaction: D/C infusion until resolution
After Resolution: Reduce dose by 50%
1st Recurrence or if Accompanied by Visual Impairment: D/C permanently
Permanently Discontinue w/ the Following:
- Grade 3 or 4 anaphylaxis
- Grade 3 or 4 serum sickness
- Grade 3 pain unresponsive to max supportive measures
- Grade 4 sensory neuropathy or Grade 3 sensory neuropathy that interferes w/ daily activities for >2 weeks
- Grade 2 peripheral motor neuropathy
- Subtotal or total vision loss
- Grade 4 hyponatremia despite appropriate fluid management

ADMINISTRATION
IV route

Administer as a diluted IV infusion only; do not administer as an IV push or bolus. Verify that patients have adequate hematologic, respiratory, hepatic, and renal function prior to initiating each course of therapy.

Preparation
Aseptically withdraw the required volume from the single-use vial and inject into a 100mL bag of 0.9% NaCl inj.
Mix by gentle inversion; do not shake.
Initiate infusion w/in 4 hrs of preparation.
Discard diluted sol 24 hrs after preparation.

STORAGE
2-8°C (36-46°F). Do not freeze or shake the vial. Protect from light.

HOW SUPPLIED
Inj: 3.5mg/mL [5mL]

CONTRAINDICATIONS
History of anaphylaxis to dinutuximab.

WARNINGS/PRECAUTIONS
Pain reported; decrease infusion rate to $0.875mg/m^2/hr$ for severe pain. Capillary leak syndrome reported; immediately interrupt or d/c therapy and institute supportive management in patients w/ symptomatic or severe capillary leak syndrome. Hypotension, infection, neurological disorders of the eye, bone marrow suppression, and electrolyte abnormalities reported. Atypical hemolytic uremic syndrome reported; permanently d/c therapy and institute supportive management for signs of hemolytic uremic syndrome. May cause fetal harm.

ADVERSE REACTIONS
Infusion reactions, neuropathy, pain, pyrexia, thrombocytopenia, lymphopenia, hypotension, hyponatremia, anemia, vomiting, diarrhea, hypokalemia, neutropenia, urticaria, hypoalbuminemia.

PREGNANCY AND LACTATION
Pregnancy: May cause fetal harm. Monoclonal antibodies are transported across the placenta as pregnancy progresses, w/ the largest amount transferred during the 3rd trimester.
Lactation: It is not known if dinutuximab is present in human milk; not for use in nursing.
Reproductive Potential: Females of reproductive potential should use effective contraception during treatment and for 2 months after the last dose of dinutuximab.

MECHANISM OF ACTION
Glycolipid disialoganglioside (GD2)-binding monoclonal antibody; binds to cell surface of GD2 and induces cell lysis of GD2-expressing cells through antibody-dependent cell-mediated cytotoxicity and complement-dependent cytotoxicity.

PHARMACOKINETICS
Absorption: C_{max}=11.5mcg/mL. **Distribution:** V_d=5.4L. **Elimination:** $T_{1/2}$=10 days.

PATIENT CONSIDERATIONS
Assessment: Assess for hematologic/respiratory/hepatic/renal dysfunction, history of anaphylaxis to drug, and pregnancy/nursing status.

Monitoring: Monitor for neuropathy, pain, capillary leak syndrome, hypotension, infection, neurological disorders of the eye, atypical hemolytic uremic syndrome, and other adverse reactions. Monitor closely for signs/symptoms of an infusion reaction during and for at least 4 hrs following completion of each infusion. Monitor serum electrolytes (daily) and peripheral blood counts.

Counseling: Inform of the risk of serious infusion reactions and anaphylaxis; severe pain and peripheral sensory and motor neuropathy; capillary leak syndrome; hypotension; infection; neurological disorders of the eye; bone marrow suppression; electrolyte abnormalities; and hemolytic uremic syndrome. Instruct to promptly report to physician if any signs/symptoms of any of these conditions develop. Advise women of reproductive potential of the potential risk to the fetus if administered during pregnancy and the need for use of effective contraception during and for at least 2 months after completing therapy.

UNIVASC — moexipril hydrochloride   Rx
Class: ACE inhibitor

> **D/C when pregnancy is detected. Drugs that act directly on the renin-angiotensin system (RAS) can cause injury/death to the developing fetus.**

ADULT DOSAGE
Hypertension

Not Receiving Diuretics:
Initial: 7.5mg qd

Titrate: Adjust dose according to BP response
If not adequately controlled, may increase or divide dose
Usual: 7.5-30mg/day given in 1 or 2 divided doses
Max: 60mg/day

Receiving Diuretics:
D/C diuretic 2-3 days prior to therapy to avoid hypotension. If BP is not controlled w/ moexipril alone, then diuretic therapy may be reinstituted
Initial: 3.75mg if diuretic therapy cannot be discontinued

PEDIATRIC DOSAGE
Pediatric use may not have been established

DOSING CONSIDERATIONS
Renal Impairment
CrCl $\leq$40mL/min/1.73m^2:
Initial: 3.75mg qd
Max: 15mg/day

Elderly
Start at lower end of dosing range

ADMINISTRATION
Oral route

Take 1 hr ac.

STORAGE
20-25°C (68-77°F). Protect from excessive moisture.

HOW SUPPLIED
Tab: 7.5mg*, 15mg* *scored

CONTRAINDICATIONS
Hypersensitivity to this product, history of ACE inhibitor-associated angioedema. Coadministration w/ aliskiren in patients w/ diabetes.

WARNINGS/PRECAUTIONS
Angioedema of the face, extremities, lips, tongue, glottis, and/or larynx reported; d/c and administer appropriate therapy if symptoms develop. Intestinal angioedema reported; monitor for abdominal pain. More reports of angioedema in blacks than nonblacks. Anaphylactoid reactions reported during desensitization w/ hymenoptera venom, dialysis w/ high-flux membranes, and LDL apheresis w/ dextran sulfate absorption. Symptomatic hypotension may occur, most likely w/ salt and volume depletion; correct depletion prior to therapy. Excessive hypotension associated w/ oliguria, azotemia, acute renal failure, or death may occur in CHF patients; monitor closely upon initiation and during first 2 weeks of therapy and whenever dose is increased. May cause agranulocytosis and bone marrow depression; monitor WBCs w/ collagen vascular disease. Rarely, associated w/ syndrome of cholestatic jaundice, fulminant hepatic necrosis, and death; d/c if jaundice or marked hepatic enzyme elevation occurs. May cause changes in renal function. Increased BUN and SrCr reported in patients w/ renal artery stenosis and w/o preexisting renal vascular disease; reduce dose and/or d/c. Hyperkalemia reported; risk factors include diabetes mellitus (DM) and renal insufficiency. Hypotension may occur w/ major surgery or during anesthesia. Persistent nonproductive cough reported. Dual blockade of the RAS is associated w/ increased risks of hypotension, hyperkalemia, and changes in renal function (including acute renal failure); closely monitor BP, renal function, and electrolytes w/ concomitant agents that also affect the RAS. Caution in elderly.

ADVERSE REACTIONS
Cough increased, dizziness, diarrhea, flu syndrome.

DRUG INTERACTIONS
See Contraindications. Avoid w/ aliskiren in patients w/ renal impairment (GFR <60mL/min). Hypotension risk and increased BUN and SrCr w/ diuretics. Increased risk of hyperkalemia w/ K$^+$-sparing diuretics (spironolactone, amiloride, triamterene), K$^+$ supplements, or K$^+$-containing salt substitutes; use w/ caution and monitor serum K$^+$. Increased lithium levels and lithium toxicity symptoms reported; use w/ caution and monitor lithium levels. Nitritoid reactions (eg, facial flushing, N/V, hypotension) reported w/ injectable gold (sodium aurothiomalate). NSAIDs, including selective COX-2 inhibitors, may deteriorate renal function. Antihypertensive effect may be attenuated by NSAIDs.

PREGNANCY AND LACTATION
Pregnancy: Category D.
Lactation: Caution in nursing.

MECHANISM OF ACTION
ACE inhibitor; reduces angiotensin II formation, decreases vasoconstriction and aldosterone secretion, and increases plasma renin.

PHARMACOKINETICS
Absorption: Incomplete. Bioavailability (13%, moexiprilat); T_{max}=1.5 hrs (moexiprilat); C_{max} and AUC reduced by 70% and 40%, respectively, w/ low-fat breakfast, or 80% and 50%, respectively, w/ high-fat breakfast. **Distribution:** V_d=183L (moexiprilat); plasma protein binding (50%, moexiprilat). **Metabolism:** Rapid via deesterification; moexiprilat (active metabolite). **Elimination:** Urine (1% unchanged, 7% moexiprilat, 5% other metabolites), feces (1% unchanged, 52% moexiprilat); $T_{1/2}$=2-9 hrs (moexiprilat).

PATIENT CONSIDERATIONS
Assessment: Assess for history of ACE inhibitor-associated angioedema, hypersensitivity to the drug, volume/salt depletion, CHF, collagen vascular disease, renal artery stenosis, DM, cerebrovascular disease, hepatic/renal function, pregnancy/nursing status, and possible drug interactions.

Monitoring: Monitor BP, hepatic/renal function, WBCs (collagen vascular disease), and serum K⁺ levels. Monitor for head/neck and intestinal angioedema, anaphylactoid reaction, and hypersensitivity reactions.

Counseling: Instruct to d/c use and to report immediately to physician if signs/symptoms of angioedema occur. Inform that lightheadedness may occur, especially during the 1st few days of therapy; instruct to d/c use and to consult physician if fainting occurs. Inform that excessive perspiration, dehydration, and other causes of volume depletion may lead to excessive fall in BP; advise to consult physician if these conditions develop. Instruct not to use K⁺ supplements or salt substitutes containing K⁺ w/o consulting physician, and to report any signs/symptoms of infection. Inform of the consequences of exposure during pregnancy and instruct to report pregnancy to physician as soon as possible.

UPTRAVI — selexipag

Class: Prostacyclin receptor agonist

Rx

ADULT DOSAGE
Pulmonary Arterial Hypertension
Treatment of pulmonary arterial HTN (WHO Group I) to delay disease progression and reduce risk of hospitalization

Initial: 200mcg bid
Titrate: Increase in increments of 200mcg bid, usually at weekly intervals
Max: 1600mcg bid

If a patient reaches a dose that cannot be tolerated, the dose should be reduced to previously tolerated dose

Missed Dose
If a dose is missed, take as soon as possible unless next dose is w/in the next 6 hrs

If treatment is missed for ≥3 days, restart at a lower dose and then retitrate

PEDIATRIC DOSAGE
Pediatric use may not have been established

DOSING CONSIDERATIONS
Hepatic Impairment
Moderate (Child-Pugh Class B):
Initial: 200mcg qd
Titrate: Increase in increments of 200mcg qd at weekly intervals, as tolerated
Severe (Child-Pugh Class C): Avoid use

ADMINISTRATION
Oral route

Tolerability may be improved when taken w/ food.
Do not split, crush, or chew tabs.

STORAGE
20-25°C (68-77°F); excursions permitted between 15-30°C (59-86°F).

HOW SUPPLIED
Tab: 200mcg, 400mcg, 600mcg, 800mcg, 1000mcg, 1200mcg, 1400mcg, 1600mcg

WARNINGS/PRECAUTIONS
Consider the possibility of associated pulmonary veno-occlusive disease if signs of pulmonary edema occur; d/c therapy if confirmed.

ADVERSE REACTIONS
Headache, diarrhea, jaw pain, N/V, myalgia, pain in extremity, flushing, arthralgia, anemia, decreased appetite, rash.

DRUG INTERACTIONS
Strong CYP2C8 inhibitors (eg, gemfibrozil) may significantly increase exposure to selexipag and its active metabolite; avoid concomitant administration.

PREGNANCY AND LACTATION
Pregnancy: There are no adequate and well-controlled studies in pregnant women.
Lactation: It is not known if selexipag is present in human milk; not for use in nursing.

MECHANISM OF ACTION
Prostacyclin receptor (IP receptor) agonist; selective for the IP receptor versus other prostanoid receptors.

PHARMACOKINETICS
Absorption: T_{max}=1-3 hrs; 3-4 hrs (active metabolite). **Distribution:** Plasma protein binding (approx 99%). **Metabolism:** Enzymatic hydrolysis of the acylsulfonamide by hepatic carboxylesterase 1, to yield the active metabolite. Oxidative metabolism via CYP3A4 and CYP2C8 leads to the formation of hydroxylated and dealkylated products. UGT1A3 and UGT2B7 are involved in the glucuronidation of the active metabolite. **Elimination:** Feces (93%); urine (12%); $T_{1/2}$=0.8-2.5 hrs; 6.2-13.5 hrs (active metabolite).

PATIENT CONSIDERATIONS
Assessment: Assess pregnancy/nursing status, and for possible drug interactions.
Monitoring: Monitor for signs of pulmonary edema and other adverse events.
Counseling: Inform not to split, crush, or chew tablets. Advise patients what to do in case of a missed dose.

URIBEL — hyoscyamine sulfate/methenamine/methylene blue/phenyl salicylate/sodium phosphate monobasic

Class: Acidifier/analgesic/antibacterial/anticholinergic/antiseptic

Rx

ADULT DOSAGE
Urinary Tract Symptoms
For treatment of symptoms of irritative voiding, relief of local symptoms that accompany lower UTIs (eg, inflammation, hypermotility, pain), and relief of urinary tract symptoms caused by diagnostic procedures

Usual: 1 cap PO qid followed by liberal fluid intake

PEDIATRIC DOSAGE
Urinary Tract Symptoms
For treatment of symptoms of irritative voiding, relief of local symptoms that accompany lower UTIs (eg, inflammation, hypermotility, pain), and relief of urinary tract symptoms caused by diagnostic procedures

>6 Years:
Individualize dose

ADMINISTRATION
Oral route

STORAGE
20-25°C (68-77°F). Keep in cool, dry place.

HOW SUPPLIED
Cap: (Methenamine/Sodium Phosphate Monobasic/Phenyl Salicylate/Methylene Blue/Hyoscyamine Sulfate) 118mg/40.8mg/36mg/10mg/0.12mg

CONTRAINDICATIONS
Hypersensitivity to any of the ingredients of Uribel is possible. Consider risk benefits with existing conditions, such as cardiac disease (especially cardiac arrhythmias, congestive heart failure, coronary heart disease, mitral stenosis), GI tract obstructive disease, glaucoma, and myasthenia gravis. Acute urinary retention may be precipitated in obstructive uropathy (eg, bladder neck obstruction due to prostatic hypertrophy).

WARNINGS/PRECAUTIONS
Do not exceed recommended dosage. D/C immediately if rapid pulse, dizziness, or blurred vision occurs. Intolerance may occur in patients intolerant to belladonna alkaloids or salicylates. Delay in gastric emptying could complicate management of gastric ulcers. Infants and young children are especially susceptible to toxic effect of belladonna alkaloids. Caution in elderly; may respond to usual doses of hyoscyamine with excitement, agitation, drowsiness, or confusion. Urine may become blue to blue-green and feces may be discolored due to excretion of methylene blue.

ADVERSE REACTIONS
Rapid pulse, flushing, blurred vision, dizziness, SOB, difficult micturition, acute urinary retention, dry mouth, N/V.

DRUG INTERACTIONS
May decrease absorption of other PO medications (eg, urinary alkalizers, thiazide diuretics, antimuscarinics, antacids/antidiarrheals, antimyasthenics, ketoconazole, MAOIs, opioids, sulfonamides). Concomitant use with antimyasthenics may reduce intestinal motility. Concomitant use with MAOIs may intensify antimuscarinic side effects. Thiazide diuretics may decrease effectiveness of methenamine. Antimuscarinic effects of hyoscyamine may be intensified with antimuscarinics. Antacids/antidiarrheals may reduce absorption of hyoscyamine and antacids may reduce effectiveness of methenamine. Space dosing by 1 hr with antacids/antidiarrheals. Take at least 2 hrs after ketoconazole intake. May increase the risk of severe constipation with opioids. Sulfonamides may precipitate with formaldehyde in the urine, increasing the danger of crystalluria.

PREGNANCY AND LACTATION
Category C, caution in nursing.

MECHANISM OF ACTION
Hyoscyamine: Parasympatholytic; relaxes smooth muscles and produces antispasmodic effect. Methenamine: Degrades in an acidic urine environment, releasing formaldehyde, providing bactericidal or bacteriostatic action. Methylene Blue: Possess weak antiseptic properties. Phenyl Salicylate: Releases salicylate that produces mild analgesia. Sodium Phosphate Monobasic: Acidifier; helps maintain an acid pH in the urine necessary for the degradation of methenamine.

PHARMACOKINETICS
Absorption: (Hyoscyamine, Methenamine, Methylene Blue): Well absorbed. **Distribution:** Plasma protein binding: Moderate (hyoscyamine), some formaldehyde bound to substances in urine and surrounding tissues (methenamine). Methenamine/Hyoscyamine: Crosses placenta; found in breast milk. **Metabolism:** Hyoscyamine: Hepatic. Methenamine: Hydrolysis to formaldehyde. Methylene Blue: Reduced to leukomethylene blue. **Elimination:** Hyoscyamine: Urine (13-50% unchanged). Methenamine: Urine (70-90% unchanged). Methylene Blue: Urine (75% unchanged).

PATIENT CONSIDERATIONS
Assessment: Assess for cardiac disease, GI tract obstructive disease, glaucoma, myasthenia gravis, obstructive uropathy, gastric ulcers, intolerance to belladonna alkaloids or salicylates, hypersensitivity, pregnancy/nursing status, and possible drug interactions.

Monitoring: Monitor for rapid pulse, dizziness, blurring of vision, delayed gastric emptying, and other adverse reactions.

Counseling: Counsel about risks and benefits of therapy. Instruct to d/c use and consult physician if rapid pulse, dizziness, or blurring of vision occurs. Advise to inform physician if taking other medications. Advise to not exceed recommended dose. Inform that urine and feces may be discolored because of methylene blue. Keep out of reach of children.

UROCIT-K — potassium citrate   Rx

Class: Urinary tract alkalinizer

ADULT DOSAGE

Urinary Alkalinization

Management of renal tubular acidosis w/ calcium stones, hypocitraturic calcium oxalate nephrolithiasis, and uric acid lithiasis w/ or w/o calcium stones

Severe Hypocitraturia (Urinary Citrate <150mg/day):
Initial: 30mEq bid or 20mEq tid w/ meals or w/in 30 min pc or after bedtime snack; measure urinary citrate and/or pH every 4 months
Max: 100mEq/day

Mild to Moderate Hypocitraturia (Urinary Citrate >150mg/day):
Initial: 15mEq bid or 10mEq tid w/in 30 min pc or after bedtime snack
Max: 100mEq/day

Use 24-hr urinary citrate and/or urinary pH measurements to determine adequacy of initial dosage and to evaluate effectiveness of any dosage change

PEDIATRIC DOSAGE

Pediatric use may not have been established

ADMINISTRATION

Oral route

Limit salt intake and encourage high fluid intake

HOW SUPPLIED

Tab, ER: 5mEq, 10mEq, 15mEq

CONTRAINDICATIONS

Hyperkalemia or conditions predisposing to hyperkalemia (eg, chronic renal failure, uncontrolled diabetes mellitus, acute dehydration, strenuous physical exercise in unconditioned individuals, adrenal insufficiency, extensive tissue breakdown, or administration of K+-sparing agent [eg, triamterene, spironolactone, amiloride]). Patients in whom there is cause for arrest or delay in tab passage through the GI tract (eg, delayed gastric emptying, esophageal compression, intestinal obstruction or stricture, or those taking anticholinergics). Peptic ulcer disease (PUD), active urinary tract infection (UTI) (with either urea-splitting or other organisms, in association with either calcium or struvite stones), and renal insufficiency (GFR <0.7mL/kg/min).

WARNINGS/PRECAUTIONS

Closely monitor for signs of hyperkalemia with periodic blood tests and ECGs. Upper GI mucosal lesions reported; d/c therapy immediately if severe vomiting, abdominal pain, or GI bleeding occurs, and investigate possibility of bowel perforation or obstruction. Monitor serum electrolytes (Na, K+, chloride, and carbon dioxide), SrCr, and CBCs every 4 months and more frequently in patients with cardiac disease, renal disease, or acidosis; d/c therapy if hyperkalemia, a significant rise in SrCr, or a significant fall in blood Hct/Hgb occurs.

ADVERSE REACTIONS

Abdominal discomfort, N/V, diarrhea, loose bowel movement.

DRUG INTERACTIONS

See Contraindications. Drugs that slow GI transit time may increase GI irritation.

PREGNANCY AND LACTATION

Category C, caution in nursing.

MECHANISM OF ACTION

Urinary tract alkalinizer; produces an alkaline load that increases urinary pH and raises urinary citrate by augmenting citrate clearance without measurably altering ultrafilterable serum citrate. Produces urine that is less conducive to crystallization of stone-forming salts.

PATIENT CONSIDERATIONS

Assessment: Assess for hyperkalemia or conditions predisposing to hyperkalemia, presence of cause for arrest or delay in tab passage through GI tract, PUD, active UTI, renal insufficiency (GFR <0.7mL/kg/min), pregnancy/nursing status, and possible drug interactions.

Monitoring: Monitor for signs of hyperkalemia and upper GI mucosal lesions. Monitor ECGs periodically, and serum electrolytes (Na, K+, chloride, and carbon dioxide), SrCr, and CBCs every 4 months or more frequently in patients with cardiac disease, renal disease, or acidosis. Measure urinary citrate and/or pH every 4 months in patients with severe hypocitraturia.

Counseling: Instruct to take drug only ud, especially with concomitant diuretics and digitalis preparations. Instruct not to crush, chew, or suck the tab. Instruct to notify physician if there is trouble swallowing tabs or if tab seems to stick in the throat, and if tarry stools or other evidence of GI bleeding is noticed. Inform that regular blood tests and ECGs will be performed to ensure safety.

UROXATRAL — alfuzosin hydrochloride   Rx

Class: Alpha₁ antagonist

ADULT DOSAGE

Benign Prostatic Hyperplasia

10mg qd

PEDIATRIC DOSAGE

Pediatric use may not have been established

ADMINISTRATION

Oral route

Take w/ food and w/ the same meal each day.
Do not chew or crush tab.

STORAGE

25°C (77°F); excursions permitted to 15-30°C (59-86°F). Protect from light and moisture.

HOW SUPPLIED

Tab, Extended-Release: 10mg

CONTRAINDICATIONS

Moderate or severe hepatic impairment (Child-Pugh categories B and C), concomitant use of potent CYP3A4 inhibitors (eg, ketoconazole, itraconazole, ritonavir), known hypersensitivity (eg, urticaria, angioedema) to alfuzosin HCl or any component of Uroxatral.

WARNINGS/PRECAUTIONS

Postural hypotension w/ or w/o symptoms (eg, dizziness) may develop w/in a few hrs following administration; caution w/ symptomatic hypotension or in those who have had a hypotensive response to other medications. Syncope may occur; caution to avoid situations in which injury could result should syncope occur. Caution w/ severe renal impairment (CrCl <30mL/min) or mild hepatic impairment. Prostate carcinoma and BPH frequently coexist; patients thought to have BPH should be examined to rule out prostate carcinoma prior to starting treatment. Intraoperative floppy iris syndrome (IFIS) observed in some patients during cataract surgery; may require modifications to surgical technique. Has been rarely associated w/ priapism. D/C if symptoms of angina pectoris appear or worsen. Caution w/ acquired or congenital QT prolongation.

ADVERSE REACTIONS

Dizziness, URTI, headache, fatigue.

DRUG INTERACTIONS

See Contraindications. Avoid use w/ other α-adrenergic antagonists. Risk of hypotension/postural hypotension and syncope may be increased w/ concomitant antihypertensives and nitrates. Caution w/ PDE-5 inhibitors; may potentially cause symptomatic hypotension. Caution w/ medications that prolong the QT interval.

PREGNANCY AND LACTATION

Pregnancy: Category B; not for use in women.

MECHANISM OF ACTION

α₁-antagonist; selectively inhibits α₁-adrenergic receptors in lower urinary tract causing smooth muscle in bladder neck and prostate to relax, resulting in an improvement in urine flow and a reduction in symptoms of BPH.

PHARMACOKINETICS

Absorption: (Fed) Absolute bioavailability (49%), C_{max}=13.6ng/mL, T_{max}=8 hrs, AUC_{0-24}=194ng•hr/mL. **Distribution:** V_d=3.2L/kg (IV); plasma protein binding (82-90%). **Metabolism:** Liver (extensive) via CYP3A4; oxidation, O-demethylation, N-dealkylation. **Elimination:** Feces (69%), urine (24%, 11% unchanged); $T_{1/2}$=10 hrs.

PATIENT CONSIDERATIONS

Assessment: Assess for hypersensitivity to drug, symptomatic hypotension, history of QT prolongation, hepatic/renal impairment, and possible drug interactions. Assess if patient is planning to undergo cataract surgery. Rule out the presence of prostate carcinoma prior to therapy.

Monitoring: Monitor for postural hypotension, syncope, hypersensitivity reactions, IFIS, QT prolongation, and other adverse reactions.

Counseling: Inform about possible occurrence of symptoms related to postural hypotension when beginning therapy; caution about driving, operating machinery, or performing hazardous tasks during this period. Instruct to inform ophthalmologist about use of the product before cataract surgery or other procedures involving the eyes, even if patient is no longer taking the medication. Advise about the possibility of priapism resulting from treatment and instruct to seek immediate medical attention if it occurs.

URSO 250 — ursodiol   Rx

Class: Bile acid

OTHER BRAND NAMES

Urso Forte

ADULT DOSAGE

Primary Biliary Cirrhosis

Usual: 13-15mg/kg/day given bid-qid

PEDIATRIC DOSAGE

Pediatric use may not have been established

ADMINISTRATION

Oral route

Take w/ food.

Urso Forte

Scored tab may be broken in halves; do not use segments broken incorrectly.
Take unchewed w/ water.

STORAGE
20-25°C (68-77°F). (Urso Forte) Half-tab: 20-25°C (68-77°F) in the current packaging for up to 28 days. Store separately from whole tabs.

HOW SUPPLIED
Tab: (Urso 250) 250mg, (Urso Forte) 500mg* *scored

CONTRAINDICATIONS
Complete biliary obstruction, known hypersensitivity or intolerance to ursodiol or any components of the formulation.

WARNINGS/PRECAUTIONS
Administer appropriate specific treatment in patients with variceal bleeding, hepatic encephalopathy, ascites, or in need of an urgent liver transplant. Monitor LFTs (gamma-glutamyl transpeptidase [GGT], alkaline phosphatase, AST, ALT) and bilirubin levels monthly for 3 months after start of therapy, and every 6 months thereafter; consider treatment discontinuation if the parameters increase to a level considered clinically significant in patients with stable historical LFT levels. Use with caution to maintain bile flow.

ADVERSE REACTIONS
Leukopenia, skin rash, peptic ulcer, blood glucose elevation, SrCr elevation, thrombocytopenia, diarrhea, abdominal pain, asthenia, nausea, dyspepsia, anorexia, esophagitis.

DRUG INTERACTIONS
Bile acid sequestering agents (eg, cholestyramine, colestipol) and aluminum-based antacids may interfere with the action of the drug by reducing its absorption. Estrogens, oral contraceptives, and clofibrate (and perhaps other lipid-lowering drugs) may counteract effectiveness.

PREGNANCY AND LACTATION
Pregnancy: Category B.
Lactation: Caution in nursing.

MECHANISM OF ACTION
Bile acid; replaces and displaces toxic concentrations of endogenous hydrophobic bile acids. In addition, produces cytoprotection of the injured bile duct epithelial cells (cholangiocytes) against toxic effects of bile acids, inhibition of apoptosis of hepatocytes, immunomodulatory effects, and stimulation of bile secretion by hepatocytes and cholangiocytes.

PHARMACOKINETICS
Absorption: Passive diffusion, incomplete. **Distribution:** Plasma protein binding (≥70%) (unconjugated). **Metabolism:** Liver via conjugation. **Elimination:** Feces (primary), urine (<1%).

PATIENT CONSIDERATIONS
Assessment: Assess for biliary obstruction, variceal bleeding, hepatic encephalopathy, ascites, need for an urgent liver transplant, hypersensitivity, intolerance, pregnancy/nursing status, and possible drug interactions.

Monitoring: Monitor for the development of adverse reactions. Monitor LFTs (GGT, alkaline phosphatase, AST, ALT) and bilirubin levels monthly for 3 months after start of therapy, and every 6 months thereafter.

Counseling: Inform that adsorption may be reduced if taking concomitant bile acid sequestering agents, aluminum-based antacids, or drugs known to alter the metabolism of cholesterol.

UTA — hyoscyamine sulfate/methenamine/methylene blue/ sodium phosphate monobasic   Rx

Class: Acidifier/antibacterial/anticholinergic/antiseptic

ADULT DOSAGE	PEDIATRIC DOSAGE
Urinary Tract Symptoms	**Urinary Tract Symptoms**
For the treatment of symptoms of irritative voiding, relief of local symptoms that accompany lower UTIs (eg, inflammation, hypermotility, pain), and relief of urinary tract symptoms caused by diagnostic procedures	For the treatment of symptoms of irritative voiding, relief of local symptoms that accompany lower UTIs (eg, inflammation, hypermotility, pain), and relief of urinary tract symptoms caused by diagnostic procedures
Usual: 1 cap qid followed by liberal fluid intake	**>6 Years:** Individualize dose

---

ADMINISTRATION
Oral route

STORAGE
15-30°C (59-86°F). Keep container tightly closed.

HOW SUPPLIED
Cap: (Hyoscyamine/Methenamine/Methylene Blue/Sodium Phosphate Monobasic) 0.12mg/120mg/10mg/40.8mg

CONTRAINDICATIONS
Hypersensitivity to any of the ingredients in this product. Consider risk-benefit with existing conditions such as cardiac disease (especially cardiac arrhythmias, congestive heart failure, coronary heart disease, mitral stenosis), GI tract obstructive disease, glaucoma, and myasthenia gravis. Acute urinary retention may be precipitated in obstructive uropathy (eg, bladder neck obstruction due to prostatic hypertrophy).

WARNINGS/PRECAUTIONS
Do not exceed recommended dosage. D/C immediately if rapid pulse, dizziness, or blurred vision occurs. Intolerance may occur in patients intolerant to

belladonna alkaloids. Delay in gastric emptying could complicate management of gastric ulcers. Infants and young children are especially susceptible to toxic effect of belladonna alkaloids. Caution in elderly; may respond to usual doses of hyoscyamine with excitement, agitation, drowsiness, or confusion. Urine may become blue to blue-green and feces may be discolored due to excretion of methylene blue.

ADVERSE REACTIONS
Rapid pulse, flushing, blurred vision, dizziness, SOB or trouble breathing, difficult micturition, acute urinary retention, dry mouth, N/V.

DRUG INTERACTIONS
May decrease absorption of other oral medications (eg, urinary alkalizers, thiazide diuretics, antimuscarinics, antacids/antidiarrheals, antimyasthenics, ketoconazole, MAOIs, opioids, sulfonamides). Concomitant use with antimyasthenics may reduce intestinal motility. Concomitant use with MAOIs may intensify antimuscarinic side effects. Thiazide diuretics may decrease effectiveness of methenamine. Antimuscarinic effects of hyoscyamine may be intensified with antimuscarinics. Antacids/antidiarrheals may reduce absorption of hyoscyamine and antacids may reduce effectiveness of methenamine. Space dosing by 1 hr with antacids/antidiarrheals. Take at least 2 hrs after ketoconazole intake. May increase the risk of severe constipation with opioids. Sulfonamides may precipitate with formaldehyde in the urine, increasing the danger of crystalluria.

PREGNANCY AND LACTATION
Category C, caution in nursing.

MECHANISM OF ACTION
Hyoscyamine: Parasympatholytic; relaxes smooth muscles and produces antispasmodic effect. Methenamine: Degrades in acidic urine environment releasing formaldehyde which provides bactericidal or bacteriostatic action. Methylene Blue: Possess weak antiseptic properties. Sodium Phosphate Monobasic: Acidifier; helps to maintain an acid pH in the urine necessary for the degradation of methenamine.

PHARMACOKINETICS
Absorption: Hyoscyamine, Methenamine, Methylene Blue: Well absorbed. **Distribution:** Hyoscyamine: Plasma Protein Binding (moderate), Methenamine: Plasma Protein Binding (some formaldehyde bound to substances in urine and surrounding tissues). Methenamine/Hyoscyamine: Found in breast milk; crosses placenta. **Metabolism:** Hyoscyamine: Hepatic. Methenamine: Hydrolysis to formaldehyde. Methylene Blue: Reduced to leukomethylene blue. **Elimination:** Hyoscyamine: Urine (13-50% unchanged). Methenamine: Urine (70-90% unchanged). Methylene Blue: Urine (75% unchanged).

PATIENT CONSIDERATIONS
Assessment: Assess for cardiac disease, GI tract obstructive disease, glaucoma, myasthenia gravis, obstructive uropathy, gastric ulcers, intolerance to belladonna alkaloids, hypersensitivity to any of the ingredients, pregnancy/nursing status, and possible drug interactions.

Monitoring: Monitor for rapid pulse, dizziness, blurring of vision, delayed gastric emptying, and other adverse reactions.

Counseling: Counsel about risks and benefits of therapy. Instruct to d/c use and consult physician if rapid pulse, dizziness, or blurring of vision occurs. Advise to not exceed recommended dose. Advise to inform physician if taking other medications. Inform that urine and feces may be discolored because of methylene blue. Instruct to keep out of reach of children.

UTIBRON NEOHALER — glycopyrrolate/indacaterol   Rx

Class: Anticholinergic/long-acting beta₂ agonist (LABA)

> Long-acting β_2-adrenergic agonists (LABAs) increase the risk of asthma-related death. Not indicated for the treatment of asthma.

ADULT DOSAGE	PEDIATRIC DOSAGE
Chronic Obstructive Pulmonary Disease	Pediatric use may not have been established
Long-Term Maint Treatment of Airflow Obstruction:	
Recommended: Orally inhale the contents of 1 cap bid using the Neohaler device	
Max: 1 cap bid	

ADMINISTRATION
Oral inh route

Use only w/ Neohaler device.
Do not swallow caps.
Administer at the same time every day.
Store caps in the blister; only remove immediately before use.

STORAGE
77°F (25°C); excursions permitted to 59-86°F (15-30°C). Store caps in the blister protected from light and moisture; remove caps from the blister immediately before use. Do not use the Neohaler device w/ any other caps. Always use the new Neohaler inhaler provided w/ each new prescription.

HOW SUPPLIED
Cap, Inh: (Indacaterol/Glycopyrrolate) 27.5mcg/15.6mcg

CONTRAINDICATIONS

Hypersensitivity to indacaterol, glycopyrrolate, or to any of the ingredients. **Indacaterol:** Asthma w/o use of a long-term asthma control medication. Not indicated for treatment of asthma.

WARNINGS/PRECAUTIONS

Do not initiate in acutely deteriorating or potentially life-threatening episodes of COPD or use for the relief of acute symptoms. D/C regular use of oral or inhaled short-acting β₂-agonists (SABAs) when beginning treatment. May produce paradoxical bronchospasm; treat immediately w/ an inhaled, short acting bronchodilator and immediately d/c Utibron Neohaler and institute alternative therapy. Immediate hypersensitivity reactions have been reported; d/c immediately and institute alternative therapy if signs suggesting an allergic reaction occur. Caution in patients w/ severe hypersensitivity to milk proteins. Caution w/ narrow-angle glaucoma and urinary retention. **Indacaterol:** Do not use more often or at higher doses than recommended; clinically significant cardiovascular (CV) effects and fatalities reported w/ excessive use. CV effects may occur; may need to d/c if such effects occur. Caution w/ CV disorders, convulsive disorders, thyrotoxicosis, diabetes mellitus (DM), ketoacidosis, and in patients who are unusually responsive to sympathomimetic amines. May produce significant hypokalemia and increases in plasma glucose.

ADVERSE REACTIONS

Nasopharyngitis, HTN.

DRUG INTERACTIONS

Indacaterol: Do not use w/ other medicines containing LABAs. Adrenergic drugs may potentiate sympathetic effects; use w/ caution. Xanthine derivatives, steroids, or diuretics may potentiate any hypokalemic effect. Caution w/ non-K⁺-sparing diuretics (eg, loop or thiazide diuretics). Extreme caution w/ MAOIs, TCAs, or other drugs known to prolong the QTc interval; action on CV system may be potentiated. Drugs known to prolong the QTc interval may be associated w/ an increased risk of ventricular arrhythmias. β-blockers and indacaterol may interfere w/ the effect of each other when administered concurrently. β-blockers may block therapeutic effects and produce severe bronchospasm in COPD patients; avoid treatment w/ β-blockers. If such therapy is needed, consider cardioselective β-blockers and use w/ caution. **Glycopyrrolate:** Avoid w/ other anticholinergic-containing drugs; may lead to an increase in anticholinergic adverse effects.

PREGNANCY AND LACTATION

Pregnancy: Category C.
Lactation: Not for use in nursing.

MECHANISM OF ACTION

Glycopyrrolate: Anticholinergic; exhibits effects through inhibition of M₃-receptors at the smooth muscle, leading to bronchodilation. **Indacaterol:** LABA; attributable to stimulation of intracellular adenyl cyclase, the enzyme that catalyzes the conversion of ATP to cAMP. Increased cAMP levels cause relaxation of bronchial smooth muscle and inhibition of release of mediators of immediate hypersensitivity from cells, especially from mast cells.

PHARMACOKINETICS

Absorption: Indacaterol: Absolute bioavailability (43-45%); T_{max}=15 min (median).Glycopyrrolate: T_{max}=5 min (median). **Distribution:** Indacaterol: (IV) V_d=2361-2557L; plasma protein binding (95.1-96.2%). Glycopyrrolate: (IV) V_d=83L (steady state); 376L (terminal phase); plasma protein binding (38-41%). **Metabolism:** Indacaterol: Via UGT1A1 to the phenolic O-glucuronide; hydroxylation via CYP3A4. Glycopyrrolate: Hydroxylation and direct hydrolysis, multiple CYP isoenzymes; M9 (carboxylic acid derivative). **Elimination:** Indacaterol: Urine (<2% unchanged), feces (54% unchanged, 23% hydroxylated indacaterol metabolites); $T_{1/2}$= 45.5-126 hrs. Glycopyrrolate: Urine (60-70%); biliary; $T_{1/2}$=33-53 hrs.

PATIENT CONSIDERATIONS

Assessment: Assess for hypersensitivity to indacaterol, glycopyrrolate, milk proteins, or any component of the product. Assess for asthma, acutely deteriorating COPD, CV disorders, convulsive disorders, thyrotoxicosis, DM, ketoacidosis, narrow-angle glaucoma, urinary retention, pregnancy/nursing status, and possible drug interactions. Evaluate use in patients unusually responsive to sympathomimetic amines.

Monitoring: Monitor for deteriorating disease, paradoxical bronchospasm, hypersensitivity reactions, CV effects, worsening of narrow-angle glaucoma, worsening of urinary retention, hypokalemia, hyperglycemia, and other adverse reactions.

Counseling: Inform that drug is not for treatment of asthma or for relief of acute symptoms of COPD. Advise that acute symptoms should be treated w/ a rescue inhaler (eg, albuterol). Instruct to seek medical attention immediately if experiencing worsening of symptoms or a need for more inhalations than usual of the rescue inhaler. Advise not to d/c therapy w/o physician guidance and not to use an additional LABA. Instruct to d/c therapy if paradoxical bronchospasm occurs. Inform about adverse effects (eg, palpitations, chest pain, rapid HR, tremor, nervousness) and other risks (eg, worsening of narrow-angle glaucoma, worsening of urinary retention) associated w/ therapy; instruct to consult physician immediately if any signs/symptoms develop. Instruct on how to correctly administer caps using the Neohaler device. Inform that the contents of the caps are for oral inhalation only and must not be swallowed. Advise to contact physician if pregnancy occurs while on therapy.

Uvadex — methoxsalen   Rx
Class: Psoralen

> Should be used only by physicians who have special competence in the diagnosis/treatment of cutaneous T-cell lymphoma and who have special training and experience in the UVAR XTS or THERAKOS CELLEX Photopheresis System.

ADULT DOSAGE	PEDIATRIC DOSAGE
Cutaneous T-Cell Lymphoma	Pediatric use may not have been established

Cutaneous T-Cell Lymphoma

Palliative Treatment of Skin Manifestations of Cutaneous T-Cell Lymphoma Unresponsive to Other Forms of Treatment:

Dosage Per Treatment Calculated According to Treatment Volume:
Treatment volume x 0.017 = mL of methoxsalen for each treatment
Inject prescribed amount into recirculation bag prior to photoactivation phase

Normal Treatment Schedule:
Give on 2 consecutive days every 4 weeks for a minimum of 7 treatment cycles (6 months)

Accelerated Treatment Schedule:
May increase frequency of treatment to 2 consecutive treatments every 2 weeks if the assessment during the 4th treatment cycle (approx 3 months) reveals an increased skin score from the baseline score

If 25% improvement in the skin score is attained after 4 consecutive weeks, may resume the regular treatment schedule

Patients maintained in the accelerated treatment schedule may receive a max of 20 cycles

---

ADMINISTRATION

Extracorporeal route

Do not dilute
Contents of vial should be injected into THERAKOS UVAR XTS or THERAKOS CELLEX photopheresis system immediately after being drawn up into syringe; do not inject directly into patients
Once drawn into plastic syringe, immediately inject into photoactivation bag; discard methoxsalen exposed to plastic syringe for >1 hr
Vials are single use only; discard any unused portion
Can adsorb onto PVC and plastics; only THERAKOS UVAR XTS or THERAKOS CELLEX photopheresis procedural kits supplied for use w/ the instrument should be used to administer this product

STORAGE
15-30°C (59-86°F).

HOW SUPPLIED
Inj: 20mcg/mL [10mL]

CONTRAINDICATIONS
Idiosyncratic or hypersensitivity reactions to methoxsalen, other psoralen compounds or any of the excipients; patients w/ aphakia; contraindications to the photopheresis procedure; or history of light sensitive disease (eg, lupus erythematosus, porphyria cutanea tarda, erythropoietic protoporphyria, variegate porphyria, xeroderma pigmentosum, albinism).

WARNINGS/PRECAUTIONS
Cutaneous squamous cell cancers reported with oral methoxsalen administration. May cause fetal harm. Sunlight/UV radiation exposure after administration may cause premature skin aging. May increase risk of skin cancers; closely monitor patients who exhibit multiple basal cell carcinomas or who have a history of basal cell carcinoma. Serious burns from either UVA/sunlight (even through window glass) can result if recommended dose is exceeded or precautions are not followed. Avoid all exposure to sunlight during the 24 hrs after treatment. Patients should wear UVA-absorbing, wrap-around sunglasses for 24 hrs after treatment to avoid cataractogenicity.

ADVERSE REACTIONS
Hypotension, cardiovascular effects, infections.

DRUG INTERACTIONS
Increased risk for photosensitivity reactions with known photosensitizing agents (eg, anthralin, coal tar and its derivatives, griseofulvin, phenothiazines, nalidixic acid, halogenated salicylanilides [bacteriostatic soaps], sulfonamides, tetracyclines, thiazides, and certain organic staining dyes [eg, methylene blue, toluidine blue, rose bengal, methyl orange]).

PREGNANCY AND LACTATION
Category D, caution in nursing.

MECHANISM OF ACTION
Psoralen; has not been established. Upon photoactivation, conjugates and forms covalent bonds with DNA, which leads to the formation of both monofunctional and bifunctional adducts. May also react with proteins. The formation of

photoadducts results in inhibition of DNA synthesis, cell division, and epidermal turnover.

PHARMACOKINETICS

Metabolism: Rapid. **Elimination:** Urine (95% metabolites).

PATIENT CONSIDERATIONS

Assessment: Assess for idiosyncratic/hypersensitivity reaction, any conditions where treatment is contraindicated or cautioned, pregnancy/nursing status, and possible drug interactions.

Monitoring: Monitor for signs/symptoms of skin burning, skin cancer (eg, cutaneous squamous cell cancers), cataracts, and premature aging of skin. Monitor closely those patients who exhibit multiple basal cell carcinomas or who have a history of basal cell carcinomas.

Counseling: Instruct emphatically to wear UVA-absorbing, wrap-around sunglasses, and cover exposed skin or use a sunblock (SP 15 or higher) for the 24-hr period following treatment, whether exposed to direct or indirect sunlight in the open or through a window glass. Advise women of childbearing potential to avoid becoming pregnant during therapy.

VAGIFEM — estradiol   Rx

Class: Estrogen

Increased risk of endometrial cancer in a woman w/ a uterus who uses unopposed estrogens. Adding a progestin to estrogen therapy reduces the risk of endometrial hyperplasia. Adequate diagnostic measures (eg, directed or random endometrial sampling) should be undertaken to rule out malignancy in postmenopausal women w/ undiagnosed, persistent or recurring abnormal genital bleeding. Should not be used for the prevention of cardiovascular (CV) disease or dementia. Increased risk of stroke and deep vein thrombosis (DVT) reported in postmenopausal women (50-79 yrs of age) treated w/ daily oral conjugated estrogens (CE) alone and when combined w/ medroxyprogesterone acetate (MPA). Increased risk of developing probable dementia reported in postmenopausal women ≥65 yrs of age treated w/ daily CE alone and when combined w/ MPA. Increased risks of pulmonary embolism (PE), MI, and invasive breast cancer reported in postmenopausal women (50-79 yrs of age) treated w/ daily oral CE combined w/ MPA. Should be prescribed at the lowest effective dose and for the shortest duration consistent w/ treatment goals and risks.

ADULT DOSAGE	PEDIATRIC DOSAGE
Atrophic Vaginitis	Pediatric use may not have been established
Due to Menopause:	
1 tab intravaginally qd for 2 weeks, followed by 1 tab intravaginally twice weekly	

ADMINISTRATION

Intravaginal route

Use supplied applicator to administer dose.
It is advisable to use the same time daily for all applications.

STORAGE

25°C (77°F); excursions permitted to 15-30°C (59-86°F). Do not refrigerate.

HOW SUPPLIED

Tab, Vaginal: 10mcg

CONTRAINDICATIONS

Undiagnosed abnormal genital bleeding, known/suspected/history of breast cancer, known/suspected estrogen-dependent neoplasia, active or history of DVT/PE/arterial thromboembolic disease (eg, stroke, MI), known anaphylactic reaction or angioedema to the medication, known liver impairment/disease, known protein C/protein S/antithrombin deficiency or other known thrombophilic disorders, known/suspected pregnancy.

WARNINGS/PRECAUTIONS

D/C immediately if stroke, DVT, PE, or MI occurs or is suspected. If feasible, d/c at least 4-6 weeks before surgery of the type associated w/ increased risk of thromboembolism, or during periods of prolonged immobilization. May increase risk of gallbladder disease requiring surgery, and ovarian cancer. May lead to severe hypercalcemia in women w/ breast cancer and bone metastases; d/c and take appropriate measures if hypercalcemia occurs. Retinal vascular thrombosis reported; if visual abnormalities or migraine occurs, d/c therapy pending examination. If examination reveals papilledema or retinal vascular lesions, d/c permanently. May elevate BP and thyroid-binding globulin levels. May be associated w/ elevations of plasma TGs, leading to pancreatitis in patients w/ preexisting hypertriglyceridemia; consider discontinuation if pancreatitis occurs. Caution w/ history of cholestatic jaundice associated w/ past estrogen use or w/ pregnancy; d/c in case of recurrence. May cause fluid retention; caution w/ cardiac/renal dysfunction. Caution w/ hypoparathyroidism; hypocalcemia may occur. Cases of malignant transformation of residual endometrial implants reported in women treated post-hysterectomy w/ estrogen-alone therapy; consider addition of progestin for these patients. May exacerbate symptoms of angioedema in women w/ hereditary angioedema. May exacerbate asthma, diabetes mellitus, epilepsy, migraine, porphyria, systemic lupus erythematosus, and hepatic hemangiomas; use w/ caution. Local abrasion induced by applicator reported, especially in women w/ severely atrophic vaginal mucosa. May affect certain endocrine and blood components in lab tests.

ADVERSE REACTIONS

Vulvovaginal mycotic infection, vulvovaginal pruritus, back pain, diarrhea.

DRUG INTERACTIONS

CYP3A4 inducers (eg, St. John's wort, phenobarbital, carbamazepine, rifampin) may decrease levels, which may decrease therapeutic effects and/or change uterine bleeding profile. CYP3A4 inhibitors (eg, erythromycin, ketoconazole, ritonavir, grapefruit juice) may increase levels, which may result in side effects. Concomitant thyroid hormone replacement therapy may require increased doses of thyroid replacement therapy.

PREGNANCY AND LACTATION

Pregnancy: Contraindicated in pregnancy.
Lactation: Not for use in nursing.

MECHANISM OF ACTION

Estrogen; binds to nuclear receptors in estrogen-responsive tissues. Circulating estrogens modulate the pituitary secretion of the gonadotropins, luteinizing hormone and follicle-stimulating hormone, through a negative feedback mechanism. Reduces elevated levels of these hormones in postmenopausal women.

PHARMACOKINETICS

Absorption: Well-absorbed. Administration of multiple doses resulted in different parameters. **Distribution:** Largely bound to sex hormone-binding globulin and albumin; found in breast milk. **Metabolism:** Liver, to estrone (metabolite) and estriol (major urinary metabolite); enterohepatic circulation via sulfate and glucuronide conjugation in the liver; biliary secretion of conjugates into the intestine; hydrolysis in the gut; reabsorption. **Elimination:** Urine (parent compound and metabolites).

PATIENT CONSIDERATIONS

Assessment: Assess for abnormal vaginal bleeding, presence/history of breast cancer, estrogen-dependent neoplasia, active or history of DVT/PE/arterial thromboembolic disease, liver impairment/disease, thrombophilic disorders, known anaphylactic reaction or angioedema to the drug, pregnancy/nursing status, other conditions where treatment is cautioned, need for progestin therapy, and possible drug interactions.

Monitoring: Monitor for signs/symptoms of CV disorders, malignant neoplasms, dementia, gallbladder disease, hypercalcemia, visual abnormalities, BP and plasma TG elevations, pancreatitis, cholestatic jaundice, hypothyroidism, fluid retention, and for other adverse events. Perform annual breast exam; schedule mammography based on age, risk factors, and prior mammogram results. Monitor thyroid function in patients on thyroid hormone replacement therapy. Perform adequate diagnostic measures (eg, endometrial sampling) in patients w/ undiagnosed persistent or recurring genital bleeding. Perform periodic evaluation to determine treatment need.

Counseling: Inform postmenopausal women of the importance of reporting vaginal bleeding to physician as soon as possible. Inform of possible adverse reactions of therapy (eg, CV disorders, malignant neoplasms, probable dementia). Advise to have yearly breast exams by a physician and perform monthly breast self-exams. Inform of possible less serious but common adverse reactions of therapy (eg, headache, breast pain and tenderness, nausea, vomiting). Instruct on how to use the applicator.

VALCHLOR — mechlorethamine   Rx

Class: Nitrogen mustard alkylating agent

ADULT DOSAGE	PEDIATRIC DOSAGE
Cutaneous T-Cell Lymphoma	Pediatric use may not have been established
Stage IA and IB Mycosis Fungoides-Type Cutaneous T-Cell Lymphoma in Patients Who Have Received Prior Skin-Directed Therapy:	
Apply a thin film qd to affected areas of the skin	

DOSING CONSIDERATIONS

Adverse Reactions

Skin Ulceration, Blistering, or Moderately-Severe or Severe Dermatitis (Marked Skin Redness with Edema):

D/C for any grade; upon improvement, restart at a reduced frequency of once every 3 days.
If reintroduction is tolerated for at least 1 week, increase frequency of application to qod for at least 1 week and then to qd application if tolerated.

ADMINISTRATION

Topical route

Caregivers must wear disposable nitrile gloves when applying gel to patients and wash hands thoroughly with soap and water after removal of gloves.
If there is accidental skin exposure to gel, caregivers must immediately wash exposed areas thoroughly with soap and water for at least 15 minutes and remove contaminated clothing.
Do not use occlusive dressings on areas of the skin where product was applied.

STORAGE

Prior to Dispensing: -25 to -15°C (-13-5°F). **Once Dispensed:** 2-8°C (36-46°F). Keep in its original box and avoid contact with food when storing in refrigerator. Discard unused product after 60 days.

HOW SUPPLIED

Gel: 0.016% [60g]

CONTRAINDICATIONS

Known severe hypersensitivity to mechlorethamine.

WARNINGS/PRECAUTIONS

Exposure to eyes causes pain, burns, inflammation, photophobia, and blurred vision; blindness and severe irreversible anterior eye injury may occur. If eye exposure occurs, immediately irrigate for at least 15 min with copious amounts of water, normal saline, or a balanced salt ophthalmic irrigating solution and obtain immediate medical (eg, ophthalmologic) consultation. Exposure of mucous membranes (eg, oral mucosa, nasal mucosa) causes pain, redness, and ulceration, which may be severe; should mucosal contact occur, immediately irrigate for at least 15 min with copious amounts of water, followed by immediate medical consultation. Avoid direct skin contact with product in individuals other than the patient; risks of secondary exposure include dermatitis, mucosal injury, and secondary cancers. Dermatitis reported; monitor for redness, swelling, inflammation, itchiness, blisters, ulceration, and secondary skin infections. Non-melanoma skin cancer reported; monitor for non-melanoma skin cancers during and after treatment. May cause fetal harm. Flammable; avoid fire, flame, and smoking until medication has dried.

ADVERSE REACTIONS
Dermatitis, pruritus, bacterial skin infection, skin ulceration/blistering, skin hyperpigmentation.

PREGNANCY AND LACTATION
Pregnancy: Category D.
Lactation: Not for use in nursing.

MECHANISM OF ACTION
Nitrogen mustard alkylating agent; inhibits rapidly proliferating cells.

PATIENT CONSIDERATIONS
Assessment: Assess for drug hypersensitivity, and pregnancy/nursing status.

Monitoring: Monitor for dermatitis (redness, swelling, inflammation, itchiness, blisters, ulceration, secondary skin infections), non-melanoma skin cancers (during and after treatment), and other adverse reactions. Monitor if eye exposure or mucosal contact occurs.

Counseling: Instruct to wash hands thoroughly with soap and water after handling or applying the product. Instruct caregivers to wear disposable nitrile gloves when applying the product to patients and to wash hands thoroughly with soap and water after removal of gloves; advise that if there is accidental skin exposure to the product, to immediately wash exposed areas thoroughly with soap and water for at least 15 min and remove contaminated clothing. Instruct not to use occlusive (air or water-tight) dressings on areas of the skin where product was applied. Advise to discard unused product, empty tubes, and used application gloves in household trash in a manner that prevents accidental application or ingestion by others, including children and pets. Advise that adherence to the recommended storage condition will ensure the product will work as expected; instruct to consult a pharmacist prior to using product that has been left at room temperature for >1 hr/day. Counsel on what to do in case of eye exposure or mucosal contact. Instruct to consult with physician if skin irritation occurs after applying the product. Instruct to notify physician of any new skin lesions and to undergo periodic assessment for signs and symptoms of skin cancer. Advise of the potential hazard to a fetus and to avoid pregnancy while using the product. Advise women to d/c nursing due to the potential for topical or systemic exposure to product. Instruct to avoid fire, flame, and smoking until medication has dried.

Valium — diazepam   CIV

Class: Benzodiazepine

ADULT DOSAGE	PEDIATRIC DOSAGE
Anxiety Disorders	**General Dosing**
Management of Disorders or for Short-Term Relief of Symptoms: 2-10mg bid-qid	**≥6 Months of Age:** **Initial:** 1-2.5mg tid or qid **Titrate:** Increase gradually prn and as tolerated
Alcohol Withdrawal	
Symptomatic Relief of Acute Withdrawal: 10mg tid or qid for first 24 hrs, then reduce to 5mg tid or qid prn	
Muscle Spasms	
Adjunctive Therapy: 2-10mg tid or qid	
Convulsive Disorders	
Adjunctive Therapy: 2-10mg bid-qid	

DOSING CONSIDERATIONS
Elderly
Elderly/Debilitated:
Initial: 2-2.5mg qd or bid
Titrate: Increase gradually prn and as tolerated

ADMINISTRATION
Oral route

STORAGE
15-30°C (59-86°F).

HOW SUPPLIED
Tab: 2mg*, 5mg*, 10mg* *scored

CONTRAINDICATIONS
Known hypersensitivity to diazepam, pediatric patients <6 months of age, myasthenia gravis, severe respiratory insufficiency, severe hepatic insufficiency, sleep apnea syndrome, acute narrow-angle glaucoma.

WARNINGS/PRECAUTIONS
May be used with treated open-angle glaucoma. Periodically reassess usefulness of drug. Not recommended for the treatment of psychotic patients. May increase frequency and/or severity of grand mal seizures and may require an increase in the dose of standard anticonvulsant medication. Abrupt withdrawal may also temporarily increase frequency and/or severity of seizures. May increase risk of congenital malformations and other developmental abnormalities. Caution during labor and delivery. Caution in the severely depressed or with evidence of latent depression or anxiety associated with depression, or suicidal tendencies; protective measures may be necessary. Psychiatric and paradoxical reactions may occur and are more likely in children and the elderly; d/c if these occur. Lower dose is recommended with chronic respiratory insufficiency. Extreme caution with history of alcohol or drug abuse. In debilitated patients, limit dose to smallest effective amount to preclude ataxia or oversedation development. Repeated use for a prolonged time may result in some loss of response to effects. Isolated reports of neutropenia and jaundice reported. Abuse and dependence reported.

ADVERSE REACTIONS
Drowsiness, fatigue, muscle weakness, ataxia.

DRUG INTERACTIONS
Mutually potentiates effects with central acting agents (eg, antipsychotics, anxiolytics/sedatives, MAOIs). Alcohol enhances sedative effects; avoid concomitant use. Slower rate of absorption with antacids. Concomitant use with compounds which inhibit certain hepatic enzymes such as CYP3A and CYP2C19 (eg, cimetidine, ketoconazole, fluvoxamine) may increase and prolong sedation. Decreased metabolic elimination of phenytoin reported.

PREGNANCY AND LACTATION
Category D, not for use in nursing.

MECHANISM OF ACTION
Benzodiazepine; exerts anxiolytic, sedative, muscle-relaxant, anticonvulsant, and amnestic effects. Thought to facilitate action of gamma aminobutyric acid, an inhibitory neurotransmitter in the CNS.

PHARMACOKINETICS
Absorption: T_{max}=1-1.5 hrs. **Distribution:** V_d=0.8-1.0L/kg; plasma protein binding (98%); crosses placenta, found in breast milk. **Metabolism:** N-demethylation via CYP3A4/2C19, hydroxylation via CYP3A4, glucuronidation; N-desmethyldiazepam and temazepam (active metabolites). **Elimination:** Urine (glucuronide conjugates); $T_{1/2}$ ≤48 hrs, ≤100 hrs (N-desmethyldiazepam).

PATIENT CONSIDERATIONS
Assessment: Assess for hypersensitivity to drug, acute narrow-angle glaucoma, myasthenia gravis, severe respiratory/hepatic insufficiency, sleep apnea syndrome, history of seizures, psychosis, depression, history of alcohol/drug abuse, debilitation, pregnancy/nursing status, and possible drug interactions.

Monitoring: Monitor for hypersensitivity reactions, withdrawal symptoms, seizures, psychiatric/paradoxical reactions, respiratory depression, loss of response during prolonged use, abuse, dependence, and other adverse reactions. Monitor CBC and LFTs periodically during long-term therapy.

Counseling: Inform of potential hazard to the fetus during pregnancy; advise to notify physician if nursing, pregnant, or intending to become pregnant during therapy. Inform that medication may produce psychological and physical dependence especially with history of alcohol/drug abuse; advise to consult physician before increasing dose or abruptly discontinuing the drug. Advise against simultaneous ingestion of alcohol and other CNS depressants during therapy. Caution against engaging in hazardous occupations requiring complete mental alertness (eg, operating machinery, driving).

Valstar — valrubicin   Rx

Class: Anthracycline

ADULT DOSAGE	PEDIATRIC DOSAGE
BCG-Refractory Bladder Carcinoma in Situ	Pediatric use may not have been established
In patients for whom immediate cystectomy would be associated w/ unacceptable morbidity/mortality	
800mg once a week for 6 weeks	
Delay administration at least 2 weeks after transurethral resection and/or fulguration	

ADMINISTRATION
Intravesical route

- Do not mix w/ other drugs.
- Prepare and store in glass, polypropylene, or polyolefin containers and tubing; use non-di(2-ethylhexyl) phthalate containing administration sets (eg, those that are polyethylene-lined).

Instillation Instructions
1. Allow four 5mL vials to warm slowly to room temperature; do not heat.
2. Withdraw 20mL from the 4 vials and dilute w/ 55mL of 0.9% NaCl inj, providing 75mL of a diluted sol; stable for 12 hrs at ≤25°C (77°F).
3. Insert a urethral catheter into the patient's bladder, drain the bladder, and slowly instill the diluted 75mL sol via gravity flow over several min.
4. Withdraw the catheter; the patient should retain the drug for 2 hrs before voiding.

5. At the end of 2 hrs, patient should void (some patients will be unable to retain the drug for the full 2 hrs).
6. Patients should maintain adequate hydration following treatment.

STORAGE
Unopened Vials: 2-8°C (36-46°F). Do not heat or freeze.

HOW SUPPLIED
Sol: 40mg/mL [5mL]

CONTRAINDICATIONS
Perforated bladder, known hypersensitivity to anthracyclines or polyoxyl castor oil, active UTI, small bladder capacity and unable to tolerate a 75mL instillation.

WARNINGS/PRECAUTIONS
Risk of metastatic bladder cancer w/ delayed cystectomy; reconsider cystectomy if there is not a complete response of carcinoma in situ (CIS) to treatment after 3 months or if CIS recurs. Avoid in patients w/ a perforated bladder or in whom the integrity of the bladder mucosa has been compromised; delay administration until bladder integrity has been restored. Evaluate the status of the bladder before instillation in patients undergoing transurethral resection of the bladder (TURB); delay administration at least two weeks after transurethral resection and/or fulguration. Caution w/ severe irritable bladder symptoms. Bladder spasm and spontaneous discharge of the intravesical instillate may occur; clamping of urinary catheter is not advised. May cause fetal harm.

ADVERSE REACTIONS
Urinary frequency, dysuria, urinary urgency, bladder spasm, hematuria, bladder pain, urinary incontinence, cystitis, UTI, nocturia, local burning symptoms, abdominal pain, nausea.

PREGNANCY AND LACTATION
Pregnancy: May cause fetal harm.
Lactation: Lactating women should not breastfeed during treatment and for 2 weeks after the final dose.
Reproduction Potential: Females of reproductive potential should use effective contraception during treatment and for 6 months after the final dose. Men w/ female partners of reproductive potential should use effective contraception during treatment and for 3 months following the final dose. May impair fertility in males of reproductive potential.

MECHANISM OF ACTION
Anthracycline; inhibits the incorporation of nucleosides into nucleic acids, causing extensive chromosomal damage, and arrests the cell cycle in G_2. Interferes w/ the normal DNA breaking-sealing action of DNA topoisomerase II.

PHARMACOKINETICS
Absorption: $AUC_{0-6\ hrs}$=78nmol/L•hr (900mg). **Metabolism:** N-trifluoroacetyladriamycin and N-trifluoroacetyladriamycinol (major metabolites). **Elimination:** Urine (98.6%, 0.4% metabolites).

PATIENT CONSIDERATIONS
Assessment: Assess for hypersensitivity to anthracyclines or polyoxyl castor oil, UTI, small bladder capacity and unable to tolerate a 75mL instillation, integrity of the bladder, perforated bladder, severe irritable bladder symptoms, and pregnancy/nursing status.
Monitoring: Monitor for bladder spasm, spontaneous discharge of the intravesical instillate, disease recurrence or progression, and other adverse reactions.
Counseling: Counsel about risks and benefits of therapy. Advise that delaying cystectomy could lead to development of metastatic bladder cancer. Inform that red-tinged urine is typical for the first 24 hrs following administration; advise to report prolonged irritable bladder symptoms or prolonged passage of red-colored urine to physician immediately. Instruct to maintain adequate hydration following treatment. Advise females of reproductive potential of the potential risk to a fetus and to use effective contraception during treatment and for 6 months after the last dose. Instruct females to inform their physician of a known or suspected pregnancy. Advise male patients w/ female partners of reproductive potential to use effective contraception during treatment and for 3 months after the last dose. Counsel females not to breastfeed during treatment and for 2 weeks after the last dose.

VALTREX — valacyclovir hydrochloride

Rx

Class: Nucleoside analogue

ADULT DOSAGE

Herpes Labialis (Cold Sores)
2g q12h for 1 day
Initiate at earliest symptom

Genital Herpes
Initial Episode: 1g bid for 10 days
Most effective when given w/in 48 hrs of onset of signs/symptoms
Recurrent Episodes: 500mg bid for 3 days
Initiate at 1st sign/symptom of episode
Suppressive Therapy:
Normal Immune Function:
1g qd
Alternative if ≤9 Recurrences/Year:
500mg qd

HIV-1 Infected Patients:
CD4+ Count ≥100 cells/mm³: 500mg bid

Reduction of Transmission:
≤9 Recurrences/Year: 500mg qd for the source partner

Herpes Zoster
1g tid for 7 days
Initiate at earliest sign/symptom; most effective if initiated w/in 48 hrs of rash onset

PEDIATRIC DOSAGE

Herpes Labialis (Cold Sores)
≥12 Years:
2g q12h for 1 day
Initiate at earliest symptom

Chickenpox
2-<18 Years:
20mg/kg tid for 5 days
Initiate at earliest sign/symptom
Max: 1g tid

DOSING CONSIDERATIONS

Renal Impairment
Herpes Labialis:
CrCl 30-49mL/min: Reduce dose to 1g q12h for 1 day
CrCl 10-29mL/min: Reduce dose to 500mg q12h for 1 day
CrCl <10mL/min: Reduce dose to 500mg single dose

Genital Herpes (Initial Episode):
CrCl 10-29mL/min: 1g q24h
CrCl <10mL/min: 500mg q24h

Genital Herpes (Recurrent Episode):
CrCl ≤29mL/min: 500mg q24h

Genital Herpes (Suppressive Therapy):
Immunocompetent Patients:
CrCl ≤29mL/min: 500mg q24h
Alternative if ≤9 Recurrences/Year:
CrCl ≤29mL/min: 500mg q48h

HIV-1 Infected Patients:
CrCl ≤29mL/min: 500mg q24h

Herpes Zoster:
CrCl 30-49mL/min: Reduce dose to 1g q12h
CrCl 10-29mL/min: Reduce dose to 1g q24h
CrCl <10mL/min: Reduce dose to 500mg q24h

Hemodialysis Patients:
Administer dose after hemodialysis

ADMINISTRATION
Oral route

Shake oral sus well before using.

Preparation of Oral Sus
Ingredients for Preparation: Valtrex caplets 500mg, cherry flavor, and Suspension Structured Vehicle USP-NF (SSV)

1. Use a pestle and mortar to grind the required number of caplets until a fine powder is produced (5 caplets for 25mg/mL sus; 10 caplets for 50mg/mL sus).
2. Add approx 5mL aliquots of SSV to the mortar and triturate the powder until a paste has been produced.
3. Continue to add approx 5mL aliquots of SSV to the mortar, mixing thoroughly between additions, until a concentrated sus is produced, to a minimum total quantity of 20mL SSV and a max total quantity of 40mL SSV for both the 25mg/mL and 50mg/mL sus.
4. Transfer the mixture to a suitable 100mL measuring flask.
5. Transfer the cherry flavor to the mortar and dissolve in approx 5mL of SSV. Once dissolved, add to the measuring flask.
6. Rinse the mortar at least 3X w/ approx 5mL aliquots of SSV, transferring the rinsing to the measuring flask between additions.
7. Make the sus to volume (100mL) w/ SSV and shake thoroughly to mix.
8. Transfer the sus to an amber glass medicine bottle w/ a child-resistant closure.

STORAGE
15-25°C (59-77°F).

HOW SUPPLIED
Tab: 500mg, 1g* *scored

CONTRAINDICATIONS
Clinically significant hypersensitivity reaction (eg, anaphylaxis) to valacyclovir, acyclovir, or any components of the formulation.

WARNINGS/PRECAUTIONS
Thrombotic thrombocytopenic purpura/hemolytic uremic syndrome (TTP/HUS) in immunocompromised patients reported at doses of 8g qd; immediately d/c if signs/symptoms occur. Acute renal failure reported. Maintain adequate hydration. CNS adverse reactions (eg, agitation, hallucinations, confusion, delirium, seizures, encephalopathy) reported in patients with or without reduced renal function and in those with underlying renal disease who received higher than recommended doses for their level of renal function; d/c if these occur. Caution in elderly and with renal impairment.

ADVERSE REACTIONS
Headache, N/V, abdominal pain, dysmenorrhea, arthralgia, nasopharyngitis, fatigue, rash, URTIs, pyrexia, decreased neutrophil counts, diarrhea, elevated ALT/AST.

DRUG INTERACTIONS
Caution with potentially nephrotoxic drugs.

PREGNANCY AND LACTATION
Pregnancy: Category B.
Lactation: Caution in nursing.

MECHANISM OF ACTION

Nucleoside analogue DNA polymerase inhibitor; rapidly converted to acyclovir, which stops replication of herpes viral DNA by competitive inhibition of viral DNA polymerase, incorporation into and termination of growing viral DNA chain, and inactivation of viral DNA polymerase.

PHARMACOKINETICS

Absorption: Rapid. Absolute bioavailability (54.5% acyclovir). Oral administration of variable doses resulted in different parameters. **Distribution:** Plasma protein binding (13.5-17.9%, 9-33% acyclovir); found in breast milk. **Metabolism:** Hepatic/ Intestinal (1st pass) to acyclovir and L-valine. **Elimination:** Urine (46%), feces (47%); $T_{1/2}$=2.5-3.3 hrs.

PATIENT CONSIDERATIONS

Assessment: Assess for hypersensitivity, immunocompromised state, renal impairment, hydration status, pregnancy/nursing status, and possible drug interactions.

Monitoring: Monitor for signs/symptoms of renal toxicity, TTP/HUS, CNS effects, and other adverse reactions.

Counseling: Advise to maintain adequate hydration. Inform that drug is not a cure for cold sores or genital herpes. For patients with cold sores, instruct to initiate treatment at earliest symptom of a cold sore; inform that treatment should not exceed 1 day (2 doses) and that doses should be taken 12 hrs apart. For patients with genital herpes, instruct to avoid contact with lesions or sexual intercourse when lesions and/or symptoms are present to avoid infecting partner(s), and to use safe sex practice in combination with suppressive therapy. For patients with herpes zoster, advise to initiate treatment as soon as possible after diagnosis. For patients with chickenpox, advise to initiate treatment at the earliest sign/ symptom.

VANCOCIN ORAL — vancomycin hydrochloride   Rx

Class: Tricyclic glycopeptide antibiotic

ADULT DOSAGE

Clostridium difficile-Associated Diarrhea

125mg qid for 10 days

Acute Enterocolitis

Staphylococcal:
500mg-2g/day in 3 or 4 divided doses for 7-10 days

PEDIATRIC DOSAGE
General Dosing

Usual: 40mg/kg/day in 3 or 4 divided doses for 7-10 days
Max: 2g/day

ADMINISTRATION
Oral route

STORAGE
15-30°C (59-86°F).

HOW SUPPLIED
Cap: 125mg, 250mg

CONTRAINDICATIONS
Known hypersensitivity to vancomycin.

WARNINGS/PRECAUTIONS

For oral use only; not systemically absorbed. Clinically significant serum concentrations reported in some patients who have taken multiple oral doses of therapy for active CDAD; significant systemic absorption may occur in some patients with inflammatory disorders of the intestinal mucosa. Monitoring of serum concentrations may be appropriate in some instances (eg, in patients with renal insufficiency and/or colitis). Nephrotoxicity reported; increased risk in patients >65 yrs of age. Ototoxicity reported mostly in patients with underlying hearing loss. Serial tests of auditory function may minimize risk of ototoxicity. May result in bacterial resistance if used in the absence of a proven or suspected bacterial infection; take appropriate measures if superinfection develops. Caution in elderly.

ADVERSE REACTIONS

N/V, abdominal pain, hypokalemia, diarrhea, pyrexia, flatulence, urinary tract infection, headache, peripheral edema, back pain, fatigue, nephrotoxicity.

DRUG INTERACTIONS

Monitor serum concentrations if used with an aminoglycoside antibiotic. Increased risk of ototoxicity with concomitant ototoxic agents (eg, aminoglycoside).

PREGNANCY AND LACTATION

Category B, not for use in nursing.

MECHANISM OF ACTION

Tricyclic glycopeptide antibiotic; inhibits cell-wall biosynthesis. Alters bacterial cell-membrane permeability and RNA synthesis.

PHARMACOKINETICS

Absorption: Poor. **Distribution:** (IV) Found in breast milk. **Elimination:** Urine, feces.

PATIENT CONSIDERATIONS

Assessment: Assess for inflammatory disorders of the intestinal mucosa, renal insufficiency, colitis, underlying hearing loss, hypersensitivity to the drug, pregnancy/nursing status, and possible drug interactions. Perform culture and susceptibility testing.

Monitoring: Monitor renal function, and for ototoxicity, superinfection, and other adverse reactions. Monitor serum concentrations when appropriate.

Counseling: Counsel that therapy should only be used to treat bacterial, not viral, infections. Instruct to take exactly ud even if patient feels better early in the course of therapy. Inform that skipping doses or not completing the full course of therapy may decrease effectiveness and increase bacterial resistance.

VANCOMYCIN INJECTION — vancomycin hydrochloride   Rx

Class: Tricyclic glycopeptide antibiotic

ADULT DOSAGE
General Dosing

Usual: 2g IV divided either as 500mg q6h or 1g q12h; administer each dose at no more than 10mg/min, or over a period of at least 60 min, whichever is longer

Streptococcus viridans/Streptococcus bovis Endocarditis:
Use alone or in combination w/ an aminoglycoside

Enterococci Endocarditis:
Use in combination w/ an aminoglycoside

Early-Onset Prosthetic Valve Endocarditis Caused by Staphylococcus epidermidis or Diphtheroids:
Use in combination w/ either rifampin, an aminoglycoside, or both

Concentrations of no more than 5mg/mL and rates of no more than 10mg/min are recommended; may use a concentration up to 10mg/mL in selected patients in need of fluid restriction

Antibiotic-Associated Pseudomembranous Colitis/ Staphylococcal Enterocolitis

Pseudomembranous Colitis Caused by Clostridium difficile/ Staphylococcal Enterocolitis: Oral Administration of Parenteral Form:
Usual: 500-2000mg/day in 3 or 4 divided doses for 7-10 days
Max: 2000mg/day

Other Indications

Treatment of the Following Infections Caused by Susceptible Strains of Microorganisms:
Serious/severe infections caused by methicillin-resistant (β-lactam-resistant) staphylococci

For penicillin-allergic patients or patients who cannot receive or have failed to respond to other drugs, including penicillins or cephalosporins

Infections caused by vancomycin-susceptible organisms that are resistant to other antimicrobial drugs

Endocarditis (eg, diphtheroid endocarditis, early-onset prosthetic valve endocarditis)
Septicemia
Bone infections
Lower respiratory tract infections
Skin and skin-structure infections

PEDIATRIC DOSAGE
General Dosing

Usual: 10mg/kg IV q6h

Total daily IV dosage may be lower in pediatric patients up to 1 month of age

Neonates:
Initial: 15mg/kg
Maint: 10mg/kg q12h for neonates in 1st week of life and q8h thereafter up to 1 month of age

Premature Infants: Longer dosing intervals may be necessary

Administer each dose over a period of at least 60 min

Antibiotic-Associated Pseudomembranous Colitis/ Staphylococcal Enterocolitis

Pseudomembranous Colitis Caused by C. difficile/Staphylococcal Enterocolitis: Oral Administration of Parenteral Form:
Usual: 40mg/kg/day in 3 or 4 divided doses for 7-10 days
Max: 2000mg/day

DOSING CONSIDERATIONS
Renal Impairment
Initial: No less than 15mg/kg, even in mild to moderate renal insufficiency
Dosage per day in mg is about 15X the GFR in mL/min; refer to PI for dosage table in patients w/ impaired renal function

Functionally Anephric Patients:
Initial: 15mg/kg
Maint: 1.9mg/kg/24h

In patients w/ marked renal impairment, may be more convenient to give maint doses of 250-1000mg once every several days rather than administering on a daily basis

Anuria:
1000mg every 7-10 days

In premature infants and the elderly, greater dosage reductions than expected may be necessary

ADMINISTRATION
IV/Oral route

Oral
May dilute appropriate dose in 1 oz of water.
Common flavoring syrup may be added to sol to improve taste.
Diluted sol may be administered via NG tube.

IV
Recommended to dilute sol to ≤5mg/mL.
Reconstitute 500mg vial w/ 10mL, 750mg vial w/ 15mL, or 1g vial w/ 20mL of sterile water for inj.
After reconstitution, vials may be stored in a refrigerator for 96 hrs w/o significant loss of potency.
Further dilute reconstituted 500mg vial, 750mg vial, or 1g vial w/ at least 100mL, 150mL, or 200mL of a suitable infusion sol, respectively.
Administer the desired dose, diluted in this manner, by intermittent IV infusion over a period of at least 60 min.

Compatibility w/ Other Drugs and IV Fluids:
The following diluents are physically and chemically compatible (w/ 4g/L vancomycin):
D5 inj
0.9% NaCl inj
D5 and 0.9% NaCl inj
Lactated Ringer's inj
Lactated Ringer's and D5 inj
Normosol-M and D5
Isolyte E

Mixtures of sol of vancomycin and β-lactam antibiotics shown to be physically incompatible; adequately flush IV lines between administration of β-lactam antibiotics.

STORAGE
20-25°C (68-77°F).

HOW SUPPLIED
Inj: 500mg, 750mg, 1g

CONTRAINDICATIONS
Known hypersensitivity to this antibiotic.

WARNINGS/PRECAUTIONS
Infusion-related events may occur. Rapid bolus administration may be associated w/ exaggerated hypotension, including shock and rarely cardiac arrest. Ototoxicity reported mostly in patients who have been given excessive doses or w/ an underlying hearing loss. Serial tests of auditory function may minimize risk of ototoxicity. Caution w/ renal insufficiency. C. difficile-associated diarrhea (CDAD) reported; may need to d/c if CDAD is suspected or confirmed. Clinically significant serum concentrations reported in some patients after multiple oral doses of therapy for active C. difficile-induced pseudomembranous colitis. May result in bacterial resistance w/ prolonged use or use in the absence of a proven or strongly suspected bacterial infection, or a prophylactic indication; take appropriate measures if superinfection develops. Rarely, pseudomembranous colitis due to C. difficile developed in patients who received IV therapy. Reversible neutropenia reported; periodically monitor leukocyte count w/ prolonged therapy. Thrombophlebitis may occur; administer slowly and rotate venous access sites. Caution in elderly.

ADVERSE REACTIONS
Infusion-related events, nephrotoxicity, pseudomembranous colitis, ototoxicity, neutropenia, inj-site inflammation.

DRUG INTERACTIONS
Concomitant use of anesthetic agents increased frequency of infusion-related events (eg, hypotension, flushing, erythema); administration as a 60-min infusion prior to anesthetic induction may minimize infusion-related events. Caution w/ concurrent and/or sequential systemic or topical use of other potentially neurotoxic and/or nephrotoxic drugs (eg, amphotericin B, aminoglycosides, bacitracin, polymyxin B, colistin, viomycin, cisplatin). Increased risk of ototoxicity w/ concomitant ototoxic agents (eg, aminoglycoside). Periodically monitor leukocyte count w/ concomitant drugs that may cause neutropenia.

PREGNANCY AND LACTATION
Pregnancy: Category C.
Lactation: Not for use in nursing.

MECHANISM OF ACTION
Tricyclic glycopeptide antibiotic; inhibits cell-wall biosynthesis. In addition, alters bacterial-cell-membrane permeability and RNA synthesis.

PHARMACOKINETICS
Absorption: (Oral) Poorly absorbed. **Distribution:** Plasma protein binding (55%); found in breast milk. **Elimination:** Urine (75%); $T_{1/2}$=4-6 hrs (normal renal function); 7.5 days (anephric patients).

PATIENT CONSIDERATIONS
Assessment: Assess for renal impairment, underlying hearing loss, drug hypersensitivity, pregnancy/nursing status, and possible drug interactions. Perform culture and susceptibility testing.

Monitoring: Monitor renal function, and for ototoxicity, CDAD, superinfection, and other adverse reactions. Periodically monitor leukocyte count w/ prolonged therapy. Closely monitor serum concentrations of therapy.

Counseling: Counsel that therapy should only be used to treat bacterial, not viral, infections. Instruct to take exactly ud even if patient feels better early in the course of therapy. Inform that skipping doses or not completing the full course

of therapy may decrease effectiveness and increase bacterial resistance. Inform that diarrhea is a common problem caused by therapy, which usually ends when therapy is discontinued. Instruct to immediately contact physician if watery and bloody stools (w/ or w/o stomach cramps and fever) occur, even as late as ≥2 months after the last dose.

VANOS — fluocinonide   Rx
Class: Corticosteroid

ADULT DOSAGE	PEDIATRIC DOSAGE
Inflammatory and Pruritic Manifestations of Corticosteroid-Responsive Dermatoses	**Inflammatory and Pruritic Manifestations of Corticosteroid-Responsive Dermatoses**
Psoriasis/Corticosteroid-Responsive Dermatoses: Apply a thin layer to affected skin area(s) qd or bid ud	**≥12 Years:** **Psoriasis/Corticosteroid-Responsive Dermatoses:** Apply a thin layer to affected skin area(s) qd or bid ud
Atopic Dermatitis: Apply a thin layer to affected skin area(s) qd ud	**Atopic Dermatitis:** Apply a thin layer to affected skin area(s) qd ud
Max: 60g/week	**Max:** 60g/week
Limit treatment to 2 consecutive weeks. D/C therapy when control is achieved. Reassess diagnosis if no improvement is seen w/in 2 weeks.	Limit treatment to 2 consecutive weeks. D/C therapy when control is achieved. Reassess diagnosis if no improvement is seen w/in 2 weeks.

ADMINISTRATION
Topical route

STORAGE
15-30°C (59-86°F).

HOW SUPPLIED
Cre: 0.1% [30g, 60g, 120g]

WARNINGS/PRECAUTIONS
For dermatologic use only; not for ophthalmic, oral, or intravaginal use. Not for use in rosacea or perioral dermatitis. Do not apply on the face, groin, or axillae. Systemic absorption may produce reversible hypothalamic-pituitary-adrenal (HPA) axis suppression w/ the potential for glucocorticosteroid insufficiency, Cushing's syndrome, hyperglycemia, and unmasking of latent diabetes mellitus (DM). Periodically evaluate for HPA axis suppression and if noted, gradually withdraw treatment, reduce frequency of application, or substitute a less potent steroid. Factors predisposing to HPA axis suppression include use of more potent steroids, use over large surface areas, prolonged use, use under occlusion, use on an altered skin barrier, and use in patients with liver failure. May suppress immune system if used for >2 weeks. Manifestations of adrenal insufficiency may require supplemental systemic corticosteroids. Pediatric patients may be more susceptible to systemic toxicity. Local adverse reactions may be more likely to occur with occlusive use, prolonged use or use of higher potency corticosteroids. Use appropriate antifungal or antibacterial agent if concomitant skin infections are present or develop; if a favorable response does not occur promptly, d/c until infection is controlled. D/C and institute appropriate therapy if irritation develops. Allergic contact dermatitis may occur; confirm by patch testing.

ADVERSE REACTIONS
Headache, application-site burning, nasopharyngitis, nasal congestion.

DRUG INTERACTIONS
Use of >1 corticosteroid-containing product at the same time may increase total systemic absorption.

PREGNANCY AND LACTATION
Pregnancy: Category C.
Lactation: Not for use in nursing.

MECHANISM OF ACTION
Corticosteroid; has not been established. Possesses anti-inflammatory and antipruritic actions. Plays a role in cellular signaling, immune function, inflammation, and protein regulation.

PHARMACOKINETICS
Absorption: Percutaneous; extent of absorption is determined by vehicle and integrity of epidermal barrier. **Distribution:** Found in breast milk (systemically administered).

PATIENT CONSIDERATIONS
Assessment: Assess for hypersensitivity to the drug, rosacea, perioral dermatitis, skin infections, liver impairment, pregnancy/nursing status, and possible drug interactions.

Monitoring: Monitor for signs/symptoms of HPA axis suppression, Cushing's syndrome, hyperglycemia, unmasking of latent DM, skin irritation, and other adverse reactions. Monitor for systemic toxicity (eg, adrenal suppression, intracranial HTN) in pediatric patients. Following withdrawal of treatment, monitor for glucocorticosteroid insufficiency. Reassess diagnosis if no improvement is seen w/in 2 weeks.

Counseling: Instruct to use externally and ud. Advise not to use for any disorder other than for which it was prescribed. Instruct to avoid contact w/ eyes and not to use on face, groin, and underarms. Instruct not to bandage, cover, or wrap treated skin, unless directed by physician. Counsel to report any signs of local adverse reactions. Advise that other corticosteroid-containing products should not be used w/o 1st consulting w/ the physician. Instruct to d/c use when control is achieved and to notify physician if no improvement seen w/in 2 weeks. Notify physician if contemplating surgery. Counsel to wash hands following application.

VANTAS — histrelin acetate   Rx

Class: Synthetic gonadotropin-releasing hormone (GnRH) analogue

ADULT DOSAGE
Advanced Prostate Cancer
Palliative Treatment:
1 implant for 12 months; implant is inserted SQ in the inner aspect of the upper arm

Remove after 12 months of therapy; at the time an implant is removed, another implant may be inserted to continue therapy

PEDIATRIC DOSAGE
Pediatric use may not have been established

ADMINISTRATION
SQ route
Refer to PI for recommended procedure for implant insertion and removal.

STORAGE
Implant: 2-8°C (36-46°F); excursions permitted to 25°C (77°F) for 7 days. Refrigerate until the day of insertion. Do not open vial until just before the time of insertion. Protect from light. Do not freeze. Implantation Kit: 20-25°C (68-77°F).

HOW SUPPLIED
Implant: 50mg

CONTRAINDICATIONS
Hypersensitivity to GnRH, GnRH agonist analogs, or any of the components in this product; women who are or may become pregnant.

WARNINGS/PRECAUTIONS
Causes a transient increase in serum concentrations of testosterone during the 1st week of treatment; may experience worsening of symptoms or onset of new symptoms (eg, bone pain, neuropathy, hematuria, ureteral or bladder outlet obstruction). Spinal cord compression, which may result in paralysis, and ureteral obstruction, which may cause renal impairment, reported; closely observe patients w/ metastatic vertebral lesions and/or w/ urinary tract obstruction during the 1st few weeks of therapy. Difficulty in locating or removing implant reported; carefully adhere to recommended procedure of implant insertion/ removal to minimize the potential for complications and for implant expulsion. Hyperglycemia and an increased risk of developing diabetes reported; monitor blood glucose and/or HbA1c periodically. Increased risk of developing MI, sudden cardiac death, and stroke reported; monitor for signs/symptoms of cardiovascular disease (CVD). Results of diagnostic tests of pituitary gonadotropic and gonadal functions conducted during and after therapy may be affected. May prolong QT/ QTc interval; caution w/ congenital long QT syndrome, CHF, frequent electrolyte abnormalities, and in patients taking drugs known to prolong the QT interval. Correct electrolyte abnormalities.

ADVERSE REACTIONS
Hot flashes, fatigue, implant-site reaction (bruising/pain/soreness/tenderness), testicular atrophy, renal impairment, gynecomastia, constipation, erectile dysfunction.

PREGNANCY AND LACTATION
Category X, not for use in nursing.

MECHANISM OF ACTION
Synthetic gonadotropin-releasing hormone analog; acts as a potent inhibitor of gonadotropin secretion when given continuously in therapeutic doses. Desensitizes responsiveness of pituitary gonadotropin, causing a reduction in testicular steroidogenesis.

PHARMACOKINETICS
Absorption: C_{max}=1.1ng/mL; T_{max}=12 hrs (median). **Distribution:** V_d=58.4L (500mcg SQ bolus). **Metabolism:** C-terminal dealkylation and hydrolysis. **Elimination:** $T_{1/2}$=3.92 hrs (SQ bolus).

PATIENT CONSIDERATIONS
Assessment: Assess for hypersensitivity to drug, metastatic vertebral lesions, urinary tract obstruction, and risk for diabetes and CVD.

Monitoring: Monitor for worsening or onset of new symptoms, signs/symptoms of spinal cord compression, ureteral obstruction, CVD, and other adverse reactions. Monitor response by measuring serum concentrations of testosterone and prostate-specific antigen periodically, especially if the anticipated clinical or biochemical response to treatment has not been achieved. Monitor blood glucose and/or HbA1c periodically. Consider periodic monitoring of ECG and electrolytes.

Counseling: Inform of risks and benefits of therapy. Instruct to refrain from wetting the inserted arm for 24 hrs and from heavy lifting or strenuous exertion of the arm for 7 days after implant insertion. Instruct to contact physician if implant was expelled from the body or if any adverse reactions develop.

VAQTA — hepatitis A vaccine, inactivated   Rx

Class: Vaccine

ADULT DOSAGE
Hepatitis A Vaccine
≥19 Years:
1mL IM, then 1mL IM booster dose 6-18 months later; administer primary dose at least 2 weeks prior to expected exposure to hepatitis A virus

Booster Immunization Following Another Manufacturer's Hepatitis A Vaccine:
A booster dose of Vaqta may be given at 6-12 months following a primary dose of Havrix

PEDIATRIC DOSAGE
Hepatitis A Vaccine
12 Months-18 Years:
0.5mL IM, then 0.5mL IM booster dose 6-18 months later; administer primary dose at least 2 weeks prior to expected exposure to hepatitis A virus

Booster Immunization Following Another Manufacturer's Hepatitis A Vaccine:
A booster dose of Vaqta may be given at 6-12 months following a primary dose of Havrix

---

ADMINISTRATION
IM route
Shake vial or syringe well to obtain a slightly opaque, white sus before withdrawal and use
Do not mix w/ any other vaccine in same syringe or vial; use separate inj sites and syringes for each vaccine
Preferred Inj Sites
Children 12-23 Months of Age: Anterolateral area of the thigh
Adults, Adolescents, and Children >2 Years: Deltoid muscle

STORAGE
2-8°C (36-46°F). Do not freeze.

HOW SUPPLIED
Inj: 25 U/0.5mL, 50 U/mL [vial, prefilled syringe]

CONTRAINDICATIONS
History of immediate and/or severe allergic or hypersensitivity reactions (eg, anaphylaxis) after a previous dose of any hepatitis A vaccine, or a previous anaphylactic reaction to any component of this vaccine, including neomycin.

WARNINGS/PRECAUTIONS
Appropriate treatment and supervision must be available for possible anaphylactic reactions. Vial stopper, syringe plunger stopper, and tip cap contain dry natural latex rubber; may cause allergic reactions in latex-sensitive individuals. Immunocompromised persons may have a diminished immune response to vaccine and may not be protected against HAV infection after vaccination. May not prevent hepatitis A infection in individuals who have an unrecognized hepatitis A infection at time of vaccination. May not protect all susceptible vaccinees.

ADVERSE REACTIONS
Inj-site pain/tenderness/soreness/warmth/swelling/erythema, headache, fever, upper respiratory tract infection, asthenia/fatigue, nausea, myalgia, irritability, diarrhea.

DRUG INTERACTIONS
Immunosuppressive therapy may reduce the immune response to vaccine.

PREGNANCY AND LACTATION
Category C, caution in nursing.

MECHANISM OF ACTION
Vaccine; presence of antibodies to HAV confers protection against hepatitis A disease.

PATIENT CONSIDERATIONS
Assessment: Assess for history of immediate and/or severe allergic/ hypersensitivity reactions to any hepatitis A vaccine or any component of the vaccine (eg, neomycin), latex sensitivity, immunosuppression, unrecognized hepatitis A infection, immunization status/vaccination history, pregnancy/nursing status, and possible drug interactions.

Monitoring: Monitor for anaphylactic/allergic/inj-site reactions, and other adverse reactions. Monitor immune response to vaccine.

Counseling: Inform of potential benefits and risks of the vaccine. Counsel about potential adverse events that have been temporally associated with the vaccination. Instruct to report any adverse events to physician.

VARIVAX — varicella virus vaccine live   Rx

Class: Vaccine

ADULT DOSAGE
Varicella Vaccine
2 doses of 0.5mL SQ; administer w/ a minimum interval of 4 weeks between doses

PEDIATRIC DOSAGE
Varicella Vaccine
12 Months-12 Years:
0.5mL SQ; if a 2nd dose is administered, there should be a minimum interval of 3 months between doses

≥13 Years:
2 doses of 0.5mL SQ; administer w/ a minimum interval of 4 weeks between doses

---

ADMINISTRATION

SQ route

Inject into the outer aspect of the upper arm (deltoid region) or anterolateral thigh

Reconstitution

Use only the sterile diluent supplied when reconstituting vaccine

Use a sterile syringe free of preservatives, antiseptics, and detergents for each reconstitution and inj

Do not freeze

Do not combine w/ any other vaccine through reconstitution or mixing

To reconstitute vaccine:

1. Withdraw total volume of provided sterile diluent into a syringe
2. Inject all of the withdrawn diluent into the vial of lyophilized vaccine; gently agitate to mix thoroughly
3. Withdraw entire contents into syringe and inject the total volume (approx 0.5mL) of reconstituted vaccine SQ
4. Administer immediately after reconstitution; discard if reconstituted vaccine is not used w/in 30 min

STORAGE

-50°C to -15°C (-58°F to +5°F). Use of dry ice may subject to temperatures colder than -50°C (-58°F). May store at 2-8°C (36-46°F) for up to 72 continuous hrs prior to reconstitution; discard if not used. Protect from light. Diluent: 20-25°C (68-77°F), or in the refrigerator.

HOW SUPPLIED

Inj: 0.5mL

CONTRAINDICATIONS

History of anaphylactic or severe allergic reaction to any component of the vaccine (eg, neomycin, gelatin) or to a previous dose of a varicella-containing vaccine, immunosuppressed or immunodeficient individuals (eg, history of primary or acquired immunodeficiency states, leukemia, lymphoma or other malignant neoplasms affecting the bone marrow or lymphatic system, AIDS, or other clinical manifestations of infection with HIV), febrile illness, active untreated tuberculosis (TB), pregnancy. Concomitant administration with immunosuppressive therapy (including immunosuppressive doses of corticosteroids).

WARNINGS/PRECAUTIONS

Do not administer IV or IM. Adequate treatment provisions, including epinephrine inj (1:1000), should be available for immediate use should anaphylaxis occur. Defer vaccination in patients with family history of congenital/hereditary immunodeficiency until immune status has been evaluated and found to be immunocompetent. The Advisory Committee for Immunization Practices has recommendations on the use of varicella vaccine in HIV-infected individuals. Transmission of vaccine virus may occur; vaccine recipients should attempt to avoid close association with susceptible high-risk individuals for up to 6 weeks following vaccination. May cause temporary depression of tuberculin skin sensitivity, leading to false negative results; perform tuberculin skin testing (with tuberculin purified protein derivative) before vaccination or on the same day, or at least 4 weeks following vaccination. Avoid pregnancy for 3 months following vaccination.

ADVERSE REACTIONS

Fever, inj-site complaints (eg, pain/soreness, swelling, erythema, rash, pruritus, hematoma, induration, stiffness, numbness), varicella-like rash.

DRUG INTERACTIONS

See Contraindications. Avoid use of salicylates (aspirin) or salicylate-containing products in patients 12 months-17 yrs of age for 6 weeks after vaccination; Reye's syndrome may occur. Defer vaccination for at least 5 months following blood/plasma transfusions, or administration of immune globulins. Do not give immune globulins for 2 months following vaccination.

PREGNANCY AND LACTATION

Contraindicated in pregnancy, caution in nursing.

MECHANISM OF ACTION

Vaccine; induces both cell-mediated and humoral immune responses to varicella zoster virus.

PATIENT CONSIDERATIONS

Assessment: Assess for previous hypersensitivity, health/immunity status, immunization history, active untreated TB, pregnancy/nursing status, possible drug interactions, and for any other conditions where treatment is contraindicated or cautioned.

Monitoring: Monitor for anaphylaxis, inj-site reactions, fever, and other adverse reactions.

Counseling: Inform of potential benefits and risks of vaccination. Advise to report any adverse reactions to physician. Inform that the vaccine may not result in protection of all vaccinees. Instruct to avoid pregnancy for 3 months after vaccination. Due to the concern for transmission of vaccine virus, instruct vaccine recipients to attempt to avoid whenever possible close association with susceptible high-risk individuals for up to 6 weeks following vaccination.

VARIZIG — varicella zoster immune globulin (human)   Rx

Class: Immune globulin

ADULT DOSAGE

Postexposure Prophylaxis of Varicella

Reduces the severity of varicella in high-risk individuals

≥40.1kg: 625 IU or 6mL
Max: (>40kg) 625 IU

PEDIATRIC DOSAGE

Postexposure Prophylaxis of Varicella

Reduces the severity of varicella in high-risk individuals

≤2kg: 62.5 IU or 0.6mL
2.1-10kg: 125 IU or 1.2mL

10.1-20kg: 250 IU or 2.4mL
20.1-30kg: 375 IU or 3.6mL
30.1-40kg: 500 IU or 4.8mL
≥40.1kg: 625 IU or 6mL

Minimum: (<2kg) 62.5 IU
Max: (>40kg) 625 IU

Consider a 2nd full dose of treatment for high-risk patients who have additional exposures to varicella >3 weeks after initial administration

Refer to pediatric dosing section for patients weighing ≤40kg

Consider a 2nd full dose of treatment for high-risk patients who have additional exposures to varicella >3 weeks after initial administration

---

ADMINISTRATION

IM route

Administer as soon as possible following varicella zoster virus exposure, ideally w/in 96 hrs

Divide the IM dose and administer in ≥2 inj sites, depending on patient size

Do not exceed 3mL/inj site

Inject into the deltoid muscle or the anterolateral aspects of the upper thigh

Due to the risk of sciatic nerve injury, do not use the gluteal region as a routine inj site

If the gluteal region is used, only use the upper, outer quadrant

STORAGE

2-8°C (36-46°F). Do not freeze.

HOW SUPPLIED

Inj: ≥125 IU/1.2mL

CONTRAINDICATIONS

Anaphylactic or severe systemic (hypersensitivity) reactions to human immune globulin preparations, IgA-deficient patients w/ antibodies against IgA and a history of hypersensitivity.

WARNINGS/PRECAUTIONS

Thrombotic events may occur during or following treatment; caution w/ a history of atherosclerosis, multiple cardiovascular (CV) risk factors, advanced age, impaired cardiac output, coagulation disorders, prolonged periods of immobilization, and/or known/suspected hyperviscosity. Consider baseline assessment of blood viscosity in patients at risk for hyperviscosity including those w/ cryoglobulins, fasting chylomicronemia/markedly high triacylglycerols (TGs), or monoclonal gammopathies. In patients who have severe thrombocytopenia or any coagulation disorder that would contraindicate IM inj, only administer if expected benefits outweigh potential risks. Severe hypersensitivity reactions may occur; d/c immediately and provide appropriate treatment if hypersensitivity occurs. Administer in a setting w/ appropriate equipment, medication, and personnel trained in the management of hypersensitivity, anaphylaxis, and shock. Made from human plasma; may carry a risk of transmitting infectious agents (eg, viruses, variant Creutzfeldt-Jakob disease agent and Creutzfeldt-Jakob disease agent). Caution in elderly who are judged to be at increased risk of thrombotic events.

ADVERSE REACTIONS

Pyrexia, N/V, inj-site pain, headache, rash.

DRUG INTERACTIONS

Passive transfer of antibodies may impair the efficacy of live attenuated virus vaccines (eg, measles, rubella, mumps, and varicella). Defer vaccination w/ live virus vaccines until approx 3 months after administration.

PREGNANCY AND LACTATION

Category C, caution in nursing.

MECHANISM OF ACTION

Immune globulin; provides passive immunization for non-immune individuals exposed to varicella zoster virus, reducing the severity of varicella infections.

PHARMACOKINETICS

Absorption: AUC_{0-28}=2472 mIU•day/mL; AUC_{0-84}=4087 mIU•day/mL; C_{max}=136 mIU/mL; T_{max}=4.5 days. **Elimination:** $T_{1/2}$=26.2 days.

PATIENT CONSIDERATIONS

Assessment: Assess for IgA-deficient patients w/ antibodies against IgA, hypersensitivity to human immune globulin preparations, severe thrombocytopenia or any coagulation disorder, risk factors for thrombotic events (eg, history of atherosclerosis, multiple CV risk factors, advanced age, impaired cardiac output, prolonged periods of immobilization, known/suspected hyperviscosity), any other conditions where treatment is contraindicated or cautioned, pregnancy/nursing status, and possible drug interactions. Consider baseline assessment of blood viscosity in patients at risk for hyperviscosity.

Monitoring: Monitor for thrombotic events, severe hypersensitivity reactions, infection, and other adverse reactions.

Counseling: Inform about the risks and benefits of treatment. Advise that treatment is intended to reduce the severity of chickenpox infections and to consult physician if signs and symptoms of varicella develop. Inform that drug may contain infectious agents such as viruses that may cause disease. Inform that persons known to have severe, potentially life-threatening reactions to human immune globulin products should not receive the drug. Instruct to notify physician immediately if any signs or symptoms of an allergic reaction develop. Inform that drug can interfere w/ immune response to live virus vaccines (eg, measles, mumps, rubella, and varicella); instruct patients to notify their immunizing physician of recent therapy.

VARUBI — rolapitant   Rx

Class: Substance P/neurokinin-1 (NK1) receptor antagonist

ADULT DOSAGE
Chemotherapy-Induced Nausea/ Vomiting

Prevention of Nausea/Vomiting Associated w/ Cisplatin-Based Highly Emetogenic Cancer Chemotherapy:

Day 1: Rolapitant 180mg 1-2 hrs prior to chemotherapy plus dexamethasone 20mg 30 min prior to chemotherapy plus 5-HT$_3$ antagonist according to the manufacturer's prescribing information

Days 2-4: Dexamethasone 8mg bid

Prevention of Nausea/Vomiting Associated w/ Moderately Emetogenic Cancer Chemotherapy and Combinations of Anthracycline and Cyclophosphamide:

Day 1: Rolapitant 180mg 1-2 hrs prior to chemotherapy plus dexamethasone 20mg 30 min prior to chemotherapy plus 5-HT$_3$ antagonist according to the manufacturer's prescribing information

Days 2-4: 5-HT$_3$ antagonist according to the manufacturer's prescribing information

PEDIATRIC DOSAGE
Pediatric use may not have been established

DOSING CONSIDERATIONS
Hepatic Impairment
Severe (Child-Pugh Class C): Avoid use; monitor for adverse reactions if use cannot be avoided

ADMINISTRATION
Oral route
Take w/o regard to meals.
Administer prior to the initiation of each chemotherapy cycle, but at no less than 2 week intervals.

STORAGE
20-25°C (68-77°F); excursions permitted to 15-30°C (59-86°F).

HOW SUPPLIED
Tab: 90mg

CONTRAINDICATIONS
Patients receiving thioridazine.

WARNINGS/PRECAUTIONS
The inhibitory effect on CYP2D6 lasts at least 7 days and may last longer after a single dose administration of rolapitant. Avoid use in patients who are receiving pimozide, a CYP2D6 substrate; increase in pimozide plasma concentrations may result in QT prolongation. Monitor for adverse reactions if concomitant use w/ other CYP2D6 substrates w/ a narrow therapeutic index cannot be avoided.

ADVERSE REACTIONS
Neutropenia, decreased appetite, dizziness, hiccups, dyspepsia, UTI, stomatitis, anemia, abdominal pain.

DRUG INTERACTIONS
See Contraindications and Warnings/Precautions. A 3-fold increase in the exposure of dextromethorphan, a CYP2D6 substrate, was observed 7 days after a single dose of rolapitant. Increased plasma concentrations of Breast Cancer Resistance Protein (BCRP) substrates (eg, methotrexate, topotecan, irinotecan) may result in potential adverse reactions; monitor for adverse reactions related to the concomitant drug if use of rolapitant cannot be avoided. Use the lowest effective dose of rosuvastatin if used concomitantly w/ rolapitant; refer to prescribing information for additional information on recommended dosing. Increased plasma concentrations of digoxin, or other P-gp substrates, may result in potential adverse reactions; monitor for adverse reactions if concomitant use w/ other P-gp substrates w/ a narrow therapeutic index cannot be avoided. Monitor for increased digoxin concentrations. Strong CYP3A4 inducers (eg, rifampin) significantly reduced plasma concentrations of rolapitant and may decrease efficacy; avoid use of rolapitant in patients who require chronic administration of such drugs.

PREGNANCY AND LACTATION
Pregnancy: There are no available data on use in pregnant women to inform any drug-associated risks. In animal reproduction studies, there were no teratogenic or embryo-fetal effects observed.
Lactation: There are no data on the presence of rolapitant in human milk, the effects of rolapitant in the breastfed infant, or the effects of rolapitant on milk production; caution in nursing.

MECHANISM OF ACTION
Selective and competitive antagonist of human substance P/NK1 receptors.

PHARMACOKINETICS
Absorption: (Healthy) C_{max}=968ng/mL; T_{max}=4 hrs. **Distribution:** Plasma protein binding (99.8%); V_d=(Healthy) 460L, (cancer patients) 387L; crosses the blood-brain barrier. **Metabolism:** Primarily via CYP3A4; M19 (C4-pyrrolidine-hydroxylated rolapitant) (major active metabolite). **Excretion:** Urine (14.2%, 8.3% as metabolites), feces (73%, 37.8% unchanged); $T_{1/2}$=169-183 hrs.

PATIENT CONSIDERATIONS
Assessment: Assess for hypersensitivity to drug, hepatic impairment, pregnancy/ nursing status, and for possible drug interactions.

Monitoring: Monitor for adverse reactions.

Counseling: Advise to inform healthcare provider when any concomitant medications are started or stopped.

VASCAZEN — omega-3-acid ethyl esters   Rx

Class: Medical food

ADULT DOSAGE
Omega-3 Deficiency
Management in Cardiovascular Disease:
4 caps/day

PEDIATRIC DOSAGE
Pediatric use may not have been established

ADMINISTRATION
Oral route
Take with or without other foods

STORAGE
15-25°C (59-77°F). Keep from freezing. Protect from direct sunlight.

HOW SUPPLIED
Cap: 1g

WARNINGS/PRECAUTIONS
Must be administered under physician supervision. Contains fish oil and soy products; avoid with known allergy to fish or soy.

ADVERSE REACTIONS
Mild reflux/aftertaste, minor leg bruising, fishy burp, flatulation, nausea.

DRUG INTERACTIONS
Caution with anticoagulants or drugs affecting coagulation; may extend bleeding time.

PREGNANCY AND LACTATION
Safety not known in pregnancy/nursing.

MECHANISM OF ACTION
Medical food; intends to restore and sustain healthy levels of eicosapentaenoic acid (EPA) and docosahexaenoic acid (DHA) in omega-3 deficient patients with CVD. Increasing dietary levels of EPA and DHA have been shown to have a host of cardio-protective benefits.

PATIENT CONSIDERATIONS
Assessment: Assess for hypersensitivity to fish or soy products, pregnancy/ nursing status, and possible drug interactions.

Monitoring: Monitor for hypersensitivity reaction and other adverse reactions. Monitor for increased bleeding time and patients receiving treatment along with drugs that affect coagulation.

Counseling: Inform of the benefits and risks of therapy. Instruct to notify physician if patient has known hypersensitivity to fish or soy products. Inform that some patients may experience a fish aftertaste/burp and taking with food may help reduce this effect. Inform of the possible adverse effects. Instruct to inform physician prior to therapy if pregnant, nursing/planning on becoming pregnant, or ≤18 yrs of age.

VASCEPA — icosapent ethyl   Rx

Class: Lipid-regulating agent

ADULT DOSAGE
Severe Hypertriglyceridemia (≥500mg/dL)
Usual: 4g/day (2 caps bid)

PEDIATRIC DOSAGE
Pediatric use may not have been established

ADMINISTRATION
Oral route
Swallow caps whole; do not break open, crush, dissolve, or chew.

STORAGE
20-25°C (68-77°F); excursions permitted to 15-30°C (59-86°F).

HOW SUPPLIED
Cap: 1g

CONTRAINDICATIONS
Known hypersensitivity (eg, anaphylactic reaction) to icosapent ethyl or any of the components of the medication.

WARNINGS/PRECAUTIONS
Contains ethyl esters of the omega-3 fatty acid, eicosapentaenoic acid (EPA), obtained from oil of fish; caution with known hypersensitivity to fish and/or shellfish. Monitor ALT and AST levels periodically during therapy in patients with hepatic impairment.

ADVERSE REACTIONS
Arthralgia, oropharyngeal pain.

DRUG INTERACTIONS
Possible prolongation of bleeding time with other drugs affecting coagulation (eg, antiplatelet agents); monitor periodically. D/C or change medications known to exacerbate hypertriglyceridemia (eg, β-blockers, thiazides, estrogens) prior to consideration of therapy.

PREGNANCY AND LACTATION
Pregnancy: Category C.
Lactation: Caution in nursing.

MECHANISM OF ACTION
Lipid-regulating agent; has not been established. EPA may reduce hepatic very low-density lipoprotein triglycerides (VLDL-TG) synthesis and/or secretion and enhances TG clearance from circulating VLDL particles.

PHARMACOKINETICS
Absorption: T_{max}=5 hrs (EPA). **Distribution:** (EPA) V_d=88L; plasma protein binding (>99%, unesterified EPA); found in breast milk. **Metabolism:** Liver via β-oxidation; EPA (active metabolite). **Elimination:** (EPA) $T_{1/2}$=89 hrs.

PATIENT CONSIDERATIONS

Assessment: Assess for drug hypersensitivity, hypersensitivity to fish and/or shellfish, hepatic impairment, pregnancy/nursing status, and possible drug interactions. Attempt to control serum lipids with appropriate diet/exercise, and control any medical problems that may contribute to lipid abnormalities (eg, diabetes mellitus, hypothyroidism, alcohol intake) prior to therapy. Assess lipid levels.

Monitoring: Monitor for allergic reactions and other adverse reactions. Monitor lipid levels. Periodically monitor ALT/AST levels with hepatic impairment.

Counseling: Instruct to notify physician if allergic to fish and/or shellfish. Inform that the use of lipid-regulating agents does not reduce the importance of appropriate nutritional intake and physical activity. Advise not to alter caps in any way and to ingest intact caps only. Instruct to take ud. If dose is missed, advise to take as soon as remembered and not to double the dose.

Vasotec — enalapril maleate   Rx

Class: ACE inhibitor

> D/C if pregnancy is detected. Drugs that act directly on the renin-angiotensin system (RAS) can cause injury/death to the developing fetus.

ADULT DOSAGE
Hypertension

Not Receiving Diuretics:
Initial: 5mg qd
Usual Range: 10-40mg/day given in single dose or 2 divided doses

May add diuretic if BP not controlled

Receiving Diuretics:
If possible, d/c diuretic 2-3 days prior to therapy. If BP is not controlled w/ enalapril alone, then diuretic therapy may be resumed
Initial: 2.5mg should be used under medical supervision for at least 2 hrs and until BP has stabilized for at least an additional hr

Heart Failure

Symptomatic CHF in Combination w/ Diuretics and Digitalis:
Initial: 2.5mg qd
Range: 2.5-20mg bid
Max: 40mg/day in divided doses

Hyponatremia (Serum Na⁺ <130mEq/L):
Initial: 2.5mg/day
Titrate: May increase to 2.5mg bid, then 5mg bid and higher prn, usually at intervals of 4 days or more
Max: 40mg/day

Asymptomatic Left Ventricular Dysfunction

Decreasing the Rate of Development of Overt Heart Failure (HF) and the Incidence of Hospitalization for HF in Clinically Stable Patients (Ejection Fraction ≤35%):
Initial: 2.5mg bid
Titrate: Increase as tolerated to 20mg/day (in divided doses)

PEDIATRIC DOSAGE
Hypertension

1 Month-16 Years:
Initial: 0.08mg/kg (up to 5mg) qd
Max: 0.58mg/kg (or 40mg/day)

DOSING CONSIDERATIONS
Renal Impairment
HTN:
CrCl ≤30mL/min:
Initial: 2.5mg qd

Dialysis Patients:
Initial: 2.5mg qd on dialysis days
Titrate: Dosage on nondialysis days should be adjusted depending on the BP response

HF:
SrCr >1.6mg/dL:
Initial: 2.5mg/day

Titrate: May increase to 2.5mg bid, then 5mg bid and higher prn, usually at intervals of 4 days or more
Max: 40mg/day

ADMINISTRATION
Oral route

Preparation of Sus (200mL of a 1.0mg/mL Sus)
1. Add 50mL of Bicitra to a polyethylene terephthalate bottle containing ten 20mg tabs; shake for at least 2 min.
2. Let concentrate stand for 60 min, then shake for additional 1 min.
3. Add 150mL of Ora-Sweet SF to concentrate and shake sus to disperse ingredients.
4. Refrigerate at 2-8°C (36-46°F) for 30 days.
5. Shake sus before each use.

STORAGE
25°C (77°F); excursions permitted to 15-30°C (59-86°F). Protect from moisture.

HOW SUPPLIED
Tab: 2.5mg*, 5mg*, 10mg*, 20mg* *scored

CONTRAINDICATIONS
Hypersensitivity to this product, history of ACE inhibitor-associated angioedema, hereditary or idiopathic angioedema, coadministration w/ aliskiren in patients w/ diabetes.

WARNINGS/PRECAUTIONS
Head/neck angioedema reported; d/c and administer appropriate therapy if angioedema occurs. Higher incidence of angioedema reported in blacks than nonblacks. Intestinal angioedema reported; monitor for abdominal pain. Effect of therapy on BP reported to be less in black patients than in nonblacks. Patients w/ history of angioedema unrelated to ACE inhibitor therapy may be at increased risk of angioedema during therapy. Anaphylactoid reactions reported during desensitization w/ hymenoptera venom, dialysis w/ high-flux membranes, and LDL apheresis w/ dextran sulfate absorption. Excessive hypotension, sometimes associated w/ oliguria and/or progressive azotemia, and rarely w/ acute renal failure and/or death, may occur; monitor patients at risk of hypotension during first 2 weeks of therapy and whenever the dose of enalapril and/or diuretic is increased. Consider dose reduction or d/c therapy or diuretic if symptomatic hypotension occurs. Neutropenia or agranulocytosis may occur; monitor WBCs in patients w/ renal disease and collagen vascular disease. Associated w/ syndrome that starts w/ cholestatic jaundice and progresses to fulminant hepatic necrosis, and sometimes death; d/c if jaundice or marked elevations of hepatic enzymes develop. Caution w/ left ventricular outflow obstruction. May cause changes in renal function; may be associated w/ oliguria and/or progressive azotemia and rarely w/ acute renal failure and/or death in severe HF patients whose renal function depends on the renin-angiotensin-aldosterone system. Increases in BUN and SrCr reported in patients w/ unilateral or bilateral renal artery stenosis; monitor renal function during the 1st few weeks of therapy in such patients. Hyperkalemia may occur; caution w/ diabetes mellitus (DM) and renal insufficiency. Persistent nonproductive cough reported. Hypotension may occur w/ major surgery or during anesthesia; may be corrected by volume expansion. Avoid in neonates and in pediatric patients w/ GFR <30mL/min.

ADVERSE REACTIONS
Fatigue, headache, dizziness.

DRUG INTERACTIONS
See Contraindications. Dual blockade of the RAS is associated w/ increased risk of hypotension, hyperkalemia, and changes in renal function (including acute renal failure); avoid combined use of RAS inhibitors. Closely monitor BP, renal function, and electrolytes w/ concomitant agents that also affect the RAS. Avoid w/ aliskiren in patients w/ renal impairment (GFR <60mL/min). Hypotension risk w/ diuretics. NSAIDs, including selective COX-2 inhibitors, may result in deterioration of renal function, including possible acute renal failure in elderly, volume depleted or patients w/ compromised renal function. K⁺-sparing diuretics, K⁺-containing salt substitutes, or K⁺ supplements may increase serum K⁺ levels; use caution and monitor serum K⁺ frequently. Avoid K⁺-sparing agents in patients w/ HF. Antihypertensive agents that cause renin release (eg, diuretics) may augment antihypertensive effect. Lithium toxicity reported w/ lithium; monitor serum lithium levels frequently. Nitritoid reactions reported rarely w/ injectable gold (eg, sodium aurothiomalate). Coadministration w/ mammalian target of rapamycin (mTOR) inhibitor (eg, temsirolimus, sirolimus, everolimus) therapy may increase risk for angioedema.

PREGNANCY AND LACTATION
Pregnancy: Category D.
Lactation: Not for use in nursing.

MECHANISM OF ACTION
ACE inhibitor; decreases plasma angiotensin II, which leads to decreased vasopressor activity and decreased aldosterone secretion.

PHARMACOKINETICS
Absorption: T_{max}=1 hr, 3-4 hrs (metabolite). **Distribution:** Crosses placenta; found in breast milk. **Metabolism:** Hydrolysis; enalaprilat (metabolite). **Elimination:** Urine and feces (94%); $T_{1/2}$=11 hrs (metabolite).

PATIENT CONSIDERATIONS

Assessment: Assess for hypersensitivity to drug, history of angioedema related to previous treatment w/ an ACE inhibitor, volume/salt depletion, renal dysfunction/disease, collagen vascular disease, renal artery stenosis, ischemic heart disease, cerebrovascular disease, left ventricular outflow obstruction, DM, pregnancy/nursing status, and possible drug interactions.

Monitoring: Monitor for hypotension, anaphylactoid reactions, angioedema, and other adverse reactions. Monitor BP, renal/hepatic function, and serum K⁺ levels. Monitor WBCs periodically in patients w/ collagen vascular disease and/or renal disease.

Counseling: Inform of pregnancy risks and instruct to notify physician as soon as possible if pregnant/planning to become pregnant; discuss treatment options in women planning to become pregnant. Instruct to d/c therapy and to immediately report signs/symptoms of angioedema. Caution about lightheadedness, especially during the 1st few days of therapy and advise to report to physician. Instruct to d/c and to consult physician if syncope occurs. Caution that excessive perspiration and dehydration may lead to excessive fall in BP; advise to consult w/ physician. Advise not to use K+ supplements or salt substitutes containing K+ w/o consulting physician. Advise patient to report any indication of infection.

Vazculep — phenylephrine hydrochloride   Rx

Class: Alpha$_1$ agonist

ADULT DOSAGE
Hypotension
Hypotension Resulting Primarily from Vasodilation in the Setting of Anesthesia:
Initial: 40-100mcg IV bolus; may administer additional boluses every 1-2 min prn
Max: 200mcg

If BP is Below Target Goal:
Initiate continuous IV infusion at a rate of 10-35mcg/min
Max: 200mcg/min

PEDIATRIC DOSAGE
Pediatric use may not have been established

DOSING CONSIDERATIONS
Renal Impairment
ESRD: Consider starting at the lower end of the recommended dose range

Hepatic Impairment
Liver Cirrhosis (Child-Pugh Class B and C): Start dosing in the recommended dose range but consider that more phenylephrine may need to be given

ADMINISTRATION
IV route
During Administration
1. Correct intravascular volume depletion
2. Correct acidosis (acidosis may reduce effectiveness of phenylephrine)

Preparation of a 100mcg/mL Sol for Bolus IV Administration
1. Withdraw 10mg (1mL of 10mg/mL) and dilute w/ 99mL of D5 Inj or 0.9% NaCl Inj
2. Withdraw an appropriate dose from the 100mcg/mL sol prior to bolus IV administration

Preparation of a Sol for Continuous IV Administration
Prepare a sol containing a final concentration of 20mcg/mL by withdrawing 10mg (1mL of 10mg/mL) and diluting w/ 500mL of D5 Inj or 0.9% NaCl Inj

STORAGE
20-25°C (68-77°F); excursions permitted to 15-30°C (59-86°F). Protect from light. Diluted Sol: Room temperature for up to 4 hrs or refrigerate for up to 24 hrs.

HOW SUPPLIED
Inj: 10mg/mL [1mL]

WARNINGS/PRECAUTIONS
Correct intravascular volume depletion and acidosis during administration. May precipitate angina in patients with severe arteriosclerosis or history of angina, exacerbate underlying HF, and increase pulmonary arterial pressure. May cause excessive peripheral and visceral vasoconstriction and ischemia to vital organs, particularly in patients with extensive peripheral vascular disease. Extravasation may cause necrosis or sloughing of tissue; check infusion site for free flow, and avoid extravasation. May cause severe bradycardia and decreased cardiac output. Contains sodium metabisulfite, which may cause allergic-type reactions, including anaphylactic symptoms and life-threatening or less severe asthmatic episodes. May increase the need for renal replacement therapy in patients with septic shock. Increasing BP response may be increased in patients with autonomic dysfunction, as may occur with spinal cord injuries. Caution in elderly.

ADVERSE REACTIONS
Reflex bradycardia, lowered cardiac output, ischemia, HTN, arrhythmias, epigastric pain, N/V, headache, blurred vision, neck pain, tremors, hypertensive crisis, dyspnea, pruritus.

DRUG INTERACTIONS
Oxytocic drugs potentiate the increasing BP effect, with the potential for hemorrhagic stroke. Increasing BP effect is increased with MAOIs, oxytocin, TCAs, angiotensin, aldosterone, atropine, steroids (eg, hydrocortisone), norepinephrine transporter inhibitors (eg, atomoxetine), and ergot alkaloids (eg, methylergonovine maleate). Increasing BP effect is decreased with α-adrenergic antagonists, PDE-5 inhibitors, mixed α- and β-receptor antagonists, calcium channel blockers (eg, nifedipine), benzodiazepines, ACE inhibitors, and centrally acting sympatholytic agents (eg, reserpine, guanfacine).

PREGNANCY AND LACTATION
Category C, caution in nursing.

MECHANISM OF ACTION
α-1 adrenergic receptor agonist; causes activation of the vascular smooth muscle cells and results in vasoconstriction.

PHARMACOKINETICS
Distribution: V$_d$=340L. **Metabolism:** Monoamine oxidase and sulfotransferase; m-hydroxymandelic acid and sulfate conjugates (major metabolites). **Elimination:** Urine (86%, 16% unchanged); T$_{1/2}$=2.5 hrs.

PATIENT CONSIDERATIONS
Assessment: Assess for arteriosclerosis, history of angina, HF, extensive peripheral vascular disease, septic shock, autonomic dysfunction, sulfite sensitivity, renal/hepatic impairment, pregnancy/nursing status, and possible drug interactions.

Monitoring: Monitor for precipitation of angina, exacerbation of HF, increased pulmonary arterial pressure, peripheral and visceral vasoconstriction and ischemia, necrosis or sloughing of tissues, bradycardia, decreased cardiac output, allergic-type reactions, and other adverse reactions. Monitor renal function. Correct intravascular volume depletion and acidosis during administration.

Counseling: Inform that certain medical conditions and medications might influence how the drug works.

Vecamyl — mecamylamine hydrochloride   Rx

Class: Ganglionic blocker

ADULT DOSAGE
Hypertension
Moderately severe to severe essential HTN and in uncomplicated cases of malignant HTN

Initial: 2.5mg bid
Titrate: May modify by increments of 2.5mg at intervals of ≥2 days
Average: 25mg/day (usually in 3 divided doses); as little as 2.5mg/day may be sufficient

PEDIATRIC DOSAGE
Pediatric use may not have been established

DOSING CONSIDERATIONS
Concomitant Medications
Other Antihypertensive Agents: Reduce dose of other antihypertensive agent and of mecamylamine; however, thiazides should be continued in their usual dose, while that of mecamylamine is decreased by ≥50%

ADMINISTRATION
Oral route

Timing of doses in relation to meals should be consistent; administration pc may cause more gradual absorption and smoother control of excessively high BP. Give the larger dose at noontime and perhaps in the evening; the morning dose should be relatively small and in some instances may be omitted.

STORAGE
20-25°C (68-77°F); excursions permitted to 15-30°C (59-86°F).

HOW SUPPLIED
Tab: 2.5mg

CONTRAINDICATIONS
Mild, moderate, labile HTN; coronary insufficiency; recent MI; uremia; glaucoma; organic pyloric stenosis; hypersensitivity to mecamylamine hydrochloride. Coadministration w/ antibiotics or sulfonamides.

WARNINGS/PRECAUTIONS
Administer w/ great discretion, if at all, when renal insufficiency is manifested by a rising or elevated BUN. CNS effects may occur; tremor, choreiform movements, mental aberrations, and convulsions occurred most often when large doses were given, especially in patients w/ cerebral or renal insufficiency. Abrupt discontinuation may cause fatal cerebral vascular accidents or acute congestive heart failure; mecamylamine should be withdrawn gradually and other antihypertensive therapy usually must be substituted. Evaluate the patient's condition carefully, especially renal and cardiovascular function. Avoid any additional impairment, which might result from added hypotension, when renal, cerebral, or coronary blood flow is deficient. Caution w/ marked cerebral and coronary arteriosclerosis or after a recent cerebral accident. Action of mecamylamine may be potentiated by excessive heat, fever, infection, hemorrhage, pregnancy, surgery, vigorous exercise, and salt depletion as a result of diminished intake or increased excretion due to diarrhea, vomiting, excessive sweating, or diuretics. Do not restrict Na+ intake during therapy; adjust dose if necessary. Urinary retention may occur; caution w/ prostatic hypertrophy, bladder neck obstruction, and urethral stricture. D/C immediately and take remedial steps if signs of paralytic ileus are present.

ADVERSE REACTIONS
Ileus, constipation, N/V, orthostatic dizziness/syncope, postural hypotension, convulsions, choreiform movements, interstitial pulmonary edema/fibrosis, urinary retention, impotence, blurred vision, weakness, fatigue.

DRUG INTERACTIONS
See Contraindications. Action of mecamylamine may be potentiated by anesthesia, other antihypertensive drugs, and alcohol.

PREGNANCY AND LACTATION
Pregnancy: Category C.
Lactation: Not for use in nursing.

MECHANISM OF ACTION
Ganglionic blocker.

PHARMACOKINETICS
Absorption: Almost complete. **Distribution:** Crosses blood-brain and placental barriers. **Excretion:** Urine (unchanged).

PATIENT CONSIDERATIONS
Assessment: Assess for hypersensitivity to drug, renal and coronary insufficiency, recent MI, uremia, glaucoma, organic pyloric stenosis, recent cerebral accident,

marked cerebral and coronary arteriosclerosis, prostatic hypertrophy, bladder neck obstruction, urethral stricture, and for any other conditions where treatment is contraindicated or cautioned. Assess pregnancy/nursing status and for possible drug interactions. Assess BP levels when patient is in the upright position.

Monitoring: Monitor for CNS effects, urinary retention, paralytic ileus, and for other adverse reactions. Monitor BP levels when patient is in the upright position.

Counseling: Inform that therapy may cause dizziness, lightheadedness, or fainting, especially when rising from a lying or sitting position. Explain that this effect may be increased by alcoholic beverages, exercise, or during hot weather. Advise that getting up slowly may help alleviate such a reaction.

VECTIBIX — panitumumab   Rx

Class: Monoclonal antibody/EGFR blocker

Dermatologic toxicities reported and were severe (NCI-CTC ≥Grade 3) in patients receiving drug monotherapy.

ADULT DOSAGE	PEDIATRIC DOSAGE
Metastatic Colorectal Cancer	Pediatric use may not have been established
Wild-Type *KRAS* (Exon 2 in Codons 12 or 13):	
As 1st line therapy in combination w/ FOLFOX, and as monotherapy following disease progression after prior treatment w/ fluoropyrimidine-, oxaliplatin-, and irinotecan-containing chemotherapy	
Usual: 6mg/kg IV infusion over 60 min, every 14 days	
If the 1st infusion is tolerated, administer subsequent infusions over 30-60 min	
Administer doses >1000mg over 90 min	

DOSING CONSIDERATIONS

Adverse Reactions

Infusion Reactions:

Mild or Moderate (Grade 1 or 2): Reduce infusion rate by 50% for the duration of that infusion

Severe: Terminate infusion; permanently d/c therapy depending on severity and/or persistence of the reaction

Dermatologic Toxicity:

Grade 3 (NCI-CTC/CTCAE) Reaction:

1st Occurrence: Withhold 1-2 doses; if reaction improves to <Grade 3, reinitiate at the original dose

2nd Occurrence: Withhold 1-2 doses; if reaction improves to <Grade 3, reinitiate at 80% of the original dose

3rd Occurrence: Withhold 1-2 doses; if reaction improves to <Grade 3, reinitiate at 60% of the original dose

4th Occurrence: Permanently d/c therapy

Grade 3 (NCI-CTC/CTCAE) Reaction Not Recovering After Withholding 1 or 2 Doses/Grade 4 Reaction: Permanently d/c therapy

ADMINISTRATION

IV infusion

Do not administer as IV push or bolus

Do not mix w/, or administer as an infusion w/, other medicinal products

Do not add other medications to sol containing panitumumab

Preparation

1. Withdraw the necessary amount of panitumumab for a dose of 6mg/kg
2. Dilute to a total volume of 100mL w/ 0.9% NaCl inj; doses >1000mg should be diluted to 150mL w/ 0.9% NaCl inj
3. Do not exceed a final concentration of 10mg/mL
4. Mix diluted sol by gentle inversion; do not shake

Administration

1. Administer using a low-protein-binding 0.2μm or 0.22μm in-line filter
2. Administer via infusion pump; flush line before and after administration w/ 0.9% NaCl inj
3. Infuse doses ≤1000mg over 60 min through a peripheral IV line or indwelling IV catheter; if 1st infusion is tolerated, administer subsequent infusions over 30-60 min
4. Administer doses >1000mg over 90 min
5. Discard any unused portion remaining in the vial

Use diluted sol w/in 6 hrs of preparation if stored at room temperature, or w/in 24 hrs of dilution if stored at 2-8°C (36-46°F)

STORAGE

2-8°C (36-46°F). Protect from direct sunlight. Do not freeze.

HOW SUPPLIED

Inj: 20mg/mL [5mL, 10mL, 20mL]

WARNINGS/PRECAUTIONS

Not indicated for treatment of patients w/ *RAS*-mutant mCRC or for whom *RAS* mutation status is unknown. Monitor for the development of inflammatory or infectious sequelae in patients who develop dermatologic or soft tissue toxicities. Life-threatening and fatal infectious complications (eg, necrotizing fasciitis,

abscesses, sepsis) and bullous mucocutaneous disease w/ blisters, erosions, and skin sloughing observed. Withhold or d/c therapy for dermatologic or soft tissue toxicity associated w/ severe or life-threatening inflammatory or infectious complications. Increased tumor progression/mortality, or lack of benefit reported in patients w/ *RAS*-mutant mCRC. Hypomagnesemia and other electrolyte disturbances reported (eg, hypokalemia); replete Mg^{2+} and other electrolytes as appropriate. Severe diarrhea and dehydration, leading to acute renal failure and other complications observed in combination w/ chemotherapy. Fatal and nonfatal pulmonary fibrosis and interstitial lung disease (ILD) reported; interrupt therapy for acute onset or worsening of pulmonary symptoms, and d/c if ILD is confirmed. Exposure to sunlight may exacerbate dermatologic toxicity; limit sun exposure during therapy. Keratitis and ulcerative keratitis reported; interrupt or d/c therapy for acute or worsening keratitis.

ADVERSE REACTIONS

Skin disorders (eg, erythema, acneiform dermatitis, pruritus, exfoliation, rash), anorexia, hypomagnesemia, paronychia, fatigue, stomatitis, N/V, diarrhea, dyspnea, cough.

DRUG INTERACTIONS

Increased mortality and toxicity in combination w/ bevacizumab and chemotherapy.

PREGNANCY AND LACTATION

Category C, not for use in nursing.

MECHANISM OF ACTION

IgG2 kappa monoclonal antibody/EGFR blocker; binds specifically to EGFR on both normal and tumor cells, and competitively inhibits binding of ligands for EGFR.

PHARMACOKINETICS

Absorption: C_{max}=213mcg/mL, AUC_{0-tau}=1306mcg•day/mL. **Elimination:** $T_{1/2}$=7.5 days.

PATIENT CONSIDERATIONS

Assessment: Assess for presence or history of interstitial pneumonitis or pulmonary fibrosis, pregnancy/nursing status, and for possible drug interactions. Obtain serum electrolyte levels (Mg^{2+}, K^+, Ca^{2+}). Assess *RAS*-mutational status in colorectal tumors and confirm the absence of a *RAS* mutation.

Monitoring: Monitor for signs/symptoms of dermatologic and soft tissue toxicities, infusion reactions, ILD, pulmonary fibrosis, keratitis/ulcerative keratitis, and other adverse reactions. Monitor electrolytes (eg, hypomagnesemia, hypocalcemia) periodically during and for up to 8 weeks after completion of therapy.

Counseling: Advise to contact physician if signs/symptoms of an infusion reaction, persistent/recurrent coughing, wheezing, dyspnea, new onset facial swelling, diarrhea, dehydration, or skin/ocular changes develop. Instruct to notify physician if pregnant or nursing. Advise of the need for adequate contraception in both males and females during and for 6 months after the last dose of therapy. Instruct to limit sun exposure (eg, use sunscreen, wear hats) during and for 2 months after the last dose of therapy.

VECTICAL — calcitriol   Rx

Class: Vitamin D analogue

ADULT DOSAGE	PEDIATRIC DOSAGE
Plaque Psoriasis	Pediatric use may not have been established
Mild to Moderate:	
Apply to affected area(s) bid (am and pm)	
Max: 200g/week	

ADMINISTRATION

Topical route

STORAGE

20-25°C (68-77°F); excursions permitted to 15-30°C (59-86°F). Do not freeze or refrigerate.

HOW SUPPLIED

Oint: 3mcg/g [5g, 100g]

WARNINGS/PRECAUTIONS

Not for oral, ophthalmic, or intravaginal use. Hypercalcemia reported; if aberrations in parameters of Ca^{2+} metabolism occur, d/c therapy until these parameters normalize. Increased absorption w/ occlusive use. Avoid excessive exposure of treated areas to natural or artificial sunlight (eg, tanning booths, sun lamps); avoid or limit phototherapy.

ADVERSE REACTIONS

Lab test abnormality, urine abnormality, psoriasis, hypercalciuria, pruritus, hypercalcemia, skin discomfort.

DRUG INTERACTIONS

Caution w/ medications known to increase serum Ca^{2+} level (eg, thiazide diuretics), Ca^{2+} supplements, or high doses of vitamin D.

PREGNANCY AND LACTATION

Category C, caution in nursing.

MECHANISM OF ACTION

Vitamin D analogue; mechanism of action in the treatment of psoriasis not established.

PATIENT CONSIDERATIONS

Assessment: Assess for known/suspected Ca^{2+} metabolism disorder, pregnancy/nursing status, and possible drug interactions.

Monitoring: Monitor for hypercalcemia, aberrations in parameters of Ca^{2+} metabolism, and other adverse reactions.

Counseling: Instruct to use ud. Instruct to apply only to areas of the skin affected by psoriasis; advise not to apply to the eyes, lips, or facial skin. Instruct to rub gently into the skin. Advise to notify their physician if adverse reactions occur. Advise to avoid excessive exposure of treated areas to sunlight, tanning booths, sun lamps, or other artificial sunlight and to inform physician about treatment if undergoing phototherapy.

VELCADE — bortezomib   Rx

Class: Proteasome inhibitor

ADULT DOSAGE

Multiple Myeloma

Initial: 1.3mg/m² IV bolus (3-5 sec) at a concentration of 1mg/mL, or SQ at a concentration of 2.5mg/mL

Previously Untreated Multiple Myeloma:
Administer in combination w/ oral melphalan and oral prednisone for nine 6-week cycles
Cycles 1-4: Administer twice weekly (Days 1, 4, 8, 11, 22, 25, 29, and 32)
Cycles 5-9: Administer once weekly (Days 1, 8, 22, and 29)

Relapsed Multiple Myeloma:
Administer twice weekly for 2 weeks (Days 1, 4, 8, and 11), followed by 10-day rest period (Days 12-21)
For extended therapy of >8 cycles, may administer on standard schedule or on a maint schedule of once weekly for 4 weeks (Days 1, 8, 15, and 22), followed by 13-day rest period (Days 23-35)

Retreatment of Relapsed Multiple Myeloma:
May start at the last tolerated dose.
Administer twice weekly (Days 1, 4, 8, and 11) every 3 weeks
Max: 8 cycles
May administer either as a single agent or in combination w/ dexamethasone

At least 72 hrs should elapse between consecutive doses

Mantle Cell Lymphoma

Initial: 1.3mg/m² IV bolus (3-5 sec) at a concentration of 1mg/mL, or SQ at a concentration of 2.5mg/mL

Previously Untreated Mantle Cell Lymphoma:
Administer in combination w/ IV rituximab, cyclophosphamide, doxorubicin, and oral prednisone (VcR-CAP) for six 3-week cycles
Administer bortezomib 1st followed by rituximab
Administer twice weekly for 2 weeks (Days 1, 4, 8, and 11), followed by a 10-day rest period on Days 12-21
For patients w/ a response 1st documented at Cycle 6, two additional VcR-CAP cycles are recommended

Relapsed Mantle Cell Lymphoma:
Administer twice weekly for 2 weeks (Days 1, 4, 8, and 11), followed by 10-day rest period (Days 12-21)
For extended therapy of >8 cycles, may administer on standard schedule

At least 72 hrs should elapse between consecutive doses

PEDIATRIC DOSAGE
Pediatric use may not have been established

DOSING CONSIDERATIONS
Hepatic Impairment
Moderate (Bilirubin >1.5-3X ULN)-Severe (Bilirubin >3X ULN): Reduce to 0.7mg/m² in the 1st cycle
Consider escalation to 1.0mg/m² or further reduction to 0.5mg/m² in subsequent cycles based on tolerability

Adverse Reactions
Combination Bortezomib, Melphalan, and Prednisone:
Prolonged Grade 4 Neutropenia or Thrombocytopenia/Thrombocytopenia w/ Bleeding Observed in Previous Cycle: Consider reduction of melphalan dose by 25% in next cycle

Platelets <30 x 10⁹/L or ANC <0.75 x 10⁹/L on a Bortezomib Dosing Day (Other Than Day 1): Withhold bortezomib dose
Several Bortezomib Doses in Consecutive Cycles Withheld Due to Toxicity:
Reduce dose by 1 dose level (from 1.3mg/m² to 1mg/m², or from 1mg/m² to 0.7mg/m²)
≥Grade 3 Nonhematological Toxicities:
Withhold therapy until symptoms resolve to Grade 1 or baseline; may be reinitiated w/ 1 dose level reduction (from 1.3mg/m² to 1mg/m², or from 1mg/m² to 0.7mg/m²)

Days 4, 8, and 11 During Cycles of Combination Bortezomib, Rituximab, Cyclophosphamide, Doxorubicin, and Prednisone Therapy:
≥Grade 3 Neutropenia, or Platelet <25 x 10⁹/L:
Withhold therapy for up to 2 weeks until the patient has an ANC ≥0.75 x 10⁹/L and platelets ≥25 x 10⁹/L
If, after bortezomib has been withheld, the toxicity does not resolve, d/c
If toxicity resolves such that the patient has an ANC ≥0.75 x 10⁹/L and platelets ≥25 x 10⁹/L, dose should be reduced by 1 dose level (from 1.3mg/m² to 1mg/m², or from 1mg/m² to 0.7mg/m²)
≥Grade 3 Nonhematological Toxicities:
Withhold therapy until symptoms of the toxicity have resolved to Grade 2 or better; may reinitiate w/ 1 dose level reduction (from 1.3mg/m² to 1mg/m², or from 1mg/m² to 0.7mg/m²)

Neuropathic Pain and/or Peripheral or Motor Neuropathy:
Grade 1 (Asymptomatic; Loss of Deep Tendon Reflexes or Paresthesia) w/o Pain or Loss of Function: No action
Grade 1 w/ Pain or Grade 2 (Moderate Symptoms; Limiting Instrumental Activities of Daily Living [ADL]): Reduce to 1mg/m²
Grade 2 w/ Pain or Grade 3 (Severe Symptoms; Limiting Self Care ADL):
Withhold therapy until toxicity resolves, then reinitiate w/ a reduced dose at 0.7mg/m² once per week
Grade 4 (Life-Threatening Consequences; Urgent Intervention Indicated): D/C therapy

Refer to PI for further dosing guidelines

ADMINISTRATION
IV/SQ route

Reconstitution
Reconstitute only w/ 0.9% NaCl; should be administered w/in 8 hrs of preparation. Different volumes of 0.9% NaCl are used to reconstitute the product for the different routes of administration.
Because each route of administration has a different reconstituted concentration, caution should be used when calculating the volume to be administered.
The reconstituted concentration for SQ administration is 2.5mg/mL when diluted w/ 1.4mL 0.9% NaCl.
The reconstituted concentration for IV administration is 1mg/mL when diluted w/ 3.5mL 0.9% NaCl.
Refer to PI for further reconstitution/preparation instructions.

STORAGE
25°C (77°F); excursions permitted to 15-30°C (59-86°F). Protect from light.
Reconstituted Sol: 25°C (77°F). May be stored in the original vial and/or the syringe prior to administration. May be stored for up to 8 hrs in a syringe; total storage time must not exceed 8 hrs when exposed to normal indoor lighting.

HOW SUPPLIED
Inj: 3.5mg

CONTRAINDICATIONS
Intrathecal administration, hypersensitivity (not including local reactions) to bortezomib, boron, or mannitol.

WARNINGS/PRECAUTIONS
Severe sensory and motor peripheral neuropathy reported; consider starting SQ therapy for patients w/ preexisting or at high risk of peripheral neuropathy. Hypotension reported. Acute development or exacerbation of CHF and new onset of decreased left ventricular ejection fraction (LVEF) reported. Isolated cases of QT interval prolongation reported. Acute respiratory distress syndrome (ARDS), acute diffuse infiltrative pulmonary disease of unknown etiology (eg, pneumonitis, interstitial pneumonia, lung infiltration), and pulmonary HTN reported; consider interrupting therapy until a prompt and comprehensive diagnostic evaluation is conducted if new or worsening cardiopulmonary symptoms develop. Posterior reversible encephalopathy syndrome (PRES) reported; d/c if PRES develops. May cause N/V, diarrhea, constipation, and ileus; antiemetic and antidiarrheal medications may be necessary. Administer fluid/electrolyte replacement therapy to prevent dehydration; interrupt for severe symptoms. Thrombocytopenia and neutropenia reported. GI and intracerebral hemorrhage occurred during thrombocytopenia; support w/ transfusions and supportive care. Tumor lysis syndrome reported. Acute liver failure reported in patients receiving multiple concomitant medications and w/ serious underlying medical conditions. Hepatic reactions, including hepatitis, increases in liver enzymes, and hyperbilirubinemia, reported; interrupt therapy to assess reversibility. Women of reproductive potential should avoid becoming pregnant while on therapy. Administer therapy after dialysis procedure. Consider retreatment in patients w/ multiple myeloma who had previously responded to treatment and have relapsed at least 6 months after completing prior therapy. Caution in elderly.

ADVERSE REACTIONS
Thrombocytopenia, neutropenia, N/V, peripheral neuropathy, diarrhea, anemia, constipation, pyrexia, anorexia, paresthesia, headache, dyspnea, leukopenia, fatigue.

DRUG INTERACTIONS
Avoid w/ St. John's wort. Efficacy may be reduced w/ strong CYP3A4 inducers (eg, rifampin); concomitant use is not recommended. Oral antidiabetic agents may

require dosage adjustment. Ketoconazole may increase exposure; monitor for signs of bortezomib toxicity and consider bortezomib dose reduction when given w/ strong CYP3A4 inhibitors (eg, ketoconazole, ritonavir). May increase exposure to drugs that are CYP2C19 substrates.

PREGNANCY AND LACTATION
Pregnancy: Category D.
Lactation: Not for use in nursing.

MECHANISM OF ACTION
Proteasome inhibitor; reversibly inhibits chymotrypsin-like activity of the 26S proteasome in cells.

PHARMACOKINETICS
Absorption: Administration via different routes resulted in different pharmacokinetic parameters. **Distribution:** V_d=498-1884L/m^2; plasma protein binding (83%). **Metabolism:** Oxidation via CYP3A4, 2C19, 1A2; 2D6, 2C9 (minor); deboronation (major pathway). **Elimination:** (IV) $T_{1/2}$ =40-193 hrs (1mg/m^2), 76-108 hrs (1.3mg/m^2).

PATIENT CONSIDERATIONS
Assessment: Assess for peripheral neuropathy, history of syncope, dehydration, risk factors for or existing heart disease, diabetes mellitus, hepatic/renal impairment, any conditions where treatment is contraindicated or cautioned, pregnancy/nursing status, and possible drug interactions. Obtain baseline BP, CBCs, and then platelet count prior to each dose.

Monitoring: Monitor for signs/symptoms of new/worsening peripheral neuropathy, hypotension, CHF, decreased LVEF, new or worsening cardiopulmonary symptoms, PRES, N/V, diarrhea, constipation, ileus, tumor lysis syndrome, hepatic toxicity, and other adverse reactions. Closely monitor patients w/ risk factors for or existing heart disease. Monitor LFTs. Monitor CBCs and blood glucose levels (in diabetics) frequently.

Counseling: Inform that therapy may cause fatigue, dizziness, syncope, orthostatic/postural hypotension; advise not to drive or operate heavy machinery if any of these symptoms develop. Advise how to avoid dehydration. Instruct to seek medical advice if symptoms of dizziness, lightheadedness, fainting spells, or muscle cramps are experienced. Advise to use effective contraceptive measures to prevent pregnancy and instruct to inform physician immediately if patient becomes pregnant. Advise that treatment should not be received while pregnant/breastfeeding. Advise to check blood sugar frequently if taking oral antidiabetic medications and instruct to notify physician if any changes in blood sugar levels occur. Instruct to contact physician if symptoms of new/worsening peripheral neuropathy, PRES or progressive multifocal leukoencephalopathy, cardiac/respiratory/hepatic toxicity, dermal reactions, an increase in BP, bleeding, fever, constipation, or decreased appetite develops.

VELETRI — epoprostenol   Rx

Class: Prostacyclin analogue

ADULT DOSAGE
Pulmonary Arterial Hypertension

Improvement of Exercise Capacity (WHO Group I):
Initial: 2ng/kg/min IV chronic infusion
Titrate: Increase in increments of 2ng/kg/min every 15 min or longer until a tolerance limit to the drug is established or further increases in the infusion rate are not clinically warranted. Use a lower dose if initial infusion rate is not tolerated

If symptoms of PAH persist or recur, adjust the infusion by 1-2ng/kg/min increments at intervals of at least 15 min

PEDIATRIC DOSAGE
Pediatric use may not have been established

DOSING CONSIDERATIONS
Elderly
Start at lower end of dosing range

Adverse Reactions
Dose-Limiting Pharmacological Effects:
Decrease gradually in 2ng/kg/min decrements every 15 min or longer until effects resolve

Other Important Considerations
Taper doses after initiation of cardiopulmonary bypass in patients receiving lung transplants

ADMINISTRATION
IV route

Administer by continuous IV infusion via a central venous catheter using an ambulatory infusion pump; may administer peripherally during initiation of treatment
Reconstitute only ud using sterile water for inj or NaCl 0.9% inj
Do not dilute reconstituted sol or administer w/ other parenteral sol or medications; consider a multi-lumen catheter if other IV therapies are routinely administered
Refer to PI for further reconstitution, administration, and infusion rate instructions

STORAGE
20-25°C (68-77°F). Do not expose to direct sunlight. Refer to PI for storage of reconstituted sol.

HOW SUPPLIED
Inj: 0.5mg, 1.5mg

CONTRAINDICATIONS
Chronic use in patients w/ CHF due to severe left ventricular systolic dysfunction, chronic use in patients who develop pulmonary edema during dose initiation, known hypersensitivity to the drug or to structurally related compounds.

WARNINGS/PRECAUTIONS
Should be used only by clinicians experienced in the diagnosis and treatment of pulmonary HTN. Initiate therapy in a setting w/ adequate personnel and equipment for physiologic monitoring and emergency care. During dose initiation, asymptomatic increases in pulmonary artery pressure coincident w/ increases in cardiac output occurred rarely; consider dose reduction in such cases. Deliver continuously on an ambulatory basis through a permanent indwelling central venous catheter during chronic use. Unless contraindicated, administer anticoagulant therapy to reduce risk of pulmonary thromboembolism or systemic embolism through a patent foramen ovale. Abrupt withdrawal (including interruptions in drug delivery) or sudden large reductions in dosage may result in symptoms associated w/ rebound pulmonary HTN (eg, dyspnea, dizziness, asthenia); avoid abrupt withdrawal or sudden large reductions in infusion rates.

ADVERSE REACTIONS
Flushing, headache, N/V, hypotension, anxiety, nervousness, agitation, chest pain, abdominal pain, dizziness, bradycardia, anorexia, musculoskeletal pain, chills/fever/sepsis/flu-like symptoms, diarrhea.

DRUG INTERACTIONS
Additional BP reductions may occur w/ diuretics, antihypertensive agents, or other vasodilators. May increase risk of bleeding w/ other antiplatelet agents or anticoagulants. May elevate levels of digoxin.

PREGNANCY AND LACTATION
Category B, caution in nursing.

MECHANISM OF ACTION
Prostacyclin analogue; causes direct vasodilation of pulmonary and systemic arterial vascular beds and inhibition of platelet aggregation.

PHARMACOKINETICS
Metabolism: Hydrolysis, enzymatic degradation; 6-keto-PGF$_1\alpha$ and 6,15-diketo-13,14-dihydro-PGF$_1\alpha$ (primary metabolites). **Elimination:** Urine (82%), feces (4%); $T_{1/2}$ ≤6 min.

PATIENT CONSIDERATIONS
Assessment: Assess for hypersensitivity to drug, CHF due to severe left ventricular systolic dysfunction, pregnancy/nursing status, and possible drug interactions. Assess patient's capacity to accept and care for permanent IV catheter and infusion pump.

Monitoring: Monitor for signs of recurrence or worsening of pulmonary HTN, pulmonary edema, and other adverse reactions. Monitor standing and supine BP and HR closely for several hrs following dose adjustments.

Counseling: Counsel about proper reconstitution and administration of the drug; advise to adhere to sterile technique in preparing the drug and in the care of the catheter. Inform that therapy will likely be needed for prolonged periods, possibly yrs.

VELPHORO — sucroferric oxyhydroxide   Rx

Class: Phosphate binder

ADULT DOSAGE
Hyperphosphatemia

Control of serum phosphorus levels in patients w/ chronic kidney disease on dialysis

Initial: 500mg tid
Titrate: Adjust in decrements or increments of 500mg/day prn until an acceptable serum phosphorous level is reached, w/ regular monitoring afterwards; titrate as often as weekly
Usual: 1500-2000mg/day; highest daily dose studied in ESRD was 3000mg/day

Distribute the total daily dose among meals

PEDIATRIC DOSAGE
Pediatric use may not have been established

ADMINISTRATION
Oral route

Take w/ meals
Tabs must be chewed; do not swallow whole
May crush tabs to aid w/ chewing and swallowing

STORAGE
25°C (77°F); excursions permitted to 15-30°C (59-86°F). Protect from moisture.

HOW SUPPLIED
Tab, Chewable: 500mg

WARNINGS/PRECAUTIONS
Monitor effect and iron homeostasis in patients with peritonitis during peritoneal dialysis, significant gastric/hepatic disorders, following major GI surgery, or with a history of hemochromatosis or other diseases with iron accumulation.

ADVERSE REACTIONS
Diarrhea, discolored feces, nausea.

DRUG INTERACTIONS

Take oral doxycycline at least 1 hr before therapy. Do not give with oral levothyroxine. Consider separating administration of therapy and an oral medication where a reduction in the bioavailability of that medication would have a clinically significant effect on its safety or efficacy. Where possible, consider monitoring for clinical response and/or blood levels of concomitant medications that have a narrow therapeutic range.

PREGNANCY AND LACTATION

Category B, safety not known in nursing.

MECHANISM OF ACTION

Phosphate binder; in the aqueous environment of the GI tract, phosphate binding takes place by ligand exchange between hydroxyl groups and/or water in sucroferric oxyhydroxide and the phosphate in the diet. The bound phosphate is eliminated with feces. Reduced dietary phosphate absorption results in reduced serum P levels and calcium-phosphorus product levels.

PATIENT CONSIDERATIONS

Assessment: Assess for GI disorders, iron accumulation disorders, pregnancy/nursing status, and possible drug interactions.

Monitoring: Monitor effect and iron homeostasis in patients with peritonitis during peritoneal dialysis, significant gastric/hepatic disorders, following major GI surgery, or with a history of hemochromatosis or other diseases with iron accumulation. Monitor serum P levels.

Counseling: Instruct to notify physician of all medications being taken. Inform that drug may cause discolored (black) stool. If ≥1 dose is missed, instruct to resume medication with the next meal; advise to not attempt to replace a missed dose.

VELTASSA — patiromer   Rx

Class: Potassium binder

> Patiromer binds to many orally administered medications, which could decrease their absorption and reduce their effectiveness. Administer other oral medications at least 6 hrs before or 6 hrs after patiromer. If adequate dosing separation is not possible, choose patiromer or the other oral medication.

ADULT DOSAGE	**PEDIATRIC DOSAGE**
Hyperkalemia	Pediatric use may not have been established
Initial: 8.4g qd	
Titrate: May increase or decrease to reach desired serum K$^+$ concentration; may increase in increments of 8.4g based on serum K$^+$ levels at 1-week or longer intervals	
Max: 25.2g qd	

ADMINISTRATION

Oral route

Administer at least 6 hrs before or 6 hrs after other oral medications.
Take w/ food.
Do not heat (eg, microwave) or add to heated foods or liquids.
Do not take medication in its dry form.
Prepare each dose immediately prior to administration.

Preparation

1. Measure 1/3 cup of water. Pour half of the water into a glass, then add patiromer and stir.
2. Add the remaining half of the water and stir thoroughly; the powder will not dissolve and the mixture will look cloudy.
3. Add more water to the mixture as needed for desired consistency.
4. Drink mixture immediately; if powder remains after drinking, add more water, stir, and drink immediately. Repeat prn to ensure the entire dose is administered.

STORAGE

2-8°C (36-46°F). If stored at room temperature 25°C (77°F), use w/in 3 months of being taken out of the refrigerator. Avoid exposure to excessive heat >40°C (104°F).

HOW SUPPLIED

Powder: 8.4g, 16.8g, 25.2g

CONTRAINDICATIONS

History of a hypersensitivity reaction to patiromer or any components of the medication.

WARNINGS/PRECAUTIONS

Not for use as an emergency treatment for life-threatening hyperkalemia. Avoid use in patients w/ severe constipation, bowel obstruction or impaction, including abnormal postoperative bowel motility disorders; may be ineffective and worsen GI conditions. May lead to hypomagnesemia; monitor serum Mg^{2+} and consider Mg^{2+} supplementation w/ low serum Mg^{2+} levels.

ADVERSE REACTIONS

Constipation, hypomagnesemia, diarrhea, nausea, abdominal discomfort, flatulence.

DRUG INTERACTIONS

See Boxed Warning.

PREGNANCY AND LACTATION

Pregnancy: Not absorbed systemically and maternal use is not expected to result in fetal risk.

Lactation: Not absorbed systemically by the mother; breastfeeding is not expected to result in risk to infant.

MECHANISM OF ACTION

Cation-exchange polymer; increases fecal K$^+$ excretion through binding of K$^+$ in the lumen of the GI tract, which reduces the concentration of free K$^+$ in the GI lumen, resulting in a reduction of serum K$^+$ levels.

PATIENT CONSIDERATIONS

Assessment: Assess for severe constipation, bowel obstruction/impaction, pregnancy/nursing status, and possible drug interactions.

Monitoring: Monitor for hypersensitivity reactions, worsening of GI motility, serum Mg^{2+} and K$^+$ levels, and other adverse reactions.

Counseling: Advise to separate dosing of other oral medications by at least 6 hrs before or after administration of therapy. Instruct to take ud w/ food and to adhere to prescribed diets. Instruct not to heat, add to heated foods or liquids, or take in its dry form.

VELTIN — clindamycin phosphate/tretinoin   Rx

Class: Lincosamide derivative/retinoid

ADULT DOSAGE	**PEDIATRIC DOSAGE**
Acne Vulgaris	**Acne Vulgaris**
Apply pea-sized amount qpm	**≥12 Years:**
	Apply pea-sized amount qpm

ADMINISTRATION

Topical route

Gently rub the medication to lightly cover the entire affected area

STORAGE

25°C (77°F); excursions permitted to 15-30°C (59-86°F). Protect from light, heat, and freezing.

HOW SUPPLIED

Gel: (Clindamycin/Tretinoin) 1.2%/0.025% [30g, 60g]

CONTRAINDICATIONS

Regional enteritis, ulcerative colitis, or history of antibiotic-associated colitis.

WARNINGS/PRECAUTIONS

Not for PO, ophthalmic, or intravaginal use. Avoid the eyes, lips, and mucous membranes. Avoid exposure to sunlight, including sunlamps. Avoid use if sunburn is present. Daily use of sunscreen products and protective apparel are recommended. Weather extremes (eg, wind, cold) may be irritating while under treatment. Clindamycin: Systemic absorption has been demonstrated following topical use. Diarrhea, bloody diarrhea, and colitis (including pseudomembranous colitis) reported; d/c if significant diarrhea occurs. Severe colitis reported following PO or parenteral administration with an onset of up to several weeks following cessation of therapy.

ADVERSE REACTIONS

Local-site reactions (eg, dryness, irritation, exfoliation, erythema).

DRUG INTERACTIONS

Avoid with erythromycin-containing products due to possible antagonism to clindamycin. May enhance action of neuromuscular-blocking agents; use with caution. Antiperistaltic agents (eg, opiates, diphenoxylate with atropine) may prolong and/or worsen severe colitis.

PREGNANCY AND LACTATION

Category C, not for use in nursing.

MECHANISM OF ACTION

Clindamycin: Lincosamide antibiotic; binds to the 50S ribosomal subunit of susceptible bacteria and prevents elongation of peptide chains by interfering with peptidyl transfer, thereby suppressing protein synthesis. Found to have in vitro activity against *Propionibacterium acnes*. Tretinoin: Retinoid; not established; suspected to decrease the cohesiveness of follicular epithelial cells with decreased microcomedone formation. Also, stimulates mitotic activity and increased turnover of follicular epithelial cells causing extrusion of the comedones.

PHARMACOKINETICS

Absorption: Clindamycin: C$_{max}$=8.73ng/mL; T$_{max}$=4 hrs. **Distribution:** Clindamycin: Found in breast milk (orally and parenterally administered).

PATIENT CONSIDERATIONS

Assessment: Assess for regional enteritis, ulcerative colitis or history of antibiotic-associated colitis, pregnancy/nursing status, and possible drug interactions. Assess use in patients whose occupations require considerable sun exposure.

Monitoring: Monitor for signs/symptoms of diarrhea, bloody diarrhea, colitis, local skin reactions, and other adverse reactions.

Counseling: Instruct to wash face gently with mild soap and water at hs and apply a thin layer over the entire face (excluding the eyes and lips) after patting the skin dry. Advise not to use more than a pea-sized amount and not to apply more than qd (at hs). Advise to avoid exposure to sunlight, sunlamps, UV light, and other medicines that may increase sensitivity to sunlight; instruct to apply sunscreen qam and reapply over the course of the day PRN. Advise that other topical medications with a strong drying effect (eg, abrasive soaps, cleansers) may cause an increase in skin irritation. Inform that medication may cause irritation (eg, erythema, scaling, itching, burning, stinging). Instruct to d/c therapy and contact physician if severe diarrhea or GI discomfort occurs.

VENCLEXTA — venetoclax

Class: BCL-2 inhibitor

Rx

ADULT DOSAGE

Chronic Lymphocytic Leukemia

Treatment of patients w/ chronic lymphocytic leukemia (CLL) w/ 17p deletion, as detected by an FDA-approved test, who have received at least 1 prior therapy

Administer according to a weekly ramp-up schedule

Week 1: 20mg qd
Week 2: 50mg qd
Week 3: 100mg qd
Week 4: 200mg qd
Week 5 and Beyond: 400mg qd

Continue until disease progression or unacceptable toxicity is observed

Missed Dose

If a dose is missed w/in 8 hrs of the time it is usually taken, take the missed dose as soon as possible and resume the normal daily dosing schedule

If a dose is missed by >8 hrs, do not take the missed dose; resume the usual dosing schedule the next day

If vomiting occurs following dosing, no additional dose should be taken; take next dose at the usual time

PEDIATRIC DOSAGE

Pediatric use may not have been established

DOSING CONSIDERATIONS

Concomitant Medications

Strong CYP3A Inhibitors:
Initiation and Ramp-Up Phase: Contraindicated
Steady Daily Dose (After Ramp-Up Phase): Avoid inhibitor use or reduce venetoclax dose by at least 75%

Moderate CYP3A Inhibitors/P-gp Inhibitors: Avoid inhibitor use or reduce venetoclax dose by at least 50%

Resume dose that was used prior to initiating CYP3A/P-gp inhibitor 2-3 days after discontinuation of the inhibitor

Renal Impairment

CrCl <80mL/min: Increased risk of tumor lysis syndrome (TLS); may require more intensive prophylaxis and monitoring to reduce the risk of TLS when initiating therapy
Severe (CrCl <30mL/min) or on Dialysis: Recommended dose has not been determined

Hepatic Impairment

Mild or Moderate: Monitor more closely for signs of toxicity during the initiation and dose ramp-up phase
Severe: Recommended dose has not been determined

Adverse Reactions

Dose Modification for Toxicity During Treatment:

Interruption at 400mg: Restart at 300mg
Interruption at 300mg: Restart at 200mg
Interruption at 200mg: Restart at 100mg
Interruption at 100mg: Restart at 50mg
Interruption at 50mg: Restart at 20mg
Interruption at 20mg: Restart at 10mg

Continue the reduced dose for 1 week before increasing the dose during the ramp-up phase

TLS:
- Withhold the next day's dose if blood chemistry changes or symptoms suggestive of TLS develop
- Resume at the same dose if resolved w/in 24-48 hrs of the last dose
- Resume at a reduced dose if blood chemistry changes require >48 hrs to resolve
- Resume at a reduced dose following resolution for any events of clinical TLS
- Consider discontinuing venetoclax for patients who require dose reductions to <100mg for more than 2 weeks

Non-Hematologic Toxicities (Grade 3 or 4):
First Occurrence: Interrupt venetoclax; once the toxicity has resolved to Grade 1 or baseline level, may resume at the same dose; no dose modification is required
Second and Subsequent Occurrences: Interrupt venetoclax; follow "dose modification for toxicity" instructions listed above when resuming treatment w/ venetoclax after resolution; a larger dose reduction may occur at the discretion of the physician

Consider discontinuing venetoclax for patients who require dose reductions to <100mg for more than 2 weeks

Hematologic Toxicities:
Grade 3 or 4 Neutropenia w/ Infection or Fever; or Grade 4 Hematologic Toxicities (Except Lymphopenia):
First Occurrence: Interrupt venetoclax. If clinically indicated, may administer granulocyte-colony stimulating factor (G-CSF) w/ venetoclax to reduce infection risk associated w/ neutropenia. May resume at the same dose once toxicity is resolved to Grade 1 or baseline
Second and Subsequent Occurrences: Interrupt venetoclax. Consider using G-CSF as clinically indicated. Follow "dose modification for toxicity" instructions listed above when resuming treatment w/ venetoclax after resolution; a larger dose reduction may occur at the discretion of the physician

Consider discontinuing venetoclax for patients who require dose reductions to <100mg for more than 2 weeks

ADMINISTRATION

Oral route

- Take w/ a meal and water at approx the same time each day.
- Swallow tab whole; do not chew, crush, or break prior to swallowing.
- Refer to prescribing information for TLS prophylaxis recommendations.

STORAGE

≤30°C (86°F).

HOW SUPPLIED

Tab: 10mg, 50mg, 100mg

CONTRAINDICATIONS

Concomitant use w/ strong CYP3A inhibitors at initiation and during ramp-up phase.

WARNINGS/PRECAUTIONS

See Dosing Considerations. Patients w/o 17p deletion at diagnosis should be retested at relapse; acquisition of 17p deletion may occur. TLS, including fatal events and renal failure requiring dialysis, reported in previously treated CLL patients w/ high tumor burden. Assess TLS risk and administer appropriate prophylaxis for TLS. Monitor blood chemistries and manage abnormalities promptly; interrupt dosing if needed. Employ more intensive measures (IV hydration, frequent monitoring, hospitalization) as overall risk increases. Grade 3 or 4 neutropenia reported; interrupt dosing or reduce dose for severe neutropenia. Consider supportive measures including antimicrobials for signs of infection and use of growth factors (eg, G-CSF). May cause embryo-fetal harm.

ADVERSE REACTIONS

Neutropenia, diarrhea, nausea, anemia, URTI, thrombocytopenia, fatigue.

DRUG INTERACTIONS

See Dosing Considerations and Contraindications. Concomitant use w/ strong (eg, ketoconazole, conivaptan, indinavir) or moderate CYP3A inhibitors (eg, erythromycin, ciprofloxacin, diltiazem) and P-gp inhibitors (eg, amiodarone, captopril, felodipine) increases exposure and may increase the risk of TLS at initiation and during ramp-up phase. Resume the venetoclax dose that was used prior to initiating the CYP3A inhibitor or P-gp inhibitor 2-3 days after discontinuing the inhibitor. Vaccinations may be less effective; do not administer live attenuated vaccines prior to, during, or after treatment until B-cell recovery occurs. Avoid grapefruit products, Seville oranges, and starfruit during treatment. Coadministration w/ multiple doses of rifampin, a strong CYP3A inducer, decreased levels; avoid w/ strong CYP3A inducers (eg, carbamazepine, phenytoin, St. John's wort) or moderate CYP3A inducers (eg, bosentan, efavirenz, modafinil) and consider alternative treatments w/ less CYP3A induction. May increase warfarin levels; closely monitor INR. Avoid P-gp substrates w/ a narrow therapeutic index (eg, digoxin, everolimus, sirolimus); take at least 6 hrs before venetoclax if coadministration must occur.

PREGNANCY AND LACTATION

Pregnancy: May cause fetal harm.
Lactation: There are no data on the presence of venetoclax in human milk, the effects on the breastfed child, or the effects on milk production; not for use in nursing.
Reproductive Potential: Females of reproductive potential should undergo pregnancy testing before initiation of therapy and use effective contraception during treatment and for at least 30 days after the last dose. Male fertility may be compromised by treatment.

MECHANISM OF ACTION

BCL-2 inhibitor; helps restore the process of apoptosis by binding directly to the BCL-2 protein, displacing pro-apoptotic proteins like BIM, triggering mitochondrial outer membrane permeabilization and the activation of caspases.

PHARMACOKINETICS

Absorption: T_{max}=5-8 hrs (fed); C_{max}=2.1µg/mL (low-fat meal), AUC=32.8µg•hr/mL (low-fat meal). **Distribution:** Highly bound to human plasma protein; V_d=256-321L. **Metabolism:** Predominantly via CYP3A4/5; M27 (major active metabolite). **Elimination:** Feces (>99.9%, 20.8% unchanged), urine (<0.1%); $T_{1/2}$=26 hrs.

PATIENT CONSIDERATIONS

Assessment: Assess for risk of TLS, renal/hepatic impairment, pregnancy/nursing status, and for possible drug interactions. Assess for the presence of 17p deletions in blood specimens.

Monitoring: Monitor for TLS, neutropenia, and any other adverse reaction. Monitor blood chemistries and CBC.

Counseling: Advise of the risk of TLS; instruct to immediately report to physician any signs/symptoms of TLS (eg, fever, chills, N/V, confusion, shortness of breath, seizure). Advise to adequately hydrate every day (approx 6-8 glasses or 56 oz of water per day) when taking therapy; instruct to drink water starting 2 days before and on the day of the first dose, and every time the dose is increased. Inform of the importance of keeping scheduled appointments for blood work or other lab tests. Inform that it may be necessary to take in the presence of a doctor to allow monitoring for TLS. Advise to contact physician immediately if a fever or any signs of infection develop. Instruct to avoid consuming grapefruit products, Seville oranges, or starfruit during treatment. Instruct to inform physician of the use of any prescription medication, OTC drugs, vitamins, and herbal products. Advise to avoid vaccination w/ live vaccines. Inform women of the potential risk to the fetus and to avoid pregnancy during treatment; instruct to contact physician if the patient becomes pregnant, or if pregnancy is suspected, during treatment. Instruct female patients of reproductive potential to use effective contraception during therapy and for at least 30 days after completing therapy. Advise not to breastfeed while taking therapy. Inform males of reproductive potential of the possibility of infertility and the possible use of sperm banking. Instruct to take ud. Advise to keep tabs in the original packaging during the first 4 weeks of treatment, and not to transfer the tabs to a different container.

VENLAFAXINE EXTENDED RELEASE TABLETS — Rx

venlafaxine hydrochloride

Class: Serotonin and norepinephrine reuptake inhibitor (SNRI)

> Antidepressants increased the risk of suicidal thinking and behavior (suicidality) in children, adolescents, and young adults in short-term studies of major depressive disorder (MDD) and other psychiatric disorders. Monitor and observe closely for clinical worsening, suicidality, or unusual changes in behavior. Not approved for use in pediatric patients.

ADULT DOSAGE

Major Depressive Disorder

Initial: 75mg qd, or 37.5mg qd for 4-7 days and then increase to 75mg qd
Titrate: May increase by increments of up to 75mg/day at ≥4-day intervals
Max: 225mg/day

Social Anxiety Disorder

Usual: 75mg qd

Conversions

Switching from Venlafaxine Immediate-Release Tabs:
May be switched to extended-release (ER) tabs at the nearest equivalent dose (mg/day); individual dose adjustments may be necessary

Dosing Considerations with MAOIs

Switching to/from an MAOI for Psychiatric Disorders:
Allow at least 14 days between discontinuation of an MAOI and initiation of treatment, and allow at least 7 days between discontinuation of treatment and initiation of an MAOI

W/ Other MAOIs (eg, Linezolid, IV Methylene Blue):
Do not start venlafaxine in patients being treated w/ linezolid or IV methylene blue
In patients already receiving venlafaxine, if acceptable alternatives are not available and benefits outweigh risks, d/c venlafaxine and administer linezolid or IV methylene blue; monitor for serotonin syndrome for 7 days or until 24 hrs after the last dose of linezolid or IV methylene blue, whichever comes first. May resume venlafaxine therapy 24 hours after the last dose of linezolid or IV methylene blue

PEDIATRIC DOSAGE

Pediatric use may not have been established

DOSING CONSIDERATIONS

Renal Impairment

GFR=10-70mL/min: Reduce total daily dose by 25-50%
Hemodialysis: Reduce total daily dose by 50%

Hepatic Impairment

Mild to Moderate: Reduce total daily dose by 50%. May be necessary to reduce the dose even more than 50% in patients w/ cirrhosis

Discontinuation

Gradually reduce dose; if intolerable symptoms occur following a decrease in dose or upon discontinuation of treatment, may consider resuming previously prescribed dose, then may continue decreasing dose at a more gradual rate

ADMINISTRATION

Oral route
Administer in a single dose w/ food at the same time each day, either in am or pm. Swallow whole w/ fluid; do not divide, crush, chew, or place in water.

STORAGE

25°C (77°F); excursions permitted to 15-30°C (59-86°F). Protect from moisture and humidity.

HOW SUPPLIED

Tab, ER: 37.5mg, 75mg, 150mg, 225mg

CONTRAINDICATIONS

Use of an MAOI for psychiatric disorders either concomitantly or w/in 7 days of stopping treatment. Treatment w/in 14 days of stopping an MAOI for psychiatric disorders. Starting treatment in patients being treated w/ other MAOIs (eg, linezolid, IV methylene blue).

WARNINGS/PRECAUTIONS

Not approved for the treatment of bipolar depression. Serotonin syndrome reported; d/c immediately if symptoms occur and initiate supportive treatment. May cause sustained HTN; consider dose reduction or discontinuation. Pupillary dilation that occurs following use may trigger an angle-closure attack in a patient w/ anatomically narrow angles who does not have a patent iridectomy. Avoid abrupt discontinuation; gradually reduce dose and monitor for withdrawal symptoms. Treatment-emergent insomnia, nervousness, weight loss, anorexia, and activation of mania/hypomania reported. Hyponatremia may occur; consider discontinuation in patients w/ symptomatic hyponatremia. Caution w/ history of mania or seizures, diseases or conditions affecting hemodynamic responses, conditions that may be compromised by increases in HR (eg, hyperthyroidism, heart failure, recent MI), renal/hepatic impairment, and in elderly. D/C if seizures occur. May increase risk of bleeding events. Elevation of cholesterol levels reported. Interstitial lung disease and eosinophilic pneumonia rarely reported; consider this diagnosis in patients w/ progressive dyspnea, cough, or chest discomfort, and consider discontinuing therapy. False (+) urine immunoassay screening tests for phencyclidine and amphetamines reported.

ADVERSE REACTIONS

Asthenia, sweating, headache, N/V, constipation, anorexia, dry mouth, dizziness, insomnia, nervousness, somnolence, abnormal ejaculation/orgasm, abnormal dreams, pharyngitis.

DRUG INTERACTIONS

See Contraindications. May cause serotonin syndrome w/ other serotonergic drugs (eg, triptans, TCAs, fentanyl), and w/ drugs that impair metabolism of serotonin; d/c immediately if serotonin syndrome occurs. Coadministration w/ weight-loss agents is not recommended. Increased risk of hyponatremia w/ diuretics. Increased risk of bleeding w/ aspirin (ASA), NSAIDs, warfarin, and other anticoagulants or drugs known to affect coagulation. Caution w/ cimetidine in elderly and in patients w/ preexisting HTN or hepatic dysfunction. May decrease clearance of haloperidol. Increased levels w/ cimetidine and ketoconazole. May increase levels of metoprolol and desipramine. May inhibit metabolism of CYP2D6 substrates. May increase exposure of risperidone. May decrease levels of indinavir. Caution w/ metoprolol, CYP3A4 inhibitors, and CNS-active drugs. Elevated clozapine levels that were temporally associated w/ adverse reactions reported following the addition of venlafaxine. Increases in PT, PTT, or INR reported w/ warfarin.

PREGNANCY AND LACTATION

Category C, not for use in nursing.

MECHANISM OF ACTION

SNRI; believed to be associated w/ its potentiation of neurotransmitter activity in CNS by inhibiting neuronal serotonin and norepinephrine reuptake.

PHARMACOKINETICS

Absorption: Well-absorbed. Absolute bioavailability (45%). 75mg ER tabs: C_{max}=26.9ng/mL, AUC=1536.3ng•hr/mL, T_{max}=6.3 hrs; (O-desmethylvenlafaxine [ODV]) C_{max}=97.9ng/mL, AUC=2926ng•hr/mL, T_{max}=11.6 hrs. **Distribution:** Plasma protein binding (27%, 30% [ODV]); found in breast milk. **Metabolism:** Extensive. Hepatic via CYP2D6; ODV (major active metabolite). **Elimination:** Urine (87%; 5% unchanged, 29% unconjugated ODV, 26% conjugated ODV); (75mg ER tabs) $T_{1/2}$=10.7 hrs, $T_{1/2}$=12.5 hrs (ODV).

PATIENT CONSIDERATIONS

Assessment: Assess for bipolar disorder risk and history of mania, seizures, MI, unstable heart disease, HTN, hyperthyroidism, susceptibility to angle-closure glaucoma, increased intraocular pressure, drug abuse, and attempted suicide. Assess for disease/condition that alters hemodynamic response, volume depletion, hepatic/renal impairment, pregnancy/nursing status, and possible drug interactions.

Monitoring: Monitor HR, BP, hepatic/renal function, weight, and ECG changes. Monitor for signs/symptoms of clinical worsening, suicidality, unusual behavior, serotonin syndrome, sustained HTN, lung disease, abnormal bleeding, angle-closure glaucoma, hyponatremia, seizures, and other adverse reactions. Measure serum cholesterol levels during long-term treatment. If discontinued abruptly, monitor for withdrawal symptoms (eg, dysphoric mood, confusion, agitation). Periodically reevaluate long-term usefulness of therapy.

Counseling: Inform about the risks and benefits of therapy. Advise to look for emergence of unusual changes in behavior, worsening of depression, and suicidal ideation, especially early during treatment and when the dose is adjusted up or down. Caution against operating hazardous machinery (including automobiles) until reasonably certain that therapy does not adversely affect ability to engage in such activities. Advise to avoid alcohol. Advise to notify physician if allergic phenomenon develops, if pregnant/breastfeeding, or if intending to become pregnant. Instruct to notify physician if taking or planning to take any prescription or OTC drugs, including herbal preparations and nutritional supplements. Caution about the risk of serotonin syndrome. Inform that concomitant use w/ ASA, NSAIDs, warfarin, or other drugs that affect coagulation may increase the risk of bleeding. Caution about the risk of angle-closure glaucoma.

VENTOLIN HFA — albuterol sulfate

Rx

Class: Short-acting beta₂ agonist (SABA)

ADULT DOSAGE	PEDIATRIC DOSAGE
Bronchospasm	**Bronchospasm**
Treatment/Prevention:	**Treatment/Prevention:**
2 inh q4-6h or 1 inh q4h	**≥4 Years:**
	2 inh q4-6h or 1 inh q4h
Exercise-Induced Bronchospasm	**Exercise-Induced Bronchospasm**
Prevention:	**Prevention:**
2 inh 15-30 min before exercise	**≥4 Years:**
	2 inh 15-30 min before exercise

DOSING CONSIDERATIONS
Elderly
Start at lower end of dosing range

ADMINISTRATION
Oral inh route

Shake well before each spray.

Priming
Before using for 1st time, if inhaler has not been used for >2 weeks, or if it has been dropped, prime inhaler by releasing 4 sprays into air, away from face. Refer to PI for further instructions on proper use.

STORAGE
20-25°C (68-77°F); excursions permitted to 15-30°C (59-86°F). Store with mouthpiece down. Do not puncture or store near heat or open flame.

HOW SUPPLIED
MDI: 90mcg of albuterol base/inh [60, 200 inhalations]

CONTRAINDICATIONS
History of hypersensitivity to any of the ingredients.

WARNINGS/PRECAUTIONS
D/C if paradoxical bronchospasm following dosing or if cardiovascular (CV) effects occur. More doses than usual may be a marker of destabilization of asthma and may require reevaluation of the patient and treatment regimen; give special consideration to the possible need for anti-inflammatory treatment (eg, corticosteroids). ECG changes and immediate hypersensitivity reactions, including anaphylaxis, may occur. Fatalities reported with excessive use. Caution with CV disorders (eg, coronary insufficiency, arrhythmias, HTN), convulsive disorders, hyperthyroidism, diabetes mellitus (DM), and in patients unusually responsive to sympathomimetic amines. Large doses of IV albuterol reported to aggravate preexisting DM and ketoacidosis. May cause significant hypokalemia. Caution in elderly.

ADVERSE REACTIONS
Throat irritation, viral respiratory infections, upper respiratory inflammation, cough, musculoskeletal pain.

DRUG INTERACTIONS
Avoid with other short-acting sympathomimetic aerosol bronchodilators; caution with additional adrenergic drugs administered by any route. Use with β-blockers may block pulmonary effects and produce severe bronchospasm in asthmatic patients; avoid concomitant use. If needed, consider cardioselective β-blockers and use with caution. ECG changes and/or hypokalemia caused by non-K⁺-sparing diuretics (eg, loop, thiazide diuretics) may be worsened. May decrease serum digoxin levels. Use extreme caution with MAOIs and TCAs, or within 2 weeks of discontinuation of such agents.

PREGNANCY AND LACTATION
Pregnancy: Category C.
Lactation: Not for use in nursing.

MECHANISM OF ACTION
β₂-agonist; activates β₂-adrenergic receptors on airway smooth muscle, leading to the activation of adenylcyclase and to an increase in the intracellular cAMP. Increased cAMP leads to the activation of protein kinase A, which inhibits the phosphorylation of myosin and lowers intracellular ionic Ca^{2+} concentrations, resulting in relaxation of the smooth muscles of all airways, from the trachea to the terminal bronchioles.

PHARMACOKINETICS
Absorption: C_{max}=3ng/mL (1080mcg of albuterol base); T_{max}=0.42 hrs.
Elimination: $T_{1/2}$=4.6 hrs.

PATIENT CONSIDERATIONS
Assessment: Assess for history of hypersensitivity to the drug, CV disorders, convulsive disorders, hyperthyroidism, DM, pregnancy/nursing status, and possible drug interactions. Assess use in patients unusually responsive to sympathomimetic amines.

Monitoring: Monitor for paradoxical bronchospasm, deterioration of asthma, CV effects, ECG changes, hypokalemia, immediate hypersensitivity reactions, and other adverse effects. Monitor BP, HR, and blood glucose levels.

Counseling: Counsel not to increase dose/frequency of doses without consulting physician. Advise to seek immediate medical attention if treatment becomes less effective for symptomatic relief, symptoms become worse, and/or there is a need to use the product more frequently than usual. Instruct on how to properly prime, clean, and use inhaler. Instruct to take concurrent inhaled drugs and asthma medications only ud by the physician. Inform of the common adverse effects of treatment. Advise to notify physician if pregnant/nursing. Instruct to avoid spraying in eyes.

VERDESO — desonide

Rx

Class: Corticosteroid

ADULT DOSAGE	PEDIATRIC DOSAGE
Atopic Dermatitis	**Atopic Dermatitis**
Mild to Moderate:	**≥3 Months of Age:**
Apply thin layer to affected area(s) bid; dispense smallest amount necessary to adequately cover affected area(s)	**Mild to Moderate:**
	Apply thin layer to affected area(s) bid; dispense smallest amount necessary to adequately cover affected area(s)
Max Duration: 4 consecutive weeks; reassess if no improvement after 4 weeks	**Max Duration:** 4 consecutive weeks; reassess if no improvement after 4 weeks
D/C when control is achieved	D/C when control is achieved

ADMINISTRATION
Topical route

Shake can before use
Invert can to dispense foam
In treating areas of the face, dispense foam in hands and gently massage into affected areas until medication disappears; for areas other than the face, foam may be dispensed directly
Avoid w/ occlusive dressings unless directed

STORAGE
20-25°C (68-77°F); excursions permitted between 15-30°C (59-86°F). Do not puncture or incinerate. Do not expose containers to heat, and/or store at temperatures above 49°C (120°F).

HOW SUPPLIED
Foam: 0.05% [100g]

WARNINGS/PRECAUTIONS
May result in systemic absorption and effects, including hypothalamic-pituitary-adrenal (HPA) axis suppression, manifestations of Cushing's syndrome, hyperglycemia, facial swelling, glycosuria, withdrawal syndrome, and growth retardation in children. May suppress immune system if used for >4 weeks. Application over large surface areas, prolonged use, or addition of occlusive dressing may augment systemic absorption. Periodic evaluation of HPA-axis suppression may be required; gradually withdraw, reduce frequency, or substitute a less potent steroid if HPA-axis suppression is noted. Pediatric patients may be more susceptible to systemic toxicity. May cause local skin adverse reactions. D/C and institute appropriate therapy if irritation develops. Institute an appropriate antifungal, antibacterial, or antiviral agent if concomitant skin infections are present or develop; if no prompt favorable response, may need to d/c until infection is controlled. Flammable; avoid fire, flame, and/or smoking during and immediately following application. Cosyntropin (adrenocorticotropic hormone₁₋₂₄) stimulation test may be helpful in evaluating for HPA-axis suppression. Avoid contact with eyes or other mucous membranes. If used during lactation, do not apply on the chest to avoid accidental ingestion by infant. Caution in elderly. Not for oral, ophthalmic, or intravaginal use.

ADVERSE REACTIONS
URTI, cough, application-site burning.

DRUG INTERACTIONS
Caution with concomitant topical corticosteroids; may produce cumulative effect.

PREGNANCY AND LACTATION
Category C, caution in nursing.

MECHANISM OF ACTION
Corticosteroid; has not been established. Plays a role in cellular signaling, immune function, inflammation, and protein regulation.

PHARMACOKINETICS
Absorption: Percutaneous; extent of absorption is determined by product formulation, integrity of the epidermal barrier, and age. **Distribution:** Found in breast milk (systemically administered). **Metabolism:** Liver. **Elimination:** Kidneys, bile.

PATIENT CONSIDERATIONS
Assessment: Assess for skin infections, pregnancy/nursing status, and for possible drug interactions.

Monitoring: Monitor for signs/symptoms of HPA-axis suppression, Cushing's syndrome, hyperglycemia, facial swelling, glycosuria, withdrawal syndrome, growth retardation, delayed weight gain, and intracranial HTN in children. Monitor for irritation, concomitant skin infections, and other adverse reactions. Perform periodic monitoring of HPA-axis suppression if medication is used over large BSA, used with occlusive dressing, or with prolonged use of drug. Reassess diagnosis if no improvement is seen within 4 weeks.

Counseling: Instruct to use externally and ud. Advise not to use for any disorder other than that for which it was prescribed. Instruct to avoid contact with eyes or other mucous membranes. Instruct to not bandage, cover, or wrap treated skin area so as to be occlusive unless directed. Counsel to report any signs of local or systemic adverse reactions. Instruct to inform physician about the treatment if surgery is contemplated. Advise to d/c therapy when control is achieved; instruct to contact physician if no improvement seen within 4 weeks. Instruct not to use other corticosteroid-containing products while on medication without consulting the physician. Inform that medication is flammable; avoid fire, flame, or smoking during and immediately after application.

VERELAN — verapamil hydrochloride   Rx

Class: Calcium channel blocker (CCB) (nondihydropyridine)

ADULT DOSAGE

Hypertension

Usual: 240mg qam
Titrate:
If inadequate response w/ 120mg, increase to 180mg qam, then 240mg qam, then 360mg qam, then 480mg qam based on therapeutic efficacy and safety evaluated approx 24 hrs after dosing

Switching from Immediate-Release Verapamil:
Use same total daily dose

PEDIATRIC DOSAGE

Pediatric use may not have been established

DOSING CONSIDERATIONS

Hepatic Impairment
Severe Liver Dysfunction: Give 30% of normal dose

Elderly/Small People
Initial: 120mg qam

ADMINISTRATION

Oral route

Take in am
Swallow whole; do not crush or chew
May sprinkle on spoonful of applesauce; swallow immediately w/o chewing; follow w/ a glass of cool water

STORAGE

20-25°C (68-77°F). Avoid excessive heat. Brief digressions >25°C, while not detrimental, should be avoided. Protect from moisture.

HOW SUPPLIED

Cap, Sustained-Release: 120mg, 180mg, 240mg, 360mg

CONTRAINDICATIONS

Severe left ventricular dysfunction, hypotension (systolic BP <90mmHg) or cardiogenic shock, sick sinus syndrome or 2nd/3rd-degree atrioventricular (AV) block (except in patients w/ a functioning artificial ventricular pacemaker), A-fib/A-flutter and an accessory bypass tract (eg, Wolff-Parkinson-White, Lown-Ganong-Levine syndromes), known hypersensitivity to verapamil hydrochloride.

WARNINGS/PRECAUTIONS

May cause CHF, pulmonary edema, hypotension, asymptomatic 1st-degree AV block, transient bradycardia, and PR interval prolongation. Marked 1st-degree block or progressive development to 2nd/3rd-degree AV block requires dose reduction, or discontinuation and institution of appropriate therapy. Elevated transaminases with and without concomitant elevation in alkaline phosphatase and bilirubin reported. Hepatocellular injury reported. Ventricular response/fibrillation has occurred in patients with paroxysmal and/or chronic A-fib/A-flutter and a coexisting accessory AV pathway. Sinus bradycardia, pulmonary edema, severe hypotension, 2nd-degree AV block, and sinus arrest reported in patients with hypertrophic cardiomyopathy. Caution with hepatic/renal impairment. May decrease neuromuscular transmission in patients with Duchenne's muscular dystrophy and may cause worsening of myasthenia gravis; decrease dose with attenuated neuromuscular transmission.

ADVERSE REACTIONS

Constipation, dizziness, headache, lethargy.

DRUG INTERACTIONS

Increased levels with CYP3A4 inhibitors (eg, erythromycin, ritonavir) and grapefruit juice. Decreased levels with CYP3A4 inducers (eg, rifampin). Hypotension, bradyarrhythmias, and lactic acidosis reported with telithromycin. May cause myopathy/rhabdomyolysis with HMG-CoA reductase inhibitors that are CYP3A4 substrates; limit dose of simvastatin to 10mg/day or lovastatin to 40mg/day, and may need to lower doses of other CYP3A4 substrates (eg, atorvastatin). Additive negative effects on HR, AV conduction, and contractility with β-blockers; avoid with ventricular dysfunction. Asymptomatic bradycardia with atrial pacemaker has been observed with concomitant use of timolol eye drops. Decreased metoprolol clearance reported. Sinus bradycardia resulting in hospitalization and pacemaker insertion has been reported with the use of clonidine; monitor HR. Chronic treatment may increase digoxin levels, which may result in digitalis toxicity. Additive effects with other antihypertensives (eg, vasodilators, ACE inhibitors, diuretics). Excessive reduction in BP with agents that attenuate α-adrenergic function (eg, prazosin). Avoid disopyramide within 48 hrs before or 24 hrs after verapamil. Additive negative inotropic effect and AV conduction prolongation with flecainide. Avoid combined therapy with quinidine with hypertrophic cardiomyopathy. May increase levels of carbamazepine, cyclosporine, and alcohol. Increased bleeding time with aspirin. Cimetidine may either reduce or not change clearance. May increase sensitivity to neurotoxic effects of lithium; monitor lithium levels. Rifampin may reduce oral bioavailability. Increased clearance with phenobarbital. Caution with inhalation anesthetics. May potentiate neuromuscular blockers; both agents may need dose reduction.

PREGNANCY AND LACTATION

Category C, not for use in nursing.

MECHANISM OF ACTION

Calcium channel blocker (nondihydropyridine); modulates the influx of Ca^{2+} across the cell membrane of arterial smooth muscle as well as in conductile and contractile myocardial cells.

PHARMACOKINETICS

Absorption: Administration of variable doses resulted in different pharmacokinetic parameters. T_{max}=7-9 hrs. (IR) Absolute bioavailability (20-35%). **Distribution:** Plasma protein binding (90%); crosses placenta, found in breast milk. **Metabolism:** Liver (extensive), norverapamil (metabolite). **Elimination:** Urine (70% metabolites, 3-4% unchanged), feces (≥16% metabolite); $T_{1/2}$=12 hrs.

PATIENT CONSIDERATIONS

Assessment: Assess for ventricular dysfunction, cardiac failure symptoms, cardiogenic shock, sick sinus syndrome, hypertrophic cardiomyopathy, Duchenne's muscular dystrophy, attenuated neuromuscular transmission, and/or any conditions where treatment is contraindicated or cautioned, pregnancy/nursing status, and possible drug interactions.

Monitoring: Monitor signs/symptoms of hypotension, CHF, heart block, ventricular fibrillation, renal/hepatic dysfunction, abnormal prolongation of PR interval, hypersensitivity reactions, and other adverse reactions. Periodically monitor LFTs, BP, ECG changes, and HR.

Counseling: Counsel to take ud. Advise to seek medical attention if any adverse reactions occur. Counsel not to breastfeed and to report immediately if pregnant.

VERELAN PM — verapamil hydrochloride   Rx

Class: Calcium channel blocker (CCB) (nondihydropyridine)

ADULT DOSAGE

Hypertension

Usual: 200mg qhs
If Inadequate Response w/ 200mg:
May titrate upward to 300mg qhs, then 400mg qhs

Upward titration should be based on the therapeutic efficacy and safety evaluated approx 24 hrs after dosing

PEDIATRIC DOSAGE

Pediatric use may not have been established

DOSING CONSIDERATIONS

Renal Impairment
Initial: 100mg qhs

Hepatic Impairment
Initial: 100mg qhs

Elderly/Low Weight
Initial: 100mg qhs

ADMINISTRATION

Oral route

Swallow whole; do not crush or chew
May sprinkle on 1 tbsp of applesauce; swallow immediately w/o chewing; follow w/ a glass of cool water

STORAGE

25°C (77°F); excursions permitted to 15-30°C (59-86°F). Protect from moisture.

HOW SUPPLIED

Cap, Extended-Release: 100mg, 200mg, 300mg

CONTRAINDICATIONS

Severe left ventricular dysfunction, hypotension (systolic BP <90mmHg), cardiogenic shock, sick sinus syndrome or 2nd/3rd-degree atrioventricular (AV) block (except in patients with a functioning artificial ventricular pacemaker), and patients with A-fib/A-flutter and an accessory bypass tract (eg, Wolff-Parkinson-White, Lown-Ganong-Levine syndromes).

WARNINGS/PRECAUTIONS

May cause CHF, pulmonary edema, hypotension, asymptomatic 1st-degree AV block, transient bradycardia, and PR interval prolongation. Marked 1st-degree block or progressive development to 2nd/3rd-degree AV block requires dose reduction, or discontinuation and institution of appropriate therapy. Elevated transaminases with and without concomitant elevations in alkaline phosphatase and bilirubin reported. Hepatocellular injury reported. Ventricular response/fibrillation has occurred in patients with paroxysmal and/or chronic A-flutter or A-fib and a coexisting accessory AV pathway with IV verapamil. Sinus bradycardia, pulmonary edema, severe hypotension, 2nd-degree AV block, and sinus arrest reported in patients with hypertrophic cardiomyopathy. Caution with hepatic/renal impairment. May decrease neuromuscular transmission in patients with Duchenne's muscular dystrophy and cause worsening of myasthenia gravis; decrease dose with attenuated neuromuscular transmission.

ADVERSE REACTIONS

Headache, infection, constipation, flu syndrome, peripheral edema, dizziness, pharyngitis, sinusitis.

DRUG INTERACTIONS

May increase levels with CYP3A4 inhibitors (eg, erythromycin, ritonavir) and grapefruit juice. May decrease levels with CYP3A4 inducers (eg, rifampin). May cause myopathy/rhabdomyolysis with HMG-CoA reductase inhibitors that are CYP3A4 substrates; limit dose of simvastatin to 10mg/day or lovastatin to 40mg/day, and may need to lower doses of other CYP3A4 substrates (eg, atorvastatin). Additive negative effects on HR, AV conduction, and/or cardiac contractility with β-blockers; avoid in patients with ventricular dysfunction treated with β-blockers. Asymptomatic bradycardia with a wandering atrial pacemaker has been observed with concomitant use of timolol eye drops. Decreased metoprolol and propranolol clearance and variable effect with atenolol reported. Chronic treatment may increase digoxin levels, which may result in digitalis toxicity.

Sinus bradycardia resulting in hospitalization and pacemaker insertion reported with the use of clonidine; monitor HR. Hypotension, bradyarrhythmias, and lactic acidosis may occur with concurrent telithromycin use. Reduced absorption with cyclophosphamide, oncovin, procarbazine, prednisone (COPP) and vindesine, adriamycin, cisplatin (VAC) cytotoxic drug regimens. May decrease clearance of paclitaxel. May increase levels of doxorubicin, carbamazepine, cyclosporine, theophylline, and alcohol. May increase bleeding time with aspirin. Additive effects with other antihypertensives (eg, vasodilators, ACE inhibitors, diuretics). Excessive reduction in BP with agents that attenuate α-adrenergic function (eg, prazosin). Avoid combined therapy with quinidine in patients with hypertrophic cardiomyopathy. Avoid disopyramide within 48 hrs before or 24 hrs after administration. Additive negative inotropic effect and AV conduction prolongation with flecainide. May increase sensitivity to neurotoxic effects of lithium with or without an increase in serum lithium levels; monitor carefully. Caution with inhalation anesthetics; titrate slowly to avoid excessive cardiovascular depression. May potentiate neuromuscular blockers (eg, curare-like and depolarizing); both agents may need dose reduction. Increased clearance with phenobarbital. Reduced oral bioavailability with rifampin. Reduced or unchanged clearance with cimetidine.

PREGNANCY AND LACTATION
Category C, not for use in nursing.

MECHANISM OF ACTION
Calcium channel blocker (nondihydropyridine); inhibits transmembrane influx of ionic Ca^{2+} into arterial smooth muscle as well as in conductile and contractile myocardial cells without altering serum Ca^{2+} concentrations.

PHARMACOKINETICS
Absorption: Administration of variable doses resulted in different pharmacokinetic parameters. T_{max}=11 hrs. (Immediate-release) Bioavailability (33-65% [R-enantiomer], 13-34% [S-enantiomer]). **Distribution:** Plasma protein binding (94% to albumin and 92% to α-1 acid glycoprotein [R-enantiomer], 88% to albumin and 86% to α-1 acid glycoprotein [S-enantiomer]); crosses placenta, found in breast milk. **Metabolism:** Liver (extensive); O-demethylation, N-dealkylation via CYP450; norverapamil (active metabolite). **Elimination:** Urine (70%, metabolites, 3-4%, unchanged), feces (≥16%, metabolites).

PATIENT CONSIDERATIONS
Assessment: Assess for ventricular dysfunction, cardiac failure symptoms, cardiogenic shock, sick sinus syndrome, hypertrophic cardiomyopathy, Duchenne's muscular dystrophy, attenuated neuromuscular transmission, any conditions where treatment is contraindicated or cautioned, pregnancy/nursing status, and possible drug interactions.

Monitoring: Monitor signs/symptoms of hypotension, CHF, heart block, ventricular fibrillation, renal/hepatic dysfunction, abnormal prolongation of PR interval, hypersensitivity, and other adverse reactions. Periodically monitor LFTs, BP, ECG changes, and HR.

Counseling: Advise to seek medical attention if any adverse reactions occur. Counsel not to breastfeed, and to report immediately if pregnant.

VERSACLOZ — clozapine   Rx
Class: Atypical antipsychotic

> Severe neutropenia, defined as an ANC <500/μL, reported; may lead to serious infection and death. Prior to initiating treatment, a baseline ANC must be ≥1500/μL for the general population, and ≥1000/μL for patients w/ documented benign ethnic neutropenia (BEN). Regularly monitor ANC during treatment. Available only through a restricted program under a Risk Evaluation and Mitigation Strategy (REMS) called the Clozapine REMS program. Orthostatic hypotension, bradycardia, syncope, and cardiac arrest reported; risk is highest during the initial titration period, particularly w/ rapid dose escalation. Caution w/ cardiovascular (CV)/cerebrovascular disease or conditions predisposing to hypotension (eg, dehydration, use of antihypertensives). Seizures reported and risk is dose related; caution w/ history of seizures or other predisposing risk factors for seizure (eg, CNS pathology, medications that lower seizure threshold, alcohol abuse). Fatal myocarditis and cardiomyopathy reported; d/c and obtain cardiac evaluation upon suspicion of these reactions. Do not rechallenge patients w/ clozapine-related myocarditis or cardiomyopathy. Elderly patients w/ dementia-related psychosis treated w/ antipsychotic drugs are at an increased risk of death. Not approved for the treatment of dementia-related psychosis.

ADULT DOSAGE
Schizophrenia

Treatment of severely ill patients w/ schizophrenia who fail to respond adequately to standard antipsychotic treatment. Risk reduction of recurrent suicidal behavior in patients w/ schizophrenia or schizoaffective disorder who are judged to be at chronic risk for reexperiencing suicidal behavior

Initial: 12.5mg qd or bid
Titrate: May increase total daily dose in increments of 25-50mg/day, if well tolerated
Target Dose: 300-450mg/day (in divided doses) by the end of 2 weeks. Subsequently, may increase dose once weekly or twice weekly, in increments of up to 100mg
Max: 900mg/day

PEDIATRIC DOSAGE
Pediatric use may not have been established

Patients responding to treatment should generally continue maint treatment on their effective dose beyond the acute episode

Reinitiation of Treatment:
When restarting in patients who have discontinued clozapine (≥2 days since last dose), reinitiate w/ 12.5mg qd or bid; if well tolerated, may increase to previous therapeutic dose more quickly than recommended for initial treatment

---

DOSING CONSIDERATIONS
Concomitant Medications
Strong CYP1A2 Inhibitors:
During coadministration, use 1/3 of clozapine dose; when discontinuing comedication, increase clozapine dose based on clinical response

Moderate or Weak CYP1A2 Inhibitors:
During coadministration, monitor for adverse reactions and consider reducing clozapine dose if necessary; when discontinuing comedication, monitor for lack of effectiveness and consider increasing clozapine dose if necessary

CYP2D6 or CYP3A4 Inhibitors:
During coadministration, monitor for adverse reactions and consider reducing clozapine dose if necessary; when discontinuing comedication, monitor for lack of effectiveness and consider increasing clozapine dose if necessary

Strong CYP3A4 Inducers:
Concomitant use is not recommended; however, if the inducer is necessary, may need to increase clozapine dose and monitor for decreased effectiveness. When discontinuing comedication, reduce clozapine dose based on clinical response

Moderate or Weak CYP1A2 or CYP3A4 Inducers:
During coadministration, monitor for decreased effectiveness and consider increasing clozapine dose if necessary; when discontinuing comedication, monitor for adverse reactions and consider reducing clozapine dose if necessary

Renal Impairment
May need to reduce dose w/ significant renal impairment

Hepatic Impairment
May need to reduce dose w/ significant hepatic impairment

Discontinuation
Method of treatment discontinuation will vary depending on patient's last ANC:
1. If abrupt treatment discontinuation is necessary due to moderate-severe neutropenia, refer to PI for appropriate ANC monitoring based on the level of neutropenia
2. If termination of therapy is planned and there is no evidence of moderate-severe neutropenia, reduce dose gradually over 1-2 weeks
3. For abrupt discontinuation for a reason unrelated to neutropenia, continue existing ANC monitoring for general population patients until ANC is ≥1500/μL and for BEN patients until ANC is ≥1000/μL or above baseline
4. During the 2 weeks after discontinuation, additional ANC monitoring is required for any patient reporting onset of fever (temperature of ≥38.5°C [≥101.3°F])

Other Important Considerations
CYP2D6 Poor Metabolizers:
May need to reduce dose

ADMINISTRATION
Oral route

Administer in divided doses.
May be taken w/ or w/o food.
Administer by the oral syringes provided (1mL or 9mL).
Shake bottle for 10 sec prior to each use.
Administer prescribed dose immediately after it is prepared; do not draw a dose and store it in the syringe for later use.

STORAGE
Store at or below 25°C (77°F). Do not refrigerate or freeze. Protect from light. Stable for 100 days after initial bottle opening.

HOW SUPPLIED
Oral Sus: 50mg/mL [100mL]

CONTRAINDICATIONS
History of serious hypersensitivity to clozapine (eg, photosensitivity, vasculitis, erythema multiforme, or Stevens-Johnson Syndrome) or any other component of this product.

WARNINGS/PRECAUTIONS
In general, do not rechallenge patients who develop severe neutropenia w/ clozapine; for some patients, the risk of serious psychiatric illness from discontinuing treatment may be greater than the risk of rechallenge. Eosinophilia may occur and may be associated w/ myocarditis, pancreatitis, hepatitis, colitis, and nephritis. Evaluate promptly for signs/symptoms of systemic reactions if eosinophilia develops and d/c immediately if clozapine-related systemic disease is suspected. QT prolongation, torsades de pointes, and other life-threatening ventricular arrhythmias, cardiac arrest, and sudden death reported. D/C if QTc interval exceeds 500 msec or symptoms consistent w/ torsades de pointes or other arrhythmias develop. Caution in patients at risk for significant electrolyte disturbance, particularly hypokalemia; correct electrolyte abnormalities before initiating treatment. Associated w/ metabolic changes (eg, hyperglycemia sometimes associated w/ ketoacidosis or hyperosmolar coma, dyslipidemia, weight gain) that may increase CV and cerebrovascular risk. Neuroleptic malignant syndrome (NMS) reported; d/c therapy immediately

and institute symptomatic treatment. Transient fever may occur and may necessitate discontinuing treatment; carefully evaluate patients to rule out severe neutropenia or infection, and consider the possibility of NMS. Pulmonary embolism (PE), deep vein thrombosis (DVT), and tardive dyskinesia (TD) reported; consider discontinuation if TD occurs. Has potent anticholinergic effects; may result in CNS and peripheral anticholinergic toxicity. Caution w/ narrow-angle glaucoma, prostatic hypertrophy, or other conditions in which anticholinergic effects can lead to significant adverse reactions. May result in GI adverse reactions (eg, constipation, intestinal obstruction, fecal impaction, paralytic ileus). May impair mental/physical abilities. Consider dose reduction if sedation, or impairment of cognitive/motor performance occurs. Caution in patients w/ risk factors for cerebrovascular adverse reactions. If abrupt discontinuation is necessary, monitor carefully for the recurrence of psychotic symptoms and adverse reactions related to cholinergic rebound (eg, profuse sweating, headache, N/V, diarrhea). Caution in elderly. Refer to PI for treatment recommendations based on ANC monitoring for the general patient population and for patients w/ BEN.

ADVERSE REACTIONS
CNS reactions (eg, sedation, dizziness/vertigo, headache, tremor), CV reactions (eg, tachycardia, hypotension, syncope), autonomic nervous system reactions (eg, hypersalivation, sweating, dry mouth, visual disturbances), GI reactions (eg, constipation, nausea), fever.

DRUG INTERACTIONS
See Boxed Warning and Dosing Considerations. Caution w/ drugs that are inducers or inhibitors of CYP1A2, CYP3A4, and CYP2D6. CYP1A2 inhibitors (eg, fluvoxamine, ciprofloxacin, oral contraceptives), CYP2D6 or CYP3A4 inhibitors (eg, cimetidine, escitalopram, erythromycin) may increase levels, potentially resulting in adverse reactions. CYP1A2 (eg, tobacco) or CYP3A4 inducers (eg, carbamazepine, phenytoin, St. John's wort) may decrease levels, resulting in decreased effectiveness. Caution w/ medications that prolong the QT interval (eg, ziprasidone, erythromycin, quinidine) or inhibit the metabolism of clozapine. Use caution when coadministering w/ other drugs metabolized by CYP2D6 (eg, phenothiazines, carbamazepine, propafenone) and may be necessary to use lower doses of such drugs; concomitant use may increase levels these CYP2D6 substrates. Caution w/ anticholinergic medications. NMS reported w/ CNS-active medications, including lithium. If used concurrently w/ an agent known to cause neutropenia (eg, some chemotherapeutic agents), consider monitoring more closely than the treatment guidelines.

PREGNANCY AND LACTATION
Pregnancy: Category B.
Lactation: Not for use in nursing.

MECHANISM OF ACTION
Atypical antipsychotic; tricyclic dibenzodiazepine derivative. Has not been established. Efficacy proposed to be mediated through antagonism of the dopamine type 2 and the serotonin type 2A receptors. Also acts as an antagonist at adrenergic, cholinergic, histaminergic, and other dopaminergic and serotonergic receptors.

PHARMACOKINETICS
Absorption: (100mg-800mg qd) C_{max}=275ng/mL; T_{max}=2.2 hrs. **Distribution:** Plasma protein binding (97%); found in breast milk. **Metabolism:** CYP1A2, CYP2D6, CYP3A4; demethylation, hydroxylation, N-oxidation. Norclozapine (limited activity). **Elimination:** Urine (50%), feces (30%); $T_{1/2}$=8 hrs (75mg single dose), 12 hrs (100mg bid).

PATIENT CONSIDERATIONS
Assessment: Assess for hypersensitivity to drug, history of seizures or other predisposing factors for seizure, risk factors for QT prolongation and serious CV reactions, narrow-angle glaucoma, prostatic hypertrophy, renal/hepatic impairment, any other conditions where treatment is cautioned, pregnancy/nursing status, and possible drug interactions. Obtain baseline ANC, lipid evaluations, ECG, and serum chemistry panel (K^+ and Mg^{2+}). Obtain baseline FPG in patients w/ diabetes mellitus (DM) or at risk for DM.

Monitoring: Monitor for signs/symptoms of severe neutropenia, orthostatic hypotension, bradycardia, syncope, cardiac arrest, seizures, myocarditis, cardiomyopathy, cognitive/motor impairment, eosinophilia, NMS, recurrence of psychosis and cholinergic rebound after abrupt discontinuation, metabolic changes (hyperglycemia, DM, dyslipidemia, weight gain), QT interval prolongation, fever, PE, DVT, TD, cerebrovascular adverse reactions, and other adverse reactions. Monitor serum electrolyte levels, glucose control in patients w/ DM and periodic FPG levels if at risk for hyperglycemia. Monitor ANC regularly to continue treatment; refer to PI for monitoring frequency.

Counseling: Inform about benefits/risks of therapy. Advise about risk of developing severe neutropenia and infection. Instruct to immediately report any sign/symptom of infection occurring at any time during therapy. Inform that drug is available only through a restricted program called the Clozapine REMS Program designed to ensure the required blood monitoring; advise of the importance of having blood tested ud. Inform about risks of orthostatic hypotension and syncope, especially during the period of initial dose titration; instruct to strictly follow the instructions of the physician for dosage and administration. Advise to consult physician immediately if patients feel faint, lose consciousness, or have signs/symptoms suggestive of bradycardia or arrhythmia. Inform about significant risk of seizure during therapy; caution about driving and any other potentially hazardous activity while taking treatment. Instruct to inform physician if taking clozapine before any new drug. Educate about the risk of metabolic changes and the need for specific monitoring. If dose was missed for >2 days, instruct not to restart medication at same dose but to contact physician for dosing instructions. Advise to notify physician if taking/planning to take any prescription or OTC drugs. Instruct to notify physician if pregnant/intending to become pregnant during therapy. Advise not to breastfeed if taking the drug.

VESICARE — solifenacin succinate   Rx
Class: Muscarinic antagonist

ADULT DOSAGE	PEDIATRIC DOSAGE
Overactive Bladder	Pediatric use may not have been established
Usual: 5mg qd	
Titrate: May increase to 10mg qd if 5mg dose is well tolerated	

DOSING CONSIDERATIONS
Concomitant Medications
Potent CYP3A4 Inhibitors:
Max: 5mg qd

Renal Impairment
CrCl <30mL/min:
Max: 5mg qd

Hepatic Impairment
Moderate (Child-Pugh B):
Max: 5mg qd
Moderate (Child-Pugh C):
Not recommended

ADMINISTRATION
Oral route

Take w/ water and swallow whole, w/ or w/o food.

STORAGE
25°C (77°F); excursions permitted from 15-30°C (59-86°F).

HOW SUPPLIED
Tab: 5mg, 10mg

CONTRAINDICATIONS
Urinary/gastric retention, uncontrolled narrow-angle glaucoma, hypersensitivity to the drug.

WARNINGS/PRECAUTIONS
Not recommended with severe hepatic impairment (Child-Pugh C). Angioedema of the face, lips, tongue, and/or larynx, and rare anaphylactic reactions reported; d/c and provide appropriate therapy. Risk of urinary retention. Caution with decreased GI motility, controlled narrow-angle glaucoma, renal/hepatic impairment, and history of QT prolongation. CNS anticholinergic effects (eg, headache, confusion, hallucinations, somnolence) reported; may impair mental/physical abilities. Monitor for signs of anticholinergic CNS effects, particularly after beginning treatment or increasing the dose; consider dose reduction or discontinuation if such effects occur.

ADVERSE REACTIONS
Dry mouth, constipation, nausea, dyspepsia, UTI, blurred vision.

DRUG INTERACTIONS
See Dosing Considerations. Ketoconazole, a potent CYP3A4 inhibitor, may increase levels. CYP3A4 inducers may decrease concentrations. Caution with medications known to prolong the QT interval.

PREGNANCY AND LACTATION
Pregnancy: Category C.
Lactation: Not for use in nursing.

MECHANISM OF ACTION
Muscarinic receptor antagonist; inhibits muscarinic receptors, which mediate contractions of urinary bladder smooth muscle and stimulation of salivary secretion.

PHARMACOKINETICS
Absorption: Absolute bioavailability (90%); C_{max}=32.3ng/mL (5mg), 62.9ng/mL (10mg); T_{max}=3-8 hrs. **Distribution:** V_d=600L; plasma protein binding (98%). **Metabolism:** Liver (extensive) via CYP3A4 (N-oxidation, 4R-hydroxylation); 4R-hydroxy solifenacin (active metabolite). **Elimination:** Urine (69.2%, <15% unchanged), feces (22.5%); $T_{1/2}$=45-68 hrs.

PATIENT CONSIDERATIONS
Assessment: Assess for hypersensitivity to the drug and for any other conditions where treatment is contraindicated or cautioned. Assess for renal/hepatic impairment, pregnancy/nursing status, and possible drug interactions.

Monitoring: Monitor for angioedema, anaphylactic reactions, signs of anticholinergic CNS effects, and other adverse reactions.

Counseling: Inform that constipation may occur; advise to contact physician if severe abdominal pain or constipation for ≥3 days occurs. Inform that blurred vision or CNS anticholinergic effects may occur; advise to exercise caution in decisions to engage in potentially dangerous activities until effects have been determined. Inform that heat prostration (due to decreased sweating) can occur when used in a hot environment. Inform that angioedema may occur and could result in fatal airway obstruction; advise to promptly d/c therapy and seek immediate attention if edema or difficulty breathing develops.

VFEND — voriconazole   Rx

Class: Azole antifungal

ADULT DOSAGE

Aspergillosis

Invasive:
LD: 6mg/kg IV q12h for the first 24 hrs
Maint:
IV: 4mg/kg q12h; may decrease to 3mg/kg q12h if unable to tolerate
Continue IV therapy for at least 7 days
PO: 200mg q12h; may increase to 300mg q12h if response is inadequate

Scedosporiosis and Fusariosis

Serious fungal infections caused by *Scedosporium apiospermum* and *Fusarium* spp. including *Fusarium solani*

LD: 6mg/kg IV q12h for the first 24 hrs
Maint:
IV: 4mg/kg q12h; may decrease to 3mg/kg q12h if unable to tolerate
Continue IV therapy for at least 7 days
PO: 200mg q12h; may increase to 300mg q12h if response is inadequate

Candida Infections

Candidemia (Non-Neutropenic Patients) and Other Deep Tissue *Candida* Infections:
LD: 6mg/kg IV q12h for the first 24 hrs
Maint:
IV: 3-4mg/kg q12h
PO: 200mg q12h; may increase to 300mg q12h if response is inadequate

Treat for at least 14 days following resolution of symptoms or last (+) culture, whichever is longer

Esophageal Candidiasis

Maint:
200mg PO q12h; may increase to 300mg q12h if response is inadequate

Treat for a minimum of 14 days and ≥7 days following resolution of symptoms

PEDIATRIC DOSAGE

Fungal Infections

Treatment of invasive aspergillosis; esophageal candidiasis; candidemia in non-neutropenic patients; and the following *Candida* infections: disseminated infections in skin and infections in abdomen, kidney, bladder wall, and wounds; serious fungal infections caused by *Scedosporium apiospermum* and *Fusarium* spp. including *Fusarium solani*, in patients intolerant of, or refractory to, other therapy

≥12 Years:
Refer to PI for dosing

DOSING CONSIDERATIONS

Concomitant Medications

Phenytoin/Efavirenz:
Increase maint dose of voriconazole

Renal Impairment

Moderate or Severe (CrCl <50mL/min):
Administer oral therapy unless an assessment of the benefit/risk to the patient justifies the use of IV therapy; monitor SrCr levels closely and consider changing to oral therapy if increases occur

Hepatic Impairment

Mild to Moderate (Child-Pugh Class A and B):
Reduce maint dose by 1/2

Adverse Reactions

If unable to tolerate 300mg PO q12h, reduce oral maint dose by 50mg steps to a minimum of 200mg q12h (or 100mg q12h for adults <40kg)

Other Important Considerations

Adults:
<40kg: Administer 1/2 the oral maint dose; may increase from 100mg q12h to 150mg q12h if response is inadequate

ADMINISTRATION

Oral/IV route

Oral

Take at least 1 hr ac or pc
Shake reconstituted sus for approx 10 sec before each use; administer using oral dispenser supplied w/ each pack
Do not mix w/ any other medication or additional flavoring agent

Sus Preparation:

Reconstitute w/ 46mL of water and shake for 1 min

IV

Requires reconstitution to 10mg/mL and subsequent dilution to ≤5mg/mL prior to administration as an infusion, at a max rate of 3mg/kg/hr over 1-2 hrs
Do not administer as an IV bolus inj
Do not infuse concomitantly w/ any blood product or short-term infusion of concentrated electrolytes, even if the 2 infusions are running in separate IV lines/ cannulas
May infuse at the same time as other IV sol containing non-concentrated electrolytes or total parenteral nutrition (TPN) through separate lines; for TPN, must administer through a different port if infused through a multiple-lumen catheter
If not used immediately, store for ≤24 hrs at 2-8°C (36-46°F)

Reconstitution:

Reconstitute w/ 19mL of water for inj to an extractable volume of 20mL containing 10mg/mL of voriconazole

Dilution:

Further dilute the required volume of the 10mg/mL voriconazole concentrate as follows:
1. Calculate required volume of 10mg/mL voriconazole concentrate based on patient's weight
2. Withdraw and discard at least an equal volume of diluent from infusion bag/ bottle to be used. Volume of diluent remaining in the bag or bottle should be such that when 10mg/mL voriconazole concentrate is added, the final concentration is not <0.5mg/mL nor >5mg/mL
3. Withdraw required volume of voriconazole concentrate from the appropriate number of vials and add to infusion bag/bottle. Discard partially used vials

Compatible IV Diluents:
9mg/mL (0.9%) NaCl, lactated Ringer's, D5 and lactated Ringer's, D5 and 0.45% NaCl, D5, D5 and 20mEq KCl, 0.45% NaCl, and D5 and 0.9% NaCl

STORAGE

Inj: Unreconstituted: 15-30°C (59-86°F). Reconstituted: 2-8°C (36-46°F) for ≤24 hrs. **Tab:** 15-30°C (59-86°F). **Oral Sus:** Unreconstituted: 2-8°C (36-46°F) for up to 18 months. Reconstituted: 15-30°C (59-86°F) for up to 14 days. Do not refrigerate or freeze.

HOW SUPPLIED

Inj: 200mg; **Sus:** 40mg/mL; **Tab:** 50mg, 200mg

CONTRAINDICATIONS

Known hypersensitivity to voriconazole or its excipients; concomitant terfenadine, astemizole, cisapride, pimozide, quinidine, sirolimus, rifampin, carbamazepine, long-acting barbiturates, efavirenz (≥400mg q24h), high-dose ritonavir (RTV) (400mg q12h), rifabutin, ergot alkaloids (ergotamine, dihydroergotamine), St. John's wort. Low-dose RTV (100mg q12h) should be avoided, unless an assessment of benefit/risk justifies the use.

WARNINGS/PRECAUTIONS

Serious hepatic reactions (eg, clinical hepatitis, cholestasis, fulminant hepatic failure) reported; if LFTs become markedly elevated compared to baseline, d/c therapy unless the medical judgment of the benefit-risk of the treatment for the patient justifies continued use. Prolonged visual adverse events (eg, optic neuritis, papilledema) reported; monitor visual function if treatment continues >28 days. May cause fetal harm. Tabs contain lactose; avoid w/ rare hereditary problems of galactose intolerance, Lapp lactase deficiency, or glucose-galactose malabsorption. May prolong QT interval, and (rare) arrhythmias (eg, torsades de pointes), cardiac arrests, and sudden deaths may occur; caution w/ proarrhythmic conditions (eg, congenital or acquired QT-prolongation, cardiomyopathy, in particular when heart failure is present, sinus bradycardia, existing symptomatic arrhythmias). Correct electrolyte disturbances prior to initiation of and during therapy. Anaphylactoid-type reactions reported w/ infusion; consider discontinuing infusion if reactions occur. Associated w/ elevations in LFTs and clinical signs of liver damage. Acute renal failure may occur. Monitor for the development of pancreatitis in patients w/ risk factors for acute pancreatitis (eg, recent chemotherapy, hematopoietic stem cell transplantation) during treatment. Serious exfoliative cutaneous reactions (eg, Stevens-Johnson syndrome) reported; d/c if exfoliative cutaneous reaction develops. Photosensitivity skin reaction reported; avoid exposure to direct sunlight during treatment. Refer to a dermatologist and consider discontinuation of therapy if phototoxic reactions occur; if therapy is continued despite the occurrence of phototoxicity-related lesions, perform dermatologic evaluation on a systematic and regular basis. Squamous cell carcinoma of the skin and melanoma reported during long-term therapy in patients w/ photosensitivity skin reactions; d/c therapy if skin lesion consistent w/ premalignant skin lesions, squamous cell carcinoma, or melanoma develops. Higher frequency of phototoxicity reactions in pediatric population. Fluorosis and periostitis reported w/ long-term therapy; d/c if skeletal pain and radiologic findings compatible w/ fluorosis and periostitis develop.

ADVERSE REACTIONS

Visual disturbances, fever, chills, rash, headache, N/V, increased alkaline phosphatase.

DRUG INTERACTIONS

See Dosing Considerations and Contraindications. Avoid w/ fluconazole and everolimus. Caution w/ concomitant medications known to prolong QT interval. Decreased exposure w/ phenytoin, low-dose RTV (100mg q12h), efavirenz, and other non-nucleoside reverse transcriptase inhibitors (NNRTIs). Decrease in AUC w/ efavirenz (300mg q24h). Increased exposure w/ fluconazole, oral contraceptives containing ethinyl estradiol and norethindrone, HIV protease inhibitors, delavirdine, and other NNRTIs. Increased exposure of alfentanil, oxycodone, tacrolimus, phenytoin, omeprazole, methadone, fentanyl, NSAIDs, oral contraceptives containing ethinyl estradiol and norethindrone, HIV protease inhibitors, NNRTIs, benzodiazepines, HMG-CoA reductase inhibitors, dihydropyridine calcium channel blockers, sulfonylurea oral hypoglycemics, vinca alkaloids, and everolimus. Increased AUC of efavirenz (300mg q24h) and cyclosporine. Decreased AUC and C_{max} of low-dose RTV (100mg q12h). Increased PT w/ warfarin. Refer to PI for further information on drug interactions.

PREGNANCY AND LACTATION

Category D, not for use in nursing.

MECHANISM OF ACTION

Azole antifungal agent; inhibits fungal CYP450-mediated 14 α-lanosterol demethylation, an essential step in fungal ergosterol biosynthesis. Accumulation of 14 α-methyl-sterols correlates w/ subsequent loss of ergosterol in fungal cell wall and may be responsible for antifungal activity of voriconazole.

PHARMACOKINETICS
Absorption: Administration of variable doses resulted in different parameters. T_{max}=1-2 hrs. **Distribution:** V_d=4.6L/kg; plasma protein binding (58%). **Metabolism:** Hepatic via CYP2C19, CYP2C9, and CYP3A4; N-oxide (major metabolite). **Elimination:** Urine (approx 80-83%, <2% unchanged).

PATIENT CONSIDERATIONS
Assessment: Assess for drug hypersensitivity, proarrhythmic conditions, hereditary problems of galactose intolerance, Lapp lactase deficiency or glucose-galactose malabsorption, electrolyte disturbances, risk factors for acute pancreatitis, photosensitivity skin reactions, hepatic/renal impairment, pregnancy/nursing status, and possible drug interactions. Obtain fungal cultures to isolate and identify causative organisms. Correct K^+, Mg^{2+}, and Ca^{2+} prior to initiating therapy.

Monitoring: Monitor for signs/symptoms of hepatotoxicity, arrhythmias, QT prolongation, cardiac arrests, infusion reactions, acute renal failure, pancreatitis, dermatological reactions, fluorosis, periostitis, electrolyte disturbances, and other adverse reactions. Monitor for drug toxicity w/ hepatic impairment. Monitor renal function. Monitor visual function (eg, acuity, visual field, color perception) if treatment continues >28 days. Monitor serum transaminase levels and bilirubin during initiation and at least weekly for the 1st month of treatment and monthly if no clinically significant changes are noted.

Counseling: Inform of the risks/benefits of therapy. Counsel to take tabs or oral sus at least 1 hr ac or pc. Inform of the potential hazards to the fetus if drug is used during pregnancy or if the patient becomes pregnant. Instruct to avoid intense or prolonged exposure to direct sunlight during therapy. Inform women of childbearing potential to use effective contraception during treatment. Inform of the signs and symptoms of hepatic reactions, allergic reactions, vision changes, and serious skin reactions; advise to contact physician if any of these conditions develop. Instruct to wear protective clothing and use sunscreen w/ high sun protection factor.

VIAGRA — sildenafil citrate   Rx

Class: Phosphodiesterase-5 (PDE-5) inhibitor

ADULT DOSAGE	PEDIATRIC DOSAGE
Erectile Dysfunction	Pediatric use may not have been established
50mg qd prn (recommended), approx 1 hr or anywhere from 30 min to 4 hrs before sexual activity	
Titrate: May increase to 100mg qd or decrease to 25mg qd, based on effectiveness and tolerance	
Max: 100mg qd	

DOSING CONSIDERATIONS
Concomitant Medications
Strong CYP3A4 Inhibitors/Erythromycin:
Initial: Consider 25mg qd

α-Blockers:
Patient should be stable on α-blocker therapy prior to initiating treatment
Initial: 25mg qd

Ritonavir:
25mg prior to sexual activity
Max: 25mg/48 hrs

Renal Impairment
CrCl <30mL/min:
Initial: Consider 25mg qd

Hepatic Impairment
Initial: Consider 25mg qd

Elderly
Initial: Consider 25mg qd

ADMINISTRATION
Oral route

May be taken w/ or w/o food.

STORAGE
25°C (77°F); excursions permitted to 15-30°C (59-86°F).

HOW SUPPLIED
Tab: 25mg, 50mg, 100mg

CONTRAINDICATIONS
Concomitant use w/ nitric oxide donors (eg, organic nitrates/nitrites) in any form, either taken regularly and/or intermittently; known hypersensitivity to sildenafil or any component of the tab; concomitant guanylate cyclase (GC) stimulators (eg, riociguat).

WARNINGS/PRECAUTIONS
Potential for cardiac risk of sexual activity in patients w/ cardiovascular disease (CVD); do not use in men for whom sexual activity is inadvisable due to underlying cardiovascular (CV) status. Has systemic vasodilatory properties that resulted in transient decreases in supine BP in clinical studies. Caution in patients w/ left ventricular outflow obstruction (eg, aortic stenosis, idiopathic hypertrophic subaortic stenosis); severely impaired autonomic control of BP; history of MI, stroke, or life-threatening arrhythmia w/in the last 6 months; resting hypotension (BP <90/50mmHg) or HTN (BP >170/110mmHg); and cardiac failure or coronary artery disease (CAD) causing unstable angina. Prolonged erection

>4 hrs and priapism reported; caution w/ anatomical penile deformation (eg, angulation, cavernosal fibrosis, Peyronie's disease), or predispositions to priapism (eg, sickle cell anemia, multiple myeloma, leukemia). Nonarteritic anterior ischemic optic neuropathy (NAION) reported. D/C if sudden loss of vision in 1 or both eyes occurs; may be a sign of NAION. Caution w/ underlying NAION risk factors; increased risk in patients w/ "crowded" optic disc and w/ previous history of NAION. D/C if sudden decrease or loss of hearing occurs. Bleeding events reported. Does not protect against STDs.

ADVERSE REACTIONS
Headache, flushing, dyspepsia, abnormal vision, nasal congestion, back pain, myalgia, nausea, dizziness, rash.

DRUG INTERACTIONS
See Dosing Considerations and Contraindications. Increased levels w/ CYP3A4 inhibitors (eg, ritonavir, erythromycin, saquinavir); stronger CYP3A4 inhibitors (eg, ketoconazole, itraconazole) may have greater effects. Potential additive BP-lowering effects w/ α-blockers and other antihypertensives (eg, amlodipine). Combination w/ other PDE-5 inhibitors or other erectile dysfunction therapies is not recommended; may further lower BP.

PREGNANCY AND LACTATION
Pregnancy: Category B, not for use in women.

MECHANISM OF ACTION
PDE-5 inhibitor; enhances effect of nitric oxide by inhibiting PDE-5, which then increases the levels of cGMP in the corpus cavernosum, resulting in smooth muscle relaxation and inflow of blood to the corpus cavernosum.

PHARMACOKINETICS
Absorption: Rapid. Absolute bioavailability (41%); T_{max}=60 min (median). **Distribution:** V_d=105L; plasma protein binding (approx 96%). **Metabolism:** Liver, via CYP3A4 (major), CYP2C9 (minor); N-desmethyl sildenafil (major active metabolite). **Elimination:** Feces (approx 80% metabolites), urine (approx 13% metabolites); $T_{1/2}$=4 hrs.

PATIENT CONSIDERATIONS
Assessment: Assess for hypersensitivity to drug; history of MI, stroke, or arrhythmia; renal/hepatic impairment; CVD; left ventricular outflow obstruction; impaired autonomic control of BP; resting hypotension or HTN; cardiac failure; CAD; anatomical penile deformation; predisposition to priapism; risk for NAION; potential underlying causes of ED; and for possible drug interactions.

Monitoring: Monitor for prolonged erection, priapism, abnormalities in vision/NAION, decrease/loss of hearing, bleeding, and other adverse reactions.

Counseling: Inform of risks and benefits of therapy. Instruct to notify physician of all prescription/nonprescription medications and supplements currently being taking and inform of the contraindication w/ regular and/or intermittent use of nitric oxide donors and if using GC stimulators. Advise patients who experience CV symptoms upon initiation of sexual activity to refrain from further activity and to discuss the episode w/ their physician. Instruct to d/c and seek medical attention if sudden loss of vision in 1 or both eyes or sudden decrease/loss of hearing occurs. Instruct to seek immediate medical assistance if erection persists >4 hrs. Counsel about protective measures necessary to guard against STDs, including HIV.

VIBATIV — telavancin   Rx

Class: Lipoglycopeptide

> Increased mortality observed in patients w/ preexisting moderate/severe renal impairment (CrCl ≤50mL/min) who were treated for hospital-acquired bacterial pneumonia/ventilator-associated bacterial pneumonia (HABP/VABP); consider therapy only when the anticipated benefit outweighs the risk. New onset or worsening renal impairment reported; monitor renal function in all patients. Women of childbearing potential should have a serum pregnancy test prior to administration. Avoid use during pregnancy unless potential benefit to the patient outweighs the potential risk to the fetus. Potential adverse developmental outcomes in humans may occur.

ADULT DOSAGE	PEDIATRIC DOSAGE
Skin and Skin Structure Infections	Pediatric use may not have been established
Complicated Gram-Positive Infections: 10mg/kg IV q24h for 7-14 days	
Pneumonia	
Hospital-Acquired/Ventilator-Associated Bacterial Pneumonia: **Susceptible Isolates of** *Staphylococcus aureus*: 10mg/kg IV q24h for 7-21 days	

DOSING CONSIDERATIONS
Renal Impairment
CrCl 30-50mL/min: 7.5mg/kg q24h
CrCl 10 to <30mL/min: 10mg/kg q48h

ADMINISTRATION
IV route

- Administer IV infusion over 60 min.

- Do not add additives or other medications to single-use vials or infuse simultaneously through the same IV line.

- If the same IV line is used for sequential infusion of additional medications, flush the line before and after infusion of therapy w/ appropriate infusion sol.

Preparation
250mg Vial: Reconstitute contents w/ 15mL of reconstitution diluent.
750mg Vial: Reconstitute contents w/ 45mL of reconstitution diluent.

- For doses of 150-800mg, reconstituted sol must be further diluted in 100-250mL of appropriate infusion sol prior to infusion.
- Doses <150mg or >800mg should be further diluted in a volume resulting in a final concentration of 0.6-8mg/mL.
- Use w/in 12 hrs when stored at room temperature or use w/in 7 days when stored under refrigeration at 2-8°C (36-46°F). Diluted sol can also be stored at -30 to -10°C (-22 to 14°F) for up to 32 days.

Appropriate Reconstitution Diluents
5% dextrose inj
Sterile water for inj
0.9% NaCl inj

Appropriate Infusion Sol
5% dextrose inj
0.9% NaCl inj
Lactated Ringer's inj

STORAGE
2-8°C (35-46°F); excursions permitted to ambient temperatures (up to 25°C [77°F]). Avoid excessive heat.

HOW SUPPLIED
Inj: 250mg, 750mg

CONTRAINDICATIONS
Use of IV unfractionated heparin sodium, known hypersensitivity to telavancin.

WARNINGS/PRECAUTIONS
Use of telavancin for the treatment of HABP/VABP should be reserved for when alternative treatments are not suitable. Decreased efficacy in patients w/ complicated skin and skin structure infection and preexisting moderate/severe renal impairment (CrCl ≤50mL/min). Renal adverse events were reported more likely to occur in patients w/ baseline comorbidities known to predispose patients to kidney dysfunction (preexisting renal disease, diabetes mellitus, CHF, or HTN). Consider alternative agent if renal toxicity is suspected. Accumulation of the solubilizer hydroxypropyl-β-cyclodextrin may occur in patients w/ renal dysfunction. May interfere w/ coagulation tests (eg, PT/INR, activated PTT [aPTT], activated clotting time, coagulation-based factor Xa assay), and urine protein tests; collect blood samples for affected coagulation tests as close as possible prior to the next dose. For patients who require aPTT monitoring while on therapy, a non-phospholipid dependent coagulation test (eg, factor Xa [chromogenic] assay) or an alternative anticoagulant not requiring aPTT monitoring may be considered. Serious and sometimes fatal hypersensitivity reactions, including anaphylactic reactions, may occur after 1st or subsequent doses; d/c at 1st sign of skin rash, or any other signs of hypersensitivity. Caution w/ known hypersensitivity to vancomycin. Infusion-related reactions (eg, "red man syndrome"-like reactions) may occur w/ rapid infusion. *Clostridium difficile*-associated diarrhea (CDAD) reported; may need to d/c if CDAD is suspected or confirmed. Use in the absence of a proven or strongly suspected bacterial infection is unlikely to provide benefit and increases the risk of development of drug-resistant bacteria. May result in overgrowth of nonsusceptible organisms; take appropriate measures if superinfection develops. QTc interval prolongation reported; avoid in patients w/ congenital long QT syndrome, known prolongation of the QTc interval, uncompensated heart failure (HF), or severe left ventricular hypertrophy (LVH). Caution in elderly patients.

ADVERSE REACTIONS
Diarrhea, taste disturbance, N/V, foamy urine.

DRUG INTERACTIONS
See Contraindications. Caution w/ drugs known to prolong the QT interval. Higher renal adverse event rates reported w/ concomitant medications known to affect kidney function (eg, NSAIDs, ACE inhibitors, loop diuretics).

PREGNANCY AND LACTATION
Pregnancy: Category C.
Lactation: Caution in nursing.

MECHANISM OF ACTION
Antibacterial agent; a lipoglycopeptide antibiotic that inhibits cell-wall biosynthesis by binding to late-stage peptidoglycan precursors, including lipid II. Binds to the bacterial membrane and disrupts membrane barrier function.

PHARMACOKINETICS
Absorption: (Multiple dose) C_{max}=108mcg/mL, AUC_{0-24}=780mcg•hr/mL.
Distribution: Plasma protein binding (90%); (Multiple dose) V_d=133mL/kg.
Elimination: Urine (76%), feces (<1%); (Multiple dose) $T_{1/2}$=8.1 hrs.

PATIENT CONSIDERATIONS
Assessment: Assess for hypersensitivity to the drug/vancomycin, renal impairment, risk of renal impairment, congenital long QT syndrome, known prolongation of the QTc interval, uncompensated HF, severe LVH, pregnancy/nursing status, and possible drug interactions. Obtain renal function values.

Monitoring: Monitor for new onset or worsening renal impairment, hypersensitivity reactions, CDAD, development of drug-resistant bacteria, overgrowth of nonsusceptible organisms, superinfection, infusion-related reactions, QTc prolongation, and other adverse reactions. Monitor renal function (eg, SrCr, CrCl) during treatment (at 48- to 72-hr intervals or more frequently, if clinically indicated), and at the end of therapy.

Counseling: Inform women of childbearing potential about the potential risk of fetal harm if drug is used during pregnancy; instruct to have a pregnancy test prior to therapy, to use effective contraceptive methods to prevent pregnancy during treatment if not pregnant, and to notify physician if pregnancy occurs.

Encourage pregnant patients to enroll in pregnancy registry. Inform that diarrhea may occur, even as late as ≥2 months after last dose of therapy; instruct to notify physician as soon as possible if watery/bloody stools (w/ or w/o stomach cramps and fever) occur. Inform that antibacterial drugs should only be used to treat bacterial, not viral, infections. Instruct to take ud; inform that skipping doses or not completing full course may decrease effectiveness and increase resistance. Counsel about common adverse effects; advise to notify physician if any unusual/known symptom persists or worsens.

VIBERZI — eluxadoline   CIV
Class: Mu-opioid receptor agonist

ADULT DOSAGE	PEDIATRIC DOSAGE
Irritable Bowel Syndrome with Diarrhea 100mg bid 75mg bid in patients who: - do not have a gallbladder - are unable to tolerate the 100mg dose - are receiving concomitant OATP1B1 inhibitors - have mild or moderate (Child-Pugh Class A or B) hepatic impairment	Pediatric use may not have been established

DOSING CONSIDERATIONS
Concomitant Medications
OATP1B1 Inhibitors: 75mg bid

Hepatic Impairment
Mild or Moderate (Child-Pugh Class A or B): 75mg bid

Adverse Reactions
D/C in patients who develop severe constipation for >4 days

ADMINISTRATION
Oral route

Take w/ food.

STORAGE
20-25°C (68-77°F); excursions permitted to 15-30°C (59-86°F).

HOW SUPPLIED
Tab: 75mg, 100mg

CONTRAINDICATIONS
Known/suspected biliary duct obstruction, or sphincter of Oddi disease/dysfunction. Alcoholism, alcohol abuse/addiction, or in patients who drink >3 alcoholic beverages per day. History of pancreatitis or structural diseases of the pancreas, including known/suspected pancreatic duct obstruction. Severe hepatic impairment (Child-Pugh Class C). History of chronic or severe constipation or sequelae from constipation, or known/suspected mechanical GI obstruction.

WARNINGS/PRECAUTIONS
Potential for increased risk of sphincter of Oddi spasm, resulting in pancreatitis or hepatic enzyme elevation; patients w/o a gallbladder are at increased risk. Consider alternative therapies in patients w/o a gallbladder and evaluate the benefits/risks of eluxadoline in these patients. Do not restart therapy in patients who developed biliary duct obstruction or sphincter of Oddi spasm while taking eluxadoline. Potential for increased risk of pancreatitis not associated w/ sphincter of Oddi spasm; majority of cases were associated w/ excessive alcohol intake. Caution in elderly.

ADVERSE REACTIONS
Constipation, N/V, abdominal pain, URTI, nasopharyngitis, abdominal distention, bronchitis, dizziness, flatulence, rash, increased ALT, fatigue, viral gastroenteritis.

DRUG INTERACTIONS
See Dosing Considerations. OATP1B1 inhibitors (eg, cyclosporine, gemfibrozil, antiretrovirals) and strong CYP inhibitors (eg, ciprofloxacin, fluconazole, clarithromycin) may increase exposure; monitor for impaired mental/physical abilities and for other eluxadoline-related adverse reactions. Increased risk for constipation-related adverse reactions w/ drugs that cause constipation (eg, alosetron, anticholinergics, opioids); avoid concomitant use. Loperamide may be used occasionally for acute management of severe diarrhea, but avoid chronic use; d/c loperamide immediately if constipation occurs. May increase exposure of OATP1B1 and BCRP substrates. Increased exposure to rosuvastatin w/ a potential for increased risk of myopathy/rhabdomyolysis; use lowest effective dose of rosuvastatin. Potential for increased exposure of CYP3A substrates w/ narrow therapeutic index (eg, alfentanil, cyclosporine, dihydroergotamine); monitor drug concentrations or other pharmacodynamic markers of drug effect when concomitant use w/ eluxadoline is initiated or discontinued.

PREGNANCY AND LACTATION
Pregnancy: There are no studies in pregnant women that inform any drug-associated risks.
Lactation: No data are available regarding the presence of eluxadoline in human milk, the effects of eluxadoline on the breastfed infant, or the effects of eluxadoline on milk production. Caution in nursing.

MECHANISM OF ACTION
Mu-opioid receptor agonist; eluxadoline is also a delta opioid receptor antagonist and a kappa opioid receptor agonist.

PHARMACOKINETICS

Absorption: C_{max}=approx 2-4ng/mL, AUC=12-22ng•hr/mL, T_{max} (median)=1.5 hrs (fed), 2 hrs (fasting). **Distribution:** Plasma protein binding (81%). **Metabolism:** Not clearly established; evidence that glucuronidation can occur to form an acyl glucuronide metabolite. **Elimination:** $T_{1/2}$=3.7-6 hrs; (300mg single dose) feces (82.2%), urine (<1%).

PATIENT CONSIDERATIONS

Assessment: Assess for hepatic impairment, known/suspected biliary duct obstruction, sphincter of Oddi disease/dysfunction, alcoholism, alcohol abuse/addiction, history of pancreatitis or structural diseases of the pancreas, history of chronic or severe constipation or sequelae from constipation, known/suspected mechanical GI obstruction, other conditions where treatment is contraindicated or cautioned, pregnancy/nursing status, and for possible drug interactions.

Monitoring: Monitor for severe constipation and new or worsening abdominal pain that may radiate to the back or shoulder, w/ or w/o N/V. If used in patients w/o a gallbladder, monitor for symptoms of sphincter of Oddi spasm (eg, elevated liver transaminases associated w/ abdominal pain or pancreatitis), especially during the 1st few weeks of treatment. Monitor patients w/ any degree of hepatic impairment for impaired mental/physical abilities.

Counseling: Instruct to d/c drug and seek medical attention if unusual or severe abdominal pain that may radiate to the back or shoulder, w/ or w/o N/V, develops or if constipation lasting >4 days is experienced. Advise to avoid chronic or acute excessive alcohol use during treatment. Instruct to take ud and to inform physician if unable to tolerate therapy. Instruct patients to not take alosetron w/ eluxadoline or not take loperamide on a chronic basis w/ eluxadoline due to the potential for constipation. Advise to avoid other medications that may cause constipation.

VIBRAMYCIN — doxycycline calcium; doxycycline hyclate; doxycycline monohydrate　　　　　　　Rx

Class: Tetracyclines

OTHER BRAND NAMES
Vibra-Tabs

ADULT DOSAGE

General Dosing

Initial: 100mg q12h on Day 1
Maint: 100mg/day
More Severe Infections (eg, Chronic UTIs): 100mg q12h

Streptococcal Infections: Continue therapy for 10 days

Gonococcal Infections

Uncomplicated Infections (Except Anorectal Infections in Men):
100mg bid for 7 days or as an alternate single visit dose, 300mg stat followed in 1 hr by a second 300mg dose

Chlamydia trachomatis Infections

Uncomplicated Urethral/Endocervical/Rectal Infections:
100mg bid for 7 days

Nongonococcal Urethritis

Caused by *C. trachomatis* and *Ureaplasma urealyticum*:
100mg bid for 7 days

Syphilis

Patients Allergic to Penicillin (PCN):

Early Syphilis:
100mg bid for 2 weeks
Syphilis of >1-Year Duration:
100mg bid for 4 weeks

Acute Epididymo-Orchitis

Caused by *Neisseria gonorrhoeae/C. trachomatis*:
100mg bid for at least 10 days

Malaria

Prophylaxis of malaria due to *Plasmodium falciparum* in short-term travelers (<4 months) to areas w/ chloroquine and/or pyrimethamine-sulfadoxine resistant strains

100mg qd; begin 1-2 days before travel and continue daily during travel and for 4 weeks after leaving malarious area

Inhalational Anthrax (Postexposure)

100mg bid for 60 days

PEDIATRIC DOSAGE

General Dosing

Severe or Life-Threatening Infections (eg, Anthrax, Rocky Mountain Spotted Fever):

<45kg:
2.2mg/kg q12h
≥45kg:
Use adult dose

Less Severe Disease:
>8 Years:
<45kg:
Initial: 4.4mg/kg divided into 2 doses on Day 1 of treatment
Maint: 2.2mg/kg (given as a qd dose or divided into bid doses)
>45kg:
Use adult dose

Streptococcal Infections: Continue therapy for 10 days

Malaria

Prophylaxis of malaria due to *P. falciparum* in short-term travelers (<4 months) to areas w/ chloroquine and/or pyrimethamine-sulfadoxine resistant strains

>8 Years:
2mg/kg qd; begin 1-2 days before travel and continue daily during travel and for 4 weeks after leaving malarious area
Max: 100mg/day

Inhalational Anthrax (Postexposure)

<45kg:
2.2mg/kg bid for 60 days
≥45kg:
Use adult dose

Other Indications
- Rocky Mountain spotted fever
- Typhus fever and the typhus group
- Q fever
- Rickettsialpox
- Tick fevers
- Respiratory tract infections
- Lymphogranuloma venereum
- Psittacosis (ornithosis)
- Trachoma
- Inclusion conjunctivitis
- Relapsing fever
- Chancroid
- Plague
- Tularemia
- Cholera
- *Campylobacter fetus* infections
- Brucellosis
- Bartonellosis
- Granuloma inguinale
- UTIs
- *Escherichia coli* infections
- *Enterobacter aerogenes* infections
- *Shigella* species infections
- *Acinetobacter* species infections
- Adjunct to amebicides in acute intestinal amebiasis
- Adjunctive therapy in severe acne

Treatment of the Following Infections When PCN is Contraindicated:
- Uncomplicated gonorrhea
- Yaws
- Listeriosis
- Vincent's infection
- Actinomycosis
- *Clostridium* species infections

ADMINISTRATION
Oral route

Administer caps/tabs w/ adequate amount of fluids; if gastric irritation occurs, administer w/ food or milk.

STORAGE
<30°C (86°F).

HOW SUPPLIED
Cap (Hyclate): 100mg; **Oral Sus (Monohydrate):** 25mg/5mL [60mL]; **Syrup (Calcium):** 50mg/5mL [473mL]; **Tab (Hyclate):** 100mg

CONTRAINDICATIONS
Hypersensitivity to any of the tetracyclines.

WARNINGS/PRECAUTIONS
May cause permanent teeth discoloration (yellow-gray-brown) if used during tooth development (last 1/2 of pregnancy to 8 yrs of age). Enamel hypoplasia reported. Use only in pediatric patients ≤8 years of age only when the potential benefits are expected to outweigh the risks in severe or life-threatening conditions (eg, anthrax, Rocky Mountain spotted fever), particularly when there are no alternative therapies. *Clostridium difficile*-associated diarrhea (CDAD) reported; may need to d/c if CDAD is suspected or confirmed. Associated w/ intracranial HTN (pseudotumor cerebri); increased risk in women of childbearing age who are overweight or have a history of intracranial HTN. Intracranial pressure can remain elevated for weeks after drug cessation; monitor patients until they stabilize. Possibility of permanent visual loss exists due to intracranial HTN; prompt ophthalmologic evaluation is needed if visual disturbance occurs during treatment. May decrease fibula growth rate in prematures or cause fetal harm during pregnancy. May increase BUN. Photosensitivity may occur; d/c at 1st evidence of skin erythema. May result in bacterial resistance if used in the absence of a proven/suspected bacterial infection or a prophylactic indication; take appropriate measures if superinfection develops. When used for malaria prophylaxis, patients may still transmit the infection to mosquitoes outside endemic areas. False elevations of urinary catecholamines may occur due to interference w/ the fluorescence test. Syrup contains sodium metabisulfite that may cause allergic-type reactions; sulfite sensitivity is seen more frequently in asthmatic patients.

ADVERSE REACTIONS
Anorexia, N/V, diarrhea, dysphagia, maculopapular rash, Stevens-Johnson syndrome, toxic epidermal necrolysis, photosensitivity, increased BUN, hypersensitivity reactions, drug rash w/ eosinophilia and systemic symptoms, hemolytic anemia, thrombocytopenia, neutropenia, eosinophilia.

DRUG INTERACTIONS
Avoid concomitant use w/ isotretinoin; may also cause pseudotumor cerebri. May depress plasma prothrombin activity; may require downward adjustment of anticoagulant dose. May interfere w/ bactericidal action of PCN; avoid concurrent use. Bismuth subsalicylate, iron-containing preparations, and antacids containing aluminum, Ca^{2+}, or Mg^{2+} may impair absorption. Barbiturates, carbamazepine, and phenytoin may decrease $T_{1/2}$. Fatal renal toxicity reported w/ methoxyflurane. May render oral contraceptives less effective.

PREGNANCY AND LACTATION

Pregnancy: Category D.
Lactation: Excreted in human milk; extent of absorption by the breastfed infant is not known. Not for use in nursing.

MECHANISM OF ACTION

Tetracycline derivative; has bacteriostatic activity. Inhibits bacterial protein synthesis by binding to the 30S ribosomal subunit.

PHARMACOKINETICS

Absorption: Complete. (200mg dose) C_{max}=2.6mcg/mL, T_{max}=2 hrs. **Distribution:** Plasma protein binding in varying degrees; found in breast milk. **Elimination:** Urine (40%/72 hrs w/ CrCl 75mL/min, 1-5%/72 hrs w/ CrCl <10mL/min), feces; $T_{1/2}$=18-22 hrs.

PATIENT CONSIDERATIONS

Assessment: Assess for previous hypersensitivity to any tetracyclines, risk of intracranial HTN, pregnancy/nursing status, and possible drug interactions. Document indications for therapy as well as culture and susceptibility testing results. Perform dark-field exam and blood serology when coexistent syphilis is suspected. Assess for sulfite sensitivity if using the syrup formulation.

Monitoring: Monitor for signs/symptoms of hypersensitivity reactions, photosensitivity, skin erythema, superinfection, CDAD, intracranial HTN, visual disturbance, and other adverse reactions. In venereal disease w/ coexistent syphilis, conduct blood serology monthly for at least 4 months. Monitor for tooth discoloration if used in pediatric patients ≤8 years of age. Perform periodic lab evaluation of organ systems, including hematopoietic, renal, and hepatic studies in long-term therapy.

Counseling: Apprise pregnant women of the potential hazard to fetus. Inform that the therapy does not guarantee protection against malaria; instruct to use measures that help avoid contact w/ mosquitoes. Instruct to avoid excessive sunlight/UV light and to d/c therapy if phototoxicity occurs; advise to consider use of sunscreen or sunblock. Instruct to drink fluids liberally. Inform that drug absorption is reduced when taking bismuth subsalicylate and when taken w/ food, especially those that contain Ca^{2+}. Inform that drug may increase the incidence of vaginal candidiasis. Instruct to take exactly ud; warn that skipping doses or not completing full course may decrease effectiveness and increase resistance. Advise that therapy should only be used to treat bacterial, not viral, infections. Inform that diarrhea may be experienced and advise to notify physician as soon as possible if watery and bloody stools (w/ or w/o stomach cramps and fever) even as late as ≥2 months after last dose occur.

VICODIN — acetaminophen/hydrocodone bitartrate CII

Class: Opioid analgesic

> Associated w/ cases of acute liver failure, at times resulting in liver transplant and death. Most of the cases of liver injury are associated w/ acetaminophen (APAP) use at doses >4000mg/day, and often involve >1 APAP-containing product.

OTHER BRAND NAMES

Vicodin HP, Vicodin ES

ADULT DOSAGE

Moderate to Moderately Severe Pain

Vicodin:
Usual: 1 or 2 tabs q4-6h prn
Max: 8 tabs/day

Vicodin ES/Vicodin HP:
Usual: 1 tab q4-6h prn
Max: 6 tabs/day

PEDIATRIC DOSAGE

Pediatric use may not have been established

DOSING CONSIDERATIONS

Elderly
Start at lower end of dosing range

ADMINISTRATION

Oral route

STORAGE

20-25°C (68-77°F).

HOW SUPPLIED

(Hydrocodone/APAP) **Tab:** (Vicodin) 5mg/300mg*; (Vicodin ES) 7.5mg/300mg*; (Vicodin HP) 10mg/300mg* *scored

CONTRAINDICATIONS

Previous hypersensitivity to hydrocodone or APAP.

WARNINGS/PRECAUTIONS

Increased risk of acute liver failure in patients w/ underlying liver disease. May cause serious skin reactions (eg, acute generalized exanthematous pustulosis, Stevens-Johnson syndrome, toxic epidermal necrolysis); d/c at the 1st appearance of skin rash or any other sign of hypersensitivity. Hypersensitivity and anaphylaxis reported; d/c immediately if signs/symptoms occur. May produce dose-related respiratory depression and irregular/periodic breathing. Respiratory depressant effects and CSF pressure elevation capacity may be markedly exaggerated in the presence of head injury, other intracranial lesions, or a preexisting increased intracranial pressure. May obscure clinical course of acute abdominal conditions and head injuries. Caution w/ hypothyroidism, Addison's disease, prostatic hypertrophy, urethral stricture, severe hepatic/renal impairment, or in the elderly/debilitated. Suppresses cough reflex; caution w/ pulmonary disease and in postoperative use. Lab test interactions may occur. May be habit-forming.

ADVERSE REACTIONS

Acute liver failure, lightheadedness, dizziness, sedation, N/V.

DRUG INTERACTIONS

Increased risk of acute liver failure w/ alcohol. Additive CNS depression w/ other narcotics, antihistamines, antipsychotics, antianxiety agents, or other CNS depressants (eg, alcohol); reduce dose of one or both agents. Concomitant use w/ MAOIs or TCAs may increase the effect of either the antidepressant or hydrocodone.

PREGNANCY AND LACTATION

Category C, not for use in nursing.

MECHANISM OF ACTION

Hydrocodone: Opioid analgesic and antitussive; not established. Action believed to be related to the existence of opiate receptors in the CNS. APAP: Nonopiate, nonsalicylate analgesic, and antipyretic; not established. Antipyretic activity is mediated through hypothalamic heat-regulating centers; inhibits prostaglandin synthetase.

PHARMACOKINETICS

Absorption: Hydrocodone: (10mg) C_{max}=23.6ng/mL; T_{max}=1.3 hrs. APAP: Rapid. **Distribution:** APAP: Found in breast milk. **Metabolism:** Hydrocodone: O-demethylation, N-demethylation, and 6-keto reduction. APAP: Liver (conjugation). **Elimination:** Hydrocodone: (10mg) $T_{1/2}$=3.8 hrs. APAP: Urine (85%, mostly glucuronide conjugate); $T_{1/2}$=1.25-3 hrs.

PATIENT CONSIDERATIONS

Assessment: Assess for history of hypersensitivity to drug, level of pain intensity, type of pain, patient's general condition and medical status, renal/hepatic impairment, pregnancy/nursing status, any other conditions where treatment is cautioned, and possible drug interactions.

Monitoring: Monitor for signs/symptoms of hypersensitivity or anaphylaxis, serious skin reactions, acute liver failure, respiratory depression, elevations in CSF pressure, drug abuse/dependence/tolerance, and other adverse reactions. In patients w/ severe hepatic/renal disease, monitor effects w/ serial hepatic and/or renal function tests.

Counseling: Instruct to look for APAP on package labels and not to use >1 APAP-containing product. Instruct to seek medical attention immediately upon ingestion of >4000mg/day of APAP, even if feeling well. Advise to d/c use and contact physician immediately if signs of allergy develop. Inform about signs of serious skin reactions. Inform that drug may impair mental/physical abilities, and to use caution if performing potentially hazardous tasks (eg, driving, operating machinery). Instruct to avoid alcohol and other CNS depressants. Inform that drug may be habit-forming; instruct to take only ud.

VICOPROFEN — hydrocodone bitartrate/ibuprofen CII

Class: Opioid analgesic

OTHER BRAND NAMES

Reprexain

ADULT DOSAGE

Acute Pain

Short-Term (Generally <10 Days) Management:
Use lowest effective dose or longest dosing interval consistent w/ individual treatment goals; adjust based on individual needs
Usual: 1 tab q4-6h prn
Max: 5 tabs/24 hrs

PEDIATRIC DOSAGE

Acute Pain

Short-Term (Generally <10 Days) Management:
≥16 Years:
Use lowest effective dose or longest dosing interval consistent w/ individual treatment goals; adjust based on individual needs
Usual: 1 tab q4-6h prn
Max: 5 tabs/24 hrs

DOSING CONSIDERATIONS

Elderly
Reduce dose

ADMINISTRATION

Oral route

STORAGE

(Vicoprofen) 25°C (77°F); excursions permitted to 15-30°C (59-86°F). (Reprexain) 20-25°C (68-77°F); excursions permitted to 15-30°C (59-86°F).

HOW SUPPLIED

(Hydrocodone/Ibuprofen) **Tab:** (Vicoprofen) 7.5mg/200mg; (Reprexain) 2.5mg/200mg, 5mg/200mg*, 10mg/200mg *scored

CONTRAINDICATIONS

Known hypersensitivity to hydrocodone or ibuprofen. History of asthma, urticaria, or other allergic-type reactions w/ aspirin (ASA) or other NSAIDs. Perioperative pain in the setting of CABG surgery.

WARNINGS/PRECAUTIONS

Not for treatment of osteoarthritis or rheumatoid arthritis. Not for treatment of corticosteroid insufficiency or substitute for corticosteroids; abrupt discontinuation of corticosteroids may lead to disease exacerbation. May diminish utility of fever and inflammation as diagnostic signs in detecting complications of presumed noninfectious, painful conditions. Not recommended w/ advanced renal disease. Ibuprofen: May increase risk of serious cardiovascular (CV) thrombotic events, MI, and stroke; increased risk w/ known CV disease or risk factors for CV disease. May cause serious GI adverse events including inflammation, bleeding, ulceration, and perforation of the stomach and intestine; extreme caution w/ history of ulcer disease or GI bleeding and caution in debilitated patients. May lead to onset of new HTN or worsening of preexisting HTN. Fluid retention and edema reported; caution in patients w/ fluid retention or heart failure (HF). Renal papillary necrosis and other renal injury reported after long-term use; caution w/ impaired renal function, HF, and liver dysfunction. Anaphylactoid reactions may occur; avoid in patients w/ ASA triad. May cause serious skin adverse events (eg, exfoliative dermatitis, Stevens-Johnson syndrome, and toxic epidermal necrolysis); d/c at 1st appearance of skin rash/hypersensitivity. Avoid in late pregnancy; may cause premature closure of ductus arteriosus. Elevations of LFTs and severe hepatic reactions (eg, jaundice, fatal fulminant hepatitis, liver necrosis, hepatic failure) reported; d/c if liver disease or systemic manifestations (eg, eosinophilia, rash) occur. Anemia reported. May inhibit platelet aggregation and prolong bleeding time. Caution w/ preexisting asthma and avoid w/ ASA-sensitive asthma. Aseptic meningitis w/ fever and coma reported. Hydrocodone: May increase risk of misuse, abuse, or diversion. May produce dose-related respiratory depression. Respiratory depressant effects and capacity to elevate CSF pressure may be markedly exaggerated in the presence of head injury, intracranial lesions, or preexisting increased intracranial pressure. May obscure diagnosis/clinical course of acute abdominal conditions or head injuries. Caution in debilitated patients, severe renal/hepatic impairment, hypothyroidism, Addison's disease, prostatic hypertrophy, or urethral stricture. Suppresses cough reflex; caution when used postoperatively and w/ pulmonary disease.

ADVERSE REACTIONS
Headache, somnolence, dizziness, constipation, dyspepsia, N/V, infection, edema, nervousness, anxiety, pruritus, diarrhea, asthenia, abdominal pain, sweating.

DRUG INTERACTIONS
ASA may increase adverse effects; concomitant administration is not recommended. Use w/ other opioid analgesics, antihistamines, antipsychotics, antianxiety agents, or other CNS depressants (eg, alcohol) may exhibit additive CNS depression; reduce dose of 1 or both agents. Ibuprofen: Increased risk of GI bleeding w/ oral corticosteroids or anticoagulants, smoking, and alcohol. May increase the risk of renal toxicity w/ diuretics and ACE inhibitors. Alterations in platelet function may occur w/ anticoagulants; monitor carefully. May diminish antihypertensive effect of ACE inhibitors. Synergistic effects on GI bleeding w/ warfarin. May decrease natriuretic effect of furosemide and loop/thiazide diuretics; monitor renal failure. May increase lithium levels; monitor for lithium toxicity. May enhance methotrexate toxicity; caution w/ coadministration. Hydrocodone: Use w/ MAOIs or TCAs may increase the effect of either the antidepressant or hydrocodone. Not recommended for patients taking MAOIs or w/in 14 days of stopping such treatment. May produce paralytic ileus w/ anticholinergics. Caution w/ concurrent agonist/antagonist analgesics (eg, pentazocine, nalbuphine, butorphanol, buprenorphine) use; may reduce analgesic effect of hydrocodone and/or precipitate withdrawal symptoms. May enhance neuromuscular blocking action of skeletal muscle relaxants and increase respiratory depression.

PREGNANCY AND LACTATION
Category C, not for use in nursing.

MECHANISM OF ACTION
Hydrocodone: Opioid analgesic and antitussive; has not been established. Suspected to be related to existence of opiate receptors in CNS. Ibuprofen: NSAID; has not been established. May be related to inhibition of cyclooxygenase activity and prostaglandin synthesis. Possesses analgesic and antipyretic activity.

PHARMACOKINETICS
Absorption: Hydrocodone: C_{max}=27ng/mL, T_{max}=1.7 hrs. Ibuprofen: C_{max}=30mcg/mL, T_{max}=1.8 hrs. **Distribution:** Hydrocodone: Plasma protein binding (19-45%). Ibuprofen: Plasma protein binding (99%). **Metabolism:** Hydrocodone: CYP2D6 via O-demethylation to hydromorphone (active metabolite); CYP3A4 via N-demethylation; 6-keto reduction. Ibuprofen: Interconversion from R-isomer to S-isomer; (+)-2-4'-(2hydroxy-2-methyl-propyl) phenyl propionic acid and (+)-2-4'-(2carboxypropyl) phenyl propionic acid (primary metabolites). **Elimination:** Hydrocodone: Urine (primary); $T_{1/2}$=4.5 hrs. Ibuprofen: Urine (50-60% metabolites, 15% unchanged drug and conjugate), $T_{1/2}$=2.2 hrs.

PATIENT CONSIDERATIONS
Assessment: Assess for history of asthma, urticaria or allergic-type reactions w/ ASA or NSAIDs, known hypersensitivity to the drug, perioperative pain in setting of CABG surgery, CV disease and its risk factors, HTN, fluid retention or HF, ulcer disease or GI bleeding, coagulation disorders, renal/hepatic impairment, any other conditions where treatment is contraindicated or cautioned, pregnancy/nursing status, and for possible drug interactions. Assess level of pain intensity, type of pain, and patient's general condition and medical status.

Monitoring: Monitor for signs/symptoms of CV thrombotic events, MI, stroke, HTN, fluid retention or edema, drug abuse and dependence, tolerance, respiratory depression, elevations in CSF, GI effects, renal/hepatic effects, anaphylactoid reactions, skin reactions, bronchospasm, aseptic meningitis, and other adverse reactions. If signs/symptoms of anemia develop, evaluate Hgb/Hct. Perform periodic monitoring of CBC and chemistry profile w/ long-term therapy. Monitor for alterations in platelet function w/ coagulation disorders or in those receiving anticoagulants.

Counseling: Caution that drug may impair mental and/or physical abilities required to perform potentially hazardous tasks (eg, operating machinery/driving). Instruct to avoid alcohol and other CNS depressants while on therapy. Warn that drug may be habit-forming; instruct to take only for as long as prescribed, in the amounts prescribed, and no more frequently than prescribed. Instruct to contact physician if CV events, GI effects, unexplained weight gain, or edema occurs. Instruct to immediately d/c therapy and contact physician if signs/symptoms of serious skin reactions or hepatotoxicity develop. Instruct to seek immediate medical attention if signs of anaphylactoid reactions develop. Instruct to report any signs of blurred vision or other eye symptoms. Instruct to avoid use in late pregnancy.

VICTOZA — liraglutide   Rx

Class: Glucagon-like peptide-1 (GLP-1) receptor agonist

> Causes dose-dependent and treatment-duration-dependent thyroid C-cell tumors at clinically relevant exposures in animal studies. It is unknown whether drug causes thyroid C-cell tumors (eg, medullary thyroid carcinoma [MTC]) in humans. Contraindicated in patients w/ a personal or family history of MTC and in patients w/ multiple endocrine neoplasia syndrome type 2 (MEN 2). Counsel patients regarding potential risk for MTC and symptoms of thyroid tumors (eg, mass in the neck, dysphagia, dyspnea, persistent hoarseness). Routine monitoring of serum calcitonin or using thyroid ultrasound is of uncertain value for early detection of MTC.

ADULT DOSAGE
Type 2 Diabetes Mellitus
Initial: 0.6mg SQ qd for 1 week
Titrate: Increase to 1.2mg qd after 1 week; if acceptable glycemic control is not achieved, increase to 1.8mg qd

Missed Dose
If a dose is missed, the once-daily regimen should be resumed w/ the next scheduled dose; if >3 days have elapsed since the last dose, reinitiate at 0.6mg, and titrate ud

PEDIATRIC DOSAGE
Pediatric use may not have been established

DOSING CONSIDERATIONS
Concomitant Medications
Consider reducing dose of concomitant insulin secretagogue or insulin when initiating therapy

ADMINISTRATION
SQ route
May be administered qd at any time of the day, independently of meals.
Inject into abdomen, thigh, or upper arm.
Inj site and timing can be changed w/o dose adjustment.

Coadministration w/ Insulin
Administer as separate inj; never mix.
May inject in the same body region but the inj should not be adjacent to each other.

STORAGE
Prior to 1st Use: 2-8°C (36-46°F). Do not freeze and do not use if it has been frozen. **After Initial Use:** 15-30°C (59-86°F) or 2-8°C (36-46°F) for 30 days. Keep the pen cap on when not in use. Always remove and safely discard the needle after each inj; store pen w/o an inj needle attached. Protect from excessive heat and sunlight.

HOW SUPPLIED
Inj: 6mg/mL [3mL prefilled multi-dose pens]

CONTRAINDICATIONS
Personal or family history of MTC, MEN 2, prior serious hypersensitivity reaction to liraglutide or to any of the product components.

WARNINGS/PRECAUTIONS
Not recommended as 1st-line therapy for patients who have inadequate glycemic control on diet and exercise. Not a substitute for insulin; do not use in type 1 diabetes mellitus (DM) or for the treatment of diabetic ketoacidosis. Further evaluate patients w/ serum calcitonin elevation or thyroid nodules. Acute pancreatitis, including fatal and nonfatal hemorrhagic or necrotizing pancreatitis, reported; observe for signs/symptoms of pancreatitis after initiation of therapy, d/c promptly if suspected, and do not restart therapy if confirmed. Consider other antidiabetic therapies in patients w/ a history of pancreatitis. Do not share pens between patients, even if the needle is changed; poses a risk for transmission of blood-borne pathogens. Acute renal failure and worsening of chronic renal failure reported; caution when initiating/escalating doses in patients w/ renal impairment. Serious hypersensitivity reactions (eg, anaphylactic reactions, angioedema) reported; d/c if a hypersensitivity reaction occurs. Use w/ caution in patients w/ a history of angioedema w/ another GLP-1 receptor agonist. Caution w/ hepatic impairment.

ADVERSE REACTIONS
N/V, diarrhea, headache, nasopharyngitis, decreased appetite, dyspepsia, URTI, constipation, back pain.

DRUG INTERACTIONS
See Dosing Considerations. Increased risk of hypoglycemia w/ insulin secretagogues (eg, sulfonylureas) or insulin. May affect the absorption of oral medications; use w/ caution.

PREGNANCY AND LACTATION
Pregnancy: Category C.
Lactation: Not for use in nursing.

MECHANISM OF ACTION
Human GLP-1 receptor agonist analogue; increases intracellular cAMP, leading to insulin release in the presence of elevated glucose concentrations. Also decreases glucagon secretion in a glucose-dependent manner and delays gastric emptying.

PHARMACOKINETICS
Absorption: Absolute bioavailability (55%), T_{max}=8-12 hrs; (0.6mg) C_{max}=35ng/mL, AUC=960ng•hr/mL. **Distribution:** Plasma protein binding (>98%); (0.6mg) V_d=13L. **Elimination:** Urine (6% metabolites), feces (5% metabolites); $T_{1/2}$=13 hrs.

PATIENT CONSIDERATIONS

Assessment: Assess for previous hypersensitivity reactions, MEN 2, personal or family history of MTC, history of pancreatitis, type of DM, diabetic ketoacidosis, renal/hepatic impairment, pregnancy/nursing status, and possible drug interactions.

Monitoring: Monitor for signs and symptoms of thyroid tumor, pancreatitis, serum calcitonin elevation, hypoglycemia, hypersensitivity reactions, and other adverse reactions. Monitor renal function, blood glucose levels, and HbA1c levels.

Counseling: Inform regarding potential risk of MTC and advise to report symptoms of thyroid tumors (eg, lump in the neck, hoarseness) to physician. Inform of the potential risk of dehydration due to GI adverse reactions and instruct to take precautions to avoid fluid depletion. Inform of the potential risk for pancreatitis and worsening renal function. Instruct to d/c therapy promptly and contact physician if persistent severe abdominal pain and/or symptoms of hypersensitivity reactions occur. Advise not to share pen w/ another person, even if the needle is changed. Advise of the potential risks/benefits of therapy and of alternative modes of therapy. Explain the importance of adhering to dietary instructions, regular physical activity, periodic blood glucose monitoring and HbA1c testing, recognition/management of hypo/hyperglycemia, and assessment for diabetes complications. Advise to seek medical advice during periods of stress (eg, fever, trauma, infection), if any unusual symptom develops, or if any known symptom persists or worsens. Instruct not to take an extra dose to make up for a missed dose and to resume as prescribed w/ the next scheduled dose.

VIDAZA — azacitidine   Rx

Class: Pyrimidine nucleoside analogue

ADULT DOSAGE

Myelodysplastic Syndromes

Treatment of the following French-American-British (FAB) myelodysplastic syndrome subtypes: refractory anemia or refractory anemia w/ ringed sideroblasts (if accompanied by neutropenia or thrombocytopenia or requiring transfusions), refractory anemia w/ excess blasts, refractory anemia w/ excess blasts in transformation, and chronic myelomonocytic leukemia

1st Treatment Cycle:
Initial: 75mg/m^2/day SQ or IV for 7 days

Subsequent Treatment Cycles:
Repeat cycle every 4 weeks
Dose may be increased to 100mg/m^2 if no beneficial effect is seen after 2 cycles and if no toxicity other than N/V has occurred

Treat for a minimum of 4-6 cycles; complete or partial response may require additional cycles

Treatment may be continued as long as the patient continues to benefit

Premedication
Premedicate for N/V

PEDIATRIC DOSAGE
Pediatric use may not have been established

DOSING CONSIDERATIONS

Adverse Reactions
Hematology Lab Values:
For patients w/ baseline WBC ≥3.0 x 10^9/L, ANC ≥1.5 x 10^9/L, and platelets ≥75.0 x 10^9/L, adjust the dose as follows, based on nadir counts for any given cycle:
ANC <0.5 x 10^9/L or Platelets <25 x 10^9/L: Administer 50% of dose in next course
ANC <0.5-1.5 x 10^9/L or Platelets 25-50 x 10^9/L: Administer 67% of dose in next course

For patients whose baseline counts are WBC <3.0 x 10^9/L, ANC<1.5 x 10^9/L, or platelets <75.0 x 10^9/L, dose adjustments should be based on nadir counts and bone marrow biopsy cellularity at the time of the nadir as noted below, unless there is clear improvement in differentiation at the time of the next cycle, in which case the dose of the current treatment should be continued
WBC or Platelet 50-75% Decrease in Counts from Baseline:
Bone Marrow Biopsy Cellularity 15-30%: Administer 50% of dose in next course
Bone Marrow Biopsy Cellularity <15%: Administer 33% of dose in next course

WBC or Platelet >75% Decrease in Counts from Baseline:
Bone Marrow Biopsy Cellularity 30-60%: Administer 75% of dose in next course
Bone Marrow Biopsy Cellularity 15-30%: Administer 50% of dose in next course
Bone Marrow Biopsy Cellularity <15%: Administer 33% of dose in next course
If a nadir as defined above has occurred, the next course of treatment should be given 28 days after the start of the preceding course, provided that both the WBC and the platelet counts are >25% above the nadir and rising
If a >25% Increase is Not Seen by Day 28: Reassess counts every 7 days
If a 25% Increase is Not Seen by Day 42: Treated w/ 50% of the scheduled dose
Serum Electrolytes and Renal Toxicity:
Unexplained Reductions in Serum Bicarbonate Levels to <20mEq/L: Reduce dose by 50% on next course

Unexplained Elevations of BUN/SrCr: Delay next cycle until values return to normal or baseline, and reduce dose by 50% on next course

ADMINISTRATION

IV/SQ route

The vial is single-use and does not contain any preservatives; discard unused portions of each vial properly.

Instructions for SQ Administration
1. Reconstitute w/ 4mL of sterile water for inj (SWFI).
2. Inject the diluents slowly into the vial.
3. Vigorously shake or roll the vial until a uniform sus is achieved; the sus will be cloudy.
4. The resulting sus will contain azacitidine 25mg/mL.
5. Do not filter the sus after reconstitution; doing so could remove the active substance.
6. To provide a homogeneous sus, the contents of the dosing syringe must be re-suspended immediately prior to administration; to re-suspend, vigorously roll the syringe between the palms until a uniform, cloudy suspension is achieved.
7. Doses >4mL should be divided equally into 2 syringes and injected into 2 separate sites; rotate sites for each inj (thigh, abdomen, or upper arm). New inj should be given ≥1 inch from an old site and never into areas where the site is tender, bruised, red, or hard.

Immediate SQ Administration:
Administer w/in 1 hr after reconstitution.

Delayed SQ Administration:
Reconstituted product may be kept in the vial or drawn into a syringe. The product must be refrigerated immediately; after removal from refrigerated conditions, the sus may be allowed to equilibrate to room temperature for up to 30 min prior to administration.

Instructions for IV Administration
1. Reconstitute the appropriate number of vials to achieve the desired dose; reconstitute each vial w/ 10mL SWFI.
2. Vigorously shake or roll the vial until all solids are dissolved.
3. The resulting sol will contain azacitidine 10mg/mL.
4. Withdraw the required amount of azacitidine sol to deliver the desired dose and inject into a 50-100mL infusion bag of either 0.9% NaCl inj or lactated Ringer's inj.
5. Administer the total dose over a period of 10-40 min; administration must be completed w/in 1 hr of reconstitution of the azacitidine vial.

IV Sol Incompatibility:
Azacitidine is incompatible w/:
1. D5 sol
2. Hespan
3. Sol containing bicarbonate

Handling Precautions
If reconstituted azacitidine comes into contact w/ the skin, immediately and thoroughly wash w/ soap and water; if it comes into contact w/ mucous membranes, flush thoroughly w/ water.

STORAGE
25°C (77°F); excursions permitted to 15-30°C (59-86°F). Reconstituted Sus: Using Non-refrigerated Water for Inj: 25°C (77°F) for up to 1 hr or 2-8°C (36-46°F) for up to 8 hrs. Using Refrigerated (2-8°C [36-46°F]) Water for Inj: 2-8°C (36-46°F) for up to 22 hrs. Reconstituted Sol: 25°C (77°F) for up to 1 hr.

HOW SUPPLIED
Inj: 100mg

CONTRAINDICATIONS
Advanced malignant hepatic tumors, hypersensitivity to azacitidine or mannitol.

WARNINGS/PRECAUTIONS
Obtain CBC, liver chemistries, and SrCr prior to 1st dose. Anemia, neutropenia, and thrombocytopenia may occur; monitor CBC frequently for response and/or toxicity (at a minimum, before each cycle). Potentially hepatotoxic in patients w/ severe preexisting hepatic impairment; caution w/ liver disease. Monitor patients w/ renal impairment for toxicity. May cause fetal harm; women of childbearing potential should avoid pregnancy, while men should not father a child during treatment. Caution in elderly.

ADVERSE REACTIONS
N/V, anemia, thrombocytopenia, pyrexia, leukopenia, diarrhea, inj-site erythema, constipation, neutropenia, ecchymosis, petechiae, rigors, weakness, hypokalemia.

DRUG INTERACTIONS
Renal toxicity reported w/ IV azacitidine in combination w/ other chemotherapeutic agents (eg, etoposide).

PREGNANCY AND LACTATION
Pregnancy: Category D.
Lactation: Not for use in nursing.

MECHANISM OF ACTION
Pyrimidine nucleoside analog; believed to cause hypomethylation of DNA and direct cytotoxicity on abnormal hematopoietic cells in the bone marrow.

PHARMACOKINETICS
Absorption: (SQ) Rapid. Absolute bioavailability (89%); C_{max}=750ng/mL; T_{max}=0.5 hr. **Distribution:** (IV) V_d=76L. **Elimination:** (IV) Urine (85%), feces (<1%). (SQ) Urine (50%); $T_{1/2}$=41 min.

PATIENT CONSIDERATIONS
Assessment: Assess for advanced malignant hepatic tumors, hypersensitivity to drug or to mannitol, renal/hepatic impairment, pregnancy/nursing status, and possible drug interactions. Obtain baseline CBC, LFTs, and SrCr.

Monitoring: Monitor CBC frequently for response and/or toxicity (at a minimum, before each cycle). Monitor LFTs, renal function, and serum electrolytes.

Counseling: Instruct to inform physician of any underlying liver or renal disease, or if pregnant/breastfeeding. Advise women of childbearing potential to avoid becoming pregnant, and men not to father a child while on therapy.

VIEKIRA PAK — dasabuvir; ombitasvir/paritaprevir/ritonavir   Rx

Class: CYP3A inhibitor/HCV NS5A inhibitor/HCV non-nucleoside NS5B palm polymerase inhibitor/ HCV NS3/4A protease inhibitor

ADULT DOSAGE

Chronic Hepatitis C (Genotype 1)
2 tabs (ombitasvir, paritaprevir, ritonavir [RTV]) qd (am) and 1 dasabuvir tab bid (am and pm)

Coadministration w/ Ribavirin (RBV):
<75kg: 1000mg/day RBV divided and administered bid w/ food
≥75kg: 1200mg/day RBV divided and administered bid w/ food

Genotype 1a, w/o Cirrhosis:
2 tabs (ombitasvir, paritaprevir, RTV) qd (am) + 1 dasabuvir tab bid (am and pm) + RBV for 12 weeks

Genotype 1a, w/ Compensated Cirrhosis (Child-Pugh A):
2 tabs (ombitasvir, paritaprevir, RTV) qd (am) + 1 dasabuvir tab bid (am and pm) + RBV for 24 weeks. 12-week treatment duration may be considered for some patients based on prior treatment history

Genotype 1b, w/ or w/o Compensated Cirrhosis (Child-Pugh A):
2 tabs (ombitasvir, paritaprevir, RTV) qd (am) + 1 dasabuvir tab bid (am and pm) for 12 weeks

Follow the genotype 1a dosing recommendations in patients w/ an unknown genotype 1 subtype or w/ mixed genotype 1 infection

Liver Transplant Recipients w/ Normal Hepatic Function and Mild Fibrosis (Metavir Fibrosis Score ≤2):
2 tabs (ombitasvir, paritaprevir, RTV) qd (am) + 1 dasabuvir tab bid (am and pm) + RBV for 24 weeks, irrespective of hepatitis C virus genotype 1 subtype. If calcineurin inhibitor used concomitantly, calcineurin inhibitor dosage adjustment is needed

PEDIATRIC DOSAGE

Pediatric use may not have been established

DOSING CONSIDERATIONS
Hepatic Impairment
Mild (Child-Pugh A): No dose adjustment needed
Moderate to Severe (Child-Pugh B and C): Contraindicated

ADMINISTRATION
Oral route

Take w/ a meal w/o regard to fat or calorie content.

STORAGE
≤30°C (86°F).

HOW SUPPLIED
Tab: (Ombitasvir/Paritaprevir/RTV) 12.5mg/75mg/50mg, (Dasabuvir) 250mg

CONTRAINDICATIONS
Moderate to severe hepatic impairment (Child-Pugh B and C). Coadministration w/ drugs that are highly dependent on CYP3A for clearance and for which elevated plasma concentrations are associated w/ serious and/or life-threatening events; coadministration w/ moderate or strong inducers of CYP3A and strong inducers of CYP2C8 that may lead to reduced efficacy of therapy; and coadministration w/ strong inhibitors of CYP2C8 that may increase dasabuvir plasma concentrations and the risk of QT prolongation. Coadministration w/ alfuzosin, ranolazine, dronedarone, carbamazepine, phenytoin, phenobarbital, colchicine, gemfibrozil, rifampin, lurasidone, ergotamine, dihydroergotamine, methylergonovine, ethinyl estradiol-containing medications (eg, combined oral contraceptives), cisapride, St. John's wort, lovastatin, simvastatin, pimozide, efavirenz, sildenafil (when used to treat pulmonary arterial HTN), triazolam, or oral midazolam. Known hypersensitivity (eg, toxic epidermal necrolysis, Stevens-Johnson syndrome) to RTV. When used w/ RBV, refer to the individual PI.

WARNINGS/PRECAUTIONS
Hepatic decompensation and hepatic failure including liver transplantation or fatal outcomes reported; monitor for signs and symptoms of hepatic decompensation and d/c if evidence of hepatic decompensation develops. Elevations of ALT to >5X ULN reported. Perform hepatic lab testing during the first 4 weeks of starting treatment and as clinically indicated thereafter. If ALT is found to be elevated above baseline levels, repeat and monitor closely. Consider discontinuing if ALT levels remain persistently >10X ULN. D/C if ALT elevation is accompanied by signs or symptoms of liver inflammation or increasing direct bilirubin, alkaline phosphatase, or INR. If coadministered w/ RBV, the warnings and precautions for RBV, in particular the pregnancy avoidance warning, apply to this combination regimen; refer to RBV PI for a full list of warnings/precautions for RBV. Any HCV/HIV-1 coinfected patients being treated should also be on a suppressive antiretroviral drug regimen to reduce the risk of HIV-1 protease inhibitor drug resistance.

ADVERSE REACTIONS
W/ RBV: Fatigue, nausea, pruritus, skin reactions, insomnia, asthenia. **W/O RBV:** Nausea, pruritus, insomnia, asthenia.

DRUG INTERACTIONS
See Contraindications. Not recommended w/ darunavir/RTV, lopinavir/RTV, rilpivirine (qd dosing), and salmeterol. Not recommended w/ voriconazole unless an assessment of the benefit-to-risk ratio justifies the use of voriconazole. Not recommended w/ metformin in patients w/ renal insufficiency or hepatic impairment. Monitor for signs of lactic acidosis (eg, respiratory distress, somnolence, non-specific abdominal distress, worsening renal function) w/ metformin. If taking quetiapine, consider alternative anti-HCV therapy. Therapeutic monitoring is recommended w/ antiarrhythmics. May increase levels of drugs that are substrates of CYP3A, UGT1A1, breast cancer resistance protein (BCRP), OATP1B1, or OATP1B3. May increase levels of ARBs, quetiapine, antiarrhythmics, calcium channel blockers (eg, amlodipine), ketoconazole, inhaled/nasal fluticasone, furosemide (C_{max}), rilpivirine, rosuvastatin, pravastatin, cyclosporine, tacrolimus, salmeterol, buprenorphine, norbuprenorphine, hydrocodone, and alprazolam. Concomitant use w/ inhaled/nasal fluticasone may reduce serum cortisol concentrations; consider alternative corticosteroids. May decrease levels of voriconazole, darunavir (C_{trough}), carisoprodol, cyclobenzaprine, norcyclobenzaprine, omeprazole, diazepam, and nordiazepam. Inhibition of P-gp, BCRP, OATP1B1, or OATP1B3 may increase levels of the various components of Viekira Pak. ALT elevation reported more frequently w/ ethinyl estradiol-containing medications (eg, combined oral contraceptives, contraceptive patches, contraceptive vaginal rings); alternative methods of contraception (eg, progestin-only contraception, nonhormonal methods) are recommended during therapy. Ethinyl estradiol-containing medications can be restarted approx 2 weeks following completion of treatment. **Paritaprevir:** Atazanavir/RTV (qd dosing), and lopinavir/RTV may increase levels. **Paritaprevir/RTV:** Strong CYP3A inhibitors may increase levels. **Dasabuvir:** CYP2C8 inhibitors may increase levels. Refer to PI for further information on drug interactions, including dosing modifications when used w/ certain concomitant therapies.

PREGNANCY AND LACTATION
Pregnancy: No adequate human data are available to establish whether or not Viekira Pak poses a risk to pregnancy outcomes.
Lactation: It is not known whether Viekira Pak and its metabolites are present in human breast milk, affect human milk production, or have effects on the breastfed infant; caution in nursing.

If administered w/ ribavirin, refer to the prescribing information of ribavirin for additional information.

MECHANISM OF ACTION
Ombitasvir: Inhibitor of HCV NS5A, which is essential for viral RNA replication and virion assembly. **Paritaprevir:** Inhibitor of HCV NS3/4A protease, which is necessary for the proteolytic cleavage of the HCV encoded polyprotein (into mature forms of the NS3, NS4A, NS4B, NS5A, and NS5B proteins) and is essential for viral replication. **Dasabuvir:** Non-nucleoside inhibitor of the HCV RNA-dependent RNA polymerase encoded by the NS5B gene, which is essential for replication of the viral genome. **RTV:** Potent CYP3A inhibitor; increases peak and trough plasma drug concentrations of paritaprevir and overall drug exposure.

PHARMACOKINETICS
Absorption: T_{max}=4-5 hrs. Dasabuvir: Absolute bioavailability (70%). C_{max}=667ng/mL (median); AUC_{0-12}=3240ng•hr/mL (median). Ombitasvir: Absolute bioavailability (48%). C_{max}=68ng/mL (median); AUC_{0-24}=1000ng•hr/mL (median). Paritaprevir: Absolute bioavailability (53%). C_{max}=262ng/mL (median); AUC_{0-24}=2220ng•hr/mL (median). RTV: C_{max}=682ng/mL (median); AUC_{0-24}=6180ng•hr/mL (median). **Distribution:** Dasabuvir: Plasma protein binding (>99.5%); V_d=149L. Ombitasvir: Plasma protein binding (99.9%); V_d=173L. Paritaprevir: Plasma protein binding (97-98.6%); V_d=103L. RTV: Plasma protein binding (>99%); V_d=21.5L (apparent). **Metabolism:** Ombitasvir: Via amide hydrolysis followed by oxidative metabolism. Paritaprevir: Via CYP3A4 (major), CYP3A5. RTV: Via CYP3A (major), CYP2D6. Dasabuvir: Via CYP2C8 (major), CYP3A. **Elimination:** Dasabuvir: Feces (94.4%, 26% unchanged), urine (~2%, 0.03% unchanged); $T_{1/2}$=5.5-6 hrs. Ombitasvir: Feces (90.2%, 87.8% unchanged), urine (1.91%, 0.03% unchanged); $T_{1/2}$=21-25 hrs. Paritaprevir: Feces (88%, 1.1% unchanged), urine (8.8%, 0.05% unchanged); $T_{1/2}$=5.5 hrs. RTV: Feces (86.4%, 33.8 unchanged), urine (11.3%, 3.5 unchanged); $T_{1/2}$=4 hrs.

PATIENT CONSIDERATIONS
Assessment: Assess for drug hypersensitivity, hepatic decompensation, hepatic impairment, pregnancy/nursing status, and possible drug interactions. Assess LFTs.

Monitoring: Monitor for hepatic decompensation, ALT elevation, and other adverse reactions. Perform hepatic lab testing (eg, direct bilirubin levels) during the first 4 weeks of starting treatment and as clinically indicated thereafter. If ALT is found to be elevated above baseline levels, repeat and monitor closely.

Counseling: Inform to watch for early warning signs of liver inflammation or failure (eg, fatigue, lack of appetite, N/V); instruct to contact physician w/o delay if such symptoms occur. Advise to avoid pregnancy during treatment w/ RBV and w/in 6 months of stopping RBV; instruct to notify physician immediately in the event of a pregnancy. Inform that therapy may interact w/ some drugs; advise to report to physician the use of any prescription, nonprescription medication, or herbal products. Inform that contraceptives containing ethinyl estradiol are contraindicated w/ therapy. Advise patients to take therapy every day at the regularly scheduled time w/ a meal w/o regard to fat or calorie content. Inform patients that it is important not to miss or skip doses and to take therapy for the duration that is recommended by physician.

VIGAMOX — moxifloxacin hydrochloride   Rx

Class: Fluoroquinolone

ADULT DOSAGE	PEDIATRIC DOSAGE
Bacterial Conjunctivitis	**Bacterial Conjunctivitis**
1 drop in the affected eye tid for 7 days	**≥1 Year:** 1 drop in the affected eye tid for 7 days

---

ADMINISTRATION
Ocular route

STORAGE
2-25°C (36-77°F).

HOW SUPPLIED
Sol: 0.5% [3mL]

CONTRAINDICATIONS
History of hypersensitivity to moxifloxacin, to other quinolones, or to any components in the medication.

WARNINGS/PRECAUTIONS
Not for inj. Do not inject subconjunctivally or introduce directly into the anterior chamber of the eye. Fatal hypersensitivity reactions reported with systemic quinolone therapy. May result in bacterial resistance with prolonged use; take appropriate measures if superinfection develops. Avoid contact lenses when signs and symptoms of bacterial conjunctivitis are present.

ADVERSE REACTIONS
Conjunctivitis, decreased visual acuity, dry eye, keratitis, ocular discomfort/ hyperemia, ocular pain/pruritus, subconjunctival hemorrhage, tearing.

PREGNANCY AND LACTATION
Category C, caution in nursing.

MECHANISM OF ACTION
Fluoroquinolone antibiotic; inhibits topoisomerase II (DNA gyrase) and topoisomerase IV.

PHARMACOKINETICS
Absorption: C_{max}=2.7ng/mL, AUC=45ng•hr/mL. **Distribution:** Presumed to be excreted in breast milk. **Elimination:** $T_{1/2}$=13 hrs.

PATIENT CONSIDERATIONS

Assessment: Assess for proper diagnosis of causative organisms (eg, slit-lamp biomicroscopy, fluorescein staining), Assess for hypersensitivity to other quinolones, and pregnancy/nursing status.

Monitoring: Monitor for signs/symptoms of hypersensitivity or anaphylactic reactions and other adverse reactions. With prolonged therapy, monitor for overgrowth of nonsusceptible organisms (eg, fungi) and for development of superinfection.

Counseling: Instruct not to touch the dropper tip to any surface to avoid contaminating the contents. Instruct to immediately d/c medication and contact physician at the 1st sign of rash or allergic reaction. Instruct not to wear contact lenses if signs and symptoms of bacterial conjunctivitis develop.

VIIBRYD — vilazodone hydrochloride   Rx

Class: Selective serotonin reuptake inhibitor (SSRI)/5-HT$_{1A}$-receptor partial agonist

> Antidepressants increased the risk of suicidal thoughts and behaviors in patients aged ≤24 yrs in short-term studies. Monitor closely for clinical worsening and for emergence of suicidal thoughts and behaviors.

ADULT DOSAGE	PEDIATRIC DOSAGE
Major Depressive Disorder	Pediatric use may not have been established
Initial: 10mg qd for 7 days	
Titrate: Increase to 20mg qd	
May increase up to 40mg qd after a minimum of 7 days between dosage increases	
Target Dose: 20-40mg qd	
Dosing Considerations with MAOIs	
Switching to/from an MAOI Antidepressant:	
Allow at least 14 days between discontinuation of an MAOI antidepressant and initiation of treatment, and allow at least 14 days after stopping treatment before starting an MAOI antidepressant	

DOSING CONSIDERATIONS
Concomitant Medications
Strong CYP3A4 Inhibitors (eg, Itraconazole, Clarithromycin, Voriconazole):
Max: 20mg qd; may resume original vilazodone dose level when CYP3A4 inhibitor is discontinued

Strong CYP3A4 Inducers (eg, Carbamazepine, Phenytoin, Rifampin) for >14 Days: Consider increasing vilazodone dose by 2-fold, up to a max of 80mg qd, over 1-2 weeks based on clinical response; gradually reduce vilazodone dosage to its original level over 1-2 weeks if CYP3A4 inducers are discontinued

Elderly
Start at lower end of dosing range

Discontinuation
Gradually reduce dose whenever possible.
Taper down from 40mg qd dose to 20mg qd for 4 days, followed by 10mg qd for 3 days.
Taper dose to 10mg qd for 7 days in patients taking 20mg qd.

ADMINISTRATION
Oral route
Take w/ food.

STORAGE
25°C (77°F); excursions permitted to 15-30°C (59-86°F).

HOW SUPPLIED
Tab: 10mg, 20mg, 40mg

CONTRAINDICATIONS
Concomitant use of MAOIs, or w/in 14 days of stopping MAOIs (eg, linezolid, IV methylene blue).

WARNINGS/PRECAUTIONS
Serotonin syndrome reported; d/c immediately if symptoms occur and initiate supportive symptomatic treatment. May increase the risk of bleeding events. May precipitate mixed/manic episode in patients w/ bipolar disorder. Avoid abrupt discontinuation. Caution w/ a seizure disorder. Pupillary dilation that occurs following use may trigger an angle closure attack in a patient w/ anatomically narrow angles who does not have a patent iridectomy; avoid use in patients w/ untreated anatomically narrow angles. Hyponatremia may occur; d/c and institute appropriate medical intervention in patients w/ symptomatic hyponatremia. Elderly patients, patients taking diuretics, and those who are volume-depleted may be at greater risk of developing hyponatremia.

ADVERSE REACTIONS
Diarrhea, N/V, insomnia.

DRUG INTERACTIONS
See Dosing Considerations and Contraindications. May cause serotonin syndrome w/ other serotonergic drugs (eg, triptans, TCAs, St. John's wort) and w/ drugs that impair metabolism of serotonin; d/c treatment and any concomitant serotonergic agents immediately if this occurs. Increased risk of bleeding w/ aspirin (ASA), NSAIDs, other antiplatelet drugs, warfarin, and other anticoagulants. Monitor coagulation indices (eg, INR) w/ warfarin when initiating/titrating/ discontinuing vilazodone. Strong CYP3A4 inhibitors may increase vilazodone exposure. Strong CYP3A4 inducers may decrease vilazodone exposure. May increase digoxin concentrations; measure digoxin concentrations before initiating concomitant use of vilazodone and continue monitoring and reduce digoxin dose as necessary.

PREGNANCY AND LACTATION
Pregnancy: There are no adequate and well-controlled studies of vilazodone in pregnant women. Consider the risks of untreated depression when discontinuing or changing treatment w/ antidepressant medication during pregnancy and postpartum. Exposure to vilazodone, in late pregnancy may lead to an increased risk for neonatal complications requiring prolonged hospitalization, respiratory support, and tube feeding, and/or persistent pulmonary HTN of the newborn. **Lactation:** There are no data on the presence of vilazodone in human milk, the effects of vilazodone on breastfed infant, or the effects of the drug on milk production. However, vilazodone is excreted in rat milk. Caution in nursing.

MECHANISM OF ACTION
SSRI and 5-HT$_{1A}$ receptor partial agonist; has not been established. Thought to enhance serotonergic activity in the CNS through selective inhibition of serotonin reuptake.

PHARMACOKINETICS
Absorption: Absolute bioavailability (72%, w/ food); C_{max}=156ng/mL (fed), AUC=1645ng•hr/mL (fed), T_{max}=4-5 hrs (median). **Distribution:** Plasma protein binding (approx 96-99%). **Metabolism:** Extensive via CYP3A4 (primary), CYP2C19, CYP2D6 (minor), and carboxylesterase. **Elimination:** Urine (1% unchanged), feces (2% unchanged); $T_{1/2}$=approx 25 hrs.

PATIENT CONSIDERATIONS

Assessment: Assess for personal/family history of bipolar disorder, mania/ hypomania, seizure disorder, untreated anatomically narrow angles, volume depletion, pregnancy/nursing status, and possible drug interactions.

Monitoring: Monitor for clinical worsening and emergence of suicidal thoughts and behaviors (especially during the initial few months of therapy and at times of dosage changes). Monitor for serotonin syndrome, angle-closure glaucoma, bleeding, activation of mania/hypomania, hyponatremia, discontinuation symptoms, and other adverse reactions. Carefully monitor the INR when initiating or discontinuing vilazodone in patients taking warfarin.

Counseling: Advise patients and caregivers to monitor for clinical worsening and to look for the emergence of suicidality, especially early during treatment and when the dose is adjusted up or down; instruct to report such symptoms to physician. Instruct to take ud. Caution about the risk of serotonin syndrome;

instruct to contact physician or report to the emergency room if patient experiences signs/symptoms of serotonin syndrome. Inform about the increased risk of bleeding w/ ASA, NSAIDs, other antiplatelet drugs, warfarin, or other anticoagulants; inform physician if taking/planning to take any prescription or OTC medications that increase the risk of bleeding. Advise patients and caregivers to observe for signs of activation of mania/hypomania; instruct to report such symptoms to physician. Instruct not to abruptly d/c therapy and to discuss any tapering regimen w/ physician. Caution about using vilazodone if patient has a history of a seizure disorder. Advise to notify physician if an allergic reaction develops. Inform physician if taking or planning to take any prescription or OTC medications.

VIMIZIM — elosulfase alfa   Rx

Class: Enzyme

> Life-threatening anaphylactic reactions observed during infusion. Anaphylaxis (eg, cough, erythema, throat tightness, urticaria, flushing, cyanosis, hypotension, rash, dyspnea, chest discomfort, GI symptoms) in conjunction with urticaria reported during infusions, regardless of duration of treatment; closely observe patients during and after administration. Inform patients of the signs/symptoms of anaphylaxis and instruct to seek immediate medical care should symptoms occur. Patients with acute respiratory illness may be at risk of serious acute exacerbation of their respiratory compromise due to hypersensitivity reactions; additional monitoring required.

ADULT DOSAGE
Mucopolysaccharidosis IVA (Morquio A Syndrome)
Usual: 2mg/kg IV over a minimum range of 3.5-4.5 hrs, based on infusion volume, once every week

Premedication
Pretreat w/ antihistamines (w/ or w/o antipyretics) 30-60 min prior to start of infusion

PEDIATRIC DOSAGE
Mucopolysaccharidosis IVA (Morquio A Syndrome)
≥5 Years:
Usual: 2mg/kg IV over a minimum range of 3.5-4.5 hrs, based on infusion volume, once every week

Premedication
Pretreat w/ antihistamines (w/ or w/o antipyretics) 30-60 min prior to start of infusion

---

DOSING CONSIDERATIONS
Adverse Reactions
Hypersensitivity Reactions: Slow, temporarily stop, or d/c infusion rate for that visit

ADMINISTRATION
IV route

Preparation Instructions
1. Determine the number of vials to be diluted based on the patient's weight and the recommended dose.
2. Dilute the calculated dose to a final volume of 100mL or 250mL using 0.9% NaCl inj; the final volume is based on the patient's weight as follows:
Patients <25kg: Final volume should be 100mL
Patients ≥25kg: Final volume should be 250mL
3. The sol should be clear to slightly opalescent and colorless to pale yellow when diluted; a sol w/ slight flocculation (eg, thin translucent fibers) is acceptable for administration.
4. Gently rotate the bag to ensure proper distribution; avoid agitation during preparation and do not shake the sol.
5. Administration should be completed w/in 48 hrs from the time of dilution.

Administration Instructions
Administer the diluted sol using a low-protein binding infusion set equipped w/ a low-protein binding 0.2µm in-line filter.

Patients <25kg:
Initial Infusion Rate: 3mL/hr for the first 15 min
Titrate: If tolerated, increase to 6mL/hr for the next 15 min; if this rate is tolerated, then the rate may be increased every 15 min in 6mL/hr increments
Max Infusion Rate: 36mL/hr
Total volume of the infusion should be delivered over a minimum of 3.5 hrs.

Patients ≥25kg:
Initial Infusion Rate: 6mL/hr for the first 15 min
Titrate: If tolerated, increase to 12mL/hr for the next 15 min; if this rate is tolerated, then the rate may be increased every 15 min in 12mL/hr increments
Max Infusion Rate: 72mL/hr
Total volume of the infusion should be delivered over a minimum of 4.5 hrs.

Do not infuse w/ other products in the infusion tubing.

Stability Information
If immediate use is not possible, store the diluted product for up to 24 hrs at 2-8°C (36-46°F), followed by up to 24 hrs at 23-27°C (73-81°F).

STORAGE
2-8°C (36-46°F). Do not freeze or shake. Protect from light. Diluted Sol: Store for up to 24 hrs at 2-8°C (36-46°F) followed by up to 24 hrs at 23-27°C (73-81°F). Complete administration within 48 hrs from the time of dilution.

HOW SUPPLIED
Inj: 1mg/mL [5mL]

WARNINGS/PRECAUTIONS
Spinal/cervical cord compression (SCC) reported. Anaphylaxis and hypersensitivity reactions reported; d/c infusion immediately and initiate appropriate treatment if severe allergic reactions occur. Caution with readministration in patients who have severe allergic reactions. Increased risk of life-threatening complications from hypersensitivity reactions in patients with acute febrile or respiratory illness at the time of infusion; consider patient's clinical status prior to administration and consider delaying the infusion. Sleep apnea is common in MPS IVA patients; evaluate airway patency prior to initiation of treatment.

ADVERSE REACTIONS
Pyrexia, N/V, headache, abdominal pain, chills, fatigue.

PREGNANCY AND LACTATION
Pregnancy: Category C.
Lactation: Caution in nursing.

MECHANISM OF ACTION
Hydrolytic lysosomal glycosaminoglycan (GAG)-specific enzyme; provides exogenous N-acetylgalactosamine-6-sulfatase that is taken up into lysosomes and increases the catabolism of GAGs KS and C6S.

PHARMACOKINETICS
Absorption: C_{max}=1.49mcg/mL (Week 0), 4.04mcg/mL (Week 22); AUC_{0-t}=238mcg•min/mL (Week 0), 577mcg•min/mL (Week 22). **Distribution:** V_d=396mL/kg (Week 0), 650mL/kg (Week 22). **Elimination:** $T_{1/2}$=7.52 min (Week 0), 35.9 min (Week 22).

PATIENT CONSIDERATIONS
Assessment: Assess for respiratory illness, clinical status, airway patency, and pregnancy/nursing status.

Monitoring: Monitor for anaphylaxis/severe allergic reactions, SCC, and other adverse reactions.

Counseling: Counsel that reactions (eg, life-threatening anaphylaxis) related to administration and infusion may occur during treatment. Inform patients of the signs and symptoms of anaphylaxis and to seek immediate medical care should symptoms occur. Inform patients and pregnant/nursing women of the Morquio A Registry and advise that their participation is voluntary and may involve long-term follow-up.

VIMOVO — esomeprazole magnesium/naproxen   Rx

Class: NSAID/proton pump inhibitor (PPI)

> NSAIDs cause an increased risk of serious cardiovascular (CV) thrombotic events, including MI and stroke, which can be fatal. This risk may occur early in treatment and may increase w/ duration of use. Contraindicated in the setting of CABG surgery. NSAIDs cause an increased risk of serious GI adverse events (eg, bleeding, ulceration, stomach/intestinal perforation), which can be fatal and can occur anytime during use and w/o warning symptoms; elderly patients and patients w/ a prior history of peptic ulcer disease and/or GI bleeding are at a greater risk.

ADULT DOSAGE
Osteoarthritis
Relief of signs/symptoms of osteoarthritis and to decrease the risk of developing gastric ulcers in patients at risk of developing NSAID-associated gastric ulcers

1 tab bid of 375mg/20mg or 500mg/20mg

Controlled studies do not extend beyond 6 months

Rheumatoid Arthritis
Relief of signs/symptoms of rheumatoid arthritis and to decrease the risk of developing gastric ulcers in patients at risk of developing NSAID-associated gastric ulcers

1 tab bid of 375mg/20mg or 500mg/20mg

Controlled studies do not extend beyond 6 months

Ankylosing Spondylitis
Relief of signs/symptoms of ankylosing spondylitis and to decrease the risk of developing gastric ulcers in patients at risk of developing NSAID-associated gastric ulcers

1 tab bid of 375mg/20mg or 500mg/20mg

Controlled studies do not extend beyond 6 months

PEDIATRIC DOSAGE
Pediatric use may not have been established

DOSING CONSIDERATIONS
Renal Impairment
Moderate to Severe (CrCl <30mL/min): Not recommended

Hepatic Impairment
Mild to Moderate: Consider possible dose reduction based on naproxen component
Severe: Avoid use

Elderly
Use lowest effective dose

Other Important Considerations

Consider a different treatment if a dose of esomeprazole lower than 40mg/day is more appropriate; Vimovo does not allow for administration of a lower daily dose of esomeprazole

ADMINISTRATION

Oral route

Swallow whole w/ liquid; do not split, chew, crush, or dissolve.
Take at least 30 min ac.

STORAGE

25°C (77°F); excursions permitted to 15-30°C (59-86°F). Protect from moisture.

HOW SUPPLIED

Tab, Delayed-Release: (Naproxen/Esomeprazole) 375mg/20mg, 500mg/20mg

CONTRAINDICATIONS

Known hypersensitivity (eg, anaphylactic reactions, serious skin reactions) to naproxen, esomeprazole magnesium, substituted benzimidazoles, or to any components of the drug product, including omeprazole. History of asthma, urticaria, or allergic-type reactions after taking aspirin (ASA) or other NSAIDs, In the setting of CABG surgery.

WARNINGS/PRECAUTIONS

Use lowest effective dose for the shortest duration possible. Not recommended for initial treatment of acute pain. Renal effects of therapy may hasten the progression of renal dysfunction in patients w/ preexisting renal disease. Monitor for changes in the signs/symptoms of asthma in patients w/ preexisting asthma (w/o known ASA sensitivity). May mask inflammation and fever. Periodically monitor Hgb in patients w/ initial Hgb ≤10g receiving long-term therapy. D/C w/ active and clinically significant bleeding from any source. **Naproxen:** Increased CV thrombotic risk w/ higher doses reported. Avoid in patients w/ a recent MI unless benefits outweigh the risks of recurrent CV thrombotic events; if used, monitor for signs of cardiac ischemia. Increased risk for GI bleeding w/ longer duration of NSAID therapy, older age, poor general health status, and advanced liver disease and/or coagulopathy; avoid use in patients at higher risk unless benefits are expected to outweigh the increased risk of bleeding. Consider alternate therapies other than NSAIDs for patients at higher risk and patients w/ active GI bleeding. Promptly initiate evaluation and treatment if a serious GI adverse event is suspected; d/c until a serious GI adverse event is ruled out. Caution in patients w/ a history of inflammatory bowel disease (ulcerative colitis, Crohn's disease); condition may be exacerbated. Hepatotoxicity reported; d/c immediately and perform a clinical evaluation if clinical signs/symptoms consistent w/ liver disease develop, or if systemic manifestations occur. May cause new onset HTN or worsen preexisting HTN. Fluid retention and edema reported. Avoid use in patients w/ severe heart failure (HF) unless benefits outweigh risks; monitor for signs of worsening HF if used. Renal papillary necrosis and other renal injury reported w/ long-term use. Renal toxicity also reported in patients in whom renal prostaglandins have a compensatory role in the maintenance of renal perfusion; increased risk w/ renal/hepatic dysfunction, dehydration, hypovolemia, and HF, and in the elderly. Correct volume status in dehydrated or hypovolemic patients prior to initiating therapy. Avoid use in patients w/ advanced renal disease unless the benefits are expected to outweigh the risk; monitor for signs of worsening renal function if used. Hyperkalemia reported. Associated w/ anaphylactic reactions in patients w/ and w/o known hypersensitivity to naproxen and in patients w/ ASA-sensitive asthma. May cause serious skin reactions (eg, exfoliative dermatitis, Stevens-Johnson syndrome, toxic epidermal necrolysis); d/c at 1st appearance of skin rash/hypersensitivity. Anemia reported. May increase the risk of bleeding events; coagulation disorders may increase this risk. **Esomeprazole:** Symptomatic response to therapy does not preclude the presence of gastric malignancy. Atrophic gastritis reported w/ long-term use of omeprazole. Acute interstitial nephritis reported; d/c if this develops. Cyanocobalamin (vitamin B12) deficiency caused by hypo- or achlorhydria may occur w/ daily long-term use (eg, >3 yrs). May increase risk of *Clostridium difficile*-associated diarrhea, especially in hospitalized patients. May be associated w/ an increased risk for osteoporosis-related fractures of the hip, wrist, or spine; increased risk w/ high dose (multiple daily doses) and long-term therapy (≥1 yr). Hypomagnesemia (symptomatic and asymptomatic) reported rarely in patients treated w/ PPIs for at least 3 months, in most cases after a year of therapy. Serum chromogranin A (CgA) levels increase secondary to PPI-induced decreases in gastric acidity and may cause false positive results in diagnostic investigations for neuroendocrine tumors; temporarily stop treatment at least 14 days before assessing CgA levels and consider repeating the test if initial CgA levels are high.

ADVERSE REACTIONS

Gastritis, diarrhea, URTI, flatulence, headache, upper abdominal pain, constipation, dizziness, peripheral edema.

DRUG INTERACTIONS

Monitor digoxin levels; digoxin dose adjustment may be needed to maintain therapeutic drug concentrations. Monitor for methotrexate (MTX) toxicity during concomitant use; may consider temporary withdrawal of Vimovo in some patients receiving high-dose MTX. **Naproxen:** Drugs that interfere w/ serotonin reuptake may potentiate the risk of bleeding. Synergistic effect on bleeding w/ anticoagulants (eg, warfarin); monitor for signs of bleeding w/ concomitant anticoagulants, antiplatelet agents (eg, ASA), SSRIs, and SNRIs. May increase risk of GI bleeding w/ use of oral corticosteroids, anticoagulants, and SSRIs; smoking; and alcohol use. ASA may increase risk of bleeding and serious GI events; concomitant use w/ analgesic doses of ASA is not recommended. Monitor patients more closely for GI bleeding w/ concomitant use of low-dose ASA for cardiac prophylaxis. May diminish antihypertensive effect of ACE inhibitors, ARBs, and β-blockers (eg, propranolol); monitor BP. Coadministration w/ ACE inhibitors or ARBs may result in deterioration of renal function (including possible acute renal failure) in patients who are elderly or volume-depleted (including those on diuretic therapy), or have renal impairment; monitor for worsening

renal function when these drugs are administered concomitantly. May reduce the natriuretic effect of loop diuretics (eg, furosemide) and thiazide diuretics; observe for signs of worsening renal function, in addition to assuring diuretic efficacy including antihypertensive effects. May increase digoxin serum concentrations and prolong the $T_{1/2}$ of digoxin. May elevate plasma lithium levels and reduce renal lithium clearance; monitor for signs of lithium toxicity. May increase the risk for MTX toxicity. May increase cyclosporine's nephrotoxicity; monitor for signs of worsening renal function. Concomitant use w/ other NSAIDs or salicylates (eg, diflunisal, salsalate) increases the risk of GI toxicity; not recommended w/ other NSAIDs or salicylates. Concomitant use w/ pemetrexed may increase the risk of pemetrexed-associated myelosuppression, renal, and GI toxicity; refer to PI for further information. Avoid w/ other naproxen-containing products. **Esomeprazole:** Increased INR and PT w/ concomitant warfarin. Concomitant use of esomeprazole 40mg resulted in reduced plasma concentrations of the active metabolite of clopidogrel and a reduction in platelet inhibition; avoid concomitant use of clopidogrel and consider use of alternative anti-platelet therapy. May decrease exposure of some antiretroviral drugs (eg, atazanavir, nelfinavir) and may reduce antiviral effect and promote the development of drug resistance. May increase exposure of other antiretroviral drugs (eg, saquinavir) and may increase toxicity. Avoid concomitant use w/ nelfinavir. Refer to the PI of atazanavir, saquinavir, and other antiretrovirals for more information. May increase exposure of cilostazol and one of its active metabolites; consider dose reduction of cilostazol. Potential for increased exposure of digoxin. Concomitant use w/ MTX (primarily at high dose) may elevate and prolong serum concentrations of MTX and/or its metabolite hydroxymethotrexate, possibly leading to MTX toxicities. May increase exposure of tacrolimus; monitor tacrolimus whole blood concentrations during concomitant treatment. May reduce the absorption of other drugs dependent on gastric pH for absorption (eg, iron salts, erlotinib, mycophenolate mofetil [MMF], ketoconazole). Caution in transplant patients receiving MMF. Increased exposure of diazepam; monitor patients for increased sedation and adjust diazepam dose as needed. CYP2C19 or CYP3A4 inducers may decrease exposure; avoid w/ St. John's wort or rifampin. Voriconazole increased esomeprazole exposure. Caution w/ digoxin or other drugs that may cause hypomagnesemia (eg, diuretics).

PREGNANCY AND LACTATION

Pregnancy: Use of NSAIDs during the 3rd trimester of pregnancy increases the risk of premature closure of the fetal ductus arteriosus. Avoid use in pregnant women starting at 30 weeks of gestation (3rd trimester).
Lactation: May be found in breast milk; caution in nursing.
Reproductive Potential: Based on the mechanism of action, NSAIDs may delay or prevent rupture of ovarian follicles that may lead to reversible infertility in some women. Small studies in women treated w/ NSAIDs have also shown a reversible delay in ovulation. Consider withdrawal of NSAIDs in women who have difficulties conceiving or who are undergoing investigation of infertility.

MECHANISM OF ACTION

Naproxen: NSAID; mechanism not completely understood but involves inhibition of COX-1 and COX-2. Has analgesic, anti-inflammatory, and antipyretic properties. May be related to prostaglandin synthetase inhibition. **Esomeprazole:** PPI; suppresses gastric acid secretion by specific inhibition of the H^+/K^+-ATPase in the gastric parietal cell. Blocks the final step in acid production, thus reducing gastric acidity.

PHARMACOKINETICS

Absorption: Naproxen: Bioavailability (95%); T_{max}=3 hrs. Esomeprazole: Rapid; T_{max}=0.43-1.2 hrs. **Distribution:** May be found in breast milk. Naproxen: V_d=0.16L/kg; plasma protein binding (>99%). Esomeprazole: V_d=16L; plasma protein binding (97%). **Metabolism:** Naproxen: Liver (extensive) via CYP2C9 and CYP1A2 into 6-0-desmethyl naproxen (metabolite). Esomeprazole: Liver (extensive) via CYP2C19 (major) into hydroxyl and desmethyl metabolites, and via CYP3A4 into esomeprazole sulphone (main metabolite). **Elimination:** Naproxen: Urine (95%, <1% unchanged, <1% 6-0-desmethyl naproxen, 66-92% conjugates), feces (≤3%); $T_{1/2}$=15 hrs. Esomeprazole: Urine (80% metabolites, <1% unchanged), feces; $T_{1/2}$=1.2-1.5 hrs.

PATIENT CONSIDERATIONS

Assessment: Assess for history of asthma, urticaria, or other allergic-type reactions w/ previous use of ASA or other NSAIDs; preexisting asthma; CV disease (CVD) or risk factors for CVD; HTN; history of peptic ulcer disease or GI bleeding; coagulation disorders; renal/hepatic impairment; pregnancy/nursing status; or any other conditions where treatment is contraindicated or cautioned. Assess volume status. Assess for possible drug interactions. Obtain baseline BP, CBC, and chemistry profile.

Monitoring: Monitor for signs/symptoms of CV thrombotic events; cardiac ischemia in patients w/ a recent MI; GI bleeding/ulceration and perforation; hepatotoxicity; new or worsening HTN; HF; edema; renal papillary necrosis and other renal injury; hyperkalemia; anaphylactic reactions; serious skin reactions; anemia; bone fractures; hypomagnesemia; and other adverse reactions. Monitor BP during initiation of therapy and throughout the course of therapy. Monitor for signs of bleeding in patients on concomitant therapy w/ anticoagulants, antiplatelet agents, SSRIs, or SNRIs. Monitor renal function in patients w/ renal/hepatic impairment, HF, dehydration, or hypovolemia. Monitor CBC and chemistry profiles periodically during long-term treatment. Monitor Mg^{2+} levels prior to and periodically during therapy w/ prolonged treatment.

Counseling: Inform of potential for CV thrombotic events, GI adverse events, and worsening CHF/edema, and advise of symptoms; instruct to report any symptoms to healthcare provider immediately. Inform of the potential for hepatotoxicity, and advise of signs/symptoms; if signs/symptoms occur, instruct to d/c and seek immediate medical therapy. Instruct to seek immediate emergency help if signs of an anaphylactic reaction occur. Advise to d/c immediately if rash develops and to contact healthcare provider as soon as possible. Advise females of reproductive potential that therapy may be associated w/ reversible infertility. Inform pregnant women to avoid use starting at 30 weeks of gestation. Instruct to report to physician if they experience a decrease in the amount they urinate or have blood in their urine. Advise patients taking therapy for long periods of time to report any weakness, tiredness, or light-headedness or rapid heartbeat and breathing or pale skin. Instruct to immediately report and seek care for diarrhea that does not improve, or any CV or neurological symptoms. Advise to report any sign/symptom of osteoporosis. Advise patient not to use other NSAIDs or salicylates concomitantly; notify of the presence of NSAIDs in OTC medications for colds, fever, or insomnia. Advise patient not to use low-dose ASA concomitantly w/o talking to healthcare provider. Instruct to report all medications being used to physician.

VIMPAT — lacosamide   CV

Class: Sodium channel inactivator

ADULT DOSAGE
Partial Onset Seizures
Monotherapy:
Initial: 100mg bid
Alternative LD: 200mg; follow 12 hrs later by 100mg bid for 1 week
Titrate: Increase by 50mg bid at weekly intervals
Maint: 150-200mg bid

Adjunctive Therapy:
Initial: 50mg bid
Alternative LD: 200mg; follow 12 hrs later by 100mg bid for 1 week
Titrate: Increase by 50mg bid at weekly intervals
Maint: 100-200mg bid
Max Maint: 200mg bid

Use IV when oral administration is temporarily not feasible

Conversions
Convert from Single Antiepileptic to Lacosamide Monotherapy:
Maintain 150-200mg bid for at least 3 days before initiating gradual withdrawal of the concomitant antiepileptic drug over at least 6 weeks

PO to IV Conversion:
Initial total daily IV dosage regimen should be equivalent to oral dosage regimen

IV to PO Conversion:
At the end of the IV treatment period, switch to oral lacosamide at the equivalent daily dosage and frequency of IV administration

PEDIATRIC DOSAGE
Partial Onset Seizures
≥17 Years:
Monotherapy:
Initial: 100mg bid
Alternative LD: 200mg; follow 12 hrs later by 100mg bid for 1 week
Titrate: Increase by 50mg bid at weekly intervals
Maint: 150-200mg bid

Adjunctive Therapy:
Initial: 50mg bid
Alternative LD: 200mg; follow 12 hrs later by 100mg bid for 1 week
Titrate: Increase by 50mg bid at weekly intervals
Maint: 100-200mg bid
Max Maint: 200mg bid

Use IV when oral administration is temporarily not feasible

Conversions
Convert from Single Antiepileptic to Lacosamide Monotherapy:
Maintain 150-200mg bid for at least 3 days before initiating gradual withdrawal of the concomitant antiepileptic drug over at least 6 weeks

PO to IV Conversion:
Initial total daily IV dosage regimen should be equivalent to oral dosage regimen

IV to PO Conversion:
At the end of the IV treatment period, switch to oral lacosamide at the equivalent daily dosage and frequency of IV administration

DOSING CONSIDERATIONS
Concomitant Medications
Strong CYP3A4 and CYP2C9 Inhibitors w/ Renal/Hepatic Impairment: Dose reduction may be necessary

Renal Impairment
Severe (CrCl ≤30mL/min)/ESRD:
Max: 300mg/day
Hemodialysis:
Consider dosage supplementation of up to 50% following a 4-hr hemodialysis treatment

Hepatic Impairment
Mild/Moderate:
Max: 300mg/day
Severe:
Not recommended

Discontinuation
Gradually withdraw over at least 1 week

ADMINISTRATION
Oral/IV route
Take w/ or w/o food.

Sol
Use a calibrated measuring device.

Inj
Infuse over 15-60 min; 30-60 min is preferable when a 15 min administration is not required.
May administer IV w/o further dilution or mixed w/ compatible diluents.
Diluted sol should not be stored for >4 hrs at room temperature.

Compatible IV Diluents
NaCl inj 0.9%
D5 inj
Lactated Ringer's inj

STORAGE
20-25°C (68-77°F); excursions permitted between 15-30°C (59-86°F). (Inj/Sol) Do not freeze. (Inj) Discard any unused portion. (Sol) Discard any unused portion after 7 weeks of 1st opening bottle.

HOW SUPPLIED
Inj: 10mg/mL [20mL]; Sol: 10mg/mL [200mL, 465mL]; Tab: 50mg, 100mg, 150mg, 200mg

WARNINGS/PRECAUTIONS
Administer LD w/ medical supervision due to increased incidence of CNS adverse reactions. May increase risk of suicidal thoughts or behavior. May cause dizziness and ataxia; may impair physical/mental abilities. Dose-dependent prolongations in PR interval reported. Caution w/ known conduction problems (eg, atrioventricular [AV] block, sick sinus syndrome w/o pacemaker), Na+ channelopathies (eg, Brugada syndrome), or w/ severe cardiac disease (eg, myocardial ischemia, heart failure, structural heart disease). IV infusion may cause bradycardia or AV block. May predispose to atrial arrhythmias, especially in patients w/ diabetic neuropathy and/or cardiovascular disease (CVD). Syncope or loss of consciousness reported in patients w/ diabetic neuropathy and those w/ a history of risk factors for cardiac disease. Multiorgan hypersensitivity reactions (also known as drug reaction w/ eosinophilia and systemic symptoms [DRESS]) may occur; d/c and start alternative treatment if suspected. Caution during dose titration in elderly. (Sol) Contains aspartame, a source of phenylalanine.

ADVERSE REACTIONS
Headache, N/V, diplopia, dizziness, fatigue, blurred vision, somnolence, tremor, nystagmus, vertigo, diarrhea, balance disorder, ataxia, dry mouth, oral hypoesthesia.

DRUG INTERACTIONS
See Dosing Considerations. Increased exposure w/ strong CYP3A4 and CYP2C9 inhibitors in patients w/ renal or hepatic impairment. Caution w/ medications that prolong PR interval (eg, β-blockers, calcium channel blockers); closely monitor if lacosamide is administered as IV route.

PREGNANCY AND LACTATION
Pregnancy: Category C.
Lactation: Not for use in nursing.

MECHANISM OF ACTION
Na+ channel inactivator; has not been established. Selectively enhances slow inactivation of voltage-gated Na+ channels, resulting in stabilization of hyperexcitable neuronal membranes and inhibition of repetitive neuronal firing.

PHARMACOKINETICS
Absorption: (Oral) Complete; absolute bioavailability (100%); T_{max}=approx 1-4 hrs. **Distribution:** V_d=0.6L/kg; plasma protein binding (<15%). **Metabolism:** CYP3A4/2C9/2C19; O-desmethyl-lacosamide (major metabolite). **Elimination:** Urine (95%), feces (<0.5%); $T_{1/2}$=approx 13 hrs.

PATIENT CONSIDERATIONS
Assessment: Assess for hepatic/renal impairment, history of depression or risk factors for cardiac disease, cardiac conduction problems and/or CVD, diabetic neuropathy, phenylketonuria, pregnancy/nursing status, and possible drug interactions. Obtain baseline ECG in patients w/ known conduction problems, Na+ channelopathies, on concomitant medications that prolong PR interval, or w/ severe cardiac disease.

Monitoring: Monitor for emergence/worsening of depression, suicidal thoughts or behavior and/or any unusual changes in mood or behavior, dizziness, ataxia, PR interval prolongation, syncope or loss of consciousness, DRESS, and other adverse reactions. Obtain an ECG after titration to steady state in patients w/ known conduction problems, Na+ channelopathies, on concomitant medications that prolong PR interval, or w/ severe cardiac disease; closely monitor these patients if administering IV. Closely monitor patients w/ hepatic/renal impairment during dose titration.

Counseling: Inform of the benefits/risks of therapy. Instruct to take ud. Counsel patients/caregivers/families about increased risk of suicidal thoughts and behavior and of the need to be alert for emergence or worsening of symptoms of depression, any unusual changes in behavior/mood, or the emergence of suicidal thoughts, behavior, or thoughts about self-harm. Instruct to report any behaviors of concern to physician immediately. Inform that dizziness, double vision, abnormal coordination and balance, and somnolence may occur; advise not to engage in hazardous activities (eg, driving/operating complex machinery) until effects of drug are known. Counsel that therapy is associated w/ ECG changes that may predispose to irregular heartbeat and syncope; if syncope develops, instruct to lay down w/ raised legs and to contact physician. Instruct to d/c if a serious hypersensitivity reaction is suspected and to promptly report any symptoms of liver toxicity. Advise to notify physician if patient becomes pregnant/intends to become pregnant, or is breastfeeding. Encourage patients to enroll in the North American Antiepileptic Drug Pregnancy Registry if they become pregnant.

VIRACEPT — nelfinavir mesylate   Rx

Class: Protease inhibitor

ADULT DOSAGE
HIV-1 Infection

Combination w/ Other Antiretrovirals:
Tab:
1250mg (five 250mg or two 625mg tabs) bid or 750mg (three 250mg tabs) tid
Max: 2500mg/day

PEDIATRIC DOSAGE
HIV-1 Infection

Combination w/ Other Antiretrovirals:
2-<13 Years:
Oral Powder:
9-<16kg: 45-55mg/kg bid or 25-35mg/kg tid
16-≥23kg: 25-35mg/kg tid

Max: 2500mg/day

250mg Tab:

10->21kg: 45-55mg/kg bid or 25-35mg/kg tid

Max: 2500mg/day

≥13 Years:

Tab:

1250mg (five 250mg or two 625mg tabs) bid or 750mg (three 250mg tabs) tid

Max: 2500mg/day

DOSING CONSIDERATIONS

Hepatic Impairment

Moderate or Severe (Child-Pugh B or C, Score ≥7): Not recommended for use

ADMINISTRATION

Oral route

Take all doses w/ meals

Patients Unable to Swallow Tabs

1. Place tab(s) in a small amount of water
2. Once dissolved, mix the liquid well and consume immediately
3. Rinse the glass w/ water and swallow the rinse to ensure entire dose is consumed

Oral Powder

1. Mix oral powder w/ a small amount of water, milk, formula, soy formula, soy milk, or dietary supplements; do not reconstitute w/ water in original container or mix w/ acidic food or juice (eg, orange juice, apple juice, apple sauce)
2. Once mixed, consume entire contents in order to obtain the full dose; if mixture is not consumed immediately, store under refrigeration for up to 6 hrs

STORAGE

15-30°C (59-86°F). (Powder) If mixture is not consumed immediately, store under refrigeration, but must not exceed 6 hrs.

HOW SUPPLIED

Powder: 50mg/g [144g]; **Tab:** 250mg, 625mg

CONTRAINDICATIONS

Concomitant use w/ drugs that are highly dependent on CYP3A for clearance and for which elevated concentrations are associated w/ serious and/or life-threatening events (eg, alfuzosin, amiodarone, quinidine, dihydroergotamine, ergotamine, methylergonovine, cisapride, lovastatin, simvastatin, pimozide, sildenafil [for treatment of pulmonary arterial HTN], triazolam, oral midazolam), and drugs that may lead to reduced efficacy of nelfinavir (eg, St. John's wort, rifampin).

WARNINGS/PRECAUTIONS

Powder contains phenylalanine; caution w/ phenylketonuria. New onset or exacerbation of diabetes mellitus (DM), hyperglycemia, and diabetic ketoacidosis reported. Increased bleeding, including spontaneous skin hematomas and hemarthrosis, in patients w/ hemophilia type A and B reported. Redistribution/accumulation of body fat reported. Immune reconstitution syndrome reported. Autoimmune disorders (eg, Graves' disease, polymyositis, and Guillain-Barre syndrome) reported in the setting of immune reconstitution and can occur many months after initiation of treatment.

ADVERSE REACTIONS

Diarrhea, nausea, flatulence, rash, abdominal pain, anorexia, leukopenia, neutropenia.

DRUG INTERACTIONS

See Contraindications. Avoid w/ colchicine in patients w/ renal/hepatic impairment. Not recommended w/ salmeterol. May increase levels of dihydropyridine calcium channel blockers, indinavir, saquinavir, trazodone, rifabutin, bosentan, colchicine, HMG-CoA reductase inhibitors (eg, atorvastatin, rosuvastatin), immunosuppressants, fluticasone, azithromycin, PDE-5 inhibitors, quetiapine, and CYP3A substrates. May decrease levels of delavirdine, phenytoin, methadone, ethinyl estradiol, and norethindrone. CYP3A or CYP2C19 inhibitors, delavirdine, indinavir, ritonavir, saquinavir, cyclosporine, tacrolimus, and sirolimus may increase levels. CYP3A or CYP2C19 inducers (eg, rifampin), omeprazole, nevirapine, carbamazepine, phenobarbital, phenytoin, and rifabutin may decrease levels. May affect warfarin concentrations; monitor INR. Give didanosine 1 hr before or 2 hrs after administration. Coadministration w/ proton pump inhibitors may lead to a loss of virologic response and development of resistance. May require initiation or dose adjustments of insulin or oral hypoglycemics for treatment of DM. Refer to PI for dosing modifications when used w/ certain concomitant therapies.

PREGNANCY AND LACTATION

Category B, not for use in nursing.

MECHANISM OF ACTION

HIV-1 protease inhibitor; prevents cleavage of gag and gag-pol polyprotein, resulting in production of immature, noninfectious virus.

PHARMACOKINETICS

Absorption: 28 days: (1250mg bid) C_{max}=4mg/L; AUC=52.8mg•hr/L. (750mg tid) C_{max}=3mg/L; AUC=43.6mg•hr/L. 14 days: (1250mg bid) C_{max}=4.7mg/L; AUC=35.3mg•hr/L. **Distribution:** V_d=2-7L/kg; plasma protein binding (>98%). **Metabolism:** Liver via CYP3A, 2C19 (oxidation). **Elimination:** Feces (78% metabolites, 22% unchanged), urine (1-2%); $T_{1/2}$=3.5-5 hrs.

PATIENT CONSIDERATIONS

Assessment: Assess for previous hypersensitivity to the drug, hepatic impairment, DM, hemophilia, pregnancy/nursing status, and possible drug interactions. Assess for phenylketonuria if planning to use the powder formulation.

Monitoring: Monitor for new onset or exacerbation of DM, hyperglycemia, diabetic ketoacidosis, immune reconstitution syndrome, autoimmune disorders, fat redistribution/accumulation, and other adverse reactions. In patients w/ hemophilia, monitor for bleeding events.

Counseling: Instruct to take ud. Inform that therapy is not a cure for HIV and that illnesses associated w/ HIV may continue. Advise to avoid doing things that can spread HIV to others. Instruct not to alter the dose or d/c therapy w/o consulting physician. Instruct to notify physician if using any other prescription/nonprescription medication, or herbal products, particularly St. John's wort. Advise to use alternative or additional contraceptive measures if taking oral contraceptives. Inform that most frequent adverse event is diarrhea, which can usually be controlled w/ nonprescription drugs (eg, loperamide). Inform that fat redistribution/accumulation may occur. Alert patients w/ phenylketonuria that powder formulation contains phenylalanine.

VIRAMUNE XR — nevirapine   Rx

Class: Non-nucleoside reverse transcriptase inhibitor (NNRTI)

> Severe, life-threatening, and in some cases fatal, hepatotoxicity (particularly in the first 18 weeks) and skin reactions (eg, Stevens-Johnson syndrome, toxic epidermal necrolysis, hypersensitivity reactions) reported. Increased risk of hepatotoxicity reported in women and patients with higher CD4+ cell counts, including pregnant women. Hepatic failure reported in patients without HIV taking nevirapine for postexposure prophylaxis (PEP). Use for occupational and non-occupational PEP is contraindicated. D/C therapy and seek medical evaluation immediately if hepatitis, transaminase elevations combined with rash or other systemic symptoms, severe skin rash, or hypersensitivity reactions develop; do not restart therapy. The 14-day lead-in period with 200mg daily dosing must be followed; may decrease the incidence of rash. Monitor intensively during the first 18 weeks of therapy, especially the first 6 weeks.

OTHER BRAND NAMES

Viramune

ADULT DOSAGE	PEDIATRIC DOSAGE
HIV-1 Infection	**HIV-1 Infection**
Combination w/ Other Antiretrovirals:	**Combination w/ Other Antiretrovirals:**
Tab (Immediate-Release [IR]):	**Tab/Oral Sus:**
Initial: 200mg qd for the first 14 days	**≥15 Days of Age:**
Maint: 200mg bid	**Initial:** 150mg/m² qd for the first 14 days
Tab, Extended-Release (ER):	**Maint:** 150mg/m² bid
Not Currently Taking IR Nevirapine:	**Max:** 400mg/day
Initial: One 200mg IR tab qd for first 14 days	**Tab, Extended-Release (ER):**
Maint: One 400mg ER tab qd	**6-<18 Years:**
Switching from IR Tab to ER Tab:	**Initial:**
Switch to 400mg ER tab qd w/o 14-day lead-in period	150mg/m² IR tab/oral sus qd for first 14 days
	Max: 200mg/day
	Maint:
	BSA 0.58-0.83m²: Two 100mg ER tabs qd
	BSA 0.84-1.16m²: Three 100mg ER tabs qd
	BSA ≥1.17m²: One 400mg ER tab qd
	Max: 400mg/day

DOSING CONSIDERATIONS

Renal Impairment

Requiring Dialysis: Administer additional 200mg IR dose after each dialysis treatment

Hepatic Impairment

Moderate or Severe (Child-Pugh Class B or C): Not recommended for use

Symptomatic Hepatic Event Occurrence: Permanently d/c; do not restart after recovery

Adverse Reactions

Severe Rash/Rash Accompanied by Constitutional Findings: D/C

Mild to Mod Rash w/o Constitutional Symptoms During Lead-In Period: Do not initiate XR therapy until rash has resolved; duration of lead-in period should not exceed 28 days, at which point an alternative regimen should be sought

Other Important Considerations

Dose Interruption for >7 Days: Restart using lead-in dosing

ADMINISTRATION

Oral route

Take w/ or w/o food

Tab, ER

Swallow whole; do not chew, crush, or divide

Oral Sus

Shake gently prior to administration

Administer the entire measured dose by using an oral dosing syringe or dosing cup

STORAGE

25°C (77°F); excursions permitted to 15-30°C (59-86°F).

HOW SUPPLIED

[IR] Sus: 50mg/5mL [240mL], **Tab:** 200mg*; **Tab, ER:** 100mg, 400mg *scored

CONTRAINDICATIONS

Moderate or severe (Child-Pugh Class B or C) hepatic impairment. Use as part of occupational and non-occupational PEP regimens.

WARNINGS/PRECAUTIONS

Not recommended for adult females with CD4+ cell counts >250 cells/mm³ or in adult males with CD4+ cell counts >400 cells/mm³. Coinfection with hepatitis B or C and/or increased transaminase elevations at the start of therapy may increase risk of later symptomatic events (≥6 weeks after starting therapy) and asymptomatic increases in AST/ALT. Caution with hepatic fibrosis/cirrhosis; monitor for drug-induced toxicity. Rhabdomyolysis reported in some patients with skin and/or liver reactions. Monitor closely if isolated rash of any severity occurs; delay in stopping treatment after the onset of rash may result in a more serious reaction. Do not use as single agent to treat HIV-1 or add on as a sole agent to a failing regimen; resistant virus emerges rapidly when administered as monotherapy. Consider potential for cross-resistance in the choice of new antiretroviral agents to be used in combination with therapy. Take into account the half-lives of the combination antiretroviral drugs when discontinuing the regimen; nevirapine has a long half-life and resistance may develop if antiretrovirals with shorter half-lives are stopped concurrently. Immune reconstitution syndrome, autoimmune disorders (eg, Graves' disease, polymyositis, Guillain-Barre syndrome) in the setting of immune reconstitution, and redistribution/accumulation of body fat reported. Caution in elderly.

ADVERSE REACTIONS

Hepatotoxicity, skin reactions, diarrhea, nausea, headache, fatigue, abdominal pain.

DRUG INTERACTIONS

Avoid with atazanavir, boceprevir, telaprevir, ketoconazole, itraconazole, and rifampin. Not recommended with fosamprenavir (without ritonavir), efavirenz, and St. John's wort or St. John's wort-containing products. May alter levels of other non-nucleoside reverse transcriptase inhibitor (NNRTI) (eg, delavirdine, etravirine, rilpivirine); avoid coadministration. Increased incidence and severity of rash with prednisone during the first 6 weeks of therapy; not recommended to prevent nevirapine-associated rash. May increase levels of 14-OH clarithromycin and rifabutin. May increase levels of antithrombotics (eg, warfarin); monitor anticoagulation levels. May decrease levels of CYP3A/2B6 substrates, clarithromycin, ethinyl estradiol, norethindrone, efavirenz, atazanavir, amprenavir, indinavir, lopinavir, methadone, nelfinavir, boceprevir, telaprevir, antiarrhythmics, anticonvulsants, ketoconazole, itraconazole, calcium channel blockers, cancer chemotherapy, ergot alkaloids, immunosuppressants, motility agents, and opiate agonists. Fluconazole may increase levels and rifampin may decrease levels. Refer to PI for further information when used with certain concomitant therapies.

PREGNANCY AND LACTATION

Category B, not for use in nursing.

MECHANISM OF ACTION

NNRTI; binds directly to reverse transcriptase and blocks RNA-dependent and DNA-dependent DNA polymerase activities by causing a disruption of the enzyme's catalytic site.

PHARMACOKINETICS

Absorption: Readily absorbed. IR: Absolute bioavailability (93%, tab), (91%, sus); C_{max}=2mcg/mL; T_{max}=4 hrs. ER (single dose): AUC=161,000ng•hr/mL; C_{max}=2060ng/mL; T_{max}=24 hrs (median). **Distribution:** V_d=1.21L/kg (IV, healthy); plasma protein binding (60%). Crosses placenta; found in breast milk. **Metabolism:** Liver (extensive); glucuronide conjugation, oxidative metabolism via CYP3A and CYP2B6. **Elimination:** $T_{1/2}$=45 hrs (single dose), 25-30 hrs (multiple dosing). IR: Urine (81.3%; <3%, parent drug), feces (10.1%).

PATIENT CONSIDERATIONS

Assessment: Assess for hepatic fibrosis/cirrhosis, hepatitis B or C coinfection, pregnancy/nursing status, and possible drug interactions. Obtain baseline LFTs. (ER) Assess the ability to swallow tabs in pediatric patients.

Monitoring: Monitor for hepatotoxicity, skin or hypersensitivity reactions, immune reconstitution syndrome, autoimmune disorders, fat redistribution/accumulation, rhabdomyolysis, and other adverse reactions. Perform intensive clinical and lab monitoring, including LFTs, during the first 18 weeks of therapy and frequently throughout treatment. Measure serum transaminases immediately if signs/symptoms of hepatitis, hypersensitivity reactions, and rash develop. Monitor anticoagulation levels with antithrombotics (eg, warfarin).

Counseling: Inform about the risks and benefits of therapy. Inform that severe liver disease/skin reactions may occur. Counsel about signs/symptoms of hepatotoxicity, skin reactions, and other adverse reactions, and advise to d/c and seek medical evaluation immediately if any occur. Inform to take drug as prescribed. Instruct not to alter the dose without consulting physician. Inform that therapy is not a cure for HIV-1 infection and that illnesses associated with HIV-1 infection, including opportunistic infections, may still occur. Advise to avoid doing things that can spread HIV-1 infection to others (eg, sharing needles or other inj equipment, sharing personal items that can have blood or body fluids on them [toothbrush, razor blades], breastfeeding). Instruct not to have any kind of sex without protection; inform to always practice safe sex by using a latex or polyurethane condom to lower the chance of sexual contact with semen, vaginal secretions, or blood. Advise to notify physician of the use of any other prescription/OTC medication, or herbal products, particularly St. John's wort. Inform women taking therapy that hormonal methods of birth control should not be used as the sole method of contraception. Inform that fat redistribution may occur. Instruct not to take IR tabs/sus and ER tabs at the same time. (ER) Advise that soft remnants of the drug may be seen in stool.

VIREAD — tenofovir disoproxil fumarate   Rx

Class: Nucleoside reverse transcriptase inhibitor (NRTI)

> Lactic acidosis and severe hepatomegaly w/ steatosis, including fatal cases, reported w/ the use of nucleoside analogues in combination w/ other antiretrovirals. Severe acute exacerbations of hepatitis reported in hepatitis B virus (HBV)-infected patients who have discontinued therapy; closely monitor hepatic function w/ both clinical and lab follow-up for at least several months. If appropriate, resumption of antihepatitis B therapy may be warranted.

ADULT DOSAGE

HIV-1 Infection

In Combination w/ Other Antiretroviral Agents:
300mg tab qd; may use oral powder (7.5 scoops) if unable to swallow tabs

Chronic Hepatitis B

300mg tab qd; may use oral powder (7.5 scoops) if unable to swallow tabs

PEDIATRIC DOSAGE

HIV-1 Infection

In Combination w/ Other Antiretroviral Agents:
2 to <12 Years:
8mg/kg qd as tabs or oral powder
Max: 300mg qd

≥12 Years (≥35kg):
300mg tab qd; may use oral powder (7.5 scoops) if unable to swallow tabs

Dosing Recommendations for Pediatric Patients ≥2 Years Using Oral Powder:
10 to <12kg: 2 scoops qd
12 to <14kg: 2.5 scoops qd
14 to <17kg: 3 scoops qd
17 to <19kg: 3.5 scoops qd
19 to <22kg: 4 scoops qd
22 to <24kg: 4.5 scoops qd
24 to <27kg: 5 scoops qd
27 to <29kg: 5.5 scoops qd
29 to <32kg: 6 scoops qd
32 to <34kg: 6.5 scoops qd
34 to <35kg: 7 scoops qd
≥35kg: 7.5 scoops qd

Dosing Recommendations for Pediatric Patients ≥2 Years and Weighing ≥17kg Using Tabs:
17 to <22kg: 150mg qd
22 to <28kg: 200mg qd
28 to <35kg: 250mg qd
≥35kg: 300mg qd

Chronic Hepatitis B

≥12 Years (≥35kg):
300mg tab qd; may use oral powder (7.5 scoops) if unable to swallow tabs

---

DOSING CONSIDERATIONS

Renal Impairment

Adults:
CrCl ≥50mL/min: 300mg tab q24h
CrCl 30-49mL/min: 300mg tab q48h
CrCl 10-29mL/min: 300mg tab q72-96h
Hemodialysis: 300mg tab every 7 days or after a total of approx 12 hrs of dialysis; administer following completion of dialysis

ADMINISTRATION

Oral route

Take tabs w/o regard to food.

Oral Powder

Measure only w/ the supplied dosing scoop.
One level scoop contains 40mg of tenofovir disoproxil fumarate.
Mix w/ 2-4 oz of soft food not requiring chewing (eg, applesauce, baby food, yogurt) and administer entire mixture immediately.
Do not administer in a liquid.

STORAGE

25°C (77°F); excursions permitted to 15-30°C (59-86°F).

HOW SUPPLIED

Oral Powder: 40mg/g [60g]; **Tab:** 150mg, 200mg, 250mg, 300mg

WARNINGS/PRECAUTIONS

Obesity and prolonged nucleoside exposure may be risk factors for lactic acidosis and severe hepatomegaly w/ steatosis. Caution w/ known risk factors for liver disease. D/C if findings suggestive of lactic acidosis or pronounced hepatotoxicity develop. Renal impairment (eg, acute renal failure, Fanconi syndrome) reported; assess CrCl prior to initiating and as clinically appropriate during therapy. In patients at risk of renal dysfunction, including patients who have previously experienced renal events while receiving adefovir dipivoxil, assess CrCl, serum phosphorus (P), urine glucose, and urine protein prior to initiation and periodically during therapy. Promptly evaluate renal function in at-risk patients w/ persistent/worsening bone pain, pain in extremities, fractures, and/or muscular pain/weakness. Use only in HIV-1 and HBV coinfected patients as part of an appropriate antiretroviral combination regimen. Before initiating therapy, offer HIV-1 antibody testing to all HBV-infected patients and test all patients w/ HIV-1 for presence of chronic hepatitis B. Decreased bone mineral density (BMD) and increased biochemical markers of bone metabolism reported; consider assessment of BMD for patients w/ history of pathologic bone fracture or other risk factors for osteoporosis or bone loss. Osteomalacia associated w/ proximal renal tubulopathy reported; consider hypophosphatemia and osteomalacia secondary to proximal renal tubulopathy in patients at risk of renal dysfunction who present w/ persistent or worsening bone or muscle symptoms. Redistribution/accumulation of body fat and immune reconstitution syndrome reported. Autoimmune disorders (eg, Graves' disease, polymyositis, Guillain-Barre syndrome) reported in the setting of immune reconstitution and can occur many months after initiation of treatment. Early virological failure and high rates of resistance substitutions reported w/ certain regimens that only contain 3 nucleoside reverse transcriptase inhibitors; use triple nucleoside regimens w/ caution. Caution in elderly.

ADVERSE REACTIONS
HIV-1 Infection: Rash, diarrhea, headache, pain, depression, asthenia, nausea.
Chronic Hepatitis B and Compensated Liver Disease: Nausea.
Chronic Hepatitis B and Decompensated Liver Disease: Abdominal pain, N/V, insomnia, pruritus, dizziness, pyrexia.

DRUG INTERACTIONS
Avoid w/ concurrent or recent use of nephrotoxic agents (eg, high-dose or multiple NSAIDs). Do not coadminister w/ tenofovir disoproxil fumarate (TDF)-containing products or w/ adefovir dipivoxil. May increase levels of didanosine; d/c didanosine if didanosine-associated adverse reactions develop. Decreases levels of atazanavir; do not coadminister w/ atazanavir w/o ritonavir. Lopinavir/ritonavir, atazanavir w/ ritonavir, and darunavir w/ ritonavir may increase levels; d/c treatment if TDF-associated adverse reactions develop. P-gp and breast cancer resistance protein transporter inhibitors may increase absorption. Coadministration w/ Harvoni may increase tenofovir exposure; monitor for TDF-associated adverse reactions w/ concomitant Harvoni w/o HIV-1 protease inhibitor/ritonavir or an HIV-1 protease inhibitor/cobicistat combination. Consider alternative hepatitis C virus or antiretroviral therapy in patients receiving concomitant Harvoni and an HIV-1 protease inhibitor/ritonavir or an HIV-1 protease inhibitor/cobicistat combination; if coadministration is necessary, monitor for TDF-associated adverse reactions. Coadministration w/ drugs that reduce renal function or compete for active tubular secretion (eg, cidofovir, acyclovir, aminoglycosides [eg, gentamicin], high-dose or multiple NSAIDs) may increase levels of tenofovir and/or the levels of other renally eliminated drugs. Refer to PI for dosing modifications when used w/ certain concomitant therapies.

PREGNANCY AND LACTATION
Pregnancy: Category B. Physicians are encouraged to register patients in the Antiretroviral Pregnancy Registry.
Lactation: Mothers should be instructed not to breastfeed due to potential for HIV-1 transmission.

MECHANISM OF ACTION
Nucleotide analogue reverse transcriptase inhibitor; inhibits activity of HIV-1 reverse transcriptase and HBV reverse transcriptase by competing w/ natural substrate deoxyadenosine 5'-triphosphate and, after incorporation into DNA, by DNA chain termination.

PHARMACOKINETICS
Absorption: Adults: (Fasted) Bioavailability (25%); (Fasted, 300mg single dose) C_{max}=0.30mcg/mL, T_{max}=1 hr, AUC=2.29mcg•hr/mL. Pediatric Patients: (12 to <18 yrs of age, 300mg tab) C_{max}=0.38mcg/mL, AUC=3.39mcg•hr/mL; (2 to <12 yrs of age, 8mg/kg oral powder) C_{max}=0.24mcg/mL, AUC=2.59mcg•hr/mL. **Distribution:** Plasma or serum protein binding (less than 0.7 and 7.2%, respectively); V_d=1.3L/kg (1mg/kg IV dose), 1.2L/kg (3mg/kg IV dose); found in breast milk. **Elimination:** (Fed, 300mg qd multiple doses) Urine (32%); (Single dose) $T_{1/2}$=17 hrs.

PATIENT CONSIDERATIONS
Assessment: Assess for risk factors for lactic acidosis or liver disease, renal dysfunction, pregnancy/nursing status, and possible drug interactions. In patients at risk of renal dysfunction, assess CrCl, serum P, urine glucose, and urine protein. Test for HIV-1 antibody (in HBV-infected patients) and presence of chronic hepatitis B (in patients w/ HIV-1). Assess BMD in patients w/ history of pathologic bone fracture or other risk factors for osteoporosis or bone loss.

Monitoring: Monitor for signs/symptoms of lactic acidosis, hepatomegaly w/ steatosis, hepatotoxicity, renal impairment, bone effects, redistribution/accumulation of body fat, immune reconstitution syndrome (eg, opportunistic infections), autoimmune disorders, and other adverse reactions. Closely monitor hepatic function w/ both clinical and lab follow-up for at least several months in HBV-infected patients who have discontinued therapy. In patients at risk of renal dysfunction, monitor CrCl, serum P, urine glucose, and urine protein periodically. Periodically monitor weight in pediatric patients to guide dose adjustment.

Counseling: Inform about risks and benefits of therapy. Inform that therapy is not a cure for HIV-1 and patients may continue to experience illness associated w/ HIV-1 infection (eg, opportunistic infections). Instruct to avoid doing things that can spread HIV or HBV to others (eg, sharing of needles/inj equipment or personal items that can have blood/body fluids on them). Advise to always practice safer sex by using latex or polyurethane condoms. Instruct not to breastfeed. Instruct not to d/c w/o 1st informing physician. Counsel about the importance of adhering to regular dosing schedule and to avoid missing doses.

VISTIDE — cidofovir   Rx
Class: Viral DNA synthesis inhibitor

> **Renal impairment is the major toxicity.** Cases of acute renal failure resulting in dialysis and/or contributing to death reported with as few as 1 or 2 doses; prehydrate with IV normal saline (NS) and administer probenecid with each dose. Monitor renal function (SrCr and urine protein) within 48 hrs prior to each dose. Modify dose with renal function changes. Contraindicated with nephrotoxic agents. Neutropenia reported; monitor neutrophil counts. Carcinogenic, teratogenic, and hypospermatic in animal studies.

ADULT DOSAGE
Cytomegalovirus Retinitis

Treatment in Patients w/ AIDS:
Initial: 5mg/kg once weekly for 2 consecutive weeks
Maint: 5mg/kg once every 2 weeks

Probenecid must be administered PO w/ each dose of cidofovir; administer 2g 3 hrs prior to cidofovir dose, and 1g at 2 hrs and again at 8 hrs after completion of the 1-hr infusion (for a total of 4g)

PEDIATRIC DOSAGE
Pediatric use may not have been established

DOSING CONSIDERATIONS
Renal Impairment
SrCr 0.3-0.4mg/dL Above Baseline: Reduce maint dose to 3mg/kg
SrCr ≥0.5mg/dL Above Baseline or Development of ≥3+ Proteinuria: D/C therapy

ADMINISTRATION
IV route

Preparation and Administration
1. Extract the appropriate volume of cidofovir from the vial and transfer the dose to an infusion bag containing 100mL 0.9% NS sol.
2. Infuse the entire volume into the patient at a constant rate over a 1-hr period; use of a standard infusion pump for administration is recommended.

Hydration
Administer at least 1L of 0.9% NS sol IV w/ each infusion of cidofovir. Infuse NS over a 1- to 2-hr period immediately before cidofovir infusion. Patients who can tolerate additional fluid load should receive a 2nd liter; if administered, the 2nd liter should be initiated either at the start of the cidofovir infusion or immediately afterwards, and infused over a 1- to 3-hr period.

STORAGE
Vial: 20-25°C (68-77°F). **Admixture:** Under refrigeration, 2-8°C (36-46°F), for no more than 24 hrs. If refrigerated, allow admixture to equilibrate to room temperature prior to use.

HOW SUPPLIED
Inj: 75mg/mL

CONTRAINDICATIONS
Initiation of therapy in patients w/ SrCr >1.5mg/dL, CrCl ≤55mL/min, or urine protein ≥100mg/dL (≥2+ proteinuria). Nephrotoxic agents (d/c at least 7 days before therapy). Direct intraocular use. Hypersensitivity to cidofovir. History of clinically severe hypersensitivity to probenecid or other sulfa-containing medications.

WARNINGS/PRECAUTIONS
Decreased intraocular pressure (IOP) and visual acuity reported; monitor IOP. Decreased serum bicarbonate associated with proximal tubule injury and renal wasting syndrome (including Fanconi's syndrome) reported. Cases of metabolic acidosis in association with liver dysfunction and pancreatitis resulting in death reported. Do not administer doses greater than recommended or exceed frequency or rate of administration. Uveitis or iritis reported; consider treatment with topical corticosteroids with or without topical cycloplegic agents. Monitor for signs and symptoms of uveitis/iritis.

ADVERSE REACTIONS
Renal toxicity, N/V, neutropenia, proteinuria, decreased IOP, uveitis/iritis, pneumonia, dyspnea, infection, fever, creatinine elevation ≥2mg/dL, decreased serum bicarbonate.

DRUG INTERACTIONS
See Contraindications.

PREGNANCY AND LACTATION
Category C, not for use in nursing.

MECHANISM OF ACTION
Viral DNA synthesis inhibitor; suppresses CMV replication by selective inhibition of viral DNA synthesis.

PHARMACOKINETICS
Absorption: Administration of variable doses (with or without probenecid) resulted in different parameters. **Distribution:** V_d=537mL/kg (without probenecid), 410mL/kg (with probenecid); plasma protein binding (<6%). **Elimination:** Urine (80-100% unchanged).

PATIENT CONSIDERATIONS
Assessment: Assess renal function (SrCr and urine protein) within 48 hrs prior to each dose, history of clinically severe hypersensitivity to probenecid or other sulfa-containing agents, pregnancy/nursing status, and possible drug interactions.

Monitoring: Monitor renal function and adjust dose as required. Give IV hydration to patients with proteinuria and repeat test as necessary. Monitor WBC counts with differential (prior to each dose), and neutrophil count. IOP, visual acuity, and ocular symptoms should be monitored periodically.

Counseling: Inform that drug does not cure CMV retinitis and that patient may continue to experience progression of retinitis during and following treatment. Advise to have regular follow-up ophthalmologic examinations. Advise to temporarily d/c zidovudine administration, or decrease zidovudine dose by 1/2, on days of cidofovir administration only. Inform of the major toxicity of the drug. Counsel on importance of completing a full course of probenecid with each cidofovir dose. Warn of potential adverse events caused by probenecid. Inform that drug may cause tumors in humans. Advise men that testes weight reduction and hypospermia may occur and may cause infertility. Inform of embryotoxicity in animal studies; advise women of childbearing potential to use effective contraception during and for 1 month following therapy and for men to practice barrier contraceptive methods during and for 3 months after therapy.

VISTOGARD — uridine triacetate   Rx

Class: Pyrimidine analog

ADULT DOSAGE	PEDIATRIC DOSAGE
Fluorouracil or Capecitabine Toxicity/Overdose	**Fluorouracil or Capecitabine Toxicity/Overdose**
Emergency treatment following a fluorouracil or capecitabine overdose regardless of the presence of symptoms, or early-onset, severe or life-threatening toxicity affecting the cardiac or central nervous system, and/or early-onset, unusually severe adverse reactions (eg, GI toxicity and/or neutropenia) w/in 96 hrs following the end of fluorouracil or capecitabine administration	Emergency treatment following a fluorouracil or capecitabine overdose regardless of the presence of symptoms, or early-onset, severe or life-threatening toxicity affecting the cardiac or central nervous system, and/or early-onset, unusually severe adverse reactions (eg, GI toxicity and/or neutropenia) w/in 96 hrs following the end of fluorouracil or capecitabine administration
10g (1 pkt) PO q6 hrs for 20 doses	6.2g/m^2 BSA (not to exceed 10g/dose) PO q6 hrs for 20 doses

---

ADMINISTRATION
Oral route
- Take w/o regard to meals.
- Administer as soon as possible after overdose or early-onset toxicity w/in 96 hrs following the end of fluorouracil or capecitabine administration.
- Measure dose using either a scale accurate to at least 0.1g, or a graduated tsp accurate to 1/4 tsp.
- Discard any unused portion of granules; do not use granules left in open packet for subsequent dosing.
- If patient vomits w/in 2 hrs of taking a dose, initiate another complete dose as soon as possible after vomiting episode; administer next dose at regularly scheduled time.
- If patient misses a dose at the scheduled time, administer that dose as soon as possible; administer the next dose at the regularly scheduled time.

Preparation
PO:
- Mix each dose w/ 3-4 oz of soft foods (eg, applesauce, pudding, yogurt) and ingest w/in 30 min. Do not chew granules. Drink at least 4 oz of water.

NG Tube/Gastrostomy (G-Tube) Tube:
- Administer via NG tube or G-Tube when necessary (eg, severe mucositis or coma).
- Prepare approximately 4 fl oz (about 100mL) of a food starch-based thickening product in water and stir briskly until thickener has dissolved.
- Crush the contents of one full 10g packet of granules to a fine powder.
- Add crushed granules to 4 oz (about 100mL) of the reconstituted food starch-based thickening product.
- For pediatric patients receiving <10g, prepare mixture at a ratio of no greater than 1g/10mL of reconstituted food starch-based thickening product and mix thoroughly.
- After administration of the mixture using the NG tube or G-Tube, flush the tube w/ water.

STORAGE
25°C (77°F); excursions permitted to 15-30°C (59-86°F).

HOW SUPPLIED
Granules: 10g/pkt [4^s 20^s]

ADVERSE REACTIONS
N/V, diarrhea.

PREGNANCY AND LACTATION
Pregnancy: Limited case reports of uridine triacetate use during pregnancy are insufficient to inform a drug-associated risk of birth defects and miscarriage.
Lactation: There are no data on the presence of uridine triacetate in human milk, the effect on the breastfed infant, or the effect on milk production; caution in nursing.

MECHANISM OF ACTION
Pyrimidine analog; deacetylated by nonspecific esterases present throughout the body, yielding uridine in the circulation. Competitively inhibits cell damage and cell death caused by fluorouracil.

PHARMACOKINETICS
Absorption: T_{max}=2-3 hrs. **Distribution:** Crosses the blood brain barrier.
Metabolism: By normal pyrimidine catabolic pathways present in most tissues.
Elimination: Urine; $T_{1/2}$=2-2.5 hrs.

PATIENT CONSIDERATIONS
Assessment: Assess for fluorouracil or capecitabine overdose/toxicity and pregnancy/nursing status.
Monitoring: Monitor for adverse reactions.
Counseling: Advise on how to properly take drug. Advise the patient or caregiver the importance of taking all 20 doses, even if they feel well. Advise that if patient

---

vomits w/in 2 hrs of taking a dose, to take another complete dose as soon as possible after vomiting; instruct to take next dose at regularly scheduled time. Advise that if a dose is missed, to take missed dose as soon as possible; instruct to take next dose at regularly scheduled time.

VITAFOL-OB — calcium carbonate/copper oxide/ferrous fumarate/folic acid/magnesium oxide/niacin (niacinamide)/vitamin A (beta carotene)/vitamin B1 (thiamine mononitrate)/vitamin B2 (riboflavin)/vitamin B6 (pyridoxine hydrochloride)/vitamin B12 (cyanocobalamin)/vitamin C (ascorbic acid)/vitamin D (cholecalciferol)/vitamin E (dl-alpha tocopheryl acetate)/zinc oxide   Rx

Class: Prenatal vitamin

> Accidental overdose of iron-containing products is a leading cause of fatal poisoning in children <6 yrs of age. Keep out of reach of children. In case of accidental overdose, call a doctor or a poison control center immediately.

ADULT DOSAGE	PEDIATRIC DOSAGE
Dietary/Nutritional Supplement	Pediatric use may not have been established
For use prior to conception, throughout pregnancy, and during postnatal period (lactating and nonlactating mothers)	
1 tab qd or ud	

ADMINISTRATION
Oral route

STORAGE
15-30°C (59-86°F). Avoid excessive heat and moisture.

HOW SUPPLIED
Tab: Ascorbic acid 70mg-Beta carotene 2700 IU-Calcium carbonate 100mg-Cholecalciferol 400 IU-Copper oxide 2mg-Cyanocobalamin 12mcg Dl-alpha tocopheryl acetate 30 IU-Ferrous fumarate 65mg-Folic acid 1 mg-Magnesium oxide 25mg-Niacinamide 18mg-Pyridoxine HCl 2.5mg-Vitamin B1 1.6mg-Vitamin B2 1.8mg-Zinc oxide 25mg

CONTRAINDICATIONS
Hypersensitivity to any of the components or color additives in this product; untreated and uncomplicated pernicious anemia; hemochromatosis and iron storage disease or the potential for iron storage disease due to chronic hemolytic anemia (eg, inherited anomalies of Hgb structure or synthesis and/or red cell enzyme deficiencies), pyridoxine responsive anemia, or cirrhosis of the liver.
Cyanocobalamin: sensitivity to cobalt.

WARNINGS/PRECAUTIONS
Caution with hypercalcemia or conditions that may lead to hypercalcemia (eg, hyperparathyroidism, those who form Ca^{2+}-containing kidney stones). High doses of vitamin D may lead to elevated levels of Ca^{2+} that reside in the blood and soft tissues; bone pain, high BP, formation of kidney stones, renal failure, and increased risk of heart disease may occur. Prolonged use of iron salts may produce iron storage disease. Folic acid, especially in doses >0.1mg daily, may obscure pernicious anemia; hematologic remission may occur while neurological manifestations remain progressive. Use of folic acid doses >1mg daily may precipitate or exacerbate the neurological damage of vitamin B12 deficiency.

ADVERSE REACTIONS
Allergic reactions.

DRUG INTERACTIONS
High doses of folic acid may decrease serum levels of anticonvulsant drugs. Avoid vitamin D supplementation with large amounts of Ca^{2+} in patients with hypercalcemia or conditions that may lead to hypercalcemia. Zinc may inhibit the absorption of certain antibiotics; take at least 2 hrs apart to minimize interactions.

MECHANISM OF ACTION
Prenatal vitamin.

PATIENT CONSIDERATIONS
Assessment: Assess for drug hypersensitivity; untreated and uncomplicated pernicious anemia; hemochromatosis; potential for iron storage disease due to chronic hemolytic anemia, pyridoxine responsive anemia, or liver cirrhosis; sensitivity to cobalt; hypercalcemia/conditions that may lead to hypercalcemia; and possible drug interactions.

Monitoring: Monitor for allergic reactions, masking of pernicious anemia, and for other adverse reactions.

Counseling: Inform of the risks/benefits of therapy. Instruct to inform physician of all concomitant medications and dietary supplements currently taking, and if any adverse reactions develop.

VITEKTA — elvitegravir   Rx

Class: HIV-integrase strand transfer inhibitor

ADULT DOSAGE

HIV-1 Infection

In combination w/ an HIV protease inhibitor coadministered w/ ritonavir (RTV) and other antiretroviral drug(s) in treatment-experienced patients

85mg Dose:
85mg qd + atazanavir 300mg qd + RTV 100mg qd
or
85mg qd + lopinavir 400mg bid + RTV 100mg bid

150mg Dose:
150mg qd + darunavir 600mg bid + RTV 100mg bid
or
150mg qd + fosamprenavir 700mg bid + RTV 100mg bid
or
150mg qd + tipranavir 500mg bid + RTV 200mg bid

PEDIATRIC DOSAGE

Pediatric use may not have been established

DOSING CONSIDERATIONS

Hepatic Impairment

Severe: Not recommended for use

ADMINISTRATION

Oral route

Take w/ food.

STORAGE

Room temperature <30°C (86°F).

HOW SUPPLIED

Tab: 85mg, 150mg

CONTRAINDICATIONS

Refer to the individual PIs for coadministered protease inhibitor and RTV.

WARNINGS/PRECAUTIONS

Immune reconstitution syndrome reported. Autoimmune disorders (eg, Graves' disease, polymyositis, Guillain-Barre syndrome) reported in the setting of immune reconstitution and can occur many months after initiation of treatment. Caution in elderly.

ADVERSE REACTIONS

Diarrhea, nausea, headache, hyperbilirubinemia, hematuria, increased serum amylase/creatine kinase/GGT, hypercholesterolemia, hypertriglyceridemia, hyperglycemia, glucosuria, neutropenia.

DRUG INTERACTIONS

Coadministration w/ HIV-1 protease inhibitors other than RTV, atazanavir, lopinavir, darunavir, fosamprenavir, or tipranavir is not recommended. Use w/ elvitegravir-containing drugs (eg, Stribild) is not recommended. Use in combination w/ a protease inhibitor and cobicistat is not recommended; may result in suboptimal levels of elvitegravir and/or the protease inhibitor, leading to loss of therapeutic effect and development of resistance. Coadministration w/ efavirenz, nevirapine, St. John's wort, rifampin, rifapentine, phenobarbital, phenytoin, carbamazepine, or oxcarbazepine is not recommended; may decrease elvitegravir levels. Coadministration w/ boceprevir is not recommended; may reduce levels of boceprevir and may alter levels of HIV protease inhibitors. CYP3A inducers may increase the clearance of elvitegravir, as well as RTV; may result in decreased plasma levels of elvitegravir and/or a concomitantly administered protease inhibitor and lead to loss of therapeutic effect and to possible resistance. Atazanavir/RTV, lopinavir/RTV, and ketoconazole may increase elvitegravir levels. Administer didanosine at least 1 hr before or 2 hrs after elvitegravir. Antacids may decrease levels; separate elvitegravir and antacid administration by at least 2 hrs. Coadministration w/ systemic dexamethasone may decrease levels; consider alternative corticosteroids. Rifabutin or bosentan may decrease levels. May increase levels of ketoconazole, bosentan, rifabutin, or 25-O-desacetylrifabutin. May increase norgestimate and decrease ethinyl estradiol levels; alternative methods of nonhormonal contraception are recommended. May increase levels of buprenorphine and norbuprenorphine and may decrease levels of naloxone and methadone. Closely monitor for sedation and cognitive effects when coadministered w/ buprenorphine/naloxone. Refer to PI for further information on drug interactions, including dose modifications required when used w/ certain concomitant therapies.

PREGNANCY AND LACTATION

Pregnancy: Category B. Physicians are encouraged to register patients in the Antiretroviral Pregnancy Registry.
Lactation: Not for use in nursing.

MECHANISM OF ACTION

HIV-1 integrase strand transfer inhibitor; prevents the integration of HIV-1 DNA into host genomic DNA, blocking the formation of the HIV-1 provirus and propagation of the viral infection.

PHARMACOKINETICS

Absorption: T_{max}=4 hrs; C_{max}=1.2mcg/mL (85mg), 1.5mcg/mL (150mg); AUC_{tau}=18mcg•hr/mL. **Distribution:** Plasma protein binding (98-99%). **Metabolism:** Oxidation via CYP3A; glucuronidation via UGT1A1/3. **Elimination:** Feces (94.8%), urine (6.7% as metabolites); $T_{1/2}$=8.7 hrs (median).

PATIENT CONSIDERATIONS

Assessment: Assess for severe hepatic impairment, pregnancy/nursing status, and for possible drug interactions.

Monitoring: Monitor for signs/symptoms of immune reconstitution syndrome, autoimmune disorders, and for other adverse reactions.

Counseling: Advise patients to remain under the care of a healthcare provider during therapy. Inform that drug is not a cure for HIV-1 infection and continuous therapy is necessary to control HIV-1 infection and decrease HIV-related illnesses. Advise to continue to practice safer sex, to use latex or polyurethane condoms, and to not reuse/share needles. Instruct to take ud, on a regular dosing schedule w/ food, and to avoid missing doses. Inform that therapy may interact w/ many drugs; advise to notify physician if using any other prescription or nonprescription medication or herbal product (eg, St. John's wort). Advise to inform physician immediately if any symptoms of infection develop.

VITUZ — chlorpheniramine maleate/hydrocodone bitartrate   CII

Class: Antihistamine/opioid antitussive

ADULT DOSAGE

Antihistamine/Cough Suppressant

Relief of cough and symptoms associated w/ upper respiratory allergies or a common cold

5mL q4h-q6h PRN
Max: 20mL/24 hrs (4 doses)

PEDIATRIC DOSAGE

Pediatric use may not have been established

DOSING CONSIDERATIONS

Elderly

Start at lower end of dosing range

ADMINISTRATION

Oral route

Measure with an accurate mL measuring device
Do not use a household tsp

STORAGE

20-25°C (68-77°F).

HOW SUPPLIED

Sol: (Hydrocodone-Chlorpheniramine) 5mg-4mg/5mL [480mL]

CONTRAINDICATIONS

Known hypersensitivity to hydrocodone bitartrate, chlorpheniramine maleate or any of the inactive ingredients of this medication; coadministration w/ MAOIs or w/in 14 days of stopping therapy; narrow-angle glaucoma; urinary retention; severe HTN; severe coronary artery disease (CAD).

WARNINGS/PRECAUTIONS

May produce dose-related respiratory depression; d/c if respiratory depression occurs and use naloxone HCl when indicated to antagonize the effect and other supportive measures as necessary. Psychic/physical dependence or tolerance may develop. Has potential for abuse. May markedly exaggerate respiratory depressant effects and elevate CSF pressure in patients with head injury, other intracranial lesions, or preexisting increase in intracranial pressure (ICP); avoid use. May impair mental/physical abilities. May obscure clinical course of head injuries and acute abdominal conditions. Caution with thyroid disease, Addison's disease, prostatic hypertrophy, urethral stricture, asthma, severe hepatic/renal impairment, and in elderly.

ADVERSE REACTIONS

Sedation, somnolence, mental clouding, lethargy, anxiety, fear, dysphoria, dizziness, nausea, psychic dependence, mood changes, blurred vision, confusion, headache, euphoria.

DRUG INTERACTIONS

Additive CNS depression with opioids, antihistamines, antipsychotics, antianxiety agents, and other CNS depressants (including alcohol); avoid use. May increase effect of either the antidepressant or hydrocodone with concomitant TCAs. May produce paralytic ileus and excessive anticholinergic effects with anticholinergics; use with caution.

PREGNANCY AND LACTATION

Category C, not for use in nursing.

MECHANISM OF ACTION

Hydrocodone: Semisynthetic narcotic antitussive/analgesic; not established. Believed to act directly on cough center. Chlorpheniramine: H_1-receptor antagonist; possesses anticholinergic and sedative activity. Prevents released histamine from dilating capillaries and causing edema of the respiratory mucosa.

PHARMACOKINETICS

Absorption: Hydrocodone: C_{max}=10.6ng/mL, T_{max}=1.4 hrs. Chlorpheniramine: C_{max}=7.20ng/mL. T_{max}=3.5 hrs. **Distribution:** Found in breast milk. **Elimination:** Hydrocodone: $T_{1/2}$=4.9 hrs. Chlorpheniramine: $T_{1/2}$=24 hrs.

PATIENT CONSIDERATIONS

Assessment: Assess for previous drug hypersensitivity, narrow-angle glaucoma, urinary retention, severe HTN/CAD, head injury, intracranial lesions, increase in ICP, acute abdominal conditions, thyroid disease, Addison's disease, prostatic hypertrophy, urethral stricture, asthma, severe renal/hepatic impairment, pregnancy/nursing status, and possible drug interactions.

Monitoring: Monitor for drug abuse/dependence, respiratory depression, elevations in CSF pressure, hypersensitivity, and other adverse reactions.

Counseling: Instruct not to increase dose/frequency. Advise to measure sol with accurate mL measuring device; inform that a household tsp is not accurate and may lead to overdosage. Instruct to avoid alcohol and other CNS depressants. Advise to avoid hazardous tasks (eg, operating machinery/driving); inform that therapy may produce marked drowsiness. Caution that therapy can cause drug dependence. Instruct not to use with an MAOI or within 14 days of stopping use.

VIVELLE-DOT — estradiol   Rx

Class: Estrogen

Estrogens increase the risk of endometrial cancer. Adding a progestin to estrogen therapy reduces the risk of endometrial hyperplasia. Adequate diagnostic measures should be undertaken to rule out malignancy with undiagnosed, persistent, or recurring abnormal genital bleeding. Should not be used for the prevention of cardiovascular (CV) disease or dementia. Increased risk of stroke and deep vein thrombosis (DVT) reported in postmenopausal women (50-79 yrs of age) treated with daily oral conjugated estrogens (CE) alone and when combined with medroxyprogesterone acetate (MPA). Increased risk of pulmonary embolism (PE), MI, and invasive breast cancer reported in postmenopausal women (50-79 yrs of age) treated with daily oral CE combined with MPA. Increased risk of developing probable dementia reported in postmenopausal women ≥65 yrs of age treated with daily CE alone and when combined with MPA. Should be prescribed at the lowest effective dose and for the shortest duration consistent with treatment goals and risks.

ADULT DOSAGE

Menopausal Vasomotor Symptoms

Moderate to Severe:
Initial: 0.0375mg/day applied 2X/week
Titrate: Dose adjustment should be guided by clinical response
Use the lowest effective dose for the shortest duration; reevaluate at 3- to 6-month intervals

Menopausal Vulvar/Vaginal Atrophy

Moderate to Severe:
Initial: 0.0375mg/day applied 2X/week
Titrate: Dose adjustment should be guided by clinical response
Use the lowest effective dose for the shortest duration; reevaluate at 3- to 6-month intervals

Postmenopausal Osteoporosis

Prevention:
Initial: 0.025mg/day 2X/week

Other Indications

Hypoestrogenism due to hypogonadism, castration, or primary ovarian failure

Conversions

In women not currently taking oral estrogens or in women switching from another estradiol transdermal therapy, treatment w/ Vivelle-Dot may be initiated at once. However, in women currently taking oral estrogens, treatment w/ Vivelle-Dot should be initiated 1 week after withdrawal of oral hormone therapy, or sooner if menopausal symptoms reappear in <1 week

PEDIATRIC DOSAGE

Pediatric use may not have been established

ADMINISTRATION
Transdermal route

Apply immediately upon removal from the protective pouch.
Apply adhesive side of patch to clean, dry area of the trunk of the body (including abdomen/buttocks); area should not be oily, damaged, or irritated.
Do not apply patch to the breasts; avoid application to waistline as tight clothing may rub the system off.
Rotate application site w/ an interval of at least 1 week between applications to a particular site.
Press the system firmly in place w/ palm of hand for about 10 sec, making sure there is good contact, especially around edges.
If the patch falls off, the same system may be reapplied; if it cannot be reapplied, a new system should be applied to another location. Continue original treatment schedule.
May be given continuously in patients who do not have an intact uterus or cyclically (eg, 3 weeks on drug followed by 1 week off drug) in patients w/ an intact uterus.

STORAGE
25°C (77°F); do not store unpouched.

HOW SUPPLIED
Patch: 0.025mg/day, 0.0375mg/day, 0.05mg/day, 0.075mg/day, 0.1mg/day [8s]

CONTRAINDICATIONS
Undiagnosed abnormal genital bleeding, known/suspected/history of breast cancer, known/suspected estrogen-dependent neoplasia, active/history of DVT/PE, active/history of arterial thromboembolic disease (eg, stroke, MI), known anaphylactic reaction or angioedema or hypersensitivity w/ the medication, known liver impairment or disease, known protein C/protein S/antithrombin deficiency or other known thrombophilic disorders, known/suspected pregnancy.

WARNINGS/PRECAUTIONS
D/C immediately if stroke, DVT, PE, or MI occurs or is suspected. If feasible, d/c at least 4-6 weeks before surgery of the type associated with an increased risk of thromboembolism, or during periods of prolonged immobilization. May increase risk of ovarian cancer, and gallbladder disease requiring surgery. May lead to severe hypercalcemia in patients with breast cancer and bone metastases; d/c and take appropriate measures if hypercalcemia occurs. Retinal vascular thrombosis reported; d/c therapy pending exam if sudden partial/complete loss of vision or sudden onset of proptosis, diplopia, or migraine occurs. D/C permanently if exam reveals papilledema or retinal vascular lesions. May elevate BP and thyroid-binding globulin levels. May elevate plasma TGs leading to pancreatitis in patients with preexisting hypertriglyceridemia; consider discontinuation if pancreatitis occurs. Caution with history of cholestatic jaundice associated with past estrogen use or with pregnancy; d/c in case of recurrence. May cause fluid retention. Caution with hypoparathyroidism as estrogen-induced hypocalcemia may occur. Cases of malignant transformation of residual endometrial implants reported in women treated post-hysterectomy with estrogen therapy alone; consider addition of progestin for patients known to have residual endometriosis post-hysterectomy. Anaphylactic/anaphylactoid reactions, and angioedema involving eye/eyelid, face, larynx, pharynx, tongue, and extremity with or without urticaria requiring medical intervention reported; do not reapply in patients who develop angioedema anytime during the course of treatment. May exacerbate symptoms of angioedema in women with hereditary angioedema. May exacerbate asthma, diabetes mellitus, epilepsy, migraine, porphyria, systemic lupus erythematosus, and hepatic hemangiomas; use with caution. May affect certain endocrine and blood components in lab tests.

ADVERSE REACTIONS
Constipation, dyspepsia, nausea, influenza-like illness, pain, nasopharyngitis, sinusitis, URTI, back pain, headache, depression, insomnia, breast tenderness, intermenstrual bleeding, sinus congestion.

DRUG INTERACTIONS
CYP3A4 inducers (eg, St. John's wort, phenobarbital, carbamazepine) may decrease levels and may decrease therapeutic effects and/or change uterine bleeding profile. CYP3A4 inhibitors (eg, erythromycin, clarithromycin, ketoconazole) may increase levels and may result in side effects. Patients concomitantly receiving thyroid replacement therapy and estrogens may require increased doses of thyroid replacement therapy; monitor thyroid function.

PREGNANCY AND LACTATION
Contraindicated in pregnancy, not for use in nursing.

MECHANISM OF ACTION
Estrogen; binds to nuclear receptors in estrogen-responsive tissues. Circulating estrogens modulate the pituitary secretion of the gonadotropins, luteinizing hormone and follicle-stimulating hormone, through a (-) feedback mechanism. Reduces elevated levels of these hormones in postmenopausal women.

PHARMACOKINETICS
Absorption: Transdermal administration of variable doses resulted in different parameters. **Distribution:** Largely bound to sex hormone-binding globulin and albumin; found in breast milk. **Metabolism:** Liver to estrone (metabolite), estriol (major urinary metabolite); sulfate and glucuronide conjugation (liver); biliary secretion of conjugates into the intestine, hydrolysis (intestine), reabsorption; CYP3A4 (partial metabolism). **Elimination:** Urine (parent compound and metabolites); $T_{1/2}$=5.9-7.7 hrs.

PATIENT CONSIDERATIONS
Assessment: Assess for undiagnosed abnormal genital bleeding, presence/history of breast cancer, estrogen-dependent neoplasia, active/history of DVT/PE/arterial thromboembolic disease, liver impairment/disease, thrombophilic disorders, drug hypersensitivity, pregnancy/nursing status, any other conditions where treatment is contraindicated or cautioned, need for progestin therapy, and for possible drug interactions.

Monitoring: Monitor for signs/symptoms of CV disorders, malignant neoplasms, dementia, gallbladder disease, hypercalcemia, visual abnormalities, BP and plasma TG elevations, cholestatic jaundice, fluid retention, anaphylactic/anaphylactoid reactions, angioedema, exacerbation of endometriosis, and other adverse reactions. Perform adequate diagnostic measures (eg, endometrial sampling) to rule out malignancy in case of undiagnosed persistent or recurring genital bleeding. Monitor thyroid function in patients on thyroid replacement therapy. Perform annual breast exam; schedule mammography based on age, risk factors, and prior mammogram results. Periodically reevaluate to determine need for therapy.

Counseling: Inform of the importance of reporting abnormal vaginal bleeding to physician as soon as possible. Inform of possible serious adverse reactions of therapy (eg, CV disorders, malignant neoplasms, probable dementia) and of possible less serious but common adverse reactions (eg, headache, breast pain and tenderness, N/V). Instruct to have yearly breast exams by a physician and to perform monthly breast self-exams.

VIVITROL — naltrexone
Class: Opioid antagonist
Rx

ADULT DOSAGE
Alcohol Dependence
Treatment of Alcohol Dependence in Patients Who are Able to Abstain from Alcohol in an Outpatient Setting Prior to Initiation of Therapy:
380mg IM every 4 weeks or once a month

Prior to initiating therapy, an opioid-free duration of a minimum of 7-10 days is recommended

Opioid Dependence
Prevention of Relapse to Opioid Dependence, Following Opioid Detoxification:
380mg IM every 4 weeks or once a month

Prior to initiating therapy, an opioid-free duration of a minimum of 7-10 days is recommended

Conversions
Switching from Buprenorphine, Buprenorphine/Naloxone, or Methadone:
Be prepared to manage withdrawal symptomatically w/ nonopioid medications

PEDIATRIC DOSAGE
Pediatric use may not have been established

ADMINISTRATION
IM route
Administer as IM gluteal inj, alternating buttocks for each subsequent inj. Must be suspended only in the diluent supplied in the carton and must be administered only w/ 1 of the administration needles supplied in the carton; do not substitute any other components for the components of the carton.
For patients w/ a larger amount of subcutaneous tissue overlying the gluteal muscle, may utilize the supplied 2-inch needle to help ensure that the injectate reaches the IM mass.
For very lean patients, the 1.5-inch needle may be appropriate to prevent the needle contacting the periosteum.
Either needle may be used for patients w/ average body habitus.
Prior to preparation, allow drug to reach room temperature (approx 45 min).
Refer to PI for further preparation and administration instructions.

STORAGE
2-8°C (36-46°F). Do not freeze. Can be stored at ≤25°C (77°F) for no more than 7 days prior administration.

HOW SUPPLIED
Inj, Extended-Release: 380mg

CONTRAINDICATIONS
Concomitant opioid analgesics; current physiologic opioid dependence; acute opioid withdrawal; failure of naloxone challenge test or positive urine screen for opioids; previous hypersensitivity to naltrexone, polylactide-co-glycolide, carboxymethylcellulose, or any other components of the diluent.

WARNINGS/PRECAUTIONS
Patients may have reduced tolerance to opioids after opioid detoxification; may result in potentially life-threatening opioid intoxication with use of previously tolerated opioid doses. Potential risk to patients attempting to overcome the antagonism by taking opioids; may lead to life-threatening opioid intoxication or fatal overdose. Inj-site reactions reported; inadvertent SQ inj may increase likelihood of severe inj-site reactions. Withdrawal syndrome, severe enough to require hospitalization, may occur when withdrawal is precipitated abruptly by the administration of an opioid antagonist to an opioid-dependent patient. Opioid-dependent patients, including those being treated for alcohol dependence, should be opioid-free before starting treatment to reduce risk of either precipitated withdrawal in patients dependent on opioids or exacerbation of a preexisting subclinical withdrawal syndrome; an opioid-free interval of a minimum of 7-10 days is recommended for patients previously dependent on short-acting opioids. May experience severe manifestations of precipitated withdrawal when being switched from opioid agonist to opioid antagonist therapy; patients transitioning from buprenorphine or methadone may be vulnerable to precipitation of withdrawal symptoms for as long as 2 weeks. A naloxone challenge test may be helpful to determine if patient is opioid-free; however, precipitated withdrawal may occur despite having negative urine toxicology screen or tolerating a naloxone challenge test. Cases of hepatitis, clinically significant liver dysfunction, and transient, asymptomatic hepatic transaminase elevations reported; d/c in the event of symptoms and/or signs of acute hepatitis. Depression and suicidality reported. In emergency situations, suggested plan for pain management is regional analgesia or use of nonopioid analgesics. If opioid therapy is required, monitor continuously in an anesthesia care setting. Cases of eosinophilic pneumonia and hypersensitivity reactions, including anaphylaxis, reported. As with any IM inj, caution with thrombocytopenia or any coagulation disorder (eg, hemophilia, severe hepatic failure). Does not eliminate or diminish alcohol withdrawal symptoms. May cross-react with certain immunoassay methods for the detection of drugs of abuse in urine. Caution with moderate to severe renal impairment.

ADVERSE REACTIONS
N/V, diarrhea, insomnia, depression, inj-site reactions, somnolence, anorexia, muscle cramps, dizziness, syncope, appetite disorder, hepatic enzyme abnormalities, nasopharyngitis, toothache, headache.

DRUG INTERACTIONS
See Contraindications. Antagonizes effects of opioid-containing medicines (eg, cough and cold remedies, antidiarrheals, opioid analgesics).

PREGNANCY AND LACTATION
Pregnancy: Category C.
Lactation: Not for use in nursing.

MECHANISM OF ACTION
Opioid antagonist; blocks the effects of opioids by competitive binding at opioid receptors, with the highest affinity for the mu opioid receptor.

PHARMACOKINETICS
Absorption: T_{max}=2 hrs (1st peak), 2-3 days (2nd peak). **Distribution:** Plasma protein binding (21%); (PO) found in breast milk. **Metabolism:** Extensive, via dihydrodiol dehydrogenase; 6β-naltrexol (primary metabolite). **Elimination:** Urine; $T_{1/2}$=5-10 days.

PATIENT CONSIDERATIONS
Assessment: Assess for opioid use, acute opioid withdrawal, thrombocytopenia, coagulation disorders, renal impairment, any other conditions where treatment is contraindicated or cautioned, pregnancy/nursing status, and possible drug interactions. Assess patients, including patients treated for alcohol dependence, for underlying opioid dependence, and for any recent use of opioids. Assess body habitus to assure that needle length is adequate.

Monitoring: Monitor for opioid intoxication/overdose, severe inj-site reactions, precipitation of opioid withdrawal, signs/symptoms of acute hepatis, depression, suicidality, hypersensitivity reactions, and other adverse reactions.

Counseling: Advise that if they previously used opioids, they may be more sensitive to lower doses of opioids and at risk of accidental overdose if they use opioids when their next dose is due, if they miss a dose, or after treatment is discontinued. Advise that patients will not perceive any effect if they attempt to self-administer heroin or any other opioid drug in small doses while on therapy. Inform that administration of large doses of heroin or any other opioid to try to bypass the blockade may lead to serious injury, coma, or death. Inform that patient may not experience the expected effects from opioid-containing analgesic, antidiarrheal, or antitussive medications. Advise that inj-site reactions may occur and instruct to seek medical attention for worsening skin reactions. Instruct to be off all opioids for a minimum of 7-10 days before starting therapy in order to avoid precipitation of opioid withdrawal. Advise not to take therapy if they have any symptoms of opioid withdrawal. Advise all patients, including those with alcohol dependence, to notify physician of any recent use of opioids or any history of opioid dependence before starting therapy. Inform that drug may cause liver injury; instruct to immediately notify physician if symptoms and/or signs of liver disease develop. Inform the patient, family members, and caregivers that the patient may experience depression while taking therapy and to contact physician if the patient becomes depressed or symptoms of depression are experienced. Instruct to carry documentation to alert medical personnel to therapy. Advise that drug may cause an allergic pneumonia; instruct to immediately notify physician if signs and symptoms of pneumonia develop. Inform that drug may cause nausea, which tends to subside within a few days post-inj. Advise that they may also experience tiredness, headache, vomiting, decreased appetite, painful joints, and muscle cramps. Advise that therapy has been shown to treat alcohol and opioid dependence only when used as part of a treatment program that includes counseling and support. Advise that dizziness may occur; instruct to avoid driving or operating heavy machinery. Advise to notify physician if pregnant or intending to become pregnant during treatment, breastfeeding, or experiencing unusual or significant side effects while on therapy.

VIVLODEX — meloxicam
Class: NSAID
Rx

> NSAIDs cause an increased risk of serious cardiovascular (CV) thrombotic events, including MI and stroke; risk may occur early in treatment and increase w/ duration of use. Contraindicated in the setting of CABG surgery. NSAIDs also cause an increased risk of serious GI adverse events, including bleeding, ulceration, and perforation of the stomach or intestines. Elderly patients and patients w/ a prior history of peptic ulcer disease and/or GI bleeding are at greater risk for serious GI events.

ADULT DOSAGE
Osteoarthritis
Initial: 5mg qd
Titrate: May increase to 10mg
Max: 10mg/day

PEDIATRIC DOSAGE
Pediatric use may not have been established

DOSING CONSIDERATIONS
Renal Impairment
Hemodialysis:
Max: 5mg/day

Other Important Considerations
Not interchangeable w/ other formulations of oral meloxicam even if the total mg strength is the same. Do not substitute similar dose strengths of other meloxicam products

ADMINISTRATION
Oral route

STORAGE
25°C (77°F); excursions permitted to 15-30°C (59-86°F). Protect from moisture.

HOW SUPPLIED
Cap: 5mg, 10mg

CONTRAINDICATIONS
Known hypersensitivity (eg, anaphylactic reactions and serious skin reactions) to meloxicam or any components of this product, history of asthma, urticaria, or other allergic-type reactions after taking aspirin (ASA) or other NSAIDs, in the setting of CABG surgery.

WARNINGS/PRECAUTIONS
Use the lowest effective dose for the shortest duration consistent w/ treatment goals. Increased CV thrombotic risk w/ higher doses reported. Avoid in patients w/ a recent MI unless benefits outweigh the risks; if used, monitor patients for signs of cardiac ischemia. Increased risk of GI bleeding w/ smoking, use of alcohol, poor general health status, advanced liver disease, and/or coagulopathy. If a serious GI adverse event is suspected, promptly initiate evaluation and treatment, and d/c until a serious GI adverse event is ruled out. May cause elevations of ALT/AST; d/c immediately and perform clinical evaluation if signs and symptoms consistent w/ liver disease develop or if systemic manifestations occur. Rare cases of severe hepatic injury, including fulminant hepatitis, liver necrosis, and hepatic failure reported. Use only if benefits outweigh risks w/ severe hepatic impairment. May lead to new onset or worsening of preexisting HTN. Fluid retention and edema reported; avoid use in patients w/ severe heart failure (HF) unless benefits outweigh risk. Long-term administration may cause renal papillary necrosis and other renal injury; increased risk w/ renal/hepatic impairment, dehydration, hypovolemia, HF, and the elderly. Avoid use in patients w/ advanced renal disease unless benefits outweigh risk. Correct volume status in dehydrated or hypovolemic patients prior to initiating therapy. May increase serum potassium concentration. May cause anaphylactic reactions and serious skin adverse reactions (eg, exfoliative dermatitis, Stevens-Johnson Syndrome, and toxic epidermal necrolysis); d/c use at 1st appearance of skin rash or any other sign of hypersensitivity. Monitor for changes in signs and symptoms of asthma when used in patients w/ preexisting asthma (w/o known ASA hypersensitivity). May cause premature closure of the fetal ductus arteriosus; avoid use in pregnant women starting at 30 weeks of gestation (3rd trimester). May cause anemia. The pharmacological activity in reducing inflammation, and possibly fever, may diminish the utility of diagnostic signs in detecting infections.

ADVERSE REACTIONS
Diarrhea, nausea, abdominal discomfort.

DRUG INTERACTIONS
Increased risk of bleeding w/ anticoagulants and drugs that interfere w/ serotonin reuptake; monitor patients w/ concomitant use of anticoagulants (eg, warfarin), antiplatelet agents (eg, aspirin), SSRIs, and SNRIs. Concomitant use w/ analgesic doses of aspirin is not generally recommended. In the setting of concomitant use of low-dose ASA for cardiac prophylaxis, monitor patients more closely for evidence of GI bleeding. Antihypertensive effect of ACE inhibitors, ARBs, or β-blockers (including propranolol) may be diminished. Coadministration w/ ACE inhibitors or ARBs may result in deterioration of renal function, including possible acute renal failure, in patients who are elderly, volume-depleted (including those on diuretic therapy), or have renal impairment. The natriuretic effect of loop diuretics (eg, furosemide) and thiazide diuretics may be reduced; monitor for efficacy and signs of worsening renal function. May increase the serum concentration and prolong the $T_{1/2}$ of digoxin; monitor serum digoxin levels. May elevate plasma lithium levels and reduce renal lithium clearance; monitor for signs of lithium toxicity. May increase the risk for methotrexate toxicity and increase cyclosporine's nephrotoxicity. Use w/ other NSAIDs or salicylates (eg, diflunisal, salsalate) increases the risk of GI toxicity; concomitant use is not recommended. May increase the risk of pemetrexed-associated myelosuppression, renal, and GI toxicity; monitor for these effects in patients w/ renal impairment whose CrCl ranges from 45-79mL/min. Interrupt meloxicam dosing for at least 5 days before, the day of, and 2 days following pemetrexed administration.

PREGNANCY AND LACTATION
Pregnancy: Use during the third trimester of pregnancy increases the risk of premature closure of the fetal ductus arteriosus; avoid use in pregnant women starting at 30 weeks of gestation.
Lactation: There are no human data available on whether meloxicam is present in human milk, or on the effects on breastfed infants, or on milk production; caution in nursing.
Reproductive Potential: Use of prostaglandin-mediated NSAIDs may delay or prevent rupture of ovarian follicles, which has been associated w/ reversible infertility in some women. Consider withdrawal of NSAIDs in women who have difficulties conceiving or who are undergoing investigation of infertility.

MECHANISM OF ACTION
NSAID; not completely understood but involves inhibition of cyclooxygenase (COX-1 and COX-2). Because meloxicam is an inhibitor of prostaglandin synthesis, its mode of action may be due to a decrease of prostaglandins in peripheral tissues.

PHARMACOKINETICS
Absorption: T_{max}=2 hrs. **Distribution:** V_d=10L; plasma protein binding (99.4%, primarily albumin). **Metabolism:** Liver (extensive); oxidation via CYP2C9 (major) and CYP3A4 (minor), 5'-carboxy meloxicam (major metabolite). **Elimination:** Urine (0.2% unchanged), feces (1.6% unchanged); $T_{1/2}$=22 hrs.

PATIENT CONSIDERATIONS
Assessment: Assess for cardiovascular disease (CVD), risk factors for CVD, history of peptic ulcer disease and/or GI bleeding, hepatic/renal dysfunction, coagulopathy, preexisting HTN, severe HF, dehydration/hypovolemia, asthma, any

other conditions where treatment is contraindicated or cautioned, pregnancy/nursing status, and possible drug interactions. Obtain baseline BP.

Monitoring: Monitor for CV thrombotic events, GI events, hepatotoxicity, HTN, HF and edema, renal toxicity, hyperkalemia, anaphylactic/skin reactions, exacerbation of ASA-sensitive asthma, and premature closure of fetal ductus arteriosus. Monitor Hgb or Hct if signs or symptoms of anemia develop. Consider periodic monitoring w/ a CBC and a chemistry profile w/ long-term treatment.

Counseling: Advise to be alert for the symptoms of CV thrombotic events and to report any of these symptoms to the healthcare provider immediately. Advise to report symptoms of GI ulcerations and bleeding to the healthcare provider. In the setting of concomitant use of low-dose ASA for cardiac prophylaxis, inform of the increased risk for and the signs and symptoms of GI bleeding. Inform of the warning signs and symptoms of hepatotoxicity and instruct to d/c therapy and seek immediate medical therapy if these occur. Advise to be alert for the symptoms of CHF and to contact healthcare provider if such symptoms occur. Inform of the signs of an anaphylactic reaction and instruct to seek immediate emergency help if these occur. Advise to d/c therapy immediately if any type of rash develops and to contact healthcare provider as soon as possible. Instruct pregnant women to avoid use of meloxicam and other NSAIDs starting at 30 weeks gestation because of the risk of the premature closing of the fetal ductus arteriosus. Instruct to avoid concomitant use of NSAIDs and low-dose ASA unless directed by healthcare provider.

VIVOTIF — typhoid vaccine live oral Ty21a   Rx

Class: Vaccine

ADULT DOSAGE	PEDIATRIC DOSAGE
Typhoid Vaccine	**Typhoid Vaccine**
Immunization Against Disease Caused by *Salmonella typhi*:	**Immunization Against Disease Caused by *Salmonella typhi*:**
1 cap 1 hr ac w/ cold or lukewarm (not to exceed body temperature) drink on alternate days (eg, days 1, 3, 5, and 7) Complete immunization (ingestion of all 4 doses) at least 1 week prior to potential exposure	**>6 Years:** 1 cap 1 hr ac w/ cold or lukewarm (not to exceed body temperature) drink on alternate days (eg, days 1, 3, 5, and 7) Complete immunization (ingestion of all 4 doses) at least 1 week prior to potential exposure
Reimmunization: 4 caps on alternate days every 5 yrs for repeated or continued exposure	**Reimmunization:** 4 caps on alternate days every 5 yrs for repeated or continued exposure

ADMINISTRATION
Oral route

Do not chew; swallow as soon after placing in the mouth as possible.

STORAGE
2-8°C (35.6-46.4°F).

HOW SUPPLIED
Cap, Delayed-Release: Single foil blister [4 doses]

CONTRAINDICATIONS
Hypersensitivity to any component of the vaccine or the enteric-coated capsule. Acute febrile illness, deficiency in ability to mount a humoral or cell-mediated immune response due to congenital or acquired immunodeficient state, including treatment w/ immunosuppressive or antimitotic drugs.

WARNINGS/PRECAUTIONS
Routine typhoid vaccination not recommended in the U.S. Do not take during acute GI illness. Postpone taking the vaccine if persistent diarrhea or vomiting is occurring. Unless a complete immunization schedule is followed, an optimum immune response may not be achieved. Not all recipients of the vaccine will be fully protected against typhoid fever. Vaccinated individuals should continue to take personal precautions against exposure to typhoid organisms (eg, avoid contact or ingestion of potentially contaminated food or water). Ensure safe and effective use of vaccine.

ADVERSE REACTIONS
Abdominal pain, nausea, headache, fever.

DRUG INTERACTIONS
See Contraindications. Do not administer w/ sulfonamides and antibiotics. Antimalaria drugs (eg, mefloquine, chloroquine, proguanil) may interfere w/ immunogenicity of vaccine; administer proguanil only if ≥10 days have elapsed since the final dose of vaccine was ingested.

PREGNANCY AND LACTATION
Pregnancy: Category C.
Lactation: Safety not known in nursing.

MECHANISM OF ACTION
Vaccine; has not been established. May evoke a local immune response in the intestinal tract; local immunity may abort infection.

PATIENT CONSIDERATIONS
Assessment: Assess for hypersensitivity to any component of the vaccine or the capsule, acute febrile illness, immunodeficiency, acute GI illness, previous immunization history, current antibiotic usage, pregnancy/nursing status, and possible drug interactions.

Monitoring: Monitor for hypersensitivity reactions and for other adverse effects. Monitor immune response to vaccine.

Counseling: Inform of the benefits and risks of the vaccine, the importance of taking all 4 caps in the correct schedule and of proper storage temperature of the caps. Advise travelers to take all necessary precautions to avoid contact or ingestion of potentially contaminated food or water, and report any adverse reactions to physician.

VOGELXO — testosterone CIII

Class: Androgen

> Virilization reported in children secondarily exposed to testosterone gel. Children should avoid contact w/ unwashed or unclothed application sites in men using testosterone gel. Advise patients to strictly adhere to recommended instructions for use.

ADULT DOSAGE	PEDIATRIC DOSAGE
Testosterone Replacement Therapy	Pediatric use may not have been established
Congenital/Acquired Primary Hypogonadism or Hypogonadotropic Hypogonadism in Males:	
Initial: 50mg (1 tube, 1 pkt, or 4 pump actuations) applied topically qd at approx the same time each day to clean, dry intact skin of shoulders and/or upper arms	
Titrate: Measure am pre-dose serum testosterone concentrations approx 14 days after initiation of therapy; if concentration is <300-1000ng/dL, may increase to 100mg (2 tubes, 2 pkts; or 8 pump actuations) qd	
Max: 100mg qd	

ADMINISTRATION
Topical route

The prescribed amount should be delivered directly into the palm of the hand and immediately applied to the shoulders and/or upper arms (area of application should be limited to the area that will be covered by a short sleeve t-shirt).
Do not apply to the genitals or to the abdomen.
Allow application site to dry completely prior to dressing.
Wash hands thoroughly w/ soap and water after application.
In order to prevent transfer to another person, clothing should be worn to cover the application sites; if direct skin-to-skin contact of the application site(s) w/ another person is anticipated, the application sites must be washed thoroughly w/ soap and water.
Avoid swimming, showering, or washing the administration site for a minimum of 2 hrs after application.
Refer to PI for further application instructions.

Unit-Dose Tubes or Pkts
50mg: Apply 1 unit-dose tube or pkt to 1 upper arm and shoulder
100mg: Apply 1 unit-dose tube or pkt to 1 upper arm and shoulder and then apply 1 unit-dose tube or pkt to the opposite upper arm and shoulder

Multidose Pump
Instruct patients to prime the pump before using it for the 1st time by fully depressing the pump mechanism (actuation) 3X and discard this portion of the product to assure precise dose delivery.
After the priming procedure, patients should completely depress the pump 1 time (actuation) for every 12.5mg of testosterone required to achieve the daily prescribed dosage.
50mg: Apply 4 pump actuations to 1 upper arm and shoulder
100mg: Apply 4 pump actuations to 1 upper arm and shoulder and then apply 4 pump actuations to the opposite upper arm and shoulder

STORAGE
20-25°C (68-77°F); excursions permitted to 15-30°C (59-86°F).

HOW SUPPLIED
Gel: 50mg [5g, tube, pkt], 12.5mg/actuation [75g, pump]

CONTRAINDICATIONS
Men w/ breast carcinoma or known/suspected prostate carcinoma; women who are or may become pregnant, or are breastfeeding.

WARNINGS/PRECAUTIONS
Topical testosterone products may have different doses, strengths, or application instructions that may result in different systemic exposure. Men w/ BPH are at an increased risk for worsening of signs and symptoms of BPH. May increase risk for prostate cancer. Increases in Hct/RBC mass may require lowering or discontinuation of therapy; may increase risk of thromboembolic events. If Hct becomes elevated, d/c therapy until Hct decreases to an acceptable concentration. Venous thromboembolic events (VTEs), including deep vein thrombosis and pulmonary embolism, reported; d/c treatment and initiate appropriate workup and management if a VTE is suspected. Increased risk of major adverse cardiovascular events (MACE) reported. Not indicated for use in women. Suppression of spermatogenesis may occur w/ large doses. Monitor for signs/symptoms of hepatic dysfunction; if these occur, promptly d/c therapy while the cause is evaluated. May promote retention of Na+ and water. Edema w/ or w/o CHF in patients w/ preexisting cardiac/renal/hepatic disease may occur; in addition to discontinuation of therapy, diuretic therapy may be required. Gynecomastia may develop and persist. May potentiate sleep apnea. Changes in serum lipid profile may occur. Caution in cancer patients at risk of hypercalcemia (and associated hypercalciuria); regularly monitor serum Ca^{2+} concentrations.

May decrease concentrations of thyroxine-binding globulins, resulting in decreased total T4 serum concentrations and increased resin uptake of T3 and T4. Flammable; avoid fire, flame, or smoking until the gel has dried.

ADVERSE REACTIONS
Application-site reactions.

DRUG INTERACTIONS
Changes in insulin sensitivity or glycemic control may occur; may decrease blood glucose, which may necessitate a decrease in the dose of antidiabetic medication. Changes in anticoagulant activity may occur; frequently monitor INR and PT in patients taking warfarin, especially at the initiation and termination of androgen therapy. Concurrent use w/ corticosteroids may result in increased fluid retention; caution in patients w/ cardiac/renal/hepatic disease.

PREGNANCY AND LACTATION
Pregnancy: Category X.
Lactation: Not for use in nursing.

MECHANISM OF ACTION
Androgen; responsible for the normal growth and development of male sex organs and for maintenance of secondary sex characteristics.

PHARMACOKINETICS
Absorption: (100mg, single dose) AUC$_{(0-24, 0-t)}$=6625ng•hr/dL, 10,425ng•hr/dL; C$_{max}$=573ng/dL. **Distribution:** Plasma protein binding (approx 40% bound to sex hormone-binding globulin). **Metabolism:** Estradiol and dihydrotestosterone (major active metabolites). **Elimination:** (IM) Urine (90%, glucuronic acid and sulfuric acid conjugates and metabolites), feces (6%, unconjugated); T$_{1/2}$=10-100 min.

PATIENT CONSIDERATIONS
Assessment: Assess for breast/prostate cancer, BPH, cardiac/renal/hepatic disease, any other conditions where treatment is contraindicated or cautioned, and possible drug interactions. Check Hct prior to therapy. Confirm diagnosis of hypogonadism by measuring testosterone levels in am on at least 2 separate days prior to initiation.

Monitoring: Monitor for worsening signs/symptoms of BPH, prostate cancer, VTE, hepatic dysfunction, Na+/water retention, gynecomastia, sleep apnea, thyroxin-binding globulin, and other adverse reactions. Monitor morning pre-dose serum testosterone concentrations approx 14 days after initiation of therapy. Monitor lipid profile periodically, particularly after starting therapy and after any dose increases. Regularly monitor serum Ca^{2+} concentrations in cancer patients at risk of hypercalcemia. Reevaluate Hct 3-6 months after starting therapy, then annually. Frequently monitor INR and PT in patients taking warfarin, especially at the initiation and termination of androgen therapy.

Counseling: Inform of the reported signs/symptoms of secondary exposure, and advise to notify physician of the possibility of secondary exposure. Inform that children and women should avoid contact w/ unwashed or unclothed application sites of men using the gel. Instruct to apply ud and strictly adhere to administration instructions to minimize the potential for secondary exposure. Inform that treatment may lead to adverse reactions (eg, changes in urinary habits, breathing disturbances, too frequent or persistent erections of the penis, N/V, changes in skin color, ankle swelling). Inform that drug is flammable; instruct to avoid fire, flame, or smoking until the gel has dried. Instruct to adhere to all recommended monitoring and report any changes in state of health (eg, changes in urinary habits, breathing, sleep, mood). Advise not to share the medication w/ anyone. Instruct to wait 2 hrs before washing or swimming following application. Inform of the possible risk of MACE when deciding whether to use or continue to use drug.

VOLTAREN GEL — diclofenac sodium Rx

Class: NSAID

> NSAIDs cause an increased risk of serious cardiovascular (CV) thrombotic events, including MI and stroke, which can be fatal. This risk may occur early in treatment and may increase w/ duration of use. Contraindicated in the setting of CABG surgery. NSAIDs cause an increased risk of serious GI adverse events (eg, bleeding, ulceration, stomach/intestinal perforation), which can be fatal and can occur anytime during use and w/o warning symptoms; elderly patients and patients w/ a prior history of peptic ulcer disease and/or GI bleeding are at a greater risk.

ADULT DOSAGE	PEDIATRIC DOSAGE
Osteoarthritis	Pediatric use may not have been established
Relief of Osteoarthritis Pain of Joints (eg, Knees, Hands):	
Lower Extremities:	
Apply 4g to affected foot, ankle, or knee qid	
Max: 16g/day to any single joint	
Upper Extremities:	
Apply 2g to affected hand, wrist, or elbow qid	
Max: 8g/day to any single joint	
Total dose should not exceed 32g/day over all affected joints	

ADMINISTRATION
Topical route

- Measure using enclosed dosing card; apply gel w/in the rectangular area of the dosing card up to the 2g or 4g line (2g for each elbow, wrist, or hand, and 4g for each knee, ankle, or foot). Use dosing card for each application.

- The dosing card containing the gel can be used to apply the gel; the hands should then be used to gently rub the gel into the skin.
- After using the dosing card, hold w/ fingertips, rinse, and dry; if treatment site is the hands, wait ≥1 hr to wash hands.
- Avoid showering or bathing for ≥1 hr after application.
- Do not apply to open wounds and avoid contact w/ eyes and mucous membranes.
- Do not apply external heat and/or occlusive dressings to treated joints.
- Avoid exposure of the treated joint(s) to natural or artificial sunlight.
- Avoid concomitant use on treated skin w/ other topical products (eg, sunscreens, cosmetics, lotions).
- Avoid wearing of clothing or gloves for at least 10 min after applying.

STORAGE
20-25°C (68-77°F). Keep from freezing. Store w/ dosing card.

HOW SUPPLIED
Gel: 1% [100g]

CONTRAINDICATIONS
Known hypersensitivity (eg, anaphylactic reactions, serious skin reactions) to diclofenac or any components of the drug product; history of asthma, urticaria, or allergic-type reactions after taking aspirin (ASA) or other NSAIDs; in the setting of CABG surgery.

WARNINGS/PRECAUTIONS
Use the lowest effective dose for the shortest duration possible. Not evaluated for use on the spine, hip, or shoulder. Increased CV thrombotic risk w/ higher doses reported. Avoid in patients w/ a recent MI unless benefits outweigh the risks of recurrent CV thrombotic events; if used, monitor for signs of cardiac ischemia. Increased risk for GI bleeding w/ longer duration of therapy, older age, poor general health status, advanced liver disease, and/or coagulopathy; avoid use in patients at higher risk unless benefits are expected to outweigh the increased risk. Consider alternate therapies other than NSAIDs for patients at higher risk and patients w/ active GI bleeding. Promptly initiate evaluation and treatment if a serious GI adverse event is suspected; d/c until a serious GI adverse event is ruled out. Hepatotoxicity reported; d/c immediately and perform a clinical evaluation if clinical signs/symptoms consistent w/ liver disease develop, if systemic manifestations occur, or if abnormal liver tests persist/worsen. May cause new onset HTN or worsen preexisting HTN. Fluid retention and edema reported. Avoid use in patients w/ severe heart failure (HF) unless benefits outweigh risks; monitor for signs of worsening HF if used. Renal papillary necrosis and other renal injury reported w/ long-term use. Renal toxicity also reported in patients in whom renal prostaglandins have a compensatory role in the maintenance of renal perfusion; increased risk w/ renal/hepatic dysfunction, dehydration, hypovolemia, and HF, and in the elderly. Correct volume status in dehydrated or hypovolemic patients prior to initiating therapy. Avoid use in patients w/ advanced renal disease unless the benefits are expected to outweigh the risk; monitor for signs of worsening renal function if used in patients w/ advanced renal disease. Hyperkalemia reported. Associated w/ anaphylactic reactions. Monitor for changes in the signs/symptoms of asthma in patients w/ preexisting asthma (w/o known ASA sensitivity). May cause serious skin reactions (eg, exfoliative dermatitis, Stevens-Johnson syndrome, toxic epidermal necrolysis); d/c at 1st appearance of skin rash/hypersensitivity. Anemia reported. May increase the risk of bleeding events; coagulation disorders may increase this risk. Monitor for signs of bleeding. May mask inflammation and fever. Minimize or avoid exposure to natural or artificial sunlight. Avoid contact w/ eyes and mucosa.

ADVERSE REACTIONS
Application-site reactions.

DRUG INTERACTIONS
Drugs that interfere w/ serotonin reuptake may potentiate the risk of bleeding. Synergistic effect on bleeding w/ anticoagulants (eg, warfarin); monitor for signs of bleeding w/ concomitant anticoagulants, antiplatelet agents, SSRIs, and SNRIs. May increase risk of GI bleeding w/ use of oral corticosteroids, anticoagulants, and SSRIs; smoking; and alcohol use. ASA may increase risk of bleeding and serious GI events; concomitant use w/ analgesic doses of ASA is not recommended. Monitor patients more closely for GI bleeding w/ concomitant use of low-dose ASA for cardiac prophylaxis. May diminish antihypertensive effect of ACE inhibitors, ARBs, and β-blockers (eg, propranolol); monitor BP. Coadministration w/ ACE inhibitors or ARBs may result in deterioration of renal function (including possible acute renal failure) in patients who are elderly or volume-depleted (including those on diuretic therapy), or have renal impairment; monitor for worsening renal function and adequately hydrate patient when these drugs are administered concomitantly. May reduce the natriuretic effect of loop diuretics (eg, furosemide) and thiazide diuretics; observe for signs of worsening renal function, in addition to assuring diuretic efficacy including antihypertensive effects. May increase digoxin serum concentrations and prolong the $T_{1/2}$ of digoxin; monitor digoxin levels. May elevate plasma lithium levels and reduce renal lithium clearance; monitor for signs of lithium toxicity. May increase the risk for methotrexate (MTX) toxicity; monitor for MTX toxicity. May increase cyclosporine's nephrotoxicity; monitor for signs of worsening renal function. Concomitant use w/ other NSAIDs or salicylates (eg, diflunisal, salsalate) increases the risk of GI toxicity; not recommended w/ other NSAIDs or salicylates. Avoid w/ oral NSAIDs unless benefit outweighs risk. Concomitant use w/ pemetrexed may increase the risk of pemetrexed-associated myelosuppression, renal, and GI toxicity; refer to prescribing information for further information.

PREGNANCY AND LACTATION
Pregnancy: Category C, prior to 30 weeks' gestation; Category D, starting at 30 weeks' gestation. Use during the 3rd trimester of pregnancy increases the risk of premature closure of the fetal ductus arteriosus; avoid use in pregnant women starting at 30 weeks of gestation (3rd trimester).
Lactation: Maybe be present in human milk; caution in nursing.

Reproductive Potential: May delay or prevent rupture of ovarian follicles, which has been associated w/ reversible infertility in some women. Small studies in women treated w/ NSAIDs have also shown a reversible delay in ovulation. Consider withdrawal of therapy in women who have difficulties conceiving or who are undergoing investigation of infertility.

MECHANISM OF ACTION
NSAID; mechanism not completely understood but involves inhibition of COX-1 and COX-2. Has analgesic, anti-inflammatory, and antipyretic properties. Mode of action may be due to a decrease of prostaglandins in peripheral tissues.

PHARMACOKINETICS
Absorption: (4g) C_{max}=15ng/mL; T_{max}=14 hrs; AUC_{0-24}=233ng•hr/mL. (12g) C_{max}=53.8ng/mL; T_{max}=10 hrs; AUC_{0-24}=807ng•hr/mL.

PATIENT CONSIDERATIONS
Assessment: Assess for history of hypersensitivity to diclofenac or to any component of this product; history of asthma, urticaria, or other allergic-type reactions w/ ASA or other NSAIDs; asthma; CV disease (CVD) or risk factors for CVD; HTN; history of peptic ulcer disease or GI bleeding; coagulation disorders; renal/hepatic impairment; pregnancy/nursing status; or any other conditions where treatment is contraindicated or cautioned. Assess volume status. Assess for possible drug interactions. Obtain baseline LFTs, BP, CBC, and chemistry profile.

Monitoring: Monitor for signs/symptoms of CV thrombotic events; cardiac ischemia in patients w/ a recent MI; GI bleeding/ulceration and perforation; hepatotoxicity; new or worsening HTN; HF; edema; renal papillary necrosis and other renal injury; hyperkalemia; anaphylactic reactions; serious skin reactions; anemia; and other adverse reactions. Monitor BP during initiation of therapy and throughout the course of therapy. Monitor for signs of bleeding in patients on concomitant therapy w/ anticoagulants, antiplatelet agents, SSRIs, or SNRIs. Monitor renal function in patients w/ renal/hepatic impairment, HF, dehydration, or hypovolemia. Monitor LFTs, CBC, and chemistry profiles periodically during long-term treatment.

Counseling: Instruct on proper use. Inform of potential for CV thrombotic events, GI adverse events, hepatotoxicity, and worsening CHF/edema, and advise of symptoms; instruct to report symptoms to healthcare provider if any occur. Instruct to seek immediate emergency help if signs of an anaphylactic reaction occur. Advise to d/c immediately if rash develops and to contact healthcare provider as soon as possible. Advise females of reproductive potential who desire pregnancy that therapy may be associated w/ a reversible delay in ovulation. Instruct pregnant women to avoid use starting at 30 weeks of gestation. Instruct patient not to use other NSAIDs or salicylates concomitantly; notify of the presence of NSAIDs in OTC medications for colds, fever, or insomnia. Inform patient not to use low-dose ASA concomitantly w/o talking to healthcare provider. Instruct to avoid contact w/ the eyes and mucosa; explain that if contact occurs, to immediately wash eye w/ water or saline and consult physician if irritation persists for >1 hr. Instruct not to apply drug to open skin wounds, infections, inflammations, or exfoliative dermatitis, as it may affect absorption and reduce tolerability of the drug. Instruct to avoid concomitant use w/ other topical products. Instruct to minimize or avoid exposure of treated areas to natural or artificial sunlight.

VOLTAREN-XR — diclofenac sodium   Rx
Class: NSAID

> NSAIDs cause an increased risk of serious cardiovascular (CV) thrombotic events, MI, and stroke, which can be fatal; risk may occur early in treatment and may increase w/ duration of use. Contraindicated in the setting of CABG surgery. May cause an increased risk of serious GI adverse events (eg, bleeding, ulceration, stomach/intestinal perforation), which can be fatal and may occur at any time during use w/o warning symptoms; elderly patients and patients w/ a prior history of peptic ulcer disease and/or GI bleeding are at greater risk.

ADULT DOSAGE	PEDIATRIC DOSAGE
Osteoarthritis 100mg qd **Rheumatoid Arthritis** 100mg qd; may increase to 100mg bid if 100mg/day is unsatisfactory	Pediatric use may not have been established

DOSING CONSIDERATIONS
Elderly
Start at lower end of dosing range if anticipated benefit outweighs potential risks

Other Important Considerations
Different formulations of diclofenac (Voltaren, Voltaren-XR, Cataflam) are not necessarily bioequivalent even if the mg strength is the same

ADMINISTRATION
Oral route

STORAGE
20-25°C (68-77°F); excursions permitted between 15-30°C (59-86°F). Protect from moisture.

HOW SUPPLIED
Tab, Extended-Release: 100mg

CONTRAINDICATIONS
Known hypersensitivity (eg, anaphylactic reactions, serious skin reactions) to diclofenac or any components of the drug product. History of asthma, urticaria, or allergic-type reactions after taking aspirin (ASA) or other NSAIDs. In the setting of CABG surgery.

WARNINGS/PRECAUTIONS

Use the lowest effective dose for the shortest duration possible. Increased CV thrombotic risk w/ higher doses reported. Avoid in patients w/ a recent MI unless benefits outweigh the risks of recurrent CV thrombotic events; if used, monitor for signs of cardiac ischemia. Increased risk for GI bleeding w/ longer duration of therapy, older age, poor general health status, and advanced liver disease and/or coagulopathy; avoid use in patients at higher risk unless benefits are expected to outweigh the increased risk, and consider alternate therapies. Promptly initiate evaluation and treatment if a serious GI adverse event is suspected; d/c until a serious GI adverse event is ruled out. Hepatotoxicity reported; d/c immediately and perform a clinical evaluation if clinical signs/symptoms consistent w/ liver disease develop, if systemic manifestations occur, or if abnormal liver tests persist/worsen. May cause new onset HTN or worsen preexisting HTN; monitor BP during initiation and throughout course of therapy. Fluid retention and edema reported. Avoid use in patients w/ severe heart failure (HF) unless benefits outweigh risks; monitor for signs of worsening HF if used. Renal papillary necrosis and other renal injury reported w/ long-term use. Renal toxicity also reported in patients in whom renal prostaglandins have a compensatory role in the maintenance of renal perfusion; increased risk w/ renal/hepatic dysfunction, dehydration, hypovolemia, and HF, and in the elderly. Correct volume status in dehydrated or hypovolemic patients prior to initiating therapy. Avoid use in patients w/ advanced renal disease unless the benefits are expected to outweigh the risk; monitor for signs of worsening renal function if used in patients w/ advanced renal disease. Hyperkalemia reported. Associated w/ anaphylactic reactions in patients w/ and w/o known hypersensitivity to diclofenac and in patients w/ ASA-sensitive asthma. Monitor for changes in the signs/symptoms of asthma in patients w/ preexisting asthma (w/o known ASA sensitivity). May cause serious skin reactions (eg, exfoliative dermatitis, Stevens-Johnson syndrome, toxic epidermal necrolysis); d/c at 1st appearance of skin rash/hypersensitivity. Anemia reported. May increase the risk of bleeding events; coagulation disorders may increase this risk. Monitor for signs of bleeding. May mask inflammation and fever.

ADVERSE REACTIONS

Abnormal renal function, anemia, dizziness, edema, elevated liver enzymes, headaches, increased bleeding time, pruritus, rashes, and tinnitus.

DRUG INTERACTIONS

Drugs that interfere w/ serotonin reuptake may potentiate the risk of bleeding. Synergistic effect on bleeding w/ anticoagulants (eg, warfarin); monitor for signs of bleeding w/ concomitant anticoagulants, antiplatelet agents (eg, ASA), SSRIs, and SNRIs. May increase risk of GI bleeding w/ use of oral corticosteroids, anticoagulants, SSRIs, smoking, and alcohol use. ASA may increase risk of bleeding and serious GI events; concomitant use w/ analgesic doses of ASA is not recommended. Monitor patients more closely for GI bleeding w/ concomitant use of low-dose ASA for cardiac prophylaxis. May diminish antihypertensive effect of ACE inhibitors, ARBs, and β-blockers (eg, propranolol); monitor BP. Coadministration w/ ACE inhibitors or ARBs may result in deterioration of renal function (including possible acute renal failure) in patients who are elderly or volume-depleted (including those on diuretic therapy), or who have renal impairment; monitor for worsening renal function and adequately hydrate patient when these drugs are administered concomitantly. May reduce the natriuretic effect of loop diuretics (eg, furosemide) and thiazide diuretics; observe for signs of worsening renal function, in addition to assuring diuretic efficacy including antihypertensive effects. May increase digoxin serum concentrations and prolong the $T_{1/2}$ of digoxin; monitor digoxin levels. May elevate plasma lithium levels and reduce renal lithium clearance; monitor for signs of lithium toxicity. May increase the risk for methotrexate (MTX) toxicity; monitor for MTX toxicity. May increase cyclosporine's nephrotoxicity; monitor for signs of worsening renal function. Concomitant use w/ other NSAIDs or salicylates (eg, diflunisal, salsalate) increases the risk of GI toxicity; not recommended w/ other NSAIDs or salicylates. Concomitant use w/ pemetrexed may increase the risk of pemetrexed-associated myelosuppression, renal, and GI toxicity; refer to prescribing information for further information. CYP2C9 inhibitors (eg, voriconazole) may enhance exposure and toxicity. CYP2C9 inducers (eg, rifampin) may lead to compromised efficacy. Dose adjustment may be warranted if administered w/ CYP2C9 inhibitors or inducers.

PREGNANCY AND LACTATION

Pregnancy: Use during the 3rd trimester of pregnancy increases the risk of premature closure of the fetal ductus arteriosus. Avoid use starting at 30 weeks of gestation (3rd trimester).
Lactation: May be present in human milk; caution in nursing.

MECHANISM OF ACTION

NSAID; mechanism not completely understood but involves inhibition of COX-1 and COX-2. Has analgesic, anti-inflammatory, and antipyretic properties. Mode of action may be due to a decrease of prostaglandins in peripheral tissues.

PHARMACOKINETICS

Absorption: Absolute bioavailability (55%); T_{max}=5.3 hrs. **Distribution:** V_d=1.4L/kg; plasma protein binding (>99%). **Metabolism:** Liver (glucuronidation and sulfation). **Elimination:** Urine (65%), bile (35%); $T_{1/2}$=2.3 hrs.

PATIENT CONSIDERATIONS

Assessment: Assess for history of hypersensitivity, history of asthma, urticaria, other allergic-type reactions w/ ASA or other NSAIDs; asthma; CV disease (CVD) or risk factors for CVD; HTN; history of peptic ulcer disease or GI bleeding; coagulation disorders; renal/hepatic impairment; pregnancy/nursing status; or any other conditions where treatment is contraindicated or cautioned. Assess volume status. Assess for possible drug interactions. Obtain baseline LFTs, BP, CBC, and chemistry profile.

Monitoring: Monitor for signs/symptoms of CV thrombotic events; cardiac ischemia in patients w/ a recent MI; GI bleeding/ulceration and perforation;

hepatotoxicity; new or worsening HTN; HF; edema; renal papillary necrosis and other renal injury; hyperkalemia; anaphylactic reactions; serious skin reactions; anemia; and other adverse reactions. Monitor BP during initiation of therapy and throughout the course of therapy. Monitor for signs of bleeding in patients on concomitant therapy w/ anticoagulants, antiplatelet agents, SSRIs, or SNRIs. Monitor renal function in patients w/ renal/hepatic impairment, HF, dehydration, or hypovolemia. Monitor LFTs, CBC and chemistry profiles periodically during long-term treatment.

Counseling: Advise patients to be alert for the symptoms of CV thrombotic events, ulcerations and bleeding, and CHF; advise to report any of these symptoms to healthcare provider immediately. Inform of the warning signs/symptoms of hepatotoxicity and anaphylactic reactions; instruct to stop treatment and seek immediate medical therapy if they occur. Advise to immediately stop treatment if rash develops and to contact healthcare provider as soon as possible. Advise females of reproductive potential who desire pregnancy that NSAIDs may be associated w/ a reversible delay in ovulation. Inform pregnant women to avoid use starting at 30 weeks of gestation. Instruct not to use other NSAIDs or salicylates concomitantly; notify of the presence of NSAIDs in OTC medications for colds, fever, or insomnia. Inform not to use low-dose ASA concomitantly w/o talking to healthcare provider.

VoSpire ER — albuterol sulfate   Rx

Class: Short-acting beta₂ agonist (SABA)

ADULT DOSAGE	PEDIATRIC DOSAGE
Bronchospasm	**Bronchospasm**
Associated w/ Reversible Obstructive Airway Disease:	**Associated w/ Reversible Obstructive Airway Disease:**
Usual: 8mg q12h; 4mg q12h may be sufficient in some patients (eg, adults of low body weight)	**6-12 Years:**
Titrate: May cautiously increase dose, if control is not achieved	**Usual:** 4mg q12h
Max: 32mg/day in divided doses (eg, q12h)	**Titrate:** May cautiously increase dose, if control is not achieved
	Max: 24mg/day in divided doses (eg, q12h)
Conversions	**>12 Years:**
Switching from Oral Albuterol Products:	**Usual:** 8mg q12h; 4mg q12h may be sufficient in some patients
Patients currently maintained on albuterol tabs/syr may be switched to albuterol extended-release (ER) tabs. Eg, the administration of one 4mg albuterol ER tab q12h is comparable to one 2mg albuterol tab q6h. Multiples of this regimen up to the max recommended daily dose also apply	**Titrate:** May cautiously increase dose, if control is not achieved
	Max: 32mg/day in divided doses (eg, q12h)
	Conversions
	Switching from Oral Albuterol Products:
	Patients currently maintained on albuterol tabs/syr may be switched to albuterol extended-release (ER) tabs. Eg, the administration of one 4mg albuterol ER tab q12h is comparable to one 2mg albuterol tab q6h. Multiples of this regimen up to the max recommended daily dose also apply

---

ADMINISTRATION
Oral route

Swallow whole w/ liquids; do not chew or crush tabs

STORAGE
20-25°C (68-77°F).

HOW SUPPLIED
Tab, Extended-Release: 4mg, 8mg

CONTRAINDICATIONS
History of hypersensitivity to albuterol or any of its components.

WARNINGS/PRECAUTIONS
Immediate hypersensitivity reactions and ECG changes may occur. D/C if paradoxical bronchospasm or cardiovascular (CV) effects occur. Caution with CV disorders (eg, coronary insufficiency, arrhythmias, HTN), convulsive disorders, hyperthyroidism, or diabetes mellitus (DM), and in patients unusually responsive to sympathomimetic amines. Reevaluate patient and treatment regimen if deterioration of asthma is observed. Consider adding anti-inflammatory agents (eg, corticosteroids) to adequately control asthma. Aggravation of preexisting DM and ketoacidosis reported with large doses of IV albuterol. May produce significant hypokalemia. Erythema multiforme and Stevens-Johnson syndrome reported with oral administration in children. Increases in selected serum chemistry values (eg, AST/ALT, serum glucose) and decreases in selected hematologic values (eg, WBC, hgb/hct) may occur in adults.

ADVERSE REACTIONS
Tremor, headache, nervousness, tachycardia, palpitations.

DRUG INTERACTIONS
Not recommended with other oral sympathomimetic agents; consider alternative therapy if regular coadministration with an aerosol bronchodilator of the adrenergic stimulant type is required. Use extreme caution with MAOIs, TCAs, or within 2 weeks of discontinuation of such agents; action of albuterol may be potentiated. Use with β-blockers may block pulmonary effects and produce

severe bronchospasm in asthmatic patients; avoid concomitant use. If needed, consider cardioselective β-blockers and use with caution. ECG changes and/or hypokalemia caused by non-K+-sparing diuretics (eg, loop or thiazide diuretics) may be worsened; use with caution. May decrease digoxin levels; monitor serum digoxin levels.

PREGNANCY AND LACTATION
Category C, not for use in nursing.

MECHANISM OF ACTION
β2-agonist; stimulates intracellular adenyl cyclase, which catalyzes conversion of adenosine triphosphate to cyclic-3',5'-adenosine monophosphate (cAMP). Increased cAMP levels are associated with relaxation of bronchial smooth muscle and inhibition of release of mediators of immediate hypersensitivity from cells, especially from mast cells.

PHARMACOKINETICS
Absorption: C_{max}=13.7ng/mL; T_{max}=6 hrs; AUC=134ng•hr/mL. **Elimination:** $T_{1/2}$=9.3 hrs.

PATIENT CONSIDERATIONS
Assessment: Assess for history of hypersensitivity to the drug, CV disorders, convulsive disorders, hyperthyroidism, DM, pregnancy/nursing status, and possible drug interactions. Assess use in patients unusually responsive to sympathomimetic amines.

Monitoring: Monitor for signs/symptoms of CV effects, ECG changes, deterioration of asthma, paradoxical bronchospasm, hypokalemia, immediate hypersensitivity reactions, and other adverse reactions.

Counseling: Instruct not to increase dose/frequency without consulting physician. Advise to seek immediate medical attention if treatment becomes less effective for symptomatic relief, symptoms become worse, and/or there is a need to use the product more frequently than usual. Instruct to take concurrent inhaled drugs and asthma medications only as directed by physician. Inform of the common adverse effects (eg, palpitations, chest pain, rapid HR, tremor, nervousness). Instruct to contact physician if pregnant/nursing.

VOTRIENT — pazopanib   Rx
Class: Kinase inhibitor

> Severe and fatal hepatotoxicity reported; monitor hepatic function and interrupt, reduce, or d/c dosing as recommended.

ADULT DOSAGE
Advanced Renal Cell Carcinoma
Initial: 800mg qd w/o food (≥1 hr ac or 2 hrs pc)
Max: 800mg

Initial Dose Reduction: 400mg
Additional Dose Decrease/Increase: Should be in 200mg steps
Advanced Soft Tissue Sarcoma
Patients Who Have Received Prior Chemotherapy:
Initial: 800mg qd w/o food (≥1 hr ac or 2 hrs pc)
Max: 800mg

Dose Decrease/Increase: Should be in 200mg steps
Missed Dose
If a dose is missed, it should not be taken if it is <12 hrs until the next dose

PEDIATRIC DOSAGE
Pediatric use may not have been established

DOSING CONSIDERATIONS
Concomitant Medications
Strong CYP3A4 Inhibitors: Avoid concomitant use; consider an alternate concomitant medication w/ no or minimal potential to inhibit CYP3A4. If coadministration is warranted, reduce pazopanib dose to 400mg; further dose reductions may be needed if adverse effects occur during therapy.
Strong CYP3A4 Inducers: Avoid concomitant use; consider an alternate concomitant medication w/ no or minimal enzyme induction potential. Do not use pazopanib if chronic use of strong CYP3A4 inducers cannot be avoided.
Hepatic Impairment
Mild: No dose adjustment is required.
Moderate: Consider alternative therapy or reduce dose to 200mg/day
Severe: Not recommended for use
ADMINISTRATION
Oral route

Do not crush tabs.
Take w/o food (≥1 hr ac or 2 hrs pc).
STORAGE
20-25°C (68-77°F); excursions permitted to 15-30°C (59-86°F).
HOW SUPPLIED
Tab: 200mg
WARNINGS/PRECAUTIONS
Patients >65 yrs of age are at greater risk for hepatotoxicity. QT prolongation and torsades de pointes reported. Cardiac dysfunction (eg, decreased left ventricular ejection fraction [LVEF], CHF) reported. Hemorrhagic events reported; avoid w/ history of hemoptysis, cerebral hemorrhage, or clinically significant GI hemorrhage in the past 6 months. Arterial thromboembolic events (ATEs) reported; caution in patients at increased risk for these events or who have had a history of these events and avoid use if an ATE has occurred w/in the past 6 months. Venous thromboembolic events (VTEs) (eg, pulmonary embolism [PE]) and GI perforation/fistula reported. Thrombotic microangiopathy (TMA), including thrombotic thrombocytopenic purpura (TTP) and hemolytic uremic syndrome (HUS), reported; permanently d/c in patients developing TMA. Interstitial lung disease (ILD)/pneumonitis reported and can be fatal; d/c therapy if ILD or pneumonitis occurs. Reversible posterior leukoencephalopathy syndrome (RPLS) reported; permanently d/c in patients developing RPLS. HTN and hypertensive crisis reported; d/c if evidence of hypertensive crisis or if HTN is severe and persistent despite antihypertensive therapy and dose reduction. May impair wound healing; d/c therapy w/ wound dehiscence and ≥7 days prior to scheduled surgery. Hypothyroidism reported. Proteinuria reported; interrupt therapy and reduce dose for 24-hr urine protein ≥3g; d/c for repeat episodes despite dose reductions. Serious infections reported; institute appropriate anti-infective therapy promptly and consider interruption or discontinuation if serious infections develop. May cause serious adverse effects on organ development in pediatric patients; not for use in pediatric patients. May cause fetal harm if used during pregnancy.

ADVERSE REACTIONS
Renal Cell Carcinoma: Diarrhea, HTN, hair color changes (depigmentation), N/V, anorexia, fatigue.
Soft Tissue Sarcoma: Fatigue, diarrhea, N/V, decreased weight/appetite, HTN, hair color changes, tumor pain, dysgeusia, headache, musculoskeletal pain, myalgia, GI pain, dyspnea, skin hypopigmentation.

DRUG INTERACTIONS
See Dosing Considerations. Concomitant use w/ proton pump inhibitors (PPIs) (eg, esomeprazole) decreased exposure; avoid concomitant use w/ drugs that raise gastric pH. If such drugs are needed, consider short-acting antacids in place of PPIs and H_2-receptor antagonists; separate antacid and pazopanib dosing by several hrs. Do not use in combination w/ other cancer therapy; increased toxicity and mortality reported w/ pemetrexed and lapatinib. Strong CYP3A4 inhibitors (eg, ketoconazole, ritonavir, clarithromycin) may increase concentrations. Avoid grapefruit or grapefruit juice. CYP3A4 inducers (eg, rifampin) may decrease plasma concentrations; consider an alternate concomitant medication w/ no or minimal enzyme induction potential. Avoid use w/ strong inhibitors of P-gp or breast cancer resistance protein (BCRP), and consider alternative concomitant medicinal products w/ no or minimal potential to inhibit P-gp or BCRP. Not recommended w/ agents w/ narrow therapeutic windows that are metabolized by CYP3A4, CYP2D6, or CYP2C8. Simvastatin may increase incidence of ALT elevations; follow pazopanib dosing guidelines or consider alternatives to pazopanib or consider discontinuing simvastatin. Caution in patients taking antiarrhythmics or other medications that may prolong the QT interval.

PREGNANCY AND LACTATION
Pregnancy: Category D.
Lactation: Not for use in nursing.
Reproductive Potential: Use effective contraception during treatment and for at least 2 weeks after last dose.

MECHANISM OF ACTION
Tyrosine kinase inhibitor; inhibits vascular endothelial growth factor receptor (VEGFR)-1, VEGFR-2, VEGFR-3, platelet-derived growth factor receptor-α and -β, fibroblast growth factor receptor-1 and -3, cytokine receptor, interleukin-2 receptor inducible T-cell kinase, leukocyte-specific protein tyrosine kinase, and transmembrane glycoprotein receptor tyrosine kinase.

PHARMACOKINETICS
Absorption: T_{max}=2-4 hrs (median); (800mg dose) AUC=1037mcg•hr/mL, C_{max}=58.1mcg/mL. **Distribution:** Plasma protein binding (>99%). **Metabolism:** CYP3A4 (major), CYP1A2/CYP2C8 (minor). **Elimination:** Feces (primary), urine (<4% administered dose); (800mg dose) $T_{1/2}$=30.9 hrs.

PATIENT CONSIDERATIONS
Assessment: Assess for history of QT interval prolongation, cardiac disease, hepatic impairment, pregnancy/nursing status, and for possible drug interactions. Assess for history of hemoptysis/cerebral hemorrhage, clinically significant GI hemorrhage, or an ATE in the past 6 months. Assess if patient is planning to undergo any surgical procedure. Assess thyroid function. Obtain baseline BP, LFTs, ECG, electrolytes, and urinalysis. Obtain baseline LVEF in patients at risk of cardiac dysfunction.

Monitoring: Monitor for signs/symptoms of hepatotoxicity, QT prolongation, torsades de pointes, cardiac dysfunction, hemorrhagic events, ATEs, VTEs, TMA, TTP, HUS, PE, RPLS, GI perforation or fistula, ILD/pneumonitis, HTN/hypertensive crisis, impaired wound healing, proteinuria, infections, and other adverse reactions. Monitor BP early after starting treatment and then frequently to ensure BP control. Perform periodic urinalysis w/ follow-up measurement of 24-hr urine protein as clinically indicated. Monitor ECG, thyroid function tests, and serum electrolytes. Monitor LFTs at Weeks 3, 5, 7, and 9, at Months 3 and 4, as clinically indicated, and periodically after Month 4. Periodically monitor LVEF in patients at risk of cardiac dysfunction.

Counseling: Advise the patient to read the FDA-approved patient labeling (Medication Guide). Advise that lab monitoring will be required prior to and while on therapy. Instruct to report any signs/symptoms of liver dysfunction, HTN, CHF, unusual bleeding, arterial thrombosis, new onset of dyspnea, chest pain, localized limb edema, GI perforation/fistula, infection, worsening of neurologic function consistent w/ RPLS, and pulmonary signs/symptoms indicative of ILD or pneumonitis. Advise to d/c treatment ≥7 days prior to a scheduled surgery.

Inform that thyroid function testing and urinalysis will be performed during treatment. Advise on how to manage diarrhea and to notify healthcare provider if moderate to severe diarrhea occurs. Advise women of childbearing potential to avoid becoming pregnant during therapy. Advise to inform healthcare provider of all concomitant medications, vitamins, or dietary and herbal supplements. Advise that depigmentation of the hair or skin may occur during treatment. Advise females of childbearing potential to use effective contraception during treatment and for at least 2 weeks after last dose.

VRAYLAR — cariprazine   Rx

Class: Atypical antipsychotic

> Elderly patients w/ dementia-related psychosis treated w/ antipsychotic drugs are at an increased risk of death: Not approved for the treatment of patients w/ dementia-related psychosis.

ADULT DOSAGE

Schizophrenia
Initial: 1.5mg qd
Titrate: Increase dose to 3mg on Day 2. Further dose adjustments can be made in 1.5mg or 3mg increments
Recommended Range: 1.5mg-6mg qd
Max: 6mg/d

Bipolar I Disorder

Acute Treatment of Manic or Mixed Episodes:
Initial: 1.5mg qd
Titrate: Increase dose to 3mg on Day 2. Further dose adjustments can be made in 1.5mg or 3mg increments
Recommended Range: 3mg-6mg qd
Max: 6mg/d

PEDIATRIC DOSAGE
Pediatric use may not have been established

DOSING CONSIDERATIONS
Concomitant Medications
Initiating a Strong CYP3A4 Inhibitor While on a Stable Dose of Cariprazine:
Reduce the current dosage of cariprazine by 1/2; reduce dose to 1.5mg or 3mg qd for patients taking 4.5mg/d. Adjust dosing regimen to qod for patients taking 1.5mg qd.
When the CYP3A4 inhibitor is withdrawn, cariprazine dosage may need to be increased.

Initiating Cariprazine While Already on a Strong CYP3A4 Inhibitor:
Administer 1.5mg cariprazine on Day 1 and on Day 3 w/ no dose administered on Day 2. From Day 4 onward, administer 1.5mg qd, then increase to a max dose of 3mg/d.
When the CYP3A4 inhibitor is withdrawn, cariprazine dosage may need to be increased.

Concomitant Use w/ CYP3A4 Inducers: Not recommended

Renal Impairment
Severe (CrCl <30mL/min): Not recommended

Hepatic Impairment
Severe (Child-Pugh Score 10-15): Not recommended

ADMINISTRATION
Oral route

May be given w/ or w/o food.

STORAGE
20-25°C (68-77°F); excursions permitted between 15-30°C (59-86°F). Protect 3mg and 4.5mg cap from light.

HOW SUPPLIED
Cap: 1.5mg, 3mg, 4.5mg, 6mg

CONTRAINDICATIONS
History of a hypersensitivity reaction to cariprazine.

WARNINGS/PRECAUTIONS
May cause neuroleptic malignant syndrome (NMS); d/c and treat immediately if this occurs. Tardive dyskinesia (TD) may develop; consider discontinuation if signs/symptoms appear. Adverse reactions (eg, extrapyramidal symptoms [EPS], akathisia) may 1st appear several weeks after initiation of therapy; monitor patient response for several weeks after initiation and after each dose increase. Consider reducing dose or discontinuing therapy. Associated w/ metabolic changes (eg, hyperglycemia, diabetes mellitus [DM], dyslipidemia, weight gain). Hyperglycemia, in some cases extreme and associated w/ ketoacidosis or hyperosmolar coma or death, reported w/ atypical antipsychotics; assess FPG before or soon after initiation of therapy and monitor periodically during long-term treatment. Leukopenia, neutropenia, and agranulocytosis reported w/ atypical antipsychotics; monitor CBC in patients w/ preexisting low WBC/ANC or history of drug-induced leukopenia/neutropenia, and consider discontinuation at 1st sign of clinically significant decline in WBC counts w/o other causative factors. D/C therapy in patients w/ absolute neutrophil count <1000/mm³ and follow their WBC until recovery. Increased risk of orthostatic hypotension and syncope during initial dose titration and when increasing dose; monitor orthostatic vital signs in patients vulnerable to hypotension, w/ known cardiovascular disease (CVD), or w/ cerebrovascular disease. May cause seizures/aspiration/esophageal dysmotility, impair mental/physical abilities, and disrupt body temperature regulation. Dysphagia reported; caution in patients at risk for aspiration.

ADVERSE REACTIONS
EPS, akathisia, dyspepsia, vomiting, somnolence, restlessness.

DRUG INTERACTIONS
See Dosing Considerations. Concomitant use of w/ strong CYP3A4 inhibitors (eg, itraconazole, ketoconazole) increases the exposures of cariprazine and its major active metabolite, didesmethyl cariprazine (DDCAR).

PREGNANCY AND LACTATION
Pregnancy: Based on animal data, therapy may cause fetal harm. Neonates exposed to antipsychotic drugs during the 3rd trimester of pregnancy are at risk for EPS and/or withdrawal symptoms following delivery; monitor neonates and manage symptoms appropriately. A pregnancy registry for atypical antipsychotics is available.
Lactation: No studies have been conducted to assess the presence of cariprazine in human milk, the effects on the breastfed infant, or the effects on milk production; caution in nursing.

MECHANISM OF ACTION
Atypical antipsychotic; mechanism not established. The efficacy of cariprazine could be mediated through a combination of partial agonist activity at central dopamine D_2 and serotonin 5-HT$_{1A}$ receptors and antagonist activity at serotonin 5-HT$_{2A}$ receptors.

PHARMACOKINETICS
Absorption: T_{max}=3-6 hrs. **Distribution:** Plasma protein binding (91-97% [cariprazine and metabolites]). **Metabolism:** Liver via CYP3A4 (extensive) and CYP2D6 (lesser extent) to desmethyl cariprazine (DCAR) and DDCAR (major active metabolites); DCAR to DDCAR via CYP3A4 and CYP2D6. **Elimination:** Urine (21%, 1.2% unchanged); $T_{1/2}$=2-4 days (cariprazine), 1-3 weeks (DDCAR).

PATIENT CONSIDERATIONS
Assessment: Assess for dementia-related psychosis, DM, risk for hypotension, history of seizures, drug hypersensitivity, or any other conditions where treatment is cautioned, hepatic/renal function, pregnancy/nursing status, and possible drug interactions. Obtain FPG.

Monitoring: Monitor for NMS, TD, EPS, akathisia, orthostatic hypotension, leukopenia, neutropenia, agranulocytosis, cognitive/motor impairment, seizures, esophageal dysmotility, aspiration, disruption of body temperature, metabolic changes, and other adverse reactions. Monitor CBC frequently during the 1st few months of therapy in patients w/ preexisting low WBC/ANC or a history of drug-induced leukopenia/neutropenia. In patients w/ clinically significant neutropenia, monitor for fever or other symptoms or signs of infection. Periodically reevaluate long-term risks and benefits of the drug.

Counseling: Counsel about risk of NMS and the signs and symptoms of TD. Advise to contact their healthcare provider if abnormal movements occur. Educate about the risk of metabolic changes, how to recognize symptoms of hyperglycemia and DM, and the need for specific monitoring (eg, blood glucose, lipids, weights). Advise patients w/ risk factors for leukopenia/neutropenia that they should have their CBC monitored while on therapy. Advise about the risk of orthostatic hypotension, especially during the period of initial dose titration. Inform that therapy has the potential to impair judgment, thinking, or motor skills; advise to use caution when operating hazardous machinery. Counsel on appropriate care in avoiding overheating and dehydration. Inform about risk for EPS and/or withdrawal symptom in neonates whose mothers were exposed to antipsychotic drugs during the 3rd trimester of pregnancy. Advise patients that there is a pregnancy exposure registry. Instruct to notify physician if pregnant/planning to become pregnant, nursing, and if taking/planning to take any prescription or OTC drugs.

VUSION — miconazole nitrate/white petrolatum/zinc oxide   Rx

Class: Antifungal agent

PEDIATRIC DOSAGE
Diaper Dermatitis

Complicated by Documented Candidiasis:
≥4 Weeks:
Apply a thin layer to diaper area with fingertips at each diaper change for 7 days. Continue treatment for full 7 days, even if there is improvement
Max Duration: 7 days

ADMINISTRATION
Topical route

Before application, gently cleanse the skin with lukewarm water and pat dry with soft towel
Avoid using any scented soaps, shampoos, or lotions on the diaper area
Do not rub into skin
Wash hands after applying

STORAGE
20-25°C (68-77°F); excursions permitted between 15-30°C (59-86°F).

HOW SUPPLIED
Oint: (Miconazole Nitrate-Zinc Oxide-White Petrolatum) 0.25%-15%-81.35% [50g]

WARNINGS/PRECAUTIONS
D/C if irritation occurs or if the disease worsens. Safety and efficacy not established in very-low-birth-weight infants, immunocompromised patients,

infants <4 weeks of age (premature or term), and in incontinent adult patients. Should not be used as a substitute for frequent diaper changes or to prevent the occurrence of diaper dermatitis (eg, in an adult institutional setting); preventative use may result in the development of drug resistance. Not for oral, ophthalmic, or intravaginal use.

ADVERSE REACTIONS
Vomiting, burning sensation, condition aggravated, administration site inflammation/pain, blister, dermatitis contact, diaper dermatitis, dry skin, erythema, pruritus, rash, skin exfoliation.

PREGNANCY AND LACTATION
Category C, safety not known in nursing.

MECHANISM OF ACTION
Miconazole: Antifungal; inhibits ergosterol biosynthesis in the cell membrane with accumulation of ergosterol precursors and toxic peroxides resulting in cytolysis of the cell. White Petrolatum/Zinc Oxide: Has not been established.

PATIENT CONSIDERATIONS
Assessment: Assess for presence of candidiasis (microscopic evidence of pseudohyphae and/or budding yeast), immunocompetence, and history of hypersensitivity.

Monitoring: Monitor for irritation or disease worsening.

Counseling: Inform that oint should be used only as prescribed. Advise not to use long term, as a substitute for frequent diaper changes, or to prevent diaper dermatitis. Instruct to use externally, as directed by the healthcare provider; not for oral, ophthalmic, or intravaginal use. Instruct to gently cleanse the diaper area with lukewarm water and pat dry with soft towel before application. Advise not to rub into the skin as this may cause additional irritation. Instruct to wash hands thoroughly after application. Instruct to see healthcare provider if symptoms have not improved by day 7.

VYTONE — hydrocortisone acetate/iodoquinol   Rx
Class: Anti-infective/corticosteroid

ADULT DOSAGE	PEDIATRIC DOSAGE
Dermatoses	**Dermatoses**
Possibly effective in contact or atopic dermatitis, impetiginized eczema, nummular eczema, endogenous chronic infectious dermatitis, stasis dermatitis, pyoderma, nuchal eczema and chronic eczematoid otitis externa, acne urticata, localized or disseminated neurodermatitis, lichen simplex chronicus, anogenital pruritus (vulvae, scroti, ani), folliculitis, bacterial dermatoses, mycotic dermatoses (eg, tinea [capitis, cruris, corporis, pedis]), moniliasis, and intertrigo	Possibly effective in contact or atopic dermatitis, impetiginized eczema, nummular eczema, endogenous chronic infectious dermatitis, stasis dermatitis, pyoderma, nuchal eczema and chronic eczematoid otitis externa, acne urticata, localized or disseminated neurodermatitis, lichen simplex chronicus, anogenital pruritus (vulvae, scroti, ani), folliculitis, bacterial dermatoses, mycotic dermatoses (eg, tinea [capitis, cruris, corporis, pedis]), moniliasis, and intertrigo
Apply to affected area(s) tid-qid or ud	**≥12 Years:** Apply to affected area(s) tid-qid or ud

---

ADMINISTRATION
Topical route

STORAGE
20-25°C (68-77°F); excursions permitted between 15-30°C (59-86°F). Brief exposure to temperatures up to 40°C (104°F) may be tolerated provided the mean kinetic temperature does not exceed 25°C (77°F); however, such exposure should be minimized. Protect from freezing and excessive heat.

HOW SUPPLIED
Cre: 2g/sachet [30^s]

CONTRAINDICATIONS
Hypersensitivity to any of the ingredients of the product.

WARNINGS/PRECAUTIONS
For external use only; avoid contact w/ eyes, lips, and mucous membranes. D/C and institute appropriate therapy if irritation develops. May stain skin, hair, or fabrics. Not for use on infants or under diapers or occlusive dressings. Hydrocortisone: Increased risk of systemic absorption if used on extensive areas or w/ occlusive dressings; take suitable precautions. Children may absorb larger amounts and thus be more susceptible to systemic toxicity. Iodoquinol: May be absorbed through the skin and interfere w/ thyroid function tests; wait at least 1 month after discontinuation to perform tests. Ferric chloride test for phenylketonuria can yield a false (+) result if drug is present in the diaper or urine. Prolonged use may result in overgrowth of nonsusceptible organisms requiring appropriate therapy.

ADVERSE REACTIONS
Burning, itching, irritation, dryness, folliculitis, hypertrichosis, acneiform eruptions, hypopigmentation, perioral dermatitis, allergic contact dermatitis, skin maceration, secondary infections, skin atrophy, striae, miliaria.

PREGNANCY AND LACTATION
Category C, caution in nursing.

MECHANISM OF ACTION
Hydrocortisone: Corticosteroid; possesses anti-inflammatory, antipruritic, and vasoconstrictive properties. Iodoquinol: Anti-infective; possesses both antifungal and antibacterial properties.

PHARMACOKINETICS
Absorption: Hydrocortisone: Extent of percutaneous absorption is determined by many factors, including the vehicle, integrity of epidermal barrier, and use of occlusive dressings. **Metabolism:** Hydrocortisone: Liver; tetrahydrocortisone and tetrahydrocortisol (metabolites). **Elimination:** Hydrocortisone: Urine (mainly as glucuronides). Iodoquinol: (Oral) Urine (3-5% as a glucuronide).

PATIENT CONSIDERATIONS
Assessment: Assess for known/suspected hypersensitivity to any ingredients of the product and pregnancy/nursing status.

Monitoring: Monitor for irritation, development of systemic toxicity in children, overgrowth of nonsusceptible organisms, and other adverse reactions. If extensive areas are treated or if occlusive dressings are used, monitor for systemic absorption of hydrocortisone.

Counseling: Instruct to use the medication ud. If irritation develops, counsel to d/c medication and contact physician. Inform that staining of the skin, hair, and fabrics may occur. Instruct caregivers of pediatric patients not to use tight-fitting diapers or plastic pants on a child being treated in the diaper area. Counsel to keep medication away from eyes, lips, and mucous membranes.

VYTORIN — ezetimibe/simvastatin   Rx
Class: Cholesterol absorption inhibitor/HMG-CoA reductase inhibitor (statin)

ADULT DOSAGE	PEDIATRIC DOSAGE
Primary Hyperlipidemia/Mixed Hyperlipidemia	Pediatric use may not have been established
Primary (Heterozygous Familial and Nonfamilial) Hyperlipidemia/Mixed Hyperlipidemia:	
Reduction of Elevated Total Cholesterol (Total-C), LDL, Apolipoprotein B, TGs, Non-HDL, and to Increase HDL:	
Initial: 10mg/10mg or 10mg/20mg qpm	
Usual: 10mg/10mg to 10mg/40mg qpm	
Titrate: After initiation or titration, analyze lipid levels after ≥2 weeks and adjust dose, if needed	
Patients Requiring Larger LDL Reduction (>55%):	
Initial: 10mg/40mg qpm	
Homozygous Familial Hypercholesterolemia	
Adjunct to Other Lipid-Lowering Treatments (eg, LDL Apheresis) or if Such Treatments are Unavailable to Reduce Elevated Total-C and LDL:	
10mg/40mg qpm	

DOSING CONSIDERATIONS
Concomitant Medications
Lomitapide:
Homozygous Familial Hypercholesterolemia:
Reduce dose by 50% if initiating lomitapide
Max: (10mg/20mg)/day (or [10mg/40mg]/day for patients who have previously taken simvastatin 80mg/day chronically [eg, for ≥12 months] w/o evidence of muscle toxicity)

Verapamil, Diltiazem, Dronedarone:
Max: 10mg/10mg qd

Amiodarone, Amlodipine, Ranolazine:
Max: 10mg/20mg qd

Bile Acid Sequestrants:
Take either ≥2 hrs before or ≥4 hrs after bile acid sequestrant

Niacin-Containing Products:
Chinese Patients Taking Lipid-Modifying Doses (≥1g/Day Niacin): Caution w/ doses >(10mg/20mg)/day; do not give 10mg/80mg dose

Renal Impairment
Chronic Kidney Disease (GFR <60mL/min/1.73m²):
Usual: 10mg/20mg qpm

Other Important Considerations
Restricted Dosing:
Use 10mg/80mg dose only in patients who have been taking 10mg/80mg dose chronically (eg, for ≥12 months) w/o evidence of muscle toxicity

If currently tolerating 10mg/80mg dose and needs to be initiated on drug that is contraindicated or is associated w/ a dose cap for simvastatin, switch to an alternative statin or statin-based regimen w/ less potential for drug-drug interaction

Do not titrate to 10mg/80mg, but place on alternative LDL lowering treatment that provides greater LDL lowering, if unable to achieve LDL goal w/ 10mg/40mg dose

ADMINISTRATION
Oral route

Take qpm w/ or w/o food.

STORAGE
20-25°C (68-77°F).

HOW SUPPLIED
Tab: (Ezetimibe/Simvastatin) 10mg/10mg, 10mg/20mg, 10mg/40mg, 10mg/80mg

CONTRAINDICATIONS
Concomitant administration of strong CYP3A4 inhibitors (eg, itraconazole, ketoconazole, posaconazole, voriconazole, HIV protease inhibitors, boceprevir, telaprevir, erythromycin, clarithromycin, telithromycin, nefazodone, cobicistat-containing products), gemfibrozil, cyclosporine, or danazol. Hypersensitivity to any component of the medication, active liver disease or unexplained persistent elevations in hepatic transaminases, women who are or may become pregnant, nursing mothers.

WARNINGS/PRECAUTIONS
Use doses >10mg/20mg w/ caution and close monitoring in patients w/ moderate to severe renal impairment. Myopathy (including immune-mediated necrotizing myopathy [IMNM]) and rhabdomyolysis reported; predisposing factors include advanced age (≥65 yrs of age), female gender, uncontrolled hypothyroidism, and renal impairment. Risk of myopathy, including rhabdomyolysis, is dose related and greater w/ simvastatin 80mg. D/C if markedly elevated CPK levels occur or myopathy is suspected/diagnosed, and temporarily withhold if experiencing an acute or serious condition predisposing to development of renal failure secondary to rhabdomyolysis. Increases in serum transaminases reported. Fatal and nonfatal hepatic failure (rare) reported; promptly interrupt therapy if serious liver injury w/ clinical symptoms and/or hyperbilirubinemia or jaundice occurs and do not restart if no alternate etiology found. Caution w/ history of liver disease, substantial alcohol consumption, and in elderly. Increases in HbA1c and FPG levels reported.

ADVERSE REACTIONS
Headache, increased ALT, myalgia, URTI, diarrhea.

DRUG INTERACTIONS
See Contraindications and Dosing Considerations. Due to the risk of myopathy/rhabdomyolysis, avoid grapefruit juice and caution w/ fenofibrates (eg, fenofibrate, fenofibric acid), lipid-modifying doses (≥1g/day) of niacin, colchicine, verapamil, diltiazem, dronedarone, lomitapide, amiodarone, amlodipine, and ranolazine. If coadministered w/ a fenofibrate, immediately d/c both agents if myopathy is suspected/diagnosed, and perform gallbladder studies/consider alternative lipid-lowering therapy if cholelithiasis is suspected. **Simvastatin:** May slightly elevate plasma digoxin concentrations; monitor patients taking digoxin when therapy is initiated. May potentiate effect of coumarin anticoagulants; determine PT before initiation and frequently during therapy. **Ezetimibe:** Reduced levels w/ cholestyramine; incremental LDL reduction may be reduced. Increased INR reported w/ warfarin.

PREGNANCY AND LACTATION
Pregnancy: Category X.
Lactation: Not for use in nursing.

MECHANISM OF ACTION
Ezetimibe: Cholesterol absorption inhibitor. Reduces blood cholesterol by inhibiting absorption of cholesterol by the small intestine. Targets the sterol transporter, Niemann-Pick C1-Like 1, which is involved in intestinal uptake of cholesterol and phytosterols. **Simvastatin:** HMG-CoA reductase inhibitor. Inhibits conversion of HMG-CoA to mevalonate, an early and rate limiting step in the biosynthetic pathway for cholesterol. Also reduces VLDL, TGs, and increases HDL.

PHARMACOKINETICS
Absorption: Simvastatin: Bioavailability (<5% as β-hydroxyacid). **Distribution:** Plasma protein binding: Ezetimibe: (>90%). Simvastatin: (95%). **Metabolism:** Ezetimibe: Small intestine, liver via glucuronide conjugation; ezetimibe-glucuronide (active metabolite). Simvastatin: Liver (extensive 1st pass), by hydrolysis via CYP3A4; β-hydroxyacid, 6'-hydroxy, 6'-hydroxymethyl, and 6'-exomethylene (major active metabolites). **Elimination:** Ezetimibe: Feces (78%, 69% ezetimibe), urine (11%, 9% ezetimibe-glucuronide); $T_{1/2}$=22 hrs. Simvastatin: Feces (60%), urine (13%).

PATIENT CONSIDERATIONS

Assessment: Assess for history of or active liver disease, unexplained persistent hepatic transaminase elevations, predisposing factors for myopathy, renal impairment, alcohol consumption, drug hypersensitivity, any other conditions where treatment is contraindicated or cautioned, pregnancy/nursing status, and possible drug interactions. Assess lipid profile and LFTs.

Monitoring: Monitor for signs/symptoms of myopathy (including IMNM), rhabdomyolysis, liver dysfunction, increases in HbA1c and FPG levels, and other adverse reactions. Monitor lipid profile, and LFTs. Check PT w/ coumarin anticoagulants.

Counseling: Inform of benefits/risks of therapy. Advise to adhere to the National Cholesterol Education Program recommended diet, a regular exercise program, and periodic testing of a fasting lipid panel. Inform about substances that should be avoided during therapy, and advise to discuss all medications, both Rx and OTC, w/ physician. Instruct to report promptly any unexplained muscle pain, tenderness, or weakness, particularly if accompanied by malaise or fever or if these muscle signs/symptoms persist after discontinuation, or any symptoms that may indicate liver injury. Inform patients using the 10mg/80mg dose that the risk of myopathy, including rhabdomyolysis, is increased. Instruct women to use an effective method of birth control to prevent pregnancy while on therapy, to d/c therapy and call physician if pregnant, and not to breastfeed while on therapy.

VYVANSE — lisdexamfetamine dimesylate   CII
Class: CNS stimulant

> CNS stimulants (amphetamines and methylphenidate-containing products) have a high potential for abuse and dependence. Assess the risk of abuse prior to prescribing and monitor for signs of abuse and dependence while on therapy.

ADULT DOSAGE	PEDIATRIC DOSAGE
Attention-Deficit Hyperactivity Disorder	**Attention-Deficit Hyperactivity Disorder**
Initial: 30mg qam	**≥6 Years:**
Titrate: May adjust in increments of 10mg or 20mg at approx weekly intervals	**Initial:** 30mg qam
Max: 70mg/day	**Titrate:** May adjust in increments of 10mg or 20mg at weekly intervals
Binge Eating Disorder	**Max:** 70mg/day
Moderate to Severe:	
Initial: 30mg qam	
Titrate: Titrate in increments of 20mg at approx weekly intervals	
Target Dose: 50-70mg/day	
Max: 70mg/day	

DOSING CONSIDERATIONS
Renal Impairment
Severe (GFR 15-<30mL/min/1.73m^2):
Max: 50mg/day
ESRD (GFR <15mL/min/1.73m^2):
Max: 30mg/day

Elderly
Start at lower end of dosing range

ADMINISTRATION
Oral route
Take in am w/ or w/o food; avoid afternoon doses.
May swallow caps whole.
Do not take anything less than 1 cap/day; do not divide a single cap.

Open Caps
1. May open caps, empty, and mix entire contents w/ yogurt, water, or orange juice; if contents of cap include any compacted powder, may use a spoon to break apart the powder.
2. Mix contents until completely dispersed.
3. Immediately consume entire mixture; do not store.
Film containing inactive ingredients may remain in glass/container once mixture is consumed.

STORAGE
20-25°C (68-77°F); excursions permitted between 15-30°C (59-86°F).

HOW SUPPLIED
Cap: 10mg, 20mg, 30mg, 40mg, 50mg, 60mg, 70mg

CONTRAINDICATIONS
Known hypersensitivity to amphetamine products or other ingredients of the medication. Concurrent use w/ an MAOI or use w/in 14 days of the last MAOI dose.

WARNINGS/PRECAUTIONS
Not indicated or recommended for weight loss. Sudden death, stroke, and MI reported in adults. Sudden death reported in children and adolescents w/ structural cardiac abnormalities and other serious heart problems. Avoid use in patients w/ known structural cardiac abnormalities, cardiomyopathy, serious heart arrhythmia, coronary artery disease, and other serious heart problems. May cause increase in BP and HR. May exacerbate symptoms of behavior disturbance and thought disorder in patients w/ a preexisting psychotic disorder. May induce a mixed/manic episode in patients w/ bipolar disorder. May cause psychotic or manic symptoms (eg, hallucinations, delusional thinking, mania) in children and adolescents w/o a prior history of psychotic illness or mania; consider discontinuation if symptoms occur. Associated w/ weight loss and slowing of growth rate in pediatric patients. Associated w/ peripheral vasculopathy, including Raynaud's phenomenon; further clinical evaluation (eg, rheumatology referral) may be appropriate for certain patients.

ADVERSE REACTIONS
Decreased appetite, insomnia, upper abdominal pain, irritability, N/V, decreased weight, dry mouth, dizziness, constipation, rash, diarrhea, anxiety, anorexia, jittery feeling, increased HR.

DRUG INTERACTIONS
See Contraindications. Urinary acidifying agents (eg, ascorbic acid) increase urinary excretion and decrease the $T_{1/2}$ of amphetamine, while urinary alkalinizing agents (eg, sodium bicarbonate) decrease urinary excretion and extend the $T_{1/2}$ of amphetamine; adjust dose accordingly.

PREGNANCY AND LACTATION
Pregnancy: Category C.
Lactation: Not for use in nursing.

MECHANISM OF ACTION
Sympathomimetic amine; CNS stimulant. Prodrug of dextroamphetamine. Blocks the reuptake of norepinephrine and dopamine into the presynaptic neuron and increases the release of these monoamines into the extraneuronal space.

PHARMACOKINETICS
Absorption: Rapid; T_{max}=1 hr (lisdexamfetamine), 3.5 hrs (dextroamphetamine). **Distribution:** Found in breast milk. **Metabolism:** Hydrolysis by RBCs; dextroamphetamine (active metabolite). **Elimination:** Urine (96%; 42% amphetamine, 25% hippuric acid, 2% unchanged), feces (0.3%); $T_{1/2}$=<1 hr.

PATIENT CONSIDERATIONS
Assessment: Assess for presence of cardiac disease, risk of abuse, risk factors for developing a manic episode, psychosis, bipolar disorder, hypersensitivity to the drug or amphetamine products, renal impairment, pregnancy/nursing status, and possible drug interactions.

Monitoring: Monitor for potential tachycardia, HTN, exacerbation of preexisting psychosis, psychotic or manic symptoms in children and adolescents, and other adverse reactions. Monitor height and weight in pediatric patients. Further evaluate patients who develop exertional chest pain, unexplained syncope, or arrhythmias. Observe carefully for signs/symptoms of peripheral vasculopathy (eg, digital changes). Monitor for signs of abuse and dependence; periodically reevaluate the need for therapy.

Counseling: Inform about drug abuse/dependence risk. Advise about serious cardiovascular risks; instruct to contact physician immediately if symptoms of cardiac disease develop. Instruct to monitor for elevations of BP and pulse rate. Inform that psychotic or manic symptoms may occur. Instruct parents or caregivers of pediatric patients that therapy may cause slowing of growth, including weight loss. Inform that therapy may impair ability to engage in potentially dangerous activities (eg, operating machinery); instruct patients to assess how the medication affects them before engaging in potentially dangerous activities. Inform about the risk of peripheral vasculopathy, including Raynaud's phenomenon; instruct to report to physician any new numbness, pain, skin color change, or sensitivity to temperature in fingers or toes, and to call physician immediately if any signs of unexplained wounds appear on fingers or toes while on therapy.

WELCHOL — colesevelam hydrochloride   Rx

Class: Bile acid sequestrant

ADULT DOSAGE
Primary Hyperlipidemia
Reduction of LDL-C in adults w/ primary hyperlipidemia (Fredrickson Type IIa) either alone or in combination w/ a statin

Tab:
Usual: 3 tabs bid or 6 tabs qd

Sus:
Usual: 3.75g qd or 1.875g bid in 4-8 oz of water, fruit juice, or diet soft drinks; stir well and drink

May be dosed at the same time as a statin or dosed apart

Type 2 Diabetes Mellitus
Tab:
Usual: 3 tabs bid or 6 tabs qd

Sus:
Usual: 3.75g qd or 1.875g bid in 4-8 oz of water, fruit juice, or diet soft drinks; stir well and drink

PEDIATRIC DOSAGE
Heterozygous Familial Hypercholesterolemia
Reduction of LDL levels in boys and postmenarchal girls as monotherapy or in combination w/ a statin after an adequate trial of diet therapy

Sus:
10-17 Years:
3.75g qd or 1.875g bid in 4-8 oz of water, fruit juice, or diet soft drinks; stir well and drink

ADMINISTRATION
Oral route
Tab
Take w/ meal and liquid.
Sus
Do not take in dry form; take w/ meals.

STORAGE
25°C (77°F); excursions permitted to 15-30°C (59-86°F). Protect from moisture. (Tab) Brief exposure to 40°C (104°F) does not adversely affect the product.

HOW SUPPLIED
Sus: 1.875g, 3.75g [pkt]; **Tab:** 625mg

CONTRAINDICATIONS
Serum TG concentrations >500mg/dL, history of hypertriglyceridemia-induced pancreatitis or bowel obstruction.

WARNINGS/PRECAUTIONS
Not for treatment of type 1 DM or diabetic ketoacidosis. Analyze lipid levels within 4-6 weeks after initiation. May increase serum TG concentrations; d/c if TG levels >500mg/dL or if hypertriglyceridemia-induced pancreatitis develops. Caution in patients with TG levels >300mg/dL or with susceptibility to deficiencies of vitamin K (eg, malabsorption syndromes, patients on warfarin) or other fat-soluble vitamins. May cause constipation; avoid with gastroparesis, GI motility disorders, those who have had major GI tract surgery, or those at risk for bowel obstruction. (Sus) Contains phenylalanine; caution with phenylketonurics. Always mix with water, fruit juice, or diet soft drinks to avoid esophageal distress; do not take in its dry form. (Tab) Caution in patients with dysphagia or swallowing disorders.

ADVERSE REACTIONS
Asthenia, constipation, dyspepsia, nausea, rhinitis, fatigue, flu syndrome, nasopharyngitis, hypoglycemia, hypertriglyceridemia, headache, influenza, pharyngitis, URTI.

DRUG INTERACTIONS
Greater increase in TG levels may occur with insulin, pioglitazone, or sulfonylureas. May decrease absorption of vitamins A, D, E, and K. May increase seizure activity or decrease phenytoin levels. May elevate TSH in patients receiving thyroid hormone replacement therapy. May increase levels of metformin extended-release. May decrease levels of cyclosporine, glimepiride, glipizide, glyburide, levothyroxine, olmesartan medoxomil, and oral contraceptives containing ethinyl estradiol and norethindrone. Administer phenytoin, cyclosporine, oral vitamin supplementation, drugs known to have reduced GI absorption when given concomitantly, or drugs that have not been tested for interaction (especially those with narrow therapeutic index) at least 4 hrs prior to colesevelam. Concomitant use with warfarin decreases INR; monitor INR.

PREGNANCY AND LACTATION
Pregnancy: Category B.
Lactation: Safety not known in nursing.

MECHANISM OF ACTION
Bile acid sequestrant; non-absorbed, lipid-lowering polymer that binds bile acids in intestine, impeding their reabsorption. Consequently, compensatory effects lead to increased LDL clearance from blood, resulting in decreased serum LDL levels. Mechanism unknown in the treatment of DM.

PHARMACOKINETICS
Absorption: Not hydrolyzed by digestive enzymes and not absorbed. **Distribution:** Limited to GI tract. **Elimination:** Urine (0.05%).

PATIENT CONSIDERATIONS
Assessment: Assess for history/risk of bowel obstruction, gastroparesis, or other GI motility disorders, history of major GI tract surgery or hypertriglyceridemia-induced pancreatitis, susceptibility to deficiencies of vitamin K or other fat-soluble vitamins, dysphagia or swallowing disorders, pregnancy/nursing status, and possible drug interactions. Obtain baseline lipid parameters (eg, TGs, non-HDL levels). Monitor INR prior to initiation in patients on warfarin therapy.

Monitoring: Monitor for hypertriglyceridemia-induced pancreatitis, hypoglycemia, dysphagia, esophageal obstruction, and other adverse events. Periodically monitor lipid profile (eg, TGs, non-HDL), blood glucose, and coadministered drug levels. Monitor INR frequently in patients on warfarin therapy.

Counseling: Instruct to take with meal and liquid. Instruct to take interacting drugs at least 4 hrs prior to colesevelam. Advise to consume diet that promotes bowel regularity. Instruct to promptly d/c and seek medical attention if severe abdominal pain/constipation or symptoms of acute pancreatitis occur. Instruct patients with primary hyperlipidemia to adhere to the recommended diet of the National Cholesterol Education Program. Instruct patients with type 2 DM to adhere to dietary instructions, regular exercise program, and regular testing of blood glucose. Advise to notify physician if dysphagia or swallowing disorders occur. (Sus) Instruct to empty entire contents of 1 pkt into a glass or cup, then add 4-8 oz of water, fruit juice, or diet-soft drinks before ingesting.

WELLBUTRIN — bupropion hydrochloride   Rx

Class: Aminoketone

> Antidepressants increased the risk of suicidal thoughts and behavior in children, adolescents, and young adults in short-term trials. Monitor closely for worsening, and for emergence of suicidal thoughts and behavior. Serious neuropsychiatric reactions reported in patients taking bupropion for smoking cessation; observe all patients for neuropsychiatric reactions. Not approved for smoking cessation.

ADULT DOSAGE
Major Depressive Disorder
Initial: 200mg/day, given as 100mg bid
Titrate: After 3 days, may increase to 300mg/day, given as 100mg tid w/ at least 6 hrs between successive doses. Increases in dose should not exceed 100mg/day in a 3-day period
Max: 450mg/day, given in divided doses of not more than 150mg each; max dose may be considered if no clinical improvement seen after several weeks of treatment at 300mg/day. Administer the 100mg tab 4X daily to not exceed the limit of 150mg in a single dose

Dosing Considerations with MAOIs

Switching to/from an MAOI Antidepressant:
Allow at least 14 days between discontinuation of an MAOI and initiation of treatment and allow at least 14 days between discontinuation of treatment and initiation of an MAOI

PEDIATRIC DOSAGE
Pediatric use may not have been established

Use w/ Reversible MAOIs (eg, Linezolid, IV Methylene Blue):
- Do not start bupropion in a patient being treated w/ linezolid or IV methylene blue.
- In patients already receiving bupropion, if acceptable alternatives are not available and benefits outweigh risks, d/c bupropion promptly and administer linezolid or IV methylene blue; monitor for 2 weeks or until 24 hrs after the last dose of linezolid or IV methylene blue, whichever comes 1st. May resume bupropion therapy 24 hrs after the last dose of linezolid or IV methylene blue.

DOSING CONSIDERATIONS

Renal Impairment
GFR <90mL/min: Consider reducing dose and/or frequency

Hepatic Impairment
Mild (Child-Pugh Score 5-6): Consider reducing dose and/or frequency
Moderate-Severe (Child-Pugh Score 7-15): Max: 75mg/day

ADMINISTRATION
Oral route

Take w/ or w/o food.
Swallow whole; do not crush, divide, or chew.

STORAGE
20-25°C (68-77°F); excursions permitted at 15-30°C (59-86°F). Protect from light and moisture.

HOW SUPPLIED
Tab: 75mg, 100mg

CONTRAINDICATIONS
Seizure disorder; current/prior diagnosis of bulimia or anorexia nervosa; patients undergoing abrupt discontinuation of alcohol, benzodiazepines, barbiturates, and antiepileptic drugs; known hypersensitivity to bupropion or other ingredients of the medication. Use of MAOIs (intended to treat psychiatric disorders) either concomitantly or w/in 14 days of discontinuing treatment. Treatment w/in 14 days of discontinuing treatment w/ an MAOI. Starting treatment in patients being treated w/ reversible MAOIs (eg, linezolid, IV methylene blue).

WARNINGS/PRECAUTIONS
Dose-related risk of seizures; increase dose gradually and do not exceed 450mg/day. D/C and do not restart treatment if a seizure occurs. Caution w/ conditions that may increase risk of seizure. May result in elevated BP and HTN. May precipitate a manic, mixed, or hypomanic manic episode; risk is increased in patients w/ bipolar disorder or who have risk factors for bipolar disorder. Screen for history of bipolar disorder and the presence of risk factors for bipolar disorder; not approved for use in treating bipolar depression. Neuropsychiatric signs and symptoms (eg, delusions, hallucinations, psychosis) reported. Pupillary dilation that occurs following use may trigger an angle-closure attack in a patient w/ anatomically narrow angles who does not have a patent iridectomy. Anaphylactoid/anaphylactic reactions reported; d/c treatment if allergic or anaphylactoid/anaphylactic reactions occur. Arthralgia, myalgia, fever w/ rash, and other serum sickness-like symptoms suggestive of delayed hypersensitivity reported. Caution in elderly. False (+) urine immunoassay screening tests for amphetamines reported.

ADVERSE REACTIONS
Agitation, dry mouth, insomnia, headache/migraine, N/V, constipation, tremor, dizziness, excessive sweating, blurred vision, tachycardia, confusion, rash, hostility, cardiac arrhythmia, auditory disturbance.

DRUG INTERACTIONS
See Contraindications. CYP2B6 inhibitors (eg, ticlopidine, clopidogrel) may increase bupropion exposure but decrease hydroxybupropion exposure; may need to adjust dose of bupropion. CYP2B6 inducers (eg, ritonavir, lopinavir, efavirenz) may decrease exposure; may need to increase bupropion dose but not to exceed max dose. Carbamazepine, phenytoin, and phenobarbital may induce metabolism and decrease exposure. If used concomitantly w/ a CYP inducer, it may be necessary to increase the dose of bupropion, but the max recommended dose should not be exceeded. May increase exposure of CYP2D6 substrates (eg, antidepressants, antipsychotics, β-blockers, type 1C antiarrhythmics [eg, propafenone, flecainide]); may need to decrease the dose of CYP2D6 substrates, particularly for drugs w/ a narrow therapeutic index. May reduce efficacy of drugs that require metabolic activation by CYP2D6 to be effective (eg, tamoxifen); may require increase doses of such drugs. Extreme caution w/ other drugs that lower seizure threshold (eg, other bupropion products, antipsychotics, antidepressants, theophylline, systemic corticosteroids); use low initial doses and increase the dose gradually. Increased risk of seizure w/ use of illicit drugs (eg, cocaine), abuse or misuse of prescription drugs (eg, CNS stimulants), use of oral hypoglycemic drugs or insulin, use of anorectic drugs, excessive use of alcohol, benzodiazepines, sedative/hypnotics, or opiates. CNS toxicity reported when coadministered w/ levodopa or amantadine; use w/ caution. Patient should minimize or avoid alcohol consumption. Increased risk of HTN w/ MAOIs or other drugs that increase dopaminergic or noradrenergic activity. Monitor for HTN w/ nicotine replacement therapy.

PREGNANCY AND LACTATION
Pregnancy: Category C.
Lactation: Found in breast milk; caution in nursing.

MECHANISM OF ACTION
Aminoketone antidepressant; has not been established. Weak inhibitor of the neuronal uptake of norepinephrine and dopamine. Presumed that action is mediated by noradrenergic and/or dopaminergic mechanisms.

PHARMACOKINETICS
Absorption: T_{max}=2 hrs, 3 hrs (hydroxybupropion). Distribution: Plasma protein binding (84%); found in breast milk. Metabolism: Extensive. Hydroxylation (CYP2B6) and reduction of carbonyl group; hydroxybupropion, threohydrobupropion, and erythrohydrobupropion (active metabolites). Elimination: Urine (87%), feces (10%), (0.5% unchanged); $T_{1/2}$=21 hrs, 20 hrs, 33 hrs, 37 hrs (bupropion, hydroxybupropion, erythrohydrobupropion, threohydrobupropion, respectively).

PATIENT CONSIDERATIONS

Assessment: Assess for bipolar disorder or risk factors for bipolar disorder, seizure disorders or conditions that may increase risk of seizure, hepatic/renal dysfunction, susceptibility to angle closure glaucoma, hypersensitivity to the drug, any other conditions where treatment is contraindicated or cautioned, pregnancy/nursing status, and possible drug interactions. Obtain baseline BP.

Monitoring: Monitor for clinical worsening, suicidality, or unusual changes in behaviors; neuropsychiatric reactions; seizures; HTN; activation of mania or hypomania; angle-closure glaucoma; anaphylactoid/anaphylactic reactions; delayed hypersensitivity; and other adverse reactions. Periodically reassess the dose and need for maint treatment.

Counseling: Inform of benefits/risks of therapy and instruct to take ud. Advise patients and caregivers of need for close observation for clinical worsening and/or suicidal risks. Educate on the symptoms of hypersensitivity and instruct to d/c if a severe allergic reaction occurs. Instruct to d/c and not restart if a seizure occurs while on therapy. Inform that excessive use or abrupt discontinuation of alcohol or sedatives may alter the seizure threshold; advise to minimize or avoid alcohol use. Inform about risk of angle-closure glaucoma. Inform that therapy may impair mental/physical abilities; advise to use caution while operating hazardous machinery/driving. Instruct to notify physician if taking/planning to take any prescription or OTC medications. Advise to contact physician if pregnant or intending to become pregnant during therapy.

WELLBUTRIN SR — bupropion hydrochloride　　　Rx
Class: Aminoketone

> Antidepressants increased the risk of suicidal thoughts and behavior in children, adolescents, and young adults in short-term trials. Monitor closely for worsening, and for emergence of suicidal thoughts and behavior. Serious neuropsychiatric reactions reported in patients taking bupropion for smoking cessation; observe all patients for neuropsychiatric reactions. Not approved for smoking cessation.

ADULT DOSAGE

Major Depressive Disorder
Initial: 150mg/day given as a single daily dose in am
Titrate: After 3 days, may increase dose to 150mg bid w/ an interval of at least 8 hrs between successive doses
Usual Target Dose: 300mg/day, given as 150mg bid
Max: May consider 400mg/day, given as 200mg bid, if no clinical improvement after several weeks of treatment at 300mg/day; do not exceed 200mg in any single dose

Dosing Considerations with MAOIs

Switching to/from an MAOI Antidepressant:
Allow at least 14 days between discontinuation of an MAOI and initiation of treatment and allow at least 14 days between discontinuation of treatment and initiation of an MAOI

Use w/ Reversible MAOIs (eg, Linezolid, IV Methylene Blue):
Do not start bupropion in a patient being treated w/ a reversible MAOI. If acceptable alternatives to linezolid or IV methylene blue treatment are not available and potential benefits of linezolid or IV methylene blue treatment are judged to outweigh risks of hypertensive reactions, bupropion should be stopped promptly, and linezolid or IV methylene blue can be administered. Monitor for 2 weeks or until 24 hrs after the last dose of linezolid or IV methylene blue, whichever comes 1st. May resume bupropion treatment 24 hrs after the last dose of linezolid or IV methylene blue.

PEDIATRIC DOSAGE
Pediatric use may not have been established

DOSING CONSIDERATIONS
Renal Impairment
GFR<90mL/min: Consider a reduced dose and/or dosing frequency
Hepatic Impairment
Mild (Child-Pugh Score 5-6): Consider reducing the dose and/or frequency of dosing
Moderate to Severe (Child-Pugh Score 7-15): Max of 100mg/day or 150mg qod

ADMINISTRATION
Oral route

Take w/ or w/o food.
Swallow whole; do not crush, divide, or chew.

STORAGE
20-25°C (68-77°F); excursions permitted at 15-30°C (59-86°F). Protect from light and moisture.

HOW SUPPLIED
Tab, Sustained-Release: 100mg, 150mg, 200mg

CONTRAINDICATIONS
Seizure disorder; current/prior diagnosis of bulimia or anorexia nervosa; undergoing abrupt discontinuation of alcohol, benzodiazepines, barbiturates, or antiepileptic drugs; known hypersensitivity to bupropion or other ingredients of the medication. Use of MAOIs (intended to treat psychiatric disorders) either concomitantly or w/in 14 days of discontinuing treatment. Treatment w/in 14 days of discontinuing treatment w/ an MAOI. Starting treatment in patients being treated w/ reversible MAOIs (eg, linezolid, IV methylene blue).

WARNINGS/PRECAUTIONS
Dose-related risk of seizures; titrate dose gradually. D/C and do not restart treatment if a seizure occurs. May result in elevated BP and HTN. Caution w/ conditions that may increase risk of seizure. May precipitate a manic, mixed, or hypomanic manic episode; not approved for use in treating bipolar depression. Neuropsychiatric signs and symptoms (eg, delusions, hallucinations, psychosis, concentration disturbance) reported. Pupillary dilation that occurs following use may trigger an angle-closure attack in a patient w/ anatomically narrow angles who does not have a patent iridectomy. D/C treatment if allergic or anaphylactoid/anaphylactic reactions occur. Arthralgia, myalgia, fever w/ rash, and other serum sickness-like symptoms suggestive of delayed hypersensitivity reported. False (+) urine immunoassay screening tests for amphetamines reported.

ADVERSE REACTIONS
Abdominal pain, dry mouth, anorexia, insomnia, dizziness, agitation, anxiety, pharyngitis, sweating, rash, tinnitus, tremor, myalgia, nausea, palpitation.

DRUG INTERACTIONS
See Contraindications. Extreme caution w/ other drugs that lower seizure threshold (eg, other bupropion products, antipsychotics, antidepressants, theophylline, systemic corticosteroids); use low initial doses and increase the dose gradually. Increased risk of seizure w/ use of illicit drugs (eg, cocaine), abuse or misuse of prescription drugs (eg, CNS stimulants), use of oral hypoglycemic drugs or insulin, use of anorectic drugs, and excessive use of alcohol, benzodiazepines, sedative/hypnotics, or opiates. Ritonavir, lopinavir, or efavirenz may decrease exposure; may need to increase bupropion dose but not to exceed max dose. May reduce efficacy of drugs that require metabolic activation by CYP2D6 to be effective (eg, tamoxifen). CNS toxicity reported when coadministered w/ levodopa or amantadine; use w/ caution. Patient should minimize or avoid alcohol consumption. Monitor BP w/ nicotine replacement therapy. Potential for drug interactions w/ CYP2B6 inducers. Increased risk of HTN w/ MAOIs or other drugs that increase dopaminergic or noradrenergic activity. May increase exposure of CYP2D6 substrates (eg, venlafaxine, nortriptyline, haloperidol, metoprolol, propafenone); may need to decrease the dose of CYP2D6 substrates, particularly for drugs w/ a narrow therapeutic index. CYP2B6 inhibitors (eg, ticlopidine, clopidogrel) may increase bupropion exposure but decrease hydroxybupropion exposure; may need to adjust bupropion dose. Carbamazepine, phenytoin, and phenobarbital may induce metabolism and decrease exposure. If used concomitantly w/ a CYP inducer, may need to increase the dose of bupropion, but not to exceed the max dose.

PREGNANCY AND LACTATION
Pregnancy: Category C.
Lactation: Found in breast milk; caution in nursing.

MECHANISM OF ACTION
Aminoketone antidepressant; has not been established. Weak inhibitor of the neuronal reuptake of norepinephrine and dopamine. Presumed that action is mediated by noradrenergic and/or dopaminergic mechanisms.

PHARMACOKINETICS
Absorption: T_{max}=3 hrs, 6 hrs (hydroxybupropion). **Distribution:** Plasma protein binding (84%); found in breast milk. **Metabolism:** Extensive. Hydroxylation (CYP2B6), reduction of carbonyl group; hydroxybupropion, threohydrobupropion, and erythrohydrobupropion (active metabolites). **Elimination:** Urine (87%), feces (10%), (0.5% unchanged); $T_{1/2}$=21 hrs, 20 hrs, 33 hrs, 37 hrs (bupropion, hydroxybupropion, erythrohydrobupropion, threohydrobupropion, respectively).

PATIENT CONSIDERATIONS
Assessment: Assess for history of bipolar disorder or presence of risk factors for bipolar disorder, hepatic/renal dysfunction, seizure disorders or conditions that may increase risk of seizure, susceptibility to angle-closure glaucoma, hypersensitivity to the drug, and any other conditions where treatment is contraindicated or cautioned, pregnancy/nursing status, and for possible drug interactions. Assess BP.

Monitoring: Monitor for clinical worsening, suicidality, unusual changes in behavior, neuropsychiatric symptoms, seizures, activation of mania or hypomania,

psychosis and other neuropsychiatric reactions, angle-closure glaucoma, anaphylactoid/anaphylactic reactions, delayed hypersensitivity, and other adverse reactions. Monitor hepatic/renal function. Monitor BP periodically. Periodically reassess the appropriate dose and the need for maint treatment.

Counseling: Inform of benefits/risks of therapy. Advise patients and caregivers of need for close observation for clinical worsening and/or suicidal risks. Educate on the symptoms of hypersensitivity and instruct to d/c if a severe allergic reaction occurs. Instruct to d/c and not restart if a seizure occurs while on therapy. Inform that therapy may impair mental/physical abilities; advise to use caution while operating hazardous machinery/driving. Inform that excessive use or abrupt discontinuation of alcohol or sedatives may alter the seizure threshold; advise to minimize or avoid alcohol use. Instruct to notify physician if taking/ planning to take any prescription or OTC medications. Advise not to use therapy in combination w/ other medicines containing bupropion hydrochloride. Advise to contact physician if pregnancy occurs or is intended during therapy. Caution about the risk of angle-closure glaucoma in susceptible patients.

WELLBUTRIN XL — bupropion hydrochloride   Rx
Class: Aminoketone

> Antidepressants increased the risk of suicidal thoughts and behavior in children, adolescents, and young adults in short-term trials. Monitor closely for worsening, and for emergence of suicidal thoughts and behaviors. Advise families and caregivers of the need for close observation and communication with the prescriber. Serious neuropsychiatric reactions reported in patients taking bupropion for smoking cessation; not approved for smoking cessation. Observe all patients for neuropsychiatric reactions.

ADULT DOSAGE	PEDIATRIC DOSAGE
Major Depressive Disorder	Pediatric use may not have been established
Initial: 150mg qd in the am	
Titrate: May increase to 300mg qd on Day 4	
Maint: Reassess periodically to determine need for maint treatment and the appropriate dose	
Seasonal Affective Disorder	
Initial: 150mg qd in the am	
Titrate: May increase to 300mg qd after 7 days	
Max: 300mg	
Prevention of Seasonal Major Depressive Disorder Episodes Associated w/ Seasonal Affective Disorder:	
Initiate in the autumn, prior to the onset of depressive symptoms. Continue through the winter season; taper and d/c in early spring	
Treated w/ 300mg/day: Decrease to 150mg qd before discontinuing	
Individualize timing of initiation and duration of treatment	
Conversions	
Switching from Wellbutrin Tab/ Wellbutrin SR Tab:	
Give same total daily dose when possible	
Dosing Considerations with MAOIs	
Switching to/from an MAOI Antidepressant:	
Allow at least 14 days between discontinuation of an MAOI and initiation of treatment, and allow at least 14 days between discontinuation of treatment and initiation of an MAOI	
W/ Other MAOIs (eg, Linezolid, IV Methylene Blue):	
Do not start bupropion in a patient being treated w/ linezolid or IV methylene blue. In patients already receiving bupropion, if acceptable alternatives are not available and benefits outweigh risks, d/c bupropion and administer linezolid or IV methylene blue; monitor for 2 weeks or until 24 hrs after the last dose of linezolid or IV methylene blue, whichever comes 1st. May resume bupropion therapy 24 hrs after the last dose of linezolid or IV methylene blue.	

DOSING CONSIDERATIONS
Renal Impairment
GFR <90mL/min: Consider reducing dose and/or frequency

Hepatic Impairment
Mild (Child-Pugh Score 5-6): Consider reducing dose and/or frequency
Moderate to Severe (Child-Pugh Score 7-15) Max Dose: 150mg qod

Discontinuation
Treated w/ 300mg qd: Decrease to 150mg qd prior to discontinuation

ADMINISTRATION
Oral route

Administer in the am, w/ or w/o food.
Swallow whole; do not crush, divide, or chew.

STORAGE
25°C (77°F); excursions permitted to 15-30°C (59-86°F).

HOW SUPPLIED
Tab, ER: 150mg, 300mg

CONTRAINDICATIONS
Seizure disorder; current/prior diagnosis of bulimia or anorexia nervosa; undergoing abrupt discontinuation of alcohol, benzodiazepines, barbiturates, and antiepileptic drugs; known hypersensitivity to bupropion or other ingredients of the medication. Use of MAOIs (intended to treat psychiatric disorders) either concomitantly or w/in 14 days of discontinuing treatment. Treatment w/in 14 days of discontinuing treatment w/ an MAOI. Starting treatment in patients being treated w/ reversible MAOIs (eg, linezolid, IV methylene blue).

WARNINGS/PRECAUTIONS
Dose-related risk of seizures; increase dose gradually, and do not exceed 300mg qd. D/C and do not restart treatment if a seizure occurs. Caution with conditions that may increase risk of seizure. May result in elevated BP and HTN. May precipitate a manic, mixed, or hypomanic manic episode; not approved for treatment of bipolar depression. Neuropsychiatric signs and symptoms (eg, delusions, hallucinations, psychosis) reported; d/c if these reactions occur. Pupillary dilation that occurs following use may trigger an angle-closure attack in a patient with anatomically narrow angles who does not have a patent iridectomy. Anaphylactoid/anaphylactic reactions reported; d/c treatment if these reactions occur. Erythema multiforme, Stevens-Johnson syndrome, and anaphylactic shock rarely reported. Arthralgia, myalgia, fever with rash, and other symptoms of serum sickness suggestive of delayed hypersensitivity reported. Caution in elderly. False (+) urine immunoassay screening tests for amphetamines reported.

ADVERSE REACTIONS
Headache, infection, dry mouth, nausea, insomnia, dizziness, agitation, tremor, anxiety, constipation, pharyngitis, sweating, tinnitus, diarrhea, anorexia, rash.

DRUG INTERACTIONS
See Contraindications. Extreme caution with drugs that lower seizure threshold (eg, other bupropion products, antipsychotics, antidepressants, theophylline, systemic corticosteroids); use low initial doses and increase the dose gradually. Increased risk of seizure with use of illicit drugs (eg, cocaine), abuse or misuse of prescription drugs (eg, CNS stimulants), use of oral hypoglycemic drugs or insulin, use of anorectic drugs, and excessive use of alcohol, benzodiazepines, sedative/hypnotics, or opiates. Potential for drug interactions with CYP2B6 inhibitors/inducers. CYP2B6 inhibitors (eg, ticlopidine, clopidogrel) may increase bupropion exposure but decrease hydroxybupropion exposure; may need to adjust bupropion dose. Ritonavir, lopinavir, and efavirenz may decrease exposure; may need to increase bupropion dose but not to exceed max dose. Carbamazepine, phenytoin, and phenobarbital may induce metabolism and decrease exposure. If used concomitantly with a CYP inducer, may need to increase bupropion dose, but not to exceed the max dose. May increase exposure of CYP2D6 substrates (eg, antidepressants, antipsychotics, β-blockers, type 1C antiarrhythmics [eg, propafenone, flecainide]); may need to decrease the dose of CYP2D6 substrates, particularly for drugs with a narrow therapeutic index. May reduce efficacy of drugs that require metabolic activation by CYP2D6 to be effective (eg, tamoxifen); may require increased doses of such drugs. CNS toxicity reported when coadministered with levodopa or amantadine; use with caution. Minimize or avoid alcohol. Increased risk of HTN with MAOIs or other drugs that increase dopaminergic or noradrenergic activity. Monitor BP with nicotine replacement therapy.

PREGNANCY AND LACTATION
Pregnancy: Category C.
Lactation: Caution in nursing.

MECHANISM OF ACTION
Aminoketone antidepressant; has not been established. Weak inhibitor of the neuronal uptake of norepinephrine and dopamine. Presumed that action is mediated by noradrenergic and/or dopaminergic mechanisms.

PHARMACOKINETICS
Absorption: T_{max}=5 hrs (median), 7 hrs (hydroxybupropion). **Distribution:** Plasma protein binding (84%); found in breast milk. **Metabolism:** Extensive. Hydroxylation (CYP2B6), reduction of carbonyl group; hydroxybupropion, threohydrobupropion, and erythrohydrobupropion (active metabolites). **Elimination:** Urine (87%), feces (10%), (0.5% unchanged); $T_{1/2}$=21 hrs, 20 hrs (hydroxybupropion), 33 hrs (erythrohydrobupropion), 37 hrs (threohydrobupropion).

PATIENT CONSIDERATIONS
Assessment: Assess for seizure disorders or conditions that may increase risk of seizure, susceptibility to angle-closure glaucoma, renal/hepatic impairment, hypersensitivity to the drug, any other conditions where treatment is contraindicated or cautioned, pregnancy/nursing status, and possible drug interactions. Obtain baseline BP and screen for risk factors/a history of bipolar disorder.

Monitoring: Monitor for clinical worsening, suicidality, unusual changes in behavior, seizures, activation of mania or hypomania, psychosis and other neuropsychiatric reactions, angle-closure glaucoma, anaphylactoid/anaphylactic reactions, delayed hypersensitivity, and other adverse reactions. Monitor BP periodically. Monitor hepatic/renal function, especially in the elderly.

Counseling: Inform of benefits/risks of therapy and counsel in its appropriate use. Advise patients and caregivers of the need for close observation for clinical worsening and/or suicidal risk. Educate on the symptoms of hypersensitivity and advise to d/c if a severe allergic reaction occurs. Instruct to d/c and not restart if a seizure occurs while on therapy. Inform that excessive use or abrupt discontinuation of alcohol or sedatives may alter the seizure threshold; advise to minimize or avoid alcohol use. Caution about the risk of angle-closure glaucoma in susceptible patients. Advise not to use therapy in combination with other medicines containing bupropion hydrochloride. Inform that therapy may impair mental/physical abilities; advise to use caution while operating hazardous machinery/driving. Instruct to notify physician if taking/planning to take any prescription or OTC medications. Advise to contact physician if pregnancy occurs or is intended during therapy. Communicate with the patient and pediatric healthcare provider regarding the infant's exposure to bupropion through human milk; instruct caregivers to immediately contact the infant's healthcare provider if they note any side effect in the infant that concerns them or is persistent.

WP THYROID — thyroid   Rx

Class: Thyroid replacement hormone

ADULT DOSAGE	PEDIATRIC DOSAGE
Hypothyroidism	**Hypothyroidism**
Initial: 32.5mg/day; 16.25mg/day is recommended in patients with longstanding myxedema, particularly if cardiovascular impairment is suspected	**Congenital:**
	0-6 Months of Age:
	4.8-6mg/kg/day (16.25-32.5mg/day)
Titrate: Increase by 16.25mg every 2-3 weeks; readjust within first 4 weeks of therapy	**6-12 Months of Age:**
	3.6-4.8mg/kg/day (32.5-48.75mg/day)
Maint: 65-130mg/day	**1-5 Years:**
	3-3.6mg/kg/day (48.75-65mg/day)
Myxedema Coma:	**6-12 Years:**
400mcg (100mcg/mL) IV of levothyroxine sodium (T4) given rapidly, followed by daily supplements of 100-200mcg given IV. Resume oral therapy when clinical situation has been stabilized and patient is able to take oral medication.	2.4-3mg/kg/day (65-97.5mg/day)
	>12 Years:
	1.2-1.8mg/kg/day (>97.5mg/day)
Pituitary TSH Suppressant	
In the treatment or prevention of various types of euthyroid goiters, including thyroid nodules, subacute, or chronic lymphocytic thyroiditis (Hashimoto's), multinodular goiter, and in the management of thyroid cancer	
1.56mg/kg/day of levothyroxine (T4) for 7-10 days	
Thyroid Cancer:	
Larger amounts of thyroid hormone than those used for replacement therapy are required	
Diagnostic Aid	
In suppression tests to differentiate suspected mild hyperthyroidism or thyroid gland anatomy	
1.56mg/kg/day of levothyroxine (T4) for 7-10 days	

DOSING CONSIDERATIONS
Elderly
Start at lower end of dosing range

Adverse Reactions
Hypothyroidism:
Angina: Appearance is an indication for dose reduction

ADMINISTRATION
Oral route

STORAGE
15-30°C (59-86°F).

HOW SUPPLIED
Tab: 16.25mg, 32.5mg, 48.75mg, 65mg, 81.25mg, 97.5mg, 113.75mg, 130mg, 146.25mg, 162.5mg, 195mg

CONTRAINDICATIONS
Uncorrected adrenal cortical insufficiency, untreated thyrotoxicosis, hypersensitivity to any of their active or extraneous constituents.

WARNINGS/PRECAUTIONS
Doses within range of daily hormonal requirements are ineffective for weight reduction in euthyroid patients; larger doses may produce serious or even life-threatening toxicity, particularly when given in association with sympathomimetic

amines. Use is unjustified for the treatment of male or female infertility unless accompanied by hypothyroidism. Caution with cardiovascular (CV) disorders (eg, angina pectoris) and in elderly with risk of occult cardiac disease; initiate at low doses and reduce dose if euthyroid state can only be reached at the expense of aggravation of CV disease. May aggravate diabetes mellitus (DM), diabetes insipidus (DI), or adrenal cortical insufficiency. Treatment of myxedema coma requires simultaneous administration of glucocorticoids. Excessive doses in infants may cause craniosynostosis. Caution in patients with strong suspicion of thyroid gland autonomy. Androgens, corticosteroids, estrogens, iodine-containing preparations, and salicylate-containing preparations may interfere with lab tests.

DRUG INTERACTIONS
Closely monitor PT in patients on oral anticoagulants; dose reduction of anticoagulant may be required. May increase insulin or oral hypoglycemic requirements. Potentially impaired absorption with cholestyramine and colestipol; space dosing by 4-5 hrs. Estrogens may decrease free T4 in patients with nonfunctioning thyroid; increase in thyroid dose may be needed.

PREGNANCY AND LACTATION
Pregnancy: Category A.
Lactation: Caution in nursing.

MECHANISM OF ACTION
Thyroid replacement hormone; not established. Enhances oxygen consumption by most tissues of the body, increases the basal metabolic rate, and the metabolism of carbohydrates, lipids, and proteins.

PHARMACOKINETICS
Absorption: (T3) 95% in 4 hrs; (T4) partial, dependent on vehicle and character of the intestinal contents, intestinal flora, including plasma protein, and soluble dietary factors. **Distribution:** Plasma protein binding (>99%), found in breast milk. **Metabolism:** (T4) Deiodination in liver, kidneys, other tissues.

PATIENT CONSIDERATIONS
Assessment: Assess for adrenal cortical insufficiency, thyrotoxicosis, hypersensitivity to the drug, CV disorders (eg, coronary artery disease, angina pectoris), DM, DI, myxedema coma, nursing status, and possible drug interactions.

Monitoring: Monitor response to treatment; urinary glucose levels in patients with DM, PT in patients receiving anticoagulants, and for aggravation of CV disease. Monitor thyroid function periodically.

Counseling: Inform that replacement therapy is taken essentially for life except in transient hypothyroidism. Instruct to immediately report to physician any signs/symptoms of thyroid hormone toxicity (eg, chest pain, increased pulse rate, palpitations, excessive sweating, heat intolerance, nervousness) or any other unusual event. Inform of the importance of frequent/close monitoring of PT and urinary glucose and the need for dose adjustment of antidiabetic and/or oral anticoagulant medication. Inform that partial loss of hair may be seen in children in 1st few months of therapy.

XALATAN — latanoprost   Rx
Class: Prostaglandin analogue

ADULT DOSAGE	PEDIATRIC DOSAGE
Elevated Intraocular Pressure	Pediatric use may not have been established
Open-Angle Glaucoma/Ocular HTN:	
1 drop in affected eye(s) qd in pm	
Max: Once-daily dosing	

DOSING CONSIDERATIONS
Concomitant Medications
Space by at least 5 min if using >1 topical ophthalmic drug

ADMINISTRATION
Ocular route

Continue w/ the next dose as normal if 1 dose is missed.

STORAGE
Protect from light. **Unopened:** 2-8°C (36-46°F). **During Shipment to Patient:** Up to 40°C (104°F) for a period not exceeding 8 days. **Opened:** Room temperature up to 25°C (77°F) for 6 weeks.

HOW SUPPLIED
Sol: 0.005% [2.5mL]

CONTRAINDICATIONS
Known hypersensitivity to latanoprost, benzalkonium chloride, or any other ingredients in the product.

WARNINGS/PRECAUTIONS
May cause changes to pigmented tissues (eg, increased pigmentation of iris [may be permanent], periorbital tissue/eyelashes [may be reversible]); regularly examine patients who develop noticeably increased iris pigmentation. May gradually change eyelashes and vellus hair in the treated eye. Caution with a history of intraocular inflammation (iritis/uveitis). Macular edema, including cystoid macular edema, reported; caution in aphakic patients, pseudophakic patients with a torn posterior lens capsule, or patients with known risk factors for macular edema. Reactivation of herpes simplex keratitis reported; caution with a history of herpetic keratitis. Avoid with active intraocular inflammation and in cases of active herpes simplex keratitis; inflammation may be exacerbated. Bacterial keratitis associated with the use of multiple-dose containers reported. Contact lenses should be removed prior to administration and may be reinserted 15 min after administration.

ADVERSE REACTIONS
Foreign body sensation, punctate epithelial keratopathy, stinging, itching, burning, conjunctival hyperemia, blurred vision, increased iris pigmentation, excessive tearing, lid discomfort/pain, dry eye, eye pain, lid crusting, lid erythema, URTI/cold/flu.

DRUG INTERACTIONS
Combined use of ≥2 prostaglandins or prostaglandin analogues is not recommended; administration of these prostaglandin drug products more than once daily may decrease the IOP-lowering effect or cause paradoxical IOP elevations. Precipitation occurs when mixed with eye drops containing thimerosal; if such drugs are used, they should be administered at least 5 min apart.

PREGNANCY AND LACTATION
Pregnancy: Category C.
Lactation: Caution in nursing.

MECHANISM OF ACTION
Prostaglandin analogue; prostanoid selective FP receptor agonist that is believed to reduce IOP by increasing outflow of aqueous humor.

PHARMACOKINETICS
Absorption: Absorbed through the cornea where the isopropyl ester prodrug is hydrolyzed to the active acid form. T_{max}=2 hrs (aqueous humor). **Distribution:** V_d=0.16L/kg. **Metabolism:** (Active acid) liver via fatty acid β-oxidation. **Elimination:** Urine (88% topical, 98% IV). (Active acid) $T_{1/2}$=17 min (IV/topical).

PATIENT CONSIDERATIONS
Assessment: Assess for hypersensitivity to drug or benzalkonium chloride, history of or active intraocular inflammation, history of herpetic keratitis, active herpes simplex keratitis, aphakia, pseudophakia with a torn posterior lens capsule, risk factors for macular edema, pregnancy/nursing status, and possible drug interactions.

Monitoring: Monitor for changes to pigmented tissues, eyelash changes, macular edema, herpetic/bacterial keratitis, and other adverse reactions.

Counseling: Inform about the possibility of increased brown pigmentation of the iris, eyelid skin darkening, and eyelash and vellus hair changes in the treated eye. Instruct to avoid allowing the tip of the dispensing container to contact the eye or surrounding structures to avoid contamination. Advise to immediately consult physician about the continued use of treatment if an intercurrent ocular condition (eg, trauma, infection) develops, if undergoing ocular surgery, or if any ocular reactions, particularly conjunctivitis and eyelid reactions, develop. Advise that contact lenses should be removed prior to administration and may be reinserted 15 min after administration. Instruct that if using >1 topical ophthalmic drug, to administer the drugs at least 5 min apart. Inform that if one dose is missed, treatment should continue with the next dose as normal.

XALKORI — crizotinib   Rx
Class: Kinase inhibitor

ADULT DOSAGE	PEDIATRIC DOSAGE
Metastatic Non-Small Cell Lung Cancer	Pediatric use may not have been established
Metastatic non-small cell lung cancer (NSCLC) w/ anaplastic lymphoma kinase (ALK)-positive tumors as detected by an FDA-approved test	
Also indicated for metastatic NSCLC w/ ROS1-positive tumors	
250mg bid until disease progression or no longer tolerated	
Missed Dose	
If a dose is missed, make up that dose unless the next dose is due w/in 6 hrs	

DOSING CONSIDERATIONS
Renal Impairment
Severe (CrCl <30mL/min) Not Requiring Dialysis: 250mg qd

Hepatic Impairment
Has not been studied; use w/ caution

Adverse Reactions
Reduce dose as below, if ≥1 dose reduction is necessary due to Grade 3 or 4 adverse reactions:
1st Dose Reduction: 200mg bid
2nd Dose Reduction: 250mg qd
Permanently D/C: If unable to tolerate 250mg qd

Hematologic Toxicities*:
CTCAE Grade 3: Withhold therapy until recovery to ≤Grade 2, then resume at the same dose schedule
CTCAE Grade 4: Withhold therapy until recovery to ≤Grade 2, then resume at next lower dose
*Except lymphopenia (unless associated w/ clinical events such as opportunistic infections)

Nonhematologic Toxicities:
ALT or AST Elevation:
>5X ULN w/ Total Bilirubin ≤1.5X ULN: Withhold therapy until recovery to baseline or ≤3X ULN, then resume at reduced dose
>3X ULN w/ Total Bilirubin >1.5X ULN (In the Absence of Cholestasis or Hemolysis): Permanently d/c therapy

Drug-Related Interstitial Lung Disease (ILD)/Pneumonitis:
Any Grade: Permanently d/c therapy

QTc Interval:
>500 msec on at Least 2 Separate ECGs: Withhold therapy until recovery to baseline or to a QTc <481 msec, then resume at reduced dose
>500 msec or ≥60 msec Change from Baseline w/ Torsades de Pointes or Polymorphic Ventricular Tachycardia or Signs/Symptoms of Serious Arrhythmia: Permanently d/c therapy

Bradycardia:
Symptomatic, May Be Severe and Medically Significant, Medical Intervention Indicated:
1. Withhold therapy until recovery to asymptomatic bradycardia or to a HR of ≥60bpm
2. Evaluate concomitant medications known to cause bradycardia, as well as anti-hypertensive medications
3. If contributing concomitant medication is identified and discontinued, or its dose is adjusted, resume at previous dose upon recovery to asymptomatic bradycardia or to a HR of ≥60bpm
4. If no contributing concomitant medication is identified, or if contributing concomitant medications are not discontinued or dose modified, resume at reduced dose upon recovery to asymptomatic bradycardia or to a HR of ≥60bpm
Life-Threatening Consequences, Urgent Intervention Indicated:
1. Permanently d/c if no contributing concomitant medication is identified
2. If contributing concomitant medication is identified and discontinued, or its dose is adjusted, resume at 250mg qd upon recovery to asymptomatic bradycardia or to a HR of ≥60bpm, w/ frequent monitoring

Visual Loss:
Grade 4 Ocular Disorder: D/C during evaluation of severe vision loss

ADMINISTRATION
Oral route

Take w/ or w/o food.
Swallow caps whole.
If vomiting occurs after taking a dose, take the next dose at the regular time.

STORAGE
20-25°C (68-77°F); excursions permitted between 15-30°C (59-86°F).

HOW SUPPLIED
Cap: 200mg, 250mg

WARNINGS/PRECAUTIONS
See Dosing Considerations. Hepatotoxicity w/ fatal outcome reported. Concurrent elevations in ALT or AST ≥3X ULN and total bilirubin ≥2X ULN, w/ normal alkaline phosphatase, reported. Elevations in ALT or AST >5X ULN reported. Severe, life-threatening, or fatal ILD/pneumonitis may occur. QTc prolongation may occur; avoid use w/ congenital long QT syndrome. Monitor ECGs and electrolytes in patients w/ CHF, bradyarrhythmias, electrolyte abnormalities, or who are taking medications known to prolong the QT interval. Symptomatic bradycardia may occur. Visual field defect w/ vision loss reported. D/C in patients w/ new onset of severe visual loss (best corrected vision <20/200 in one or both eyes); perform an ophthalmological evaluation consisting of best corrected visual acuity, retinal photographs, visual fields, optical coherence tomography (OCT) and other evaluations as appropriate for new onset of severe visual loss. Can cause fetal harm if used during pregnancy.

ADVERSE REACTIONS
Vision disorders, N/V, diarrhea, edema, constipation, elevated transaminases, fatigue, decreased appetite, URI, dizziness, neuropathy.

DRUG INTERACTIONS
Increased plasma concentrations w/ strong CYP3A inhibitors (eg, clarithromycin, ketoconazole, ritonavir) and grapefruit/grapefruit juice; avoid use. Caution w/ moderate CYP3A inhibitors. Decreased plasma concentrations w/ strong CYP3A inducers (eg, carbamazepine, phenytoin, rifampin); avoid use. Avoid w/ CYP3A substrates w/ narrow therapeutic range (eg, cyclosporine, fentanyl, tacrolimus); may require dose reductions of the CYP3A substrates if concomitant use is required. Avoid w/ other agents known to cause bradycardia (eg, β-blockers, nondihydropyridine calcium channel blockers, clonidine, digoxin) to the extent possible.

PREGNANCY AND LACTATION
Pregnancy: Can cause fetal harm.
Lactation: Do not breastfeed during therapy and for 45 days after the final dose.
Reproductive Potential: Females of reproductive potential should use effective contraception during therapy and for at least 45 days after the final dose. Males w/ female partners of reproductive potential should use condoms during therapy and for at least 90 days after the final dose. May cause reduced fertility in females and males of reproductive potential.

MECHANISM OF ACTION
Tyrosine kinase inhibitor; inhibits receptor tyrosine kinases, including ALK, hepatocyte growth factor receptor, ROS1, and recepteur d'origine nantais.

PHARMACOKINETICS
Absorption: Absolute bioavailability (43%); T_{max}=4-6 hrs (median). **Distribution:** V_d=1772L (IV); plasma protein binding (91%). **Metabolism:** Liver (extensive) via CYP3A4/5; oxidation and O-dealkylation (primary), and conjugation. **Elimination:** Feces (63%, 53% unchanged), urine (22%, 2.3% unchanged); $T_{1/2}$=42 hrs.

PATIENT CONSIDERATIONS

Assessment: Assess for congenital long QT syndrome, CHF, bradyarrhythmias, electrolyte abnormalities, hepatic/renal impairment, pregnancy/nursing status, and possible drug interactions. Assess for presence of ALK or ROS1 positivity in tumor specimens.

Monitoring: Monitor for signs/symptoms of ILD, pneumonitis, QTc prolongation, bradycardia, visual loss, and other adverse reactions. Monitor LFTs including ALT and total bilirubin every 2 weeks during the first 2 months, then once a month and as clinically indicated, w/ more frequent repeat testing if transaminase elevations develop. Monitor ECGs and electrolytes in patients w/ CHF, bradyarrhythmias, electrolyte abnormalities, or who are taking medications known to prolong the QT interval. Monitor HR and BP regularly. Monitor CBCs including differential WBC counts monthly and as clinically indicated, w/ more frequent repeat testing if Grade 3 or 4 abnormalities are observed, or if fever or infection occurs. Perform an ophthalmological evaluation consisting of best corrected visual acuity, retinal photographs, visual fields, OCT, and other evaluations as appropriate for new onset of severe visual loss.

Counseling: Instruct to immediately report symptoms of hepatotoxicity or any new or worsening pulmonary symptoms. Advise to report symptoms of bradycardia and to inform physician about the use of any heart or BP medications. Inform of potential risk of severe visual loss and to immediately contact physician if severe visual loss develops. Inform that visual changes (eg, perceived flashes of light, blurry vision, light sensitivity, floaters) are commonly reported adverse events and may occur while driving or operating machinery. Instruct to avoid grapefruit or grapefruit juice while on therapy; advise to inform physician of all concomitant medications, including prescription medicines, OTC drugs, vitamins, and herbal products. Advise on what to do if a dose is missed or if vomiting occurs after taking a dose. Inform of potential risk to a fetus. Advise to inform physician of known/suspected pregnancy, and not to breastfeed during therapy and for 45 days after the final dose. Advise females of reproductive potential and males w/ female partners of reproductive potential on effective contraception use. Advise females and males of reproductive potential of potential for reduced fertility.

XANAX — alprazolam   CIV
Class: Benzodiazepine

ADULT DOSAGE	**PEDIATRIC DOSAGE**
Anxiety Disorders	Pediatric use may not have been established
Management of Disorders or Short-Term Relief of Symptoms:	
Initial: 0.25-0.5mg tid	
Titrate: May increase at intervals of 3-4 days	
Max: 4mg/day in divided doses	
Panic Disorder	
W/ or w/o Agoraphobia:	
Initial: 0.5mg tid	
Titrate: May increase by ≤1mg/day every 3-4 days; slower titration to doses >4mg/day	
Range: 1-10mg/day	

DOSING CONSIDERATIONS
Hepatic Impairment
Advanced Liver Disease:
Initial: 0.25mg bid-tid
Titrate: May increase gradually prn

Elderly
Elderly/Debilitated:
Initial: 0.25mg bid-tid
Titrate: May increase gradually prn

Discontinuation
Reduce dose gradually when discontinuing therapy or when decreasing daily dosage. Decrease daily dose by no more than 0.5mg every 3 days; some patients may require an even slower dosage reduction

ADMINISTRATION
Oral route

STORAGE
20-25°C (68-77°F).

HOW SUPPLIED
Tab: 0.25mg*, 0.5mg*, 1mg*, 2mg* *scored

CONTRAINDICATIONS
Known sensitivity to this drug or other benzodiazepines, acute narrow-angle glaucoma, concomitant ketoconazole or itraconazole.

WARNINGS/PRECAUTIONS
May be used with treated open-angle glaucoma. Increased risk of dependence with doses >4mg/day, treatment for >12 weeks, and in panic disorder patients. Seizures, including status epilepticus, reported with dose reduction or abrupt discontinuation. Early am anxiety and emergence of anxiety symptoms between doses reported; give same total daily dose divided as more frequent administrations. Withdrawal reactions may occur; reduce dose or d/c therapy gradually. May impair mental/physical abilities. May cause fetal harm; avoid use during 1st trimester. Hypomania/mania reported in patients with depression. Caution with severe depression, suicidal ideation/plans, impaired renal/hepatic/pulmonary function, elderly, and debilitated patients. Has a weak uricosuric effect. Decreased systemic elimination rate with alcoholic liver disease/obesity.

ADVERSE REACTIONS
Drowsiness, lightheadedness, fatigue/tiredness, irritability, depression, headache, confusion, insomnia, dry mouth, constipation, diarrhea, N/V, tachycardia/palpitations, blurred vision, nasal congestion.

DRUG INTERACTIONS

See Contraindications. Not recommended with azole antifungals. Avoid with very potent CYP3A inhibitors. Caution with alcohol, other CNS depressants, diltiazem, isoniazid, macrolides (eg, erythromycin, clarithromycin), grapefruit juice, sertraline, paroxetine, ergotamine, cyclosporine, amiodarone, nicardipine, nifedipine, and other CYP3A inhibitors. Additive CNS depressant effects with psychotropics, anticonvulsants, antihistaminics, ethanol, and other drugs that produce CNS depression. Increased digoxin concentrations reported (especially in patients >65 yrs of age); monitor for signs/symptoms of digoxin toxicity. May increase plasma concentrations of imipramine and desipramine. Fluoxetine, fluvoxamine, nefazodone, cimetidine, and oral contraceptives may increase concentrations. CYP3A inducers (eg, carbamazepine), propoxyphene, and smoking may decrease levels. May require dose adjustment or discontinuation with HIV protease inhibitors (eg, ritonavir).

PREGNANCY AND LACTATION

Pregnancy: Category D.
Lactation: Not for use in nursing.

MECHANISM OF ACTION

Benzodiazepine; has not been established. Presumed to bind at stereo specific receptors at several sites within the CNS.

PHARMACOKINETICS

Absorption: Readily absorbed; T_{max}=1-2 hrs; C_{max}=8-37ng/mL (0.5-3mg). **Distribution:** Plasma protein binding (80%); found in breast milk; crosses the placenta. **Metabolism:** Liver (extensive) via CYP3A4; 4-hydroxyalprazolam and α-hydroxyalprazolam (major metabolites). **Elimination:** Urine; $T_{1/2}$=11.2 hrs.

PATIENT CONSIDERATIONS

Assessment: Assess for drug hypersensitivity, acute narrow-angle glaucoma, depression, suicidal ideation, renal/hepatic/pulmonary function, debilitation, history of alcohol/substance abuse, history of seizures/epilepsy, pregnancy/nursing status, and possible drug interactions. Assess for risk of dependence among panic disorder patients.

Monitoring: Monitor for dependence, rebound/withdrawal symptoms, early am anxiety and emergence of anxiety symptoms, CNS depression, episodes of hypomania/mania, suicidality, other treatment-emergent symptoms, and adverse reactions. Monitor CBC, urinalysis, and blood chemistry periodically. Periodically reassess usefulness of therapy.

Counseling: Advise to inform physician about any alcohol consumption and medicines taken and if nursing, pregnant, planning to be pregnant, or if pregnancy occurs while on therapy. Advise to avoid alcohol during treatment. Advise not to drive or operate dangerous machinery until becoming familiar with the effects of therapy. Advise not to increase/decrease dose or abruptly d/c therapy without consultation; instruct to follow gradual dosage-tapering schedule. Inform of risks associated with doses >4mg/day.

XANAX XR — alprazolam   CIV

Class: Benzodiazepine

ADULT DOSAGE
Panic Disorder

W/ or w/o Agoraphobia:

Initial: 0.5-1mg qd, preferably in the am
Titrate: May increase at intervals of 3-4 days in increments of ≤1mg/day
Usual: 3-6mg/day; some patients may require doses >6mg/day
Maint: 1-10mg/day

Conversions
Switching from Immediate-Release (IR) Tabs to Extended-Release (ER) Tabs:
Patients who are currently being treated w/ divided doses of IR alprazolam tabs may be switched to ER tabs at the same total daily dose taken qd. If therapeutic response after switching is inadequate, may titrate dose as recommended

PEDIATRIC DOSAGE
Pediatric use may not have been established

DOSING CONSIDERATIONS
Hepatic Impairment
Advanced Liver Disease:
Initial: 0.5mg qd
Titrate: May increase gradually if needed and tolerated
Elderly
Elderly/Debilitated:
Initial: 0.5mg qd
Titrate: May increase gradually if needed and tolerated

Discontinuation
Reduce dose gradually when discontinuing therapy or when decreasing daily dosage. Decrease daily dose by no more than 0.5mg every 3 days; some patients may require an even slower dosage reduction

ADMINISTRATION
Oral route

May be administered qd, preferably in the am.
Tabs should be taken intact; do not chew, crush, or break.

STORAGE
25°C (77°F); excursions permitted to 15-30°C (59-86°F).

HOW SUPPLIED
Tab, ER: 0.5mg, 1mg, 2mg, 3mg

CONTRAINDICATIONS
Known sensitivity to this drug or other benzodiazepines, acute narrow-angle glaucoma, concomitant ketoconazole or itraconazole.

WARNINGS/PRECAUTIONS
May be used with treated open-angle glaucoma. Increased risk of dependence with doses >4mg/day, treatment for >12 weeks, and in panic disorder patients. Seizures, including status epilepticus, reported with dose reduction or abrupt discontinuation. Early am anxiety/emergence of anxiety symptoms between doses reported. Withdrawal reactions may occur; reduce dose or d/c therapy gradually. May impair mental/physical abilities. May cause fetal harm; avoid use during 1st trimester. Caution with severe depression, suicidal ideation/plans, impaired renal/hepatic/pulmonary function, elderly, and debilitated patients. Hypomania/mania reported in patients with depression. Has a weak uricosuric effect. Decreased systemic elimination rate with alcoholic liver disease/obesity.

ADVERSE REACTIONS
Sedation, somnolence, memory impairment, dysarthria, abnormal coordination, fatigue, depression, constipation, mental impairment, ataxia, dry mouth, nausea, decreased libido, increased/decreased appetite/weight.

DRUG INTERACTIONS
See Contraindications. Not recommended with azole antifungals. Avoid with very potent CYP3A inhibitors. Caution with alcohol, other CNS depressants, diltiazem, isoniazid, macrolides (eg, erythromycin, clarithromycin), grapefruit juice, sertraline, paroxetine, ergotamine, cyclosporine, amiodarone, nicardipine, nifedipine, and other CYP3A inhibitors. Additive CNS depressant effects with psychotropics, anticonvulsants, antihistaminics, ethanol, and other drugs that produce CNS depression. Increased digoxin concentrations reported (especially in patients >65 yrs of age); monitor for signs/symptoms of digoxin toxicity. May increase plasma concentrations of imipramine and desipramine. Fluoxetine, fluvoxamine, nefazodone, cimetidine, and oral contraceptives may increase concentrations. CYP3A inducers (eg, carbamazepine), propoxyphene, and smoking may decrease levels. May require dose adjustment or discontinuation with HIV protease inhibitors (eg, ritonavir).

PREGNANCY AND LACTATION
Pregnancy: Category D.
Lactation: Not for use in nursing.

MECHANISM OF ACTION
Benzodiazepine; has not been established. Presumed to bind at stereo specific receptors at several sites within the CNS.

PHARMACOKINETICS
Absorption: Readily absorbed (IR); absolute bioavailability (90%); refer to PI for additional parameters. **Distribution:** Plasma protein binding (80%); crosses the placenta; found in breast milk. **Metabolism:** Liver (extensive), via CYP3A4; 4-hydroxyalprazolam and α-hydroxyalprazolam (major metabolites). **Elimination:** Urine; $T_{1/2}$=10.7-15.8 hrs.

PATIENT CONSIDERATIONS
Assessment: Assess for drug hypersensitivity, acute narrow-angle glaucoma, depression, suicidal ideation, renal/hepatic/pulmonary function, debilitation, history of alcohol/substance abuse, history of seizures/epilepsy, pregnancy/nursing status, and possible drug interactions. Assess for risk of dependence among panic disorder patients.

Monitoring: Monitor for dependence, relapse, rebound or withdrawal symptoms, early am anxiety and emergence of anxiety symptoms, CNS depression, episodes of hypomania/mania, suicidality, other treatment-emergent symptoms, and other adverse reactions. Monitor CBC, urinalysis, and blood chemistry periodically. Periodically reassess usefulness of therapy.

Counseling: Advise to take in the am and not crush or chew tabs. Advise to inform physician about any alcohol consumption and medicines taken and if nursing, pregnant, planning to be pregnant, or if pregnancy occurs while on therapy. Advise to avoid alcohol during treatment. Advise not to drive or operate dangerous machinery until becoming familiar with the effects of the medication. Advise not to increase/decrease dose or abruptly d/c therapy without consultation; instruct to follow gradual dosage-tapering schedule. Inform of risks associated with doses >4mg/day.

XARELTO — rivaroxaban   Rx

Class: Selective factor Xa inhibitor

> **Premature discontinuation increases the risk of thrombotic events. If therapy is discontinued for a reason other than pathological bleeding or completion of a course of therapy, consider coverage w/ another anticoagulant. Epidural or spinal hematomas have occurred in patients treated w/ rivaroxaban who are receiving neuraxial anesthesia or undergoing spinal puncture; long-term or permanent paralysis may result. Use of indwelling epidural catheters, concomitant use of other drugs that affect hemostasis (eg, NSAIDs, platelet inhibitors, other anticoagulants), history of traumatic or repeated epidural or spinal punctures, history of spinal deformity or spinal surgery, or unknown optimal timing between the administration of therapy and neuraxial procedure may increase the risk of developing epidural or spinal hematomas. Monitor frequently for signs/symptoms of neurological impairment; urgent treatment is necessary if neurological compromise occurs. Consider benefits and risks before neuraxial intervention in patients anticoagulated or to be anticoagulated for thromboprophylaxis.**

ADULT DOSAGE

Reduce Risk of Stroke and Systemic Embolism in Nonvalvular Atrial Fibrillation
20mg qd w/ pm meal

Deep Vein Thrombosis/Pulmonary Embolism

Prophylaxis:
Give initial dose 6-10 hrs after surgery provided that hemostasis has been established
Following Hip Replacement Surgery:
10mg qd for 35 days
Following Knee Replacement Surgery: 10mg qd for 12 days

Treatment:
15mg bid w/ food for the first 21 days, then 20mg qd w/ food, at approx the same time each day

Reduction in Risk of Recurrence Following Initial 6 Months of Treatment:
20mg qd w/ food at approx the same time each day

Conversions

Switching from Warfarin:
D/C warfarin and start therapy as soon as INR is <3.0

Switching to Warfarin:
No clinical data available to guide conversion; d/c rivaroxaban and begin both a parenteral anticoagulant and warfarin at the time the next dose of rivaroxaban would have been taken

Switching to Other Anticoagulants Other Than Warfarin:
If switching to rapid onset anticoagulant, d/c rivaroxaban and give 1st dose of other anticoagulant (oral or parenteral) at the time that the next dose would have been taken

Switching from Other Anticoagulants Other Than Warfarin:
Start rivaroxaban 0-2 hrs prior to next scheduled pm dose of drug (eg, low molecular weight heparin or non-warfarin oral anticoagulant) and omit administration of other anticoagulant. For continuous IV infusion of unfractionated heparin, stop infusion and start rivaroxaban at the same time.

Missed Dose

Receiving 15mg BID:
Take rivaroxaban immediately to ensure intake of 30mg/day; may take two 15mg tabs at once.
Continue w/ regular 15mg bid as recommended on following day.

Receiving 20mg, 15mg, or 10mg QD:
Take missed dose immediately

PEDIATRIC DOSAGE

Pediatric use may not have been established

- -

DOSING CONSIDERATIONS

Renal Impairment
Reduction in Risk of Stroke in Nonvalvular A-Fib:
CrCl 15-50mL/min: 15mg qd w/ pm meal

Hepatic Impairment
Moderate (Child-Pugh B) and Severe (Child-Pugh C): Avoid use

Other Important Considerations
Surgery/Intervention:
If anticoagulation must be discontinued w/ surgery or other procedures, d/c therapy at least 24 hrs before procedure to reduce the risk of bleeding. Weigh risk of bleeding against urgency of intervention to decide whether procedure should be delayed until 24 hrs after last dose.
After procedure, restart therapy as soon as adequate hemostasis has been established.

ADMINISTRATION

Oral route

15mg and 20mg tabs should be taken w/ food, while 10mg tabs can be taken w/ or w/o food.

Unable to Swallow Whole Tabs
Tabs may be crushed and mixed w/ applesauce immediately prior to use. After administering crushed 15mg or 20mg tabs, immediately follow dose w/ food.

Administration via NG Tube/Gastric Feeding Tube
Tabs may be crushed and suspended in 50mL of water after confirming gastric placement of tube.

Avoid administration distal to the stomach.
After administration of 15mg or 20mg tabs, immediately follow dose w/ enteral feeding.

Stability
Crushed tabs are stable in water and applesauce for up to 4 hrs.

STORAGE
25°C (77°F); excursions permitted to 15-30°C (59-86°F).

HOW SUPPLIED

Tab: 10mg, 15mg, 20mg; (Starter Pack) 15mg [42ˢ], 20mg [9ˢ]

CONTRAINDICATIONS

Active pathological bleeding, severe hypersensitivity reaction to rivaroxaban (eg, anaphylactic reactions).

WARNINGS/PRECAUTIONS

May increase risk of bleeding and cause serious or fatal bleeding; risk of thrombotic events should be weighed against risk of bleeding before initiation of treatment. Promptly evaluate any signs/symptoms of blood loss and consider the need for blood replacement; d/c in patients w/ active pathological hemorrhage. Specific antidote for rivaroxaban is not available; not expected to be dialyzable because of high plasma protein binding. An epidural catheter should not be removed earlier than 18 hrs after last administration of therapy. The next dose should not be administered earlier than 6 hrs after catheter removal. If traumatic puncture occurs, delay administration for 24 hrs. Periodically assess renal function and adjust therapy accordingly in patients w/ nonvalvular A-fib; consider dose adjustment or discontinuation in patients who develop acute renal failure while on therapy. Avoid use in the treatment of deep vein thrombosis (DVT)/pulmonary embolism (PE), reduction in risk of recurrence of DVT/PE, and for prophylaxis of DVT following hip or knee replacement surgery in patients w/ CrCl <30mL/min. Monitor for signs/symptoms of blood loss in patients w/ CrCl 30-50mL/min in prophylaxis of DVT following hip or knee replacement surgery. D/C if acute renal failure develops while on therapy for DVT prophylaxis. Avoid w/ any hepatic disease associated w/ coagulopathy. Should only be used in pregnant women if the potential benefit justifies the potential risk to the mother and fetus; promptly evaluate any signs/symptoms suggesting blood loss. Not recommended in patients w/ prosthetic heart valves. Initiation of treatment is not recommended acutely as an alternative to unfractionated heparin in patients w/ PE who present w/ hemodynamic instability or who may receive thrombolysis or pulmonary embolectomy.

ADVERSE REACTIONS

Bleeding complications.

DRUG INTERACTIONS

See Boxed Warning. May result in changes in exposure w/ inhibitors/inducers of CYP3A4/5, CYP2J2, and P-gp and ATP-binding cassette G2 transporters. Increased exposure w/ combined P-gp and CYP3A4 inhibitors (eg, ketoconazole, ritonavir, clarithromycin) may increase bleeding risk; avoid w/ combined P-gp and strong CYP3A4 inhibitors (eg, ketoconazole, itraconazole, lopinavir/ritonavir). Avoid w/ combined P-gp and strong CYP3A4 inducers (eg, carbamazepine, phenytoin, rifampin); may decrease exposure and efficacy. Concomitant single dose of enoxaparin resulted in an additive effect on anti-factor Xa activity. Concomitant single dose of warfarin resulted in an additive effect on factor Xa inhibition and PT. Concomitant use of other drugs that impair hemostasis (eg, P2Y12 platelet inhibitors, other antithrombotic agents, fibrinolytic therapy, NSAIDs/aspirin, SSRIs, SNRIs) increases the risk of bleeding. May increase bleeding time w/ clopidogrel. Avoid concurrent use w/ other anticoagulants due to increased bleeding risk unless benefit outweighs risk. May increase exposure and may increase bleeding risk w/ combined P-gp and moderate CYP3A4 inhibitors (eg, diltiazem, dronedarone, erythromycin) in renally impaired patients; avoid use in patients w/ CrCl 15-80mL/min who are receiving concomitant combined P-gp and moderate CYP3A4 inhibitors unless potential benefit justifies risk.

PREGNANCY AND LACTATION

Pregnancy: Category C.
Lactation: Not for use in nursing.

MECHANISM OF ACTION

Selective factor Xa inhibitor; inhibits free factor Xa and prothrombinase activity. Has no direct effect on platelet aggregation, but indirectly inhibits platelet aggregation induced by thrombin. By inhibiting factor Xa, rivaroxaban decreases thrombin generation. Does not require a cofactor for activity.

PHARMACOKINETICS

Absorption: Absolute bioavailability (80-100% [10mg], 66% [20mg, fasted]); T_{max}=2-4 hrs. **Distribution:** V_d=50L; plasma protein binding (92-95%). **Metabolism:** Oxidative degradation via CYP3A4/5 and CYP2J2; hydrolysis. **Elimination:** Urine (36% unchanged), feces (7% unchanged); $T_{1/2}$=5-9 hrs (20-45 yrs of age), 11-13 hrs (elderly).

PATIENT CONSIDERATIONS

Assessment: Assess for known hypersensitivity, active pathological bleeding, risk factors for developing epidural or spinal hematomas, conditions that may increase risk of bleeding, renal/hepatic impairment, prosthetic heart valves, PE w/ hemodynamic instability or patients who may receive thrombolysis or pulmonary embolectomy, pregnancy/nursing status, and possible drug interactions.

Monitoring: Monitor for signs/symptoms of bleeding, stroke, thrombotic events, and other adverse reactions. In patients undergoing neuraxial anesthesia or spinal puncture, monitor for epidural or spinal hematomas and neurological impairment. Monitor renal function periodically.

Counseling: Instruct to take only ud. Advise to follow missed dosing instructions. Advise not to d/c w/o consulting physician. Advise to report any unusual bleeding or bruising. Inform that it may take longer than usual to stop bleeding, and that patients may bruise and/or bleed more easily. Advise patients who had neuraxial anesthesia or spinal puncture to watch for signs and symptoms of spinal/epidural hematoma, especially if concomitantly taking NSAIDs or platelet inhibitors; instruct to contact physician immediately if symptoms occur. Instruct to inform physician about therapy before any invasive procedure. Instruct to inform physicians and dentists if taking, or planning to take, any prescription or OTC drugs or herbals. Advise to inform physician immediately if nursing/pregnant or intending to nurse or become pregnant. Advise pregnant women receiving therapy to immediately report to the physician any bleeding or symptoms of blood loss.

Xartemis XR — acetaminophen/oxycodone hydrochloride   CII

Class: Opioid analgesic

> Exposes users to the risk of opioid addiction, abuse, and misuse, leading to overdose and death; assess each patient's risk prior to prescribing, and monitor regularly for development of these behaviors/conditions. Serious, life-threatening, or fatal respiratory depression may occur; monitor for respiratory depression, especially during initiation or following a dose increase. Accidental ingestion, especially in children, can result in a fatal overdose of oxycodone. Prolonged use during pregnancy can result in neonatal opioid withdrawal syndrome; advise pregnant women of the risk and ensure availability of appropriate treatment. Associated with cases of acute liver failure, at times resulting in liver transplant and death. Most cases of liver injury are associated with acetaminophen (APAP) use at doses that exceed the max daily limit, and often involve >1 APAP-containing product.

ADULT DOSAGE

Acute Pain

Use when alternative treatment options are inadequate

1st Opioid Analgesic:
Usual: 2 tabs q12h
May administer 2nd dose of 2 tabs as early as 8 hrs after initial dose, if needed
Subsequent doses are to be administered 2 tabs q12h
Max: Do not exceed 4000mg of acetaminophen

PEDIATRIC DOSAGE

Pediatric use may not have been established

DOSING CONSIDERATIONS

Renal Impairment
Initial: 1 tab and adjust prn
Hepatic Impairment
Initial: 1 tab and adjust prn

Discontinuation
Use a gradual downward titration of the dose of 50% every 2-4 days to prevent signs/symptoms of withdrawal.
Do not abruptly d/c.

ADMINISTRATION

Oral route

Swallow tab whole, one at a time w/ enough water to ensure complete swallowing.
Do not break, chew, crush, cut, dissolve, or split.
May take w/ or w/o food.

STORAGE

25°C (77°F); excursions permitted to 15-30°C (59-86°F).

HOW SUPPLIED

Tab, Extended-Release: (Oxycodone/APAP) 7.5mg/325mg

CONTRAINDICATIONS

Known hypersensitivity to oxycodone, acetaminophen, or any other component of this product, significant respiratory depression, acute or severe bronchial asthma or hypercarbia, known/suspected paralytic ileus.

WARNINGS/PRECAUTIONS

Reserve for use in patients for whom alternative treatment options (eg, nonopioid analgesics) are ineffective, not tolerated, or would be otherwise inadequate. Not interchangeable with other oxycodone/APAP products. Overestimating dose when converting from another opioid product may result in fatal overdose with 1st dose. Life-threatening respiratory depression is more likely to occur in elderly, cachectic, or debilitated patients. Consider alternative nonopioid analgesics in patients with significant chronic obstructive pulmonary disease or cor pulmonale, and in patients having a substantially decreased respiratory reserve, hypoxia, hypercarbia, or preexisting respiratory depression. Increased risk of acute liver failure in patients with underlying liver disease. May cause serious skin reactions (eg, acute generalized exanthematous pustulosis, Stevens-Johnson syndrome, toxic epidermal necrolysis), which can be fatal; d/c at the 1st appearance of skin rash or any other sign of hypersensitivity. Respiratory depressant effects and CSF pressure elevation capacity may be markedly exaggerated in the presence of head injury, other intracranial lesions, or preexisting increased intracranial pressure (ICP). May obscure clinical course of head injury and acute abdominal conditions. May cause severe hypotension; caution with circulatory shock. May produce orthostatic hypotension in ambulatory patients. APAP use associated with hypersensitivity and anaphylaxis; avoid in patients with APAP allergy. Consider use of an alternative analgesic in patients who have difficulty swallowing and in patients at risk for underlying GI disorders resulting in a small GI lumen. Monitor for decreased bowel motility in postoperative patients. May cause spasm of the sphincter of Oddi; monitor patients with biliary tract disease, including

acute pancreatitis. May impair mental/physical abilities. Physical dependence and tolerance may occur; do not stop therapy abruptly. Not recommended for use during or immediately prior to labor. Caution with renal/hepatic impairment and in elderly.

ADVERSE REACTIONS

Respiratory depression, acute liver failure, N/V, dizziness, headache, constipation, somnolence.

DRUG INTERACTIONS

Oxycodone: Concomitant use with alcohol or other CNS depressants (eg, sedatives, anxiolytics, hypnotics, neuroleptics, other opioids) may cause hypotension, profound sedation, coma, respiratory depression, and death; reduce dose of 1 or both agents. CYP3A4 inhibitors (eg, macrolides, azole antifungals, protease inhibitors) may increase plasma levels and prolong opioid effects; these effects could be more pronounced with concomitant use of CYP2D6 (amiodarone, quinidine, antidepressants) and 3A4 inhibitors. CYP450 inducers (eg, rifampin, carbamazepine, phenytoin) may induce metabolism, leading to a decrease in plasma concentration and efficacy. Caution when initiating treatment in patients currently taking or discontinuing CYP3A4 inhibitors or inducers; evaluate these patients at frequent intervals and consider dose adjustments until stable drug effects are achieved. May enhance the neuromuscular blocking action of skeletal muscle relaxants and produce an increased degree of respiratory depression. MAOIs reported to intensify effects causing anxiety, confusion, and significant respiratory depression or coma; not recommended with MAOIs or within 14 days of stopping such treatment. Caution with agonist/antagonist analgesics (eg, pentazocine, nalbuphine, butorphanol, buprenorphine); may reduce analgesic effect and/or may precipitate withdrawal symptoms. Concurrent use with anticholinergics or other medications with anticholinergic activity may result in increased risk of urinary retention and/or severe constipation, which may lead to paralytic ileus. **APAP:** Increased risk of acute liver failure with alcohol. Do not use concomitantly with other APAP-containing products.

PREGNANCY AND LACTATION

Pregnancy: Category C.
Lactation: Not for use in nursing.

MECHANISM OF ACTION

Oxycodone: Opioid analgesic; opioid agonist whose principal therapeutic action is analgesia. **APAP:** Nonopioid, nonsalicylate analgesic and antipyretic; site and mechanism for the analgesic effect not established. Antipyretic effect is accomplished through inhibition of endogenous pyrogen action on the hypothalamic heat-regulating centers.

PHARMACOKINETICS

Absorption: Oxycodone: Oral bioavailability (60-87%). Oxycodone and APAP: Administration of variable doses resulted in different parameters. **Distribution:** Found in breastmilk. Oxycodone: V_d=2.6L/kg (IV); plasma protein binding (45%); crosses placenta. APAP: V_d=0.9L/kg; plasma protein binding (20%). **Metabolism:** Oxycodone: Extensive; CYP2D6 to oxymorphone; noroxycodone (major metabolite). APAP: Liver via CYP2E1, CYP1A2, CYP3A4; conjugation and oxidation. **Elimination:** Oxycodone: Urine (≤19% free oxycodone, ≤50% conjugated oxycodone, ≤14% conjugated oxymorphone); $T_{1/2}$=4.5 hrs. APAP: Urine (<9% unchanged); $T_{1/2}$=5.8 hrs.

PATIENT CONSIDERATIONS

Assessment: Assess for risks for opioid abuse, addiction, or misuse, pain type/severity, prior opioid therapy, patient's general condition and medical status, respiratory depression, COPD, cor pulmonale, decreased respiratory reserve, hypoxia, hypercapnia, renal/hepatic impairment, paralytic ileus, acute/severe bronchial asthma, biliary tract disease, increased ICP, history of hypersensitivity to drug, any other conditions where treatment is contraindicated or cautioned, pregnancy/nursing status, and possible drug interactions.

Monitoring: Monitor for development of addiction, abuse, or misuse, physical dependence, tolerance, acute liver failure, respiratory depression, hypotension, skin/hypersensitivity/anaphylactic reactions, decreased bowel motility in postoperative patients, biliary tract disease, acute pancreatitis, and other adverse reactions. Periodically reevaluate therapy.

Counseling: Inform that medication is not interchangeable with other forms of oxycodone/APAP, that it is a narcotic pain reliever, and that it must be taken only ud. Instruct not to take >2 tabs at once unless instructed by physician. Instruct not to adjust dose without consulting physician. Instruct not to take >4000mg of APAP/day and to call physician if more than the recommended dose was taken. Inform that use of medication, even when taken ud, may result in addiction, abuse, and misuse. Instruct not to share with others and to take steps to protect from theft or misuse. Inform of the risk of life-threatening respiratory depression; advise how to recognize respiratory depression and when to seek medical attention. Inform that accidental exposure, especially in children, may result in respiratory depression or death. Instruct to dispose of unused tab by flushing down the toilet. Instruct females of reproductive potential who become or are planning to become pregnant to consult a physician prior to initiating or continuing therapy; inform that prolonged use during pregnancy can result in neonatal opioid withdrawal syndrome. Advise women not to breastfeed during therapy. Inform that potentially serious additive effects may occur if used with alcohol or other CNS depressants; instruct not to use such drugs unless supervised by a physician. Inform that drug may cause drowsiness, dizziness, or lightheadedness, and may impair mental and/or physical abilities; advise to refrain from any potentially dangerous activity until it is established that they are not adversely affected. Counsel patients on the possibility of withdrawal symptoms with cessation of therapy. Advise of the potential for severe constipation and other adverse reactions.

XELJANZ — tofacitinib   Rx
Class: Kinase inhibitor

Increased risk for developing serious infections (eg, active tuberculosis [TB], invasive fungal infections, bacterial/viral infections due to opportunistic pathogens) that may lead to hospitalization or death. Most patients who developed these infections were taking concomitant immunosuppressants (eg, methotrexate [MTX], corticosteroids). If a serious infection develops, interrupt treatment until infection is controlled. Test for latent TB prior to and during therapy; initiate latent TB treatment prior to therapy. Consider risks and benefits prior to initiating therapy in patients w/ chronic or recurrent infection. Monitor for development of signs and symptoms of infection during and after treatment. Lymphoma and other malignancies reported. Increased rate of Epstein-Barr virus-associated post-transplant lymphoproliferative disorder observed in renal transplant patients w/ concomitant immunosuppressive medications.

OTHER BRAND NAMES
Xeljanz XR

ADULT DOSAGE
Rheumatoid Arthritis
As monotherapy or in combination w/ methotrexate (MTX) or other nonbiologic disease-modifying antirheumatic drugs (DMARDs) for moderately to severely active rheumatoid arthritis in patients who have had an inadequate response or intolerance to MTX

Tab:
5mg bid

Tab, Extended-Release (ER):
11mg qd

Conversions
Switching From Tab to Tab, ER:
Patients treated w/ Xeljanz 5mg bid may be switched to Xeljanz XR 11mg qd following the last dose of Xeljanz 5mg

PEDIATRIC DOSAGE
Pediatric use may not have been established

DOSING CONSIDERATIONS
Concomitant Medications
Potent CYP3A4 Inhibitors:
Tab: Reduce dose to 5mg qd

≥1 Concomitant Medication Resulting in Both Moderate CYP3A4 Inhibition and Potent CYP2C19 Inhibition:
Tab: Reduce dose to 5mg qd

Potent CYP3A4 Inducers:
Tab/Tab, ER: Not recommended for use

Renal Impairment
Moderate or Severe:
Tab: Reduce dose to 5mg qd

Hepatic Impairment
Moderate:
Tab: Reduce dose to 5mg qd

Severe:
Tab/Tab, ER: Not recommended for use

Adverse Reactions
Lymphopenia:
Absolute Lymphocyte Count <500 cells/mm³: Do not initiate treatment
Absolute Lymphocyte Count ≥500 cells/mm³: Maintain dose
Absolute Lymphocyte Count <500 cells/mm³ (Confirmed by Repeat Testing): D/C treatment

Neutropenia:
ANC <1000 cells/mm³: Do not initiate treatment
ANC >1000 cells/mm³: Maintain dose
ANC 500-1000 cells/mm³: For persistent decreases in this range, interrupt dosing until ANC is >1000; when ANC is >1000, resume at Xeljanz 5mg bid/Xeljanz XR 11mg qd
ANC <500 cells/mm³ (Confirmed by Repeat Testing): D/C treatment

Anemia:
Hgb <9g/dL: Do not initiate treatment
Hgb ≤2g/dL Decrease and ≥9g/dL: Maintain dose
Hgb >2g/dL Decrease or <8g/dL (Confirmed by Repeat Testing): Interrupt administration until Hgb values have normalized

ADMINISTRATION
Oral route

Take w/ or w/o food.
Swallow ER tabs whole and intact; do not crush, split, or chew.

STORAGE
20-25°C (68-77°F).

HOW SUPPLIED
Tab: (Xeljanz) 5mg; **Tab, ER:** (Xeljanz XR) 11mg

WARNINGS/PRECAUTIONS
See Dosing Considerations. Avoid w/ active, serious infection, including localized infections. Caution in patients w/ chronic/recurrent infections, who have been exposed to TB, w/ a history of a serious/opportunistic infection, who have resided in/traveled to areas of endemic TB/mycoses, or w/ predisposing factors to infection. Interrupt treatment if an opportunistic infection or sepsis occurs. Viral reactivation, including herpes virus reactivation (eg, herpes zoster), reported; screen for viral hepatitis before starting therapy. Increased risk of herpes zoster; risk appears to be higher in patients treated in Japan. Consider risks and benefits of treatment in patients w/ a known malignancy other than a successfully treated non-melanoma skin cancer or when considering continuing treatment in patients who develop a malignancy. Non-melanoma skin cancers reported; periodic skin examination is recommended for patients at increased risk for skin cancer. GI perforation reported; caution in patients w/ increased risk for GI perforation (eg, history of diverticulitis). Promptly evaluate for early identification of GI perforation in patients presenting w/ new onset of abdominal symptoms. Associated w/ initial lymphocytosis, neutropenia, increases in lipid parameters, and liver enzyme elevations. Interrupt treatment if drug-induced liver injury is suspected until this diagnosis has been excluded. Caution in elderly and diabetes patients. **Tab, ER:** Caution w/ preexisting severe GI narrowing (pathologic or iatrogenic).

ADVERSE REACTIONS
Infections (eg, URTIs, nasopharyngitis), diarrhea, headache.

DRUG INTERACTIONS
See Boxed Warning and Dosing Considerations. Avoid w/ live vaccines. Increased immunosuppression w/ potent immunosuppressive drugs (eg, azathioprine, tacrolimus, cyclosporine); concurrent use w/ potent immunosuppressants (eg, azathioprine, cyclosporine) or biologic DMARDs is not recommended. Increased exposure w/ potent CYP3A4 inhibitors (eg, ketoconazole), and drugs that are both moderate CYP3A4 inhibitors and potent CYP2C19 inhibitors (eg, fluconazole). Decreased exposure resulting in loss of or reduced clinical response to treatment w/ potent CYP3A4 inducers (eg, rifampin).

PREGNANCY AND LACTATION
Pregnancy: Category C. Physicians are encouraged to register pregnant patients in the pregnancy registry.
Lactation: Not for use in nursing.

MECHANISM OF ACTION
Kinase inhibitor; inhibits Janus kinase, which transmits signals arising from cytokine or growth factor-receptor interactions on the cellular membrane to influence cellular processes of hematopoiesis and immune cell function.

PHARMACOKINETICS
Absorption: (Tab) Absolute bioavailability (74%); T_{max}=0.5-1 hr. (Tab, ER) T_{max}=4 hrs. **Distribution:** (IV) V_d=87 L; plasma protein binding (40%). **Metabolism:** Liver via CYP3A4 (primary) and CYP2C19 (minor). **Elimination:** Urine (30% unchanged); $T_{1/2}$=3 hrs (Tab), 6 hrs (Tab, ER).

PATIENT CONSIDERATIONS
Assessment: Assess for infections (eg, bacteria, fungi, viruses), including latent or active TB, predisposing factors to infection, active hepatic disease or impairment, known malignancy, risk of GI perforation, diabetes, preexisting GI narrowing, pregnancy/nursing status, and possible drug interactions. Obtain baseline absolute lymphocyte count, ANC, and lipid and Hgb levels.

Monitoring: Monitor for TB (active, reactivation, or latent), invasive fungal infections, or bacterial, viral, and other opportunistic infections during and after therapy. Monitor for viral reactivation, lymphoma, malignancy, lymphoproliferative disorders, GI perforations, and other adverse reactions. Monitor absolute lymphocyte counts every 3 months. Monitor neutrophil counts and Hgb after 4-8 weeks of treatment and every 3 months thereafter. Routinely monitor LFTs. Monitor lipid parameters approx 4-8 weeks following initiation. Perform periodic skin examination in patients at increased risk of skin cancer.

Counseling: Advise about potential risks/benefits of therapy. Inform that therapy may lower resistance to infection; advise patients not to start taking medication if they have an active infection. Instruct to contact physician immediately if symptoms suggesting an infection appear during treatment to ensure rapid evaluation and appropriate treatment. Advise that the risk of herpes zoster is increased in patients treated w/ therapy. Inform that medication may increase risk of lymphoma and other cancers; instruct to inform physician of any type of cancer that they have ever had. Inform that certain lab tests may be affected and that blood tests are required before and during treatment. Inform that medication should not be used during pregnancy unless clearly necessary; advise to inform physician right away if pregnant. Advise to enroll in the pregnancy registry for pregnant women who have taken medication during pregnancy. **Tab, ER:** Inform that an inert tablet shell may pass in the stool or via colostomy and that the active medication has already been absorbed by the time the inert tablet shell is seen.

XELODA — capecitabine   Rx
Class: Fluoropyrimidine carbamate

Altered coagulation parameters and/or bleeding, including death, reported w/ concomitant coumarin-derivative anticoagulants (eg, warfarin, phenprocoumon). Monitor PT and INR frequently in order to adjust anticoagulant dose accordingly. Postmarketing reports showed clinically significant increases in PT and INR in patients who were stabilized on anticoagulants at start of therapy. Age >60 yrs and a diagnosis of cancer independently predispose to an increased risk of coagulopathy.

ADULT DOSAGE
Metastatic Colorectal Cancer
1st-line treatment of metastatic colorectal carcinoma and as a single agent for adjuvant treatment in patients w/ Dukes' C colon cancer who have undergone complete

PEDIATRIC DOSAGE
Pediatric use may not have been established

resection of the primary tumor when treatment w/ fluoropyrimidine therapy alone is preferred

Monotherapy:
Usual: $1250mg/m^2$ bid for 2 weeks followed by a 1-week rest period, given as 3-week cycles

Adjuvant to Dukes' C Colon Cancer:
$1250mg/m^2$ bid for 2 weeks followed by 1-week rest period, given as 3-week cycles for total of 8 cycles (24 weeks)

Refer to PI for dose calculations based on BSA

Metastatic Breast Cancer

Treatment of metastatic breast cancer in combination w/ docetaxel after failure of prior anthracycline-containing chemotherapy. Monotherapy treatment of metastatic breast cancer in patients resistant to both paclitaxel and anthracycline-containing chemotherapy regimen or resistant to paclitaxel and for whom further anthracycline therapy is not indicated

Monotherapy:
$1250mg/m^2$ bid for 2 weeks followed by a 1-week rest period, given as 3-week cycles

Combination w/ Docetaxel:
Usual: $1250mg/m^2$ bid for 2 weeks followed by 1-week rest period, combined w/ docetaxel at $75mg/m^2$ as a 1-hr IV infusion every 3 weeks
Premedication:
Start prior to docetaxel administration

Refer to PI for dose calculations based on BSA

DOSING CONSIDERATIONS
Concomitant Medications
Phenytoin and Coumarin-Derivative Anticoagulants: May need to reduce dose of phenytoin and coumarin-derivative anticoagulants

Renal Impairment
Moderate (CrCl 30-50mL/min): Reduce to 75% of starting dose when used as monotherapy or in combination w/ docetaxel (from $1250mg/m^2$ to $950mg/m^2$ bid)

Adverse Reactions
Toxicity NCIC Grade 2:
1st Appearance: Interrupt until resolved to Grade 0-1, then give 100% of dose
2nd Appearance: Interrupt until resolved to Grade 0-1, then give 75% of dose
3rd Appearance: Interrupt until resolved to Grade 0-1, then give 50% of dose
4th Appearance: D/C treatment permanently

Toxicity NCIC Grade 3:
1st Appearance: Interrupt until resolved to Grade 0-1, then give 75% of dose
2nd Appearance: Interrupt until resolved to Grade 0-1, then give 50% of dose
3rd Appearance: D/C treatment permanently

Toxicity NCIC Grade 4:
1st Appearance: D/C permanently or if physician deems it to be in the best interest to continue, interrupt until resolved to Grade 0-1, then give 50% of dose

Refer to PI for docetaxel dose reductions when used in combination w/ capecitabine

ADMINISTRATION
Oral route

Swallow tabs whole w/ water w/in 30 min pc; do not cut or crush.

STORAGE
$25°C$ ($77°F$); excursions permitted to $15-30°C$ ($59-86°F$). Keep tightly closed.

HOW SUPPLIED
Tab: 150mg, 500mg

CONTRAINDICATIONS
Severe renal impairment (CrCl <30mL/min); known hypersensitivity to capecitabine, any components of the medication, or 5-fluorouracil (5-FU).

WARNINGS/PRECAUTIONS
May induce diarrhea; give fluid and electrolyte replacement w/ severe diarrhea. Cardiotoxicity (eg, MI/ischemia, angina) observed; may be more common in patients w/ a prior history of coronary artery disease (CAD). Increased risk for acute early-onset of toxicity and severe, life-threatening, or fatal adverse reactions (eg, mucositis, diarrhea, neutropenia, neurotoxicity) in patients w/ certain homozygous or certain compound heterozygous mutations in the dihydropyrimidine dehydrogenase (DPD) gene that results in complete or near complete absence of DPD activity; withhold or permanently d/c therapy based on clinical assessment of the onset, duration, and severity of the observed toxicities. Patients w/ partial DPD activity may also have increased risk of severe,

life-threatening, or fatal adverse reactions. Dehydration reported and may cause acute renal failure; patients w/ preexisting compromised renal function are at higher risk. Patients w/ anorexia, asthenia, N/V, or diarrhea may rapidly become dehydrated; monitor during administration and do not restart treatment until patient is rehydrated and any precipitating causes have been corrected or controlled. Caution w/ mild and moderate renal impairment. Severe mucocutaneous reactions (eg, Stevens-Johnson syndrome, toxic epidermal necrolysis) may occur; permanently d/c in patients who experience a severe mucocutaneous reaction possibly attributable to treatment. Hand-and-foot syndrome may occur. Hyperbilirubinemia reported; interrupt therapy if drug-related Grade 3 or 4 elevations in bilirubin occur until the hyperbilirubinemia decreases to ≤3X ULN. Necrotizing enterocolitis, neutropenia, thrombocytopenia, anemia, and decreases in Hgb reported. Avoid w/ baseline neutrophil counts of $<1.5 \times 10^9$/L and/or thrombocyte counts of $<100 \times 10^9$/L. Caution in elderly; patients ≥80 yrs of age may experience greater incidence of Grade 3 or 4 adverse events. Caution w/ mild to moderate hepatic dysfunction due to liver metastases. May cause fetal harm.

ADVERSE REACTIONS
Diarrhea, hand-and-foot syndrome, asthenia, pyrexia, anemia, N/V, fatigue, dermatitis, thrombocytopenia, constipation, taste disturbance, stomatitis, alopecia, abdominal pain, decreased appetite.

DRUG INTERACTIONS
See Boxed Warning and Dosing Considerations. Higher risk of dehydration w/ known nephrotoxic agents. May increase the mean AUC of S-warfarin. May increase phenytoin levels. Leucovorin may increase levels and toxicity of 5-FU. Caution w/ CYP2C9 substrates.

PREGNANCY AND LACTATION
Pregnancy: Category D.
Lactation: Not for use in nursing.

MECHANISM OF ACTION
Fluoropyrimidine carbamate; binds to thymidylate synthase to form a covalently bound ternary complex that inhibits the formation of thymidylate from 2'-deoxyuridylate, which inhibits DNA synthesis/cell division, and interferes w/ RNA processing and protein synthesis.

PHARMACOKINETICS
Absorption: T_{max}=1.5 hrs. **Distribution:** Plasma protein binding (<60%); primarily bound to human albumin (approx 35%). **Metabolism:** Extensive enzymatic conversion to 5-FU; hydrogenated to the much less toxic 5-fluoro-5, 6-dihydro-fluorouracil by DPD; cleavage of the pyrimidine ring to 5-fluoro-ureido-propionic acid; cleavage to α-fluoro-β-alanine. **Elimination:** Urine (95.5%, 3% unchanged), feces (2.6%); $T_{1/2}$=0.75 hr.

PATIENT CONSIDERATIONS
Assessment: Assess for hypersensitivity to drug or to 5-FU, complete or near complete absence of DPD activity, partial DPD activity, renal/hepatic dysfunction, history of CAD, pregnancy/nursing status, and possible drug interactions. Obtain baseline neutrophil/thrombocyte counts.

Monitoring: Monitor for severe diarrhea, necrotizing enterocolitis, cardiotoxicity, acute early-onset of toxicity, severe/life-threatening/fatal adverse reactions, hand-and-foot syndrome, hyperbilirubinemia, neutropenia, thrombocytopenia, anemia, decreases in Hgb, severe toxicity, dehydration, acute renal failure, severe mucocutaneous reactions, and other adverse reactions. Monitor PT and INR frequently w/ concomitant oral coumarin-derivative anticoagulant therapy.

Counseling: Instruct to d/c therapy and contact physician immediately if moderate/severe toxicity, Grade ≥2 diarrhea/stomatitis, or severe bloody diarrhea w/ severe abdominal pain and fever is experienced. Advise to notify physician if patient has known DPD deficiency; inform that patient is at an increased risk of acute early-onset of toxicity and severe, life-threatening, or fatal adverse reactions if patient has complete or near complete absence of DPD activity. Instruct to d/c therapy immediately in patients experiencing Grade ≥2 dehydration/nausea/vomiting/hand-and-foot syndrome. Instruct to contact physician immediately if fever or infection occurs. Counsel about pregnancy risks; instruct to avoid pregnancy during therapy.

XENICAL — orlistat   Rx

Class: Lipase inhibitor

ADULT DOSAGE	PEDIATRIC DOSAGE
Obesity	**Obesity**
Obesity management in patients w/ an initial BMI $≥30kg/m^2$ or $≥27kg/m^2$ in the presence of other risk factors	Obesity management in patients w/ an initial BMI $≥30kg/m^2$ or $≥27kg/m^2$ in the presence of other risk factors
120mg tid w/ each main meal containing fat **Max:** 120mg tid	**≥12 Years:** 120mg tid w/ each main meal containing fat **Max:** 120mg tid

------

ADMINISTRATION
Oral route

Administer during or up to 1 hr after the meal.
Use w/ nutritionally balanced, reduced-calorie diet that contains approx 30% of calories from fat; distribute daily intake of fat, carbohydrate, and protein over 3 main meals. Omit dose if a meal is missed or contains no fat.
Patients should take a multivitamin containing fat-soluble vitamins to ensure adequate nutrition; the vitamin supplement should be taken at least 2 hrs before or after the administration of orlistat (eg, hs).

STORAGE
25°C (77°F); excursions permitted to 15-30°C (59-86°F).

HOW SUPPLIED
Cap: 120mg

CONTRAINDICATIONS
Pregnancy, chronic malabsorption syndrome, cholestasis, known hypersensitivity to orlistat or to any component of the product.

WARNINGS/PRECAUTIONS
Weight loss may affect glycemic control in patients w/ diabetes mellitus. Severe liver injury w/ hepatocellular necrosis or acute hepatic failure reported, w/ some cases resulting in liver transplant or death; d/c therapy and other suspect medications immediately and obtain LFTs. May increase levels of urinary oxalate; caution w/ a history of hyperoxaluria or calcium oxalate nephrolithiasis. Cases of oxalate nephrolithiasis and oxalate nephropathy w/ renal failure reported; monitor renal function. May increase risk of cholelithiasis due to substantial weight loss. Exclude organic causes of obesity (eg, hypothyroidism). GI events may increase w/ a high-fat diet (>30% total daily calories from fat).

ADVERSE REACTIONS
Oily spotting, flatus w/ discharge, fecal urgency, fatty/oily stool, oily evacuation, increased defecation, fecal incontinence.

DRUG INTERACTIONS
Reduced cyclosporine plasma levels reported; administer cyclosporine 3 hrs after administration of orlistat. Reduced absorption of β-carotene supplement and inhibited absorption of vitamin E acetate supplement reported. Hypothyroidism reported w/ levothyroxine; administer at least 4 hrs apart and monitor for thyroid function changes. Vitamin K absorption may be decreased. Decreased prothrombin, increased INR, and unbalanced anticoagulant treatment resulting in change of hemostatic parameters reported in patients treated w/ anticoagulants; monitor closely for changes in coagulation parameters w/ chronic stable doses of warfarin or other anticoagulants. Reduced exposure of amiodarone and its metabolite reported; may reduce therapeutic effect of amiodarone. Convulsions reported w/ antiepileptic drugs; monitor for possible changes in the frequency and/or severity of convulsions. Loss of virological control reported in HIV-infected patients taking orlistat w/ antiretroviral drugs; monitor HIV RNA levels frequently in patients being treated for HIV infection and d/c orlistat if there is a confirmed increase in HIV viral load. May require reduction in dosage of oral hypoglycemic agents (eg, sulfonylureas) or insulin in diabetics.

PREGNANCY AND LACTATION
Pregnancy: Category X.
Lactation: Caution in nursing.

MECHANISM OF ACTION
Lipase inhibitor; exerts therapeutic activity in the lumen of the stomach and small intestine by forming a covalent bond w/ the active serine residue site of gastric and pancreatic lipases. The inactivated enzymes are thus unavailable to hydrolyze dietary fats in the form of TGs into absorbable free fatty acids and monoglycerides.

PHARMACOKINETICS
Absorption: Minimal. T_{max}=8 hrs (360mg dose). **Distribution:** Plasma protein binding (>99%). **Metabolism:** M1 and M3 (primary and secondary metabolites). **Elimination:** (360mg single dose) Feces (97%, 83% unchanged), urine (<2%); $T_{1/2}$=1-2 hrs, 3 hrs (M1), 13.5 hrs (M3).

PATIENT CONSIDERATIONS
Assessment: Assess for hypersensitivity to the drug, chronic malabsorption syndrome, cholestasis, history of hyperoxaluria or calcium oxalate nephrolithiasis, organic causes of obesity (eg, hypothyroidism), pregnancy/nursing status, and possible drug interactions. Obtain baseline weight, FPG, and lipid profile.

Monitoring: Monitor for hepatic dysfunction, cholelithiasis, signs/symptoms of hypersensitivity reactions, GI events, and other adverse events. Monitor renal function in patients at risk for renal insufficiency. Monitor closely for changes in coagulation parameters w/ chronic stable doses of warfarin.

Counseling: Advise to inform physician if taking cyclosporine, β-carotene or vitamin E supplements, levothyroxine, warfarin, antiepileptic drugs, amiodarone, or antiretroviral drugs due to potential interactions. Inform of the common adverse events (eg, oily spotting, flatus w/ discharge, fecal urgency) associated w/ the use of the drug. Inform of the potential risks that include lowered absorption of fat-soluble vitamins and potential liver injury, increased urinary oxalate, and cholelithiasis. Inform of the potential benefits that therapy may result in, such as weight loss and improvement in obesity-related risk factors. Instruct to report any symptoms of hepatic dysfunction while on therapy. Instruct patient to take drug ud w/ meals or up to 1 hr pc. Advise to take a multivitamin qd at least 2 hrs before or after administration, or at hs. Instruct to adhere to dietary guidelines.

XERESE — acyclovir/hydrocortisone   Rx

Class: Anti-infective/corticosteroid

ADULT DOSAGE	**PEDIATRIC DOSAGE**
Herpes Labialis (Cold Sores)	**Herpes Labialis (Cold Sores)**
Early treatment of recurrent herpes labialis to reduce the likelihood of ulcerative cold sores and to shorten the lesion healing time	Early treatment of recurrent herpes labialis to reduce the likelihood of ulcerative cold sores and to shorten the lesion healing time
Apply a quantity sufficient to cover the affected area (including outer margin) 5X/day for 5 days	**≥6 Years:** Apply a quantity sufficient to cover the affected area (including outer margin) 5X/day for 5 days
Initiate therapy as early as possible after the 1st signs/symptoms (eg, during the prodrome or when lesions appear)	Initiate therapy as early as possible after the 1st signs/symptoms (eg, during the prodrome or when lesions appear)

ADMINISTRATION
Topical route

STORAGE
20-25°C (68-77°F); excursions permitted to 15-30°C (59-86°F). Do not freeze.

HOW SUPPLIED
Cre: (Acyclovir/Hydrocortisone) 5%/1% [5g]

WARNINGS/PRECAUTIONS
For cutaneous use only. Do not use in the eye, inside the mouth or nose, or on the genitals. Other orofacial lesions may be difficult to distinguish from a cold sore; monitor for cold sores that fail to heal within 2 weeks. Has a potential for irritation and contact sensitization.

ADVERSE REACTIONS
Application-site reactions (eg, drying/flaking of skin, burning/tingling, erythema, pigmentation changes, inflammation).

PREGNANCY AND LACTATION
Category B, caution in nursing.

MECHANISM OF ACTION
Acyclovir: Anti-infective (synthetic purine nucleoside analogue); stops herpes viral DNA replication by competitive inhibition of viral DNA polymerase, by incorporation into and termination of the growing viral DNA chain, and by inactivation of viral DNA polymerase. Hydrocortisone: Corticosteroid; possesses anti-inflammatory effects that suppress the clinical manifestations of disease in a wide range of disorders where inflammation is a prominent feature.

PHARMACOKINETICS
Absorption: Hydrocortisone: Percutaneous; extent of absorption is determined by many factors (eg, vehicle, integrity of epidermal barrier, use of occlusive dressings). **Metabolism:** Hydrocortisone: Liver. **Elimination:** Hydrocortisone: Kidneys, bile.

PATIENT CONSIDERATIONS
Assessment: Assess for type of lesions (eg, bacterial, fungal infections), and pregnancy/nursing status.

Monitoring: Monitor for clinical response, irritation, contact sensitization, and other adverse reactions.

Counseling: Inform that medication is not a cure for cold sores and it is for cutaneous use only for herpes labialis of the lips and around the mouth. Advise not to use in the eye, inside the mouth/nose, or on genitals. Counsel to use ud. Advise to avoid unnecessary rubbing of the affected area to avoid aggravating or transferring the infection. Instruct to seek medical advice when a cold sore fails to heal within 2 weeks. Encourage immunocompromised patients to consult a physician concerning the treatment of any infection.

XGEVA — denosumab   Rx

Class: IgG$_2$ monoclonal antibody

ADULT DOSAGE	**PEDIATRIC DOSAGE**
Bone Metastasis from Solid Tumors	**Giant Cell Tumor of Bone**
Prevention of Skeletal-Related Events: 120mg SQ every 4 weeks	Treatment of tumor that is unresectable or where surgical resection is likely to result in severe morbidity
Giant Cell Tumor of Bone	
Treatment of tumor that is unresectable or where surgical resection is likely to result in severe morbidity	**Adolescents (Skeletally Mature):** 120mg SQ every 4 weeks w/ additional 120mg doses on Days 8 and 15 of the 1st month of therapy
120mg SQ every 4 weeks w/ additional 120mg doses on Days 8 and 15 of the 1st month of therapy	
Hypercalcemia of Malignancy	
Refractory to Bisphosphonate Therapy: 120mg SQ every 4 weeks w/ additional 120mg doses on Days 8 and 15 of the 1st month of therapy	

ADMINISTRATION
SQ route
Administer in the upper arm, upper thigh, or abdomen.
Remove from refrigerator and bring to room temperature (up to 25°C [77°F]) prior to administration; do not warm any other way.
Avoid vigorous shaking.
Use 27-gauge needle to withdraw and inject entire vial contents.
Do not re-enter vial; discard vial after single-use or entry.

STORAGE
2-8°C (36-46°F). Do not freeze. Once removed from the refrigerator, do not expose to >25°C (77°F) or direct light; use w/in 14 days. Protect from direct light and heat.

HOW SUPPLIED
Inj: 120mg/1.7mL

CONTRAINDICATIONS
Hypocalcemia, known clinically significant hypersensitivity to denosumab.

WARNINGS/PRECAUTIONS
Do not give w/ other drugs that contain the same active ingredient (eg, Prolia). Hypersensitivity, including anaphylaxis, reported; initiate appropriate treatment and d/c therapy permanently if an anaphylactic or other clinically significant allergic reaction occurs. May cause severe symptomatic hypocalcemia, and fatal cases reported; increased risk in patients w/ increasing renal dysfunction, and w/ inadequate/no Ca^{2+} supplementation. Correct preexisting hypocalcemia prior to treatment, monitor Ca^{2+} levels throughout therapy especially in 1st weeks of initiation, and administer Ca^{2+}, Mg^{2+}, and vitamin D as necessary. Osteonecrosis of the jaw (ONJ) may occur; perform an oral exam and appropriate preventive dentistry prior to initiation of therapy and periodically during therapy. Avoid invasive dental procedures during therapy; consider temporary discontinuation of therapy if an invasive dental procedure must be performed. Atypical femoral fractures reported; evaluate patients w/ thigh/groin pain to rule out an incomplete femur fracture and consider interruption of therapy. Clinically significant hypercalcemia reported in patients w/ growing skeletons weeks to months following treatment discontinuation. May cause fetal harm.

ADVERSE REACTIONS
Fatigue/asthenia, hypophosphatemia, nausea.

DRUG INTERACTIONS
Monitor Ca^{2+} levels more frequently w/ other drugs that can lower Ca^{2+} levels.

PREGNANCY AND LACTATION
Pregnancy: Category D. Effects are likely to be greater during the 2nd and 3rd trimesters of pregnancy. Report pregnancies to Amgen.
Lactation: Not for use in nursing.
Reproductive Potential: Females of reproductive potential should use highly effective contraception during therapy, and for at least 5 months after the last dose of therapy. There is potential for fetal exposure when a male treated w/ therapy has unprotected sexual intercourse w/ a pregnant partner.

MECHANISM OF ACTION
IgG_2 monoclonal antibody; binds to RANK ligand (RANKL), a transmembrane or soluble protein essential for the formation, function, and survival of osteoclasts (cells responsible for bone resorption), thereby modulating Ca^{2+} release from bone. It prevents RANKL from activating its receptor, RANK, on the surface of osteoclasts, their precursors, and osteoclast-like giant cells.

PHARMACOKINETICS
Absorption: Bioavailability (62%). **Distribution:** Crosses placenta. **Elimination:** $T_{1/2}$=28 days.

PATIENT CONSIDERATIONS
Assessment: Assess for preexisting or risk of hypocalcemia, drug hypersensitivity, pregnancy/nursing status, and possible drug interactions. Perform an oral exam and appropriate preventive dentistry.

Monitoring: Monitor for anaphylactic/hypersensitivity reaction, ONJ, atypical femoral fracture, and other adverse reactions. Monitor Ca^{2+} levels. Perform an oral exam and appropriate preventive dentistry periodically.

Counseling: Advise to contact physician if experiencing symptoms of hypersensitivity reaction, hypocalcemia, ONJ, or atypical femoral fracture; persistent pain or slow healing of the mouth or jaw after dental surgery; or if pregnant/nursing. Advise to contact physician if symptoms of hypercalcemia following treatment discontinuation in patients w/ growing skeletons occur. Advise of the need for proper oral hygiene and routine dental care, to inform dentist that patient is receiving the drug, and to avoid invasive dental procedures during treatment. Advise females of reproductive potential to use highly effective contraception during and for at least 5 months after treatment. Advise that denosumab is also marketed as Prolia; instruct to inform physician if taking Prolia.

XIAFLEX — collagenase clostridium histolyticum   Rx

Class: Collagenase

> Corporal rupture (penile fracture), penile ecchymoses or hematoma, sudden penile detumescence, and/or a penile "popping" sound or sensation reported. Promptly evaluate signs/symptoms to assess for corporal rupture or severe penile hematoma that may require surgical intervention. Available for the treatment of Peyronie's disease only through a restricted program under a Risk Evaluation and Mitigation Strategy (REMS) called the Xiaflex REMS Program.

ADULT DOSAGE
Dupuytren's Contracture

W/ a Palpable Cord:
0.58mg per inj administered into a palpable cord w/ a contracture of a metacarpophalangeal (MP) joint or a proximal interphalangeal (PIP) joint

Approx 24-72 hrs after inj, perform a finger extension procedure if a contracture persists to facilitate cord disruption; refer to PI for instructions

4 weeks after inj and finger extension procedure, if a MP or PIP contracture remains, the cord may be re-injected w/ a single dose of 0.58mg and the

PEDIATRIC DOSAGE
Pediatric use may not have been established

finger extension procedure may be repeated (approx 24-72 hrs after inj); inj and finger extension procedures may be administered up to 3X per cord at approx 4-week intervals

Perform up to 2 inj in the same hand according to the inj procedure during a treatment visit; 2 palpable cords affecting 2 joints may be injected or 1 palpable cord affecting 2 joints in the same finger may be injected at 2 locations during a treatment visit

If patient has other palpable cords w/ contractures of MP or PIP joints, these cords may be injected at other treatment visits approx 4 weeks apart

Peyronie's Disease
Treatment of adult men w/ a palpable plaque and curvature deformity of at least 30° at the start of therapy

0.58mg per inj administered into a Peyronie's plaque; if >1 plaque is present, inject into the plaque causing the curvature deformity

A treatment course consists of a max of 4 treatment cycles; each treatment cycle consists of 2 inj procedures. The 2nd inj procedure is performed 1-3 days after the 1st

The penile modeling procedure is performed 1-3 days after the 2nd inj of the treatment cycle; refer to PI for instructions

The interval between treatment cycles is approx 6 weeks. The treatment course, therefore, consists of a max of 8 inj procedures and 4 modeling procedures

If the curvature deformity is <15° after the 1st, 2nd, or 3rd treatment cycle, or if further treatment is not clinically indicated, then the subsequent treatment cycles should not be administered

---

ADMINISTRATION
Intralesional route

Dupuytren's Contracture
Each vial and sterile diluent should only be used for a single inj; if 2 joints on the same hand are to be treated during a treatment visit, separate vials and syringes should be used for each reconstitution and inj.

Reconstitution of Lyophilized Powder:
1. Before use, allow the vial containing the lyophilized powder and the vial containing the diluent for reconstitution to stand at room temperature for at least 15 min and no longer than 60 min.
2. Use only the supplied diluent for reconstitution; the diluent contains Ca^{2+}, which is required for the activity of Xiaflex.
3. Using a 1mL syringe w/ 0.01mL graduations and a 27-gauge 1/2-inch needle (not supplied), withdraw a volume of the diluent supplied, as follows:
For Cords Affecting a MP Joint: 0.39mL
For Cords Affecting a PIP Joint: 0.31mL
4. Inject the diluent slowly into the sides of the vial containing the lyophilized powder.
5. Slowly swirl the sol to ensure that all of the lyophilized powder has gone into sol; do not invert the vial or shake the sol.
6. The reconstituted sol can be kept at room temperature for up to 1 hr or refrigerated for up to 4 hrs prior to administration; if the sol is refrigerated, allow it to return to room temperature for approx 15 min before use.
7. Discard the syringe and needle used for reconstitution and the diluent vial.

Preparation Prior to Inj:
1. Administration of a local anesthetic agent prior to inj is not recommended, as it may interfere w/ proper placement of the Xiaflex inj.
2. If injecting into a cord affecting the PIP joint of the 5th finger, care should be taken to inject as close to the palmar digital crease as possible (as far proximal to the digital PIP joint crease), and the needle insertion should not be >2-3mm in depth. Tendon ruptures occurred after inj near the digital PIP joint crease.
3. Reconfirm the cord(s) to be injected; the site chosen for each inj should be the area where the contracting cord is maximally separated from the underlying flexor tendons and where the skin is not intimately adhered to the cord.
4. Apply an antiseptic at the inj site and allow the skin to dry.

Inj Procedure:
1. Using a new 1mL hubless syringe that contains 0.01mL graduations w/ a permanently fixed, 27-gauge 1/2-inch needle (not supplied), withdraw a volume of reconstituted sol (containing 0.58mg of Xiaflex) as follows:
For Cords Affecting a MP Joint: 0.25mL
For Cords Affecting a PIP Joint: 0.20mL

2. W/ your non-dominant hand, secure the patient's hand to be treated while simultaneously applying tension to the cord, and w/ your dominant hand, place the needle into the cord, using caution to keep the needle w/in the cord.

3. Avoid having needle tip pass completely through the cord to help minimize the potential for inj into tissues other than the cord.

4. After needle placement, if there is any concern that the needle is in the flexor tendon, apply a small amount of passive motion at the distal interphalangeal joint.

5. If insertion of the needle into a tendon is suspected or paresthesia is noted by the patient, withdraw the needle and reposition it into the cord; if the needle is in the proper location, there will be some resistance noted during the inj procedure.

6. After confirming that the needle is correctly placed in the cord, inject approx 1/3 of the dose.

7. Withdraw the needle tip from the cord and reposition it in a slightly more distal location (approx 2-3mm) to the initial inj in the cord and inject another 1/3 of the dose.

8. Again withdraw the needle tip from the cord and reposition it a 3rd time proximal to the initial inj (approx 2-3mm) and inject the final portion of the dose into the cord.

9. When administering 2 inj in the same hand during a treatment visit, use a new syringe and separate vial of reconstituted sol for each inj. Repeat steps 1-9.

10. When administering 2 inj in the same hand during a treatment visit, begin w/ the affected finger in the most lateral aspect of the hand and continue toward the medial aspect (eg, 5th finger to index finger).

11. When administering 2 inj in a cord affecting 2 joints in the same finger, begin w/ the affected joint in the most proximal aspect of the finger and continue toward the distal aspect (eg, MP to PIP).

12. Wrap the patient's treated hand w/ a soft, bulky, gauze dressing.

13. Instruct the patient to limit motion of the treated finger(s) and to keep the injected hand elevated until hs.

14. Instruct the patient not to attempt to disrupt the injected cord(s) by self-manipulation and to return to the healthcare provider's office the next day for follow-up and a finger extension procedure(s), if needed.

15. Discard the unused portion of the reconstituted sol and diluent after inj; do not store, pool, or use any vials containing unused reconstituted sol or diluent.

Peyronie's Disease
Reconstitution of Lyophilized Powder:

1. Before use, allow the vial containing the lyophilized powder and the vial containing the diluent for reconstitution to stand at room temperature for at least 15 min and no longer than 60 min.

2. Use only the supplied diluent for reconstitution; the diluent contains Ca^{2+}, which is required for the activity of Xiaflex.

3. Using a 1mL syringe w/ 0.01mL graduations and a 27-gauge 1/2-inch needle (not supplied), withdraw a volume of 0.39mL of the diluent supplied.

4. Inject the diluent slowly into the sides of the vial containing the lyophilized powder.

5. Slowly swirl the sol to ensure that all of the lyophilized powder has gone into sol; do not invert the vial or shake the sol.

6. The reconstituted sol can be kept at room temperature for up to 1 hr or refrigerated for up to 4 hrs prior to administration; if the sol is refrigerated, allow it to return to room temperature for approx 15 min before use.

7. Discard the syringe and needle used for reconstitution and the diluent vial.

Identification of Treatment Area:
Prior to each treatment cycle, identify the treatment area as follows:

1. Induce a penile erection; a single intracavernosal inj of 10 or 20mcg of alprostadil may be used for this purpose. Apply antiseptic at inj site and allow the skin to dry prior to intracavernosal inj.

2. Locate the plaque at the point of max concavity (or focal point) in bend of the penis.

3. Mark the point w/ a surgical marker; this indicates target area in the plaque for Xiaflex deposition.

Inj Procedure:

1. Apply antiseptic at the inj site and allow the skin to dry.

2. Administer suitable local anesthetic, if desired.

3. Using a new hubless syringe containing 0.01mL graduations w/ a permanently fixed 27-gauge 1/2-inch needle (not supplied), withdraw a volume of 0.25mL of reconstituted sol (containing 0.58mg of Xiaflex).

4. The penis should be in a flaccid state before inj.

5. Place the needle tip on the side of the target plaque in alignment w/ the point of maximal concavity.

6. Orient the needle so that it enters the edge of the plaque and advance the needle into the plaque itself from the side; do not advance the needle beneath the plaque nor perpendicularly towards the corpora cavernosum.

7. Insert and advance the needle transversely through the width of the plaque, towards the opposite side of the plaque w/o passing completely through it.

8. Proper needle position is tested and confirmed by carefully noting resistance to minimal depression of the syringe plunger.

9. W/ the tip of the needle placed w/in the plaque, initiate inj, maintaining steady pressure to slowly inject Xiaflex into the plaque.

10. Withdraw the needle slowly so as to deposit the full dose along the needle track w/in the plaque; for plaques that are only a few mm in width, the distance of withdrawal of the syringe may be very minimal.

11. Upon complete withdrawal of the needle, apply gentle pressure at the inj site.

12. Apply a dressing as necessary.

13. Discard the unused portion of the reconstituted sol and diluent after each inj; do not store, pool, or use any vials containing unused reconstituted sol or diluent.

14. The 2nd inj of each treatment cycle should be made approx 2-3mm apart from the 1st inj.

STORAGE
2-8°C (36-46°F). Do not freeze. **Reconstituted Sol:** May keep at room temperature of 20-25°C (68-77°F) for up to 1 hr or refrigerate at 2-8°C (36-46°F) for up to 4 hrs.

HOW SUPPLIED
Inj: 0.9mg

CONTRAINDICATIONS
Treatment of Peyronie's plaques that involve the penile urethra, history of hypersensitivity to the medication or to collagenase used in any other therapeutic application or application method.

WARNINGS/PRECAUTIONS
Should be administered by a healthcare provider experienced in inj procedures of the hand and treatment of Dupuytren's contracture, or experienced in treatment of male urological diseases who has completed required training for use of collagenase clostridium histolyticum in the treatment of Peyronie's disease. Inj into collagen-containing structures (eg, tendons/ligaments of the hand, corpora cavernosa of the penis) may result in damage to those structures and possible permanent injury (eg, tendon rupture, ligament damage). Avoid injecting into the urethra, corpora cavernosa, tendons, nerves, blood vessels, or other collagen-containing structures. Other serious local reactions (eg, pulley rupture, ligament injury, complex regional pain syndrome, sensory abnormality of the hand) reported. Severe allergic reactions (eg, anaphylaxis) may occur. Avoid in patients w/ coagulation disorders.

ADVERSE REACTIONS
Dupuytren's Contracture: Peripheral edema, contusion, injection-site hemorrhage, injection-site reaction, pain in the injected extremity.
Peyronie's Disease: Penile hematoma, penile swelling, penile pain.

DRUG INTERACTIONS
Avoid in patients receiving concomitant anticoagulants, except low-dose aspirin (eg, ≤150mg/day).

PREGNANCY AND LACTATION
Pregnancy: Category B.
Lactation: Caution in nursing.

MECHANISM OF ACTION
Collagenase; hydrolyzes collagen, resulting in lysis of collagen deposits.

PHARMACOKINETICS
Absorption: (Peyronie's Disease) C_{max}= <29ng/mL (collagenase AUX-I), <71ng/mL (collagenase AUX-II); T_{max}=10 min.

PATIENT CONSIDERATIONS
Assessment: Assess for history of hypersensitivity to drug or to collagenase in other therapeutic applications, Peyronie's plaque involving the penile urethra, coagulation disorders, pregnancy/nursing status, and possible drug interactions.

Monitoring: Monitor for signs/symptoms of hypersensitivity reactions, tendon rupture, ligament damage, corporal rupture, penile ecchymoses/hematoma, sudden penile detumescence, penile "popping" sound or sensation, and other adverse reactions.

Counseling: Dupuytren's Contracture: Advise of serious complications that may result in inability to fully bend finger and may require surgery. Inform that inj is likely to result in swelling, bruising, bleeding, and/or pain of injected site and surrounding tissue. After inj, instruct not to flex/extend the fingers of injected hand, not to disrupt injected cord(s) by self-manipulation, to elevate injected hand until hs, and to promptly contact physician if there is evidence of infection, sensory changes in treated finger(s), trouble bending finger(s) after the swelling goes down, or skin laceration. Instruct to return for follow up 1-3 days after the inj visit. Instruct not to perform strenuous activity w/ injected hand until advised to do so, to wear splint at hs for up to 4 months, and to perform a series of finger flexion and extension exercises each day. **Peyronie's Disease:** Advise of serious complications that may require surgery to correct. Inform that penis may appear bruised and/or swollen, and that they may have mild to moderate penile pain that can be relieved by taking OTC medications. Instruct to promptly contact physician if they have severe pain, swelling, purple bruising/swelling of the penis, difficulty urinating or blood in the urine, or sudden loss of ability to maintain an erection; inform that these may be accompanied by a popping or cracking sound from the penis. Instruct to return to physician's office when directed for further inj(s) and/or penile modeling procedure(s), and to wait 2 weeks after 2nd inj of a treatment cycle before resuming sexual activity, provided pain and swelling have subsided. Advise not to have sex between the 1st and 2nd inj of a treatment cycle.

XIFAXAN — rifaximin   Rx

Class: Semisynthetic rifampin analogue

ADULT DOSAGE	PEDIATRIC DOSAGE
Traveler's Diarrhea	**Traveler's Diarrhea**
Noninvasive Strains of *Escherichia coli*:	**Noninvasive Strains of *E. coli*:**
200mg tid for 3 days	**≥12 Years:**
Hepatic Encephalopathy	200mg tid for 3 days
Reduction in Risk of Overt Recurrence:	
550mg bid	
Irritable Bowel Syndrome	
W/ Diarrhea:	
550mg tid for 14 days	
May retreat up to 2X w/ the same dosage regimen in patients who have recurrence of symptoms	

ADMINISTRATION
Oral route

Take w/ or w/o food.

STORAGE
20-25°C (68-77°F); excursions permitted to 15-30°C (59-86°F).

HOW SUPPLIED
Tab: 200mg, 550mg

CONTRAINDICATIONS
Hypersensitivity to rifaximin, any of the rifamycin antimicrobial agents, or any of the components in this medication.

WARNINGS/PRECAUTIONS
Should not be used in patients w/ diarrhea complicated by fever and/or blood in the stool or diarrhea due to pathogens other than *E. coli*. D/C if diarrhea symptoms worsen or persist >24-48 hrs; consider alternative antibiotic therapy. *Clostridium difficile*-associated diarrhea (CDAD) reported; may need to d/c if CDAD suspected or confirmed. Use in the absence of a proven or strongly suspected bacterial infection or a prophylactic indication may increase the risk of development of bacterial resistance. Caution w/ severe hepatic impairment (Child-Pugh Class C); may increase systemic exposure.

ADVERSE REACTIONS
Headache, peripheral edema, nausea, dizziness, fatigue, ascites, muscle spasms, pruritus, abdominal pain, anemia, depression, nasopharyngitis, arthralgia, dyspnea, pyrexia.

DRUG INTERACTIONS
Caution w/ P-gp inhibitors (eg, cyclosporine); may increase systemic exposure.

PREGNANCY AND LACTATION
Pregnancy: In rabbits, ocular, oral and maxillofacial, cardiac, and lumbar spine malformations were observed. Ocular malformations were observed in both rats and rabbits at doses that caused reduced maternal body weight gain.
Lactation: There is no information regarding the presence of rifaximin in human milk, the effects of rifaximin on the breastfed infant, or the effects of rifaximin on milk production. The developmental and health benefits of breastfeeding should be considered along w/ the mother's clinical need for therapy and any potential adverse effects on the breastfed infant from therapy or from the underlying maternal condition.

MECHANISM OF ACTION
Semisynthetic rifampin analogue; binds to β-subunit of bacterial DNA-dependent RNA polymerase blocking 1 of the steps in transcription, resulting in inhibition of bacterial protein synthesis and consequently inhibition of the growth of bacteria.

PHARMACOKINETICS
Absorption: Administration of variable doses resulted in different pharmacokinetic parameters. **Distribution:** Plasma protein binding (67.5%, healthy), (62%, hepatic impairment). **Metabolism:** Mainly by CYP3A4 (in vitro). **Elimination:** (400mg, healthy) Feces (96.62% mostly unchanged), urine (0.32% mostly metabolites, 0.03% unchanged). $T_{1/2}$=5.6 hrs (healthy); 6 hrs (irritable bowel syndrome w/ diarrhea).

PATIENT CONSIDERATIONS
Assessment: If diarrhea is present, assess for causative organisms and assess if diarrhea is complicated by fever or blood in stool. Assess for drug hypersensitivity, hepatic impairment, pregnancy/nursing status, and possible drug interactions.

Monitoring: Monitor for signs/symptoms of a hypersensitivity reaction, CDAD, development of drug-resistant bacteria, worsening of symptoms, and other adverse reactions.

Counseling: If being treated for traveler's diarrhea, instruct to d/c therapy and contact physician if diarrhea persists for >24-48 hrs or worsens. Advise to seek medical care for fever and/or blood in the stool. Inform that watery and bloody stools (w/ or w/o stomach cramps and fever) may occur even as late as ≥2 months after last dose; advise to contact physician as soon as possible. Inform that drug only treats bacterial, not viral, infections. Inform that skipping doses or not completing full course of therapy may decrease the effectiveness of treatment and increase resistance. Inform that there is an increase systemic exposure to therapy in patients w/ severe hepatic impairment (Child-Pugh Class C).

XIGDUO XR — dapagliflozin/metformin hydrochloride　　Rx

Class: Biguanide/sodium-glucose cotransporter 2 (SGLT2) inhibitor

---

Cases of metformin-associated lactic acidosis resulting in death, hypothermia, hypotension, and resistant bradyarrhythmias reported. Risk factors include renal impairment; concomitant use of certain drugs (eg, cationic drugs such as topiramate); age ≥65 years; having a radiological study w/ contrast media; surgery and other procedures; hypoxic states (eg, acute CHF); excessive alcohol intake; and hepatic impairment. D/C therapy immediately and institute general supportive measures in a hospital setting if metformin-associated lactic acidosis is suspected. Prompt hemodialysis is recommended.

ADULT DOSAGE
Type 2 Diabetes Mellitus
When treatment w/ both dapagliflozin and metformin is appropriate

Initial: Individualize dose based on current treatment
Titrate: Adjust dose based on effectiveness and tolerability.

PEDIATRIC DOSAGE
Pediatric use may not have been established

Dose escalations should be gradual to reduce GI side effects
Max: (10mg/2000mg)/day

Patients taking pm dose of metformin XR should skip their last dose before starting Xigduo XR

DOSING CONSIDERATIONS
Renal Impairment
eGFR <60mL/min/1.73m²: Contraindicated
eGFR ≥60mL/min/1.73m²: No dose adjustment necessary

Hepatic Impairment
Not recommended

Other Important Considerations
Patients w/ Volume-Depletion:
Correct this condition before initiating treatment

Iodinated Contrast Imaging Procedures:
D/C therapy at the time of, or prior to, an iodinated contrast imaging procedure in patients w/ a history of liver disease, alcoholism, or heart failure; or in patients who will be administered intra-arterial iodinated contrast. Reevaluate eGFR 48 hrs after the imaging procedure and restart therapy if renal function is stable

ADMINISTRATION
Oral route

Take qam w/ food.
Swallow tabs whole; do not crush, cut, or chew.

STORAGE
20-25°C (68-77°F); excursions permitted between 15-30°C (59-86°F).

HOW SUPPLIED
Tab: (Dapagliflozin/Metformin Extended-Release) 5mg/500mg, 5mg/1000mg, 10mg/500mg, 10mg/1000mg

CONTRAINDICATIONS
Moderate to severe renal impairment (eGFR <60mL/min/1.73m²), ESRD, or patients on dialysis. Acute or chronic metabolic acidosis, including diabetic ketoacidosis w/ or w/o coma. History of a serious hypersensitivity reaction to dapagliflozin or hypersensitivity to metformin.

WARNINGS/PRECAUTIONS
See Dosing Considerations. Not recommended for patients w/ type 1 diabetes mellitus or diabetic ketoacidosis. Obtain an eGFR at least annually; renal function should be assessed more frequently in patients at increased risk for the development of renal impairment (eg, elderly). **Dapagliflozin:** Causes intravascular volume contraction and can cause renal impairment. Symptomatic hypotension may occur after initiating therapy, particularly in patients w/ impaired renal function (eGFR <60mL/min/1.73m²), elderly patients, or patients on loop diuretics; assess and correct volume status before initiating treatment in patients w/ ≥1 of these characteristics. Ketoacidosis (including fatal cases) reported; if suspected, d/c and institute prompt treatment. Assess for ketoacidosis in patients presenting w/ signs/symptoms consistent w/ severe metabolic acidosis regardless of presenting blood glucose levels. Consider temporarily discontinuing therapy in clinical situations known to predispose to ketoacidosis (eg, prolonged fasting due to acute illness or surgery). Acute kidney injury reported; consider factors that may predispose to acute kidney injury before initiating therapy. Consider temporarily discontinuing in any setting of reduced oral intake or fluid losses; monitor for acute kidney injury. D/C therapy promptly and institute treatment if acute kidney injury occurs. May increase SrCr and decrease eGFR; elderly patients and patients w/ impaired renal function may be more susceptible. Serious UTIs (eg, urosepsis, pyelonephritis), requiring hospitalization, reported; evaluate for signs/symptoms of UTIs and treat promptly, if indicated. Increases risk of genital mycotic infections; monitor and treat appropriately. Increase in LDL levels reported. Cases of bladder cancer reported; do not use in patients w/ active bladder cancer and caution in patients w/ prior history of bladder cancer. Monitoring glycemic control w/ urine glucose tests or 1,5-anhydroglucitol assay is not recommended. **Metformin:** Withholding of food and fluids during surgical or other procedures may increase the risk for volume depletion, hypotension, and renal impairment; temporarily d/c while patient has restricted food and fluid intake. D/C if a condition associated w/ hypoxemia occurs (eg, cardiovascular collapse, acute MI, sepsis). Hypoglycemia may occur when caloric intake is deficient or when strenuous exercise is not compensated by caloric supplementation; elderly, debilitated, or malnourished patients and those w/ adrenal or pituitary insufficiency or alcohol intoxication are particularly susceptible to hypoglycemic effects. Hypoglycemia may be difficult to recognize in the elderly. May decrease vitamin B12 levels to subnormal levels; monitor hematologic parameters annually.

ADVERSE REACTIONS
Female genital mycotic infection, nasopharyngitis, UTI, diarrhea, headache.

DRUG INTERACTIONS
Concomitant use w/ topiramate or other carbonic anhydrase inhibitors (eg, zonisamide, acetazolamide, dichlorphenamide) may increase risk for lactic acidosis; consider more frequent monitoring of these patients. **Dapagliflozin:** May increase risk of hypoglycemia when combined w/ insulin or an insulin secretagogue; lower dose of insulin or insulin secretagogue may be required. **Metformin:** Hypoglycemia may occur during concomitant use w/ other glucose-lowering agents (eg, sulfonylureas, insulin) or ethanol. Alcohol potentiates the effect of metformin on lactate metabolism; avoid excessive alcohol intake. May be difficult to recognize hypoglycemia w/ β-adrenergic blocking drugs. Drugs that are eliminated by renal tubular secretion (eg, cationic drugs such as cimetidine), impair renal function, result in significant hemodynamic change, interfere w/ acid-base balance, or increase metformin accumulation may increase the risk

of metformin-associated lactic acidosis; consider more frequent monitoring of these patients. Thiazides and other diuretics, corticosteroids, phenothiazines, thyroid products, estrogens, oral contraceptives, phenytoin, nicotinic acid, sympathomimetics, calcium channel blockers, and isoniazid may produce hyperglycemia and lead to loss of glycemic control; monitor for loss of glycemic control when such drugs are administered and monitor for hypoglycemia when such drugs are withdrawn.

PREGNANCY AND LACTATION
Pregnancy: Category C.
Lactation: Not for use in nursing.

MECHANISM OF ACTION
Dapagliflozin: SGLT2 inhibitor; reduces reabsorption of filtered glucose and lowers the renal threshold for glucose, and thereby increases urinary glucose excretion. **Metformin:** Biguanide; decreases hepatic glucose production, decreases intestinal absorption of glucose, and improves insulin sensitivity by increasing peripheral glucose uptake and utilization.

PHARMACOKINETICS
Absorption: Dapagliflozin: Absolute oral bioavailability (78%, 10mg); T_{max}=2 hrs (fasted). Metformin: T_{max}=7 hrs (median). **Distribution:** Dapagliflozin: Plasma protein binding (91%). Metformin: V_d=654L (850mg immediate-release). **Metabolism:** Dapagliflozin: Primarily mediated by UGT1A9; CYP-mediated metabolism (minor). **Elimination:** Dapagliflozin: Urine (75%, <2% unchanged), feces (21%, 15% unchanged); $T_{1/2}$=12.9 hrs (10mg). Metformin: Urine (90%); $T_{1/2}$=6.2 hrs (plasma); 17.6 hrs (blood).

PATIENT CONSIDERATIONS
Assessment: Assess for hypersensitivity, acute/chronic metabolic acidosis (including diabetic ketoacidosis), risk factors for lactic acidosis, hypoxemia, alcoholism, presence of malnourishment or debilitation, adrenal/pituitary insufficiency, predisposition to developing subnormal vitamin B12 levels, risk for genital mycotic infections, history of bladder cancer, volume status, renal/hepatic impairment, any other conditions where treatment is contraindicated or cautioned, pregnancy/nursing status, and possible drug interactions. Assess if patient is planning to undergo any surgical procedure or any radiologic studies w/ intravascular iodinated contrast materials. Obtain baseline LFTs, FPG, HbA1c, eGFR, and hematologic parameters.

Monitoring: Monitor for signs/symptoms of lactic acidosis, hypotension, ketoacidosis, UTIs, genital mycotic infections, bladder cancer, and other adverse reactions. Monitor for changes in clinical status. Monitor renal function, at least annually; monitor more frequently in patients in whom development of renal impairment is anticipated (eg, elderly). Monitor hematologic parameters annually. Perform routine serum vitamin B12 measurements at 2- to 3-yr intervals in patients predisposed to developing subnormal vitamin B12 levels. Monitor FPG, HbA1c, and LDL levels.

Counseling: Inform of the potential risks and benefits of therapy; alternative modes of therapy; and the importance of adherence to dietary instructions, regular physical activity, periodic blood glucose monitoring and HbA1c testing, recognition and management of hypo/hyperglycemia, and assessment of diabetes complications. Advise to seek medical advice promptly during periods of stress (eg, fever, trauma, infection, surgery), as medication requirements may change. Counsel against excessive alcohol intake. Inform about the importance of regular testing of renal function and hematological parameters while on therapy. Inform that the incidence of hypoglycemia may be increased when added to an insulin secretagogue (eg, sulfonylurea) or insulin. Instruct to immediately report to physician if pregnant/breastfeeding, if experiencing symptoms of hypotension, or any signs of macroscopic hematuria or any other symptoms potentially related to bladder cancer. Inform that the inactive ingredients may occasionally be eliminated in the feces as a soft mass that may resemble the original tab. Inform of the risks of lactic acidosis, its symptoms, and conditions that predispose to its development; instruct to d/c immediately and notify physician if unexplained hyperventilation, myalgias, malaise, unusual somnolence, dizziness, slow or irregular heartbeat, sensation of feeling cold (especially in the extremities), or other nonspecific symptoms occur. Instruct to have adequate fluid intake. Instruct to d/c and seek medical advice immediately if symptoms of ketoacidosis occur. Counsel on the signs/symptoms of vaginal yeast infections, balanitis, balanoposthitis, and UTIs; inform of treatment options and when to seek medical advice. Instruct to d/c therapy and consult physician if any signs/symptoms suggesting an allergic reaction or angioedema develop. Inform that acute kidney injury has been reported and instruct to seek medical advice immediately if they have reduced oral intake or increased fluid losses.

XOFIGO — radium Ra 223 dichloride **Rx**
Class: Radiopharmaceutical agent

ADULT DOSAGE
Prostate Carcinoma

Use in patients w/ castration-resistant prostate cancer, symptomatic bone metastases and no known visceral metastatic disease

55kBq (1.49 microcurie)/kg by slow IV inj over 1 min given at 4-week intervals for 6 inj

Use the following to calculate the volume to be administered:
1. Patient's body weight (kg)

PEDIATRIC DOSAGE
Pediatric use may not have been established

2. Dosage level 55kBq/kg body weight or 1.49 microcurie/kg body weight
3. Radioactivity concentration of the product (1100kBq/mL; 30 microcurie/mL) at the reference date
4. Decay correction factor to correct for physical decay of radium-223

Volume to be administered (mL) = (Body weight in kg x 55kBq/kg body weight)/(Decay factor x 1100kBq/mL)

or

Volume to be administered (mL) = (Body weight in kg x 1.49 microcurie/kg body weight)/(Decay factor x 30 microcurie/mL)

Refer to PI for decay correction factor table

ADMINISTRATION
IV route

Do not dilute or mix w/ any sol.
Flush IV access line or cannula w/ isotonic saline before and after inj.
Use proper radiation protection when handling the drug.
Refer to PI for further information on instructions for use/handling.

STORAGE
Room temperature <40°C (104°F) in the original container or equivalent radiation shielding.

HOW SUPPLIED
Inj: 1100kBq/mL (30 microcurie/mL) [6mL]

CONTRAINDICATIONS
Pregnancy, women of childbearing potential.

WARNINGS/PRECAUTIONS
Bone marrow failure and myelosuppression (eg, thrombocytopenia, neutropenia, pancytopenia, leukopenia) reported; perform hematologic evaluation at baseline and prior to every dose. Before the 1st administration, the ANC should be ≥1.5 x 10^9/L, the platelet count ≥100 x 10^9/L and Hgb ≥10g/dL. Before subsequent administrations, the ANC should be ≥1 x 10^9/L and the platelet count ≥50 x 10^9/L. D/C therapy if there is no recovery to these values w/in 6-8 weeks after the last administration. Monitor closely and provide supportive care measures in patients w/ compromised bone marrow reserve; d/c in patients who experience life-threatening complications despite supportive care for bone marrow failure. Caution in elderly.

ADVERSE REACTIONS
N/V, diarrhea, peripheral edema, anemia, lymphocytopenia, leukopenia, thrombocytopenia, neutropenia.

DRUG INTERACTIONS
Concomitant use w/ chemotherapy is not recommended due to the potential for additive myelosuppression; d/c therapy if chemotherapy, other systemic radioisotopes, or hemibody external radiotherapy is administered during the treatment period.

PREGNANCY AND LACTATION
Pregnancy: Category X.
Lactation: It is not known whether radium-223 dichloride is excreted in human milk; not for use in nursing.
Reproductive Potential: Men who are sexually active should use condoms and their female partners of reproductive potential should use a highly effective contraceptive method during and for 6 months after completing treatment. There is a potential risk that radiation by Xofigo could impair human fertility.

MECHANISM OF ACTION
Radiopharmaceutical agent; α particle-emitting isotope radium-223, which mimics Ca^{2+} and forms complexes w/ the bone mineral hydroxyapatite at areas of increased bone turnover, such as bone metastases. The high linear energy transfer of α emitters leads to a high frequency of double-strand DNA breaks in adjacent cells, resulting in an antitumor effect on bone metastases.

PHARMACOKINETICS
Distribution: Distributed primarily into bone. **Elimination:** Urine (minimal), feces.

PATIENT CONSIDERATIONS
Assessment: Assess for compromised bone marrow reserve. Perform hematologic evaluation at baseline.

Monitoring: Monitor for bone marrow failure, myelosuppression, and other adverse reactions. Perform hematologic evaluation prior to every dose.

Counseling: Advise patients to be compliant w/ blood cell count monitoring appointments, to stay well hydrated, and to monitor oral intake, fluid status, and urine output while on therapy. Explain the importance of routine blood cell counts. Instruct to report signs of bleeding or infections, dehydration, hypovolemia, urinary retention, or renal failure/insufficiency. Inform that there is no restriction regarding contact w/ other people after receiving therapy. Advise to follow good hygiene practices while on therapy and for at least 1 week after the last inj in order to minimize radiation exposure from bodily fluids to household members and caregivers. Instruct caregivers to use universal precautions for patient care (eg, gloves and barrier gowns when handling bodily fluids). Advise patients who are sexually active to use condoms and their female partners of reproductive potential to use a highly effective method of birth control during therapy and for 6 months following completion of treatment.

XOLAIR — omalizumab   Rx

Class: Monoclonal antibody/IgE blocker

> Anaphylaxis, presenting as bronchospasm, hypotension, syncope, urticaria, and/or angioedema of throat or tongue, reported as early as after the 1st dose and beyond 1 yr of therapy; closely observe patients. Inform of the signs/symptoms of anaphylaxis and instruct to seek immediate medical care should symptoms occur.

ADULT DOSAGE

Asthma

Moderate to Severe Persistent Asthma w/ a (+) Skin Test or In Vitro Reactivity to a Perennial Aeroallergen and Inadequately Controlled w/ Inhaled Corticosteroids:
75-375mg SQ every 2 or 4 weeks, based on body weight (kg) and pretreatment serum total IgE level (IU/mL)

Periodically reassess the need for continued therapy based upon the patient's disease severity and level of asthma control

Refer to PI for dose determination charts and further information

Chronic Idiopathic Urticaria

Symptomatic Despite H1 Antihistamine Treatment:
150mg or 300mg SQ every 4 weeks

Periodically reassess the need for continued therapy

PEDIATRIC DOSAGE

Asthma

Moderate to Severe Persistent Asthma w/ a (+) Skin Test or In Vitro Reactivity to a Perennial Aeroallergen and Inadequately Controlled w/ Inhaled Corticosteroids:
≥6 Years:
75-375mg SQ every 2 or 4 weeks, based on body weight (kg) and pretreatment serum total IgE level (IU/mL)

Periodically reassess the need for continued therapy based upon the patient's disease severity and level of asthma control

Refer to PI for dose determination charts and further information

Chronic Idiopathic Urticaria

Symptomatic Despite H1 Antihistamine Treatment:
≥12 Years:
150mg or 300mg SQ every 4 weeks

Periodically reassess the need for continued therapy.

ADMINISTRATION
SQ route
The inj may take 5-10 sec to administer.
Do not administer more than 150mg (contents of one vial) per inj site.

Number of Inj and Total Inj Volume
75mg inj involves 1 inj (0.6mL total volume inj).
150mg inj involves 1 inj (1.2mL total volume inj).
225mg inj involves 2 inj (1.8mL total volume inj).
300mg inj involves 2 inj (2.4mL total volume inj).
375mg inj involves 3 inj (3.0mL total volume inj).

Reconstitution for Single Vial
Before reconstitution, determine the number of vials that will need to be reconstituted.
1. Reconstitute w/ sterile water for inj (SWFI).
2. Draw 1.4mL of SWFI into a 3mL syringe equipped w/ a 1-inch, 18-gauge needle.
3. Insert the needle and inject the SWFI directly onto the product.
4. Gently swirl the upright vial for approx 1 min; do not shake.
5. Gently swirl the vial for 5-10 sec approx every 5 min in order to dissolve any remaining solids. The lyophilized product takes 15-20 min to dissolve.
6. If it takes longer than 20 min to dissolve completely, gently swirl the vial for 5-10 sec approx every 5 min until there are no visible gel-like particles in the sol. Do not use if the contents of the vial do not dissolve completely by 40 min.
7. Invert the vial for 15 sec in order to allow the sol to drain toward the stopper.
8. Using a new 3mL syringe equipped w/ a 1-inch, 18-gauge needle, draw the sol into the syringe.
9. Replace the 18-gauge needle w/ a 25-gauge needle for SQ inj.

STORAGE
2-8°C (36-46°F). **Reconstituted:** 2-8°C (36-46°F) for up to 8 hrs, or 4 hrs at room temperature. Protect from direct sunlight.

HOW SUPPLIED
Inj: 150mg

CONTRAINDICATIONS
Severe hypersensitivity reaction to omalizumab or any ingredient of this medication.

WARNINGS/PRECAUTIONS
Not indicated for treatment of other forms of urticaria, relief of acute bronchospasm or status asthmaticus, or other allergic conditions. Administer only in a healthcare setting prepared to manage anaphylaxis and observe patients for an appropriate period after administration. D/C if a severe hypersensitivity reaction occurs. Malignant neoplasms reported. Do not abruptly d/c systemic or inhaled corticosteroids when initiating therapy. Eosinophilic conditions reported; be alert to eosinophilia, vasculitic rash, worsening pulmonary symptoms, cardiac complications, and/or neuropathy, especially upon reduction of oral corticosteroids. Monitor patients at high risk for geohelminth infections (eg, roundworm, hookworm). Signs/symptoms similar to those seen in patients w/ serum sickness, including arthritis/arthralgia, rash, fever, and lymphadenopathy, reported; d/c if these symptoms develop. Serum total IgE levels increase due to formation of Xolair:IgE complexes and may persist for up to 1 yr following discontinuation of therapy; do not use serum total IgE levels obtained <1 yr following discontinuation to reassess dosing regimen for asthma patients.

ADVERSE REACTIONS
Asthma: ≥12 Years: Arthralgia, pain (general), leg pain, fatigue, dizziness, fracture, arm pain, pruritus, dermatitis, earache.
Asthma: 6 to <12 Years: Nasopharyngitis, headache, pyrexia, upper abdominal pain, pharyngitis streptococcal, otitis media, viral gastroenteritis, arthropod bites, epistaxis.
Chronic Idiopathic Urticaria (CIU): Nausea, nasopharyngitis, sinusitis, URTI, viral URTI, arthralgia, headache, cough.

PREGNANCY AND LACTATION
Pregnancy: The data w/ Xolair use in pregnant women are insufficient to inform on drug-associated risk. Monoclonal antibodies (eg, omalizumab) are transported across the placenta in a linear fashion as pregnancy progresses; potential effects on a fetus are likely to be greater during the 2nd and 3rd trimesters of pregnancy.
Lactation: Caution in nursing.

MECHANISM OF ACTION
Monoclonal antibody/IgE blocker; (asthma) inhibits binding of IgE to the high-affinity IgE receptor on the surface of mast cells and basophils, limiting the degree of release of mediators of allergic response. CIU: Has not been established; binds to IgE and lowers free IgE levels; IgE receptors on cells down-regulate.

PHARMACOKINETICS
Absorption: Slow. Absolute bioavailability (62%); T_{max}=7-8 days. **Distribution:** V_d=78mL/kg. **Elimination:** $T_{1/2}$=26 days (asthma), 24 days (CIU).

PATIENT CONSIDERATIONS
Assessment: Assess for acute bronchospasm or status asthmaticus, malignancies, hypersensitivity reaction to drug or any of its ingredients, risk of geohelminth infections, and pregnancy/nursing status. Obtain baseline body weight and serum IgE levels.

Monitoring: Monitor for anaphylaxis, hypersensitivity reactions, inj-site reactions, malignancies, viral/geohelminth infections, URTIs, eosinophilia, vasculitic rash, worsening pulmonary symptoms, cardiac complications, neuropathy, arthritis/arthralgia, rash, fever, lymphadenopathy, and other adverse reactions. Periodically reassess need for continued therapy. Monitor body weight, CBC, and IgE levels prn.

Counseling: Instruct to read the medication guide before treatment. Inform of the risk of life-threatening anaphylaxis; instruct to seek immediate medical care if symptoms of anaphylaxis occur. Instruct not to decrease dose of or stop taking any other asthma or CIU medications unless otherwise instructed. Inform that immediate improvement of asthma or CIU symptoms may not be seen after beginning therapy. Instruct to notify physician if pregnant or breastfeeding.

XOLEGEL — ketoconazole   Rx

Class: Azole antifungal

ADULT DOSAGE

Seborrheic Dermatitis
Apply qd to affected area for 2 weeks

PEDIATRIC DOSAGE

Seborrheic Dermatitis
≥12 Years:
Apply qd to affected area for 2 weeks

ADMINISTRATION
Topical route

STORAGE
25°C (77°F); excursions permitted to 15-30°C (59-86°F).

HOW SUPPLIED
Gel: 2% [45g]

WARNINGS/PRECAUTIONS
Not for oral, ophthalmic, or intravaginal use. Flammable; avoid fire, flame, or smoking during and immediately following application. May cause local irritation at application site; d/c if irritation occurs or if disease worsens. If used during lactation and applied to chest, use caution to avoid accidental ingestion by infant. Hepatitis, lowered testosterone, and adrenocorticotropic hormone-induced corticosteroid serum levels reported with orally administered ketoconazole.

ADVERSE REACTIONS
Application-site burning.

DRUG INTERACTIONS
Coadministration of oral ketoconazole with CYP3A4 metabolized HMG-CoA reductase inhibitors (eg, simvastatin, lovastatin, atorvastatin) may increase risk of skeletal muscle toxicity, including rhabdomyolysis.

PREGNANCY AND LACTATION
Category C, caution in nursing.

MECHANISM OF ACTION
Azole antifungal; not established.

PHARMACOKINETICS
Absorption: Day 7: C_{max}=1.35ng/mL; T_{max}=8 hrs (median); AUC_{0-24}=20.8ng•hr/mL. Day 14: C_{max}=0.80ng/mL; T_{max}=7 hrs (median); AUC_{0-24}=15.6ng•hr/mL.

PATIENT CONSIDERATIONS
Assessment: Assess pregnancy/nursing status.

Monitoring: Monitor for irritation and worsening of seborrheic dermatitis.

Counseling: Inform that drug is for external use only. Instruct to use ud and to avoid contact with eyes, nostrils, and mouth. Advise to wash hands after application. Instruct not to use for any disorder other than that for which it has been prescribed. Advise to report any signs of adverse reactions to physician.

XOPENEX — levalbuterol hydrochloride   Rx

Class: Short-acting beta₂ agonist (SABA)

ADULT DOSAGE	PEDIATRIC DOSAGE
Bronchospasm	**Bronchospasm**
Treatment or Prevention of Bronchospasm Associated w/ Reversible Obstructive Airway Disease:	**Treatment or Prevention of Bronchospasm Associated w/ Reversible Obstructive Airway Disease:**
Initial: 0.63mg tid (q6-8h) by nebulization	**6-11 Years:**
Titrate: May increase to 1.25mg tid in patients w/ inadequate response to initial dose or w/ more severe asthma	**Usual:** 0.31mg tid by nebulization **Max:** 0.63mg tid
For doses <1.25mg, must use the non-concentrate formulation	**≥12 Years:**
	Initial: 0.63mg tid (q6-8h) by nebulization
	Titrate: May increase to 1.25mg tid in patients w/ inadequate response to initial dose or w/ more severe asthma
	For doses <1.25mg, must use the non-concentrate formulation

ADMINISTRATION
Oral inh route

Administer using a standard jet nebulizer (w/ face mask or mouthpiece) connected to an air compressor
Do not mix w/ other drugs in a nebulizer

Concentrate
Dilute w/ sterile normal saline before administration

STORAGE
20-25°C (68-77°F). Store in protective foil pouch at all times. Protect from light and excessive heat. Discard if sol is not colorless. (Non-Concentrate) Use w/in 2 weeks once foil pouch is opened; once removed from pouch, use w/in 1 week. (Concentrate) Use immediately once foil pouch is opened.

HOW SUPPLIED
Sol, Inhalation: 0.31mg/3mL, 0.63mg/3mL, 1.25mg/3mL [24⁵]; (Concentrate) 1.25mg/0.5mL [30⁵]

CONTRAINDICATIONS
History of hypersensitivity to levalbuterol or racemic albuterol.

WARNINGS/PRECAUTIONS
Reevaluate patient and treatment regimen if a previously effective dose regimen fails to provide relief, or there is a need for more doses than usual; anti-inflammatory treatment (eg, corticosteroids) may be needed. Not a substitute for corticosteroids. May produce paradoxical bronchospasm; d/c immediately and institute alternative therapy. May produce clinically significant cardiovascular (CV) effects (eg, changes in HR or BP); may need to d/c if this occurs. ECG changes and immediate hypersensitivity reactions may occur. Fatalities reported w/ excessive use; do not exceed recommended dose. Caution w/ CV disorders (eg, coronary insufficiency, arrhythmias, HTN), convulsive disorders, hyperthyroidism, or diabetes mellitus (DM), and in patients unusually responsive to sympathomimetic amines. Changes in blood glucose may occur; large doses of IV racemic albuterol reported to aggravate preexisting DM and ketoacidosis. May produce significant hypokalemia. Caution w/ renal impairment.

ADVERSE REACTIONS
Nervousness, tremor, rhinitis, increased cough, diarrhea, flu syndrome, viral infection, sinusitis, fever, headache, pharyngitis, rash, asthenia, pain.

DRUG INTERACTIONS
Avoid w/ other short-acting sympathomimetic bronchodilators or epinephrine; caution w/ additional adrenergic drugs administered by any route. Use w/ β-blockers may block pulmonary effects and produce severe bronchospasm in asthmatic patients; avoid concomitant use, but if needed, consider cardioselective β-blockers and use w/ caution. ECG changes and/or hypokalemia caused by non-K⁺-sparing diuretics (eg, loop/thiazide diuretics) may be worsened; use w/ caution and consider monitoring K⁺ levels. May decrease serum digoxin levels; monitor serum digoxin levels w/ concomitant use. Use extreme caution w/ MAOIs or TCAs, or w/in 2 weeks of discontinuation of such agents, or consider alternative therapy in patients taking MAOIs or TCAs.

PREGNANCY AND LACTATION
Category C, not for use in nursing.

MECHANISM OF ACTION
β₂-agonist; activates β₂-adrenergic receptors on airway smooth muscle, leading to the activation of adenylate cyclase and to an increase in intracellular cAMP. Increased cAMP leads to the activation of protein kinase A, which inhibits the phosphorylation of myosin and lowers intracellular ionic Ca^{2+} concentrations, resulting in relaxation of the smooth muscles of all airways, from the trachea to the terminal bronchioles.

PHARMACOKINETICS
Absorption: Administration of variable doses in different age groups resulted in different pharmacokinetic parameters. **Metabolism:** GI tract via SULT1A3 (sulfotransferase). **Elimination:** Urine (80-100%, unchanged or primary metabolite), feces (<20%); $T_{1/2}$=3.3 hrs (1.25mg, ≥12 yrs of age).

PATIENT CONSIDERATIONS
Assessment: Assess for history of hypersensitivity to the drug or racemic albuterol, CV disorders, convulsive disorders, hyperthyroidism, DM, ketoacidosis, renal impairment, pregnancy/nursing status, and possible drug interactions. Assess use in patients unusually responsive to sympathomimetic amines.

Monitoring: Monitor for paradoxical bronchospasm, deterioration of asthma, CV effects, ECG changes, hypokalemia, immediate hypersensitivity reactions, and other adverse effects. Monitor BP, HR, and blood glucose levels. Monitor renal function in the elderly.

Counseling: Instruct to report any hypersensitivity reactions to physician. Advise not to increase dose/frequency of doses w/o consulting physician. Advise to seek immediate medical attention if treatment becomes less effective for symptomatic relief, symptoms become worse, and/or there is a need to use the product more frequently than usual. Inform that product may produce paradoxical bronchospasm; instruct to d/c if this occurs. Instruct to take concurrent inhaled drugs and asthma medications only ud by the physician. Inform of the common adverse reactions of treatment (eg, chest pain, palpitations, fast HR). Advise to notify physician if pregnant/nursing.

XOPENEX HFA — levalbuterol tartrate   Rx

Class: Short-acting beta₂ agonist (SABA)

ADULT DOSAGE	PEDIATRIC DOSAGE
Bronchospasm	**Bronchospasm**
Associated w/ Reversible Obstructive Airway Disease:	**Associated w/ Reversible Obstructive Airway Disease:**
2 inh (90mcg) q4-6h	**≥4 Years:**
1 inh (45mcg) q4h may be sufficient in some patients	2 inh (90mcg) q4-6h
	1 inh (45mcg) q4h may be sufficient in some patients

DOSING CONSIDERATIONS
Elderly
Start at lower end of dosing range

ADMINISTRATION
Oral inh route

Shake well before use.
Avoid spraying in the eyes.
Wash actuator w/ warm water and air dry thoroughly at least once a week.
Discard canister after 200 actuations have been used from the 15g canister and 80 actuations from the 8.4g canister.

Priming
Prime inhaler before use for the 1st time or if not used for >3 days by releasing 4 test sprays into the air, away from face.

STORAGE
20-25°C (68-77°F). Store w/ mouthpiece down. Protect from freezing and direct sunlight. Contents under pressure; do not puncture or incinerate. Exposure to temperatures >49°C (120°F) may cause bursting.

HOW SUPPLIED
MDI: 45mcg/inh [80, 200 inhalations]

CONTRAINDICATIONS
History of hypersensitivity to levalbuterol, racemic albuterol, or any other component of the medication.

WARNINGS/PRECAUTIONS
If a previously effective dose regimen fails to provide the usual response or if more doses than usual are needed, this may be a marker of destabilization of asthma and may require reevaluation of the patient and treatment regimen; anti-inflammatory treatment (eg, corticosteroids) may be needed. D/C if paradoxical bronchospasm occur. ECG changes and immediate hypersensitivity reactions may occur. May need to d/c if cardiovascular (CV) effects occur. Fatalities reported w/ excessive use; do not exceed recommended dose. Caution w/ CV disorders (eg, coronary insufficiency, arrhythmias, HTN), convulsive disorders, hyperthyroidism, or diabetes mellitus (DM), and in patients unusually responsive to sympathomimetic amines. May produce significant hypokalemia. Caution w/ renal impairment.

ADVERSE REACTIONS
Pharyngitis, rhinitis, pain, vomiting, dizziness, asthma, bronchitis.

DRUG INTERACTIONS
Avoid w/ other short-acting sympathomimetic aerosol bronchodilators or epinephrine; caution w/ additional adrenergic drugs administered by any route. Use w/ β-blockers may block pulmonary effects and produce severe bronchospasm in asthmatic patients; avoid concomitant use. If needed, consider cardioselective β-blockers and use w/ caution. ECG changes and/or hypokalemia caused by non-K⁺-sparing diuretics (eg, loop or thiazide diuretics) may be worsened; use w/ caution and consider monitoring K⁺ levels. May decrease digoxin levels; monitor serum digoxin levels. Use extreme caution w/ MAOIs or TCAs, or w/in 2 weeks of discontinuation of such agents.

PREGNANCY AND LACTATION
Pregnancy: Category C.
Lactation: Not for use in nursing.

MECHANISM OF ACTION
β₂-agonist; activates β₂-adrenergic receptors on airway smooth muscle, leading to activation of adenylate cyclase and to an increase in cAMP. Increased cAMP leads to the activation of protein kinase A, which inhibits the phosphorylation of myosin and lowers intracellular ionic Ca^{2+} concentrations, resulting in relaxation of the smooth muscles of all airways, from the trachea to the terminal bronchioles.

PHARMACOKINETICS
Absorption: Administration of variable doses in different age groups resulted in different pharmacokinetic parameters. **Metabolism:** GI tract via SULT1A3 (sulfotransferase). **Elimination:** Urine (80-100%), feces (<20%).

PATIENT CONSIDERATIONS
Assessment: Assess for history of hypersensitivity to drug or racemic albuterol, CV disorders, convulsive disorders, hyperthyroidism, DM, renal impairment, pregnancy/nursing status, and possible drug interactions. Assess use in patients unusually responsive to sympathomimetic amines.

Monitoring: Monitor for paradoxical bronchospasm, deterioration of asthma, CV effects, ECG changes, hypokalemia, immediate hypersensitivity reactions, and other adverse effects. Monitor BP, HR, and ECG changes.

Counseling: Counsel not to increase dose or frequency of doses w/o consulting physician. Advise to seek immediate medical attention if treatment becomes less effective for symptomatic relief, symptoms become worse, and/or there is a need to use the product more frequently than usual. Inform that drug may cause paradoxical bronchospasm; instruct to d/c if this occurs. Instruct to take concurrent inhaled drugs and other asthma medications only ud. Inform of the common side effects (eg, chest pain, palpitations, rapid HR, tremor, nervousness). Instruct to notify physician if pregnant/nursing. Advise to discard after 200 actuations have been released from the 15g canister or 80 actuations have been released from the 8.4g canister.

XTAMPZA ER — oxycodone   CII
Class: Opioid analgesic

> Exposes patients and other users to the risks of opioid addiction, abuse, and misuse, which can lead to overdose and death; assess risk prior to prescribing and regularly monitor for these behavior conditions. Serious, life-threatening, or fatal respiratory depression may occur; monitor for respiratory depression, especially during initiation or following a dose increase. Accidental ingestion, especially by children, can result in a fatal overdose. Prolonged use during pregnancy can result in neonatal opioid withdrawal syndrome and requires management; if prolonged use is required, advise patient of the risk and ensure that appropriate treatment is available. Concomitant CYP3A4 inhibitors may increase oxycodone plasma concentrations. Discontinuation of a concomitant CYP3A4 inducer may result in an increase in oxycodone plasma concentration. Monitor patients receiving any CYP3A4 inhibitor or inducer.

ADULT DOSAGE
Severe Pain (Daily, Around-the-Clock Management)

Use when alternative treatments are inadequate

First Opioid Analgesic (Opioid-Naive):
Initial: 9mg q12h

Not Opioid Tolerant:
Initial: 9mg q12h

Titrate: Adjust to dose that provides adequate analgesia and minimizes adverse reactions. If pain increases after dose stabilization, identify source of increased pain before increasing dose. Dose may be adjusted q1-2 days.

Max: 288mg/day

Use lowest effective dose for the shortest duration consistent w/ individual treatment goals

Conversions
Oral Oxycodone to Xtampza ER:
Give 1/2 of total daily oral oxycodone dose as Xtampza ER q12h; monitor for dosage adjustment

Other Opioids to Xtampza ER:
Initial: 9mg q12h; d/c all other around-the-clock opioids

Methadone to Xtampza ER:
Closely monitor; conversion ratio may vary widely

Transdermal Fentanyl to Xtampza ER:
Substitute 25mcg/hr patch for 9mg q12h cap; monitor closely
Start Xtampza ER 18 hrs after removal of last transdermal patch

Oxycodone HCl=Xtampza ER (Oxycodone Base):
10mg=9mg
15mg=13.5mg
20mg=18mg
30mg=27mg
40mg=36mg

PEDIATRIC DOSAGE
Pediatric use may not have been established

DOSING CONSIDERATIONS
Renal Impairment
CrCl <60mL/min:
Use conservative approach to dose initiation and adjust according to the clinical situation
Use alternate analgesics for patients who require <9mg of Xtampza ER

Hepatic Impairment
Initial: 1/3 to 1/2 usual starting dose followed by careful dose titration; monitor closely for adverse events
Use alternate analgesics for patients who require <9mg of Xtampza ER

Elderly
Use w/ caution; start at low end of dosing range.

Adverse Reactions
Unacceptable Opioid-Related Adverse Reactions: May reduce subsequent doses

Discontinuation
Gradually titrate downwards; do not d/c abruptly

ADMINISTRATION
Oral route

- Must be taken w/ food; take w/ approx same amount of food for every dose in order to ensure consistent plasma levels.
- Single doses >36mg or total daily dose >72mg are to be administered only to patients in whom tolerance to an opioid of comparable potency has been established.

Patients Unable to Swallow Cap
1. Open the cap and sprinkle contents (microspheres) onto a small amount of soft food (eg, applesauce, pudding, yogurt) or into a cup and then administer directly into mouth and swallow immediately.
2. Rinse mouth to ensure all contents have been swallowed.
3. Discard cap shells after contents have been sprinkled.

NG Tube or Gastrostomy Tube
1. Flush tube w/ water.
2. Open cap and carefully pour microspheres directly into tube. Do not premix cap contents w/ the liquid that you will be using to flush them through the tube.
3. Draw up 15mL of water into a syringe, insert the syringe into tube, and flush microspheres through tube.
4. Repeat flushing 2 more times, each w/ 10mL of water.

Milk or liquid nutritional supplement may be used as vehicles for flush and administration through feeding tubes.

STORAGE
25°C (77°F); excursions permitted between 15-30°C (59-86°F).

HOW SUPPLIED
Cap, Extended-Release: 9mg, 13.5mg, 18mg, 27mg, 36mg

CONTRAINDICATIONS
Significant respiratory depression, acute or severe bronchial asthma in an unmonitored setting or in the absence of resuscitative equipment, known or suspected GI obstruction, (eg, paralytic ileus), hypersensitivity (eg, anaphylaxis) to oxycodone.

WARNINGS/PRECAUTIONS
Increased risk of decreased respiratory drive in patients w/ significant COPD or cor pulmonale, and those w/ a substantially decreased respiratory reserve, hypoxia, hypercapnia, or preexisting respiratory depression. Life-threatening respiratory depression is more likely to occur in elderly, cachectic, or debilitated patients; monitor closely, particularly when initiating/titrating and w/ concomitant use w/ other respiratory depressants. Consider use of non-opioid analgesics in these patients. Adrenal insufficiency reported w/ opioid use; wean patient off opioid and treat w/ corticosteroids until adrenal function recovers. May cause severe hypotension (eg, orthostatic hypotension, syncope) in ambulatory patients. Increased risk in patients whose ability to maintain BP has been compromised by a reduced blood volume or concurrent administration of certain CNS depressant drugs (eg, phenothiazines, general anesthetics); monitor signs of hypotension after initiating or titrating. Avoid use w/ circulatory shock. May reduce respiratory drive, and resultant CO_2 retention may further increase intracranial pressure in patients who are susceptible to the intracranial effects of CO_2 retention (eg, increased intracranial pressure, brain tumors); monitor for signs of sedation and respiratory depression, especially at initiation. May obscure clinical course in a patient w/ a head injury. Avoid use w/ impaired consciousness or coma. May cause spasm of the sphincter of Oddi and increases in serum amylase. Monitor patients w/ biliary tract disease, including acute pancreatitis, for worsening symptoms. May increase frequency of seizures in patients w/ seizure disorders, and may increase risk of seizures in other clinical settings associated w/ seizures; monitor patients w/ a history of seizure disorders for worsened seizure control therapy. May impair the mental or physical abilities.

ADVERSE REACTIONS
N/V, headache, constipation, somnolence, pruritus, dizziness.

DRUG INTERACTIONS
CYP3A4 inhibitors (eg, erythromycin, ketoconazole, ritonavir) may increase plasma concentration; consider dosage reduction of Xtampza ER until stable drug effects are achieved. If CYP3A4 inhibitor is discontinued, consider increasing the Xtampza ER dose until stable drug effects are achieved; monitor for signs of opioid withdrawal. CYP3A4 inducers (eg, rifampin, carbamazepine, phenytoin) may decrease plasma concentration; consider increasing the Xtampza ER dosage until stable drug effects are achieved. If CYP3A4 inducer is discontinued, consider Xtampza ER dosage reduction and monitor for signs of respiratory depression. Concomitant use of CNS depressants can increase risk of hypotension, respiratory depression, profound sedation, coma, and death; consider dose reduction of one or both drugs and monitor for signs of respiratory depression, sedation,

and hypotension. May cause serotonin syndrome w/ other drugs that affect the serotonergic neurotransmitter system (eg, SSRIs, SNRIs, TCAs); carefully observe and d/c Xtampza ER if serotonin syndrome is suspected. Mixed agonist/antagonist (eg, pentazocine, nalbuphine, butorphanol) and partial agonist opioid analgesics (eg, buprenorphine) may reduce the analgesic effect of Xtampza ER and/or precipitate withdrawal symptoms; avoid concomitant use. May enhance neuromuscular blocking action of skeletal muscle relaxants and produce an increased degree of respiratory depression; monitor for signs of respiratory depression that may be greater than otherwise expected and decrease the dosage of Xtampza ER and/or the muscle relaxant as necessary. May reduce efficacy of diuretics by inducing the release of antidiuretic hormone; monitor for signs of diminished diuresis and/or effects on BP and increase the dosage of the diuretic as needed. Anticholinergics may increase risk of urinary retention and/or severe constipation, which may lead to paralytic ileus; monitor for signs of urinary retention or reduced gastric motility.

PREGNANCY AND LACTATION
Pregnancy: There are no available data in pregnant women to inform a drug-associated risk for major birth defects and miscarriage. Prolonged use during pregnancy may cause neonatal opioid withdrawal syndrome. Monitor neonates during labor for signs of excess sedation and respiratory depression.
Lactation: Present in breast milk; not for use in nursing.
Females and Males of Reproductive Potential: Chronic use may cause reduced fertility.

MECHANISM OF ACTION
Opioid analgesic; precise mechanism of the analgesic action is unknown. Specific CNS opioid receptors for endogenous compounds w/ opioid-like activity have been identified throughout the brain and spinal cord and are thought to play a role in the analgesic effects of this drug.

PHARMACOKINETICS
Absorption: T_{max}=4.5 hrs (fed); C_{max}=55.3ng/mL (fed, intact cap); AUC=540hr•ng/mL (fed, intact cap). Refer to PI for sprinkled cap parameters. **Distribution:** V_d=2.6L/kg; plasma protein binding (approx 45%); crosses the placenta; found in the breast milk. **Metabolism:** Extensive via CYP3A4 and CYP2D6 to noroxycodone (major metabolite), oxymorphone (metabolite), and noroxymorphone (major metabolite). **Elimination:** Urine; $T_{1/2}$=5.6 hrs.

PATIENT CONSIDERATIONS
Assessment: Assess for risks for opioid abuse, addiction, or misuse, patient's general condition and medical status, severity and type of pain, respiratory depression, bronchial asthma, COPD, cor pulmonale, hypercarbia, GI obstruction, drug hypersensitivity, renal/hepatic impairment, pregnancy/nursing status, any other conditions where treatment is contraindicated or cautioned, and possible drug interactions.

Monitoring: Monitor for development of addiction, abuse, or misuse, physical dependence, tolerance, respiratory depression, impaired consciousness, adrenal insufficiency, hypotension, seizures, and other adverse reactions. Monitor serum amylase levels. Monitor patients w/ biliary tract disease. Carefully monitor during initiation or when titrating the dose.

Counseling: Inform of risks/benefits of therapy. Instruct on proper administration. Inform that use can result in addiction, abuse, and misuse, which can lead to overdose and death. Instruct not to share w/ others and advise to take steps to protect from theft or misuse. Advise how to recognize respiratory depression and to seek medical attention if breathing difficulties develop. Inform that accidental ingestion, especially by children, may result in respiratory depression or death. Instruct to take steps to store securely and to dispose of unused caps by flushing down the toilet. Inform that potentially serious additive effects may occur if Xtampza ER is used w/ other CNS depressants and advise not to use such drugs unless supervised by a healthcare provider. Inform that serotonin syndrome may occur w/ concomitant use of serotonergic drugs; warn of the symptoms of serotonin syndrome and advise to seek medical attention right away if symptoms develop. Inform that treatment may cause adrenal insufficiency and advise to seek medical attention if experiencing a constellation of adrenal insufficiency symptoms. Instruct how to recognize symptoms of low BP and how to reduce the risk of serious consequences should hypotension occur. Inform that anaphylaxis may occur and advise how to recognize such a reaction and when to seek medical attention. Inform female patients of reproductive potential that prolonged use during pregnancy can result in neonatal opioid withdrawal syndrome and that treatment can cause fetal harm; instruct to inform healthcare provider of a known or suspected pregnancy. Advise that breastfeeding is not recommended during treatment. Inform that chronic use of opioids may cause reduced fertility. Inform that treatment may impair the ability to perform potentially hazardous activities (eg, driving a car, operating heavy machinery); advise not to perform such tasks until the patient knows how he or she will react to treatment. Advise of the potential for severe constipation, including management instructions and when to seek medical attention.

Xtandi — enzalutamide
Class: Antiandrogen

Rx

ADULT DOSAGE	PEDIATRIC DOSAGE
Metastatic Castration-Resistant Prostate Cancer	Pediatric use may not have been established
160mg (four 40mg caps) qd	

DOSING CONSIDERATIONS
Concomitant Medications
Strong CYP2C8 Inhibitors: Avoid concomitant use; if coadministration is necessary, reduce enzalutamide dose to 80mg qd. If coadministration of the strong inhibitor is discontinued, return to enzalutamide dose used prior to initiation of the strong CYP2C8 inhibitor
Strong CYP3A4 Inducers: Avoid concomitant use; if coadministration is necessary, increase enzalutamide dose from 160mg to 240mg qd. If coadministration of the strong inducer is discontinued, return to enzalutamide dose used prior to initiation of the strong CYP3A4 inducer

Adverse Reactions
≥Grade 3 Toxicity/Intolerable Side Effect: Withhold dosing for 1 week or until symptoms improve to ≤Grade 2, then resume at the same or a reduced dose (120mg or 80mg), if warranted

ADMINISTRATION
Oral route

Take w/ or w/o food.
Swallow caps whole; do not chew, dissolve, or open.

STORAGE
20-25°C (68-77°F); excursions permitted from 15-30°C (59-86°F). Store in a dry place; keep container tightly closed.

HOW SUPPLIED
Cap: 40mg

CONTRAINDICATIONS
Women who are or may become pregnant.

WARNINGS/PRECAUTIONS
Seizures reported; caution in engaging in any activity where sudden loss of consciousness could cause serious harm to patient or to others. D/C permanently if seizures develop during treatment. Posterior reversible encephalopathy syndrome (PRES) reported; d/c if PRES develops. Caution in elderly.

ADVERSE REACTIONS
Asthenia/fatigue, back pain, decreased appetite, constipation, arthralgia, diarrhea, hot flush, URTI, peripheral edema, dyspnea, musculoskeletal pain, decreased weight, headache, HTN, dizziness/vertigo.

DRUG INTERACTIONS
See Dosing Considerations. Coadministration of a strong CYP2C8 inhibitor (gemfibrozil) increased exposure of enzalutamide. Coadministration of rifampin (strong CYP3A4 inducer and moderate CYP2C8 inducer) decreased exposure. St John's wort may decrease exposure and should be avoided. May reduce plasma exposure of midazolam (CYP3A4 substrate), warfarin (CYP2C9 substrate), and omeprazole (CYP2C19 substrate). Avoid concomitant use w/ narrow therapeutic index drugs that are metabolized by CYP3A4 (eg, alfentanil, cyclosporine, dihydroergotamine, sirolimus), CYP2C9 (eg, phenytoin, warfarin), and CYP2C19 (eg, S-mephenytoin); enzalutamide may decrease their exposure. If coadministration w/ warfarin cannot be avoided, conduct additional INR monitoring.

PREGNANCY AND LACTATION
Pregnancy: Category X.
Lactation: Not for use in nursing.

MECHANISM OF ACTION
Nonsteroidal antiandrogen; acts on different steps in the androgen receptor signaling pathway. Competitively inhibits androgen binding to androgen receptors and inhibits androgen receptor nuclear translocation and interaction w/ DNA.

PHARMACOKINETICS
Absorption: C_{max}=16.6mcg/mL, 12.7mcg/mL (major active metabolite); T_{max}=1 hr (median). **Distribution:** V_d=110L; plasma protein binding (97-98%, 95% active metabolite). **Metabolism:** Hepatic via CYP2C8 and CYP3A4; N-desmethyl enzalutamide (major active metabolite). **Elimination:** Urine (71%), feces (14%, 0.4% unchanged, 1% active metabolite); $T_{1/2}$=5.8 days, 7.8-8.6 days (major active metabolite).

PATIENT CONSIDERATIONS
Assessment: Assess pregnancy/nursing status and for possible drug interactions.

Monitoring: Monitor for seizures, PRES, and other adverse reactions. Conduct additional INR monitoring if coadministration w/ warfarin cannot be avoided.

Counseling: Instruct to take dose at the same time each day. Inform those receiving a gonadotropin-releasing hormone analogue to maintain such treatment during the course of therapy. Inform that therapy has been associated w/ increased risk of seizures; discuss conditions that may predispose to seizures and medications that may lower seizure threshold. Advise of risk of engaging in any activity where sudden loss of consciousness could cause serious harm to self or others. Inform patients to contact physician right away if they have loss of consciousness or seizures. Inform to contact physician right away if rapidly worsening symptoms possibly indicative of PRES are experienced. Instruct not to interrupt, modify dose, or d/c therapy w/o 1st consulting physician. Instruct not to take more than the prescribed dose per day. Apprise of the common side effects associated w/ therapy. Inform that drug may cause infections, falls and fall-related injuries, and HTN. Instruct to use a condom if having intercourse w/ a pregnant woman, and to use a condom and another effective birth control method if having intercourse w/ a woman of childbearing potential; advise that these measures are required during and for 3 months after treatment.

XULANE — ethinyl estradiol/norelgestromin   Rx
Class: Estrogen/progestogen combination

> Cigarette smoking increases risk of serious cardiovascular (CV) events from hormonal contraceptive use. Risk increases w/ age, particularly in women >35 years of age, and w/ the number of cigarettes smoked. Should not be used by women who are >35 yrs of age and smoke. May increase risk of venous thromboembolism (VTE) among users of norelgestromin and ethinyl estradiol transdermal system compared to women who use certain oral contraceptives. Has higher steady state concentrations and a lower peak concentration than oral contraceptives.

OTHER BRAND NAMES
Ortho Evra (Discontinued)

ADULT DOSAGE
Contraception

Apply 1st patch during the first 24 hrs of menstrual period or on the 1st Sunday after menstrual period begins. Apply patch each week on the same day for 3 weeks (21 total days). Week 4 is patch-free. On the day after Week 4 ends, a new 4-week cycle is started by applying a new patch. There should not be more than a 7-day patch-free interval between dosing cycles

Conversions
Switching From the Pill or Vaginal Contraceptive Ring:
Complete current pill/ring cycle and apply 1st patch on the day patient would have normally started next pill or inserted next vaginal ring; if patch is applied >1 week after taking last active pill or removal of last vaginal ring, use nonhormonal contraceptive concurrently for the first 7 days of patch use

PEDIATRIC DOSAGE
Contraception
Not indicated for use premenarche; refer to adult dosing

DOSING CONSIDERATIONS
Other Important Considerations
Use After Childbirth:
Start no sooner than 4 weeks after childbirth in women who elect not to breastfeed. If use is begun postpartum, and patient has not yet had a period, consider the possibility of ovulation and conception occurring prior to use; use an additional method of contraception, (eg, condom and spermicide, diaphragm and spermicide) for the first 7 days.

Use After Abortion/Miscarriage:
1st Trimester: May start patch use immediately; additional method of contraception is not needed. If patch use is not started w/in 5 days following a 1st trimester abortion, follow instructions for starting patch for the 1st time and use non-hormonal contraceptive method in the meantime
2nd Trimester: Start no earlier than 4 weeks after a 2nd trimester abortion/miscarriage

ADMINISTRATION
Transdermal route

Apply immediately upon removal from protective pouch.
Only 1 patch should be worn at a time; make sure to remove old patch prior to applying the new patch.
Do not cut, damage, or alter patch in any way.
Apply to clean and dry skin on upper outer arm, abdomen, buttock, or back in a place where it will not be rubbed by tight clothing; do not place on breasts, on cut/irritated skin, or on the same location as previous patch.
Do not reapply patch if it is no longer sticky, if it has become stuck to itself or another surface, or if it has other material stuck to it.
Refer to PI for further administration instructions.

Sunday Start Regimen
Use a non-hormonal backup method of birth control (eg, condom and spermicide, diaphragm and spermicide) for the first 7 days of the 1st cycle only. If period starts on a Sunday, the 1st patch should be applied that day, and no backup contraception is needed.

STORAGE
20-25°C (68-77°F). Store patches in their protective pouches. Do not store in the refrigerator or freezer.

HOW SUPPLIED
Patch: (Ethinyl Estradiol [EE]/Norelgestromin [NGMN]) (35mcg/150mcg)/day [1^s, 3^s]

CONTRAINDICATIONS
High risk of arterial/venous thrombotic diseases (eg, smoking if >35 yrs of age, history/presence of deep vein thrombosis/pulmonary embolism, inherited or acquired hypercoagulopathies, cerebrovascular disease, coronary artery disease, thrombogenic valvular or thrombogenic rhythm diseases of the heart [eg, subacute bacterial endocarditis w/ valvular disease, A-fib], uncontrolled HTN; diabetes mellitus w/ vascular disease, headaches w/ focal neurological symptoms or migraine headaches w/ aura [women >35 yrs of age w/ any migraine headaches]), benign or malignant liver tumors, liver disease, undiagnosed abnormal uterine bleeding, pregnancy, current or history of breast cancer or other estrogen- or progestin-sensitive cancer.

WARNINGS/PRECAUTIONS
May be less effective in preventing pregnancy in women who weigh ≥198 lbs (90kg). Increased risk of thromboembolic/thrombotic disease, and arterial thromboses. Risk of VTE is highest during the 1st year of use of combination hormonal contraceptives (CHCs) and when restarting hormonal contraception after a break of ≥4 weeks. D/C if an arterial or deep venous thrombotic event occurs. D/C if unexplained loss of vision, proptosis, diplopia, papilledema, or retinal vascular lesions develop; evaluate for retinal vein thrombosis immediately. If feasible, d/c at least 4 weeks before and through 2 weeks after major surgery or other surgeries associated w/ an elevated risk of VTE. D/C during prolonged immobilization. Start use no earlier than 4 weeks after delivery in women who are not breastfeeding. D/C if jaundice develops. Hepatic adenomas and increased risk of hepatocellular carcinoma reported. Increase in BP reported. Monitor BP in women w/ well-controlled HTN; d/c if BP rises significantly. Increased risk of cervical cancer or intraepithelial neoplasia, and gallbladder disease. Women w/ a history of pregnancy-related cholestasis may be at an increased risk for CHC-related cholestasis. May decrease glucose tolerance; monitor prediabetic and diabetic women. Consider alternative contraception w/ uncontrolled dyslipidemia. May increase risk of pancreatitis w/ hypertriglyceridemia or a family history thereof. Evaluate the cause of new headaches that are recurrent, persistent, or severe, and d/c if indicated; consider discontinuation in case of increased frequency or severity of migraine during use. Unscheduled bleeding and spotting reported. Consider non-hormonal causes and take adequate diagnostic measures to rule out malignancy, other pathology, or pregnancy in the event of unscheduled bleeding. Consider possibility of pregnancy in the event of amenorrhea. Amenorrhea or oligomenorrhea may occur after discontinuation of therapy. Administration of therapy should not be used as a test for pregnancy. Caution w/ history of depression; d/c if depression recurs to a serious degree. May raise the serum concentrations of sex hormone-binding globulin. Exogenous estrogens may induce or exacerbate symptoms of angioedema in patients w/ hereditary angioedema. Chloasma may occur, especially in women w/ a history of chloasma gravidarum; women w/ a tendency to chloasma should avoid exposure to sun or UV radiation. May influence the results of certain laboratory tests.

ADVERSE REACTIONS
Breast symptoms, N/V, headache, application-site disorder, abdominal pain, dysmenorrhea, vaginal bleeding, menstrual disorders, mood/affect/anxiety disorders.

DRUG INTERACTIONS
Drugs or herbal products that induce certain enzymes, including CYP3A4 (eg, phenytoin, barbiturates, products containing St. John's wort), may decrease levels and potentially diminish effectiveness or increase breakthrough bleeding; use an alternative method of contraception or a backup method when used concomitantly w/ enzyme inducers, and continue backup contraception for 28 days after discontinuing the enzyme inducer. Atorvastatin or rosuvastatin may increase EE exposure; ascorbic acid and acetaminophen (APAP) may increase EE levels. CYP3A4 inhibitors (eg, itraconazole, voriconazole, grapefruit juice) may increase plasma hormone levels. Significant changes (decreased/increased) sometimes noted in estrogen and/or progestin levels when coadministered w/ HIV/hepatitis C virus protease inhibitors or w/ non-nucleoside reverse transcriptase inhibitors. May inhibit the metabolism of other compounds (eg, cyclosporine, prednisolone, theophylline) and increase their plasma concentrations. May decrease concentrations of APAP, clofibric acid, morphine, salicylic acid, and temazepam. May decrease levels of lamotrigine and reduce seizure control; dosage adjustments of lamotrigine may be necessary. May raise the serum concentrations of thyroxine-binding globulin and cortisol-binding globulin; dose of replacement thyroid hormone or cortisol therapy may need to be increased.

PREGNANCY AND LACTATION
Pregnancy: Contraindicated in pregnancy.
Lactation: Not for use in nursing. May reduce milk production. Small amounts of contraceptive steroids and/or metabolites are present in breast milk.

MECHANISM OF ACTION
Estrogen/progestogen combination; acts by suppression of gonadotropins. Although the primary mechanism of this action is inhibition of ovulation, other alterations include changes in the cervical mucus (which increase the difficulty of sperm entry into the uterus) and the endometrium (which reduce the likelihood of implantation).

PHARMACOKINETICS
Absorption: Administration of therapy in various cycles resulted in different parameters; refer to PI for additional parameters. **Distribution:** Found in breast milk. EE: Serum albumin binding (extensive). NGMN: Serum protein binding (>97%) (NGMN and norgestrel). **Metabolism:** EE: Hydroxylated, glucuronide, and sulfate conjugates (metabolites). NGMN: Hepatic; hydroxylated and conjugated metabolites, norgestrel (metabolite). **Elimination:** Urine, feces (metabolites); $T_{1/2}$=17 hrs (EE), 28 hrs (NGMN).

PATIENT CONSIDERATIONS
Assessment: Assess for risk of arterial or venous thrombotic diseases, benign or malignant liver tumors, liver disease, undiagnosed abnormal uterine bleeding, presence or history of breast cancer or other estrogen- or progestin-sensitive cancer, pregnancy/nursing status, smoking status, and any other conditions where treatment is contraindicated/cautioned. Assess for possible drug interactions.

Monitoring: Monitor for arterial thrombotic or VTE events, hepatic adenomas, hepatocellular carcinoma, gallbladder disease, and other adverse effects. Monitor lipid levels w/ hyperlipidemia, BP w/ history of HTN, serum glucose levels in diabetic and prediabetic patients, for signs of worsening depression w/ previous history. Conduct a yearly visit w/ patient for a BP check and for other indicated healthcare.

Counseling: Inform of risks and benefits of therapy. Inform that cigarette smoking increases risk of serious CV events, and that women who are >35 yrs of age and smoke should not use CHCs. Advise that use of CHCs increases risk of VTE; inform that risk is highest during 1st year of use of CHCs and when restarting hormonal contraception after a break of ≥4 weeks. Inform that therapy does not protect against HIV infection (AIDS) and other sexually transmitted infections. Instruct to d/c if pregnancy occurs during use. Instruct to apply a single patch on the same day every week (Weeks 1-3). Instruct on what to do in the event a patch is missed. Instruct women who start CHC postpartum, and who have not yet had a period, to use an additional method of contraception until they have used patch for 7 consecutive days. Instruct to use a backup or alternative method of contraception when enzyme inducers are concomitantly used. Inform that breast milk production may be reduced w/ use. Inform that amenorrhea may occur. Advise that pregnancy should be ruled out in the event of amenorrhea in 2 or more consecutive cycles. Advise that insufficient drug delivery occurs when patch becomes partially or completely detached and remains detached.

XURIDEN — uridine triacetate   Rx

Class: Pyrimidine analog

ADULT DOSAGE	**PEDIATRIC DOSAGE**
Hereditary Orotic Aciduria	**Hereditary Orotic Aciduria**
Initial: 60mg/kg qd	**Initial:** 60mg/kg qd
Titrate: Increase dose to 120mg/kg for insufficient efficacy (eg, orotic acid levels remaining above normal or increasing above usual/expected range, worsening of other signs/symptoms of the disease)	**Titrate:** Increase dose to 120mg/kg for insufficient efficacy (eg, orotic acid levels remaining above normal or increasing above usual/expected range, worsening of other signs/symptoms of the disease)
Max: 8g/day	**Max:** 8g/day
Refer to PI for further dosing information	Refer to PI for further dosing information

ADMINISTRATION
Oral route

Measure dose using either a balance accurate to at least 0.1g, or a graduated tsp, accurate to the fraction of the dose to be administered.
Discard unused portion of granules once the measured dose has been removed from the packet.
A 2g pkt contains approx 3/4 tsp of the drug; for patients requiring doses in multiples of 2g (3/4 tsp), an entire pkt(s) may be administered w/o weighing/measuring.

Administration w/ Food
1. Mix measured amount of granules in 3-4 oz of applesauce, pudding, or yogurt.
2. Swallow the applesauce/pudding/yogurt immediately; do not chew the granules and do not save the applesauce/pudding/yogurt for later use.
3. Drink at least 4 oz of water.

May be mixed w/ milk or infant formula instead of soft foods, as described above; refer to PI for further details.

STORAGE
25°C (77°F); excursions permitted to 15-30°C (59-86°F).

HOW SUPPLIED
Oral Granules: 2g/pkt [30ˢ]

PREGNANCY AND LACTATION
Pregnancy: There are no available data on uridine use in pregnant women to inform a drug-associated risk.
Lactation: There are no data on the presence of uridine in human milk, the effect on the breastfed infant, or the effect on milk production; caution in nursing.

MECHANISM OF ACTION
Pyrimidine analogue; deacetylated by nonspecific esterases present throughout the body, yielding uridine in the systemic circulation.

PHARMACOKINETICS
Absorption: T_{max}=2-3 hrs; administration of variable doses resulted in different pharmacokinetic parameters. **Distribution:** Crosses the blood-brain barrier.
Metabolism: Via normal pyrimidine catabolic pathways present in most tissues.
Elimination: Kidneys; $T_{1/2}$=2-2.5 hrs.

PATIENT CONSIDERATIONS
Assessment: Assess pregnancy/nursing status. Assess baseline lab values affected by hereditary orotic aciduria.

Monitoring: Monitor for signs/symptoms of worsening hereditary orotic aciduria. Monitor urine levels of orotic acid and monitor lab values (eg, RBC or WBC indices) affected by hereditary orotic aciduria.

Counseling: Instruct on how to administer medication. Advise to measure the prescribed dose using either a balance accurate to at least 0.1g, or a graduated tsp, accurate to the fraction of the dose to be administered. Instruct to discard unused portion of granules after measuring out the dose. Advise that medication can be taken mixed in applesauce, pudding, yogurt, milk, or infant formula. Instruct to notify physician if condition worsens or if pregnant/nursing.

XYNTHA — antihemophilic factor (recombinant)   Rx

Class: Antihemophilic factor (recombinant)

OTHER BRAND NAMES
Xyntha Solofuse

ADULT DOSAGE	**PEDIATRIC DOSAGE**
Congenital Hemophilia A	**Congenital Hemophilia A**
Dosage (IU) = Body weight (kg) x desired factor VIII (FVIII) rise (IU/dL or % of normal) x 0.5 (IU/kg per IU/dL)	Dosage (IU) = Body weight (kg) x desired factor VIII (FVIII) rise (IU/dL or % of normal) x 0.5 (IU/kg per IU/dL)
Control and Prevention of Bleeding Episodes:	**Control and Prevention of Bleeding Episodes:**
Minor Bleed: Dose to maintain plasma FVIII activity at 20-40 IU/dL, given q12-24h for at least 1 day, depending upon the severity of the bleeding episode	**Minor Bleed:** Dose to maintain plasma FVIII activity at 20-40 IU/dL, given q12-24h for at least 1 day, depending upon the severity of the bleeding episode
Moderate Bleed: Dose to maintain plasma FVIII activity at 30-60 IU/dL, given q12-24h for 3-4 days or until adequate local hemostasis is achieved	**Moderate Bleed:** Dose to maintain plasma FVIII activity at 30-60 IU/dL, given q12-24h for 3-4 days or until adequate local hemostasis is achieved
Major Bleed: Dose to maintain plasma FVIII activity at 60-100 IU/dL, given q8-24h until bleeding is resolved	**Major Bleed:** Dose to maintain plasma FVIII activity at 60-100 IU/dL, given q8-24h until bleeding is resolved
Perioperative Management:	**Perioperative Management:**
Minor Operations: Dose to maintain plasma FVIII activity at 30-60 IU/dL, given q12-24h for 3-4 days or until adequate local hemostasis is achieved; a single infusion + oral antifibrinolytic therapy w/in 1 hr may be sufficient for a tooth extraction	**Minor Operations:** Dose to maintain plasma FVIII activity at 30-60 IU/dL, given q12-24h for 3-4 days or until adequate local hemostasis is achieved; a single infusion + oral antifibrinolytic therapy w/in 1 hr may be sufficient for a tooth extraction
Major Operations: Dose to maintain plasma FVIII activity at 60-100 IU/dL, given q8-24h until threat is resolved, or in the case of surgery, until adequate local hemostasis and wound healing are achieved	**Major Operations:** Dose to maintain plasma FVIII activity at 60-100 IU/dL, given q8-24h until threat is resolved, or in the case of surgery, until adequate local hemostasis and wound healing are achieved

ADMINISTRATION
IV route

Do not administer in the same tubing or container as other medications.
If using 1 vial of Xyntha w/ 1 Xyntha Solofuse, use a separate ≥10mL luer lock syringe to draw back the reconstituted contents of the vial and the syringe.
If using multiple syringes/vials of the medication, reconstitute each syringe/vial according to the instructions using a separate ≥10mL luer lock syringe to draw back the reconstituted contents of each syringe/vial.
Administer w/in 3 hrs after reconstitution or after removal of grey rubber tip cap from Solofuse.

Refer to PI for further details on administration, preparation, and reconstitution

STORAGE
2-8°C (36-46°F) for up to 36 months from the date of manufacture until the expiration date. May also store at room temperature not to exceed 25°C (77°F) for up to 3 months. Avoid freezing. Avoid prolonged exposure to light. (Solofuse) At the end of 3-month period, immediately use or discard the product. Do not put back into the refrigerator. (Xyntha) At the end of 3-month period, immediately use, discard, or return product to refrigerated storage. May return to the refrigerator until the expiration date after room temperature storage. Do not store at room temperature and return it to the refrigerator more than once. Diluent Syringe: 2-25°C (36-77°F).

HOW SUPPLIED
Inj: 250 IU, 500 IU, 1000 IU, 2000 IU; (Solofuse) 250 IU, 500 IU, 1000 IU, 2000 IU; 3000 IU

CONTRAINDICATIONS
Life-threatening immediate hypersensitivity reactions, including anaphylaxis, to the product or its components, including hamster proteins.

WARNINGS/PRECAUTIONS
Not indicated in patients w/ von Willebrand's disease. Initiate therapy under the supervision of a physician experienced in the treatment of hemophilia A. Allergic-type hypersensitivity reactions, including anaphylaxis, reported; d/c if symptoms occur and administer emergency treatment. FVIII inhibitors reported; perform an assay that measures FVIII inhibitor concentration if expected FVIII activity levels are not attained or if bleeding is not controlled w/ an appropriate dose.

ADVERSE REACTIONS
Headache, arthralgia, N/V, diarrhea, asthenia, pyrexia, cough.

PREGNANCY AND LACTATION
Category C, caution in nursing.

MECHANISM OF ACTION
Antihemophilic factor (recombinant); temporarily replaces the missing clotting FVIII that is needed for effective hemostasis.

PHARMACOKINETICS
Absorption: (Initial visit) C_{max}=1.08 IU/mL; AUC=13.5 IU•hr/mL. (Month 6) C_{max}=1.24 IU/mL; AUC=15 IU•hr/mL. (Pre-surgery) C_{max}=1.08 IU/mL; AUC=16 IU•hr/mL. (Adolescents) C_{max}=0.97 IU/mL; AUC=8.5 IU•hr/mL. (Young Children)

C_{max}=0.78 IU/mL; AUC=12.2 IU·hr/mL. **Distribution:** V_d= 66.1mL/kg (initial visit), 67.4mL/kg (month 6), 69mL/kg (pre-surgery), 67.1mL/kg (adolescents), 66.9mL/kg (young children). **Elimination:** $T_{1/2}$=11.2 hrs (initial visit), 11.8 hrs (month 6), 16.7 hrs (pre-surgery), 6.9 hrs (adolescents), 8.3 hrs (young children).

PATIENT CONSIDERATIONS

Assessment: Assess for hypersensitivity to drug or hamster proteins or other constituents of the product, location and extent of bleeding, patient's clinical condition, and pregnancy/nursing status. Assess plasma FVIII activity levels.

Monitoring: Monitor for development of FVIII inhibitors, plasma FVIII activity levels, clinical response, signs/symptoms of hypersensitivity reactions, and other adverse reactions.

Counseling: Advise to report physician if any adverse reactions develop, if pregnant or intending to become pregnant, or if breastfeeding. Inform about early signs/symptoms of hypersensitivity reactions (eg, hives, generalized urticaria, chest tightness) and anaphylaxis; instruct to d/c use and contact physician if symptoms occur. Advise to contact physician if lack of clinical response to FVIII replacement therapy is experienced. Advise to consult physician prior to travel and to bring adequate supply based on patient's current regimen of treatment when traveling. (Solofuse) Inform that local irritation may occur.

XYREM — sodium oxybate   CIII
Class: CNS depressant

> Obtundation and clinically significant respiratory depression occurred at recommended doses; almost all patients in trials were receiving CNS stimulants. Sodium oxybate is the Na⁺ salt of gamma hydroxybutyrate (GHB); abuse of GHB, alone or in combination w/ other CNS depressants, is associated w/ CNS adverse reactions, including seizure, respiratory depression, decreased level of consciousness, coma, and death. Available only through a restricted distribution program (Xyrem REMS Program).

ADULT DOSAGE
Narcolepsy

Treatment of Cataplexy and Excessive Daytime Sleepiness:
Initial: 4.5g/night administered in 2 equally divided doses (2.25g qhs and 2.25g taken 2.5-4 hrs later)
Titrate: Increase by 1.5g/night at weekly intervals (additional 0.75g qhs and 0.75g taken 2.5-4 hrs later)
Effective Dose Range: 6-9g/night
Max: 9g/night

PEDIATRIC DOSAGE
Pediatric use may not have been established

DOSING CONSIDERATIONS
Concomitant Medications
Divalproex Sodium:
Patients Already Stabilized on Xyrem: Addition of divalproex sodium should be accompanied by an initial reduction in the nightly dose of Xyrem by at least 20%
Patients Already Taking Divalproex Sodium: Use lower starting dose of Xyrem; monitor patient response and adjust dose accordingly

Hepatic Impairment
Initial: 2.25g/night administered in 2 equally divided doses (approx 1.13g qhs and approx 1.13g taken 2.5-4 hrs later)

Elderly
Start at lower end of dosing range

ADMINISTRATION
Oral route
Take 1st dose at least 2 hrs after eating
Prepare both doses prior to bedtime
Prior to ingestion, dilute each dose w/ approx 1/4 cup (approx 60mL) of water in the empty pharmacy vials provided
Take both doses while in bed and lie down immediately after dosing
Remain in bed following ingestion of the 1st and 2nd doses; an alarm may need to be set to awaken for 2nd dose

STORAGE
25°C (77°F); excursions permitted to 15-30°C (59-86°F).

HOW SUPPLIED
Oral Sol: 0.5g/mL [180mL]

CONTRAINDICATIONS
Concomitant use w/ sedative hypnotic agents and alcohol. Succinic semialdehyde dehydrogenase deficiency.

WARNINGS/PRECAUTIONS
May impair physical/mental abilities. Evaluate for history of drug abuse and monitor closely for signs of misuse/abuse. May impair respiratory drive, especially in patients w/ compromised respiratory function. Increased central apneas, oxygen desaturation events, and sleep-related breathing disorders may occur. Sleep-related breathing disorders tend to be more prevalent in obese patients, postmenopausal women not on hormone replacement therapy, and narcolepsy patients. Caution w/ history of depressive illness and/or suicide attempt; monitor for emergence of depressive symptoms. Confusion, anxiety, and other neuropsychiatric reactions (eg, hallucinations, paranoia) reported; carefully evaluate emergence of confusion, thought disorders, and/or behavior abnormalities. Parasomnias reported; fully evaluate episodes of sleepwalking. Contains high salt content; consider amount of daily Na⁺ intake in each dose in patients sensitive to salt intake.

ADVERSE REACTIONS
N/V, dizziness, diarrhea, somnolence, enuresis, tremor, attention disturbance, pain, sleep paralysis, paresthesia, disorientation, irritability, hyperhidrosis.

DRUG INTERACTIONS
See Dosing Considerations and Contraindications. Concurrent use w/ other CNS depressants (eg, opioid analgesics, sedating antidepressants/antipsychotics/antiepileptic drugs, muscle relaxants) may increase risk of respiratory depression, hypotension, profound sedation, syncope, and death; consider dose reduction or discontinuation of ≥1 CNS depressants (including sodium oxybate) if combination therapy is required. Consider interruption of treatment w/ sodium oxybate if short-term use of an opioid (eg, post- or perioperative) is required. Concomitant use w/ divalproex sodium resulted in a 25% mean increase in systemic exposure to sodium oxybate; monitor response closely and adjust dose accordingly if concomitant use is warranted.

PREGNANCY AND LACTATION
Category C, caution in nursing.

MECHANISM OF ACTION
CNS depressant; has not been established. Hypothesized that the therapeutic effects are mediated through $GABA_B$ actions at noradrenergic, dopaminergic, and thalamocortical neurons.

PHARMACOKINETICS
Absorption: Rapid; absolute bioavailability (88%); T_{max}=0.5-1.25 hr.
Distribution: V_d=190-384mL/kg; plasma protein binding (<1%). **Metabolism:** GHB dehydrogenase catalyzes the conversion of sodium oxybate to succinic semialdehyde, which is biotransformed to succinic acid by succinic semialdehyde dehydrogenase. Succinic acid enters the Krebs cycle. β-oxidation (secondary).
Elimination: Lungs, urine (<5% unchanged); $T_{1/2}$=0.5-1 hr.

PATIENT CONSIDERATIONS
Assessment: Assess for succinic semialdehyde dehydrogenase deficiency, alcohol intake, history of drug abuse, compromised respiratory function, history of depressive illness and/or suicide attempt, hepatic impairment, sensitivity to salt intake, pregnancy/nursing status, and possible drug interactions.

Monitoring: Monitor for obtundation, respiratory depression, CNS depression, signs of abuse/misuse, sleep-disordered breathing, depression and suicidality, confusion, anxiety, other neuropsychiatric reactions, parasomnias, and other possible adverse reactions.

Counseling: Inform about the Xyrem REMS Program. Instruct to see prescriber frequently (every 3 months) to review therapy. Instruct to store drug in a secure place, out of reach of children/pets. Inform that patients are likely to fall asleep quickly (w/in 5-15 min) after taking the drug; instruct to remain in bed after taking 1st and 2nd doses. Advise not to drink alcohol or take other sedative hypnotics while on therapy. Inform that therapy can be associated w/ respiratory depression. Instruct to avoid operating hazardous machinery until patients are reasonably certain that therapy does not affect them adversely and for at least 6 hrs after the 2nd nightly dose. Advise to contact physician if depressed mood, markedly diminished interest or pleasure in usual activities, significant change in weight and/or appetite, psychomotor agitation or retardation, increased fatigue, feelings of guilt or worthlessness, slowed thinking or impaired concentration, or suicidal ideation develops. Inform that sleepwalking may occur; instruct to notify physician if this occurs. Inform patients who are sensitive to salt intake that the drug contains a significant amount of Na⁺ and they should limit their Na⁺ intake.

YASMIN — drospirenone/ethinyl estradiol   Rx
Class: Estrogen/progestogen combination

> Cigarette smoking increases the risk of serious cardiovascular (CV) events. Risk increases w/ age (>35 yrs of age) and w/ the number of cigarettes smoked. Should not be used by women who are >35 yrs of age and smoke.

OTHER BRAND NAMES
Ocella, Syeda

ADULT DOSAGE
Contraception

1 tab qd at the same time each day for 28 days, then repeat

Start either on 1st day of menses or on 1st Sunday after onset of menses

Conversions

Switching from a Different Birth Control Pill:
Start on the same day that a new pack of the previous oral contraceptive would have been started

Switching from a Method Other Than a Birth Control Pill:
Transdermal Patch/Vaginal Ring/Inj:
Start when the next application or dose would have been due
Intrauterine Contraceptive/Implant:
Start on day of removal

PEDIATRIC DOSAGE
Contraception

Not indicated for use premenarche; refer to adult dosing

DOSING CONSIDERATIONS

Adverse Reactions

GI Disturbances: In case of severe vomiting/diarrhea, absorption may not be complete and additional contraceptive measures should be taken; if vomiting occurs w/in 3-4 hrs after taking tab, may regard as missed dose

Other Important Considerations

Postpartum Women Who Elect Not to Breastfeed/After a 2nd Trimester Abortion:

Start therapy no earlier than 4 weeks postpartum. If patient initiates therapy postpartum and has not yet had a period, evaluate for possible pregnancy and instruct to use an additional method of contraception until patient has taken 7 consecutive days of therapy

ADMINISTRATION

Oral route

Take tabs in the order directed on the package, preferably after pm meal or at hs w/ some liquid, prn.

Take w/o regard to meals.

If 1st taken later than the 1st day of menstrual cycle, use a nonhormonal contraceptive as back-up during the first 7 days of therapy.

Take single missed pills as soon as remembered.

STORAGE

(Syeda) 20-25°C (68-77°F). (Yasmin, Ocella) 25°C (77°F); excursions permitted to 15-30°C (59-86°F).

HOW SUPPLIED

Tab: (Drospirenone [DRSP]/Ethinyl Estradiol [EE]) 3mg/0.03mg

CONTRAINDICATIONS

Renal impairment, adrenal insufficiency, high risk of arterial/venous thrombotic diseases (eg, smoking if >35 yrs of age, presence/history of deep vein thrombosis/pulmonary embolism, cerebrovascular disease, coronary artery disease, thrombogenic valvular or thrombogenic rhythm diseases of the heart [eg, subacute bacterial endocarditis w/ valvular disease, or A-fib], inherited/acquired hypercoagulopathies, uncontrolled HTN, diabetes mellitus w/ vascular disease, headache w/ focal neurological symptoms or migraine w/ or w/o aura if >35 yrs of age), undiagnosed abnormal uterine bleeding, presence/history of breast cancer or other estrogen/progestin-sensitive cancer, benign/malignant liver tumors, liver disease, pregnancy.

WARNINGS/PRECAUTIONS

Increased risk of venous thromboembolism (VTE) and arterial thromboses (eg, stroke, MI). D/C if an arterial/venous thrombotic event occurs. If feasible, d/c at least 4 weeks before and through 2 weeks after major surgery or other surgeries known to have an elevated risk of thromboembolism. D/C if there is unexplained loss of vision, proptosis, diplopia, papilledema, or retinal vascular lesions; evaluate for retinal vein thrombosis immediately. Potential for hyperkalemia in high-risk patients; contraindicated in patients predisposed to hyperkalemia. May increase risk of cervical cancer or intraepithelial neoplasia, and gallbladder disease. D/C if jaundice develops. May increase risk of hepatic adenomas and hepatocellular carcinoma. Cholestasis may occur w/ history of pregnancy-related cholestasis. Women w/ a history of combination oral contraceptive (COC)-related cholestasis may have the condition recur w/ subsequent COC use. Increased BP reported; d/c if BP rises significantly. May decrease glucose tolerance; monitor prediabetic and diabetic women. Consider alternative contraception w/ uncontrolled dyslipidemia. May increase risk of pancreatitis w/ hypertriglyceridemia or family history thereof. Evaluate the cause and d/c if indicated, if new headaches that are recurrent, persistent, or severe develop. Increase in frequency/severity of migraines may be a reason for immediate discontinuation of therapy. Unscheduled bleeding and spotting may occur; rule out pregnancy or malignancy. Post-pill amenorrhea or oligomenorrhea may occur. Caution w/ history of depression; d/c if depression recurs to a serious degree. May change results of some lab tests (eg, coagulation factors, binding proteins). Exogenous estrogens may induce/exacerbate angioedema in women w/ hereditary angioedema. Chloasma may occur, especially w/ a history of chloasma gravidarum; avoid sun or UV radiation exposure in women w/ a tendency to chloasma.

ADVERSE REACTIONS

Premenstrual syndrome, headache/migraine, breast pain/tenderness/discomfort, N/V, irregular uterine bleeding.

DRUG INTERACTIONS

Potential for an increase in serum K⁺ concentration w/ other drugs that may increase serum K⁺ concentration (eg, ACE inhibitors, heparin, aldosterone antagonists, NSAIDs); monitor serum K⁺ concentrations during 1st treatment cycle in women receiving daily, long-term treatment for chronic conditions or diseases w/ medications that may increase serum K⁺ concentration. Consider monitoring serum K⁺ concentration in high-risk patients who take a strong CYP3A4 inhibitor long-term and concomitantly. Drugs or herbal products that induce certain enzymes, including CYP3A4 (eg, phenytoin, bosentan, products containing St. John's wort) may decrease effectiveness or increase breakthrough bleeding; use an alternative method of contraception or a back-up method when enzyme inducers are used, and continue back-up contraception for 28 days after discontinuing the enzyme inducer to ensure contraceptive reliability. Atorvastatin may increase EE exposure; ascorbic acid and acetaminophen may increase EE levels. Moderate or strong CYP3A4 inhibitors (eg, itraconazole, clarithromycin, diltiazem, grapefruit juice) may increase plasma concentrations of estrogen or progestin or both. Significant changes (increase/decrease) in plasma estrogen and progestin levels noted in some cases w/ HIV/hepatitis C virus protease inhibitors or non-nucleoside reverse transcriptase inhibitors. Pregnancy reported w/ antibiotics. May decrease levels of lamotrigine and reduce seizure control; dosage adjustments of lamotrigine may be necessary. May need to increase dose of thyroid hormone in patients on thyroid hormone replacement therapy due to increased levels of thyroid-binding globulin. May increase plasma levels of CYP3A4 substrates (eg, midazolam), CYP2C19 substrates (eg, omeprazole, voriconazole), and CYP1A2 substrates (eg, theophylline, tizanidine).

PREGNANCY AND LACTATION

Contraindicated in pregnancy, not for use in nursing.

MECHANISM OF ACTION

Estrogen/progestogen oral contraceptive; acts primarily by suppressing ovulation. Also causes cervical mucus changes that inhibit sperm penetration and endometrial changes that reduce the likelihood of implantation.

PHARMACOKINETICS

Absorption: DRSP: Absolute bioavailability (76%); (Cycle 13/Day 21) C_{max}=78.7ng/mL; T_{max}=1.6 hrs; AUC=968ng•h/mL. EE: Absolute bioavailability (40%); (Cycle 13/Day 21) C_{max}=90.5pg/mL; T_{max}=1.6 hrs; AUC=469pg•h/mL. **Distribution:** Found in breast milk. DRSP: V_d=4L/kg, plasma protein binding (97%). EE: V_d=4-5L/kg; plasma protein binding (98.5%). **Metabolism:** DRSP: Reduction, subsequent sulfation, oxidation catalyzed by CYP3A4. EE: Gut and liver (1st-pass), conjugation w/ glucuronide or sulfate, hydroxylation (via CYP3A4). **Elimination:** DRSP: Urine, feces; $T_{1/2}$=30 hrs. EE: Urine, feces; $T_{1/2}$=24 hrs.

Refer to PI for additional parameters.

PATIENT CONSIDERATIONS

Assessment: Assess for renal impairment, abnormal uterine bleeding, adrenal insufficiency, pregnancy/nursing status, any other conditions where treatment is contraindicated or cautioned, and possible drug interactions.

Monitoring: Monitor for bleeding irregularities, venous/arterial thrombotic events, cervical cancer or intraepithelial neoplasia, retinal vein thrombosis or any other ophthalmic changes, jaundice, new/worsening headaches or migraines, depression, cholestasis w/ history of pregnancy-related cholestasis, pancreatitis, and other adverse reactions. Monitor thyroid function if receiving thyroid replacement therapy, glucose levels in diabetic or prediabetic patients, lipid levels w/ dyslipidemia, and BP in patients w/ HTN. Monitor serum K⁺ levels during the 1st treatment cycle in women receiving daily, long-term treatment for chronic conditions or diseases w/ medications that may increase serum K⁺ concentration. Conduct a yearly visit in all patients for a BP check and for other indicated healthcare.

Counseling: Inform of risk/benefits of therapy. Counsel that cigarette smoking increases the risk of serious CV events. Inform of the risk of VTE. Advise that drug does not protect against HIV infection and other STDs. Instruct to take ud. Counsel on what to do if pills are missed or if vomiting occurs w/in 3-4 hrs after taking tab. Advise to inform physician of all concomitant medications and herbal supplements currently being taken. Inform that amenorrhea may occur and pregnancy should be ruled out if amenorrhea occurs in ≥2 consecutive cycles. Counsel to use a back-up or alternative method of contraception when enzyme inducers are used w/ therapy. Inform that therapy may reduce breast milk production. Counsel women who start therapy postpartum and have not yet had a period to use an additional method of contraception until drug is taken for 7 consecutive days. Instruct to d/c if pregnancy occurs during treatment.

YAZ — drospirenone/ethinyl estradiol   Rx

Class: Estrogen/progestogen combination

> Cigarette smoking increases the risk of serious cardiovascular (CV) events. Risk increases w/ age (>35 yrs of age) and w/ number of cigarettes smoked. Should not be used by women who are >35 yrs of age and smoke.

OTHER BRAND NAMES

Loryna

ADULT DOSAGE

Contraception

1 tab qd at the same time each day for 28 days, then repeat

Start either on 1st day of menses or on 1st Sunday after onset of menses

Premenstrual Dysphoric Disorder

In Women Who Desire Oral Contraception:

Yaz:

1 tab qd at the same time each day for 28 days, then repeat

Start either on 1st day of menses or on 1st Sunday after onset of menses

Acne Vulgaris

Moderate Acne in Women Who Desire Oral Contraception:

1 tab qd at the same time each day for 28 days, then repeat

Start either on 1st day of menses or on 1st Sunday after onset of menses

Conversions

Switching from a Different Birth Control Pill: Start on the same day that a new pack of the previous oral contraceptive would have been started

PEDIATRIC DOSAGE

Contraception

Not indicated for use premenarche; refer to adult dosing

Premenstrual Dysphoric Disorder

In Women Who Desire Oral Contraception:

Yaz:

Not indicated for use premenarche; refer to adult dosing

Acne Vulgaris

Moderate Acne in Postpubertal Women ≥14 Years Who Desire Oral Contraception:

1 tab qd at the same time each day for 28 days, then repeat

Start either on 1st day of menses or on 1st Sunday after onset of menses

Switching from a Method Other Than a Birth Control Pill:
Transdermal Patch/Vaginal Ring/Inj: Start when the next application or dose would have been due
Intrauterine Contraceptive/Implant: Start on day of removal

DOSING CONSIDERATIONS
Adverse Reactions
GI Disturbances: In case of severe vomiting/diarrhea, absorption may not be complete and additional contraceptive measures should be taken; if vomiting occurs w/in 3-4 hrs after taking tab, may regard as missed tab

Other Important Considerations
Postpartum Women Who Elect Not to Breastfeed/After 2nd Trimester Abortion: Start therapy no earlier than 4 weeks postpartum. If patient initiates therapy postpartum and has not yet had a period, evaluate for possible pregnancy and instruct to use an additional method of contraception until patient has taken 7 consecutive days of therapy

ADMINISTRATION
Oral route

Take tabs in the order directed on the package, preferably after pm meal or hs w/ some liquid, prn.
May be taken w/o regard to meals.
If 1st taken later than the 1st day of menstrual cycle, use a nonhormonal contraceptive as backup during the first 7 days of therapy.
Take single missed pills as soon as remembered.

STORAGE
(Yaz) 25°C (77°F); excursions permitted to 15-30°C (59-86°F). (Loryna) 20-25°C (68-77°F).

HOW SUPPLIED
Tab: (Drospirenone [DRSP]/Ethinyl Estradiol [EE]) 3mg/0.02mg

CONTRAINDICATIONS
Renal impairment, adrenal insufficiency, high risk of arterial/venous thrombotic disease (eg, smoking if >35 yrs of age, active or history of deep vein thrombosis/pulmonary embolism, cerebrovascular disease, coronary artery disease, thrombogenic valvular/thrombogenic rhythm diseases of the heart [eg, subacute bacterial endocarditis w/ valvular disease, or A-fib], inherited/acquired hypercoagulopathies, uncontrolled HTN, diabetes mellitus [DM] w/ vascular disease, headache w/ focal neurological symptoms or migraine w/ or w/o aura if >35 yrs of age), undiagnosed abnormal uterine bleeding, presence/history of breast cancer or other estrogen/progestin-sensitive cancer, benign/malignant liver tumors, liver disease, pregnancy.

WARNINGS/PRECAUTIONS
Increased risk of venous thromboembolism (VTE) and arterial thromboses (eg, stroke, MI); d/c if an arterial or venous thrombotic event occurs. D/C if unexplained loss of vision, proptosis, diplopia, papilledema, or retinal vascular lesions occur; evaluate for retinal vein thrombosis immediately. If feasible, d/c at least 4 weeks before and through 2 weeks after major surgery or other surgeries known to have an elevated risk of thromboembolism. Potential for hyperkalemia in high-risk patients; contraindicated in patients w/ conditions that predispose to hyperkalemia. May increase risk of cervical cancer or intraepithelial neoplasia and gallbladder disease. D/C if jaundice develops. May increase risk of hepatic adenomas and hepatocellular carcinoma. Cholestasis may occur in women w/ a history of pregnancy-related cholestasis. Women w/ a history of combination oral contraceptive (COC)-related cholestasis may have the condition recur w/ subsequent COC use. Increased BP reported; d/c if BP rises significantly. May decrease glucose tolerance; monitor prediabetic and diabetic women. Consider alternative contraception for women w/ uncontrolled dyslipidemias. May increase risk of pancreatitis in women w/ hypertriglyceridemia or family history thereof. Evaluate the cause and d/c if indicated, if new headaches that are recurrent, persistent, or severe develop. Increase in frequency/severity of migraines may be a reason for immediate discontinuation of therapy. Unscheduled bleeding and spotting may occur; rule out pregnancy or malignancy. Post-pill amenorrhea or oligomenorrhea may occur. Caution w/ history of depression; d/c if depression recurs to serious degree. May change the results of some lab tests (eg, coagulation factors, binding proteins). Exogenous estrogens may induce/exacerbate angioedema in women w/ hereditary angioedema. Chloasma may occur, especially w/ a history of chloasma gravidarum; avoid sun or UV radiation exposure in women w/ a tendency to chloasma.

ADVERSE REACTIONS
Menstrual irregularities, N/V, headache/migraine, breast pain/tenderness.

DRUG INTERACTIONS
Drugs or herbal products that induce certain enzymes, including CYP3A4 (eg, phenytoin, barbiturates, carbamazepine), may decrease effectiveness or increase breakthrough bleeding; use an alternative or back-up method of contraception when enzyme inducers are used, and continue back-up contraception for 28 days after discontinuing the enzyme inducer. Atorvastatin may increase EE exposure; ascorbic acid and acetaminophen may increase EE levels. Moderate or strong CYP3A4 inhibitors (eg, itraconazole, verapamil, clarithromycin, diltiazem, grapefruit juice) may increase plasma concentrations of estrogen or progestin or both. Significant changes (increase or decrease) in estrogen and progestin levels noted in some cases w/ HIV/hepatitis C virus protease inhibitors or w/ non-nucleoside reverse transcriptase inhibitors. Pregnancy reported while taking hormonal contraceptives and antibiotics. Potential for an increase in serum K^+ concentration w/ use of other drugs that may increase serum K^+ concentration (eg, ACE inhibitors, heparin, aldosterone antagonists, NSAIDs); monitor serum

K^+ concentrations during first treatment cycle in patients receiving concomitant daily, long-term treatment for chronic conditions or diseases. Consider monitoring serum K^+ concentration in high-risk patients who take a strong CYP3A4 inhibitor long-term and concomitantly. May decrease levels of lamotrigine and reduce seizure control; may need to adjust dose of lamotrigine. May increase plasma levels of CYP3A4 substrates (eg, midazolam), CYP2C19 substrates (eg, omeprazole, voriconazole), and CYP1A2 substrates (eg, theophylline, tizanidine). May increase levels of thyroid-binding globulin; may need to increase dose of thyroid hormone in patients on thyroid hormone replacement therapy.

PREGNANCY AND LACTATION
Contraindicated in pregnancy, not for use in nursing.

MECHANISM OF ACTION
Estrogen/progestogen oral contraceptive; acts by primarily suppressing ovulation. Also causes cervical mucus changes that inhibit sperm penetration and endometrial changes that reduce the likelihood of implantation.

PHARMACOKINETICS
Absorption: DRSP: Absolute bioavailability (76%); (Cycle 1/Day 21) C_{max}=70.3ng/mL; T_{max}=1.5 hrs; AUC=763ng•hr/mL. EE: Absolute bioavailability (40%); (Cycle 1/Day 21) C_{max}=45.1pg/mL; T_{max}=1.5 hrs; AUC=220pg•hr/mL. Refer to PI for additional parameters. **Distribution:** Found in breast milk; DRSP: V_d=4L/kg; serum protein binding (97%). EE: V_d=4-5L/kg; serum albumin binding (98.5%). **Metabolism:** DRSP: Reduction, subsequent sulfation, oxidation catalyzed by CYP3A4. EE: Gut and liver (1st-pass), conjugation w/ glucuronide or sulfate, hydroxylation (via CYP3A4). **Elimination:** DRSP: Urine, feces; $T_{1/2}$=30 hrs. EE: Urine, feces; $T_{1/2}$=24 hrs.

PATIENT CONSIDERATIONS
Assessment: Assess for renal impairment, abnormal uterine bleeding, adrenal insufficiency, pregnancy/nursing status, any other conditions where treatment is cautioned or contraindicated, and for possible drug interactions.

Monitoring: Monitor for bleeding irregularities, venous/arterial thrombotic events, cervical cancer or intraepithelial neoplasia, retinal vein thrombosis or any other ophthalmic changes, jaundice, new/worsening headaches or migraines, depression, cholestasis w/ history of pregnancy-related cholestasis, pancreatitis, and other adverse reactions. Monitor thyroid function if receiving thyroid replacement therapy, glucose levels in diabetic or prediabetic women, lipid levels w/ dyslipidemia, and BP in patients w/ HTN. Monitor serum K^+ levels during the 1st treatment cycle in women receiving daily, long-term treatment for chronic conditions or diseases w/ medications that may increase serum K^+ concentrations. Conduct a yearly visit in all patients for a BP check and for other indicated healthcare.

Counseling: Inform of risk/benefits of therapy. Counsel that cigarette smoking increases the risk of serious CV events. Inform of the risk of VTE. Inform that drug does not protect against HIV infection and other STDs. Instruct to take ud. Advise to inform physician of all concomitant medications and herbal supplements currently taking. Instruct to take therapy at the same time every day. Advise on what to do if pills are missed or vomiting occurs w/in 3-4 hrs after taking therapy. Counsel to use a back-up or alternative method of contraception when enzyme inducers are used concomitantly. Inform that therapy may reduce breast milk production. Inform that amenorrhea may occur and pregnancy should be ruled out if amenorrhea occurs in ≥2 consecutive cycles. Counsel women who start therapy postpartum and have not yet had a period, to use an additional method of contraception until an active pill has been taken for 7 consecutive days. Instruct to d/c therapy if pregnancy occurs during treatment.

YERVOY — ipilimumab   Rx
Class: Monoclonal antibody/CTLA-4 blocker

> Can result in severe and fatal immune-mediated adverse reactions, and may involve any organ system; the most common reactions are enterocolitis, hepatitis, dermatitis (eg, toxic epidermal necrolysis (TEN)), neuropathy, and endocrinopathy. The majority of these reactions initially manifested during treatment; however, a minority occurred weeks to months after discontinuation of therapy. Permanently d/c therapy and initiate systemic high-dose corticosteroid therapy for severe immune-mediated reactions. Assess for signs/symptoms of enterocolitis, dermatitis, neuropathy, and endocrinopathy, and evaluate clinical chemistries (eg, LFTs, ACTH level, thyroid function tests) at baseline and before each dose.

ADULT DOSAGE	PEDIATRIC DOSAGE
Unresectable or Metastatic Melanoma	Pediatric use may not have been established
3mg/kg IV over 90 min every 3 weeks for a max of 4 doses	
In the event of toxicity, doses may be delayed, but all treatment must be administered w/in 16 weeks of the first dose	
Cutaneous Melanoma	
Adjuvant treatment of patients w/ pathologic involvement of regional lymph nodes of >1mm who have undergone complete resection, including total lymphadenectomy	
10mg/kg IV over 90 min every 3 weeks for 4 doses followed by 10mg/kg every 12 weeks for up to 3 years	
In the event of toxicity, doses are omitted, not delayed	

DOSING CONSIDERATIONS

Hepatic Impairment

Mild (Total Bilirubin >1-1.5X ULN or AST >ULN): No dose adjustment needed
Moderate (Total Bilirubin >1.5-3X ULN and Any AST) or Severe (Total Bilirubin >3X ULN and Any AST): Not studied

Adverse Reactions

Endocrine:

Symptomatic Endocrinopathy: Withhold therapy; resume in patients w/ complete or partial resolution of adverse reactions (Grade 0 to 1) and who are receiving <7.5mg prednisone or equivalent per day.
Symptomatic Reactions Lasting ≥6 Weeks: Permanently d/c.
Inability to Reduce Corticosteroid Dose to 7.5mg Prednisone or Equivalent per Day: Permanently d/c.

Ophthalmologic:

Grade 2 through 4 Reactions Not Improving to Grade 1 w/in 2 Weeks While Receiving Topical Therapy: Permanently d/c.
Grade 2 through 4 Reactions Requiring Systemic Treatment: Permanently d/c.

All Other:

Grade 2: Withhold therapy; resume in patients w/ complete or partial resolution of adverse reactions (Grade 0 to 1) and who are receiving <7.5mg prednisone or equivalent per day.
Grade 2 Reactions Lasting ≥6 Weeks: Permanently d/c.
Inability to Reduce Corticosteroid Dose to 7.5mg Prednisone or Equivalent per Day: Permanently d/c.
Grade 3 or 4: Permanently d/c.

ADMINISTRATION

IV route

Administer diluted sol over 90 min through an IV line containing a sterile, non-pyrogenic, low-protein-binding in-line filter.
Flush the IV line w/ 0.9% NaCl inj or D5 inj after each dose.
Do not mix w/, or administer as an infusion w/, other medicinal products.

Preparation of Sol

1. Allow the vials to stand at room temperature for approx 5 min prior to preparation of infusion.
2. Withdraw the required volume of ipilimumab and transfer into an IV bag.
3. Dilute w/ 0.9% NaCl inj or D5 inj to prepare a diluted sol, w/ a final concentration ranging from 1-2mg/mL.
4. Mix diluted sol by gentle inversion; do not shake.
5. Store diluted sol for no more than 24 hrs at 2-8°C (36-46°F) or at 20-25°C (68-77°F).
6. Discard partially used vials or empty vials.

STORAGE

2-8°C (36-46°F). Do not freeze. Protect from light.

HOW SUPPLIED

Inj: 5mg/mL [10mL, 40mL]

WARNINGS/PRECAUTIONS

Refer to Dosing Considerations for recommendations to withhold or d/c therapy for the following adverse reactions. Refer to PI for corticosteroid dose in the management of the following adverse reactions. Immune-mediated enterocolitis, including fatal cases, can occur. Permanently d/c in patients w/ severe enterocolitis and initiate corticosteroids; initiate corticosteroid taper upon improvement to ≤Grade 1. Withhold therapy for moderate enterocolitis; administer antidiarrheal treatment and, if persistent for >1 week, initiate corticosteroids. Immune-mediated hepatitis, including fatal cases, can occur. Permanently d/c in patients w/ Grade 3 or 4 hepatotoxicity and administer corticosteroids; when LFTs show sustained improvement or return to baseline, initiate corticosteroid taper. Withhold therapy in patients w/ Grade 2 hepatotoxicity. Immune-mediated dermatitis, including fatal cases, can occur. Permanently d/c in patients w/ Stevens-Johnson syndrome, TEN, or rash complicated by full thickness dermal ulceration, or necrotic, bullous, or hemorrhagic manifestations. Administer corticosteroids; when dermatitis is controlled, initiate corticosteroid taper. Withhold in patients w/ moderate to severe signs/symptoms. Immune-mediated neuropathies, including fatal cases, can occur. Permanently d/c in patients w/ severe neuropathy (eg, Guillain-Barre-like syndromes). Consider initiation of corticosteroids. Withhold in patients w/ moderate neuropathy (not interfering w/ daily activities). Immune-mediated endocrinopathies, including life-threatening cases, can occur. Withhold in symptomatic patients; initiate corticosteroids and appropriate hormone replacement therapy. Permanently d/c for clinically significant or severe immune-mediated adverse reactions; initiate corticosteroids for severe immune-mediated adverse reactions. Administer corticosteroid eye drops to patients who develop uveitis, iritis, or episcleritis; permanently d/c for immune-mediated ocular disease that is unresponsive to local immunosuppressive therapy. Can cause fetal harm.

ADVERSE REACTIONS

Unresectable/Metastatic Melanoma: Diarrhea, colitis, pruritus, rash, fatigue.
Adjuvant Treatment of Melanoma: Rash, pruritus, diarrhea, N/V, colitis, weight decreased, fatigue, pyrexia, headache, decreased appetite, insomnia.

DRUG INTERACTIONS

Increased transaminases w/ or w/o concomitant increases in total bilirubin reported in patients who received concurrent vemurafenib (960mg bid or 720mg bid).

PREGNANCY AND LACTATION

Pregnancy: Ipilimumab can cause fetal harm based on its mechanism of action and data from animal studies. Human IgG1 is known to cross the placental barrier; therefore, ipilimumab has the potential to be transmitted from the mother to the developing fetus. Effects are likely to be greater during the 2nd and 3rd trimesters. Advise pregnant women of potential risk to fetus. A Pregnancy Safety Surveillance Study has been established to collect information about pregnancies in women who have received ipilimumab; advise pregnant women to enroll.
Lactation: D/C nursing during treatment and for 3 months following the final dose.
Reproductive Potential: Females of reproductive potential should use effective contraception during treatment and for 3 months following the last dose.

MECHANISM OF ACTION

Human monoclonal antibody/CTLA-4 blocker; binds to CTLA-4 and blocks its interaction w/ its ligands, CD80/CD86. Blockade of CTLA-4 has been shown to augment T-cell activation and proliferation, including the activation and proliferation of tumor infiltrating T-effector cells and reduction of T-regulatory cell function, which may contribute to a general increase in T-cell responsiveness, including the antitumor immune response.

PHARMACOKINETICS

Distribution: Crosses placenta. **Elimination:** $T_{1/2}$=15.4 days.

PATIENT CONSIDERATIONS

Assessment: Assess pregnancy/nursing status. Evaluate clinical chemistries, including LFTs, ACTH level, and thyroid function tests, at baseline.
Monitoring: Monitor for signs/symptoms of immune-mediated enterocolitis, hepatitis, dermatitis, motor or sensory neuropathy, hypophysitis, adrenal insufficiency, hypo/hyperthyroidism, and other adverse reactions. Monitor clinical chemistries, including LFTs, ACTH level, and thyroid function tests before each dose, and as clinically indicated based on symptoms.
Counseling: Inform of the potential risk of immune-mediated adverse reactions. Advise female patients that therapy can cause fetal harm. Instruct females of reproductive potential to use effective contraception during treatment and for 3 months after the last dose. Advise to contact physician if pregnant or if pregnancy is suspected. Advise females who may have been exposed to drug during pregnancy to contact Bristol-Myers Squibb; advise pregnant women to enroll in the Pregnancy Safety Surveillance Study. Advise women not to breastfeed during treatment and for 3 months after the last dose.

YONDELIS — trabectedin   Rx

Class: Alkylating agent

ADULT DOSAGE	PEDIATRIC DOSAGE
Unresectable or Metastatic Liposarcoma or Leiomyosarcoma	Pediatric use may not have been established
In patients who received a prior anthracycline-containing regimen	
Recommended: 1.5mg/m² as an IV infusion every 21 days, until disease progression or unacceptable toxicity, in patients w/ normal bilirubin and AST or ALT ≤2.5X ULN	
Premedication	
Administer dexamethasone 20mg IV 30 min prior to each dose	

DOSING CONSIDERATIONS

Renal Impairment

Mild (CrCl 60-89mL/min) or Moderate (CrCl 30-59mL/min): No dose adjustment recommended
Severe (CrCl <30mL/min) or ESRD: Has not been evaluated

Hepatic Impairment

Moderate (Bilirubin Levels 1.5X to 3X ULN, and AST and ALT <8X ULN): Recommended Dose: 0.9mg/m²
Severe (Bilirubin Levels >3X ULN, and Any AST and ALT): Do not administer

Adverse Reactions

Permanently D/C For:

- Persistent adverse reactions requiring a delay in dosing of >3 weeks
- Adverse reactions requiring dose reduction following trabectedin administered at 1mg/m² for patients w/ normal hepatic function or at 0.3mg/m² for patients w/ preexisting moderate hepatic impairment
- Severe liver dysfunction (all of the following: bilirubin 2X ULN and AST/ALT 3X ULN w/ alkaline phosphatase <2X ULN) in the prior treatment cycle for patients w/ normal liver function at baseline
- Exacerbation of liver dysfunction in patients w/ preexisting moderate hepatic impairment

Delay Next Dose for Up to 3 Weeks:

- Platelets <100,000 platelets/µL
- ANC <1500 neutrophils/µL
- Total bilirubin >ULN
- AST/ALT >2.5X ULN
- Alkaline phosphatase >2.5X ULN
- Creatine phosphokinase >2.5X ULN
- Decreased left ventricular ejection fraction (LVEF): less than lower limit of normal or clinical evidence of cardiomyopathy
- Other nonhematologic Grade 3 or 4 adverse reactions

Reduce Next Dose by One Dose Level for Adverse Reaction(s) During Prior Cycle:

- Platelets <25,000 platelets/µL
- ANC <1000 neutrophils/µL w/ fever/infection or <500 neutrophils/µL lasting >5 days

- Total bilirubin >ULN
- AST/ALT >5X ULN
- Alkaline phosphatase >2.5X ULN
- Creatine phosphokinase >5X ULN
- Decreased LVEF: absolute decrease of ≥10% from baseline and less than lower limit of normal or clinical evidence of cardiomyopathy
- Other nonhematologic Grade 3 or 4 adverse reactions

Dose Reductions for Patients w/ Normal Hepatic Function or Mild Hepatic Impairment (Including Patients w/ Bilirubin 1 to 1.5X ULN, and Any AST or ALT) Prior to Initiation of Treatment:
1st Dose Reduction: $1.2mg/m^2$ every 3 weeks
2nd Dose Reduction: $1mg/m^2$ every 3 weeks
Dose Reductions for Patients w/ Moderate Hepatic Function Prior to Initiation of Treatment:
1st Dose Reduction: $0.6mg/m^2$ every 3 weeks
2nd Dose Reduction: $0.3mg/m^2$ every 3 weeks
The dose should not be increased in subsequent treatment cycles once the dose is reduced for adverse reactions

ADMINISTRATION
IV route

Infuse reconstituted, diluted sol over 24 hrs through a central venous line using an infusion set w/ a 0.2 micron polyethersulfone in-line filter.
Complete infusion w/in 30 hrs of initial reconstitution; discard any unused portion of the product or of the infusion sol.
Do not mix w/ other drugs.
Discard any remaining sol w/in 30 hrs of reconstituting the lyophilized powder.

Preparation:
1. Inject 20mL of sterile water for inj into the vial; shake the vial until complete dissolution.
2. Immediately following reconstitution, withdraw the calculated volume of drug and further dilute in 500mL of 0.9% NaCl and D5 inj.

Compatibility:
Type 1 colorless glass vials
PVC and polyethylene bags and tubing
Polyethylene and polypropylene mixture bags
Polyethersulfone in-line filters
Titanium, platinum, or plastic ports
Silicone and polyurethane catheters
Pumps having contact surfaces made of PVC, polyethylene, or polyethylene/polypropylene

STORAGE
2-8°C (36-46°F).

HOW SUPPLIED
Inj: (Powder) 1mg

CONTRAINDICATIONS
Severe hypersensitivity (eg, anaphylaxis) to trabectedin.

WARNINGS/PRECAUTIONS
See Dosing Considerations. Neutropenic sepsis, rhabdomyolysis, musculoskeletal toxicity, hepatotoxicity, and cardiomyopathy can occur. Extravasation, resulting in tissue necrosis requiring debridement, can occur. Can cause fetal harm.

ADVERSE REACTIONS
N/V, fatigue, constipation, decreased appetite, diarrhea, peripheral edema, dyspnea, headache.

DRUG INTERACTIONS
Ketoconazole may increase systemic exposure; avoid use of strong CYP3A inhibitors (eg, oral ketoconazole, itraconazole, clarithromycin). Avoid grapefruit or grapefruit juice. If a strong CYP3A inhibitor for short-term use (eg, <14 days) must be used, administer the strong CYP3A inhibitor 1 week after infusion, and d/c the day prior to the next infusion. Rifampin may decrease systemic exposure; avoid strong CYP3A inducers (eg, rifampin, phenobarbital, St. John's wort).

PREGNANCY AND LACTATION
Pregnancy: Can cause fetal harm based on mechanism of action.
Lactation: There are no data on the presence of trabectedin in human milk, the effects on the breastfed infant, or the effects on milk production; not for use during nursing.
Reproductive Potential: Female patients of reproductive potential should use effective contraception during and for 2 months after the last dose of therapy. Males w/ a female sexual partner of reproductive potential should use effective contraception during and for 5 months after the last dose of therapy. May result in decreased fertility in males and females.

MECHANISM OF ACTION
Alkylating agent; binds guanine residues in the minor groove of DNA, forming adducts and resulting in a bending of the DNA helix towards the major groove. Adduct formation triggers a cascade of events that can affect the subsequent activity of DNA binding proteins, including some transcription factors, and DNA repair pathways, resulting in perturbation of the cell cycle and eventual cell death.

PHARMACOKINETICS
Distribution: V_d >5000L; plasma protein binding (approx 97%). **Metabolism:** Hepatic metabolism via CYP3A (extensive). **Elimination:** Urine (6%), feces (58%). $T_{1/2}$=approx 175 hrs.

PATIENT CONSIDERATIONS
Assessment: Assess for drug hypersensitivity, LVEF, pregnancy/nursing status, and for possible drug interactions. Assess neutrophil count, creatine phosphokinase levels, and LFTs prior to each dose.

Monitoring: Monitor for rhabdomyolysis, hepatotoxicity, extravasation, and for other adverse reactions. Monitor neutrophil count periodically, and LVEF at 2- to 3-month intervals.

Counseling: Inform of the risks of myelosuppression; instruct to contact physician immediately for fever or unusual bruising, bleeding, tiredness, or paleness. Advise to contact physician immediately if experiencing symptoms of rhabdomyolysis, hepatotoxicity, cardiomyopathy, hypersensitivity, or extravasation. Inform pregnant women of the potential risk to fetus and advise to contact physician if pregnant or suspected to be pregnant during treatment. Advise females of reproductive potential to use effective contraception during treatment and for at least 2 months after last dose. Advise males w/ female partners of reproductive potential to use effective contraception during treatment and for at least 5 months after last dose. Advise females not to breastfeed during treatment.

ZALTRAP — ziv-aflibercept   Rx
Class: Vascular endothelial growth factor (VEGF) inhibitor

> Severe and sometimes fatal hemorrhage, including GI hemorrhage, reported in combination w/ 5-fluorouracil, leucovorin, and irinotecan (FOLFIRI). Monitor for signs and symptoms of GI bleeding and other severe bleeding. Do not administer in patients w/ severe hemorrhage. Nonfatal/fatal GI perforation may occur; d/c therapy in patients who experience GI perforation. Severe compromised wound healing may occur in combination w/ FOLFIRI; d/c in patients w/ compromised wound healing. Suspend for at least 4 weeks prior to elective surgery; do not resume for at least 4 weeks following major surgery and until the surgical wound is fully healed.

ADULT DOSAGE
Metastatic Colorectal Cancer
In combination w/ FOLFIRI for patients w/ cancer that is resistant to or has progressed following an oxaliplatin-containing regimen

4mg/kg IV infusion over 1 hr every 2 weeks until disease progression or unacceptable toxicity

Administer prior to any component of the FOLFIRI regimen on day of treatment

PEDIATRIC DOSAGE
Pediatric use may not have been established

DOSING CONSIDERATIONS
Discontinuation
D/C Therapy For:
- Severe hemorrhage
- GI perforation
- Compromised wound healing
- Fistula formation
- Hypertensive crisis or hypertensive encephalopathy
- Arterial thromboembolic events
- Nephrotic syndrome or thrombotic microangiopathy
- Reversible posterior leukoencephalopathy syndrome (RPLS)

Temporarily Suspend Therapy:
- At least 4 weeks prior to elective surgery
- For recurrent or severe hypertension, until controlled; upon resumption, permanently reduce dose to 2mg/kg
- For proteinuria of 2g/24 hrs; resume when proteinuria is <2g/24 hrs. For recurrent proteinuria, suspend therapy until proteinuria is <2g/24 hrs and then permanently reduce dose to 2mg/kg

ADMINISTRATION
IV route

Preparation
- Do not re-enter the vial after the initial puncture; discard any unused portion left in the vial.
- Withdraw the prescribed dose and dilute in 0.9% NaCl sol or 5% dextrose sol for inj; final concentration is 0.6-8mg/mL.
- Use polyvinyl chloride (PVC) infusion bags containing bis (2-ethylhexyl) phthalate (DEHP) or polyolefin infusion bags.

Administration
- Administer through a 0.2µm polyethersulfone filter.
- Do not use filters made of polyvinylidene fluoride or nylon.
- Do not administer as an IV push or bolus.
- Do not combine w/ other drugs in the same infusion bag or IV line.
- Store diluted sol at 2-8°C (36-46°F) for up to 24 hrs, or at 20-25°C (68-77°F) for up to 8 hrs.

Administer using an infusion set made of 1 of the following materials:
- PVC containing DEHP
- DEHP-free PVC containing trioctyl-trimellitate
- Polypropylene
- Polyethylene-lined PVC
- Polyurethane

STORAGE
2-8°C (36-46°F). Keep vials in original carton to protect from light.

HOW SUPPLIED
Inj: 25mg/mL [4mL, 8mL]

WARNINGS/PRECAUTIONS
For minor surgery (eg, central venous access port placement, biopsy, tooth extraction), may initiate/resume therapy once surgical wound is fully healed.

Fistula formation, involving GI and non-GI sites, reported; d/c in patients who develop fistula. Increased risk of Grade 3-4 HTN; treat w/ appropriate antihypertensives and continue monitoring BP regularly. Arterial thromboembolic events (ATEs) (eg, transient ischemic attack, cerebrovascular accident, angina pectoris); severe proteinuria; nephrotic syndrome; and thrombotic microangiopathy (TMA) reported. Higher incidence of neutropenic complications (eg, febrile neutropenia, neutropenic infection) reported; delay therapy until neutrophil count is ≥1.5 x 10^9/L. Diarrhea and dehydration reported; closely monitor elderly for diarrhea and dehydration. RPLS reported; confirm diagnosis of RPLS w/ MRI and d/c if RPLS develops.

ADVERSE REACTIONS
Leukopenia, diarrhea, neutropenia, proteinuria, increased AST, stomatitis, fatigue, thrombocytopenia, increased ALT, hypertension, decreased weight, decreased appetite, epistaxis, abdominal pain, dysphonia, increased SrCr, headache.

PREGNANCY AND LACTATION
Pregnancy: Category C.
Lactation: Not for use in nursing.
Reproduction Potential: Male and female reproductive function and fertility may be compromised during treatment; females and males of reproductive potential should use highly effective contraception during and up to a minimum of 3 months after the last dose.

MECHANISM OF ACTION
VEGF inhibitor; binds to human VEGF-A, to human VEGF-B, and to human PlGF, and thereby inhibits the binding and activation of their cognate receptors. This inhibition can result in decreased neovascularization and decreased vascular permeability.

PHARMACOKINETICS
Elimination: $T_{1/2}$=6 days.

PATIENT CONSIDERATIONS
Assessment: Assess for recent surgery, severe hemorrhage, compromised wound healing, HTN, proteinuria, history of ATEs, neutropenia, and pregnancy/nursing status. Obtain baseline CBC w/ differential count.

Monitoring: Monitor for signs/symptoms of bleeding, GI perforation, fistula formation, compromised wound healing, hypertensive crisis/encephalopathy, ATEs, nephrotic syndrome, TMA, diarrhea, dehydration, RPLS, and other adverse reactions. Monitor BP every 2 weeks or more frequently as indicated. Monitor proteinuria by urine dipstick analysis and/or urinary protein creatinine ratio (UPCR) for the development or worsening of proteinuria; obtain a 24-hr urine collection in patients w/ a dipstick of ≥2+ for protein or UPCR >1. Monitor CBC w/ differential count prior to initiation of each cycle.

Counseling: Advise to contact physician if bleeding/symptoms of bleeding, elevated BP/symptoms from HTN, severe diarrhea, vomiting, severe abdominal pain, or fever or other signs of infection occur. Inform of the increased risk of compromised wound healing and instruct not to undergo surgery or procedures, including tooth extractions, w/o discussing 1st w/ the physician. Inform of an increased risk of ATEs. Inform of the potential risks to the fetus or neonate during pregnancy or nursing; instruct to use highly effective contraception in both males and females during and for at least 3 months following last dose of therapy; advise to immediately contact physician if patient or their partner becomes pregnant during treatment.

ZARAH — drospirenone/ethinyl estradiol   Rx
Class: Estrogen/progestogen combination

> Cigarette smoking increases the risk of serious cardiovascular (CV) side effects from oral contraceptive use. Risk increases with age (>35 yrs of age) and with heavy smoking (≥15 cigarettes/day). Women who use oral contraceptives should be strongly advised not to smoke.

ADULT DOSAGE	PEDIATRIC DOSAGE
Contraception	**Contraception**
1 blue tab qd for 21 consecutive days, followed by 1 peach tab for 7 days	Not indicated for use premenarche; refer to adult dosing
Start 1st Sunday after menses begins or 1st day of menses	
Conversions	
Switching from Another Oral Contraceptive:	
Start on the same day that a new pack of the previous oral contraceptive would have been started	

DOSING CONSIDERATIONS
Other Important Considerations
Non-Lactating Postpartum Women:
Start therapy 4 weeks postpartum

ADMINISTRATION
Oral route

Take dose at the exact same time every day (preferably after the evening meal or hs) at intervals not exceeding 24 hrs
Do not consider as effective contraception until after first 7 consecutive days of product administration; instruct to use a nonhormonal contraceptive as backup during the first 7 days

STORAGE
20-25°C (68-77°F).

HOW SUPPLIED
Tab: (Ethinyl Estradiol [EE]/Drospirenone [DRSP]) 0.03mg/3mg

CONTRAINDICATIONS
Renal or adrenal insufficiency, hepatic dysfunction, thrombophlebitis, thromboembolic disorders, history of deep vein thrombophlebitis or thromboembolic disorders, cerebrovascular or coronary artery disease (CAD), valvular heart disease with thrombogenic complications, severe HTN, diabetes with vascular involvement, headaches with focal neurological symptoms, known or suspected breast carcinoma, endometrial carcinoma or other known or suspected estrogen-dependent neoplasia, undiagnosed abnormal genital bleeding, cholestatic jaundice of pregnancy or jaundice with prior pill use, liver tumor (benign or malignant) or active liver disease, pregnancy, heavy smoking (>15 cigarettes daily) and >35 yrs of age.

WARNINGS/PRECAUTIONS
May cause hyperkalemia in high-risk patients; avoid use in patients predisposed to hyperkalemia (eg, renal insufficiency, hepatic dysfunction, adrenal insufficiency). Monitor K^+ levels during 1st treatment cycle with conditions predisposed to hyperkalemia. Increased risk of myocardial infarction (MI), thromboembolism, stroke, gallbladder disease, vascular disease, and hepatic neoplasia. Increased risk of morbidity and mortality in patients with HTN, hyperlipidemia, obesity, and diabetes mellitus (DM). May increase risk of breast cancer and cervical intraepithelial neoplasia. Retinal thrombosis reported; d/c use if unexplained partial or complete loss of vision, onset of proptosis or diplopia, papilledema, or retinal vascular lesions develop. May cause glucose intolerance; monitor prediabetic and diabetic patients. May cause fluid retention. May increase BP; monitor closely with HTN and d/c if significant elevation of BP occurs. D/C with onset or exacerbation of migraine or development of headache with new pattern which is persistent, recurrent, and severe. Breakthrough bleeding and spotting reported; rule out malignancy or pregnancy. Monitor closely with hyperlipidemias. D/C if jaundice develops. Monitor closely with depression and d/c if depression recurs to serious degree. Contact lens wearers who develop visual changes or changes in lens tolerance should be assessed by an ophthalmologist. Should not be used to induce withdrawal bleeding as a test for pregnancy or to treat threatened or habitual abortion during pregnancy. May affect certain endocrine, LFTs, and blood components in lab tests. Does not protect against HIV infection (AIDS) and other STDs.

ADVERSE REACTIONS
N/V, breakthrough bleeding, spotting, amenorrhea, migraine, depression, vaginal candidiasis, edema, weight changes, breast changes, GI symptoms (abdominal cramps and bloating), menstrual flow changes.

DRUG INTERACTIONS
Concomitant use with rifampin, anticonvulsants (eg, phenobarbital, phenytoin, carbamazepine), or phenylbutazone may reduce contraceptive effectiveness and increase menstrual irregularities. Pregnancy reported with antimicrobials (eg, ampicillin, tetracycline, griseofulvin). St. John's wort may reduce contraceptive effectiveness and cause breakthrough bleeding. Increased levels with atorvastatin, ascorbic acid, and acetaminophen (APAP). Risk of hyperkalemia with ACE inhibitors, angiotensin-II receptor antagonists, K^+-sparing diuretics, heparin, aldosterone antagonists, and NSAIDs; monitor K^+ levels during 1st cycle. May increase levels of cyclosporine, prednisolone, and theophylline. May decrease APAP levels and increase clearance of temazepam, salicylic acid, morphine, and clofibric acid.

PREGNANCY AND LACTATION
Category X, not for use in nursing.

MECHANISM OF ACTION
Estrogen/progestogen oral contraceptive; suppresses gonadotropins. Inhibits ovulation and produces changes in cervical mucus (increasing difficulty of sperm entry into uterus) and endometrium (reducing likelihood of implantation).

PHARMACOKINETICS
Absorption: DRSP: Absolute bioavailability (76%); (Cycle 13/Day 21) C_{max}=78.7ng/mL; T_{max}=1.6 hrs; AUC=968ng•h/mL. EE: Absolute bioavailability (40%); (Cycle 13/Day 21) C_{max}=90.5pg/mL; T_{max}=1.6 hrs; AUC=469.5pg•h/mL. **Distribution:** Found in breast milk; DRSP: V_d=4L/kg; serum protein binding (97%). EE: V_d=4-5L/kg; serum albumin binding (98.5%). **Metabolism:** DRSP: Liver, via CYP3A4 (minor). EE: Hydroxylation (via CYP3A4), conjugation (glucuronidation and sulfation). **Elimination:** DRSP: Urine, feces; $T_{1/2}$=30 hrs. EE: Urine, feces; $T_{1/2}$=24 hrs.

PATIENT CONSIDERATIONS
Assessment: Assess for current or history of thrombophlebitis or thromboembolic disorders, cerebrovascular disorders, or any other conditions where treatment is contraindicated or cautioned. Assess for pregnancy/nursing status and for possible drug interactions. Assess use in patients with contact lenses, HTN, DM, hyperlipidemia, and who are obese.

Monitoring: Monitor for signs/symptoms of MI, thromboembolism, cerebrovascular disease, carcinoma of the breast, cervical intraepithelial neoplasia, hepatic neoplasia, onset or exacerbation of a migraine headache, gallbladder disease, ocular lesions, hypertriglyceridemia, HTN, bleeding irregularities, jaundice, and for fluid retention. Monitor for signs of worsening depression in patients with a history of depression. Monitor lipid levels in patients with a history of hyperlipidemia. Monitor blood glucose levels in patients with DM. Monitor BP in patients with HTN. Perform annual history and physical exam. Monitor K^+ levels in patients at risk for hyperkalemia. Refer patients with contact lenses to an ophthalmologist if visual changes or changes in contact lens tolerance occur.

Counseling: Inform that drug does not protect against HIV infection (AIDS) and other STDs. Inform of potential risks/benefits of oral contraceptives. Counsel not to smoke while on treatment. Instruct to take medication at the same time daily. Inform that there may be spotting, light bleeding, or nausea during first 1-3 packs; advise not to d/c medication and if symptoms persist, notify physician. Inform that if started later than the 1st day of the menstrual cycle, it should not be considered effective as a contraceptive until after first 7 consecutive days of administration. Instruct what to do in the event pills are missed.

ZARONTIN — ethosuximide   Rx
Class: Succinimide

ADULT DOSAGE	PEDIATRIC DOSAGE
Absence Seizures	**Absence Seizures**
Control of Absence (Petit Mal) Epilepsy:	**Control of Absence (Petit Mal) Epilepsy:**
Initial: 500mg qd	**3-6 Years:**
Titrate: Increase dose by small increments. May increase daily dose by 250mg every 4-7 days until control is achieved w/ minimal side effects	**Initial:** 250mg qd
	Titrate: Increase dose by small increments. May increase daily dose by 250mg every 4-7 days until control is achieved w/ minimal side effects
Dosages >1.5g/day, in divided doses, should be administered only under the strictest supervision of physician	**≥6 Years:**
	Initial: 500mg qd
May be coadministered w/ other anticonvulsants when other forms of epilepsy coexist	**Titrate:** Increase dose by small increments. May increase daily dose by 250mg every 4-7 days until control is achieved w/ minimal side effects
	Optimal dose for most pediatric patients is 20mg/kg/day; subsequent dose schedules may be based on effectiveness and plasma level determinations
	Dosages >1.5g/day, in divided doses, should be administered only under the strictest supervision of physician
	May be coadministered w/ other anticonvulsants when other forms of epilepsy coexist

ADMINISTRATION
Oral route

STORAGE
Cap: 25°C (77°F); excursions permitted to 15-30°C (59-86°F). **Oral Sol:** 20-25°C (68-77°F). Preserve in tight containers. Protect from freezing and light.

HOW SUPPLIED
Cap: 250mg; **Oral Sol:** 250mg/5mL [474mL]

CONTRAINDICATIONS
History of hypersensitivity to succinimides.

WARNINGS/PRECAUTIONS
Blood dyscrasias, including some w/ fatal outcome, reported; perform blood counts if signs/symptoms of infection develop. Abnormal renal/liver function studies reported; extreme caution w/ known liver/renal disease. Systemic lupus erythematosus (SLE) reported. May increase risk of suicidal thoughts or behavior. Serious dermatologic reactions, including Stevens-Johnson syndrome (SJS), reported; d/c at the 1st sign of a rash unless rash is clearly not drug-related. Do not resume therapy and consider alternative therapy if signs/symptoms suggest SJS. Drug reaction w/ eosinophilia and systemic symptoms (DRESS), also known as multi organ hypersensitivity, reported; evaluate immediately if signs/symptoms are present, and d/c if an alternative etiology cannot be established. Cases of birth defects reported. May increase frequency of grand mal seizures when used alone in mixed types of epilepsy. Proceed slowly when increasing/decreasing dosage, and when adding or eliminating other medications. Abrupt withdrawal may precipitate absence (petit mal) status.

ADVERSE REACTIONS
DRESS, GI symptoms (eg, anorexia, vague gastric upset, N/V, epigastric/abdominal pain), leukopenia, drowsiness, headache, sleep disturbances, urticaria, pruritic erythematous rashes, myopia, vaginal bleeding, microscopic hematuria.

DRUG INTERACTIONS
May interact w/ other antiepileptic drugs (eg, may increase phenytoin levels; increased/decreased levels w/ valproic acid); periodic serum level determinations of these drugs may be necessary.

PREGNANCY AND LACTATION
Pregnancy: Cases of birth defects reported; cannot be regarded as adequate to prove a definite cause and effect relationship. Consider discontinuation prior to and during pregnancy in individual cases where the severity and frequency of the seizure disorder are such that the removal of medication does not pose a serious threat to the patient. Physicians are advised to recommend pregnant patients to enroll in the North American Antiepileptic Drug (NAAED) Pregnancy Registry. **Lactation:** Excreted in breast milk; caution in nursing.

MECHANISM OF ACTION
Succinimide; suppresses the paroxysmal 3 cycle/sec spike and wave activity associated w/ lapses of consciousness that is common in absence (petit mal) seizures. Frequency of attacks is reduced by depression of motor cortex and elevation of the CNS threshold to convulsive stimuli.

PHARMACOKINETICS
Distribution: Crosses placenta; found in breast milk.

PATIENT CONSIDERATIONS
Assessment: Assess for history of hypersensitivity to succinimides, depression, suicidal thoughts or behavior, known liver/renal disease, mixed type epilepsy, pregnancy/nursing status, and possible drug interactions. Obtain baseline CBC.

Monitoring: Monitor for blood dyscrasias, signs and/or symptoms of infection, SLE, serious dermatologic reactions, emergence/worsening of depression, suicidal thoughts or behavior, unusual changes in mood or behavior, and other adverse reactions. Monitor for occurrence of grand mal seizures in patients w/ mixed types of epilepsy who are on monotherapy. Perform periodic blood counts, urinalysis, and LFTs.

Counseling: Instruct to take only ud. Inform that therapy may impair mental/physical abilities; caution against performance of potentially hazardous tasks. Inform of the importance of strictly adhering to prescribed dosage regimen. Instruct to promptly contact physician if any signs/symptoms of infection develop. Advise of the need to be alert for the emergence or worsening of depression, any unusual changes in mood or behavior, or emergence of suicidal thoughts/behavior or thoughts about self-harm, and to immediately report to physician any behaviors of concern. Instruct that a rash may herald a serious medical event and to report to physician immediately if rash occurs. Encourage to enroll in the NAAED Pregnancy Registry if pregnant.

ZARXIO — filgrastim-sndz   Rx
Class: Granulocyte colony-stimulating factor (G-CSF)

ADULT DOSAGE	PEDIATRIC DOSAGE
Chemotherapy-Associated Neutropenia	**General Dosing**
Decreases incidence of infection, as manifested by febrile neutropenia, in patients w/ nonmyeloid malignancies receiving myelosuppressive anticancer drugs associated w/ a significant incidence of severe neutropenia w/ fever. Also reduces the time to neutrophil recovery and duration of fever, following induction or consolidation chemotherapy treatment of patients w/ acute myeloid leukemia (AML)	Refer to prescribing information for information on pediatric dosing
Receiving Myelosuppressive Chemotherapy or Induction and/or Consolidation Chemotherapy for AML:	
Initial: 5mcg/kg/day qd	
Titrate: May increase in increments of 5mcg/kg for each chemotherapy cycle, according to duration and severity of ANC nadir	
D/C if ANC increases beyond 10,000/mm³	
To reduce the duration of neutropenia and neutropenia-related clinical sequelae in patients w/ nonmyeloid malignancies undergoing myeloablative chemotherapy followed by marrow transplantation	
Receiving Bone Marrow Transplant: 10mcg/kg/day by IV infusion no longer than 24 hrs	
Titrate:	
When ANC >1000/mm³ for 3 Consecutive Days: Reduce to 5mcg/kg/day, then	
If ANC Remains >1000/mm³ for 3 More Consecutive Days: D/C therapy, then	
If ANC Decreases to <1000/mm³: Resume at 5mcg/kg/day	
If ANC decreases to <1000/mm³ at any time during the 5mcg/kg/day administration, increase to 10mcg/kg/day, and retitrate following the above steps	
Hematopoietic Progenitor Cell Mobilization	
Mobilizes autologous hematopoietic progenitor cells into the peripheral blood for collection by leukapheresis	
10mcg/kg/day SQ for ≥4 days before the 1st leukapheresis procedure and continued until the last leukapheresis	

Monitor neutrophil counts after 4 days of therapy, and d/c if WBC count rises to >100,000/mm³

Administration of therapy for 6-7 days w/ leukapheresis on Days 5, 6, and 7 was found to be safe and effective

Severe Chronic Neutropenia
Reduces incidence and duration of sequelae

Initial:
Congenital: 6mcg/kg SQ bid
Idiopathic/Cyclic: 5mcg/kg SQ qd
Titrate: Adjust dose based on clinical course and ANC

ADMINISTRATION
SQ/IV route

- Direct administration to patients requiring doses <0.3mL (180mcg) is not recommended due to potential for dosing errors.
- Avoid administration of prefilled syringe in persons w/ latex allergies; needle cap contains natural rubber latex.
- Prior to use, remove prefilled syringe from the refrigerator and allow therapy to reach room temperature for a minimum of 30 min and a max of 24 hrs.
- Discard any prefilled syringe left at room temperature for >24 hrs.

SQ Administration
- Inject in the outer area of upper arms, abdomen, thighs, or upper outer areas of buttocks.

Chemotherapy-Associated Neutropenia
Cancer Patients Receiving Myelosuppressive Chemotherapy or Induction and/or Consolidation Chemotherapy for Acute Myeloid Leukemia:
- May administer by SQ inj, by short IV infusion (15-30 min), or by continuous IV infusion.
- Administer at least 24 hrs after cytotoxic chemotherapy.
- Do not administer w/in the 24-hr period prior to chemotherapy.
- Administer daily for up to 2 weeks or until ANC has reached 10,000/mm³ following the expected chemotherapy-induced neutrophil nadir.

Cancer Patients Receiving Bone Marrow Transplant:
- Administer 1st dose at least 24 hrs after cytotoxic chemotherapy and at least 24 hrs after bone marrow infusion.

Dilution
- May dilute in D5 to concentrations between 5-15mcg/mL.
- Protect diluted concentrations between 5-15mcg/mL from adsorption to plastic materials by the addition of albumin (human) to a final concentration of 2mg/mL.
- When diluted in D5 or D5 plus albumin (human), compatible w/ glass bottles, polyvinylchloride, polyolefin, and polypropylene.
- Do not dilute w/ saline; product may precipitate.
- May store at room temperature for up to 24 hrs; the 24-hr time period includes the time during room temperature storage of the infusion sol and the duration of the infusion.

STORAGE
2-8°C (36-46°F). Protect from light. Do not shake. Avoid freezing; if frozen, thaw in the refrigerator before administration. Discard if frozen more than once.

HOW SUPPLIED
Inj: 300mcg/0.5mL, 480mcg/0.8mL

CONTRAINDICATIONS
History of serious allergic reactions to human granulocyte colony-stimulating factors such as filgrastim or pegfilgrastim products.

WARNINGS/PRECAUTIONS
Splenic rupture, including fatal cases, reported. Acute respiratory distress syndrome (ARDS) reported; d/c in patients w/ ARDS. Serious allergic-type reactions, including anaphylaxis, reported; permanently d/c in patients w/ serious allergic reactions. Sickle cell crisis, in some cases fatal, reported in patients w/ sickle cell trait/disease. Glomerulonephritis reported; evaluate for cause if glomerulonephritis is suspected, and consider dose reduction or interruption of therapy if causality is likely. Not approved for peripheral blood progenitor cell collection mobilization in healthy donors; alveolar hemorrhage manifesting as pulmonary infiltrates and hemoptysis reported. Capillary leak syndrome (CLS) reported. Myelodysplastic syndrome (MDS) and AML reported to occur in the natural history of congenital neutropenia w/o cytokine therapy. Cytogenetic abnormalities, transformation to MDS, and AML observed in patients treated for severe chronic neutropenia (SCN); carefully consider the risks and benefits of continuing therapy if a patient w/ SCN develops abnormal cytogenetics or myelodysplasia. Thrombocytopenia and leukocytosis reported. Cutaneous vasculitis reported; hold therapy w/ cutaneous vasculitis and may start therapy at a reduced dose when the symptoms resolve and the ANC has decreased. May act as a growth factor for any tumor type. Consider transient positive bone-imaging changes when interpreting bone-imaging results.

ADVERSE REACTIONS
Nonmyeloid Malignancies Receiving Myelosuppressive Anti-Cancer Drugs: Pyrexia, pain, rash, cough, dyspnea.
AML: Pain, epistaxis, rash.
Nonmyeloid Malignancies Undergoing Myeloablative Chemotherapy Followed by Bone Marrow Transplantation: Rash.
Undergoing Peripheral Blood Progenitor Cell Mobilization and Collection: Bone pain, pyrexia, headache.
Severe Chronic Neutropenia: Pain, anemia, epistaxis, diarrhea, hypoesthesia, alopecia.

DRUG INTERACTIONS
Do not use in the period 24 hrs before through 24 hours after the administration of cytotoxic chemotherapy. Avoid simultaneous use w/ chemotherapy and radiation therapy.

PREGNANCY AND LACTATION
Pregnancy: Category C.
Lactation: Caution in nursing.

MECHANISM OF ACTION
Granulocyte colony-stimulating factor; acts on hematopoietic cells by binding to specific cell surface receptors and stimulating proliferation, differentiation commitment, and some end-cell functional activation.

PHARMACOKINETICS
Absorption: (SQ) Absolute Bioavailability (60-70%); C_{max}=4ng/mL (3.45mcg/kg), 49ng/mL (11.5mcg/kg); T_{max}=2-8 hrs. **Distribution:** (IV) V_d=150mL/kg; crosses placenta. **Elimination:** $T_{1/2}$=3.5 hrs (IV), 231 min (34.5mcg/kg IV), 210 min (3.45mcg/kg SQ).

PATIENT CONSIDERATIONS
Assessment: Assess for hypersensitivity to the drug, latex allergy, sickle cell disorder, pregnancy/nursing status, and possible drug interactions. Confirm diagnosis of SCN prior to therapy. Obtain baseline CBC and platelet count in patients receiving myelosuppressive chemotherapy/induction, and/or consolidation chemotherapy for AML.

Monitoring: Monitor for serious allergic-type reactions, splenic rupture, ARDS, sickle cell crisis, glomerulonephritis, CLS, cutaneous vasculitis, thrombocytopenia, leukocytosis, and other adverse reactions. Monitor for cytogenetic abnormalities, transformation to MDS, and AML in patients w/ SCN. In patients receiving myelosuppressive chemotherapy/induction, and/or consolidation chemotherapy for AML, monitor CBC and platelet count twice weekly. In patients w/ SCN, monitor CBC w/ differential and platelet counts during the initial 4 weeks of therapy and during the 2 weeks following any dose adjustment, and, once patient is clinically stable, monthly during the 1st yr of treatment; thereafter, if clinically stable, less frequent routine monitoring is recommended. Frequently monitor CBCs and platelet counts following marrow transplantation.

Counseling: Instruct patient and caregiver on direct patient administration, including how to measure the required dose, particularly if on a dose other than the entire syringe. Inform that rupture or enlargement of the spleen may occur; advise to immediately report to physician if symptoms develop. Advise to seek immediate medical attention if signs/symptoms of a hypersensitivity reaction occur. Advise to immediately report to physician if dyspnea or signs/symptoms of vasculitis develop. Discuss potential risks and benefits for patients w/ sickle cell disease prior to administration. Advise female of reproductive potential that therapy should be used during pregnancy only if the potential benefit justifies the potential risk to the fetus.

ZAVESCA — miglustat   Rx
Class: Glucosylceramide synthase inhibitor

ADULT DOSAGE	PEDIATRIC DOSAGE
Type 1 Gaucher Disease As monotherapy for mild to moderate type 1 Gaucher disease when enzyme replacement therapy is not a therapeutic option **Recommended Dose:** 100mg tid at regular intervals	Pediatric use may not have been established

DOSING CONSIDERATIONS
Renal Impairment
Mild (CrCl 50-70mL/min):
Initial: 100mg bid
Moderate (CrCl 30-50mL/min):
Initial: 100mg qd
Severe (CrCl <30mL/min):
Not recommended for use
Elderly
Start at lower end of dosing range

Adverse Reactions
Tremor, Diarrhea, Other: May be necessary reduce dose to one 100mg cap qd or bid in some patients

ADMINISTRATION
Oral route

Therapy should be directed by physicians who are knowledgeable in the management of Gaucher disease.

STORAGE
20-25°C (68-77°F); brief exposure to 15-30°C (59-86°F) permitted.

HOW SUPPLIED
Cap: 100mg

WARNINGS/PRECAUTIONS
Peripheral neuropathy reported; perform baseline and repeat neurological evaluations at 6-month intervals. Reassess risks/benefits of therapy if symptoms of peripheral neuropathy develop; may consider cessation of treatment. Tremor or exacerbation of existing tremor reported; reduce dose to ameliorate tremor or d/c if tremor does not resolve w/in days of dose reduction. Diarrhea and weight

loss commonly reported; avoid high carbohydrate content foods if diarrhea occurs. Evaluate for significant underlying GI disease in patients w/ persistent GI events that continue during treatment, and in those who do not respond to usual interventions. Caution w/ significant GI disease (eg, inflammatory bowel disease), and in elderly. Mild reductions in platelet counts may occur.

ADVERSE REACTIONS
Diarrhea, weight decrease, abdominal pain/distention, flatulence, N/V, tremor, dizziness, headache, leg cramps, unsteady gait, back pain, generalized weakness, constipation, dry mouth.

DRUG INTERACTIONS
May increase clearance of imiglucerase.

PREGNANCY AND LACTATION
Pregnancy: Category C.
Lactation: Not for use in nursing.

MECHANISM OF ACTION
Glucosylceramide synthase inhibitor; helps reduce the rate of glycosphingolipid biosynthesis so that the amount of glycosphingolipid substrate is reduced to a level which allows the residual activity of the deficient glucocerebrosidase enzyme to be more effective (substrate reduction therapy). Can reduce the synthesis of glucosylceramide-based glycosphingolipids.

PHARMACOKINETICS
Absorption: T_{max}=2-2.5 hrs. **Distribution:** V_d=83-105L. **Elimination:** Urine (83%, 67% unchanged), feces (12%); $T_{1/2}$=6-7 hrs.

PATIENT CONSIDERATIONS
Assessment: Assess for renal impairment, existing tremor, GI disease, pregnancy/nursing status, and possible drug interactions. Obtain baseline neurological evaluation.

Monitoring: Monitor for signs/symptoms of peripheral neuropathy, tremor/exacerbation of tremor, diarrhea, weight loss, and other adverse reactions. Perform neurological evaluations at 6-month intervals. Monitor platelet counts.

Counseling: Instruct to promptly report any signs/symptoms of peripheral neuropathy (eg, numbness, tingling, pain, burning in hands/feet), and the development of tremor or worsening in an existing tremor. Advise that diarrhea and weight loss may occur; instruct to adhere to dietary instructions, and to avoid high carbohydrate content foods during treatment if diarrhea occurs. Inform of the potential risks and benefits of therapy and of alternative modes of therapy.

ZEBETA — bisoprolol fumarate   Rx

Class: Selective beta₁ blocker

ADULT DOSAGE	PEDIATRIC DOSAGE
Hypertension	Pediatric use may not have been established
Initial: 5mg qd	
Titrate: May increase to 10mg and then, if necessary, to 20mg qd	

DOSING CONSIDERATIONS
Renal Impairment
CrCl <40mL/min:
Initial: 2.5mg qd; use caution w/ dose titration

Hepatic Impairment
Initial: 2.5mg qd; use caution w/ dose titration

Other Important Considerations
Patients w/ Bronchospastic Disease:
Initial: 2.5mg qd

ADMINISTRATION
Oral route

STORAGE
20-25°C (68-77°F). Protect from moisture.

HOW SUPPLIED
Tab: 5mg*, 10mg *scored

CONTRAINDICATIONS
Cardiogenic shock, overt cardiac failure, 2nd- or 3rd-degree atrioventricular (AV) block, marked sinus bradycardia.

WARNINGS/PRECAUTIONS
Avoid abrupt withdrawal; exacerbation of angina pectoris, MI, and ventricular arrhythmia in patients with coronary artery disease, and exacerbation of symptoms of hyperthyroidism or precipitation of thyroid storm reported. Reinstitute temporary therapy if withdrawal symptoms occur. May mask manifestations of hypoglycemia or clinical signs of hyperthyroidism (eg, tachycardia). Caution with compensated cardiac failure, diabetes mellitus, bronchospastic disease, and hepatic/renal impairment. May precipitate cardiac failure; d/c at the 1st signs/symptoms of heart failure (HF) or continue therapy while HF is treated with other drugs. Caution with peripheral vascular disease; may precipitate or aggravate symptoms of arterial insufficiency. Caution with history of severe anaphylactic reaction to a variety of allergens; reactivity may increase with repeated challenge.

ADVERSE REACTIONS
Headache, URI, peripheral edema, fatigue, ALT/AST elevation.

DRUG INTERACTIONS
Patients with a history of severe anaphylactic reaction to a variety of allergens taking β-blockers may be unresponsive to usual doses of epinephrine. D/C several days before withdrawal of clonidine. Excessive reduction of sympathetic activity with catecholamine-depleting drugs (eg, reserpine, guanethidine); monitor closely. Avoid with other β-blockers. Caution with myocardial depressants or inhibitors of AV conduction, such as calcium antagonists (eg, verapamil, diltiazem) or antiarrhythmics (eg, disopyramide). Increased risk of bradycardia with digitalis glycosides. Increased clearance with rifampin. Caution with insulin or oral hypoglycemic agents. Reversed effects with bronchodilator therapy. Additive BP lowering effects in mild to moderate HTN with HCTZ.

PREGNANCY AND LACTATION
Category C, caution in nursing.

MECHANISM OF ACTION
β₁-selective adrenoreceptor blocking agent; not established. May decrease cardiac output, inhibit renin release by the kidneys, and diminution of tonic sympathetic outflow from the vasomotor centers in the brain.

PHARMACOKINETICS
Absorption: (10mg) Absolute bioavailability (80%); C_{max}=(5mg) 16ng/mL, (20mg) 70ng/mL; (5-20mg) T_{max}=2-4 hrs. **Distribution:** Plasma protein binding (30%). **Elimination:** Urine (50%, unchanged), feces (<2%); $T_{1/2}$=9-12 hrs.

PATIENT CONSIDERATIONS
Assessment: Assess for conditions where treatment is contraindicated or cautioned, pregnancy/nursing status, and possible drug interactions.

Monitoring: Monitor for hypoglycemia, hyperthyroidism, hepatic/renal function, signs/symptoms of HF, withdrawal, and arterial insufficiency. Monitor HR, ECG, CBC with platelet and differential count.

Counseling: Instruct not to interrupt or d/c therapy without consulting physician. Notify physician if difficulty in breathing, signs/symptoms of CHF or excessive bradycardia develop. Educate about signs/symptoms of drug's potential adverse effects. Advise to exercise caution while driving, operating machinery, or engaging in other tasks requiring alertness.

ZECUITY — sumatriptan   Rx

Class: 5-HT₁ᵦ/₁ᴅ agonist (triptans)

ADULT DOSAGE	PEDIATRIC DOSAGE
Migraine	Pediatric use may not have been established
Acute Treatment w/ or w/o Aura: Apply 1 patch for 4 hrs or until red light emitting diode light goes off. If headache relief is incomplete, a 2nd patch may be applied ≥2 hrs after activation of the 1st patch to a different site	
Max: 1 patch/dose or 2 patches/24 hrs	
The safety of using >4 patches in 1 month has not been established	

DOSING CONSIDERATIONS
Elderly
Start at lower end of dosing range

ADMINISTRATION
Transdermal route

Apply to dry intact, non-irritated skin on upper arm or thigh on a site that is relatively hair free and w/o scars, tattoos, abrasions, or other skin conditions; may secure the system w/ medical tape if needed.
Do not apply to a previous application site until the site remains erythema free for at least 3 days.
Once applied, push the activation button to turn on the red light emitting diode (LED) w/in 15 min.
When the LED light turns off, dosing is complete and the system can be removed. After use, fold the system so the adhesive side sticks to itself and safely discard away from children and pets.

STORAGE
20-25°C (68-77°F); excursions permitted to 15-30°C (59-86°F). Do not refrigerate or freeze. Contains lithium-manganese dioxide batteries; dispose in accordance with state and local regulations.

HOW SUPPLIED
Iontophoretic Transdermal System: 6.5mg/4 hrs

CONTRAINDICATIONS
Ischemic coronary artery disease (CAD) (eg, angina pectoris, history of MI, documented silent ischemia), coronary artery vasospasm (eg, Prinzmetal's angina), Wolff-Parkinson-White syndrome or arrhythmias associated with other cardiac accessory conduction pathway disorders, history of stroke, transient ischemic attack, history of hemiplegic or basilar migraine, peripheral vascular disease, ischemic bowel disease, uncontrolled HTN, severe hepatic impairment, or allergic contact dermatitis to sumatriptan. Recent (within 24 hrs) use of ergotamine-containing medication, ergot-type medication (eg, dihydroergotamine, methysergide) or another 5-hydroxytryptamine₁ agonist. Concurrent administration of an MAO-A inhibitor or recent (within 2 weeks) use of an MAO-A inhibitor. Known hypersensitivity to sumatriptan or components of this medication.

WARNINGS/PRECAUTIONS
For transdermal use only. Use only if a clear diagnosis of migraine has been established. Reconsider the diagnosis of migraine before giving a 2nd dose if

patient does not respond to the 1st dose of therapy. No evidence of benefit for the use of a 2nd transdermal system (TDS) to treat headache recurrence or incomplete headache relief during a migraine attack. Contains metal parts; remove before an MRI procedure. Do not apply in areas near or over electrically-active implantable or body-worn medical devices (eg, implantable cardiac pacemaker, body-worn insulin pump, implantable deep brain stimulator). May lead to allergic contact dermatitis; d/c if suspected. Systemic sensitization or other systemic reactions may develop if other sumatriptan-containing products are taken via other routes (eg, PO, SQ); administer 1st subsequent dose under close medical supervision. May cause coronary artery vasospasm (Prinzmetal's angina) and sensations of tightness, pain, pressure, and heaviness in the chest, throat, neck, and jaw, usually of noncardiac origin. Perform cardiovascular (CV) evaluation in triptan-naive patients who have multiple CV risk factors before treatment; if negative, consider 1st administration in a medically supervised setting and perform an ECG upon activation of TDS. Consider periodic CV evaluation in intermittent long-term users. Life-threatening cardiac rhythm disturbances reported; d/c if these occur. Cerebral hemorrhage, subarachnoid hemorrhage, and stroke may occur; exclude other potentially serious neurological conditions prior to therapy in patients not previously diagnosed as migraineurs, and in migraineurs who present with atypical symptoms. May cause noncoronary vasospastic reactions (eg, peripheral vascular ischemia, GI vascular ischemia/infarction, splenic infarction, Raynaud's syndrome). Transient/permanent blindness and significant partial vision loss reported. Overuse may lead to exacerbation of headache; detoxification including drug withdrawal, and treatment of withdrawal symptoms may be necessary. Serotonin syndrome may occur; d/c if suspected. Significant elevation in BP, including hypertensive crisis with acute impairment of organ systems, reported. Anaphylactic/anaphylactoid reactions may occur. Seizures reported; caution in patients with a history of epilepsy or conditions associated with a lowered seizure threshold.

ADVERSE REACTIONS
Application-site reactions (pain, paresthesia, pruritus, warmth, discomfort, irritation, discoloration, vesicles).

DRUG INTERACTIONS
See Contraindications. Serotonin syndrome reported with SSRIs, SNRIs, TCAs, or MAOIs.

PREGNANCY AND LACTATION
Category C, not for use in nursing.

MECHANISM OF ACTION
Selective 5-HT$_{1B/1D}$ agonist; thought to be due to the agonist effects at the 5HT$_{1B/1D}$ receptors on intracranial blood vessels (including arteriovenous anastomoses) and sensory nerves of the trigeminal system, which result in cranial vessel constriction and inhibition of proinflammatory neuropeptide release.

PHARMACOKINETICS
Absorption: C_{max}=22ng/mL, AUC_{0-inf}=110 hr•ng/mL, T_{max} =1.1 hrs (median). **Distribution:** (Healthy) V_d=2.4L/kg; plasma protein binding (14-21%). **Metabolism:** via MAO-A; indole acetic acid (IAA) (major metabolite). **Elimination:** Urine (11%, unchanged, 69% IAA), $T_{1/2}$=3.1 hrs.

PATIENT CONSIDERATIONS

Assessment: Assess for cardiovascular disease, HTN, hemiplegic/basilar migraine, ECG changes, and any other conditions where treatment is cautioned or contraindicated, hepatic function, pregnancy/nursing status, and for possible drug interactions. Confirm diagnosis of migraine and exclude other potentially serious neurologic conditions prior to therapy. Perform CV evaluation in patients who have CV risk factors.

Monitoring: Monitor for signs/symptoms of cardiac events, cerebrovascular events, peripheral vascular ischemia, GI vascular ischemia/infarction, serotonin syndrome, allergic contact dermatitis, anaphylactic/anaphylactoid reactions, visual disturbances, HTN, and other adverse reactions. Perform ECG immediately after administration of therapy and monitor CV function in intermittent long-term users. Monitor for medication overuse; exacerbation of headache may occur.

Counseling: Instruct to use TDS ud; instruct not to bathe, shower, or swim while wearing TDS. Inform that most patients experience some skin redness under the TDS upon removal, which usually disappears within 24 hrs. Inform patients that the TDS contains metal parts and must be removed before an MRI procedure. Inform that treatment may cause serious CV adverse reactions (eg, MI or stroke) that may result in hospitalization and even death. Instruct patients to be alert for signs/symptoms of chest pain, SOB, weakness, and slurring of speech; instruct to notify physician if these symptoms and other symptoms of vasospastic reactions occur. Inform patients of the signs and symptoms of allergic contact dermatitis, and instruct to seek medical advice if skin lesions suggestive of allergic contact dermatitis develop. Counsel about the possible drug interactions and the risk of anaphylactic/anaphylactoid reactions. Inform patients that the use of therapy ≥10 days per month may lead to exacerbation of headache; encourage to record headache frequency and drug use. Advise to notify physician if pregnant/nursing or planning to become pregnant. Instruct patients to evaluate their ability to perform complex tasks during migraine attacks and after using therapy.

ZEGERID — omeprazole/sodium bicarbonate   Rx
Class: Proton pump inhibitor (PPI)/antacid

ADULT DOSAGE	PEDIATRIC DOSAGE
	Pediatric use may not have been established

ADULT DOSAGE

Gastroesophageal Reflux Disease

Symptomatic GERD (w/ No Esophageal Erosions):
20mg qd for up to 4 weeks

Erosive Esophagitis (Diagnosed by Endoscopy):
20mg qd for 4-8 weeks

May give up to an additional 4 weeks if no response to 8 weeks of therapy. May consider additional 4- to 8-week courses if there is recurrence of erosive esophagitis or GERD symptoms

Maint of Healing of Erosive Esophagitis:
20mg qd; controlled studies do not extend beyond 12 months

Recommended doses are based upon omeprazole

Upper GI Bleeding

Risk Reduction in Critically Ill Patients:
Sus, 40mg/1680mg:
Initial: 40mg, followed by 40mg after 6-8 hrs
Maint: 40mg qd for 14 days

Recommended doses are based upon omeprazole

Duodenal Ulcers

Active:
20mg qd for 4-8 weeks

Recommended doses are based upon omeprazole

Gastric Ulcers

Active Benign:
40mg qd for 4-8 weeks

Recommended doses are based upon omeprazole

PEDIATRIC DOSAGE
Pediatric use may not have been established

DOSING CONSIDERATIONS
Hepatic Impairment
Consider dose reduction, particularly for maint of healing of erosive esophagitis

Other Important Considerations
Asian Population: Recommended dose reduction, particularly for maint of healing of erosive esophagitis

ADMINISTRATION
Oral route

Both the 20mg and 40mg oral sus packets contain the same amount of sodium bicarbonate (1680mg). Two packets of 20mg are not equivalent to one packet of 40mg; do not substitute two 20mg packets for one packet of 40mg.
Both the 20mg and 40mg caps contain the same amount of sodium bicarbonate (1100mg). Two caps of 20mg are not equivalent to one cap of 40mg; do not substitute two 20mg caps for one cap of 40mg.

Take on an empty stomach at least 1 hr ac.

Administration of Cap
Swallow intact w/ water; do not use other liquids.
Do not open cap and sprinkle contents into food.

Preparation and Administration of Sus
Empty pkt contents into a small cup containing 1-2 tbsp of water; do not use other liquids or foods.
Stir well and drink immediately.
Refill cup w/ water and drink.

Administration Through NG or Orogastric Tube:
Suspend enteral feeding approx 3 hrs before and 1 hr after administration of sus.
Constitute the sus w/ approx 20mL of water; do not use other liquids or foods.
Stir well and administer immediately.
Use an appropriately sized syringe to instill sus in tube.
Wash sus through the tube w/ 20mL of water.

STORAGE
25°C (77°F); excursions permitted to 15-30°C (59-86°F). Protect from light and moisture.

HOW SUPPLIED
(Omeprazole/Sodium Bicarbonate) **Cap:** 20mg/1100mg, 40mg/1100mg; **Sus:** (20mg/1680mg)/pkt, (40mg/1680mg)/pkt

CONTRAINDICATIONS
Known hypersensitivity to any components of the formulation.

WARNINGS/PRECAUTIONS

Omeprazole: Symptomatic response does not preclude the presence of gastric malignancy. Atrophic gastritis reported w/ long-term use. Acute interstitial nephritis reported; d/c if this develops. Cyanocobalamin (vitamin B12) deficiency may occur w/ daily long-term treatment (eg, >3 yrs) w/ any acid-suppressing medications. May increase risk of *Clostridium difficile*-associated diarrhea (CDAD), especially in hospitalized patients. May increase risk of osteoporosis-related fractures of the hip, wrist, or spine, especially w/ high-dose and long-term therapy. Use lowest dose and shortest duration appropriate to the condition being treated. Hypomagnesemia reported and may require Mg^{2+} replacement and discontinuation of therapy; consider monitoring Mg^{2+} levels prior to and periodically during therapy w/ prolonged treatment. Drug-induced decrease in gastric acidity results in enterochromaffin-like cell hyperplasia and increased chromogranin A (CgA) levels, which may interfere w/ investigations for neuroendocrine tumors; temporarily d/c treatment before assessing CgA levels and consider repeating the test if initial CgA levels are high. **Sodium Bicarbonate:** Consider the Na^+ content when administering to patients on a Na^+-restricted diet. Caution w/ Bartter's syndrome, hypokalemia, hypocalcemia, and problems w/ acid-base balance. Chronic use may lead to systemic alkalosis, and increased Na^+ intake may produce edema and weight increase.

ADVERSE REACTIONS

Headache, abdominal pain, N/V, diarrhea.

DRUG INTERACTIONS

Monitor for the need to adjust dose of drugs metabolized via CYP450 (eg, cyclosporine, disulfiram, benzodiazepines). **Omeprazole:** Reduces pharmacological activity of clopidogrel; avoid concomitant use, and consider alternative antiplatelet therapy. Caution w/ digoxin or drugs that may cause hypomagnesemia (eg, diuretics). May elevate and prolong levels of methotrexate (MTX) and/or its metabolite, possibly leading to MTX toxicities; consider temporary withdrawal of therapy w/ high-dose MTX. May reduce the absorption of drugs where gastric pH is an important determinant of bioavailability; ketoconazole, atazanavir, iron salts, erlotinib, and mycophenolate mofetil (MMF) absorption may decrease, while digoxin absorption may increase. Monitor when digoxin is taken concomitantly. Caution in transplant patients receiving MMF. May prolong elimination of drugs metabolized by hepatic oxidation (eg, diazepam, warfarin, phenytoin). Increased INR and PT reported w/ warfarin. Voriconazole (combined inhibitor of CYP2C19 and CYP3A4) may increase levels. May decrease levels of atazanavir and nelfinavir; coadministration not recommended. May increase levels of saquinavir and tacrolimus; consider dose reduction of saquinavir. CYP2C19 or CYP3A4 inducers may decrease levels; avoid w/ St. John's wort or rifampin. **Sodium Bicarbonate:** Long-term use of bicarbonate w/ Ca^{2+} or milk can cause milk-alkali syndrome.

PREGNANCY AND LACTATION

Pregnancy: Category C.
Lactation: Not for use in nursing.

MECHANISM OF ACTION

Omeprazole: Proton pump inhibitor; substituted benzimidazoles that suppresses gastric acid secretion by specific inhibition of the (H^+/K^+)-ATPase enzyme system at the secretory surface of the gastric parietal cell. Blocks the final step of acid production. **Sodium Bicarbonate:** Antacid; raises gastric pH, thus protecting omeprazole from acid degradation.

PHARMACOKINETICS

Absorption: Omeprazole: Rapid; T_{max}=30 min. (Sus) Absolute bioavailability (30-40%); C_{max}=1954ng/mL; $AUC_{(0-inf)}$=1665ng•hr/mL (after Dose 1 of 40mg/1680mg), 3356ng•hr/mL (after Dose 2 of 40mg/1680mg). (Cap) C_{max}=1526ng/mL.
Distribution: Omeprazole: Plasma protein binding (95%); found in breast milk.
Metabolism: Omeprazole: Hydroxyomeprazole and corresponding carboxylic acid (metabolites). **Elimination:** Omeprazole: Urine (77% as metabolites), feces; $T_{1/2}$=1 hr.

PATIENT CONSIDERATIONS

Assessment: Assess for risk of osteoporosis-related fractures, Na^+-restricted diet, Bartter's syndrome, hypokalemia, hypocalcemia, acid-base balance problems, hypersensitivity to the drug, pregnancy/nursing status, and possible drug interactions. Obtain baseline Mg^{2+} levels in patients expected to be on prolonged therapy.

Monitoring: Monitor for signs/symptoms of atrophic gastritis, acute interstitial nephritis, cyanocobalamin deficiency, CDAD, bone fractures, systemic alkalosis, hypersensitivity reactions, and other adverse reactions. Monitor Mg^{2+} levels periodically in patients expected to be on prolonged therapy. Monitor INR and PT when given w/ warfarin.

Counseling: Inform that different formulations are not bioequivalent; do not substitute one for the other. Inform patients on a Na^+-restricted diet of the Na^+ content in product. Inform that increased Na^+ intake may cause swelling and weight gain; instruct to contact physician if these occur. Inform that the most frequent adverse reactions associated w/ therapy include headache, abdominal pain, N/V, diarrhea, and flatulence. Advise that harmful effect of therapy on the fetus cannot be ruled out. Advise to use w/ caution if regularly taking Ca^{2+} supplements. Advise to immediately report and seek care for diarrhea that does not improve and for any cardiovascular/neurological symptoms (eg, palpitations, dizziness, seizures, tetany).

ZELAPAR — selegiline hydrochloride   Rx

Class: Monoamine oxidase inhibitor (MAOI) (type B)

ADULT DOSAGE	PEDIATRIC DOSAGE
Parkinson's Disease	Pediatric use may not have been established
Adjunct in the Management of Patients Being Treated w/ Levodopa/Carbidopa Who Exhibit Deterioration in the Quality of Response to this Therapy:	
Initial: 1.25mg qd for at least 6 weeks	
Titrate: After 6 weeks, may increase to 2.5mg qd if a desired benefit has not been achieved and the patient is tolerating therapy	
Max: 2.5mg qd	
Maint: 1.25mg or 2.5mg qd, depending on individual clinical response	

DOSING CONSIDERATIONS

Renal Impairment
Severe/ESRD (CrCl <30mL/min): Not recommended

Hepatic Impairment
Mild-Moderate (Child-Pugh Score 5-9): Reduce daily dose (from 2.5mg to 1.25mg qd), depending on clinical response
Severe (Child-Pugh Score >9): Not recommended

ADMINISTRATION

Oral route
Take in the am before breakfast and w/o liquid; avoid ingesting food or liquids for 5 min before and after taking the drug
Do not attempt to push through the foil backing; peel back the backing w/ dry hands, and gently remove tab(s)
Immediately place on top of the tongue

STORAGE

25°C (77°F); excursions permitted to 15-30°C (59-86°F). Use within 3 months of opening pouch and immediately upon opening individual blister.

HOW SUPPLIED

Tab, Disintegrating: 1.25mg

CONTRAINDICATIONS

Concomitant use with any other MAOI, meperidine, tramadol, methadone, or propoxyphene; at least 14 days should elapse between discontinuation of selegiline and initiation of treatment with these medications. Concomitant use with St. John's wort, cyclobenzaprine, or dextromethorphan.

WARNINGS/PRECAUTIONS

Not recommended with severe hepatic impairment (Child-Pugh score >9), severe renal impairment, and end-stage renal disease (CrCl <30mL/min). Do not use at doses >2.5mg/day due to risks associated with nonselective inhibition of MAO. Monitor for new onset HTN or exacerbation of HTN that is not adequately controlled. Falling asleep during activities of daily living and somnolence reported; d/c therapy if daytime sleepiness or episodes of falling asleep during activities that require active participation (eg, conversations, eating) develop. May impair mental/physical abilities. Orthostatic hypotension reported; increased risk in the period after increasing the daily dose from 1.25mg to 2.5mg, and in geriatric patients. May potentiate dopaminergic side effects of levodopa and may cause/exacerbate dyskinesia; decreasing the dose of levodopa may lessen dyskinesia. Hallucinations reported. New/worsening mental status and behavioral changes, which may be severe, including psychotic-like behavior, may occur; do not use in patients with a major psychotic disorder. Increased sexual urges, binge eating, intense urges to gamble or spend money, and/or other intense urges, and the inability to control these urges may occur; consider dose reduction or discontinuation if such urges develop. A symptom complex resembling neuroleptic malignant syndrome reported with rapid dose reduction, withdrawal of, or changes in antiparkinsonian therapy. Patients with Parkinson's disease may have a higher risk of developing melanoma. Mild oropharyngeal abnormality reported. Contains phenylalanine. Caution in elderly.

ADVERSE REACTIONS

Constipation, skin disorders, vomiting, dizziness, dyskinesia, insomnia, dyspnea, myalgia, rash.

DRUG INTERACTIONS

See Contraindications. Hypertensive reactions reported in patients who ingested tyramine-containing consumables (food or drink) while receiving swallowed selegiline at the recommended dose. Uncontrolled HTN reported when taking the recommended dose of swallowed selegiline and a sympathomimetic medication (ephedrine). Avoid with any antidepressant; serotonin syndrome and hyperpyrexia reported. At least 14 days should elapse between discontinuation of therapy and initiation of an SSRI, SNRI, TCA, tetracyclic, or triazolopyridine antidepressant. Allow at least 5 weeks (longer with chronic/high-dose fluoxetine) to elapse between discontinuation of fluoxetine and initiation of selegiline due to the long $T_{1/2}$ of fluoxetine and its active metabolite. Caution with CYP3A4 inducers (eg, phenytoin, carbamazepine, nafcillin). Dopamine antagonists (eg, antipsychotics, metoclopramide) may diminish effectiveness.

PREGNANCY AND LACTATION
Category C, caution in nursing.

MECHANISM OF ACTION
MAOI (Type B); irreversibly inhibits MAO-B activity (by blocking the catabolism of dopamine), which may result in increased dopamine levels. May act through other mechanisms to increase dopaminergic activity.

PHARMACOKINETICS
Absorption: Rapid. T_{max}=10-15 min; C_{max}=3.34ng/mL (1.25mg), 4.47ng/mL (2.5mg). **Distribution:** Plasma protein binding (up to 85%). **Metabolism:** Liver via CYP2B6 and CYP3A4; l-methamphetamine, N-desmethylselegiline, and l-amphetamine (metabolites). **Elimination:** Urine (metabolites, mainly as l-methamphetamine), feces (small amount); (1.25mg) $T_{1/2}$ (median)=1.3 hrs (single dose), 10 hrs (steady state).

PATIENT CONSIDERATIONS
Assessment: Assess for hepatic/renal impairment, HTN, dyskinesia, major psychotic disorder, phenylketonuria, pregnancy/nursing status, and possible drug interactions.

Monitoring: Monitor for HTN, drowsiness/sleepiness, hypotension, dyskinesia, hallucinations, new/worsening mental status and behavioral changes, psychotic-like behavior, intense urges, mild oropharyngeal abnormalities, and other adverse reactions. Monitor for melanomas frequently and on a regular basis.

Counseling: Inform of the risk of using higher daily doses; provide a brief description of the hypertensive tyramine reaction. Instruct to immediately report severe headache or other atypical/unusual symptoms not previously experienced, or very high BP. Advise to avoid certain foods (eg, aged cheese) containing a very large amount of tyramine while on therapy. Instruct to inform physician if taking or planning to take any prescription or OTC drugs. Instruct not to drive a car or engage in other potentially dangerous activities until patient has gained sufficient experience with therapy. Inform that symptomatic (or asymptomatic) hypotension may develop; caution against rising rapidly after sitting or lying down for prolonged periods and at the initiation of treatment. Instruct to contact physician if discontinuation of therapy is desired, or if hallucinations/psychotic-like behavior, new/increased gambling urges, increased sexual urges, or other intense urges develop. Advise to have periodic skin examinations. Inform that drug may cause irritation of the buccal mucosa, and that it contains aspartame, which could cause problems in patients with phenylketonuria. Instruct to take drug as prescribed.

ZELBORAF — vemurafenib   Rx

Class: Kinase inhibitor

ADULT DOSAGE
Unresectable or Metastatic Melanoma with BRAF V600E Mutation

960mg q12h until disease progression or unacceptable toxicity occurs

Missed Dose

Missed dose can be taken up to 4 hrs prior to next dose

PEDIATRIC DOSAGE
Pediatric use may not have been established

DOSING CONSIDERATIONS
Adverse Reactions
Permanently D/C If:
Grade 4 adverse reaction, 1st appearance (if clinically appropriate) or 2nd appearance
QTc prolongation >500 msec and increased by >60 msec from pretreatment values

Withhold for:
NCI CTCAE Grade 2 or greater adverse reactions

Upon Recovery to Grade 0-1, Restart at a Reduced Dose as Follows:
720mg bid for 1st appearance of intolerable Grade 2 or Grade 3 adverse reactions
480mg bid for 2nd appearance of Grade 2 (if intolerable) or Grade 3 adverse reactions or for 1st appearance of Grade 4 adverse reaction (if clinically appropriate)
Do not reduce dose to below 480mg bid

ADMINISTRATION
Oral route
Take w/ or w/o meal.
Do not crush or chew.
Do not take an additional dose if vomiting occurs after therapy; continue w/ the next scheduled dose.

STORAGE
20-25°C (68-77°F); excursions permitted between 15-30°C (59-86°F).

HOW SUPPLIED
Tab: 240mg

WARNINGS/PRECAUTIONS
See Dosing Considerations. Not indicated for wild-type BRAF melanoma. Cutaneous malignancies (eg, cutaneous squamous cell carcinoma [SCC], keratoacanthoma, melanoma) reported and non-cutaneous SCC of the head and neck may occur; monitor closely for signs or symptoms of new non-cutaneous SCC or other malignancies. Potential risk factors associated w/ cutaneous SCC include ≥65 yrs of age, prior skin cancer, and chronic sun exposure. May promote malignancies associated w/ activation of renin-angiotensin system through

mutation or other mechanisms. Increased cell proliferation in BRAF wild-type cells can occur w/ BRAF inhibitors; confirm evidence of BRAF V600E mutation in tumor specimens prior to initiating therapy. Anaphylaxis and other serious hypersensitivity/dermatological reactions may occur; d/c permanently if severe hypersensitivity/dermatological reactions occur. QT prolongation leading to an increased risk of ventricular arrhythmias (eg, torsades de pointes) may occur. Do not initiate therapy in patients w/ uncorrectable electrolyte abnormalities, QTc >500 msec, long QT syndrome, or who are taking medicines known to prolong the QT interval. Liver injury leading to functional hepatic impairment (eg, coagulopathy or other organ dysfunction) may occur. Uveitis, blurred vision, photophobia, and mild to severe photosensitivity may occur. May cause fetal harm. Radiation sensitization and recall reported in patients treated w/ radiation prior to, during, or subsequent to therapy; fatal cases have been reported in patients w/ visceral organ involvement. Renal failure (eg, acute interstitial nephritis, acute tubular necrosis) may occur.

ADVERSE REACTIONS
Arthralgia, rash, alopecia, fatigue, photosensitivity reaction, nausea, pruritus, skin papilloma.

DRUG INTERACTIONS
Strong CYP3A4 inhibitors (eg, ketoconazole, nefazodone, clarithromycin) and inducers (eg, phenytoin, carbamazepine, rifampin) may alter vemurafenib concentrations; avoid concomitant use and replace these drugs w/ alternative drugs when possible. Administration w/ tizanidine (a sensitive CYP1A2 substrate) increased tizanidine systemic exposure; avoid w/ drugs w/ a narrow therapeutic window that are predominantly metabolized by CYP1A2. If coadministration cannot be avoided, closely monitor and consider dose reduction of concomitant CYP1A2 substrates. Increases in transaminases and bilirubin occurred w/ concurrent ipilimumab. Administration w/ digoxin (a sensitive P-gp substrate) increased digoxin systemic exposure; avoid concurrent use of P-gp substrates known to have narrow therapeutic indices. If use is unavoidable, consider dose reduction of P-gp substrates w/ narrow therapeutic indices.

PREGNANCY AND LACTATION
Pregnancy: Category D. Women of childbearing age and men should use contraception during and for at least 2 months after discontinuation of therapy. **Lactation:** Not for use in nursing.

MECHANISM OF ACTION
Kinase inhibitor; inhibits some mutated forms of BRAF serine-threonine kinase (eg, BRAF V600E). BRAF V600E can cause cell proliferation in the absence of growth factors that would normally be required for proliferation.

PHARMACOKINETICS
Absorption: T_{max}=3 hrs (median); C_{max}=62mcg/mL; AUC_{0-12}=601mcg•hr/mL. **Distribution:** Plasma protein binding (>99%); V_d=106L. **Elimination:** Feces (approx 94%), urine (approx 1%); $T_{1/2}$=57 hrs (median).

PATIENT CONSIDERATIONS
Assessment: Assess for BRAF V600E mutation, prior skin cancer, chronic sun exposure, electrolyte abnormality, long QT syndrome, prior treatment w/ radiation, pregnancy/nursing status, and possible drug interactions. Perform dermatologic evaluation and obtain baseline ECG, electrolyte levels, LFTs, and SrCr.

Monitoring: Monitor for development of new primary malignancies, new non-cutaneous SCC, other malignancies, severe dermatologic and hypersensitivity reactions, photosensitivity, uveitis, renal failure, and other adverse reactions. Perform dermatologic evaluation every 2 months during treatment and consider for 6 months after discontinuation. Monitor for QTc prolongation during treatment and after dose modification of therapy; evaluate ECG and electrolytes after 15 days, monthly during the first 3 months, then every 3 months thereafter, or as clinically indicated. Monitor LFTs monthly or as clinically needed. Monitor closely when administered concomitantly or sequentially w/ radiation treatment. Periodically monitor SrCr levels.

Counseling: Inform about the potential benefits and risks of treatment. Inform that BRAF V600E mutation assessment is required for patient selection. Inform about the increased risk of developing new primary cutaneous malignancies and advise on the importance of immediately reporting any skin changes. Inform about the risk of QT prolongation, which may result in ventricular arrhythmias; advise on the importance of monitoring ECG and electrolytes during treatment. Inform about the risk of photosensitivity and advise to avoid sun exposure and to wear protective clothing, sunscreen, and lip balm w/ SPF ≥30 when outdoors. Inform that anaphylaxis, other serious hypersensitivity reactions, and severe dermatologic reactions can occur. Advise to stop taking therapy and to seek immediate medical attention/contact healthcare provider if these occur. Inform that liver injury can occur, and advise of the importance of laboratory monitoring of their liver during treatment. Advise to contact healthcare provider immediately for ophthalmologic symptoms. Advise of risk of fetal harm; instruct women of childbearing age and men to use contraception during and for at least 2 months after ending therapy. Advise patients to inform healthcare provider if they have had or are planning to receive radiation therapy. Inform that renal failure may occur; inform about the importance of monitoring SrCr prior to and during treatment.

ZEMPLAR IV — paricalcitol   Rx

Class: Vitamin D analogue

ADULT DOSAGE	PEDIATRIC DOSAGE
Secondary Hyperparathyroidism	**Secondary Hyperparathyroidism**
Prevention and treatment of secondary hyperparathyroidism associated w/ chronic kidney disease Stage 5	Prevention and treatment of secondary hyperparathyroidism associated w/ chronic kidney disease Stage 5
	≥5 Years:
Initial: 0.04-0.1mcg/kg (2.8-7mcg) as a bolus dose no more frequently than qod at any time during dialysis	**Initial:** 0.04-0.1mcg/kg (2.8-7mcg) as a bolus dose no more frequently than qod at any time during dialysis
Titrate: Increase by 2-4mcg at 2- to 4-week intervals if satisfactory response is not observed	**Titrate:** Increase by 2-4mcg at 2- to 4-week intervals if satisfactory response is not observed
If an elevated Ca^{2+} level or a Ca^{2+} x P product >75 is noted, immediately reduce dose or interrupt until these parameters are normalized; then, reinitiate at a lower dose	If an elevated Ca^{2+} level or a Ca^{2+} x P product >75 is noted, immediately reduce dose or interrupt until these parameters are normalized; then, reinitiate at a lower dose
Patients on a Ca^{2+}-Based Phosphate Binder: Decrease or withhold dose, or switch to a non-Ca^{2+}-based phosphate binder	**Patients on a Ca^{2+}-Based Phosphate Binder:** Decrease or withhold dose, or switch to a non-Ca^{2+}-based phosphate binder
Dose Titration Based on Parathyroid Hormone (PTH) Levels: **PTH Levels the Same/Increasing:** Increase dose	**Dose Titration Based on Parathyroid Hormone (PTH) Levels:** **PTH Levels the Same/Increasing:** Increase dose
PTH Levels Decreasing by <30%: Increase dose	**PTH Levels Decreasing by <30%:** Increase dose
PTH Levels Decreasing by >30%, <60%: Maintain dose	**PTH Levels Decreasing by >30%, <60%:** Maintain dose
PTH Levels Decreasing by >60%: Decrease dose	**PTH Levels Decreasing by >60%:** Decrease dose
PTH Levels 1.5-3X ULN: Maintain dose	**PTH Levels 1.5-3X ULN:** Maintain dose

ADMINISTRATION
IV route

STORAGE
25°C (77°F); excursions permitted between 15-30°C (59-86°F). Multidose Vial: Room temperature for up to 7 days, after initial use.

HOW SUPPLIED
Inj: 2mcg/mL [1mL], 5mcg/mL [1mL, 2mL]

CONTRAINDICATIONS
Vitamin D toxicity, hypercalcemia. Hypersensitivity to any ingredient in this product.

WARNINGS/PRECAUTIONS
Acute overdose may cause hypercalcemia. Closely monitor serum Ca^{2+} and P levels (eg, twice weekly) during dose adjustment; reduce or interrupt dose if clinically significant hypercalcemia develops. Chronic administration may place patients at risk of hypercalcemia, elevated Ca x P product, and metastatic calcification; chronic hypercalcemia can lead to generalized vascular calcification and other soft-tissue calcification. Adynamic bone lesions may develop if PTH levels are suppressed to abnormal levels.

ADVERSE REACTIONS
N/V, GI hemorrhage, edema, pneumonia, sepsis, influenza, pyrexia, chills, palpitations, dry mouth, arthralgia, malaise.

DRUG INTERACTIONS
May increase risk of hypercalcemia with high doses of Ca^{2+}-containing preparations or thiazide diuretics. High intake of Ca^{2+} and phosphate may lead to serum abnormalities requiring more frequent patient monitoring and individualized dose titration. Withhold prescription-based doses of vitamin D and its derivatives during treatment to avoid hypercalcemia. Do not administer aluminum-containing preparations (eg, antacids, phosphate binders) chronically with paricalcitol, as increased blood levels of aluminum and aluminum bone toxicity may occur. Caution with digitalis compounds. Caution with ketoconazole and other strong CYP3A inhibitors (eg, atazanavir, clarithromycin, indinavir, itraconazole, nefazodone, nelfinavir, ritonavir, saquinavir, telithromycin, voriconazole).

PREGNANCY AND LACTATION
Category C, not for use in nursing.

MECHANISM OF ACTION
Vitamin D analog; binds to vitamin D receptor, which results in selective activation of vitamin D responsive pathways. Shown to reduce PTH levels by inhibiting PTH synthesis and secretion.

PHARMACOKINETICS
Absorption: C_{max}=1.680ng/mL (hemodialysis), 1.832ng/mL (peritoneal dialysis); AUC=14.51ng•hr/mL (hemodialysis), 16.01ng•hr/mL (peritoneal dialysis). **Distribution:** V_d=30.8L (hemodialysis), 34.9L (peritoneal dialysis); plasma protein binding (≥99.8%). **Metabolism:** Liver (extensive) via hydroxylation and glucuronidation, by CYP24, CYP3A4, and UGT1A4; 24(R)-hydroxy paricalcitol (minor metabolite). **Elimination:** Feces (63%; 2% unchanged), urine (19%); $T_{1/2}$=13.9 hrs (hemodialysis), 15.4 hrs (peritoneal dialysis).

PATIENT CONSIDERATIONS
Assessment: Assess for vitamin D toxicity, hypercalcemia, drug hypersensitivity, pregnancy/nursing status, and possible drug interactions.

Monitoring: Monitor for hypercalcemia, elevated Ca x P product, metastatic calcification, adynamic bone lesions, and other adverse reactions. Monitor serum Ca^{2+} and P frequently (eg, twice weekly) during initial phase, and at least monthly once dosage has been established. Monitor serum/plasma PTH every 3 months. Frequently monitor laboratory tests during dose adjustment.

Counseling: Inform about the importance of adherence to a dietary regimen of Ca^{2+} supplementation and P restriction. Advise that appropriate types of phosphate-binding compounds may be needed to control serum P levels, but excessive use of aluminum-containing compounds should be avoided. Inform about signs/symptoms of hypercalcemia (eg, feeling tired, difficulty thinking clearly, loss of appetite, N/V, constipation, increased thirst and urination, weight loss).

ZEMPLAR ORAL — paricalcitol   Rx

Class: Vitamin D analogue

ADULT DOSAGE	PEDIATRIC DOSAGE
Secondary Hyperparathyroidism	Pediatric use may not have been established
Associated w/ Chronic Kidney Disease (CKD) Stages 3 and 4:	
Initial:	
Baseline Intact Parathyroid Hormone (iPTH) Level:	
≤500pg/mL: 1mcg qd or 2mcg 3X/week	
>500pg/mL: 2mcg qd or 4mcg 3X/week	
Titrate:	
Individualize dose and base dose on serum/plasma iPTH levels, w/ monitoring of serum Ca^{2+} and serum phosphorus (P)	
Adjust dose at 2- to 4-week intervals	
iPTH Level Relative to Baseline: Same, Increased, or Decreased by <30%: Increase dose by 1mcg qd or 2mcg 3X/week	
Decreased by ≥30% and ≤60%: Maintain dose	
Decreased by >60% or iPTH <60pg/mL: Decrease dose by 1mcg qd or 2mcg 3X/week	
Do not administer the 3X/week dose more often than qod	
If patient is taking the lowest dose on the daily regimen (1mcg qd) and a dose reduction is needed, the dose can be decreased to 1mcg 3X/week; if further dose reduction is required, withhold therapy prn and restart at a lower dosing frequency	
Associated w/ CKD Stage 5: Administer 3X/week, not more frequently than qod	
Initial: Base dose on a baseline iPTH level (pg/mL)/80	
Treat only after baseline serum Ca^{2+} has been adjusted to ≤9.5mg/dL	
Titrate: Individualize and base dose on iPTH, serum Ca^{2+}, and P levels; Titration Dose (mcg) = Most Recent iPTH Level (pg/mL)/80	

DOSING CONSIDERATIONS
Concomitant Medications
On a Ca^{2+}-Based Phosphate Binder:
CKD Stages 3 and 4: May decrease or withhold the phosphate-binder dose, or switch to a non-Ca^{2+}-based phosphate binder. If hypercalcemia is observed, reduce or withhold paricalcitol dose until these parameters are normalized
CKD Stage 5: If an elevated serum Ca^{2+} observed, and on a Ca^{2+}-based phosphate binder, may decrease or withhold the binder dose, or switch to a non-Ca^{2+}-based phosphate binder. If serum Ca^{2+} is elevated, decrease paricalcitol dose by 2-4mcg lower than that calculated by the most recent iPTH/80. If further adjustment is required, reduce or withhold paricalcitol dose until these parameters are normalized

Other Important Considerations
Closely monitor serum Ca^{2+} and P levels after initiation, during dose titration periods, and w/ coadministration of strong CYP3A inhibitors

ADMINISTRATION
Oral route

May be taken w/o regard to food.

STORAGE
25°C (77°F); excursions permitted between 15-30°C (59-86°F).

HOW SUPPLIED
Cap: 1mcg, 2mcg

CONTRAINDICATIONS
Hypercalcemia, vitamin D toxicity.

WARNINGS/PRECAUTIONS
Excessive administration may cause over suppression of PTH, hypercalcemia, hypercalciuria, hyperphosphatemia, and adynamic bone disease. Acute hypercalcemia may exacerbate tendencies for cardiac arrhythmias and seizures. Chronic hypercalcemia can lead to generalized vascular calcification and other soft-tissue calcification. May increase SrCr and therefore decrease the estimated GFR in predialysis patients.

ADVERSE REACTIONS
Headache, hypotension, HTN, diarrhea, N/V, constipation, edema, arthritis, dizziness, insomnia, nasopharyngitis, viral infection, hypersensitivity, peritonitis, fluid overload.

DRUG INTERACTIONS
May increase risk of hypercalcemia w/ high doses of Ca^{2+}-containing preparations or thiazide diuretics. Concomitant high intake of Ca^{2+} and phosphate may lead to serum abnormalities requiring more frequent patient monitoring and individualized dose titration. Withhold prescription-based doses of vitamin D and its derivatives during treatment to avoid hypercalcemia. Digitalis toxicity is potentiated by hypercalcemia of any cause; caution w/ digitalis compounds. Do not coadminister aluminum-containing preparations (eg, antacids, phosphate binders) chronically; increased blood levels of aluminum and aluminum bone toxicity may occur. Increased exposure w/ strong CYP3A inhibitors (eg, ketoconazole, atazanavir, clarithromycin); may need to adjust paricalcitol dose, and closely monitor iPTH and serum Ca^{2+} concentrations if a patient initiates or discontinues therapy w/ a strong CYP3A4 inhibitor. Drugs that impair intestinal absorption of fat-soluble vitamins (eg, cholestyramine) may interfere w/ absorption. Mineral oil or other substances that may affect absorption of fat may influence absorption.

PREGNANCY AND LACTATION
Pregnancy: Category C.
Lactation: Not for use in nursing.

MECHANISM OF ACTION
Vitamin D analogue; binds to vitamin D receptor, which results in the selective activation of vitamin D responsive pathways. Shown to reduce PTH levels by inhibiting PTH synthesis and secretion.

PHARMACOKINETICS
Absorption: Absolute bioavailability (72-86%) (healthy, CKD Stage 5 patients on hemodialysis, CKD Stage 5 patients on peritoneal dialysis). Refer to PI for pharmacokinetic characteristics in CKD patients. **Distribution:** V_d=44-46L (CKD Stages 3 and 4); plasma protein binding ($\geq$99.8%). **Metabolism:** Liver (extensive) via hydroxylation and glucuronidation, by CYP24, CYP3A4, and UGT1A4. **Elimination:** Feces (70%; 2% unchanged), urine (18%); $T_{1/2}$=14-20 hrs (CKD Stages 3, 4, and 5).

PATIENT CONSIDERATIONS
Assessment: Assess for hypercalcemia, vitamin D toxicity, pregnancy/nursing status, and possible drug interactions.

Monitoring: Monitor for hypercalcemia and other adverse reactions. During the initial dosing or following any dose adjustment, monitor serum Ca^{2+}, serum P, and serum/plasma iPTH at least every 2 weeks for 3 months, then monthly for 3 months, and every 3 months thereafter.

Counseling: Inform of the most common adverse reactions (eg, diarrhea, HTN, dizziness, vomiting). Advise to adhere to instructions regarding diet and P restriction, and to return for routine monitoring. Instruct to contact physician if symptoms of elevated Ca^{2+} (eg, feeling tired, difficulty thinking clearly, loss of appetite) develop. Advise to inform physician of all medications (eg, prescription and nonprescription drugs, supplements, herbal preparations) being taken and any change to medical condition.

ZENPEP — pancrelipase

Class: Pancreatic enzyme supplement

Rx

ADULT DOSAGE
Exocrine Pancreatic Insufficiency

Due to Cystic Fibrosis or Other Conditions:
Start at the lowest recommended dose and increase gradually
Initial: 500 lipase U/kg/meal
Max: 2500 lipase U/kg/meal (or $\leq$10,000 lipase U/kg/day) or <4000 lipase U/g fat ingested/day

PEDIATRIC DOSAGE
Exocrine Pancreatic Insufficiency

Due to Cystic Fibrosis or Other Conditions:
Start at the lowest recommended dose and increase gradually
$\leq$12 Months of Age:
3000 lipase U per 120mL of formula or per breastfeeding immediately prior to each feeding

>12 Months-<4 Years:
Initial: 1000 lipase U/kg/meal
Max: 2500 lipase U/kg/meal (or $\leq$10,000 lipase U/kg/day) or <4000 lipase U/g fat ingested/day

$\geq$4 Years:
Initial: 500 lipase U/kg/meal
Max: 2500 lipase U/kg/meal (or $\leq$10,000 lipase U/kg/day) or <4000 lipase U/g fat ingested/day

ADMINISTRATION
Oral route
Take during meals or snacks, w/ sufficient fluid.
Half of the dose used for meals should be given w/ each snack.
Swallow whole; do not crush/chew cap or cap contents.
If necessary, the cap contents can be sprinkled on soft acidic foods (eg, applesauce, commercial preparations of bananas or pears).
Contents of the cap may also be given directly to the mouth.
Do not mix directly into formula or breast milk.

STORAGE
Avoid excessive heat. Protect from moisture. (Original glass container) 20-25°C (68-77°F); brief excursions permitted to 15-40°C (59-104°F). (Repackaged HDPE container) Store up to 30°C (86°F) for up to 6 months; brief excursions permitted to 15-40°C (59-104°F) for up to 30 days.

HOW SUPPLIED
Cap, Delayed-Release: (Lipase/Protease/Amylase) 3000 U/10,000 U/14,000 U; 5000 U/17,000 U/24,000 U; 10,000 U/32,000 U/42,000 U; 15,000 U/47,000 U/63,000 U; 20,000 U/63,000 U/84,000 U; 25,000 U/79,000 U/105,000 U; 40,000 U/126,000 U/168,000 U

WARNINGS/PRECAUTIONS
Not interchangeable with other pancrelipase products. Fibrosing colonopathy reported; monitor closely for progression to stricture formation. Colonic strictures have been associated with doses >6000 lipase U/kg/meal in children <12 yrs of age. Caution with doses >2500 lipase U/kg/meal (or >10,000 lipase U/kg/day); use only if these doses are documented to be effective by 3-day fecal fat measures indicating significant improvement. Examine patients receiving >6000 lipase U/kg/meal; immediately decrease or titrate dose downward to a lower range. Ensure that no drug is retained in the mouth. Should not be crushed or chewed, or mixed in foods with pH >4.5; may disrupt enteric coating of cap, resulting in early release of enzymes, irritation of oral mucosa, and/or loss of enzyme activity. Caution in patients with gout, renal impairment, or hyperuricemia; may increase blood uric acid levels. Risk for transmission of viral diseases. Caution with known allergy to proteins of porcine origin; severe allergic reactions reported.

ADVERSE REACTIONS
GI disorders (eg, abdominal pain, flatulence), headache, cough, weight decreased, early satiety, contusion.

PREGNANCY AND LACTATION
Pregnancy: Category C.
Lactation: Caution in nursing.

MECHANISM OF ACTION
Pancreatic enzyme supplement; catalyzes the hydrolysis of fats to monoglycerides, glycerol, and free fatty acids, proteins into peptides and amino acids, and starch into dextrins and short-chain sugars (eg, maltose, maltriose) in the duodenum and proximal small intestine, thereby acting like digestive enzymes physiologically secreted by the pancreas.

PATIENT CONSIDERATIONS
Assessment: Assess for gout, renal impairment, hyperuricemia, allergy to porcine proteins, and pregnancy/nursing status.

Monitoring: Monitor for fibrosing colonopathy, stricture formation, oral mucosa irritation, viral diseases, allergic reactions, and other adverse reactions. Monitor serum uric acid levels.

Counseling: Instruct to take ud, with food and sufficient fluids. Inform that if a dose is missed, take the next dose with the next meal/snack ud; instruct not to double doses. Inform that cap contents can be mixed with soft acidic foods (eg, applesauce), if necessary. Advise to contact physician immediately if allergic reactions develop. Instruct to notify physician if pregnant/breastfeeding or planning to become pregnant/breastfeed during treatment. Instruct to notify physician before initiating treatment if patient has a history of abnormal glucose levels.

ZENTRIP — meclizine hydrochloride

Class: Antihistamine

OTC

ADULT DOSAGE
Motion Sickness

Usual: Dissolve 1-2 strips on tongue qd or ud
For prevention, take at least 1 hr before travel starts

PEDIATRIC DOSAGE
Motion Sickness

$\geq$12 Years:
Usual: Dissolve 1-2 strips on tongue qd or ud
For prevention, take at least 1 hr before travel starts

ADMINISTRATION
Oral route

STORAGE
20-30°C (68-86°F). Protect from light.

HOW SUPPLIED
Strip, Oral: 25mg

WARNINGS/PRECAUTIONS
Avoid use in children <12 yrs of age. Caution with glaucoma, breathing problems (eg, emphysema, chronic bronchitis), and difficulty in urination due to an enlarged prostate gland. D/C use and consult physician if rash, redness, itching, or difficulty in urination occurs, or if symptoms of dry mouth continue or increase. Drowsiness may occur and may impair mental/physical abilities.

ADVERSE REACTIONS
Drowsiness.

DRUG INTERACTIONS
Alcohol, sedatives, and tranquilizers may increase drowsiness. Avoid alcohol use.

PREGNANCY AND LACTATION
Safety not known in pregnancy and nursing.

MECHANISM OF ACTION
Antihistamine.

PATIENT CONSIDERATIONS
Assessment: Assess for breathing problems (eg, emphysema, chronic bronchitis), glaucoma, difficulty in urination due to an enlarged prostate gland, pregnancy/nursing status, and possible drug interactions.

Monitoring: Monitor for drowsiness, rash, redness, itching, difficulty in urination and increased/continued symptoms of dry mouth.

Counseling: Inform that drowsiness may occur; caution when driving a vehicle or operating machinery. Instruct to avoid alcohol use. Instruct to d/c and consult physician if rash, redness, itching, or difficulty in urination occurs, or if symptoms of dry mouth continue or increase. Advise to consult physician before use if taking sedatives or tranquilizers and if pregnant/nursing.

Zenzedi — dextroamphetamine sulfate CII
Class: CNS stimulant

> High potential for abuse. Prolonged use may lead to drug dependence and must be avoided. Misuse may cause sudden death and serious cardiovascular adverse events.

ADULT DOSAGE
Narcolepsy

Initial: 10mg/day
Titrate: May increase daily dose in increments of 10mg at weekly intervals until optimal response is obtained
Usual: 5-60mg/day in divided doses

Give 1st dose on awakening; additional doses (1 or 2) at intervals of 4-6 hrs

PEDIATRIC DOSAGE
Narcolepsy

Usual: 5-60mg/day in divided doses

Give 1st dose on awakening; additional doses (1 or 2) at intervals of 4-6 hrs

6-12 Years:
Initial: 5mg/day
Titrate: May increase daily dose in increments of 5mg at weekly intervals until optimal response is obtained

≥12 Years:
Initial: 10mg/day
Titrate: May increase daily dose in increments of 10mg at weekly intervals until optimal response is obtained

Attention-Deficit Hyperactivity Disorder

3-5 Years:
Initial: 2.5mg qd
Titrate: May increase daily dose in increments of 2.5mg at weekly intervals until optimal response is obtained

≥6 Years:
Initial: 5mg qd or bid
Titrate: May increase daily dose in increments of 5mg at weekly intervals until optimal response is obtained. Only in rare cases will it be necessary to exceed a total of 40mg/day

Give 1st dose on awakening; additional doses (1 or 2) at intervals of 4-6 hrs

DOSING CONSIDERATIONS
Adverse Reactions
Narcolepsy Patients:
Reduce dose if bothersome adverse reactions appear (eg, insomnia, anorexia)

ADMINISTRATION
Oral route

Avoid late pm doses

STORAGE
20-25°C (68-77°F); excursions permitted to 15-30°C (59-86°F).

HOW SUPPLIED
Tab: 2.5mg, 5mg*, 7.5mg, 10mg*, 15mg, 20mg, 30mg *scored

CONTRAINDICATIONS
Advanced arteriosclerosis, symptomatic cardiovascular disease (CVD), moderate to severe HTN, hyperthyroidism, known hypersensitivity or idiosyncrasy to the sympathomimetic amines, glaucoma, agitated states, and history of drug abuse. During or w/in 14 days following MAOI use.

WARNINGS/PRECAUTIONS
Avoid with known serious structural cardiac abnormalities, cardiomyopathy, serious heart rhythm abnormalities, coronary artery disease, or other serious cardiac problems. Sudden death reported in children and adolescents with structural cardiac abnormalities or other serious heart problems. Sudden deaths, stroke, and MI reported in adults. May cause a modest increase in average BP and HR. Promptly perform cardiac evaluation if symptoms of cardiac disease develop. May exacerbate symptoms of behavior disturbance and thought disorder in patients with preexisting psychotic disorder. Caution in patients with comorbid bipolar disorder; may induce mixed/manic episodes. May cause treatment-emergent psychotic or manic symptoms in children and adolescents without prior history of psychotic illness or mania; consider discontinuation if such symptoms occur. Aggressive behavior or hostility reported in children and adolescents with ADHD. May cause long-term suppression of growth in children; may need to interrupt treatment in patients not growing or gaining height or weight as expected. May lower convulsive threshold; d/c if seizures occur. Associated with peripheral vasculopathy, including Raynaud's phenomenon. Difficulties with accommodation and blurring of vision reported. May exacerbate motor and phonic tics, and Tourette's syndrome. May elevate plasma corticosteroid levels and interfere with urinary steroid determinations.

ADVERSE REACTIONS
Palpitations, tachycardia, BP elevation, dizziness, insomnia, euphoria, dyskinesia, tremor, headache, dryness of mouth, diarrhea, constipation, urticaria, impotence, changes in libido.

DRUG INTERACTIONS
See Contraindications. GI acidifying agents (eg, guanethidine, reserpine, glutamic acid HCl) and urinary acidifying agents (eg, ammonium chloride, sodium acid phosphate) lower blood levels and efficacy. Inhibits adrenergic blockers. GI alkalinizing agents (eg, sodium bicarbonate) and urinary alkalinizing agents (eg, acetazolamide, some thiazides) increase blood levels and potentiate actions. May enhance activity of TCAs or sympathomimetic agents. Desipramine or protriptyline and possibly other TCAs cause striking and sustained increases in the concentration of *d*-amphetamine in the brain; cardiovascular effects can be potentiated. May counteract sedative effects of antihistamines. May antagonize hypotensive effects of antihypertensives. Chlorpromazine and haloperidol blocks dopamine and norepinephrine reuptake, thus inhibiting central stimulant effects. May delay intestinal absorption of ethosuximide, phenobarbital, and phenytoin; coadministration with phenobarbital or phenytoin may produce a synergistic anticonvulsant action. Lithium carbonate may inhibit stimulatory effects. Potentiates analgesic effect of meperidine. Acidifying agents used in methenamine therapy increase urinary excretion and reduce efficacy. Enhances adrenergic effect of norepinephrine. In cases of propoxyphene overdosage, CNS stimulation is potentiated and fatal convulsions can occur. Inhibits hypotensive effect of veratrum alkaloids.

PREGNANCY AND LACTATION
Category C, not for use in nursing.

MECHANISM OF ACTION
Sympathomimetic amine; has not been established. Has CNS stimulant activity.

PHARMACOKINETICS
Absorption: C_{max}=36.6ng/mL; T_{max}=3 hrs. **Distribution:** Found in breast milk.
Elimination: $T_{1/2}$=12 hrs.

PATIENT CONSIDERATIONS
Assessment: Assess for hypersensitivity/idiosyncrasy to sympathomimetic amines, advanced arteriosclerosis, symptomatic CVD, moderate to severe HTN, hyperthyroidism, glaucoma, agitated states, history of drug abuse, tics, Tourette's syndrome, preexisting psychotic disorder, risk for/comorbid bipolar disorder, medical conditions that might be compromised by increases in BP or HR, any other conditions where treatment is cautioned, pregnancy/nursing status, and possible drug interactions.

Monitoring: Monitor for changes in HR and BP, signs/symptoms of cardiac disease, exacerbation of symptoms of behavior disturbance and thought disorder, psychosis, mania, appearance of or worsening of aggressive behavior or hostility, seizures, peripheral vasculopathy (eg, digital changes), visual disturbances, exacerbation of motor and phone tics or Tourette's syndrome, and other adverse reactions. In pediatric patients, monitor growth.

Counseling: Inform about benefits and risks of treatment. Counsel that drug has high potential for abuse. Caution against engaging in potentially hazardous activities (eg, operating machinery/vehicles). Inform about risk of peripheral vasculopathy, including Raynaud's phenomenon. Instruct to report signs/symptoms of peripheral vasculopathy to physician. Instruct to call physician immediately with any signs of unexplained wounds appearing on fingers or toes.

Zepatier — elbasvir/grazoprevir Rx
Class: HCV NS5A inhibitor/HCV NS3/4A protease inhibitor

ADULT DOSAGE
Chronic Hepatitis C

Treatment of Chronic Hepatitis C Virus (HCV) Genotypes 1 or 4 Infection w/ or w/o Ribavirin (RBV):
1 tab qd

Treatment Regimen and Duration of Therapy in Patients w/ or w/o Cirrhosis:
Test patients w/ HCV genotype 1a infection for presence of virus w/ NS5A resistance-associated polymorphisms prior to initiation of treatment to determine dosage regimen and duration

PEDIATRIC DOSAGE
Pediatric use may not have been established

Genotype 1a: Treatment-Naive or Peginterferon Alfa (PegIFN)/RBV-Experienced w/o Baseline NS5A Polymorphisms:
Zepatier for 12 weeks

Genotype 1a: Treatment-Naive or PegIFN/RBV-Experienced w/ Baseline NS5A Polymorphisms:
Zepatier + RBV for 16 weeks

Genotype 1b: Treatment-Naive or PegIFN/RBV-Experienced:
Zepatier for 12 weeks

Genotype 1a or 1b: PegIFN/RBV/ Protease Inhibitor-Experienced:
Zepatier + RBV for 12 weeks

Genotype 4: Treatment-Naive:
Zepatier for 12 weeks

Genotype 4: PegIFN/RBV-Experienced:
Zepatier + RBV for 16 weeks

ADMINISTRATION
Oral route

Take w/ or w/o food.
Refer to RBV labeling for dosing and administration instructions.

STORAGE
20-25°C (68-77°F); excursions permitted between 15-30°C (59-86°F). Protect from moisture.

HOW SUPPLIED
Tab: (Elbasvir/Grazoprevir) 50mg/100mg

CONTRAINDICATIONS
Moderate or severe hepatic impairment (Child-Pugh B or C). Coadministration w/ OATP1B1/3 inhibitors or w/ strong CYP3A inducers. Coadministration w/ phenytoin, carbamazepine, rifampin, St. John's wort, efavirenz, atazanavir, darunavir, lopinavir, saquinavir, tipranavir, or cyclosporine. If administered w/ RBV, refer to the RBV prescribing information for a list of contraindications for RBV.

WARNINGS/PRECAUTIONS
ALT elevations reported; perform hepatic laboratory testing prior to therapy, at treatment week 8, and as clinically indicated. Additional hepatic laboratory testing should be performed at treatment week 12 in patients receiving 16 weeks of therapy. Consider discontinuing therapy if ALT levels remain persistently >10X ULN. D/C if ALT elevation is accompanied by signs/symptoms of liver inflammation or increasing conjugated bilirubin, alkaline phosphatase, or INR. Refer to the RBV prescribing information for a full list of warnings and precautions for RBV.

ADVERSE REACTIONS
Zepatier for 12 Weeks: Fatigue, headache, nausea.
Zepatier + Ribavirin for 16 Weeks: Anemia, headache.

DRUG INTERACTIONS
See Contraindications. Moderate or strong CYP3A inducers may decrease levels and therapeutic effect; not recommended w/ moderate CYP3A inducers. Strong CYP3A inhibitors may increase levels. Not recommended w/ nafcillin, ketoconazole, bosentan, etravirine, modafinil, or elvitegravir/cobicistat/ emtricitabine/tenofovir (disoproxil fumarate or alafenamide). Nafcillin, bosentan, etravirine, and modafinil may decrease levels. Systemic ketoconazole may increase levels and may increase the overall risk of hepatotoxicity. Coadministration w/ systemic tacrolimus may increase tacrolimus levels; upon initiation of coadministration w/ Zepatier, frequently monitor tacrolimus whole blood concentrations, changes in renal function, and for tacrolimus-associated adverse events. Elvitegravir/cobicistat/ emtricitabine/tenofovir disoproxil (fumarate or alafenamide) may increase levels. May increase atorvastatin levels; atorvastatin dose should not exceed 20mg/day. May increase rosuvastatin levels; rosuvastatin dose should not exceed 10mg/day. May increase fluvastatin, lovastatin, and simvastatin levels; monitor for statin-associated adverse events and use lowest necessary dose. **Grazoprevir:** OATP1B1/3 inhibitors may increase levels.

PREGNANCY AND LACTATION
Pregnancy: No adequate human data are available to establish whether or not Zepatier poses a risk to pregnancy outcomes. If Zepatier is administered w/ RBV, the combination regimen is contraindicated in pregnant women and in men whose female partners are pregnant; refer to the RBV prescribing information for more information on use in pregnancy.
Lactation: It is not known whether Zepatier is present in human breast milk, affects human milk production, or has effects on the breastfed infant; caution in nursing. If Zepatier is administered w/ RBV, the information for RBV w/ regard to nursing mothers also applies to this combination regimen; refer to the RBV prescribing information for information on use during lactation.
Females and Males of Reproductive Potential: If Zepatier is administered w/ RBV, the information for RBV w/ regard to pregnancy testing, contraception, and infertility also applies to this combination regimen; refer to RBV prescribing information for additional information.

MECHANISM OF ACTION
Elbasvir: Inhibitor of HCV NS5A, which is essential for viral RNA replication and virion assembly. **Grazoprevir:** An inhibitor of the HCV NS3/4A protease which is necessary for the proteolytic cleavage of the HCV encoded polyprotein (into mature forms of the NS3, NS4A, NS4B, NS5A, and NS5B proteins) and is essential for viral replication.

PHARMACOKINETICS
Absorption: Elbasvir: T_{max}=3 hrs (median); AUC_{0-24}=1920ng•hr/mL; C_{max}=121ng/ mL. Grazoprevir: T_{max}=2 hrs (median); AUC_{0-24}=1420ng•hr/mL; C_{max}=165ng/mL.
Distribution: Elbasvir: Plasma protein binding (>99.9%); V_d=680L. Grazoprevir: Plasma protein binding (>98.8%); V_d=1250L. **Metabolism:** Oxidative metabolism via CYP3A (partial). **Excretion:** Feces (>90%), urine (<1%). Elbasvir: $T_{1/2}$=24 hrs. Grazoprevir: $T_{1/2}$=31 hrs.

PATIENT CONSIDERATIONS
Assessment: Assess for hypersensitivity to drug, pregnancy/nursing status, and for possible drug interactions. Test patients w/ HCV genotype 1a infection for the presence of virus w/ NS5A resistance-associated polymorphisms. Perform baseline hepatic laboratory testing.

Monitoring: Monitor for ALT elevations and for any other adverse reaction. Perform hepatic laboratory testing at treatment week 8, and as clinically indicated; perform additional hepatic laboratory testing at treatment week 12 for patients receiving 16 weeks of therapy.

Counseling: Instruct to observe for warning signs of liver inflammation (eg, fatigue, weakness, lack of appetite, N/V, jaundice, discolored feces) and to contact physician w/o delay if such symptoms occur. Advise to notify physician if pregnant or nursing. Advise to report the use of any prescription, non-prescription medication, or herbal products to physician. Inform that therapy should be taken every day at the regularly scheduled time w/ or w/o food.

ZERBAXA — ceftolozane/tazobactam　　　Rx
Class: Beta-lactamase inhibitor/cephalosporin

ADULT DOSAGE	PEDIATRIC DOSAGE
Intra-Abdominal Infections	Pediatric use may not have been established
Complicated Infections: 1.5g (1g/0.5g) q8h for 4-14 days, in conjunction w/ metronidazole 500mg IV q8h	
Urinary Tract Infections	
Complicated Infections, Including Pyelonephritis: 1.5g (1g/0.5g) q8h for 7 days	

DOSING CONSIDERATIONS
Renal Impairment
CrCl 30-50mL/min: 750mg (500mg/250mg) q8h
CrCl 15-29mL/min: 375mg (250mg/125mg) q8h
ESRD on Hemodialysis:
LD: 750mg (500mg/250mg)
Maint: 150mg (100mg/50mg) q8h for remainder of treatment period (on hemodialysis days, administer dose at earliest possible time following completion of dialysis)

ADMINISTRATION
IV route

Infuse over 1 hr.
Do not mix w/ other drugs or physically add to sol containing other drugs. Reconstituted sol may be held for 1 hr prior to transfer and dilution in a suitable infusion bag.
Following dilution of sol, may store for 24 hrs when stored at room temperature or 7 days when stored under refrigeration at 2-8°C (36-46°F); do not freeze constituted sol or diluted infusion.

Preparation
Constitute vial w/ 10mL of sterile water for inj or 0.9% NaCl for inj (final vol is approx 11.4mL); shake gently to dissolve.
Withdraw appropriate volume from reconstituted vial and add to an infusion bag containing 100mL of 0.9% NaCl for inj or D5 inj.

Preparation of Doses:
1.5g (1g/0.5g) Dose: Withdraw 11.4mL (entire vial contents)
750mg (500mg/250mg) Dose: Withdraw 5.7mL
375mg (250mg/125mg) Dose: Withdraw 2.9mL
150mg (100mg/50mg) Dose: Withdraw 1.2mL

STORAGE
2-8°C (36-46°F). Protect from light.

HOW SUPPLIED
Inj: (Ceftolozane/Tazobactam) 1g/0.5g

CONTRAINDICATIONS
Serious hypersensitivity to the components of Zerbaxa (ceftolozane and tazobactam), piperacillin/tazobactam, or other members of the beta-lactam class.

WARNINGS/PRECAUTIONS
Serious and occasionally fatal hypersensitivity (anaphylactic) reactions reported; d/c therapy and institute appropriate therapy if an anaphylactic reaction occurs. Caution w/ cephalosporin, penicillin (PCN), or other β-lactam allergy; cross sensitivity may occur. *Clostridium difficile*-associated diarrhea (CDAD) reported; d/c if CDAD is confirmed. Use in the absence of a proven or strongly suspected bacterial infection is unlikely to provide benefit and increases the risk of the development of drug-resistant bacteria. Caution in elderly.

ADVERSE REACTIONS
N/V, headache, diarrhea, pyrexia, constipation, insomnia, hypokalemia.

PREGNANCY AND LACTATION
Pregnancy: Category B.
Lactation: Caution in nursing.

MECHANISM OF ACTION
Ceftolozane: Cephalosporin; inhibits cell-wall biosynthesis, and is mediated through binding to PCN-binding proteins. **Tazobactam:** β-lactamase inhibitor; binds covalently to some chromosomal and plasmid-mediated bacterial β-lactamases.

PHARMACOKINETICS
Absorption: Ceftolozane: (Day 1) C_{max}=69.1mcg/mL, T_{max}=1.02 hrs, AUC=172mcg•hr/mL; (Day 10) C_{max}=74.4mcg/mL, T_{max}=1.07 hrs, AUC=182mcg•hr/mL. Tazobactam: (Day 1) C_{max}=18.4mcg/mL, T_{max}=1.02 hrs, AUC=24.4mcg•hr/mL; (Day 10) C_{max}=18mcg/mL, T_{max}=1.01 hrs, AUC=25mcg•hr/mL. **Distribution:** Plasma protein binding (16-21% [ceftolozane], 30% [tazobactam]); V_d=13.5L (ceftolozane), 18.2L (tazobactam). **Metabolism:** Tazobactam: Hydrolysis. **Elimination:** Ceftolozane: Urine (>95% as unchanged parent drug); $T_{1/2}$=2.77 hrs (Day 1), 3.12 hrs (Day 10). Tazobactam: Urine (>80% as parent compound); $T_{1/2}$=0.91 hr (Day 1), 1.03 hrs (Day 10).

PATIENT CONSIDERATIONS
Assessment: Assess for hypersensitivity/allergy to drug, piperacillin/tazobactam, cephalosporin, PCN, or other β-lactams, renal impairment, pregnancy/nursing status, and possible drug interactions.

Monitoring: Monitor for signs and symptoms of hypersensitivity reactions, CDAD, and other adverse reactions. Monitor CrCl daily in patients w/ changing renal function.

Counseling: Advise that allergic reactions, including serious allergic reactions, may occur and require immediate treatment. Advise that diarrhea is a common problem caused by antibacterial drugs and sometimes, frequent watery or bloody diarrhea may occur and may be a sign of a more serious intestinal infection; if severe watery and bloody diarrhea develops, instruct to contact physician. Inform that therapy should only be used to treat bacterial, not viral, infections. Instruct to take exactly ud even if the patient feels better early in the course of therapy. Inform that skipping doses or not completing the full course of therapy may decrease effectiveness and increase risk of bacterial resistance.

ZERIT — stavudine   Rx
Class: Nucleoside reverse transcriptase inhibitor (NRTI)

> Lactic acidosis and severe hepatomegaly with steatosis, including fatal cases, reported with nucleoside analogues. Fatal lactic acidosis reported in pregnant women who received the combination of stavudine and didanosine with other antiretroviral agents; use with caution. Fatal and nonfatal pancreatitis reported when used as part of a combination regimen that included didanosine.

ADULT DOSAGE	PEDIATRIC DOSAGE
HIV-1 Infection	**HIV-1 Infection**
Combination with Other Antiretrovirals:	**Combination with Other Antiretrovirals:**
<60kg: 30mg q12h	**Birth-13 Days of Age:**
≥60kg: 40mg q12h	0.5mg/kg q12h
	≥14 Days of Age:
	<30kg: 1mg/kg q12h
	≥30kg: Use adult dose

DOSING CONSIDERATIONS
Renal Impairment
CrCl 26-50mL/min:
<60kg: 15mg q12h
≥60kg: 20mg q12h

CrCl 10-25mL/min or on Hemodialysis:
<60kg: 15mg q24h
≥60kg: 20mg q24h
Administer after completion of hemodialysis on dialysis days and at the same time of day on non-dialysis days

ADMINISTRATION
Oral route

Take with or without food
Shake oral sol vigorously prior to measuring each dose

STORAGE
25°C (77°F); excursions permitted between 15-30°C (59-86°F). (Sol) Protect from excessive moisture. After Constitution: 2-8°C (36-46°F). Discard any unused portion after 30 days.

HOW SUPPLIED
Cap: 15mg, 20mg, 30mg, 40mg; **Sol:** 1mg/mL [200mL]

CONTRAINDICATIONS
Clinically significant hypersensitivity to stavudine or to any components contained in the formulation.

WARNINGS/PRECAUTIONS
Female gender, obesity, and prolonged nucleoside exposure may be risk factors for lactic acidosis and severe hepatomegaly with steatosis. Caution in patients with known risk factors for liver disease. Suspend treatment if findings suggestive of symptomatic hyperlactatemia, lactic acidosis, or pronounced hepatotoxicity develop; consider permanent discontinuation with confirmed lactic acidosis. Increased frequency of liver function abnormalities, including severe

and potentially fatal hepatic adverse events in patients with preexisting liver dysfunction; monitor accordingly and consider interruption or discontinuation if worsening of liver disease is evident. Motor weakness reported rarely; d/c if this develops. Dose-related peripheral sensory neuropathy reported; occurs more frequently in patients with advanced HIV-1 disease, history of peripheral neuropathy, or receiving other drugs associated with neuropathy (eg, didanosine). Consider permanent discontinuation if peripheral neuropathy develops. Redistribution/accumulation of body fat reported; monitor for signs/symptoms of lipoatrophy or lipodystrophy. Immune reconstitution syndrome reported. Autoimmune disorders (eg, Graves' disease, polymyositis, Guillain-Barre syndrome) reported in the setting of immune reconstitution and can occur many months after initiation of treatment. Caution with renal impairment and in elderly.

ADVERSE REACTIONS
Lactic acidosis, severe hepatomegaly with steatosis, peripheral neurologic symptoms/neuropathy, headache, diarrhea, rash, N/V, increased AST/ALT/amylase.

DRUG INTERACTIONS
See Boxed Warning. Suspend combination of stavudine and didanosine and any other agents that are toxic to the pancreas in patients with suspected pancreatitis; caution with reinstitution of stavudine and avoid use in combination with didanosine if pancreatitis is confirmed. Avoid with zidovudine or hydroxyurea with or without didanosine. Hepatic decompensation may occur in combination with interferon and ribavirin in HIV-1/HCV coinfected patients; monitor for clinical toxicities and consider discontinuation if this occurs. Caution with doxorubicin or ribavirin.

PREGNANCY AND LACTATION
Category C, not for use in nursing.

MECHANISM OF ACTION
Synthetic thymidine nucleoside analogue; inhibits activity of HIV-1 reverse transcriptase by competing with natural substrate thymidine triphosphate and by causing DNA chain termination following its incorporation into viral DNA. Inhibits cellular DNA polymerases β and gamma and markedly reduces synthesis of mitochondrial DNA.

PHARMACOKINETICS
Absorption: Rapid. Oral bioavailability (86.4%) (adults), (76.9%) (pediatrics); C_{max}=536ng/mL (adults); T_{max}=1 hr; AUC_{0-24}=2568ng•hr/mL. **Distribution:** (IV) V_d=46L (adults), 0.73L/kg (pediatrics). **Metabolism:** Oxidized stavudine, glucuronide conjugates, and N-acetylcysteine conjugate (minor metabolites). **Elimination:** Urine (42%) (IV, adults), (34%) (pediatrics); $T_{1/2}$=1.6 hrs (adults), 0.96 hr (pediatrics).

PATIENT CONSIDERATIONS
Assessment: Assess for drug hypersensitivity, risk factors for lactic acidosis or liver disease, renal/hepatic impairment, history of peripheral neuropathy, pregnancy/nursing status, and possible drug interactions.

Monitoring: Monitor for signs/symptoms of lactic acidosis, hepatotoxicity, worsening of liver disease, motor weakness, peripheral neuropathy, pancreatitis, fat redistribution/accumulation, lipoatrophy/lipodystrophy, immune reconstitution syndrome (eg, opportunistic infections), and autoimmune disorders.

Counseling: Inform that therapy is not a cure for HIV and patients may continue to experience illnesses associated with HIV. Advise to avoid doing things that can spread HIV to others (eg, sharing needles, other inj equipment, or personal items that can have blood or body fluids on them; sex without protection; breastfeeding). Advise diabetic patients that oral sol contains 50mg of sucrose/mL. Advise to seek medical attention immediately if symptoms of hyperlactatemia or lactic acidosis syndrome (eg, unexplained weight loss, abdominal discomfort, N/V, fatigue, dyspnea, motor weakness) develop. Instruct to report symptoms of peripheral neuropathy to physician. Advise to avoid alcohol while on therapy. Inform that fat redistribution/accumulation may occur.

ZESTORETIC — hydrochlorothiazide/lisinopril   Rx
Class: ACE inhibitor/thiazide diuretic

> D/C when pregnancy is detected. Drugs that act directly on the renin-angiotensin system (RAS) can cause injury/death to the developing fetus.

ADULT DOSAGE	PEDIATRIC DOSAGE
Hypertension	Pediatric use may not have been established
BP Uncontrolled w/ Lisinopril/HCTZ Monotherapy:	
10mg/12.5mg or 20mg/12.5mg qd, depending on current monotherapy dose	
May increase HCTZ dose after 2-3 weeks	
If BP is controlled w/ HCTZ 25mg/day, but significant K+ loss is experienced, similar or greater BP control w/o electrolyte disturbance may be achieved by switching to 10mg/12.5mg qd	
Replacement Therapy: Combination may be substituted for the titrated individual components	

DOSING CONSIDERATIONS
Elderly
Start at lower end of dosing range

ADMINISTRATION
Oral route

STORAGE
20-25°C (68-77°F). Protect from excessive light and humidity.

HOW SUPPLIED
Tab: (Lisinopril/HCTZ) 10mg/12.5mg, 20mg/12.5mg, 20mg/25mg

CONTRAINDICATIONS
Hypersensitivity to this product; history of ACE inhibitor-associated angioedema; hereditary or idiopathic angioedema; anuria; or hypersensitivity to other sulfonamide-derived drugs. Coadministration w/ aliskiren in patients w/ diabetes.

WARNINGS/PRECAUTIONS
Not for initial therapy of HTN. Not recommended w/ severe renal impairment (CrCl ≤30mL/min). Caution in elderly. **Lisinopril:** Head/neck angioedema reported; promptly d/c and administer appropriate therapy. Higher rate of angioedema in blacks than nonblacks. Intestinal angioedema reported; monitor for abdominal pain. Patients w/ a history of angioedema unrelated to ACE inhibitor therapy may be at increased risk of angioedema during therapy. Anaphylactoid reactions reported during desensitization w/ hymenoptera venom, dialysis w/ high-flux membranes, and LDL apheresis w/ dextran sulfate absorption. Excessive hypotension may occur in salt/volume-depleted persons (eg, patients treated vigorously w/ diuretics or on dialysis). Excessive hypotension, which may be associated w/ oliguria and/or progressive azotemia, and rarely w/ acute renal failure and/or death, may occur in patients w/ severe CHF; monitor closely during first 2 weeks of therapy and whenever dose is increased. Caution w/ ischemic heart or cerebrovascular disease in whom an excessive fall in BP could result in a MI or cerebrovascular accident. Leukopenia/neutropenia and bone marrow depression may occur. Associated w/ a syndrome that starts w/ cholestatic jaundice or hepatitis and progresses to fulminant hepatic necrosis and sometimes death (rare); d/c if jaundice or marked elevations of hepatic enzymes develop. Caution w/ left ventricular outflow obstruction. May cause changes in renal function; in patients w/ severe CHF whose renal function is dependent on the RAS, oliguria and/or progressive azotemia, and (rare) acute renal failure and/or death may occur. May increase BUN/SrCr in hypertensive patients; monitor renal function during the 1st few weeks of therapy in patients w/ renal artery stenosis. Dosage reduction of lisinopril and/or discontinuation of the diuretic may be required if BUN/SrCr increase occurs. Hyperkalemia and persistent nonproductive cough reported. Hypotension may occur w/ major surgery or during anesthesia. **HCTZ:** May cause idiosyncratic reaction, resulting in acute transient myopia and acute angle-closure glaucoma; d/c as rapidly as possible. May precipitate azotemia in patients w/ renal disease. Caution w/ hepatic dysfunction or progressive liver disease; may precipitate hepatic coma. Sensitivity reactions may occur. May cause exacerbation or activation of systemic lupus erythematosus (SLE), hyperuricemia or precipitation of frank gout, manifestation of latent diabetes mellitus (DM), hypomagnesemia, and hypercalcemia. Observe for signs of fluid or electrolyte imbalance. Hypokalemia may sensitize or exaggerate the response of the heart to toxic effects of digitalis. Enhanced effects in postsympathectomy patients. D/C or withhold if progressive renal impairment becomes evident. D/C before testing for parathyroid function. Increased cholesterol and TG levels reported.

ADVERSE REACTIONS
Dizziness, headache, cough, fatigue, orthostatic effects.

DRUG INTERACTIONS
See Contraindications. NSAIDs, including selective COX-2 inhibitors, may reduce effects of diuretics and ACE inhibitors. Increased risk of lithium toxicity; avoid w/ lithium. Nitritoid reactions reported w/ injectable gold. **Lisinopril:** NSAIDs, including selective COX-2 inhibitors, may deteriorate renal function in patients who are elderly, volume depleted, or w/ compromised renal function. NSAIDs may attenuate the antihypertensive effects. Dual blockade of the RAS is associated w/ increased risks of hypotension, hyperkalemia, and changes in renal function (including acute renal failure); avoid combined use of RAS inhibitors, or closely monitor BP, renal function, and electrolytes w/ concomitant agents that also affect the RAS. Avoid w/ aliskiren in patients w/ renal impairment (GFR <60mL/min). Hypotension risk and increased BUN and SrCr w/ diuretics. Increased risk of hyperkalemia w/ K+-sparing diuretics (eg, spironolactone, eplerenone, triamterene, amiloride), K+ supplements, or K+-containing salt substitutes; use w/ caution and monitor serum K+. Coadministration w/ mTOR inhibitors (eg, temsirolimus, sirolimus, everolimus) may increase risk for angioedema. **HCTZ:** Potentiation of orthostatic hypotension may occur w/ alcohol, barbiturates, or narcotics. Dosage adjustment of antidiabetic drugs (oral agents, insulin) may be required. Additive effect or potentiation w/ other antihypertensives. Anionic exchange resins (cholestyramine, colestipol) may impair absorption. Corticosteroids and adrenocorticotropic hormone may intensify electrolyte depletion, particularly hypokalemia. May decrease response to pressor amines (eg, norepinephrine). May increase responsiveness to nondepolarizing skeletal muscle relaxants (eg, tubocurarine).

PREGNANCY AND LACTATION
Pregnancy: Category D.
Lactation: Not for use in nursing.

MECHANISM OF ACTION
Lisinopril: ACE inhibitor; decreases plasma angiotensin II, which leads to decreased vasopressor activity and decreased aldosterone secretion. **HCTZ:** Thiazide diuretic; not established. Affects distal renal tubular mechanism of electrolyte reabsorption. Increases excretion of Na+ and Cl-.

PHARMACOKINETICS
Absorption: Lisinopril: T_{max}=7 hrs. **Distribution:** Crosses placenta. HCTZ: Found in breast milk. **Elimination:** Lisinopril: Urine (unchanged); $T_{1/2}$=12 hrs. HCTZ: Kidneys (≥61% unchanged); $T_{1/2}$=5.6-14.8 hrs.

PATIENT CONSIDERATIONS
Assessment: Assess for hereditary/idiopathic angioedema, anuria, DM, volume/salt depletion, CHF, ischemic heart or cerebrovascular disease, collagen vascular disease, left ventricular outflow obstruction, SLE, history of ACE inhibitor-associated angioedema, hypersensitivity to drug or sulfonamide-derived drugs, renal/hepatic dysfunction, postsympathectomy status, pregnancy/nursing status, and possible drug interactions.

Monitoring: Monitor for signs/symptoms of angioedema, anaphylactoid/idiosyncratic/hypersensitivity reactions, exacerbation/activation of SLE, hyperuricemia or precipitation of gout, latent DM, fluid/electrolyte imbalance, and other adverse reactions. Monitor BP, renal/hepatic function, serum electrolytes, cholesterol, and TG levels. Consider periodic monitoring of WBCs in patients w/ collagen vascular disease and renal disease.

Counseling: Inform about fetal risks if taken during pregnancy and discuss treatment options in women planning to become pregnant; instruct to report pregnancy to physician as soon as possible. Instruct to d/c therapy and to immediately report signs/symptoms of angioedema. Instruct to report lightheadedness, especially during the 1st few days of therapy; advise to d/c therapy and consult w/ a physician if actual syncope occurs. Inform that excessive perspiration, dehydration, and other causes of volume depletion (eg, diarrhea, vomiting) may lead to a fall in BP; advise to consult w/ physician. Advise not to use salt substitutes containing K+ w/o consulting physician. Advise to promptly report any indication of infection (eg, sore throat, fever).

ZESTRIL — lisinopril   Rx
Class: ACE inhibitor

> D/C when pregnancy is detected. Drugs that act directly on the renin-angiotensin system (RAS) can cause injury and death to the developing fetus.

ADULT DOSAGE
Hypertension
Initial: 10mg qd; 5mg qd in patients taking diuretics
Usual Range: 20-40mg qd
Max: 80mg

May add a low-dose diuretic (eg, HCTZ 12.5mg) if BP is not controlled

Heart Failure
Adjunct w/ Diuretics and (Usually) Digitalis to Reduce Signs and Symptoms of Systolic Heart Failure (HF):
Initial: 5mg qd; 2.5mg qd w/ hyponatremia (serum Na+ <130mEq/L)
Max: 40mg qd

Diuretic dose may need to be adjusted to help minimize hypovolemia

Acute Myocardial Infarction
Reduction of Mortality in Hemodynamically Stable Patients w/ in 24 Hrs of Acute MI (AMI):
5mg w/in 24 hrs of onset of symptoms, followed by 5mg after 24 hrs, 10mg after 48 hrs, and then 10mg qd for at least 6 weeks

In patients w/ low systolic BP (SBP) (≤120mmHg and >100mmHg) during the first 3 days after infarct, initiate w/ 2.5mg; consider doses of 2.5mg or 5mg if hypotension occurs (SBP ≤100mmHg). D/C therapy if prolonged hypotension occurs (SBP <90mmHg for >1 hr)

PEDIATRIC DOSAGE
Hypertension
≥6 Years:
GFR >30mL/min/1.73m²:
Initial: 0.07mg/kg qd (up to 5mg total)
Max: 0.61mg/kg (up to 40mg) qd

DOSING CONSIDERATIONS
Renal Impairment
CrCl 10-30mL/min: Reduce initial dose to 1/2 the usual recommended dose (eg, HTN, 5mg; systolic HF/AMI, 2.5mg); titrate up as tolerated to a max of 40mg qd
Hemodialysis or CrCl <10mL/min: Initiate at 2.5mg qd

ADMINISTRATION
Oral route

STORAGE
20-25°C (68-77°F). Protect from moisture, freezing, and excessive heat.

HOW SUPPLIED
Tab: 2.5mg, 5mg*, 10mg, 20mg, 30mg, 40mg *scored

CONTRAINDICATIONS

History of ACE inhibitor-associated angioedema or hypersensitivity, hereditary or idiopathic angioedema, coadministration w/ aliskiren in patients w/ diabetes.

WARNINGS/PRECAUTIONS

Not recommended in pediatric patients w/ GFR <30mL/min/1.73m^2. Head/neck angioedema reported; d/c promptly and administer appropriate therapy. Intestinal angioedema reported; monitor for abdominal pain. Patients w/ history of angioedema unrelated to ACE inhibitor therapy may be at increased risk of angioedema during therapy. Less effect on BP and higher rates of angioedema in blacks than nonblacks. Anaphylactoid reactions reported during desensitization w/ hymenoptera venom, dialysis w/ high-flux membranes, and LDL apheresis w/ dextran sulfate absorption; consider using a different type of dialysis membrane or a different class of antihypertensives. May cause changes in renal function, including acute renal failure, especially in patients whose renal function depends on the RAS; consider withholding or discontinuing therapy if a clinically significant decrease in renal function develops. May cause symptomatic hypotension, sometimes complicated by oliguria, progressive azotemia, acute renal failure, or death; closely monitor patients at risk of excessive hypotension during first 2 weeks of treatment and whenever therapy and/or diuretic dose is increased. Avoid in patients who are hemodynamically unstable after AMI. Symptomatic hypotension may occur in patients w/ severe aortic stenosis or hypertrophic cardiomyopathy. Hypotension may occur w/ major surgery or during anesthesia. May cause hyperkalemia; monitor serum K$^+$ periodically. Associated w/ a syndrome that starts w/ cholestatic jaundice or hepatitis and progresses to fulminant hepatic necrosis, and sometimes death; d/c if jaundice or marked hepatic enzyme elevations occur.

ADVERSE REACTIONS

HTN: Headache, dizziness, cough.
HF: Hypotension, chest pain.
AMI: Hypotension, renal dysfunction.

DRUG INTERACTIONS

See Contraindications. Initiation of therapy in patients on diuretics may result in excessive reduction of BP. Decrease or d/c diuretic or increase the salt intake prior to initiation of therapy; if this is not possible, reduce the starting dose of lisinopril. Attenuates K$^+$ loss caused by thiazide-type diuretics. Increased risk of hyperkalemia w/ K$^+$-sparing diuretics, K$^+$-containing salt substitutes, or K$^+$ supplements; monitor serum K+ periodically. Increased hypoglycemic risk w/ insulin or oral hypoglycemics. NSAIDs, including selective COX-2 inhibitors, may cause deterioration of renal function in the elderly, volume-depleted, or w/ compromised renal function. Antihypertensive effect of therapy may be attenuated by NSAIDs. Dual blockade of the RAS is associated w/ increased risks of hypotension, hyperkalemia, and changes in renal function (including acute renal failure); avoid combined use of RAS inhibitors, or closely monitor BP, renal function, and electrolytes w/ concomitant agents that also affect the RAS. Avoid w/ aliskiren in patients w/ renal impairment (GFR <60mL/min). Lithium toxicity reported; monitor serum lithium levels during concurrent use. Nitritoid reactions reported w/ injectable gold (sodium aurothiomalate). Concomitant mTOR inhibitors (eg, temsirolimus, sirolimus, everolimus) may increase risk for angioedema.

PREGNANCY AND LACTATION

Pregnancy: May cause fetal harm. Use of drugs that act on the RAS during the 2nd and 3rd trimesters of pregnancy reduces fetal renal function and increases fetal and neonatal morbidity and death.
Lactation: Not for use in nursing.

MECHANISM OF ACTION

ACE inhibitor; decreases plasma angiotensin II, which leads to decreased vasopressor activity and aldosterone secretion.

PHARMACOKINETICS

Absorption: T_{max}=7 hrs (adults), 6 hrs (pediatric patients). **Elimination:** Urine (unchanged); $T_{1/2}$=12 hrs.

PATIENT CONSIDERATIONS

Assessment: Assess for hypersensitivity to the drug, history of ACE inhibitor-associated angioedema, hereditary/idiopathic angioedema, diabetes mellitus, risk factors for hyperkalemia, risk for excessive hypotension, severe aortic stenosis or hypertrophic cardiomyopathy, renal impairment, pregnancy/nursing status, and possible drug interactions.

Monitoring: Monitor for angioedema, anaphylactoid reactions, and other adverse reactions. Monitor BP, LFTs, serum K$^+$, and renal function.

Counseling: Inform of pregnancy risks and discuss treatment options for women planning to become pregnant; instruct to report pregnancy to physician as soon as possible. Instruct to immediately report signs/symptoms of angioedema and to avoid drug until they have consulted w/ prescribing physician. Instruct to report lightheadedness, especially during 1st few days of therapy; if syncope occurs, advise to d/c therapy until physician is consulted. Advise that excessive perspiration, dehydration, and other causes of volume depletion may lead to excessive fall in BP; instruct to consult w/ a physician. Advise not to use salt substitutes containing K$^+$ w/o consulting physician. Advise diabetic patients treated w/ oral antidiabetic agents or insulin to closely monitor for hypoglycemia, especially during the 1st month of combined use. Instruct to report promptly any indication of infection, which may be a sign of leukopenia/neutropenia.

ZETIA — ezetimibe   Rx

Class: Cholesterol absorption inhibitor

ADULT DOSAGE	PEDIATRIC DOSAGE
Primary Hyperlipidemia	Pediatric use may not have been established
Heterozygous familial and nonfamilial hyperlipidemia, alone or in combination w/ a statin; mixed hyperlipidemia in combination w/ fenofibrate	
10mg qd	
Homozygous Familial Hypercholesterolemia	
10mg qd in combination w/ atorvastatin or simvastatin	
Homozygous Sitosterolemia	
10mg qd	

- -

DOSING CONSIDERATIONS

Concomitant Medications
Bile Acid Sequestrant:
Give either ≥2 hrs before or ≥4 hrs after bile acid sequestrant

Renal Impairment
Moderate to Severe (GFR <60mL/min):
Use caution and monitor closely w/ simvastatin doses >20mg

Hepatic Impairment
Moderate to Severe: Not recommended

ADMINISTRATION

Oral route
Take w/ or w/o food.

STORAGE

25°C (77°F); excursions permitted to 15-30°C (59-86°F). Protect from moisture.

HOW SUPPLIED

Tab: 10mg

CONTRAINDICATIONS

Active liver disease or unexplained persistent elevations in hepatic transaminase levels, women who are or may become pregnant, and nursing mothers when used with statins. Known hypersensitivity to any component of this product.

WARNINGS/PRECAUTIONS

Not recommended with moderate to severe hepatic impairment. Should be used in accordance with the product labeling for the concurrently administered drug (eg, specific statin or fenofibrate). Liver enzyme elevations reported with statins. Consider withdrawal of therapy and/or statin if an increase in ALT or AST ≥3X ULN persists. Myopathy and rhabdomyolysis reported; immediately d/c therapy and any concomitant statin or fibrate, if myopathy is diagnosed/suspected. Increased risk for skeletal muscle toxicity with higher doses of statin, advanced age (>65 yrs of age), hypothyroidism, renal impairment, depending on the statin used, and concomitant use of other drugs. Caution and close monitoring when used with simvastatin >20mg in patients with moderate to severe renal impairment.

ADVERSE REACTIONS

URTI, diarrhea, arthralgia, sinusitis, pain in extremity.

DRUG INTERACTIONS

Caution with cyclosporine; monitor cyclosporine levels. May increase cholesterol excretion into the bile, leading to cholelithiasis with fibrates; avoid with fibrates (except fenofibrate). Consider alternative lipid-lowering therapy if cholelithiasis occurs with fenofibrate. Decreased levels with cholestyramine; incremental LDL-C reduction may be reduced. Monitor INR levels when used with warfarin.

PREGNANCY AND LACTATION

Pregnancy: Category C.
Lactation: Caution in nursing.

MECHANISM OF ACTION

Cholesterol absorption inhibitor; localizes at the brush border of the small intestine and inhibits the absorption of cholesterol, leading to a decrease delivery of intestinal cholesterol to the liver. Targets the sterol transporter, Niemann-Pick C1-like 1, which is involved in intestinal uptake of cholesterol and phytosterols.

PHARMACOKINETICS

Absorption: (Fasted) C_{max}=3.4-5.5ng/mL, 45-71ng/mL (metabolite); T_{max}=4-12 hrs, 1-2 hrs (metabolite). **Distribution:** Plasma protein binding (>90%). **Metabolism:** Small intestine and liver via glucuronide conjugation; ezetimibe-glucuronide (active metabolite). **Elimination:** Feces (78%, 69% unchanged drug), urine (11%, 9% metabolite); $T_{1/2}$=22 hrs.

PATIENT CONSIDERATIONS

Assessment: Assess for hepatic impairment, pregnancy/nursing status, and possible drug interactions. Obtain baseline lipid profile. Assess for conditions where treatment is contraindicated and risk factors for skeletal muscle toxicity. Obtain baseline LFTs when used with statin.

Monitoring: Monitor for signs/symptoms of elevated liver enzymes, myopathy, rhabdomyolysis, and other adverse reactions. Perform periodic monitoring of lipid profile. Periodically monitor LFTs during concomitant statin therapy.

Counseling: Advise to adhere to the National Cholesterol Education Program recommended diet, a regular exercise program, and periodic testing of a fasting lipid panel. Counsel about risk of myopathy; instruct to promptly report to the physician if any unexplained muscle pain, tenderness, or weakness occurs. Advise to discuss with physician about all medications, both prescription and OTC, currently being taken. Counsel women of childbearing age to use an effective method of birth control while using added statin therapy and instruct to d/c combination therapy and contact physician if they become pregnant. Instruct breastfeeding women not to take the medication if concomitantly using statins; advise patients who have lipid disorder and are breastfeeding to discuss the options with their physician.

ZETONNA — ciclesonide   Rx

Class: Non-halogenated glucocorticoid

ADULT DOSAGE	PEDIATRIC DOSAGE
Seasonal/Perennial Allergic Rhinitis	**Seasonal/Perennial Allergic Rhinitis**
Usual: 1 actuation/nostril qd (37mcg/actuation)	**≥12 Years:**
Max: 1 actuation in each nostril (74mcg/day)	**Usual:** 1 actuation/nostril qd (37mcg/actuation)
	Max: 1 actuation in each nostril (74mcg/day)

ADMINISTRATION
Intranasal route

Tilt head back slightly and insert the end of the nose piece into 1 nostril, pointing it slightly toward the outside nostril wall away from the nasal septum (the wall between the 2 nostrils), while holding the other nostril closed with 1 finger
Press down on the canister to release 1 spray and at the same time breathe in gently through the nostril, hold breath for a few sec then breathe out slowly through the mouth
Repeat steps for 2nd spray in other nostril

Priming
Prime pump by actuating 3 times prior to initial use or if not used for 10 consecutive days

STORAGE
25°C (77°F); excursions permitted to 15-30°C (59-86°F). Contents under pressure; do not puncture or use or store near heat or open flame. Exposure to >49°C (120°F) may cause bursting. Never throw into fire or incinerator.

HOW SUPPLIED
Aerosol: 37mcg/actuation [60 actuations]

CONTRAINDICATIONS
Known hypersensitivity to ciclesonide or any of the ingredients of this medication.

WARNINGS/PRECAUTIONS
Epistaxis, nasal ulceration, and nasal septal perforation reported; d/c if any of these reactions occur. Avoid spraying directly onto nasal septum. Localized *Candida albicans* infections of nose or pharynx may occur; discontinuation of therapy and treatment may be required if infection develops. May impair wound healing; avoid in patients with recent nasal septal ulcers, nasal surgery, or nasal trauma until healed. Glaucoma and cataracts may develop; monitor patients with vision changes, history of increased intraocular pressure (IOP), glaucoma, or cataracts. Hypersensitivity reactions reported. Caution with active or quiescent tuberculosis (TB) infections, untreated local/systemic fungal/bacterial infections, systemic viral or parasitic infections, or ocular herpes simplex. Risk for more serious/fatal course of infections (eg, chickenpox, measles); avoid exposure in patients who have not had these diseases or been properly immunized. Risk of acute adrenal insufficiency and withdrawal symptoms when replacing systemic corticosteroids with topical corticosteroids. Hypercorticism and adrenal suppression may occur; d/c slowly if symptoms of hypercorticism and adrenal suppression occur. May exacerbate symptoms of asthma and other conditions requiring long-term systemic corticosteroid use with rapid dose decrease. May cause reduced growth velocity in pediatric patients. Caution in elderly patients.

ADVERSE REACTIONS
Headache, epistaxis, nasal discomfort, nasopharyngitis, back pain, oropharyngeal pain, sinusitis, upper respiratory tract infection, influenza, bronchitis, urinary tract infection, cough.

DRUG INTERACTIONS
Oral ketoconazole may increase levels of active metabolite des-ciclesonide.

PREGNANCY AND LACTATION
Category C, caution in nursing.

MECHANISM OF ACTION
Non-halogenated glucocorticoid; has not been established. Shown to have a wide range of effects on multiple cell types (eg, mast cells, eosinophils, neutrophils, macrophages, lymphocytes) and mediators (eg, histamine, eicosanoids, leukotrienes, cytokines) involved in allergic inflammation.

PHARMACOKINETICS
Absorption: Oral bioavailability (<1%). Des-ciclesonide: C_{max}=59pg/mL.
Distribution: (IV) V_d=2.9L/kg (ciclesonide), 12.1L/kg (des-ciclesonide); plasma protein binding (≥99%). **Metabolism:** Hydrolyzed to des-ciclesonide (active metabolite); further metabolism in liver, via CYP3A4, CYP2D6. **Elimination:** (IV) Feces (66%), urine (≤20%).

PATIENT CONSIDERATIONS
Assessment: Assess patients who have not been immunized or exposed to infections (eg, measles, chickenpox). Assess for drug hypersensitivity, TB, any infections, ocular herpes simplex, history of increased IOP, glaucoma, cataracts, recent nasal septal ulcers, nasal surgery/trauma, use of other inhaled or systemic corticosteroids, pregnancy/nursing status, and possible drug interactions.

Monitoring: Monitor for hypercorticism, adrenal suppression, TB, infections, ocular herpes simplex, chickenpox, measles, epistaxis, nasal septal perforation, growth velocity in children, wound healing, visual changes, hypoadrenalism in infants born to mothers receiving corticosteroids during pregnancy, hypersensitivity reactions, and other adverse reactions. Monitor for signs of adrenal insufficiency and withdrawal symptoms in the event of replacing systemic with topical corticosteroids.

Counseling: Counsel on appropriate priming and administration. Advise to take ud at regular intervals and not to exceed prescribed dosage. Counsel about risks of nasal septal perforation, epistaxis, nasal ulceration, and other adverse reactions. Contact physician if symptoms do not improve by a reasonable time or if condition worsens. Inform that glaucoma and cataracts may develop; inform physician if change in vision occurs. Instruct to avoid exposure to chickenpox or measles and to consult physician without delay if exposed. Inform that worsening of existing TB infections, fungal/bacterial/viral/parasitic infections, or ocular herpes simplex may occur. Instruct to avoid spraying in eyes or directly on the nasal septum.

ZIAC — bisoprolol fumarate/hydrochlorothiazide   Rx

Class: Selective beta₁ blocker/thiazide diuretic

ADULT DOSAGE	PEDIATRIC DOSAGE
Hypertension	Pediatric use may not have been established
Uncontrolled BP on 2.5mg-20mg/day Bisoprolol or Controlled BP on 50mg/day HCTZ w/ Hypokalemia:	
Initial: 2.5mg/6.25mg qd	
Titrate: May increase at 14-day intervals	
Max: 20mg/12.5mg (two 10mg/6.25mg tab) qd, as appropriate	
Replacement Therapy: May substitute for titrated individual components	
Cessation of Therapy: Withdrawal should be achieved gradually over a period of 2 weeks	

ADMINISTRATION
Oral route

STORAGE
20-25°C (68-77°F).

HOW SUPPLIED
Tab: (Bisoprolol/HCTZ) 2.5mg/6.25mg, 5mg/6.25mg, 10mg/6.25mg

CONTRAINDICATIONS
Cardiogenic shock, overt cardiac failure, 2nd- or 3rd-degree atrioventricular (AV) block, marked sinus bradycardia, anuria, hypersensitivity to either component of this product or to other sulfonamide-derived drugs.

WARNINGS/PRECAUTIONS
Caution with impaired hepatic function/progressive liver disease. **Bisoprolol:** Caution with compensated cardiac failure. May precipitate cardiac failure; consider discontinuation at 1st signs/symptoms of heart failure (HF). Exacerbations of angina pectoris, MI, and ventricular arrhythmia with coronary artery disease (CAD) reported upon abrupt discontinuation; caution against interruption or discontinuation without physician's advice. May precipitate or aggravate symptoms of arterial insufficiency with peripheral vascular disease (PVD); exercise caution. Avoid with bronchospastic disease, but may use with caution if unresponsive/intolerant of other antihypertensives. Chronically administered therapy should not be routinely withdrawn prior to major surgery; however, may augment risks of general anesthesia and surgical procedures. Caution with diabetes mellitus (DM); may mask tachycardia occurring with hypoglycemia. May mask hyperthyroidism and precipitate thyroid storm with abrupt discontinuation. **HCTZ:** May precipitate azotemia with impaired renal function. D/C if progressive renal impairment becomes apparent. May precipitate hepatic coma with hepatic impairment. May cause idiosyncratic reaction, resulting in acute transient myopia and acute angle-closure glaucoma; d/c as rapidly as possible. Monitor for fluid/electrolyte disturbances (eg, hyponatremia, hypochloremic alkalosis, hypokalemia, hypomagnesemia). Decreased Ca^{2+} excretion and altered parathyroid glands, with hypercalcemia and hypophosphatemia, observed on prolonged therapy. Precipitation of hyperuricemia/gout and sensitivity reactions may occur. Photosensitivity reactions and exacerbation/activation of systemic lupus erythematosus (SLE) reported. Enhanced effects in postsympathectomy patient. D/C prior to parathyroid function test.

ADVERSE REACTIONS
Hyperuricemia, dizziness, fatigue, headache, diarrhea.

DRUG INTERACTIONS
May potentiate other antihypertensive agents. Avoid with other β-blockers. Excessive reduction of sympathetic activity with catecholamine-depleting drugs (eg, reserpine, guanethidine); monitor closely. D/C for several days prior to clonidine withdrawal. Caution with myocardial depressants or inhibitors of AV conduction (eg, certain calcium antagonists [particularly phenylalkylamine and benzothiazepine classes], antiarrhythmic agents [eg, disopyramide]). **Bisoprolol:** Digitalis glycosides may increase risk of bradycardia. Rifampin may increase clearance. May be unresponsive to usual doses of epinephrine. **HCTZ:** Alcohol, barbiturates, or narcotics may potentiate orthostatic hypotension.

Antidiabetic drugs (eg, oral agents, insulin) may require dosage adjustments. Impaired absorption with cholestyramine and colestipol resins. Corticosteroids and adrenocorticotropic hormone may intensify electrolyte depletion, particularly hypokalemia. May decrease response to pressor amines (eg, norepinephrine). May increase response to nondepolarizing skeletal muscle relaxants (eg, tubocurarine). Do not give with lithium; increased risk of lithium toxicity. NSAIDs may reduce diuretic, natriuretic, and antihypertensive effects.

PREGNANCY AND LACTATION
Pregnancy: Category C.
Lactation: Not for use in nursing.

MECHANISM OF ACTION
Bisoprolol: β_1-selective adrenoreceptor blocking agent; not established. May decrease cardiac output, inhibit renin release by the kidneys, and decrease tonic sympathetic outflow from vasomotor centers in the brain. **HCTZ:** Thiazide diuretic; not established. Affects renal tubular mechanisms of electrolyte reabsorption and increases excretion of Na^+ and Cl^-.

PHARMACOKINETICS
Absorption: Well-absorbed. Bisoprolol: Absolute bioavailability (80%); C_{max}=9ng/mL (2.5mg-6.25mg), 19ng/mL (5mg-6.25mg), 36ng/mL (10mg-6.25mg); T_{max}=3 hrs. HCTZ: C_{max}=30ng/mL; T_{max}=2.5 hrs. **Distribution:** Bisoprolol: Plasma protein binding (30%). HCTZ: Plasma protein binding (40-68%); crosses placenta; found in breast milk. **Elimination:** Bisoprolol: Urine (55% unchanged); feces (<2%); $T_{1/2}$=7-15 hrs. HCTZ: Urine (60% unchanged); $T_{1/2}$=4-10 hrs.

PATIENT CONSIDERATIONS

Assessment: Assess for cardiogenic shock, overt/compensated cardiac failure, 2nd- or 3rd-degree AV block, marked sinus bradycardia, anuria, sulfonamide hypersensitivity, CAD, PVD, bronchospastic disease, DM, hyperthyroidism, renal/hepatic impairment, history of sulfonamide/penicillin allergy, parathyroid disease, SLE, pregnancy/nursing status, and possible drug interactions. Obtain baseline serum electrolytes.

Monitoring: Monitor for signs/symptoms of HF, withdrawal, hypoglycemia, hyperthyroidism, renal/hepatic impairment, idiosyncratic reaction, fluid or electrolyte disturbances, precipitation of hyperuricemia or gout, and hypersensitivity reactions. Perform periodic monitoring of serum electrolytes.

Counseling: Instruct not to d/c therapy without physician's supervision, especially in patients with CAD. Advise to consult physician if any difficulty in breathing occurs, or other signs/symptoms of CHF or excessive bradycardia develop. Inform that hypoglycemia may be masked in patients subject to spontaneous hypoglycemia, or diabetic patients receiving insulin or oral hypoglycemic agents; instruct to use with caution. Advise to avoid driving, operating machinery, or engaging in other tasks requiring alertness until reaction to drug is known. Advise that photosensitivity reactions may occur.

ZIAGEN — abacavir   Rx

Class: Nucleoside reverse transcriptase inhibitor (NRTI)

> Serious and sometimes fatal hypersensitivity reactions w/ multiple organ involvement reported; d/c immediately if a hypersensitivity reaction is suspected and never restart therapy or any other abacavir-containing product. Patients who carry the HLA-B*5701 allele are at a higher risk of a hypersensitivity reaction; screen all patients for HLA-B*5701 allele prior to initiating or reinitiating therapy, unless patient has a previously documented HLA-B*5701 allele assessment. Lactic acidosis and severe hepatomegaly w/ steatosis, including fatal cases, reported w/ the use of nucleoside analogues and other antiretrovirals. D/C if clinical or lab findings suggestive of lactic acidosis or pronounced hepatotoxicity occur.

ADULT DOSAGE
HIV-1 Infection

Combination w/ Other Antiretrovirals:
300mg bid or 600mg qd

PEDIATRIC DOSAGE
HIV-1 Infection

Combination w/ Other Antiretrovirals:
≥3 Months of Age:
Sol:
8mg/kg bid or 16 mg/kg qd
Max: 600mg/day

Tab:
14 to <20kg:
QD Dosing:
300mg (1 tab)
BID Dosing:
AM Dose: 150mg (1/2 tab)
PM Dose: 150mg (1/2 tab)

≥20 to <25kg:
QD Dosing:
450mg (1 1/2 tabs)
BID Dosing:
AM Dose: 150mg (1/2 tab)
PM Dose: 300mg (1 tab)

≥25kg:
QD Dosing:
600mg (2 tabs)
BID Dosing:
AM Dose: 300mg (1 tab)
PM Dose: 300mg (1 tab)

DOSING CONSIDERATIONS
Hepatic Impairment
Mild (Child-Pugh Class A): 200mg (10mL) bid

ADMINISTRATION
Oral route

Take w/ or w/o food.
Screen for the HLA-B*5701 allele prior to initiating therapy.

STORAGE
20-25°C (68-77°F). **Sol:** Do not freeze. May be refrigerated.

HOW SUPPLIED
Sol: (Abacavir Sulfate) 20mg/mL [240mL]; **Tab:** (Abacavir Sulfate) 300mg* *scored

CONTRAINDICATIONS
Prior hypersensitivity reaction to abacavir, moderate or severe hepatic impairment, patients w/ HLA-B*5701 allele.

WARNINGS/PRECAUTIONS
Obesity and prolonged nucleoside exposure may be risk factors for lactic acidosis and severe hepatomegaly w/ steatosis; caution w/ known risk factors for liver disease. Suspend therapy if clinical or lab findings suggestive of lactic acidosis or pronounced hepatotoxicity develop. Immune reconstitution syndrome reported. Autoimmune disorders (eg, Graves' disease, polymyositis, Guillain-Barre syndrome) reported to occur in the setting of immune reconstitution and can occur many months after initiation of treatment. Redistribution/accumulation of body fat reported. Consider the underlying risk of coronary heart disease when prescribing therapy. Caution in elderly.

ADVERSE REACTIONS
Dreams/sleep disorders, drug hypersensitivity, N/V, headache/migraine, malaise, fatigue, diarrhea, rashes, abdominal pain, gastritis, depressive disorders, dizziness, fever.

DRUG INTERACTIONS
Not recommended w/ other products containing abacavir. Ethanol decreases elimination, causing an increase in overall exposure. May increase oral methadone clearance; an increased methadone dose may be required in a small number of patients.

PREGNANCY AND LACTATION
Pregnancy: Physicians are encouraged to register patients in the Antiretroviral Pregnancy Registry. Fetal harm has been seen in animal studies; relevance to human pregnancy registry data is unknown.
Lactation: Mothers should be instructed not to breastfeed due to potential for HIV-1 transmission.

MECHANISM OF ACTION
Carbocyclic nucleoside analogue; inhibits HIV-1 reverse transcriptase activity by competing w/ the natural substrate deoxyguanosine-5'-triphosphate and by its incorporation into viral DNA.

PHARMACOKINETICS
Absorption: Rapid and extensive. Absolute bioavailability (83%) (tab). (300mg bid) C_{max}=3mcg/mL; AUC_{0-12h}=6.02mcg•hr/mL. (600mg qd) C_{max}=4.26mcg/mL; AUC=11.95mcg•hr/mL. **Distribution:** (IV) V_d=0.86L/kg; plasma protein binding (50%). **Metabolism:** Via alcohol dehydrogenase and glucuronyl transferase; carbovir triphosphate (active metabolite). **Elimination:** Urine (1.2% unchanged, 81% metabolites), feces (16%); $T_{1/2}$=1.54 hrs.

PATIENT CONSIDERATIONS

Assessment: Assess for previous hypersensitivity to the drug, hepatic impairment, risk factors for lactic acidosis or liver disease, risk of coronary heart disease, pregnancy/nursing status, and possible drug interactions. Screen for HLA-B*5701 allele prior to initiation of therapy. Assess medical history for prior exposure to any abacavir-containing product.

Monitoring: Monitor for hypersensitivity reactions, lactic acidosis, hepatotoxicity, immune reconstitution syndrome, autoimmune disorders, fat redistribution/accumulation, MI, and other adverse reactions.

Counseling: Inform about the risk of hypersensitivity reactions; instruct to contact physician immediately if symptoms develop, and not to restart therapy or any other abacavir-containing product w/o medical consultation. Inform that lactic acidosis (w/ liver enlargement) and fat redistribution/accumulation may occur. Inform that drug is not a cure for HIV-1 infection and that illnesses associated w/ HIV-1 may still be experienced. Advise to avoid doing things that can spread HIV-1 to others (eg, sharing needles, other inj equipment, or personal items that can have blood or body fluids on them; having sex w/o protection; breastfeeding). Instruct to take all HIV medications exactly as prescribed.

ZIANA — clindamycin phosphate/tretinoin   Rx

Class: Lincosamide derivative/retinoid

ADULT DOSAGE
Acne Vulgaris

Apply at hs, a pea-sized amount onto 1 fingertip; dot onto the chin, cheeks, nose, and forehead; then gently rub over entire face

PEDIATRIC DOSAGE
Acne Vulgaris

≥12 Years:
Apply at hs, a pea-sized amount onto 1 fingertip; dot onto the chin, cheeks, nose, and forehead; then gently rub over entire face

ADMINISTRATION
Topical route

STORAGE
25°C (77°F); excursions permitted to 15-30°C (59-86°F). Protect from light and freezing. Keep away from heat. Keep tube tightly closed.

HOW SUPPLIED
Gel: (Clindamycin/Tretinoin) 1.2%/0.025% [30g, 60g]

CONTRAINDICATIONS
Regional enteritis, ulcerative colitis, or history of antibiotic-associated colitis.

WARNINGS/PRECAUTIONS
Not for oral, ophthalmic, or intravaginal use. Keep away from eyes, mouth, angles of the nose, and mucous membranes. Avoid exposure to sunlight, including sunlamps. Avoid use if sunburn is present. Daily use of sunscreen products and protective apparel are recommended. Weather extremes (eg, wind, cold) may be irritating while under treatment. Clindamycin: Systemic absorption has been demonstrated following topical use. Diarrhea, bloody diarrhea, and colitis (including pseudomembranous colitis) reported; d/c if significant diarrhea occurs. Severe colitis reported following PO or parenteral administration with an onset of up to several weeks following cessation of therapy.

ADVERSE REACTIONS
Nasopharyngitis, local skin reactions (erythema, scaling, itching, burning), GI symptoms.

DRUG INTERACTIONS
Caution with topical medications, medicated/abrasive soaps and cleansers, soaps/cosmetics with strong drying effect, products with high concentrations of alcohol, astringents, spices, or lime because skin irritation may be increased. Avoid with erythromycin-containing products. May enhance action of neuromuscular blocking agents; use with caution. Antiperistaltic agents (eg, opiates, diphenoxylate with atropine) may prolong and/or worsen severe colitis.

PREGNANCY AND LACTATION
Category C, not for use in nursing.

MECHANISM OF ACTION
Clindamycin: Lincosamide antibiotic; binds to 50S ribosomal subunits of susceptible bacteria and prevents elongation of peptide chains by interfering with peptidyl transfer, thereby suppressing bacterial protein synthesis. Found to have (in vitro) activity against *Propionibacterium acnes*. Tretinoin: Retinoid; not established. Suspected to decrease cohesiveness of follicular epithelial cells with decreased microcomedo formation. Also, stimulates mitotic activity and increased turnover of follicular epithelial cells, causing extrusion of comedones.

PHARMACOKINETICS
Absorption: Tretinoin: Percutaneous (minimal). **Distribution:** Orally and parenterally administered clindamycin found in breast milk. **Metabolism:** Tretinoin: 13-cis-retinoic acid and 4-oxo-13-cis-retinoic acid (metabolites).

PATIENT CONSIDERATIONS
Assessment: Assess for regional enteritis, ulcerative colitis, or history of antibiotic-associated colitis, pregnancy/nursing status, and possible drug interactions. Assess use in patients whose occupations require considerable sun exposure.

Monitoring: Monitor for signs/symptoms of diarrhea, bloody diarrhea, colitis, local skin reactions, and other adverse reactions.

Counseling: Instruct to wash face gently with mild soap and warm water at hs and apply a thin layer over the entire face (excluding the eyes and lips) after patting the skin dry. Advise not to use more than recommended amount and not to apply more than qd (at hs). Instruct to apply sunscreen qam and reapply over the course of the day PRN. Advise to avoid exposure to sunlight, sunlamp, UV light, and other medicines that may increase sensitivity to sunlight. Inform that medication may cause irritation (eg, erythema, scaling, itching, burning, stinging). Instruct to d/c therapy and contact physician if severe diarrhea or GI discomfort occurs.

ZIDOVUDINE — zidovudine   Rx
Class: Nucleoside reverse transcriptase inhibitor (NRTI)

> Associated w/ hematologic toxicity (eg, neutropenia, severe anemia), particularly w/ advanced HIV-1 disease. Symptomatic myopathy associated w/ prolonged use. Lactic acidosis and severe hepatomegaly w/ steatosis, including fatal cases, reported w/ nucleoside analogues; suspend treatment if lactic acidosis or pronounced hepatotoxicity occurs.

OTHER BRAND NAMES
Retrovir

ADULT DOSAGE
Prevention of Maternal-Fetal HIV Transmission
>14 Weeks of Pregnancy:
PO:
100mg 5X/day until start of labor
During Labor and Delivery:
IV:
2mg/kg over 1 hr followed by continuous infusion of 1mg/kg/hr until clamping of umbilical cord

PEDIATRIC DOSAGE
HIV-1 Infection
Combination w/ Other Antiretrovirals:
4 Weeks-<18 Years:
Weight Based:
4-<9kg: 12mg/kg bid or 8mg/kg tid (24mg/kg/day)
≥9-<30kg: 9mg/kg bid or 6mg/kg tid (18mg/kg/day)
≥30kg: 300mg bid or 200mg tid (600mg/day)

HIV-1 Infection
Combination w/ Other Antiretrovirals:
PO:
300mg bid
IV:
1mg/kg at a constant rate over 1 hr q4h

BSA Based:
240mg/m² bid or 160mg/m² tid (480mg/m²/day)
Prevention of Maternal-Fetal HIV Transmission
Neonates:
Start w/in 12 hrs after birth and continue through 6 weeks of age
PO: 2mg/kg q6h (8mg/kg/day)
IV: 1.5mg/kg over 30 min q6h (6mg/kg/day)

DOSING CONSIDERATIONS
Renal Impairment
Hemodialysis/Peritoneal Dialysis/CrCl <15mL/min:
PO: 100mg q6-8h
IV: 1mg/kg q6-8h
Adverse Reactions
Significant Anemia (Hgb <7.5g/dL or Reduction >25% of Baseline)/Neutropenia (Granulocyte Count <750 cells/mm³ or Reduction >50% from Baseline):
May require dose interruption until evidence of marrow recovery occurs; if marrow recovery occurs following dose interruption, may resume dose using adjunctive measures (eg, epoetin alfa), depending on hematologic indices and patient tolerance

ADMINISTRATION
Oral/IV route

Administer IV infusion only until oral therapy can be administered

PO
Take w/ or w/o food

IV
Avoid rapid infusion and bolus inj
Infusion must be diluted prior to administration

Dilution Instructions
1. Remove calculated dose from the 20mL vial and add to D5 inj sol to a concentration ≤4mg/mL
2. Administer diluted sol w/in 8 hrs if stored at 25°C (77°F) or 24 hrs if stored at 2-8°C (36-46°F), to minimize contamination

STORAGE
(Tab) 20-25°C (68-77°F). (Retrovir) 15-25°C (59-77°F). (Cap) Protect from moisture. (Inj) Protect from light. Diluted Sol: Stable for 24 hrs at room temperature and for 48 hrs if refrigerated at 2-8°C (36-46°F).

HOW SUPPLIED
Tab: 300mg; **(Retrovir) Cap:** 100mg; **Inj:** 10mg/mL [20mL]; **Syrup:** 10mg/mL [240mL]

CONTRAINDICATIONS
Life-threatening hypersensitivity reaction (eg, anaphylaxis, Stevens-Johnson syndrome) to any of the components of the formulation.

WARNINGS/PRECAUTIONS
Caution w/ granulocyte count <1000 cells/mm³ or Hgb <9.5g/dL; monitor blood counts frequently in patients w/ poor bone marrow reserve, particularly w/ advanced HIV-1 disease and periodically w/ other HIV-infected patients and w/ asymptomatic/early HIV-1 disease. Vial stoppers for inj contain natural rubber latex which may cause allergic reactions in latex-sensitive individuals. Obesity and prolonged nucleoside exposure may be risk factors for lactic acidosis and severe hepatomegaly w/ steatosis. Caution w/ any known risk factors for liver disease and in elderly. Pancytopenia and immune reconstitution syndrome reported. Autoimmune disorders (eg, Graves' disease, polymyositis, Guillain-Barre syndrome) reported to occur in the setting of immune reconstitution and can occur many months after initiation of treatment. May cause redistribution/accumulation of body fat.

ADVERSE REACTIONS
Hematologic toxicity, myopathy, lactic acidosis, severe hepatomegaly w/ steatosis, headache, N/V, malaise, anorexia, asthenia, constipation, abdominal pain/cramps, arthralgia, chills.

DRUG INTERACTIONS
Avoid w/ stavudine, nucleoside analogues affecting DNA replication (eg, ribavirin), doxorubicin, and other combination products containing zidovudine. Hepatic decompensation may occur in HIV/hepatitis C virus (HCV) coinfected patients receiving interferon alfa w/ or w/o ribavirin; closely monitor for treatment-associated toxicities. May increase risk of hematologic toxicities w/ ganciclovir, interferon alfa, ribavirin, and other bone marrow suppressive or cytotoxic agents.

PREGNANCY AND LACTATION
Category C, not for use in nursing.

MECHANISM OF ACTION
Synthetic nucleoside analogue; inhibits reverse transcriptase via DNA chain termination after incorporation of the nucleotide analogue.

PHARMACOKINETICS
Absorption: (Oral) Rapid. Bioavailability (64%); T_{max}=0.5-1.5 hrs. (IV) C_{max}=1.1mcg/mL. **Distribution:** V_d=1.6L/kg; plasma protein binding (<38%); crosses the placenta; found in breast milk. **Metabolism:** Hepatic. 3'-azido-3'-deoxy-5'-O-β-D-glucopyranuronosylthymidine (major metabolite). **Elimination:** Urine (14% unchanged, 74% metabolite [oral]; 18% unchanged, 60% metabolite [IV]); $T_{1/2}$=0.5-3 hrs. Refer to PI for pediatric patients and patients w/ renal impairment pharmacokinetic parameters.

PATIENT CONSIDERATIONS

Assessment: Assess for previous hypersensitivity reaction to the drug, advanced HIV disease, latex sensitivity, risk factors for lactic acidosis/liver disease, bone marrow compromise, renal/hepatic impairment, pregnancy/nursing status, and possible drug interactions. (Oral) Assess ability to swallow cap/tab in children.

Monitoring: Monitor for signs/symptoms of hematologic toxicity, lactic acidosis, hepatomegaly w/ steatosis, myopathy, immune reconstitution syndrome, autoimmune disorders, fat redistribution/accumulation, and other adverse reactions. Monitor blood counts/hematologic indices periodically and the need for dosage adjustment.

Counseling: Inform that potentially life-threatening hypersensitivity reactions can occur; instruct to immediately contact physician if rash develops. Inform about risk for hematologic toxicities and advise on importance of close blood count monitoring while on therapy. Counsel about the possible occurrence of myopathy and myositis w/ pathological changes during prolonged use and that therapy may cause a rare but serious condition called lactic acidosis w/ liver enlargement (hepatomegaly). Inform that hepatic decompensation has occurred in HIV-1/HCV coinfected patients receiving combination antiretroviral therapy and interferon alfa w/ or w/o ribavirin. Inform that immune reconstitution syndrome may occur; advise to inform physician immediately of any symptoms of infection. Inform that redistribution/accumulation of body fat may occur. Instruct to report any other adverse events that occur. Instruct not to breastfeed to prevent postnatal transmission. Inform that drug is not a cure for HIV-1 infection and that illness associated w/ HIV-1 may still be experienced. Inform to take all HIV medications exactly as prescribed. Advise to avoid doing things that can spread HIV-1 infection to others; instruct to continue to practice safe sex.

ZINACEF — cefuroxime   Rx

Class: Cephalosporin (2nd generation)

ADULT DOSAGE

General Dosing
Usual: 750mg-1.5g q8h for 5-10 days

Severe/Complicated Infections:
1.5g q8h

Life-Threatening Infections/ Infections Due to Less Susceptible Organisms:
1.5g q6h

Urinary Tract Infections
Uncomplicated:
750mg q8h

Skin and Skin Structure Infections
750mg q8h

Gonococcal Infections
Disseminated:
750mg q8h

Uncomplicated:
Single 1.5g IM dose, given at 2 different sites + 1g oral probenecid

Pneumonia
Uncomplicated:
750mg q8h

Bone/Joint Infections
1.5g q8h

Bacterial Meningitis
Max: 3g q8h

Prophylaxis of Postoperative Infections
1.5g IV just before surgery (approx 0.5-1 hr before initial incision), then 750mg IM/IV q8h w/ prolonged procedure

Open Heart Surgery (Perioperative):
1.5g IV at induction of anesthesia and q12h thereafter, for total of 6g

Treatment Duration
Continue therapy for a minimum of 48-72 hrs after the patient becomes asymptomatic or after evidence of bacterial eradication has been obtained

Streptococcus pyogenes **Infections:**
Treat for ≥10 days

Other Indications
- Lower respiratory tract infections
- Septicemia

PEDIATRIC DOSAGE

General Dosing
>3 Months of Age:
50-100mg/kg/day in equally divided doses q6-8h

Severe/Serious Infections: 100mg/kg/day (not to exceed max adult dose)

Bone/Joint Infections
>3 Months of Age:
150mg/kg/day in divided doses q8h (not to exceed max adult dose)

Bacterial Meningitis
>3 Months of Age:
200-240mg/kg/day IV in divided doses q6-8h

Treatment Duration
Continue therapy for a minimum of 48-72 hrs after the patient becomes asymptomatic or after evidence of bacterial eradication has been obtained

Streptococcus pyogenes **Infections:**
Treat for ≥10 days

DOSING CONSIDERATIONS

Renal Impairment
Adults:
CrCl >20mL/min: 750mg-1.5g q8h
CrCl 10-20mL/min: 750mg q12h
CrCl <10mL/min: 750mg q24h
Hemodialysis: Give a further dose at the end of the dialysis

Pediatrics:
Modify dosing frequency consistent w/ adult recommendations

ADMINISTRATION
IM/IV routes

IM
Reconstitute 750mg vial w/ 3.0mL sterile water for inj (SWFI); withdraw the resulting sus completely for inj.
Administer by deep IM inj into a large muscle mass (eg, gluteus or lateral part of thigh).
Avoid inadvertent inj into a blood vessel.

IV
Reconstitute 750mg and 1.5g vial w/ 8.3mL and 16mL, respectively, w/ SWFI.
Reconstitute 7.5g pharmacy bulk vial w/ 77mL of SWFI.
Continuous IV Infusion:
May add sol to an IV infusion pack containing compatible IV sol.
Do not add to sol of aminoglycoside.
Direct Intermittent IV Administration:
Slowly inject over 3-5 min into vein or give through the tubing system if also receiving other IV sol.
Intermittent IV Infusion w/ a Y-Type Administration Set:
Temporarily d/c administration of any other sol at the same site while infusing therapy.
TwistVial:
Reconstitute w/ 50 or 100mL of D5 inj, 0.9% NaCl inj, or 0.45% NaCl inj in compatible flexible diluent containers.
Frozen Galaxy Plastic Container:
Thaw container at room temperature or under refrigeration.
Do not force thaw by immersion in water baths or by microwave irradiation; do not refreeze.
Do not add supplementary medications and must not be used in series connections.
Refer to PI for additional administration procedures, use of frozen plastic container, compatibility, and stability.

STORAGE
(Dry State) 15-30°C (59-86°F). Protect from light. **Frozen Premixed Sol:** Do not store above -20°C (-4°F).

HOW SUPPLIED
Inj: 750mg, 1.5g, 1.5g/50mL

CONTRAINDICATIONS
Allergy to the cephalosporin group of antibiotics.

WARNINGS/PRECAUTIONS
Caution in penicillin (PCN)-sensitive patients; determine whether patient has had previous hypersensitivity reactions to cephalosporins, PCN, or other drugs. D/C if an allergic reaction occurs. *Clostridium difficile*-associated diarrhea (CDAD) reported; may need to d/c if CDAD is suspected or confirmed. May result in overgrowth of nonsusceptible organisms w/ prolonged use; take appropriate measures if superinfection develops. Use in the absence of a proven or strongly suspected bacterial infection or a prophylactic indication is unlikely to provide benefit and increases the risk of the development of drug-resistant bacteria. Hearing loss reported in pediatric patients treated for meningitis. Risk of decreased prothrombin activity in patients w/ renal/hepatic impairment, poor nutritional state, protracted course of therapy, and patients previously stabilized on anticoagulant therapy. Lab test interactions may occur. Caution w/ impaired renal function, history of GI disease (particularly colitis), and in elderly.

ADVERSE REACTIONS
Local reactions, decreased Hgb and Hct, eosinophilia, ALT/AST elevation.

DRUG INTERACTIONS
Caution w/ potent diuretics; may adversely affect the renal function. Nephrotoxicity reported w/ concomitant aminoglycosides. May decrease prothrombin activity; caution w/ anticoagulants. May affect the gut flora, leading to lower estrogen reabsorption and reduced efficacy of combined estrogen/progesterone oral contraceptives.

PREGNANCY AND LACTATION
Category B, caution in nursing.

MECHANISM OF ACTION
Cephalosporin (2nd generation); bactericidal; inhibits bacterial cell-wall synthesis.

PHARMACOKINETICS
Absorption: C_{max}=(750mg) 27mcg/mL (IM), 50mcg/mL (IV). (1.5g) 100mcg/mL (IV); T_{max}(750mg)=45 min (IM), 15 min (IV). **Distribution:** Plasma protein binding (50%); found in breast milk. **Elimination:** Urine (89%); $T_{1/2}$=80 min.

PATIENT CONSIDERATIONS
Assessment: Assess for known allergy to cephalosporins, PCN, or other drugs, renal/hepatic impairment, nutritional status, history of GI disease (eg, colitis), pregnancy/nursing status, and possible drug interactions. Obtain baseline culture and susceptibility tests.

Monitoring: Monitor for signs/symptoms of an allergic reaction, CDAD, and development of superinfection. In pediatric patients w/ meningitis, monitor for hearing loss. Monitor renal function and PT.

Counseling: Inform that drug only treats bacterial, not viral, infections. Instruct to take exactly ud; explain that skipping doses or not completing full course of therapy may decrease effectiveness and increase the likelihood of bacterial resistance. Inform that diarrhea may occur and will usually end if therapy is discontinued. Instruct to contact physician as soon as possible if watery/bloody stools (w/ or w/o stomach cramps, fever) develop even as late as ≥2 months after last dose of therapy, and if other adverse reactions occur.

ZINBRYTA — daclizumab   Rx

Class: Monoclonal antibody/interleukin-2R (IL-2R) alpha (CD25) blocker

> May cause severe liver injury including life-threatening events, liver failure, and autoimmune hepatitis; can occur at any time during treatment and seen up to 4 months after last dose. Contraindicated in patients w/ preexisting hepatic disease or hepatic impairment. Obtain ALT, AST, and bilirubin levels prior to initiation of therapy. Test transaminase levels and total bilirubin monthly and assess before the next dose. Follow transaminase levels and total bilirubin monthly for 6 months after the last dose. In case of elevation in transaminases or total bilirubin, treatment interruption or discontinuation may be required. Immune-mediated disorders (eg, skin reactions, lymphadenopathy, noninfectious colitis) reported. Reported that some patients required systemic corticosteroids or other immunosuppressant treatment for autoimmune hepatitis/immune-mediated disorders and continued this treatment after the last dose of therapy. Only available through a restricted program under a Risk Evaluation and Mitigation Strategy (REMS) called the Zinbryta REMS Program.

ADULT DOSAGE	PEDIATRIC DOSAGE
Multiple Sclerosis	Pediatric use may not have been established
Relapsing forms of multiple sclerosis (MS) in patients who have had an inadequate response to ≥2 drugs indicated for the treatment of MS	
150mg once monthly	

DOSING CONSIDERATIONS
Hepatic Impairment
ALT or AST >5X ULN or Total Bilirubin >2X ULN or ALT or AST ≥3 but <5X ULN and Total Bilirubin >1.5 but <2X ULN:
- Interrupt therapy and investigate for other etiologies of abnormal lab values
- If no other etiologies are identified, then d/c
- If other etiologies are identified, reassess overall risk-benefit profile of treatment and consider whether to resume daclizumab when both AST or ALT are <2X ULN and total bilirubin is ≤ULN

Other Dosing Considerations
- Evaluate patients at high risk for tuberculosis (TB) infection prior to initiating treatment
- If positive for TB, treat tuberculosis by standard medical practice prior to therapy
- Avoid initiating in patients w/ TB or other severe active infection
- Prior to initiation, screen for hepatitis B and C
- Consider any necessary immunization w/ live vaccines prior to treatment; live vaccines are not recommended during treatment and up to 4 months after discontinuation of treatment

ADMINISTRATION
SQ route
- Remove from the refrigerator 30 min before administration, to allow drug to warm to room temperature. Do not use external heat sources. Do not place back into refrigerator after allowing it to warm to room temperature.
- Inject into thigh, abdomen, or back of the upper arm.
- Use each prefilled syringe one time and then discard appropriately.

STORAGE
2-8°C (36-46°F). Store in the original carton to protect from light. Do not freeze or expose to temperatures >30°C (86°F). Discard if frozen. If refrigeration is unavailable, may store protected from light up to 30°C (86°F) for a period up to 30 days. Discard after 30 days w/o refrigeration.

HOW SUPPLIED
Inj: 150mg/mL

CONTRAINDICATIONS
Preexisting hepatic disease or hepatic impairment, including ALT or AST at least 2X ULN; history of autoimmune hepatitis or other autoimmune condition involving the liver; history of hypersensitivity to daclizumab or any other components of the formulation.

WARNINGS/PRECAUTIONS
See Dosing Considerations. If clinical signs or symptoms suggestive of hepatic dysfunction develop (eg, unexplained N/V, abdominal pain, fatigue, anorexia, jaundice, dark urine), promptly measure serum transaminases and total bilirubin and interrupt or d/c treatment. D/C if autoimmune hepatitis is suspected. Ensure adequate evaluation to confirm etiology or to exclude other causes if immune-mediated disorders are suspected; consider discontinuing treatment and refer to an appropriate specialist for further evaluation and treatment if a serious immune-mediated disorder develops. May cause anaphylaxis, angioedema, and urticaria after the first dose or at any time during treatment; d/c and do not restart treatment if anaphylaxis or other allergic reactions occur. Increases the risk for infections. Avoid initiating in patients w/ severe active infection until the infection is fully controlled. If serious infection develops, consider withholding treatment until the infection resolves. Depression-related events (eg, suicidal ideation, suicide attempt) reported; caution w/ previous or current depressive disorders. Consider discontinuing therapy if severe depression and/or suicidal ideation develops.

ADVERSE REACTIONS
Nasopharyngitis, URTI, rash, influenza, dermatitis, oropharyngeal pain, bronchitis, eczema, lymphadenopathy, depression, pharyngitis, increased ALT.

DRUG INTERACTIONS
See Dosing Considerations. Caution w/ hepatotoxic drugs; carefully consider need for herbal products or dietary supplements that can cause hepatotoxicity.

PREGNANCY AND LACTATION
Pregnancy: Administration to monkeys during gestation resulted in embryofetal death and reduced fetal growth at maternal exposures >30X than expected clinically. In monkeys administered 50mg/kg weekly from gestation day 50 to birth, there were no effects on pre- or postnatal development for up to 6 months after birth.
Lactation: There are no data on the presence of daclizumab in human milk, the effects on the breastfed child, or the effects of the drug on milk production; caution in nursing.

MECHANISM OF ACTION
Monoclonal antibody; precise mechanism unknown but presumed to involve modulation of IL-2 mediated activation of lymphocytes through binding to CD25, a subunit of the high-affinity IL-2 receptor.

PHARMACOKINETICS
Absorption: Absolute bioavailability (approx 90%); T_{max}=5-7 days; C_{max}=30μg/mL; AUC=640μg-days/mL. **Distribution:** V_d=6.34L. **Metabolism:** Undergoes catabolism to peptides and amino acids w/o renal elimination. **Elimination:** $T_{1/2}$=21 days.

PATIENT CONSIDERATIONS
Assessment: Assess for history of hypersensitivity to daclizumab or any other components of the formulation, hepatitis B and C, preexisting hepatic disease or hepatic impairment, history of autoimmune hepatitis or other autoimmune condition involving the liver, TB or other severe active infection, previous or current depressive disorders, pregnancy/nursing status, and for possible drug interactions. Obtain baseline ALT, AST, and bilirubin levels.

Monitoring: Monitor for hepatic injury, immune-mediated disorders, anaphylaxis, angioedema, urticaria, infections, new or worsening depression, suicidal ideation, and other adverse reactions. Monitor transaminase levels and total bilirubin monthly and assess before the next dose. Monitor transaminase levels and total bilirubin monthly for 6 months after the last dose.

Counseling: Advise of symptoms of allergic reactions/anaphylaxis, hepatic dysfunction, lymphadenopathy, GI reactions (eg, colitis), and dermatologic reactions; instruct to report such symptoms to healthcare provider immediately. Discuss the importance of monitoring hepatic lab values monthly and for up to 6 months after the last dose of therapy. Inform patients that they will be given a Zinbryta Patient Wallet Card that they should carry w/ them at all times; advise to show card to other treating healthcare providers. Advise that therapy can cause the immune system to attack healthy cells in the body and this can affect any organ system. Inform that treatment is only available through a REMS program and that the patient must enroll in the program and comply w/ ongoing monitoring requirements. Inform that there is an increased risk of developing infections during treatment; instruct to contact healthcare provider if symptoms of infection develop. Advise of the symptoms of depression and suicidal ideation and instruct to report symptoms of depression or thoughts of suicide to healthcare provider immediately. Provide appropriate instruction for methods of self-inj.

ZINECARD — dexrazoxane   Rx

Class: EDTA derivative

ADULT DOSAGE	PEDIATRIC DOSAGE
Doxorubicin-Induced Cardiomyopathy	Pediatric use may not have been established
For reducing the incidence and severity of cardiomyopathy associated w/ doxorubicin administration in women w/ metastatic breast cancer who have received a cumulative doxorubicin dose of 300 mg/m² and who will continue to receive doxorubicin therapy to maintain tumor control. Do not use w/ the initiation of doxorubicin therapy	
Usual: 10:1 ratio of dexrazoxane:doxorubicin (eg, 500mg/m²:50mg/m²)	

DOSING CONSIDERATIONS
Renal Impairment
Moderate to Severe (CrCl <40mL/min): Reduce dexrazoxane dose by 50% (5:1 ratio of dexrazoxane:doxorubicin)

Hepatic Impairment
Reduce dose proportionately (maintaining the 10:1 ratio)

Elderly
Start at lower end of dosing range

ADMINISTRATION
IV route

Do not administer via IV push
Do not mix w/ other drugs
Administer via IV infusion over 15 min
Give doxorubicin w/in 30 min after completion of dexrazoxane infusion

Preparation and Handling of Infusion Sol
Reconstitute w/ 25mL of sterile water for inj for a 250mg vial and 50mL for a 500mg vial
Dilute the reconstituted sol further w/ lactated Ringer's inj to a concentration of 1.3 to 3.0 mg/mL in IV infusion bags for IV infusion

STORAGE
25°C (77°F); excursions permitted to 15-30°C (59-86°F). Reconstituted Sol: Stable for 30 min at room temperature or 2-8°C (36-46°F) for up to 3 hrs. Diluted Infusion Sol: Stable for 1 hr at room temperature or 2-8°C (36-46°F) for up to 4 hrs.

HOW SUPPLIED
Inj: 250mg, 500mg

CONTRAINDICATIONS
Concomitant use with non-anthracycline chemotherapy regimens.

WARNINGS/PRECAUTIONS
Do not use with the initiation of doxorubicin therapy. Treatment does not completely eliminate the risk of anthracycline-induced cardiac toxicity. Monitor cardiac function before and periodically during therapy to assess left ventricular ejection fraction (LVEF); if results indicate deterioration in cardiac function associated with doxorubicin, carefully evaluate the benefit of continued therapy against the risk of irreversible cardiac damage. Secondary malignancies (eg, acute myeloid leukemia, myelodysplastic syndrome) reported in combination with chemotherapy. May cause fetal harm. Caution in elderly.

ADVERSE REACTIONS
Alopecia, N/V, fatigue, anorexia, stomatitis, fever, infection, diarrhea, pain on inj, sepsis, neurotoxicity, streaking/erythema, phlebitis, esophagitis, dysphagia.

DRUG INTERACTIONS
See Contraindications. Avoid during initiation of fluorouracil, doxorubicin, and cyclophosphamide therapy; may interfere with the antitumor efficacy of the regimen. May add to myelosuppression caused by chemotherapeutic agents; obtain CBC prior to and during each course of therapy, and administer dexrazoxane and chemotherapy only when adequate hematologic parameters are met.

PREGNANCY AND LACTATION
Category D, not for use in nursing.

MECHANISM OF ACTION
EDTA derivative; not established. Suspected to interfere with iron-mediated free radical generation thought to be responsible, in part, for anthracycline-induced cardiomyopathy.

PHARMACOKINETICS
Absorption: (500mg/m^2) C_{max}=36.5mcg/mL, T_{max}=15 min. **Distribution:** (500mg/m^2) V_d=22.4L/m^2; (600mg/m^2) V_d=22L/m^2. **Elimination:** (500mg/m^2) Urine (42%); $T_{1/2}$=2.5 hrs. (600mg/m^2) $T_{1/2}$=2.1 hrs.

PATIENT CONSIDERATIONS
Assessment: Assess for renal/hepatic impairment, pregnancy/nursing status, and possible drug interactions. Monitor cardiac function to assess LVEF. Obtain baseline CBC.

Monitoring: Monitor for secondary malignancies and other adverse reactions. Obtain CBC during each course of chemotherapy. Monitor cardiac function periodically during therapy to assess LVEF.

Counseling: Inform about the risks/benefits of therapy. Advise women of reproductive potential that drug may cause fetal harm; instruct to use highly effective contraception during treatment.

ZIOPTAN — tafluprost   Rx

Class: Prostaglandin analogue

ADULT DOSAGE	PEDIATRIC DOSAGE
Elevated Intraocular Pressure	Pediatric use may not have been established
Open-Angle Glaucoma/Ocular HTN: 1 drop in the conjunctival sac of the affected eye(s) qpm	

DOSING CONSIDERATIONS
Concomitant Medications
Space by at least 5 min if using >1 topical ophthalmic drug

ADMINISTRATION
Ocular route

STORAGE
2-8°C (36-46°F). Store in the original pouch. After the pouch is opened, store in the opened foil pouch for up to 28 days at 20-25°C (68-77°F). Protect from moisture.

HOW SUPPLIED
Sol: 0.0015% [0.3mL]

WARNINGS/PRECAUTIONS
May cause changes to pigmented tissues (eg, increased pigmentation of the iris [may be permanent], eyelid and eyelashes [may be reversible]). Regularly examine patients with noticeably increased iris pigmentation. May gradually change eyelashes and vellus hair (eg, increased length, color, thickness, shape, and number of lashes) in the treated eye. Caution with active intraocular inflammation (eg, iritis/uveitis); inflammation may be exacerbated. Macular edema, including cystoid macular edema, reported; caution in aphakic patients, pseudophakic patients with a torn posterior lens capsule, or patients with risk factors for macular edema.

ADVERSE REACTIONS
Conjunctival hyperemia, ocular stinging/irritation, ocular pruritus, cataract formation, dry eye, ocular pain, blurred vision, headache, common cold, cough, urinary tract infection.

PREGNANCY AND LACTATION
Category C, caution in nursing.

MECHANISM OF ACTION
Prostaglandin analog; exact mechanism unknown. Selective FP prostanoid receptor agonist believed to reduce IOP by increasing uveoscleral outflow.

PHARMACOKINETICS
Absorption: Tafluprost Acid: C_{max}=26pg/mL (Day 1), 27pg/mL (Day 8); T_{max}=10 min (median, Days 1 and 8); AUC=394pg•min/mL (Day 1), 432pg•min/mL (Day 8). **Metabolism:** Hydrolyzed to tafluprost acid (active metabolite); further metabolized via fatty acid β-oxidation and phase II conjugation.

PATIENT CONSIDERATIONS
Assessment: Assess for active intraocular inflammation, risk factors for macular edema, aphakic patients, pseudophakic patients with a torn posterior lens capsule, and pregnancy/nursing status.

Monitoring: Monitor for changes to pigmented tissues, changes in eyelashes and vellus hair, macular edema, and other adverse reactions.

Counseling: Advise not to exceed qd dosing; inform that more frequent administration may decrease IOP lowering effect of the medication. Inform that the medication does not contain a preservative; instruct to use immediately after opening for administration. Inform about risk of increased brown pigmentation of the iris (may be permanent) and darkening of eyelid skin (may be reversible after discontinuation). Inform about the possibility of eyelash and vellus hair changes in the treated eye. Advise to consult physician immediately if a new ocular condition (eg, trauma, infection) or any ocular reactions (eg, conjunctivitis, eyelid reactions) develop, if a sudden decrease in visual acuity is experienced, or if patient has ocular surgery. Instruct to administer at least 5 min apart if using >1 topical ophthalmic drug. Instruct on proper storage of cartons and opened/unopened foil pouches.

ZIPSOR — diclofenac potassium   Rx

Class: NSAID

> NSAIDs cause an increased risk of serious cardiovascular (CV) thrombotic events (eg, MI, stroke), which can be fatal; risk may occur early in treatment and may increase w/ duration of use. Contraindicated in the setting of CABG surgery. NSAIDs cause an increased risk of serious GI adverse events (eg, bleeding, ulceration, stomach/intestinal perforation), which can be fatal and may occur at any time during use w/o warning symptoms; elderly patients and patients w/ a prior history of peptic ulcer disease and/or GI bleeding are at greater risk.

ADULT DOSAGE	PEDIATRIC DOSAGE
Mild to Moderate Pain	Pediatric use may not have been established
Acute Pain: 25mg qid	
Use lowest effective dose for the shortest duration of time	

DOSING CONSIDERATIONS
Hepatic Impairment
Start treatment at the lowest dose; if efficacy is not achieved w/ lowest dose, d/c use
Elderly
If the anticipated benefit outweighs the potential risks, start at lower end of dosing range; monitor for adverse effects

ADMINISTRATION
Oral route

Different dose strengths and formulations of oral diclofenac are not interchangeable.

STORAGE
20-25°C (68-77°F); excursions permitted between 15-30°C (59-86°F) Protect from moisture.

HOW SUPPLIED
Cap: 25mg

CONTRAINDICATIONS
Known hypersensitivity (eg, anaphylactic reactions, serious skin reactions) to diclofenac, any other component of the drug product, or to bovine protein; history of asthma, urticaria, or allergic-type reactions after taking aspirin (ASA) or other NSAIDs; in the setting of CABG surgery.

WARNINGS/PRECAUTIONS
Use the lowest effective dose for the shortest duration possible. Avoid in patients w/ a recent MI unless benefits outweigh the risks of recurrent CV thrombotic events; if used, monitor for signs of cardiac ischemia. Increased risk for GI bleeding w/ longer duration of therapy, older age, poor general health status, and advanced liver disease and/or coagulopathy; avoid use in patients at higher risk unless benefits are expected to outweigh the increased risk. Consider alternate

therapies other than NSAIDs for patients at higher risk and patients w/ active GI bleeding. Promptly initiate evaluation and treatment if a serious GI adverse event is suspected; d/c until a serious GI adverse event is ruled out. Hepatotoxicity reported; d/c immediately and perform a clinical evaluation if clinical signs/ symptoms consistent w/ liver disease develop, if systemic manifestations occur, or if abnormal liver tests persist or worsen. May cause new onset HTN or worsen preexisting HTN. Fluid retention and edema reported. Avoid use in patients w/ severe heart failure (HF) unless benefits outweigh risks; monitor for signs of worsening HF if used. Renal papillary necrosis and other renal injury reported w/ long-term use. Renal toxicity also reported in patients in whom renal prostaglandins have a compensatory role in the maintenance of renal perfusion; increased risk w/ renal/hepatic dysfunction, dehydration, hypovolemia, and HF, and in the elderly. Correct volume status in dehydrated or hypovolemic patients prior to initiating therapy. Avoid use in patients w/ advanced renal disease unless the benefits are expected to outweigh the risk; monitor for signs of worsening renal function if used in patients w/ advanced renal disease. Hyperkalemia reported. Associated w/ anaphylactic reactions in patients w/ and w/o known hypersensitivity to diclofenac and in patients w/ ASA-sensitive asthma. Monitor for changes in the signs/symptoms of asthma in patients w/ preexisting asthma (w/o known ASA sensitivity). May cause serious skin reactions (eg, exfoliative dermatitis, Stevens-Johnson syndrome, toxic epidermal necrolysis); d/c at 1st appearance of skin rash/hypersensitivity. Anemia reported. May increase the risk of bleeding events; coagulation disorders may increase this risk. Monitor for signs of bleeding. May mask inflammation and fever.

ADVERSE REACTIONS
Abdominal pain, constipation, diarrhea, dyspepsia, N/V, dizziness, headache, somnolence, pruritus, increased sweating.

DRUG INTERACTIONS
Drugs that interfere w/ serotonin reuptake may potentiate the risk of bleeding. Synergistic effect on bleeding w/ anticoagulants (eg, warfarin); monitor for signs of bleeding w/ concomitant anticoagulants, antiplatelet agents (eg, ASA), SSRIs, and SNRIs. May increase risk of GI bleeding w/ use of oral corticosteroids, anticoagulants, and SSRIs; smoking; and alcohol use. ASA may increase risk of bleeding and serious GI events; concomitant use w/ analgesic doses of ASA is not recommended. Not a substitute for ASA for CV prophylaxis; monitor patients more closely for GI bleeding w/ concomitant use of low-dose ASA for cardiac prophylaxis. May diminish antihypertensive effect of ACE inhibitors, ARBs, and β-blockers (eg, propranolol); monitor BP. Coadministration w/ ACE inhibitors or ARBs may result in deterioration of renal function (including possible acute renal failure) in patients who are elderly or volume-depleted (including those on diuretic therapy), or have renal impairment; monitor for worsening renal function and adequately hydrate patient when these drugs are administered concomitantly. May reduce the natriuretic effect of loop diuretics (eg, furosemide) and thiazide diuretics; observe for signs of worsening renal function, in addition to assuring diuretic efficacy including antihypertensive effects. May increase digoxin serum concentrations and prolong the $T_{1/2}$ of digoxin; monitor digoxin levels. May elevate plasma lithium levels and reduce renal lithium clearance; monitor for signs of lithium toxicity. May increase the risk for methotrexate toxicity. May increase cyclosporine's nephrotoxicity; monitor for signs of worsening renal function. Concomitant use w/ other NSAIDs or salicylates (eg, diflunisal, salsalate) increases the risk of GI toxicity; not recommended w/ other NSAIDs or salicylates. Concomitant use w/ pemetrexed may increase the risk of pemetrexed-associated myelosuppression, renal, and GI toxicity; refer to prescribing information for further information. CYP2C9 inhibitors (eg, voriconazole) may enhance exposure and toxicity. CYP2C9 inducers (eg, rifampin) may lead to compromised efficacy. Dose adjustment may be warranted if administered w/ CYP2C9 inhibitors or inducers. Caution w/ concomitant drugs known to be potentially hepatotoxic (eg, acetaminophen, antibiotics, anti-epileptics).

PREGNANCY AND LACTATION
Pregnancy: Category C, prior to 30 weeks' gestation; Category D, starting at 30 weeks' gestation. Use during the 3rd trimester of pregnancy increases the risk of premature closure of the fetal ductus arteriosus. Avoid use starting at 30 weeks of gestation (3rd trimester).
Lactation: It is not known whether Zipsor is excreted in human milk; however, there is a case report indicating that diclofenac can be detected at low levels in breast milk; not for use in nursing.
Reproductive Potential: May delay or prevent rupture of ovarian follicles, which has been associated w/ reversible infertility in some women. Small studies in women treated w/ NSAIDs have also shown a reversible delay in ovulation. Consider withdrawal of therapy in women who have difficulties conceiving or who are undergoing investigation of infertility.

MECHANISM OF ACTION
NSAID; mechanism is not completely understood but involves inhibition of COX-1 and COX-2. Has analgesic, anti-inflammatory, and antipyretic properties.

PHARMACOKINETICS
Absorption: Bioavailability (50%), C_{max}=1087ng/mL, AUC=597ng•hr/mL, T_{max}=0.47 hr. Distribution: V_d=1.3L/kg; plasma protein binding (>99%); may be found in breast milk. Metabolism: Via CYP2C9 to 4'-hydroxy-diclofenac (major metabolite), glucuronidation/sulfation. Elimination: Urine (approx 65%), bile (approx 35%); $T_{1/2}$=1.07 hr (unchanged).

PATIENT CONSIDERATIONS
Assessment: Assess for history of hypersensitivity to diclofenac or to any component of this product; history of asthma, urticaria, or other allergic-type reactions w/ ASA or other NSAIDs; asthma; CV disease (CVD) or risk factors for CVD; HTN; history of peptic ulcer disease or GI bleeding; coagulation disorders; renal/hepatic impairment; pregnancy/nursing status; or any other conditions where treatment is contraindicated or cautioned. Assess volume status. Assess

for possible drug interactions. Obtain baseline LFTs, BP, CBC, and chemistry profile.

Monitoring: Monitor for signs/symptoms of CV thrombotic events; cardiac ischemia in patients w/ a recent MI; GI bleeding/ulceration and perforation; hepatotoxicity; new or worsening HTN; HF; edema; renal papillary necrosis and other renal injury; hyperkalemia; anaphylactic reactions; serious skin reactions; anemia; and other adverse reactions. Monitor BP during initiation of therapy and throughout the course of therapy. Monitor for signs of bleeding in patients on concomitant therapy w/ anticoagulants, antiplatelet agents, SSRIs, or SNRIs. Monitor renal function in patients w/ renal/hepatic impairment, HF, dehydration, or hypovolemia. Monitor LFTs, CBC, and chemistry profiles periodically during long-term treatment.

Counseling: Inform of potential for CV thrombotic events, GI adverse events, and worsening HF/edema, and advise of symptoms; instruct to report any symptoms to healthcare provider immediately. Inform of the potential for hepatotoxicity, and advise of signs/symptoms; if signs/symptoms occur, instruct to d/c and seek immediate medical therapy. Instruct to seek immediate emergency help if signs of an anaphylactic reaction occur. Advise to d/c immediately if rash develops and to contact healthcare provider as soon as possible. Advise females of reproductive potential who desire pregnancy that therapy may be associated w/ a reversible delay in ovulation. Advise pregnant women to avoid use starting at 30 weeks of gestation. Advise patient not to use other NSAIDs or salicylates concomitantly; notify of the presence of NSAIDs in OTC medications for colds, fever, or insomnia. Advise patient not to use low-dose ASA concomitantly w/o talking to healthcare provider.

ZIRGAN — ganciclovir   Rx

Class: Guanosine derivative

ADULT DOSAGE	PEDIATRIC DOSAGE
Acute Herpetic Keratitis	**Acute Herpetic Keratitis**
1 drop in the affected eye 5X/day (approx q3h while awake) until corneal ulcer heals, then 1 drop 3X/day for 7 days	**≥2 Years:** 1 drop in the affected eye 5X/day (approx q3h while awake) until corneal ulcer heals, then 1 drop 3X/day for 7 days

ADMINISTRATION
Ocular route

STORAGE
15-25°C (59-77°F). Do not freeze.

HOW SUPPLIED
Ophthalmic Gel: 0.15% [5g]

WARNINGS/PRECAUTIONS
For topical ophthalmic use only. Avoid wearing contact lenses during the course of treatment or if signs and symptoms of herpetic keratitis are present.

ADVERSE REACTIONS
Blurred vision, eye irritation, punctate keratitis, conjunctival hyperemia.

PREGNANCY AND LACTATION
Category C, caution in nursing.

MECHANISM OF ACTION
Guanosine derivative; competitively inhibits viral DNA-polymerase and directly incorporates into viral primer strand DNA, resulting in DNA chain termination and prevention of replication.

PATIENT CONSIDERATIONS
Assessment: Assess for signs and symptoms of herpetic keratitis, and pregnancy/ nursing status.

Monitoring: Monitor for eye pain, redness, itching or inflammation, and for other adverse reactions.

Counseling: Advise that dropper tip should not touch any surface, as this may contaminate the gel. Advise to consult physician if pain develops, or if redness, itching, or inflammation becomes aggravated. Instruct not to wear contact lenses during treatment.

ZITHROMAX 250MG, 500MG TABLETS AND ORAL SUSPENSION — azithromycin   Rx

Class: Macrolide

ADULT DOSAGE	PEDIATRIC DOSAGE
Nongonococcal Urethritis	**Community-Acquired Pneumonia**
1g single dose	**≥6 Months of Age:**
Nongonococcal Cervicitis	10mg/kg single dose on Day 1, followed by 5mg/kg qd on Days 2-5
1g single dose	Refer to PI for dosage guidelines
Gonococcal Infections	**Acute Otitis Media**
Urethritis and Cervicitis:	**≥6 Months of Age:**
2g single dose	30mg/kg single dose or 10mg/kg qd for 3 days or 10mg/kg single dose on Day 1 followed by 5mg/kg/day on Days 2-5.
Community-Acquired Pneumonia	Refer to PI for dosage guidelines
500mg single dose on Day 1, then 250mg qd on Days 2-5	

Pharyngitis/Tonsillitis
2nd-Line Therapy:
500mg single dose on Day 1, then
250mg qd on Days 2-5

Skin and Skin Structure Infections
Uncomplicated:
500mg single dose on Day 1, then
250mg qd on Days 2-5

Acute Bacterial Exacerbation of Chronic Bronchitis
500mg qd for 3 days or 500mg as
a single dose on Day 1, followed by
250mg qd on Days 2-5

Acute Bacterial Sinusitis
500mg qd for 3 days

Genital Ulcers
Chancroid:
1g single dose

Acute Bacterial Sinusitis
≥6 Months of Age:
10mg/kg qd for 3 days
Refer to PI for dosage guidelines

Pharyngitis/Tonsillitis
2nd-Line Therapy:
≥2 Years:
12mg/kg qd for 5 days
Refer to PI for dosage guidelines

ADMINISTRATION
Oral route
Take tab/sus w/ or w/o food.
Shake sus well before each use.

Sus (100mg/5mL, 200mg/5mL)
Reconstitution:
Add 9mL of water to 300mg or 600mg sus bottle, 12mL of water to 900mg sus bottle, or 15mL of water to 1200mg sus bottle.
After mixing, store at 5-30°C (41-86°F) and use w/in 10 days; discard after full dosing is completed.

STORAGE
Tab: 15-30°C (59-86°F). **Sus:** (Dry Powder) <30°C (86°F). (Constituted) 5-30°C (41-86°F).

HOW SUPPLIED
Oral Sus: 100mg/5mL, 200mg/5mL; **Tab:** 250mg, 500mg

CONTRAINDICATIONS
History of cholestatic jaundice/hepatic dysfunction associated w/ prior use of therapy; known hypersensitivity to azithromycin, erythromycin, or any macrolide or ketolide drug.

WARNINGS/PRECAUTIONS
Serious allergic reactions (eg, angioedema, anaphylaxis), dermatologic reactions (eg, Stevens-Johnson syndrome, toxic epidermal necrolysis), and cases of drug reaction w/ eosinophilia and systemic symptoms (DRESS) reported; d/c if an allergic reaction occurs and institute appropriate therapy. Abnormal liver function, hepatitis, cholestatic jaundice, hepatic necrosis, and hepatic failure reported; d/c immediately if signs and symptoms of hepatitis occur. Prolonged cardiac repolarization and QT interval, and torsades de pointes, reported. Consider risk of QT prolongation that can be fatal for at-risk groups, including patients w/ known QT interval prolongation, history of torsades de pointes, congenital long QT syndrome, bradyarrhythmias, uncompensated heart failure, ongoing proarrhythmic conditions (eg, uncorrected hypokalemia/hypomagnesemia), and clinically significant bradycardia. The elderly may be more susceptible to drug-associated effects on the QT interval. *Clostridium difficile*-associated diarrhea (CDAD) reported; may need to d/c if CDAD is suspected or confirmed. Exacerbation of myasthenia gravis symptoms and new onset of myasthenic syndrome reported. Should not be relied upon to treat syphilis; may mask or delay the symptoms of incubating syphilis. All patients w/ sexually transmitted urethritis or cervicitis should have a serologic test for syphilis and appropriate testing for gonorrhea performed at the time of diagnosis. May result in bacterial resistance if used in the absence of proven or strongly suspected bacterial infection or a prophylactic indication. Do not use in patients w/ pneumonia who are judged to be inappropriate for oral therapy due to moderate to severe illness or risk factors (eg, cystic fibrosis, nosocomial infections, known/suspected bacteremia).

ADVERSE REACTIONS
Adult Patients: Diarrhea/loose stools, nausea, abdominal pain.
Pediatric Patients: (Acute Otitis Media/Community-Acquired Pneumonia) Diarrhea, abdominal pain, N/V, rash. (Pharyngitis/Tonsillitis) Diarrhea, N/V, abdominal pain, headache.

DRUG INTERACTIONS
Caution w/ drugs known to prolong the QT interval and w/ Class IA (eg, quinidine, procainamide) and Class III (eg, dofetilide, amiodarone, sotalol) antiarrhythmic agents. Nelfinavir increases levels; closely monitor for known adverse reactions (eg, liver enzyme abnormalities, hearing impairment). May potentiate effects of oral anticoagulants (eg, warfarin); monitor PT. Monitor carefully when coadministered w/ digoxin or phenytoin.

PREGNANCY AND LACTATION
Pregnancy: Category B. Should be used during pregnancy only if clearly needed.
Lactation: Excreted in human breast milk in small amounts; caution in nursing.

MECHANISM OF ACTION
Macrolide; acts by binding to the 50S ribosomal subunit of susceptible microorganisms and interferes w/ bacterial protein synthesis.

PHARMACOKINETICS
Absorption: (250mg cap) Absolute bioavailability (38%). **Distribution:** Found in breast milk in small amounts. **Elimination:** Biliary (major route, predominantly unchanged), urine (6% unchanged); $T_{1/2}$=68 hrs (single 500mg dose).

Administration of variable doses resulted in different parameters.

PATIENT CONSIDERATIONS
Assessment: Assess for hypersensitivity to azithromycin, erythromycin, any macrolide, or ketolide drug; history of cholestatic jaundice/hepatic dysfunction associated w/ prior use of therapy; risk for QT prolongation; myasthenia gravis; pregnancy/nursing status; and possible drug interactions. Perform appropriate culture and susceptibility testing. In patients w/ sexually transmitted urethritis or cervicitis, perform serologic test for syphilis and appropriate testing for gonorrhea at the time of diagnosis. Assess for patients w/ pneumonia judged to be inappropriate for oral therapy due to moderate to severe illness or risk factors (eg, cystic fibrosis, nosocomial infections, known/suspected bacteremia).

Monitoring: Monitor for signs/symptoms of serious allergic/dermatologic reactions, DRESS, hepatotoxicity, CDAD, QT prolongation, new onset of myasthenic syndrome or exacerbation of myasthenia gravis, and other adverse reactions.

Counseling: Inform that diarrhea may occur and will usually end if therapy is discontinued. Instruct to contact physician as soon as possible if watery and bloody stools (w/ or w/o stomach cramps and fever) develop even as late as ≥2 months after the last dose. Instruct to d/c therapy immediately and contact physician if any signs of an allergic reaction occur. Instruct not to take the medication simultaneously w/ aluminum- and Mg²⁺-containing antacids. Explain that therapy should only be used to treat bacterial, not viral, infections. Instruct to take exactly ud; inform that skipping doses or not completing the full course of therapy may decrease effectiveness of immediate treatment and increase bacterial resistance.

ZITHROMAX 600MG TABLETS AND ORAL SUSPENSION — azithromycin   Rx

Class: Macrolide

ADULT DOSAGE

Nongonococcal Urethritis
Due to *Chlamydia trachomatis*:
Sus:
1g single dose

Nongonococcal Cervicitis
Due to *C. trachomatis*:
Sus:
1g single dose

Mycobacterial Infections
Disseminated *Mycobacterium avium* Complex Disease:
Tab:
Prevention: 1200mg once weekly; may combine w/ approved dosage regimen of rifabutin
Treatment: 600mg/day in combination w/ 15mg/kg/day ethambutol

PEDIATRIC DOSAGE
Pediatric use may not have been established

ADMINISTRATION
Oral route
Take tab/sus w/ or w/o food.

Sus (Single-Dose Pkt)
Do not use to administer doses other than 1000mg.
Not for pediatric use.

Reconstitution:
Mix entire contents of pkt w/ 2 oz (approx 60mL) of water.
Drink entire contents immediately and add an additional 2 oz of water, mix, and drink to ensure complete consumption of dosage.

STORAGE
Tab: ≤30°C (86°F). **Sus:** 5-30°C (41-86°F).

HOW SUPPLIED
Sus: 1g [single-dose pkt]; **Tab:** 600mg

CONTRAINDICATIONS
History of cholestatic jaundice/hepatic dysfunction associated w/ prior use of therapy. Known hypersensitivity to azithromycin, erythromycin, any macrolide, or ketolide drug.

WARNINGS/PRECAUTIONS
Serious allergic reactions (eg, angioedema, anaphylaxis), dermatologic reactions (eg, Stevens Johnson syndrome, toxic epidermal necrolysis), and cases of drug reaction w/ eosinophilia and systemic symptoms (DRESS) reported; d/c if an allergic reaction occurs and institute appropriate therapy. Allergic symptoms may recur, despite initial successful symptomatic treatment, w/o further therapy exposure. Abnormal liver function, hepatitis, cholestatic jaundice, hepatic necrosis, and hepatic failure reported; d/c immediately if signs and symptoms of hepatitis occur. Prolonged cardiac repolarization and QT interval, and torsades de pointes reported. Consider risk of QT prolongation that can be fatal for at-risk groups, including patients w/ known QT interval prolongation, history of torsades de pointes, congenital long QT syndrome, bradyarrhythmias, uncompensated heart failure, ongoing proarrhythmic conditions (eg, uncorrected hypokalemia/hypomagnesemia), and clinically significant bradycardia. The elderly may be more susceptible to drug-associated effects on the QT interval. *Clostridium difficile*-associated diarrhea (CDAD) reported; may

need to d/c if CDAD is suspected or confirmed. Exacerbation of myasthenia gravis symptoms and new onset of myasthenic syndrome reported. Should not be relied upon to treat gonorrhea or syphilis; may mask or delay the symptoms of incubating gonorrhea or syphilis. All patients w/ sexually transmitted urethritis or cervicitis should have a serologic test for syphilis and appropriate cultures for gonorrhea performed at the time of diagnosis. May result in bacterial resistance if used in the absence of proven or strongly suspected bacterial infection or a prophylactic indication.

ADVERSE REACTIONS
Diarrhea/loose stools, nausea, abdominal pain.

DRUG INTERACTIONS
Caution w/ drugs known to prolong the QT interval and w/ Class IA (eg, quinidine, procainamide) and Class III (eg, dofetilide, amiodarone, sotalol) antiarrhythmic agents. Nelfinavir increases levels; closely monitor for known adverse reactions (eg, liver enzyme abnormalities, hearing impairment). May potentiate effects of oral anticoagulants (eg, warfarin); monitor PT. Monitor carefully when coadministered w/ digoxin or phenytoin.

PREGNANCY AND LACTATION
Pregnancy: Category B. Should be used during pregnancy only if clearly needed.
Lactation: Excreted in breast milk in small amounts; caution in nursing.

MECHANISM OF ACTION
Macrolide; acts by binding to the 50S ribosomal subunit of susceptible microorganisms and interferes w/ bacterial protein synthesis.

PHARMACOKINETICS
Absorption: (Two 600mg tabs) Absolute bioavailability (34%). **Distribution:** Found in breast milk in small amounts; V_d=31.1L/kg. **Elimination:** Biliary (major route, predominantly unchanged), urine (6% unchanged); $T_{1/2}$=68 hrs (single 500mg dose).
Administration of variable doses resulted in different parameters.

PATIENT CONSIDERATIONS
Assessment: Assess for hypersensitivity to azithromycin, erythromycin, any macrolide, or ketolide drug; history of cholestatic jaundice/hepatic dysfunction associated w/ prior use of therapy; risk for QT prolongation; myasthenia gravis; pregnancy/nursing status; and possible drug interactions. Perform appropriate culture and susceptibility testing. In patients w/ sexually transmitted urethritis or cervicitis, perform serologic test for syphilis and appropriate testing for gonorrhea at the time of diagnosis.

Monitoring: Monitor for signs/symptoms of serious allergic/dermatologic reactions, DRESS, hepatotoxicity, CDAD, QT prolongation, new onset of myasthenic syndrome or exacerbation of myasthenia gravis, and other adverse reactions.

Counseling: Advise that there may be increased tolerability when tabs are taken w/ food. Inform that diarrhea may occur and will usually end if therapy is discontinued. Instruct to contact physician as soon as possible if watery and bloody stools (w/ or w/o stomach cramps and fever) develop even as late as ≥2 months after the last dose. Instruct to d/c therapy immediately and contact physician if any signs of an allergic reaction occur. Instruct not to take the medication simultaneously w/ aluminum- and Mg^{2+}-containing antacids. Explain that therapy should only be used to treat bacterial, not viral, infections. Instruct to take exactly ud; inform that skipping doses or not completing the full course of therapy may decrease effectiveness of immediate treatment and increase bacterial resistance.

ZITHROMAX INJECTION — azithromycin
Class: Macrolide   Rx

ADULT DOSAGE
Community-Acquired Pneumonia
500mg as a single dose IV qd for at least 2 days, then 500mg PO (two 250mg tabs) qd to complete a 7- to 10-day course

Acute Pelvic Inflammatory Disease
500mg as a single dose IV qd for 1-2 days, followed by 250mg qd PO to complete a 7-day course

PEDIATRIC DOSAGE
Pediatric use may not have been established

ADMINISTRATION
IV route
Infusate concentration and rate of infusion should be either 1mg/mL over 3 hrs or 2mg/mL over 1 hr.
Infuse over at least 60 min.
Do not add other IV substances, additives, or other medications or infuse simultaneously through same IV line.

Reconstitution
Reconstitute initial sol by adding 4.8mL of sterile water for injection to the 500mg vial using a standard 5mL (non-automated) syringe.
Reconstituted sol is stable for 24 hrs when stored <30°C (86°F).
Dilute further prior to administration.

Dilution
Transfer 5mL of the 100mg/mL sol into the appropriate amount of any compatible diluent.

Diluted inj is stable for 24 hrs at ≤30°C (86°F) or for 7 days if stored under refrigeration (5°C [41°F]).

Compatible Diluents:
0.9% NaCl, 0.45% NaCl, D5W, lactated Ringer's sol, D5 in 0.45% NaCl w/ 20mEq KCl, D5 in lactated Ringer's sol, D5 in 0.3% NaCl, D5 in 0.45% NaCl, Normosol-M in D5, Normosol-R in D5.

STORAGE
Diluted inj is stable for 24 hrs at ≤30°C (86°F) or for 7 days if stored under refrigeration (5°C [41°F]).

HOW SUPPLIED
Inj: 500mg

CONTRAINDICATIONS
History of cholestatic jaundice/hepatic dysfunction associated w/ prior use of therapy or known hypersensitivity to azithromycin, erythromycin, or any macrolide or ketolide drug.

WARNINGS/PRECAUTIONS
Serious allergic reactions (eg, angioedema, anaphylaxis) and dermatologic reactions (eg, Stevens-Johnson syndrome, toxic epidermal necrolysis, drug reaction w/ eosinophilia and systemic symptoms) reported; d/c if an allergic reaction occurs and institute appropriate therapy. Allergic symptoms may reappear after symptomatic therapy has been discontinued. Abnormal liver function, hepatitis, cholestatic jaundice, hepatic necrosis, and hepatic failure reported; d/c immediately if signs and symptoms of hepatitis occur. Prolonged cardiac repolarization and QT interval, and torsades de pointes reported. Consider risk of QT prolongation that can be fatal for at-risk groups, including patients w/ known QT interval prolongation, history of torsades de pointes, congenital long QT syndrome, bradyarrhythmias, uncompensated heart failure, ongoing proarrhythmic conditions (eg, uncorrected hypokalemia/hypomagnesemia), and clinically significant bradycardia. Elderly may be more susceptible to drug-associated effects on the QT interval. *Clostridium difficile*-associated diarrhea (CDAD) reported; may need to d/c if CDAD is suspected or confirmed. Exacerbation of myasthenia gravis symptoms and new onset of myasthenic syndrome reported. Use in the absence of a proven or strongly suspected bacterial infection may result in bacterial resistance. Local IV-site reactions reported; avoid higher concentrations (>2mg/mL).

ADVERSE REACTIONS
Community-Acquired Pneumonia (CAP): Diarrhea/loose stools, N/V, abdominal pain, pain at inj site, local inflammation.
Pelvic Inflammatory Disease: Diarrhea, nausea, vaginitis, abdominal pain, anorexia, rash/pruritus.

DRUG INTERACTIONS
Caution w/ drugs known to prolong the QT interval and w/ Class IA (eg, quinidine, procainamide) and Class III (eg, dofetilide, amiodarone, sotalol) antiarrhythmic agents. Increased levels w/ nelfinavir; closely monitor for known adverse reactions (eg, liver enzyme abnormalities, hearing impairment). May potentiate effects of oral anticoagulants (eg, warfarin); monitor PT. Monitor carefully when coadministered w/ digoxin or phenytoin.

PREGNANCY AND LACTATION
Pregnancy: Category B.
Lactation: Excreted in human breast milk in small amounts; caution in nursing.

MECHANISM OF ACTION
Macrolide; acts by binding to the 50S ribosomal subunit of susceptible microorganisms and interferes w/ microbial protein synthesis.

PHARMACOKINETICS
Absorption: (CAP Patients) C_{max}=3.63mcg/mL, AUC=9.60mcg•h/mL.
Distribution: Found in breast milk. **Elimination:** Urine (11% after 1st dose), (14%, 5th dose); $T_{1/2}$=68 hrs.

PATIENT CONSIDERATIONS
Assessment: Assess for hypersensitivity to drug, history of cholestatic jaundice/hepatic dysfunction associated w/ prior use of therapy, risk for QT prolongation, myasthenia gravis, pregnancy/nursing status, and possible drug interactions. Perform appropriate culture and susceptibility testing.

Monitoring: Monitor for signs/symptoms of serious allergic/dermatologic reactions, hepatotoxicity, CDAD, QT prolongation, new onset of myasthenic syndrome or exacerbation of myasthenia gravis, and other adverse reactions. Monitor for local IV-site reactions.

Counseling: Inform that diarrhea may occur and will usually end if therapy is discontinued. Instruct to contact physician as soon as possible if watery and bloody stools (w/ or w/o stomach cramps, fever) develop even as late as 2 or more months after the last dose.

ZMAX — azithromycin
Class: Macrolide   Rx

ADULT DOSAGE
Acute Bacterial Sinusitis
2g single dose

Community-Acquired Pneumonia
2g single dose

PEDIATRIC DOSAGE
Community-Acquired Pneumonia
≥6 Months of Age:
60mg/kg (27mg/lb) single dose; dose in mL is equivalent to weight in lb (1mL/lb dose)

If ≥34kg, administer 2g single dose

ADMINISTRATION
Oral route
Take on an empty stomach, at least 1 hr ac or 2 hrs pc.
Constitute w/ 60mL of water; shake well before using.
Consume reconstituted sus w/in 12 hrs.

Pediatrics
Use a dosing spoon, medicine syringe, or cup for patients <34kg.
Discard any remaining sus after dosing in pediatric patients.

Additional Treatment After Vomiting
If vomiting occurs w/in 5 min of administration, consider additional antibiotic treatment.
If vomiting occurs 5-60 min following administration or in patients w/ delayed gastric emptying, consider alternative therapy.
If vomiting occurs ≥60 min following therapy, a 2nd dose or alternative treatment is not warranted.

STORAGE
Dry Powder: ≤30°C (86°F). **Reconstituted Sus:** 25°C (77°F); excursions permitted to 15-30°C (59-86°F). Do not refrigerate or freeze.

HOW SUPPLIED
Oral Sus, Extended-Release: 2g

CONTRAINDICATIONS
Known hypersensitivity to azithromycin, erythromycin or any macrolide or ketolide drug, history of cholestatic jaundice/hepatic dysfunction associated w/ prior use of azithromycin.

WARNINGS/PRECAUTIONS
Not recommended in patients w/ pneumonia judged to be inappropriate for oral therapy due to moderate to severe illness or risk factors (eg, cystic fibrosis, nosocomial infections, known/suspected bacteremia). Serious allergic reactions (eg, angioedema, anaphylaxis, Stevens Johnson syndrome, toxic epidermal necrolysis, drug reaction w/ eosinophilia and systemic symptoms) reported. Allergic symptoms may recur after initial successful symptomatic treatment w/o further azithromycin exposure. Abnormal liver function, hepatitis, cholestatic jaundice, hepatic necrosis, and hepatic failure reported, some of which resulted in death; d/c immediately if signs/symptoms of hepatitis occur. Prolonged cardiac repolarization and QT interval, and torsades de pointes reported. Consider the risk of QT prolongation for at-risk groups including patients w/ known QT interval prolongation, history of torsades de pointes, congenital long QT syndrome, bradyarrhythmias, uncompensated heart failure, ongoing proarrhythmic conditions (eg, uncorrected hypokalemia/hypomagnesemia), or clinically significant bradycardia. Elderly patients may be more susceptible to drug-associated effects on the QT interval. *Clostridium difficile*-associated diarrhea (CDAD) reported; may need to d/c if CDAD is confirmed or suspected. Exacerbation of symptoms of myasthenia gravis and new onset of myasthenic syndrome reported. Caution w/ GFR <10mL/min; higher incidence of GI adverse events reported. May result in bacterial resistance if used in the absence of a proven/suspected bacterial infection.

ADVERSE REACTIONS
Diarrhea/loose stools, N/V, abdominal pain, headache.

DRUG INTERACTIONS
Caution w/ drugs known to prolong QT interval and Class IA (eg, quinidine, procainamide) or Class III (eg, dofetilide, amiodarone, sotalol) antiarrhythmic agents. Nelfinavir may increase levels; closely monitor for adverse reactions (eg, liver enzyme abnormalities, hearing impairment). May potentiate effects of oral anticoagulants (eg, warfarin); monitor PT. Monitor carefully when digoxin or phenytoin are used concomitantly w/ azithromycin.

PREGNANCY AND LACTATION
Pregnancy: Category B.
Lactation: Excreted in human breast milk in small amounts; caution in nursing.

MECHANISM OF ACTION
Macrolide; binds to the 23S rRNA of the 50S ribosomal subunit and interferes w/ bacterial protein synthesis by impeding the assembly of the 50S ribosomal subunit.

PHARMACOKINETICS
Absorption: (Healthy adults) C_{max}=0.821mcg/mL; T_{max}=5 hrs (median); AUC=20mcg•hr/mL. **Distribution:** V_d=31.1L/kg; plasma protein binding (51% at 0.02mcg/mL, 7% at 2mcg/mL); found in breast milk in small amounts. **Elimination:** Bile (major, unchanged), urine (6%, unchanged); $T_{1/2}$=59 hrs.

PATIENT CONSIDERATIONS

Assessment: Assess for previous hypersensitivity to the drug, erythromycin, or any macrolide/ketolide antibiotic, risk for QT interval prolongation, myasthenia gravis, delayed gastric emptying, history of cholestatic jaundice/hepatic dysfunction associated w/ prior use of azithromycin, renal/hepatic dysfunction, pregnancy/nursing status, and possible drug interactions. Perform appropriate culture and susceptibility tests prior to treatment.

Monitoring: Monitor for signs/symptoms of allergic/skin reactions, CDAD, GI adverse effects, cardiac repolarization or QT prolongation, torsades de pointes, exacerbation of myasthenia gravis, new onset of myasthenic syndrome, hepatotoxicity, and other adverse reactions.

Counseling: Inform that drug needs time to work and that patient may not feel better right away. Instruct to contact physician if symptoms do not improve in a few days, if any signs of allergic reaction occur, or if watery and bloody stools (w/ or w/o stomach cramps) develop even as late as ≥2 months after dosing. Instruct to contact physician for further treatment if vomiting occurs w/in 1st hr of administration. Inform that therapy treats bacterial, not viral, infections.

Instruct to take ud; advise that not taking the complete dose may decrease effectiveness and increase the likelihood of bacterial resistance. Advise to take w/o regard to antacids containing magnesium hydroxide and/or aluminum hydroxide.

ZOCOR — simvastatin   Rx
Class: HMG-CoA reductase inhibitor (statin)

ADULT DOSAGE	PEDIATRIC DOSAGE
Hyperlipidemia	**Heterozygous Familial Hypercholesterolemia**
Initial: 10mg or 20mg qpm	
Usual Range: 5-40mg/day	**10-17 Years (At Least 1 Year Postmenarche):**
High Risk for Coronary Heart Disease Events:	**Initial:** 10mg qpm
Initial: 40mg/day	**Range:** 10-40mg/day
	Titrate: Adjust at ≥4-week intervals
Lipid determinations should be performed after 4 weeks of therapy and periodically thereafter	**Max:** 40mg/day
Homozygous Familial Hypercholesterolemia	
40mg/day qpm	
Lipid determinations should be performed after 4 weeks of therapy and periodically thereafter	

DOSING CONSIDERATIONS
Concomitant Medications
Verapamil, Diltiazem, or Dronedarone:
Max: 10mg/day

Amiodarone, Amlodipine, or Ranolazine:
Max: 20mg/day

Lomitapide:
Homozygous Familial Hypercholesterolemia:
Reduce dose by 50% if initiating lomitapide
Max: 20mg/day (or 40mg/day for patients who have previously taken simvastatin 80mg/day chronically [eg, ≥12 months] w/o evidence of muscle toxicity)

Niacin-Containing Products:
Chinese Patients Taking Lipid-Modifying Doses (≥1g/day Niacin):
Caution w/ doses >20mg/day; do not give 80mg dose

Renal Impairment
Severe:
Initial: 5mg/day; use caution and monitor closely

Other Important Considerations
Restricted Dosing:
Use 80mg dose only in patients who have been taking simvastatin 80mg chronically (eg, ≥12 months) w/o evidence of muscle toxicity

If currently tolerating 80mg dose and needs to be initiated on a drug that is contraindicated or is associated w/ a dose cap for simvastatin, switch to an alternative statin w/ less potential for drug-drug interaction

In patients unable to achieve LDL goal utilizing the 40mg dose, place on alternative LDL-lowering treatment that provides greater LDL lowering; do not titrate therapy to 80mg dose

ADMINISTRATION
Oral route

STORAGE
5-30°C (41-86°F).

HOW SUPPLIED
Tab: 5mg, 10mg, 20mg, 40mg, 80mg

CONTRAINDICATIONS
Concomitant administration of strong CYP3A4 inhibitors (eg, itraconazole, ketoconazole, posaconazole, voriconazole, HIV protease inhibitors, boceprevir, telaprevir, erythromycin, clarithromycin, telithromycin, nefazodone, cobicistat-containing products), gemfibrozil, cyclosporine, or danazol; hypersensitivity to any component of this medication; active liver disease, which may include unexplained persistent elevations in hepatic transaminases; women who are or may become pregnant; nursing mothers.

WARNINGS/PRECAUTIONS
Myopathy (including immune-mediated necrotizing myopathy [IMNM]) and rhabdomyolysis reported; predisposing factors include advanced age (≥65 yrs of age), female gender, uncontrolled hypothyroidism, and renal impairment. Risk of myopathy, including rhabdomyolysis, is dose related and greater w/ 80mg doses. D/C if markedly elevated CPK levels occur or myopathy is diagnosed/suspected, and temporarily withhold in any patient experiencing an acute or serious condition predisposing to development of renal failure secondary to rhabdomyolysis. Persistent increases in serum transaminases reported. Fatal and nonfatal hepatic failure (rare) reported; promptly interrupt therapy if serious liver injury w/ clinical symptoms and/or hyperbilirubinemia or jaundice occurs and do not restart if no alternate etiology found. Increases in HbA1c and FPG levels reported. Caution w/ substantial alcohol consumption, history of liver disease, and in the elderly.

ADVERSE REACTIONS
Abdominal pain, headache, myalgia, constipation, nausea, atrial fibrillation, gastritis, diabetes mellitus, insomnia, vertigo, bronchitis, eczema, URTI, UTI(s).

DRUG INTERACTIONS

See Contraindications and Dosing Considerations. Due to the risk of myopathy/rhabdomyolysis, avoid grapefruit juice and caution w/ fibrates, lipid-modifying doses (≥1g/day) of niacin, colchicine, verapamil, diltiazem, dronedarone, lomitapide, amiodarone, amlodipine, and ranolazine. May slightly elevate digoxin concentrations; monitor patients taking digoxin when therapy is initiated. May potentiate effect of coumarin anticoagulants; determine PT before initiation and frequently during therapy.

PREGNANCY AND LACTATION

Category X, not for use in nursing.

MECHANISM OF ACTION

HMG-CoA reductase inhibitor; specific inhibitor of HMG-CoA reductase, the enzyme that catalyzes the conversion of HMG-CoA to mevalonate, an early and rate-limiting step in the biosynthetic pathway for cholesterol. Reduces VLDL and TG and increases HDL.

PHARMACOKINETICS

Absorption: T_{max}=1.3-2.4 hrs. **Distribution:** Plasma protein binding (95%). **Metabolism:** Liver (extensive 1st pass), by hydrolysis via CYP3A4; β-hydroxyacid, 6'-hydroxy, 6'-hydroxymethyl, and 6'-exomethylene derivatives (major active metabolites). **Elimination:** Feces (60%), urine (13%).

PATIENT CONSIDERATIONS

Assessment: Assess for history of or active liver disease, unexplained persistent hepatic transaminase elevations, predisposing factors for myopathy, renal impairment, alcohol consumption, drug hypersensitivity, any other conditions where treatment is contraindicated or cautioned, pregnancy/nursing status, and possible drug interactions. Assess lipid profile and LFTs.

Monitoring: Monitor for signs/symptoms of myopathy (including IMNM), rhabdomyolysis, liver dysfunction, increases in HbA1c and FPG levels, and other adverse reactions. Monitor lipid profile, LFTs when clinically indicated, and CPK levels.

Counseling: Inform of benefits/risks of therapy. Advise to adhere to the National Cholesterol Education Program recommended diet, a regular exercise program, and periodic testing of a fasting lipid panel. Inform about substances that should be avoided during therapy, and advise to discuss all medications, both prescription and OTC, w/ physician. Instruct to report promptly any unexplained muscle pain, tenderness, or weakness, particularly if accompanied by malaise or fever or if these muscle signs or symptoms persist after discontinuation, or any symptoms that may indicate liver injury. Inform patients using the 80mg dose that the risk of myopathy, including rhabdomyolysis, is increased. Instruct women of childbearing age to use an effective method of birth control to prevent pregnancy while on therapy, to d/c therapy and call physician if pregnant, and not to breastfeed while on therapy.

ZOHYDRO ER — hydrocodone bitartrate   CII

Class: Opioid analgesic

> Exposes users to risks of addiction, abuse, and misuse, leading to overdose and death; assess each patient's risk prior to prescribing, and monitor regularly for development of these behaviors/conditions. Serious, life-threatening, or fatal respiratory depression may occur; monitor during initiation or following a dose increase. Swallow cap whole; crushing, dissolving, or chewing cap can cause rapid release and absorption of potentially fatal dose. Accidental ingestion, especially in children, can result in a fatal overdose. Prolonged use during pregnancy can result in neonatal opioid withdrawal syndrome; advise pregnant women of the risk and ensure availability of appropriate treatment. Avoid alcohol consumption or medication that contains alcohol; may result in increased plasma levels and a potentially fatal overdose of hydrocodone. Concomitant use w/ all CYP3A4 inhibitors and discontinuation of a concomitantly administered CYP3A4 inducer may increase plasma concentrations and potentially cause fatal respiratory depression; monitor patients during concomitant therapy.

ADULT DOSAGE

Severe Pain (Daily, Around-the-Clock Management)

1st Opioid Analgesic/Not Opioid Tolerant:
Initial: 10mg q12h

Titration and Maint:
Individually titrate to a dose that provides adequate analgesia and minimizes adverse reactions
Adjust in increments of 10mg q12h every 3-7 days
If breakthrough pain is experienced, patient may require a dose increase or need rescue medication w/ an appropriate dose of an immediate-release analgesic

50mg capsules, a single dose >40mg, or total daily dose >80mg are only for use in patients in whom tolerance to an opioid of comparable potency has been established

Conversions

From Other Oral Opioids:
D/C all other around-the-clock opioids when therapy is initiated

PEDIATRIC DOSAGE

Pediatric use may not have been established

Conversion Factors to Zohydro ER (Prior Oral Opioid: Approx Oral Conversion Factor):
Hydrocodone 10mg: 1
Oxycodone 10mg: 1
Methadone 10mg: 1
Oxymorphone 5mg: 2
Hydromorphone 3.75mg: 2.67
Morphine 15mg: 0.67
Codeine 100mg: 0.10

Calculation for Estimated Daily Dose for Zohydro ER:
Always round dose down, if necessary, to appropriate strengths available

Currently on Single Opioid: Sum the current total daily dose of opioid, then multiply total daily dose by the conversion factor to calculate the approx oral hydrocodone daily dose, then divide the daily dose in half for q12h administration

Currently on >1 Opioid: Calculate approx oral hydrocodone dose for each opioid and sum totals to obtain approx total hydrocodone daily dose, then divide the daily dose in half for q12h administration

Currently on Fixed-Ratio Opioid/Non-Opioid Analgesic Products: Use only the opioid component of these products in the conversion

From Methadone:
Closely monitor; ratio between methadone and other opioid agonists may vary widely as a function of previous dose exposure. Methadone has a long $T_{1/2}$ and tends to accumulate in the plasma

From Transdermal Fentanyl:
May initiate therapy 18 hrs following removal of fentanyl patch
Initial: Substitute 10mg q12h for each 25mcg/h fentanyl patch

DOSING CONSIDERATIONS

Elderly
Use caution; start at lower end of the dosing range

Renal Impairment
Initial: Start w/ low dose; monitor closely for respiratory depression and sedation

Hepatic Impairment
Severe:
Initial: 10mg q12h; monitor closely for adverse events (eg, respiratory depression)

Discontinuation
Gradually titrate dose downwards every 2-4 days
Taper Schedule:
20-30mg q12h: 10mg q12h on Days 1 and 2, stop on Day 3
40-70mg q12h: 40mg q12h on Days 1 and 2, 20mg q12h on Days 3 and 4, 10mg q12h on Days 5 and 6, stop on Day 7
80-100mg q12h: 80mg q12h on Days 1 and 2, 60mg q12h on Days 3 and 4, 40mg q12h on Days 5 and 6, 20mg q12h on Days 7 and 8, 10mg q12h on Days 9 and 10, stop on day 11
>100mg q12h: Avoid abrupt discontinuation; use a gradual downward titration every 2-4 days

ADMINISTRATION

Oral route
Swallow cap whole; do not crush, dissolve, or chew.

STORAGE

25°C (77°F); excursions permitted to 15-30°C (59-86°F).

HOW SUPPLIED

Cap, Extended-Release: 10mg, 15mg, 20mg, 30mg, 40mg, 50mg

CONTRAINDICATIONS

Significant respiratory depression, acute or severe bronchial asthma in an unmonitored setting or in the absence of resuscitative equipment, known/suspected paralytic ileus, hypersensitivity (eg, anaphylaxis) to hydrocodone or to any other component of the medication.

WARNINGS/PRECAUTIONS

Reserve for use in patients for whom alternative treatment options are ineffective, not tolerated, or would be otherwise inadequate to provide sufficient management of pain. Should only be prescribed by healthcare professionals knowledgeable in the use of potent opioids for the management of chronic pain. Overestimating the dose when converting from another opioid product may result in fatal overdose w/ the 1st dose. Life-threatening respiratory depression is more likely to occur in elderly, cachectic, or debilitated patients. Consider alternative nonopioid analgesics in patients w/ significant COPD or cor pulmonale, and in patients having a substantially decreased respiratory reserve, hypoxia, hypercapnia, or preexisting respiratory depression. May cause severe hypotension, including orthostatic hypotension and syncope in ambulatory patients; increased risk in patients whose ability to maintain BP has been compromised by depleted blood volume, or after concurrent administration w/ drugs such as phenothiazines or other agents which compromise vasomotor tone. Monitor patients who may be susceptible to intracranial effects of carbon dioxide retention (eg, those w/ evidence of increased intracranial pressure, brain tumors) for signs of sedation and respiratory depression, particularly when initiating therapy. May obscure clinical course in patients w/ head injury, and acute abdominal conditions. Avoid w/ circulatory shock, impaired consciousness, or coma. May cause spasm of the sphincter of Oddi. May aggravate convulsions and induce/aggravate seizures. May impair mental/physical abilities. Not recommended for use during and immediately prior to labor.

ADVERSE REACTIONS
Constipation, N/V, somnolence, fatigue, headache, dizziness, dry mouth, pruritus, abdominal pain, peripheral edema, URTI, UTI, muscle spasms, back pain, tremor.

DRUG INTERACTIONS
See Boxed Warning. Concomitant use w/ other CNS depressants (eg, sedatives, anxiolytics, neuroleptics) may increase the risk of respiratory depression, profound sedation, hypotension, coma, and death; if coadministration is considered, reduce dose of one or both agents. Monitor use in elderly, cachectic, and debilitated patients when coadministered w/ other drugs that depress respiration. CYP3A4 inhibitors (eg, erythromycin, ketoconazole, ritonavir) may increase plasma levels and prolong opioid effects; these effects could be more pronounced w/ concomitant use of CYP2D6 and 3A4 inhibitors; if coadministration is necessary, monitor for respiratory depression and sedation at frequent intervals and consider dose adjustments until stable drug effects are achieved. CYP3A4 inducers (eg, rifampin, carbamazepine, phenytoin) may decrease levels and cause lack of efficacy or development of a withdrawal syndrome; if coadministration is necessary, monitor for signs of opioid withdrawal and consider dose adjustments until stable drug effects are achieved. Mixed agonist/antagonist (eg, pentazocine, nalbuphine, butorphanol) and partial agonist (buprenorphine) analgesics may reduce analgesic effect or precipitate withdrawal symptoms; avoid coadministration. Severe and unpredictable potentiation by MAOIs reported; not recommended for use in patients who have received MAOIs w/in 14 days. Anticholinergics or other medications w/ anticholinergic activity may increase the risk of urinary retention or severe constipation, which may lead to paralytic ileus; monitor for signs of urinary retention and constipation in addition to respiratory and CNS depression when used concurrently.

PREGNANCY AND LACTATION
Pregnancy: Prolonged use of opioid analgesics during pregnancy may cause neonatal opioid withdrawal syndrome. Based on animal data, advise pregnant women of potential risks to fetus. Crosses placenta. Not recommended for use in women during and immediately prior to labor; opioid analgesics can prolong labor.
Lactation: Present in human milk; not for use in nursing.

MECHANISM OF ACTION
Opioid analgesic; semi-synthetic opioid agonist w/ relative selectivity for the μ-opioid receptor, although it can interact w/ other opioid receptors at higher doses. Acts as a full agonist, binding to and activating opioid receptors at sites in the periaquaductal and periventricular gray matter, the ventro-medial medulla, and the spinal cord to produce analgesia.

PHARMACOKINETICS
Absorption: T_{max}=5 hrs. **Distribution:** Crosses placenta; found in breast milk. **Metabolism:** N-demethylation, O-demethylation, and 6-keto reduction; norhydrocodone, hydromorphone (metabolites). **Elimination:** Kidneys; $T_{1/2}$=8 hrs.

PATIENT CONSIDERATIONS
Assessment: Assess for abuse/addiction risk, pain type/severity, prior opioid therapy, opioid tolerance, respiratory depression, COPD or other respiratory complications, head injury, paralytic ileus, convulsive disorders, renal/hepatic impairment, drug hypersensitivity, pregnancy/nursing status, possible drug interactions, and any other conditions where treatment is contraindicated or cautioned.

Monitoring: Monitor for respiratory depression (especially w/in first 24-72 hrs of initiation), decreased bowel motility in postoperative patients, biliary tract disease, acute pancreatitis, seizures/convulsions, and other adverse reactions. Monitor for hypotension after initiating or titrating dose. Monitor renal function, particularly in elderly. Monitor for development of addiction, abuse, or misuse. Periodically reassess the continued need for therapy.

Counseling: Inform that use of drug can result in addiction, abuse, and misuse; instruct not to share w/ others and to take steps to protect from theft or misuse. Inform of the risk of life-threatening respiratory depression; advise how to recognize respiratory depression and to seek medical attention if experiencing breathing difficulties. Inform that accidental ingestion, especially in children, may result in respiratory depression or death. Advise to store securely and dispose unused cap by flushing down toilet. Advise female patients that drug may cause fetal harm and neonatal opioid withdrawal syndrome; instruct to inform physician w/ a known/suspected pregnancy. Advise that breastfeeding is not recommended during treatment. Inform that potentially serious additive effects may occur if used w/ alcohol or other CNS depressants, and not to use such drugs unless supervised by a healthcare provider. Inform that drug may cause orthostatic hypotension and syncope; instruct how to recognize symptoms of low BP. Advise not to perform hazardous activities until the patient knows how he or she will react to the medication. Advise of potential for severe constipation, including management instructions. Advise how to recognize anaphylaxis and when to seek medical attention.

ZOLADEX 3.6 MG — goserelin acetate

Rx

Class: Synthetic gonadotropin-releasing hormone (GnRH) analogue

ADULT DOSAGE

B₂-C Prostate Carcinoma

Combination w/ Flutamide for Locally Confined Stage T2b-T4 Prostate Carcinoma:
One 3.6mg implant SQ, followed in 28 days by one 10.8mg implant SQ

Start 8 weeks prior to initiating radiotherapy and continue during radiation therapy

Alternative Therapy:
4 SQ injections of 3.6mg implant at 28-day intervals (2 implants preceding and 2 during radiotherapy)

Prostate Carcinoma

Palliative Treatment for Advanced Prostate Carcinoma:
One 3.6mg implant SQ every 28 days

Endometriosis

Management of Endometriosis, Including Pain Relief and Reduction of Endometriotic Lesions:
One 3.6mg implant SQ every 28 days for 6 months

Endometrial Thinning

Prior to Endometrial Ablation for Dysfunctional Uterine Bleeding:
One or two 3.6mg implants SQ (each depot given 4 weeks apart)

Advanced Breast Cancer

Palliative Treatment in Pre- and Perimenopausal Women:
One 3.6mg implant SQ every 28 days

PEDIATRIC DOSAGE
Pediatric use may not have been established

ADMINISTRATION
SQ route

Endometrial Thinning
Perform surgery after 4 weeks after administration of 1 implant or w/in 2-4 weeks after administration of 2nd implant when 2 implants are administered

Administration Instructions
1. Place patient in comfortable position w/ upper part of body slightly raised; prepare an area of anterior abdominal wall below navel line w/ alcohol swab
2. Removed syringe from foil pouch and grasp the red safety tab and pull away from syringe; do not attempt to remove air bubbles from syringe like liquid inj
3. Hold syringe around protective sleeve, pinch skin of anterior wall below navel line and insert needle, bevel side up, at a 30-45° angle into skin in one continuous motion until protective sleeve touches skin of patient
4. Depress barrel until the protective sleeve clicks; sleeve will automatically begin to slide to cover needle.

STORAGE
Room temperature; do not exceed 25°C (77°F).

HOW SUPPLIED
Implant: 3.6mg

CONTRAINDICATIONS
Known hypersensitivity to GnRH, GnRH agonist analogues, or any components in the medication; pregnancy (unless used for palliative treatment of advanced breast cancer).

WARNINGS/PRECAUTIONS
May cause fetal harm. Premenopausal women should use effective nonhormonal contraception during therapy and for 12 weeks following discontinuation of therapy. Initially, may cause transient increase in serum testosterone levels in men and estrogen in women; worsening of symptoms or onset of additional signs/symptoms may occur during the 1st few weeks of treatment. May experience temporary increase in bone pain; manage symptomatically. Ureteral obstruction and spinal cord compression reported w/ prostate cancer; institute standard treatment if spinal cord compression or renal impairment secondary to ureteral obstruction develops, and in extreme cases in prostate cancer patients, consider an immediate orchiectomy. Hyperglycemia and increased risk of developing diabetes reported in men. Increased risk of developing MI, sudden cardiac death, and stroke reported in men. Hypercalcemia reported in patients w/ bone metastases. Hypersensitivity, antibody formation, and acute anaphylactic reactions reported. May cause an increase in cervical resistance; caution when dilating the cervix for endometrial ablation. Androgen deprivation therapy may prolong QT/QTc interval; consider whether benefits outweigh the potential risks in patients w/ congenital long QT syndrome, CHF, frequent electrolyte abnormalities, and in patients taking drugs known to prolong the QT interval. Correct electrolyte abnormalities. Inj-site injury and vascular injury (eg, pain, hematoma, hemorrhage, hemorrhagic shock) requiring blood transfusions and surgical intervention reported; caution w/ low BMI and/or in patients receiving full dose anticoagulation. Retreatment is not recommended for management of endometriosis; consider monitoring bone mineral density (BMD) if further

treatment is contemplated. Addition of hormone replacement therapy is effective in reducing bone mineral loss and occurrence of vasomotor symptoms and vaginal dryness associated w/ hypoestrogenism. Lab test interactions may occur. Intended for long-term administration for the management of advanced prostate/breast cancer unless clinically inappropriate.

ADVERSE REACTIONS

Hot flushes, sexual dysfunction, decreased erections, seborrhea, vasodilatation, breast atrophy, tumor flare, vaginitis, emotional lability, decreased libido, sweating, depression, headache, acne, peripheral edema.

PREGNANCY AND LACTATION

Category X (w/ endometriosis and endometrial thinning) or Category D (w/ advanced breast cancer), not for use in nursing.

MECHANISM OF ACTION

Synthetic gonadotropin-releasing hormone analogue; acts as an inhibitor of pituitary gonadotropin secretion. In males, causes initial increase in serum luteinizing hormone and follicle-stimulating hormone levels, w/ subsequent increases in serum testosterone levels; chronic administration suppresses pituitary gonadotropins, causing a fall in testosterone levels to post-castration levels. In females, chronic exposure causes decrease in serum estradiol to levels consistent w/ postmenopausal state, leading to reduction of ovarian size and function, reduction in size of uterus and mammary gland, and regression of sex hormone-responsive tumors.

PHARMACOKINETICS

Absorption: Rapid. (Males) C_{max}=2.84ng/mL, T_{max}=12-15 days, AUC=27.8ng•day/mL; (Females) C_{max}=1.46ng/mL, T_{max}=8-22 days, AUC=18.5ng•day/mL. **Distribution:** (Sol) (250mcg SQ dose) V_d=44.1L (males), 20.3L (females); plasma protein binding (27.3%). **Metabolism:** Hydrolysis of C-terminal amino acids. **Elimination:** Urine (>90%, 20% unchanged).

PATIENT CONSIDERATIONS

Assessment: Assess for hypersensitivity to the drug, cardiovascular (CV) risk factors, diabetes, congenital long QT syndrome, CHF, electrolyte abnormalities, low BMI, and pregnancy/nursing status. Obtain baseline serum testosterone, estrogen, blood glucose, and/or HbA1c levels. Assess if patient is receiving full dose anticoagulation.

Monitoring: Monitor for occurrence or worsening of signs/symptoms of prostate/breast cancer, ureteral obstruction, spinal cord compression, renal impairment, hypersensitivity/acute anaphylactic reactions, antibody formation, bone pain, CV disease, hypercalcemia, inj-site/vascular injury, and other adverse reactions. Periodically monitor BMD, serum testosterone, estrogen, blood glucose, and/or HbA1c levels. Consider periodic monitoring of ECGs and electrolytes.

Counseling: Inform of risks and benefits of therapy. Inform men of the risk of developing ureteral obstruction, spinal cord compression, reduction in BMD, diabetes or loss of glycemic control in patients w/ preexisting diabetes, MI, sudden cardiac death, and stroke. Advise to contact physician if experiencing any symptoms of inj-site injury or if any adverse events develop. Inform women that menstruation should stop w/ effective doses; instruct to notify physician if regular menstruation persists. Inform that patient may experience persistent amenorrhea. Inform that drug may cause fetal harm and increase risk for pregnancy loss. Advise against pregnancy and/or breastfeeding except for palliative treatment of advanced breast cancer. Advise premenopausal women to use nonhormonal contraception during and for 12 weeks after treatment ends. Instruct to avoid initiating treatment if the patient has undiagnosed abnormal vaginal bleeding or is allergic to the drug. Inform of the most frequent side effects associated w/ hypoestrogenism and that the addition of hormone replacement therapy may decrease vasomotor symptoms and vaginal dryness associated w/ hypoestrogenism. Inform that drug may cause a reduction in BMD in women.

ZOLINZA — vorinostat   Rx

Class: Histone deacetylase (HDAC) inhibitor

ADULT DOSAGE	PEDIATRIC DOSAGE
Cutaneous T-Cell Lymphoma	Pediatric use may not have been established
Cutaneous Manifestations in Progressive, Persistent or Recurrent Disease on or Following 2 Systemic Therapies: 400mg qd	
Intolerant to Therapy: May reduce to 300mg qd; may further reduce to 300mg qd for 5 consecutive days each week, as necessary	
Treatment may be continued as long as there is no evidence of progressive disease or unacceptable toxicity	

DOSING CONSIDERATIONS

Hepatic Impairment

Mild to Moderate (Bilirubin 1-3X ULN/AST>ULN): Reduce starting dose to 300mg qd

Severe (Bilirubin>3X ULN): There is insufficient evidence to recommend a starting dose for patients w/ severe hepatic impairment; patients w/ severe hepatic impairment have not been treated at doses >200mg/day

ADMINISTRATION

Oral route

Take w/ food.

Do not open or crush cap.

Avoid direct contact of powder w/ skin or mucous membranes; wash thoroughly if such contact occurs.

Avoid exposure to crushed and/or broken cap.

STORAGE

20-25°C (68-77°F); excursions permitted between 15-30°C (59-86°F).

HOW SUPPLIED

Cap: 100mg

WARNINGS/PRECAUTIONS

Pulmonary embolism (PE) and deep vein thrombosis (DVT) reported; monitor for signs and symptoms of these events, particularly w/ prior history of thromboembolic events. Dose-related thrombocytopenia and anemia may occur; adjust dosage or d/c treatment as clinically appropriate. GI disturbances (eg, N/V, diarrhea) reported. Adequately control preexisting N/V and diarrhea before beginning therapy. Hyperglycemia observed. Monitor blood cell counts and chemistry tests, including serum electrolytes, Mg^{2+}, Ca^{2+}, glucose, and SrCr every 2 weeks during the first 2 months of therapy and monthly thereafter. Correct hypokalemia and hypomagnesemia prior to therapy. Monitor K^+ and Mg^{2+} more frequently in symptomatic patients (eg, patients w/ N/V, diarrhea, fluid imbalance, cardiac symptoms). May cause fetal harm. Caution w/ renal/hepatic impairment and in elderly.

ADVERSE REACTIONS

Diarrhea, fatigue, N/V, thrombocytopenia, anemia, anorexia, dysgeusia, decreased weight, dry mouth, increased blood creatinine, chills, constipation, dizziness.

DRUG INTERACTIONS

Prolongation of PT and INR observed w/ coumarin-derivative anticoagulants; monitor PT and INR more frequently. Severe thrombocytopenia and GI bleeding reported w/ concomitant w/ other histone deacetylase inhibitors (eg, valproic acid); monitor platelet counts every 2 weeks for the first 2 months.

PREGNANCY AND LACTATION

Pregnancy: Category D.

Lactation: Not for use in nursing.

MECHANISM OF ACTION

Histone deacetylase (HDAC) inhibitor; inhibits HDAC enzymes, HDAC1, HDAC2, HDAC3, and HDAC6, which catalyze the removal of acetyl groups from the lysine residues of proteins, including histones and transcription factors. HDAC inhibition results in accumulation of acetyl groups on the histone lysine residues resulting in an open chromatin structure and transcriptional activation; cell growth is terminated and apoptosis occurs.

PHARMACOKINETICS

Absorption: (Fasted, single 400mg dose) C_{max}=1.2µM, T_{max}=1.5 hrs (median), AUC=4.2µM•hr; (High-fat meal, single 400mg dose) C_{max}=1.2µM, T_{max}=4 hrs (median), AUC=5.5µM•hr. (Fed, multiple 400mg doses) C_{max}=1.2µM, T_{max}=4 hrs (median), AUC=6.0µM•hr. **Distribution:** Plasma protein binding (71%). **Metabolism:** Liver via glucuronidation, hydrolysis, and β-oxidation. **Elimination:** Urine (<1% unchanged); $T_{1/2}$=2 hrs.

PATIENT CONSIDERATIONS

Assessment: Assess for renal/hepatic impairment, history of thromboembolic events, GI disturbances, fluid imbalance, cardiac symptoms, diabetes, hypokalemia, hypomagnesemia, pregnancy/nursing status, and possible drug interactions.

Monitoring: Monitor for signs/symptoms of PE and DVT, thrombocytopenia, anemia, GI disturbances, dehydration, hyperglycemia, and other adverse reactions. Monitor blood cell counts, chemistry tests, electrolytes, serum glucose, and SrCr every 2 weeks for the first 2 months and monthly thereafter. Monitor K^+ and Mg^{2+} more frequently in symptomatic patients.

Counseling: Inform about risks and benefits of therapy. Instruct to drink at least 2L/day of fluids to prevent dehydration. Advise to promptly report to physician if excessive vomiting or diarrhea, unusual bleeding, signs of DVT, or any other adverse events develop.

ZOLOFT — sertraline hydrochloride   Rx

Class: Selective serotonin reuptake inhibitor (SSRI)

> Antidepressants increased the risk of suicidal thinking and behavior (suicidality) in children, adolescents, and young adults in short-term studies of major depressive disorder (MDD) and other psychiatric disorders. Monitor and observe closely for clinical worsening, suicidality, or unusual changes in behavior in patients who are started on antidepressant therapy. Not approved for use in pediatric patients except for patients w/ obsessive-compulsive disorder.

ADULT DOSAGE	PEDIATRIC DOSAGE
Premenstrual Dysphoric Disorder	**Obsessive Compulsive Disorder**
Initial: 50mg qd throughout menstrual cycle or limited to luteal phase	**6-12 Years:** **Initial:** 25mg qd
Titrate: If unresponsive to initial dose, may increase at 50mg increments/cycle up to 150mg/day when dosing daily throughout menstrual cycle or 100mg/day when dosing during luteal phase.	**13-17 Years:** **Initial:** 50mg qd
	Titrate: Adjust dose at intervals ≥1 week
	Max: 200mg/day
	Periodically reassess to determine need for maint treatment

If 100mg/day has been established w/ luteal phase dosing, use a 50mg/day titration step for 3 days at the beginning of each luteal phase dosing period.

Adjust to maintain patient on the lowest effective dose; periodically reassess to determine need for continued treatment

Major Depressive Disorder
Usual: 50mg qd
Max: 200mg/day

Periodically reassess to determine need for maint treatment

Obsessive Compulsive Disorder
Usual: 50mg qd
Titrate: Adjust dose at intervals ≥1 week
Max: 200mg/day

Periodically reassess to determine need for maint treatment

Panic Disorder
Initial: 25mg qd
Titrate: Increase to 50mg qd after 1 week; adjust dose at intervals ≥1 week
Max: 200mg/day

Periodically reassess to determine need for maint treatment

Social Anxiety Disorder
Initial: 25mg qd
Titrate: Increase to 50mg qd after 1 week; adjust dose at intervals ≥1 week
Max: 200mg/day

Dose adjustments may be needed to maintain patient on the lowest effective dose; periodically reassess to determine need for long-term treatment

Post-traumatic Stress Disorder
Initial: 25mg qd
Titrate: Increase to 50mg qd after 1 week; adjust dose at intervals ≥1 week
Max: 200mg/day

Periodically reassess to determine need for maint treatment

Dosing Considerations with MAOIs
Switching to/from an MAOI for Psychiatric Disorders:
Allow at least 14 days between discontinuation of an MAOI and initiation of treatment, and allow at least 14 days between discontinuation of treatment and initiation of an MAOI

Use w/ Other MAOIs (eg, Linezolid, IV Methylene Blue):
Do not start sertraline in patients being treated w/ linezolid or IV methylene blue.
If acceptable alternatives are not available and benefits outweigh risks, d/c sertraline promptly and administer linezolid or IV methylene blue; monitor for serotonin syndrome for 2 weeks or until 24 hrs after the last dose of linezolid or IV methylene blue, whichever comes 1st. May resume sertraline therapy 24 hrs after the last dose of linezolid or IV methylene blue.

- - - - - - - - - - - - - - - - - - -

DOSING CONSIDERATIONS
Hepatic Impairment
Use lower or less frequent dose
Pregnancy
During 3rd Trimester: Consider potential risks/benefits of treatment
Discontinuation
A gradual reduction in dose rather than abrupt cessation is recommended whenever possible
May consider resuming previously prescribed dose if intolerable symptoms occur following a dose decrease or upon discontinuation of treatment. May continue decreasing the dose subsequently but at a more gradual rate

ADMINISTRATION
Oral route
Administer qam or qpm.

Dosing Considerations with MAOIs
Switching to/from an MAOI for Psychiatric Disorders:
Allow at least 14 days between discontinuation of an MAOI and initiation of treatment, and allow at least 14 days between discontinuation of treatment and initiation of an MAOI

Use w/ Other MAOIs (eg, Linezolid, IV Methylene Blue):
Do not start sertraline in patients being treated w/ linezolid or IV methylene blue.
If acceptable alternatives are not available and benefits outweigh risks, d/c sertraline promptly and administer linezolid or IV methylene blue; monitor for serotonin syndrome for 2 weeks or until 24 hrs after the last dose of linezolid or IV methylene blue, whichever comes 1st. May resume sertraline therapy 24 hrs after the last dose of linezolid or IV methylene blue.

Sol
Must be diluted before use
Mix dose w/ 4 oz of water, ginger ale, lemon/lime soda, lemonade, or orange juice only; do not mix w/ any other liquids
Take dose immediately after mixing; do not mix in advance

STORAGE
25°C (77°F); excursions permitted to 15-30°C (59-86°F).

HOW SUPPLIED
Sol: 20mg/mL [60mL]; **Tab:** 25mg*, 50mg*, 100mg* *scored

CONTRAINDICATIONS
Hypersensitivity to sertraline or any of the inactive ingredients in this medication. Use of an MAOI for psychiatric disorders either concomitantly or w/in 14 days of stopping treatment. Treatment w/in 14 days of stopping an MAOI for psychiatric disorders. Starting treatment in a patient being treated w/ other MAOIs (eg, linezolid, IV methylene blue). Concomitant use w/ pimozide. (Sol) Concomitant use w/ disulfiram.

WARNINGS/PRECAUTIONS
Not approved for treatment of bipolar depression. May precipitate mixed/manic episode in patients at risk for bipolar disorder; screen for risk of bipolar disorder prior to initiating treatment. Serotonin syndrome reported; d/c immediately and initiate supportive symptomatic treatment. Pupillary dilation that occurs following use may trigger an angle-closure attack in a patient w/ anatomically narrow angles who does not have a patent iridectomy. Activation of mania/hypomania, altered platelet function and/or abnormal lab results, decreased serum uric acid, and weight loss reported. Adverse events reported upon discontinuation, particularly when abrupt; reduce dose gradually whenever possible. May increase the risk of bleeding events. Seizures reported; caution w/ seizure disorder. Caution w/ diseases/conditions that could affect metabolism or hemodynamic responses. Hyponatremia may occur; caution in elderly and volume-depleted patients. Consider discontinuation in patients w/ symptomatic hyponatremia and institute appropriate medical intervention. Caution in 3rd trimester of pregnancy due to risk of serious neonatal complications. False (+) urine immunoassay screening tests for benzodiazepines reported. (Sol) Dropper dispenser contains dry natural rubber; caution w/ latex sensitivity.

ADVERSE REACTIONS
Ejaculation failure, dry mouth, increased sweating, somnolence, fatigue, tremor, anorexia, dizziness, headache, diarrhea, dyspepsia, nausea, constipation, agitation, insomnia.

DRUG INTERACTIONS
See Dosage and Contraindications. May cause serotonin syndrome w/ other serotonergic drugs (eg, triptans, TCAs, fentanyl, lithium, tramadol, tryptophan, buspirone, St. John's wort) and w/ drugs that impair metabolism of serotonin; d/c immediately if this occurs. May cause a shift in plasma concentrations resulting in an adverse effect w/ other tightly protein bound drugs (eg, warfarin, digitoxin), and conversely adverse effects may result from displacement of sertraline. Caution w/ other CNS active drugs. Monitor lithium, phenytoin, and valproate levels w/ appropriate dose adjustments. May increase levels of drugs metabolized by CYP2D6, especially those w/ a narrow therapeutic index (eg, TCAs for treatment of MDD, propafenone, flecainide); concomitant use of a drug metabolized by CYP2D6 may require lower doses, and an increase of the coadministered drug may be required when sertraline is withdrawn. Weakness, hyperreflexia, and incoordination reported (rare) w/ sumatriptan. May induce metabolism of cisapride. Increased risk of bleeding w/ aspirin (ASA), NSAIDs, warfarin, and other anticoagulants or other drugs known to affect platelet function. Altered anticoagulant effects reported w/ warfarin; carefully monitor PT when therapy is initiated or stopped. Avoid w/ alcohol. Increased risk of hyponatremia w/ diuretics. Cimetidine may increase levels and $T_{1/2}$. May reduce clearance of diazepam and tolbutamide.

PREGNANCY AND LACTATION
Pregnancy: Category C.
Lactation: Caution in nursing.

MECHANISM OF ACTION
SSRI; presumed to be linked to inhibition of CNS neuronal uptake of serotonin.

PHARMACOKINETICS
Absorption: T_{max}=4.5-8.4 hrs. **Distribution:** Plasma protein binding (98%). **Metabolism:** Liver (extensive); N-demethylation, oxidative deamination, reduction, hydroxylation, glucuronide conjugation; N-desmethylsertraline (metabolite). **Elimination:** Urine (40-45%), feces (40-45%, 12-14% unchanged); $T_{1/2}$=26 hrs (sertraline), 62-104 hrs (N-desmethylsertraline).

PATIENT CONSIDERATIONS
Assessment: Assess for presence/risk for bipolar disorder, susceptibility to angle-closure glaucoma, conditions where treatment is contraindicated or cautioned, pregnancy/nursing status, and possible drug interactions.

Monitoring: Monitor for clinical worsening of depression, suicidality, or unusual changes in behavior, serotonin syndrome, hyponatremia, abnormal bleeding, angle-closure glaucoma, activation of mania/hypomania, seizures, and other adverse reactions. Periodically monitor height and weight of pediatric patients w/ long-term therapy. Periodically reevaluate long-term usefulness of therapy. Carefully monitor PT when therapy is initiated or stopped w/ warfarin.

Counseling: Counsel about benefits, risks, and appropriate use of therapy. Encourage families and caregivers to be alert for emergence of unusual changes in behavior, worsening of depression, and suicidal ideation, especially early during treatment and when dose is adjusted up or down; instruct to report symptoms to physician, especially if severe, abrupt in onset, or not part of presenting symptoms. Caution about risk of serotonin syndrome w/ concomitant triptans, tramadol, or other serotonergic agents. Caution about risk of angle-closure glaucoma. Advise patients to use caution when driving or operating machinery until they learn how they respond to medication. Inform that concomitant use w/ NSAIDs, ASA, warfarin, and other drugs that affect coagulation may increase the risk of bleeding. Counsel to avoid alcohol and to use caution when using OTC products. Advise to notify physician if pregnant, intending to become pregnant, or if breastfeeding.

ZOLPIMIST — zolpidem tartrate   CIV

Class: GABA$_A$ agonist

ADULT DOSAGE
Insomnia
Short-Term Treatment of Insomnia Characterized by Difficulties w/ Sleep Initiation:
Initial: 5mg (women), and either 5mg or 10mg (men), taken qhs
Titrate: May increase to 10mg if the 5mg dose is not effective
Max: 10mg qhs

PEDIATRIC DOSAGE
Pediatric use may not have been established

DOSING CONSIDERATIONS
Concomitant Medications
CNS Depressants: May need to adjust dose of zolpidem and concomitant CNS depressant

Hepatic Impairment
5mg qhs

Elderly
Elderly/Debilitated: 5mg qhs

ADMINISTRATION
Oral route
Take immediately before hs w/ at least 7-8 hrs remaining before the planned time of awakening.
Must be primed before use for the 1st time.
To prime, point the black spray opening away from face and other people and spray 5X.
For administration, hold container upright w/ the black spray opening pointed directly into the mouth; fully press down on the pump to make sure a full dose (5mg) is sprayed directly into the mouth over the tongue. If a 10mg dose is prescribed, a 2nd spray should be administered.
If not used for at least 14 days, must be primed again w/ 1 spray.
Do not take w/ or immediately after a meal.

STORAGE
25°C (77°F); excursions permitted to 15-30°C (59-86°F). Store upright. Do not freeze. Avoid prolonged exposure to temperatures >30°C (86°F).

HOW SUPPLIED
Spray: 5mg/actuation [30 actuations, 60 actuations]

CONTRAINDICATIONS
Hypersensitivity to zolpidem.

WARNINGS/PRECAUTIONS
Increased risk of next-day psychomotor impairment if taken w/ less than a full night of sleep remaining (7-8 hrs). May impair mental/physical abilities. Initiate only after careful evaluation; failure of insomnia to remit after 7-10 days of treatment may indicate presence of a primary psychiatric and/or medical illness. Cases of angioedema involving the tongue, glottis, or larynx reported; do not rechallenge if angioedema develops. Abnormal thinking, behavioral changes, and visual/auditory hallucinations reported. Complex behaviors (eg, sleep-driving) reported; consider discontinuation if a sleep-driving episode occurs. Amnesia, anxiety, and other neuropsychiatric symptoms may occur. Worsening of depression and suicidal thoughts and actions (including completed suicides) reported in primarily depressed patients; prescribe the least amount of drug that is feasible at any one time. Caution w/ compromised respiratory function, including sleep apnea and myasthenia gravis. Withdrawal signs and symptoms reported following rapid dose decrease or abrupt discontinuation; monitor for tolerance, abuse, and dependence.

ADVERSE REACTIONS
Short-Term Treatment (up to 10 Nights): Drowsiness, dizziness, diarrhea.
Long-Term Treatment (28-35 Nights): Dizziness, drugged feelings.

DRUG INTERACTIONS
See Dosing Considerations. Increased risk of CNS depression and complex behaviors w/ other CNS depressants (eg, benzodiazepines, opioids, TCAs, alcohol). Use w/ other sedative-hypnotics (eg, other zolpidem products) at hs or in the middle of the night is not recommended. Increased risk of next-day psychomotor impairment w/ other CNS depressants or drugs that increase zolpidem levels. May decrease peak levels of imipramine. Additive effect of decreased alertness w/ imipramine and chlorpromazine. Additive adverse effect on decreased psychomotor performance w/ chlorpromazine. Additive adverse effect on psychomotor performance reported between alcohol and oral zolpidem. Concurrent use of oral zolpidem w/ sertraline reported to increase C_{max} and decrease T_{max} of zolpidem. Fluoxetine may increase $T_{1/2}$ of zolpidem. CYP3A inhibitors may increase zolpidem exposure. Itraconazole may increase exposure of zolpidem. Rifampin, a CYP3A4 inducer, may significantly reduce the exposure to and the pharmacodynamic effects of zolpidem; concurrent use w/ rifampin may decrease the efficacy of zolpidem. Concomitant use w/ ketoconazole, a potent CYP3A4 inhibitor, may increase the pharmacodynamic effects of zolpidem; consider using a lower dose of zolpidem when coadministered w/ ketoconazole.

PREGNANCY AND LACTATION
Pregnancy: Category C.
Lactation: Found in breast milk; caution in nursing.

MECHANISM OF ACTION
Imidazopyridine, nonbenzodiazepine hypnotic; interacts w/ a gamma-aminobutyric acid-BZ receptor complex. Binds the BZ$_1$ receptor preferentially w/ a high affinity ratio of the α_1/α_5 subunits.

PHARMACOKINETICS
Absorption: Rapid from oral mucosa and GI tract. C_{max}=114ng/mL (5mg), 210ng/mL (10mg); T_{max}=0.9 hrs (5mg, 10mg). **Distribution:** Plasma protein binding (92.5%); found in breast milk. **Elimination:** Renal; $T_{1/2}$=2.7 hrs (5mg), 3 hrs (10mg).

PATIENT CONSIDERATIONS
Assessment: Assess for physical and/or psychiatric disorder, compromised respiratory function, myasthenia gravis, hepatic impairment, history of drug/alcohol addiction or abuse, hypersensitivity to the drug, pregnancy/nursing status, and possible drug interactions.

Monitoring: Monitor for CNS depression, angioedema, abnormal thinking, behavioral changes, visual/auditory hallucinations, complex behaviors, worsening of depression, suicidal thoughts/actions, respiratory depression, and other adverse reactions. Monitor for withdrawal signs/symptoms following rapid dose decrease or abrupt discontinuation.

Counseling: Inform about the benefits and risks of treatment. Instruct to take only as prescribed; advise to wait at least 8 hrs after dosing before driving or engaging in other activities requiring full mental alertness. Instruct to contact physician immediately if any adverse reactions (eg, severe anaphylactic/anaphylactoid reactions, sleep-driving and other complex behaviors, suicidal thoughts) develop. Advise not to use the drug if patient drank alcohol that evening. Instruct patients not to increase the dose and to inform physician if it is believed that the drug does not work.

ZOLVIT — acetaminophen/hydrocodone bitartrate   CIII

Class: Opioid analgesic

> Associated with cases of acute liver failure, at times resulting in liver transplant and death. Most of the cases of liver injury are associated with acetaminophen (APAP) use at doses >4000mg/day, and often involve >1 APAP-containing product.

ADULT DOSAGE
Moderate to Severe Pain
Usual: 2.25 tsp every 4-6 hrs prn
Max: 13.5 tsp/day

PEDIATRIC DOSAGE
Moderate to Severe Pain
12-15kg (2-3 Years):
Usual: 2.8mL every 4-6 hrs prn
Max: 16.8mL/day

16-22kg (4-6 Years):
Usual: 3.75mL every 4-6 hrs prn
Max: 22.5mL/day

23-31kg (7-9 Years):
Usual: 5.6mL every 4-6 hrs prn
Max: 33.6mL/day

32-45kg (10-13 Years):
Usual: 7.5mL every 4-6 hrs prn
Max: 45mL/day

≥46kg (≥14 Years):
Usual: 11.25mL every 4-6 hrs prn
Max: 67.5mL/day

DOSING CONSIDERATIONS
Elderly
Start at lower end of dosing range

ADMINISTRATION
Oral route
Administer dose accurately; use a calibrated measuring device

STORAGE
20-25°C (68-77°F).

HOW SUPPLIED
Sol: (Hydrocodone/APAP) (10mg/300mg)/15mL [16 fl oz]

CONTRAINDICATIONS
Hypersensitivity to hydrocodone, APAP, or any other component of this product.

WARNINGS/PRECAUTIONS
May be habit-forming. Increased risk of acute liver failure in patients with underlying liver disease. May cause serious skin reactions (eg, acute generalized exanthematous pustulosis, Stevens-Johnson syndrome, toxic epidermal necrolysis); d/c at the first appearance of skin rash or any other sign of hypersensitivity. Hypersensitivity and anaphylaxis reported; d/c if signs/symptoms occur. May produce dose-related respiratory depression, and irregular and periodic breathing. Infants may have increased sensitivity to the respiratory depressant effects of opioids; if use is contemplated, administer cautiously, in substantially reduced initial doses, by personnel experienced in administering opioids to infants, with intensive monitoring. Respiratory depressant effects and CSF pressure elevation capacity may be markedly exaggerated in the presence of head injury, other intracranial lesions, or preexisting increased intracranial pressure. May obscure clinical course of head injuries and acute abdominal

conditions. Potential for abuse. Caution with hypothyroidism, Addison's disease, prostatic hypertrophy, urethral stricture, severe hepatic/renal impairment, or in elderly/debilitated. Suppresses cough reflex; caution with pulmonary disease and in postoperative use. Physical dependence and tolerance may develop.

ADVERSE REACTIONS
Acute liver failure, bradycardia, cardiac arrest, anxiety, dizziness, drowsiness, hypoglycemic coma, abdominal pain, constipation, spasm of vesical sphincters, agranulocytosis, hemolytic anemia, skeletal muscle flaccidity, acute airway obstruction, apnea.

DRUG INTERACTIONS
Additive CNS depression with other narcotics, antihistamines, antipsychotics, antianxiety agents, or other CNS depressants (eg, alcohol); reduce dose of one or both agents. Concomitant use with MAOIs or TCAs may increase the effect of either the antidepressant or hydrocodone. Increased risk of acute liver failure with alcohol.

PREGNANCY AND LACTATION
Category C, not for use in nursing.

MECHANISM OF ACTION
Hydrocodone: Opioid analgesic; not established. Action believed to be related to the existence of opiate receptors in the CNS. APAP: Nonopiate, nonsalicylate analgesic and antipyretic; not established. Antipyretic activity is mediated through hypothalamic heat regulating centers; inhibits prostaglandin synthetase.

PHARMACOKINETICS
Absorption: Hydrocodone: (10mg) C_{max}=23.6ng/mL; T_{max}=1.3 hrs. APAP: Rapid.
Distribution: Hydrocodone: Crosses placenta. APAP: Found in breast milk.
Metabolism: Hydrocodone: O-demethylation, N-demethylation, and 6-keto reduction. APAP: Liver (conjugation). **Elimination:** Hydrocodone: (10mg) $T_{1/2}$=3.8 hrs. APAP: Urine (85%); $T_{1/2}$=1.25-3 hrs.

PATIENT CONSIDERATIONS
Assessment: Assess for history of hypersensitivity, level of pain intensity, type of pain, patient's general condition and medical status, renal/hepatic impairment, pregnancy/nursing status, any other conditions where treatment is contraindicated or cautioned, and for possible drug interactions.

Monitoring: Monitor for signs/symptoms of hypersensitivity or anaphylaxis, serious skin reactions, respiratory depression, elevations in CSF pressure, drug abuse, tolerance, dependence, and other adverse reactions. In patients with severe hepatic/renal disease, monitor effects with serial hepatic and/or renal function tests.

Counseling: Instruct to look for APAP on package labels and not to use >1 APAP-containing product. Instruct to seek medical attention immediately upon ingestion of >4000mg/day APAP, even if feeling well. Advise to d/c and contact physician if signs of allergy (eg, rash, difficulty breathing) develop. Inform that drug may impair mental/physical abilities; instruct to avoid performing potentially hazardous tasks (eg, driving, operating machinery) while taking the medication. Instruct to avoid alcohol and other CNS depressants. Inform that drug may be habit-forming; instruct to take only ud.

ZOMACTON — somatropin (rDNA origin)   Rx
Class: Recombinant human growth hormone (hGH)

PEDIATRIC DOSAGE
Growth Hormone Deficiency

Due to Inadequate Secretion of Endogenous Growth Hormone:
Up to 0.1mg/kg SQ 3X/week (up to 0.3mg/kg/week)

ADMINISTRATION
SQ route

Reconstitution
- Reconstitute 5mg vial w/ 1-5mL of bacteriostatic 0.9% NaCl for inj (benzyl alcohol preserved); reconstitute w/ sterile normal saline for inj and use only one dose per vial when administering to newborns.
- Reconstitute 10mg vial w/ 1mL syringe of bacteriostatic water for inj containing 0.33% metacresol.
- Swirl vial w/ a gentle rotary motion until contents are completely dissolved and the sol is clear.
- Do not shake; shaking or vigorous mixing will cause sol to be cloudy.
- Some cloudiness may occur after refrigeration; allow product to warm to room temperature and do not use if cloudiness persists or particulate matter is noted.
- May be administered using a standard sterile disposable syringe or a Zoma-Jet Needle-Free inj device.
- For proper use, refer to user's manual provided w/ administration device.

STORAGE
2-8°C (36-46°F). Avoid freezing the accompanying diluent. **Reconstituted Sol:** 2-8°C (36-46°F) for up to 14 days when reconstituted w/ bacteriostatic 0.9% NaCl and for up to 28 days when reconstituted w/ bacteriostatic water for inj. Do not freeze.

HOW SUPPLIED
Inj: 5mg, 10mg

CONTRAINDICATIONS
Hypersensitivity to somatropin or to any of the excipients, closed epiphyses, active proliferative or severe nonproliferative diabetic retinopathy, active

malignancy or evidence of progression or recurrence of an underlying intracranial tumor. Acute critical illness due to complications following open heart surgery, abdominal surgery or multiple accidental trauma, or w/ acute respiratory failure. Prader-Willi syndrome (PWS) w/ severe obesity or w/ severe respiratory impairment. Growth failure due to genetically confirmed PWS. Known sensitivity to benzyl alcohol (found in bacteriostatic 0.9% NaCl diluent) or allergy to metacresol (found in bacteriostatic water for inj diluent).

WARNINGS/PRECAUTIONS
Evaluate patients w/ PWS for signs of upper airway obstruction (eg, new/increased snoring) and sleep apnea before treatment and interrupt therapy if these signs occur. Implement effective weight control in patients w/ PWS and treat respiratory infections aggressively. Pancreatitis reported rarely. Bacteriostatic 0.9% NaCl diluent contains benzyl alcohol, which has been associated w/ serious adverse events and death, particularly in pediatric patients; reconstitute w/ sterile normal saline for inj when administering the 5mg inj to newborns. Carry out therapy under the guidance of a physician experienced in the diagnosis and management of pediatric patients w/ growth hormone deficiency (GHD). Monitor all patients w/ a history of GHD secondary to an intracranial neoplasm routinely while on therapy for progression/recurrence of the tumor. Increased risk of developing malignancies in children w/ certain rare genetic causes of short stature; monitor for development of neoplasms. Monitor for increased growth or potential malignant changes of preexisting nevi. May decrease insulin sensitivity and unmask undiagnosed impaired glucose tolerance and overt diabetes mellitus (DM). New onset type 2 DM reported. Monitor standard hormonal replacement therapy in patients w/ hypopituitarism. Undiagnosed/untreated hypothyroidism may prevent optimal response. Central (secondary) hypothyroidism may become evident or worsen during treatment; may need to initiate thyroid hormone replacement therapy. Increased incidence of slipped capital femoral epiphysis and progression of scoliosis may occur. Intracranial HTN w/ papilledema, visual changes, headache, and/or N/V reported; d/c therapy if papilledema is observed by funduscopy. Monitor bone age, especially in patients who are pubertal and/or receiving thyroid hormone replacement therapy. Tissue atrophy may occur when administered at the same site over a long period; rotate inj site. Local/systemic allergic reactions may occur. Serum levels of inorganic phosphorus, alkaline phosphatase, and insulin-like growth factor-1 (IGF-1) may increase after therapy.

ADVERSE REACTIONS
Headache, gynecomastia, inj-site reactions (eg, pain, bruise), pancreatitis.

DRUG INTERACTIONS
May need to adjust dose of antihyperglycemic agents (eg, insulin, oral agents), and thyroid hormone replacement therapy. May inhibit 11β-hydroxysteroid dehydrogenase type 1, resulting in reduced serum cortisol concentrations; may need glucocorticoid replacement or dose adjustments of glucocorticoid therapy. Glucocorticoid therapy may attenuate growth-promoting effects in children; carefully adjust glucocorticoid replacement dosing. May increase clearance of antipyrine. May alter clearance of compounds metabolized by CYP450 liver enzymes (eg, corticosteroids, sex steroids, anticonvulsants, cyclosporine); monitor carefully.

PREGNANCY AND LACTATION
Pregnancy: Category C.
Lactation: Caution in nursing.

MECHANISM OF ACTION
Recombinant human growth hormone; stimulates linear growth in children who lack adequate levels of endogenous growth hormone. Produces increased growth rates and IGF-1 concentrations that are similar to those seen after therapy w/ human growth hormone of pituitary origin.

PHARMACOKINETICS
Absorption: Absolute bioavailability (approx 70%); C_{max}=80ng/mL; T_{max}=approx 7 hrs. **Elimination:** $T_{1/2}$=approx 2.7 hrs.

PATIENT CONSIDERATIONS
Assessment: Assess for PWS, preexisting DM or impaired glucose tolerance, hypothyroidism, hypopituitarism, history of scoliosis, hypersensitivity to drug/benzyl alcohol/metacresol, any other conditions where treatment is contraindicated or cautioned, pregnancy/nursing status, and possible drug interactions. Perform funduscopic exam.

Monitoring: Monitor for neoplasms, respiratory infection (patients w/ PWS), increased growth or malignant changes of preexisting nevi, slipped capital femoral epiphysis, progression of scoliosis, intracranial HTN, allergic reactions, pancreatitis, and other adverse reactions. Routinely monitor all patients w/ a history of GHD secondary to an intracranial neoplasm for progression or recurrence of the tumor. Perform periodic thyroid function tests, funduscopic exam, and monitoring of glucose levels and bone age. Monitor growth of patient.

Counseling: Inform about potential benefits and risks of therapy. Instruct on proper administration and disposal of therapy.

ZOMETA — zoledronic acid   Rx
Class: Bisphosphonate

ADULT DOSAGE
Hypercalcemia of Malignancy

Albumin-Corrected Serum Ca²⁺ ≥12mg/dL (3.0mmol/L):
Max: 4mg as a single-dose; infuse IV over no less than 15 min

PEDIATRIC DOSAGE
Pediatric use may not have been established

May consider retreatment if serum Ca^{2+} does not return to normal or remain normal after initial treatment; wait for a minimum of 7 days before retreatment

Vigorous saline hydration should be initiated promptly and an attempt should be made to restore the urine output to about 2L/day throughout treatment; adequately hydrate patients throughout treatment, but avoid overhydration, especially in patients w/ cardiac failure

Multiple Myeloma and Metastatic Bone Lesions of Solid Tumors

In Conjunction w/ Standard Antineoplastic Therapy:
4mg IV infusion over no less than 15 min every 3-4 weeks

Prostate cancer should have progressed after treatment w/ at least 1 hormonal therapy

DOSING CONSIDERATIONS
Renal Impairment
Multiple Myeloma and Metastatic Bone Lesions of Solid Tumors:
CrCl >60mL/min: 4mg
CrCl 50-60mL/min: 3.5mg
CrCl 40-49mL/min: 3.3mg
CrCl 30-39mL/min: 3mg
Withhold treatment for renal deterioration

Other Important Considerations
Multiple Myeloma and Metastatic Bone Lesions of Solid Tumors:
Administer oral Ca^{2+} supplement of 500mg and a multiple vitamin containing 400 IU of vitamin D daily

ADMINISTRATION
IV route

Infuse IV over no less than 15 min.
Do not mix w/ Ca^{2+} or other divalent cation-containing infusion sol (eg, lactated Ringer's sol), and administer as a single IV sol in a line separate from all other drugs.

4mg/100mL Single-Use Ready-to-Use Bottle
This sol is ready-to-use and may be administered directly to the patient w/o further preparation.

Preparation of Reduced Doses from Ready-to-Use Bottle (4mg/100mL):
- Remove 12mL, 18mL, or 25mL from bottle and replace w/ an equal volume of sterile 0.9% NaCl or D5 inj for a dose of 3.5mg, 3.3mg, or 3mg, respectively.
- If not used immediately after dilution, refrigerate sol at 2-8°C (36-46°F).
- Equilibrate refrigerated sol to room temperature prior to administration; total time between dilution, storage in refrigerator, and end of administration must not exceed 24 hrs.

4mg/5mL Single-Use Vial
This concentrate should immediately be diluted in 100mL of sterile 0.9% NaCl or D5 inj. Do not store undiluted concentrate in a syringe, to avoid inadvertent inj.

Preparation of Reduced Doses from Single-Use Vial (4mg/5mL):
- Remove 4.4mL (3.5mg), 4.1mL (3.3mg), or 3.8mL (3mg) from vial and immediately dilute in 100mL of sterile 0.9% NaCl or D5 inj.
- If not used immediately after dilution, refrigerate sol at 2-8°C (36-46°F).
- Equilibrate refrigerated sol to room temperature prior to administration; total time between dilution, storage in refrigerator, and end of administration must not exceed 24 hrs.

STORAGE
25°C (77°F); excursions permitted to 15-30°C (59-86°F).

HOW SUPPLIED
Inj: 4mg/5mL, 4mg/100mL

CONTRAINDICATIONS
Hypersensitivity to zoledronic acid or any components of Zometa.

WARNINGS/PRECAUTIONS
Contains same active ingredient as Reclast; do not treat concomitantly w/ Reclast or other bisphosphonates. Adequately rehydrate patients w/ hypercalcemia of malignancy prior to administration and throughout treatment. Carefully monitor standard hypercalcemia-related metabolic parameters (eg, serum levels of Ca^{2+}, phosphate, and Mg^{2+}) as well as SrCr, following initiation of therapy; if hypocalcemia, hypophosphatemia, or hypomagnesemia occur, short-term supplemental therapy may be necessary. Caution in patients w/ hypercalcemia of malignancy w/ severe renal impairment. Not recommended in patients w/ bone metastases w/ severe renal impairment. Osteonecrosis of the jaw (ONJ) reported; risk may increase w/ duration of exposure to drug. Perform dental examination w/ preventive dentistry prior to treatment and if possible, avoid invasive dental procedures while on treatment. Severe and occasionally incapacitating bone, joint, and/or muscle pain reported; d/c if severe symptoms develop. Atypical subtrochanteric and diaphyseal femoral fractures reported; examine contralateral femur in patients who have sustained femoral shaft fracture. Any patient w/ a history of bisphosphonate exposure who presents w/ thigh/groin pain in the absence of trauma should be suspected of having an atypical fracture and should be evaluated; consider discontinuation in patients suspected to have an atypical femur fracture. Bronchoconstriction may occur in aspirin-sensitive patients. May cause fetal harm. Hypocalcemia and cardiac arrhythmias/neurologic adverse events secondary to cases of severe hypocalcemia reported; correct hypocalcemia before initiating treatment and adequately supplement w/ Ca^{2+} and vitamin D. Caution in elderly.

ADVERSE REACTIONS
Bone pain, N/V, insomnia, fatigue, pyrexia, anemia, constipation, dyspnea, diarrhea, weakness, myalgia, cough, arthralgia, edema (lower limb).

DRUG INTERACTIONS
Caution w/ aminoglycosides or calcitonin; may have an additive effect to lower serum Ca^{2+} level for prolonged periods. Caution w/ drugs known to cause hypocalcemia; severe hypocalcemia may develop. Caution w/ loop diuretics due to an increased risk of hypocalcemia; do not use in patients w/ hypercalcemia of malignancy until patient is adequately rehydrated. Caution w/ other potentially nephrotoxic drugs.

PREGNANCY AND LACTATION
Pregnancy: Category D. May cause fetal harm when administered to a pregnant woman.
Lactation: Not for use in nursing.

MECHANISM OF ACTION
Bisphosphonate; not established. Inhibits bone resorption by inhibiting osteoclastic activity and inducing osteoclast apoptosis. Also blocks osteoclastic resorption of mineralized bone and cartilage through its binding to bone.

PHARMACOKINETICS
Elimination: Urine (39%); $T_{1/2}$=146 hrs.

PATIENT CONSIDERATIONS
Assessment: Assess for hypocalcemia, risk factors for ONJ, hypersensitivity to drug, aspirin sensitivity, renal impairment, pregnancy/nursing status, and possible drug interactions. Assess hydration status and SrCr prior to each treatment. Perform dental exam w/ preventive dentistry. Measure serum Ca^{2+}.

Monitoring: Monitor renal function, standard hypercalcemia-related metabolic parameters (eg, serum Ca^{2+}, phosphate, Mg^{2+}), and hydration status. Monitor for ONJ, musculoskeletal pain, atypical femur fracture, bronchoconstriction, hypocalcemia, and other adverse reactions.

Counseling: Instruct to notify physician of kidney problems, if pregnant/planning to become pregnant, if breastfeeding, or if aspirin-sensitive. Inform of the importance of getting blood tests during the course of therapy. Advise to have dental exam prior to treatment and avoid invasive dental procedures during treatment. Inform of the importance of good dental hygiene, routine dental care, and regular dental check-ups. Advise to immediately notify physician about any oral symptoms (eg, loosening of a tooth, pain, swelling, or non-healing of sores or discharge) during treatment. Advise patients w/ multiple myeloma or bone metastasis of solid tumors to take an oral Ca^{2+} supplement of 500mg and a multiple vitamin containing 400 IU of vitamin D daily. Instruct to report any thigh, hip, or groin pain. Inform of the most common side effects that may develop.

ZOMIG — zolmitriptan   Rx
Class: 5-$HT_{1B/1D}$ agonist (triptans)

OTHER BRAND NAMES
Zomig-ZMT

ADULT DOSAGE	PEDIATRIC DOSAGE
Migraine	**Migraine**
W/ or w/o Aura:	**W/ or w/o Aura:**
Nasal Spray:	**≥12 Years:**
Initial: 2.5mg	**Nasal Spray:**
May give another dose at least 2 hrs after the previous dose if migraine is not resolved by 2 hrs or returns after transient improvement	**Initial:** 2.5mg
Max: 5mg/dose or 10mg/24 hrs	May give another dose at least 2 hrs after the previous dose if migraine is not resolved by 2 hrs or returns after transient improvement
Safety of treating an average of >4 migraines in a 30-day period has not been established	**Max:** 5mg/dose or 10mg/24 hrs
Tabs:	Safety of treating an average of >4 migraines in a 30-day period has not been established
Initial: 1.25mg or 2.5mg	
May give another dose at least 2 hrs after the previous dose if migraine is not resolved by 2 hrs or returns after transient improvement	
Max: 5mg/dose or 10mg/24 hrs	
Safety of treating an average of >3 migraines in a 30-day period has not been established	

DOSING CONSIDERATIONS
Concomitant Medications
Cimetidine:
Max: 2.5mg/dose or 5mg/24 hrs
Hepatic Impairment
Nasal Spray:
Moderate to Severe: Not recommended

Tabs:
Moderate to Severe: 1.25mg (1/2 of one 2.5mg tab)
Severe: Max: 5mg/day

Tab, Disintegrating:
Moderate to Severe: Not recommended

ADMINISTRATION
Oral/nasal routes

Spray
Refer to PI for proper administration instructions.

Tab, Disintegrating
Do not remove from blister until just prior to dosing.
Place tab on the tongue until dissolved, then swallow w/ saliva.

STORAGE
20-25°C (68-77°F). (Tab/Tab, Disintegrating) Protect from light and moisture.

HOW SUPPLIED
Spray: 2.5mg, 5mg [100µL]; **Tab:** 2.5mg*, 5mg; **Tab, Disintegrating:** (ZMT) 2.5mg, 5mg *scored

CONTRAINDICATIONS
Ischemic coronary artery disease (angina pectoris, history of MI, or documented silent ischemia), other significant underlying cardiovascular (CV) disease, or coronary artery vasospasm, including Prinzmetal's angina. Wolff-Parkinson-White syndrome, arrhythmias associated w/ other cardiac accessory conduction pathway disorders, history of stroke, transient ischemic attack (TIA), history of hemiplegic/basilar migraine, peripheral vascular disease, ischemic bowel disease, and uncontrolled HTN. Recent use of another 5-HT₁-agonist, ergotamine-containing medication, or ergot-type medication (eg, dihydroergotamine, methysergide), hypersensitivity to zolmitriptan. Concurrent MAOI-A or recent use/discontinuation of an MAOI-A (w/in 2 weeks).

WARNINGS/PRECAUTIONS
If no treatment response for the 1st migraine attack, reconsider diagnosis before treating any subsequent attacks. Not for prevention of migraine attacks. Serious cardiac adverse reactions, including MI reported. May cause coronary artery vasospasm (Prinzmetal's angina). Perform CV evaluation in triptan-naive patients who have multiple CV risk factors (eg, increased age, diabetes, HTN, strong family history of coronary artery disease [CAD]) prior to therapy; consider administering 1st dose in a medically supervised setting and performing an ECG immediately following administration if CV evaluation is negative. Consider periodic CV evaluation in patients who are intermittent long-term users who have multiple CV risk factors and a negative CV evaluation. Life-threatening cardiac rhythm disturbances, including ventricular tachycardia and ventricular fibrillation, reported; d/c if these disturbances occur. Sensations of tightness, pain, and pressure in the chest, throat, neck, and jaw commonly occur (usually of noncardiac origin). Cerebral/subarachnoid hemorrhage and stroke reported; exclude other potentially serious neurological conditions before treating headaches in patients not previously diagnosed w/ migraine, and in migraine patients w/ atypical migraine symptoms. May cause noncoronary vasospastic reactions (eg, peripheral vascular ischemia, GI vascular ischemia and infarction, Raynaud's syndrome, splenic infarction). Transient and permanent blindness and significant partial vision loss reported. Overuse of acute migraine drugs may lead to exacerbation of headache; detoxification may be necessary. Serotonin syndrome may occur; d/c if suspected. HTN reported. Caution in elderly. (Tab, Disintegrating) Caution w/ phenylketonuria; each 2.5mg and 5mg ODT contains 2.81mg and 5.62mg phenylalanine. (Tab, Disintegrating; Spray) Not recommended in patients w/ moderate or severe hepatic impairment. (Spray) D/C if a cerebrovascular event occurs.

ADVERSE REACTIONS
Dizziness, paresthesia, nausea. (Tab) Neck/throat/jaw pain, asthenia, somnolence, warm/cold sensation, heaviness sensation, dry mouth. (Spray) Unusual taste, hyperesthesia, dysgeusia, nasal discomfort, oropharyngeal pain.

DRUG INTERACTIONS
See Contraindications. Ergot-containing drugs may prolong vasospastic reactions. Increased exposure w/ MAOI-A. Risk of vasospastic reactions w/ 5-HT₁ᵦ/₁ᴅ-agonists (eg, triptans). Serotonin syndrome may occur, particularly during coadministration w/ SSRIs, SNRIs, TCAs, and MAOIs. $T_{1/2}$ and blood levels reported to double w/ cimetidine.

PREGNANCY AND LACTATION
Pregnancy: Category C.
Lactation: Not for use in nursing.

MECHANISM OF ACTION
5-HT₁ᴅ/₁ᴮ-agonist. Suspected to be due to the agonist effects at the 5-HT₁ᴮ/₁ᴅ receptors on intracranial blood vessels (including arteriovenous anastomoses) and sensory nerves of the trigeminal system, which results in cranial vessel constriction and inhibition of pro-inflammatory neuropeptide release.

PHARMACOKINETICS
Absorption: (PO) Well-absorbed, (Spray) rapid; absolute bioavailability (40%); T_{max}=(Tab, Disintegrating/Spray) 3 hrs, (Tab) 1.5 hrs. **Distribution:** V_d=(PO) 7L/kg, (Spray) 8.4L/kg; plasma protein binding (25%). **Metabolism:** N-desmethyl (active metabolite). **Elimination:** (PO) Urine (65%, 8% unchanged), feces (30%); $T_{1/2}$=(Spray) 3 hrs.

PATIENT CONSIDERATIONS
Assessment: Confirm diagnosis of migraine before therapy. Assess for ischemic CAD, HTN, history of hemiplegic/basilar migraine, hypersensitivity to drug, or any other conditions where treatment is contraindicated or cautioned. Assess for hepatic impairment, pregnancy/nursing status, and possible drug interactions. Perform a CV evaluation for patients who have multiple CV risk factors.

Monitoring: Monitor for signs/symptoms of cardiac adverse reactions; cerebrovascular events; vasospastic reactions; tightness/pain/pressure sensations in the chest, throat, neck, and jaw; peripheral vascular ischemia; serotonin syndrome; increased BP; and other adverse reactions. Perform ECG immediately after administration of therapy and monitor CV function in intermittent long-term users who have multiple CV risk factors.

Counseling: Instruct to take ud. Inform that treatment may cause serious CV events that may result in hospitalization and even death. Instruct patients to be alert for signs/symptoms of chest pain, SOB, weakness, and slurring of speech; advise to notify physician if any of these signs/symptoms are observed. Inform that the use of therapy ≥10 days per month may lead to exacerbation of headache; encourage to record headache frequency and drug use. Counsel about the possible drug interactions. Advise to notify physician if pregnant/nursing or planning to become pregnant. (Tab, Disintegrating) Inform patients w/ phenylketonuria that it contains phenylalanine. (Spray) Counsel on proper administration technique for nasal spray; advise to avoid spraying contents in the eyes.

ZONISAMIDE — zonisamide   Rx

Class: Sulfonamide anticonvulsant

OTHER BRAND NAMES
Zonegran

ADULT DOSAGE	PEDIATRIC DOSAGE
Partial Seizures **As Adjunctive Therapy in Patients w/ Epilepsy:** **>16 Years:** Give qd or bid **Initial:** 100mg/day **Titrate:** After 2 weeks, may increase to 200mg/day for at least 2 weeks. May then increase to 300mg/day and 400mg/day, w/ the dose stable for at least 2 weeks to achieve steady state at each level. Evidence suggests that doses of 100-600mg/day are effective, but there is no suggestion of increasing response above 400mg/day	Pediatric use may not have been established

DOSING CONSIDERATIONS
Renal Impairment
May require slower titration and more frequent monitoring

Hepatic Impairment
May require slower titration and more frequent monitoring

Elderly
Start at lower end of dosing range

Discontinuation
D/C gradually

ADMINISTRATION
Oral route

Take w/ or w/o food.
Swallow caps whole.

STORAGE
25°C (77°F); excursions permitted to 15-30°C (59-86°F). Store in a dry place and protect from light.

HOW SUPPLIED
Cap: 50mg; (Zonegran) 25mg, 100mg

CONTRAINDICATIONS
Hypersensitivity to sulfonamides or zonisamide.

WARNINGS/PRECAUTIONS
Potentially fatal reactions to sulfonamides (eg, Stevens-Johnson syndrome, toxic epidermal necrolysis, fulminant hepatic necrosis, agranulocytosis, aplastic anemia, other blood dyscrasias) reported; d/c immediately if signs of hypersensitivity or other serious reactions occur. Consider discontinuation if unexplained rash develops; if the drug is not discontinued, observe frequently. Drug reaction w/ eosinophilia and systemic symptoms (DRESS)/multiorgan hypersensitivity reported; evaluate immediately if signs/symptoms present and d/c if an alternative etiology cannot be established. Oligohydrosis and hyperthermia reported in pediatric patients; not approved for use in pediatric patients. Increased risk of suicidal thoughts/behavior. May cause metabolic acidosis (generally dose-dependent); conditions or therapies that predispose to acidosis may be additive to the bicarbonate-lowering effects of zonisamide. Consider dose reduction or discontinuation of therapy if metabolic acidosis develops and persists; if the decision is to continue therapy, consider alkali treatment. Abrupt withdrawal may precipitate increased seizure frequency or status epilepticus; reduce dose or d/c gradually. May cause serious fetal adverse effects. May cause CNS-related adverse events (eg, psychiatric symptoms, psychomotor slowing, somnolence, fatigue). May impair mental/physical abilities. Caution w/ hepatic dysfunction. Nephrolithiasis and increased SrCr/BUN reported; d/c if acute renal failure or a clinically significant sustained increase in SrCr/BUN develops. Do not use in patients w/ renal failure (estimated GFR <50mL/min). Status epilepticus reported. Increases serum Cl⁻ and alkaline phosphatase and decreases serum bicarbonate, phosphorus, Ca^{2+}, and albumin. Caution in elderly.

ADVERSE REACTIONS

Somnolence, anorexia, dizziness, ataxia, agitation/irritability, difficulty w/ memory and/or concentration.

DRUG INTERACTIONS

Caution when starting or stopping zonisamide or changing the zonisamide dose in patients who are also receiving drugs that are P-gp substrates (eg, digoxin, quinidine). CYP3A4 inducers (eg, phenytoin, carbamazepine, phenobarbital) may increase metabolism/clearance and decrease $T_{1/2}$ of zonisamide. These effects are unlikely to be of clinical significance when zonisamide is added to existing therapy; however, since changes in zonisamide concentrations may occur if concomitant CYP3A4-inducing antiepileptic or other drugs are withdrawn, dose adjusted, or introduced, an adjustment of the zonisamide dose may be required. Patient should be closely monitored and dose of zonisamide and other drugs that are CYP3A4 substrates may need to be adjusted if coadministration w/ a potent CYP3A4 inducer (eg, rifampicin) is necessary. Caution w/ alcohol or other CNS depressants. Concomitant use w/ other carbonic anhydrase inhibitors (eg, topiramate, acetazolamide, dichlorphenamide) may increase the severity of metabolic acidosis and may also increase the risk of kidney stone formation; monitor for the appearance or worsening of metabolic acidosis w/ concomitant use. Concomitant medications that can induce or inhibit N-acetyl-transferases may affect the pharmacokinetics of zonisamide. Caution w/ other drugs that predispose patients to heat-related disorders (eg, carbonic anhydrase inhibitors, anticholinergics).

PREGNANCY AND LACTATION

Pregnancy: May cause serious adverse fetal effects. Women of childbearing potential should use effective contraception. Monitor pregnant patients and newborns of mothers treated w/ zonisamide for metabolic acidosis. Physicians are advised to recommend that pregnant patients enroll in the North American Antiepileptic Drug (NAAED) Pregnancy Registry.
Lactation: Found in breast milk; not for use in nursing.

MECHANISM OF ACTION

Sulfonamide anticonvulsant; mechanism has not been established. Blocks Na^+ channels and reduces voltage-dependent, transient inward currents (T-type Ca^{2+} currents), consequently stabilizing neuronal membranes and suppressing neuronal hypersynchronization.

PHARMACOKINETICS

Absorption: C_{max}=2-5mcg/mL; T_{max}=2-6 hrs (fasted), 4-6 hrs (fed). **Distribution:** V_d=1.45L/kg; plasma protein binding (40%); found in breast milk. **Metabolism:** Liver via reduction by CYP3A4 and acetylation; 2-sulfamoylacetyl phenol, N-acetyl zonisamide (metabolites). **Elimination:** Urine (62%, unchanged and metabolite), feces (3%); $T_{1/2}$=63 hrs.

PATIENT CONSIDERATIONS

Assessment: Assess for hypersensitivity to sulfonamides or the drug, depression, conditions or therapies that predispose to acidosis, renal/hepatic impairment, pregnancy/nursing status, and possible drug interactions. Obtain baseline serum bicarbonate level.

Monitoring: Monitor for signs/symptoms of severe reactions (eg, skin reactions, hematologic events, DRESS/multiorgan hypersensitivity), decreased sweating, increased body temperature, emergence/worsening of depression, suicidal thoughts/behavior, any unusual changes in mood/behavior, metabolic acidosis, seizures (upon abrupt withdrawal), CNS-related adverse events, and other adverse reactions. Monitor renal function and serum bicarbonate levels periodically.

Counseling: Inform about risks/benefits of therapy and instruct to take only as prescribed. Advise not to drive or operate other complex machinery until patient gains sufficient experience on therapy to determine whether it affects performance. Instruct to immediately contact physician if patient experiences skin rash; worsening of seizures; signs/symptoms of kidney stone formation, hematological complications, or metabolic acidosis; emergence/worsening of depression symptoms; any unusual changes in mood/behavior; suicidal thoughts/ behavior; or thoughts about self-harm. Inform that increasing fluid intake and urine output may reduce risk of kidney stone formation, particularly in those w/ predisposing risk factors for stones. Advise women of childbearing potential to use effective contraception while on therapy. Instruct to notify physician if pregnant/breastfeeding or if intending to become pregnant or to breastfeed during therapy; encourage to enroll in the NAAED Pregnancy Registry if patient becomes pregnant.

ZONTIVITY — vorapaxar   Rx

Class: Protease-activated receptor-1 (PAR-1) antagonist

> **Do not use in patients w/ a history of stroke, transient ischemic attack (TIA), intracranial hemorrhage (ICH), or active pathological bleeding. May increase the risk of bleeding, including ICH and fatal bleeding.**

ADULT DOSAGE	PEDIATRIC DOSAGE
Reduction of Thrombotic Cardiovascular Events	Pediatric use may not have been established
In Patients w/ a History of MI or w/ Peripheral Arterial Disease:	
1 tab (2.08mg) qd; use w/ aspirin and/or clopidogrel according to their indications or standard of care	

DOSING CONSIDERATIONS
Hepatic Impairment
Severe: Not recommended

ADMINISTRATION
Oral route

Take w/ or w/o food.

STORAGE
20-25°C (68-77°F); excursions permitted to 15-30°C (59-86°F). Protect from moisture.

HOW SUPPLIED
Tab: 2.08mg

CONTRAINDICATIONS
Active pathological bleeding (eg, ICH, peptic ulcer). History of stroke, TIA, or ICH.

WARNINGS/PRECAUTIONS
Increases the risk of bleeding in proportion to the patient's underlying bleeding risk. Suspect bleeding in any patient who is hypotensive and has recently undergone coronary angiography, percutaneous coronary intervention, CABG surgery, or other surgical procedures. Withholding therapy for a brief period will not be useful in managing an acute bleeding event; has no known treatment to reverse the antiplatelet effect of therapy; significant inhibition of platelet aggregation remains 4 weeks after discontinuation of therapy.

ADVERSE REACTIONS
Bleeding, anemia.

DRUG INTERACTIONS
May increase risk of bleeding w/ anticoagulants, fibrinolytic therapy, chronic NSAIDs, SSRIs, and SNRIs; avoid concomitant use of warfarin or other anticoagulants. Avoid concomitant use w/ strong CYP3A inhibitors (eg, ketoconazole, clarithromycin, ritonavir) or strong CYP3A inducers (eg, rifampin, carbamazepine, St. John's wort).

PREGNANCY AND LACTATION
Pregnancy: Category B.
Lactation: Not for use in nursing.

MECHANISM OF ACTION
PAR-1 antagonist; inhibits thrombin-induced and thrombin receptor agonist peptide-induced platelet aggregation.

PHARMACOKINETICS
Absorption: Absolute bioavailability (approx 100%); T_{max}=1 hr (fasted). **Distribution:** V_d=approx 424L; plasma protein binding (≥99%). **Metabolism:** Via CYP3A4 and CYP2J2; M20 (major circulating active metabolite). **Elimination:** Urine (25%), feces (58%); $T_{1/2}$=8 days.

PATIENT CONSIDERATIONS
Assessment: Assess for history of stroke, TIA, or ICH; active pathological bleeding, risk factors for bleeding, hepatic impairment, pregnancy/nursing status, and for possible drug interactions.

Monitoring: Monitor for signs/symptoms of bleeding and other adverse reactions.

Counseling: Inform about the benefits and risks of therapy. Instruct to take exactly ud and not to d/c w/o discussing it w/ the prescribing physician. Inform that may bleed and bruise more easily. Advise to report any unanticipated, prolonged, or excessive bleeding, or blood in stool or urine. Instruct to notify physicians or dentists about therapy before any surgery or dental procedure. Advise to inform physician of all medications currently taking/planning to take.

ZORBTIVE — somatropin (rDNA origin)   Rx

Class: Human growth hormone (hGH)

ADULT DOSAGE	PEDIATRIC DOSAGE
Short Bowel Syndrome	Pediatric use may not have been established
In Patients Receiving Specialized Nutritional Support:	
0.1mg/kg qd SQ for 4 weeks	
Max: 8mg/day	

DOSING CONSIDERATIONS
Concomitant Medications
Changes to concomitant medications should be avoided
Elderly
Start at a lower dose

Adverse Reactions
Treat moderate fluid retention and arthralgias symptomatically or reduce dose by 50%
D/C for up to 5 days for severe toxicities; upon resolution of symptoms, resume at 50% of original dose
Permanently d/c if severe toxicity recurs or does not disappear w/in 5 days

ADMINISTRATION
SQ route

Rotate inj site

Reconstitution
Each vial of 8.8mg is reconstituted in 1-2mL of bacteriostatic water for inj (0.9% benzyl alcohol)
Approx 10% mechanical loss can be associated w/ reconstitution and administration from multidose vials

Inject the diluent into the vial aiming the liquid against the glass vial wall to reconstitute
Swirl the vial w/ a gentle rotary motion until contents are dissolved completely
The sol should be clear immediately after reconstitution. Do not inject if the reconstituted product is cloudy immediately after reconstitution or after refrigeration
The reconstituted sol can be refrigerated for up to 14 days. Allow refrigerated sol to come to room temperature prior to administration
A standard insulin-type SQ syringe is recommended for administration

STORAGE
Before Reconstitution: 15-30°C (59-86°F). After Reconstitution with Bacteriostatic Water for Inj: 2-8°C (36-46°F) for up to 14 days. Avoid freezing.

HOW SUPPLIED
Inj: 8.8mg

CONTRAINDICATIONS
Acute critical illness due to complications following open heart or abdominal surgery, multiple accidental trauma, or acute respiratory failure; active neoplasia (either newly diagnosed or recurrent); benzyl alcohol sensitivity; known hypersensitivity to growth hormone.

WARNINGS/PRECAUTIONS
Benzyl alcohol associated with toxicity in newborns. If sensitivity occurs, may reconstitute with sterile water for inj; use immediately and discard any unused portion. Allergic reactions may occur. Associated with acute pancreatitis. Cases of new-onset impaired glucose intolerance, new-onset type 2 diabetes mellitus (DM), exacerbation of preexisting DM, diabetic ketoacidosis, and diabetic coma reported. Syndrome of intracranial HTN with papilledema, visual changes, headache, and N/V reported in small number of children with growth failure treated with growth hormone products; perform funduscopic evaluation at the initiation and periodically during therapy. Increased tissue turgor and musculoskeletal discomfort may occur during therapy but may resolve spontaneously with analgesic therapy, or after reducing the frequency of dosing. Carpal tunnel syndrome may occur; d/c if symptoms do not resolve after reducing the dose or frequency. Caution in elderly.

ADVERSE REACTIONS
Edema, melena, rectal hemorrhage, arthritis, fungal infection, inflammation at the inj site, paresthesia, phantom pain, bronchospasm, dyspnea, purpura, skin disorder, insomnia, hypomagnesemia, dysuria.

DRUG INTERACTIONS
May impact cortisol and cortisone metabolism. May unmask previously undiagnosed primary (and secondary) hypoadrenalism requiring glucocorticoid therapy. Use of glucocorticoid replacement therapy for previously diagnosed hypoadrenalism, especially cortisone acetate or prednisone, may require an increase in maint or stress doses. Dose adjustment of antidiabetics may be required.

PREGNANCY AND LACTATION
Category B, caution in nursing.

MECHANISM OF ACTION
Human growth hormone; anabolic and anticatabolic agent that exerts influence by interacting with specific receptors on a variety of cell types. On gut, actions may be direct or mediated via local or systemic production of insulin-like growth factor-1; also enhances transmucosal transport of water, electrolytes, and nutrients.

PHARMACOKINETICS
Absorption: Absolute bioavailability (70-90%). **Distribution:** (IV) V_d=12L. **Metabolism:** Liver, kidneys. **Elimination:** $T_{1/2}$=3.94 hrs (SQ), 0.58 hrs (IV).

PATIENT CONSIDERATIONS
Assessment: Assess for acute critical illness, active neoplasia, hypersensitivity to benzyl alcohol, pregnancy/nursing status, and possible drug interactions. Perform baseline funduscopic examination.

Monitoring: Monitor for hypersensitivity/allergic reactions, acute pancreatitis, impaired glucose intolerance, new-onset type 2 DM, exacerbation of preexisting DM, diabetic ketoacidosis, diabetic coma, carpal tunnel syndrome, increased tissue turgor, musculoskeletal discomfort, and other adverse reactions. Perform funduscopic examination periodically.

Counseling: Inform about the risks and benefits associated with the treatment. Instruct to notify physician if they experience any side effects or discomfort during treatment. Advise to properly dispose the needles and syringes using an appropriate container; advise not to reuse the needles and syringes. Instruct to rotate inj sites to avoid localized tissue atrophy.

ZORTRESS — everolimus   Rx
Class: Immunosuppressant

Should only be prescribed by physicians experienced in immunosuppressive therapy and management of organ transplant patients. Immunosuppression may lead to increased susceptibility to infection and possible development of malignancies (eg, lymphoma, skin cancer). Increased risk of kidney arterial and venous thrombosis leading to graft loss was reported, mostly w/in the first 30 days post-transplantation. Increased nephrotoxicity may occur in combination w/ standard doses of cyclosporine; reduce dose of cyclosporine to reduce renal dysfunction, and monitor cyclosporine and everolimus whole blood trough concentrations. Increased mortality w/in the first 3 months post-transplantation in heart transplant patients on immunosuppressive regimens w/ or w/o induction therapy; not recommended in heart transplantation.

ADULT DOSAGE
Renal Transplant
Prophylaxis of Organ Rejection in Kidney Transplant:
Initial: 0.75mg bid, in combination w/ basiliximab induction and concurrently w/ reduced dose of cyclosporine; give as soon as possible after transplantation.
Initiate oral prednisone once oral medication is tolerated.
Titrate: May require dose adjustment based on blood concentrations achieved, tolerability, individual response, change in concomitant medications, and clinical situation; optimal dose adjustments should be based on trough levels obtained 4 or 5 days after a previous dosing change

Recommended Therapeutic Range: 3-8ng/mL (based on LC/MS/MS assay method); if trough level is <3ng/mL, double total daily dose, or if trough level is >8ng/mL on 2 consecutive measures, decrease by 0.25mg bid

Refer to PI for further drug monitoring instructions and for cyclosporine therapeutic drug monitoring parameters

Hepatic Transplant
Prophylaxis of Allograft Rejection w/ a Liver Transplant:
Initial: 1mg bid, in combination w/ reduced dose of tacrolimus; start at least 30 days post-transplant
Titrate: May require dose adjustment based on blood concentrations achieved, tolerability, individual response, change in concomitant medications, and clinical situation; optimal dose adjustments should be based on trough levels obtained 4 or 5 days after a previous dosing change

Recommended Therapeutic Range: 3-8ng/mL (based on LC/MS/MS assay method); if trough level is <3ng/mL, double total daily dose, or if trough level is >8ng/mL on 2 consecutive measures, decrease by 0.25mg bid

Refer to PI for further drug monitoring instructions and for tacrolimus therapeutic drug monitoring parameters

---

DOSING CONSIDERATIONS
Hepatic Impairment
Mild (Child-Pugh Class A): Reduce initial daily dose by 1/3 of normal daily dose
Moderate or Severe (Child-Pugh Class B or C): Reduce initial daily dose to 1/2 of the normal daily dose

ADMINISTRATION
Oral route

Do not crush; swallow whole w/ water.
Administer consistently approx 12 hrs apart w/ or w/o food and at the same time as cyclosporine or tacrolimus.

STORAGE
25°C (77°F); excursions permitted to 15-30°C (59-86°F). Protect from light and moisture.

HOW SUPPLIED
Tab: 0.25mg, 0.5mg, 0.75mg

CONTRAINDICATIONS
Known hypersensitivity to everolimus, sirolimus, or to components of the drug product.

WARNINGS/PRECAUTIONS
Limit exposure to sunlight and UV light. Prophylaxis for *Pneumocystis jiroveci (carinii)* pneumonia and CMV recommended. Increased risk of hepatic artery thrombosis (HAT), which may lead to graft loss or death; do not give earlier than 30 days after liver transplant. Consider switching to other immunosuppressive therapies if renal function does not improve after dose adjustments or if dysfunction is thought to be drug related. Angioedema, increased risk of delayed wound healing, increased occurrence of wound-related complications, and generalized fluid accumulation reported. Interstitial lung disease (ILD), implying lung intraparenchymal inflammation (pneumonitis) and/or fibrosis of noninfectious etiology, some w/ pulmonary HTN as a secondary event reported; resolution may occur upon drug interruption w/ or w/o glucocorticoid therapy. Consider diagnosis of ILD for symptoms of infectious pneumonia that

PEDIATRIC DOSAGE
Pediatric use may not have been established

do not respond to antibiotic therapy and in whom non-drug causes have been ruled out. Increased risk of hyperlipidemia and proteinuria w/ higher whole blood trough concentrations; use of anti-lipid therapy may not normalize lipid levels. Reevaluate the risk/benefit of continuing therapy in patients w/ severe refractory hyperlipidemia. Increased risk of polyoma virus infections, including polyoma virus-associated nephropathy (PVAN) and progressive multiple leukoencephalopathy (PML), may occur; consider reductions in immunosuppression if evidence of PVAN or PML develops. Concomitant use w/ cyclosporine may increase risk of thrombotic microangiopathy/TTP/hemolytic uremic syndrome. May increase risk of new-onset diabetes mellitus (DM) after transplant. Azoospermia or oligospermia may be observed. Avoid w/ rare hereditary problems of galactose intolerance (Lapp lactase deficiency, glucose-galactose malabsorption); diarrhea and malabsorption may occur.

ADVERSE REACTIONS
Kidney Transplantation: Peripheral edema, constipation, HTN, nausea, anemia, urinary tract infection, hyperlipidemia.
Liver Transplantation: Diarrhea, headache, peripheral edema, HTN, nausea, pyrexia, abdominal pain, leukopenia.

DRUG INTERACTIONS
See Boxed Warning. Caution w/ drugs known to impair renal function. May increase risk of angioedema w/ drugs known to cause angioedema (eg, ACE inhibitors). Monitor for development of rhabdomyolysis w/ HMG-CoA reductase inhibitors and/or fibrates; use of simvastatin and lovastatin are strongly discouraged in patients receiving everolimus w/ cyclosporine. Coadministration w/ strong CYP3A4 inhibitors (eg, ketoconazole, clarithromycin, ritonavir) and strong CYP3A4 inducers (eg, rifampin, rifabutin) is not recommended w/o close monitoring of everolimus whole blood trough concentrations. Avoid w/ live vaccines, grapefruit, and grapefruit juice. Inhibitors of P-gp (eg, digoxin, cyclosporine), moderate inhibitors of CYP3A4 and P-gp (eg, fluconazole, macrolide antibiotics, nicardipine), and verapamil may increase levels. If coadministered w/ erythromycin or verapamil, monitor everolimus blood concentrations and if necessary, make a dose adjustment. Caution w/ CYP3A4 and CYP2D6 substrates w/ a narrow therapeutic index. Increased levels w/ cyclosporine; dose adjustment may be needed if cyclosporine dose is altered. CYP3A4 inducers (eg, St. John's wort, carbamazepine, phenobarbital) may decrease levels. Combination immunosuppressant therapy should be used w/ caution. May increase octreotide C_{min} levels.

PREGNANCY AND LACTATION
Pregnancy: Category C.
Lactation: Not for use in nursing.

MECHANISM OF ACTION
Macrolide immunosuppressant; inhibits antigenic and interleukin (IL-2 and IL-15) stimulated activation and proliferation of T and B lymphocytes. Binds to a cytoplasmic protein, the FK506 binding protein-12 (FKBP-12), to form an immunosuppressive complex (everolimus: FKBP-12) that binds to and inhibits the mammalian target of rapamycin, a key regulatory kinase in cells.

PHARMACOKINETICS
Absorption: (0.75mg bid) AUC=75ng•hr/mL, C_{max}=11.1ng/mL, T_{max}=1-2 hrs. **Distribution:** Plasma protein binding (74%); (0.75mg bid) V_d=110L. **Metabolism:** Via CYP3A4 and P-gp. **Elimination:** Feces (80%), urine (5%). (0.75mg bid) $T_{1/2}$=30 hrs.

PATIENT CONSIDERATIONS
Assessment: Assess for hereditary problems of galactose intolerance, hepatic impairment, hypersensitivity to the drug or to sirolimus, pregnancy/nursing status, and possible drug interactions. Obtain baseline lipid and glucose levels.

Monitoring: Monitor for infections, angioedema, thrombosis, wound-related complications, fluid accumulation, lymphomas and other malignancies, hyperlipidemia, hepatic impairment, proteinuria, PVAN, HAT, ILD, pneumonitis, and other adverse reactions. Monitor everolimus and cyclosporine or tacrolimus whole blood trough concentrations, lipid profile, blood glucose concentrations, renal function, and hematologic parameters.

Counseling: Counsel to avoid grapefruit and grapefruit juice. Inform of the risk of developing lymphomas and other malignancies, particularly of the skin; instruct to limit exposure to sunlight and UV light. Advise that therapy has been associated w/ an increased risk of kidney arterial and venous thrombosis, resulting in graft loss, usually occurring w/in the first 30 days post-transplantation. Inform of the risks of impaired kidney function w/ concomitant cyclosporine as well as the need for routine blood concentration monitoring for both drugs; advise of the importance of SrCr monitoring. Inform of risk of hyperlipidemia and the importance of lipid profile monitoring. Advise women to avoid pregnancy throughout treatment and for 8 weeks after discontinuation. Instruct to notify physician of all medications and herbal/dietary supplements being taken. Inform that therapy has been associated w/ impaired or delayed wound healing, and fluid accumulation. Inform of increased risk of proteinuria, DM, infections, noninfectious pneumonitis, and angioedema; advise to contact physician if symptoms develop. Instruct to avoid receiving live vaccines.

ZORVOLEX — diclofenac   Rx
Class: NSAID

ADULT DOSAGE
Mild to Moderate Pain
Acute:
18mg or 35mg tid
Osteoarthritis
35mg tid

PEDIATRIC DOSAGE
Pediatric use may not have been established

DOSING CONSIDERATIONS
Hepatic Impairment
Start at lowest dose; d/c use if efficacy is not achieved w/ lowest dose
Elderly
If the anticipated benefit outweighs the potential risks, start at lower end of dosing range; monitor for adverse effects

ADMINISTRATION
Oral route
- Taking w/ food may cause a reduction in effectiveness compared to taking on an empty stomach.
- Not interchangeable w/ other formulations of oral diclofenac even if the mg strength is the same.

STORAGE
20-25°C (68-77°F); excursions permitted to 15-30°C (59-86°F). Protect from moisture.

HOW SUPPLIED
Cap: 18mg, 35mg

CONTRAINDICATIONS
Known hypersensitivity to diclofenac or any components of the drug product; history of asthma, urticaria, or other allergic-type reactions w/ aspirin (ASA) or other NSAIDs; in the setting of CABG surgery.

WARNINGS/PRECAUTIONS
Use lowest effective dose for shortest duration possible. Avoid in patients w/ a recent MI unless benefits outweigh the risks; if used, monitor for signs of cardiac ischemia. Increased risk for GI bleeding w/ longer duration of therapy, older age, poor general health status, and advanced liver disease and/or coagulopathy; avoid use in patients at higher risk unless benefits are expected to outweigh the increased risk and consider alternate therapies. Promptly initiate evaluation and treatment if a serious GI adverse event is suspected; d/c until a serious GI adverse event is ruled out. Hepatotoxicity reported; d/c immediately and perform a clinical evaluation if clinical signs/symptoms consistent w/ liver disease develop, if systemic manifestations occur, or if abnormal liver tests persist or worsen. May cause new onset HTN or worsen preexisting HTN. Fluid retention and edema reported. Avoid use in patients w/ severe heart failure (HF) unless benefits outweigh risks; monitor for signs of worsening HF if used. Renal papillary necrosis and other renal injury reported w/ long-term use. Renal toxicity also reported in patients in whom renal prostaglandins have a compensatory role in the maintenance of renal perfusion; increased risk w/ renal/hepatic dysfunction, dehydration, hypovolemia, and HF, and in the elderly. Correct volume status in dehydrated or hypovolemic patients prior to initiating therapy. Avoid use in patients w/ advanced renal disease unless the benefits are expected to outweigh the risk; monitor for signs of worsening renal function if used in patients w/ advanced renal disease. Hyperkalemia reported. Associated w/ anaphylactic reactions. Monitor for changes in the signs/symptoms of asthma in patients w/ preexisting asthma (w/o known ASA sensitivity). May cause serious skin reactions (eg, exfoliative dermatitis, Stevens-Johnson syndrome, toxic epidermal necrolysis); d/c at 1st appearance of skin rash/hypersensitivity. Anemia reported. May increase the risk of bleeding events; coagulation disorders may increase this risk. May mask inflammation and fever.

ADVERSE REACTIONS
Edema, N/V, headache, dizziness, constipation, pruritus, diarrhea, flatulence, pain in extremity, abdominal pain, sinusitis, increased ALT, increased blood creatinine, HTN, dyspepsia.

DRUG INTERACTIONS
Drugs that interfere w/ serotonin reuptake may potentiate the risk of bleeding. Synergistic effect on bleeding w/ anticoagulants (eg, warfarin); monitor for signs of bleeding w/ concomitant anticoagulants, antiplatelet agents, SSRIs, and SNRIs. May increase risk of GI bleeding w/ use of oral corticosteroids, anticoagulants, and SSRIs; smoking; and alcohol use. ASA may increase risk of bleeding and serious GI events; concomitant use w/ analgesic doses of ASA is not recommended. Monitor patients more closely for GI bleeding w/ concomitant use of low-dose ASA for cardiac prophylaxis. May diminish antihypertensive effect of ACE inhibitors, ARBs, or β-blockers (eg, propranolol); monitor BP. Coadministration w/ ACE inhibitors or ARBs may result in deterioration of renal function (including possible acute renal failure) in patients who are elderly or volume-depleted (including those on diuretic therapy), or who have renal impairment; monitor for worsening renal function. Adequately hydrate and assess renal function at the beginning of the concomitant treatment and periodically thereafter. May reduce natriuretic effect of loop diuretics (eg, furosemide) and thiazide diuretics; observe for signs of worsening renal function, in addition to assuring diuretic efficacy including antihypertensive effects. May increase serum concentration and prolong $T_{1/2}$ of digoxin; monitor serum digoxin levels. May cause elevations in plasma lithium levels and reductions in renal lithium clearance; monitor for signs of lithium toxicity. May increase risk for methotrexate toxicity. May increase cyclosporine's nephrotoxicity; monitor for signs of worsening renal function. Use w/ other NSAIDs or salicylates (eg, diflunisal, salsalate) increases risk of GI toxicity; concomitant use not recommended. May increase the risk of pemetrexed-associated myelosuppression, renal, and GI toxicity; refer to prescribing information for further information. CYP2C9 inhibitors (eg, voriconazole) may enhance exposure and toxicity of diclofenac whereas

coadministration w/ CYP2C9 inducers (eg, rifampin) may lead to compromised efficacy of diclofenac; a dosage adjustment may be warranted.

PREGNANCY AND LACTATION

Pregnancy: Category C, prior to 30 weeks' gestation; Category D, starting at 30 weeks' gestation. Use during the 3rd trimester of pregnancy increases the risk of premature closure of the fetal ductus arteriosus; avoid use in pregnant women starting at 30 weeks of gestation (3rd trimester).
Lactation: May be present in human milk; caution in nursing.
Reproductive Potential: May delay or prevent rupture of ovarian follicles. Consider withdrawal of therapy in women who have difficulties conceiving or who are undergoing investigation of infertility.

MECHANISM OF ACTION

NSAID; has not been established. May involve inhibition of the COX-1 and COX-2 pathways. May also be related to prostaglandin synthetase inhibition. Exhibits anti-inflammatory, analgesic, and antipyretic activities.

PHARMACOKINETICS

Absorption: T_{max}=1 hr (fasted), 3.32 hrs (fed). **Distribution:** V_d=1.3L/kg (diclofenac potassium); serum protein binding (>99%). May be found in breast milk.
Metabolism: Via CYP2C9 (major metabolite), glucuronidation/sulfation, CYP3A4 (minor metabolites), acylglucuronidation via UGT2B7 and oxidation via CYP2C8 may also play a role; 4'-hydroxy-diclofenac (major metabolite). **Elimination:** Urine (65%), bile (35%); $T_{1/2}$=2 hrs.

PATIENT CONSIDERATIONS

Assessment: Assess for hypersensitivity to diclofenac or to any component of this product; history of asthma, urticaria, or other allergic-type reactions after taking ASA or other NSAIDs; asthma; CV disease (CVD) or risk factors for CVD; HTN; history of peptic ulcer disease or GI bleeding; coagulation disorders; renal/hepatic impairment; pregnancy/nursing status; or any other conditions where treatment is contraindicated or cautioned. Assess volume status. Assess for possible drug interactions. Obtain baseline BP, CBC, and chemistry profile.

Monitoring: Monitor for signs/symptoms of CV thrombotic events; cardiac ischemia in patients w/ a recent MI; GI bleeding/ulceration and perforation; hepatotoxicity; new or worsening HTN; HF; edema; renal papillary necrosis and other renal injury; hyperkalemia; anaphylactic reactions; serious skin reactions; anemia; and other adverse reactions. Monitor BP during initiation of therapy and throughout the course of therapy. Monitor for signs of bleeding in patients on concomitant therapy w/ anticoagulants, antiplatelet agents, SSRIs, or SNRIs. Monitor renal function in patients w/ renal/hepatic impairment, HF, dehydration, or hypovolemia. Periodically monitor CBC and chemistry profiles including LFTs in patients receiving long-term treatment.

Counseling: Advise to be alert for the symptoms of CV thrombotic events and to report symptoms immediately. Advise to report symptoms of ulcerations and bleeding. Inform of the increased risk for and the signs and symptoms of GI bleeding w/ ASA. Inform of the warning signs and symptoms of hepatotoxicity; instruct to d/c and seek immediate medical therapy. Advise to be alert for the symptoms of CHF and to contact healthcare provider if such symptoms occur. Inform of the signs of an anaphylactic reaction and instruct to seek immediate emergency help if these occur. Advise to d/c immediately if any type of rash develops, and to contact healthcare provider as soon as possible. Advise females of reproductive potential who desire pregnancy that NSAIDs may be associated w/ a reversible delay in ovulation. Inform pregnant women to avoid use of diclofenac and other NSAIDs starting at 30 weeks' gestation. Inform patients that the concomitant use w/ other NSAIDs or salicylates is not recommended. Alert patients that NSAIDs may be present in OTC medications for treatment of colds, fever, or insomnia. Advise not to use low-dose ASA w/o consultation.

ZOSTAVAX — zoster vaccine live   Rx

Class: Vaccine

ADULT DOSAGE	PEDIATRIC DOSAGE
Herpes Zoster	Pediatric use may not have been established
Prevention:	
≥50 Years: 0.65mL SQ in the deltoid region of the upper arm	

ADMINISTRATION

SQ route

Inject in the deltoid region of the upper arm.
Do not inject IV or IM.

Preparation/Reconstitution

- Should be reconstituted immediately upon removal from the freezer.
- Use only the diluent supplied.
- Withdraw entire contents of the diluent into the syringe.
- To avoid excessive foaming, slowly inject all of the diluent in the syringe into vial of lyophilized vaccine and gently agitate to mix thoroughly.
- Withdraw the entire contents of reconstituted vaccine into a syringe and inject total volume SQ.
- Administer immediately after reconstitution; discard reconstituted vaccine if not used w/in 30 min.
- Do not freeze reconstituted vaccine.

STORAGE

Before Reconstitution: -50°C to -15°C (-58°F to 5°F). May store and/or transport at 2-8°C (36-46°F) for up to 72 continuous hrs prior to reconstitution; discard if

not used w/in 72 hrs of removal from -15°C (5°F). Protect from light. **Diluent:** 20-25°C (68-77°F) or 2-8°C (36-46°F). **After Reconstitution:** Administer immediately; discard if not used w/in 30 min. Do not freeze.

HOW SUPPLIED

Inj: Minimum of 19,400 PFU/0.65mL

CONTRAINDICATIONS

History of anaphylactic/anaphylactoid reaction to gelatin, neomycin, or any other component of the vaccine; immunosuppression or immunodeficiency, including history of primary or acquired immunodeficiency states, leukemia, lymphoma or other malignant neoplasms affecting the bone marrow or lymphatic system, AIDS or other clinical manifestations of infection w/ HIV, and those on immunosuppressive therapy; pregnancy.

WARNINGS/PRECAUTIONS

Avoid pregnancy for 3 months following administration. Serious adverse reactions, including anaphylaxis, reported; adequate treatment provisions (eg, epinephrine inj [1:1000]) should be available for immediate use. Transmission of vaccine virus may occur between vaccinees and susceptible contacts. Consider deferral in acute illness (eg, fever) or in patients w/ active untreated tuberculosis (TB). Duration of protection >4 yrs after vaccination is unknown. May not protect all vaccine recipients.

ADVERSE REACTIONS

Inj-site reactions (erythema, pain, tenderness, swelling, pruritus, warmth), headache.

DRUG INTERACTIONS

See Contraindications. Reduced immune response to Zostavax reported when administered concurrently w/ Pneumovax 23; consider separating administration of the 2 vaccines by at least 4 weeks.

PREGNANCY AND LACTATION

Pregnancy: Contraindicated in pregnancy.
Lactation: Caution in nursing.

MECHANISM OF ACTION

Vaccine; boosts varicella zoster virus-specific immunity and protects against zoster and its complications.

PATIENT CONSIDERATIONS

Assessment: Assess for history of anaphylactic/anaphylactoid reaction to gelatin, neomycin, or any other component of the vaccine; immunosuppression/ immunodeficiency; acute illness; active untreated TB; pregnancy/nursing status; and possible drug interactions.

Monitoring: Monitor for anaphylactic/anaphylactoid reactions and other adverse reactions.

Counseling: Inform of benefits and risks of vaccine, including potential risk of transmitting vaccine virus to susceptible individuals (eg, immunosuppressed/ immunodeficient individuals, pregnant women who have not had chickenpox). Advise patients to inform physician about reactions to previous vaccines and instruct to notify physician if any adverse reactions or any symptoms of concern develop.

ZOSYN — piperacillin/tazobactam   Rx

Class: Beta-lactamase inhibitor/broad-spectrum penicillin (PCN)

ADULT DOSAGE	PEDIATRIC DOSAGE
General Dosing	**Peritonitis**
Usual: 3.375g q6h for 7-10 days; administer by IV infusion over 30 min	**2-9 Months of Age:** (80mg/10mg)/kg q8h
Nosocomial Pneumonia	**≥9 Months of Age: ≤40kg:** (100mg/12.5mg)/kg q8h
Moderate to Severe:	**>40kg:** Use adult dose
Initial: 4.5g q6h plus an aminoglycoside for 7-14 days; administer Zosyn by IV infusion over 30 min	Administer by IV infusion over 30 min
	Appendicitis
Aminoglycoside treatment should be continued in patients from whom *Pseudomonas aeruginosa* is isolated	**2-9 Months of Age:** (80mg/10mg)/kg q8h
	≥9 Months of Age: ≤40kg: (100mg/12.5mg)/kg q8h
Other Indications	**>40kg:** Use adult dose
- Appendicitis (complicated by rupture or abscess)	Administer by IV infusion over 30 min
- Peritonitis	
- Uncomplicated/complicated skin and skin structure infections (eg, cellulitis, cutaneous abscess, ischemic/diabetic foot infections)	
- Postpartum endometritis	
- Pelvic inflammatory disease	
- Moderate community-acquired pneumonia	

DOSING CONSIDERATIONS

Renal Impairment
Adults:
All Indications (Except Nosocomial Pneumonia):
CrCl >40mL/min: 3.375g q6h
CrCl 20-40mL/min: 2.25g q6h
CrCl <20mL/min (Not Receiving Hemodialysis): 2.25g q8h

Hemodialysis: 2.25g q12h (max: 2.25g q12h); administer an additional 0.75g dose following each hemodialysis session on hemodialysis days
Continuous Ambulatory Peritoneal Dialysis: 2.25g q12h
Nosocomial Pneumonia:
CrCl >40mL/min: 4.5g q6h
CrCl 20-40mL/min: 3.375g q6h
CrCl <20mL/min (Not Receiving Hemodialysis): 2.25g q6h
Hemodialysis: 2.25g q8h (max: 2.25g q8h); administer an additional 0.75g dose following each hemodialysis session on hemodialysis days
Continuous Ambulatory Peritoneal Dialysis: 2.25g q8h
Elderly
Start at lower end of dosing range

ADMINISTRATION
IV route

Infuse over 30 min.
During the infusion it is desirable to d/c the primary infusion sol.

Single-Dose Vials
- Reconstitute 2.25g, 3.375g, and 4.5g vials w/ 10mL, 15mL, and 20mL, respectively w/ a compatible reconstitution diluent; swirl until dissolved.
- Further dilute reconstituted sol in a compatible IV sol (recommended volume per dose of 50-150mL).
- Use immediately after reconstitution; discard any unused portion after 24 hrs if stored at 20-25°C (68-77°F) or after 48 hrs if stored at 2-8°C (36-46°F). Do not freeze vials after reconstitution.

- Do not mix w/ other drugs in a syringe or infusion bottle.
- Not chemically stable in sol that contain only sodium bicarbonate and sol that significantly alter the pH.
- Do not add to blood products or albumin hydrolysates.

Compatible Reconstitution Diluents:
- 0.9% NaCl for inj
- Sterile water for inj (SWFI)
- D5
- Bacteriostatic saline/parabens
- Bacteriostatic water/parabens
- Bacteriostatic saline/benzyl alcohol
- Bacteriostatic water/benzyl alcohol

Compatible IV Sol:
- 0.9% NaCl for inj
- SWFI (max recommended volume per dose of SWFI is 50mL)
- Dextran 6% in saline
- D5
- Lactated Ringer's sol (compatible only w/ reformulated Zosyn containing EDTA and is compatible for co-administration via a Y-site)

Galaxy Containers
- Administer using sterile equipment, after thawing to room temperature.
- Zosyn containing EDTA is compatible for co-administration via a Y-site IV tube w/ Lactated Ringer's inj.
- Do not add supplementary medication.
- Discard unused portions.
- Do not use plastic containers in series connections.

Thawing of Plastic Container:
- Thaw frozen container at 20-25°C (68-77°F) or 2-8°C (36-46°F); do not force thaw by immersion in water baths or by microwave irradiation.
- Thawed solution is stable for 14 days at 2-8°C (36-46°F) or 24 hrs at 20-25°C (68-77°F); do not refreeze.

Refer to PI for further stability information and for compatibility w/ aminoglycosides.

STORAGE
Vials: 20-25°C (68-77°F). **Galaxy Containers:** At or below -20°C (-4°F).

HOW SUPPLIED
Inj: (Piperacillin/Tazobactam) 2g/0.25g (2.25g), 3g/0.375g (3.375g), 4g/0.5g (4.5g) [vial]; (2g/0.25g [2.25g])/50mL, (3g/0.375g [3.375g])/50mL, (4g/0.5g [4.5g])/100mL [Galaxy]. Also available as a Pharmacy Bulk Package.

CONTRAINDICATIONS
History of allergic reactions to any of the penicillins, cephalosporins, or β-lactamase inhibitors.

WARNINGS/PRECAUTIONS
See Dosing Considerations. Use w/ care in patients w/ renal impairment or on hemodialysis. Serious and occasionally fatal hypersensitivity (anaphylactic/anaphylactoid) reactions, including shock, reported; d/c and institute appropriate therapy if an allergic reaction occurs. Severe cutaneous adverse reactions (eg, Stevens-Johnson syndrome, toxic epidermal necrolysis, drug reaction w/ eosinophilia and systemic symptoms, acute generalized exanthematous pustulosis) may occur; monitor closely if a skin rash develops and d/c if lesions progress. *Clostridium difficile*-associated diarrhea (CDAD) reported; may need to d/c if CDAD is suspected or confirmed. Bleeding manifestations, sometimes associated w/ abnormalities of coagulation tests, reported; d/c and institute appropriate therapy if bleeding manifestations occur. Leukopenia/neutropenia may occur and is most frequently associated w/ prolonged administration. May cause neuromuscular excitability or convulsions w/ higher than recommended doses, particularly in the presence of renal failure. Caution in patients w/ restricted salt intake. Monitor electrolytes periodically in patients w/ low K+ reserves. May result in bacterial resistance w/ use in the absence of a proven/suspected bacterial infection. Associated w/ increased incidence of fever and rash in cystic fibrosis patients. Lab test interactions may occur.

ADVERSE REACTIONS
Diarrhea, headache, constipation, N/V, rash, pruritus, dyspepsia, insomnia.

DRUG INTERACTIONS
Piperacillin may inactivate aminoglycosides. May decrease serum concentrations of tobramycin; monitor aminoglycoside levels in patients w/ ESRD. Probenecid prolongs $T_{1/2}$; avoid coadministration unless the benefit outweighs the risk. Test coagulation parameters more frequently w/ high doses of heparin, oral anticoagulants, or other drugs that may affect blood coagulation system or thrombocyte function. Caution w/ cytotoxic therapy or diuretics; consider possibility of hypokalemia. **Piperacillin:** May prolong neuromuscular blockade of vecuronium or any nondepolarizing muscle relaxant. May reduce methotrexate (MTX) clearance; frequently monitor MTX levels as well as for the signs/symptoms of MTX toxicity. Increased incidence of acute kidney injury reported w/ concomitant vancomycin as compared to vancomycin alone; monitor kidney function.

PREGNANCY AND LACTATION
Pregnancy: Category B.
Lactation: Caution in nursing.

MECHANISM OF ACTION
Piperacillin: Broad-spectrum penicillin (PCN); exerts bactericidal activity by inhibiting septum formation and cell-wall synthesis of susceptible bacteria.
Tazobactam: β-lactamase enzyme inhibitor.

PHARMACOKINETICS
Distribution: Plasma protein binding (30%); crosses the placenta. Piperacillin: Found in breast milk in low concentrations. **Metabolism:** Piperacillin: Desethyl metabolite (minor microbiologically active). **Elimination:** Kidneys. $T_{1/2}$=0.7-1.2 hrs. Piperacillin: Urine (68% unchanged), bile. Tazobactam: Urine (80% unchanged), bile.

Refer to PI for additional pharmacokinetic parameters.

PATIENT CONSIDERATIONS
Assessment: Assess for previous hypersensitivity reaction to PCN, cephalosporins, or β-lactamase inhibitors; salt intake restriction; cystic fibrosis; low K+ reserves; renal impairment; pregnancy/nursing status; and possible drug interactions.

Monitoring: Monitor hematopoietic function (especially w/ prolonged therapy [≥21 days]), renal function, and serum electrolytes periodically. Monitor for hypersensitivity reactions, CDAD, severe cutaneous reactions, leukopenia/neutropenia, bleeding manifestations, and for neuromuscular excitability or convulsions. Monitor for rash and fever in cystic fibrosis patients.

Counseling: Inform about risks/benefits of therapy. Counsel that drug only treats bacterial, not viral, infections. Instruct to take ud; inform that skipping doses or not completing full course may decrease effectiveness and increase bacterial resistance. Advise to d/c and notify physician if experiencing watery/bloody diarrhea (w/ or w/o stomach cramps and fever) even as late as ≥2 months after the last dose, or an allergic reaction. Instruct to notify physician if pregnant/nursing. Inform that serious hypersensitivity reactions may occur which may require immediate treatment.

ZOVIRAX ORAL — acyclovir   Rx

Class: Nucleoside analogue

ADULT DOSAGE
Herpes Zoster
800mg q4h, 5X/day for 7-10 days
Genital Herpes
Initial:
200mg q4h, 5X/day for 10 days
Recurrent Disease:
Chronic Suppressive Therapy: 400mg bid up to 12 months
Alternative: 200mg 3-5X/day
Intermittent Therapy:
200mg q4h, 5X/day for 5 days
Initiate at earliest sign/symptom of recurrence
Chickenpox
800mg qid for 5 days
Initiate at earliest sign/symptom

PEDIATRIC DOSAGE
Chickenpox
≥2 Years:
≤40kg: 20mg/kg qid for 5 days
>40kg: 800mg qid for 5 days
Initiate at earliest sign/symptom

- -

DOSING CONSIDERATIONS
Renal Impairment
Genital Herpes (Initial/Intermittent Therapy):
CrCl ≤10mL/min: Reduce dose to 200mg q12h

Genital Herpes (Chronic Suppressive Therapy):
CrCl ≤10mL/min: Reduce dose to 200mg q12h

Herpes Zoster/Chickenpox:
CrCl 10-25mL/min: 800mg q8h
CrCl ≤10mL/min: 800mg q12h

Hemodialysis: Adjust dosing schedule so that an additional dose is administered after each dialysis

ADMINISTRATION
Oral route

Bioequivalence of Dosage Forms
Sus shown to be bioequivalent to caps.
One 800mg tab shown to be bioequivalent to four 200mg caps.

STORAGE
15-25°C (59-77°F); protect from moisture.

HOW SUPPLIED
Cap: 200mg; **Sus:** 200mg/5mL [473mL]; **Tab:** 400mg, 800mg

CONTRAINDICATIONS
Hypersensitivity to acyclovir or valacyclovir.

WARNINGS/PRECAUTIONS
Renal failure sometimes resulting in death reported. Thrombotic thrombocytopenic purpura/hemolytic uremic syndrome (TTP/HUS) in immunocompromised patients reported. Maintain adequate hydration. Caution in elderly.

ADVERSE REACTIONS
N/V, diarrhea, malaise.

DRUG INTERACTIONS
Probenecid may increase levels and $T_{1/2}$ of IV formulation. May increase risk of renal impairment and/or CNS symptoms with nephrotoxic agents; use caution.

PREGNANCY AND LACTATION
Pregnancy: Category B.
Lactation: Caution in nursing.

MECHANISM OF ACTION
Synthetic purine nucleoside analogue; stops replication of herpes viral DNA by competitive inhibition of viral DNA polymerase, incorporation into and termination of growing viral DNA chain, and inactivation of viral DNA polymerase.

PHARMACOKINETICS
Absorption: Oral administration of variable doses resulted in different parameters. **Distribution:** Plasma protein binding (9-33%); found in breast milk. **Elimination:** $T_{1/2}$=2.5-3.3 hrs.

PATIENT CONSIDERATIONS
Assessment: Assess for immunocompromised state, hypersensitivity to valacyclovir, renal impairment, nursing status, and possible drug interactions.
Monitoring: Monitor for signs/symptoms of TTP/HUS. Monitor BUN and SrCr.
Counseling: Instruct to consult physician if experiencing severe or troublesome adverse reactions, if pregnant/intending to become pregnant, or intending to breastfeed. Advise to maintain adequate hydration. Inform that therapy is not a cure for genital herpes; advise to avoid contact with lesions or intercourse when lesions/symptoms are present.

ZUBSOLV — buprenorphine/naloxone   CIII

Class: Partial opioid agonist/opioid antagonist

ADULT DOSAGE

Opioid Dependence

Used as part of a complete treatment plan to include counseling and psychosocial support

Administer as single daily dose for maint treatment or in divided doses for induction treatment

One Zubsolv 5.7mg/1.4mg SL tab provides equivalent buprenorphine exposure to one Suboxone 8mg/2mg SL tab

Prior to Induction:
Consider type of opioid dependence (eg, long- or short-acting opioid products), the time since last opioid use, and degree or level of opioid dependence. The 1st dose of therapy should be started only when objective and clear signs of moderate withdrawal are evident

Induction:
Day 1:
Up to 5.7mg/1.4mg is recommended, given as:
Initial: 1.4mg/0.36mg
Remainder of Day 1: Dose of up to 4.2mg/1.08mg should be divided into doses of 1-2 tabs of 1.4mg/0.36mg at 1.5- to 2-hr intervals; some patients (eg, those w/ recent exposure to buprenorphine) may tolerate up to 3 x 1.4mg/0.36mg tabs as a single, second dose

Day 2:
Recommended: Single daily dose of up to 11.4mg/2.9mg

Patients Dependent on Methadone or Long-Acting Opioid Products:
Buprenorphine monotherapy is recommended in patients taking

PEDIATRIC DOSAGE
Pediatric use may not have been established

long-acting opioids when used according to approved administration instructions. Following induction, may transition patient to Zubsolv SL tab qd

Patients Dependent on Heroin or Other Short-Acting Opioid Products:
May be induced w/ Zubsolv SL tab or w/ SL buprenorphine monotherapy. At treatment initiation, Zubsolv dose should be administered when moderate objective signs of opioid withdrawal appear, not <6 hrs after the patient last used opioids

Maint:
Target Dose: 11.4mg/2.9mg as single daily dose
Titrate: Adjust dose progressively in increments/decrements of 1.4mg/0.36mg or 2.9mg/0.71mg to maintain treatment and suppress opioid withdrawal signs and symptoms
Range: 2.9mg/0.71mg to 17.2mg/4.2mg per day, based on individual needs

Conversions

Switching Between Zubsolv and Other Buprenorphine/Naloxone Combination Products:
Dose adjustments may be necessary Monitor for signs of over-medication or under-dosing (eg, withdrawal)
Corresponding Dosage Strengths When Switching Between Suboxone SL Tabs (Including Generic Equivalents) and Zubsolv:
One 2mg/0.5mg Buprenorphine/ Naloxone SL Tab:
One 1.4mg/0.36mg Zubsolv SL tab
4mg/1mg Buprenorphine/Naloxone (Two 2mg/0.5mg SL Tabs):
One 2.9mg/0.71mg Zubsolv SL tab
One 8mg/2mg Buprenorphine/ Naloxone SL Tab:
One 5.7mg/1.4mg Zubsolv SL tab
12mg/3mg Buprenorphine/Naloxone (One 8mg/2mg SL Tab and Two 2mg/0.5mg SL Tabs):
One 8.6mg/2.1mg Zubsolv SL tab
16mg/4mg Buprenorphine/Naloxone (Two 8mg/2mg SL Tabs):
One 11.4mg/2.9mg Zubsolv SL tab

DOSING CONSIDERATIONS
Hepatic Impairment
Moderate: Use may not be appropriate
Severe: Avoid use

Elderly
Start at low end of dosing range

Discontinuation
Should be made as part of a comprehensive treatment plan

ADMINISTRATION
SL route

Do not cut, crush, break, chew, or swallow; SL tab should be placed under tongue until dissolved.
For dosages requiring more than one SL tab, place all tabs in different places under tongue at same time.
Advise patients not to eat or drink anything until tab is completely dissolved. Follow the same manner of dosing w/ continued use to ensure consistency in bioavailability.
If sequential mode of administration is preferred, follow the same manner of dosing w/ continued use to ensure consistency in bioavailability.

STORAGE
20-25°C (68-77°F); excursions permitted to 15-30°C (59-86°F).

HOW SUPPLIED
Tab, SL: (Buprenorphine/Naloxone) 1.4mg/0.36mg, 2.9mg/0.71mg, 5.7mg/1.4mg, 8.6mg/2.1mg, 11.4mg/2.9mg

CONTRAINDICATIONS
Hypersensitivity to buprenorphine or naloxone.

WARNINGS/PRECAUTIONS
Hypersensitivity reactions, bronchospasm, angioneurotic edema, and anaphylactic shock reported. May precipitate opioid withdrawal signs and symptoms if administered before the agonist effects of the opioid have subsided. Not appropriate as an analgesic. Avoid w/ severe hepatic impairment; may be used w/ caution for maintenance treatment in patients w/ moderate hepatic

impairment who have initiated treatment on a buprenorphine product w/o naloxone. May impair mental/physical abilities. May produce orthostatic hypotension in ambulatory patients. Caution w/ debilitated patients, myxedema or hypothyroidism, adrenal cortical insufficiency (eg, Addison's disease), CNS depression or coma, toxic psychoses, prostatic hypertrophy, urethral stricture, acute alcoholism, delirium tremens, kyphoscoliosis, and in elderly. **Buprenorphine:** Potential for abuse. Significant respiratory depression reported; caution w/ compromised respiratory function. To manage overdose, higher than normal doses and repeated administration of naloxone may be necessary. Accidental pediatric exposure can cause fatal respiratory depression. Chronic use produces physical dependence. Cytolytic hepatitis and hepatitis w/ jaundice reported. If a hepatic event is suspected, biological and etiological evaluation is recommended; careful discontinuation may be needed depending on the case. Neonatal abstinence syndrome reported when used during pregnancy. May elevate CSF pressure; caution w/ head injury, intracranial lesions, and other circumstances when CSF pressure may be increased. May produce miosis and changes in consciousness level that may interfere w/ patient evaluation. May increase intracholedochal pressure; caution w/ biliary tract dysfunction. May obscure diagnosis or clinical course of patients w/ acute abdominal conditions.

ADVERSE REACTIONS
Headache, withdrawal syndrome, pain, N/V, sweating, constipation, abdominal pain, vasodilation.

DRUG INTERACTIONS
May cause respiratory depression, coma, and death w/ benzodiazepines or other CNS depressants (eg, alcohol); caution when used concurrently. May cause increased CNS depression w/ opioid analgesics, general anesthetics, benzodiazepines, phenothiazines, other tranquilizers, sedative/hypnotics, or other CNS depressants (eg, alcohol); consider dose reduction of one or both agents if used concomitantly. Concomitant use w/ CYP3A4 inhibitors (eg, ketoconazole, erythromycin, HIV protease inhibitors) should be monitored and may require dose reduction of one or both agents. Monitor for signs/symptoms of opioid withdrawal w/ CYP3A4 inducers (eg, efavirenz, phenobarbital, carbamazepine). Monitor buprenorphine dose in patients on chronic buprenorphine treatment if non-nucleoside reverse transcriptase inhibitors are added to treatment regimen. Atazanavir and atazanavir/ritonavir may increase levels; monitor and consider dose reduction of buprenorphine.

PREGNANCY AND LACTATION
Pregnancy: Category C.
Lactation: Caution in nursing.

MECHANISM OF ACTION
Buprenorphine: Partial agonist at the μ-opioid receptor and antagonist at the kappa-opioid receptor. **Naloxone:** Potent antagonist at the μ-opioid receptor.

PHARMACOKINETICS
Distribution: Plasma protein binding (96%, buprenorphine; 45%, naloxone); found in breast milk (buprenorphine and norbuprenorphine). **Metabolism:** Buprenorphine: N-dealkylation (by CYP3A4) and glucuronidation; norbuprenorphine (major metabolite). Naloxone: Glucuronidation, N-dealkylation, and reduction; naloxone-3-glucuronide (metabolite). **Elimination:** Buprenorphine: Urine (30%), feces (69%); $T_{1/2}$=24-42 hrs. Naloxone: $T_{1/2}$=2-12 hrs.

PATIENT CONSIDERATIONS
Assessment: Assess for history of hypersensitivity reactions, debilitation, myxedema, hypothyroidism, acute alcoholism, adrenal cortical insufficiency (eg, Addison's disease), CNS depression or coma, toxic psychoses, prostatic hypertrophy, urethral stricture, delirium tremens, kyphoscoliosis, biliary tract dysfunction, hepatic impairment, compromised respiratory function, hepatitis B or C infection, head injury, intracranial lesions and other circumstances in which CSF pressure may be increased, acute abdominal conditions, pregnancy/nursing status, and possible drug interactions. Obtain baseline LFTs.
Monitoring: Monitor for hypersensitivity reactions, signs/symptoms of opioid withdrawal, impaired mental/physical ability, orthostatic hypotension, respiratory depression, drug abuse/dependence, cytolytic hepatitis, hepatitis w/ jaundice, elevation of CSF pressure, miosis, changes in consciousness levels, and other adverse reactions. Monitor LFTs periodically. Monitor for over-medication as well as withdrawal or other signs of under-dosing when switching between other buprenorphine/naloxone products.
Counseling: Warn about danger of self-administration of benzodiazepines and other CNS depressants, including alcohol, while on therapy. Advise that the drug contains an opioid that can be a target for abuse; instruct to keep tabs in safe place protected from theft and children. Instruct to seek medical attention immediately if a child is exposed to the drug. Caution that drug may impair mental/physical abilities and cause orthostatic hypotension. Advise to take tab qd after induction and not to change dose w/o consulting physician. Counsel about instructions for missed dose. Inform that treatment can cause dependence and withdrawal syndrome may occur upon discontinuation. Advise patients seeking to d/c treatment w/ buprenorphine for opioid dependence to work closely w/ physician on a tapering schedule, and apprise of the potential to relapse to illicit drug use associated w/ discontinuation of treatment. Advise to report to physician all medications prescribed or currently being used. Advise women regarding possible effects during pregnancy. Advise women who are breastfeeding to monitor the infant for drowsiness and difficulty breathing. Advise to instruct family members that, in event of emergency, the treating physician or staff should be informed that patient is physically dependent on an opioid. Advise to dispose of unused drugs as soon as they are no longer needed by flushing the tabs down the toilet.

ZUPLENZ — ondansetron   Rx
Class: 5-HT₃ receptor antagonist

ADULT DOSAGE
Chemotherapy-Induced Nausea/Vomiting
Prevention of N/V Associated w/ Highly Emetogenic Cancer Chemotherapy (Including Cisplatin ≥50mg/m²):
24mg given successively as three 8mg films administered 30 min before start of single-day chemotherapy
Prevention of N/V Associated w/ Initial and Repeat Courses of Moderately Emetogenic Cancer Chemotherapy:
8mg bid; give 1st dose 30 min before start of chemotherapy, w/ a subsequent dose 8 hrs after 1st dose, then administer 8mg q12h for 1-2 days after completion of chemotherapy

Radiotherapy Associated Nausea/Vomiting
Prevention of N/V Associated w/ Radiotherapy in Patients Receiving Either Total Body Irradiation, Single High-Dose Fraction to the Abdomen, or Daily Fractions to the Abdomen:
8mg tid
Total Body Irradiation:
8mg given 1-2 hrs before each fraction of radiotherapy administered each day
Single High-Dose Fraction Radiotherapy to Abdomen:
8mg given 1-2 hrs before radiotherapy, w/ subsequent doses q8h after 1st dose for 1-2 days after completion of radiotherapy
Daily Fractionated Radiotherapy to Abdomen:
8mg given 1-2 hrs before radiotherapy, w/ subsequent doses q8h after 1st dose for each day radiotherapy is given

Postoperative Nausea/Vomiting
Prevention:
16mg given successively as two 8mg films 1 hr before induction of anesthesia

PEDIATRIC DOSAGE
Chemotherapy-Induced Nausea/Vomiting
Prevention of N/V Associated w/ Initial and Repeat Courses of Moderately Emetogenic Cancer Chemotherapy:
4-11 Years:
4mg tid; give 1st dose 30 min before start of chemotherapy, w/ subsequent doses 4 and 8 hrs after 1st dose, then administer q8h for 1-2 days after completion of chemotherapy
≥12 Years:
8mg bid; give 1st dose 30 min before start of chemotherapy, w/ a subsequent dose 8 hrs after 1st dose, then administer 8mg q12h for 1-2 days after completion of chemotherapy

DOSING CONSIDERATIONS
Hepatic Impairment
Severe (Child-Pugh ≥10):
Max: 8mg/day
ADMINISTRATION
Oral route
1. W/ dry hands, fold pouch along the dotted line to expose the tear notch
2. While still folded, tear the pouch carefully along the edge and remove the oral soluble film from pouch
3. Immediately place film on top of the tongue where it dissolves in 4-20 seconds
4. Once oral soluble film is dissolved, swallow w/ or w/o liquid. Allow each film to dissolve completely before administering the next film
5. Wash hands after administration
STORAGE
20-25°C (68-77°F).
HOW SUPPLIED
Film, Oral: 4mg, 8mg
CONTRAINDICATIONS
Concomitant use with apomorphine, known hypersensitivity to ondansetron.
WARNINGS/PRECAUTIONS
Hypersensitivity reactions reported in patients hypersensitive to other selective 5-HT₃ receptor antagonists; d/c immediately at the 1st sign of hypersensitivity. ECG changes, including QT interval prolongation and torsades de pointes, reported; avoid in patients with congenital long QT syndrome. Serotonin syndrome reported with 5-HT₃ receptor antagonists; d/c and initiate supportive treatment if symptoms occur. Use in patients following abdominal surgery or with chemotherapy-induced N/V may mask a progressive ileus and/or gastric distension. Does not stimulate gastric/intestinal peristalsis; do not use instead of NG suction.
ADVERSE REACTIONS
Headache, diarrhea, malaise/fatigue, constipation, hypoxia, pyrexia, dizziness, gynecological disorder, anxiety/agitation, urinary retention, pruritus.

DRUG INTERACTIONS

See Contraindications. Potent CYP3A4 inducers (eg, phenytoin, carbamazepine, rifampicin) may significantly increase clearance and decrease blood levels. May reduce analgesic activity of tramadol. Serotonin syndrome reported with concomitant use of other serotonergic drugs (eg, SSRIs, SNRIs, MAOIs, mirtazapine, fentanyl).

PREGNANCY AND LACTATION

Category B, caution in nursing.

MECHANISM OF ACTION

Selective 5-HT$_3$ receptor antagonist; has not been established. Blocks 5-HT$_3$ receptors from serotonin. Released serotonin may stimulate the vagal afferents through 5-HT$_3$ receptors and initiate the vomiting reflex.

PHARMACOKINETICS

Absorption: Well-absorbed from GI tract. (Single 8mg dose, fasted, healthy) T_{max}=1.3 hrs; AUC=225ng•hr/mL, C_{max}=37.28ng/mL. **Distribution:** Plasma protein binding (70-76%). **Metabolism:** Extensive via CYP3A4, 1A2, 2D6; hydroxylation (primary), glucuronide/sulfate conjugation. **Elimination:** Urine (5% parent compound); (Single 8mg dose, fasted, healthy) $T_{1/2}$=4.6 hrs.

PATIENT CONSIDERATIONS

Assessment: Assess for previous hypersensitivity to the drug, congenital long QT syndrome, electrolyte abnormalities, congestive heart failure (CHF), bradyarrhythmias, hepatic impairment, pregnancy/nursing status, and possible drug interactions.

Monitoring: Monitor for QT interval prolongation, torsades de pointes, emergence of serotonin syndrome, hypersensitivity reactions, and other adverse reactions. Monitor ECG in patients with electrolyte abnormalities, CHF, bradyarrhythmias, and in patients taking other medications that lead to QT prolongation. In patients who recently underwent abdominal surgery or in patients with chemotherapy-induced N/V, monitor for masking of a progressive ileus and/or gastric distension.

Counseling: Inform about potential benefits/risks of therapy. Inform that drug may cause serious cardiac arrhythmias; instruct patients to contact physician if they perceive a change in their HR, feel lightheaded, or have a syncopal episode. Inform that chances of developing severe cardiac arrhythmias are higher in patients with a personal/family history of abnormal heart rhythms, in patients taking medications that may cause electrolyte abnormalities, and in patients with hypokalemia or hypomagnesemia. Advise of the possibility of serotonin syndrome with concomitant use of other serotonergic agents; instruct to seek immediate medical attention if changes in mental status, autonomic instability, or neuromuscular symptoms with or without GI symptoms occur. Inform that drug may cause headache, malaise/fatigue, constipation, and diarrhea; instruct to report the use of all medications, especially apomorphine or any drug of the 5-HT$_3$ antagonist class, to physician. Inform that drug may cause hypersensitivity reactions, some as severe as anaphylaxis and bronchospasm; instruct to report any hypersensitivity reactions to physician. Instruct on how to use drug.

ZURAMPIC — lesinurad   Rx

Class: Uric acid transporter 1 (URAT1) inhibitor

> Acute renal failure reported; more common when given alone. Use in combination w/ a xanthine oxidase inhibitor.

ADULT DOSAGE	PEDIATRIC DOSAGE
Hyperuricemia	Pediatric use may not have been established
Use w/ a xanthine oxidase inhibitor (eg, allopurinol, febuxostat) for treatment of hyperuricemia associated w/ gout in patients who have not achieved target serum uric acid levels w/ a xanthine oxidase inhibitor alone	
200mg qd	
Not recommended for patients taking daily doses of allopurinol <300mg (or <200mg w/ CrCl <60mL/min)	

DOSING CONSIDERATIONS

Renal Impairment

CrCl <45mL/min: Do not initiate

CrCl Persistently <45mL/min: D/C use

Hepatic Impairment

Severe: Not studied; not recommended

Other Important Considerations

Do not d/c for gout flares; manage as appropriate. Gout flare prophylaxis is recommended when starting treatment

ADMINISTRATION

Oral route

- Take in am w/ food and water; stay well hydrated.
- Take at the same time as morning dose of xanthine oxidase inhibitor.
- Interrupt therapy if treatment w/ xanthine oxidase inhibitor is interrupted.

STORAGE

20-25°C (68-77°F); excursions permitted from 15-30°C (59-86°F). Protect from light.

HOW SUPPLIED

Tab: 200mg

CONTRAINDICATIONS

Severe renal impairment (CrCl <30mL/min), ESRD, kidney transplant recipients, patients on dialysis, tumor lysis syndrome or Lesch-Nyhan syndrome.

WARNINGS/PRECAUTIONS

See Dosing Considerations. Not recommended for treatment of asymptomatic hyperuricemia. Do not use as monotherapy. SrCr elevations reported when used w/ a xanthine oxidase inhibitor. Renal adverse reactions reported after initiation of therapy; evaluate renal function prior to initiation and periodically thereafter. Monitor more frequently if CrCl is <60mL/min or w/ SrCr elevations 1.5-2X the pre-treatment value. Interrupt treatment if SrCr is elevated to >2X the pre-treatment value. Interrupt treatment and measure SrCr promptly if symptoms that may indicate acute uric acid nephropathy (eg, flank pain, N/V) occur. Do not restart w/o another explanation for SrCr abnormalities. Major adverse cardiovascular events observed; relationship w/ treatment has not been established.

ADVERSE REACTIONS

Headache, influenza, increased blood creatinine, GERD.

DRUG INTERACTIONS

Increased exposure w/ CYP2C9 inhibitors, and in CYP2C9 poor metabolizers; use w/ caution w/ moderate CYP2C9 inhibitors (eg, fluconazole, amiodarone), and in CYP2C9 poor metabolizers. Decreased exposure when co-administered w/ moderate CYP2C9 inducers (eg, rifampin, carbamazepine). Possible reduced efficacy of concomitant CYP3A substrates (eg, HMG-CoA inhibitors, sildenafil, amlodipine); monitor efficacy (eg, BP, cholesterol levels). Do not administer w/ epoxide hydrolase inhibitors (eg, valproic acid); may interfere w/ metabolism. Hormonal contraceptives, (eg, oral, injectable, transdermal, implantable forms) may not be reliable; use additional methods of contraception. Aspirin at doses >325mg/day may decrease efficacy of lesinurad in combination w/ allopurinol.

PREGNANCY AND LACTATION

Pregnancy: No teratogenicity or effects on fetal development were observed in embryo-fetal development studies w/ oral administration to pregnant rats and rabbits.

Lactation: Present in the milk of rats; caution in nursing.

MECHANISM OF ACTION

Uric acid transporter 1 (URAT1) inhibitor; reduces serum uric acid levels by inhibiting the function of transporter proteins involved in uric acid reabsorption in the kidney. Inhibits the function of two apical transporters responsible for uric acid reabsorption, URAT1, and organic anion transporter 4.

PHARMACOKINETICS

Absorption: Rapid; absolute bioavailability (approx 100%); T_{max}=1-4 hrs. **Distribution:** Plasma protein binding (>98%); V_d=20L. **Metabolism:** Oxidative metabolism mainly via CYP2C9. **Elimination:** Urine (63%, 30% unchanged), feces (32%); $T_{1/2}$=5 hrs.

PATIENT CONSIDERATIONS

Assessment: Assess tumor lysis syndrome or Lesch-Nyhan syndrome and pregnancy/nursing status. Assess renal function.

Monitoring: Monitor renal function; monitor more frequently if CrCl <60mL/min. Monitor for gout flares and other adverse reactions.

Counseling: Advise on proper use; instruct not to take a missed dose later in the day, to wait to take dose on the next day, and not to double the dose. Advise to stay well hydrated. Inform that renal events have been reported; advise that periodic monitoring of blood creatinine levels are recommended. Inform that gout flares may occur after initiation and of the importance of taking gout flare prophylaxis medication to help prevent gout flares. Advise not to d/c if a gout flare occurs during treatment.

ZUTRIPRO — chlorpheniramine maleate/hydrocodone bitartrate/ pseudoephedrine hydrochloride   CII

Class: Antihistamine/antitussive/decongestant

ADULT DOSAGE	PEDIATRIC DOSAGE
Antihistamine/Cough Suppressant/ Nasal Decongestant	Pediatric use may not have been established
Relief of cough and nasal congestion associated with common cold and symptoms, including nasal congestion associated with upper respiratory allergies	
5mL q4-6 hrs prn	
Max: 4 doses (20mL) in 24 hrs	

DOSING CONSIDERATIONS

Elderly

Start at lower end of dosing range

ADMINISTRATION

Oral route

Measure w/ an accurate mL measuring device; do not use a household tsp to measure dose

STORAGE

20-25°C (68-77°F).

HOW SUPPLIED

Sol: (Hydrocodone bitartrate-Chlorpheniramine maleate-Pseudoephedrine HCl) 5mg-4mg-60mg/5mL [480mL]

CONTRAINDICATIONS

Known hypersensitivity to hydrocodone bitartrate, pseudoephedrine hydrochloride, chlorpheniramine maleate, or any of the inactive ingredients of this medication; coadministration w/ MAOI therapy or w/in 14 days of stopping such therapy; narrow-angle glaucoma; urinary retention; severe HTN; severe coronary artery disease (CAD).

WARNINGS/PRECAUTIONS

Caution with diabetes, thyroid disease, Addison's disease, prostatic hypertrophy or urethral stricture, asthma, severe renal/hepatic impairment, and in elderly. Hydrocodone: May produce dose-related respiratory depression; d/c if it occurs; use naloxone HCl, and other supportive measures when indicated. Risk of psychic/physical dependence, tolerance, and potential for abuse. May elevate CSF pressure in presence of head injury, other intracranial lesions or a preexisting increase in intracranial pressure; avoid use. May obscure clinical course of head injuries and acute abdominal conditions. Hydrocodone/Chlorpheniramine: May impair mental/physical abilities. Pseudoephedrine: May produce cardiovascular (CV) and CNS effects (eg, insomnia, dizziness, weakness, tremor, arrhythmias); caution with CV disorders. CNS stimulation with convulsions or CV collapse with accompanying hypotension reported.

ADVERSE REACTIONS

Sedation, somnolence, mental clouding, lethargy, impairment of mental and physical performance, anxiety, dysphoria, dizziness, psychic dependence, mood changes, nervousness, sleeplessness, visual disturbances, headache.

DRUG INTERACTIONS

See Contraindications. Additive CNS depressant effects with opioids, antihistamines, antipsychotics, anti-anxiety agents, or other CNS depressants (including alcohol); avoid use. Hydrocodone: Coadministration with TCAs may increase the effect of either the antidepressant or hydrocodone. Additive cholinergic blockade may occur with anticholinergics. Hydrocodone/Chlorpheniramine: Anticholinergics may produce paralytic ileus; caution with concomitant use.

PREGNANCY AND LACTATION

Category C, not for use in nursing.

MECHANISM OF ACTION

Hydrocodone: Semisynthetic narcotic antitussive/analgesic; not established, believed to act directly on the cough center. Chlorpheniramine: Antihistamine (H_1-receptor antagonist); possesses anticholinergic and sedative activity. Prevents released histamine from dilating capillaries and causing edema of the respiratory mucosa. Pseudoephedrine: Orally active sympathomimetic amine; exerts decongestant action on the nasal mucosa.

PHARMACOKINETICS

Absorption: Hydrocodone: C_{max}=10.6ng/mL, T_{max}=1.4 hrs. Chlorpheniramine: C_{max}=7.2ng/mL, T_{max}=3.5 hrs. Pseudoephedrine: C_{max}=212ng/mL, T_{max}=1.8 hrs. **Distribution:** Found in breast milk. **Metabolism:** Liver (Pseudoephedrine). **Elimination:** Hydrocodone: $T_{1/2}$=4.9 hrs. Chlorpheniramine: $T_{1/2}$=24 hrs. Pseudoephedrine: Urine (unchanged); $T_{1/2}$=5.6 hrs.

PATIENT CONSIDERATIONS

Assessment: Assess for drug hypersensitivity, narrow-angle glaucoma, urinary retention, severe HTN/CAD, head injury, acute abdominal conditions, CV disorders, diabetes, thyroid disease, asthma, severe renal/hepatic impairment, or any other conditions where treatment is contraindicated or cautioned, pregnancy/nursing status, and for possible drug interactions.

Monitoring: Monitor for drug abuse/dependence, respiratory depression, elevations in CSF pressure, hypersensitivity, and other adverse reactions.

Counseling: Instruct to take as prescribed; counsel not to exceed recommended dose/frequency. Advise to measure sol with accurate mL measuring device; inform that a household tsp is not accurate and could lead to overdosage. Instruct to avoid alcohol and other CNS depressants. Advise to avoid hazardous tasks (eg, operating machinery/driving); inform that therapy may produce drowsiness and impair mental/physical abilities. Caution that therapy can cause drug dependence.

ZYBAN — bupropion hydrochloride   Rx

Class: Aminoketone

> Serious neuropsychiatric reactions reported in patients taking bupropion for smoking cessation. Weigh risks against benefits of use. Antidepressants increased the risk of suicidal thoughts and behavior in children, adolescents, and young adults in short-term trials. Monitor closely for worsening, and for emergence of suicidal thoughts and behavior.

ADULT DOSAGE

Smoking Cessation Aid

Initiate treatment while patient is still smoking.
Patients should set a "target quit date" w/in the first 2 weeks of treatment.
Initial: 150mg qd for first 3 days
Titrate: Increase to 300mg/day, given as 150mg bid w/ an interval of at least 8 hrs between each dose
Max: 300mg/day

Continue treatment for 7-12 weeks; if patient has not quit smoking after 7-12 weeks, should d/c and reassess treatment plan.

PEDIATRIC DOSAGE

Pediatric use may not have been established

May consider continuing therapy in patients who successfully quit smoking after 12 weeks of treatment but do not feel ready to d/c treatment; base longer treatment on individual patient benefits/risks.

Dosing Considerations with MAOIs

Switching to/from an MAOI:
Allow at least 14 days between discontinuation of an MAOI and initiation of treatment and allow at least 14 days between discontinuation of treatment and initiation of an MAOI

Reversible MAOIs (eg, Linezolid, IV Methylene Blue):
Do not start bupropion in patients being treated w/ reversible MAOIs. If acceptable alternatives are not available, d/c bupropion and administer linezolid or IV methylene blue; monitor for 2 weeks or until 24 hrs after the last dose of linezolid or IV methylene blue, whichever comes 1st. May resume bupropion 24 hrs after the last dose of linezolid or IV methylene blue.

DOSING CONSIDERATIONS

Renal Impairment
GFR <90mL/min: Consider reducing dose and/or frequency

Hepatic Impairment
Mild (Child-Pugh Score: 5-6): Consider reducing dose and/or frequency
Moderate to Severe (Child-Pugh Score: 7-15) Max Dose: 150mg qod

ADMINISTRATION

Oral route

Swallow tab whole; do not crush, divide, or chew.
Take w/ or w/o food.
Avoid hs dosing to minimize insomnia.
May be used w/ a nicotine transdermal system.

STORAGE

20-25°C (68-77°F); excursions permitted between 15-30°C (59-86°F). Protect from light and moisture.

HOW SUPPLIED

Tab, Sustained-Release: 150mg

CONTRAINDICATIONS

Seizure disorder. Current/prior diagnosis of bulimia or anorexia nervosa. Undergoing abrupt discontinuation of alcohol, benzodiazepines, barbiturates, or antiepileptic drugs. Use of MAOIs (intended to treat psychiatric disorders) either concomitantly or w/in 14 days of discontinuing treatment. Treatment w/ in 14 days of discontinuing treatment w/ an MAOI. Starting treatment in patients being treated w/ reversible MAOIs (eg, linezolid, IV methylene blue). Known hypersensitivity to bupropion or other ingredients of this medication.

WARNINGS/PRECAUTIONS

Dose-related risk of seizures; do not exceed 300mg/day and titrate gradually. D/C and do not restart treatment if a seizure occurs. May result in elevated BP and HTN. May precipitate a manic, mixed, or hypomanic episode; risk appears to be increased in patients w/ bipolar disorder or who have risk factors for bipolar disorder. Not approved for use in treating bipolar depression. Pupillary dilation that occurs following use may trigger an angle-closure attack in a patient w/ anatomically narrow angles who does not have a patent iridectomy. D/C if an allergic or anaphylactoid/anaphylactic reaction occurs. Arthralgia, myalgia, fever w/ rash, and other serum sickness-like symptoms suggestive of delayed hypersensitivity reported. False (+) urine immunoassay screening tests for amphetamines reported. Caution in the elderly.

ADVERSE REACTIONS

Insomnia, rhinitis, dry mouth, dizziness, disturbed concentration, anxiety, nausea, constipation, arthralgia.

DRUG INTERACTIONS

See Contraindications. CYP2B6 inhibitors (eg, ticlopidine, clopidogrel) may increase bupropion exposure but decrease hydroxybupropion exposure; may need to adjust bupropion dose. CYP2B6 inducers (eg, ritonavir, lopinavir, efavirenz) may decrease exposure; may need to increase bupropion dose but not to exceed max dose. Carbamazepine, phenytoin, and phenobarbital may induce metabolism and decrease exposure; may be necessary to increase dose of bupropion, but not to exceed max dose if used w/ a CYP inducer. May increase exposure of CYP2D6 substrates (eg, venlafaxine, haloperidol, metoprolol, propafenone); may need to decrease dose of CYP2D6 substrate, particularly for drugs w/ a narrow therapeutic index. May reduce efficacy of drugs that require metabolic activation by CYP2D6 to be effective (eg, tamoxifen); may require increased doses of the drug. Use extreme caution w/ other drugs that lower seizure threshold (eg, antipsychotics, theophylline, systemic corticosteroids); use low initial doses and increase gradually. Increased risk of seizure w/ illicit drugs (eg, cocaine), abuse or misuse of prescription drugs (eg, CNS stimulants), oral hypoglycemic drugs, insulin, anorectic drugs, excessive use of alcohol, benzodiazepines, sedative/hypnotics, or opiates. CNS toxicity reported w/ levodopa or amantadine; use w/ caution. Minimize or avoid alcohol. Increased risk of HTN w/ MAOIs or other drugs that increase dopaminergic or noradrenergic activity. Higher incidence of treatment-emergent HTN reported w/ nicotine replacement therapy; monitor BP. Physiological changes resulting from smoking cessation, w/ or w/o bupropion, may alter the pharmacokinetics or pharmacodynamics of certain drugs (eg, theophylline, warfarin, insulin) for which dosage adjustment may be necessary.

PREGNANCY AND LACTATION
Pregnancy: Category C.
Lactation: Caution in nursing.

MECHANISM OF ACTION
Aminoketone; has not been established. Weak inhibitor of the neuronal reuptake of norepinephrine and dopamine. Presumed that action is related to noradrenergic and/or dopaminergic mechanisms.

PHARMACOKINETICS
Absorption: T_{max}=3 hrs; 6 hrs (hydroxybupropion). **Distribution:** Plasma protein binding (84%); found in breast milk. **Metabolism:** Liver (extensive); hydroxylation (CYP2B6), hydroxybupropion (active metabolite). Reduction of carbonyl group, threohydrobupropion, and erythrohydrobupropion (active metabolites). **Elimination:** Urine (87%) and feces (10%), (0.5% unchanged); $T_{1/2}$=21 hrs (bupropion), 20 hrs (hydroxybupropion), 33 hrs (erythrohydrobupropion), 37 hrs (threohydrobupropion).

PATIENT CONSIDERATIONS
Assessment: Assess for bipolar disorder, hepatic/renal dysfunction, susceptibility to angle-closure glaucoma, seizure disorder or conditions that may increase the risk of seizure, hypersensitivity to the drug, any other conditions where treatment is contraindicated or cautioned, pregnancy/nursing status, and possible drug interactions. Assess BP.

Monitoring: Monitor for clinical worsening, suicidality, unusual changes in behavior, seizures, activation of mania or hypomania, neuropsychiatric reactions, angle-closure glaucoma, anaphylactoid/anaphylactic reactions, delayed hypersensitivity, and other adverse reactions. Monitor hepatic/renal function and BP.

Counseling: Inform about benefits/risks of therapy. Advise patients and caregivers to observe for clinical worsening, suicidal risks, and unusual changes in behavior. Inform that quitting smoking may be associated w/ nicotine withdrawal symptoms or exacerbation of preexisting psychiatric illness. Advise to notify physician immediately if agitation, hostility, depressed mood, changes in thinking or behavior, or suicidal ideation/behavior occurs. Educate on the symptoms of hypersensitivity and to d/c if a severe allergic reaction occurs. Instruct to d/c and not restart if a seizure occurs while on therapy. Inform that excessive use or abrupt discontinuation of alcohol, benzodiazepines, antiepileptic drugs, or sedatives/hypnotics can increase the risk of seizure; advise to minimize or avoid alcohol use. Caution about the risk of angle-closure glaucoma. Inform that therapy may impair mental/physical abilities; advise to use caution while operating hazardous machinery/driving. Counsel to notify physician if taking/planning to take any prescription or OTC medications. Advise not to use in combination w/ any other medications that contain bupropion. Advise to notify physician if pregnant, intending to become pregnant, or if nursing. If taking >150mg/day, instruct to take in 2 doses at least 8 hrs apart, to minimize the risk of seizures. Inform that tab may have an odor.

Zyclara — imiquimod   Rx

Class: Immune response modifier

ADULT DOSAGE	PEDIATRIC DOSAGE
Actinic Keratosis	**External Genital and Perianal Warts**
Clinically typical visible or palpable, actinic keratoses of the full face or balding scalp in immunocompetent patients	**≥12 Years:**
	3.75%:
2.5%, 3.75%:	Apply as a thin layer to warts qd before hs until total clearance or for up to 8 weeks; may use up to 0.25g (1 pkt or 1 full pump actuation) at each application.
Apply as a thin film qd to affected area before hs for two 2-week treatment cycles separated by a 2-week no treatment period; may apply up to 0.5g (2 pkts or 2 full pump actuations) to treatment area at each application.	Leave cre on skin for approx 8 hrs, and then remove by washing the area w/ mild soap and water.
Leave cre on skin for approx 8 hrs, and then remove by washing the area w/ mild soap and water.	Prescribe up to 56 pkts or two 7.5g pumps for total treatment course
Prescribe no more than 56 pkts or two 7.5g pumps for total 2-cycle treatment course	
External Genital and Perianal Warts	
3.75%:	
Apply as a thin layer to warts qd before hs until total clearance or for up to 8 weeks; may use up to 0.25g (1 pkt or 1 full pump actuation) at each application.	
Leave cre on skin for approx 8 hrs, and then remove by washing the area w/ mild soap and water.	
Prescribe up to 56 pkts or two 7.5g pumps for total treatment course	

DOSING CONSIDERATIONS
Adverse Reactions
Local Skin Reactions:

Actinic Keratosis:
May take rest period of several days if required
Neither 2-week treatment cycle should be extended due to missed dose or rest periods

External Genital and Perianal Warts:
May need rest period of several days; resume once reaction subsides
May use non-occlusive dressings in management of skin reactions

ADMINISTRATION
Topical route

Wash hands before and after application.
Prime pumps before 1st use by repeatedly depressing the actuator until cre is dispensed.
Rub in until no longer visible.

Actinic Keratosis
Avoid use in or on lips and nostrils or in or near eyes.

STORAGE
25°C (77°F); excursions permitted to 15-30°C (59-86°F). Avoid freezing.

HOW SUPPLIED
Cre: 2.5% [7.5g pump], 3.75% [7.5g pump, 28$]

WARNINGS/PRECAUTIONS
Not for oral, ophthalmic, intra-anal, or intravaginal use. Intense local skin reactions (eg, skin weeping, erosion) may occur; may require dosing interruption. May exacerbate inflammatory skin conditions, including chronic graft-versus-host disease. Severe local inflammatory reactions of the female external genitalia may lead to severe vulvar swelling, which may lead to urinary retention; interrupt or d/c if severe vulvar swelling occurs. Administration not recommended until the skin is healed from any previous drug or surgical treatment. Flu-like signs and symptoms may accompany or precede local skin reactions; consider dosing interruption and assessment of the patient. Lymphadenopathy reported. Avoid or minimize natural or artificial sunlight exposure (including sunlamps). Avoid w/ sunburn until fully recovered. Caution in patients who may have considerable sun exposure (eg, due to their occupation) or w/ inherent sensitivity to sunlight. Avoid use of any other imiquimod products in the same treatment area; may increase risk for and severity of local skin/systemic reactions. Caution w/ preexisting autoimmune conditions.

ADVERSE REACTIONS
Local skin reactions (erythema, scabbing/crusting, flaking/scaling/dryness, edema, erosion/ulceration, exudate), application-site pruritus/pain/irritation, headache, fatigue, influenza-like illness, nausea.

PREGNANCY AND LACTATION
Pregnancy: Category C.
Lactation: Caution in nursing.

MECHANISM OF ACTION
Immune response modifier; mechanism not established. Toll-like receptor 7 agonist that activates immune cells; associated w/ increases in markers for cytokines and immune cells.

PHARMACOKINETICS
Absorption: (Actinic Keratoses) C_{max}=0.323ng/mL, T_{max} (median)=9 hrs. (External Genital and Perianal Warts) C_{max}=0.488ng/mL, T_{max} (median)=12 hrs. **Elimination:** (Actinic Keratoses) $T_{1/2}$=29.3 hrs. (External Genital and Perianal Warts) $T_{1/2}$=24.1 hrs.

PATIENT CONSIDERATIONS
Assessment: Assess for inflammatory skin conditions, sunburn, inherent sensitivity to sunlight, preexisting autoimmune conditions, sunlight exposure, and pregnancy/nursing status.

Monitoring: Monitor for local skin reactions, severe vulvar swelling, flu-like signs/symptoms, other adverse reactions, and response to treatment.

Counseling: Instruct to use ud by physician, wash hands before and after application, and avoid contact w/ eyes, lips, nostrils, anus, and vagina. Advise not to bandage or otherwise occlude treatment area, not to reuse partially used pkts, and to discard pkts after full treatment course completion. Inform that local skin and systemic reactions may occur; instruct to contact physician if these occur. Instruct not to extend treatment cycle >2 weeks (actinic keratoses) or treatment >8 weeks (external genital and perianal warts) due to missed doses or rest periods. **Actinic Keratosis:** Instruct to continue treatment for the full treatment course even if all actinic keratoses appear to be gone. Instruct to wash treatment area w/ mild soap and water before and 8 hrs after application. Instruct to allow treatment area to dry thoroughly before application. Instruct to avoid or minimize exposure to natural or artificial sunlight (tanning beds or UVA/B treatment); encourage to use sunscreen and protective clothing (eg, hat). Inform that additional lesions may become apparent in the treatment area during treatment. **External Genital and Perianal Warts:** Instruct to wash treatment area w/ mild soap and water 8 hrs after application. Instruct to avoid sexual (genital, anal, oral) contact while cre is on the skin. Advise female patients to take special care during application at the vaginal opening. Instruct uncircumcised males treating warts under the foreskin to retract the foreskin and clean the area daily. Inform that new warts may develop during therapy. Inform that drug may weaken condoms and vaginal diaphragms; explain that concurrent use is not recommended. Instruct to remove cre by washing treatment area w/ mild soap and water if severe local skin reaction occurs.

ZYDELIG — idelalisib ℞

Class: Kinase inhibitor

> Fatal and/or serious hepatotoxicity reported; monitor hepatic function prior to and during treatment; interrupt and then reduce or d/c as recommended. Fatal and/or serious and severe diarrhea or colitis reported; monitor for the development of severe diarrhea or colitis; interrupt and then reduce or d/c as recommended. Fatal and serious pneumonitis may occur; monitor for pulmonary symptoms and bilateral interstitial infiltrates; interrupt or d/c as recommended. Fatal and serious intestinal perforation may occur; d/c therapy for intestinal perforation.

ADULT DOSAGE

Relapsed Small Lymphocytic Lymphoma

In Patients Who Have Received at Least 2 Prior Systemic Therapies:
Max Initial: 150mg bid

Relapsed Chronic Lymphocytic Leukemia

Combination w/ Rituximab:
Max Initial: 150mg bid

Relapsed Follicular B-cell Non-Hodgkin Lymphoma

In Patients Who Have Received at Least 2 Prior Systemic Therapies:
Max Initial: 150mg bid

PEDIATRIC DOSAGE
Pediatric use may not have been established

DOSING CONSIDERATIONS
Adverse Reactions
Pneumonitis:
D/C in patients w/ any severity of symptomatic pneumonitis
ALT/AST:
>3-5X ULN: Maintain dose; monitor at least weekly until ≤1X ULN
>5-20X ULN: Withhold treatment; monitor at least weekly until ≤1X ULN, then resume at 100mg bid
>20X ULN: D/C permanently
Bilirubin:
>1.5-3X ULN: Maintain dose; monitor at least weekly until ≤1X ULN
>3-10X ULN: Withhold treatment; monitor at least weekly until ≤1X ULN, then resume at 100mg bid
>10X ULN: D/C permanently
Diarrhea:
Moderate (Increase of 4-6 stools/day): Maintain dose; monitor at least weekly until resolved
Severe (Increase of ≥7 stools/day)/Hospitalization: Withhold treatment; monitor at least weekly until resolved, then resume at 100mg bid
Life-Threatening: D/C permanently
Neutropenia:
ANC 1-<1.5 Gi/L: Maintain dose
ANC 0.5-<1 Gi/L: Maintain dose; monitor at least weekly
ANC <0.5 Gi/L: Interrupt treatment; monitor at least weekly until ANC >0.5 Gi/L, then resume at 100mg bid
Thrombocytopenia:
Platelets 50-<75 Gi/L: Maintain dose
Platelets 25-<50 Gi/L: Maintain dose; monitor at least weekly
Platelets >25 Gi/L: Interrupt treatment; monitor at least weekly, then resume at 100mg bid when platelets ≥25 Gi/L

ADMINISTRATION
Oral route
Swallow tab whole.
Take w/ or w/o food.

STORAGE
20-30°C (68-86°F); excursions permitted to 15-30°C (59-86°F).

HOW SUPPLIED
Tab: 100mg, 150mg

CONTRAINDICATIONS
History of serious allergic reactions, including anaphylaxis and toxic epidermal necrolysis (TEN).

WARNINGS/PRECAUTIONS
TEN reported with rituximab and bendamustine; other severe or life-threatening (Grade ≥3) cutaneous reactions (eg, exfoliative dermatitis, erythematous rash, maculopapular rash, skin disorder) reported in idelalisib-treated patients; monitor for development of severe cutaneous reactions and d/c therapy. Serious allergic reactions (eg, anaphylaxis) reported; d/c permanently and institute appropriate therapy if serious allergic reactions develop. Treatment-emergent Grade 3 or 4 neutropenia reported; monitor blood counts at least every 2 weeks for the first 3 months, and at least weekly while neutrophil counts are <1 Gi/L. May cause fetal harm. If contraceptive methods are being considered, females of reproductive potential should use effective contraception during treatment, and for at least 1 month after the last dose. Monitor for signs of idelalisib toxicity in patients with baseline hepatic impairment.

ADVERSE REACTIONS
Hepatotoxicity, colitis, diarrhea, pneumonitis, intestinal perforation, pyrexia, sepsis, febrile neutropenia, N/V, GERD, stomatitis, headache, chills, pain, rash.

DRUG INTERACTIONS
Avoid with drugs that may cause liver toxicity and drugs that cause diarrhea. Decreased exposure with strong CYP3A inducers (eg, rifampin, phenytoin, St. John's wort, carbamazepine); avoid coadministration. May increase exposure of a sensitive CYP3A substrate; avoid with CYP3A substrates. Increased exposure with strong CYP3A inhibitors; monitor for signs of idelalisib toxicity.

PREGNANCY AND LACTATION
Pregnancy: Category D.
Lactation: Not for use in nursing.

MECHANISM OF ACTION
Phosphatidylinositol 3-kinase inhibitor; induces apoptosis and inhibits proliferation in cell lines derived from malignant B-cells and in primary tumor cells. Inhibits several cell signaling pathways, including B-cell receptor signaling and the CXCR4 and CXCR5 signaling, which are involved in trafficking and homing of B-cells to the lymph nodes and bone marrow. Treatment of lymphoma cells resulted in inhibition of chemotaxis and adhesion, and reduced cell viability.

PHARMACOKINETICS
Absorption: T_{max}=1.5 hrs (fasted, median). **Distribution:** V_d=23L; plasma protein binding (>84%). **Metabolism:** Via aldehyde oxidase and CYP3A, GS-563117 (major metabolite); UGT1A4 (minor metabolism). **Elimination:** (150mg single dose) Urine (14%, 49% [GS-563117]), feces (78%, 44% [GS-563117]); $T_{1/2}$=8.2 hrs.

PATIENT CONSIDERATIONS
Assessment: Assess for history of serious allergic reactions, pregnancy/nursing status, and possible drug interactions. Assess hepatic function.

Monitoring: Monitor for diarrhea, colitis, pulmonary symptoms and bilateral interstitial infiltrates, intestinal perforation, neutropenia, thrombocytopenia, new/worsening abdominal pain, chills, fever, N/V, severe cutaneous reactions, serious allergic reactions, and other adverse reactions. Monitor ALT and AST every 2 weeks for the first 3 months of treatment, every 4 weeks for the next 3 months, then every 1-3 months thereafter. Monitor weekly for liver toxicity if the ALT or AST rises above 3X ULN until resolved. Monitor blood counts at least every 2 weeks for the first 3 months of therapy, and at least weekly in patients while neutrophil counts are <1.0 Gi/L. Monitor for signs of idelalisib toxicity in patients with baseline hepatic impairment.

Counseling: Advise that significant elevations in liver enzymes may occur, and that serial testing of serum liver tests (ALT, AST, bilirubin) are recommended while taking the drug. Instruct to report liver dysfunction symptoms to physician. Advise that severe diarrhea or colitis may occur and to notify physician immediately if bowel movements increase by ≥6/day. Advise of the possibility of pneumonitis, intestinal perforation, severe cutaneous reactions, and anaphylaxis; instruct to contact physician if any signs/symptoms of these conditions develop. Advise of the need for periodic monitoring of blood counts; instruct to notify physician if fever or any signs of infection develop. Advise women of the potential hazard to fetus and to avoid pregnancy during therapy; instruct to use adequate contraception during therapy and for at least 1 month after completing therapy. Advise not to breastfeed during treatment. Instruct to take exactly as prescribed and not to change dose or stop therapy unless told to do so by physician. Advise that if a dose is missed by <6 hrs, to take missed dose right away and take next dose as usual. If a dose is missed by >6 hrs, advise to wait and take next dose at the usual time.

ZYFLO CR — zileuton ℞

Class: 5-lipoxygenase (5-LOX) inhibitor

OTHER BRAND NAMES
Zyflo

ADULT DOSAGE
Asthma

Prophylaxis and Chronic Treatment:
Tab:
600mg qid

Tab, ER:
1200mg bid

PEDIATRIC DOSAGE
Asthma

Prophylaxis and Chronic Treatment:
≥12 Years:
Tab:
600mg qid

Tab, ER:
1200mg bid

ADMINISTRATION
Oral route

Tab
May take w/ meals and hs

Tab, ER
Do not chew, cut, or crush
Take w/in 1 hr after am and pm meals

STORAGE
20-25°C (68-77°F); (Tab, ER) excursions permitted to 15-30°C (59-86°F). Protect from light.

HOW SUPPLIED
Tab: 600mg*; **Tab, Extended-Release (ER):** 600mg *scored

CONTRAINDICATIONS
Active liver disease or transaminase elevations (≥3X ULN), history of allergic reaction to zileuton or any of its inactive ingredients.

WARNINGS/PRECAUTIONS
Not for use in reversal of bronchospasm in acute asthma attacks and status asthmaticus. Elevations of serum ALT/bilirubin may occur; increased risk for

ALT elevation in females >65 yrs of age and those with preexisting transaminase elevations. Symptomatic hepatitis with jaundice may develop. D/C and follow transaminase levels until normal if signs of liver dysfunction or serum transaminase ≥5X ULN occur. Caution in patients who consume substantial quantities of alcohol and/or have a past history of liver disease. Neuropsychiatric events, including sleep disorders and behavior changes, reported; evaluate risks and benefits of continuing treatment.

ADVERSE REACTIONS
Headache, elevation of ALT/bilirubin, nausea, myalgia, upper respiratory tract infection, sinusitis, pharyngolaryngeal pain, diarrhea.

DRUG INTERACTIONS
May increase theophylline and propranolol concentrations; monitor levels and reduce dose as necessary. Monitor use with other β-blockers. May increase warfarin levels; monitor PT or other coagulation tests and adjust dose appropriately. (Tab) Not recommended for use with terfenadine. Monitor use with certain drugs metabolized by CYP3A4 (eg, dihydropyridine calcium channel blockers, cyclosporine, cisapride, astemizole). (Tab, ER) Monitor use with CYP3A4 inhibitors such as ketoconazole.

PREGNANCY AND LACTATION
Category C, not for use in nursing.

MECHANISM OF ACTION
Leukotriene inhibitor; antiasthmatic agent, inhibits leukotriene (LTB$_4$, LTC$_4$, LTD$_4$, and LTE$_4$) formation by inhibiting the enzyme 5-lipoxygenase.

PHARMACOKINETICS
Absorption: (Tab) Rapid; T_{max}=1.7 hrs, C_{max}=4.98mcg/mL, AUC=19.2mcg•hr/mL; (Tab, ER) T_{max}=2.1 hrs (fasting), T_{max}=4.3 hrs (fed). **Distribution:** V_d=1.2L/kg; plasma protein binding (93%). **Metabolism:** Liver, via oxidation by CYP1A2, CYP2C9, CYP3A4. **Elimination:** Urine (94.5%; <0.5% unchanged, <0.5% metabolites), feces (2.2%); (Tab) $T_{1/2}$=2.5 hrs; (Tab, ER) $T_{1/2}$=3.2 hrs.

PATIENT CONSIDERATIONS
Assessment: Assess for active/history of liver disease, acute asthma attacks, status asthmaticus, preexisting transaminase elevation, neuropsychiatric events, alcohol use, previous hypersensitivity, pregnancy/nursing status, and possible drug interactions.

Monitoring: Monitor serum bilirubin level. Monitor serum ALT prior to therapy, once a month for first 3 months, every 2-3 months for remainder of 1st yr, and periodically thereafter. Monitor for signs/symptoms of hepatitis, jaundice, liver dysfunction, neuropsychiatric events (eg, sleep disorders, behavior changes). Monitor alcohol consumption and worsening of asthma.

Counseling: Inform that drug is indicated for chronic treatment, not for acute episodes, of asthma. Instruct to take regularly as prescribed. Advise not to reduce dose or d/c other antiasthma medications unless instructed. Instruct to notify healthcare provider if signs/symptoms of liver dysfunction or neuropsychiatric events occur. Advise to consult physician before starting or discontinuing any prescription or OTC medications. Counsel about potential for liver damage and need for liver enzyme monitoring on regular basis. (Tab, ER) Instruct to take within 1 hr after am and pm meals. Do not cut, crush, or chew.

ZYKADIA — ceritinib   Rx

Class: Kinase inhibitor

ADULT DOSAGE
Metastatic Non-Small Cell Lung Cancer

W/ anaplastic lymphoma kinase-positive metastatic non-small cell lung cancer who have progressed on or are intolerant to crizotinib

750mg qd until disease progression or unacceptable toxicity

Missed Dose

If a dose is missed, make up that dose unless the next dose is due w/in 12 hrs

PEDIATRIC DOSAGE
Pediatric use may not have been established

DOSING CONSIDERATIONS
Concomitant Medications
Strong CYP3A Inhibitors:
Avoid concurrent use; if unavoidable, reduce ceritinib dose by approx 1/3, rounded to the nearest 150mg dose strength
After discontinuation of a strong CYP3A inhibitor, resume ceritinib dose that was taken prior to initiating the strong CYP3A4 inhibitor

Adverse Reactions
Unable to Tolerate 300mg/day: D/C therapy

ALT or AST Elevation:
>5X ULN w/ Total Bilirubin ≤2X ULN: Withhold therapy until recovery to baseline or ≤3X ULN, then resume w/ a 150mg dose reduction
>3X ULN w/ Total Bilirubin >2X ULN (In the Absence of Cholestasis or Hemolysis): Permanently d/c therapy

Treatment-Related Interstitial Lung Disease/Pneumonitis:
Any Grade: Permanently d/c therapy

QTc Interval:
>500 msec on ≥2 Separate ECGs: Withhold therapy until QTc interval is <481 msec or recovery to baseline if baseline QTc is ≥481 msec, then resume w/ a 150mg dose reduction

Prolongation w/ Torsades de Pointes or Polymorphic Ventricular Tachycardia or Signs/Symptoms of Serious Arrhythmia: Permanently d/c therapy
Severe or Intolerable N/V or Diarrhea (Despite Optimal Antiemetic/Antidiarrheal Therapy):
Withhold therapy until improved, then resume w/ a 150mg dose reduction
Persistent Hyperglycemia >250mg/dL (Despite Optimal Antihyperglycemic Therapy):
1. Withhold therapy until hyperglycemia is adequately controlled, then resume w/ a 150mg dose reduction
2. D/C therapy if adequate hyperglycemic control cannot be achieved w/ optimal medical management

Bradycardia:
Symptomatic, Not Life Threatening:
1. Withhold therapy until recovery to asymptomatic bradycardia or to a HR of ≥60 bpm
2. Evaluate concomitant medications known to cause bradycardia and adjust ceritinib dose
Clinically Significant, Requiring Intervention or Life Threatening in Patients Taking a Concomitant Medication Also Known to Cause Bradycardia or Hypotension:
1. Withhold therapy until recovery to asymptomatic bradycardia or to a HR of ≥60 bpm
2. If concomitant medication can be adjusted or discontinued, resume ceritinib w/ a 150mg dose reduction, w/ frequent monitoring
Life Threatening in Patients Not Taking a Concomitant Medication Also Known to Cause Bradycardia or Hypotension:
Permanently d/c therapy

Lipase/Amylase Elevation:
>2X ULN: Withhold and monitor serum lipase and amylase; resume w/ a 150mg dose reduction after recovery to <1.5X ULN

ADMINISTRATION
Oral route

Take on an empty stomach (do not administer w/in 2 hrs of a meal).
If vomiting occurs during treatment, do not administer an additional dose and continue w/ the next scheduled dose.

STORAGE
25°C (77°F); excursions permitted between 15-30°C (59-86°F).

HOW SUPPLIED
Cap: 150mg

WARNINGS/PRECAUTIONS
Diarrhea, N/V, and abdominal pain reported; monitor and manage appropriately. Drug-induced hepatotoxicity reported; monitor LFTs including ALT, AST, and total bilirubin once a month and as clinically indicated, w/ more frequent testing if transaminase elevations occur. Severe, life-threatening, or fatal interstitial lung disease (ILD)/pneumonitis may occur; monitor for pulmonary symptoms. Exclude other potential causes and d/c therapy permanently w/ treatment-related ILD/pneumonitis. QTc interval prolongation may occur; avoid use w/ congenital long QT syndrome. Conduct periodic monitoring w/ ECGs and electrolytes in patients w/ congestive heart failure (CHF), bradyarrhythmias, and electrolyte abnormalities. Hyperglycemia may occur; initiate or optimize anti-hyperglycemic medications. Bradycardia may occur; monitor HR and BP regularly. Pancreatitis reported. May cause fetal harm.

ADVERSE REACTIONS
Increased ALT/AST, N/V, diarrhea, abdominal pain, constipation, esophageal disorder, fatigue, decreased appetite, rash, ILD/pneumonitis, decreased hemoglobin, increased creatinine/glucose/lipase.

DRUG INTERACTIONS
See Dosing Considerations. Caution w/ medications known to prolong QTc interval. Avoid w/ other agents known to cause bradycardia (eg, β-blockers, non-dihydropyridine calcium channel blockers, clonidine). Increased systemic exposure w/ ketoconazole. Avoid w/ strong CYP3A inhibitors. Decreased systemic exposure w/ rifampin. Avoid w/ strong CYP3A inducers (eg, carbamazepine, phenytoin, rifampin). Avoid w/ grapefruit and grapefruit juice. Avoid concurrent use of CYP3A substrates (eg, alfentanil, cyclosporine, tacrolimus) and CYP2C9 substrates (eg, phenytoin, warfarin) w/ narrow therapeutic indices; consider dose reduction of substrates if concomitant use is unavoidable.

PREGNANCY AND LACTATION
Category D, not for use in nursing.

MECHANISM OF ACTION
Tyrosine kinase inhibitor; inhibits anaplastic lymphoma kinase, insulin-like growth factor 1 receptor, insulin receptor, and ROS1.

PHARMACOKINETICS
Absorption: T_{max}=4-6 hrs. **Distribution:** V_d=4230L (single 750mg dose); plasma protein binding (97%). **Metabolism:** Liver via CYP3A. **Elimination:** (single 750mg dose) Feces (92.3%, 68% unchanged), urine (1.3%); $T_{1/2}$=41 hrs.

PATIENT CONSIDERATIONS
Assessment: Assess for congenital long QT syndrome, CHF, bradyarrhythmias, electrolyte abnormalities, hepatic impairment, pregnancy/nursing status, and possible drug interactions. Obtain baseline LFTs, fasting serum glucose, ECG, and lipase and amylase levels.

Monitoring: Monitor for signs/symptoms of GI toxicity, ILD, pneumonitis, QTc interval prolongation, and other adverse reactions. Monitor LFTs once a month and as clinically indicated. Conduct periodic monitoring of ECGs and electrolytes in patients w/ CHF, bradyarrhythmias, electrolyte abnormalities, or who are taking medications known to prolong the QTc interval. Monitor lipase, amylase, and glucose levels, HR, and BP regularly.

Counseling: Inform that diarrhea, N/V, and abdominal pain are the most commonly reported adverse reactions; advise to contact physician for severe or persistent GI symptoms and inform of supportive care options (eg, antiemetics, antidiarrheal medications). Instruct to contact physician immediately for signs/symptoms of hepatotoxicity and hyperglycemia. Inform of the risks of severe or fatal ILD/pneumonitis; advise to immediately report new or worsening respiratory symptoms. Inform of the risks of QTc interval prolongation and bradycardia; advise to contact physician immediately to report new signs/symptoms or changes in/new use of heart/BP medications. Inform of the signs/symptoms of pancreatitis. Advise to inform physician if pregnant. Inform females of reproductive potential of the risk to fetus; advise to use effective contraception during treatment and for at least 2 weeks following completion of therapy. Advise not to breastfeed and not to consume grapefruit and grapefruit juice during treatment.

ZYLET — loteprednol etabonate/tobramycin　　Rx

Class: Aminoglycoside/corticosteroid

ADULT DOSAGE	PEDIATRIC DOSAGE
Steroid-Responsive Inflammatory Ocular Conditions	Pediatric use may not have been established
Instill 1 or 2 drops q4-6h into the conjunctival sac of the affected eye; may increase frequency to q1-2h during the initial 24-48 hrs	
Reduce frequency gradually as condition improves	
Not more than 20mL should be prescribed initially	

ADMINISTRATION
Ocular route

STORAGE
15-25°C (59-77°F). Protect from freezing; store upright.

HOW SUPPLIED
Sus: (Loteprednol Etabonate-Tobramycin) 0.5%-0.3% [5mL, 10mL]

CONTRAINDICATIONS
Most viral diseases of the cornea and conjunctiva, including epithelial herpes simplex keratitis (dendritic keratitis), vaccinia, and varicella; mycobacterial infection of the eye; fungal diseases of ocular structures.

WARNINGS/PRECAUTIONS
Prolonged use may result in glaucoma with optic nerve damage, visual acuity and fields of vision defects; caution with glaucoma and monitor intraocular pressure (IOP) if used for ≥10 days. May result in posterior subcapsular cataract formation. May delay healing and increase incidence of bleb formation if used after cataract surgery, or cause perforations in diseases that cause thinning of the cornea or sclera; initial and renewal of prescription should be made only after examination with aid of magnification (eg, slit-lamp biomicroscopy, fluorescein staining). Prolonged use may suppress host response and thus increase the hazard of secondary ocular infections. May mask infection or enhance existing infection in acute purulent conditions of the eye. Reevaluate if signs and symptoms fail to improve after 2 days. May prolong the course and exacerbate the severity of many viral infections of the eye (including herpes simplex); caution with history of herpes simplex. Fungal infections of the cornea may develop with long-term application; consider fungal invasion in any persistent corneal ulceration where steroid has been used or is in use. Sensitivity to topically applied aminoglycosides may occur; d/c if hypersensitivity develops and institute appropriate therapy. Do not d/c therapy prematurely.

ADVERSE REACTIONS
Superficial punctuate keratitis, increased IOP, burning/stinging upon instillation, headache, vision disorders, discharge, itching, lacrimation disorder, photophobia, corneal deposits, ocular discomfort, eyelid disorder.

PREGNANCY AND LACTATION
Category C, caution in nursing.

MECHANISM OF ACTION
Loteprednol Etabonate: Corticosteroid; has not been established. Suspected to act by induction of phospholipase A_2 inhibitory proteins (lipocortins), which control the biosynthesis of potent inflammatory mediators by inhibiting the release of arachidonic acid. Tobramycin: Aminoglycoside antibiotic; provides action against susceptible organisms.

PHARMACOKINETICS
Distribution: Loteprednol Etabonate: (Systemic) Found in breast milk.

PATIENT CONSIDERATIONS
Assessment: Assess for viral diseases of cornea and conjunctiva (eg, dendritic keratitis, vaccinia, varicella), mycobacterial infection of the eye, fungal diseases of ocular structures, glaucoma, diseases that cause thinning of the cornea or sclera, recent cataract surgery, history of herpes simplex, and pregnancy/nursing status.

Monitoring: Monitor for signs/symptoms of hypersensitivity reactions, glaucoma, defects in visual acuity and fields of vision, posterior subcapsular cataract formation, delayed wound healing, incidence of bleb formation, ocular perforations, exacerbation of viral infections of the eye, secondary infection, and fungal infection of the cornea. Monitor IOP if used ≥10 days.

Counseling: Instruct not to allow dropper tip to touch any surface to avoid contamination. Counsel not to wear soft contact lenses during therapy. Advise to consult physician if pain develops, if redness, itching, or inflammation becomes aggravated, or if signs/symptoms fail to improve after 2 days. Instruct to use ud.

ZYLOPRIM — allopurinol　　Rx

Class: Xanthine oxidase inhibitor

ADULT DOSAGE	PEDIATRIC DOSAGE
Recurrent Calcium Oxalate Calculi	**Secondary Hyperuricemia with Malignancies**
Uric Acid Excretion >800mg/day (Males) and >750mg/day (Females): 200-300mg/day in divided doses or as single equivalent	**<6 Years:** 150mg/day
Titrate: Adjusted up or down depending upon the resultant control of the hyperuricosuria based upon subsequent 24-hr urinary urate determinations	**6-10 Years:** 300mg/day
Gout	Evaluate response after 48 hrs and adjust dose if necessary
Management of signs and symptoms of primary or secondary gout (acute attacks, tophi, joint destruction, uric acid lithiasis, and/or nephropathy)	
Mild Gout: 200-300mg/day **Max:** 800mg/day	
Moderately Severe Tophaceous Gout: 400-600mg/day **Max:** 800mg/day	
Reduction of Flare-Up of Acute Gouty Attacks: **Initial:** 100mg/day **Titrate:** Increase by 100mg/week until serum uric acid level is ≤6mg/dL **Max:** 800mg/day	
Divide dose if >300mg/day	
Uric Acid Nephropathy	
Management of elevated serum and urinary uric acid levels in patients w/ leukemia, lymphoma, and malignancies receiving cancer therapy.	
600-800mg/day for 2-3 days w/ high fluid intake **Max:** 800mg/day	
Divide dose if >300mg/day	
Conversions	
Conversion from a Uricosuric Agent: Gradually reduce dose of uricosuric agent over several weeks while gradually increasing allopurinol to the required dose	

DOSING CONSIDERATIONS
Concomitant Medications
Colchicine/Anti-Inflammatory Agents: While adjusting dose of allopurinol, continue therapy until serum uric acid is normal and no acute gouty attacks occur for months

Renal Impairment
CrCl 10-20mL/min: 200mg/day

CrCl <10mL/min:
Max: 100mg/day

CrCl <3mL/min: Lengthen dosing intervals

ADMINISTRATION
Oral route

Better tolerated if taken following meal
Recommend sufficient fluid intake to yield a daily urinary output of at least 2L; maintain neutral or slightly alkaline urine

STORAGE
15-25°C (59-77°F) in dry place. (300mg) Protect from light.

HOW SUPPLIED
Tab: 100mg*, 300mg* *scored

WARNINGS/PRECAUTIONS
Not for treatment of asymptomatic hyperuricemia. D/C at 1st appearance of skin rash or other signs which indicate an allergic reaction. Hepatotoxicity, elevated serum alkaline phosphatase/transaminase, and bone marrow suppression reported. Monitor LFTs during early stages of therapy with preexisting liver disease. May impair mental/physical abilities. Acute gouty attacks increase during early stages of therapy reported; give colchicine or anti-inflammatory agents. Maintain sufficient fluid intake to yield a daily urinary output of at least 2L and maintain neutral or slightly alkaline urine. Renal failure reported with hyperuricemia secondary to neoplastic diseases; caution with multiple myeloma and congestive myocardial disease. Caution with renal impairment or concurrent illnesses affecting renal function such as HTN and diabetes mellitus (DM); monitor renal function periodically.

ADVERSE REACTIONS
Acute gout attacks, rash, diarrhea, SGOT/SGPT increase, alkaline phosphatase increase, nausea.

DRUG INTERACTIONS

Inhibits oxidation of mercaptopurine; reduce mercaptopurine or azathioprine to 1/3 or 1/4 of usual dose with concomitant use. Prolongs half-life of dicumarol and chlorpropamide. Decreased effects with uricosuric agents. Increased toxicity with thiazide diuretics; monitor renal function. May increase cyclosporine levels; monitor cyclosporine levels and consider possible adjustment of cyclosporine dose. Increased skin rash with ampicillin and amoxicillin. Enhanced bone marrow suppression with cyclophosphamide and other cytotoxic agents among patients with neoplastic disease, except leukemia.

PREGNANCY AND LACTATION

Category C, caution in nursing.

MECHANISM OF ACTION

Xanthine oxidase inhibitor; acts on purine catabolism; reduces production of uric acid by inhibiting biochemical reactions immediately preceding its formation.

PHARMACOKINETICS

Absorption: C_{max}=3mcg/mL (allopurinol), 6.5mcg/mL (oxipurinol); T_{max}=1.5 hrs (allopurinol), 4.5 hrs (oxipurinol). **Distribution:** Found in breast milk. **Metabolism:** Oxidation; oxipurinol (active metabolite). **Elimination:** Kidneys, feces (20%); $T_{1/2}$=1-2 hrs (allopurinol), 15 hrs (oxipurinol).

PATIENT CONSIDERATIONS

Assessment: Assess for renal/hepatic function or preexisting disease, concurrent illnesses affecting renal function (eg, HTN, DM, multiple myeloma, congestive myocardial disease), pregnancy/nursing status, and possible drug interactions. Obtain serum uric acid to provide correct dosage and schedule.

Monitoring: Monitor LFTs, serum uric acid, and renal function periodically. Monitor for signs/symptoms of hepatotoxicity, bone marrow depression, renal dysfunction, hypersensitivity/allergic reaction, and other adverse reactions.

Counseling: Advise to seek medical attention immediately at 1st sign of skin rash, painful urination, blood in urine, irritation of eyes, or swelling of the lips/mouth. Inform that optimal benefit may be delayed for 2-6 weeks of therapy. Encourage to increase fluid intake during therapy to prevent renal stones. Counsel not to double the dose at the next scheduled time if a dose is missed. Inform about certain risks associated when used concomitantly with other drugs (eg, dicumarol, sulfinpyrazone, mercaptopurine). Inform that drowsiness may occur and physical/mental abilities may be impaired. Instruct to take after meals to minimize gastric irritation.

ZYMAXID — gatifloxacin　　　Rx

Class: Fluoroquinolone

ADULT DOSAGE	PEDIATRIC DOSAGE
Bacterial Conjunctivitis	**Bacterial Conjunctivitis**
Day 1: 1 drop in the affected eye(s) q2h while awake, up to 8X/day	**≥1 Year:**
Days 2-7: 1 drop bid-qid while awake	**Day 1:** 1 drop in the affected eye(s) q2h while awake, up to 8X/day
	Days 2-7: 1 drop bid-qid while awake

ADMINISTRATION

Ocular route

STORAGE

15-25°C (59-77°F). Protect from freezing.

HOW SUPPLIED

Sol: 0.5% [2.5mL]

WARNINGS/PRECAUTIONS

For ophthalmic use only; should not be introduced directly into the anterior chamber of the eye. Overgrowth of nonsusceptible organisms, including fungi, may result with prolonged use. D/C use and institute alternative therapy if superinfection occurs. Avoid wearing contact lenses if there are signs and symptoms of bacterial conjunctivitis or during the course of therapy.

ADVERSE REACTIONS

Worsening of the conjunctivitis, eye irritation, dysgeusia, eye pain.

PREGNANCY AND LACTATION

Category C, caution in nursing.

MECHANISM OF ACTION

Fluoroquinolone antibiotic; inhibition of DNA gyrase and topoisomerase IV. DNA gyrase is an essential enzyme involved in replication, transcription, and repair of bacterial DNA. Topoisomerase IV is an enzyme known to play a key role in partitioning of chromosomal DNA during bacterial cell division.

PATIENT CONSIDERATIONS

Assessment: Assess for conjunctivitis, proper diagnosis of causative organisms (eg, slit-lamp biomicroscopy, fluorescein staining), and pregnancy/nursing status.

Monitoring: Monitor for adverse events and overgrowth of nonsusceptible organisms (eg, fungi) with prolonged therapy.

Counseling: Inform that sol is for ophthalmic use only and should not be introduced directly into the anterior chamber of the eye. Advise not to wear contact lenses if there are signs and symptoms of bacterial conjunctivitis and during course of therapy. Instruct to avoid contaminating the applicator tip with material from the eyes, fingers, or other sources.

ZYPREXA — olanzapine　　　Rx

Class: Atypical antipsychotic

> Elderly patients w/ dementia-related psychosis treated w/ antipsychotic drugs are at an increased risk of death; most deaths appeared to be cardiovascular (eg, heart failure, sudden death) or infectious (eg, pneumonia) in nature. Not approved for the treatment of patients w/ dementia-related psychosis. When used w/ fluoxetine, refer to the Boxed Warning section of the PI for Symbyax.

OTHER BRAND NAMES

Zyprexa Zydis

ADULT DOSAGE

Bipolar I Disorder

Oral:
Manic or Mixed Episodes (Monotherapy):
Initial: 10mg or 15mg qd
Titrate: Adjust by increments/decrements of 5mg qd at intervals of not <24 hrs
Max: 20mg/day
Maint: 5-20mg/day

Manic or Mixed Episodes (w/ Lithium or Valproate):
Initial: 10mg qd
Max: 20mg/day

Depressive Episodes (w/ Fluoxetine):
Initial: 5mg w/ 20mg fluoxetine qpm
Range: 5-12.5mg w/ 20-50mg fluoxetine
Max: 18mg w/ 75mg fluoxetine

Agitation

Acute Agitation Associated w/ Schizophrenia and Bipolar I Mania:
IM:
10mg; consider 5mg or 7.5mg when clinical factors warrant
Range: 2.5-10mg. Assess for orthostatic hypotension prior to any subsequent dosing
Max: 3 doses of 10mg 2-4 hrs apart
May initiate PO therapy in a range of 5-20mg/day as soon as clinically appropriate, if ongoing therapy is indicated

Depression

Treatment-Resistant Depression (w/ Fluoxetine):
Oral:
Initial: 5mg w/ 20mg fluoxetine qpm
Range: 5-20mg w/ 20-50mg fluoxetine
Max: 18mg w/ 75mg fluoxetine

Schizophrenia

Oral:
Initial: 5-10mg qd
Target Dose: 10mg/day w/in several days. Adjust dose by increments/decrements of 5mg qd at intervals of not <1 week
Max: 20mg/day
Maint: 10-20mg/day

PEDIATRIC DOSAGE

Schizophrenia

13-17 Years:
Oral:
Initial: 2.5mg or 5mg qd
Target Dose: 10mg/day. Adjust dose by increments/decrements of 2.5mg or 5mg
Max: 20mg/day
Maint: Use lowest dose needed to maintain remission

Bipolar I Disorder

Oral:
Manic or Mixed Episodes:
13-17 Years:
Initial: 2.5mg or 5mg qd
Target Dose: 10mg/day. Adjust dose by increments/decrements of 2.5mg or 5mg
Max: 20mg/day
Maint: Use lowest dose needed to maintain remission

Depressive Episodes (w/ Fluoxetine):
10-17 Years:
Initial: 2.5mg w/ 20mg fluoxetine qpm
Max: 12mg w/ 50mg fluoxetine

DOSING CONSIDERATIONS

Hepatic Impairment

Zyprexa and Fluoxetine in Combination: Starting dose of oral olanzapine 2.5-5mg w/ fluoxetine 20mg

Elderly

IM Dosing: 5mg/inj

Other Important Considerations

Debilitated/Predisposed to Hypotension/Slower Metabolizers/Sensitive to Olanzapine:
Schizophrenia: 5mg as a starting dose; when indicated, escalate dose w/ caution
IM Dosing: 2.5mg/inj

Predisposed to Hypotension/Slow Metabolizers of Olanzapine or Fluoxetine/Sensitive to Olanzapine:
Zyprexa and Fluoxetine in Combination: Starting dose of oral olanzapine 2.5-5mg w/ fluoxetine 20mg

ADMINISTRATION

Oral/IM routes

Tab; Tab, Disintegrating
Take w/o regard to meals.

Inj
Do not administer IV or SQ. Inject IM slowly, deep into the muscle mass.

Dissolve the contents of the vial using 2.1mL of sterile water for inj to provide approx 5mg/mL of olanzapine.
Use immediately (w/in 1 hr) after reconstitution.
Do not combine in a syringe w/ diazepam inj or w/ haloperidol inj.
Do not reconstitute w/ lorazepam inj.

Tab, Disintegrating
After opening sachet, peel back foil on blister.
Do not push tab through foil.
Upon opening the blister, remove tab and place entire tab in the mouth using dry hands.
Disintegration occurs rapidly in saliva so it can be easily swallowed w/ or w/o liquid.

STORAGE
20-25°C (68-77°F); excursions permitted between 15-30°C (59-86°F). **Reconstituted Inj:** 20-25°C (68-77°F) for up to 1 hr; excursions permitted between 15-30°C (59-86°F). **Tab/Tab, Disintegrating:** Protect from light and moisture. **Inj:** Protect from light. Do not freeze.

HOW SUPPLIED
Inj: 10mg; **Tab:** 2.5mg, 5mg, 7.5mg, 10mg, 15mg, 20mg; **Tab, Disintegrating:** (Zydis) 5mg, 10mg, 15mg, 20mg

CONTRAINDICATIONS
When used w/ fluoxetine, refer to the Symbyax PI. When used w/ lithium or valproate, refer to the individual PIs.

WARNINGS/PRECAUTIONS
Supervision should accompany therapy in patients at high risk of attempted suicide. Neuroleptic malignant syndrome (NMS) reported; d/c and instill intensive symptomatic treatment and monitoring. Associated w/ metabolic changes including hyperglycemia, dyslipidemia, and weight gain; may be associated w/ increased cardiovascular/cerebrovascular risk. Hyperglycemia, in some cases extreme and associated w/ ketoacidosis or hyperosmolar coma or death, reported; caution in patients w/ diabetes mellitus or borderline increased blood glucose levels. Dose-related hyperprolactinemia reported. Tardive dyskinesia (TD) may develop; consider discontinuation if signs/symptoms develop unless treatment is required despite the presence of the syndrome. May induce orthostatic hypotension; caution w/ known cardiovascular disease (CVD), cerebrovascular disease, and conditions that would predispose to hypotension. Leukopenia, neutropenia, and agranulocytosis reported; consider discontinuing at 1st sign of a clinically significant decline in WBC count in the absence of other causative factors. D/C if severe neutropenia (ANC <1000/mm³) develops. May cause esophageal dysmotility and aspiration, and disruption of body temperature regulation. Seizures reported; caution w/ history of seizures or w/ conditions that potentially lower the seizure threshold. Not approved for treatment of patients w/ Alzheimer's disease. May impair mental/physical abilities. Caution in patients w/ clinically significant prostatic hypertrophy, narrow-angle glaucoma, history of paralytic ileus or related conditions, cardiac patients, and in the elderly.

ADVERSE REACTIONS
Postural hypotension, constipation, dry mouth, weight gain, somnolence, dizziness, personality disorder, akathisia, asthenia, dyspepsia, tremor, increased appetite, abdominal pain, headache, insomnia.

DRUG INTERACTIONS
May potentiate orthostatic hypotension w/ diazepam and alcohol. Increased clearance w/ carbamazepine (CYP1A2 inducer), and omeprazole and rifampin (CYP1A2 inducers or glucuronyl transferase inducers). Decreased clearance w/ fluoxetine (CYP2D6 inhibitor) and fluvoxamine (CYP1A2 inhibitor); consider lower dose of olanzapine w/ concomitant fluvoxamine. Caution w/ other centrally acting drugs, alcohol, and drugs whose effects can induce hypotension, bradycardia, or respiratory/CNS depression. May enhance effects of certain antihypertensives. May antagonize effects of levodopa and dopamine agonists. Caution w/ anticholinergic drugs; may contribute to an elevation in core body temperature. **IM:** Not recommended w/ parenteral benzodiazepines. IM lorazepam may potentiate somnolence. **Oral:** Decreased levels w/ activated charcoal.

PREGNANCY AND LACTATION
Pregnancy: Category C.
Lactation: Not for use in nursing.

MECHANISM OF ACTION
Thienobenzodiazepine; not established. Proposed that efficacy in schizophrenia is mediated through a combination of dopamine and serotonin type 2 ($5HT_2$) antagonism.

PHARMACOKINETICS
Absorption: (PO) Well-absorbed, T_{max}=6 hrs; (IM) Rapid, T_{max}=15-45 min. **Distribution:** Found in breast milk. (PO) V_d=1000L; plasma protein binding (93%). **Metabolism:** Via direct glucuronidation and CYP450-mediated oxidation; 10-N-glucuronide and 4'-N-desmethyl olanzapine (major metabolites). **Elimination:** (PO) Urine (57%, 7% unchanged), feces (30%); $T_{1/2}$=21-54 hrs.

PATIENT CONSIDERATIONS
Assessment: Assess for CVD, cerebrovascular disease, risk of hypotension, history of seizures or conditions that could lower the seizure threshold, prostatic hypertrophy, narrow-angle glaucoma, history of paralytic ileus, hepatic impairment, risk factors for leukopenia/neutropenia, pregnancy/nursing status, and possible drug interactions. Assess for dementia-related psychosis and Alzheimer's disease in the elderly. Obtain baseline lipid profile, CBC, and FPG levels.

Monitoring: Monitor for signs/symptoms of NMS, TD, orthostatic hypotension, seizures, disruption of body temperature regulation, hyperprolactinemia, and other adverse reactions. Periodically monitor FPG, lipid levels, CBC, and weight of patient. In patients w/ clinically significant neutropenia, monitor for fever or

other symptoms/signs of infection. Periodically reassess to determine the need for maintenance treatment.

Counseling: Advise of potential benefits and risks of therapy. Counsel about the signs and symptoms of NMS. Inform of potential risk of hyperglycemia-related adverse events. Inform that medication may cause dyslipidemia and weight gain. Inform that medication may cause orthostatic hypotension; instruct to contact physician if dizziness, fast or slow heartbeat, or fainting occurs. Inform that medication may impair judgment, thinking, or motor skills; instruct to use caution when operating hazardous machinery, including automobiles. Instruct to avoid overheating and dehydration and to contact physician if severely ill and have symptoms of dehydration. Instruct to notify physician if taking, planning to take, or have stopped taking any prescription or OTC products, including herbal supplements. Instruct to avoid alcohol. Inform that orally disintegrating tab contains phenylalanine. Advise to notify physician if pregnant or planning to become pregnant during treatment. Advise to avoid breastfeeding during therapy.

ZYPREXA RELPREVV — olanzapine   Rx
Class: Atypical antipsychotic

> Adverse events w/ signs and symptoms consistent w/ overdose, in particular, sedation (including coma) and/or delirium reported following inj. Must be administered in a registered healthcare facility w/ ready access to emergency response services. Observe patient for at least 3 hrs after each inj. Available only through a restricted distribution program called Zyprexa Relprevv Patient Care Program and requires prescriber, healthcare facility, patient, and pharmacy enrollment. Elderly patients w/ dementia-related psychosis treated w/ antipsychotic drugs are at an increased risk of death; most deaths appeared to be cardiovascular (eg, heart failure, sudden death) or infectious (eg, pneumonia) in nature. Not approved for the treatment of patients w/ dementia-related psychosis.

ADULT DOSAGE
Schizophrenia
Establish tolerability w/ oral olanzapine prior to initiating treatment
Range: 150-300mg IM every 2 weeks or 405mg IM every 4 weeks
Max: 405mg IM every 4 weeks or 300mg IM every 2 weeks

Conversions
10mg/day Oral Olanzapine:
Initial: 210mg every 2 weeks or 405mg every 4 weeks for the first 8 weeks
Maint: 150mg every 2 weeks or 300mg every 4 weeks

15mg/day Oral Olanzapine:
Initial: 300mg every 2 weeks for the first 8 weeks
Maint: 210mg every 2 weeks or 405mg every 4 weeks

20mg/day Oral Olanzapine:
Initial/Maint: 300mg every 2 weeks

PEDIATRIC DOSAGE
Pediatric use may not have been established

DOSING CONSIDERATIONS
Elderly
Consider lower starting dose

Other Important Considerations
Debilitated/Predisposition to Hypotension/Slow Metabolizers/Sensitive to Olanzapine:
Initial: 150mg IM every 4 weeks
Titrate: When indicated, escalate dose w/ caution

ADMINISTRATION
IM route
Use gloves when reconstituting; flush w/ water if contact is made w/ skin.
Must be suspended using only the diluent supplied in the convenience kit.

Reconstitution
1. Determine amount of diluent to be added to powder for reconstitution of each vial strength; refer to PI.
2. Inject diluent into the powder vial. Shake the vial vigorously until the sus appears smooth and is consistent in color and texture; suspended product will be yellow and opaque.
3. If foam forms, let vial stand to allow foam to dissipate.
4. If not used right away, shake product vigorously to re-suspend; reconstituted product remains stable for up to 24 hrs in the vial.

Injecting
1. Before administering, confirm there will be someone to accompany the patient after the 3-hr observation period. If this cannot be confirmed, do not give the inj.
2. Refer to PI to determine the final volume to inject. Sus concentration is 150mg/mL.
3. For administration, select the 19-gauge, 1.5-inch (38mm) Hypodermic Needle-Pro needle w/ needle protection device. For obese patients, a 2-inch (50mm), 19-gauge or larger needle (not included in convenience kit) may be used. To help prevent clogging, a 19-gauge or larger needle must be used.
4. Once the sus has been removed from the vial, it should be injected immediately.
5. Administer by deep IM gluteal inj only; do not administer IV or SQ.
6. After insertion of the needle into the muscle, aspirate for several sec to ensure

that no blood appears. If any blood is drawn into the syringe, discard the syringe and the dose and begin w/ a new convenience kit. The inj should be performed w/ steady, continuous pressure.

7. Do not massage the inj site.

STORAGE
Room temperature ≤30°C (86°F). **Reconstituted Sol:** May store at room temperature for 24 hrs. Use immediately once withdrawn into the syringe.

HOW SUPPLIED
Inj, Extended-Release: 210mg, 300mg, 405mg

WARNINGS/PRECAUTIONS
Supervision should accompany therapy in patients at high risk for attempted suicide. Neuroleptic malignant syndrome (NMS) reported; d/c and instill intensive symptomatic treatment and monitoring. Associated w/ metabolic changes, including hyperglycemia, dyslipidemia, and weight gain, which may be associated w/ increased cardiovascular/cerebrovascular risk. Hyperglycemia, in some cases extreme and associated w/ ketoacidosis or hyperosmolar coma or death, reported; caution in patients w/ diabetes mellitus or borderline increased blood glucose levels. Dose-related hyperprolactinemia reported. Tardive dyskinesia (TD) may develop; consider discontinuation if signs/symptoms develop unless treatment is required despite the presence of the syndrome. May induce orthostatic hypotension; caution w/ known cardiovascular disease (CVD), cerebrovascular disease, and conditions that would predispose to hypotension. Leukopenia, neutropenia, and agranulocytosis reported; consider discontinuation at 1st sign of clinically significant decline in WBC count in the absence of other causative factors. D/C if severe neutropenia (ANC <1000/mm^3) develops. May cause esophageal dysmotility and aspiration, and disruption of body temperature regulation. Seizures reported; caution w/ history of seizures or w/ conditions that potentially lower the seizure threshold. Not approved for use in patients w/ Alzheimer's disease. May impair mental/physical abilities. Caution in patients w/ clinically significant prostatic hypertrophy, narrow-angle glaucoma, history of paralytic ileus or related conditions, cardiac patients, and in the elderly.

ADVERSE REACTIONS
Headache, sedation, diarrhea, cough, back pain, N/V, nasal congestion, dry mouth, nasopharyngitis, weight gain, abdominal pain, somnolence, increased appetite.

DRUG INTERACTIONS
May potentiate orthostatic hypotension w/ diazepam and alcohol. Increased clearance w/ carbamazepine (CYP1A2 inducer), and omeprazole and rifampin (CYP1A2 inducers or glucuronyl transferase inducers). Decreased clearance w/ fluoxetine (CYP2D6 inhibitor) and fluvoxamine (CYP1A2 inhibitor); consider lower dose of olanzapine w/ concomitant fluvoxamine. Caution w/ other centrally acting drugs, alcohol, and drugs whose effects can induce hypotension, bradycardia, or respiratory/CNS depression. May enhance effects of certain antihypertensive agents. May antagonize effects of levodopa and dopamine agonists. Caution w/ anticholinergic drugs; may contribute to an elevation in core body temperature. IM lorazepam may potentiate somnolence. Monitor for excessive sedation and cardiorespiratory depression w/ parenteral benzodiazepines.

PREGNANCY AND LACTATION
Pregnancy: Category C.
Lactation: Not for use in nursing.

MECHANISM OF ACTION
Thienobenzodiazepine; not established. Proposed that efficacy in schizophrenia is mediated through a combination of dopamine and serotonin type 2 (5HT$_2$) antagonism.

PHARMACOKINETICS
Absorption: (Zyprexa IntraMuscular) Rapid, T_{max}=15-45 min. **Distribution:** V_d=1000L; plasma protein binding (93%); (PO) found in breast milk. **Metabolism:** Via direct glucuronidation and CYP450 mediated oxidation; 10-N-glucuronide, 4'-N-desmethyl olanzapine (major metabolites). **Elimination:** (PO) Urine (57%, 7% unchanged), feces (30%); $T_{1/2}$=30 days.

PATIENT CONSIDERATIONS
Assessment: Assess for tolerability w/ oral olanzapine, CVD, cerebrovascular disease, risk of hypotension, history of seizures or conditions that could lower the seizure threshold, prostatic hypertrophy, narrow-angle glaucoma, history of paralytic ileus, risk factors for leukopenia/neutropenia, pregnancy/nursing status, and possible drug interactions. Assess for dementia-related psychosis and Alzheimer's disease in the elderly. Obtain baseline lipid profile, CBC, and FPG levels.

Monitoring: Monitor for sedation and/or delirium for at least 3 hrs post-inj. Monitor for signs/symptoms of NMS, TD, orthostatic hypotension, seizures, disruption of body temperature regulation, hyperprolactinemia, and other adverse reactions. In patients w/ clinically significant neutropenia, monitor for fever or other symptoms/signs of infection. In high-risk patients, monitor closely for a suicide attempt. Perform periodic monitoring of FPG, lipid levels, and weight of patient. Perform frequent monitoring of CBC in patients w/ a history of a clinically significant low WBC count or drug-induced leukopenia/neutropenia.

Counseling: Advise of potential benefits and risks of therapy. Advise of the risk of post-inj delirium/sedation syndrome following administration; advise not to drive or operate heavy machinery for rest of the day. Counsel about the signs/symptoms of NMS. Inform of potential risk of hyperglycemia-related adverse events. Counsel that medication may cause dyslipidemia and weight gain. Inform that medication may cause orthostatic hypotension; instruct to contact physician if dizziness, fast or slow heartbeat, or fainting occurs. Inform that medication may impair judgment, thinking, or motor skills; instruct to use caution when operating hazardous machinery, including automobiles. Instruct to avoid overheating and dehydration. Instruct to notify physician if taking, planning to take, or have stopped taking any prescription or OTC drugs, including herbal supplements. Instruct to avoid alcohol. Advise to notify physician if pregnant/planning to become pregnant during treatment. Advise to avoid breastfeeding during therapy.

ZYTIGA — abiraterone acetate   Rx
Class: Antiandrogen

ADULT DOSAGE	PEDIATRIC DOSAGE
Metastatic Castration-Resistant Prostate Cancer 1000mg qd w/ prednisone 5mg PO bid	Pediatric use may not have been established

DOSING CONSIDERATIONS
Concomitant Medications
Strong CYP3A4 Inducers (eg, Phenytoin, Carbamazepine, Rifampin):
Avoid concomitant strong CYP3A4 inducers during treatment
If a strong CYP3A4 inducer must be coadministered, increase the abiraterone dosing frequency to bid only during the coadministration period (eg, from 1000mg qd to 1000mg bid); reduce dose back to the previous dose/frequency if inducer is discontinued

Hepatic Impairment
Moderate (Child-Pugh Class B): Reduce dose to 250mg qd
Severe (Child-Pugh Class C): Not recommended

Adverse Reactions
Elevations in ALT and/or AST >5X ULN or Total Bilirubin >3X ULN w/ Baseline Moderate Hepatic Impairment:
D/C use and do not retreat

Development of Hepatotoxicity During Treatment (ALT and/or AST >5X ULN or Total Bilirubin >3X ULN):
Interrupt treatment; may restart at a reduced dose of 750mg qd following return of LFTs to baseline or to AST and ALT ≤2.5X ULN and total bilirubin ≤1.5X ULN
If hepatotoxicity recurs at 750mg qd, may restart retreatment at 500mg qd, following return of LFTs to baseline or to AST and ALT ≤2.5X ULN and total bilirubin ≤1.5X ULN
If hepatotoxicity recurs at 500mg qd, d/c treatment
Permanently d/c for patients who develop a concurrent elevation of ALT >3X ULN and total bilirubin >2X ULN in the absence of biliary obstruction or other causes responsible for the concurrent elevation

ADMINISTRATION
Oral route

Swallow tab whole w/ water; do not crush or chew.
Take on an empty stomach; no food should be consumed for at least 2 hrs before and 1 hr after the dose is taken.
Women who are pregnant or may be pregnant should not handle drug w/o protection (eg, gloves).

STORAGE
20-25°C (68-77°F); excursions permitted from 15-30°C (59-86°F).

HOW SUPPLIED
Tab: 250mg

CONTRAINDICATIONS
Women who are or may become pregnant.

WARNINGS/PRECAUTIONS
See Dosing Considerations. May cause HTN, hypokalemia, and fluid retention; caution w/ history of cardiovascular disease (CVD) or w/ underlying medical conditions that might be compromised by increases in BP, hypokalemia, or fluid retention. Adrenocortical insufficiency reported in patients receiving abiraterone in combination w/ prednisone, following interruption of daily steroids and/or w/ concurrent infection or stress; use caution and monitor for signs/symptoms, particularly if patients are withdrawn from prednisone, have prednisone dose reductions, or experience unusual stress. Signs/symptoms of adrenocortical insufficiency may be masked by adverse reactions associated w/ mineralocorticoid excess. Increased dosage of corticosteroids may be indicated before, during, and after stressful situations. ALT/AST increases, severe hepatic toxicity, including fulminant hepatitis, acute liver failure and deaths reported; promptly measure serum total bilirubin, AST, and ALT if signs/symptoms suggestive of hepatotoxicity develop. Safety of retreatment of patients who develop AST or ALT ≥20X ULN and/or bilirubin ≥10X ULN is unknown.

ADVERSE REACTIONS
Fatigue, joint swelling/discomfort, edema, hot flush, diarrhea, vomiting, cough, HTN, dyspnea, UTI, contusion, hypertriglyceridemia, elevated AST/ALT.

DRUG INTERACTIONS
See Dosing Considerations. Rifampin (strong CYP3A4 inducer) reported to decrease exposure. Increased levels of dextromethorphan (CYP2D6 substrate) reported. Avoid coadministration w/ CYP2D6 substrates w/ narrow therapeutic index (eg, thioridazine); if alternative treatments cannot be used, exercise caution and consider dose reduction of the concomitant CYP2D6 substrate. Increased exposure of pioglitazone (CYP2C8 substrate) reported; monitor closely for signs of toxicity related to a CYP2C8 substrate w/ narrow therapeutic index if used concomitantly.

PREGNANCY AND LACTATION
Pregnancy: Category X, may cause fetal harm.
Lactation: Not for use in nursing.

MECHANISM OF ACTION
Androgen biosynthesis inhibitor; inhibits 17 α-hydroxylase/C17,20-lyase (CYP17), an enzyme expressed in testicular, adrenal, and prostatic tumor tissues and required for androgen biosynthesis.

PHARMACOKINETICS
Absorption: T_{max}=2 hrs (median); C_{max}=226ng/mL; AUC=993ng•hr/mL.
Distribution: V_d=19,669L; plasma protein binding (>99%). **Metabolism:** Hydrolysis via esterase to abiraterone (active metabolite). **Elimination:** Feces (approx 88%, approx 55% unchanged), urine (approx 5%); $T_{1/2}$=12 hrs.

PATIENT CONSIDERATIONS
Assessment: Assess for hepatic impairment, history of CVD and underlying medical conditions that might be compromised by increases in BP, hypokalemia, or fluid retention, and for possible drug interactions. Obtain baseline AST, ALT, and bilirubin levels. Control HTN and correct hypokalemia before treatment.

Monitoring: Monitor for HTN, hypokalemia, and fluid retention at least monthly, signs/symptoms of adrenocortical insufficiency, and other adverse reactions. Monitor ALT, AST, and bilirubin levels every 2 weeks for the first 3 months (or weekly for the 1st month, then every 2 weeks for the following 2 months in patients w/ baseline moderate hepatic impairment), and monthly thereafter. For patients who resume treatment after development of hepatotoxicity, monitor serum transaminases and bilirubin at a minimum of every 2 weeks for 3 months, and monthly thereafter.

Counseling: Inform that drug is used together w/ prednisone and instruct to take ud and not to interrupt or stop either of these medications w/o consulting a physician. Inform those receiving gonadotropin-releasing hormone agonists to maintain such treatment during therapy. Instruct that if a daily dose is missed, to take the normal dose the following day, but if >1 daily dose is skipped, advise to inform physician. Counsel about the common side effects (eg, peripheral edema, hypokalemia, HTN, elevated LFTs, UTI). Inform that liver function will be monitored using blood tests. Advise that drug may harm a developing fetus and that women who are pregnant or may be pregnant should not handle the drug w/o protection (eg, gloves). Instruct to use a condom if having sex w/ a pregnant woman, and to use a condom and another effective method of birth control if having sex w/ a woman of childbearing potential; advise that these measures are required during and for 1 week after treatment.

Zyvox — linezolid   Rx

Class: Oxazolidinone class antibacterial

ADULT DOSAGE

Pneumonia

Nosocomial/Community-Acquired Pneumonia, Including Concurrent Bacteremia:
600mg IV/PO q12h for 10-14 consecutive days

Vancomycin-Resistant *Enterococcus faecium* Infections

Including Concurrent Bacteremia:
600mg IV/PO q12h for 14-28 consecutive days

Skin and Skin Structure Infections

Complicated:
IV/Oral:
600mg q12h for 10-14 consecutive days

Uncomplicated:
Oral:
400mg q12h for 10-14 consecutive days

PEDIATRIC DOSAGE

Skin and Skin Structure Infections

Preterm Neonates <7 Days of Age:
Initial: 10mg/kg q12h
Titrate: Increase to 10mg/kg q8h if clinical response is suboptimal. All neonates should receive 10mg/kg q8h by 7 days of life
Treatment Duration: 10-14 consecutive days

Complicated:
IV/Oral:
Birth-11 Years:
10mg/kg q8h for 10-14 consecutive days
≥12 Years:
600mg q12h for 10-14 consecutive days

Uncomplicated:
Oral:
<5 Years:
10mg/kg q8h for 10-14 consecutive days
5-11 Years:
10mg/kg q12h for 10-14 consecutive days
≥12 Years:
600mg q12h for 10-14 consecutive days

Pneumonia

Nosocomial/Community-Acquired Pneumonia, Including Concurrent Bacteremia:

IV/PO:
Preterm Neonates <7 Days of Age:
Initial: 10mg/kg q12h
Titrate: Increase to 10mg/kg q8h if clinical response is suboptimal. All neonates should receive 10mg/kg q8h by 7 days of life
Treatment Duration: 10-14 consecutive days

Birth-11 Years:
10mg/kg q8h for 10-14 consecutive days

≥12 Years:
600mg q12h for 10-14 consecutive days

Vancomycin-Resistant *Enterococcus faecium* Infections

Including Concurrent Bacteremia:

IV/PO:
Neonates <7 Days of Age:
Initial: 10mg/kg q12h
Titrate: Increase to 10mg/kg q8h if clinical response is suboptimal. All neonates should receive 10mg/kg q8h by 7 days of life
Treatment Duration: 14-28 consecutive days

Birth-11 Years:
10mg/kg q8h for 14-28 consecutive days

≥12 Years:
600mg q12h for 14-28 consecutive days

ADMINISTRATION
Oral/IV route

May be administered w/o regard to the timing of meals.
No dose adjustment is necessary when switching from IV to oral administration.

IV
May exhibit a yellow color that can intensify over time w/o adversely affecting potency.
Infuse over 30-120 min.
Do not use infusion bag in series connections.
Do not introduce additives into linezolid inj sol; if given concomitantly w/ another drug, give each drug separately.
Flush line before and after infusion if the same IV line is used for sequential infusion of several drugs.

Compatible IV Sol:
0.9% NaCl
D5 inj
Lactated Ringer's inj
Refer to PI for incompatibilities.

Sus
Reconstitute w/ 123mL distilled water in 2 portions; shake vigorously after each portion.
After constitution, before using, gently mix by inverting the bottle 3-5X.
Do not shake.
Store reconstituted sus at room temperature; use w/in 21 days.

STORAGE
25°C (77°F). Protect from light. Keep bottles tightly closed to protect from moisture. Keep infusion bags in the overwrap until ready to use. Protect infusion bags from freezing.

HOW SUPPLIED
Inj: 2mg/mL [100mL, 200mL, 300mL]; **Oral Sus:** 100mg/5mL [150mL]; **Tab:** 600mg

CONTRAINDICATIONS
Hypersensitivity to linezolid or any of the other product components, concomitant use w/ MAOIs A or B (eg, phenelzine, isocarboxazid) or w/in 2 weeks of taking such drugs,

WARNINGS/PRECAUTIONS
Myelosuppression (eg, anemia, leukopenia, pancytopenia, thrombocytopenia) reported; monitor CBCs weekly, particularly in those who receive treatment for >2 weeks, w/ preexisting myelosuppression, receiving concomitant drugs that produce bone marrow suppression, or w/ a chronic infection who have received previous or concomitant antibiotic therapy. Consider discontinuation if myelosuppression develops or worsens. Peripheral and optic neuropathies and visual blurring reported; prompt ophthalmic evaluation is recommended if patient experiences visual impairment symptoms. Monitor visual function if used for extended periods (≥3 months) or if new visual symptoms develop. Weigh continued use against potential risk if peripheral/optic neuropathy occurs. Do not administer w/ carcinoid syndrome. Not approved and should not be used for the treatment of catheter-related bloodstream infections or catheter-site infections. Not indicated for the treatment of gram-negative infections; initiate specific gram-negative therapy immediately if a concomitant gram-negative pathogen is documented or suspected. *Clostridium difficile*-associated diarrhea (CDAD) reported; may need to d/c if CDAD is suspected or confirmed. Do not administer w/ uncontrolled HTN, pheochromocytoma, or thyrotoxicosis, unless patients are monitored for potential increases in BP. Lactic acidosis reported; evaluate immediately if recurrent N/V, unexplained acidosis, or a low bicarbonate level develops. Convulsions reported. May result in bacterial resistance if used in the absence of a proven or suspected bacterial infection or a prophylactic indication.

ADVERSE REACTIONS
Diarrhea, headache, N/V, anemia, thrombocytopenia, abnormal Hgb/WBCs/neutrophils, serum AST/ALT/alkaline phosphatase/lipase/total bilirubin elevations.

DRUG INTERACTIONS
See Contraindications. Serotonin syndrome reported w/ serotonergic agents, including antidepressants such as SSRIs; do not administer in patients taking

serotonin reuptake inhibitors, TCAs, 5-HT$_1$ receptor agonists (triptans), meperidine, bupropion, or buspirone, unless clinically appropriate and patients are carefully observed for signs/symptoms of serotonin syndrome or neuroleptic malignant syndrome (NMS)-like reactions. If alternatives to linezolid are not available and the potential benefits of linezolid outweigh the risks of serotonin syndrome or NMS-like reactions, promptly d/c the serotonergic antidepressant and administer linezolid; monitor for 2 weeks (5 weeks if fluoxetine was taken) or until 24 hrs after the last dose of linezolid, whichever comes 1st. Do not administer w/ directly and indirectly acting sympathomimetic agents (eg, pseudoephedrine), vasopressive agents (eg, epinephrine, norepinephrine), or dopaminergic agents (eg, dopamine, dobutamine), unless patients are monitored for potential increases in BP. Symptomatic hypoglycemia reported in patients w/ diabetes mellitus (DM) receiving insulin or oral hypoglycemic agents when treated w/ linezolid; may need to decrease dose of insulin or oral hypoglycemic agent, or d/c the oral hypoglycemic agent, insulin, or linezolid, if hypoglycemia occurs.

PREGNANCY AND LACTATION
Pregnancy: Category C.
Lactation: Caution in nursing.

MECHANISM OF ACTION
Oxazolidinone antibacterial; binds to a site on the bacterial 23S ribosomal RNA of the 50S subunit and prevents the formation of a functional 70S initiation complex, which is essential for bacterial reproduction.

PHARMACOKINETICS
Absorption: (PO) Extensive. Absolute bioavailability (100%). **Distribution:** V$_d$=40-50L; plasma protein binding (31%). **Metabolism:** Oxidation of the morpholine ring. **Elimination:** Urine (30% unchanged), feces (as metabolites).

Administration of variable doses resulted in different pharmacokinetic parameters.

PATIENT CONSIDERATIONS
Assessment: Assess for hypersensitivity to drug, catheter-related bloodstream/catheter-site infections, uncontrolled HTN, pheochromocytoma, thyrotoxicosis, carcinoid syndrome, other conditions where treatment is contraindicated or cautioned, pregnancy/nursing status, and possible drug interactions.

Monitoring: Monitor for myelosuppression, peripheral/optic neuropathy, CDAD, lactic acidosis, convulsions, potential increases in BP, and other adverse reactions. Monitor CBCs weekly. Monitor visual function if used for extended periods (≥3 months) or if new visual symptoms develop.

Counseling: Explain that therapy should only be used to treat bacterial, not viral, infections. Instruct to take exactly ud even if the patient feels better early in the course of therapy. Inform that skipping doses or not completing the full course of therapy may decrease effectiveness of treatment and increase bacterial resistance. Instruct to notify physician if patient has a history of HTN or seizures, is taking medications containing pseudoephedrine or phenylpropanolamine (eg, cold remedies, decongestants) or antidepressants, or is experiencing visual changes. Instruct to avoid large quantities of foods or beverages w/ high tyramine content. Inform phenylketonurics that oral sus contains phenylalanine. Advise that diarrhea is a common problem caused by therapy that usually ends when therapy is discontinued. Instruct to immediately contact physician if watery and bloody stools (w/ or w/o stomach cramps and fever) occur, even as late as ≥2 months after having taken the last dose. Inform patients, particularly those w/ DM, that hypoglycemia may occur; instruct to contact physician if this occurs.

SECTION 10

SPECIALTY DRUG SUMMARIES

In addition to the new Drug Summaries section, PDR has elected to provide a section devoted specifically to specialty drugs.* This new section provides quick reference to concise information for the latest updated and newly approved FDA-regulated drugs considered to be in a specialty category. Each alphabetically ordered specialty drug summary provides easy access to key details from current FDA-approved labeling, including: brand and generic names; pharmacological class; boxed warning; indications/dosage (organized by adult and pediatric patients in a streamlined, two-column format); dosing considerations; administration information; specifics on safe storage and handling; how supplied details; contraindications; relevant warnings and precautions; key adverse reactions; drug interactions; pregnancy and lactation details; mechanism of action; pharmacokinetics; and information on assessment, monitoring, and counseling.

Abbreviations used within these specialty drug summaries are defined in the *Abbreviations, Acronyms, and Symbols* table on page S-1449.

This section may not include every available specialty drug. Additionally, specialty designation may differ from one specialty formulary to another and may be specific to benefit plans.

For additional detailed information, please refer to full FDA-approved labeling. Visit PDR.net® for further drug listings.

PDR® invites its readership to provide input on what section content would be most relevant to you. To share your preferences for future content, please call 800-232-7379.

8-MOP — methoxsalen   Rx
Class: Psoralen

> Should be used only by physicians who have special competence in the diagnosis/treatment of psoriasis and vitiligo and who have special training and experience in photochemotherapy. The use of methoxsalen and ultraviolet (UV) radiation therapy should be under constant supervision of such a physician. Photochemotherapy should be restricted to patients with severe, recalcitrant, disabling psoriasis that is not adequately responsive to other forms of therapy, and only when the diagnosis is certain. Because of the risks of ocular damage, aging skin, and skin cancer (eg, melanoma), inform patients about the risks inherent in this therapy. May not be interchanged with Oxsoralen-Ultra without retitration.

ADULT DOSAGE
Psoriasis

For symptomatic control of severe, recalcitrant, disabling psoriasis not adequately responsive to other forms of therapy and when the diagnosis has been supported by biopsy in conjunction w/ controlled doses of long wave UVA radiation

Dose should be taken 2 hours before UVA exposure

Initial:
<30kg: 10mg
30-50kg: 20mg
51-65kg: 30mg
66-80kg: 40mg
81-90kg: 50mg
91-115kg: 60mg
<115kg: 70mg

Titrate: May increase by 10mg after 15 treatments if no response or only minimal response obtained

Max: Do not treat more often than once qod; number of doses per week determined by the patient's schedule of UVA exposures

Vitiligo
Repigmentation of Idiopathic Vitiligo in conjunction w/ Controlled Doses of long Wave UV Radiation:
20mg 2-4hrs before UV exposure

Therapy should be on alternate days and never 2 consecutive days

Light Exposure (Based on Skin Color):
Initial Exposure:
Light: 15 min
Medium: 20 min
Dark: 25 min

Second Exposure:
Light: 20 min
Medium: 25 min
Dark: 30 min

Third Exposure:
Light: 25 min
Medium: 30 min
Dark: 35 min

Fourth Exposure:
Light: 30 min
Medium: 35 min
Dark: 40 min

Subsequent Exposure:
Gradually increase exposure based on erythema and tenderness of the amelanotic skin

Other Indications
For use with UVAR system in palliative treatment of skin manifestations of cutaneous T-cell lymphoma unresponsive to other therapies in conjunction w/ long wave UV radiation of WBCs

---

ADMINISTRATION
Oral route
Take w/ food or milk
STORAGE
25°C (77°F); excursions permitted to 15-30°C (59-86°F).
HOW SUPPLIED
Cap: 10mg
CONTRAINDICATIONS
Idiosyncratic reactions to psoralen compounds, history of light sensitive diseases (eg, lupus erythematosus, porphyria cutanea tarda, erythropoietic protoporphyria,

PEDIATRIC DOSAGE
Pediatric use may not have been established

---

variegate porphyria, xeroderma pigmentosum, albinism), history/active melanoma, invasive squamous cell carcinoma, aphakia.

WARNINGS/PRECAUTIONS
May cause serious skin burns if exceed recommended dose or exposure. Increased risk of squamous cell carcinoma reported; caution in patients who are fair skinned or those who had pre-PUVA exposure to prolonged tar and UVB treatment, ionizing radiation, or arsenic. Should wear UVA-absorbing, wrap-around sunglasses for 24 hrs following methoxsalen ingestion to avoid cataractogenicity. Sunlight/UV radiation exposure may cause premature skin aging. Diligently observe and treat basal cell carcinomas. Monitor for carcinomas with history of previous x-ray, grenz ray, or arsenic therapy. Caution with hepatic impairment. Avoid vertical UVA chamber with cardiac disease or if unable to tolerate prolonged standing or exposure to heat stress. Safety of total cumulative dose of UVA that can be given over long periods of time not established. Avoid sunbathing 24 hrs before or 48 hrs post treatment. Avoid sun exposure for at least 8 hrs after ingestion; if cannot be avoided, wear protective devices (eg, hat, gloves) and/or apply sunscreens that contain ingredients that filter out UVA radiation. Do not apply sunscreens to areas affected by psoriasis until after treatment in the UVA chamber. Protect eyes, abdominal skin, breasts, genitalia, and other sensitive areas for approximately 1/3 of the initial exposure time until tanning occurs. Unless affected by disease, shield male genitalia. Perform ophthalmologic exam before therapy, then yearly. Obtain CBC, anti-nuclear antibody test, LFTs, and renal function tests before therapy, then 6-12 months subsequently.

ADVERSE REACTIONS
Nausea, nervousness, insomnia, psychological depression, pruritus, erythema.

DRUG INTERACTIONS
Caution with photosensitizers such as anthralin, coal tar and its derivatives, griseofulvin, phenothiazines, nalidixic acid, fluoroquinolone antibiotics, halogenated salicylanilides (bacteriostatic soaps), sulfonamides, tetracyclines, thiazides, and certain organic staining dyes (eg, methylene blue, toluidine blue, rose bengal, methyl orange).

PREGNANCY AND LACTATION
Category C, caution in nursing.

MECHANISM OF ACTION
Psoralen; not established. Upon photoactivation, conjugates and forms covalent bonds with DNA, which leads to the formation of both monofunctional and bifunctional adducts. May also react with proteins. Acts as photosensitizer. In the treatment of vitiligo, suggested that the melanocytes in the hair follicle are stimulated to move up the follicle and repopulate the epidermis. In the treatment of psoriasis, mechanism suspected to be DNA photodamage, which causes a decrease in cell proliferation but other vascular, leukocyte, or cell regulatory mechanisms may also play a minor role.

PHARMACOKINETICS
Elimination: Urine (95%).

PATIENT CONSIDERATIONS
Assessment: Assess for conditions where treatment is contraindicated or cautioned, history of previous x-ray, grenz ray or arsenic therapy, pregnancy/nursing status, and possible drug interactions. Perform ophthalmological exam and obtain baseline for CBC (Hgb, Hct, WBC), anti-nuclear antibodies, LFTs, and renal function tests (eg, SrCr, BUN).

Monitoring: Monitor for signs/symptoms of skin burning, development of cancers (eg, basal cell carcinomas, squamous cell carcinoma), cataracts, and premature aging of skin. Perform annual ophthalmologic exam. Every 6-12 months, monitor CBC (Hgb, Hct, WBC), anti-nuclear antibodies, LFTs, and renal function tests.

Counseling: Inform of potential risks/benefits of therapy. Instruct to wear special wrap-around sunglasses that totally block or absorb UV light; instruct to put them on immediately after taking medication and to continue wearing them for 24 hours if any light is present. Advise to not allow exposure of skin and lips to sunlight for 8 hours after treatment. Instruct to not expose skin to either sunlight or sun lamps within 24 hours of a scheduled treatment. Instruct to wear protective clothing (hat, gloves) to cover as much of body as possible after treatment as well as use a sunscreen product having a protection factor of at least 15. Notify physician if pregnant/nursing or planning to become pregnant.

ABRAXANE — paclitaxel protein-bound   Rx
Class: Antimicrotubule agent

> Do not administer to patients who have baseline neutrophil counts of <1500 cells/mm³. Perform frequent peripheral blood cell counts to monitor occurrence of bone marrow suppression, primarily neutropenia. Do not substitute for or w/ other paclitaxel formulations.

ADULT DOSAGE
Non-Small Cell Lung Cancer
Locally Advanced or Metastatic:
100mg/m² IV infusion over 30 min on Days 1, 8, and 15 of each 21-day cycle Give carboplatin on Day 1 of each 21-day cycle immediately after paclitaxel

Do not administer on Day 1 of a cycle until ANC is at least 1500 cells/mm³ and platelet count is at least 100,000 cells/mm³

PEDIATRIC DOSAGE
Pediatric use may not have been established

Metastatic Pancreatic Adenocarcinoma

125mg/m^2 IV infusion over 30-40 min on Days 1, 8, and 15 of each 28-day cycle

Give gemcitabine immediately after paclitaxel on Days 1, 8, and 15 of each 28-day cycle

Metastatic Breast Cancer

After failure of combination chemotherapy or relapse w/in 6 months of adjuvant chemotherapy

260mg/m^2 IV over 30 min every 3 weeks

DOSING CONSIDERATIONS

Hepatic Impairment

Metastatic Breast Cancer:

Moderate (AST <10X ULN and Bilirubin >1.5 to ≤3X ULN):
Initial: 200mg/m^2 for the 1st course of therapy
Titrate: May increase up to 260mg/m^2 in subsequent courses if reduced dose tolerated for 2 cycles

Severe (AST <10X ULN and Bilirubin >3 to ≤5X ULN):
Initial: 200mg/m^2 for the 1st course of therapy
Titrate: May increase up to 260mg/m^2 in subsequent courses if reduced dose tolerated for 2 cycles

AST >10X ULN or Bilirubin >5X ULN: Not recommended

Non-Small Cell Lung Cancer:

Moderate (AST <10X ULN and Bilirubin >1.5 to ≤3X ULN):
Initial: 80mg/m^2 for the 1st course of therapy
Titrate: May increase up to 100mg/m^2 in subsequent courses if reduced dose tolerated for 2 cycles
Severe (AST <10X ULN and Bilirubin >3 to ≤5X ULN):
Initial: 80mg/m^2 for the 1st course of therapy
Titrate: May increase up to 100mg/m^2 in subsequent courses if reduced dose tolerated for 2 cycles

AST >10X ULN or Bilirubin >5X ULN: Not recommended

Adverse Reactions

Metastatic Breast Cancer:

Severe Neutropenia (Neutrophil <500 cells/mm^3 for ≥1 Week) or Severe Sensory Neuropathy: Reduce to 220mg/m^2
Recurrence of Severe Neutropenia or Severe Sensory Neuropathy: Reduce to 180mg/m^2
Grade 3 Sensory Neuropathy: Hold treatment until resolution to Grade 1 or 2, followed by a dose reduction for all subsequent courses

Non-Small Cell Lung Cancer:

Severe Neutropenia or Thrombocytopenia: Withhold treatment until ANC at least 1500 cells/mm^3 and platelet count at least 100,000 cells/mm^3 on Day 1 or to ANC of at least 500 cells/mm^3 and platelet count of at least 50,000 cells/mm^3 on Days 8 or 15 of the cycle; upon resumption of dosing, permanently reduce as outlined below
Grade 3-4 Peripheral Neuropathy: Withhold; resume at reduced dose w/ improvement to Grade 1 or complete resolution

Neutropenic Fever (ANC <500/mm^3 w/ Fever >38°C) or Delay of Next Cycle by >7 Days for ANC <1500/mm^3 or ANC <500/mm^3 for >7 Days:
1st Occurrence: Reduce to 75mg/m^2 weekly
2nd Occurrence: Reduce to 50mg/m^2 weekly
3rd Occurrence: D/C treatment

Platelet Count <50,000/mm^3:
1st Occurrence: Reduce to 75mg/m^2 weekly
2nd Occurrence: D/C treatment

Severe Sensory Neuropathy (Grade 3 or 4):
1st Occurrence: Reduce to 75mg/m^2 weekly
2nd Occurrence: Reduce to 50mg/m^2 weekly
3rd Occurrence: D/C treatment

Pancreatic Adenocarcinoma:
Dose Level Reductions:
1st Dose Reduction: 100mg/m^2
2nd Dose Reduction: 75mg/m^2
Additional Dose Reduction Required: D/C

Febrile Neutropenia (Grade 3 or 4): Withhold until fever resolves and ANC ≥1500; resume at next lower dose level
Peripheral Neuropathy (Grade 3 or 4): Withhold until improvement to ≤Grade 1; resume at next lower dose level
Cutaneous Toxicity (Grade 2 or 3): Reduce to next lower dose level; d/c treatment if toxicity persists
GI Toxicity (Grade 3 Mucositis or Diarrhea): Withhold until improvement to ≤Grade 1; resume at next lower level
Neutropenia and/or Thrombocytopenia at the Start of a Cycle or w/in a Cycle: Refer to PI

ADMINISTRATION

IV route

If paclitaxel (lyophilized cake or reconstituted sus) contacts the skin, wash the skin immediately and thoroughly w/ soap and water; if contact occurs w/ mucous membranes, flush the membranes thoroughly w/ water.
Limit the infusion to 30 min to reduce infusion-related reactions.

Preparation

Reconstitute each vial by slowly injecting 20mL of 0.9% NaCl inj onto the inside wall of the vial over a minimum of 1 min.
Allow vial to sit for a minimum of 5 min after inj into vial; gently swirl and/or invert the vial slowly for at least 2 min.
If foaming/clumping occurs, stand sol for at least 15 min until foam subsides.
Reconstituted sus should be milky and homogenous. Inj the appropriate amount of reconstituted sus into an empty, sterile IV bag.
Discard reconstituted sus if proteinaceous strands are observed.

Stability

Reconstituted paclitaxel in the vial should be used immediately, but may be refrigerated at 2-8°C (36-46°F) for a max of 24 hrs if necessary.
If not used immediately, each vial of reconstituted sus should be replaced in the original carton to protect it from bright light.
The sus for infusion when prepared in an infusion bag should be used immediately but may be refrigerated at 2-8°C (36-46°F) and protected from light for a max of 24 hrs.
Total combined refrigerated storage time of sus and in the infusion bag is 24 hrs; this may be followed by storage in the infusion bag at ambient temperature (approx 25°C [77°F]) and lighting conditions for a maximum of 4 hrs.
Discard any unused portion.

STORAGE

20-25°C (68-77°F). Retain in original packaging to protect from bright light.

HOW SUPPLIED

Inj: 100mg

CONTRAINDICATIONS

Patients w/ baseline neutrophil counts of <1500 cells/mm^3. Severe hypersensitivity reaction to this product should not be rechallenged w/ the drug.

WARNINGS/PRECAUTIONS

Bone marrow suppression (primarily neutropenia) is dose-dependent and a dose-limiting toxicity. Withhold therapy if ANC <500 cells/mm^3 and platelets are <50,000 cells/mm^3 and delay initiation of the next cycle if ANC is <1500 cells/mm^3 or platelets are <100,000 cells/mm^3 on Day 1 of the cycle in patients w/ pancreatic adenocarcinoma. Sensory neuropathy is dose- and schedule-dependent. Sepsis reported; initiate treatment w/ broad-spectrum antibiotics if patient becomes febrile (regardless of ANC). Pneumonitis reported; interrupt treatment and gemcitabine during evaluation of suspected pneumonitis. After ruling out infectious etiology and upon making a diagnosis of pneumonitis, permanently d/c combination therapy. Severe and sometimes fatal hypersensitivity reactions, including anaphylactic reactions, reported. Caution w/ hepatic impairment; not recommended in patients who have total bilirubin >5X ULN or AST >10X ULN and in patients w/ metastatic adenocarcinoma of the pancreas who have moderate to severe hepatic impairment (total bilirubin >1.5X ULN and AST ≤10X ULN). Contains human albumin; may carry a remote risk for transmission of viral diseases. May cause fetal harm. Men should be advised not to father a child while receiving treatment.

ADVERSE REACTIONS

Alopecia, neutropenia, thrombocytopenia, sensory/peripheral neuropathy, abnormal ECG, fatigue/asthenia, myalgia/arthralgia, AST elevation, alkaline phosphatase elevation, anemia, nausea, infections, diarrhea.

DRUG INTERACTIONS

Caution w/ medicines known to inhibit (eg, ketoconazole and other imidazole antifungals, erythromycin, fluoxetine, gemfibrozil, ritonavir) or induce (eg, rifampicin, carbamazepine, phenytoin, efavirenz, nevirapine) either CYP2C8 or CYP3A4.

PREGNANCY AND LACTATION

Category D, not for use in nursing.

MECHANISM OF ACTION

Antimicrotubule agent; promotes assembly of microtubules from tubulin dimers and stabilizes microtubules by preventing depolymerization. This stability results in inhibition of the normal dynamic reorganization of the microtubule network that is essential for vital interphase and mitotic cellular functions.

PHARMACOKINETICS

Distribution: V_d=1741L; plasma protein binding (94%). **Metabolism:** Liver via CYP2C8 to 6α-hydroxypaclitaxel (major metabolite), and CYP3A4. **Elimination:** Urine (4% unchanged, <1% metabolites), feces (20%); $T_{1/2}$=13-27 hrs.

PATIENT CONSIDERATIONS

Assessment: Assess for previous hypersensitivity reactions to drug, hepatic impairment, pregnancy/nursing status, and possible drug interactions. Obtain baseline CBC, including neutrophil counts, and LFTs.

Monitoring: Monitor for bone marrow suppression, sensory neuropathy, sepsis, pneumonitis, hypersensitivity reactions, and other adverse reactions. Frequently monitor CBC (including neutrophil counts); perform prior to dosing on Day 1 (for metastatic breast cancer) and Days 1, 8, and 15 (for non-Small cell lung cancer and pancreatic cancer).

Counseling: Inform that drug may cause fetal harm; advise women of childbearing potential to avoid becoming pregnant. Advise men not to father a child while on therapy. Inform of the risk of low blood cell counts and severe and life-threatening infections; instruct to contact physician immediately for fever or evidence of infection. Advise to contact physician for persistent vomiting, diarrhea, or signs of dehydration. Inform that sensory neuropathy occurs frequently and instruct to report to physician any numbness, tingling, pain, or weakness involving the extremities. Inform that alopecia, fatigue/asthenia, and myalgia/arthralgia occur frequently w/ therapy. Instruct to contact physician for signs of an allergic reaction and for sudden onset of dry, persistent cough or SOB.

ACTEMRA — tocilizumab   Rx

Class: Monoclonal antibody/interleukin-6 (IL-6) receptor antagonist

> Increased risk for developing serious infections (eg, active tuberculosis (TB), invasive fungal infections, bacterial/viral infections due to opportunistic pathogens) that may lead to hospitalization or death. Most patients who developed these infections were taking concomitant immunosuppressants (eg, methotrexate [MTX], corticosteroids). If serious infection develops, interrupt treatment until infection is controlled. Test for latent TB prior to and during therapy; initiate latent TB treatment prior to therapy. Consider risks and benefits prior to initiating therapy in patients w/ chronic or recurrent infection. Monitor for development of signs/symptoms of infection during and after treatment.

ADULT DOSAGE

Rheumatoid Arthritis

Moderately to Severely Active:

IV:
4mg/kg every 4 weeks; may increase to 8mg/kg every 4 weeks based on clinical response
Max: 800mg/infusion

SQ:
<100kg: 162mg every other week, followed by an increase to every week based on response
≥100kg: 162mg every week

Transition from IV to SQ:
Administer 1st SQ dose instead of the next scheduled IV dose

May be used alone or in combination w/ methotrexate or other nonbiologic disease-modifying antirheumatic drugs

PEDIATRIC DOSAGE

Juvenile Idiopathic Arthritis

≥2 Years:

IV:
Active Polyarticular Juvenile Idiopathic Arthritis:
<30kg: 10mg/kg every 4 weeks
≥30kg: 8mg/kg every 4 weeks

Active Systemic Juvenile Idiopathic Arthritis:
<30kg: 12mg/kg every 2 weeks
≥30 kg: 8mg/kg every 2 weeks

May be used alone or in combination w/ methotrexate

Do not change dose based on a single visit body weight measurement

---

DOSING CONSIDERATIONS

Adverse Reactions

Rheumatoid Arthritis:

Liver Enzyme Abnormalities:

>1-3X ULN: Modify dose of concomitant disease-modifying antirheumatic drugs if appropriate. For persistent increases in this range, reduce dose to 4mg/kg or hold until ALT or AST have normalized if receiving IV. If receiving SQ, reduce inj frequency to every other week or hold dosing until ALT/AST have normalized and resume at every other week and increase frequency

<3-5X ULN: Hold until <3X ULN and follow recommendations above for >1-3X ULN. If persistent increases in this range, d/c therapy

<5X ULN: D/C

Low ANC:

ANC <500/mm³: D/C

ANC 500-1000/mm³: Hold dosing until ANC >1000/mm³. If receiving IV, resume at 4mg/kg and increase to 8mg/kg; if receiving SQ, resume at every other week and increase to every week

Low Platelet Counts:

<50,000/mm³: D/C

50,000-100,000/mm³: Hold until >100,000/mm³. If receiving IV, resume at 4mg/kg and increase to 8mg/kg. If receiving SQ, resume at every other week and increase to every week

Polyarticular/Systemic Juvenile Idiopathic Arthritis:
Dose reduction recommended for liver enzyme abnormalities, low neutrophil counts, and low platelet counts at levels similar to patients w/ rheumatoid arthritis
If appropriate, modify dose or stop methotrexate and/or other medications and hold therapy until clinical situation has been evaluated
Decision to d/c for a lab abnormality should be based on medical assessment of patient

ADMINISTRATION

IV/SQ route

Do not initiate therapy in patients w/ an ANC <2000/mm³, platelet count <100,000/mm³, or who have ALT or AST >1.5X ULN.
Do not administer as IV bolus/push.

IV

Preparation:

Polyarticular and Systemic Juvenile Idiopathic Arthritis:
<30kg: Use a 50mL infusion bag/bottle of 0.9% NaCl
≥30kg: Use a 100mL infusion bag/bottle of 0.9% NaCl

Rheumatoid Arthritis:
≥30kg: Use a 100mL infusion bag/bottle of 0.9% NaCl

Dilution:
Withdraw a volume of 0.9% NaCl inj, equal to volume of tocilizumab inj required for patient's dose from infusion bag/bottle.
Withdraw amount of tocilizumab for IV infusion from vial(s) and add slowly into NaCl infusion bag/bottle; gently invert bag to avoid foaming to mix sol.

Administration:
Administer infusion over 60 min, and must be administered w/ an infusion set.
Do not infuse concomitantly in same IV line w/ other drugs.
Fully diluted sol are compatible w/ polypropylene, polyethylene and polyvinyl chloride infusion bags and polypropylene, polyethylene, and glass infusion bottles.

SQ

Inject full amount in syringe (0.9mL), which provides 162mg of tocilizumab.
Rotate inj sites w/ each inj and never inj into moles, scars, or areas where the skin is tender, bruised, red, hard, or not intact.

STORAGE

2-8°C (36-46°F). Do not freeze. Protect from light; store in original package until time of use. Keep syringes dry. Diluted Sol for Infusion: 2-8°C (36-46°F) or room temperature for up to 24 hrs. Protect from light. Discard unused portion.

HOW SUPPLIED

Inj: 20mg/mL [4mL, 10mL, 20mL vials]; 162mg/0.9mL [prefilled syringe]

CONTRAINDICATIONS

Known hypersensitivity to tocilizumab.

WARNINGS/PRECAUTIONS

Avoid w/ active infection, including localized infections. Caution in patients who have been exposed to TB, w/ history of serious/opportunistic infection, who resided or traveled in areas of endemic TB/mycoses, or w/ underlying conditions that may predispose them to infection. Viral reactivation and herpes zoster exacerbation observed. GI perforation reported; caution in patients at risk for GI perforation. Neutropenia, thrombocytopenia, elevation of liver enzymes, and increase in lipid parameters reported; do not initiate treatment if ANC <2000/mm³, platelets <100,000/mm³, or ALT/AST >1.5X ULN. D/C treatment w/ ANC <500/mm³, platelets <50,000/mm³, or ALT/AST >5X ULN. May increase risk of malignancies. Hypersensitivity reactions, including anaphylaxis and death, reported; d/c immediately and permanently if anaphylaxis or other hypersensitivity reaction occurs. Should only be infused IV by a healthcare professional w/ appropriate medical support to manage anaphylaxis. MS and chronic inflammatory demyelinating polyneuropathy reported rarely in RA studies; caution w/ preexisting or recent onset demyelinating disorders. Not recommended in patients w/ active hepatic disease or hepatic impairment. Caution in elderly.

ADVERSE REACTIONS

URTIs, nasopharyngitis, headache, HTN, increased ALT/AST, dizziness, bronchitis, infusion reaction, neutropenia, diarrhea, inj-site reaction, total cholesterol elevation, increased LDL.

DRUG INTERACTIONS

See Boxed Warning. Avoid w/ live vaccines. May increase metabolism of CYP450 substrates (eg, 1A2, 2B6, 2C9, 2C19, 2D6, 3A4). Upon initiation or discontinuation of tocilizumab, monitor therapeutic effect (eg, warfarin) or drug concentrations (eg, cyclosporine, theophylline) and adjust dose prn. Caution w/ CYP3A4 substrates where decrease in effectiveness is undesirable (eg, oral contraceptives, lovastatin, atorvastatin). Avoid w/ biological DMARDs (eg, TNF antagonists, interleukin [IL]-1R antagonists, anti-CD20 monoclonal antibodies, selective costimulation modulators) due to increased immunosuppression and risk of infection. Increased frequency and magnitude of transaminase elevations w/ hepatotoxic drugs (eg, MTX). Decreased exposure of simvastatin and omeprazole.

PREGNANCY AND LACTATION

Category C, not for use in nursing.

MECHANISM OF ACTION

IL-6 receptor antagonist monoclonal antibody; binds specifically to both soluble and membrane-bound IL-6 receptors (sIL-6R and mIL-6R) and inhibits IL-6-mediated signaling through these receptors.

PHARMACOKINETICS

Absorption: Administration of variable doses resulted in different pharmacokinetic parameters. **Distribution:** V_d=6.4L (RA), 4.08L (PJIA), 2.54L (SJIA). **Elimination:** (RA) $T_{1/2}$=Up to 11 days (4mg/kg IV); up to 13 days (8mg/kg IV, 162mg every week); 5 days (162mg every other week SQ). (SJIA) $T_{1/2}$=Up to 23 days. (PJIA) $T_{1/2}$= Up to 16 days.

PATIENT CONSIDERATIONS

Assessment: Assess for infections (eg, bacteria, fungi, viruses), including latent TB. Assess for demyelinating disorders, risk of GI perforation, active hepatic disease or impairment, hypersensitivity to drug, pregnancy/nursing status, and possible drug interactions. Obtain baseline lipid levels and platelet, liver transaminases, and neutrophil counts.

Monitoring: Monitor for signs/symptoms of TB and other infections. Monitor for hypersensitivity reactions, GI perforation, malignancies, and demyelinating disorders. Monitor neutrophil counts, platelet counts, and LFTs, after 4-8 weeks after initiation and every 3 months thereafter in RA patients, or at the time of 2nd infusion and every 4-8 weeks thereafter in PJIA patients, or every 2-4 weeks thereafter in SJIA patients. Monitor lipid levels 4-8 weeks after initiation then at approx 24-week intervals.

Counseling: Advise of the potential risks/benefits of therapy. Inform that therapy may lower resistance to infections and may cause serious GI side effects; instruct to contact physician if symptoms of infection or severe, persistent abdominal pain appear. Advise to inform physician of travel history, especially to places that are endemic for TB/mycoses. Inform that some patients have developed serious allergic reactions, including anaphylaxis. Advise to seek immediate medical attention if any symptoms of serious allergic reactions develop. Inform of inj techniques and procedures. Advise not to reuse needles/syringes and instruct on proper disposal procedures.

ACTIMMUNE — interferon gamma-1b   Rx

Class: Biological response modifier

ADULT DOSAGE

Chronic Granulomatous Disease

Reduces frequency and severity of serious infections associated w/ chronic granulomatous disease

BSA >0.5m^2: 50mcg/m^2 SQ 3X weekly
BSA ≤0.5m^2: 1.5mcg/kg/dose SQ 3X weekly

Severe Malignant Osteopetrosis

Delays time to disease progression

BSA >0.5m^2: 50mcg/m^2 SQ 3X weekly
BSA ≤0.5m^2: 1.5mcg/kg/dose SQ 3X weekly

PEDIATRIC DOSAGE

Chronic Granulomatous Disease

Reduces frequency and severity of serious infections associated w/ chronic granulomatous disease

≥1 Year:
BSA >0.5m^2: 50mcg/m^2 SQ 3X weekly
BSA ≤0.5m^2: 1.5mcg/kg/dose SQ 3X weekly

Severe Malignant Osteopetrosis

Delays time to disease progression

≥1 Month of Age:
BSA >0.5m^2: 50mcg/m^2 SQ 3X weekly
BSA ≤0.5m^2: 1.5mcg/kg/dose SQ 3X weekly

DOSING CONSIDERATIONS

Elderly
Start at lower end of dosing range

Adverse Reactions
If severe reactions occur, reduce dose by 50% or interrupt therapy until the adverse reaction abates

ADMINISTRATION
SQ route

Optimum inj sites are the right and left deltoid and anterior thigh.
For single use only; discard any unused portion.
Do not mix w/ other drugs in same syringe.
May be administered using either sterilized glass or plastic disposable syringes.
Avoid excessive or vigorous agitation; do not shake.

STORAGE
2-8°C (36-46°F). Do not freeze. May store an unused vial at room temperature up to 12 hrs prior to use. Discard vials if not used w/in the 12-hr period; do not return to the refrigerator.

HOW SUPPLIED
Inj: 100mcg (2 million IU)/0.5mL

CONTRAINDICATIONS
Hypersensitivity to interferon gamma, *Escherichia coli* derived products, or any component of the product.

WARNINGS/PRECAUTIONS
Acute/transient flu-like symptoms (eg, fever, chills) induced by high doses may exacerbate preexisting cardiac conditions; monitor patients w/ preexisting cardiac conditions (eg, ischemia, CHF, arrhythmia) for signs/symptoms of exacerbation. Some of the flu-like symptoms may be minimized by hs administration; may also use acetaminophen (APAP) to ameliorate these effects. Decreased mental status, gait disturbances, and dizziness reported, particularly w/ doses >250mcg/m^2/day; monitor patients w/ seizure disorders or compromised CNS function. Reversible neutropenia and thrombocytopenia reported; may be severe and dose related. Monitor neutrophil and platelet counts in patients w/ myelosuppression during treatment. Repeated administration to patients w/ advanced hepatic disease or severe renal insufficiency may result in drug accumulation; monitor liver and renal function regularly. Elevations in AST and/or ALT reported; modify dose if severe hepatic enzyme elevations develop. Acute serious hypersensitivity reactions may occur; d/c immediately and institute appropriate therapy if an acute reaction develops. Transient cutaneous rashes reported. Renal toxicity reported. Stopper of the glass vial contains natural rubber (a derivative of latex) which may cause allergic reactions.

ADVERSE REACTIONS
Fever, headache, rash, chills, inj-site erythema or tenderness, fatigue, diarrhea, N/V, myalgia, arthralgia.

DRUG INTERACTIONS
Monitor neutrophil and platelet counts when administered in combination w/ other potentially myelosuppressive agents. Concurrent use of drugs having neurotoxic (including effects on the CNS), hematotoxic, or cardiotoxic effects may increase toxicity in these systems. Hepatotoxic and/or nephrotoxic drugs may have an effect on Actimmune clearance. Avoid simultaneous administration w/ other heterologous serum protein preparations or immunological preparations (eg, vaccines); risk of an unexpected or amplified immune response. May lead to a depression of the hepatic metabolism of certain drugs that utilize CYP450 pathway.

PREGNANCY AND LACTATION
Pregnancy: There are no adequate and well-controlled studies in pregnant women. Actimmune should be used during pregnancy only if the potential benefit justifies the potential risk to the fetus.
Lactation: It is not known whether Actimmune is excreted in human milk; not for use in nursing.
Reproductive Potential: It cannot be excluded that the presence of higher levels of interferon gamma may impair male fertility and that in certain cases of female infertility increased levels of interferon gamma may have played a role.

MECHANISM OF ACTION
Biological response modifier; exact mechanism not established. Enhances the oxidative metabolism of macrophages, antibody dependent cellular cytotoxicity, activation of natural killer cells, and the expression of Fc receptors and major histocompatibility antigens.

PHARMACOKINETICS
Absorption: Slow. C_{max}=0.6ng/mL; T_{max}=7 hrs. **Elimination:** $T_{1/2}$=5.9 hrs (100mcg/m^2).

PATIENT CONSIDERATIONS

Assessment: Assess for hypersensitivity to the drug and to *E. coli* derived products, preexisting cardiac conditions, seizure disorders, compromised CNS function, myelosuppression, pregnancy/nursing status, and possible drug interactions. Obtain baseline CBC, differential and platelet counts, renal and liver function tests, and urinalysis.

Monitoring: Monitor for flu-like symptoms, decreased mental status, gait disturbances, dizziness, hypersensitivity reactions, neutropenia, thrombocytopenia, and other adverse reactions. Monitor CBC, differential and platelet counts, renal and liver function tests, and urinalysis at 3-month intervals during treatment. In patients <1 yr of age, monitor LFTs monthly.

Counseling: Inform of potential benefits and risks of therapy. Instruct on appropriate use if home use is desirable. Inform of importance of proper disposal and caution against any reuse of needles and syringes. Instruct to dispose full container according to the directions provided by the physician. Inform that the most common adverse reactions are flu-like or constitutional symptoms (eg, fever, headache, chills, myalgia, fatigue) may decrease in severity as treatment continues. Explain that some of the flu-like symptoms may be minimized by hs administration. Inform that APAP may be used to prevent or partially alleviate fever and headache. Advise that undesirable effects (eg, fatigue, convulsion, confusional state, disorientation, hallucination) may be experienced during treatment; inform that these effects may be enhanced by alcohol. Instruct to use caution when driving a car or operating machinery.

ADAGEN — pegademase bovine   Rx

Class: Enzyme

PEDIATRIC DOSAGE

Adenosine Deaminase Deficiency

Enzyme replacement for adenosine deaminase deficiency in patients w/ severe combined immunodeficiency disease who are not suitable candidates for, or who have failed, bone marrow transplantation

Use in infants from birth or in children of any age at the time of diagnosis

Administer IM every 7 days

Recommended Dosing Schedule:
1st Dose: 10 U/kg
2nd Dose: 15 U/kg
3rd Dose: 20 U/kg

Maint: 20 U/kg/week
Titrate: May further increase by 5 U/kg/week if necessary
Max Single Dose: 30 U/kg

ADMINISTRATION
IM route

Do not dilute or mix w/ any other drug prior to administration

STORAGE
2-8°C (36-46°F). Do not freeze; do not use if there are any indications that it may have been frozen.

HOW SUPPLIED
Inj: 250 U/mL [1.5mL]

CONTRAINDICATIONS
Severe thrombocytopenia.

WARNINGS/PRECAUTIONS
Not for IV use. Caution with thrombocytopenia. Report immediately to manufacturer any laboratory or clinical indication of a decrease in potency of therapy. Determine plasma ADA activity and RBC deoxyadenosine triphosphate (dATP) prior to treatment. A desirable range of plasma ADA activity should be 15-35µmol/hr/mL. Refer to PI for details in monitoring plasma ADA activity and RBC dATP levels. Improvement in the general clinical status may be gradual but should be apparent by the end of the 1st yr of therapy. Antibody to drug may develop and may result in more rapid clearance of the drug. If a persistent fall in pre-inj levels of plasma ADA to <10µmol/hr/mL occurs, antibody formation should be suspected; if other causes for a decline in plasma ADA levels can be ruled out, perform a specific assay for antibody to ADA and the drug (ELISA, enzyme inhibition). Consider dose adjustment and other measures to induce tolerance and restore adequate ADA activity if antibody to ADA or drug is found to be the cause of a persistent fall in plasma ADA activity. Failure to maintain adequate levels of plasma ADA activity may result in a decline in immune function, with increased risk of opportunistic infections and complications of infection; closely monitor immune function and clinical status and take precautions to minimize risk of infection if a persistent decline in plasma ADA activity occurs.

ADVERSE REACTIONS

Headache, inj-site pain/erythema, hemolytic anemia, autoimmune hemolytic anemia, thrombocythemia, thrombocytopenia, autoimmune thrombocytopenia, urticaria, lymphomas.

DRUG INTERACTIONS

Activities of vidarabine (substrate for ADA), 2'-deoxycoformycin (potent inhibitor of ADA), and pegademase bovine may be substantially altered if used in combination with one another.

PREGNANCY AND LACTATION

Category C, caution in nursing.

MECHANISM OF ACTION

Enzyme; provides specific and direct replacement of the deficient enzyme. Eliminates the toxic metabolites of ADA deficiency, and results in improved immune function.

PHARMACOKINETICS

Absorption: T_{max}=2-3 days. **Elimination:** $T_{1/2}$=3->6 days.

PATIENT CONSIDERATIONS

Assessment: Assess for thrombocytopenia, immunologic status, pregnancy/nursing status, and possible drug interactions. Determine plasma ADA activity and RBC dATP.

Monitoring: Monitor immune function, clinical status, and for antibody development. Monitor plasma ADA activity levels and biochemical markers of ADA deficiency (primarily RBC dATP content).

Counseling: Inform caregivers of the benefits and risks of the treatment and the importance of measuring plasma ADA activity and RBC dATP levels.

ADCETRIS — brentuximab vedotin   Rx

Class: CD30-directed antibody-drug conjugate

> JC virus infection resulting in progressive multifocal leukoencephalopathy (PML) and death may occur.

ADULT DOSAGE	PEDIATRIC DOSAGE
Hodgkin Lymphoma	Pediatric use may not have been established

Hodgkin Lymphoma

Treatment of patients w/ classical Hodgkin lymphoma after failure of autologous hematopoietic stem cell transplant (auto-HSCT) or after failure of ≥2 prior multi-agent chemotherapy regimens in patients who are not auto-HSCT candidates

Initial: 1.8mg/kg IV (up to 180mg) over 30 min every 3 weeks until disease progression or unacceptable toxicity

Hodgkin Lymphoma Post-auto-HSCT Consolidation

Treatment of patients w/ classical Hodgkin lymphoma at high risk of relapse or progression as post-auto-HSCT consolidation

Initial: 1.8mg/kg IV (up to 180mg) over 30 min every 3 weeks

Initiate treatment w/in 4-6 weeks post-auto-HSCT or upon recovery from auto-HSCT; continue treatment until a max of 16 cycles, disease progression, or unacceptable toxicity

Systemic Anaplastic Large Cell Lymphoma

Use after failure of ≥1 prior multi-agent chemotherapy regimen

Initial: 1.8mg/kg IV (up to 180mg) over 30 min every 3 weeks until disease progression or unacceptable toxicity

---

DOSING CONSIDERATIONS

Renal Impairment
Severe (CrCl <30mL/min): Avoid use

Hepatic Impairment
Mild (Child-Pugh A):
Initial: 1.2mg/kg up to 120mg
Moderate (Child-Pugh B)/Severe (Child-Pugh C): Avoid use

Adverse Reactions
Peripheral Neuropathy:
New or Worsening Grade 2 or 3: Hold dosing until neuropathy improves to Grade 1 or baseline, then restart at 1.2mg/kg
Grade 4: D/C therapy

Neutropenia:
Grade 3 or 4: Hold dose until resolution to baseline or Grade 2 or lower; consider granulocyte colony-stimulating factor (G-CSF) prophylaxis for subsequent cycles if Grade 3 or 4 neutropenia was experienced in the previous cycle

Recurrent Grade 4 Neutropenia Despite G-CSF Prophylaxis: Consider discontinuation or reduce dose to 1.2mg/kg

ADMINISTRATION

IV route

For IV infusion only.
Do not mix w/, or administer as an infusion w/, other medicinal products.
If sol is not diluted/used immediately, store at 2-8°C (36-46°F) and use w/in 24 hrs of reconstitution. Do not freeze.

Reconstitution
1. Reconstitute each 50mg vial w/ 10.5mL sterile water for inj to yield 5mg/mL.
2. Direct the stream toward vial wall and not directly at the cake or powder.
3. Swirl the vial gently to aid dissolution; do not shake.
4. Dilute immediately into an infusion bag following reconstitution.

Dilution
1. Withdraw required calculated reconstituted amount of sol from the vial and immediately add it to an infusion bag containing a minimum volume of 100mL of 0.9% NaCl, D5 or lactated Ringer's inj to a final concentration of 0.4mg/mL to 1.8mg/mL.
2. Invert the bag gently to mix sol.
3. Infuse sol immediately following dilution.

STORAGE

2-8°C (36-46°F). Protect from light.

HOW SUPPLIED

Inj: 50mg

CONTRAINDICATIONS

Concomitant bleomycin due to pulmonary toxicity.

WARNINGS/PRECAUTIONS

See Dosing Considerations. Peripheral neuropathy (sensory and motor) reported. Infusion-related reactions, including anaphylaxis, reported; d/c immediately and permanently and institute appropriate therapy if anaphylaxis occurs. Interrupt treatment if an infusion-related reaction occurs and institute appropriate medical management; patients who have experienced a prior infusion-related reaction should be premedicated for subsequent infusions. Prolonged (≥1 week) severe neutropenia, Grade 3 or 4 thrombocytopenia, anemia, or febrile neutropenia reported; monitor CBCs prior to each dose and consider more frequent monitoring for patients w/ Grade 3 or 4 neutropenia. Serious infections and opportunistic infections (eg, pneumonia, bacteremia, sepsis, septic shock) reported; closely monitor during treatment for the emergence of possible bacterial, fungal, or viral infections. Increased risk of tumor lysis syndrome in patients w/ rapidly proliferating tumor and high tumor burden; monitor closely and take appropriate measures. Increased risk of ≥Grade 3 adverse reactions and deaths in patients w/ severe renal impairment and w/ moderate or severe hepatic impairment. Serious hepatotoxicity, including fatal outcomes, may occur after the 1st dose or after rechallenge; preexisting liver disease, elevated baseline LFTs, and concomitant medications may increase risk. Patients experiencing new/worsening/recurrent hepatotoxicity may require a delay, change in dose, or discontinuation of therapy. Hold dosing for any suspected case of PML and d/c if diagnosis is confirmed. Events of noninfectious pulmonary toxicity (eg, pneumonitis, interstitial lung disease, acute respiratory distress syndrome) reported; in the event of new/worsening pulmonary symptoms, hold dosing during evaluation and until symptomatic improvement. Stevens-Johnson syndrome (SJS) and toxic epidermal necrolysis (TEN) reported; d/c and administer appropriate therapy if SJS or TEN occurs. Fatal and serious GI complications (eg, perforation, hemorrhage, intestinal obstruction) reported; in the event of new/worsening GI symptoms, perform a prompt diagnostic evaluation and treat appropriately. May cause fetal harm.

ADVERSE REACTIONS

Classical Hodgkin Lymphoma: Neutropenia, peripheral sensory neuropathy, fatigue, URTI, N/V, diarrhea, anemia, pyrexia, thrombocytopenia, rash, abdominal pain, cough.
Classical Hodgkin Lymphoma Post-auto-HSCT Consolidation: Neutropenia, peripheral sensory neuropathy, thrombocytopenia, anemia, URTI, fatigue, peripheral motor neuropathy, nausea, cough, diarrhea.
Systemic Anaplastic Large Cell Lymphoma: Neutropenia, anemia, peripheral sensory neuropathy, fatigue, nausea, pyrexia, rash, diarrhea, pain.

DRUG INTERACTIONS

See Contraindications. Concomitant ketoconazole (potent CYP3A4 inhibitor) or P-gp inhibitors may increase exposure to monomethyl auristatin E (MMAE); monitor closely for adverse reactions when given concomitantly w/ strong CYP3A4 or P-gp inhibitors. Coadministration w/ rifampin (potent CYP3A4 inducer) may decrease exposure to MMAE.

PREGNANCY AND LACTATION

Pregnancy: Can cause fetal harm based on the findings from animal studies and the drug's mechanism of action.
Lactation: Not for use in nursing.
Reproductive Potential: Verify pregnancy status of females of reproductive potential prior to initiating therapy. Females of reproductive potential should avoid pregnancy during treatment and for at least 6 months after the final dose of therapy; females should immediately report pregnancy. May damage spermatozoa and testicular tissue, resulting in possible genetic abnormalities. Males w/ female sexual partners of reproductive potential should use effective contraception during treatment and for at least 6 months after the final dose of therapy. Male fertility may be compromised by treatment.

MECHANISM OF ACTION

CD30-directed antibody-drug conjugate (ADC); binds to CD30-expressing cells, followed by internalization of ADC-CD30 complex, and release of MMAE via proteolytic cleavage. Binding of MMAE to tubulin disrupts the microtubule network w/in the cell, inducing cell cycle arrest and apoptotic death of the cell.

PHARMACOKINETICS

Absorption: (MMAE) T_{max}=1-3 days. **Distribution:** (MMAE) Plasma protein binding (68-82%); (ADC) V_d=6-10L. **Metabolism:** (MMAE) Oxidation via CYP3A4/5. **Elimination:** (MMAE) Urine, feces (24%); $T_{1/2}$=4-6 days (ADC).

PATIENT CONSIDERATIONS

Assessment: Assess for history of infusion-related reactions, renal/hepatic impairment, pregnancy/nursing status, and for possible drug interactions. Assess for rapidly proliferating tumors and high tumor burden. Obtain baseline CBC, liver enzymes, and bilirubin.

Monitoring: Monitor for peripheral neuropathy, anaphylaxis, infusion reactions, tumor lysis syndrome, SJS, TEN, fever, opportunistic infections, PML, pulmonary toxicity, GI complications, and other adverse reactions. Monitor CBCs prior to each dose and perform more frequent monitoring w/ Grade 3 or 4 neutropenia. Monitor liver enzymes and bilirubin.

Counseling: Inform that therapy may cause peripheral neuropathy; advise to report to physician any numbness/tingling of hands or feet, or any muscle weakness. Advise to contact physician if a fever of ≥38.05°C (100.5°F) or other evidence of potential infection develops; if signs/symptoms of infusion reactions w/in 24 hrs of infusion are experienced; or if severe abdominal pain, chills, fever, N/V, or diarrhea develop. Advise to report symptoms that may indicate liver injury/hepatotoxicity, or pulmonary toxicity. Instruct to immediately report changes in mood/usual behavior; confusion, thinking problems, or loss of memory; changes in vision, speech, or walking; or decreased strength or weakness on 1 side of the body. Inform that therapy can cause fetal harm. Advise women to avoid pregnancy during treatment and for at least 6 months after the final dose; advise males w/ female sexual partners of reproductive potential to use effective contraception during treatment and for at least 6 months after the final dose. Instruct to report pregnancy immediately; advise to avoid breastfeeding while receiving therapy.

ADCIRCA — tadalafil   Rx

Class: Phosphodiesterase-5 (PDE-5) inhibitor

ADULT DOSAGE	PEDIATRIC DOSAGE
Pulmonary Arterial Hypertension	Pediatric use may not have been established
Treatment of pulmonary arterial HTN (WHO Group 1) to improve exercise ability	
40mg (two 20mg tabs) qd	

DOSING CONSIDERATIONS

Concomitant Medications

Patients on Ritonavir (RTV) for at Least 1 Week:
Initial: 20mg qd
Titrate: Increase to 40mg qd based on individual tolerability

Adding RTV:
Avoid use of tadalafil during the initiation of RTV
Stop tadalafil at least 24 hrs prior to starting RTV
After at least 1 week following RTV initiation, resume tadalafil at 20mg qd
Increase to 40mg qd based on individual tolerability

Renal Impairment

Mild (CrCl 51-80mL/min) or Moderate (CrCl 31-50mL/min):
Initial: 20mg qd
Titrate: Increase to 40mg qd based on individual tolerability
Severe (CrCl <30mL/min and on Hemodialysis): Avoid use

Hepatic Impairment

Mild or Moderate Hepatic Cirrhosis (Child-Pugh Class A or B):
Initial: Consider 20mg qd
Severe Hepatic Cirrhosis (Child-Pugh Class C): Avoid use

ADMINISTRATION

Oral route

Take w/ or w/o food
Dividing the dose (40mg) over the course of the day is not recommended

STORAGE

25°C (77°F); excursions permitted to 15-30°C (59-86°F).

HOW SUPPLIED

Tab: 20mg

CONTRAINDICATIONS

Patients using any form of organic nitrate, either regularly or intermittently, or guanylate cyclase (GC) stimulator (eg, riociguat), known serious hypersensitivity to tadalafil (Adcirca or Cialis).

WARNINGS/PRECAUTIONS

Patients who experience anginal chest pain after taking tadalafil should seek immediate medical attention. May cause a transient decrease in BP; caution w/ underlying cardiovascular disease (CVD). Patients w/ severely impaired autonomic control of BP or w/ left ventricular outflow obstruction may be particularly sensitive to vasodilatory effects. May significantly worsen cardiovascular status of patients w/ pulmonary veno-occlusive disease (PVOD); not recommended w/ veno-occlusive disease. Consider PVOD if signs of pulmonary edema occur. Nonarteritic anterior ischemic optic neuropathy (NAION) reported; seek immediate medical attention if sudden loss of vision in 1 or both eyes occurs. Not recommended in patients w/ hereditary degenerative retinal disorders (eg, retinitis pigmentosa). Seek immediate medical attention in the event of sudden decrease or loss of hearing. Prolonged erections >4 hrs and priapism reported rarely; caution w/ conditions that might predispose to priapism (eg, sickle cell anemia, multiple myeloma, leukemia) or in patients w/ anatomical penile deformation (eg, angulation, cavernosal fibrosis, Peyronie's disease). Caution w/ bleeding disorders or significant active peptic ulceration.

ADVERSE REACTIONS

Headache, myalgia, nasopharyngitis, flushing, respiratory tract infection, pain in extremity, nausea, back pain, dyspepsia, nasal congestion.

DRUG INTERACTIONS

See Contraindications and Dosing Considerations. If nitrate administration is deemed medically necessary in a life-threatening situation, at least 48 hrs should elapse after the last dose of tadalafil before nitrate administration is considered; administer nitrates only under close medical supervision w/ appropriate hemodynamic monitoring. Additive hypotensive effects w/ α-adrenergic blockers, antihypertensives (eg, amlodipine, ARBs, bendroflumethiazide, enalapril, metoprolol), and alcohol. Avoid w/ potent CYP3A inhibitors (eg, ketoconazole, itraconazole) or chronic therapy of potent CYP3A inducers (eg, rifampin). Do not give w/ Cialis or other PDE-5 inhibitors.

PREGNANCY AND LACTATION

Category B, caution in nursing.

MECHANISM OF ACTION

PDE-5 inhibitor; increases the concentrations of cGMP, resulting in relaxation of pulmonary vascular smooth muscle cells and vasodilation of the pulmonary vascular bed.

PHARMACOKINETICS

Absorption: T_{max}=4 hrs (median). **Distribution:** V_d=77L; plasma protein binding (94%). **Metabolism:** Liver via CYP3A to a catechol metabolite, which undergoes extensive methylation and glucuronidation; methylcatechol glucuronide (major circulating metabolite). **Elimination:** Feces (61%), urine (36%); $T_{1/2}$=35 hrs.

PATIENT CONSIDERATIONS

Assessment: Assess for CVD, PVOD, renal/hepatic impairment, history of NAION, hereditary degenerative retinal disorders, conditions that might predispose to priapism, anatomical deformation of the penis, bleeding disorders, active peptic ulceration, hypersensitivity to drug, pregnancy/nursing status, and possible drug interactions.

Monitoring: Monitor for signs/symptoms of anginal chest pain, pulmonary edema, NAION, hearing loss, prolonged erections >4 hrs, priapism, and other adverse reactions. Monitor BP.

Counseling: Inform of contraindication of treatment w/ any use of organic nitrates or GC stimulators. Instruct not to take Cialis or other PDE-5 inhibitors. Advise to seek immediate medical attention if sudden loss of vision in 1 or both eyes, sudden decrease/loss of hearing, or erection lasting >4 hrs occurs. Counsel about appropriate action to take if anginal chest pain requiring nitroglycerin occurs following intake of therapy.

ADEMPAS — riociguat   Rx

Class: Soluble guanylate cyclase (sGC) stimulator

> Do not administer to a pregnant female; may cause fetal harm. Exclude pregnancy before the start of treatment, monthly during treatment, and 1 month after stopping treatment. Prevent pregnancy during and for 1 month after stopping treatment; use acceptable methods of contraception. For all female patients, available only through a restricted program called the Adempas Risk Evaluation and Mitigation Strategy (REMS) Program.

ADULT DOSAGE	PEDIATRIC DOSAGE
Chronic-Thromboembolic Pulmonary Hypertension	Pediatric use may not have been established
Treatment of persistent/recurrent chronic thromboembolic pulmonary hypertension (CTEPH) WHO Group 4 after surgical treatment, or inoperable CTEPH, to improve exercise capacity and WHO functional class	
Initial: 1mg tid; consider 0.5mg tid for patients who may not tolerate the hypotensive effect	
Titrate: Increase by 0.5mg tid if systolic BP remains >95mmHg and patient has no signs/symptoms of hypotension	
Dose increases should be no sooner than 2 weeks apart	
Max: 2.5mg tid; if patient has symptoms of hypotension, decrease the dose by 0.5mg tid	
Dose Interruption: Retitrate if treatment is interrupted for ≥3 days	
Pulmonary Arterial Hypertension	
Treatment of pulmonary arterial HTN, (WHO Group 1), to improve exercise capacity, WHO functional class, and to delay clinical worsening	

Initial: 1mg tid; consider 0.5mg tid for patients who may not tolerate the hypotensive effect
Titrate: Increase by 0.5mg tid if systolic BP remains >95mmHg and patient has no signs/symptoms of hypotension

Dose increases should be no sooner than 2 weeks apart
Max: 2.5mg tid; if patient has symptoms of hypotension, decrease the dose by 0.5mg tid
Dose Interruption:
Retitrate if treatment is interrupted for ≥3 days

DOSING CONSIDERATIONS
Concomitant Medications
Strong CYP and P-gp/Breast Cancer Resistance Protein (P-gp/BCRP) Inhibitors (eg, Azole Antimycotics, HIV Protease Inhibitors):
Initial: 0.5mg tid

Other Important Considerations
Patients Who Smoke:
Consider titrating to dosages >2.5mg tid, if tolerated
May require a dose decrease in patients who stop smoking

ADMINISTRATION
Oral route
Take PO w/ or w/o food

STORAGE
25°C (77°F); excursions permitted from 15-30°C (59-86°F).

HOW SUPPLIED
Tab: 0.5mg, 1mg, 1.5mg, 2mg, 2.5mg

CONTRAINDICATIONS
Pregnancy. Coadministration with nitrates or nitric oxide (NO) donors (eg, amyl nitrite) in any form, specific PDE-5 inhibitors (eg, sildenafil, tadalafil, vardenafil), or nonspecific PDE inhibitors (eg, dipyridamole, theophylline).

WARNINGS/PRECAUTIONS
Reduces BP; consider the potential for symptomatic hypotension or ischemia in patients with hypovolemia, severe left ventricular outflow obstruction, resting hypotension, or autonomic dysfunction. Serious bleeding/hemoptysis/hemorrhagic events reported. May significantly worsen the cardiovascular status of patients with pulmonary veno-occlusive disease (PVOD); administration to such patients is not recommended. If signs of pulmonary edema occur, consider possibility of associated PVOD and, if confirmed, d/c treatment. Caution in elderly.

ADVERSE REACTIONS
Headache, dyspepsia, gastritis, dizziness, N/V, diarrhea, hypotension, anemia, gastroesophageal reflux disease, constipation.

DRUG INTERACTIONS
See Contraindications and Dosage. Consider the potential for symptomatic hypotension or ischemia with concomitant antihypertensives. Smoking may reduce concentrations. Strong CYP inhibitors and P-gp/BCRP inhibitors increase exposure and may result in hypotension. Strong CYP3A inducers (eg, rifampin, phenytoin, carbamazepine) may significantly reduce exposure. Antacids (eg, aluminum hydroxide, magnesium hydroxide) decrease absorption and should not be taken within 1 hr of taking riociguat.

PREGNANCY AND LACTATION
Category X, not for use in nursing.

MECHANISM OF ACTION
sGC stimulator; sensitizes sGC to endogenous NO by stabilizing the NO-sGC binding. Also, directly stimulates sGC via a different binding site, independently of NO. Stimulates the NO-sGC-cGMP pathway and leads to increased generation of cGMP with subsequent vasodilation.

PHARMACOKINETICS
Absorption: Absolute bioavailability (94%); T_{max}=1.5 hrs. **Distribution:** V_d=30L; plasma protein binding (95%). **Metabolism:** CYP1A1, CYP3A, CYP2C8, CYP2J2; M1 (major active metabolite) (catalyzed by CYP1A1). **Elimination:** Urine (40%), feces (53%); $T_{1/2}$=12 hrs.

PATIENT CONSIDERATIONS
Assessment: Assess for hypovolemia, severe left ventricular outflow obstruction, resting hypotension, autonomic dysfunction, PVOD, pregnancy/nursing status, and possible drug interactions.

Monitoring: Monitor for signs/symptoms of hypotension, bleeding, pulmonary edema, and other adverse reactions. Obtain pregnancy tests monthly during treatment and 1 month after discontinuation of treatment.

Counseling: Counsel on the risk of fetal harm when used during pregnancy; instruct females of reproductive potential to use effective contraception during therapy and for 1 month after stopping treatment. Instruct to contact physician immediately if pregnancy is suspected. Inform female patients that they must enroll in the Adempas REMS Program. Advise about the potential risks/signs of hemoptysis and to report any potential signs of hemoptysis to physician. Instruct to report all current and new medications, and smoking history to physician. Advise that antacids should not be taken within 1 hr of taking the drug. Inform that drug can cause dizziness, which can affect the ability to drive and use machines.

ADRUCIL — fluorouracil
Class: Antimetabolite

Rx

> To be given only by or under the supervision of a qualified physician experienced in cancer chemotherapy and well versed in the use of potent antimetabolites. Because of the possibility of severe toxic reactions, patients should be hospitalized at least during initial course of therapy.

ADULT DOSAGE
Carcinoma
Palliative Management of Colon/Rectum/Breast/Stomach/Pancreas Carcinoma:

12mg/kg qd for Days 1-4; if no toxicity is observed, administer 6mg/kg on Day 6, 8, 10, and 12 unless toxicity occurs
Max: 800mg/day

Poor-Risk Patients/Inadequate Nutritional State:
6mg/kg/day for Days 1-3; if no toxicity is observed, administer 3mg/kg on Day 5, 7, and 9 unless toxicity occurs
Max: 400mg/day

Maint:
If toxicity has not been a problem:
- May repeat 1st course every 30 days after last day of previous course, or
- Give 10-15mg/kg/week as a single dose when toxic signs from initial course subside; do not exceed 1g/week

Determine and adjust dose based on patient's reaction to previous course

PEDIATRIC DOSAGE
Pediatric use may not have been established

DOSING CONSIDERATIONS
Important Modifications
Obese Patients/Spurious Weight Gain: Use estimated lean body mass (dry weight)

ADMINISTRATION
IV route

No dilution required.
If precipitate occurs due to low temperature exposure, resolubilize by heating to 60°C (140°F) and shaking vigorously; allow to cool to body temperature before use.

STORAGE
20-25°C (68-77°F). Protect from light. Retain in carton until time of use.

HOW SUPPLIED
Inj: 50mg/mL [10mL]

CONTRAINDICATIONS
Poor nutritional state, depressed bone marrow function, potentially serious infections, or known hypersensitivity to fluorouracil.

WARNINGS/PRECAUTIONS
Highly toxic drug w/ a narrow margin of safety. Extreme caution in poor-risk patients w/ a history of high-dose pelvic irradiation or previous use of alkylating agents, those w/ a widespread bone marrow involvement by metastatic tumors, or hepatic/renal impairment. Dipyrimidine dehydrogenase deficiency prolongs 5-fluorouracil clearance; may cause severe toxicity (eg, stomatitis, diarrhea, neutropenia, neurotoxicity). May cause fetal harm during pregnancy. Severe hematological toxicity, GI hemorrhage, and death reported. D/C if stomatitis, esophagopharyngitis, leukopenia (WBCs <3500) or rapidly falling WBC count, intractable vomiting, diarrhea, GI ulceration/bleeding, thrombocytopenia (platelets <100,000), or hemorrhage from any site occurs. Palmar-plantar erythrodysesthesia syndrome (hand-foot syndrome) reported; may gradually resolves over 5-7 days following discontinuation.

ADVERSE REACTIONS
Stomatitis, esophagopharyngitis, diarrhea, anorexia, nausea, emesis, leukopenia, alopecia, dermatitis.

DRUG INTERACTIONS
Leucovorin calcium or any form of therapy that adds to the stress of the patient, interferes w/ nutrition, or depresses bone marrow function may increase toxicity.

PREGNANCY AND LACTATION
Pregnancy: Category D. May cause fetal harm.
Lactation: Not for use in nursing.

MECHANISM OF ACTION
Antimetabolite; blocks the methylation reaction of deoxyuridylic acid to thymidylic acid, thereby interfering w/ the synthesis of DNA and to a lesser extent inhibiting the formation of RNA.

PHARMACOKINETICS
Distribution: Crosses blood-brain barrier. **Metabolism:** Liver. **Elimination:** Urine (7-20% unchanged); $T_{1/2}$=16 min.

PATIENT CONSIDERATIONS
Assessment: Assess for known hypersensitivity to the drug, nutritional state, bone marrow function or involvement of bone marrow by metastatic tumors,

presence of serious infections, history of high-dose pelvic irradiation, previous use of alkylating agents, hepatic/renal impairment, dipyrimidine dehydrogenase deficiency, pregnancy/nursing status, and possible drug interactions. Assess WBC counts w/ differential before each dose.

Monitoring: Monitor for signs and symptoms of stomatitis, esophagopharyngitis, leukopenia, thrombocytopenia, or rapidly falling WBC count, intractable vomiting, diarrhea, GI ulceration/bleeding, hemorrhage, palmar-plantar erythrodysesthesia syndrome, and other adverse reactions.

Counseling: Inform of the expected toxic effects, particularly oral manifestations. Alert patients to the possibility of alopecia and inform that it is usually a transient effect. Advise women of childbearing potential to avoid becoming pregnant.

ADVATE — antihemophilic factor (recombinant)   Rx

Class: Antihemophilic factor (recombinant)

ADULT DOSAGE

Hemophilia A

Control/Prevention of Bleeding Episodes:
Minor Bleed:
Required Factor VIII (FVIII) Level 20-40 IU/dL: 10-20 IU/kg IV; repeat q12-24h until bleeding is resolved (approx 1-3 days)

Moderate Bleed:
Required FVIII Level 30-60 IU/dL: 15-30 IU/kg IV; repeat q12-24h until bleeding is resolved (approx ≥3 days)

Major Bleed:
Required FVIII Level 60-100 IU/dL: 30-50 IU/kg IV; repeat q8-24h until resolution of bleeding episode has occurred

Perioperative Management:
Minor Surgery:
Required FVIII Level 60-100 IU/dL: 30-50 IU/kg single dose w/in 1 hr of the operation. Repeat after 12-24 hrs for optional additional dosing prn to control bleeding. Consider adjunctive therapy for dental procedures

Major Surgery:
Required FVIII Level 80-120 IU/dL
Pre-/Post-Operative: One 40-60 IU/kg IV dose preoperatively to achieve 100% activity; repeat q8-24h, depending on desired level of FVIII/state of wound healing. Give until healing is complete

Routine Prophylaxis:
20-40 IU/kg IV qod (3-4X/week) or an every 3rd-day dosing regimen to maintain FVIII trough levels ≥1%. Adjust dose based on response

Dosing Equation:
IU/dL (or % of Normal) = [Total Dose (IU)/Body Weight (kg)] x 2 [IU/dL]/[IU/kg]
or
Required Dose (IU) = Body Weight (kg) x Desired FVIII Rise (IU/dL or % of Normal) x 0.5 (IU/kg per IU/dL)

PEDIATRIC DOSAGE

Hemophilia A

Control/Prevention of Bleeding Episodes:
Minor Bleed:
Required Factor VIII (FVIII) Level 20-40 IU/dL: 10-20 IU/kg IV; repeat q12-24h (q8-24h for <6 yrs of age) until bleeding is resolved (approx 1-3 days)

Moderate Bleed:
Required FVIII Level 30-60 IU/dL: 15-30 IU/kg IV; repeat q12-24h (q8-24h for <6 yrs of age) until bleeding is resolved (approx ≥3 days)

Major Bleed:
Required FVIII Level 60-100 IU/dL: 30-50 IU/kg IV; repeat q8-24h (q6-12h for <6 yrs of age) until resolution of bleeding episode has occurred

Perioperative Management:
Minor Surgery:
Required FVIII Level 60-100 IU/dL: 30-50 IU/kg single dose w/in 1 hr of the operation. Repeat after 12-24 hrs for optional additional dosing prn to control bleeding. Consider adjunctive therapy for dental procedures

Major Surgery:
Required FVIII Level 80-120 IU/dL
Pre-/Postoperative: One 40-60 IU/kg IV dose preoperatively to achieve 100% activity; repeat q8-24h (q6-24h for <6 yrs of age), depending on desired level of FVIII/state of wound healing. Give until healing is complete

Routine Prophylaxis:
20-40 IU/kg IV qod (3-4X/week) or an every 3rd-day dosing regimen to maintain FVIII trough levels ≥1%. Adjust dose based on response

Dosing Equation:
IU/dL (or % of Normal) = [Total Dose (IU)/Body Weight (kg)] x 2 [IU/dL]/[IU/kg]
OR
Required Dose (IU) = Body Weight (kg) x Desired FVIII Rise (IU/dL or % of Normal) x 0.5 (IU/kg per IU/dL)

ADMINISTRATION
IV route

Preparation/Reconstitution/Administration
1. Allow package to reach room temperature, then open package.
2. Place product vial on flat surface and w/ 1 hand holding housing system, press down firmly on diluent vial w/ other hand until system is fully collapsed and diluent flows down into product vial; do not tilt system until transfer is complete.
3. Once diluent transfer is complete, swirl gently until powder is dissolved; do not shake or refrigerate after reconstitution.
4. Remove blue cap from housing and connect syringe to system; do not inject air into the system.
5. Turn system upside down (factor concentrate vial now on top) and draw factor concentrate into syringe slowly.
6. Disconnect syringe, attach a suitable needle, and inject as instructed; if a patient is to receive >1 Advate-Baxject III system or a combination of Advate-Baxject II and an Advate-Baxject III system, contents may be drawn into the same syringe.

Administer over a period of ≤5 min (max infusion rate of 10mL/min) w/in 3 hrs after reconstitution.

Determine pulse rate before and during administration; should a significant increase in pulse rate occur, reducing rate of administration/temporarily halting inj usually allows symptoms to disappear promptly.
Use plastic syringes w/ this product.

STORAGE
2-8°C (36-46°F) in powder form. May be stored at room temperature up to 30°C (86°F) for ≤6 months not to exceed the expiration date; must not be returned to refrigerated temperature. Do not freeze.

HOW SUPPLIED
Inj: 250 IU, 500 IU, 1000 IU, 1500 IU, 2000 IU, 3000 IU, 4000 IU

CONTRAINDICATIONS
Life-threatening hypersensitivity reactions (eg, anaphylaxis) to mouse or hamster protein or other constituents of the product (eg, mannitol, trehalose, sodium chloride, histidine, Tris, calcium chloride, polysorbate 80, and/or glutathione).

WARNINGS/PRECAUTIONS
Not indicated for the treatment of von Willebrand disease. Allergic-type hypersensitivity reactions, including anaphylaxis, reported; d/c if symptoms occur and administer emergency treatment. Monitor plasma FVIII activity levels by the one-stage clotting assay to confirm the adequate FVIII levels have been achieved and maintained when clinically indicated. Neutralizing antibodies (inhibitors) reported, predominantly in previously untreated and previously minimally treated patients. Monitor for the development of FVIII inhibitors by appropriate clinical observation and lab testing. If expected plasma FVIII activity levels are not attained, or if bleeding is not controlled with an expected dose, perform Bethesda assay that measures FVIII inhibitor concentration. If inhibitor titer <10 Bethesda Units (BU)/mL, additional antihemophilic factor concentrate may neutralize inhibitor and may permit appropriate hemostatic response. If inhibitor titer is >10 BU/mL, adequate hemostasis may not be achieved; inhibitor titer may rise following infusion; use alternative therapeutic approaches and agents.

ADVERSE REACTIONS
Pyrexia, headache, cough, nasopharyngitis, arthralgia, vomiting, upper respiratory tract infection, limb injury, nasal congestion, diarrhea.

PREGNANCY AND LACTATION
Pregnancy: Category C.
Lactation: Caution in nursing.

MECHANISM OF ACTION
Antihemophilic factor (recombinant); temporarily replaces the missing coagulation FVIII that is needed for effective hemostasis.

PHARMACOKINETICS
Absorption: C_{max}=128 IU/dL (>16 Yrs of Age). **Distribution:** V_d= 0.4dL/kg (>16 yrs of age). **Elimination:** $T_{1/2}$=12 hrs (adults). Refer to PI for pediatric parameters.

PATIENT CONSIDERATIONS
Assessment: Assess for life threatening hypersensitivity reactions including anaphylaxis to mouse/hamster protein or other constituents of the product, location and extent of bleeding, patient's clinical condition, and pregnancy/nursing status. Assess FVIII activity levels. Obtain baseline pulse rate prior to administration.

Monitoring: Monitor for signs/symptoms of hypersensitivity reactions and other adverse reactions. Monitor plasma FVIII activity levels, clinical response, development of FVIII inhibitors, and pulse rate.

Counseling: Advise to report any adverse reactions or problems following administration of therapy to physician. Inform of the early signs of hypersensitivity reactions (eg, hives, pruritus, urticaria); instruct to d/c and seek immediate emergency treatment if symptoms develop. Inform that inhibitor formation may occur; advise to contact physician/treatment center if there is lack of clinical response. Advise to consult physician prior to travel and to bring an adequate supply of therapy based on current treatment regimen while traveling.

ADYNOVATE — antihemophilic factor (recombinant), pegylated   Rx

Class: Antihemophilic factor (recombinant)

ADULT DOSAGE

Congenital Hemophilia A

On-demand Treatment and Control of Bleeding Episodes:
Minor Bleed:
Target Factor VIII (FVIII) Level 20-40 IU/dL: 10-20 IU/kg q12-24h until bleeding is resolved

Moderate Bleed:
Target FVIII Level 30-60 IU/dL: 15-30 IU/kg q12-24h until bleeding is resolved

Major Bleed:
Target FVIII Level 60-100 IU/dL: 30-50 IU/kg q8-24h until bleeding is resolved

Routine Prophylaxis to Reduce Frequency of Bleeding Episodes: 40-50 IU/kg 2X/week; adjust based on clinical response

PEDIATRIC DOSAGE

Congenital Hemophilia A

≥12 Years:
On-demand Treatment and Control of Bleeding Episodes:
Minor Bleed:
Target FVIII Level 20-40 IU/dL: 10-20 IU/kg q12-24h until bleeding is resolved

Moderate Bleed:
Target FVIII Level 30-60 IU/dL: 15-30 IU/kg q12-24h until bleeding is resolved

Major Bleed:
Target FVIII Level 60-100 IU/dL: 30-50 IU/kg q8-24h until bleeding is resolved

Routine Prophylaxis to Reduce Frequency of Bleeding Episodes: 40-50 IU/kg 2X/week; adjust based on clinical response

Dosing Equation:
IU/dL (or % of Normal) = [Total Dose (IU)/Body Weight (kg)] x 2 (IU/dL per IU/kg)

or

Dose (IU) = Body Weight (kg) x Desired FVIII Rise (IU/dL or % of Normal) x 0.5 (IU/kg per IU/dL)

Dosing Equation:
IU/dL (or % of Normal) = [Total Dose (IU)/Body Weight (kg)] x 2 (IU/dL per IU/kg)

or

Dose (IU) = Body Weight (kg) x Desired FVIII Rise (IU/dL or % of Normal) x 0.5 (IU/kg per IU/dL)

ADMINISTRATION
IV route
Administer as soon as possible, but no later than 3 hrs after reconstitution.

Reconstitution
1. Allow vials and diluent to reach room temperature before use.
2. Remove plastic caps from vials.
3. Open Baxject II Hi-Flow device package by peeling lid, w/o touching inside; do not remove the device from package.
4. Turn package over and press straight down to fully insert clear plastic spike through diluent vial stopper.
5. Grip the Baxject II Hi-Flow package at its edge and pull package off device. Do not remove the blue cap from the Baxject II Hi-Flow device. Do not touch the exposed purple plastic spike.
6. Turn system over so that diluent vial is on top. Quickly insert purple plastic spike fully into the Adynovate vial stopper by pushing straight down; vacuum will draw diluent into the Adynovate vial.
7. Swirl gently until completely dissolved; do not refrigerate after reconstitution.
8. If dose requires more than one vial of drug, reconstitute each vial using the above steps. Use a different Baxject II Hi-Flow device to reconstitute each vial of Adynovate and diluent.

Administration Steps
1. Remove the blue cap from the Baxject II Hi-Flow device. Connect the syringe to the Baxject II Hi-Flow device. Use of a Luer-lock syringe is recommended. Do not inject air.
2. Turn the system upside down (drug vial now on top). Draw factor concentrate into the syringe by pulling the plunger back slowly.
3. If patient is to receive more than one vial, contents of multiple vials may be drawn into the same syringe.
4. Disconnect the syringe; attach a suitable needle.
5. Inject intravenously over a period of ≤5 min (max infusion rate 10mL/min).

STORAGE
2-8°C (36-46°F) in powder form. May be stored at room temperature up to 30°C (86°F) for ≤1 month not to exceed the expiration date; must not be returned to refrigerated temperature. Do not freeze. Store vials in their original box and protect them from extreme exposure to light.

HOW SUPPLIED
Inj: 250 IU, 500 IU, 1000 IU, 2000 IU

CONTRAINDICATIONS
Prior anaphylactic reaction to Adynovate, to the parent molecule Advate, mouse or hamster protein, or excipients of the product (eg, Tris, mannitol, trehalose, glutathione, polysorbate 80).

WARNINGS/PRECAUTIONS
Not indicated for the treatment of von Willebrand disease. Initiate treatment under the supervision of a physician experienced in the treatment of hemophilia A. May cause allergic-type hypersensitivity reactions, including anaphylaxis; immediately d/c and initiate appropriate treatment if hypersensitivity reactions occur. Formation of neutralizing antibodies (inhibitors) to FVIII may occur; monitor for the development of FVIII inhibitors by appropriate clinical observation and lab tests. If expected plasma FVIII activity levels are not attained, or if bleeding is not controlled w/ an expected dose, perform Bethesda assay that measures FVIII inhibitor concentration. Monitor plasma factor VIII activity by performing a validated one-stage clotting assay to confirm the adequate FVIII levels have been achieved and maintained.

ADVERSE REACTIONS
Headache, nausea.

PREGNANCY AND LACTATION
Pregnancy: There are no data for use in pregnant women to inform a drug-associated risk. It is unknown whether treatment can cause fetal harm when administered to a pregnant woman or can affect reproduction capacity.
Lactation: There is no information regarding the presence in human milk, the effect on the breastfed infant, or the effects on milk production.

MECHANISM OF ACTION
Antihemophilic factor (recombinant); temporarily replaces the missing coagulation FVIII that is needed for effective hemostasis.

PHARMACOKINETICS
Absorption: C_{max}=95 IU/dL (12 to <18 years), 122 IU/dL (≥18 years); T_{max}=0.26 hrs (12 to <18 years), 0.46 hrs (≥18 years); AUC_{0-Inf}=1642 IU•h/dL (12 to <18 years), 2264 IU•h/dL (≥18 years). **Distribution:** V_d=0.56dL/kg (12 to <18 years), 0.43dL/kg (≥18 years). **Elimination:** $T_{1/2}$=13.43 hrs (12 to <18 years), 14.69 hrs (≥18 years).

PATIENT CONSIDERATIONS
Assessment: Assess for history of prior anaphylaxis to Adynovate, to the parent molecule Advate, mouse or hamster protein, or excipients of the product; location and extent of bleeding; patient's clinical condition; and pregnancy/nursing status. Assess FVIII activity levels.

Monitoring: Monitor for signs/symptoms of hypersensitivity reactions and other adverse reactions. Monitor plasma FVIII activity levels, clinical response, and development of FVIII inhibitors.

Counseling: Advise to report any adverse reactions or problems following administration of therapy to physician. Inform of the early signs of hypersensitivity reactions (eg, hives, pruritus, urticaria); instruct to d/c and seek immediate emergency treatment if symptoms develop.

AFINITOR — everolimus   Rx
Class: Kinase inhibitor

OTHER BRAND NAMES
Afinitor Disperz

ADULT DOSAGE

Breast Cancer
Treatment of postmenopausal women w/ advanced hormone receptor (HR)-positive, HER2-negative breast cancer in combination w/ exemestane, after failure of treatment w/ letrozole or anastrozole
Tab:
10mg qd; continue until disease progression or unacceptable toxicity occurs

Advanced Neuroendocrine Tumors
Treatment of progressive neuroendocrine tumors of pancreatic origin w/ unresectable, locally advanced or metastatic disease; also indicated for progressive, well-differentiated, non-functional neuroendocrine tumors of GI or lung origin w/ unresectable, locally advanced or metastatic disease
Tab:
10mg qd; continue until disease progression or unacceptable toxicity occurs

Advanced Renal Cell Carcinoma
After Failure of Treatment w/ Sunitinib or Sorafenib:
Tab:
10mg qd; continue until disease progression or unacceptable toxicity occurs

Renal Angiomyolipoma with Tuberous Sclerosis Complex
In Patients Not Requiring Immediate Surgery:
Tab:
10mg qd; continue until disease progression or unacceptable toxicity occurs

Subependymal Giant Cell Astrocytoma with Tuberous Sclerosis Complex
Requiring Therapeutic Intervention but Cannot Be Curatively Resected: Tab/Tab for Oral Sus:
Initial: 4.5mg/m² qd
Adjust dose at 2-week intervals prn to achieve/maintain trough concentrations of 5-15ng/mL
Continue until disease progression or unacceptable toxicity occurs

Therapeutic Drug Monitoring:
Assess trough levels 2 weeks after initiation, a change in dose, a change in coadministration of CYP3A4/P-gp inducers/inhibitors, a change in hepatic function, or a change in dosage form.
Once a stable dose is attained, monitor trough levels every 3-6 months in patients w/ changing BSA or every 6-12 months in patients w/ stable BSA.
Titrate (Based on Trough Levels):
<5ng/mL: Increase daily dose by 2.5mg (tab) or 2mg (tab for oral sus)
<15ng/mL: Reduce daily dose by 2.5mg (tab) or 2mg (tab for oral sus)
If dose reduction is required for patients receiving the lowest available strength, administer qod

PEDIATRIC DOSAGE

Subependymal Giant Cell Astrocytoma with Tuberous Sclerosis Complex
Requiring Therapeutic Intervention but Cannot Be Curatively Resected: Tab/Tab for Oral Sus:
≥1 Year:
Initial: 4.5mg/m² qd
Adjust dose at 2-week intervals prn to achieve/maintain trough concentrations of 5-15ng/mL.
Continue until disease progression or unacceptable toxicity occurs

Therapeutic Drug Monitoring:
Assess trough levels 2 weeks after initiation, a change in dose, a change in coadministration of CYP3A4/P-gp inducers/inhibitors, a change in hepatic function, or a change in dosage form.
Once a stable dose is attained, monitor trough levels every 3-6 months in patients w/ changing BSA or every 6-12 months in patients w/ stable BSA.
Titrate (Based on Trough Levels):
<5ng/mL: Increase daily dose by 2.5mg (tab) or 2mg (tab for oral sus)
<15ng/mL: Reduce daily dose by 2.5mg (tab) or 2mg (tab for oral sus)
If dose reduction is required for patients receiving the lowest available strength, administer qod

DOSING CONSIDERATIONS
Concomitant Medications
Advanced HR-Positive, HER2-Negative Breast Cancer, Advanced Neuroendocrine Tumors (NET), Advanced Renal Cell Carcinoma (RCC), Renal Angiomyolipoma w/ Tuberous Sclerosis Complex (TSC):

Strong CYP3A4/P-gp Inhibitors: Avoid use
Moderate CYP3A4/P-gp Inhibitors (If Coadministration Is Necessary):
- Reduce to 2.5mg qd; may increase to 5mg if tolerated
- 2-3 days after discontinuation of the moderate inhibitor, return to dose used prior to initiating the inhibitor

Avoid grapefruit, grapefruit juice, and other foods known to inhibit CYP450 and P-gp activity during treatment

Strong CYP3A4/P-gp Inducers: Avoid use
If Coadministration Is Required:
- Consider doubling daily dose by increments of ≤5mg
- 3-5 days after discontinuation of the strong inducer, return to dose used prior to initiating the inducer

Avoid St. John's wort during treatment

Subependymal Giant Cell Astrocytoma (SEGA) w/ TSC:

Strong CYP3A4/P-gp Inhibitors: Avoid use
Moderate CYP3A4/P-gp Inhibitors (If Coadministration Is Necessary):
Initial: 2.5mg/m² qd (reduce dose by approx 50%); administer qod if receiving the lowest available strength
- 2-3 days after discontinuation of the moderate inhibitor, return to dose used prior to initiating the inhibitor

Avoid ingestion of foods or nutritional supplements (eg, grapefruit, grapefruit juice) known to inhibit CYP450 or P-gp activity

Strong CYP3A4/P-gp Inducers: Avoid use
If Necessary: Double the dose and assess tolerability
Initial: 9mg/m² qd
Return to dose used prior to initiating the inducer if the strong inducer is discontinued

Avoid ingestion of foods or nutritional supplements (eg, St. John's wort) known to induce CYP450 activity

Hepatic Impairment
Advanced HR-Positive, HER2-Negative Breast Cancer, Advanced NET, Advanced RCC, Renal Angiomyolipoma w/ TSC:
Mild (Child-Pugh Class A): 7.5mg qd; reduce to 5mg qd if not tolerated
Moderate (Child-Pugh Class B): 5mg qd; reduce to 2.5mg qd if not tolerated
Severe (Child-Pugh Class C): 2.5mg qd if benefit outweighs the risk

SEGA w/ TSC:
Severe (Child-Pugh Class C):
Initial: 2.5mg/m² qd (reduce starting dose by approx 50%)

Adverse Reactions
Advanced HR-Positive, HER2-Negative Breast Cancer, Advanced NET, Advanced RCC, Renal Angiomyolipoma w/ TSC:
If dose reduction is required, administer approx 50% lower than the previously administered daily dose
Noninfectious Pneumonitis:
Grade 1 (Asymptomatic, Radiographic Findings Only):
- Initiate appropriate monitoring
Grade 2 (Symptomatic, Not Interfering w/ Activities of Daily Living [ADL]):
- Consider interrupting therapy, rule out infection, and consider treatment w/ corticosteroids until symptoms improve to Grade ≤1
- Reinitiate at a lower dose
- D/C if failure to recover w/in 4 weeks
Grade 3 (Symptomatic, Interfering w/ ADL; O₂ Indicated):
- Interrupt therapy until symptoms resolve to Grade ≤1, rule out infection, and consider treatment w/ corticosteroids
- Consider reinitiating at a lower dose
- Consider discontinuation if toxicity recurs at Grade 3
Grade 4 (Life-Threatening, Ventilator Support Indicated):
- D/C, rule out infection, and consider treatment w/ corticosteroids
Stomatitis:
Grade 1 (Minimal Symptoms, Normal Diet):
- Manage w/ nonalcoholic or salt water (0.9%) mouthwash several times a day
Grade 2 (Symptomatic but Can Eat and Swallow Modified Diet):
- Temporarily interrupt dose until recovery to Grade ≤1; reinitiate at the same dose
- If stomatitis recurs at Grade 2, interrupt dose until recovery to Grade ≤1; reinitiate at a lower dose
- Manage w/ topical analgesic mouth treatments (eg, benzocaine, butyl aminobenzoate, tetracaine, menthol, phenol) ± topical corticosteroids (eg, triamcinolone oral paste); avoid agents w/ alcohol, hydrogen peroxide, iodine, and thyme derivatives
Grade 3 (Symptomatic and Unable to Aliment or Hydrate Orally):
- Temporarily interrupt dose until recovery to Grade ≤1
- Reinitiate at a lower dose
- Manage w/ topical analgesic mouth treatments (eg, benzocaine, butyl aminobenzoate, tetracaine, menthol, phenol) ± topical corticosteroids (eg, triamcinolone oral paste); avoid agents w/ alcohol, hydrogen peroxide, iodine, and thyme derivatives
Grade 4 (Symptoms Associated w/ Life-Threatening Consequences):
- D/C and treat appropriately
Other Nonhematologic Toxicities (Excluding Metabolic Events):
Grade 1:
- If toxicity is tolerable, no dose adjustment required; initiate appropriate medical therapy and monitor

Grade 2:
- If toxicity is tolerable, no dose adjustment required; initiate appropriate medical therapy and monitor
- If toxicity becomes intolerable, temporarily interrupt dose until recovery to Grade ≤1; reinitiate at same dose
- If toxicity recurs at Grade 2, interrupt until recovery to Grade ≤1; reinitiate at lower dose
Grade 3:
- Temporarily interrupt dose until recovery to Grade ≤1
- Initiate appropriate therapy and monitor
- Consider reinitiating at a lower dose
- If toxicity recurs at Grade 3, consider discontinuation
Grade 4:
- D/C and treat appropriately
Metabolic Events (eg, Hyperglycemia, Dyslipidemia):
Grade 1:
- Initiate appropriate medical therapy and monitor
Grade 2:
- Manage w/ appropriate medical therapy and monitor
Grade 3:
- Temporarily interrupt dose
- Reinitiate at a lower dose
- Manage w/ appropriate therapy and monitor
Grade 4:
- D/C and treat appropriately
SEGA w/ TSC:
- Temporarily interrupt or permanently d/c for severe or intolerable adverse reactions
- If dose reduction is required when reinitiating therapy, reduce dose by 50%
- If dose reduction is required for patients receiving the lowest available strength, administer qod

ADMINISTRATION
Oral route

Take qd at the same time every day.
Take consistently either w/ or w/o food.
Do not combine the 2 dosage forms to achieve the desired total dose.
Do not break or crush.

Tab
Swallow whole w/ a glass of water.

Tab for Oral Sus
Wear gloves to avoid possible contact w/ drug when preparing sus for another person.
Administer as sus only.
Administer sus immediately after preparation and discard if not given w/in 60 min after preparation.
Prepare sus in water only.

Preparation Using an Oral Syringe:
1. Place prescribed dose into a 10mL syringe; do not exceed a total of 10mg/syringe and if higher doses are required, prepare an additional syringe.
2. Draw approx 5mL of water and 4mL of air into syringe.
3. Place the filled syringe into a container (tip up) for 3 min, until the tabs are in sus.
4. Gently invert the syringe 5X immediately prior to administration.
5. After administration of the prepared sus, draw approx 5mL of water and 4mL of air into the same syringe, and swirl the contents to suspend remaining particles; administer entire contents of the syringe.

Preparation Using a Small Drinking Glass:
1. Place prescribed dose into a small drinking glass (max size 100mL) containing approx 25mL of water; do not exceed a total of 10mg/glass and if higher doses are required, prepare an additional glass.
2. Allow 3 min for sus to occur.
3. Stir contents gently w/ a spoon, immediately prior to drinking.
4. After administration of the prepared sus, add 25mL of water and stir w/ the same spoon to resuspend remaining particles; administer entire contents of glass.

STORAGE
25°C (77°F); excursions permitted between 15-30°C (59-86°F). Protect from light and moisture.

HOW SUPPLIED
Tab for Oral Sus: (Afinitor Disperz) 2mg, 3mg, 5mg; **Tab:** (Afinitor) 2.5mg, 5mg, 7.5mg, 10mg

CONTRAINDICATIONS
Hypersensitivity to the active substance, to other rapamycin derivatives, or to any of the excipients of this product.

WARNINGS/PRECAUTIONS
See Dosing Considerations. Not indicated for the treatment of functional carcinoid tumors in NET. Noninfectious pneumonitis reported; some cases reported w/ pulmonary HTN as a secondary event. Immunosuppressive properties may predispose patients to infections, including infections w/ opportunistic pathogens. Localized and systemic infections, including reactivation of hepatitis B, reported. Complete treatment of preexisting invasive fungal infections prior to therapy. Institute appropriate treatment if diagnosis of an infection is made and consider interruption or discontinuation of therapy. If a diagnosis of invasive systemic fungal infection is made, d/c therapy. *Pneumocystis jiroveci* pneumonia (PJP) reported; consider prophylaxis of PJP when concomitant use of corticosteroids or other immunosuppressive agents are required. Mouth ulcers, stomatitis, and oral mucositis reported. Cases of

renal failure (including acute renal failure), some w/ fatal outcome, observed. May delay wound healing and increase the occurrence of wound-related complications (eg, wound dehiscence, wound infection, incisional hernia); use caution in the perisurgical period. Elevated SrCr, proteinuria, hyperglycemia, hyperlipidemia, hypertriglyceridemia, and decreased Hgb, lymphocytes, neutrophils, and platelets reported. Exposure is increased in patients w/ hepatic impairment. Avoid close contact w/ those who have received live vaccines during treatment. In pediatric patients w/ SEGA who do not require immediate treatment, complete the recommended childhood series of live virus vaccinations prior to therapy; an accelerated vaccination schedule may be appropriate. Can cause fetal harm; advise females of reproductive potential to avoid becoming pregnant and to use effective contraception during and for 8 weeks after ending treatment. Caution in elderly.

ADVERSE REACTIONS
Advanced HR-Positive, HER2-Negative Breast Cancer/Advanced NET/Advanced RCC: Stomatitis, infections, rash, fatigue, diarrhea, edema, abdominal pain, nausea, fever, asthenia, cough, headache, decreased appetite.
Renal Angiomyolipoma w/ TSC: Stomatitis.
SEGA w/ TSC: Stomatitis, respiratory tract infection.

DRUG INTERACTIONS
See Dosing Considerations. ACE inhibitors may increase risk for angioedema. Avoid use of live vaccines while on therapy. More frequent monitoring is recommended when coadministered w/ other drugs that may induce hyperglycemia. Significant increases in everolimus exposure reported when coadministered w/ ketoconazole (a strong CYP3A4 inhibitor and a P-gp inhibitor), erythromycin (a moderate CYP3A4 inhibitor and a P-gp inhibitor), and verapamil (a moderate CYP3A4 inhibitor and a P-gp inhibitor). Decreased everolimus levels reported when coadministered w/ rifampin (a strong inducer of CYP3A4 and an inducer of P-gp). St. John's wort may decrease everolimus exposure unpredictably. May increase levels of midazolam, octreotide, and exemestane.

PREGNANCY AND LACTATION
Pregnancy: May cause fetal harm.
Lactation: Do not breastfeed during treatment and for 2 weeks after the last dose.
Reproductive Potential: Females of reproductive potential should use effective contraception during and for 8 weeks after ending treatment. Menstrual irregularities, secondary amenorrhea, and increases in luteinizing hormone and follicle-stimulating hormone reported. Female fertility may be compromised. May impair male fertility.

MECHANISM OF ACTION
Kinase inhibitor; inhibitor of mammalian target of rapamycin (mTOR), a serine-threonine kinase, downstream of the PI3K/AKT pathway. Binds to an intracellular protein, FKBP-12, resulting in an inhibitory complex formation w/ mTOR complex 1, inhibiting mTOR kinase activity. Inhibition of mTOR has been shown to reduce cell proliferation, angiogenesis, and glucose uptake. Also, inhibits the expression of hypoxia-inducible factor and reduces the expression of vascular endothelial growth factor.

PHARMACOKINETICS
Absorption: T_{max}=1-2 hrs. **Distribution:** Plasma protein binding (74%). **Metabolism:** CYP3A4 and P-gp. **Elimination:** (3mg single dose) Urine (5%), feces (80%); $T_{1/2}$=30 hrs.

PATIENT CONSIDERATIONS
Assessment: Assess for hypersensitivity, preexisting fungal infections, pregnancy/nursing status, and possible drug interactions. Assess hepatic function and renal function, including measurement of BUN, urinary protein, or SrCr. Obtain FPG, lipid profile, and CBC prior to start of therapy. Assess vaccination history in pediatric patients w/ SEGA.

Monitoring: Monitor for signs/symptoms of hypersensitivity reactions, noninfectious pneumonitis, infections, mouth ulcers, stomatitis, oral mucositis, and other adverse reactions. Monitor FPG, lipid profile, CBC count, and renal function, including measurement of BUN, urinary protein, or SrCr, periodically. Routine therapeutic drug monitoring is recommended in SEGA w/ TSC.

Counseling: Inform that noninfectious pneumonitis or infections may develop; advise to report new or worsening respiratory symptoms or any signs or symptoms of infection. Inform patients that they are more susceptible to angioedema if concomitantly taking ACE inhibitors; advise to be aware of any signs/symptoms of angioedema and to seek prompt medical attention. Inform of the possibility of developing mouth ulcers, stomatitis, and oral mucositis; instruct to use topical treatments and mouthwashes (w/o alcohol, peroxide, iodine, or thyme) in such cases. Inform of the possibility of developing kidney failure and the need to monitor kidney function. Inform of the possibility of impaired wound healing or dehiscence during therapy. Inform of the need to monitor blood chemistry and hematology prior to therapy and periodically thereafter. Advise to notify healthcare provider of all concomitant medications, including OTC medications and dietary supplements. Advise to avoid the use of live vaccines and close contact w/ those who have received live vaccines. Advise of risk of fetal harm. Advise female patients of reproductive potential to use effective contraception during treatment and for 8 weeks after the last dose. Advise not to breastfeed during treatment and for 2 weeks after the last dose. Advise males and females of reproductive potential of the potential risk for impaired fertility. Instruct to follow the dosing instructions ud; inform that missed doses may be taken up to 6 hrs after scheduled time but that if >6 hrs have elapsed, dose should be skipped and resumed at next scheduled time. Advise to read and carefully follow the FDA-approved "Instructions for Use."

ALDURAZYME — laronidase Rx
Class: Alpha-L-iduronidase

> Life-threatening anaphylactic reactions observed during infusion. Appropriate medical support should be readily available when administered. Patients with compromised respiratory function or acute respiratory disease may be at risk of serious acute exacerbation of their respiratory compromise due to infusion reactions; additional monitoring required.

ADULT DOSAGE
Mucopolysaccharidosis I
Patients w/ Hurler and Hurler-Scheie forms, and for patients w/ the Scheie form who have moderate to severe symptoms

Usual: 0.58mg/kg once weekly as an IV infusion over 3-4 hrs

Infusion Rate:
Initial: 10mcg/kg/hr
Titrate: Increase every 15 min during 1st hr as tolerated
Max: 200mcg/kg/hr. Maintain at max rate for the remainder of the infusion (2-3 hrs)
≥20kg: Give total volume of 250mL
≤20kg: Give total volume of 100mL

Premedication
Recommended 60 min prior to the start of the infusion and may include antihistamines, antipyretics, or both

PEDIATRIC DOSAGE
Mucopolysaccharidosis I
Patients w/ Hurler and Hurler-Scheie forms, and for patients w/ the Scheie form who have moderate to severe symptoms

≥6 Months of Age:
Usual: 0.58mg/kg once weekly as an IV infusion over 3-4 hrs

Infusion Rate:
Initial: 10mcg/kg/hr
Titrate: Increase every 15 min during 1st hr as tolerated
Max: 200mcg/kg/hr. Maintain at max rate for the remainder of the infusion (2-3 hrs)
≥20kg: Give total volume of 250mL
≤20kg: Give total volume of 100mL

Premedication
Recommended 60 min prior to the start of the infusion and may include antihistamines, antipyretics, or both

---

ADMINISTRATION
IV route
Vial is intended for single use only; do not use more than 1 time
Use infusion bag immediately after dilution w/ saline; if immediate use is not possible, refrigerate the diluted sol at 2-8°C (36-46°F) for up to 36 hrs
Do not administer w/ other medicinal products in the same infusion

Preparation and Administration Instructions
1. Prepare using low-protein-binding containers
2. Determine the number of vials to be diluted; refer to PI for equation
3. Round up to the next whole vial and remove the required number of vials from the refrigerator to allow them to reach room temperature; do not heat or microwave vials
4. Withdraw and discard a volume of the 0.9% NaCl inj from the infusion bag, equal to the volume of laronidase concentrate to be added
5. Slowly withdraw the calculated volume of laronidase from the appropriate number of vials, using caution to avoid excessive agitation; do not use a filter needle, as this may cause agitation
6. Slowly add the laronidase sol to the 0.9% NaCl inj using care to avoid agitation of the sol; do not use a filter needle
7. Gently rotate the infusion bag to ensure proper distribution; do not shake the sol
8. The entire infusion volume (100mL for patients weighing ≤20kg and 250mL for patients weighing >20kg) should be delivered over approx 3-4 hrs
9. The initial infusion rate of 10μg/kg/hr may be incrementally increased every 15 min during the 1st hr, as tolerated, until a max infusion rate of 200μg/kg/hr is reached; refer to PI for incremental rates for infusion
10. The max rate is then maintained for the remainder of the infusion (2-3 hrs)
11. Administer the diluted sol using a low-protein-binding infusion set equipped w/ a low-protein-binding 0.2μm in-line filter

Patients w/ Underlying Cardiac/Respiratory Compromise and Weighing ≤30kg: Consider diluting the sol in a volume of 100mL and administering at a decreased infusion rate

STORAGE
2-8°C (36-46°F). Do not freeze or shake. Protect from light. Diluted Sol: 2-8°C (36-46°F) for up to 36 hrs.

HOW SUPPLIED
Inj: 2.9mg/5mL

WARNINGS/PRECAUTIONS
D/C infusion immediately and initiate appropriate treatment if anaphylactic or other severe allergic reactions occur. Caution if epinephrine is consider in patients with MPS I due to increased prevalence of coronary artery disease. Caution with readministration in patients who have experienced anaphylactic or severe allergic reactions. Increased risk of infusion reactions in patients with acute febrile or respiratory illness at the time of infusion; consider patient's clinical status prior to administration and consider delaying the infusion. Sleep apnea is common in MPS I patients; evaluate airway patency prior to initiation of treatment. Caution in patients susceptible to fluid overload, or with acute underlying respiratory illness or compromised cardiac and/or respiratory function for whom fluid restriction is indicated; may be at risk of serious exacerbation of cardiac or respiratory status during infusions. If infusion reactions occur, regardless of pretreatment, decreasing the infusion rate, temporarily stopping the infusion, or administering additional antipyretics and/or antihistamines may ameliorate the symptoms.

ADVERSE REACTIONS

Anaphylactic reactions, infusion reactions (eg, flushing, pyrexia, headache, rash), abdominal pain/discomfort, inj-site reaction, upper respiratory tract infection, hyperreflexia, paresthesia, poor venous access, otitis media, chills, BP increased, tachycardia.

PREGNANCY AND LACTATION

Category B, caution in nursing.

MECHANISM OF ACTION

α-L-iduronidase enzyme variant; provides exogenous enzyme for uptake into lysosomes and increase catabolism of glycosaminoglycan.

PHARMACOKINETICS

Absorption: C_{max}=1.2-1.7mcg/mL, AUC=4.5-6.9mcg•hr/mL. **Distribution:** V_d=0.24-0.6L/kg. **Elimination:** $T_{1/2}$=1.5-3.6 hrs.

PATIENT CONSIDERATIONS

Assessment: Assess for susceptibility to fluid overload, respiratory illness, compromised cardiac and/or respiratory function, clinical status, and pregnancy/nursing status. Evaluate airway patency prior to initiation of treatment.

Monitoring: Monitor for anaphylaxis/severe allergic reactions (eg, respiratory failure, respiratory distress, stridor, tachypnea, bronchospasm, obstructive airway disorder, hypoxia, hypotension, bradycardia, urticaria), infusion-related reactions, exacerbation of cardiac or respiratory status, and other adverse reactions. Monitor closely during readministration.

Counseling: Counsel that allergic reactions may occur during treatment, including life-threatening anaphylaxis. Advise to report any adverse reactions experienced while on treatment. Encourage patients and pregnant/nursing women with MPS I to enroll in the MPS I Registry.

ALECENSA — alectinib   Rx

Class: Kinase inhibitor

ADULT DOSAGE

Metastatic Non-Small Cell Lung Cancer

W/ anaplastic lymphoma kinase (ALK)-positive, metastatic non-small cell lung cancer (NSCLC) who have progressed on or are intolerant to crizotinib

600mg bid until disease progression or unacceptable toxicity

Missed Dose

If a dose is missed or vomiting occurs after taking a dose, take the next dose at the scheduled time

PEDIATRIC DOSAGE

Pediatric use may not have been established

DOSING CONSIDERATIONS

Adverse Reactions

Dose Reduction Schedule:
Starting Dose: 600mg bid
1st Dose Reduction: 450mg bid
2nd Dose Reduction: 300mg bid
D/C if patients are unable to tolerate the 300mg twice daily dose

ALT or AST >5X ULN w/ Total Bilirubin ≤2X ULN: Temporarily withhold until recovery to baseline or to ≤3X ULN, then resume at reduced dose as per dose reduction schedule

ALT or AST >3X ULN w/ Total Bilirubin >2X ULN in the Absence of Cholestasis or Hemolysis: Permanently d/c
Total Bilirubin Elevation of >3X ULN: Temporarily withhold until recovery to baseline or to ≤1.5X ULN, then resume at reduced dose as per dose reduction schedule

Any Grade Treatment-Related Interstitial Lung Disease (ILD)/Pneumonitis: Permanently d/c

Symptomatic Bradycardia: Withhold until recovery to asymptomatic bradycardia or to a HR ≥60 bpm
- If contributing concomitant medication is identified and discontinued, or its dose is adjusted, resume alectinib at previous dose upon recovery to asymptomatic bradycardia or to a HR ≥60 bpm
- If no contributing concomitant medication is identified, or if contributing concomitant medications are not discontinued or dose modified, resume alectinib at reduced dose as per dose reduction schedule upon recovery to asymptomatic bradycardia or to HR ≥60 bpm

Bradycardia (Life-Threatening Consequences, Urgent Intervention Indicated): Permanently d/c alectinib if no contributing concomitant medication is identified
- If contributing concomitant medication is identified and discontinued, or its dose is adjusted, resume alectinib at reduced dose upon recovery to asymptomatic bradycardia or to a HR ≥60 bpm w/ frequent monitoring as clinically indicated; permanently d/c in case of recurrence

Creatine Phosphokinase (CPK) Elevation>5X ULN: Temporarily withhold until recovery to baseline or to ≤2.5X ULN, then resume at same dose
CPK Elevation >10X ULN or 2nd Occurrence of CPK Elevation of >5X ULN: Temporarily withhold until recovery to baseline or ≤2.5X ULN, then resume at reduced dose as per dose reduction schedule

ADMINISTRATION

Oral route

Take w/ food.

Do not open or dissolve the contents of the capsule.

STORAGE

≤30°C (86°F); protect from light and moisture.

HOW SUPPLIED

Cap: 150mg

WARNINGS/PRECAUTIONS

See Dosing Considerations. Elevations of AST >5X ULN, ALT >5X ULN, and bilirubin >3X ULN reported; monitor LFTs including ALT, AST, and total bilirubin q2 weeks during the first 2 months of treatment, then periodically, w/ more frequent testing if transaminase/ bilirubin elevations occur. Severe ILD reported; promptly investigate for ILD/pneumonitis in any patient who presents w/ worsening of respiratory symptoms (eg, dyspnea, cough, fever). Immediately withhold treatment in patients diagnosed w/ ILD/pneumonitis and permanently d/c if no other potential causes of ILD/pneumonitis have been identified. Symptomatic bradycardia may occur; monitor HR and BP regularly. Myalgia or musculoskeletal pain and elevations of CPK levels reported. Assess CPK levels q2 weeks during 1st month of treatment and in patients reporting unexplained muscle pain, tenderness, or weakness. May cause fetal harm.

ADVERSE REACTIONS

Fatigue, constipation, edema, myalgia, cough, rash, N/V, headache, diarrhea, dyspnea, back pain, increased weight, vision disorder.

PREGNANCY AND LACTATION

Pregnancy: Can cause fetal harm.
Lactation: Do not breastfeed during treatment and for 1 week after the final dose.
Reproductive Risk Potential:
Females: Use effective contraception during treatment and for 1 week after the final dose.
Males: Males w/ female partners of reproductive potential should use effective contraception during treatment and for 3 months following the final dose.

MECHANISM OF ACTION

Tyrosine kinase inhibitor; targets ALK and RET. Inhibits ALK phosphorylation and ALK-mediated activation of the downstream signaling proteins STAT3 and AKT, and decreases tumor cell viability in multiple cell lines harboring ALK fusions, amplifications, or activating mutations.

PHARMACOKINETICS

Absorption: Absolute bioavailability (37%), T_{max}=4 hrs, AUC: 7430ng•h/mL; 2810ng•h/mL (M4). **Distribution:** V_d=4016L, 10,093L (M4); plasma protein binding (>99%, parent drug and M4). **Metabolism:** Via CYP3A4 to M4 (major active metabolite). **Elimination:** Urine (<0.5%), Feces (98%; 84% unchanged, 6% M4). $T_{1/2}$=33 hrs, 31 hrs (M4).

PATIENT CONSIDERATIONS

Assessment: Assess for hepatic impairment, pregnancy/nursing status, and possible drug interactions.

Monitoring: Monitor LFTs including ALT, AST, and total bilirubin q2 weeks during the first 2 months of treatment, then periodically w/ more frequent testing in patients who develop transaminase and bilirubin elevations. Monitor for worsening of respiratory symptoms indicative of ILD/pneumonitis (eg, dysphea, cough, fever) and monitor for unexplained muscle pain, tenderness, or weakness. Assess CPK levels q2 weeks for the 1st month of treatment and as clinically indicated in patients reporting symptoms. Monitor HR and BP regularly.

Counseling: Advise about the signs/symptoms of bilirubin and hepatic transaminase elevations. Inform about the risks of severe ILD/pneumonitis. Instruct to report new or worsening respiratory symptoms, symptoms of bradycardia (eg, dizziness, lightheadedness, syncope), and to report about the use of any heart or BP medications. Advise of signs/symptoms of myalgia and instruct to report new or worsening symptoms of muscle pain or weakness. Advise to avoid prolonged sun exposure while taking this medication and for at least 7 days after discontinuation. Advise to use a broad spectrum UVA/UVB sunscreen and lip balm (SPF ≥50) to help protect against potential sunburn. Inform that therapy may cause fetal harm; advise females of reproductive potential to use effective contraception during treatment and for at least 1 week after the last dose. Advise male patients w/ female partners of reproductive potential to use effective contraception during treatment and for 3 months after the last dose. Advise women not to breastfeed during treatment and for 1 week after the last dose. Instruct to take alectinib twice a day w/ food, and to swallow whole. Advise that if a dose is missed or if the patient vomits after taking a dose, not to take an extra dose, but to take the next dose at the regular time.

ALFERON N — interferon alfa-n3 (human leukocyte derived)   Rx

Class: Biological response modifier

ADULT DOSAGE

Refractory/Recurring External Condylomata Acuminata

0.05mL (250,000 IU)/wart into base of the wart 2X/week up to 8 weeks

Large Warts:
Inject at several points around periphery of the wart

Max:
0.5mL (2.5 million IU)/session

PEDIATRIC DOSAGE

Pediatric use may not have been established

ADMINISTRATION
Intralesional route

30 gauge needle preferable

STORAGE
2-8°C (36-46°F). Do not freeze or shake.

HOW SUPPLIED
Inj: 5,000,000 IU/1mL

CONTRAINDICATIONS
Known hypersensitivity to human interferon alpha proteins or any component of the product; anaphylactic sensitivity to mouse immunoglobulin, egg protein, or neomycin.

WARNINGS/PRECAUTIONS
Caution with cardiovascular disease (CVD) (eg, unstable angina, uncontrolled congestive heart failure), severe pulmonary disease (eg, chronic obstructive pulmonary disease), coagulation disorders (eg, thrombophlebitis, pulmonary embolism, hemophilia), diabetes mellitus (DM) with ketoacidosis, severe myelosuppression, and seizure disorders. D/C and institute appropriate medical therapy if acute and serious hypersensitivity reactions occur. Risk of transmitting infectious agents (eg, viruses, Creutzfeldt Jakob disease agent). Caution in fertile men and women; use contraception while on therapy. Changes in menstrual cycle and decreased estradiol/progesterone levels may occur.

ADVERSE REACTIONS
Fever, myalgia, headache, chills, fatigue, dizziness, malaise, arthralgia, back pain, N/V, dyspepsia/heartburn.

PREGNANCY AND LACTATION
Category C, not for use in nursing.

MECHANISM OF ACTION
Biological response modifier; naturally occurring proteins with antiviral, antiproliferative, and immunoregulatory properties. Binds to specific membrane receptors on cell surface, initiating induction of protein synthesis, promoting inhibition of viral replication, suppression of cell proliferation, and/or immunomodulating activities.

PATIENT CONSIDERATIONS
Assessment: Assess for cardiovascular CVD, severe pulmonary diseases, DM, coagulation disorders, severe myelosuppression, seizure disorders, and pregnancy/nursing status.

Monitoring: Monitor for flu-like symptoms, hypersensitivity reactions, and other adverse reactions.

Counseling: Counsel about early signs of hypersensitivity reactions; notify physician if symptoms occur. Inform of the risks/benefits of therapy. Caution not to change brands of interferon without medical consultation.

ALIMTA — pemetrexed disodium   **Rx**

Class: Antifolate

ADULT DOSAGE

Nonsquamous Non-Small Cell Lung Cancer
Initial treatment of locally advanced or metastatic nonsquamous non-small cell lung cancer (NSCLC) in combination w/ cisplatin. Maint treatment of patients w/ locally advanced or metastatic nonsquamous NSCLC whose disease has not progressed after 4 cycles of platinum-based first-line chemotherapy. Single-agent for the treatment of patients w/ locally advanced or metastatic nonsquamous NSCLC after prior chemotherapy

Combination w/ Cisplatin:
$500mg/m^2$ IV infused over 10 min on Day 1 of each 21-day cycle
Give cisplatin $75mg/m^2$ infused over 2 hrs beginning 30 min after the end of administration

Single Agent:
$500mg/m^2$ IV infused over 10 min on Day 1 of each 21-day cycle

Malignant Pleural Mesothelioma
Patients whose disease is unresectable or who are otherwise not candidates for curative surgery in combination w/ cisplatin

Combination w/ Cisplatin:
$500mg/m^2$ IV infused over 10 min on Day 1 of each 21-day cycle
Give cisplatin $75mg/m^2$ infused over 2 hrs beginning 30 min after the end of administration

PEDIATRIC DOSAGE
Pediatric use may not have been established

Premedication
Initiate folic acid (400-1000mcg) PO qd beginning 7 days before the 1st dose; continue during the full course of therapy and for 21 days after the last dose of therapy. Administer vitamin B12 1mg IM 1 week prior to the 1st dose and every 3 cycles thereafter. Subsequent vitamin B12 inj may be given the same day as treatment. Give dexamethasone 4mg PO bid the day before, the day of, and the day after administration of therapy.

DOSING CONSIDERATIONS
Adverse Reactions
As a Single Agent or in Combination:
Hematologic Toxicities:
Nadir ANC <500/mm^3 and Nadir Platelets ≥50,000/mm^3: 75% of previous dose (pemetrexed and cisplatin)
Nadir Platelets <50,000/mm^3 w/o Bleeding Regardless of Nadir ANC: 75% of previous dose (pemetrexed and cisplatin)
Nadir Platelets <50,000/mm^3 w/ Bleeding Regardless of Nadir ANC: 50% of previous dose (pemetrexed and cisplatin)
Nonhematologic Toxicities:
≥Grade 3 (Excluding Neurotoxicity): Withhold treatment until resolution to ≤pre-therapy value
Any Grade 3 or 4 Toxicities Except Mucositis: 75% of previous dose (pemetrexed and cisplatin)
Any Diarrhea Requiring Hospitalization (Irrespective of Grade) or Grade 3 or 4 Diarrhea: 75% of previous dose (pemetrexed and cisplatin)
Grade 3 or 4 Mucositis: 50% of previous pemetrexed dose, 100% of previous cisplatin dose
Neurotoxicity:
CTC Grade 1: 100% of previous pemetrexed and cisplatin dose
CTC Grade 2: 100% of previous pemetrexed dose, 50% of previous cisplatin dose
Discontinuation
For Any of the Following:
1. Experiences any hematologic or nonhematologic Grade 3 or 4 toxicity after 2 dose reductions
2. Grade 3 or 4 neurotoxicity is observed

ADMINISTRATION
IV route

Preparation
1. Calculate dose and determine the number of vials needed.
2. Reconstitute each 100mg vial w/ 4.2mL of 0.9% NaCl (preservative free). Reconstitute each 500mg vial w/ 20mL of 0.9% NaCl (preservative free).
3. Gently swirl each vial until the powder is completely dissolved. The resulting sol is clear and ranges in color from colorless to yellow or green-yellow w/o adversely affecting product quality.
4. An appropriate quantity of the reconstituted sol must be further diluted into a sol of 0.9% NaCl (preservative free), so that the total volume of sol is 100mL.
5. Administered as an IV infusion over 10 min.

Compatibility and Stability
Compatible w/ standard polyvinyl chloride administration sets and IV sol bags. Stable for up to 24 hrs following initial reconstitution, when refrigerated.

Handling Precautions
If sol contacts the skin, wash the skin immediately and thoroughly w/ soap and water. If sol contacts the mucous membranes, flush thoroughly w/ water.

STORAGE
Unreconstituted: 25°C (77°F); excursions permitted to 15-30°C (59-86°F).
Reconstituted and Infusion Sol: Stable at 2-8°C (36-46°F) for up to 24 hrs.

HOW SUPPLIED
Inj: 100mg, 500mg

CONTRAINDICATIONS
History of severe hypersensitivity reaction to pemetrexed.

WARNINGS/PRECAUTIONS
Not indicated for the treatment of patients with squamous cell NSCLC. Premedicate with folic acid and vitamin B12 to reduce hematologic/GI toxicity, and with dexamethasone. Do not substitute oral vitamin B12 for IM vitamin B12. Bone marrow suppression may occur; myelosuppression is usually the dose-limiting toxicity. Caution with renal/hepatic impairment and in elderly. Avoid in patients with CrCl <45mL/min. D/C if hematologic or nonhematologic Grade 3 or 4 toxicity after two dose reductions or immediately if Grade 3 or 4 neurotoxicity is observed. Do not start a cycle of treatment unless CrCl is ≥45mL/min, ANC is ≥1500 cells/mm^3, and platelet count is ≥100,000 cells/mm^3; obtain CBC and renal function tests at the beginning of each cycle and prn. May cause fetal harm; use effective contraception to prevent pregnancy.

ADVERSE REACTIONS
Anemia, anorexia, fatigue, leukopenia, N/V, stomatitis, neutropenia, rash/desquamation, thrombocytopenia, constipation, pharyngitis, diarrhea.

DRUG INTERACTIONS
Reduced clearance with ibuprofen. In patients with mild to moderate renal insufficiency (CrCl 45-79mL/min), caution with NSAIDs; avoid NSAIDs with short

$T_{1/2}$ (eg, diclofenac, indomethacin) for 2 days before, the day of, and 2 days following therapy. Interrupt dosing of NSAIDs with longer $T_{1/2}$ (eg, meloxicam, nabumetone) for at least 5 days before, the day of, and 2 days following therapy. If concomitant NSAID administration is necessary, monitor for toxicity. Delayed clearance with nephrotoxic or tubularly secreted drugs (eg, probenecid).

PREGNANCY AND LACTATION
Category D, not for use in nursing.

MECHANISM OF ACTION
Antifolate; disrupts folate-dependent metabolic processes essential for cell replication. Inhibits thymidylate synthase, dihydrofolate reductase, and glycinamide ribonucleotide formyltransferase.

PHARMACOKINETICS
Distribution: V_d=16.1L; plasma protein binding (81%). **Elimination:** Urine (70-90% unchanged); $T_{1/2}$=3.5 hrs (normal renal function).

PATIENT CONSIDERATIONS
Assessment: Assess for drug hypersensitivity, renal/hepatic impairment, pregnancy/nursing status, and possible drug interactions. Obtain CBC and renal function tests at the beginning of each cycle.

Monitoring: Monitor for signs and symptoms of hematologic/nonhematologic toxicities, bone marrow suppression (eg, neutropenia, thrombocytopenia, anemia), GI toxicity, neurotoxicity, and other adverse events. Monitor CBC with platelet counts and for nadir and recovery. Perform renal and hepatic function tests periodically.

Counseling: Inform about benefits and risks of therapy. Instruct on the need for folic acid and vitamin B12 supplementation to reduce treatment-related hematological and GI toxicities, and of the need for corticosteroids to reduce treatment-related dermatologic toxicity. Inform about risks of low blood cell counts and instruct to contact physician immediately if signs of infection (eg, fever, bleeding or symptoms of anemia) occur. Instruct to contact physician if persistent vomiting, diarrhea, or signs of dehydration appear. Instruct to inform physician of all concomitant prescription or OTC medications (eg, NSAIDs). Inform female patients of the potential hazard to fetus; advise to avoid pregnancy and to use effective contraceptive measures to prevent pregnancy during treatment.

ALKERAN — melphalan   Rx
Class: Nitrogen mustard alkylating agent

> Administer under the supervision of a qualified physician experienced in the use of cancer chemotherapeutic agents. Severe bone marrow suppression with resulting infection/bleeding may occur. Potentially mutagenic and leukemogenic. Inj has shown more myelosuppression than oral melphalan. (Inj) Hypersensitivity reactions (eg, anaphylaxis) reported.

ADULT DOSAGE
Multiple Myeloma

Inj:
Palliative treatment of patients for whom oral therapy is not appropriate

Usual: 16mg/m², administered as a single infusion over 15-20 min

Administer at 2-week intervals for 4 doses, then, after adequate recovery from toxicity, at 4-week intervals

PO:
Palliative treatment

Usual: 6mg/day (3 tabs/day); entire dose may be given at one time

After 2-3 weeks of treatment, d/c for up to 4 weeks; when the WBC and platelet counts are rising, a maint dose of 2mg/day may be instituted

Refer to PI for other oral dosage regimes used by various investigators

Epithelial Ovarian Cancer

PO:
Palliation of non-resectable epithelial carcinoma of the ovary

Usual: 0.2mg/kg/day for 5 days as a single course

Repeat courses every 4-5 weeks depending upon hematologic tolerance

PEDIATRIC DOSAGE
Pediatric use may not have been established

DOSING CONSIDERATIONS
Renal Impairment
Inj:
BUN ≥30mg/dL: Consider dose reduction of up to 50%
PO:
Moderate to Severe: May be prudent to use a reduced dose initially
Elderly
Start at lower end of dosing range

ADMINISTRATION
IV/Oral route

IV Route
Preparation for Administration/Stability:
1. Reconstitute melphalan for inj by rapidly injecting 10mL of the supplied diluent directly into the vial of lyophilized powder using a sterile needle (≥20-gauge needle diameter) and syringe
2. Immediately shake vial vigorously until a clear sol is obtained; this provides a 5mg/mL sol of melphalan. Rapid addition of the diluent followed by immediate vigorous shaking is important for proper dissolution
3. Immediately dilute the dose to be administered in 0.9% NaCl inj, to a concentration ≤0.45mg/mL
4. Administer the diluted product over a minimum of 15 min
5. Complete administration w/in 60 min of reconstitution

The time between reconstitution/dilution and administration should be kept to a minimum because reconstituted and diluted sol melphalan are unstable

Administration Precautions:
If the sol contacts the skin or mucosa, immediately wash the skin or mucosa thoroughly w/ soap and water
Care should be taken to avoid possible extravasation of melphalan and in cases of poor peripheral venous access, consideration should be given to use of a central venous line

STORAGE
Protect from light. (Inj): 15-30°C (59-86°F). Reconstituted Sol: Administer within 60 min. Do not refrigerate. (Tab): 2-8°C (36-46°F).

HOW SUPPLIED
Inj: 50mg; **Tab:** 2mg

CONTRAINDICATIONS
Prior resistance to agent, hypersensitivity to melphalan.

WARNINGS/PRECAUTIONS
Obtain platelet count, Hgb, WBCs, and differential count at the start of therapy and prior to each subsequent course. If thrombocytopenia and/or leukopenia occurs, withhold therapy until blood counts have sufficiently recovered. Frequently monitor blood counts to determine optimal dosage and to avoid toxicity. Consider dose adjustments on the basis of blood counts at the nadir and day of treatment. Do not readminister if hypersensitivity occurs. Secondary malignancies reported (some received other chemotherapeutic agents or radiation therapy). The potential benefits from therapy must be weighed against possible risk of the induction of a second malignancy. Causes chromatid/chromosome damage, ovary function suppression in premenopausal women (resulting in amenorrhea), and fetal harm. Reversible and irreversible testicular suppression reported. Extreme caution in patients whose bone marrow reserve may have been compromised by prior irradiation or chemotherapy, or whose marrow function is recovering from previous cytotoxic therapy. Avoid live vaccines in immunocompromised patients. Caution in elderly. (Inj) May cause local tissue damage if extravasation occurs; do not inject directly into a peripheral vein. (Tab) If leukocyte count falls <3000 cells/mcL or platelets <100,000 cells/mcL, d/c until peripheral blood counts recover. Caution with azotemia.

ADVERSE REACTIONS
Bone marrow suppression, infection, bleeding, leukopenia, thrombocytopenia, anemia, hypersensitivity reactions, anaphylaxis.

DRUG INTERACTIONS
(Inj) Severe renal failure reported with oral cyclosporine. Cisplatin may affect melphalan kinetics by inducing renal dysfunction and subsequently altering melphalan clearance. May reduce the threshold for BCNU lung toxicity. Nalidixic acid may increase incidence of severe hemorrhagic necrotic enterocolitis in pediatric patients.

PREGNANCY AND LACTATION
Category D, not for use in nursing.

MECHANISM OF ACTION
Nitrogen mustard alkylating agent (phenylalanine derivative); cytotoxic action appears to be related to the extent of its interstrand cross-linking with DNA by probable binding at the N^7 position of guanine; active against both resting and rapidly dividing tumor cells.

PHARMACOKINETICS
Absorption: (Tab) Absolute bioavailability (56-93%). (0.2-0.25mg/kg) C_{max}=212ng/mL, T_{max}=1 hr (median), AUC=498ng•hr/mL. (IV) C_{max}=1.2mcg/mL (10mg/m²), 2.8mcg/mL (20mg/m²). **Distribution:** V_d=0.5L/kg; plasma protein binding (53-92%). **Metabolism:** Hydrolysis. **Elimination:** (IV) $T_{1/2}$=75 min. (Tab) Urine (10%), $T_{1/2}$=1.5 hrs (0.6mg/kg). $T_{1/2}$=1 hr (0.2-0.25mg/kg).

PATIENT CONSIDERATIONS
Assessment: Assess for prior resistance to the drug, prior irradiation or chemotherapy, previous cytotoxic therapy, renal insufficiency, azotemia, pregnancy/nursing status, drug hypersensitivity, and possible drug interactions. Obtain baseline CBC with differential count.

Monitoring: Monitor for induction of a second malignancy, amenorrhea, testicular suppression, renal impairment, bone marrow suppression (severe infections, bleeding, symptomatic anemia), hypersensitivity reactions, and other adverse events. Obtain CBC with differential count prior to each subsequent course.

Counseling: Inform about major acute toxicities related to bone marrow suppression, hypersensitivity reactions, GI and pulmonary toxicity, and major long-term toxicities related to infertility and secondary malignancy. Instruct patients to never take the drug without close medical supervision and advise to seek medical attention if skin rash, vasculitis, bleeding, fever, persistent cough, N/V, amenorrhea, weight loss, and unusual lumps or masses develop. Advise to avoid becoming pregnant.

ALPHANATE — antihemophilic factor/von Willebrand factor complex (human)   Rx

Class: Antihemophilic agent

ADULT DOSAGE

Hemophilia A

Treatment and Prevention of Bleeding Episodes and Excess Bleeding During and After Surgery:
Dose Calculation:
Expected In Vivo Peak Increase in FVIII Level (IU/dL or % of Normal):
Dosage (IU) = Body Weight (kg) x Desired FVIII Rise (IU/dL or % of normal) x 0.5 (IU/kg per IU/dL)
or
IU/dL (or % of Normal) = [Total Dose (IU)/Body Weight (kg)] x 2

Dosing should aim at maintaining a plasma factor VIII activity level at or above the plasma levels (in IU/dL or in % of normal) outlined below

Minor Bleeding:
Required FVIII:C Level 30% of Normal: 15 IU/kg bid for 1-2 days, until hemorrhage stops and healing is achieved

Moderate Bleeding:
Required FVIII:C Level 50% of Normal: 25 IU/kg bid for 2-7 days, on average, until healing is achieved

Major Bleeding:
Required FVIII:C Level 80-100% of Normal:
Initial: 40-50 IU/kg bid for at least 3-5 days; bring FVIII:C levels to 80-100%
Maint: 25 IU/kg bid until healing is achieved for up to 10 days; intracranial hemorrhage may require prophylaxis therapy for up to 6 months

Surgery:
Prior to Surgery:
Required FVIII:C Level 80-100% of Normal: 40-50 IU/kg once
After Surgery:
Required FVIII:C Level 60-100% of Normal: 30-50 IU/kg bid for the next 7-10 days or until healing is achieved

von Willebrand's Disease

Treatment and Prevention of Excess Bleeding During and After Surgery or Other Invasive Procedure:
In patients w/ von Willebrand Disease (VWD) in whom desmopressin is either ineffective or contraindicated

Minor Surgery/Bleeding:
Preoperative/Preprocedure: 60 IU von Willebrand factor (VWF):RCo/kg
Maint: 40-60 IU VWF:RCo/kg at 8- to 12-hr intervals prn for 1-3 days
Target FVIII:C Activity Levels: 40-50 IU/dL
Therapeutic Goal (Trough):
>50 IU/dL
Max: 150 IU/dL

Major Surgery/Bleeding:
Preoperative/Preprocedure: 60 IU VWF:RCo/kg
Maint: 40-60 IU VWF:RCo/kg at 8- to 12-hr intervals prn for at least 3-7 days
Target FVIII:C Activity Levels: 100 IU/dL
Therapeutic Goal (Trough):
>50 IU/dL
Max: 150 IU/dL

PEDIATRIC DOSAGE

von Willebrand's Disease

Treatment and Prevention of Excess Bleeding During and After Surgery or Other Invasive Procedure:
In patients w/ VWD in whom desmopressin is either ineffective or contraindicated

Minor Surgery/Bleeding:
Preoperative/Preprocedure: 75 IU VWF:RCo/kg
Maint: 50-75 IU VWF:RCo/kg at 8- to 12-hr intervals prn for 1-3 days
Target FVIII:C Activity Levels: 40-50 IU/dL
Therapeutic Goal (Trough):
>50 IU/dL
Max: 150 IU/dL

Major Surgery/Bleeding:
Preoperative/Preprocedure: 75 IU VWF:RCo/kg
Maint: 50-75 IU VWF:RCo/kg at 8- to 12-hr intervals prn for at least 3-7 days
Target FVIII:C Activity Levels: 100 IU/dL
Therapeutic Goal (Trough): >50 IU/dL
Max: 150 IU/dL

Hemophilia A

Treatment and Prevention of Bleeding Episodes and Excess Bleeding During and After Surgery:
Dose Calculation:
Expected In Vivo Peak Increase in FVIII Level (IU/dL or % of Normal):
Dosage (IU) = Body Weight (kg) x Desired FVIII Rise (IU/dL or % of normal) x 0.5 (IU/kg per IU/dL)
or
IU/dL (or % of Normal) = [Total Dose (IU)/Body Weight (kg)] x 2

Dosing should aim at maintaining a plasma factor VIII activity level at or above the plasma levels (in IU/dL or in % of normal) outlined below

Minor Bleeding:
Required FVIII:C Level 30% of Normal: 15 IU/kg bid for 1-2 days, until hemorrhage stops and healing is achieved

Moderate Bleeding:
Required FVIII:C Level 50% of Normal: 25 IU/kg bid for 2-7 days, on average, until healing is achieved

Major Bleeding:
Required FVIII:C Level 80-100% of Normal:
Initial: 40-50 IU/kg bid for at least 3-5 days; bring FVIII:C levels to 80-100%
Maint: 25 IU/kg bid until healing is achieved for up to 10 days; intracranial hemorrhage may require prophylaxis therapy for up to 6 months

Surgery:
Prior to Surgery:
Required FVIII:C Level 80-100% of Normal: 40-50 IU/kg once
After Surgery:
Required FVIII:C Level 60-100% of Normal: 30-50 IU/kg bid for the next 7-10 days or until healing is achieved

ADMINISTRATION

IV route

Refer to PI for reconstitution instructions; do not refrigerate after reconstitution. Store reconstituted product at room temperature (not to exceed 30°C [86°F]) prior to administration; administer w/in 3 hrs.
Use plastic disposable syringes.
Do not administer at a rate exceeding 10mL/min.

STORAGE

≤25°C (77°F). Do not freeze.

HOW SUPPLIED

Inj: 250 IU FVIII/5mL, 500 IU FVIII/5mL, 1000 IU FVIII/10mL, 1500 IU FVIII/10mL, 2000 IU FVIII/10mL

CONTRAINDICATIONS

Life-threatening immediate hypersensitivity reactions, including anaphylaxis, to this product or its components.

WARNINGS/PRECAUTIONS

Not indicated for patients w/ severe VWD (type 3) undergoing major surgery. Anaphylaxis and severe hypersensitivity reactions may occur; d/c if symptoms occur and initiate appropriate treatment. Procoagulant activity-neutralizing antibodies (inhibitors) may develop. If expected plasma FVIII activity levels are not attained, or if bleeding is not controlled w/ an appropriate dose, perform an appropriate assay that measures FVIII inhibitor concentration. Thromboembolic events reported in VWD patients; consider antithrombotic measures in VWD patients at risk for thrombosis. Monitor plasma levels of VWF:RCo and FVIII activities to avoid sustained excessive VWF and FVIII activity levels (>150 IU/dL), which may increase risk of thrombotic events, during continued treatment. Contains blood group specific isoagglutinins. Monitor patients for signs of intravascular hemolysis and decreasing Hct when large and/or frequent doses are required in patients of blood groups A, B, or AB; cases of acute hemolytic anemia, increased bleeding tendency or hyperfibrinogenemia reported. Consider alternative therapy should this condition worsen despite discontinuation of therapy. Rapid administration may result in vasomotor reactions; do not administer at a rate >10mL/min. May carry a risk of transmitting infectious agents (eg, viruses, Creutzfeldt-Jakob disease agent).

ADVERSE REACTIONS

Pruritus, headache, back pain, paresthesia, respiratory distress, facial edema, pain, rash, chills.

PREGNANCY AND LACTATION

Pregnancy: Category C.
Lactation: No human or animal data; use only if clearly needed.

MECHANISM OF ACTION

Antihemophilic agent; temporarily replaces the missing coagulation factor VIII and VWF needed for effective hemostasis. FVIII is an essential cofactor in activation of factor X leading to formation of thrombin and fibrin. VWF promotes platelet aggregation and platelet adhesion on damaged vascular endothelium; also serves as a stabilizing carrier protein for the procoagulant protein FVIII.

PHARMACOKINETICS

Elimination: Hemophilia A: FVIII: $T_{1/2}$=17.9 hrs. VWD: VWF:RCo: $T_{1/2}$=7.67 hrs; FVIII:C: $T_{1/2}$=21.58 hrs; VWF:Ag: $T_{1/2}$=13.06 hrs.

PATIENT CONSIDERATIONS

Assessment: Assess for VWD type, severity of the deficiency/hemorrhage, risk factors for thrombosis, blood type, hypersensitivity to drug, and pregnancy/nursing status. Assess plasma FVIII levels.

Monitoring: Monitor for anaphylaxis, hypersensitivity reactions, thromboembolic events, intravascular hemolysis, vasomotor reactions, infections, and other adverse reactions. Monitor for development of FVIII and VWF inhibitors. Perform appropriate assays to determine if FVIII and/or VWF inhibitor(s) are present if bleeding is not controlled w/ expected dose of therapy. Monitor plasma levels of VWF:RCo and FVIII activities, and clinical response.

Counseling: Advise to contact physician or go to the emergency department right away if a hypersensitivity reaction occurs; inform of the early signs of hypersensitivity reactions. Instruct to contact physician or treatment center for further treatment and/or assessment if patients experience a lack of clinical response to therapy. Advise to contact physician or go to emergency department right away if a thromboembolic event occurs. Advise patients, especially pregnant women and immunocompromised individuals, to immediately report any signs/symptoms of fever, rash, joint pain, or sore throat, to physician.

ALPHANINE SD — coagulation factor IX (human)   Rx

Class: Antihemophilic agent

ADULT DOSAGE

Hemophilia B

<16 Years:
Prevention/Control of Bleeding:
Minor Hemorrhages:
Raise factor IX (FIX) levels to at least 20-30% (20-30 IU/kg bid) until hemorrhage stops and healing achieved (1-2 days)
Moderate Hemorrhages:
Raise FIX levels to 25-50% (25-50 IU/kg bid) until healing is achieved (2-7 days)
Major Hemorrhages:
Raise FIX levels to 50% for at least 3-5 days (30-50 IU/kg bid) and maintain at 20% (20 IU/kg bid) until healing is achieved (up to 10 days)

PEDIATRIC DOSAGE

Pediatric use may not have been established

Surgery:
Prior to surgery, raise FIX levels to 50-100% of normal (50-100 IU/kg bid). Maintain at 50-100% FIX levels (50-100 IU/kg bid) for the next 7-10 days, or until healing is achieved

Calculation of Number of FIX IU Required:
Number of FIX (IU) Required = Weight (kg) x Desired Increase in Plasma FIX (%) x 1.0 IU/kg

ADMINISTRATION
IV route
Use w/in 3 hrs after reconstitution
Do not exceed administration rate of 10mL/min

Reconstitution
Warm diluent (sterile water for inj) and concentrate to at least room temperature (but not >37°C [98°F])
If the same patient is to receive >1 vial of concentrate, contents of 2 vials may be drawn into the same syringe through separate unused Mix2Vial sets

STORAGE
2-8°C (36-46°F); stable for 3 yrs, up to the expiration date. Do not freeze. May store at room temperature ≤30°C (86°F) for 1 month.

HOW SUPPLIED
Inj: 500 IU, 1000 IU, 1500 IU [10mL]

WARNINGS/PRECAUTIONS
May carry risk of transmitting infectious agents (eg, viruses, Creutzfeldt-Jakob disease [CJD]). Thrombosis or disseminated intravascular coagulation (DIC) reported. Observe closely for signs or symptoms of DIC in surgery patients or individuals with known liver disease. Allergic-type hypersensitivity reactions, including anaphylaxis, may occur; closely observe patients with major deletions of the FIX gene and d/c if any symptoms occur. Nephrotic syndrome reported following attempted immune tolerance induction with FIX products in hemophilia B patients with FIX inhibitors and history of severe allergic reactions to FIX; safety and efficacy in attempted immune tolerance induction has not been established. Anaphylaxis may occur in previously untreated patients after median exposure of 11 days; monitor closely between the 10th and 20th exposure days. Strictly follow dosing guidelines to minimize possibility of thrombogenic complications. Avoid exceeding administration rate of 10mL/min to prevent vasomotor reactions. Handle cautiously due to risk of exposure to viral infection. Discard unused contents and equipment after use into appropriate safety container; do not resterilize.

ADVERSE REACTIONS
Allergic reactions, mild chills, nausea, stinging at infusion site, thrombosis, DIC.

PREGNANCY AND LACTATION
Category C, safety not known in nursing.

MECHANISM OF ACTION
Antihemophilic agent; provides hemostatic protection during and after surgery and bleeding episodes.

PHARMACOKINETICS
Elimination: $T_{1/2}$=21 hrs.

PATIENT CONSIDERATIONS
Assessment: Assess for hypersensitivity to the drug, severity of bleeding, liver disease, recent surgery, history of severe allergic reactions, pregnancy/nursing status, and known FIX gene deletion mutations. Assess FIX levels.

Monitoring: Monitor for thrombosis, DIC, viral infection, hypersensitivity reactions, and other adverse reactions. Monitor previously untreated patients for anaphylactic reactions between the 10th and 20th exposure days. Monitor FIX levels.

Counseling: Inform of the early signs/symptoms of hypersensitivity reactions (eg, hives, urticaria, chest tightness, dyspnea, wheezing, faintness, hypotension, anaphylaxis); advise to d/c and notify physician or seek immediate emergency care, depending on the severity of the reactions. Inform that drug is made from human plasma and may contain infectious agents that can cause disease (eg, viruses, CJD agent).

ALPROLIX — coagulation factor IX (recombinant), Fc fusion protein Rx
Class: Antihemophilic factor (recombinant)

ADULT DOSAGE	PEDIATRIC DOSAGE
Hemophilia B	**Hemophilia B**

ADULT DOSAGE
Hemophilia B

Bleeding Episodes:
1 IU/kg increases the circulating level of factor IX (FIX) by 1% IU/dL

Control/Treatment of Bleeding Episodes:
Minor and Moderate Bleeding:
Required FIX Level 30-60 IU/dL:
Repeat q48h if there is further evidence of bleeding

PEDIATRIC DOSAGE
Hemophilia B

Bleeding Episodes:
<12 Years:
Higher dose/kg body weight or more frequent dosing may be needed

≥12 Years:
1 IU/kg increases the circulating level of FIX by 1% IU/dL

Major Bleeding:
Required FIX Level 80-100 IU/dL:
Consider a repeat dose after 6-10 hrs and then q24h for the first 3 days; the dose may be reduced and frequency of dosing may be extended after day 3 to q48h or longer until bleeding stops and healing is achieved

Perioperative Management:
Minor Surgery:
Required FIX Level 50-80 IU/dL:
Single infusion may be sufficient; repeat as needed after 24-48 hrs until bleeding stops and healing is achieved

Major Surgery:
Required FIX Level 60-100 IU/dL:
Consider repeat dose after 6-10 hours and then q24h for the first 3 days

Due to its long $T_{1/2}$, the dose may be reduced and frequency of dosing in the post-surgical setting may be extended after day 3 to q48h or longer until bleeding stops and healing is achieved

Routine Prophylaxis:
Initial: 50 IU/kg IV once weekly or 100 IU/kg IV once every 10 days

Dosing Formulas:
IU/dL (or % of normal) = [Total Dose (IU)/Body Weight (kg)] x Recovery (IU/dL per IU/kg) or
Dose (IU) = Body Weight (kg) x Desired FIX Rise (IU/dL or, % of normal) x Reciprocal of Recovery (IU/kg per IU/dL)

Control/Treatment of Bleeding Episodes:
Minor and Moderate Bleeding:
Required FIX Level 30-60 IU/dL: Repeat q48h if there is further evidence of bleeding

Major Bleeding:
Required FIX Level 80-100 IU/dL:
Consider a repeat dose after 6-10 hrs and then q24h for the first 3 days; the dose may be reduced and frequency of dosing may be extended after day 3 to q48h or longer until bleeding stops and healing is achieved

Perioperative Management:
Minor Surgery:
Required FIX Level 50-80 IU/dL:
Single infusion may be sufficient; repeat as needed after 24-48 hrs until bleeding stops and healing is achieved

Major Surgery:
Required FIX Level 60-100 IU/dL:
Consider repeat dose after 6-10 hrs and then q24h for the first 3 days

Due to its long $T_{1/2}$, the dose may be reduced and frequency of dosing in the post-surgical setting may be extended after day 3 to q48h or longer until bleeding stops and healing is achieved

Routine Prophylaxis:
Initial: 50 IU/kg IV once weekly or 100 IU/kg IV once every 10 days

Dosing Formulas:
IU/dL (or % of normal) = [Total Dose (IU)/Body Weight (kg)] x Recovery (IU/dL per IU/kg) or
Dose (IU) = Body Weight (kg) x Desired FIX Rise (IU/dL or, % of normal) x Reciprocal of Recovery (IU/kg per IU/dL)

ADMINISTRATION
IV route
- Administer as bolus infusion.
- Rate of administration should not be faster than 10mL/min.
- Do not administer reconstituted sol in the same tubing or container w/ other medications.
- Allow the vial and prefilled diluent syringe to reach room temperature before use; use reconstituted sol as soon as possible, no later than 3 hrs after reconstitution.

STORAGE
2-8°C (36-46°F). Protect from light. Do not freeze. May store at room temperature ≤30°C (86°F) for a single 6-month period; record the date when the product was removed from refrigeration. Do not place the product back into refrigerator after warming to room temperature. **Reconstituted Sol:** May store at room temperature ≤30°C (86°F) for not >3 hrs. Discard any product not used w/in 3 hrs after reconstitution. Protect from direct sunlight. Do not refrigerate after reconstitution.

HOW SUPPLIED
Inj: 250 IU, 500 IU, 1000 IU, 2000 IU, 3000 IU

CONTRAINDICATIONS
Known history of hypersensitivity reactions, including anaphylaxis, to this product or its excipients.

WARNINGS/PRECAUTIONS
Not indicated for induction of immune tolerance in patients w/ hemophilia B. Initiate treatment under the supervision of a qualified physician experienced in the treatment of hemophilia B. Allergic-type hypersensitivity reactions, including anaphylaxis, reported; d/c use and initiate appropriate treatment if hypersensitivity symptoms occur. Formation of neutralizing antibodies (inhibitors) to FIX reported; monitor regularly for the development of inhibitors by appropriate clinical observations and lab tests. Association between occurrence of FIX inhibitor and allergic reactions reported; evaluate patients experiencing allergic reactions for the presence of an inhibitor. Increased risk of anaphylaxis upon subsequent challenge in individuals w/ FIX inhibitors. Associated w/ the development of thromboembolic complications, especially in individuals receiving continuous infusion through a central venous catheter.

ADVERSE REACTIONS
Headache, oral paresthesia.

PREGNANCY AND LACTATION
Pregnancy: Category C.
Lactation: Caution in nursing.

MECHANISM OF ACTION
Recombinant antihemophilic factor; temporarily replaces the missing coagulation FIX needed for effective hemostasis. Contains the Fc region of human IgG_1, which

binds to the neonatal Fc receptor (FcRn). FcRn is part of a naturally occurring pathway that delays lysosomal degradation of immunoglobulins by cycling them back into circulation, and prolonging their plasma $T_{1/2}$.

PHARMACOKINETICS
Absorption: AUC_{inf}=1619.1 hr•IU/dL; C_{max}=46.04 IU/dL. **Distribution:** V_d=327mL/kg. **Elimination:** $T_{1/2}$=86.52 hrs. Refer to PI for pediatric and adolescent pharmacokinetic parameters.

PATIENT CONSIDERATIONS
Assessment: Assess for known hypersensitivity to drug or to its excipients; severity of bleeding; presence of FIX inhibitors; and pregnancy/nursing status.

Monitoring: Monitor for hypersensitivity reactions, thromboembolic complications, and other adverse reactions. Monitor plasma FIX activity. Monitor for the development of FIX inhibitors if expected FIX activity plasma levels are not attained, or if bleeding is not controlled w/ the recommended dose.

Counseling: Advise to report to physician any adverse reactions or problems following administration. Advise to contact physician or treatment facility for further treatment and/or assessment if experiencing a lack of clinical response to FIX therapy. Inform of the early signs of hypersensitivity reactions and anaphylaxis; instruct to d/c use and contact physician if these symptoms occur.

AMIFOSTINE — amifostine   Rx
Class: Thiophosphate protective agent

ADULT DOSAGE	PEDIATRIC DOSAGE
Renal Toxicity	Pediatric use may not have been established

ADULT DOSAGE

Renal Toxicity

Reduces cumulative renal toxicity associated w/ repeated administration of cisplatin in patients w/ advanced ovarian cancer

Initial: 910mg/m² qd as a 15-min IV infusion, starting 30 min prior to chemotherapy

Interrupt infusion if systolic BP decreases significantly from baseline; may restart infusion if BP returns to normal w/in 5 min and patient is asymptomatic

If full dose cannot be administered, give 740mg/m² for subsequent chemotherapy cycles
Administer antiemetic medication, including dexamethasone 20mg IV and a serotonin 5-HT₃ receptor antagonist prior to and w/ amifostine; additional antiemetics may be required

Xerostomia

Reduces incidence of moderate to severe xerostomia in patients undergoing postoperative radiation treatment for head and neck cancer, where the radiation port includes a substantial portion of parotid glands

200mg/m² qd as a 3-min IV infusion, starting 15-30 min prior to standard fraction radiation therapy

Administer antiemetic medication prior to and w/ amifostine; oral 5-HT₃ receptor antagonists have been effective

---

ADMINISTRATION
IV route
Adequately hydrate patient prior to infusion and keep in supine position during infusion.

Reconstitution
- Reconstitute w/ 9.7mL of sterile 0.9% NaCl; use w/ other sol is not recommended.
- Stable for up to 5 hrs at approx 25°C (77°F) or up to 24 hrs at 2-8°C (36-46°F).

STORAGE
20-25°C (68-77°F).

HOW SUPPLIED
Inj: 500mg

CONTRAINDICATIONS
Known hypersensitivity to aminothiol compounds.

WARNINGS/PRECAUTIONS
Do not administer in other settings where chemotherapy can produce a significant survival benefit or cure, or in patients receiving definitive radiotherapy, except in the context of a clinical study. Do not give in patients who are hypotensive, in a state of dehydration, or taking antihypertensives that cannot be stopped for 24 hrs preceding treatment. Monitor BP every 5 min during infusion, and thereafter as clinically indicated. Do not exceed 15 min for 910mg/m² infusion.

Place patient in Trendelenburg position and infuse normal saline if hypotension occurs. May cause serious cutaneous reactions (especially when used as a radioprotectant) that may require permanent discontinuation or urgent dermatologic consultation and biopsy; carefully monitor for cutaneous reactions prior to, during, and after administration. Allergic manifestations (eg, anaphylaxis) reported; d/c immediately and permanently in case of severe acute allergic reactions. Administer antiemetic(s) (eg, dexamethasone 20mg IV, 5-HT₃ receptor antagonist) prior to and in conjunction w/ therapy; carefully monitor fluid balance when administered w/ highly emetogenic chemotherapy. Monitor serum Ca^{2+} levels if at risk for hypocalcemia (eg, nephrotic syndrome, receiving multiple doses of amifostine); administer Ca^{2+} supplements if necessary. Caution in elderly, or in patients w/ preexisting cardiovascular (CV) or cerebrovascular conditions.

ADVERSE REACTIONS
Hypotension, N/V, cutaneous eruptions.

DRUG INTERACTIONS
Caution w/ antihypertensives or other drugs that could cause or potentiate hypotension. Interrupt antihypertensive therapy 24 hrs preceding administration in patients receiving amifostine doses recommended for chemotherapy.

PREGNANCY AND LACTATION
Pregnancy: Embryotoxic in rabbits; should be used during pregnancy only if the potential benefit justifies the potential risk to the fetus.
Lactation: Not for use in nursing.

MECHANISM OF ACTION
Thiophosphate protective agent; dephosphorylated to the active free thiol metabolite, which reduces cumulative renal toxicity of cisplatin and toxic effects of radiation on normal oral tissues. The higher concentration of the thiol metabolite in normal tissues is available to bind to and detoxify reactive metabolites of cisplatin. Can also scavenge reactive oxygen species generated by exposure to either cisplatin or radiation.

PHARMACOKINETICS
Metabolism: Dephosphorylation by alkaline phosphatase; free thiol, disulfide (active metabolites). **Elimination:** Renal; $T_{1/2}$=8 min.

PATIENT CONSIDERATIONS
Assessment: Assess for hypersensitivity to aminothiol compounds, hydration status, cutaneous reactions, CV or cerebrovascular conditions, risk for hypocalcemia, pregnancy/nursing status, and possible drug interactions. Obtain baseline BP.

Monitoring: Monitor for cutaneous/allergic reactions, and other adverse reactions. Monitor fluid balance when administered w/ highly emetogenic chemotherapy, and serum Ca^{2+} levels if at risk for hypocalcemia. Monitor BP every 5 min during infusion, and thereafter as clinically indicated. If infusion duration is <5 min, monitor BP at least before and immediately after infusion, and thereafter as clinically indicated.

Counseling: Inform about the risks and benefits of therapy. Inform physician if pregnant, planning to become pregnant, or nursing. Instruct to report to physician if any adverse reactions develop.

AMPYRA — dalfampridine   Rx
Class: Potassium channel blocker

ADULT DOSAGE	PEDIATRIC DOSAGE
Multiple Sclerosis **To Improve Walking:** **Max:** 10mg bid (approx 12 hrs apart)	Pediatric use may not have been established

ADMINISTRATION
Oral route
Take w/ or w/o food
Take tab whole; do not divide, crush, chew, or dissolve

STORAGE
25°C (77°F); excursions permitted to 15-30°C (59-86°F).

HOW SUPPLIED
Tab, Extended-Release: 10mg

CONTRAINDICATIONS
History of seizure, moderate or severe renal impairment (CrCl ≤50mL/min), history of hypersensitivity to this medication or 4-aminopyridine.

WARNINGS/PRECAUTIONS
May cause seizures; d/c and do not restart in patients who experience a seizure while on therapy. Caution with mild renal impairment (CrCl 51-80mL/min). Avoid with other forms of 4-aminopyridine; d/c use of any product containing 4-aminopyridine prior to initiating therapy. May cause anaphylaxis and severe allergic reactions; d/c if signs and symptoms occur. Urinary tract infections (UTIs) reported; evaluate and treat patients as clinically indicated.

ADVERSE REACTIONS
UTI, insomnia, dizziness, headache, nausea, asthenia, back pain, balance disorder, MS relapse, paresthesia, nasopharyngitis, constipation.

PREGNANCY AND LACTATION
Category C, not for use in nursing.

MECHANISM OF ACTION
Broad-spectrum K^+ channel blocker; has not been established. Has been shown to increase conduction of action potentials in demyelinated axons through inhibition of K^+ channels.

PHARMACOKINETICS

Absorption: Rapid and complete. C_{max}=17.3-21.6ng/mL (fasted), T_{max}=3-4 hrs (fasted). **Distribution:** Plasma protein binding (1-3%); V_d=2.6L/kg. **Metabolism:** Hydroxylation; CYP2E1 (major). **Elimination:** Urine (95.9%, 90.3% parent drug), feces (0.5%); $T_{1/2}$=5.2-6.5 hrs.

PATIENT CONSIDERATIONS

Assessment: Assess for hypersensitivity to the drug or 4-aminopyridine, history of seizures, and pregnancy/nursing status. Obtain baseline CrCl.

Monitoring: Monitor for seizures, anaphylaxis, severe allergic reactions, UTIs, and other adverse reactions. Monitor CrCl at least annually.

Counseling: Inform that therapy may cause seizures and to d/c treatment if seizure is experienced. Instruct to take exactly ud and not take a double dose if a dose is missed. Instruct not to take more than 2 tabs in a 24-hr period and to make sure that there is an approximate 12-hr interval between doses. Inform of the signs/symptoms of anaphylaxis; instruct to d/c therapy and seek medical care if anaphylaxis develops.

APOKYN — apomorphine hydrochloride   Rx

Class: Dopamine receptor agonist

ADULT DOSAGE

Parkinson's Disease

Acute, intermittent treatment of hypomobility, "off" episodes ("end-of-dose wearing off" and unpredictable "on/off" episodes) in patients w/ advanced Parkinson's disease

Initial Test Dose:
0.2mL (2mg); begin dosing when patients are in an "off" state
Check both supine and standing BP and pulse predose and at 20, 40, and 60 min postdose (and after 60 min, if there is significant hypotension at 60 min)
If significant orthostatic hypotension develops in response to test dose, do not consider patients candidates for treatment

If Initial Test Dose Tolerated:
Initial: 0.2mL (2mg) prn to treat recurring "off" episodes
Titrate: Increase in increments of 0.1mL (1mg) every few days, if needed, on an outpatient basis

Subsequent Dosing:
Determine that patient needs and tolerates a higher test dose (0.3mL [3mg] or 0.4mL [4mg]), under close medical supervision; outpatient dosing trial may follow using a dose 0.1mL (1mg) lower than the tolerated test dose

If Patient Tolerates 0.2mL (2mg) Test Dose but Responds Inadequately:
May administer 0.4mL (4mg) at the next observed "off" period (at least 2 hrs after initial test dose)

If Patient Tolerates and Responds to 0.4mL (4mg) Test Dose:
Initial Maint: 0.3mL (3mg) prn to treat recurring "off" episodes
Titrate: May increase in 0.1mL (1mg) increments every few days, if needed, on an outpatient basis

If Patient Does Not Tolerate 0.4mL (4mg) Test Dose:
May administer 0.3mL (3mg) during a separate "off" period (at least 2 hrs after the previous dose)

If Patient Tolerates 0.3mL (3mg) Test Dose:
Initial Maint: 0.2mL (2mg) prn to treat existing "off" episodes
Titrate: May increase to 0.3mL (3mg) after a few days, if needed and if the 0.2mL (2mg) dose is tolerated; do not increase to 0.4mL (4mg) on an outpatient basis in such patients

Max: 0.6mL (6mg)/dose

Re-treatment and Interruption in Therapy:
If a single dose of therapy is ineffective for a particular "off"

PEDIATRIC DOSAGE

Pediatric use may not have been established

---

period, do not give a 2nd dose for that "off" episode
Do not administer a repeat dose sooner than 2 hrs after last dose
If therapy is interrupted for >1 week, restart on 0.2mL (2mg) dose and gradually titrate to effect and tolerability

Premedication

Initiate therapy w/ a concomitant antiemetic; oral trimethobenzamide (300mg tid) should be started 3 days prior to initial dose and continued at least during the first 2 months of therapy

---

DOSING CONSIDERATIONS

Renal Impairment
Mild/Moderate: Reduce test dose and starting dose to 0.1mL (1mg)

Hepatic Impairment
Mild/Moderate: Closely monitor

ADMINISTRATION
SQ route
Administer only by a multiple-dose pen w/ supplied cartridges
Initial dose and dose titrations should be performed by a healthcare provider
Rotate inj site

STORAGE
25°C (77°F); excursions permitted to 15-30°C (59-86°F).

HOW SUPPLIED
Inj: 10mg/mL [3mL]

CONTRAINDICATIONS
Concomitant use w/ 5HT3 antagonists, including antiemetics (eg, ondansetron, granisetron, dolasetron, palonosetron) and alosetron; hypersensitivity to apomorphine and its excipients, including sulfite (eg, sodium metabisulfite).

WARNINGS/PRECAUTIONS
Serious adverse reactions (eg, thrombus formation, pulmonary embolism) following IV use reported; not for IV administration. N/V, syncope, orthostatic hypotension, and falling reported. Falling asleep during activities of daily living may occur; d/c if daytime sleepiness or episodes of falling asleep develop. May impair mental/physical abilities. Hallucinations/psychotic-like behavior reported; avoid w/ major psychotic disorder. May cause or worsen dyskinesias. May cause intense urges to gamble, increased sexual urges, intense urges to spend money uncontrollably, and other intense urges and the inability to control these urges while on therapy; consider dose reduction or discontinuation of therapy. Coronary events (eg, angina, MI, cardiac arrest, sudden death) reported; caution w/ known cardiovascular (CV)/cerebrovascular disease. May prolong the QT interval and increase potential for proarrhythmic effects; caution w/ hypokalemia, hypomagnesemia, bradycardia, or genetic predisposition (eg, congenital prolongation of the QT interval). Monitor for withdrawal-emergent hyperpyrexia and confusion, fibrotic complications (eg, retroperitoneal fibrosis, pulmonary infiltrates, pleural effusion/thickening, cardiac valvulopathy), and melanoma. May cause priapism. Potential for abuse.

ADVERSE REACTIONS
Yawning, dyskinesia, N/V, somnolence, dizziness, rhinorrhea, hallucinations, edema, chest pain, inj-site reaction, fall, arthralgia, insomnia, headache, depression.

DRUG INTERACTIONS
See Contraindications. Antihypertensives and vasodilators may increase risk of hypotension, MI, serious pneumonia, serious falls, and bone and joint injuries. Dopamine antagonists, such as neuroleptics (eg, phenothiazines, butyrophenones, thioxanthenes) or metoclopramide, may diminish effectiveness. Caution w/ drugs that prolong QT/QTc interval. May increase drowsiness w/ sedating medications. Avoid w/ alcohol.

PREGNANCY AND LACTATION
Category C, not for use in nursing.

MECHANISM OF ACTION
Non-ergoline dopamine agonist; not established, suspected to stimulate postsynaptic dopamine D_2-type receptors w/in the caudate-putamen in the brain.

PHARMACOKINETICS
Absorption: Rapid; T_{max}=10-60 min. **Distribution:** V_d=218L. **Metabolism:** Sulfation, N-demethylation, glucuronidation, and oxidation. **Elimination:** $T_{1/2}$=40 min.

PATIENT CONSIDERATIONS
Assessment: Assess for hypersensitivity to the drug, sulfite sensitivity, asthma, risk for QT prolongation, history of psychotic disorders, CV/cerebrovascular disease, dyskinesia, hepatic/renal impairment, pregnancy/nursing status, and possible drug interactions. Obtain baseline BP (supine and standing position).

Monitoring: Monitor for N/V, syncope, QT/QTc interval prolongation and other proarrhythmic effects, hypotension, hallucinations/psychotic-like behavior, coronary/cerebral ischemia, dyskinesia (or exacerbation), impulse control/compulsive behaviors, hepatic/renal impairment, withdrawal-emergent hyperpyrexia and confusion, fibrotic complications, priapism, and other adverse reactions. Perform periodic skin exams to monitor for melanomas. Monitor BP closely.

Counseling: Instruct to use only as prescribed. Instruct to rotate the inj site and observe proper aseptic technique. Inform of the potential risks and benefits of therapy. Inform that hypersensitivity/allergic reaction may occur; advise patients to avoid taking the drug again if a reaction occurs. Advise not to drive a car or engage in any other potentially dangerous activities while on treatment. Advise to limit alcohol intake. Alert patients that they may have increased risk for falling when using the drug. Inform of the potential for hallucinations, psychotic-like behavior, hypotension, sedating effects including somnolence and the possibility of falling asleep, coronary events, dyskinesias, and other adverse events. Instruct to rise slowly after sitting or lying down after taking the drug. Advise to inform physician if new or increased gambling urges, increased sexual urges, or other intense urges develop while on treatment. Instruct to notify physician if pregnancy occurs, or if intending to become pregnant and/or breastfeed.

APTIVUS — tipranavir   Rx

Class: Protease inhibitor

> Both fatal and nonfatal intracranial hemorrhage (ICH) reported. Clinical hepatitis and hepatic decompensation, including some fatalities, reported. Extra vigilance is warranted in patients w/ chronic hepatitis B or hepatitis C coinfection due to an increased risk of hepatotoxicity.

ADULT DOSAGE	PEDIATRIC DOSAGE
HIV-1 Infection	**HIV-1 Infection**
Coadministered w/ ritonavir (RTV) in treatment-experienced patients infected w/ HIV-1 strains resistant to >1 protease inhibitor	Coadministered w/ ritonavir (RTV) in treatment-experienced patients infected w/ HIV-1 strains resistant to >1 protease inhibitor
Cap:	**2-18 Years:**
Usual: 500mg (two 250mg caps) + 200mg RTV bid	**Usual:** 14mg/kg + 6mg/kg RTV (or 375mg/m² + 150mg/m² RTV) bid
Sol:	**Max:** 500mg + 200mg RTV bid
Usual: 500mg (5mL) + 200mg RTV bid	

DOSING CONSIDERATIONS
Adverse Reactions
Pediatrics:
Development of Intolerance/Toxicity: Decrease dose to 12mg/kg + 5mg/kg ritonavir (RTV) (or 290mg/m² + 115mg/m² RTV) bid

ADMINISTRATION
Oral route

Coadministered w/ Ritonavir (RTV) Caps/Sol
May be taken w/ or w/o meals

Coadministered w/ RTV Tabs
Must only be taken w/ meals

STORAGE
Must be used w/in 60 days after 1st opening the bottle. (Cap) Prior to Opening the Bottle: 2-8°C (36-46°F). After Opening the Bottle: 25°C (77°F); excursions permitted to 15-30°C (59-86°F). (Sol) 25°C (77°F); excursions permitted to 15-30°C (59-86°F). Do not refrigerate or freeze.

HOW SUPPLIED
Cap: 250mg; **Sol:** 100mg/mL [95mL]

CONTRAINDICATIONS
Moderate or severe (Child-Pugh Class B or C) hepatic impairment. Coadministration w/ drugs that are highly dependent on CYP3A for clearance or are potent CYP3A inducers (eg, amiodarone, bepridil, flecainide, propafenone, quinidine, rifampin, dihydroergotamine, ergonovine, ergotamine, methylergonovine, cisapride, St. John's wort, lovastatin, simvastatin, pimozide, oral midazolam, triazolam, alfuzosin, and sildenafil [for treatment of pulmonary arterial HTN]). Refer to the individual monograph for RTV.

WARNINGS/PRECAUTIONS
Not recommended for treatment-naive patients. Caution w/ elevated transaminases, hepatitis B or C coinfection, mild hepatic impairment (Child-Pugh Class A), supplemental high doses of vitamin E, known sulfonamide allergy, patients at risk of increased bleeding from trauma, surgery, or other medical conditions, and in elderly. D/C if signs and symptoms of clinical hepatitis develop. D/C if asymptomatic elevations in AST or ALT >10X the ULN or if asymptomatic elevations in AST or ALT between 5-10X the ULN and increases in total bilirubin >2.5X the ULN occur. Rash (eg, urticarial, maculopapular, possible photosensitivity) accompanied by joint pain/stiffness, throat tightness, or generalized pruritus reported; d/c and initiate appropriate treatment if severe skin rash develops. New onset diabetes mellitus (DM), exacerbation of preexisting DM, hyperglycemia, and diabetic ketoacidosis reported. Increased total cholesterol and TG levels reported. Immune reconstitution syndrome reported; autoimmune disorders (eg, Graves' disease, polymyositis, and Guillain-Barre syndrome) have also been reported in the setting of immune reconstitution. Redistribution/accumulation of body fat may occur. Increased bleeding in patients w/ hemophilia type A and B reported; additional factor VIII may be given. (Sol) Avoid supplemental vitamin E greater than a standard multivitamin as oral sol contains 116 IU/mL of vitamin E, which is higher than the Reference Daily Intake (adults 30 IU, pediatrics approx 10 IU). Refer to individual monograph for RTV.

ADVERSE REACTIONS
ICH, clinical hepatitis, hepatic decompensation, diarrhea, N/V, abdominal pain, pyrexia, fatigue, headache, cough, rash, anemia, weight decreased, hypertriglyceridemia, bleeding.

DRUG INTERACTIONS
See Contraindications. Not recommended w/ other protease inhibitors, boceprevir, telaprevir, salmeterol, and fluticasone. Concomitant colchicine is contraindicated in renally/hepatically impaired patients. Avoid w/ atorvastatin and etravirine. Caution w/ medications known to increase the risk of bleeding (eg, antiplatelets, anticoagulants, or high doses of vitamin E). May increase levels of rilpivirine, SSRIs (eg, fluoxetine, paroxetine, sertraline), atorvastatin, rosuvastatin, trazodone, desipramine, colchicine, bosentan, itraconazole, ketoconazole, clarithromycin, rifabutin, quetiapine, parenteral midazolam, normeperidine, and PDE-5 inhibitors. May decrease levels of etravirine, abacavir, atazanavir, didanosine, zidovudine, amprenavir, lopinavir, saquinavir, raltegravir, valproic acid, methadone, meperidine, and omeprazole. Increased levels w/ fluconazole, enfuvirtide, clarithromycin, and atazanavir. Decreased levels w/ buprenorphine/naloxone, carbamazepine, phenobarbital, and phenytoin. May alter levels of voriconazole, calcium channel blockers, and immunosuppressants. May decrease levels of ethinyl estradiol by 50%; use alternative methods of nonhormonal contraception. Monitor glucose w/ hypoglycemic agents. Monitor INR w/ warfarin. (Cap) May produce disulfiram-like reactions w/ disulfiram or other drugs that produce the reaction (eg, metronidazole). See Prescribing Information for detailed information.

PREGNANCY AND LACTATION
Category C, not for use in nursing.

MECHANISM OF ACTION
Protease inhibitor; inhibits virus-specific processing of viral Gag and Gag-Pol polyproteins in HIV-1 infected cells, thus preventing formation of mature virions.

PHARMACOKINETICS
Absorption: Tipranavir/RTV: (Female) C_{max}=94.8µM, T_{max}=2.9 hrs, AUC_{0-12h}=851µM•hr; (Male) C_{max}=77.6µM, T_{max}=3 hrs, AUC_{0-12h}=710µM•hr. Refer to Prescribing Information for pediatric parameters by age. **Distribution:** Plasma protein binding (>99.9%). **Metabolism:** Liver via CYP3A4. **Elimination:** Tipranavir/RTV: Feces (82.3% [median], 79.9% unchanged), urine (4.4%, 0.5% unchanged); $T_{1/2}$=5.5 hrs (females), 6 hrs (males).

PATIENT CONSIDERATIONS
Assessment: Assess for hepatitis B or C infection, hepatic impairment, increased bleeding risk, hemophilia, sulfonamide allergy, DM, pregnancy/nursing status, and possible drug interactions. Assess LFTs and lipid levels. Assess the ability to swallow caps in pediatric patients.

Monitoring: Monitor for signs and symptoms of clinical hepatitis, hepatic decompensation, ICH, rash, DM, hyperglycemia, diabetic ketoacidosis, bleeding, immune reconstitution syndrome, autoimmune disorders, fat redistribution, and other adverse reactions. Monitor for LFTs and lipid levels periodically during treatment. Monitor INR w/ warfarin.

Counseling: Inform of the risks and benefits of therapy. Advise to seek medical attention for symptoms of hepatitis (eg, fatigue, malaise, anorexia, nausea), any unusual/unexplained bleeding, and rash. Advise to report use of all medications, including prescription or nonprescription medications (eg, St. John's wort). Instruct to avoid vitamin E supplements greater than a standard multivitamin when taking oral sol. Instruct to report any history of sulfonamide allergy. Instruct to use additional or alternative contraceptive measures for patients taking estrogen-based hormonal contraceptives. Inform that redistribution/accumulation of body fat may occur. Instruct to take medication ud. Inform that therapy is not a cure for HIV-1 infection and that illness associated w/ HIV-1 infection may continue, including opportunistic infection; advise to remain under the care of a physician during therapy. Advise to avoid doing things that can spread HIV-1 infection to others.

ARALAST NP — alpha1-proteinase inhibitor (human)   Rx

Class: Alpha₁-proteinase inhibitor (A₁PI)

ADULT DOSAGE	PEDIATRIC DOSAGE
Alpha₁-Antitrypsin Deficiency	Pediatric use may not have been established
Chronic Augmentation Therapy in Patients w/ Clinically Evident Emphysema Due to Severe Congenital Deficiency of Alpha₁-Proteinase Inhibitor:	
60mg/kg once weekly by IV infusion. Administer at a rate ≤0.2mL/kg/min as determined by response and comfort of patient	

DOSING CONSIDERATIONS
Adverse Reactions
Reduce infusion rate or halt infusion if adverse reactions occur; resume at a tolerable rate after symptoms subside

ADMINISTRATION
IV route

Reconstitution
1. Allow product and diluent to reach room temperature before reconstitution
2. Remove cover from 1 end of the double-ended transfer needle; insert exposed end of the needle through the center of the stopper in the diluent vial
3. Remove plastic cap from the other end of the double-ended transfer needle now seated in the stopper of the diluent vial. Invert diluent vial and insert exposed end of the needle through the center of the stopper in the product vial at an

angle, making certain that diluent vial is always above product vial. The angle of insertion directs flow of diluent against the side of the product vial. Vacuum in the vial is sufficient to allow transfer of all of the diluent

4. Disconnect the 2 vials from the transfer needle; next, remove double-ended transfer needle from product vial

5. Let vial stand until most of contents is in sol, then gently swirl until powder is completely dissolved; do not shake content of vial. Do not invert vial until ready to withdraw content

6. A few small, visible particles may remain in the reconstituted product. These will be removed by sterile 20-micron filter

Administration

1. Several vials may be pooled into an empty, sterile IV sol container using aseptic technique and a sterile 20-micron filter
2. Administer w/in 3 hrs after reconstitution; administer alone, w/o mixing w/ other agents or diluting sol

STORAGE

≤25°C (77°F). Do not freeze. Store in original carton to protect from light. Discard any unused contents.

HOW SUPPLIED

Inj: 0.5g, 1g

CONTRAINDICATIONS

IgA deficient patients with antibodies against IgA.

WARNINGS/PRECAUTIONS

For IV use only. May contain trace amounts of IgA; increased risk of developing severe hypersensitivity and anaphylactic reactions in patients with selective/severe IgA deficiency. D/C infusion if symptoms of hypersensitivity occur and administer appropriate emergency treatment. May carry risk of transmitting infectious agents (eg, viruses, variant Creutzfeldt-Jakob disease [CJD], CJD agent).

ADVERSE REACTIONS

Headache, musculoskeletal discomfort, vessel puncture site bruise, nausea, rhinorrhea, respiratory tract infections, aminotransferase (ALT/AST) elevations.

PREGNANCY AND LACTATION

Category C, caution in nursing.

MECHANISM OF ACTION

α_1-PI (α_1-antitrypsin); inhibits serine proteases such as neutrophil elastase, which is capable of degrading protein components of the alveolar walls, and chronically present in the lung.

PHARMACOKINETICS

Absorption: C_{max}=1.6mg/mL, $AUC_{0-35d/dose}$=0.0837days•kg/mL. **Elimination:** $T_{1/2}$=4.7 days.

PATIENT CONSIDERATIONS

Assessment: Assess for IgA deficiency, severe congenital α_1-PI deficiency, and pregnancy/nursing status.

Monitoring: Monitor for hypersensitivity/anaphylactic reactions, infections and other adverse reactions. Monitor vital signs continuously and closely monitor patient and infusion rate.

Counseling: Inform of the early signs of hypersensitivity reactions; advise to d/c use and contact physician and/or seek immediate emergency care, depending on the severity of reaction, if these symptoms occur. Inform that product is made from human plasma and the possibility of transmitting infectious agents cannot be totally excluded.

ARANESP — darbepoetin alfa   Rx

Class: Erythropoiesis-stimulating agent (ESA)

> Increased risk of death, MI, stroke, venous thromboembolism, thrombosis of vascular access, and tumor progression or recurrence. Use the lowest dose sufficient to reduce/avoid the need for RBC transfusions. **Chronic Kidney Disease (CKD):** Greater risks for death, serious adverse cardiovascular (CV) reactions, and stroke when administered ESAs to target Hgb level of >11g/dL. **Cancer:** Shortened overall survival and/ or increased risk of tumor progression or recurrence in patients w/ breast, non-small cell lung, head and neck, lymphoid, and cervical cancers. Must enroll in and comply w/ the ESA APPRISE Oncology Program to prescribe and/or dispense drug to patients. Use only for anemia from myelosuppressive chemotherapy. Not indicated for patients receiving myelosuppressive chemotherapy when anticipated outcome is cure. D/C following completion of chemotherapy course.

ADULT DOSAGE

Anemia Due to Chronic Kidney Disease

On Dialysis:
Initiate when Hgb is <10g/dL
Initial: 0.45mcg/kg IV/SQ weekly or 0.75mcg/kg IV/SQ once every 2 weeks; IV route is recommended for hemodialysis patients
Titrate: Adjust dose based on Hgb levels. If Hgb approaches or exceeds 11g/dL, reduce or interrupt dose

Not on Dialysis:
Initiate when Hgb is <10g/dL, the rate of Hgb decline indicates likelihood of a RBC transfusion, and when reducing the risk of alloimmunization and/or other RBC transfusion-related risks is a goal

Initial: 0.45mcg/kg IV/SQ once every 4 weeks
Titrate: Adjust dose based on Hgb levels. If Hgb exceeds 10g/dL, reduce or interrupt dose and use lowest dose sufficient to reduce RBC transfusion

All Patients:
Titrate:
Do not increase dose more frequently than once every 4 weeks; dose decreases may occur more frequently
Rapid Increase in Hgb (>1g/dL in Any 2-Week Period): Reduce by ≥25% prn to reduce rapid responses
Hgb Has Not Increased by >1g/dL After 4 Weeks of Therapy: Increase by 25%
No Adequate Response Over a 12-Week Escalation Period: Further dose increase is unlikely to improve response and may increase risks. Use lowest dose to maintain Hgb level sufficient to reduce the need of RBC transfusion; d/c if responsiveness does not improve

Anemia Due to Chemotherapy

Anemia in Patients w/ Nonmyeloid Malignancies:
Initiate when Hgb is <10g/dL and if there is a minimum of 2 additional months of chemotherapy

Initial: 2.25mcg/kg SQ weekly or 500mcg SQ every 3 weeks until completion of chemotherapy course
Titrate:
Hgb Increases >1g/dL in Any 2-Week Period/Hgb Reaches a Level Needed to Avoid RBC Transfusion: Reduce dose by 40%
Hgb Exceeds Level Needed to Avoid RBC Transfusion: Withhold until Hgb approaches a level where RBC transfusions may be required; reinitiate at a dose 40% below previous dose
Hgb Increases by <1g/dL and Remains <10g/dL After 6 Weeks of Therapy: Increase dose to 4.5mcg/kg/week (weekly schedule) or no dose adjustment (3-week schedule)
No Response in Hgb Levels/Still Require RBC Transfusions After 8 Weeks of Therapy/Following Completion of Chemotherapy Course: D/C therapy

Conversions

On Dialysis:
Conversion from Epoetin Alfa:
Administer less frequently than epoetin alfa; administer once weekly or every 2 weeks in patients who were receiving epoetin alfa 2-3X weekly or once weekly, respectively

Estimate the starting weekly dose based on weekly epoetin alfa dose at the time of substitution
Epoetin Alfa Dose (U/Week):
<1500: 6.25mcg/week
1500-2499: 6.25mcg/week
2500-4999: 12.5mcg/week
5000-10,999: 25mcg/week
11,000-17,999: 40mcg/week
18,000-33,999: 60mcg/week
34,000-89,999: 100mcg/week
≥90,000: 200mcg/week
Maintain the route of administration

Not on Dialysis:
The dose conversion above does not accurately estimate the once monthly dose of darbepoetin alfa

----

ADMINISTRATION
IV/SQ route
Do not shake.
Do not use if it has been frozen or shaken.
Do not dilute and do not administer in conjunction w/ other drug sol.
Discard any unused portion in vials or prefilled syringes; do not re-enter vial.

PEDIATRIC DOSAGE

Anemia Due to Chronic Kidney Disease

Initiate when Hgb is <10g/dL
Initial: 0.45mcg/kg IV/SQ weekly; patients not receiving dialysis may be initiated at a dose of 0.75mcg/kg once every 2 weeks
Titrate:
Adjust dose based on Hgb levels. If Hgb approaches or exceeds 12g/dL, reduce or interrupt dose.
Do not increase dose more frequently than once every 4 weeks; dose decreases may occur more frequently.
Rapid Increase in Hgb (>1g/dL in Any 2-Week Period): Reduce by ≥25% prn to reduce rapid responses

Hgb Has Not Increased by >1g/dL After 4 Weeks of Therapy: Increase by 25%
No Adequate Response Over a 12-Week Escalation Period: Further dose increase is unlikely to improve response and may increase risks. Use lowest dose to maintain Hgb level sufficient to reduce the need of RBC transfusion; d/c if responsiveness does not improve

Conversions

On Dialysis:
Conversion from Epoetin Alfa:
Administer less frequently than epoetin alfa; administer once weekly or every 2 weeks in patients who were receiving epoetin alfa 2-3X weekly or once weekly, respectively

Estimate the starting weekly dose based on weekly epoetin alfa dose at the time of substitution
Epoetin Alfa Dose (U/Week):
1500-2499: 6.25mcg/week
2500-4999: 10mcg/week
5000-10,999: 20mcg/week
11,000-17,999: 40mcg/week
18,000-33,999: 60mcg/week
34,000-89,999: 100mcg/week
≥90,000: 200mcg/week
Maintain the route of administration

Not on Dialysis:
The dose conversion above does not accurately estimate the once monthly dose of darbepoetin alfa

Self-Administration of Prefilled Syringe

If patient or caregiver is unable to demonstrate successful measuring of dose and administration of product, consider whether patient is an appropriate candidate for self-administration or whether patient would benefit from a different darbepoetin alfa presentation.

STORAGE

2-8°C (36-46°F). Do not freeze. Protect from light.

HOW SUPPLIED

Inj: 25mcg/mL, 40mcg/mL, 60mcg/mL, 100mcg/mL, 150mcg/0.75mL, 200mcg/mL, 300mcg/mL [single-dose vial]; 10mcg/0.4mL, 25mcg/0.42mL, 40mcg/0.4mL, 60mcg/0.3mL, 100mcg/0.5mL, 150mcg/0.3mL, 200mcg/0.4mL, 300mcg/0.6mL, 500mcg/mL [single-dose prefilled syringe]

CONTRAINDICATIONS

Uncontrolled HTN, pure red cell aplasia (PRCA) that begins after treatment w/ darbepoetin alfa or other erythropoietin protein drugs, serious allergic reactions to darbepoetin alfa.

WARNINGS/PRECAUTIONS

Not indicated for use in patients w/ cancer receiving hormonal agents, biologic products, or radiotherapy, unless also receiving concomitant myelosuppressive chemotherapy, nor indicated as a substitute for RBC transfusions in patients requiring immediate correction of anemia. Evaluate transferrin saturation and serum ferritin prior to and during treatment; administer supplemental iron when serum ferritin is <100mcg/L or serum transferrin saturation is <20%. Correct/exclude other causes of anemia (eg, vitamin deficiency, metabolic/chronic inflammatory conditions, bleeding) before initiating therapy. Caution in patients w/ coexistent CV disease and stroke. Not approved for reduction of RBC transfusions in patients scheduled for surgical procedures. Hypertensive encephalopathy reported in patients w/ CKD. Appropriately control HTN prior to initiation of and during treatment; reduce/withhold therapy if BP becomes difficult to control. Increased risk of seizures. Cases of PRCA and severe anemia, w/ or w/o other cytopenias that arise following development of neutralizing antibodies to erythropoietin, reported. Withhold and evaluate for neutralizing antibodies to erythropoietin if severe anemia and low reticulocyte count develop; d/c permanently if PRCA develops, and do not switch to other ESAs. Serious allergic reactions may occur; immediately and permanently d/c treatment and administer appropriate therapy if a serious allergic/anaphylactic reaction occurs. Patients may require adjustments in dialysis prescriptions after initiation of therapy, or may require increased anticoagulation w/ heparin to prevent clotting of extracorporeal circuit during hemodialysis. Needle cover of the prefilled syringe contains dry natural rubber (a derivative of latex), which may cause allergic reactions.

ADVERSE REACTIONS

Patients w/ CKD: (Adults) HTN, dyspnea, peripheral edema, cough, procedural hypotension. (Pediatrics) HTN, inj-site pain, rash, convulsions.
Patients w/ Cancer Receiving Chemotherapy: Abdominal pain, edema, thrombovascular events.

PREGNANCY AND LACTATION

Pregnancy: Category C.
Lactation: It is not known if darbepoetin alfa is present in human milk; caution in nursing.

MECHANISM OF ACTION

Erythropoiesis-stimulating protein; stimulates erythropoiesis by the same mechanism as endogenous erythropoietin.

PHARMACOKINETICS

Absorption: Adults w/ CKD: (SQ) Slow. Bioavailability (37%) (on dialysis); T_{max}=48 hrs. Pediatric Patients w/ CKD: (SQ) Bioavailability (54%). Adults w/ Cancer: (SQ, 6.75mcg/kg) T_{max}=71 hrs. **Elimination:** Adults w/ CKD: (IV) $T_{1/2}$=21 hrs (on dialysis). (SQ) $T_{1/2}$=46 hrs (on dialysis), 70 hrs (not on dialysis). Adults w/ Cancer: (SQ, 6.75mcg/kg) $T_{1/2}$=74 hrs.

PATIENT CONSIDERATIONS

Assessment: Assess for uncontrolled HTN, previous hypersensitivity to the drug, latex allergy, causes of anemia, pregnancy/nursing status, and other conditions where treatment is cautioned/contraindicated. Obtain baseline Hgb levels, transferrin saturation, and serum ferritin.

Monitoring: Monitor for signs/symptoms of an allergic reaction, CV/thromboembolic events, stroke, PRCA, severe anemia, progression/recurrence of tumor, HTN, and other adverse reactions. Monitor BP, transferrin saturation, and serum ferritin. Monitor closely for premonitory neurologic symptoms during the 1st several months following initiation of treatment. Following initiation of therapy and after each dose adjustment, monitor Hgb weekly until Hgb is stable and sufficient to minimize need for RBC transfusion, and then monitor Hgb less frequently (at least monthly in CKD patients), provided Hgb levels remain stable.

Counseling: Inform of the risks/benefits of therapy, including the increased risks of mortality, serious CV reactions, thromboembolic reactions, stroke, and tumor progression. Advise of the need to have regular lab tests for Hgb. Inform cancer patients that they must sign the patient-healthcare provider acknowledgment form prior to the start of each treatment course. Instruct to undergo regular BP monitoring, adhere to prescribed antihypertensive regimen, and follow recommended dietary restrictions. Advise to contact healthcare provider for new-onset neurologic symptoms or change in seizure frequency. Instruct patients who self-administer regarding proper disposal; dangers of reusing needles, syringes, or unused portions of single-dose vials; and the importance of informing healthcare provider if difficulty occurs when measuring or administering partial doses from the prefilled syringe.

ARCALYST — rilonacept   Rx

Class: Interleukin-1 (IL-1) receptor antagonist

ADULT DOSAGE
Cryopyrin-Associated Periodic Syndromes

Including familial cold autoinflammatory syndrome and Muckle-Wells syndrome

LD: 320mg, administered as two 2mL SQ inj of 160mg each given on the same day at 2 different sites
Maint: Once-weekly inj of 160mg, administered as a single 2mL, SQ inj

PEDIATRIC DOSAGE
Cryopyrin-Associated Periodic Syndromes

Including familial cold autoinflammatory syndrome and Muckle-Wells syndrome

12-17 Years:
LD: 4.4mg/kg (max: 320mg), administered as one or two SQ inj w/ a max single-inj volume of 2mL
Maint: Once-weekly inj of 2.2mg/kg (max: 160mg), administered as a single SQ inj, up to 2mL

If initial (loading) dose is given as 2 inj, administer them on the same day at 2 different sites

---

ADMINISTRATION

SQ route

Do not administer more often than once weekly
Rotate inj sites (eg, abdomen, thigh, upper arm); never inject at sites that are bruised, red, tender, or hard
Use each vial for a single dose only; discard the vial after withdrawal of drug

Preparation and Administration

1. Withdraw 2.3mL of preservative-free sterile water for inj through a 27-gauge, 1/2-inch needle attached to a 3mL syringe and inject into the drug product vial for reconstitution
2. Discard the needle and syringe used for reconstitution; do not use for SQ inj
3. Reconstitute the vial contents by shaking the vial for approx 1 min and then allowing it to sit for 1 min; the resulting 80mg/mL sol is sufficient to allow a withdrawal volume of up to 2mL for SQ inj
4. Withdraw the recommended dose volume, up to 2mL (160mg), of the sol w/ a new 27-gauge 1/2-inch needle attached to a new 3mL syringe

Use reconstituted sol w/in 3 hrs

STORAGE

2-8°C (36-46°F). Store inside original carton to protect from light. (Reconstituted Sol) Keep at room temperature and use w/in 3 hrs of reconstitution. Protect from light.

HOW SUPPLIED

Inj: 220mg

WARNINGS/PRECAUTIONS

May increase risk of infection; d/c if serious infection develops. Do not initiate w/ active or chronic infection. May increase risk of tuberculosis (TB) or other atypical/opportunistic infections; evaluate and treat possible latent TB infection before initiating therapy. May increase risk of malignancies. All recommended vaccinations (eg, pneumococcal and inactivated influenza vaccine) should be received by patients as appropriate before initiation of therapy. Monitor for changes in lipid profiles. Hypersensitivity reactions reported (rare); d/c and initiate appropriate therapy if occurs.

ADVERSE REACTIONS

Inj-site reactions, URTI, sinusitis, cough, hypoesthesia, nausea, diarrhea, stomach discomfort, UTI, *Mycobacterium intracellulare* infection, GI bleeding, colitis, bronchitis, *Streptococcus pneumoniae* meningitis.

DRUG INTERACTIONS

Avoid live vaccines. Increased risk of serious infections and neutropenia w/ tumor necrosis factor (TNF) inhibitors; coadministration not recommended. Not recommended w/ other interleukin-1 (IL-1) blockers. Monitor effect or concentration of CYP450 substrates w/ narrow therapeutic index (eg, warfarin); adjust dose prn.

PREGNANCY AND LACTATION

Category C, caution in nursing.

MECHANISM OF ACTION

IL-1 blocker; acts as a soluble decoy receptor that binds IL-1β and prevents its interaction w/ cell surface receptors. Also binds IL-1α and IL-1 receptor antagonist w/ reduced affinity.

PATIENT CONSIDERATIONS

Assessment: Assess for active or chronic infection, vaccination history, latent TB, pregnancy/nursing status, and possible drug interactions.

Monitoring: Monitor for development of serious infection, malignancies, and hypersensitivity reactions, reactivation of latent TB, changes in lipid profile, and other adverse reactions.

Counseling: Instruct on aseptic reconstitution, inj technique, preparation, and disposal if to be administered by the patient or caregiver. Inform that inj-site reactions (eg, pain, erythema, swelling, pruritus, bruising, etc.) may occur; instruct to notify physician if reaction persists. Advise to avoid injecting at already swollen/red area. Inform that serious/life-threatening infections may occur; instruct to notify physician if an infection develops. Instruct not to take w/ drugs that block TNF or other IL-1 blockers (eg, anakinra).

ARESTIN — minocycline hydrochloride   Rx

Class: Tetracyclines

ADULT DOSAGE

Periodontitis

Adjunct to scaling and root planing procedures for reduction of pocket depth

Dose varies depending on the size, shape, and number of pockets being treated

Up to 122 unit-dose cartridges have been used in a single visit and up to 3 treatments, at 3-month intervals, have been administered in pockets w/ pocket depth of ≥5mm

PEDIATRIC DOSAGE

Pediatric use may not have been established

ADMINISTRATION

Subgingival route
Administration does not require local anesthesia
Sterilize the handle mechanism between patients

Preparation and Administration

1. Remove the disposable cartridge from its pouch and connect it to the handle mechanism
2. Insert the unit-dose cartridge to the base of the periodontal pocket
3. Press the thumb ring in the handle mechanism to expel the powder while gradually withdrawing the tip from the base of the pocket
4. Arestin does not have to be removed, as it is bioresorbable, nor is an adhesive or dressing required

STORAGE

20-25°C (68-77°F)/60% RH; excursions permitted to 15-30°C (59-86°F). Avoid exposure to excessive heat.

HOW SUPPLIED

Microsphere Delivery System: 1mg

CONTRAINDICATIONS

Known sensitivity to minocycline or tetracyclines.

WARNINGS/PRECAUTIONS

May cause permanent discoloration of the teeth (yellow-gray brown) if used during tooth development (last half of pregnancy, infancy, childhood to 8 yrs of age); do not use in this age group, or in pregnant or nursing women, unless potential benefits outweigh potential risks. Enamel hypoplasia reported. Photosensitivity, manifested by an exaggerated sunburn reaction, reported; d/c at the 1st evidence of skin erythema. Hypersensitivity reactions (eg, anaphylaxis) reported. Serious skin reactions (eg, Stevens-Johnson syndrome, erythema multiforme) reported with oral therapy. Oral therapy associated with the development of autoimmune syndromes including a lupus-like syndrome; in symptomatic patients, perform LFTs, antinuclear antibodies (ANA), CBC, and other appropriate tests, and do not administer further treatment to the patient. Not recommended in an acutely abscessed periodontal pocket. May result in overgrowth of nonsusceptible microorganisms including fungi; take appropriate measures if superinfection is suspected. Caution with a history of predisposition to oral candidiasis.

ADVERSE REACTIONS

Headache, infection, flu syndrome, pain, periodontitis, tooth disorder, tooth caries, dental pain, gingivitis, stomatitis, mouth ulceration, pharyngitis, dyspepsia, mucous membrane disorder.

PREGNANCY AND LACTATION

Category D, not for use in nursing.

MECHANISM OF ACTION

Tetracycline derivative; not established. Bacteriostatic and exerts antimicrobial activity by inhibiting protein synthesis.

PHARMACOKINETICS

Distribution: Found in breast milk.

PATIENT CONSIDERATIONS

Assessment: Assess for hypersensitivity to drug or tetracyclines, history of predisposition to oral candidiasis, and pregnancy/nursing status.

Monitoring: Monitor for photosensitivity, hypersensitivity reactions, skin reactions, autoimmune syndromes, superinfection, and other adverse reactions. If symptomatic of autoimmune syndrome, perform LFTs, ANA, and CBC.

Counseling: Apprise of the potential hazard to the fetus if used during pregnancy, or if the patient becomes pregnant while on therapy. Advise that photosensitivity manifested by an exaggerated sunburn reaction can occur; instruct to d/c treatment at the 1st evidence of skin erythema. Instruct to avoid chewing hard, crunchy, or sticky foods (carrots, taffy, and gum) with the treated teeth for 1 week and avoid touching treated areas. Advise not to use interproximal cleaning devices around the treated sites for 10 days after administration. Instruct to notify dentist promptly if pain, swelling, itching, rash, papules, reddening, difficulty breathing, other signs and symptoms of hypersensitivity, or other problems occur.

ARRANON — nelarabine   Rx

Class: Deoxyguanosine analogue

> Severe neurologic adverse reactions reported, including altered mental states (eg, severe somnolence), CNS effects (eg, convulsions), and peripheral neuropathy, ranging from numbness and paresthesias to motor weakness and paralysis. Adverse reactions associated with demyelination and ascending peripheral neuropathies similar in appearance to Guillain-Barre syndrome also reported. Close monitoring for neurologic adverse reactions is strongly recommended. D/C if neurologic adverse reactions of NCI Common Toxicity Criteria ≥Grade 2 occur.

ADULT DOSAGE

T-Cell Acute Lymphoblastic Leukemia

In patients whose disease has not responded to or has relapsed following treatment w/ ≥2 chemotherapy regimens

1500mg/m^2 IV over 2 hrs on Days 1, 3, and 5, repeated every 21 days

T-Cell Lymphoblastic Lymphoma

In patients whose disease has not responded to or has relapsed following treatment w/ ≥2 chemotherapy regimens

1500mg/m^2 IV over 2 hrs on Days 1, 3, and 5, repeated every 21 days

PEDIATRIC DOSAGE

T-Cell Acute Lymphoblastic Leukemia

In patients whose disease has not responded to or has relapsed following treatment w/ ≥2 chemotherapy regimens

650mg/m^2/day IV over 1 hr for 5 consecutive days, repeated every 21 days

T-Cell Lymphoblastic Lymphoma

In patients whose disease has not responded to or has relapsed following treatment w/ ≥2 chemotherapy regimens

650mg/m^2/day IV over 1 hr for 5 consecutive days, repeated every 21 days

DOSING CONSIDERATIONS

Adverse Reactions

Neurologic Reactions ≥Grade 2: D/C treatment
Dosage may be delayed for other toxicity including hematologic toxicity

ADMINISTRATION

IV route

Preparation

Do not dilute nelarabine prior to administration
Transfer the appropriate dose of nelarabine into polyvinylchloride infusion bags or glass containers for administration

STORAGE

25°C (77°F); excursions permitted to 15-30°C (59-86°F). Stable in polyvinylchloride infusion bags or glass containers for up to 8 hrs at up to 30°C.

HOW SUPPLIED

Inj: 5mg/mL [50mL]

WARNINGS/PRECAUTIONS

Leukopenia, thrombocytopenia, anemia, and neutropenia, including febrile neutropenia, reported; regularly monitor CBC including platelets. May cause fetal harm. IV hydration should be given for the management of hyperuricemia in patients at risk for tumor lysis syndrome; may also consider giving allopurinol in patients at risk for hyperuricemia. Closely monitor for toxicities in patients with moderate or severe renal impairment (CrCl ≤50mL/min) or severe hepatic impairment (total bilirubin >3X ULN). Caution in elderly.

ADVERSE REACTIONS

Altered mental status, CNS effects, peripheral neuropathy, anemia, thrombocytopenia, neutropenia, leukopenia, N/V, diarrhea, constipation, fatigue, pyrexia, cough, headache.

DRUG INTERACTIONS

Use with adenosine deaminase inhibitors (eg, pentostatin) is not recommended. Patients treated previously or concurrently with intrathecal chemotherapy or previously with craniospinal irradiation may be at increased risk for neurologic adverse events. Avoid administration of live vaccines to immunocompromised patients.

PREGNANCY AND LACTATION

Category D, not for use in nursing.

MECHANISM OF ACTION

Deoxyguanosine analogue; nucleoside metabolic inhibitor; demethylated by adenosine deaminase to ara-G, mono-phosphorylated by deoxyguanosine kinase and deoxycytidine kinase, and subsequently converted to the active 5'-triphosphate, ara-GTP. Accumulation of ara-GTP in leukemic blasts allows for incorporation into DNA, leading to inhibition of DNA synthesis and cell death.

PHARMACOKINETICS

Absorption: C$_{max}$=5µg/mL, 31.4µg/mL (ara-G); AUC=4.4µg•hr/mL, 162µg•hr/mL (ara-G). **Distribution:** Plasma protein binding (<25%). (Adults) V$_{ss}$=197L/m^2, 50L/m^2 (ara-G); (Pediatrics) V$_{ss}$=213L/m^2, 33L/m^2 (ara-G). **Metabolism:** O-demethylation via adenosine deaminase; ara-G (metabolite). **Elimination:** Urine (6.6%, 27% ara-G); (Adults) T$_{1/2}$=18 min, 3.2 hrs (ara-G), (Pediatrics) T$_{1/2}$=13 min, 2 hrs (ara-G).

PATIENT CONSIDERATIONS

Assessment: Assess for renal/hepatic impairment, risk of tumor lysis syndrome or hyperuricemia, pregnancy/nursing status, and possible drug interactions.

Monitoring: Monitor for signs/symptoms of neurotoxicity (eg, somnolence, confusion, convulsions, ataxia, peripheral neuropathy, hypoesthesia), hyperuricemia, leukopenia, thrombocytopenia, anemia, neutropenia, and other adverse reactions. Perform regular monitoring of CBC, including platelets.

Counseling: Inform that therapy may cause somnolence and therefore caution should be taken when operating hazardous machinery or driving. Instruct to contact physician if new or worsening symptoms of peripheral neuropathy develop (eg, tingling or numbness in fingers, hands, toes or feet; difficulty with fine motor coordination tasks; unsteadiness while walking, weakness arising from a low chair/climbing stairs, increased tripping). Instruct to contact physician if seizures, fever, or signs of infection develop. Advise to use effective contraceptive measures to prevent pregnancy and to avoid breastfeeding during treatment.

ARZERRA — ofatumumab   Rx

Class: Monoclonal antibody/CD20 blocker

> Hepatitis B virus (HBV) reactivation may occur, in some cases resulting in fulminant hepatitis, hepatic failure, and death. Progressive multifocal leukoencephalopathy (PML) resulting in death may occur.

ADULT DOSAGE
Chronic Lymphocytic Leukemia

Previously Untreated Chronic Lymphocytic Leukemia (CLL):
In combination w/ chlorambucil, for the treatment of patients for whom fludarabine-based therapy is considered inappropriate
Cycle 1: 300mg on Day 1, followed 1 week later by 1000mg on Day 8, followed by
Subsequent 28-Day Cycles: 1000mg on Day 1 for a minimum of 3 cycles until best response or a max of 12 cycles

Relapsed CLL:
In combination w/ fludarabine and cyclophosphamide
Cycle 1: 300mg on Day 1, followed 1 week later by 1000mg on Day 8, followed by
Subsequent 28-Day Cycles: 1000mg on Day 1 for a max of 6 cycles

Extended Treatment in CLL:
As a single agent for patients who are in complete or partial response after at least 2 lines of therapy for recurrent or progressive CLL
Day 1: 300mg
Day 8: 1000mg
Subsequent Doses: 1000mg 7 weeks later and every 8 weeks thereafter for up to a max of 2 yrs

Refractory CLL:
Treatment of patients refractory to fludarabine and alemtuzumab
Recommended: 300mg initially on Day 1, followed 1 week later by 2000mg weekly for 7 doses (Infusions 2 through 8), followed 4 weeks later by 2000mg every 4 weeks for 4 doses (Infusions 9 through 12)

Infusion Rates:
Previously Untreated CLL, Relapsed CLL, and Extended Treatment in CLL:
Initial 300mg Dose: Initiate at a rate of 3.6mg/hr (12mL/hr)
Subsequent Infusions of 1000mg: Initiate at a rate of 25mg/hr (25mL/hr); initiate at a rate of 12mg/hr if a Grade ≥3 infusion-related adverse event occurred during the previous infusion

Refractory CLL:
Infusion 1 (300mg Dose): Initiate at a rate of 3.6mg/hr (12mL/hr)
Infusion 2 (2000mg Dose): Initiate at a rate of 24mg/hr (12mL/hr)
Infusions 3 Through 12 (2000mg Doses): Initiate at a rate of 50mg/hr (25mL/hr)

The rate of infusion may be increased every 30 min in the absence of an infusion-related adverse event; refer to PI for further infusion rate information

Premedication
Administer 30 min to 2 hrs prior to each infusion

PEDIATRIC DOSAGE
Pediatric use may not have been established

Previously Untreated CLL, Relapsed CLL, or Extended Treatment in CLL:
Infusions 1 and 2:
IV corticosteroid (prednisolone or equivalent) 50mg + oral acetaminophen (APAP) 1000mg + oral/IV antihistamine (diphenhydramine 50mg, cetirizine 10mg, or equivalent)
Infusion 3 and Beyond (Up to 13 Infusions [Previously Untreated CLL]; Up to 7 Infusions [Relapsed CLL]; Up to 14 Infusions [Extended Treatment in CLL]):
IV corticosteroid (prednisolone or equivalent) 0-50mg (may be reduced/omitted for subsequent infusions if a Grade ≥3 infusion-related adverse event did not occur w/ the preceding infusion[s]) + oral APAP 1000mg + oral/IV antihistamine (diphenhydramine 50mg, cetirizine 10mg, or equivalent)

Refractory CLL:
Infusions 1, 2, and 9:
IV corticosteroid (prednisolone or equivalent) 100mg + oral APAP 1000mg + oral/IV antihistamine (diphenhydramine 50mg, cetirizine 10mg, or equivalent)
Infusions 3 Through 8:
IV corticosteroid (prednisolone or equivalent) 0-100mg (may be reduced/omitted for subsequent infusions if a Grade ≥3 infusion-related adverse event did not occur w/ the preceding infusion[s]) + oral APAP 1000mg + oral/IV antihistamine (diphenhydramine 50mg, cetirizine 10mg, or equivalent)
Infusions 10 Through 12:
IV corticosteroid (prednisolone or equivalent) 50-100mg (prednisolone may be reduced to 50-100mg [or equivalent] if a Grade ≥3 infusion-related adverse event did not occur w/ Infusion 9) + oral APAP 1000mg + oral/IV antihistamine (diphenhydramine 50mg, cetirizine 10mg, or equivalent)

DOSING CONSIDERATIONS
Adverse Reactions
Infusion Reactions:
Interrupt infusion for reactions of any severity. Treatment can be resumed at the discretion of the treating physician; the following infusion rate modifications can be used as a guide.
If infusion reaction resolves/remains ≤Grade 2, resume infusion according to initial grade of reaction:
- **Grade 1 or 2:** Infuse at 1/2 of the previous infusion rate.
- **Grade 3 or 4:** Infuse at a rate of 12mL/hr.
After resuming infusion, may increase infusion rate as specified in the PI, based on patient tolerance.
Consider permanent discontinuation if severity of infusion reaction does not resolve to ≤Grade 2 despite adequate clinical intervention; permanently d/c therapy if anaphylactic reaction develops.

ADMINISTRATION
IV route
Dilute and administer as an IV infusion; do not administer as IV push or bolus, or as SQ inj.
Do not shake.

Preparation of Sol
300mg Dose:
1. Withdraw and discard 15mL from a 1000mL bag of 0.9% NaCl inj.
2. Withdraw 5mL from each of 3 single-use 100mg vials and add to the bag.
3. Mix diluted sol by gentle inversion.

1000mg Dose:
1. Withdraw and discard 50mL from a 1000mL bag of 0.9% NaCl inj.
2. Withdraw 50mL from 1 single-use 1000mg vial and add to the bag.
3. Mix diluted sol by gentle inversion.

2000mg Dose:
1. Withdraw and discard 100mL from a 1000mL bag of 0.9% NaCl inj.
2. Withdraw 50mL from each of 2 single-use 1000mg vials and add to the bag.
3. Mix diluted sol by gentle inversion.

Store diluted sol at 2-8°C (36-46°F).
No incompatibilities between therapy and polyvinylchloride or polyolefin bags and administration sets have been observed.

Administration Instructions

- Do not mix w/, or administer as an infusion w/, other medicinal products.
- Administer using an infusion pump and an administration set.
- Flush the IV line w/ 0.9% NaCl inj before and after each dose.
- Start infusion w/in 12 hrs of preparation.
- Discard prepared sol after 24 hrs.

STORAGE

2-8°C (36-46°F). Do not freeze. Protect from light.

HOW SUPPLIED

Inj: 20mg/mL [5mL, 50mL]

WARNINGS/PRECAUTIONS

Administer in an environment where facilities to adequately monitor and treat infusion reactions are available. May cause serious, including fatal, infusion reactions; interrupt for infusion reactions of any severity and institute medical management for severe reactions. Permanently d/c if an anaphylactic reaction occurs. Screen for HBV infection before initiating treatment. Monitor patients w/ evidence of current or prior HBV infection for clinical and laboratory signs of hepatitis or HBV reactivation during and for several months following treatment. Immediately d/c therapy and any concomitant chemotherapy, and institute appropriate treatment if HBV reactivation develops. Fatal infection due to hepatitis B in patients who have not been previously infected reported. Consider PML in any patient w/ new onset of or changes in preexisting neurological signs/symptoms; if PML is suspected, d/c therapy and initiate evaluation for PML. Tumor lysis syndrome (TLS), including the need for hospitalization, reported; increased risk w/ high tumor burden and/or high circulating lymphocyte counts (>25 x 10^9/L). Consider tumor lysis prophylaxis w/ antihyperuricemics and hydration beginning 12-24 hrs prior to infusion. Severe cytopenias, including neutropenia, thrombocytopenia, and anemia, may occur; monitor CBC at regular intervals during and after conclusion of therapy, and at increased frequency in patients who develop Grade 3 or 4 cytopenias.

ADVERSE REACTIONS

Previously Untreated CLL: Infusion reactions, neutropenia.
Relapsed CLL: Infusion reactions, neutropenia, leukopenia, febrile neutropenia.
Extended Treatment in CLL: Infusion reactions, neutropenia, URTIs.
Refractory CLL: Neutropenia, pneumonia, pyrexia, cough, diarrhea, anemia, fatigue, dyspnea, rash, nausea, bronchitis, URTIs.

DRUG INTERACTIONS

Pancytopenia, agranulocytosis, and fatal neutropenic sepsis reported w/ chlorambucil. Do not administer live viral vaccines to recently treated patients.

PREGNANCY AND LACTATION

Pregnancy: There are no data on the use of therapy in pregnant women to inform a drug-associated risk. May cause fetal B-cell depletion; avoid administering live vaccines to neonates and infants exposed to ofatumumab in utero until B-cell recovery occurs.
Lactation: There is no information regarding the presence of ofatumumab in human milk, the effects on the breastfed infant, or the effects on milk production. Human IgG is known to be present in human milk. Published data suggest that antibodies in breast milk do not enter the neonatal and infant circulations in substantial amounts. Caution in nursing.

MECHANISM OF ACTION

CD20-directed cytolytic monoclonal antibody; binds specifically to both the small and large extracellular loops of CD20 molecule. The Fab domain of ofatumumab binds to the CD20 molecule and the Fc domain mediates immune effector functions to result in B-cell lysis in vitro. Possible mechanisms of cell lysis include complement-dependent cytotoxicity and antibody-dependent, cell-mediated cytotoxicity.

PHARMACOKINETICS

Distribution: V_d=6.1L. **Elimination:** $T_{1/2}$=17.6 days.

PATIENT CONSIDERATIONS

Assessment: Assess for current/prior HBV infection, risk for TLS, pregnancy/nursing status, and possible drug interactions.
Monitoring: Monitor for signs/symptoms of HBV reactivation, hepatitis, PML, infusion reactions, TLS, and other adverse reactions. Monitor CBC at regular intervals during and after conclusion of therapy, and at increased frequency in patients who develop Grade 3 or 4 cytopenias.
Counseling: Instruct to inform physician of signs/symptoms of infusion reactions (eg, chills, rash, breathing problems w/in 24 hrs of infusion); symptoms of hepatitis (eg, worsening fatigue, yellow discoloration of skin/eyes); new neurological symptoms (eg, confusion, dizziness, loss of balance); bleeding, easy bruising, petechiae, pallor, worsening weakness, or fatigue; or signs of infections (eg, fever, cough). Advise to notify physician if pregnant/nursing. Advise of the need for monitoring and possible need for treatment if patient has a history of hepatitis B infection, for periodic monitoring of blood counts, and for avoiding vaccination w/ live viral vaccines.

ASTAGRAF XL — tacrolimus

Rx

Class: Calcineurin-inhibitor immunosuppressant

> Increased risk for developing serious infections and malignancies w/ tacrolimus extended-release (ER) caps or other immunosuppressants that may lead to hospitalization or death. Increased mortality in female liver transplant patients reported; not approved for use in liver transplantation.

ADULT DOSAGE

Organ Rejection Prophylaxis

Kidney Transplant:
To be used in combination w/ other immunosuppressants

≥16 Years:
Initial:
W/ Mycophenolate Mofetil (MMF), Steroids, and Basiliximab Induction: 0.15-0.2mg/kg administered prior to reperfusion or w/in 48 hrs of the completion of the transplant procedure (timing may be delayed until renal function has recovered)

W/ MMF and Steroids w/o Basiliximab Induction:
First Dose (Preoperative): 0.1mg/kg administered as a single dose w/in 12 hrs prior to reperfusion
Second Dose (Postoperative): 0.2mg/kg administered at least 4 hrs after the preoperative dose and w/in 12 hrs after reperfusion

Titrate:
Adjust dosing based on clinical assessments of rejection and tolerability, and to achieve trough concentration ranges as follows:

Target Tacrolimus Whole Blood Trough Concentrations:
During Month 1 Post Transplant:
W/ Basiliximab Induction:
7-15ng/mL
W/O Basiliximab Induction:
10-15ng/mL
Months 2-6 Post Transplant:
5-15ng/mL
<6 Months Post Transplant:
5-10ng/mL

African-American patients may need to be titrated to higher doses to attain comparable trough concentrations compared to Caucasian patients.

Therapeutic Drug Monitoring:
Measure tacrolimus whole blood trough concentrations at least 2X on separate days during the first week after initiation of dosing and after a change in dosage, after a change in coadministration of CYP3A4 inducers and/or inhibitors, or after a change in renal or hepatic function

Missed Dose

If a dose is missed, the dose may be taken up to 14 hrs after the scheduled time (eg, for a missed 8:00 am dose, take by 10:00 pm)

Beyond the 14-hr time frame, the patient should wait until the usual scheduled time the following morning to take the next regular daily dose

---

DOSING CONSIDERATIONS

Hepatic Impairment

Severe (Child Pugh ≥10): Lower doses may be required

Elderly

Start at lower end of dosing range

ADMINISTRATION

Oral route

Not interchangeable or substitutable w/ other tacrolimus ER or immediate-release (IR) products.
Take consistently qam at the same time, on an empty stomach at least 1 hr ac or at least 2 hrs pc.
Swallow whole w/ liquid; do not chew, divide, or crush.
Avoid eating grapefruit or drinking grapefruit juice or alcoholic beverages while taking tacrolimus ER caps.

STORAGE

25°C (77°F); excursions permitted to 15-30°C (59-86°F).

HOW SUPPLIED

Cap, ER: 0.5mg, 1mg, 5mg

CONTRAINDICATIONS

Known hypersensitivity to tacrolimus.

PEDIATRIC DOSAGE

Pediatric use may not have been established

WARNINGS/PRECAUTIONS

Increases risk of developing lymphomas and other malignancies, particularly of the skin. Avoid or limit exposure to sunlight and UV light. Post-transplant lymphoproliferative disorder, associated w/ Epstein-Barr virus (EBV), reported in immunosuppressed organ transplant patients; risk appears greatest in those individuals who are EBV seronegative. Monitor EBV serology during treatment. Increases risk of developing bacterial, viral (eg, polyomavirus-associated nephropathy, JC virus-associated progressive multifocal leukoencephalopathy, CMV infections), fungal, and protozoal infections, including opportunistic infections; monitor for the development of infection and adjust immunosuppressive regimen to balance the risk of rejection w/ risk of infection. Graft rejection and other serious adverse reactions due to medication errors reported; not interchangeable or substitutable w/ other tacrolimus ER or IR products. New onset diabetes reported after transplant. May cause acute or chronic nephrotoxicity; consider dosage reduction in patients w/ elevated SrCr and tacrolimus whole blood trough concentrations greater than the recommended range. May cause a spectrum of neurotoxicities; consider dosage reduction or discontinuation if neurotoxicity occurs. Mild to severe hyperkalemia reported and treatment may be required. HTN may occur and antihypertensive therapy may be required. May prolong the QT/QTc interval and cause torsades de pointes; avoid in patients w/ congenital long QT syndrome. Consider obtaining ECG and monitoring electrolytes (Mg^{2+}, K^+, Ca^{2+}) periodically during treatment in patients w/ CHF, bradyarrhythmias, those taking certain antiarrhythmic medications or other products that lead to QT prolongation, and those w/ electrolyte disturbances. Whenever possible, administer the complete complement of vaccines before transplantation and therapy. Cases of pure red cell aplasia (PRCA) reported; consider discontinuation of therapy if PRCA is diagnosed.

ADVERSE REACTIONS

Diarrhea, constipation, nausea, peripheral edema, tremor, anemia.

DRUG INTERACTIONS

See Administration. Risk for nephrotoxicity may increase when concomitantly administered w/ CYP3A inhibitors or drugs associated w/ nephrotoxicity (eg, aminoglycosides, ganciclovir, amphotericin B); monitor renal function and consider dosage reduction if nephrotoxicity occurs. Agents associated w/ hyperkalemia (eg, K^+-sparing diuretics, ACE inhibitors, ARBs) may increase risk for hyperkalemia. Avoid use of live attenuated vaccines during treatment. Inactivated vaccines noted to be safe for administration after transplantation may not be sufficiently immunogenic during treatment w/ tacrolimus ER caps. Increases exposure to mycophenolic acid (MPA) products; monitor for MPA-associated adverse reactions and reduce dose of concomitantly administered MPA products as needed. Grapefruit or grapefruit juice may increase tacrolimus whole blood trough concentrations and increase risk of serious adverse reactions. Alcohol may increase the rate of tacrolimus release and increase the risk of serious adverse reactions. Strong CYP3A inducers (eg, rifampin, phenytoin, St. John's wort) may decrease tacrolimus whole blood trough concentrations and increase risk of rejection; increase tacrolimus ER caps dose and monitor tacrolimus whole blood trough concentrations. Strong CYP3A inhibitors (eg, nelfinavir, boceprevir, voriconazole, posaconazole) may increase tacrolimus whole blood trough concentrations and increase the risk of serious adverse reactions; reduce tacrolimus ER caps dose (for voriconazole and posaconazole, give 1/3 of the original dose) and adjust dose based on tacrolimus whole blood trough concentrations. Mild or moderate CYP3A inhibitors (eg, clotrimazole, erythromycin, calcium channel blockers) and other drugs (eg, Mg^{2+} and aluminum hydroxide antacids, metoclopramide) may increase tacrolimus whole blood trough concentrations and increase the risk of serious adverse reactions; monitor tacrolimus whole blood trough concentrations and reduce tacrolimus ER caps dose if needed. Mild or moderate CYP3A inducers (eg, methylprednisolone, prednisone) may decrease tacrolimus concentrations; monitor tacrolimus whole blood trough concentrations and adjust tacrolimus ER caps dose if needed.

PREGNANCY AND LACTATION

Pregnancy: Category C.
Lactation: Present in breast milk; not for use in nursing.

MECHANISM OF ACTION

Macrolide immunosuppressant; binds to FKBP-12, forming a complex of tacrolimus-FKBP-12, Ca^{2+}, calmodulin, and calcineurin, and inhibiting phosphatase activity of calcineurin. Inhibits the expression and/or production of several cytokines that include interleukin (IL)-1 β, IL-2, IL-3, IL-4, IL-5, IL-6, IL-8, IL-10, gamma interferon, TNF-α, and granulocyte macrophage colony stimulating factor. Also inhibits IL-2 receptor expression and nitric oxide release, and induces apoptosis and production of transforming growth factor-β that can lead to immunosuppressive activity. Net result is inhibition of T-lymphocyte activation and proliferation as well as T-helper-cell-dependent B-cell response.

PHARMACOKINETICS

Absorption: Administration of variable doses in different populations resulted in different pharmacokinetic parameters. **Distribution:** Plasma protein binding (99%); crosses placenta; found in breast milk. **Metabolism:** Liver (extensive), via CYP3A (demethylation and hydroxylation); 13-demethyl tacrolimus (major metabolite); 31-demethyl metabolite (active metabolite). **Elimination:** Feces (92.6%), urine (2.3%); $T_{1/2}$=38 hrs (4mg daily for 10 days).

PATIENT CONSIDERATIONS

Assessment: Assess for congenital long QT syndrome, CHF, bradyarrhythmias, electrolyte disturbances, renal/hepatic impairment, hypersensitivity to the drug, pregnancy/nursing status, and possible drug interactions.

Monitoring: Monitor for lymphomas and other malignancies (eg, skin changes), infections (including opportunistic infections), nephrotoxicity, neurotoxicity, HTN, QT prolongation, PRCA, and for other adverse reactions. Measure tacrolimus whole blood trough concentrations at least 2X on separate days during the first week after initiation of dosing and after any change in dosage, after a change in coadministration of CYP3A4 inducers and/or inhibitors, or after a change in renal or hepatic function. Monitor serum K^+ periodically and glucose concentrations. Monitor EBV serology. Consider obtaining ECG and monitoring electrolytes (Mg^{2+}, K^+, Ca^{2+}) periodically during treatment in patients w/ CHF, bradyarrhythmias, those taking certain antiarrhythmic medications or other products that lead to QT prolongation, and those w/ electrolyte disturbances.

Counseling: Inform of the risks and benefits of therapy. Instruct to inspect the medicine when a new prescription is received and before taking it; advise to contact healthcare provider if there are any changes. Instruct to take exactly ud. Advise to avoid alcoholic beverages, grapefruit, and grapefruit juice while on therapy. Instruct to take a missed dose as soon as possible but not more than 14 hrs after the scheduled time; beyond the 14-hr timeframe, instruct to wait until the usual scheduled time the following am to take the next scheduled dose. Inform of increased risk of developing lymphomas and other malignancies. Advise to limit exposure to sunlight and UV light by wearing protective clothing and using sunscreen w/ a high protection factor. Instruct to contact physician if any symptoms of infection, frequent urination, increased thirst or hunger, vision changes, delirium, or tremors develop. Inform that drug can cause hyperkalemia and that monitoring of K^+ levels may be necessary. Inform that therapy can cause high BP that may require treatment w/ antihypertensive therapy. Advise that drug can interfere w/ the usual response to immunizations and that patient should avoid live vaccines. Instruct to attend all visits and complete all blood tests ordered by medical team. Instruct to inform physician if planning to become pregnant or to breastfeed, or if starting or stopping any concomitant medications.

ATGAM — lymphocyte immune globulin, anti-thymocyte globulin (equine)   **Rx**

Class: Lymphocyte-selective immunosuppressant

> Antithymocyte globulins can cause anaphylaxis when injected IV. Physicians should be prepared for the potential risk of anaphylaxis and monitor patients for signs/symptoms during infusion.

ADULT DOSAGE

Renal Allograft Rejection

10-15mg/kg/day for 14 days

Additional alternate-day therapy up to a total of 21 doses may be given

Aplastic Anemia

Moderate to severe aplastic anemia in patients who are unsuitable for bone marrow transplantation

10-20mg/kg/day for 8-14 days; may administer additional alternate-day therapy up to a total of 21 doses

Patients may need prophylactic platelet transfusions to maintain platelets at clinically acceptable levels

PEDIATRIC DOSAGE

Renal Allograft Rejection

10-15mg/kg/day for 14 days

Additional alternate-day therapy up to a total of 21 doses may be given

Aplastic Anemia

Moderate to severe aplastic anemia in patients who are unsuitable for bone marrow transplantation

10-20mg/kg/day for 8-14 days; may administer additional alternate-day therapy up to a total of 21 doses

Patients may need prophylactic platelet transfusions to maintain platelets at clinically acceptable levels

---

DOSING CONSIDERATIONS

Elderly
Start at lower end of dosing range

ADMINISTRATION

IV route

Preparation of Sol

1. Atgam may be transparent to slightly opalescent, colorless to faintly pink or brown, and may develop a slight granular or flaky deposit during storage.
2. Dilute in an inverted bottle of sterile vehicle so the undiluted Atgam does not contact air inside.
3. Add the total daily dose to the sterile vehicle; do not exceed a concentration of 4mg/mL.
4. Gently rotate or swirl diluted sol to effect thorough mixing; do not shake Atgam (diluted or undiluted).

Administration

1. Allow the diluted sol to reach room temperature before infusion.
2. Administer into a vascular shunt, arterial venous fistula, or a high-flow central vein through an in-line filter w/ a pore size of 0.2-1μm; use the in-line filter w/ all infusions of Atgam.
3. Use high-flow veins to minimize the occurrence of phlebitis and thrombosis.
4. Do not infuse a dose in <4 hrs.

Compatibility and Stability

Once diluted, Atgam has been shown to be physically and chemically stable for up to 24 hrs at concentrations of up to 4mg/mL in the following diluents:
0.9% NaCl inj
D5 and 0.225% NaCl inj
D5 and 0.45% NaCl inj

Do not dilute in dextrose inj, as low salt concentrations may cause precipitation. Do not use highly acidic infusion sol since these sol may contribute to physical instability over time.
Store diluted product in a refrigerator if it is prepared prior to the time of infusion; do not exceed a total time in dilution of 24 hrs (including infusion time).

STORAGE

2-8°C (36-46°F). Do not freeze.

HOW SUPPLIED
Inj: 50mg/mL [5mL]

CONTRAINDICATIONS
History of a systemic reaction (eg, anaphylactic reaction) during prior administration of this product or any other equine gamma globulin preparation.

WARNINGS/PRECAUTIONS
Serious immune-mediated reactions reported. Clinical signs associated w/ anaphylaxis, other infusion-associated reactions, and serum sickness reported; d/c if anaphylaxis occurs. A systemic reaction (eg, generalized rash, tachycardia, dyspnea, hypotension, anaphylaxis) precludes any additional administration of drug. Skin testing is strongly recommended before starting treatment in order to identify those at greatest risk of systemic anaphylaxis. Allergic reactions (eg, anaphylaxis) reported in patients whose skin test is negative. Skin testing will not predict for later development of serum sickness. Seriously consider alternative forms of therapy in the presence of a locally positive skin test. If use of therapy is deemed appropriate following a locally positive skin test, administer treatment in a setting where intensive life support facilities are immediately available and a physician familiar w/ the treatment of potentially life-threatening allergic reactions is in attendance. May carry a risk of transmitting infectious agents (eg, viruses, and theoretically, the Creutzfeldt-Jakob disease agent). Abnormal tests of liver function and renal function reported in patients w/ aplastic anemia and other hematologic abnormalities. May increase incidence of cytomegalovirus infection.

ADVERSE REACTIONS
Pyrexia, chills, rash, thrombocytopenia, leukopenia, arthralgia, urticaria, headache, N/V, infection, thrombophlebitis.

DRUG INTERACTIONS
Do not administer live vaccines to patients about to receive, receiving, or after treatment w/ Atgam; concomitant administration w/ live virus vaccines carries a potential of uncontrolled viral replication in the immunosuppressed patient. If administered, live viruses may interfere w/ treatment. Previously masked reactions to therapy may appear when the dose of corticosteroids and other immunosuppressants is being reduced.

PREGNANCY AND LACTATION
Pregnancy: Not known whether Atgam can cause fetal harm when administered to a pregnant woman or can affect reproduction capacity; should be used during pregnancy only if the potential benefit justifies the potential risk to the fetus. **Lactation:** Not known whether Atgam is excreted in human milk; not for use in nursing.

MECHANISM OF ACTION
Lymphocyte-selective immunosuppressant; mechanism of drug induced immunosuppression has not been determined. Primary mechanism may be depletion of circulating lymphocytes, with greatest effect on T lymphocytes. Lymphocyte depletion may be caused by complement dependent lysis and/ or activation-induced apoptosis. Also, immunosuppression may be mediated by the binding of antibodies to lymphocytes, which results in partial activation and induction of T lymphocyte anergy. Mechanism for aplastic anemia is attributed to drug's immunosuppressive actions. Also, directly stimulates growth of hematopoietic stem cells and release of hematopoietic growth factors (eg, interleukin-3, granulocyte/macrophage colony stimulating factor).

PHARMACOKINETICS
Elimination: $T_{1/2}$=1.5-13 days.

PATIENT CONSIDERATIONS
Assessment: Assess for history of any systemic reaction during prior administration of Atgam or any equine gamma globulin preparation, pregnancy/ nursing status, and possible drug interactions. Perform skin testing before the 1st infusion. In patients w/ aplastic anemia and other hematologic abnormalities, assess LFTs and renal function.

Monitoring: Monitor for anaphylaxis/allergic reactions, immune-mediated reactions, infection, and other adverse reactions. Monitor LFTs and renal function in patients w/ aplastic anemia and other hematologic abnormalities.

Counseling: Inform of the risks/benefits of therapy. Advise patients receiving therapy that they will be monitored in a facility equipped and staffed w/ adequate laboratory and supportive medical resources. Inform that therapy may cause serious allergic reactions, infection, or abnormal liver or renal function. Advise to d/c and seek immediate medical attention if any signs/symptoms of an allergic or immune reaction occur. Explain that therapy may carry a risk of transmitting infectious agents (eg, viruses). Instruct to d/c therapy and report any sign/ symptoms of leukopenia, thrombocytopenia, or infection (eg, fever, sweating, chills, muscle aches, cough, SOB, diarrhea, or stomach pain) to physician.

ATRIPLA — efavirenz/emtricitabine/tenofovir disoproxil fumarate   Rx

Class: Non-nucleoside reverse transcriptase inhibitor (NNRTI)/nucleoside reverse transcriptase inhibitor (NRTI) combination

> Lactic acidosis and severe hepatomegaly w/ steatosis, including fatal cases, reported w/ the use of nucleoside analogues. Not approved for the treatment of chronic hepatitis B virus (HBV) infection and safety and efficacy have not been established in patients coinfected w/ HBV and HIV. Severe acute exacerbations of hepatitis B reported in patients coinfected w/ HBV upon discontinuation of emtricitabine or tenofovir disoproxil fumarate (TDF); closely monitor hepatic function for at least several months after stopping therapy. If appropriate, initiation of antihepatitis B therapy may be warranted.

ADULT DOSAGE
HIV-1 Infection
Alone/Combination w/ Other Antiretrovirals:
1 tab qd

PEDIATRIC DOSAGE
HIV-1 Infection
Alone/Combination w/ Other Antiretrovirals:
≥12 Years and ≥40kg:
1 tab qd

DOSING CONSIDERATIONS
Concomitant Medications
Rifampin:
≥50kg: Additional 200mg/day of efavirenz is recommended
Renal Impairment
Moderate or Severe (CrCl <50mL/min): Not recommended for use
Hepatic Impairment
Moderate or Severe: Not recommended for use

ADMINISTRATION
Oral route

Take on an empty stomach.
Bedtime dosing may improve tolerability of nervous system symptoms.

STORAGE
25°C (77°F); excursions permitted to 15-30°C (59-86°F).

HOW SUPPLIED
Tab: (Efavirenz/Emtricitabine/TDF) 600mg/200mg/300mg

CONTRAINDICATIONS
Hypersensitivity to efavirenz. Coadministration w/ voriconazole.

WARNINGS/PRECAUTIONS
Hepatic failure reported; monitor liver enzymes w/ underlying hepatic diseases. In patients w/ persistent elevations of serum transaminases >5X ULN, weigh benefit of continued therapy against risks of significant liver toxicity. Immune reconstitution syndrome and autoimmune disorders (eg, Graves' disease, polymyositis, Guillain-Barre syndrome) in the setting of immune reconstitution reported. Redistribution/accumulation of body fat has been observed. Caution in elderly. **Efavirenz:** Serious psychiatric adverse events and CNS symptoms reported; if serious psychiatric adverse events occur, evaluate to assess if they are related to therapy and determine risks and benefits of continued therapy. May impair mental/physical abilities. May cause fetal harm if administered during 1st trimester of pregnancy; avoid pregnancy during use. Use adequate contraceptive measures for 12 weeks after discontinuation. Skin rash reported; d/c if severe rash associated w/ blistering, desquamation, mucosal involvement, or fever develops. Consider alternative therapy in patients who have had a life-threatening cutaneous reaction (eg, Stevens-Johnson syndrome). Consider appropriate antihistamine prophylaxis in pediatric patients before initiating therapy. Convulsions reported; caution w/ history of seizures. **TDF:** Obesity and prolonged nucleoside exposure may be risk factors for lactic acidosis and severe hepatomegaly w/ steatosis. Caution w/ known risk factors for liver disease. D/C if lactic acidosis or pronounced hepatotoxicity occurs. Renal impairment, including acute renal failure and Fanconi syndrome, reported. Decreased bone mineral density (BMD), increased biochemical markers of bone metabolism, and osteomalacia reported; consider assessment of BMD in patients w/ a history of pathologic bone fracture or other risk factors for osteoporosis or bone loss. Arthralgias and muscle pain/weakness reported in cases of proximal renal tubulopathy. Consider hypophosphatemia and osteomalacia secondary to proximal renal tubulopathy in patients at risk of renal dysfunction who present w/ persistent or worsening bone or muscle symptoms.

ADVERSE REACTIONS
Diarrhea, nausea, fatigue, headache, dizziness, depression, insomnia, abnormal dreams, rash.

DRUG INTERACTIONS
See Contraindications. Avoid w/ adefovir dipivoxil, drugs which contain the same active components as Atripla, atazanavir, drugs containing same component or lamivudine, other NNRTIs, boceprevir, posaconazole, or nephrotoxic agents (eg, high-dose or multiple NSAIDs). Potential additive CNS effects w/ alcohol or psychoactive drugs. May increase levels of didanosine and ritonavir (RTV). May decrease levels of amprenavir, indinavir, lopinavir, saquinavir, maraviroc, raltegravir, simeprevir, carbamazepine, anticonvulsants, bupropion, sertraline, itraconazole, ketoconazole, clarithromycin, rifabutin, diltiazem or other calcium channel blockers, atorvastatin, pravastatin, simvastatin, norelgestromin, levonorgestrel, etonogestrel, immunosuppressants, and methadone. May decrease levels of artemether, dihydroartemisinin, and/or lumefantrine resulting in a decrease antimalarial efficacy of artemether/lumefantrine; use w/ caution. **Efavirenz:** RTV may increase levels. Avoid w/ simeprevir. Carbamazepine, anticonvulsants, rifabutin, and rifampin may decrease levels. CYP3A substrates, inhibitors, or inducers may alter levels. May alter plasma levels of warfarin or drugs metabolized by CYP3A or CYP2B6. **TDF/ Emtricitabine:** Coadministration of drugs that reduce renal function or compete for active tubular secretion (eg, acyclovir, adefovir dipivoxil, cidofovir, ganciclovir, valacyclovir, valganciclovir, aminoglycosides [eg, gentamicin], and high-dose or multiple NSAIDs) may increase levels of emtricitabine, TDF, and/or other renally eliminated drugs. Monitor closely for didanosine-associated adverse reactions w/ TDF. Atazanavir, darunavir w/ RTV, and lopinavir/RTV may increase TDF levels. An increase in absorption may be observed when TDF is coadministered w/ an inhibitor of P-gp or breast cancer resistance protein. Refer to PI for further information on drug interactions.

PREGNANCY AND LACTATION
Pregnancy: Category D. Physicians are encouraged to register patients who become pregnant in the Antiretroviral Pregnancy Registry.
Lactation: Excreted in human milk; not for use in nursing.

MECHANISM OF ACTION

Efavirenz: NNRTI; noncompetitive inhibition of HIV-1 reverse transcriptase (RT). **Emtricitabine:** Nucleoside analogue of cytidine; inhibits activity of HIV-1 RT by competing w/ natural substrate deoxycytidine 5'-triphosphate and incorporating into nascent viral DNA, resulting in chain termination. **TDF:** Acyclic nucleoside phosphonate diester analogue of adenosine monophosphate; inhibits activity of HIV-1 RT by competing w/ the natural substrate deoxyadenosine 5'-triphosphate and, after incorporation into the DNA, by DNA chain termination.

PHARMACOKINETICS

Absorption: Efavirenz: C_{max}=12.9µM, T_{max}=3-5 hrs, AUC=184µM•hr. Emtricitabine: Rapid; absolute bioavailability (93%), C_{max}=1.8mcg/mL, T_{max}=1-2 hrs, AUC=10mcg•hr/mL. TDF: Bioavailability (25%, fasted), C_{max}=296ng/mL, T_{max}=1 hr, AUC=2287ng•hr/mL. **Distribution:** Efavirenz: Plasma protein binding (99.5-99.75%); found in breast milk. Emtricitabine: Plasma protein binding (<4%); found in breast milk. TDF: Plasma protein binding (<0.7%); found in breast milk. **Metabolism:** Efavirenz: Via CYP3A and CYP2B6. Emtricitabine: 3'-sulfoxide diastereomers and glucuronic acid conjugate (metabolites). **Elimination:** Efavirenz: Urine (14-34% mostly metabolites), feces (16-61% mostly unchanged); $T_{1/2}$=52-76 hrs (single dose), 40-55 hrs (multiple doses). Emtricitabine: Urine (86%, 13% metabolites); $T_{1/2}$=10 hrs (single dose). TDF: (IV) Urine (70-80% unchanged); $T_{1/2}$=17 hrs (single dose).

PATIENT CONSIDERATIONS

Assessment: Assess for obesity, prolonged nucleoside exposure, liver dysfunction or risk factors for liver disease, renal dysfunction, HBV infection, psychiatric history, history of injection drug use/seizures/cutaneous reaction, drug hypersensitivity, pregnancy/nursing status, and possible drug interactions. Assess BMD in patients w/ a history of pathological bone fracture or w/ other risk factors for osteoporosis or bone loss. Assess estimated CrCl, serum P, urine glucose and urine protein in patients at risk for renal dysfunction.

Monitoring: Monitor for signs/symptoms of lactic acidosis, severe hepatomegaly w/ steatosis, psychiatric/nervous system symptoms, new onset/worsening renal impairment, decreased BMD, increased biochemical markers for bone metabolism, osteomalacia, convulsions, immune reconstitution syndrome (eg, opportunistic infections), fat redistribution/accumulation, skin rash, and other adverse reactions. Monitor for acute exacerbations of hepatitis B in patients w/ coinfection upon discontinuation of therapy. Monitor LFTs. Monitor estimated CrCl, serum P, urine glucose, and urine protein periodically in patients at risk for renal dysfunction.

Counseling: Inform that therapy is not a cure for HIV-1 infection and illnesses associated w/ HIV-1 infection may still be experienced. Advise to practice safe sex, use latex or polyurethane condoms, not to share personal items (eg, toothbrush, razor blades), needles, or other inj equipment, and not to breastfeed. Inform that lactic acidosis, severe hepatomegaly w/ steatosis, and renal impairment have occurred. Instruct to avoid potentially hazardous tasks such as driving or operating machinery if CNS symptoms occur. Instruct to contact physician if severe psychiatric adverse experiences or a rash occur. Advise that fat redistribution/accumulation and decreases in BMD may occur. Advise to avoid pregnancy while on therapy and to use adequate contraceptive measures for 12 weeks after discontinuation; instruct that barrier contraception must always be used in combination w/ other methods of contraception. Advise to avoid potentially hazardous tasks if experiencing CNS/psychiatric symptoms or taking alcohol or psychoactive drugs. Advise that severe acute exacerbation of hepatitis B may occur if coinfected. Advise to report use of any prescription, nonprescription medication, vitamins, and herbal supplements.

AUBAGIO — teriflunomide   Rx

Class: Pyrimidine synthesis inhibitor

> Severe liver injury, including fatal liver failure, reported in patients treated w/ leflunomide; similar risk would be expected because recommended doses of teriflunomide and leflunomide result in a similar range of plasma concentrations of teriflunomide. Concomitant use w/ other potentially hepatotoxic drugs may increase risk of severe liver injury. Obtain transaminase and bilirubin levels w/in 6 months before initiation of therapy. Monitor ALT levels at least monthly for 6 months after starting therapy. D/C therapy and start an accelerated elimination procedure w/ cholestyramine or charcoal if drug-induced liver injury is suspected. Contraindicated in patients w/ severe hepatic impairment. Increased risk of developing elevated serum transaminases in patients w/ preexisting liver disease. May cause major birth defects if used during pregnancy. Pregnancy must be excluded before initiation; contraindicated in pregnant women or women of childbearing potential who are not using reliable contraception. Avoid pregnancy during treatment or before completion of an accelerated elimination procedure after treatment.

ADULT DOSAGE
Multiple Sclerosis
Relapsing Forms:
Usual: 7mg or 14mg qd

PEDIATRIC DOSAGE
Pediatric use may not have been established

ADMINISTRATION
Oral route
May take w/ or w/o food.

STORAGE
20-25°C (68-77°F); excursions permitted between 15-30°C (59-86°F).

HOW SUPPLIED
Tab: 7mg, 14mg

CONTRAINDICATIONS
Severe hepatic impairment, women who are pregnant or of childbearing potential not using reliable contraception, concomitant use of leflunomide, history of hypersensitivity reaction to teriflunomide, leflunomide, or to any of its inactive ingredients.

WARNINGS/PRECAUTIONS
Not for use w/ preexisting acute or chronic liver disease, or those w/ serum ALT >2X ULN before initiating therapy. Consider discontinuing therapy if serum transaminase >3X ULN. Consider resumption of therapy if liver injury is not drug induced. Consider additional monitoring if given w/ other potentially hepatotoxic drugs. Eliminated slowly from the plasma. An accelerated elimination procedure can be used at any time after discontinuation of therapy; refer to PI. Decrease in WBC count and platelet count reported; obtain CBC w/in 6 months before initiation of treatment, and base further monitoring on signs and symptoms of bone marrow suppression. Avoid starting treatment until active acute or chronic infections are resolved. Consider suspending treatment and using an accelerated elimination procedure if serious infection develops. Not recommended w/ severe immunodeficiency, bone marrow disease, or severe, uncontrolled infections. May cause immunosuppression and increased susceptibility to infections. Screen patients for latent tuberculosis (TB) infection; if positive treat by standard medical practice prior to initiating therapy w/ teriflunomide. May increase risk of malignancy. May cause anaphylaxis and severe allergic reactions (eg, Stevens-Johnson syndrome, toxic epidermal necrolysis, drug reaction w/ eosinophilia and systemic symptoms); d/c treatment and begin accelerated elimination process immediately if reactions are clearly drug related. Do not re-expose after such reactions. Peripheral neuropathy reported; increased risk w/ >60 yrs of age, concomitant neurotoxic medications, and diabetes. Consider discontinuing and performing an accelerated elimination procedure if peripheral neuropathy symptoms develop. HTN was reported. Interstitial lung disease (ILD) (eg, acute interstitial pneumonitis) and worsening of preexisting ILD reported. New onset or worsening of pulmonary symptoms, w/ or w/o associated fever, may be a reason for discontinuation; consider initiation of an accelerated elimination procedure. Monitor for hematologic toxicity if switching to another agent w/ a known potential for hematologic suppression.

ADVERSE REACTIONS
Headache, diarrhea, nausea, alopecia, increase in ALT.

DRUG INTERACTIONS
See Boxed Warning and Contraindications. May increase exposure of drugs metabolized by CYP2C8 (eg, paclitaxel, pioglitazone, rosiglitazone. May decrease exposure of drugs metabolized by CYP1A2 (eg, alosetron, duloxetine, theophylline). May increase exposure of OAT3 substrates (eg, cefaclor, cimetidine, ciprofloxacin). Monitor and adjust the dose of OAT3 substrates and drugs metabolized by CYP2C8/CYP1A2 as required. Vaccination w/ live vaccines is not recommended. Coadministration w/ warfarin requires close monitoring of the INR; may decrease peak INR. May increase the systemic exposures of ethinyl estradiol and levonorgestrel; consider the type or dose of contraceptives to be used. Inhibits activity of breast cancer resistance protein (BCRP) and OATP1B1/1B3; do not exceed rosuvastatin dose of 10mg qd if used concomitantly. Consider reducing the dose of other BCRP substrates (eg, mitoxantrone) and drugs in the OATP family (eg, methotrexate, rifampin), especially HMG-CoA reductase inhibitors (eg, atorvastatin, nateglinide, pravastatin); monitor closely for signs and symptoms of increased exposures.

PREGNANCY AND LACTATION
Pregnancy: Category X. Detected in human semen; men should use reliable contraception. Men wishing to father a child should d/c treatment and undergo an accelerated elimination procedure.
Lactation: Not for use in nursing.

MECHANISM OF ACTION
Pyrimidine synthesis inhibitor; immunomodulatory agent w/ anti-inflammatory properties that inhibits dihydroorotate dehydrogenase. Exact mechanism is unknown but may involve a reduction in the number of activated lymphocytes in CNS.

PHARMACOKINETICS
Absorption: T_{max}=1-4 hrs (median). **Distribution:** V_d=11L (IV); plasma protein binding (>99%). **Metabolism:** Hydrolysis (primary), oxidation (minor), N-acetylation, sulfate conjugation. **Elimination:** Urine (22.6%), feces (37.5%).

PATIENT CONSIDERATIONS
Assessment: Assess for previous hypersensitivity, severe immunodeficiency, bone marrow disease, severe uncontrolled infections, ILD, hepatic impairment, diabetes, any other conditions where treatment is cautioned or contraindicated, pregnancy/nursing status, and for possible drug interactions. Obtain transaminase levels, bilirubin levels, and CBC w/in 6 months before initiation of therapy. Obtain BP. Screen for latent TB infection w/ a tuberculin skin test or blood test for mycobacterium TB infection.

Monitoring: Monitor for signs/symptoms of hypersensitivity and skin reactions, immunosuppression and infections, bone marrow suppression, severe liver injury, peripheral neuropathy, skin reactions, ILD, new onset or worsening of pulmonary symptoms, malignancy, and other adverse reactions. Monitor ALT levels at least monthly for 6 months after starting therapy. Monitor BP periodically thereafter.

Counseling: Instruct to contact physician if unexplained N/V, abdominal pain, fatigue, anorexia, jaundice, dark urine, or symptoms of infection develop. Advise women of childbearing potential and men and their female partners to use effective contraception during treatment and until completion of an accelerated elimination procedure. Instruct to immediately report pregnancy if suspected or confirmed. Advise that therapy may stay in the blood for up to 2 yrs after the last dose and that an accelerated elimination procedure may be used if needed. Instruct to avoid some vaccines during treatment and for at least 6 months after discontinuation. Advise to contact physician if symptoms of peripheral neuropathy develop. Inform that treatment may increase BP. Advise to either d/c breastfeeding or d/c therapy. Advise to d/c and seek immediate medical attention if signs/symptoms of a hypersensitivity reaction occur.

AVASTIN — bevacizumab   Rx

Class: Vascular endothelial growth factor (VEGF) inhibitor

> GI perforation reported; d/c w/ GI perforation. Increased incidence of wound-healing and surgical complications; d/c at least 28 days prior to elective surgery. Do not initiate for at least 28 days after surgery and until surgical wound is fully healed. D/C in patients w/ wound dehiscence. Severe or fatal hemorrhage, including hemoptysis, GI bleeding, CNS hemorrhage, epistaxis, and vaginal bleeding, may occur; do not administer to patients w/ serious hemorrhage or recent hemoptysis.

ADULT DOSAGE

Metastatic Colorectal Cancer

1st- or 2nd-line treatment in combination w/ IV 5-fluorouracil-based chemotherapy; 2nd-line treatment in combination w/ fluoropyrimidine-irinotecan- or fluoropyrimidine-oxaliplatin-based chemotherapy, in patients who have progressed on a 1st-line bevacizumab-containing regimen

In Combination w/ Bolus-IFL:
5mg/kg every 2 weeks

In Combination w/ FOLFOX4:
10mg/kg every 2 weeks

In Combination w/ Fluoropyrimidine-Irinotecan- or Fluoropyrimidine-Oxaliplatin-Based Chemotherapy:
5mg/kg every 2 weeks or 7.5mg/kg every 3 weeks

Nonsquamous Non-Small Cell Lung Cancer

1st-line treatment of unresectable, locally advanced, recurrent, or metastatic nonsquamous non-small cell lung cancer in combination w/ carboplatin and paclitaxel

15mg/kg every 3 weeks

Glioblastoma

W/ progressive disease following prior therapy as a single agent

10mg/kg every 2 weeks

Metastatic Renal Cell Carcinoma

10mg/kg every 2 weeks w/ Interferon Alfa

Cervical Cancer

Treatment of persistent, recurrent, or metastatic carcinoma of the cervix in combination w/ paclitaxel and cisplatin or paclitaxel and topotecan

15mg/kg every 3 weeks

Ovarian, Fallopian Tube, or Peritoneal Cancer

Treatment of patients w/ platinum-resistant recurrent epithelial ovarian, fallopian tube, or primary peritoneal cancer who received no more than 2 prior chemotherapy regimens in combination w/ paclitaxel, pegylated liposomal doxorubicin, or topotecan

10mg/kg every 2 weeks w/ 1 of the following IV chemotherapy regimens: paclitaxel, pegylated liposomal doxorubicin, or topotecan (weekly); or 15mg/kg every 3 weeks in combination w/ topotecan (every 3 weeks)

PEDIATRIC DOSAGE

Pediatric use may not have been established

DOSING CONSIDERATIONS

Discontinuation

D/C For:
1. GI perforations, fistula formation in the GI tract or involving an internal organ, intra-abdominal abscess
2. Wound dehiscence and wound healing complications requiring medical intervention
3. Serious hemorrhage (requiring medical intervention)
4. Severe arterial thromboembolic events
5. Life-threatening (Grade 4) venous thromboembolic events, including pulmonary embolism
6. Hypertensive crisis or hypertensive encephalopathy
7. Posterior reversible encephalopathy syndrome
8. Nephrotic syndrome

Temporarily Suspend For:
1. At least 4 weeks prior to elective surgery
2. Severe HTN not controlled w/ medical management
3. Moderate to severe proteinuria
4. Severe infusion reactions

ADMINISTRATION

IV route

Do not administer as an IV push/bolus; administer only as an IV infusion.
Do not initiate until ≥28 days following major surgery and after surgical incision has fully healed.
Give 1st infusion over 90 min.
Give 2nd infusion over 60 min if 1st infusion is tolerated.
Give all subsequent infusions over 30 min if infusion over 60 min is tolerated.

Preparation

Withdraw necessary amount and dilute in a total volume of 100mL of 0.9% NaCl inj.
Discard any unused portion left in a vial, as the product contains no preservatives.
Do not administer or mix w/ dextrose sol.

STORAGE

2-8°C (36-46°F). Protect from light. Do not freeze or shake. **Diluted Sol:** May be stored at 2-8°C (36-46°F) for up to 8 hrs. Store in original carton until time of use.

HOW SUPPLIED

Inj: 100mg/4mL, 400mg/16mL

WARNINGS/PRECAUTIONS

Not indicated for adjuvant treatment of colon cancer. Avoid use in patients w/ ovarian cancer w/ evidence of recto-sigmoid involvement by pelvic examination or bowel involvement on CT scan or clinical symptoms of bowel obstruction. GI fistula reported. Serious and sometimes fatal non-GI fistula formation involving tracheoesophageal (TE), bronchopleural, biliary, vaginal, renal, and bladder sites may occur; d/c permanently in patients w/ TE fistula or any Grade 4 fistula. Necrotizing fasciitis, usually secondary to wound-healing complications, GI perforation, or fistula formation, reported; d/c therapy if necrotizing fasciitis develops. Arterial thromboembolic events (ATEs) (eg, cerebral infarction, transient ischemic attacks, MI, angina) reported; increased risk w/ history of arterial thromboembolism, diabetes, or age >65 yrs. May increase risk of venous thromboembolic events (VTEs) in patients treated for persistent, recurrent, or metastatic cervical cancer. Increased incidence of severe HTN. Posterior reversible encephalopathy syndrome (PRES) reported. Increased incidence and severity of proteinuria; suspend therapy for ≥2g proteinuria/24 hrs and resume when proteinuria is <2g/24 hrs. Nephrotic syndrome may occur. Infusion reactions reported. May cause fetal harm. Increases the risk of ovarian failure.

ADVERSE REACTIONS

Epistaxis, headache, HTN, rhinitis, proteinuria, taste alteration, dry skin, rectal hemorrhage, lacrimation disorder, back pain, exfoliative dermatitis.

DRUG INTERACTIONS

May decrease paclitaxel exposure w/ paclitaxel/carboplatin.

PREGNANCY AND LACTATION

Pregnancy: May cause fetal harm; animal models link angiogenesis, VEGF and VEGF Receptor 2 to critical aspects of female reproduction, embryofetal development, and postnatal development. Advise pregnant women of the potential risk to a fetus.
Lactation: No data are available regarding the presence of bevacizumab in human milk; not for use in nursing.
Reproductive Potential: Females of reproductive potential should use effective contraception during treatment and for 6 months following the last dose of therapy. Increases the risk of ovarian failure and may impair fertility.

MECHANISM OF ACTION

VEGF inhibitor; binds VEGF and prevents the interaction of VEGF to its receptors (Flt-1, KDR) on the surface of endothelial cells. The interaction of VEGF w/ its receptors leads to endothelial cell proliferation and new blood vessel formation.

PHARMACOKINETICS

Elimination: $T_{1/2}$=20 days.

PATIENT CONSIDERATIONS

Assessment: Assess for recent hemoptysis, serious hemorrhage, HTN, proteinuria, history of ATEs, diabetes, pregnancy/nursing status, and possible drug interactions. Assess for prior surgical history and for any scheduled elective surgeries. Assess for evidence of recto-sigmoid involvement in patients w/ ovarian cancer.

Monitoring: Monitor for GI perforation, fistula formation, wound-healing complications, hemorrhage, ATEs, VTEs, hypertensive crisis, hypertensive encephalopathy, PRES, nephrotic syndrome, severe infusion reactions, and other adverse reactions. Monitor BP every 2-3 weeks, treat w/ appropriate anti-hypertensive therapy, and monitor BP regularly; continue to monitor BP at regular intervals w/ drug-induced or -exacerbated HTN after drug discontinuation. Monitor for proteinuria by dipstick urine analysis for the development or worsening of proteinuria w/ serial urinalyses.

Counseling: Advise to undergo routine BP monitoring and to contact physician if BP is elevated. Instruct to immediately seek medical attention for unusual bleeding, high fever, rigors, sudden onset of worsening neurological function, persistent/severe abdominal pain, severe constipation, or vomiting. Inform of the increased risk of wound-healing complications, ovarian failure, and ATE. Advise females of reproductive potential to use effective contraception during treatment and for 6 months after therapy, and to inform physician of a known/suspected pregnancy. Advise nursing women that breastfeeding is not recommended during treatment.

AVEED — testosterone undecanoate   CIII

Class: Androgen

> Serious pulmonary oil microembolism (POME) reactions, involving urge to cough, dyspnea, throat tightening, chest pain, dizziness, and syncope; and episodes of anaphylaxis, including life-threatening reactions, reported to occur during or immediately after administration. Following each inj, observe patients in healthcare setting for 30 min. Available only through a restricted program under a Risk Evaluation and Mitigation Strategy (REMS) called the Aveed REMS Program.

ADULT DOSAGE

Testosterone Replacement Therapy

Congenital/Acquired Primary Hypogonadism or Hypogonadotropic Hypogonadism in Males:
Usual: 3mL (750mg) IM, followed by 3mL (750mg) after 4 weeks, then 3mL (750mg) every 10 weeks thereafter

PEDIATRIC DOSAGE
Pediatric use may not have been established

ADMINISTRATION
IM route

Inject deeply into the gluteal muscle (gluteus medius); avoid intravascular inj. Between consecutive inj, alternate the inj site between left and right buttock. Following each inj, observe patients for 30 min in order to provide appropriate medical treatment in the event of serious POME reactions or anaphylaxis.

Preparation and Administration Instructions
1. Remove only the gray plastic cap while leaving the aluminum metal ring and clamp seal in place
2. Withdraw 3mL (750mg) of sol from the vial
3. Replace the syringe needle used to draw up the sol from the vial w/ a new IM needle to inj
4. Discard any unused portion of the vial
5. Enter the muscle and maintain the syringe at a 90° angle w/ the needle in its deeply imbedded position
6. Aspirate for several sec to ensure that no blood appears
7. If no blood is aspirated, reinforce the current needle position to avoid any movement of the needle and slowly (over 60-90 sec) depress the plunger carefully and at a constant rate, until all the medication has been delivered

STORAGE
25°C (77°F); excursions permitted to 15-30°C (59-86°F).

HOW SUPPLIED
Inj: 750mg/3mL

CONTRAINDICATIONS
Men w/ breast carcinoma or known/suspected prostate carcinoma; women who are or may become pregnant, or who are breastfeeding; men w/ known hypersensitivity to this product or any of its ingredients (eg, testosterone undecanoate, refined castor oil, benzyl benzoate).

WARNINGS/PRECAUTIONS
Patients w/ BPH and geriatric patients are at an increased risk of worsening of signs and symptoms of BPH. May increase risk for prostate cancer. Increases in Hct/RBC mass, may require discontinuation; may increase the risk of thromboembolic events. If Hct becomes elevated, d/c therapy until Hct decreases to an acceptable level. Venous thromboembolic events (VTEs), including deep vein thrombosis and pulmonary embolism, reported; d/c treatment and initiate appropriate workup and management if a VTE is suspected. Increased risk of major adverse cardiovascular events (MACE) reported. Not indicated for use in women. Suppression of spermatogenesis may occur w/ large doses. Monitor for signs/symptoms of hepatic dysfunction; if these occur, promptly d/c therapy while the cause is evaluated. May promote retention of Na^+ and water. Edema w/ or w/o CHF in patients w/ preexisting cardiac/renal/hepatic disease may occur; in addition to discontinuation of therapy, diuretic therapy may be required. Gynecomastia may develop and persist. May potentiate sleep apnea. Changes in serum lipid profile may require dose adjustment of lipid lowering drugs or discontinuation of testosterone therapy. Caution in cancer patients at risk of hypercalcemia (and associated hypercalciuria); regularly monitor serum Ca^{2+} concentrations. May decrease concentrations of thyroxine-binding globulin (TBG), resulting in decreased total T4 serum concentrations and increased resin uptake of T3 and T4.

ADVERSE REACTIONS
POME, anaphylaxis, acne, inj-site pain, prostate specific antigen increased.

DRUG INTERACTIONS
Changes in insulin sensitivity or glycemic control may occur; may decrease blood glucose, which may necessitate a decrease in the dose of antidiabetic medication in diabetic patients. Changes in anticoagulant activity may occur; frequently monitor INR and PT in patients taking warfarin, especially at the initiation and termination of androgen therapy. Concurrent use w/ corticosteroids may result in increased fluid retention; caution in patients w/ cardiac/renal/hepatic disease.

PREGNANCY AND LACTATION
Category X, not for use in nursing.

MECHANISM OF ACTION
Androgen; responsible for the normal growth and development of male sex organs and for maintenance of secondary sex characteristics.

PHARMACOKINETICS
Absorption: T_{max}=7 days (median); C_{max}=90.9ng/dL. **Distribution:** Plasma protein binding (40%, sex hormone-binding globulin). **Metabolism:** Via ester cleavage of the undecanoate group; estradiol and dihydrotestosterone (major active metabolites). **Elimination:** Urine (90%, glucuronic and sulfuric acid-conjugates or metabolites), feces (6%, unconjugated); $T_{1/2}$=10-100 min.

PATIENT CONSIDERATIONS
Assessment: Assess for breast/prostate cancer, BPH, cardiac/renal/hepatic disease, obesity, chronic lung diseases, any other conditions where treatment is contraindicated or cautioned, and possible drug interactions. Check Hct prior to therapy. Confirm diagnosis of hypogonadism by measuring testosterone levels in am on at least 2 separate days prior to initiation.

Monitoring: Monitor for worsening signs/symptoms of BPH, prostate cancer, VTE, MACE, hepatic dysfunction, Na^+/water retention, gynecomastia, sleep apnea, and other adverse reactions. Monitor serum lipid profile and TBG. Regularly monitor serum Ca^{2+} concentrations in cancer patients at risk of hypercalcemia. Reevaluate Hct 3-6 months after starting therapy, then annually. Frequently monitor INR and PT in patients taking warfarin, especially at the initiation and termination of androgen therapy.

Counseling: Advise of the risks of serious POME and anaphylaxis; instruct to remain at the healthcare setting for 30 min after each inj. Inform that treatment may lead to adverse reactions (eg, changes in urinary habits, breathing disturbances, too frequent or persistent erections of the penis, N/V, changes in skin color, ankle swelling). Instruct to adhere to all recommended monitoring and report any changes in state of health (eg, changes in urinary habits, breathing, sleep, mood). Inform of the possible risk of MACE when deciding whether to use or continue to use drug.

AVONEX — interferon beta-1a   Rx

Class: Biological response modifier

ADULT DOSAGE

Multiple Sclerosis

Treatment of relapsing forms to slow the accumulation of physical disability and decrease the frequency of clinical exacerbations

30mcg once a week

Reduce the Incidence and Severity of Flu-Like Symptoms:
Initial: 7.5mcg
Titrate: Increase by 7.5mcg each week for the next 3 weeks until the recommended dose is achieved (30mcg/week)

Premedication for Flu-Like Symptoms:
Analgesics/antipyretics on treatment days may help ameliorate flu-like symptoms

PEDIATRIC DOSAGE
Pediatric use may not have been established

ADMINISTRATION
IM route

Rotate inj site to minimize inj-site reactions.
Do not inject into skin that is irritated, reddened, bruised, infected, or scarred in any way.
If deemed appropriate, may substitute a 25-gauge/1-inch needle for the 23-gauge/1.25-inch needle for prefilled syringe or inj of reconstituted sol.
Use only the supplied needle w/ the autoinjector.
Reconstitute lyophilized powder w/ supplied diluent (10mL of sterile water for inj).
Refer to PI for further administration instructions.

STORAGE
Do not freeze or expose to high temperatures. Protect from light. Discard product and do not use if exposed to conditions other than recommended. **Lyophilized Powder:** 2-8°C (36-46°F) or 25°C (77°F) for up to 30 days if refrigeration is unavailable. **Reconstituted Sol:** 2-8°C (36-46°F); use w/in 6 hrs. **Prefilled Syringe/Autoinjector:** 2-8°C (36-46°F) or ≤25°C (77°F) for up to 7 days if refrigeration is unavailable. After removing from refrigeration, allow to warm to room temperature (about 30 min). Once removed from refrigerator, do not store >25°C (77°F).

HOW SUPPLIED
Inj: 30mcg [vial], 30mcg/0.5mL [prefilled syringe, prefilled autoinjector]

CONTRAINDICATIONS
History of hypersensitivity to natural or recombinant interferon beta, or any other component of the formulation. **Vial:** History of hypersensitivity to albumin (human).

WARNINGS/PRECAUTIONS
Depression, suicidal ideation, and/or development of new or worsening of other preexisting psychiatric disorders, including psychosis, reported; consider discontinuation if depression or other severe psychiatric symptoms develop. Severe hepatic injury, including cases of hepatic failure (rare) and asymptomatic elevation of hepatic transaminases, reported. Anaphylaxis (rare) and other allergic reactions (eg, dyspnea, orolingual edema, skin rash, urticaria) reported; d/c if these occur. Cases of CHF, cardiomyopathy, and cardiomyopathy w/ CHF reported. Decreased peripheral blood counts, including rare pancytopenia and thrombocytopenia, and seizures, reported. Thrombotic microangiopathy (TMA), including thrombotic thrombocytopenic purpura and hemolytic uremic syndrome, reported; d/c if clinical symptoms and lab findings consistent w/ TMA occur, and manage as clinically indicated. Autoimmune disorders of multiple target organs, including idiopathic thrombocytopenia, hyper/hypothyroidism, and rare cases of autoimmune hepatitis reported; consider discontinuing therapy if a new autoimmune disorder develops.

ADVERSE REACTIONS
Headache, flu-like symptoms, myalgia, asthenia, nausea, pain, fever, chills, depression, UTI, dizziness, URTI, sinusitis, arthralgia, abdominal pain.

DRUG INTERACTIONS

Consider the potential risk of interferon beta-1a when used in combination w/ known hepatotoxic drugs or other products (eg, alcohol) prior to starting interferon beta-1a or before starting hepatotoxic drugs.

PREGNANCY AND LACTATION

Pregnancy: Category C.

Lactation: It is not known whether interferon beta-1a is excreted in human milk.

MECHANISM OF ACTION

Biological response modifier; not established. Exerts biological effects by binding to specific receptors on the surface of human cells, initiating a complex cascade of intracellular events that leads to the expression of numerous interferon-induced gene products and markers.

PHARMACOKINETICS

Absorption: T_{max}=15 hrs. **Elimination:** $T_{1/2}$=19 hrs.

PATIENT CONSIDERATIONS

Assessment: Assess for history of hypersensitivity to the drug or to human albumin, psychiatric disorders, CHF, myelosuppression, thyroid dysfunction, pregnancy/nursing status, and possible drug interactions. Obtain baseline CBC, differential WBCs, platelet counts, and blood chemistries including LFTs.

Monitoring: Monitor for depression, suicidal ideation, new or worsening of preexisting psychiatric disorders, autoimmune disorders, allergic reactions, anaphylaxis, signs of hepatic injury, TMA, seizures, and other adverse reactions. Monitor for worsening of cardiac condition during initiation of and continued treatment in patients w/ preexisting CHF. Monitor CBC, differential WBCs, platelet counts, and blood chemistries including LFTs. Monitor thyroid function periodically.

Counseling: Caution not to change dosage or schedule of administration w/o medical consultation. Inform that prefilled syringe tip cap of this product contains natural rubber latex, which may cause allergic reactions. Instruct on self-inj technique and procedures. Advise to notify physician if pregnant/planning to become pregnant. Instruct to notify physician if any adverse reactions (eg, hepatic dysfunction, allergic reactions, anaphylaxis, worsening cardiac condition, seizures) occur. Inform that symptoms of depression, suicidal ideation, or psychotic disorders may occur; instruct to report these immediately to physician if they occur. Inform that flu-like symptoms are common following initiation of therapy.

BARACLUDE — entecavir   Rx

Class: Nucleoside reverse transcriptase inhibitor (NRTI)

> Severe acute exacerbations of hepatitis B reported upon discontinuation of therapy; monitor liver function for at least several months after discontinuation. If appropriate, may initiate antihepatitis B therapy. Potential for development of resistance to HIV nucleoside reverse transcriptase inhibitors if entecavir is used to treat chronic hepatitis B virus (HBV) infection in patients with untreated HIV infection. Not recommended for HIV/HBV coinfected patients not receiving highly active antiretroviral therapy (HAART). Lactic acidosis and severe hepatomegaly with steatosis, including fatal cases, have been reported with the use of nucleoside analogue inhibitors.

ADULT DOSAGE

Chronic Hepatitis B

In patients w/ evidence of active viral replication and either evidence of persistent elevations in serum aminotransferases (ALT/AST) or histologically active disease

Compensated Liver Disease: Nucleoside-Inhibitor Treatment-Naive:
0.5mg qd

History of Hepatitis B Viremia While Receiving Lamivudine or Known Lamivudine- or Telbivudine-Resistant Substitutions:
1mg qd

Decompensated Liver Disease:
1mg qd

PEDIATRIC DOSAGE

Chronic Hepatitis B

In patients w/ evidence of active viral replication and either evidence of persistent elevations in serum aminotransferases (ALT/AST) or histologically active disease

≥2 Years:
Treatment-Naive:
10-11kg: 3mL qd
<11-14kg: 4mL qd
<14-17kg: 5mL qd
<17-20kg: 6mL qd
<20-23kg: 7mL qd
<23-26kg: 8mL qd
<26-30kg: 9mL qd
<30kg: 10mL or 0.5mg tab qd

Lamivudine-Experienced:
10-11kg: 6mL qd
<11-14kg: 8mL qd
<14-17kg: 10mL qd
<17-20kg: 12mL qd
<20-23kg: 14mL qd
<23-26kg: 16mL qd
<26-30kg: 18mL qd
<30kg: 20mL or 1mg tab qd

Compensated Liver Disease: Nucleoside-Inhibitor Treatment-Naive:
≥16 Years:
0.5mg qd

History of Hepatitis B Viremia While Receiving Lamivudine or Known Lamivudine- or Telbivudine-Resistant Substitutions:
≥16 Years:
1mg qd

DOSING CONSIDERATIONS
Renal Impairment
CrCl 30-<50mL/min:
Usual: 0.25mg qd or 0.5mg q48h
Lamivudine-Refractory or Decompensated Liver Disease: 0.5mg qd or 1mg q48h
CrCl 10-<30mL/min:
Usual: 0.15mg qd or 0.5mg q72h
Lamivudine-Refractory or Decompensated Liver Disease: 0.3mg qd or 1mg q72h
CrCl <10mL/min or CAPD:
Usual: 0.05mg qd or 0.5mg every 7 days
Lamivudine-Refractory or Decompensated Liver Disease: 0.1mg qd or 1mg every 7 days
Hemodialysis:
Usual: 0.05mg qd or 0.5mg every 7 days (after session if administered on hemodialysis day)
Lamivudine-Refractory or Decompensated Liver Disease: 0.1mg qd or 1mg every 7 days (after session if administered on hemodialysis day)

ADMINISTRATION
Oral route

Take on an empty stomach (at least 2 hrs pc and 2 hrs before the next meal)

STORAGE
25°C (77°F); excursions permitted between 15-30°C (59-86°F). Protect from light.

HOW SUPPLIED
Sol: 0.05mg/mL [210mL]; **Tab:** 0.5mg, 1mg

WARNINGS/PRECAUTIONS
Dosage adjustment is recommended in renal dysfunction (CrCl <50mL/min), including patients on hemodialysis or continuous ambulatory peritoneal dialysis. May require HIV antibody testing prior to treatment. Caution with known risk factors for liver disease. D/C if lactic acidosis or pronounced hepatotoxicity occurs. Caution in elderly.

ADVERSE REACTIONS
Hepatitis B exacerbation, lactic acidosis, hepatomegaly, headache, fatigue, dizziness, nausea, ALT/lipase/total bilirubin elevation, hyperglycemia, glycosuria, hematuria.

DRUG INTERACTIONS
May increase levels of either entecavir or concomitant drugs that reduce renal function or compete for active tubular secretion; closely monitor for adverse events.

PREGNANCY AND LACTATION
Category C, not for use in nursing.

MECHANISM OF ACTION
Guanosine nucleoside analogue; inhibits base priming, reverse transcription of negative strand from pregenomic mRNA, and synthesis of positive strand of HBV DNA.

PHARMACOKINETICS
Absorption: C_{max}=4.2ng/mL (0.5mg), 8.2ng/mL (1mg); T_{max}=0.5-1.5 hrs. **Distribution:** Serum protein binding (13%). **Metabolism:** Glucuronidation and sulfate conjugation. **Elimination:** Urine (62-73% unchanged); $T_{1/2}$=128-149 hrs.

PATIENT CONSIDERATIONS
Assessment: Assess for hepatic/renal impairment, pregnancy/nursing status, and possible drug interactions. Perform HIV antibody testing before initiating therapy.

Monitoring: Monitor for signs/symptoms of lactic acidosis, hepatotoxicity, renal/hepatic impairment, and other adverse reactions.

Counseling: Advise to remain under care of physician during therapy and report any new symptoms or concurrent medications. Advise that treatment has not been shown to reduce risk of transmission of HBV to others through sexual contact or blood contamination. Advise to take the missed dose as soon as remembered unless it is almost time for the next dose and not to take 2 doses at the same time. Inform that treatment may lower the amount of HBV in the body and improve the condition of the liver, but will not cure HBV. Counsel that it is not known whether treatment will reduce risk of liver cancer or cirrhosis. Inform that deterioration of liver disease may occur in some cases if treatment is discontinued, and instruct to discuss any change in regimen with physician. Inform that drug may increase the chance of HIV resistance to HIV medication if HIV-infected patient is not receiving effective HIV treatment.

BCG VACCINE — BCG live   Rx

Class: Attenuated live BCG culture

ADULT DOSAGE
Prevention of Tuberculosis

Not Previously Infected w/ Mycobacterium tuberculosis and at High Risk for Exposure:
0.2-0.3mL

Conduct tuberculin test 2-3 months after administration of therapy; repeat vaccination for those who remain tuberculin (-) to 5 tuberculin units of tuberculin after 2-3 months

PEDIATRIC DOSAGE
Prevention of Tuberculosis

Not Previously Infected w/ Mycobacterium tuberculosis and at High Risk for Exposure:
<1 Month of Age:
Reduce dose by 1/2 (by using 2mL of sterile water for inj when reconstituting); if a vaccinated infant remains tuberculin (-) to 5 tuberculin units on skin testing, and if indications for vaccination persist, infant should receive a full dose after 1 yr of age

≥1 Month of Age:
0.2-0.3mL
Conduct tuberculin test 2-3 months after administration of therapy; repeat vaccination for those who remain tuberculin (-) to 5 tuberculin units of tuberculin after 2-3 months

ADMINISTRATION
Percutaneous route
Administer in the deltoid region using a sterile multiple puncture device
Perform a Mantoux skin-test prior to vaccination to demonstrate absence of tuberculous infection

Preparation
Add 1mL of sterile water for inj at 4-25°C (39-77°F) to 1 vial of vaccine
Gently swirl vial until homogenous sus is obtained; avoid forceful agitation
Keep reconstituted vaccine refrigerated and use w/in 2 hrs; do not freeze
Do not filter contents of vaccine vial
Avoid exposing to direct sunlight
Avoid bacteriostatic sol

<1 Month of Age:
Use 2mL of sterile water for inj at 4-25°C (39-77°F) when reconstituting

Administration
Drop immunizing dose from syringe and needle onto the cleansed surface of the skin; spread over a 1-inch by 2-inch area using the edge of the multiple puncture device
Firmly grasp arm from underneath, tensing the skin, and center the multiple puncture device over the vaccine; apply firm downward pressure such that the device points are well buried in the skin
Maintain pressure for 5 sec, then release pressure underneath arm and remove the device; do not "rock" device
Repeat procedure if points do not puncture the skin
After successful puncture, spread vaccine as evenly as possible over the puncture area w/ the edge of the device; may add an additional 1-2 drops of vaccine to ensure a very wet vaccination site
Loosely cover site and keep dry for 24 hrs

STORAGE
2-8°C (36-46°F). Protect from direct sunlight.

HOW SUPPLIED
Inj: 1-8 x 10^8 colony-forming units

CONTRAINDICATIONS
Active TB; persons whose immunologic responses are impaired because of HIV infections, congenital immunodeficiency (eg, chronic granulomatous disease, interferon gamma receptor deficiency), leukemia, lymphoma, generalized malignancy, or whose immunologic responses have been suppressed by steroids, alkylating agents, antimetabolites, or radiation; allergy to any component of this vaccine or an anaphylactic or allergic reaction to a previous dose of this vaccine; severe immune deficiency syndromes; children w/ family history of immune deficiency disease.

WARNINGS/PRECAUTIONS
May not protect 100% of susceptible individuals. Moderate axillary/cervical lymphadenopathy and induration and subsequent pustule formation at inj site may occur and persist for as long as 3 months after vaccination. More severe local reactions (eg, ulceration at the vaccination site, regional suppurative lymphadenitis with draining sinuses, caseous lesions or purulent drainage at the puncture site) may occur within 5 months after vaccination and could persist for several weeks. Acute, localized irritative toxicities may be accompanied by systemic manifestations, consistent with a flu-like syndrome. Consider evaluation for serious infectious complication if symptoms such as fever ≥39.4°C (103°F), or acute localized inflammation persisting for >2-3 days occur. Start treatment without delay if the Bacillus of Calmette-Guerin (BCG) infection is suspected; ≥2 antimycobacterial agents should be administered while diagnostic evaluation, including cultures, is conducted in patients who develop persistent fever or experience an acute febrile illness consistent with BCG infection. Negative cultures do not necessarily rule out infection. Most serious complication of vaccination is disseminated BCG infection; BCG osteitis may occur 4 months to 2 yrs after vaccination and fatal disseminated BCG disease may occur. Epinephrine inj must be available should an acute anaphylactic reaction occur. Recommended only for those who are tuberculin (-) to a recent skin test with 5 TU. Following vaccination, usually not possible to clearly distinguish between a tuberculin reaction caused by persistent post-vaccination sensitivity and one caused by a virulent suprainfection after vaccination. Caution in attributing a positive skin test to vaccination; further investigate a sharp rise in the tuberculin reaction since the latest test (except in immediate post-vaccination period). Caution in elderly, vaccinated infants exposed to persons with active TB, and persons in groups at high risk for HIV infection.

ADVERSE REACTIONS
Moderate axillary or cervical lymphadenopathy and induration and subsequent pustule formation at inj site, ulceration at the vaccination site, regional suppurative lymphadenitis with draining sinuses, caseous lesions/purulent draining at the puncture site.

DRUG INTERACTIONS
Antimicrobials or immunosuppressive agents may interfere with the development of immune response; use only under medical supervision. Immune response to vaccine may be impaired if administered within 30 days of another live vaccine; whenever possible, live vaccines administered on different days should be administered at least 30 days apart.

PREGNANCY AND LACTATION
Category C, not for use in nursing.

MECHANISM OF ACTION
Vaccine.

PATIENT CONSIDERATIONS
Assessment: Assess for previous hypersensitivity to vaccine or any of its components, active TB, immunosuppression, any other conditions where treatment is contraindicated or cautioned, pregnancy/nursing status, and possible drug interactions. Review immunization history.

Monitoring: Monitor for systemic BCG infection, fever, acute localized inflammation, and other adverse reactions.

Counseling: Inform of benefits/risks of therapy. Advise that vaccine contains live organisms and that infection of others is possible. Inform that may experience flu-like symptoms for 24-48 hrs following vaccination; instruct to consult physician immediately if experiencing fever ≥39.4°C (103°F), or if acute local reactions persisting for >2-3 days occur. Instruct to report any unusual adverse reactions to physician.

BEBULIN — factor IX complex　　　　Rx
Class: Antihemophilic agent

ADULT DOSAGE	PEDIATRIC DOSAGE
Hemophilia B	Pediatric use may not have been established

ADULT DOSAGE

Hemophilia B

Prevention/Control of Bleeding:
Minor Bleeding:
Desired Factor IX (FIX) Level 20% of Normal:
Initial: 25-35 IU/kg once. May repeat after 24 hrs

Moderate Bleeding:
Desired FIX Level 40% of Normal:
Initial: 50-65 IU/kg q24h for 2 days or until adequate wound healing

Major Bleeding:
Desired FIX Level ≥60% of Normal:
Initial: 75-90 IU/kg q24h for 2-3 days or until adequate wound healing
Maint: 2/3 of initial dose

Surgical Procedures:
Preoperative LD:
Administer 1 hr prior to surgery. Depending on type of surgery, continue replacement therapy over 1 to several weeks until adequate wound healing is achieved. Average treatment interval for the initial and late post-operative period is 12 hrs and 24 hrs, respectively.

Minor Surgery/Tooth Extraction:
Day of Operation:
FIX Levels 40-60% of Normal:
50-75 IU/kg

Initial Postoperative Period:
FIX Levels 20-40% of Normal:
25-65 IU/kg for 1-2 weeks. Extraction of several teeth may require use for up to 1 week

Major Surgery:
Day of Operation:
FIX Levels ≥60% of Normal:
75-90 IU/kg

Initial Postoperative Period:
FIX Levels 20-60% of Normal:
25-75 IU/kg for 1-2 weeks

Late Postoperative Period:
FIX Levels 20% of Normal: 25-35 IU/kg from 3rd week onwards

ADMINISTRATION
IV route

Reconstitution
Do not mix w/ other medicinal products or solvents, other than the enclosed sterilized water for inj
Warm unopened vials of both diluent and concentrate to room temperature (not to exceed 37°C [98°F])
Gently agitate or rotate the concentrate vial until all material is dissolved
Administer w/in 3 hrs after reconstitution as the sol does not contain a preservative. Do not refrigerate after reconstitution

STORAGE
2-8°C (35-46°F). Do not freeze.

HOW SUPPLIED
Inj: 20mL [vial]

CONTRAINDICATIONS

Known history of hypersensitivity reactions to the product, known allergy to heparin and known history of heparin-induced thrombocytopenia.

WARNINGS/PRECAUTIONS

Not for use in the treatment of Factor VII deficiency. Thromboembolic events (deep vein thrombosis, pulmonary embolism, thrombotic stroke) as well as disseminated intravascular coagulation (DIC) reported. Higher risk of thromboembolic complications including DIC and hyperfibrinolysis in patients with congenital or acquired coagulation disorders, with repeated dosing or high doses. Monitor closely for signs/symptoms of intravascular coagulation or thrombosis. Monitor FIX level in patients predisposed to thromboembolic complications (eg, history of coronary artery disease, liver disease, pre- or post-operative patients, neonates). D/C infusion immediately and initiate appropriate diagnostic and therapeutic measures at the 1st signs/symptoms of thrombosis or embolism. Hypersensitivity reactions including anaphylactic/anaphylactoid reactions reported; d/c infusion immediately and administer appropriate emergency treatment if an anaphylactic/anaphylactoid reaction develops. Formation of circulating antibodies inhibiting FIX reported. Nephrotic syndrome reported following attempted immune tolerance induction; safety and efficacy for immune tolerance induction have not been established. May carry risk of transmitting infectious agents (eg, viruses, Creutzfeldt-Jakob disease). Contains heparin; take heparin content into account when performing clotting tests sensitive to heparin.

ADVERSE REACTIONS

Hypotension, dizziness, urticaria, erythema, pyrexia, chills.

DRUG INTERACTIONS

Effect of vitamin K antagonists (eg, warfarin) can be temporarily overcome by the administration of human prothrombin complex products, which provides increased plasma levels of functional vitamin-K dependent coagulation Factors (II, IX and X).

PREGNANCY AND LACTATION

Category C, safety not known in nursing.

MECHANISM OF ACTION

Antihemophilic agent; increases plasma levels of FIX and temporarily corrects the coagulation defect in FIX deficiency.

PATIENT CONSIDERATIONS

Assessment: Assess for hypersensitivity to the drug, allergy to heparin, history of heparin-induced thrombocytopenia, congenital/acquired coagulation disorders, predisposition to thromboembolic complications, and pregnancy/nursing status. Assess FIX level.

Monitoring: Monitor for DIC, thrombosis or embolism, hypersensitivity reactions, nephrotic syndrome, and other adverse reactions. Monitor FIX levels.

Counseling: Instruct to d/c use and notify physician if signs/symptoms of an immediate hypersensitivity reaction (eg, fever, urticaria/hives, rash, nausea, retching, angioedema, laryngeal edema, stridor, dysphonia, bronchospasm, hypotension, dizziness, lightheadedness, loss of consciousness) occur. Inform of all signs/symptoms of parvovirus B19 infection (eg, fever, drowsiness, chills, and runny nose followed about 2 weeks later by a rash and joint pain) and the seriousness of it in pregnant women and immune-compromised individuals.

BELEODAQ — belinostat   Rx

Class: Histone deacetylase (HDAC) inhibitor

ADULT DOSAGE	**PEDIATRIC DOSAGE**
Peripheral T-Cell Lymphoma	Pediatric use may not have been established
Relapsed or Refractory:	
1000mg/m² IV infusion over 30 min qd on Days 1-5 of a 21-day cycle	
May repeat cycles every 21 days until disease progression or unacceptable toxicity	
Dosing Based on Genotype Consideration	
Patients Homozygous for the UGT1A1*28 Allele: Reduce starting dose to 750mg/m²	

DOSING CONSIDERATIONS
Adverse Reactions
Hematologic Toxicities:
Nadir ANC <0.5 x 10⁹/L (Any Platelet Count): Decrease dose by 25% (750mg/m²)
Platelet Count <25 x 10⁹/L (Any Nadir ANC): Decrease dose by 25% (750mg/m²)
Recurrent Nadir ANC <0.5 x 10⁹/L and/or Recurrent Platelet Count <25 x 10⁹/L After 2 Dosage Reductions: D/C therapy
Nonhematologic Toxicities:
Any CTCAE Grade 3 or 4 Adverse Reaction: Decrease dose by 25% (750mg/m²); for N/V, and diarrhea, only dose modify if the duration is >7 days w/ supportive management
Recurrence of CTCAE Grade 3 or 4 Adverse Reaction After 2 Dosage Reductions: D/C therapy

ADMINISTRATION
IV route

Reconstitution and Infusion Instructions
1. Add 9mL of sterile water for inj into the vial w/ a suitable syringe to achieve a concentration of 50mg/mL
2. Swirl the contents of the vial until there are no visible particles in the resulting sol
3. Withdraw the volume needed for the required dosage (based on the 50mg/mL concentration and the patient's BSA) and transfer to an infusion bag containing 250mL of 0.9% NaCl inj
4. Connect the infusion bag containing drug sol to an infusion set w/ a 0.22μm in-line filter for administration
5. Infuse over 30 min; may extend to 45 min if infusion-site pain or other symptoms potentially attributable to the infusion occur

STORAGE
20-25°C (68-77°F); excursions permitted between 15-30°C (59-86°F). Retain in original package until use. Reconstituted Sol: 15-25°C (59-77°F) for up to 12 hrs. Infusion Bag with Drug Sol: 15-25°C (59-77°F) for up to 36 hrs including infusion time.

HOW SUPPLIED
Inj: 500mg

WARNINGS/PRECAUTIONS
May cause thrombocytopenia, leukopenia (neutropenia and lymphopenia), and/or anemia. Serious and sometimes fatal infections, including pneumonia and sepsis, reported; do not administer to patients with an active infection. Patients with a history of extensive or intensive chemotherapy may be at higher risk of life-threatening infections. May cause fatal hepatotoxicity and LFT abnormalities. Tumor lysis syndrome (TLS) reported; caution with advanced stage disease and/or high tumor burden. N/V and diarrhea reported and may require the use of antiemetic and antidiarrheal medications. May cause fetal harm.

ADVERSE REACTIONS
N/V, fatigue, pyrexia, anemia, constipation, diarrhea, dyspnea, rash, peripheral edema, cough, thrombocytopenia, pruritus, chills, increased blood lactate dehydrogenase, decreased appetite.

DRUG INTERACTIONS
Avoid with strong UGT1A1 inhibitors.

PREGNANCY AND LACTATION
Category D, not for use in nursing.

MECHANISM OF ACTION
Histone deacetylase inhibitor; causes the accumulation of acetylated histones and other proteins, inducing cell cycle arrest and/or apoptosis of some transformed cells. Shows preferential cytotoxicity towards tumor cells compared to normal cells.

PHARMACOKINETICS
Distribution: Plasma protein binding (92.9-95.8%). **Metabolism:** Liver by UGT1A1 (primary); belinostat amide and belinostat acid (by CYP2A6, CYP2C9, and CYP3A4), methyl belinostat, 3-(anilinosulfonyl)-benzenecarboxylic acid, and belinostat glucuronide (major metabolites). **Elimination:** Urine (<2%, unchanged); $T_{1/2}$=1.1 hrs.

PATIENT CONSIDERATIONS

Assessment: Assess for active infection, history of extensive or intensive chemotherapy, advanced stage disease and/or high tumor burden, reduced UGT1A1 activity, pregnancy/nursing status, and possible drug interactions. Obtain baseline CBCs. Perform serum chemistry tests, including renal and hepatic functions, prior to the start of the 1st dose of each cycle.

Monitoring: Monitor for signs/symptoms of hematologic/hepatic/GI toxicity, infections, TLS, and other adverse reactions. Monitor CBCs weekly.

Counseling: Instruct to report symptoms of N/V, diarrhea, thrombocytopenia, leukopenia, anemia, and infection. Inform of the potential risk to the fetus and for women to avoid pregnancy while receiving therapy. Advise to understand the importance of monitoring LFT abnormalities and to immediately report potential symptoms of liver injury.

BENDEKA — bendamustine hydrochloride   Rx

Class: Alkylating agent

ADULT DOSAGE	**PEDIATRIC DOSAGE**
Chronic Lymphocytic Leukemia	Pediatric use may not have been established
100mg/m² IV over 10 min on Days 1 and 2 of a 28-day cycle, up to 6 cycles	
B-Cell Non-Hodgkin Lymphoma	
Indolent B-cell non-Hodgkin lymphoma that has progressed during or w/in 6 months of treatment w/ rituximab or a rituximab-containing regimen	
120mg/m² IV over 10 min on Days 1 and 2 of a 21-day cycle, up to 8 cycles	

DOSING CONSIDERATIONS
Renal Impairment
CrCl <40mL/min: Not recommended for use

Hepatic Impairment
Moderate (AST or ALT 2.5-10X ULN and Total Bilirubin 1.5-3X ULN): Not recommended for use
Severe (Total Bilirubin >3X ULN): Not recommended for use

Adverse Reactions
Treatment Delay:
Grade 4 Hematologic Toxicity: Delay administration
Clinically Significant ≥Grade 2 Nonhematologic Toxicity: Delay administration
May reinitiate once nonhematologic toxicity has recovered to ≤Grade 1 and/or blood counts have improved (ANC ≥1 x 10^9/L, platelets ≥75 x 10^9/L); dose reduction may be warranted

Chronic Lymphocytic Leukemia (CLL):
Hematologic Toxicity:
≥Grade 3: Reduce to 50mg/m² on Days 1 and 2 of each cycle; if ≥Grade 3 toxicity recurs, reduce to 25mg/m² on Days 1 and 2 of each cycle

Nonhematologic Toxicity:
≥Grade 3: Reduce to 50mg/m² on Days 1 and 2 of each cycle

May consider dose re-escalation in subsequent cycles

B-Cell Non-Hodgkin Lymphoma:
Hematologic Toxicity:
Grade 4: Reduce to 90mg/m² on Days 1 and 2 of each cycle; if Grade 4 toxicity recurs, reduce dose to 60mg/m² on Days 1 and 2 of each cycle

Nonhematologic Toxicity:
≥Grade 3: Reduce to 90mg/m² on Days 1 and 2 of each cycle; if ≥Grade 3 toxicity recurs, reduce to 60mg/m² on Days 1 and 2 of each cycle

ADMINISTRATION
IV route
Cytotoxic drug; follow applicable special handling and disposal procedures.

Preparation
Allow vial to reach room temperature (15-30°C or 59-86°F) prior to use.
Contents may partially freeze when refrigerated; if particulate matter is observed after achieving room temperature, do not use.
Aseptically withdraw the volume needed for the required dose from the 25mg/mL sol and immediately transfer the sol to a 50mL infusion bag of 0.9% NaCl inj, or 2.5% dextrose/0.45% NaCl inj, or D5 inj.
After transferring, thoroughly mix the contents of the infusion bag; the resulting final concentration should be w/in 1.85-5.6mg/mL.

Admixture Stability
Contains no antimicrobial preservative; prepare admixture as close as possible to the time of administration.
If diluted w/ 0.9% NaCl or 2.5% dextrose/0.45% NaCl inj, the final admixture is stable for 24 hrs when stored at 2-8°C (36-46°F) or for 6 hrs when stored at 15-30°C (59-86°F) and room light; administration must be completed w/in this period of time.
If diluted w/ D5 inj, the final admixture is stable for 24 hrs when stored at 2-8°C (36-46°F) or for 3 hrs when stored at 15-30°C (59-86°F) and room light; administration must be completed w/in this period of time.

Stability of Partially Used Vials
Stable for up to 28 days when stored in original carton at 2-8°C (36-46°F); each vial is not recommended for >6 dose withdrawals.

Refer to PI for further administration instructions.

STORAGE
2-8°C (36-46°F). Protect from light.

HOW SUPPLIED
Inj: 100mg/4mL

CONTRAINDICATIONS
Known hypersensitivity (eg, anaphylactic and anaphylactoid reactions) to bendamustine, polyethylene glycol 400, propylene glycol, or monothioglycerol.

WARNINGS/PRECAUTIONS
Severe myelosuppression reported; may require dose delays and/or subsequent dose reductions if recovery to the recommended values has not occurred by the 1st day of the next scheduled cycle. Frequently monitor CBC, including leukocytes, platelets, Hgb, and neutrophils. Infection (eg, pneumonia, sepsis, septic shock, hepatitis) and death reported. Increased risk for reactivation of infections (eg, hepatitis B, cytomegalovirus, mycobacterium tuberculosis, herpes zoster); perform appropriate measures for infection and infection reactivation prior to administration. Infusion reactions and severe anaphylactic/anaphylactoid reactions reported; monitor clinically and d/c for severe reactions. Consider measures to prevent severe reactions (eg, antihistamines, antipyretics, corticosteroids) in subsequent cycles in patients who have experienced Grade 1 or 2 infusion reactions. Consider discontinuation for Grade 3 infusion reactions as clinically appropriate; d/c for Grade 4 infusion reactions. Patients who experience ≥Grade 3 allergic-type reactions were not typically rechallenged. Tumor lysis syndrome reported; preventive measures include vigorous hydration and close monitoring of blood chemistry, particularly K⁺ and uric acid levels. Skin reactions (eg, rash, toxic skin reactions, bullous exanthema) reported; monitor closely and withhold or d/c if skin reactions are severe or progressive. Premalignant and malignant diseases (eg, myelodysplastic syndrome, myeloproliferative disorders, acute myeloid leukemia, bronchial carcinoma) reported. Extravasations reported; assure good venous access prior to starting infusion and monitor for infusion-site redness, swelling, pain, infection, and necrosis during and after administration. May cause fetal harm. Caution w/ mild/moderate renal impairment and w/ mild hepatic impairment.

ADVERSE REACTIONS
CLL: Pyrexia, N/V.
Non-Hodgkin Lymphoma: N/V, fatigue, diarrhea, pyrexia.

DRUG INTERACTIONS
CYP1A2 inhibitors (eg, fluvoxamine, ciprofloxacin) may increase plasma concentrations of bendamustine and may decrease plasma concentrations of active metabolites. CYP1A2 inducers (eg, omeprazole, smoking) may decrease plasma concentrations of bendamustine and may increase plasma concentrations of active metabolites. Use caution or consider alternative treatments if treatment w/ CYP1A2 inhibitors/inducers is needed. May increase risk of severe skin toxicity w/ allopurinol.

PREGNANCY AND LACTATION
Pregnancy: Category D. Avoid becoming pregnant during treatment and for 3 months after therapy has stopped; men should use reliable contraception for the same time period.
Lactation: Not for use in nursing.

MECHANISM OF ACTION
Alkylating agent; has not been established. Bifunctional mechlorethamine derivative containing a purine-like benzimidazole ring; forms electrophilic alkyl groups that form covalent bonds w/ electron-rich nucleophilic moieties, resulting in interstrand DNA crosslinks. Bifunctional covalent linkage can lead to cell death via several pathways. Active against both quiescent and dividing cells.

PHARMACOKINETICS
Absorption: C_{max}=35µg/mL. **Distribution:** Plasma protein binding (94-96%); V_d=20-25L. **Metabolism:** Extensive via hydrolytic (primary), oxidative, and conjugative pathways; gamma-hydroxy-bendamustine (M3), N-desmethyl-bendamustine (M4) (active minor metabolites) via CYP1A2. **Elimination:** Urine (50%, 3.3% unchanged, <1% as M3 and M4), feces (25%); $T_{1/2}$=40 min, 3 hrs (M3), 30 min (M4).

PATIENT CONSIDERATIONS
Assessment: Assess for renal/hepatic impairment, hypersensitivity to bendamustine and components of the product, pregnancy/nursing status, and possible drug interactions. Obtain baseline CBC and ANC should be ≥1 x 10^9/L and platelet count should be ≥75 x 10^9/L.

Monitoring: Monitor for signs/symptoms of myelosuppression, infections, anaphylaxis/infusion reactions, tumor lysis syndrome, skin reactions, premalignant/malignant diseases, extravasation, lab abnormalities, and other adverse reactions. Monitor CBCs and blood chemistry, particularly K⁺ and uric acid levels.

Counseling: Inform of the possibility of mild/serious allergic reactions and instruct to immediately report such symptoms. Inform that therapy may cause a decrease in WBC counts, platelets, and RBC counts, and of the need for frequent monitoring of blood counts; instruct to report SOB, significant fatigue, bleeding, fever, or other signs of infection. Advise that therapy may cause tiredness; instruct to avoid driving or operating dangerous tools or machinery if tiredness occurs. Inform that therapy may cause N/V, diarrhea, and mild rash or itching; instruct to report any adverse reactions immediately to physician. Advise women to avoid becoming pregnant and to use reliable contraception throughout treatment and for 3 months after discontinuation of therapy; instruct to immediately report pregnancy and to avoid nursing while on therapy. Advise men to use reliable contraception throughout treatment and for 3 months after discontinuation of therapy.

BENEFIX — coagulation factor IX (recombinant)   **Rx**

Class: Antihemophilic factor (recombinant)

ADULT DOSAGE	**PEDIATRIC DOSAGE**
Hemophilia B	**Hemophilia B**
Dosing Formula:	**<15 Years:**
Number of Factor IV IU Required (IU) = Body Weight (kg) x Desired Factor IX Increase (% or IU/dL) x Reciprocal of Observed Recover (IU/kg per IU/dL)	**Dosing Formula:** Number of Factor IV IU Required (IU) = Body Weight (kg) x Desired Factor IX Increase (% or IU/dL) x Reciprocal of Observed Recover (IU/kg per IU/dL)
Control/Prevention of Bleeding Episodes/Perioperative Management: **Minor Bleeding (Required Factor IX Level 20-30 IU/dL):** q12-24 hrs for 1-2 days	**Control/Prevention of Bleeding Episodes/Perioperative Management:** **Minor Bleeding (Required Factor IX Level 20-30 IU/dL):** q12-24 hrs for 1-2 days
Moderate Bleeding (Required Factor IX Level 25-50 IU/dL): q12-24 hrs until bleeding stops and healing begins (about 2-7 days)	**Moderate Bleeding (Required Factor IX Level 25-50 IU/dL):** q12-24 hrs until bleeding stops and healing begins (about 2-7 days)
Major Bleeding (Required Factor IX Level 50-100 IU/dL): q12-24 hrs for 7-10 days	**Major Bleeding (Required Factor IX Level 50-100 IU/dL):** q12-24 hrs for 7-10 days
Average Recovery: One IU/kg increased the circulating activity of Factor IX by 0.8+/-0.2 IU/dL	**Average Recovery:** One IU/kg increased the circulating activity of Factor IX by 0.7+/-0.3 IU/dL

ADMINISTRATION
IV route

Administer w/in 3 hrs of reconstitution.
Use all components in the reconstitution and administration of this product as soon as possible after opening their sterile containers to minimize unnecessary exposure to the atmosphere.
A dose may be administered over a period of several minutes; rate of administration should be adapted to the comfort level of each individual patient.
Do not mix or administer in the same tubing or container w/ other medicinal products.

If red blood cell agglutination is observed in the tubing or syringe, discard all material (tubing, syringe and sol) and resume administration w/ a new package.

STORAGE
2-30°C (36-86°F). Do not freeze. **Following Reconstitution:** Use w/in 3 hrs.

HOW SUPPLIED
Inj: 250 IU, 500 IU, 1000 IU, 2000 IU, 3000 IU

CONTRAINDICATIONS
Life-threatening immediate hypersensitivity reactions, including anaphylaxis, to the product or its components, including hamster proteins.

WARNINGS/PRECAUTIONS
Initiate therapy under the supervision of a physician experienced in the treatment of hemophilia B. Hypersensitivity reactions (eg, anaphylaxis) reported; d/c if symptoms occur. Contains trace amounts of hamster proteins; may develop hypersensitivity to these nonhuman mammalian proteins. Thrombotic events reported in patients receiving continuous infusion through a central venous catheter. Nephrotic syndrome reported following immune tolerance induction in hemophilia B patients w/ FIX inhibitors and a history of allergic reactions to FIX. May develop FIX inhibitors; perform an assay that measures FIX inhibitor concentration if expected plasma FIX activity levels are not attained, or if bleeding is not controlled w/ an expected dose. Determine FIX inhibitor levels in Bethesda Units. Not indicated for treatment of other factor deficiencies (eg, factors II, VII, VIII, and X), hemophilia A patients w/ inhibitors to factor VIII, reversal of coumarin-induced anticoagulation, and treatment of bleeding due to low levels of liver-dependent coagulation factors.

ADVERSE REACTIONS
Nausea, altered taste, injection-site reaction/pain, hypotension, bronchospastic reactions, headache, dizziness, rash, hives, flushing, fever, dyspnea, FIX inhibition.

PREGNANCY AND LACTATION
Pregnancy: Category C.
Lactation: Caution in nursing.

MECHANISM OF ACTION
Recombinant antihemophilic factor; temporarily replaces the missing clotting FIX that is needed for effective hemostasis.

PHARMACOKINETICS
Absorption: (Initial Visit) C_{max}=54.5 IU/dL; AUC=940 IU•hr/dL. (Month 6) C_{max}=57.3 IU/dL; AUC=923 IU•hr/dL. **Elimination:** $T_{1/2}$=22.4 hrs (initial visit), 23.8 hrs (Month 6), 19.8 hrs (children, ≥2 yrs-<12 yrs), 21.1 hrs (adolescents, ≥12 yrs-≤15 yrs).

PATIENT CONSIDERATIONS
Assessment: Assess for hypersensitivity to drug or its components, including hamster proteins; presence of FIX inhibitors; and pregnancy/nursing status.

Monitoring: Monitor for signs/symptoms of hypersensitivity reactions, thromboembolic complications, nephrotic syndrome, and for other adverse reactions. Monitor FIX activity plasma levels. Monitor for the development of FIX inhibitors if expected plasma FIX activity levels are not attained.

Counseling: Inform about early signs/symptoms of hypersensitivity (eg, hives, generalized urticaria, angioedema, chest tightness, dyspnea, wheezing); advise to d/c use and contact physician if symptoms occur. Instruct to inform physician if experiencing a lack of clinical response to FIX replacement therapy.

BENLYSTA — belimumab

Rx

Class: Monoclonal antibody/BLyS blocker

ADULT DOSAGE	PEDIATRIC DOSAGE
Systemic Lupus Erythematosus	Pediatric use may not have been established
Treatment of Patients w/ Active, Autoantibody-Positive, Systemic Lupus Erythematosus Receiving Standard Therapy:	
10mg/kg at 2-week intervals for the first 3 doses, and at 4-week intervals thereafter	
Infuse IV over a period of 1 hr	
Premedication	
Consider administering premedication for prophylaxis against infusion reactions and hypersensitivity reactions	

DOSING CONSIDERATIONS
Adverse Reactions
May slow or interrupt the infusion rate if patient develops an infusion reaction. D/C infusion immediately if patient experiences a serious hypersensitivity reaction

ADMINISTRATION
IV route

Administer by IV infusion only; do not administer as an IV push or bolus.
Must be reconstituted and diluted prior to administration.
Do not infuse concomitantly in the same IV line w/ other agents.

Reconstitution Instructions
1. Remove vial from the refrigerator and allow to stand for 10-15 min to reach room temperature.
2. Reconstitute the 120mg vial w/ 1.5mL sterile water for inj (SWFI) and the 400mg vial w/ 4.8mL SWFI; reconstituted sol will contain a concentration of 80mg/mL belimumab.

3. Direct the stream of sterile water toward the side of the vial to minimize foaming.
4. Gently swirl the vial for 60 sec.
5. Allow the vial to sit at room temperature during reconstitution, gently swirling the vial for 60 sec every 5 min until the powder is dissolved; do not shake.
6. Reconstitution is typically complete w/in 10-15 min after the sterile water has been added, but it may take up to 30 min. Protect the reconstituted sol from sunlight.
7. If a mechanical reconstitution device (swirler) is used to reconstitute belimumab, it should not exceed 500 rpm and the vial swirled for no longer than 30 min.
8. Once reconstitution is complete, the sol should be opalescent and colorless to pale yellow, and w/o particles; small air bubbles, however, are expected and acceptable.

Dilution Instructions
9. Dilute the reconstituted product to 250mL in 0.9% NaCl inj (normal saline) for IV infusion. From a 250mL infusion bag or bottle of normal saline, withdraw and discard a volume equal to the volume of the reconstituted sol required for the patient's dose, then add the required volume of the reconstituted sol into the infusion bag or bottle.
10. Gently invert the bag or bottle to mix the sol; any unused sol in the vials must be discarded.
11. If reconstituted sol is not used immediately, it should be stored protected from direct sunlight at 2-8°C (36-46°F); sol diluted in normal saline may be stored at 2-8°C (36-46°F) or room temperature. The total time from reconstitution of belimumab to completion of infusion should not exceed 8 hrs.
12. No incompatibilities between belimumab and polyvinylchloride or polyolefin bags have been observed.

STORAGE
2-8°C (36-46°F). Do not freeze. Protect from light and store vials in original carton until use. Avoid exposure to heat.

HOW SUPPLIED
Inj: 120mg [5mL], 400mg [20mL]

CONTRAINDICATIONS
History of anaphylaxis w/ belimumab.

WARNINGS/PRECAUTIONS
Deaths reported; etiologies included infection, cardiovascular disease, and suicide. Serious and sometimes fatal infections reported; caution w/ chronic infections and consider interrupting therapy if a new infection develops while undergoing treatment. Patients receiving any therapy for chronic infection should not begin therapy. JC virus-associated progressive multifocal leukoencephalopathy (PML) resulting in neurological deficits, including fatal cases, reported. Consider diagnosis of PML in any patient presenting w/ new-onset or deteriorating neurological signs/symptoms. Consider stopping therapy in patients w/ confirmed PML. Malignancies (including non-melanoma skin cancers), infusion reactions, psychiatric events (eg, depression) reported. Hypersensitivity reactions, including anaphylaxis and death, reported; d/c immediately if serious hypersensitivity reactions occur. Monitor patients during and for an appropriate period of time after administration. Caution in elderly and in black/African-American patients. Not recommended w/ severe active lupus nephritis or severe active CNS lupus.

ADVERSE REACTIONS
Serious infections, nausea, diarrhea, pyrexia, nasopharyngitis, bronchitis, insomnia, pain in extremity, depression, migraine, pharyngitis, cystitis, leukopenia, viral gastroenteritis.

DRUG INTERACTIONS
Not recommended w/ other biologics or IV cyclophosphamide. Live vaccines should not be given for 30 days before or concurrently w/ therapy; may interfere w/ the response to immunizations.

PREGNANCY AND LACTATION
Pregnancy: Category C. Women of childbearing potential should use adequate contraception during treatment and for ≥4 months after the final treatment. A pregnancy registry has been established; physicians are encouraged to register patients and pregnant women are encouraged to enroll themselves.
Lactation: Not for use in nursing.

MECHANISM OF ACTION
Monoclonal antibody/BLyS blocker; blocks binding of soluble human BLyS, a B-cell survival factor, to its receptors on B cells. Inhibits survival of B cells, including autoreactive B cells, and reduces the differentiation of B cells into immunoglobulin-producing plasma cells.

PHARMACOKINETICS
Absorption: AUC=3083mcg•day/mL; C_{max}=313mcg/mL. **Distribution:** V_d=5.29L; crosses placenta. **Elimination:** $T_{1/2}$=19.4 days.

PATIENT CONSIDERATIONS
Assessment: Assess for chronic infection, history of depression or other serious psychiatric disorders, previous anaphylaxis w/ the drug, history of multiple drug allergies or significant hypersensitivity, pregnancy/nursing status, and possible drug interactions.

Monitoring: Monitor for infusion and hypersensitivity reactions, infections, PML, malignancy, psychiatric events, and other adverse reactions.

Counseling: Inform about risks/benefits of therapy. Advise that drug may decrease ability to fight infections; instruct to notify physician if signs/symptoms of an infection develop. Advise to contact physician if new or worsening neurological symptoms (eg, memory loss, confusion, dizziness/loss of balance, difficulty talking/walking, vision problems) are experienced. Educate on the signs/symptoms of hypersensitivity and infusion reactions; instruct to immediately report symptoms of an allergic reaction during or after the administration of therapy. Instruct to contact physician if new or worsening depression, suicidal thoughts, or other mood changes develop. Inform patients that they should not receive live vaccines while on therapy. Instruct to notify physician if pregnant/ planning on becoming pregnant or breastfeeding; encourage pregnant patients to enroll in the pregnancy registry.

administration if self-administration is deemed appropriate. Given the potential for airway obstruction during acute laryngeal HAE attacks, advise patients self-administering the drug to immediately seek medical attention in an appropriate healthcare facility after treatment. Advise self-administering patients to contact physician after treating suspected abdominal HAE attacks. Instruct to record the lot number from vial label every time medication is used.

BERINERT — C1 esterase inhibitor (human)   Rx

Class: C1 esterase inhibitor

ADULT DOSAGE	PEDIATRIC DOSAGE
Hereditary Angioedema	**Hereditary Angioedema**
Treatment of Acute Abdominal, Facial, or Laryngeal Hereditary Angioedema (HAE) Attacks: 20 IU/kg by slow IV inj at a rate of approx 4mL/min	**Treatment of Acute Abdominal, Facial, or Laryngeal HAE Attacks:** 20 IU/kg by slow IV inj at a rate of approx 4mL/min

---

ADMINISTRATION
IV route
Do not mix w/ other medicinal products; administer by a separate infusion line.
Use either the Mix2Vial transfer set provided or a commercially available double-ended needle and vented filter spike.

Reconstitution
Ensure that drug and diluent vials are at room temperature.
Reconstitute w/ 10mL of sterile water for inj.
Gently swirl drug vial, until fully dissolved; do not shake.
Pool contents of multiple vials into 1 syringe, if patient requires >1 vial; use a new unused Mix2Vial transfer set for each drug vial.
Use reconstituted sol w/in 8 hrs; do not refrigerate or freeze. Reconstituted product should only be stored in the vial.
Use a silicone-free syringe for reconstitution and administration.

STORAGE
2-25°C (36-77°F). Do not freeze. Protect from light.

HOW SUPPLIED
Inj: 500 IU

CONTRAINDICATIONS
Prior life-threatening hypersensitivity reactions, including anaphylaxis, to C1 esterase inhibitor preparations.

WARNINGS/PRECAUTIONS
Severe hypersensitivity reactions may occur; d/c therapy immediately and institute appropriate treatment. Serious arterial and venous thromboembolic events reported; caution in patients w/ risk factors (eg, presence of an indwelling venous catheter/access device, prior history of thrombosis, underlying atherosclerosis, use of oral contraceptives or certain androgens, morbid obesity, immobility). Monitor patients w/ known risk factors for thromboembolic events during and after administration. Drug is made from human blood; may contain infectious agents (eg, viruses, Creutzfeldt-Jakob disease [CJD] agent) that can cause disease.

ADVERSE REACTIONS
Dysgeusia.

PREGNANCY AND LACTATION
Pregnancy: In a retrospective case collection study of 20 pregnant women who received Berinert w/ repeated doses up to 3,500 IU per attack, there were no complications reported during delivery and no harmful effects were reported on these women's 34 neonates. Should be given to a pregnant woman only if clearly needed.
Lactation: Caution in nursing.

MECHANISM OF ACTION
C1 esterase inhibitor; regulates the complement system, intrinsic coagulation (contact) system, fibrinolytic system, and the coagulation cascade by forming complexes between the proteinase and the inhibitor, resulting in inactivation of both and consumption of C1 esterase inhibitor. Suppression of contact system activation is thought to modulate the vascular permeability, which induces the HAE attacks, by preventing the generation of bradykinin.

PHARMACOKINETICS
Absorption: (15 IU/kg) AUC=27.5hr•IU/mL. **Distribution:** V_d=18.6mL/kg.
Elimination: $T_{1/2}$=21.9 hrs.
Refer to PI for additional parameters (eg, adjusted for baseline levels, pediatric patients).

PATIENT CONSIDERATIONS
Assessment: Assess for previous hypersensitivity reactions to drug, risk factors for thromboembolic events, and pregnancy/nursing status.
Monitoring: Monitor for hypersensitivity reactions, thromboembolic events, infections, and other adverse reactions.
Counseling: Counsel about risks and benefits of therapy. Instruct to immediately report signs/symptoms of allergic hypersensitivity reactions and thromboembolic events to physician. Advise to notify physician if pregnant/intending to become pregnant or if breastfeeding/planning to breastfeed. Advise to consult physician prior to travel and to bring adequate supply of medication when traveling. Advise to bring medication when visiting physician/healthcare facility for an acute HAE attack. Inform that medication is made from human blood and may carry a risk of transmitting infectious agents (eg, viruses, CJD agent). Instruct on proper

---

BETASERON — interferon beta-1b   Rx

Class: Biological response modifier

ADULT DOSAGE	PEDIATRIC DOSAGE
Multiple Sclerosis	Pediatric use may not have been established
Treatment of Relapsing Forms:	
Initial: 0.0625mg (0.25mL) qod	
Titrate: Increase over a 6-week period to 0.25mg (1mL) qod	
Dose Titration Schedule:	
Weeks 1-2: 0.0625mg (0.25mL) qod	
Weeks 3-4: 0.125mg (0.5mL) qod	
Weeks 5-6: 0.1875mg (0.75mL) qod	
Weeks ≥7: 0.25mg (1mL) qod	
Premedication	
For Flu-Like Symptoms: Concurrent use of analgesics and/or antipyretics on treatment days may help ameliorate flu-like symptoms	
Missed Dose	
Take it as soon as possible; do not take therapy on 2 consecutive days. The next inj should be taken about 48 hrs (2 days) after that dose.	

ADMINISTRATION
SQ route
Rotate inj sites.
Do not reuse needles or syringes.

Preparation
Attach prefilled syringe containing the diluent (NaCl, 0.54% sol) to vial using the vial adapter.
Slowly inject 1.2mL of diluent into vial and gently swirl; do not shake.
If not used immediately after reconstitution, refrigerate sol at 2-8°C (35-46°F) and use w/in 3 hrs; do not freeze.
Refer to PI for additional administration instructions.

STORAGE
20-25°C (68-77°F); excursions of 15-30°C (59-86°F) are permitted for up to 3 months.

HOW SUPPLIED
Inj: 0.3mg

CONTRAINDICATIONS
History of hypersensitivity to natural or recombinant interferon beta, albumin (human), or any other component of the formulation.

WARNINGS/PRECAUTIONS
Severe hepatic injury, including cases of hepatic failure (rare) and asymptomatic elevation of serum transaminases reported; monitor for signs/symptoms of hepatic injury and consider discontinuing therapy if serum transaminase levels significantly increase, or if associated w/ clinical symptoms (eg, jaundice). Anaphylaxis (rare) and other allergic reactions reported; d/c if anaphylaxis occurs. Depression and suicide reported; consider discontinuation of therapy if depression develops. Monitor for worsening of cardiac condition during initiation of and continued treatment in patients w/ preexisting CHF; cases of CHF, cardiomyopathy, and cardiomyopathy w/ CHF reported. Consider discontinuation of therapy if worsening of CHF occurs w/ no other etiology. Inj-site necrosis/reactions reported; avoid administration into affected area until fully healed in patients who continue therapy after inj-site necrosis has occurred. If multiple lesions occur, d/c until healed. Leukopenia reported; monitor CBC and differential WBC counts. May require more intensive monitoring of CBC, w/ differential and platelet counts in patients w/ myelosuppression. Cases of thrombotic microangiopathy (TMA), including thrombotic thrombocytopenic purpura and hemolytic uremic syndrome, reported; d/c if symptoms and findings consistent w/ TMA occur and manage as clinically indicated. May cause seizures. Cases of drug-induced lupus erythematosus reported; d/c if signs/symptoms characteristic of this syndrome develop.

ADVERSE REACTIONS
Inj-site reaction, lymphopenia, flu-like symptoms, myalgia, leukopenia, neutropenia, increased liver enzymes, headache, hypertonia, pain, rash, insomnia, abdominal pain, asthenia.

DRUG INTERACTIONS
Potential risk for hepatic injury w/ other products associated w/ hepatic injury (eg, hepatotoxic drugs, alcohol).

PREGNANCY AND LACTATION
Pregnancy: Category C.
Lactation: Not for use in nursing.

MECHANISM OF ACTION
Biological response modifier; has not been established. Believed that interferon β-1b receptor binding induces expression of proteins responsible for its pleiotropic

bioactivities. Immunomodulatory effects include enhancement of suppressor T-cell activity, reduction of proinflammatory cytokine production, down-regulation of antigen presentation, and inhibition of lymphocyte trafficking into the CNS.

PHARMACOKINETICS
Absorption: (0.5mg, SQ) Bioavailability (50%); C_{max}=40 IU/mL; T_{max}=1-8 hrs.
Distribution: (0.006-2mg, IV) V_d=0.25-2.88L/kg. **Elimination:** (0.006-2mg, IV) $T_{1/2}$=8 min-4.3 hrs

PATIENT CONSIDERATIONS

Assessment: Assess for hypersensitivity to the drug or human albumin, preexisting CHF, myelosuppression, pregnancy/nursing status, and possible drug interactions. Obtain baseline CBC, differential WBC counts, platelet counts, and blood chemistries including LFTs.

Monitoring: Monitor for hepatic injury, anaphylaxis, depression, suicidal ideation, worsening of CHF, inj-site reactions, leukopenia, TMA, flu-like symptom complex, seizures, drug-induced erythematosus, and other adverse reactions. Monitor CBC and differential WBC counts, platelet counts, and blood chemistries, including LFTs, at regular intervals (1, 3, 6 months) following initiation and periodically thereafter in the absence of clinical symptoms. Periodically evaluate patient understanding and use of aseptic self-inj techniques and procedures, particularly if inj-site necrosis has occurred.

Counseling: Caution not to change dosage or schedule of administration w/o medical consultation. Instruct patients on proper aseptic technique and procedures. Advise not to reuse needles/syringes and instruct on safe disposal procedures. Inform of the importance of rotating inj sites w/ each dose. Instruct to notify physician if pregnant, planning to become pregnant, or if any adverse reactions (eg, hepatic dysfunction, allergic reactions, anaphylaxis, worsening of cardiac condition, inj-site necrosis, seizures) occur. Inform that symptoms of depression or suicidal ideation may occur and instruct to notify physician immediately if these occur. Inform that flu-like symptoms are common following initiation of therapy. Instruct to take missed dose as soon as possible, but not to take on 2 consecutive days; instruct patient to consult w/ physician if taken on 2 consecutive days.

BETHKIS — tobramycin
Rx

Class: Aminoglycoside

ADULT DOSAGE	PEDIATRIC DOSAGE
Pseudomonas aeruginosa Infections	*Pseudomonas aeruginosa* Infections
In Cystic Fibrosis Patients:	**In Cystic Fibrosis Patients:**
300mg bid by oral inh (as close to 12 hrs apart as possible; not <6 hrs apart) in repeated cycles of 28 days on drug, followed by 28 days off drug	**≥6 Years:**
	300mg bid by oral inh (as close to 12 hrs apart as possible; not <6 hrs apart) in repeated cycles of 28 days on drug, followed by 28 days off drug

---

ADMINISTRATION
Oral inh route

Administer by using a hand-held Pari LC Plus reusable nebulizer w/ a Pari Vios air compressor over approx 15 min and until sputtering from the output of the nebulizer has occurred for at least 1 min
Do not mix w/ other medicines in the nebulizer
Administer other inhaled medicines (eg, bronchodilators) before administration of therapy
Refer to PI for further preparation and administration instructions

STORAGE
2-8°C (36-46°F). Upon removal from the refrigerator, or if refrigeration is unavailable, may be stored at room temperature (up to 25°C [77°F]) for up to 28 days. Do not expose to intense light.

HOW SUPPLIED
Sol, Inhalation: 300mg/4mL

CONTRAINDICATIONS
Known hypersensitivity to any aminoglycoside.

WARNINGS/PRECAUTIONS
Ototoxicity (eg, tinnitus) may occur; caution with auditory or vestibular dysfunction. Nephrotoxicity may occur; caution with renal dysfunction. If nephrotoxicity occurs, d/c therapy until serum concentrations fall <2mcg/mL. If an increase in SrCr develops, closely monitor renal function. May aggravate muscle weakness; caution with muscular disorders (eg, myasthenia gravis, Parkinson's disease). Bronchospasm and wheezing reported. Consider an audiogram for patients with any evidence of or at increased risk for auditory dysfunction. May cause fetal harm.

ADVERSE REACTIONS
Decreased forced expiratory volume, rales, increased RBC sedimentation rate, dysphonia, wheezing, epistaxis, pharyngolaryngeal pain, bronchitis.

DRUG INTERACTIONS
Avoid concurrent and/or sequential use with other drugs with neurotoxic or ototoxic potential. Some diuretics may enhance toxicity by altering concentrations in serum and tissue; do not administer with ethacrynic acid, furosemide, urea, or mannitol.

PREGNANCY AND LACTATION
Category D; not for use in nursing.

MECHANISM OF ACTION
Aminoglycoside; acts primarily by disrupting protein synthesis in the bacterial cell, which eventually leads to death of the cell.

PHARMACOKINETICS
Distribution: Crosses placenta. **Elimination:** Expectorated sputum (unabsorbed); $T_{1/2}$=4.4 hrs.

PATIENT CONSIDERATIONS

Assessment: Assess for auditory, vestibular, or renal dysfunction, muscular disorders, drug hypersensitivity, pregnancy/nursing status, and possible drug interactions. Consider a baseline audiogram for patients at increased risk for auditory dysfunction.

Monitoring: Monitor for ototoxicity, nephrotoxicity, muscle weakness, bronchospasm, wheezing, and other adverse reactions. Consider an audiogram for patients who show any evidence of auditory dysfunction.

Counseling: Instruct to take drug ud, and to complete a full 28-day course of therapy even if feeling better. Inform of the adverse reactions associated with therapy, such as ototoxicity, bronchospasm, nephrotoxicity, and neuromuscular disorders. Inform of the need to monitor hearing, serum concentrations, and renal function during treatment. Advise to inform physician if pregnant/nursing or planning to become pregnant. Counsel on proper storage of the drug.

BiCNU — carmustine
Rx

Class: Nitrosourea alkylating agent

> Bone marrow suppression, thrombocytopenia, and leukopenia reported. Monitor blood counts weekly for at least 6 weeks after a dose. Do not give more frequently than every 6 weeks. Base dose adjustments on nadir blood counts from prior dose. Pulmonary toxicity appears to be dose related (>1400mg/m² cumulative dose are at greater risk) and can occur yrs after treatment. Administer only under supervision of a physician experienced in the use of antineoplastic agents.

ADULT DOSAGE	PEDIATRIC DOSAGE
General Dosing	Pediatric use may not have been established
As palliative therapy as a single agent or in established combination therapy w/ other approved chemotherapeutic agents	
Single Agent in Previously Untreated Patients:	
150-200mg/m² IV every 6 weeks, as a single dose or divided into daily inj (eg, 75-100mg/m² on 2 successive days)	
When used in combination w/ other myelosuppressive drugs or in patients in whom bone marrow reserve is depleted, adjust dose accordingly	
Brain Tumors	
Used for glioblastoma, brainstem glioma, medulloblastoma, astrocytoma, ependymoma, and metastatic brain tumors	
Multiple Myeloma	
Used in combination w/ prednisone	
Hodgkin's Disease	
As secondary therapy in combination w/ other approved drugs in patients who relapse while being treated w/ primary therapy, or who fail to respond to primary therapy	
Non-Hodgkin's Lymphoma	
As secondary therapy in combination w/ other approved drugs for patients who relapse while being treated w/ primary therapy, or who fail to respond to primary therapy	

DOSING CONSIDERATIONS
Elderly
Start at lower end of dosing range

Adverse Reactions
Dose Reductions:
Leukocytes 2000-2999/mm³ and Platelets 25,000-74,999/mm³: Administer 70% of prior dose
Leukocytes <2000/mm³ and Platelets <25,000/mm³: Administer 50% of previous dose

Do not administer a repeat course until circulating blood elements have returned to acceptable levels (platelets >100,000/mm³, leukocytes >4000/mm³), and this is usually in 6 weeks

ADMINISTRATION
IV route

Only administer by slow IV infusion; administration over a period of <2 hrs can lead to pain and burning at the inj site
Not intended for use as a multiple dose vial
Only use glass containers for administration

Preparation of IV Sol
1. Dissolve carmustine w/ 3mL of the supplied sterile diluent (dehydrated alcohol inj)
2. Add 27mL sterile water for inj
3. Each mL of resulting sol contains 3.3mg of carmustine in 10% ethanol
4. The reconstituted sol may be further diluted w/ D5 inj

Handling Precautions
If lyophilized material or sol contacts the skin or mucosa, immediately wash the skin or mucosa thoroughly w/ soap and water

STORAGE
2-8°C (36-46°F). Unopened Vial: Stable for ≤3 yrs. Reconstituted: Stable for 24 hrs. If crystals are seen, redissolve by warming vial to room temperature with agitation. Reconstituted and Further Diluted: Room temperature; protect from light; use within 8 hrs.

HOW SUPPLIED
Inj: 100mg

CONTRAINDICATIONS
Previous hypersensitivity to carmustine.

WARNINGS/PRECAUTIONS
Long-term use may be associated with secondary malignancies. Avoid pregnancy; may cause fetal harm. Inj-site reactions may occur; monitor infusion site for possible infiltration. Reduce dose or d/c when toxic effects or adverse reactions occur; caution with reinstitution. Conduct baseline and periodic pulmonary function tests. May cause liver dysfunction. Monitor LFTs and renal function periodically. Do not give a repeat course until platelets and leukocytes have returned to acceptable levels. Caution in elderly patients.

ADVERSE REACTIONS
Delayed myelosuppression, pulmonary infiltrates/fibrosis, N/V, hepatic toxicity, progressive azotemia, renal failure, local soft tissue toxicity, neuroretinitis, chest pain, headache, allergic reaction, hypotension, tachycardia.

DRUG INTERACTIONS
Greater myelotoxicity reported with cimetidine. Adjust dose accordingly when given with other myelosuppressive drugs.

PREGNANCY AND LACTATION
Category D, not for use in nursing.

MECHANISM OF ACTION
Nitrosourea; alkylates DNA and RNA. May inhibit several key enzymatic processes by carbamoylation of amino acids in proteins.

PHARMACOKINETICS
Elimination: Urine (60-70%) and respiration (10%).

PATIENT CONSIDERATIONS
Assessment: Assess for drug hypersensitivity, history of lung disease, other concomitant diseases, pregnancy/nursing status, and possible drug interactions. Obtain baseline CBC, renal/hepatic function, and pulmonary function. Assess for need of antiemetics.

Monitoring: Monitor liver/renal function periodically, pulmonary function frequently, and blood counts weekly for at least 6 weeks after dose. Monitor for possible bone marrow suppression, pulmonary toxicity, secondary malignancy development, and infiltration at infusion site.

Counseling: Inform of benefits and risks of the treatment. Advise to avoid pregnancy/nursing; apprise women of potential hazard to fetus. Instruct to notify physician if any adverse reactions develop.

BIVIGAM — immune globulin intravenous (human)   Rx

Class: Immune globulin

> Thrombosis may occur. Renal dysfunction, acute renal failure, osmotic nephrosis, and death reported w/ immune globulin intravenous (IGIV) products, particularly those containing sucrose; this product does not contain sucrose. For patients at risk of thrombosis (eg, advanced age, prolonged immobilization, hypercoagulable conditions, history of venous/arterial thrombosis, use of estrogens, indwelling central vascular catheters, hyperviscosity, cardiovascular risk factors), renal dysfunction, or renal failure (eg, preexisting renal insufficiency, diabetes mellitus, age >65 yrs, volume depletion, sepsis, paraproteinemia, or receiving known nephrotoxic drugs), administer at the minimum dose and infusion rate practicable. Ensure adequate hydration before administration. Monitor for signs/symptoms of thrombosis and assess blood viscosity if at risk for hyperviscosity.

ADULT DOSAGE	PEDIATRIC DOSAGE
Primary Humoral Immunodeficiency	Pediatric use may not have been established
Replacement Therapy:	
Recommended Dose: 300-800mg/kg every 3-4 weeks	
Titrate: May adjust to achieve desired trough levels and clinical response	
Initial Infusion Rate:	
0.5mg/kg/min (0.005mL/kg/min) for the first 10 min	
Maint Infusion Rate:	
Increase every 20 min (if tolerated) by 0.8mg/kg/min up to 6mg/kg/min	

DOSING CONSIDERATIONS
Elderly
Do not exceed recommended doses; administer at minimum infusion rate practicable

Adverse Reactions
Slow or stop the infusion if adverse reactions occur; may resume at a lower rate if symptoms subside

ADMINISTRATION
IV route
Allow refrigerated product to come to room temperature before use and maintain at room temperature during administration.
Do not freeze or heat; do not use any sol that has been frozen or heated.
Do not shake.
Do not mix w/ other IGIV products or other IV medications.
If large doses are to be administered, several vials may be pooled using aseptic technique into sterile infusion bags and infused.
Do not dilute.

STORAGE
2-8°C (36-46°F). Do not freeze or heat; do not use any sol that has been frozen or heated.

HOW SUPPLIED
Inj: 10% [50mL, 100mL]

CONTRAINDICATIONS
History of an anaphylactic or severe systemic reaction to the administration of human immune globulin, IgA-deficient patients w/ antibodies to IgA and a history of hypersensitivity.

WARNINGS/PRECAUTIONS
Contains trace amounts of IgA; severe hypersensitivity reactions may occur. D/C infusion immediately and institute appropriate treatment if hypersensitivity develops. Consider discontinuation if renal function deteriorates. Hyperproteinemia, increased serum viscosity, and hyponatremia may occur. Distinguish true hyponatremia from pseudohyponatremia that is associated w/ or related to hyperproteinemia w/ concomitant decreased calculated serum osmolality or elevated osmolar gap; treatment aimed at decreasing serum free water in patients w/ pseudohyponatremia may lead to volume depletion, a further increase in serum viscosity, and a possible predisposition to thrombotic events. Aseptic meningitis syndrome (AMS) may occur; may occur more frequently w/ high doses (eg, 2g/kg) and/or rapid infusion; rule out other causes of meningitis. Delayed hemolytic anemia may develop and acute hemolysis reported. Noncardiogenic pulmonary edema may occur; if transfusion-related acute lung injury (TRALI) is suspected, perform tests for presence of antineutrophil antibodies in both the product and patient's serum. May carry a risk of transmitting infectious agents (eg, viruses, Creutzfeldt-Jakob disease agent). May interfere w/ some serological tests.

ADVERSE REACTIONS
Headache, fatigue, infusion-site reaction, nausea, sinusitis, BP increased, diarrhea, dizziness, lethargy.

DRUG INTERACTIONS
See Boxed Warning. Passive transfer of antibodies may transiently interfere w/ the immune response to live virus vaccines (eg, measles, mumps, rubella, varicella).

PREGNANCY AND LACTATION
Pregnancy: Category C.
Lactation: Caution in nursing.

MECHANISM OF ACTION
Immune globulin; not established. Replacement therapy in patients w/ primary humoral immunodeficiency. The broad spectrum of neutralizing IgG antibodies against bacterial and viral pathogens and their toxins helps to avoid recurrent serious opportunistic infections.

PHARMACOKINETICS
Absorption: C_{max}=2137mg/dL; T_{max}=3.5 hrs; AUC=33,592 day•mg/dL. **Distribution:** V_d=0.626dL/kg. **Elimination:** $T_{1/2}$=30 days.

PATIENT CONSIDERATIONS
Assessment: Assess for history of anaphylactic or severe systemic reactions to human immune globulin, IgA deficiency, risk of thrombosis/renal dysfunction/renal failure, pregnancy/nursing status, and possible drug interactions. Assess renal function. Consider baseline assessment of blood viscosity in patients at risk for hyperviscosity, including those w/ cryoglobulins, fasting chylomicronemia/markedly high TGs, or monoclonal gammopathies.

Monitoring: Monitor for thrombosis, hypersensitivity reactions, hyperproteinemia, increased serum viscosity, hyponatremia, hemolytic anemia, pulmonary adverse reactions, infection, and other adverse reactions. Monitor renal function and urine output periodically. Perform neurological exam, including CSF studies, if AMS is suspected. Perform confirmatory lab testing if signs/symptoms of hemolysis are present after an infusion. Perform tests for the presence of antineutrophil antibodies in both product and patient's serum if TRALI is suspected. Monitor vital signs throughout the infusion.

Counseling: Instruct to immediately report signs/symptoms of acute renal dysfunction/failure, thrombosis, AMS, hemolysis, TRALI, and infection. Inform that drug is made from human plasma and may contain infectious agents that can cause disease. Inform that product can interfere w/ immune response to live viral vaccines; instruct to notify physician of this potential interaction when receiving vaccinations.

BLEOMYCIN — bleomycin sulfate   Rx
Class: Cytotoxic glycopeptide antibiotic

> Pulmonary fibrosis is the most severe toxicity reported (presenting as pneumonitis occasionally progressing to pulmonary fibrosis); higher occurrence in elderly and those receiving >400 U total dose. A severe idiosyncratic reaction consisting of hypotension, mental confusion, fever, chills, and wheezing reported in lymphoma patients. Administer only under supervision of a physician experienced in the use of antineoplastic agents.

ADULT DOSAGE
Squamous Cell Carcinoma
Head and neck (including mouth, tongue, tonsil, nasopharynx, oropharynx, sinus, palate, lip, buccal mucosa, gingivae, epiglottis, skin, larynx), penis, cervix, and vulva

0.25-0.5 U/kg (10-20 U/m²) IV/IM/SQ weekly or twice weekly

Non-Hodgkin's Lymphoma
0.25-0.5 U/kg (10-20 U/m²) IV/IM/SQ weekly or twice weekly

Treat w/ ≤2 U for the first 2 doses; follow regular dosage schedule if no acute reaction occurs

Hodgkin Lymphoma
0.25-0.5 U/kg (10-20 U/m²) IV/IM/SQ weekly or twice weekly
Maint: After 50% response, administer 1 U/day or 5 U weekly IV/IM

Treat w/ ≤2 U for the first 2 doses; follow regular dosage schedule if no acute reaction occurs

Testicular Carcinoma
Embryonal Cell/Choriocarcinoma/Teratocarcinoma:
0.25-0.5 U/kg (10-20 U/m²) IV/IM/SQ weekly or twice weekly

Malignant Pleural Effusions
Sclerosing agent for the treatment of malignant pleural effusion and prevention of recurrent pleural effusions

60 U as a single dose bolus intrapleural inj

PEDIATRIC DOSAGE
Pediatric use may not have been established

DOSING CONSIDERATIONS
Renal Impairment
CrCl 40-50mL/min: 70% of dose
CrCl 30-40mL/min: 60% of dose
CrCl 20-30mL/min: 55% of dose
CrCl 10-20mL/min: 45% of dose
CrCl 5-10mL/min: 40% of dose

ADMINISTRATION
IM, IV, SQ, and intrapleural routes

IM/SQ Administration
15-U Vial: Reconstitute w/ 1-5mL of sterile water for inj (SWFI), 0.9% NaCl for inj, or sterile bacteriostatic water for inj
30-U Vial: Reconstitute w/ 2-10mL of SWFI, 0.9% NaCl for inj, or sterile bacteriostatic water for inj

IV Administration
15-U Vial: Dissolve contents in 5mL of 0.9% NaCl for inj and administer slowly over 10 min
30-U Vial: Dissolve contents in 10mL of 0.9% NaCl for inj and administer slowly over 10 min

Intrapleural Administration
Dissolve 60 U in 50-100mL of 0.9% NaCl for inj, and administer through a thoracostomy tube following drainage of excess pleural fluid and confirmation of complete lung expansion; refer to PI for additional information

Handling Precautions
If bleomycin for inj contacts the skin, immediately wash the skin thoroughly w/ soap and water
If contact w/ mucous membranes occurs, flush the membranes immediately and thoroughly w/ water

STORAGE
2-8°C (36-46°F); Solution reconstituted in NaCl 0.9% is stable for 24 hrs at room temperature.

HOW SUPPLIED
Inj: 15 U, 30 U

CONTRAINDICATIONS
Hypersensitivity or idiosyncratic reaction to bleomycin injection.

WARNINGS/PRECAUTIONS
Extreme caution with significant renal impairment or compromised pulmonary function. Pulmonary toxicity may occur; dose and age related, more common in >70 yrs and >400 U total dose. Frequent roentgenograms are recommended; d/c if pulmonary changes noted or pulmonary diffusion capacity for carbon monoxide (DL$_{CO}$) <30-35% of pretreatment value. Monitor for severe idiosyncratic reactions, especially after 1st and 2nd doses. Renal and hepatic toxicity reported. Caution with CrCl <50mL/min; monitor renal function carefully. Caution in elderly.

ADVERSE REACTIONS
Pulmonary toxicity (pneumonitis, pulmonary fibrosis), idiosyncratic reactions, erythema, rash, striae, vesiculation, hyperpigmentation, skin tenderness.

DRUG INTERACTIONS
Pulmonary toxicities may occur at lower doses when coadministered with other antineoplastics. Vascular toxicities reported when coadministered with other antineoplastics. Renal clearance may be affected when coadministered with nephrotoxic drugs (eg, cisplatin). Increased risk of pulmonary toxicity with G-CSF (filgrastim) or other cytokines. Reports of Raynaud's phenomenon in combination with vinblastine with/without cisplatin.

PREGNANCY AND LACTATION
Category D, not for use in nursing.

MECHANISM OF ACTION
Cytotoxic glycopeptide antibiotic; has not been established. Suspected to inhibit DNA, RNA, and protein synthesis.

PHARMACOKINETICS
Absorption: Rapid. T$_{max}$=30-60 min. Bioavailability (100% IM, 70% SQ, 45% intraperitoneal [IP]/intrapleural [IPL]). **Distribution:** V$_d$=17.5L/m². **Metabolism:** Bleomycin hydrolase. **Elimination:** Urine (65% IV, 40% IPL); T$_{1/2}$=2 hrs (IV).

PATIENT CONSIDERATIONS
Assessment: Assess pregnancy/nursing status, renal/hepatic/pulmonary function, and possible drug interactions. Obtain baseline DL$_{CO}$.

Monitoring: Monitor renal function periodically, DL$_{CO}$ monthly. Perform chest x-ray every 1-2 weeks. Monitor signs/symptoms of severe idiosyncratic reaction (hypotension, mental confusion, fever, chills, wheezing), onset of pulmonary toxicity (dyspnea, fine rales, pneumonitis, pulmonary fibrosis, pulmonary function test changes), and liver function.

Counseling: Inform of pregnancy risks. Seek medical attention if symptoms of severe idiosyncratic reaction (hypotension, mental confusion, fever, chills, wheezing) or deterioration of pulmonary function (eg, dyspnea) occurs.

BLINCYTO — blinatumomab   Rx
Class: CD19-directed CD3 T-cell engager

> Cytokine release syndrome (CRS), which may be life-threatening or fatal, reported; interrupt or d/c therapy as recommended. Neurological toxicities, which may be severe, life-threatening, or fatal, reported; interrupt or d/c therapy as recommended.

ADULT DOSAGE
Acute Lymphoblastic Leukemia
Philadelphia Chromosome-Negative: Relapsed or Refractory B-Cell Precursor:

>45kg:
Cycle 1: 9mcg/day on Days 1-7, and 28mcg/day on Days 8-28
Subsequent Cycles: 28mcg/day on Days 1-28

Single cycle of treatment consists of 4 weeks of continuous IV infusion followed by a 2-week treatment-free interval
Treatment course consists of up to 2 cycles for induction followed by 3 additional cycles for consolidation treatment (up to a total of 5 cycles)

PEDIATRIC DOSAGE
Acute Lymphoblastic Leukemia
Philadelphia Chromosome-Negative: Relapsed or Refractory B-Cell Precursor:

Limited experience in pediatric patients

Evaluated in a dose-escalation study of 41 pediatric patients with relapsed or refractory B-precursor acute lymphoblastic leukemia (median age was 6 yrs [range: 2-17 yrs]). Administered at doses of 5-30mcg/m²/day. Recommended phase 2 regimen was 5mcg/m²/day on Days 1-7 and 15mcg/m²/day on Days 8-28 for cycle 1, and 15mcg/m²/day on Days 1-28 for subsequent cycles

Steady-state concentrations were comparable in adult and pediatric patients at the equivalent dose levels based on BSA-based regimens

DOSING CONSIDERATIONS
Adverse Reactions
If interruption after an adverse event is no longer than 7 days, continue same cycle to a total of 28 days of infusion inclusive of days before and after the interruption in that cycle. If an interruption due to an adverse event is >7 days, start a new cycle

Cytokine Release Syndrome:
Grade 3: Withhold until resolved, then restart at 9mcg/day. Escalate to 28mcg/day after 7 days if the toxicity does not recur
Grade 4: D/C permanently

Neurological Toxicity:
Seizure: D/C permanently if >1 seizure occurs
Grade 3: Withhold until no more than Grade 1 (mild) for at least 3 days, then restart at 9mcg/day. Escalate to 28mcg/day after 7 days if the toxicity does not recur. If the toxicity occurred at 9mcg/day, or if the toxicity takes >7 days to resolve, d/c permanently
Grade 4: D/C permanently

Other Clinically Relevant Adverse Reactions:
Grade 3: Withhold until no more than Grade 1 (mild), then restart at 9mcg/day. Escalate to 28mcg/day after 7 days if the toxicity does not recur. If the toxicity takes >14 days to resolve, d/c permanently
Grade 4: Consider discontinuing permanently

ADMINISTRATION
IV route

Premedicate with dexamethasone 20mg IV 1 hr prior to the 1st dose of each cycle, prior to a step dose (eg, Cycle 1 day 8), or when restarting an infusion after an interruption of ≥4 hrs.

Administer as a continuous IV infusion at a constant flow rate using an infusion pump that is programmable, lockable, non-elastomeric, and has an alarm.

Infusion bags should be infused over 24 hrs or 48 hrs.

Infuse the total 240mL sol according to the instructions on the pharmacy label on the bag at 1 of the following constant infusion rates:
Infusion rate of 10mL/hr for a duration of 24 hrs, or 5mL/hr for a duration of 48 hrs.

Refer to PI for further administration, reconstitution, and preparation instructions.

STORAGE
2-8°C (36-46°F). Protect from light until time of use. Do not freeze. May store lyophilized vial and IV sol stabilizer for a max of 8 hrs at room temperature.
Reconstituted Vial: 23-27°C (73-81°F) for 4 hrs, or 2-8°C (36-46°F) for 24 hrs. Protect from light. **Prepared IV Bag Containing Sol for Infusion:** 23-27°C (73-81°F) for 48 hrs (storage time includes infusion time; if not administered within the time frames and temperatures indicated, discard and do not refrigerate again), or 2-8°C (36-46°F) for 8 days. Ship in packaging that has been validated to maintain temperature of the contents at 2-8°C (36-46°F). Do not freeze.

HOW SUPPLIED
Inj: 35mcg

CONTRAINDICATIONS
Known hypersensitivity to blinatumomab or to any component of the product formulation.

WARNINGS/PRECAUTIONS
Hospitalization is recommended for the first 9 days of the 1st cycle and the first 2 days of the 2nd cycle. For all subsequent cycle starts and reinitiation (eg, if treatment is interrupted for ≥4 hrs), supervision by a healthcare professional or hospitalization is recommended. Infusion reactions may occur and may be clinically indistinguishable from manifestations of CRS. Disseminated intravascular coagulation (DIC), capillary leak syndrome (CLS), and hemophagocytic lymphohistiocytosis/macrophage activation syndrome (HLH/MAS) reported in the setting of CRS. Serious infections (eg, sepsis, pneumonia, bacteremia, opportunistic infections, catheter-site infections) reported; administer prophylactic antibiotics and employ surveillance testing during treatment as appropriate. Tumor lysis syndrome (TLS) reported; use appropriate prophylactic measures, including pretreatment nontoxic cytoreduction and on-treatment hydration; may require either temporary interruption or discontinuation of therapy. Neutropenia and febrile neutropenia, including life-threatening cases, reported; interrupt therapy if prolonged neutropenia occurs. Risk for loss of consciousness. Associated with transient elevations in liver enzymes; interrupt therapy if the transaminases rise to >5X ULN or if bilirubin rises to >3X ULN. Cranial magnetic resonance imaging changes showing leukoencephalopathy observed, especially in patients with prior treatment with cranial irradiation and antileukemic chemotherapy (including systemic high-dose methotrexate or intrathecal cytarabine); clinical significance of this is unknown. Preparation and administration errors reported; follow instructions strictly to minimize medication errors. Potential for immunogenicity. Caution in elderly.

ADVERSE REACTIONS
CRS, neurological toxicities, pyrexia, headache, peripheral edema, febrile neutropenia, nausea, hypokalemia, constipation, anemia, diarrhea, fatigue, bacterial infections, tremor, cough.

DRUG INTERACTIONS
May suppress CYP450 enzymes; highest risk during the first 9 days of the 1st cycle and the first 2 days of the 2nd cycle in patients receiving concomitant CYP450 substrates, particularly those with a narrow therapeutic index; monitor for toxicity (eg, warfarin) or drug concentrations (eg, cyclosporine) and adjust dose of concomitant drug PRN.

PREGNANCY AND LACTATION
Category C, not for use in nursing.

MECHANISM OF ACTION
Bispecific CD19-directed CD3 T-cell engager; binds to CD19 expressed on the surface of cells of B-lineage origin and CD3 expressed on the surface of T cells. Activates endogenous T cells by connecting CD3 in the T-cell receptor complex with CD19 on benign and malignant B cells. Mediates formation of a synapse between the T cell and the tumor cell, up-regulation of cell adhesion molecules, production of cytolytic proteins, release of inflammatory cytokines, and proliferation of T cells, resulting in redirected lysis of CD19+ cells.

PHARMACOKINETICS
Distribution: V_d=4.52L. **Elimination:** $T_{1/2}$=2.11 hrs.

PATIENT CONSIDERATIONS
Assessment: Assess for known hypersensitivity to drug or to any component of the formulation, prior treatment with cranial irradiation and antileukemic chemotherapy, pregnancy/nursing status, and possible drug interactions. Obtain baseline WBC count, absolute neutrophil count (ANC), ALT, AST, gamma-glutamyl transferase (GGT), and total bilirubin.

Monitoring: Monitor for signs/symptoms of CRS, DIC, CLS, HLH/MAS, neurological toxicities, infections, TLS, loss of consciousness, and other adverse reactions. Monitor for neutropenia/febrile neutropenia; monitor lab parameters (eg, WBC count, ANC) during infusion. Monitor ALT, AST, GGT, and total blood bilirubin during therapy.

Counseling: Advise to contact physician for any signs/symptoms of CRS or infusion reactions, neurological toxicities, or infections (eg, pneumonia). Advise to refrain from driving and engaging in hazardous occupations/activities (eg, operating heavy/potentially dangerous machinery) while on therapy and inform that neurological events may be experienced. Inform that it is very important to keep area around the IV catheter clean to reduce the risk of infection. Advise to not adjust setting on the infusion pump; inform that any changes to pump function may result in dosing errors. Instruct to contact physician or nurse immediately if there is a problem with the infusion pump or the pump alarms.

BOSULIF — bosutinib   Rx
Class: Kinase inhibitor

ADULT DOSAGE	PEDIATRIC DOSAGE
Chronic Myelogenous Leukemia	Pediatric use may not have been established
Chronic, accelerated, or blast phase Philadelphia chromosome-positive chronic myelogenous leukemia w/ resistance or intolerance to prior therapy	
500mg qd until disease progression or patient intolerance	
Titrate: Consider escalation to 600mg qd in patients who do not reach complete hematological response by Week 8 or a complete cytogenetic response by Week 12, who did not have Grade 3 or higher adverse reactions, and who are currently taking 500mg qd	

DOSING CONSIDERATIONS
Concomitant Medications
CYP3A Strong or Moderate Inducers/Inhibitors: Avoid use

Renal Impairment
CrCl 30-50mL/min:
Initial: 400mg qd

CrCl <30mL/min:
Initial: 300mg qd

Declining Renal Function/Not Tolerating 500mg: Follow recommendations for toxicity

Hepatic Impairment
Mild (Child-Pugh A), Moderate (Child-Pugh B), or Severe (Child-Pugh C): 200mg qd

Adverse Reactions
Elevated Liver Transaminases:
≥3X ULN w/ Bilirubin elevations >2X ULN and Alkaline Phosphatase <2X ULN: D/C therapy
>5X ULN: Withhold therapy until recovery to ≤2.5X ULN and resume at 400mg qd thereafter; if recovery takes longer than 4 weeks, d/c therapy

Diarrhea:
Grade 3-4: Withhold therapy until recovery to Grade ≤1; may resume at 400mg qd

Other Significant, Moderate/Severe Nonhematologic Toxicity:
Withhold until toxicity has resolved, then consider 400mg qd; if clinically appropriate, consider re-escalating to 500mg qd

Myelosuppression:
ANC <1000 x 10⁶/L or Platelets <50,000 x 10⁶/L:
Withhold therapy until ANC ≥1000 x 10^6/L and platelets ≥50,000 x 10^6/L; resume therapy at the same dose if recovery occurs w/in 2 weeks
If blood counts remain low for >2 weeks, upon recovery, reduce dose by 100mg and resume treatment
If cytopenia recurs, reduce dose by an additional 100mg upon recovery and resume treatment

Doses less than 300 mg/day have not been evaluated

ADMINISTRATION
Oral route

Take w/ food.
Do not crush or cut tab; do not touch or handle crushed or broken tabs.

STORAGE
20-25°C (68-77°F); excursions permitted to 15-30°C (59-86°F).

HOW SUPPLIED
Tab: 100mg, 500mg

CONTRAINDICATIONS
Hypersensitivity to bosutinib.

WARNINGS/PRECAUTIONS
Diarrhea, N/V, and abdominal pain reported; monitor and manage patients using standards of care. Thrombocytopenia, anemia, and neutropenia reported; withhold, reduce dose, or d/c therapy as necessary. Hepatic toxicity reported.

Fluid retention reported and may manifest as pericardial effusion, pleural effusion, pulmonary edema, and/or peripheral edema; monitor and manage patients using standards of care. Consider dose adjustment w/ baseline and treatment emergent renal impairment. May cause fetal harm.

ADVERSE REACTIONS
Diarrhea, N/V, thrombocytopenia, abdominal pain, rash, anemia, pyrexia, fatigue, neutropenia, edema, asthenia, respiratory tract infection, decreased appetite, headache, dyspnea.

DRUG INTERACTIONS
See Dosing Considerations. Lansoprazole may decrease levels; consider using short-acting antacids or H_2-blockers instead of proton pump inhibitors, but separate dosing by >2 hrs. May increase concentrations of drugs that are P-gp substrates (eg, digoxin).

PREGNANCY AND LACTATION
Category D, not for use in nursing.

MECHANISM OF ACTION
Tyrosine kinase inhibitor; inhibits the Bcr-Abl kinase that promotes CML. Also inhibits Src-family kinases, including Src, Lyn, and Hck.

PHARMACOKINETICS
Absorption: (500mg, Multiple-dose) C_{max}=200ng/mL; AUC=3650ng•hr/mL. (500mg, Single-dose) T_{max}=4-6 hrs (median). **Distribution:** Plasma protein binding (94%, in vitro; 96%, ex vivo [healthy]); (500mg, Single-dose) V_d=6080L. **Metabolism:** Via CYP3A4; oxydechlorinated bosutinib and N-desmethylated bosutinib (major circulating metabolites). **Elimination:** (Healthy) Feces (91.3%), urine (3%); (500mg, Single-dose) $T_{1/2}$=22.5 hrs.

PATIENT CONSIDERATIONS
Assessment: Assess for hypersensitivity to drug, hepatic/renal impairment, pregnancy/nursing status, and possible drug interactions.

Monitoring: Monitor for signs/symptoms of GI toxicity, fluid retention, and other adverse reactions. Perform CBC weekly for the 1st month and then monthly thereafter, or as clinically indicated. Perform monthly LFTs for the first 3 months and as clinically indicated; monitor more frequently in patients w/ transaminase elevations. Monitor renal function during therapy w/ particular attention to patients w/ preexisting renal impairment or risk factors for renal dysfunction.

Counseling: Instruct to take medication exactly as prescribed and not to change the dose or d/c unless directed by physician. Instruct that if a dose is missed beyond 12 hrs, to skip the dose and take the usual prescribed dose on the following day. Advise to seek medical attention promptly if symptoms of GI problems or fluid retention develop, developing renal problems or if symptoms of other adverse reactions (eg, respiratory tract infections, rash, fatigue) are significant. Instruct to immediately report fever, any suggestion of infection, signs/symptoms of bleeding or easy bruising, or jaundice. Inform that drug may cause fetal harm; counsel females of reproductive potential to use effective contraceptive measures to prevent pregnancy during and for at least 30 days after completing treatment. Instruct to contact physician immediately if pregnancy occurs during treatment. Advise not to breastfeed or provide breast milk to infants while on therapy; if a patient wishes to restart breastfeeding after treatment, advise to discuss the appropriate timing w/ physician. Inform that drug and certain other medicines, including OTC drugs and herbal supplements (eg, St. John's wort), can interact w/ each other and may alter the effects of treatment.

BOTOX — onabotulinumtoxinA   Rx
Class: Acetylcholine release inhibitor

> Effects may spread from the area of inj to produce symptoms consistent w/ botulinum toxin effects (eg, asthenia, generalized muscle weakness, diplopia, ptosis, dysphagia, dysphonia, dysarthria, urinary incontinence, breathing difficulties). Symptoms have been reported hrs to weeks after inj. Swallowing and breathing difficulties can be life threatening and there have been reports of death. Risk of symptoms is probably greatest in children treated for spasticity but can also occur in adults treated for spasticity and other conditions, particularly in patients who have an underlying condition that would predispose them to these symptoms. In unapproved uses and approved indications, cases of spread of effect have been reported at doses comparable to those used to treat cervical dystonia and spasticity and at lower doses.

ADULT DOSAGE
Bladder Dysfunction
Overactive Bladder (OAB):
W/ symptoms of urge urinary incontinence, urgency, and frequency, in patients who have an inadequate response to or are intolerant of an anticholinergic medication

100 U; recommended dilution is 100 U/10mL w/ preservative-free 0.9% NaCl inj
Max: 100 U

Detrusor Overactivity:
Treatment of urinary incontinence due to detrusor overactivity associated w/ a neurologic condition in patients who have an inadequate response to or are intolerant of an anticholinergic medication

200 U per treatment; do not exceed

Consider for reinjection when the clinical effect of the previous inj

PEDIATRIC DOSAGE
Blepharospasm and Strabismus
Associated w/ dystonia, including benign essential blepharospasm or VII nerve disorders

≥12 Years:
Blepharospasm:
Initial: 1.25-2.5 U (0.05-0.1mL at each site)
Dose may be increased up to 2-fold if response from initial treatment does not last longer than 2 months; little benefit obtainable from injecting >5 U/site
Max: 200 U in a 30-day period

Recommended Dilution:
For 1.25 U: 100 U/8mL
For 2.5 U: 100 U/4mL

Strabismus:
Inject between 0.05-0.15mL/muscle

---

has diminished, but no sooner than 12 weeks from the prior bladder inj

Refer to PI for further dosing and administration instructions

Migraine
Prophylaxis of headaches in patients w/ chronic migraine (≥15 days per month w/ headache lasting ≥4 hrs/day)

155 U IM using a sterile 30-gauge, 0.5-inch needle as 0.1mL (5 U) inj per each site; recommended dilution is 200 U/4mL or 100 U/2mL, w/ a final concentration of 5 U/0.1mL

Inj should be divided across 7 specific head/neck muscle areas as follows:
Frontalis: 20 U divided in 4 sites
Corrugator: 10 U divided in 2 sites
Procerus: 5 U in 1 site
Occipitalis: 30 U divided in 6 sites
Temporalis: 40 U divided in 8 sites
Trapezius: 30 U divided in 6 sites
Cervical Paraspinal: 20 U divided in 4 sites

Recommended re-treatment schedule is every 12 weeks

Refer to PI for further dosing and administration instructions

Spasticity
Recommended Dilution: 200 U/4mL or 100 U/2mL w/ preservative-free 0.9% NaCl inj

Tailor dosing based on individual size, number, and location of muscles involved, severity of spasticity, presence of local muscle weakness, patient's previous response, or adverse event history w/ therapy. Repeat treatment may be administered when the effect of a previous inj has diminished, but generally no sooner than 12 weeks after the previous inj

Upper Limb:
To decrease the severity of increased muscle tone in elbow flexors (biceps), wrist flexors (flexor carpi radialis and flexor carpi ulnaris), finger flexors (flexor digitorum profundus and flexor digitorum sublimis), and thumb flexors (adductor pollicis and flexor pollicis longus)

Dosing by Muscle for Upper Limb:
Biceps Brachii: 100-200 U divided in 4 sites
Flexor Carpi Radialis: 12.5-50 U in 1 site
Flexor Carpi Ulnaris: 12.5-50 U in 1 site
Flexor Digitorum Profundus: 30-50 U in 1 site
Flexor Digitorum Sublimis: 30-50 U in 1 site
Adductor Pollicis: 20 U in 1 site
Flexor Pollicis Longus: 20 U in 1 site
Max: 50 U/site

Lower Limb:
To decrease the severity of increased muscle tone in ankle and toe flexors (gastrocnemius, soleus, tibialis posterior, flexor hallucis longus, and flexor digitorum longus)

Dosing by Muscle for Lower Limb:
Gastrocnemius Medial Head: 75 U divided in 3 sites
Gastrocnemius Lateral Head: 75 U divided in 3 sites
Soleus: 75 U divided in 3 sites
Tibialis Posterior: 75 U divided in 3 sites
Flexor Hallucis Longus: 50 U divided in 2 sites
Flexor Digitorum Longus: 50 U divided in 2 sites

Refer to PI for further dosing and administration instructions

---

Initial Doses in Units:
Use the lower listed doses for treatment of small deviations. Use the larger doses only for large deviations
Vertical Muscles and Horizontal Strabismus <20 Prism Diopters: 1.25-2.5 U in any 1 muscle
Horizontal Strabismus of 20-50 Prism Diopters: 2.5-5 U in any 1 muscle
Persistent VI Nerve Palsy of ≥1 Month Duration: 1.25-2.5 U in the medial rectus muscle

Subsequent Doses for Residual/ Recurrent Strabismus:
1. Reexamine patients 7-14 days after each inj to assess the effect of that dose
2. Patients experiencing adequate paralysis of the target muscle that require subsequent inj should receive a dose comparable to the initial dose
3. Subsequent doses for patients experiencing incomplete paralysis of the target muscle may be increased up to 2-fold compared to the previously administered dose
4. Do not administer subsequent inj until effects of the previous dose have dissipated as evidenced by substantial function in the injected and adjacent muscles

Max: 25 U single inj for any 1 muscle

Refer to PI for further dosing and administration instructions

Cervical Dystonia

To reduce the severity of abnormal head position and neck pain associated w/ cervical dystonia

≥16 Years:
Tailor dose based on patient's head and neck position, localization of pain, muscle hypertrophy, patient response, and adverse event history
Initial: Start at a lower dose for a patient w/o prior use of Botox
Recommended Dilution: 200 U/2mL, 200 U/4mL, 100 U/1mL, or 100 U/2mL w/ preservative-free 0.9% NaCl inj, depending on volume and number of inj sites desired to achieve treatment objectives; refer to PI for dilution instructions for Botox vials
Max: 50 U/site
Refer to PI for further dosing and administration instructions

Hyperhidrosis

Severe Primary Axillary Hyperhidrosis Inadequately Managed w/ Topical Agents:
50 U/axilla; recommended dilution is 100 U/4mL w/ 0.9% preservative-free sterile saline

Administer repeat inj when the clinical effect of previous inj diminishes

Refer to PI for further dosing and administration instructions

Blepharospasm and Strabismus

Associated w/ dystonia, including benign essential blepharospasm or VII nerve disorders

Blepharospasm:
Initial: 1.25-2.5 U (0.05-0.1mL at each site)
Dose may be increased up to 2-fold if response from initial treatment does not last longer than 2 months; little benefit obtainable from injecting >5 U/site
Max: 200 U in a 30-day period

Recommended Dilution:
For 1.25 U: 100 U/8mL
For 2.5 U: 100 U/4mL

Strabismus:
Inject between 0.05-0.15mL/muscle

Initial Doses in Units:
Use the lower listed doses for treatment of small deviations. Use the larger doses only for large deviations
Vertical Muscles and Horizontal Strabismus <20 Prism Diopters: 1.25-2.5 U in any 1 muscle
Horizontal Strabismus of 20-50 Prism Diopters: 2.5-5 U in any 1 muscle
Persistent VI Nerve Palsy of ≥1 Month Duration: 1.25-2.5 U in the medial rectus muscle

Subsequent Doses for Residual/ Recurrent Strabismus:
1. Reexamine patients 7-14 days after each inj to assess the effect of that dose
2. Patients experiencing adequate paralysis of the target muscle that require subsequent inj should receive a dose comparable to the initial dose
3. Subsequent doses for patients experiencing incomplete paralysis of the target muscle may be increased up to 2-fold compared to the previously administered dose
4. Do not administer subsequent inj until effects of the previous dose have dissipated as evidenced by substantial function in the injected and adjacent muscles

Max: 25 U single inj for any 1 muscle
Refer to PI for further dosing and administration instructions

DOSING CONSIDERATIONS

Elderly
Start at lower end of dosing range

Other Important Considerations
In treating adult patients for ≥1 indication, the max cumulative dose should not exceed 400 U in a 3-month interval

ADMINISTRATION

Intradermal/IM/Intradetrusor route

Refer to PI for further administration instructions.

Preparation/Dilution
1. Prior to inj, reconstitute each vial w/ only sterile, preservative-free 0.9% NaCl inj.
2. Draw up the proper amount of diluent in the appropriate size syringe; refer to PI for dilution instructions for Botox vials.
3. Slowly inject the diluent into the vial.
4. Discard the vial if a vacuum does not pull the diluent into the vial.
5. Gently mix w/ the saline by rotating the vial.
6. Draw into an appropriately sized sterile syringe an amount of the reconstituted toxin slightly greater than the intended dose.
7. Expel air bubbles in the syringe barrel.
8. Attach the syringe to an appropriate inj needle; confirm patency of the needle.
9. A new, sterile needle and syringe should be used to enter the vial on each occasion for removal.
10. Reconstituted Botox should be stored at 2-8°C (36-46°F) and should be administered w/in 24 hrs.

Overactive Bladder
Administration Instructions:
1. Fill (prime) inj needle w/ approx 1mL of reconstituted Botox prior to the start of inj (depending on the needle length) to remove any air.
2. Insert the needle approx 2mm into the detrusor, and space 20 inj of 0.5mL each (total volume of 10mL) approx 1cm apart.
3. For the final inj, inject approx 1mL of sterile normal saline so that the remaining Botox in the needle is delivered to the bladder.
4. After the inj are given, patients should demonstrate their ability to void prior to leaving the clinic; observe patient for at least 30 min post-inj and until a spontaneous void has occurred.

Detrusor Overactivity
200 U Vial of Botox:
1. Reconstitute a 200 U vial w/ 6mL of preservative-free 0.9% NaCl inj and mix vial gently.
2. Draw 2mL from the vial into each of three 10mL syringes.
3. Complete reconstitution by adding 8mL of preservative-free 0.9% NaCl inj into each of 10mL syringes, and mix gently; this will result in three 10mL syringes each containing 10mL (approx 67 U in each), for a total of 200 U of reconstituted Botox.
4. Use immediately after reconstitution in the syringe; dispose of any unused saline.

100 U Vial of Botox:
1. Reconstitute two 100 U vials, each w/ 6mL of preservative-free 0.9% NaCl inj and mix vials gently.
2. Draw 4mL from each vial into each of two 10mL syringes; draw the remaining 2mL from each vial into a third 10mL syringe for a total of 4mL in each syringe.
3. Complete reconstitution by adding 6mL of preservative-free 0.9% NaCl inj into each of the 10mL syringes, and mix gently; this will result in three 10mL syringes each containing 10mL (approx 67 U in each), for a total of 200 U of reconstituted Botox.
4. Use immediately after reconstitution in the syringe; dispose of any unused saline.

Administration Instructions:
1. Fill (prime) inj needle w/ approx 1mL of reconstituted Botox prior to the start of inj (depending on the needle length) to remove any air.
2. Insert the needle approx 2mm into the detrusor, and space 30 inj of 1mL each (total volume of 30mL) approx 1cm apart.
3. For the final inj, inject approx 1mL of sterile normal saline so that the remaining Botox in the needle is delivered to the bladder.
4. After the inj are given, the saline used for bladder wall visualization should be drained; observe patient for at least 30 min post-inj.

Migraine
A 1-inch needle may be needed in the neck region for patients w/thick neck muscles. W/ the exception of the procerus muscle, which should be injected at 1 site (midline), all muscles should be injected bilaterally w/ half the number of inj sites administered to the left, and half to the right side of the head and neck.

Spasticity
An appropriately sized needle (eg, 25-30 gauge) may be used for superficial muscles, and a longer 22-gauge needle may be used for deeper musculature; localization of the involved muscles w/ techniques such as needle electromyographic guidance or nerve stimulation is recommended.

Cervical Dystonia
Use a sterile needle (eg, 25-30 gauge) of an appropriate length; localization of the involved muscles w/ electromyographic guidance may be useful.

Primary Axillary Hyperhidrosis
Define the hyperhidrotic area to be injected using standard staining techniques (eg, Minor's Iodine-Starch Test); refer to PI for instructions.
Using a 30-gauge needle, inject 50 U (2mL) intradermally in 0.1-0.2mL aliquots to each axilla evenly distributed in multiple sites (10-15) approx 1-2cm apart.
Each inj site has a ring of effect of up to approx 2cm in diameter; evenly space inj sites to minimize the area of no effect.
Inject each dose to a depth of approx 2mm and at a 45° angle to the skin surface, w/ the bevel side up to minimize leakage and to ensure the inj remain intradermal; if inj sites are marked in ink, do not inject Botox directly through the ink mark to avoid a permanent tattoo effect.

Blepharospasm

Use a sterile, 27- to 30-gauge needle w/o electromyographic guidance to inject into the medial and lateral pre-tarsal orbicularis oculi of upper lid and into the lateral pre-tarsal orbicularis oculi of the lower lid.
Avoiding inj near levator palpebrae superioris may reduce complication of ptosis.
Avoiding medial lower lid inj, and thereby reducing diffusion into inferior oblique, may reduce the complication of diplopia.
Ecchymosis occurs easily in soft eyelid tissues; prevent by applying pressure at inj site immediately after inj.

Strabismus

Inject into extraocular muscles utilizing electrical activity recorded from tip of inj needle as a guide to placement w/in the target muscle; inj w/o surgical exposure or electromyographic guidance should not be attempted.
To prepare the eye for inj, it is recommended that several drops of a local anesthetic and an ocular decongestant be given several min prior to inj.

STORAGE

Unopened Vials: 2-8°C (36-46°F) for up to 36 months. Administer w/in 24 hrs of reconstitution; during this time period, store reconstituted sol at 2-8°C (36-46°F).

HOW SUPPLIED

Inj: 100 U, 200 U

CONTRAINDICATIONS

Infection at the proposed inj site(s). Intradetrusor inj is contraindicated in patients w/ OAB or detrusor overactivity associated w/ a neurologic condition who have a UTI, in patients w/ urinary retention, and in patients w/ post-void residual (PVR) urine volume >200mL who are not routinely performing clean intermittent self-catheterization (CIC). Hypersensitivity to any botulinum toxin preparation or to any of the components in the medication.

WARNINGS/PRECAUTIONS

Not interchangeable w/ other botulinum toxin products; cannot be compared to nor converted into U of any other botulinum toxin products. Serious adverse reactions reported w/ unapproved uses. Serious and/or immediate hypersensitivity reactions reported; d/c and institute appropriate medical therapy immediately. Patients w/ neuromuscular disorders may be at increased risk of clinically significant effects; monitor patients w/ peripheral motor neuropathic diseases, amyotrophic lateral sclerosis, or neuromuscular junction disorders. May cause swallowing or breathing difficulties; increased risk of dysphagia in patients w/ smaller neck muscle mass and in those who require bilateral inj into the sternocleidomastoid muscle for treatment of cervical dystonia. Inj into levator scapulae may increase risk of URI and dysphagia. Closely monitor patients w/ compromised respiratory status being treated for spasticity. Reduced blinking from inj of orbicularis muscle may lead to corneal exposure, persistent epithelial defect, and corneal ulceration, especially in patients w/ VII nerve disorders; employ vigorous treatment for any epithelial defect. Retrobulbar hemorrhages sufficient to compromise retinal circulation reported in patients being treated for strabismus; appropriate instruments to decompress the orbit should be accessible. Bronchitis was reported more frequently in patients being treated for upper limb spasticity and URTIs were reported more frequently in patients being treated for upper/lower limb spasticity. Autonomic dysreflexia associated w/ intradetrusor inj may occur in patients treated for detrusor overactivity associated w/ a neurological condition. Increases the incidence of UTI in patients w/ OAB. In patients who are not catheterizing, assess PVR urine volume w/in 2 weeks post-treatment and periodically as medically appropriate up to 12 weeks, particularly in patients w/ multiple sclerosis (MS) or diabetes mellitus (DM). Depending on patient symptoms, institute catheterization if PVR urine volume exceeds 200mL and continue until PVR falls to <200mL. Contains albumin; carries an extremely remote risk for transmission of viral diseases and Creutzfeldt-Jakob disease.

ADVERSE REACTIONS

OAB: UTI, dysuria, urinary retention, bacteriuria, residual urine volume.
Detrusor Overactivity Associated w/ a Neurologic Condition: UTI, urinary retention, hematuria, constipation, muscular weakness, dysuria, gait disturbance.
Chronic Migraine: Neck pain, headache, migraine, eyelid ptosis, musculoskeletal stiffness, muscular weakness, myalgia, inj-site pain, bronchitis, musculoskeletal pain.
Upper Limb Spasticity: Nausea, fatigue, bronchitis, pain in extremity, muscular weakness.
Lower Limb Spasticity: Arthralgia, back pain.
Cervical Dystonia: Dysphagia, URI, neck pain, headache.
Primary Axillary Hyperhidrosis: Inj-site pain/hemorrhage, non-axillary sweating, infection, pharyngitis, flu syndrome, headache, fever, neck/back pain, pruritus, anxiety.

DRUG INTERACTIONS

Potentiation of toxin effect may occur w/ aminoglycosides or other agents interfering w/ neuromuscular transmission (eg, curare-like compounds).
Use of anticholinergic drugs after administration may potentiate systemic anticholinergic effects. Excessive neuromuscular weakness may be exacerbated by administration of another botulinum toxin prior to the resolution of the effects of a previously administered botulinum toxin. Use of a muscle relaxant before/after administration may exaggerate excessive weakness.

PREGNANCY AND LACTATION

Pregnancy: Category C.
Lactation: Caution in nursing.

MECHANISM OF ACTION

Purified neurotoxin complex; blocks neuromuscular transmission by binding to acceptor sites on motor or sympathetic nerve terminals, entering the nerve terminals, and inhibiting release of acetylcholine.

PATIENT CONSIDERATIONS

Assessment: Assess for infection at proposed inj site(s), muscle weakness/hypertrophy, neuromuscular disorders, compromised swallowing or respiratory function, increased risk for dysphagia, VII nerve disorders, MS, DM, potential

causes of secondary hyperhidrosis (eg, hyperthyroidism), hypersensitivity, pregnancy/nursing status, and possible drug interactions. In patients undergoing intradetrusor inj, assess for UTI, urinary retention, and if PVR urine volume is >200mL and not routinely performing CIC.
Monitoring: Monitor for spread of toxin effects, hypersensitivity reactions, weakening of neck muscles, swallowing/speech/respiratory disorders, UTI, and other adverse reactions. Monitor patients w/ peripheral motor neuropathic diseases, amyotrophic lateral sclerosis, neuromuscular junction disorders, or compromised respiratory status. In patients w/ strabismus, monitor for retrobulbar hemorrhages. Monitor for bronchitis and URTIs in patients w/ spasticity. Monitor PVR urine volume (in patients who are not catheterizing) w/in 2 weeks post-treatment and periodically as medically appropriate up to 12 weeks, particularly in patients w/ MS or DM.
Counseling: Advise to inform physician if unusual symptoms (eg, swallowing, speaking, breathing difficulty) develop, or if any existing symptom worsens. Instruct to avoid driving or engaging in other potentially hazardous activities if loss of strength, muscle weakness, blurred vision, or drooping eyelids occur. Advise to contact physician if experiencing difficulties in voiding or burning sensation upon voiding after bladder inj for urinary incontinence.

BRAVELLE — urofollitropin   Rx

Class: Follicle-stimulating hormone (FSH)

ADULT DOSAGE	PEDIATRIC DOSAGE
Ovulation Induction	Pediatric use may not have been established
In Women Who Have Previously Received Pituitary Suppression:	
1st Cycle of Treatment:	
Initial: 150 IU per day for 5 days	
Subsequent Cycles:	
Initial/Titrate: Based on history of the ovarian response to therapy Do not make adjustments more frequently than once every 2 days Do not exceed >75-150 IU per adjustment	
Max: 450 IU per day	
Max Duration: Do not exceed 12 days of treatment	
When pre-ovulatory conditions are reached, administer human chorionic gonadotropin (hCG) to induce final oocyte maturation and ovulation Withhold hCG in cases where the ovarian monitoring on the last day of treatment suggests an increased risk of ovarian hyperstimulation syndrome (OHSS) Encourage woman and her partner to have intercourse daily, beginning on the day prior to the administration of hCG and until ovulation becomes apparent Discourage intercourse when the risk of OHSS is increased	
Assisted Reproductive Technology	
Development of multiple follicles as part of an assisted reproductive technology cycle in ovulatory women who previously received pituitary suppression	
Initial: 225 IU/day starting on cycle day 2 or 3 and continued until sufficient follicular development; should not exceed 12 days May be administered together w/ menotropins for inj; total initial dose for combined therapy should not exceed 225 IU (150 IU of urofollitropin and 75 IU of menotropins or 75 IU of urofollitropin and 150 IU of menotropins)	
Titrate: Adjust dose after 5 days based on ovarian response Do not make additional dose adjustments more frequently than every 2 days or by more than 75-150 IU/ per adjustment	
Max: 450 IU (w/ or w/o menotropins)	
Continue treatment until adequate follicular development is evident, then administer human chorionic gonadotropin (hCG) Withhold hCG if, on the last day of therapy, ovarian monitoring suggests an increased risk of ovarian hyperstimulation syndrome	

ADMINISTRATION
SQ/IM route
Administer SQ in the abdomen

STORAGE
3-25°C (37-77°F). Protect from light. Use immediately after reconstitution.

HOW SUPPLIED
Inj: 75 IU

CONTRAINDICATIONS
Hypersensitivity to urofollitropins, high follicle stimulating hormone (FSH) levels indicating primary ovarian failure, presence of uncontrolled non-gonadal endocrinopathies (eg, thyroid, adrenal, pituitary disorders), sex hormone dependent tumors of the reproductive tract and accessory organ, tumors of pituitary gland or hypothalamus, abnormal uterine bleeding of undetermined origin, ovarian cysts or enlargement of undetermined origin not due to polycystic ovary syndrome, pregnancy.

WARNINGS/PRECAUTIONS
Should only be used by physicians who are experienced in infertility treatment. May cause OHSS with or without pulmonary/vascular complications and multiple births. Hypersensitivity/anaphylactic reactions reported. Abnormal ovarian enlargement may occur; use lowest effective dose. Prohibit intercourse in women with significant ovarian enlargement; hemoperitoneum resulting from rupture of ovarian cysts may occur. Transient LFT abnormalities suggestive of hepatic dysfunction reported in association with OHSS. Withhold hCG if ovaries are abnormally enlarged on the last day of therapy; monitor patients for at least 2 weeks after hCG administration. D/C therapy and consider whether patient needs to be hospitalized if severe OHSS occurs. Serious pulmonary conditions (eg, atelectasis, acute respiratory distress syndrome), thromboembolic events, ovarian torsion, and multi-fetal gestation/births reported. Risk of congenital malformations or ectopic pregnancy may be increased in women undergoing ART. May increase risk of spontaneous abortions and ovarian neoplasms.

ADVERSE REACTIONS
OHSS, headache, nausea, vaginal hemorrhage, ovarian disorder, pelvic pain/cramps, respiratory disorder, hot flashes, abdominal pain/cramps/fullness/enlargement, inj-site reaction, pain.

PREGNANCY AND LACTATION
Category X, not for use in nursing.

MECHANISM OF ACTION
FSH; produces ovarian follicular growth in women who do not have primary ovarian failure.

PHARMACOKINETICS
Absorption: Multiple Dose (150 IU for 7 days): C_{max}=14.8 mIU/mL (SQ), 11.5 mIU/mL (IM); T_{max}=9.6 hrs (SQ), 11.3 hrs (IM); AUC=234.7 mIU•hr/mL (SQ), 192.1 mIU•hr/mL (IM). **Elimination:** Multiple Dose (150 IU for 7 days): $T_{1/2}$=20.6 hrs (SQ), 15.2 hrs (IM).

PATIENT CONSIDERATIONS
Assessment: Assess for previous hypersensitivity to the drug, primary ovarian failure, uncontrolled non-gonadal endocrinopathies, tumors of pituitary gland or hypothalamus, pregnancy/nursing status, and any other conditions where treatment is contraindicated or cautioned. Perform a complete gynecologic/endocrinologic evaluation, and diagnose the cause of infertility.

Monitoring: Monitor for hypersensitivity/anaphylactic reactions, OHSS, ovarian enlargement, ovarian torsion, pulmonary conditions, thromboembolic events, and other adverse reactions. Monitor for signs of ovulation and ovarian response. Monitor serum estradiol levels and perform vaginal ultrasound.

Counseling: Instruct on the correct usage and dosing of therapy; caution not to change dosage or the schedule of administration unless instructed to do so by physician. Prior to therapy, inform about the time commitment and monitoring procedures necessary for treatment. Instruct to contact physician if dose is missed and not to double next dose. Inform of the risks of OHSS, OHSS-associated symptoms, ovarian torsion, and multi-fetal gestation/birth with the use of the drug.

BUPHENYL — sodium phenylbutyrate   Rx

Class: Urea cycle disorder agent

ADULT DOSAGE
Urea Cycle Disorders

Adjunctive therapy in the chronic management of urea cycle disorders involving deficiencies of carbamylphosphate synthetase (CPS), ornithine transcarbamylase (OTC), or argininosuccinic acid synthetase (AS), in all patients w/ neonatal-onset deficiency, or in patients w/ late-onset disease who have a history of hyperammonemic encephalopathy

Tab:
Usual: 9.9-13g/m²/day
Max: 20g/day (40 tabs/day)

Take in equally divided amounts w/ each meal or feeding (eg, 3-6X/day)

PEDIATRIC DOSAGE
Urea Cycle Disorders

Adjunctive therapy in the chronic management of urea cycle disorders involving deficiencies of CPS, OTC, or AS, in all patients w/ neonatal-onset deficiency, or in patients w/ late-onset disease who have a history of hyperammonemic encephalopathy

Powder:
<20kg:
Usual: 450-600mg/kg/day
Max: 20g/day

Powder/Tab:
<20kg:
Usual: 9.9-13g/m²/day
Max: 20g/day (40 tabs/day)

Take in equally divided amounts w/ each meal or feeding (eg, 3-6X/day)

ADMINISTRATION
Oral route (powder/tab); NG or gastrostomy tube (powder)

Powder
Mix w/ food (solid or liquid) for immediate use; however, when dissolved in water, the powder is stable for up to 1 week at room temperature or refrigerated. When powder is added to liquid, only sodium phenylbutyrate will dissolve, the excipients will not.
Shake lightly before use.

STORAGE
15-30°C (59-86°F). Keep bottle tightly closed.

HOW SUPPLIED
Powder: 250g; **Tab:** 500mg

CONTRAINDICATIONS
Management of acute hyperammonemia.

WARNINGS/PRECAUTIONS
Each tab contains 62mg of Na^+ and the powder contains 11.7g of Na^+ per 100g of powder; use w/ great care, if at all, in patients w/ CHF, severe renal insufficiency, and in states of Na^+ retention w/ edema. Caution w/ hepatic/renal insufficiency or inborn errors of β oxidation. Maintain plasma levels of ammonia, arginine, branched-chain amino acids, and serum proteins w/in normal limits, and maintain plasma glutamine levels at <1000μmol/L. Use of tabs for neonates, infants, and children <20kg is not recommended.

ADVERSE REACTIONS
Amenorrhea/menstrual dysfunction, decreased appetite, body odor, bad taste/taste aversion, hypoalbuminemia, metabolic acidosis/alkalosis, anemia, hyperchloremia, hypophosphatemia, decreased total protein, increased alkaline phosphatase, increased liver transaminase, leukopenia/leukocytosis, thrombocytopenia.

DRUG INTERACTIONS
Probenecid may affect renal excretion of the conjugated product of sodium phenylbutyrate, as well as its metabolite. Hyperammonemia induced by haloperidol and by valproic acid reported. Use of corticosteroids may cause the breakdown of body protein and increase plasma ammonia levels.

PREGNANCY AND LACTATION
Pregnancy: Category C.
Lactation: It is not known whether this drug is excreted in human milk; caution in nursing.

MECHANISM OF ACTION
Prodrug of phenylacetate; rapidly metabolized to phenylacetate, which conjugates w/ glutamine via acetylation to form phenylacetylglutamine. Decreases elevated plasma ammonia glutamine levels and increases waste nitrogen excretion in the form of phenylacetylglutamine.

PHARMACOKINETICS
Absorption: Phenylbutyrate: (Tab) T_{max}= 1.35 hrs, C_{max}=218mcg/mL; (Powder) T_{max}=1 hr, C_{max}=195mcg/mL. Phenylacetate: (Tab) T_{max}=3.74 hrs, C_{max}=48.5mcg/mL; (Powder) T_{max}=3.55 hrs, C_{max}=45.3mcg/mL. **Metabolism:** Liver, kidney. **Elimination:** Kidneys (approx 80-100%, as phenylacetylglutamine); $T_{1/2}$= Phenylbutyrate: (Tab) 0.77 hr; (Powder) 0.76 hr. Phenylacetate: (Tab) 1.15 hrs; (Powder) 1.29 hrs.

PATIENT CONSIDERATIONS
Assessment: Assess for acute hyperammonemia, CHF, hepatic/renal insufficiency, inborn errors of β oxidation, Na^+ retention w/ edema, hypersensitivity to drug, pregnancy/nursing status, and possible drug interactions.

Monitoring: Monitor for hypersensitivity reactions and other adverse reactions. Monitor serum levels of phenylbutyrate and its metabolites, phenylacetate, and phenylacetylglutamine periodically. Routinely perform urinalysis, blood chemistry profiles, and hematologic tests.

Counseling: Instruct to take drug exactly as prescribed and to follow the prescribed diet. If a dose is missed, instruct to take it as soon as possible that same day. Inform that the total daily dose should be taken in equally divided amounts w/ meals. Instruct to inform physician of other medications being taken and when symptoms of sleepiness and lightheadedness occur.

BUSULFEX — busulfan   Rx

Class: Alkylating agent

> Causes severe and prolonged myelosuppression at the recommended dosage. Hematopoietic progenitor cell transplantation is required to prevent potentially fatal complications of the prolonged myelosuppression.

ADULT DOSAGE
Chronic Myeloid Leukemia

In Combination w/ Cyclophosphamide as a Conditioning Regimen Prior to Allogeneic Hematopoietic Progenitor Cell Transplantation:

Initial:
<12kg: 0.8mg/kg (ideal body weight [IBW] or actual body weight [whichever is lower]) q6h IV for 4 days for a total of 16 doses (Days -7, -6, -5, and -4)

PEDIATRIC DOSAGE
Pediatric use may not have been established

Obese/Severely Obese: Dose based on adjusted IBW; refer to PI for calculation

Give 60mg/kg of cyclophosphamide IV as a 1-hr infusion on each of the 2 days beginning no sooner than 6 hrs following the 16th dose of treatment (Days -3 and -2)

Premedication

Administer anticonvulsants (eg, benzodiazepines, phenytoin, valproic acid, or levetiracetam) 12 hrs prior to treatment to 24 hrs after the last dose of treatment.

Administer antiemetics prior to 1st dose of treatment and continue on a fixed schedule throughout treatment.

ADMINISTRATION

IV route

Use an administration set w/ minimal residual hold-up volume (2-5mL) for product administration.

Use gloves when preparing; if sol contacts the skin/mucosa, wash thoroughly w/ water.

Dilute w/ 0.9% NaCl or D5W; final concentration should be approx 0.5mg/mL.

Do not put into an IV bag or large-volume syringe that does not contain NaCl or D5W.

Always add busulfan to the diluent, not the diluent to the busulfan; mix thoroughly by inverting several times.

Use infusion pumps to administer diluted sol.

Set flow rate of the pump to deliver the entire prescribed dose over 2 hrs; rapid infusion not tested/not recommended.

Prior to and following each infusion, flush indwelling catheter line w/ approx 5mL of NaCl or D5W.

Do not infuse concomitantly w/ another IV sol of unknown compatibility.

STORAGE

Unopened: 2-8°C (36-46°F). **Diluted in 0.9% NaCl or D5W:** 25°C (77°F) for up to 8 hrs; complete the infusion w/in that time. **Diluted in 0.9% NaCl:** 2-8°C (36-46°F) for up to 12 hrs; complete the infusion w/in that time.

HOW SUPPLIED

Inj: 6mg/mL [10mL]

CONTRAINDICATIONS

History of hypersensitivity to any of its components.

WARNINGS/PRECAUTIONS

Use antibiotic therapy and platelet and RBC support when medically indicated. Seizures reported; caution in patients w/ history of a seizure disorder or head trauma. May be associated w/ increased risk of developing hepatic veno-occlusive disease; increased risk in patients who have received prior radiation therapy, ≥3 cycles of chemotherapy, or a prior progenitor cell transplant. Can cause fetal harm. Cardiac tamponade reported in pediatric patients w/ thalassemia; monitor for signs/symptoms and promptly evaluate/treat if suspected. Bronchopulmonary dysplasia w/ pulmonary fibrosis may occur following chronic therapy. May cause cellular dysplasia in many organs.

ADVERSE REACTIONS

N/V, stomatitis (mucositis), anorexia, insomnia, diarrhea, fever, hypomagnesemia, anxiety, abdominal pain, headache, hyperglycemia, hypokalemia, rash, asthenia, chills.

DRUG INTERACTIONS

Itraconazole decreases clearance. Phenytoin increases clearance. Use of acetaminophen prior to (<72 hrs) or concurrent w/ therapy may result in reduced busulfan clearance. Caution w/ other potentially epileptogenic drugs.

PREGNANCY AND LACTATION

Pregnancy: Can cause fetal harm based on animal data.
Lactation: It is not known if busulfan is present in human milk; d/c breastfeeding during treatment.
Reproductive Potential: Females of reproductive potential and males w/ female partners of reproductive potential should use effective contraception during and after treatment. Ovarian suppression and amenorrhea reported in premenopausal women. Sterility, azoospermia, and testicular atrophy reported in males.

MECHANISM OF ACTION

Alkylating agent; hydrolyzes to release the methanesulfonate groups, producing reactive carbonium ions that can alkylate DNA.

PHARMACOKINETICS

Absorption: C_{max}=1222ng/mL; AUC=1167µM•min. **Distribution:** Plasma protein binding (32.4%). **Metabolism:** Conjugation w/ glutathione; conjugate undergoes extensive oxidative metabolism in liver. **Elimination:** Urine (30%).

PATIENT CONSIDERATIONS

Assessment: Assess for history of hypersensitivity to any of the components, history of seizure disorder or head trauma, risk of developing hepatic veno-occlusive disease, pregnancy/nursing status, and possible drug interactions.
Monitoring: Monitor for seizures, hepatic veno-occlusive disease, cardiac tamponade, bronchopulmonary/cellular dysplasia, and other adverse reactions. Monitor CBCs, including WBC differentials, and quantitative platelet counts daily during treatment and until engraftment is demonstrated. Monitor serum

transaminases, alkaline phosphatase, and bilirubin daily through bone marrow transplant Day +28 to detect hepatotoxicity.
Counseling: Inform of the possibility of developing low blood cell counts and the need for hematopoietic progenitor cell infusion; instruct to immediately report to physician if fever develops. Inform of the risks associated w/ therapy (eg, veno-occlusive liver disease) as well as the plan for regular blood monitoring during therapy. Advise females of reproductive potential of the potential risk to a fetus and to inform physician w/ a known or suspected pregnancy. Advise females and males of reproductive potential to use effective contraception during and after treatment. Instruct to d/c breastfeeding during treatment. Advise females and males of reproductive potential that drug may cause temporary or permanent infertility.

CABOMETYX — cabozantinib

Class: Kinase inhibitor

Rx

ADULT DOSAGE	PEDIATRIC DOSAGE
Advanced Renal Cell Carcinoma	Pediatric use may not have been established
Use in patients who have received prior anti-angiogenic therapy	
60mg qd until patient no longer experiences clinical benefit or experiences unacceptable toxicity	
Missed Dose	
Do not take a missed dose w/in 12 hrs of next dose	

DOSING CONSIDERATIONS

Concomitant Medications

Strong CYP3A4 Inhibitor:
Reduce daily Cabometyx dose by 20mg; resume dose that was used prior to initiating CYP3A4 inhibitor 2-3 days after discontinuation of the strong inhibitor
Do not ingest foods (eg, grapefruit, grapefruit juice) or nutritional supplements that are known to inhibit CYP450 during treatment

Strong CYP3A4 Inducer:
Increase daily Cabometyx dose by 20mg as tolerated; resume dose that was used prior to initiating CYP3A4 inducer 2-3 days after discontinuation of the strong inducer
Max: 80mg

Renal Impairment

Mild or Moderate: No dosage adjustment is required
Severe: There is no experience in patients w/ severe renal impairment

Hepatic Impairment

Mild/Moderate (Child-Pugh Score A or B): Initial: 40mg qd
Severe: Not recommended for use

Adverse Reactions

Withhold for NCI CTCAE Grade 4 adverse reactions, and for Grade 3 or intolerable Grade 2 adverse reactions that cannot be managed w/ a dose reduction or supportive care

Upon resolution/improvement (eg, return to baseline or resolution to Grade 1), reduce dose as follows:
- If previously receiving 60mg qd, resume at 40mg qd
- If previously receiving 40mg qd, resume at 20mg qd
- If previously receiving 20mg qd, resume at 20mg if tolerated, otherwise, d/c

Discontinuation

Permanently d/c for any of the following:
- Development of unmanageable fistula or GI perforation
- Severe hemorrhage
- Arterial thromboembolic event (eg, MI, cerebral infarction)
- Hypertensive crisis or severe hypertension despite optimal medical management
- Nephrotic syndrome
- Reversible posterior leukoencephalopathy syndrome (RPLS)

Other Important Modifications

Stop treatment at least 28 days prior to scheduled surgery, including dental surgery

ADMINISTRATION

Oral route

- Do not substitute Cabometyx tabs w/ cabozantinib caps.
- Do not administer w/ food; do not eat for at least 2 hrs before and at least 1 hr after taking tab.
- Swallow tab whole; do not crush.

STORAGE

20-25°C (68-77°F); excursions permitted from 15-30°C (59-86°F).

HOW SUPPLIED

Tab: 20mg, 40mg, 60mg

WARNINGS/PRECAUTIONS

See Dosing Considerations. Severe hemorrhage reported; do not administer to patients that have or are at risk for severe hemorrhage. GI perforations/fistulas reported; monitor for symptoms and d/c use in patients who experience a fistula which cannot be appropriately managed or a GI perforation. Increased incidence of thrombotic events; d/c if acute MI or any other arterial thromboembolic complication develops. Increased incidence of treatment-emergent HTN; monitor BP prior to initiation and regularly during treatment. Withhold for HTN that is not adequately controlled w/ medical management; when controlled, resume at reduced dose. Diarrhea reported; withhold in patients who develop intolerable Grade 2 diarrhea or Grade 3-4 diarrhea that cannot be managed w/ standard antidiarrheal treatments until improvement to Grade 1; resume at a reduced dose. Palmar-plantar erythrodysesthesia syndrome (PPES) reported; withhold in patients who develop intolerable Grade 2 PPES or Grade 3 PPES until improvement to Grade 1; resume at a reduced dose. RPLS reported; perform an evaluation for RPLS if presenting w/ seizures, headache, visual disturbances, confusion, or altered mental function. May cause fetal harm.

ADVERSE REACTIONS
Diarrhea, fatigue, N/V, decreased appetite, PPES, HTN, decreased weight, constipation.

DRUG INTERACTIONS
See Dosing Considerations. Strong CYP3A4 inhibitors (eg, boceprevir, clarithromycin, saquinavir) may increase exposure and may increase the risk of exposure-related toxicity. Strong CYP3A4 inducers (eg, rifampin, phenytoin, carbamazepine) may decrease exposure and this may lead to reduced efficacy.

PREGNANCY AND LACTATION
Pregnancy: May cause fetal harm.
Lactation: Not for use in nursing.
Females and Males of Reproductive Potential: Females of reproductive potential should use effective contraception during treatment and for 4 months after final dose. May impair fertility in females and males.

MECHANISM OF ACTION
Kinase inhibitor; inhibits the tyrosine kinase activity of MET, VEGFR-1, -2, and -3, AXL, RET, ROS1, TYRO3, MER, KIT, TRKB, FLT-3, and TIE-2. These receptor tyrosine kinases are involved in both normal cellular function and pathologic processes (eg, oncogenesis, metastasis, tumor angiogenesis, drug resistance, maintenance of tumor microenvironment).

PHARMACOKINETICS
Absorption: T_{max}=2-3 hrs (median). **Distribution:** V_d=319L; plasma protein binding (≥99.7%). **Metabolism:** Via CYP3A4. **Elimination:** Urine (27%), feces (54%, 43% unchanged); $T_{1/2}$=99 hrs.

PATIENT CONSIDERATIONS
Assessment: Assess for risk for severe hemorrhage, hepatic impairment, pregnancy/nursing status, and possible drug interactions. Assess BP.

Monitoring: Monitor for severe hemorrhage, fistulas, GI perforations, thrombotic events, diarrhea, PPES, RPLS, and other adverse reactions. Monitor BP.

Counseling: Instruct on proper use. Instruct to contact healthcare provider to seek immediate medical attention for signs or symptoms of unusual severe bleeding/hemorrhage. Instruct to contact healthcare provider at the first signs of poorly formed or loose stool or an increased frequency of bowel movements; for progressive or intolerable rash; before any planned surgeries, including dental surgery; and if significant weight loss occurs. Advise to inform healthcare provider of all prescription or nonprescription medication or herbal products that the patient is taking. Advise females of reproductive potential of the potential risk to a fetus and instruct to contact healthcare provider if pregnancy occurs or is suspected during treatment. Advise patients of reproductive potential to use effective contraception during treatment and for at least 4 months after the final dose. Advise not to breastfeed during treatment and for 4 months following the last dose.

CAMPATH — alemtuzumab   Rx
Class: Monoclonal antibody/CD52 blocker

> Serious, including fatal, pancytopenia/marrow hypoplasia, autoimmune idiopathic thrombocytopenia, and autoimmune hemolytic anemia may occur; single doses >30mg or cumulative doses >90mg/week increase the incidence of pancytopenia. May result in serious, including fatal, infusion reactions; monitor during infusion and withhold therapy for Grade 3 or 4 infusion reactions. Gradually escalate therapy to the recommended dose at the initiation of therapy and after interruption of therapy for ≥7 days. Serious, including fatal, bacterial, viral, fungal, and protozoan infections may occur; administer prophylaxis against *Pneumocystis jiroveci* pneumonia (PCP) and herpes virus infections.

ADULT DOSAGE
B-Cell Chronic Lymphocytic Leukemia

Recommended Dosing Regimen:
Gradually escalate to max recommended single dose of 30mg
Escalation ordinarily accomplished in 3-7 days

Escalation Strategy:
1. Administer 3mg/day until infusion reactions are ≤Grade 2
2. Then administer 10mg/day until infusion reactions are ≤Grade 2
3. Then administer 30mg/day 3X/ week on alternate days

Total duration of therapy, including escalation, is 12 weeks

Premedication
50mg diphenhydramine and 500-1000mg acetaminophen 30 min prior to first infusion and each dose escalation

PEDIATRIC DOSAGE
Pediatric use may not have been established

DOSING CONSIDERATIONS
Concomitant Medications
Pneumocystis jiroveci Pneumonia Prophylaxis:
Trimethoprim/sulfamethoxazole DS bid 3X/week
Herpetic Prophylaxis:
Famciclovir 250mg bid or equivalent

Adverse Reactions
ANC <250/μL and/or Platelets ≤25,000/μL:
1st Occurrence: Withhold therapy, then resume at 30mg when ANC ≥500/μL and platelets ≥50,000/μL
2nd Occurrence: Withhold therapy, then resume at 10mg when ANC ≥500/μL and platelets ≥50,000/μL
3rd Occurrence: D/C therapy

≥50% Decrease From Baseline in Patients Initiating Therapy with Baseline ANC ≤250/μL and/or Baseline Platelets ≤25,000/μL:
1st Occurrence: Withhold therapy, then resume at 30mg upon return to baseline value(s)
2nd Occurrence: Withhold therapy, then resume at 10mg upon return to baseline value(s)
3rd Occurrence: D/C therapy

ADMINISTRATION
IV route
Administer as an IV infusion over 2 hrs
Do not administer as IV push or bolus
Do not add or simultaneously infuse other drugs through the same IV line
Refer to PI for further preparation and administration instructions

STORAGE
2-8°C (36-46°F). Do not freeze. If accidentally frozen, thaw at 2-8°C (36-46°F) before administration. Protect from direct sunlight. Diluted Sol: 2-8°C (36-46°F) or 15-30°C (59-86°F). Protect from light. Use within 8 hrs.

HOW SUPPLIED
Inj: 30mg/mL [1mL]

WARNINGS/PRECAUTIONS
Prolonged myelosuppression and pure red cell/bone marrow aplasia reported; withhold therapy for severe cytopenias (except lymphopenia) and d/c for autoimmune cytopenias or recurrent/persistent severe cytopenias (except lymphopenia). Severe and prolonged lymphopenia with increased incidence of opportunistic infections reported; administer PCP and herpes viral prophylaxis during therapy and for a minimum of 2 months after completion of therapy or until the CD4+ count is ≥200 cells/μL, whichever occurs later. Monitor for cytomegalovirus (CMV) infection during treatment and for at least 2 months after completion of treatment; withhold therapy for serious infections and during CMV infection treatment or confirmed CMV viremia. Administer only irradiated blood products to avoid transfusion-associated graft versus host disease unless emergent circumstances dictate immediate transfusion.

ADVERSE REACTIONS
Cytopenias, infusion reactions, CMV and other infections, immunosuppression, nausea, emesis, abdominal pain, insomnia, anxiety, cardiac dysrhythmias, HTN, headache, dyspnea, diarrhea.

DRUG INTERACTIONS
Do not administer live viral vaccines to patients who have recently received therapy.

PREGNANCY AND LACTATION
Category C, not for use in nursing.

MECHANISM OF ACTION
Monoclonal antibody/CD52-blocker; binds to CD52 antigen. Proposed mechanism of action is antibody-dependent cellular-mediated lysis following cell surface binding to the leukemic cells.

PHARMACOKINETICS
Distribution: V_d=0.18L/kg; crosses placenta. **Elimination:** $T_{1/2}$=11 hrs (after first 30mg dose), 6 days (after last 30mg dose).

PATIENT CONSIDERATIONS
Assessment: Assess pregnancy/nursing status and for possible drug interactions. Obtain baseline CBCs and platelet counts.

Monitoring: Monitor CBCs weekly and more frequently if worsening anemia, neutropenia, or thrombocytopenia occurs. Assess CD4+ counts after treatment until recovery to ≥200 cells/μL. Monitor for CMV infection during treatment and for at least 2 months after completion of treatment. Monitor for cytopenias, infusion reactions, immunosuppression, infection, and other adverse reactions.

Counseling: Advise to report any signs/symptoms of cytopenias, infusion reactions, and infection. Counsel of the need to take premedications and prophylactic anti-infectives as prescribed. Advise that irradiation of blood products is required. Inform not to be immunized with live viral vaccines if recently treated with the drug. Advise to use effective contraceptive methods during treatment and for a minimum of 6 months following therapy.

CAMPTOSAR — irinotecan hydrochloride   Rx
Class: Topoisomerase I inhibitor

> Early and late forms of diarrhea can occur. Early diarrhea may be accompanied by cholinergic symptoms; may be prevented or ameliorated by atropine. Late diarrhea can be life-threatening; treat properly w/ loperamide. Monitor patients w/ diarrhea; give fluid/electrolytes PRN or institute antibiotic therapy if ileus, fever, or severe neutropenia develops. Interrupt therapy and reduce subsequent doses if severe diarrhea occurs. Severe myelosuppression may occur.

ADULT DOSAGE

Metastatic Carcinoma of the Colon/Rectum

1st-line therapy in combination w/ 5-fluorouracil (5-FU) and leucovorin (LV) for metastatic carcinoma of the colon or rectum, and for patients w/ metastatic carcinoma of the colon or rectum whose disease has recurred or progressed following initial 5-FU therapy

Combination w/ 5-FU and LV: Administer as 90-min infusion followed by LV and 5-FU

Regimen 1 (6-Week Cycle w/ Bolus 5-FU/LV): 125mg/m^2 IV over 90 min on Days 1, 8, 15, and 22

Modified Dose Levels:
Starting Dose: 125mg/m^2
Dose Level-1: 100mg/m^2
Dose Level-2: 75mg/m^2

Regimen 2 (6-Week Cycle w/ Infusional 5-FU/LV): 180mg/m^2 IV over 90 min on Days 1, 15, and 29

Modified Dose Levels:
Starting Dose: 180mg/m^2
Dose Level-1: 150mg/m^2
Dose Level-2: 120mg/m^2

Both Regimens:
Begin next cycle on Day 43
Refer to PI for doses of 5-FU/LV

Single Therapy:
Regimen 1 (Weekly): 125mg/m^2 IV over 90 min on Days 1, 8, 15, and 22 followed by 2-week rest

Titrate: Subsequent doses may be adjusted as high as 150mg/m^2 or to as low as 50mg/m^2 in 25-50mg/m^2 decrements, depending upon individual tolerance

Modified Dose Levels:
Starting Dose: 125mg/m^2
Dose Level-1: 100mg/m^2
Dose Level-2: 75mg/m^2

Regimen 2 (Every 3 Weeks): 350mg/m^2 IV over 90 min once every 3 weeks

Titrate: Subsequent doses may be adjusted as low as 200mg/m^2 in 50mg/m^2 decrements, depending upon individual tolerance

Modified Dose Levels:
Starting Dose: 350mg/m^2
Dose Level-1: 300mg/m^2
Dose Level-2: 250mg/m^2

DOSING CONSIDERATIONS

Renal Impairment
Dialysis: Not recommended

Other Important Considerations
Reduced UGT1A1 Activity
Consider reducing starting dose by at least one level for known homozygous UGT1A1*28 allele
Subsequent dose modifications are based on individual tolerance; refer to PI

Prior Pelvic or Abdominal Radiotherapy/Performance Status of 2/Increased Bilirubin
Consider reducing starting dose by one level

Refer to PI for Subsequent Dose Modifications for Single-Agent Schedules
All dose modifications should be based on worst preceding toxicity

Elderly
In patients ≥70 yrs, the once-every-3-week-dosage schedule should be 300mg/m^2

ADMINISTRATION
IV route

Dilute in D5 inj or 0.9% NaCl inj to a final concentration of 0.12-2.8mg/mL
Do not add other drugs to the infusion sol

Stability
Use immediately after reconstitution, since it contains no antibacterial preservative
Use admixture prepared w/ D5 Inj w/in 24 hrs if refrigerated (2-8°C or 36-46°F)
Use admixture prepared w/ D5 Inj or NaCl w/in 4 hrs if kept at room temperature
If reconstitution and dilution are performed under strict aseptic conditions (eg, Laminar Air Flow bench), use sol w/in 12 hrs at room temperature or 24 hrs if refrigerated (2-8°C or 36-46°F)

STORAGE
15-30°C (59-86°F). Protect from light. Keep in carton until time of use. Avoid freezing.

PEDIATRIC DOSAGE
Pediatric use may not have been established

HOW SUPPLIED
Inj: 20mg/mL [2mL, 5mL, 15mL]

WARNINGS/PRECAUTIONS
Not recommended in patients on dialysis or w/ bilirubin >2mg/dL. If late diarrhea occurs, delay subsequent weekly therapy until return of pretreatment bowel function for at least 24 hrs w/o antidiarrheals; decrease subsequent doses if late diarrhea is Grade 2, 3, or 4. Avoid diuretics or laxatives in patients w/ diarrhea. Deaths due to sepsis following severe neutropenia reported; d/c if neutropenic fever occurs, or if ANC <1000/mm^3. Increased risk for neutropenia in patients homozygous for the UGT1A1*28 allele. Severe anaphylactic/anaphylactoid reactions reported; d/c if anaphylactic reaction occurs. Renal impairment/acute renal failure reported, usually in patients who became volume depleted from severe vomiting and/or diarrhea. Interstitial pulmonary disease (IPD) events reported; d/c therapy if IPD is diagnosed and institute appropriate treatment. Should not be used w/ a regimen of 5-FU/LV administered for 4-5 consecutive days every 4 weeks due to increased toxicity. Increased toxicity in patients w/ performance status 2 at baseline. May cause fetal harm. Caution to avoid extravasation and monitor for inflammation at infusion site. Premedicate w/ antiemetics at least 30 min prior to therapy. Consider prophylactic/therapeutic administration of atropine if cholinergic symptoms develop. Caution in patients w/ deficient glucuronidation of bilirubin (eg, Gilbert's syndrome), renal/hepatic impairment, previous pelvic/abdominal irradiation, and in elderly. Avoid in unresolved bowel obstruction.

ADVERSE REACTIONS
N/V, diarrhea, neutropenia, abdominal pain, anemia, asthenia, anorexia, alopecia, fever, constipation, leukopenia, decreased body weight.

DRUG INTERACTIONS
Avoid concurrent irradiation therapy. Greater incidence of akathisia reported w/ prochlorperazine. Exposure is substantially reduced w/ CYP3A4 enzyme-inducing anticonvulsants phenytoin, phenobarbital, carbamazepine, or St. John's wort; consider substituting non-enzyme-inducing therapies at least 2 weeks prior to initiation of treatment. Ketoconazole (a CYP3A4 and UGT1A1 inhibitor) increased exposure; coadministration w/ other inhibitors of CYP3A4 (eg, clarithromycin, lopinavir, itraconazole) or UGT1A1 (eg, atazanavir, gemfibrozil, indinavir) may increase exposure. D/C strong CYP3A4 inhibitors at least 1 week prior to starting therapy. Do not administer w/ strong CYP3A4 inducers or strong CYP3A4 or UGT1A1 inhibitors unless there are no therapeutic alternatives. May prolong neuromuscular-blocking effects of suxamethonium, and the neuromuscular blockade of nondepolarizing drugs may be antagonized.

PREGNANCY AND LACTATION
Category D, not for use in nursing.

MECHANISM OF ACTION
Topoisomerase I inhibitor; binds to topoisomerase I-DNA complex and prevents religation of single-strand breaks.

PHARMACOKINETICS
Absorption: Irinotecan: C_{max}=1660ng/mL (125mg/m^2), 3392ng/mL (340mg/m^2); AUC_{0-24}=10,200ng•h/mL (125mg/m^2), 20,604ng•h/mL (340mg/m^2). SN-38: C_{max}=26.3ng/mL (125mg/m^2), 56ng/mL (340mg/m^2); AUC_{0-24}=229ng•h/mL (125mg/m^2), 474ng•h/mL (340mg/m^2). **Distribution:** Irinotecan: V_d=110L/m^2 (125mg/m^2), 234L/m^2 (340mg/m^2); plasma protein binding (30-68%). SN-38: Plasma protein binding (95%). **Metabolism:** Irinotecan: Liver (extensive) by esterases to SN-38 (active metabolite), and by CYP3A4-mediated oxidation. SN-38: UGT1A1 mediating glucuronidation. **Elimination:** Irinotecan: Urine (11-20%); $T_{1/2}$=5.8 hrs (125mg/m^2), 11.7 hrs (340mg/m^2). SN-38: Urine (<1%); $T_{1/2}$=10.4 hrs (125mg/m^2), 21 hrs (340mg/m^2).

PATIENT CONSIDERATIONS

Assessment: Assess for unresolved bowel obstruction, UGT1A1 status, deficient glucuronidation of bilirubin (Gilbert's syndrome), pelvic/abdominal irradiation, preexisting lung disease, renal/hepatic impairment, pregnancy/nursing status, and possible drug interactions. Obtain baseline CBC.

Monitoring: Monitor for diarrhea, signs/symptoms of neutropenia, neutropenic complications (eg, neutropenic fever), ileus, respiratory symptoms, inflammation and/or extravasation of infusion site, cholinergic symptoms, hypersensitivity reactions, and other adverse reactions. For patients w/ diarrhea, monitor for signs/symptoms of dehydration, electrolyte imbalance, ileus, fever, or severe neutropenia. Monitor CBC w/ differential.

Counseling: Instruct to seek medical attention if experiencing diarrhea for 1st time during treatment, black or bloody stools, dehydration, inability to take fluids by mouth due to N/V, or inability to get diarrhea under control w/in 24 hrs. Inform about potential for dizziness or visual disturbances, which may occur w/in 24 hrs. Explain importance of routine blood cell counts. Instruct to report any occurrence of fever or infection. Inform that therapy may cause fetal harm, and advise to avoid becoming pregnant while on therapy. Explain about the possibility of alopecia. Inform that the product contains sorbitol.

CAPRELSA — vandetanib

Class: Kinase inhibitor

Rx

> May prolong the QT interval. Torsades de pointes and sudden death reported. Avoid w/ hypocalcemia, hypokalemia, hypomagnesemia, or long QT syndrome; correct hypocalcemia, hypokalemia, and/or hypomagnesemia prior to therapy. Monitor electrolytes periodically. Avoid drugs known to prolong QT interval. Only prescribers and pharmacies certified w/ the restricted distribution program are able to prescribe and dispense this therapy.

ADULT DOSAGE

Medullary Thyroid Cancer

Symptomatic or progressive cancer in patients w/ unresectable locally advanced or metastatic disease

300mg qd until disease progression or unacceptable toxicity occurs

Missed Dose

Do not take a missed dose w/in 12 hrs of the next dose

PEDIATRIC DOSAGE

Pediatric use may not have been established

DOSING CONSIDERATIONS

Renal Impairment

Moderate (CrCl ≥30 to <50mL/min) and Severe (CrCl <30mL/min):

Initial: 200mg qd

Hepatic Impairment

Moderate and Severe: Not recommended for use

Adverse Reactions

Corrected QT Interval, Fridericia (QTcF) >500 ms:

Interrupt therapy, then resume at a reduced dose when the QTcF returns to <450 ms

CTCAE Grade ≥3 Toxicities:

Interrupt therapy, then resume at 200mg (two 100mg tabs) when toxicity resolves or improves to CTCAE Grade 1

For recurrent toxicities, reduce the dose to 100mg after resolution or improvement to CTCAE Grade 1 severity, if continued treatment is warranted

ADMINISTRATION

Oral route

Take w/ or w/o food.
Do not crush tabs.
May disperse in 2 oz of water by stirring for approx 10 min (will not completely dissolve); do not use other liquids for dispersion. Swallow immediately and mix any remaining residue w/ additional 4 oz of water and swallow. The dispersion can also be administered through nasogastric or gastrostomy tubes.

STORAGE

25°C (77°F); excursions permitted to 15-30°C (59-86°F).

HOW SUPPLIED

Tab: 100mg, 300mg

CONTRAINDICATIONS

Congenital long QT syndrome.

WARNINGS/PRECAUTIONS

See Dosing Considerations. Caution in patients w/ indolent, asymptomatic, or slowly progressing disease. Do not start therapy w/ QTcF interval >450 ms. Avoid w/ history of torsades de pointes, bradyarrhythmias, or uncompensated heart failure (HF). Severe and sometimes fatal skin reactions (eg, Stevens-Johnson syndrome, toxic epidermal necrosis) reported; permanently d/c and refer the patient for urgent medical evaluation. Photosensitivity reactions may occur during treatment and up to 4 months after discontinuation. Interstitial lung disease (ILD) or pneumonitis reported; interrupt treatment for acute/worsening pulmonary symptoms and d/c if ILD is confirmed. Ischemic cerebrovascular events and serious hemorrhagic events reported; d/c if severe. Avoid w/ recent history of hemoptysis of ≥1/2 tsp of red blood. HF reported; monitor for signs/symptoms of HF and consider discontinuation in patients w/ HF. Diarrhea of ≥Grade 3 reported; interrupt therapy for severe diarrhea and resume at a reduced dose upon improvement. HTN, including hypertensive crisis, may occur; monitor for HTN. Reduce dose or interrupt therapy if HTN occurs; do not resume therapy if BP cannot be controlled. Reversible posterior leukoencephalopathy syndrome (RPLS) reported; d/c in patients w/ RPLS. Increased exposure w/ impaired renal function. May cause fetal harm.

ADVERSE REACTIONS

Diarrhea/colitis, rash, acneiform dermatitis, HTN, nausea, headache, URTIs, decreased appetite, abdominal pain.

DRUG INTERACTIONS

See Boxed Warning. Rifampicin, a strong CYP3A4 inducer, decreases levels. Avoid use w/ strong CYP3A4 inducers, St. John's wort, antiarrhythmic drugs (eg, amiodarone, disopyramide, procainamide), and other drugs that may prolong QT interval (eg, chloroquine, clarithromycin, dolasetron). Increased plasma levels of metformin that is transported by organic cation transporter type 2 (OCT2); use caution and closely monitor for toxicities when administering w/ drugs that are transported by OCT2. Increases digoxin levels; use w/ caution and closely monitor for toxicities. May require dose increase of thyroid replacement therapy; if signs or symptoms of hypothyroidism occur, examine thyroid hormone levels and adjust thyroid replacement therapy accordingly.

PREGNANCY AND LACTATION

Pregnancy: Category D.
Lactation: Not for use in nursing.
Reproductive Potential: Females of reproductive potential should avoid pregnancy. Use effective contraception during treatment and up to 4 months after the last dose.

MECHANISM OF ACTION

Multikinase inhibitor; inhibits the tyrosine kinase activity of the epidermal growth factor receptor and vascular endothelial growth factor receptor families, RET, BRK, TIE2, and members of the EPH receptor and Src kinase families, which are involved in both normal cellular function and pathologic processes such as oncogenesis, metastasis, tumor angiogenesis, and maintenance of the tumor microenvironment.

PHARMACOKINETICS

Absorption: Slow; T_{max}=6 hrs (median). **Distribution:** V_d=7450L; plasma protein binding (90% in vitro). **Metabolism:** Via CYP3A4; vandetanib N-oxide and N-desmethyl vandetanib (metabolites). **Elimination:** Urine (25%), feces (44%); $T_{1/2}$=19 days (median).

PATIENT CONSIDERATIONS

Assessment: Assess for congenital long QT syndrome, history of torsades de pointes or hemoptysis, bradyarrhythmias, uncompensated HF, renal/hepatic impairment, pregnancy/nursing status, and possible drug interactions. Obtain baseline ECG, serum K^+, Ca^{2+}, Mg^{2+}, and TSH levels.

Monitoring: Monitor for QT interval prolongation, torsades de pointes, skin/photosensitivity reactions, ILD, ischemic cerebrovascular events, hemorrhage, HF, diarrhea, hypothyroidism, HTN, RPLS, and other adverse reactions. Monitor ECG, serum K^+, Ca^{2+}, Mg^{2+}, and TSH levels at 2-4 weeks and 8-12 weeks after initial therapy, every 3 months thereafter, and following any dose reduction for QT prolongation, or any dose interruptions >2 weeks. Monitor renal function.

Counseling: Advise to take ud. Instruct to contact physician in the event of syncope, pre-syncopal symptoms, and cardiac palpitations. Inform patients that the physician will monitor electrolytes and ECGs during treatment. Advise to contact physician in the event of skin reactions or rash, sudden onset or worsening of breathlessness, persistent cough or fever, diarrhea, seizures, headaches, visual disturbances, confusion, or difficulty thinking. Advise patients of reproductive potential to use effective contraception during therapy and for at least 4 months after the last dose and to immediately contact physician if pregnancy is suspected or confirmed. Advise to d/c nursing while on therapy. Instruct to use appropriate sun protection due to the increased susceptibility to sunburn while on therapy and for at least 4 months after drug discontinuation.

CARBAGLU — carglumic acid   **Rx**

Class: Carbamoyl phosphate synthetase 1 activator

ADULT DOSAGE

Hyperammonemia

Divide total daily dose into 2-4 doses and round to the nearest 100mg

Acute Hyperammonemia:

Adjunctive therapy for acute hyperammonemia due to the deficiency of the hepatic enzyme N-acetylglutamate synthase (NAGS)

Initial: 100-250mg/kg/day
Titrate: Adjust dose based on plasma ammonia levels and clinical symptoms

During acute episodes, concomitant administration w/ other ammonia-lowering therapies (eg, alternate pathway medications), hemodialysis, and dietary protein restriction are recommended

Chronic Hyperammonemia:

Maint therapy for chronic hyperammonemia due to the deficiency of the hepatic enzyme NAGS

Titrate to target normal plasma ammonia level for age; maint doses usually is <100mg/kg/day

During maint therapy, concomitant use of other ammonia-lowering therapies and protein restriction may be reduced or discontinued based on plasma ammonia levels

PEDIATRIC DOSAGE

Hyperammonemia

Divide total daily dose into 2-4 doses

Acute Hyperammonemia:

Adjunctive therapy for acute hyperammonemia due to the deficiency of the hepatic enzyme NAGS

Initial: 100-250mg/kg/day
Titrate: Adjust dose based on plasma ammonia levels and clinical symptoms

During acute episodes, concomitant administration w/ other ammonia-lowering therapies (eg, alternate pathway medications), hemodialysis, and dietary protein restriction are recommended

Chronic Hyperammonemia:

Maint therapy for chronic hyperammonemia due to the deficiency of the hepatic enzyme NAGS

Titrate to target normal plasma ammonia level for age; maint doses usually is <100mg/kg/day

During maint therapy, concomitant use of other ammonia-lowering therapies and protein restriction may be reduced or discontinued based on plasma ammonia levels

---

ADMINISTRATION

Oral/NG route

Do not swallow whole or crush tabs.

Preparation for Oral Administration

Adults:

1. Disperse each 200mg tab in a minimum of 2.5mL of water and administer immediately; tabs do not dissolve completely in water and undissolved particles of the tab may remain in the mixing container.
2. To ensure complete delivery of dose, rinse the mixing container w/ additional volumes of water and swallow the contents immediately.
3. Do not use in other foods and liquids.

Pediatrics (Using an Oral Syringe):

1. Mix each 200mg tab in 2.5mL of water to yield a concentration of 80mg/mL in a mixing container.
2. Shake gently to allow for quick dispersal.
3. Draw up the appropriate volume of dispersion in an oral syringe and administer immediately; discard the unused portion.
4. Refill the oral syringe w/ a minimum volume of water (1-2mL) and administer immediately.

Preparation for NG Tube Administration

Adults:
1. Mix each 200mg tab in a minimum of 2.5mL of water.
2. Shake gently to allow for quick dispersal.
3. Administer the dispersion immediately through the NG tube.
4. Flush w/ additional water to clear the NG tube.

Pediatrics:
1. Mix each 200mg tab in 2.5mL of water to yield a concentration of 80mg/mL in a mixing container.
2. Shake gently to allow for quick dispersal.
3. Draw up the appropriate volume of dispersion and administer immediately through a NG tube; discard the unused portion.
4. Flush w/ additional water to clear the NG tube.

STORAGE
Before Opening: 2-8°C (36-46°F). **After Opening:** Do not refrigerate or store >30°C (86°F). Protect from moisture. Discard 1 month after 1st opening.

HOW SUPPLIED
Tab: 200mg* *scored

WARNINGS/PRECAUTIONS
Any episode of acute symptomatic hyperammonemia should be treated as a life-threatening emergency; treatment may require dialysis, preferably hemodialysis. Uncontrolled hyperammonemia can rapidly result in brain injury/damage or death; promptly use all therapies necessary to reduce plasma ammonia levels. Monitor plasma ammonia levels, neurological status, lab tests, and clinical responses during treatment. Maintain plasma ammonia levels w/in normal range for age via individual dose adjustment. Maintain complete protein restriction for 24-48 hrs and maximize caloric supplementation to reverse catabolism and nitrogen turnover.

ADVERSE REACTIONS
Infections, vomiting, abdominal pain, pyrexia, tonsillitis, anemia, ear infection, diarrhea, nasopharyngitis, headache.

PREGNANCY AND LACTATION
Pregnancy: Category C.
Lactation: Not for use in nursing.

MECHANISM OF ACTION
Carbamoyl phosphate synthetase 1 (CPS 1) activator; a synthetic analogue of N-acetylglutamate (NAG). Acts as a replacement for NAG in NAGS deficiency patients by activating CPS 1, the enzyme that converts ammonia into urea.

PHARMACOKINETICS
Absorption: T_{max}=3 hrs (median). **Distribution:** V_d=2657L. **Metabolism:** Via intestinal bacterial flora. **Elimination:** Urine (9%, unchanged), feces (up to 60%, unchanged), lungs; $T_{1/2}$=5.6 hrs (median).

PATIENT CONSIDERATIONS
Assessment: Assess plasma ammonia levels and pregnancy/nursing status.

Monitoring: Monitor plasma ammonia levels, neurological status, lab tests, and clinical responses.

Counseling: Advise that when plasma ammonia levels have normalized, dietary protein intake can usually be increased w/ the goal of unrestricted protein intake. Instruct not to breastfeed while on therapy. Inform of the most common adverse reactions (eg, vomiting, abdominal pain, pyrexia).

CARBOPLATIN — carboplatin   Rx

Class: Platinum analogue

Administer under the supervision of a qualified physician experienced in the use of cancer chemotherapeutic agents. Appropriate management of therapy and complications is possible only when adequate treatment facilities are readily available. Bone marrow suppression is dose-related and may be severe, resulting in infection and/or bleeding. Anemia may be cumulative and may require transfusion support. Vomiting may also occur frequently. Anaphylactic-like reactions reported and may occur within minutes of administration; epinephrine, corticosteroids, and antihistamines have been employed to alleviate symptoms.

ADULT DOSAGE
Ovarian Carcinoma

Do not repeat intermittent courses until neutrophil count is ≥2000 and platelet count is ≥100,000

Single Agent:
360mg/m² every 4 weeks

Combination with Cyclophosphamide:
Carboplatin: 300mg/m² every 4 weeks for 6 cycles
Cyclophosphamide: 600mg/m² every 4 weeks for 6 cycles

Alternative Formula Dosing:
Total Dose (mg) = (target AUC) x (GFR + 25)

PEDIATRIC DOSAGE
Pediatric use may not have been established

DOSING CONSIDERATIONS
Renal Impairment
CrCl 41-59mL/min: Administer 250mg/m² on Day 1
CrCl 16-40mL/min: Administer 200mg/m² on Day 1

Adverse Reactions
Platelets >100,000 and Neutrophils >2000: Administer 125% of dose
Platelets <50,000 and Neutrophils <500: Administer 75% of dose
Refer to PI for formula dosing

Elderly
Use formula dosing

ADMINISTRATION
IV route

Administer by an infusion lasting ≥15 min
Avoid preparing or administering inj with needles or IV sets containing aluminum parts

Preparation of IV Sol
1. Sol may be further diluted to concentrations as low as 0.5mg/mL with 5% Dextrose in Water or 0.9% Sodium Chloride Injection, USP
2. When prepared as directed, sol is stable for 8 hrs at room temperature (25°C)

STORAGE
Unopened Vials: 20-25°C (68-77°F). Protect from light. Opened Vials: 25°C (77°F) for up to 14 days following multiple needle entries. Further Diluted Sol: 25°C (77°F) for 8 hrs. Refer to PI for handling and disposal instructions.

HOW SUPPLIED
Inj: 10mg/mL [5mL, 15mL, 45mL, 60mL]

CONTRAINDICATIONS
History of severe allergic reactions to cisplatin or other platinum-containing compounds, or mannitol; severe bone marrow depression; significant bleeding.

WARNINGS/PRECAUTIONS
Frequently monitor peripheral blood counts during treatment and, when appropriate, until recovery is achieved. Increased bone marrow suppression in patients who have received prior therapy, especially regimens with cisplatin, and with renal impairment. May induce emesis; may be more severe in patients previously receiving emetogenic therapy. Increased incidence of peripheral neurotoxicity in patients >65 yrs of age and in patients previously treated with cisplatin. Loss of vision, which can be complete for light and colors, reported with higher than recommended doses. High doses (>4X the recommended dose) resulted in severe LFT abnormalities. May cause fetal harm. Aluminum may react with drug, causing precipitate formation and loss of potency.

ADVERSE REACTIONS
N/V, thrombocytopenia, neutropenia, leukopenia, anemia, pain, asthenia, central neurotoxicity, electrolyte loss, SrCr/BUN/Bilirubin/AST/alkaline phosphatase elevations.

DRUG INTERACTIONS
Bone marrow depression may be more severe with other bone marrow suppressing drugs or with radiotherapy; use with other bone marrow suppressing drugs must be carefully managed with respect to dosage and timing to minimize additive effects. Increased renal and/or audiologic toxicity with aminoglycosides; use with caution. May potentiate renal effects of nephrotoxic compounds.

PREGNANCY AND LACTATION
Category D, not for use in nursing.

MECHANISM OF ACTION
Platinum coordination compound; produces predominantly interstrand DNA cross-links.

PHARMACOKINETICS
Distribution: V_d=16L. **Elimination:** Urine (65% unchanged within 12 hrs; 71% unchanged within 24 hrs); $T_{1/2}$=5 days (platinum).

PATIENT CONSIDERATIONS
Assessment: Assess for severe bone marrow depression, significant bleeding, history of severe allergic reactions to drug, other platinum-containing compounds, or mannitol, renal impairment, pregnancy/nursing status, and possible drug interactions.

Monitoring: Monitor for bone marrow suppression, anemia, anaphylactic-like reactions, and other adverse reactions. Monitor peripheral blood counts.

Counseling: Instruct to inform physician if pregnant/breastfeeding or intending to become pregnant; advise women of childbearing potential to avoid becoming pregnant. Inform of the possible side effects and instruct to contact physician should any occur.

CARIMUNE NF — immune globulin intravenous (human)   Rx

Class: Immune globulin

Thrombosis may occur. Renal dysfunction, acute renal failure, osmotic nephrosis, and death may occur in predisposed patients with immune globulin intravenous (IGIV) products. Renal dysfunction and acute renal failure occur more commonly with IGIV products containing sucrose; this product contains sucrose. For patients at risk of thrombosis (eg, using estrogens), renal dysfunction (eg, receiving known nephrotoxic drugs), or acute renal failure, administer at the minimum dose and infusion rate practicable. Ensure adequate hydration before administration. Monitor for signs/symptoms of thrombosis and assess blood viscosity if at risk for hyperviscosity.

ADULT DOSAGE
Primary Immunodeficiency
Maint Treatment:
Usual: 0.4-0.8g/kg IV infusion once every 3-4 weeks
Infusion Rates:
Initial: 0.5mg/kg/min
Titrate: If tolerated, after 30 min, may increase to 1mg/kg/min for the next 30 min; thereafter, may gradually increase in a stepwise manner as tolerated
Max: 3mg/kg/min
Previously Untreated Agammaglobulinemic/ Hypogammaglobulinemic Patients:
Give 1st infusion as a 3% sol; may give subsequent infusions at a higher concentration if patient shows good tolerance

Immune Thrombocytopenic Purpura
Acute and Chronic:

Induction:
Usual: 0.4g/kg on 2-5 consecutive days; give as 6% sol
Infusion Rates:
Initial: 0.5mg/kg/min
Titrate: If tolerated, after 30 min, may increase to 1mg/kg/min for the next 30 min; thereafter, may gradually increase in a stepwise manner as tolerated
Max: 3mg/kg/min
Maint:
Chronic Immune Thrombocytopenic Purpura:
If after induction, platelet count falls to <30,000/μL and/or patient manifests clinically significant bleeding, may give 0.4g/kg as a single IV infusion
If an adequate response does not result, may increase to 0.8-1g/kg as a single infusion

PEDIATRIC DOSAGE
Primary Immunodeficiency
Maint Treatment:
Usual: 0.4-0.8g/kg IV infusion once every 3-4 weeks
Infusion Rates:
Initial: 0.5mg/kg/min
Titrate: If tolerated, after 30 min, may increase to 1mg/kg/min for the next 30 min; thereafter, may gradually increase in a stepwise manner as tolerated
Max: 3mg/kg/min
Previously Untreated Agammaglobulinemic/ Hypogammaglobulinemic Patients:
Give 1st infusion as a 3% sol; may give subsequent infusions at a higher concentration if patient shows good tolerance

Immune Thrombocytopenic Purpura
Acute and Chronic:

Induction:
Usual: 0.4g/kg on 2-5 consecutive days; give as 6% sol
Infusion Rates:
Initial: 0.5mg/kg/min
Titrate: If tolerated, after 30 min, may increase to 1mg/kg/min for the next 30 min; thereafter, may gradually increase in a stepwise manner as tolerated
Max: 3mg/kg/min
In acute immune thrombocytopenic purpura of childhood, if initial platelet count response to first 2 doses is adequate (30,000-50,000/μL), may d/c therapy after 2nd day of the 5-day course
Maint:
Chronic Immune Thrombocytopenic Purpura:
If after induction, platelet count falls to <30,000/μL and/or patient manifests clinically significant bleeding, may give 0.4g/kg as a single IV infusion
If an adequate response does not result, may increase to 0.8-1g/kg as a single infusion

DOSING CONSIDERATIONS
Renal Impairment
Risk of Renal Dysfunction:
Infuse at a rate <2mg/kg/min
Elderly
Infuse at a rate <2mg/kg/min
Adverse Reactions
Stop or slow infusion if side effects occur, until symptoms subside
Other Important Considerations
Risk for Thrombosis:
Max Infusion Rate: <2mg/kg/min

ADMINISTRATION
IV route

Do not dilute w/ other infusible drugs or mix w/ other medications or fluids; give by a separate infusion line
Begin administration promptly when reconstitution occurs outside of sterile laminar air flow conditions; when reconstitution is carried out in a sterile laminar flow hood using aseptic technique, may begin administration w/in 24 hours provided the sol has been refrigerated during that time

Reconstitution
1. Remove protective cover from 1 end of the transfer set and insert the exposed needle through the rubber stopper into diluent bottle
2. Remove 2nd protective cover from the other end of the transfer set. Quickly plunge diluent bottle onto the lyophilisate bottle and bring the bottles into an upright position. Allow the diluent to flow into the lyophilisate bottle
3. Once the appropriate amount of diluent is transferred, lift diluent bottle off the spike to release vacuum and remove the spike
4. Swirl vigorously; do not shake

May pool several reconstituted vials of identical concentration and diluent in an empty sterile glass or plastic IV infusion container if large doses are to be administered
Filtering is acceptable but not required; antibacterial filters (0.2 microns) may be used
Do not freeze sol

Refer to PI for infusion rates based on concentrations, and required diluent volumes if reconstituted from individual vial package or when using other diluents/higher concentrations

STORAGE
Room temperature ≤30°C (86°F). Do not freeze reconstituted sol.

HOW SUPPLIED
Inj: 3g, 6g, 12g

CONTRAINDICATIONS
History of an anaphylactic or severe systemic reaction to the administration of human immune globulin; IgA deficiency, especially w/ known antibody against IgA.

WARNINGS/PRECAUTIONS
May carry a risk of transmitting infectious agents (eg, viruses, and theoretically, the Creutzfeldt-Jakob disease agent). Patients with agamma- or extreme hypogammaglobulinemia who have never before received immunoglobulin substitution treatment or whose time from last treatment is >8 weeks, may be at risk of developing inflammatory reactions on rapid infusion (>2mg/kg/min); epinephrine and other appropriate resuscitative drugs and equipment should be available for treatment of an acute anaphylactic reaction. Patients should not be volume depleted prior to initiation of infusion. Consider discontinuation if renal function deteriorates. Aseptic meningitis syndrome (AMS) reported and may occur more frequently with high doses (2g/kg); rule out other causes of meningitis. Hemolytic anemia may develop due to enhanced RBC sequestration; monitor for clinical signs and symptoms of hemolysis. Noncardiogenic pulmonary edema/transfusion-related acute lung injury (TRALI) reported; if TRALI is suspected, perform tests for presence of antineutrophil antibodies in both the product and patient serum. D/C infusion immediately if anaphylaxis or other severe reactions occur. Caution in patients >65 yrs of age and judged to be at increased risk of developing renal insufficiency.

ADVERSE REACTIONS
Thrombosis, renal dysfunction, acute renal failure, osmotic nephrosis, flushing of face, tightness in chest, chills, fever, dizziness, nausea, diaphoresis, hypotension, HTN, arthralgia, myalgia.

DRUG INTERACTIONS
See Boxed Warning. May impair efficacy of live attenuated viral vaccines (eg, measles, mumps, rubella).

PREGNANCY AND LACTATION
Category C, safety not known in nursing.

MECHANISM OF ACTION
Immune globulin; mechanism in ITP not established. Contains a broad spectrum of antibody specificities against bacterial, viral, parasitic, and mycoplasma antigens, that are capable of both opsonization and neutralization of microbes and toxins.

PHARMACOKINETICS
Absorption: T_{max}=2-5 days (IM). **Distribution:** Crosses placenta. **Elimination:** $T_{1/2}$=3 weeks.

PATIENT CONSIDERATIONS
Assessment: Assess for history of anaphylactic or severe systemic reactions to human immune globulin, IgA deficiency, risk of thrombosis/renal dysfunction/ acute renal failure, volume status, pregnancy/nursing status, and possible drug interactions. Assess renal function. Consider baseline assessment of blood viscosity in patients at risk for hyperviscosity, including those with cryoglobulins, fasting chylomicronemia/markedly high TGs, or monoclonal gammopathies.

Monitoring: Monitor for thrombosis, infection, inflammatory/anaphylactic reactions, hemolysis, pulmonary adverse reactions, and other adverse reactions. Monitor renal function and urine output periodically. Perform neurological exam, including CSF studies, if AMS is suspected. Perform tests for presence of antineutrophil antibodies in both the product and patient serum if TRALI is suspected. Monitor vital signs continuously.

Counseling: Instruct to immediately report symptoms of decreased urine output, sudden weight gain, fluid retention/edema, and/or SOB, and symptoms of thrombosis to physician. Inform that drug is made from human plasma and may contain infectious agents that can cause disease. Inform that product may impair efficacy of live attenuated viral vaccines; instruct to inform immunizing physician of recent therapy with this product.

CAYSTON — aztreonam   Rx
Class: Monobactam

ADULT DOSAGE
Cystic Fibrosis

To Improve Respiratory Symptoms in Patients w/ *Pseudomonas aeruginosa*:
75mg tid via nebulizer for a 28-day course (followed by 28 days off therapy); take doses at least 4 hrs apart

PEDIATRIC DOSAGE
Cystic Fibrosis

To Improve Respiratory Symptoms in Patients w/ *Pseudomonas aeruginosa*:
≥7 Years:
75mg tid via nebulizer for a 28-day course (followed by 28 days off therapy); take doses at least 4 hrs apart

---

ADMINISTRATION
Inh route

Do not mix w/ any other drugs
Use bronchodilator before administration

Reconstitution

Administer immediately after reconstitution; do not reconstitute until ready to administer a dose

To open the glass vial, carefully remove the metal ring by lifting or pulling the tab and remove the gray rubber stopper

Twist the tip off the diluent ampule and squeeze the liquid into the glass vial

Replace the rubber stopper, then gently swirl the vial until contents have completely dissolved

Administration

Administer only using an Altera nebulizer system

Pour reconstituted sol into the handset of the nebulizer system

Turn the unit on and place the mouthpiece of the handset in the mouth and breathe normally only through the mouth

Administration typically takes between 2-3 min

Refer to PI for further instructions on how to test and clean the nebulizer

STORAGE

2-8°C (36-46°F). Once removed from refrigerator, store at room temperature up to 25°C (77°F) for up to 28 days. Protect from light.

HOW SUPPLIED

Sol, Inhalation: 75mg/vial

CONTRAINDICATIONS

Known allergy to aztreonam.

WARNINGS/PRECAUTIONS

Severe allergic reactions reported; d/c and initiate treatment as appropriate if allergic reaction occurs. Caution with history of β-lactam allergy (eg, penicillins [PCNs], cephalosporins, carbapenems); cross-reactivity may occur. Treatment is associated with bronchospasm. Decrease in forced expiratory volume in 1 sec (FEV_1) after treatment course reported; assess baseline FEV_1 and other pulmonary symptoms prior to therapy. May result in bacterial resistance with use in the absence of known *P. aeruginosa* infection.

ADVERSE REACTIONS

Cough, nasal congestion, wheezing, pharyngolaryngeal pain, pyrexia, chest discomfort, abdominal pain, vomiting, bronchospasm.

PREGNANCY AND LACTATION

Category B, safe in nursing.

MECHANISM OF ACTION

Monobactam; binds to PCN-binding proteins of susceptible bacteria, which leads to inhibition of bacterial cell-wall synthesis and death of the cell.

PHARMACOKINETICS

Absorption: C_{max}=0.55mcg/mL, 0.67mcg/mL, 0.65mcg/mL (Days 0, 14, and 28, respectively). **Distribution:** Serum protein binding (56%); (IV) found in breast milk, crosses the placenta. **Metabolism:** Hydrolysis. **Elimination:** Urine (10%, unchanged), (IV) feces (12%); $T_{1/2}$=2.1 hrs.

PATIENT CONSIDERATIONS

Assessment: Assess for previous hypersensitivity to the drug, history of β-lactam allergy, presence of pulmonary symptoms, and pregnancy/nursing status. Obtain baseline FEV_1.

Monitoring: Monitor for signs/symptoms of allergic reactions, bronchospasm, and other adverse reactions. Monitor for pulmonary exacerbations.

Counseling: Counsel that therapy should only be used to treat bacterial, not viral, infections. Instruct to take exactly ud; inform that skipping doses or not completing full course of therapy may decrease effectiveness and increase resistance. Advise that therapy is for inhalation use and only using an Altera nebulizer system. Inform that if a dose is missed, all 3 daily doses should be taken as long as doses are at least 4 hrs apart. Advise to contact physician if allergic reaction or new/worsening symptoms develop. Advise to use a bronchodilator prior to administration. Instruct patients taking several medications to administer drugs in the following order: bronchodilator, mucolytics, and lastly, aztreonam.

CELLCEPT — mycophenolate mofetil   Rx

Class: Inosine monophosphate dehydrogenase (IMPDH) inhibitor

> Use during pregnancy is associated w/ increased risks of 1st trimester pregnancy loss and congenital malformations; counsel females of reproductive potential regarding pregnancy prevention and planning. Immunosuppression may lead to increased susceptibility to infection and possible development of lymphoma. Should only be prescribed by physicians experienced in immunosuppressive therapy and management of organ transplant patients. Manage patients in facilities equipped and staffed w/ adequate lab and supportive medical resources.

ADULT DOSAGE
Renal Transplant

Prophylaxis of organ rejection in patients receiving allogeneic renal transplants; use concomitantly w/ cyclosporine and corticosteroids

1g PO/IV bid

Cardiac Transplant

Prophylaxis of organ rejection in patients receiving allogeneic cardiac transplants; use concomitantly w/ cyclosporine and corticosteroids

1.5g PO/IV bid

PEDIATRIC DOSAGE
Renal Transplant

Prophylaxis of organ rejection in patients receiving allogeneic renal transplants; use concomitantly w/ cyclosporine and corticosteroids

3 Months-18 Years:

Sus:
600mg/m² bid
Max Daily Dose: 2g/10mL

Cap:
BSA 1.25-1.5m²: 750mg bid

Cap/Tab:
BSA >1.5m²: 1g bid

Hepatic Transplant

Prophylaxis of organ rejection in patients receiving allogeneic hepatic transplants; use concomitantly w/ cyclosporine and corticosteroids

1.5g PO bid or 1g IV bid

DOSING CONSIDERATIONS
Renal Impairment
Renal Transplant:
Severe Chronic Renal Impairment (GFR <25mL/min) Outside the Immediate Post-Transplant Period: Avoid doses >1g bid

No dose adjustments needed in renal transplant patients experiencing delayed graft function postoperatively

Adverse Reactions
Neutropenia (ANC <1.3 x 10³/μL): Interrupt or reduce dose

ADMINISTRATION
Oral/IV route

Exercise caution in handling; refer to PI.

Oral
Give initial dose as soon as possible after transplant.

Administer on an empty stomach; may administer w/ food if necessary in stable renal transplant patients.

Do not crush tab; do not open or crush cap.

Sus may be given via NG tube (minimum size of 8 French).

IV
Administer w/in 24 hrs following transplant.

Administer by slow IV infusion over no less than 2 hrs by either peripheral or central vein.

May administer for up to 14 days; switch to oral therapy as soon as patient can tolerate oral medication.

Start administration w/in 4 hrs from reconstitution and dilution.

Do not mix or administer concurrently via same infusion catheter w/ other IV drugs or infusion admixtures.

Preparation
Sus:
1. Measure 94mL of water in a graduated cylinder.
2. Add approx 1/2 the total amount of water to bottle and shake closed bottle well for about 1 min.
3. Add remainder of water and shake closed bottle well for about 1 min.
4. Remove child-resistant cap and push bottle adapter into neck of bottle; close bottle w/ child-resistant cap tightly.

IV Reconstitution:
2 vials are needed to prepare a 1g dose; 3 vials are needed for a 1.5g dose. Reconstitute contents of each vial by injecting 14mL of D5 inj; gently shake vials to dissolve.

IV Dilution:
For a 1g dose, further dilute contents of the 2 reconstituted vials into 140mL of D5 inj.
For a 1.5g dose, further dilute contents of the 3 reconstituted vials into 210mL of D5 inj.
Final concentration of both sol is 6mg/mL.

STORAGE
25°C (77°F); excursions permitted to 15-30°C (59-86°F). Constituted Sus: Stable up to 60 days; may also be refrigerated at 2-8°C (36-46°F). Do not freeze.

HOW SUPPLIED
Cap: 250mg; **Inj:** 500mg/20mL; **Sus:** 200mg/mL; **Tab:** 500mg

CONTRAINDICATIONS
Hypersensitivity to mycophenolate mofetil, mycophenolic acid, or any component of the medication. **Inj:** Allergy to Polysorbate 80.

WARNINGS/PRECAUTIONS
Do not administer IV sol by rapid or bolus inj. May increase risk of developing malignancies, particularly of the skin; limit exposure to sunlight and UV light in patients w/ increased risk for skin cancer. Polyomavirus-associated nephropathy (PVAN), JC virus-associated progressive multifocal leukoencephalopathy (PML), cytomegalovirus infections, and reactivation of hepatitis B virus (HBV) or hepatitis C virus (HCV) reported; consider dose reduction if new or reactivated viral infection develops. PVAN, especially due to BK virus infection, may lead to deteriorating renal function and renal graft loss. Consider PML in differential diagnosis in patients reporting neurological symptoms and consider consultation w/ a neurologist. Severe neutropenia reported; interrupt or reduce dose if neutropenia develops. Cases of pure red cell aplasia (PRCA) reported when used w/ other immunosuppressive agents. Acceptable birth control must be used during therapy and for 6 weeks after discontinuation. GI bleeding, ulceration, and perforation reported; caution w/ active serious digestive system disease. Avoid doses >1g bid in renal transplant patients w/ severe chronic renal impairment (GFR <25mL/min); caution w/ delayed renal graft function post-transplant. More reports of opportunistic/herpes virus infections in cardiac transplant patients in comparison w/ azathioprine. Avoid w/ rare hereditary deficiency of hypoxanthine-guanine phosphoribosyl-transferase (HGPRT) (eg, Lesch-Nyhan and Kelley-Seegmiller syndromes). Oral sus contains 0.56mg phenylalanine/mL; caution w/ phenylketonurics. Caution in elderly.

ADVERSE REACTIONS
Infection, diarrhea, leukopenia, sepsis, N/V, HTN, peripheral edema, abdominal pain, fever, headache, constipation, hyperglycemia, anemia, insomnia.

DRUG INTERACTIONS

Avoid w/ azathioprine, drugs that interfere w/ enterohepatic recirculation (eg, cholestyramine), and norfloxacin-metronidazole combination. Vaccinations may be less effective; avoid live, attenuated vaccines. Decreased exposure w/ rifampin; concomitant use not recommended unless benefit outweighs risk. Increased levels of both drugs w/ drugs that compete w/ renal tubular secretion (eg, acyclovir/ valacyclovir, ganciclovir/valganciclovir, probenecid). Oral ciprofloxacin and amoxicillin plus clavulanic acid may decrease levels. Mean mycophenolic acid (MPA) exposure may be 30-50% greater when mycophenolate mofetil is administered w/o cyclosporine compared to when coadministered w/ cyclosporine. Expect changes in exposure when switching from cyclosporine A to an immunosuppressant that does not interfere w/ the enterohepatic cycle (eg, tacrolimus, belatacept). Telmisartan decreases levels. May decrease levels and effectiveness of hormonal contraceptives; use w/ caution and must use additional barrier contraceptive methods. Drugs that alter GI flora may reduce levels available for absorption. Decreased levels w/ proton pump inhibitors (eg, lansoprazole, pantoprazole), Mg^{2+}- and aluminum-containing antacids, and Ca^{2+} free phosphate binders (eg, sevelamer). Do not administer simultaneously w/ antacids containing aluminum and magnesium hydroxides. Do not administer Ca^{2+} free phosphate binders simultaneously; may give 2 hrs after intake. Combination immunosuppressant therapy should be used w/ caution.

PREGNANCY AND LACTATION

Pregnancy: Category D.
Lactation: Not for use in nursing.

MECHANISM OF ACTION

Inosine monophosphate dehydrogenase inhibitor; inhibits the de novo pathway of guanosine nucleotide synthesis w/o incorporation into deoxyribonucleic acid.

PHARMACOKINETICS

Absorption: Rapid and complete; (oral) absolute bioavailability (94%). Refer to PI for parameters in different populations. **Distribution:** V_d=3.6L/kg (IV), 4L/ kg (oral); plasma albumin binding (97% MPA, 82% phenolic glucuronide of MPA [MPAG]). **Metabolism:** Complete hydrolysis to MPA (active metabolite). MPA is metabolized by glucuronyl transferase to MPAG, which is converted to MPA via enterohepatic recirculation. **Elimination:** (Oral) Urine (93%; <1% MPA, 87% MPAG), feces (6%); MPA: $T_{1/2}$=17.9 hrs (oral), 16.6 hrs (IV).

PATIENT CONSIDERATIONS

Assessment: Assess for hypersensitivity to the drug or its components, hepatic/ renal impairment, delayed renal graft function post-transplant, phenylketonuria, hereditary deficiency of HGPRT (eg, Lesch-Nyhan and Kelley-Seegmiller syndromes), active digestive disease, vaccination history, nursing status, and possible drug interactions. Assess pregnancy status using serum or urine test of at least 25 mIU/mL sensitivity, immediately before starting therapy.

Monitoring: Monitor for signs/symptoms of lymphomas, skin cancer, and other malignancies, infections, HCV/HBV reactivation, neutropenia, PRCA, GI bleeding/ perforation/ulceration, and other adverse reactions. Monitor CBC weekly during the 1st month, twice monthly for the 2nd and 3rd months of therapy, and then monthly through the 1st yr. Monitor pregnancy status by obtaining pregnancy test 8-10 days after initiation of therapy and repeatedly during follow-up visits.

Counseling: Inform that use during pregnancy is associated w/ an increased risk of 1st trimester pregnancy loss and congenital malformations; discuss pregnancy testing, prevention (including acceptable contraception methods), and planning. Discuss appropriate alternative immunosuppressants w/ less potential for embryofetal toxicity if patient is considering pregnancy. Advise of complete dosage instructions and inform about increased risk of lymphoproliferative disease and certain other malignancies. Inform of the need for repeated appropriate lab tests during therapy. Instruct patients to report immediately any evidence of infection, unexpected bruising, bleeding, or any other manifestation of bone marrow depression. Advise not to breastfeed during therapy. Encourage to enroll in the pregnancy registry if patient becomes pregnant while on medication.

CEPROTIN — protein C concentrate (human)   Rx

Class: Anticoagulant protein

ADULT DOSAGE	PEDIATRIC DOSAGE
Severe Congenital Protein C Deficiency	**Severe Congenital Protein C Deficiency**
Prevention and Treatment of Venous Thrombosis and Purpura Fulminans: Acute Episodes/Short-Term Prophylaxis:	**Prevention and Treatment of Venous Thrombosis and Purpura Fulminans: Acute Episodes/Short-Term Prophylaxis:**
Initial: 100-120 IU/kg	**Initial:** 100-120 IU/kg
Subsequent 3 Doses: 60-80 IU/kg q6h; adjust dose to maintain target peak protein C activity of 100%	**Subsequent 3 Doses:** 60-80 IU/kg q6h; adjust dose to maintain target peak protein C activity of 100%
Maint: 45-60 IU/kg q6h or q12h After resolution of acute episode, continue on same dose to maintain trough protein C activity level >25% for duration of treatment	**Maint:** 45-60 IU/kg q6h or q12h After resolution of acute episode, continue on same dose to maintain trough protein C activity level >25% for duration of treatment
Long-Term Prophylaxis: **Maint:** 45-60 IU/kg q12h	**Long-Term Prophylaxis:** **Maint:** 45-60 IU/kg q12h
Dose, frequency, and duration of treatment depends on the severity of the protein C deficiency, age, clinical condition, and plasma level of protein C; adjust the dose regimen according	Dose, frequency, and duration of treatment depend on the severity of the protein C deficiency, age, clinical condition, and plasma level of protein C; adjust the dose regimen according

to the pharmacokinetic profile for each patient

In patients receiving prophylactic administration, higher peak protein C activity levels may be warranted in situations of increased risk of thrombosis

Maintenance of trough protein C activity levels >25% is recommended

Protein C Activity Monitoring: Measurement using a chromogenic assay is recommended for the determination of the patient's plasma level of protein C before and during treatment

In the case of an acute thrombotic event, perform measurements immediately before the next inj until patient is stabilized; after patient is stabilized, continue monitoring to maintain trough protein C level >25%

to the pharmacokinetic profile for each patient

In patients receiving prophylactic administration, higher peak protein C activity levels may be warranted in situations of increased risk of thrombosis

Maintenance of trough protein C activity levels >25% is recommended

Protein C Activity Monitoring: Measurement using a chromogenic assay is recommended for the determination of the patient's plasma level of protein C before and during treatment

In the case of an acute thrombotic event, perform measurements immediately before the next inj until patient is stabilized; after patient is stabilized, continue monitoring to maintain trough protein C level >25%

DOSING CONSIDERATIONS
Concomitant Medications
Initiation of Vitamin K Antagonists:
If switched to oral anticoagulants, protein C replacement must be continued until stable anticoagulation is obtained. Start w/ low dose of anticoagulant and adjust incrementally, rather than using a standard loading dose of the anticoagulant

ADMINISTRATION

IV route

Administer by infusion at max inj rate of 2mL/min; for children w/ body weight of <10kg, inj rate should not exceed 0.2mL/kg/min.
Administer at room temperature not more than 3 hrs after reconstitution.

Preparation
Bring drug and sterile water for inj (SWFI) to room temperature. Reconstitute w/ the supplied SWFI.
Gently swirl the vial until all powder is completely dissolved.
Use reconstituted sol w/in 3 hrs of reconstitution.

STORAGE
2-8°C (36-46°F); stable for 3 yrs. Store vial in the original carton to protect from light. Do not freeze.

HOW SUPPLIED
Inj: 500 IU, 1000 IU

WARNINGS/PRECAUTIONS
Therapy should be initiated under supervision of a physician experienced in replacement therapy w/ coagulation factors/inhibitors where monitoring of protein C activity is feasible. May contain traces of mouse protein and/or heparin; d/c inj/infusion if symptoms of hypersensitivity/allergic reactions occur. May carry a risk of transmitting infectious agents (eg, viruses, and theoretically, the Creutzfeldt-Jakob disease agent). Bleeding episodes reported. Heparin-induced thrombocytopenia may occur; determine platelet count immediately and consider discontinuation of therapy. Contains Na^+ (>200mg in max daily dose); closely monitor patients w/ renal impairment for Na^+ overload.

ADVERSE REACTIONS
Hypersensitivity or allergic reactions, lightheadedness.

DRUG INTERACTIONS
Concurrent use of anticoagulants may cause bleeding episodes; simultaneous administration w/ tissue plasminogen activator (tPA) may further increase the risk of bleeding from tPA. When starting treatment w/ oral anticoagulants belonging to class of vitamin K antagonists, a transient hypercoagulable state may arise before the desired anticoagulant effect becomes apparent; start w/ a low dose of anticoagulant and adjust incrementally.

PREGNANCY AND LACTATION
Pregnancy: Category C.
Lactation: Not studied for use in nursing mothers; use only if clearly needed.

MECHANISM OF ACTION
Anticoagulant protein; protein C is the precursor of a vitamin K-dependent anticoagulant glycoprotein (serine protease). It is converted by thrombin/ thrombomodulin-complex on the endothelial cell surface to activated Protein C (APC). APC exerts its effect by inactivation of the activated forms of factors V and VIII, leading to a decrease in thrombin formation. APC has also shown to have profibrinolytic effects.

PHARMACOKINETICS
Absorption: C_{max}=110 IU/dL (median); AUC=1500 IU•h/dL (median); T_{max}=0.5 hr (median). **Distribution:** V_d=0.74dL/kg (median). **Elimination:** $T_{1/2}$ (non-compartmental approach)=9.8 hrs (median).

PATIENT CONSIDERATIONS

Assessment: Assess for hypersensitivity/allergy to mouse protein and/or heparin, Na^+ restricted diet, renal impairment, pregnancy/nursing status, and possible drug interactions. Determine plasma level of protein C.

Monitoring: Monitor for hypersensitivity/allergic reactions, bleeding episodes, infections, heparin-induced thrombocytopenia, and Na^+ overload in patients w/ renal impairment. Monitor platelet count, plasma level of protein C, and coagulation parameters.

Counseling: Inform patients of the early signs of hypersensitivity reactions (eg, hives, generalized urticaria, chest tightness, wheezing, hypotension, anaphylaxis). Inform that the drug may contain traces of mouse protein or heparin as a result of manufacturing process. Advise to immediately d/c and inform physician if symptoms of hypersensitivity/allergic reaction occur.

CERDELGA — eliglustat   Rx

Class: Glucosylceramide synthase inhibitor

ADULT DOSAGE

Type 1 Gaucher Disease

Long-term treatment of patients who are CYP2D6 extensive metabolizers (EMs), intermediate metabolizers (IMs), or poor metabolizers (PMs) as detected by an FDA-cleared test

Usual:
CYP2D6 EMs/IMs: 84mg bid
CYP2D6 PMs: 84mg qd

PEDIATRIC DOSAGE

Pediatric use may not have been established

DOSING CONSIDERATIONS
Concomitant Medications
Strong/Moderate CYP2D6 Inhibitors:
CYP2D6 EMs/IMs: Reduce dose to 84mg qd
Strong/Moderate CYP3A Inhibitors:
Grapefruit/Grapefruit Juice: Avoid
CYP2D6 EMs: Reduce dose to 84mg qd
Renal Impairment
Moderate to Severe Impairment/ESRD: Use not recommended
Hepatic Impairment
All Stages/Cirrhosis: Use not recommended
Other Important Considerations
Administer therapy 24 hrs after the last dose of the previous enzyme replacement therapy (eg, imiglucerase, velaglucerase alfa, taliglucerase alfa)

ADMINISTRATION
Oral route
Swallow caps whole, preferably w/ water; do not crush, dissolve, or open
May be taken w/ or w/o food

STORAGE
20-25°C (68-77°F); excursions permitted between 15-30°C (59-86°F).

HOW SUPPLIED
Cap: 84mg

CONTRAINDICATIONS
EMs or IMs taking a strong or moderate CYP2D6 inhibitor concomitantly with a strong or moderate CYP3A inhibitor. IMs or PMs taking a strong CYP3A inhibitor.

WARNINGS/PRECAUTIONS
May cause increases in ECG intervals (PR, QTc, and QRS) at substantially elevated eliglustat plasma concentrations; not recommended in patients with preexisting cardiac disease (congestive heart failure, recent acute myocardial infarction, bradycardia, heart block, ventricular arrhythmia) or long QT syndrome. Not recommended with moderate to severe renal impairment, end-stage renal disease, and in all stages of hepatic impairment or cirrhosis. Patients who are CYP2D6 ultra-rapid metabolizers may not achieve adequate concentrations of eliglustat to achieve a therapeutic effect.

ADVERSE REACTIONS
Fatigue, headache, nausea, diarrhea, back pain, pain in extremities, upper abdominal pain, flatulence, oropharyngeal pain, dizziness, asthenia, cough, dyspepsia, gastroesophageal reflux disease, constipation.

DRUG INTERACTIONS
See Dosing Considerations and Contraindications. Avoid consumption of grapefruit or grapefruit juice. For patients currently treated with imiglucerase, velaglucerase alfa, or taliglucerase alfa, eliglustat may be administered 24 hrs after the last dose of the previous enzyme replacement therapy (ERT). Not recommended with class IA (eg, quinidine, procainamide) and class III (eg, amiodarone, sotalol) antiarrhythmic medications. CYP2D6 and CYP3A inhibitors may significantly increase exposure and result in prolongation of the PR, QTc, and/or QRS cardiac interval which could result in cardiac arrhythmias; not recommended with moderate CYP3A inhibitors (eg, fluconazole) in IMs and PMs, or weak CYP3A inhibitors (eg, ranitidine) in PMs. Strong CYP3A inducers (eg, rifampin, carbamazepine, St. John's wort) significantly decrease exposure; coadministration is not recommended in EMs, IMs, and PMs. May increase concentrations of P-glycoprotein (eg, digoxin, phenytoin, colchicine, dabigatran etexilate) or CYP2D6 (eg, metoprolol, nortriptyline, perphenazine) substrates; monitor therapeutic drug concentrations, as indicated, or consider reducing the dosage of the concomitant drug and titrate to clinical effect. Measure serum digoxin concentrations before initiating eliglustat, reduce digoxin dose by 30%, and continue monitoring.

PREGNANCY AND LACTATION
Category C, not for use in nursing.

MECHANISM OF ACTION
Glucosylceramide synthase inhibitor; acts as a substrate reduction therapy for GD1.

PHARMACOKINETICS
Absorption: Administration to patients with different CYP2D6 metabolizer statuses resulted in different parameters. **Distribution:** Plasma protein binding (76-83%); (IV) V_d=835L (EMs). **Metabolism:** Extensive via CYP2D6 (major) and CYP3A4 (minor); sequential oxidation of the octanoyl moiety followed by oxidation of the 2,3-dihydro-1,4-benzodioxane moiety, or a combination of the two pathways. **Elimination:** (PO) Urine (41.8%), feces (51.4%). $T_{1/2}$=6.5 hrs (EMs), 8.9 hrs (PMs).

PATIENT CONSIDERATIONS
Assessment: Assess for preexisting cardiac disease, long QT syndrome, renal/hepatic impairment, CYP2D6 metabolizer status, pregnancy/nursing status, and possible drug interactions.

Monitoring: Monitor for ECG changes and other adverse reactions.

Counseling: Advise to discuss all the medications being taken, including any herbal supplements or vitamins, with physician. Advise to inform physician if new symptoms (eg, palpitations, fainting, dizziness) develop. Instruct to avoid consumption of grapefruit or its juice. Inform patients currently treated with imiglucerase, velaglucerase alfa, or taliglucerase alfa, that drug may be administered 24 hrs after the last dose of the previous ERT.

CEREZYME — imiglucerase   Rx

Class: Enzyme

ADULT DOSAGE

Type 1 Gaucher Disease

For long-term enzyme replacement therapy for patients w/ confirmed Type 1 Gaucher disease that results in anemia, thrombocytopenia, bone disease, and/or hepatomegaly or splenomegaly

Initial: Doses range from 2.5 U/kg 3X a week to 60 U/kg once every 2 weeks

Titrate: Adjust dose based on achievement of therapeutic goals

Administer by IV infusion over 1-2 hrs

PEDIATRIC DOSAGE

Type 1 Gaucher Disease

2-16 Years:
For long-term enzyme replacement therapy for patients w/ confirmed Type 1 Gaucher disease that results in anemia, thrombocytopenia, bone disease, and/or hepatomegaly or splenomegaly

Initial: Doses range from 2.5 U/kg 3X a week to 60 U/kg once every 2 weeks

Titrate: Adjust dose based on achievement of therapeutic goals

Administer by IV infusion over 1-2 hrs

ADMINISTRATION
IV Route
May filter the diluted sol through an inline low protein binding 0.2μm filter

Reconstitution Instructions
1. Determine the correct amount to be administered
2. Reconstitute the appropriate number of vials w/ sterile water for inj; the final concentrations and administration volumes are as follows:
Sterile Water for Reconstitution:
200 U Vial: 5.1mL
400 U Vial: 10.2mL
Final Volume of Reconstituted Product:
200 U Vial: 5.3mL
400 U Vial: 10.6mL
Concentration After Reconstitution:
200 U Vial: 40 U/mL
400 U Vial: 40 U/mL
Withdrawal Volume:
200 U Vial: 5mL
400 U Vial: 10mL
Units of Enzyme w/in Final Volume:
200 U Vial: 200 U
400 U Vial: 400 U
3. Dilute the appropriate amount w/ 0.9% NaCl inj to a final volume of 100-200mL
4. Dilute promptly after reconstitution and do not store for subsequent use

The dosage administered in individual infusions may be slightly increased or decreased to utilize fully each vial as long as the monthly administered dose remains substantially unaltered

STORAGE
2-8°C (36-46°F). Reconstituted: Stable for up to 12 hrs at 25°C (77°F) and at 2-8°C (36-46°F). Diluted: 2-8°C (36-46°F) for up to 24 hrs.

HOW SUPPLIED
Inj: 200 U, 400 U

WARNINGS/PRECAUTIONS
Development of IgG antibody to drug during the 1st yr of therapy reported; higher risk of a hypersensitivity reaction in patients w/ IgG antibody. Caution w/ previous hypersensitivity to the product. Anaphylactoid reactions reported; conduct further treatment w/ caution. Pulmonary HTN and pneumonia reported; evaluate patients w/ respiratory symptoms in the absence of fever for presence of pulmonary HTN. Caution in patients who have developed antibodies or hypersensitivity reactions to alglucerase.

ADVERSE REACTIONS
Inj-site reactions, pruritus, flushing, urticaria, angioedema, chest discomfort, dyspnea, coughing, cyanosis, hypotension, N/V, rash, headache, fever.

PREGNANCY AND LACTATION
Category C, caution in nursing.

MECHANISM OF ACTION
Human enzyme β-glucocerebrosidase analog; catalyzes hydrolysis of glucocerebroside to glucose and ceramide.

PHARMACOKINETICS
Distribution: V_d=0.09-0.15L/kg. **Elimination:** $T_{1/2}$=3.6-10.4 min.

PATIENT CONSIDERATIONS
Assessment: Assess for previous hypersensitivity to drug or alglucerase, and pregnancy/nursing status.

Monitoring: Monitor for pulmonary HTN, pneumonia, hypersensitivity reactions, and other adverse reactions. Monitor periodically for IgG antibody formation during 1st yr of treatment.

Counseling: Counsel about possible adverse effects and instruct to report to physician should any develop.

CETROTIDE — cetrorelix acetate   Rx
Class: Gonadotropin-releasing hormone (GnRH) antagonist

ADULT DOSAGE	PEDIATRIC DOSAGE
Ovarian Stimulation	Pediatric use may not have been established
Inhibition of premature luteinizing hormone surges in women undergoing controlled ovarian stimulation	
Ovarian stimulation therapy w/ gonadotropins (follicle-stimulating hormone [FSH], human menopausal gonadotropin) is started on cycle Day 2 or 3; adjust gonadotropins dose according to individual response	
Usual: 0.25mg SQ once daily administered on either stimulation Day 5 (am or pm) or Day 6 (am) and continued daily until the day of hCG administration	
No hCG should be administered if the ovaries show an excessive response to treatment	

ADMINISTRATION
SQ route
1. Twist the inj needle w/ the yellow mark (20 gauge) on the prefilled syringe
2. Push the needle through the center of the rubber stopper of the vial and slowly inj the solvent into the vial
3. Leaving the syringe in the vial, gently swirl the vial until the sol is clear w/o residue; avoid forming bubbles
4. Draw total contents of the vial into the syringe
5. Replace the needle w/ the yellow mark by the inj needle w/ the grey mark (27 gauge)
6. Invert the syringe and push the plunger until all air bubbles have been expelled
7. Choose an inj site in the lower abdominal area, 1 inch away from the navel; rotate inj site each day
8. Clean the inj site and gently pinch up the skin surrounding the site of inj
9. Dispose syringe and needles properly after use

STORAGE
2-8°C (36-46°F). Store packaged tray in the outer carton to protect from light.

HOW SUPPLIED
Inj: 0.25mg

CONTRAINDICATIONS
Hypersensitivity to cetrorelix acetate, extrinsic peptide hormones, mannitol, GnRH, or any other GnRH analogues; known/suspected pregnancy; lactation; severe renal impairment.

WARNINGS/PRECAUTIONS
Should be prescribed by physicians who are experienced in fertility treatment. Pregnancy must be excluded before starting treatment. Cases of hypersensitivity reactions, including anaphylactoid reactions reported; caution with signs and symptoms of active allergic conditions or known history of allergic predisposition. Not recommended with severe allergic conditions.

ADVERSE REACTIONS
Ovarian hyperstimulation syndrome.

PREGNANCY AND LACTATION
Category X, not for use in nursing.

MECHANISM OF ACTION
GnRH antagonist; competes with natural GnRH for binding to membrane receptors on pituitary cells and thus controls the release of LH and FSH in a dose-dependent manner.

PHARMACOKINETICS
Absorption: Rapid. Absolute bioavailability (85%); (Multiple dose, 0.25mg) C_{max}=6.42ng/mL, T_{max}=1 hr, AUC=44.5ng•hr/mL. **Distribution:** (IV, single dose of 3mg) V_d=1L/kg; plasma protein binding (86%). **Metabolism:** Peptidases; 1-4 peptide (predominant metabolite). **Elimination:** (10mg dose) Urine (2-4% unchanged), bile (5-10% unchanged and metabolites); $T_{1/2}$=20.6 hrs (multiple dose, 0.25mg).

PATIENT CONSIDERATIONS
Assessment: Assess for hypersensitivity to the drug, GnRH, GnRH analogs, mannitol, or extrinsic peptide hormones. Assess for severe renal impairment, allergic conditions or history of allergic predisposition, and pregnancy/nursing status.

Monitoring: Monitor for hypersensitivity reactions and other adverse reactions.

Counseling: Inform about the duration of treatment, the required monitoring procedures, and the risk of possible adverse reactions. Inform that the medication should not be taken if pregnant. Instruct on proper inj technique for self-administration.

CHOLBAM — cholic acid   Rx
Class: Bile acid

ADULT DOSAGE	PEDIATRIC DOSAGE
Bile Acid Synthesis Disorders	**Bile Acid Synthesis Disorders**
Treatment of bile acid synthesis disorders due to single enzyme defects	Treatment of bile acid synthesis disorders due to single enzyme defects
Usual: 10-15mg/kg qd, or in 2 divided dose	**≥3 Weeks of Age:** **Usual:** 10-15mg/kg qd, or in 2 divided doses
Peroxisomal Disorders	**Peroxisomal Disorders**
Adjunctive treatment of peroxisomal disorders including Zellweger spectrum disorders in patients who exhibit manifestations of liver disease, steatorrhea, or complications from decreased fat soluble vitamin absorption	Adjunctive treatment of peroxisomal disorders including Zellweger spectrum disorders in patients who exhibit manifestations of liver disease, steatorrhea, or complications from decreased fat soluble vitamin absorption
Usual: 10-15mg/kg qd, or in 2 divided doses	**≥3 Weeks of Age:** **Usual:** 10-15mg/kg qd, or in 2 divided doses

---

DOSING CONSIDERATIONS
Discontinuation
D/C if liver function does not improve w/in 3 months of the start of treatment or complete biliary obstruction develops

D/C at any time if there are persistent clinical or lab indicators of worsening liver function or cholestasis. Concurrent elevations of serum gamma glutamyltransferase and serum ALT may indicate overdose. Continue to monitor lab parameters of liver function and consider restarting dose when the parameters return to baseline

Other Important Considerations
Familial Hypertriglyceridemia:
Patients w/ newly diagnosed, or a family history of, familial hypertriglyceridemia may have a poor absorption of therapy from the intestine and require a 10% increase in the recommended dosage
Usual: 11-17mg/kg qd, or in 2 divided doses

Monitor clinical response including steatorrhea, and lab values including transaminases, bilirubin, and PT/INR to determine the adequacy of the dosage regimen

Administer the lowest dose of therapy that effectively maintains liver function

ADMINISTRATION
Oral route

Take w/ food
Take at least 1 hr before or 4-6 hrs (or at as great an interval as possible) after a bile acid binding resin or aluminum-based antacid
Do not crush or chew the caps
Refer to PI for number of caps needed to achieve dosage of 10mg/kg/day and 15mg/kg/day

Patients Unable to Swallow Caps
Caps can be opened and the contents mixed w/ either infant formula or expressed breast milk (for younger children), or soft food such as mashed potatoes or apple puree (for older children and adults) in order to mask any unpleasant taste:
1. Hold the cap over the prepared liquid/food, gently twist open, and allow the contents to fall into the liquid/food
2. Mix the entire cap contents w/ 1 or 2 tbsp (15-30mL) of infant formula, expressed breast milk, or soft food
3. Stir for 30 sec
4. Cap contents will remain as fine granules in the milk or food, and will not dissolve
5. Administer the mixture immediately

STORAGE
20-25°C (68-77°F); excursions permitted between 15-30°C (59-86°F).

HOW SUPPLIED
Cap: 50mg, 250mg

WARNINGS/PRECAUTIONS
Should be initiated and monitored by an experienced hepatologist or pediatric gastroenterologist. Monitor liver function and d/c in patients who develop worsening of liver function while on treatment.

ADVERSE REACTIONS
Diarrhea, reflux esophagitis, malaise, jaundice, skin lesion, nausea, abdominal pain, intestinal polyp, UTI, peripheral neuropathy.

DRUG INTERACTIONS

Concomitant medications that inhibit canalicular membrane bile acid transporters such as bile salt efflux pump (eg, cyclosporine) may exacerbate accumulation of conjugated bile salts in the liver and result in clinical symptoms; avoid concomitant use, and if concomitant use is necessary, monitor serum transaminases and bilirubin. Bile acid binding resins (eg, cholestyramine, colestipol, colesevelam) adsorb and reduce bile acid absorption and may reduce efficacy of cholic acid; take cholic acid at least 1 hr before or 4-6 hrs (or at as great an interval as possible) after a bile acid binding resin. Aluminum-based antacids may reduce the bioavailability of cholic acid; take cholic acid at least 1 hr before or 4-6 hrs (or at as great an interval as possible) after an aluminum-based antacid.

PREGNANCY AND LACTATION

Pregnancy: There is a pregnancy surveillance program that monitors pregnancy outcomes in women exposed to cholic acid during pregnancy (COCOA Registry [Cholbam: Child and mother's health]); women who become pregnant during treatment are encouraged to enroll. Limited published case reports discuss pregnancies in women taking cholic acid for 3β-hydroxysteroid dehydrogenase deficiency resulting in healthy infants; these reports may not adequately inform the presence or absence of drug-associated risk w/ the use of cholic acid during pregnancy.

Lactation: Endogenous cholic acid is present in human milk. Caution in nursing.

MECHANISM OF ACTION

Bile acid; has not been established. It is known that cholic acid and its conjugates are endogenous ligands of the nuclear receptor, farnesoid X receptor (FXR). FXR regulates enzymes and transporters that are involved in bile acid synthesis and in the enterohepatic circulation to maintain bile acid homeostasis under normal physiologic conditions.

PHARMACOKINETICS

Absorption: Passive diffusion along the length of the GI tract. **Metabolism:** Liver; conjugated w/ glycine or taurine by bile acid-CoA synthetase and bile acid-CoA: amino acid N-acetyltransferase. Conjugated cholic acid is secreted into bile, reabsorbed in the ileum, and enters another cycle of enterohepatic circulation. **Elimination:** Feces.

PATIENT CONSIDERATIONS

Assessment: Assess for newly diagnosed or a family history of familial hypertriglyceridemia, hepatic impairment, pregnancy/nursing status, and possible drug interactions. Assess serum or urinary bile acid levels using mass spectrometry.

Monitoring: Monitor for worsening liver function or cholestasis, complete biliary obstruction, and other adverse reactions. Monitor serum AST/ALT/gamma-glutamyl transpeptidase, alkaline phosphatase, bilirubin, and INR every month for the first 3 months, every 3 months for the next 9 months, every 6 months during the subsequent 3 yrs, and annually thereafter. Monitor liver function more frequently during periods of rapid growth, concomitant disease, and pregnancy. Monitor clinical response to therapy.

Counseling: Advise the need to undergo lab testing periodically while on treatment to assess liver function. Advise that therapy may worsen liver impairment; instruct to immediately report to physician any symptoms associated w/ liver impairment (eg, skin or the whites of eyes turn yellow, urine turns dark or brown [tea colored], pain on the right side of stomach, bleeding or bruising occurs more easily than normal, increased lethargy). Instruct to take exactly ud. Advise that there is a pregnancy surveillance program that monitors pregnancy outcomes in women exposed to cholic acid during pregnancy.

CIMZIA — certolizumab pegol

Rx

Class: Tumor necrosis factor (TNF) blocker

> Increased risk for developing serious infections (eg, active tuberculosis [TB], latent TB reactivation, invasive fungal infections, bacterial/viral and other opportunistic infections) leading to hospitalization or death, mostly w/ concomitant use w/ immunosuppressants (eg, methotrexate or corticosteroids). D/C if serious infection or sepsis develops. Active TB/reactivation of latent TB may present w/ disseminated or extrapulmonary disease; test for latent TB before and during therapy and initiate treatment for latent TB prior to therapy. Invasive fungal infections reported; consider empiric antifungal therapy in patients at risk who develop severe systemic illness. Consider risks and benefits prior to therapy in patients w/ chronic or recurrent infection. Monitor patients for development of infection during and after treatment, including development of TB in patients who tested (-) for latent TB infection prior to therapy. Lymphoma and other malignancies, some fatal, reported in children and adolescents. Not indicated for pediatric patients.

ADULT DOSAGE

Crohn's Disease

Moderately to Severely Active Disease w/ Inadequate Response to Conventional Therapy:
Initial: 400mg (given as 2 SQ inj of 200mg) initially, and at Weeks 2 and 4
Maint: 400mg every 4 weeks

Rheumatoid Arthritis

Moderately to Severely Active:
Recommended: 400mg (given as 2 SQ inj of 200mg) initially and at Weeks 2 and 4, followed by 200mg every other week
Maint: Consider 400mg every 4 weeks

PEDIATRIC DOSAGE

Pediatric use may not have been established

Psoriatic Arthritis

Active:
Recommended: 400mg (given as 2 SQ inj of 200mg) initially and at Weeks 2 and 4, followed by 200mg every other week
Maint: Consider 400mg every 4 weeks

Ankylosing Spondylitis

Active:
Recommended: 400mg (given as 2 SQ inj of 200mg) initially and at Weeks 2 and 4, followed by 200mg every 2 weeks or 400mg every 4 weeks

---

DOSING CONSIDERATIONS

Concomitant Medications

Not recommended in combination w/ biological disease-modifying anti-rheumatic drugs (DMARDs) or other TNF blocker therapy

ADMINISTRATION

SQ route

Rotate inj sites; avoid areas where the skin is tender, bruised, red, or hard. Once reconstituted, can store in the vials for up to 24 hrs between 2-8°C (36-46°F) prior to inj; do not freeze.

Lyophilized Powder for Inj
Preparation:
1. Bring to room temperature for 30 min before reconstituting; do not warm the vial in any other way.
2. Reconstitute vial(s) w/ 1mL of sterile water for inj (SWFI) using 20-gauge needle provided; direct SWFI at the vial wall rather than directly on the product.
3. Gently swirl each vial for 1 min w/o shaking, assuring that all of the powder comes in contact w/ SWFI.
4. Continue swirling every 5 min as long as non-dissolved particles are observed; full reconstitution may take as long as 30 min.
5. Final reconstituted sol contains 200mg/mL.

Administration:
1. Prior to injecting, reconstituted sol should be at room temperature (but not for >2 hrs prior to administration).
2. Withdraw reconstituted sol into a separate syringe for each vial using a new 20-gauge needle for each vial so that each syringe contains 1mL of sol (200mg of certolizumab pegol).
3. Replace 20-gauge needle(s) on syringes w/ a 23-gauge(s) for administration.
4. Inject full contents of syringe(s) SQ by pinching the skin of the thigh or abdomen; when a 400mg dose is needed (given as 2 SQ inj of 200mg), inj should occur at separate sites in the thigh or abdomen.

Prefilled Syringe
After proper training in SQ inj technique, a patient may self-inject w/ a prefilled syringe if appropriate.
Patients using prefilled syringes should be instructed to inject full amount in syringe (1mL), according to the directions provided in Instructions for Use booklet.

STORAGE

2-8°C (36-46°F). Do not freeze. Protect sol from light.

HOW SUPPLIED

Inj: 200mg/mL [prefilled syringe, vial]

WARNINGS/PRECAUTIONS

May be used as monotherapy or concomitantly w/ non-biological DMARDs. Do not initiate w/ an active infection. Increased risk of infection in elderly patients and in patients w/ comorbid conditions; consider the risks prior to therapy for those who have been exposed to TB, w/ a history of an opportunistic infection, who have resided or traveled in areas of endemic TB or mycoses, or w/ any underlying conditions predisposing to infection. Postmarketing cases of aggressive and fatal hepatosplenic T-cell lymphoma (HSTCL) reported; the majority of cases occurred in adolescent and young adult males w/ Crohn's disease or ulcerative colitis. Acute and chronic leukemia, melanoma, and Merkel cell carcinoma reported. Perform periodic skin examination, particularly in patients w/ risk factors for skin cancer. New onset and worsening of CHF reported; caution in patients w/ heart failure (HF) and monitor carefully. Hypersensitivity reactions reported (rare); d/c and institute appropriate therapy if such reactions occur. Hepatitis B virus (HBV) reactivation reported; if reactivation occurs, d/c and initiate antiviral therapy w/ appropriate supportive treatment. Monitor patients closely and exercise caution when considering resumption of therapy. Associated w/ rare cases of new onset or exacerbation of clinical symptoms and/or radiographic evidence of CNS and peripheral demyelinating disease; caution w/ preexisting or recent-onset central or peripheral nervous system demyelinating disorders. Rare cases of neurological disorders (eg, seizure disorder, optic neuritis, peripheral neuropathy) reported. Hematological reactions (eg, leukopenia, pancytopenia, thrombocytopenia) reported; caution in patients w/ ongoing, or a history of, significant hematologic abnormalities, and consider discontinuation in patients w/ confirmed significant hematologic abnormalities. May result in the formation of autoantibodies and rarely, in the development of a lupus-like syndrome; d/c if lupus-like syndrome develops. Lab test interactions may occur.

ADVERSE REACTIONS

URTIs, rash, UTIs.

DRUG INTERACTIONS

See Boxed Warning and Dosing Considerations. Avoid concurrent use w/ live (eg, attenuated) vaccines. Not recommended w/ anakinra, abatacept, rituximab, or natalizumab; may increase risk of serious infections. Carefully consider the potential risk of HSTCL w/ the combination of azathioprine or 6-mercaptopurine.

PREGNANCY AND LACTATION

Pregnancy: Category B; may be eliminated at a slower rate in exposed infants than in adult patients. There is a pregnancy exposure registry that monitors pregnancy outcomes in women exposed to the drug during pregnancy. **Lactation:** Not for use in nursing.

MECHANISM OF ACTION

TNF-blocker; binds to and selectively neutralizes TNF-α, which has a central role in inflammatory processes.

PHARMACOKINETICS

Absorption: C_{max}=approx 43-49mcg/mL; T_{max}=54-171 hrs; bioavailability (approx 80%). **Distribution:** V_d=6-8L. **Elimination:** $T_{1/2}$=approx 14 days.

PATIENT CONSIDERATIONS

Assessment: Assess for active/chronic/recurrent infection (eg, TB, HBV), TB exposure, history of an opportunistic infection, recent travel to areas of endemic TB or endemic mycoses, underlying conditions that may predispose to infection, HF, presence or history of significant hematologic abnormalities, neurologic disorders, risk factors for skin cancer, pregnancy/nursing status, and possible drug interactions. Perform test for latent TB infection.

Monitoring: Monitor for sepsis, TB (active, reactivation, or latent), invasive fungal infections, bacterial/viral/other infections, lymphoma/other malignancies, new onset/worsening of CHF, active HBV infection, hematological events, hypersensitivity reactions, CNS demyelinating disorders, lupus-like syndrome, and other adverse reactions. Perform periodic skin examination, particularly in patients w/ risk factors for skin cancer and test for latent TB infection.

Counseling: Advise of potential risks and benefits of therapy. Inform that therapy may lower the ability of the immune system to fight infections; instruct to immediately contact physician if any signs/symptoms of an infection develop, including TB and HBV reactivation. Inform about the risks of lymphoma and other malignancies while on therapy. Advise to seek immediate medical attention if any symptoms of severe allergic reactions occur. Advise to report to physician signs of new or worsening medical conditions (eg, heart disease, neurological diseases, autoimmune disorders) and symptoms of cytopenia (eg, bruising, bleeding, persistent fever). Instruct about proper administration techniques.

CINRYZE — C1 esterase inhibitor (human)   Rx

Class: C1 esterase inhibitor

ADULT DOSAGE	PEDIATRIC DOSAGE
Hereditary Angioedema	**Hereditary Angioedema**
Routine Prophylaxis Against Angioedema Attacks:	**Routine Prophylaxis Against Angioedema Attacks:**
1000 U IV every 3 or 4 days at an infusion rate of 1mL/min (10 min)	**Adolescents:**
	1000 U IV every 3 or 4 days at an infusion rate of 1mL/min (10 min)

ADMINISTRATION

IV route

Use either the Mix2Vial transfer device or a commercially available double-ended needle.

Preparation/Handling

A silicone-free syringe is recommended for reconstitution/administration.
Each vial is for single use only.
Do not mix w/ other materials.
Do not use if frozen.

Reconstitution

1. Two vials of reconstituted drug are combined for a single dose; sterile water for inj (SWFI) is required.
2. Bring the powder and SWFI (diluent) to room temperature if refrigerated.
3. Remove protective covering from top of the Mix2Vial transfer device package; do not remove device from package.
4. Must access diluent vial prior to the drug vial to prevent loss of vacuum.
5. Place diluent on a flat surface and insert the blue end of the device into the diluent vial, pushing down until the spike penetrates through the center of the diluent vial stopper and the device snaps in place. The Mix2Vial transfer device must be positioned completely vertical prior to penetrating the stopper closure.
6. Remove and discard plastic package; do not touch the exposed end of the device.
7. Place drug vial on a flat surface, invert diluent vial containing 5mL SWFI, and insert the clear end into the drug vial, pushing down until the spike penetrates the rubber stopper and the device snaps into place. The Mix2Vial transfer device must be positioned completely vertical prior to penetrating the stopper closure. The SWFI will automatically flow into drug vial, because the vacuum in the vial will draw in the diluent; do not use if there is no vacuum in the vial.
8. Gently swirl drug vial until all powder is dissolved; do not shake.
9. Disconnect the SWFI vial by turning it counterclockwise; do not remove the clear end of the Mix2Vial transfer device from drug vial.

Administration

1. Two reconstituted drug vials are combined for a single dose.
2. Utilizing a sterile, disposable 10mL syringe, draw back plunger to admit 5mL air into the syringe.
3. Attach the syringe onto the top of the clear end of the Mix2Vial transfer device by turning it clockwise.

4. Invert the vial and inject air into the sol and then slowly withdraw reconstituted product into syringe.
5. Detach the syringe from the vial by turning it counterclockwise and releasing it from the clear end of the Mix2Vial transfer device.
6. Using the same syringe, repeat steps 2-5 w/ a 2nd vial to make the complete dose; administer promptly after preparation in syringe.
7. Attach a suitable needle or infusion set w/ winged adapter, and inject IV.
Administer at room temperature w/in 3 hrs after reconstitution.

STORAGE

2-25°C (36-77°F). Do not freeze. Protect from light.

HOW SUPPLIED

Inj: 500 U

CONTRAINDICATIONS

Life-threatening immediate hypersensitivity reactions, including anaphylaxis to the product.

WARNINGS/PRECAUTIONS

Severe hypersensitivity reactions may occur; d/c infusion and institute appropriate treatment. Serious arterial and venous thromboembolic (TE) events reported; weigh benefits against the risks in patients w/ risk factors (eg, presence of an indwelling venous catheter/access device, prior history of thrombosis, underlying atherosclerosis, use of oral contraceptives or certain androgens, morbid obesity, immobility). Monitor patients w/ known risk factors for TE events during and after administration. Drug is made from human blood; may carry a risk of transmitting infectious agents (eg, viruses, Creutzfeldt-Jakob disease [CJD] agent).

ADVERSE REACTIONS

Headache, rash, N/V.

PREGNANCY AND LACTATION

Pregnancy: No adequate and well-controlled studies in pregnant women. It is not known whether drug can cause fetal harm or affect reproduction capacity. Give to a pregnant woman only if clearly needed. **Lactation:** It is not known whether drug is excreted in human milk; caution in nursing.

MECHANISM OF ACTION

C1 esterase inhibitor; regulates the activation of the complement and intrinsic coagulation (contact system) pathway and the fibrinolytic system by forming complexes between the proteinases and the inhibitor, resulting in inactivation of both and consumption of the C1 inhibitor. It is thought by some that increased vascular permeability and the clinical manifestations of hereditary angioedema attacks are primarily mediated through contact system activation. Suppression of contact system activation through inactivation of plasma kallikrein and factor XIIa is thought to modulate this vascular permeability by preventing the generation of bradykinin.

PHARMACOKINETICS

Absorption: C_{max}=0.68 U/mL (single dose), 0.85 U/mL (double dose); T_{max}=3.9 hrs (single dose), 2.7 hrs (double dose); $AUC_{(0-t)}$=74.5 U•hr/mL (single dose), 95.9 U•hr/mL (double dose). **Elimination:** $T_{1/2}$=56 hrs (single dose), 62 hrs (double dose).

PATIENT CONSIDERATIONS

Assessment: Assess for previous hypersensitivity reactions to drug, risk factors for TE events, and pregnancy/nursing status.

Monitoring: Monitor for hypersensitivity reactions, TE events, infection, and other adverse reactions.

Counseling: Counsel about risks and benefits of therapy. Instruct to immediately report signs of allergic-type hypersensitivity reactions and TE events to physician; advise to d/c therapy if symptoms of allergic-type hypersensitivity reactions occur. Advise to notify physician if pregnant/intending to become pregnant or if breastfeeding/planning to breastfeed. Advise to bring an adequate supply of therapy for routine prevention when traveling. Inform that medication is made from human blood and may carry a risk of transmitting infectious agents (eg, viruses, CJD agent).

CISPLATIN — cisplatin   Rx

Class: Platinum analogue

Should be administered under the supervision of a qualified physician experienced in the use of cancer chemotherapeutic agents. Cumulative renal toxicity associated w/ therapy is severe. Myelosuppression and N/V are also major dose-related toxicities. Ototoxicity, manifested by tinnitus, and/or loss of high frequency hearing, and occasionally deafness, is significant. Anaphylactic-like reactions reported. Exercise caution to prevent inadvertent overdose; avoid inadvertent overdose due to confusion w/ carboplatin or prescribing practices that fail to differentiate daily doses from total dose per cycle. Doses >100mg/m²/cycle once every 3-4 weeks are rarely used.

ADULT DOSAGE	PEDIATRIC DOSAGE
Testicular Tumor	Pediatric use may not have been established
Combination therapy w/ other chemotherapeutic agents in patients w/ metastatic tumors who have already received surgical/ radiotherapeutic procedures	
Usual: 20mg/m² IV daily for 5 days per cycle	
Repeat Courses: Do not give until SrCr <1.5mg/100mL, and/or BUN <25mg/100mL	
Do not give until circulating blood elements are at an acceptable level (platelets ≥100,000/mm³, WBCs ≥4000/mm³)	

Subsequent doses should not be given until an audiometric analysis indicates that auditory acuity is w/in normal limits

Ovarian Tumor

Combination therapy w/ other chemotherapeutic agents in patients w/ metastatic tumors who have already received surgical/ radiotherapeutic procedures

Usual: 75-100mg/m² IV per cycle once every 4 weeks in combination w/ 600mg/m² IV cyclophosphamide once every 4 weeks; administer sequentially

Secondary therapy in patients refractory to standard chemotherapy who have not previously received cisplatin inj

Monotherapy: 100mg/m² IV per cycle once every 4 weeks

Repeat Courses:
Do not give until SrCr <1.5mg/100mL, and/or BUN <25mg/100mL
Do not give until circulating blood elements are at an acceptable level (platelets ≥100,000/mm³, WBCs ≥4000/mm³)
Subsequent doses should not be given until an audiometric analysis indicates that auditory acuity is w/in normal limits

Bladder Cancer

Advanced Transitional Cell Bladder Cancer No Longer Amenable to Local Treatments:
50-70mg/m² IV per cycle once every 3-4 weeks depending on extent of prior exposure to radiation and/or prior chemotherapy

Heavily Pretreated Patients:
Initial: 50mg/m² per cycle every 4 weeks

Repeat Courses:
Do not give until SrCr <1.5mg/100mL, and/or BUN <25mg/100mL
Do not give until circulating blood elements are at an acceptable level (platelets ≥100,000/mm³, WBCs ≥4000/mm³)
Subsequent doses should not be given until an audiometric analysis indicates that auditory acuity is w/in normal limits

ADMINISTRATION

IV route

Administer by slow IV infusion; do not give by rapid IV inj.
Pretreatment hydration w/ 1-2L of fluid infused for 8-12 hrs prior to dose recommended.
Dilute in 2L of D5 in 1/2 or 1/3 normal saline containing 37.5g of mannitol; infuse over a 6- to 8-hr period.
Protect diluted sol from light if not to be used w/in 6 hrs.
Maintain adequate hydration and urinary output during the following 24 hrs.
Always wear impervious gloves when handling vials and IV sets containing cisplatin; immediately and thoroughly wash the skin w/ soap and water, and flush the mucosa w/ water if contact occurs.

STORAGE

20-25°C (68-77°F). Do not refrigerate. Protect from light. Contents remaining in the amber vial following initial entry is stable for 28 days protected from light or for 7 days under fluorescent room light.

HOW SUPPLIED

Inj: 1mg/mL [50mL, 100mL, 200mL]

CONTRAINDICATIONS

Preexisting renal impairment, myelosuppression, hearing impairment, history of allergic reactions to cisplatin or other platinum-containing compounds.

WARNINGS/PRECAUTIONS

Avoid aluminum-containing needles or IV sets; may cause precipitate formation and loss of potency. Severe neuropathies reported w/ higher doses or greater frequencies than those recommended. Loss of motor function reported. Elderly patients may be more susceptible to nephrotoxicity and peripheral neuropathy. Can cause fetal harm; avoid becoming pregnant. Development of acute leukemia coincident w/ therapy reported. Inj-site reactions may occur; closely monitor the infusion site for possible infiltration during administration. Monitor peripheral blood counts weekly.

ADVERSE REACTIONS

Nephrotoxicity, ototoxicity, anaphylactic-like reactions, myelosuppression, N/V, diarrhea, vascular toxicities, serum electrolyte disturbances, hyperuricemia, neurotoxicity, ocular toxicity, hepatotoxicity.

DRUG INTERACTIONS

Cumulative nephrotoxicity potentiated by aminoglycosides. Acute leukemia may develop when given in combination w/ leukemogenic agents. Anticonvulsant levels may become subtherapeutic. Response duration adversely affected when pyridoxine was used in combination w/ altretamine and cisplatin. Increased risk of ototoxicity by prior or simultaneous cranial irradiation, and may be more severe w/ other ototoxic drugs (eg, aminoglycosides, vancomycin). Vascular toxicities coincident w/ the use of cisplatin in combination w/ other antineoplastic agents have been reported.

PREGNANCY AND LACTATION

Pregnancy: Category D. Can cause fetal harm; patients should be advised to avoid becoming pregnant.
Lactation: Reported to be found in human milk; not for use in nursing.

MECHANISM OF ACTION

Heavy metal platinum complex.

PHARMACOKINETICS

Distribution: V_d=11-12L/m²; plasma platinum protein binding (90%); found in breast milk. **Excretion:** Urine (13-17%, unchanged [1 hr after administration of 50mg/m²]); $T_{1/2}$=20-30 min (cisplatin), ≥5 days (albumin-platinum complex).

PATIENT CONSIDERATIONS

Assessment: Assess for history of allergic reaction to the drug or other platinum-containing compounds, preexisting renal impairment, hearing impairment, myelosuppression, pregnancy/nursing status, and possible drug interactions. Assess SrCr, BUN, CrCl, Mg²⁺, Na⁺, K⁺, and Ca²⁺ levels and perform audiometric test prior to therapy.

Monitoring: Monitor for nephrotoxicity, neuropathies, ototoxicity, myelosuppression, N/V, vascular toxicities, serum electrolyte disturbances, hyperuricemia, neurotoxicity, ocular toxicity, and anaphylactic-like reactions and other adverse reactions. Monitor peripheral blood counts weekly, and LFTs periodically. Monitor for motor function and infusion site for possible infiltration. Perform neurologic exam regularly. Assess SrCr, BUN, CrCl, Mg²⁺, Na⁺, K⁺, and Ca²⁺ levels prior to each subsequent course. Perform audiometric testing prior to each subsequent dose, and for several years post therapy in children.

Counseling: Inform about possible adverse effects and instruct to report any adverse effects. Advise to avoid pregnancy/nursing.

CLADRIBINE — cladribine   Rx

Class: Chlorinated purine nucleoside analogue

> Administer under the supervision of a qualified physician experienced in the use of antineoplastic therapy. Suppression of bone marrow function should be anticipated; usually is reversible and appears to be dose dependent. Serious neurological toxicity and acute nephrotoxicity reported with high doses (4-9X the recommended dose). Acute nephrotoxicity observed, especially when given with other nephrotoxic agents/therapies.

ADULT DOSAGE

Active Hairy Cell Leukemia

Usual: 0.09mg/kg/day as a single course given by continuous infusion for 7 consecutive days

If patient does not respond to initial course of treatment, it is unlikely that they will benefit from additional courses

PEDIATRIC DOSAGE

Pediatric use may not have been established

DOSING CONSIDERATIONS

Adverse Reactions

Neurotoxicity/Renal Toxicity: Consider delaying or discontinuing the drug

ADMINISTRATION

IV route

Vials are for single-use only; discard any unused portion
Do not mix sol containing cladribine inj w/ other IV drugs or additives or infuse simultaneously via a common IV line
A precipitate may occur during the exposure of cladribine inj to low temperatures; it may be resolubilized by allowing the sol to warm naturally to room temperature and by shaking vigorously. Do not heat or microwave

Preparation and Administration

To Prepare a Single Daily Dose:
Pass through a sterile 0.22μm disposable hydrophilic syringe filter prior to introduction into the infusion bag, prior to each daily infusion
1. Add the calculated dose (0.09mg/kg or 0.09mL/kg) of cladribine inj through the sterile filter to an infusion bag containing 500mL of 0.9% NaCl inj
2. Infuse continuously over 24 hrs
3. Repeat daily for a total of 7 consecutive days

To Prepare a 7-Day Infusion:
The 7-day infusion sol should only be prepared w/ bacteriostatic 0.9% NaCl inj (0.9% benzyl alcohol preserved); sol prepared w/ bacteriostatic NaCl inj for individuals weighing >85kg may have reduced preservative effectiveness due to greater dilution of the benzyl alcohol preservative

Pass both cladribine inj and the diluent through a sterile 0.22μm disposable hydrophilic syringe filter as each sol is being introduced into the infusion reservoir
1. Add the calculated dose of cladribine inj (7 days x 0.09mg/kg or 0.09mL/kg) to the infusion reservoir through the sterile filter
2. Add a calculated amount of bacteriostatic 0.9% NaCl inj (0.9% benzyl alcohol preserved) also through the filter to bring the total volume of the sol to 100mL
3. After completing sol preparation, clamp off the line, disconnect and discard the filter
4. Aspirate air bubbles from the reservoir as necessary using the syringe and a dry 2nd sterile filter or a sterile vent filter assembly
5. Reclamp the line and discard the syringe and filter assembly
6. Infuse continuously over 7 days

Stability
Once diluted, administer sol of cladribine inj promptly or store in the refrigerator (2-8°C) for ≤8 hrs prior to start of administration

Handling Precautions
If cladribine inj contacts the skin or mucous membranes, wash the involved surface immediately w/ copious amounts of water

STORAGE
Unopened Vials: 2-8°C (36-46°F). Protect from light. Do not refreeze, heat, or microwave. Diluted Sol: 2-8°C (36-46°F); stable for 8 hrs.

HOW SUPPLIED
Inj: 1mg/mL [10mL]

CONTRAINDICATIONS
Hypersensitivity to this drug or any of its components.

WARNINGS/PRECAUTIONS
Fever with/without neutropenia reported; initiate empiric antibiotics as clinically indicated. Serious and fatal infections (eg, respiratory/viral skin infections, sepsis) reported. Caution with active infections, known or suspected renal/hepatic insufficiency, or severe bone marrow impairment; monitor for signs of hematologic and nonhematologic toxicity. Tumor lysis syndrome reported (rare). Can cause fetal harm. Caution in elderly. Recommended diluent contains benzyl alcohol which has been associated with gasping syndrome in premature infants.

ADVERSE REACTIONS
Bone marrow suppression, neutropenia, fever, anemia, thrombocytopenia, infection, administration site reactions, rash, headache, decreased appetite, cough, diarrhea, N/V, fatigue, dizziness.

DRUG INTERACTIONS
See Boxed Warning. Not recommended with live attenuated vaccines; may increase risk of infection. Caution with drugs known to cause immunosuppression or myelosuppression.

PREGNANCY AND LACTATION
Category D, not for use in nursing.

MECHANISM OF ACTION
Chlorinated purine nucleoside analogue; inhibits DNA synthesis and repair in both actively dividing and quiescent lymphocytes and monocytes.

PHARMACOKINETICS
Distribution: V_d=9L/kg; plasma protein binding (20%). **Elimination:** Urine (18%); $T_{1/2}$=6.7 hrs.

PATIENT CONSIDERATIONS
Assessment: Assess for previous hypersensitivity to the drug, hematologic impairment, renal/hepatic dysfunction, active infection, pregnancy/nursing status, and possible drug interactions.

Monitoring: Monitor for signs/symptoms of bone marrow suppression, tumor lysis syndrome, fever, infection, neurological toxicity, hypersensitivity reactions, and other adverse reactions. Monitor peripheral blood counts, especially during the first 4-8 weeks after treatment. Perform bone marrow aspiration and biopsy after peripheral counts have normalized to assess response. Monitor renal/hepatic function periodically.

Counseling: Inform of the risks and benefits of treatment. Inform that therapy can cause fetal harm; advise females of reproductive potential to use highly effective contraception during treatment. Advise to inform physician of any infections.

CLOLAR – clofarabine   Rx
Class: Antimetabolite

PEDIATRIC DOSAGE
Acute Lymphoblastic Leukemia
- Treatment of relapsed or refractory acute lymphoblastic leukemia after at least 2 prior regimens

1-21 Years:
52mg/m² IV infusion over 2 hrs daily for 5 consecutive days
- Repeat treatment cycles following recovery or return to baseline organ function, approx every 2-6 weeks
- Consider prophylactic antiemetic medications and steroids

DOSING CONSIDERATIONS
Concomitant Medications
Drugs w/ Known Renal Toxicity: Minimize exposure to these during the 5 days of clofarabine administration
Drugs Known to Induce Hepatic Toxicity: Consider avoiding concomitant use

Renal Impairment
CrCl 30-60mL/min: Reduce dose by 50%

Adverse Reactions
Hypotension: D/C therapy if hypotension develops during the 5 days of administration
Hematologic Toxicity:
Administer subsequent cycles no sooner than 14 days from the starting day of the previous cycle and provided the patient's ANC is ≥0.75 x 10⁹/L
Grade 4 Neutropenia (ANC <0.5 x 10⁹/L) Lasting ≥4 Weeks: Reduce dose by 25% for the next cycle
Non-Hematologic Toxicity:
Clinically Significant Infection: Withhold until infection is controlled, then restart at full dose
Grade 3 Non-Infectious Toxicity (Excluding Transient Elevations in Serum Transaminases and/or Serum Bilirubin and/or N/V Controlled by Antiemetic Therapy): Withhold, then reinstitute at a 25% dose reduction when resolution or return to baseline
Grade 4 Non-Infectious Toxicity: D/C administration
Early Signs/Symptoms of Systemic Inflammatory Response Syndrome/Capillary Leak: D/C administration and provide appropriate supportive measures
≥Grade 3 Increase in Creatinine/Bilirubin: D/C administration, then reinstitute w/ a 25% dose reduction when patient is stable and organ function has returned to baseline. If hyperuricemia is anticipated (tumor lysis), initiate measures to control uric acid

ADMINISTRATION
IV route
Do not administer any other medications through the same IV line.
Provide supportive care (eg, IV fluids, antihyperuricemic treatment, alkalinization of urine) throughout the 5 days of clofarabine administration to reduce the effects of tumor lysis and other adverse events.

Preparation
1. Filter clofarabine through sterile 0.2 micron syringe filter.
2. Dilute w/ D5 inj or 0.9% NaCl inj prior to IV infusion to a final concentration between 0.15mg/mL and 0.4mg/mL.
3. Use w/in 24 hrs of preparation.

STORAGE
Undiluted: 25°C (77°F); excursions permitted to 15-30°C (59-86°F). **Diluted:** Room temperature; must be used w/in 24 hrs of preparation.

HOW SUPPLIED
Inj: 20mg/20mL

WARNINGS/PRECAUTIONS
Causes myelosuppression, which may be severe and prolonged. Serious and fatal hemorrhage, including cerebral, GI, and pulmonary hemorrhage, reported; majority of cases were associated w/ thrombocytopenia. Increases the risk of infection (eg, severe and fatal sepsis, opportunistic infections); monitor for signs/symptoms of infection, d/c therapy, and treat promptly. May result in tumor lysis syndrome; monitor and initiate preventive measures including adequate IV fluids and measures to control uric acid. May cause a cytokine release syndrome (eg, tachypnea, tachycardia, hypotension, pulmonary edema) that may progress to systemic inflammatory response syndrome (SIRS) w/ capillary leak syndrome and organ impairment, which may be fatal; d/c immediately and provide appropriate supportive measures. Consider prophylactic steroids to mitigate SIRS or capillary leak syndrome; consider use of diuretics and/or albumin. Patients who have previously received hematopoietic stem cell transplant may be at higher risk for veno-occlusive disease (VOD) of the liver following administration of therapy in combination w/ etoposide and cyclophosphamide; monitor and d/c therapy if suspected. Severe and fatal hepatotoxicity, including hepatitis and hepatic failure, reported; monitor hepatic function and for signs/symptoms of hepatitis and hepatic failure, and d/c therapy for ≥Grade 3 liver enzyme elevations and/or bilirubin elevations. Elevated creatinine, acute renal failure, and hematuria reported; monitor patients for renal toxicity and interrupt or d/c therapy as necessary. Fatal and serious cases of enterocolitis (eg, neutropenic colitis, cecitis, *Clostridium difficile* colitis) reported; monitor for signs/symptoms and treat promptly. Serious and fatal cases of Stevens-Johnson syndrome (SJS) and toxic epidermal necrolysis (TEN) reported; d/c for exfoliative or bullous rash, or if SJS or TEN is suspected. May cause fetal harm. Monitor cardiac function during administration and monitor patients taking medications known to affect BP. Moderately emetogenic; consider prophylactic antiemetic medications.

ADVERSE REACTIONS
N/V, diarrhea, febrile neutropenia, headache, rash, pruritus, pyrexia, fatigue, palmar-plantar erythrodysesthesia syndrome, anxiety, flushing, mucosal inflammation.

DRUG INTERACTIONS
Minimize exposure to drugs w/ known renal toxicity during the 5 days of therapy; risk of renal toxicity may be increased. Consider avoiding concomitant use of medications known to induce hepatic toxicity.

PREGNANCY AND LACTATION
Pregnancy: Category D. May cause fetal harm. Women of childbearing potential should avoid becoming pregnant while receiving treatment; all patients should use effective contraceptive measures to prevent pregnancy.
Lactation: Not for use in nursing.

MECHANISM OF ACTION

Antimetabolite; purine nucleoside metabolic inhibitor. Inhibits DNA synthesis by decreasing cellular deoxynucleotide triphosphate pools through an inhibitory action on ribonucleotide reductase, and by terminating DNA chain elongation and inhibiting repair through incorporation into DNA chain by competitive inhibition of DNA polymerases. Also disrupts the integrity of mitochondrial membrane, leading to release of the pro-apoptotic mitochondrial proteins, cytochrome C and apoptosis-inducing factor, leading to programmed cell death.

PHARMACOKINETICS

Distribution: V_d=172L/m²; plasma protein binding (47%). **Metabolism:** 5'-triphosphate clofarabine (active metabolite). **Elimination:** Urine (49-60%, unchanged); $T_{1/2}$=5.2 hrs.

PATIENT CONSIDERATIONS

Assessment: Assess for renal impairment, pregnancy/nursing status, and possible drug interactions.

Monitoring: Monitor for signs and symptoms of infection, myelosuppression, hemorrhage, tumor lysis syndrome, cytokine release syndrome, SIRS, capillary leak syndrome, VOD, hepatotoxicity, enterocolitis, SJS, TEN, exfoliative or bullous rash, and other adverse reactions. Monitor CBCs, platelets and coagulation parameters, cardiac function, and renal/hepatic function.

Counseling: Advise to return for regular blood counts and to report any symptoms associated w/ hematological toxicity to physician. Inform to report to physician immediately if signs or symptoms of infection occur. Advise of the signs/symptoms of SIRS. Instruct to avoid medications, including OTC and herbal medications, that may be hepatotoxic or nephrotoxic, during the 5 days of treatment. Advise patients of the possibility of developing liver function abnormalities and to immediately report signs/symptoms of jaundice. Advise male and female patients w/ reproductive potential to use effective contraceptive measures to prevent pregnancy. Instruct female patients to avoid breastfeeding during treatment. Advise patients that N/V, diarrhea, or skin rash may be experienced, and to seek medical attention if these symptoms are significant.

COAGADEX — coagulation factor X (human)   Rx

Class: Coagulation factor X (human)

ADULT DOSAGE

Hereditary Factor X Deficiency

Indicated for hereditary factor X deficiency for on-demand treatment and control of bleeding episodes, and for perioperative management of bleeding in patients w/ mild hereditary factor X deficiency

Dose and duration of the treatment depend on the severity of the Factor X deficiency, location and extent of the bleeding, and on the patient's clinical condition

Base dose and frequency on the individual clinical response; do not administer >60 IU/kg daily

Each vial of therapy is labeled w/ the actual Factor X potency/content in IU

Estimate the expected in vivo peak increase in Factor X level expressed as IU/dL (or % of normal) using the following formula:
Estimated Increment of Factor X (IU/dL or % of normal) = [Total Dose (IU)/Body Weight (kg)] x 2

Dose to achieve a desired in vivo peak increase in Factor X level may be calculated using the following formula:
Dose (IU) = Body Weight (kg) x Desired Factor X Rise (IU/dL) x 0.5

Desired Factor X rise is the difference between the patient's plasma Factor X level and the desired level. The dosing formula is based on the observed recovery of 2 IU/dL per IU/kg

On-Demand Treatment and Control of Bleeding Episodes:

Infuse 25 IU/kg when the first sign of bleeding occurs; repeat at intervals of 24 hrs until bleed stops

Perioperative Management of Bleeding:

To ensure that hemostatic levels are obtained and maintained, measure post-infusion plasma Factor X levels before and after surgery

PEDIATRIC DOSAGE

Hereditary Factor X Deficiency

Indicated for hereditary factor X deficiency for on-demand treatment and control of bleeding episodes, and for perioperative management of bleeding in patients w/ mild hereditary factor X deficiency

≥12 Years:

Dose and duration of the treatment depend on the severity of the Factor X deficiency, location and extent of the bleeding, and on the patient's clinical condition

Base dose and frequency on the individual clinical response; do not administer >60 IU/kg daily

Each vial of therapy is labeled w/ the actual Factor X potency/content in IU

Estimate the expected in vivo peak increase in Factor X level expressed as IU/dL (or % of normal) using the following formula:
Estimated Increment of Factor X (IU/dL or % of normal) = [Total Dose (IU)/Body Weight (kg)] x 2

Dose to achieve a desired in vivo peak increase in Factor X level may be calculated using the following formula:
Dose (IU) = Body Weight (kg) x Desired Factor X Rise (IU/dL) x 0.5

Desired Factor X rise is the difference between the patient's plasma Factor X level and the desired level. The dosing formula is based on the observed recovery of 2 IU/dL per IU/kg

On-Demand Treatment and Control of Bleeding Episodes:

Infuse 25 IU/kg when the first sign of bleeding occurs; repeat at intervals of 24 hrs until bleed stops

Perioperative Management of Bleeding:

To ensure that hemostatic levels are obtained and maintained, measure post-infusion plasma Factor X levels before and after surgery

Presurgery: Calculate the dose to raise plasma Factor X levels to 70-90 IU/dL using the following formula:
Required dose (IU) = Body Weight (kg) x Desired Factor X Rise (IU/dL) x 0.5

Postsurgery: Repeat dose as necessary to maintain plasma Factor X levels at a minimum of 50 IU/dL until the patient is no longer at risk of bleeding due to surgery

Presurgery: Calculate the dose to raise plasma Factor X levels to 70-90 IU/dL using the following formula:
Required dose (IU) = Body Weight (kg) x Desired Factor X Rise (IU/dL) x 0.5

Postsurgery: Repeat dose as necessary to maintain plasma Factor X levels at a minimum of 50 IU/dL until the patient is no longer at risk of bleeding due to surgery

ADMINISTRATION

IV route

Administer by IV infusion at a rate of 10mL/min, but no more than 20mL/min. Refer to PI for preparation and reconstitution instructions.

STORAGE

Store in a refrigerator or at room temperature (2-30°C [36-86°F]). Do not freeze. Protect from light. Use reconstituted sol w/in 1 hr of reconstitution.

HOW SUPPLIED

Inj: 250 IU, 500 IU

CONTRAINDICATIONS

Life-threatening hypersensitivity reactions to Coagadex or any of the components.

WARNINGS/PRECAUTIONS

Allergic-type hypersensitivity reactions, including anaphylaxis, are possible; d/c immediately and administer appropriate emergency treatment if hypersensitivity symptoms occur. Contains traces of human proteins other than Factor X. Formation of neutralizing antibodies (inhibitors) to Factor X may occur; perform an assay that measures Factor X inhibitor concentration if expected Factor X activity levels are not attained, or if bleeding is not controlled w/ an expected dose. May carry a risk of transmitting infectious agents (eg, viruses, the variant Creutzfeldt-Jakob disease agent and, theoretically, the Creutzfeldt-Jakob disease agent).

ADVERSE REACTIONS

Infusion-site erythema, infusion-site pain, fatigue, back pain.

DRUG INTERACTIONS

Caution in patients who are receiving other plasma products that may contain Factor X (eg, fresh frozen plasma, prothrombin complex concentrates). Likely to be counteracted by direct and indirect Factor Xa inhibitors.

PREGNANCY AND LACTATION

Pregnancy: It is not known whether therapy can cause fetal harm; give only if clearly needed.
Lactation: There is no information regarding the presence of drug in human milk; caution in nursing.

MECHANISM OF ACTION

Plasma-derived human blood coagulation factor; temporarily replaces the missing Factor X needed for effective hemostasis.

PHARMACOKINETICS

Absorption: C_{max}=0.504 IU/mL; AUC_{0-144h}=17.1 IU•hr/mL. **Distribution:** V_d=56.3 mL/kg. **Elimination:** $T_{1/2}$=30.3 hrs.

PATIENT CONSIDERATIONS

Assessment: Assess for life threatening hypersensitivity reactions to any constituent of the product, location and extent of bleeding, patient's clinical condition, pregnancy/nursing status, and for possible drug interactions.

Monitoring: Monitor for signs/symptoms of hypersensitivity reactions, transmission of infectious agents, and other adverse reactions. Monitor plasma Factor X activity by performing a validated test (eg, one-stage clotting assay), to confirm that adequate Factor X levels have been achieved and maintained. Monitor for the development of Factor X inhibitors. Perform a Nijmegen-Bethesda inhibitor assay if expected Factor X plasma levels are not attained or if bleeding is not controlled w/ the expected dose of therapy.

Counseling: Instruct to immediately report to healthcare professional the early signs/symptoms of a hypersensitivity reaction (eg, burning, stinging, erythema, chills, cough, dizziness, fever, generalized urticaria, headache, hives, hypotension, lethargy, N/V, tightness of the chest). Inform that the development of inhibitors to Factor X is a possible complication of treatment; advise to contact healthcare provider for further treatment and/or assessment if a lack of clinical response to therapy is experienced. Inform that therapy is made from human plasma and may contain infectious agents that can cause diseases; instruct to report any symptoms that concern the patient.

COMBIVIR — lamivudine/zidovudine   Rx

Class: Nucleoside reverse transcriptase inhibitor (NRTI) combination

Lactic acidosis and severe hepatomegaly w/ steatosis, including fatal cases, reported w/ nucleoside analogues; d/c treatment if lactic acidosis or pronounced hepatotoxicity occurs. Severe acute exacerbations of hepatitis B reported in patients coinfected w/ hepatitis B virus (HBV) upon discontinuation of therapy; closely monitor hepatic function for at least several months. If appropriate, initiation of antihepatitis B therapy may be warranted. **Zidovudine:** Associated w/ hematologic toxicity (eg, neutropenia, anemia), particularly w/ advanced HIV-1 disease. Symptomatic myopathy associated w/ prolonged use.

ADULT DOSAGE

HIV-1 Infection

Combination w/ Other Antiretrovirals:
1 tab bid

PEDIATRIC DOSAGE

HIV-1 Infection

Combination w/ Other Antiretrovirals:
≥30kg:
1 tab bid

DOSING CONSIDERATIONS

Renal Impairment
CrCl <50mL/min: Not recommended for use

Hepatic Impairment
Not recommended for use

ADMINISTRATION
Oral route
If child is unable to swallow tab, the liquid oral formulations should be prescribed: Epivir (lamivudine) oral sol and Retrovir (zidovudine) syr.

STORAGE
2-30°C (36-86°F).

HOW SUPPLIED
Tab: (Lamivudine/Zidovudine) 150mg/300mg* *scored

CONTRAINDICATIONS
History of hypersensitivity reaction to lamivudine or zidovudine.

WARNINGS/PRECAUTIONS
Not recommended due to lack of dosage adjustment in pediatrics weighing <30 kg, or inpatients requiring dosage adjustment (eg, renal impairment [CrCl <50mL/min], hepatic impairment, or those experiencing dose-limiting adverse reactions). Caution w/ history or known risk factors for pancreatitis; d/c if pancreatitis occurs. Immune reconstitution syndrome reported. Autoimmune disorders (eg, Graves' disease, polymyositis, Guillain-Barre syndrome) reported to occur in the setting of immune reconstitution and can occur many months after initiation of treatment. May cause redistribution/accumulation of body fat. Caution w/ any known risk factors for liver disease and in elderly. **Lamivudine:** Emergence of lamivudine-resistant HBV reported. **Zidovudine:** Caution w/ granulocyte count <1000 cells/mm³ or Hgb <9.5g/dL; monitor blood counts frequently w/ advanced HIV-1 and periodically w/ other HIV-1 infected patients. Interrupt therapy if anemia or neutropenia develops.

ADVERSE REACTIONS
Headache, malaise, fatigue, fever, chills, N/V, diarrhea, anorexia, insomnia, nasal signs and symptoms, cough.

DRUG INTERACTIONS
Avoid w/ other lamivudine-, zidovudine-, and/or emtricitabine-containing products. **Lamivudine:** Avoid w/ zalcitabine. Hepatic decompensation may occur in HIV/hepatitis C virus (HCV) coinfected patients receiving interferon-alfa w/ or w/o ribavirin. Nelfinavir and trimethoprim/sulfamethoxazole may increase levels. **Zidovudine:** Avoid w/ stavudine, doxorubicin, and nucleoside analogues (eg, ribavirin). May increase risk of hematologic toxicities w/ ganciclovir, interferon alfa, ribavirin, bone marrow suppressors, or cytotoxic agents. Atovaquone, fluconazole, methadone, probenecid, and valproic acid may increase levels. Clarithromycin, nelfinavir, rifampin, and ritonavir may decrease levels.

PREGNANCY AND LACTATION
Pregnancy: Category C
Lactation: Not for use in nursing.

MECHANISM OF ACTION
Nucleoside analogue combination; inhibits reverse transcriptase via DNA chain termination after incorporation of the nucleotide analogue.

PHARMACOKINETICS
Absorption: Lamivudine: Rapid; bioavailability (86%). Zidovudine: Rapid; bioavailability (64%). **Distribution:** Lamivudine: V_d=1.3L/kg; plasma protein binding (<36%); found in breast milk. Zidovudine: V_d=1.6L/kg; plasma protein binding (<38%); crosses the placenta; found in breast milk. **Metabolism:** Lamivudine: Trans-sulfoxide (metabolite). Zidovudine: Hepatic; 3'-azido-3'-deoxy-5'-O-β-D-glucopyranuronosylthymidine (GZDV) (major metabolite). **Elimination:** Lamivudine: (IV) Urine (70% unchanged); $T_{1/2}$=5-7 hrs. Zidovudine: Urine (14% unchanged, 74% GZDV); $T_{1/2}$=0.5-3 hrs.

PATIENT CONSIDERATIONS
Assessment: Assess for advanced HIV disease, bone marrow compromise, liver function and risk factors for liver disease, hepatitis B infection, history of pancreatitis and risk factors for its development, renal function, hypersensitivity to drug, pregnancy/nursing status, and possible drug interactions. Children should be assessed for the ability to swallow tablets. Obtain baseline weight and CBCs.

Monitoring: Monitor signs/symptoms that suggest pancreatitis, lactic acidosis, hepatotoxicity, myopathy and myositis, immune reconstitution syndrome (eg, opportunistic infections), autoimmune disorders, and hypersensitivity reactions. Monitor CBCs and renal/hepatic function.

Counseling: Inform about risk for hematologic toxicities and advise on importance of close blood count monitoring while on therapy. Counsel about the possible occurrence of myopathy and myositis w/ pathological changes during prolonged use and that therapy may cause a rare but serious condition called lactic acidosis w/ hepatomegaly. Inform that deterioration of liver disease has occurred in patients coinfected w/ HBV w/ treatment discontinuation. Instruct to discuss w/ physician any changes in regimen. Caution patients about the use of other medication and instruct to avoid use w/ other lamivudine-, zidovudine-, and/or emtricitabine-containing products. Inform that hepatic decompensation has been reported in patients coinfected w/ HCV receiving interferon alfa w/ or w/o ribavirin. Inform that fat redistribution/accumulation may occur. Inform that therapy is not a cure for HIV-1 infection and patients may continue to experience illnesses associated w/ HIV-1. Advise to avoid doing things that can spread HIV-1 infection to others (eg, sharing of needles/inj equipment/personal items that can have blood or body fluids on them, having sex w/o protection, breastfeeding). Advise to take exactly as prescribed.

COMETRIQ — cabozantinib   Rx

Class: Kinase inhibitor

> GI perforations and fistulas reported; d/c if perforation or fistula develops. Severe, sometimes fatal, hemorrhage (eg, hemoptysis, GI hemorrhage) reported; monitor for signs and symptoms of bleeding. Do not administer w/ severe hemorrhage.

ADULT DOSAGE

Medullary Thyroid Cancer

Progressive, Metastatic:
140mg (one 80mg and three 20mg caps) qd until disease progression or unacceptable toxicity occurs

PEDIATRIC DOSAGE
Pediatric use may not have been established

DOSING CONSIDERATIONS

Concomitant Medications
Strong CYP3A4 Inhibitors:
Reduce the daily dose by 40mg (eg, from 140mg to 100mg qd).
Resume the dose that was used prior to initiating the CYP3A4 inhibitor 2-3 days after discontinuation of the strong inhibitor.

Strong CYP3A4 Inducers:
Increase the daily dose by 40mg (eg, from 140mg to 180mg qd) as tolerated. Resume the dose that was used prior to initiating the CYP3A4 inducer 2-3 days after discontinuation of the strong inducer.
Max: 180mg/day

Hepatic Impairment
Mild to Moderate:
Initial: 80mg
Severe: Not recommended

Adverse Reactions
Withhold for Any of the Following:
- NCI CTCAE Grade 4 hematologic adverse reactions
- Grade ≥3 nonhematologic adverse reactions
- Intolerable Grade 2 adverse reactions

Upon Improvement (eg, Return to Baseline or Resolution to Grade 1), Reduce as Follows:
- If previously receiving 140mg qd, resume at 100mg qd (one 80mg and one 20mg cap)
- If previously receiving 100mg qd, resume at 60mg qd (three 20mg caps)
- If previously receiving 60mg qd, resume at 60mg if tolerated, otherwise d/c

Permanently D/C for Any of the Following:
- Development of visceral perforation or fistula formation
- Severe hemorrhage
- Serious arterial thromboembolic event (eg, MI, cerebral infarction)
- Nephrotic syndrome
- Malignant HTN, hypertensive crisis, persistent uncontrolled HTN despite optimal medical management
- Osteonecrosis of the jaw (ONJ)
- Reversible posterior leukoencephalopathy syndrome (RPLS)

Other Important Considerations
Do not ingest foods (eg, grapefruit, grapefruit juice) or nutritional supplements that are known to inhibit CYP450 while on therapy

ADMINISTRATION
Oral route

Do not substitute Cometriq caps w/ cabozantinib tabs.
Do not take w/ food; do not eat for at least 2 hrs before and at least 1 hr after taking the dose.
Take w/ a full glass (at least 8 fl oz) of water.
Do not take a missed dose w/in 12 hrs of the next dose.
Swallow caps whole; do not open or crush the caps.

STORAGE
20-25°C (68-77°F); excursions are permitted from 15-30°C (59-86°F).

HOW SUPPLIED
Cap: 20mg, 80mg

WARNINGS/PRECAUTIONS
See Dosing Considerations. Avoid w/ recent history of hemorrhage or hemoptysis. Increased incidence of thrombotic events reported; d/c if an acute MI, cerebral infarction, or any other clinically significant arterial thromboembolic complication occurs. Wound complications reported; d/c at least 28 days prior to scheduled surgery; may resume therapy after surgery if wound healing is adequate. Withhold therapy in patients w/ dehiscence or wound healing complications requiring medical intervention. Increased incidence of HTN reported; withhold w/ uncontrolled HTN then resume at reduced dose when controlled. ONJ reported; d/c if ONJ occurs and withhold at least 28 days prior to invasive dental procedures. Palmar-plantar erythrodysesthesia syndrome (PPES) reported; withhold w/ intolerable Grade 2 PPES or Grade 3 PPES until improvement to

Grade 1; resume at reduced dose. Proteinuria reported. RPLS reported; evaluate for RPLS in patients presenting w/ seizures, headache, visual disturbances, confusion, or altered mental function. May cause fetal harm; use effective contraception during and up to 4 months after completion of therapy.

ADVERSE REACTIONS
Diarrhea, stomatitis, PPES, decreased weight, decreased appetite, nausea, fatigue, oral pain, hair color changes, dysgeusia, HTN, abdominal pain, constipation, increased AST, increased ALT.

DRUG INTERACTIONS
See Dosing Considerations. Strong CYP3A4 inhibitors (eg, ketoconazole, itraconazole, clarithromycin) may increase exposure; avoid coadministration or reduce dose of cabozantinib if concomitant use cannot be avoided. Strong CYP3A4 inducers (eg, dexamethasone, phenytoin, carbamazepine) may decrease exposure; avoid chronic coadministration or increase dose of cabozantinib if concomitant use cannot be avoided. Avoid w/ foods (eg, grapefruits, grapefruit juice) or nutritional supplements known to inhibit CYP450 activity. MRP2 inhibitors (eg, abacavir, cidofovir, furosemide) may increase exposure; monitor for increased toxicity w/ concomitant MRP2 inhibitors.

PREGNANCY AND LACTATION
Pregnancy: May cause fetal harm.
Lactation: Not for use in nursing during treatment and for 4 months after the final dose.
Reproductive Potential: Females of reproductive potential should use effective contraception during treatment and for 4 months after the final dose. May impair fertility in females and males of reproductive potential.

MECHANISM OF ACTION
Kinase inhibitor; inhibits the tyrosine kinase activity of RET, MET, VEGFR-1, -2, and -3, KIT, TRKB, FLT-3, AXL, ROS1, TYRO3, MER, and TIE-2, involved in both normal cellular function and pathologic processes such as oncogenesis, metastasis, tumor angiogenesis, drug resistance, and maintenance of the tumor microenvironment.

PHARMACOKINETICS
Absorption: T_{max}=2-5 hrs. **Distribution:** V_d=349L; plasma protein binding (≥99.7%). **Metabolism:** Via CYP3A4. **Elimination:** Urine (27%), feces (54%; 43% unchanged); $T_{1/2}$=55 hrs.

PATIENT CONSIDERATIONS
Assessment: Assess for history of hemorrhage/hemoptysis, scheduled/recent surgery or invasive dental procedure, wounds, HTN, hepatic impairment, pregnancy/nursing status, and possible drug interactions. Obtain baseline BP and perform an oral examination.

Monitoring: Monitor for signs and symptoms of GI perforations and fistulas, hemorrhage, thrombotic events, dehiscence, wound healing complications, ONJ, PPES, nephrotic syndrome, RPLS (eg, seizures, headache, visual disturbances), and other adverse reactions. Monitor BP and urine protein regularly, and perform oral examinations periodically.

Counseling: Advise to notify physician if severe diarrhea, progressive or intolerable rash, mouth sores, oral pain, changes in taste, N/V, weight loss, or other adverse reactions occur. Instruct to contact physician prior to any planned surgeries, including dental procedures. Advise females of reproductive potential of the potential risk to fetus and instruct to contact physician if pregnancy occurs or is suspected during treatment. Instruct to use effective contraception during therapy and for at least 4 months after the last dose. Advise women not to breastfeed during treatment and for 4 months following the last dose. Instruct not to consume grapefruits or grapefruit juice while taking treatment.

COMPLERA — emtricitabine/rilpivirine/tenofovir disoproxil fumarate

Rx

Class: Non-nucleoside reverse transcriptase inhibitor (NNRTI)/nucleoside reverse transcriptase inhibitor (NRTI) combination

> Lactic acidosis and severe hepatomegaly w/ steatosis, including fatal cases, reported w/ the use of nucleoside analogues in combination w/ other antiretrovirals. Not approved for the treatment of chronic hepatitis B virus (HBV) infection. Severe acute exacerbations of hepatitis B reported in patients coinfected w/ HBV upon discontinuation of therapy; closely monitor hepatic function for at least several months. If appropriate, initiation of antihepatitis B therapy may be warranted.

ADULT DOSAGE
HIV-1 Infection

As a complete regimen for the treatment of HIV-1 infection in patients w/ no antiretroviral treatment history and w/ HIV-1 RNA ≤100,000 copies/mL at the start of therapy, and in certain virologically-suppressed (HIV-1 RNA <50 copies/mL) patients on a stable antiretroviral regimen at start of therapy

Recommended Dose: 1 tab qd

PEDIATRIC DOSAGE
HIV-1 Infection

As a complete regimen for the treatment of HIV-1 infection in patients w/ no antiretroviral treatment history and w/ HIV-1 RNA ≤100,000 copies/mL at the start of therapy, and in certain virologically-suppressed (HIV-1 RNA <50 copies/mL) patients on a stable antiretroviral regimen at start of therapy

≥12 Years:
≥35kg:
Recommended Dose: 1 tab qd

DOSING CONSIDERATIONS
Concomitant Medications
W/ Rifabutin: Additional 25mg tab of rilpivirine qd recommended to be taken concomitantly w/ Complera

Renal Impairment
Moderate or Severe (CrCl <50mL/min): Not recommended for use

ADMINISTRATION
Oral route
Take w/ food.

STORAGE
25°C (77°F); excursions permitted to 15-30°C (59-86°F).

HOW SUPPLIED
Tab: (Emtricitabine/Rilpivirine/Tenofovir Disoproxil Fumarate [TDF]) 200mg/25mg/300mg

CONTRAINDICATIONS
Coadministration w/ CYP3A inducers or agents that increase gastric pH causing decreased plasma concentrations, which may result in loss of virologic response and possible resistance (eg, carbamazepine, oxcarbazepine, phenobarbital, phenytoin, rifampin, rifapentine, proton pump inhibitors [eg, dexlansoprazole, esomeprazole, lansoprazole, omeprazole, pantoprazole, rabeprazole], systemic dexamethasone [more than a single dose], St. John's wort).

WARNINGS/PRECAUTIONS
When considering replacing the current regimen in virologically-suppressed patients, patients should have no history of virologic failure, have been stably suppressed for at least 6 months prior to switching therapy, currently be on the 1st or 2nd antiretroviral regimen prior to switching therapy, and have no current/past history of resistance to any of the 3 drug components. Additional monitoring of HIV-1 RNA and regimen tolerability is recommended after replacing therapy to assess for potential virologic failure or rebound. Immune reconstitution syndrome, autoimmune disorders (eg, Graves' disease, polymyositis, Guillain-Barre syndrome) in the setting of immune reconstitution, and redistribution/accumulation of body fat reported. Caution in elderly. **Rilpivirine:** Severe skin and hypersensitivity reactions reported, including cases of drug reaction w/ eosinophilia and systemic symptoms; d/c immediately and initiate appropriate therapy if signs/symptoms develop. Depressive disorders reported; immediate medical evaluation is recommended if severe depressive symptoms occur. Hepatic adverse events reported; increased risk for worsening/development of liver-associated test elevations in patients w/ underlying hepatitis B or C, or marked liver-associated test elevations prior to treatment. Consider liver-associated test monitoring for patients w/o preexisting hepatic dysfunction or other risk factors. **TDF:** Caution w/ known risk factors for liver disease. D/C if lactic acidosis or pronounced hepatotoxicity occurs. Renal impairment (eg, acute renal failure, Fanconi syndrome) reported. Decreased bone mineral density (BMD), increased biochemical markers of bone metabolism, and osteomalacia reported. Consider assessment of BMD in patients w/ history of pathologic bone fracture or other risk factors for osteoporosis or bone loss. Arthralgias and muscle pain/weakness reported in cases of proximal renal tubulopathy. Consider hypophosphatemia and osteomalacia secondary to proximal renal tubulopathy in patients at risk of renal dysfunction who present w/ persistent or worsening bone or muscle symptoms.

ADVERSE REACTIONS
Rilpivirine w/ Emtricitabine/TDF: Nausea, headache, dizziness, depressive disorders, insomnia, abnormal dreams, rash.
Emtricitabine/TDF: Diarrhea, nausea, fatigue, headache, dizziness, depression, insomnia, abnormal dreams, rash.

DRUG INTERACTIONS
See Dosing Considerations and Contraindications. Avoid w/ concurrent or recent use of nephrotoxic agents (eg, high-dose or multiple NSAIDs). Avoid administration w/ other antiretrovirals, adefovir dipivoxil, or drugs containing any of the same active components or lamivudine. Avoid w/ rilpivirine unless needed for dose adjustment (eg, w/ rifabutin). **Rilpivirine:** Caution w/ drugs that may reduce exposure or drugs w/ a known risk of torsades de pointes. Decreased levels, loss of virologic response, and possible resistance w/ CYP3A inducers or drugs increasing gastric pH (eg, antacids, H_2-receptor antagonists [H_2-RAs]). Administer antacids at least 2 hrs before or at least 4 hrs after dosing, and H_2-RAs at least 12 hrs before or at least 4 hrs after dosing. Decreased levels w/ rifabutin. CYP3A inhibitors, azole antifungals, clarithromycin, erythromycin, or telithromycin may increase levels. May decrease levels of ketoconazole and methadone. **Emtricitabine and TDF:** Drugs that reduce renal function or compete for active tubular secretion (eg, acyclovir, aminoglycosides [eg, gentamicin], high-dose or multiple NSAIDs) may increase levels of emtricitabine, TDF, and/or other renally eliminated drugs. **TDF:** Cases of acute renal failure after initiation of high-dose or multiple NSAIDs reported in HIV-infected patients w/ risk factors for renal dysfunction who appeared stable on TDF; consider alternatives to NSAIDs, if needed. Increased levels w/ ledipasvir/sofosbuvir; monitor for adverse reactions.

PREGNANCY AND LACTATION
Pregnancy: Category B. An Antiretroviral Pregnancy Registry has been established to monitor fetal outcomes of pregnant women.
Lactation: Emtricitabine and TDF are found in breast milk. Not for use in nursing.

MECHANISM OF ACTION
Emtricitabine: Nucleoside analogue of cytidine; inhibits activity of HIV-1 reverse transcriptase (RT) by competing w/ natural substrate deoxycytidine 5'-triphosphate and being incorporated into nascent viral DNA, resulting in chain termination. **Rilpivirine:** Non-nucleoside reverse transcriptase inhibitor;

inhibits HIV-1 replication by noncompetitive inhibition of HIV-1 RT. **TDF:** Acyclic nucleoside phosphonate diester analogue of adenosine monophosphate; inhibits activity of HIV-1 RT by competing w/ the natural substrate deoxyadenosine 5'-triphosphate and, after incorporation into DNA, by DNA chain termination.

PHARMACOKINETICS

Absorption: Emtricitabine: Absolute bioavailability (93%), C_{max}=1.8mcg/mL, T_{max}=1-2 hrs, AUC=10mcg•hr/mL. Rilpivirine: T_{max}=4-5 hrs, AUC=2235ng•hr/mL. TDF: Bioavailability (25%, fasted), C_{max}=0.30mcg/mL, T_{max}=1 hr, AUC=2.29mcg•hr/mL. **Distribution:** Emtricitabine: Plasma protein binding (<4%); found in breast milk. Rilpivirine: Plasma protein binding (99.7%). TDF: Plasma protein binding (<0.7%); found in breast milk. **Metabolism:** Emtricitabine: 3'-sulfoxide diastereomers, glucuronic acid conjugate (metabolites). Rilpivirine: Oxidative metabolism by CYP3A system. **Elimination:** Emtricitabine: Feces (14%), urine (86%, 13% metabolites); $T_{1/2}$=10 hrs. Rilpivirine: Feces (85%, 25% unchanged), urine (6.1%, <1% unchanged); $T_{1/2}$=50 hrs. TDF: (IV) Urine (70-80% unchanged); $T_{1/2}$=17 hrs.

PATIENT CONSIDERATIONS

Assessment: Assess for history of virologic failure, current/past history of resistance to any of the drug components, obesity, prolonged nucleoside exposure, liver dysfunction or risk factors for liver disease, renal impairment, HBV infection, pregnancy/nursing status, and possible drug interactions. Assess BMD in patients w/ a history of pathological bone fracture or w/ other risk factors for osteoporosis/bone loss. Assess estimated CrCl, serum phosphorus (P), urine glucose, and urine protein in patients at risk for renal dysfunction.

Monitoring: Monitor for signs/symptoms of lactic acidosis, severe skin and hypersensitivity reactions, severe hepatomegaly w/ steatosis, depressive symptoms, hepatotoxicity, decreased BMD, increased biochemical markers for bone metabolism, osteomalacia, fat redistribution/accumulation, immune reconstitution syndrome (eg, opportunistic infections), autoimmune disorders, renal impairment, and other adverse reactions. Monitor patients coinfected w/ HBV and HIV-1 w/ clinical and lab follow-up for acute exacerbations of hepatitis B for at least several months upon discontinuation of therapy. Monitor estimated CrCl, serum P, urine glucose, and urine protein periodically in patients at risk for renal dysfunction. Additional monitoring of HIV-1 RNA and regimen tolerability is recommended after replacing therapy to assess for potential virologic failure or rebound.

Counseling: Inform that therapy is not a cure for HIV infection; advise that continuous therapy is necessary to control HIV infection and decrease HIV-related illnesses. Advise to practice safer sex and use latex or polyurethane condoms. Inform that there is a pregnancy exposure registry to monitor outcomes in women exposed to therapy during pregnancy. Instruct to never reuse or share needles. Advise not to breastfeed. Advise to take on a regular dosing schedule w/ food and avoid missing doses. Inform that a protein drink is not a substitute for food. Advise on missed dose instructions. Instruct to contact physician if symptoms of lactic acidosis or severe hepatomegaly w/ steatosis, depression, or infection occurs. Inform that hepatotoxicity has been reported during treatment. Instruct to immediately stop taking therapy and seek medical attention if patient develops a rash associated w/ any of the following symptoms: fever; blisters; mucosal involvement; eye inflammation (conjunctivitis); severe allergic reaction causing swelling of the face, eyes, lips, mouth, tongue, or throat; and any signs/symptoms of liver problems. Inform that laboratory tests will be performed and appropriate therapy will be initiated if severe rash occurs. Inform that fat redistribution/accumulation, renal impairment, and decreases in BMD may occur. Advise to inform physician if taking any other prescription/nonprescription medications or herbal products (eg, St. John's wort).

COPAXONE — glatiramer acetate   Rx
Class: Immunomodulatory agent

ADULT DOSAGE	PEDIATRIC DOSAGE
Multiple Sclerosis	Pediatric use may not have been established
Relapsing Forms:	
20mg/mL: Administer SQ qd	
40mg/mL: Administer SQ 3X/week and at least 48 hrs apart	
20mg/mL and 40mg/mL are not interchangeable	

ADMINISTRATION
SQ route
Allow to stand at room temperature for 20 min before administration.
Areas for SQ self-inj include arms, abdomen, hips, and thighs.

STORAGE
2-8°C (36-46°F). If needed, may store at 15-30°C (59-86°F) for up to 1 month, but refrigeration is preferred; avoid exposure to higher temperatures or intense light. Do not freeze; discard if frozen.

HOW SUPPLIED
Inj: 20mg/mL, 40mg/mL

CONTRAINDICATIONS
Known hypersensitivity to glatiramer acetate or mannitol.

WARNINGS/PRECAUTIONS
Immediate post-inj reaction (eg, flushing, chest pain, palpitations, anxiety, dyspnea, throat constriction, urticaria) reported. Transient chest pain reported. Localized lipoatrophy at inj sites and inj-site skin necrosis may occur; follow proper inj technique and rotate inj sites w/ each inj. May interfere w/ immune functions. Continued alteration of cellular immunity due to chronic treatment may result in untoward effects.

ADVERSE REACTIONS
Inj-site reactions, vasodilatation, rash, dyspnea, chest pain.

PREGNANCY AND LACTATION
Pregnancy: Category B.
Lactation: Caution in nursing.

MECHANISM OF ACTION
Immunomodulatory agent; not established. Thought to act by modifying immune processes that are believed to be responsible for the pathogenesis of multiple sclerosis (MS).

PATIENT CONSIDERATIONS
Assessment: Assess for hypersensitivity to drug or mannitol, and pregnancy/nursing status.

Monitoring: Monitor for immediate post-inj reactions, chest pain, lipoatrophy, inj-site skin necrosis, and other adverse reactions.

Counseling: Advise to inform physician if pregnant, planning to become pregnant, or breastfeeding. Inform that drug may cause an immediate post-inj reaction and that symptoms are generally transient and self-limited and do not require specific treatment; inform that these symptoms may occur early or may have their onset several months after treatment initiation. Inform that transient chest pain (either as part of the immediate post-inj reaction or in isolation) may occur; advise to seek medical attention if chest pain of unusual duration or intensity occurs. Instruct to follow proper inj technique and to rotate inj areas and sites w/ each inj to help minimize localized lipoatrophy and inj-site necrosis. Inform that 20mg/mL and 40mg/mL are not interchangeable. Advise to use aseptic technique. Caution against the reuse of needles or syringes. Inform of safe disposal procedures.

COPEGUS — ribavirin   Rx
Class: Nucleoside analogue

> Not for monotherapy treatment of chronic hepatitis C (CHC) virus infection. Primary toxicity is hemolytic anemia. Anemia associated w/ therapy may result in worsening of cardiac disease and lead to fatal and nonfatal MI. Avoid w/ history of significant or unstable cardiac disease. Contraindicated in women who are pregnant and male partners of pregnant women. Extreme care must be taken to avoid pregnancy during therapy and for 6 months after completion of therapy. Use at least 2 reliable forms of effective contraception during therapy and for 6 months after discontinuation.

ADULT DOSAGE	PEDIATRIC DOSAGE
Chronic Hepatitis C with Compensated Liver Disease	**Chronic Hepatitis C with Compensated Liver Disease**
Combination w/ Peginterferon Alfa-2a:	**Combination w/ Peginterferon Alfa-2a:**
Not Previously Treated w/ Interferon Alfa:	**Not Previously Treated w/ Interferon Alfa:**
Monoinfection:	**Monoinfection:**
Genotypes 1, 4:	**≥5 Years:**
<75kg: 1000mg/day in 2 divided doses	**23kg-33kg:** 200mg qam and 200mg qpm
≥75kg: 1200mg/day in 2 divided doses	**34kg-46kg:** 200mg qam and 400mg qpm
Duration: 48 weeks	**47kg-59kg:** 400mg qam and 400mg qpm
Genotypes 2, 3: 800mg/day in 2 divided doses	**60kg-74kg:** 400mg qam and 600mg qpm
Duration: 24 weeks	**≥75kg:** 600mg qam and 600mg qpm
HIV Coinfection:	**Duration:**
800mg/day in 2 divided doses	**Genotypes 2, 3:** 24 weeks
Duration: 48 weeks (regardless of genotype)	**Other Genotypes:** 48 weeks
	Maintain pediatric dosing through the completion of therapy if initiating treatment prior to 18th birthday

---

DOSING CONSIDERATIONS
Renal Impairment
CrCl 30-50mL/min: Alternating doses, 200mg and 400mg qod
CrCl <30mL/min and/or Hemodialysis: 200mg/day

Adverse Reactions
W/O Cardiac Disease:
Hgb <10g/dL:
Adults:
200mg qam and 400mg qpm
Pediatrics: ≥5 Years:
23kg-33kg: 200mg qam
34kg-59kg: 200mg qam and 200mg qpm
≥60kg: 200mg qam and 400mg qpm

Hgb <8.5g/dL:
Adults and Pediatrics: ≥5 Years:
D/C Copegus

W/ History of Stable Cardiac Disease:
Hgb Decrease of ≥2g/dL During Any 4-Week Treatment Period:
Adults:
200mg qam and 400mg qpm
Pediatrics: ≥5 Years:
23kg-33kg: 200mg qam
34kg-59kg: 200mg qam and 200mg qpm
≥60kg: 200mg qam and 400mg qpm
Hgb <12g/dL After 4 Weeks at Reduced Dose:
Adults and Pediatrics: ≥5 Years:
D/C Copegus

Adults: May restart at 600mg/day and further increase to 800mg/day once therapy has been withheld due to clinical adverse event or lab abnormality. Increasing to original dose (1000-1200mg/day) is not recommended

Peds: May attempt to increase to original dose once lab abnormalities or clinical adverse events resolve. Restart at 50% of full dose if therapy has been withheld due to clinical adverse event or lab abnormality

Discontinuation
Consider if at least a 2 log$_{10}$ HCV RNA reduction from baseline by Week 12 is not reached
Consider if HCV RNA levels remain detectable after Week 24
D/C if hepatic decompensation develops during treatment

ADMINISTRATION
Oral route

Take w/ food.
Refer to peginterferon alfa-2a labeling for dosing and administration instructions.

STORAGE
25°C (77°F); excursions permitted between 15-30°C (59-86°F).

HOW SUPPLIED
Tab: 200mg

CONTRAINDICATIONS
Women who are or may become pregnant and men whose female partners are pregnant, hemoglobinopathies (eg, thalassemia major, sickle cell anemia), and in combination w/ didanosine. When used w/ Pegasys, refer to the individual monograph.

WARNINGS/PRECAUTIONS
Not for the treatment of adenovirus, respiratory syncytial virus, parainfluenza or influenza infections. Combination therapy is associated w/ significant adverse reactions (eg, severe depression and suicidal ideation, hemolytic anemia, suppression of bone marrow function, autoimmune/infectious/ophthalmologic/cerebrovascular disorders, pulmonary dysfunction, colitis, pancreatitis, diabetes). A negative pregnancy test is necessary prior to initiation. Caution w/ baseline risk of severe anemia (eg, spherocytosis, history of GI bleeding). Risk of hepatic decompensation and death in CHC patients w/ cirrhosis. Severe acute hypersensitivity reactions and serious skin reactions reported. D/C w/ hepatic decompensation, confirmed pancreatitis, severe hypersensitivity, or if signs/symptoms of severe skin reactions develop. Pulmonary disorders (eg, dyspnea, pulmonary infiltrates, pneumonitis, pulmonary HTN) reported; closely monitor and, if appropriate, d/c therapy if pulmonary infiltrates/function impairment develops. Caution w/ preexisting cardiac disease; d/c if cardiovascular status deteriorates. Decreases in height and weight reported in pediatric patients. Suspend therapy w/ signs and symptoms of pancreatitis.

ADVERSE REACTIONS
Fatigue, asthenia, neutropenia, headache, pyrexia, myalgia, irritability, anxiety, nervousness, insomnia, alopecia, rigors, N/V, diarrhea.

DRUG INTERACTIONS
See Contraindications. Closely monitor for toxicities (eg, hepatic decompensation) w/ nucleoside reverse transcriptase inhibitors; consider dose reduction or discontinuation. May reduce phosphorylation of lamivudine, stavudine, and zidovudine. Severe neutropenia and severe anemia reported w/ zidovudine; consider discontinuation of zidovudine if appropriate. Severe pancytopenia, bone marrow suppression, and myelotoxicity reported w/ azathioprine; d/c peginterferon alfa-2a, ribavirin, and azathioprine if pancytopenia develops.

PREGNANCY AND LACTATION
Pregnancy: Category X. A Ribavirin Pregnancy Registry has been established to monitor maternal-fetal outcomes or pregnancies of female patients and female partners of male patients exposed to ribavirin during treatment and for 6 months following cessation of treatment.
Lactation: Not for use in nursing.

MECHANISM OF ACTION
Nucleoside analogue; not established. Has direct antiviral activity in tissue culture against many RNA viruses; increases mutation frequency in the genomes of several RNA viruses and ribavirin triphosphate inhibits HCV polymerase in a biochemical reaction.

PHARMACOKINETICS
Absorption: C$_{max}$=2748ng/mL; T$_{max}$=2 hrs; AUC$_{0-12h}$=25,361ng•hr/mL. **Elimination:** T$_{1/2}$=120-170 hrs.

PATIENT CONSIDERATIONS
Assessment: Assess for hemoglobinopathies, autoimmune hepatitis, hepatic decompensation, baseline risk of severe anemia, history of or preexisting cardiac disease, renal impairment, hypersensitivity to drug, nursing status, and possible drug interactions. Conduct pregnancy test (including in female partners of male patients), standard hematological and biochemical lab tests, ECG in patients w/ preexisting cardiac abnormalities, thyroid function test, and CD4 count in HIV/AIDS patients.

Monitoring: Monitor for hepatic decompensation, pancreatitis, hypersensitivity/skin reactions, pulmonary infiltrates/function impairment, and other adverse reactions. Monitor growth in pediatrics, cardiac status, TSH, and HCV RNA. Perform hematological tests at Weeks 2 and 4 and biochemical tests at Week 4; perform additional testing periodically. Perform pregnancy testing monthly and for 6 months after discontinuation (including female partners of male patients).

Counseling: Counsel on risks/benefits associated w/ treatment. Inform of pregnancy risks; instruct to use 2 forms of effective contraception during therapy and for 6 months after discontinuation of therapy (including female partners of male patients). Advise to notify physician in the event of pregnancy. Advise that lab evaluations are required prior to starting therapy and periodically thereafter. Advise to be well hydrated, especially during the initial stages of treatment. Caution to avoid driving/operating machinery if dizziness, somnolence, or fatigue develops. Advise to take w/ food, and instruct not to drink alcohol; inform that alcohol may exacerbate CHC infection. Inform to take missed doses as soon as possible during the same day; advise not to double the next dose. Inform to take appropriate precautions to prevent HCV transmission or in the event of treatment failure.

CORIFACT — factor XIII concentrate (human)   Rx
Class: Plasma glycoprotein

ADULT DOSAGE	PEDIATRIC DOSAGE
Congenital FXIII Deficiency	**Congenital FXIII Deficiency**
Routine prophylactic treatment and perioperative management of surgical bleeding	Routine prophylactic treatment and perioperative management of surgical bleeding
40 IU/kg at a rate not to exceed 4mL/min. Adjust dose ± 5 IU/kg to maintain 5-20% trough level of FXIII activity	40 IU/kg at a rate not to exceed 4mL/min. Adjust dose ± 5 IU/kg to maintain 5-20% trough level of FXIII activity
Routine Prophylaxis: Administer every 28 days	**Routine Prophylaxis:** Administer every 28 days
Perioperative Management: Individualize dose based on FXIII activity level, type of surgery, and clinical response. Monitor FXIII activity levels during and after surgery	**Perioperative Management:** Individualize dose based on FXIII activity level, type of surgery, and clinical response. Monitor FXIII activity levels during and after surgery
Dose Adjustment Using the Berichrom Activity Assay:	**Dose Adjustment Using the Berichrom Activity Assay:**
One Trough Level of <5%: Increase by 5 IU/kg	**One Trough Level of <5%:** Increase by 5 IU/kg
Trough Level of 5% to 20%: No change	**Trough Level of 5% to 20%:** No change
Two Trough Levels of >20%: Decrease by 5 IU/kg	**Two Trough Levels of >20%:** Decrease by 5 IU/kg
One Trough Level of >25%: Decrease by 5 IU/kg	**One Trough Level of >25%:** Decrease by 5 IU/kg
Dose Adjustment for Perioperative Management:	**Dose Adjustment for Perioperative Management:**
If Time Since Last Dose is w/in 7 Days: Additional dose may not be needed	**If Time Since Last Dose is w/in 7 Days:** Additional dose may not be needed
If Time Since Last Dose is 8-21 Days: Additional partial or full dose may be needed based on FXIII activity level	**If Time Since Last Dose is 8-21 Days:** Additional partial or full dose may be needed based on FXIII activity level
If Time Since Last Dose is 21-28 Days: Full prophylactic dose	**If Time Since Last Dose is 21-28 Days:** Full prophylactic dose

ADMINISTRATION
IV route

Use w/in 4 hrs after reconstitution; refer to prescribing information for further information on reconstitution.

STORAGE
2-8°C (36-46°F) up to 36 months. May store at room temperature ≤25°C (77°F) for up to 6 months; do not return to the refrigerator after it is stored at room temperature. Protect from light. Do not freeze. **Reconstituted Sol:** Use w/in 4 hrs after reconstitution. Do not refrigerate or freeze.

HOW SUPPLIED
Inj: 1000-1600 U

CONTRAINDICATIONS
Known anaphylactic or severe systemic reactions to human plasma-derived products.

WARNINGS/PRECAUTIONS
Hypersensitivity reactions reported; d/c administration immediately and institute appropriate treatment if signs/symptoms of anaphylaxis or hypersensitivity

reactions occur. Development of inhibitory antibodies against FXIII detected; monitor for such development. Presence of inhibitory antibodies may manifest as an inadequate response to treatment; perform an assay that measures FXIII inhibitory antibody concentrations if expected plasma FXIII activity levels are not attained, or if breakthrough bleeding occurs. Thromboembolic complications reported; monitor patients w/ known risk factors for thrombotic events. May carry a risk of transmitting infectious agents (eg, viruses, and theoretically, Creutzfeldt-Jakob disease agent).

ADVERSE REACTIONS
Joint inflammation, hypersensitivity, rash, pruritus, erythema, hematoma, arthralgia, headache, elevated thrombin-antithrombin levels, increased blood lactate dehydrogenase.

PREGNANCY AND LACTATION
Pregnancy: Category C.
Lactation: Caution in nursing.

MECHANISM OF ACTION
Plasma glycoprotein; consists of two A-subunits and two B-subunits. FXIIIa promotes cross-linking of fibrin during coagulation and is essential to the physiological protection of the clot against fibrinolysis. FXIIIa catalyzes the cross-linking of fibrin α- and gamma-chains for fibrin stabilization and renders the fibrin clot more elastic and resistant to fibrinolysis. FXIIIa also crosslinks α_2-plasmin inhibitor to the α-chain of fibrin, resulting in protection of the fibrin clot from degradation by plasmin. The B-subunits function as carrier molecules for A-subunits; stabilize the structure of A-subunits and protect them from proteolysis.

PHARMACOKINETICS
Absorption: AUC=184 U•hr/mL; C_{max}=0.9 U/mL; T_{max}=1.7 hrs. **Distribution:** V_d=51.1mL/kg. **Elimination:** $T_{1/2}$=6.6 days.

PATIENT CONSIDERATIONS
Assessment: Assess for risk factors for thrombotic events, hypersensitivity to drug, and pregnancy/nursing status.

Monitoring: Monitor for hypersensitivity reactions, thromboembolic complications, infections, and other adverse reactions. Monitor trough FXIII activity level. If breakthrough bleeding occurs, or if expected peak plasma FXIII activity levels are not attained, perform an investigation to determine the presence of FXIII inhibitory antibodies.

Counseling: Inform of the signs/symptoms of allergic hypersensitivity reactions (eg, urticaria, rash, tightness of the chest, wheezing, hypotension and/or anaphylaxis), immunogenicity (eg, breakthrough bleeding), and thrombosis (eg, limb or abdomen swelling and/or pain, chest pain, SOB, loss of sensation or motor power, altered consciousness, vision, or speech). Inform that medication is made from human blood, and thus may carry a risk of transmitting infectious agents.

COSENTYX – secukinumab
Rx

Class: Monoclonal antibody/IL-17A antagonist

ADULT DOSAGE
Plaque Psoriasis

In Patients Who Are Candidates for Systemic/Phototherapy:

Moderate to Severe:
300mg at Weeks 0, 1, 2, 3, and 4, followed by 300mg every 4 weeks; a dose of 150mg may be acceptable for some patients

Each 300mg dose is given as two 150mg inj

Psoriatic Arthritis

W/ Coexistent Moderate to Severe Plaque Psoriasis:
Use the dosing recommendations for plaque psoriasis

Other Psoriatic Arthritis:
Administer w/ or w/o a LD
W/ a LD: 150mg at Weeks 0, 1, 2, 3, and 4 and every 4 weeks thereafter
W/O a LD: 150mg every 4 weeks
If active psoriatic arthritis continues, consider a dosage of 300mg

May administer w/ or w/o methotrexate

Ankylosing Spondylitis

Administer w/ or w/o a LD

W/ a LD: 150mg at Weeks 0, 1, 2, 3, and 4 and every 4 weeks thereafter
W/O a LD: 150mg every 4 weeks

PEDIATRIC DOSAGE
Pediatric use may not have been established

ADMINISTRATION
SQ route
Administer each inj at a different anatomic location (eg, upper arms, thighs, any quadrant of abdomen) than previous inj.
Do not inject into areas where the skin is tender, bruised, erythematous, indurated, or affected by psoriasis.

Preparation
Pen and Prefilled Syringe:
Before inj, remove from refrigerator and allow to reach room temperature (15-30 min) w/o removing needle cap.
Administer w/in 1 hr after removal from refrigerator and discard any unused product remaining in the pen/prefilled syringe.

Single-Use Vial:
Preparation time from piercing the stopper until end of reconstitution should not exceed 90 min.
1. Remove vial from refrigerator and allow to stand for 15-30 min to reach room temperature; ensure sterile water for inj (SWFI) is at room temperature.
2. Slowly inject 1mL of SWFI into vial.
3. Tilt vial at a 45° angle and gently rotate between fingertips for 1 min; do not shake/invert vial.
4. Allow to stand for 10 min at room temperature, then tilt vial at a 45° angle and gently rotate between fingertips for 1 min; do not shake/invert vial.
5. Allow vial to stand undisturbed at room temperature for approx 5 min.
6. Prepare the required number for vials and use immediately or store in refrigerator at 2-8°C (36-46°F) for up to 24 hrs. Do not freeze. After refrigeration, allow reconstituted sol to reach room temperature (15-30 min) before administration; administer w/in 1 hr after removal from 2-8°C (36-46°F) storage.

STORAGE
2-8°C (36-46°F). Protect from light. Do not freeze. To avoid foaming, do not shake.

HOW SUPPLIED
Inj: 150mg/mL [prefilled syringe, Sensoready pen], 150mg [vial]

CONTRAINDICATIONS
Previous serious hypersensitivity reaction to secukinumab or any components of the medication.

WARNINGS/PRECAUTIONS
May increase risk of infections; exercise caution when considering use in patients w/ a chronic infection or a history of recurrent infection. If serious infection develops, closely monitor and d/c until infection resolves. Evaluate for tuberculosis (TB) infection prior to initiating treatment; do not administer to patients w/ active TB infection. Initiate treatment of latent TB prior to administering therapy; consider anti-TB therapy prior to initiation in patients w/ a past history of latent or active TB in whom an adequate course of treatment cannot be confirmed. Caution w/ inflammatory bowel disease; exacerbations and new onset reported. Trend towards greater disease activity and increased adverse events seen w/ active Crohn's disease. Anaphylaxis and urticaria reported; d/c immediately and initiate appropriate therapy if an anaphylactic or other serious allergic reaction occurs. Removable cap of the Sensoready pen and prefilled syringe contains natural rubber latex, which may cause an allergic reaction in latex-sensitive individuals. Prior to initiating therapy, consider completion of all age appropriate immunizations according to current immunization guidelines.

ADVERSE REACTIONS
Ankylosing Spondylitis: Nasopharyngitis, nausea, URTI, infections.
Plaque Psoriasis: Nasopharyngitis, diarrhea, URTI, infections.
Psoriatic Arthritis: Nasopharyngitis, URTI, headache, nausea, hypercholesterolemia, infections.

DRUG INTERACTIONS
Avoid w/ live vaccines. Non-live vaccinations received during a course of therapy may not elicit an immune response sufficient to prevent disease. May normalize formation of CYP450 enzymes; upon initiation or discontinuation of therapy in patients who are receiving concomitant CYP450 substrates, particularly those w/ a narrow therapeutic index, consider monitoring for therapeutic effect (eg, warfarin) or drug concentration (eg, cyclosporine) and consider dosage modification of the CYP450 substrate.

PREGNANCY AND LACTATION
Pregnancy: Category B.
Lactation: Caution in nursing.

MECHANISM OF ACTION
Monoclonal antibody/interleukin-17A (IL-17A) antagonist; selectively binds to the IL-17A cytokine and inhibits its interaction w/ the IL-17 receptor. Inhibits the release of proinflammatory cytokines and chemokines.

PHARMACOKINETICS
Absorption: Bioavailability (55-77%); C_{max}=13.7mcg/mL (150mg), 27.3mcg/mL (300mg); T_{max}=6 days. **Distribution:** V_d=7.10-8.60L (IV). **Elimination:** $T_{1/2}$=22-31 days.

PATIENT CONSIDERATIONS
Assessment: Assess for previous hypersensitivity to the drug, chronic infection or history of recurrent infection, TB infection, inflammatory bowel disease, latex sensitivity, immunization status, pregnancy/nursing status, and possible drug interactions.

Monitoring: Monitor for signs/symptoms of infection, inflammatory bowel disease, anaphylactic/allergic reactions, and other adverse reactions. Monitor for signs/symptoms of active TB during and after treatment.

Counseling: Advise of the potential benefits and risks of therapy. Inform that drug may lower the ability of immune system to fight infections; instruct to contact physician if any symptoms of infection develop. Advise to seek immediate medical attention if any symptoms of a serious hypersensitivity reaction occur. Instruct in inj techniques, as well as proper syringe and needle disposal, and caution against reuse of needles and syringes.

COSMEGEN — dactinomycin

Rx

Class: Actinomycin antibiotic

> Administer only under supervision of a physician experienced in the use of cancer chemotherapeutic agents. Highly toxic; handle and administer with care. Avoid inhalation of dust or vapors and contact with skin or mucous membranes (especially eyes). Avoid exposure during pregnancy. Review and follow special handling procedures prior to handling. Extremely corrosive to soft tissue. Severe damage to soft tissue may occur with extravasation during IV use; may lead to contracture of the arms.

ADULT DOSAGE

Wilms' Tumor/Childhood Rhabdomyosarcoma/Ewing's Sarcoma

15mcg/kg/day for 5 days

Metastatic Nonseminomatous Testicular Cancer

1000mcg/m² on Day 1 of combination therapy

Gestational Trophoblastic Neoplasia

Monotherapy:
12mcg/kg/day for 5 days

Combination Therapy:
500mcg on Days 1 and 2

Regional Perfusion in Locally Recurrent/Locoregional Solid Malignancies

50mcg/kg for lower extremity or pelvis
35mcg/kg for upper extremity

Dose intensity per 2-week cycle should not exceed 15mcg/kg/day or 400-600mcg/m²/day for 5 days

PEDIATRIC DOSAGE

Wilms' Tumor/Childhood Rhabdomyosarcoma/Ewing's Sarcoma

<6 Months of Age:
15mcg/kg/day for 5 days

Metastatic Nonseminomatous Testicular Cancer

<6 Months of Age:
1000mcg/m² on Day 1 of combination therapy

Gestational Trophoblastic Neoplasia

<6 Months of Age:
Monotherapy:
12mcg/kg/day for 5 days

Combination Therapy:
500mcg on Days 1 and 2

Regional Perfusion in Locally Recurrent/Locoregional Solid Malignancies

<6 Months of Age:
50mcg/kg for lower extremity or pelvis 35mcg/kg for upper extremity

Dose intensity per 2-week cycle should not exceed 15mcg/kg/day or 400-600mcg/m²/day for 5 days

---

DOSING CONSIDERATIONS
Other Important Considerations
See PI for agents used in combination therapy
Calculate dose for obese or edematous patients based on BSA
May need lower dose in obese patients, or with previous chemotherapy/radiation use

Elderly
Start at lower end of dosing range

ADMINISTRATION
IV route
Refer to PI for preparation, administration, management of extravasation, and special handling instructions as well as accidental contact measures

STORAGE
20-25°C (68-77°F). Protect from light and humidity. Reconstituted Sol: Must be used within 4 hrs of initial reconstitution when stored at room temperature.

HOW SUPPLIED
Inj: 0.5mg

CONTRAINDICATIONS
Hypersensitivity to any component of this product, during or about the time of chickenpox or herpes zoster infection.

WARNINGS/PRECAUTIONS
May affect hematopoietic system resulting in myelosuppression; monitor frequently for adverse reactions. Possible anaphylactoid reaction may occur. Observe daily for toxic side effects with combination chemotherapy; d/c if stomatitis, diarrhea, or severe hematopoietic depression occurs until patient has recovered. Veno-occlusive disease (primarily hepatic) reported particularly in children <48 months. Complications of perfusion technique reported. Renal, hepatic, and bone marrow function abnormalities reported in patients with neoplastic diseases; monitor frequently. Caution in elderly. Perform careful calculation of dosage prior to administration of each dose.

ADVERSE REACTIONS
Contracture of the arms, damage to soft tissues, extravasation, N/V, sepsis, infection, malaise, fatigue, lethargy, fever, myalgia, proctitis, hypocalcemia, growth retardation.

DRUG INTERACTIONS
Do not administer live virus vaccines. Increased incidence of GI toxicity, marrow suppression, and 2nd primary tumors with radiation. Normal skin and buccal and pharyngeal mucosa may show early erythema with radiation. May reactivate erythema from previous radiation therapy. Severe oropharyngeal mucositis may occur with irradiation directed toward nasopharynx. Caution

if used within 2 months of irradiation for treatment of right-sided Wilms' tumor; hepatomegaly and elevated AST levels reported. Do not administer with radiotherapy for Wilms' tumor unless the benefit outweighs risks. May be necessary to decrease the usual dose with additional/previous chemotherapy or radiation therapy.

PREGNANCY AND LACTATION
Category D, not for use in nursing.

MECHANISM OF ACTION
Actinomycin antibiotic; believed to produce its cytotoxic effects by binding to DNA and inhibiting RNA synthesis.

PHARMACOKINETICS
Elimination: Urine and feces (30%); $T_{1/2}$=36 hrs.

PATIENT CONSIDERATIONS

Assessment: Assess for infection with chickenpox or herpes zoster, obesity, edema, other disease/conditions, pregnancy/nursing status, history of radiotherapy, immunization history, and possible drug interactions.

Monitoring: Monitor for myelosuppression, anaphylactoid reaction, stomatitis, diarrhea, severe hematopoietic depression, veno-occlusive disease, complications of perfusion technique, toxic effects, and other adverse reactions. Frequently monitor renal, hepatic, and bone marrow functions.

Counseling: Advise women of childbearing potential to avoid becoming pregnant; apprise of the potential hazard to the fetus if used during pregnancy or become pregnant while on therapy. Instruct to report any toxic or adverse effects.

COTELLIC — cobimetinib

Rx

Class: Kinase inhibitor

ADULT DOSAGE

Unresectable or Metastatic Melanoma with BRAF V600E or V600K Mutations

60mg qd for the first 21 days of each 28-day cycle in combination w/ vemurafenib

Continue therapy until disease progression or unacceptable toxicity

Missed Dose
If a dose is missed or if vomiting occurs when the dose is taken, resume dosing w/ the next scheduled dose

PEDIATRIC DOSAGE
Pediatric use may not have been established

DOSING CONSIDERATIONS
Concomitant Medications
Do not take strong or moderate CYP3A inhibitors. If concurrent short-term (≤14 days) use of moderate CYP3A inhibitors is unavoidable, reduce cobimetinib dose to 20mg; after discontinuation of a moderate CYP3A inhibitor, resume previous dose of cobimetinib 60mg. Use an alternative to a strong or moderate CYP3A inhibitor in patients who are taking a reduced dose of cobimetinib (40 or 20mg daily).

Renal Impairment
Moderate (CrCl 30-89mL/min): Dose adjustment is not recommended
Severe: A recommended dose has not been established

Adverse Reactions
Recommended Dose Reductions for Cobimetinib:
1st Dose Reduction: 40mg qd
2nd Dose Reduction: 20mg qd
Subsequent Modification: Permanently d/c if unable to tolerate 20mg qd

Hemorrhage:
Grade 3: Withhold for ≤4 weeks. If improved to Grade 0 or 1, resume at the next lower dose level. If not improved w/in 4 weeks, permanently d/c.
Grade 4: Permanently d/c

Cardiomyopathy:
Asymptomatic, Absolute Decrease in Left Ventricular Ejection Fraction (LVEF) from Baseline of >10% and <Lower Limit of Normal (LLN): Withhold for 2 weeks; repeat LVEF. Resume at next lower dose if LVEF is ≥LLN and absolute decrease from baseline LVEF is ≤10%. Permanently d/c if LVEF is <LLN or absolute decrease from baseline LVEF is >10%.
Symptomatic LVEF Decrease from Baseline: Withhold for ≤4 weeks; repeat LVEF. Resume at next lower dose if symptoms resolve, LVEF is ≥LLN, and absolute decrease from baseline LVEF is ≤10%. Permanently d/c if symptoms persist, LVEF is <LLN, or absolute decrease from baseline LVEF is >10%.

Dermatologic Reactions:
Grade 2 (Intolerable), Grade 3 or 4: Withhold or reduce dose

Serous Retinopathy or Retinal Vein Occlusion:
Serous Retinopathy: Withhold for ≤4 weeks. If signs and symptoms improve, resume at the next lower dose level. If not improved or symptoms recur at the lower dose w/in 4 weeks, permanently d/c.
Retinal Vein Occlusion: Permanently d/c

Liver Lab Abnormalities and Hepatotoxicity:
1st Occurrence Grade 4: Withhold for ≤4 weeks. If improved to Grade 0 or 1, then resume at the next lower dose level. If not improved to Grade 0 or 1 w/in 4 weeks, permanently d/c.
Recurrent Grade 4: Permanently d/c

Rhabdomyolysis and Creatine Phosphokinase (CPK) Elevations:
Grade 4 CPK Elevation/Any CPK Elevation and Myalgia: Withhold for ≤4 weeks. If improved to Grade 3 or lower, resume at the next lower dose level. If not improved w/in 4 weeks, permanently d/c.

Photosensitivity:
Grade 2 (Intolerable), Grade 3 or Grade 4: Withhold for ≤4 weeks. If improved to Grade 0 or 1, resume at the next lower dose level. If not improved w/in 4 weeks, permanently d/c.

Other:
Grade 2 (Intolerable)/Any Grade 3 Adverse Reactions: Withhold for ≤4 weeks. If improved to Grade 0 or 1, resume at the next lower dose level. If not improved w/in 4 weeks, permanently d/c.

1st Occurrence of Any Grade 4 Adverse Reaction: Withhold until adverse reaction improves to Grade 0 or 1. Then resume at the next lower dose level, or permanently d/c.

Recurrent Grade 4 Adverse Reaction: Permanently d/c

ADMINISTRATION
Oral route

Take w/ or w/o food.

STORAGE
<30°C (86°F).

HOW SUPPLIED
Tab: 20mg

WARNINGS/PRECAUTIONS
See Dosing Considerations. New primary malignancies, cutaneous and non-cutaneous, may occur; monitor patients for signs or symptoms of non-cutaneous malignancies. Perform dermatologic evaluations prior to initiation of therapy and every 2 months during therapy, and monitor for 6 months following discontinuation. Hemorrhage (including major hemorrhages), severe rash and other skin reactions, and photosensitivity (including severe cases) may occur. Cardiomyopathy may occur; evaluate LVEF prior to initiation, 1 month after initiation, and every 3 months thereafter until discontinuation. If restarting treatment after a dose reduction/interruption, evaluate LVEF at approx 2 weeks, 4 weeks, 10 weeks, and 16 weeks, and then as clinically indicated. Ocular toxicities, including serous retinopathy, may occur; perform an ophthalmological evaluation at regular intervals and any time a patient reports new or worsening visual disturbances. Hepatotoxicity may occur; monitor liver lab tests before initiation and monthly during treatment, or more frequently as clinically indicated. Rhabdomyolysis may occur; obtain baseline serum CPK and creatinine levels prior to initiation, periodically during treatment, and as clinically indicated. May cause fetal harm.

ADVERSE REACTIONS
Diarrhea, photosensitivity reaction, N/V, pyrexia.

DRUG INTERACTIONS
See Dosing Considerations. Strong CYP3A4 inhibitors (itraconazole) may increase systemic exposure. Strong CYP3A inducers may decrease systemic exposure and reduce efficacy; avoid concurrent use w/ strong or moderate CYP3A inducers (eg, carbamazepine, efavirenz, phenytoin).

PREGNANCY AND LACTATION
Pregnancy: Can cause fetal harm when administered to a pregnant woman.
Lactation: There is no information regarding the presence of cobimetinib in human milk, effects on the breastfed infant, or effects on milk production; advise not to breastfeed during treatment and for 2 weeks after the final dose.
Reproductive Potential: May reduce fertility in females and males. Females of reproductive potential should use effective contraception during treatment and for 2 weeks after the final dose.

MECHANISM OF ACTION
Kinase inhibitor; reversible inhibitor of mitogen-activated protein kinase/extracellular signal regulated kinase 1 (MEK1) and MEK2, which promotes cellular proliferation. BRAF V600E mutations result in constitutive activation of the BRAF pathway, which includes MEK1 and MEK2. Inhibits tumor cell growth (tumor cell lines expressing BRAF V600E); coadministration w/ vemurafenib resulted in increased apoptosis in vitro and reduced tumor growth. Also prevented vemurafenib-mediated growth enhancement of a wild-type BRAF tumor cell line.

PHARMACOKINETICS
Absorption: Absolute bioavailability (46%); T_{max}=2.4 hrs (median); C_{max}=273ng/mL; AUC_{0-24h}=4340ng•h/mL. **Distribution:** Plasma protein binding (95%); V_d=806L. **Metabolism:** CYP3A oxidation and UGT2B7 glucuronidation. **Elimination:** Feces (76%, 6.6% unchanged); urine (17.8%, 1.6% unchanged); $T_{1/2}$=44 hrs.

PATIENT CONSIDERATIONS
Assessment: Confirm the presence of BRAF V600E or V600K mutation in tumor specimens and evaluate LVEF, liver lab tests, and baseline serum CPK and creatinine levels prior to initiation. Perform dermatologic evaluations. Assess pregnancy/nursing status.

Monitoring: Monitor for signs or symptoms of non-cutaneous malignancies, hemorrhage, photosensitivity, pregnancy, and other adverse reactions. Perform dermatologic evaluations every 2 months during therapy and monitor for 6 months following discontinuation. Monitor LVEF 1 month after initiation, and every 3 months thereafter until discontinuation. If restarting treatment after a dose reduction/interruption, evaluate LVEF at approx 2 weeks, 4 weeks, 10 weeks, and 16 weeks, and then as clinically indicated. Perform ophthalmological evaluations at regular intervals and any time a patient reports new or worsening visual disturbances. Monitor liver lab tests monthly during treatment or as indicated. Obtain serum CPK and creatinine levels periodically.

Counseling: Advise to contact healthcare provider immediately for change in or development of new skin lesions, severe skin changes, any changes in vision, muscle pain or weakness, and any signs/symptoms of unusual severe bleeding/hemorrhage, left ventricular dysfunction, or liver dysfunction. Advise to report any history of cardiac disease and of the requirement for cardiac monitoring prior to and during treatment. Advise that treatment requires monitoring of their liver function. Advise to avoid sun exposure, wear protective clothing, and use broad-spectrum UVA/UVB sunscreen and lip balm (SPF ≥30) when outdoors. Advise females of reproductive potential of the potential risk to a fetus and to use effective contraception during treatment and for at least 2 weeks after the final dose; advise to contact healthcare provider if they become pregnant, or if pregnancy is suspected, during treatment. Advise not to breastfeed during treatment and for 2 weeks after the final dose.

CRINONE — progesterone   Rx

Class: Progesterone

ADULT DOSAGE	PEDIATRIC DOSAGE
Assisted Reproductive Technology	Pediatric use may not have been established
For Infertile Women w/ Progesterone Deficiency:	
8%:	
Women Who Require Progesterone Supplementation:	
90mg once daily	
Women w/ Partial or Complete Ovarian Failure Who Require Progesterone Replacement:	
90mg bid	
If pregnancy occurs, may continue treatment until placental autonomy is achieved, up to 10-12 weeks	
Secondary Amenorrhea	
4%:	
Administer qod up to a total of 6 doses	
In Women Who Fail to Respond to	
4%:	
8%:	
Administer qod up to a total of 6 doses	

ADMINISTRATION
Intravaginal route

STORAGE
20-25°C (68-77°F).

HOW SUPPLIED
Gel: 4% [45mg], 8% [90mg]

CONTRAINDICATIONS
Known sensitivity to this product (progesterone or any of the other ingredients), undiagnosed vaginal bleeding, liver dysfunction or disease, known/suspected malignancy of breast or genital organs, missed abortion, active thrombophlebitis or thromboembolic disorders, history of hormone-associated thrombophlebitis or thromboembolic disorders.

WARNINGS/PRECAUTIONS
A dosage increase from 4% gel can only be accomplished by using the 8% gel; increasing the volume of gel administered does not increase the amount of progesterone absorbed. D/C immediately if signs of thrombotic disorders (eg, thrombophlebitis, cerebrovascular disorders, pulmonary embolism, retinal thrombosis) occur or are suspected. Include special reference to breast and pelvic organs as well as Papanicolaou smear in pretreatment exam. Consider nonfunctional causes in cases of breakthrough bleeding. Adequate diagnostic measures should be taken in cases of undiagnosed vaginal bleeding. May cause fluid retention; carefully observe patients with epilepsy, migraine, asthma, or cardiac/renal dysfunction. Pathologist should be advised of progesterone therapy when relevant specimens are submitted. Caution with history of psychic depression; d/c if depression recurs to a serious degree. May decrease glucose tolerance; carefully observe diabetic patients while on therapy.

ADVERSE REACTIONS
Bloating, abdominal pain/cramps, breast pain, depression, headache, nausea, perineal pain, constipation, diarrhea, arthralgia, libido decreased, nervousness, somnolence, breast enlargement, nocturia.

PREGNANCY AND LACTATION
Safety not known in pregnancy/nursing.

MECHANISM OF ACTION
Progesterone; transforms a proliferative endometrium into a secretory endometrium to increase endometrial receptivity for implantation of embryo. Helps maintain pregnancy.

PHARMACOKINETICS
Absorption: Administration of variable doses resulted in different parameters.
Distribution: Plasma protein binding (96-99% albumin and corticosteroid binding globulin); found in breast milk. **Metabolism:** (PO) 5β-pregnan-3α, 20α-diol glucuronide (major urinary metabolite); 5β-pregnan-3α-ol-20-one

(5β-pregnanolone), 5α-pregnan-3α-ol-20-one (5α-pregnanolone) (plasma metabolites). **Elimination:** Kidney (50-60%, metabolites); bile and feces (10%). Refer to PI for information on additional PK parameters.

PATIENT CONSIDERATIONS

Assessment: Assess for known sensitivity to the product, undiagnosed vaginal bleeding, liver dysfunction or disease, known/suspected malignancy of breast or genital organs, missed abortion, active thrombophlebitis or thromboembolic disorders, history of hormone-associated thrombophlebitis or thromboembolic disorders, epilepsy, migraine, asthma, cardiac/renal dysfunction, history of psychic depression, diabetes, pregnancy/nursing status, and use of other vaginal products. Perform Papanicolaou smear.

Monitoring: Monitor for signs/symptoms of thrombotic disorders, breakthrough bleeding, decrease in glucose tolerance, recurrence of depression, fluid retention, and other adverse reactions.

Counseling: Counsel about risks and benefits of treatment. Instruct not to use with other local intravaginal therapy; if used concurrently, advise that there should be at least a 6-hr period before or after gel administration. Inform that small, white globules may appear as a vaginal discharge possibly due to gel accumulation, even several days after usage.

CRIXIVAN — indinavir sulfate   Rx

Class: Protease inhibitor

ADULT DOSAGE	PEDIATRIC DOSAGE
HIV-1 Infection	Pediatric use may not have been established
Combination w/ Other Antiretrovirals: 800mg q8h	

DOSING CONSIDERATIONS
Concomitant Medications
Delavirdine:
Consider dose reduction to 600mg q8h when administering delavirdine 400mg tid
Didanosine:
Administer at least 1 hr apart on an empty stomach
Itraconazole:
Reduce dose to 600mg q8h when administering itraconazole 200mg bid
Ketoconazole:
Reduce dose to 600mg q8h when administering ketoconazole 200mg bid
Rifabutin:
Reduce rifabutin dose to half the standard dose and increase indinavir dose to 1000mg q8h

Hepatic Impairment
Mild-to-Moderate Hepatic Insufficiency Due to Cirrhosis:
Reduce dose to 600mg q8h

Adverse Reactions
Nephrolithiasis/Urolithiasis:
May temporarily interrupt (eg, 1-3 days) or d/c therapy

ADMINISTRATION
Oral route

Administer w/o food but w/ water 1 hr ac or 2 hrs pc.
May administer w/ other liquids (eg, skim milk, juice, coffee, tea) or w/ a light meal.
Drink at least 1.5L of liquids during the course of 24 hrs to ensure adequate hydration.

STORAGE
15-30°C (59-86°F). Protect from moisture.

HOW SUPPLIED
Cap: 200mg, 400mg

CONTRAINDICATIONS
Coadministration w/ CYP3A4 substrates for which elevated concentrations potentially cause serious or life-threatening reactions (eg, alfuzosin, amiodarone, dihydroergotamine, ergonovine, ergotamine, methylergonovine, cisapride, lovastatin, simvastatin, pimozide, sildenafil [for treatment of pulmonary arterial HTN], oral midazolam, triazolam, alprazolam). Clinically significant hypersensitivity to any of its components.

WARNINGS/PRECAUTIONS
Nephrolithiasis/urolithiasis reported. Ensure adequate hydration in all patients. Acute hemolytic anemia, including cases resulting in death, reported; once a diagnosis is apparent, institute appropriate measures, including discontinuation of therapy. Hepatitis, including cases resulting in hepatic failure and death, reported. New onset or exacerbation of diabetes mellitus (DM), hyperglycemia, and diabetic ketoacidosis reported; initiation or dose adjustments of insulin or oral hypoglycemic agents may be required. Indirect hyperbilirubinemia reported frequently during treatment, and infrequently associated w/ increases in serum transaminases. Tubulointerstitial nephritis w/ medullary calcification and cortical atrophy observed in patients w/ asymptomatic severe leukocyturia (>100 cells/high power field); closely follow patients w/ asymptomatic severe leukocyturia and monitor frequently w/ urinalyses. Consider discontinuation of therapy in all patients w/ severe leukocyturia. Immune reconstitution syndrome reported. Autoimmune disorders (eg, Graves' disease, polymyositis, Guillain-Barre syndrome) reported in the setting of immune reconstitution and can occur

many months after initiation of treatment. Spontaneous bleeding in patients w/ hemophilia A and B reported. Redistribution/accumulation of body fat reported. Caution in elderly.

ADVERSE REACTIONS
Nephrolithiasis/urolithiasis, hyperbilirubinemia, abdominal pain, headache, N/V, dizziness, pruritus, diarrhea, back pain.

DRUG INTERACTIONS
See Contraindications and Dosing Considerations. Caution w/ atorvastatin, rosuvastatin, parenteral midazolam, sildenafil (for treatment of erectile dysfunction), tadalafil, or vardenafil. Do not coadminister w/ rifampin. Not recommended w/ St. John's wort, atazanavir, salmeterol, or fluticasone (when indinavir is coadministered w/ a potent CYP3A4 inhibitor [eg, ritonavir]). Avoid w/ colchicine in patients w/ renal/hepatic impairment. May increase levels of CYP3A/CYP3A4 substrates, ritonavir, saquinavir, antiarrhythmics, trazodone, colchicine, quetiapine, dihydropyridine calcium channel blockers, clarithromycin, bosentan, atorvastatin, rosuvastatin, immunosuppressants, salmeterol, fluticasone, parenteral midazolam, rifabutin, sildenafil, tadalafil, and vardenafil. CYP3A/CYP3A4 inducers, St. John's wort, efavirenz, nevirapine, anticonvulsants, rifabutin, and venlafaxine may decrease levels. CYP3A/CYP3A4 inhibitors, delavirdine, nelfinavir, ritonavir, clarithromycin, itraconazole, and ketoconazole may increase levels. Refer to PI for dosing modifications when used w/ certain concomitant therapies.

PREGNANCY AND LACTATION
Pregnancy: Category C.
Lactation: Not for use in nursing.

MECHANISM OF ACTION
HIV-1 protease inhibitor; binds to the protease active site and inhibits the activity of the enzyme. This inhibition prevents cleavage of the viral polyproteins resulting in the formation of immature noninfectious viral particles.

PHARMACOKINETICS
Absorption: Rapid (fasted). C_{max}=12,617nM; T_{max}=0.8 hrs; AUC=30,691nM•hr.
Distribution: Plasma protein binding (60%). **Metabolism:** Oxidation (via CYP3A4 [major]) and glucuronide conjugation. **Elimination:** Urine (<20%, unchanged); $T_{1/2}$=1.8 hrs.

PATIENT CONSIDERATIONS
Assessment: Assess for hypersensitivity to drug, hepatic insufficiency, DM, hemophilia, pregnancy/nursing status, and possible drug interactions.

Monitoring: Monitor for nephrolithiasis/urolithiasis, hemolytic anemia, hepatitis, new onset or exacerbation of DM, hyperglycemia, diabetic ketoacidosis, hyperbilirubinemia, serum transaminase elevations, immune reconstitution syndrome, autoimmune disorders, fat redistribution/accumulation, and other adverse reactions. Closely follow patients w/ asymptomatic severe leukocyturia and monitor frequently w/ urinalyses. In patients w/ hemophilia, monitor for bleeding events.

Counseling: Instruct to take drug ud. Inform that drug is not a cure for HIV-1 infection and that illnesses associated w/ HIV may continue. Advise to avoid doing things that can spread HIV to others. Instruct not to modify or d/c therapy w/o consulting physician. Instruct to report to physician the use of any other prescription/nonprescription medication or herbal products (eg, St. John's wort). Inform that fat redistribution/accumulation may occur. Instruct to notify physician if pregnant or nursing.

CYCLOPHOSPHAMIDE CAPSULES — cyclophosphamide   Rx

Class: Nitrogen mustard alkylating agent

ADULT DOSAGE	PEDIATRIC DOSAGE
Malignant Diseases	**Malignant Diseases**
Malignant lymphomas (Stages III and IV of the Ann Arbor staging system), Hodgkin's disease, lymphocytic lymphoma (nodular or diffuse), mixed-cell type lymphoma, histiocytic lymphoma, Burkitt's lymphoma; multiple myeloma; chronic lymphocytic leukemia, chronic granulocytic leukemia (usually ineffective in acute blastic crisis), acute myelogenous and monocytic leukemia, acute lymphoblastic (stem-cell) leukemia (cyclophosphamide given during remission is effective in prolonging its duration); mycosis fungoides (advanced disease); neuroblastoma (disseminated disease); adenocarcinoma of the ovary; retinoblastoma; and carcinoma of the breast	Malignant lymphomas (Stages III and IV of the Ann Arbor staging system), Hodgkin's disease, lymphocytic lymphoma (nodular or diffuse), mixed-cell type lymphoma, histiocytic lymphoma, Burkitt's lymphoma; multiple myeloma; chronic lymphocytic leukemia, chronic granulocytic leukemia (usually ineffective in acute blastic crisis), acute myelogenous and monocytic leukemia, acute lymphoblastic (stem-cell) leukemia (cyclophosphamide given during remission is effective in prolonging its duration); mycosis fungoides (advanced disease); neuroblastoma (disseminated disease); adenocarcinoma of the ovary; retinoblastoma; and carcinoma of the breast
1-5mg/kg/day; adjust in accord w/ evidence of antitumor activity and/or leukopenia	1-5mg/kg/day; adjust in accord w/ evidence of antitumor activity and/or leukopenia

As Part of Combined Cytotoxic Regimens:

May be necessary to reduce dose of cyclophosphamide as well as that of the other drugs

As Part of Combined Cytotoxic Regimens:

May be necessary to reduce dose of cyclophosphamide as well as that of the other drugs

Nephrotic Syndrome

Biopsy proven minimal change nephrotic syndrome in patients who failed to adequately respond to or are unable to tolerate adrenocorticosteroid therapy

2mg/kg/day for 8-12 weeks
Max Cumulative Dose: 168mg/kg

DOSING CONSIDERATIONS

Elderly

Start at lower end of dosing range

ADMINISTRATION

Oral route

Take in am; during or immediately after administration, adequate amounts of fluid should be ingested or infused to force diuresis.

Swallow whole; do not open, chew, or crush.

Handling Precautions

Handle and dispose of cyclophosphamide in a manner consistent w/ other cytotoxic drugs.

If contact w/ broken caps occurs, wash hands immediately and thoroughly.

STORAGE

20-25°C (68-77°F).

HOW SUPPLIED

Cap: 25mg, 50mg

CONTRAINDICATIONS

Hypersensitivity to this medication, urinary outflow obstruction.

WARNINGS/PRECAUTIONS

May cause myelosuppression, bone marrow failure, and severe immunosuppression that may lead to serious and sometimes fatal infections. May reactivate latent infections. Do not administer to patients w/ neutrophils ≤1500/mm^3 and platelets <50,000/mm^3. Treatment may not be indicated, or should be interrupted, or the dose reduced, in patients who have or who develop a serious infection. Granulocyte colony-stimulating factor (G-CSF) may be administered to reduce the risks of neutropenia complications associated w/ cyclophosphamide use. Hemorrhagic cystitis, pyelitis, ureteritis, and hematuria reported; d/c therapy if severe hemorrhagic cystitis occurs. Urotoxicity (bladder ulceration, necrosis, fibrosis, contracture, secondary cancer) may occur and may require interruption of treatment or cystectomy. Exclude or correct any urinary tract obstructions before starting treatment. Caution w/ active UTIs. Myocarditis, myopericarditis, pericardial effusion including cardiac tamponade, CHF, and supraventricular/ventricular arrhythmias reported; caution w/ risk factors for cardiotoxicity and w/ preexisting cardiac disease. Pneumonitis, pulmonary fibrosis, pulmonary veno-occlusive disease (VOD) and other forms of pulmonary toxicity leading to respiratory failure reported during and following treatment. Secondary malignancies (urinary tract cancer, myelodysplasia, acute leukemias, lymphomas, thyroid cancer, sarcomas) reported. Liver VOD, including fatal outcome, reported. May cause fetal harm. Male and female reproductive function and fertility may be impaired. May interfere w/ normal wound healing. Hyponatremia associated w/ increased total body water, acute water intoxication, and a syndrome resembling syndrome of inappropriate secretion of antidiuretic hormone reported. Caution w/ severe renal impairment (CrCl 10-24mL/min). In patients requiring dialysis, consider use of a consistent interval between therapy and dialysis.

ADVERSE REACTIONS

Neutropenia, fever, N/V, anorexia, alopecia, skin pigmentation, changes in nails.

DRUG INTERACTIONS

Severe myelosuppression may be expected particularly in patients pretreated w/ and/or receiving concomitant chemotherapy and/or radiation therapy. Protease inhibitors may increase concentration of cytotoxic metabolites and may increase incidence of infections and neutropenia. Increased hematotoxicity and/or immunosuppression w/ ACE inhibitors, natalizumab, paclitaxel, thiazide diuretics, and zidovudine. Increased cardiotoxicity w/ anthracyclines, cytarabine, pentostatin, radiation therapy of the cardiac region, and trastuzumab. Increased pulmonary toxicity w/ amiodarone and G-CSF or granulocyte macrophage colony-stimulating factor. Increased nephrotoxicity w/ amphotericin B. Acute water intoxication reported w/ indomethacin. Increased risk of hepatotoxicity w/ azathioprine. Increased incidence of liver VOD and mucositis w/ busulfan. Increased incidence of mucositis w/ protease inhibitors. Increased risk of hemorrhagic cystitis w/ past or concomitant radiation treatment. Higher incidence of noncutaneous malignant solid tumors w/ etanercept in patients w/ Wegener's granulomatosis. Acute encephalopathy reported w/ metronidazole. Concomitant use of tamoxifen may increase the risk of thromboembolic complications. Both increased and decreased warfarin effect reported. May lower concentrations of cyclosporine, which may result in an increased incidence of graft-versus-host disease. Prolonged apnea may occur w/ concurrent depolarizing muscle relaxants (eg, succinylcholine); caution if patient has been treated w/in 10 days of general anesthesia.

PREGNANCY AND LACTATION

Pregnancy: Category D. Exposure to cyclophosphamide during pregnancy may cause fetal malformations, miscarriage, fetal growth retardation, and toxic effects in the newborn.

Lactation: Not for use in nursing.

Reproductive Potential: Female patients of reproductive potential should use highly effective contraception during and for up to 1 year after completion of treatment. Male patients who are sexually active w/ female partners who are or may become pregnant should use a condom during and for at least 4 months after treatment. Amenorrhea (transient or permanent) and oligomenorrhea reported in women. Men may develop oligospermia or azoospermia.

MECHANISM OF ACTION

Nitrogen mustard alkylating agent; thought to involve cross-linking of tumor cell DNA.

PHARMACOKINETICS

Absorption: T_{max}=1 hr. **Distribution:** V_d=30-50L; plasma protein binding (20%; >60%, metabolites); found in breast milk. **Metabolism:** Liver to active alkylating metabolites by a mixed function microsomal oxidase system. **Elimination:** (IV) Urine (10-20%, unchanged), bile (4%); $T_{1/2}$=3-12 hrs.

PATIENT CONSIDERATIONS

Assessment: Assess for urinary outflow obstruction, active UTI, infections, risk for neutropenia complications and cardiotoxicity, preexisting cardiac disease, renal impairment, drug hypersensitivity, pregnancy/nursing status, and possible drug interactions. Obtain baseline CBCs.

Monitoring: Monitor for myelosuppression, bone marrow failure, immunosuppression, infections, hemorrhagic cystitis, urinary tract/renal/cardiac/pulmonary toxicity, secondary malignancies, VOD, hyponatremia, and other adverse reactions. Monitor CBCs. Regularly check urinary sediment for presence of erythrocytes and other signs of urotoxicity and/or nephrotoxicity.

Counseling: Inform of the possibility of myelosuppression, immunosuppression, and infections; explain the need for routine blood cell counts. Instruct patients to monitor their temperature frequently and to immediately report any occurrence of fever. Advise to report urinary symptoms and the need for increasing fluid intake and frequent voiding. Advise to contact physician immediately for any of the following: new onset or worsening SOB, cough, swelling of the ankles/legs, palpitations, weight gain of >5 lbs in 24 hrs, dizziness, or loss of consciousness. Advise to report promptly any new or worsening respiratory symptoms. Advise female patients of reproductive potential to use highly effective contraception during treatment and for up to 1 yr after completion of therapy. Advise male patients who are sexually active w/ a female partner who is or may become pregnant to use condoms during treatment and for up to 4 months after completion of therapy. Instruct to immediately contact physician if pregnancy occurs or is suspected. Inform of the possible side effects associated w/ cyclophosphamide administration and of other undesirable effects that could affect the ability to drive or use machines. Instruct patients to swallow cyclophosphamide capsules whole and not to open, chew, or crush the capsules. Advise caregivers to wear gloves when handling containers and caps and to avoid exposure to broken caps; instruct to wash hands immediately and thoroughly if contact w/ broken caps occurs.

CYCLOPHOSPHAMIDE INJECTION — cyclophosphamide   **Rx**

Class: Nitrogen mustard alkylating agent

ADULT DOSAGE	PEDIATRIC DOSAGE
Malignant Diseases	**Malignant Diseases**
No Hematologic Deficiency:	**No Hematologic Deficiency:**
IV:	**IV:**
Monotherapy:	**Monotherapy:**
Initial: 40-50mg/kg in divided doses over 2-5 days	**Initial:** 40-50mg/kg in divided doses over 2-5 days
Other Regimens: 10-15mg/kg every 7-10 days OR 3-5mg/kg twice weekly	**Other Regimens:** 10-15mg/kg every 7-10 days OR 3-5mg/kg twice weekly
Oral:	**Oral:**
Initial/Maint: 1-5mg/kg/day	**Initial/Maint:** 1-5mg/kg/day
Adjust IV/Oral doses in accord with evidence of antitumor activity and/or leukopenia	Adjust IV/Oral doses in accord with evidence of antitumor activity and/or leukopenia
Combined Cytotoxic Regimens:	**Combined Cytotoxic Regimens:**
May need to reduce dose of cyclophosphamide as well as that of the other drugs	May need to reduce dose of cyclophosphamide as well as that of the other drugs
	Nephrotic Syndrome
	Biopsy Proven Minimal Change:
	Oral:
	2 mg/kg/day for 8 to 12 weeks
	Max Cumulative Dose: 168mg/kg

DOSING CONSIDERATIONS

Elderly

Start at lower end of dosing range

ADMINISTRATION

IV/Oral route

During or immediately after administration, adequate amounts of fluid should be ingested or infused to force dieresis; administer in the morning

Preparation and Administration
Reconstitution Instructions:
For Direct IV Inj:
500mg: Reconstitute with 25mL 0.9% NaCl
1g: Reconstitute with 50mL 0.9% NaCl
2g: Reconstitute with 100mL 0.9% NaCl

For IV Infusion:
500mg: Reconstitute with 25mL 0.9% NaCl or SWFI
1g: Reconstitute with 50mL 0.9% NaCl or SWFI
2g: Reconstitute with 100mL 0.9% NaCl or SWFI

Dilution Instructions:
Dilute the reconstituted sol to a minimum concentration of 2mg/mL with any of the following:
5% Dextrose Inj
5% Dextrose and 0.9% NaCl Inj
0.45% NaCl Inj

Storage of Reconstituted/Diluted Sol:
Reconstituted Sol (Without Further Dilution):
0.9% NaCl Inj: Up to 24 hrs at room temperature; up to 6 days refrigerated
SWFI: Do not store; use immediately

Diluted Sol:
0.45% NaCl Inj: Up to 24 hrs at room temperature; up to 6 days refrigerated
5% Dextrose Inj: Up to 24 hrs at room temperature; up to 36 hrs refrigerated
5% Dextrose and 0.9% NaCl Inj: Up to 24 hrs at room temperature; up to 36 hrs refrigerated

Use of Reconstituted Sol for Oral Administration:
Prepare by dissolving cyclophosphamide for inj in Aromatic Elixir, National Formulary
Store under refrigeration in glass containers and use within 14 days

STORAGE
≤25°C (77°F).

HOW SUPPLIED
Inj: 500mg, 1g, 2g

CONTRAINDICATIONS
Hypersensitivity to this medication, urinary outflow obstruction.

WARNINGS/PRECAUTIONS
May cause myelosuppression, bone marrow failure, and severe immunosuppression that may lead to serious and sometimes fatal infections. May reactivate latent infections. Do not administer to patients with neutrophils ≤1500/mm³ and platelets <50,000/mm³. Interrupt therapy or reduce dose if serious infection develops. Consider primary and secondary prophylaxis with granulocyte colony-stimulating factor (G-CSF) in patients at increased risk for neutropenia complications. Hemorrhagic cystitis, pyelitis, ureteritis, and hematuria reported; d/c therapy if severe hemorrhagic cystitis occurs. Urotoxicity (bladder ulceration, necrosis, fibrosis, contracture, secondary cancer) may require interruption of treatment or cystectomy. Exclude or correct any urinary tract obstructions before starting treatment. Caution with active urinary tract infections (UTIs). Myocarditis, myopericarditis, pericardial effusion including cardiac tamponade, congestive heart failure, and supraventricular/ventricular arrhythmias reported; caution with risk factors for cardiotoxicity and with preexisting cardiac disease. Pneumonitis, pulmonary fibrosis, pulmonary veno-occlusive disease (VOD), and other forms of pulmonary toxicity leading to respiratory failure reported during and following treatment. Secondary malignancies (urinary tract cancer, myelodysplasia, acute leukemias, lymphomas, thyroid cancer, sarcomas) reported. Liver VOD, including fatal outcome, reported. May cause fetal harm. Male and female reproductive function and fertility may be impaired. May interfere with normal wound healing. Hyponatremia associated with increased total body water, acute water intoxication, and a syndrome resembling syndrome of inappropriate secretion of antidiuretic hormone reported. Caution with severe renal impairment (CrCl 10-24mL/min) and in elderly. In patients requiring dialysis, consider use of a consistent interval between therapy and dialysis.

ADVERSE REACTIONS
Neutropenia, N/V, anorexia, alopecia, fever, skin pigmentation, changes in nails.

DRUG INTERACTIONS
Severe myelosuppression may be expected, particularly in patients pretreated with and/or receiving concomitant chemotherapy and/or radiation therapy. Protease inhibitors may increase the concentration of cytotoxic metabolites and may increase the incidence of infections, neutropenia, and mucositis. Increased hematotoxicity and/or immunosuppression with ACE inhibitors, natalizumab, paclitaxel, thiazide diuretics, and zidovudine. Increased cardiotoxicity with anthracyclines, cytarabine, pentostatin, radiation therapy of the cardiac region, and trastuzumab. Increased pulmonary toxicity with amiodarone and G-CSF or granulocyte macrophage colony-stimulating factor. Increased nephrotoxicity with amphotericin B. Acute water intoxication reported with indomethacin. Increased risk of hepatotoxicity with azathioprine. Increased incidence of liver VOD and mucositis with busulfan. Increased risk of hemorrhagic cystitis with past or concomitant radiation treatment. Higher incidence of noncutaneous malignant solid tumors with etanercept in patients with Wegener's granulomatosis. Acute encephalopathy reported with metronidazole. Concomitant use of tamoxifen may increase the risk of thromboembolic complications. Both increased and decreased warfarin effect reported. May lower concentrations of cyclosporine, which may result in an increased incidence of graft-versus-host disease. Prolonged apnea may occur with concurrent depolarizing muscle relaxants (eg, succinylcholine); caution if patient has been treated within 10 days of general anesthesia.

PREGNANCY AND LACTATION
Category D, not for use in nursing.

MECHANISM OF ACTION
Nitrogen mustard alkylating agent; thought to involve cross-linking of tumor cell DNA.

PHARMACOKINETICS
Absorption: (Oral) T_{max}=1 hr. **Distribution:** V_d=30-50L; plasma protein binding (20%; >60%, metabolites); found in breast milk. **Metabolism:** Liver to active alkylating metabolites by a mixed function microsomal oxidase system. **Elimination:** (IV) Urine (10-20%, unchanged); bile (4%); $T_{1/2}$=3-12 hrs.

PATIENT CONSIDERATIONS

Assessment: Assess for urinary outflow obstruction, active UTI, infections, risk for neutropenia complications and cardiotoxicity, preexisting cardiac disease, renal impairment, drug hypersensitivity, pregnancy/nursing status, and possible drug interactions. Obtain baseline CBCs.

Monitoring: Monitor for myelosuppression, bone marrow failure, immunosuppression, infections, hemorrhagic cystitis, urinary tract/renal/cardiac/pulmonary toxicity, secondary malignancies, VOD, hyponatremia, and other adverse reactions. Monitor CBCs. Regularly check urinary sediment for presence of erythrocytes and other signs of urotoxicity and/or nephrotoxicity.

Counseling: Inform of the possibility of myelosuppression, immunosuppression, and infections; explain the need for routine blood cell counts. Instruct patients to monitor their temperature frequently and to immediately report any occurrence of fever. Advise to report urinary symptoms and the need for increasing fluid intake and frequent voiding. Advise to contact physician immediately for any of the following: new onset or worsening SOB, cough, swelling of the ankles/legs, palpitations, weight gain of >5 lbs in 24 hrs, dizziness, or loss of consciousness. Advise to report promptly any new or worsening respiratory symptoms. Advise female patients of reproductive potential to use highly effective contraception during treatment and for up to 1 yr after completion of therapy. Advise male patients who are sexually active with a female partner who is or may become pregnant to use condoms during treatment and for up to 4 months after completion of therapy. Instruct to immediately contact physician if pregnancy occurs or is suspected. Inform of the possible side effects and of other undesirable effects that could affect ability to drive or use machines.

CYCLOPHOSPHAMIDE TABLETS — cyclophosphamide   Rx

Class: Nitrogen mustard alkylating agent

ADULT DOSAGE	PEDIATRIC DOSAGE
Malignant Diseases	**Malignant Diseases**
Malignant lymphomas (Stages III and IV of the Ann Arbor staging system), Hodgkin's disease, lymphocytic lymphoma (nodular or diffuse), mixed-cell type lymphoma, histiocytic lymphoma, Burkitt's lymphoma; multiple myeloma; chronic lymphocytic leukemia, chronic granulocytic leukemia (usually ineffective in acute blastic crisis), acute myelogenous and monocytic leukemia, acute lymphoblastic (stem-cell) leukemia in children (cyclophosphamide given during remission is effective in prolonging its duration); mycosis fungoides (advanced disease); neuroblastoma (disseminated disease); adenocarcinoma of the ovary; retinoblastoma; and carcinoma of the breast	Malignant lymphomas (Stages III and IV of the Ann Arbor staging system), Hodgkin's disease, lymphocytic lymphoma (nodular or diffuse), mixed-cell type lymphoma, histiocytic lymphoma, Burkitt's lymphoma; multiple myeloma; chronic lymphocytic leukemia, chronic granulocytic leukemia (usually ineffective in acute blastic crisis), acute myelogenous and monocytic leukemia, acute lymphoblastic (stem-cell) leukemia in children (cyclophosphamide given during remission is effective in prolonging its duration); mycosis fungoides (advanced disease); neuroblastoma (disseminated disease); adenocarcinoma of the ovary; retinoblastoma; and carcinoma of the breast
1-5mg/kg/day; adjust in accord w/ evidence of antitumor activity and/or leukopenia	1-5mg/kg/day; adjust in accord w/ evidence of antitumor activity and/or leukopenia
As Part of Combined Cytotoxic Regimens:	**As Part of Combined Cytotoxic Regimens:**
May be necessary to reduce dose of cyclophosphamide as well as that of the other drugs	May be necessary to reduce dose of cyclophosphamide as well as that of the other drugs
	Nephrotic Syndrome
	Biopsy proven minimal change nephrotic syndrome in patients whose disease fails to respond adequately to appropriate adrenocorticosteroid therapy or in whom the adrenocorticosteroid therapy produces or threatens to produce intolerable side effects
	2.5-3mg/kg/day for 60-90 days
	Adrenocorticosteroid therapy may be tapered and discontinued during the course of cyclophosphamide therapy

DOSING CONSIDERATIONS
Elderly
Start at lower end of dosing range

ADMINISTRATION
Oral route

STORAGE
≤25°C (77°F); product will withstand brief exposure to temperatures up to 30°C (86°F). Protect from temperatures >30°C (86°F).

HOW SUPPLIED
Tab: 25mg, 50mg

CONTRAINDICATIONS
Severely depressed bone marrow function, prior hypersensitivity to this medication.

WARNINGS/PRECAUTIONS
Second malignancies (eg, urinary bladder, myeloproliferative, lymphoproliferative) reported. May cause fetal harm. Interferes with oogenesis and spermatogenesis. May cause sterility in both sexes; development of sterility appears to depend on the dose, duration of therapy, and the state of gonadal function at the time of treatment. Amenorrhea associated with decreased estrogen and increased gonadotropin secretion reported. Ovarian fibrosis with apparently complete loss of germ cells after prolonged treatment in late prepubescence reported. Testicular atrophy may occur. Hemorrhagic cystitis and/or urinary bladder fibrosis may develop; d/c if severe hemorrhagic cystitis occurs. Cardiac toxicity reported. May cause significant suppression of immune responses. Serious infections may develop in severely immunosuppressed patients; interrupt or reduce dose in patients who have or who develop viral, bacterial, fungal, protozoan, or helminthic infections. Anaphylactic reactions and possible cross-sensitivity with other alkylating agents reported. Caution with leukopenia, thrombocytopenia, tumor cell infiltration of bone marrow, previous x-ray therapy, previous therapy with other cytotoxic agents, and hepatic/renal impairment. May need to adjust dose in adrenalectomized patients. May interfere with normal wound healing. Caution in elderly.

ADVERSE REACTIONS
Leukopenia/neutropenia, N/V, anorexia, alopecia, skin pigmentation, changes in nails, hemorrhagic ureteritis, renal tubular necrosis, syndrome of inappropriate antidiuretic hormone secretion.

DRUG INTERACTIONS
May potentiate doxorubicin-induced cardiotoxicity. Chronic administration of high doses of phenobarbital increases rate of metabolism and leukopenic activity of cyclophosphamide. Potentiates effect of succinylcholine chloride. Caution if patient has been treated with cyclophosphamide within 10 days of general anesthesia.

PREGNANCY AND LACTATION
Category D, not for use in nursing.

MECHANISM OF ACTION
Nitrogen mustard alkylating agent; thought to involve cross-linking of tumor cell DNA.

PHARMACOKINETICS
Absorption: Well absorbed. Bioavailability (>75%). (IV) T_{max}=2-3 hrs (metabolites).
Distribution: Plasma protein binding (>60%, metabolites); found in breast milk.
Metabolism: Liver to active alkylating metabolites by a mixed function microsomal oxidase system. **Elimination:** Urine (5-25%, unchanged); $T_{1/2}$=3-12 hrs.

PATIENT CONSIDERATIONS
Assessment: Assess for bone marrow depression, immunosuppression, infections, hepatic/renal impairment, adrenalectomy, drug hypersensitivity, any other conditions where treatment is cautioned, pregnancy/nursing status, and possible drug interactions.

Monitoring: Monitor for second malignancies, reproductive dysfunction, hemorrhagic cystitis, urinary bladder fibrosis, cardiac dysfunction/toxicity, immunosuppression, infections, anaphylactic reactions, and other adverse reactions. Monitor hematologic profile (particularly neutrophils and platelets), and examine urine for red cells regularly.

Counseling: Inform of the risks and benefits of therapy. Advise women of childbearing potential to avoid becoming pregnant.

CYRAMZA — ramucirumab   Rx
Class: Monoclonal antibody/VEGFR2 blocker

> **Increased risk of hemorrhage and GI hemorrhage, including severe and sometimes fatal hemorrhagic events; permanently d/c if severe bleeding occurs. May increase risk of GI perforation; permanently d/c if this occurs. Impaired wound healing may occur; d/c therapy in patients w/ impaired wound healing. Withhold therapy prior to surgery and d/c therapy if wound healing complications develop.**

ADULT DOSAGE
Advanced or Metastatic, Gastric or Gastroesophageal Junction Adenocarcinoma

W/ Disease Progression on or After Prior Fluoropyrimidine- or Platinum-Containing Chemotherapy:
As a Single Agent, or in Combination w/ Paclitaxel:

Usual: 8mg/kg every 2 weeks administered as an IV infusion over 60 min. Continue until disease progression or unacceptable toxicity

PEDIATRIC DOSAGE
Pediatric use may not have been established

When given in combination, administer prior to administration of paclitaxel

Metastatic Non-Small Cell Lung Cancer

W/ Disease Progression:
On or After Platinum-Based Chemotherapy:

Usual: 10mg/kg IV over 60 min on Day 1 of a 21-day cycle prior to docetaxel infusion. Continue until disease progression or unacceptable toxicity

Metastatic Colorectal Cancer

W/ Disease Progression:
On or After Prior Therapy w/ Bevacizumab, Oxaliplatin, and a Fluoropyrimidine:

Usual: 8mg/kg IV over 60 min every 2 weeks prior to FOLFIRI (irinotecan, folinic acid, and 5-fluorouracil) administration. Continue until disease progression or unacceptable toxicity

Premedication

Prior to each infusion, premedicate all patients w/ an IV histamine H_1 antagonist (eg, diphenhydramine) For patients who have experienced a Grade 1 or 2 infusion-related reaction, also premedicate w/ dexamethasone (or equivalent) and acetaminophen prior to each infusion

---

DOSING CONSIDERATIONS
Adverse Reactions
Infusion Related Reactions (IRRs):
- Reduce infusion rate by 50% for Grade 1 or 2 IRRs
- Permanently d/c for Grade 3 or 4 IRRs

HTN:
- Interrupt for severe HTN until controlled w/ medical management
- Permanently d/c for severe HTN that cannot be controlled w/ antihypertensive therapy

Proteinuria:
- Interrupt for urine protein levels ≥2g/24 hrs
- Reinitiate at a reduced dose (6mg/kg, if initial dose was 8mg/kg; or 8mg/kg, if initial dose was 10mg/kg) once the urine protein level returns to <2g/24 hrs. If protein level ≥2g/24 hrs reoccurs, interrupt and reduce dose (5mg/kg, if initial dose was 8mg/kg; or 6mg/kg, if initial dose was 10mg/kg) once the urine protein level returns to <2g/24 hrs
- Permanently d/c for urine protein level >3g/24 hrs or in the setting of nephrotic syndrome

Wound Healing Complications:
Interrupt prior to scheduled surgery until the wound is fully healed

Arterial Thromboembolic Events, GI Perforation, or Grade 3 or 4 Bleeding:
Permanently d/c

ADMINISTRATION
IV route

Calculate dose and required volume of ramucirumab needed to prepare the infusion sol.
Withdraw required volume of ramucirumab and further dilute w/ only 0.9% NaCl Inj in an IV infusion container to a final volume of 250mL.
Do not use dextrose containing sol.
Gently invert container to ensure adequate mixing.
Do not dilute w/ other sol or coinfuse w/ other electrolytes or medications.
Administer diluted ramucirumab infusion via infusion pump over 60 min through a separate infusion line. Use of a protein sparing 0.22-micron filter is recommended.
Flush line w/ sterile NaCl 0.9% sol for inj at the end of infusion.
Do not administer as an IV push or bolus.

Refer to PI for further administration and preparation instructions.

STORAGE
2-8°C (36-46°F). Protect from light. Do not freeze or shake. **Diluted Sol:** 2-8°C (36-46°F) for no >24 hrs or <25°C (77°F) for 4 hrs. Do not freeze or shake.

HOW SUPPLIED
Inj: 10mg/mL [10mL, 50mL]

WARNINGS/PRECAUTIONS
Serious, sometimes fatal, arterial thromboembolic events (ATEs) (eg, MI, cardiac arrest, cerebrovascular accident) reported. Increased incidence of severe HTN reported; control HTN prior to initiation of treatment. Permanently d/c treatment in patients w/ hypertensive crisis or hypertensive encephalopathy. IRRs reported; monitor during infusion for signs and symptoms of IRRs in a setting w/ available resuscitation equipment. Clinical deterioration, manifested by new onset or worsening encephalopathy, ascites, or hepatorenal syndrome, reported in patients w/ Child-Pugh B or C cirrhosis. Use in patients w/ Child-Pugh B or C cirrhosis

only if potential benefits of treatment are judged to outweigh risks of clinical deterioration. Reversible posterior leukoencephalopathy syndrome (RPLS) reported; confirm diagnosis of RPLS w/ MRI and d/c if RPLS develops. Severe proteinuria and hypothyroidism reported. May cause fetal harm.

ADVERSE REACTIONS
Hemorrhage, GI hemorrhage/perforation, impaired wound healing, HTN, diarrhea, hyponatremia, headache, neutropenia, epistaxis, proteinuria, fatigue/asthenia, stomatitis/mucosal inflammation.

PREGNANCY AND LACTATION
Pregnancy: Based on its mechanism of action, ramucirumab can cause fetal harm; animal models link angiogenesis, vascular endothelial growth factor (VEGF) and VEGF Receptor 2 (VEGFR2) to critical aspects of female reproduction, embryofetal development, and postnatal development. Advise pregnant women of the potential risk to a fetus.
Lactation: There is no information on the presence of ramucirumab in human milk; not for use in nursing.
Reproductive Potential: Females of reproductive potential should use effective contraception during treatment and for at least 3 months after the last dose of therapy. May impair fertility of female patients.

MECHANISM OF ACTION
Monoclonal antibody/VEGF receptor 2 antagonist; specifically binds to VEGF receptor 2 and blocks binding of VEGF receptor ligands, VEGF-A, VEGF-C, and VEGF-D. As a result, ramucirumab inhibits ligand-stimulated activation of VEGF receptor 2, thereby inhibiting ligand-induced proliferation, and migration of human endothelial cells.

PHARMACOKINETICS
Elimination: $T_{1/2}$=14 days.

PATIENT CONSIDERATIONS
Assessment: Assess for HTN, presence of wound, upcoming surgery, Child-Pugh B or C cirrhosis, and pregnancy/nursing status.
Monitoring: Monitor for hemorrhage, ATEs, IRRs, GI perforation, wound healing complications, clinical deterioration in patients w/ Child-Pugh B or C cirrhosis patients, RPLS, and other adverse reactions. Monitor BP (every 2 weeks or more frequently as indicated). Monitor proteinuria by urine dipstick and/or urinary protein creatinine ratio for the development of worsening of proteinuria. Monitor thyroid function.
Counseling: Inform of the risks and benefits of therapy. Instruct to contact physician for bleeding or symptoms of bleeding, BP elevation or symptoms of HTN, severe diarrhea, vomiting, or severe abdominal pain. Advise to undergo routine BP monitoring. Inform that drug has the potential to impair wound healing; instruct not to undergo surgery w/o first discussing this potential risk w/ physician. Advise females of reproductive potential regarding potential infertility effects of therapy, and to use effective contraception during treatment and for at least 3 months after the last dose of treatment. Counsel not to breastfeed during treatment.

CYSTADANE — betaine anhydrous
Class: Methylating agent

Rx

ADULT DOSAGE
Homocystinuria
Usual: 3g bid
Titrate: Gradually increase dose until plasma total homocysteine is undetectable or present only in small amounts
Max: 20g/day

PEDIATRIC DOSAGE
Homocystinuria
<3 Years:
Initial: 100mg/kg/day, divided bid doses
Titrate: Increase weekly by 50mg/kg increments
≥3 Years:
Usual: 3g bid
Titrate: Gradually increase dose until plasma total homocysteine is undetectable or present only in small amounts
Max: 20g/day

ADMINISTRATION
Oral Route
Preparation
1. Measure the prescribed amount w/ the provided measuring scoop (1 level 1.7mL scoop is equal to 1g of betaine anhydrous powder)
2. Dissolve in 4-6 oz (120-180mL) of water, juice, milk, or formula, or mix w/ food for immediate ingestion

STORAGE
15-30°C (59-86°F). Protect from moisture.

HOW SUPPLIED
Sol (Powder): 180g

WARNINGS/PRECAUTIONS
May elevate methionine concentrations. Cerebral edema reported w/ hypermethioninemia. Plasma methionine concentrations should be kept <1,000µmol/L through dietary modification and, if necessary, through a reduction in betaine anhydrous dose.

ADVERSE REACTIONS
Hypermethioninemia, cerebral edema, nausea, GI distress.

PREGNANCY AND LACTATION
Category C, caution in nursing.

MECHANISM OF ACTION
Methylating agent; acts as a methyl group donor in the remethylation of homocysteine to methionine in patients w/ homocystinuria.

PATIENT CONSIDERATIONS
Assessment: Assess for homocystinuria, CBS deficiency, MTHFR deficiency, cbl defect, and pregnancy/nursing status.
Monitoring: Monitor for hypermethioninemia, cerebral edema and other adverse reactions. Monitor blood homocysteine levels to measure response to therapy. Monitor plasma methionine concentrations w/ CBS deficiency.
Counseling: Instruct patients and caregivers that drug should only be taken ud by their physician. Instruct to shake bottle before removing cap. Advise to measure prescribed amount w/ scoop provided. Counsel to mix w/ 4-6 oz of water, juice, milk, or formula until completely dissolved, or mix w/ food, then ingest immediately.

CYSTAGON — cysteamine bitartrate

Rx

Class: Cystine-depleting agent

ADULT DOSAGE
Nephropathic Cystinosis
Initial: 1/4 to 1/6 of the maint dose
Maint: 2g/day divided qid; dose should be reached after 4-6 weeks of incremental dosage increases
Titrate: Increase dose if the leukocyte cystine level remains >2nmol/ 1/2 cystine/mg protein
Max: 1.95g/m²/day

Measure white cell cystine level 5-6 hrs after administration in new patients after the maint dose is achieved

Transfer from Cysteamine HCl/ Phosphocysteamine Sol:
Patients may be transferred to equimolar doses of Cystagon caps

Patients being transferred should have their white cell cystine levels measured in 2 weeks, and thereafter every 3 months to assess optimal dosage

Missed Dose
If it is w/in 2 hrs of the next dose, skip the missed dose and go back to the regular dosing schedule

PEDIATRIC DOSAGE
Nephropathic Cystinosis
≤12 Years:
Initial: 1/4 to 1/6 of the maint dose
Maint: 1.3g/m²/day of the free base, divided qid
Max: 1.95g/m²/day

<12 Years and >110 lbs:
Initial: 1/4 to 1/6 of the maint dose
Maint: 2g/day divided qid; dose should be reached after 4-6 weeks of incremental dosage increases
Titrate: Increase dose if the leukocyte cystine level remains >2nmol/ 1/2 cystine/mg protein
Max: 1.95g/m²/day

Measure white cell cystine level 5-6 hrs after administration in new patients after the maint dose is achieved

Transfer from Cysteamine HCl/ Phosphocysteamine Sol:
Patients may be transferred to equimolar doses of Cystagon caps

Patients being transferred should have their white cell cystine levels measured in 2 weeks, and thereafter every 3 months to assess optimal dosage

Missed Dose
If it is w/in 2 hrs of the next dose, skip the missed dose and go back to the regular dosing schedule

---

DOSING CONSIDERATIONS
Adverse Reactions
Poor Tolerability Initially Due to GI Tract Symptoms/Transient Skin Rashes:
Temporarily stop therapy, then reinstitute at a lower dose and gradually increase to the proper dose

ADMINISTRATION
Oral route

Children <6 Years
Administer by sprinkling the cap contents over food; do not administer intact caps due to risk of aspiration

STORAGE
20-25°C (68-77°F). Protect from light and moisture.

HOW SUPPLIED
Cap: 50mg, 150mg

CONTRAINDICATIONS
Hypersensitivity to cysteamine bitartrate or penicillamine.

WARNINGS/PRECAUTIONS
If skin rash develops, d/c therapy until rash clears; may restart at a lower dose and slowly titrate to therapeutic dose. Do not readminister if severe skin rash develops. CNS symptoms (eg, seizures, lethargy, somnolence, depression, encephalopathy) may occur; evaluate and adjust dose as necessary. May impair mental/physical abilities. GI tract symptoms (eg, N/V, anorexia, abdominal pain), GI ulceration, and bleeding reported; may have to interrupt therapy and adjust dose if such things develop. Interstitial nephritis with early renal failure reported. Dose of 1.95g/m²/day was associated with increased number of treatment withdrawals due to intolerance and adverse events. Reversible leukopenia and abnormal LFTs may occur; monitor blood counts and LFTs. Benign intracranial HTN (or pseudotumor cerebri) and/or papilledema reported; perform periodic eye examination. Serious skin lesions, skin striae, bone lesions along with leg pain and joint hyperextension reported with high doses; reduce dose if occurs.

ADVERSE REACTIONS

Vomiting, anorexia, fever, diarrhea, lethargy, rash.

PREGNANCY AND LACTATION

Category C, not for use in nursing.

MECHANISM OF ACTION

Cystine depleting agent; participates within lysosomes in a thiol-disulfide interchange reaction converting cystine into cysteine and cysteine-cysteamine mixed disulfide, both of which can exit the lysosome in patients with cystinosis.

PHARMACOKINETICS

Absorption: (Pediatrics) T_{max}=1.4 hrs, C_{max}=2.6µg/mL, AUC=6.3µg•hr/mL.
Distribution: (Pediatrics) V_d=156L; plasma protein binding (52%).

PATIENT CONSIDERATIONS

Assessment: Assess for skin rash, hypersensitivity to the drug or penicillamine, and pregnancy/nursing status.

Monitoring: Monitor for skin rash, CNS symptoms, GI ulceration/bleeding, GI tract symptoms, interstitial nephritis, benign intracranial HTN and/or papilledema, skin/bone lesions, and skin striae. Monitor blood counts and LFTs. Perform periodic eye exam. For new patients, measure leukocyte cystine levels 5-6 hrs after dose administration after the maint dose is achieved. Patients being transferred from cysteamine hydrochloride or phosphocysteamine sol to caps should have their leukocyte cystine levels measured in 2 weeks, and thereafter every 3 months to assess optimal dosage.

Counseling: Inform about the signs/symptoms of serious GI toxicity and what steps to take if they occur. Instruct to contact physician if any of the following develop: headache, tinnitus, dizziness, nausea, diplopia, blurry vision, loss of vision, pain behind the eye, or pain with eye movement. Advise to sprinkle cap contents over food for children <6 yrs. Advise if missed dose is within 2 hrs of the next dose, to skip missed dose and go back to regular dosing schedule.

CYSTARAN — cysteamine   Rx

Class: Cystine-depleting agent

ADULT DOSAGE	PEDIATRIC DOSAGE
Cystinosis	**Cystinosis**
Corneal Cystine Crystal Accumulation w/ Cystinosis:	**Corneal Cystine Crystal Accumulation w/ Cystinosis:**
Usual: 1 drop ou, every waking hr	**Usual:** 1 drop ou, every waking hr

ADMINISTRATION

Ocular route

STORAGE

-25 to -15°C (-13 to 5°F). Thaw for approximately 24 hrs before use. Thawed Bottle: 2-25°C (36-77°F) for up to 1 week. Do not refreeze. Discard after 1 week of use. Keep bottle tightly closed when not in use.

HOW SUPPLIED

Sol: 0.44% [15mL]

WARNINGS/PRECAUTIONS

For topical ophthalmic use only. Caution not to touch the eyelids or surrounding areas with the dropper tip to minimize contaminating the dropper tip and sol. Benign intracranial HTN (or pseudotumor cerebri) reported in patients concurrently using oral cysteamine. Contains benzalkonium chloride, which may be absorbed by soft contact lenses; remove contact lenses prior to application and may reinsert 15 min following administration.

ADVERSE REACTIONS

Sensitivity to light, redness, eye pain/irritation, headache, visual field defects.

PREGNANCY AND LACTATION

Category C, not for use in nursing.

MECHANISM OF ACTION

Cystine depleting agent; converts cystine to cysteine and cysteine-cysteamine mixed disulfides and reduces corneal cystine crystal accumulation.

PATIENT CONSIDERATIONS

Assessment: Assess for contact lens use and pregnancy/nursing status.

Monitoring: Monitor for benign intracranial HTN and other adverse reactions.

Counseling: Counsel on proper storage of bottles. Advise not to touch the eyelid or surrounding areas with the dropper tip of the bottle and that the cap should remain on the bottle when not in use. Advise to remove contact lenses prior to application and that lenses may be reinserted 15 min following administration. Inform that medication is for topical ophthalmic use only.

CYTARABINE — cytarabine   Rx

Class: Antimetabolite

> Should only be used by physicians experienced in cancer chemotherapy. For induction therapy, treat in a facility w/ lab and supportive resources sufficient to monitor drug tolerance and protect and maintain a patient compromised by drug toxicity. The main toxic effect of therapy is bone marrow suppression w/ leukopenia, thrombocytopenia, and anemia. Less serious toxicity includes N/V, diarrhea and abdominal pain, oral ulceration, and hepatic dysfunction. The physician must judge possible benefit against the known toxic effects of the drug in considering the advisability of therapy.

ADULT DOSAGE

Acute Non-Lymphocytic Leukemia

Used in combination w/ other approved anticancer drugs for remission induction in acute non-lymphocytic leukemia

Usual: 100mg/m²/day by continuous IV infusion (Days 1-7) or 100mg/m² IV q12h (Days 1-7)

Meningeal Leukemia

Prophylaxis and treatment of meningeal leukemia via intrathecal administration

100mg/mL Inj (Preservative-Free Only):
5-75mg/m²; frequency of administration may vary from qd for 4 days to once every 4 days

Most Frequently Used Dose:
30mg/m² every 4 days until CSF findings are normal, followed by 1 additional treatment

Dose schedule is usually governed by type and severity of CNS manifestations and response to previous therapy

Other Indications

Treatment of acute lymphocytic leukemia and the blast phase of chronic myelocytic leukemia

PEDIATRIC DOSAGE

Acute Non-Lymphocytic Leukemia

Used in combination w/ other approved anticancer drugs for remission induction in acute non-lymphocytic leukemia

Usual: 100mg/m²/day by continuous IV infusion (Days 1-7) or 100mg/m² IV q12h (Days 1-7)

DOSING CONSIDERATIONS

Renal Impairment

Use w/ caution; may need to reduce dose

Hepatic Impairment

Use w/ caution; may need to reduce dose

ADMINISTRATION

Intrathecal (preservative-free only)/IV/SQ route

20mg/mL Inj: Contains benzyl alcohol; do not use intrathecally

Chemical Stability in Infusion Sol

100mg/mL Inj:
94-96% of cytarabine is present after 192 hrs storage at room temperature when added to the following:
1. Water for inj
2. D5 in water
3. NaCl inj

If a precipitate has formed as a result of exposure to low temperatures, redissolve by warming up to 55°C (131°F) for no longer than 30 min and shake until the precipitate has dissolved; allow to cool prior to use

20mg/mL Inj:
97-100% of cytarabine is present after 8 days storage at room temperature when diluted w/ the following:
1. Water for inj
2. D5 inj
3. NaCl inj

STORAGE

15-30°C (59-86°F). Protect from light.

HOW SUPPLIED

Inj: 20mg/mL [25mL], 100mg/mL [20mL]

CONTRAINDICATIONS

Hypersensitivity to this drug.

WARNINGS/PRECAUTIONS

Intrathecal administration may cause systemic toxicity; monitor hemopoietic system carefully. Paraplegia, necrotizing leukoencephalopathy, isolated neurotoxicity, and blindness reported w/ intrathecal administration. Increased risk of spinal cord toxicity when administered both intrathecally and IV w/in a few days. Anaphylaxis resulting in acute cardiopulmonary arrest reported immediately after IV administration. Severe and at times fatal CNS, GI, and pulmonary toxicity (different from that seen w/ conventional therapy regimens of cytarabine) reported following some experimental dose schedules; complete alopecia is more commonly seen w/ experimental high-dose therapy. Severe skin rash, leading to skin desquamation reported rarely. May cause fetal harm when administered to a pregnant woman. A syndrome of sudden respiratory distress, rapidly progressing to pulmonary edema and radiographically pronounced cardiomegaly reported following experimental high-dose therapy used for the treatment of relapsed leukemia. Delayed progressive ascending paralysis resulting in death reported in patients w/ childhood acute myelogenous leukemia who received intrathecal and IV therapy at conventional doses. Monitor platelet/leukocyte counts daily during induction therapy and perform bone marrow exams frequently once blasts have disappeared from peripheral blood; consider suspending or modifying therapy when drug-induced marrow depression has resulted in a platelet count <50,000/mm³ or a polymorphonuclear granulocyte count <1000/mm³. When indicated, restart therapy when definite signs of marrow recovery appear. Caution w/ preexisting drug-induced bone marrow suppression and hepatic/renal impairment. May induce hyperuricemia secondary to rapid lysis of neoplastic cells. Acute pancreatitis reported in patients receiving continuous infusion. **20mg/mL:** Contains benzyl alcohol; benzyl alcohol has been reported to be associated w/ fatal "gasping syndrome" in premature infants. Do not use preparation containing benzyl alcohol if experimental high-dose therapy is used or if therapy is given intrathecally.

ADVERSE REACTIONS

Anorexia, N/V, diarrhea, oral/anal inflammation or ulceration, hepatic dysfunction, fever, rash, thrombophlebitis, bleeding (all sites).

DRUG INTERACTIONS

May inhibit efficacy of fluorocytosine. Reversible decreases in digoxin levels and renal glycoside excretion reported w/ β-acetyldigoxin and chemotherapy regimens containing cyclophosphamide, vincristine, and prednisone w/ or w/o cytarabine or procarbazine; monitoring of digoxin levels may be indicated. A study between gentamicin and cytarabine showed a cytarabine related antagonism for the susceptibility of *Klebsiella pneumoniae* strains; lack of a prompt therapeutic response may indicate the need for reevaluation of antibacterial therapy in patients on cytarabine being treated w/ gentamicin for a *K. pneumoniae* infection. Acute pancreatitis reported in patients receiving prior L-asparaginase treatment. Cardiomyopathy w/ subsequent death reported following experimental high-dose therapy in combination w/ cyclophosphamide when used for bone marrow transplant preparation.

PREGNANCY AND LACTATION

Pregnancy: Category D.
Lactation: Not for use in nursing.

MECHANISM OF ACTION

Antimetabolite; not established. Appears to act through inhibition of DNA polymerase. Also incorporates into both DNA and RNA.

PHARMACOKINETICS

Absorption: (SQ/IM) T_{max}=20-60 min. **Metabolism:** Rapid; 1-β-D-.arabinofuranosyluracil (inactive metabolite). **Elimination:** Urine (80%, approx 90% as metabolite); $T_{1/2}$=1-3 hrs.

PATIENT CONSIDERATIONS

Assessment: Assess for preexisting drug-induced bone marrow suppression, hepatic/renal impairment, hypersensitivity to the drug, pregnancy/nursing status, and possible drug interactions.

Monitoring: Monitor for anaphylaxis, bone marrow suppression, skin rash, alopecia, syndrome of sudden respiratory distress, acute pancreatitis, and other adverse reactions. Monitor leukocyte/platelet counts and perform bone marrow examinations frequently. Monitor hepatic and renal function periodically. Monitor blood uric acid levels.

Counseling: Inform of the risks and benefits of therapy. Advise women of childbearing potential to avoid becoming pregnant during therapy. Instruct to notify physician if pregnant or nursing, or if any adverse reactions develop.

CYTOGAM — cytomegalovirus immune globulin
intravenous (human)   Rx
Class: Immune globulin

ADULT DOSAGE
Cytomegalovirus Disease

Prophylaxis of Cytomegalovirus Disease Associated w/ Kidney, Lung, Liver, Pancreas, and Heart Transplantation:

Kidney Transplant:
150mg/kg w/in 72 hrs of transplant, then 100mg/kg at 2, 4, 6, and 8 weeks post-transplant, then 50mg/kg at 12 and 16 weeks post-transplant

Liver/Pancreas/Lung/Heart Transplant:
150mg/kg w/in 72 hrs of transplant, then 150mg/kg at 2, 4, 6, and 8 weeks post-transplant, then 100mg/kg at 12 and 16 weeks post-transplant

Max: 150mg/kg/infusion

Initial Dose:
Administer at 15mg/kg/hr IV; may increase rate to 30mg/kg/hr if no adverse reactions after 30 min, then may increase to max rate of 60mg/kg/hr if no adverse reactions after a subsequent 30 min (volume not to exceed 75mL/hr)

Subsequent Doses:
Administer at 15mg/kg/hr for 15 min; increase to 30mg/kg/hr for 15 min, then increase to max rate of 60mg/kg/hr if no adverse reactions (volume not to exceed 75mL/hr)

Monitor vital signs preinfusion, mid-way, and post-infusion as well as before any rate increase

PEDIATRIC DOSAGE
Pediatric use may not have been established

DOSING CONSIDERATIONS
Adverse Reactions
Minor Side Effect (eg, Nausea, Back Pain, Flushing): Slow rate or temporarily interrupt infusion
Anaphylaxis or Drop in BP: D/C infusion and use antidote (eg, diphenhydramine, adrenalin)

ADMINISTRATION
IV route

Do not shake vial; avoid foaming

Infusion Instructions
Begin infusion w/in 6 hrs after entering vial and complete w/in 12 hrs of entering vial
Administer through an IV line using an administration set that contains an in-line filter (pore size 15µ) and a constant infusion pump (eg, IVAC pump or equivalent); smaller in-line filter (0.2µ) is also acceptable
Pre-dilution before infusion not recommended
Administer through a separate IV line; if not possible, may be piggybacked into a preexisting line if that line contains either NaCl inj, or 1 of the following dextrose sol (w/ or w/o NaCl added): D2.5W, D5W, D10W, D20W
Do not dilute >1:2 w/ any of the above-named sol if a preexisting line must be used

STORAGE
2-8°C (36-46°F); use ≤6 hrs after entering vial.

HOW SUPPLIED
Inj: 50mL

CONTRAINDICATIONS
Selective immunoglobulin A deficiency, history of a prior severe reaction associated w/ the administration of this or other human immunoglobulin preparations.

WARNINGS/PRECAUTIONS
Consider use with ganciclovir for transplantation other than kidney from CMV seropositive donors into seronegative recipients. Risk of transmission of blood-borne viral agents and Creutzfeldt-Jakob disease agent. Renal dysfunction, acute renal failure, osmotic nephrosis and death reported; caution in patients with pre-existing renal impairment, diabetes mellitus (DM), volume depletion, sepsis, paraproteinemia, or who are >65 yrs. Monitor vital signs continuously and observe carefully for any symptoms throughout the infusion. Allergic reactions may occur; d/c therapy and institute appropriate therapy if hypotension or anaphylaxis occurs. Monitor urine output, renal function, including BUN and SrCr, before and during therapy; d/c therapy if renal function deteriorates. Aseptic meningitis syndrome (AMS) reported; perform a thorough neurological exam and CSF studies. Monitor for clinical signs and symptoms of hemolysis; hemolytic anemia may occur. Noncardiogenic pulmonary edema or Transfusion-Related Acute Lung Injury (TRALI) reported; monitor for pulmonary adverse reactions. Thrombotic events reported; increased risk with history of atherosclerosis, multiple cardiovascular (CV) risk factors, advanced age, impaired cardiac output, and/or known or suspected hyperviscosity.

ADVERSE REACTIONS
Flushing, chills, muscle cramps, back pain, fever, N/V, arthralgia, wheezing, increased BUN and SrCr.

DRUG INTERACTIONS
Defer live virus vaccines (eg, measles, mumps, rubella) for 3 months after therapy; may interfere with immune response. Caution with nephrotoxic drugs; may predispose to acute renal failure.

PREGNANCY AND LACTATION
Category C, safety not known in nursing.

MECHANISM OF ACTION
Immune globulin; contains relatively high concentrations of antibodies directed against CMV; can raise the relevant antibodies to levels sufficient to attenuate or reduce the incidence of serious CMV disease.

PATIENT CONSIDERATIONS
Assessment: Assess for IgA deficiency, renal impairment, volume depletion, DM, age, sepsis, paraproteinemia, atherosclerosis, multiple CV risk factors, impaired cardiac output, hypersensitivity to the drug or other human immunoglobulin preparations, pregnancy/nursing status, and possible drug interactions. Obtain baseline renal function (eg, SrCr, BUN). Assess baseline assessment of blood viscosity in patients at risk for hyperviscosity, including those with cryoglobulins, fasting chylomicronemia/markedly high TG, or monoclonal gammopathies. Obtain vital signs.

Monitoring: Monitor for hemolysis, hemolytic anemia, pulmonary adverse reactions, and thrombotic events. Monitor vital signs, renal function and urine output periodically. Perform neurological exam and CSF studies if signs and symptoms of AMS develop. Perform tests for presence of anti-neutrophil antibodies in both product and patient serum if TRALI is suspected.

Counseling: Instruct to report all infections to the physician. Inform about potential benefits/risks. Instruct to immediately report symptoms of decreased urine output, sudden weight gain, and/or SOB to the physician.

CYTOVENE — ganciclovir sodium   Rx

Class: Synthetic guanine derivative nucleoside analogue

> Clinical toxicity includes granulocytopenia, anemia, and thrombocytopenia. In animal studies, ganciclovir was carcinogenic and teratogenic, and caused aspermatogenesis. Use only for the treatment of cytomegalovirus (CMV) retinitis in immunocompromised patients, and prevention of CMV disease in transplant patients at risk for CMV disease.

ADULT DOSAGE

Cytomegalovirus Retinitis

Treatment in Immunocompromised Patients (Including Patients w/ AIDS):
Initial: 5mg/kg q12h for 14-21 days
Maint: 5mg/kg qd, 7 days per week or 6mg/kg qd, 5 days per week

CMV Progression During Maint Treatment:
Reinduction treatment is recommended

Cytomegalovirus Disease

Prevention in Transplant Recipients:
Initial: 5mg/kg q12h for 7-14 days
Maint: 5mg/kg qd, 7 days per week or 6mg/kg qd, 5 days per week

PEDIATRIC DOSAGE

Pediatric use may not have been established

DOSING CONSIDERATIONS

Renal Impairment

CrCl 50-69mL/min:
Initial: 2.5mg/kg q12h
Maint: 2.5mg/kg q24h

CrCl 25-49mL/min:
Initial: 2.5mg/kg q24h
Maint: 1.25mg/kg q24h

CrCl 10-24mL/min:
Initial: 1.25mg/kg q24h
Maint: 0.625mg/kg q24h

CrCl <10mL/min:
Initial: 1.25mg/kg 3X/week, following hemodialysis
Maint: 0.625mg/kg 3X/week, following hemodialysis

Patients Undergoing Hemodialysis:
Max: 1.25mg/kg 3X/week, following each hemodialysis session

Adverse Reactions

Neutropenia, Anemia, and/or Thrombocytopenia: Consider dosage reductions; ganciclovir should not be administered in patients w/ severe neutropenia (ANC <500/μL) or severe thrombocytopenia (platelets <25,000/μL)

ADMINISTRATION

IV route
Do not administer by rapid or bolus IV inj.
Administer at constant rate over 1 hr.

Preparation

Reconstituted Sol:
1. Reconstitute by injecting 10mL of sterile water for inj into the vial; do not use bacteriostatic water for inj containing parabens.
2. Shake the vial to dissolve the drug.

Infusion Sol:
- Based on patient weight, the appropriate volume of the reconstituted sol should be removed from the vial and added to an acceptable infusion fluid (typically 100mL) for delivery over the course of 1 hr; infusion concentrations >10mg/mL are not recommended.
- Compatible w/ 0.9% NaCl, D5, Ringer's inj, and lactated Ringer's inj.
- Further dilute w/ 0.9% NaCl inj when reconstituted w/ sterile water for inj.

Handling

Sol are alkaline (pH 11); avoid direct contact of the skin or mucous membranes w/ sol. If such contact occurs, wash thoroughly w/ soap and water; rinse eyes thoroughly w/ plain water.

STORAGE

25°C (77°F); excursions permitted to 15-30°C (59-86°F). **Reconstituted Sol in Vial:** Stable at room temperature for 12 hrs. Do not refrigerate. **Diluted Infusion Sol:** Refrigerate; do not freeze. Use w/in 24 hrs of dilution.

HOW SUPPLIED

Inj: 500mg

CONTRAINDICATIONS

Hypersensitivity to ganciclovir or acyclovir.

WARNINGS/PRECAUTIONS

Do not administer if the ANC is <500 cells/μL or the platelet count is <25,000 cells/μL. Caution w/ preexisting cytopenias or history of cytopenic reactions to other drugs, chemicals, or irradiation. May cause inhibition of spermatogenesis in men. May cause suppression of fertility in women. Women of childbearing potential should use effective contraception during treatment and men should practice barrier contraception during and for at least 90 days following therapy. Caution in the elderly and in patients w/ renal impairment. Larger doses and more rapid infusions increase toxicity. SQ/IM inj may cause severe tissue irritation. Administration should be accompanied by adequate hydration. Phlebitis and/or pain may occur at the site of IV infusion. Administer only into veins w/ adequate blood flow. Do not administer by rapid or bolus IV inj.

ADVERSE REACTIONS

Fever, diarrhea, leukopenia, anemia, sepsis, anorexia, vomiting, infection, sweating, chills, neuropathy, catheter infection, catheter sepsis, thrombocytopenia, pruritus.

DRUG INTERACTIONS

May increase levels/exposure of didanosine. Concomitant use of oral ganciclovir w/ zidovudine reported to decrease ganciclovir exposure and increase zidovudine exposure. Both zidovudine and ganciclovir have the potential to cause neutropenia and anemia; some patients may not tolerate concomitant therapy w/ these drugs at full dosage. Concomitant use of oral ganciclovir w/ probenecid reported to increase ganciclovir exposure and decrease renal clearance of ganciclovir. Avoid w/ imipenem-cilastatin unless potential benefits outweigh the risk; generalized seizures have been reported. May have additive toxicity w/ drugs that inhibit replication of rapidly dividing cell populations (eg, dapsone, pentamidine, flucytosine, vincristine, vinblastine, doxorubicin); consider benefits/risks of concomitant use w/ ganciclovir. Concomitant use w/ nephrotoxic agents (eg, cyclosporine, amphotericin B) may increase SrCr levels.

PREGNANCY AND LACTATION

Pregnancy: Category C.
Lactation: Not for use in nursing.

MECHANISM OF ACTION

Synthetic guanine derivative nucleoside analogue; believed to inhibit viral DNA synthesis by competitive inhibition of viral DNA polymerases and incorporation into viral DNA, resulting in eventual termination of viral DNA elongation.

PHARMACOKINETICS

Absorption: C_{max}=8.27-9mcg/mL; AUC=22.1-26.8mcg•hr/mL. **Distribution:** Plasma protein binding (1-2%); V_d=0.74L/kg. **Elimination:** Urine (91.3%, unchanged); $T_{1/2}$=3.5 hrs.

PATIENT CONSIDERATIONS

Assessment: Assess for hypersensitivity to ganciclovir or acyclovir; preexisting cytopenias or history of cytopenic reactions to other drugs, chemicals, or irradiation; renal impairment; pregnancy/nursing status; and possible drug interactions. Obtain baseline CBC, platelet count, and ANC.

Monitoring: Monitor for granulocytopenia, anemia, thrombocytopenia, phlebitis/pain at the inj site, and other adverse reactions. Perform frequent monitoring of CBC and platelet counts, especially in patients in whom ganciclovir or other nucleoside analogues have previously resulted in leukopenia, or in whom neutrophil counts are <1000 cells/μL at the beginning of treatment. Monitor SrCr or CrCl, and for retinitis progression.

Counseling: Inform that major toxicities of therapy are granulocytopenia (neutropenia), anemia, and thrombocytopenia and that dose modification may be required, including discontinuation. Advise of the importance of close monitoring of blood counts while on therapy. Inform that therapy has been associated w/ SrCr elevations and that therapy may cause infertility. Advise women of childbearing potential that therapy should not be used during pregnancy and that effective contraception should be used during therapy. Advise men to practice barrier contraception during and for at least 90 days following treatment. Inform that therapy may be a potential carcinogen. Advise that drug is not a cure for CMV retinitis and that immunocompromised patients may continue to experience progression of retinitis during and after treatment; instruct to have ophthalmologic follow-up examinations at a minimum of every 4-6 weeks during treatment. Counsel transplant recipients regarding the high frequency of impaired renal function reported in transplant recipients who received ganciclovir in controlled clinical trials, particularly in patients receiving concomitant administration of nephrotoxic agents (eg, cyclosporine, amphotericin B).

DACARBAZINE — dacarbazine   Rx

Class: Alkylating agent

> Administer under the supervision of a qualified physician experienced in the use of cancer chemotherapeutic agents. Hemopoietic depression is the most common toxicity. Hepatic necrosis reported. Carcinogenic and teratogenic in animals. Weigh carefully the possibility of achieving therapeutic benefit against the risk of toxicity.

ADULT DOSAGE

Metastatic Malignant Melanoma

2-4.5mg/kg/day for 10 days; may repeat every 4 weeks

Alternative:
250mg/m²/day IV for 5 days, may repeat every 3 weeks

Hodgkin Lymphoma

Secondary Line Therapy When Used w/ Other Agents:
150mg/m²/day for 5 days; may repeat every 4 weeks

Alternative:
375mg/m² on Day 1, to be repeated every 15 days

PEDIATRIC DOSAGE

Pediatric use may not have been established

ADMINISTRATION
IV route

Reconstitution
Reconstitute 200mg/vial and 500mg/vial w/ 19.7mL and 49.25mL of sterile water for inj to resulting sol containing 10mg/mL
Reconstituted sol may be further diluted w/ D5 or NaCl and administered as IV infusion
Use w/in 8 hrs of reconstitution

STORAGE
2-8°C (36-46°F). Protect from light. Reconstituted sol maybe stored at 4°C (39.2°F) for up to 72 hrs or at normal room conditions (temperature and light) for up to 8 hrs. Diluted reconstituted sol may be stored 4°C (39.2°F) for up to 24 hrs or at normal room conditions for up to 8 hrs.

HOW SUPPLIED
Inj: 200mg [20mL]

CONTRAINDICATIONS
Prior hypersensitivity to dacarbazine injection.

WARNINGS/PRECAUTIONS
Hemopoietic toxicity may warrant temporary suspension or cessation of therapy. Hepatic toxicity w/ hepatic vein thrombosis and hepatocellular necrosis reported. Anaphylaxis may occur. Extravasation of the drug SQ during IV administration may result in tissue damage and severe pain. Local pain, burning sensation, and irritation at the site of inj may occur.

ADVERSE REACTIONS
Hemopoietic depression, hepatic necrosis, anorexia, N/V.

DRUG INTERACTIONS
Hepatic toxicity w/ hepatic vein thrombosis and hepatocellular necrosis may occur w/ concomitant antineoplastics.

PREGNANCY AND LACTATION
Category C, not for use in nursing.

MECHANISM OF ACTION
Alkylating agent; has not been established. Suspected to inhibit DNA synthesis by acting as a purine analogue, due to action as an alkylating agent, and interaction w/ SH groups.

PHARMACOKINETICS
Metabolism: Extensive; 5-aminoimidazole-4-carboxamide (major metabolite).
Elimination: Urine (40% unchanged), $T_{1/2}$=5 hrs.

PATIENT CONSIDERATIONS
Assessment: Assess for hepatic/renal/bone marrow function, hypersensitivity, and pregnancy/nursing status.

Monitoring: Monitor for signs/symptoms of hemopoietic depression/toxicity, hepatic necrosis/toxicity, anaphylaxis, and inj-site reaction. Monitor WBCs, RBCs, and platelet levels for possible bone marrow depression.

Counseling: Inform of potential adverse events, including N/V and anorexia. Advise not to eat for 4-6 hrs prior to treatment. Inform of the signs/symptoms of hemopoietic depression, hepatic toxicity, or allergic reactions and instruct to tell physician if any of these occur.

DACOGEN — decitabine   Rx

Class: DNA methyltransferase inhibitor

ADULT DOSAGE
Myelodysplastic Syndromes

Including previously treated and untreated, de novo and secondary myelodysplastic syndromes of all French-American-British subtypes and intermediate-1, intermediate-2, and high-risk International Prognostic Scoring System groups

Treat for a minimum of 4 cycles

Treatment Regimen 1:
15mg/m² by continuous IV infusion over 3 hrs repeated q8h for 3 days; repeat cycle every 6 weeks

If hematologic recovery (ANC ≥1000/µL and platelets ≥50,000/µL) from a previous treatment cycle requires >6 weeks, delay the next cycle of therapy and reduce dose temporarily by following this algorithm:
Recovery Requiring >6, but <8 Weeks: Delay dosing for up to 2 weeks and temporarily reduce dose to 11mg/m² q8h (33mg/m²/day, 99mg/m²/cycle) upon restarting therapy
Recovery Requiring >8, but <10 Weeks: Assess for disease progression (by bone marrow aspirates); in the absence of progression, delay dosing up to

PEDIATRIC DOSAGE
Pediatric use may not have been established

2 more weeks and reduce dose to 11mg/m² q8h (33mg/m²/day, 99mg/m²/cycle) upon restarting therapy, then maintain or increase in subsequent cycles as clinically indicated

Treatment Regimen 2:
20mg/m² by continuous IV infusion over 1 hr repeated daily for 5 days; repeat cycle every 4 weeks

If myelosuppression is present, delay subsequent treatment cycles until there is hematologic recovery (ANC ≥1000/µL and platelets ≥50,000/µL)

Premedication
Treatment Regimen 1 and 2:
May premedicate w/ standard antiemetic therapy

DOSING CONSIDERATIONS
Adverse Reactions
Following the 1st cycle of treatment, if any of the following nonhematologic toxicities are present, do not restart treatment until the toxicity is resolved:
1. SrCr ≥2mg/dL
2. ALT, total bilirubin ≥2X ULN
3. Active or uncontrolled infection

ADMINISTRATION
IV route

Preparation
1. Reconstitute w/ 10mL of sterile water for inj; upon reconstitution, each mL contains approx 5mg of decitabine at pH 6.7-7.3
2. Immediately after reconstitution, further dilute the sol w/ 0.9% NaCl inj, or D5 inj to a final drug concentration of 0.1-1mg/mL
3. Unless used w/in 15 min of reconstitution, the diluted sol must be prepared using cold (2-8°C [36-46°F]) infusion fluids

STORAGE
25°C (77°F); excursions permitted to 15-30°C (59-86°F). Diluted Sol: 2-8°C (36-46°F) for up to a max of 4 hrs until administration if not use w/in 15 min of reconstitution.

HOW SUPPLIED
Inj: 50mg

WARNINGS/PRECAUTIONS
Neutropenia and thrombocytopenia may occur; perform CBC and platelet counts prn to monitor response and toxicity. Myelosuppression and worsening neutropenia may occur more frequently in the 1st or 2nd treatment cycles; consider the need for early institution of growth factors and/or antimicrobial agents for the prevention or treatment of infections. May cause fetal harm; women of childbearing potential should avoid becoming pregnant during and for 1 month following completion of treatment. Men should not father a child during and for 2 months following completion of treatment. Use effective contraception in women and men w/ female partners of childbearing potential during and following therapy. Caution w/ renal and hepatic impairment.

ADVERSE REACTIONS
Neutropenia, thrombocytopenia, anemia, fatigue, pyrexia, N/V, cough, petechiae, constipation, diarrhea, hyperglycemia, dyspnea, leukopenia, headache, insomnia.

PREGNANCY AND LACTATION
Category D, not for use in nursing.

MECHANISM OF ACTION
DNA methyltransferase inhibitor; causes hypomethylation of DNA and cellular differentiation or apoptosis.

PHARMACOKINETICS
Absorption: (15mg/m²) C_{max}=73.8ng/mL, AUC=163ng•hr/mL; (20mg/m²) C_{max}=147ng/mL, AUC=115ng•hr/mL. **Metabolism:** Deamination by cytidine deaminase in liver, granulocytes, intestinal epithelium, and whole blood.
Elimination: $T_{1/2}$=0.62 hr (15mg/m²), 0.54 hr (20mg/m²).

PATIENT CONSIDERATIONS
Assessment: Assess for renal/hepatic impairment and pregnancy/nursing status. Obtain baseline liver chemistries, SrCr, CBC, and platelet counts.

Monitoring: Monitor for signs/symptoms of neutropenia, thrombocytopenia, myelosuppression, renal/hepatic impairment, infections, and other adverse reactions. Monitor CBC and platelet counts prior to each dosing cycle.

Counseling: Advise women of childbearing potential to avoid becoming pregnant during therapy and for 1 month afterwards and men not to father a child during therapy and for 2 months afterwards; counsel to use effective contraception. Advise to monitor and report any symptoms of neutropenia, thrombocytopenia, or fever to physician as soon as possible.

DAKLINZA — daclatasvir   Rx

Class: HCV NS5A inhibitor

ADULT DOSAGE
Chronic Hepatitis C

Indicated for use w/ sofosbuvir, w/ or w/o ribavirin, for the treatment of patients w/ chronic hepatitis C virus (HCV) genotype 1 or genotype 3 infection

Recommended Daclatasvir Dose:
60mg qd

Recommended Treatment Regimen and Duration:
Genotype 1:
W/O Cirrhosis or w/ Compensated (Child-Pugh A) Cirrhosis: Daclatasvir + sofosbuvir for 12 weeks
Decompensated (Child-Pugh B or C) Cirrhosis or Post-Transplant: Daclatasvir + sofosbuvir + ribavirin for 12 weeks

Genotype 3:
W/O Cirrhosis: Daclatasvir + sofosbuvir for 12 weeks
Compensated (Child-Pugh A) or Decompensated (Child-Pugh B or C) Cirrhosis, or Post-Transplant: Daclatasvir + sofosbuvir + ribavirin for 12 weeks

The recommended treatment durations are also applicable to patients w/ HCV/HIV-1 coinfection

For specific sofosbuvir and ribavirin dosage recommendations, refer to the individual PIs

PEDIATRIC DOSAGE
Pediatric use may not have been established

DOSING CONSIDERATIONS
Concomitant Medications
Strong CYP3A Inhibitors and Certain HIV Antiviral Agents:
Reduce daclatasvir dose to 30mg qd

Moderate CYP3A Inducers and Nevirapine:
Increase daclatasvir dose to 90mg qd

Discontinuation
D/C daclatasvir if sofosbuvir is permanently discontinued

ADMINISTRATION
Oral route

Take w/ or w/o food.

STORAGE
25°C (77°F); excursions permitted between 15-30°C (59-86°F).

HOW SUPPLIED
Tab: 30mg, 60mg, 90mg

CONTRAINDICATIONS
In combination w/ strong CYP3A inducers (eg, phenytoin, carbamazepine, rifampin, St. John's wort). When used w/ sofosbuvir and ribavirin, refer to the individual PIs.

WARNINGS/PRECAUTIONS
Consider screening for the presence of NS5A polymorphisms at amino acid positions M28, Q30, L31, and Y93 in patients w/ cirrhosis who are infected w/ HCV genotype 1a prior to treatment initiation. Symptomatic bradycardia and cases requiring pacemaker intervention have been reported when amiodarone is coadministered w/ sofosbuvir in combination w/ another chronic HCV direct-acting antiviral, including daclatasvir. Patients also taking β-blockers or those w/ underlying cardiac comorbidities and/or advanced liver disease may be at increased risk for symptomatic bradycardia w/ coadministration of amiodarone. Coadministration of amiodarone w/ daclatasvir in combination w/ sofosbuvir is not recommended; if coadministration is required, cardiac monitoring in an inpatient setting for the first 48 hrs of coadministration is recommended, after which outpatient or self-monitoring of HR should occur on a daily basis through at least the first 2 weeks of treatment. Patients discontinuing amiodarone just prior to starting sofosbuvir in combination w/ daclatasvir should also undergo similar cardiac monitoring. Immediately evaluate patients who develop signs/symptoms of bradycardia. If administered w/ ribavirin, refer to the ribavirin PI for a full list of the warnings and precautions for ribavirin.

ADVERSE REACTIONS
Daclatasvir in Combination w/ Sofosbuvir: Headache, fatigue.
Daclatasvir in Combination w/ Sofosbuvir and Ribavirin: Headache, anemia, fatigue, nausea.

DRUG INTERACTIONS
See Dosing Considerations, Contraindications, and Warnings/Precautions. Strong CYP3A inducers or moderate CYP3A inducers (eg, bosentan, dexamethasone, nafcillin) may decrease levels and therapeutic effect. Strong CYP3A inhibitors (eg, clarithromycin, itraconazole, nefazodone) may increase levels. May increase systemic exposure to medicinal products that are substrates of P-gp, OATP 1B1 or 1B3, or breast cancer resistance protein, which could increase or prolong their therapeutic effect or adverse reactions. HIV protease inhibitors (eg, atazanavir w/ ritonavir, indinavir, nelfinavir, saquinavir) may increase levels; decrease daclatasvir dose to 30mg qd. Cobicistat-containing antiretroviral regimens (eg, atazanavir/cobicistat, elvitegravir/cobicistat/emtricitabine/tenofovir disoproxil fumarate) may increase levels; decrease daclatasvir dose to 30mg qd except w/ darunavir combined w/ cobicistat. Non-nucleoside reverse transcriptase inhibitors (eg, efavirenz, etravirine, nevirapine) may decrease levels; increase daclatasvir dose to 90mg qd. May increase levels of dabigatran. Use w/ dabigatran is not recommended in specific renal impairment groups, depending on the indication; refer to dabigatran PI for specific recommendations. May increase digoxin levels; monitor digoxin levels. May increase levels of HMG-CoA reductase inhibitors (eg, atorvastatin, rosuvastatin, simvastatin); monitor for HMG-CoA reductase inhibitor-associated adverse events (eg, myopathy). May increase levels of buprenorphine and norbuprenorphine; monitor for buprenorphine-associated adverse events. Refer to PI for further information on drug interactions.

PREGNANCY AND LACTATION
Pregnancy: No adequate human data are available to determine whether or not daclatasvir poses a risk to pregnancy outcomes.
Lactation: It is not known whether daclatasvir is present in human milk, affects human milk production, or has effects on the breastfed infant; caution in nursing.

If administered w/ ribavirin, refer to ribavirin PI for additional information.

MECHANISM OF ACTION
HCV NS5A inhibitor; binds to the N-terminus of NS5A and inhibits both viral RNA replication and virion assembly.

PHARMACOKINETICS
Absorption: T_{max}=2 hrs; AUC=10,973ng•hr/mL; absolute bioavailability (67%).
Distribution: Plasma protein binding (approx 99%); V_d=47L. **Metabolism:** Primarily via CYP3A. **Elimination:** Feces (88%, 53% unchanged), urine (6.6%, primarily unchanged); $T_{1/2}$=12-15 hrs.

PATIENT CONSIDERATIONS
Assessment: Assess for hypersensitivity to drug, pregnancy/nursing status, and possible drug interactions. Perform cardiac monitoring in patients discontinuing amiodarone just prior to starting daclatasvir. Consider screening for the presence of NS5A polymorphisms at amino acid positions M28, Q30, L31, and Y93 in patients w/ cirrhosis who are infected w/ HCV genotype 1a prior to treatment initiation.

Monitoring: Monitor for bradycardia if coadministering daclatasvir w/ sofosbuvir and amiodarone. Monitor for other adverse reactions.

Counseling: Inform that therapy may interact w/ other drugs; advise to report to physician the use of any other medication or herbal products. Advise to seek medical evaluation immediately for symptoms of bradycardia (eg, fainting, dizziness, lightheadedness, weakness). Inform that therapy should not be used alone and that it should be used in combination w/ sofosbuvir w/ or w/o ribavirin. Advise to avoid pregnancy during combination treatment w/ daclatasvir and sofosbuvir w/ ribavirin for 6 months after completion of treatment; instruct to notify physician immediately in the event of a pregnancy.

DARZALEX — daratumumab   Rx

Class: Monoclonal antibody/CD38 blocker

ADULT DOSAGE
Multiple Myeloma

Patients w/ multiple myeloma who have received at least 3 prior lines of therapy including a proteasome inhibitor (PI) and an immunomodulatory agent or who are double-refractory to a PI and an immunomodulatory agent

Recommended Dose: 16mg/kg IV
Weeks 1-8: Administer weekly
Weeks 9-24: Administer every 2 weeks
Week 25 Onwards Until Disease Progression: Administer every 4 weeks

Infusion Rates:
1st Infusion:
Dilution Volume: 1000mL
Initial Rate (1st hr): 50mL/hr
Rate Increment: 50mL/hr every hr
Max Rate: 200mL/hr

2nd Infusion:
Dilution Volume: 500mL
Initial Rate (1st hr): 50mL/hr
Rate Increment: 50mL/hr every hr
Max Rate: 200mL/hr

Escalate infusion rate only if there were no Grade 1 or greater infusion reactions during the first 3 hrs of the 1st infusion

PEDIATRIC DOSAGE
Pediatric use may not have been established

Subsequent Infusions:
Dilution Volume: 500mL
Initial Rate (1st hr): 100mL/hr
Rate Increment: 50mL/hr every hr
Max Rate: 200mL/hr

Escalate infusion rate only if there were no Grade 1 or greater infusion reactions during a final infusion rate of ≥100 mL/hr in the first 2 infusions

Premedication

IV corticosteroid (methylprednisolone 100mg, or equivalent dose of an intermediate-acting or long-acting corticosteroid) + oral antipyretics (acetaminophen 650-1000mg) + oral or IV antihistamine (diphenhydramine 25-50mg or equivalent)

Administer to all patients 1 hr prior to every infusion; following 2nd infusion, may reduce the corticosteroid dose (methylprednisolone 60mg IV)

Post-Infusion Medication

Administer to all patients oral corticosteroid (20mg methylprednisolone or equivalent dose of a corticosteroid in accordance w/ local standards) on the 1st and 2nd day after all infusions

For patients w/ a history of obstructive pulmonary disorder, consider prescribing post-infusion medications (eg, short and long-acting bronchodilators, inhaled corticosteroids). Following the first 4 infusions, if patient experiences no major infusion reactions, may d/c additional inhaled post-infusion medications

Missed Dose

If a planned dose is missed, administer the dose as soon as possible and adjust dosing schedule accordingly, maintaining the treatment interval

----

DOSING CONSIDERATIONS

Adverse Reactions
Infusion Reactions:

Immediately interrupt infusion and manage symptoms if an infusion reaction of any grade/severity develops

Grade 1-2: Once reaction symptoms resolve, resume the infusion at no more than 1/2 the rate at which the reaction occurred; may resume infusion rate escalation at increments and intervals as appropriate if patient does not experience any further reaction symptoms

Grade 3: Consider restarting infusion at no more than 1/2 the rate at which the reaction occurred if the intensity of the reaction decreases to Grade 2 or lower. Resume infusion rate escalation if the patient does not experience additional symptoms. Repeat these steps in the event of recurrence of Grade 3 symptoms; permanently d/c upon the 3rd occurrence of a Grade 3 or greater infusion reaction

Grade 4: Permanently d/c treatment

Other Important Considerations
Prophylaxis for Herpes Zoster Reactivation:

Initiate antiviral prophylaxis to prevent herpes zoster reactivation w/in 1 week of starting daratumumab and continue for 3 months following treatment

ADMINISTRATION

IV route

Administer only as an IV infusion after dilution.

Administer diluted sol using an infusion set fitted w/ a flow regulator and w/ an in-line, sterile, non-pyrogenic, low protein-binding polyethersulfone filter (pore size 0.22 or 0.2μm).

Must use polyurethane, polybutadiene, polyvinyl chloride (PVC), polypropylene (PP), or polyethylene (PE) administration sets.

Infusion should be completed w/in 15 hrs.

Do not store any unused portion of the infusion sol for reuse.

Do not infuse concomitantly in the same IV line w/ other agents.

Preparation

1. Calculate the dose (mg), total volume (mL) of daratumumab sol required, and the number of daratumumab vials needed based on patient actual body weight.
2. Aseptically, remove a volume of 0.9% NaCl inj from the infusion bag/container that is equal to the required volume of daratumumab sol.
3. Withdraw the necessary amount of daratumumab sol and dilute to the appropriate volume by adding to the infusion bag/container containing 0.9% NaCl inj; infusion bags/containers must be made of PVC, PP, PE, or polyolefin blend (PE+PP).
4. Gently invert the bag/container to mix the sol; do not shake.

Following dilution, may store the infusion bag/container for up to 24 hrs in a refrigerator at 2-8°C (36-46°F), protected from light; do not freeze.
Use immediately after allowing the bag/container to come to room temperature. Diluted sol may develop very small, translucent to white proteinaceous particles; do not use if visibly opaque particles, discoloration, or foreign particles are observed.

STORAGE
2-8°C (36-46°F). Do not freeze or shake. Protect from light.

HOW SUPPLIED
Inj: 20mg/mL [5mL, 20mL]

WARNINGS/PRECAUTIONS

See Dosing Considerations. Should be administered by a healthcare professional, w/ immediate access to emergency equipment and appropriate medical support. Severe infusion reactions (eg, bronchospasm, hypoxia, dyspnea, HTN) reported; interrupt infusion for reactions of any severity and institute medical management as needed. Binds to CD38 on RBCs and results in a positive Indirect Antiglobulin Test (Coombs test); may persist for up to 6 months after the last infusion. Daratumumab bound to RBCs masks detection of antibodies to minor antigens in the patient's serum; determination of a patient's ABO and Rh blood type are not impacted. Notify blood transfusion centers of this interference w/ serological testing and inform blood banks that a patient has received daratumumab. Type and screen patients prior to starting therapy. If an emergency transfusion is required, non-cross-matched ABO/RhD-compatible RBCs can be given per local blood bank practices. Daratumumab may be detected on both, the serum protein electrophoresis and immunofixation assays used for the clinical monitoring of endogenous M-protein; this interference may impact the determination of complete response and of disease progression in some patients w/ IgG kappa myeloma protein; consider other methods to evaluate the depth of response in patients w/ persistent very good partial response.

ADVERSE REACTIONS

Infusion reaction, fatigue, N/V, pyrexia, back pain, cough, URTI, arthralgia, nasal congestion, diarrhea, dyspnea, pain in extremity, nasopharyngitis, decreased appetite, constipation.

PREGNANCY AND LACTATION

Pregnancy: May cause fetal myeloid or lymphoid-cell depletion and decrease bone density; defer administering live vaccines to neonates and infants exposed to daratumumab in utero until a hematology evaluation is completed.
Lactation: Caution in nursing.
Reproductive Potential: Women of reproductive potential should use effective contraception during treatment and for 3 months after cessation of treatment.

MECHANISM OF ACTION

Human CD38-directed monoclonal antibody; binds to CD38 and inhibits the growth of CD38 expressing tumor cells by inducing apoptosis directly through Fc mediated cross linking as well as by immune-mediated tumor cell lysis through complement dependent cytotoxicity, antibody dependent cell mediated cytotoxicity, and antibody dependent cellular phagocytosis.

PHARMACOKINETICS

Absorption: C_{max}=915μg/mL. **Distribution:** V_d=4.7L. **Elimination:** $T_{1/2}$=18 days.

PATIENT CONSIDERATIONS

Assessment: Assess for hypersensitivity to drug, history of an obstructive pulmonary disorder, history of herpes zoster, and pregnancy/nursing status. Type and screen patient's blood.

Monitoring: Monitor for infusion reactions, lab test interactions, and for other adverse reactions.

Counseling: Advise to seek immediate medical attention if any signs/symptoms of an infusion reaction develop. Advise patients to inform healthcare providers including blood transfusion centers/personnel that they are taking daratumumab, in the event of a planned transfusion.

DAUNORUBICIN — daunorubicin hydrochloride   Rx

Class: Anthracycline

Give into a rapidly flowing IV infusion and never give by IM/SQ route; extravasation may cause severe local tissue necrosis. Myocardial toxicity manifested in its most severe form by potentially fatal congestive heart failure may occur during therapy or months to yrs after termination of therapy; incidence increases after a total cumulative dose >400-550mg/m² in adults, >300mg/m² in children >2 yrs of age, or >10mg/kg in children <2 yrs of age. Severe myelosuppression occurs; may lead to infection or hemorrhage. Should be administered only by physicians experienced in leukemia chemotherapy and in facilities with laboratory and supportive resources adequate to monitor drug tolerance and protect and maintain a patient compromised by drug toxicity. Reduce dosage in patients with hepatic/renal impairment.

ADULT DOSAGE

Acute Non-Lymphocytic Leukemia

Remission Induction in Myelogenous, Monocytic, Erythroid Leukemia:
<60 Years:
Daunorubicin HCl 45mg/m²/day IV on Days 1-3 of 1st course and on Days 1 and 2 of subsequent courses + cytosine arabinoside 100mg/m²/day IV infusion for 7 days for the 1st course and for 5 days for subsequent courses

PEDIATRIC DOSAGE

Acute Lymphocytic Leukemia

Remission Induction:
Daunorubicin HCl 25mg/m² IV on Day 1 every week + vincristine 1.5mg/m² IV on Day 1 every week + prednisone 40mg/m²/day PO

If remission is partial after 4 courses, may give additional 1 or 2 courses

<2 Years or <0.5m² BSA:
Calculate dose based on weight (1mg/kg) instead of BSA

≥60 Years:
Daunorubicin HCl 30mg/m²/day IV on Days 1-3 of 1st course and on Days 1 and 2 of subsequent courses + cytosine arabinoside 100mg/m²/day IV infusion for 7 days for the 1st course and for 5 days for subsequent courses

Acute Lymphocytic Leukemia

Remission Induction:
Daunorubicin HCl 45mg/m²/day IV on Days 1-3 + vincristine 2mg IV on Days 1, 8, and 15 + prednisone 40mg/m²/day PO on Days 1-22 (tapered between Days 22-29) + L-asparaginase 500 IU/kg/day for 10 days IV on Days 22-32

DOSING CONSIDERATIONS
Renal Impairment
SrCr >3mg/dL: Reduce dose by 50%

Hepatic Impairment
Serum Bilirubin:
1.2-3mg/dL: Reduce dose by 25%
<3mg/dL: Reduce dose by 50%

ADMINISTRATION
IV route

Do not mix w/ other drugs or heparin

Preparation and Administrations
1. Withdraw desired dose into a syringe containing 10-15mL of 0.9% NaCl inj
2. Inject into the tubing or sidearm in a rapidly flowing IV infusion of D5 inj or 0.9% NaCl inj

STORAGE
Unopened: 2-8°C (36-46°F). Prepared Sol for Infusion: 20-25°C (68-77°F) for up to 24 hrs. Protect from light.

HOW SUPPLIED
Inj: 5mg/mL [4mL]

CONTRAINDICATIONS
Hypersensitivity to daunorubicin hydrochloride.

WARNINGS/PRECAUTIONS
Do not start in patients with preexisting drug-induced bone marrow suppression unless treatment benefit warrants risk. Increased risk of drug-induced cardiac toxicity in patients with preexisting heart disease and previous therapy with doxorubicin; do not use in patients who have previously received the recommended max cumulative doses of doxorubicin or daunorubicin. Total dose administered should take into account any previous or concomitant therapy with other potentially cardiotoxic agents or related compounds (eg, doxorubicin). Significant hepatic/renal impairment may enhance toxicity of recommended doses. May cause fetal harm. Control any systemic infection before beginning therapy. May transiently impart red coloration to urine. May induce hyperuricemia secondary to rapid lysis of leukemic cells; may begin allopurinol administration prior to initiating therapy. Initiate appropriate therapy if hyperuricemia develops. Caution in elderly.

ADVERSE REACTIONS
Myocardial toxicity, myelosuppression, alopecia, N/V, hyperuricemia, mucositis.

DRUG INTERACTIONS
Increased cardiotoxicity with cyclophosphamide or thoracic irradiation. May require dose reduction of daunorubicin when used concurrently with other myelosuppressive agents. Hepatotoxic drugs (eg, high-dose methotrexate) may increase risk of toxicity. Secondary leukemias reported with other antineoplastics or radiation therapy.

PREGNANCY AND LACTATION
Category D, not for use in nursing.

MECHANISM OF ACTION
Anthracycline; has antimitotic and cytotoxic activity. Inhibits topoisomerase II activity by stabilizing the DNA-topoisomerase II complex, preventing the religation portion of the ligation-religation reaction that topoisomerase II catalyzes, resulting in single-strand and double-strand DNA breaks. Also, may inhibit polymerase activity, affect regulation of gene expression, and produce free radical damage to DNA.

PHARMACOKINETICS
Distribution: Crosses placenta. **Metabolism:** Liver and other tissues (extensive), by cytoplasmic aldo-keto reductases; daunorubicinol (active metabolite). **Elimination:** Urine (25% active form), bile (40%); $T_{1/2}$=18.5 hrs, 26.7 hrs (daunorubicinol).

PATIENT CONSIDERATIONS
Assessment: Assess for drug-induced bone marrow suppression, previous doxorubicin therapy, systemic infection, cardiac/hepatic/renal function, hypersensitivity to drug, pregnancy/nursing status, and possible drug interactions. Evaluate peripheral blood and bone marrow.

Monitoring: Monitor for myocardial toxicity, myelosuppression, infection, hemorrhage, extravasation, and other adverse events. Monitor CBC frequently, hepatic/renal function prior to each course, and blood uric acid levels. Perform ECG and/or determination of systolic ejection fraction before each course of therapy.

Counseling: Inform that drug may cause fetal harm; advise women of childbearing potential to avoid becoming pregnant. Inform that drug may transiently impart a red coloration to urine. Instruct that if product contacts the skin or mucosa, to wash the area thoroughly with soap and water.

DepoCyt – cytarabine liposome ℞

Class: Antimetabolite

> Chemical arachnoiditis, a syndrome manifested primarily by N/V, headache, and fever, was a common adverse event reported in all clinical studies, and may be fatal if left untreated. Treat concurrently w/ dexamethasone to mitigate the symptoms of chemical arachnoiditis.

ADULT DOSAGE	PEDIATRIC DOSAGE
Lymphomatous Meningitis	Pediatric use may not have been established
Induction: 50mg every 14 days for 2 doses (Weeks 1 and 3)	
Consolidation: 50mg every 14 days for 3 doses (Weeks 5, 7, and 9) followed by 1 additional dose at Week 13	
Maint: 50mg every 28 days for 4 doses (Weeks 17, 21, 25, and 29)	
Give dexamethasone 4mg bid PO/IV for 5 days beginning on day of therapy	

DOSING CONSIDERATIONS
Adverse Reactions
Drug-Related Neurotoxicity: Reduce to 25mg. D/C if neurotoxicity persists

ADMINISTRATION
Intrathecal (intraventricular or lumbar puncture) route

Allow vial to warm to room temperature and gently agitate or invert to resuspend particles immediately prior to withdrawal from vial
Avoid aggressive agitation
Should be withdrawn from vial immediately before administration
If drug contacts skin, wash immediately w/ soap and water. If drug contacts mucous membranes, flush thoroughly w/ water
Do not mix w/ any other medications
Do not use in-line filters when administering
Administer directly into CSF via an intraventricular reservoir or by direct inj into the lumbar sac
Inject slowly over a period of 1-5 min

Following administration by lumbar puncture, instruct patient to lie flat for 1 hr. Patients should be observed by physician for immediate toxic reactions

STORAGE
2-8°C (36-46°F). Protect from freezing and avoid aggressive agitation. Use w/in 4 hrs of withdrawal from vial.

HOW SUPPLIED
Inj: 10mg/mL [5mL]

CONTRAINDICATIONS
Hypersensitivity to cytarabine or any component of the formulation, active meningeal infection.

WARNINGS/PRECAUTIONS
Hydrocephalus reported. May cause myelopathy and other neurologic toxicity and can rarely lead to a permanent neurologic deficit. Blockage to CSF flow may result in increased free cytarabine concentrations in the CSF and an increased risk of neurotoxicity; consider assessment of CSF flow before treatment is started. CNS toxicity reported. In some cases, a combination of neurological signs and symptoms has been reported as cauda equina syndrome. Toxic effects may occur at any time during therapy; monitor continuously for the development of neurotoxicity. Transient elevations in CSF protein and WBCs reported. May cause fetal harm.

ADVERSE REACTIONS
Chemical arachnoiditis, headache, pyrexia, N/V, confusion, abnormal gait, convulsions, weakness, lethargy, fatigue, constipation, pain, dizziness, memory impairment, UTI.

DRUG INTERACTIONS
May increase risk of neurotoxicity w/ other chemotherapeutic agents or w/ cranial/spinal irradiation. Enhanced neurotoxicity w/ other intrathecal cytotoxic agents reported.

PREGNANCY AND LACTATION
Category D, not for use in nursing.

MECHANISM OF ACTION
Antimetabolite; not established. Appears to act primarily through inhibition of DNA polymerase. Also incorporates into DNA and RNA.

PHARMACOKINETICS
Absorption: C_{max}=30-50mcg/mL; T_{max}=1 hr. **Metabolism:** Cytarabine-5-triphosphate (active metabolite). **Elimination:** Urine; $T_{1/2}$=5.9-82.4 hrs.

PATIENT CONSIDERATIONS
Assessment: Assess for drug hypersensitivity, active meningeal infection, CSF flow, pregnancy/nursing status, and possible drug interactions.

Monitoring: Monitor for chemical arachnoiditis, neurotoxicity, and other adverse reactions.

Counseling: Inform about the expected adverse events (eg, headache, N/V, fever) and the early signs/symptoms of neurotoxicity. Emphasize the importance of concurrent dexamethasone administration at the initiation of each cycle of treatment. Instruct to seek medical attention if signs/symptoms of neurotoxicity develop or if oral dexamethasone is not well tolerated. Advise women of childbearing potential that therapy may cause fetal harm if used during pregnancy.

DESFERAL — deferoxamine mesylate   Rx

Class: Iron-chelating agent

ADULT DOSAGE	**PEDIATRIC DOSAGE**
Acute Iron Toxicity	**Acute Iron Toxicity**
Due to Transfusion-Dependent Anemias:	**Due to Transfusion-Dependent Anemias:**
IM/IV:	**≥3 Years:**
Initial: 1000mg, then 500mg q4h for 2 doses; give subsequent 500mg doses q4-12h depending upon clinical response	**IM/IV:**
Max: 6000mg/24 hrs	**Initial:** 1000mg, then 500mg q4h for 2 doses; give subsequent 500mg doses q4-12h depending upon clinical response
IM is preferred and should be used for all patients not in shock	**Max:** 6000mg/24 hrs
IV is only for patients in a state of cardiovascular collapse; as soon as clinical condition of the patient permits, d/c IV administration and administer IM	IM is preferred and should be used for all patients not in shock
	IV is only for patients in a state of cardiovascular collapse; as soon as clinical condition of the patient permits, d/c IV administration and administer IM
Chronic Iron Overload	
Due to Transfusion-Dependent Anemias:	**Chronic Iron Overload**
IM:	**Due to Transfusion-Dependent Anemias:**
Usual: 500-1000mg/day	**≥3 Years:**
Max: 1000mg/day	**IM:**
IV:	**Usual:** 500-1000mg/day
Usual: 40-50mg/kg/day over 8-12 hrs for 5-7 days per week	**Max:** 1000mg/day
Max: 60mg/kg/day	**IV:**
In patients who are poorly compliant, may administer prior to or following same day blood transfusion (eg, 1g over 4 hrs on the day of transfusion)	**Usual:** 20-40mg/kg/day over 8-12 hrs for 5-7 days per week
	Max: 40mg/kg/day
SQ:	In patients who are poorly compliant, may administer prior to or following same day blood transfusion (eg, 1g over 4 hrs on the day of transfusion)
Initial: 1000-2000mg/day (20-40mg/kg/day) over 8-24 hrs using a small pump for continuous infusion	**SQ:**
	Initial: 1000-2000mg/day (20-40mg/kg/day) over 8-24 hrs using a small pump for continuous infusion

---

DOSING CONSIDERATIONS

Elderly
Start at lower end of dosing range

ADMINISTRATION
IM/IV/SQ route

For single use only; use immediately after reconstitution (commencement of treatment w/in 3 hrs)
Reconstituted sol may be stored at room temperature for a max of 24 hrs before use

IM Preparation
For a final concentration of 213mg/mL, add 2mL of sterile water for inj (SWFI) to the 500mg vial or 8mL of SWFI to the 2g vial

IV
Acute Iron Toxicity:
Slow IV infusion; do not exceed 15mg/kg/hr for 1st 1000mg; subsequent IV dosing should not exceed 125mg/hr
Preparation:
For a final concentration of 95mg/mL, add 5mL of SWFI to the 500mg vial or 8mL of SWFI to the 2g vial

SQ Preparation
For a final concentration of 95mg/mL, add 5mL of SWFI to the 500mg vial or 8mL of SWFI to the 2g vial

STORAGE
≤25°C (77°F). After reconstitution, may store at room temperature for a max period of 24 hrs before use. Do not refrigerate reconstituted sol. Do not use turbid sol.

HOW SUPPLIED
Inj: 500mg, 2g

CONTRAINDICATIONS
Known hypersensitivity to the active substance in this product, severe renal disease, anuria.

WARNINGS/PRECAUTIONS
Ocular and auditory disturbances reported with prolonged use, high doses, or low ferritin levels. Perform periodic visual acuity tests, slit-lamp exams, funduscopy, and audiometry with prolonged treatment. Increases in serum creatinine (possibly dose-related), acute renal failure, and renal tubular disorders reported; monitor for changes in renal function. High doses with low ferritin levels have been associated with growth retardation. Adult respiratory distress syndrome, also in children, reported after high IV doses in acute iron intoxication or thalassemia. Give via IM, slow SQ, or IV infusion; skin flushing, urticaria, hypotension, and shock reported with rapid IV injection. May cause mucormycosis and enhance susceptibility to *Yersinia* infections; d/c if infections occur. May cause neurological dysfunction in patients with aluminum-related encephalopathy and receiving dialysis and may precipitate onset of dialysis dementia. Presence of aluminum overload may decrease serum calcium and aggravate hyperparathyroidism. Monitor pediatrics body weight and growth every 3 months. Caution in elderly patients.

ADVERSE REACTIONS
Inj-site reactions, hypersensitivity reactions, tachycardia, hypotension, shock, abdominal discomfort, diarrhea, N/V, blood dyscrasia, growth retardation, bone changes, dysuria.

DRUG INTERACTIONS
Cardiac dysfunction reported with high-dose vitamin C (>500mg/day in adults) in patients with severe chronic iron overload; avoid vitamin C supplements in cardiac failure patients. Only give vitamin C after 1 month of regular deferoxamine therapy. Concurrent prochlorperazine may lead to temporary impairment of consciousness. May distort imaging results with gallium-67; d/c deferoxamine 48 hrs before scintigraphy.

PREGNANCY AND LACTATION
Category C, caution in nursing.

MECHANISM OF ACTION
Iron chelating agent; chelates iron by forming a stable complex that prevents iron from entering into further chemical reactions.

PHARMACOKINETICS
Metabolism: Primarily by plasma enzymes. **Elimination:** Urine, feces.

PATIENT CONSIDERATIONS

Assessment: Assess for previous hypersensitivity to the drug, history of severe renal disease or anuria, pregnancy/nursing status, and possible drug interactions.

Monitoring: Monitor for signs/symptoms of ocular disturbances (eg, blurring of vision, cataracts, visual loss, visual defects, scotoma, impaired peripheral or color or night vision, optic neuritis, corneal opacities, retinal pigmentary abnormalities), auditory disturbances (eg, tinnitus, hearing loss), and for infection. Monitor for changes in renal function. Perform periodic visual acuity tests, slit-lamp exams, funduscopy, and audiometry in patients on prolonged therapy. In pediatric patients, monitor for signs of growth retardation; monitor body weight and growth every 3 months.

Counseling: Inform that vitamin C supplements should not be given during therapy in patients with cardiac failure. Inform that urine may occasionally show reddish discoloration. Advise to refrain from driving or operating machines if experiencing dizziness or other nervous system disturbances or impairment of vision or hearing. Instruct to notify physician if pregnant or nursing, experiencing vision or hearing disturbances, or an allergic reaction develops.

DOCEFREZ — docetaxel   Rx

Class: Antimicrotubule agent

> Increased incidence of treatment-related mortality with abnormal liver function, at higher doses, and in patients with non-small cell lung carcinoma (NSCLC) and a history of prior treatment with platinum-based chemotherapy who receive docetaxel as a single agent at 100mg/m². Should not be given to patients with bilirubin >ULN, or with AST/ALT >1.5X ULN concomitant with alkaline phosphatase >2.5X ULN; increased risk of grade 4 neutropenia, febrile neutropenia, infections, severe thrombocytopenia, severe stomatitis, severe skin toxicity, and toxic death. Obtain LFTs prior to each treatment cycle. Should not be given if neutrophils <1500 cells/mm³; perform frequent blood cell counts. Severe hypersensitivity reactions reported in patients who received a 3-day dexamethasone premedication; d/c immediately and administer appropriate therapy. Contraindicated with history of severe hypersensitivity reactions to other drugs formulated with polysorbate 80. Severe fluid retention reported despite dexamethasone premedication.

ADULT DOSAGE	**PEDIATRIC DOSAGE**
Breast Cancer	Pediatric use may not have been established
Locally advanced or metastatic breast cancer after failure of prior chemotherapy	
60-100mg/m² IV over 1 hr every 3 weeks	
Non-Small Cell Lung Cancer	
Single Agent:	
Locally advanced or metastatic non-small cell lung cancer after failure of prior platinum-based chemotherapy	
75mg/m² IV over 1 hr every 3 weeks	
Combination w/ Cisplatin:	
Unresectable, locally advanced or metastatic non-small cell lung cancer in patients who have not previously	

received chemotherapy for this condition

75mg/m² IV over 1 hr immediately, followed by cisplatin 75mg/m² over 30-60 min every 3 weeks

Metastatic Prostate Cancer
Combination w/ prednisone for androgen independent (hormone refractory) metastatic prostate cancer

75mg/m² IV over 1 hr every 3 weeks + prednisone 5mg PO bid

Premedication
Breast Cancer/Non-Small Cell Lung Cancer:
PO corticosteroids (eg, dexamethasone 8mg bid) for 3 days starting 1 day prior to docetaxel administration

Metastatic Prostate Cancer:
PO dexamethasone 8mg, at 12 hrs, 3 hrs, and 1 hr before docetaxel infusion

- -

DOSING CONSIDERATIONS
Concomitant Medications
Strong CYP3A4 Inhibitors: Avoid concomitant use; if coadministration required, consider a 50% dose reduction

Hepatic Impairment
Bilirubin >ULN: Not recommended for use
AST and/or ALT >1.5X ULN w/ Alkaline Phosphatase >2.5X ULN: Not recommended for use

Adverse Reactions
Breast Cancer:
Initial Dose 100mg/m²:
Experience Febrile Neutropenia, Neutrophils <500 cells/mm³ for >1 Week, or Severe/Cumulative Cutaneous Reactions: Reduce dose to 75mg/m²; if patient continues to experience these reactions, either decrease dose to 55mg/m² or d/c treatment
Initial Dose 60mg/m²:
Do not Experience Febrile Neutropenia, Neutrophils <500 cells/mm³ for >1 Week, Severe/Cumulative Cutaneous Reactions, or Severe Peripheral Neuropathy During Therapy: May tolerate higher doses
Develop ≥Grade 3 Peripheral Neuropathy: D/C treatment

Non-Small Cell Lung Cancer:
Monotherapy:
Experience Febrile Neutropenia, Neutrophils <500 cells/mm³ for >1 Week, Severe/Cumulative Cutaneous Reactions, or Other Grade 3/4 Non-Hematological Toxicities: Withhold treatment until toxicity resolves, then resume at 55mg/m²
Develop ≥Grade 3 Peripheral Neuropathy: D/C treatment

Combination w/ Cisplatin:
Nadir of Platelet Count During Previous Course of Therapy is <25,000 cells/mm³ or Febrile Neutropenia/Serious Non-Hematologic Toxicities Experienced: Reduce dose in subsequent cycles to 65mg/m²; if further dose reduction is required, reduce to 50mg/m²

Prostate Cancer:
Experience Febrile Neutropenia, Neutrophils <500 cells/mm³ for >1 Week, Severe/Cumulative Cutaneous Reactions, or Moderate Neurosensory Signs and/or Symptoms: Reduce dose to 60mg/m²; if patient continues to experience these reactions, d/c treatment

ADMINISTRATION
IV route
Administration Precautions
Contact of reconstituted sol w/ plasticized PVC equipment or devices used to prepare sol for infusion is not recommended; store the infusion sol in bottles (glass, polypropylene) or plastic bags (polypropylene, polyolefin) and administer through polyethylene-lined administration sets

Preparation of Reconstituted Sol
1. Allow the appropriate number of docetaxel vials and diluent (35.4% ethanol in polysorbate 80) vials to stand at room temperature for approx 5 min
2. **For Docetaxel 20:** Use 1mL syringe w/ needle of 18- to 21-gauge, 1 1/2 inch for withdrawing diluent
   For Docetaxel 80: Use 4mL syringe w/ needle of 18- to 21-gauge, 1 1/2 inch for withdrawing diluent
3. **For Docetaxel 20:** Withdraw 1mL from diluent vial into a syringe by partially inverting the vial, and transfer it to the docetaxel vial
   For Docetaxel 80: Withdraw 4mL from diluent vial into a syringe by partially inverting the vial, and transfer it to the docetaxel vial
4. Shake the reconstituted vial well in order to completely dissolve the docetaxel powder present in the vial
   For the 20mg Vial: Resultant concentration is 20mg/0.8mL
   For the 80mg Vial: Resultant concentration is 24mg/mL
5. Some air bubbles may be present in the sol due to the polysorbate 80; allow the sol to stand for a few min to allow any air bubbles to dissipate

Preparation of Infusion Sol
1. Withdraw the required amount of reconstituted docetaxel sol w/ a calibrated syringe and inject into a 250mL infusion bag or bottle of either 0.9% NaCl sol or

D5 sol to produce a final concentration of 0.3-0.74mg/mL; if a dose >200mg is required, use a larger volume of the infusion vehicle so that a concentration of 0.74mg/mL is not exceeded
2. Thoroughly mix the infusion by manual rotation
3. Docetaxel reconstituted sol is supersaturated, therefore may crystallize over time; if crystals appear, the sol must no longer be used and shall be discarded

Handling Precautions
If lyophilized powder, reconstituted sol, or infusion sol comes in contact w/ the skin, wash w/ soap and water immediately and thoroughly
If lyophilized powder, reconstituted sol, or infusion sol comes in contact w/ mucosa, wash w/ water immediately and thoroughly

STORAGE
2-8°C (36-46°F). Protect from bright light. Reconstituted Sol: Use immediately or store either in the refrigerator or at room temperature for a max of 8 hrs. Infusion Sol (in either 0.9% NaCl or D5W): Stable at 2-25°C (36-77°F) for 6 hrs; use within 6 hrs including the 1 hr IV administration. Infusion sol is stable in non-PVC bags up to 48 hrs at 2-8°C (36-46°F).

HOW SUPPLIED
Inj: 20mg, 80mg

CONTRAINDICATIONS
History of severe hypersensitivity reactions to docetaxel or to other drugs formulated with polysorbate 80, neutrophils <1500 cells/mm³.

WARNINGS/PRECAUTIONS
Avoid retreatment with subsequent cycles until neutrophils recover to a level >1500 cells/mm³ and platelets recover to a level >100,000 cells/mm³. Fatal GI bleeding associated with severe drug-induced thrombocytopenia reported in BC patients with severe liver impairment. Do not rechallenge patients with a history of severe hypersensitivity reactions to therapy. Monitor from the 1st dose for possible exacerbation of preexisting effusions. Acute myeloid leukemia or myelodysplasia reported in patients given anthracyclines and/or cyclophosphamide, including use in adjuvant therapy for BC. Localized erythema of extremities with edema followed by desquamation reported; adjust dose if severe skin toxicity occurs. Severe neurosensory symptoms (eg, paresthesia, dysesthesia, pain) may develop; adjust dose if symptoms occur and d/c treatment if symptoms persist. Cystoid macular edema (CME) reported; d/c and initiate appropriate treatment if CME is diagnosed, and consider alternative non-taxane cancer treatment. Intoxication reported with some formulations of docetaxel due to the alcohol content. Alcohol content of the drug may affect CNS; caution in whom alcohol intake should be avoided or minimized. Alcohol content of the drug may impair physical/mental abilities. Severe asthenia reported. May cause fetal harm. Caution in elderly.

ADVERSE REACTIONS
Neutropenia, hypersensitivity, fluid retention, asthenia, dysgeusia, thrombocytopenia, constipation, nail disorders, skin reactions, N/V, alopecia, myalgia, neuropathy.

DRUG INTERACTIONS
Avoid with CYP3A4 inhibitors; consider a 50% docetaxel dose reduction if coadministration with a strong CYP3A4 inhibitor (eg, ketoconazole, clarithromycin, atazanavir) cannot be avoided. Protease inhibitors, particularly ritonavir, may increase exposure. CYP3A4 inducers or substrates may alter metabolism.

PREGNANCY AND LACTATION
Category D, not for use in nursing.

MECHANISM OF ACTION
Antimicrotubule agent; acts by disrupting the microtubular network in cells that is essential for mitotic and interphase cellular functions. Binds to free tubulin and promotes assembly of tubulin into stable microtubules while simultaneously inhibiting their disassembly, which results in the inhibition of mitosis in cells.

PHARMACOKINETICS
Distribution: V_d=113L; plasma protein binding (94%). **Metabolism:** Via CYP3A4. **Elimination:** Urine (6%, within 7 days), feces (75%, within 7 days); $T_{1/2}$=11.1 hrs.

PATIENT CONSIDERATIONS
Assessment: Assess for history of severe hypersensitivity reactions to the drug or other drugs formulated with polysorbate 80, preexisting effusion, hepatic impairment, pregnancy/nursing status, and possible drug interactions. Obtain baseline CBC and LFTs. Perform a comprehensive ophthalmologic examination in patients with impaired vision.

Monitoring: Monitor for neutropenia, hypersensitivity reactions, fluid retention, acute myeloid leukemia, hematologic effects, cutaneous reactions, exacerbation of effusions, neurosensory symptoms, asthenia, CME, and other adverse reactions. Monitor CBC frequently and LFTs prior to each cycle of therapy.

Counseling: Inform about risks and benefits of therapy. Inform that drug may cause fetal harm; advise women of childbearing potential to avoid becoming pregnant and use effective contraceptives. Explain the significance of oral corticosteroid administration to help facilitate compliance; instruct to report if not compliant. Instruct to immediately report signs of hypersensitivity reactions, fluid retention, myalgia, or cutaneous/neurologic reactions. Counsel about the side effects associated with the drug. Explain the significance of routine blood cell counts. Instruct to monitor temperature frequently and immediately report any occurrence of fever. Explain about the possible side effects of the alcohol content in the drug, including possible side effects on the CNS. Advise patients in whom alcohol should be avoided or minimized to consider the alcohol content of the drug; inform that alcohol could impair their ability to drive or use machines immediately after infusion.

DOCETAXEL — docetaxel

Class: Antimicrotubule agent

Rx

> Increased incidence of treatment-related mortality reported in patients w/ hepatic dysfunction, in patients receiving higher-doses, and in patients w/ non-small cell lung cancer (NSCLC) and a history of prior treatment w/ platinum-based chemotherapy who receive docetaxel as a single agent at a dose of 100mg/m². Avoid if bilirubin >ULN, or AST/ALT >1.5X ULN concomitant w/ alkaline phosphatase >2.5X ULN; may increase risk for the development of Grade 4 neutropenia, febrile neutropenia, infections, severe thrombocytopenia, severe stomatitis, severe skin toxicity, and toxic death. Patients w/ isolated elevations of transaminase >1.5X ULN reported to have a higher rate of febrile neutropenia Grade 4 but did not have an increased incidence of toxic death. Obtain bilirubin, AST or ALT, and alkaline phosphatase values prior to each cycle. Avoid therapy if neutrophils <1500 cells/mm³. Monitor for the occurrence of neutropenia; perform frequent blood cell counts on all patients. Severe hypersensitivity reactions reported w/ dexamethasone premedication; d/c immediately if symptoms occur. Contraindicated w/ history of severe hypersensitivity reactions to docetaxel or other drugs formulated w/ polysorbate 80. Severe fluid retention may occur despite dexamethasone premedication.

OTHER BRAND NAMES
Taxotere

ADULT DOSAGE

Breast Cancer

Locally advanced or metastatic breast cancer after failure of prior chemotherapy

60-100mg/m² IV over 1 hr every 3 weeks

Combination w/ Doxorubicin and Cyclophosphamide:

Adjuvant treatment of operable node-positive breast cancer

75mg/m² 1 hr after doxorubicin 50mg/m² and cyclophosphamide 500mg/m² every 3 weeks for 6 courses

Prophylactic G-CSF may be used to mitigate risk of hematological toxicities

Non-Small Cell Lung Cancer

Single Agent:

Locally advanced or metastatic NSCLC after failure of prior platinum-based chemotherapy

75mg/m² IV over 1 hr every 3 weeks

Combination w/ Cisplatin:

Unresectable, locally advanced or metastatic NSCLC in chemotherapy-naive patients

75mg/m² IV over 1 hr immediately followed by cisplatin 75mg/m² over 30-60 min every 3 weeks

Metastatic Prostate Cancer

Combination w/ prednisone for androgen-independent (hormone refractory) metastatic prostate cancer

75mg/m² IV over 1 hr every 3 weeks + prednisone 5mg PO bid

Gastric Adenocarcinoma

Combination w/ cisplatin and fluorouracil for advanced gastric adenocarcinoma, including adenocarcinoma of the gastroesophageal junction, in chemotherapy-naive patients

75mg/m² IV over 1 hr, followed by cisplatin 75mg/m² IV over 1-3 hrs (both on Day 1 only), followed by fluorouracil 750mg/m²/day IV over 24 hrs x 5 days, starting at end of cisplatin infusion

Repeat treatment every 3 weeks

Squamous Cell Carcinoma of the Head and Neck

Combination w/ cisplatin and fluorouracil for induction treatment of locally advanced squamous cell carcinoma of the head and neck (SCCHN)

Administer prophylaxis for neutropenic infections

Induction Followed by Radiotherapy:

Locally advanced inoperable SCCHN

75mg/m² IV over 1 hr, followed by cisplatin 75mg/m² IV over 1 hr, on Day 1, followed by fluorouracil as a

PEDIATRIC DOSAGE

Pediatric use may not have been established

---

continuous IV infusion at 750mg/m²/day x 5 days

Administer every 3 weeks for 4 cycles; following chemotherapy, patients should receive radiotherapy

Induction Followed by Chemoradiotherapy:

Locally advanced (unresectable, low surgical cure, or organ preservation) SCCHN

75mg/m² IV over 1 hr on Day 1, followed by cisplatin 100mg/m² IV over 30 min to 3 hrs, followed by fluorouracil 1000mg/m²/day as a continuous IV infusion from Day 1 to Day 4

Administer every 3 weeks for 3 cycles; following chemotherapy, patients should receive chemoradiotherapy

Premedication

All Patients:
Oral corticosteroids (see below for prostate cancer) such as dexamethasone 16mg/day (8mg bid) for 3 days starting 1 day prior to docetaxel administration

Prostate Cancer:
Given the concurrent use of prednisone, the recommended regimen is dexamethasone 8mg PO, at 12 hrs, 3 hrs, and 1 hr before docetaxel infusion

Gastric Adenocarcinoma/Head and Neck Cancer:
Patients must receive antiemetics and appropriate hydration for cisplatin administration

---

DOSING CONSIDERATIONS

Concomitant Medications
Strong CYP3A4 Inhibitors: Avoid use; consider a 50% docetaxel dose reduction if patients require coadministration of a strong CYP3A4 inhibitor

Hepatic Impairment
AST/ALT >2.5 to ≤5X ULN and Alkaline Phosphatase ≤2.5X ULN, or AST/ALT >1.5 to ≤5X ULN and Alkaline Phosphatase >2.5 to ≤5X ULN: Reduce docetaxel dose by 20%
AST/ALT >5X ULN and/or Alkaline Phosphatase >5X ULN: D/C treatment

Adverse Reactions
Breast Cancer:
Initial Dose 100mg/m²:
Experience Febrile Neutropenia, Neutrophils <500 cells/mm³ for >1 Week, or Severe/Cumulative Cutaneous Reactions: Reduce dose to 75mg/m²; if reactions continue, either reduce dose to 55mg/m² or d/c treatment
Initial Dose 60mg/m²:
Do Not Experience Febrile Neutropenia, Neutrophils <500 cells/mm³ for >1 Week, Severe/Cumulative Cutaneous Reactions, or Severe Peripheral Neuropathy: May tolerate higher doses
≥Grade 3 Peripheral Neuropathy: D/C treatment

Combination Therapy in Adjuvant Treatment of Breast Cancer:
Febrile Neutropenia: Administer G-CSF in all subsequent cycles; if reaction continues, continue G-CSF and reduce docetaxel dose to 60mg/m²
Grade 3 or 4 Stomatitis: Reduce docetaxel dose to 60mg/m²
Severe/Cumulative Cutaneous Reactions or Moderate Neurosensory Signs and/or Symptoms: Reduce docetaxel dose to 60mg/m²; if reactions continue at 60mg/m², d/c treatment

NSCLC:
Monotherapy:
Experience Febrile Neutropenia, Neutrophils <500 cells/mm³ for >1 Week, or Severe/Cumulative Cutaneous Reactions, or Other Grade 3-4 Nonhematological Toxicities: Withhold treatment until toxicity resolves, then resume at 55mg/m²
≥Grade 3 Peripheral Neuropathy: D/C treatment

Combination Therapy:
Nadir of Platelet Count During Previous Course of Therapy is <25,000 cells/mm³ w/ Febrile Neutropenia/Serious Nonhematologic Toxicities: Reduce docetaxel dose in subsequent cycles to 65mg/m²; if further dose reduction is required, 50mg/m² is recommended

Prostate Cancer:
Experience Febrile Neutropenia, Neutrophils <500 cells/mm³ for >1 Week, Severe/Cumulative Cutaneous Reactions, or Moderate Neurosensory Signs and/or Symptoms: Reduce docetaxel dose to 60mg/m²; if reactions continue at 60mg/m², d/c treatment

Gastric Adenocarcinoma/Head and Neck Cancer:
Experience Episode of Febrile Neutropenia or Prolonged Neutropenia/ Neutropenic Infection Occurs Despite G-CSF Use: Reduce docetaxel dose to 60mg/m^2; if subsequent episodes of complicated neutropenia occur, reduce docetaxel dose to 45mg/m^2. D/C if toxicities persist
Grade 4 Thrombocytopenia: Reduce docetaxel dose to 60mg/m^2; do not retreat w/ subsequent cycles until neutrophils recover to >1500 cells/mm^3 and platelets recover to >100,000 cells/mm^3. D/C if toxicities persist

Toxicities w/ Docetaxel in Combination w/ Cisplatin and Fluorouracil:
Grade 3 Diarrhea:
1st Episode: Reduce fluorouracil dose by 20%
2nd Episode: Reduce docetaxel dose by 20%

Grade 4 Diarrhea:
1st Episode: Reduce docetaxel and fluorouracil doses by 20%
2nd Episode: D/C treatment

Grade 3 Stomatitis/Mucositis:
1st Episode: Reduce fluorouracil dose by 20%
2nd Episode: Stop fluorouracil only, at all subsequent cycles
3rd Episode: Reduce docetaxel dose by 20%

Grade 4 Stomatitis/Mucositis:
1st Episode: Stop fluorouracil only, at all subsequent cycles
2nd Episode: Reduce docetaxel dose by 20%

Refer to PI for cisplatin and fluorouracil dose modifications

ADMINISTRATION
IV route

Administration Precautions
Contact of the docetaxel inj w/ plasticized PVC equipment or devices used to prepare sol for infusion is not recommended; store the final docetaxel dilution for infusion in bottles (glass, polypropylene) or plastic bags (polypropylene, polyolefin) and administer through polyethylene-lined administration sets.

Preparation
Requires no prior dilution w/ a diluent and is ready to add to the infusion sol.

Docetaxel Inj Concentrate (20mg/mL):
Do not use the two-vial formulation (inj concentrate and diluent) w/ the one-vial formulation.
Refer to PI for further administration instructions.

STORAGE
20-25°C (68-77°F), (Taxotere) 2-25°C (36-77°F). Multi-use vials are stable for up to 28 days when stored at 2-8°C (36-46°F) after use. Protect from light.
Reconstituted Sol: 0.9% NaCl or D5: Stable at 2-25°C (36-77°F) for 4 hrs or (Taxotere) 6 hrs. (Taxotere) Infusion sol is stable in non-PVC bags up to 48 hrs at 2-8°C (36-46°F).

HOW SUPPLIED
Inj: 10mg/mL [2mL, 8mL, 16mL], (Taxotere) 20mg/mL [1mL, 4mL]

CONTRAINDICATIONS
History of severe hypersensitivity reactions to docetaxel or to other drugs formulated w/ polysorbate 80. Neutrophils <1500 cells/mm^3.

WARNINGS/PRECAUTIONS
Avoid subsequent cycles until neutrophils recover to level >1500 cells/mm^3 and platelets to >100,000 cells/mm^3. Severe fluid retention reported; monitor from the 1st dose for possible exacerbation of preexisting effusions. Acute myeloid leukemia or myelodysplasia may occur in adjuvant therapy (eg, adjuvant therapy in breast cancer). Localized erythema of the extremities w/ edema followed by desquamation reported; adjust dose if severe skin toxicity occurs. Severe neurosensory symptoms (eg, paresthesia, dysesthesia, pain) may develop; adjust dose if symptoms occur and d/c treatment if symptoms persist. Cystoid macular edema (CME) reported; d/c and initiate appropriate treatment if CME is diagnosed, and/or consider alternative non-taxane cancer treatment. Severe asthenia reported. May cause fetal harm. Caution in elderly. Intoxication reported due to alcohol content. Alcohol content of the drug may affect CNS; caution in whom alcohol intake should be avoided or minimized. Alcohol content of the drug may impair physical/mental abilities.

ADVERSE REACTIONS
Infections, neutropenia, anemia, febrile neutropenia, hypersensitivity, thrombocytopenia, neuropathy, dysgeusia, dyspnea, constipation, anorexia, nail disorders, fluid retention, asthenia, pain.

DRUG INTERACTIONS
See Dosing Considerations. Avoid w/ CYP3A4 inhibitors (eg, ketoconazole, clarithromycin, atazanavir); may increase docetaxel exposure. CYP3A4 inducers and substrates may alter metabolism. Protease inhibitors (eg, ritonavir) may increase exposure. Renal insufficiency and renal failure reported w/ concomitant nephrotoxic drugs. Radiation pneumonitis may occur in patients receiving concomitant radiotherapy (rare).

PREGNANCY AND LACTATION
Pregnancy: Category D.
Lactation: Not for use in nursing.

MECHANISM OF ACTION
Antimicrotubule agent; acts by disrupting the microtubular network in cells that is essential for mitotic and interphase cellular functions.

PHARMACOKINETICS
Distribution: V_d=113L; plasma protein binding (94-97%). **Metabolism:** CYP3A4.
Elimination: Urine (6%), feces (75%); $T_{1/2}$=11.1 hrs.

PATIENT CONSIDERATIONS
Assessment: Assess for history of severe hypersensitivity reactions to the drug or other drugs w/ polysorbate 80, preexisting effusion, hepatic impairment, pregnancy/nursing status, and possible drug interactions. Obtain baseline weight, CBC w/ platelets, and differential count. Obtain bilirubin, AST or ALT, and alkaline phosphatase values prior to each cycle of therapy.

Monitoring: Monitor for fluid retention, acute myeloid leukemia, hematologic effects, skin toxicities, exacerbation of effusions, neurosensory symptoms, hepatic impairment, hypersensitivity reactions, asthenia, CME, and other adverse reactions. Monitor weight, CBC w/ platelets, and differential count. Perform a comprehensive ophthalmologic examination in patients w/ impaired vision.

Counseling: Inform about risks and benefits of therapy. Inform that drug may cause fetal harm; advise to avoid pregnancy and to use effective contraceptives. Explain the significance of oral corticosteroid administration to help facilitate compliance; instruct to report if not compliant. Instruct to report signs of hypersensitivity reactions, fluid retention, myalgia, or cutaneous/neurologic reactions. Counsel about side effects that are associated w/ the drug. Explain the significance of routine blood cell counts. Instruct to monitor temperature frequently and to immediately report any occurrence of fever. Explain about the possible side effects of the alcohol content in the drug, including possible side effects on the CNS. Advise patients in whom alcohol should be avoided or minimized to consider the alcohol content of the drug; inform that alcohol could impair their ability to drive or use machines immediately after infusion.

DOXIL — doxorubicin hydrochloride liposome   **Rx**

Class: Anthracycline

> May cause myocardial damage, including CHF, as the total cumulative dose approaches 550mg/m^2; include prior use of other anthracyclines or anthracenediones in total cumulative dose calculations. Risk of cardiomyopathy may be increased at lower cumulative doses w/ prior mediastinal irradiation. Acute infusion-related reactions occurred in patients w/ solid tumors. Serious, life-threatening, and fatal infusion reactions reported.

ADULT DOSAGE
Ovarian Carcinoma

Progressed/Recurred After Platinum-Based Therapy:
50mg/m^2 IV over 60 min every 28 days until disease progression or unacceptable toxicity

AIDS-Related Kaposi's Sarcoma

After Failure of Prior Systemic Chemotherapy or Intolerance to Such Therapy:
20mg/m^2 IV over 60 min every 21 days until disease progression or unacceptable toxicity

Multiple Myeloma

In combination w/ bortezomib in patients who have not previously received bortezomib and have received at least 1 prior therapy

30mg/m^2 IV over 60 min on Day 4 of each 21-day cycle for 8 cycles or until disease progression or unacceptable toxicity

Administer therapy after bortezomib on Day 4 of each cycle

PEDIATRIC DOSAGE
Pediatric use may not have been established

DOSING CONSIDERATIONS
Hepatic Impairment
Serum Bilirubin ≥1.2mg/dL: Reduce dose

Adverse Reactions
Hand-Foot Syndrome (HFS):
Grade 1:
If previous Grade 3 or 4 HFS, delay dose up to 2 weeks, then decrease dose by 25%
Grade 2:
Delay dosing up to 2 weeks or until resolved to Grade 0-1
If resolved to Grade 0-1 w/in 2 weeks, continue treatment at previous dose if no previous Grade 3 or 4 HFS, or decrease dose by 25% if previous Grade 3 or 4 toxicity
D/C if no resolution after 2 weeks
Grade 3 or 4:
Delay dosing up to 2 weeks or until resolved to Grade 0-1, then decrease dose by 25%
D/C if no resolution after 2 weeks

Stomatitis:
Grade 1:
If previous Grade 3 or 4 toxicity, delay dose up to 2 weeks, then decrease by 25%
Grade 2:
Delay dosing up to 2 weeks or until resolved to Grade 0-1
If resolved to Grade 0-1 w/in 2 weeks, resume treatment at previous dose if no previous Grade 3 or 4 stomatitis, or decrease dose by 25% if previous Grade 3 or 4 toxicity
D/C if no resolution after 2 weeks

Grade 3 or 4:
Delay dosing up to 2 weeks or until resolved to Grade 0-1; decrease dose by 25% and return to original dose interval
D/C if no resolution after 2 weeks

Neutropenia/Thrombocytopenia:
Grade 2 or 3:
Delay until ANC ≥1500 and platelet count ≥75,000; resume treatment at previous dose
Grade 4:
Delay until ANC ≥1500 and platelet count ≥75,000; resume at 25% dose reduction or continue previous dose w/ prophylactic granulocyte growth factor

Toxicities When Administered in Combination w/ Bortezomib:
Fever ≥38°C and ANC <1000/mm³: Withhold dose for this cycle if before Day 4; decrease dose by 25% if after Day 4 of previous cycle
On any Day of Administration After Day 1 of Each Cycle:
Platelet Count <25,000/mm³ or Hgb <8g/dL or ANC <500/mm³: Withhold dose for this cycle if before Day 4; decrease dose by 25% if after Day 4 of previous cycle and if bortezomib is reduced for hematologic toxicity
Grade 3 or 4 Nonhematologic Toxicity: Do not dose until recovered to Grade <2, then reduce dose by 25%

Suspected Extravasation:
D/C for burning or stinging sensation or other evidence indicating perivenous infiltration or extravasation
Manage confirmed or suspected extravasation as follows:
1. Do not remove the needle until attempts are made to aspirate extravasated fluid
2. Do not flush the line; avoid applying pressure to the site
3. Apply ice to the site intermittently for 15 min qid for 3 days
4. Elevate extremity if extravasation is in an extremity

ADMINISTRATION
IV route

Do not substitute for doxorubicin HCl inj.
Administer 1st dose at an initial rate of 1mg/min; if no infusion-related adverse reactions are observed, increase infusion rate to complete the administration of the drug over 1 hr.
Do not administer as an undiluted sus or as an IV bolus.
Do not use w/ in-line filters.
Do not rapidly flush the IV line.
Do not mix w/ other drugs.

Preparation
Dilute doses up to 90mg in 250mL of D5 inj prior to administration.
Dilute doses >90mg in 500mL of D5 inj prior to administration.
Refrigerate diluted Doxil at 2-8°C (36-46°F) and administer w/in 24 hrs.

STORAGE
Unopened Vials: 2-8°C (36-46°F). Do not freeze.

HOW SUPPLIED
Inj: 20mg/10mL, 50mg/25mL

CONTRAINDICATIONS
History of severe hypersensitivity reactions, including anaphylaxis, to doxorubicin HCl.

WARNINGS/PRECAUTIONS
Do not substitute for doxorubicin HCl inj. Administer only when potential benefits outweigh the risk in patients w/ a history of cardiovascular disease (CVD). Temporarily stop therapy in the event of an infusion-related reaction until resolution, then resume at a reduced infusion rate; d/c infusion for serious or life-threatening infusion-related reactions. HFS reported; d/c if HFS is severe and debilitating. Secondary oral cancers, primarily squamous cell carcinoma, reported w/ long-term (>1 yr) exposure; malignancies were diagnosed both during treatment and up to 6 yrs after last dose. Examine patients at regular intervals for the presence of oral ulceration or w/ any oral discomfort that may be indicative of secondary oral cancer. May cause fetal harm.

ADVERSE REACTIONS
Asthenia, fatigue, fever, N/V, stomatitis, diarrhea, constipation, anorexia, HFS, rash, neutropenia, thrombocytopenia, anemia.

PREGNANCY AND LACTATION
Pregnancy: Can cause fetal harm.
Lactation: It is not known whether Doxil is present in human milk; not for use in nursing.
Reproductive Potential: May damage spermatozoa and testicular tissue, resulting in possible genetic fetal abnormalities. Females and males w/ female partners of reproductive potential should use effective contraception during and for 6 months after treatment. May cause infertility and result in amenorrhea in females; premature menopause can occur. May result in oligospermia, azoospermia, and permanent loss of fertility in males.

MECHANISM OF ACTION
Anthracycline topoisomerase II inhibitor; suspected to bind DNA and inhibit nucleic acid synthesis.

PHARMACOKINETICS
Absorption: (10mg/m²) C_{max}=4.12mcg/mL, AUC=277mcg/mL•hr. (20mg/m²) C_{max}=8.34mcg/mL, AUC=590mcg/mL•hr. **Distribution:** (10mg/m²) V_d=2.83L/m²; (20mg/m²) V_d=2.72L/m². **Metabolism:** Doxorubicinol (major metabolite). **Elimination:** 1st Phase: $T_{1/2}$=4.7 hrs (10mg/m²), 5.2 hrs (20mg/m²). 2nd Phase: $T_{1/2}$=52.3 hrs (10mg/m²), 55 hrs (20mg/m²).

PATIENT CONSIDERATIONS

Assessment: Assess for drug hypersensitivity, history of CVD, hepatic dysfunction, pregnancy/nursing status. Assess left ventricular cardiac function (eg, multigated acquisition, echocardiogram) prior to initiation of therapy.

Monitoring: Monitor for signs/symptoms of myocardial damage, infusion-related reactions, HFS, secondary oral cancers, and other adverse reactions. Monitor cardiac function.
Counseling: Instruct to contact physician if a new onset of fever, symptoms of an infection, or symptoms of HF develop. Advise about the symptoms of infusion-related reactions and instruct to seek immediate medical attention if any of these symptoms develop. Instruct to notify physician if symptoms of HFS or stomatitis develop. Advise females of reproductive potential of the potential risk to a fetus and to inform physician w/ a known or suspected pregnancy. Advise females and males of reproductive potential to use effective contraception during and for 6 months following treatment, and inform that therapy may cause temporary or permanent infertility. Instruct females not to breastfeed during treatment. Inform that a reddish-orange color may appear in urine and other body fluids.

DOXORUBICIN — doxorubicin hydrochloride   Rx
Class: Anthracycline

> Myocardial damage (eg, acute left ventricular failure) may occur; risk of cardiomyopathy is proportional to the cumulative exposure and is further increased with concomitant cardiotoxic therapy. Assess left ventricular ejection fraction (LVEF) before and regularly during and after treatment. Secondary acute myelogenous leukemia (AML) and myelodysplastic syndrome (MDS) reported at a higher incidence. Extravasation may result in severe local tissue injury and necrosis requiring wide excision of the affected area and skin grafting; immediately terminate the drug and apply ice to the affected area. Severe myelosuppression resulting in serious infection, septic shock, requirement for transfusions, hospitalization, and death may occur.

OTHER BRAND NAMES
Adriamycin

ADULT DOSAGE
Breast Cancer

As a component of multi-agent adjuvant chemotherapy for treatment of women w/ axillary lymph node involvement following resection of primary breast cancer

60mg/m² IV bolus on Day 1 of each 21-day treatment cycle, in combination w/ cyclophosphamide, for a total of 4 cycles

Other Indications

Treatment of acute lymphoblastic/myeloblastic leukemia, Hodgkin/non-Hodgkin lymphoma, and metastatic disease (breast cancer, Wilms' tumor, neuroblastoma, soft tissue/bone sarcoma, ovarian carcinoma, transitional cell bladder carcinoma, thyroid carcinoma, gastric carcinoma, bronchogenic carcinoma)

Single Agent:
60-75mg/m² IV every 21 days

Combination w/ Other Chemotherapy Drugs:
40-75mg/m² IV every 21-28 days

Consider use of the lower dose in the recommended dose range or longer intervals between cycles for heavily pretreated, elderly, or obese patients; cumulative doses above 550mg/m² are associated w/ an increased risk of cardiomyopathy

PEDIATRIC DOSAGE
Breast Cancer

As a component of multi-agent adjuvant chemotherapy for treatment of women w/ axillary lymph node involvement following resection of primary breast cancer

60mg/m² IV bolus on Day 1 of each 21-day treatment cycle, in combination w/ cyclophosphamide, for a total of 4 cycles

Other Indications

Treatment of acute lymphoblastic/myeloblastic leukemia, Hodgkin/non-Hodgkin lymphoma, and metastatic disease (breast cancer, Wilms' tumor, neuroblastoma, soft tissue/bone sarcoma, ovarian carcinoma, transitional cell bladder carcinoma, thyroid carcinoma, gastric carcinoma, bronchogenic carcinoma)

Single Agent:
60-75mg/m² IV every 21 days

Combination w/ Other Chemotherapy Drugs:
40-75mg/m² IV every 21-28 days

Consider use of the lower dose in the recommended dose range or longer intervals between cycles for heavily pretreated or obese patients; cumulative doses above 550mg/m² are associated w/ an increased risk of cardiomyopathy

----

DOSING CONSIDERATIONS
Hepatic Impairment
Serum Bilirubin:
1.2-3mg/dL: Reduce dose by 50%
3.1-5mg/dL: Reduce dose by 75%
<5mg/dL: D/C therapy
Other Important Considerations
Cardiac Impairment: D/C therapy if signs/symptoms of cardiomyopathy develop.
ADMINISTRATION
IV route

Do not admix w/ other drugs

IV Inj
Preparation:
1. Reconstitute w/ 0.9% NaCl inj to obtain a final concentration of 2mg/mL as follows:
5mL 0.9% NaCl inj: To reconstitute 10mg doxorubicin HCl vial
10mL 0.9% NaCl inj: To reconstitute 20mg doxorubicin HCl vial
25mL 0.9% NaCl inj: To reconstitute 50mg doxorubicin HCl vial
75mL 0.9% NaCl inj: To reconstitute 150mg doxorubicin HCl vial
2. Gently shake vial until the contents have dissolved

Administration:
1. Administer through a central IV line or a secure and free-flowing peripheral venous line containing 0.9% NaCl inj, 0.45% NaCl inj, or D5 inj

2. Administer over 3-10 min; decrease rate of administration if erythematous streaking along the vein proximal to the site of infusion or facial flushing occurs

Continuous IV Infusion

Preparation:
Dilute sol or reconstituted sol in 0.9% NaCl inj or D5 inj

Administration:
1. Infuse through a central catheter only; decrease rate of administration if erythematous streaking along the vein proximal to the site of infusion or facial flushing occurs
2. Protect from light from preparation for infusion until completion of infusion

Management of Suspected Extravasation

D/C therapy if burning/stinging sensation or other evidence indicating perivenous infiltration or extravasation occurs

Manage Confirmed/Suspected Extravasation as Follows:
1. Do not remove needle until attempts are made to aspirate extravasated fluid
2. Do not flush the line
3. Avoid applying pressure to the site
4. Apply ice to the site immediately for 15 min qid for 3 days
5. If extravasation is in an extremity, elevate the extremity
6. Consider administration of dexrazoxane in adults

Incompatibilities

1. Precipitate may form if mixed w/ heparin or fluorouracil
2. Avoid contact w/ alkaline sol as it can lead to hydrolysis of doxorubicin HCl

Proper Handling Procedures

Treat accidental contact w/ skin or eyes immediately by copious lavage w/ water, soap and water, or sodium bicarbonate sol and seek medical attention; do not abrade skin by using a scrub brush

STORAGE

(Sol) 2-8°C (36-46°F). Protect from light. Storage under refrigerated conditions may result in the formation of a gelled product; place gelled product at 15-30°C (59-86°F) for 2-4 hrs to return the product to a slightly viscous, mobile sol, (Powder) 15-30°C (59-86°F). Protect from light.

HOW SUPPLIED

Inj: (Powder) 10mg, 20mg, 50mg, 150mg; (Sol) 2mg/mL [5mL, 10mL, 25mL, 75mL, 100mL]

CONTRAINDICATIONS

Severe myocardial insufficiency, recent (occurring w/in the past 4-6 weeks) myocardial infarction (MI), severe persistent drug-induced myelosuppression, severe hepatic impairment (Child-Pugh Class C or serum bilirubin level >5mg/dL), severe hypersensitivity reaction to doxorubicin hydrochloride (eg, anaphylaxis).

WARNINGS/PRECAUTIONS

Cumulative doses >550mg/m^2 are associated with an increased risk of cardiomyopathy; include prior doses of other anthracyclines or anthracenediones in total cumulative dosage calculations. Cardiomyopathy may develop during treatment or up to several years after completion of treatment. Additive or potentially synergistic increase in the risk of cardiomyopathy in patients who have received radiotherapy to the mediastinum. Pericarditis/myocarditis reported. Consider the use of dexrazoxane to reduce the incidence and severity of cardiomyopathy due to therapy in patients who have received a cumulative dose of 300mg/m^2 and who will continue to receive therapy. Arrhythmias (eg, tachyarrhythmias, bradycardia) and ECG changes may occur. May induce tumor lysis syndrome in patients with rapidly growing tumors. May increase radiation-induced toxicity to the myocardium, mucosa, skin, and liver. Radiation recall (eg, cutaneous and pulmonary toxicity) may occur in patients who receive treatment after prior radiation therapy. May cause fetal harm. May damage spermatozoa and testicular tissue, resulting in possible genetic fetal abnormalities. Use highly effective contraception during treatment and for 6 months after treatment. May cause infertility and result in amenorrhea in females of reproductive potential. Premature menopause may occur; recovery of menses and ovulation is related to age at treatment. May result in oligospermia, azoospermia, and permanent loss of fertility. Pediatric patients are at risk for developing late cardiovascular (CV) dysfunction. May contribute to prepubertal growth failure and gonadal impairment in pediatric patients.

ADVERSE REACTIONS

Myocardial damage, secondary AML/MDS, myelosuppression, extravasation, tissue necrosis, alopecia, vomiting.

DRUG INTERACTIONS

See Boxed Warning. Increased levels and clinical effect with inhibitors of CYP3A4, CYP2D6, and/or P-glycoprotein (P-gp) (eg, verapamil); avoid concurrent use. Inducers of CYP3A4 (eg, phenobarbital, phenytoin, St. John's wort) and P-gp inducers may decrease levels; avoid concurrent use. Increased risk of cardiac dysfunction with trastuzumab; avoid concurrent use. Paclitaxel, when given prior to therapy, increases the levels of doxorubicin and its metabolites; administer therapy prior to paclitaxel if used concomitantly. Do not administer dexrazoxane as a cardioprotectant at the initiation of doxorubicin-containing chemotherapy regimens. May potentiate 6-mercaptopurine-induced hepatotoxicity.

PREGNANCY AND LACTATION

Category D, not for use in nursing.

MECHANISM OF ACTION

Anthracycline; thought to be related to nucleotide base intercalation and cell membrane lipid binding activities of the drug. Intercalation inhibits nucleotide replication and action of DNA and RNA polymerases. The interaction with topoisomerase II to form DNA-cleavable complexes appears to be an important mechanism of doxorubicin cytocidal activity.

PHARMACOKINETICS

Distribution: V_d=809-1214L/m^2; plasma protein binding (75%); found in breast milk. **Metabolism:** Enzymatic reduction; doxorubicinol (major metabolite). **Elimination:** Bile (40%), urine (5-12%, <3% doxorubicinol); T$_{1/2}$=20-48 hrs.

PATIENT CONSIDERATIONS

Assessment: Assess for severe myocardial insufficiency, recent MI, hepatic impairment, hypersensitivity to the drug, obesity, any other conditions where treatment is contraindicated or cautioned, pregnancy/nursing status, and possible drug interactions. Obtain baseline blood counts and LFTs. Assess LVEF and left ventricular cardiac function (eg, multigated acquisition, echocardiogram).

Monitoring: Monitor for signs/symptoms of cardiomyopathy, arrhythmias, AML, MDS, extravasation, tissue necrosis, complications due to myelosuppression, tumor lysis syndrome, radiation sensitization, radiation recall, and other adverse reactions. Perform long-term periodic CV monitoring in pediatric patients. Monitor LVEF and LFTs. Evaluate blood uric acid levels, K$^+$, Ca^{2+}, phosphate, and creatinine after initial treatment. Assess left ventricular cardiac function during treatment and after treatment; increase frequency of assessments as the cumulative dose exceeds 300mg/m^2.

Counseling: Inform of the risks and benefits of therapy. Advise to contact physician for symptoms of heart failure during or after treatment, new onset fever, or symptoms of infection. Inform about an increased risk of treatment-related leukemia. Inform that therapy may cause fetal harm when administered during pregnancy; instruct to contact physician if patient becomes pregnant, or if pregnancy is suspected, while on therapy. Advise females of reproductive potential and males with female sexual partners of reproductive potential to use effective contraception during treatment and for 6 months after treatment. Inform that therapy may cause premature menopause in females and loss of fertility in males. Instruct to d/c nursing while receiving therapy. Inform that N/V, diarrhea, mouth/oral pain, and sores may occur; advise to contact physician if any severe symptoms that prevent patient from eating and drinking develop. Inform that alopecia may develop, and urine may appear red for 1-2 days after administration.

DUOPA — carbidopa/levodopa   Rx

Class: Dopa-decarboxylase inhibitor/dopamine precursor

ADULT DOSAGE	PEDIATRIC DOSAGE
Parkinson's Disease	Pediatric use may not have been established

ADULT DOSAGE

Parkinson's Disease

Prior to initiation of therapy, convert patient from all other forms of levodopa to oral immediate-release (IR) carbidopa-levodopa (1:4 ratio)

Initial:

Step 1: Calculate/Administer Morning Dose for Day 1:
a. Determine total amount of levodopa (in mg) in the 1st dose of oral IR carbidopa-levodopa that was taken on the previous day
b. Convert the levodopa dose from mg to mL by multiplying the oral dose by 0.8 and dividing by 20mg/mL (Morning Dose)
c. Add 3mL to the Morning Dose to prime the intestinal tube (Total Morning Dose)
d. Administer Total Morning Dose over 10-30 min

Step 2: Calculate/Administer Continuous Dose for Day 1:
a. Determine amount of oral IR levodopa the patient received from the oral IR carbidopa-levodopa doses throughout the previous day (16 waking hrs) in mg; do not include doses taken at night when calculating the levodopa amount
b. Subtract 1st oral levodopa dose taken by the patient on the previous day (determined in Step 1 (a)) from total oral levodopa dose (determined in Step 2 (a)) and divide the result by 20mg/mL to get the Continuous Dose (in mL) over 16 hrs
c. The hourly infusion rate (mL/hr) is obtained by dividing the Continuous Dose by 16 (hrs)
d. If persistent/numerous "Off" periods occur during the 16-hr infusion, consider increasing the Continuous Dose or using the Extra Dose function. If dyskinesia/levodopa-related adverse reactions occur, consider decreasing the Continuous Dose or stopping infusion until adverse reactions subside

Titrate:
Morning Dose:
Inadequate Response w/in 1 hr of Morning Dose on Preceding Day:
Morning Dose on Preceding Day
≤6mL: Increase Morning Dose by 1 mL

PEDIATRIC DOSAGE

Pediatric use may not have been established

Morning Dose on Preceding Day
>6mL: Increase Morning Dose by 2mL
Exclude the 3mL to prime tube
Continuous Dose Adjustment:
Consider increasing dose based on clinical response and on the number/volume of Extra Doses that was needed for the previous day
Max: 2g of levodopa component (eg, 1 cassette/day) over 16 hrs
Extra Doses:
Initial: 1mL (20mg of levodopa)
Titrate: Increase in 0.2mL increments
Limit frequency to 1 extra dose q2h

- -

DOSING CONSIDERATIONS
Adverse Reactions
Dyskinesia/Therapy-Related Adverse Reactions on Preceding Day:
Morning Dose: If patient experienced dyskinesias or therapy-related adverse reactions w/in 1 hr of Morning Dose on preceding day, then decrease morning dose by 1mL
Continuous Dose:
Troublesome Adverse Reactions Lasting for a Period of ≥1 hr: Decrease dose by 0.3mL/hr
Troublesome Adverse Reactions Lasting for 2 or More Periods of ≥1 hr: Decrease dose by 0.6mL/hr
Discontinuation
Avoid sudden discontinuation/rapid dose reduction; if patients need to d/c therapy, taper dose or switch to oral IR carbidopa-levodopa tabs.
When using a PEG-J tube, may d/c by withdrawing tube and letting the stoma heal.
ADMINISTRATION
Naso-jejunal/PEG-J route
- Bring to room temperature before administration; 20 min prior to use, take 1 cassette out of the refrigerator/carton.
- Deliver as 16-hr infusion either through a naso-jejunal tube (short-term administration) or through a PEG-J tube (long-term administration).
- Do not use cassettes for longer than 16 hrs; do not reuse an opened cassette.
- At the end of daily infusion, disconnect PEG-J tube from the pump, flush w/ room temperature potable water using a syringe, and take night-time dose of oral IR carbidopa-levodopa.
- Cassettes are specifically designed to be connected to the CADD-Legacy 1400 pump.
Morning of PEG-J Procedure
- Ensure patients take their oral Parkinson's disease medications.
Refer to PI for tubing sets recommendations for long-term and short-term administration.
STORAGE
-20°C (-4°F). Thaw at 2-8°C (36-46°F) prior to dispensing; refer to PI for thawing instructions. Protect from light.
HOW SUPPLIED
Sus: (Carbidopa/Levodopa) (4.63mg/20mg)/mL [100mL]
CONTRAINDICATIONS
Patients who are currently taking a nonselective MAOI (eg, phenelzine, tranylcypromine) or who have recently (w/in 2 weeks) taken a nonselective MAOI.
WARNINGS/PRECAUTIONS
GI complications may occur and may result in serious outcomes (eg, need for surgery, death). Orthostatic hypotension reported; monitor especially after starting or increasing dose. Hallucinations, psychosis, and confusion reported; hallucinations may be responsive to a dose reduction of levodopa. Do not use in patients w/ a major psychotic disorder. Intense urges to gamble, increased sexual urges, intense urges to spend money, binge or compulsive eating, and/or other intense urges, and the inability to control these urges, may occur; consider dose reduction or discontinuation if such urges develop. Depression reported. A symptom complex resembling neuroleptic malignant syndrome (hyperpyrexia and confusion) reported in association w/ rapid dose reduction, withdrawal of, or changes in dopaminergic therapy; avoid sudden discontinuation/rapid dose reduction and taper dose if discontinuing therapy. May cause or exacerbate dyskinesias; may require dose reduction of therapy or other medications used to treat Parkinson's disease. Polyneuropathy reported; monitor periodically for signs of neuropathy after starting therapy, especially in patients w/ preexisting neuropathy and in patients taking medications or those who have medical conditions associated w/ neuropathy. MI and arrhythmia reported; monitor for symptoms, especially those w/ a history of MI or cardiac arrhythmias. Perform periodic skin examinations to monitor for melanoma. May increase risk for elevated BUN and CPK. May increase levels of catecholamines and metabolites in plasma and urine, giving false-positive results suggesting the diagnosis of pheochromocytoma. May cause increased IOP in patients w/ glaucoma.
Levodopa: Falling asleep during activities of daily living and somnolence reported; consider discontinuation if significant daytime sleepiness or episodes of falling asleep during activities that require active participation occur.
ADVERSE REACTIONS
Complication of device insertion, nausea, depression, peripheral edema, HTN, URTI, oropharyngeal pain, incision-site erythema, atelectasis.

DRUG INTERACTIONS
See Contraindications. Selective MAO-B inhibitors (eg, rasagiline, selegiline) may be associated w/ orthostatic hypotension; monitor patients. Antihypertensive medications may cause symptomatic postural hypotension; may need a dose reduction of antihypertensive medication after starting or increasing the dose of Duopa. Iron salts or multivitamins containing iron salts may form chelates and may reduce bioavailability; monitor for worsening Parkinson's symptoms. **Levodopa:** Caution w/ concomitant use of sedating medications; may increase the risk for somnolence. Dopamine D2 receptor antagonists (eg, phenothiazines, butyrophenones, risperidone, metoclopramide, papaverine) and isoniazid may reduce the effectiveness of levodopa; monitor for worsening Parkinson's symptoms. Absorption may be decreased in patients on a high-protein diet.
PREGNANCY AND LACTATION
Pregnancy: Category C.
Lactation: Caution in nursing.
MECHANISM OF ACTION
Dopa-decarboxylase inhibitor/dopamine precursor. **Carbidopa:** Inhibits decarboxylation of peripheral levodopa, making more levodopa available for delivery to the brain. **Levodopa:** Crosses blood-brain barrier and presumably is converted to dopamine in the brain.
PHARMACOKINETICS
Absorption: Levodopa: Bioavailability (97%); T_{max}=2.5 hrs. **Distribution:** Carbidopa: Plasma protein binding (36%). Levodopa: Plasma protein binding (10-30%); crosses the placenta; found in breast milk. **Metabolism:** Carbidopa: α-methyl-3-methoxy-4-hydroxyphenylpropionic acid and α-methyl-3,4-dihydroxyphenylpropionic acid (main metabolites). Levodopa: Decarboxylation, O-methylation, transamination, and oxidation. **Elimination:** Carbidopa: Urine (30% unchanged); $T_{1/2}$=2 hrs. Levodopa: $T_{1/2}$=1.5 hrs (in the presence of carbidopa).

PATIENT CONSIDERATIONS
Assessment: Assess for major psychotic disorder, risk factors that may increase risk for somnolence (eg, presence of sleep disorders), peripheral neuropathy, history of MI or cardiac arrhythmias, glaucoma, pregnancy/nursing status, and possible drug interactions.
Monitoring: Monitor for GI complications, drowsiness or falling asleep during activities of daily living, orthostatic hypotension, hallucinations/psychosis/confusion, impulse control/compulsive behaviors, depression w/ suicidal tendencies, dyskinesias, neuropathy, ischemic heart disease, arrhythmia, and other adverse reactions. Monitor for hyperpyrexia and confusion if sudden discontinuation or rapid dose reduction occurs. Perform periodic skin examinations to monitor for melanoma. Monitor IOP in patients w/ glaucoma after starting therapy.
Counseling: Inform of risks and benefits of therapy. Instruct to inform physician of any previous surgery in the upper part of the abdomen. Advise that foods that are high in protein may reduce the effectiveness of therapy. Instruct to contact physician if experiencing symptoms of GI complications, depression or worsening of depression, suicidal thoughts, hallucinations, abnormal thinking, psychotic behavior, confusion, new/increased gambling urges, sexual urges, uncontrolled spending, binge/compulsive eating, or other urges, or if any symptoms or features suggesting neuropathy develop. Inform of the potential sedating effects caused by therapy. Advise not to drive a car, operate machinery, or engage in other potentially dangerous activities until effects of therapy are known. Advise of possible additive effects when taking other sedating medications, alcohol, or other CNS depressants in combination w/ therapy. Inform that syncope and hypotension w/ or w/o symptoms may develop; caution against standing rapidly after sitting or lying down, especially if patient has been doing so for prolonged periods and especially at the initiation of treatment. Advise to contact physician before stopping therapy and to notify physician if withdrawal symptoms develop. Inform that therapy may cause or exacerbate preexisting dyskinesia. Advise to have a regular skin examination by a qualified healthcare provider.

DYSPORT — abobotulinumtoxinA   Rx
Class: Acetylcholine release inhibitor

> **Distant spread of toxin effects (eg, asthenia, generalized muscle weakness, diplopia) reported hrs to weeks after inj. Swallowing and breathing difficulties can be life threatening and there have been reports of death. Risk of symptoms is greatest in children treated for spasticity but can also occur in adults. In unapproved uses and approved indications, cases of spread of effect have been reported at doses comparable to or lower than the max recommended total dose.**

ADULT DOSAGE
Cervical Dystonia
Initial: 500 U IM as a divided dose among affected muscles in patients w/ or w/o a history of prior treatment w/ botulinum toxin
Titrate: Adjustments can be made in 250 U steps according to response; total dose administered in a single treatment should be between 250 U and 1000 U
Max: 1000 U
Retreatment, if needed, should not occur in intervals of <12 weeks

PEDIATRIC DOSAGE
Lower Limb Spasticity
≥2 Years:
Dosing by Muscle:
Gastrocnemius: 6-9 U/kg (≤4 inj)
Soleus: 4-6 U/kg (≤2 inj)
Total: 10-15 U/kg divided across both muscles (≤6 inj)
Individual doses to be injected can be used w/in range mentioned w/o exceeding 15 U/kg total dose for unilateral inj or 30 U/kg for bilateral inj or 1000 U, whichever is lower

Glabellar Lines

Temporary improvement in the appearance of moderate to severe glabellar lines associated w/ procerus and corrugator muscle activity

<65 Years:
Total of 50 U IM in 5 equal aliquots of 10 U each

Inject into each of 5 sites: 2 in each corrugator muscle, and 1 in the procerus muscle

Administer no more frequently than every 3 months

When used for retreatment, reconstitute and inject using the same techniques as initial treatment

Spasticity

To decrease the severity of increased muscle tone in elbow flexors, wrist flexors, and finger flexors

Dosing by Muscle:
Flexor Carpi Radialis: 100-200 U (1-2 inj)
Flexor Carpi Ulnaris: 100-200 U (1-2 inj)
Flexor Digitorum Profundus: 100-200 U (1-2 inj)
Flexor Digitorum Superficialis: 100-200 U (1-2 inj)
Brachialis: 200-400 U (1-2 inj)
Brachioradialis: 100-200 U (1-2 inj)
Biceps Brachii: 200-400 U (1-2 inj)
Pronator Teres: 100-200 U (1 inj)

Although actual location of inj sites can be determined by palpation, use of inj guiding technique (eg, electromyography, electrical stimulation) is recommended

Generally, no more than 1mL should be administered at any single inj site

Repeat treatment should be administered when the effect of a previous inj has diminished, but no sooner than 12 weeks after the previous inj

Although actual location of inj sites can be determined by palpation, use of inj guiding technique is recommended

ADMINISTRATION
IM route

- Supplied as a single-use vial.
- Once reconstituted, store in the original container at 2-8°C (36-46°F); do not freeze. Protect from light. Use w/in 24 hrs.

Cervical Dystonia
Preparation and Administration:
Reconstitute each 500 U vial w/ 1mL of preservative-free 0.9% NaCl inj to yield a sol of 50 U/0.1mL.
Reconstitute each 300 U vial w/ 0.6 mL of preservative-free 0.9% NaCl inj to yield a sol equivalent to 50 U/0.1mL.

Glabellar Lines
Preparation and Administration:
Reconstitute each 300 U vial w/ 2.5mL of preservative-free 0.9% NaCl inj prior to inj; concentration of resulting sol will be 10 U/0.08mL (12 U/0.1mL) to be delivered in 5 equally divided aliquots of 0.08mL each.
AbobotulinumtoxinA may also be reconstituted w/ 1.5mL of preservative-free 0.9% NaCl inj for a sol of 10 U/0.05mL (20 U/0.1mL) to be delivered in 5 equally divided aliquots of 0.05mL each.
Use a 30-gauge needle when administering.

Inj Technique:
In order to reduce the complication of ptosis, the following steps should be taken:
1. Avoid inj near the levator palpebrae superioris, particularly in patients w/ larger brow depressor complexes.
2. Medial corrugator inj should be placed at least 1cm above the bony supraorbital ridge.
3. Ensure the injected volume/dose is accurate and where feasible kept to a minimum.
4. Do not inject toxin closer than 1cm above the central eyebrow.

To inject abobotulinumtoxinA, advance the needle through the skin into the underlying muscle while applying finger pressure on superior medial orbital rim.

Upper Limb Spasticity
Preparation and Administration:
- Reconstitute to a recommended concentration of 100 U/mL or 200 U/mL w/ preservative-free 0.9% NaCl inj.

Lower Limb Spasticity
Preparation and Administration:
- Reconstitute 500 U vial w/ 2.5mL of preservative-free 0.9% NaCl.
- Reconstitute 500 U vial w/ 1.5mL of preservative-free 0.9% NaCl.
- Resulting sol will be 20 U/0.1 mL; further dilution may be required to achieve the final volume for inj.
- No more than 0.5mL should be administered in any single inj site.
- Use immediately after reconstitution in the syringe.
Refer to PI for more detailed information on preparation/administration.

STORAGE
2-8°C (36-46°F). Protect from light.

HOW SUPPLIED
Inj: 300 U, 500 U

CONTRAINDICATIONS
Allergy to cow's milk protein, infection at the proposed inj site(s), known hypersensitivity to any botulinum toxin preparation or to any of the components in the formulation.

WARNINGS/PRECAUTIONS
Not interchangeable w/ other botulinum toxin products; cannot be compared or converted into U of any other botulinum toxin products. May weaken neck muscles that serve as accessory muscles of ventilation. May require immediate medical attention if problems w/ swallowing, speech, or respiratory disorders develop. Caution w/ surgical alterations to facial anatomy, excessive weakness or atrophy in the target muscle(s), marked facial asymmetry, inflammation at the inj site(s), ptosis, excessive dermatochalasis, deep dermal scarring, thick sebaceous skin, or the inability to substantially lessen glabellar lines by physically spreading them apart. Increased incidence of eyelid ptosis w/ higher doses. Closely monitor patients w/ peripheral motor neuropathic diseases, amyotrophic lateral sclerosis, neuromuscular junction disorders (eg, myasthenia gravis or Lambert-Eaton syndrome); may increase risk of clinically significant effects including severe dysphagia and respiratory compromise from typical doses. Contains albumin; carries remote risk of transmitting viral diseases and Creutzfeldt-Jakob disease. Caution in elderly.

ADVERSE REACTIONS
Cervical Dystonia: Muscular weakness, dysphagia, dry mouth, inj-site discomfort, fatigue, headache, musculoskeletal pain, dysphonia, inj-site pain, eye disorders.
Glabellar Lines: Nasopharyngitis, headache, inj-site pain, inj-site reaction, URTI, eyelid edema, eyelid ptosis, sinusitis, nausea, blood present in urine.
Upper Limb Spasticity: UTI, nasopharyngitis, muscular weakness, musculoskeletal pain, dizziness, fall, depression.
Lower Limb Spasticity: URTI, nasopharyngitis, influenza, pharyngitis, cough, pyrexia.

DRUG INTERACTIONS
Potentiation of toxin effect may occur w/ aminoglycosides or w/ other agents interfering w/ neuromuscular transmission (eg, curare-like agents); monitor closely. Use of anticholinergic drugs after administration may potentiate systemic anticholinergic effects. Excessive weakness may be exacerbated if another botulinum toxin is administered before effects resolve from the previous botulinum toxin inj administration. Use of a muscle relaxant before/after administration may exaggerate excessive weakness.

PREGNANCY AND LACTATION
Pregnancy: Produced embryo-fetal toxicity in relation to maternal toxicity in animal studies; should only be used during pregnancy if the potential benefit justifies the potential risk to the fetus.
Lactation: There are no data on the presence of abobotulinumtoxinA in human or animal milk, the effects on the breastfed child, or the effects on milk production; caution in nursing.
Reproductive Potential: Produced adverse effects on mating behavior and fertility in animal studies.

MECHANISM OF ACTION
Acetylcholine release inhibitor; inhibits release of acetylcholine from peripheral cholinergic nerve endings. Binds to specific surface receptors on nerve endings and internalizes by receptor mediated endocytosis, leading to intracellular blockage of neurotransmitter exocytosis into the neuromuscular junction.

PATIENT CONSIDERATIONS
Assessment: Assess for allergy to cow's milk protein, infection/inflammation at proposed inj site(s), preexisting swallowing/breathing difficulties, surgical facial alterations, excessive weakness or atrophy in the target muscle(s), marked facial asymmetry, ptosis, excessive dermatochalasis, deep dermal scarring, thick sebaceous skin, inability to substantially lessen glabellar lines by physically spreading them apart, preexisting neuromuscular disorders, pregnancy/nursing status, and possible drug interactions.

Monitoring: Monitor for spread of the toxin effects, weakening of neck muscles, and swallowing/speech/respiratory disorders. Monitor patients w/ peripheral motor neuropathic diseases, amyotrophic lateral sclerosis, or neuromuscular junction disorders.

Counseling: Advise to notify physician if any unusual symptoms develop (eg, difficulty w/ swallowing, speaking, or breathing) or if any known symptom persists or worsens. Instruct to avoid driving or engaging in potentially hazardous activities if loss of strength, muscle weakness, blurred vision, or drooping eyelids occur.

EDURANT — rilpivirine

Rx

Class: Non-nucleoside reverse transcriptase inhibitor (NNRTI)

ADULT DOSAGE	PEDIATRIC DOSAGE
HIV-1 Infection	**HIV-1 Infection**
In combination w/ other antiretrovirals, in antiretroviral treatment-naive patients w/ HIV-1 RNA ≤100,000 copies/mL at the start of therapy	In combination w/ other antiretrovirals, in antiretroviral treatment-naive patients w/ HIV-1 RNA ≤100,000 copies/mL at the start of therapy
25mg qd	**≥12 Years:**
	≥35kg:
	25mg qd

DOSING CONSIDERATIONS
Concomitant Medications
W/ Rifabutin: Increase Edurant dose to 50mg qd; when coadministration is stopped, decrease dose to 25mg qd

ADMINISTRATION
Oral route
Take w/ a meal.

STORAGE
25°C (77°F); excursions permitted to 15-30°C (59-86°F). Protect from light.

HOW SUPPLIED
Tab: 25mg

CONTRAINDICATIONS
Concomitant use w/ carbamazepine, oxcarbazepine, phenobarbital, phenytoin, rifampin, rifapentine, proton pump inhibitors (eg, esomeprazole, lansoprazole, omeprazole, pantoprazole, rabeprazole), systemic dexamethasone (more than a single dose), and St. John's wort.

WARNINGS/PRECAUTIONS
Severe skin and hypersensitivity reactions reported, including cases of drug reaction w/ eosinophilia and systemic symptoms; d/c immediately and initiate appropriate therapy if signs/symptoms develop. Depressive disorders reported; immediate medical evaluation is recommended if severe depressive symptoms occur. Hepatotoxicity reported; underlying hepatitis B or C, or marked elevation in transaminases prior to treatment may increase risk for worsening or development of transaminase elevations. Consider liver enzyme monitoring in patients w/o preexisting hepatic dysfunction or other risk factors. Immune reconstitution syndrome, redistribution/accumulation of body fat, and autoimmune disorders (eg, Graves' disease, polymyositis, Guillain-Barre syndrome) in the setting of immune reconstitution reported. Caution w/ severe renal impairment or ESRD; monitor for adverse effects. Caution in elderly.

ADVERSE REACTIONS
Lab abnormalities (increased SrCr, AST/ALT, total bilirubin, total cholesterol, LDL), depressive disorders, insomnia, headache, rash, somnolence, N/V, dizziness, abdominal pain.

DRUG INTERACTIONS
See Dosing Considerations and Contraindications. Caution w/ drugs that may reduce exposure. Coadministration w/ CYP3A inducers or drugs that increase gastric pH may result in decreased levels, loss of virologic response, and possible resistance to rilpivirine or to the class of non-nucleoside reverse transcriptase inhibitors (NNRTIs). CYP3A inhibitors may increase levels. Not recommended w/ delavirdine and other NNRTIs (eg, efavirenz, etravirine, nevirapine). Concomitant didanosine should be given on an empty stomach and at least 2 hrs before or at least 4 hrs after therapy. Darunavir/ritonavir (RTV), lopinavir/RTV, unboosted protease inhibitors (PIs) or other boosted PIs may increase levels. Azole antifungals may increase levels; monitor for breakthrough fungal infections w/ azole antifungals. May decrease ketoconazole levels. Clarithromycin, erythromycin, or telithromycin may increase levels; consider alternatives (eg, azithromycin) when possible. Rifabutin may decrease levels. Antacids and H₂-receptor antagonists may significantly decrease levels. Administer antacids either at least 2 hrs before or at least 4 hrs after therapy. Administer H₂-receptor antagonists at least 12 hrs before or at least 4 hrs after therapy. Clinical monitoring is recommended w/ methadone as methadone maintenance therapy may need to be adjusted in some patients. Caution w/ drugs that have a known risk of torsades de pointes.

PREGNANCY AND LACTATION
Pregnancy: Category B. Physicians are encouraged to register patients in the Antiretroviral Pregnancy Registry.
Lactation: Mothers should be instructed not to breastfeed due to potential for HIV-1 transmission.

MECHANISM OF ACTION
NNRTI; inhibits HIV-1 replication by noncompetitive inhibition of HIV-1 reverse transcriptase.

PHARMACOKINETICS
Absorption: AUC_{24h}=2235ng•hr/mL, T_{max}=4-5 hrs. **Distribution:** Plasma protein binding (approx 99.7%). **Metabolism:** Liver via CYP3A oxidation. **Elimination:** Feces (85%, 25% unchanged), urine (6.1%, <1% unchanged); $T_{1/2}$=approx 50 hrs.

PATIENT CONSIDERATIONS
Assessment: Assess for severe renal impairment or ESRD, underlying hepatic disease, marked transaminase elevations, pregnancy/nursing status, and possible drug interactions. Perform appropriate lab testing in patients w/ underlying hepatic disease or w/ marked transaminase elevations.

Monitoring: Monitor for severe skin and hypersensitivity reactions, depressive disorders, immune reconstitution syndrome, autoimmune disorders, fat redistribution/accumulation, hepatotoxicity, and other adverse reactions.

Counseling: Inform that product is not a cure for HIV infection; advise that continuous therapy is necessary to control HIV infection and decrease HIV-related illnesses. Advise to continue to practice safer sex and to use latex or polyurethane condoms. Instruct never to reuse or share needles. Inform mothers to avoid nursing to reduce risk of transmission of HIV to their baby. Advise to take medication ud. Advise not to alter the dose or d/c therapy w/o consulting physician. If a dose is missed w/in 12 hrs of the time it is usually taken, instruct to take as soon as possible w/ a meal and then to take the next dose at the regular scheduled time. If dose is missed by >12 hrs of the time it is usually taken, instruct not to take the missed dose, but resume the usual dosing schedule. Advise to report to physician the use of any other prescription/nonprescription or herbal products (eg, St. John's wort). Inform of the signs/symptoms of severe skin and hypersensitivity reactions and instruct to immediately stop taking therapy and seek medical attention if a rash develops associated w/ such symptoms. Inform patients that lab tests will be performed and appropriate therapy will be initiated if severe rash occurs. Instruct to seek medical evaluation if depressive symptoms are experienced. Inform that hepatotoxicity has been reported and redistribution/accumulation of body fat may occur.

EGRIFTA — tesamorelin

Rx

Class: Growth hormone (GH)-releasing factor

ADULT DOSAGE	PEDIATRIC DOSAGE
Lipodystrophy	Pediatric use may not have been established
Reduction of Excess Abdominal Fat in HIV-Infected Patients:	
2mg SQ in the abdomen qd	

ADMINISTRATION
SQ route
Rotate inj sites to different areas of the abdomen
Do not inject into scar tissue, bruises, or the navel
Administer immediately following reconstitution

Reconstitution
Two vials of tesamorelin must be reconstituted w/ the diluent provided
1. Reconstitute the first vial w/ 2.2mL of diluent
2. Mix by rolling the vial gently in hands for 30 sec; do not shake
3. Reconstitute the second vial w/ the entire sol from the first vial
4. Mix by rolling the vial gently in hands for 30 sec; do not shake

STORAGE
Unreconstituted: 2-8°C (36-46°F). Reconstituted: Do not freeze or refrigerate. Diluent/Syringes/Needles: 20-25°C (68-77°F). Protect from light. Keep in the original box until use.

HOW SUPPLIED
Inj: 1mg

CONTRAINDICATIONS
Pregnancy, newly diagnosed or recurrent active malignancy, disruption of hypothalamic-pituitary axis due to hypophysectomy, hypopituitarism, pituitary tumor/surgery, head irradiation or head trauma, known hypersensitivity to tesamorelin and/or mannitol (an excipient).

WARNINGS/PRECAUTIONS
Carefully consider whether to continue treatment in patients who do not show clear efficacy response. Not indicated for weight loss management (weight neutral effect). Initiate therapy after careful evaluation of the potential benefit of treatment for patients with history of nonmalignant neoplasms or history of treated and stable malignancies. Carefully consider the increased background risk of malignancies in HIV-positive patients before initiation of therapy. Stimulates growth hormone (GH) production and increases serum insulin growth factor-1 (IGF-1); monitor IGF-1 levels closely and consider discontinuation of therapy in patients with persistent elevations of IGF-1 levels (eg, >3 standard deviation scores), particularly if the efficacy response is not robust. Fluid retention may occur. May cause glucose intolerance and increase the risk for developing diabetes. Hypersensitivity reactions may occur; d/c treatment immediately when suspected. May cause inj-site reactions. Consider discontinuation in critically ill patients; increased mortality in patients with acute critical illness due to complications following open heart surgery, abdominal surgery, or multiple accidental trauma, or those with acute respiratory failure.

ADVERSE REACTIONS
Arthralgia, pain in extremity, peripheral edema, inj-site reactions (eg, erythema, pruritus, pain), myalgia, paresthesia, hypoesthesia, nausea, rash.

DRUG INTERACTIONS
May modulate CYP450 mediated antipyrine clearance; monitor carefully in combination with other drugs known to be metabolized by CYP450 liver enzymes. May require an increase in maintenance or stress doses of glucocorticoids following initiation of therapy, particularly in patients treated with cortisone acetate and prednisone.

PREGNANCY AND LACTATION
Category X, not for use in nursing.

MECHANISM OF ACTION
Human GH-releasing factor synthetic analogue; acts on pituitary somatotroph cells to stimulate the synthesis and pulsatile release of endogenous GH, which is both anabolic and lipolytic. GH exerts its effects by interacting with specific

receptors on a variety of target cells, including chondrocytes, osteoblasts, myocytes, hepatocytes, and adipocytes, resulting in a host of pharmacodynamic effects.

PHARMACOKINETICS
Absorption: Absolute bioavailability (<4%); AUC=852.8pg•hr/mL, C_{max}=2822.3pg/mL, T_{max}=0.15 hr. **Distribution:** V_d=10.5L/kg. **Elimination:** $T_{1/2}$=38 min (14 consecutive days of administration).

PATIENT CONSIDERATIONS
Assessment: Assess for hypersensitivity to the drug and/or mannitol, hypothalamic-pituitary axis disruption due to hypophysectomy, hypopituitarism, pituitary tumor/surgery, head irradiation or head trauma, active malignancy, history of nonmalignant neoplasms or treated and stable malignancies, diabetes, acute critical illness, pregnancy/nursing status, and possible drug interactions. Evaluate glucose status.

Monitoring: Monitor for fluid retention, hypersensitivity/inj-site reactions, and other adverse reactions. Monitor for response and IGF-1 levels. Monitor for changes in glucose metabolism periodically in patients who develop impaired glucose tolerance or diabetes and for potential development or worsening of retinopathy in patients with diabetes.

Counseling: Advise that treatment may cause symptoms consistent with fluid retention. Instruct to seek prompt medical attention and to d/c therapy immediately when hypersensitivity reactions occur. Advise to rotate inj site to reduce incidence of inj-site reactions. Counsel not to share syringe with another person, even if the needle is changed. Instruct women to d/c treatment if pregnant and not to breastfeed.

ELAPRASE — idursulfase   Rx
Class: Enzyme

> Life-threatening anaphylactic reactions observed during and up to 24 hrs after infusion. Anaphylaxis, presenting as respiratory distress, hypoxia, hypotension, urticaria, and/or angioedema of throat or tongue reported during and after infusions, regardless of duration of the course of treatment; closely observe patients. Inform patients of the signs/symptoms of anaphylaxis and instruct to seek immediate medical care should symptoms occur. Patients with compromised respiratory function or acute respiratory disease may be at risk of serious acute exacerbation of their respiratory compromise due to hypersensitivity reactions; additional monitoring required.

ADULT DOSAGE	PEDIATRIC DOSAGE
Hunter Syndrome (Mucopolysaccharidosis II)	**Hunter Syndrome (Mucopolysaccharidosis II)**
Usual: 0.5mg/kg once weekly as an IV infusion over 3 hrs; gradually reduce infusion to 1 hr if no hypersensitivity reactions are observed	**≥5 Years:** **Usual:** 0.5mg/kg once weekly as an IV infusion over 3 hrs; gradually reduce infusion to 1 hr if no hypersensitivity reactions are observed
Patients may require longer infusion times if hypersensitivity reactions occur; however, infusion times should not exceed 8 hrs	Patients may require longer infusion times if hypersensitivity reactions occur; however, infusion times should not exceed 8 hrs
Infusion Rate: **Initial:** 8mL/hr for the first 15 min **Titrate:** May increase rate by 8mL/hr increments every 15 min if well tolerated **Max:** 100mL/hr	**Infusion Rate:** **Initial:** 8mL/hr for the first 15 min **Titrate:** May increase rate by 8mL/hr increments every 15 min if well tolerated **Max:** 100mL/hr
Infusion rate may be slowed, temporarily stopped, or discontinued for that visit in the event of hypersensitivity reactions	Infusion rate may be slowed, temporarily stopped, or discontinued for that visit in the event of hypersensitivity reactions

ADMINISTRATION
IV Route

Preparation Instructions
1. Determine the total volume of idursulfase to be administered and the number of vials needed based on the patient's weight and the recommended dose; refer to PI for calculation
2. Round up to the next whole vial to determine the total number of vials needed
3. Remove the required number of vials from the refrigerator to allow them to reach room temperature; do not shake the idursulfase sol
4. Withdraw the calculated volume of idursulfase from the appropriate number of vials
5. Add the calculated volume of idursulfase sol to a 100mL bag of 0.9% NaCl inj for IV infusion
6. Mix gently; do not shake the sol

Administration Instructions
Administer the diluted idursulfase sol using a low-protein-binding infusion set equipped w/ a low-protein-binding 0.2μm in-line filter
Do not infuse w/ other products in the infusion tubing

Stability
If immediate use is not possible, store the diluted sol in the refrigerator at 2-8°C (36-46°F) for up to 24 hrs

STORAGE
Vial: 2-8°C (36-46°F). Diluted Sol: 2-8°C (36-46°F) for ≤24 hrs. Protect from light. Do not freeze or shake.

HOW SUPPLIED
Inj: 2mg/mL [3mL]

WARNINGS/PRECAUTIONS
Immediately d/c if anaphylactic or other acute reactions occur and initiate appropriate treatment; medical support should be readily available upon administration. Risk of hypersensitivity, serious adverse reactions, and antibody development in Hunter syndrome patients with severe genetic mutations. Consider delaying infusion in patients with compromised respiratory function or acute febrile or respiratory illness. Caution in patients susceptible to fluid overload, or patients with acute underlying respiratory illness or compromised cardiac and/or respiratory function for whom fluid restriction is indicated; may be at risk of serious exacerbation of cardiac or respiratory status during infusions.

ADVERSE REACTIONS
Anaphylactic/hypersensitivity reactions, rash, urticaria, pruritus, flushing, pyrexia, headache, diarrhea, musculoskeletal pain, cough, fatigue, tachycardia, chills, erythema.

PREGNANCY AND LACTATION
Category C, caution in nursing.

MECHANISM OF ACTION
Hydrolytic lysosomal glycosaminoglycan-specific enzyme; provides exogenous enzyme for uptake into cellular lysosomes.

PHARMACOKINETICS
Absorption: C_{max}=1.5mcg/mL (Week 1), 1.1mcg/mL (Week 27); AUC=206 min•mcg/mL (Week 1), 169 min•mcg/mL (Week 27). **Distribution:** V_d=213mL/kg (Week 1), 254mL/kg (Week 27). **Elimination:** $T_{1/2}$= 44 min (Week 1), 48 min (Week 27).

PATIENT CONSIDERATIONS
Assessment: Assess for compromised respiratory function, genetic mutations, susceptibility to fluid overload, fluid restriction, respiratory/febrile illness, clinical status, and pregnancy/nursing status.

Monitoring: Monitor for anaphylactic/hypersensitivity reactions (eg, respiratory distress, hypoxia, hypotension, urticaria, angioedema of the throat/tongue), respiratory disease exacerbations, and other adverse events.

Counseling: Advise that life-threatening anaphylactic reactions have occurred during and after infusion. Advise that patients who have experienced anaphylactic reactions may require prolonged observation. Inform that patients with compromised respiratory function or acute respiratory disease may be at risk of serious acute exacerbation of their respiratory compromise due to hypersensitivity reactions. Encourage patients to participate in the Hunter Outcome Survey program.

ELELYSO — taliglucerase alfa   Rx
Class: Enzyme

ADULT DOSAGE	PEDIATRIC DOSAGE
Type 1 Gaucher Disease	**Type 1 Gaucher Disease**
Treatment-Naive Patients: 60 U/kg every other week as a 60-120 min IV infusion	**≥4 Years:** **Treatment-Naive Patients:** 60 U/kg every other week as a 60-120 min IV infusion
Switching from Imiglucerase: Patients previously treated on a stable dose of imiglucerase should be switched to taliglucerase alfa at that same dose	**Switching from Imiglucerase:** Patients previously treated on a stable dose of imiglucerase should be switched to taliglucerase alfa at that same dose
Infusion Rate: **Initial:** 1.2mL/min **Titrate:** After tolerability is established, the infusion rate may be increased, but should not exceed the max recommended infusion rate **Max:** 2.2mL/min	**Infusion Rate:** **Initial:** 1mL/min **Titrate:** After tolerability is established, the infusion rate may be increased, but should not exceed the max recommended infusion rate **Max:** 2mL/min

ADMINISTRATION
IV route

For single use only; do not use the vial more than one time.
Therapy should be reconstituted, diluted, and administered under the supervision of a healthcare professional.

Preparation Instructions
1. Determine the number of vials to be reconstituted based on the patient's weight and the recommended dose of 60 U/kg; refer to PI for calculation.
2. Remove the required number of vials from the refrigerator; do not heat/microwave these vials or leave them at room temperature longer than 24 hrs prior to reconstitution.
3. Reconstitute each vial w/ 5.1mL of sterile water for inj to yield a reconstituted product w/ a concentration of 40 U/mL and an extractable volume of 5mL.
4. Upon reconstitution, mix vials gently; do not shake.
5. Withdraw the calculated dose of drug from the appropriate number of vials and dilute w/ 0.9% NaCl inj, to a final volume of 100-200mL as follows:
Adults: May use a final volume of 130-150mL; however, if the volume of reconstituted product alone is ≥130-150mL, then the final volume should not exceed 200mL.
Pediatrics: Use final volume of 100-120mL.
6. Mix gently; do not shake. Since this is a protein sol, slight flocculation (described as translucent fibers) occurs occasionally after dilution.

Administration Instructions
After reconstitution and dilution, administer the preparation via IV infusion and filter through an in-line low protein-binding 0.2µm filter.

Stability
If immediate use is not possible, may store the reconstituted product for up to 24 hrs at 2-8°C (36-46°F) under protection from light or up to 4 hrs at 20-25°C (68-77°F) w/o protection from light.

STORAGE
2-8°C (36-46°F). Do not freeze. Protect from light. **Reconstituted/Diluted Sol Under Protection from Light:** 2-8°C (36-46°F) for up to 24 hrs. **Reconstituted Sol w/o Protection from Light:** 20-25°C (68-77°F) for up to 4 hrs. Do not freeze.

HOW SUPPLIED
Inj: 200 U/vial

WARNINGS/PRECAUTIONS
Serious hypersensitivity reactions, including anaphylaxis, reported; have appropriate medical support readily available. If anaphylaxis or severe hypersensitivity reactions occur, d/c infusion immediately and initiate appropriate medical treatment. Manage hypersensitivity reactions based on the severity of the reaction; include slowing or temporary interruption of infusion and/or administration of antihistamines, antipyretics, and/or corticosteroids for mild reactions. Pretreatment w/ antihistamines and/or corticosteroids may prevent subsequent hypersensitivity reactions. Consider the risks and benefits of readministering treatment in patients who have experienced a severe reaction associated w/ therapy and use caution upon rechallenge.

ADVERSE REACTIONS
Treatment-Naive Adults: Headache, arthralgia, fatigue, N/V, urticaria, dizziness, abdominal pain, pruritus, flushing, anti-drug antibodies (ADAs).
Patients Switched from Imiglucerase: Arthralgia, headache, pain in extremity, ADAs.

PREGNANCY AND LACTATION
Pregnancy: The limited available data on use of therapy in pregnant women are not sufficient to inform a drug-associated risk.
Lactation: There are no data on the presence of taliglucerase in human milk, the effects on the breast fed infant, or the effects on milk production; caution in nursing.

MECHANISM OF ACTION
Hydrolytic lysosomal glucocerebroside-specific enzyme; catalyzes the hydrolysis of glucocerebroside to glucose and ceramide, reducing the amount of accumulated glucocerebroside.

PHARMACOKINETICS
Absorption: 60 U/kg (Median): AUC=2984ng•h/mL (Pediatric Patients), 6459ng•h/mL (Adults). **Distribution:** 60 U/kg (Median): V_d=8.8L (Pediatric Patients), V_d=10.7L (Adults). **Elimination:** 60 U/kg (Median): $T_{1/2}$=32.5 min (Pediatric Patients), 28.7 min (Adults).

PATIENT CONSIDERATIONS
Assessment: Assess for previous hypersensitivity to the drug and pregnancy/nursing status.

Monitoring: Monitor for signs/symptoms of hypersensitivity reactions (eg, anaphylaxis) and other adverse reactions. Monitor for ADAs in ADA-positive patients or in patients who experienced hypersensitivity reactions to taliglucerase alfa or other enzyme replacement therapies.

Counseling: Inform patients and caregivers that reactions related to administration and infusion, including life-threatening anaphylaxis and severe hypersensitivity reactions, may occur during and after treatment; instruct to report signs/symptoms and to seek immediate medical care should these occur. Inform that patients should be carefully reevaluated for treatment w/ the drug if serious hypersensitivity reactions occur.

ELIGARD — leuprolide acetate   Rx

Class: Synthetic gonadotropin-releasing hormone (GnRH) analogue

ADULT DOSAGE	PEDIATRIC DOSAGE
Advanced Prostate Cancer	Pediatric use may not have been established
Palliative Treatment:	
7.5mg: 1 inj every month	
22.5mg: 1 inj every 3 months	
30mg: 1 inj every 4 months	
45mg: 1 inj every 6 months	

ADMINISTRATION
SQ route

Inj site should vary periodically; avoid areas w/ brawny or fibrous SQ tissue or locations that could be rubbed or compressed (eg, w/ a belt or clothing waistband). Use gloves during mixing and administration.
Allow the product to reach room temperature before mixing.
Once mixed, administer w/in 30 min; refer to PI for mixing procedure.

Administration Procedure
1. Choose an inj site on the abdomen, upper buttocks, or anywhere w/ adequate amounts of SQ tissue that does not have excessive pigment, nodules, lesions, or hair; choose an area that has not recently been used.
2. Cleanse the inj-site area w/ an alcohol swab.
3. Using the thumb and forefinger of your non-dominant hand, grab and bunch the area of skin around the inj site.

4. Using your dominant hand, insert the needle quickly at a 90° angle to the skin surface; after the needle is inserted, release the skin w/ your non-dominant hand.
5. Inject the drug using a slow, steady push. Press down on the plunger until the syringe is empty.
6. Withdraw the needle quickly at the same 90° angle used for insertion.
7. Immediately following the withdrawal of the needle, activate the safety shield on the needle.

STORAGE
2-8°C (35.6-46.4°F). Once outside the refrigerator, store in its original packaging at 15-30°C (59-86°F) for up to 8 weeks prior to mixing and administration.

HOW SUPPLIED
Inj: 7.5mg, 22.5mg, 30mg, 45mg

CONTRAINDICATIONS
Patients w/ hypersensitivity to GnRH, GnRH agonist analogues, or any of the components of the medication. Women who are or may become pregnant.

WARNINGS/PRECAUTIONS
Transient increase in serum concentrations of testosterone and worsening of symptoms or onset of new signs/symptoms (eg, bone pain, neuropathy, hematuria) during the 1st few weeks of therapy may occur. Cases of ureteral obstruction and/or spinal cord compression reported; institute standard treatment if these complications occur. Closely monitor patients w/ metastatic vertebral lesions and/or urinary tract obstruction during 1st few weeks of therapy. Suppresses pituitary-gonadal system; may affect results of diagnostic tests of pituitary gonadotropic and gonadal functions conducted during and after therapy. Hyperglycemia and increased risk of developing diabetes, MI, sudden cardiac death, and stroke reported. May prolong QT/QTc interval; consider whether the benefits outweigh the potential risks in patients w/ congenital long QT syndrome, CHF, frequent electrolyte abnormalities, and in patients taking drugs known to prolong the QT interval.

ADVERSE REACTIONS
Hot flashes/sweats, inj-site reactions (eg, transient burning/stinging, pain, erythema), malaise/fatigue, testicular atrophy, weakness, gynecomastia, myalgia, arthralgia, dizziness, decreased libido, clamminess, night sweats, nausea.

PREGNANCY AND LACTATION
Pregnancy: Category X.
Lactation: Not for use in nursing.

MECHANISM OF ACTION
Synthetic GnRH analogue; acts as a potent inhibitor of gonadotropin secretion when given continuously.

PHARMACOKINETICS
Absorption: Administration of variable doses resulted in different parameters.
Distribution: (IV bolus dose) V_d=27L; plasma protein binding (43-49%).
Metabolism: Pentapeptide (M-1) metabolite (major metabolite). **Elimination:** (1mg IV bolus dose) $T_{1/2}$=3 hrs.

PATIENT CONSIDERATIONS
Assessment: Assess for hypersensitivity to drug, metastatic vertebral lesions, urinary tract obstructions, congenital long QT syndrome, CHF, electrolyte abnormalities, and diabetes mellitus. Obtain baseline serum testosterone levels and prostate specific antigen (PSA) levels. Obtain baseline blood glucose and/or HbA1c levels. Correct electrolyte abnormalities.

Monitoring: Monitor for worsening/occurrence of signs/symptoms of prostate cancer, spinal cord compression, ureteral obstruction, signs/symptoms suggestive of cardiovascular disease development, and other adverse reactions. Periodically monitor blood glucose, HbA1c, testosterone, and PSA levels. Consider periodic monitoring of ECG and electrolytes.

Counseling: Inform that hot flashes may be experienced. Advise that increased bone pain, difficulty in urinating, and onset or aggravation of weakness or paralysis may be experienced during the 1st few weeks of therapy. Instruct to notify physician if new or worsened symptoms develop after beginning treatment. Inform about inj-site related adverse reactions (eg, transient burning/stinging, pain, bruising, redness); instruct to notify physician if such reactions do not resolve. Advise to contact physician immediately if an allergic reaction develops.

ELITEK — rasburicase   Rx

Class: Recombinant urate-oxidase enzyme

> May cause serious and fatal hypersensitivity reactions including anaphylaxis; immediately and permanently d/c in patients who experience a serious hypersensitivity reaction. Do not administer w/ G6PD deficiency. Prior to initiation, screen patients at higher risk for G6PD deficiency (eg, African/Mediterranean ancestry). Immediately and permanently d/c in patients developing hemolysis or methemoglobinemia. Enzymatically degrades uric acid in blood samples left at room temperature. Collect blood samples in pre-chilled tubes containing heparin and immediately immerse and maintain sample in an ice water bath; assay plasma samples w/in 4 hrs of collection.

ADULT DOSAGE	PEDIATRIC DOSAGE
Hyperuricemia	**Hyperuricemia**
Initial management of expected plasma uric acid elevation due to tumor lysis syndrome in patients w/ leukemia/lymphoma/solid tumor malignancies receiving anticancer therapy	Initial management of expected plasma uric acid elevation due to tumor lysis syndrome in patients w/ leukemia/lymphoma/solid tumor malignancies receiving anticancer therapy
Recommended Dose: 0.2mg/kg IV over 30 min qd for up to 5 days	**1 Month-17 Years:** **Recommended Dose:** 0.2mg/kg IV over 30 min qd for up to 5 days

ADMINISTRATION
IV route

Preparation
Reconstitute 1.5mg vial w/ 1mL diluent or the 7.5mg vial w/ 5mL diluent.
Mix by swirling gently; do not shake or vortex.
Inject reconstituted sol into infusion bag containing 0.9% sterile NaCl to make 50mL.

Do not administer as a bolus inj.
Infuse over 30 min through separate line or flush line w/ at least 15mL of normal saline prior to and after infusion.
Do not use filters during reconstitution or infusion.
Discard unused sol 24 hrs following reconstitution.

STORAGE
2-8°C (36-46°F). Do not freeze. Protect from light.

HOW SUPPLIED
Inj: 1.5mg, 7.5mg

CONTRAINDICATIONS
History of anaphylaxis or severe hypersensitivity to rasburicase, G6PD deficiency, development of hemolytic reactions or methemoglobinemia w/ rasburicase.

WARNINGS/PRECAUTIONS
Use only for a single course of treatment. Institute appropriate monitoring and support measures (eg, transfusion support for hemolysis/methemoglobinemia, methylene-blue administration for methemoglobinemia).

ADVERSE REACTIONS
N/V, fever, peripheral edema, anxiety, headache, abdominal pain, constipation, diarrhea, hypophosphatemia, pharyngolaryngeal pain, increased ALT, mucositis, rash.

PREGNANCY AND LACTATION
Pregnancy: Category C.
Lactation: Not for use in nursing.

MECHANISM OF ACTION
Recombinant urate-oxidase enzyme; catalyzes enzymatic oxidation of poorly soluble uric acid into an inactive and soluble metabolite (allantoin).

PHARMACOKINETICS
Distribution: V_d=110-127mL/kg (pediatric patients), 75.8-138mL/kg (adults).
Elimination: $T_{1/2}$=15.7-22.5 hrs.

PATIENT CONSIDERATIONS
Assessment: Assess for G6PD deficiency, history of anaphylaxis or severe hypersensitivity to rasburicase, history of hemolytic reactions or methemoglobinemia w/ rasburicase, and pregnancy/nursing status.

Monitoring: Monitor for hypersensitivity reactions (eg, anaphylaxis), hemolysis, methemoglobinemia, and other adverse reactions.

Counseling: Instruct to notify physician immediately if any of the following occur: allergic reactions, bronchospasm, chest pain/tightness, dyspnea, hypoxia, hypotension, shock, or urticaria.

ELLENCE — epirubicin hydrochloride   Rx
Class: Anthracycline

> Severe local tissue necrosis may occur with extravasation during administration; do not give IM or SQ. Cardiac toxicity, including fatal congestive heart failure (CHF), may occur either during or months to yrs after termination of therapy. Use extreme caution if cumulative dose of 900mg/m² is exceeded. Increased risk of cardiac toxicity with active/dormant cardiovascular disease (CVD), prior or concomitant radiotherapy to the mediastinal/pericardial area, previous therapy with other anthracyclines or anthracenediones, or concomitant use of other cardiotoxic drugs. Secondary acute myelogenous leukemia (AML) reported in patients with breast cancer treated with anthracyclines. More common occurrence of refractory secondary leukemia when given with DNA-damaging antineoplastic agents, heavy pretreatment with cytotoxic drugs, or when doses of anthracyclines have been escalated. Severe myelosuppression may occur.

ADULT DOSAGE
Breast Cancer

Adjuvant Therapy:
Axillary Node Tumor Involvement Following Resection:
100-120mg/m² in repeated 3- or 4-week cycles as follows:
CEF-120 Regimen:
60mg/m² on Days 1 and 8 every 28 days for 6 cycles
FEC-100 Regimen:
100mg/m² on Day 1 every 21 days for 6 cycles

Give prophylactic antibiotic therapy if administering the 120mg/m² regimen

PEDIATRIC DOSAGE
Pediatric use may not have been established

DOSING CONSIDERATIONS
Renal Impairment
Severe (SrCr >5mg/dL): Consider lower doses

Hepatic Impairment
Bilirubin 1.2-3mg/dL or AST 2-4X Upper Limit of Normal:
Administer 1/2 of recommended starting dose

Bilirubin >3mg/dL or AST >4X Upper Limit of Normal:
Administer 1/4 of recommended starting dose

Adverse Reactions
Hematologic and Nonhematologic Toxicities:
Reduce Day 1 dose in subsequent cycles to 75% of the Day 1 dose given in the current cycle
Delay Day 1 chemo in subsequent courses until platelet counts are ≥100,000/mm³, ANC ≥1500/mm³, and nonhematologic toxicities have recovered to ≤Grade 1
Bone Marrow Dysfunction:
Heavily Pretreated Patients/Preexisting Bone Marrow Depression/Neoplastic Bone Marrow Infiltration:
Consider lower starting dose (75-90mg/m²)
Patients Receiving a Divided Dose:
Day 8 dose should be 75% of Day 1 if platelet counts are 75,000-100,000/mm³ and ANC is 1000-1499/mm³
Day 8 Platelet Counts are <75,000/mm³, ANC <1000/mm³, or Grades 3/4 Nonhematologic Toxicity Occurred:
Omit Day 8 dose

ADMINISTRATION
IV route

Do not administer IM/SQ
Consider prophylactic use of antiemetics

Preparation and Administration Precautions
Storage of the sol for inj at refrigerated conditions can result in the formation of a gelled product. This gelled product will return to a slightly viscous to mobile sol after 2 to a max of 4 hrs equilibration at controlled room temperature (15-25°C)

Take the following protective measures when handling Ellence:
1. Train personnel in appropriate techniques for reconstitution and handling
2. Exclude pregnant staff from working with this drug
3. Wear protective clothing (goggles, gowns, and disposable gloves) and masks when handling Ellence
4. Define a designated area for syringe preparation (preferably under a laminar flow system), with the work surface protected by disposable, plastic-backed, absorbent paper
5. Place all items used for reconstitution, administration, or cleaning (including gloves) in high-risk, waste-disposal bags for high temperature incineration
6. Treat spillage or leakage with dilute sodium hypochlorite (1% available chlorine) sol, preferably by soaking, and then water. Place all contaminated and cleaning materials in high-risk, waste-disposal bags for incineration. Treat accidental contact with the skin or eyes immediately by copious lavage with water, or soap and water, or sodium bicarbonate sol. However, do not abrade the skin by using a scrub brush. Seek medical attention. Always wash hands after removing gloves

Incompatibilities:
1. Avoid prolonged contact with any sol of an alkaline pH as it will result in hydrolysis of the drug. Do not mix Ellence with heparin or fluorouracil due to chemical incompatibility that may lead to precipitation
2. Ellence can be used in combination with other antitumor agents, but do not mix with other drugs in the same syringe

Preparation of Infusion Sol:
1. Administer Ellence into the tubing of a freely flowing IV infusion (0.9% sodium chloride or 5% glucose sol)
2. Patients receiving initial therapy at the recommended starting doses of 100-120mg/m² should generally have Ellence infused over 15-20 min. For patients who require lower starting doses due to organ dysfunction or who require modification of Ellence doses during therapy, the infusion time may be proportionally decreased, but should not be less than 3 min
3. A direct push injection is not recommended due to the risk of extravasation, which may occur even in the presence of adequate blood return upon needle aspiration. Venous sclerosis may result from inj into small vessels or repeated inj into the same vein
4. Use Ellence within 24 hrs of first penetration of the rubber stopper. Discard any unused sol

STORAGE
2-8°C (36-46°F). Use sol within 24 hrs after removal from refrigeration. Do not freeze. Protect from light.

HOW SUPPLIED
Inj: 2mg/mL [25mL, 100mL]

CONTRAINDICATIONS
Cardiomyopathy, heart failure, recent myocardial infarction, severe arrhythmias, previous treatment w/ max cumulative dose of anthracyclines, hypersensitivity to epirubicin, other anthracyclines, or anthracenediones.

WARNINGS/PRECAUTIONS
Administer only under the supervision of qualified physicians experienced in the use of cytotoxic therapy. Allow patients to recover from acute toxicities (eg, stomatitis, neutropenia, thrombocytopenia, generalized infections) of prior cytotoxic treatment before initiation of therapy. Venous sclerosis may result from inj into a small vessel or from repeated inj into the same vein; administer slowly into the tubing of a freely running IV infusion. If possible, avoid veins over joints or in extremities with compromised venous or lymphatic drainage; terminate infusion immediately and restart in another vein if a burning or stinging sensation indicates perivenous infiltration. Excessively rapid administration may cause facial flushing as well as local erythematous streaking along the vein. Regularly monitor left ventricular ejection fraction (LVEF) with prompt discontinuation at the 1st sign of impaired function. Avoid with severe hepatic impairment. May induce hyperuricemia and tumor lysis syndrome; consider monitoring serum uric acid, K⁺, Ca²⁺, phosphate, and creatinine immediately after initial chemotherapy administration. Hydration, urine alkalinization, and prophylaxis with allopurinol

to prevent hyperuricemia may minimize potential complications of tumor lysis syndrome. Emetogenic; consider prophylactic antiemetics. Thrombophlebitis and thromboembolic phenomena reported. May cause fetal harm; women of childbearing potential should use effective contraception. Males with female sexual partners of childbearing potential should use contraception during and after cessation of therapy; may damage testicular tissue and spermatozoa. Caution in female patients ≥70 yrs of age.

ADVERSE REACTIONS
Cardiac toxicity, AML, alopecia, amenorrhea, anemia, N/V, diarrhea, infection, lethargy, leukopenia, mucositis, neutropenia, thrombocytopenia, hot flashes.

DRUG INTERACTIONS
See Boxed Warning. Avoid with other cardiotoxic agents unless cardiac function is closely monitored. Caution with calcium channel blockers. Avoid with live vaccines; may diminish response to killed/inactivated vaccines. Cimetidine may increase exposure; d/c cimetidine during treatment. Concomitant use with other cytotoxic drugs (eg, paclitaxel, docetaxel) may show additive toxicity, especially hematologic and GI effects. Increased exposure when administered immediately prior to or after paclitaxel. Changes in hepatic function induced by concomitant therapies may affect metabolism, pharmacokinetics, therapeutic efficacy, and/or toxicity. Administration after previous radiation therapy may induce an inflammatory recall reaction at irradiation site.

PREGNANCY AND LACTATION
Category D, not for use in nursing.

MECHANISM OF ACTION
Anthracycline; not established. Forms a complex with DNA by intercalation between nucleotide base pairs, with consequent inhibition of nucleic acid (DNA and RNA) and protein synthesis. This triggers DNA cleavage by topoisomerase II, resulting in cytocidal activity. Also inhibits DNA helicase activity, preventing the enzymatic separation of double-stranded DNA and interfering with replication and transcription. Also involved in oxidation/reduction reactions by generating cytotoxic free radicals.

PHARMACOKINETICS
Absorption: Administration of multiple doses resulted in different parameters. **Distribution:** Plasma protein binding (77%). **Metabolism:** Liver (extensive and rapid), other organs and cells; reduction, conjugation, hydrolytic, and redox processes; epirubicinol (metabolite). **Elimination:** Feces (34%), urine (27%). Refer to PI for additional pharmacokinetic information.

PATIENT CONSIDERATIONS
Assessment: Assess for CVD, acute toxicities from prior cytotoxic treatment, hepatic/renal impairment, risk factors for cardiac toxicities, hypersensitivity to drug, pregnancy/nursing status, possible drug interactions, and other conditions where treatment is contraindicated or cautioned. Obtain baseline CBC, total bilirubin, AST, creatinine, and cardiac function (LVEF).

Monitoring: Monitor for cardiotoxicity, AML, myelosuppression, hypersensitivity reactions, tumor lysis syndrome, extravasation, thrombophlebitis/thromboembolic phenomena, and other adverse reactions. Monitor LVEF regularly, especially in patients with risk factors for increased cardiac toxicity. Monitor total and differential WBCs, RBCs, platelet counts, creatinine, AST, total bilirubin, and cardiac function before and during each cycle.

Counseling: Inform patients of the expected adverse effects, including GI symptoms, alopecia, and potential neutropenic complications. Advise about the risk of leukemia and irreversible myocardial damage. Instruct to consult physician if vomiting, dehydration, fever, evidence of infection, symptoms of CHF, or inj-site pain occurs. Inform that urine may appear red for 1-2 days; advise not to be alarmed. Advise men undergoing treatment to use effective contraceptive methods. Inform that women may develop irreversible amenorrhea or premature menopause.

ELOCTATE — antihemophilic factor (recombinant), fc fusion protein   Rx
Class: Antihemophilic factor (recombinant)

ADULT DOSAGE
Hemophilia A
Dosing Calculations:
Dose (IU) = body weight (kg) x desired Factor VIII (FVIII) rise (IU/dL or % of normal) x 0.5 (IU/kg per IU/dL)Estimated increment of FVIII (IU/dL or % of normal) = [Total Dose (IU)/body weight (kg)] x 2 (IU/dL per IU/kg)Dose and duration of therapy depend on the severity of the FVIII deficiency, the location and extent of the bleeding, and clinical condition

On-Demand Treatment/Control of Bleeding Episodes:
Minor and Moderate Bleeding:
40-60 IU/dL or % of Normal FVIII Level Required: 20-30 IU/kg q24-48h until bleeding is resolved

Major Bleeding:
80-100 IU/dL or % of Normal FVIII Level Required: 40-50 IU/kg q12-24h until bleeding is resolved (approx 7-10 days)

PEDIATRIC DOSAGE
Hemophilia A
Dosing Calculations:
Dose (IU) = body weight (kg) x desired FVIII rise (IU/dL or % of normal) x 0.5 (IU/kg per IU/dL)

Estimated increment of FVIII (IU/dL or % of normal) = [Total Dose (IU)/body weight (kg)] x 2 (IU/dL per IU/kg)

Dose and duration of therapy depend on the severity of the FVIII deficiency, the location and extent of the bleeding, and clinical condition

On-Demand Treatment/Control of Bleeding Episodes:
Minor and Moderate Bleeding:
40-60 IU/dL or % of Normal FVIII Level Required: 20-30 IU/kg q24-48h (q12-24h if <6 yrs of age) until bleeding is resolved

Perioperative Management:
Minor Surgery:
50-80 IU/dL or % of Normal FVIII Level Required: 25-40 IU/kg q24h for at least 1 day until healing is achieved
Major Surgery:
80-120 IU/dL or % of Normal FVIII Level Required (Pre- and Post-Operative): 40-60 IU/kg followed by a repeat dose of 40-50 IU/kg after 8-24 hrs and then q24h to maintain FVIII activity w/in the target range; continue until adequate wound healing, then continue therapy for at least 7 days to maintain a FVIII activity w/in the target range
Prophylaxis:
Initial: 50 IU/kg every 4 days
Titrate: Adjust based on patient response w/ dosing in the range of 25-65 IU/kg at 3- to 5-day intervals

Major Bleeding:
80-100 IU/dL or % of Normal FVIII Level Required: 40-50 IU/kg q12-24h (q8-24h if <6 yrs of age) until bleeding is resolved (approx 7-10 days)
Perioperative Management:
Minor Surgery:
50-80 IU/dL or % of Normal FVIII Level Required: 25-40 IU/kg q24h (q12-24h if <6 yrs of age) for at least 1 day until healing is achieved
Major Surgery:
80-120 IU/dL or % of Normal FVIII Level Required (Pre- and Post-Operative): 40-60 IU/kg followed by a repeat dose of 40-50 IU/kg after 8-24 hrs (6-24 hrs if <6 yrs of age) and then q24h to maintain FVIII activity w/in the target range; continue until adequate wound healing, then continue therapy for at least 7 days to maintain a FVIII activity w/in the target range
Prophylaxis:
<6 Years:
Initial: 50 IU/kg administered twice weekly
Titrate: Adjust based on patient response w/ dosing in the range of 25-65 IU/kg at 3- to 5-day intervals; more frequent or higher doses up to 80 IU/kg may be required
≥6 Years:
Initial: 50 IU/kg every 4 days
Titrate: Adjust based on patient response w/ dosing in the range of 25-65 IU/kg at 3- to 5-day intervals

---

ADMINISTRATION
IV route

Do not administer reconstituted sol in the same tubing or container w/ other medications.
Perform IV bolus infusion; rate of administration should be determined by comfort level, and no faster than 10mL/min.
Use the reconstituted sol as soon as possible, but no later than 3 hrs after reconstitution; protect from direct sunlight.
Do not refrigerate after reconstitution.

Reconstitution
1. Allow vial and pre-filled diluent syringe to reach room temperature before use.
2. Using supplied adapter and syringe, slowly depress the plunger rod to inject all of the diluent into the vial.
3. With the syringe still connected to the adapter, gently swirl until product is completely dissolved; do not shake.
4. Turn the vial upside down and slowly draw the sol into the syringe.
5. Gently unscrew the syringe from the adapter and dispose of the vial w/ the adapter still attached.

Refer to PI for combining 2 or more vials.

STORAGE
2-8°C (36-46°F). Protect from light. Do not freeze. May store at room temperature ≤30°C (86°F) for a single period of up to 6 months; record the date that product is removed from refrigeration on the carton in the area provided. Do not return the product to the refrigerator after storage at room temperature. **Reconstituted Sol:** May store at room temperature ≤30°C (86°F) for up to 3 hrs. Discard any product not used w/in 3 hrs after reconstitution. Protect from direct sunlight. Do not refrigerate after reconstitution.

HOW SUPPLIED
Inj: 250 IU, 500 IU, 750 IU, 1000 IU, 1500 IU, 2000 IU, 3000 IU

CONTRAINDICATIONS
Life-threatening hypersensitivity reactions to Eloctate or other constituents of the product.

WARNINGS/PRECAUTIONS
Not indicated for the treatment of von Willebrand disease. Hypersensitivity reactions, including anaphylaxis, may occur; immediately d/c administration and initiate appropriate treatment if hypersensitivity reactions occur. Formation of neutralizing antibodies (inhibitors) to FVIII reported; monitor for the development of FVIII inhibitors by appropriate clinical observations and lab tests. If plasma FVIII level fails to increase as expected or if bleeding is not controlled after administration of therapy, suspect presence of an inhibitor; perform a Bethesda inhibitor assay.

ADVERSE REACTIONS
Arthralgia, malaise, myalgia, headache, rash.

PREGNANCY AND LACTATION
Pregnancy: There are no studies in pregnant women to inform a drug-associated risk. It is not known whether therapy can cause fetal harm when administered to a pregnant woman, or whether it can affect reproduction capacity.

Lactation: There is no information regarding the presence in human milk, the effect on the breastfed infant, or the effects on milk production; caution in nursing.

MECHANISM OF ACTION
Recombinant antihemophilic factor; temporarily replaces the missing coagulation FVIII needed for effective hemostasis. Contains the Fc region of human IgG$_1$, which binds to the neonatal Fc receptor.

PHARMACOKINETICS
Absorption: AUC/Dose=54.1 IU•hr/dL per IU/kg. **Distribution:** V$_d$=49.5mL/kg. **Elimination:** T$_{1/2}$=19.7 hrs. Refer to PI for pediatric and adolescent pharmacokinetic parameters.

PATIENT CONSIDERATIONS

Assessment: Assess for hypersensitivity to drug, location and severity of bleeding, and pregnancy/nursing status. Assess FVIII activity levels.

Monitoring: Monitor for hypersensitivity reactions, and other adverse reactions. Monitor plasma FVIII activity. Monitor for the development of FVIII inhibitors.

Counseling: Instruct to contact physician or go to the emergency department right away if a hypersensitivity reaction occurs. Advise to report any adverse reactions or problems following administration to physician. Advise to contact physician or treatment facility for further treatment and/or assessment if experiencing a lack of clinical response to FVIII therapy.

Eloxatin — oxaliplatin   Rx

Class: Platinum analogue

> Anaphylactic reactions reported, and may occur w/in min of administration. Epinephrine, corticosteroids, and antihistamines have been employed to alleviate symptoms of anaphylaxis.

ADULT DOSAGE	PEDIATRIC DOSAGE
Colon Cancer	Pediatric use may not have been established
Stage III:	

Colon Cancer

Stage III:

In combination w/ 5-fluorouracil (5-FU)/leucovorin (LV) for adjuvant treatment in patients who have undergone complete resection of the primary tumor

Day 1: Oxaliplatin 85mg/m^2 IV infusion + LV 200mg/m^2 IV infusion; both given over 120 min at the same time in separate bags using a Y-line, followed by 5-FU 400mg/m^2 IV bolus given over 2-4 min, followed by 5-FU 600mg/m^2 IV infusion as a 22-hr continuous infusion

Day 2: LV 200 mg/m^2 IV infusion over 120 min, followed by 5-FU 400mg/m^2 IV bolus given over 2-4 min, followed by 5-FU 600 mg/m^2 IV infusion as a 22-hr continuous infusion

Administer every 2 weeks; treatment is recommended for a total of 6 months (12 cycles)

Advanced Colorectal Cancer

Combination w/ 5-FU/LV:

Day 1: Oxaliplatin 85mg/m^2 IV infusion + LV 200mg/m^2 IV infusion; both given over 120 min at the same time in separate bags using a Y-line, followed by 5-FU 400mg/m^2 IV bolus given over 2-4 min, followed by 5-FU 600mg/m^2 IV infusion as a 22-hr continuous infusion

Day 2: LV 200 mg/m^2 IV infusion over 120 min, followed by 5-FU 400mg/m^2 IV bolus given over 2-4 min, followed by 5-FU 600 mg/m^2 IV infusion as a 22-hr continuous infusion

Administer every 2 weeks. Continue treatment until disease progression or unacceptable toxicity

Premedication

Antiemetics, including 5-HT$_3$ blockers w/ or w/o dexamethasone, are recommended

---

DOSING CONSIDERATIONS

Renal Impairment
Severe:
Initial: 65mg/m^2

Adverse Reactions

Adjuvant Therapy in Stage III Colon Cancer:
Persistent Grade 2 Neurosensory Events That Do Not Resolve:
Consider reducing dose to 75mg/m^2; 5-FU/LV regimen need not be altered

Persistent Grade 3 Neurosensory Events:
Consider discontinuing; 5-FU/LV regimen need not be altered
After Recovery from Grade 3/4 GI (Despite Prophylactic Treatment), or Grade 4 Neutropenia, or Febrile Neutropenia, or Grade 3/4 Thrombocytopenia:
Reduce oxaliplatin dose to 75mg/m^2 and 5-FU to 300mg/m^2 bolus and 500mg/m^2 22-hr infusion; delay next dose until neutrophils ≥1.5 x 10^9/L and platelets ≥75 x 10^9/L

Advanced Colorectal Cancer (Previously Treated/Untreated):
Persistent Grade 2 Neurosensory Events That Do Not Resolve:
Consider reducing dose to 65mg/m^2; 5-FU/LV regimen need not be altered
Persistent Grade 3 Neurosensory Events:
Consider discontinuing therapy; 5-FU/LV regimen need not be altered
After Recovery from Grade 3/4 GI (Despite Prophylactic Treatment), or Grade 4 Neutropenia, or Febrile Neutropenia, or Grade 3/4 Thrombocytopenia:
Reduce oxaliplatin dose to 65mg/m^2 and 5-FU by 20% (300mg/m^2 bolus and 500mg/m^2 22-hr infusion); delay next dose until neutrophils ≥1.5 x 10^9/L and platelets ≥75 x 10^9/L

ADMINISTRATION

IV route

Incompatible in sol w/ alkaline medications or media (eg, basic sol of 5-FU); do not mix w/ these or administer simultaneously through the same infusion line. Flush the infusion line w/ D5 inj prior to administration of any concomitant medication.
Do not use needles or IV administration sets containing aluminum parts to prepare or mix the drug; aluminum has been reported to cause degradation of platinum compounds.
Prolongation of infusion time for oxaliplatin from 2 hrs to 6 hrs may mitigate acute toxicities; infusion times for 5-FU and LV do not need to be changed.

Preparation of Infusion Sol
The sol must be further diluted in an infusion sol of 250-500mL of D5 inj; never perform a final dilution w/ a NaCl sol or other Cl⁻ containing sol.
After dilution, the shelf life is 6 hrs at 20-25°C (68-77°F) or up to 24 hrs at 2-8°C (36-46°F).
After final dilution, protection from light is not required.

STORAGE
25°C (77°F); excursions permitted to 15-30°C (59-86°F). Do not freeze and protect from light (keep in original outer carton).

HOW SUPPLIED
Inj: 5mg/mL [50mg, 100mg]

CONTRAINDICATIONS
History of known allergy to oxaliplatin or other platinum compounds.

WARNINGS/PRECAUTIONS
Should be administered under the supervision of a physician experienced in the use of cancer chemotherapeutic agents. An early onset, acute, reversible, primarily peripheral, sensory neuropathy and a persistent (>14 days), primarily peripheral, sensory neuropathy, reported. Cold temperature/objects may precipitate or exacerbate acute neurological symptoms; avoid ice for mucositis prophylaxis during infusion. Reversible posterior leukoencephalopathy syndrome (RPLS), also known as posterior reversible encephalopathy syndrome (PRES), reported. Grade 3 or 4 neutropenia reported in patients w/ colorectal cancer treated w/ oxaliplatin in combination w/ 5-FU and LV. Sepsis, neutropenic sepsis, and septic shock reported; withhold oxaliplatin for sepsis or septic shock. Potentially fatal pulmonary fibrosis reported. If unexplained respiratory symptoms develop, d/c until further pulmonary investigation excludes interstitial lung disease or pulmonary fibrosis. Hepatotoxicity observed; consider hepatic vascular disorders, and if appropriate, investigate in case of abnormal LFT results or portal HTN, which cannot be explained by liver metastases. QT prolongation and ventricular arrhythmias including fatal torsades de pointes reported; correct hypokalemia or hypomagnesemia prior to initiating therapy and monitor these electrolytes periodically during therapy. Avoid in patients w/ congenital long QT syndrome. ECG monitoring is recommended if therapy is initiated in patients w/ CHF, bradyarrhythmias, drugs known to prolong the QT interval (eg, Class Ia and III antiarrhythmics), and electrolyte abnormalities. Rhabdomyolysis, including fatal cases reported; d/c if any signs/symptoms of rhabdomyolysis occur. May cause fetal harm. Caution w/ renal impairment.

ADVERSE REACTIONS
Peripheral sensory neuropathy, neutropenia, thrombocytopenia, anemia, N/V, increased transaminases/alkaline phosphatase, diarrhea, fatigue, stomatitis, abdominal pain, fever, skin disorder, anorexia, dyspnea.

DRUG INTERACTIONS
Increased 5-FU plasma levels reported w/ doses of 130mg/m^2 oxaliplatin dosed every 3 weeks. Potentially nephrotoxic agents may decrease clearance. Prolonged PT and INR occasionally associated w/ hemorrhage reported in patients who concomitantly received oxaliplatin plus 5-FU/LV and anticoagulants; monitor patients requiring oral anticoagulants closely.

PREGNANCY AND LACTATION
Pregnancy: Category D.
Lactation: Not for use in nursing.

MECHANISM OF ACTION
Organoplatinum complex; inhibits deoxyribonucleic acid replication and transcription.

PHARMACOKINETICS
Absorption: C$_{max}$=0.814mcg/mL. **Distribution:** V$_d$=440L; plasma protein binding (>90%). **Metabolism:** Rapid, extensive nonenzymatic biotransformation. **Elimination:** Urine (54%), feces (2%); T$_{1/2}$=391 hrs.

PATIENT CONSIDERATIONS

Assessment: Assess for history of known allergy to the drug or other platinum compounds, renal impairment, congenital long QT syndrome, hypokalemia, hypomagnesemia, pregnancy/nursing status, and possible drug interactions. Assess LFTs, WBC count w/ differential, Hgb, platelet count, and blood chemistries before each cycle.

Monitoring: Monitor for signs/symptoms of anaphylactic reactions, neurosensory toxicity, pulmonary toxicity, hepatotoxicity, RPLS, neutropenia, sepsis, septic shock, QT prolongation, ventricular arrhythmias, rhabdomyolysis, and other adverse reactions. Monitor patients w/ renal impairment closely and monitor patients requiring oral anticoagulants closely. Monitor Mg^{2+} and K^+ levels periodically. Perform ECG monitoring in patients w/ CHF, bradyarrhythmias, patients taking drugs known to prolong the QT interval, and in patients w/ electrolyte abnormalities.

Counseling: Inform of pregnancy risks. Advise to expect side effects, particularly neurologic effects, both the acute, reversible effects and the persistent neurosensory toxicity. Inform that acute neurosensory toxicity may be precipitated or exacerbated by exposure to cold or cold objects. Instruct to avoid cold drinks and ice, and to cover exposed skin prior to exposure to cold temperature or cold objects. Inform of the risk of low blood cell counts and to contact physician immediately if fever, particularly if associated w/ persistent diarrhea, or evidence of infection develops. Advise to contact physician if persistent vomiting, diarrhea, fever, signs of dehydration, cough or breathing difficulties, or signs of an allergic reaction occur. Advise of the potential effects of vision abnormalities; instruct to use caution when driving and using machines.

EMPLICITI — elotuzumab   Rx

Class: Monoclonal antibody/SLAMF7-directed

ADULT DOSAGE
Multiple Myeloma

Use in combination w/ lenalidomide and dexamethasone for the treatment of patients w/ multiple myeloma who have received 1-3 prior therapies

Recommended Dose: 10mg/kg IV every week for the first 2 cycles and every 2 weeks thereafter; each cycle consists of 28 days

Continue treatment until disease progression or unacceptable toxicity

Dexamethasone:
Administer 28mg PO 3-24 hrs before elotuzumab plus 8mg IV 45-90 min before elotuzumab, on days that elotuzumab is administered. Administer 40mg PO on days that elotuzumab is not administered but a dose of dexamethasone is scheduled (Days 8 and 22 of cycle 3 and all subsequent cycles).

Lenalidomide:
25mg PO qd on Days 1-21 of a 28-day treatment cycle

Infusion Rate:
Cycle 1, Dose 1:
0-30 min: 0.5mL/min
30-60 min: 1mL/min
≥60 min: 2mL/min

Cycle 1, Dose 2:
0-30 min: 1mL/min
≥30 min: 2mL/min

Cycle 1, Dose 3 and 4 and All Subsequent Cycles:
2mL/min

Max: 2mL/min; 5mL/min in patients who have received 4 cycles of treatment

Premedication
Premedicate w/ the Following 45-90 min Prior to Each Elotuzumab Infusion:
- 8mg IV dexamethasone;
- 25-50mg PO or IV diphenhydramine or equivalent H1 blocker;
- 50mg IV or 150mg oral ranitidine or equivalent H2 blocker;
- 650-1000mg oral acetaminophen

PEDIATRIC DOSAGE
Pediatric use may not have been established

DOSING CONSIDERATIONS
Adverse Reactions
Infusion Reactions:
≥Grade 2: Interrupt elotuzumab infusion and institute appropriate medical/ supportive measures. Upon resolution to ≤Grade 1, restart at 0.5mL/min and

---

gradually increase at a rate of 0.5mL/min every 30 min as tolerated to the rate at which the infusion reaction occurred; resume escalation regimen if there is no recurrence of the infusion reaction. Monitor vital signs every 30 min for 2 hrs after end of infusion, in patients who experience an infusion reaction; if infusion reaction recurs, d/c elotuzumab infusion and do not restart on that day
Severe: May require permanent discontinuation and emergency treatment
Other Important Considerations
If the dose of 1 drug in the regimen is delayed, interrupted, or discontinued, treatment w/ the other drugs may continue as scheduled. If dexamethasone is delayed or discontinued, base decision whether to administer elotuzumab on clinical judgment (ie, risk of hypersensitivity)

ADMINISTRATION
IV route
Administer w/ an infusion set and sterile, nonpyrogenic, low-protein-binding filter (w/ a pore size of 0.2-1.2µm) using an automated infusion pump.
Do not mix w/, or administer as an infusion w/, other medicinal products.

Reconstitution
- Reconstitute 300mg vial w/ 13mL sterile water for inj (SWFI) and 400mg vial w/ 17mL SWFI; post-reconstitution concentration is 25mg/mL.
- Use a syringe of adequate size and ≤18-gauge needle.
- Dissolve by swirling/inverting vial; avoid vigorous agitation/shaking. The lyophilized powder should dissolve in <10 min.
- Allow reconstituted sol to stand for 5-10 min.

Dilution
- Once the reconstitution is completed, withdraw necessary volume for calculated dose from each vial, up to a max of 16mL from 400mg vial and 12mL from 300mg vial.
- Further dilute w/ 230mL of either 0.9% NaCl inj or D5 inj into an infusion bag made of polyvinyl chloride or polyolefin.
- Volume of 0.9% NaCl inj or D5 inj can be adjusted so as not to exceed 5mL/kg of patient weight at any given dose.

Complete infusion w/in 24 hrs of reconstitution. If not used immediately, may store at 2-8°C (36-46°F) and protect from light for up to 24 hrs (max of 8 hrs of the total 24 hrs can be at 20-25°C [68-77°F] and room light).

STORAGE
2-8°C (36-46°F). Protect from light. Do not freeze or shake.

HOW SUPPLIED
Inj: 300mg, 400mg

CONTRAINDICATIONS
Refer to the individual monographs for lenalidomide and dexamethasone.

WARNINGS/PRECAUTIONS
See Dosing Considerations. May cause infusion reactions. Infections reported; monitor and treat promptly. Invasive second primary malignancies (SPMs) reported; monitor for development of SPMs. Elevations in liver enzymes consistent w/ hepatotoxicity reported; monitor liver enzymes periodically. D/C treatment upon ≥Grade 3 elevation of liver enzymes; may consider treatment continuation after return to baseline values. Can be detected on both serum protein electrophoresis and immunofixation assays used for the clinical monitoring of endogenous M-protein; may impact determination of complete response and possibly relapse from complete response in patients w/ IgG kappa myeloma protein.

ADVERSE REACTIONS
Fatigue, diarrhea, pyrexia, constipation, cough, peripheral neuropathy, nasopharyngitis, URTI, decreased appetite, pneumonia.

PREGNANCY AND LACTATION
Pregnancy: There are no studies w/ pregnant women to inform any drug-associated risks.
Lactation: Not for use in nursing.
Refer to the individual monographs for lenalidomide and dexamethasone.

MECHANISM OF ACTION
IgG1 monoclonal antibody that specifically targets the SLAMF7 protein. Directly activates natural killer cells through both the SLAMF7 pathway and Fc receptors. Also targets SLAMF7 on myeloma cells and facilitates the interaction w/ natural killer cells to mediate the killing of myeloma cells through antibody-dependent cellular cytotoxicity. The combination of elotuzumab and lenalidomide resulted in enhanced activation of natural killer cells that was greater than the effects of either agent alone and increased anti-tumor activity.

PATIENT CONSIDERATIONS
Assessment: Assess baseline liver enzyme values and pregnancy/nursing status.
Monitoring: Monitor for infusion reactions, infections, SPMs, hepatotoxicity, and other adverse reactions. Monitor liver enzymes periodically.
Counseling: Inform of risks/benefits of therapy. Advise to contact physician if experiencing signs/symptoms of infusion reactions w/in 24 hrs of infusion. Inform that oral premedication is necessary prior to infusion to reduce the risk of infusion reaction. Advise that lenalidomide has the potential to cause fetal harm and has specific requirements regarding contraception, pregnancy testing, blood and sperm donation, and transmission in sperm. Inform of the risk of developing infections and SPMs during treatment; instruct to report any symptoms of infection. Inform of the risk of hepatotoxicity and instruct to report any signs/ symptoms associated w/ this event.

EMTRIVA — emtricitabine Rx

Class: Nucleoside reverse transcriptase inhibitor (NRTI)

> Lactic acidosis and severe hepatomegaly with steatosis, including fatal cases, reported with the use of nucleoside analogues alone or in combination with other antiretrovirals. Not approved for the treatment of chronic hepatitis B virus (HBV) infection. Severe acute exacerbations of hepatitis B reported in patients who have discontinued therapy. Closely monitor hepatic function with both clinical and lab follow-up for at least several months in patients who are coinfected with HIV-1 and HBV and d/c therapy. If appropriate, initiation of antihepatitis B therapy may be warranted.

ADULT DOSAGE

HIV-1 Infection

Combination w/ Other Antiretrovirals:
Cap:
200mg qd
Sol:
240mg (24mL) qd

PEDIATRIC DOSAGE

HIV-1 Infection

Combination w/ Other Antiretrovirals
0-3 Months of Age:
Sol:
3mg/kg qd

3 Months-17 Years:
Cap:
<33kg: 200mg qd
Sol:
6mg/kg qd
Max: 240mg (24mL) qd

DOSING CONSIDERATIONS

Renal Impairment

CrCl 30-49mL/min:
Cap: 200mg q48h
Sol: 120mg (12mL) q24h

CrCl 15-29mL/min:
Cap: 200mg q72h
Sol: 80mg (8mL) q24h

CrCl <15mL/min or on Hemodialysis:
Cap: 200mg q96h; give dose after dialysis, if dosing on day of dialysis
Sol: 60mg (6mL) q24h; give dose after dialysis, if dosing on day of dialysis

ADMINISTRATION

Oral route

Take w/o regard to food

STORAGE

(Cap) 25°C (77°F); excursions permitted to 15-30°C (59-86°F). (Sol) 2-8°C (36-46°F). Use within 3 months if stored at 25°C (77°F).

HOW SUPPLIED

Cap: 200mg; **Sol:** 10mg/mL [170mL]

CONTRAINDICATIONS

Prior hypersensitivity to any of the components in this product.

WARNINGS/PRECAUTIONS

Obesity and prolonged nucleoside exposure may be risk factors for lactic acidosis and severe hepatomegaly with steatosis. Caution with known risk factors for liver disease. D/C if lactic acidosis or pronounced hepatotoxicity develops. Test for chronic HBV before initiating therapy. Reduce dose and closely monitor clinical response and renal function with renal impairment. Redistribution/accumulation of body fat and immune reconstitution syndrome reported. Autoimmune disorders (eg, Graves' disease, polymyositis, Guillain-Barre syndrome) in the setting of immune reconstitution reported. Caution in elderly.

ADVERSE REACTIONS

Lactic acidosis, severe hepatomegaly with steatosis, headache, diarrhea, nausea, fatigue, dizziness, depression, insomnia, abnormal dreams, rash, abdominal pain, asthenia, increased cough, rhinitis.

DRUG INTERACTIONS

Do not coadminister with emtricitabine- or lamivudine-containing products.

PREGNANCY AND LACTATION

Category B, not for use in nursing.

MECHANISM OF ACTION

Nucleoside reverse transcriptase inhibitor; inhibits the activity of the HIV-1 reverse transcriptase by competing with the natural substrate deoxycytidine 5'-triphosphate and by being incorporated into nascent viral DNA, which results in chain termination.

PHARMACOKINETICS

Absorption: Rapid and extensive. T_{max}=1-2 hrs. (Cap) Absolute bioavailability (93%); C_{max}=1.8mcg/mL; AUC=10mcg•hr/mL. (Sol) Absolute bioavailability (75%). **Distribution:** Plasma protein binding (<4%); found in breast milk. **Metabolism:** Oxidation and conjugation; 3'-sulfoxide diastereomers and 2'-O-glucuronide (metabolites). **Elimination:** Urine (86%), feces (14%); $T_{1/2}$=10 hrs.

PATIENT CONSIDERATIONS

Assessment: Assess for previous hypersensitivity, risk factors for lactic acidosis and liver disease, HBV infection, renal impairment, pregnancy/nursing status, and possible drug interactions.

Monitoring: Monitor for signs/symptoms of lactic acidosis, severe hepatomegaly with steatosis, hepatotoxicity, redistribution/accumulation of body fat, immune reconstitution syndrome, autoimmune disorders, and other adverse reactions. Closely monitor hepatic function with both clinical and lab follow-up for at least several months in patients who are coinfected with HIV-1 and HBV and d/c therapy. Closely monitor clinical response and renal function with renal impairment.

Counseling: Inform that therapy is not a cure for HIV-1 infection and illnesses associated with HIV-1 infection, including opportunistic infections, may continue. Instruct not to breastfeed, and not to share needles or other injection equipment and personal items that can have blood or body fluids on them (eg, toothbrushes, razor blades). Advise to always practice safer sex by using a latex or polyurethane condom to lower the chance of sexual contact with semen, vaginal secretions, or blood. Inform that it is important to take drug with combination therapy on a regular dosing schedule to avoid missing doses. Instruct to notify physician if symptoms suggestive of lactic acidosis or pronounced hepatotoxicity (eg, N/V, unusual or unexpected stomach discomfort, weakness) develop.

ENBREL — etanercept Rx

Class: Tumor necrosis factor (TNF) blocker

> Increased risk for developing serious infections (eg, active tuberculosis [TB], latent TB reactivation, invasive fungal infections, bacterial/viral infections, opportunistic infections) leading to hospitalization or death, mostly w/ concomitant use w/ immunosuppressants (eg, methotrexate [MTX], corticosteroids). D/C if serious infection or sepsis develops. Active/latent reactivation of TB may present w/ disseminated or extrapulmonary disease; test for latent TB before and during therapy and initiate treatment for latent TB prior to therapy. Consider empiric antifungal therapy in patients at risk for invasive fungal infections who develop severe systemic illness. Monitor for development of infection during and after treatment, including development of TB in patients who tested (-) for latent TB infection prior to therapy. Lymphoma and other malignancies, some fatal, reported in children and adolescents.

ADULT DOSAGE

Plaque Psoriasis

Initial: 50mg twice weekly for 3 months; initial doses of 25mg or 50mg/week were also shown to be efficacious
Maint: 50mg once weekly

Rheumatoid Arthritis

50mg weekly
Max: 50mg/week

May continue MTX, glucocorticoids, salicylates, NSAIDs, or analgesics during treatment

Psoriatic Arthritis

50mg weekly
Max: 50mg/week

May continue MTX, glucocorticoids, salicylates, NSAIDs, or analgesics during treatment

Ankylosing Spondylitis

50mg weekly
Max: 50mg/week

May continue MTX, glucocorticoids, salicylates, NSAIDs, or analgesics during treatment

PEDIATRIC DOSAGE

Juvenile Idiopathic Arthritis

Moderately to Severely Active:
≥2 Years:
<63kg: 0.8mg/kg weekly
≥63kg: 50mg weekly

May continue glucocorticoids, NSAIDs, or analgesics during treatment

ADMINISTRATION

SQ route

Do not mix contents of 1 vial of Enbrel sol w/ the contents of another vial of Enbrel.
Do not add any other medications to sol containing Enbrel.
Do not reconstitute Enbrel w/ other diluents.
Do not filter reconstituted sol during preparation or administration.

Preparation Using the Single-Use Prefilled Syringe

Leave at room temperature for about 15-30 min before injecting.
Check to see if the amount of liquid in the prefilled syringe falls between the 2 purple fill level indicator lines; do not use if the syringe does not have the right amount of liquid.

Preparation Using the SureClick Autoinjector

Leave at room temperature for at least 30 min before injecting.

Preparation Using the Multiple-Use Vial

Reconstitute w/ 1mL of sterile bacteriostatic water for inj (0.9% benzyl alcohol). Do not use vial adaptor if multiple doses are to be withdrawn from the vial; use a 25-gauge needle if the vial will be used for multiple doses.
Reconstituted sol must be refrigerated at 2-8°C (36-46°F) and used w/in 14 days; discard reconstituted sol after 14 days.
Leave at room temperature for about 15-30 min before injecting.

If Using Vial Adapter:

1. Twist adapter onto the diluents syringe.
2. Place vial adapter over Enbrel vial and insert vial adapter into vial stopper.
3. Push down on plunger to inject diluent into Enbrel vial; inject the diluent very slowly into the Enbrel vial if using a 25-gauge needle.
4. Keeping the diluent syringe in place, gently swirl the contents of the Enbrel vial during dissolution.
5. Withdraw the correct dose of reconstituted sol into the syringe.
6. Remove the syringe from the vial adapter or remove the 25-gauge needle from the syringe.
7. Attach a 27-gauge needle to inject Enbrel.

STORAGE

2-8°C (36-46°F). Do not shake. Protect from light or physical damage. Storage at room temperature at 20-25°C (68-77°F) for a max single period of 14 days is permissible, w/ protection from light, sources of heat, and (vial) humidity; once the product has been stored at room temperature, do not place back into the refrigerator. Discard if not used w/in 14 days at room temperature. Do not store in extreme heat or cold. Do not freeze. (Vial) **Reconstituted Sol:** Use immediately or may refrigerate for up to 14 days.

HOW SUPPLIED

Inj: 25mg [multiple-use vial, single-use prefilled syringe], 50mg [single-use prefilled syringe, single-use prefilled SureClick autoinjector]

CONTRAINDICATIONS

Sepsis.

WARNINGS/PRECAUTIONS

Do not initiate in patients w/ an active infection. Increased risk of infection in patients >65 yrs of age and in patients w/ comorbid conditions. New onset or exacerbation of CNS and peripheral nervous system demyelinating disorders, acute and chronic leukemia, new onset and worsening of CHF, melanoma and non-melanoma skin cancer, and Merkel cell carcinoma reported; consider periodic skin examinations for all patients at increased risk for skin cancer. Pancytopenia, including aplastic anemia, reported; consider discontinuation of therapy in patients w/ confirmed significant hematologic abnormalities. Reactivation of hepatitis B in patients who were previously infected w/ hepatitis B virus (HBV) reported; closely monitor for signs of active HBV infection during and for several months after therapy. Consider discontinuing therapy and initiating antiviral therapy w/ appropriate supportive treatment if HBV reactivation develops. Allergic reactions reported; d/c immediately and initiate appropriate therapy if an anaphylactic or other serious allergic reaction occurs. Needle cover of prefilled syringe and needle cover w/in the needle cap of autoinjector contain dry natural rubber; may cause allergic reactions in latex-sensitive individuals. If possible, pediatric patients should be brought up-to-date w/ all immunizations in agreement w/ current immunization guidelines prior to initiating therapy. May result in the formation of autoantibodies and in the development of a lupus-like syndrome or autoimmune hepatitis; d/c and evaluate patient if a lupus-like syndrome or autoimmune hepatitis develops. Caution w/ moderate to severe alcoholic hepatitis and in the elderly. Patients w/ a significant exposure to varicella virus should temporarily d/c therapy and be considered for prophylactic treatment w/ varicella zoster immune globulin.

ADVERSE REACTIONS

Infections, sepsis, malignancies, inj-site reactions, diarrhea, rash, pyrexia, pruritus.

DRUG INTERACTIONS

See Boxed Warning. Avoid w/ live vaccines. Not recommended w/ anakinra or abatacept; may increase risk of serious infections. Not recommended in patients w/ Wegener's granulomatosis receiving immunosuppressive agents; increased incidence of noncutaneous solid malignancies when added to standard therapy (eg, cyclophosphamide). Not recommended w/ cyclophosphamide. Mild decrease in mean neutrophil counts reported w/ sulfasalazine. Hypoglycemia reported following initiation of therapy in patients receiving antidiabetic medication; reduction in antidiabetic medication may be necessary.

PREGNANCY AND LACTATION

Category B, caution in nursing.

MECHANISM OF ACTION

TNF-blocker; inhibits binding of TNF-α and TNF-β (lymphotoxin alpha [LT-α]) to cell surface TNF-receptors, rendering TNF biologically inactive.

PHARMACOKINETICS

Absorption: C_{max}=2.4mcg/mL (50mg once weekly), 2.6mcg/mL (25mg twice weekly); T_{max}=69 hrs (single 25mg dose). **Distribution:** Found in breast milk; crosses the placenta. **Elimination:** $T_{1/2}$=102 hrs (single 25mg dose).

PATIENT CONSIDERATIONS

Assessment: Assess for sepsis, active/chronic/recurrent infection, history of an opportunistic infection, recent travel in areas of endemic TB or endemic mycoses, underlying conditions that may predispose to infection, central or peripheral nervous system demyelinating disorders, CHF, history of significant hematologic abnormalities, latex sensitivity, alcoholic hepatitis, risk for skin cancer, pregnancy/nursing status, and possible drug interactions. Test for latent TB infection and for HBV infection. Assess immunization history in pediatric patients.

Monitoring: Monitor for development of infection during and after treatment. Monitor for sepsis, central or peripheral nervous system demyelinating disorders, malignancies, new or worsening CHF, hematologic abnormalities, allergic reactions, lupus-like syndrome, autoimmune hepatitis, and other adverse reactions. Monitor for active TB and periodically test for latent TB. Monitor for HBV reactivation during therapy and for several months following termination of therapy. Consider periodic skin examinations for all patients at increased risk for skin cancer.

Counseling: Advise of the potential risks and benefits of therapy. Inform that therapy may lower the ability of immune system to fight infections; instruct to contact physician if any symptoms of infection, TB, or HBV develop. Advise to report any signs of new/worsening medical conditions (eg, CNS demyelinating disorders, CHF, autoimmune disorders) or any symptoms suggestive of pancytopenia. Counsel about the risk of lymphoma and other malignancies. Instruct to seek immediate medical attention if any symptoms of a severe allergic reaction develop. Advise that the needle cover of prefilled syringe and the needle cover w/in the needle cap of the autoinjector contain dry natural rubber (a derivative of latex), which may cause allergic reactions in individuals sensitive to latex. Instruct in inj technique, as well as proper syringe and needle disposal, and caution against reuse of needles and syringes. Advise to inform physician if pregnant/breastfeeding.

ENTYVIO — vedolizumab

Rx

Class: Monoclonal antibody/integrin receptor antagonist

ADULT DOSAGE

Ulcerative Colitis

Moderately to Severely Active:
For inducing/maintaining clinical response and remission, improving endoscopic appearance of the mucosa, and achieving corticosteroid-free remission in patients who have had an inadequate response w/, lost response to, or were intolerant to a TNF blocker or immunomodulator; or had an inadequate response w/, were intolerant to, or demonstrated dependence on corticosteroids

300mg IV infusion over 30 min at 0, 2, and 6 weeks and then every 8 weeks thereafter

D/C if no evidence of therapeutic benefit seen by Week 14

Crohn's Disease

Moderately to Severely Active:
For achieving clinical response and remission, and achieving corticosteroid-free remission in patients who have had an inadequate response w/, lost response to, or were intolerant to a TNF blocker or immunomodulator; or had an inadequate response w/, were intolerant to, or demonstrated dependence on corticosteroids

300mg IV infusion over 30 min at 0, 2, and 6 weeks and then every 8 weeks thereafter

D/C if no evidence of therapeutic benefit seen by Week 14

PEDIATRIC DOSAGE

Pediatric use may not have been established

ADMINISTRATION

IV route

Do not administer as an IV push or bolus.
Lyophilized powder must be reconstituted w/ sterile water for inj (SWFI) and diluted in 250mL of sterile 0.9% NaCl inj prior to administration.
After infusion is complete, flush w/ 30mL of sterile 0.9% NaCl inj.

Reconstitution

1. Reconstitute vial containing lyophilized powder w/ 4.8mL of SWFI using a syringe w/ a 21- to 25- gauge needle.
2. Insert the syringe needle into the vial through the center of the stopper and direct the stream of SWFI to the glass wall of the vial to avoid excessive foaming.
3. Gently swirl vial for at least 15 sec; do not vigorously shake or invert.
4. Allow sol to sit for up to 20 min at room temperature to allow for reconstitution and for any foam to settle; may swirl and inspect for dissolution during this time. If not fully dissolved after 20 min, allow another 10 min for dissolution; do not use vial if the drug product is not dissolved w/in 30 min.
5. Prior to withdrawing the reconstituted sol from vial, gently invert vial 3X.
6. Withdraw 5mL (300mg) of reconstituted sol using a syringe w/ a 21- to 25- gauge needle.

Dilution

Add the 5mL (300mg) of reconstituted sol to 250mL of 0.9% NaCl and gently mix infusion bag; once reconstituted and diluted, use infusion sol as soon as possible. Do not add other medicinal products to the prepared infusion sol or IV infusion set. May store infusion sol for up to 4 hrs at 2-8°C (36-46°F), if necessary; do not freeze.

STORAGE

2-8°C (36-46°F). Protect from light. **Infusion Sol:** 2-8°C (36-46°F) for up to 4 hrs. Do not freeze.

HOW SUPPLIED

Inj: 300mg

CONTRAINDICATIONS

Known serious or severe hypersensitivity reaction to vedolizumab or any of the excipients (eg, dyspnea, bronchospasm, urticaria, flushing, rash, increased HR).

WARNINGS/PRECAUTIONS

Hypersensitivity reactions reported; d/c immediately and initiate appropriate treatment if anaphylaxis or other serious allergic reactions occur. Increased risk for developing infections; not recommended in patients with active, severe infections until the infections are controlled. Consider withholding treatment if a severe infection develops. Consider screening for tuberculosis according to the local practice. Progressive multifocal leukoencephalopathy (PML) may occur; monitor for any new onset, or worsening, of neurological signs and symptoms. If PML is suspected, withhold dosing and refer to a neurologist; if confirmed, d/c dosing permanently. Elevations of transaminase and/or bilirubin reported; d/c if jaundice or other evidence of significant liver injury develops. Prior to initiating treatment, all patients should be brought up to date with all immunizations according to current immunization guidelines.

ADVERSE REACTIONS

Nasopharyngitis, headache, arthralgia, nausea, pyrexia, upper respiratory tract infection, fatigue, cough, bronchitis, influenza, back pain, rash, pruritus, sinusitis, oropharyngeal pain, pain in extremities.

DRUG INTERACTIONS

Avoid with natalizumab; potential for increased risk of PML and other infections. Avoid with TNF blockers; potential for increased risk of infections. Live vaccines may be administered concurrently with therapy only if the benefits outweigh the risks.

PREGNANCY AND LACTATION

Category B, caution in nursing.

MECHANISM OF ACTION

Monoclonal antibody/integrin receptor antagonist; specifically binds to the α4β7 integrin and blocks the interaction of α4β7 integrin with mucosal addressin cell adhesion molecule-1 and inhibits the migration of memory T-lymphocytes across the endothelium into inflamed GI parenchymal tissue.

PHARMACOKINETICS

Distribution: V_d=5L; crosses placenta. **Elimination:** $T_{1/2}$=25 days.

PATIENT CONSIDERATIONS

Assessment: Assess for hypersensitivity to drug, infections, history of recurring severe infections, pregnancy/nursing status, and possible drug interactions. Assess immunization history.

Monitoring: Monitor for infusion/hypersensitivity reactions, infections, PML, liver injury, and other adverse reactions.

Counseling: Instruct to report immediately if symptoms consistent with a hypersensitivity reaction occur during or following infusion. Advise to notify physician if any signs/symptoms of infection develop. Instruct to report immediately any symptoms that may indicate PML (new onset or worsening of neurological signs/symptoms) and/or liver injury (eg, fatigue, anorexia, right upper abdominal discomfort, dark urine, jaundice).

ENVARSUS XR — tacrolimus   Rx

Class: Calcineurin-inhibitor immunosuppressant

> Increased risk for developing serious infections and malignancies w/ tacrolimus extended-release (ER) or other immunosuppressants that may lead to hospitalization or death.

ADULT DOSAGE

Organ Rejection Prophylaxis

Prophylaxis of organ rejection in kidney transplant patients converted from tacrolimus immediate-release (IR) formulations, in combination w/ other immunosuppressants

Conversion from Tacrolimus IR Formulations:

Administer an Envarsus XR qd dose that is 80% of the total daily dose of the tacrolimus IR product

Monitor tacrolimus whole blood trough concentrations and titrate dose to achieve target whole blood trough concentration ranges of 4-11ng/mL

African-American patients, compared to Caucasian patients, may need to be titrated to higher doses to attain comparable trough concentrations

Therapeutic Drug Monitoring:

Measure tacrolimus whole blood trough concentrations at least 2X on separate days during the first week after initiation of dosing and after any change in dosage, after a change in coadministration of CYP3A inducers and/or inhibitors, or after a change in renal or hepatic function

When interpreting measured concentrations, consider that the time to achieve tacrolimus steady state is approx 7 days after initiating or changing the dose

Missed Dose

If a dose is missed, the dose should be taken as soon as possible w/in 15 hrs after missing the dose

Beyond the 15-hr time frame, the patient should wait until the usual scheduled time to take the next regular daily dose; it is not recommended to double the next dose to make up for the missed dose

PEDIATRIC DOSAGE

Pediatric use may not have been established

DOSING CONSIDERATIONS

Hepatic Impairment

Severe (Child-Pugh >10): May require lower doses

ADMINISTRATION

Oral route

Take on an empty stomach at the same time of the day, preferably in the am. Swallow whole w/ fluid (preferably water); do not chew, divide, or crush. Not interchangeable or substitutable w/ other tacrolimus ER or IR products. Avoid eating grapefruit or drinking grapefruit juice or alcoholic beverages.

STORAGE

25°C (77°F); excursions permitted to 15-30°C (59-86°F).

HOW SUPPLIED

Tab, ER: 0.75mg, 1mg, 4mg

CONTRAINDICATIONS

Known hypersensitivity to tacrolimus.

WARNINGS/PRECAUTIONS

Increases risk of developing lymphomas and other malignancies, particularly of the skin. Post-transplant lymphoproliferative disorder (PTLD), associated w/ Epstein-Barr virus (EBV), has been reported in immunosuppressed organ transplant patients; risk of PTLD appears greatest in those individuals who are EBV seronegative; monitor EBV serology during treatment. Increases risk of developing bacterial, viral (eg, polyomavirus-associated nephropathy, JC virus-associated progressive multifocal leukoencephalopathy, CMV infection), fungal, and protozoal infections, including opportunistic infections; monitor for the development of infection and adjust immunosuppressive regimen to balance the risk of rejection w/ risk of infection. Graft rejection and other serious adverse reactions due to medication errors reported; not interchangeable or substitutable w/ other tacrolimus ER or IR products. New onset diabetes reported after transplant. Can cause acute or chronic nephrotoxicity; consider dosage reduction in patients w/ elevated SrCr and tacrolimus whole blood trough concentrations greater than the recommended range. May cause a spectrum of neurotoxicities; consider dosage reduction or discontinuation if neurotoxicity occurs. Mild to severe hyperkalemia reported. HTN may occur and antihypertensive therapy may be required. May prolong the QT/QTc interval and cause torsades de pointes; avoid in patients w/ congenital long QT syndrome. Consider obtaining ECG and monitoring electrolytes (Mg^{2+}, K^+, Ca^{2+}) periodically during treatment in patients w/ CHF, bradyarrhythmias, those taking certain antiarrhythmic medications or other products that lead to QT prolongation, and those w/ electrolyte disturbances. Whenever possible, administer the complete complement of vaccines before transplantation and therapy. Cases of pure red cell aplasia (PRCA) reported; consider discontinuation of therapy if PRCA is diagnosed.

ADVERSE REACTIONS

Diarrhea, increased blood creatinine, UTI, nasopharyngitis, headache, URTI, peripheral edema, HTN.

DRUG INTERACTIONS

See Administration. Risk for nephrotoxicity may increase when concomitantly administered w/ CYP3A inhibitors or drugs associated w/ nephrotoxicity (eg, aminoglycosides, ganciclovir, amphotericin B, cisplatin, protease inhibitors); monitor renal function and consider dosage reduction if nephrotoxicity occurs. Agents associated w/ hyperkalemia (eg, K^+-sparing diuretics, ACE inhibitors, ARB[s]) may increase risk for hyperkalemia. Avoid use of live attenuated vaccines during treatment. Inactivated vaccines noted to be safe for administration after transplantation may not be sufficiently immunogenic during treatment w/ Envarsus XR. Increases exposure to mycophenolic acid (MPA) products; monitor for MPA associated adverse reactions and reduce dose of concomitantly administered MPA products as needed. Grapefruit or grapefruit juice may increase tacrolimus whole blood trough concentrations and increase risk of serious adverse reactions. Alcohol may modify rate of tacrolimus release. Strong CYP3A inducers (eg, rifampin, phenytoin, St. John's wort) may decrease tacrolimus whole blood trough concentrations and increase risk of rejection; increase Envarsus XR dose and monitor tacrolimus whole blood trough concentrations. Strong CYP3A inhibitors (eg, nelfinavir, telaprevir, voriconazole, posaconazole) may increase tacrolimus whole blood trough concentrations and increase the risk of serious adverse reactions; reduce Envarsus XR (for voriconazole and posaconazole, give 1/3 of the original dose) and adjust dose based on tacrolimus whole blood trough concentrations. Mild or moderate CYP3A inhibitors (eg, clotrimazole, erythromycin, verapamil, amiodarone) and other drugs (eg, Mg^{2+} and aluminum hydroxide antacids, metoclopramide) may increase tacrolimus whole blood trough concentrations and increase the risk of serious adverse reactions; monitor tacrolimus whole blood trough concentrations and reduce Envarsus XR dose if needed. Mild or moderate CYP3A inducers (eg, methylprednisolone, prednisone) may decrease tacrolimus concentrations; monitor tacrolimus whole blood trough concentrations and adjust Envarsus XR dose if needed.

PREGNANCY AND LACTATION

Pregnancy: Category C.
Lactation: Present in breast milk; not for use in nursing.

MECHANISM OF ACTION

Macrolide immunosuppressant; binds to FKBP-12, forming a complex of tacrolimus-FKBP-12, Ca^{2+}, calmodulin, and calcineurin, and inhibiting phosphatase activity of calcineurin. Inhibits the expression and/or production of several cytokines that include interleukin (IL)-1 beta, IL-2, IL-3, IL-4, IL-5, IL-6, IL-8, IL-10, gamma interferon, TNF-α, and granulocyte macrophage colony stimulating factor. Also inhibits IL-2 receptor expression and nitric oxide release, induces apoptosis and production of transforming growth factor-β that can lead to immunosuppressive activity. Net result is inhibition of T-lymphocyte activation and proliferation as well as T-helper-cell-dependent B-cell response.

PHARMACOKINETICS

Absorption: Administration of variable doses in different populations resulted in different pharmacokinetic parameters. **Distribution:** Plasma protein binding (99%); crosses placenta; found in breast milk. **Metabolism:** Liver (extensive), via CYP3A (demethylation and hydroxylation); 13-demethyl tacrolimus (major metabolite); 31-demethyl metabolite (active metabolite). **Excretion:** Feces (92.6%), urine (2.3%); $T_{1/2}$=31 hrs (2mg qd).

PATIENT CONSIDERATIONS

Assessment: Assess for congenital long QT syndrome, CHF, bradyarrhythmias, electrolyte disturbances, renal/hepatic impairment, hypersensitivity to the drug, pregnancy/nursing status, and possible drug interactions.

Monitoring: Monitor for lymphomas and other malignancies, infections (including opportunistic infections), nephrotoxicity, neurotoxicity, HTN, QT prolongation, PRCA, and for other adverse reactions. Measure tacrolimus whole blood trough concentrations at least 2X on separate days during the first week after initiation of dosing and after any change in dosage, after a change in coadministration of CYP3A inducers and/or inhibitors, or after a change in renal or hepatic function. Monitor serum K^+ and glucose concentrations. Monitor EBV serology. Consider obtaining ECG and monitoring electrolytes (Mg^{2+}, Ca^{2+}) periodically during treatment in patients w/ CHF, bradyarrhythmias, those taking certain antiarrhythmic medications or other products that lead to QT prolongation, and those w/ electrolyte disturbances.

Counseling: Inform of the risks and benefits of therapy. Instruct to inspect the medicine when a new prescription is received and before taking it. Advise to avoid alcohol, grapefruit, or grapefruit juice while on therapy. Instruct to take a missed dose as soon as remembered but not more than 15 hrs after the scheduled time; beyond the 15-hr timeframe, instruct to wait until the usual scheduled time the following am to take the next scheduled dose. Advise to limit exposure to sunlight and UV light by wearing protective clothing and using sunscreen w/ a high protection factor. Instruct to contact physician if any symptoms of infection, frequent urination, increased thirst or hunger, vision changes, delirium, or tremors develop. Inform that therapy can cause high BP that may require treatment w/ antihypertensive therapy. Inform that drug can cause hyperkalemia and that monitoring of K^+ levels may be necessary. Advise that drug can interfere w/ the usual response to immunizations and that patient should avoid live vaccines. Instruct to attend all visits and complete all blood tests ordered by medical team. Instruct to inform physician if planning to become pregnant or to breastfeed, or if starting or stopping any concomitant medications.

EPCLUSA — sofosbuvir/velpatasvir   Rx

Class: HCV NS5A inhibitor/HCV nucleotide analogue NS5B polymerase inhibitor

ADULT DOSAGE	PEDIATRIC DOSAGE
Chronic Hepatitis C	Pediatric use may not have been established
Genotype 1, 2, 3, 4, 5, or 6:	
W/O Cirrhosis or w/ Compensated Cirrhosis (Child-Pugh A):	
1 tab qd for 12 weeks	
W/ Decompensated Cirrhosis (Child-Pugh B or C):	
1 tab qd + ribavirin for 12 weeks	
For further information on ribavirin dosing and dosing modifications, refer to the ribavirin PI	

DOSING CONSIDERATIONS

Renal Impairment
Mild/Moderate: No dosage adjustment required
Severe (eGFR <30mL/min/1.73m²)/ESRD: No dosage recommendation can be given due to higher exposures of the predominant sofosbuvir metabolite

ADMINISTRATION

Oral route
Take w/ or w/o food.

STORAGE

<30°C (86°F).

HOW SUPPLIED

Tab: (Sofosbuvir/Velpatasvir) 400mg/100mg

CONTRAINDICATIONS

Combination therapy w/ ribavirin is contraindicated in patients for whom ribavirin is contraindicated; refer to ribavirin PI.

WARNINGS/PRECAUTIONS

Serious symptomatic bradycardia reported when amiodarone is coadministered w/ sofosbuvir and another HCV direct-acting antiviral. Fatal cardiac arrest reported in a patient taking amiodarone who was coadministered a sofosbuvir-containing regimen. Patients also taking β-blockers, or those w/ underlying cardiac comorbidities and/or advanced liver disease, may be at increased risk for symptomatic bradycardia w/ coadministration of amiodarone. Not recommended w/ amiodarone. If coadministration is required, cardiac monitoring in an in-patient setting for the first 48 hrs of coadministration is recommended, after which outpatient or self-monitoring of HR should occur on a daily basis through at least the first 2 weeks of therapy. Patients discontinuing amiodarone just prior to starting therapy should also undergo similar cardiac monitoring. P-gp inducers and/or moderate to potent CYP2B6,

CYP2C8, or CYP3A4 inducers (eg, rifampin, St. John's wort, carbamazepine) may significantly decrease plasma concentrations; concomitant use not recommended. If administered w/ ribavirin, refer to the ribavirin PI for the warnings and precautions for ribavirin.

ADVERSE REACTIONS

Monotherapy: Headache, fatigue.
W/ Ribavirin: Fatigue, anemia, nausea, headache, insomnia, diarrhea.

DRUG INTERACTIONS

See Warnings/Precautions. May increase topotecan, rosuvastatin, and atorvastatin levels; coadministration w/ topotecan not recommended. Monitor for HMG-CoA reductase inhibitor-associated adverse reactions. May increase digoxin levels; monitor digoxin levels. Do not exceed rosuvastatin dose of 10mg. Decreased levels w/ carbamazepine, phenytoin, phenobarbital, oxcarbazepine, rifabutin, rifampin, rifapentine, tipranavir/ritonavir, and St. John's wort; coadministration not recommended. May increase tenofovir levels when coadministered w/ tenofovir disoproxil fumarate-containing regimens; monitor for tenofovir-associated adverse reactions. **Velpatasvir:** Inhibits drug transporters P-gp, BCRP, OATP1B1, OATP1B3, and OATP2B1; may increase exposure of substrates of these transporters. Decreased concentrations w/ drugs that increase gastric pH (eg, antacids, H_2-receptor antagonists, proton pump inhibitor [PPIs]). Separate antacid administration by 4 hrs. H_2-receptor antagonists may be administered simultaneously w/ or 12 hrs apart from Epclusa at a dose that does not exceed doses comparable to famotidine 40mg bid. Coadministration w/ PPIs not recommended. If necessary, administer Epclusa w/ food 4 hrs before omeprazole 20mg; use w/ other PPIs has not been studied. Decreased levels w/ efavirenz; coadministration w/ efavirenz-containing regimens not recommended. Refer to PI for further dosing modifications when used w/ certain concomitant medications.

PREGNANCY AND LACTATION

Pregnancy: No adequate human data are available to establish whether or not Epclusa poses a risk to pregnancy outcomes.
Lactation: It is not known whether the components of Epclusa and its metabolites are present in human breast milk, affect human milk production, or have effects on the breastfed infant; caution in nursing.

If administered w/ ribavirin, refer to the PI of ribavirin for additional information.

MECHANISM OF ACTION

Sofosbuvir: HCV nucleotide analogue NS5B polymerase inhibitor; undergoes intracellular metabolism to form the pharmacologically active uridine analogue triphosphate (GS-461203), which can be incorporated into HCV RNA by the NS5B polymerase and acts as a chain terminator. **Velpatasvir:** HCV NS5A protein inhibitor; HCV NS5A protein is required for viral replication.

PHARMACOKINETICS

Absorption: Sofosbuvir: T_{max}=0.5-1 hrs. C_{max}=567ng/mL, 898ng/mL (GS-331007). AUC=1268ng•hr/mL, 14,372ng•hr/mL (GS-331007). Velpatasvir: T_{max}=3 hrs. C_{max}=259ng/mL. AUC=2980ng•hr/mL. **Distribution:** Sofosbuvir: Plasma protein binding (61-65% sofosbuvir). Velpatasvir: Plasma protein binding (>99.5% velpatasvir). **Metabolism:** Sofosbuvir: Via Cathepsin A, CES1, and HINT1. Prodrug that undergoes intracellular metabolism to form GS-461203. GS-331007 is the primary circulating metabolite. Velpatasvir: Via CYP2B6, CYP2C8, CYP3A4. **Elimination:** Sofosbuvir: Urine (80%, predominantly as GS-331007), feces (14%); $T_{1/2}$=0.5 hrs, 25 hrs (GS-331007) (median). Velpatasvir: Urine (0.4%), feces (94%); $T_{1/2}$=15 hrs (median).

PATIENT CONSIDERATIONS

Assessment: Assess for hypersensitivity to drug, cardiac comorbidities, renal impairment, pregnancy/nursing status, and for potential drug interactions.

Monitoring: Monitor for bradycardia if coadministering w/ amiodarone or if discontinuing amiodarone just prior to starting therapy; perform cardiac monitoring in an in-patient setting for the first 48 hrs of coadministration, after which outpatient or self-monitoring of the HR should occur on a daily basis through at least the first 2 weeks of treatment. Perform clinical and hepatic lab monitoring for patients w/ decompensated cirrhosis receiving concomitant treatment w/ ribavirin. Monitor for other adverse reactions.

Counseling: Advise to take ud. Inform that it is important not to miss or skip doses and to continue therapy for the recommended duration. Advise to seek medical evaluation immediately for symptoms of bradycardia. Inform that treatment may interact w/ other drugs and advise to report to healthcare provider the use of any other prescription or nonprescription medication or herbal products. Advise to avoid pregnancy during combination treatment w/ ribavirin and for 6 months after completion of treatment. Instruct to notify healthcare provider immediately in the event of a pregnancy.

EPIVIR — lamivudine   Rx

Class: Nucleoside reverse transcriptase inhibitor (NRTI)

Lactic acidosis and severe hepatomegaly w/ steatosis, including fatal cases, reported w/ nucleoside analogues; d/c treatment if lactic acidosis or pronounced hepatotoxicity occurs. Severe acute exacerbations of hepatitis B reported in patients coinfected w/ hepatitis B virus (HBV) upon discontinuation of therapy; closely monitor hepatic function for at least several months. If appropriate, initiation of antihepatitis B therapy may be warranted. Epivir tabs and oral sol (used to treat HIV-1 infection) contain a higher dose of lamivudine than Epivir-HBV tabs and oral sol (used to treat chronic HBV infection); patients w/ HIV-1 infection should only receive dosage forms appropriate for HIV-1 treatment.

ADULT DOSAGE
HIV-1 Infection
In Combination w/ Other Antiretrovirals:
150mg bid or 300mg qd

If lamivudine is administered to a patient infected w/ HIV-1 and HBV, the dosage indicated for HIV-1 therapy should be used as part of an appropriate combination regimen

PEDIATRIC DOSAGE
HIV-1 Infection
In Combination w/ Other Antiretrovirals:
≥3 Months of Age:
Oral Sol:
4mg/kg bid or 8mg/kg qd
Max: 300mg/day

Tab:
QD Dosing Regimen:
14 to <20kg: 150mg
≥20 to <25kg: 225mg
≥25kg: 300mg

Data regarding the efficacy of qd dosing is limited to subjects who transitioned from bid dosing to qd dosing after 36 weeks of treatment

BID Dosing Regimen (Using Scored 150mg Tab):
14 to <20kg:
AM Dose: 75mg
PM Dose: 75mg
Total Daily Dose: 150mg

≥20 to <25kg:
AM Dose: 75mg
PM Dose: 150mg
Total Daily Dose: 225mg

≥25kg:
AM Dose: 150mg
PM Dose: 150mg
Total Daily Dose: 300mg

DOSING CONSIDERATIONS
Renal Impairment
Adults and Adolescents (≥25kg):
CrCl ≥50mL/min: 150mg bid or 300mg qd
CrCl 30-49mL/min: 150mg qd
CrCl 15-29mL/min: 150mg 1st dose, then 100mg qd
CrCl 5-14mL/min: 150mg 1st dose, then 50mg qd
CrCl <5mL/min: 50mg 1st dose, then 25mg qd
No additional dosing is required after routine (4-hr) hemodialysis or peritoneal dialysis
Pediatric Patients:
Consider dose reduction and/or increase in dosing interval

ADMINISTRATION
Oral route

Take w/ or w/o food.
Pediatric Patients
Epivir scored tab is the preferred formulation for HIV-1 infected pediatric patients who weigh ≥14kg and for whom a solid dosage form is appropriate.
Assess ability to swallow tabs before prescribing; for patients unable to safely and reliably swallow tabs, oral sol should be prescribed.

STORAGE
Tab: 25°C (77°F); excursions permitted to 15-30°C (59-86°F). **Oral Sol:** 25°C (77°F).

HOW SUPPLIED
Oral Sol: 10mg/mL [240mL]; **Tab:** 150mg*, 300mg *scored

CONTRAINDICATIONS
Previous hypersensitivity reaction to lamivudine.

WARNINGS/PRECAUTIONS
Obesity and prolonged nucleoside exposure may be risk factors for lactic acidosis and severe hepatomegaly w/ steatosis. Caution w/ known risk factors for liver disease. Emergence of lamivudine-resistant HBV reported. Caution in pediatric patients w/ a history of prior antiretroviral nucleoside exposure, history of pancreatitis, or other significant risk factors for development of pancreatitis; d/c if pancreatitis develops. Immune reconstitution syndrome reported. Autoimmune disorders (eg, Graves' disease, polymyositis, Guillain-Barre syndrome) reported to occur in the setting of immune reconstitution and can occur many months after initiation of treatment. Redistribution/accumulation of body fat may occur. Lower virologic suppression rates, lower plasma lamivudine exposure, and viral resistance reported more frequently in pediatric patients who received oral sol than those who received tabs; consider more frequent monitoring of HIV-1 viral load w/ oral sol. Consider HIV-1 viral load and CD4+ cell count/percentage when selecting the dosing interval for patients initiating treatment w/ oral sol. Caution in elderly.

ADVERSE REACTIONS
Adults: Headache, nausea, malaise, fatigue, nasal signs/symptoms, diarrhea, cough.
Pediatric Patients: Fever, cough.

DRUG INTERACTIONS
Hepatic decompensation reported in HIV-1/hepatitis C virus coinfected patients receiving antiretroviral therapy for HIV-1 and interferon-alfa w/ or w/o ribavirin; closely monitor for treatment-associated toxicities during coadministration and consider discontinuation of lamivudine as medically appropriate. Possible interaction w/ drugs whose main route of elimination is active renal secretion via the organic cationic transport system (eg, trimethoprim).

PREGNANCY AND LACTATION
Pregnancy: Physicians are encouraged to register patients in the Antiretroviral Pregnancy Registry. Embryonic toxicity produced in rabbits at a dose that produced similar human exposures as the recommended clinical dose; relevance to human pregnancy registry data is unknown.
Lactation: Mothers should be instructed not to breastfeed due to potential for HIV-1 transmission.

MECHANISM OF ACTION
Nucleoside analogue. Lamivudine is phosphorylated to its active 5'-triphosphate metabolite, lamivudine triphosphate (3TC-TP); 3TC-TP inhibits HIV-1 reverse transcriptase via DNA chain termination after incorporation of the nucleotide analogue into viral DNA.

PHARMACOKINETICS
Absorption: Rapid; absolute bioavailability (86% [150mg tab], 87% [oral sol]); $AUC_{(0-12)}$=5.53mcg•h/mL; C_{max}=1.4mcg/mL; T_{max}=0.9 hrs (fasting), 3.2 hrs (fed). **Distribution:** V_d=1.3L/kg (IV); plasma protein binding (<36%); crosses placenta. **Metabolism:** Trans-sulfoxide (metabolite). **Elimination:** Urine (majority unchanged); $T_{1/2}$=5-7 hrs.

PATIENT CONSIDERATIONS
Assessment: Assess for renal impairment, risk factors for lactic acidosis and liver disease, HIV-1 and HBV coinfection, previous hypersensitivity, pregnancy/nursing status, and possible drug interactions. In pediatric patients, assess for a history of prior antiretroviral nucleoside exposure, a history of pancreatitis, or risk factors for pancreatitis. Consider HIV-1 viral load and CD4+ cell count/percentage when selecting the dosing interval for patients initiating treatment w/ oral sol.
Monitoring: Monitor for signs/symptoms of pancreatitis, immune reconstitution syndrome, autoimmune disorders, fat redistribution/accumulation, lactic acidosis, hepatomegaly w/ steatosis, hepatitis B exacerbation, renal dysfunction, and hypersensitivity reactions. Monitor hepatic function closely for several months in patients w/ HIV/HBV coinfection who d/c therapy.
Counseling: Inform about risks/benefits of therapy. Advise that lactic acidosis and severe hepatomegaly w/ steatosis have been reported w/ use of nucleoside analogues; instruct to d/c if symptoms suggestive of lactic acidosis or pronounced hepatotoxicity develop. Advise to discuss any changes in regimen w/ physician. Advise parents/guardians of pediatric patients to monitor for signs and symptoms of pancreatitis. Instruct to inform physician immediately of any signs/symptoms of infection. Inform that redistribution/accumulation of body fat may occur. Advise diabetic patients that each 15mL dose of oral sol contains 3g of sucrose. Advise that there is a pregnancy exposure registry that monitors pregnancy outcomes in women exposed to therapy during pregnancy. Instruct women w/ HIV-1 infection not to breastfeed.

EPIVIR-HBV — lamivudine   Rx
Class: Nucleoside reverse transcriptase inhibitor (NRTI)

> Lactic acidosis and severe hepatomegaly with steatosis, including fatal cases, reported with nucleoside analogues. Suspend treatment if lactic acidosis or pronounced hepatotoxicity occurs. Severe acute exacerbations of hepatitis B reported upon discontinuation of therapy; closely monitor hepatic function for at least several months. If appropriate, initiation of antihepatitis B therapy may be warranted. Not approved for treatment of HIV infection. Lamivudine dosage in Epivir-HBV is subtherapeutic and monotherapy is inappropriate for treatment of HIV infection. HIV-1 resistance may emerge in chronic hepatitis B-infected patients with unrecognized/untreated HIV infection. Offer HIV counseling and testing to all patients prior to therapy and periodically thereafter.

ADULT DOSAGE
Chronic Hepatitis B
100mg qd

PEDIATRIC DOSAGE
Chronic Hepatitis B
2-17 Years:
3mg/kg qd
Max: 100mg/day

DOSING CONSIDERATIONS
Renal Impairment
CrCl 30-49mL/min: 100mg 1st dose, then 50mg qd
CrCl 15-29mL/min: 100mg 1st dose, then 25mg qd
CrCl 5-14mL/min: 35mg 1st dose, then 15mg qd
CrCl <5mL/min: 35mg 1st dose, then 10mg qd

ADMINISTRATION
Oral route

Take w/ or w/o food.
Tabs and oral sol are interchangeable.
Use oral sol for doses <100mg.
Do not use w/ other medications that contain lamivudine or emtricitabine.
Refer to PI for assessing patients during treatment.

STORAGE
Tab: 25°C (77°F); excursions permitted to 15-30°C (59-86°F). **Sol:** 20-25°C (68-77°F); store in tightly closed bottles.

HOW SUPPLIED
Oral Sol: 5mg/mL [240mL]; **Tab:** 100mg

CONTRAINDICATIONS
Previous hypersensitivity reaction (eg, anaphylaxis) to lamivudine or to any component of the tabs or oral sol.

WARNINGS/PRECAUTIONS

Consider initiation of treatment only when use of an alternative antiviral agent with a higher genetic barrier to resistance is not available/appropriate. Obesity and prolonged nucleoside exposure may be risk factors for lactic acidosis and severe hepatomegaly with steatosis. Caution with known risk factors for liver disease. Emergence of resistance-associated HBV substitutions reported; monitor ALT and HBV DNA levels if suspected. Not approved for patients dually infected with HBV and HIV. Epivir HBV contains a lower lamivudine dose than Epivir, Combivir, Epzicom, and Trizivir. If a decision is made to administer lamivudine to such coinfected patients, use the higher dosage indicated for HIV therapy as part of an appropriate combination regimen and refer to PI of such drugs. Caution in elderly patients.

ADVERSE REACTIONS

Lactic acidosis, severe hepatomegaly with steatosis, exacerbations of hepatitis B, ear/nose/throat infections, sore throat, diarrhea, serum lipase increase, CPK increase, ALT increase, thrombocytopenia.

DRUG INTERACTIONS

Avoid with other lamivudine- and emtricitabine-containing products. Possible interaction with other drugs whose main route of elimination is active renal secretion via the organic cationic transport system (eg, trimethoprim).

PREGNANCY AND LACTATION

Category C, not for use in nursing.

MECHANISM OF ACTION

Nucleoside analogue; inhibits HBV reverse transcriptase via DNA chain termination after incorporation of the nucleotide analogue into viral DNA.

PHARMACOKINETICS

Absorption: Absolute bioavailability (86% tab, 87% sol); AUC=4.7mcg•hr/mL (repeated daily doses); C_{max}=1.28mcg/mL; T_{max}=0.5-2.0 hrs. **Distribution:** V_d=1.3L/kg (IV); plasma protein binding (<36%); found in breast milk. **Metabolism:** Transsulfoxide (metabolite). **Elimination:** Urine (unchanged); $T_{1/2}$=5-7 hrs.

PATIENT CONSIDERATIONS

Assessment: Assess for hepatic/renal impairment, previous nucleoside exposure, risk factors for liver disease, HIV infection, hypersensitivity to drug, pregnancy/nursing status, and possible drug interactions. Perform HIV counseling and testing. Obtain baseline ALT and HBV DNA levels.

Monitoring: Monitor for renal/hepatic dysfunction, loss of therapeutic response (eg, persistent ALT elevation, increasing HBV DNA levels after an initial decline below assay limit, progression of clinical signs/symptoms of hepatic disease, worsening of hepatic necroinflammatory findings), signs/symptoms of lactic acidosis, hepatomegaly with steatosis, emergence of resistant HIV, hepatitis B exacerbation, and hypersensitivity reactions. Monitor hepatic function closely for several months in patients who d/c therapy.

Counseling: Advise to remain under the care of a physician during therapy and to report any new symptoms or concurrent medications. Inform that drug is not a cure for hepatitis B and that long-term benefits and relationship of initial treatment response to outcomes (eg, hepatocellular carcinoma, decompensated cirrhosis) are unknown. Inform that liver disease deterioration may occur upon discontinuation. Instruct to discuss any changes in regimen with physician. Inform that emergence of resistant HBV and worsening of disease can occur; advise to report any new symptoms to physician. Counsel on importance of HIV testing to avoid inappropriate therapy and development of resistant HIV. Inform that drug contains a lower dose of lamivudine than Epivir, Combivir, Epzicom, and Trizivir; instruct not to take concurrently with these products. Instruct not to take concurrently with emtricitabine-containing products (eg, Atripla, Complera, Emtriva, Stribild, Truvada). Inform that therapy has not been shown to reduce the risk of HBV transmission through sexual contact/blood contamination. Instruct to avoid doing things that can spread HBV infection to others. Inform diabetics that each 20mL dose of oral sol contains 4g of sucrose.

EPOGEN — epoetin alfa

Rx

Class: Erythropoiesis-stimulating agent (ESA)

> Increased risk of death, MI, stroke, venous thromboembolism (VTE), thrombosis of vascular access, and tumor progression or recurrence. Use the lowest dose sufficient to reduce/avoid the need for RBC transfusions. Chronic Kidney Disease (CKD): Greater risks for death, serious adverse cardiovascular (CV) reactions, and stroke when administered to target Hgb level >11g/dL. Cancer: Shortened overall survival and/or increased risk of tumor progression or recurrence in patients with breast, non-small cell lung, head and neck, lymphoid, and cervical cancers. Must enroll in and comply with the ESA APPRISE Oncology Program to prescribe and/or dispense drug to patients. Use only for anemia from myelosuppressive chemotherapy. Not indicated for patients receiving myelosuppressive chemotherapy when anticipated outcome is cure. D/C following completion of a chemotherapy course. Perisurgery: Due to increased risk of deep venous thrombosis (DVT), DVT prophylaxis is recommended.

ADULT DOSAGE

Anemia

Chronic Kidney Disease Associated Anemia:
Initiate When:
On Dialysis: Hgb <10g/dL
Not On Dialysis: Hgb <10g/dL, the rate of Hgb decline indicates likelihood of requiring a RBC transfusion, and reducing the risk of alloimmunization and/or other RBC transfusion-related risks is a goal
Initial: 50-100 U/kg IV/SQ 3X/week

PEDIATRIC DOSAGE

Anemia

Chronic Kidney Disease Associated Anemia:
1 Month-16 Years:
On Dialysis:
Initial: 50 U/kg IV/SQ 3X weekly
Titrate: When Hgb approaches/exceeds 11g/dL, reduce or interrupt dose
Do not increase dose more frequently than once every 4 weeks; decreases in dose may occur more frequently

Titrate:
On Dialysis: When Hgb approaches/exceeds 11g/dL, reduce or interrupt dose
Not On Dialysis: When Hgb approaches/exceeds 10g/dL, reduce or interrupt dose
All Chronic Kidney Disease Patients:
Do not increase dose more frequently than once every 4 weeks; decreases in dose may occur more frequently
If Hgb rises rapidly (eg, >1g/dL in any 2-week period), decrease dose by 25% or more prn to reduce rapid responses
If Hgb has not increased by >1g/dL after 4 weeks, increase dose by 25%
If no response after 12-week escalation period, use lowest dose to maintain sufficient Hgb level to reduce need for RBC transfusions and evaluate other causes of anemia

Zidovudine (≤4200mg) Associated Anemia in HIV-Infected Patients w/ Endogenous Serum Erythropoietin Levels of ≤500 mU/mL:
Initial: 100 U/kg IV/SQ 3X/week
Titrate:
Hgb Does Not Increase After 8 Weeks of Therapy: Increase by 50-100 U/kg at 4- to 8-week intervals until Hgb reaches a level needed to avoid RBC transfusions or 300 U/kg
Hgb >12g/dL: Withhold dose. When Hgb <11g/dL, resume at 25% below the previous dose
D/C if increase in Hgb is not achieved at a dose of 300 U/kg for 8 weeks

Chemotherapy Associated Anemia:
Initiate when Hgb <10g/dL and if there is a minimum of 2 additional months of planned chemotherapy
Initial: 150 U/kg SQ 3X/week or 40,000 U SQ weekly until completion of a chemotherapy course
Titrate:
Dose Reduction: Reduce by 25% if Hgb increases >1g/dL in any 2-week period or reaches a level needed to avoid RBC transfusions. Withhold if Hgb exceeds level needed to avoid RBC transfusions; reinitiate at 25% below previous dose when Hgb approaches a level where RBC transfusions may be required
Dose Increase: If Hgb increases by <1g/dL and remains below 10g/dL after initial 4 weeks, increase dose to 300 U/kg 3X/week or 60,000 U/week
D/C therapy if there is no response in Hgb levels or if RBC transfusions are still required after 8 weeks

Surgery Patients:
Used to reduce the need for allogeneic RBC transfusions among patients w/ perioperative Hgb >10-≤13g/dL who are at high risk for perioperative blood loss from elective, noncardiac, nonvascular surgery
Usual: 300 U/kg/day SQ qd for 10 days before, on the day of, and for 4 days after surgery; or 600 U/kg SQ in 4 doses administered 21, 14, and 7 days before surgery and on the day of surgery. Deep vein thrombosis prophylaxis is recommended

If Hgb rises rapidly (eg, >1g/dL in any 2-week period), decrease dose by 25% or more prn to reduce rapid responses
If Hgb has not increased by >1g/dL after 4 weeks, increase dose by 25%
If no response after 12-week escalation period, use lowest dose to maintain sufficient Hgb level to reduce need for RBC transfusions and evaluate other causes of anemia

Chemotherapy Associated Anemia: 5-18 Years:
Initial: 600 U/kg IV weekly until completion of a chemotherapy course
Titrate:
Dose Reduction: Reduce by 25% if Hgb increases >1g/dL in any 2-week period or Hgb reaches a level needed to avoid RBC transfusions. Withhold if Hgb exceeds level needed to avoid RBC transfusions; reinitiate at 25% below previous dose when Hgb approaches a level where RBC transfusions may be required
Dose Increase: If Hgb increases by <1g/dL and remains below 10g/dL after initial 4 weeks, increase dose to 900 U/kg weekly
D/C therapy if there is no response in Hgb levels or if RBC transfusions are still required after 8 weeks
Max: 60,000 U/week

DOSING CONSIDERATIONS

Elderly
Individualize dose selection and adjustment to achieve and maintain target Hgb

ADMINISTRATION

IV/SQ route

IV route is recommended for chronic kidney disease patients on hemodialysis.

Preparation/Administration
Do not shake; do not use if shaken or frozen.
Preservative-free single-use vials may be admixed in a syringe w/ bacteriostatic 0.9% NaCl inj, w/ benzyl alcohol 0.9% in a 1:1 ratio.
Do not dilute or mix w/ other drug sol.

Do not re-enter preservative-free vials; discard unused portions.
Store unused portions of multidose vials at 2-8°C (36-46°F); discard after 21 days after initial entry.

STORAGE
2-8°C (36-46°F). Do not freeze; do not use if it has been frozen. Protect from light. Discard unused portions of multidose vials 21 days after initial entry.

HOW SUPPLIED
Inj: (Single-dose vial) 2000 U/mL, 3000 U/mL, 4000 U/mL, 10,000 U/mL; (multidose vial) 10,000 U/mL [2mL], 20,000 U/mL [1mL]

CONTRAINDICATIONS
Uncontrolled HTN, pure red cell aplasia (PRCA) that begins after treatment with epoetin alfa or other erythropoietin protein drugs, serious allergic reactions to epoetin alfa. **Multidose Vials:** Neonates, infants, pregnant women, and nursing mothers.

WARNINGS/PRECAUTIONS
Not indicated for use in patients with cancer receiving hormonal agents, biologic products, or radiotherapy, unless also receiving concomitant myelosuppressive chemotherapy; in patients scheduled for surgery who are willing to donate autologous blood; in patients undergoing cardiac/vascular surgery; or as a substitute for RBC transfusions in patients requiring immediate correction of anemia. Evaluate transferrin saturation and serum ferritin prior to and during treatment; administer supplemental iron when serum ferritin is <100mcg/L or serum transferrin saturation is <20%. Correct/exclude other causes of anemia (eg, vitamin deficiency, metabolic/chronic inflammatory conditions, bleeding) before initiating therapy. Hypertensive encephalopathy and seizures reported in patients with CKD; increases risk of seizures in CKD patients. Appropriately control HTN prior to initiation of and during treatment; reduce/withhold therapy if BP becomes difficult to control. PRCA and severe anemia, with or without other cytopenias that arise following the development of neutralizing antibodies to erythropoietin, reported. Withhold and evaluate for neutralizing antibodies to erythropoietin if severe anemia and low reticulocyte count develop; d/c permanently if PRCA develops, and do not switch to other erythropoiesis-stimulating agents. Serious allergic reactions may occur; immediately and permanently d/c therapy. Contains albumin; may carry an extremely remote risk for transmission of viral diseases or Creutzfeldt-Jakob disease. Patients may require adjustments in their dialysis prescriptions after initiation of therapy, or require increased anticoagulation with heparin to prevent clotting of extracorporeal circuit during hemodialysis. Multidose vial contains benzyl alcohol; benzyl alcohol is associated with serious adverse events and death, particularly in pediatric patients.

ADVERSE REACTIONS
MI, stroke, VTE, thrombosis of vascular access, tumor progression/recurrence, pyrexia, N/V, HTN, cough, arthralgia, dizziness, pruritus, rash, headache.

PREGNANCY AND LACTATION
Category C, caution in nursing (single-dose vial).

MECHANISM OF ACTION
Erythropoiesis-stimulating glycoprotein; stimulates erythropoiesis by the same mechanism as endogenous erythropoietin.

PHARMACOKINETICS
Absorption: Adults and Pediatrics with CKD: (SQ) T_{max}=5-24 hrs. Anemic Cancer Patients: (SQ) T_{max}=13.3 hrs (150 U/kg 3X weekly), 38 hrs (40,000 U weekly). **Elimination:** Adults and Pediatrics with CKD: (IV) $T_{1/2}$=4-13 hrs. Anemic Cancer Patients: (SQ) $T_{1/2}$=16-67 hrs.

PATIENT CONSIDERATIONS
Assessment: Assess for uncontrolled HTN, previous hypersensitivity to the drug, causes of anemia, pregnancy/nursing status, and other conditions where treatment is contraindicated or cautioned. Obtain baseline Hgb levels, transferrin saturation, and serum ferritin.

Monitoring: Monitor for signs/symptoms of an allergic reaction, CV/thromboembolic events, stroke, premonitory neurologic symptoms, PRCA, severe anemia, progression/recurrence of tumor, and other adverse reactions. Monitor BP, transferrin saturation, and serum ferritin. Following initiation of therapy and after each dose adjustment, monitor Hgb weekly until Hgb is stable, then at least monthly, and to maintain Hgb sufficient to minimize need for RBC transfusions.

Counseling: Inform of the risks and benefits of therapy, and of the increased risks of mortality, serious CV reactions, thromboembolic reactions, stroke, and tumor progression. Advise of the need to have regular lab tests for Hgb. Inform cancer patients that they must sign the patient-physician acknowledgment form prior to therapy. Instruct to undergo regular BP monitoring, adhere to prescribed antihypertensive regimen, and follow recommended dietary restrictions. Advise to contact physician for new-onset neurologic symptoms or change in seizure frequency. Instruct regarding proper disposal and caution against reuse of needles, syringes, or unused portions of single-dose vials.

Epzicom — abacavir sulfate/lamivudine   Rx
Class: Nucleoside reverse transcriptase inhibitor (NRTI) combination

---

Lactic acidosis and severe hepatomegaly w/ steatosis, including fatal cases, reported w/ nucleoside analogues and other antiretrovirals; d/c if clinical or laboratory findings suggestive of lactic acidosis or pronounced hepatotoxicity occur. **Abacavir:** Serious and sometimes fatal hypersensitivity reactions w/ multiple organ involvement reported; d/c immediately if a hypersensitivity reaction is suspected and never restart therapy or any other abacavir-containing product because more severe symptoms, including death, can occur w/in hours. Patients who carry the HLA-B*5701 allele are at a higher risk of a hypersensitivity reaction; screen all patients for HLA-B*5701 allele prior to initiating or reinitiating therapy, unless patient has a previously documented HLA-B*5701 allele assessment. **Lamivudine:** Severe acute exacerbations of hepatitis B reported in patients coinfected w/ hepatitis B virus (HBV) and have discontinued therapy; closely monitor hepatic function for at least several months in patients who d/c therapy and are coinfected w/ HBV. If appropriate, initiation of antihepatitis B therapy may be warranted.

ADULT DOSAGE	PEDIATRIC DOSAGE
HIV-1 Infection	**HIV-1 Infection**
Combination w/ Other Antiretrovirals: 1 tab qd	**Combination w/ Other Antiretrovirals:** ≥25kg: 1 tab qd

DOSING CONSIDERATIONS
Renal Impairment
CrCl <50mL/min: Not recommended

Hepatic Impairment
Mild (Child-Pugh Class A): Not recommended
Moderate (Child-Pugh Class B) or Severe (Child-Pugh Class C): Contraindicated

ADMINISTRATION
Oral route

Take w/ or w/o food.
Screen for the HLA-B*5701 allele prior to initiating therapy.

STORAGE
25°C (77°F); excursions permitted to 15-30°C (59-86°F).

HOW SUPPLIED
Tab: (Abacavir sulfate/Lamivudine) 600mg/300mg

CONTRAINDICATIONS
Patients w/ HLA-B*5701 allele, prior hypersensitivity reaction to abacavir or lamivudine, moderate or severe hepatic impairment.

WARNINGS/PRECAUTIONS
Immune reconstitution syndrome reported. Autoimmune disorders (eg, Graves' disease, polymyositis, Guillain-Barre syndrome) reported to occur in the setting of immune reconstitution and can occur many months after initiation of treatment. Redistribution/accumulation of body fat reported. Caution in elderly. **Abacavir:** May increase risk of MI. Consider the underlying risk of coronary heart disease when prescribing therapy. **Lamivudine:** Emergence of lamivudine-resistant HBV reported.

ADVERSE REACTIONS
Drug hypersensitivity, insomnia, depression/depressed mood, headache/migraine, fatigue/malaise, dizziness/vertigo, nausea, diarrhea.

DRUG INTERACTIONS
Avoid w/ other abacavir-, lamivudine-, and/or emtricitabine-containing products. **Abacavir:** May increase oral methadone clearance; an increased methadone dose may be required in a small number of patients. **Lamivudine:** Closely monitor for treatment-associated toxicities, especially hepatic decompensation, in patients receiving interferon alfa w/ or w/o ribavirin and Epzicom; consider discontinuation of Epzicom and dose reduction/discontinuation of interferon alfa, ribavirin, or both.

PREGNANCY AND LACTATION
Pregnancy: Physicians are encouraged to register patients in the Antiretroviral Pregnancy Registry. Fetal harm has been seen in animal studies; relevance to human pregnancy registry data is unknown.
Lactation: Mothers should be instructed not to breastfeed due to potential for HIV-1 transmission.

MECHANISM OF ACTION
Abacavir: Carbocyclic nucleoside analogue; inhibits HIV-1 reverse transcriptase (RT) activity by competing w/ natural substrate dGTP and by its incorporation into viral DNA. **Lamivudine:** Nucleoside analogue; inhibits RT via DNA chain termination after incorporation of the nucleotide analogue.

PHARMACOKINETICS
Absorption: Rapid. Abacavir: Oral bioavailability (86%), C_{max}=4.26mcg/mL, AUC=11.95mcg•hr/mL. Lamivudine: Oral bioavailability (86%), C_{max}=2.04mcg/mL, AUC=8.87mcg•hr/mL. **Distribution:** Abacavir: V_d=0.86L/kg; plasma protein binding (50%). Lamivudine: V_d=1.3L/kg; crosses placenta. **Metabolism:** Abacavir: Via alcohol dehydrogenase and glucuronyl transferase; 5'-carboxylic acid and 5'-glucuronide (metabolites). Lamivudine: Trans-sulfoxide (metabolite). **Elimination:** Abacavir: $T_{1/2}$=1.45 hrs. Lamivudine: Urine (70%, unchanged) (IV); $T_{1/2}$=5-7 hrs.

PATIENT CONSIDERATIONS
Assessment: Assess medical history for prior exposure to any abacavir-containing product. Assess for HBV infection, history of hypersensitivity reactions, HLA-B*5701 status (including patients of unknown HLA-B*5701 status who have previously tolerated abacavir), hepatic/renal impairment, risk factors for coronary heart disease, pregnancy/nursing status, and possible drug interactions.

Monitoring: Monitor for signs/symptoms of hypersensitivity reactions, lactic acidosis, hepatomegaly w/ steatosis, immune reconstitution syndrome, autoimmune disorders, fat redistribution/accumulation, MI, and other adverse reactions. Monitor hepatic/renal function. Closely monitor hepatic function for several months after discontinuing therapy in patients coinfected w/ HIV-1 and HBV.

Counseling: Inform patients regarding hypersensitivity reactions w/ abacavir; instruct to contact physician immediately if symptoms develop and not to restart or replace w/ any other abacavir-containing products w/o medical consultation. Inform that the drug may cause lactic acidosis w/ hepatomegaly. Inform patients coinfected w/ HIV-1 and HBV that worsening of liver disease has occurred in some cases when treatment w/ lamivudine was discontinued; instruct to discuss any changes in regimen w/ the physician. Inform that hepatic decompensation has occurred in HIV-1/hepatitis C virus coinfected patients receiving combination antiretroviral therapy for HIV-1 and interferon alfa w/ or w/o ribavirin. Inform that redistribution/accumulation of body fat may occur. Advise that drug is not a cure for HIV-1 infection and continuous therapy is necessary to control HIV-1 infection and decrease HIV-related illness. Instruct patients to take all HIV medications exactly as prescribed. Advise not to re-use or share needles/other inj equipment and not to share personal items (eg, toothbrush, razor blades), to continue to practice safer sex by using latex or polyurethane condoms, and not to breastfeed.

ERBITUX — cetuximab   Rx

Class: Monoclonal antibody/EGFR blocker

> Serious infusion reactions, some fatal, reported; immediately interrupt and permanently d/c infusion if these reactions occur. Cardiopulmonary arrest and/or sudden death occurred in patients w/ squamous cell carcinoma of the head and neck (SCCHN) treated w/ cetuximab in combination w/ radiation therapy or w/ European Union-approved cetuximab in combination w/ platinum-based therapy w/ 5-fluorouracil (5-FU); closely monitor serum electrolytes during and after therapy.

ADULT DOSAGE

Squamous Cell Carcinoma of the Head and Neck

W/ Radiation Therapy for the Initial Treatment of Locally or Regionally Advanced Squamous Cell Carcinoma of the Head and Neck (SCCHN):
Initial: $400mg/m^2$ administered 1 week prior to initiation of a course of radiation therapy as a 120 min IV infusion
Maint: $250mg/m^2$ infused over 60 min weekly for the duration of radiation therapy (6-7 weeks)
Max Infusion Rate: 10mg/min
Complete administration 60 min prior to radiation therapy

W/ Platinum-Based Therapy w/ 5-fluorouracil (5-FU) for the 1st-Line Treatment of Patients w/ Recurrent Locoregional Disease or Metastatic SCCHN:
Initial: $400mg/m^2$ administered on the day of initiation of platinum-based therapy w/ 5-FU as a 120 min IV infusion
Maint: $250mg/m^2$ infused over 60 min weekly until disease progression or unacceptable toxicity
Max Infusion Rate: 10mg/min
Complete administration 60 min prior to platinum-based therapy w/ 5-FU

As Monotherapy in Patients w/ Recurrent/Metastatic SCCHN for Whom Prior Platinum-Based Therapy Failed:
Initial: $400mg/m^2$ administered as a 120 min IV infusion
Maint: $250mg/m^2$ infused over 60 min weekly until disease progression or unacceptable toxicity
Max Infusion Rate: 10mg/min

Metastatic Colorectal Cancer

Treatment of *K-Ras* wild-type, epidermal growth factor receptor-expressing, metastatic colorectal cancer in combination w/ FOLFIRI (irinotecan, 5-fluorouracil, leucovorin) for 1st-line treatment, in combination w/ irinotecan in patients who are refractory to irinotecan-based chemotherapy, and as monotherapy in patients who have failed oxaliplatin- and irinotecan-based chemotherapy or are intolerant to irinotecan

Initial: $400mg/m^2$ administered as a 120-min IV infusion; complete administration 60 min prior to FOLFIRI
Maint: $250mg/m^2$ infused over 60 min weekly until disease progression or unacceptable toxicity; complete administration 60 min prior to FOLFIRI
Max Infusion Rate: 10mg/min

Premedication

H_1-antagonist (eg, 50mg diphenhydramine) IV 30-60 min prior to 1st dose; premedication for subsequent doses should be based on clinical judgment and presence/severity of prior infusion reactions

PEDIATRIC DOSAGE

Pediatric use may not have been established

DOSING CONSIDERATIONS

Adverse Reactions

NCI CTC Grade 1 or 2 and Non-Serious NCI CTC Grade 3 Infusion Reaction:
Reduce infusion rate by 50%; immediately and permanently d/c for serious infusion reactions, requiring medical intervention and/or hospitalization

Severe Acneiform Rash (NCI CTC Grade 3 or 4):
1st Occurrence: Delay infusion 1-2 weeks
W/ Improvement: Continue at $250mg/m^2$
No Improvement: D/C treatment

2nd Occurrence: Delay infusion 1-2 weeks
W/ Improvement: Reduce to $200mg/m^2$
No Improvement: D/C treatment

3rd Occurrence: Delay infusion 1-2 weeks
W/ Improvement: Reduce to $150mg/m^2$
No Improvement: D/C treatment

4th Occurrence: D/C treatment

ADMINISTRATION

IV route
Do not administer as IV push or bolus.
Administer via infusion pump or syringe pump.
Administer through low protein binding 0.22μm in-line filter.
Do not shake or dilute.

STORAGE

Vials: 2-8°C (36-46°F). Do not freeze. **Infusion Containers:** Stable for up to 12 hrs at 2-8°C (36-46°F) and up to 8 hrs at 20-25°C (68-77°F).

HOW SUPPLIED

Inj: 2mg/mL [50mL, 100mL]

WARNINGS/PRECAUTIONS

Caution when used in combination w/ radiation therapy or platinum-based therapy w/ 5-FU in head and neck cancer patients w/ history of coronary artery disease (CAD), CHF, or arrhythmias. Interstitial lung disease (ILD) reported; interrupt for acute onset or worsening of pulmonary symptoms and permanently d/c if ILD is confirmed. Dermatologic toxicities (eg, acneiform rash, skin drying/fissuring, paronychial inflammation, infectious sequelae, hypertrichosis) reported. Life-threatening and fatal bullous mucocutaneous disease w/ blisters, erosions, and skin sloughing has also been observed; limit sun exposure during therapy. Addition of cetuximab to radiation and cisplatin inpatients reported to increase incidence of Grade 3-4 mucositis, radiation recall syndrome, acneiform rash, cardiac events, and electrolyte disturbances compared to radiation and cisplatin alone; addition of cetuximab did not improve progression-free survival. Hypomagnesemia and electrolyte abnormalities reported; replete electrolytes as necessary. Do not resume nursing earlier than 60 days following the last dose of therapy if nursing is interrupted. Not indicated for the treatment of *Ras* mutant colorectal cancer or when *Ras* mutation test results are unknown, or for the treatment of patients w/ colorectal cancer that harbor somatic mutations in exon 2 (codons 12 and 13), exon 3 (codons 59 and 61), and exon 4 (codons 117 and 146) of either *K-ras* or *N-ras*.

ADVERSE REACTIONS

Cardiopulmonary arrest, infusion reactions, cutaneous reactions (eg, rash, pruritus, nail changes), headache, diarrhea, infection, sepsis, asthenia, nausea, emesis, fatigue, fever, pain, dyspnea, cough.

PREGNANCY AND LACTATION

Category C, not for use in nursing.

MECHANISM OF ACTION

EGFR antagonist (human/mouse chimeric monoclonal antibody); binds specifically to EGFR on both normal and tumor cells and competitively inhibits the binding of epidermal growth factor and other ligands, such as transforming growth factor-α.

PHARMACOKINETICS

Absorption: C_{max}=168-235mcg/mL. **Distribution:** V_d=2-3L/m^2; may cross the placenta. **Elimination:** $T_{1/2}$=112 hrs.

PATIENT CONSIDERATIONS

Assessment: Assess for history of CAD, CHF, arrhythmias, pulmonary disorders, pregnancy/nursing status, and possible drug interactions. Obtain serum electrolyte levels (including Mg^{2+}, K^+, Ca^{2+}). Determine EGFR-expression status and confirm the absence of a *Ras* mutation in colorectal tumors using FDA-approved tests.

Monitoring: Monitor for signs/symptoms of infusion reactions, cardiopulmonary arrest, acute onset or worsening of pulmonary symptoms, dermatologic toxicities and infectious sequelae, and for other adverse reactions. Monitor patients for 1 hr after infusion in a setting w/ resuscitation equipment and other agents necessary to treat anaphylaxis; monitor longer to confirm resolution of the event in patients requiring treatment for infusion reactions. Periodically monitor for hypomagnesemia, hypocalcemia, and hypokalemia during and for at least 8 weeks after therapy.

Counseling: Advise to report to physician signs/symptoms of infusion reactions. Inform of pregnancy/nursing risks; advise to use adequate contraception during and for 6 months after last dose for both males and females. Inform that nursing is not recommended during and for 2 months following last dose of therapy. Instruct to limit sun exposure (eg, use of sunscreen, wear hats) during and for 2 months after last dose of therapy.

ERIVEDGE — vismodegib Rx

Class: Hedgehog pathway inhibitor

> May cause embryo-fetal death or severe birth defects when administered to pregnant woman. Verify pregnancy status of females of reproductive potential w/in 7 days prior to initiating therapy. Advise females of reproductive potential to use effective contraception during and after therapy. Advise males of the potential risk of exposure through semen and to use condoms w/ a pregnant partner or a female partner of reproductive potential. Advise pregnant women of the potential risks to a fetus.

ADULT DOSAGE
Basal Cell Carcinoma

Metastatic basal cell carcinoma, or locally advanced basal cell carcinoma that has recurred following surgery or in patients who are not candidates for surgery, and who are not candidates for radiation

150mg qd until disease progression or until unacceptable toxicity

PEDIATRIC DOSAGE

Pediatric use may not have been established

ADMINISTRATION
Oral route

Take w/ or w/o food
Swallow caps whole; do not open or crush caps

STORAGE
20-25°C (68-77°F); excursions permitted between 15-30°C (59-86°F).

HOW SUPPLIED
Cap: 150mg

WARNINGS/PRECAUTIONS
Do not donate blood or blood products while on therapy and for 7 months after the final dose. Vismodegib is present is semen; males should not donate semen during and for 3 months after the final dose of therapy.

ADVERSE REACTIONS
Muscle spasm, alopecia, dysgeusia, weight loss, fatigue, N/V, diarrhea, decreased appetite, constipation, arthralgia, ageusia.

PREGNANCY AND LACTATION
Pregnancy: May cause fetal harm.
Lactation: No data are available regarding the presence of vismodegib in human milk. Breastfeeding is not recommended during therapy and for 7 months after the final dose.
Reproductive Potential: Females of reproductive potential should use effective contraception during therapy and for 7 months after the final dose of therapy. Amenorrhea may occur in females of reproductive potential.
Vismodegib is present in semen. Males should use condoms, even after vasectomy, to avoid exposure to pregnant partners and female partners of reproductive potential, and should not donate semen, during therapy and for 3 months after the final dose of therapy.

MECHANISM OF ACTION
Hedgehog pathway inhibitor; binds to and inhibits Smoothened, a transmembrane protein involved in Hedgehog signal transduction.

PHARMACOKINETICS
Absorption: Absolute bioavailability (31.8%). **Distribution:** V_d=16.4-26.6L; plasma protein binding (>99%). **Metabolism:** Oxidation, glucuronidation, and pyridine ring cleavage. **Elimination:** Feces (82%), urine (4.4%); $T_{1/2}$=4 days (continuous qd dosing), 12 days (single dose).

PATIENT CONSIDERATIONS
Assessment: Assess pregnancy status w/in 7 days prior to initiating therapy. Assess nursing status and for possible drug interactions.

Monitoring: Monitor for disease progression, toxicities, and other adverse reactions.

Counseling: Inform pregnant women of the potential risk to a fetus; advise females of reproductive potential to use effective contraception during therapy and for 7 months after the final dose of therapy. Advise males, even those w/ prior vasectomy, to use condoms to avoid potential drug exposure in both pregnant partners and female partners of reproductive potential during therapy and for 3 months after the final dose. Advise female patients and female partners of male patients to contact their healthcare provider w/ a known/suspected pregnancy. Advise males not to donate semen during therapy and for 3 months after the final dose. Advise women that breastfeeding is not recommended during therapy and for 7 months after final dose. Advise not to donate blood or blood products while on therapy and for 7 months after the final dose.

ERWINAZE — asparaginase erwinia chrysanthemi Rx

Class: Enzyme

ADULT DOSAGE
Acute Lymphoblastic Leukemia

As a component of multiagent chemotherapeutic regimen in patients who have developed hypersensitivity to *Escherichia coli*-derived asparaginase

PEDIATRIC DOSAGE
Acute Lymphoblastic Leukemia

As a component of multiagent chemotherapeutic regimen in patients who have developed hypersensitivity to *E. coli*-derived asparaginase

To Substitute for a Dose of Pegaspargase:
Usual: 25,000 IU/m² IM/IV 3X/week (M/W/F) for 6 doses for each planned pegaspargase dose

To Substitute for a Dose of Native *E. coli* Asparaginase:
Usual: 25,000 IU/m² IM/IV for each scheduled *E. coli* asparaginase dose

To Substitute for a Dose of Pegaspargase:
Usual: 25,000 IU/m² IM/IV 3X/week (M/W/F) for 6 doses for each planned pegaspargase dose

To Substitute for a Dose of Native *E. coli* Asparaginase:
Usual: 25,000 IU/m² IM/IV for each scheduled *E. coli* asparaginase dose

ADMINISTRATION
IM/IV route

Preparation
Reconstitute the contents of each vial by slowly injecting 1mL or 2mL of preservative free sterile NaCl (0.9%) Inj against the inner vial wall
Dissolve contents by gentle mixing or swirling
Withdraw the volume containing the calculated dose from the vial into a polypropylene syringe w/in 15 min of reconstitution

IM
Limit volume to 2mL/single inj site
If >2mL dose, use multiple inj sites

IV
Slowly inject the reconstituted asparaginase into an IV infusion bag containing 100mL of normal saline acclimatized to room temperature
Do not shake or squeeze the IV bag
Infuse in 100mL of normal saline over 1 hr
Do not infuse other IV drugs through the same IV line while infusing asparaginase

STORAGE
2-8°C (36-46°F). Protect from light. Do not freeze or refrigerate reconstituted sol. Administer w/in 4 hrs or discard.

HOW SUPPLIED
Inj: 10,000 IU

CONTRAINDICATIONS
History of serious hypersensitivity reactions to this medication (eg, anaphylaxis), history of serious thrombosis, pancreatitis, or hemorrhagic events w/ prior L-asparaginase therapy.

WARNINGS/PRECAUTIONS
Grade 3 and 4 hypersensitivity reactions and serious thrombotic events, including sagittal sinus thrombosis and PE, reported; d/c if any of these occur. Pancreatitis reported; d/c for severe or hemorrhagic pancreatitis manifested by abdominal pain >72 hrs and amylase elevation ≥2.0X ULN. W/ mild pancreatitis, hold until signs/symptoms subside and amylase levels return to normal. May resume treatment after resolution of mild pancreatitis or symptoms of thrombotic/hemorrhagic event. Irreversible glucose intolerance may occur. Administer insulin therapy as necessary in patients w/ hyperglycemia. Consider monitoring nadir (predose) serum asparaginase activity (NSAA) levels w/ IV administration and switching to IM administration if desired NSAA levels are not achieved.

ADVERSE REACTIONS
Systemic hypersensitivity, pancreatitis, local reactions, abnormal transaminases, N/V, fever, hyperglycemia.

PREGNANCY AND LACTATION
Category C, not for use in nursing.

MECHANISM OF ACTION
Enzyme; catalyzes the deamidation of asparagine to aspartic acid and ammonia, resulting in a reduction in circulating levels of asparagine. Thought to be based on the inability of leukemic cells to synthesize asparagine, resulting in cytotoxicity specific for leukemic cells that depend on an exogenous source of amino acid asparagine for their protein metabolism and survival.

PATIENT CONSIDERATIONS
Assessment: Assess for history of serious hypersensitivity reactions, pancreatitis, thrombosis, or hemorrhagic events w/ prior L-asparaginase therapy, and pregnancy/nursing status. Obtain baseline serum glucose and coagulation parameters.

Monitoring: Monitor for hypersensitivity reactions, thrombotic or hemorrhagic events, symptoms of pancreatitis, and other adverse reactions. Monitor serum glucose periodically and coagulation parameters. Monitor NSAA levels w/ IV administration.

Counseling: Inform patients of the risk of allergic reactions, pancreatitis, hyperglycemia, glucose intolerance, thrombosis, and hemorrhage, and instruct to seek medical advice immediately if signs/symptoms of these conditions occur. Inform to notify physician if pregnant or nursing.

ESBRIET — pirfenidone Rx

Class: Pyridone

ADULT DOSAGE
Idiopathic Pulmonary Fibrosis

Days 1-7: 1 cap tid
Days 8-14: 2 caps tid
Day 15 Onward: 3 caps tid
Maint/Max: 2403mg/day (9 caps/day)

PEDIATRIC DOSAGE
Pediatric use may not have been established

DOSING CONSIDERATIONS
Concomitant Medications
Strong CYP1A2 Inhibitors (eg, Fluvoxamine, Enoxacin):
Reduce to 1 cap tid
Moderate CYP1A2 Inhibitors (eg, Ciprofloxacin 750mg bid):
Reduce to 2 caps tid

Adverse Reactions
Significant (eg, GI, Photosensitivity, Rash):
Consider temporary dosage reductions or interruptions to allow for resolution of symptoms

Elevated Liver Enzymes:
ALT and/or AST >3 but ≤5X ULN w/o Symptoms or Hyperbilirubinemia:
1. D/C confounding medications, exclude other causes, and monitor patient closely
2. Repeat LFTs as clinically indicated
3. Full daily dosage may be maintained, if clinically appropriate, or reduced or interrupted (eg, until LFTs are w/in normal limits) w/ subsequent retitration to full dosage as tolerated

ALT and/or AST >3 but ≤5X ULN w/ Symptoms or Hyperbilirubinemia:
D/C permanently and do not rechallenge

ALT and/or AST >5X ULN:
D/C permanently and do not rechallenge

Other Important Considerations
Treatment Interruption ≥14 Days:
Reinitiate by undergoing the initial 2-week titration regimen up to full maint dose
Treatment Interruption <14 Days:
Resume w/ dosage prior to the interruption

ADMINISTRATION
Oral route
Take at the same time each day w/ food.

STORAGE
25°C (77°F); excursions permitted to 15-30°C (59-86°F).

HOW SUPPLIED
Cap: 267mg

WARNINGS/PRECAUTIONS
Increases in ALT and AST >3X ULN reported; rarely associated w/ concomitant bilirubin elevations. Photosensitivity reactions reported. GI events (eg, N/V, diarrhea, dyspepsia, GERD, abdominal pain) reported. Caution w/ mild (Child-Pugh Class A) to moderate (Child-Pugh Class B) hepatic impairment, or mild (CrCl 50-80mL/min)/moderate (CrCl 30-50mL/min)/severe (CrCl <30mL/min) renal impairment. Not recommended w/ severe (Child-Pugh Class C) hepatic impairment or ESRD requiring dialysis.

ADVERSE REACTIONS
N/V, rash, abdominal pain, URTI, diarrhea, fatigue, headache, dyspepsia, dizziness, anorexia, GERD, sinusitis, insomnia, weight decreased, arthralgia.

DRUG INTERACTIONS
See Dosing Considerations. Fluvoxamine or other strong CYP1A2 inhibitors (eg, enoxacin) significantly increase exposure; d/c use of such agents prior to treatment, and avoid during treatment. If such agents are the only drug of choice, dosage reductions are recommended; monitor for adverse reactions and consider discontinuation of pirfenidone prn. Ciprofloxacin (moderate CYP1A2 inhibitor) moderately increases exposure; if ciprofloxacin at the dosage of 750mg bid cannot be avoided, dosage reductions are recommended. Monitor closely when ciprofloxacin is used at a dosage of 250mg or 500mg qd. Agents or combinations of agents that are moderate or strong inhibitors of both CYP1A2 and ≥1 other CYP isoenzymes involved in the metabolism of pirfenidone (CYP2C9, 2C19, 2D6, 2E1) should be discontinued prior to and avoided during treatment. CYP1A2 inducers may decrease exposure, which may lead to loss of efficacy; d/c use of strong CYP1A2 inducers prior to treatment and avoid concomitant use. Avoid concomitant medications known to cause photosensitivity. Smoking causes decreased exposure, which may alter the efficacy profile; stop smoking prior to treatment and avoid smoking during treatment.

PREGNANCY AND LACTATION
Pregnancy: Category C
Lactation: Not for use in nursing.

MECHANISM OF ACTION
Pyridone; has not been established.

PHARMACOKINETICS
Absorption: C_{max} (median, 801mg single dose)=0.5 hrs. T_{max} (median)=0.5 hrs, 3 hrs (w/ food). **Distribution:** Plasma protein binding (58%); V_d=59-71L. **Metabolism:** Primarily in liver via CYP1A2, CYP2C9, 2C19, 2D6, and 2E1; 5-carboxy-pirfenidone (metabolite). **Elimination:** Urine (80% [approx 99.6% as metabolite]); $T_{1/2}$=3 hrs.

PATIENT CONSIDERATIONS
Assessment: Assess for renal/hepatic impairment, smoking, pregnancy/nursing status, and possible drug interactions. Conduct LFTs.

Monitoring: Monitor for photosensitivity reaction, rash, GI events, and other adverse reactions. Conduct LFTs monthly for the first 6 months and every 3 months thereafter.

Counseling: Inform that periodic monitoring of LFTs may be required. Instruct to immediately report any symptoms of a liver problem, photosensitivity reaction, rash, or persistent GI effects to physician. Advise to avoid or minimize exposure to sunlight (eg, sunlamps) during therapy; instruct to use a sunblock (SPF ≥50) and to wear clothing that protects against sun exposure. Encourage to stop smoking prior to treatment and to avoid smoking while on therapy.

ETOPOPHOS — etoposide phosphate   Rx
Class: Podophyllotoxin derivative

> Administer under the supervision of a qualified physician experienced in the use of cancer chemotherapeutic agents. Severe myelosuppression w/ resulting infection or bleeding may occur.

ADULT DOSAGE	PEDIATRIC DOSAGE
Testicular Tumor	Pediatric use may not have been established
Combination therapy w/ other approved chemotherapeutic agents in patients w/ refractory testicular tumors who have already received appropriate surgical, chemotherapeutic, and radiotherapeutic therapy	
Usual: 50-100mg/m³/day IV on Days 1-5 to 100mg/m²/day IV on Days 1, 3, and 5	
After adequate recovery from any toxicity, repeat chemotherapy courses at 3- to 4-week intervals	
Small Cell Lung Cancer	
Combination w/ other approved chemotherapeutic agents as first-line treatment in patients w/ small cell lung cancer	
35mg/m²/day IV for 4 days to 50mg/m²/day IV for 5 days	
After adequate recovery from any toxicity, repeat chemotherapy courses at 3- to 4-week intervals	

DOSING CONSIDERATIONS
Concomitant Medications
Dosage should be modified to take into account the myelosuppressive effect of other drugs in the combination or the effects of prior x-ray therapy or chemotherapy which may have compromised bone marrow reserve

Renal Impairment
CrCl 15-50mL/min:
Initial: 75% of dose; base subsequent dosing on tolerance and clinical effect
CrCl <15mL/min: Consider further dose reduction

ADMINISTRATION
IV route
Do not give by bolus IV inj.
May be administered at infusion rates from 5-210 min.

Preparation
1. Reconstitute w/ sterile water for inj (SWFI), D5W inj, 0.9% NaCl inj, bacteriostatic water for inj w/ benzyl alcohol, or bacteriostatic NaCl for inj w/ benzyl alcohol to 20mg/mL or 10mg/mL etoposide (22.7 or 11.4mg/mL etoposide phosphate, respectively).
2. Can be further diluted to 0.1mg/mL etoposide w/ either D5W inj or 0.9% NaCl inj.

STORAGE
Unopened Vials: 2-8°C (36-46°F). Protect from light. **Reconstituted Sol:** 2-8°C (36-46°F) for 7 days; at 20-25°C (68-77°F) for 24 hrs following reconstitution w/ SWFI, D5W, or 0.9% NaCl; stable for 48 hours at 20-25°C (68-77°F) following reconstitution w/ bacteriostatic water for inj w/ benzyl alcohol, or bacteriostatic NaCl for inj w/ benzyl alcohol. **Diluted Sol:** 2-8°C (36-46°F) or 20-25°C (68-77°F) for 24 hrs.

HOW SUPPLIED
Inj: 100mg

CONTRAINDICATIONS
Prior hypersensitivity to etoposide, etoposide phosphate, or any other component of the formulation.

WARNINGS/PRECAUTIONS
Frequently observe for myelosuppression during and after therapy. If platelet count <50,000/mm³ or ANC <500/mm³ occurs, withhold further therapy until the blood counts have sufficiently recovered. Anaphylactic reactions and inj-site reactions may occur; closely monitor the infusion site for possible infiltration during administration. May cause fetal harm; females of reproductive potential should use effective contraception during treatment and for at least 6 months after the final dose. May cause infertility and result in amenorrhea in females of reproductive potential. Premature menopause may occur; recovery of menses and ovulation is related to age at treatment. May cause oligospermia, azoospermia, and permanent loss of fertility in male patients. May damage spermatozoa and testicular tissue, resulting in possible genetic fetal abnormalities; males w/ female sexual partners of reproductive potential should use condoms during treatment and for at least 4 months after the final dose. May be carcinogenic in humans; acute leukemia w/ or w/o a preleukemic phase reported rarely. Reduce dose or d/c if severe reactions occur; reinstitution of therapy should be carried out w/ caution, and w/ adequate consideration of further need for the drug and alertness as to possible recurrence of toxicity. Patients w/ low serum albumin may be at increased risk for drug-associated toxicities. Caution in elderly.

ADVERSE REACTIONS

Leukopenia, neutropenia, thrombocytopenia, anemia, asthenia/malaise, N/V, alopecia, chills, fever, anorexia, mucositis, constipation, abdominal pain.

DRUG INTERACTIONS

Caution w/ drugs known to inhibit phosphatase activities (eg, levamisole HCl). Decreased total body clearance and increased exposure of oral etoposide when coadministered w/ high-dose cyclosporin A. Antiepileptic medications (eg, phenytoin, phenobarbital, carbamazepine, valproic acid) is associated w/ increased clearance and reduced efficacy of etoposide. Concomitant warfarin therapy may result in elevated INR; closely monitor INR.

PREGNANCY AND LACTATION

Pregnancy: Category D.
Lactation: Not for use in nursing.

MECHANISM OF ACTION

Podophyllotoxin derivative; induces DNA strand breaks by interacting w/ DNA-topoisomerase II or forming free radicals.

PHARMACOKINETICS

Absorption: (150mg/m^2 w/ a 3.5-hr infusion time) AUC=168.3mcg•hr/mL, C_{max}=20mcg/mL. (90mg/m^2, 100mg/m^2, and 110mg/m^2 w/ a 60-min infusion time) AUC=96.1mcg•hr/mL, C_{max}=20.1mcg/mL. **Distribution:** V_d=7-17L/m^2; plasma protein binding (97%). **Metabolism:** Dephosphorylation to etoposide (active). **Elimination:** Biliary excretion; feces (44%), urine (56%, 45% unchanged); $T_{1/2}$=4-11 hrs.

PATIENT CONSIDERATIONS

Assessment: Assess for renal impairment, low serum albumin, drug hypersensitivity, pregnancy/nursing status, and possible drug interactions. Obtain platelet count, Hgb, WBC count, and differential at the start of therapy and prior to each subsequent cycle.

Monitoring: Monitor for signs/symptoms of myelosuppression, anaphylactic/inj-site/severe reactions, acute leukemia, and other adverse reactions. Perform periodic CBC at appropriate intervals during and after therapy. Closely monitor INR in patients on concomitant therapy w/ warfarin.

Counseling: Inform of benefits and risks of therapy. Counsel on pregnancy risks; advise females of reproductive potential to use effective contraception during treatment and for at least 6 months after the final dose. Instruct male patients who have female sexual partners of reproductive potential to use condoms during treatment and for at least 4 months after the final dose.

ETOPOSIDE CAPSULES — etoposide   Rx

Class: Podophyllotoxin derivative

> Administer under the supervision of a qualified physician experienced in the use of cancer chemotherapeutic agents. Severe myelosuppression w/ resulting infection or bleeding may occur.

ADULT DOSAGE	**PEDIATRIC DOSAGE**
Small Cell Lung Cancer	Pediatric use may not have been established
Combination w/ other approved chemotherapeutic agents as first line treatment	
Recommended: 2X the IV dose rounded to nearest 50mg	
Dosage should be modified to take into account the myelosuppressive effects of other drugs in the combination or the effects of prior x-ray therapy or chemotherapy which may have compromised bone marrow reserve	

DOSING CONSIDERATIONS
Renal Impairment
CrCl 15-50mL/min:
Initial: 75% of dose; base subsequent dosing on tolerance and clinical effect
CrCl <15mL/min: Consider further dose reduction
ADMINISTRATION
Oral route
STORAGE
2-8°C (36-46°F). Protect from freezing and from light.
HOW SUPPLIED
Cap: 50mg
CONTRAINDICATIONS
Previous hypersensitivity to etoposide or any component of the formulation.
WARNINGS/PRECAUTIONS
Frequently observe for myelosuppression during and after therapy. Withhold further therapy until the blood counts have sufficiently recovered if platelet count <50,000/mm^3 or if ANC <500/mm^3. Anaphylactic-like reactions reported. May cause fetal harm during pregnancy. May be carcinogenic in humans; acute leukemia w/ or w/o a preleukemic phase reported rarely. D/C or reduce dose if severe reactions occur; reinstitution of therapy should be carried out w/ caution, and w/ adequate consideration of further need for the drug and alertness as to possible recurrence of toxicity. Patients w/ low serum albumin may be at an increased risk for etoposide-associated toxicities. Caution in elderly.

ADVERSE REACTIONS

Myelosuppression, N/V, alopecia.

DRUG INTERACTIONS

High-dose cyclosporine A reduces total body clearance and increases exposure of etoposide.

PREGNANCY AND LACTATION

Pregnancy: Category D.
Lactation: Not for use in nursing.

MECHANISM OF ACTION

Podophyllotoxin derivative; induces DNA strand breaks by interacting w/ DNA-topoisomerase II or formation of free radicals.

PHARMACOKINETICS

Absorption: (Cap) Bioavailability (50%). **Distribution:** V_d=7-17L/m^2; plasma protein binding (97%). **Metabolism:** Liver (O-demethylation) via CYP3A4; hydroxy acid (metabolite). **Elimination:** Biliary excretion. (IV) (100-124mg/m^2) Feces (44%), urine (56%, 45% unchanged); $T_{1/2}$=4-11 hrs.

PATIENT CONSIDERATIONS

Assessment: Assess for drug hypersensitivity, low serum albumin, renal impairment, pregnancy/nursing status, and possible drug interactions. Obtain platelet count, Hgb, WBC count, and differential at start of therapy and prior to each subsequent cycle.

Monitoring: Monitor for signs/symptoms of myelosuppression, anaphylactic/severe reactions, and other adverse reactions. Monitor tolerance and clinical effect in patients w/ renal impairment. Perform periodic CBCs at appropriate intervals during and after therapy.

Counseling: Inform of benefits and risks of therapy. Inform of pregnancy risks; instruct to avoid pregnancy and nursing while on therapy.

EVOMELA — melphalan   Rx

Class: Alkylating agent

> Severe bone marrow suppression w/ resulting infection/bleeding may occur; monitor hematologic lab parameters. IV melphalan has shown more myelosuppression than oral melphalan. Hypersensitivity reactions (eg, anaphylaxis) reported; d/c treatment for serious hypersensitivity reactions. Produces chromosomal aberrations and should be considered potentially leukemogenic.

ADULT DOSAGE	**PEDIATRIC DOSAGE**
Multiple Myeloma	Pediatric use may not have been established
High-dose Conditioning Treatment Prior to Hematopoietic Progenitor (Stem) Cell Transplantation: 100mg/m^2/day IV for 2 consecutive days (Day 3 and Day 2) prior to autologous stem cell transplantation (ASCT, Day 0); administer prophylactic antiemetics	
For patients weighing >130% of their ideal body weight, body surface area should be calculated based on adjusted ideal body weight	
Palliative Treatment When Oral Therapy Is Not Appropriate: 16mg/m^2 IV at 2-week intervals for 4 doses, then, after adequate recovery from toxicity, at 4-week intervals; administer prophylactic antiemetics	

DOSING CONSIDERATIONS
Renal Impairment
Conditioning Treatment: No dose adjustment is necessary
Palliative Treatment (BUN ≥30mg/dL): Consider dose reduction of up to 50%
ADMINISTRATION
IV route
Cytotoxic drug; follow applicable special handling and disposal procedures. Do not mix w/ other melphalan for inj drug products.
Reconstitution/Infusion
1. Use 8.6mL of normal saline to reconstitute and make a 50mg/10mL (5mg/mL) nominal concentration.
2. Calculate the required volume needed for dose and withdraw from vial.
3. Add required volume to appropriate volume of 0.9% NaCl inj to a final concentration of 0.45mg/mL.
4. Infuse over 30 min (conditioning treatment) or as a single IV infusion over 15-20 min (palliative treatment). May cause local tissue damage should extravasation occur; do not administer by direct inj into a peripheral vein. Administer by injecting slowly into a fast-running IV infusion via a central venous access line.
Stability
- Reconstituted drug product is stable for 24 hrs at 5°C w/o any precipitation, due to high solubility.
- Reconstituted drug product is stable for 1 hr at room temperature.
- Admixture sol is stable for 4 hrs at room temperature in addition to the 1 hr following reconstitution.

STORAGE
25°C (77°F); excursions permitted between 15-30°C (59-86°F). Protect from light; retain in original carton until use.

HOW SUPPLIED
Inj: 50mg

CONTRAINDICATIONS
History of serious allergic reaction to melphalan.

WARNINGS/PRECAUTIONS
Hepatic disorders (eg, abnormal LFTs, hepatitis, jaundice) and hepatic veno-occlusive disease reported; monitor liver chemistries. Acute hypersensitivity reactions, (eg, anaphylaxis) reported; d/c treatment for serious hypersensitivity reactions. Chromatid or chromosome damage and secondary malignancies (eg, myeloproliferative syndrome or acute leukemia) reported; consider potential benefit against possible risk. May cause fetal harm. May cause reversible/irreversible testicular suppression or suppression of ovarian function in premenopausal women. **Conditioning Regimen:** Myeloablation occurs in all patients receiving conditioning treatment; do not begin if a stem cell product is not available for rescue. Monitor CBC, and provide supportive care for infections, anemia, and thrombocytopenia until there is adequate hematopoietic recovery. May cause N/V, mucositis, and diarrhea; provide supportive care. Provide nutritional support and analgesics for patients w/ severe mucositis. **Palliative Treatment:** Risk of severe myelosuppression is increased in patients w/ compromised bone marrow (by prior irradiation, prior chemotherapy, or recovering from chemotherapy); perform periodic CBC during course of treatment and provide supportive care for infections, bleeding, and symptomatic anemia. N/V, diarrhea, and oral ulceration may occur; provide supportive care.

ADVERSE REACTIONS
Diarrhea, N/V, fatigue, hypokalemia, anemia, decrease in neutrophil, WBC, lymphocyte, and platelet counts.

DRUG INTERACTIONS
Severe renal impairment reported w/ oral cyclosporine. May reduce the threshold for BCNU lung toxicity. Nalidixic acid may increase incidence of severe hemorrhagic necrotic enterocolitis in pediatric patients.

PREGNANCY AND LACTATION
Pregnancy: Can cause fetal harm.
Lactation: It is not known whether melphalan is present in human milk. Not for use in nursing.
Reproductive Potential: Avoid pregnancy; females of reproductive potential should use effective contraception methods during and after treatment. May damage spermatozoa and testicular tissue, resulting in possible genetic fetal abnormalities; males w/ female sexual partners of reproductive potential should use effective contraception during and after treatment.

MECHANISM OF ACTION
Alkylating agent; cytotoxicity appears to be related to the extent of its interstrand cross-linking w/ DNA, probably by binding at the N^7 position of guanine. Active against both resting and rapidly dividing tumor cells.

PHARMACOKINETICS
Absorption: C_{max}=1.2mcg/mL (10mg/m^2), 2.8mcg/mL (20mg/m^2). **Distribution:** V_d=0.5L/kg; plasma protein binding (50-90%). **Metabolism:** Hydrolysis. **Elimination:** $T_{1/2}$=75 min. Urine (5.8-21.3%).

PATIENT CONSIDERATIONS
Assessment: Assess for prior irradiation or chemotherapy, renal impairment, pregnancy/nursing status, drug hypersensitivity, and possible drug interactions. Obtain baseline hematological parameters.

Monitoring: Monitor for GI toxicity, hepatotoxicity, induction of a second malignancy, amenorrhea, testicular suppression, bone marrow suppression, hypersensitivity reactions, and other adverse events. Monitor CBC and other hematologic lab parameters.

Counseling: Advise to report any signs or symptoms of thrombocytopenia, leukopenia, and anemia; inform of the need for routine blood counts. Inform of signs/symptoms of mucositis; instruct on ways to reduce risk of development, and on ways to maintain nutrition and control discomfort if it occurs. Advise to report symptoms of N/V and diarrhea. Advise to immediately report symptoms of hypersensitivity reactions. Inform of the potential long-term risks related to secondary malignancy. Advise of the potential risk to a fetus. Advise females of reproductive potential to avoid pregnancy, which may include use of effective contraception during and after treatment. Advise females to contact their healthcare provider if they become pregnant, or if pregnancy is suspected. Inform about the risk for infertility. Advise not to breastfeed. Advise males w/ female sexual partners of reproductive potential that effective contraception should be used during and after treatment.

EVOTAZ — atazanavir/cobicistat   Rx
Class: CYP3A inhibitor/protease inhibitor

ADULT DOSAGE
HIV-1 Infection
In Combination w/ Other Antiretroviral Agents in Treatment Naive/Experienced Patients:
1 tab qd

PEDIATRIC DOSAGE
Pediatric use may not have been established

DOSING CONSIDERATIONS
Concomitant Medications
Dose separation may be required when coadministered w/ H$_2$-receptor antagonists (H$_2$RAs) or proton-pump inhibitors (PPIs)

Renal Impairment
CrCl <70mL/min: Coadministration w/ tenofovir disoproxil fumarate (TDF) is not recommended
ESRD on Hemodialysis (Treatment-Experienced Patients): Not recommended

Hepatic Impairment
Not recommended

ADMINISTRATION
Oral route

Take w/ food.

STORAGE
25°C (77°F); excursions permitted to 15-30°C (59-86°F).

HOW SUPPLIED
Tab: (Atazanavir [ATV]/Cobicistat) 300mg/150mg

CONTRAINDICATIONS
Prior significant hypersensitivity (eg, Stevens-Johnson syndrome, erythema multiforme, or toxic skin eruptions) to any of the components of this product. Coadministration w/ drugs that are highly dependent on CYP3A or UGT1A1 for clearance, and for which elevated plasma concentrations of the interacting drugs are associated w/ serious and/or life-threatening events, and w/ strong CYP3A inducers that may lead to lower exposure and loss of efficacy of therapy (alfuzosin, ranolazine, dronedarone, carbamazepine, phenobarbital, phenytoin, colchicine, rifampin, irinotecan, lurasidone, triazolam, oral midazolam, dihydroergotamine, ergotamine, methylergonovine, cisapride, St. John's wort, lovastatin, simvastatin, pimozide, nevirapine, sildenafil [when used for the treatment of pulmonary HTN], indinavir).

WARNINGS/PRECAUTIONS
Use in treatment-experienced patients should be guided by the number of baseline primary protease inhibitor resistance substitutions. Patients w/ underlying hepatitis B or C infections or marked elevations in transaminases may be at increased risk for developing further transaminase elevations or hepatic decompensation. Redistribution/accumulation of body fat reported. Caution in elderly. **ATV:** May prolong the PR interval. 2nd-degree atrioventricular block and other conduction abnormalities reported; consider ECG monitoring in patients w/ preexisting conduction system disease. Cases of Stevens-Johnson syndrome, erythema multiforme, mild-to-moderate maculopapular skin eruptions, and toxic skin eruptions, including drug rash eosinophilia and systemic symptoms (DRESS) syndrome, reported; d/c if severe rash develops. Cases of nephrolithiasis and/or cholelithiasis reported; consider temporary interruption or discontinuation of therapy if signs/symptoms occur. Asymptomatic elevations in indirect (unconjugated) bilirubin may occur. Hepatic transaminase elevations that occur w/ hyperbilirubinemia should be evaluated for alternative etiologies. Consider alternative therapy if jaundice or scleral icterus associated w/ bilirubin elevations presents cosmetic concerns for patients. Immune reconstitution syndrome and autoimmune disorders (eg, Graves' disease, polymyositis, Guillain-Barre syndrome) in the setting of immune reconstitution reported. New-onset or exacerbation of diabetes mellitus (DM), hyperglycemia, and diabetic ketoacidosis reported; may require either initiation or dose adjustments of insulin or oral hypoglycemic agents. Increased bleeding in patients w/ hemophilia A and B reported. **Cobicistat:** Decreases estimated CrCl w/o affecting actual renal glomerular function; consider effect when interpreting changes in estimated CrCl in patients initiating therapy, particularly w/ medical conditions or receiving drugs needing monitoring w/ estimated CrCl. Closely monitor patients w/ confirmed increase in SrCr >0.4mg/dL from baseline for renal safety. Consider alternative medications that do not require dosage adjustments in patients w/ renal impairment.

ADVERSE REACTIONS
Jaundice, ocular icterus, nausea.

DRUG INTERACTIONS
See Dosing Considerations and Contraindications. Coadministration of therapy w/ TDF in combination w/ concomitant or recent use of a nephrotoxic agent is not recommended. Not recommended w/ products containing the individual components of Evotaz, ritonavir (RTV) or products containing RTV, other antiretroviral drugs that require CYP3A inhibition to achieve adequate exposures (eg, other HIV protease inhibitors, elvitegravir), efavirenz, etravirine, boceprevir, telaprevir, simeprevir, voriconazole, apixaban, rivaroxaban, dabigatran etexilate (in specific renal impairment groups), salmeterol, inhaled/nasal corticosteroids that are metabolized by CYP3A, or avanafil. Not recommended w/ drugs highly dependent on CYP2C8 for clearance w/ narrow therapeutic indices (eg, paclitaxel, repaglinide). Coadministration w/ TDF and H$_2$RA in treatment-experienced patients is not recommended; administer either at the same time or at a minimum of 10 hrs after H$_2$RA dose. Coadministration w/ PPIs in treatment-experienced patients is not recommended; give therapy a minimum of 12 hrs after PPI administration in treatment-naive patients. CYP3A4 inhibitors may increase levels. Clarithromycin, erythromycin, telithromycin, ketoconazole, and itraconazole may increase levels; consider alternative antibiotics. Bosentan may decrease levels. CYP3A4 inducers may decrease levels and reduce the therapeutic effect leading to development of resistance to ATV. Anticonvulsants that induce CYP3A (eg, oxcarbazepine) may decrease levels; consider alternative anticonvulsant or antiretroviral therapy, if coadministration is necessary, monitor for lack/loss of virologic response and clinical monitoring of anticonvulsants is recommended. May increase levels of maraviroc, antiarrhythmics, digoxin, clarithromycin, erythromycin, telithromycin, dasatinib, nilotinib, vinblastine, vincristine, anticonvulsants metabolized by CYP3A (eg, clonazepam), TCAs,

trazodone, ketoconazole, itraconazole, colchicine, rifabutin, quetiapine, β-blockers, calcium channel blockers, corticosteroids, bosentan, atorvastatin, fluvastatin, pravastatin, rosuvastatin, immunosuppressants (eg, cyclosporine, everolimus, sirolimus, tacrolimus), fentanyl, tramadol, neuroleptics, PDE-5 inhibitors, and sedatives/hypnotics (eg, buspirone, diazepam, zolpidem). May increase levels of drugs that are primarily metabolized by CYP3A, UGT1A1 and/or CYP2D6 or substrates of P-gp, BCRP, OATP1B1, and/or OATP1B3, increasing/prolonging their therapeutic effects and adverse reactions, and requiring dose adjustments and/or additional monitoring of these drugs. Monitor for tenofovir-associated adverse reactions w/ TDF. Monitor INR w/ warfarin. Caution w/ antidepressants (eg, SSRIs, TCAs) and w/ narcotics used for treatment of opioid dependence (buprenorphine, naloxone, methadone). Coadministration w/ corticosteroids that are metabolized by CYP3A, particularly long-term use, may increase the risk for development of systemic corticosteroid effects. Coadministration w/ dexamethasone or other corticosteroids that induce CYP3A may result in loss of therapeutic effect and development of resistance to ATV. Consider alternative nonhormonal forms of contraception if taking hormonal contraceptives. Coadministration w/ parenteral midazolam should be done in a setting that ensures close clinical monitoring and appropriate medical management in case of respiratory depression and/or prolonged sedation. **ATV:** Reduced levels w/ PPIs, antacids, buffered medications, or H$_2$RAs. Administer a minimum of 2 hrs apart w/ concomitant use of antacids. Coadministration w/ didanosine buffered tabs may decrease atazanavir exposure. Simultaneous coadministration w/ didanosine enteric coated caps and atazanavir w/ food, may decrease didanosine exposure. **Cobicistat:** Renal impairment, including cases of acute renal failure and Fanconi syndrome, reported when used in an antiretroviral regimen containing TDF. Refer to PI for further detailed information on drug interactions, including dosing modifications required when used w/ certain concomitant therapies.

PREGNANCY AND LACTATION
Pregnancy: Category B. Do not use in treatment-experienced pregnant patients taking an H$_2$RA and/or TDF during the 2nd or 3rd trimester. Physicians are encouraged to register patients who become pregnant in the Antiretroviral Pregnancy Registry.
Lactation: Mothers should be instructed not to breastfeed due to potential for HIV-1 transmission.

MECHANISM OF ACTION
ATV: Protease inhibitor; selectively inhibits the virus-specific processing of viral Gag and Gag-Pol polyproteins in HIV-1 infected cells, thus preventing formation of mature virions. **Cobicistat:** CYP3A inhibitor; increases the systemic exposure of the CYP3A substrate ATV by inhibiting its metabolism.

PHARMACOKINETICS
Absorption: ATV: Rapid. T$_{max}$=3.5 hrs (median). Cobicistat: (Fed) C$_{max}$=1.5μg/mL, AUC$_{tau}$=11.1μg•hr/mL, T$_{max}$=3 hrs (median). **Distribution:** ATV: Plasma protein binding (86%). Cobicistat: Plasma protein binding (97-98%). **Metabolism:** ATV: Extensive via CYP3A; glucuronidation, N-dealkylation, hydrolysis, and oxygenation w/ dehydrogenation (minor). Cobicistat: CYP3A, CYP2D6 (minor). **Elimination:** ATV: T$_{1/2}$=approx 7.5 hrs (w/ light meal). Cobicistat: Feces (86.2%), urine (8.2%); T$_{1/2}$=approx 3-4 hrs (median).

PATIENT CONSIDERATIONS
Assessment: Assess for previous hypersensitivity to the drug, preexisting conduction system disease, hemophilia, preexisting DM, renal/hepatic impairment, pregnancy/nursing status, and possible drug interactions. Assess estimated CrCl. Assess for primary protease inhibitor resistance substitutions in treatment-experienced patients. When coadministering w/ TDF, assess estimated CrCl, urine glucose, and urine protein at baseline. Perform baseline hepatic laboratory testing in patients w/ underlying hepatitis B or C infections or marked transaminase elevations.

Monitoring: Monitor for fat redistribution/accumulation, cardiac conduction abnormalities, rash, Stevens-Johnson syndrome, DRESS syndrome, nephrolithiasis, cholelithiasis, hyperbilirubinemia, new onset or exacerbation of DM, hyperglycemia, diabetic ketoacidosis, immune reconstitution syndrome, autoimmune disorders, and other adverse reactions. Monitor for bleeding in patients w/ hemophilia. Perform routine monitoring of estimated CrCl, urine glucose, and urine protein when used w/ TDF. Monitor serum phosphorus levels in patients at risk for renal impairment when used w/ TDF. Perform hepatic laboratory testing in patients w/ underlying hepatitis B or C infections or marked transaminase elevations.

Counseling: Inform that therapy is not a cure for HIV and that illnesses associated w/ HIV may continue. Advise to remain under the care of a physician during therapy. Advise to avoid activities that can spread HIV infection to others. Instruct to take ud and not to d/c therapy w/o consulting physician. Advise not to miss a dose, but if a dose is missed by ≤12 hrs, instruct to take the missed dose right away and take next dose at the usual time, or if missed by >12 hrs, instruct to wait and take next dose at the usual time and not to double next dose. Inform of the potential for serious drug interactions, and explain that some drugs should not be taken concomitantly, or some drugs may need a change in dose. Advise to report use of any prescription/nonprescription medication or herbal products, particularly St. John's wort. Instruct patients receiving hormonal contraceptives to use additional or alternative nonhormonal contraceptive measures during therapy. Inform that therapy may produce ECG changes; advise to consult physician if symptoms (eg, dizziness, lightheadedness) are experienced. Inform that mild rashes w/o other symptoms and severe skin reactions have been reported; advise to immediately contact physician if signs/symptoms of severe skin/hypersensitivity reactions develop. Inform that kidney stones and/or gallstones, and fat redistribution/accumulation have been reported. Inform that asymptomatic elevations in indirect bilirubin accompanied by yellowing of the skin or whites of the eyes have occurred and that alternative antiretroviral therapy may be considered if patients have cosmetic concerns.

EXJADE — deferasirox   Rx
Class: Iron-chelating agent

> May cause acute renal failure and death, particularly in patients w/ comorbidities and those w/ advanced stages of hematologic disorders. Measure SrCr and determine CrCl in duplicate prior to initiation of therapy and monitor renal function at least monthly thereafter. Monitor creatinine weekly for the 1st month, then at least monthly for patients w/ baseline renal impairment or increased risk of acute renal failure. Consider dose reduction, interruption, or discontinuation based on increases in SrCr. May cause hepatic injury, including hepatic failure and death. Measure serum transaminases and bilirubin prior to initiating treatment, every 2 weeks during the 1st month, and at least monthly thereafter. Avoid in patients w/ severe (Child-Pugh C) hepatic impairment and reduce dose w/ moderate (Child-Pugh B) hepatic impairment. May cause GI hemorrhages, which may be fatal, especially in elderly who have advanced hematologic malignancies and/or low platelet counts. Monitor patients and d/c therapy if GI ulceration or hemorrhage suspected.

ADULT DOSAGE
Chronic Iron Overload

Transfusional Iron Overload:
Only consider when a patient has evidence of chronic transfusional iron overload, which should include the transfusion of at least 100mL/kg of packed RBCs (eg, at least 20 U of packed RBCs for a 40kg person or more in those >40kg) and a serum ferritin consistently >1000mcg/L

Initial: 20mg/kg qd; calculate doses (mg/kg/day) to nearest whole tab
Maint: May adjust dose every 3-6 months based on serum ferritin trends. Make dose adjustments in steps of 5 or 10mg/kg and tailor adjustments to individual response and therapeutic goals. If inadequately controlled w/ doses of 30mg/kg (eg, serum ferritin persistently >2500mcg/L and not showing a decreasing trend over time), doses up to 40mg/kg may be considered. If serum ferritin falls consistently <500mcg/L, consider interrupting therapy temporarily.
Max: 40mg/kg

In Non-Transfusion-Dependent Thalassemia (NTDT) Syndromes:
Only consider in a patient w/ a liver iron concentration (LIC) of at least 5mg of iron/g of liver dry weight (mg Fe/g dw) and a serum ferritin >300mcg/L

Initial: 10mg/kg qd; calculate doses (mg/kg/day) to nearest whole tab. If baseline LIC >15mg Fe/g dw, consider increasing dose to 20mg/kg/day after 4 weeks.
Maint: Interrupt treatment when serum ferritin is <300mcg/L and obtain LIC to determine whether it has fallen to <3mg Fe/g dw. After 6 months of therapy, if LIC remains >7mg Fe/g dw, increase to a max of 20mg/kg/day. If after 6 months of therapy LIC is 3-7mg Fe/g dw, continue treatment at no more than 10mg/kg/day. When LIC is <3mg Fe/g dw, interrupt treatment and continue to monitor LIC. Restart treatment when LIC rises again to >5mg Fe/g dw.
Max: 20mg/kg/day

PEDIATRIC DOSAGE
Chronic Iron Overload

Transfusional Iron Overload:
Only consider when a patient has evidence of chronic transfusional iron overload, which should include the transfusion of at least 100mL/kg of packed RBCs (eg, at least 20 U of packed RBCs for a 40kg person or more in those >40kg) and a serum ferritin consistently >1000mcg/L

≥2 Years:
Initial: 20mg/kg qd; calculate doses (mg/kg/day) to nearest whole tab
Maint: May adjust dose every 3-6 months based on serum ferritin trends. Make dose adjustments in steps of 5 or 10mg/kg and tailor adjustments to individual response and therapeutic goals. If inadequately controlled w/ doses of 30mg/kg (eg, serum ferritin persistently >2500mcg/L and not showing a decreasing trend over time), doses up to 40mg/kg may be considered. If serum ferritin falls consistently <500mcg/L, consider interrupting therapy temporarily.
Max: 40mg/kg

In NTDT Syndromes:
Only consider in a patient w/ an LIC of at least 5mg Fe/g dw and a serum ferritin >300mcg/L

≥10 Years:
Initial: 10mg/kg qd; calculate doses (mg/kg/day) to nearest whole tab. If baseline LIC >15mg Fe/g dw, consider increasing dose to 20mg/kg/day after 4 weeks.
Maint: Interrupt treatment when serum ferritin is <300mcg/L and obtain LIC to determine whether it has fallen to <3mg Fe/g dw. After 6 months of therapy, if LIC remains >7mg Fe/g dw, increase to a max of 20mg/kg/day. If after 6 months of therapy LIC is 3-7mg Fe/g dw, continue treatment at no more than 10mg/kg/day. When LIC is <3mg Fe/g dw, interrupt treatment and continue to monitor LIC. Restart treatment when LIC rises again to >5mg Fe/g dw.
Max: 20mg/kg/day

- - - - - - - - - -

DOSING CONSIDERATIONS
Concomitant Medications
Bile Acid Sequestrants/Potent UDP-Glucuronosyltransferase (UGT) Inducers:
Avoid w/ bile acid sequestrants (eg, cholestyramine, colesevelam, colestipol) or potent UGT inducers (eg, rifampicin, phenytoin, phenobarbital, ritonavir). If concomitant use is necessary w/ 1 of these agents, consider increasing initial dose of deferasirox by 50%, and monitor serum ferritin levels and clinical responses for further dose modification.

Renal Impairment
Baseline Renal Impairment:
CrCl 40-60mL/min: Reduce starting dose by 50%
SrCr >2X ULN or CrCl <40mL/min: Contraindicated

Increases in SrCr During Therapy:
All Patients: D/C therapy for SrCr >2X age-appropriate ULN or for CrCl <40mL/min

Transfusional Iron Overload:
2-15 Years: Reduce dose by 10mg/kg if SrCr increases to >33% above average baseline measurement and greater than age-appropriate ULN
≥16 Years: If SrCr increases by ≥33% above average baseline measurement, repeat SrCr w/in 1 week, and if still elevated by ≥33%, reduce dose by 10mg/kg

NTDT Syndromes:
10-15 Years: Reduce dose by 5mg/kg if SrCr increases to >33% above average baseline measurement and greater than age-appropriate ULN
≥16 Years: If SrCr increases by ≥33% above the average baseline measurement, repeat SrCr w/in 1 week, and if still elevated by ≥33%, interrupt therapy if dose is 5mg/kg, or reduce by 50% if the dose is 10mg/kg or 20mg/kg

Hepatic Impairment
Baseline Hepatic Impairment:
Mild (Child-Pugh A): No dose adjustment necessary
Moderate (Child-Pugh B): Reduce starting dose by 50%
Severe (Child-Pugh C): Avoid use

Elderly
Start at lower end of dosing range

ADMINISTRATION
Oral route

Do not chew tabs or swallow whole.
Take qd on an empty stomach at least 30 min before food, preferably at the same time each day.
Completely disperse tabs by stirring in water, orange juice, or apple juice until a fine sus is obtained.
Disperse doses of <1g in 3.5 oz of liquid and doses of ≥1g in 7 oz of liquid.
After swallowing sus, resuspend any residue in a small volume of liquid and swallow.

STORAGE
25°C (77°F); excursions permitted to 15-30°C (59-86°F). Protect from moisture.

HOW SUPPLIED
Tab: 125mg, 250mg, 500mg

CONTRAINDICATIONS
SrCr >2X age-appropriate ULN or CrCl <40mL/min, poor performance status, high-risk myelodysplastic syndrome (MDS), advanced malignancies, platelet counts <50 x 10⁹/L, known hypersensitivity to deferasirox or any component of this medication.

WARNINGS/PRECAUTIONS
Renal tubular damage including Fanconi's syndrome reported, most commonly in children and adolescents w/ β-thalassemia and serum ferritin levels <1500mcg/L. Intermittent proteinuria reported; monitor for proteinuria monthly. Hepatic toxicity appears to be more common in patients >55 yrs of age. Hepatic failure was more common in patients w/ significant comorbidities, including liver cirrhosis and multiorgan failure. Consider dose modifications or interruption of treatment for severe or persistent elevations in serum transaminases and bilirubin. Patients w/ mild (Child-Pugh A) or moderate (Child-Pugh B) hepatic impairment may be at higher risk for hepatic toxicity. Nonfatal upper GI irritation, ulceration, and hemorrhage reported. There have been reports of ulcers complicated w/ GI perforation (including fatal outcome). Neutropenia, agranulocytosis, worsening anemia, and thrombocytopenia, including fatal events, reported; risk may increase w/ preexisting hematologic disorders. Interrupt treatment in patients who develop cytopenias until the cause has been determined. Increased risk of toxicity in elderly; monitor more frequently. May cause serious hypersensitivity reactions (eg, anaphylaxis, angioedema); d/c and institute appropriate medical intervention if reactions are severe. Do not reintroduce in patients who have experienced previous hypersensitivity reactions on deferasirox products. Severe skin reactions, including Stevens-Johnson syndrome (SJS), toxic epidermal necrolysis (TEN), and erythema multiforme, reported. Cannot exclude risk of other skin reactions (eg, drug reaction w/ eosinophilia and systemic symptoms). D/C immediately and do not reintroduce if severe skin reactions are suspected. Rashes may occur; interrupt treatment in severe cases and may consider reintroduction at a lower dose w/ escalation after resolution of rash. Auditory and ocular disturbances reported. Perform auditory and ophthalmic testing every 12 months; monitor more frequently if disturbances are noted and consider dose reduction or interruption. Measure serum ferritin monthly for possible overchelation of iron for patients w/ transfusional iron overload. For patients w/ NTDT, measure serum ferritin monthly and measure LIC by liver biopsy or by using an FDA-cleared/approved method for monitoring patients receiving therapy every 6 months on treatment.

ADVERSE REACTIONS
Transfusional Iron Overload: Abdominal pain, N/V, diarrhea, skin rashes, increases in SrCr.
NTDT Syndromes: Nausea, rash, diarrhea.

DRUG INTERACTIONS
See Dosing Considerations. Avoid w/ aluminum-containing antacid preparations. May induce CYP3A4, resulting in a decrease in CYP3A4 substrate concentration; closely monitor for signs of reduced effectiveness w/ drugs metabolized by CYP3A4 (eg, cyclosporine, fentanyl, quetiapine). Inhibits CYP2C8 and CYP1A2, resulting in an increase in CYP2C8 (eg, repaglinide, paclitaxel) and CYP1A2 (eg, duloxetine, theophylline, tizanidine) substrate concentration; closely monitor for signs of exposure-related toxicity. Consider decreasing the dose of repaglinide and monitor blood glucose levels carefully. Avoid w/ theophylline or other CYP1A2 substrates w/ a narrow therapeutic index (eg, tizanidine); monitor theophylline concentrations and consider theophylline dose modification if theophylline must be coadministered. Increased risk of GI hemorrhage w/ drugs that have ulcerogenic or hemorrhagic potential (eg, NSAIDs, corticosteroids, oral bisphosphonates, anticoagulants).

PREGNANCY AND LACTATION
Pregnancy: Category C.
Lactation: Not for use in nursing.

MECHANISM OF ACTION
Iron-chelating agent; a tridentate ligand that binds iron w/ high affinity in a 2:1 ratio.

PHARMACOKINETICS
Absorption: Absolute bioavailability (70%); T_{max}=1.5-4 hrs (median). **Distribution:** V_d=14.37L (adults); plasma protein binding (99%). **Metabolism:** Glucuronidation via UGT1A1 (major) and UGT1A3 (minor) followed by deconjugation in the intestine and reabsorption (enterohepatic recycling); oxidation via CYP450 (minor). **Elimination:** Feces (84%), urine (8%); $T_{1/2}$=8-16 hrs.

PATIENT CONSIDERATIONS
Assessment: Assess for high-risk MDS, performance status, renal/hepatic impairment, advanced malignancies, hematological disorders, comorbidities, hypersensitivity to the drug, pregnancy/nursing status, and possible drug interactions. Perform baseline auditory and ophthalmic examinations. Obtain baseline SrCr in duplicate, serum transaminases, bilirubin, and blood counts. Determine CrCl (Cockcroft-Gault method). In patients w/ transfusional iron overload, obtain baseline serum ferritin level. In patients w/ iron overload in NTDT syndromes, obtain LIC by liver biopsy or by an FDA-cleared/approved method for identifying patients for treatment w/ deferasirox therapy and obtain baseline serum ferritin level on at least 2 measurements 1 month apart.

Monitoring: Monitor for acute renal failure, hepatic failure, GI ulceration/hemorrhage, neutropenia, agranulocytosis, worsening anemia, thrombocytopenia, hypersensitivity reactions, rashes, SJS, TEN, erythema multiforme, and other adverse reactions. Monitor blood counts. Perform auditory and ophthalmic tests every 12 months. Monitor closely for efficacy and adverse reactions that may require dose titration in patients w/ mild or moderate hepatic impairment. Monitor serum transaminases and bilirubin every 2 weeks during the 1st month of therapy and at least monthly thereafter. Monitor SrCr weekly during the 1st month after initiation or modification of therapy and at least monthly thereafter. Monitor SrCr and/or CrCl more frequently if creatinine levels are increasing. Monitor serum ferritin and for proteinuria monthly. In patients w/ iron overload in NTDT syndromes, monitor LIC every 6 months. Monitor elderly more frequently for toxicity.

Counseling: Instruct to take ud. Instruct not to take the medication simultaneously w/ aluminum-containing antacids. Inform of the importance of auditory and ophthalmic testing before starting treatment and thereafter at regular intervals. Caution patients experiencing dizziness to avoid driving or operating machinery. Inform about drug interactions including potential for GI ulcers/bleeding and loss of effectiveness due to drug interactions. Advise that blood tests will be performed every month or more frequently if patient is at increased risk of complications. Inform that severe kidney and liver problems, blood disorders, stomach hemorrhage, and death have been reported. Inform that skin rash and serious allergic reactions have been reported; advise to d/c therapy and contact physician immediately if severe reactions occur.

Exondys 51 — eteplirsen   Rx

Class: Antisense oligonucleotide

ADULT DOSAGE	PEDIATRIC DOSAGE
Duchenne Muscular Dystrophy	**Duchenne Muscular Dystrophy**
Treatment of Duchenne muscular dystrophy (DMD) in patients who have a confirmed mutation of the DMD gene that is amenable to exon 51 skipping	Treatment of DMD in patients who have a confirmed mutation of the DMD gene that is amenable to exon 51 skipping
30mg/kg once weekly	30mg/kg once weekly
Missed Dose	**Missed Dose**
Administered as soon as possible after the scheduled time	Administered as soon as possible after the scheduled time

DOSING CONSIDERATIONS
Renal Impairment
Has not been studied

Hepatic Impairment
Has not been studied

ADMINISTRATION
IV route

- Administer as a 35- to 60-min IV infusion.
- Flush IV access line w/ 0.9% NaCl prior to and after infusion.
- Do not mix w/ other medications or infuse other medications concomitantly via the same IV access line.
- May apply topical anesthetic cream to infusion site prior to administration.

Preparation
1. Determine volume needed and the correct number of vials to supply full calculated dose.
2. Allow vials to warm to room temperature. Mix contents of each vial by gently inverting 2-3X; do not shake.
3. Withdraw calculated volume w/ a syringe fitted w/ a 21-gauge or smaller non-coring needle.
4. Dilute in 0.9% NaCl, to make a total volume of 100-150mL; visually inspect diluted sol for particulates.
5. Contains no preservatives and should be administered immediately after dilution.
6. Complete infusion of diluted sol w/in 4 hrs of dilution; if immediate use is not possible, diluted sol may be stored for up to 24 hrs at 2-8°C (36-46°F). Do not freeze. Discard unused sol.

STORAGE
2-8°C (36-46°F). Do not freeze. Protect from light.

HOW SUPPLIED
Inj: 100mg/2mL, 500mg/10mL

WARNINGS/PRECAUTIONS
Approved under accelerated approval based on an increase in dystrophin in skeletal muscle observed in some patients; clinical benefit of eteplirsen has not been established. Continued approval for this indication may be contingent upon verification of a clinical benefit in confirmatory trials.

ADVERSE REACTIONS
Balance disorder, vomiting.

PREGNANCY AND LACTATION
Pregnancy: No human/animal data available to assess use during pregnancy.
Lactation: No human/animal data to assess the effect on milk production, the presence of eteplirsen in milk, or the effects on the breastfed infant; caution in nursing.

MECHANISM OF ACTION
Antisense oligonucleotide; designed to bind to exon 51 of dystrophin pre-mRNA, resulting in exclusion of this exon during mRNA processing in patients w/ genetic mutations that are amenable to exon 51 skipping.

PHARMACOKINETICS
Distribution: Plasma protein binding (6-17%); V_d=600mL/kg. **Elimination:** Urine; $T_{1/2}$=3-4 hrs.

PATIENT CONSIDERATIONS
Assessment: Assess for renal/hepatic impairment.
Monitoring: Monitor for adverse events.
Counseling: Instruct to notify physician if any adverse reactions develop.

EXTAVIA — interferon beta-1b   Rx

Class: Biological response modifier

ADULT DOSAGE	**PEDIATRIC DOSAGE**
Multiple Sclerosis	Pediatric use may not have been
Relapsing Forms:	established
Initial: 0.0625mg (0.25mL) SQ qod	
Titrate: Increase over a 6-week period to 0.25mg (1mL) SQ qod	
Titration Schedule:	
Weeks 1-2: 0.0625mg (0.25mL) qod	
Weeks 3-4: 0.125mg (0.5mL) qod	
Weeks 5-6: 0.1875mg (0.75mL) qod	
Week 7 and After: 0.25mg (1mL) qod	
Premedication	
For Flu-Like Symptoms:	
Concurrent use of analgesics and/or antipyretics on treatment days may help ameliorate flu-like symptoms	
Missed Dose	
Take it as soon as possible; do not take therapy on 2 consecutive days. The next inj should be taken about 48 hrs (2 days) after that dose	

ADMINISTRATION
SQ route
Rotate inj sites.
Do not reuse needles or syringes.
After reconstitution, if not used immediately, refrigerate reconstituted sol at 2-8°C (35-46°F) and use w/in 3 hrs; do not freeze.

Reconstitution
1. Attach the prefilled syringe containing the diluent (NaCl, 0.54% sol) to vial using the vial adapter. The removable rubber cap of the diluent prefilled syringe contains natural latex, which may cause allergic reactions and should not be handled by latex-sensitive individuals.
2. Slowly inject 1.2mL of diluent into vial.
3. Gently swirl vial to dissolve drug completely; do not shake. If foaming occurs, allow the vial to sit undisturbed until the foam settles.
4. Keeping syringe and vial adapter in place, turn assembly over so that vial is on top; withdraw appropriate dose.
5. Remove the vial from the vial adapter before injecting.

STORAGE
20-25°C (68-77°F); excursions of 15-30°C (59-86°F) are permitted for up to 3 months. After reconstitution, if not used immediately, refrigerate and use w/in 3 hrs. Do not freeze.

HOW SUPPLIED
Inj: 0.3mg

CONTRAINDICATIONS
Hypersensitivity to natural or recombinant interferon beta, albumin (human), mannitol, or any other component of the formulation.

WARNINGS/PRECAUTIONS
Severe hepatic injury including hepatic failure (rare) and asymptomatic elevation of serum transaminases reported; consider discontinuing therapy if serum transaminase levels significantly increase, or if associated w/ clinical symptoms (eg, jaundice). Anaphylaxis (rare) and other allergic reactions reported; d/c if anaphylaxis occurs. The removable rubber cap of the diluent prefilled syringe contains natural rubber latex, which may cause allergic reactions and should not be handled by latex-sensitive individuals. Depression and suicide reported; consider discontinuation of therapy if depression develops. CHF, cardiomyopathy, and cardiomyopathy w/ CHF reported; monitor for worsening of cardiac condition during initiation of and continued treatment in patients w/ preexisting CHF. Consider discontinuation of therapy if worsening of CHF occurs w/ no other etiology. Inj-site necrosis/reactions reported; avoid administration into affected area until fully healed in patients who continue therapy after inj-site necrosis has occurred. If multiple lesions occur, d/c until healed. Leukopenia reported; patients w/ myelosuppression may require more intensive monitoring of CBC, w/ differential and platelet counts. Cases of thrombotic microangiopathy (TMA), including thrombotic thrombocytopenic purpura and hemolytic uremic syndrome, reported; d/c if clinical symptoms and lab findings consistent w/ TMA occur and manage as clinically indicated. May cause seizures. Drug-induced lupus erythematosus reported; d/c therapy in patients developing new signs/symptoms characteristic of this syndrome.

ADVERSE REACTIONS
Inj-site reaction, lymphopenia, flu-like symptoms, myalgia, leukopenia, neutropenia, increased liver enzymes, headache, hypertonia, pain, rash, insomnia, abdominal pain, asthenia.

DRUG INTERACTIONS
Potential risk for hepatic injury w/ known hepatotoxic drugs or other products (eg, alcohol).

PREGNANCY AND LACTATION
Pregnancy: Category C. Spontaneous abortions while on treatment were reported in four patients participating in the interferon beta-1b RRMS clinical trial.
Lactation: Not for use in nursing.

MECHANISM OF ACTION
Biological response modifier; has not been established. Believed that interferon β-1b receptor binding induces expression of proteins that are responsible for pleiotropic bioactivities. Immunomodulatory effects include the enhancement of suppressor T-cell activity, reduction of proinflammatory cytokine production, down-regulation of antigen presentation, and inhibition of lymphocyte trafficking into the CNS.

PHARMACOKINETICS
Absorption: (0.5mg, SQ) Bioavailability (50%); C_{max}=40 IU/mL; T_{max}=1-8 hrs.
Distribution: (0.006-2mg, IV) V_d=0.25-2.88L/kg. **Elimination:** (0.006-2mg, IV) $T_{1/2}$=8 min-4.3 hrs.

PATIENT CONSIDERATIONS
Assessment: Assess for hypersensitivity to the drug or human albumin, preexisting CHF, myelosuppression, latex sensitivity, pregnancy/nursing status, and possible drug interactions. Obtain baseline CBC, differential WBC counts, platelet counts, and blood chemistries, including LFTs.

Monitoring: Monitor for hepatic injury, anaphylaxis, depression, suicidal ideation, worsening of CHF, inj-site necrosis/reactions, leukopenia, TMA, flu-like symptom complex, seizures, drug-induced lupus erythematosus, and other adverse reactions. Monitor CBC and differential WBC count, platelet counts, and blood chemistries, including LFTs, at regular intervals (1, 3, and 6 months) following introduction, and then periodically thereafter in the absence of clinical symptoms. Periodically evaluate patient understanding and use of aseptic self-inj techniques and procedures, particularly if inj-site necrosis occurred.

Counseling: Instruct on proper aseptic technique and procedures. Advise not to reuse needles/syringes and instruct on safe disposal procedures. Inform of the importance of rotating inj sites w/ each dose. Instruct to notify physician if pregnant, planning to become pregnant, or if any adverse reactions (eg, hepatic dysfunction, allergic reactions, anaphylaxis, worsening of cardiac condition, inj-site necrosis, seizures, drug-induced lupus erythematosus) occur. Inform latex-sensitive individuals that the removable rubber cap of the diluent prefilled syringe contains natural rubber latex. Inform that symptoms of depression or suicidal ideation may occur and instruct to notify physician immediately if these occur. Inform that flu-like symptoms are common following initiation of therapy. Instruct to take missed dose as soon as possible, but not to take on 2 consecutive days.

EYLEA — aflibercept   Rx

Class: Vascular endothelial growth factor (VEGF) inhibitor

ADULT DOSAGE	**PEDIATRIC DOSAGE**
Neovascular (Wet) Age-Related Macular Degeneration	Pediatric use may not have been established
2mg (0.05mL) every 4 weeks for first 12 weeks, followed by 2mg once every 8 weeks; some patients may need every 4 week dosing after the first 12 weeks	
Macular Edema	
Following Retinal Vein Occlusion:	
2mg (0.05mL) once every 4 weeks	
Diabetic Macular Edema	
2mg (0.05mL) every 4 weeks for first 5 inj, followed by 2mg once every 8 weeks; some patients may need every	

4 week dosing after the first 20 weeks (5 months)

Diabetic Retinopathy
In Patients w/ Diabetic Macular Edema:
2mg (0.05mL) every 4 weeks for first 5 inj, followed by 2mg once every 8 weeks; some patients may need every 4 week dosing after the first 20 weeks (5 months)

ADMINISTRATION
Intravitreal route

Intravitreal inj should be performed w/ a 30-gauge x 1/2-inch inj needle.

Preparation for Administration
1. Attach the 19-gauge x 1.5-inch, 5-micron, filter needle to the 1-mL syringe.
2. Push the filter needle into the center of the vial stopper until the needle is completely inserted into the vial and the tip touches the bottom or bottom edge of the vial.
3. Withdraw all of the vial contents into the syringe, keeping the vial in an upright position, slightly inclined to ease complete withdrawal. To deter the introduction of air, ensure the bevel of the filter needle is submerged into the liquid. Continue to tilt the vial during withdrawal keeping the bevel of the filter needle submerged in the liquid.
4. Ensure that the plunger rod is drawn sufficiently back when emptying the vial in order to completely empty the filter needle.
5. Remove the filter needle from the syringe and properly dispose of the filter needle; do not use the filter needle for intravitreal inj.
6. Attach the 30-gauge x 1/2-inch inj needle to the syringe.
7. Holding the syringe w/ the needle pointing up, check for bubbles. If there are bubbles, gently tap the syringe w/ finger until the bubbles rise to the top.
8. To eliminate all of the bubbles and to expel excess drug, slowly depress plunger so that the plunger tip aligns w/ the line that marks 0.05mL on the syringe.

Injection Procedure
Adequate anesthesia and a topical broad-spectrum microbicide should be given prior to the inj.
Each vial should only be used for the treatment of a single eye; if the contralateral eye requires treatment, use a new vial and change the sterile field, syringe, gloves, drapes, eyelid speculum, filter, and inj needles before administering to the other eye. After inj, discard any unused product.

STORAGE
2-8°C (36-46°F). Do not freeze. Protect from light.

HOW SUPPLIED
Inj: 40mg/mL [0.05mL]

CONTRAINDICATIONS
Ocular/periocular infections, active intraocular inflammation. Known hypersensitivity to aflibercept or any of the excipients in this medication.

WARNINGS/PRECAUTIONS
Endophthalmitis and retinal detachments may occur. Acute increases in IOP noted w/in 60 min of inj. Sustained increases in IOP reported after repeated dosing. Monitor IOP and perfusion of the optic nerve head and manage appropriately. Potential risk of arterial thromboembolic events (ATEs) (nonfatal stroke, nonfatal MI, vascular death).

ADVERSE REACTIONS
Conjunctival hemorrhage, eye pain, cataract, vitreous floaters, intraocular pressure increased, vitreous detachment.

PREGNANCY AND LACTATION
Pregnancy: Category C.
Lactation: Not for use in nursing.
Reproductive Potential: Females of reproductive potential should use effective contraception prior to the initial dose, during treatment, and for at least 3 months after the last inj.

MECHANISM OF ACTION
VEGF inhibitor; acts as a soluble decoy receptor that binds VEGF-A and placental growth factor, and thereby can inhibit the binding and activation of these cognate VEGF receptors.

PHARMACOKINETICS
Absorption: C_{max}=0.02mcg/mL (wet age-related macular degeneration), 0.05mcg/mL (retinal vein occlusion), 0.03mcg/mL (diabetic macular edema); T_{max}=1-3 days. **Distribution:** (IV) V_d=6L. **Metabolism:** Proteolysis. **Elimination:** (IV, 2-4mg/kg) $T_{1/2}$=5-6 days.

PATIENT CONSIDERATIONS
Assessment: Assess for hypersensitivity to the drug, ocular/periocular infections, active intraocular inflammation, and pregnancy/nursing status.
Monitoring: Monitor for signs/symptoms of endophthalmitis, retinal detachment, ATEs, and other adverse reactions. Monitor IOP and perfusion of the optic nerve head.
Counseling: Advise to seek immediate care from an ophthalmologist if eye becomes red, sensitive to light, painful, or patient develops a change in vision in the days following administration. Inform that temporary visual disturbances may be experienced after inj and the associated eye examinations; advise not to drive or use machinery until visual function has recovered sufficiently.

FABRAZYME — agalsidase beta
Class: Enzyme

Rx

ADULT DOSAGE
Fabry Disease
Usual: 1mg/kg IV infusion every 2 weeks

Infusion Rate:
Initial: ≤0.25mg/min (15mg/hr); rate may be slowed if infusion reactions occur
Titrate: After tolerance is well established, rate may be increased in increments of 0.05-0.08mg/min (3-5mg/hr) w/ each subsequent infusion based on tolerance

Patients <30kg: Max rate should remain at 0.25mg/min (15mg/hr)
Patients ≥30kg: Administration duration should not be <1.5 hrs

Re-Challenge:
For patients who have had a positive skin test to Fabrazyme or who have tested positive for anti-Fabrazyme IgE

Initial Re-Challenge: Administration should be a low dose at a lower infusion rate (eg, 1/2 the therapeutic dose [0.5mg/kg] at 1/25 the initial standard recommended rate [0.01mg/min])

Titrate: Once the infusion is tolerated, the dose may be increased to reach the approved dose of 1mg/kg and the infusion rate may be increased by slowly titrating upwards (doubled every 30 min up to a max rate of 0.25mg/min), as tolerated

Premedication
Administer antipyretics prior to infusion

PEDIATRIC DOSAGE
Fabry Disease
≥8 Years:
Usual: 1mg/kg IV infusion every 2 weeks

Infusion Rate:
Initial: ≤0.25mg/min (15mg/hr); rate may be slowed if infusion reactions occur
Titrate: After tolerance is well established, rate may be increased in increments of 0.05-0.08mg/min (3-5mg/hr) w/ each subsequent infusion based on tolerance

Patients <30kg: Max rate should remain at 0.25mg/min (15mg/hr)
Patients ≥30kg: Administration duration should not be <1.5 hrs

Re-Challenge:
For patients who have had a positive skin test to Fabrazyme or who have tested positive for anti-Fabrazyme IgE

Initial Re-Challenge: Administration should be a low dose at a lower infusion rate (eg, 1/2 the therapeutic dose [0.5mg/kg] at 1/25 the initial standard recommended rate [0.01mg/min])

Titrate: Once the infusion is tolerated, the dose may be increased to reach the approved dose of 1mg/kg and the infusion rate may be increased by slowly titrating upwards (doubled every 30 min up to a max rate of 0.25mg/min), as tolerated

Premedication
Administer antipyretics prior to infusion

ADMINISTRATION
IV route

Vials are for single use only; discard any unused product

Reconstitution and Dilution
1. Allow vials and diluent to reach room temperature prior to reconstitution (approx 30 min); the number of 35mg and 5mg vials needed is based on the patient's body weight and the recommended dose of 1mg/kg
2. Select a combination of 35mg and 5mg vials so that the total number of mg is equal to or greater than the patient's number of kg of body weight
3. Reconstitute each 35mg vial by slowly injecting 7.2mL of sterile water for inj (SWFI) down the inside wall of each vial. Roll and tilt each vial gently; each vial will yield a 5mg/mL sol (total extractable amount per vial is 35mg, 7mL)
4. Reconstitute each 5mg vial by slowly injecting 1.1mL of SWFI down the inside wall of each vial. Roll and tilt each vial gently; each vial will yield a 5mg/mL sol (total extractable amount per vial is 5mg, 1mL)
5. The reconstituted sol should be further diluted w/ 0.9% NaCl inj to a total volume based on patient weight as follows:
≤35kg: Minimum total volume of 50mL
35.1-70kg: Minimum total volume of 100mL
70.1-100kg: Minimum total volume of 250mL
<100kg: Minimum total volume of 500mL
6. Prior to adding the volume of reconstituted Fabrazyme required for the patient dose, remove an equal volume of 0.9% NaCl inj from the infusion bag
7. Slowly withdraw the reconstituted sol from each vial up to the total volume required for the patient dose
8. Inject the reconstituted sol directly into the NaCl sol; do not inject in the airspace w/in the infusion bag. Discard any vial w/ unused reconstituted sol
9. Gently invert infusion bag to mix the sol, avoiding vigorous shaking and agitation

Administration
Do not use filter needles during the preparation of the infusion
Do not infuse Fabrazyme in the same IV line w/ other products
Administer using an in-line low protein binding 0.2 µm filter

STORAGE
2-8°C (36-46°F). Reconstituted and Diluted Sol: 2-8°C (36-46°F) for up to 24 hrs.

HOW SUPPLIED
Inj: 5mg, 35mg

WARNINGS/PRECAUTIONS
Life-threatening anaphylactic reactions and severe allergic reactions observed; d/c immediately if such severe reactions occur and initiate necessary emergency treatment. Appropriate medical support should be readily available during administration. Infusion reactions reported; decrease infusion rate, temporarily stop infusion, and/or administer additional antipyretics, antihistamines, and/or steroids to ameliorate symptoms. Consider immediately discontinuing therapy

if a severe infusion reaction occurs. Pretreat w/ an antipyretic and antihistamine in patients experiencing infusion reactions. Use extreme caution when readministering in patients who have experienced an anaphylactic/severe allergic or infusion reaction. Higher risk of severe complications from infusion reactions in patients w/ compromised cardiac function. Consider testing for IgE antibodies in patients who experienced suspected allergic reactions and consider the risks and benefits of continued treatment in patients w/ anti-agalsidase beta IgE antibodies. Rechallenge of patients who have had a positive skin test to agalsidase beta or who have tested positive for agalsidase beta-specific IgE antibody should only occur under the direct supervision of qualified personnel, w/ appropriate medical support measures readily available.

ADVERSE REACTIONS
URTI, chills, pyrexia, headache, cough, paresthesia, fatigue, peripheral edema, dizziness, rash, nasal congestion, pain in extremity, back pain, myalgia, HTN.

PREGNANCY AND LACTATION
Category B, caution in nursing.

MECHANISM OF ACTION
Recombinant human α-galactosidase A enzyme; catalyzes the hydrolysis of glycosphingolipids, including globotriaosylceramide, reducing their deposition in capillary endothelium of the kidney, heart, and skin.

PHARMACOKINETICS
Administration of variable doses/infusion length in adults and pediatric patients resulted in different pharmacokinetic parameters; refer to PI.

PATIENT CONSIDERATIONS

Assessment: Assess for anaphylactic, allergic, infusion, and/or immune-mediated reactions from previous dose, cardiac function, and pregnancy/nursing status.

Monitoring: Monitor for anaphylactic, allergic, and infusion reactions, immunogenicity, and other adverse reactions.

Counseling: Inform of the importance of participating in the Fabry Registry. Instruct to notify physician if any adverse reaction develops.

FARYDAK — panobinostat   **Rx**

Class: Histone deacetylase (HDAC) inhibitor

> Severe diarrhea reported; monitor for symptoms, institute antidiarrheal treatment, interrupt panobinostat, and then reduce dose or d/c panobinostat. Severe and fatal cardiac ischemic events, severe arrhythmias, and ECG changes reported. Arrhythmias may be exacerbated by electrolyte abnormalities. Obtain ECG and electrolytes at baseline and periodically during treatment as clinically indicated.

ADULT DOSAGE
Multiple Myeloma
In combination w/ bortezomib (BTZ) and dexamethasone for the treatment of patients w/ multiple myeloma who have received at least 2 prior regimens, including BTZ and an immunomodulatory agent

Initial: 20mg once qod for 3 doses/week in Weeks 1 and 2 of each 21-day cycle for up to 8 cycles

Consider continuing treatment for an additional 8 cycles for patients w/ clinical benefit who do not experience unresolved severe or medically significant toxicity; total duration of treatment may be up to 16 cycles (48 weeks)

Recommended Dosing Schedule w/ BTZ and Dexamethasone:
Cycles 1-8:
- Panobinostat on Days 1, 3, 5, 8, 10, 12, and then rest for 1 week
- BTZ (1.3mg/m² inj) on Days 1, 4, 8, 11, and then rest for 1 week
- Dexamethasone (20mg PO) on Days 1, 2, 4, 5, 8, 9, 11, 12, and then rest for 1 week

Cycles 9-16:
- Panobinostat on Days 1, 3, 5, 8, 10, 12, and then rest for 1 week
- BTZ (1.3mg/m² inj) on Days 1, 8, and then rest for 1 week
- Dexamethasone (20mg PO) on Days 1, 2, 8, 9, and then rest for 1 week

Missed Dose
- If a dose is missed it can be taken up to 12 hrs after the specified time
- If vomiting occurs, patient should not repeat the dose but should take the next usual scheduled dose

PEDIATRIC DOSAGE
Pediatric use may not have been established

DOSING CONSIDERATIONS
Concomitant Medications
Strong CYP3A Inhibitors:
Reduce starting dose to 10mg

Hepatic Impairment
Mild: Reduce starting dose to 15mg
Moderate: Reduce starting dose to 10mg
Severe: Avoid use

Adverse Reactions
Management of adverse reactions may require treatment interruption and/or dose reductions.
If dose reduction is required, the dose of panobinostat should be reduced in increments of 5mg.
If the dosing of panobinostat is reduced <10mg given 3X per week, d/c panobinostat. Keep the same treatment schedule (3-week treatment cycle) when reducing dose.

Thrombocytopenia:
Platelets <50 x 10⁹/L (CTCAE Grade 3): Maintain panobinostat dose; monitor platelet counts at least weekly.
Maintain BTZ dose.
Platelets <50 x 10⁹/L w/ Bleeding (CTCAE Grade 3) or Platelets <25 x 10⁹/L (CTCAE Grade 4): Interrupt panobinostat; monitor platelet counts at least weekly until ≥50 x 10⁹/L, then restart at reduced dose.
Interrupt BTZ until thrombocytopenia resolves to ≥50 x 10⁹/L.
If only 1 dose was omitted prior to correction to these levels, restart BTZ at same dose.
If ≥2 doses were omitted consecutively, or w/in the same cycle, BTZ should be restarted at a reduced dose.

Neutropenia:
ANC 0.75-1.0 x 10⁹/L (CTCAE Grade 3): Maintain panobinostat dose.
Maintain BTZ dose.
ANC 0.5-0.75 x 10⁹/L (CTCAE Grade 3) (2 or More Occurrences): Interrupt panobinostat until ANC ≥1.0 x 10⁹/L, then restart at same dose.
Maintain BTZ dose.
ANC <1.0 x 10⁹/L (CTCAE Grade 3) w/ Febrile Neutropenia (Any Grade):
Interrupt panobinostat until febrile neutropenia resolves and ANC ≥1.0 x 10⁹/L, then restart at reduced dose.
Interrupt BTZ until febrile neutropenia resolves and ANC ≥1.0 x 10⁹/L.
If only 1 dose was omitted prior to correction to these levels, restart BTZ at same dose.
If ≥2 doses were omitted consecutively, or w/in the same cycle, BTZ should be restarted at a reduced dose.
ANC <0.5 x 10⁹/L (CTCAE Grade 4): Interrupt panobinostat until ANC ≥1.0 x 10⁹/L, then restart at reduced dose.
Interrupt BTZ until febrile neutropenia resolves and ANC ≥1.0 x 10⁹/L.
If only 1 dose was omitted prior to correction to these levels, restart BTZ at same dose.
If ≥2 doses were omitted consecutively, or w/in the same cycle, BTZ should be restarted at a reduced dose.

Anemia:
Hgb <8g/dL (CTCAE Grade 3): Interrupt panobinostat until Hgb ≥10g/dL. Restart at reduced dose.

Diarrhea:
Moderate Diarrhea, 4-6 Stools/Day (CTCAE Grade 2): Interrupt panobinostat until resolved, then restart at same dose.
Consider interruption of BTZ until resolved; restart at same dose.
Severe Diarrhea (≥7 Stools/Day) IV Fluids or Hospitalization Required (CTCAE Grade 3): Interrupt panobinostat until resolved, then restart at reduced dose.
Interrupt BTZ until resolved, then restart at reduced dose.
Life-Threatening Diarrhea (CTCAE Grade 4): Permanently d/c panobinostat. Permanently d/c BTZ.

N/V:
Severe Nausea (CTCAE Grade 3/4) or Severe/Life-Threatening Vomiting (CTCAE Grade 3/4): Interrupt panobinostat until resolved, then restart at reduced dose

Myelosuppression:
Interrupt or reduce dose of panobinostat in patients who have thrombocytopenia, neutropenia, or anemia according to instructions listed above.
Consider platelet transfusions in patients w/ severe thrombocytopenia.
D/C panobinostat treatment if thrombocytopenia does not improve despite the recommended treatment modifications or if repeated platelet transfusions are required.
Consider dose reduction and/or use of growth factors (eg, granulocyte colony-stimulating factor) in the event of Grade 3 or 4 neutropenia.
D/C panobinostat if neutropenia does not improve despite dose modifications, colony-stimulating factors, or in case of severe infection.

GI Toxicity:
May require treatment interruption or dose reduction if diarrhea, nausea, or vomiting occurs.
Treat w/ antidiarrheal medication (eg, loperamide) at 1st sign of abdominal cramping, loose stools, or onset of diarrhea.
Consider and administer prophylactic antiemetics as clinically indicated.

Other Adverse Drug Reactions:
Patients Experiencing Grade 3/4 Adverse Drug Reactions Other Than Thrombocytopenia, Neutropenia, or GI Toxicity:
CTC Grade 2 Toxicity Recurrence and CTC Grade 3 and 4: Omit dose until recovery to CTC ≤Grade 1 and restart treatment at a reduced dose.
CTC Grade 3 or 4 Toxicity Recurrence: May consider further dose reduction once the adverse events have resolved to CTC ≤Grade 1

ADMINISTRATION
Oral route

Take on each scheduled day at about the same time, either w/ or w/o food.
Swallow cap whole w/ a cup of water; do not open, crush, or chew.
Direct contact of the powder in cap w/ skin or mucous membranes should be avoided; wash thoroughly if such contact occurs.

STORAGE
20-25°C (68-77°F); excursions permitted between 15-30°C (59-86°F). Protect from light.

HOW SUPPLIED
Cap: 10mg, 15mg, 20mg

WARNINGS/PRECAUTIONS
Do not initiate in patients w/ history of recent MI or unstable angina. May prolong cardiac ventricular repolarization (QT interval); do not initiate in patients w/ a QTcF >450 msec or clinically significant baseline ST-segment or T-wave abnormalities. If during therapy the QTcF increases to ≥480 msec, interrupt therapy. If QT prolongation does not resolve, d/c therapy permanently. Fatal and serious hemorrhage reported. Myelosuppression (eg, severe thrombocytopenia, neutropenia, anemia) may occur. Localized and systemic infections (eg, pneumonia, bacterial infections, invasive fungal infections, viral infections) reported; if diagnosis of infection is made, institute appropriate anti-infective treatment promptly and consider interruption or discontinuation of therapy. Should not be initiated in patients w/ active infections. Hepatic dysfunction reported; if abnormal LFTs are observed, may consider dose adjustment until values return to normal or pretreatment levels. May cause fetal harm.

ADVERSE REACTIONS
Diarrhea, fatigue, N/V, peripheral edema, decreased appetite, pyrexia, hypophosphatemia, hypokalemia, hyponatremia, increased creatinine, thrombocytopenia, lymphopenia, leukopenia, neutropenia, anemia.

DRUG INTERACTIONS
See Dosing Considerations. Avoid w/ strong CYP3A inducers. Increased levels w/ strong CYP3A inhibitors; avoid star fruit, pomegranate or pomegranate juice, and grapefruit or grapefruit juice. Avoid coadministration w/ sensitive CYP2D6 substrates (eg, atomoxetine, metoprolol, venlafaxine) or CYP2D6 substrates that have a narrow therapeutic index (eg, thioridazine, pimozide); if concomitant use of CYP2D6 substrates is unavoidable, monitor patients frequently for adverse reactions. Not recommended w/ antiarrhythmics (eg, amiodarone, disopyramide, procainamide) and other drugs known to prolong the QT interval (eg, chloroquine, halofantrine, clarithromycin). Antiemetic drugs w/ known QT prolonging risk (eg, dolasetron, ondansetron, tropisetron) can be used w/ frequent ECG monitoring.

PREGNANCY AND LACTATION
Pregnancy: May cause fetal harm.
Lactation: It is not known if panobinostat is present in human milk; not for use in nursing.
Reproductive Potential: Females of reproductive potential should avoid becoming pregnant while on therapy. Sexually active females of reproductive potential should use effective contraception while taking therapy and for at least 3 months after the last dose of therapy. Sexually active men should use condoms while on treatment and for 6 months after last dose of therapy.

MECHANISM OF ACTION
Histone deacetylase inhibitor (HDAC); inhibits the enzymatic activity of HDACs at nanomolar concentrations, resulting in increased acetylation of histone proteins, an epigenetic alteration that results in a relaxing of chromatin and leads to transcriptional activation.

PHARMACOKINETICS
Absorption: Absolute bioavailability (approx 21%); T_{max}=2 hrs. **Distribution:** Plasma protein binding (90%). **Metabolism:** Extensive; reduction, hydrolysis, oxidation, and glucuronidation; CYP3A; 2D6, 2C19 (minor). **Elimination:** Urine (29-51%, <2.5% unchanged), feces (44-77%, <3.5% unchanged); $T_{1/2}$=37 hrs.

PATIENT CONSIDERATIONS
Assessment: Assess for history of recent MI or unstable angina, active infection, pregnancy/nursing status, and possible drug interactions. Obtain baseline CBC, LFTs, ECG, and electrolyte levels (including K^+, Mg^{2+}, and phosphate). Assess hydration status.

Monitoring: Monitor for signs/symptoms of diarrhea, cardiac ischemic events, arrhythmias, hemorrhage, infection, and other adverse reactions. Monitor ECG periodically as clinically indicated. Monitor CBC, hydration status, and electrolyte blood levels weekly (or more frequently if clinically indicated). Monitor LFTs regularly. Monitor for toxicity more frequently in patients >65 yrs of age, especially for GI toxicity, myelosuppression, and cardiac toxicity.

Counseling: Instruct to take exactly ud. If a dose is missed, advise to take dose as soon as possible and up to 12 hrs after the specified dose time. If vomiting occurs, advise not to repeat dose, but to take the next usual prescribed dose on schedule. Instruct to avoid star fruit, pomegranate/pomegranate juice, and grapefruit/grapefruit juice while on therapy. Advise to report to physician if any signs/symptoms of a heart problem develop while on therapy (eg, chest pain/discomfort, changes in heartbeat, palpitations). Inform about risk of thrombocytopenia; advise to contact physician right away if any signs of bleeding occur. Explain the need to perform laboratory tests prior to start of therapy and while on therapy. Inform about the risk of neutropenia and severe, life-threatening infections; instruct to contact physician immediately if fever and/or any sign of infection develops. Inform that drug may cause severe N/V and diarrhea that may require medication for treatment; advise to contact physician at the start of diarrhea, if persistent vomiting develops, or if any signs of dehydration develop. Instruct to consult w/ physician prior to using medications w/ laxative properties. Inform that drug may cause fetal harm. Advise women of reproductive potential to use effective contraception while taking therapy

and for at least 3 months after the last dose of the drug. Counsel sexually active men to use condoms while receiving therapy and for at least 6 months following the last dose of the drug. Instruct not to breastfeed during therapy.

FASLODEX — fulvestrant   Rx
Class: Estrogen receptor antagonist

ADULT DOSAGE
Breast Cancer

Monotherapy:
For hormone receptor (HR)-positive metastatic breast cancer in postmenopausal women w/ disease progression following antiestrogen therapy

500mg IM into buttocks slowly (1-2 min/inj) as two 5mL inj, 1 in each buttock, on Days 1, 15, 29, and once monthly thereafter

Combination Therapy w/ Palbociclib:
For HR-positive, HER2-negative advanced or metastatic breast cancer in women w/ disease progression after endocrine therapy

500mg IM into buttocks slowly (1-2 min/inj) as two 5mL inj, 1 in each buttock, on Days 1, 15, 29, and once monthly thereafter + 125mg palbociclib PO qd for 21 consecutive days followed by 7 days off treatment to complete a 28-day cycle. Refer to the PI of palbociclib

Pre/perimenopausal patients treated on combination therapy w/ palbociclib should be treated w/ luteinizing hormone-releasing hormone agonists according to current clinical practice standards

When used in combination w/ palbociclib, refer to the PI for its dose modification, management of toxicities, and for use w/ concomitant medications

PEDIATRIC DOSAGE
Pediatric use may not have been established

DOSING CONSIDERATIONS
Hepatic Impairment
Moderate (Child-Pugh Class B): 250mg IM into buttock slowly (1-2 min) as one 5mL inj on Days 1, 15, 29, and once monthly thereafter
Severe (Child-Pugh Class C): Has not been evaluated

ADMINISTRATION
IM route

Administer the inj according to the local guidelines for performing large volume IM inj. Use caution if administering fulvestrant at the dorsogluteal inj site due to the proximity of the underlying sciatic nerve.
Refer to PI for further administration instructions.

STORAGE
2-8°C (36-46°F). Store in original carton until time of use to protect from light.

HOW SUPPLIED
Inj: 50mg/mL [5mL]

CONTRAINDICATIONS
Known hypersensitivity to fulvestrant or to any of the components.

WARNINGS/PRECAUTIONS
Caution w/ bleeding diatheses and thrombocytopenia. Increased exposure w/ moderate hepatic impairment. Inj site related events including sciatica, neuralgia, neuropathic pain, and peripheral neuropathy reported. May cause fetal harm during pregnancy. May interfere w/ estradiol measurement by immunoassay, resulting in falsely elevated estradiol levels.

ADVERSE REACTIONS
Monotherapy: (500mg) Inj-site pain, nausea, bone pain; (250mg) nausea, back pain, inj-site pain.
Combination Therapy w/ Palbociclib: Neutropenia, leukopenia, infections, fatigue, N/V, anemia, stomatitis, headache, diarrhea, thrombocytopenia, constipation, alopecia, rash, decreased appetite, pyrexia.

DRUG INTERACTIONS
Caution w/ anticoagulant use.

PREGNANCY AND LACTATION
Pregnancy: May cause fetal harm.
Lactation: There is no information regarding the presence of fulvestrant in human milk, nor of its effects on milk production or breastfed infant. Do not breastfeed during therapy and for 1 year after the final dose.
Reproductive Potential: Pregnancy testing is recommended w/in 7 days prior to initiating therapy for females of reproductive potential. Females of reproductive potential should use effective contraception during treatment and for 1 year after the last dose. May impair fertility in females and males of reproductive potential.

MECHANISM OF ACTION

Estrogen receptor (ER) antagonist; binds to the ER in a competitive manner and downregulates ER protein in human breast cancer cells.

PHARMACOKINETICS

Absorption: (Single dose) C_{max}=25.1ng/mL; AUC=11,400ng•hr/mL. (Multiple dose) C_{max}=28ng/mL; AUC=13,100ng•hr/mL. **Distribution:** V_d=3-5L/kg; plasma protein binding (99%). **Metabolism:** Oxidation (via CYP3A4), aromatic hydroxylation, conjugation. **Elimination:** Feces (approx 90%), urine (<1%); $T_{1/2}$=40 days (250mg).

PATIENT CONSIDERATIONS

Assessment: Assess for bleeding diatheses, thrombocytopenia, hepatic impairment, hypersensitivity to the drug, pregnancy/nursing status, and possible drug interactions.

Monitoring: Monitor for inj-site reactions and other adverse reactions.

Counseling: Advise females of reproductive potential of the potential fetal risk and instruct to use effective contraception during treatment and for 1 year after the last dose. Advise females to inform their healthcare provider of a known or suspected pregnancy. Instruct women not to breastfeed during treatment and for 1 year after the last dose. Inform of adverse reactions and instruct to seek medical attention if any adverse reactions develop.

FEIBA NF — anti-inhibitor coagulant complex Rx

Class: Antihemophilic agent

> Thrombotic and thromboembolic events reported, particularly following administration of high doses and/or in patients with thrombotic risk factors.

ADULT DOSAGE	PEDIATRIC DOSAGE
Hemophilia	Pediatric use may not have been established
Control of Spontaneous Bleeding Episodes and Cover Surgical Interventions in Hemophilia A and Hemophilia B w/ Inhibitors:	
Usual: 50-100 U/kg	
Max: 200 U/kg/day	
Joint Hemorrhage:	
Initial: 50 U/kg q12h	
Titrate: May increase to 100 U/kg q12h if hemorrhage does not stop. Continue treatment until clear signs of clinical improvement appear	
Mucous Membrane Bleeding:	
Initial: 50 U/kg q6h	
Titrate: May increase to 100 U/kg q6h if hemorrhage does not stop. Examine for visible bleeding cessation and perform repeated Hgb/Hct measurements	
Soft Tissue Hemorrhage:	
100 U/kg q12h	
Other Severe Hemorrhage:	
100 U/kg q6-12h. May be indicated at 6-hr intervals until clear clinical improvement is achieved. Do not exceed single doses of 100 U/kg and a daily dose of 200 U/kg unless severity of bleeding warrants and justifies use of higher doses	

ADMINISTRATION

IV route

Do not exceed 2 U/kg/min infusion rate
Do not mix w/ other medicinal products or solvents

Reconstitution
1. Allow the unopened vials and sterile water for inj (diluent) to reach room temperature (not above 37°C, 98°F)
2. After adding diluent, swirl gently until sol is completely dissolved
3. Do not refrigerate after reconstitution

STORAGE

Room temperature ≤25°C (77°F). Avoid freezing. Protect from light. Reconstituted Sol: Do not refrigerate.

HOW SUPPLIED

Inj: 500 U, 1000 U, 2500 U

CONTRAINDICATIONS

Patients with known normal coagulation mechanism, significant signs of disseminated intravascular coagulation (DIC), or acute thrombosis or embolism (including myocardial infarction). Treatment of bleeding episodes resulting from coagulation factor deficiencies in the absence of inhibitors to coagulation factor VIII or coagulation factor IX.

WARNINGS/PRECAUTIONS

Should be initiated and supervised by a physician experienced in the management of hemophilia. D/C administration immediately and initiate diagnostic/therapeutic measures at 1st sign or symptom of an infusion/hypersensitivity reaction or thrombotic/thromboembolic event. Monitor patients receiving >100 U/kg for DIC development and/or acute coronary ischemia symptoms; give high doses only as long as absolutely necessary to stop bleeding. Caution in patients at risk of DIC, arterial or venous thrombosis, or with increased risk of thromboembolic complications; weigh potential benefit of treatment against risk of these complications. May carry a risk of transmitting infectious agents (eg, viruses, Creutzfeldt-Jakob disease); consider appropriate vaccination against hepatitis A and B virus of patients who receive therapy. Response to bypassing agents may vary due to patient-specific factors. Anamnestic responses with rise in factor VIII inhibitor titer observed. Perform platelet count at the time of initial use and if anticipated treatment responses are not achieved. Attempts at normalizing whole blood clotting time, activated PTT (aPTT) and thrombelastography values by increasing the dose may not be successful and are strongly discouraged because of the potential hazard of producing DIC by overdose.

ADVERSE REACTIONS

Thrombotic/thromboembolic events, allergic-type hypersensitivity reactions, infusion reactions, somnolence, dizziness, dysgeusia, hypoesthesia, dyspnea, nausea, chills, pyrexia, chest pain/discomfort, anamnestic response.

DRUG INTERACTIONS

Consider possibility of thrombotic events with systemic antifibrinolytics (eg, tranexamic acid, aminocaproic acid); avoid use of antifibrinolytics until 12 hrs after administration.

PREGNANCY AND LACTATION

Category C, caution in nursing.

MECHANISM OF ACTION

Antihemophilic agent; shortens the aPTT of plasma containing factor VIII inhibitor.

PATIENT CONSIDERATIONS

Assessment: Assess for normal coagulation mechanism, significant signs of DIC, acute thrombosis or embolism, risk of DIC or arterial/venous thrombosis, increased risk of thromboembolic complications, hypersensitivity to drug, pregnancy/nursing status, and possible drug interactions.

Monitoring: Monitor for signs/symptoms of DIC, acute coronary ischemia, thrombotic/thromboembolic events, infusion/hypersensitivity reactions, infections, and other adverse events. Perform platelet count at the time of initial use and if anticipated treatment responses are not achieved. Monitor for visible bleeding cessation and perform repeated Hgb/Hct measurements when dosing patients with mucous membrane bleeding.

Counseling: Inform about risks and benefits of treatment. Advise about the early signs of hypersensitivity reactions and instruct to d/c use and seek immediate emergency treatment if symptoms occur. Inform pregnant women and immune-compromised individuals about symptoms of parvovirus B19 (fever, drowsiness, chills, and runny nose followed about 2 weeks later by rash, and joint pain). Inform about symptoms of hepatitis A (dark urine, yellowed complexion, several days to weeks of poor appetite, tiredness, and low-grade fever followed by N/V, and upper abdominal pain) infection. Instruct to record the batch number of the product if administered outside a healthcare setting. Advise to report any adverse reactions following administration.

FERRIPROX ORAL SOLUTION — deferiprone Rx

Class: Iron-chelating agent

> May cause agranulocytosis that can lead to serious infections and death; neutropenia may precede development of agranulocytosis. Measure ANC before starting therapy and monitor ANC weekly while on therapy; interrupt therapy if neutropenia develops. Interrupt therapy if infection develops, and monitor ANC more frequently. Advise patients to report immediately any symptoms indicative of infection.

ADULT DOSAGE	PEDIATRIC DOSAGE
Transfusional Iron Overload	Pediatric use may not have been established
Due to thalassemia syndromes when current chelation therapy is inadequate	
Initial: 25mg/kg tid	
Titrate: Adjust dose based on individual patient's response and therapeutic goals. Monitor serum ferritin concentration every 2-3 months; consider temporarily interrupting therapy if serum ferritin is consistently <500mcg/L until serum ferritin rises >500mcg/L	
Max: 33mg/kg tid	
Round dose to the nearest 2.5mL. Refer to PI for volume of sol required to achieve a 25mg/kg and 33mg/kg dose	

DOSING CONSIDERATIONS

Concomitant Medications

Other Medications or Supplements Containing Polyvalent Cations (eg, Iron, Aluminum, Zinc): Allow at least a 4-hr interval

UGT1A6 Inhibitors (eg, Diclofenac, Probenecid, Silymarin [Milk Thistle]): Avoid concomitant use

ADMINISTRATION

Oral route

Use w/in 35 days after first opening of the bottle; discard the contents of the bottle after 35 days.

Store in the original container and carton to protect from light.
Store at 20-25°C (68-77°F); excursions permitted to 15-30°C (59-86°F).
Refer to PI for instructions for use.

STORAGE
20-25°C (68-77°F); excursions permitted to 15-30°C (59-86°F). Store in original package to protect from light.

HOW SUPPLIED
Oral Sol: 100mg/mL [500mL]

CONTRAINDICATIONS
Known hypersensitivity to deferiprone or to any of the excipients in the formulation.

WARNINGS/PRECAUTIONS
Implement a plan to monitor for and to manage agranulocytosis/neutropenia prior to initiating therapy. Immediately d/c therapy and all other medications w/ a potential to cause neutropenia if neutropenia (ANC <1.5 x 10^9/L and >0.5 x 10^9/L) develops; obtain a CBC, including a WBC count corrected for the presence of nucleated red blood cells, an ANC, and a platelet count daily until recovery (ANC ≥1.5 x 10^9/L). Consider hospitalization and other management as clinically appropriate if agranulocytosis (ANC <0.5 x 10^9/L) develops; do not resume therapy in patients who have developed agranulocytosis and do not rechallenge patients who develop neutropenia, unless potential benefits outweigh potential risks. Can cause fetal harm; avoid pregnancy while on therapy. Increased ALT/AST values reported; monitor serum ALT values monthly during therapy and consider interruption of therapy if there is a persistent increase in serum transaminase levels. Decreased plasma zinc concentrations reported; monitor plasma zinc, and supplement in the event of a deficiency.

ADVERSE REACTIONS
Chromaturia, N/V, abdominal pain, alanine aminotransferase increased, arthralgia, neutropenia.

DRUG INTERACTIONS
See Dosing Considerations. Avoid w/ other drugs known to be associated w/ neutropenia/agranulocytosis; if not possible, monitor ANC more frequently. Potential to bind polyvalent cations (eg, iron, aluminum, zinc).

PREGNANCY AND LACTATION
Pregnancy: Category D.
Lactation: It is not known whether deferiprone is excreted in human milk; not for use in nursing.

MECHANISM OF ACTION
Iron-chelating agent; binds w/ ferric ions to form neutral 3:1 (deferiprone:iron) complexes that are stable over a wide range of pH values.

PHARMACOKINETICS
Absorption: Rapid. T_{max}=1 hr (fasted), ≤2 hrs (fed). (1500mg, fasted) C_{max}=20mcg/mL, AUC=50mcg•hr/mL. **Metabolism:** UGT1A6; 3-O-glucuronide (major metabolite). **Elimination:** Urine (75-90%) (primarily as metabolite); $T_{1/2}$=2 hrs.

PATIENT CONSIDERATIONS
Assessment: Assess for hypersensitivity to the drug, pregnancy/nursing status, and possible drug interactions. Obtain baseline ANC.

Monitoring: Monitor for signs/symptoms of agranulocytosis, neutropenia, infection, and other adverse reactions. Monitor ANC weekly, serum ferritin concentration every 2-3 months, ALT values monthly, and plasma zinc concentrations.

Counseling: Inform of the risks of developing agranulocytosis and instruct to immediately interrupt therapy and report to physician if experiencing any symptoms of infection (eg, fever, sore throat, flu-like symptoms). Advise to take 1st dose in the morning, the 2nd at midday, and the 3rd in the evening. Advise that administration w/ meals may reduce nausea. Instruct to contact physician in case of an overdose. Inform that urine might show a reddish/brown discoloration, which is not harmful. Advise women of reproductive potential to avoid pregnancy while on therapy; advise to notify physician if pregnant or planning to become pregnant. Instruct not to breastfeed while on therapy. Inform that drug is light sensitive, and advise to store in the originally supplied bottle and carton.

FERRIPROX TABLETS — deferiprone   Rx

Class: Iron-chelating agent

> May cause agranulocytosis that can lead to serious infections and death; neutropenia may precede development of agranulocytosis. Measure ANC before starting therapy and monitor weekly on therapy; interrupt therapy if neutropenia develops. Interrupt therapy if infection develops; monitor ANC more frequently. Advise patients to report immediately any symptoms indicative of infection.

ADULT DOSAGE	PEDIATRIC DOSAGE
Transfusional Iron Overload	Pediatric use may not have been established
Due to thalassemia syndromes when current chelation therapy is inadequate	
Initial: 25mg/kg tid	
Titrate: Adjust dose based on individual patient's response and therapeutic goals	
Max: 33mg/kg tid	
Round dose to the nearest 250mg (1/2 tab)	
Refer to PI for tab requirement to achieve a 25mg/kg and 33mg/kg dose level	

ADMINISTRATION
Oral route

Monitor serum ferritin concentration every 2-3 months
Consider temporarily interrupting therapy if serum ferritin falls consistently <500mcg/L

STORAGE
20-25°C (68-77°F); excursions permitted to 15-30°C (59-86°F).

HOW SUPPLIED
Tab: 500mg* *scored

CONTRAINDICATIONS
Known hypersensitivity to deferiprone or to any of the excipients in the formulation.

WARNINGS/PRECAUTIONS
Implement a plan to monitor for and to manage agranulocytosis/neutropenia prior to initiating therapy. Immediately d/c therapy and all other medications w/ a potential to cause neutropenia if neutropenia (ANC <1.5 x 10^9/L and >0.5 x 10^9/L) develops; obtain a CBC, including a WBC count corrected for the presence of nucleated red blood cells, an ANC, and a platelet count daily until recovery (ANC ≥1.5 x 10^9/L). Consider hospitalization and other management as clinically appropriate if agranulocytosis (ANC <0.5 x 10^9/L) develops; do not resume therapy in patients who have developed agranulocytosis and do not rechallenge patients who develop neutropenia, unless potential benefits outweigh potential risks. May cause fetal harm in pregnant women; avoid pregnancy while on therapy. Increased ALT/AST values reported; monitor serum ALT values monthly during therapy and consider interruption of therapy if there is a persistent increase in serum transaminase levels. Decreased plasma zinc concentrations reported; monitor plasma zinc, and supplement in the event of a deficiency.

ADVERSE REACTIONS
Agranulocytosis, neutropenia, chromaturia, N/V, abdominal pain, ALT increased, arthralgia, diarrhea, increased appetite.

DRUG INTERACTIONS
Avoid w/ other drugs known to be associated w/ neutropenia/agranulocytosis; if not possible, closely monitor ANC. Closely monitor for adverse reactions that may require downward dose titration or interruption when deferiprone is concomitantly administered w/ a UGT1A6 inhibitor. Potential to bind polyvalent cations (eg, iron, aluminum, zinc); allow at least a 4-hr interval between deferiprone and other medications (eg, antacids), or supplements containing polyvalent cations.

PREGNANCY AND LACTATION
Category D; not for use in nursing.

MECHANISM OF ACTION
Iron-chelating agent; binds w/ ferric ions to form neutral 3:1 (deferiprone:iron) complexes that are stable over a wide range of pH values.

PHARMACOKINETICS
Absorption: Rapid. T_{max}=1 hr (fasted), ≤2 hrs (fed). (1500mg, fasted) C_{max}=20mcg/mL, AUC=53mcg•hr/mL. **Distribution:** V_d=1.6L/kg; plasma protein binding (<10%). **Metabolism:** UGT 1A6; 3-O-glucuronide (major metabolite). **Elimination:** Urine (75-90%) (primarily as metabolite); $T_{1/2}$=1.9 hrs.

PATIENT CONSIDERATIONS
Assessment: Assess for hypersensitivity to the drug, pregnancy/nursing status, and possible drug interactions. Obtain baseline ANC.

Monitoring: Monitor for signs/symptoms of agranulocytosis, neutropenia, infection, arrhythmia, hypersensitivity reaction, and other adverse reactions. Monitor ANC weekly, serum ferritin concentration every 2-3 months, ALT values monthly, and plasma zinc concentrations.

Counseling: Instruct to immediately d/c therapy and contact physician if any symptoms of an infection occur. Advise to take 1st dose in the morning, the 2nd at midday, and the 3rd in the evening. Advise that administration w/ meals may reduce nausea. Advise to contact physician in case of an overdose. Inform that urine might show a reddish/brown discoloration, which is not harmful. Counsel women of reproductive potential to avoid pregnancy while on therapy; advise to notify physician if pregnant, or planning to become pregnant. Instruct not to breastfeed while on therapy.

FIRAZYR — icatibant   Rx

Class: Bradykinin B_2-receptor antagonist

ADULT DOSAGE	PEDIATRIC DOSAGE
Hereditary Angioedema	Pediatric use may not have been established
Treatment of Acute Attacks:	
30mg SQ in the abdominal area; may give additional doses at intervals of at least 6 hrs if response is inadequate or if symptoms recur	
Max: 3 doses/24 hrs	

ADMINISTRATION
SQ route

Inject in the abdominal area over at least 30 sec.
Attach provided 25-gauge needle to syringe hub and screw on securely; do not use a different needle.

STORAGE
2-25°C (36-77°F). Do not freeze.

HOW SUPPLIED
Inj: 30mg [prefilled syringe]

WARNINGS/PRECAUTIONS
Given the potential for airway obstruction during acute laryngeal hereditary angioedema (HAE) attacks, advise patients to immediately seek medical attention in an appropriate healthcare facility in addition to treatment w/ icatibant.

ADVERSE REACTIONS
Inj-site reaction, pyrexia, increased transaminase, dizziness.

DRUG INTERACTIONS
May attenuate the antihypertensive effect of ACE inhibitors.

PREGNANCY AND LACTATION
Pregnancy: Category C.
Lactation: Caution in nursing.

MECHANISM OF ACTION
Bradykinin B_2 receptor antagonist; inhibits bradykinin from binding the B_2 receptor and thereby treats the clinical symptoms of an acute, episodic attack of HAE.

PHARMACOKINETICS
Absorption: Absolute bioavailability (97%); C_{max}=974ng/mL; AUC=2165ng•hr/mL; T_{max}=0.75 hrs. **Distribution:** V_d=29L. **Metabolism:** Extensive by proteolytic enzymes. **Elimination:** Urine (<10% unchanged); $T_{1/2}$=1.4 hrs.

PATIENT CONSIDERATIONS

Assessment: Assess for airway obstruction, pregnancy/nursing status, and possible drug interactions.

Monitoring: Monitor for airway obstruction during acute laryngeal HAE attacks, and possible adverse reactions.

Counseling: Instruct to administer as prescribed. Advise that therapy may be self-administered upon recognition of an HAE attack after training under the guidance of a healthcare professional. Instruct patients w/ laryngeal symptoms to immediately seek medical attention in an appropriate healthcare facility after administration. Inform patient of possible adverse reactions (eg, inj-site reactions, drowsiness). Advise not to drive or use machinery if feeling tired or dizzy.

FIRMAGON — degarelix   Rx

Class: Gonadotropin-releasing hormone (GnRH) antagonist

ADULT DOSAGE	**PEDIATRIC DOSAGE**
Advanced Prostate Cancer	Pediatric use may not have been established
Initial: 240mg (given as 2 SQ inj of 120mg) at a concentration of 40mg/mL	
Maint: 80mg (given as 1 SQ inj) at a concentration of 20mg/mL; administer every 28 days Administer 1st maint dose 28 days after initial dose	

ADMINISTRATION
SQ route

Inject into abdominal region in areas that will not be exposed to pressure (eg, not close to waistband, belt, or ribs).
Perform a slow, deep SQ inj over 30 sec; do not rub the inj site after retracting the needle.
Inj site should vary periodically.
Administer reconstituted sol w/in 1 hr after addition of sterile water for inj (SWFI); reconstitute just prior to administration.
Do not shake the vials.

Starting Dose
One starting dose comprises 240mg given as two 3mL inj of 120mg each.
Reconstitute each 120mg vial w/ a prefilled syringe containing 3mL of SWFI.

Maint Dose
One maint dose comprises 80mg given as one 4mL inj.
Reconstitute each 80mg vial w/ a prefilled syringe containing 4.2mL of SWFI.

Reconstitution Instructions
1. Attach the vial adapter to the vial by pressing the adapter down until it snaps in place.
2. Assemble the syringe by inserting the plunger rod into the prefilled syringe containing SWFI.
3. Transfer the sterile water from the syringe to the vial by unscrewing the gray syringe plug and twisting the prefilled syringe onto the vial adapter.
4. With the syringe still attached, gently swirl until the liquid is clear w/ no powder or visible particles; do not shake.
5. Transfer the reconstituted liquid from the vial to the syringe.

STORAGE
25°C (77°F); excursions permitted to 15-30°C (59-86°F).

HOW SUPPLIED
Inj: 80mg, 120mg

CONTRAINDICATIONS
Known hypersensitivity to degarelix or to any of the product components, women who are or may become pregnant.

WARNINGS/PRECAUTIONS
Hypersensitivity reactions, including anaphylaxis, urticaria, and angioedema reported; d/c immediately if serious hypersensitivity reaction occurs, and manage as clinically indicated. Do not rechallenge w/ the drug in patients who have a known history of serious hypersensitivity reactions to the drug. Androgen deprivation therapy may prolong the QT interval; consider whether the benefits outweigh potential risks in patients w/ congenital long QT syndrome, CHF, frequent electrolyte abnormalities, and in patients taking drugs known to prolong the QT interval. Correct electrolyte abnormalities; consider periodically monitoring of ECGs and electrolytes. May cause suppression of pituitary gonadal system. Caution in patients w/ CrCl <50mL/min and w/ severe hepatic dysfunction.

ADVERSE REACTIONS
Inj-site reactions (eg, pain, erythema, swelling, induration), hot flashes, weight gain, fatigue, increased serum gamma-glutamyltransferase and transaminases levels.

PREGNANCY AND LACTATION
Pregnancy: Category X.
Lactation: Not for use in nursing.

MECHANISM OF ACTION
GnRH receptor antagonist; binds reversibly to the pituitary GnRH receptors, thereby reducing the release of gonadotropins and consequently, testosterone.

PHARMACOKINETICS
Absorption: AUC=1054ng•day/mL, C_{max}=26.2ng/mL, T_{max}=2 days. **Distribution:** V_d>1L/kg (IV), >1000L (SQ);plasma protein binding (approx 90%). **Metabolism:** Peptide hydrolysis. **Elimination:** Renal (approx 20-30%), hepatobiliary (approx 70-80%); (SQ) $T_{1/2}$=approx 53 days (median).

PATIENT CONSIDERATIONS

Assessment: Assess for previous hypersensitivity reactions, congenital long QT syndrome, electrolyte abnormalities, CHF, renal/hepatic impairment, and for possible drug interactions. Obtain baseline prostate specific antigen (PSA) levels.

Monitoring: Monitor for hypersensitivity reactions, QT interval prolongation, and other adverse reactions. Perform periodic measurements of PSA levels; if PSA levels are elevated, measure serum testosterone levels. In patients w/ hepatic impairment, monitor testosterone concentrations monthly until medical castration is achieved, then consider every other month testosterone monitoring approach.

Counseling: Inform about possible side effects of androgen deprivation therapy (eg, hot flashes, flushing of skin, weight gain). Advise about possible side effects related to therapy (eg, redness, swelling, itching at inj site).

FLEBOGAMMA 10% DIF — immune globulin
intravenous (human)   Rx

Class: Immune globulin

> Thrombosis may occur; administer at the minimum dose and infusion rate practicable for patients at risk (eg, advanced age, prolonged immobilization, hypercoagulable conditions, history of venous or arterial thrombosis, use of estrogens, indwelling central vascular catheters, hyperviscosity, cardiovascular [CV] risk factors). Ensure adequate hydration before administration. Monitor for signs/symptoms of thrombosis and assess blood viscosity if at risk for hyperviscosity. Renal dysfunction, acute renal failure, osmotic nephrosis, and death have been related to immune globulin intravenous (IGIV) products. Patients predisposed to acute renal failure include those w/ preexisting renal insufficiency, diabetes mellitus (DM), age >65 yrs, volume depletion, sepsis, paraproteinemia, or receiving known nephrotoxic drugs. Reports of renal dysfunction and acute renal failure occur more commonly w/ IGIV products, particularly those containing sucrose; this product does not contain sucrose.

ADULT DOSAGE	**PEDIATRIC DOSAGE**
Primary Immunodeficiency	**Chronic Primary Immune Thrombocytopenia**
Replacement therapy in PI including the humoral immune defects in common variable immunodeficiency, x-linked agammaglobulinemia, severe combined immunodeficiency, and Wiskott-Aldrich syndrome.	**≥2 Years:** 1g/kg (10mL/kg) qd for 2 days **Titrate:** Adjust to achieve desired serum trough levels and clinical response
300-600mg/kg (3-6mL/kg) every 3-4 weeks **Titrate:** Adjust to achieve desired serum trough IgG levels and clinical response	
Chronic Primary Immune Thrombocytopenia	
1g/kg (10mL/kg) qd for 2 days **Titrate:** Adjust to achieve desired serum trough IgG levels and clinical response	

DOSING CONSIDERATIONS
Elderly
≥65 Years and at Risk for Developing Thrombosis or Renal Insufficiency:
Infuse at the minimum infusion rate practicable and <0.04mL/kg/min (4mg/kg/min)

Adverse Reactions
Slow or stop infusion, or administer IGIV at 5% concentration, if adverse reactions occur; may resume at a lower rate if symptoms subside

ADMINISTRATION

IV route

- May pool several vials into an empty sterile sol container if large doses are to be administered.
- Do not dilute w/ IV fluids.
- Infuse through a separate IV line; do not add any medications or IV fluids to the infusion container. Do not mix IGIV products of different formulations or from different manufacturers.
- Discard unused contents and administration devices after use.
- Discard partially used vials; sol contains no preservative.
- Use promptly any vial that has been entered.
- Do not use sol that has been frozen or is turbid.

Initial Infusion Rate:
0.01mL/kg/min (1mg/kg/min) for the first 30 min.

Maint Dose Rate:
May increase gradually to 0.04mL/kg/min (4mg/kg/min) and if tolerated, gradually to a max of 0.08mL/kg/min (8mg/kg/min).

For the first 2-3 infusions, may administer at infusion rates slower than recommended rates; if after administration of the 1st few infusions no adverse drug reactions are observed, may slowly increase infusion rate for subsequent infusions to max rate.

STORAGE

2-25°C (36-77°F) for up to 24 months. Do not freeze; do not use if sol has been frozen. Keep in original carton to protect from light.

HOW SUPPLIED

Inj: 10% [50mL, 100mL, 200mL]

CONTRAINDICATIONS

History of anaphylactic or severe systemic hypersensitivity reactions to the administration of human immune globulin. IgA deficient patients w/ antibodies to IgA and a history of hypersensitivity.

WARNINGS/PRECAUTIONS

Contains trace amounts of IgA; severe hypersensitivity and anaphylactic reactions w/ a fall in BP may occur. D/C infusion immediately and institute appropriate treatment if hypersensitivity develops. Consider discontinuation if renal function deteriorates. Hyperproteinemia, increased serum viscosity, and hyponatremia may occur. Distinguish true hyponatremia from pseudohyponatremia related to hyperproteinemia w/ concomitant decreased calculated serum osmolarity or elevated osmolar gap; treatment aimed at decreasing serum free water in patients w/ pseudohyponatremia may lead to volume depletion, a further increase in serum viscosity, and a higher risk of thrombosis. Aseptic meningitis syndrome (AMS) reported and may occur more frequently w/ high dose (eg, >2g/kg) and/or rapid infusion; rule out other causes of meningitis. May contain blood group antibodies that may act as hemolysins and induce in vivo coating of RBCs w/ immunoglobulin, causing a positive direct antiglobulin test (Coombs' test) and hemolysis. Delayed hemolytic anemia may develop. Monitor for clinical signs/symptoms of hemolysis, particularly patients w/ risk factors (eg, high doses [>2g/kg], given either as a single administration or divided over several days, non-O blood group, underlying inflammatory state); measure hemoglobin or hematocrit prior to infusion and w/in 36-96 hrs post infusion in higher risk patients. If clinical signs/symptoms of hemolysis or a significant drop in hemoglobin or hematocrit have been observed, perform appropriate confirmatory laboratory testing. If transfusion is required, perform adequate cross-matching to avoid exacerbating on-going hemolysis. Noncardiogenic pulmonary edema reported; if transfusion-related acute lung injury (TRALI) is suspected, perform tests for presence of antineutrophil and anti-HLA antibodies in both the product and patient's serum. Higher risk for development of fever, chills, and N/V in patients who receive drug for the 1st time or are being restarted on the product after a treatment hiatus of >8 weeks; monitor carefully. May carry risk of transmitting infectious agents (eg, viruses, Creutzfeldt-Jakob disease agent). May interfere w/ some serological tests. Contains sorbitol; avoid in patients w/ hereditary fructose intolerance (HFI).

ADVERSE REACTIONS

Primary Immunodeficiency: Headache, fever/pyrexia, shaking, tachycardia, hypotension, back pain, myalgia, hypertension, chest pain, pain, nausea, infusion-site reactions, pain in extremities.

Chronic Primary Immune Thrombocytopenia: Headache, pyrexia, N/V, chills, increased body temperature, dizziness, back pain, hypotension, HTN, increased HR, diarrhea.

DRUG INTERACTIONS

See Boxed Warning. Passive transfer of antibodies may transiently impair the immune response to live attenuated virus vaccines (eg, measles, mumps, rubella).

PREGNANCY AND LACTATION

Pregnancy: It is not known whether Flebogamma 10% DIF can cause fetal harm when administered to a pregnant woman or can affect reproduction capacity; should be given to a pregnant woman only if clearly needed.
Lactation: There is no information regarding presence in human milk, effects on the breastfed infant, or effects on milk production; caution in nursing.

MECHANISM OF ACTION

Immune globulin; not established. Supplies a broad spectrum of opsonizing and neutralizing immunoglobulin G antibodies against a wide variety of bacterial and viral agents. Also contains a spectrum of antibodies capable of reacting w/ cells (eg, erythrocytes).

PHARMACOKINETICS

Absorption: (3-Week Dosing Interval) C_{max}=19.5mg/mL, AUC=339.51 day•mg/mL; (4-Week Dosing Interval) C_{max}=20.92mg/mL, AUC=342.37 day•mg/mL.
Distribution: Crosses placenta. **Elimination:** $T_{1/2}$=34 days (3-week dosing interval), 37 days (4-week dosing interval).

PATIENT CONSIDERATIONS

Assessment: Assess for history of anaphylactic or severe systemic hypersensitivity reactions to human immunoglobulin, IgA deficiency, HFI, DM, volume depletion, sepsis, paraproteinemia, CV risk factors, advanced age, history of venous/arterial thrombosis, hypercoagulable conditions, presence of prolonged immobilization, use of indwelling central vascular catheters, pregnancy/nursing status, and possible drug interactions. Assess renal function (eg, BUN, SrCr, urine output) prior to initial infusion. Consider baseline assessment of blood viscosity in patients at risk for hyperviscosity, including those w/ cryoglobulins, fasting chylomicronemia/markedly high TGs, or monoclonal gammopathies.

Monitoring: Monitor for hypersensitivity/anaphylactic reactions, thrombosis, hemolytic anemia, hyperproteinemia, hyperviscosity, hyponatremia, pulmonary adverse reactions, infection, and other adverse reactions. Monitor renal function and urine output periodically. Perform neurological exam, including CSF studies if AMS is suspected. Perform confirmatory lab testing if signs/symptoms of hemolysis are present after an infusion. Perform tests for the presence of antineutrophil and anti-HLA antibodies in both product and patient's serum if TRALI is suspected. Monitor vital signs throughout the infusion.

Counseling: Instruct to immediately report to physician signs/symptoms of decreased urine output, sudden weight gain, fluid retention/edema, SOB, severe headache, neck stiffness, drowsiness, fever, sensitivity to light, painful eye movements, N/V, increased HR, fatigue, yellowing of skin or eyes, dark-colored urine, trouble breathing, chest pain, or blue lips or extremities. Instruct to immediately report symptoms of thrombosis (eg, pain and/or swelling of an arm or leg w/ warmth over affected area, discoloration of an arm or leg, unexplained SOB, chest pain/discomfort that worsens on deep breathing, unexplained rapid pulse, numbness or weakness on one side of the body) to physician. Inform that drug is made from human plasma and may contain infectious agents that can cause disease; instruct to report to physician any symptoms that might be caused by infections. Inform that product can interfere w/ immune response to live viral vaccines (eg, measles, mumps, rubella); instruct to notify physician of this potential interaction when patient is receiving vaccinations.

FLEBOGAMMA 5% DIF — immune globulin intravenous (human)

Rx

Class: Immune globulin

> Thrombosis may occur; administer at the minimum dose and infusion rate practicable for patients at risk (eg, advanced age, prolonged immobilization, hypercoagulable conditions, history of venous/arterial thrombosis, use of estrogens, indwelling central vascular catheters, hyperviscosity, cardiovascular [CV] risk factors). Ensure adequate hydration before administration. Monitor for signs/symptoms of thrombosis and assess blood viscosity if at risk for hyperviscosity. Renal dysfunction, acute renal failure, osmotic nephrosis, and death reported w/ immune globulin intravenous (IGIV) products, particularly those containing sucrose; this product does not contain sucrose. Patients predisposed to acute renal failure include those w/ preexisting renal insufficiency, diabetes mellitus (DM), age >65 yrs, volume depletion, sepsis, paraproteinemia, or receiving known nephrotoxic drugs; administer at the minimum dose and rate of infusion practicable.

ADULT DOSAGE	PEDIATRIC DOSAGE
Primary Immunodeficiency	**Primary Immunodeficiency**
Humoral immune defects in common variable immunodeficiency, X-linked agammaglobulinemia, severe combined immunodeficiency, Wiskott-Aldrich syndrome, etc.	Humoral immune defects in common variable immunodeficiency, X-linked agammaglobulinemia, severe combined immunodeficiency, Wiskott-Aldrich syndrome, etc.
Usual Dose: 300-600mg/kg (6-12mL/kg) every 3-4 weeks	**>2 Years:** **Usual Dose:** 300-600mg/kg (6-12mL/kg) every 3-4 weeks
Initial Infusion Rate: 0.01mL/kg/min (0.5mg/kg/min)	**Initial Infusion Rate:** 0.01mL/kg/min (0.5mg/kg/min)
Titrate: May increase rate of infusion gradually if well-tolerated during first 30 min	**Titrate:** May increase rate of infusion gradually if well-tolerated during first 30 min
Maint/Max Infusion Rate: 0.10mL/kg/min (5mg/kg/min)	**Maint/Max Infusion Rate:** 0.10mL/kg/min (5mg/kg/min)
Adjust dose according to the clinical response	Adjust dose according to the clinical response
Adjust dosage over time to achieve the desired trough IgG levels and clinical responses	Adjust dosage over time to achieve the desired trough IgG levels and clinical responses

- - - - - - - - - - - -

DOSING CONSIDERATIONS

Renal Impairment
Administer at the minimum dose and infusion rate practicable

Elderly
>65 Years and at Risk for Developing Thrombosis or Renal Insufficiency:
Administer at the minimum dose and infusion rate practicable, and at <0.06mL/kg/min (3mg/kg/min)

ADMINISTRATION

IV route

If large doses are to be administered, may pool several vials of Flebogamma 5% DIF into an empty sterile sol container.
Do not dilute w/ IV fluids.
Do not inject other medications into IV tubing being used for Flebogamma 5% DIF.
Infuse through a separate IV line.

Do not add any medications or IV fluids to infusion container.
Do not mix IGIV products of different formulations or from different
manufacturers.
Use promptly any vial that has been entered.
Do not use sol that has been frozen.

STORAGE
2-25°C (36-77°F) for 24 months. Do not freeze; do not use if sol has been frozen.
Keep in original carton to protect from light.

HOW SUPPLIED
Inj: 5% [10mL, 50mL, 100mL, 200mL, 400mL]

CONTRAINDICATIONS
History of anaphylactic or severe systemic hypersensitivity reaction to human
immune globulin. Immunoglobulin A (IgA) deficient patients w/ antibodies to IgA
and a history of hypersensitivity.

WARNINGS/PRECAUTIONS
Contains trace amounts of IgA; severe hypersensitivity and anaphylactic
reactions w/ a fall in BP may occur, even in patients who had tolerated previous
treatment w/ IGIV. D/C infusion immediately and institute appropriate treatment
if hypersensitivity reaction develops. Consider discontinuation if renal function
deteriorates. Hyperproteinemia, increased serum viscosity, and hyponatremia
may occur. Distinguish true hyponatremia from pseudohyponatremia related to
hyperproteinemia w/ concomitant decreased calculated serum osmolarity or
elevated osmolar gap; treatment aimed at decreasing serum free water in patients
w/ pseudohyponatremia may lead to volume depletion, a further increase in
serum viscosity, and a higher risk of thrombosis. Aseptic meningitis syndrome
(AMS) reported and may occur more frequently w/ high dose (>1g/kg) or rapid
infusion; rule out other causes of meningitis. Delayed hemolytic anemia may
develop and acute hemolysis reported. If transfusion is indicated for patients who
develop hemolysis w/ clinically compromising anemia, perform adequate cross-
matching to avoid exacerbating on-going hemolysis. Noncardiogenic pulmonary
edema reported; if transfusion-related acute lung injury (TRALI) is suspected,
perform tests for presence of antineutrophil and anti-HLA antibodies in both the
product and patient's serum. Higher risk for development of fever, chills, and
N/V in patients who receive drug for the 1st time or are being restarted on the
product after a treatment hiatus of >8 weeks; monitor carefully. May carry risk
of transmitting infectious agents (eg, viruses, variant Creutzfeldt-Jakob disease
(CJD) agent and, theoretically, the CJD agent). Caution in elderly. May interfere
w/ some serological tests.

ADVERSE REACTIONS
Thrombosis, renal dysfunction, acute renal failure, osmotic nephrosis, headache,
pyrexia, pain, diarrhea, rigors, urticaria, hypotension, tachycardia, abdominal pain,
infusion-site reactions, N/V.

DRUG INTERACTIONS
See Boxed Warning. Passive transfer of antibodies may transiently impair the
immune response to live attenuated virus vaccines (eg, measles, mumps, rubella).

PREGNANCY AND LACTATION
Pregnancy: Category C.
Lactation: Safety not known in nursing.

MECHANISM OF ACTION
Immune globulin; not established. Supplies a broad spectrum of opsonizing
and neutralizing IgG antibodies against a wide variety of bacterial and viral
agents. Also contains a spectrum of antibodies capable of reacting w/ cells (eg,
erythrocytes).

PHARMACOKINETICS
Absorption: (3-Week Dosing Interval) C_{max}=1,929mg/dL, AUC_{0-last}=31,159 day•mg/
dL; (4-Week Dosing Interval) C_{max}=2,069mg/dL, AUC_{0-last}=32,894 day•mg/dL.
Distribution: Crosses placenta. **Elimination:** $T_{1/2}$=30 days (3-week dosing interval),
32 days (4-week dosing interval).

PATIENT CONSIDERATIONS
Assessment: Assess for history of anaphylactic or severe systemic hypersensitivity
reactions to human immune globulin, IgA deficiency, volume depletion, CV/
thrombosis/renal failure/hemolysis risk factors, pregnancy/nursing status, and
possible drug interactions. Assess renal function (eg, BUN, SrCr, urine output)
prior to initial infusion. Consider baseline assessment of blood viscosity in
patients at risk for hyperviscosity, including those w/ cryoglobulins, fasting
chylomicronemia/markedly high TGs, or monoclonal gammopathies. Consider
appropriate lab testing, including measurement of Hgb or Hct prior to infusion, in
patients at risk for hemolysis.
Monitoring: Monitor for hypersensitivity/anaphylactic reactions, thrombosis,
hemolytic anemia, hyperproteinemia, hyperviscosity, hyponatremia, pulmonary
adverse reactions, infection, and other adverse reactions. Monitor renal function
and urine output periodically. Perform neurological exam, including CSF studies, if
AMS is suspected. Perform tests for the presence of antineutrophil and anti-HLA
antibodies in both the product and patient's serum if TRALI is suspected. Monitor
vital signs throughout the infusion. Consider appropriate lab testing (eg, Hgb,
Hct) w/in 36-96 hrs post infusion in patients at risk for hemolysis, and appropriate
confirmatory lab testing if signs/symptoms of hemolysis develop or a significant
drop in Hgb/Hct is observed.
Counseling: Instruct to immediately report signs/symptoms of decreased urine
output, sudden weight gain, fluid retention/edema, SOB, severe headache, neck
stiffness, drowsiness, fever, sensitivity to light, painful eye movements, N/V,
increased HR, fatigue, yellowing of skin or eyes, dark-colored urine, trouble
breathing, chest pain, or blue lips/extremities to physician. Instruct to immediately
report symptoms of thrombosis (eg, pain and/or swelling of an arm or leg w/
warmth over affected area, discoloration of an arm or leg, unexplained SOB)
to physician. Inform that drug is made from human plasma and may contain

infectious agents that can cause disease; instruct to report any symptoms of
concern and might be caused by infections to physician. Inform that product can
interfere w/ immune response to live viral vaccines (eg, measles, mumps, rubella);
instruct patients to notify their physician of this potential interaction when they
are receiving vaccinations.

FLOLAN — epoprostenol sodium   **Rx**
Class: Prostacyclin analogue

ADULT DOSAGE	PEDIATRIC DOSAGE
Pulmonary Arterial Hypertension	Pediatric use may not have been
Treatment of pulmonary arterial HTN (WHO Group I) to improve exercise capacity	established
Initial: 2ng/kg/min IV infusion; consider reducing the dose if asymptomatic increases in pulmonary artery pressure coincident w/ increases in cardiac output occur	
Titrate: Alter the infusion by 1-2ng/kg/min increments at intervals of at least 15 min	

DOSING CONSIDERATIONS
Elderly
Start at lower end of dosing range
Adverse Reactions
Dose-Related Adverse Reactions:
Decrease gradually in 2ng/kg/min decrements every 15 min or longer until the
dose-limiting effects resolve
Other Important Considerations
Taper doses after initiation of cardiopulmonary bypass in patients receiving lung
transplants

ADMINISTRATION
IV route

Administer continuous chronic infusion through a central venous catheter;
temporary peripheral IV infusion may be used until central access is established
Do not administer as bolus inj
Do not administer or dilute reconstituted sol w/ other parenteral sol or medications;
consider a multi-lumen catheter if other IV therapies are routinely administered

Reconstitution
Reconstitute only w/ sterile diluent for Flolan or pH 12 sterile diluent for Flolan
Final Concentration of 3000ng/mL:
Dissolve contents of one 0.5mg vial w/ 5mL of sterile diluent. Then withdraw 3mL
and add to sufficient sterile diluent to make a total of 100mL
Final Concentration of 5000ng/mL:
Dissolve contents of one 0.5mg vial w/ 5mL of sterile diluent. Then withdraw
entire vial contents and add to sufficient sterile diluent to make a total of 100mL
Final Concentration of 10,000ng/mL:
Dissolve contents of two 0.5mg vials w/ 5mL of sterile diluent. Then withdraw
entire vial contents and add to sufficient sterile diluent to make a total of 100mL
Final Concentration of 15,000ng/mL:
Dissolve contents of one 1.5mg vial w/ 5mL of sterile diluent. Then withdraw entire
vial contents and add to sufficient sterile diluent to make a total of 100mL

Refer to PI for further administration and infusion rate instructions

STORAGE
15-25°C (59-77°F). Protect from light. Unopened Vials of Sterile Diluent and pH
12 Sterile Diluent: 15-25°C (59-77°F). Do not freeze. Refer to PI for storage of
reconstituted sol.

HOW SUPPLIED
Inj: 0.5mg, 1.5mg

CONTRAINDICATIONS
Heart failure (HF) caused by reduced left ventricular ejection fraction,
hypersensitivity to epoprostenol or any of its ingredients.

WARNINGS/PRECAUTIONS
D/C therapy and do not readminister if pulmonary edema develops during
initiation; consider the possibility of associated pulmonary veno-occlusive disease.
Symptoms associated w/ rebound pulmonary HTN (eg, dyspnea, dizziness,
asthenia) may occur; avoid abrupt withdrawal (including interruptions in drug
delivery) or sudden large reductions in dosage. May cause hypotension and other
reactions (eg, flushing, N/V, dizziness, headache); monitor BP and symptoms
regularly during initiation and after dose change. Increased risk for hemorrhagic
complications, particularly for patients w/ other risk factors for bleeding.

ADVERSE REACTIONS
Flushing, headache, N/V, jaw pain, diarrhea, tachycardia, chills/fever/sepsis/
flu-like symptoms, hypotension, anxiety/hyperkinesias/nervousness/tremor,
hyperesthesia/hypesthesia/paresthesia, dizziness, anorexia, eczema/rash/
urticaria, myalgia, nonspecific musculoskeletal pain.

PREGNANCY AND LACTATION
Category B, not for use in nursing.

MECHANISM OF ACTION
Prostacyclin analogue; causes direct vasodilation of pulmonary and systemic
arterial vascular beds and inhibition of platelet aggregation.

PHARMACOKINETICS

Metabolism: Hydrolysis, enzymatic degradation; 6-keto-PGF$_1\alpha$ and 6,15-diketo-13,14-dihydro-PGF$_1\alpha$ (primary metabolites). **Elimination:** Urine (82%), feces (4%); $T_{1/2} \leq 6$ min.

PATIENT CONSIDERATIONS

Assessment: Assess for HF caused by reduced left ventricular ejection fraction, risk factors for bleeding, hypersensitivity to drug, and pregnancy/nursing status. Assess patients receiving lung transplants.

Monitoring: Monitor for pulmonary edema, rebound pulmonary HTN, vasodilation, hypotension, hemorrhagic complications, and other adverse reactions. Measure standing and supine BP for several hrs following establishment of a new chronic infusion rate.

Counseling: Counsel about proper reconstitution and administration of the drug. Inform that therapy will likely be needed for prolonged periods, possibly yrs. Advise to adjust infusion rates only under the direction of a physician. Instruct to have access to a backup infusion pump and IV infusion sets to avoid interruptions in drug delivery. Advise to contact physician if any unusual bruising or bleeding develops.

FLOXURIDINE — floxuridine   Rx

Class: Antimetabolite

> Should be given only by or under supervision of a qualified physician. Due to possibility of severe toxic reactions, all patients should be hospitalized for initiation of 1st course of therapy.

OTHER BRAND NAMES
FUDR (Discontinued)

ADULT DOSAGE	PEDIATRIC DOSAGE
Gastrointestinal Adenocarcinoma	Pediatric use may not have been established
Palliative management of GI adenocarcinoma metastatic to the liver in carefully selected patients who are considered incurable by surgery or other means	
Usual: 0.1-0.6mg/kg/day by continuous arterial infusion	
Higher dose ranges (0.4-0.6mg) are usually employed for hepatic artery infusion	
Therapy can be given until adverse reactions appear; may resume when reactions subside	
Maintain on therapy as long as response continues	

ADMINISTRATION
Intra-arterial route
Each vial must be reconstituted w/ 5mL sterile water for inj to yield sol containing approx 100mg/mL
Calculated daily dose(s) is then diluted w/ D5 or 0.9% NaCl inj to a volume appropriate for infusion apparatus to be used
Administration is best achieved w/ use of an appropriate pump to overcome pressure in large arteries and to ensure a uniform rate of infusion

STORAGE
Powder: 20-25°C (68-77°F). Reconstituted: 2-8°C (36-46°F) for ≤2 weeks.

HOW SUPPLIED
Inj: 500mg

CONTRAINDICATIONS
Poor nutritional state, depressed bone marrow function, potentially serious infections.

WARNINGS/PRECAUTIONS
Highly toxic drug w/ narrow margin of safety. Use extreme caution in poor risk patients w/ renal/hepatic dysfunction, history of high-dose pelvic irradiation, or previous use of alkylating agents. Not intended as an adjuvant to surgery. May cause fetal harm when administered during pregnancy. May cause severe hematological toxicity, GI hemorrhage, and death. D/C promptly if myocardial ischemia, stomatitis/esophagopharyngitis (at 1st visible sign), leukopenia (WBC <3500) or rapidly falling WBC, intractable vomiting, diarrhea, frequent bowel movements/watery stools, GI ulceration and bleeding, thrombocytopenia (platelets <100,000), or hemorrhage from any site occurs.

ADVERSE REACTIONS
N/V, diarrhea, enteritis, stomatitis, localized erythema, anemia, leukopenia, thrombocytopenia, elevations of alkaline phosphatase, serum transaminase, serum bilirubin, lactic dehydrogenase.

DRUG INTERACTIONS
Any form of therapy that adds to the stress of patient, interferes with nutrition or depresses bone marrow function will increase toxicity of floxuridine.

PREGNANCY AND LACTATION
Category D, not for use in nursing.

MECHANISM OF ACTION
Antimetabolite; interferes w/ the synthesis of deoxyribonucleic acid and, to a lesser extent, inhibits formation of ribonucleic acid.

PHARMACOKINETICS
Metabolism: Liver; 5-fluorouracil (active metabolite). **Elimination:** Urine (parent drug and metabolites).

PATIENT CONSIDERATIONS

Assessment: Assess nutritional state, and for bone marrow depression, serious infections, hepatic/renal impairment, history of high-dose pelvic irradiation, previous use of alkylating agents, pregnancy/nursing status, and possible drug interactions.

Monitoring: Monitor for myocardial ischemia, stomatitis, esophagopharyngitis, intractable vomiting, diarrhea, frequent bowel movements/watery stools, GI ulceration/bleeding, leukopenia, thrombocytopenia, hemorrhage from any site, and for any other adverse reaction. Monitor platelet and WBC counts.

Counseling: Counsel about expected toxic effects of therapy, particularly oral manifestations. Alert patients to the possibility of alopecia and inform that it is usually a transient effect. Apprise pregnant women of the potential hazard to the fetus if drug is used during pregnancy; advise women of childbearing potential to avoid becoming pregnant while on drug. Advise mothers not to nurse while receiving this drug.

FLUDARABINE — fludarabine phosphate   Rx

Class: Antimetabolite

> Should be administered under the supervision of a qualified physician experienced in the use of antineoplastic therapy. May severely suppress bone marrow function. Severe neurologic effects (eg, blindness, coma, death) occurred with doses 4X greater than the recommended dose; similar severe CNS toxicity reported with recommended dose. Life-threatening and sometimes fatal autoimmune phenomena (eg, hemolytic anemia) reported; evaluate and closely monitor for hemolysis. Unacceptably high incidence of fatal pulmonary toxicity reported in combination with pentostatin (deoxycoformycin); concomitant use is not recommended.

OTHER BRAND NAMES
Fludara (Discontinued)

ADULT DOSAGE	PEDIATRIC DOSAGE
B-Cell Chronic Lymphocytic Leukemia	Pediatric use may not have been established
B-cell chronic lymphocytic leukemia unresponsive to or progressed during treatment w/ at least 1 standard alkylating agent-containing regimen	
Usual: 25mg/m² IV over 30 min qd for 5 consecutive days, commence each 5-day course every 28 days	
Administer 3 additional cycles following achievement of maximal response, and then d/c therapy	

DOSING CONSIDERATIONS
Renal Impairment
Moderate (CrCl 30-70mL/min): Reduce by 20%

Adverse Reactions
May decrease or delay dose based on evidence of hematologic or nonhematologic toxicity

ADMINISTRATION
IV route

Reconstitution of Powder
Reconstitute w/ 2mL of sterile water for inj; each mL of the sol will then contain 25mg of drug
Can further be diluted in 100cc or 125cc of D5 inj or 0.9% NaCl inj
Use w/in 8 hrs of reconstitution
Do not mix w/ other drugs

STORAGE
(Inj Sol) 2-8°C (36-46°F). Use within 8 hrs of opening. (Powder for Inj) 20-25°C (68-77°F). Reconstituted Sol: Use within 8 hrs.

HOW SUPPLIED
Inj: 50mg/2mL

CONTRAINDICATIONS
Hypersensitivity to fludarabine or its components.

WARNINGS/PRECAUTIONS
Consider delaying or discontinuing therapy if neurotoxicity occurs. Caution in patients with advanced age, renal insufficiency, bone marrow impairment, immunodeficiency, and history of opportunistic infection. Do not use in patients with severe renal impairment (CrCl <30mL/min). Infection and disease progression/transformation reported. Tumor lysis syndrome (TLS) reported in patients with large tumor burdens. Transfusion-associated graft-versus-host disease reported after transfusion of nonirradiated blood; consider the use of irradiated blood products in those patients requiring transfusions while undergoing treatment. May cause fetal harm. May impair mental/physical abilities.

ADVERSE REACTIONS
Myelosuppression, CNS toxicity, hemolytic anemia, fever, chills, infection, N/V, pneumonia, fatigue, cough, weakness, malaise, anorexia, pain, edema.

DRUG INTERACTIONS
See Boxed Warning. Avoid live vaccines during and after treatment.

PREGNANCY AND LACTATION
Category D, not for use in nursing.

MECHANISM OF ACTION
Antimetabolite; not established. Appears to act by inhibiting DNA polymerase-α, ribonucleotide reductase, and DNA primase, thus inhibiting DNA synthesis.

PHARMACOKINETICS
Distribution: Plasma protein binding (19-29%). **Metabolism:** Rapid dephosphorylation to 2-fluoro-ara-A (active metabolite), then intracellular phosphorylation by deoxycytidine kinase to 2-fluoro-ara-ATP. **Elimination:** $T_{1/2}$=20 hrs (2-fluoro-ara-A).

PATIENT CONSIDERATIONS
Assessment: Assess for renal/bone marrow impairment, immunodeficiency, history/risk of opportunistic infections, risk of TLS, hypersensitivity to drug, pregnancy/nursing status, and possible drug interactions.

Monitoring: Monitor for bone marrow suppression, CNS toxicity, autoimmune phenomena, hemolysis, infection, disease progression/transformation, TLS, and other adverse events. Periodically monitor peripheral blood counts/hematologic profile.

Counseling: Inform of the risks and benefits of therapy. Inform of the importance of periodic assessment of blood count to detect the development of anemia, neutropenia, and thrombocytopenia. Instruct to notify physician if pregnant, planning to become pregnant, or breastfeeding. Advise women of childbearing potential to avoid becoming pregnant. Inform that drug may reduce ability to drive or use machines. Advise to avoid vaccination with live vaccines during and after treatment. Instruct to consult physician if any adverse events develop.

FLUOROPLEX — fluorouracil Rx

Class: Antimetabolite

ADULT DOSAGE	PEDIATRIC DOSAGE
Multiple Actinic or Solar Keratoses Apply sufficient medication to cover the entire face or other affected areas bid for 2-6 weeks When the inflammatory reaction reaches the erosion, ulceration, and necrosis stage, d/c use Increasing the frequency of application and a longer period of administration may be required on areas other than the head and neck	Pediatric use may not have been established

ADMINISTRATION
Topical route

Apply w/ fingertips; wash hands following application.

STORAGE
15-30°C (59-86°F). Avoid freezing.

HOW SUPPLIED
Cre: 1% [30g]

CONTRAINDICATIONS
Women who are or may become pregnant. Allergy to any component of this product.

WARNINGS/PRECAUTIONS
Delayed hypersensitivity reaction may occur. Occlusive dressings may increase the incidence of inflammatory reactions in the adjacent normal skin. Avoid prolonged exposure to sunlight or other forms of UV irradiation during treatment. May increase absorption w/ ulcerated or inflamed skin. Conduct biopsy to areas failing to respond to treatment or recurring after treatment to rule out frank neoplasm.

ADVERSE REACTIONS
Pain, pruritus, burning, irritation, inflammation, allergic contact dermatitis, telangiectasia, hyperpigmentation, scarring.

PREGNANCY AND LACTATION
Pregnancy: Category X.
Lactation: Not for use in nursing.

MECHANISM OF ACTION
Keratoses agent; blocks the methylation reaction of deoxyuridylic acid to thymidylic acid, thereby interfering w/ synthesis of DNA and, to a lesser extent, inhibiting formation of RNA.

PATIENT CONSIDERATIONS
Assessment: Assess for drug hypersensitivity, inflamed/ulcerated skin, and pregnancy/nursing status.

Monitoring: Monitor for delayed hypersensitivity reaction, inflammatory reactions in adjacent normal skin, and other adverse effects. Perform a biopsy of areas failing to respond to treatment or recurring after treatment.

Counseling: Instruct to apply w/ care near eyes, nose, and mouth. Counsel to apply medication w/ the fingers and wash hands immediately after. Inform that reaction in treated areas may be unsightly during therapy and, in some cases, for several weeks following cessation of therapy.

FOLLISTIM AQ — follitropin beta Rx

Class: Follicle-stimulating hormone (FSH)

ADULT DOSAGE

Ovulation Induction

Induction of ovulation and pregnancy in anovulatory infertile women in whom the cause of infertility is functional and not due to primary ovarian failure

Vial:
Initial: 75 IU qd for at least the first 7 days
Titrate: Make subsequent dose adjustments at weekly intervals based on ovarian response; if needed, increase dose by 25-50 IU at weekly intervals until follicular growth and/or serum estradiol levels indicate adequate ovarian response
Max: 300 IU/day

Cartridge:
Initial: 50 IU qd for at least the first 7 days
Titrate: Make subsequent dose adjustments at weekly intervals based on ovarian response; if needed, increase dose by 25-50 IU at weekly intervals until follicular growth and/or serum estradiol levels indicate adequate ovarian response
Max: 250 IU/day

Continue treatment until ultrasonic visualizations/serum estradiol determinations approximate pre-ovulatory conditions seen in normal individuals

Ovarian Stimulation

Pregnancy in normal ovulatory women undergoing controlled ovarian stimulation as part of an in vitro fertilization or intracytoplasmic sperm inj cycle

Cartridge:
Initial: 200 IU qd for at least the first 7 days of treatment
Titrate: Adjust subsequent doses up or down based on ovarian response
Dose reduction in high responders can be considered from the 6th day onward
Maint:
Normal Responders: Daily starting dose can be continued until pre-ovulatory conditions are achieved (7-12 days)
Low or Poor Responders: Increase daily dose according to ovarian response; max of 500 IU/day
High Responders (At Risk of Abnormal Ovarian Enlargement and/or Ovarian Hyperstimulation Syndrome): Decrease or temporarily d/c the daily dose or d/c the cycle, depending on response

Perform oocyte retrieval 34-36 hrs following human chorionic gonadotropin administration

Assisted Reproductive Technology

Development of multiple follicles in ovulatory women

Vial:
Initial: 150-225 IU qd for at least the first 4 days of treatment
Titrate: Adjust subsequent dosing based on ovarian response
Maint:
Normal Responders: Daily starting dose can be continued until pre-ovulatory conditions are achieved (6-12 days)
Low or Poor Responders: Increase daily dose according to ovarian response; max of 600 IU/day
High Responders (At Risk of Abnormal Ovarian Enlargement and/or Ovarian Hyperstimulation Syndrome): Decrease or temporarily d/c the daily dose or d/c the cycle, depending on response

PEDIATRIC DOSAGE
Pediatric use may not have been established

Perform oocyte retrieval 34-36 hrs following human chorionic gonadotropin administration

Induction of Spermatogenesis

In men w/ primary and secondary hypogonadotropic hypogonadism in whom the cause of infertility is not due to primary testicular failure

Pretreatment w/ human chorionic gonadotropin (hCG) is required
Usual: 450 IU/week (given as 225 IU twice weekly or 150 IU 3X/week) w/ hCG; consider lower dose w/ Follistim AQ cartridge
Continue concomitant therapy for at least 3-4 months before any improvement can be expected

Conversions

When administering Follistim AQ Cartridge, a lower starting dose and lower dose adjustments (as compared to reconstituted Follistim) should be considered

Follistim AQ Cartridge w/ the pen injector device delivers on average an 18% higher amount of follitropin beta when compared to reconstituted Follistim delivered w/ a conventional syringe and needle; refer to PI for conversion chart

ADMINISTRATION

(Cartridge) SQ route, (Vial) SQ/IM route

Cartridge
Do not add any other medicines into the cartridge

Vial
Do not mix w/ any other medicines in the same vial or in the same syringe

STORAGE

2-8°C (36-46°F). Upon Dispensing: 2-8°C (36-46°F) until expiration date, or 25°C (77°F) (cartridge)/≤25°C (77°F) (vial) for 3 months or until expiration date, whichever occurs 1st. Protect from light. Do not freeze. (Cartridge) Once Used: 2-25°C (36-77°F) for a max of 28 days.

HOW SUPPLIED

Inj: (Cartridge) 150 IU, 300 IU, 600 IU, 900 IU; (Vial) 75 IU/0.5mL, 150 IU/0.5mL

CONTRAINDICATIONS

Prior hypersensitivity to recombinant FSH products, FSH levels indicating primary gonadal failure, presence of uncontrolled nongonadal endocrinopathies (eg, thyroid, adrenal, or pituitary disorders), tumor of the ovary, breast, uterus, testis, hypothalamus, or pituitary gland, pregnancy, heavy or irregular vaginal bleeding of undetermined origin, ovarian cysts or enlargement not due to polycystic ovary syndrome. Hypersensitivity to streptomycin or neomycin.

WARNINGS/PRECAUTIONS

Should be used only by physicians experienced in infertility treatment. May cause ovarian hyperstimulation syndrome (OHSS) with or without pulmonary/vascular complications and multiple births. Use lowest effective dose to minimize hazards associated with abnormal ovarian enlargement. Do not administer HCG if ovaries are abnormally enlarged on the last day of therapy; prohibit intercourse with significant ovarian enlargement after ovulation. Hepatic dysfunction reported in association with OHSS. Withhold HCG if there is a risk for OHSS evident prior to HCG administration. Monitor for OHSS development for at least 2 weeks after HCG administration; d/c therapy, including HCG, and consider hospitalization if serious OHSS occurs. OHSS increases the risk of injury to the ovary; avoid pelvic examination. Serious pulmonary conditions (eg, atelectasis, acute respiratory distress syndrome), thromboembolic reactions (both in association with, and separate from, OHSS), ovarian torsion, multifetal gestation and births, ectopic pregnancies, ovarian neoplasms, and increased risk of spontaneous abortions reported. Incidence of congenital malformations after IVF/ICSI or ART may be slightly higher than after spontaneous conception. Increased risk of venous/arterial thromboembolic events in women with recognized risk factors for thrombosis; caution in such patients. Women who are undergoing ovulation induction should be encouraged with their partners to have intercourse daily, beginning on the day prior to the administration of hCG and until ovulation becomes apparent. (Cartridge) Not recommended for the blind or visually impaired without the assistance of an individual with good vision who is trained in the proper use of the inj device.

ADVERSE REACTIONS

Headache, OHSS, inj-site reaction/pain, dermoid cyst, acne, rash, gynecomastia, pelvic pain.

PREGNANCY AND LACTATION

Category X, not for use in nursing.

MECHANISM OF ACTION

FSH; stimulates ovarian follicular growth in women who do not have primary ovarian failure. Stimulates spermatogenesis in men with hypogonadotropic hypogonadism when administered with HCG.

PHARMACOKINETICS

Absorption: Administration of variable doses resulted in different parameters.
Distribution: (IV) V_d=8L. **Elimination:** (IM, Single 300 IU Dose): $T_{1/2}$=43.9 hrs. 7-Day Treatment: $T_{1/2}$=26.9 hrs (75 IU), 30.1 hrs (150 IU), 28.9 hrs (225 IU). (SQ, Cartridge, Single 150 IU Dose): $T_{1/2}$=33.4 hrs.

PATIENT CONSIDERATIONS

Assessment: Assess for hypersensitivity to drug or to streptomycin or neomycin, high FSH levels indicating primary gonadal failure, uncontrolled nongonadal endocrinopathies, heavy/irregular vaginal bleeding, ovarian cysts/enlargement, pregnancy/nursing status, risk factors for thrombosis, and tumors of the ovary, breast, uterus, testis, hypothalamus, or pituitary gland. Obtain complete gynecologic, medical, and endocrinologic evaluation. Evaluate the fertility status of the female or male partner.

Monitoring: Monitor for OHSS, abnormal ovarian enlargement, pulmonary/vascular complications, ovarian torsion, and other adverse reactions. Monitor for ovulation and spermatogenesis. Monitor for signs of excessive ovarian stimulation at least qod during treatment and during a 2-week post-treatment period.

Counseling: Prior to beginning therapy, inform about the time commitment and monitoring procedures necessary to undergo treatment. Counsel about risk of multifetal gestations, OHSS, and other possible side effects. Inform not to double the next dose if a dose is missed and to contact physician for further dosing instructions.

FOLOTYN — pralatrexate　　　　　　　　　Rx

Class: Dihydrofolic acid reductase inhibitor

ADULT DOSAGE	PEDIATRIC DOSAGE
Peripheral T-Cell Lymphoma	Pediatric use may not have been established
Relapsed or Refractory: 30mg/m² IV push over 3-5 min once weekly for 6 weeks in 7-week cycles until progressive disease or unacceptable toxicity	
Pretreatment Vitamin Supplementation: **Folic Acid:** 1.0-1.25mg PO qd beginning 10 days before 1st dose of Folotyn; continue during the full course of therapy and for 30 days after the last dose **Vitamin B12:** 1mg IM w/in 10 weeks prior to 1st dose of Folotyn and every 8-10 weeks thereafter; subsequent inj may be given the same day as treatment w/ Folotyn	

DOSING CONSIDERATIONS

Renal Impairment
Mild to Moderate: No dose reduction necessary
Severe (eGFR 15 to <30mL/min/1.73m²): 15mg/m²

Hepatic Impairment
Not studied

Adverse Reactions
Prior to Any Dose:
- Mucositis should be ≤Grade 1
- Platelet count should be ≥100,000/mcL for 1st dose and ≥50,000/mcL for all subsequent doses
- ANC should be ≥1000/mcL

Mucositis on Day of Treatment:
Grade 2: Omit dose; continue prior dose upon recovery to ≤Grade 1
Grade 2 Recurrence: Omit dose; administer 20mg/m² upon recovery to ≤Grade 1 (10mg/m² upon recovery in patients w/ severe renal impairment)
Grade 3: Omit dose; administer 20mg/m² upon recovery to ≤Grade 1 (10mg/m² upon recovery in patients w/ severe renal impairment)
Grade 4: Stop therapy

Blood Count on Day of Treatment:
Platelet Count <50,000/mcL for:
1 Week: Omit dose; continue prior dose upon restart
2 Weeks: Omit dose; administer 20mg/m² upon restart (10mg/m² upon recovery in patients w/ severe renal impairment)
3 Weeks: Stop therapy

ANC 500-1000/mcL and No Fever for:
1 Week: Omit dose; continue prior dose upon restart

ANC 500-1000/mcL w/ Fever or ANC <500/mcL for:
1 Week: Omit dose and give G-CSF or GM-CSF support; continue prior dose w/ G-CSF or GM-CSF support upon restart
2 Weeks or Recurrence: Omit dose and give G-CSF or GM-CSF support; administer 20mg/m² w/ G-CSF or GM-CSF support upon restart (10mg/m² w/ G-CSF or GM-CSF support upon recovery in patients w/ severe renal impairment)
3 Weeks or 2nd Recurrence: Stop therapy

Toxicity Grade on Day of Treatment for Other Treatment-Related Toxicities:
Grade 3: Omit dose; administer 20mg/m² upon recovery to ≤Grade 2 (10mg/m² upon recovery in patients w/ severe renal impairment)
Grade 4: Stop therapy

ADMINISTRATION

IV route

Do not dilute.

Administer via the side port of a free-flowing 0.9% NaCl inj, IV line.

Vials contain no preservatives and are intended for single use only; after withdrawal of dose, discard vial including any unused portion.

Special Handling Instructions

Use of gloves and other protective clothing is recommended.

If contact w/ skin occurs, immediately and thoroughly wash w/ soap and water.

If contact w/ mucous membranes occurs, flush thoroughly w/ water.

STORAGE

2-8°C (36-46°F) in original carton to protect from light. **Unopened Vials:** Stable at room temperature for 72 hrs in original carton; discard if left at room temperature for >72 hrs. Discard any unused portion remaining after inj.

HOW SUPPLIED

Inj: 20mg/mL [1mL, 2mL]

WARNINGS/PRECAUTIONS

May cause bone marrow suppression, manifested by thrombocytopenia, neutropenia, and/or anemia. May cause mucositis. Supplement w/ folic acid and vitamin B12 to reduce the risk of treatment-related hematological toxicity and mucositis. May cause severe dermatologic reactions, including death, and it may be progressive and increase in severity w/ further treatment; withhold or d/c if severe reactions occur. May cause tumor lysis syndrome (TLS); monitor patients who are at increased risk of TLS and treat promptly. May cause hepatic toxicity and LFT abnormalities; omit dose until recovery and adjust or d/c therapy based on the severity of the hepatic toxicity. Greater risk for increased exposure and toxicity in patients w/ moderate to severe renal impairment; monitor for renal function and systemic toxicity and adjust dosing accordingly. Serious adverse drug reactions, including toxic epidermal necrolysis and mucositis, reported in patients w/ end-stage renal disease (ESRD) undergoing dialysis; avoid in patients w/ ESRD, including those undergoing dialysis unless the potential benefit justifies the potential risk. May cause fetal harm during pregnancy. Caution in elderly.

ADVERSE REACTIONS

Mucositis, thrombocytopenia, N/V, fatigue, pyrexia, sepsis, febrile neutropenia, dehydration, dyspnea, anemia, constipation, edema, cough, epistaxis.

DRUG INTERACTIONS

Increasing doses of probenecid may delay clearance and increase exposure; monitor closely for signs of systemic toxicity due to increased drug exposure w/ probenecid or other drugs that may affect relevant transporter systems (eg, NSAIDs).

PREGNANCY AND LACTATION

Pregnancy: Category D.
Lactation: Not for use in nursing.

MECHANISM OF ACTION

Folate analogue metabolic inhibitor; competitively inhibits dihydrofolate reductase. Also a competitive inhibitor for polyglutamylation by the enzyme folylpolyglutamyl synthetase. This inhibition results in the depletion of thymidine and other biological molecules, the synthesis of which depends on single carbon transfer.

PHARMACOKINETICS

Distribution: V_d=105L (*S*-diastereomer), 37L (*R*-diastereomer); plasma protein binding (67%). **Elimination:** Urine (39%), feces (34%), respiratory (10%); $T_{1/2}$=12-18 hrs.

PATIENT CONSIDERATIONS

Assessment: Assess for severity of mucositis, pregnancy/nursing status, and for possible drug interactions. Perform serum chemistry tests (eg, renal and hepatic function) prior to the start of therapy. Obtain baseline CBC.

Monitoring: Monitor for bone marrow suppression, mucositis, dermatologic reactions, TLS, systemic toxicity, and for other adverse reactions. Perform serum chemistry tests (eg, renal and hepatic function) prior to the start of the 1st and 4th dose of each cycle. Monitor CBC and severity of mucositis weekly.

Counseling: Advise to take folic acid and vitamin B12 as a prophylactic measure to reduce the risk of possible side effects. Inform of the risk of low blood cell counts and to contact physician immediately if any signs of infection (eg, fever), bleeding, or symptoms of anemia occur. Inform of signs/symptoms of mucositis, ways to reduce the risk of development, and ways to maintain nutrition and control discomfort from mucositis if it occurs. Advise about the risks for and the signs/symptoms of dermatologic reactions and instruct to notify physician immediately if any skin reactions occur. Inform about the risk of and the signs/symptoms of TLS and instruct to notify physician if symptoms occur. Advise to inform physician if taking any concomitant medications, including prescription and nonprescription drugs. Instruct to notify physician if pregnant, planning to be pregnant, or if nursing.

FORTEO — teriparatide (rDNA origin)   Rx

Class: Recombinant human parathyroid hormone

ADULT DOSAGE

Osteoporosis

High Risk for Fracture:

Postmenopausal Women w/ Osteoporosis:
20mcg qd

Primary or Hypogonadal Osteoporosis in Men:
20mcg qd

Glucocorticoid-Induced Osteoporosis in Men and Women:
20mcg qd

Use for >2 yrs during a patient's lifetime is not recommended

PEDIATRIC DOSAGE

Pediatric use may not have been established

ADMINISTRATION

SQ route

Inject into the thigh or abdominal wall.

Administer initially under circumstances where the patient can sit or lie down if symptoms of orthostatic hypotension occur.

STORAGE

2-8°C (36-46°F). Recap pen when not in use. Minimize time out of the refrigerator during the use period; may deliver dose immediately following removal from the refrigerator. Do not freeze; do not use if it has been frozen. Discard after the 28-day use period.

HOW SUPPLIED

Inj: 20mcg/dose [28 doses]

CONTRAINDICATIONS

Hypersensitivity to teriparatide or to any of its excipients.

WARNINGS/PRECAUTIONS

Use for >2 yrs during a patient's lifetime is not recommended. Do not give in patients w/ bone metastases or history of skeletal malignancies, metabolic bone diseases other than osteoporosis, preexisting hypercalcemia, or underlying hypercalcemic disorder (eg, primary hyperparathyroidism). Transiently increases serum Ca^{2+}. Consider measurement of urinary Ca^{2+} excretion if active urolithiasis or preexisting hypercalciuria are suspected; caution w/ active or recent urolithiasis. Transient episodes of symptomatic orthostatic hypotension reported w/ administration of initial doses; administer initially under circumstances where the patient can sit or lie down if symptoms of orthostatic hypotension occur.

ADVERSE REACTIONS

Pain, arthralgia, rhinitis, asthenia, N/V, dizziness, headache, HTN, increased cough, pharyngitis, constipation, dyspepsia, diarrhea, rash, insomnia.

DRUG INTERACTIONS

Hypercalcemia may predispose to digitalis toxicity; caution if taking digoxin concomitantly.

PREGNANCY AND LACTATION

Category C, not for use in nursing.

MECHANISM OF ACTION

Recombinant human parathyroid hormone; binds to specific high-affinity cell-surface receptors. Stimulates new bone formation on trabecular and cortical (periosteal and/or endosteal) bone surfaces by preferential stimulation of osteoblastic activity over osteoclastic activity. Produces an increase in skeletal mass, markers of bone formation and resorption, and bone strength.

PHARMACOKINETICS

Absorption: Rapid. Absolute bioavailability (approx 95%); T_{max}=30 min.
Distribution: (IV) V_d=approx 0.12L/kg. **Metabolism:** Liver (nonspecific enzymatic mechanisms). **Elimination:** Kidneys; $T_{1/2}$=approx 1 hr.

PATIENT CONSIDERATIONS

Assessment: Assess for increased baseline risk for osteosarcoma, bone metastases or history of skeletal malignancies, metabolic bone disease other than osteoporosis, hypercalcemia, hypercalcemic disorder, hypercalciuria, active or recent urolithiasis, hypersensitivity to drug, pregnancy/nursing status, and possible drug interactions. Consider measurement of urinary Ca^{2+} excretion if active urolithiasis or preexisting hypercalciuria are suspected.

Monitoring: Monitor for signs/symptoms of osteosarcoma, orthostatic hypotension, and other adverse reactions.

Counseling: Inform of potential risk of osteosarcoma and encourage to enroll in the voluntary Forteo Patient Registry. Instruct to sit or lie down if lightheadedness or palpitations following inj develop; if symptoms persist or worsen, advise to consult physician before continuing treatment. Instruct to contact physician if persistent symptoms of hypercalcemia (eg, N/V, constipation, lethargy, muscle weakness) develop. Counsel on roles of supplemental Ca^{2+} and/or vitamin D, weight-bearing exercise, and modification of certain behavioral factors (eg, smoking, alcohol consumption). Instruct on proper use of delivery device (pen) and proper disposal of needles; advise not to share pen w/ other patients and not to transfer contents to a syringe.

FUSILEV — levoleucovorin Rx

Class: Cytoprotective agent

ADULT DOSAGE

Rescue Therapy

After High Dose Methotrexate (MTX) Therapy in Osteosarcoma:

Normal MTX Elimination:
7.5mg (5mg/m^2) IV q6h for 10 doses starting 24 hrs after the beginning of MTX infusion

Delayed Late MTX Elimination:
Continue 7.5mg IV q6h, until MTX level is <0.05μm

Delayed Early MTX Elimination and/ or Evidence of Acute Renal Injury:
75mg IV q3h until MTX level is <1μm; then 7.5mg IV q3h until MTX level is <0.05μm. Continue therapy, hydration and urinary alkalinization until MTX level is <0.05μm and resolution of renal failure
If significant clinical toxicity w/ less severe abnormalities in MTX elimination/renal function is observed, extend rescue therapy for an additional 24 hrs in subsequent courses of therapy

Methotrexate Toxicity

Used to diminish the toxicity and counteract the effects of impaired MTX elimination and of inadvertent overdosage of folic acid antagonists

7.5mg (5mg/m^2) IV q6h until serum MTX is <10^{-8}M

Titrate: Increase to 50mg/m^2 IV q3h until MTX level is <10^{-8}M if 24-hr SrCr is 50% over baseline, or if 24-hr MTX level is >5 x 10^{-6}M, or 48-hr level is >9 x 10^{-7}M

Employ concurrent hydration (3L/ day) and urinary alkalinization w/ Na bicarbonate; adjust bicarbonate dose to maintain urine pH at ≥7

Start rescue therapy as soon as possible after overdose and w/in 24 hrs of MTX administration when there is delayed excretion

Metastatic Colorectal Cancer

Palliative Treatment in Combination w/ 5-Fluorouracil (5-FU):
Usual: 100mg/m^2 slow IV over a minimum of 3 min, followed by 370mg/m^2 5-FU IV, daily for 5 days, or
10mg/m^2 IV, followed by 425mg/m2 5-FU IV, daily for 5 days

May repeat at 4-week intervals for 2 courses, then at 4- to 5-week intervals provided that patient has completely recovered from toxic effects of prior treatment course

May increase 5-FU dose by 10% if no toxicity. Reduce 5-FU daily dose by 20% w/ moderate GI/hematologic toxicity and by 30% w/ severe toxicity

PEDIATRIC DOSAGE
Pediatric use may not have been established

DOSING CONSIDERATIONS

Renal Impairment
Rescue Therapy: Higher doses or prolonged administration may be indicated

Other Important Considerations
3rd Space Fluid Collection/Inadequate Hydration:
Rescue Therapy: Higher doses or prolonged administration may be indicated

ADMINISTRATION
IV route

Do not administer intrathecally
Do not administer w/ other agents in the same admixture
Administer 5-FU and levoleucovorin separately
No more than 16mL (160mg) of reconstituted sol should be injected IV per min

Preparation
Reconstitute 50mg vial w/ 5.3mL of 0.9% NaCl inj to yield a levoleucovorin concentration 10mg/mL
May further dilute, immediately, to concentrations of 0.5mg/mL in 0.9% NaCl inj or D5 inj

STORAGE
(Powder) 25°C (77°F); excursions permitted from 15-30°C (59-86°F). Protect from light. Reconstitution/Dilution with 0.9% NaCl: Room temperature for ≤12 hrs. Dilution with D5W: Room temperature for ≤4 hrs. (Sol) 2-8°C (36-46°F). Protect from light. Dilution with 0.9% NaCl or D5W: Room temperature for ≤4 hrs.

HOW SUPPLIED
Inj: 50mg, 10mg/mL [17.5mL, 25mL]

WARNINGS/PRECAUTIONS
Do not inject >16mL/min. Do not administer intrathecally. Not approved for pernicious anemia and megaloblastic anemias secondary to the lack of vitamin B12; improper use may cause a hematologic remission while neurologic manifestations continue to progress. Do not initiate or continue therapy with 5-FU in patients with symptoms of GI toxicity until symptoms have completely resolved; caution in elderly and/or debilitated. Monitor patients with diarrhea until it has resolved, as rapid clinical deterioration leading to death can occur. Seizures and/or syncope reported in cancer patients, most commonly in those with CNS metastases or other predisposing factors.

ADVERSE REACTIONS
Stomatitis, N/V, diarrhea, dyspepsia, typhlitis, dyspnea, dermatitis, confusion, neuropathy, abnormal renal function, taste perversion.

DRUG INTERACTIONS
May enhance 5-FU toxicity. Seizures and/or syncope reported with fluoropyrimidine. Increased treatment failure and morbidity rates in trimethoprim-sulfamethoxazole-treated HIV patients with *Pneumocystis carinii* pneumonia. Folic acid in large amounts may counteract antiepileptic effect of phenobarbital, phenytoin, and primidone, and increase seizure frequency in children; use with caution when taken with anticonvulsants.

PREGNANCY AND LACTATION
Category C, not for use in nursing.

MECHANISM OF ACTION
Folate analog; counteracts the therapeutic and toxic effects of folic acid antagonists, which act by inhibiting dihydrofolate reductase. Enhances therapeutic effects of fluoropyrimidines used in cancer therapy (eg, 5-FU).

PHARMACOKINETICS
Absorption: (Total-Tetrahydrofolate [THF]) C_{max}=1722ng/mL; (5-methyl-THF) C_{max}=275ng/mL, T_{max}=0.9 hrs. **Metabolism:** 5-methyl-THF (metabolite). **Elimination:** $T_{1/2}$=5.1 hrs (total-THF), 6.8 hrs (5-methyl-THF).

PATIENT CONSIDERATIONS

Assessment: Assess for previous allergic reactions to folic acid or folinic acid, pernicious anemia and megaloblastic anemias secondary to the lack of vitamin B12, GI toxicity, third-space fluid accumulation (eg, ascites, pleural effusion), renal impairment, inadequate hydration, CNS metastases, pregnancy/nursing status, and possible drug interactions.

Monitoring: Monitor for GI toxicity, seizures, syncope, and hypersensitivity reactions. Monitor patients with diarrhea until it has resolved. Monitor fluid and electrolytes in patients with abnormalities in MTX excretion. Monitor SrCr and MTX levels at least qd.

Counseling: Inform about risks and benefits of therapy. Advise to notify physician if any adverse reaction occurs. Instruct to inform physician if pregnant/nursing.

FUZEON — enfuvirtide Rx

Class: Fusion inhibitor

ADULT DOSAGE

HIV-1 Infection

In Combination w/ Other Antiretrovirals:
90mg bid

PEDIATRIC DOSAGE

HIV-1 Infection

In Combination w/ Other Antiretrovirals:
6-16 Years:
2mg/kg bid
Max: 90mg bid

Refer to PI for pediatric dosing guidelines based on body weight

ADMINISTRATION
SQ route

Inject in upper arm, anterior thigh, or abdomen.
Give each inj at a site different from the previous inj site, and only where there is no current inj-site reaction from an earlier dose.
Do not inject near areas where large nerves course close to the skin, directly over a blood vessel, into moles, scar tissue, bruises, or near the navel, surgical scars, tattoos, or burn sites.

Directions for Use
1. Reconstitute w/ 1mL of sterile water for inj.
2. Gently tap the vial for 10 sec, and then gently roll between the hands to avoid foaming and to ensure all particles of drug are in contact w/ the liquid and no drug remains on the vial wall.
3. Allow to stand until the powder goes completely into sol (which could take up to 45 min); may reduce reconstitution time by gently rolling the vial between the hands until product is completely dissolved. Allow more time to dissolve if drug is foamy or jelled.
4. Once reconstituted, inject immediately or store at 2-8°C (36-46°F) and use w/in 24 hrs. If refrigerated, bring to room temperature before inj.
Refer to PI for further instructions.

STORAGE
25°C (77°F); excursions permitted to 15-30°C (59-86°F).

HOW SUPPLIED
Inj: 90mg/mL

CONTRAINDICATIONS
Known hypersensitivity to enfuvirtide or to any of its components.

WARNINGS/PRECAUTIONS
Local inj-site reactions reported; monitor for signs/symptoms of cellulitis or local infection. Administration w/ Biojector 2000 may result in neuralgia and/or paresthesia, bruising, and hematomas. Patients w/ hemophilia or other coagulation disorders may have a higher risk of post-inj bleeding. May cause bacterial pneumonia; monitor for signs/symptoms of pneumonia, especially those predisposed to pneumonia (eg, low initial CD4 cell count, high initial viral load, IV drug use, smoking, prior history of lung disease). Associated w/ systemic hypersensitivity reactions; d/c immediately if signs/symptoms develop. May lead to anti-enfuvirtide antibody production, which cross-reacts w/ HIV gp41 and could result in false-positive HIV test w/ an ELISA assay. Immune reconstitution syndrome reported. Autoimmune disorders (eg, Graves' disease, polymyositis, Guillain-Barre syndrome) reported in the setting of immune reconstitution and can occur many months after initiation of treatment.

ADVERSE REACTIONS
Local inj-site reactions, diarrhea, fatigue, nausea.

DRUG INTERACTIONS
May result in a higher risk of post-inj bleeding w/ anticoagulants.

PREGNANCY AND LACTATION
Pregnancy: Category B. An antiretroviral pregnancy registry has been established to monitor maternal-fetal outcomes of pregnant women.
Lactation: Not for use in nursing.

MECHANISM OF ACTION
Fusion inhibitor; interferes w/ the entry of HIV-1 into cells by inhibiting fusion of viral and cellular membranes. Binds to the first heptad-repeat in the gp41 subunit of the viral envelope glycoprotein and prevents the conformational changes required for the fusion of viral and cellular membranes.

PHARMACOKINETICS
Absorption: Absolute bioavailability (84.3%); C_{max}=5mcg/mL; AUC_{0-12h}=48.7mcg•hr/mL; T_{max}=4 hrs. **Distribution:** (IV)V_d=5.5L. Plasma protein binding (92%). **Metabolism:** Liver via hydrolysis; M_3 (metabolite). **Elimination:** $T_{1/2}$=3.8 hrs.

PATIENT CONSIDERATIONS
Assessment: Assess for risk factors for pneumonia (eg, history of lung disease, decreased CD4 cell count, increased viral load, IV drug use, smoking), infections, hemophilia, history of coagulation disorders, pregnancy/nursing status, and possible drug interactions.

Monitoring: Monitor for signs/symptoms of cellulitis or local inj-site reactions, pneumonia, immune reconstitution syndrome, autoimmune disorders, post-inj bleeding, nerve pain/paresthesia, hypersensitivity reactions, and other adverse reactions.

Counseling: Inform that therapy is not a cure for HIV-1 infection and patients may continue to experience illnesses associated w/ HIV-1 infection, including opportunistic infections. Advise to avoid doing things that can spread HIV-1 infection to others (eg, sharing needles or personal items that can have blood fluids on them, having sex w/o protection, breastfeeding). Inform of risk for inj-site reactions; instruct to monitor for signs/symptoms of cellulitis and local infections. Advise to seek medical attention if experiencing signs/symptoms of pneumonia (eg, cough w/ fever, rapid breathing, SOB) and systemic hypersensitivity (eg, rash, fever, N/V). Advise that the drug must be taken as a part of a combination antiretroviral regimen. Advise to inform physician if pregnant, planning to become pregnant, or breastfeeding. Instruct not to change dosage or schedule w/o consulting physician.

GAMASTAN S/D — immune globulin (human)   Rx

Class: Immune globulin

> Thrombosis may occur and it may occur in the absence of known risk factors (eg, advanced age, prolonged immobilization, hypercoagulable conditions, history of venous or arterial thrombosis, use of estrogens, indwelling central vascular catheters, hyperviscosity, cardiovascular risk factors). For patients at risk of thrombosis, do not exceed the recommended dose of therapy. Ensure adequate hydration before administration. Monitor for signs/symptoms of thrombosis and assess blood viscosity in patients at risk for hyperviscosity.

ADULT DOSAGE
Hepatitis A Prophylaxis
Prophylaxis Before or Soon After Exposure:
Household and Institutional Hepatitis A Case Contacts: 0.02mL/kg (0.01mL/lb) IM
Traveling to Areas Where Hepatitis A is Common:
<3-Month Stay:
0.02mL/kg IM
≥3-Month Stay:
0.06mL/kg IM; repeat every 4-6 months
Measles (Rubeola)
To Prevent or Modify Measles (Rubeola) in Susceptible Persons Exposed <6 Days Previously:
0.25mL/kg (0.11mL/lb) IM

PEDIATRIC DOSAGE
Measles (Rubeola)
Prophylaxis Before or Soon After Exposure:
Immunocompromised:
0.5mL/kg IM immediately postexposure
Max: 15mL

Varicella
To Modify Varicella if Varicella-Zoster Immune Globulin (Human) is Unavailable:
0.6-1.2mL/kg IM
Rubella
To Lessen the Likelihood of Infection and Fetal Damage in Susceptible Women Exposed to Rubella Who Will Not Consider a Therapeutic Abortion:
0.55mL/kg IM

DOSING CONSIDERATIONS
Other Important Considerations
Varicella:
Risk of Thrombosis: Administer at the lower range of recommended dose

ADMINISTRATION
IM route
Administer preferably in the anterolateral aspect of the upper thigh or deltoid muscle of the upper arm; avoid in the gluteal region
Doses >10mL should be divided and injected into several muscle sites
Do not inject into a blood vessel

STORAGE
2-8°C (36-46°F). Do not freeze.

HOW SUPPLIED
Inj: 2mL, 10mL

CONTRAINDICATIONS
Isolated immunoglobulin A (IgA) deficiency, severe thrombocytopenia or any coagulation disorder that would contraindicate IM inj.

WARNINGS/PRECAUTIONS
Not indicated in persons with clinical manifestations of hepatitis A or in those exposed >2 weeks previously. If susceptible, immunocompromised child is exposed to measles; immediately give therapy; do not administer measles vaccine or any other live viral vaccine to immunocompromised children. Caution with history of prior systemic allergic reactions following the administration of human immunoglobulin preparations. May carry a risk of transmitting infectious agents (eg, viruses, and theoretically, the Creutzfeldt-Jakob disease agent). Do not administer SQ or IV because of the potential for serious reactions (eg, renal dysfunction/failure/hemolysis, transfusion-related acute lung injury). Do not perform skin tests; intradermal inj of concentrated gamma globulin sol with its buffers causes a localized area of inflammation, which can be misinterpreted as a positive allergic reaction. True allergic responses to IM human gamma globulin reported rarely; have epinephrine available to treat acute allergic symptoms.

ADVERSE REACTIONS
Thrombosis, pain and tenderness at inj site, urticaria, angioedema.

DRUG INTERACTIONS
Should not be given at the same time with measles vaccine. If child is >12 months and received therapy; measles vaccine should be given about 3 months later when measles antibody titer will have disappeared. Passive transfer of antibodies may transiently impair the immune responses to live attenuated virus vaccines (eg, mumps, rubella, varicella) for up to 6 months and for ≥1 yr to measles (rubeola).

PREGNANCY AND LACTATION
Category C, safety not known in nursing.

MECHANISM OF ACTION
Immune globulin.

PHARMACOKINETICS
Absorption: T_{max}=2 days. **Elimination:** $T_{1/2}$=23 days.

PATIENT CONSIDERATIONS
Assessment: Assess for isolated IgA deficiency, severe thrombocytopenia or any coagulation disorder that would contraindicate IM inj, history of prior systemic allergic reactions to human immunoglobulin preparations, pregnancy/nursing status, possible drug interactions, and for any other conditions where treatment is cautioned or contraindicated. Assess baseline blood viscosity in patients at risk for hyperviscosity.

Monitoring: Monitor for thrombosis, allergic reactions, transmission of infectious disease, and other adverse reactions.

Counseling: Inform of the risks/benefits of therapy. Instruct to contact physician if any signs/symptoms of infection, symptoms of thrombosis or any other adverse reaction develop. Inform that product may transiently impair the immune responses to live attenuated virus vaccines; instruct to notify immunizing physician of therapy with immune globulin (human).

GAMMAGARD LIQUID — immune globulin infusion (human)   Rx

Class: Immune globulin

> Thrombosis may occur; administer at the minimum dose and infusion rate practicable for patients at risk (eg, advanced age, prolonged immobilization, hypercoagulable conditions, history of venous/arterial thrombosis, use of estrogens, indwelling vascular catheters, hyperviscosity, cardiovascular [CV] risk factors). Ensure adequate hydration before administration. Monitor for signs/symptoms of thrombosis and assess blood viscosity if at risk of hyperviscosity. Renal dysfunction, acute renal failure, osmotic nephrosis, and death may occur w/ immune globulin intravenous (IGIV) products in predisposed patients. Patients predisposed to renal dysfunction include those w/ preexisting renal insufficiency, diabetes mellitus [DM], age >65 yrs, volume depletion, sepsis, paraproteinemia, or those receiving known nephrotoxic drugs. Renal dysfunction and acute renal failure occur more commonly w/IGIV products containing sucrose; this product does not contain sucrose.

ADULT DOSAGE

Primary Humoral Immunodeficiency

Replacement therapy for primary humoral immunodeficiency, including but not limited to, common variable immunodeficiency, X-linked agammaglobulinemia, congenital agammaglobulinemia, Wiskott-Aldrich syndrome, and severe combined immunodeficiencies

IV:
Usual: 300-600mg/kg every 3-4 weeks based on clinical response
Initial Infusion Rate:
0.5mL/kg/hr (0.8mg/kg/min) for 30 min
Maint Infusion Rate:
Increase every 30 min (if tolerated) up to 5mL/kg/hr (8mg/kg/min)
Adjust dose according to IgG levels and clinical response

Missed Dose:
Administer missed dose as soon as possible, and then resume scheduled treatments every 3 or 4 weeks, as applicable

Switching from IV to SQ:
Obtain serum IgG trough level before initiation to guide subsequent dose adjustments
Start initial SQ dose approx 1 week after last IV infusion

SQ:
Initial: 1.37 x previous IV dose divided by number of weeks between IV doses
Maint: Based on clinical response and target IgG trough level
Initial Infusion Rate:
<40kg:
20mL/site at 15mL/hr/site
>40kg:
30mL/site at 20mL/hr/site
Maint Infusion Rate:
<40kg:
20mL/site at 15-20mL/hr/site
>40kg:
30mL/site at 20-30mL/hr/site
Refer to PI for dose adjustment guidelines

Multifocal Motor Neuropathy

As a maint therapy to improve muscle strength and disability in patients w/ multifocal motor neuropathy
Usual: 0.5-2.4g/kg/month IV based on clinical response
Initial Infusion Rate: 0.5mL/kg/hr (0.8mg/kg/min)
Maint Infusion Rate: May increase infusion rate if tolerated up to 5.4mL/kg/hr (9mg/kg/min)

PEDIATRIC DOSAGE

Primary Humoral Immunodeficiency

Replacement therapy for primary humoral immunodeficiency, including but not limited to, common variable immunodeficiency, X-linked agammaglobulinemia, congenital agammaglobulinemia, Wiskott-Aldrich syndrome, and severe combined immunodeficiencies

>2 Years:
IV:
Usual: 300-600mg/kg every 3-4 weeks based on clinical response
Initial Infusion Rate:
0.5mL/kg/hr (0.8mg/kg/min) for 30 min
Maint Infusion Rate:
Increase every 30 min (if tolerated) up to 5mL/kg/hr (8mg/kg/min)
Adjust dose according to IgG levels and clinical response

Missed Dose:
Administer missed dose as soon as possible, and then resume scheduled treatments every 3 or 4 weeks, as applicable

Switching from IV to SQ:
Obtain serum IgG trough level before initiation to guide subsequent dose adjustments
Start initial SQ dose approx 1 week after last IV infusion

SQ:
Initial: 1.37 x previous IV dose divided by number of weeks between IV doses
Maint: Based on clinical response and target IgG trough level
Initial Infusion Rate:
<40kg:
20mL/site at 15mL/hr/site
>40kg:
30mL/site at 20mL/hr/site
Maint Infusion Rate:
<40kg:
20mL/site at 15-20mL/hr/site
>40kg:
30mL/site at 20-30mL/hr/site
Refer to PI for dose adjustment guidelines

DOSING CONSIDERATIONS
Other Important Considerations
Receiving Immune Globulin for the 1st Time, Upon Switching Brands or if There Has Been a Long Interval Since Previous Infusion:
Adverse reactions may occur more frequently; start at lower infusion rates and gradually increase as tolerated

Risk of Renal Dysfunction/Thrombotic Events or >65 Years:
Administer at min infusion rate practicable. Maximal infusion rate should be <3.3mg/kg/min (<2mL/kg/hr); consider d/c if renal function deteriorates

ADMINISTRATION
IV/SQ route

Preparation and Handling
Any vial that has been entered should be used promptly
Allow refrigerated product to come to room temperature before use. Do not microwave
Do not shake
Do not mix w/ other products
Do not use normal saline as a diluent. If dilution is desired, use D5W as diluent
May flush infusion line w/ normal saline. An in-line filter is optional
Record name and lot number of the product in the recipient's record

Administration
IV:
Monitor vital signs throughout infusion
Slow or stop infusion if adverse reactions occur. If symptoms subside promptly, may resume infusion at a lower rate that does not result in recurrence of the symptoms
Ensure that patients w/ preexisting renal insufficiency are not volume depleted
SQ:
Rotate sites each week

1. Attach sterile syringe to needle and draw air into syringe barrel equal to amount of product to be withdrawn; inject air into vial and withdraw desired volume; if multiple vials are required to achieve required dose, repeat this step
2. Follow manufacturer's instructions for preparing pump and administration tubing, if needed. Be sure to prime pump tubing to ensure that no air is left in tubing and needle
3. Select the number of infusion sites depending on volume of the total dose. Potential sites for infusion include back of arms, abdomen, thighs, and lower back. Ensure sites are at least 2 inches apart; avoid bony prominences
4. Grasp skin and pinch at least 1 inch of skin between 2 fingers; insert needle at a 90° angle w/ darting motion into SQ tissue. Secure the needle
5. Prior to start of infusion, check each needle for correct placement to make sure that a blood vessel has not been punctured; gently pull back on the attached syringe plunger and monitor for any blood return in the needle set; if you see any blood, remove and discard needle set, repeating priming and needle insertion steps in a different infusion site w/ a new needle set
6. Secure needle(s) in place to skin by applying sterile protective dressing over site
7. Start infusion; follow manufacturer's instructions to turn pump on
8. Document infusion; remove peel-off label w/ product lot number and expiration date from vial and place in treatment diary/log book to keep track of product lots used; keep treatment diary/log book current by recording time, date, dose, product label and any reactions after each infusion

Refer to PI for further administration instructions

STORAGE
2-8°C (36-46°F) for up to 36 months, or room temperature up to 25°C (77°F) for up to 24 months. Do not freeze.

HOW SUPPLIED
Inj: 10% [10mL, 25mL, 50mL, 100mL, 200mL, 300mL]

CONTRAINDICATIONS
History of anaphylactic or severe systemic hypersensitivity reactions to Immune Globulin (Human). IgA-deficient patients w/ antibodies to IgA and a history of hypersensitivity.

WARNINGS/PRECAUTIONS
Contains trace amounts of IgA; severe hypersensitivity and anaphylactic reactions may occur. D/C infusion immediately and institute appropriate treatment in case of hypersensitivity. Consider discontinuation if renal function deteriorates. Hyperproteinemia, increased serum viscosity, and hyponatremia, may occur. Aseptic meningitis syndrome (AMS) reported w/ IV use and may occur more frequently w/ high dose (2g/kg) therapy and/or rapid infusion; rule out other causes of meningitis. Contains blood group antibodies that may cause positive direct antiglobulin test. Delayed hemolytic anemia may develop and acute intravascular hemolysis reported. If transfusion is indicated for patients who develop hemolysis w/ clinically compromising anemia, perform adequate cross-matching to avoid exacerbating on-going hemolysis. Noncardiogenic pulmonary edema (transfusion-related acute lung injury [TRALI]) reported; perform tests for presence of antineutrophil and anti-HLA antibodies in both the product and patient's serum if TRALI is suspected. May carry a risk of transmitting infectious agents (eg, viruses, Creutzfeldt-Jakob disease agent). May cause false positive serological testing results; potential for misinterpretation.

ADVERSE REACTIONS
Primary Humoral Immunodeficiency: (IV) Headache, fatigue, pyrexia, N/V, chills, rigors, pain in extremity, diarrhea, migraine, dizziness, cough, urticaria, asthma, pharyngolaryngeal pain, rash, arthralgia, myalgia, peripheral edema, pruritus, cardiac murmur. (SQ) Infusion site (local) event, headache, fatigue, HR increased, pyrexia, upper abdominal pain, N/V, asthma, systolic BP increased, diarrhea, ear pain, aphthous stomatitis, migraine, oropharyngeal pain, pain in extremity.
Multifocal Motor Neuropathy: Headache, chest discomfort, muscle spasms, muscular weakness, nausea, oropharyngeal pain, pain in extremity.

DRUG INTERACTIONS
See Boxed Warning. Passive transfer of antibodies may transiently impair immune response to live attenuated virus vaccines (eg, mumps, rubella, varicella [up to 6 months]; measles [≥1 yr]).

PREGNANCY AND LACTATION
Category C, caution in nursing.

MECHANISM OF ACTION
Immune globulin; not established. Supplies a broad spectrum of opsonizing and neutralizing IgG antibodies against a wide variety of bacterial and viral agents.

Also contains a spectrum of antibodies capable of interacting w/ and altering the activity of cells of the immune system as well as antibodies capable of reacting w/ cells such as erythrocytes.

PHARMACOKINETICS
Absorption: C_{max}=2240mg/dL (IV), 1393mg/dL (SQ); T_{max}=2.9 days (SQ); AUC=9958mg•days/dL (IV), 9176mg•days/dL (SQ). **Distribution:** Crosses the placenta. **Elimination:** $T_{1/2}$=35 days (IV).

PATIENT CONSIDERATIONS

Assessment: Assess for history of anaphylactic or severe hypersensitivity to human immunoglobulin, IgA deficiency, thrombosis/CV/renal dysfunction/ hemolysis risk factors, pregnancy/nursing status, and possible drug interactions. Assess renal function (eg, BUN, SrCr, urine output) prior to initial infusion. Consider baseline assessment of blood viscosity in patients at risk for hyperviscosity, including those w/ cryoglobulins, fasting chylomicronemia/ markedly high TGs, or monoclonal gammopathies. Consider appropriate lab testing, including measurement of Hgb or Hct in patients at risk for hemolysis.

Monitoring: Monitor for signs and symptoms of hypersensitivity/anaphylactic reactions, hemolysis, hemolytic anemia, pulmonary adverse reactions, hyperproteinemia, increased serum viscosity, hyponatremia, local infusion reactions (SQ), thrombosis, and other adverse reactions. Monitor renal function and urine output periodically. Monitor vital signs throughout the infusion. Consider appropriate lab testing (eg, Hgb/Hct) w/in 36-96 hrs post infusion in patients at risk for hemolysis, and appropriate confirmatory lab testing if signs/ symptoms of hemolysis develop or a significant drop in Hgb/Hct is observed. Perform neurological exam, including CSF studies, if AMS is suspected. Perform tests for presence of anti-neutrophil antibodies and anti-human leukocyte antigen antibodies in both product and patient serum if TRALI is suspected.

Counseling: Instruct to immediately report signs/symptoms of decreased urine output, sudden weight gain, fluid retention/edema, SOB, severe headache, neck stiffness, drowsiness, fever, sensitivity to light, painful eye movements, N/V, increased HR, fatigue, yellowing of skin/eyes, dark-colored urine, trouble breathing, chest pain, blue lips/extremities, or fever that can occur 1-6 hrs after infusion to physician. Instruct to immediately report symptoms of thrombosis (eg, pain and/or swelling of an arm or leg w/ warmth over affected area, discoloration of an arm/leg, chest pain/discomfort that worsens on deep breathing, unexplained rapid pulse). Inform that product is made from human plasma and may contain infectious agents that can cause disease; instruct to report any symptoms that might be caused by infections to physician. Inform that product can interfere w/ immune response to live virus vaccines (eg, measles, mumps, rubella); instruct to notify immunizing physician of this potential interaction when they are receiving vaccinations. (IV) If a patient misses a dose, administer missed dose as soon as possible, and then resume scheduled treatments every 3 or 4 weeks as applicable. (SQ) If self-administration is deemed appropriate, instruct and train patients/ caregivers on SQ infusion and document demonstration of ability to administer infusions. Counsel on the importance of consistent weekly SQ infusion. Instruct to keep a treatment diary/log book. Inform that mild to moderate local infusion-site reactions (eg, swelling, redness) may occur; instruct to contact physician if a local reaction increases in severity or persists for more than a few days.

GAMMAGARD S/D — immune globulin intravenous (human)   Rx

Class: Immune globulin

> Thrombosis may occur; administer at the minimum dose and infusion rate practicable for patients at risk (eg, advanced age, prolonged immobilization, hypercoagulable conditions, history of venous or arterial thrombosis, use of estrogens, indwelling vascular catheters, hyperviscosity and cardiovascular [CV] risk factors). Ensure adequate hydration before administration. Monitor for signs/symptoms of thrombosis and assess blood viscosity if at risk for hyperviscosity. Renal dysfunction, acute renal failure, osmotic nephropathy, and death reported with immune globulin intravenous (IGIV) products, particularly those containing sucrose; this product does not contain sucrose. Patients at risk for acute renal failure include those with preexisting renal insufficiency, diabetes mellitus (DM), advanced age (>65 yrs of age), volume depletion, sepsis, paraproteinemia, or those receiving known nephrotoxic drugs.

ADULT DOSAGE

Primary Immunodeficiency

Associated w/ Defects in Humoral Immunity:
Usual: 300-600mg/kg infused at 3- to 4-week intervals
Titrate: Adjust dose according to clinical response; frequency/dose may vary

B-Cell Chronic Lymphocytic Leukemia

Prevention of Bacterial Infections in Patients w/ Hypogammaglobulinemia and/or Recurrent Bacterial Infections:
Usual: 400mg/kg infused at every 3- to 4-week intervals

Idiopathic Thrombocytopenic Purpura

Treatment of Chronic Idiopathic Thrombocytopenic Purpura to Increase Platelet Count and to Prevent and/or Control Bleeding:

PEDIATRIC DOSAGE

Primary Immunodeficiency

Associated w/ Defects in Humoral Immunity:
≥2 Years:
Usual: 300-600mg/kg infused at 3- to 4-week intervals
Titrate: Adjust dose according to clinical response; frequency/dose may vary

B-Cell Chronic Lymphocytic Leukemia

Prevention of Bacterial Infections in Patients w/ Hypogammaglobulinemia and/or Recurrent Bacterial Infections:
Usual: 400mg/kg infused at every 3- to 4-week intervals

Kawasaki Syndrome

Prevention of Coronary Artery Aneurysms Associated w/ Kawasaki Syndrome:

Usual: 1g/kg
Need for additional doses can be determined by clinical response and platelet count; may give up to 3 separate doses on alternate days if required

Usual: 1g/kg as single dose or 400mg/kg for 4 consecutive days beginning w/in 7 days of onset of fever
Administer concomitantly w/ appropriate aspirin therapy (80-100mg/kg/day in 4 divided doses)

DOSING CONSIDERATIONS
Renal Impairment
Risk of Renal Dysfunction:
Administer at the minimum allowable rate of infusion and gradually titrate up to a more conservative maximal rate of <3.3mg/kg/min (<2mL/kg/hr of a 10% sol or <4mL/kg/hr of a 5% sol)

Elderly
Administer at the minimum infusion rate practicable

Adverse Reactions
Slow or stop infusion if adverse reactions occur; may resume at a lower rate if symptoms subside promptly

Other Important Considerations
Risk of Thrombotic Complications:
Administer at the minimum allowable rate of infusion and gradually titrate up to a more conservative maximal rate of <3.3mg/kg/min (<2mL/kg/hr of a 10% sol or <4mL/kg/hr of a 5% sol)

ADMINISTRATION
IV route

Administer as soon as possible after reconstitution and at room temperature
Begin administration as soon as possible w/in 2 hrs if reconstitution is performed aseptically outside of a sterile laminar air flow hood
Administer w/in 24 hrs if reconstitution is performed aseptically inside of a sterile laminar flow hood and stored in original glass container or pooled into ViaFlex bags under constant refrigeration (2-8°C)
Use the antecubital veins, if possible, especially for 10% sol
Administer separately from other medications; do not mix w/ human immune globulin IV products from other manufacturers

Infusion Rates
5% Sol:
Initial: 0.5mL/kg/hr
Max: 4mL/kg/hr
10% Sol:
May infuse w/ the 10% concentration if tolerating 5% concentration at 4mL/kg/hr
Initial: 0.5mL/kg/hr
Max: 8mL/kg/hr

Reconstitution
1. Allow drug and diluent to reach room temperature if refrigerated
2. To make a 5% sol, use full volume of diluent bottle; to make a 10% sol, use 1/2 of volume of diluent bottle (25mL from 2.5g bottle, 48mL from 5g bottle, and 96mL from 10g bottle)
3. Remove spike cap from 1 end of transfer device; do not touch spike
4. Use exposed end of transfer device to spike diluent bottle perpendicularly through center of stopper
5. Ensure collar collapses fully into device by pushing down on transfer device firmly; while holding onto transfer device, remove remaining spike cover from other end of transfer device; do not touch spike
6. Spike concentrate bottle through center of stopper while quickly inverting diluent bottle to minimize spilling out diluents
7. Ensure that collar collapses fully into device by pushing down on diluent bottle firmly
8. After transfer of diluent is complete, remove transfer device and empty diluent bottle
9. Immediately swirl concentrate bottle gently to thoroughly mix contents. Do not shake

STORAGE
≤25°C (77°F) for 24 months. Do not freeze.

HOW SUPPLIED
Inj: IgA <1µg/mL in 5% sol [5g, 10g], IgA ≤2.2µg/mL in 5% sol [2.5g, 5g, 10g]

CONTRAINDICATIONS
History of anaphylactic or severe systemic hypersensitivity reactions to the administration of human immunoglobulin, IgA deficient patients w/ antibodies to IgA and a history of hypersensitivity.

WARNINGS/PRECAUTIONS
Contains trace amounts of IgA; severe hypersensitivity/anaphylactic reactions with a fall in BP reported. D/C infusion immediately and institute appropriate treatment if hypersensitivity develops. Consider discontinuation if renal function deteriorates. Aseptic meningitis syndrome (AMS) reported and may occur more frequently with high dose (2g/kg) therapy; rule out other causes of meningitis. Hemolytic anemia may develop subsequent to therapy; monitor for signs/ symptoms of hemolysis and perform appropriate confirmatory lab testing if this occurs. Noncardiogenic pulmonary edema may occur; if transfusion-related acute lung injury (TRALI) is suspected, test for presence of anti-neutrophil and anti-HLA antibodies in both the product and patient's serum. May carry risk of transmitting infectious agents (eg, viruses, Creutzfeldt-Jakob disease agent). Hyperproteinemia and increased serum viscosity may occur. The amount of Na^{2+} in product may add materially to recommended daily allowance of dietary sodium for patients on a low sodium diet; calculate the amount of Na^{2+} from the product

and use it when determining dietary sodium intake. Certain components used in packaging of product contain natural rubber latex; caution with sensitivity to rubber latex. Adverse reactions may occur in patients who receive drug for the 1st time, upon switching brands, or if there has been a long hiatus since previous infusion; start at lower rate and gradually increase as tolerated. Administer at the minimum infusion rate practicable in patients ≥65 yrs of age. May interfere with some serological tests.

ADVERSE REACTIONS
Thrombosis, renal dysfunction, acute renal failure, osmotic nephropathy, headache, nausea, chills, asthenia, pyrexia, upper abdominal pain, diarrhea, back pain, hyperhidrosis, flushing, dizziness.

DRUG INTERACTIONS
See Boxed Warning. Passive transfer of antibodies may transiently impair the immune responses to live attenuated vaccines (eg, measles, mumps, rubella, and varicella).

PREGNANCY AND LACTATION
Category C, caution in nursing.

MECHANISM OF ACTION
Immune globulin; not established. Supplies a broad spectrum of opsonizing and neutralizing immunoglobulin G antibodies against bacterial and viral agents. Also contains a spectrum of antibodies capable of reacting with cells (eg, erythrocytes).

PHARMACOKINETICS
Absorption: C_{max}=1859mg/dL (previously untreated); T_{max}=30 min. **Elimination:** $T_{1/2}$=37.7 days (previously treated), 17.7-37.6 days (immunodeficient).

PATIENT CONSIDERATIONS
Assessment: Assess for history of anaphylactic or severe systemic hypersensitivity reactions to human immunoglobulin, IgA deficiency, DM, advanced age, history of venous/arterial thrombosis, volume depletion, sepsis, paraproteinemia, CV risk factors, hypercoagulable conditions, presence of prolonged immobilization, use of indwelling vascular catheters, sensitivity to rubber latex, pregnancy/ nursing status, and possible drug interactions. Assess renal function (eg, BUN, SrCr) prior to initial infusion. Consider baseline assessment of blood viscosity in patients at risk for hyperviscosity, including those with cryoglobulins, fasting chylomicronemia/markedly high TGs, or monoclonal gammopathies.

Monitoring: Monitor for hypersensitivity/anaphylactic reactions, thrombosis, pulmonary adverse reactions, infection, hemolytic anemia, hyperviscosity, hyperproteinemia, hypernatremia, and other adverse reactions. Monitor renal function and urine output periodically. Perform neurological exam, including CSF studies if AMS is suspected. Monitor for signs/symptoms of hemolysis and perform appropriate confirmatory lab testing if these occur. Perform appropriate tests for anti-neutrophil and anti-HLA antibodies in both the product and patient serum if TRALI is suspected. Monitor vital signs throughout the infusion.

Counseling: Instruct to immediately report signs/symptoms of decreased urine output, sudden weight gain, fluid retention/edema, SOB, severe headache, neck stiffness, drowsiness, fever, sensitivity to light, painful eye movements, N/V, increased HR, fatigue, yellowing of skin or eyes, dark-colored urine, trouble breathing, chest pain, or blue lips or extremities to physician. Instruct to immediately report symptoms of thrombosis (eg, pain and/or swelling of an arm or leg with warmth over affected area, discoloration of an arm or leg, unexplained SOB, chest pain/discomfort that worsens on deep breathing, unexplained rapid pulse, numbness or weakness on one side of the body) to physician. Inform that drug is made from human plasma and may contain infectious agents that can cause disease; instruct to report any symptoms that might be caused by infections to physician. Inform that product can interfere with immune response to live viral vaccines (eg, measles, mumps, rubella); instruct to inform immunizing physician of recent therapy with immunoglobulin so that appropriate precautions can be taken.

GAMMAKED — immune globulin injection (human)   Rx
Class: Immune globulin

Thrombosis may occur; administer at the minimum dose and infusion rate practicable for patients at risk (eg, advanced age, prolonged immobilization, hypercoagulable conditions, history of venous or arterial thrombosis, use of estrogens, indwelling central vascular catheters, hyperviscosity, cardiovascular risk factors). Ensure adequate hydration before administration. Monitor for signs/symptoms of thrombosis and assess blood viscosity if at risk for hyperviscosity. Renal dysfunction, acute renal failure, osmotic nephrosis, and death may occur with immune globulin intravenous (IGIV) products. Patients predisposed to renal dysfunction include those with preexisting renal insufficiency, diabetes mellitus, >65 yrs of age, volume depletion, sepsis, paraproteinemia, or those receiving known nephrotoxic drugs; administer at the minimum concentration available and minimum infusion rate practicable.

ADULT DOSAGE
Primary Humoral Immunodeficiency
Replacement Therapy:
IV:
Usual: 300-600mg/kg (3-6mL/kg) every 3-4 weeks
Titrate: Adjust dose over time to achieve desired trough levels and clinical responses

Infusion Rate:
Initial: 1mg/kg/min (0.01mL/kg/min) for first 30 min
Max: 8mg/kg/min (0.08mL/kg/min)

PEDIATRIC DOSAGE
Primary Humoral Immunodeficiency
Replacement Therapy:
IV:
Usual: 300-600mg/kg (3-6mL/kg) every 3-4 weeks
Titrate: Adjust dose over time to achieve desired trough levels and clinical responses

Infusion Rate:
Initial: 1mg/kg/min (0.01mL/kg/min) for first 30 min
Max: 8mg/kg/min (0.08mL/kg/min)

Risk of Measles Exposure:
Administer a dose of at least 400mg/kg (4mL/kg) just prior to expected measles exposure, if receiving a dose of <400mg/kg every 3-4 weeks and at risk of measles exposure

If exposed to measles, administer a dose of 400mg/kg as soon as possible after exposure

SQ:
Individualize dose based on clinical response and serum IgG trough levels; start treatment 1 week after last immune globulin IV infusion
Initial Weekly Dose: 1.37 x previous immune globulin IV dose (in grams)/ Number of weeks between immune globulin IV doses
Dose Adjustment: Refer to PI

Infusion Rate:
Usual: 20mL/hr per infusion site (max number of infusion sites is 8)

Idiopathic Thrombocytopenic Purpura
To Raise Platelet Counts to Prevent Bleeding or to Allow Patient to Undergo Surgery:
2g/kg IV (total dose) divided in 2 doses of 1g/kg (10mL/kg) on 2 consecutive days (if fluid volume is not a concern) or into 5 doses of 0.4g/kg on 5 consecutive days

May withhold 2nd dose of 1g/kg if adequate platelet count is observed at 24 hrs after the 1st dose

Infusion Rate:
Initial: 1mg/kg/min for first 30 min
Max: 8mg/kg/min

Chronic Inflammatory Demyelinating Polyneuropathy
Treatment to Improve Neuromuscular Disability/Impairment and Maint Therapy to Prevent Relapse:
LD: 2g/kg (20mL/kg) IV in divided doses over 2-4 consecutive days
Maint: 1g/kg IV over 1 day or divided into 2 doses of 0.5g/kg on 2 consecutive days, every 3 weeks

Infusion Rate:
Initial: 2mg/kg/min for first 30 min
Max: 8mg/kg/min

Risk of Measles Exposure:
Administer a dose of at least 400mg/kg (4mL/kg) just prior to expected measles exposure, if receiving a dose of <400mg/kg every 3-4 weeks and at risk of measles exposure

If exposed to measles, administer a dose of 400mg/kg as soon as possible after exposure

Idiopathic Thrombocytopenic Purpura
To Raise Platelet Counts to Prevent Bleeding or to Allow Patient to Undergo Surgery:
2g/kg IV (total dose) divided in 2 doses of 1g/kg (10mL/kg) on 2 consecutive days (if fluid volume is not a concern) or into 5 doses of 0.4g/kg on 5 consecutive days

May withhold 2nd dose of 1g/kg if adequate platelet count is observed at 24 hrs after the 1st dose

Infusion Rate:
Initial: 1mg/kg/min for first 30 min
Max: 8mg/kg/min

DOSING CONSIDERATIONS
Elderly
Administer at the minimum infusion rate practicable

Adverse Reactions
Slow or stop infusion if adverse reactions occur; may resume at a lower rate if symptoms subside promptly

ADMINISTRATION
IV/SQ route

Administer at room temperature
Avoid simultaneous administration w/ heparin through a single lumen delivery device; flush heparin lock through which therapy was administered w/ D5W or 0.9% NaCl for inj, and do not flush w/ heparin
Do not mix w/ immune globulin IV products from other manufacturers

IV
Use only 18-gauge needles to penetrate the stopper for dispensing product from the 10mL vial
Use 16-gauge needles or dispensing pins only w/ ≥25mL vial sizes

SQ
Do not shake
Using a sterile syringe/needle, prepare to withdraw by 1st injecting air into vial that is equivalent to the amount of drug to be withdrawn, then withdraw the desired volume
Follow manufacturer's instructions for filling pump reservoir and preparing the pump, administration tubing, and Y-site connection tubing, if needed
Prime administration tubing by filling tubing/needle w/ drug, to ensure that no air is left in tubing/needle
Inj sites should be clean, dry, and at least 2 inches apart
Grasp the skin between 2 fingers and insert the needle into the SQ tissue
Repeat priming and needle insertion steps using a new needle, administration tubing, and a new infusion site
If using multiple, simultaneous inj sites, use Y-site connection tubing and secure to the administration tubing
Infuse following manufacturer's instructions for the pump

Preparation and Handling
Do not freeze; do not use if sol has been frozen
Infuse using a separate line, w/o mixing w/ other IV fluids or medications; infusion line can be flushed w/ D5W or 0.9% NaCl for inj
If dilution is required, may dilute w/ D5W; do not dilute w/ saline
Content of vials may be pooled under aseptic conditions into sterile infusion bags and infused w/in 8 hrs after pooling

STORAGE
2-8°C (36-46°F) for 36 months from date of manufacture. May be stored at ≤25°C (77°F) for up to 6 months anytime during the 36 month shelf life; discard if not used. Do not freeze.

HOW SUPPLIED
Inj: 1g/10mL [10mL, 25mL, 50mL, 100mL, 200mL]

CONTRAINDICATIONS
History of anaphylactic or severe systemic reaction to human immune globulin, IgA deficient patients w/ antibodies against IgA and history of hypersensitivity.

WARNINGS/PRECAUTIONS
Contains trace amounts of IgA; severe hypersensitivity/anaphylactic reactions may occur. D/C infusion immediately and institute appropriate treatment if hypersensitivity develops. Consider discontinuation if renal function deteriorates. Hyperproteinemia, increased serum viscosity, and hyponatremia may occur. Distinguish true hyponatremia from pseudohyponatremia with concomitant decreased calculated serum osmolality or elevated osmolar gap; treatment aimed at decreasing serum free water in patients with pseudohyponatremia may lead to volume depletion, a further increase in serum viscosity, and a possible predisposition to thrombosis. Aseptic meningitis syndrome (AMS) reported and may occur more frequently with high doses (2g/kg) and/or rapid infusion; rule out other causes of meningitis. Delayed hemolytic anemia may develop and acute hemolysis reported. Noncardiogenic pulmonary edema may occur; if transfusion-related acute lung injury (TRALI) is suspected, perform appropriate tests for presence of anti-neutrophil and anti-HLA antibodies in both the product and patient's serum. High dose regimen (1g/kg for 1-2 days) is not recommended for individuals with expanded fluid volumes or where fluid volume may be a concern. May carry a risk of transmitting infectious agents (eg, viruses, Creutzfeldt-Jakob disease agent). Risk of hematoma formation in ITP patients; do not administer SQ. Administer at minimum infusion rate practicable in elderly. May interfere with some serological tests.

ADVERSE REACTIONS
Thrombosis, renal dysfunction, acute renal failure, osmotic nephrosis, headache, pyrexia, chills, HTN, rash, nausea, asthenia.

DRUG INTERACTIONS
See Boxed Warning. Passive transfer of antibodies may transiently interfere with immune response to live virus vaccines (eg, measles, mumps, rubella, varicella).

PREGNANCY AND LACTATION
Category C, safety not known in nursing.

MECHANISM OF ACTION
Immune globulin; not established. Supplies a broad spectrum of opsonic and neutralizing IgG antibodies against bacteria, viral, parasitic, mycoplasma agents, and their toxins.

PHARMACOKINETICS
Absorption: (IV) C_{max}=19.04mg/mL, AUC=6746.48mg•hr/mL. (SQ) AUC=1947mg•hr/mL. **Distribution:** Crosses the placenta. **Elimination:** (IV) $T_{1/2}$=35.74 days.

PATIENT CONSIDERATIONS
Assessment: Assess for history of anaphylactic or severe systemic reactions to human immune globulin, IgA deficiency, risk of thrombosis/renal dysfunction, pregnancy/nursing status, volume depletion, and possible drug interactions. Assess renal function (eg, BUN, SrCr, urine output) prior to initial infusion. Obtain baseline Hgb/Hct in patients at risk for hemolysis. Consider baseline assessment of blood viscosity in patients at risk for hyperviscosity, including those with cryoglobulins, fasting chylomicronemia/markedly high TGs, or monoclonal gammopathies.

Monitoring: Monitor for hypersensitivity/anaphylactic reactions, thrombosis, hemolytic anemia, hyperproteinemia, hyperviscosity, hyponatremia, pulmonary adverse reactions, infection, and other adverse reactions. Monitor renal function and urine output periodically. Perform neurological exam, including CSF studies, if AMS is suspected. Perform appropriate lab testing (eg, Hgb, Hct) prior to infusion and within approximately 36-96 hrs post infusion in patients at risk for hemolysis, and additional testing if signs/symptoms of hemolysis develop or a significant drop in Hgb/Hct is observed. Perform test for presence of antineutrophil and anti-HLA antibodies in both the product and patient's serum if TRALI is suspected. Monitor vital signs throughout the infusion.

Counseling: Instruct to immediately report any signs/symptoms of decreased urine output, sudden weight gain, fluid retention/edema, SOB, severe headache, neck stiffness, drowsiness, fever, sensitivity to light, painful eye movements, N/V, increased HR, fatigue, yellowing of skin or eyes, dark-colored urine, trouble breathing, chest pain, or blue lips/extremities to physician. Instruct to immediately report symptoms of thrombosis to physician. Inform that drug is made from human plasma and may contain infectious agents that can cause disease; instruct to report any symptoms of concern. Inform that product can interfere with immune response to live viral vaccines; instruct to notify physician of this potential interaction when receiving vaccinations. Instruct on SQ infusion for home treatment, including measures to be taken in case of adverse reactions.

GAMMAPLEX — immune globulin intravenous (human)   **Rx**
Class: Immune globulin

> Thrombosis may occur. Renal dysfunction, acute renal failure, osmotic nephrosis, and death may occur in predisposed patients who receive immune globulin intravenous (IGIV) products. Renal dysfunction and acute renal failure occur more commonly w/ IGIV products containing sucrose; this product does not contain sucrose. For patients at risk of thrombosis (eg, using estrogens), renal dysfunction (eg, receiving known nephrotoxic drugs), or acute renal failure, administer at the minimum dose and infusion rate practicable. Ensure adequate hydration before administration. Monitor for signs/symptoms of thrombosis and assess blood viscosity if at risk for hyperviscosity.

ADULT DOSAGE
Primary Humoral Immunodeficiency
Replacement Therapy:
300-800mg/kg (6-16mL/kg) every 3-4 weeks
Titrate: Adjust to achieve desired serum trough levels and clinical response
Initial Infusion Rate for First 15 Min:
0.5mg/kg/min (0.01mL/kg/min)
Maint Infusion Rate (If Tolerated):
Increase gradually every 15 min to 4mg/kg/min (0.08mL/kg/min)

Chronic Immune Thrombocytopenic Purpura
Usual: 1g/kg (20mL/kg) on 2 consecutive days (total dose of 2g/kg)
Initial Infusion Rate for First 15 Min:
0.5mg/kg/min (0.01mL/kg/min) IV
Maint Infusion Rate (If Tolerated):
Increase gradually every 15 min to 4mg/kg/min (0.08mL/kg/min)

PEDIATRIC DOSAGE
Primary Humoral Immunodeficiency
≥2 Years:
Replacement Therapy:
300-800mg/kg (6-16mL/kg) every 3-4 weeks
Titrate: Adjust to achieve desired serum trough levels and clinical response
Initial Infusion Rate for First 15 Min:
0.5mg/kg/min (0.01mL/kg/min)
Maint Infusion Rate (If Tolerated):
Increase gradually every 15 min to 4mg/kg/min (0.08mL/kg/min)

DOSING CONSIDERATIONS
Elderly
Do not exceed recommended doses; administer at minimum infusion rate practicable

Adverse Reactions
Slow or stop infusion if adverse reactions occur; may resume at lower rate if symptoms subside

ADMINISTRATION
IV route

Do not shake.
Do not mix w/ other IV medications (including normal saline) or other IGIV products; infuse using separate infusion line.
An infusion pump may be used to control rate of administration.
If large doses are to be administered, several vials may be pooled using aseptic technique; begin infusion w/in 2 hrs after pooling.
Promptly administer after piercing cap.
Should be at room temperature (up to 25°C [77°F]) at the time of administration.

STORAGE
2-25°C (35.6-77°F). Stable for 24 months. Protect from light. Do not freeze. Do not use if sol has been frozen.

HOW SUPPLIED
Inj: 5% [50mL, 100mL, 200mL, 400mL]

CONTRAINDICATIONS
History of anaphylactic or severe systemic reaction to human immune globulin. Hereditary intolerance to fructose, infants/neonates for whom sucrose or fructose tolerance has not been established. IgA-deficient patients w/ antibodies to IgA and a history of hypersensitivity.

WARNINGS/PRECAUTIONS
Ensure that patients w/ preexisting renal insufficiency are not volume depleted; consider discontinuation if renal function deteriorates. Contains trace amounts of IgA; severe hypersensitivity reactions may occur. D/C infusion immediately and institute appropriate treatment in case of hypersensitivity. Hyperproteinemia, increased serum viscosity, and hyponatremia may occur. Distinguish true hyponatremia from pseudohyponatremia that is associated w/ or related to hyperproteinemia w/ concomitant decreased calculated serum osmolality or elevated osmolar gap; treatment aimed at decreasing serum free water in patients w/ pseudohyponatremia may lead to volume depletion, a further increase in serum viscosity, and a possible predisposition to thrombotic events. Aseptic meningitis syndrome (AMS) may occur and may occur more frequently in association w/ high doses (2g/kg) and/or rapid infusion of IGIV; rule out other causes of meningitis. Delayed hemolytic anemia may develop; acute hemolysis reported. Noncardiogenic pulmonary edema may occur; if transfusion-related acute lung injury (TRALI) is suspected, perform appropriate tests for presence of antineutrophil antibodies in both the product and patient's serum. Caution w/ high-dose regimen (for chronic immune thrombocytopenic purpura [ITP]) in patients at increased risk of thrombosis, hemolysis, acute kidney injury, or volume overload. May carry a risk of transmitting infectious agents (eg, viruses, and, theoretically, the Creutzfeldt-Jakob disease agent). May interfere w/ some serological tests. May cause a positive direct or indirect antiglobulin (Coombs') test. Caution in elderly.

ADVERSE REACTIONS

Headache, pyrexia, fatigue, N/V, HTN, chills, myalgia, pain, arthralgia, dehydration, pruritus, nasal congestion/edema, URTI, rash.

DRUG INTERACTIONS

See Boxed Warning. May transiently interfere w/ immune response to live virus vaccines (eg, measles, mumps, rubella, varicella).

PREGNANCY AND LACTATION

Pregnancy: Category C.
Lactation: Safety not known in nursing.

MECHANISM OF ACTION

Immune globulin. Chronic ITP: Has not been established. Primary Humoral Immunodeficiency (PI): Acts through a broad spectrum of opsonic and neutralizing IgG antibodies against pathogens and their toxins involving antigen binding and effector functions.

PHARMACOKINETICS

Absorption: PI: (Adult, 21-Day Dosing Interval) C_{max}=1060mg/dL; AUC=6280 days•mg/mL; T_{max}=3.33 hrs; (Adult, 28-Day Dosing Interval) C_{max}=1190mg/dL; AUC=8770 days•mg/dL; T_{max}=3.30 hrs. **Distribution:** PI: (Adult, 21-Day Dosing Interval) V_d=0.60dL/kg; (Adult, 28-Day Dosing Interval) V_d=0.43dL/kg. **Elimination:** PI: (Adult, 21-Day Dosing Interval) $T_{1/2}$=6.06 days; (Adult, 28-Day Dosing Interval) $T_{1/2}$=5.79 days. Refer to PI for information on pediatrics.

PATIENT CONSIDERATIONS

Assessment: Assess for history of anaphylactic or severe systemic hypersensitivity reactions to human immunoglobulin, IgA deficiency, risk of thrombosis/renal dysfunction/renal failure/hemolysis/volume overload, any other conditions where treatment is contraindicated or cautioned, pregnancy/nursing status, and possible drug interactions. Assess renal function (eg, BUN, SrCr) prior to initial infusion. Consider baseline assessment of blood viscosity in patients at risk for hyperviscosity, including those w/ cryoglobulins, fasting chylomicronemia/markedly high TGs, or monoclonal gammopathies. Consider appropriate lab testing in patients at higher risk for hemolysis, including measurement of Hgb/Hct prior to infusion.

Monitoring: Monitor for thrombosis, hemolytic anemia, hypersensitivity/anaphylactic reactions, pulmonary adverse reactions, hyperproteinemia, increased serum viscosity, hyponatremia, and other adverse reactions. Monitor renal function and urine output periodically. Perform neurological exam, including CSF studies if AMS is suspected. Consider testing in patients at higher risk for hemolysis, including measurement of Hgb/Hct w/in approx. 36-96 hrs post infusion. Perform appropriate confirmatory lab testing if signs/symptoms of hemolysis or a significant drop in Hgb/Hct have been observed. Perform appropriate tests for presence of antineutrophil antibodies in both the product and the patient's serum if TRALI is suspected. Monitor clinical response and vital signs throughout the infusion.

Counseling: Inform about potential risks/benefits of therapy. Instruct to immediately report signs/symptoms of acute renal dysfunction/failure, thrombosis, AMS, hemolysis, and TRALI. Inform that drug is made from human plasma and may contain infectious agents that can cause disease. Inform that product can interfere w/ immune response to live viral vaccines; instruct to inform immunizing physician of recent therapy w/ this product.

GAMUNEX-C — immune globulin injection (human)   Rx

Class: Immune globulin

> Thrombosis may occur; administer at the minimum dose and infusion rate practicable for patients at risk (eg, advanced age, prolonged immobilization, hypercoagulable conditions, history of venous or arterial thrombosis, use of estrogens, indwelling central vascular catheters, hyperviscosity, cardiovascular risk factors). Ensure adequate hydration before administration. Monitor for signs/symptoms of thrombosis and assess blood viscosity if at risk for hyperviscosity. Renal dysfunction, acute renal failure, osmotic nephrosis, and death may occur with immune globulin intravenous (IGIV) products, particularly those containing sucrose; this product does not contain sucrose. Patients predisposed to renal dysfunction include those with preexisting renal insufficiency, diabetes mellitus, age >65 yrs, volume depletion, sepsis, paraproteinemia, or those receiving known nephrotoxic drugs.

ADULT DOSAGE

Primary Humoral Immunodeficiency

Replacement Therapy:
IV:
Usual: 300-600mg/kg (3-6mL/kg) every 3-4 weeks
Titrate: Adjust dose over time to achieve desired trough levels and clinical responses

Infusion Rate:
Initial: 1mg/kg/min (0.01mL/kg/min) for first 30 min
Max: 8mg/kg/min (0.08mL/kg/min)

Risk of Measles Exposure:
Administer a dose of at least 400mg/kg (4mL/kg) just prior to expected measles exposure, if receiving a dose of <400mg/kg every 3-4 weeks and at risk of measles exposure

If exposed to measles, administer a dose of 400mg/kg as soon as possible after exposure

PEDIATRIC DOSAGE

Primary Humoral Immunodeficiency

Replacement Therapy:
IV:
Usual: 300-600mg/kg (3-6mL/kg) every 3-4 weeks
Titrate: Adjust dose over time to achieve desired trough levels and clinical responses

Infusion Rate:
Initial: 1mg/kg/min (0.01mL/kg/min) for first 30 min
Max: 8mg/kg/min (0.08mL/kg/min)

Risk of Measles Exposure:
Administer a dose of at least 400mg/kg (4mL/kg) just prior to expected measles exposure, if receiving a dose of <400mg/kg every 3-4 weeks and at risk of measles exposure

If exposed to measles, administer a dose of 400mg/kg as soon as possible after exposure

SQ:

Individualize dose based on clinical response and serum IgG trough levels; start dose 1 week after last immune globulin IV infusion
Initial Weekly Dose: 1.37 x previous immune globulin IV dose (in grams)/Number of weeks between immune globulin IV doses
Dose Adjustment: Refer to PI

Infusion Rate:
Usual: 20mL/hr per infusion site (max number of infusion sites is 8)

Idiopathic Thrombocytopenic Purpura

To Raise Platelet Counts to Prevent Bleeding or to Allow Patient to Undergo Surgery:
2g/kg IV (total dose) divided in 2 doses of 1g/kg (10mL/kg) on 2 consecutive days (if fluid volume is not a concern) or into 5 doses of 0.4g/kg on 5 consecutive days

May withhold 2nd dose of 1g/kg if adequate platelet count is observed at 24 hrs after the 1st dose

Infusion Rate:
Initial: 1mg/kg/min for first 30 min
Max: 8mg/kg/min

Chronic Inflammatory Demyelinating Polyneuropathy

Treatment to Improve Neuromuscular Disability/Impairment and Maint Therapy to Prevent Relapse:
LD: 2g/kg (20mL/kg) IV in divided doses over 2-4 consecutive days
Maint: 1g/kg IV over 1 day or divided into 2 doses of 0.5g/kg on 2 consecutive days, every 3 weeks

Infusion Rate:
Initial: 2mg/kg/min for first 30 min
Max: 8mg/kg/min

Idiopathic Thrombocytopenic Purpura

To Raise Platelet Counts to Prevent Bleeding or to Allow Patient to Undergo Surgery:
2g/kg IV (total dose) divided in 2 doses of 1g/kg (10mL/kg) on 2 consecutive days (if fluid volume is not a concern) or into 5 doses of 0.4g/kg on 5 consecutive days

May withhold 2nd dose of 1g/kg if adequate platelet count is observed at 24 hrs after the 1st dose

Infusion Rate:
Initial: 1mg/kg/min for first 30 min
Max: 8mg/kg/min

DOSING CONSIDERATIONS

Elderly
Administer at the minimum infusion rate practicable

Adverse Reactions
Slow or stop infusion if adverse reactions occur; may resume at a lower rate if symptoms subside promptly

ADMINISTRATION

IV/SQ route

Administer at room temperature
Avoid simultaneous administration w/ heparin through a single lumen delivery device; flush heparin lock through which therapy was administered w/ D5W or 0.9% NaCl for inj, and do not flush w/ heparin
Do not mix w/ immune globulin IV products from other manufacturers

IV
Use only 18-gauge needles to penetrate the stopper for dispensing product from the 10mL vial
Use 16-gauge needles or dispensing pins only w/ ≥25mL vial sizes

SQ
Do not shake
Using a sterile syringe/needle, prepare to withdraw by 1st injecting air into vial that is equivalent to the amount of drug to be withdrawn, then withdraw the desired volume
Follow manufacturer's instructions for filling pump reservoir and preparing the pump, administration tubing, and Y-site connection tubing, if needed
Prime administration tubing by filling tubing/needle w/ drug, to ensure that no air is left in tubing/needle
Inj sites should be clean, dry, and at least 2 inches apart
Grasp the skin between 2 fingers and insert the needle into the SQ tissue
Repeat priming and needle insertion steps using a new needle, administration tubing, and a new infusion site
If using multiple, simultaneous inj sites, use Y-site connection tubing and secure to the administration tubing
Infuse following manufacturer's instructions for the pump

Preparation and Handling
Do not freeze; do not use if sol has been frozen
Infuse using a separate line, w/o mixing w/ other IV fluids or medications; infusion line can be flushed w/ D5W or 0.9% NaCl for inj
If dilution is required, may dilute w/ D5W; do not dilute w/ saline
Content of vials may be pooled under aseptic conditions into sterile infusion bags and infused w/in 8 hrs after pooling

STORAGE
2-8°C (36-46°F) for 36 months from date of manufacture. May be stored at ≤25°C (77°F) for up to 6 months anytime during the 36 month shelf life; discard if not used. Do not freeze; do not use if sol has been frozen.

HOW SUPPLIED
Inj: 1g/10mL [10mL, 25mL, 50mL, 100mL, 200mL, 400mL]

CONTRAINDICATIONS
History of anaphylactic or severe systemic reaction to human immune globulin, IgA deficient patients w/ antibodies to IgA and history of hypersensitivity.

WARNINGS/PRECAUTIONS
Contains trace amounts of IgA; severe hypersensitivity/anaphylactic reactions may occur. D/C infusion immediately and institute appropriate treatment if hypersensitivity develops. Consider discontinuation if renal function deteriorates. Hyperproteinemia, increased serum viscosity, and hyponatremia may occur. Distinguish true hyponatremia from pseudohyponatremia with concomitant decreased calculated serum osmolarity or elevated osmolar gap; treatment aimed at decreasing serum free water in patients with pseudohyponatremia may lead to volume depletion, a further increase in serum viscosity, and a possible predisposition to thrombosis. Aseptic meningitis syndrome (AMS) reported and may occur more frequently with high dose (2g/kg) therapy and/or rapid infusion; rule out other causes of meningitis. Delayed hemolytic anemia may develop and acute hemolysis reported. Noncardiogenic pulmonary edema may occur; if transfusion-related acute lung injury (TRALI) is suspected, perform tests for presence of antineutrophil and anti-HLA antibodies in both the product and patient's serum. The high dose regimen (1g/kg for 1-2 days) is not recommended for individuals with expanded fluid volumes or where fluid volume may be a concern. May carry risk of transmitting infectious agents (eg, viruses, Creutzfeldt-Jakob disease agent). Risk of hematoma formation in ITP patients; do not administer SQ. Administer at minimum infusion rate in elderly and those at risk for renal dysfunction. May interfere with some serological tests.

ADVERSE REACTIONS
Thrombosis, renal dysfunction, acute renal failure, osmotic nephrosis, increased cough, rhinitis, pharyngitis, headache, fever, diarrhea, N/V, asthma, asthenia, ear pain, inj-site reaction.

DRUG INTERACTIONS
See Boxed Warning. Passive transfer of antibodies may transiently interfere with immune response to live virus vaccines (eg, measles, mumps, rubella, varicella).

PREGNANCY AND LACTATION
Category C, safety not known in nursing.

MECHANISM OF ACTION
Immune globulin; not established. Supplies a broad spectrum of opsonic and neutralizing IgG antibodies against bacteria, viral, parasitic, mycoplasma agents, and their toxins.

PHARMACOKINETICS
Absorption: (IV) C_{max}=19.04mg/mL, AUC=6746.48mg•hr/mL. (SQ) AUC=1947mg•hr/mL. **Distribution:** Crosses placenta. **Elimination:** (IV) $T_{1/2}$=35.74 days.

PATIENT CONSIDERATIONS
Assessment: Assess for history of anaphylactic or severe systemic hypersensitivity reactions to human immunoglobulin, IgA deficiency, risk factors for renal dysfunction or thrombosis, pregnancy/nursing status, and possible drug interactions. Assess renal function (eg, BUN, SrCr, urine output) prior to initial infusion. Obtain baseline Hgb/Hct in patients at risk for hemolysis. Consider baseline assessment of blood viscosity in patients at risk for hyperviscosity, including those with cryoglobulins, fasting chylomicronemia/markedly high TGs, or monoclonal gammopathies.

Monitoring: Monitor for hypersensitivity/anaphylactic reactions, thrombosis, hemolytic anemia, hyperproteinemia, hyperviscosity, hyponatremia, pulmonary adverse reactions, infection, and other adverse reactions. Monitor renal function and urine output periodically. Perform neurological exam, including CSF studies, if AMS is suspected. Perform appropriate lab testing (eg, Hgb, Hct) within approximately 36-96 hrs post infusion in patients at risk for hemolysis, and additional testing if signs/symptoms of hemolysis or a significant drop in Hgb/Hct is observed. Perform tests for the presence of antineutrophil and anti-HLA antibodies in both the product and patient's serum if TRALI is suspected. Monitor vital signs throughout the infusion.

Counseling: Instruct to immediately report any signs/symptoms of decreased urine output, sudden weight gain, fluid retention/edema, SOB, severe headache, neck stiffness, drowsiness, fever, sensitivity to light, painful eye movements, N/V, increased HR, fatigue, yellowing of skin or eyes, dark-colored urine, trouble breathing, chest pain, or blue lips/extremities to physician. Instruct to immediately report symptoms of thrombosis to physician. Inform that drug is made from human plasma and may contain infectious agents that can cause disease; instruct to report any symptoms of concern. Inform that product can interfere with immune response to live viral vaccines; instruct to notify physician of this potential interaction when receiving vaccinations. Instruct on SQ infusion for home treatment, including measures to be taken in case of adverse reactions.

GANIRELIX — ganirelix acetate   Rx
Class: Gonadotropin-releasing hormone (GnRH) antagonist

ADULT DOSAGE	**PEDIATRIC DOSAGE**
Ovarian Stimulation	Pediatric use may not have been established
Inhibition of premature luteinizing hormone surges in women undergoing controlled ovarian hyperstimulation	
250mcg qd during the mid to late portion of the follicular phase; continue treatment daily until the day of human chorionic gonadotropin administration	

ADMINISTRATION
SQ route

Directions for Inj
1. Swab and clean w/ a disinfectant about 2 inches around the point where the needle will be inserted and allow to dry for at least 1 min.
2. Inj in the abdomen around the navel or upper thigh; vary the injection site w/ each inj.
3. Insert needle at the base of the pinched-up skin at an angle of 45-90 degrees to the skin surface.
4. Pull syringe out quickly and apply pressure to the site w/ a swab containing disinfectant.

STORAGE
25°C (77°F); excursions permitted to 15-30°C (59-86°F). Protect from light.

HOW SUPPLIED
Inj: 250mcg/0.5mL

CONTRAINDICATIONS
Known hypersensitivity to ganirelix acetate or to any of its components, or to GnRH or any other GnRH analog; known/suspected pregnancy.

WARNINGS/PRECAUTIONS
Should be prescribed by physicians who are experienced in infertility treatment. Pregnancy must be excluded before starting treatment. Cases of hypersensitivity reactions, including anaphylactoid reactions, reported; caution w/ signs and symptoms of active allergic conditions. Not recommended w/ severe allergic conditions. Packaging contains natural rubber latex, which may cause allergic reactions.

ADVERSE REACTIONS
Abdominal pain (gynecological), headache.

PREGNANCY AND LACTATION
Pregnancy: Contraindicated in pregnancy.
Lactation: Not for use in nursing.

MECHANISM OF ACTION
GnRH antagonist; acts by competitively blocking the GnRH receptors on the pituitary gonadotroph and subsequent transduction pathway. It induces a rapid, reversible suppression of gonadotropin secretion.

PHARMACOKINETICS
Absorption: Rapid. Absolute bioavailability (91.1%); T_{max}=1.1 hr; AUC=96ng•h/mL (single dose), 77.1ng•h/mL (multiple dose); C_{max}=14.8ng/mL (single dose), 11.2ng/mL (multiple dose). **Distribution:** V_d=43.7L (IV, single dose), 76.5L (multiple dose); plasma protein binding (81.9%). **Metabolism:** 1-4 peptide and 1-6 peptide (primary metabolites). **Elimination:** (IV) Feces (75.1%), urine (22.1%); $T_{1/2}$=12.8 hrs (single dose), 16.2 hrs (multiple dose).

PATIENT CONSIDERATIONS
Assessment: Assess for hypersensitivity to the drug, allergic conditions, pregnancy/nursing status, and for possible drug interactions.

Monitoring: Monitor for hypersensitivity and other adverse reactions.

Counseling: Instruct on proper injection technique. Inform about the duration of treatment, the required monitoring procedures, and the risk of possible adverse reactions. Inform that the medication should not be taken if pregnant; instruct to notify physician if pregnant.

GATTEX — teduglutide (rDNA origin)   Rx
Class: Glucagon-like peptide-2 (GLP-2)

ADULT DOSAGE	**PEDIATRIC DOSAGE**
Short Bowel Syndrome	Pediatric use may not have been established
Treatment in Patients Dependent on Parenteral Support: 0.05mg/kg SQ qd	

DOSING CONSIDERATIONS
Renal Impairment
Moderate and Severe (CrCl <50mL/min)/ESRD: Reduce dose by 50%

ADMINISTRATION
SQ route
Alternate inj sites, which can include thighs, arms, and quadrants of abdomen.

Preparation for Administration
- Reconstitute each drug vial by slowly injecting the 0.5mL of preservative-free sterile water for inj provided in the prefilled syringe.
- Allow vial containing drug and water to stand for approx 30 sec and then gently roll the vial between palms for about 15 sec; do not shake.
- Allow the mixed contents to stand for about 2 min; if undissolved powder is observed, gently roll vial again until all material is dissolved. If the product remains undissolved after the 2nd attempt, do not use.
- Use product w/in 3 hrs after reconstitution.

STORAGE
Prior to Dispensing: 2-8°C (36-46°F) for cartons of drug vials and one-vial kits. Do not freeze. Store at room temperature up to 25°C (77°F) for cartons of ancillary supplies. **After Dispensing:** Room temperature up to 25°C (77°F) for 90 days. Do not freeze.

HOW SUPPLIED
Inj: 5mg [vial]

WARNINGS/PRECAUTIONS
May cause hyperplastic changes including neoplasia; consider risks and benefits in patients at increased malignancy risk and patients w/ active non-GI malignancy. D/C in patients w/ active GI malignancy (GI tract, hepatobiliary, pancreatic). Colorectal polyps reported; perform colonoscopy of entire colon w/ removal of polyps w/in 6 months prior to therapy. Perform colonoscopy (or alternate imaging) at the end of 1 yr of therapy, and subsequently every 5 yrs or more often as needed. If polyp is found, adhere to current polyp follow-up guidelines. Monitor for small bowel neoplasia and remove benign neoplasm. D/C in case of colorectal cancer or small bowel cancer. If intestinal or stomal obstruction develops, temporarily d/c and manage; may restart therapy when obstructive presentation resolves. Cholecystitis, cholangitis, cholelithiasis, and pancreatitis reported; to identify onset/worsening of gallbladder/biliary/pancreatic disease, assess bilirubin, alkaline phosphatase, lipase, and amylase w/in 6 months prior to therapy, and at least every 6 months while on therapy, or more frequently if needed. Evaluate further if clinically meaningful changes are seen (eg, imaging of gallbladder, biliary tract, pancreas) and reassess the need for continued treatment. Fluid overload and CHF reported; adjust parenteral support and reassess therapy if fluid overload occurs, especially in patients w/ underlying cardiovascular disease (CVD). Reassess the need for continued treatment if significant cardiac deterioration develops. Discontinuation may result in fluid/electrolyte imbalance; monitor fluid/electrolyte status carefully.

ADVERSE REACTIONS
Abdominal pain, inj-site reactions, nausea, headache, abdominal distension, URTI.

DRUG INTERACTIONS
Altered mental status reported w/ benzodiazepines; concomitant oral drugs (eg, benzodiazepines, phenothiazines) requiring titration or w/ narrow therapeutic index may require dose adjustment due to potential for increased absorption.

PREGNANCY AND LACTATION
Pregnancy: Category B. Only use during pregnancy if clearly needed.
Lactation: Not for use in nursing.

MECHANISM OF ACTION
Human glucagon-like peptide-2 (GLP-2) analogue; binds to GLP-2 receptors located in intestinal subpopulations of enteroendocrine cells, subepithelial myofibroblasts, and enteric neurons of submucosal and myenteric plexus resulting in local release of multiple mediators, including insulin-like growth factor-1, nitric oxide, and keratinocyte growth factor.

PHARMACOKINETICS
Absorption: (Healthy) Absolute bioavailability (88%), T_{max}=3-5 hrs. (Short bowel syndrome [SBS]) C_{max}=36ng/mL (median), AUC=0.15µg•hr/mL (median). **Distribution:** V_d=103mL/kg (healthy). **Metabolism:** Catabolic pathways into small peptides and amino acids. **Elimination:** $T_{1/2}$=2 hrs (healthy), 1.3 hrs (SBS).

PATIENT CONSIDERATIONS
Assessment: Assess for malignancy risks, active GI and non-GI malignancy, intestinal/stomal obstruction, gallbladder/biliary/pancreatic disease, CVD, pregnancy/nursing status, and possible drug interactions. Obtain baseline bilirubin, alkaline phosphatase, lipase, and amylase levels and perform colonoscopy of the entire colon w/ removal of polyps w/in 6 months prior to therapy.

Monitoring: Monitor for hyperplastic changes, colorectal polyps, colorectal cancer, small bowel neoplasia, intestinal obstruction, cholecystitis, cholangitis, cholelithiasis, pancreatitis, fluid overload, CHF, cardiac deterioration, and other adverse reactions. Monitor fluid/electrolyte status upon discontinuation. Perform follow-up colonoscopy (or alternate imaging) at the end of 1 yr of therapy and subsequently every 5 yrs or more often as needed. Perform lab assessments of bilirubin, alkaline phosphatase, lipase, and amylase at least every 6 months or more frequently if needed.

Counseling: Inform of the risks/benefits of therapy. Advise patients w/ active GI malignancy that therapy should be discontinued. Inform of the importance of having a colonoscopy (or alternate imaging) done before and after treatment. Advise that patients should be monitored for small bowel neoplasia. Advise to tell physician if any signs/symptoms suggestive of intestinal obstruction are experienced. Inform that lab assessments should be done prior to and then every 6 months while on therapy to monitor pancreas/gallbladder/biliary function. Advise to report all signs/symptoms suggestive of cholecystitis, cholangitis, cholelithiasis, and of pancreatic disease while on therapy. Instruct patients w/ CVD to report to physician any signs of fluid overload or cardiac decompensation while on therapy. Instruct to report to physician any concomitant oral medications that are currently being taken. Inform that inj-site reactions may occur; instruct to contact physician if severe reaction is experienced. Inform that abdominal pain and swelling may occur; advise to contact physician if symptoms of intestinal obstruction develop.

GAZYVA — obinutuzumab   Rx
Class: Monoclonal antibody/CD20 blocker

> Hepatitis B virus (HBV) reactivation may occur, in some cases resulting in fulminant hepatitis, hepatic failure, and death; screen all patients for HBV infection before treatment initiation. Monitor HBV-positive patients during and after treatment. D/C therapy and concomitant medications in the event of HBV reactivation. Progressive multifocal leukoencephalopathy (PML), including fatal PML, may occur.

ADULT DOSAGE
Chronic Lymphocytic Leukemia
In combination w/ chlorambucil for the treatment of patients w/ previously untreated chronic lymphocytic leukemia (CLL)

Recommended Dose: Each dose is 1000mg IV, w/ the exception of the 1st infusions in Cycle 1, which are administered on Day 1 (100mg) and Day 2 (900mg)

Dose to Be Administered During 6 Treatment Cycles, Each of 28 Days Duration:

Cycle 1 (LD):
Day 1: 100mg administered at 25mg/hr over 4 hrs; do not increase the infusion rate
Day 2: 900mg administered at 50mg/hr; may escalate infusion rate in increments of 50mg/hr every 30 min to a max rate of 400mg/hr
Days 8 and 15: 1000mg; if no infusion reaction occurred during the previous infusion and the final infusion rate was 100mg/hr or faster, infusions can be started at a rate of 100mg/hr and increased every 30 min to a max of 400mg/hr

Cycles 2-6:
Day 1: 1000mg; if no infusion reaction occurred during the previous infusion and the final infusion rate was 100mg/hr or faster, infusions can be started at a rate of 100mg/hr and increased by 100mg/hr increments every 30 min to a max of 400mg/hr

Follicular Lymphoma
In combination w/ bendamustine followed by obinutuzumab monotherapy for the treatment of patients w/ follicular lymphoma who relapsed after, or are refractory to, a rituximab-containing regimen

Recommended Dose: 1000mg IV

Dose to Be Administered During 6 Treatment Cycles, Each of 28 Days Duration, Followed by Obinutuzumab Monotherapy:

Cycle 1 (LD):
Day 1: 1000mg administered at 50mg/hr; may escalate in 50mg/hr increments every 30 min to a max of 400mg/hr
Days 8 and 15: 1000mg. If no infusion reaction occurred during the previous infusion and the final infusion rate was 100mg/hr or faster, infusions can be started at a rate of 100mg/hr and increased by 100mg/hr increments every 30 min to a max of 400mg/hr

Cycles 2-6:
Day 1: 1000mg. If no infusion reaction occurred during the previous infusion and the final infusion rate was 100mg/hr or faster, infusions can be started at a rate of 100mg/hr and increased by 100mg/hr increments every 30 min to a max of 400mg/hr

Monotherapy:
1000mg every 2 months for 2 years. If no infusion reaction occurred during the previous infusion and the final infusion rate was 100mg/hr or faster, infusions can be started at a rate of 100mg/hr and increased by 100mg/hr increments every 30 min to a max of 400mg/hr

PEDIATRIC DOSAGE
Pediatric use may not have been established

Physicians' Desk Reference®, the trusted drug reference for over 70 years

Premedication

Tumor Lysis Syndrome (TLS):
Patients w/ high tumor burden, high circulating absolute lymphocyte counts (>25 x 10⁹/L), or renal impairment are considered at risk of TLS and should receive prophylaxis. Premedicate w/ antihyperuricemics (eg, allopurinol or rasburicase) and ensure adequate hydration prior to start of therapy; continue prophylaxis prior to each subsequent infusion, prn.

Infusion Related Reactions (IRR):
Cycle 1:
CLL Days 1 and 2; Follicular Lymphoma (FL) Day 1:
All Patients: 20mg IV dexamethasone or 80mg IV methylprednisolone completed at least 1 hr before obinutuzumab infusion, 650-1000mg acetaminophen and an antihistamine (eg, 50mg diphenhydramine) at least 30 min before obinutuzumab infusion

All Subsequent Infusions:
All Patients: 650-1000mg acetaminophen at least 30 min before obinutuzumab infusion.

Patients w/ IRR (Grade 1-2) w/ Previous Infusion: 650-1000mg acetaminophen and an antihistamine (eg, 50mg diphenhydramine) at least 30 min before obinutuzumab infusion.

Patients w/ Grade 3 IRR w/ Previous Infusion or Lymphocyte Count >25 x 10⁹/L Prior to Next Treatment: 20mg IV dexamethasone or 80mg IV methylprednisolone completed at least 1 hr prior to obinutuzumab infusion, and 650-1000mg acetaminophen and an antihistamine (eg, 50mg diphenhydramine) at least 30 min before obinutuzumab infusion

Antimicrobial Prophylaxis:
Patients w/ Grade 3-4 neutropenia lasting >1 week are strongly recommended to receive antimicrobial prophylaxis until resolution of neutropenia to Grade 1 or 2. Consider antiviral and antifungal prophylaxis

Missed Dose

If a planned dose is missed, administer as soon as possible

CLL: Adjust dosing schedule accordingly. If appropriate, patients who do not complete the Day 1 Cycle 1 dose may proceed to the Day 2 Cycle 1 dose

FL: During Gazyva and bendamustine treatment, adjust the dosing schedule accordingly. During monotherapy, maintain the original dosing schedule for subsequent doses

DOSING CONSIDERATIONS
Adverse Reactions
Infusion Reaction:
Grade 1-2 (Mild to Moderate):
Reduce infusion rate or interrupt infusion and treat symptoms; once symptoms resolve, continue/resume infusion.
If no further symptoms, infusion rate escalation may resume at the increments and intervals as appropriate for the treatment cycle dose.
CLL Patients Only: Day 1 infusion rate may be increased back up to 25mg/hr after 1 hr but not increased further

Grade 3 (Severe):
Interrupt infusion and manage symptoms; once symptoms resolve, consider restarting infusion at no more than 1/2 the previous rate.
If no further symptoms, infusion rate escalation may resume at the increments and intervals as appropriate for the treatment cycle dose.
Permanently d/c treatment if a Grade 3 infusion-related symptom occurs at re-challenge.
CLL Patients Only: Day 1 infusion rate may be increased back up to 25mg/hr after 1 hr but not increased further

Grade 4 (Life Threatening):
Stop infusion immediately and permanently d/c therapy

Interruption for Toxicity:
Infection, Grade 3 or 4 Cytopenia, or a ≥Grade 2 Nonhematologic Toxicity:
Consider treatment interruption

ADMINISTRATION
IV route

Administer only as an IV infusion through a dedicated line.
Do not administer as IV push or bolus.
Do not mix w/ other drugs.
Should only be administered by a healthcare professional w/ appropriate medical support to manage severe infusion reactions.

Preparation
Dilute into a 0.9% NaCl PVC or non-PVC polyolefin infusion bag; do not use other diluents (eg, D5).
Mix diluted sol by gentle inversion.
Do not shake or freeze.

CLL:
Preparation of Sol for Infusion on Day 1/Day 2 of Cycle 1:
1. Withdraw 40mL of obinutuzumab sol and dilute 4mL into a 100mL infusion bag for immediate administration.
2. Dilute remaining 36mL into a 250mL infusion bag at the same time for use on Day 2. Store at 2-8°C (36-46°F) for up to 24 hrs. Use immediately once the diluted bag comes to room temperature.

Preparation of Sol for Infusion on Day 8/Day 15 of Cycle 1 and Day 1 of Cycles 2-6:
Withdraw 40mL of obinutuzumab sol and dilute into a 250mL infusion bag.

FL:
Preparation of Sol for Infusion:
Withdraw 40mL of obinutuzumab sol and dilute 40mL into a 250mL infusion bag.

Can be administered at final concentration of 0.4-4mg/mL.

Stability
Use diluted infusion sol immediately.
If not used immediately, store in refrigerator at 2-8°C (36-46°F) for up to 24 hrs prior to use.

STORAGE
2-8°C (36-46°F). Protect from light. Do not freeze. **Diluted Sol:** Stable in 0.9% NaCl at 0.4-20mg/mL for 24 hrs at 2-8°C (36-46°F) followed by 48 hrs (including infusion time) at room temperature ≤30°C (86°F).

HOW SUPPLIED
Inj: 1000mg/40mL

WARNINGS/PRECAUTIONS
See Dosing Considerations. Consider diagnosis of PML in any patient presenting w/ new onset or changes to preexisting neurologic manifestations; d/c therapy and consider discontinuation or reduction of any concomitant chemotherapy or immunosuppressive therapy in patients who develop PML. May cause severe and life-threatening infusion reactions; institute medical management for infusion reactions prn. Monitor patients w/ preexisting cardiac/pulmonary conditions more frequently throughout infusion and postinfusion period. Hypotension may occur as part of an infusion reaction; consider withholding antihypertensive treatments for 12 hrs prior to and during each infusion, and for the 1st hr after administration until BP is stable. TLS, including fatal cases, reported; monitor lab parameters of patients at risk for TLS, during the initial days of treatment. Correct electrolyte abnormalities, monitor renal function and fluid balance, and administer supportive care to treat TLS. Serious bacterial, fungal, and new/reactivated viral infections may occur during and following therapy; fatal infections reported. Do not administer to patients w/ active infection; patients w/ a history of recurring/chronic infections may be at increased risk of infection. Severe, life-threatening neutropenia (eg, febrile neutropenia) reported; consider granulocyte colony-stimulating factors or dose delays w/ Grade 3 or 4 neutropenia. Severe and life-threatening thrombocytopenia and fatal hemorrhagic events reported; monitor for thrombocytopenia and hemorrhagic events, especially during the 1st cycle. Monitor platelet counts more frequently in patients w/ Grade 3 or 4 thrombocytopenia until resolution and consider subsequent dose delays of obinutuzumab and chemotherapy or dose reductions of chemotherapy.

ADVERSE REACTIONS
CLL: Infusion reactions, neutropenia, thrombocytopenia, anemia, pyrexia, cough, nausea, diarrhea.
Non-Hodgkin Lymphoma: Cough, URTIs, neutropenia, sinusitis, diarrhea, infusion related reactions, nausea, fatigue, bronchitis, arthralgia, pyrexia, nasopharyngitis, UTIs.

DRUG INTERACTIONS
Immunization w/ live virus vaccines is not recommended during treatment and until B-cell recovery. Consider withholding concomitant medications, which may increase bleeding risk (platelet inhibitors, anticoagulants), especially during the 1st cycle.

PREGNANCY AND LACTATION
Pregnancy: Likely to cause fetal B-cell depletion based on findings from animal studies and the drug's mechanism of action. Avoid administering live vaccines to neonates and infants exposed to therapy in utero until B-cell recovery occurs.
Lactation: There is no information regarding the presence of obinutuzumab in human milk, the effects on the breastfed infant, or the effects on milk production; caution in nursing.

MECHANISM OF ACTION
Monoclonal antibody/CD20-blocker; binds to CD20 antigen expressed on the surface of pre B- and mature B-lymphocytes, mediating B-cell lysis through engagement of immune effector cells, by directly activating intracellular death signaling pathways, and/or activation of the complement cascade.

PHARMACOKINETICS

Distribution: V_d=4.1L (CLL). V_d=4.3L (Non-Hodgkin Lymphoma). Crosses placenta.
Elimination: $T_{1/2}$=26.4 days (CLL). $T_{1/2}$=36.8 days (Non-Hodgkin Lymphoma).

PATIENT CONSIDERATIONS

Assessment: Assess for active/history of chronic/recurring infection, preexisting cardiac/pulmonary conditions, preexisting neurologic manifestations, any other conditions where treatment is cautioned, pregnancy/nursing status, and possible drug interactions. Assess for HBV infection by measuring HBsAg and anti-HBc. Obtain baseline blood counts.

Monitoring: Monitor for signs/symptoms of bacterial/fungal/viral infections, PML, infusion reactions, TLS, neutropenia, thrombocytopenia, hemorrhagic events, and other adverse reactions. Monitor blood counts at regular intervals. Closely monitor patients during entire infusion. Monitor patients w/ evidence of current or prior HBV infection for clinical and lab signs of hepatitis or HBV reactivation during and for several months following treatment. Monitor patients w/ preexisting cardiac/pulmonary conditions more frequently throughout the infusion and the postinfusion period. Monitor renal function and fluid balance in patients w/ TLS.

Counseling: Instruct to seek immediate medical attention for signs/symptoms of infusion reactions, symptoms of TLS, signs of infections, symptoms of hepatitis, and new or changes in neurological symptoms. Advise of the need for periodic monitoring of blood counts and instruct to avoid vaccination w/ live viral vaccines. Inform patients w/ a history of HBV infection that they should be monitored and sometimes treated for their hepatitis. Advise pregnant women of potential fetal B-cell depletion.

GEMCITABINE — gemcitabine   Rx

Class: Nucleoside metabolic inhibitor

OTHER BRAND NAMES
Gemzar

ADULT DOSAGE

Ovarian Carcinoma

In combination w/ carboplatin for advanced ovarian cancer that has relapsed ≥6 months after completion of platinum-based therapy

$1000mg/m^2$ IV infusion over 30 min on Days 1 and 8 of each 21-day cycle + carboplatin AUC 4 IV after gemcitabine administration on Day 1 of each 21-day cycle

Metastatic Breast Cancer

In combination w/ paclitaxel for 1st-line treatment of metastatic breast cancer after failure of prior anthracycline-containing adjuvant chemotherapy, unless anthracyclines were clinically contraindicated

$1250mg/m^2$ IV over 30 min on Days 1 and 8 of each 21-day cycle; administer paclitaxel at $175mg/m^2$ on Day 1 as a 3-hr IV infusion before gemcitabine administration

Non-Small Cell Lung Cancer

In combination w/ cisplatin for 1st-line treatment of patients w/ inoperable, locally advanced (Stage IIIA or IIIB), or metastatic (Stage IV) non-small cell lung cancer

Every 4-Week Schedule:
$1000mg/m^2$ IV over 30 min on Days 1, 8, and 15; administer cisplatin IV at $100mg/m^2$ on Day 1 after gemcitabine infusion

Every 3-Week Schedule:
$1250mg/m^2$ IV over 30 min on Days 1 and 8; administer cisplatin IV at $100mg/m^2$ on Day 1 after gemcitabine infusion

Pancreatic Adenocarcinoma

1st-line treatment for patients w/ locally advanced (nonresectable Stage II or Stage III) or metastatic (Stage IV) adenocarcinoma of the pancreas; for patients previously treated w/ 5-FU

$1000mg/m^2$ IV over 30 min

Treatment Schedule:
Weeks 1-8: Weekly dosing for the first 7 weeks, followed by 1-week rest
After Week 8: Weekly dosing on Days 1, 8, and 15 of 28-day cycles

PEDIATRIC DOSAGE

Pediatric use may not have been established

DOSING CONSIDERATIONS

Adverse Reactions

Ovarian Cancer:
Myelosuppression on Treatment Day 1:
Absolute Granulocyte Count (AGC) $<1500 \times 10^6/L$ or Platelet Count $<100,000 \times 10^6/L$: Delay treatment cycle

Myelosuppression on Treatment Day 8:
AGC $1000\text{-}1499 \times 10^6/L$ or Platelet Count $75,000\text{-}99,999 \times 10^6/L$: Administer 50% of full dose
AGC $<1000 \times 10^6/L$ or Platelet Count $<75,000 \times 10^6/L$: Hold therapy

Myelosuppression in Previous Cycle:
Permanently reduce dose to $800mg/m^2$ on Days 1 and 8 for initial occurrence of any of the following:
- AGC $<500 \times 10^6/L$ for >5 days
- AGC $<100 \times 10^6/L$ for >3 days
- Febrile neutropenia
- Platelets $<25,000 \times 10^6/L$
- Cycle delay of >1 week due to toxicity

If any of the above toxicities occur after initial dose reduction, permanently reduce dose to $800mg/m^2$ on Day 1 only

Breast Cancer:
Myelosuppression on Treatment Day 1:
AGC $<1500 \times 10^6/L$ or Platelet Count $<100,000 \times 10^6/L$: Hold therapy

Myelosuppression on Treatment Day 8:
AGC $1000\text{-}1199 \times 10^6/L$ or Platelet Count $50,000\text{-}75,000 \times 10^6/L$: Administer 75% of full dose
AGC $700\text{-}999 \times 10^6/L$ and Platelet Count $\geq50,000 \times 10^6/L$: Administer 50% of full dose
AGC $<700 \times 10^6/L$ or Platelet Count $<50,000 \times 10^6/L$: Hold therapy

Non-Small Cell Lung Cancer/Pancreatic Cancer:
Myelosuppression:
AGC $500\text{-}999 \times 10^6/L$ or Platelet Count $50,000\text{-}99,999 \times 10^6/L$: Administer 75% of full dose
AGC $<500 \times 10^6/L$ or Platelet Count $<50,000 \times 10^6/L$: Hold therapy

Nonhematologic Toxicities in Any Indication:
Permanently d/c gemcitabine for any of the following:
- Unexplained dyspnea or other evidence of severe pulmonary toxicity
- Severe hepatic toxicity
- Hemolytic-uremic syndrome
- Capillary leak syndrome
- Posterior reversible encephalopathy syndrome

Other Severe (Grade 3 or 4) Nonhematologic Toxicities: Hold therapy or reduce dose by 50% until toxicity resolves; no dose modifications are recommended for alopecia, nausea, or vomiting

ADMINISTRATION

IV route.

Preparation for IV Infusion
Reconstitute the vials w/ 0.9% NaCl inj w/o preservatives:
200mg Vial: Add 5mL
1g Vial: Add 25mL
2g Vial: Add 50mL
These dilutions yield a gemcitabine concentration of 38mg/mL.
Prior to administration, dilute the appropriate amount of drug w/ 0.9% NaCl inj; final concentrations may be as low as 0.1mg/mL.
Sol is stable for 24 hrs at controlled room temperature of 20-25°C (68-77°F); do not refrigerate.

Handling Precautions
Wear gloves when preparing therapy.
Immediately wash the skin thoroughly or rinse the mucosa w/ copious amounts of water if gemcitabine for inj contacts the skin or mucus membranes.

STORAGE
20-25°C (68-77°F); excursions permitted between 15-30°C (59-86°F).

HOW SUPPLIED
Inj: 2g; (Gemzar) 200mg, 1g

CONTRAINDICATIONS
Known hypersensitivity to gemcitabine.

WARNINGS/PRECAUTIONS
Prolongation of infusion time beyond 60 min or more frequent than weekly dosing resulted in an increased incidence of clinically significant hypotension, severe flu-like symptoms, myelosuppression, and asthenia. Myelosuppression manifested by neutropenia, thrombocytopenia, and anemia occurs w/ monotherapy; increased risk when combined w/ other cytotoxic drugs. Pulmonary toxicity (eg, interstitial pneumonitis, pulmonary fibrosis/edema, adult respiratory distress syndrome) reported; may lead to fatal respiratory failure despite discontinuation of therapy. D/C if unexplained dyspnea (w/ or w/o bronchospasm) or any evidence of pulmonary toxicity develops. Hemolytic-uremic syndrome (HUS), including fatalities from renal failure or the requirement for dialysis, may occur; consider the diagnosis of HUS if anemia (w/ evidence of microangiopathic hemolysis, elevation of bilirubin/lactate dehydrogenase, or reticulocytosis), severe thrombocytopenia, or evidence of renal failure (SrCr/BUN elevation) develops. Permanently d/c therapy in patients w/ HUS or severe renal impairment. Liver injury, including liver failure and death, reported alone or in combination w/ other potentially hepatotoxic drugs; administration in patients w/ concurrent liver metastases or a preexisting history of hepatitis, alcoholism, or liver cirrhosis may lead to exacerbation of the underlying hepatic insufficiency. D/C if severe liver injury develops. May cause fetal harm. Capillary leak syndrome (CLS) w/ severe

consequences reported; d/c if CLS develops. Posterior reversible encephalopathy syndrome (PRES) reported; confirm the diagnosis of PRES w/ MRI and d/c if PRES develops.

ADVERSE REACTIONS
N/V, anemia, increased ALT/AST/alkaline phosphatase, neutropenia, proteinuria, fever, hematuria, rash, thrombocytopenia, dyspnea, edema.

DRUG INTERACTIONS
Not indicated for use in combination w/ radiation therapy; life-threatening mucositis, especially esophagitis and pneumonitis occurred w/ concurrent thoracic radiation (given together or ≤7 days apart). Radiation recall reported in patients who received gemcitabine after prior radiation (given >7 days apart).

PREGNANCY AND LACTATION
Pregnancy: Category D.
Lactation: Not for use in nursing.

MECHANISM OF ACTION
Nucleoside metabolic inhibitor; kills cells undergoing DNA synthesis and blocks the progression of cells through the G1/S-phase boundary.

PHARMACOKINETICS
Distribution: V_d=50L/m². **Metabolism:** Via nucleoside kinases to diphosphate and triphosphate nucleosides; gemcitabine triphosphate (active metabolite). **Elimination:** Urine (92-98%, <10% unchanged); $T_{1/2}$=42-94 min.

PATIENT CONSIDERATIONS
Assessment: Assess for hypersensitivity to drug, renal/hepatic dysfunction, pregnancy/nursing status, and possible drug interactions. Obtain CBC, including differential and platelet count, prior to each dose.

Monitoring: Monitor for signs/symptoms of myelosuppression, pulmonary toxicity, HUS, CLS, PRES, and other adverse reactions. Periodically monitor renal/hepatic function.

Counseling: Inform of the risks and benefits of therapy. Advise of the potential need for blood transfusions and increased susceptibility to infections. Instruct to immediately contact physician if any signs/symptoms of infection, fever, prolonged/unexpected bleeding, bruising, SOB, wheezing, cough, changes in the color/volume of urine output, jaundice, or pain/tenderness in the right upper abdominal quadrant develops. Inform that drug may cause fetal harm; instruct to notify physician if pregnant or nursing.

GENGRAF — cyclosporine   Rx
Class: Calcineurin-inhibitor immunosuppressant

> Should only be prescribed by physicians experienced in the management of systemic immunosuppressive therapy for indicated diseases. Manage patients in facilities equipped and staffed w/ adequate lab and supportive medical resources. Increased susceptibility to infection and development of neoplasia (eg, lymphoma) may result from immunosuppression. May be coadministered w/ other immunosuppressive agents in kidney, liver, and heart transplant patients. Not bioequivalent to Sandimmune and cannot be used interchangeably w/o physician supervision. Caution in switching from Sandimmune. Monitor cyclosporine blood levels in transplant and rheumatoid arthritis (RA) patients to avoid toxicity due to high levels. Dose adjustments should be made in transplant patients to minimize possible organ rejection due to low levels. (Psoriasis) Increased risk of developing skin malignancies in psoriasis patients previously treated w/ PUVA, methotrexate (MTX) or other immunosuppressive agents, UVB, coal tar, or radiation therapy. May cause systemic HTN and nephrotoxicity; risk increases w/ increasing dose and duration. Monitor for renal dysfunction, including structural kidney damage, during therapy.

ADULT DOSAGE
Organ Rejection Prophylaxis

Kidney, Liver, and Heart Allogeneic Transplants:
Newly Transplanted Patients:
Initial dose may be given 4-12 hrs prior to transplant or postoperatively; dose varies depending on transplanted organ and other immunosuppressive agents included in protocol

Suggested Initial Doses:
Renal Transplant: 9mg/kg/day ± 3mg/kg/day
Liver Transplant: 8mg/kg/day ± 4mg/kg/day
Heart Transplant: 7mg/kg/day ± 3mg/kg/day

Always administer daily dose in 2 divided doses (bid) and adjust subsequent dose to achieve a predefined cyclosporine blood concentration

Adjunct therapy w/ adrenal corticosteroids is recommended initially

Conversion from Sandimmune:
Start w/ the same daily dose as was previously used w/ Sandimmune (1:1 dose conversion); dose should subsequently be adjusted to attain the pre-conversion blood trough concentration

PEDIATRIC DOSAGE
Organ Rejection Prophylaxis

Kidney, Liver, and Heart Allogeneic Transplants:
Transplant recipients as young as 1 year of age have received cyclosporine (MODIFIED) w/ no unusual adverse effects

---

It is strongly recommended that the blood trough concentration be monitored every 4-7 days after conversion to Gengraf, until the blood trough concentration attains the pre-conversion value

Patients w/ Poor Absorption of Sandimmune:
Due to the increase in bioavailability of cyclosporine following conversion to Gengraf, the blood trough concentration may exceed the target range; caution when converting patients at doses >10mg/kg/day

Titrate dose individually based on trough levels, tolerability, and clinical response; measure blood trough concentrations more frequently, at least 2X a week (daily, if initial dose >10mg/kg/day) until the concentration stabilizes w/in the desired range

Has been used in combination w/ azathioprine and corticosteroids

Rheumatoid Arthritis
Severe active rheumatoid arthritis where the disease has not adequately responded to MTX

Initial: 2.5mg/kg/day, taken in 2 divided doses
Titrate: May increase by 0.5-0.75mg/kg/day after 8 weeks and again after 12 weeks
Max: 4mg/kg/day

Salicylates, NSAIDs, and oral corticosteroids may be continued

D/C if no benefit is seen by 16 weeks of therapy

Combination w/ MTX:
Use same initial dose and dosage range; most patients can be treated w/ Gengraf doses of ≤3mg/kg/day when combined w/ MTX doses of up to 15mg/week

Plaque Psoriasis
In immunocompetent patients w/ severe, recalcitrant, plaque psoriasis who failed to respond to at least 1 systemic therapy (eg, PUVA, retinoids, MTX) or in patients for whom other systemic therapies are contraindicated, or cannot be tolerated

Initial: 2.5mg/kg/day, taken in 2 divided doses for at least 4 weeks
Titrate: If significant clinical improvement does not occur, increase the dose at 2-week intervals by approx 0.5mg/kg/day
Max: 4mg/kg/day

D/C if satisfactory response cannot be achieved after 6 weeks at 4mg/kg/day or the patient's max tolerated dose

Once a patient is adequately controlled and appears stable, the dose should be lowered, and the patient treated w/ the lowest dose that maintains an adequate response

---

DOSING CONSIDERATIONS
Renal Impairment
In Kidney, Liver, and Heart Transplant: Reduce dose if indicated
In Rheumatoid Arthritis/Psoriasis: Not recommended for use

Hepatic Impairment
Severe: Dose reduction may be necessary

Elderly
Start at lower end of dosing range

Adverse Reactions
Rheumatoid Arthritis/Psoriasis: Decrease dose by 25-50% at any time to control adverse events or clinically significant lab abnormalities; d/c if dose reduction is not effective in controlling abnormalities or if the adverse event or abnormality is severe

Other Important Considerations
Avoid consumption of grapefruit or grapefruit juice during therapy

ADMINISTRATION
Oral route

Always administer daily dose in 2 divided doses (bid).
Administer on a consistent schedule w/ regard to time of day and relation to meals.

Sol
To make the sol more palatable, dilute w/ room temperature orange or apple juice; avoid switching diluents frequently.

Instructions:
1. Take the prescribed amount of sol from the container using the dosing syringe supplied, and transfer the sol to a glass of orange or apple juice; use a glass container, not plastic.
2. Stir well and drink at once; do not allow diluted sol to stand before drinking.
3. Rinse the glass w/ more diluent to ensure that the total dose is consumed.
4. After use, dry the outside of the dosing syringe w/ a clean towel and store in a clean, dry place; do not rinse the dosing syringe w/ water or other cleaning agents.
5. If the syringe requires cleaning, it must be completely dry before resuming use.

STORAGE
20-25°C (68-77°F). **Sol:** Do not refrigerate. Use w/in 2 months once opened. May form gel at <20°C (68°F); light flocculation, or formation of light sediment may occur. Allow to warm to 25°C (77°F) to reverse these changes.

HOW SUPPLIED
Cap: 25mg, 50mg, 100mg; **Sol:** 100mg/mL [50mL]

CONTRAINDICATIONS
Hypersensitivity to cyclosporine or to any components of the medication.
RA/Psoriasis: Abnormal renal function, uncontrolled HTN, malignancies. **Psoriasis:** Concomitant PUVA or UVB therapy, MTX or other immunosuppressants, coal tar or radiation therapy.

WARNINGS/PRECAUTIONS
Elevations in SrCr and BUN may occur and reflect a reduction in GFR; impaired renal function at any time requires close monitoring, and frequent dose adjustment may be indicated. Elevations in SrCr and BUN levels in renal transplant patients do not necessarily indicate rejection; evaluate patient before initiating dose adjustment. Thrombocytopenia and microangiopathic hemolytic anemia, resulting in graft failure, reported. Significant hyperkalemia (sometimes associated w/ hyperchloremic metabolic acidosis) and hyperuricemia reported. May cause hepatotoxicity and liver injury (eg, cholestasis, jaundice, hepatitis, liver failure). Avoid excessive UV light exposure. Oversuppression of the immune system may result in an increased risk of infection/malignancy; caution when using a treatment regimen containing multiple immunosuppressants. Increased risk of developing bacterial, viral, fungal, protozoal, and opportunistic infections (eg, polyoma virus infections). JC virus-associated progressive multifocal leukoencephalopathy and polyomavirus-associated nephropathy, especially due to BK virus infection, reported; consider reduction in immunosuppression if either develops. Convulsions and encephalopathy including posterior reversible encephalopathy syndrome, and rarely, optic disc edema, reported. HTN may occur and persist, and may require antihypertensive therapy. **Cap:** Consider the alcohol content of the drug when giving to patients in whom alcohol intake should be avoided or minimized (eg, pregnant or breastfeeding women, patients presenting w/ liver disease or epilepsy, alcoholic patients, pediatric patients).

ADVERSE REACTIONS
Kidney, Liver, and Heart Transplantation: Renal dysfunction, tremor, hirsutism, HTN, gum hyperplasia.
RA: Renal dysfunction, HTN, headache, GI disturbances, hirsutism/hypertrichosis.
Psoriasis: Renal dysfunction, headache, HTN, hypertriglyceridemia, hirsutism/hypertrichosis, paresthesia/hyperesthesia, influenza-like symptoms, N/V, diarrhea, abdominal discomfort, lethargy, musculoskeletal/joint pain.

DRUG INTERACTIONS
See Boxed Warning, Dosing Considerations, and Contraindications. Avoid w/ K+-sparing diuretics, aliskiren, bosentan, dabigatran, and compounds that decrease drug absorption (eg, orlistat). Vaccination may be less effective; avoid live vaccines during therapy. Caution w/ rifabutin, nephrotoxic drugs, HIV protease inhibitors, K+-sparing drugs (eg, ACE inhibitors, ARBs), K+-containing drugs, and K+-rich diet. Ciprofloxacin, gentamicin, tobramycin, vancomycin, trimethoprim w/ sulfamethoxazole, melphalan, amphotericin B, ketoconazole, azapropazone, colchicine, diclofenac, naproxen, sulindac, cimetidine, ranitidine, tacrolimus, fibric acid derivatives (eg, bezafibrate, fenofibrate), MTX, and NSAIDs may potentiate renal dysfunction; closely monitor renal function and reduce dose of coadministered drug or consider alternative treatment if a significant impairment of renal function occurs. CYP3A4 and/or P-gp inducers/inhibitors may alter levels; adjust cyclosporine dose appropriately. Diltiazem, nicardipine, verapamil, fluconazole, itraconazole, ketoconazole, voriconazole, azithromycin, clarithromycin, erythromycin, quinupristin/dalfopristin, methylprednisolone, allopurinol, amiodarone, bromocriptine, colchicine, danazol, imatinib, metoclopramide, nefazodone, oral contraceptives, HIV protease inhibitors, grapefruit, grapefruit juice, boceprevir, and telaprevir may increase levels. St. John's wort, nafcillin, rifampin, carbamazepine, oxcarbazepine, phenobarbital, phenytoin, bosentan, octreotide, sulfinpyrazone, terbinafine, and ticlopidine may decrease levels. May increase plasma levels of bosentan, dabigatran, and substrates of CYP3A4, P-gp, or organic anion transporter proteins. May increase levels of ambrisentan; do not titrate ambrisentan dose to the recommended max daily dose when coadministering w/ cyclosporine. May reduce clearance of digoxin, colchicine, prednisolone, HMG-CoA reductase inhibitors (statins), aliskiren, bosentan, dabigatran, repaglinide, NSAIDs, sirolimus, and etoposide.

Digitalis toxicity reported; monitor digoxin levels. May increase levels and enhance toxic effects of colchicine; reduce colchicine dose. Myotoxicity cases seen w/ statins; temporarily withhold or d/c statin therapy if signs of myopathy develop or w/ risk factors predisposing to severe renal injury. May increase levels of repaglinide and thereby increase the risk of hypoglycemia; closely monitor blood glucose levels. High doses of cyclosporine may increase the exposure to anthracycline antibiotics (eg, doxorubicin, mitoxantrone, daunorubicin) in cancer patients. May double diclofenac blood levels; dose of diclofenac should be in the lower end of the therapeutic range. May increase MTX levels and decrease levels of MTX metabolite. Concomitant use w/ sirolimus increases levels of sirolimus and causes elevations of SrCr; give sirolimus 4 hrs after cyclosporine. Frequent gingival hyperplasia reported w/ nifedipine; avoid concomitant use w/ nifedipine in patients in whom gingival hyperplasia develops as a side effect of cyclosporine. Convulsions reported w/ high-dose methylprednisolone. Calcium antagonists may interfere w/ cyclosporine metabolism.

PREGNANCY AND LACTATION
Pregnancy: Category C.
Lactation: Not for use in nursing.

MECHANISM OF ACTION
Cyclic polypeptide immunosuppressant; specific and reversible inhibition of immunocompetent lymphocytes in the G_0- and G_1-phase of the cell cycle. T-lymphocytes are preferentially inhibited w/ T-helper cell as main target, although T-suppressor cell may also be suppressed. Also inhibits lymphokine production and release (eg, interleukin-2).

PHARMACOKINETICS
Absorption: Incomplete; T_{max}=1.5-2 hrs. Pharmacokinetic parameters varied w/ different indications (renal/liver transplant, RA, and/or psoriasis). **Distribution:** V_d=3-5L/kg (IV, solid organ transplant recipients); plasma protein binding (90%); found in breast milk. **Metabolism:** (Extensive) Liver via CYP3A and less in the GI tract and kidneys. Oxidation and demethylation pathways; M1, M9, M4N (major metabolites). **Elimination:** Bile (primary), urine (6%, 0.1% unchanged); $T_{1/2}$=8.4 hrs.

PATIENT CONSIDERATIONS
Assessment: Assess for hypersensitivity to the drug, renal dysfunction, uncontrolled HTN, presence of malignancies, pregnancy/nursing status, and for possible drug interactions. **RA:** Before initiating treatment, assess BP (on at least 2 occasions) and obtain 2 SrCr levels. **Psoriasis:** Prior to treatment, perform a dermatological and physical examination, including measuring BP (on at least 2 occasions). Assess for presence of occult infection and for the presence of tumors. Assess for atypical skin lesions and biopsy them. Obtain baseline SrCr (on 2 occasions), BUN, CBC, Mg^{2+}, K+, uric acid, and lipid levels.

Monitoring: Monitor for signs/symptoms of hepatotoxicity, liver injury, nephrotoxicity, thrombocytopenia, microangiopathic hemolytic anemia, HTN, hyperkalemia, lymphomas and other malignancies, serious/opportunistic/polyomavirus infections, convulsions and other neurotoxicities, and other adverse reactions. Monitor cyclosporine blood levels routinely in transplant patients and periodically in RA patients. **RA:** Monitor BP and SrCr every 2 weeks during the initial 3 months of therapy and then monthly if patient is stable. Monitor SrCr and BP after an increase of the dose of NSAIDs and after initiation of new NSAID therapy. If coadministered w/ MTX, monitor CBC and LFTs monthly. **Psoriasis:** Monitor for occult infection and for the presence of tumors. Monitor SrCr, BUN, BP, CBC, uric acid, K+, lipids, and Mg^{2+} every 2 weeks during first 3 months of treatment, then monthly if stable, or more frequently during dose adjustments.

Counseling: Instruct to contact physician before changing formulations of cyclosporine, which may require dose changes. Inform that repeated lab tests are required while on therapy. Advise of the potential risks if used during pregnancy and inform of the increased risk of neoplasia, HTN, and renal dysfunction. Inform that vaccinations may be less effective and instruct to avoid live vaccines during therapy. Advise to avoid grapefruit/grapefruit juice and excessive sun exposure.

GENOTROPIN — somatropin (rDNA origin)   Rx

Class: Recombinant human growth hormone (hGH)

OTHER BRAND NAMES
Genotropin MiniQuick

ADULT DOSAGE	PEDIATRIC DOSAGE
Growth Hormone Deficiency	**Growth Hormone Deficiency**
Adult or Childhood-Onset Etiology: Divide weekly dose into 6-7 SQ inj	Due to an inadequate secretion of endogenous growth hormone
Non Weight-Based:	Individualize dose
Initial: 0.2mg/day (range, 0.15-0.30mg/day)	0.16-0.24mg/kg/week; divide weekly dose into 6-7 SQ inj
Titrate: May increase gradually every 1-2 months by increments of 0.1-0.2mg/day based on clinical response and insulin-like growth factor-I (IGF-I) concentrations	**Prader-Willi Syndrome**
Maint: Individualize dose	Individualize dose
Weight-Based:	0.24mg/kg/week; divide weekly dose into 6-7 SQ inj
Initial: Up to 0.04mg/kg/week	**Turner Syndrome**
Titrate: May increase up to 0.08mg/kg/week at 4- to 8-week intervals based on clinical response, side effects, and determination of age- and gender-adjusted serum IGF-I concentrations	Individualize dose
	0.33mg/kg/week; divide weekly dose into 6-7 SQ inj
	Idiopathic Short Stature
	Treatment of idiopathic short stature, defined by height standard deviation

score ≤-2.25, and associated w/ growth rates unlikely to permit attainment of adult height in the normal range, in pediatric patients whose epiphyses are not closed and for whom diagnostic evaluation excludes other causes associated w/ short stature that should be observed or treated by other means

Individualize dose

Up to 0.47mg/kg/week; divide weekly dose into 6-7 SQ inj

Small for Gestational Age

Treatment of growth failure in children born small for gestational age who fail to manifest catch-up growth by age 2 years

Individualize dose

Up to 0.48mg/kg/week; divide weekly dose into 6-7 SQ inj

DOSING CONSIDERATIONS
Concomitant Medications
Oral Estrogen: May increase the dose requirements in women

Elderly
Consider lower starting dose and smaller dose increments

ADMINISTRATION
SQ route

May be given in the thigh, buttocks, or abdomen; the site of SQ inj should be rotated daily to help prevent lipoatrophy.

STORAGE
(Pen cartridge) 2-8°C (36-46°F). Do not freeze. Protect from light. After reconstitution, refrigerate for up to 28 days. (MiniQuick) Refrigerate prior to dispensing, but may be stored at or below 25°C (77°F) for up to 3 months after dispensing. After reconstitution, refrigerate for up to 24 hrs before use.

HOW SUPPLIED
Inj: (Pen cartridge) 5mg, 12mg; (MiniQuick) 0.2mg, 0.4mg, 0.6mg, 0.8mg, 1mg, 1.2mg, 1.4mg, 1.6mg, 1.8mg, 2mg [0.25mL]

CONTRAINDICATIONS
Acute critical illness due to complications following open heart surgery, abdominal surgery, multiple accidental trauma, or w/ acute respiratory failure. Pediatric patients w/ Prader-Willi syndrome (PWS) who are severely obese, have a history of upper airway obstruction or sleep apnea, or have severe respiratory impairment. Active malignancy, or evidence of progression or recurrence of an underlying intracranial tumor. Active proliferative or severe nonproliferative diabetic retinopathy. Growth promotion in pediatric patients w/ closed epiphyses. Known hypersensitivity to somatropin or any of its excipients, known sensitivity to m-cresol (pen cartridge).

WARNINGS/PRECAUTIONS
Reevaluate adults who were treated w/ somatropin for growth hormone deficiency (GHD) in childhood and whose epiphyses are closed. Treatment for short stature should be discontinued when epiphyses are fused. Implement effective weight control in patients w/ PWS and treat respiratory infections aggressively; interrupt therapy if patient shows signs of upper airway obstruction and/or new onset sleep apnea. Increased risk of a second neoplasm in childhood cancer survivors reported. Increased risk of developing malignancies in children w/ certain rare genetic causes of short stature; monitor for development of neoplasms if treatment is initiated. Monitor for increased growth, or potential malignant changes, of preexisting nevi. Undiagnosed impaired glucose tolerance and overt diabetes mellitus (DM) may be unmasked, and new-onset type 2 DM reported. Intracranial HTN (IH) w/ papilledema, visual changes, headache, N/V reported; d/c if papilledema is observed. If somatropin-induced IH is diagnosed, treatment can be restarted at a lower dose after IH-associated signs and symptoms have resolved. Fluid retention in adults may occur. Monitor other hormonal replacement treatments in patients w/ hypopituitarism. Undiagnosed/untreated hypothyroidism may prevent optimal response. Hypothyroidism may become evident or worsen. Slipped capital femoral epiphyses and progression of scoliosis may occur in pediatric patients. Increased risk of ear/hearing disorders and cardiovascular (CV) disorders in Turner syndrome (TS) patients. Tissue atrophy may occur when administered at the same site over a long period; rotate inj site. Allergic reactions may occur. Serum levels of inorganic phosphorus, alkaline phosphatase, parathyroid hormone, and IGF-I may increase. Pancreatitis rarely reported. Obese patients may manifest adverse effects when treated w/ a weight-based regimen.

ADVERSE REACTIONS
Peripheral swelling/edema, arthralgia, URI, pain/stiffness in extremities, paresthesia, headache, fatigue, myalgia, inj-site reactions/rashes, glucose intolerance, unmasking of latent central hypothyroidism.

DRUG INTERACTIONS
May inhibit 11β-hydroxysteroid dehydrogenase type 1, resulting in reduced serum cortisol concentrations; may need glucocorticoid replacement or dose adjustments of glucocorticoid therapy. Glucocorticoid therapy may attenuate growth-promoting effects in children; carefully adjust glucocorticoid replacement dosing. May increase clearance of antipyrine. May alter clearance of compounds metabolized by CYP450 liver enzymes (eg, corticosteroids, sex steroids, anticonvulsants, cyclosporine); monitor carefully. May require larger doses w/ oral estrogen replacement. May need to adjust dose of insulin and/or oral/injectable hypoglycemic agents, and thyroid hormone replacement therapy.

PREGNANCY AND LACTATION
Category B, caution in nursing.

MECHANISM OF ACTION
Recombinant hGH; stimulates linear growth in pediatrics. Normalizes concentrations of IGF-I/Somatomedin C in patients w/ GHD or PWS. Reduces fat mass, increases lean body mass, and causes metabolic alterations that include beneficial changes in lipid metabolism, and normalization of IGF-I concentrations in adults w/ GHD.

PHARMACOKINETICS
Absorption: Absolute bioavailability (80%). Administration of variable doses resulted in different parameters. **Distribution:** V_d=1.3L/kg. **Metabolism:** Liver and kidneys (protein catabolism). **Elimination:** $T_{1/2}$=3 hrs (adults).

PATIENT CONSIDERATIONS
Assessment: Assess for signs of upper airway obstruction and sleep apnea, preexisting DM or impaired glucose tolerance, history of scoliosis, hypothyroidism, hypopituitarism, otitis media or other ear disorders in TS patients, hypersensitivity to drug or m-cresol, any other conditions where treatment is contraindicated/cautioned, pregnancy/nursing status, and possible drug interactions. Perform funduscopic exam.

Monitoring: Monitor growth, for clinical response, neoplasms, increased growth or malignant changes of preexisting nevi, IH, fluid retention, allergic reactions, pancreatitis, slipped capital femoral epiphyses and progression of scoliosis in pediatric patients (eg, onset of limp, hip or knee pain), and other adverse reactions. Perform periodic thyroid function tests, funduscopic exam, and monitoring of glucose levels. In patients w/ PWS, monitor weight as well as for signs of respiratory infections, sleep apnea, and upper airway obstruction. Monitor patients w/ history of GHD secondary to an intracranial neoplasm routinely while on therapy for progression/recurrence of tumor. In patients w/ TS, monitor for ear/CV disorders.

Counseling: Inform about potential benefits and risks of therapy, proper administration, usage, and disposal, and caution against any reuse of needles and syringes.

GENVOYA — cobicistat/elvitegravir/emtricitabine/tenofovir alafenamide   **Rx**

Class: CYP3A inhibitor/HIV integrase strand transfer inhibitor/nucleoside reverse transcriptase inhibitor (NRTI) combination

> Lactic acidosis and severe hepatomegaly w/ steatosis, including fatal cases, reported w/ the use of nucleoside analogues in combination w/ other antiretrovirals. Not approved for the treatment of chronic hepatitis B virus (HBV) infection. Severe acute exacerbations of hepatitis B reported in patients who are coinfected w/ HBV and HIV-1 and have discontinued products containing emtricitabine and/or tenofovir disoproxil fumarate (TDF); closely monitor hepatic function w/ both clinical and lab follow-up for at least several months in patients who are coinfected w/ HIV-1 and HBV and d/c therapy. If appropriate, initiation of anti-hepatitis B therapy may be warranted.

ADULT DOSAGE
HIV-1 Infection

For use as a complete regimen in adults who have no antiretroviral treatment history or to replace the current antiretroviral regimen in those who are virologically-suppressed (HIV-1 RNA <50 copies/mL) on a stable antiretroviral regimen for at least 6 months w/ no history of treatment failure and no known substitutions associated w/ resistance to the individual components of the drug

≥35kg:
1 tab qd

PEDIATRIC DOSAGE
HIV-1 Infection

For use as a complete regimen in pediatrics who have no antiretroviral treatment history or to replace the current antiretroviral regimen in those who are virologically-suppressed (HIV-1 RNA <50 copies/mL) on a stable antiretroviral regimen for at least 6 months w/ no history of treatment failure and no known substitutions associated w/ resistance to the individual components of the drug

≥12 Years and ≥35kg:
1 tab qd

DOSING CONSIDERATIONS
Renal Impairment
CrCl <30mL/min: Not recommended for use

Hepatic Impairment
Severe (Child-Pugh Class C): Not recommended for use

ADMINISTRATION
Oral route

Take w/ food.

STORAGE
<30°C (86°F).

HOW SUPPLIED
Tab: (Cobicistat/Elvitegravir/Emtricitabine/Tenofovir Alafenamide [TAF]) 150mg/150mg/200mg/10mg

CONTRAINDICATIONS
Concomitant use w/ drugs that are highly dependent on CYP3A for clearance and for which elevated plasma concentrations are associated w/ serious and/or life-threatening events (eg, alfuzosin, carbamazepine, phenobarbital, phenytoin,

rifampin, dihydroergotamine, ergotamine, methylergonovine, cisapride, St. John's wort, lovastatin, simvastatin, pimozide, sildenafil [when dosed as Revatio for the treatment of pulmonary arterial HTN], triazolam, oral midazolam).

WARNINGS/PRECAUTIONS

Test for HBV infection prior to initiation of therapy. Redistribution/accumulation of body fat reported. Not recommended in patients w/ estimated CrCl <30mL/min. **Emtricitabine and TAF:** Obesity and prolonged nucleoside exposure may be risk factors for lactic acidosis and severe hepatomegaly. Caution in any patient w/ known risk factors for liver disease. **Emtricitabine:** Immune reconstitution syndrome and autoimmune disorders (eg, Graves' disease, polymyositis, Guillain-Barre syndrome) in the setting of immune reconstitution reported. **TAF:** Renal impairment, including cases of acute renal failure and Fanconi syndrome, reported w/ tenofovir prodrugs; d/c in patients who develop clinically significant decreases in renal function or evidence of Fanconi syndrome. Decreased bone mineral density (BMD) and increased biochemical markers of bone metabolism reported. Osteomalacia associated w/ proximal renal tubulopathy reported in association w/ the use of TDF-containing products. Hypophosphatemia and osteomalacia secondary to proximal renal tubulopathy have occurred in patients at risk of renal dysfunction who present w/ persistent or worsening bone or muscle symptoms while receiving products containing TDF. **Cobicistat:** May produce elevations of SrCr.

ADVERSE REACTIONS

Nausea.

DRUG INTERACTIONS

See Contraindications. Avoid w/ elvitegravir, cobicistat, emtricitabine, TDF, lamivudine, adefovir dipivoxil, ritonavir, other antiretrovirals, rifabutin, rifapentine, or salmeterol. CYP3A inducers may decrease plasma concentration of cobicistat, elvitegravir, and TAF and may lead to loss of therapeutic effect and development of resistance. Coadministration w/ drugs that reduce renal function or compete for active tubular secretion (eg, acyclovir, cidofovir, ganciclovir, valacyclovir, valganciclovir, aminoglycosides [eg, gentamicin]) may increase concentrations of emtricitabine, tenofovir, and other renally eliminated drugs and this may increase the risk of adverse reactions. May increase levels of antiarrhythmics (eg, digoxin), itraconazole, ketoconazole, voriconazole, colchicine, quetiapine, ethosuximide, β-blockers, calcium channel blockers, inhaled or nasal fluticasone, bosentan, atorvastatin, immunosuppressants, salmeterol, neuroleptics, PDE-5 inhibitors, and sedatives/hypnotics. May increase levels of clarithromycin and telithromycin; reduce clarithromycin dose by 50% in patients w/ CrCl 50-60mL/min. Monitor INR upon coadministration w/ warfarin. Ethosuximide and oxcarbazepine may decrease elvitegravir, cobicistat, and TAF levels; consider alternative anticonvulsants w/ oxcarbazepine and monitor upon coadministration w/ ethosuximide. May increase levels of antidepressants (eg, SSRIs [except sertraline], TCAs, trazodone); carefully titrate antidepressant dose and monitor response. Ketoconazole, itraconazole, and voriconazole may increase levels of elvitegravir and cobicistat. Avoid w/ colchicine in patients w/ renal or hepatic impairment. Rifabutin and rifapentine may decrease elvitegravir, cobicistat, and TAF levels. Consider alternative antiretroviral therapy w/ quetiapine if initiating therapy while on quetiapine. Dexamethasone may decrease elvitegravir and cobicistat levels; consider an alternative corticosteroid. May increase levels of diazepam and parenterally administered midazolam; consider dose reduction for midazolam. May increase norgestimate and decrease ethinyl estradiol levels; consider alternative (nonhormonal) methods of contraception. Cyclosporine may increase elvitegravir and cobicistat levels. May increase levels of buprenorphine and norbuprenorphine and may decrease levels of naloxone. **TAF:** Patients taking nephrotoxic agents (eg, NSAIDs) are at increased risk of developing renal-related adverse reactions. P-gp inducers may decrease levels. **Cobicistat:** May increase levels of CYP3A substrates or CYP2D6 substrates, and substrates of P-gp, BCRP, OATP1B1, or OATP1B3. CYP3A inhibitors may increase levels. Clarithromycin and telithromycin may increase levels. **Elvitegravir:** May decrease plasma levels of CYP2C9 substrates. Antacids (eg, aluminum and magnesium hydroxide) may decrease levels; separate administration by at least 2 hrs. Refer to PI for dosing modifications when used w/ certain concomitant therapies.

PREGNANCY AND LACTATION

Pregnancy: Category B. An antiretroviral pregnancy registry has been established to monitor fetal outcomes of pregnant women.
Lactation: Emtricitabine is secreted in human milk. Not for use in nursing.

MECHANISM OF ACTION

Elvitegravir: HIV-1 integrase strand inhibitor; inhibits the strand transfer activity of HIV-1 integrase, preventing the integration of HIV-1 DNA into host genomic DNA, blocking the formation of HIV-1 provirus and propagation of the viral infection. **Cobicistat:** CYP3A inhibitor; inhibits CYP3A-mediated metabolism that leads to enhancement of systemic exposure of CYP3A substrates (eg, elvitegravir). **Emtricitabine:** Nucleoside analogue of cytidine; inhibits the activity of HIV-1 reverse transcriptase by competing w/ the natural substrate deoxycytidine 5'-triphosphate and by being incorporated into nascent viral DNA, resulting in chain termination. **TAF:** Acyclic nucleoside phosphonate (nucleotide) analogue of adenosine 5'-monophosphate; inhibits HIV replication through incorporation into viral DNA by the HIV reverse transcriptase, which results in DNA chain-termination.

PHARMACOKINETICS

Absorption: Elvitegravir: C_{max}=2.1mcg/mL, AUC=22.8mcg•hr/mL, T_{max}=4 hrs. Cobicistat: C_{max}=1.5mcg/mL, AUC=9.5mcg•hr/mL, T_{max}=3 hrs. Emtricitabine: C_{max}=2.1mcg/mL, AUC=11.7mcg•hr/mL, T_{max}=3 hrs. TAF: C_{max}=0.16mcg/mL, AUC=0.21mcg•hr/mL, T_{max}=1 hr. **Distribution:** Elvitegravir: Plasma protein binding (99%). Cobicistat: Plasma protein binding (98%). Emtricitabine: Plasma protein binding (<4%); found in breast milk. TAF: Plasma protein binding (80%). **Metabolism:** Elvitegravir: CYP3A (major); UGT1A1/3 (minor). Cobicistat: CYP3A (major), CYP2D6 (minor). TAF: Hydrolysis, tenofovir (major metabolite),

phosphorylation, tenofovir diphosphate (active metabolite). **Elimination:** Elvitegravir: Feces (94.8%), urine (6.7%); $T_{1/2}$=12.9 hrs (median). Cobicistat: Feces (86.2%), urine (8.2%); $T_{1/2}$=3.5 hrs (median). Emtricitabine: Urine (70%), feces (13.7%); $T_{1/2}$=10 hrs (median). TAF: Feces (31.7%), urine (<1%); $T_{1/2}$=0.51 hrs (median).

PATIENT CONSIDERATIONS

Assessment: Assess for obesity, prolonged nucleoside exposure, risk factors for liver disease, renal/hepatic impairment, pregnancy/nursing status, and possible drug interactions. Assess BMD in patients who have a history of pathological bone fracture or w/ other risk factors for osteoporosis or bone loss. Obtain baseline estimated CrCl, urine glucose, urine protein, and SrCr. Perform test for HBV infection prior to therapy.

Monitoring: Monitor for signs/symptoms of lactic acidosis, severe hepatomegaly w/ steatosis, new onset/worsening renal impairment, immune reconstitution syndrome, autoimmune disorders, fat redistribution/accumulation, decreased BMD, increased biochemical markers for bone metabolism, osteomalacia, and other adverse reactions. Monitor for exacerbations of hepatitis B in patients w/ coinfection for at least several months upon discontinuation of therapy. Monitor BMD, estimated CrCl, urine glucose, urine protein, and SrCr. Monitor serum phosphorus levels in patients w/ chronic kidney disease. Monitor INR upon coadministration w/ warfarin.

Counseling: Instruct to take on a regular dosing schedule w/ food and to avoid missing doses. Advise to report use of any prescription or nonprescription medication or herbal products, including St. John's wort. Instruct to contact physician if symptoms of lactic acidosis/pronounced hepatotoxicity or any symptoms of infection occur. Inform that hepatitis B testing is recommended prior to initiating therapy. Advise that fat redistribution/accumulation, renal impairment, and decreases in BMD may occur. Inform that there is an antiretroviral pregnancy registry to monitor fetal outcomes of pregnant women exposed to the drug. Instruct mothers not to breastfeed.

GILENYA — fingolimod   Rx

Class: Sphingosine 1-phosphate receptor modulator

ADULT DOSAGE	PEDIATRIC DOSAGE
Multiple Sclerosis	Pediatric use may not have been established
Treatment of relapsing forms of multiple sclerosis (MS) to reduce the frequency of clinical exacerbations and to delay the accumulation of physical disability	
0.5mg qd	

ADMINISTRATION

Oral route

Take w/ or w/o food.
Patients who initiate therapy and those who reinitiate treatment after discontinuation for >14 days require 1st dose monitoring.

First Dose Monitoring

Administer the 1st dose in a setting in which resources to appropriately manage symptomatic bradycardia are available. Observe all patients for 6 hrs for signs/symptoms of bradycardia w/ hourly pulse and BP measurement. Obtain an ECG prior to dosing and at the end of the observation period.

Additional observation should be instituted until the finding has resolved in the following situations:
1. HR 6 hrs post-dose is <45 bpm.
2. HR 6 hrs post-dose is at the lowest value post-dose (suggesting that the max pharmacodynamic effect on the heart may not have occurred).
3. ECG 6 hrs post-dose shows new onset 2nd degree or higher atrioventricular (AV) block.

Should post-dose symptomatic bradycardia occur, initiate appropriate management, begin continuous ECG monitoring, and continue observation until the symptoms have resolved.

Should a patient require pharmacologic intervention for symptomatic bradycardia, continuous overnight ECG monitoring in a medical facility should be instituted, and the 1st dose monitoring strategy should be repeated after the 2nd dose.

Reinitiation of Therapy Following Discontinuation

If therapy is discontinued for >14 days, after the 1st month of treatment, the same precautions (1st dose monitoring) as for initial dosing should apply. W/in the first 2 weeks of treatment, 1st dose procedures are recommended after interruption of ≥1 day; during weeks 3 and 4 of treatment, 1st dose procedures are recommended after treatment interruption of >7 days.

STORAGE

25°C (77°F); excursions permitted to 15-30°C (59-86°F). Protect from moisture.

HOW SUPPLIED

Cap: 0.5mg

CONTRAINDICATIONS

Patients who in the last 6 months experienced MI, unstable angina, stroke, transient ischemic attack (TIA), decompensated heart failure (HF) requiring hospitalization, or Class III/IV HF. History/presence of Mobitz Type II 2nd- or 3rd-degree AV block or sick sinus syndrome (unless w/ functioning pacemaker), baseline QTc interval ≥500 msec, treatment w/ Class IA/III anti-arrhythmic drugs, hypersensitivity reaction to fingolimod or any of the excipients of the formulation.

WARNINGS/PRECAUTIONS

Bradyarrhythmia and AV blocks may occur; monitor during treatment initiation. Cases of syncope reported after 1st dose. May increase risk of infections; consider suspending treatment if a serious infection develops. Do not start treatment in patients w/ active acute/chronic infections until the infection(s) is resolved. Include disseminated herpetic infections in the differential diagnosis of patients receiving therapy and present w/ an atypical MS relapse or multiorgan failure. Cases of Kaposi's sarcoma reported. Cryptococcal infections reported; initiate prompt diagnostic evaluation and treatment if signs/symptoms occur. Caution when switching to fingolimod from immune-modulating or immunosuppressive medications to avoid unintended additive effects. Test for antibodies to varicella zoster virus (VZV) prior to commencing treatment in patients w/o a healthcare professional confirmed history of chickenpox or w/o a documentation of a full course of vaccination against VZV. Give VZV vaccination to antibody-negative patients; initiate therapy 1 month after vaccination. Progressive multifocal leukoencephalopathy (PML) reported; withhold therapy and perform appropriate diagnostic evaluation at the 1st sign/symptom suggestive of PML. May increase risk of macular edema; patients w/ history of uveitis or w/ diabetes mellitus (DM) are at increased risk. Posterior reversible encephalopathy syndrome (PRES) reported rarely; d/c if suspected. Dose-dependent reductions in forced expiratory volume over 1 sec and diffusion lung capacity for carbon monoxide (DLCO) reported. Liver transaminase elevations and liver injury w/ hepatocellular and/or cholestatic hepatitis reported; d/c if significant liver impairment confirmed. May cause fetal harm; women of childbearing potential should use effective contraception during and for 2 months after stopping therapy. May cause HTN and decreased lymphocyte counts. Basal cell carcinoma associated w/ therapy; promptly evaluate suspicious skin lesions. Hypersensitivity reactions (eg, rash, urticaria, angioedema) reported. Caution w/ severe hepatic impairment and in elderly.

ADVERSE REACTIONS

Headache, liver transaminase elevations, influenza, abdominal/back pain, diarrhea, cough, pain in extremity, sinusitis.

DRUG INTERACTIONS

See Contraindications. Monitor patients on QT prolonging drugs w/ known risk of torsades de pointes (eg, citalopram, methadone, erythromycin) overnight w/ continuous ECG in a medical facility. Severe bradycardia or heart block may occur w/ drugs that slow the HR or AV conduction (eg, β-blockers, digoxin, HR-slowing calcium channel blockers). Increased blood levels w/ ketoconazole. May reduce the immune response to vaccination. Vaccination may be less effective during and for up to 2 months after discontinuation of treatment; avoid live attenuated vaccines during and for 2 months after treatment. Antineoplastic, immune-modulating, or immunosuppressive therapies (eg, corticosteroids) may increase the risk of immunosuppression; consider the risk of additive immune system effects if these therapies are coadministered w/ fingolimod. Consider the duration and mode of action when switching from drugs w/ prolonged immune effects (eg, natalizumab, teriflunomide, mitoxantrone) to avoid unintended additive immunosuppressive effects.

PREGNANCY AND LACTATION

Pregnancy: Category C. A pregnancy registry has been established to collect information about the effect of this drug during pregnancy.
Lactation: It is not known whether this drug is excreted in human milk. Not for use in nursing.

MECHANISM OF ACTION

Sphingosine 1-phosphate receptor modulator. Fingolimod is metabolized to the active metabolite, fingolimod-phosphate. Fingolimod-phosphate binds w/ high affinity to sphingosine 1-phosphate receptors 1, 3, 4, and 5 and blocks the capacity of lymphocytes to egress from lymph nodes, reducing the number of lymphocytes in peripheral blood. The mechanism by which fingolimod exerts its effects in MS is unknown, but may involve reduction of lymphocyte migration into the CNS.

PHARMACOKINETICS

Absorption: Absolute oral bioavailability (93%); T_{max}=12-16 hrs. **Distribution:** V_d=1200L; protein binding (>99.7%). **Metabolism:** Reversible stereoselective phosphorylation; oxidative biotransformation catalyzed by CYP4F2 and possibly other CYP4F isoenzymes; formation of inactive non-polar ceramide analogues. **Elimination:** Urine (81%, inactive metabolites), feces (<2.5%, parent drug and fingolimod-phosphate); $T_{1/2}$=6-9 days.

PATIENT CONSIDERATIONS

Assessment: Assess if MI, unstable angina, stroke, TIA, decompensated HF requiring hospitalization, or Class III/IV HF was experienced in the last 6 months. Assess for history or presence of Mobitz Type II 2nd- or 3rd-degree AV block or sick sinus syndrome, pregnancy/nursing status, any other conditions where treatment is cautioned or contraindicated, and for drug interactions. Assess ECG, CBC, and LFTs. Perform an examination of the fundus including the macula.

Monitoring: Monitor for signs/symptoms of bradyarrhythmia, AV blocks, hepatic dysfunction, infection, PML, macular edema, PRES, and other adverse reactions. Monitor BP and lymphocyte counts. Perform spirometric evaluation of respiratory function and evaluation of DLCO if clinically indicated. Perform an examination of the fundus including the macula 3-4 months after starting therapy, at any time after a patient reports visual disturbances while on therapy, and regularly in patients w/ DM or history of uveitis.

Counseling: Instruct not to d/c w/o 1st consulting the prescribing physician. Advise to contact physician if patient accidently takes more drug than prescribed. Advise that decreased HR may occur upon initiation of treatment and that observation in the clinic or other facility for at least 6 hrs after the 1st dose will be required. Instruct to contact physician if symptoms of infection, new onset/worsening of dyspnea, unexplained N/V, abdominal pain, fatigue, anorexia, jaundice, dark urine, and/or any changes in vision develop. Instruct to delay treatment w/ fingolimod until after VZV vaccination if patient has

not had chickenpox or a previous VZV vaccination. Inform on the importance of contacting the physician if symptoms suggestive of PML develop; explain that typical symptoms are diverse, progress over days to weeks, and include progressive weakness on one side of the body or clumsiness of limbs, disturbance of vision, and changes in thinking, memory, and orientation leading to confusion and personality changes. Advise women of childbearing age to use effective contraception during and for 2 months after stopping treatment. Inform that drug remains in the blood and continues to have effects for up to 2 months following the last dose. Advise that basal cell carcinoma is associated w/ therapy, and that suspicious skin lesions should be promptly evaluated. Advise that drug may cause hypersensitivity reactions, and to contact physician if any symptoms occur.

GILOTRIF — afatinib   Rx

Class: Kinase inhibitor

ADULT DOSAGE	PEDIATRIC DOSAGE
Metastatic Non-Small Cell Lung Cancer	Pediatric use may not have been established
1st-line Treatment for Tumors Which Have Epidermal Growth Factor Receptor (EGFR) Exon 19 Deletions or Exon 21 (L858R) Substitution Mutations: 40mg qd until disease progression or no longer tolerated	
Metastatic Squamous Non-Small Cell Lung Cancer (NSCLC) Progressing After Platinum-Based Chemotherapy: 40mg qd until disease progression or no longer tolerated	
Missed Dose Do not take a missed dose w/in 12 hrs of the next dose	

DOSING CONSIDERATIONS

Concomitant Medications

If P-gp Inhibitor is Required:
Reduce afatinib daily dose by 10mg if not tolerated; resume previous dose after discontinuation of the P-gp inhibitor as tolerated

If Chronic Therapy w/ a P-gp Inducer is Required:
Increase afatinib daily dose by 10mg as tolerated; resume previous dose 2-3 days after discontinuation of the P-gp inducer

Renal Impairment
Severe (GFR 15-29mL/min/1.73m²):
Initial: 30mg qd

Hepatic Impairment
Severe (Child-Pugh C): Closely monitor and adjust dose if not tolerated

Adverse Reactions

Withhold for Any Adverse Reactions Of:
1. NCI CTCAE Grade ≥3
2. Diarrhea of Grade ≥2 persisting for ≥2 consecutive days while taking antidiarrheal medication
3. Cutaneous reactions of Grade 2 that are prolonged (lasting >7 days) or intolerable
4. Renal impairment of ≥Grade 2

Resume treatment when adverse reaction fully resolves, returns to baseline, or improves to Grade 1; reinstitute at a reduced dose (eg, 10mg/day less than the dose at which the adverse reaction occurred)

Permanently D/C For:
1. Life-threatening bullous, blistering, or exfoliative skin lesions
2. Confirmed interstitial lung disease (ILD)
3. Severe drug-induced hepatic impairment
4. Persistent ulcerative keratitis
5. Symptomatic left ventricular dysfunction
6. Severe or intolerable adverse reaction occurring at a dose of 20mg/day

ADMINISTRATION

Oral route

Take at least 1 hr ac or 2 hrs pc.

STORAGE

25°C (77°F); excursions permitted to 15-30°C (59-86°F). Protect from exposure to high humidity and light.

HOW SUPPLIED

Tab: 20mg, 30mg, 40mg

WARNINGS/PRECAUTIONS

See Dosing Considerations. Select patients for first-line treatment of metastatic NSCLC based on the presence of EGFR exon 19 deletions or exon 21 (L858R) substitution mutations in tumor specimens. May cause diarrhea that results in dehydration w/ or w/o renal impairment; provide an antidiarrheal agent (eg, loperamide) for administration at onset of diarrhea and continue anti-diarrheal therapy until loose bowel movements cease for 12 hrs. Bullous and exfoliative skin disorders (eg, toxic epidermal necrolysis, Stevens-Johnson syndrome) reported. ILD or ILD-like adverse reactions (eg, lung infiltration, pneumonitis, acute respiratory distress syndrome) reported; withhold therapy during evaluation of patients w/ suspected ILD and d/c in patients w/ confirmed ILD. Liver test abnormalities reported; withhold therapy in patients who develop worsening liver function and d/c in patients who develop severe hepatic impairment while on therapy. Keratitis reported; withhold during evaluation of patients w/ suspected keratitis. Interrupt or d/c therapy if diagnosis of ulcerative keratitis is confirmed. Caution w/ a history of keratitis, ulcerative keratitis, or severe dry eye. May cause fetal harm.

ADVERSE REACTIONS
Diarrhea, rash/acneiform dermatitis, stomatitis, paronychia, dry skin, decreased appetite, N/V, pruritus.

DRUG INTERACTIONS
See Dosing Considerations. P-gp inhibitors (eg, ritonavir, ketoconazole, verapamil) may increase exposure. P-gp inducers (eg, rifampicin, carbamazepine, phenytoin) may decrease exposure.

PREGNANCY AND LACTATION
Pregnancy: May cause fetal harm.
Lactation: Lactating woman should not breastfeed during treatment and for 2 weeks after the final dose.
Reproductive Potential: Females of reproductive potential should use effective contraception during treatment and for at least 2 weeks after the last dose. May reduce fertility in females and males of reproductive potential.

MECHANISM OF ACTION
Tyrosine kinase inhibitor; covalently binds to the kinase domains of EGFR (ErbB1), HER2 (ErbB2), and HER4 (ErbB4) and irreversibly inhibits tyrosine kinase autophosphorylation, resulting in downregulation of ErbB signaling.

PHARMACOKINETICS
Absorption: T_{max}=2-5 hrs. **Distribution:** Plasma protein binding (approx 95%). **Metabolism:** Covalent adducts to proteins (major circulating metabolites); enzymatic metabolism (minimal). **Elimination:** Feces (85%), urine (4%); $T_{1/2}$=37 hrs.

PATIENT CONSIDERATIONS

Assessment: Assess for history of keratitis, ulcerative keratitis, severe dry eye, renal/hepatic impairment, pregnancy/nursing status, and possible drug interactions. Assess for presence of EGFR exon 19 deletions or exon 21 (L858R) substitution mutations in tumor specimens in patients receiving treatment for EGFR mutation-positive metastatic NSCLC.

Monitoring: Monitor for diarrhea, cutaneous reactions, renal dysfunction, ILD, hepatic toxicity, keratitis, symptomatic left ventricular dysfunction, and other adverse reactions. Obtain periodic liver testing during treatment.

Counseling: Advise to notify physician if diarrhea develops and instruct to seek medical attention promptly for severe/persistent diarrhea. Advise to minimize sun exposure w/ protective clothing and to use sunscreen while taking therapy. Instruct to immediately report any new/worsening lung symptoms, or any combination of the following symptoms: trouble breathing or SOB, cough, or fever. Advise to immediately report any symptoms of a liver problem, eye problems, and for any of the following: new onset or worsening SOB or exercise intolerance, cough, fatigue, swelling of the ankles/legs, palpitations, or sudden weight gain. Advise not to take a missed dose w/in 12 hrs of the next dose. Advise females of reproductive potential to use highly effective contraception during treatment, and for at least 2 weeks after taking the last dose. Advise to d/c nursing while taking therapy and for 2 weeks after the last dose.

GLASSIA — alpha1-proteinase inhibitor (human)   Rx
Class: Alpha₁-proteinase inhibitor (A₁PI)

ADULT DOSAGE	PEDIATRIC DOSAGE
Alpha₁-Antitrypsin Deficiency	Pediatric use may not have been established
Chronic Augmentation and Maint Therapy in Individuals w/ Clinically Evident Emphysema Due to Severe Congenital Deficiency of Alpha₁-Proteinase Inhibitor:	
60mg/kg once weekly by IV infusion. Administer at a rate ≤0.2mL/kg/min and as determined by response and comfort of patient	

DOSING CONSIDERATIONS
Adverse Reactions
If infusion related adverse reactions occur, reduce rate or interrupt infusion as appropriate until symptoms subside; resume infusion at a rate tolerated by patient, except in the case of severe reaction

ADMINISTRATION
IV route
Preparation
1. Allow product to reach room temperature prior to infusing
2. Infuse directly from vial or, alternatively for large dose, pool vials into an empty, sterile container for IV infusion using the supplied filter needle. In the latter case, use a vented filter spike to withdraw the material from vial and then use the supplied 5 micron filter needle to transfer the product into the IV infusion container
Administration
1. Administer alone; do not mix w/ other agents or diluting sol

2. When infusing directly from the vials, use a vented filter spike. If the contents of vials have been pooled to a sterile IV container, use an appropriate IV administration set
3. Always use a 5 micron in-line filter during infusion
4. Administer at room temperature w/in 3 hrs of entering vials

STORAGE
2-8°C (36-46°F). Do not freeze. May be stored at room temperatures not >25°C (77°F) for up to 1 month.

HOW SUPPLIED
Inj: 1g [50mL]

CONTRAINDICATIONS
IgA-deficient patients w/ antibodies against IgA, individuals w/ a history of severe immediate hypersensitivity reactions (eg, anaphylaxis) to Alpha₁-PI products.

WARNINGS/PRECAUTIONS
May contain trace amounts of IgA. D/C infusion if hypersensitivity symptoms occur and administer appropriate emergency treatment. May carry a risk of transmitting infectious agents (eg, viruses, variant Creutzfeldt-Jakob disease [CJD], CJD agent).

ADVERSE REACTIONS
Cough, upper respiratory tract infection, headache, sinusitis, chest discomfort, dizziness, increased hepatic enzyme, exacerbation of chronic obstructive pulmonary disease, urticaria.

PREGNANCY AND LACTATION
Category C, caution in nursing.

MECHANISM OF ACTION
α₁-PI; inhibits serine proteases such as neutrophil elastase, which is capable of degrading protein components of the alveolar walls and which is chronically present in the lung.

PHARMACOKINETICS
Absorption: $AUC_{(0-168\ hr)}$=89mg•hr/mL. **Distribution:** V_d=3.2L. **Elimination:** $T_{1/2}$=111 hrs.

PATIENT CONSIDERATIONS

Assessment: Assess for drug hypersensitivity, α₁-PI deficiency, IgA deficiency, and pregnancy/nursing status.

Monitoring: Monitor for signs/symptoms of infusion-related reactions, hypersensitivity reactions, infections, and other adverse reactions. Monitor vital signs continuously. Closely monitor the infusion rate during administration.

Counseling: Inform of the early signs of hypersensitivity reactions; advise to d/c and contact physician and/or seek immediate emergency care if these symptoms occur. Inform that the product is made from human plasma and may carry risk of transmitting infectious agents.

GLEEVEC — imatinib mesylate   Rx
Class: Kinase inhibitor

ADULT DOSAGE	PEDIATRIC DOSAGE
Hypereosinophilic Syndrome/Chronic Eosinophilic Leukemia	**Ph+ Chronic Myeloid Leukemia**
In patients who have the FIP1L1-PDGFRα fusion kinase (mutational analysis or FISH demonstration of CHIC2 allele deletion) and for patients who are FIP1L1-PDGFRα fusion kinase negative or unknown	**Newly Diagnosed Patients in Chronic Phase:** ≥1 Year: 340mg/m²/day Max: 600mg/day
400mg/day	Dose can be given qd or split in 2 (am and pm)
Demonstrated FIP1L1-PDGFRα Fusion Kinase:	**Ph+ Acute Lymphoblastic Leukemia**
Initial: 100mg qd	**In Combination w/ Chemotherapy for Newly Diagnosed Patients:**
Titrate: May increase to 400mg qd in the absence of adverse reactions if response is insufficient	≥1 Year: 340mg/m² qd Max: 600mg qd
Dermatofibrosarcoma Protuberans	
Unresectable, Recurrent, and/or Metastatic:	
800mg/day (as 400mg bid)	
Kit (CD117)-Positive Gastrointestinal Stromal Tumors	
Unresectable and/or Metastatic Malignant:	
400mg qd	
Titrate: May increase up to 800mg/day (as 400mg bid) as clinically indicated	
Adjuvant Treatment Following Complete Gross Resection:	
400mg qd; optimal treatment duration unknown	
Ph+ Chronic Myeloid Leukemia	
Newly diagnosed patients in chronic phase and patients in blast crisis, accelerated phase, or in chronic phase after failure of interferon-alpha therapy	

Chronic Phase:
400mg qd
Titrate: May increase to 600mg qd

Accelerated Phase/Blast Crisis:
600mg qd
Titrate: May increase to 800mg/day
(as 400mg bid)

A dose increase may be considered in the absence of severe adverse reaction and severe non-leukemia related neutropenia or thrombocytopenia in the following circumstances: disease progression (at any time), failure to achieve a satisfactory hematologic response after at least 3 months of treatment, failure to achieve a cytogenetic response after 6-12 months of treatment, or loss of a previously achieved hematologic or cytogenetic response

Ph+ Acute Lymphoblastic Leukemia

Relapsed/Refractory:
600mg qd

Myelodysplastic/Myeloproliferative Diseases

Associated w/ PDGFR Gene Re-Arrangements:
400mg qd

Determine PDGFRb gene rearrangements status prior to initiating treatment w/ an FDA-approved test

Aggressive Systemic Mastocytosis

Determine D816V c-Kit mutation status prior to initiating treatment w/ an FDA-approved test

W/O D816V c-Kit Mutation:
400mg qd

c-Kit Mutational Status Unknown/Unavailable:
400mg qd may be considered for patients not responding satisfactorily to other therapies

Associated w/ Eosinophilia:
Initial: 100mg qd
Titrate: May increase to 400mg qd in the absence of adverse reactions if response is insufficient

---

DOSING CONSIDERATIONS
Concomitant Medications
Strong CYP3A4 Inducers: Avoid use; if necessary, increase imatinib dose by at least 50% and carefully monitor clinical response

Renal Impairment
Mild (CrCl 40-59mL/min):
Max: 600mg

Moderate (CrCl 20-39mL/min):
Initial: Reduce dose by 50%; future doses can be increased as tolerated
Max: 400mg

Severe (CrCl <20mL/min): Use w/ caution; a dose of 100mg/day was tolerated in 2 patients w/ severe renal impairment

Hepatic Impairment
Mild and Moderate: Dose adjustment is not required

Severe: Reduce dose by 25%

Adverse Reactions
Bilirubin >3X Institutional ULN (IULN) or Liver Transaminases >5X IULN:
1. Withhold therapy until bilirubin levels return to <1.5X IULN and transaminase levels to <2.5X IULN
2. Continue treatment at a reduced daily dose:
Adults: 400mg to 300mg, 600mg to 400mg, or 800mg to 600mg
Pediatrics: 340mg/m²/day to 260mg/m²/day

Severe Nonhematologic (eg, Severe Hepatotoxicity, Severe Fluid Retention):
Withhold therapy until the event has resolved; resume treatment as appropriate depending on initial severity of event

Neutropenia/Thrombocytopenia:
ANC <1.0 x 10⁹/L and/or Platelets <50 x 10⁹/L:
Adults:
Initial Dose 100mg:
1. Withhold treatment until ANC ≥1.5 x 10⁹/L and platelets ≥75 x 10⁹/L
2. Resume treatment at previous dose (dose before severe adverse reaction)

Initial Dose 400mg:
1. Withhold treatment until ANC ≥1.5 x 10⁹/L and platelets ≥75 x 10⁹/L

2. Resume treatment at the original starting dose of 400mg
3. If recurrence of ANC <1.0 x 10⁹/L and/or platelets <50 x 10⁹/L, repeat step 1 and resume at a reduced dose of 300mg

Initial Dose 800mg:
1. Withhold treatment until ANC ≥1.5 x 10⁹/L and platelets ≥75 x 10⁹/L
2. Resume treatment at 600mg
3. In the event of recurrence of ANC <1.0 x 10⁹/L and/or platelets <50 x 10⁹/L, repeat step 1 and resume at reduced dose of 400mg

Pediatrics:
Initial Dose 340mg/m²:
1. Withhold treatment until ANC ≥1.5 x 10⁹/L and platelets ≥75 x 10⁹/L
2. Resume treatment at previous dose (dose before severe adverse reaction)
3. In the event of recurrence of ANC <1.0 x 10⁹/L and/or platelets <50 x 10⁹/L, repeat step 1 and resume at reduced dose of 260mg/m²

ANC <0.5 x 10⁹/L and/or Platelets <10 x 10⁹/L:
Adults:
Initial Dose 600mg:
1. Check if cytopenia is related to leukemia (marrow aspirate or biopsy)
2. If cytopenia is unrelated to leukemia, reduce dose to 400mg
3. If cytopenia persists 2 weeks, reduce further to 300mg
4. If cytopenia persists 4 weeks and is still unrelated to leukemia, withhold treatment until ANC ≥1 x 10⁹/L and platelets ≥20 x 10⁹/L and then resume treatment at 300mg

ADMINISTRATION
Oral route
Take w/ a meal and a large glass of water.
Do not crush tabs.
Doses of 400mg or 600mg should be administered qd, whereas a dose of 800mg should be administered as 400mg bid. Doses ≥800mg/day should be accomplished using the 400mg tab to reduce iron exposure.
Treatment may be continued as long as there is no evidence of progressive disease or unacceptable toxicity.

Patients Unable to Swallow Tabs
1. Disperse tabs in a glass of water or apple juice.
2. Required number of tabs should be placed in the appropriate volume of beverage (approx 50mL for a 100mg tab and 200mL for a 400mg tab).
3. Stir w/ a spoon and administer immediately after complete disintegration of tab.

STORAGE
25°C (77°F); excursions permitted to 15-30°C (59-86°F). Protect from moisture.

HOW SUPPLIED
Tab: 100mg*, 400mg* *scored

WARNINGS/PRECAUTIONS
Edema and serious fluid retention reported. Hematologic toxicity (eg, anemia/neutropenia/thrombocytopenia) reported; perform CBCs weekly for the 1st month, biweekly for the 2nd month, and periodically thereafter as clinically indicated (eg, every 2-3 months). CHF and left ventricular dysfunction reported; carefully monitor patients w/ cardiac disease or risk factors for cardiac failure or history of renal failure, and evaluate/treat any patient w/ cardiac or renal failure. Hepatotoxicity may occur. Cases of fatal liver failure and severe liver injury requiring liver transplants reported. Grade 3/4 hemorrhages in clinical studies in patients w/ newly diagnosed CML and w/ GIST reported. GI tumor sites may be the source of GI hemorrhages; GI hemorrhage in patients w/ newly diagnosed Ph+ CML reported, and gastric antral vascular ectasia reported. GI irritation/perforation reported. In patients w/ HES w/ occult infiltration of HES cells w/in the myocardium, cases of cardiogenic shock/left ventricular dysfunction have been associated w/ HES cell degranulation upon initiation of therapy; reversible w/ administration of systemic steroids, circulatory support measures, and temporarily withholding treatment. Consider echocardiogram and determination of serum troponin in patients w/ HES/CEL, MDS/MPD, or ASM associated w/ high eosinophil levels; if either is abnormal, consider prophylactic use of systemic steroids (1-2mg/kg) for 1-2 weeks concomitantly at initiation of therapy. Bullous dermatologic reactions, including erythema multiforme and Stevens-Johnson syndrome, reported. May cause fetal harm; sexually active female patients of reproductive potential should use highly effective contraception during treatment and for 14 days after stopping therapy. Growth retardation reported in children and preadolescents; closely monitor growth. Tumor lysis syndrome (TLS) reported in patients w/ CML, GIST, ALL, and eosinophilic leukemia; caution in patients at risk of TLS (those w/ tumors w/ high proliferative rate or high tumor burden prior to treatment), and correct dehydration and treat high uric acid levels prior to initiation of treatment. May impair mental/physical abilities.

ADVERSE REACTIONS
N/V, edema, muscle cramps, musculoskeletal pain, diarrhea, rash, fatigue, headache, abdominal pain.

DRUG INTERACTIONS
See Dosing Considerations. Concomitant administration w/ strong CYP3A4 inducers may reduce total exposure of imatinib; consider alternative agents. Concomitant administration w/ strong CYP3A4 inhibitors may significantly increase imatinib exposure. Grapefruit juice may increase levels; avoid grapefruit juice. Imatinib will increase levels of CYP3A4 substrates (eg, triazolo-benzodiazepines, dihydropyridine calcium channel blockers, certain HMG-CoA reductase inhibitors); caution when administering w/ CYP3A4 substrates that have a narrow therapeutic window. Because warfarin is metabolized by CYP2C9 and CYP3A4, use low-molecular weight or standard heparin instead of warfarin in patients who require anticoagulation. Use caution when administering w/ CYP2D6

substrates that have a narrow therapeutic window. When concomitantly used w/ chemotherapy, liver toxicity reported; monitor hepatic function. Hypothyroidism reported in thyroidectomy patients undergoing levothyroxine replacement; closely monitor TSH levels.

PREGNANCY AND LACTATION
Pregnancy: May cause fetal harm when administered to a pregnant woman. Women should avoid pregnancy during therapy.
Lactation: Imatinib and its active metabolite are excreted into human milk. Not for use in nursing.
Reproductive Potential: Test pregnancy status in females w/ reproductive potential prior to the initiation of treatment. Females of reproductive potential should use effective contraception (methods that result in <1% pregnancy rates) during treatment and for 14 days after stopping treatment.

MECHANISM OF ACTION
Protein-tyrosine kinase inhibitor; inhibits the BCR-ABL tyrosine kinase, the constitutive abnormal tyrosine kinase created by the Philadelphia chromosome abnormality in CML. Inhibits proliferation and induces apoptosis in BCR-ABL positive cell lines as well as fresh leukemic cells from Ph+ CML. Inhibits the receptor tyrosine kinases for PDGF and SCF, c-Kit, and inhibits PDGF- and SCF-mediated cellular events. Inhibits proliferation and induces apoptosis in GIST cells, which express an activating c-Kit mutation, in vitro.

PHARMACOKINETICS
Absorption: Well-absorbed. Absolute bioavailability (98%); T_{max}=2-4 hrs.
Distribution: Plasma protein binding (95%); found in breast milk. **Metabolism:** Liver via CYP3A4 (major), CYP1A2, CYP2D6, CYP2C9, CYP2C19 (minor); N-demethylated piperazine derivative (major active metabolite). **Elimination:** Feces (68%, 20% unchanged), urine (13%, 5% unchanged); $T_{1/2}$=18 hrs (imatinib), 40 hrs (active metabolite).

PATIENT CONSIDERATIONS
Assessment: Assess for cardiac disease, renal impairment, dehydration, high uric acid levels, pregnancy/nursing status, and possible drug interactions. Perform echocardiogram and determine troponin levels in patients w/ HES/CEL and w/ MDS/MPD or ASM associated w/ high eosinophil levels. Obtain baseline CBC and LFTs.

Monitoring: Monitor for signs and symptoms of fluid retention, CHF, left ventricular dysfunction, hemorrhage, GI disorders, TLS, bullous dermatologic reactions, and other adverse events. Perform CBCs weekly for the 1st month, biweekly for the 2nd month, and periodically thereafter. Monitor LFTs monthly or as clinically indicated. Monitor growth in children, and TSH levels in thyroidectomy patients undergoing levothyroxine replacement.

Counseling: Instruct to take drug exactly as prescribed and not to change the dose or to stop taking the medication unless told to do so by physician. Inform of the possibility of developing edema and fluid retention; instruct to contact physician if unexpected rapid weight gain occurs. Inform of the possibility of developing liver function abnormalities and serious hepatic toxicity; instruct to immediately contact physician if signs of liver failure occur (eg, jaundice, anorexia, bleeding, bruising). Advise women of reproductive potential to avoid becoming pregnant and instruct to notify physician if pregnant. Instruct females of reproductive potential to use highly effective contraception during treatment and for 14 days after stopping treatment. Instruct to avoid breastfeeding during treatment and for 1 month after the last dose. Inform that the drug and certain other medicines can interact w/ each other; advise to inform physician if taking/planning to take iron supplements. Advise to avoid grapefruit juice and other foods known to inhibit CYP3A4 while on therapy. Advise that growth retardation has been reported in children and preadolescents, and that growth should be monitored. Caution about driving a car or operating machinery.

GONAL-F — follitropin alfa   Rx
Class: Follicle-stimulating hormone (FSH)

ADULT DOSAGE
Ovulation Induction

Infertile Women w/ Oligo-Anovulation:
Initial: 75 IU/day
Titrate: Incremental adjustments of up to 37.5 IU may be considered after 14 days; may further increase dose, if necessary, every 7 days
Treatment duration should not exceed 35 days unless E2 rise indicates imminent follicular development
Individualize initial dose administered in subsequent cycles based on response of preceding cycle
Max: 300 IU/day

Administer 5000 U of human chorionic gonadotropin (hCG) 1 day after the last dose of Gonal-f; withhold if serum estradiol is >2000pg/mL
D/C therapy if ovaries are abnormally enlarged or abdominal pain occurs

Assisted Reproductive Technology
For development of multiple follicles in ovulatory women

PEDIATRIC DOSAGE
Pediatric use may not have been established

Initial: 150 IU/day starting in the early follicular phase (cycle Day 2 or 3) until sufficient follicular development achieved (should not exceed 10 days)

Suppressed Endogenous Gonadotropin Levels:
Initial: 225 IU/day
Continue treatment until adequate follicular development is indicated
Titrate: Consider dose adjustments after 5 days based on response; do not adjust more frequently than every 3-5 days and by no more than 75-150 IU additionally at each adjustment
Max: 450 IU/day

Administer 5000-10000 U of human chorionic gonadotropin (hCG) once adequate follicular development is evident; withhold in cases where ovaries are abnormally enlarged on the last day of therapy

Induction of Spermatogenesis

In men w/ primary and secondary hypogonadotropic hypogonadism in whom the cause of infertility is not due to primary testicular failure

Pretreatment:
Human Chorionic Gonadotropin (hCG): 1000-2250 U 2-3X per week; continue for a period sufficient to achieve serum testosterone levels w/in the normal range (may require 3-6 months and may need to increase dose)
After normal serum testosterone levels are reached, administer Gonal-f

Usual: 150 IU w/ 1000 U of hCG (or dose required to maintain normal testosterone levels) 3X a week
Duration: May need to administer for up to 18 months
Max: 300 IU 3X a week

ADMINISTRATION
SQ route

Multidose 450 IU Vial:
Dissolve contents w/ 1mL bacteriostatic water for inj (0.9% benzyl alcohol) for a concentration of 600 IU/mL

Multidose 1050 IU Vial:
Dissolve contents w/ 2mL bacteriostatic water for inj (0.9% benzyl alcohol) for a concentration of 600 IU/mL

STORAGE
Before/After Reconstitution: 2-25°C (36-77°F). Protect from light. Discard unused reconstituted sol after 28 days.

HOW SUPPLIED
Inj: 450 IU, 1050 IU [vial]

CONTRAINDICATIONS
Prior hypersensitivity to recombinant FSH preparations or one of their excipients, high follicle-stimulating hormone (FSH) levels indicating primary gonadal failure, uncontrolled thyroid or adrenal dysfunction, sex-hormone-dependent tumors of the reproductive tract and accessory organs, organic intracranial lesions (eg, pituitary tumor). (Women) Abnormal uterine bleeding of undetermined origin, ovarian cyst or enlargement of undetermined origin, pregnancy.

WARNINGS/PRECAUTIONS
Should only be used by physicians thoroughly familiar with infertility problems and management. Uncomplicated ovarian enlargement with abdominal distention and/or abdominal pain may occur; d/c treatment, do not administer hCG, and advise patient not to have intercourse. May cause ovarian hyperstimulation syndrome (OHSS) with or without pulmonary or vascular complications. Hepatic dysfunction reported in association with OHSS. Withhold hCG if evidence of OHSS develops prior to hCG administration. Monitor patients for at least 2 weeks after hCG administration; d/c treatment and hospitalize patient if severe OHSS occurs. Serious pulmonary conditions (eg, atelectasis, acute respiratory distress syndrome, exacerbation of asthma), thromboembolic events (both in association with, and separate from, OHSS), and multiple births reported. In infertile patients with oligo-anovulation, the couple should be encouraged to have intercourse daily, beginning on the day prior to administration of hCG until ovulation becomes apparent. Patients with tubal obstruction should receive therapy only if enrolled in an in vitro fertilization program. Evaluation of partner's fertility potential must be conducted prior to initiation.

ADVERSE REACTIONS
Breast pain, acne, inj-site pain, fatigue. (Women) Intermenstrual bleeding, ovarian hyperstimulation, abdominal pain, nausea, diarrhea, flatulence, headache, ovarian cysts, pain, upper respiratory tract infection. (Men) Gynecomastia.

PREGNANCY AND LACTATION
Category X, not for use in nursing.

MECHANISM OF ACTION
FSH; stimulates ovarian follicular growth in women who do not have primary ovarian failure. Stimulates spermatogenesis in men with hypogonadotropic hypogonadism when administered with hCG.

PHARMACOKINETICS
Absorption: Administration of variable doses resulted in different parameters.

PATIENT CONSIDERATIONS
Assessment: Assess for prior hypersensitivity to drug, primary gonadal/testicular failure, uncontrolled thyroid or adrenal dysfunction, sex-hormone-dependent tumors of the reproductive tract and accessory organs, organic intracranial lesions, abnormal uterine bleeding, ovarian cysts or enlargement, tubal obstruction, partner's fertility potential, pregnancy/nursing status, and any conditions where drug is cautioned. Perform thorough gynecologic/endocrinologic/medical evaluation, including pelvic anatomy assessment. Obtain baseline FSH, gonadotropin, and serum testosterone levels. Refer to PI for patient selection process.

Monitoring: Monitor for OHSS, pulmonary/vascular complications, ovarian enlargement, abdominal pain, and other adverse reactions. Monitor ovarian response with serum estradiol and vaginal ultrasound regularly. A follow-up visit should be conducted in the luteal phase. Confirm ovulation by direct and indirect indices of progesterone production and by sonographic visualization of the ovaries.

Counseling: Inform about duration of treatment and the required monitoring of the condition. Counsel about possibility of multiple births, risk of OHSS, and other adverse reactions. In infertile patients with oligo-anovulation, encourage to have intercourse daily, beginning on the day prior to administration of hCG until ovulation becomes apparent. If ovaries become abnormally enlarged or abdominal pain occurs, advise patient not to have intercourse and to consult physician.

GONAL-F RFF — follitropin alfa   Rx

Class: Follicle-stimulating hormone (FSH)

ADULT DOSAGE

Ovulation Induction

Infertile Women w/ Oligo-Anovulation:
Initial: 75 IU/day for 1st cycle
Titrate: Incremental adjustments of up to 37.5 IU may be considered after 14 days; may further increase dose, if necessary, every 7 days
Treatment duration should not exceed 35 days unless E2 rise indicates imminent follicular development
Administer human chorionic gonadotropin (hCG) after the last dose of follitropin alfa; withhold if serum estradiol is >2000pg/mL
Do not administer hCG and d/c therapy if ovaries are abnormally enlarged or abdominal pain occurs
Max: 300 IU/day

Assisted Reproductive Technology

For development of multiple follicles in ovulatory women

Initial: 150 IU/day starting in the early follicular phase (cycle day 2 or 3) until sufficient follicular development is attained (should not exceed 10 days)
<35 Years w/ Suppressed Endogenous Gonadotropin Levels:
Initial: 150 IU/day
≥35 Years w/ Suppressed Endogenous Gonadotropin Levels:
Initial: 225 IU/day
Continue treatment until adequate follicular development is indicated

Titrate: Adjust dose after 5 days based on response; do not adjust more frequently than every 3-5 days and by no more than 75-150 IU additionally at each adjustment
Max: 450 IU/day

Administer human chorionic gonadotropin once adequate follicular development is evident; withhold in cases where ovaries are abnormally enlarged on the last day of therapy

PEDIATRIC DOSAGE
Pediatric use may not have been established

ADMINISTRATION
SQ route

Pen
Administer SQ in the abdomen

Inj
Dissolve contents of ≥1 single-dose vials in 1mL of sterile water for inj; concentration should not exceed 450 IU/mL
Administer SQ immediately
Discard any unused reconstituted material

STORAGE
Pen: Prior To Dispensing: 2-8°C (36-46°F). Upon Dispensing: 2-8°C (36-46°F) until expiration date or 20-25°C (68-77°F) for up to 3 months or until expiration date, whichever comes first. After 1st Inj: 2-8°C (36-46°F) or 20-25°C (68-77°F) for up to 28 days. Protect from light. Do not freeze. Discard unused material after 28 days. Vial: 2-25°C (36-77°F). Protect from light. Use immediately after reconstitution. Discard unused material.

HOW SUPPLIED
Inj: 75 IU [vial]; 300 IU/0.5mL, 450 IU/0.75mL, 900 IU/1.5mL [prefilled pen]

CONTRAINDICATIONS
High follicle-stimulating hormone (FSH) levels indicating primary gonadal failure, uncontrolled thyroid or adrenal dysfunction, sex-hormone-dependent tumors of the reproductive tract and accessory organs, organic intracranial lesion (eg, pituitary tumor), abnormal uterine bleeding of undetermined origin, ovarian cyst or enlargement of undetermined origin, pregnancy.

WARNINGS/PRECAUTIONS
Should only be used by physicians thoroughly familiar with infertility problems and their management. Uncomplicated ovarian enlargement with abdominal distention and/or abdominal pain may occur; d/c treatment, do not administer hCG, and advise patient not to have intercourse. May cause ovarian hyperstimulation syndrome (OHSS) with or without pulmonary or vascular complications. Hepatic dysfunction reported in association with OHSS. Withhold hCG if evidence of OHSS develops prior to hCG administration. Monitor patients for at least 2 weeks after hCG administration; d/c treatment and hospitalize patient if severe OHSS occurs. Serious pulmonary conditions (eg, atelectasis, acute respiratory distress syndrome, and exacerbation of asthma), thromboembolic events (both associated with and separate from OHSS), and multiple births reported. In infertile patients with oligo-anovulation, the couple should be encouraged to have intercourse daily, beginning on the day prior to administration of hCG until ovulation becomes apparent from the indices employed for determination of progestational activity. Patients with tubal obstruction should receive therapy only if enrolled in an in vitro fertilization program. Evaluation of partner's fertility potential must be conducted prior to initiation of therapy.

ADVERSE REACTIONS
Vaginal hemorrhage, abdomen enlargement, ovarian cyst, ovarian hyperstimulation, abdominal pain, breast pain, diarrhea, flatulence, headache, pharyngitis, rhinitis, sinusitis, nausea, inj-site bruising/pain.

PREGNANCY AND LACTATION
Category X, not for use in nursing.

MECHANISM OF ACTION
FSH; stimulates ovarian follicular growth in women who do not have primary ovarian failure.

PHARMACOKINETICS
Absorption: C_{max}=9.83 IU/L; T_{max}=15.5 hrs; AUC=884 IU•hr/L. **Elimination:** $T_{1/2}$=53 hrs.

PATIENT CONSIDERATIONS
Assessment: Assess for prior hypersensitivity to drug, primary gonadal failure, uncontrolled thyroid or adrenal dysfunction, sex-hormone-dependent tumors of the reproductive tract and accessory organs, organic intracranial lesions, abnormal uterine bleeding or other signs of endometrial abnormalities, ovarian cysts or enlargement, tubal obstruction, and for any other conditions where treatment is contraindicated or cautioned. Assess pregnancy/nursing status and partner's fertility potential. Perform thorough gynecologic/endocrinologic evaluation, including pelvic anatomy assessment. Obtain baseline FSH and gonadotropin levels.

Monitoring: Monitor for OHSS, pulmonary/vascular complications, ovarian enlargement, abdominal pain, and other adverse reactions. Monitor ovarian response with serum estradiol and vaginal ultrasound regularly. In infertile patients with oligo-anovulation, conduct a follow-up visit in the luteal phase. Confirm ovulation by direct and indirect indices of progesterone production and by sonographic visualization of the ovaries.

Counseling: Inform about duration of treatment and the required monitoring of the condition. Counsel about possibility of multiple births, risk of OHSS, and other adverse reactions. In infertile patients with oligo-anovulation, encourage to have intercourse daily, beginning on the day prior to administration of hCG until ovulation becomes apparent. If ovaries become abnormally enlarged or abdominal pain occurs, advise patient not to have intercourse and to consult physician.

GONAL-F RFF REDI-JECT — follitropin alfa   Rx

Class: Follicle-stimulating hormone (FSH)

ADULT DOSAGE

Ovulation Induction

Initial: (1st Cycle) 75 IU/day SQ for 14 days. Individualize initial dose in subsequent cycles based on history of ovarian response to therapy
Titrate: If indicated by ovarian response, an incremental dose adjustments of up to 37.5 IU may be considered after initial 14 days. If indicated by the ovarian response, make additional incremental adjustments in dose, up to 37.5 IU, every 7 days
Max: 300 IU/day. Do not exceed 35 days of treatment

Continue treatment until follicular growth and/or serum estradiol levels indicate an adequate ovarian response. When pre-ovulatory conditions are reached, administer human chorionic gonadotropin (hCG) to induce final oocyte maturation and ovulation. Withhold hCG in cases where the ovarian monitoring suggests an increased risk of ovarian hyperstimulation syndrome on the last day of therapy

Assisted Reproductive Technology

Initial: 150 IU/day SQ on cycle Day 2 or 3 until sufficient follicular development is attained. Do not exceed 10 days

Suppressed Endogenous Gonadotropin Levels:

Initial:
<35 Years: 150 IU/day SQ
≥35 Years: 225 IU/day SQ

Titrate: Adjust after 5 days based on ovarian response. Do not make additional dose adjustments more frequently than every 3-5 days or by more than 75-150 IU at each adjustment

Continue treatment until adequate follicular development is evident, and then administer hCG. Administration of hCG should be withheld in cases where ovarian monitoring suggests increased risk of ovarian hyperstimulation syndrome on last day of therapy
Max: 450 IU/day

PEDIATRIC DOSAGE
Pediatric use may not have been established

ADMINISTRATION
SQ route

Inject in the abdomen
Do not attempt to mix any other medications inside of the device
Do not shake
Remove from refrigerator at least 30 min prior to use

STORAGE
Prior to Dispensing: 2-8°C (36-46°F). Upon Dispensing: 2-8°C (36-46°F) until expiration date, or 20-25°C (68-77°F) for up to 3 months or until expiration date, whichever comes 1st. After 1st Inj: 2-8°C (36-46°F) or 20-25°C (68-77°F) for up to 28 days. Protect from light. Do not freeze. Discard unused material after 28 days.

HOW SUPPLIED
Inj: 300 IU/0.5mL, 450 IU/0.75mL, 900 IU/1.5mL

CONTRAINDICATIONS
Prior hypersensitivity to recombinant FSH products, high follicle-stimulating hormone (FSH) levels indicating primary gonadal failure, pregnancy, presence of uncontrolled non-gonadal endocrinopathies (eg, thyroid, adrenal, pituitary disorders), sex hormone dependent tumors of the reproductive tract and accessory organs, tumors of pituitary gland or hypothalamus, abnormal uterine bleeding of undetermined origin, ovarian cyst or enlargement of undetermined origin (not due to polycystic ovary syndrome).

WARNINGS/PRECAUTIONS
Should only be used by physicians who are experienced in infertility treatment. Serious systemic hypersensitivity reactions (eg, anaphylaxis) reported; d/c if an anaphylactic or other serious allergic reaction occurs and initiate appropriate therapy. Abnormal ovarian enlargement may occur; individualize treatment and use lowest effective dose. Prohibit intercourse in women with significant ovarian enlargement after ovulation because of danger of hemoperitoneum resulting from rupture of ovarian cysts. May cause ovarian hyperstimulation syndrome (OHSS). Transient liver function test abnormalities suggestive of hepatic dysfunction with or without morphologic changes on liver biopsy reported in association with OHSS. Withhold hCG if evidence of OHSS develops prior to hCG administration. Assess for the development of OHSS for at least 2 weeks after hCG administration; d/c and consider hospitalizing patient if serious OHSS occurs. Serious pulmonary conditions (eg, atelectasis, acute respiratory distress syndrome, exacerbation of asthma), thromboembolic events, ovarian torsion, and multi-fetal gestation/births reported. Incidence of congenital malformations after some ART may be slightly higher than after spontaneous conception. Incidence of ectopic pregnancy may be increased in women undergoing ART; early confirmation of intrauterine pregnancy should be determined by β-hCG testing and transvaginal ultrasound. Increased risk of spontaneous abortion. Infrequent reports of ovarian neoplasms, both benign and malignant, reported in women who have had multiple drug therapy for controlled ovarian stimulation.

ADVERSE REACTIONS
Headache, abdominal pain, nausea, flatulence, diarrhea, ovarian cyst, ovarian hyperstimulation, inj-site pain/bruising/inflammation/reaction, abdominal enlargement.

PREGNANCY AND LACTATION
Category X, not for use in nursing.

MECHANISM OF ACTION
FSH; stimulates ovarian follicular growth in women who do not have primary ovarian failure.

PHARMACOKINETICS
Absorption: C_{max}=9.83 IU/L; T_{max}=15.5 hrs; AUC_{last}=884 IU•hr/L. **Elimination:** $T_{1/2}$=53 hrs.

PATIENT CONSIDERATIONS

Assessment: Assess for prior hypersensitivity to recombinant FSH products, primary gonadal failure, uncontrolled non-gonadal endocrinopathies, sex hormone dependent tumors of the reproductive tract and accessory organs, tumors of pituitary gland/hypothalamus, abnormal uterine bleeding of undetermined origin, ovarian cysts or enlargement of undetermined origin, pregnancy status, any other conditions where treatment is contraindicated or cautioned, nursing status, and male partner's fertility potential. Perform complete gynecologic/endocrinologic evaluation, and diagnose the cause of infertility.

Monitoring: Monitor for hypersensitivity, ovarian enlargement, OHSS, pulmonary conditions, thromboembolic events, ovarian torsion, multi-fetal gestation/births, congenital malformations, ectopic pregnancy, spontaneous abortion, ovarian neoplasms, and other adverse reactions. Monitor for signs of ovulation and ovarian response.

Counseling: Instruct on the correct usage and dosing of therapy; caution not to change dosage or the schedule of administration unless instructed by the physician. Prior to beginning therapy, inform about the time commitment and monitoring procedures necessary for treatment. Advise not to double the next dose if the dose is missed, and to contact healthcare provider for further dosing instructions. Inform about the risks of OHSS and OHSS-associated symptoms including lung and blood vessel problems, and the possibility of multi-fetal gestation and birth. Encourage patients being treated for ovulation induction, to have intercourse daily, beginning on the day prior to administration of hCG and until ovulation becomes apparent. Advise not to have intercourse if ovaries become abnormally enlarged or when the risk for OHSS is increased.

GRANIX — tbo-filgrastim   Rx

Class: Granulocyte colony-stimulating factor (G-CSF)

ADULT DOSAGE

Chemotherapy-Associated Neutropenia

Reducing the Duration of Severe Neutropenia in Patients w/ Non-Myeloid Malignancies Receiving Myelosuppressive Anticancer Drugs:
5mcg/kg/day SQ

Continue daily dosing until the expected neutrophil nadir is passed and the neutrophil count has recovered to the normal range

PEDIATRIC DOSAGE
Pediatric use may not have been established

ADMINISTRATION
SQ route

Administer the 1st dose no earlier than 24 hrs following myelosuppressive chemotherapy; do not administer w/in 24 hrs prior to chemotherapy.
Prefilled syringes are for single use only; discard unused portions.
Recommended sites of administration include abdomen (except for the 2-inch area around the navel), the front of the middle thighs, the upper outer areas of the buttocks, or the upper back portion of the upper arms.
Vary inj site daily.
Do not inject into an area that is tender, red, bruised, hard, or that has scars or stretch marks.
Avoid shaking syringe.

STORAGE
2-8°C (36-46°F). Protect from light. May be removed from 2-8°C (36-46°F) storage for a single period of up to 5 days between 23-27°C (73-81°F); if not used w/in 5 days, may be returned to 2-8°C (36-46°F).

HOW SUPPLIED
Inj: 300mcg/0.5mL, 480mcg/0.8mL

WARNINGS/PRECAUTIONS
May be administered by either a healthcare professional or by a patient/caregiver; before a decision is made to allow therapy to be administered by a patient/caregiver, ensure that the patient is an appropriate candidate for self-administration or administration by a caregiver. Splenic rupture, including fatal cases, may occur; d/c therapy and evaluate for an enlarged spleen or splenic rupture if upper abdominal or shoulder pain occurs. Acute respiratory distress syndrome (ARDS) may occur; evaluate for ARDS if fever and lung infiltrates or respiratory distress develops, and d/c if ARDS occurs. Serious allergic reactions may occur; permanently d/c if such reactions occur. Severe and sometimes fatal sickle cell crises may occur in patients w/ sickle cell disease; d/c in patients undergoing a sickle cell crisis. Capillary leak syndrome (CLS) may occur; closely monitor and give standard symptomatic treatment if symptoms develop. May act as a growth factor for any tumor type. Increased hematopoietic activity of the bone marrow in response to therapy has been associated w/ transient positive bone imaging changes; consider this when interpreting bone-imaging results.

ADVERSE REACTIONS
Bone pain.

DRUG INTERACTIONS
Caution w/ drugs that may potentiate the release of neutrophils (eg, lithium).

PREGNANCY AND LACTATION
Pregnancy: Category C.
Lactation: Caution in nursing.

MECHANISM OF ACTION
Granulocyte colony-stimulating factor (G-CSF); binds to G-CSF receptors and stimulates proliferation of neutrophils. Known to stimulate differentiation commitment and some end-cell functional activation, which increases neutrophil counts and activity.

PHARMACOKINETICS
Absorption: Absolute bioavailability (33%); T_{max}=4-6 hrs (median). **Elimination:** $T_{1/2}$=3.2-3.8 hrs (median).

PATIENT CONSIDERATIONS

Assessment: Assess for history of hypersensitivity to the drug, history of serious allergic reactions to filgrastim or pegfilgrastim, sickle cell disease, pregnancy/nursing status, and possible drug interactions. Assess CBC prior to chemotherapy.

Monitoring: Monitor for enlarged spleen/splenic rupture, ARDS, serious allergic reactions, sickle cell crisis (in patients w/ sickle cell disease), CLS, and other adverse reactions. Monitor CBC twice per week until recovery.

Counseling: Instruct patient or caregivers on the proper storage, preparation, and administration technique once it is determined that a patient is an appropriate candidate for self-administration or administration by a caregiver. Instruct to report any symptoms of adverse reactions to physician. Inform that bone pain is common and analgesics may be necessary. Counsel to be alert for signs of infection and to report these findings to physician immediately. Inform not to become pregnant while on therapy; advise of the possibility of fetal harm if pregnancy occurs.

H.P. Acthar Gel — *corticotropin*   Rx

Class: Corticosteroid

ADULT DOSAGE

Multiple Sclerosis

Acute Exacerbations:
80-120 U/day IM/SQ for 2-3 weeks

May be necessary to taper dose and increase inj interval to gradually d/c

Other Indications

Usual: 40-80 U IM/SQ q24-72h
May be necessary to taper dose and increase inj interval to gradually d/c

Rheumatic Disorders:
Adjunctive therapy for short-term administration in psoriatic arthritis, rheumatoid arthritis (including juvenile), and ankylosing spondylitis

Collagen Diseases:
Treatment during an exacerbation or as maint in cases of systemic lupus erythematosus and polymyositis

Dermatologic Diseases:
Severe erythema multiforme and Stevens-Johnson syndrome

Allergic States:
Serum sickness

Ophthalmic Diseases:
Treatment of severe acute and chronic allergic and inflammatory processes (eg, keratitis, iritis, iridocyclitis, diffuse posterior uveitis and choroiditis, optic neuritis, chorioretinitis, anterior segment inflammation)

Respiratory Diseases:
Symptomatic sarcoidosis

Edematous State:
Induces a diuresis or a remission of proteinuria in the nephrotic syndrome w/o uremia of the idiopathic type or that is due to lupus erythematosus

PEDIATRIC DOSAGE

Infantile Spasms

<2 Years:
75 U/m² bid IM for 2 weeks
Gradually taper dose over a 2-week period

Tapering Schedule:
30 U/m² qam for 3 days; 15 U/m² qam for 3 days; 10 U/m² qam for 3 days; and 10 U/m² every other am for 6 days

Other Indications

<2 Years:
Usual: 40-80 U IM/SQ q24-72h
May be necessary to taper dose and increase inj interval to gradually d/c

Rheumatic Disorders:
Adjunctive therapy for short-term administration in psoriatic arthritis, rheumatoid arthritis (including juvenile), and ankylosing spondylitis

Collagen Diseases:
Treatment during an exacerbation or as maint in cases of systemic lupus erythematosus and polymyositis

Dermatologic Diseases:
Severe erythema multiforme and Stevens-Johnson syndrome

Allergic States:
Serum sickness

Ophthalmic Diseases:
Treatment of severe acute and chronic allergic and inflammatory processes (eg, keratitis, iritis, iridocyclitis, diffuse posterior uveitis and choroiditis, optic neuritis, chorioretinitis, anterior segment inflammation)

Respiratory Diseases:
Symptomatic sarcoidosis

Edematous State:
Induces a diuresis or a remission of proteinuria in the nephrotic syndrome w/o uremia of the idiopathic type or that is due to lupus erythematosus

---

ADMINISTRATION
IM/SQ route
Warm to room temperature before use.
Do not over-pressurize vial prior to withdrawing.

STORAGE
2-8°C (36-46°F).

HOW SUPPLIED
Inj: 80 U/mL [5mL]

CONTRAINDICATIONS
IV administration; administration of live or live attenuated vaccines in patients receiving immunosuppressive doses; suspected congenital infection in infants; patients w/ scleroderma, osteoporosis, systemic fungal infections, ocular herpes simplex, recent surgery, history or presence of a peptic ulcer, CHF, uncontrolled HTN, primary adrenocortical insufficiency, adrenocortical hyperfunction, or sensitivity to proteins of porcine origin.

WARNINGS/PRECAUTIONS
May increase risks of infection (eg, viral, bacterial, fungal, protozoan/helminthic); monitor patients w/ latent tuberculosis (TB) or tuberculin reactivity closely, and institute chemoprophylaxis if therapy is prolonged. May cause hypothalnegativeamic-pituitary-axis (HPA) suppression and Cushing's syndrome; monitor w/ chronic use. HPA suppression may occur following prolonged therapy w/ the potential for adrenal insufficiency after withdrawal; symptoms of adrenal insufficiency in infants treated for infantile spasms may be difficult to identify. Taper dose upon discontinuation of treatment to minimize adrenal insufficiency. May cause BP elevation, salt and water retention, and increased K⁺ and Ca²⁺ excretion; dietary salt restriction and K⁺ supplementation may be necessary. Caution w/ HTN, CHF, or renal insufficiency. Killed or inactivated vaccines may be administered; however, response to such vaccines cannot be predicted. Caution w/ other immunization procedures, especially if on high doses; possible hazards of neurological complications and a lack of antibody response. May mask symptoms of other diseases/disorders w/o altering the course of other disease/disorder. May cause GI bleeding and gastric ulcer. Increased risk for perforation in patients w/ certain GI disorders; caution where there is the possibility of impending perforation, abscess or other pyogenic infections, diverticulitis, fresh intestinal anastomoses, and active or latent peptic ulcer. May be associated w/ CNS effects (eg, euphoria, insomnia, mood swings, personality changes, severe depression, frank psychotic manifestations). May aggravate existing emotional instability and psychotic tendencies. May cause worsening of comorbid disease; caution w/ diabetes and myasthenia gravis. Prolonged use may produce posterior subcapsular cataracts, glaucoma w/ possible damage to optic nerves, and enhance establishment of secondary ocular infections. Potential for immunogenicity; prolonged use may increase the risk of a hypersensitivity reaction. Enhanced effect in patients w/ hypothyroidism or liver cirrhosis. Long-term use may have negative effects on growth and physical development in children, and may change their appetite. May decrease bone formation, increase bone resorption, and inhibit osteoblast function, which may lead to inhibition of bone growth in pediatrics and adolescents and development of osteoporosis at any age; caution w/ increased risk of osteoporosis (eg, postmenopausal women). Shown to have an embryocidal effect.

ADVERSE REACTIONS
Fluid retention, alteration in glucose tolerance, BP elevation, behavioral and mood changes, increased appetite, weight gain.

DRUG INTERACTIONS
See Contraindications. May accentuate the electrolyte loss associated w/ diuretic therapy.

PREGNANCY AND LACTATION
Category C, not for use in nursing.

MECHANISM OF ACTION
Adrenocorticotropic hormone; mechanism in treatment of infantile spasms is unknown. Stimulates the adrenal cortex to secrete cortisol, corticosterone, aldosterone, and a number of weakly androgenic substances. Also reported to bind to melanocortin receptors.

PHARMACOKINETICS
Elimination: (IV) $T_{1/2}$=15 min.

PATIENT CONSIDERATIONS

Assessment: Assess for congenital infection in infants, scleroderma, osteoporosis, systemic fungal infections, ocular herpes simplex, recent surgery, history or presence of a peptic ulcer, CHF, uncontrolled HTN, primary adrenocortical insufficiency, adrenocortical hyperfunction, sensitivity to proteins of porcine origin, latent TB or tuberculin reactivity, renal insufficiency, pregnancy/nursing status, and for any other conditions where treatment is contraindicated or cautioned. Assess for possible drug interactions.

Monitoring: Monitor during and for a period following discontinuation of therapy for signs of infection, abnormal cardiac function, HTN, hyperglycemia, change in body weight, and fecal blood loss. Monitor for signs/symptoms HPA suppression, Cushing's syndrome, adrenal insufficiency, hypokalemia, GI bleeding and perforation, behavioral and mood disturbances, aggravation of emotional instability or psychotic tendencies, cataracts, glaucoma, worsening of comorbid diseases, hypersensitivity reactions, for other adverse reactions. Monitor growth and physical development of pediatric patients on prolonged therapy. Monitor bone density in patients on long-term therapy.

Counseling: Instruct to take medication as prescribed and not to d/c suddenly unless instructed by physician. Inform of the importance of careful monitoring while on therapy and during treatment titration. Advise to contact physician if infection or fever, BP elevation, blood in the stool, or a change in color of the stool develops. Instruct to limit contact w/ other people w/ infections while on therapy. Inform caregivers and families of infants and children that irritability and sleep disturbances may occur, but are reversible once therapy is discontinued. Inform patient, caregivers, and families that changes in appetite may occur, but are reversible once therapy is discontinued. Instruct patient, parents, and caregivers to monitor for signs/symptoms of adrenal insufficiency after treatment discontinuation, and to observe for and recognize these symptoms in infants. Advise patients not to be vaccinated w/ live or live attenuated vaccines, and that other immunization procedures in patient or in a family member who will be in contact w/ the patient, should be undertaken w/ caution during therapy. Advise patients, their caregivers, and families that prolonged use in children may result in Cushing's syndrome and associated adverse reactions, may inhibit skeletal growth, and may cause osteoporosis and decreased bone density. Inform that therapy may mask symptoms of other diseases/disorders w/o altering the course of the other disease/disorder. Instruct parents and caregivers of infants treated for infantile spasms to notify physician of any new onset of seizures. Apprise women of potential harm to the fetus.

Halaven — eribulin mesylate   Rx

Class: Antimicrotubule agent

ADULT DOSAGE	PEDIATRIC DOSAGE
Metastatic Breast Cancer	Pediatric use may not have been established
Treatment of patients who have previously received at least 2 chemotherapeutic regimens (anthracycline and a taxane in adjuvant/metastatic setting) for the treatment of metastatic disease	
Recommended: 1.4mg/m²	
Administer IV over 2-5 min on Days 1 and 8 of a 21-day cycle	
Unresectable or Metastatic Liposarcoma	
Treatment of patients who have received a prior anthracycline-containing regimen	
Recommended: 1.4mg/m²	
Administer IV over 2-5 min on Days 1 and 8 of a 21-day cycle	

DOSING CONSIDERATIONS

Renal Impairment
Moderate to Severe (CrCl 15-49mL/min):
1.1mg/m²

Hepatic Impairment
Mild (Child-Pugh A):
1.1mg/m²

Moderate (Child-Pugh B):
0.7mg/m²

Adverse Reactions
Do Not Administer on Day 1 or Day 8 for Any of the Following:
ANC <1000/mm³
Platelets <75,000/mm³
Grade 3 or 4 nonhematological toxicities

The Day 8 Dose May Be Delayed for a Maximum of 1 Week:
If toxicities do not resolve or improve to <Grade 2 severity by Day 15, omit the dose.
If toxicities resolve or improve to <Grade 2 severity by Day 15, administer at a reduced dose and initiate the next cycle no sooner than 2 weeks later.

Permanently Reduce to 1.1mg/m² for Any of the Following:
ANC <500/mm³ for >7 days

ANC <1000/mm³ w/ fever or infection
Platelets <25,000/mm³
Platelets <50,000/mm³ requiring transfusion
Nonhematologic Grade 3 or 4 toxicities
Omission or delay of Day 8 dose in previous cycle for toxicity

Reduce to 0.7mg/m² If:
Occurrence of any event requiring permanent dose reduction while receiving 1.1mg/m²

D/C If:
Occurrence of any event requiring permanent dose reduction while receiving 0.7mg/m²

If a dose has been delayed for toxicity and toxicities have recovered to <Grade 2, resume at a reduced dose.
Do not re-escalate dose after it has been reduced.

ADMINISTRATION
IV route

Withdraw required amount of eribulin from the single use vial and administer undiluted or diluted in 100mL of 0.9% NaCl inj.
Do not dilute in or administer through an IV line containing sol w/ dextrose.
Do not administer in the same IV line concurrent w/ other medicinal products.
Store undiluted eribulin in the syringe for up to 4 hrs at room temperature or for up to 24 hrs under refrigeration (4°C [40°F]).
Store diluted sol of eribulin for up to 4 hrs at room temperature or up to 24 hrs under refrigeration.

STORAGE
25°C (77°F); excursions permitted to 15-30°C (59-86°F). Do not freeze.

HOW SUPPLIED
Inj: 0.5mg/mL [2mL]

WARNINGS/PRECAUTIONS
See Dosing Considerations. Severe neutropenia (ANC <500/mm³) reported. Peripheral neuropathy reported. Can cause fetal harm. QT prolongation reported; monitor ECG in patients w/ CHF, bradyarrhythmias, and electrolyte abnormalities. Correct hypokalemia or hypomagnesemia prior to therapy. Avoid w/ congenital long QT syndrome.

ADVERSE REACTIONS
Metastatic Breast Cancer: Neutropenia, anemia, asthenia/fatigue, alopecia, peripheral neuropathy, nausea, constipation.
Liposarcoma: Fatigue, nausea, alopecia, constipation, peripheral neuropathy, abdominal pain, pyrexia.

DRUG INTERACTIONS
Monitor ECG w/ drugs known to prolong the QT interval (eg, Class IA and III antiarrhythmics).

PREGNANCY AND LACTATION
Pregnancy: Can cause fetal harm based on findings from an animal reproduction study and mechanism of action. Advise pregnant women of the potential risk to fetus.
Lactation: There is no information regarding the presence of eribulin or its metabolites in human milk, the effects on the breastfed infant, or the effects on milk production. Advise women not to breastfeed during treatment and for 2 weeks after the final dose.
Reproductive Potential: Advise females of reproductive potential to use effective contraception during treatment and for at least 2 weeks following the final dose. Advise males w/ female partners of reproductive potential to use effective contraception during treatment and for 3.5 months following the final dose. May result in damage to male reproductive tissues leading to impaired fertility of unknown duration.

MECHANISM OF ACTION
Antimicrotubule agent; inhibits the growth phase of microtubules via a tubulin-based antimitotic mechanism leading to G_2/M cell-cycle block, disruption of mitotic spindles, and, ultimately, apoptotic cell death after prolonged mitotic blockage.

PHARMACOKINETICS
Distribution: V_d=43-114L/m²; plasma protein binding (49-65%). **Elimination:** Urine (9%, 91% unchanged), feces (82%, 88% unchanged); $T_{1/2}$=40 hrs.

PATIENT CONSIDERATIONS
Assessment: Assess for renal/hepatic impairment, CHF, bradyarrhythmias, congenital long QT syndrome, electrolyte abnormalities, pregnancy/nursing status, and possible drug interactions. Correct hypokalemia or hypomagnesemia prior to initiating therapy. Assess for peripheral neuropathy and obtain CBC prior to each dose.

Monitoring: Monitor for severe neutropenia, peripheral motor and sensory neuropathy, and other adverse reactions. Monitor ECG in patients w/ CHF, bradyarrhythmias, and electrolyte abnormalities. Monitor K^+ and Mg^{2+} levels periodically. Increase frequency of CBC monitoring if Grade 3 or 4 cytopenias develop.

Counseling: Advise to contact physician for a fever ≥38.1°C (100.5°F) or other signs/symptoms of infection (eg, chills, cough, burning/pain on urination). Advise to inform physician of new/worsening numbness, tingling, and pain in the extremities. Advise females of reproductive potential of the potential risk to a fetus, to inform physician of known/suspected pregnancy, and to use effective contraception during treatment and for at least 2 weeks after the final dose. Advise males w/ female partners of reproductive potential to use effective contraception during treatment and for 3.5 months following the final dose. Advise women not to breastfeed during treatment and for 2 weeks after the final dose.

HARVONI — ledipasvir/sofosbuvir   Rx

Class: HCV NS5A inhibitor/HCV nucleotide analogue NS5B polymerase inhibitor

ADULT DOSAGE

Chronic Hepatitis C

Chronic HCV Genotype 1, 4, 5, or 6 Infection:
1 tab qd w/ or w/o ribavirin

Treatment Duration:

Genotype 1:
Treatment-Naive w/o Cirrhosis or w/ Compensated Cirrhosis (Child-Pugh A): 12 weeks; may consider treatment duration of 8 weeks in patients w/o cirrhosis who have pre-treatment HCV RNA <6 mIU/mL
Treatment-Experienced w/o Cirrhosis: 12 weeks
Treatment-Experienced w/ Compensated Cirrhosis: 24 weeks; may consider Harvoni + ribavirin for 12 weeks in patients w/ cirrhosis who are eligible for ribavirin
Treatment-Naive and Treatment-Experienced w/ Decompensated Cirrhosis (Child-Pugh B or C): Harvoni + ribavirin for 12 weeks

Genotype 1 or 4:
Treatment-Naive and Treatment-Experienced Liver Transplant Recipients w/o Cirrhosis, or w/ Compensated Cirrhosis: Harvoni + ribavirin for 12 weeks

Genotype 4, 5, or 6:
Treatment-Naive and Treatment-Experienced w/o Cirrhosis or w/ Compensated Cirrhosis: 12 weeks

The recommended treatment durations are also applicable to patients w/ HCV/HIV-1 coinfection

For further information on ribavirin dosing and dosing modifications, refer to the ribavirin PI

PEDIATRIC DOSAGE
Pediatric use may not have been established

DOSING CONSIDERATIONS
Renal Impairment
Mild/Moderate: No dosage adjustment required
Severe/ESRD: No dosage recommendation can be given due to higher exposures of the predominant sofosbuvir metabolite

ADMINISTRATION
Oral route
Take w/ or w/o food.

STORAGE
Room temperature <30°C (86°F).

HOW SUPPLIED
Tab: (Ledipasvir/Sofosbuvir) 90mg/400mg

CONTRAINDICATIONS
If administered w/ ribavirin, refer to the ribavirin prescribing information for a list of contraindications for ribavirin.

WARNINGS/PRECAUTIONS
Symptomatic bradycardia, as well as fatal cardiac arrest and cases requiring pacemaker intervention, reported when coadministered w/ amiodarone. Patients also taking β-blockers, or those w/ underlying cardiac comorbidities and/or advanced liver disease, may be at increased risk for symptomatic bradycardia w/ coadministration of amiodarone. Not recommended w/ amiodarone. If coadministration is required, cardiac monitoring in an in-patient setting for the first 48 hrs of coadministration is recommended, after which outpatient or self-monitoring of HR should occur on a daily basis through at least the first 2 weeks of therapy. Patients discontinuing amiodarone just prior to starting therapy should also undergo similar cardiac monitoring. P-gp inducers (eg, rifampin, St. John's wort) may decrease levels and may lead to a reduced therapeutic effect; not recommended w/ P-gp inducers. Not recommended w/ other products containing sofosbuvir. If administered w/ ribavirin, refer to the ribavirin prescribing information for the warnings and precautions for ribavirin.

ADVERSE REACTIONS
Fatigue, headache, asthenia.

DRUG INTERACTIONS
See Warnings/Precautions. Not recommended w/ carbamazepine, phenytoin, phenobarbital, oxcarbazepine, rifabutin, rifapentine, or tipranavir/ritonavir (RTV); may decrease levels. Not recommended w/ rosuvastatin; may increase rosuvastatin levels and consequently increase risk of myopathy, including rhabdomyolysis. May increase digoxin levels; monitor digoxin levels. Monitor for tenofovir-associated adverse reactions in patients receiving concomitant therapy w/ a regimen containing tenofovir disoproxil fumarate (TDF) w/o an HIV protease inhibitor/RTV or cobicistat. Coadministration w/ regimens containing TDF and an HIV protease inhibitor/RTV or cobicistat may increase tenofovir levels; consider alternative HCV or antiretroviral therapy to avoid increases in tenofovir exposures; if coadministration is necessary, monitor for tenofovir-associated adverse reactions. Coadministration w/ combination of elvitegravir, cobicistat, emtricitabine, and TDF is not recommended; may increase tenofovir levels. **Ledipasvir:** May increase intestinal absorption of coadministered substrates of P-gp or breast cancer resistance protein. Drugs that increase gastric pH may decrease levels. Separate administration w/ antacids by 4 hrs. May administer H$_2$-receptor antagonists (eg, famotidine) simultaneously or 12 hrs apart from Harvoni at a dose that does not exceed doses comparable to famotidine 40mg bid. Proton-pump inhibitor doses comparable to omeprazole ≤20mg can be administered simultaneously under fasted conditions. Not recommended w/ simeprevir; may increase levels. Refer to PI for further information on drug interactions.

PREGNANCY AND LACTATION
Pregnancy: No adequate human data are available to establish whether or not Harvoni poses a risk to pregnancy outcomes.
Lactation: It is not known whether Harvoni and its metabolites are present in human breast milk, affect human milk production, or have effects on the breastfed infant; caution in nursing.

If administered w/ ribavirin, refer to the prescribing information of ribavirin for additional information.

MECHANISM OF ACTION
Ledipasvir: Inhibits HCV NS5A protein, which is required for viral replication.
Sofosbuvir: Inhibits HCV NS5B RNA-dependent RNA polymerase, which is required for viral replication.

PHARMACOKINETICS
Absorption: Ledipasvir: C_{max}=323ng/mL; T_{max}=4-4.5 hrs (median); AUC_{0-24}=7290ng•hr/mL. Sofosbuvir: C_{max}=618ng/mL, 707ng/mL (GS-331007); T_{max}=0.8-1 hr (median), 3.5-4 hrs (GS-331007, median); AUC_{0-24}=1320ng•hr/mL, 12,000ng•hr/mL (GS-331007). **Distribution:** Ledipasvir: Plasma protein binding (>99.8%). Sofosbuvir: Plasma protein binding (61-65%). **Metabolism:** Ledipasvir: Slow oxidative metabolism via an unknown mechanism. Sofosbuvir: Liver (extensive) to pharmacologically active nucleoside analogue triphosphate GS-461203; dephosphorylation to GS-331007 (inactive metabolite). **Elimination:** Ledipasvir: Urine (1%), feces (86%; 70% unchanged, 2.2% metabolite); $T_{1/2}$=47 hrs (median). Sofosbuvir: Urine (80%; 78% GS-331007, 3.5% unchanged), feces (14%), expired air (2.5%); $T_{1/2}$=0.5 hr (median), 27 hrs (GS-331007, median).

PATIENT CONSIDERATIONS
Assessment: Assess for hypersensitivity to drug, pregnancy/nursing status, and possible drug interactions.

Monitoring: Monitor for bradycardia if coadministering w/ amiodarone or if discontinuing amiodarone just prior to starting therapy; perform cardiac monitoring in an in-patient setting for the first 48 hrs of coadministration, after which outpatient or self-monitoring of the HR should occur on a daily basis through at least the first 2 weeks of treatment. Perform clinical and hepatic lab monitoring for patients w/ decompensated cirrhosis receiving concomitant treatment w/ ribavirin. Monitor for other adverse reactions.

Counseling: Advise to seek medical evaluation immediately for symptoms of bradycardia. Inform that therapy may interact w/ other drugs; advise to report to physician the use of any other medication or herbal products. Advise to avoid pregnancy during combination treatment w/ ribavirin and for 6 months after completion of treatment; instruct to notify physician immediately in the event of a pregnancy. Advise to take therapy at the regularly scheduled time w/ or w/o food.

HELIXATE FS — antihemophilic factor (recombinant)   Rx

Class: Antihemophilic factor (recombinant)

ADULT DOSAGE
Hemophilia A

Dose Calculation:
Dosage (Units) = Body Weight (kg) x Desired Factor VIII (FVIII) Rise (IU/dL or % of Normal) x 0.5 (IU/kg per IU/dL), or
IU/dL (or % Normal) = Total Dose (IU)/Body Weight (kg) x 2 (IU/dL per IU/kg)

Dose and duration of therapy depend on the severity of the FVIII deficiency, the location and extent of the bleeding, and clinical condition

Control and Prevention of Bleeding Episodes:

Minor Bleeding:
20-40 IU/dL of FVIII Level Required:
10-20 IU/kg IV; repeat if there is evidence of further bleeding until bleeding is resolved

Moderate Bleeding:
30-60 IU/dL of FVIII Level Required:
15-30 IU/kg IV q12-24h until bleeding is resolved

PEDIATRIC DOSAGE
Hemophilia A

Dose Calculation:
Dosage (Units) = Body Weight (kg) x Desired Factor VIII (FVIII) Rise (IU/dL or % of Normal) x 0.5 (IU/kg per IU/dL), or
IU/dL (or % Normal) = Total Dose (IU)/ Body Weight (kg) x 2 (IU/dL per IU/kg)

Dose and duration of therapy depend on the severity of the FVIII deficiency, the location and extent of the bleeding, and clinical condition

Control and Prevention of Bleeding Episodes:

Minor Bleeding:
20-40 IU/dL of FVIII Level Required:
10-20 IU/kg IV; repeat if there is evidence of further bleeding until bleeding is resolved

Major Bleeding:
80-100 IU/dL of FVIII Level Required: 40-50 IU/kg IV initially; repeat 20-25 IU/kg q8-12h until bleeding is resolved

Perioperative Management:

Minor Surgery:
30-60 IU/dL FVIII Level Required: 15-30 IU/kg IV q12-24h until bleeding is resolved

Major Surgery:
100 IU/dL FVIII Level Required: 50 IU/kg IV preoperatively to achieve 100% activity; give q6-12h until healing is complete

Routine Prophylaxis:
25 U/kg IV 3X/week

Moderate Bleeding:
30-60 IU/dL of FVIII Level Required: 15-30 IU/kg IV q12-24h until bleeding is resolved

Major Bleeding:
80-100 IU/dL of FVIII Level Required: 40-50 IU/kg IV initially; repeat 20-25 IU/kg q8-12h until bleeding is resolved

Perioperative Management:

Minor Surgery:
30-60 IU/dL FVIII Level Required: 15-30 IU/kg IV q12-24h until bleeding is resolved

Major Surgery:
100 IU/dL FVIII Level Required: 50 IU/kg IV preoperatively to achieve 100% activity; give q6-12h until healing is complete

Routine Prophylaxis:
25 U/kg IV qod

DOSING CONSIDERATIONS
Elderly
Individualize dose selection

ADMINISTRATION
IV route

Warm unopened diluent and concentrate to a temperature not to exceed 37°C (99°F) before preparing.
Administer over a period of 1-15 min w/in 3 hrs after reconstitution.
Adapt rate of administration to response of individual patient.
Determine pulse rate before and during administration; if there is a significant increase in pulse rate, reduce the rate of administration/temporarily halt infusion to allow symptoms to disappear.
Refer to PI for vacuum transfer and reconstitution directions.

STORAGE
2-8°C (36-46°F) for up to 30 months from the date of manufacture; may store for up to 12 months at ≤25°C (77°F) w/in this period. Do not return to the refrigerator once stored at room temperature. Do not freeze. Protect from extreme exposure to light and store lyophilized powder in the carton prior to use.
After Reconstitution: Store at room temperature and administer w/in 3 hrs.

HOW SUPPLIED
Inj: 250 IU, 500 IU, 1000 IU, 2000 IU, 3000 IU

CONTRAINDICATIONS
Life-threatening hypersensitivity reactions, including anaphylaxis to mouse or hamster protein or other constituents of product (sucrose, glycine, histidine, sodium, calcium chloride, polysorbate 80, imidazole, tri-n-butyl phosphate, and copper).

WARNINGS/PRECAUTIONS
Not indicated for the treatment of von Willebrand disease. Hypersensitivity reactions, including anaphylaxis, reported; d/c if symptoms occur and seek immediate emergency treatment. Neutralizing antibodies (inhibitors) reported, predominantly in previously untreated patients. If expected plasma FVIII activity levels are not attained or if bleeding is not controlled w/ expected dose, perform an assay that measures FVIII inhibitor concentration; use Bethesda Units (BU) to titer inhibitors. Hemophilic patients w/ cardiovascular (CV) risk factors or diseases may be at the same risk to develop CV events as nonhemophilic patients when clotting has been normalized by treatment w/ FVIII. Monitor plasma FVIII activity levels and for development of FVIII inhibitors; adequate hemostasis may not be achieved if inhibitor titers are >10 BU/mL.

ADVERSE REACTIONS
Skin related hypersensitivity reactions (eg, rash, pruritus), infusion-site reactions (eg, inflammation, pain), central venous access device associated infections.

PREGNANCY AND LACTATION
Pregnancy: Category C.
Lactation: Caution in nursing.

MECHANISM OF ACTION
Antihemophilic factor (recombinant); temporarily replaces the missing clotting FVIII that is needed for effective hemostasis.

PHARMACOKINETICS
Absorption: (12-33 yrs of age) Initial: C_{max}=114.95 IU/dL, AUC=1588.05 IU•hr/dL; Week 24: C_{max}=109.42 IU/dL, AUC=1487.08 IU•hr/dL. (Children) AUC=1320 IU•hr/dL.
Elimination: $T_{1/2}$=13.74 hrs (12-33 yrs of age, initial), 14.6 hrs (12-33 yrs of age, Week 24), 10.7 hrs (children).

PATIENT CONSIDERATIONS
Assessment: Assess for known hypersensitivity to mouse or hamster protein or other constituents of the product, location and extent of bleeding, patient's clinical condition, CV risk factors, and pregnancy/nursing status. Assess plasma FVIII activity levels. Obtain baseline pulse rate prior to administration.

Monitoring: Monitor for signs/symptoms of hypersensitivity reactions, CV events, and other adverse reactions. Monitor plasma FVIII activity levels, clinical response, development of FVIII inhibitors, and pulse rate during administration.

Counseling: Advise to report any adverse reactions or problems to physician. Inform about early signs of hypersensitivity reactions and anaphylaxis; instruct

to d/c therapy and seek immediate emergency treatment if signs/symptoms develop. Instruct to contact physician if lack of clinical response to FVIII replacement therapy is experienced. Advise to consult physician prior to travel and to bring an adequate supply based on patient's current treatment regimen while traveling.

HEMOFIL M — antihemophilic factor (human)   Rx

Class: Antihemophilic agent

ADULT DOSAGE	PEDIATRIC DOSAGE
Hemophilia A	Pediatric use may not have been established
Prevention/Control of Hemorrhagic Episodes:	
Early Hemarthrosis/Muscle Bleed/ Oral Bleed:	
Required Antihemophilic Factor (AHF) Activity: 20-40 IU/dL: Begin infusion q12-24h for 1-3 days until bleeding episode is resolved or healing is achieved	
More Extensive Hemarthrosis/Muscle Bleed/Hematoma:	
Required AHF Activity: 30-60 IU/dL: Repeat infusion q12-24h for usually 3 days or more until pain and disability are resolved	
Life-Threatening Bleeds:	
Required AHF Activity: 60-100 IU/ dL: Repeat infusion q8-24h until threat is resolved	
Surgery:	
Minor Surgery (eg, Tooth Extraction): Required AHF Activity: 60-80 IU/dL: A single infusion plus oral antifibrinolytic therapy w/in 1 hr	
Major Surgery:	
Required AHF Activity: 80-100 IU/ dL (Pre- and Post-Operative): Repeat infusion q8-24h depending on state of healing	
Dose Calculation:	
Expected in vivo Peak AHF (or % of Normal) = [Dose (IU)/Body Weight (kg)] × 2	

DOSING CONSIDERATIONS
Other Important Considerations
Presence of a Low Titer Inhibitor: Doses larger than those recommended may be necessary as per standard care

ADMINISTRATION
IV route

Administer at room temperature; do not administer >3 hrs after reconstitution
May be administered at a rate of up to 10mL/min
Plastic syringes are recommended for use w/ this product

Reconstitution/Administration
1. Bring dry concentrate and diluent (sterile water for inj) to room temperature
2. If patient is to receive >1 bottle of concentrate, contents of 2 bottles may be drawn into the same syringe by drawing up each bottle through separate unused filter needles; filter needles are intended to filter the contents of a single bottle only
3. Do not refrigerate after reconstitution

STORAGE
2-8°C (36-46°F) or at room temperature not exceeding 30°C (86°F). Avoid freezing. Reconstituted Sol: Do not refrigerate.

HOW SUPPLIED
Inj: 250 IU, 500 IU, 1000 IU, 1700 IU

CONTRAINDICATIONS
Known hypersensitivity to active substance, excipients, or to mouse proteins.

WARNINGS/PRECAUTIONS
Allergic-type hypersensitivity reactions, including anaphylaxis, reported. Neutralizing antibodies (inhibitors) to FVIII may develop; risk factors include type of FVIII gene mutation, family history, and ethnicity. If expected plasma FVIII activity levels are not attained or if bleeding is not controlled with an appropriate dose, evaluate for the development of FVIII inhibitors. May not be effective in patients with high titer FVIII inhibitors; consider other therapeutic options. Made from human plasma; may contain infectious agents (eg, viruses, Creutzfeldt-Jakob disease agent) that can cause disease. Consider appropriate vaccination (against hepatitis A and B) for patients in regular/repeated receipt of plasma-derived products. Identification of the clotting defect as a FVIII deficiency is essential prior to initiation of therapy. May develop hypersensitivity to mouse proteins. Determine pulse rate before and during administration; reduce rate of administration or temporarily halt inj if significant increase occurs. Certain components used in packaging contain natural rubber latex; caution in patients with sensitivity to natural rubber latex.

ADVERSE REACTIONS
FVIII inhibition.

PREGNANCY AND LACTATION
Category C, caution in nursing.

MECHANISM OF ACTION
Antihemophilic agent; increases plasma levels of AHF and temporarily corrects the coagulation defect in hemophilia A.

PHARMACOKINETICS
Elimination: $T_{1/2}$=14.8 hrs (FVIII deficient).

PATIENT CONSIDERATIONS

Assessment: Assess for FVIII deficiency, hypersensitivity to drug, mouse protein or latex, and pregnancy/nursing status. Determine pulse rate prior to administration.

Monitoring: Monitor for development of FVIII inhibitors, infections, hypersensitivity reactions, and other adverse reactions. Monitor pulse rate during administration. Perform appropriate laboratory tests at suitable intervals to assure that adequate AHF levels are reached and maintained.

Counseling: Inform of risks and benefits of therapy. Advise to report any adverse reactions or problems following administration to the physician. Advise pregnant women or immune compromised individuals of the effects of parvovirus B19 (eg, fever, drowsiness, chills, runny nose, followed about 2 weeks later by rash and joint pain). Inform of the signs/symptoms of hepatitis A (eg, several days to weeks of poor appetite, tiredness, low grade fever followed by N/V and pain in the belly, dark urine, and a yellowed complexion); instruct to consult physician if such symptoms appear. Inform about early signs of hypersensitivity reactions (eg, hives, generalized urticaria, facial edema, flushing, nausea, chest tightness, wheezing, dyspnea, hypotension, anaphylaxis); instruct to d/c therapy and contact physician if these occur.

HEPAGAM B — hepatitis B immune globulin intravenous (human) Rx

Class: Immune globulin

ADULT DOSAGE

Prevention of Hepatitis B Recurrence Following Liver Transplantation

In HBsAg-Positive Patients:
Usual: 20,000 IU/dose IV according to the following regimen
Infusion Rate: 2mL/min

Dosing Regimen:
Anhepatic Phase: 1st dose
Week 1 Postoperative: Daily from Day 1-7
Weeks 2-12 Postoperative: Every 2 weeks from Day 14
Month 4 Onwards: Monthly

May need to adjust dose if anti-HBs levels of 500 IU/L are not reached w/in 1st week post-liver transplantation

Postexposure Prophylaxis

Acute Exposure to Blood Containing HBsAg:
0.06mL/kg IM as soon as possible after exposure
Give 2nd dose 1 month after the 1st dose in patients who refuse hepatitis B vaccine or are known non-responders to vaccine

Sexual Exposure to HBsAg-Positive Persons:
0.06mL/kg IM + hepatitis B vaccine series; give w/in 14 days of sexual contact or if sexual contact w/ infected person will continue

Household Exposure to Person w/ Acute Hepatitis B Virus Infection:
Prophylaxis not indicated unless there is an identifiable blood exposure to the index patient (eg, by sharing toothbrushes/razors); treat such exposures like sexual exposures

PEDIATRIC DOSAGE

Postexposure Prophylaxis

Perinatal Exposure of Infants Born to HBsAg-Positive Mothers:
0.5mL IM administered after physiologic stabilization of infant and preferably w/in 12 hrs of birth
Administer concurrently w/ hepatitis B vaccine

Household Exposure to Person w/ Acute Hepatitis B Virus Infection:
<12 Months of Age:
0.5mL IM + hepatitis B vaccine

≥12 Months of Age:
Prophylaxis not indicated unless there is an identifiable blood exposure to the index patient (eg, by sharing toothbrushes/razors); treat such exposures like sexual exposures

---

DOSING CONSIDERATIONS
Elderly
Start at lower end of dosing range

Adverse Reactions
Prevention of Hepatitis B Recurrence Following Liver Transplantation:
If discomfort or infusion-related adverse reaction develops, decrease to 1mL/min or slower

Other Important Considerations
Prevention of Hepatitis B Recurrence Following Liver Transplantation:
Surgical Bleeding, Abdominal Fluid Drainage (>500mL), or Undergoing

Plasmapheresis:
May increase to 1/2 dose IV (10,000 IU) q6h until the target anti-HBs is reached

ADMINISTRATION
IV/IM route
May be administered at the same time (but at a different site), or ≤1 month preceding hepatitis B vaccination
Do not shake vials during preparation
Promptly use any vial that has been entered; do not reuse or save for future use
For IV administration, administer through a separate IV line using an infusion pump
Use normal saline as diluent if dilution is preferred prior to IV administration; do not use D5W

STORAGE
2-8°C (36-46°F). Do not freeze. Use within 6 hrs after vial has been entered.

HOW SUPPLIED
Inj: >312 IU/mL [1mL, 5mL]

CONTRAINDICATIONS
Immunoglobulin A (IgA) deficient patients with the potential to develop anti-IgA antibodies and have an anaphylactoid reaction. Patients with severe thrombocytopenia or any coagulation disorder that would contraindicate IM inj.

WARNINGS/PRECAUTIONS
Severe hypersensitivity reactions may occur; d/c infusion immediately and begin appropriate emergency treatment. Administer in a setting with appropriate equipment, medication, and personnel trained in the management of hypersensitivity, anaphylaxis, and shock. Contains maltose that may interfere with some types of blood glucose monitoring systems (eg, those based on the glucose dehydrogenase pyrroloquinoline quinone method); may result in falsely elevated glucose readings and, consequently, inappropriate administration of insulin, resulting in life-threatening hypoglycemia. Monitor liver transplant patients regularly for serum anti-HBs antibody levels using a quantitative assay to ensure that adequate protective levels are maintained. Monitor for any symptoms of an infusion reaction throughout the infusion period and immediately following an infusion; follow recommended infusion rate closely. Made from human plasma; may carry a risk of transmitting infectious agents (eg, viruses, Creutzfeldt-Jakob disease agent). Thrombotic events may occur during or following treatment; caution with a history of atherosclerosis, multiple cardiovascular (CV) risk factors, advanced age, impaired cardiac output, coagulation disorders, prolonged periods of immobilization, and/or known/suspected hyperviscosity. Consider baseline assessment of blood viscosity in patients at risk for hyperviscosity, including those with cryoglobulins, fasting chylomicronemia/markedly high triglycerides, or monoclonal gammopathies. Administer at the min rate of infusion practicable in patients at risk of thrombotic events. May interfere with some serological tests. Caution in elderly.

ADVERSE REACTIONS
Hypotension, nausea.

DRUG INTERACTIONS
May impair efficacy of live attenuated virus vaccines (eg, measles, rubella, mumps, varicella); if patient received hepatitis B immune globulin <14 days after live virus vaccination, revaccinate 3 months after administration of the immune globulin, unless serologic test results indicate that antibodies were produced.

PREGNANCY AND LACTATION
Category C, caution in nursing.

MECHANISM OF ACTION
Immune globulin; provides passive immunization for individuals exposed to HBV, by binding to the surface antigen and reducing the rate of hepatitis B infection.

PHARMACOKINETICS
Absorption: (IM) T_{max}=4-5 days (healthy). **Distribution:** (IM) V_d=7.5L (healthy). **Elimination:** (IM) $T_{1/2}$=22-25 days (healthy).

PATIENT CONSIDERATIONS

Assessment: Assess for history of anaphylactic or severe systemic reactions to parenteral administration of human globulin preparations, IgA deficiency, thrombocytopenia or any coagulation disorder, risk factors for thrombotic events (eg, history of atherosclerosis, multiple CV risk factors, advanced age, impaired cardiac output, prolonged periods of immobilization, hyperviscosity), any other conditions where treatment is contraindicated or cautioned, pregnancy/nursing status, and for possible drug interactions. Consider baseline assessment of blood viscosity in patients at risk for hyperviscosity.

Monitoring: Monitor for hypersensitivity reactions, infection, thrombotic events, and for other adverse reactions. Monitor for infusion reactions throughout the infusion period and immediately following an infusion. Monitor serum anti-HBs antibody levels regularly in liver transplant patients.

Counseling: Inform about the risks and benefits of treatment. Inform that the drug may contain infectious agents such as viruses that may cause disease. Inform that persons known to have severe, life-threatening reactions to human globulin products should not receive the drug. Instruct to notify physician immediately if any signs or symptoms of an allergic reaction develop. Advise liver transplant patients about the potential interference with non-glucose specific monitoring systems.

HEPSERA — adefovir dipivoxil   Rx

Class: Nucleotide analogue reverse transcriptase inhibitor

> Lactic acidosis and severe hepatomegaly with steatosis, including fatal cases, reported with the use of nucleoside analogues alone or in combination with other antiretrovirals. Severe acute exacerbations of hepatitis reported in patients who have discontinued therapy. Closely monitor hepatic function with both clinical and lab follow-up for at least several months in patients who d/c therapy. If appropriate, resumption of antihepatitis B therapy may be warranted. Chronic use may result in nephrotoxicity in patients at risk of or having underlying renal dysfunction; monitor renal function and adjust dose if required. HIV resistance may occur in patients with unrecognized or untreated HIV infection.

ADULT DOSAGE	PEDIATRIC DOSAGE
Chronic Hepatitis B	Chronic Hepatitis B
10mg qd	≥12 Years:
	10mg qd

DOSING CONSIDERATIONS
Renal Impairment
CrCl 30-49mL/min: 10mg q48h
CrCl 10-29mL/min: 10mg q72h
Hemodialysis: 10mg every 7 days following dialysis

ADMINISTRATION
Oral route

Take without regard to food

STORAGE
25°C (77°F); excursions permitted to 15-30°C (59-86°F).

HOW SUPPLIED
Tab: 10mg

CONTRAINDICATIONS
Hypersensitivity to any of the components of the product.

WARNINGS/PRECAUTIONS
Caution in adolescents with underlying renal dysfunction; monitor renal function closely. Offer HIV antibody testing before initiating therapy. Obesity and prolonged nucleoside exposure may be risk factors for lactic acidosis and severe hepatomegaly with steatosis. Caution with known risk factors for liver disease. D/C if findings suggestive of lactic acidosis or pronounced hepatotoxicity develop. Resistance to the drug can result in viral load rebound, which may result in exacerbation of hepatitis B, and in the setting of diminished hepatic function, lead to liver decompensation and possible fatal outcome. To reduce risk of resistance in patients with lamivudine-resistant hepatitis B virus (HBV), use adefovir dipivoxil in combination with lamivudine and not as monotherapy. To reduce risk of resistance in patients receiving monotherapy, consider modification of treatment if serum HBV DNA remains >1000 copies/mL with continued treatment. Caution in elderly.

ADVERSE REACTIONS
Nephrotoxicity, lactic acidosis, severe hepatomegaly with steatosis, asthenia, headache, abdominal pain, nausea, flatulence, diarrhea, dyspepsia.

DRUG INTERACTIONS
Avoid with tenofovir disoproxil fumarate (TDF) or TDF-containing products. Coadministration with drugs that reduce renal function or compete for active tubular secretion may increase levels of either adefovir and/or these coadministered drugs. Caution with nephrotoxic agents (eg, cyclosporine, tacrolimus, aminoglycosides, vancomycin, NSAIDs).

PREGNANCY AND LACTATION
Category C, not for use in nursing.

MECHANISM OF ACTION
Nucleotide analogue reverse transcriptase inhibitor; inhibits HBV DNA polymerase (reverse transcriptase) by competing with natural substrate deoxyadenosine triphosphate and by causing DNA chain termination after incorporation into viral DNA.

PHARMACOKINETICS
Absorption: Bioavailability (59%); C_{max}=18.4ng/mL; T_{max}=1.75 hrs (median); AUC=220ng•h/mL. Refer to PI for pharmacokinetic parameters in pediatric patients and in patients with varying degrees of renal function. **Distribution:** V_d=392mL/kg (IV, 1mg/kg/day), 352mL/kg (IV, 3mg/kg/day); plasma protein binding (≤4%). **Elimination:** Urine (45%); $T_{1/2}$=7.48 hrs.

PATIENT CONSIDERATIONS
Assessment: Assess for renal dysfunction, risk factors for lactic acidosis and liver disease, hypersensitivity, pregnancy/nursing status, and possible drug interactions. Perform HIV antibody testing and assess CrCl.

Monitoring: Monitor for signs/symptoms of lactic acidosis, hepatotoxicity, nephrotoxicity, clinical resistance, and other adverse reactions. Monitor hepatic function (in patients who d/c therapy) and renal function.

Counseling: Inform of risks, benefits, and alternative modes of therapy. Instruct to follow a regular dosing schedule to avoid missing doses. Advise to immediately report any severe abdominal pain, muscle pain, yellowing of the eyes, dark urine, pale stools, and/or loss of appetite. Instruct to notify physician if any unusual/known symptom develops, persists, or worsens. Advise not to d/c therapy without informing physician. Advise that routine lab monitoring and follow-up is important during therapy. Inform of importance of obtaining HIV antibody testing prior to starting therapy. Counsel women of childbearing age about risks of drug exposure during pregnancy, and to notify physician if the patient becomes pregnant while on therapy. Inform pregnant patients about the pregnancy registry.

HERCEPTIN — trastuzumab   Rx

Class: Monoclonal antibody/HER2 blocker

> May result in cardiac failure; incidence and severity were highest w/ anthracycline-containing chemotherapy regimens. Evaluate left ventricular function prior to and during treatment; d/c in patients receiving adjuvant therapy and withhold in patients w/ metastatic disease for clinically significant decrease in left ventricular function. May result in serious and fatal infusion reactions and pulmonary toxicity; interrupt infusion for dyspnea or clinically significant hypotension, and monitor until symptoms completely resolve. D/C for anaphylaxis, angioedema, interstitial pneumonitis, or acute respiratory distress syndrome. Exposure during pregnancy may result in oligohydramnios and oligohydramnios sequence manifesting as pulmonary hypoplasia, skeletal abnormalities, and neonatal death.

ADULT DOSAGE	PEDIATRIC DOSAGE
HER2 Overexpressing Node Positive or Node Negative Breast Cancer	Pediatric use may not have been established

Adjuvant Treatment:
During and Following Paclitaxel, Docetaxel, or Docetaxel/Carboplatin:
Initial: 4mg/kg IV infusion over 90 min, then at 2mg/kg IV infusion over 30 min weekly during chemotherapy for the first 12 weeks (paclitaxel or docetaxel) or 18 weeks (docetaxel/carboplatin)
Subsequent Doses: 1 week following the last weekly dose, give 6mg/kg IV infusion over 30-90 min every 3 weeks

Single Agent w/in 3 Weeks Following Completion of Multimodality Anthracycline-Based Chemotherapy Regimens:
Initial: 8mg/kg IV infusion over 90 min
Subsequent Doses: 6mg/kg IV infusion over 30-90 min every 3 weeks

Administer for a total of 52 weeks; extending adjuvant treatment >1 yr is not recommended

HER2 Overexpressing Metastatic Breast Cancer

Alone or in Combination w/ Paclitaxel:
Initial: 4mg/kg IV infusion over 90 min
Subsequent Doses: 2mg/kg IV infusion over 30 min once a week until disease progression

HER2 Overexpressing Metastatic Gastric or Gastroesophageal Junction Adenocarcinoma

Patients Who Have Not Received Prior Treatment for Metastatic Disease:
Initial: 8mg/kg IV infusion over 90 min
Subsequent Doses: 6mg/kg IV infusion over 30-90 min every 3 weeks until disease progression

Give in combination w/ cisplatin and capecitabine or 5-fluorouracil

Missed Dose

Dose Missed by ≤1 Week:
- Administer the usual maint dose (weekly schedule: 2mg/kg; 3-weekly schedule: 6mg/kg) as soon as possible; do not wait until the next planned cycle
- Administer subsequent maint doses 7 days or 21 days later according to the weekly or 3-weekly schedules, respectively

Dose Missed by >1 Week:
- Administer a reloading dose over approx 90 min (weekly schedule: 4mg/kg; 3-weekly schedule: 8mg/kg) as soon as possible
- Administer subsequent maint doses (weekly schedule: 2mg/kg; 3-weekly schedule: 6mg/kg) 7 days or 21 days later according to the weekly or 3-weekly schedules, respectively

DOSING CONSIDERATIONS
Adverse Reactions
Infusion Reactions:
Mild or Moderate: Decrease rate of infusion
Dyspnea/Clinically Significant Hypotension: Interrupt infusion
Severe/Life-threatening: D/C therapy
Cardiomyopathy:
Withhold Therapy for at Least 4 Weeks for Either of the Following:
1. ≥16% absolute decrease in left ventricular ejection fraction (LVEF) from pretreatment values
2. LVEF below institutional limits of normal and ≥10% absolute decrease in LVEF from pretreatment values
May Resume Therapy If:
LVEF returns to normal limits and absolute decrease from baseline is ≤15% w/in 4-8 weeks
Permanently D/C Therapy For:
Persistent (>8 weeks) LVEF decline or for suspension of dosing on more than 3 occasions for cardiomyopathy

ADMINISTRATION
IV route
Do not administer as IV push or bolus.
Do not mix w/ other drugs.
Do not substitute for or w/ ado-trastuzumab emtansine.
Reconstitution
Reconstitute each 440mg vial w/ 20mL of bacteriostatic water for inj, containing 1.1% benzyl alcohol as a preservative to yield a multidose sol containing 21mg/mL. In patients w/ known hypersensitivity to benzyl alcohol, reconstitute w/ 20mL of sterile water for inj (SWFI) w/o preservative to yield a single-use sol.
Swirl vial gently; do not shake.
Allow vial to stand undisturbed for approx 5 min after reconstitution.
If reconstituted w/ SWFI w/o preservative, use immediately and discard any unused portion.
Store reconstituted product at 2-8°C (36-46°F); discard any unused product after 28 days.
Dilution
1. Determine the dose (mg) and calculate the volume of the 21mg/mL reconstituted sol needed.
2. Withdraw this amount from the vial and add it to an infusion bag containing 250mL of 0.9% NaCl inj; do not use D5 sol.
3. Gently invert the bag to mix the sol.

STORAGE
2-8°C (36-46°F). Do not freeze following reconstitution/dilution. **Diluted in Polyvinylchloride or Polyethylene Bags Containing 0.9% NaCl Inj:** 2-8°C (36-46°F) for no more than 24 hrs prior to use.

HOW SUPPLIED
Inj: 440mg

WARNINGS/PRECAUTIONS
See Dosing Considerations. Patients w/ symptomatic intrinsic lung disease or extensive tumor involvement of the lungs, resulting in dyspnea at rest, may have more severe pulmonary toxicity. Detection of HER2 protein overexpression is necessary for appropriate patient selection; use FDA-approved tests for the specific tumor type to assess HER2 protein overexpression and HER2 gene amplification.

ADVERSE REACTIONS
Adjuvant and Metastatic Breast Cancer: Fever, N/V, infusion reactions, diarrhea, infections, increased cough, headache, fatigue, dyspnea, rash, neutropenia, anemia, myalgia.
Metastatic Gastric Cancer: Neutropenia, diarrhea, fatigue, anemia, stomatitis, weight loss, URTIs, fever, thrombocytopenia, mucosal inflammation, nasopharyngitis, dysgeusia.

DRUG INTERACTIONS
See Boxed Warning. Higher incidence of neutropenia w/ myelosuppressive chemotherapy. Increased risk of cardiac dysfunction in patients who receive anthracycline after stopping trastuzumab; if possible, avoid anthracycline-based therapy for up to 7 months after stopping trastuzumab, but if anthracyclines are used, carefully monitor cardiac function.

PREGNANCY AND LACTATION
Pregnancy: May cause fetal harm; cases of oligohydramnios and of oligohydramnios sequence reported. Monitor women who received trastuzumab during pregnancy or w/in 7 months prior to conception for oligohydramnios. There is a pregnancy exposure registry and a pregnancy pharmacovigilance program for women who become pregnant during treatment or w/in 7 months following the last dose.
Lactation: It is not known if trastuzumab is excreted in human milk; caution in nursing.
Reproductive Potential: Verify the pregnancy status of females of reproductive potential prior to the initiation of therapy. Advise females of reproductive potential to use effective contraception during treatment and for 7 months following the last dose of trastuzumab.

MECHANISM OF ACTION
Monoclonal antibody (IgG1 kappa)/HER2 blocker; inhibits proliferation of human tumor cells that overexpress HER2.

PHARMACOKINETICS
Absorption: Administration of various doses resulted in different pharmacokinetic parameters.

PATIENT CONSIDERATIONS
Assessment: Assess cardiac function, including baseline LVEF. Assess HER2 protein overexpression and HER2 gene amplification. Assess for symptomatic intrinsic lung disease or extensive tumor involvement of lungs, pregnancy/nursing status, and possible drug interactions.
Monitoring: Monitor for infusion reactions, pulmonary toxicity, neutropenia, and other adverse reactions. Monitor LVEF every 3 months during and upon completion of therapy, and every 6 months for at least 2 yrs following completion of therapy as a component of adjuvant therapy. Repeat LVEF measurement at 4-week intervals if therapy is withheld for significant left ventricular cardiac dysfunction.
Counseling: Advise to contact physician immediately for any symptoms of cardiomyopathy (eg, new onset/worsening SOB, cough, swelling of ankles/legs). Advise women that exposure to trastuzumab during pregnancy or w/in 7 months prior to conception may result in fetal harm. Advise to contact physician w/ a known/suspected pregnancy. Advise women who may be exposed to therapy during pregnancy or w/in 7 months of conception to enroll in the MotHER Pregnancy Registry and to report pregnancy to manufacturer. Advise females of reproductive potential to use effective contraception during treatment and for at least 7 months following the last dose of therapy.

HETLIOZ — tasimelteon   **Rx**
Class: Melatonin receptor agonist

ADULT DOSAGE	PEDIATRIC DOSAGE
Non-24-Hour Sleep-Wake Disorder 20mg/day before hs, at the same time every night	Pediatric use may not have been established

----

DOSING CONSIDERATIONS
Hepatic Impairment
Severe (Child-Pugh Class C): Not recommended

ADMINISTRATION
Oral route
Take w/o food.
Swallow cap whole.

STORAGE
25°C (77°F); excursions permitted to 15-30°C (59-86°F). Protect from exposure to light and moisture.

HOW SUPPLIED
Cap: 20mg

WARNINGS/PRECAUTIONS
Effects of therapy may not occur for weeks or months because of individual differences in circadian rhythms. May cause somnolence; limit activity before going to bed. May impair mental/physical abilities. Not recommended w/ severe hepatic impairment.

ADVERSE REACTIONS
Headache, increased ALT, nightmare/abnormal dreams, URTI, UTI.

DRUG INTERACTIONS
Large increase in exposure w/ fluvoxamine or other strong CYP1A2 inhibitors; avoid concomitant use. Decreased exposure w/ reduced efficacy w/ rifampin or other CYP3A4 inducers; avoid concomitant use. Efficacy may be reduced in smokers due to induction of CYP1A2 levels.

PREGNANCY AND LACTATION
Category C, caution in nursing.

MECHANISM OF ACTION
Melatonin receptor agonist; not established. Activity at MT_1 and MT_2 receptors thought to be involved in the control of circadian rhythms.

PHARMACOKINETICS
Absorption: Absolute bioavailability (38.3%); T_{max}=0.5-3 hrs (fasted). **Distribution:** V_d=59-126L; plasma protein binding (90%). **Metabolism:** Extensive. Oxidation at multiples sites and oxidative dealkylation via CYP1A2 and CYP3A4. Phenolic glucuronidation (major phase II metabolic route). **Elimination:** Urine (80%, <1% unchanged), feces (4%); $T_{1/2}$=1.3 hrs, 1.3-3.7 hrs (metabolites).

PATIENT CONSIDERATIONS
Assessment: Assess for severe hepatic impairment, smoking, pregnancy/nursing status, and possible drug interactions.
Monitoring: Monitor for somnolence, impairment of mental/physical abilities, and other adverse reactions.
Counseling: Inform about the potential risks and benefits of therapy. Advise to take therapy before hs at the same time every night; advise to skip dose if unable to take at scheduled time. Instruct to limit activity before going to bed after taking drug. Inform that daily use for several weeks or months may be necessary before benefit from therapy is observed.

HIZENTRA — immune globulin subcutaneous (human)   Rx
Class: Immune globulin

Thrombosis may occur; administer at the minimum dose and infusion rate practicable for patients at risk (eg, advanced age, prolonged immobilization, hypercoagulable conditions, history of venous or arterial thrombosis, use of estrogens, indwelling central vascular catheters, hyperviscosity, cardiovascular risk factors). Ensure adequate hydration before administration. Monitor for signs/symptoms of thrombosis and assess blood viscosity if at risk for hyperviscosity.

ADULT DOSAGE
Primary Humoral Immunodeficiency

Individualize dose based on clinical response and immunoglobulin G (IgG) trough levels

Before treatment, ensure that patients have received Immune Globulin Intravenous (IGIV) (Human) treatment at regular intervals for at least 3 months

Refer to PI for dose calculations when switching to Hizentra from IGIV or Immune Globulin Subcutaneous (IGSC)

Weekly/Frequent Dose:
Start 1 week after last IGIV infusion or Hizentra/IGSC infusion

Biweekly Dose:
Start 1 or 2 weeks after the last IGIV infusion or 1 week after the last IGIV infusion or 1 week after the last weekly Hizentra/IGSC infusion

Risk of Measles Exposure:
If exposed to measles, give minimum dose as soon as possible after exposure

Weekly Dose: Administer a minimum of 200mg/kg for 2 consecutive weeks

Biweekly Dose: One infusion of a minimum of 400mg/kg

Dose Adjustment:
Determine if dose adjustment should be considered by measuring serum IgG trough level 2-3 months after switching to Hizentra

Weekly Dosing:
When switching from IGIV to weekly dosing, target serum IgG trough level is projected to be approx 16% higher than last trough level during prior IGIV therapy

Biweekly dosing:
When switching from IGIV to biweekly dosing, target serum trough level is projected to be approx 10% higher than last IGIV trough level

When switching from weekly to biweekly dosing, the target trough is projected to be approx 5% lower than the last trough level on weekly therapy

Frequent dosing:
When switching from weekly dosing to more frequent dosing, the target serum IgG trough level is projected to be approx 3-4% higher than the last trough level on weekly therapy

Refer to PI for dose adjustments based on trough levels

PEDIATRIC DOSAGE
Primary Humoral Immunodeficiency
≥2 Years:

Individualize dose based on clinical response and immunoglobulin G (IgG) trough levels

Before treatment, ensure that patients have received Immune Globulin Intravenous (IGIV) (Human) treatment at regular intervals for at least 3 months

Refer to PI for dose calculations when switching to Hizentra from IGIV or Immune Globulin Subcutaneous (IGSC)

Weekly/Frequent Dose:
Start 1 week after last IGIV infusion or Hizentra/IGSC infusion

Biweekly Dose:
Start 1 or 2 weeks after the last IGIV infusion or 1 week after the last weekly Hizentra/IGSC infusion

Risk of Measles Exposure:
If exposed to measles, give minimum dose as soon as possible after exposure

Weekly Dose: Administer a minimum of 200mg/kg for 2 consecutive weeks

Biweekly Dose: One infusion of a minimum of 400mg/kg

Dose Adjustment:
Determine if dose adjustment should be considered by measuring serum IgG trough level 2-3 months after switching to Hizentra

Weekly Dosing:
When switching from IGIV to weekly dosing, target serum IgG trough level is projected to be approx 16% higher than last trough level during prior IGIV therapy

Biweekly dosing:
When switching from IGIV to biweekly dosing, target serum trough level is projected to be approx 10% higher than last IGIV trough level

When switching from weekly to biweekly dosing, the target trough is projected to be approx 5% lower than the last trough level on weekly therapy

Frequent dosing:
When switching from weekly dosing to more frequent dosing, the target serum IgG trough level is projected to be approx 3-4% higher than the last trough level on weekly therapy

Refer to PI for dose adjustments based on trough levels

ADMINISTRATION
SQ route

SQ infusion only using an infusion pump; do not inject into a blood vessel
Infuse in the abdomen, thigh, upper arm, and/or lateral hip
May use up to 4 inj sites simultaneously or up to 12 sites consecutively/infusion; inj sites should be ≥2 inches apart
Change the actual inj site w/ each administration
Do not exceed a volume of 15mL/inj site for the 1st infusion; volume may be increased to 20mL/site for the 5th infusion and then to 25mL/site, as tolerated
Recommended flow rate is 15mL/h/site for the 1st infusion then increased to 25mL/h/site for subsequent infusions
Do not mix w/ other products
Do not shake
Single-use only; discard all used administration supplies and any unused product immediately after each infusion in accordance w/ local requirements
Refer to PI for further administration instructions

STORAGE
Room temperature (up to 25°C [77°F]); stable for up to 30 months. Do not freeze; do not use if product has been frozen. Keep in original carton to protect from light.

HOW SUPPLIED
Inj: 0.2g/mL [5mL, 10mL, 20mL, 50mL]

CONTRAINDICATIONS
History of an anaphylactic or severe systemic reaction to the administration of human immune globulin or to components of this product, such as polysorbate 80. Hyperprolinemia (type I or II). Immunoglobulin A (IgA)-deficient patients w/ antibodies against IgA and a history of hypersensitivity.

WARNINGS/PRECAUTIONS
Contains ≤50mcg/mL of IgA; severe hypersensitivity reactions may occur. If hypersensitivity reaction occurs; d/c infusion immediately and institute appropriate treatment. Aseptic meningitis syndrome (AMS) reported and may occur more frequently w/ high doses (≥2g/kg) and/or rapid infusion; rule out other causes of meningitis. Acute renal dysfunction/failure, acute tubular necrosis, proximal tubular nephropathy, osmotic nephrosis and death may occur w/ human immune globulin products, especially those containing sucrose; this product does not contain sucrose. Ensure patients are not volume depleted before administering therapy. If renal function deteriorates; consider discontinuation of therapy. May contain blood group antibodies that may cause hemolysis and a positive Coombs' test result. Noncardiogenic pulmonary edema may occur; if transfusion-related acute lung injury (TRALI) is suspected, test for the presence of antineutrophil antibodies in both product and patient's serum. Made from human plasma; may carry risk of transmitting infectious agents (eg, viruses, Creutzfeldt-Jakob disease agent). May lead to misinterpretation of results of serological testing.

ADVERSE REACTIONS
Thrombosis, local reactions, headache, diarrhea, fatigue, back pain, N/V, pain in extremity, cough, rash, pruritus, abdominal pain (upper), migraine, pain.

DRUG INTERACTIONS
See Boxed Warning. Caution w/ nephrotoxic drugs; may increase risk of renal dysfunction/failure. May interfere w/ response to live virus vaccines (eg, measles, mumps, rubella, varicella).

PREGNANCY AND LACTATION
Category C, safety not known in nursing.

MECHANISM OF ACTION
Immune globulin; has not been fully established. Supplies broad spectrum of opsonizing and neutralizing IgG antibodies against a wide variety of bacterial and viral agents.

PHARMACOKINETICS
Absorption: C_{max}=1616mg/dL; AUC=10,560 day•mg/dL; T_{max}=2.9 days. Refer to PI for additional pharmacokinetic parameters.

PATIENT CONSIDERATIONS
Assessment: Assess for hypersensitivity reaction to human immune globulin, IgA deficiency, hyperprolinemia, risk factors for thrombosis/renal dysfunction, blood viscosity, volume-depletion, pregnancy/nursing status, and for possible drug interactions. Assess renal function (eg, BUN, SrCr) before the initial infusion.

Monitoring: Monitor for signs/symptoms of severe hypersensitivity reactions, thrombosis, hemolysis, pulmonary adverse reactions, infections, hyperviscosity, and other adverse reactions. Monitor renal function and urine output periodically. Perform neurological exam, including CSF studies, if AMS is suspected. Test for presence of antineutrophil antibodies in both product and patient's serum if TRALI is suspected.

Counseling: Instruct patients on self administration, if appropriate. Ensure the patient understands the importance of adhering to prescribed administration schedule. Advise that patient should be tested regularly to ensure correct levels of drug in the blood. Inform that therapy may interfere w/ the response to live virus vaccines. Advise to report immediately to physician if any signs/symptoms of hypersensitivity reactions, thrombosis, AMS, renal dysfunction, hemolysis, or TRALI occur. Inform patients to interrupt or terminate infusion if a hypersensitivity reaction occurs. Inform that drug is made from human blood and may carry a risk of transmitting infectious agents.

HUMATE-P — antihemophilic factor/von Willebrand factor complex (human)   Rx
Class: Antihemophilic agent

ADULT DOSAGE
Hemophilia A

Treatment/Prevention of Bleeding:
Minor Hemorrhage:
LD: 15 IU factor VIII (FVIII):C/kg to achieve a FVIII:C plasma level of approx 30% of normal; 1 infusion may be sufficient
May give 1/2 of LD qd or bid for 1-2 days if needed

Moderate Hemorrhage:
LD: 25 IU FVIII:C/kg to achieve a FVIII:C level of 50% of normal, followed by 15 IU FVIII:C/kg q8-12h for

PEDIATRIC DOSAGE
von Willebrand's Disease

Treatment of spontaneous and trauma-induced bleeding episodes, and prevention of excessive bleeding during and after surgery patients w/ severe VWD as well as patients w/ mild to moderate VWD where use of desmopressin is known or suspected to be inadequate

Dosing is based on VWF:RCo IU

the first 1-2 days to maintain FVIII:C level at 30% of normal
Continue same dose qd or bid for up to 7 days or until adequate wound healing is achieved

Life-Threatening Hemorrhage:
Initial: 40-50 IU FVIII:C/kg, followed by 20-25 IU FVIII:C/kg q8h to maintain FVIII:C level at 80-100% of normal for 7 days
Continue same dose qd or bid for another 7 days to maintain FVIII:C level at 30-50% of normal

von Willebrand's Disease

Treatment of spontaneous and trauma-induced bleeding episodes, and prevention of excessive bleeding during and after surgery patients w/ severe von Willebrand disease (VWD) as well as patients w/ mild to moderate VWD where use of desmopressin is known or suspected to be inadequate

Dosing is based on von Willebrand factor (VWF):ristocetin cofactor (RCo) IU

40-80 IU VWF:RCo/kg q8-12h; adjust dose based on extent and location of bleeding. Repeat dose prn based on appropriate monitoring of clinical and laboratory measures

Type 1 Mild (Baseline VWF:RCo >30%):
Minor (When Desmopressin is Inadequate)/Major Hemorrhage:
LD: 40-60 IU/kg. Then 40-50 IU/kg q8-12h for 3 days to keep VWF:RCo trough level >50%, then 40-50 IU/kg/day for up to 7 days

Type 1 Moderate/Severe (Baseline VWF:RCo <30%):
Minor Hemorrhage:
40-50 IU/kg (1 or 2 doses)
Major Hemorrhage:
LD: 50-75 IU/kg. Then 40-60 IU/kg q8-12h for 3 days to keep VWF:RCo trough level >50%, then 40-60 IU/kg/day for up to 7 days

Type 2 (All Variants) and Type 3:
Minor Hemorrhage:
40-50 IU/kg (1 or 2 doses)
Major Hemorrhage:
LD: 60-80 IU/kg. Then 40-60 IU/kg q8-12h for 3 days to keep VWF:RCo trough level >50%, then 40-60 IU/kg/day for up to 7 days

For major bleeds in all types of VWD where repeated dosing is required, monitor and maintain the FVIII level according to the guidelines for hemophilia A therapy

Prevention of Excessive Bleeding During and After Surgery:
Emergency:
LD: 50-60 IU VWF:RCo/kg
Non-Emergency:
LD: Refer to PI for guidelines for calculating the LD
Maint: 1/2 of LD initially. Refer to PI for treatment recommendations for subsequent maintenance doses based on type of surgery, target VWF:RCo and FVIII plasma trough level, and minimum duration of treatment

Usual: 40-80 IU VWF:RCo/kg q8-12h
Titrate: Adjust dose based on extent and location of bleeding. Repeat dose prn based on appropriate monitoring of clinical and laboratory measures

Type 1 Mild (Baseline VWF:RCo >30%):
Major/Minor Hemorrhage:
LD: 40-60 IU/kg. Then 40-50 IU/kg q8-12h for 3 days to keep VWF:RCo trough level >50%, then 40-50 IU/kg/day for up to 7 days

Type 1 Moderate/Severe (Baseline VWF:RCo <30%):
Minor Hemorrhage:
40-50 IU/kg (1 or 2 doses)
Major Hemorrhage:
LD: 50-75 IU/kg. Then 40-60 IU/kg q8-12h for 3 days to keep VWF:RCo trough level >50%, then 40-60 IU/kg/day for up to 7 days

Type 2 (All Variants) and Type 3:
Minor Hemorrhage:
40-50 IU/kg (1 or 2 doses)
Major Hemorrhage:
LD: 60-80 IU/kg. Then 40-60 IU/kg q8-12h for 3 days to keep VWF:RCo trough level >50%, then 40-60 IU/kg/day for up to 7 days

For major bleeds in all types of VWD where repeated dosing is required, monitor and maintain the FVIII level according to the guidelines for hemophilia A therapy

Prevention of Excessive Bleeding During and After Surgery:
Emergency:
LD: 50-60 IU VWF:RCo/kg
Non-Emergency:
LD: Refer to PI for guidelines for calculating the LD
Maint: 1/2 of LD initially. Refer to PI for treatment recommendations for subsequent maintenance doses based on type of surgery, target VWF:RCo and FVIII plasma trough level, and minimum duration of treatment

ADMINISTRATION
IV route
- Slowly infuse the sol (max 4mL/min) w/ a suitable IV administration set.
- Discard administration equipment and any unused product after use.

Reconstitution
- Ensure product vial and diluent vial are at room temperature before reconstitution.
- If a single patient is to receive >1 vial, pool the contents of multiple vials into 1 syringe; use separate unused Mix2Vial for each product vial.
- Use plastic disposable syringes.
- Do not refrigerate after reconstitution; administer w/in 3 hrs of reconstitution.

STORAGE
≤25°C (77°F); stable for 36 months up to the expiration date on its label. Do not freeze. **Reconstituted Sol:** Use w/in 3 hrs after reconstitution. Do not refrigerate.
HOW SUPPLIED
Inj: (FVIII/VWF:RCo) 250 IU/600 IU, 500 IU/1200 IU, 1000 IU/2400 IU
CONTRAINDICATIONS
History of anaphylactic or severe systemic reaction to antihemophilic factor or VWF preparations.
WARNINGS/PRECAUTIONS
Thromboembolic events reported especially w/ known risk factors for thrombosis; caution and consider antithrombotic measures in all at-risk VWD patients. Monitor patients w/ blood groups A, B, and AB for signs of intravascular hemolysis and decreasing Hct, and treat appropriately when doses are very large or need to be repeated frequently. Monitor VWF:RCo and FVIII levels of VWD patients using standard coagulation tests at least qd in order to adjust the dosage prn and to avoid excessive accumulation of coagulation factors. Made from human plasma; may contain infectious agents (eg, viruses [parvovirus B19 virus (B19V), hepatitis A virus (HAV)], Creutzfeldt-Jakob disease [CJD] agent) that can cause disease. Consider administration of hepatitis A and B vaccines to individuals receiving plasma derivatives.
ADVERSE REACTIONS
Allergic-anaphylactic reactions, postoperative wound bleeding, inj-site bleeding, epistaxis.
PREGNANCY AND LACTATION
Pregnancy: Category C.
Lactation: Caution in nursing.
MECHANISM OF ACTION
Antihemophilic agent; FVIII is an essential cofactor in activation of factor X, leading to the formation of thrombin and, subsequently, fibrin. VWF promotes platelet aggregation and platelet adhesion on damaged vascular endothelium; activated platelets interact w/ clotting proteins to form a clot. VWF also serves as a stabilizing carrier protein for the procoagulant protein FVIII.
PHARMACOKINETICS
Distribution: VWD: V_d=53mL/kg. **Elimination:** Hemophilia A: $T_{1/2}$=12.2 hrs. VWD: $T_{1/2}$=11 hrs (median).

PATIENT CONSIDERATIONS

Assessment: Assess for history of anaphylactic or severe systemic reaction to antihemophilic factor or VWF preparations, severity of hemorrhage, risk factors for thrombosis, presence of VWF inhibitors, blood type, VWD type, baseline VWF:RCo/FVIII level, and pregnancy/nursing status.

Monitoring: Monitor for thromboembolic events, anaphylactic or severe systemic reactions, infections, presence of FVIII inhibitors, and other adverse reactions. Monitor for signs of intravascular hemolysis and decreasing Hct levels when large or frequent doses are required w/ blood groups A, B, and AB. Monitor VWF:RCo and FVIII trough levels at least once a day in VWD patients, especially those undergoing surgery.

Counseling: Inform that drug is made from human plasma and may contain infectious agents that can cause disease (eg, viruses, CJD agent). Explain that the risk that it may transmit an infectious agent has been reduced by screening plasma donors, by testing the donated plasma for certain virus infections, and by inactivating and/or removing certain viruses during manufacturing. Inform that some viruses (eg, B19V, HAV), may be difficult to remove or inactivate. Advise patients, especially pregnant and immune-compromised individuals, to report low-grade fever, rash, joint pain, anorexia, N/V, fatigue, jaundice, or any other adverse reactions.

HUMATROPE — somatropin (rDNA origin)　　Rx

Class: Recombinant human growth hormone (hGH)

ADULT DOSAGE
Growth Hormone Deficiency

Adult or Childhood-Onset Etiology: Non-Weight Based:
Initial: 0.2mg/day SQ (range, 0.15-0.30mg/day)
Titrate: May increase gradually every 1-2 months by increments of 0.1-0.2mg/day based on clinical response and serum insulin-like growth factor-I (IGF-I) concentrations
Maint: Individualize dose

Weight-Based:
Initial: ≤0.006mg/kg/day SQ
Titrate: May increase based on individual requirements
Max: 0.0125mg/kg/day

Clinical response, side effects, and determination of age- and gender-adjusted serum IGF-I concentrations should be used as guidance in dose titration

PEDIATRIC DOSAGE
Growth Hormone Deficiency

Due to an inadequate secretion of endogenous growth hormone

Individualize dose
Usual: 0.026-0.043mg/kg/day SQ (0.18-0.30mg/kg/week)

The calculated weekly dose should be divided into equal doses given either 6 or 7 days/week

Turner Syndrome

Treatment of short stature associated w/ Turner syndrome

Individualize dose
Usual: Up to 0.054mg/kg/day SQ (0.375mg/kg/week)

The calculated weekly dose should be divided into equal doses given either 6 or 7 days/week

Idiopathic Short Stature

Treatment of idiopathic short stature defined by height standard deviation score (SDS) ≤-2.25 and associated w/ growth rates unlikely to permit attainment of adult height in the normal range, in pediatric patients for whom diagnostic evaluation excludes other causes of short stature that should be observed or treated by other means

Individualize dose
Usual: Up to 0.053mg/kg/day SQ (0.37mg/kg/week)

The calculated weekly dose should be divided into equal doses given either 6 or 7 days/week

Small for Gestational Age
Treatment of growth failure in children born small for gestational age (SGA) who fail to demonstrate catch-up growth by age 2-4 yrs

Individualize dose
Usual: Up to 0.067mg/kg/day SQ (0.47mg/kg/week)

The calculated weekly dose should be divided into equal doses given either 6 or 7 days/week

Short Stature Homeobox-Containing Gene (SHOX) Deficiency
Individualize dose
Usual: 0.050mg/kg/day SQ (0.35mg/kg/week)
The calculated weekly dose should be divided into equal doses given either 6 or 7 days/week

DOSING CONSIDERATIONS
Concomitant Medications
Oral Estrogen: May increase the dose requirements in women

Elderly
Consider lower starting dose and smaller dose increments

ADMINISTRATION
SQ route

Rotate inj sites to avoid lipoatrophy
For pediatric patients, the calculated weekly dosage should be divided into equal doses given either 6 or 7 days/week.
For adult patients, the prescribed dose should be administered daily

Reconstitution
Vial:
1. Each 5mg vial should be reconstituted w/ 1.5-5mL of diluent
2. Following reconstitution, swirl the vial w/ a gentle rotary motion until contents are completely dissolved; do not shake, and use it only if it is clear
3. If sensitivity to the diluent occurs, may reconstitute w/ bacteriostatic water for inj (benzyl alcohol preserved), or sterile water for inj; the reconstituted sol should be used immediately and any unused sol should be discarded
4. If it is reconstituted w/ bacteriostatic water for inj, the sol should be kept refrigerated at 36-46°F (2-8°C) and used w/in 14 days
5. When administered to a newborn infant, it should be reconstituted w/ the diluent provided or, if the infant is sensitive to the diluent, sterile water for inj
6. When reconstituted w/ sterile water for inj, the sol should be kept refrigerated at 36-46°F (2-8°C) and used w/in 24 hrs

Cartridge:
1. The cartridge has been designed for use only w/ the Humatrope inj device
2. Each cartridge should be reconstituted using only the diluent syringe that accompanies the cartridge and should not be reconstituted w/ the diluent for Humatrope provided w/ the vials
3. The reconstituted sol should be clear. If the sol is cloudy or contains particulate matter, the contents must not be injected
4. Cartridges should not be used if the patient is allergic to metacresol or glycerin

STORAGE
2-8°C (36-46°F). Avoid freezing diluent. (Vial) After Reconstitution with Diluent for Humatrope or Bacteriostatic Water for Inj: 2-8°C (36-46°F) for up to 14 days. Avoid freezing. After Reconstitution with Sterile Water: 2-8°C (36-46°F); used within 24 hrs. Discard unused portion. (Cartridge) After Reconstitution with Diluent for Humatrope: 2-8°C (36-46°F) for up to 28 days. Avoid freezing.

HOW SUPPLIED
Inj: 5mg [vial]; 6mg, 12mg, 24mg [cartridge]

CONTRAINDICATIONS
Acute critical illness due to complications following open heart surgery, abdominal surgery, multiple accidental trauma, or w/ acute respiratory failure. Pediatric patients w/ Prader-Willi syndrome (PWS) who are severely obese, have a history of upper airway obstruction or sleep apnea, or have severe respiratory impairment. Pediatric patients who have growth failure due to genetically confirmed PWS. Active malignancy or evidence of progression or recurrence of an underlying intracranial tumor. Active proliferative or severe nonproliferative diabetic retinopathy. Growth promotion in pediatric patients w/ closed epiphyses. Known hypersensitivity to somatropin or diluent.

WARNINGS/PRECAUTIONS
Reevaluate adults who were treated with somatropin for GHD in childhood and whose epiphyses are closed. Implement effective weight control in patients with PWS and treat respiratory infections aggressively. Increased risk of a second neoplasm in childhood cancer survivors reported. Increased risk of developing malignancies in children with certain rare genetic causes of short stature; monitor for development of neoplasms if treatment is initiated. Monitor for increased growth, or potential malignant changes, of preexisting nevi. Undiagnosed impaired glucose tolerance and overt diabetes mellitus (DM) may be unmasked, and new onset type 2 DM reported. Intracranial HTN with papilledema, visual changes, headache, N/V reported; d/c if papilledema occurs. Fluid retention in adults may occur. Monitor other hormonal replacement treatments in patients with hypopituitarism. Undiagnosed/untreated hypothyroidism may prevent optimal response. Hypothyroidism may become evident or worsen. Slipped capital femoral epiphysis (SCFE) and progression of scoliosis may occur in pediatric patients. Increased risk of ear/hearing disorders and cardiovascular (CV) disorders in TS patients. Pancreatitis reported rarely. Tissue atrophy may occur; rotate inj site. Allergic reactions may occur. Serum levels of inorganic phosphorus, alkaline phosphatase, parathyroid hormone, and IGF-I may increase. Obese individuals are more likely to manifest adverse effects when treated w/ a weight-based regimen. Estrogen replete women may need higher doses than men. Caution in the elderly.

ADVERSE REACTIONS
Otitis media, ear disorder, arthrosis, pain, edema, arthralgia, myalgia, HTN, paresthesia, gynecomastia, scoliosis, hyperlipidemia, rhinitis, flu syndrome, AST increased.

DRUG INTERACTIONS
May inhibit 11β-hydroxysteroid dehydrogenase type 1, resulting in reduced serum cortisol concentrations; may need glucocorticoid replacement or dose adjustments of glucocorticoid therapy. Glucocorticoid therapy may attenuate growth-promoting effects in children; carefully adjust glucocorticoid replacement dosing. May increase clearance of antipyrine. May alter clearance of compounds metabolized by CYP450 liver enzymes (eg, corticosteroids, sex steroids, anticonvulsants, cyclosporine); monitor carefully. May require greater dose with oral estrogen replacement. May need to adjust dose of insulin and/or other hypoglycemic agents, and thyroid hormone replacement therapy.

PREGNANCY AND LACTATION
Category C, caution in nursing.

MECHANISM OF ACTION
Recombinant human GH; binds to dimeric GH receptors located within the cell membranes of target tissue cells, resulting in intracellular signal transduction and subsequent induction of transcription and translation of GH-dependent proteins, including IGF-I, IGF BP-3, and acid labile subunit.

PHARMACOKINETICS
Absorption: Absolute bioavailability (75%); C_{max}=63.3ng/mL; AUC=585ng•hr/mL. **Distribution:** V_d=0.957L/kg. **Metabolism:** Liver and kidneys (protein catabolism). **Elimination:** Urine; $T_{1/2}$=3.81 hrs.

PATIENT CONSIDERATIONS
Assessment: Assess for PWS, preexisting DM or impaired glucose tolerance, hypothyroidism, hypopituitarism, history of scoliosis, hypersensitivity to drug or diluent, pregnancy/nursing status, any other conditions where treatment is contraindicated or cautioned, and possible drug interactions. Perform funduscopic exam.

Monitoring: Monitor for SCFE and progression of scoliosis in pediatric patients (eg, onset of limp, hip or knee pain), growth, clinical response, compliance, neoplasm, increased growth or malignant changes of preexisting nevi, intracranial HTN, pancreatitis, fluid retention, allergic reactions, and other adverse reactions. In patients with PWS, monitor weight as well as for signs of respiratory infection, sleep apnea, and upper airway obstruction. Monitor patients with a history of GHD secondary to an intracranial neoplasm for progression/recurrence of the tumor. Perform periodic thyroid function tests, funduscopic exam, and monitoring glucose levels. In patients with TS, monitor for ear/CV disorders.

Counseling: Inform of the potential benefits and risks of therapy, proper administration, and usage and disposal. Caution against any reuse of needles and syringes.

HUMIRA — adalimumab   Rx
Class: Monoclonal antibody/TNF blocker

Increased risk of serious infections (eg, active tuberculosis [TB], including latent TB reactivation; invasive fungal infections; and bacterial, viral, and other infections due to opportunistic pathogens) that may lead to hospitalization or death, mostly w/ concomitant use of immunosuppressants (eg, methotrexate [MTX], corticosteroids). D/C if serious infection or sepsis develops. TB patients have frequently presented w/ disseminated or extrapulmonary disease; test for latent TB before and during therapy and initiate treatment for latent TB prior to adalimumab use. Consider empiric antifungal therapy in patients at risk for invasive fungal infections who develop severe systemic illness. Monitor patients closely for development of infection during and after treatment, including development of TB in patients who tested negative for latent TB infection prior to therapy. Lymphoma and other malignancies, some fatal, reported in children and adolescents. Postmarketing cases of aggressive and fatal hepatosplenic T-cell lymphoma reported; the majority of cases occurred in patients w/ Crohn's disease (CD) or ulcerative colitis (UC) and the majority were in adolescent and young adult males. Almost all of these patients were treated concomitantly w/ azathioprine or 6-mercaptopurine.

ADULT DOSAGE

Rheumatoid Arthritis

To reduce signs/symptoms, induce major clinical response, inhibit progression of structural damage, and improve physical function in patients w/ moderately to severely active rheumatoid arthritis

40mg every other week; may increase to 40mg every week in patients not taking concomitant MTX

May be used alone or in combination w/ MTX or other nonbiologic DMARDs

Psoriatic Arthritis

To reduce signs/symptoms, inhibit progression of structural damage, and improve physical function in patients w/ active psoriatic arthritis

40mg every other week

May be used alone or in combination w/ nonbiologic disease-modifying anti-rheumatic drugs

Ankylosing Spondylitis

To reduce signs/symptoms in patients w/ active ankylosing spondylitis

40mg every other week

Crohn's Disease

To reduce signs/symptoms and induce/maintain clinical remission in patients w/ moderately to severely active CD who have had an inadequate response to conventional therapy and/or lost response to or are intolerant to infliximab

Day 1: 160mg (given as four 40mg inj in 1 day or as two 40mg inj/day for 2 consecutive days)
Day 15: 80mg
Day 29 and Onward: 40mg every other week

Use beyond 1 year has not been evaluated

Plaque Psoriasis

Treatment of moderate to severe chronic plaque psoriasis in candidates for systemic therapy or phototherapy when other systemic therapies are medically less appropriate

Initial: 80mg
Maint: 40mg every other week starting 1 week after initial dose

Ulcerative Colitis

To induce and sustain clinical remission in patients w/ moderately to severely active UC who have had an inadequate response to immunosuppressants

Day 1: 160mg (given as four 40mg inj in 1 day or as two 40mg inj/day for 2 consecutive days)
Day 15: 80mg
Day 29 and Onward: 40mg every other week

Only continue if clinical remission is evident by 8 weeks (Day 57) of therapy

Hidradenitis Suppurativa

Treatment of moderate to severe hidradenitis suppurativa
Day 1: 160mg (given as four 40mg inj on Day 1 or as two 40mg inj/day for 2 consecutive days)
Day 15: 80mg
Day 29 and Onward: 40mg every week

Uveitis

Treatment of non-infectious intermediate, posterior and panuveitis

Initial: 80mg
Maint: 40mg every other week starting 1 week after initial dose

PEDIATRIC DOSAGE

Juvenile Idiopathic Arthritis

To reduce signs/symptoms of moderately to severely active polyarticular juvenile idiopathic arthritis

≥2 Years:
10 to <15kg: 10mg every other week
15 to <30kg: 20mg every other week
≥30kg: 40mg every other week

May be used alone or in combination w/ MTX

Crohn's Disease

To reduce signs/symptoms and induce/maintain clinical remission in patients w/ moderately to severely active CD who have had an inadequate response to corticosteroids or immunomodulators

≥6 Years:
17 to <40kg:
Day 1: 80mg (given as two 40mg inj in 1 day)
Day 15: 40mg
Day 29 and Onward: 20mg every other week

≥40kg:
Day 1: 160mg (given as four 40mg inj in 1 day or as two 40mg inj/day for 2 consecutive days)
Day 15: 80mg (given as two 40mg inj in 1 day)
Day 29 and Onward: 40mg every other week

ADMINISTRATION

SQ route
May be left at room temperature for about 15-30 min before injecting; do not remove the cap or cover while allowing it to reach room temperature.
Inject at separate sites in the thigh or abdomen. Rotate inj sites; avoid areas where skin is tender, bruised, red, or hard.

STORAGE

2-8°C (36-46°F). Do not freeze; do not use if frozen, even if it has been thawed. Store in original carton until time of administration to protect from light. May be stored up to a max of 25°C (77°F) for up to 14 days, if needed. Do not store in extreme heat or cold.

HOW SUPPLIED

Inj: 10mg/0.2mL, 20mg/0.4mL [prefilled syringe]; 40mg/0.4mL, 40mg/0.8mL [prefilled syringe, prefilled pen]; 40mg/0.8mL [vial]

WARNINGS/PRECAUTIONS

Do not initiate in patients w/ an active infection. Increased risk of infection in patients >65 yrs of age and in patients w/ comorbid conditions. Malignancies, including acute and chronic leukemia, lymphoma, and nonmelanoma skin cancer (NMSC), reported in adults. Anaphylaxis and angioneurotic edema reported; d/c immediately and institute appropriate therapy if an anaphylactic or other serious allergic reaction occurs. May increase risk of HBV reactivation in chronic carriers; closely monitor for signs of active HBV infection during and for several months after therapy termination. D/C if HBV reactivation develops and start effective antiviral therapy w/ appropriate supportive treatment. Caution in considering the use in patients w/ new onset or exacerbation of central or peripheral nervous system demyelinating disorders; D/C if these disorders develop. New or worsening congestive heart failure (CHF), and hematologic system adverse reactions, including significant cytopenia (eg, thrombocytopenia, leukopenia), reported. May result in the formation of autoantibodies and development of a lupus-like syndrome; d/c if symptoms suggestive of a lupus-like syndrome develop. If possible, pediatric patients should be brought up to date w/ all immunizations in agreement w/ current immunization guidelines prior to initiating therapy. Avoid having latex-sensitive patients handle the needle cover of the prefilled syringe; it contains dry rubber (latex). Caution in elderly.

ADVERSE REACTIONS

URTI, sinusitis, inj-site reactions, headache, rash, nausea, flu syndrome, abdominal pain, hyperlipidemia, hypercholesterolemia, back pain, hematuria, increased alkaline phosphatase, UTI, HTN.

DRUG INTERACTIONS

See Boxed Warning. Reduced clearance w/ MTX. Concomitant administration w/ other biologic DMARDs (eg, anakinra, abatacept) or other TNF blockers is not recommended due to possible increased risk for infections and other potential pharmacological interactions. Avoid w/ live vaccines. Upon initiation or discontinuation of adalimumab in patients being treated w/ CYP450 substrates w/ a narrow therapeutic index, monitor therapeutic effect (eg, warfarin) or drug concentration (eg, cyclosporine, theophylline) and adjust individual dose of the drug product prn.

PREGNANCY AND LACTATION

Pregnancy: Limited clinical data available from the Humira Pregnancy Registry. Monoclonal antibodies are increasingly transported across the placenta as pregnancy progresses w/ the largest amount transferred during the 3rd trimester. Consider risks and benefits prior to administering live or live-attenuated vaccines to infants exposed to Humira in utero.
Lactation: Low amount (0.1-1%) found in human milk. No reports of adverse effects on infant and no effects on milk production. Caution in nursing.

MECHANISM OF ACTION

Monoclonal antibody/TNF-α receptor blocker; binds specifically to TNF-α and blocks its interaction w/ the p55 and p75 cell surface TNF receptors. Also lyses surface TNF-expressing cells in vitro in the presence of complement.

PHARMACOKINETICS

Absorption: (40mg SQ single dose) Absolute bioavailability (64%), C_{max}=4.7mcg/mL, T_{max}=131 hrs. **Distribution:** Found in breast milk; (0.25-10mg/kg IV dose) V_d=4.7-6L. **Elimination:** (0.25-10mg/kg IV dose) $T_{1/2}$=2 weeks.

PATIENT CONSIDERATIONS

Assessment: Assess for active/chronic/recurrent infection, history of an opportunistic infection, recent travel in areas of endemic TB or endemic mycoses, underlying conditions that may predispose to infection, central or peripheral nervous system demyelinating disorders, CHF, latex sensitivity, drug hypersensitivity, pregnancy/nursing status, and for possible drug interactions. Test for latent TB infection and for HBV infection. Assess immunization history in pediatric patients. Perform a skin examination, particularly in patients w/ a medical history of prior prolonged immunosuppressant therapy or in psoriasis patients w/ a history of psoralen plus ultraviolet light (PUVA) treatment for the presence of NMSC.
Monitoring: Monitor for development of infection during and after treatment. Monitor for malignancies, hypersensitivity reactions, neurological reactions, hematological reactions, worsening/new-onset CHF, lupus-like syndrome, and other adverse reactions. Monitor for active TB and periodically test for latent TB. Monitor for HBV reactivation during therapy and for several months following termination of therapy. Perform periodic skin examinations, particularly in patients w/ a medical history of prior prolonged immunosuppressant therapy or in psoriasis patients w/ a history of PUVA treatment for the presence of NMSC.
Counseling: Inform about the potential benefits/risks of therapy. Inform that therapy may lower the ability of the immune system to fight infections; instruct to contact physician if any symptoms of infection, including TB, invasive fungal infections, or reactivation of HBV infections, develop. Counsel about the risk of

malignancies. Advise to seek immediate medical attention if any symptoms of a severe allergic reaction develop. Advise latex-sensitive patients that the needle cap of the prefilled syringe contains latex. Advise to report to physician any signs of new/worsening medical conditions (eg, CHF, neurological disease, autoimmune disorders) or any symptoms suggestive of a cytopenia (eg, bleeding, bruising, persistent fever). Instruct on proper inj technique, as well as proper syringe and needle disposal.

Hycamtin Capsules — topotecan   Rx

Class: Topoisomerase I inhibitor

> May cause severe myelosuppression. Administer only to patients with neutrophil counts of ≥1500 cells/mm^3 and platelet counts ≥100,000 cells/mm^3. Monitor blood cell counts.

ADULT DOSAGE	**PEDIATRIC DOSAGE**
Relapsed Small Cell Lung Cancer	Pediatric use may not have been established
In patients w/ a prior complete or partial response and who are ≥45 days from the end of 1st-line chemotherapy	
2.3mg/m^2/day qd for 5 consecutive days, repeated every 21 days	
Round dose to nearest 0.25mg, and prescribe the minimum number of 1mg and 0.25mg caps; prescribe the same number of caps for each of the 5 dosing days	

DOSING CONSIDERATIONS
Renal Impairment
Moderate (CrCl 30-49mL/min): 1.5mg/m^2/day
Severe (CrCl <30mL/min): 0.6mg/m^2/day

Dose can be increased after the 1st course by 0.4mg/m^2/day if no severe hematologic or GI toxicities occur

Adverse Reactions
Diarrhea:
Grade 3 or 4: Do not administer
After Recovery ≤Grade 1: Reduce dose by 0.4mg/m^2/day for subsequent courses
Hematologic Toxicities:
Do not administer subsequent courses until neutrophils recover to >1000 cells/mm^3, platelets recover to >100,000 cells/mm^3, Hgb levels recover to ≥9.0g/dL (w/ transfusion if necessary)
Reduce Dose by 0.4mg/m^2/day for:
1. Neutrophil counts <500 cells/mm^3 associated w/ fever or infection or lasting for ≥7 days
2. Neutrophil counts 500-1000 cells/mm^3 lasting beyond Day 21 of the treatment course
3. Platelet counts <25,000 cells/mm^3

ADMINISTRATION
Oral route

Take w/ or w/o food
Swallow whole; do not chew, crush, or divide
Do not prescribe a replacement dose for emesis

STORAGE
2-8°C (36-46°F). Protect from light.

HOW SUPPLIED
Cap: 0.25mg, 1mg

CONTRAINDICATIONS
History of severe hypersensitivity reactions to topotecan.

WARNINGS/PRECAUTIONS
Do not give a replacement dose for emesis. May cause fatal typhlitis (neutropenic enterocolitis); consider the possibility of typhlitis in patients presenting with fever, neutropenia, and abdominal pain. Diarrhea, including severe and life-threatening diarrhea requiring hospitalization reported; manage diarrhea aggressively and avoid with Grade 3 or 4 diarrhea. Interstitial lung disease (ILD), including fatalities, reported; monitor for pulmonary symptoms indicative of ILD (eg, cough, fever, dyspnea, and/or hypoxia) and d/c therapy if a new diagnosis of ILD is confirmed. May cause fetal harm during pregnancy. May have acute and long-term effects on fertility in females. May damage spermatozoa in males, resulting in possible genetic and fetal abnormalities.

ADVERSE REACTIONS
Severe myelosuppression, anemia, neutropenia, thrombocytopenia, N/V, diarrhea, alopecia, fatigue, anorexia, pyrexia, asthenia.

DRUG INTERACTIONS
P-glycoprotein inhibitors (eg, azithromycin, ketoconazole, ritonavir) and breast cancer resistance protein inhibitors (eg, cyclosporine, eltrombopag) may increase the systemic exposure to oral topotecan; avoid concomitant use.

PREGNANCY AND LACTATION
Category D, not for use in nursing.

MECHANISM OF ACTION
Topoisomerase I inhibitor; binds to the topoisomerase I-DNA complex and prevents religation of these single strand breaks.

PHARMACOKINETICS
Absorption: Rapid. T_{max}=1-2 hrs; oral bioavailability (40%). **Distribution:** Plasma protein binding (35%). **Metabolism:** Reversible pH dependent hydrolysis; N-desmethyl topotecan (metabolite). **Elimination:** Urine (20%, 2% N-desmethyl topotecan), feces (33%, 1.5% N-desmethyl topotecan); $T_{1/2}$=3-6 hrs.

PATIENT CONSIDERATIONS
Assessment: Assess for history of severe hypersensitivity reactions to drug, Grade 3 or 4 diarrhea, risk factors for ILD, pregnancy/nursing status, renal impairment, and possible drug interactions. Assess baseline neutrophil and platelet counts.

Monitoring: Monitor for signs/symptoms of myelosuppression, typhlitis, ILD, diarrhea, and other adverse reactions. Monitor peripheral blood cell counts frequently.

Counseling: Inform that therapy decreases blood cell counts and frequent blood tests will be performed while on therapy to monitor for bone marrow suppression. Instruct to notify physician promptly if fever or other signs of infection develop. Advise patients on pregnancy planning and prevention. Advise females of reproductive potential to use highly effective contraception during therapy and for 1 month following treatment and for men with female sexual partners of reproductive potential to use effective contraception during therapy and for 3 months following therapy. Advise to d/c nursing during treatment. Advise male and female patients of the potential risk for impaired fertility and possible family planning options. Inform that therapy may cause diarrhea, which may be severe and life-threatening; instruct patients how to manage and/or prevent diarrhea and to inform physician if severe diarrhea occurs during treatment.

Hycamtin for Injection — topotecan   Rx

Class: Topoisomerase I inhibitor

> May cause severe myelosuppression. Administer only to patients w/ baseline neutrophil counts of ≥1500 cells/mm^3 and platelet counts ≥100,000 cells/mm^3. Monitor blood cell counts.

ADULT DOSAGE	**PEDIATRIC DOSAGE**
Ovarian Carcinoma	Pediatric use may not have been established
Treatment of metastatic carcinoma after disease progression on or after initial or subsequent chemotherapy, as a single agent	
1.5mg/m^2 by IV infusion over 30 min daily for 5 consecutive days, starting on Day 1 of a 21-day course **Max:** 4mg IV	
Small Cell Lung Cancer	
Treatment of patients w/ platinum-sensitive disease who progressed at least 60 days after initiation of 1st-line chemotherapy, as a single agent	
1.5mg/m^2 by IV infusion over 30 min daily for 5 consecutive days, starting on Day 1 of a 21-day course **Max:** 4mg IV	
Cervical Cancer	
Stage IV-B, recurrent, or persistent carcinoma of the cervix not amenable to curative treatment	
0.75mg/m^2 by IV infusion over 30 min daily on Days 1, 2, and 3 in combination w/ cisplatin 50mg/m^2 on Day 1, repeated every 21 days **Max:** 4mg IV	

DOSING CONSIDERATIONS
Renal Impairment
Moderate (CrCl 20-39mL/min): Reduce dose to 0.75mg/m^2 for single-agent use

Adverse Reactions
Hematologic Toxicities:
For single-agent use, reduce dose to 1.25mg/m^2 for:
1. Neutrophil counts <500 cells/mm^3, or administer granulocyte colony-stimulating factor (G-CSF) starting no sooner than 24 hrs following the last dose of topotecan
2. Platelet counts <25,000 cells/mm^3 during previous cycle

For combination use w/ cisplatin, reduce dose to 0.60mg/m^2 (and further to 0.45mg/m^2 if necessary) for:
1. Febrile neutropenia (neutrophil counts <1000 cells/mm^3 w/ temperature of ≥38°C [100.4°F]), or administer G-CSF starting no sooner than 24 hrs following the last dose of topotecan
2. Platelet counts <25,000 cells/mm^3 during previous cycle

ADMINISTRATION
IV route

Preparation
1. Reconstitute each 4mg vial w/ 4mL sterile water for inj
2. Dilute the appropriate volume of reconstituted sol in either 0.9% NaCl IV infusion or D5W inj prior to administration

Use immediately after reconstitution
Reconstituted vials of topotecan diluted for infusion are stable at approx 20-25°C (68-77°F) and ambient lighting conditions for 24 hrs

STORAGE
20-25°C (68-77°F). Protect from light.

HOW SUPPLIED
Inj: 4mg

CONTRAINDICATIONS
History of severe hypersensitivity reactions to topotecan.

WARNINGS/PRECAUTIONS
Bone marrow suppression (primarily neutropenia) is the dose-limiting toxicity; neutropenia is not cumulative over time. Do not treat w/ subsequent courses until neutrophils recover to >1000 cells/mm³, platelets recover to >100,000 cells/mm³, and Hgb levels recover to 9g/dL (w/ transfusion if necessary). May cause fatal typhlitis (neutropenic enterocolitis); consider the possibility of typhlitis in patients presenting w/ fever, neutropenia, and abdominal pain. Interstitial lung disease (ILD), including fatalities, reported; monitor for pulmonary symptoms indicative of ILD (eg, cough, fever, dyspnea, hypoxia), and d/c therapy if a new diagnosis of ILD is confirmed. Embryofetal toxicity may occur. Extravasation reported; immediately d/c administration and institute recommended management procedures if signs/symptoms occur.

ADVERSE REACTIONS
Severe myelosuppression, neutropenia, pneumonia, anemia, diarrhea, abdominal pain, thrombocytopenia, N/V, fatigue, asthenia, dyspnea, stomatitis-pharyngitis, constipation, sepsis, pain.

DRUG INTERACTIONS
Concomitant administration w/ G-CSF may prolong duration of neutropenia; if G-CSF is used, it should be started no sooner than 24 hrs following last dose of therapy. Severe myelotoxicity reported when used in combination w/ cisplatin.

PREGNANCY AND LACTATION
Pregnancy: May cause fetal harm.
Lactation: It is not known whether topotecan is present in human milk; not for use in nursing.
Reproductive Potential: Females of reproductive potential should use effective contraception during treatment and for 1 month after the last dose. Males w/ a female sexual partner of reproductive potential should use effective contraception during and for 3 months after treatment. May damage spermatozoa, resulting in possible genetic and fetal abnormalities in males. May have both acute and long-term effects on fertility in females.

MECHANISM OF ACTION
Topoisomerase I inhibitor; binds to topoisomerase I-DNA complex and prevents re-ligation of DNA single-strand breaks.

PHARMACOKINETICS
Distribution: Plasma protein binding (approx 35%). **Metabolism:** Reversible pH-dependent hydrolysis; N-desmethyl topotecan (metabolite). **Elimination:** (IV) Feces (17.9% total topotecan, 1.7% N-desmethyl topotecan), urine (50.8% total topotecan, 3.1% N-desmethyl topotecan); $T_{1/2}$=2-3 hrs.

PATIENT CONSIDERATIONS
Assessment: Assess for previous hypersensitivity to drug, renal impairment, risk factors of ILD, pregnancy/nursing status, and possible drug interactions. Assess baseline neutrophil and platelet counts.

Monitoring: Monitor for signs/symptoms of myelosuppression, typhlitis, ILD, extravasation, and other adverse reactions. Perform frequent monitoring of peripheral blood counts.

Counseling: Inform that therapy decreases blood cell counts and that frequent blood tests will be performed while on therapy to monitor for the occurrence of bone marrow suppression. Instruct to promptly notify physician if fever, other signs of infection (eg, chills, cough, burning pain on urination), or bleeding develops. Advise pregnant women of the potential risk to a fetus and advise to contact physician if pregnant, or if pregnancy is suspected during treatment. Instruct females of reproductive potential to use effective contraception during treatment and for 1 month after the last dose. Instruct males w/ a female sexual partner of reproductive potential to use effective contraception during treatment and for 3 months after the last dose. Advise nursing mothers to d/c nursing during treatment. Inform male and female patients of the potential risk for impaired fertility and possible family planning options. Advise that therapy may cause asthenia or fatigue; inform that these symptoms may impair ability to safely drive or operate machinery.

HyperHEP B SD — hepatitis B immune globulin (human)   Rx

Class: Immune globulin

ADULT DOSAGE
Postexposure Prophylaxis

Acute Exposure to Blood Containing HBsAg:
0.06mL/kg IM as soon as possible after exposure and w/in 24 hrs, if possible; give a 2nd dose 1 month after 1st dose if hepatitis B vaccine is refused

Refer to PI for recommendations following percutaneous or permucosal exposure

Sexual Exposure to HBsAg-Positive Person:
0.06mL/kg IM single dose w/ hepatitis B vaccine series; give w/in 14 days of last sexual contact or if sexual contact w/ infected person will continue

Household Exposure to Persons w/ Acute Hepatitis B Virus Infection:
Prophylaxis not indicated unless there is an identifiable blood exposure to the index patient (eg, by sharing toothbrushes/razors); treat such exposures like sexual exposures

PEDIATRIC DOSAGE
Postexposure Prophylaxis

Safety/effectiveness not established

Perinatal Exposure of Infants Born to HBsAg and HBeAg Positive Mothers:
0.5mL IM after physiologic stabilization of infant and preferably w/in 12 hrs of birth; administer hepatitis B vaccine in 3 doses of 0.5mL IM (1st dose w/in 7 days of birth, then 1 month and 6 months after 1st dose)

Repeat dose at 3 months if 1st dose of hepatitis B vaccine is delayed for as long as 3 months, or repeat at 3 and 6 months if hepatitis B vaccine is refused

Household Exposure to Persons w/ Acute Hepatitis B Virus Infection: <12 Months of Age:
0.5mL IM along w/ hepatitis B vaccine

ADMINISTRATION
IM route

May be administered at the same time (but at a different site), or ≤1 month preceding hepatitis B vaccination
Administer preferably in the deltoid muscle of the upper arm or lateral thigh muscle; do not use the gluteal region

STORAGE
2-8°C (36-46°F). Do not freeze.

HOW SUPPLIED
Inj: 0.5mL, 1mL (syringe); 1mL, 5mL (vial)

WARNINGS/PRECAUTIONS
May contain infectious agents (eg, viruses, Creutzfeldt-Jakob disease agent) that can cause disease. Caution with a history of prior systemic allergic reactions to human immune globulin preparations; epinephrine should be available. Administer only when benefits outweigh the risks in patients with severe thrombocytopenia or any coagulation disorder that would contraindicate IM inj. Do not administer IV.

ADVERSE REACTIONS
Pain and tenderness at the inj site, urticaria, angioedema, anaphylactic reactions.

DRUG INTERACTIONS
May interfere with live virus vaccines; defer vaccination until approximately 3 months after hepatitis B immune globulin administration.

PREGNANCY AND LACTATION
Category C, safety not known in nursing.

MECHANISM OF ACTION
Immune globulin; provides passive immunization for individuals exposed to HBV as evidenced by a reduction in the attack rate of hepatitis B.

PHARMACOKINETICS
Elimination: $T_{1/2}$= 17.5-25 days.

PATIENT CONSIDERATIONS
Assessment: Assess for history of allergic reactions to human immune globulin preparations, severe thrombocytopenia or any coagulation disorder, pregnancy/nursing status, and possible drug interactions.

Monitoring: Monitor for allergic reactions, transmission of infectious disease, and other adverse reactions.

Counseling: Inform of the risks/benefits of therapy. Instruct to contact physician if any signs/symptoms of infection or if any other adverse reactions develop.

HyperRho S/D Full Dose — rho(D) immune globulin (human)   Rx

Class: Immune globulin

ADULT DOSAGE
Suppression of Rh Isoimmunization

Pregnancy and Other Obstetric Conditions:
Prevention of Rh hemolytic disease of newborn by administration to Rho(D) negative mother w/in 72 hrs after birth of Rho(D) positive infant, provided that mother is Rho(D) negative and not already sensitized to the Rho(D) factor, and her child is Rho(D) positive and has a negative direct antiglobulin test

Postpartum Prophylaxis:
Give 1 full dose syringe preferably w/in 72 hrs of delivery if volume of RBCs that has entered circulation is ≤15mL

Perform a fetal red cell count to determine required dose in instances where a large fetomaternal hemorrhage is suspected (>30mL of whole blood or 15mL RBCs); divide RBC volume of calculated fetomaternal hemorrhage by 15mL to obtain number of syringes to give; if >15mL of red cells is suspected or if dose calculation results in a fraction, administer the next higher whole number of syringes

PEDIATRIC DOSAGE
Pediatric use may not have been established

Antenatal Prophylaxis:
Give 1 full dose syringe at approx 28 weeks' gestation; must be followed by another full dose, w/in 72 hrs following delivery, if infant is Rh positive

Following Threatened Abortion (Any Stage of Gestation w/ Continuation of Pregnancy):
Give a full dose, and if >15mL of red cells is suspected due to fetomaternal hemorrhage, same dose modification in postpartum prophylaxis applies

Miscarriage, Abortion, or Termination of Ectopic Pregnancy (≥13 Weeks' Gestation):
Give a full dose, and if >15mL of red cells is suspected due to fetomaternal hemorrhage, same dose modification in postpartum prophylaxis applies; if pregnancy is terminated prior to 13 weeks' gestation, may use a single mini-dose instead of full-dose

Following Amniocentesis (Either 15-18 Weeks' Gestation or During 3rd Trimester)/Abdominal Trauma (2nd/3rd Trimester):
Give a full dose, and if there is a fetomaternal hemorrhage in excess of 15mL of red cells, same dose modification in postpartum prophylaxis applies

If abdominal trauma, amniocentesis, or other adverse event requires administration of full dose at 13-18 weeks' gestation, give another full dose at 26-28 weeks

Give therapy w/in 72 hrs after delivery if baby is Rh positive; if delivery occurs w/in 3 weeks after last dose, the postpartum dose may be withheld unless there is fetomaternal hemorrhage >15mL of RBCs

Transfusion:
Prevention of isoimmunization in Rho(D) negative individuals who have been transfused w/ Rho(D) positive RBCs or blood components containing RBCs

Multiply volume of Rh positive whole blood given by Hct of donor unit to give volume of RBCs transfused. Divide volume of RBCs by 15mL to provide number of syringes to be given; if dose calculation results in a fraction, administer the next higher whole number of syringes
Administer w/in 72 hrs after an incompatible transfusion, but preferably as soon as possible

ADMINISTRATION
IM route

Administer in the deltoid muscle of the upper arm or lateral thigh muscle; do not inject into the gluteal region

Multiple Syringe Dose
Calculate number of full dose syringes to be given; total volume can be given in divided doses at different sites at 1 time or total dose may be divided and injected at intervals, provided total dosage is given w/in 72 hrs of fetomaternal hemorrhage or transfusion

STORAGE
2-8°C (36-46°F). Do not freeze.

HOW SUPPLIED
Inj: ≥1500 IU

WARNINGS/PRECAUTIONS
Never administer to neonates. Made from human plasma; may contain infectious agents (eg, viruses, Creutzfeldt-Jakob disease agent) that can cause disease. Caution with history of prior systemic allergic reactions following administration of human immunoglobulin preparations. Must weigh the benefits/risks of hypersensitivity reactions in patients with isolated immunoglobulin A (IgA) deficiency; increased potential for developing antibodies to IgA and could have anaphylactic reactions to subsequent administration of blood products that contain IgA. Bleeding complications may be encountered in patients with thrombocytopenia or other bleeding disorders. Large fetomaternal hemorrhage late in pregnancy or following delivery may cause a weak mixed field positive D^u test result; if there is any doubt about the mother's Rh type, give $Rh_o(D)$

immune globulin (human). Although systemic reactions to human immunoglobulin preparations are rare, epinephrine should be available for treatment of acute anaphylactic reactions. Babies born of women treated antepartum may have a weakly positive direct antiglobulin test at birth. Passively acquired anti-Rh_o(D) may be detected in maternal serum if antibody screening tests are performed subsequent to antepartum/postpartum administration.

ADVERSE REACTIONS
Slight soreness at inj site, slight temperature elevation, elevated bilirubin levels.

DRUG INTERACTIONS
Other antibodies in the preparation may interfere with response to live vaccines (eg, measles, mumps, polio, rubella); avoid immunization with live vaccines within 3 months after therapy.

PREGNANCY AND LACTATION
Category C, safety not known in nursing.

MECHANISM OF ACTION
Immune globulin; prevents isoimmunization in Rh_o(D) negative individual exposed to Rh_o(D) positive blood by suppressing immune response of Rh_o(D) negative individuals to Rh_o(D) positive RBCs.

PATIENT CONSIDERATIONS

Assessment: Assess for history of prior systemic allergic reactions to human immunoglobulin preparations, IgA deficiency, thrombocytopenia or other bleeding disorders, Rh status of mother/father/fetus, pregnancy/nursing status, and possible drug interactions.

Monitoring: Monitor for inj-site/anaphylactic reactions, signs/symptoms of infection, and other adverse reactions.

Counseling: Inform of risks/benefits of therapy. Advise to consult physician if signs/symptoms of infection, inj-site reactions, or anaphylactic reactions occur.

HYPERRHO S/D MINI-DOSE — rho(D) immune globulin (human)

Class: Immune globulin   **Rx**

ADULT DOSAGE	**PEDIATRIC DOSAGE**
Suppression of Rh Isoimmunization	Pediatric use may not have been established
Prevention of isoimmunization of Rho(D)-negative women at the time of spontaneous or induced abortion of up to 12 weeks' gestation, provided that the mother must be Rho(D) negative and must not already be sensitized to the Rho(D) antigen, the father is not known to be Rho(D) negative, and gestation is not more than 12 weeks at termination	
Postabortion or Postmiscarriage of Up to 12 Weeks' Gestation: 1 mini dose syringe IM w/in 3 hrs or as soon as possible following spontaneous/induced abortion; if prompt administration is not possible, give w/in 72 hrs following termination of pregnancy	

ADMINISTRATION
IM route

Administer in deltoid muscle of upper arm or lateral thigh muscle; do not use gluteal region

STORAGE
2-8°C (36-46°F). Do not freeze.

HOW SUPPLIED
Inj: 250 IU [syringe]

WARNINGS/PRECAUTIONS
For IM administration only. Never administer IV. Do not administer to neonates. May carry a risk of transmitting infectious agents (eg, viruses, Creutzfeldt-Jakob disease agent). Signs/symptoms of viral infections, particularly hepatitis C, may develop in patients receiving blood or plasma products; report all infections possibly transmitted by the product to manufacturer. Must weigh the benefits against potential risks of hypersensitivity reactions in patients with isolated immunoglobulin A (IgA) deficiency. Caution with history of prior systemic allergic reactions following the administration of human Ig preparations. Caution with thrombocytopenia or other bleeding disorders; bleeding complications may be encountered. Acute anaphylactic symptoms may occur; have epinephrine available.

ADVERSE REACTIONS
Slight soreness at inj site, slight temperature elevation, sensitization.

DRUG INTERACTIONS
May interfere with the response to live vaccines (eg, measles, mumps, polio, or rubella); avoid immunization with live vaccines within 3 months after administration.

PREGNANCY AND LACTATION
Category C, safety not known in nursing.

MECHANISM OF ACTION

Immune globulin; prevents formation of anti-Rh$_o$(D) antibody in Rh$_o$(D)-negative women who are exposed to the Rh$_o$(D) antigen at the time of spontaneous or induced abortion (up to 12 weeks' gestation); suppresses the stimulation of active immunity by Rh$_o$(D)-positive fetal erythrocytes that may enter the maternal circulation at the time of termination of the pregnancy.

PATIENT CONSIDERATIONS

Assessment: Assess for history of prior systemic allergic reactions, IgA deficiency, thrombocytopenia or other bleeding disorder, Rh status of woman and man, gestational age, pregnancy/nursing status, and possible drug interactions.

Monitoring: Monitor for inj-site reactions, anaphylactic reactions, signs/symptoms of viral infection, and other adverse reactions.

Counseling: Inform of risks/benefits of therapy.

HYQVIA — immune globulin infusion (human) with recombinant human hyaluronidase

Rx

Class: Immune globulin

> Thrombosis may occur in the absence of known risk factors. For patients at risk of thrombosis (eg, advanced age, prolonged immobilization, hypercoagulable conditions, history of venous or arterial thrombosis, use of estrogens, indwelling vascular catheters, hyperviscosity, cardiovascular risk factors), administer at the minimum dose and infusion rate practicable. Ensure adequate hydration before administration. Monitor for signs/symptoms of thrombosis and assess blood viscosity if at risk for hyperviscosity.

ADULT DOSAGE

Primary Immunodeficiency

Treatment Initiation:
For patients previously on another IgG treatment, administer 1st dose approx 1 week after the last infusion of previous treatment

Increase dose and frequency from a 1-week dose to a 3- or 4-week dose; refer to PI for initial treatment interval/dosage ramp-up schedule

Switching from Immune Globulin IV (Human) Therapy:
Administer at the same dose and frequency as previous IV treatment, after initial dose ramp-up

Naive to IgG Therapy or Switching from Immune Globulin SQ (Human) Therapy:
300-600mg/kg at 3- to 4-week intervals, after initial ramp-up

Individualization of Dose:
If administered at the same dose and frequency, serum IgG levels from Hyqvia should be comparable to serum IgG levels from IV treatment

Dose Adjustment:
Calculate the difference between patient's serum IgG trough level during Hyqvia treatment and the IgG trough level during previous IV treatment, then refer to PI for individualization in volume administered per dosing interval for intended change in IgG trough level

PEDIATRIC DOSAGE

Pediatric use may not have been established

ADMINISTRATION

SQ route

Use an infusion pump capable of infusing dose at rates up to 300mL/hr/site; use a SQ needle set that is 24 gauge and labeled for high flow rates.

Infuse the 2 components of Hyqvia sequentially, beginning w/ the recombinant human hyaluronidase.

Initiate the infusion of the full dose of the immune globulin infusion 10% (human) through the same SQ needle set w/in approx 10 min of the recombinant human hyaluronidase infusion.

For each full or partial vial of immune globulin infusion 10% (human) used, administer the entire contents of the recombinant human hyaluronidase vial.

Selection of Infusion Site(s)

The suggested site(s) for infusion are the abdomen and thighs.

If 2 sites are used, the 2 infusion sites should be on opposite sides of the body. Avoid bony prominences, or areas that are scarred, inflamed, or infected.

Volume per Site

Administer up to 600mL/site for patients ≥40kg and up to 300mL/site for patients <40kg.

A 2nd site can be used at the discretion of the physician and patient based on tolerability and total volume.

If a 2nd site is used, administer half of total volume of the recombinant human hyaluronidase of Hyqvia in each site.

Rate of Infusion

Administer the recombinant human hyaluronidase of Hyqvia at an initial rate per site of approx 1-2mL/min, or as tolerated.

Refer to PI for immune globulin infusion 10% (human) infusion rates.

If infusions at the full dose and maximum rate are tolerated, adjust both the time intervals and number of rate changes of the ramp-up used for successive infusions at the discretion of the physician and patient.

Preparation and Handling

Allow refrigerated product to come to room temperature before use; do not apply heat or place in microwave.

Do not shake; do not mix the recombinant human hyaluronidase and the immune globulin infusion 10% (human) of Hyqvia into the same container prior to administration.

Do not mix or administer components of Hyqvia w/ other products; administer components sequentially.

Do not use either component alone.

Flush the infusion line w/ normal saline or D5W if required.

Refer to PI for further instructions for administration.

STORAGE

2-8°C (36-46°F) for up to 36 months; or up to 25°C (77°F) for up to 3 months during the first 24 months from the manufacturing date. Do not return to the refrigerator after it has been stored at room temperature. Do not freeze. Protect from light.

HOW SUPPLIED

Inj: (Immune Globulin Infusion 10% [Human] [vial 1]-Recombinant Human Hyaluronidase [vial 2]) 2.5g/25mL-200 U/1.25mL, 5g/50mL-400 U/2.5mL, 10g/100mL-800 U/5mL, 20g/200mL-1600 U/10mL, 30g/300mL-2400 U/15mL

CONTRAINDICATIONS

History of anaphylactic or severe systemic reaction to IgG; IgA-deficient patients w/ antibodies to IgA and a history of hypersensitivity; known systemic hypersensitivity to hyaluronidase or recombinant human hyaluronidase.

WARNINGS/PRECAUTIONS

Do not infuse into or around an infected area due to potential risk of spreading a localized infection. **Immune Globulin Infusion 10% (Human):** Contains trace amount of IgA; severe hypersensitivity reactions may occur. D/C infusion immediately and institute appropriate treatment if hypersensitivity develops. Aseptic meningitis syndrome (AMS) reported and may occur more frequently w/ high doses; rule out other causes of meningitis. Acute intravascular hemolysis reported following IV administration, and delayed hemolytic anemia may develop. Acute renal dysfunction/failure reported w/ IV administration; ensure that patients are not volume depleted prior to the initiation of infusion. In patients at risk of developing renal dysfunction because of preexisting renal insufficiency or predisposition to acute renal failure (eg, diabetes mellitus, age >65, receiving known nephrotoxic drugs), monitor renal function and consider lower, more frequent dosing. Consider discontinuation if renal function deteriorates. Non-cardiogenic pulmonary edema/transfusion-related acute lung injury (TRALI) reported w/ IV administration; if TRALI is suspected, conduct an evaluation, including tests for presence of anti-neutrophil and anti-HLA antibodies in both the product and patient serum. May carry a risk of transmitting infectious agents (eg, viruses, the variant Creutzfeldt-Jakob disease (CJD), theoretically, the classic CJD agent). May interfere w/ some serological tests. **Recombinant Human Hyaluronidase:** Development of non-neutralizing antibodies to the recombinant human hyaluronidase component reported; may cross-react w/ endogenous PH20.

ADVERSE REACTIONS

Local reactions, headache, antibody formation against recombinant human hyaluronidase, fatigue, N/V, pyrexia.

DRUG INTERACTIONS

Passive transfer of antibodies may transiently impair immune responses to live attenuated virus vaccines (eg, mumps, rubella, varicella) for up to 6 months and for a year or more to measles.

PREGNANCY AND LACTATION

Pregnancy: Category C. Women who become pregnant are encouraged to enroll in the pregnancy registry.
Lactation: The effects of antibodies that bind to recombinant human hyaluronidase transferred during human lactation are unknown; caution in nursing.

MECHANISM OF ACTION

Immune Globulin Infusion 10% (Human): Immune globulin; has not been established. Supplies a broad spectrum of opsonizing and neutralizing IgG antibodies against a wide variety of bacterial and viral agents. Also contains a spectrum of antibodies capable of interacting w/ and altering the activity of cells of the immune system as well as antibodies capable of reacting w/ cells (eg, erythrocytes). **Recombinant Human Hyaluronidase:** Increases dispersion and absorption of immune globulin infusion 10% (human) and increases permeability of the SQ tissue by temporarily depolymerizing hyaluronan.

PHARMACOKINETICS

Absorption: Absolute bioavailability (93.3%); C_{max}=1607mg/dL; AUC=91.4g•days/L; T_{max}=5 days (median). **Elimination:** $T_{1/2}$=59.3 days.

PATIENT CONSIDERATIONS

Assessment: Assess for history of anaphylactic or severe systemic reactions to IgG administration, IgA deficiency, risk of thrombosis/renal dysfunction, hydration status, infection at infusion site, hypersensitivity to drug, pregnancy/nursing status, and possible drug interactions. Assess renal function, including BUN and SrCr. Consider baseline assessment of blood viscosity in patients at risk for hyperviscosity (eg, those w/ cryoglobulins, fasting chylomicronemia/markedly high TGs, monoclonal gammopathies).

Monitoring: Monitor for thrombosis, hypersensitivity reactions, hemolytic anemia, pulmonary adverse reactions, infection, and other adverse reactions. Monitor renal function and urine output periodically. Conduct a thorough neurological examination on patients exhibiting signs/symptoms of AMS, including CSF studies, to rule out other causes of meningitis. Perform confirmatory lab testing if signs/symptoms of hemolysis are present after an infusion. Perform tests for the presence of anti-neutrophil and anti-HLA antibodies in both the product and patient serum if TRALI is suspected.

Counseling: Instruct to immediately report to physician any signs/symptoms of hypersensitivity, thrombosis, AMS, hemolysis, renal dysfunction/failure, TRALI, and infection. Inform that drug is made from human plasma and may contain infectious agents that can cause disease. Inform female patient of the possibility of participating in the pregnancy registry. Inform that product can interfere w/ immune response to live viral vaccines; instruct to notify physician of this potential interaction when receiving vaccinations. If self-administration is deemed appropriate, instruct on how to administer therapy. Counsel about the importance of following regularly scheduled infusions to maintain appropriate steady IgG levels. Instruct to keep a treatment infusion log. Inform that mild to moderate local infusion-site reactions (eg, swelling, redness) may occur; instruct to contact physician if a local reaction increases in severity or persists for more than a few days. Instruct on the importance of following the directions for the pump for infusion of the drug.

IBRANCE — palbociclib

Rx

Class: Kinase inhibitor

ADULT DOSAGE

HR Positive, HER2 Negative Advanced or Metastatic Breast Cancer

Initial Endocrine-Based Therapy in Postmenopausal Women:
125mg qd for 21 consecutive days followed by 7 days off treatment + 2.5mg letrozole qd continuously throughout the 28-day cycle

Women w/ Disease Progression Following Endocrine Therapy:
125mg qd for 21 consecutive days followed by 7 days off treatment + 500mg fulvestrant on Days 1, 15, 29, and once monthly thereafter

Pre/perimenopausal should be treated w/ luteinizing hormone-releasing hormone agonists according to current clinical practice standards

Missed Dose

If patient vomits/misses dose, patient should not take an additional dose that day; patient should take next prescribed dose at usual time

PEDIATRIC DOSAGE
Pediatric use may not have been established

DOSING CONSIDERATIONS
Concomitant Medications
Strong CYP3A Inhibitors:
Avoid concomitant use and consider alternative concomitant medication w/ no/ minimal CYP3A inhibition
If Concomitant Use Cannot Be Avoided: Reduce palbociclib dose to 75mg qd. If strong inhibitor is discontinued, increase dose (after 3-5 half lives of the inhibitor) to the dose used prior to initiating the strong inhibitor

Adverse Reactions
Recommended Starting Dose: 125mg/day
1st Dose Reduction: 100mg/day
2nd Dose Reduction: 75mg/day
If further dose reduction below 75mg/day is required, d/c treatment
Hematologic Toxicities (Except Lymphopenia Unless Associated w/ Clinical Events):
Monitor CBC prior to start of therapy, at the beginning of each cycle, as well as on Day 14 of the first 2 cycles, and as clinically indicated
Grade 1 or 2: No dose adjustment required
Grade 3:
Day 1 of Cycle:
Withhold, repeat CBC monitoring w/in 1 week. When recovered to Grade ≤2, start the next cycle at the same dose
Day 14 of First 2 Cycles:
Continue at current dose to complete cycle. Repeat CBC on Day 21
Consider dose reduction in cases of prolonged (>1 week) recovery from Grade 3 neutropenia or recurrent Grade 3 neutropenia in subsequent cycles
Grade 3 Neutropenia w/ Fever ≥38.5°C and/or Infection:
Withhold until recovery to Grade ≤2; resume at the next lower dose
Grade 4:
Withhold until recovery to Grade ≤2; resume at the next lower dose
Nonhematologic Toxicities:
Grade 1 or 2: No dose adjustment required

Grade ≥3: If persisting despite medical treatment, withhold until symptoms resolve to Grade ≤1 or Grade ≤2 (if not considered a safety risk for patient). Resume at next lower dose

ADMINISTRATION
Oral route

Take w/ food at the same time each day.
Swallow whole; do not chew, crush, or open prior to swallowing.

STORAGE
20-25°C (68-77°F); excursions permitted between 15-30°C (59-86°F).

HOW SUPPLIED
Cap: 75mg, 100mg, 125mg

WARNINGS/PRECAUTIONS
Decreased neutrophil counts and febrile neutropenia reported; dose interruption, reduction, or delay in starting treatment cycles is recommended for patients who develop Grade 3 or 4 neutropenia. Pulmonary embolism (PE) reported; monitor and treat as medically appropriate. May cause fetal harm.

ADVERSE REACTIONS
Neutropenia, leukopenia, infections, fatigue, nausea, anemia, stomatitis, headache, diarrhea, thrombocytopenia, constipation, alopecia, vomiting, rash, decreased appetite.

DRUG INTERACTIONS
See Dosing Considerations. Increased plasma exposure w/ strong CYP3A inhibitors (itraconazole). Avoid grapefruit or grapefruit juice. Decreased plasma exposure w/ strong CYP3A inducers (eg, rifampin); avoid concomitant use w/ strong CYP3A inducers (eg, phenytoin, carbamazepine, St John's wort). Multiple doses increased midazolam plasma exposure. May need to reduce dose of sensitive CYP3A substrate w/ a narrow therapeutic index (eg, alfentanil, cyclosporine, ergotamine) as therapy may increase their exposure.

PREGNANCY AND LACTATION
Pregnancy: Can cause fetal harm.
Lactation: It is not known if palbociclib is present in human milk; not for use in nursing.
Reproductive Potential: Females of reproductive potential should use effective contraception during and for at least 3 weeks after last dose. Male fertility may be compromised.

MECHANISM OF ACTION
Kinase inhibitor; reduces cellular proliferation of estrogen receptor-positive breast cancer cell lines by blocking progression of the cell from G1 into S phase of the cell cycle.

PHARMACOKINETICS
Absorption: Absolute bioavailability (46%) (125mg); T_{max}=6-12 hrs. **Distribution:** Plasma protein binding (approx 85%); V_d=2583L. **Metabolism:** Hepatic (extensive); oxidation, sulfonation, acylation, glucuronidation; glucuronide conjugate (major circulating metabolite). **Elimination:** Feces (2.3% unchanged, 26% [sulfamic acid conjugate]), urine (6.9% unchanged); $T_{1/2}$=29 hrs.

PATIENT CONSIDERATIONS
Assessment: Assess for pregnancy/nursing status and possible drug interactions. Obtain baseline CBC.

Monitoring: Monitor for signs/symptoms of PE, and other adverse reactions. Monitor CBC at the beginning of each cycle, as well as on Day 14 of the first 2 cycles, and as clinically indicated.

Counseling: Advise to immediately report any signs/symptoms of myelosuppression/infection, or PE. Instruct not to consume grapefruit products while on therapy. Inform patients to avoid strong CYP3A inhibitors/inducers. Advise to inform physician of all concomitant medications, including prescription medicines, OTC drugs, vitamins, and herbal products. Instruct not to take additional dose if the patient vomits or misses a dose and to take the next dose at the usual time. Advise females of reproductive potential to use effective contraception during therapy and for at least 3 weeks after the last dose. Advise women not to breastfeed during treatment and for 3 weeks after the last dose. Advise to contact physician if patient becomes pregnant, or if pregnancy is suspected, during treatment.

ICLUSIG — ponatinib

Rx

Class: Kinase inhibitor

> Arterial and venous thrombosis and occlusions, including fatal MI, stroke, stenosis of large arterial vessels of the brain, severe peripheral vascular disease, and the need for urgent revascularization procedures, reported; monitor for evidence of thromboembolism and vascular occlusion, and interrupt or d/c immediately for vascular occlusion. Heart failure (HF), including fatalities, reported; monitor cardiac function and interrupt or d/c therapy for new/worsening HF. Hepatotoxicity, liver failure, and death reported; monitor hepatic function and interrupt therapy if hepatotoxicity is suspected.

ADULT DOSAGE
Chronic Myeloid Leukemia

Chronic/Accelerated/Blast Phase: In Patients for Whom No Other Tyrosine Kinase Inhibitor is Indicated or Who are T315I-Positive:
Initial: 45mg qd
Titrate: Consider dose reduction for patients in chronic or accelerated phase who have achieved a major cytogenetic response

PEDIATRIC DOSAGE
Pediatric use may not have been established

Chronic Myeloid Leukemia

Chronic/Accelerated/Blast Phase:
In Patients for Whom No Other Tyrosine Kinase Inhibitor is Indicated or Who are T315I-Positive:
Initial: 45mg qd
Titrate: Consider dose reduction for patients in chronic or accelerated phase who have achieved a major cytogenetic response

Ph+ Acute Lymphoblastic Leukemia

In Patients for Whom No Other Tyrosine Kinase Inhibitor is Indicated or Who are T315I-Positive:
Initial: 45mg qd

Ph+ Acute Lymphoblastic Leukemia

In Patients for Whom No Other Tyrosine Kinase Inhibitor is Indicated or Who are T315I-Positive:
Initial: 45mg qd

DOSING CONSIDERATIONS

Concomitant Medications
Strong CYP3A Inhibitors: Reduce ponatinib dose to 30mg qd

Hepatic Impairment
Child-Pugh A, B, or C:
Initial: 30mg qd

Adverse Reactions
Myelosuppression:
ANC <1 x 10^9/L or Platelet Count <50 x 10^9/L:
First Occurrence:
Interrupt therapy and resume at 45mg after recovery to ANC ≥1.5 x 10^9/L and platelet ≥75 x 10^9/L
Second Occurrence:
Interrupt therapy and resume at 30mg after recovery to ANC ≥1.5 x 10^9/L and platelet ≥75 x 10^9/L
Third Occurrence:
Interrupt therapy and resume at 15mg after recovery to ANC ≥1.5 x 10^9/L and platelet ≥75 x 10^9/L

Serious Non-Hematologic:
Modify the dose or interrupt treatment
Arterial/Venous Occlusion:
Do not restart unless the potential benefit outweighs the risk of recurrence and the patient has no other treatment options
Reactions Other Than Arterial/Venous Occlusion:
Do not restart until the serious event has resolved or the potential benefit of resuming therapy outweighs the risk

Hepatic Toxicity:
Liver Transaminase >3X ULN (≥Grade 2):
Occurrence at 45mg:
Interrupt therapy and resume at 30mg after recovery to ≤Grade 1 (<3X ULN)
Occurrence at 30mg:
Interrupt therapy and resume at 15mg after recovery to ≤Grade 1
Occurrence at 15mg:
D/C therapy
AST/ALT ≥3X ULN w/ Bilirubin >2X ULN and Alkaline Phosphatase <2X ULN:
D/C therapy

Pancreatitis/Lipase Elevation:
Asymptomatic Grade 1 or 2 Lipase Elevation:
Consider therapy interruption or dose reduction

Asymptomatic Grade 3 or 4 Lipase Elevation (>2X ULN)/Asymptomatic Radiologic Pancreatitis (Grade 2 Pancreatitis):
Occurrence at 45mg:
Interrupt therapy and resume at 30mg after recovery to ≤Grade 1 (<1.5X ULN)
Occurrence at 30mg:
Interrupt therapy and resume at 15mg after recovery to ≤Grade 1
Occurrence at 15mg:
D/C therapy
Symptomatic Grade 3 Pancreatitis:
Occurrence at 45mg:
Interrupt therapy and resume at 30mg after complete resolution of symptoms and recovery of lipase elevation to ≤Grade 1
Occurrence at 30mg:
Interrupt therapy and resume at 15mg after complete resolution of symptoms and recovery of lipase elevation to ≤Grade 1
Occurrence at 15mg:
D/C therapy

Grade 4 Pancreatitis:
D/C therapy

Discontinuation
Consider if response has not occurred by 3 months of therapy

ADMINISTRATION
Oral route

Take w/ or w/o food.
Swallow whole; do not crush or dissolve.

STORAGE
20-25°C (68-77°F); excursions permitted to 15-30°C (59-86°F).

HOW SUPPLIED
Tab: 15mg, 30mg, 45mg

WARNINGS/PRECAUTIONS
Not indicated and not recommended for the treatment of patients w/ newly diagnosed chronic phase chronic myeloid leukemia. Venous thromboembolic events reported; consider dose modification or discontinuation if serious venous thromboembolism (VTE) develops. HTN reported; interrupt, reduce dose, or d/c therapy if HTN is not medically controlled. Interrupt treatment and consider evaluating for renal artery stenosis in the event of significant worsening, labile, or treatment-resistant HTN. Pancreatitis reported; check serum lipase every 2 weeks for the first 2 months and then monthly thereafter or as clinically indicated. Consider additional serum lipase monitoring in patients w/ a history of pancreatitis or alcohol abuse. Peripheral and cranial neuropathy reported; consider interrupting therapy and evaluate if neuropathy is suspected. Serious ocular toxicities leading to blindness or blurred vision reported. Serious bleeding events reported; interrupt therapy for serious or severe hemorrhage and evaluate. Fluid retention reported; interrupt, reduce, or d/c therapy as clinically indicated. Symptomatic bradyarrhythmias and supraventricular tachyarrhythmias reported; interrupt therapy and evaluate. Severe (Grade 3 or 4) myelosuppression reported; adjust the dose as recommended. Tumor lysis syndrome may occur in patients w/ advanced disease; ensure adequate hydration and treat high uric acid levels prior to initiating therapy. May compromise wound healing. Serious GI perforation (fistula) reported in 1 patient 38 days postcholecystectomy. Interrupt therapy for at least 1 week prior to major surgery; base decision when to resume therapy after surgery on clinical judgment of adequate wound healing. May cause fetal harm. Caution in elderly.

ADVERSE REACTIONS
HTN, rash, abdominal pain, fatigue, headache, dry skin, constipation, arthralgia, nausea, pyrexia, thrombocytopenia, neutropenia, leukopenia, anemia, lymphopenia.

DRUG INTERACTIONS
See Dosing Considerations. Ketoconazole may increase levels; reduce ponatinib starting dose when administering w/ strong CYP3A inhibitors (eg, boceprevir, clarithromycin, conivaptan, grapefruit juice). Avoid w/ strong CYP3A inducers (eg, carbamazepine, phenytoin, rifampin, St. John's wort) unless the benefit outweighs the risk of decreased ponatinib exposure; monitor for reduced efficacy. Lansoprazole may decrease exposure minimally.

PREGNANCY AND LACTATION
Pregnancy: Category D. Based on its mechanism of action and findings in animals, ponatinib can cause fetal harm when administered to a pregnant woman; pregnancy should be avoided while taking therapy.
Lactation: Not for use in nursing.

MECHANISM OF ACTION
Kinase inhibitor; inhibits the tyrosine kinase activity of ABL and T315I mutant ABL. Inhibits the activity of additional kinases including members of the VEGFR, PDGFR, FGFR, EPH receptors and SRC families of kinases, and KIT, RET, TIE2, and FLT3. Inhibits the viability of cells expressing native or mutant BCR-ABL, including T315I.

PHARMACOKINETICS
Absorption: C_{max}=73ng/mL; AUC=1253ng•hr/mL; T_{max}=6 hrs. **Distribution:** V_d=1223L; plasma protein binding (>99%). **Metabolism:** Phase I (via CYP3A4, and to a lesser extent CYP2C8, CYP2D6, and CYP3A5) and phase II; also by esterases and/or amidases. **Elimination:** Feces (87%), urine (5%); $T_{1/2}$=24 hrs.

PATIENT CONSIDERATIONS
Assessment: Assess for history of pancreatitis or alcohol abuse, upcoming surgery, pregnancy/nursing status, and possible drug interactions. Assess hydration status and uric acid levels. Obtain baseline LFTs. Conduct comprehensive eye exams at baseline.

Monitoring: Monitor for signs/symptoms of thromboembolism, vascular occlusion, HF, hepatotoxicity, VTE, HTN, pancreatitis, neuropathy, ocular toxicity, hemorrhage, fluid retention, cardiac arrhythmias, myelosuppression, tumor lysis syndrome, compromised wound healing, GI perforation, and other adverse reactions. Monitor cardiac function. Monitor LFTs at least monthly or as clinically indicated. Monitor serum lipase every 2 weeks for the first 2 months and monthly thereafter or as clinically indicated. Conduct comprehensive eye exams periodically. Monitor CBC every 2 weeks for the first 3 months and then monthly or as clinically indicated.

Counseling: Inform of the risks and benefits of therapy. Instruct to immediately contact physician w/ any signs/symptoms suggestive of a blood clot, HF, slow/fast HR, liver failure, HTN, pancreatitis, neuropathy, ocular toxicity, hemorrhage, fluid retention, or if fever develops, particularly in association w/ any suggestion of infection. Advise to inform physician if patient is planning to undergo or recently had a surgical procedure. Inform that cases of GI perforation have been reported. Advise women of the potential hazard to a fetus and to avoid becoming pregnant. Instruct to take drug exactly as prescribed and not to change dose or stop taking the drug w/o physician's advice. Inform that drug contains 121mg of lactose monohydrate in a 45mg daily dose.

IDAMYCIN PFS — idarubicin hydrochloride

Rx

Class: Anthracycline

> Give slowly into a freely flowing IV infusion and never give by IM/SQ route; extravasation may cause severe local tissue necrosis. May cause myocardial toxicity leading to congestive heart failure. Severe myelosuppression occurs when used at effective therapeutic doses. Administer only under the supervision of a physician experienced in leukemia chemotherapy and in facilities with laboratory and supportive resources adequate to monitor drug tolerance and protect and maintain a patient compromised by drug toxicity. Reduce dose with hepatic/renal impairment.

ADULT DOSAGE	PEDIATRIC DOSAGE
Acute Myeloid Leukemia	Pediatric use may not have been established
In Combination with Other Antileukemic Drugs:	
Induction: 12mg/m^2/day for 3 days by slow (10-15 min) IV inj in combo with cytarabine as 100mg/m^2/day by continuous infusion x 7 days or as 25mg/m^2 IV bolus followed by 200mg/m^2/day x 5 days continuous infusion	
May give a 2nd course in patients that have unequivocal evidence of leukemia after the 1st induction course	

DOSING CONSIDERATIONS
Renal Impairment
Consider dose reduction

Hepatic Impairment
Consider dose reduction
Bilirubin >5 mg%: Do not administer

Adverse reactions
Severe mucositis: Delay 2nd course until recovery and reduce dose by 25%

ADMINISTRATION
IV route

Do not mix with other drugs; precipitation occurs with heparin
Administer slowly (over 10 to 15 minutes) into the tubing of a freely running IV infusion of NaCl Inj (0.9%) or D5 Inj
The tubing should be attached to a Butterfly needle or other suitable device and inserted preferably into a large vein

STORAGE
2-8°C (36-46°F). Protect from light.

HOW SUPPLIED
Inj: 1mg/mL [5mL, 10mL, 20mL]

WARNINGS/PRECAUTIONS
Avoid with preexisting bone marrow suppression induced by previous drug therapy or radiotherapy unless the benefit warrants the risk. Increased risk of drug-induced cardiac toxicity with preexisting heart disease, previous therapy with anthracyclines at high cumulative doses or other potentially cardiotoxic agents, concomitant or previous radiation to the mediastinal-pericardial area, or in patients with anemia, bone marrow suppression, infections, leukemic pericarditis and/or myocarditis, active/dormant cardiovascular disease, or previous therapy with other anthracyclines or anthracenediones; monitor cardiac function during treatment. May induce hyperuricemia secondary to rapid lysis of leukemic cells; take appropriate measures to prevent hyperuricemia and to control any systemic infection before starting therapy. D/C inj/infusion immediately if signs/symptoms of extravasation occur, and restart in another vein.

ADVERSE REACTIONS
Myocardial toxicity, severe myelosuppression, infection, N/V, hair loss, abdominal cramps, diarrhea, hemorrhage, mucositis, headache, fever, mental status changes, dermatologic and pulmonary effects.

DRUG INTERACTIONS
Increased risk of drug-induced cardiac toxicity with concomitant use of drugs with the ability to suppress cardiac contractility or cardiotoxic drugs (eg, trastuzumab, cyclophosphamide, paclitaxel). Avoid with other cardiotoxic agents unless the patient's cardiac function is monitored frequently. Patients receiving anthracyclines after stopping treatment with other cardiotoxic agents, especially those with long T$_{1/2}$, may also be at an increased risk of developing cardiotoxicity; avoid use of therapy for at least 5 half-lives after discontinuation of the cardiotoxic agent; if therapy is used before this time, carefully monitor cardiac function.

PREGNANCY AND LACTATION
Category D, not for use in nursing.

MECHANISM OF ACTION
Anthracycline; DNA-intercalating analog of daunorubicin that has an inhibitory effect on nucleic acid synthesis and interacts with the enzyme topoisomerase II.

PHARMACOKINETICS
Distribution: Plasma protein binding (97%, 94% idarubicinol). **Metabolism:** Extrahepatic (extensive); idarubicinol (active metabolite). **Elimination:** Bile (major), renal (minor); T$_{1/2}$=22 hrs (monotherapy), 20 hrs (with cytarabine), >45 hrs (idarubicinol).

PATIENT CONSIDERATIONS
Assessment: Assess for preexisting bone marrow suppression, risk of drug-induced cardiac toxicity, hepatic/renal function, pregnancy/nursing status, and possible drug interactions.

Monitoring: Monitor for signs/symptoms of extravasation, hyperuricemia, other toxicities, and other adverse reactions. Monitor CBCs and cardiac/hepatic/renal function.

Counseling: Inform of benefits and risks of therapy. Advise women of childbearing potential to avoid becoming pregnant.

IFEX — ifosfamide

Rx

Class: Cyclophosphamide analogue

> Myelosuppression can be severe and lead to fatal infections; monitor blood counts prior to and at intervals after each treatment cycle. CNS toxicities can be severe and result in encephalopathy and death; monitor for CNS toxicity and d/c treatment for encephalopathy. Nephrotoxicity can be severe and result in renal failure. Hemorrhagic cystitis can be severe and can be reduced by prophylactic use of mesna.

ADULT DOSAGE	PEDIATRIC DOSAGE
Germ Cell Testicular Cancer	Pediatric use may not have been established
In Combination w/ Certain Other Antineoplastic Agents for 3rd-line Chemotherapy:	
1.2g/m^2/day for 5 consecutive days; administer as a slow IV infusion lasting a minimum of 30 min	
Repeat treatment every 3 weeks or after recovery from hematologic toxicity	

ADMINISTRATION
IV route

Use in combination w/ mesna to reduce incidence of hemorrhagic cystitis
Give w/ at least 2L of oral or IV fluid per day to prevent bladder toxicity

Preparation
1g Vial: Add 20mL of SWFI or bacteriostatic water for inj (benzyl alcohol or parabens preserved) for a final concentration of 50mg/mL
3g Vial: Add 60mL of SWFI or bacteriostatic water for inj (benzyl alcohol or parabens preserved) for a final concentration of 50mg/mL

Sol may be further diluted to achieve concentrations of 0.6-20mg/mL in the following fluids:
1. D5 inj
2. 0.9% NaCl inj
3. Lactated ringer's inj
4. SWFI

STORAGE
20-25°C (68-77°F). Protect from temperatures >30°C (86°F). Constituted/Constituted and Further Diluted Sol: Refrigerate and use within 24 hrs.

HOW SUPPLIED
Inj: 1g, 3g

CONTRAINDICATIONS
Known hypersensitivity to administration of ifosfamide, urinary outflow obstruction.

WARNINGS/PRECAUTIONS
Increased risk of myelosuppression in patients with reduced renal function. Infections reported and latent infections can be reactivated; close hematologic monitoring is recommended. Avoid with WBC count <2000/µL and/or a platelet count <50,000/µL, unless clinically essential. Caution in patients with infection, severe immunosuppression, or compromised bone marrow reserve, as indicated by leukopenia, granulocytopenia, extensive bone marrow metastases, prior radiation therapy, or prior therapy with other cytotoxic agents. May impair mental/physical abilities. Renal parenchymal, tubular necrosis, and other renal function disorders reported; caution with preexisting renal impairment or reduced nephron reserve. Exclude or correct any urinary tract obstructions before starting treatment. Obtain a urinalysis prior to each dose; if microscopic hematuria (>10 RBCs/high power field) is present, withhold subsequent administration until complete resolution. Caution with active urinary tract infections. Cardiotoxicity, interstitial pneumonitis, pulmonary fibrosis, and other forms of pulmonary toxicity, leading to respiratory failure, reported. Secondary malignancies may develop several yrs after therapy is discontinued. Veno-occlusive liver disease reported. May cause fetal harm. Interferes with oogenesis and spermatogenesis; amenorrhea, azoospermia, and sterility in both sexes reported. Anaphylactic/anaphylactoid reactions, and cross-sensitivity between oxazaphosphorine cytotoxic agents reported. May interfere with normal wound healing. Caution with renal/hepatic impairment and in elderly.

ADVERSE REACTIONS
Myelosuppression, infections, CNS toxicities, encephalopathy, nephrotoxicity, renal failure, hemorrhagic cystitis, N/V, alopecia, hematuria/macrohematuria.

DRUG INTERACTIONS
Severe myelosuppression frequently observed when used with other chemotherapeutic/hematotoxic agents and/or radiation therapy. Potential for additive effects with drugs acting on the CNS (eg, antiemetics, sedatives, narcotics, antihistamines); use such agents with caution or, if necessary, d/c in case of ifosfamide-induced encephalopathy. Increased risk of hemorrhagic cystitis with past or concomitant radiation of the bladder or busulfan treatment. Increased risk of cardiotoxic effects with prior or concomitant treatment with other cardiotoxic agents or radiation of the cardiac region. CYP3A4 inducers (eg, carbamazepine, phenytoin, fosphenytoin, phenobarbital, rifampin, St. John's wort)

may increase metabolism of ifosfamide to its active alkylating metabolites and formation of the neurotoxic/nephrotoxic metabolite, chloroacetaldehyde; closely monitor for toxicities and consider dose adjustment. CYP3A4 inhibitors (eg, ketoconazole, fluconazole, itraconazole, sorafenib, aprepitant, fosaprepitant, grapefruit, grapefruit juice) may decrease metabolism of ifosfamide to its active alkylating metabolites, perhaps decreasing the effectiveness of treatment.

PREGNANCY AND LACTATION
Category D, not for use in nursing.

MECHANISM OF ACTION
Cyclophosphamide analogue; not established. Prodrug that requires metabolic activation by CYP450 isoenzymes to exert its cytotoxic activity; action is primarily through DNA crosslinks caused by alkylation by the isophosphoramide mustard at guanine N-7 positions. The formation of inter- and intra-strand cross-links in the DNA results in cell death.

PHARMACOKINETICS
Distribution: $(1.5g/m^2)$ V_d (median)=0.64L/kg (Day 1), 0.72L/kg (Day 5); found in breast milk. **Metabolism:** Liver (extensive) via ring oxidation to form 4-hydroxy-ifosfamide (active metabolite), and side-chain oxidation. **Elimination:** $(5g/m^2)$ Urine (70-86% metabolites, 61% unchanged. $(1.6-2.4g/m^2)$ Urine (12-18% unchanged). $(1.5g/m^2)$ $T_{1/2}$=7 hrs $(1.6-2.4g/m^2)$, 15 hrs $(3.8-5g/m^2)$.

PATIENT CONSIDERATIONS
Assessment: Assess for hypersensitivity to drug, urinary outflow obstruction, infection, risk of cardiotoxicity, hepatic impairment, any other conditions where treatment is cautioned, pregnancy/nursing status, and possible drug interactions. Obtain WBC count, platelet count, Hgb, and a urinalysis prior to each dose. Evaluate glomerular and tubular kidney function.

Monitoring: Monitor for signs/symptoms of myelosuppression, CNS/renal/cardiac/pulmonary toxicity, hemorrhagic cystitis, infection, secondary malignancies, veno-occlusive liver disease, anaphylactic/anaphylactoid reactions, and other adverse reactions. Monitor blood counts (WBC, platelet, Hgb) at intervals after each treatment cycle. Evaluate glomerular and tubular kidney function during and after treatment. Monitor urinary sediment regularly for the presence of erythrocytes and other signs of uro/nephrotoxicity. Monitor serum and urine chemistries (eg, K^+, phosphorus) regularly.

Counseling: Inform of the risks associated with therapy as well as the plan for regular blood monitoring during therapy. Instruct to report fever or other symptoms of infection, and preexisting cardiac disease. Counsel about the need to increase fluid intake and frequent voiding to prevent accumulation in the bladder. Inform of the potential hazard to fetus if patient becomes pregnant or fathers a child during therapy and for up to 6 months after therapy; instruct to use effective methods of contraception. Inform of the potential for serious adverse reactions and tumorigenicity when children are breastfed during therapy. Advise that drug may cause GI disorders and that alcohol may increase N/V. Counsel about the importance of proper oral hygiene.

ILARIS — canakinumab   Rx

Class: Monoclonal antibody/interleukin-1 (IL-1) beta blocker

ADULT DOSAGE
Cryopyrin-Associated Periodic Syndromes

Including familial cold autoinflammatory syndrome and Muckle-Wells syndrome

15-40kg: 2mg/kg
<40kg: 150mg
Administer every 8 weeks as a single dose via SQ inj

PEDIATRIC DOSAGE
Cryopyrin-Associated Periodic Syndromes

Including familial cold autoinflammatory syndrome and Muckle-Wells syndrome

≥4 Years:
15-40kg: 2mg/kg; may increase to 3mg/kg if response is inadequate
<40kg: 150mg

Administer every 8 weeks as a single dose via SQ inj

Systemic Juvenile Idiopathic Arthritis

≥2 Years:
≥7.5kg: 4mg/kg SQ every 4 weeks
Max: 300mg/dose

ADMINISTRATION
SQ route

Supplied in a single-use vial; discard any unused product or waste material. Avoid inj into scar tissue as this may result in insufficient exposure.

Preparation and Administration
1. Reconstitute each vial by slowly injecting 1mL of preservative-free sterile water for inj w/ a 1mL syringe and an 18-gauge x 2-inch needle.
2. Swirl the vial slowly at an angle of about 45° for approx 1 min and allow to stand for 5 min; do not shake. Then gently turn the vial upside down and back again 10X.
3. Allow to stand for 15 min at room temperature to obtain a clear sol. The reconstituted sol has a final concentration of 150mg/mL. Tap the side of the vial to remove any residual liquid from the stopper; the reconstituted sol should be essentially free from particulates, and clear to opalescent. The sol may be colorless or may have a slight brownish-yellow tint; if the sol has a distinctly brown discoloration it should not be used. Slight foaming of the product upon reconstitution is not unusual.
4. Using a sterile syringe and needle, carefully withdraw the required volume depending on the dose to be administered (0.2-1mL) and SQ inject using a 27-gauge x 0.5-inch needle.

STORAGE
2-8°C (36-46°F). Do not freeze. Protect from light. **Reconstituted Sol:** Room temperature if used w/in 60 min of reconstitution, or 2-8°C (36-46°F) and use w/in 4 hrs of reconstitution. Protect from light.

HOW SUPPLIED
Inj: 180mg

CONTRAINDICATIONS
Confirmed hypersensitivity to the active substance or to any of the excipients.

WARNINGS/PRECAUTIONS
Associated w/ an increased risk of serious infections; caution in patients w/ infections or history of recurring infections or underlying conditions that may predispose to infections, and do not administer during an active infection requiring medical intervention. D/C if serious infection develops. May increase risk of tuberculosis (TB) reactivation or of opportunistic infections (eg, aspergillosis, atypical mycobacterial infections, cytomegalovirus). Evaluate for active and latent TB infection prior to treatment initiation; perform appropriate screening tests in all patients, and treat those testing positive according to standard medical practice prior to therapy. May increase risk of malignancies. Hypersensitivity reactions reported. Prior to initiation of therapy, patients should receive all recommended vaccinations, as appropriate, including pneumococcal vaccine and inactivated influenza vaccine. Macrophage activation syndrome (MAS) reported in systemic juvenile idiopathic arthritis (SJIA) patients.

ADVERSE REACTIONS
Cryopyrin-Associated Periodic Syndromes (CAPS): Nasopharyngitis, diarrhea, influenza, headache, nausea.
SJIA: Infections (nasopharyngitis and URTI), abdominal pain, inj-site reactions.

DRUG INTERACTIONS
Increased risk of serious infections w/ TNF inhibitors; coadministration is not recommended. Not recommended w/ other agents that block interleukin-1 (IL-1) or its receptors. Do not give w/ live vaccines. May alter effect or concentration of drugs metabolized by CYP450 enzymes; monitor effect or concentration and adjust dose of CYP450 substrates w/ a narrow therapeutic index (eg, warfarin) as needed.

PREGNANCY AND LACTATION
Pregnancy: The limited human data from postmarketing reports are not sufficient to inform a drug-associated risk. Transported across the placenta in a linear fashion as pregnancy progresses; therefore, potential fetal exposure is likely to be greater during the 2nd and 3rd trimesters.
Lactation: There is no information regarding the presence of canakinumab in human milk, the effects on the breastfed infant, or the effects on milk production. Caution in nursing.

MECHANISM OF ACTION
Monoclonal anti-human IL-1β antibody of the IgG1/kappa isotype; binds to human IL-1β and neutralizes its activity by blocking its interaction w/ IL-1 receptors.

PHARMACOKINETICS
Absorption: Adults w/ CAPS: Absolute bioavailability (66%); C_{max}=16mcg/mL; T_{max}=7 days. Pediatric Patients w/ CAPS: T_{max}=2-7 days. **Distribution:** CAPS, 70kg Patients: V_d=6.01L. SJIA, 33kg Patients: V_d=3.2L. **Elimination:** Adults w/ CAPS: $T_{1/2}$=26 days. Pediatric Patients w/ CAPS: $T_{1/2}$=22.9-25.7 days.

PATIENT CONSIDERATIONS
Assessment: Assess for drug hypersensitivity, infections, history of recurring infections or underlying conditions that may predispose to infections, active/latent TB, vaccination history, pregnancy/nursing status, and possible drug interactions.

Monitoring: Monitor for serious infections, signs/symptoms of TB, malignancies, hypersensitivity reactions, MAS or triggers for MAS, and other adverse reactions.

Counseling: Advise of the potential benefits and risks of therapy. Advise that healthcare providers should perform administration of drug. Instruct to immediately contact physician if an infection, signs of an allergic reaction, persistent inj-site reaction, or signs/symptoms or high-risk exposure suggestive of TB (eg, persistent cough, weight loss, subfebrile temperature) develop. Advise female patients of the potential risk to a fetus.

ILUVIEN — fluocinolone acetonide   Rx

Class: Corticosteroid

ADULT DOSAGE
Diabetic Macular Edema

Previously Treated with Corticosteroids without a Significant Rise in Intraocular Pressure:
0.19mg (1 implant) in the affected eye

PEDIATRIC DOSAGE
Pediatric use may not have been established

ADMINISTRATION
Intravitreal route

Inj Procedure
1. Remove the applicator from the tray with sterile gloved hands touching only the sterile interior tray surface and applicator
2. Prior to injection, the applicator tip must be kept above the horizontal plane to ensure that the implant is properly positioned within the applicator
3. Before inserting the needle into the eye, push the applicator button down and slide it to the first stop (at the curved black marks alongside the button track). At the first stop, release the button and it should move to the UP position. If the button does not rise to the UP position, do not proceed with this unit

4. Optimal placement of the implant is inferior to the optic disc and posterior to the equator of the eye

5. Measure 4 millimeters inferotemporal from the limbus with the aid of calipers for point of entry into the sclera

6. Remove the protective cap from the needle and inspect the tip to ensure it is not bent

7. Gently displace the conjunctiva so that after withdrawing the needle, the conjunctival and scleral needle entry sites will not align

8. Insert the needle through the conjunctiva and sclera. To release the implant, while the button is in the UP position, advance the button by sliding it forward to the end of the button track and remove the needle. Ensure that the button reaches the end of the track before removing the needle

STORAGE
15-30°C (59-86°F).

HOW SUPPLIED
Implant: 0.19mg

CONTRAINDICATIONS
Glaucoma w/ cup to disc ratios of >0.8; active or suspected ocular or periocular infections including most viral diseases of the cornea and conjunctiva, including active epithelial herpes simplex keratitis (dendritic keratitis), vaccinia, varicella, mycobacterial infections, and fungal diseases; known hypersensitivity to any components of this product.

WARNINGS/PRECAUTIONS
Intravitreal inj has been associated with endophthalmitis, eye inflammation, increased IOP, and retinal detachments. May produce posterior subcapsular cataracts, increased IOP, and glaucoma, and may enhance the establishment of secondary ocular infections due to bacteria, fungi, or viruses. Not recommended in patients with history of ocular herpes simplex; potential for reactivation of the viral infection. Risk of implant migration into the anterior chamber in patients whose posterior lens capsule is absent or has a tear.

ADVERSE REACTIONS
Cataract, myodesopsia, eye pain, conjunctival hemorrhage, posterior capsule opacification, eye irritation, conjunctivitis, corneal edema, foreign body sensation in eyes, eye pruritus, ocular hyperemia, anemia, headache, renal failure, pneumonia.

PREGNANCY AND LACTATION
Category C, caution in nursing.

MECHANISM OF ACTION
Corticosteroid; inhibits inflammatory responses to a variety of inciting agents. Inhibits edema, fibrin deposition, capillary dilation, leukocyte migration, capillary proliferation, fibroblast proliferation, deposition of collagen, and scar formation associated with inflammation.

PHARMACOKINETICS
Distribution: Found in breast milk (systemically administered).

PATIENT CONSIDERATIONS

Assessment: Assess for hypersensitivity to product components, glaucoma with cup to disc ratios of >0.8, active or suspected ocular or periocular infections, history of ocular herpes simplex, absent or torn posterior lens capsule, and pregnancy/nursing status.

Monitoring: Monitor for eye inflammation, retinal detachment, posterior subcapsular cataracts, glaucoma, secondary ocular infections, and other adverse reactions. Monitor for elevation of IOP and for endophthalmitis by checking for perfusion of the optic nerve head immediately after inj, tonometry within 30 min following inj, and biomicroscopy between 2-7 days after inj.

Counseling: Advise that a cataract may occur after treatment; if this occurs, inform that vision will decrease and that an operation to remove the cataract and restore vision will be needed. Advise that increased IOP may develop, which may need to be managed with eye drops or surgery. Inform that in the days following intravitreal inj, patients are at risk for potential complications including development of endophthalmitis or elevated IOP; instruct to report any symptoms suggestive of endophthalmitis without delay. Advise to seek immediate care from an ophthalmologist if the eye becomes red, sensitive to light, painful, or if a change in vision develops. Inform that temporary visual blurring after receiving an intravitreal inj may be experienced; instruct to avoid driving/using machines until this has resolved.

IMBRUVICA — ibrutinib
Rx

Class: Kinase inhibitor

ADULT DOSAGE

Mantle Cell Lymphoma

Patients Who Have Received at Least 1 Prior Therapy:
560mg qd until disease progression or unacceptable toxicity occurs

Chronic Lymphocytic Leukemia/ Small Lymphocytic Lymphoma

Patients w/ or w/o 17p Deletion:
420mg qd until disease progression or unacceptable toxicity occurs

Combination w/ Bendamustine and Rituximab:
Bendamustine and rituximab administered every 28 days for up to 6 cycles + 420mg ibrutinib qd until disease progression or unacceptable toxicity occurs

PEDIATRIC DOSAGE
Pediatric use may not have been established

Waldenstrom's Macroglobulinemia
420mg qd until disease progression or unacceptable toxicity occurs

Missed Dose
If a dose is not taken at the scheduled time, it can be taken as soon as possible on the same day w/ a return to the normal schedule the following day; extra capsules of ibrutinib should not be taken to make up for the missed dose

----

DOSING CONSIDERATIONS
Concomitant Medications
Avoid coadministration w/ strong or moderate CYP3A inhibitors and consider alternative agents w/ less CYP3A inhibition

Strong CYP3A Inhibitors Taken Chronically (eg, Ritonavir, Indinavir, Nelfinavir): Concomitant use is not recommended
Short-term Use (for ≤7 Days) of Strong CYP3A Inhibitors (eg, Antifungals, Antibiotics): Consider interrupting ibrutinib therapy until the CYP3A inhibitor is no longer needed
If Moderate CYP3A Inhibitor (eg, Fluconazole, Darunavir, Erythromycin) Is Necessary: Reduce ibrutinib dose to 140mg

Hepatic Impairment
Mild (Child-Pugh Class A): 140mg qd
Moderate or Severe (Child-Pugh Classes B and C): Avoid use

Adverse Reactions
Interrupt Therapy For:
- Any Grade ≥3 nonhematological toxicities
- Grade ≥3 neutropenia w/ infection or fever
- Grade 4 hematological toxicities

1st Toxicity Occurrence:
Mantle Cell Lymphoma (MCL): Restart at 560mg qd once symptoms of the toxicity have resolved to Grade 1 or baseline (recovery)
Chronic Lymphocytic Leukemia (CLL), Small Lymphocytic Lymphoma (SLL) and Waldenstrom's Macroglobulinemia (WM): Restart at 420mg qd after recovery

2nd Toxicity Occurrence:
MCL: Restart at 420mg qd after recovery
CLL, SLL and WM: Restart at 280mg qd after recovery

3rd Toxicity Occurrence:
MCL: Restart at 280mg qd after recovery
CLL, SLL and WM: Restart at 140mg qd after recovery

4th Toxicity Occurrence:
MCL, CLL, SLL, and WM: D/C ibrutinib

ADMINISTRATION
Oral route

Take at approx the same time each day.
Swallow caps whole w/ water; do not open, break, or chew.

STORAGE
20-25°C (68-77°F); excursions permitted between 15-30°C (59-86°F). Retain in original package until dispensing.

HOW SUPPLIED
Cap: 140mg

WARNINGS/PRECAUTIONS
See Dosing Considerations. Fatal and ≥Grade 3 bleeding events reported. Consider the benefit-risk of withholding therapy for at least 3-7 days pre- and post-surgery depending upon the type of surgery and the risk of bleeding. Fatal and nonfatal infections reported. Cases of progressive multifocal leukoencephalopathy (PML) reported. Evaluate patients for fever and infections and treat appropriately. Treatment-emergent Grade 3 or 4 cytopenias reported; monitor CBC monthly. A-fib and A-flutter reported, particularly in patients w/ cardiac risk factors, HTN, acute infections, and a previous history of A-fib; perform ECG if arrhythmic symptoms (eg, palpitations, lightheadedness) or new onset dyspnea develop. Manage A-fib appropriately and if it persists, consider the risks and benefits of treatment and follow dose modification guidelines. HTN reported; monitor for new onset HTN or HTN that is not adequately controlled after starting therapy. Secondary primary malignancies (eg, nonmelanoma skin cancer, non-skin carcinomas) reported. Tumor lysis syndrome (TLS) reported. Assess baseline risk (eg, high tumor burden) and take appropriate precautions; monitor patients closely and treat as appropriate. May cause fetal harm. Management of hyperviscosity in patients w/ WM may include plasmapheresis before and during treatment; modifications to ibrutinib dosing are not required.

ADVERSE REACTIONS
Neutropenia, thrombocytopenia, diarrhea, anemia, musculoskeletal pain, rash, nausea, bruising, fatigue, hemorrhage, pyrexia.

DRUG INTERACTIONS
See Dosing Considerations. Risk of bleeding may be increased in patients receiving antiplatelet or anticoagulant therapies. Ketoconazole (a strong CYP3A inhibitor) increased levels. Closely monitor patients taking concomitant strong or moderate CYP3A inhibitors for signs of ibrutinib toxicity. Avoid grapefruit and Seville oranges during treatment. Rifampin (a strong CYP3A inducer) decreased levels; avoid use w/ strong CYP3A inducers (eg, carbamazepine, rifampin, St. John's wort) and consider alternative agents w/ less CYP3A induction.

PREGNANCY AND LACTATION

Pregnancy: Can cause fetal harm based on findings from animal studies.
Lactation: There is no information regarding the presence of ibrutinib or its metabolites in human milk, the effects on the breastfed infant, or the effects on milk production. Caution in nursing.
Reproductive Potential: Verify the pregnancy status of females of reproductive potential prior to initiating therapy. Females of reproductive potential should avoid pregnancy while taking ibrutinib and for up to 1 month after ending treatment. Men should avoid fathering a child while receiving ibrutinib, and for 1 month following the last dose of therapy.

MECHANISM OF ACTION

Bruton's tyrosine kinase (BTK) inhibitor; forms a covalent bond w/ a cysteine residue in the BTK active site, leading to inhibition of BTK enzymatic activity. BTK is a signaling molecule of the B-cell antigen receptor and cytokine receptor pathways. BTK's role in signaling through the B-cell surface receptors results in activation of pathways necessary for B-cell trafficking, chemotaxis, and adhesion.

PHARMACOKINETICS

Absorption: Absolute bioavailability (2.9%, fasted condition); T_{max}=1-2 hrs (median); AUC=953ng•hr/mL (560mg), 680ng•hr/mL (420mg). **Distribution:** Plasma protein binding (97.3%); V_d=10,000L. **Metabolism:** Liver via CYP3A (primary), CYP2D6 (minor); PCI-45227 (a dihydrodiol metabolite) (active). **Elimination:** Feces (80%, 1% unchanged), urine (<10%); $T_{1/2}$=4-6 hrs.

PATIENT CONSIDERATIONS

Assessment: Assess for cardiac risk factors, acute infections, HTN, history of A-fib, planned/recent surgery, hepatic impairment, pregnancy/nursing status, and possible drug interactions.

Monitoring: Monitor for signs of bleeding, fever, infections, PML, A-fib, HTN, secondary primary malignancies, TLS, and other adverse reactions. Monitor CBC monthly. Perform ECG in patients who develop arrhythmic symptoms (eg, palpitations, lightheadedness) or new onset dyspnea.

Counseling: Inform of the possibility of bleeding, and instruct to report any signs/symptoms of bleeding (eg, blood in stools or urine, prolonged or uncontrolled bleeding) to physician. Advise that therapy may need to be interrupted for medical or dental procedures. Inform of the possibility of serious infection, and instruct to report any signs/symptoms of infection (eg, fever, chills, weakness, confusion) to physician. Counsel to report any signs of A-Fib (eg, palpitations, lightheadedness, fainting, SOB, chest discomfort) to physician. Inform that high blood pressure may occur, which may require treatment w/ anti-hypertensive therapy. Inform that other malignancies (eg, skin cancers) may occur. Advise of the potential risk of TLS and instruct to report any signs/symptoms associated w/ this event to physician. Inform women of the potential hazard of therapy to a fetus and instruct to avoid becoming pregnant during treatment and for 1 month after the last dose. Inform of the common side effects associated w/ therapy. Advise to inform physician of all concomitant medications, including prescription medicines, OTC drugs, vitamins, and herbal products. Inform that loose stools or diarrhea may occur and instruct to contact physician if diarrhea persists. Counsel to maintain adequate hydration.

IMLYGIC — talimogene laherparepvec   Rx

Class: Oncolytic viral therapy

ADULT DOSAGE

Melanoma

Local treatment of unresectable cutaneous, subcutaneous, and nodal lesions in patients w/ melanoma recurrent after initial surgery

The total inj volume for each treatment visit should not exceed 4mL for all injected lesions combined

Initial Treatment:
Up to 4mL at a concentration of 10^6 (1 million) plaque-forming units (PFU)/mL

Second Treatment (3 Weeks After Initial Treatment):
Up to 4mL at a concentration of 10^8 (100 million) PFU/mL

All Subsequent Treatments Including Reinitiation (2 Weeks After Previous Treatment):
Up to 4mL at a concentration of 10^8 (100 million) PFU/mL

Continue treatment for at least 6 months unless other treatment is required or until there are no injectable lesions to treat

Reinitiate treatment if new unresectable cutaneous, subcutaneous, or nodal lesions appear after a complete response

PEDIATRIC DOSAGE

Pediatric use may not have been established

ADMINISTRATION

Intralesional route

Administer by inj into cutaneous, subcutaneous, and/or nodal lesions that are visible, palpable, or detectable by ultrasound guidance.

Prioritization of Lesions to be Injected

Initial Treatment:
-Inject largest lesion(s) first.
-Prioritize inj of remaining lesion(s) based on lesion size until max inj volume is reached or until all injectable lesion(s) have been treated.

Second and All Subsequent Treatments:
-Inject any new lesion(s) (lesions that have developed since initial or previous treatment) first.
-Prioritize inj of remaining lesion(s) based on lesion size until max inj volume is reached or until all injectable lesion(s) have been treated.

Inj Volume Determination (Per Lesion)

<5cm Lesion: Up to 4mL inj
<2.5-5cm Lesion: Up to 2mL inj
<1.5-2.5cm Lesion: Up to 1mL inj
<0.5-1.5cm Lesion: Up to 0.5mL inj
≤0.5cm Lesion: Up to 0.1mL inj

When lesions are clustered together, inject them as a single lesion according to above.

Preparation and Handling

Healthcare providers who are immunocompromised or pregnant should not prepare or administer talimogene laherparepvec and should not come into direct contact w/ the inj sites, dressings, or body fluids of treated patients.
Avoid accidental exposure and follow universal biohazard precautions for preparation, administration, and handling.

1. Determine the total volume required for inj, up to 4mL.
2. Thaw frozen vials at room temperature (20-25°C [68-77°F]) until talimogene laherparepvec is liquid (approx 30 min). Do not expose the vial to higher temperatures. Keep the vial in original carton during thawing.
3. Swirl gently. Do not shake.
4. After thawing, administer immediately or store in original vial and carton, protected from light in a refrigerator (2-8°C [36-46°F]) for no longer than the following:
10^6 (1 million) PFU/mL: 12 hrs
10^8 (100 million) PFU/mL: 48 hrs
NOTE: Do not refreeze after thawing. Discard any vial left in the refrigerator longer than the specified times.
5. Prepare sterile syringes and needles. A detachable needle of 18-26G may be used for withdrawal and a detachable needle of 22-26G may be used for inj. Small unit syringes (eg, 0.5mL insulin syringes) are recommended for better inj control.
6. Using aseptic technique, remove the vial cap and withdraw the product from the vial into the syringe(s), noting the total volume. Avoid generating aerosols when loading syringes w/ product, and use a biologic safety cabinet if available.

Administration

1. Treat the inj site w/ a topical or local anesthetic agent, if necessary. Do not inject anesthetic agent directly into the lesion. Inject anesthetic agent around the periphery of the lesion.
2. Using a single insertion point, inject talimogene laherparepvec along multiple tracks as far as the radial reach of the needle allows w/in the lesion to achieve even and complete dispersion. Multiple insertion points may be used if a lesion is larger than the radial reach of the needle.
3. Inject talimogene laherparepvec evenly and completely w/in the lesion by pulling the needle back w/o exiting the lesion. Redirect the needle as many times as necessary while injecting the remainder of the dose. Continue until the full dose is evenly and completely dispersed.
4. When removing the needle, withdraw it from the lesion slowly to avoid leakage of talimogene laherparepvec at the insertion point.
5. Repeat steps 1-4 for other lesions to be injected.
6. Use a new needle any time the needle is completely removed from a lesion and each time a different lesion is injected.

Post-Inj

1. Apply pressure to the inj site(s) w/ sterile gauze for at least 30 sec.
2. Swab the inj site(s) and surrounding area w/ alcohol.
3. Change gloves and cover the injected lesion(s) w/ an absorbent pad and dry occlusive dressing.
4. Wipe the exterior of occlusive dressing w/ alcohol.
5. Advise patients to:
-Keep the inj site(s) covered for at least the 1st week after each treatment visit or longer if the inj site is weeping or oozing.
-Replace the dressing if it falls off.

STORAGE

Store at -90 to -70°C (-130 to -94°F). Protect from light and store in the carton until use.

HOW SUPPLIED

Inj: 10^6 (1 million) PFU/mL, 10^8 (100 million) PFU/mL [1mL]

CONTRAINDICATIONS

Immunocompromised patients, including those w/ a history of primary or acquired immunodeficient states, leukemia, lymphoma, AIDS or other clinical manifestations of infection w/ HIV, and those on immunosuppressive therapy. Pregnant patients,

WARNINGS/PRECAUTIONS

Accidental exposure may lead to transmission of talimogene laherparepvec and herpetic infection. Healthcare providers, close contacts (household members, caregivers, sex partners, or persons sharing the same bed), pregnant women, and newborns should avoid direct contact w/ injected lesions, dressings, or body fluids of treated patients. Caregivers should wear protective gloves when assisting patients in applying or changing occlusive dressings and observe safety precautions for disposal of used dressings, gloves, and cleaning materials. In the event of an accidental exposure, exposed individuals should clean the affected area thoroughly w/ soap and water and/or a disinfectant. If signs or symptoms of herpetic infection develop, the exposed individuals should contact their healthcare provider for appropriate treatment. Patients should avoid touching or scratching inj sites or their occlusive dressings. Patients who develop suspicious herpes-like lesions should follow standard hygienic practices to prevent viral transmission. Patients or close contacts w/ suspected herpetic infections should also contact their healthcare provider to evaluate the lesions. Necrosis or ulceration of tumor tissue may occur; careful wound care and infection precautions are recommended, particularly if tissue necrosis results in open wounds. Impaired healing at the inj site reported. May increase the risk of impaired healing in patients w/ underlying risk factors (eg, previous radiation at the inj site or lesions in poorly vascularized areas); consider risks and benefits of continuing treatment if there is persistent infection or delayed healing of the inj site(s). Immune-mediated events, including glomerulonephritis, vasculitis, pneumonitis, worsening psoriasis, and vitiligo, reported; consider risks and benefits before initiating treatment in patients who have underlying autoimmune disease or before continuing treatment in patients who develop immune-mediated events. Plasmacytoma reported in proximity to the inj site after administration in a patient w/ smoldering multiple myeloma. Consider risks and benefits of treatment in patients w/ multiple myeloma or in whom plasmacytoma develops during treatment.

ADVERSE REACTIONS
Fatigue, chills, pyrexia, nausea, influenza-like illness, inj-site pain.

DRUG INTERACTIONS
Acyclovir or other antiherpetic viral agents may interfere w/ effectiveness; consider the risks and benefits before administering antiviral agents to manage herpetic infection.

PREGNANCY AND LACTATION
Pregnancy: Women of childbearing potential should use an effective method of contraception to prevent pregnancy during treatment. If a pregnant woman has an infection w/ wild-type herpes simplex virus type 1 (primary or reactivation), there is potential for the virus to cross the placental barrier and also a risk of transmission during birth due to viral shedding. While there are no clinical data to date on talimogene laherparepvec infections in pregnant women, there could be a risk to the fetus or neonate if this drug were to act in the same manner.
Lactation: There is no information regarding the presence in human milk, the effects on the breastfed infant, or the effects on milk production. Not for use in nursing.

MECHANISM OF ACTION
Genetically modified oncolytic viral therapy; replicates w/in tumors to produce the immune stimulatory protein GM-CSF. Causes lysis of tumors, followed by release of tumor-derived antigens, which together w/ virally derived GM-CSF may promote an antitumor immune response; exact mechanism is unknown.

PATIENT CONSIDERATIONS
Assessment: Assess for history of primary or acquired immunodeficient states, leukemia, lymphoma, AIDS or other clinical manifestations of infection w/ HIV, immunosuppressive therapy, underlying autoimmune disease, multiple myeloma, pregnancy/nursing status, and possible drug interactions.

Monitoring: Monitor for accidental exposure, herpetic infection, inj-site complications, immune-mediated events, and plasmacytoma at the inj site.

Counseling: Advise to avoid direct contact w/ inj sites, dressings, or body fluids; wear gloves when changing dressing; and avoid touching or scratching inj sites. Advise to keep inj sites covered for at least the first week after each treatment visit or longer if the inj site is weeping or oozing. Advise to dispose of used dressings and cleaning materials in household waste in a sealed plastic bag. Instruct females of childbearing potential to use an effective method of contraception during treatment. Advise that close contacts who are pregnant or immunocompromised should not change dressings or clean inj sites. In case of accidental exposure, instruct to clean the exposed area w/ soap and water and/or a disinfectant.

IMOGAM RABIES-HT — rabies immune globulin (human)   Rx

Class: Immune globulin

OTHER BRAND NAMES
HyperRAB S/D

ADULT DOSAGE
Postexposure Prophylaxis
Usual: 20 IU/kg (0.133mL/kg) IM; give at time of 1st vaccine dose

If anatomically feasible, use full dose to thoroughly infiltrate area around wound and any remaining volume should be administered IM

Administer to all persons suspected of rabies exposure, except persons who have been previously immunized w/ rabies vaccine and have confirmed adequate rabies antibody titer; administer as promptly as possible after exposure, but may be administered through the 7th day after the 1st dose of vaccine is given

PEDIATRIC DOSAGE
Pediatric use may not have been established

ADMINISTRATION
IM route
Never administer in the same syringe or needle or in the same anatomical site as rabies vaccine
Administer in the deltoid muscle of the upper arm or lateral thigh muscle; do not use gluteal region as an inj site

STORAGE
2-8°C (35-46°F). Do not freeze.

HOW SUPPLIED
Inj: 150 IU/mL (HyperRAB S/D) [2mL, 10mL]; (Imogam Rabies-HT) [2mL]

CONTRAINDICATIONS
(Imogam Rabies-HT) Repeated doses once vaccine treatment has been initiated.

WARNINGS/PRECAUTIONS
May contain infectious agents (eg, viruses, variant Creutzfeldt-Jakob disease agent, Creutzfeldt-Jakob disease agent) that can cause disease. Increased potential for developing antibodies to IgA and for anaphylactic reactions to subsequent administration of IgA-containing blood products in persons with IgA deficiency. Do not administer IV. Epinephrine inj (1:1000) must be immediately available should an acute anaphylactic reaction occur. Caution in patients with history of prior systemic allergic reactions to human immunoglobulin preparations. (HyperRAB S/D) Bleeding complications may occur in patients with thrombocytopenia or other bleeding disorders. (Imogam Rabies-HT) Administration of rabies postexposure prophylaxis is a medical urgency, not a medical emergency, but decisions must not be delayed. Postexposure vaccine failures reported abroad when some deviation was made from the recommended postexposure treatment protocol or when less than the currently recommended amount of antirabies sera was administered.

ADVERSE REACTIONS
(HyperRAB S/D) Soreness at inj site, mild temperature elevations. (Imogam Rabies-HT) Erythema, induration, pruritus, regional adenopathy, pain or tenderness at inj site, headache, and malaise.

DRUG INTERACTIONS
May interfere with the response to live vaccines (eg, measles, mumps, polio, or rubella); immunization of live vaccines should not be given within 3 months after rabies immune globulin (human) administration. (HyperRAB S/D) Do not repeat dose once rabies vaccine treatment has been initiated.

PREGNANCY AND LACTATION
Category C, caution in nursing. (HyperRAB S/D) safety not known in nursing.

MECHANISM OF ACTION
Immune globulin; provides passive protection from rabies virus exposure.

PATIENT CONSIDERATIONS
Assessment: Assess for history of allergic reactions to human immunoglobulin preparations, IgA deficiency, thrombocytopenia or other bleeding disorders, pregnancy/nursing status, and for possible drug interactions.

Monitoring: Monitor for allergic reactions, transmission of infectious disease, and other adverse reactions.

Counseling: Inform of the risks/benefits of therapy. Instruct to contact physician about any signs/symptoms of infection or if any other adverse reactions develop.

IMOVAX RABIES — rabies vaccine   Rx

Class: Vaccine

ADULT DOSAGE
Rabies Vaccine

Preexposure:
Primary:
3 doses of 1mL IM on Days 0, 7, and on either 21 or 28
Booster:
1mL IM in high-risk patients to maintain minimum 1:5 serum dilution by rapid fluorescent focus inhibition test
Test serum sample for rabies antibodies every 6 months in patients in the continuous risk category (eg, rabies research lab workers, rabies biologics production workers) and every 2 yrs in the frequent risk category (eg, rabies diagnostic lab workers, cavers, veterinarians and staff)

Postexposure:
Previously Unimmunized:
5 doses of 1mL IM; 1 dose immediately after exposure on Day 0, and on Days 3, 7, 14, and 28
Administer 1st vaccine dose w/ rabies immune globulin (RIG) 20 IU/kg on Day 0
Previously Immunized:
2 doses of 1mL IM; 1 dose immediately after exposure and 1 dose 3 days later (no RIG needed)

PEDIATRIC DOSAGE
Rabies Vaccine

Preexposure:
Primary:
3 doses of 1mL IM on Days 0, 7, and on either 21 or 28
Booster:
1mL IM in high-risk patients to maintain minimum 1:5 serum dilution by rapid fluorescent focus inhibition test
Test serum sample for rabies antibodies every 6 months in patients in the continuous risk category (eg, rabies research lab workers, rabies biologics production workers) and every 2 yrs in the frequent risk category (eg, rabies diagnostic lab workers, cavers, veterinarians and staff)

Postexposure:
Previously Unimmunized:
5 doses of 1mL IM; 1 dose immediately after exposure on Day 0, and on Days 3, 7, 14, and 28
Administer 1st vaccine dose w/ rabies immune globulin (RIG) 20 IU/kg on Day 0
Previously Immunized:
2 doses of 1mL IM; 1 dose immediately after exposure and 1 dose 3 days later (no RIG needed)

If the immune status of a previously vaccinated person who did not receive the recommended rabies vaccine is not known, full primary postexposure antirabies treatment (RIG + 5 doses of vaccine) may be needed

Refer to PI for pre/postexposure prophylaxis guides

If the immune status of a previously vaccinated person who did not receive the recommended rabies vaccine is not known, full primary postexposure antirabies treatment (RIG + 5 doses of vaccine) may be needed

Refer to PI for pre/postexposure prophylaxis guides

ADMINISTRATION
IM route

Inject into the deltoid muscle (adults and older children) or in anterolateral aspect of thigh (infants and small children)
If possible, use full calculated dose of RIG to infiltrate the wound(s); if it is not possible, administer any remaining portion of the dose IM at a site different from the site used to administer the vaccine
Do not mix w/ any other vaccine; use immediately

Reconstitution
Do not remove the stopper or the metal seal holding it in place
Attach the plunger and reconstitution needle to the syringe, inject the diluent into the vaccine vial; gently swirl the contents
Remove the reconstitution needle and discard
Attach a sterile needle of your choice, suitable for IM inj

STORAGE
2-8°C (35-46°F). Do not freeze.

HOW SUPPLIED
Inj: 1mL

WARNINGS/PRECAUTIONS
Avoid injection into or near blood vessels and nerves. Avoid use of the gluteal area. Do not use as a multidose vial for intradermal inj. Serum sickness type reactions reported with booster doses in preexposure prophylaxis. Neurologic illness resembling Guillain-Barre syndrome reported. All serious systemic neuroparalytic/ anaphylactic reactions to a rabies vaccine should be immediately reported to the state health department or the manufacturer. May give antihistamines in patients with history of hypersensitivity. Anaphylactic reactions may occur; have epinephrine (1:1000) available. Persons with known hypersensitivity to any of the contained antibiotics could manifest an allergic reaction. Immunosuppressive illnesses can interfere with the development of active immunity and predispose the patient to developing rabies. Contains albumin; remote risk of viral diseases and variant Creutzfeldt-Jakob disease transmission.

ADVERSE REACTIONS
Inj-site reactions (eg, pain, erythema, swelling, itching), headache, nausea, abdominal pain, muscle aches, dizziness.

DRUG INTERACTIONS
Corticosteroids and other immunosuppressive agents can interfere with the development of active immunity and predispose the patient to developing rabies; test serum for rabies antibody when rabies postexposure prophylaxis is administered to persons receiving corticosteroids or other immunosuppressive therapy to ensure that an adequate response has developed. Avoid immunosuppressive agents during postexposure therapy, unless essential.

PREGNANCY AND LACTATION
Category C, caution in nursing.

MECHANISM OF ACTION
Vaccine; stimulates the immune system to produce antibodies that may protect against rabies.

PATIENT CONSIDERATIONS
Assessment: Assess current health status, immunization history, hypersensitivity, immunosuppression, pregnancy/nursing status, and possible drug interactions.

Monitoring: Monitor serum sickness type reactions, neurologic illness resembling Guillain-Barre syndrome, systemic neuroparalytic/anaphylactic reactions, hypersensitivity reactions, transmission of infectious agents, and other adverse reactions. Test for antibody development in postexposure prophylaxis.

Counseling: Inform of potential benefits/risks of vaccination and possible adverse reactions. Instruct to report any adverse reactions to physician.

INCRELEX — mecasermin (rDNA origin)   Rx
Class: Insulin-like growth factor-1 (IGF-1)

PEDIATRIC DOSAGE
Severe Primary Insulin-Like Growth Factor-1 Deficiency

For the treatment of growth failure in children w/ severe primary insulin-like growth factor-1 (IGF-1) deficiency or w/ growth hormone (GH) gene deletion who have developed neutralizing antibodies to GH

≥2 Years:
Initial: 0.04-0.08mg/kg SQ bid
Titrate: If well tolerated for at least 1 week, may increase by 0.04mg/kg/ dose to the max dose

Max: 0.12mg/kg bid
Reduce dose if hypoglycemia occurs w/ recommended dose despite adequate food intake

ADMINISTRATION
SQ route

Administer shortly before or after (± 20 min) a meal or snack; withhold dose if patient is unable to eat shortly before or after a dose.
Rotate inj sites to a different site (upper arm, thigh, buttock, or abdomen) w/ each inj.
Do not increase subsequent doses to make up for ≥1 omitted dose.

STORAGE
Avoid freezing. Protect from direct light. **Before Opening:** 2-8°C (35-46°F). **After Opening:** Stable for 30 days after initial vial entry at 2-8°C (35-46°F).

HOW SUPPLIED
Inj: 10mg/mL [40mg]

CONTRAINDICATIONS
Active or suspected malignancy; allergy to mecasermin (rhIGF-1) or any of the inactive ingredients in this product; any experience of severe hypersensitivity to this product; growth promotion in patients w/ closed epiphyses; IV administration.

WARNINGS/PRECAUTIONS
Not a substitute to GH for approved GH indications. Treatment w/ therapy should be supervised by a physician who is experienced in the diagnosis and management of pediatric patients w/ short stature associated w/ severe primary IGF-1 deficiency or w/ GH gene deletion and who have developed neutralizing antibodies to GH. Correct thyroid and nutritional deficiencies before initiating therapy. D/C if malignancy develops. Hypoglycemia may occur; avoid engaging in any high-risk activities w/in 2-3 hrs after dosing, particularly during initiation of therapy until tolerability and a stable dose have been established. Allergic reactions reported; interrupt treatment and initiate prompt medical attention. Intracranial HTN (IH) w/ papilledema, visual changes, headache, nausea, and/ or vomiting reported; funduscopic examination is recommended at initiation of treatment and periodically thereafter. Lymphoid tissue hypertrophy associated w/ complications (eg, snoring, sleep apnea, chronic middle ear effusions) reported. Slipped capital femoral epiphysis can occur in patients who experience rapid growth; carefully evaluate any pediatric patient w/ onset of a limp or complaints of hip or knee pain. Progression of scoliosis may occur in patients who experience rapid growth. Contains benzyl alcohol; gasping syndrome associated w/ benzyl alcohol dosages >99mg/kg/day in neonates and low-birth weight neonates.

ADVERSE REACTIONS
Hypoglycemia, tonsillar hypertrophy.

PREGNANCY AND LACTATION
Pregnancy: Category C.
Lactation: Caution in nursing.

MECHANISM OF ACTION
IGF-1; activates the type 1 IGF-1 receptor in target tissues, leading to intracellular signaling which stimulates multiple processes resulting in statural growth.

PHARMACOKINETICS
Absorption: Absolute bioavailability (close to 100%); (0.12mg/kg in children) C_{max}=234ng/mL, T_{max}=2 hrs, AUC_{0-8}=2932 hr•ng/mL. **Distribution:** V_d=0.257L/ kg; plasma protein binding (>80%). **Metabolism:** Liver and kidney. **Elimination:** $T_{1/2}$=5.8 hrs (0.12mg/kg in children).

PATIENT CONSIDERATIONS
Assessment: Assess for active/suspected malignancy, hypersensitivity to drug, closed epiphyses, thyroid deficiency, nutritional deficiency, and scoliosis. Perform funduscopic examination and obtain preprandial glucose levels.

Monitoring: Monitor for hypoglycemia, IH, allergic reactions, lymphoid tissue hypertrophy, slipped capital femoral epiphysis, progression of scoliosis, and other adverse reactions. Monitor preprandial glucose levels and perform funduscopic examination periodically.

Counseling: Instruct about the proper administration of the drug. Educate patients and caregivers on the identification of signs/symptoms of hypoglycemia and serious allergic reactions and instruct to seek prompt medical attention if such events occur. Inform that therapy should be discontinued if a serious allergic reaction occurs. Instruct about proper needle disposal and not reusing needles and syringes.

INFERGEN — interferon alfacon-1   Rx
Class: Biological response modifier

> May cause or aggravate fatal or life-threatening neuropsychiatric, autoimmune, ischemic, and infectious disorders. Monitor closely with periodic clinical and lab evaluations. D/C in patients with persistently severe or worsening signs/symptoms of these conditions. When used with ribavirin, refer to the individual monograph.

ADULT DOSAGE
Chronic Hepatitis C with Compensated Liver Disease
Monotherapy:
Initial: 9mcg as a single inj 3X/week x 24 weeks
Retreatment: 15mcg as a single inj 3X/week up to 48 weeks

PEDIATRIC DOSAGE
Pediatric use may not have been established

Combination Treatment with Ribavirin:
15mcg as a single inj with weight-based ribavirin at 1000mg-1200mg (<75kg and ≥75kg) PO in 2 divided doses up to 48 weeks

DOSING CONSIDERATIONS
Renal Impairment
CrCl <50mL/min: Not recommended for use

Adverse Reactions
Serious:
Monotherapy: Dose reduction to 7.5mcg may be needed
Combination with Ribavirin: Stepwise reduction from 15mcg to 9mcg and from 9mcg to 6mcg may be needed.
Depression:
Moderate: Decrease dose from 15mcg to 9mcg; or from 9mcg to 6mcg, no change to ribavirin dose
Severe: D/C treatment
Refer to PI for visit schedule
Hematologic Toxicities:
ANC <0.75 x 10⁹/L or Platelets <50 x 10⁹/L: Reduce dose from 15mcg to 9mcg, or 9mcg to 6mcg; maintain ribavirin dose at 1200mg or 1000mg
ANC <0.50 x 10⁹/L: Suspend treatment until ANC values return to >1000/mm³
Platelets <25 x 10⁹/L: D/C treatment
Anemia:
Hgb <10g/dL with History of Cardiac or Cerebrovascular Disease: Reduce dose from 15mcg to 9mcg or 9 mcg to 6mcg and the ribavirin dose by 200 mg/day
Hgb <8.5g/dL: D/C treatment

Discontinuation
Patients who fail to achieve at least a 2 log₁₀ drop at 12 weeks or undetectable HCV-RNA at week 24
Ribavirin should be discontinued in any patient who temporarily or permanently discontinues Infergen

ADMINISTRATION
SQ route

STORAGE
2-8°C (36-46°F). Do not freeze; avoid vigorous shaking and exposure to direct sunlight. May allow to reach room temperature prior to inj. Discard unused portion.

HOW SUPPLIED
Inj: 9mcg/0.3mL, 15mcg/0.5mL

CONTRAINDICATIONS
Hepatic decompensation (Child-Pugh score >6 [Class B and C]), autoimmune hepatitis, known hypersensitivity to interferon alphas or to any component of the product. When used with ribavirin, refer to the individual monograph.

WARNINGS/PRECAUTIONS
Use of monotherapy for the treatment of hepatitis C is not recommended unless a patient is unable to take ribavirin. Patients with response of <1 log₁₀ drop HCV RNA on previous treatment, Genotype 1, high viral load (≥850,000 IU/mL), African American race, and/or presence of cirrhosis are less likely to benefit from retreatment with combination therapy. May cause severe psychiatric adverse events; extreme caution with history of depression. If patients develop psychiatric problems, monitor during treatment and in the 6-month follow-up period; d/c if psychiatric symptoms persist/worsen, or suicidal ideation/aggressive behavior towards others are identified. Cardiovascular (CV) events (eg, hypotension, arrhythmia, tachycardia, angina pectoris, cardiomyopathy, myocardial infarction [MI]) reported. Caution with CV disease; monitor with history of MI and arrhythmic disorder. Dyspnea, pulmonary infiltrates, pneumonia, bronchiolitis obliterans, interstitial pneumonitis, pulmonary HTN, and sarcoidosis, some resulting in respiratory failure and/or deaths, may be induced or aggravated; d/c if persistent or unexplained pulmonary infiltrates/pulmonary function impairment develops. Risk of hepatic decompensation in CHC patients with cirrhosis; d/c if symptoms of hepatic decompensation occur. Increases in SrCr levels, including renal failure, reported; evaluate renal function in all patients. Monitor for signs/symptoms of toxicity in patients with renal impairment. Ischemic and hemorrhagic cerebrovascular events reported. May suppress bone marrow function, resulting in severe cytopenias; d/c if severe decreases in neutrophil (<0.5 x 10⁹/L) or platelet counts (<25 x 10⁹/L). Caution with abnormally low peripheral blood cell counts and in transplantation or chronically immunosuppressed patients. Development or exacerbation of autoimmune disorders reported; caution with other autoimmune disorders. Hemorrhagic/ischemic colitis, pancreatitis, serious acute hypersensitivity reactions, and ophthalmologic disorders reported; d/c therapy if these occur. Caution with history of endocrine disorders. Perform periodic ophthalmologic exams in patients with preexisting ophthalmologic disorders (eg, diabetic retinopathy, hypertensive retinopathy). Hyperthyroidism/hypothyroidism occurrence/aggravation, hyperglycemia, and diabetes mellitus (DM) reported; d/c if uncontrollable. Neutropenia, thrombocytopenia, hypertriglyceridemia, and thyroid disorders reported; perform lab tests prior to therapy, 2 weeks after initiation, and periodically thereafter. Caution in elderly. Use with ribavirin: Caution in patients with low baseline neutrophil counts (<1500 cells/mm³). Avoid with history of significant/unstable cardiac disease.

ADVERSE REACTIONS
Neuropsychiatric/autoimmune/ischemic/infectious disorders, depression, insomnia, headache, fatigue, fever, myalgia, rigors, body pain, increased sweating, nausea, abdominal pain.

DRUG INTERACTIONS
Peripheral neuropathy reported with telbivudine. Caution with agents that are known to cause myelosuppression. When used with ribavirin, refer to the individual monograph.

PREGNANCY AND LACTATION
Category C, Category X (with ribavirin); caution in nursing, not for use in nursing (with ribavirin).

MECHANISM OF ACTION
Type-I interferon; binds to the interferon cell-surface receptor leading to the production of several interferon-stimulated gene products.

PATIENT CONSIDERATIONS
Assessment: Assess for hypersensitivity reactions, neuropsychiatric/autoimmune/ischemic/infectious disorders, cardiac/CV/pulmonary disease, transplantation or chronically immunosuppressed patients, autoimmune disorder, renal/hepatic dysfunction, preexisting ophthalmologic disorders, endocrine disorders, or any other condition where treatment is contraindicated or cautioned. Assess pregnancy/nursing status and for possible drug interactions. Obtain baseline CBCs with platelet count, SrCr/CrCl, serum albumin, bilirubin, TSH/T4, and eye exam. Obtain ECG with preexisting cardiac abnormalities before combination therapy.

Monitoring: Monitor for occurrence or aggravation of neuropsychiatric/autoimmune/ischemic/infectious disorders, depression, psychiatric symptoms, CV events, persistent or unexplained pulmonary infiltrates, pulmonary function impairment, hepatic/renal impairment, ischemic/hemorrhagic cerebrovascular events, bone marrow suppression, development/exacerbation of autoimmune disorders, colitis, pancreatitis, serious acute hypersensitivity reactions, ophthalmologic disorders, neutropenia, thrombocytopenia, hypertriglyceridemia, thyroid disorders, DM, hyperglycemia, and other adverse reactions. Monitor for signs/symptoms of interferon toxicity, including increases in SrCr with impaired renal function. Perform periodic ophthalmologic exam in patients with preexisting ophthalmologic disorder. Monitor lab tests (eg, CBCs with platelet count, SrCr/CrCl, serum albumin, bilirubin, TSH, T4) 2 weeks after initiation of therapy and periodically thereafter.

Counseling: Inform about the benefits and risks associated with therapy. Instruct to avoid pregnancy during and for 6 months post-treatment with combination therapy; recommend monthly pregnancy tests during this period. Inform that therapy should only be initiated when a negative pregnancy test has been obtained. Inform that there are no data regarding whether therapy will prevent transmission of HCV infection to others. Inform of the most common/common adverse reactions occurring during therapy; inform that non-narcotic analgesics and bedtime administration may be used to prevent or lessen some of these symptoms. Advise to rule out other possible causes of persistent fever. Instruct about the importance of proper disposal procedures and caution against the reuse of needles, syringes, or re-entry of the vial. Advise to report signs/symptoms of depression or suicidal ideation to the physician. Inform that lab evaluations are required before and during therapy. Instruct patients to keep well hydrated.

INLYTA — axitinib   Rx
Class: Kinase inhibitor

ADULT DOSAGE	PEDIATRIC DOSAGE
Advanced Renal Cell Carcinoma	Pediatric use may not have been established
Initial: 5mg bid (q12h)	

DOSING CONSIDERATIONS
Hepatic Impairment
Moderate (Child-Pugh Class B): Reduce dose by half
Titrate: Increase or decrease dose based on individual safety and tolerability

Adverse Reactions
May require temporary interruption or permanent discontinuation, and/or dose reduction to 3mg bid
May further reduce to 2mg bid if needed

Concomitant Medications
Strong CYP3A4/5 Inhibitors:
Avoid coadministration, but if needed, decrease dose by half and increase or decrease subsequent doses based on individual safety and tolerability
Strong CYP3A4/5 Inhibitors Discontinuation:
Allow 3-5 half-lives of CYP3A4/5 inhibitor to elapse after discontinuation before returning to dose used prior to coadministration

Other Important Considerations
Normotensive/No Concomitant Antihypertensive/Tolerated for ≥2 Consecutive Weeks w/ No Adverse Reaction >Grade 2:
May increase to 7mg bid, and further to 10mg bid (using the same criteria)

ADMINISTRATION
Oral route

Take w/ or w/o food
Swallow whole w/ a glass of water

STORAGE
20-25°C (68-77°F); excursions permitted to 15-30°C (59-86°F).

HOW SUPPLIED
Tab: 1mg, 5mg

WARNINGS/PRECAUTIONS
HTN/Hypertensive crisis reported; treat prn with standard antihypertensive therapy. Reduce dose if persistent HTN occurs despite antihypertensive therapy; d/c if HTN is severe and persistent or if hypertensive crisis develops. Arterial/venous thromboembolic events reported; caution with history of or risk for arterial/venous thromboembolic events. Hemorrhagic events reported; do not use in patients with evidence of untreated brain metastasis or recent active GI bleeding. Temporarily interrupt treatment if any bleeding requiring medical intervention occurs. Cardiac failure reported; management may require permanent discontinuation of therapy. GI perforation/fistulas, hypothyroidism, and hyperthyroidism reported. Treat thyroid dysfunction according to standard medical practice to maintain euthyroid state. D/C treatment at least 24 hrs prior to surgery; resume therapy after surgery based on clinical judgment of adequate wound healing. D/C if reversible posterior leukoencephalopathy (RPLS) occurs. Proteinuria reported; reduce dose or interrupt temporarily if moderate to severe proteinuria develops. Increased ALT reported. Caution with moderate hepatic impairment and with end-stage renal disease (CrCl <15mL/min). May cause fetal harm.

ADVERSE REACTIONS
Diarrhea, HTN, fatigue, decreased appetite, N/V, dysphonia, palmar-plantar erythrodysesthesia syndrome, weight decrease, asthenia, constipation, hypothyroidism, cough, mucosal inflammation, arthralgia, stomatitis.

DRUG INTERACTIONS
See Dosage. Avoid with grapefruit, grapefruit juice, and strong CYP3A4/5 inducers (eg, rifampin, dexamethasone, phenytoin, St. John's wort). Moderate CYP3A4/5 inducers (eg, bosentan, efavirenz, etravirine) may reduce exposure; avoid use if possible.

PREGNANCY AND LACTATION
Category D, not for use in nursing.

MECHANISM OF ACTION
Kinase inhibitor; inhibits receptor tyrosine kinases, including vascular endothelial growth factor receptors (VEGFR)-1, VEGFR-2, and VEGFR-3, resulting in inhibition of VEGF-mediated endothelial cell proliferation, cell survival, and tumor growth.

PHARMACOKINETICS
Absorption: (Single 5mg dose) Absolute bioavailability (58%); C_{max}=27.8ng/mL, AUC=265ng•hr/mL, T_{max}=2.5-4.1 hrs (median). **Distribution:** V_d=160L; plasma protein binding (>99%). **Metabolism:** Liver via CYP3A4/5 (primary), CYP1A2, 2C19, and UGT1A1 (lesser extent). **Elimination:** Feces (41%, 12% unchanged), urine (23%, metabolites); $T_{1/2}$=2.5-6.1 hrs.

PATIENT CONSIDERATIONS
Assessment: Assess for HTN, risk for/history of arterial/venous thromboembolic events, untreated brain metastasis, recent active GI bleeding, thyroid dysfunction, proteinuria, renal/hepatic impairment, pregnancy/nursing status, and possible drug interactions. Obtain baseline AST, ALT, and bilirubin levels. Control BP prior to initiation of treatment.

Monitoring: Monitor for HTN/hypertensive crisis, thromboembolic events, hemorrhage, symptoms of GI perforation/fistula, thyroid dysfunction, RPLS, proteinuria, signs/symptoms of cardiac failure, and other adverse events. Monitor AST, ALT, and bilirubin levels periodically.

Counseling: Inform about benefits/risks of therapy. Inform that HTN may develop; instruct to have BP monitored regularly during treatment. Instruct to inform physician if experiencing symptoms suggestive of thromboembolic events, abnormal thyroid function, any bleeding episodes, or persistent/severe abdominal pain. Advise that cardiac failure may develop during therapy and that signs/symptoms should be monitored regularly during treatment. Advise to inform physician if patient has an unhealed wound or has surgery scheduled. Advise to inform physician if patient has worsening of neurological function consistent with RPLS (eg, headache, seizure, lethargy, confusion, blindness, other visual and neurologic disturbances). Advise to avoid becoming pregnant while on therapy and counsel both male and female patients to use effective birth control. Instruct female patients not to breastfeed while receiving treatment. Advise to inform physician about all concomitant medications, vitamins, or dietary and herbal supplements. Instruct not to take additional dose if the patient vomits or misses a dose and to take the next dose at the usual time.

INTELENCE — etravirine   Rx

Class: Non-nucleoside reverse transcriptase inhibitor (NNRTI)

ADULT DOSAGE	PEDIATRIC DOSAGE
HIV-1 Infection	**HIV-1 Infection**
Combination w/ Other Antiretrovirals Treatment-Experienced: Evidence of Viral Replication and HIV-1 Strains Resistant to an NNRTI and Other Antiretrovirals: 200mg bid	**Combination w/ Other Antiretrovirals Treatment-Experienced:** Evidence of Viral Replication and HIV-1 Strains Resistant to an NNRTI and Other Antiretrovirals: **6 to <18 Years:** ≥16 to <20kg: 100mg bid ≥20 to <25kg: 125mg bid ≥25 to <30kg: 150mg bid ≥30kg: 200mg bid

---

ADMINISTRATION
Oral route
Take after a meal.
Swallow whole w/ liquid.
May be dispersed in a glass of water if unable to swallow whole.

Dispersion Instructions
- Place the tablet(s) in 5mL (1 tsp) of water, or at least enough liquid to cover the medication, stir well until the water looks milky.
- If desired, add more water or alternatively orange juice or milk (Do not place the tablets in orange juice or milk w/out first adding water). The use of grapefruit juice or warm (>40°C) or carbonated beverages should be avoided.
- Drink it immediately, rinse the glass several times w/ water, orange juice, or milk and completely swallow the rinse each time to takes the entire dose.

STORAGE
25°C (77°F); excursions permitted to 15-30°C (59-86°F). Store in the original bottle. Protect from moisture.

HOW SUPPLIED
Tab: 25mg*, 100mg, 200mg *scored

WARNINGS/PRECAUTIONS
Severe, potentially life-threatening, and fatal skin reactions (eg, erythema multiforme, toxic epidermal necrolysis, Stevens-Johnson syndrome) and hypersensitivity reactions including drug rash with eosinophilia and systemic symptoms reported; d/c immediately if these occur and initiate appropriate therapy. Immune reconstitution syndrome, autoimmune disorders (eg, Graves' disease, polymyositis, Guillain-Barre syndrome) in the setting of immune reconstitution, and redistribution/accumulation of body fat reported. Caution in elderly.

ADVERSE REACTIONS
Rash, peripheral neuropathy.

DRUG INTERACTIONS
May alter therapeutic effect and adverse reaction profile with drugs that induce, inhibit, or are substrates of CYP3A, CYP2C9, and CYP2C19, or are transported by P-glycoprotein. Avoid with other NNRTIs, delavirdine, rilpivirine, atazanavir (ATV) without low-dose ritonavir (RTV), fosamprenavir (FPV) without low-dose RTV, FPV/RTV, tipranavir/RTV, indinavir without low-dose RTV, nelfinavir without low-dose RTV, RTV (600mg bid), carbamazepine, phenobarbital, phenytoin, rifampin, rifapentine, and St. John's wort. Coadministration with boceprevir is not recommended in the presence of other drugs which may further decrease etravirine exposure (eg, darunavir/RTV, lopinavir/RTV, saquinavir/RTV, tenofovir disoproxil fumarate, or rifabutin). Caution with digoxin; use lowest dose initially. May increase levels of nelfinavir without RTV, digoxin, warfarin (monitor INR), anticoagulants, 14-OH-clarithromycin, voriconazole, diazepam, boceprevir, fluvastatin, and pitavastatin. May increase maraviroc levels in the presence of a potent CYP3A inhibitor (eg, RTV boosted protease inhibitor). May decrease levels of maraviroc, antiarrhythmics, itraconazole, ketoconazole, rifabutin, telaprevir, atorvastatin, lovastatin, simvastatin, immunosuppressant, and clopidogrel (active) metabolite. May decrease dolutegravir levels; should only be used with dolutegravir when coadministered with ATV/RTV, darunavir/RTV, or lopinavir/RTV. Fluconazole and voriconazole may increase exposure. Posaconazole, itraconazole, or ketoconazole may increase levels. May decrease clarithromycin exposure. Caution with artemether/lumefantrine. Efavirenz, nevirapine, rifabutin, systemic dexamethasone, and boceprevir may decrease levels. Darunavir/RTV, lopinavir/RTV, and saquinavir/RTV may decrease exposure. Consider alternatives to clarithromycin, such as azithromycin, for treatment of *Mycobacterium avium* complex. Monitor for withdrawal symptoms when coadministered with methadone, buprenorphine, buprenorphine/naloxone. May need to alter sildenafil dose. Refer to PI for additional drug interaction information.

PREGNANCY AND LACTATION
Category B, not for use in nursing.

MECHANISM OF ACTION
NNRTI; binds directly to reverse transcriptase and blocks the RNA-dependent and DNA-dependent DNA polymerase activities by causing a disruption of the enzyme's catalytic site.

PHARMACOKINETICS
Absorption: T_{max}=2.5-4 hrs; AUC_{12h}=4522ng•hr/mL (adults), 3742ng•hr/mL (pediatric patients). **Distribution:** Plasma protein binding (99.9%). **Metabolism:** Liver via CYP3A, CYP2C9, and CYP2C19; methyl hydroxylation. **Elimination:** Feces (93.7%, 81.2-86.4% unchanged), urine (1.2%); $T_{1/2}$=41 hrs.

PATIENT CONSIDERATIONS
Assessment: Assess treatment history, pregnancy/nursing status, and for possible drug interactions. Perform resistance testing where possible.

Monitoring: Monitor for signs/symptoms of severe skin/hypersensitivity reactions, body fat redistribution/accumulation, immune reconstitution syndrome (eg, opportunistic infections), autoimmune disorders, and other adverse reactions. Monitor clinical status, including liver transaminases. Monitor INR when combined with warfarin.

Counseling: Inform that product is not a cure for HIV infection and patients may continue to develop opportunistic infections and other complications associated with HIV disease. Advise to avoid doing things that can spread HIV-1 infection to others. Advise to take medication ud. Instruct to always use in combination with other antiretrovirals. Advise not to alter dose or d/c therapy without consulting physician. If a dose is missed within 6 hrs of time usually taken, instruct to take as soon as possible following a meal. If scheduled time exceeds 6 hrs, instruct not to take the missed dose and resume the usual dosing schedule. Advise to report to physician the use of any other prescription/nonprescription or herbal products (eg, St. John's wort). Counsel to d/c and notify physician if severe rash develops. Advise that redistribution or accumulation of body fat may occur.

INTRON A — interferon alfa-2b, recombinant Rx
Class: Biological response modifier

> May cause or aggravate fatal or life-threatening neuropsychiatric, autoimmune, ischemic, and infectious disorders. Monitor closely w/ periodic clinical and lab evaluations. D/C in patients w/ persistently severe or worsening signs/symptoms of these conditions.

ADULT DOSAGE

Malignant Melanoma
Adjuvant to surgical treatment in patients w/ malignant melanoma who are free of disease but at high risk for systemic recurrence, w/in 56 days of surgery

Induction: 20 million IU/m² IV, over 20 min, 5 consecutive days/week for 4 weeks
Maint: 10 million IU/m² SQ 3X/week for 48 weeks

Follicular Lymphoma
Initial treatment of clinically aggressive follicular non-Hodgkin's lymphoma w/ anthracycline-containing combination chemotherapy

5 million IU SQ 3X/week for up to 18 months

Chronic Hepatitis B
Treatment in patients w/ compensated liver disease and those who are serum hepatitis B surface antigen (HBsAg) positive for at least 6 months and have evidence of hepatitis B virus replication (serum hepatitis B e antigen [HBeAg] positive) w/ elevated serum ALT

5 million IU IM/SQ qd or 10 million IU IM/SQ 3X/week for 16 weeks

AIDS-Related Kaposi's Sarcoma
30 million IU/m²/dose IM/SQ 3X/ week until disease progression or maximal response has been achieved after 16 weeks of treatment

Condylomata Acuminata
1 million IU/lesion 3X/week alternating days for 3 weeks
Max: 5 lesions/course
An additional course may be administered at 12-16 weeks

Chronic Hepatitis C
Treatment in patients w/ compensated liver disease who have a history of blood or blood-product exposure and/or are hepatitis C virus (HCV) antibody positive; treatment in combination w/ ribavirin in patients w/ compensated liver disease previously untreated w/ α-interferon therapy; treatment in combination w/ ribavirin in patients who have relapsed following α-interferon therapy

3 million IU IM/SQ 3X/week

In patients tolerating therapy w/ normalization of ALT at 16 weeks of treatment, extend therapy for 18-24 months

In patients who do not normalize their ALTs or have persistently high levels of HCV RNA after 16 weeks of therapy, consider discontinuing therapy

Hairy Cell Leukemia
2 million IU/m² IM/SQ 3X/week for up to 6 months

PEDIATRIC DOSAGE

Chronic Hepatitis C
Treatment in combination w/ ribavirin in patients w/ compensated liver disease previously untreated w/ α-interferon therapy

≥3 Years:
3 million IU IM/SQ 3X/week

In patients tolerating therapy w/ normalization of ALT at 16 weeks of treatment, extend therapy for 18-24 months

In patients who do not normalize their ALTs or have persistently high levels of hepatitis C virus RNA after 16 weeks of therapy, consider discontinuing therapy

Chronic Hepatitis B
Treatment in patients w/ compensated liver disease and those who are serum HBsAg positive for at least 6 months and have evidence of hepatitis B virus replication (serum HBeAg positive) w/ elevated serum ALT

≥1 Year:
3 million IU/m² SQ 3X/week for the 1st week, then 6 million IU/m² SQ 3X/ week for total duration of 16-24 weeks
Max: 10 million IU3X/week

DOSING CONSIDERATIONS

Concomitant Medications
Doses of myelosuppressive drugs were reduced by 25% from a full-dose CHOP regimen, and cycle length increased by 33% (eg, from 21 to 28 days) when alpha interferon was added to the regimen

Adverse Reactions
Hairy Cell Leukemia:
If severe adverse reactions develop, reduce dose by 50% or temporarily withhold therapy until adverse reactions abate, then resume at 50%; permanently d/c if

severe adverse reactions persist or recur following dose adjustment.
D/C for progressive disease or failure to respond after 6 months of treatment.
Malignant Melanoma:
Severe (Including Granulocytes >250/mm³ but <500/mm³ or ALT/AST >5-10X ULN): Withhold until adverse reactions abate, then restart at 50% of the previous dose
Permanently D/C for:
1. Toxicity that does not abate after withholding treatment
2. Severe adverse reactions which recur in patients receiving reduced doses
3. Granulocytes <250/mm³ or ALT/AST >10X ULN
Follicular Lymphoma:
Neutrophils <1000/mm³ or Platelets <50,000/mm³: Withhold therapy
Neutrophils >1000/mm³, but <1500/mm³: Reduce dose by 50%; may re-escalate to starting dose after resolution of hematologic toxicity (ANC >1500/mm³)
Neutrophils <1500/mm³ or Platelets <75,000/mm³: Delay chemotherapy cycle
AST >5X ULN or SrCr >2mg/dL: Permanently d/c therapy
AIDS-Related Kaposi's Sarcoma:
Severe: Reduce dose by 50% or withhold; resume at a reduced dose if adverse reactions abate w/ interruption of dosing. Permanently d/c if adverse reactions persist or recur in patients receiving a reduced dose
Chronic Hepatitis C:
Severe: Reduce dose by 50% or d/c temporarily until adverse reactions abate; d/c therapy if intolerance persists after dose adjustment
Chronic Hepatitis B:
Severe or Lab Abnormalities: Reduce dose by 50% or d/c if appropriate, until the adverse reactions abate; d/c therapy if intolerance persists after dose adjustment
WBCs <1.5 x 10⁹/L or Granulocytes <0.75 x 10⁹/L or Platelets <50 x 10⁹/L: Reduce dose by 50%
WBCs <1.0 x 10⁹/L or Granulocytes <0.5 x 10⁹/L or Platelets <25 x 10⁹/L: Permanently d/c

ADMINISTRATION
IM/SQ/IV/Intralesional route

Administer in the pm when possible.
May administer acetaminophen at the time of inj to reduce the incidence of certain adverse reactions.
Allow sol to come to room temperature before using.
Refer to PI for dosage forms/strengths selection for each indication.

Preparation
Powder for Inj:
Reconstitute w/ 1mL sterile water for inj (SWFI).
Do not re-enter vial after withdrawing dose; discard unused portion.
IM, SQ, or Intralesional Administration:
Inject 1mL diluent (SWFI) into vial; swirl gently.
Withdraw appropriate dose and inject IM, SQ, or intralesionally.
IV Infusion:
Prepare infusion sol immediately prior to use.
Inject 1mL diluent (SWFI) into vial; swirl gently.
Withdraw and inject appropriate dose into a 100mL bag of 0.9% NaCl inj; final concentration should not be <10 million IU/100mL.

Sol for Inj:
Reconstitution prior to administration is not required.
Withdraw appropriate dose from vial and inject IM, SQ, or intralesionally; not recommended for IV administration.

Administration
Hairy Cell Leukemia:
Administer by SQ route in patients w/ platelet counts <50,000/mm³; do not administer IM.

Condylomata Acuminata:
Administer inj intralesionally using a tuberculin or similar syringe and a 25- to 30-gauge needle.
Needle should be directed at the center of the base of the wart and at an angle almost parallel to the plane of the skin (approx that in the commonly used PPD test); caution not to go beneath the lesion too deeply.
Avoid SQ inj; do not inject too superficially.

STORAGE
2-8°C (36-46°F). **Powder:** Use immediately after reconstitution; may store up to 24 hrs at 2-8°C (36-46°F). **Sol:** Do not freeze. Keep away from heat.

HOW SUPPLIED
Inj: 10 million IU, 18 million IU, 50 million IU [powder]; 18 million IU, 25 million IU [sol]

CONTRAINDICATIONS
Hypersensitivity to interferon alpha or any component of the product, autoimmune hepatitis, decompensated liver disease. When used w/ Rebetol, refer to the individual monograph.

WARNINGS/PRECAUTIONS
Caution w/ coagulation disorders (eg, thrombophlebitis, pulmonary embolism), severe myelosuppression, and debilitating medical conditions (eg, history of pulmonary disease, diabetes mellitus [DM] prone to ketoacidosis). Cardiovascular (CV) adverse experiences (eg, arrhythmia, cardiomyopathy, MI), and ischemic and hemorrhagic cerebrovascular events reported; caution w/ history of CV disease (CVD). Depression and suicidal behavior reported; d/c if severe psychiatric disorder develops, or if psychiatric symptoms persist/worsen, or suicidal/homicidal ideation or aggressive behavior towards others is identified. Obtundation, coma, and encephalopathy may occur in some patients, usually in elderly, treated w/ higher doses. May be associated w/ exacerbated symptoms

of psychiatric disorders in patients w/ co-occurring psychiatric and substance use disorders. May suppress bone marrow function and may result in severe cytopenias; d/c if severe decreases in neutrophil (<0.5 x 10^9/L) or platelet counts (<25 x 10^9/L) occur. Ophthalmologic disorders may be induced or aggravated; conduct baseline eye exam and monitor periodically w/ preexisting ophthalmologic disorders. D/C if new or worsening ophthalmologic disorders develop. Thyroid abnormalities and DM reported; d/c if these conditions develop and cannot be normalized by medication. Hepatotoxicity and autoimmune disorders reported; monitor and d/c if appropriate. May increase risk of hepatic decompensation and death in patients w/ cirrhosis; permanently d/c for evidence of severe (Grade 3) hepatic injury/decompensation (Child-Pugh score >6 [class B and C]). D/C if signs/symptoms of liver failure develop. Avoid in patients w/ a history of autoimmune disease and in patients who are immunosuppressed transplant recipients. Pulmonary disorders may be induced or aggravated. Closely monitor if the chest x-ray shows pulmonary infiltrates or there is evidence of pulmonary function impairment and d/c if appropriate. Powder formulation contains albumin; carries an extremely remote risk for transmission of viral diseases and Creutzfeldt-Jakob disease. Should not be used w/ rapidly progressive visceral disease. Acute serious hypersensitivity reactions reported; d/c immediately if an acute reaction develops. Transient rashes occurred in some patients following inj. New or exacerbated sarcoidosis, exacerbated psoriasis, and hypertriglyceridemia reported. Consider discontinuation if persistently elevated TG levels associated w/ symptoms of potential pancreatitis occur. Hemolytic anemia, dental, and periodontal disorders reported when used in combination w/ ribavirin. Variations in dosage, routes of administration, and adverse reactions exist among different brands of interferon; do not use different brands of interferon in any single treatment regimen. Caution in elderly.

ADVERSE REACTIONS
Flu-like symptoms, fatigue, fever, chills, neutropenia, myalgia, anorexia, N/V, rigors, headache, GI disorders.

DRUG INTERACTIONS
May increase theophylline levels. Caution w/ other potentially myelosuppressive agents (eg, zidovudine). Higher incidence of neutropenia w/ zidovudine. Peripheral neuropathy may occur when used in combination w/ telbivudine.

PREGNANCY AND LACTATION
Pregnancy: Category C, Category X (w/ ribavirin). A Ribavirin Pregnancy Registry has been established to monitor maternal-fetal outcomes of pregnancies in female patients and female partners of male patients exposed to ribavirin during treatment and for 6 months following cessation of treatment.
Lactation: It is not known whether this drug is excreted in human milk. Not for use in nursing.

MECHANISM OF ACTION
α-interferon; binds to specific membrane receptors on cell surface, initiating induction of certain enzymes, suppression of cell proliferation, immunomodulating activities, and inhibition of virus replication in virus-infected cells.

PHARMACOKINETICS
Absorption: (IM/SQ) C_{max}=18-116 IU/mL, T_{max}=3-12 hrs; (IV) C_{max}=135-273 IU/mL.
Elimination: (IM/SQ) $T_{1/2}$=2-3 hrs; (IV) $T_{1/2}$=2 hrs.

PATIENT CONSIDERATIONS

Assessment: Assess for history of psychiatric disorders, CVD, autoimmune, and ophthalmologic disorders, hepatic/renal impairment, hypersensitivity reactions, or any other condition where treatment is contraindicated or cautioned. Assess pregnancy/nursing status and for possible drug interactions. Obtain baseline chest x-ray, standard hematologic tests (including Hgb, complete and differential WBC counts, and platelet count), blood chemistries (electrolytes, LFTs, and TSH), and eye exam. Perform ECG in patients w/ preexisting cardiac abnormalities and/or in advanced stages of cancer. Perform liver biopsy in patients w/ chronic hepatitis B and chronic hepatitis C. Test for presence of HCV antibody in patients w/ chronic hepatitis C.

Monitoring: Monitor for occurrence or aggravation of neuropsychiatric, autoimmune, ischemic, and infectious disorders; hypersensitivity reactions; exacerbation of preexisting psoriasis or sarcoidosis; development of new sarcoidosis; renal/hepatic dysfunction; and other adverse reactions. Closely monitor patients w/ a history of MI or arrhythmic disorder, liver/pulmonary function abnormalities, and WBC counts in myelosuppressed patients and in those receiving other myelosuppressive medications. Monitor hepatic function w/ serum bilirubin, ALT, AST, alkaline phosphatase, and lactate dehydrogenase at 2, 8, and 12 weeks following initiation, then every 6 months while receiving therapy. Monitor LFTs, PT, alkaline phosphatase, albumin, and bilirubin levels periodically and at approx 2-week intervals during ALT flare. Monitor TGs, LFTs, electrolytes, chest x-ray, complete and differential WBC count, and platelet count periodically. Perform ECG in patients w/ preexisting cardiac abnormalities and/or in advanced stages of cancer. Repeat TSH testing at 3 and 6 months during therapy. Perform periodic ophthalmologic exams in patients who have a preexisting ophthalmologic disorder. Perform complete eye exam if any ocular symptoms develop. If psychiatric problems develop, including clinical depression, monitor during treatment and in the 6-month follow-up period. (Chronic hepatitis B) Monitor CBCs, platelet counts, LFTs (including serum ALT, albumin, bilirubin) at treatment Weeks 1, 2, 4, 8, 12, and 16. Evaluate HBeAg, HBsAg, and ALT at the end of therapy, then at 3 and 6 months post-therapy. (Hepatitis C) Monitor CBC and platelet counts at Weeks 1 and 2 following initiation of therapy and monthly thereafter. Evaluate serum ALT at approx 3-month intervals to assess response to treatment. (Malignant Melanoma) Monitor differential WBC counts and LFTs weekly during induction phase and monthly during maintenance phase of therapy.

Counseling: Inform of risks/benefits associated w/ treatment. Instruct on proper use of product. Advise to seek medical attention if symptoms indicative of a serious adverse reaction associated w/ therapy develops (eg, suicidal ideation, chest pain, decrease in/or loss of vision, severe abdominal pain, high persistent fever, bruising, dyspnea). Inform that some side effects, such as fatigue and decreased concentration, may interfere w/ the ability to perform certain tasks. Advise to remain well hydrated during the initial stages of treatment; inform that use of an antipyretic may ameliorate some of the flu-like symptoms. Instruct self-administering patients on the importance of site selection and rotating inj site, proper disposal of needles/syringes, and caution against reuse of needles/syringes. Inform of the risks to the fetus when therapy is used in combination w/ ribavirin during pregnancy; encourage to report to Ribavirin Pregnancy Registry to monitor maternal-fetal outcomes. Instruct female patients and female partners of male patients to use 2 forms of birth control during treatment and for 6 months after therapy is discontinued. Instruct to brush teeth thoroughly bid and to have regular dental exam. Inform that some patients may experience vomiting. Advise to rinse out the mouth thoroughly afterwards if vomiting occurs.

INVIRASE — saquinavir mesylate   Rx
Class: Protease inhibitor

ADULT DOSAGE	PEDIATRIC DOSAGE
HIV-1 Infection	Pediatric use may not have been established
In Combination w/ Ritonavir (RTV) and Other Antiretroviral Agents:	
>16 Years:	
Standard Dose: 1000mg bid + 100mg RTV bid	
Treatment-Naive Patients: **Initial:** 500mg bid + 100mg RTV bid for the first 7 days of treatment **Maint:** After 7 days, 1000mg bid + 100mg RTV bid	
Switching Immediately (No Washout Period) from Another RTV-Containing Regimen or a Non-Nucleoside Reverse Transcriptase Inhibitor-Based Regimen (Excluding Delavirdine, Rilpivirine): Initiate and continue at 1000mg bid + 100mg RTV bid	
Switching from a Regimen Containing Delavirdine/Rilpivirine: 500mg bid + 100mg RTV bid for the first 7 days of treatment When already taking RTV 100mg bid as part of an antiretroviral regimen, no additional RTV is recommended	

DOSING CONSIDERATIONS
Concomitant Medications
Treatment w/ Medications That Have the Potential to Increase QT Interval and Concomitant Saquinavir/RTV:
Use only if no alternative therapy is available. Perform ECG prior to initiation and do not initiate in patients w/ a QT interval >450 msec. If baseline QT interval is <450 msec, perform ECG after 3-4 days of therapy. D/C saquinavir/RTV or the concomitant therapy or both if a subsequent increase in QT interval by >20 msec after commencing concomitant therapy occurs.

Renal Impairment
Severe or ESRD: Has not been studied; use w/caution

ADMINISTRATION
Oral route

Cobicistat is not interchangeable w/ RTV to increase systemic exposure of saquinavir.
Take RTV at the same time as saquinavir, w/in 2 hrs pc.
Refer to RTV labeling for additional dosage and administration for RTV.

Patients Unable to Swallow Caps
1. Open the caps and place contents into an empty container.
2. Add 15mL of either sugar syrup or sorbitol syrup (for patients w/ type 1 diabetes or glucose intolerance) or 3 tsp of jam to the contents of the caps in the container.
3. Stir w/ a spoon for 30-60 sec.
4. Administer the full amount prepared for each dose.
5. Sus should be at room temperature before administering.

STORAGE
25°C (77°F); excursions permitted to 15-30°C (59-86°F).

HOW SUPPLIED
Cap: 200mg; **Tab:** 500mg

CONTRAINDICATIONS
Congenital long QT syndrome, refractory hypokalemia or hypomagnesemia, complete atrioventricular (AV) block w/o implanted pacemakers, high risk of complete AV block, severe hepatic impairment (when administered w/ RTV), and w/ drugs that both increase saquinavir plasma levels and prolong the QT interval. Clinically significant hypersensitivity (eg, anaphylactic reaction, Stevens-Johnson syndrome) to saquinavir, saquinavir mesylate, or any of its ingredients. Coadministration of saquinavir/RTV w/ CYP3A substrates for which increased plasma levels may result in serious or life-threatening reactions (eg, alfuzosin,

amiodarone, bepridil, dofetilide, flecainide, lidocaine [systemic], propafenone, quinidine, trazodone, clarithromycin, erythromycin, halofantrine, pentamidine, rifampin, dihydroergotamine, ergonovine, ergotamine, methylergonovine, cisapride, atazanavir, lovastatin, simvastatin, tacrolimus, pimozide, chlorpromazine, sertindole, clozapine, haloperidol, mesoridazine, phenothiazines, thioridazine, ziprasidone, sildenafil for treatment of pulmonary arterial HTN, triazolam, oral midazolam, dapsone, disopyramide, quinine).

WARNINGS/PRECAUTIONS

See Dosing Considerations. Refer to the individual monograph of RTV. Must be used in combination w/ RTV. Interrupt therapy if serious or severe toxicity occurs until etiology is identified or toxicity resolves. May prolong the PR and QT intervals in a dose-dependent fashion. 2nd- or 3rd-degree AV block and torsades de pointes reported. Monitor ECG w/ underlying structural heart disease, preexisting conduction system abnormalities, cardiomyopathies, ischemic heart disease, CHF, bradyarrhythmias, hepatic impairment, and electrolyte abnormalities. Correct hypokalemia/hypomagnesemia prior to therapy and monitor periodically. Do not initiate treatment if QT interval ≥450 msec. For a baseline QT interval <450 msec, monitor ECG after approx 10 days; d/c if QT interval is increased >20 msec over pretreatment. New onset or exacerbation of diabetes mellitus (DM), hyperglycemia, diabetic ketoacidosis, immune reconstitution syndrome, autoimmune disorders (eg, Graves' disease, polymyositis, Guillain-Barre syndrome) in the setting of immune reconstitution, redistribution/accumulation of body fat, and spontaneous bleeding w/ hemophilia A and B reported. Worsening liver disease in patients w/ underlying hepatitis B or C, cirrhosis, chronic alcoholism, and/or other underlying liver abnormalities reported. Elevated cholesterol and/or TG levels observed; marked elevation in TGs is a risk factor for pancreatitis. Caps contain lactose; should not induce symptoms of intolerance. Various degrees of cross-resistance among protease inhibitors have been observed. Caution in elderly.

ADVERSE REACTIONS

N/V, diarrhea, abdominal pain, fatigue, pneumonia, lipodystrophy, DM/hyperglycemia, fever, bronchitis, influenza, sinusitis, rash, pruritus.

DRUG INTERACTIONS

See Contraindications. May significantly increase the exposure of drugs primarily metabolized by CYP3A. Drugs that affect CYP3A and/or P-gp may modify pharmacokinetics. Not recommended w/ delavirdine, efavirenz, nevirapine, indinavir, nelfinavir, tipranavir/RTV, ibutilide, sotalol, carbamazepine, phenobarbital, phenytoin, fusidic acid, ketoconazole or itraconazole >200mg/day, dexamethasone, salmeterol, fluticasone, and garlic caps. Caution w/ lopinavir/RTV; additive effects on QT and/or PR interval prolongation may occur. May increase warfarin levels; monitor INR. Increases colchicine levels; avoid colchicine w/ renal/hepatic impairment. Streptogramin antibiotics (eg, quinupristin/dalfopristin) may increase levels; use w/ caution due to possible cardiac arrhythmias. Increases quetiapine levels; consider alternative antiretroviral therapy. May decrease methadone levels; use w/ caution due to additive effects on QT and/or PR interval prolongation. Decreases ethinyl estradiol levels; use alternative or additional contraceptive measures. Increases levels of sildenafil, vardenafil, and tadalafil; avoid tadalafil during initiation of therapy. St. John's wort decreases levels; avoid use. Increases levels of indinavir, maraviroc, fusidic acid, ketoconazole, rifabutin, benzodiazepines, IV midazolam, calcium channel blockers, digoxin, bosentan, salmeterol, fluticasone, atorvastatin, cyclosporine, rapamycin, TCAs, fentanyl, alfentanil, and IV vincamine. Delavirdine, indinavir, nelfinavir, fusidic acid, nefazodone, and omeprazole may increase levels. Efavirenz, nevirapine, tipranavir/RTV, dexamethasone, garlic capsules, and potent CYP3A inducers (eg, phenobarbital, phenytoin, carbamazepine) may decrease levels. May require initiation or adjustments of insulin or oral hypoglycemics for treatment of DM. Refer to PI for further information, including information on dosing modifications when used w/ certain concomitant therapies.

PREGNANCY AND LACTATION

Pregnancy: Category B. Physicians are encouraged to register pregnant patients in the Antiretroviral Pregnancy Registry.
Lactation: Not for use in nursing.

MECHANISM OF ACTION

HIV-1 protease inhibitor; binds to the protease active site and inhibits activity of the enzyme, preventing cleavage of the viral polyproteins, and resulting in the formation of immature, noninfectious viral particles.

PHARMACOKINETICS

Absorption: Administration of variable doses and combinations resulted in different parameters. **Distribution:** Plasma protein binding (approx 98%). (12mg IV) V_d=700L. **Metabolism:** Hepatic via CYP3A4. **Elimination:** (600mg PO) Urine (1%), feces (88%). (10.5mg IV) Urine (3%), feces (81%).

PATIENT CONSIDERATIONS

Assessment: Assess for congenital long QT syndrome; refractory hypokalemia or hypomagnesemia; clinically significant hypersensitivity to saquinavir, saquinavir mesylate, or any of the ingredients in the cap or tab; hepatic/renal impairment; and for any other conditions where treatment is contraindicated or cautioned. Assess pregnancy/nursing status and for possible drug interactions. Obtain baseline serum K^+, Mg^{2+}, TG, and cholesterol levels, and an ECG.

Monitoring: Monitor for signs/symptoms of AV block, PR/QT interval prolongation, torsades de pointes, bleeding in hemophilia patients, immune reconstitution syndrome, autoimmune disorders, fat redistribution/accumulation, new onset/exacerbation of DM, and other adverse reactions. Monitor for worsening liver disease in patients w/ underlying hepatitis B or C, cirrhosis, chronic alcoholism, and/or other underlying liver abnormalities. Periodically monitor ECG results, serum K^+ and Mg^{2+} levels, TG and cholesterol levels, and hepatic/renal function.

Counseling: Inform that therapy is not a cure for HIV-1 infection and that illnesses associated w/ HIV-1 infection may continue, including opportunistic infections. Advise to avoid doing things that can spread HIV-1 infection to others. Inform that changes in the ECG (PR interval or QT interval prolongation) may occur; instruct to consult physician if experiencing dizziness, lightheadedness, or palpitations. Advise to report the use of any other prescription/nonprescription medications or herbal products (eg, St. John's wort). Inform that redistribution or accumulation of body fat may occur. Advise that therapy must be used in combination w/ RTV. Inform about the importance of taking medication every day; instruct not to alter dose or d/c therapy w/o consulting physician.

IRESSA — gefitinib   Rx

Class: Kinase inhibitor

ADULT DOSAGE	PEDIATRIC DOSAGE
Metastatic Non-Small Cell Lung Cancer 1st-line treatment of patients whose tumors have EGFR exon 19 deletions or exon 21 (L858R) substitution mutations as detected by an FDA-approved test 250mg qd until disease progression or unacceptable toxicity **Missed Dose** Do not take a missed dose w/in 12 hrs of the next dose	Pediatric use may not have been established

---

DOSING CONSIDERATIONS
Concomitant Medications
Strong CYP3A4 inducers:
Increase Iressa to 500mg/day in the absence of severe adverse drug reaction; resume at 250mg seven days after discontinuation of the strong CYP3A4 inducer

Adverse Reactions
Withhold Therapy (for up to 14 Days) for Any of the Following:
1. Acute onset or worsening of pulmonary symptoms (dyspnea, cough, fever)
2. NCI CTCAE ≥Grade 2 in ALT and/or AST elevations
3. NCI CTCAE ≥Grade 3 diarrhea
4. Signs/symptoms of severe or worsening ocular disorders including keratitis
5. NCI CTCAE ≥Grade 3 skin reactions

Resume treatment when the adverse reaction fully resolves or improves to NCI CTCAE Grade 1

Permanently D/C for:
1. Confirmed interstitial lung disease (ILD)
2. Severe hepatic impairment
3. GI perforation
4. Persistent ulcerative keratitis

ADMINISTRATION
Oral route

Take w/ or w/o food.

Patients w/ Difficulty Swallowing Solids
1. Immerse tabs in 4-8 oz of water by dropping the tab in water, and stir for approx 15 min.
2. Immediately drink the liquid or administer through a NG tube.
3. Rinse the container w/ 4-8 oz of water and immediately drink or administer through the NG tube.

STORAGE
20-25°C (68-77°F).

HOW SUPPLIED
Tab: 250mg

WARNINGS/PRECAUTIONS
Select patients for treatment based on the presence of EGFR exon 19 deletion or exon 21 (L858R) substitution mutations in their tumor. ILD or ILD-like adverse reactions reported; withhold therapy and promptly investigate in any patient w/ worsening of respiratory symptoms, and permanently d/c therapy if ILD is confirmed. Liver test abnormalities reported; withhold therapy in patients w/ worsening liver function and d/c in patients w/ severe hepatic impairment. GI perforation reported; permanently d/c therapy if GI perforation occurs. Grade 3 or 4 diarrhea reported; withhold therapy for severe/persistent (up to 14 days) diarrhea. Ocular disorders including keratitis reported; interrupt or d/c therapy for severe/worsening ocular disorders. Bullous conditions including toxic epidermal necrolysis, Stevens-Johnson syndrome, and erythema multiforme reported; interrupt or d/c therapy if the patient develops severe bullous, blistering, or exfoliating conditions. May cause fetal harm.

ADVERSE REACTIONS
Skin reactions, diarrhea, decreased appetite, N/V, asthenia, pyrexia, stomatitis, conjunctivitis/blepharitis/dry eye, nail disorders, alopecia, hemorrhage (including epistaxis and hematuria).

DRUG INTERACTIONS
See Dosing Considerations. Strong CYP3A4 inducers (eg, rifampicin, phenytoin, TCA) increase metabolism and decrease levels of gefitinib. Strong CYP3A4 inhibitors (eg, ketoconazole, itraconazole) decrease metabolism and increase levels of gefitinib; monitor adverse reactions during coadministration. Drugs that

elevate gastric pH may reduce gefitinib levels; avoid concomitant use w/ PPIs, if possible. If treatment w/ a PPI is required, take gefitinib 12 hrs after the last dose or 12 hrs before the next dose of the PPI. Take gefitinib 6 hrs after or 6 hrs before an H_2-receptor antagonist or an antacid. INR elevations and/or hemorrhage reported during coadministration w/ warfarin; regularly monitor patients taking warfarin for changes in prothrombin time or INR.

PREGNANCY AND LACTATION
Pregnancy: May cause fetal harm.
Lactation: Not for use in nursing.
Reproductive Potential: Females of reproductive potential should use effective contraception during treatment, and for at least 2 weeks following completion of therapy. Therapy may result in reduced fertility in females of reproductive potential.

MECHANISM OF ACTION
Kinase inhibitor; reversibly inhibits the kinase activity of wild-type and certain activating mutations of EGFR, preventing autophosphorylation of tyrosine residues associated w/ the receptor, thereby inhibiting further downstream signaling and blocking EGFR-dependent proliferation.

PHARMACOKINETICS
Absorption: Bioavailability (60%); T_{max}=3-7 hrs. **Distribution:** V_d=1400L (IV); plasma protein binding (90%; albumin and α1-acid glycoprotein). **Metabolism:** Extensive via CYP3A4; O-desmethyl gefitinib (major active component) produced by CYP2D6. **Elimination:** Feces (86%), urine (<4%); (IV) $T_{1/2}$=48 hrs.

PATIENT CONSIDERATIONS
Assessment: Assess for hepatic impairment, pregnancy/nursing status, and possible drug interactions. Assess for presence of EGFR exon 19 deletions or exon 21 (L858R) substitution mutations in tumors.

Monitoring: Monitor for ILD, hepatotoxicity, GI perforation, diarrhea, ocular disorders, bullous and exfoliative skin disorders, and other adverse reactions. Obtain periodic liver function testing.

Counseling: Advise to immediately contact physician for new onset/worsening of pulmonary symptoms. Instruct to contact physician to report any new symptoms indicating hepatic toxicity. Advise that therapy can increase the risk of GI perforation and to seek immediate medical attention for severe abdominal pain. Instruct to contact physician for severe/persistent diarrhea. Counsel to promptly contact physician if eye symptoms, lacrimation, light sensitivity, blurred vision, eye pain, red eye, or changes in vision develop. Advise that therapy can increase the risk of bullous and exfoliative skin disorders and to seek immediately medical attention for severe skin reactions. Inform pregnant women of the potential risk to a fetus or potential risk for loss of the pregnancy. Advise females of reproductive potential to use effective contraception during treatment, and for at least 2 weeks following completion of therapy. Advise to d/c nursing during treatment.

ISENTRESS — raltegravir   Rx
Class: HIV-integrase strand transfer inhibitor

ADULT DOSAGE	PEDIATRIC DOSAGE
HIV-1 Infection	**HIV-1 Infection**
Combination w/ Other Antiretrovirals:	**Combination w/ Other Antiretrovirals:**
Tab:	**≥4 Weeks of Age:**
400mg bid	**Tab:**
	≥25kg: 400mg bid
In Combination w/ Rifampin:	**Tab, Chewable:**
800mg bid	**11-<14kg:** 75mg bid
	14-<20kg: 100mg bid
	20-<28kg: 150mg bid
	28-<40kg: 200mg bid
	≥40kg: 300mg bid
	Max: 300mg bid
	Sus:
	3-<4kg: 1mL (20mg) bid
	4-<6kg: 1.5mL (30mg) bid
	6-<8kg: 2mL (40mg) bid
	8-<11kg: 3mL (60mg) bid
	11-<14kg: 4mL (80mg) bid
	14-<20kg: 5mL (100mg) bid
	Max: 100mg bid

ADMINISTRATION
Oral route
Take w/ or w/o food.

Tab
Swallow whole.

Tab, Chewable
Chew or swallow whole.

Sus
1. Pour sus pack contents into mixing cup, add 5mL of water, and mix.
2. To mix, swirl mixing cup w/ a gentle circular motion for 30-60 sec; do not turn mixing cup upside down.
3. Measure the recommended dose w/ provided syringe and administer w/in 30 min of mixing.
4. Discard any remaining sus.

STORAGE
20-25°C (68-77°F); excursions permitted to 15-30°C (59-86°F). **Tab, Chewable:** Protect from moisture. **Sus:** Do not open foil pkt until ready for use.

HOW SUPPLIED
Sus (Powder): 100mg/pkt; **Tab:** 400mg; **Tab, Chewable:** 25mg, 100mg* *scored

WARNINGS/PRECAUTIONS
Do not substitute chewable tabs or oral sus for the 400mg film-coated tab; not bioequivalent. Severe, potentially life-threatening, and fatal skin reactions (eg, Stevens-Johnson syndrome, toxic epidermal necrolysis), and hypersensitivity reactions reported; d/c therapy and other suspect agents immediately if signs/symptoms develop. Immune reconstitution syndrome reported. Autoimmune disorders (eg, Graves' disease, polymyositis, Guillain-Barre syndrome) reported in the setting of immune reconstitution and can occur many months after initiation of treatment. Caution in patients at increased risk of myopathy or rhabdomyolysis and in elderly. Avoid dosing before a dialysis session. **Tab, Chewable:** Contains phenylalanine.

ADVERSE REACTIONS
Insomnia, headache, nausea, hyperglycemia, ALT/AST elevation, hyperbilirubinemia, low ANC, serum lipase/creatine kinase/pancreatic amylase increase, thrombocytopenia.

DRUG INTERACTIONS
See Dosage. UGT1A1 inhibitors may increase levels. UGT1A1 inducers (eg, rifampin) may decrease levels. Coadministration or staggered administration w/ aluminum- and/or magnesium hydroxide-containing antacids is not recommended.

PREGNANCY AND LACTATION
Category C, not for use in nursing.

MECHANISM OF ACTION
HIV-1 integrase strand transfer inhibitor; inhibits the catalytic activity of HIV-1 integrase thus preventing the formation of HIV-1 provirus, resulting in the prevention of propagation of the viral infection.

PHARMACOKINETICS
Absorption: Adults: (Tab) T_{max}=3 hrs (fasted); AUC_{0-12h}=14.3μM•hr. Pediatrics: AUC_{0-12h}=14.1μM•hr (tab), 22.1μM•hr (tab, chewable; ≥25kg patient), 18.6μM•hr (tab, chewable; 11-<25kg patient), 24.5μM•hr (sus). **Distribution:** Adults: Plasma protein binding (83%). **Metabolism:** Glucuronidation via UGT1A1; raltegravir-glucuronide (metabolite). **Elimination:** Adults: Urine (9% unchanged, 23% raltegravir-glucuronide), feces (51% unchanged); $T_{1/2}$=9 hrs.

PATIENT CONSIDERATIONS
Assessment: Assess for risk of myopathy or rhabdomyolysis, previous hypersensitivity to the drug, pregnancy/nursing status, and possible drug interactions. Assess if patient is undergoing dialysis session. **Tab, Chewable:** Assess for phenylketonuria.

Monitoring: Monitor for signs/symptoms of severe skin/hypersensitivity reactions, immune reconstitution syndrome, autoimmune disorders, and other adverse reactions. If a severe skin reaction or hypersensitivity reaction develops, monitor clinical status, including liver aminotransferases.

Counseling: Instruct to inform physician if any unusual symptom develops, or if any known symptom persists or worsens. Inform that drug is not a cure for HIV-1 infection and that illnesses associated w/ HIV-1 may still be experienced. Advise to avoid doing things that can spread HIV-1 to others. Instruct to always practice safe sex by using a latex or polyurethane condom. Instruct to immediately d/c therapy and seek medical attention if rash develops w/ signs/symptoms of a more serious skin reaction. Instruct to immediately report to physician if any unexplained muscle pain, tenderness, or weakness occurs. Instruct to avoid taking aluminum- and/or magnesium hydroxide-containing antacids. **Tab, Chewable:** Inform patients w/ phenylketonuria that product contains phenylalanine. **Sus:** Instruct to administer w/in 30 min of mixing.

ISTODAX — romidepsin   Rx
Class: Histone deacetylase (HDAC) inhibitor

ADULT DOSAGE	PEDIATRIC DOSAGE
Cutaneous T-Cell Lymphoma	Pediatric use may not have been established
Use in patients that have received at least 1 prior systemic therapy	
14mg/m² over 4 hrs on Days 1, 8, and 15 of a 28-day cycle	
Repeat cycle every 28 days provided that patient continues to benefit from and tolerates the drug	
Peripheral T-Cell Lymphoma	
Use in patients that have received at least 1 prior therapy	
14mg/m² over 4 hrs on Days 1, 8, and 15 of a 28-day cycle	
Repeat cycle every 28 days provided that patient continues to benefit from and tolerates the drug	

DOSING CONSIDERATIONS
Renal Impairment
ESRD: Use w/ caution

Hepatic Impairment
Moderate/Severe: Use w/ caution

Adverse Reactions

Nonhematologic Toxicities (Except Alopecia):

Grade 2 or 3: Delay treatment until toxicity returns to ≤Grade 1 or baseline, then restart at 14mg/m². If Grade 3 toxicity recurs, delay treatment until toxicity returns to ≤Grade 1 or baseline, then permanently reduce dose to 10mg/m²

Grade 4: Delay treatment until toxicity returns to ≤Grade 1 or baseline, then permanently reduce dose to 10mg/m²

Recurrence of Grade 3 or 4 Toxicities After Dose Reduction: D/C therapy

Hematologic Toxicities:

Grade 3 or 4 Neutropenia or Thrombocytopenia: Delay treatment until specific cytopenia returns to ANC ≥1.5 x 10⁹/L and platelet count ≥75 x 10⁹/L or baseline, then restart at 14mg/m²

Grade 4 Febrile (≥38.5°C [101.3°F]) Neutropenia or Thrombocytopenia Requiring Platelet Transfusion: Delay treatment until specific cytopenia returns to ≤Grade 1 or baseline, then permanently reduce dose to 10mg/m²

ADMINISTRATION

IV route

Preparation and Administration

1. Withdraw 2.2mL from the supplied diluent vial, and slowly inject it into the 10mg single-use vial. The reconstituted sol will contain 5mg/mL and is stable for up to 8 hrs at room temperature.
2. Before infusion, further dilute romidepsin in 500mL 0.9% NaCl inj.
3. Infuse over 4 hrs.

The diluted sol is compatible w/ polyvinyl chloride, ethylene vinyl acetate, and polyethylene infusion bags as well as glass bottles, and is chemically stable for up to 24 hrs at room temperature. However, it should be administered as soon after dilution as possible

STORAGE

Carton: 20-25°C (68-77°F); excursions permitted between 15-30°C (59-86°F).

HOW SUPPLIED

Inj: 10mg

WARNINGS/PRECAUTIONS

May cause thrombocytopenia, leukopenia (neutropenia/lymphopenia), and anemia. Serious/fatal infections (eg, pneumonia, sepsis, and viral reactivation, including Epstein Barr and hepatitis B viruses) reported; increased risk w/ history of prior treatment w/ monoclonal antibodies directed against lymphocyte antigens and in patients w/ disease involvement of the bone marrow. Consider monitoring for reactivation and antiviral prophylaxis in patients w/ evidence of prior hepatitis B infection. ECG changes reported; caution w/ congenital long QT syndrome and history of significant cardiovascular disease (CVD). Confirm that K⁺/Mg²⁺ levels are w/in the normal range prior to administration. Tumor lysis syndrome (TLS) reported; increased risk in patients w/ advanced stage disease and/or high tumor burden. May cause fetal harm.

ADVERSE REACTIONS

Neutropenia, lymphopenia, thrombocytopenia, infections, N/V, fatigue, anorexia, anemia, ECG T-wave changes.

DRUG INTERACTIONS

Avoid w/ rifampin and other potent CYP3A4 inducers (eg, dexamethasone, phenytoin, rifapentine, St. John's wort). Caution w/ antiarrhythmics or drugs that prolong QT. Strong CYP3A4 inhibitors (eg, ketoconazole, clarithromycin, indinavir, nelfinavir) may increase concentrations. Prolongation of PT and elevation of INR w/ warfarin; monitor PT and INR more frequently w/ warfarin. Caution w/ P-gp inhibitors; may increase levels of romidepsin.

PREGNANCY AND LACTATION

Pregnancy: Category D.
Lactation: Not for use in nursing.

MECHANISM OF ACTION

Histone deacetylase inhibitor; catalyzes the removal of acetyl groups from acetylated lysine residues in histones, resulting in the modulation of gene expression.

PHARMACOKINETICS

Absorption: C_{max}=377ng/mL; AUC_{0-inf}=1549ng•hr/mL. **Distribution:** Plasma protein binding (92-94%). **Metabolism:** Extensive. CYP3A4 (primary); CYP3A5, CYP1A1, CYP2B6, and CYP2C19 (minor). **Elimination:** $T_{1/2}$=3 hrs.

PATIENT CONSIDERATIONS

Assessment: Assess for normal K⁺/Mg²⁺ levels, history of hepatitis B, history of prior treatment w/ monoclonal antibodies directed against lymphocyte antigens, disease involvement of the bone marrow, hepatic/renal function, congenital long QT syndrome/history of CVD, pregnancy/nursing status, and possible drug interactions. Obtain baseline ECG.

Monitoring: Monitor for myelosuppression, infections, reactivation of viral infection, and other adverse reactions. Closely monitor for TLS w/ advanced stage disease and/or high tumor burden. Monitor PT/INR w/ warfarin. Perform ECGs periodically and monitor blood counts regularly.

Counseling: Inform that N/V, low blood counts, and infections may occur; instruct to report symptoms of N/V, fever or other signs of infection, significant fatigue, SOB, bleeding, cough, burning on urination, flu-like symptoms, muscle aches, or worsening skin problems. Advise to report any previous history of hepatitis B prior to therapy. Advise of the risk of TLS (especially those w/ advanced stage disease and/or high tumor burden) and to maintain high fluid intake for at least 72 hrs after each dose. Advise to seek medical counseling if pregnancy occurs during treatment.

IXEMPRA — ixabepilone

Class: Antimicrotubule agent

Rx

> In combination with capecitabine, contraindicated in patients with AST/ALT >2.5X ULN or bilirubin >1X ULN due to increased risk of toxicity and neutropenia-related death.

ADULT DOSAGE

Breast Cancer

Combination w/ Capecitabine:
Metastatic or locally advanced breast cancer resistant to treatment w/ an anthracycline and a taxane, or in patients whose cancer is taxane resistant and for whom further anthracycline therapy is contraindicated

40mg/m² IV over 3 hrs every 3 weeks
BSA >2.2m²: Calculate dose based on 2.2m²

Monotherapy:
Metastatic or locally advanced breast cancer in patients whose tumors are resistant or refractory to anthracyclines, taxanes, and capecitabine

40mg/m² IV over 3 hrs every 3 weeks
BSA >2.2m²: Calculate dose based on 2.2m²

Retreatment Criteria:
Do not begin a new cycle of treatment unless neutrophil count is ≥1500 cells/mm³, platelet count is ≥100,000 cells/mm³, and nonhematologic toxicities have improved to Grade 1 (mild) or resolved

Premedication

All patients must be premedicated approx 1 hr before infusion w/:

An H₁ antagonist (eg, diphenhydramine 50mg PO or equivalent) and an H₂ antagonist (eg, ranitidine 150-300mg PO or equivalent)

Patients who experienced a hypersensitivity reaction require premedication w/ corticosteroids (eg, dexamethasone 20mg IV, 30 min before infusion or PO, 60 min before infusion) in addition to pretreatment w/ H₁ and H₂ antagonists

PEDIATRIC DOSAGE

Pediatric use may not have been established

DOSING CONSIDERATIONS

Concomitant Medications

Strong CYP3A4 Inhibitors (Including Grapefruit Juice): Avoid concomitant use; if coadministration is necessary, reduce dose to 20mg/m². If the strong inhibitor is discontinued, allow a washout period of approx 1 week before adjusting the dose upward to the indicated dose

Strong CYP3A4 Inducers: Avoid concomitant use; if coadministration is necessary, gradually increase dose to 60mg/m² IV over 4 hrs once patient has been maintained on a strong CYP3A4 inducer. If the strong inducer is discontinued, return to the dose used prior to initiation of the strong inducer

Hepatic Impairment

Monotherapy:
AST and ALT ≤10X ULN and Bilirubin ≤1.5X ULN: 32mg/m²
AST and ALT ≤10X ULN and Bilirubin >1.5-≤3X ULN: 20-30mg/m²

Recommendations are for 1st course of therapy; further decreases in subsequent courses should be based on individual tolerance

Adverse Reactions

Monotherapy or Combination Therapy:
Nonhematologic Toxicities:
Grade 2 Neuropathy (Moderate) Lasting ≥7 Days: Decrease dose by 20%
Grade 3 Neuropathy (Severe) Lasting <7 Days: Decrease dose by 20%
Grade 3 Neuropathy (Severe) Lasting ≥7 Days or Disabling Neuropathy: D/C treatment
Any Grade 3 Toxicity (Severe) Other Than Neuropathy: Decrease dose by 20%
Any Grade 4 Toxicity (Disabling): D/C treatment

Hematologic Toxicities:
Neutrophil <500 cells/mm³ for ≥7 Days: Decrease dose by 20%
Febrile Neutropenia: Decrease dose by 20%
Platelets <25,000/mm³ or Platelets <50,000/mm³ w/ Bleeding: Decrease dose by 20%

Refer to PI for capecitabine dose modifications

ADMINISTRATION

IV route

Preparation and Administration

Prior to constituting ixabepilone for inj, remove the kit from the refrigerator and allowed to stand at room temperature for approx 30 min. When the vials are 1st removed from the refrigerator, a white precipitate may be observed in the diluents vial. This precipitate will dissolve to form a clear sol once the diluents warms to room temperature. After constituting w/ the diluent, the concentration of ixabepilone is 2mg/mL

To Constitute:

1. W/ a suitable syringe, withdraw the diluents and slowly inject it into the ixabepilone for inj vial:

15mg Ixempra: Constitute w/ 8mL of diluent
45mg Ixempra: Constitute w/ 23.5mL of diluent

2. Gently swirl and invert the vial until the powder is completely dissolved

To Dilute:

Before administration, the constituted sol must be further diluted w/ 1 of the specified infusion fluids listed below. The infusion must be prepared in a DEHP [di-(2-ethylhexyl) phthalate] free bag
The following infusion fluids have been qualified for use:

1. Lactated Ringer's inj
2. 0.9% NaCl inj (pH adjusted w/ sodium bicarbonate inj)
When using a 250mL or a 500mL bag of 0.9% NaCl inj to prepare the infusion, the pH must be adjusted to a pH between 6.0 and 9.0 by adding 2mEq (eg, 2mL of an 8.4% w/v sol or 4mL of a 4.2% w/v sol) of sodium bicarbonate inj, prior to the addition of the constituted sol
3. PLASMA-LYTE A inj pH 7.4

For most doses, a 250mL bag of infusion fluid is sufficient. However, it is necessary to check the final infusion concentration of each dose based on the volume of infusion fluid to be used. The final concentration for infusion must be between 0.2mg/mL and 0.6mg/mL; refer to PI for how to calculate the final infusion concentration

1. Withdraw the appropriate volume of constituted sol containing 2mg/mL
2. Transfer to an IV bag containing an appropriate volume of infusion fluid to achieve the final desired concentration
3. Thoroughly mix the infusion bag by manual rotation

The infusion sol must be administered through an appropriate in-line filter w/ a microporous membrane of 0.2-1.2μm. DEHP-free infusion containers and administration sets must be used. Any remaining sol should be discarded according to institutional procedures for antineoplastics

STORAGE

2-8°C (36-46°F). Protect from light. Constituted Sol: Dilute as soon as possible or store in the vial (not the syringe) for a max of 1 hr at room temperature and room light. Diluted with Infusion Fluid: Stable at room temperature and room light for a max of 6 hrs.

HOW SUPPLIED

Inj: 15mg, 45mg

CONTRAINDICATIONS

History of a severe (CTC Grade 3/4) hypersensitivity reaction to agents containing Cremophor EL or its derivatives (eg, polyoxyethylated castor oil). Neutrophil count <1500 cells/mm³ or platelet count <100,000 cells/mm³. In combination with capecitabine, patients with AST/ALT >2.5X ULN or bilirubin >1X ULN.

WARNINGS/PRECAUTIONS

Peripheral neuropathy reported; caution with diabetes mellitus (DM) or preexisting peripheral neuropathy. Myelosuppression, which is dose-dependent and primarily manifested as neutropenia, reported; frequently monitor peripheral blood cell counts. Monotherapy is not recommended in patients with AST/ALT >10X ULN or bilirubin >3X ULN, and should be used with caution in patients with AST/ALT >5X ULN. Observe for hypersensitivity reactions; d/c infusion and start aggressive supportive treatment if severe hypersensitivity reactions occur. May cause fetal harm. Cardiac adverse reactions (eg, myocardial ischemia, ventricular dysfunction) reported during combination therapy; caution with history of cardiac disease, and consider discontinuation of ixabepilone if cardiac ischemia or impaired cardiac function develops. Contains dehydrated alcohol USP; consider possibility of CNS and other effects of alcohol.

ADVERSE REACTIONS

Peripheral sensory neuropathy, fatigue/asthenia, myalgia/arthralgia, alopecia, N/V, stomatitis/mucositis, diarrhea, musculoskeletal pain, palmar-plantar erythrodysesthesia (hand-foot) syndrome, anorexia, abdominal pain, nail disorder, constipation, hematologic abnormalities.

DRUG INTERACTIONS

Strong CYP3A4 inhibitors (eg, ketoconazole, itraconazole, clarithromycin, atazanavir, grapefruit juice) may increase levels; avoid, or if must be coadministered, reduce dose of ixabepilone. Caution with mild/moderate CYP3A4 inhibitors (eg, erythromycin, fluconazole, verapamil). Monitor closely for acute toxicities in patients receiving CYP3A4 inhibitors during treatment. Strong CYP3A4 inducers (eg, rifampin, dexamethasone) may decrease levels; avoid, or if must be coadministered, consider gradual dose adjustment of ixabepilone. St. John's wort may decrease levels unpredictably; avoid concomitant use.

PREGNANCY AND LACTATION

Category D, not for use in nursing.

MECHANISM OF ACTION

Microtubule inhibitor; semi-synthetic analog of epothilone B. Binds directly to β-tubulin subunits on microtubules, leading to suppression of microtubule dynamics. Blocks cells in the mitotic phase of the cell division cycle, leading to cell death.

PHARMACOKINETICS

Absorption: C_{max}=252ng/mL; T_{max}=3 hrs; AUC=2143ng•hr/mL. **Distribution:** V_d>1000L; plasma protein binding (67-77%). **Metabolism:** Liver (extensive); oxidation via CYP3A4. **Elimination:** Feces (65%, 1.6% unchanged); urine (21%, 5.6% unchanged); $T_{1/2}$=52 hrs.

PATIENT CONSIDERATIONS

Assessment: Assess for history of a severe hypersensitivity reaction to Cremophor EL or its derivatives (eg, polyoxyethylated castor oil), DM, preexisting peripheral neuropathy, history of cardiac disease, pregnancy/nursing status, and possible drug interactions. Obtain CBC and LFTs.

Monitoring: Monitor for signs/symptoms of neuropathy, myelosuppression, hypersensitivity reactions, cardiac ischemia/impairment, and other adverse reactions. Perform periodic clinical observation and lab tests (eg, CBC, LFTs).

Counseling: Advise to report to physician any numbness and tingling of the hands or feet, chest pain, difficulty breathing, palpitations, or unusual weight gain. Instruct to contact physician if a fever of ≥100.5°F or other evidence of potential infection (eg, chills, cough, burning or pain on urination) develops, or if experiencing urticaria, pruritus, rash, flushing, swelling, dyspnea, chest tightness, or other hypersensitivity-related symptoms following an infusion. Advise to use effective contraceptive measures to prevent pregnancy and to avoid nursing during treatment.

IXINITY — coagulation factor IX (recombinant)   Rx

Class: Antihemophilic factor (recombinant)

ADULT DOSAGE

Hemophilia B

Initial Dose:
Initial Dose = body weight (kg) x desired factor IX (FIX) increase (% of normal or IU/dL) x reciprocal of observed recovery (IU/kg per IU/dL)

Incremental Recovery in Previously Treated Patients (PTPs):
For an incremental recovery of 0.98 IU/dL, calculate the dose as follows:
Dose (IU) = body weight (kg) x desired FIX increase (% of normal or IU/dL) x 1.02dL/kg

Control and Prevention of Bleeding Episodes:
Minor Bleeding:
Dose to achieve peak FIX level of 30-60 IU/dL, given q24h for 1-3 days, until healing is achieved

Moderate Bleeding:
Dose to achieve peak FIX level of 40-60 IU/dL, given q24h for 2-7 days, until healing is achieved

Major or Life-Threatening Bleeding:
Dose to achieve peak FIX level of 60-100 IU/dL, given q12-24h for 2-14 days, until healing is achieved

Perioperative Management:
Minor Surgery (eg, Uncomplicated Dental Extractions):
Preoperative:
Dose to achieve peak FIX level of 50-80 IU/dL

Postoperative:
Dose to achieve peak FIX level of 30-80 IU/dL q24h for 1-5 days, depending on type of procedure

Major Surgery:
Preoperative:
Dose to achieve peak FIX level of 60-80 IU/dL

Postoperative:
Refer to PI for desired peak FIX level, dosing interval, and duration of therapy

PEDIATRIC DOSAGE

Hemophilia B

≥12 Years:
Initial Dose:
Initial Dose = body weight (kg) x desired FIX increase (% of normal or IU/dL) x reciprocal of observed recovery (IU/kg per IU/dL)

Incremental Recovery in PTPs:
For an incremental recovery of 0.98 IU/dL, calculate the dose as follows:
Dose (IU) = body weight (kg) x desired FIX increase (% of normal or IU/dL) x 1.02 dL/kg

Control and Prevention of Bleeding Episodes:
Minor Bleeding:
Dose to achieve peak FIX level of 30-60 IU/dL, given q24h for 1-3 days, until healing is achieved

Moderate Bleeding:
Dose to achieve peak FIX level of 40-60 IU/dL, given q24h for 2-7 days, until healing is achieved

Major or Life-Threatening Bleeding:
Dose to achieve peak FIX level of 60-100 IU/dL, given q12-24h for 2-14 days, until healing is achieved

Perioperative Management:
Minor Surgery (eg, Uncomplicated Dental Extractions):
Preoperative:
Dose to achieve peak FIX level of 50-80 IU/dL

Postoperative:
Dose to achieve peak FIX level of 30-80 IU/dL q24h for 1-5 days, depending on type of procedure

Major Surgery:
Preoperative:
Dose to achieve peak FIX level of 60-80 IU/dL

Postoperative:
Refer to PI for desired peak FIX level, dosing interval, and duration of therapy

---

ADMINISTRATION

IV route

Preparation and Reconstitution

1. Allow Ixinity and the Pre-filled Syringe to reach room temperature before use.
2. Connect the Pre-filled Syringe to the vial adapter by pushing the syringe tip down onto the Luer-Lok in the center of the vial adapter, and screw until the syringe is secured.
3. In a continuous motion, place the vial adapter over the Ixinity vial; firmly push the filter spike of the vial adapter through the center of Ixinity vial's rubber circle until the clear plastic cap snaps onto the Ixinity vial. Push the plunger down to complete the transfer of all liquid from the syringe to the Ixinity vial.

4. W/ the syringe and the vial still attached, gently swirl, in a circular motion, the Ixinity vial until the product is fully dissolved/reconstituted.

5. Remove the Pre-filled Syringe (now empty) from the vial adapter by turning it counterclockwise until it is completely detached.

5. Leave the vial adapter attached to the vial and attach the Administration Syringe to the vial adapter by turning clockwise until it is securely attached.

6. Keeping the Administration Syringe plunger pressed, turn the Ixinity vial upside down. Draw the sol from the vial through the filter spike in the vial adapter by pulling the plunger back slowly until all sol is transferred into the Administration Syringe.

7. Keep the Administration Syringe plunger facing downwards and unscrew the syringe from the vial adapter.

8. If only dosing w/ a single vial, proceed to administer Ixinity via IV infusion; otherwise proceed to Pooling Instructions.

Pooling Instructions

1. If ≥2 vials are required to achieve the required dose, remove the Pre-filled Syringe from the vial adapter on the reconstituted 2nd vial by turning it counterclockwise until it is completely detached.

2. Leave the vial adapter attached to the vial and attach the Administration Syringe containing the reconstituted Ixinity from the 1st vial by turning it clockwise until it is securely in place.

3. Turn the Ixinity vial upside down and slowly pull on the plunger rod to draw the sol into the Administration Syringe. The Administration Syringe provided w/ Ixinity may be used to pool up to 3 vials. If pooling is complete, proceed to administer Ixinity via IV infusion.

4. If >3 vials are required, use a larger (ie, >20mL) sterile Luer-Lok syringe and repeat Steps 1-3 above for all required vials of Ixinity. Once reconstituted product is pooled from all required vials, proceed to administer Ixinity via IV infusion.

Infuse reconstituted sol immediately or w/in 3 hrs of storage at room temperature after reconstitution. Do not refrigerate after reconstitution.

Administration Instructions

Do not mix w/ other medicinal products for infusion.

1. Attach the Administration Syringe containing the reconstituted Ixinity sol to a sterile infusion set.

2. Adapt the infusion rate to the comfort level of each patient, not exceeding 10mL/min.

STORAGE

2-25°C (36-77°F). Do not freeze. Protect from light. Infuse reconstituted sol immediately or w/in 3 hrs of storage at room temperature after reconstitution. Do not refrigerate after reconstitution.

HOW SUPPLIED

Inj: 500 IU, 1000 IU, 1500 IU

CONTRAINDICATIONS

Known hypersensitivity to product or its excipients, including hamster protein.

WARNINGS/PRECAUTIONS

Not indicated for induction of immune tolerance in patients w/ hemophilia B. Hypersensitivity reactions, including anaphylaxis, may occur; immediately d/c and initiate appropriate treatment if allergic/anaphylactic-type reactions occur. Contains trace amounts of Chinese hamster ovary proteins; patients may develop hypersensitivity to these proteins. May develop FIX inhibitors; perform an assay that measures FIX inhibitor concentration if expected FIX activity plasma levels are not attained, or if bleeding is not controlled as expected w/ the calculated dose. Patients w/ FIX inhibitors are at an increased risk of severe hypersensitivity reactions or anaphylaxis if reexposed to therapy. Nephrotic syndrome reported following attempted immune tolerance induction in hemophilia B patients w/ FIX inhibitors and a history of allergic reactions. Thromboembolism may occur; monitor for early signs of thromboembolism and consumptive coagulopathy in patients w/ liver disease, fibrinolysis, perioperative status, or risk for thromboembolic events or disseminated intravascular coagulation (DIC).

ADVERSE REACTIONS

Headache.

PREGNANCY AND LACTATION

Pregnancy: Category C.
Lactation: Caution in nursing.

MECHANISM OF ACTION

Recombinant antihemophilic factor; replaces FIX, thereby enabling a temporary correction of the factor deficiency and correction of the bleeding tendencies.

PHARMACOKINETICS

Absorption: (75 IU/kg in PTPs) AUC_{0-inf}=1573 IU/dL/hr; C_{max}=73 IU/dL.
Distribution: (75 IU/kg in PTPs) V_d=175mL/kg. **Elimination:** (75 IU/kg in PTPs) $T_{1/2}$=24 hrs.
Refer to PI for additional pharmacokinetic parameters.

PATIENT CONSIDERATIONS

Assessment: Assess for known hypersensitivity to drug or its excipients (including hamster protein), severity of FIX deficiency, location and extent of bleeding, presence of FIX inhibitors, liver disease, fibrinolysis, perioperative status, risk for thromboembolic events or DIC, and pregnancy/nursing status.

Monitoring: Monitor for hypersensitivity reactions, nephrotic syndrome, thromboembolism, and other adverse reactions. Monitor for FIX inhibitors if expected FIX activity plasma levels are not attained, or if bleeding is not controlled as expected w/ the calculated dose. Monitor for FIX activity levels w/ the one-stage clotting assay to confirm that adequate FIX levels have been achieved and maintained, when clinically indicated.

Counseling: Advise to report any adverse reactions or problems following administration to physician. Inform of the early signs of hypersensitivity reactions

and anaphylaxis; instruct to d/c and contact physician if symptoms occur. Advise to contact physician or treatment facility for further treatment and/or assessment if experiencing a lack of clinical response to FIX replacement therapy. Instruct to follow the specific preparation and administration procedures provided by physician.

JADENU — deferasirox   Rx
Class: Iron-chelating agent

> May cause acute renal failure and death, particularly in patients w/ comorbidities and those in the advanced stages of their hematologic disorders. Measure SrCr and determine CrCl in duplicate prior to initiation of therapy and monitor renal function at least monthly thereafter. Monitor creatinine weekly for the 1st month, then at least monthly for patients w/ baseline renal impairment or increased risk of acute renal failure. Consider dose reduction, interruption, or discontinuation based on increases in SrCr. May cause hepatic injury, including hepatic failure and death. Measure serum transaminases and bilirubin prior to initiating treatment, every 2 weeks during the 1st month, and at least monthly thereafter. Avoid in patients w/ severe (Child-Pugh C) hepatic impairment and reduce dose w/ moderate (Child-Pugh B) hepatic impairment. May cause GI hemorrhages, which may be fatal, especially in elderly who have advanced hematologic malignancies and/or low platelet counts. Monitor patients and d/c therapy if GI ulceration or hemorrhage is suspected.

ADULT DOSAGE
Chronic Iron Overload

Transfusional Iron Overload:
Only consider when a patient has evidence of chronic transfusional iron overload, which should include the transfusion of at least 100mL/kg of packed RBCs (eg, at least 20 U of packed RBCs for a 40kg person or more in individuals weighing >40kg), and a serum ferritin consistently >1000mcg/L

Initial: 14mg/kg qd; calculate doses (mg/kg/day) to the nearest whole tab
Maint: May adjust dose every 3-6 months based on serum ferritin trends. Make dose adjustments in steps of 3.5 or 7mg/kg and tailor adjustments to individual response and therapeutic goals. If inadequately controlled w/ doses of 21mg/kg (eg, serum ferritin levels persistently >2500mcg/L and not showing a decreasing trend over time), doses of up to 28mg/kg may be considered. Consider temporarily interrupting therapy if serum ferritin falls consistently <500mcg/L.
Max: 28mg/kg

In Non-Transfusion-Dependent Thalassemia (NTDT) Syndromes:
Only consider in a patient w/ a liver iron concentration (LIC) of at least 5mg of iron per gram of liver dry weight (mg Fe/g dw) and a serum ferritin >300mcg/L

Initial: 7mg/kg qd; calculate doses (mg/kg/day) to the nearest whole tab. Consider increasing dose to 14mg/kg/day after 4 weeks if baseline LIC is >15mg Fe/g dw.
Maint: Interrupt treatment when serum ferritin is <300mcg/L and obtain an LIC to determine whether LIC has fallen to <3mg Fe/g dw. After 6 months of therapy, if LIC remains >7mg Fe/g dw, increase dose to a max of 14mg/kg/day. If after 6 months of therapy, LIC is 3-7mg Fe/g dw, continue treatment at no more than 7mg/kg/day. When LIC is <3mg Fe/g dw, interrupt treatment and continue to monitor LIC. Restart treatment when LIC rises again to >5mg Fe/g dw.
Max: 14mg/kg/day

Conversions

Converting from Exjade to Jadenu:
Jadenu dose should be about 30% lower, rounded to nearest whole tab

Transfusion-Dependent Iron Overload:
Initial: 14mg/kg/day (for 20mg/kg/day Exjade)
Titration Increments: 3.5-7mg/kg (for 5-10mg/kg Exjade)
Max: 28mg/kg/day (for 40mg/kg/day Exjade)

PEDIATRIC DOSAGE
Chronic Iron Overload

Transfusional Iron Overload:
Only consider when a patient has evidence of chronic transfusional iron overload, which should include the transfusion of at least 100mL/kg of packed RBCs (eg, at least 20 U of packed RBCs for a 40kg person or more in individuals weighing >40kg), and a serum ferritin consistently >1000mcg/L

≥2 Years:
Initial: 14mg/kg qd; calculate doses (mg/kg/day) to the nearest whole tab
Maint: May adjust dose every 3-6 months based on serum ferritin trends. Make dose adjustments in steps of 3.5 or 7mg/kg and tailor adjustments to individual response and therapeutic goals. If inadequately controlled w/ doses of 21mg/kg (eg, serum ferritin levels persistently >2500mcg/L and not showing a decreasing trend over time), doses of up to 28mg/kg may be considered. Consider temporarily interrupting therapy if serum ferritin falls consistently <500mcg/L.
Max: 28mg/kg

In NTDT Syndromes:
Only consider in a patient w/ an LIC of at least 5mg Fe/g dw and a serum ferritin >300mcg/L

≥10 Years:
Initial: 7mg/kg qd; calculate doses (mg/kg/day) to the nearest whole tab. Consider increasing dose to 14mg/kg/day after 4 weeks if baseline LIC is >15mg Fe/g dw.
Maint: Interrupt treatment when serum ferritin is <300mcg/L and obtain an LIC to determine whether LIC has fallen to <3mg Fe/g dw. After 6 months of therapy, if LIC remains >7mg Fe/g dw, increase dose to a max of 14mg/kg/day. If after 6 months of therapy, LIC is 3-7mg Fe/g dw, continue treatment at no more than 7mg/kg/day. When LIC is <3mg Fe/g dw, interrupt treatment and continue to monitor LIC. Restart treatment when LIC rises again to >5mg Fe/g dw.
Max: 14mg/kg/day

Conversions

Converting from Exjade to Jadenu:
Jadenu dose should be about 30% lower, rounded to nearest whole tab

Transfusion-Dependent Iron Overload:
Initial: 14mg/kg/day (for 20mg/kg/day Exjade)
Titration Increments: 3.5-7mg/kg (for 5-10mg/kg Exjade)
Max: 28mg/kg/day (for 40mg/kg/day Exjade)

NTDT Syndromes:
Initial: 7mg/kg/day (for 10mg/kg/day Exjade)
Titration Increments: 3.5-7mg/kg (for 5-10mg/kg Exjade)
Max: 14mg/kg/day (for 20mg/kg/day Exjade)

NTDT Syndromes:
Initial: 7mg/kg/day (for 10mg/kg/day Exjade)
Titration Increments: 3.5-7mg/kg (for 5-10mg/kg Exjade)
Max: 14mg/kg/day (for 20mg/kg/day Exjade)

DOSING CONSIDERATIONS
Concomitant Medications
Bile Acid Sequestrants/Potent UDP-Glucuronosyltransferase (UGT) Inducers:
Avoid w/ bile acid sequestrants (eg, cholestyramine, colesevelam, colestipol) or potent UGT inducers (eg, rifampicin, phenytoin, phenobarbital, ritonavir). If concomitant use is necessary w/ 1 of these agents, consider increasing initial deferasirox dose by 50%, and monitor serum ferritin levels and clinical responses for further dose modification.

Renal Impairment
Baseline Renal Impairment:
CrCl 40-60mL/min: Reduce initial dose by 50%
SrCr >2X ULN or CrCl <40mL/min: Contraindicated

Increases in SrCr During Therapy:
All Patients: D/C therapy for SrCr >2X the age-appropriate ULN or for CrCl <40mL/min

Transfusional Iron Overload:
2-15 Years: Reduce dose by 7mg/kg if SrCr increases to >33% above the average baseline measurement and greater than the age-appropriate ULN
≥16 Years: If SrCr increases by ≥33% above the average baseline measurement, repeat SrCr w/in 1 week, and if still elevated by ≥33%, reduce dose by 7mg/kg

NTDT Syndromes:
10-15 Years: Reduce dose by 3.5mg/kg if SrCr increases to >33% above the average baseline measurement and greater than the age-appropriate ULN
≥16 Years: If SrCr increases by ≥33% above the average baseline measurement, repeat SrCr w/in 1 week, and if still elevated by ≥33%, interrupt therapy if the dose is 3.5mg/kg, or reduce by 50% if the dose is 7 or 14mg/kg

Hepatic Impairment
Baseline Hepatic Impairment:
Mild (Child-Pugh A): No dose adjustment necessary
Moderate (Child-Pugh B): Reduce initial dose by 50%
Severe (Child-Pugh C): Avoid therapy

Elderly
Start at lower end of dosing range

ADMINISTRATION
Oral route
Swallow tab w/ water or other liquids, preferably at the same time each day. May be taken on an empty stomach or w/ a light meal (containing <7% fat content and approx 250 calories).
For patients who have difficulty swallowing whole tabs, may crush tabs and mix w/ soft foods (eg, yogurt, applesauce) immediately prior to use; dose should be immediately and completely consumed and not stored for future use. Avoid commercial crushers w/ serrated surfaces for crushing a single 90mg tab.

STORAGE
25°C (77°F); excursions permitted to 15-30°C (59-86°F). Protect from moisture.

HOW SUPPLIED
Tab: 90mg, 180mg, 360mg

CONTRAINDICATIONS
SrCr >2X the age-appropriate ULN or CrCl <40mL/min, poor performance status, high-risk myelodysplastic syndrome (MDS), advanced malignancies, platelet counts <50 x 10⁹/L, known hypersensitivity to deferasirox or any component of this medication.

WARNINGS/PRECAUTIONS
Renal tubular damage including Fanconi's syndrome reported, most commonly in children and adolescents w/ β-thalassemia and serum ferritin levels <1500mcg/L: Intermittent proteinuria reported; monitor for proteinuria monthly. Hepatic toxicity appears to be more common in patients >55 yrs of age. Hepatic failure was more common in patients w/ significant comorbidities, including liver cirrhosis and multiorgan failure. Consider dose modifications or interruption of treatment for severe or persistent elevations in serum transaminases and bilirubin. Patients w/ mild (Child-Pugh A) or moderate (Child-Pugh B) hepatic impairment may be at higher risk for hepatic toxicity. Nonfatal upper GI irritation, ulceration, and hemorrhage reported. There have been reports of ulcers complicated w/ GI perforation (including fatal outcome). Neutropenia, agranulocytosis, worsening anemia, and thrombocytopenia, including fatal events, reported; risk may increase w/ preexisting hematologic disorders. Interrupt treatment in patients who develop cytopenias until the cause has been determined. Increased risk of toxicity in elderly; monitor more frequently. May cause serious hypersensitivity reactions (eg, anaphylaxis, angioedema); d/c and institute appropriate medical intervention if reactions are severe. Do not reintroduce in patients who have experienced previous hypersensitivity reactions on deferasirox products. Severe skin reactions, including Stevens-Johnson syndrome (SJS), toxic epidermal necrolysis (TEN), and erythema multiforme, reported. Cannot exclude risk of other skin reactions (eg, drug reaction w/ eosinophilia and systemic symptoms). D/C immediately and do not reintroduce if severe skin reactions are suspected. Rashes may occur; interrupt treatment in severe cases and may consider reintroduction

at a lower dose w/ escalation after resolution of rash. Auditory and ocular disturbances reported. Perform auditory and ophthalmic testing every 12 months; monitor more frequently if disturbances are noted and consider dose reduction or interruption. Measure serum ferritin monthly for possible overchelation of iron for patients w/ transfusional iron overload. For patients w/ NTDT, measure serum ferritin monthly and measure LIC by liver biopsy or by using an FDA-cleared/approved method for monitoring patients receiving therapy every 6 months on treatment.

ADVERSE REACTIONS
Transfusional Iron Overload: Abdominal pain, N/V, diarrhea, skin rashes, increases in SrCr.
NTDT Syndromes: Nausea, rash, diarrhea.

DRUG INTERACTIONS
See Dosing Considerations. Avoid w/ aluminum-containing antacid preparations. May induce CYP3A4, resulting in a decrease in CYP3A4 substrate concentration; closely monitor for signs of reduced effectiveness w/ drugs metabolized by CYP3A4 (eg, cyclosporine, fentanyl, quetiapine). Inhibits CYP2C8 and CYP1A2, resulting in an increase in CYP2C8 (eg, repaglinide, paclitaxel) and CYP1A2 (eg, duloxetine, theophylline, tizanidine) substrate concentration; closely monitor for signs of exposure-related toxicity. Consider decreasing the dose of repaglinide and monitor blood glucose levels carefully. Avoid w/ theophylline or other CYP1A2 substrates w/ a narrow therapeutic index (eg, tizanidine); monitor theophylline concentrations and consider theophylline dose modification if theophylline must be coadministered. Increased risk of GI hemorrhage w/ drugs that have ulcerogenic or hemorrhagic potential (eg, NSAIDs, corticosteroids, oral bisphosphonates, anticoagulants).

PREGNANCY AND LACTATION
Pregnancy: There are no adequate or well-controlled studies in pregnant women. Administration to animals during pregnancy and lactation resulted in decreased offspring viability and an increase in renal anomalies in male offspring at exposures that were less than the recommended human exposure. Use during pregnancy only if potential benefit justifies the potential risk to the fetus.
Lactation: Not for use in nursing.

MECHANISM OF ACTION
Iron-chelating agent; a tridentate ligand that binds iron w/ high affinity in a 2:1 ratio.

PHARMACOKINETICS
Absorption: Absolute bioavailability (tab for oral sus: 70%, tab: 36% greater than tab for oral sus); T_{max}=1.5-4 hrs (median). **Distribution:** V_d=14.37L (adults); plasma protein binding (99%). **Metabolism:** Glucuronidation via UGT1A1 (major) and UGT1A3 (minor) followed by deconjugation in the intestine and reabsorption (enterohepatic recycling); oxidation via CYP450 (minor). **Elimination:** Feces (84%), urine (8%); $T_{1/2}$=8-16 hrs.

PATIENT CONSIDERATIONS
Assessment: Assess for high-risk MDS, performance status, renal/hepatic impairment, advanced malignancies, hematological disorders, comorbidities, hypersensitivity to the drug, pregnancy/nursing status, and possible drug interactions. Perform baseline auditory and ophthalmic examinations. Obtain baseline SrCr in duplicate, serum transaminases, bilirubin, and blood counts. Determine CrCl (Cockcroft-Gault method). In patients w/ transfusional iron overload, obtain baseline serum ferritin level. In patients w/ iron overload in NTDT syndromes, obtain LIC by liver biopsy or by an FDA-cleared/approved method for identifying patients for treatment w/ deferasirox therapy, and obtain baseline serum ferritin level on at least 2 measurements 1 month apart.

Monitoring: Monitor for acute renal failure, hepatic failure, GI ulceration/hemorrhage, neutropenia, agranulocytosis, worsening anemia, thrombocytopenia, hypersensitivity reactions, rashes, SJS, TEN, erythema multiforme, and other adverse reactions. Monitor blood counts. Perform auditory and ophthalmic tests every 12 months. Monitor closely for efficacy and adverse reactions that may require dose titration in patients w/ mild or moderate hepatic impairment. Monitor serum transaminases and bilirubin every 2 weeks during the 1st month of therapy and at least monthly thereafter. Monitor SrCr weekly during the 1st month after initiation or modification of therapy and at least monthly thereafter. Monitor SrCr and/or CrCl more frequently if creatinine levels are increasing. Monitor serum ferritin and for proteinuria monthly. In patients w/ iron overload in NTDT syndromes, monitor LIC every 6 months. Monitor elderly more frequently for toxicity.

Counseling: Instruct to take ud. Instruct not to take the medication simultaneously w/ aluminum-containing antacids. Inform of the importance of auditory and ophthalmic testing before starting treatment and thereafter at regular intervals. Caution patients experiencing dizziness to avoid driving or operating machinery. Inform about drug interactions including potential for GI ulcers/bleeding and loss of effectiveness due to drug interactions. Advise that blood tests will be performed every month or more frequently if patient is at increased risk of complications. Inform that severe kidney and liver problems, blood disorders, stomach hemorrhage, and death have been reported. Inform that skin rash and serious allergic reactions have been reported; advise to d/c therapy and contact physician immediately if severe reactions occur.

JAKAFI — ruxolitinib   **Rx**
Class: Kinase inhibitor

ADULT DOSAGE

Intermediate or High-Risk Myelofibrosis

Including Primary Myelofibrosis, Post-Polycythemia Vera Myelofibrosis, Post-Essential Thrombocythemia Myelofibrosis:

Initial:
Platelet Count >200 x 10⁹/L: 20mg bid
Platelet Count 100-200 x 10⁹/L: 15mg bid
Platelet Count 50 to <100 x 10⁹/L: 5mg bid
Titrate: Based on safety and efficacy

Polycythemia Vera

In Patients Who Have Had an Inadequate Response to or Are Intolerant of Hydroxyurea:

Initial: 10mg bid
Titrate: Based on safety and efficacy

PEDIATRIC DOSAGE
Pediatric use may not have been established

DOSING CONSIDERATIONS

Dose Reductions
Myelofibrosis:
Starting Treatment w/ Platelet Count of 50 to <100 x 10⁹/L:
Platelet Count <25 x 10⁹/L or ANC <0.5 x 10⁹/L: Interrupt treatment; may restart after recovery of platelet count to >35 x 10⁹/L and ANC to >0.75 x 10⁹/L
Starting Treatment w/ Platelet Count of ≥100 x 10⁹/L:
Platelet Count <50 x 10⁹/L or ANC <0.5 x 10⁹/L: Interrupt treatment and may restart after recovery of platelet count to >50 x 10⁹/L and ANC to >0.75 x 10⁹/L

Refer to PI for further information on restarting treatment

Polycythemia Vera:
Hgb <8g/dL or Platelet Count <50 x 10⁹/L or ANC <1.0 x 10⁹/L: Interrupt dosing; may restart after recovery of hematologic parameters to acceptable levels
Hgb 8 to <10g/dL or Platelet Count 50 to <75 x 10⁹/L: Reduce dose by 5mg bid; if on 5mg bid, decrease to 5mg qd
Hgb 10 to <12g/dL and Platelet Count 75 to <100 x 10⁹/L: Consider dose reductions w/ the goal of avoiding dose interruptions for anemia and thrombocytopenia

Refer to PI for further information on restarting treatment

Concomitant Medications
Strong CYP3A4 Inhibitors or Fluconazole Doses ≤200mg:
Initial Dose:

Myelofibrosis:
Platelet Count 50 to <100 x 10⁹/L: 5mg qd
Platelet Count ≥100 x 10⁹/L: 10mg bid

Polycythemia Vera: 5mg bid

Maint Dose:
5mg QD: Avoid concomitant use or interrupt treatment for the duration of strong CYP3A4 inhibitor or fluconazole use
5mg BID: Reduce to 5mg qd
≥10mg BID: Reduce dose by 50% (round up to the closest available tab strength)

Daily Fluconazole Doses >200mg: Avoid concomitant use

Renal Impairment
Initial Dose:

Myelofibrosis w/ Moderate or Severe (CrCl 15-59mL/min) Impairment:
Platelet Count <50 x 10⁹/L: Avoid use
Platelet Count 50 to <100 x 10⁹/L: 5mg/day
Platelet Count 100-150 x 10⁹/L: 10mg bid
ESRD on Dialysis:
Platelet Count 100-200 x 10⁹/L: 15mg once after a dialysis session
Platelet Count >200 x 10⁹/L: 20mg once after a dialysis session

Polycythemia Vera w/ Moderate or Severe (CrCl 15-59mL/min) Impairment:
Any Platelet Count: 5mg bid
ESRD on Dialysis: 10mg

Hepatic Impairment
Initial Dose:

Myelofibrosis w/ Mild, Moderate, or Severe (Child-Pugh Categories A, B, C) Impairment:
Platelet Count <50 x 10⁹/L: Avoid use
Platelet Count 50 to <100 x 10⁹/L: 5mg/day
Platelet Count 100-150 x 10⁹/L: 10mg bid

Polycythemia Vera w/ Mild, Moderate, or Severe (Child-Pugh Categories A, B, C) Impairment:
Any Platelet Count: 5mg bid

Adverse Reactions
Hematologic Toxicity and Thrombocytopenia:
Refer to PI for further modifications for myelofibrosis and polycythemia vera

Bleeding:
- Interrupt treatment for bleeding requiring intervention regardless of platelet count
- Once bleeding event has resolved, consider resuming treatment at prior dose if underlying cause of bleeding has been controlled
- If bleeding event has resolved but underlying cause persists, consider resuming treatment at a lower dose

Discontinuation
When discontinuing for reasons other than thrombocytopenia, consider gradual tapering (eg, 5mg bid each week)

Other Important Considerations
Insufficient Response:
- Doses should not be increased during the first 4 weeks of therapy and not more frequently than every 2 weeks
- D/C if no spleen size reduction or symptom improvement after 6 months of therapy

Myelofibrosis:
Starting Treatment w/ Platelet Count 50 to <100 x 10⁹/L:
May increase by increments of 5mg/day to a max of 10mg bid if:
1. Platelet count has remained at least 40 x 10⁹/L, and
2. Platelet count has not fallen by more than 20% in the prior 4 weeks, and
3. ANC is >1 x 10⁹/L, and
4. Dose has not been reduced or interrupted for an adverse event or hematological toxicity in the prior 4 weeks

Continuation of treatment for >6 months should be limited to when the benefits outweigh the potential risks

Starting Treatment w/ Platelet Count ≥100 x 10⁹/L:
If platelet and neutrophil counts are adequate, may increase in 5mg bid increments to a max of 25mg bid if:
1. Failure to achieve a reduction from pretreatment baseline in either palpable spleen length of 50% or a 35% reduction in spleen volume measured by CT or MRI;
2. Platelet count >125 x 10⁹/L at 4 weeks and platelet count never <100 x 10⁹/L;
3. ANC levels >0.75 x 10⁹/L

Long-term maintenance at 5mg bid should be limited to when the benefits outweigh the potential risks

Polycythemia Vera:
If platelet, Hgb, and neutrophil counts are adequate, may increase in 5mg bid increments to a max of 25mg bid if:
1. Inadequate efficacy demonstrated by one or more of the following:
a. Continued need for phlebotomy
b. WBC count greater than ULN range
c. Platelet count greater than ULN range
d. Palpable spleen that is reduced by <25% from baseline
2. Platelet count ≥140 x 10⁹/L
3. Hgb ≥12g/dL
4. ANC ≥1.5 x 10⁹/L

ADMINISTRATION
Oral route

Take w/ or w/o food.

NG Tube (8 French or Greater) Alternative
Use if unable to ingest tabs.
Suspend one tab in approx 40mL of water w/ stirring for approx 10 min. W/IN 6 hrs after tab has dispersed, the sus can be administered using an appropriate syringe.

STORAGE
20-25°C (68-77°F); excursions permitted between 15-30°C (59-86°F).

HOW SUPPLIED
Tab: 5mg, 10mg, 15mg, 20mg, 25mg

WARNINGS/PRECAUTIONS
See Dosing Considerations. Avoid in ESRD (CrCl <15mL/min) not requiring dialysis. May cause thrombocytopenia, anemia, and neutropenia. Manage thrombocytopenia by reducing the dose or temporarily interrupting treatment; platelet transfusions may be necessary. May require blood transfusions and/or dose modifications in patients developing anemia. Withhold treatment until recovery of severe neutropenia (ANC <0.5 x 10⁹/L). Serious bacterial, mycobacterial, fungal, and viral infections may occur; active serious infections should be resolved before starting therapy. Tuberculosis (TB) reported; test for latent infection in those at higher risk prior to treatment initiation. Observe for signs/symptoms of active TB and manage promptly. Progressive multifocal leukoencephalopathy (PML) reported; d/c and evaluate if PML is suspected. Hepatitis B viral load (HBV-DNA titer) increases, w/ or w/o associated elevations in ALT and AST reported in patients w/ chronic HBV infections; patients w/ chronic HBV infection should be treated and monitored according to clinical guidelines. Symptoms from myeloproliferative neoplasms may return to pretreatment levels over a period of 1 week following discontinuation of therapy. Fever, respiratory distress, hypotension, disseminated intravascular coagulation, or multiorgan failure may occur after discontinuation; evaluate for and treat any intercurrent illness and consider restarting or increasing dose if one or more of these adverse events occur. Non-melanoma skin cancers (eg, basal cell, squamous cell, Merkel cell carcinoma) reported. Increases in lipid parameters including total cholesterol, LDL cholesterol, and TGs reported; assess lipid parameters approx 8-12 weeks following initiation of therapy and monitor and treat according to clinical guidelines.

ADVERSE REACTIONS
Bruising, dizziness, headache, UTIs, weight gain, flatulence, thrombocytopenia, anemia, neutropenia, ALT/AST/cholesterol elevations, abdominal pain, diarrhea, fatigue, pruritus.

DRUG INTERACTIONS
See Dosing Considerations. Strong CYP3A4 inhibitor ketoconazole may increase levels and exposure. Concomitant use w/ combined CYP3A4 and CYP2C9 inhibitor fluconazole at doses of 100-400mg qd may increase exposure of ruxolitinib. Strong CYP3A4 inducer rifampin may decrease levels and exposure; monitor patients frequently and adjust ruxolitinib dose based on safety and efficacy.

PREGNANCY AND LACTATION
Pregnancy: Category C.
Lactation: Not for use in nursing.

MECHANISM OF ACTION
Kinase inhibitor; inhibits Janus associated kinases (JAKs) JAK1 and JAK2 which mediate the signaling of a number of cytokines and growth factors that are important for hematopoiesis and immune function.

PHARMACOKINETICS
Absorption: Rapid; T_{max}=1-2 hrs. **Distribution:** V_d=72L (myelofibrosis), 75L (polycythemia vera); plasma protein binding (97%). **Metabolism:** Via CYP3A4 and CYP2C9 (lesser extent). **Elimination:** Urine (74%), feces (22%); $T_{1/2}$=3 hrs (ruxolitinib), 5.8 hrs (ruxolitinib and metabolites).

PATIENT CONSIDERATIONS
Assessment: Assess for risk factors for TB, renal/hepatic impairment, pregnancy/nursing status, and possible drug interactions. Resolve active serious infections prior to therapy. Perform CBC and platelet count before initiating therapy. Assess baseline lipid levels.

Monitoring: Monitor for thrombocytopenia, anemia, neutropenia, infections, PML, TB, exacerbation of symptoms from myeloproliferative neoplasms following discontinuation of therapy, non-melanoma skin cancers, and other adverse reactions. Monitor CBCs and platelet counts every 2-4 weeks until doses are stabilized, and then as clinically indicated. Perform periodic skin examinations. Monitor HBV-DNA titer levels in patients w/ HBV. Monitor lipid levels approx 8-12 weeks following initiation of therapy.

Counseling: Inform that therapy is associated w/ thrombocytopenia, anemia, and neutropenia and of the need to monitor CBC before and during treatment; advise to observe for and report bleeding to the physician. Inform of the signs/symptoms of infection, herpes zoster, and PML; instruct to report and seek medical advice if such symptoms are observed. Inform that after discontinuation of therapy, signs/symptoms from myeloproliferative neoplasms are expected to return; instruct not to interrupt or d/c therapy w/o consulting physician. Inform that drug may increase the risk of certain non-melanoma skin cancers; advise to inform physician if patient has have ever had any type of skin cancer or if the patient observes any new or changing skin lesions. Inform that therapy may increase blood cholesterol, and advise of the need to monitor blood cholesterol levels. Advise to inform physician of all medications, including OTC medications, herbal products, and dietary supplements, that are being taken. Instruct patients on dialysis not to take their dose before dialysis but only following dialysis. Advise patients to continue taking the medication every day ud and not to change the dose or stop therapy w/o consulting their physician.

JETREA — ocriplasmin   Rx
Class: Enzyme

ADULT DOSAGE	PEDIATRIC DOSAGE
Vitreomacular Adhesion	Pediatric use may not have been established
Symptomatic:	
0.125mg (0.1mL of the diluted sol) by intravitreal inj to the affected eye once as a single dose	

ADMINISTRATION
Intravitreal route

Must dilute before use.
Adequate anesthesia and broad spectrum microbiocide should be administered.
Insert inj needle 3.5-4mm posterior to limbus aiming towards center of vitreous cavity, avoiding horizontal meridian; inj volume of 0.1mL is then delivered into mid-vitreous.
Each vial should only be used to provide a single inj for a single eye. If contralateral eye requires treatment, use new vial; treatment of the other eye is not recommended w/in 7 days of the initial inj.
Repeated administration in the same eye is not recommended.

Preparation
1. Remove vial from freezer and allow to thaw at room temperature (w/in a few min).
2. Add 0.2mL of 0.9% w/v NaCl inj (sterile, preservative-free) into vial and gently swirl until mixed.
3. Withdraw all of diluted sol using a sterile #19 gauge needle and discard needle after withdrawal of vial contents; do not use this needle for intravitreal inj.
4. Replace the needle w/ a sterile #30 gauge needle, carefully expel air bubbles and excess drug from syringe and adjust dose to the 0.1mL mark on syringe; use sol immediately.

STORAGE
Store frozen at ≤-20°C (-4°F). Protect from light.

HOW SUPPLIED
Inj: 2.5mg/mL [0.2mL]

WARNINGS/PRECAUTIONS
Must only be administered by a qualified physician. Monitor for IOP elevation immediately following inj. Decreased vision reported; majority were due to progression of the condition w/ traction and many required surgical intervention. Intraocular inflammation/infection/hemorrhage, increased IOP, retinal detachment/tear, and dyschromatopsia (electroretinographic changes reported in approx half of these cases) reported; monitor appropriately. Lens subluxation reported in a premature infant who received a dose 1.4X higher than the recommended dose.

ADVERSE REACTIONS
Vitreous floaters, conjunctival hemorrhage, eye pain, photopsia, blurred vision, macular hole, reduced visual acuity, visual impairment, retinal edema.

PREGNANCY AND LACTATION
Pregnancy: Category C.
Lactation: Not known if excreted in human milk; caution in nursing.

MECHANISM OF ACTION
Proteolytic enzyme; has proteolytic activity against protein components of the vitreous body and the vitreoretinal interface (eg, laminin, fibronectin, collagen), thereby dissolving the protein matrix responsible for the vitreomacular adhesion.

PATIENT CONSIDERATIONS
Assessment: Assess pregnancy/nursing status.

Monitoring: Monitor for decreased vision, increased IOP (eg, check for perfusion of the optic nerve head, tonometry), lens subluxation, retinal detachment/tear, dyschromatopsia, and other adverse reactions.

Counseling: Advise to seek immediate care from an ophthalmologist if the eye becomes red, sensitive to light, painful, or develops a change in vision. Inform that temporary visual impairment may be experienced; instruct patients not to drive or operate heavy machinery until visual impairment has resolved, and advise to seek care from an ophthalmologist if visual impairment persists or decreases further.

JEVTANA — cabazitaxel   Rx
Class: Antimicrotubule agent

> Neutropenic deaths reported. Perform frequent blood cell counts to monitor for neutropenia. Contraindicated in patients w/ neutrophil counts of ≤1500 cells/mm³. Severe hypersensitivity reactions may occur; may include generalized rash/erythema, hypotension, and bronchospasm. D/C infusion immediately if a severe hypersensitivity reaction occurs and administer appropriate therapy. Patients should receive premedication. Contraindicated in patients who have a history of severe hypersensitivity reactions to cabazitaxel or other drugs formulated w/ polysorbate 80.

ADULT DOSAGE	PEDIATRIC DOSAGE
Metastatic Prostate Cancer	Pediatric use may not have been established
Treatment of patients w/ hormone-refractory metastatic prostate cancer previously treated w/ a docetaxel-containing treatment regimen	
25mg/m² as a 1-hr IV infusion every 3 weeks in combination w/ oral prednisone 10mg administered daily throughout treatment	
Premedication	
Premedicate at least 30 min prior to each dose w/ the following IV medications:	
Antihistamine: Dexchlorpheniramine 5mg, diphenhydramine 25mg, or equivalent	
Corticosteroid: Dexamethasone 8mg or equivalent	
H₂ Antagonist: Ranitidine 50mg or equivalent	
Antiemetic prophylaxis is recommended and may be given PO or IV prn	

DOSING CONSIDERATIONS
Concomitant Medications
Strong CYP3A Inhibitors: Avoid coadministration w/ these drugs; if coadministration is required, consider a 25% cabazitaxel dose reduction

Hepatic Impairment
Mild (Total Bilirubin >1 to ≤1.5X ULN or AST >1.5X ULN): Reduce dose to 20mg/m²
Moderate (Total Bilirubin >1.5 to ≤3X ULN and AST=Any): Reduce dose to 15mg/m²

Adverse Reactions
Prolonged Grade ≥3 Neutropenia (>1 Week) Despite Appropriate Medication (Including G-CSF): Delay treatment until neutrophil count is >1500 cells/mm³, then reduce dose to 20mg/m²; use G-CSF for secondary prophylaxis
Febrile Neutropenia/Neutropenic Infections: Delay treatment until improvement or resolution, and until neutrophil count is >1500 cells/mm³, then reduce dose to 20mg/m²; use G-CSF for secondary prophylaxis
Grade ≥3 Diarrhea or Persisting Diarrhea Despite Appropriate Medication, Fluid, and Electrolyte Replacement: Delay treatment until improvement or resolution, then reduce dose to 20mg/m²

Grade 2 Peripheral Neuropathy: Delay treatment until improvement or resolution, then reduce dose to 20mg/m²
Grade ≥3 Peripheral Neuropathy: D/C therapy

D/C therapy if patient continues to experience any of the above reactions at 20mg/m²

ADMINISTRATION
IV route

Do not mix w/ any other drugs
Do not use PVC infusion containers or polyurethane infusion sets for preparation and administration of infusion sol
Use an in-line filter of 0.22μm nominal pore size (also referred to as 0.2μm) during administration

Preparation Instructions
Cabazitaxel requires 2 dilutions prior to administration

Step 1 - First Dilution:
1. Mix each vial of cabazitaxel 60mg/1.5mL w/ entire contents of supplied diluent; once reconstituted, the resultant sol contains 10mg/mL cabazitaxel
2. When transferring the diluent, direct the needle onto the inside wall of cabazitaxel vial and inject slowly to limit foaming
3. Remove syringe/needle and gently mix the initial diluted sol by repeated inversions for at least 45 sec to assure full mixing of drug and diluent; do not shake
4. Let the sol stand for a few min to allow any foam to dissipate, and check that the sol is homogeneous and contains no visible particulate matter; it is not required that all foam dissipate prior to continuing the preparation process
5. The resulting initial diluted sol (cabazitaxel 10mg/mL) requires further dilution before administration; the 2nd dilution should be done immediately (w/in 30 min) to obtain the final infusion

Step 2 - Second (Final) Dilution:
1. Withdraw the recommended dose from the cabazitaxel sol containing 10mg/mL using a calibrated syringe and further dilute into a sterile 250mL PVC-free container of either 0.9% NaCl sol or D5 sol for infusion; if a dose >65mg of cabazitaxel is required, use a larger volume of the infusion vehicle so that a concentration of 0.26mg/mL is not exceeded
2. The concentration of final infusion sol should be between 0.10mg/mL and 0.26mg/mL
3. Remove syringe and thoroughly mix the final infusion sol by gently inverting the bag or bottle
4. As the final infusion sol is supersaturated, it may crystallize over time; do not use if this occurs and discard

Fully prepared cabazitaxel infusion sol (in either 0.9% NaCl sol or D5 sol) should be used w/in 8 hrs at ambient temperature (including the 1-hr infusion), or for a total of 24 hrs under refrigeration (including the 1-hr infusion)

If cabazitaxel 1st diluted sol, or 2nd (final) dilution for IV infusion should come into contact w/ skin or mucosae, immediately and thoroughly wash w/ soap and water

STORAGE
25°C (77°F); excursions permitted to 15-30°C (59-86°F). Do not refrigerate.

HOW SUPPLIED
Inj: 60mg/1.5mL

CONTRAINDICATIONS
Neutrophil counts ≤1500/mm³, severe hepatic impairment (total bilirubin >3X ULN), history of severe hypersensitivity reactions to cabazitaxel or to other drugs formulated with polysorbate 80.

WARNINGS/PRECAUTIONS
Bone marrow suppression manifested as neutropenia, anemia, thrombocytopenia, and/or pancytopenia may occur. G-CSF may be administered to reduce risks of neutropenia complications; consider primary prophylaxis w/ G-CSF in patients w/ high-risk clinical features (eg, >65 yrs of age, poor performance status, previous episodes of febrile neutropenia, extensive prior radiation ports, poor nutritional status, or other serious comorbidities) that predispose them to increased complications from prolonged neutropenia. Caution in patients w/ Hgb <10g/dL. Observe patients closely for hypersensitivity reactions, especially during the 1st and 2nd infusions. N/V and severe diarrhea may occur. Death related to diarrhea and electrolyte imbalance reported; intensive measures may be required for severe diarrhea and electrolyte imbalance. GI hemorrhage and perforation, ileus, enterocolitis, neutropenic enterocolitis, including fatal outcome, reported; risk may be increased w/ neutropenia, age, steroid use, concomitant use of NSAIDs, antiplatelet therapy, or anticoagulants, and prior history of pelvic radiotherapy, adhesions, ulceration, and GI bleeding. Abdominal pain/tenderness, fever, persistent constipation, diarrhea (w/ or w/o neutropenia), may be early manifestations of serious GI toxicity and should be evaluated and treated promptly; treatment delay or discontinuation may be necessary. Renal failure, including cases w/ fatal outcome, reported; identify causes and treat aggressively. Carefully monitor patients w/ ESRD (CrCl <15mL/min). Caution in elderly. Not indicated for use in female patients; may cause fetal harm when administered to a pregnant woman.

ADVERSE REACTIONS
Hypersensitivity reactions, neutropenia, anemia, leukopenia, thrombocytopenia, diarrhea, fatigue, N/V, constipation, asthenia, abdominal pain, anorexia, back pain, hematuria, dyspnea.

DRUG INTERACTIONS
See Dosing Considerations. Strong CYP3A inhibitors (eg, ketoconazole, clarithromycin, atazanavir) may increase levels.

PREGNANCY AND LACTATION
Category D, not for use in nursing.

MECHANISM OF ACTION
Antimicrotubule agent; binds to tubulin and promotes its assembly into microtubules while simultaneously inhibiting disassembly, which results in the inhibition of mitotic and interphase cellular functions.

PHARMACOKINETICS
Absorption: C_{max}=226ng/mL; AUC=991ng•hr/mL; T_{max}=1 hr. **Distribution:** V_d=4864L; plasma protein binding (89-92%). **Metabolism:** Liver (extensive) via CYP3A4/5, and to a lesser extent, CYP2C8. **Elimination:** Urine (3.7%, 2.3% unchanged), feces (76%); $T_{1/2}$=95 hrs.

PATIENT CONSIDERATIONS
Assessment: Assess for history of hypersensitivity to drug or to other drugs formulated w/ polysorbate 80, hepatic/renal impairment, risk of developing GI complications, pregnancy/nursing status, and possible drug interactions. Assess for high-risk clinical features that may predispose to increased complications from prolonged neutropenia. Obtain baseline CBC, including neutrophil count.

Monitoring: Monitor for signs/symptoms of neutropenia, infections, hypersensitivity reactions, severe diarrhea, dehydration, N/V, electrolyte imbalance, renal failure, serious GI toxicity, and other adverse reactions. Monitor CBCs, including neutrophil count, on a weekly basis during cycle 1 and before each treatment cycle thereafter.

Counseling: Counsel about the risk of potential hypersensitivity; instruct to immediately report signs of a hypersensitivity reaction. Inform that drug decreases blood count (eg, WBCs, platelets, and RBCs), and thus it is important that periodic assessment of their blood count be performed to detect the development of neutropenia, thrombocytopenia, anemia, and/or pancytopenia. Instruct to frequently monitor temperature and to immediately report any occurrence of fever to physician. Explain that it is important to take the oral prednisone as prescribed; instruct to report to physician if not compliant w/ oral corticosteroid regimen. Instruct to immediately report to physician any occurrence of fever, significant vomiting or diarrhea, decreased urinary output, or hematuria. Counsel about side effects associated w/ exposure, such as severe and fatal infections, dehydration, and renal failure. Inform about importance of providing a list of prescription and non-prescription drugs to physician. Inform elderly patients that certain side effects may be more frequent or severe.

JUXTAPID — lomitapide   Rx
Class: Lipid-regulating agent

> May cause elevations in transaminases; measure ALT, AST, alkaline phosphatase, and total bilirubin prior to therapy, and then ALT/AST regularly as recommended. Adjust dose if ALT/AST is ≥3X ULN. D/C for clinically significant liver toxicity. May increase hepatic fat w/ or w/o increases in transaminases. Hepatic steatosis associated w/ lomitapide treatment may be a risk factor for progressive liver disease, including steatohepatitis and cirrhosis. Available only through a restricted program under a Risk Evaluation and Mitigation Strategy (REMS) because of the risk of hepatotoxicity. Prescribe only to patients w/ a clinical or laboratory diagnosis consistent w/ homozygous familial hypercholesterolemia.

ADULT DOSAGE
Homozygous Familial Hypercholesterolemia

Prior to treatment, initiate a low-fat diet supplying <20% of energy from fat

Initial: 5mg qd
Titrate: After ≥2 weeks, may increase dose to 10mg qd; and then at ≥4-week intervals, may increase to 20mg qd, then 40mg qd, and then up to a max of 60mg qd
Max: 60mg qd

PEDIATRIC DOSAGE
Pediatric use may not have been established

- - - - - - - - - - - - - - - - - - - -

DOSING CONSIDERATIONS
Concomitant Medications
W/ Moderate and Strong CYP3A4 Inhibitors: Contraindicated

W/ Weak CYP3A4 Inhibitors:
Max: 30mg/day

W/ Oral Contraceptives:
Max: 40mg/day

Initiating Weak CYP3A4 Inhibitor in Patients Already Taking Lomitapide 10mg qd or More:
Decrease dose of lomitapide by half; patients taking lomitapide 5mg qd may continue w/ same dosage. May carefully titrate to a max of 30mg qd except when coadministered w/ oral contraceptives, in which case the max recommended lomitapide dosage is 40mg qd

Renal Impairment
ESRD Receiving Dialysis:
Max: 40mg/day

Hepatic Impairment
Mild (Child-Pugh A):
Max: 40mg/day

Adverse Reactions
ALT/AST ≥3X and <5X ULN:
- Confirm elevation w/ repeat measurement w/in 1 week.
- If confirmed, reduce dose and obtain additional liver-related tests if not already measured (eg, alkaline phosphatase, total bilirubin, INR).

- Repeat tests weekly and withhold dosing if signs of abnormal liver function (increase in bilirubin/INR) are present, if transaminase levels rise above 5X ULN, or if transaminase levels do not fall below 3X ULN w/in approx 4 weeks; investigate to identify probable cause in these cases of persistent or worsening abnormalities.
- Consider reducing dose and monitor liver-related tests more frequently if resuming therapy after transaminases resolve to <3X ULN.

ALT/AST ≥5X ULN:
- Withhold dosing, obtain additional liver-related tests if not already measured (eg, alkaline phosphatase, total bilirubin, INR), and investigate to identify probable cause.
- Reduce dose and monitor liver-related tests more frequently if resuming therapy after transaminases resolve to <3X ULN.

If transaminase elevations are accompanied by clinical symptoms of liver injury, increases in bilirubin ≥2X ULN, or active liver disease, d/c treatment and investigate to identify probable cause

ADMINISTRATION
Oral route

Take qd w/ a glass of water, w/o food, at least 2 hrs after pm meal. Swallow cap whole; do not open, crush, dissolve, or chew. Take daily supplements containing 400 IU vitamin E and at least 200mg linoleic acid, 210mg α-linolenic acid, 110mg eicosapentaenoic acid, and 80mg docosahexaenoic acid.

STORAGE
20-25°C (68-77°F); excursions permitted to 15-30°C (59-86°F). May tolerate brief exposure up to 40°C (104°F), provided the mean kinetic temperature does not exceed 25°C (77°F); however, such exposure should be minimized. Protect from moisture.

HOW SUPPLIED
Cap: 5mg, 10mg, 20mg, 30mg, 40mg, 60mg

CONTRAINDICATIONS
Pregnancy, moderate or severe hepatic impairment (based on Child-Pugh category B or C), active liver disease including unexplained persistent elevations of serum transaminases, concomitant moderate or strong CYP3A4 inhibitors.

WARNINGS/PRECAUTIONS
See Contraindications and Dosing Considerations. If baseline LFTs are abnormal, consider initiating therapy after an appropriate work-up and the baseline abnormalities are explained or resolved. May cause fetal harm. May reduce absorption of fat-soluble nutrients, especially in patients w/ chronic bowel or pancreatic diseases that predispose to malabsorption. GI adverse reactions reported; absorption of concomitant oral medications may be affected in patients who develop diarrhea or vomiting. Severe diarrhea reported; monitor patients who are more susceptible to complications from diarrhea and consider reducing the dose or suspending therapy. Avoid in patients w/ rare hereditary problems of galactose intolerance, Lapp lactase deficiency, or glucose-galactose malabsorption; may result in diarrhea and malabsorption. Caution in elderly.

ADVERSE REACTIONS
Diarrhea, N/V, dyspepsia, abdominal pain.

DRUG INTERACTIONS
See Dosing Considerations and Contraindications. Not recommended w/ other LDL-lowering agents that can increase hepatic fat. Avoid grapefruit juice. Alcohol may increase levels of hepatic fat and induce/exacerbate liver injury; avoid consumption of >1 alcoholic drink/day. Caution w/ other medications known to have potential for hepatotoxicity (eg, isotretinoin, amiodarone, acetaminophen [>4g/day for ≥3 days/week]). Increased exposure w/ weak CYP3A4 inhibitors (eg, alprazolam, atorvastatin, cimetidine). May increase INR and plasma concentrations of both R(+)-warfarin and S(-)-warfarin; regularly monitor INR (particularly after any changes in lomitapide dosage) and adjust dose of warfarin as clinically indicated. May double the exposure of simvastatin; refer to simvastatin PI for dosing recommendations. May increase the exposure of lovastatin; consider reducing the dose of lovastatin when initiating therapy. May increase the absorption of P-gp substrates (eg, aliskiren, colchicine, digoxin); consider dose reduction of the P-gp substrate. Separate dosing by at least 4 hrs w/ bile acid sequestrants.

PREGNANCY AND LACTATION
Pregnancy: Category X. There is a pregnancy exposure registry that monitors pregnancy outcomes in women exposed to drug during pregnancy.
Lactation: Not for use in nursing.
Reproductive Potential: Females of reproductive potential should have a negative pregnancy test before starting therapy, and should use effective contraception during therapy.

MECHANISM OF ACTION
Lipid-regulating agent; directly binds and inhibits microsomal TG transfer protein, which resides in the lumen of the endoplasmic reticulum, thereby preventing the assembly of apolipoprotein B-containing lipoproteins in enterocytes and hepatocytes. This inhibits the synthesis of chylomicrons and VLDL. The inhibition of the synthesis of VLDL leads to reduced levels of plasma LDL.

PHARMACOKINETICS
Absorption: Absolute bioavailability (7%); T_{max}=6 hrs. **Distribution:** V_d=985-1292L; plasma protein binding (99.8%). **Metabolism:** Liver (extensive) via oxidation, oxidative N-dealkylation, glucuronide conjugation, piperidine ring opening. CYP3A4; M1 and M3 (major metabolites). **Elimination:** Feces (33.4-35.1%, mostly unchanged), urine (52.9-59.5%, mostly M1); $T_{1/2}$=39.7 hrs.

PATIENT CONSIDERATIONS
Assessment: Assess for active liver disease, including unexplained persistent elevations of serum transaminases, bowel/pancreatic disease, galactose intolerance, renal dysfunction, pregnancy/nursing status, and possible drug

interactions. Measure ALT/AST, alkaline phosphatase, and serum bilirubin prior to therapy.

Monitoring: Monitor for hepatic steatosis, hepatotoxicity, and GI and other adverse reactions. Monitor renal/hepatic function. During the 1st yr, perform hepatic-related tests (eg, ALT, AST) prior to each increase in dose or monthly, whichever occurs 1st. After the 1st yr, perform these tests at least every 3 months and before any dose increase. Monitor INR w/ warfarin.

Counseling: Inform to take ud. Encourage to participate in the registry to monitor/evaluate long-term effects and inform that participation is voluntary. Advise that medication is only available from certified pharmacies enrolled in the REMS program. Discuss the importance of liver-related tests before initiation, prior to each dose escalation, and periodically thereafter. Advise of the potential for increased risk of liver injury if alcohol is consumed and instruct to limit alcohol consumption to not >1 drink/day. Advise to report any symptoms of possible liver injury (eg, fever, jaundice, lethargy, flu-like symptoms). Advise females of reproductive potential to have a negative pregnancy test before starting treatment and to use effective contraception while on therapy. Discuss the importance of taking daily supplements. Inform that GI adverse reactions are common and that strict adherence to a low-fat diet (<20% of total calories from fat) may reduce these reactions. Instruct to d/c therapy and contact physician if severe diarrhea occurs or if symptoms such as lightheadedness, decreased urine output, or tiredness occur. Inform that absorption of oral medications may be affected in patients who develop diarrhea or vomiting; instruct to seek physician's advice if symptoms develop. Instruct to omit grapefruit juice from diet; advise to inform physician about all medications, nutritional supplements, and vitamins taken. If a dose is missed, instruct to take the normal dose at the usual time the next day; if dose is interrupted for more than a week, advise to contact physician before restarting treatment.

KADCYLA — ado-trastuzumab emtansine   **Rx**

Class: Monoclonal antibody/HER2 blocker/antimicrotubule agent

> Do not substitute for or w/ trastuzumab. Serious hepatotoxicity, including liver failure and death, reported; monitor serum transaminases and bilirubin prior to initiation of therapy and prior to each dose. Reduce dose or d/c as appropriate in cases of increased serum transaminases/total bilirubin. May lead to reductions in left ventricular ejection fraction (LVEF). Evaluate left ventricular function prior to and during treatment; withhold treatment for clinically significant decrease in left ventricular function. Exposure during pregnancy may result in embryo-fetal harm; advise patients of these risks and the need for effective contraception.

ADULT DOSAGE	PEDIATRIC DOSAGE
HER2-Positive Metastatic Breast Cancer	Pediatric use may not have been established
As a single agent for patients who previously received trastuzumab and a taxane, separately or in combination; patients should have either received prior therapy for metastatic disease, or developed disease recurrence during or w/in 6 months of completing adjuvant therapy	
3.6mg/kg IV infusion every 3 weeks (21-day cycle) until disease progression or unacceptable toxicity **Max:** 3.6mg/kg/dose	
1st Infusion: Administer over 90 min; observe during infusion and for at least 90 min following the initial dose **Subsequent Infusions:** Administer over 30 min if prior infusions were well tolerated; observe during infusion and for at least 30 min after infusion	
Missed Dose If a planned dose is delayed or missed, administer as soon as possible; do not wait until the next planned cycle. Adjust the schedule of administration to maintain a 3-week interval between doses; administer at the dose and rate the patient tolerated in the most recent infusion.	

- -

DOSING CONSIDERATIONS
Renal Impairment
Mild (CrCl 60-89mL/min): Dose adjustment not needed
Moderate (CrCl 30-59mL/min): Dose adjustment not needed
Severe (CrCl <30mL/min): Limited data available; no dose adjustment can be recommended

Hepatic Impairment
Mild or Moderate: No adjustment to the starting dose is required
Severe: Not studied

Adverse Reactions
Infusion-Related Reactions: Slow or interrupt infusion rate
Life-Threatening Infusion-Related Reactions: Permanently d/c

Dose Reduction Schedule:
1st Reduction: 3mg/kg
2nd Reduction: 2.4mg/kg
Requirement for Further Reduction: D/C treatment
Do not re-escalate after a dose reduction is made

Increased Serum Transaminases (AST/ALT):
Grade 2 (>2.5 to ≤5X ULN): Treat at same dose level
Grade 3 (>5 to ≤20X ULN): Do not administer until AST/ALT recovers to Grade ≤2, then reduce 1 dose level
Grade 4 (>20X ULN): Permanently d/c treatment

Hyperbilirubinemia:
Grade 2 (>1.5 to ≤3X ULN): Do not administer until total bilirubin recovers to Grade ≤1, then treat at same dose level
Grade 3 (>3 to ≤10X ULN): Do not administer until total bilirubin recovers to Grade ≤1, then reduce 1 dose level
Grade 4 (>10X ULN): Permanently d/c treatment

Serum Transaminases >3X ULN w/ Total Bilirubin >2X ULN: Permanently d/c treatment
Nodular Regenerative Hyperplasia: Permanently d/c treatment

Left Ventricular Dysfunction:
Symptomatic CHF: D/C treatment
LVEF <40%: Do not administer. Repeat LVEF assessment w/in 3 weeks; if LVEF <40% is confirmed, d/c treatment
LVEF 40% to ≤45% and Decrease is ≥10% Points from Baseline: Do not administer. Repeat LVEF assessment w/in 3 weeks; if LVEF has not recovered to w/in 10% points from baseline, d/c treatment
LVEF 40% to ≤45% and Decrease is <10% Points from Baseline: Continue treatment and repeat LVEF assessment w/in 3 weeks
LVEF >45%: Continue treatment

Thrombocytopenia:
Grade 3 (Platelets 25,000/mm³ to <50,000/mm³): Do not administer until platelet count recovers to ≤Grade 1 (≥75,000/mm³), then treat at same dose level
Grade 4 (Platelets <25,000/mm³): Do not administer until platelet count recovers to ≤Grade 1, then reduce 1 dose level
Pulmonary Toxicity: Permanently d/c in patients diagnosed w/ interstitial lung disease or pneumonitis
Peripheral Neuropathy: Temporarily d/c w/ Grade 3 or 4 until resolution to ≤Grade 2

ADMINISTRATION
IV route

Do not substitute for or w/ trastuzumab.
Do not administer as an IV push or bolus.
Do not mix or administer as an infusion w/ other medicinal products.
Administer as an IV infusion only w/ a 0.2 or 0.22 micron in-line polyethersulfone filter. Reconstituted product contains no preservative and is intended for single use only.

Reconstitution
1. Slowly inject 5mL of sterile water for inj (SWFI) into the 100mg vial, or 8mL of SWFI into the 160mg vial to yield a sol containing 20mg/mL.
2. Swirl the vial gently until completely dissolved; do not shake.
3. The reconstituted lyophilized vials should be used immediately following reconstitution; if not used immediately, may store the reconstituted vials for up to 24 hrs at 2-8°C (36-46°F). Discard unused reconstituted vials after 24 hrs. Do not freeze.

Dilution
1. Calculate the volume of the 20mg/mL reconstituted sol needed.
2. Withdraw this amount from the vial and add it to an infusion bag containing 250mL of 0.9% NaCl inj; do not use D5 sol.
3. Gently invert the bag to mix the sol; do not shake.
4. The diluted infusion sol should be used immediately; if not used immediately, may store at 2-8°C (36-46°F) for up to 24 hrs prior to use (this storage time is additional to the time allowed for the reconstituted vials). Do not freeze or shake.

STORAGE
2-8°C (36-46°F) until time of reconstitution. Do not freeze or shake.

HOW SUPPLIED
Inj: 100mg, 160mg

WARNINGS/PRECAUTIONS
See Dosing Considerations. Serious hepatobiliary disorders and nodular regenerative hyperplasia of the liver reported. Increased risk of developing left ventricular dysfunction. Cases of interstitial lung disease, including pneumonitis, some leading to acute respiratory distress syndrome or fatal outcome, reported. Patients w/ dyspnea at rest due to complications of advanced malignancy and co-morbidities may be at increased risk of pulmonary toxicity. Not recommended for patients who had trastuzumab permanently discontinued due to infusion-related reactions and/or hypersensitivity. Infusion-related reactions reported. Serious, allergic/anaphylactic-like reaction reported; medications/emergency equipment should be available for immediate use. Cases of hemorrhagic events, including CNS, respiratory, and GI hemorrhage, reported. Thrombocytopenia and peripheral neuropathy reported. Detection of HER2 protein overexpression or gene amplification is necessary for selection of patients appropriate for therapy; assessment of HER2 status should be performed by laboratories w/ demonstrated proficiency in the specific technology being utilized. Reactions secondary to extravasation reported; closely monitor the infusion site for possible subcutaneous infiltration during drug administration. May cause fetal harm.

ADVERSE REACTIONS
Fatigue, nausea, musculoskeletal pain, hemorrhage, thrombocytopenia, headache, increased transaminases, constipation, epistaxis.

DRUG INTERACTIONS
Avoid w/ strong CYP3A4 inhibitors (eg, ketoconazole, clarithromycin, atazanavir) due to the potential for increase in exposure and toxicity; consider alternate medication w/ no or minimal potential to inhibit CYP3A4. If unavoidable, consider delaying treatment until the strong CYP3A4 inhibitors have cleared from circulation. If a strong CYP3A4 inhibitor is coadministered and treatment cannot be delayed, closely monitor for adverse reactions. Caution w/ anticoagulant or antiplatelet therapy; consider additional monitoring when concomitant use is medically necessary.

PREGNANCY AND LACTATION
Pregnancy: Can cause fetal harm when administered to a pregnant woman. Monitor women who received Kadcyla during pregnancy or w/in 7 months prior to conception for oligohydramnios; if oligohydramnios occurs, perform fetal testing that is appropriate for gestational age and consistent w/ community standards of care. There is a pregnancy exposure registry that monitors pregnancy outcomes in women exposed to Kadcyla during pregnancy; women who received Kadcyla during pregnancy or w/in 7 months prior to conception should enroll in the MotHER Pregnancy Registry. In addition, there is a pregnancy pharmacovigilance program; if Kadcyla is administered during pregnancy, or if a patient becomes pregnant while receiving Kadcyla or w/in 7 months following the last dose of Kadcyla, immediately report exposure to Genentech.
Lactation: There is no information regarding the presence of Kadcyla in human milk, the effects on the breastfed infant, or the effects on milk production. DM1, the cytotoxic component of Kadcyla, may cause serious adverse reactions in breastfed infants based on its mechanism of action. Avoid breastfeeding during treatment and for 7 months following the last dose of Kadcyla.
Reproductive Potential: Females of reproductive potential should use effective contraception during treatment and for 7 months following the last dose. Verify pregnancy status prior to initiation of therapy. Male patients w/ female partners of reproductive potential should use effective contraception during treatment and for 4 months following the last dose. May impair fertility in females and males of reproductive potential.

MECHANISM OF ACTION
Monoclonal antibody (IgG1)/HER2 blocker/Antimicrotubule agent (DM1); the HER2-targeted antibody-drug conjugate binds to HER2 receptor and intracellularly releases DM1-containing cytotoxic catabolites. Binding of DM1 to tubulin disrupts microtubule networks, resulting in cell cycle arrest and apoptotic death. Also inhibits HER2 receptor signaling, mediates antibody-dependent cell-mediated cytotoxicity, and inhibits shedding of the HER2 extracellular domain in human breast cancer cells that overexpress HER2.

PHARMACOKINETICS
Absorption: C_{max}=83.4mg/mL (ado-trastuzumab emtansine conjugate [ADC]); 4.61ng/mL (DM1). **Distribution:** ADC: V_d=3.13L. DM1: Plasma protein binding (93%). **Metabolism:** DM1: Liver via CYP3A4/5. **Elimination:** $T_{1/2}$=4 days (ADC).

PATIENT CONSIDERATIONS
Assessment: Assess for history of trastuzumab-induced infusion-related reactions, left ventricular dysfunction, dyspnea at rest, pregnancy/nursing status, and for possible drug interactions. Assess HER2 status. Assess LVEF prior to initiation of therapy. Assess platelet counts, serum transaminases, and bilirubin at baseline.

Monitoring: Monitor for signs/symptoms of neurotoxicity, hepatotoxicity, nodular regenerative hyperplasia, left ventricular dysfunction, interstitial lung disease (eg, pneumonitis), peripheral neuropathy, hemorrhage, thrombocytopenia, infusion-related reactions, allergic/anaphylactic reactions, and other adverse reactions. Monitor LVEF at regular intervals (eg, every 3 months). Repeat LVEF assessment w/in approx 3 weeks in patients whose treatment was withheld due to significant decrease in left ventricular function. Monitor platelet counts, serum transaminases, and bilirubin prior to each dose.

Counseling: Inform of the possibility of severe liver injury and advise to immediately seek medical attention if symptoms of acute hepatitis occur. Advise to contact physician immediately if new onset/worsening SOB, cough, ankles/legs swelling, weight gain (>5 lbs in 24 hrs), dizziness, loss of consciousness, or palpitations occur. Inform pregnant women/females of reproductive potential that drug exposure during pregnancy or w/in 7 months prior to conception can result in fetal harm; advise to use effective contraception during therapy and for 7 months following last dose. Advise women exposed to therapy during pregnancy or who become pregnant w/in 7 months following last dose that there is a pregnancy exposure registry and a pregnancy pharmacovigilance program that monitors pregnancy outcomes. Advise to enroll in the MotHER Pregnancy Registry and report pregnancy to Genentech. Advise male patients w/ female partners of reproductive potential to use effective contraception during treatment and for 4 months following the last dose. Advise women not to breastfeed during treatment and for 7 months after the last dose.

KALBITOR — ecallantide   Rx
Class: Plasma kallikrein inhibitor

> Anaphylaxis reported. Should only be administered by a healthcare professional with appropriate medical support to manage anaphylaxis and hereditary angioedema (HAE). Healthcare professionals should be aware of the similarity of symptoms between hypersensitivity reactions and HAE; monitor patients closely.

ADULT DOSAGE	PEDIATRIC DOSAGE
Hereditary Angioedema	**Hereditary Angioedema**
Treatment of Acute Attacks:	**Treatment of Acute Attacks:**
Usual: 30mg (3mL) SQ in three 10mg (1mL) inj; if attack persists, may administer an additional 30mg dose w/in 24 hrs	**≥12 Years:**
	Usual: 30mg (3mL) SQ in three 10mg (1mL) inj; if attack persists, may administer an additional 30mg dose w/in 24 hrs

DOSING CONSIDERATIONS
Elderly
Start at lower end of dosing range

ADMINISTRATION
SQ route

Using aseptic technique, withdraw 1mL (10mg) from vial using a large bore needle
Change needle on the syringe to a needle suitable for SQ inj; recommended needle size is 27 gauge
Inject into the skin of the abdomen, thigh, or upper arm
Repeat procedure for each of the 3 vials comprising the dose. Inj site for each inj may be in the same or in different anatomic locations (abdomen, thigh, upper arm); no need for site rotation
Separate inj sites by at least 2 inches (5cm) and away from anatomical site of attack

STORAGE
2-8°C (36-46°F). Protect from light. Vials Removed From Refrigeration: <30°C (86°F). Use within 14 days or return to refrigeration until use.

HOW SUPPLIED
Inj: 10mg/mL

CONTRAINDICATIONS
Known clinical hypersensitivity to ecallantide.

WARNINGS/PRECAUTIONS
Potentially serious hypersensitivity reactions reported. Caution in elderly.

ADVERSE REACTIONS
Anaphylaxis, headache, N/V, fatigue, diarrhea, upper respiratory tract infection, inj-site reactions, nasopharyngitis, pruritus, upper abdominal pain, pyrexia, immunogenicity.

PREGNANCY AND LACTATION
Category C, caution in nursing.

MECHANISM OF ACTION
Plasma kallikrein inhibitor; binds to plasma kallikrein and blocks its binding site, inhibiting the conversion of high molecular weight kininogen to bradykinin.

PHARMACOKINETICS
Absorption: C_{max}=586ng/mL; T_{max}=2-3 hrs; AUC=3017ng•hr/mL. **Distribution:** V_d=26.4L. **Elimination:** Urine; $T_{1/2}$=2 hrs.

PATIENT CONSIDERATIONS
Assessment: Assess for clinical hypersensitivity to drug, and pregnancy/nursing status.

Monitoring: Monitor for anaphylaxis, hypersensitivity reactions, and other adverse reactions.

Counseling: Advise that drug may cause anaphylaxis and other hypersensitivity reactions.

KALETRA — lopinavir/ritonavir   Rx

Class: Protease inhibitor

ADULT DOSAGE
HIV-1 Infection

In Combination w/ Other Antiretrovirals:

<3 Lopinavir Resistance-Associated Substitutions:
400mg/100mg bid or 800mg/200mg qd

≥3 Resistance-Associated Substitutions:
400mg/100mg bid

PEDIATRIC DOSAGE
HIV-1 Infection

In Combination w/ Other Antiretrovirals:

14 Days-6 Months of Age:
Sol:
Weight-Based: (16mg/4mg)/kg bid
BSA-Based: (300mg/75mg)/m² bid
Therapy is not recommended in combination w/ efavirenz, nevirapine, or nelfinavir in patients <6 months or age

6 Months-18 Years:
W/O Concomitant Efavirenz, Nevirapine, or Nelfinavir:

Sol:

Weight-Based:
<15kg: (12mg/3mg)/kg bid
≥15-40kg: (10mg/2.5mg)/kg bid
Max: 400mg/100mg bid
BSA-Based:
(230mg/57.5mg)/m² bid
Max: 400mg/100mg bid

Tab:
Weight-Based:
15-25kg: 200mg/50mg bid
<25-35kg: 300mg/75mg bid
<35kg: 400mg/100mg bid
BSA-Based:
≥0.6 to <0.9m²: 200mg/50mg bid
≥0.9 to <1.4m²: 300mg/75mg bid
≥1.4m²: 400mg/100mg bid

DOSING CONSIDERATIONS
Concomitant Medications
Combination w/ Efavirenz, Nevirapine, or Nelfinavir:
6 Months-18 Years:
Sol:
Weight-Based:
<15kg: (13mg/3.25mg)/kg bid

<15-45kg: (11mg/2.75mg)/kg bid
Max: 533mg/133mg bid
BSA-Based:
(300mg/75mg)/m² bid
Max: 533mg/133mg bid
Tab:
Weight-Based:
15-20kg: 200mg/50mg bid
<20-30kg: 300mg/75mg bid
<30-45kg: 400mg/100mg bid
<45kg: 500mg/125mg bid
BSA-Based:
≥0.6 to <0.8m²: 200mg/50mg bid
≥0.8 to <1.2m²: 300mg/75mg bid
≥1.2 to <1.7m²: 400mg/100mg bid
≥1.7m²: 500mg/125mg bid

Adults:
Sol: 520mg/130mg bid
Tab: 500mg/125mg bid

Hepatic Impairment
Caution w/ use

Other Important Considerations
Use in Pregnancy:
No Documented Lopinavir-Associated Resistance Substitutions:
Tab:
400/100mg bid

ADMINISTRATION
Oral route

Tab
Take w/ or w/o food.
Swallow whole; do not crush, break, or chew.

Sol
Take w/ food.

STORAGE
Tab: 20-25°C (68-77°F); excursions permitted to 15-30°C (59-86°F). **Sol:** 2-8°C (36-46°F). Avoid exposure to excessive heat. If stored at room temperature up to 25°C (77°F), sol should be used w/in 2 months.

HOW SUPPLIED
(Lopinavir/Ritonavir) **Sol:** (80mg/20mg)/mL [160mL]; **Tab:** 100mg/25mg, 200mg/50mg

CONTRAINDICATIONS
Previously demonstrated clinically significant hypersensitivity (eg, toxic epidermal necrolysis, Stevens-Johnson syndrome, erythema multiforme, urticaria, angioedema) to Kaletra or any of its components. Coadministration w/ CYP3A substrates for which elevated plasma concentrations are associated w/ serious and/or life-threatening reactions and w/ potent CYP3A inducers where significantly reduced lopinavir levels may be associated w/ the potential for loss of virologic response and possible resistance and cross-resistance (eg, alfuzosin, rifampin, lurasidone, pimozide, dihydroergotamine, ergotamine, methylergonovine, cisapride, St. John's wort, lovastatin, simvastatin, sildenafil [when used to treat pulmonary arterial HTN], triazolam, oral midazolam).

WARNINGS/PRECAUTIONS
Pancreatitis reported; evaluate and suspend therapy if clinically appropriate. Hepatotoxicity reported; conduct appropriate lab testing prior to therapy and monitor closely during treatment. Patients w/ underlying hepatitis B or C or marked serum transaminase elevations prior to treatment may be at increased risk for developing or worsening of transaminase elevations or hepatic decompensation. PR and QT interval prolongation, torsades de pointes, and cases of 2nd- and 3rd-degree atrioventricular block reported; caution w/ underlying structural heart disease, preexisting conduction system abnormalities, ischemic heart disease, or cardiomyopathies. Avoid use w/ congenital long QT syndrome or hypokalemia. New onset or exacerbation of diabetes mellitus (DM), hyperglycemia, diabetic ketoacidosis, immune reconstitution syndrome, autoimmune disorders (eg, Graves' disease, polymyositis, Guillain-Barre syndrome) in the setting of immune reconstitution, redistribution/accumulation of body fat, and increased bleeding w/ hemophilia A and B reported. Elevated cholesterol and TG levels reported; marked elevation in TGs is a risk factor for pancreatitis. QD regimen is not recommended for adults w/ ≥3 lopinavir resistance-associated substitutions, in pregnant women, or in pediatric patients <18 yrs. Caution w/ hepatic impairment and in elderly. **Sol:** Contains alcohol and propylene glycol. Avoid use of sol during pregnancy and in preterm neonates in the immediate postnatal period; preterm neonates may be at increased risk of propylene glycol-associated adverse events and other toxicities. If benefit of treating infants immediately after birth outweighs potential risk, monitor closely for increases in serum osmolality and SrCr, and for drug-related toxicity.

ADVERSE REACTIONS
Diarrhea, N/V, hypertriglyceridemia, hypercholesterolemia.

DRUG INTERACTIONS
See Contraindications and Dosing Considerations. Caution w/ drugs that prolong the PR interval (eg, calcium channel blockers [CCBs], β-adrenergic blockers, digoxin, atazanavir). Avoid w/ colchicine in patients w/ renal/hepatic impairment, tadalafil during initiation, tipranavir/ritonavir combination, and drugs that prolong the QT interval. Not recommended w/ voriconazole, high doses of itraconazole or ketoconazole, boceprevir, avanafil, salmeterol, and simeprevir. Not recommended w/ fluticasone or other glucocorticoids that are metabolized by CYP3A unless benefit outweighs the risk of systemic corticosteroid effects. May increase levels of CYP3A substrates, colchicine, fentanyl, tenofovir, indinavir, nelfinavir, M8 metabolite of nelfinavir, saquinavir, maraviroc, antiarrhythmics, vincristine, vinblastine,

dasatinib, nilotinib, trazodone, itraconazole, ketoconazole, bedaquiline, rifabutin and rifabutin metabolite, clarithromycin in patients w/ renal impairment, IV midazolam, dihydropyridine CCBs, bosentan, atorvastatin, rosuvastatin, immunosuppressants, salmeterol, rivaroxaban, glucocorticoids, avanafil, sildenafil, tadalafil, vardenafil, rilpivirine, simeprevir, and quetiapine. May decrease levels of methadone, phenytoin, bupropion, hydroxybupropion (active metabolite of bupropion), atovaquone, abacavir, zidovudine, lamotrigine, valproate, voriconazole, boceprevir, amprenavir, and etravirine. Delavirdine, ritonavir, and CYP3A inhibitors may increase levels. May decrease levels of ethinyl estradiol; alternative methods of nonhormonal contraception are recommended. May alter concentrations of warfarin; monitor INR. Efavirenz, nevirapine, nelfinavir, carbamazepine, phenobarbital, and phenytoin may decrease levels; not for qd dosing regimen. Rifampin, fosamprenavir/ritonavir, systemic corticosteroids, and CYP3A inducers may decrease levels. May require initiation or dose adjustments of insulin or oral hypoglycemics for treatment of DM. **Sol:** Contains alcohol; may produce disulfiram-like reactions w/ disulfiram or metronidazole. Didanosine should be given 1 hr before or 2 hrs after sol. Refer to PI for further information and dosing modifications when used w/ certain concomitant therapies.

PREGNANCY AND LACTATION

Pregnancy: Physicians are encouraged to register patients in the Antiretroviral Pregnancy Registry. There are insufficient data to recommend dosing for pregnant patients w/ lopinavir-associated resistance substitutions. QD dosing is not recommended in pregnancy. Avoid use of oral sol during pregnancy due to alcohol content.
Lactation: Not for use in nursing.

MECHANISM OF ACTION

Lopinavir: HIV-1 protease inhibitor; prevents cleavage of the Gag-Pol polyprotein, resulting in the production of immature, noninfectious viral particles. **Ritonavir:** HIV-1 protease inhibitor; CYP3A inhibitor that inhibits metabolism of lopinavir, increasing its plasma levels.

PHARMACOKINETICS

Absorption: Lopinavir: (400mg/100mg bid) C_{max}=9.8µg/mL, T_{max}=4 hrs, AUC=92.6µg•h/mL. Refer to PI for pediatric parameters. **Distribution:** Lopinavir: Plasma protein binding (98-99%). **Metabolism:** Lopinavir: Hepatic via CYP3A (extensive). Ritonavir: Induces own metabolism. **Elimination:** Unchanged Lopinavir: Urine (2.2%), feces (19.8%).

PATIENT CONSIDERATIONS

Assessment: Assess for history of hypersensitivity reactions, history of pancreatitis, hepatitis B or C, cirrhosis, DM or hyperglycemia, dyslipidemia, hemophilia type A or B, structural heart disease, preexisting conduction system abnormalities, ischemic heart disease or cardiomyopathies, congenital long QT syndrome, hypokalemia, renal/hepatic impairment, pregnancy/nursing status, and for possible drug interactions. Assess children for the ability to swallow intact tab.

Monitoring: Monitor for signs/symptoms of pancreatitis, hyperglycemia, hepatic dysfunction, immune reconstitution syndrome, autoimmune disorders, fat redistribution/accumulation, hypersensitivity reactions, and other adverse reactions. Monitor lipid profile, glucose levels, total bilirubin levels, ECG changes, serum lipase levels, and serum amylase levels. Monitor infants for increase in serum osmolality, SrCr, and other toxicities.

Counseling: Instruct to take prescribed dose ud. Advise to inform physician if weight changes in children occur. Inform that if a dose is missed, a dose should be taken as soon as possible and to return to normal schedule; instruct not to double the next dose. Advise that therapy is not a cure for HIV; opportunistic infections may still occur. Instruct to avoid doing things that can spread HIV-1 infection to others. Instruct not to have any kind of sex w/o protection; advise to practice safe sex by always using a latex or polyurethane condom to lower the chance of sexual contact w/ semen, vaginal secretions, or blood. Instruct to notify physician if using other prescription/OTC or herbal products, particularly St. John's wort. Inform that skin rashes, liver function changes, ECG changes, redistribution/accumulation of body fat, new onset or worsening of preexisting diabetes, and hyperglycemia may occur. Instruct to seek medical attention if symptoms of worsening liver disease (eg, loss of appetite, abdominal pain, jaundice, itchy skin), dizziness, abnormal heart rhythm, loss of consciousness, or any other adverse reactions develop.

KALYDECO — ivacaftor   Rx

Class: CFTR potentiator

ADULT DOSAGE

Cystic Fibrosis

W/ G551D, G1244E, G1349D, G178R, G551S, S1251N, S1255P, S549N, S549R, or R117H mutation in the cystic fibrosis transmembrane conductance regulator gene

Usual: 150mg tab q12h

PEDIATRIC DOSAGE

Cystic Fibrosis

W/ G551D, G1244E, G1349D, G178R, G551S, S1251N, S1255P, S549N, S549R, or R117H mutation in the cystic fibrosis transmembrane conductance regulator gene

Granules:
2-<6 Years:
<14kg:
Usual: 50mg pkt q12h
≥14kg:
Usual: 75mg pkt q12h

Tab:
≥6 Years:
Usual: 150mg tab q12h

DOSING CONSIDERATIONS

Concomitant Medications
Moderate CYP3A Inhibitors: Reduce dose to 1 tab or 1 pkt of granules qd
Strong CYP3A Inhibitors: Reduce dose to 1 tab or 1 pkt of granules 2X/week
Avoid food containing grapefruit or Seville oranges

Hepatic Impairment
Moderate (Child-Pugh Class B): Reduce dose to 1 tab or 1 pkt of granules qd
Severe (Child-Pugh Class C): Use w/ caution at 1 tab or 1 pkt of granules qd or less frequently

ADMINISTRATION

Oral route

Take w/ fat-containing food (eg, eggs, butter, whole-milk dairy products)

Granules
Mix the entire contents of each pkt w/ 1 tsp (5mL) of age-appropriate soft food or liquid (eg, pureed fruits or vegetables, yogurt, applesauce, water, milk, juice) and consume completely
Food or liquid should be at or below room temperature
Once mixed, the product has been shown to be stable for 1 hr, and therefore should be consumed during this period
Administer each dose just before or just after fat-containing food

STORAGE

20-25°C (68-77°F); excursions permitted to 15-30°C (59-86°F).

HOW SUPPLIED

Granules: 50mg/pkt, 75mg/pkt; **Tab:** 150mg

WARNINGS/PRECAUTIONS

Elevated transaminases reported. Monitor closely if increased transaminase levels develop until abnormalities resolve and interrupt dosing w/ ALT or AST >5X ULN; consider benefits and risks of resuming dosing. Consider more frequent monitoring of LFTs w/ history of transaminase elevations. Caution w/ severe renal impairment (CrCl ≤30mL/min), or ESRD. Non-congenital lens opacities/cataracts reported in pediatric patients. Use FDA-cleared CF mutation test to detect the presence of CFTR mutation followed by verification w/ bidirectional sequencing when recommended by the mutation test instructions for use if patient's genotype is unknown. Not effective in patients w/ CF who are homozygous for the F508del mutation in the CFTR gene.

ADVERSE REACTIONS

Headache, oropharyngeal pain, URTI, nasal congestion, abdominal pain, nasopharyngitis, diarrhea, rash, nausea, dizziness, rhinitis, arthralgia, bacteria in sputum, wheezing, acne.

DRUG INTERACTIONS

See Dosing Considerations. Not recommended w/ strong CYP3A inducers (eg, rifampin, phenytoin, St. John's wort); these drugs may substantially decrease exposure. Strong CYP3A inhibitors (eg, ketoconazole, itraconazole, clarithromycin), moderate CYP3A inhibitors (eg, fluconazole, erythromycin), and grapefruit juice may increase levels. May increase levels of sensitive CYP3A substrates (eg, midazolam) and/or P-gp substrates (eg, digoxin, cyclosporine, tacrolimus); use w/ caution and monitor appropriately.

PREGNANCY AND LACTATION

Category B, caution in nursing.

MECHANISM OF ACTION

CFTR potentiator; facilitates increased Cl⁻ transport by potentiating the channel-open probability (or gating) of the CFTR protein.

PHARMACOKINETICS

Absorption: Administration of variable doses resulted in different parameters in pediatric patients. (150mg) C_{max}=768ng/mL, AUC=10,600ng•hr/mL, T_{max}=approx 4 hrs (median). **Distribution:** V_d=353L (150mg); plasma protein binding (approx 99%); likely found in breast milk. **Metabolism:** Extensive via CYP3A; M1 and M6 (major metabolites). **Elimination:** Feces (87.8%, approx 65% metabolites), urine (negligible as unchanged drug); $T_{1/2}$=approx 12 hrs.

PATIENT CONSIDERATIONS

Assessment: Assess for history of transaminase elevations, renal/hepatic impairment, patients who are homozygous for the F508del mutation in the CFTR gene, pregnancy/nursing status, and possible drug interactions. If genotype is unknown, perform FDA-cleared CF mutation test to detect the presence of the CFTR mutation followed by verification w/ bidirectional sequencing when recommended by the mutation test instructions for use. Obtain baseline ophthalmological examinations in pediatric patients.

Monitoring: Monitor for adverse reactions. Monitor ALT/AST levels every 3 months during the 1st yr of therapy and annually thereafter. Perform follow-up ophthalmological examinations in pediatric patients.

Counseling: Inform that elevation in liver tests have occurred and LFTs will be performed prior to initiating therapy, every 3 months during the 1st yr, and annually thereafter. Instruct to inform physician of all medications that are currently being taken, including any herbal supplements or vitamins. Instruct to avoid food containing grapefruit or Seville oranges. Instruct to take exactly ud. In case a dose of drug is missed w/in 6 hrs of the time it is usually taken, instruct to take the prescribed dose w/ fat-containing food as soon as possible. If >6 hrs have passed since drug is usually taken, instruct not to take the missed dose, and to resume the usual dosing schedule. Advise to contact physician if patients have questions about missed dose. Inform that abnormality of the eye lens has been noted in children and adolescents receiving therapy.

KANUMA — sebelipase alfa   Rx

Class: Enzyme

ADULT DOSAGE
Lysosomal Acid Lipase Deficiency
1mg/kg IV infusion once every other week

PEDIATRIC DOSAGE
Lysosomal Acid Lipase Deficiency
Rapidly Progressive Lysosomal Acid Lipase (LAL) Deficiency Presenting w/in First 6 Months of Life:
Initial: 1mg/kg IV infusion once weekly
Titrate: Increase to 3mg/kg once weekly if optimal response is not achieved

Pediatric Patients w/ LAL Deficiency: 1mg/kg IV infusion once every other week

ADMINISTRATION
IV route
Vials are for single-use only; discard any unused product.
Use immediately after dilution; if immediate use is not possible, store ≤24 hrs at 2-8°C (36-46°F).
Do not freeze or shake.
Protect from light.

Preparation
1. Determine the number of vials needed based on the patient's weight and the recommended dose of 1mg/kg or 3mg/kg.
2. Round to the next whole vial and remove required number of vials from refrigerator and allow to reach room temperature.
3. Mix gently by inversion; do not shake vials or prepared infusion.

Administration
Administer sol as an IV infusion using a low-protein binding infusion set w/ an in-line, low-protein binding 0.2 micron filter.
Infuse over ≥2 hrs; consider further prolonging the infusion time for patients receiving 3mg/kg dose or those who have experienced hypersensitivity reactions.
A 1-hr infusion may be considered for patients receiving 1mg/kg dose who tolerate the infusion.

STORAGE
2-8°C (36-46°F) in original carton to protect from light. Do not shake or freeze vials.

HOW SUPPLIED
Inj: 20mg/10mL

WARNINGS/PRECAUTIONS
Hypersensitivity reactions, including anaphylaxis, reported; immediately d/c infusion and initiate appropriate medical treatment if anaphylaxis occurs. Management of hypersensitivity reactions should be based on severity of the reaction and may include temporarily interrupting infusion, lowering infusion rate, and/or treatment w/ antihistamines, antipyretics, and/or corticosteroids. If interrupted, infusion may resume at a slower rate w/ increases as tolerated. Pretreatment w/ antipyretics and/or antihistamines may prevent subsequent reactions. Immediately d/c infusion and initiate appropriate medical treatment if a severe hypersensitivity reaction occurs; consider risks/benefits of readministration following a severe reaction. Observe closely during and after infusion. Produced in the egg whites of genetically engineered chickens; caution w/ known systemic hypersensitivity reactions to eggs or egg products.

ADVERSE REACTIONS
Rapidly Progressive Disease Presenting w/in First 6 Months of Life: Diarrhea, vomiting, fever, rhinitis, anemia, cough, nasopharyngitis, urticaria.
Pediatrics and Adults: Headache, fever, oropharyngeal pain, nasopharyngitis, asthenia, constipation, nausea.

PREGNANCY AND LACTATION
Pregnancy: There are no available data on sebelipase alfa in pregnant women to inform any drug-associated risk.
Lactation: There are no data on the presence of sebelipase alfa in human milk, the effects on the breastfed infant, or the effects on milk production; caution in nursing.

MECHANISM OF ACTION
Recombinant human LAL; binds to cell surface receptors via glycans expressed on the protein and is subsequently internalized into lysosomes. Catalyzes the lysosomal hydrolysis of cholesteryl esters and triglycerides to free cholesterol, glycerol, and free fatty acids.

PHARMACOKINETICS
Absorption: AUC=942ng•hr/mL (4-11 yrs), 1454ng•hr/mL (12-17 yrs), 1861ng•hr/mL (≥18 yrs); C_{max}=490ng/mL (4-11 yrs), 784ng/mL (12-17 yrs), 957ng/mL (≥18 yrs); T_{max}=1.3 hr (4-11 yrs), 1.1 hr (12-17 yrs), 1.3 hr (≥18 yrs). **Distribution:** 3.6L (4-11 yrs), 5.4L (12-17 yrs), 5.3L (≥18 yrs). **Elimination:** $T_{1/2}$=5.4 min (4-11 yrs), 6.6 min (12-17 yrs), 6.6 min (≥18 yrs).

PATIENT CONSIDERATIONS
Assessment: Assess for known systemic hypersensitivity reactions to eggs or egg products.
Monitoring: Monitor for hypersensitivity/anaphylactic reactions.
Counseling: Advise that hypersensitivity/anaphylactic reactions may occur during and after treatment. Inform of the signs/symptoms of anaphylaxis/hypersensitivity reactions, and advise to seek immediate medical care should signs/symptoms occur.

KCENTRA — prothrombin complex concentrate (human)   Rx

Class: Prothrombin complex concentrate (human)

> Patients being treated w/ vitamin K antagonists (VKA) therapy have underlying disease states that predispose them to thromboembolic events. Weigh potential benefits of reversing VKA against potential risks of thromboembolic events, especially in patients w/ history of a thromboembolic event. Carefully consider resumption of anticoagulation as soon as risk of thromboembolic events outweighs risk of acute bleeding. Both fatal and nonfatal arterial and venous thromboembolic complications reported; monitor for signs/symptoms of thromboembolic events. May not be suitable in patients w/ thromboembolic events in the prior 3 months.

ADULT DOSAGE
Vitamin K Antagonist Reversal
Urgent reversal of acquired coagulation factor deficiency induced by vitamin K antagonist therapy in patients w/ acute major bleeding or need for an urgent surgery/invasive procedure
Individualize dose based on current predose INR value and body weight

Pretreatment INR of 2-<4:
25 IU of factor IX/kg
Max: 2500 U of factor IX
Pretreatment INR of 4-6:
35 IU of factor IX/kg
Max: 3500 U of factor IX
Pretreatment INR of >6:
50 IU of factor IX/kg
Max: 5000 U of factor IX

PEDIATRIC DOSAGE
Pediatric use may not have been established

ADMINISTRATION
IV route
Administer vitamin K concurrently
Actual potency per vial of factors II, VII, IX and X, proteins C and S is stated on the carton

Reconstitution
1. Ensure that drug vial and diluent vial are at room temperature
2. Remove drug and diluent vial caps and open Mix2Vial transfer set package by peeling away lid; leave Mix2Vial transfer set in clear package
3. Place diluent vial on a flat surface and hold vial tightly; grip Mix2Vial transfer set together w/ clear package and push plastic spike at blue end of Mix2Vial transfer set firmly through center of stopper of diluent vial
4. Carefully remove clear package from Mix2Vial transfer set; make sure to pull up only clear package, not Mix2Vial transfer set
5. W/ drug vial placed firmly on flat surface, invert diluent vial w/ Mix2Vial transfer set attached and push plastic spike of transparent adapter firmly through center of stopper of drug vial; diluent will automatically transfer into drug vial
6. W/ diluent and drug vial still attached to Mix2Vial transfer set, gently swirl drug vial to ensure that drug is fully dissolved; do not shake vial
7. W/ 1 hand, grasp drug side of Mix2Vial transfer set and w/ other hand grasp blue diluent-side of Mix2Vial transfer set, and unscrew set into 2 pieces
8. Draw air into an empty, sterile syringe; while drug vial is upright, screw syringe to Mix2Vial transfer set; inject air into drug vial; while keeping syringe plunger pressed, invert system upside down and draw concentrate into syringe by pulling plunger back slowly
9. Now that concentrate has been transferred into syringe, firmly grasp barrel of syringe (keeping plunger facing down) and unscrew syringe from Mix2Vial transfer set; attach syringe to a suitable IV administration set
10. After reconstitution, administration should begin promptly or w/in 4 hrs
11. If same patient is to receive >1 vial, may pool contents of multiple vials; use a separate unused Mix2Vial transfer set for each product vial

Administration
Do not mix w/ other medicinal products; administer through a separate infusion line
Administer at room temperature
Administer by IV infusion at a rate of 0.12mL/kg/min (approx 3 U/kg/min), up to a max rate of 8.4mL/min (approx 210 U/min)
No blood should enter syringe, as there is possibility of fibrin clot formation

STORAGE
2-25°C (36-77°F). Do not freeze. Protect from light. Reconstituted Sol: 2-25°C (36-77°F). If cooled, warm sol to 20-25°C (68-77°F) prior to administration. Do not freeze. Use w/in 4 hrs following reconstitution.

HOW SUPPLIED
Inj: 500 U, 1000 U

CONTRAINDICATIONS
Disseminated intravascular coagulation (DIC), heparin-induced thrombocytopenia (HIT).

WARNINGS/PRECAUTIONS
Repeat dosing is not recommended. Hypersensitivity reactions observed; d/c immediately and institute appropriate treatment if a severe allergic reaction or anaphylactic-type reaction occurs. DIC reported. May carry a risk of transmitting infectious agents (eg, viruses, the variant Creutzfeldt-Jakob disease agent, and theoretically, the Creutzfeldt-Jakob disease agent).

ADVERSE REACTIONS
Arterial and venous thromboembolic complications, headache, N/V, hypotension, anemia, pleural effusion, tachycardia, A-fib, insomnia.

PREGNANCY AND LACTATION
Category C, caution in nursing.

MECHANISM OF ACTION
Prothrombin complex concentrate (human); rapidly increases plasma levels of the vitamin K-dependent coagulation factors II, VII, IX, and X as well as the antithrombotic proteins C and S.

PHARMACOKINETICS
Absorption: AUC=1850.8 IU/dL x h, 7282.2 IU/dL x h, 512.9 IU/dL x h, 6921.5 IU/dL x h, 5397.5 IU/dL x h, 3651.6 IU/dL x h (factor IX, factor II, factor VII, factor X, protein C, protein S). **Distribution:** V_d=114.3mL/kg, 71.4mL/kg, 45mL/kg, 55.5mL/kg, 62.2mL/kg, 78.8mL/kg (factor IX, factor II, factor VII, factor X, protein C, protein S). **Elimination:** $T_{1/2}$=42.4 hrs, 60.4 hrs, 5 hrs, 31.8 hrs, 49.6 hrs, 50.4 hrs (factor IX, factor II, factor VII, factor X, protein C, protein S).

PATIENT CONSIDERATIONS
Assessment: Assess for known anaphylactic/severe systemic reactions to the drug, DIC, HIT, history of a thromboembolic event, and pregnancy/nursing status. Measure INR prior to treatment and close to time of dosing.

Monitoring: Monitor for signs/symptoms of thromboembolic events, hypersensitivity reactions, DIC, infection, and other adverse reactions. Monitor INR and clinical response during and after treatment.

Counseling: Inform of the signs/symptoms of allergic hypersensitivity reactions and thrombosis. Inform that, because drug is made from human blood, it may carry a risk of transmitting infectious agents.

KEDBUMIN — albumin (human)   Rx

Class: Human albumin

ADULT DOSAGE

Hypovolemia
Initial: 25g

Hypoalbuminemia
Due to Illness or Active Bleeding:
Usual: 50-75g

Cirrhotic Ascites
Maint of cardiovascular function following the removal of large volumes of ascitic fluid due to cirrhosis
Usual: 6-8g for every 1000mL of ascitic fluid removed

Ovarian Hyperstimulation Syndrome
Usual: 50-100g over 4 hrs and repeated at 4- to 12-hr intervals as necessary, or 10-50g single infusion

Adult Respiratory Distress Syndrome
Usual: 25g over 30 min and repeated at 8 hrs for 3 days if necessary; use in conjunction w/ diuretics

Hemodialysis
Use in patients undergoing long term dialysis or for those patients who are fluid-overloaded and cannot tolerate substantial volumes of salt sol for therapy of shock or hypotension
Usual: 100mL

Cardiopulmonary Bypass
Part of Priming Fluids:
Estimate dose from the difference between the desired and actual total serum protein concentration multiplied by the estimated plasma volume (approx 40mL/kg) x 2

PEDIATRIC DOSAGE

Hypovolemia
12-16 Years:
Adjust dose based on age, weight, and clinical conditions

Hypoalbuminemia
12-16 Years:
Usual: 50-75g

Hemodialysis
Use in patients undergoing long term dialysis or for those patients who are fluid-overloaded and cannot tolerate substantial volumes of salt sol for therapy of shock or hypotension
12-16 Years:
Usual: 100mL

Cardiopulmonary Bypass
Part of Priming Fluids:
12-16 Years:
Estimate dose from the difference between the desired and actual total serum protein concentration multiplied by the estimated plasma volume (approx 40mL/kg) x 2

General Dosing
<12 Years:
Use in children <12 yrs of age has not been clinically evaluated; individualize dose based on clinical state and body weight
Usual: 1/4-1/2 of the adult dose

ADMINISTRATION
IV route

May dilute w/ 5% glucose or 0.9% NaCl
Adjust infusion rate to the rate of removal in plasma exchange
Warm product to room temperature if large volumes are to be administered
Do not begin administration >4 hrs after container has been entered; discard unused material
Do not mix w/ other medicinal products, including blood and blood components; may administer concomitantly w/ other parenteral infusions (eg, whole blood, plasma, saline, glucose, sodium lactate)
Do not mix w/ protein hydrolysates or sol containing alcohol
Usual rate of administration in children should be 1/4 the adult rate

STORAGE
≤30°C (86°F). Protect from light. Do not freeze.

HOW SUPPLIED
Inj: 25% [50mL, 100mL, vial]

CONTRAINDICATIONS
History of hypersensitivity to albumin, excipients used in its formulation, or components of the container; severe anemia; heart failure (HF).

WARNINGS/PRECAUTIONS
Hypersensitivity or allergic reactions reported; d/c infusion and initiate appropriate treatment if a severe reaction (eg, shock, anaphylaxis) occurs. Use with caution in conditions where hypervolemia and its consequences or hemodilution could represent a special risk (eg, arterial HTN, esophageal varices, pulmonary edema, hemorrhagic diathesis, renal and post-renal anuria). Risk of potentially fatal hemolysis and acute renal failure from use of Sterile Water for Inj as a diluent; do not dilute with Sterile Water for Inj. Ensure adequate substitution of other blood constituents (eg, coagulation factors, electrolytes, platelets, erythrocytes) when replacing comparatively large volumes of albumin. Ensure adequate hydration of the patient and carefully monitor to avoid circulatory overload. Regularly monitor hemodynamic performance. May carry a risk of transmitting infectious agents (eg, viruses, Creutzfeldt-Jakob disease agent).

ADVERSE REACTIONS
Flushing, urticaria, fever, chills, N/V, tachycardia, hypotension.

PREGNANCY AND LACTATION
Category C, safety not known in nursing.

MECHANISM OF ACTION
Human albumin; has a role in osmotic regulation. Responsible for 75% of normal oncotic pressure within the intravascular space. Other physiological functions include binding and transport of molecules (hormones, enzymes, drugs, and toxins), free radical scavenging, hemostatic effects (platelet function inhibition and antithrombotic effects), and capillary membrane permeability.

PHARMACOKINETICS
Elimination: $T_{1/2}$=19 days.

PATIENT CONSIDERATIONS
Assessment: Assess for severe anemia, HF, conditions where hypervolemia and its consequences or hemodilution could represent a special risk, history of hypersensitivity to drug, and pregnancy/nursing status.

Monitoring: Monitor for hypersensitivity/allergic reactions, circulatory overload, infection, and other adverse reactions. Regularly monitor hemodynamic performance (eg, arterial BP and pulse rate, central venous pressure, pulmonary artery occlusion pressure, urine output, electrolyte levels, Hct/Hgb).

Counseling: Inform about potential risks and benefits of therapy. Inform about the possibility of transmitting infectious agents (eg, viruses).

KEVEYIS — dichlorphenamide   Rx

Class: Carbonic anhydrase inhibitor

ADULT DOSAGE

Periodic Paralysis

Primary Hyperkalemic Periodic Paralysis, Primary Hypokalemic Periodic Paralysis, and Related Variants:
Initial: 50mg bid
Titrate: Increase or decrease at weekly intervals based on response
Max: 200mg/day
Evaluate therapy after 2 months of treatment

PEDIATRIC DOSAGE
Pediatric use may not have been established

ADMINISTRATION
Oral route

STORAGE
20-25°C (68-77°F).

HOW SUPPLIED
Tab: 50mg* *scored

CONTRAINDICATIONS
Hypersensitivity to dichlorphenamide or other sulfonamides; hepatic insufficiency; severe pulmonary disease, limiting compensation to metabolic acidosis caused by dichlorphenamide; and concomitant use w/ high-dose aspirin (ASA).

WARNINGS/PRECAUTIONS
Fatalities associated w/ sulfonamides have occurred due to adverse reactions (eg, Stevens-Johnson syndrome, toxic epidermal necrolysis, fulminant hepatic necrosis, agranulocytosis, aplastic anemia, other blood dyscrasias); d/c at first appearance of skin rash or any sign of immune-mediated or idiosyncratic adverse reaction. Increases K^+ excretion and can cause hypokalemia; risk is greater when given to patients w/ conditions associated w/ hypokalemia, and in patients receiving other drugs that may cause hypokalemia. May cause hyperchloremic non-anion gap metabolic acidosis; concomitant use w/ other drugs that cause metabolic acidosis may increase the severity of metabolic acidosis. Baseline and periodic measurement of serum K^+ and serum bicarbonate are recommended. If hypokalemia or metabolic acidosis develops/persists, consider reducing dose or discontinuing dichlorphenamide. Increases risk of falls; risk is greater in elderly and w/ higher doses. Consider dose reduction/discontinuation in patients who experience falls while on therapy.

ADVERSE REACTIONS
Paresthesia, cognitive disorder, dysgeusia, confusional state, headache, hypoesthesia, lethargy, fatigue, muscle spasms, rash, diarrhea, nausea, malaise, decreased weight, dyspnea.

DRUG INTERACTIONS
See Contraindications. Anorexia, tachypnea, lethargy, and coma reported w/ high-dose ASA. Caution w/ low-dose ASA.

PREGNANCY AND LACTATION
Pregnancy: Category C.
Lactation: Caution in nursing.
MECHANISM OF ACTION
Carbonic anhydrase inhibitor; precise mechanism unknown.

PATIENT CONSIDERATIONS
Assessment: Assess for hypersensitivity to drug or other sulfonamides, hepatic insufficiency, severe pulmonary disease, conditions associated w/ hypokalemia, ASA use, and pregnancy/nursing status. Obtain baseline serum K+ and serum bicarbonate levels.

Monitoring: Monitor for skin rash or any sign of immune-mediated or idiosyncratic adverse reaction. Evaluate patient's response to therapy after 2 months of treatment. Monitor serum K+ and serum bicarbonate levels.

Counseling: Advise to notify physician if experiencing worsening symptoms of periodic paralysis. Inform that treatment may cause drowsiness/fatigue and may impair ability to drive and operate machinery.

KEYTRUDA — pembrolizumab   Rx

Class: Monoclonal antibody/programmed death receptor-1 (PD-1) blocker

ADULT DOSAGE	PEDIATRIC DOSAGE
Unresectable or Metastatic Melanoma	Pediatric use may not have been established
2mg/kg every 3 weeks until disease progression or unacceptable toxicity	
Metastatic Non-Small Cell Lung Cancer	
Treatment of metastatic non-small cell lung cancer (NSCLC) in patients whose tumors express PD-L1 as determined by an FDA-approved test w/ disease progression on or after platinum-containing chemotherapy	
Patients w/ epidermal growth factor receptor or anaplastic lymphoma kinase genomic tumor aberrations should have disease progression on FDA-approved therapy for these aberrations prior to receiving pembrolizumab	
2mg/kg every 3 weeks until disease progression or unacceptable toxicity	
Squamous Cell Carcinoma of the Head and Neck	
Treatment of recurrent or metastatic head and neck squamous cell carcinoma (HNSCC) w/ disease progression on or after platinum-containing chemotherapy	
200mg every 3 weeks until disease progression, unacceptable toxicity, or up to 24 months in patients w/o disease progression	

DOSING CONSIDERATIONS
Adverse Reactions
Withhold for the Following:
- Grade 2 pneumonitis
- Grade 2 or 3 colitis
- Grade 3 or 4 endocrinopathies
- Grade 2 nephritis
- AST/ALT >3 and up to 5X ULN or total bilirubin >1.5 and up to 3X ULN
- Any other severe or Grade 3 treatment-related adverse reaction

Resume Therapy:
In patients whose adverse reactions recover to Grade 0-1

Permanently D/C for the Following:
- Any life-threatening adverse reaction (excluding endocrinopathies controlled w/ hormone replacement therapy)
- Grade 3 or 4 pneumonitis or recurrent pneumonitis of Grade 2 severity
- Grade 3 or 4 nephritis
- AST/ALT >5X ULN or total bilirubin >3X ULN; for patients w/ liver metastasis who begin treatment w/ Grade 2 AST/ALT, if AST/ALT increases by ≥50% relative to baseline and lasts for at least 1 week
- Grade 3 or 4 infusion-related reactions
- Inability to reduce corticosteroid dose to ≤10mg/day of prednisone (or equivalent) w/in 12 weeks
- Persistent Grade 2 or 3 adverse reactions (excluding endocrinopathies controlled w/ hormone replacement therapy) that do not recover to Grade 0-1 w/in 12 weeks after last dose of therapy
- Any severe or Grade 3 treatment-related adverse reaction that recurs

ADMINISTRATION
IV route
Administer as an IV infusion over 30 min through an IV line containing a sterile, non-pyrogenic, low-protein binding 0.2-5 micron in-line/add-on filter.
Do not coadminister other drugs through the same infusion line.

Preparation
- Add 2.3mL of sterile water for inj for a resulting concentration of 25mg/mL; inject the water along the walls of the vial, not directly on lyophilized powder.
- Slowly swirl vial and allow up to 5 min for bubbles to clear; do not shake.
- Dilute inj sol or reconstituted powder prior to IV administration by withdrawing required volume from vial(s) and transferring into an IV bag containing 0.9% NaCl inj or D5 inj.
- Mix diluted sol by gentle inversion; final concentration should be 1-10mg/mL.

Reconstituted/Diluted Sol from 50mg Vial
Store at room temperature for ≤6 hrs from the time of reconstitution, or at 2-8°C (36-46°F) for ≤24 hrs from the time of reconstitution. If refrigerated, allow the diluted sol to come to room temperature prior to administration. Do not freeze.

Diluted Sol from 25mg/mL Vial
Store at room temperature for ≤6 hrs from the time of dilution, or at 2-8°C (36-46°F) for ≤24 hrs from the time of dilution. If refrigerated, allow the diluted sol to come to room temperature prior to administration. Do not freeze.

STORAGE
2-8°C (36-46°F). **Sol:** Protect from light. Do not freeze. Do not shake.

HOW SUPPLIED
Inj: (Powder) 50mg; (Sol) 25mg/mL [4mL]

WARNINGS/PRECAUTIONS
Immune-mediated pneumonitis, colitis, hepatitis, and nephritis reported; administer corticosteroids for ≥Grade 2. Hypophysitis reported; administer corticosteroids and hormone replacement as clinically indicated. Thyroid disorders can occur at any time during treatment. Administer replacement hormones for hypothyroidism and manage hyperthyroidism w/ thionamides and beta-blockers as appropriate. Type 1 diabetes mellitus (DM), including diabetic ketoacidosis, reported; administer insulin for type 1 DM, and withhold therapy and administer antihyperglycemics in patients w/ severe hyperglycemia. Other clinically important immune-mediated reactions may occur; evaluate and administer corticosteroids based on severity of the adverse reaction. Upon improvement to ≤Grade 1, initiate corticosteroid taper and continue to taper over at least 1 month. Severe and life-threatening infusion-related reactions reported. Can cause fetal harm.

ADVERSE REACTIONS
Melanoma: Fatigue, diarrhea.
NSCLC: Fatigue, decreased appetite, dyspnea, cough.
HNSCC: Fatigue, decreased appetite, dyspnea.

PREGNANCY AND LACTATION
Pregnancy: Can cause fetal harm based on its mechanism of action.
Lactation: D/C nursing during treatment and for 4 months after the final dose.
Reproductive Potential: Females of reproductive potential should use effective contraception during treatment and for at least 4 months following the final dose.

MECHANISM OF ACTION
Human PD-1-blocking antibody; binds to PD-1 receptor on T cells and blocks its interaction w/ PD-L1 and PD-L2, releasing PD-1 pathway-mediated inhibition of the immune response, including the anti-tumor immune response.

PHARMACOKINETICS
Distribution: V_d=7.38L. **Elimination:** $T_{1/2}$=27 days.

PATIENT CONSIDERATIONS
Assessment: Assess pregnancy/nursing status. Obtain baseline liver/renal/thyroid function.

Monitoring: Monitor for signs/symptoms of pneumonitis, colitis, hypophysitis, changes in liver/renal function, hyperglycemia/type 1 DM, infusion-related reactions, and other adverse reactions. Evaluate patients w/ suspected pneumonitis w/ radiographic imaging. Monitor for changes in thyroid function (periodically during treatment, and as indicated based on clinical evaluation) and for signs/symptoms of thyroid disorders. Monitor for immune-mediated adverse reactions; ensure adequate evaluation to confirm etiology or exclude other causes.

Counseling: Inform of the risk of immune-mediated adverse reactions that may require corticosteroid treatment and interruption or discontinuation of therapy (eg, pneumonitis, colitis, hepatitis, hypophysitis, nephritis, hyper/hypothyroidism, type 1 DM); instruct to immediately contact physician if signs/symptoms of an immune-mediated adverse reaction occur. Advise to contact physician immediately for signs/symptoms of infusion-related reactions. Advise of the importance of keeping scheduled appointments for blood work or other lab tests. Advise women that drug may cause fetal harm; instruct women of reproductive potential to use highly effective contraception during and for 4 months after the last dose of therapy. Advise nursing mothers not to breastfeed while taking therapy.

KINERET — anakinra   Rx

Class: Interleukin-1 (IL-1) receptor antagonist

ADULT DOSAGE	PEDIATRIC DOSAGE
Rheumatoid Arthritis	**Cryopyrin-Associated Periodic Syndromes**
For the reduction in signs and symptoms and slowing the progression of structural damage in moderately to severely active rheumatoid arthritis in patients who have failed 1 or more disease modifying antirheumatic drugs	**NOMID:**
	Initial: 1-2mg/kg
100mg/day at approx the same time every day	**Titrate:** Adjust in 0.5-1mg/kg increments

Cryopyrin-Associated Periodic Syndromes

Neonatal-Onset Multisystem Inflammatory Disease (NOMID):
Initial: 1-2mg/kg
Titrate: Adjust in 0.5-1mg/kg increments
Max: 8mg/kg/day

QD administration is generally recommended, but the dose may be split into bid administrations

Max: 8mg/kg/day
QD administration is generally recommended, but the dose may be split into bid administrations

---

DOSING CONSIDERATIONS
Renal Impairment
Severe/ESRD (CrCl <30mL/min): Consider qod administration

ADMINISTRATION
SQ route

Each syringe is intended for a single use; a new syringe must be used for each dose and any unused portion after each dose should be discarded.

STORAGE
2-8°C (36-46°F). Do not freeze or shake. Protect from light.

HOW SUPPLIED
Inj: 100mg/0.67mL

CONTRAINDICATIONS
Hypersensitivity to *Escherichia coli*-derived proteins, anakinra, or to any component of product.

WARNINGS/PRECAUTIONS
Associated w/ an increased incidence of serious infections in rheumatoid arthritis (RA) patients; d/c administration in RA if a serious infection develops. In NOMID patients, weigh the risk of a NOMID flare when discontinuing treatment against the potential risk of continued treatment. Do not initiate in patients w/ active infections. May increase risk of tuberculosis (TB) or other atypical or opportunistic infections; follow current CDC guidelines both to evaluate for and to treat possible latent TB infections before initiating therapy. Hypersensitivity reactions, including anaphylactic reactions and angioedema, reported; d/c administration and initiate appropriate therapy if a severe hypersensitivity reaction occurs. May cause a decrease in neutrophil counts; assess neutrophil counts prior to initiating treatment, during treatment, monthly for 3 months, and thereafter quarterly for up to 1 yr. Caution in elderly.

ADVERSE REACTIONS
Inj-site reaction, worsening of RA, URTI, headache, nausea, diarrhea, sinusitis, arthralgia, flu like-symptoms, abdominal pain.

DRUG INTERACTIONS
Neutropenia and higher rate of serious infections reported w/ etanercept; use in combination w/ TNF-blocking agents is not recommended. Do not give w/ live vaccines.

PREGNANCY AND LACTATION
Pregnancy: Category B.
Lactation: Caution in nursing.

MECHANISM OF ACTION
Interleukin-1 (IL-1) receptor antagonist; blocks the biologic activity of IL-1 α and β by competitively inhibiting IL-1 binding to the IL-1 type I receptor, which is expressed in a wide variety of tissues and organs.

PHARMACOKINETICS
Absorption: Absolute bioavailability (95%) (healthy); T_{max}=3-7 hrs (RA); C_{max}=3628ng/mL (median) (NOMID). **Elimination:** $T_{1/2}$=4-6 hrs (RA), 5.7 hrs (median) (NOMID).

PATIENT CONSIDERATIONS
Assessment: Assess for hypersensitivity to *E. coli*-derived proteins or to drug, active infections, latent TB, latex sensitivity, renal impairment, pregnancy/nursing status, and possible drug interactions. Assess neutrophil counts.

Monitoring: Monitor for serious infections, TB or other atypical/opportunistic infections, hypersensitivity reactions, and other adverse reactions. Monitor neutrophil counts monthly for 3 months, and thereafter quarterly for up to 1 yr.

Counseling: Instruct on the proper dosage and administration. Instruct on the importance of proper disposal, and caution against the reuse of needles, syringes, and drug product. Inform that drug may lower the ability of immune system to fight infections; advise to contact physician if any symptoms of infection develop. Inform that inj-site reactions may occur; caution to avoid injecting into an area that is already swollen or red, and advise to consult physician if any persistent reaction develops. Counsel about the signs/symptoms of allergic and other adverse drug reactions and the appropriate actions to be taken if experiencing any of these signs/symptoms.

KITABIS PAK — tobramycin   Rx
Class: Aminoglycoside

ADULT DOSAGE
Cystic Fibrosis

Patients w/ *Pseudomonas aeruginosa*:
1 single-use ampule (300mg/5mL) bid by oral inh in alternating periods of 28 days on drug followed by 28 days off drug

PEDIATRIC DOSAGE
Cystic Fibrosis

Patients w/ *Pseudomonas aeruginosa*:
>6 Years:
1 single-use ampule (300mg/5mL) bid by oral inh in alternating periods of 28 days on drug followed by 28 days off drug

---

ADMINISTRATION
Oral inh route

Take doses as close to 12 hrs apart as possible; not <6 hrs apart
Administer using only the Pari LC Plus Reusable Nebulizer with a DeVilbiss Pulmo-Aide air compressor
Entire treatment should take approximately 15 min to complete; continue treatment until all inh sol has been delivered and there is no longer any mist being produced
Do not dilute/mix inh sol with other drugs in the nebulizer, including dornase alfa

STORAGE
2-8°C (36-46°F). Upon removal from the refrigerator, or if refrigeration is unavailable, may be stored at room temperature (up to 25°C [77°F]) for up to 28 days. Do not expose to intense light.

HOW SUPPLIED
Sol, Inhalation: 300mg/5mL

CONTRAINDICATIONS
Known hypersensitivity to any aminoglycoside.

WARNINGS/PRECAUTIONS
Bronchospasm, ototoxicity (eg, tinnitus), and nephrotoxicity may occur. If ototoxicity is noted, or nephrotoxicity develops, patient should be managed as medically appropriate, including potentially discontinuing tobramycin inh sol. May aggravate muscle weakness because of a potential curare-like effect on neuromuscular function. If neuromuscular blockade occurs, it may be reversed by administration of Ca^{2+} salts but mechanical assistance may be necessary. May cause fetal harm.

ADVERSE REACTIONS
Cough, pharyngitis, increased sputum, dyspnea, hemoptysis, decreased lung function, voice alteration, taste perversion, rash.

DRUG INTERACTIONS
Avoid concurrent and/or sequential use with other drugs with neurotoxic, nephrotoxic, or ototoxic potential. Some diuretics may enhance aminoglycoside toxicity by altering aminoglycoside concentrations in serum and tissue; do not administer with ethacrynic acid, furosemide, urea, or IV mannitol. Monitor for toxicities associated with aminoglycosides if used concomitantly with parenteral aminoglycosides; monitor serum tobramycin levels.

PREGNANCY AND LACTATION
Category D, not for use in nursing.

MECHANISM OF ACTION
Aminoglycoside; acts primarily by disrupting protein synthesis, leading to altered cell membrane permeability, progressive disruption of the cell envelope, and eventual cell death.

PHARMACOKINETICS
Distribution: Crosses placenta. **Elimination:** Expectorated sputum (Unabsorbed); $T_{1/2}$=2 hrs (IV).

PATIENT CONSIDERATIONS
Assessment: Assess for auditory or vestibular dysfunction, renal dysfunction, neuromuscular disorders, drug hypersensitivity, pregnancy/nursing status, and possible drug interactions.

Monitoring: Monitor for bronchospasm, ototoxicity, nephrotoxicity, neuromuscular effects, and other adverse reactions.

Counseling: Advise to inform physician if SOB or wheezing occurs soon after administration, or if ringing in the ears, dizziness, or any changes in hearing develop. Instruct to notify physician if planning to become pregnant or if nursing. Instruct patients on multiple therapies to take their medications prior to inhaling the tobramycin inh sol, or ud by physician.

KOATE-DVI — antihemophilic factor (human)   Rx
Class: Antihemophilic agent

ADULT DOSAGE
Hemophilia A
Individualize dose

Mild Hemorrhage:
10 IU/kg (approx 20% rise in [factor VIII] FVIII level)
May repeat if there is evidence of further bleeding

Moderate Hemorrhage (Approx 30-40% Rise in FVIII Level Needed):
15-25 IU/kg
May give repeated doses of 10-15 IU/kg q8-12h if further therapy is required

Severe Hemorrhage (Approx 80-100% Rise in FVIII Level Needed):
Initial: 40-50 IU/kg
Maint: 20-25 IU/kg q8-12h

Major Surgical Procedures (Approx 100% Rise in FVIII Level Needed):
50 IU/kg preoperative dose; check FVIII levels throughout the perioperative course to ensure adequate replacement therapy

PEDIATRIC DOSAGE
Pediatric use may not have been established

May repeat infusion prn q6-12h initially, and for a total of 10-14 days until healing is complete

Prophylaxis of Bleeding:
May administer on a regular schedule

Calculation of Dosage:
Expected % FVIII Increase (% of Normal) = (# of Units Administered x 2%/IU/kg)/Body Weight in kg

---

ADMINISTRATION
IV route

Administer IV by either direct syringe inj or drip infusion
Must administer w/in 3 hrs after reconstitution
Rate of administration should be adapted to the response of the individual patient; administration of the entire dose in 5-10 min is generally well tolerated

Preparation
1. Warm sterile water (diluent) to room temperature
2. Immediately after adding diluent, agitate vigorously for 10-15 sec, then swirl continuously until completely dissolved
3. If the same patient is using >1 vial, contents of multiple vials may be drawn into the same syringe through the filter needles provided

STORAGE
2-8°C (36-46°F); may store lyophilized powder at room temperature up to 25°C (77°F) for 6 months. Avoid freezing. Reconstituted Sol: Do not refrigerate.

HOW SUPPLIED
Inj: 250 IU, 500 IU, 1000 IU

WARNINGS/PRECAUTIONS
May carry a risk of transmitting infectious agents (eg, viruses, Creutzfeldt-Jakob disease); consider appropriate vaccination against hepatitis A and B virus of patients who receive therapy. Monitor patients of blood groups A, B, or AB by means of Hct for signs of progressive anemia, as well as by direct Coombs' tests, when large or frequently repeated doses are required.

ADVERSE REACTIONS
Allergic-type reactions, blurred vision, headache, nausea, abdominal pain, jittery feeling.

PREGNANCY AND LACTATION
Category C, safety not known in nursing.

MECHANISM OF ACTION
Antihemophilic agent; provides an increase in plasma levels of FVIII and can temporarily correct coagulation defect.

PHARMACOKINETICS
Elimination: $T_{1/2}$=16.12 hrs.

PATIENT CONSIDERATIONS
Assessment: Assess for drug hypersensitivity and pregnancy/nursing status.

Monitoring: Monitor clinical response, FVIII levels, for infection, and other adverse reactions. Monitor patients of blood groups A, B, or AB by means of Hct for signs of progressive anemia, as well as by direct Coombs' tests, when large or frequently repeated doses are required.

Counseling: Advise to consult physician if symptoms of parvovirus B19 infection (eg, fever, drowsiness, chills, and runny nose followed about 2 weeks later by a rash and joint pain) or hepatitis A (eg, several days to weeks of poor appetite, tiredness, and low-grade fever followed by N/V and pain in the belly) appear.

KOGENATE FS — antihemophilic factor (recombinant)   Rx

Class: Antihemophilic factor (recombinant)

ADULT DOSAGE
Hemophilia A

On-Demand Treatment and Control of Bleeding Episodes:
Minor Bleeding:
Required Factor VIII (FVIII) Level 20-40 IU/dL: 10-20 IU/kg IV; repeat dose if there is evidence of further bleeding until bleeding is resolved

Moderate Bleeding:
Required FVIII Level 30-60 IU/dL: 15-30 IU/kg IV q12-24h until bleeding is resolved

Major Bleeding:
Required FVIII Level 80-100 IU/dL: **Initial:** 40-50 IU/kg IV; repeat 20-25 IU/kg IV q8-12h until bleeding is resolved

Perioperative Management:
Minor Surgery:
Required FVIII Level 30-60 IU/dL: 15-30 IU/kg IV q12-24h until bleeding is resolved

Major Surgery:
Required FVIII Level 100 IU/dL: 50

PEDIATRIC DOSAGE
Hemophilia A

On-Demand Treatment and Control of Bleeding Episodes:
Minor Bleeding:
Required FVIII Level 20-40 IU/dL: 10-20 IU/kg IV; repeat dose if there is evidence of further bleeding until bleeding is resolved

Moderate Bleeding:
Required FVIII Level 30-60 IU/dL: 15-30 IU/kg IV q12-24h until bleeding is resolved

Major Bleeding:
Required FVIII Level 80-100 IU/dL: **Initial:** 40-50 IU/kg IV; repeat 20-25 IU/kg IV q8-12h until bleeding is resolved

Perioperative Management:
Minor Surgery:
Required FVIII Level 30-60 IU/dL: 15-30 IU/kg IV q12-24h until bleeding is resolved

Major Surgery:
Required FVIII Level 100 IU/dL: 50

IU/kg IV preoperatively to achieve 100% activity; give q6-12h until healing is complete

Routine Prophylaxis:
25 U/kg IV 3X/week

Dose Calculation:
Dosage (Units) = Body Weight (kg) x Desired FVIII Rise (IU/dL or % Normal) x 0.5 (IU/kg per IU/dL), or
IU/dL (or % Normal) = Total Dose (IU)/ Body Weight (kg) x 2 (IU/dL per IU/kg)

IU/kg IV preoperatively to achieve 100% activity; give q6-12h until healing is complete

Routine Prophylaxis:
25 U/kg IV qod

Dose Calculation:
Dosage (Units) = Body Weight (kg) x Desired FVIII Rise (IU/dL or % Normal) x 0.5 (IU/kg per IU/dL), or
IU/dL (or % Normal) = Total Dose (IU)/ Body Weight (kg) x 2 (IU/dL per IU/kg)

ADMINISTRATION
IV route

Reconstitute and administer w/ the components provided w/ each package. Administer using the provided administration set over 1-15 min; adapt the rate of administration to the response of the patient.
Determine pulse rate before and during administration; if there is a significant increase in pulse rate, reduce rate of administration/temporarily halt infusion to allow the symptoms to disappear promptly.
After reconstitution, store sol at room temperature and administer w/in 3 hrs.
Refer to PI for vacuum transfer and reconstitution instructions.

STORAGE
2-8°C (36-46°F) for up to 30 months from the date of manufacture. During this period, may store for up to 12 months at temperatures up to 25°C (77°F); do not return product to the refrigerator once stored at room temperature. Do not freeze. Protect from extreme exposure to light and store lyophilized powder in the carton prior to use.

HOW SUPPLIED
Inj: 250 IU, 500 IU, 1000 IU, 2000 IU, 3000 IU

CONTRAINDICATIONS
Life-threatening hypersensitivity reactions (eg, anaphylaxis) to mouse or hamster proteins, or other constituents of the product (eg, sucrose, glycine, histidine, sodium, calcium chloride, polysorbate 80, imidazole, tri-n-butyl phosphate, and copper).

WARNINGS/PRECAUTIONS
Not indicated for the treatment of von Willebrand disease. Hypersensitivity reactions including anaphylaxis reported; d/c if symptoms occur and seek emergency treatment. Contains trace amounts of mouse immunoglobulin G and hamster proteins; may develop hypersensitivity to these non-human mammalian proteins. Neutralizing antibodies (inhibitors) reported, predominantly in previously untreated patients. If expected plasma FVIII activity levels are not attained or if bleeding is not controlled w/ expected dose, perform an assay that measures FVIII inhibitor concentration. Hemophilic patients w/ cardiovascular (CV) risk factors or diseases may be at the same risk to develop CV events as non-hemophilic patients when clotting has been normalized by treatment w/ FVIII. Monitor plasma FVIII activity levels and for development of FVIII inhibitors. If inhibitor titers <10 BU/mL, administration of additional Kogenate FS may neutralize the inhibitor and may permit an appropriate hemostatic response. If inhibitor titers >10 BU/mL, adequate hemostasis may not be achieved.

ADVERSE REACTIONS
Inhibitor formation in previously untreated and minimally treated patients, skin-associated hypersensitivity reactions, infusion site reactions, central venous access device associated infections.

PREGNANCY AND LACTATION
Pregnancy: Category C.
Lactation: Caution in nursing.

MECHANISM OF ACTION
Antihemophilic factor (recombinant); temporarily replaces the missing clotting FVIII that is needed for effective hemostasis.

PHARMACOKINETICS
Absorption: 12-33 Years of Age: C_{max}=114.95 IU/dL (initial), 109.42 IU/dL (Week 24); AUC=1588.05 IU•hr/dL (initial), 1487.08 IU•hr/dL (Week 24). Children: AUC=1320 IU•hr/dL. **Elimination:** $T_{1/2}$=13.74 hrs (12-33 yrs of age, initial), 14.6 hrs (12-33 yrs of age, Week 24), 10.7 hrs (children).

PATIENT CONSIDERATIONS
Assessment: Assess for known hypersensitivity to mouse or hamster proteins, or other constituents of the product, location and extent of bleeding, patient's clinical condition, CV risk factors, and pregnancy/nursing status. Assess plasma FVIII activity levels. Obtain baseline pulse rate prior to administration.

Monitoring: Monitor for signs/symptoms of hypersensitivity reactions, CV events, and other adverse reactions. Monitor plasma FVIII activity levels, clinical response, development of FVIII inhibitors, and pulse rate.

Counseling: Advise to report any adverse reactions to physician. Counsel about early signs of hypersensitivity reactions (eg, hives, generalized urticaria, chest tightness) and anaphylaxis; instruct to d/c therapy and seek immediate emergency treatment if signs/symptoms develop. Instruct to contact physician if lack of clinical response to FVIII replacement therapy is experienced. Advise to consult physician prior to travel and to bring an adequate supply based on patient's current regimen of treatment while traveling.

KORLYM — mifepristone

Class: Glucocorticoid receptor antagonist

Rx

A potent antagonist of progesterone and cortisol. Antiprogestational effect will result in termination of pregnancy; pregnancy must be excluded before initiation of treatment and prevented during treatment and for 1 month after stopping treatment by the use of a nonhormonal medically acceptable method of contraception, unless patient has had surgical sterilization. Pregnancy must be excluded if treatment is interrupted for >14 days in females of reproductive potential.

ADULT DOSAGE

Hyperglycemia Secondary to Hypercortisolism

In patients w/ endogenous Cushing's syndrome who have type 2 diabetes mellitus or glucose intolerance and have failed surgery or are not candidates for surgery

Initial: 300mg qd
Titrate: May increase dose by 300mg/day; do not increase dose more frequently than once every 2-4 weeks
Max: 1200mg qd (not to exceed 20mg/kg/day)

If Treatment is Interrupted:
Reinitiate at lowest dose (300mg); if interrupted because of adverse reactions, titration should aim for a dose lower than the one that resulted in treatment interruption

PEDIATRIC DOSAGE

Pediatric use may not have been established

DOSING CONSIDERATIONS
Renal Impairment
Max: 600mg/day

Hepatic Impairment
Mild to Moderate:
Max: 600mg/day

ADMINISTRATION
Oral route

Take as a single daily dose w/ a meal
Swallow tab whole; do not split, crush, or chew
STORAGE
25°C (77°F); excursions permitted to 15-30°C (59-86°F).
HOW SUPPLIED
Tab: 300mg
CONTRAINDICATIONS
Pregnancy, endometrial hyperplasia w/ atypia or endometrial carcinoma, or history of unexplained vaginal bleeding. Concomitant simvastatin, lovastatin, CYP3A substrates w/ narrow therapeutic ranges (eg, cyclosporine, dihydroergotamine, ergotamine, fentanyl, pimozide, quinidine, sirolimus, tacrolimus), or systemic corticosteroids for serious medical conditions/illnesses (eg, immunosuppression after organ transplantation), prior hypersensitivity reactions to mifepristone or to any of the product components.
WARNINGS/PRECAUTIONS
May experience adrenal insufficiency; if suspected, d/c immediately and administer glucocorticoids without delay. Hypokalemia reported; correct hypokalemia prior to treatment. Treat hypokalemia with IV/PO K⁺-supplementation based on severity; consider adding mineralocorticoid antagonists if hypokalemia persists. May cause vaginal bleeding and endometrial changes; caution with hemorrhagic disorders or if receiving concurrent anticoagulant therapy. Refer to a gynecologist if vaginal bleeding occurs. May prolong QT interval; always use the lowest effective dose. Risk for opportunistic infections (eg, *Pneumocystis jiroveci* pneumonia); perform appropriate diagnostic tests and consider treatment for *P. jiroveci*. Caution in patients with underlying heart conditions (eg, heart failure, coronary vascular disease). Avoid with severe hepatic impairment.
ADVERSE REACTIONS
N/V, fatigue, headache, decreased blood K⁺, arthralgia, peripheral edema, HTN, dizziness, decreased appetite, endometrial hypertrophy, vaginal bleeding, dry mouth, diarrhea, myalgia.
DRUG INTERACTIONS
See Contraindications. Avoid with CYP3A inducers (eg, rifampin, rifabutin, rifapentine, phenobarbital, phenytoin, carbamazepine, St. John's wort). Increases levels of drugs whose metabolism is largely or solely mediated by CYP3A; discontinuation/dose reduction or therapeutic drug monitoring may be necessary. Increased levels with ketoconazole and other strong CYP3A inhibitors (eg, itraconazole, nefazodone, ritonavir, nelfinavir, indinavir, atazanavir, amprenavir, fosamprenavir, boceprevir, clarithromycin, conivaptan, lopinavir, mibefradil, posaconazole, saquinavir, telaprevir, telithromycin, voriconazole); when use is necessary, use extreme caution and limit dose of mifepristone to 300mg/day. Caution with moderate CYP3A inhibitors (eg, amprenavir, aprepitant, atazanavir, ciprofloxacin, darunavir/ritonavir, diltiazem, erythromycin, fluconazole, fosamprenavir, grapefruit juice, imatinib, verapamil). May increase levels of CYP2C8/2C9 substrates (eg, NSAIDs, warfarin, repaglinide); use the smallest recommended dose of these drugs and closely monitor for adverse effects. May significantly increase fluvastatin exposure. Caution with drugs that are metabolized by CYP2B6 (eg, bupropion, efavirenz); may significantly increase exposure of these drugs. May interfere with the effectiveness of hormonal

contraceptives; use nonhormonal contraceptive methods. Use in patients who receive corticosteroids for other conditions (eg, autoimmune disorders) may lead to exacerbation or deterioration of such conditions; antagonizes the desired effects of glucocorticoid in these clinical settings. Use lowest effective dose with other QT prolonging drugs or K⁺-channel variants resulting in a long QT interval.
PREGNANCY AND LACTATION
Category X, not for use in nursing.
MECHANISM OF ACTION
Glucocorticoid receptor antagonist; selective antagonist of progesterone receptor at low doses and blocks glucocorticoid receptor at higher doses.
PHARMACOKINETICS
Absorption: T_{max}=1-2 hrs (single dose), 1-4 hrs (multiple 600mg doses).
Distribution: Plasma protein binding (99.2%); found in breast milk. **Metabolism:** Liver; demethylation and hydroxylation; CYP3A4. **Elimination:** Feces (90%); $T_{1/2}$=85 hrs (multiple 600mg doses).
PATIENT CONSIDERATIONS

Assessment: Assess for drug hypersensitivity, immunosuppression after organ transplant and autoimmune disorders treated with corticosteroids, history of unexplained vaginal bleeding and endometrial hyperplasia with atypia or endometrial carcinoma, women with hemorrhagic disorders, underlying heart conditions, renal/hepatic impairment, pregnancy/nursing status, and for possible drug interactions. Evaluate for precipitating causes of hypoadrenalism (eg, infection, trauma).

Monitoring: Monitor for adrenal insufficiency, hypokalemia, vaginal bleeding, endometrial changes, QT interval prolongation, infection, hypersensitivity reactions, and other adverse reactions. Monitor serum K⁺ 1-2 weeks after starting or increasing dose and periodically thereafter.

Counseling: Advise females of reproductive potential that drug will cause termination of pregnancy; counsel regarding pregnancy prevention and planning with a nonhormonal contraceptive prior to therapy and up to 1 month after the end of treatment. Instruct to contact physician immediately if pregnancy is suspected or confirmed.

KOVALTRY — antihemophilic factor (recombinant)

Class: Antihemophilic factor (recombinant)

Rx

ADULT DOSAGE
Congenital Hemophilia A
Dose:
Required dose (IU) = body weight (kg) x desired Factor VIII (FVIII) rise (% of normal or IU/dL) x reciprocal of expected/observed recovery (eg, 0.5 for a recovery of 2 IU/dL per IU/kg)

Treatment/Control of Bleeding Episodes:
Minor Bleed:
Required FVIII Level 20-40 IU/dL:
Repeat q12-24h for at least 1 day, until bleeding episode as indicated by pain is resolved or healing is achieved

Moderate Bleed:
Required FVIII Level 30-60 IU/dL:
Repeat q12-24h for 3-4 days or more until pain and acute disability are resolved

Major Bleed:
Required FVIII Level 60-100 IU/dL:
Repeat q8-24h until bleeding is resolved

Perioperative Management:
Minor Surgery:
Required FVIII Level 30-60 IU/dL (Pre- and Post-Operative): Repeat q24h for at least 1 day until healing is achieved

Major Surgery:
Required FVIII Level 80-100 IU/dL (Pre- and Post-Operative): Repeat q8-24h until adequate wound healing is complete, then continue therapy for at least another 7 days to maintain FVIII activity of 30-60 IU/dL

Routine Prophylaxis:
20-40 IU/kg IV 2-3X/week; adjust dose based on response

PEDIATRIC DOSAGE
Congenital Hemophilia A
Dose:
Required dose (IU) = body weight (kg) x desired FVIII rise (% of normal or IU/dL) x reciprocal of expected/observed recovery (eg, 0.5 for a recovery of 2 IU/dL per IU/kg)

Treatment/Control of Bleeding Episodes:
Minor Bleed:
Required FVIII Level 20-40 IU/dL:
Repeat q12-24h for at least 1 day, until bleeding episode as indicated by pain is resolved or healing is achieved

Moderate Bleed:
Required FVIII Level 30-60 IU/dL:
Repeat q12-24h for 3-4 days or more until pain and acute disability are resolved

Major Bleed:
Required FVIII Level 60-100 IU/dL:
Repeat q8-24h until bleeding is resolved

Perioperative Management:
Minor Surgery:
Required FVIII Level 30-60 IU/dL (Pre- and Post-Operative): Repeat q24h for at least 1 day until healing is achieved

Major Surgery:
Required FVIII Level 80-100 IU/dL (Pre- and Post-Operative): Repeat q8-24h until adequate wound healing is complete, then continue therapy for at least another 7 days to maintain FVIII activity of 30-60 IU/dL

Routine Prophylaxis:
Adolescents: 20-40 IU/kg 2-3X/week; adjust dose based on response
≤12 Years: 25-50 IU/kg 2-3X/week or qod according to individual requirements

ADMINISTRATION
IV route

- Refer to PI for reconstitution instructions.
- Administer as soon as possible; if not, store at room temperature for <3 hrs.

- Infuse IV over a period of 1-15 min; adapt rate of administration to response of each individual patient.

STORAGE
2-8°C (36-46°F) for up to 30 months from the date of manufacture; may be stored for a single period of up to 12 months at temperatures up to 25°C (77°F). Do not freeze. Record starting date of room temperature storage on the unopened product carton. Once stored at room temperature, do not return to refrigerator. Protect from extreme light exposure. Store vial w/ lyophilized powder in carton prior to use.

HOW SUPPLIED
Inj: 250 IU, 500 IU, 1000 IU, 2000 IU, 3000 IU

CONTRAINDICATIONS
History of hypersensitivity reactions to the active substance, to any of the excipients, or to mouse or hamster proteins.

WARNINGS/PRECAUTIONS
Not indicated for the treatment of von Willebrand disease. Hypersensitivity reactions, including anaphylaxis, are possible w/ treatment; d/c if symptoms occur and seek emergency treatment. Formation of neutralizing antibodies (inhibitors) can occur; greater risk in previously untreated patients. Carefully monitor for development of FVIII inhibitors. If expected plasma FVIII activity levels are not attained, or if bleeding is not controlled as expected w/ administered dose, perform Bethesda assay that measures FVIII inhibitor concentration. Hemophilic patients w/ cardiovascular (CV) risk factors/diseases may be at the same risk to develop CV events as non-hemophilic patients when clotting has been normalized by treatment. Catheter-related infections may be observed when administered via central venous access devices. Monitor plasma FVIII activity levels using a validated test to confirm that adequate FVIII levels have been achieved and maintained.

ADVERSE REACTIONS
Headache, pyrexia, pruritus.

PREGNANCY AND LACTATION
Pregnancy: There are no data for use in pregnant women to inform on drug-associated risk.
Lactation: There is no information regarding the presence of drug in human milk, the effects on the breastfed infant, or the effects on milk production; caution in nursing.

MECHANISM OF ACTION
Antihemophilic factor (recombinant); temporarily replaces the missing coagulation FVIII that is needed for effective hemostasis.

PHARMACOKINETICS
Absorption: C_{max}=99.7 IU/dL; AUC=1601.3 IU•h/dL. **Distribution:** V_d=0.63dL/kg. **Elimination:** $T_{1/2}$=14.3 hrs. Refer to PI for pediatric parameters.

PATIENT CONSIDERATIONS
Assessment: Assess for hypersensitivity reactions including anaphylaxis to mouse/hamster protein or other constituents of the product, location and extent of bleeding, patient's clinical condition, and pregnancy/nursing status. Assess FVIII activity levels.

Monitoring: Monitor for signs/symptoms of hypersensitivity reactions and other adverse reactions. Monitor plasma FVIII activity levels, clinical response, and development of FVIII inhibitors.

Counseling: Warn of the early signs of hypersensitivity reaction; advise to d/c use and seek immediate emergency treatment if symptoms occur. Advise to contact physician or treatment center for further treatment and/or assessment if experiencing a lack of clinical response, as this may be a manifestation of an inhibitor. Advise to discard all equipment, including any unused product, in an appropriate container. Advise to consult w/ healthcare provider prior to travel; advise to bring an adequate supply while traveling based on current regimen.

KRYSTEXXA — pegloticase   Rx
Class: Recombinant urate-oxidase enzyme

> Anaphylaxis and infusion reactions reported during and after administration. Anaphylaxis may occur w/ any infusion, including a 1st infusion, and generally manifests w/in 2 hrs of infusion; delayed-type hypersensitivity reactions also reported. Should be administered in a healthcare setting and by a healthcare provider prepared to manage anaphylaxis and infusion reactions. Premedicate w/ antihistamines and corticosteroids. Closely monitor for an appropriate period of time for anaphylaxis after administration. Monitor serum uric acid levels prior to infusions and consider discontinuing treatment if levels increase to >6mg/dL, particularly when 2 consecutive levels >6mg/dL are observed.

ADULT DOSAGE	PEDIATRIC DOSAGE
Chronic Gout	Pediatric use may not have been established
In Patients Refractory to Conventional Therapy: 8mg given as an IV infusion every 2 weeks	
Premedication	
Patients should receive pre-infusion medications (eg, antihistamines, corticosteroids) to minimize the risk of anaphylaxis and infusion reactions	

- -

DOSING CONSIDERATIONS
Concomitant Medications
Oral Urate-Lowering Medications: Before starting pegloticase, d/c oral urate-lowering medications and do not institute therapy w/ oral urate-lowering agents while patient is receiving pegloticase therapy

Adverse Reactions
If an infusion reaction occurs during administration, the infusion may be slowed, or stopped and restarted at a slower rate

ADMINISTRATION
IV route

Preparation
1. Withdraw 1mL of pegloticase from the vial into a sterile syringe; discard any unused portion of product remaining in the 2mL vial.
2. Inject into a single 250mL bag of 0.9% NaCl inj or 0.45% NaCl inj for IV infusion; do not mix or dilute w/ other drugs.
3. Invert the infusion bag containing the dilute pegloticase sol a number of times to ensure thorough mixing; do not shake.
4. Pegloticase diluted in infusion bags is stable for 4 hrs at 2-8°C (36-46°F) and at 20-25°C (68-77°F); however, recommended to be stored under refrigeration, not frozen, protected from light, and used w/in 4 hrs of dilution.
5. Before administration, allow diluted sol to reach room temperature; never subject pegloticase in a vial or in an IV infusion fluid to artificial heating (eg, hot water, microwave).

Administration
Use diluted sol w/in 4 hrs of dilution.
Administer only by IV infusion over no less than 120 min via gravity feed, syringe-type pump, or infusion pump.
Do not administer as an IV push or bolus.
Consider observing patients for approx 1 hr post-infusion, since infusion reactions may occur after completion of infusion.

STORAGE
2-8°C (36-46°F). Protect from light. Do not shake or freeze.

HOW SUPPLIED
Inj: 8mg/mL

CONTRAINDICATIONS
G6PD deficiency.

WARNINGS/PRECAUTIONS
Not recommended for the treatment of asymptomatic hyperuricemia. Gout flares may occur after initiation of therapy; gout flare prophylaxis w/ an NSAID or colchicine is recommended starting at least 1 week before initiation of therapy and lasting at least 6 months, unless medically contraindicated or not tolerated. Therapy does not need to be discontinued because of a gout flare; manage the gout flare concurrently as appropriate for the individual patient. CHF exacerbation reported; caution w/ CHF and monitor closely following infusion. Risk of anaphylaxis and infusion reactions may increase during retreatment due to immunogenicity; carefully monitor patients receiving retreatment after a drug-free interval.

ADVERSE REACTIONS
Anaphylaxis, infusion reactions, gout flares, N/V, contusion/ecchymosis, nasopharyngitis, constipation, chest pain.

DRUG INTERACTIONS
See Dosing Considerations. Potential for anti-PEG antibody development that may bind to other pegylated drugs; impact on response to other PEG-containing therapeutics is unknown.

PREGNANCY AND LACTATION
Pregnancy: Category C.
Lactation: Not for use in nursing unless clear benefit can overcome unknown risk.

MECHANISM OF ACTION
Recombinant urate-oxidase enzyme; catalyzes the oxidation of uric acid to allantoin, thereby lowering serum uric acid.

PATIENT CONSIDERATIONS
Assessment: Assess for G6PD deficiency, CHF, and pregnancy/nursing status. Assess serum uric acid levels prior to infusion.

Monitoring: Monitor for signs/symptoms of anaphylaxis, infusion reactions, gout flares, CHF exacerbation, and other adverse reactions.

Counseling: Inform that anaphylaxis and infusion reactions may occur at any infusion while on therapy; counsel on the importance of adhering to any prescribed medications to help prevent or lessen the severity of these reactions. Advise to seek medical care immediately if patient experiences any symptoms of an allergic reaction during or at any time after infusion. Advise to d/c any oral urate-lowering agents before therapy and not to take any oral urate-lowering agents while on therapy. Inform that gout flares may initially increase when starting therapy, and that medications to help reduce flares may need to be taken regularly for the 1st few months after therapy is started; advise not stop therapy if a flare occurs.

KUVAN — sapropterin dihydrochloride   Rx
Class: Synthetic tetrahydrobiopterin

ADULT DOSAGE	PEDIATRIC DOSAGE
Hyperphenylalaninemia	**Hyperphenylalaninemia**
Used in conjunction w/ a phenylalanine (Phe)-restricted diet to reduce blood Phe levels in patients w/ hyperphenylalaninemia due to tetrahydrobiopterin (BH4)-responsive phenylketonuria (PKU)	Used in conjunction w/ a Phe-restricted diet to reduce blood Phe levels in patients w/ hyperphenylalaninemia due to BH4-responsive PKU
Initial: 10-20mg/kg qd	**Initial:**
Titrate: Check blood Phe levels after 1 week of treatment and periodically for up to a month	**1 Month-6 Years:** 10mg/kg qd **≥7 Years:** 10-20mg/kg qd
	Titrate: Check blood Phe levels after 1 week of treatment and periodically for up to a month

10mg/kg/day Initial Dose:
If blood Phe does not decrease from baseline, the dose may be increased to 20mg/kg/day; d/c treatment if blood Phe does not decrease after 1 month of treatment at 20mg/kg/day

20mg/kg/day Initial Dose:
D/C treatment in patients who do not respond after 1 month of treatment

May adjust dose w/in the range of 5-20mg/kg/day once responsiveness to therapy has been established.

10mg/kg/day Initial Dose:
If blood Phe does not decrease from baseline, the dose may be increased to 20mg/kg/day; d/c treatment if blood Phe does not decrease after 1 month of treatment at 20mg/kg/day

20mg/kg/day Initial Dose:
D/C treatment in patients who do not respond after 1 month of treatment

May adjust dose w/in the range of 5-20mg/kg/day once responsiveness to therapy has been established.

ADMINISTRATION
Oral route

Take w/ a meal, preferably at the same time each day.

Instructions for Use
Tabs:
Swallow whole or dissolve in 120-240mL of water or apple juice and take w/in 15 min of dissolution.
May stir or crush tabs to make them dissolve faster.
Patients may see small pieces floating on top of the water or apple juice; this is normal and safe for patients to swallow.
If after drinking the medicine patients still see pieces of the tab in the container, more water or apple juice can be added to make sure all of the medicine is consumed.
Tabs may also be crushed and then mixed in a small amount of soft foods (eg, applesauce or pudding).

Powder for Oral Sol:
Dissolve in 120-240mL of water or apple juice and take w/in 30 min of dissolution or stir in a small amount of soft foods (eg, applesauce, pudding).
Empty the contents of the packet(s) in water, apple juice, or a small amount of soft foods and mix thoroughly; the powder should dissolve completely.
Infants ≤10kg: Kuvan may be dissolved in as little as 5mL of water or apple juice and a portion of this sol corresponding to a 10mg/kg dose may be administered via an oral dosing syringe; refer to PI for additional dosing information for infants at the recommended starting dose of 10mg/kg/day or 20mg/kg/day.

STORAGE
20-25°C (68-77°F); excursions allowed between 15-30°C (59-86°F). Protect from moisture.

HOW SUPPLIED
Powder: 100mg, 500mg; **Tab:** 100mg

WARNINGS/PRECAUTIONS
Hypersensitivity reactions (eg, anaphylaxis, rash) reported; d/c therapy, initiate appropriate treatment, and continue dietary Phe restrictions in patients who experience anaphylaxis. Gastritis and hyperactivity reported. Increased risk for low levels of blood Phe in children <7 yrs of age treated w/ doses of 20mg/kg/day. Treatment should be directed by physicians knowledgeable in the management of PKU. Active management of dietary Phe intake is required to ensure adequate Phe control and nutritional balance. Monitor blood Phe levels during treatment to ensure adequate blood Phe control; frequent blood monitoring is recommended in pediatric patients. Not all patients w/ PKU respond to therapy; response to treatment cannot be pre-determined by lab testing, and can only be determined by therapeutic trial of sapropterin. Monitor LFTs in patients w/ liver impairment. Carefully monitor patients who have renal impairment.

ADVERSE REACTIONS
Headache, rhinorrhea, pharyngolaryngeal pain, diarrhea, vomiting, cough, nasal congestion.

DRUG INTERACTIONS
May require more frequent monitoring of blood Phe levels w/ drugs known to affect folate metabolism (eg, methotrexate) and their derivatives. Monitor BP w/ drugs that affect nitric oxide-mediated vasorelaxation (eg, PDE-5 inhibitors). Caution w/ levodopa; monitor for change in neurologic status. Potential for sapropterin to inhibit P-gp and breast cancer resistance protein (BCRP) in the gut at the therapeutic doses; co-administration may increase systemic exposure to drugs that are substrates for P-gp or BCRP.

PREGNANCY AND LACTATION
Pregnancy: Category C; a patient registry has been established.
Lactation: It is not known whether sapropterin is present in human milk; use caution in nursing.

MECHANISM OF ACTION
Synthetic BH4; activates residual phenylalanine hydroxylase enzyme, improves the normal oxidative metabolism of Phe, and decreases Phe levels.

PHARMACOKINETICS
Metabolism: Converted to quinoid dihydrobiopterin and metabolized to dihydrobiopterin and biopterin; enzymes dihydrofolate reductase and dihydropteridine reductase are responsible for the metabolism and recycling of BH4. **Elimination:** $T_{1/2}$=6.7 hrs.

PATIENT CONSIDERATIONS
Assessment: Assess for history of hypersensitivity to the drug, hepatic/renal impairment, pregnancy/nursing status, and possible drug interactions. Obtain baseline blood Phe levels.

Monitoring: Monitor for signs/symptoms of hypersensitivity reactions, gastritis, hyperactivity, and other adverse reactions. Monitor for response to treatment and dietary Phe intake. Monitor blood Phe levels; perform frequent blood monitoring

in pediatric patients. Monitor LFTs in patients w/ liver impairment. Monitor patients w/ renal impairment carefully.

Counseling: Inform of the risks/benefits of therapy. Advise that therapy may cause low blood Phe levels. Instruct to use in conjunction w/ a Phe-restricted diet. Inform that not all patients w/ PKU may respond to therapy and that response can only be determined by a therapeutic trial. Advise to have frequent blood Phe measurements and nutritional counseling w/ physician or healthcare team knowledgeable in the management of PKU. Instruct not to modify existing dietary Phe intake during the evaluation of therapy period. Instruct not to continue treatment if determined to be a non-responder during the evaluation of therapy period. Inform that therapy may cause hypersensitivity reactions and hyperactivity. Instruct to contact physician if symptoms of severe gastritis occur. Inform that blood Phe levels that are too high for prolonged periods of time can result in neurologic impairment. Advise that close monitoring is recommended to ensure maintenance of adequate blood Phe control, and that the dose of Kuvan should be adjusted if necessary. Inform that BioMarin has a product registry for PKU patients to collect data on women who become pregnant while receiving treatment. Inform that this drug may interact with other drugs. Advise to report the use of any other prescription or nonprescription medication.

KYNAMRO — mipomersen sodium
Class: Lipid-regulating agent

Rx

> May cause elevations in transaminases; measure ALT, AST, alkaline phosphatase, and total bilirubin prior to therapy, and then ALT/AST regularly as recommended. Withhold dose if ALT/AST is ≥3X ULN. D/C for clinically significant liver toxicity. May increase hepatic fat, w/ or w/o concomitant increases in transaminases. Available only through a restricted program under a Risk Evaluation and Mitigation Strategy (REMS) because of the risk of hepatotoxicity. Prescribe only to patients w/ a clinical or laboratory diagnosis consistent w/ homozygous familial hypercholesterolemia.

ADULT DOSAGE
Homozygous Familial Hypercholesterolemia

200mg SQ once weekly; give on the same day every week, but if dose is missed, give at least 3 days from the next weekly dose

PEDIATRIC DOSAGE
Pediatric use may not have been established

DOSING CONSIDERATIONS
Renal Impairment
W/ Severe Renal Impairment, Clinically Significant Proteinuria, or On Renal Dialysis: Not recommended

Hepatic Impairment
Moderate or Severe (Child-Pugh B or C) or Active Liver Disease (eg, Unexplained Persistent Elevations of Serum Transaminases): Contraindicated

Adverse Reactions
Transaminase Elevations:
ALT/AST ≥3X and <5X ULN:
- Confirm elevation w/ repeat measurement w/in 1 week
- If confirmed, withhold dosing, and obtain additional liver-related tests if not already measured (eg, total bilirubin, alkaline phosphatase, INR) and investigate to identify probable cause
- If resuming therapy after transaminases resolve to <3X ULN, consider monitoring liver-related tests more frequently

ALT/AST ≥5X ULN:
- Withhold dosing, obtain additional liver-related tests if not already measured (eg, total bilirubin, alkaline phosphatase, INR) and investigate to identify probable cause
- If resuming therapy after transaminases resolve to <3X ULN, monitor liver-related tests more frequently

If transaminase elevations are accompanied by clinical symptoms of liver injury, increases in bilirubin ≥2X ULN, or active liver disease, d/c therapy and investigate to identify probable cause.

ADMINISTRATION
SQ route

Remove from refrigerated storage and allow to reach room temperature for at least 30 min prior to administration.
Inject into abdomen, thigh region, or outer area of the upper arm.
Do not inject in areas of active skin disease or injury; avoid areas of tattooed skin and scarring.

STORAGE
2-8°C (36-46°F). Protect from light and keep in the original carton until time of use. If refrigeration is unavailable, may store at ≤30°C (86°F), away from heat sources, for up to 14 days.

HOW SUPPLIED
Inj: 200mg/mL [1mL]

CONTRAINDICATIONS
Moderate or severe hepatic impairment (Child-Pugh B or C); active liver disease, including unexplained persistent elevations of serum transaminases; known hypersensitivity to any component of this product.

WARNINGS/PRECAUTIONS
See Dosing Considerations and Contraindications. Not recommended as an adjunct to LDL apheresis. If baseline LFTs are abnormal, consider initiating therapy after an appropriate work-up and the baseline abnormalities are explained or resolved. During the 1st year, measure liver-related tests monthly;

after the 1st year, measure liver-related tests at least every 3 months. At any time during treatment, d/c for persistent/clinically significant elevations. Inj-site reactions (eg, erythema, pain, tenderness) reported; follow proper technique for SQ administration. Flu-like symptoms (eg, influenza-like illness, pyrexia, chills) reported.

ADVERSE REACTIONS
Inj-site reactions, flu-like symptoms, nausea, headache, elevations in serum transaminases (specifically ALT).

DRUG INTERACTIONS
Not recommended w/ other LDL-lowering agents that can increase hepatic fat. Alcohol may increase levels of hepatic fat and induce/exacerbate liver injury; avoid consumption of >1 alcoholic drink/day. Caution w/ other medications known to have potential for hepatotoxicity (eg, isotretinoin, amiodarone, acetaminophen [>4g/day for ≥3 days/week], methotrexate, tetracyclines, tamoxifen); more frequent monitoring of liver-related tests may be warranted.

PREGNANCY AND LACTATION
Pregnancy: Category B. May cause fetal harm.
Lactation: Not for use in nursing.
Reproductive Potential: Females of reproductive potential should use effective contraception during therapy.

MECHANISM OF ACTION
Lipid-regulating agent; an antisense oligonucleotide targeted to human messenger ribonucleic acid (mRNA) for Apo B-100, the principal apolipoprotein of LDL and its metabolic precursor, VLDL. Complementary to the coding region of the mRNA for Apo B-100, and binds by Watson and Crick base pairing. The hybridization to the cognate mRNA results in RNase H-mediated degradation of the cognate mRNA, thus inhibiting translation of the Apo B-100 protein.

PHARMACOKINETICS
Absorption: T_{max}=3-4 hrs. **Distribution:** Plasma protein binding (≥90%).
Metabolism: In tissues via endonucleases to form shorter oligonucleotides that are then substrates for additional metabolism by exonucleases. **Elimination:** Urine (<4%); $T_{1/2}$=1-2 months.

PATIENT CONSIDERATIONS
Assessment: Assess for hepatic/renal impairment, drug hypersensitivity, pregnancy/nursing status, and possible drug interactions. Obtain baseline lipid levels, ALT/AST, alkaline phosphatase, and total bilirubin.

Monitoring: Monitor for inj-site reactions, flu-like symptoms, and other adverse reactions. Monitor LFTs monthly during 1st yr and at least every 3 months after 1st yr of therapy. Monitor lipid levels at least every 3 months for the 1st yr of therapy. Evaluate LDL level after 6 months to determine if LDL reduction achieved is sufficiently robust to warrant the potential risk of liver toxicity.

Counseling: Inform that transaminase elevations and hepatic steatosis may occur; inform of the importance of monitoring LFTs prior to therapy and periodically thereafter. Advise of the potential for increased risk of liver injury if alcohol is consumed; instruct to limit alcohol consumption to ≤1 drink/day. Advise to report any symptoms of possible liver injury (eg, N/V, fever, anorexia). Inform that inj-site reactions and flu-like symptoms have been reported. Instruct patient or caregiver on the proper technique of administration and safe disposal procedures. Instruct females of reproductive potential to use effective contraception during therapy.

KYPROLIS — carfilzomib   Rx

Class: Proteasome inhibitor

ADULT DOSAGE	PEDIATRIC DOSAGE
Relapsed or Refractory Multiple Myeloma	Pediatric use may not have been established

ADULT DOSAGE (continued)

In Combination w/ Lenalidomide + Dexamethasone in Patients Who Have Received 1-3 Lines of Therapy:
Each 28-day period is considered 1 treatment cycle; treatment may be continued until disease progression or unacceptable toxicity occurs

Lenalidomide: 25mg PO on Days 1-21 of each cycle
Dexamethasone: 40mg PO or IV on Days 1, 8, 15, and 22 of each cycle

Cycle 1:
Administer 20mg/m² carfilzomib on Days 1 and 2. If tolerated, escalate to a target dose of 27mg/m² on Day 8; continue w/ tolerated dose on Days 9, 15, and 16

Cycles 2-12:
Administer 27mg/m² carfilzomib on Days 1, 2, 8, 9, 15, and 16

Cycles 13 and Thereafter:
Administer 27mg/m² carfilzomib on Days 1, 2, 15, and 16. D/C carfilzomib after Cycle 18

In Combination w/ Dexamethasone in Patients Who Have Received 1-3 Lines of Therapy:
Each 28-day period is considered 1 treatment cycle; treatment may be continued until disease progression or unacceptable toxicity occurs

Dexamethasone: 20mg PO or IV on Days 1, 2, 8, 9, 15, 16, 22, and 23 of each cycle

Cycle 1:
Administer 20mg/m² carfilzomib on Days 1 and 2. If tolerated, escalate to a target dose of 56mg/m² starting on Day 8; continue w/ tolerated dose on Days 9, 15, and 16

Cycles 2 and Thereafter:
Administer 56mg/m² carfilzomib on Days 1, 2, 8, 9, 15, and 16

Single Agent in Patients Who Have Received ≥1 Line of Therapy:
Each 28-day period is considered 1 treatment cycle; treatment may be continued until disease progression or unacceptable toxicity occurs

20/27mg/m² Regimen:
Cycle 1:
Administer 20mg/m² carfilzomib on Days 1 and 2. If tolerated, escalate to a target dose of 27mg/m² starting on Day 8; continue w/ tolerated dose on Days 9, 15, and 16

Cycles 2-12:
Administer 27mg/m² carfilzomib on Days 1, 2, 8, 9, 15, and 16

Cycles 13 and Thereafter:
Administer 27mg/m² carfilzomib on Days 1, 2, 15, and 16

20/56mg/m² Regimen:
Cycle 1:
Administer 20mg/m² carfilzomib on Days 1 and 2. If tolerated, escalate to a target dose of 56mg/m² starting on Day 8; continue w/ tolerated dose on Days 9, 15, and 16

Cycles 2-12:
Administer 56mg/m² carfilzomib on Days 1, 2, 8, 9, 15, and 16

Cycles 13 and Thereafter:
Administer 56mg/m² carfilzomib on Days 1, 2, 15, and 16

Premedication

Hydration and Fluid Monitoring:
Prior to Each Dose in Cycle 1: Give both oral (30mL/kg at least 48 hrs before Cycle 1, Day 1) and IV fluids (250-500mL of appropriate IV fluid prior to each dose in Cycle 1); if needed, give an additional 250-500mL of IV fluids following administration
Subsequent Cycles: Continue oral and/or IV hydration prn

Dexamethasone:
Administer recommended dexamethasone 30 min to 4 hrs prior to all doses of carfilzomib during Cycle 1 to reduce the incidence and severity of infusion reactions; reinstate dexamethasone premedication if these symptoms occur during subsequent cycles
20/27mg/m² Regimen: 4mg PO or IV
20/56mg/m² Regimen: 8mg PO or IV

Thromboprophylaxis:
Recommended for patients being treated w/ combination of carfilzomib w/ dexamethasone or w/ lenalidomide + dexamethasone; base regimen on underlying risks

Infection Prophylaxis:
Consider antiviral prophylaxis to decrease the risk of herpes zoster reactivation

DOSING CONSIDERATIONS

Adverse Reactions
Dose Level Reductions:
27mg/m^2 Dose:
First Dose Reduction: 20mg/m^2
Second Dose Reduction: 15mg/m^2; d/c if toxicity persists
56mg/m^2 Dose:
First Dose Reduction: 45mg/m^2
Second Dose Reduction: 36mg/m^2
Third Dose Reduction: 27mg/m^2; d/c if toxicity persists

Hematologic Toxicity:
ANC <0.5 x 10^9/L:
- Withhold dose
- If recovered to ≥0.5 x 10^9/L, continue at same dose level
- For subsequent drops to <0.5 x 10^9/L, follow same recommendations as above and consider 1 dose level reduction when restarting carfilzomib

Febrile Neutropenia (ANC <0.5 x 10^9/L and an Oral Temperature >38.5°C (101.3°F) or 2 Consecutive Readings of >38.0°C (100.4°F) for 2 Hrs):
- Withhold dose
- If ANC returns to baseline grade and fever resolves, resume at the same dose level

Platelets <10 x 10^9/L or Evidence of Bleeding w/ Thrombocytopenia:
- Withhold dose; if recovered to ≥10 x 10^9/L and/or bleeding is controlled, continue at same dose level
- For subsequent drops to <10 x 10^9/L, follow the same recommendations as above and consider 1 dose level reduction when restarting carfilzomib

Renal Toxicity:
SrCr ≥2X Baseline, or CrCl <15mL/min or CrCl Decreases to ≤50% of Baseline, or Need for Dialysis:
- Withhold dose and continue monitoring renal function (SrCr or CrCl)
- If attributable to carfilzomib, resume when renal function has recovered to w/in 25% of baseline; start at 1 dose level reduction
- If not attributable to carfilzomib, dosing may be resumed at the discretion of the physician
- For patients on dialysis, administer the dose after dialysis

Other Non-Hematologic Toxicity:
All Other Severe or Life-Threatening (CTCAE Grades 3 and 4) Non-Hematological Toxicities:
- Withhold until resolved or returned to baseline
- Consider restarting the next scheduled treatment at 1 dose level reduction

ADMINISTRATION
IV route
- Calculate dose based on actual BSA at baseline; patients w/ BSA >2.2m^2 should receive a dose based on a BSA of 2.2m^2.
- Dose does not need to be adjusted for weight change of ≤20%.
- Do not mix w/ or administer as an infusion w/ other medicinal products.
- Flush IV line w/ normal saline or D5 inj immediately before and after administration.
- Do not administer as a bolus.

Infusion Times
W/ Lenalidomide and Dexamethasone: 10 min
W/ Dexamethasone: 30 min
20/27mg/m^2 Monotherapy Regimen: 10 min
20/56mg/m^2 Monotherapy Regimen: 30 min

Reconstitution/Preparation
1. Slowly inject 29mL (for 60mg vial) or 15mL (for 30mg vial) of sterile water for inj, directing the sol onto the inside wall of the vial to minimize foaming.
2. Gently swirl and/or invert vial slowly for about 1 min, or until complete dissolution; do not shake. If foaming occurs, allow sol to settle in the vial until foaming subsides (approx 5 min) and the sol is clear.
3. When administering in an IV bag, withdraw calculated dose from vial and dilute into 50mL or 100mL D5 inj IV bag.
4. Discard any unused portion left in the vial; do not administer more than one dose from a vial.

Stability of Reconstituted Carfilzomib
Total time from reconstitution to administration should not exceed 24 hrs.
Stable for 24 hrs at 2-8°C (36-46°F).
Stable for 4 hrs at 15-30°C (59-86°F).

STORAGE
Unopened Vials: 2-8°C (36-46°F). Protect from light.

HOW SUPPLIED
Inj: 30mg, 60mg

WARNINGS/PRECAUTIONS
See Dosing Considerations. New onset/worsening of preexisting cardiac failure, restrictive cardiomyopathy, myocardial ischemia, and MI including fatalities reported following administration. Death due to cardiac arrest has occurred w/in a day of administration. Renal insufficiency adverse events reported; acute renal failure was reported more frequently in patients w/ advanced relapsed and refractory multiple myeloma who received carfilzomib monotherapy. Cases of tumor lysis syndrome (TLS), including fatal outcomes, reported; monitor for evidence of TLS during treatment and manage promptly, including interruption of therapy until TLS is resolved. Consider uric acid-lowering drugs in patients at risk for

TLS. Acute respiratory distress syndrome, acute respiratory failure, and acute diffuse infiltrative pulmonary disease reported; d/c in the event of drug-induced pulmonary toxicity. Pulmonary arterial HTN (PAH) reported; withhold therapy until resolved or returned to baseline and consider whether to restart therapy based on a benefit/risk assessment. Dyspnea reported; evaluate dyspnea to exclude cardiopulmonary conditions. HTN, including hypertensive crisis and hypertensive emergency, reported; withhold carfilzomib and evaluate if HTN cannot be adequately controlled. Venous thromboembolic events (eg, deep venous thrombosis, pulmonary embolism) reported; consider an alternative method of contraception during treatment w/ carfilzomib in combination w/ dexamethasone or lenalidomide + dexamethasone in patients using oral contraceptives or a hormonal method of contraception associated w/ a risk of thrombosis. Infusion reactions may occur immediately following or up to 24 hrs after treatment. Fatal or serious cases of hemorrhage, including GI, pulmonary, and intracranial hemorrhage and epistaxis, have been reported; promptly evaluate signs/symptoms of blood loss and reduce or withhold dose as appropriate. Thrombocytopenia reported; reduce or withhold dose as appropriate. Hepatic failure, including fatal cases, reported. May increase serum transaminases; reduce or withhold dose as appropriate. Thrombotic microangiopathy, including thrombotic thrombocytopenic purpura/hemolytic uremic syndrome (TTP/HUS), reported; if diagnosis is suspected, d/c therapy and evaluate. If diagnosis of TTP/HUS is excluded, therapy can be restarted. Posterior reversible encephalopathy syndrome (PRES) reported; d/c if suspected and evaluate. May cause fetal harm.

ADVERSE REACTIONS
Monotherapy: Anemia, fatigue, thrombocytopenia, nausea, pyrexia, dyspnea, diarrhea, headache, cough, peripheral edema.
Combination Therapy: Anemia, neutropenia, diarrhea, dyspnea, fatigue, thrombocytopenia, pyrexia, insomnia, muscle spasm, cough, URTI, hypokalemia.

PREGNANCY AND LACTATION
Pregnancy: Can cause fetal harm based on animal studies and the drug's mechanism of action.
Lactation: There is no information regarding the presence of carfilzomib in human milk, the effects on the breastfed infant, or the effects on milk production; caution in nursing.
Females and Males of Reproductive Potential: Females of reproductive potential should use effective contraceptive measures or abstain from sexual activity to prevent pregnancy during therapy and for at least 30 days following completion of therapy. Males of reproductive potential should use effective contraceptive measures or abstain from sexual activity to prevent pregnancy during therapy and for at least 90 days following completion of therapy.

MECHANISM OF ACTION
Proteasome inhibitor; irreversibly binds to the N-terminal threonine-containing active sites of the 20S proteasome, the proteolytic core particle w/in the 26S proteasome.

PHARMACOKINETICS
Absorption: (27mg/m^2 single dose) AUC=379ng•hr/mL; C$_{max}$=4232ng/mL; (56mg/m^2 single dose) AUC=948ng•hr/mL; C$_{max}$=2079ng/mL. **Distribution:** (20mg/m^2) V$_d$=28L; plasma protein binding (97%). **Metabolism:** Rapid and extensive; peptidase cleavage and epoxide hydrolysis (major); CYP450 (minor). **Elimination:** (Doses ≥15mg/m^2) T$_{1/2}$≤1 hr.

PATIENT CONSIDERATIONS
Assessment: Assess for dehydration, hypersensitivity to drug, preexisting cardiac failure, hepatic dysfunction, renal impairment, and pregnancy/nursing status. Obtain baseline CBC, LFTs, SrCr, and weight. Consider antiviral prophylaxis therapy.

Monitoring: Monitor for signs/symptoms of cardiac toxicities, acute renal failure, TLS, dehydration, pulmonary toxicity, PAH, dyspnea, HTN, venous thromboembolic events, infusion reactions, hemorrhage, TTP/HUS, PRES, hepatic failure, and other adverse reactions. Monitor CBC, LFTs, and SrCr.

Counseling: Inform of the risks and symptoms of cardiac failure and ischemia. Advise on appropriate measures to take to avoid dehydration and instruct to notify physician if dehydration symptoms develop. Inform that patient may experience cough or SOB and instruct to contact physician if SOB occurs. Inform of the risk of venous thromboembolism and counsel on the options for prophylaxis. Advise to seek immediate medical attention for symptoms of venous thrombosis or embolism. Inform about the common signs/symptoms of infusion reactions. Advise patients that they may bruise or bleed more easily or that it may take longer to stop bleeding; inform of the signs of occult bleeding and instruct to report to physician any prolonged, unusual, or excessive bleeding. Inform about the risk of developing hepatic failure and advise to contact physician if jaundice develops. Instruct to contact physician if neurologic symptoms (eg, headaches, confusion, seizures, visual loss) develop. Instruct not to drive or operate machinery if fatigue, dizziness, fainting, and/or drop in BP are experienced. Advise females of reproductive potential to use effective contraceptive measures to prevent pregnancy during and for at least 30 days after treatment and instruct to inform physician immediately if pregnant. Advise males of reproductive potential to use effective contraceptive measures to prevent pregnancy during and for at least 90 days after treatment. Instruct not to breastfeed while on therapy. Advise to notify physician if using or planning to take other prescription or OTC drugs.

LEMTRADA — alemtuzumab

Rx

Class: Monoclonal antibody/CD52 blocker

> May cause serious, sometimes fatal, autoimmune conditions such as immune thrombocytopenia (ITP) and anti-glomerular basement membrane disease; monitor CBCs with differential, SrCr levels, and urinalysis with urine cell counts at periodic intervals for 48 months after the last dose. May cause serious and life threatening infusion reactions; administer in a setting with appropriate equipment and personnel to manage anaphylaxis or serious infusion reactions. Monitor patients for 2 hrs after each infusion. Serious infusion reactions can also occur after the 2-hr monitoring period. May cause an increased risk of malignancies, including thyroid cancer, melanoma, and lymphoproliferative disorders; perform baseline and yearly skin exams. Available only through a restricted distribution program, Lemtrada Risk Evaluation Mitigation Strategy (REMS).

ADULT DOSAGE
Multiple Sclerosis
Relapsing Forms:

Usual: 12mg/day for 2 treatment courses

First Treatment Course:
12mg/day on 5 consecutive days (60mg total dose)

Second Treatment Course:
12mg/day on 3 consecutive days (36mg total dose) administered 12 months after the first treatment course

Corticosteroids:
Premedicate with high dose corticosteroids (1000mg methylprednisolone or equivalent) immediately prior to infusion and for the first 3 days of each treatment course

Herpes Prophylaxis:
Administer antiviral prophylaxis for herpetic viral infections starting on the first day of each treatment course and continue for at least 2 months following treatment or until CD4+ lymphocyte count is ≥200 cells/μL, whichever occurs later

PEDIATRIC DOSAGE
Pediatric use may not have been established

ADMINISTRATION
IV route

Preparation and Infusion
Withdraw 1.2mL from the vial into a syringe and inject into a 100mL bag of 0.9% NaCl or D5W.
Invert the bag to mix the sol.
Infuse Lemtrada over 4 hrs starting within 8 hrs after dilution.
Do not add or simultaneously infuse other drug substances through the same IV line.
Do not give as an IV push or bolus.

STORAGE
2-8°C (36-46°F). Do not freeze or shake. Store in original carton to protect from light. Diluted Sol: Store for as long as 8 hrs either at 15-25°C (59-77°F) or at 2-8°C (36-46°F). Protect from light.

HOW SUPPLIED
Inj: 10mg/mL

CONTRAINDICATIONS
Human immunodeficiency virus (HIV).

WARNINGS/PRECAUTIONS
Reserve for patients who have had an inadequate response to two or more drugs indicated for the treatment of MS. Determine whether patient has a history of varicella or if has been vaccinated for varicella zoster virus (VZV) prior to treatment; if not, test patient for antibodies to VZV and consider vaccination for those who are antibody-negative. Complete any necessary immunizations at least 6 weeks prior to treatment. Therapy can result in the formation of autoantibodies; autoantibodies may be transferred from the mother to the fetus during pregnancy. Case of transplacental transfer of anti-thyrotropin receptor antibodies resulting in neonatal Graves' disease occurred after alemtuzumab treatment in the mother. May cause cytokinase release syndrome resulting in infusion reactions; consider pretreatment with antihistamines and/or antipyretics prior to therapy. Caution when initiating therapy in patients with preexisting or ongoing malignancies. Immediately obtain CBC if ITP is suspected and promptly initiate appropriate medical intervention if confirmed. Glomerular nephropathies reported. Perform further evaluation for nephropathies if significant changes from baseline in SrCr, unexplained hematuria, or proteinuria are observed. Autoimmune thyroid disorders reported; administer only if potential benefit justifies potential risks in patients with an ongoing thyroid disorder. Autoimmune cytopenias such as neutropenia, hemolytic anemia, and pancytopenia reported; use CBC results to monitor for cytopenias and prompt medical intervention is indicated if a cytopenia is confirmed. Infections (eg, urinary tract infection, appendicitis, gastroenteritis, pneumonia, tooth infection) reported. Consider delaying administration in patients with active infection until the infection is fully controlled. Herpes viral infection, cervical human papilloma virus (HPV) (eg, cervical dysplasia) infection, active/latent tuberculosis (TB), fungal infections (oral and vaginal candidiasis), and Listeria meningitis reported. Avoid or adequately heat foods that are potential sources of *Listeria monocytogenes*. Caution in patients identified as carriers of hepatitis B virus (HBV) and/or hepatitis C virus (HCV) as these patients may be at risk of irreversible liver damage relative to a potential virus reactivation as a consequence of their preexisting status. Hypersensitivity pneumonitis and pneumonitis with fibrosis reported. Contains same active ingredient (alemtuzumab) found in Campath; exercise increased vigilance for additive and long-lasting effects on the immune system if use is considered in a patient who has previously received Campath.

ADVERSE REACTIONS
Autoimmune conditions, infusion reactions, malignancies, rash, headache, pyrexia, nasopharyngitis, N/V, urinary tract infection, fatigue, insomnia, upper respiratory tract infection, herpes viral infection, urticaria, pruritus.

DRUG INTERACTIONS
Do not administer live viral vaccines following a course of therapy; may increase the risk of infection. Concomitant use with antineoplastic or immunosuppressive therapies could increase risk of immunosuppression.

PREGNANCY AND LACTATION
Category C; not for use in nursing.

MECHANISM OF ACTION
Monoclonal antibody/CD52-blocker; has not been established. Presumed to involve binding to CD52. Following cell surface binding to T and B lymphocytes, results in antibody-dependent cellular cytolysis and complement-mediated lysis.

PHARMACOKINETICS
Absorption: C_{max}=3014ng/mL (Day 5, 1st treatment course), 2276ng/mL (Day 3, 2nd treatment course). **Distribution:** V_d= 14.1 L. **Elimination:** $T_{1/2}$= 2 weeks.

PATIENT CONSIDERATIONS
Assessment: Assess for HIV, history of varicella, thyroid disorder, HBV, HBC, any other conditions where treatment is cautioned, pregnancy/nursing status, and possible drug interactions. Obtain CBC with differential, SrCr levels, and urinalysis with urine cell counts. Perform a test of thyroid function (eg, thyroid-stimulating hormone level). Perform TB screening according to local guidelines. Perform baseline skin examination. Assess vital signs and immunization history.

Monitoring: Monitor for autoimmune conditions (eg, ITP, anti-glomerular basement membrane disease), malignancies (eg, thyroid cancer, melanoma, lymphoproliferative disorders, lymphoma), glomerular nephropathies, infusion reactions, thyroid disorders, autoimmune cytopenias, infections, TB, and other adverse reactions. Monitor CBCs with differential, SrCr levels, and urinalysis with urine cell counts monthly for 48 months after the last dose; perform testing after 48 months based on clinical findings. Monitor vital signs periodically during infusion. Monitor for infusion reactions during and for at least 2 hrs after each infusion. Perform thyroid function test every 3 months until 48 months after the last infusion; continue to test thyroid function after 48 months if clinically indicated. Consider additional monitoring in patients with medical conditions that may predispose to cardiovascular or pulmonary compromise. Perform yearly skin examination. Perform annual HPV screening in female patients.

Counseling: Inform of benefits and risks of therapy. Instruct to contact physician promptly if experience any symptoms of potential autoimmune disease (eg, bleeding, easy bruising, petechiae). Advise of the importance of monthly blood and urine tests for 48 months following the last course of therapy; inform that monitoring may need to continue past 48 months if there are signs/symptoms of autoimmunity. Instruct to contact physician if experience symptoms reflective of a potential thyroid disorder. Inform that infusion reactions can occur after patient leaves the infusion center; instruct to report symptoms that occur during and after each infusion to physician. Inform that must enroll in the Lemtrada REMS Program. Instruct to carry the Lemtrada REMS patient safety information card in case of an emergency. Advise of the risk of malignancies, including thyroid cancer and melanoma; instruct to have yearly skin examinations. Instruct to take prescribed medication for herpes prophylaxis ud. Advise that yearly screening for HPV is recommended. Advise to avoid, or adequately heat foods that are potential sources of *L. monocytogenes* if have had a recent course of therapy. Instruct to notify physician if pregnant, breastfeeding, or if any adverse reactions develop. Instruct patients to inform physician if they have taken Campath.

LENVIMA — lenvatinib

Rx

Class: Kinase inhibitor

ADULT DOSAGE
Differentiated Thyroid Carcinoma

Locally Recurrent or Metastatic, Progressive, Radioactive Iodine-Refractory Differentiated Thyroid Cancer (DTC):
24mg (two 10mg caps and one 4mg cap) qd

Continue until disease progression or until unacceptable toxicity

Advanced Renal Cell Carcinoma

In Combination w/ Everolimus for the Treatment of Advanced Renal Cell Carcinoma (RCC) Following 1 Prior Anti-Angiogenic Therapy:
18mg (one 10mg cap and two 4mg caps) in combination w/ 5mg everolimus qd

PEDIATRIC DOSAGE
Pediatric use may not have been established

Continue lenvatinib plus everolimus until disease progression or until unacceptable toxicity

Missed Dose

If a dose is missed and cannot be taken w/in 12 hrs, skip that dose and take the next dose at the usual time of administration

DOSING CONSIDERATIONS
Renal Impairment
Severe (CrCl <30mL/min):
DTC: 14mg qd
RCC: 10mg qd

Mild or Moderate: No dose adjustment is recommended
ESRD: Not studied
Hepatic Impairment
Severe (Child-Pugh C):
DTC: 14mg qd
RCC: 10mg qd

Mild or Moderate: No dose adjustment is recommended
Adverse Reactions
HTN:
- **Grade 3 (Despite Optimal Antihypertensive Therapy):** Withhold; resume at a reduced dose after resolution to Grade 0, 1, or 2
- **Grade 4:** D/C therapy; do not resume

Cardiac Dysfunction:
- **Grade 3:** Withhold; resume at a reduced dose after resolution to Grade 0, 1, or baseline
- **Grade 4:** D/C therapy; do not resume

Arterial Thrombotic Event:
- **Any Grade:** D/C therapy; do not resume

Hepatotoxicity:
- **Grade 3 or 4:** Withhold or d/c; consider resuming at reduced dose if resolves to Grade 0-1 or baseline

Hepatic Failure:
- **Grade 3 or 4:** D/C therapy; do not resume

Proteinuria:
- **Greater Than or Equal to 2g/24 hrs:** Withhold; resume at reduced dose after resolution to <2g/24 hrs

Nephrotic Syndrome:
D/C therapy; do not resume

Nausea, Vomiting, and Diarrhea:
- **Grade 3:** Withhold; resume at reduced dose after resolution to Grade 0, 1, or baseline. Initiate prompt medical management for N/V or diarrhea

Vomiting and Diarrhea:
- **Grade 4 (Despite Medical Management):** D/C therapy; do not resume

Renal Failure or Impairment:
- **Grade 3 or 4:** Withhold or d/c; consider resuming at reduced dose if resolves to Grade 0-1 or baseline

GI Perforation:
- **Any Grade:** D/C therapy; do not resume

Fistula:
- **Grade 3 or 4:** D/C therapy; do not resume

QTc Prolongation:
- **Greater Than 500 ms:** Withhold; resume at reduced dose after resolution to <480 ms or baseline

Reversible Posterior Leukoencephalopathy Syndrome (RPLS):
- **Any Grade:** Withhold or d/c; consider resuming at reduced dose if resolves to Grade 0 to 1

Hemorrhage:
- **Grade 3:** Withhold; resume at reduced dose after resolution to Grade 0 to 1
- **Grade 4:** D/C therapy; do not resume

Manage other adverse reactions according to the instructions below for DTC or RCC

Persistent and Intolerable Grade 2 or 3 Adverse Reactions or Grade 4 Lab Abnormalities in DTC:
1st Occurrence: Interrupt until resolved to Grade 0-1 or baseline; decrease dose to 20mg (two 10mg caps) qd
2nd Occurrence: Interrupt until resolved to Grade 0-1 or baseline; decrease dose to 14mg (one 10mg cap + one 4mg cap) qd
3rd Occurrence: Interrupt until resolved to Grade 0-1 or baseline; decrease dose to 10mg (one 10mg cap) qd
- Initiate medical management for N/V or diarrhea prior to interruption or dose reduction
- Reduce dose in succession based on the previous daily dose level (24mg/day, 20mg/day, or 14mg/day)
- 2nd or 3rd occurrence may refer to either the same or a different adverse reaction that requires dose modification

Persistent and Intolerable Grade 2 or 3 Adverse Reactions or Grade 4 Lab Abnormalities in RCC:
1st Occurrence: Interrupt until resolved to Grade 0-1 or baseline; decrease dose to 14mg (one 10mg cap + one 4mg cap) qd

2nd Occurrence: Interrupt until resolved to Grade 0-1 or baseline; decrease dose to 10mg (one 10mg cap) qd
3rd Occurrence: Interrupt until resolved to Grade 0-1 or baseline; decrease dose to 8mg (two 4 mg cap) qd
- Initiate medical management for N/V or diarrhea prior to interruption or dose reduction
- Reduce dose in succession based on the previous daily dose level (18mg/day, 14mg/day, 10mg/day, or 8mg/day)
- 2nd or 3rd occurrence may refer to either the same or a different adverse reaction that requires dose modification

Refer to the full prescribing information for everolimus for recommended dose modifications. For toxicities thought to be related to everolimus alone, d/c, interrupt, or use alternate day dosing. For toxicities thought to be related to both lenvatinib and everolimus, 1st reduce lenvatinib and then everolimus

ADMINISTRATION
Oral route

Take w/ or w/o food.
Take at the same time each day.
Swallow caps whole.
Alternatively, may dissolve caps in a small glass of liquid.
- Measure 1 tbsp of water or apple juice and put caps into the liquid w/o breaking or crushing them.
- Leave caps in the liquid for at least 10 min, stir for at least 3 min, and then drink mixture.
- After drinking, add the same amount (1 tbsp) of water or apple juice to the glass, swirl the contents a few times, and then swallow the additional liquid.

STORAGE
25°C (77°F); excursions permitted to 15-30°C (59-86°F).

HOW SUPPLIED
Cap: 4mg, 10mg

WARNINGS/PRECAUTIONS
See Dosing Considerations. HTN, cardiac dysfunction, arterial thromboembolic events, increases in AST/ALT, hepatic failure (including fatal events), acute hepatitis, renal failure/impairment, GI perforation or fistula, and RPLS reported. Proteinuria reported; obtain a 24-hr urine protein if urine dipstick proteinuria ≥2+ is detected. Diarrhea reported; initiate prompt medical management for the development of diarrhea and monitor for dehydration. QT interval prolongation reported; monitor ECG in patients w/ congenital long QT syndrome, CHF, bradyarrhythmias, or in patients taking drugs known to prolong the QT interval (eg, Class Ia and III antiarrhythmics). Hypocalcemia reported; monitor blood Ca^{2+} levels at least monthly and replace Ca^{2+} as necessary. Hemorrhagic events including fatal events and serious tumor related bleeds reported; consider the risk of severe or fatal hemorrhage associated w/ tumor invasion/infiltration of major blood vessels (eg, carotid artery). Impairment of exogenous thyroid suppression and thyroid dysfunction may occur; monitor thyroid function before initiation of, and at least monthly throughout, treatment. Treat hypothyroidism accordingly to maintain a euthyroid state. May cause fetal harm.

ADVERSE REACTIONS
DTC: HTN, fatigue, diarrhea, arthralgia/myalgia, decreased appetite, weight decreased, N/V, stomatitis, headache, proteinuria, palmar-plantar erythrodysesthesia syndrome, abdominal pain, dysphonia.
RCC: Diarrhea, fatigue, arthralgia/myalgia, decreased appetite, N/V, stomatitis/oral inflammation, HTN, peripheral edema, cough, abdominal pain, dyspnea, rash, weight decreased, hemorrhagic events, proteinuria.

PREGNANCY AND LACTATION
Pregnancy: May cause fetal harm.
Lactation: Not for use in nursing.
Reproductive Potential: Females of reproductive potential should use effective contraception during treatment and for at least 2 weeks following completion of therapy. May result in reduced fertility in females of reproductive potential. May result in damage to male reproductive tissues leading to reduced fertility of unknown duration.

MECHANISM OF ACTION
Kinase inhibitor; inhibits the kinase activities of vascular endothelial growth factor (VEGF) receptors VEGFR1 (FLT1), VEGFR2 (KDR), and VEGFR3 (FLT4). Also inhibits other receptor tyrosine kinases that have been implicated in pathogenic angiogenesis, tumor growth, and cancer progression in addition to their normal cellular functions, including fibroblast growth factor (FGF) receptors FGFR 1, 2, 3, and 4; the platelet derived growth factor receptor alpha, KIT, and RET.

PHARMACOKINETICS
Absorption: T_{max}=1-4 hrs. **Distribution:** Plasma protein binding (98-99%).
Metabolism: Enzymatic (CYP3A and aldehyde oxidase) and non-enzymatic processes. **Elimination:** Feces (64%), urine (25%); $T_{1/2}$=28 hrs.

PATIENT CONSIDERATIONS
Assessment: Assess for proteinuria, congenital long QT syndrome, CHF, bradyarrhythmias, electrolyte abnormalities, renal/hepatic impairment, pregnancy/nursing status, and if taking drugs known to prolong the QT interval. Assess BP and control prior to treatment.

Monitoring: Monitor for signs/symptoms of cardiac decompensation, arterial thromboembolic events, renal failure/impairment, GI perforation and fistula formation, proteinuria, diarrhea, RPLS, hemorrhagic events, QT interval prolongation, and other adverse reactions. Monitor BP after 1 week, then every 2 weeks for the first 2 months, and then at least monthly thereafter. Monitor LFTs every 2 weeks for the first 2 months, and at least monthly thereafter. Monitor and correct electrolyte abnormalities. Monitor ECG in patients w/ congenital long QT syndrome, CHF, bradyarrhythmias, and in patients taking drugs known to prolong QT interval. Monitor blood Ca^{2+} levels at least monthly. Monitor thyroid function at least monthly.

Counseling: Advise to undergo regular BP monitoring and to contact physician if BP is elevated. Inform that therapy may cause cardiac dysfunction; instruct to immediately contact physician if any clinical symptoms of cardiac dysfunction are experienced. Advise to seek immediate medical attention for new onset chest pain or acute neurologic symptoms consistent w/ MI or stroke. Inform of the need to undergo lab tests to monitor for kidney function, protein in the urine, and liver function; instruct to report any new symptoms indicating hepatic toxicity or failure. Advise when to start standard anti-diarrheal therapy and to maintain adequate hydration; instruct to contact physician if unable to maintain adequate hydration. Advise that therapy may increase the risk of GI perforation or fistula; instruct to seek immediate medical attention for severe abdominal pain. Inform patients who are at risk for QTc prolongation that they will need to undergo regular ECGs; advise all patients of the need to undergo laboratory tests to monitor electrolytes. Explain that therapy may increase the risk of severe bleeding; instruct to contact physician for bleeding or symptoms of severe bleeding. Inform females of reproductive potential of the potential risk to a fetus and instruct to inform physician of a known or suspected pregnancy. Instruct females of reproductive potential to use effective contraception during treatment and for at least 2 weeks following completion of therapy. Advise nursing women to d/c breastfeeding during treatment.

LETAIRIS — ambrisentan   **Rx**

Class: Endothelin receptor antagonist

> Do not administer to a pregnant female; may cause serious birth defects. Exclude pregnancy before initiation of treatment. Females of reproductive potential must use acceptable methods of contraception during and for 1 month after treatment; obtain monthly pregnancy tests during and 1 month after discontinuation of treatment. Females can only receive the drug through a restricted program called the Letairis Risk Evaluation and Mitigation Strategy (REMS) program.

ADULT DOSAGE	**PEDIATRIC DOSAGE**
Pulmonary Arterial Hypertension	Pediatric use may not have been established
Treatment of pulmonary arterial HTN (PAH) (WHO Group 1) to improve exercise ability and delay clinical worsening; can be used w/ tadalafil to reduce the risks of disease progression and hospitalization for worsening PAH, and to improve exercise ability	
Initial: 5mg qd w/ or w/o tadalafil 20mg qd **Titrate:** At 4 wk intervals, either dose of ambrisentan or tadalafil can be increased to ambrisentan 10mg or tadalafil 40mg	

DOSING CONSIDERATIONS
Hepatic Impairment
Elevation of Liver Transaminases:
D/C if elevations of ALT/AST >5X ULN or if elevations are accompanied by bilirubin >2X ULN, or by signs/symptoms of liver dysfunction and other causes are excluded

ADMINISTRATION
Oral route
Do not split, crush, or chew tabs.

STORAGE
25°C (77°F); excursions permitted to 15-30°C (59-86°F).

HOW SUPPLIED
Tab: 5mg, 10mg

CONTRAINDICATIONS
Pregnancy, idiopathic pulmonary fibrosis (IPF), including IPF patients w/ pulmonary HTN (WHO Group 3).

WARNINGS/PRECAUTIONS
May cause peripheral edema; more common w/ concomitant tadalafil and in the elderly. If clinically significant fluid retention develops, evaluate further to determine the cause and the possible need for specific treatment or discontinuation of therapy. If acute pulmonary edema develops during initiation of therapy, consider the possibility of pulmonary veno-occlusive disease (PVOD); d/c if confirmed. May decrease sperm counts. Decreases in Hgb concentration and Hct reported and may result in anemia requiring transfusion. Initiation of therapy is not recommended w/ clinically significant anemia. Consider discontinuation if a clinically significant Hgb decrease is observed and other causes have been excluded. Avoid w/ preexisting moderate/severe hepatic impairment. Fully investigate the cause of liver injury if hepatic impairment develops.

ADVERSE REACTIONS
W/O Tadalafil: peripheral edema, nasal congestion, flushing, sinusitis.
W/ Tadalafil: peripheral edema, headache, nasal congestion, cough, anemia, dyspepsia, bronchitis.

DRUG INTERACTIONS
Cyclosporine may increase exposure; limit dose of ambrisentan to 5mg qd when coadministered w/ cyclosporine.

PREGNANCY AND LACTATION
Pregnancy: Category X.
Lactation: Not for use in nursing.

MECHANISM OF ACTION
Endothelin receptor antagonist; highly selective for endothelin type-A (ET_A) receptor versus endothelin type-B (ET_B) receptor. ET_A and ET_B help mediate effects of endothelin-1 (ET-1) in the vascular smooth muscle and endothelium. Primary actions of ET_A are vasoconstriction and cell proliferation. Predominant actions of ET_B are vasodilation, antiproliferation, and ET-1 clearance.

PHARMACOKINETICS
Absorption: T_{max}=2 hrs. **Distribution:** Plasma protein binding (99%). **Metabolism:** Liver via CYP3A, 2C19, and UGTs 1A9S, 2B7S, and 1A3S. **Elimination:** $T_{1/2}$=9 hrs.

PATIENT CONSIDERATIONS

Assessment: Assess for IPF, anemia, hepatic impairment, pregnancy/nursing status, and possible drug interactions. Obtain baseline Hgb level.

Monitoring: Monitor for fluid retention, pulmonary edema, PVOD, hepatic impairment, and other adverse reactions. Obtain monthly pregnancy tests in females of reproductive potential during therapy and 1 month after discontinuation of treatment. Measure Hgb at 1 month after initiating therapy and periodically thereafter.

Counseling: Instruct on the risk of fetal harm when used in pregnancy and instruct to immediately contact physician if pregnancy is suspected. Inform female patients that drug is only available through a restricted program called the Letairis REMS program. Inform female patients that they must sign an enrollment form and that female patients of reproductive potential must comply w/ pregnancy testing and contraception requirements. Educate and counsel females of reproductive potential on the use of emergency contraception in the event of unprotected sex or known or suspected contraceptive failure. Advise prepubertal females to immediately report to physician any reproductive status changes. Instruct to contact physician if any symptoms of liver injury occur. Advise of the importance of Hgb testing and of other risks associated w/ therapy (eg, decreases in Hgb, Hct, and sperm count; fluid overload).

LEUKINE — sargramostim   **Rx**

Class: Granulocyte-macrophage colony stimulating factor (GM-CSF)

ADULT DOSAGE	**PEDIATRIC DOSAGE**
Acute Myelogenous Leukemia	Pediatric use may not have been established
Use following induction chemotherapy in older adult patients to shorten time to neutrophil recovery and to reduce the incidence of severe and life-threatening infections and infections resulting in death	
≥55 Years: **Usual:** 250mcg/m²/day IV over a 4-hr period starting approx on Day 11 or 4 days following completion of induction chemotherapy, if Day 10 bone marrow is hypoplastic w/ <15% blasts If 2nd cycle of induction chemotherapy is necessary, give 4 days after completion of chemotherapy if bone marrow is hypoplastic w/ <5% blasts Continue until ANC >1500 cells/mm³ for 3 consecutive days or max of 42 days D/C immediately if leukemic regrowth occurs	
Hematopoietic Progenitor Cell Mobilization **Mobilization into Peripheral Blood for Collection by Leukapheresis:** **Usual:** 250mcg/m²/day IV over 24 hrs or SQ qd; continue dosing at the same dose through the collection period Reduce dose by 50% if WBC >50,000 cells/mm³ Consider other mobilization therapy if adequate numbers of progenitor cells are not collected	
Post Peripheral Blood Progenitor Cell Transplantation: **Usual:** 250mcg/m²/day IV over 24 hrs or SQ qd beginning immediately following infusion of progenitor cells Continue until ANC >1500 cells/mm³ for 3 consecutive days is attained	
Myeloid Reconstitution Acceleration of myeloid recovery in patients w/ non-Hodgkin's lymphoma, acute lymphoblastic	

leukemia and Hodgkin's disease undergoing autologous bone marrow transplantation (BMT) or allogeneic BMT

Usual: 250mcg/m²/day IV over 2-hr period beginning 2-4 hrs after bone marrow infusion and not <24 hrs after last dose of chemotherapy/radiotherapy

Do not give until post marrow infusion ANC is <500 cells/mm³

Continue until ANC >1500 cells/mm³ for 3 consecutive days is attained

D/C immediately if blast cells appear or disease progression occurs

Bone Marrow Transplantation

Delayed or Failed Engraftment of Allogeneic or Autologous BMT:

Usual: 250mcg/m²/day IV over 2 hrs for 14 days; may repeat after 7 days off therapy if engraftment has not occurred

May give 500mcg/m²/day IV for 14 days after another 7 days off therapy if engraftment still has not occurred

D/C immediately if blast cells appear or disease progression occurs

------

DOSING CONSIDERATIONS

Adverse Reactions

Severe: Reduce dose by 50% or temporarily d/c until reaction abates if severe adverse reaction occurs

ADMINISTRATION

IV/SQ route

Preparation

1. Should be reconstituted aseptically w/ 1mL of diluent; contents of vials reconstituted w/ different diluents should not be mixed together
2. Lyophilized Leukine vials contain no antibacterial preservative, and therefore sol prepared w/ sterile water for inj should be administered as soon as possible, and w/in 6 hrs following reconstitution and/or dilution for IV infusion. The vial should not be reentered or reused. Do not save any unused portion for administration more than 6 hrs following reconstitution
3. Reconstituted sol prepared w/ bacteriostatic water for inj (0.9% benzyl alcohol) may be stored for up to 20 days at 2-8°C prior to use. Discard reconstituted sol after 20 days. Previously reconstituted sol mixed w/ freshly reconstituted sol must be administered w/in 6 hrs following mixing. Preparations containing benzyl alcohol should not be used in neonates
4. During reconstitution of lyophilized Leukine the diluent should be directed at the side of the vial and the contents gently swirled to avoid foaming during dissolution. Avoid excessive or vigorous agitation; do not shake
5. Should be used for SQ inj w/o further dilution. Dilution for IV infusion should be performed in 0.9% NaCl inj. If the final concentration is below 10mcg/mL, Albumin (Human) at a final concentration of 0.1% should be added to the saline prior to addition of drug to prevent adsorption to the components of the drug delivery system
6. To obtain a final concentration of 0.1% Albumin (Human), add 1mg Albumin (Human) per 1mL 0.9%NaCl inj (eg, use 1mL 5% Albumin [Human] in 50mL 0.9% NaCl inj
7. An inline membrane filter should not be used for IV infusion
8. In the absence of compatibility and stability information, no other medication should be added to infusion sol containing Leukine. Use only 0.9% NaCl inj to prepare IV infusion sol

STORAGE

2-8°C (36-46°F). Do not freeze/shake.

HOW SUPPLIED

Inj: 250mcg, 500mcg/mL

CONTRAINDICATIONS

Excessive leukemic myeloid blasts in bone marrow or peripheral blood (≥10%); hypersensitivity to GM-CSF, yeast-derived products or any component of the product; concomitant use w/ chemotherapy or radiotherapy.

WARNINGS/PRECAUTIONS

Contains benzyl alcohol, which has been associated with a fatal "gasping syndrome" in premature infants; avoid with neonates. Edema, capillary leak syndrome, pleural and/or pericardial effusion reported. May aggravate fluid retention in patients with preexisting pleural and pericardial effusions; caution with preexisting fluid retention, pulmonary infiltrate, and congestive heart failure (CHF). Monitor for respiratory symptoms during or immediately following infusion, especially with preexisting lung disease; reduce infusion rate by half if dyspnea occurs and d/c if respiratory symptoms worsen despite infusion rate reduction. Caution in patients with hypoxia. Occasional transient supraventricular arrhythmia reported; caution with preexisting cardiac disease. May induce elevation of SrCr or bilirubin and hepatic enzymes in patients with preexisting renal or hepatic dysfunction. Serious allergic or anaphylactic reactions reported; d/c immediately and initiate appropriate therapy. A syndrome characterized by respiratory distress, hypoxia, flushing, hypotension, syncope, and/or tachycardia reported following the 1st administration of therapy in a particular cycle. Interrupt or reduce

dose by 50% if ANC >20,000 cells/mm³ or if platelet count >500,000/mm³. Caution when used in any malignancy with myeloid characteristics due of the possibility of tumor growth potentiation. Effective in accelerating myeloid recovery in patients receiving bone marrow purged by anti-B lymphocyte monoclonal antibodies. Tumor cells may be released and reinfused into the patient in the leukapheresis product when used to mobilize PBPC.

ADVERSE REACTIONS

Fever, N/V, diarrhea, alopecia, rash, headache, stomatitis, anorexia, mucous membrane disorder, asthenia, malaise, abdominal pain, edema, HTN.

DRUG INTERACTIONS

See Contraindications. Caution with drugs that may potentiate myeloproliferative effects (eg, lithium, corticosteroids).

PREGNANCY AND LACTATION

Category C, caution in nursing.

MECHANISM OF ACTION

Granulocyte-macrophage colony stimulating factor; induces partially committed progenitor cells to divide and differentiate in the granulocyte-macrophage pathways which include neutrophils, monocytes/macrophages and myeloid-derived dendritic cells. Capable of activating mature granulocytes and macrophages and promoting the proliferation of megakaryocytic and erythroid progenitors.

PHARMACOKINETICS

Absorption: IV: (Liquid) C_{max}=5ng/mL, AUC=640ng/mL•min; (Lyophilized) C_{max}=5.4ng/mL, AUC=677ng/mL•min. SQ: C_{max}=1.5ng/mL, T_{max}=1-3 hrs; AUC=549ng/mL•min (liquid), 501ng/mL•min (lyophilized). **Elimination:** $T_{1/2}$=60 min (IV); 162 min (SQ).

PATIENT CONSIDERATIONS

Assessment: Assess for known hypersensitivity to the drug or yeast-derived products, excessive leukemic myeloid blasts in bone marrow/peripheral blood, fluid retention, pulmonary infiltrate, CHF, lung disease, any malignancy with myeloid characteristics, hypoxia, cardiac disease, pregnancy status, and possible drug interactions. Assess renal and hepatic function.

Monitoring: Monitor for edema, capillary leak syndrome, pleural/pericardial effusion, fluid retention aggravation, dyspnea or respiratory symptoms, supraventricular arrhythmia, allergic/anaphylactic reactions, and other adverse reactions. Monitor CBC with differential (including examination for the presence of blast cells) twice weekly and renal/hepatic function at least biweekly. Monitor body weight and hydration status carefully.

Counseling: Inform the person who will administer therapy of the proper dose, method of reconstitution, and administration if the medication is to be given outside the hospital. Instruct on the importance of proper disposal and caution against reuse of needles, syringes, drug product, and diluent if home use is prescribed. Inform of serious/common adverse reactions associated with therapy. Advise female patients of childbearing potential of the possible risks of therapy to the fetus.

LEUPROLIDE — leuprolide acetate   **Rx**

Class: Synthetic gonadotropin-releasing hormone (GnRH) analogue

OTHER BRAND NAMES

Lupron (Discontinued)

ADULT DOSAGE	PEDIATRIC DOSAGE
Advanced Prostate Cancer	Pediatric use may not have been established
Palliative Treatment of Advanced Prostatic Cancer:	
1mg (0.2mL or 20-unit mark) SQ qd	

ADMINISTRATION

SQ route

Rotate inj site periodically

Follow the pictorial directions on the administering the inj

STORAGE

<25°C (77°F). Do not freeze. Protect from light.

HOW SUPPLIED

Inj: 5mg/mL [2.8mL]

CONTRAINDICATIONS

Known hypersensitivity to GnRH, GnRH agonist analogs, or any of the excipients in leuprolide acetate inj; women who are or may become pregnant.

WARNINGS/PRECAUTIONS

Anaphylactic reactions reported. Suppresses pituitary-gonadal system at therapeutic doses. Contains benzyl alcohol; monitor for symptoms of hypersensitivity, usually local, at the inj site. Serum levels of testosterone increase initially; transient worsening of symptoms or occurrence of additional signs/symptoms of prostate cancer may develop during the 1st few weeks of treatment. May experience temporary increase in bone pain. Isolated cases of ureteral obstruction and spinal cord compression have been observed, which may contribute to paralysis with or without fatal complications. Closely monitor patients with metastatic vertebral lesions and/or urinary tract obstruction during 1st few weeks of therapy. Hyperglycemia, increased risk of developing diabetes/myocardial infarction, sudden cardiac death, and stroke reported. May prolong QT/QTc interval; consider benefits of therapy versus potential risks in patients with congenital long QT syndrome, congestive heart failure, frequent electrolyte abnormalities, and in patients taking drugs known to prolong the QT interval.

ADVERSE REACTIONS
Hot flashes, ECG changes/ischemia, general pain, peripheral edema, asthenia, high BP, constipation, headache, insomnia/sleep disorders, anorexia, urinary frequency/urgency, hematuria, N/V, anemia, bone pain.

PREGNANCY AND LACTATION
Category X, not for use in nursing.

MECHANISM OF ACTION
Synthetic gonadotropin-releasing hormone agonist; potent inhibitor of gonadotropin secretion. Following an initial stimulation of gonadotropins, chronic administration results in suppression of ovarian and testicular steroidogenesis.

PHARMACOKINETICS
Distribution: V_d=27L (IV bolus); plasma protein binding (43-49%). (M-I) T_{max}=2-6 hrs. **Metabolism:** M-I (major metabolite). **Elimination:** (3.75mg Depot Sus) Urine (<5% as parent and M-I); (1mg IV Bolus) $T_{1/2}$=3 hrs.

PATIENT CONSIDERATIONS
Assessment: Assess for previous hypersensitivity to drug, hypersensitivity to benzyl alcohol, metastatic vertebral lesions, urinary tract obstruction, cardiovascular disease (CVD), electrolyte abnormalities, and diabetes mellitus. Assess for drugs known to prolong QT interval, and pregnancy/nursing status. Correct electrolyte abnormalities. Obtain baseline serum testosterone, prostate-specific antigen (PSA) levels, and blood glucose levels.

Monitoring: Monitor for response to therapy. Monitor for signs/symptoms of a hypersensitivity reaction. Monitor for signs/symptoms of worsening prostate cancer, ureteral obstruction, spinal cord compression, signs/symptoms suggestive of CVD, and other adverse reactions. Periodically monitor serum testosterone, PSA levels, blood glucose and/or HbA1c, and changes in bone density. Monitor ECG and electrolytes periodically.

Counseling: Instruct to notify physician if any type of hypersensitivity reaction occurs. Advise not to d/c therapy even if feeling better. Instruct to contact physician if symptoms of hot flashes or new or worsening symptoms (eg, bone pain, increased difficulty in urinating, onset or aggravation of nerve symptoms) occur.

LEUPROLIDE PEDIATRIC — leuprolide acetate   Rx

Class: Synthetic gonadotropin-releasing hormone (GnRH) analogue

OTHER BRAND NAMES
Lupron (Discontinued)

PEDIATRIC DOSAGE
Central Precocious Puberty
Confirm clinical diagnosis prior to initiation of therapy
Initial: 50mcg/kg/day, administered as a single SQ inj
Titrate: Increase by 10mcg/kg/day if total downregulation is not achieved; this dose will be considered the maint dose

---

DOSING CONSIDERATIONS
Discontinuation
Consider before age 11 for females and age 12 for males

ADMINISTRATION
SQ route
Rotate inj site periodically

STORAGE
<25°C (77°F). Do not freeze. Protect from light.

HOW SUPPLIED
Inj: 5mg/mL [2.8mL]

CONTRAINDICATIONS
Known hypersensitivity to GnRH, GnRH agonist analogs, or any of the excipients in leuprolide acetate inj; women who are or may become pregnant.

WARNINGS/PRECAUTIONS
Anaphylactic reactions reported. An increase in clinical signs and symptoms may be observed during the early phase of therapy. Noncompliance/inadequate dosing may result in inadequate control of the pubertal process and the return of pubertal signs (eg, menses, breast development, testicular growth). Long-term consequences of inadequate control may include a further compromise of adult stature. Suppresses pituitary-gonadal system at therapeutic dose. Contains benzyl alcohol; monitor for symptoms of hypersensitivity, usually local, at the inj site.

ADVERSE REACTIONS
Inj-site reactions including abscess, emotional lability, vaginitis/vaginal bleeding/vaginal discharge, acne/seborrhea, general pain, rash including erythema multiforme, headache, vasodilation.

PREGNANCY AND LACTATION
Category X, not for use in nursing.

MECHANISM OF ACTION
Synthetic GnRH agonist; potent inhibitor of gonadotropin secretion. Following an initial stimulation of gonadotropins, chronic administration results in suppression of ovarian and testicular steroidogenesis.

PHARMACOKINETICS
Distribution: V_d=27L (IV bolus, adult male); plasma protein binding (43-49%). (M-I) T_{max}=2-6 hrs. **Metabolism:** M-I (major metabolite). **Elimination:** (3.75mg Depot Sus) Urine (<5% as parent and M-I) (adults); (1mg IV Bolus) $T_{1/2}$=3 hrs (adult male).

PATIENT CONSIDERATIONS
Assessment: Assess for previous hypersensitivity to drug and for hypersensitivity to benzyl alcohol. Assess pregnancy status. Confirm clinical diagnosis of CPP by a pubertal response to a GnRH stimulation test and bone age advanced 1 yr beyond the chronological age. Obtain baseline height and weight, sex steroid levels, adrenal steroid level, β human chorionic gonadotropin level, pelvic/adrenal/testicular ultrasound, and computerized tomography of the head.

Monitoring: Monitor for signs/symptoms of noncompliance. Monitor for signs/symptoms of a hypersensitivity reaction and for other adverse reactions.

Counseling: Instruct to notify physician if any type of a hypersensitivity reaction occurs. Inform parent/guardian of the importance of continuous therapy and that irregular dosing could restart the maturation process. Inform that a female patient may experience menses/spotting during the first 2 months of therapy and instruct to notify the physician immediately if bleeding continues beyond the 2nd month. Instruct to report any unusual signs/symptoms (eg, continued pubertal changes, substantial mood swings, behavioral changes).

LEXIVA — fosamprenavir calcium   Rx

Class: Protease inhibitor

ADULT DOSAGE
HIV-1 Infection

Combination w/ Other Antiretrovirals:
Therapy-Naive:
1400mg bid w/o ritonavir (RTV)
1400mg qd + RTV 200mg qd
1400mg qd + RTV 100mg qd
700mg bid + RTV 100mg bid
Protease Inhibitor-Experienced:
700mg bid + RTV 100mg bid

PEDIATRIC DOSAGE
HIV-1 Infection

Combination w/ Other Antiretrovirals:

Sus:
Protease Inhibitor-Naive (≥4 Weeks of Age) and Protease Inhibitor-Experienced (≥6 Months of Age):
<11kg: 45mg/kg bid + RTV 7mg/kg bid
11 to <15kg: 30mg/kg bid + RTV 3mg/kg bid
15 to <20kg: 23mg/kg bid + RTV 3mg/kg bid
≥20kg: 18mg/kg bid + RTV 3mg/kg bid
Max: 700mg bid + RTV 100mg bid

Protease Inhibitor-Naive (≥2 Years of Age):
30mg/kg bid w/o RTV

Tab:
Administering w/o RTV:
≥47kg: 1400mg bid

DOSING CONSIDERATIONS
Hepatic Impairment
Mild (Child-Pugh Score 5-6):
Therapy-Naive: Reduce dose to 700mg bid w/o RTV
Therapy-Naive/Protease Inhibitor-Experienced: Reduce dose to 700mg bid + RTV 100mg qd

Moderate (Child-Pugh Score 7-9):
Therapy-Naive: Reduce dose to 700mg bid w/o RTV
Therapy-Naive/Protease Inhibitor-Experienced: Reduce dose to 450mg bid + RTV 100mg qd

Severe (Child-Pugh Score 10-15):
Therapy-Naive: Reduce dose to 350mg bid w/o RTV
Therapy-Naive/Protease Inhibitor-Experienced: Reduce dose to 300mg bid + RTV 100mg qd

Other Important Considerations
Pediatrics:
Only administer to infants ≥38 weeks gestation and who have attained a postnatal age of 28 days
RTV Combination Treatment:
Tabs: May be used for patients ≥39kg
RTV Caps: May be used for patients ≥33kg

ADMINISTRATION
Oral route

Tab
Take w/ or w/o food.

Sus
Shake vigorously before using.
Adults: Take w/o food.
Pediatrics: Take w/ food.
Re-dose if emesis occurs w/in 30 min after dosing.

STORAGE
(Tab) 25°C (77°F); excursions permitted to 15-30°C (59-86°F). (Sus) 5-30°C (41-86°F). Do not freeze.

HOW SUPPLIED
Sus: 50mg/mL [225mL]; **Tab:** 700mg

CONTRAINDICATIONS

Clinically significant hypersensitivity (eg, Stevens-Johnson syndrome) to any of the components of this product or to amprenavir. Concomitant use w/ drugs that are highly dependent on CYP3A4 for clearance and for which elevated concentrations are associated w/ serious and/or life-threatening events (eg, alfuzosin, flecainide, propafenone, rifampin, dihydroergotamine, ergonovine, ergotamine, methylergonovine, cisapride, St. John's wort, lovastatin, simvastatin, lurasidone, pimozide, delavirdine, sildenafil when used for pulmonary arterial HTN, midazolam, triazolam). When used w/ RTV, refer to the individual monograph.

WARNINGS/PRECAUTIONS

Severe/life-threatening skin reactions, including Stevens-Johnson syndrome, reported; d/c if severe/life-threatening rashes or moderate rashes w/ systemic symptoms occur. Caution w/ known sulfonamide allergy. Use w/ RTV at higher-than-recommended doses should not be used due to possible transaminase elevations. May increase risk for transaminase elevations in patients w/ hepatitis B or C or marked transaminase elevations prior to treatment. New onset or exacerbation of diabetes mellitus (DM), hyperglycemia, and diabetic ketoacidosis reported. Immune reconstitution syndrome, autoimmune disorders (eg, Graves' disease, polymyositis, and Guillain-Barre syndrome) in the setting of immune reconstitution, redistribution/accumulation of body fat, and lipid elevations reported. Acute hemolytic anemia reported w/ amprenavir. Spontaneous bleeding w/ hemophilia A and B reported. Nephrolithiasis reported; consider temporarily interrupting or discontinuing therapy if signs/symptoms occur. Caution in the elderly. Not recommended for qd administration w/ RTV for adult protease inhibitor-experienced patients or any pediatric patients. Not recommended w/ or w/o RTV for protease inhibitor-experienced pediatric patients <6 months of age.

ADVERSE REACTIONS

Adults: Diarrhea, rash, N/V, headache.

DRUG INTERACTIONS

See Contraindications. Not recommended w/ CYP3A4 substrates w/ narrow therapeutic windows, nevirapine (w/o RTV), simeprevir, and salmeterol. Fosamprenavir/RTV is not recommended w/ boceprevir, fluticasone, paritaprevir/RTV/ombitasvir/dasabuvir, and high doses of ketoconazole or itraconazole. Avoid (w/ RTV) concomitant colchicine in patients w/ renal/hepatic impairment. May increase levels of simeprevir (w/ RTV), nevirapine, maraviroc, antiarrhythmics, trazodone, ketoconazole, itraconazole, colchicine, rifabutin, quetiapine (w/ RTV), benzodiazepines, calcium channel blockers, bosentan, atorvastatin, immunosuppressants, salmeterol, fluticasone, PDE-5 inhibitors, TCAs, and esomeprazole. May decrease levels of boceprevir, lopinavir, raltegravir, dolutegravir, methadone, ethinyl estradiol, atazanavir (w/ RTV), phenytoin, and paroxetine. May alter levels of warfarin; monitor INR. CYP3A4 inhibitors, indinavir, nelfinavir, and phenytoin (w/ RTV) may increase levels. CYP3A4 inducers (eg, rifampin), boceprevir, efavirenz, nevirapine, lopinavir/RTV, saquinavir, raltegravir, maraviroc, carbamazepine, phenobarbital, phenytoin, dexamethasone, H₂-receptor antagonists, and ethinyl estradiol/norethindrone may decrease levels. May require initiation or dose adjustments of insulin or oral hypoglycemics for treatment of DM. Refer to prescribing information for dosing modifications when used w/ certain concomitant therapies.

PREGNANCY AND LACTATION

Pregnancy: Category C.
Lactation: Not for use in nursing.

MECHANISM OF ACTION

HIV protease inhibitor; prodrug that is rapidly hydrolyzed to amprenavir. Binds to active site of HIV-1 protease and thereby prevents the processing of viral Gag and Gag-Pol polyprotein precursors, resulting in the formation of immature noninfectious viral particles.

PHARMACOKINETICS

Absorption: Administration of variable doses resulted in different parameters.
Distribution: Amprenavir: Plasma protein binding (90%). **Metabolism:** Gut, rapid hydrolysis to amprenavir and inorganic phosphate. Amprenavir: Liver via CYP3A4. **Elimination:** Amprenavir: Urine (14%, metabolites), (1%, unchanged), feces (75%, metabolites); $T_{1/2}$=7.7 hrs.

PATIENT CONSIDERATIONS

Assessment: Assess for hypersensitivity to the drug, sulfonamide allergy, hepatitis B or C, hepatic impairment, preexisting DM, hemophilia, lipid disorder, pregnancy/nursing status, and possible drug interactions. Obtain serum transaminase, TG, and cholesterol levels.

Monitoring: Monitor for signs/symptoms of skin reactions, hepatic toxicity, new onset or exacerbation of DM, hyperglycemia, diabetic ketoacidosis, immune reconstitution syndrome, autoimmune disorders, redistribution/accumulation of body fat, lipid elevations, nephrolithiasis, hemolytic anemia, and other adverse effects. In patients w/ hemophilia A or B, monitor for spontaneous bleeding events. Monitor TG, cholesterol, and serum transaminase levels periodically.

Counseling: Advise to report to physician the use of other prescription, OTC, or herbal products, particularly St. John's wort. Inform that use w/ PDE-5 inhibitors may increase risk of hypotension, visual changes, and priapism; instruct to contact physician if any of these symptoms occur. Advise patients taking hormonal contraceptives to use alternate contraceptive measures during therapy. Instruct to notify physician of any sulfa allergy. Inform that redistribution or accumulation of body fat may occur during therapy. Inform that therapy is not a cure for HIV-1 infection and that illnesses associated w/ HIV-1 infection may continue, including opportunistic infections. Advise to avoid doing things that can spread HIV-1 infection to others. Instruct not to breastfeed to prevent postnatal transmission. Advise not to alter the dose or d/c therapy w/o consulting physician. (Sus) Instruct to shake vigorously before each use and inform that refrigeration may improve the taste.

LONSURF — tipiracil/trifluridine

Rx

Class: Thymidine phosphorylase inhibitor/nucleoside metabolic inhibitor

ADULT DOSAGE

Metastatic Colorectal Cancer

Treatment of patients who have been previously treated w/ fluoropyrimidine-, oxaliplatin- and irinotecan-based chemotherapy, an anti-VEGF biological therapy, and if RAS wild-type, an anti-EGFR therapy

Initial: 35mg/m²/dose bid on Days 1-5 and Days 8-12 of each 28-day cycle until disease progression or unacceptable toxicity
Max: 80mg/dose (based on the trifluridine component)
Round dose to the nearest 5mg increment

PEDIATRIC DOSAGE

Pediatric use may not have been established

DOSING CONSIDERATIONS

Obtain CBC counts prior to and on Day 15 of each cycle

Do Not Initiate the Cycle Until:
ANC ≥1500/mm³ or febrile neutropenia is resolved
Platelets are ≥75,000/mm³
Grade 3 or 4 nonhematological adverse reactions are resolved to Grade 0 or 1

W/in a Treatment Cycle, Withhold for Any of the Following:
ANC <500/mm³ or febrile neutropenia
Platelets <50,000/mm³
Grade 3 or 4 nonhematological adverse reactions

After Recovery, Resume Therapy After Reducing the Dose by 5mg/m²/dose from the Previous Dose Level, if the Following Occur:
Febrile neutropenia
Uncomplicated Grade 4 neutropenia (which has recovered to ≥1500/mm³) or thrombocytopenia (which has recovered to ≥75,000/mm³) that results in >1 week delay in start of next cycle
Nonhematologic Grade 3 or Grade 4 adverse reaction except for Grade 3 nausea and/or vomiting controlled by antiemetic therapy or Grade 3 diarrhea responsive to antidiarrheal medication

Max of 3 dose reductions are permitted to a minimum dose of 20mg/m² bid. Do not escalate dose after it has been reduced.

ADMINISTRATION

Oral route
Take w/in 1 hr of completion of morning and evening meals.

STORAGE

20-25°C (68-77°F); excursions permitted to 15-30°C (59-86°F). If stored outside original bottle, discard after 30 days.

HOW SUPPLIED

Tab: (Trifluridine/Tipiracil) 15mg/6.14mg, 20mg/8.19mg.

WARNINGS/PRECAUTIONS

Severe and life-threatening myelosuppression consisting of anemia, neutropenia, thrombocytopenia, and febrile neutropenia reported; obtain CBC counts prior to and on Day 15 of each cycle of therapy and more frequently as clinically indicated. May cause fetal harm. Females of reproductive potential should use effective contraception during treatment.

ADVERSE REACTIONS

Anemia, neutropenia, asthenia/fatigue, N/V, thrombocytopenia, decreased appetite, diarrhea, abdominal pain, pyrexia.

PREGNANCY AND LACTATION

Pregnancy: Based on animal data and the drug's mechanism of action, therapy may cause fetal harm.
Lactation: There are no data to assess effects of drug or its metabolites on the breastfed infant or the effects on milk production. Due to the potential for serious adverse reactions in breastfeeding infants, women should not breastfeed during treatment and for 1 day following the final dose.
Reproductive Potential: Females of reproductive potential should use effective contraception during treatment. Males w/ female partners of reproductive potential should use condoms during treatment and for at least 3 months after the final dose.

MECHANISM OF ACTION

Tipiracil: Thymidine phosphorylase inhibitor; increases trifluridine exposure by inhibiting its metabolism by thymidine phosphorylase. **Trifluridine:** Nucleoside metabolic inhibitor; following uptake into cancer cells, trifluridine is incorporated into DNA, interferes w/ DNA synthesis and inhibits cell proliferation.

PHARMACOKINETICS

Absorption: Trifluridine: T_{max}=2 hrs. **Distribution:** Trifluridine: Plasma protein binding (>96%). Tipiracil: Plasma protein binding (<8%). **Metabolism:** Trifluridine: Mainly via thymidine phosphorylase. **Elimination:** Trifluridine: Urine (1.5% unchanged, 19.2% metabolite); $T_{1/2}$=2.1 hrs. Tipiracil: Urine (29.3% unchanged); $T_{1/2}$=2.4 hrs.

PATIENT CONSIDERATIONS

Assessment: Assess pregnancy/nursing status. Obtain CBC counts prior to each cycle.
Monitoring: Monitor for adverse reactions. Obtain CBC counts on Day 15 of each cycle and more frequently as clinically indicated.

Counseling: Advise to immediately contact healthcare provider if patients experience signs/symptoms of infection and advise to keep all appointments for blood tests. Advise not to take additional doses to make up for missed or held doses. Instruct to contact healthcare provider for severe or persistent N/V, diarrhea, or abdominal pain. Instruct to take w/in 1 hr after eating am and pm meals. Inform patient that anyone else who handles the medication should wear gloves. Advise pregnant women of the potential risk to the fetus. Instruct females of reproductive potential to use effective contraception during treatment. Instruct males w/ female partners of reproductive potential to use condoms during treatment and for at least 3 months after the final dose. Advise women not to breastfeed during treatment and for 1 day following the final dose.

LUCENTIS — ranibizumab   Rx

Class: Monoclonal antibody/vascular endothelial growth factor (VEGF)-A blocker

ADULT DOSAGE	PEDIATRIC DOSAGE
Neovascular (Wet) Age-Related Macular Degeneration	Pediatric use may not have been established
0.5mg (0.05mL of 10mg/mL sol) once a month (approx 28 days)	
May administer 3 monthly doses followed by less frequent dosing (eg, 4-5 doses on average in 9 months)	
May also administer 1 dose every 3 months after 4 monthly doses	
Macular Edema	
Following Retinal Vein Occlusion:	
0.5mg (0.05mL of 10mg/mL sol) once a month (approx 28 days)	
Diabetic Macular Edema	
0.3mg (0.05mL of 6mg/mL sol) once a month (approx 28 days)	
Diabetic Retinopathy	
Non-Proliferative/Proliferative Diabetic Retinopathy w/ Diabetic Macular Edema:	
0.3mg (0.05mL of 6mg/mL sol) once a month (approx 28 days)	

ADMINISTRATION
Intravitreal route

Preparation
1. All of vial contents are withdrawn through a 5-micron, 19-gauge filter needle attached to a 1-cc tuberculin syringe.
2. Discard filter needle after withdrawal of the vial contents and do not use for intravitreal inj.
3. Replace filter needle w/ a sterile 30-gauge x 1/2-inch needle for intravitreal inj.
4. Contents should be expelled until plunger tip is aligned w/ line that marks 0.05mL on the syringe.

Administration
1. Adequate anesthesia and a broad-spectrum microbicide should be given prior to inj.
2. Each vial should only be used for treatment of a single eye; if contralateral eye requires treatment, a new vial should be used and the sterile field, syringe, gloves, drapes, eyelid speculum, filter, and inj needles should be changed before administration to other eye.

STORAGE
2-8°C (36-46°F). Do not freeze. Protect from light. Store in the original carton until time of use.

HOW SUPPLIED
Inj: 6mg/mL, 10mg/mL

CONTRAINDICATIONS
Ocular or periocular infections. Known hypersensitivity to ranibizumab or any of the excipients in the medication.

WARNINGS/PRECAUTIONS
Endophthalmitis and retinal detachments may occur; always use proper aseptic inj technique. Increases in IOP reported both preinj and postinj (at 60 min); monitor IOP prior to/following inj and manage appropriately. Potential risk of arterial thromboembolic events (ATEs) (eg, nonfatal stroke, nonfatal MI, vascular death). Fatal events may occur in patients w/ DME and DR at baseline.

ADVERSE REACTIONS
Conjunctival hemorrhage, eye pain, vitreous floaters/detachment, increased IOP, intraocular inflammation, cataract, nasopharyngitis, foreign body sensation in eyes, eye irritation, lacrimation increased, visual disturbance/vision blurred, ocular hyperemia, dry eye, influenza, headache.

DRUG INTERACTIONS
Serious intraocular inflammation may develop when used adjunctively w/ verteporfin photodynamic therapy (PDT); incidence reported when drug was administered 7 days after verteporfin PDT.

PREGNANCY AND LACTATION
Pregnancy: Fetal harm has been seen in animal studies. Treatment may pose a risk to embryo-fetal development and reproductive capacity. Give to a pregnant woman only if clearly needed.

Lactation: It is not known if ranibizumab is present in human milk; caution in nursing.

MECHANISM OF ACTION
Monoclonal antibody/human vascular endothelial growth factor A (VEGF-A) blocker; binds to receptor-binding site of VEGF-A and prevents the interaction of VEGF-A w/ its receptors (VEGFR1 and VEGFR2) on the surface of endothelial cells, reducing endothelial cell proliferation, vascular leakage, and new blood vessel formation.

PHARMACOKINETICS
Absorption: (Neovascular Age-Related Macular Degeneration) C_{max}=1.7ng/mL, T_{max}=1 day. **Elimination:** $T_{1/2}$=9 days.

PATIENT CONSIDERATIONS
Assessment: Assess for ocular or periocular infections, hypersensitivity to the drug, pregnancy/nursing status, and possible drug interactions.

Monitoring: Monitor for signs/symptoms of endophthalmitis, retinal detachments, ATEs, hypersensitivity reactions, and other adverse reactions. Monitor IOP prior to and 30 min following inj using tonometry. Check for perfusion of the optic nerve head immediately after inj. Monitor following inj to permit early treatment should an infection occur.

Counseling: Inform about the risk of developing endophthalmitis following administration. Instruct to seek immediate care from an ophthalmologist if the eye becomes red, sensitive to light, painful, or develops a change in vision.

LUMIZYME — alglucosidase alfa   Rx

Class: Enzyme

> Life-threatening anaphylactic/severe hypersensitivity reactions occurred during and after infusions. Immune-mediated reactions presenting as proteinuria, nephrotic syndrome, and necrotizing skin lesions occurred following treatment. Closely observe patients during and after administration and be prepared to manage anaphylaxis and hypersensitivity reactions. Inform patients of the signs/symptoms of anaphylaxis and hypersensitivity/immune-mediated reactions and have them seek immediate medical care should any occur. Risk of serious acute exacerbation of cardiac or respiratory compromise due to fluid overload in infantile-onset Pompe disease patients with compromised cardiac or respiratory function; additional monitoring required.

ADULT DOSAGE	PEDIATRIC DOSAGE
Pompe Disease	**Pompe Disease**
Acid α-Glucosidase Deficiency:	**Acid α-Glucosidase Deficiency:**
Usual: 20mg/kg every 2 weeks as a 4-hr IV infusion	**Usual:** 20mg/kg every 2 weeks as a 4-hr IV infusion
Administer infusions in a step-wise manner using an infusion pump; refer to PI for recommended infusion volumes and rates at each step	Administer infusions in a step-wise manner using an infusion pump; refer to PI for recommended infusion volumes and rates at each step
Infusion Rate:	**Infusion Rate:**
Initial: ≤1mg/kg/hr	**Initial:** ≤1mg/kg/hr
Titrate: May increase by 2mg/kg/hr every 30 min, after tolerance is established	**Titrate:** May increase by 2mg/kg/hr every 30 min, after tolerance is established
Max: 7mg/kg/hr	**Max:** 7mg/kg/hr
Infusion rate may be slowed or temporarily stopped in the event of mild to moderate hypersensitivity reactions; in the event of anaphylaxis/severe hypersensitivity reaction, immediately d/c administration of alglucosidase alfa, and initiate appropriate medical treatment	Infusion rate may be slowed or temporarily stopped in the event of mild to moderate hypersensitivity reactions; in the event of anaphylaxis/severe hypersensitivity reaction, immediately d/c administration of alglucosidase alfa, and initiate appropriate medical treatment

ADMINISTRATION
IV route

For single use only; discard any unused product

Preparation Instructions
1. Determine the number of vials to be reconstituted based on the patient's weight and the recommended dose of 20mg/kg; refer to PI for calculation
2. Round up to the next whole vial to determine the total number of vials needed
3. Remove the required number of vials from the refrigerator and allow them to reach room temperature prior to reconstitution (approx 30 min)
4. Reconstitute each alglucosidase alfa vial by slowly injecting 10.3mL of sterile water for inj to the inside wall of each vial; each vial will yield a concentration of 5mg/mL. The total extractable dose per vial is 50mg/10mL
5. Avoid forceful impact of the water for inj on the powder and avoid foaming; this is done by slow drop-wise addition of the water for inj down the inside of the vial and not directly onto the lyophilized cake
6. Tilt and roll each vial gently; do not invert, swirl, or shake
7. Protect the reconstituted alglucosidase alfa sol from light
8. The reconstituted sol may occasionally contain some alglucosidase alfa particles (typically <10/vial) in the form of thin white strands or translucent fibers subsequent to the initial inspection and/or following dilution for infusion. These particles have been shown to contain alglucosidase alfa and may appear after the initial reconstitution step and increase over time. Studies have shown that these particles are removed via in-line filtration w/o having a detectable effect on the purity or strength

9. Dilute alglucosidase alfa in 0.9% NaCl for inj immediately after reconstitution, to a final concentration of 0.5-4mg/mL; refer to PI for recommended total infusion volume based on patient weight

10. Slowly withdraw the reconstituted sol from each vial; avoid foaming in the syringe

11. Remove airspace from the infusion bag to minimize particle formation due to the sensitivity of alglucosidase alfa to air-liquid interfaces

12. Add the reconstituted alglucosidase alfa sol slowly and directly into the NaCl sol; do not add directly into airspace that may remain w/in the infusion bag. Avoid foaming in the infusion bag

13. Gently invert or massage the infusion bag to mix; do not shake

Administration Instructions
Administer alglucosidase alfa using an in-line low-protein-binding 0.2μm filter
Do not infuse alglucosidase alfa in the same IV line w/ other product

Stability
If immediate use is not possible, the reconstituted and diluted sol is stable for up to 24 hrs at 2-8°C (36-46°F)

STORAGE
2-8°C (36-46°F). Reconstituted and Diluted Sol: 2-8°C (36-46°F); stable for up to 24 hrs. Protect from light. Do not freeze or shake.

HOW SUPPLIED
Inj: 50mg

WARNINGS/PRECAUTIONS
Anaphylaxis and hypersensitivity reactions observed up to 3 hrs after infusion. Immune-mediated reactions occurred several weeks to 3 yrs after initiation of infusion. Nephrotic syndrome secondary to membranous glomerulonephritis reported in patients who had persistently positive anti-rhGAA IgG antibody titers; perform periodic urinalysis. Consider discontinuation and initiate appropriate medical treatment if immune-mediated reactions occur. Risk of serious exacerbation of cardiac or respiratory compromise during infusion in patients with acute underlying respiratory illness or compromised cardiac and/or respiratory function; appropriate medical support and monitoring measures should be readily available. Ventricular arrhythmias and bradycardia, resulting in cardiac arrest or death, or requiring cardiac resuscitation or defibrillation reported in infantile-onset Pompe disease patients with cardiac hypertrophy during general anesthesia for central venous catheter placement; use caution when administering general anesthesia. Use extreme caution if readministering in patients who have experienced anaphylaxis or hypersensitivity reactions. Potential for immunogenicity.

ADVERSE REACTIONS
Anaphylactic/severe hypersensitivity/immune-mediated reactions, vomiting, rash, pyrexia, urticaria, HTN, decreased oxygen saturation, cough, tachypnea, tachycardia, hyperhidrosis, flushing, chest discomfort.

PREGNANCY AND LACTATION
Category C, caution in nursing.

MECHANISM OF ACTION
Enzyme; provides exogenous source of GAA. Binds to mannose-6-phosphate receptors on the cell surface, and is internalized and transported into lysosomes, where it undergoes proteolytic cleavage that results in increased enzymatic activity.

PHARMACOKINETICS
Absorption: C_{max}=162mcg/mL, AUC=811mcg•hr/mL. **Distribution:** Found in breast milk. **Elimination:** $T_{1/2}$=2.3 hrs.

PATIENT CONSIDERATIONS
Assessment: Assess for acute underlying respiratory illness or compromised cardiac and/or respiratory function, previous hypersensitivity, pregnancy/nursing status, and for any drug interactions. Obtain baseline vital signs.

Monitoring: Monitor for anaphylactic/severe hypersensitivity/immune-mediated reactions, exacerbation of cardiac/respiratory compromise, and other adverse reactions. Perform periodic urinalysis. Monitor for IgG antibody formation every 3 months for 2 yrs then annually thereafter. Monitor vital signs following every infusion rate increase and following the infusion.

Counseling: Advise that reactions related to administration and infusion, including life-threatening anaphylaxis and hypersensitivity/immune mediated reactions, may occur during and after treatment; inform of their signs/symptoms and instruct to seek medical care if any occur. Advise patients and caregivers that patients with underlying respiratory illness or compromised cardiac/respiratory function may be at risk of acute cardiorespiratory failure and may require close observation during and after administration. Encourage patients and caregivers to participate in the Pompe Registry.

LUPANETA PACK — leuprolide acetate/norethindrone acetate   Rx
Class: Progestin/synthetic gonadotropin-releasing hormone (GnRH) analogue

ADULT DOSAGE	PEDIATRIC DOSAGE
Endometriosis	Pediatric use may not have been established

Endometriosis

Initial management of painful symptoms and for management of symptom recurrence

Premenopausal Women and Women ≤65 Years:
3.75mg:
Leuprolide: 3.75mg IM once a month for up to 6 inj (6 months of therapy)
Norethindrone: 5mg PO qd for up to 6 months of therapy

11.25mg:
Leuprolide: 11.25mg IM once every 3 months for up to 2 inj (6 months of therapy)
Norethindrone: 5mg PO qd for up to 6 months of therapy

Initial course of treatment is not to exceed 6 months; if symptoms recur after initial course, consider retreatment for up to another 6 months

Max: Two 6-month courses

DOSING CONSIDERATIONS
Other Important Considerations
Different Formulations:
Do not administer 3 doses of the 3.75mg 1-month formulation simultaneously to mimic the pharmacological profile of the 11.25mg 3-month formulation. A fractional dose of the 3-month formulation is not equivalent to the same dose of the monthly formulation and should not be given

ADMINISTRATION
IM/Oral route

Reconstitution and Administration
Reconstitute and administer as a single IM inj; inject immediately or discard if not used w/in 2 hrs
Instructions:
1. Screw the white plunger into the end stopper until the stopper begins to turn
2. Holding the syringe upright, release the diluent by slowly pushing (6-8 sec) the plunger until the 1st middle stopper is at the blue line in the middle of the barrel
3. Keep the syringe upright and mix the microspheres (powder) thoroughly by gently shaking the syringe until the powder forms a uniform sus; the sus will appear milky
4. If the powder adheres to the stopper or caking/clumping is present, tap the syringe w/ finger to disperse; do not use if any of the powder has not gone into sus
5. Keeping the syringe upright, w/ the opposite hand pull the needle cap upward w/o twisting. Keep the syringe upright and advance the plunger to expel the air from the syringe; now the syringe is ready for inj
6. Administer IM into the gluteal area, anterior thigh, or deltoid; alternate inj sites
7. Once the syringe has been withdrawn, immediately activate the LuproLoc safety device by pushing the arrow on the lock upward towards the needle tip w/ the thumb or finger, until the needle cover of the safety device over the needle is fully extended and a click is heard or felt

If a blood vessel is accidentally penetrated, aspirated blood will be visible just below the luer lock and can be seen through the transparent LuproLoc safety device. If blood is present, remove the needle immediately; do not inj the medication

STORAGE
25°C (77°F); excursions permitted to 15-30°C (59-86°F).

HOW SUPPLIED
Inj: (Leuprolide) 3.75mg (1-Month), 11.25mg (3-Month); **Tab:** (Norethindrone) 5mg

CONTRAINDICATIONS
Hypersensitivity to GnRH, GnRH agonist analogs, any of the excipients in leuprolide acetate for depot suspension, or norethindrone acetate; undiagnosed abnormal uterine bleeding; known/suspected or planned pregnancy during the course of therapy; lactating women; known/suspected or history of breast cancer or other hormone-sensitive cancer; current or history of thrombotic or thromboembolic disorder; liver tumors or liver disease.

WARNINGS/PRECAUTIONS
Use for total of >12 months is not recommended. Retreatment w/ leuprolide alone is not recommended. Leuprolide induces a hypoestrogenic state that results in loss of decreased bone mineral density (BMD), some of which may not be reversible; concurrent use of norethindrone is effective in reducing the loss of BMD. May pose additional risk in women w/ major risk factors for decreased BMD (eg, chronic alcohol [>3 U/day] or tobacco use, strong family history of osteoporosis, or chronic use of drugs that can decrease BMD, such as anticonvulsants or corticosteroids); weigh risks and benefits carefully. Exclude pregnancy before initiating therapy. Leuprolide inhibits ovulation and stops menstruation, but contraception is not ensured; use nonhormonal methods of contraception. D/C norethindrone, pending examination, if a sudden partial or complete loss of vision or sudden onset of proptosis, diplopia, or migraine occurs. D/C Lupaneta Pack if examination reveals papilledema or retinal vascular lesions. Depression may occur or worsen; caution w/ history of clinical depression and d/c if depression recurs to a serious degree. Adverse events of asthma reported in women w/ preexisting histories of asthma, sinusitis, and environmental or drug allergies. Symptoms consistent w/ an anaphylactoid or asthmatic process reported. Assess and manage risk factors for cardiovascular (CV) disease before initiating treatment; closely monitor patients w/ risk factors for arterial vascular disease and/or venous thromboembolism (VTE). Increase in symptoms associated w/ endometriosis may be observed during initial days of therapy; should dissipate w/ continued therapy. Norethindrone may cause some degree of fluid retention; caution w/ conditions that might be influenced by this effect (eg, epilepsy, migraine, cardiac/renal dysfunctions). Convulsions reported w/ leuprolide. Suppresses pituitary-gonadal system; may affect diagnostic tests for pituitary gonadotropic and gonadal functions conducted during treatment and up to 3 months after discontinuation.

ADVERSE REACTIONS

Hot flashes, headache, asthenia, pain, altered bowel function, N/V, GI disturbance, weight gain, depression, dizziness, insomnia, decreased libido, nervousness, skin reactions, vaginitis.

DRUG INTERACTIONS

Drugs or herbal products that induce or inhibit certain enzymes, including CYP3A4, may decrease or increase the serum levels of norethindrone.

PREGNANCY AND LACTATION

Category X, not for use in nursing.

MECHANISM OF ACTION

Leuprolide: Synthetic gonadotropin-releasing hormone analogue; initial elevation followed by a prolonged suppression of pituitary gonadotropins. Repeated dosing at quarterly intervals results in decreased secretion of gonadal steroids, causing gonadal steroid-dependent tissues and functions to become quiescent. Norethindrone: Progestogen; induces secretory changes in an estrogen-primed endometrium.

PHARMACOKINETICS

Absorption: Norethindrone: C_{max}=26.19ng/mL, T_{max}=1.83 hrs, AUC=166.9ng/mL•hr.
Distribution: Leuprolide: Plasma protein binding (43-49%), V_d=27L (IV). Norethindrone: Sex hormone-binding globulin (36%), and albumin (61%); V_d=4L/kg; found in breast milk. **Metabolism:** Leuprolide; M-I (metabolite). Norethindrone: Extensive via reduction, followed by sulfate and glucuronide conjugation. **Elimination:** Leuprolide: (3.75mg) Urine (<5% as parent and M-I metabolite); $T_{1/2}$=3 hrs (1mg IV). Norethindrone: Urine and feces (primarily as metabolites); $T_{1/2}$=9 hrs.

PATIENT CONSIDERATIONS

Assessment: Assess for hypersensitivity to the drug, risk factors for decreased BMD, CV disease risk factors, risk factors for arterial vascular disease and/or VTE, any other conditions where treatment is contraindicated or cautioned, pregnancy/nursing status, and possible drug interactions. Assess if patient is using a nonhormonal method of contraception.

Monitoring: Monitor for symptoms of anaphylactoid reactions, asthmatic episodes, loss of vision, sudden onset of proptosis/diplopia/migraine, papilledema or retinal vascular lesions, convulsions, and other adverse reactions. Closely monitor w/ risk factors for arterial vascular disease and/or VTE. Evaluate BMD before retreatment.

Counseling: Inform of risks and benefits of therapy. Instruct not to use if allergic to drug, pregnant, planning a pregnancy, suspected to be pregnant, or if breastfeeding. Inform about the risk of loss of BMD and about limitation of treatment to two 6-month courses. Counsel about the risk to an exposed fetus and the need to use nonhormonal contraception. Instruct to d/c norethindrone if sudden loss of vision, double vision, or sudden migraine develops. Counsel on the possibility of development or worsening of depression during treatment. Counsel about the need for close monitoring if patient has CV risk factors, or conditions like epilepsy, migraine, or renal dysfunction. Instruct to notify physician if new or worsened symptoms develop after beginning therapy.

LUPRON DEPOT (GYN) — leuprolide acetate   Rx

Class: Synthetic gonadotropin-releasing hormone (GnRH) analogue

ADULT DOSAGE

Endometriosis

Including pain relief and reduction of endometriotic lesions

Women ≤65 Years:

3.75mg:
3.75mg leuprolide IM once a month for 6 months, alone or in combination w/ norethindrone acetate

11.25mg:
11.25mg leuprolide IM once every 3 months for 6 months, alone or in combination w/ norethindrone acetate

Symptom Recurrence After a Course of Therapy:

3.75mg:
Consider retreatment w/ a 6-month course of leuprolide administered monthly and norethindrone acetate 5mg/day; retreatment beyond this one 6-month course cannot be recommended

11.25mg:
Consider retreatment w/ a 6-month course of leuprolide administered every 3 months and norethindrone acetate 5mg/day; retreatment beyond this one 6-month course cannot be recommended

Leuprolide alone is not recommended for retreatment; if norethindrone acetate is contraindicated, then retreatment is not recommended

Uterine Leiomyomata (Fibroids)

Used concomitantly w/ iron therapy for the preoperative hematologic

PEDIATRIC DOSAGE

Pediatric use may not have been established

---

improvement of patients w/ anemia caused by uterine leiomyomata

Women ≤65 Years:
3.75mg:
3.75mg leuprolide IM once a month for up to 3 months

11.25mg:
Recommended dose is 1 inj

ADMINISTRATION

IM route

Different Formulations

Due to different release characteristics, a fractional dose of the 3-month depot formulation is not equivalent to the same dose of the monthly formulation and should not be given

Reconstitution and Administration

Reconstitute the lyophilized microspheres and administer as a single IM inj; inject immediately or discard if not used w/in 2 hrs

Instructions:

1. Screw the white plunger into the end stopper until the stopper begins to turn
2. Holding the syringe upright, release the diluent by slowly pushing (6-8 sec) the plunger until the 1st stopper is at the blue line in the middle of the barrel
3. Keep the syringe upright and mix the microspheres (powder) thoroughly by gently shaking the syringe until the powder forms a uniform sus; the sus will appear milky
4. If the powder adheres to the stopper or caking/clumping is present, tap the syringe w/ your finger to disperse; do not use if any of the powder has not gone into sus
5. Holding the syringe upright, w/ the opposite hand pull the needle cap upward w/o twisting
6. Keep the syringe upright and advance the plunger to expel the air from the syringe; now the syringe is ready for inj
7. After cleaning the inj site w/ an alcohol swab, administer the IM inj by inserting the needle at a 90° angle into the gluteal area, anterior thigh, or deltoid; alternate inj sites
NOTE: Aspirated blood would be visible just below the luer lock connection if a blood vessel is accidentally penetrated and can be seen through the transparent LuproLoc safety device. If blood is present, remove the needle immediately; do not inj the medication
8. Inject the entire contents of the syringe IM
9. Once the syringe has been withdrawn, immediately activate the LuproLoc safety device by pushing the arrow on the lock upward towards the needle tip w/ the thumb or finger, until the needle cover of the safety device over the needle is fully extended and a click is heard or felt

STORAGE

25°C (77°F); excursions permitted to 15-30°C (59-86°F). Reconstituted Sol: Discard if not used within 2 hrs.

HOW SUPPLIED

Inj: 3.75mg, (3-Month) 11.25mg

CONTRAINDICATIONS

Undiagnosed abnormal vaginal bleeding, women who are or may become pregnant, nursing women. When used with norethindrone acetate, refer to the individual monograph. Known hypersensitivity to GnRH, GnRH agonist analogues, or any of the excipients in leuprolide acetate inj.

WARNINGS/PRECAUTIONS

Exclude pregnancy before therapy. Use 11.25mg formulation only if hormonal suppression is required for at least 3 months; exposure should be limited to 6 months of therapy. Usually inhibits ovulation and menstruation but contraception is not insured; use nonhormonal methods of contraception. Increase in clinical signs and symptoms may occur during initial days of therapy. Symptoms consistent with an anaphylactoid or asthmatic process reported rarely. Use of therapy may pose an additional risk in patients with major risk factors for decreased bone mineral content (eg, chronic alcohol and/or tobacco use, strong family history of osteoporosis, chronic use of drugs that can reduce bone mass [eg, anticonvulsants, corticosteroids]); weigh risks and benefits before leuprolide acetate alone is instituted and consider concomitant therapy with norethindrone acetate 5mg/day; retreatment not advisable in patients with major risk factors for loss of bone mineral content. Retreatment of endometriosis beyond one 6-month course and use of drug alone for retreatment not recommended. Convulsions reported. Suppresses pituitary-gonadal system; may affect diagnostic tests for pituitary gonadotropic and gonadal functions during treatment and up to 3 months after discontinuation. With Norethindrone Acetate: D/C norethindrone acetate treatment if sudden partial or complete loss of vision or sudden onset of proptosis, diplopia, or migraine occurs. Thrombophlebitis and pulmonary embolism may occur. Caution with risk factors for cardiovascular disease (CVD) (eg, lipid abnormalities, cigarette smoking). Caution with a history of depression; d/c if severe depression occurs. May cause some degree of fluid retention; caution with conditions which might be influenced by this factor (eg, epilepsy, migraine, asthma, cardiac or renal dysfunction).

ADVERSE REACTIONS

Hot flashes, headache, dizziness, nervousness, weight changes, asthenia, joint disorder, vaginitis, depression, insomnia, N/V, pain, GI disturbances, skin reactions, edema.

PREGNANCY AND LACTATION

Category X, not for use in nursing.

MECHANISM OF ACTION

Synthetic gonadotropin-releasing hormone analog; initial stimulation followed by a prolonged suppression of pituitary gonadotropins. Repeated dosing results in decreased secretion of gonadal steroids, causing gonadal steroid-dependent tissues and functions to become quiescent.

PHARMACOKINETICS

Absorption: (3.75mg) C_{max}=4.6-10.2ng/mL, T_{max}=4 hrs. **Distribution:** Plasma protein binding (43-49%), V_d=27L (IV). **Metabolism:** M-I (major metabolite). **Elimination:** (3.75mg) Urine (<5% as parent and metabolite); $T_{1/2}$=3 hrs (1mg IV).

PATIENT CONSIDERATIONS

Assessment: Assess for hypersensitivity to the drug, abnormal vaginal bleeding, risk factors for decreased bone mineral density (BMD), pregnancy/nursing status, and possible drug interactions. Prior to concomitant therapy with norethindrone acetate, assess for risk factors for CVD, conditions which might be influenced by fluid retention, and for a history of depression.

Monitoring: Monitor for symptoms of anaphylactoid reactions, asthmatic episodes, loss of vision, sudden onset of proptosis/diplopia/migraine, thrombophlebitis, pulmonary embolism, worsening depression, convulsions, and other adverse reactions. Evaluate BMD prior to retreatment.

Counseling: Inform of risks and benefits of therapy. Instruct to notify physician if regular menstruation persists during therapy. Advise of pregnancy risks; instruct to use nonhormonal method of contraception. Instruct to avoid breastfeeding during use. Inform that if successive doses are missed, breakthrough bleeding or ovulation may occur with the potential for conception. Instruct to d/c therapy and consult physician if pregnancy occurs during treatment. Inform of the possibility of development or worsening of depression and occurrence of memory disorders. Inform of adverse events associated with hypoestrogenism and loss in BMD during therapy.

LUPRON DEPOT (ONCOLOGY) — leuprolide acetate   Rx

Class: Synthetic gonadotropin-releasing hormone (GnRH) analogue

ADULT DOSAGE	PEDIATRIC DOSAGE
Advanced Prostate Cancer	Pediatric use may not have been established
Palliative Treatment:	
7.5mg for 1-Month Administration: 1 inj every 4 weeks	
22.5mg for 3-Month Administration: 1 inj every 12 weeks	
30mg for 4-Month Administration: 1 inj every 16 weeks	
45mg for 6-Month Administration: 1 inj every 24 weeks	
Treatment is usually continued upon development of metastatic castration-resistant prostate cancer	

ADMINISTRATION

IM route

Do not use concurrently a fractional dose, or a combination of doses of any depot formulation due to different release characteristics.

Preparation and Administration

1. Screw the white plunger into the end stopper until stopper begins to turn.
2. Hold syringe upright and release diluent by slowly pushing (6-8 sec) plunger until 1st middle stopper is at the blue line in the middle of the barrel.
3. Keeping the syringe upright, mix the microspheres (powder) thoroughly by gently shaking the syringe until a uniform sus forms; the sus will appear milky.
4. Tap syringe w/ finger if powder adheres to the stopper or if caking/clumping is present; do not use if any powder has not gone into sus.
5. Keeping the syringe upright, pull the needle cap upward w/o twisting and advance the plunger to expel air from the syringe.
6. After cleaning the inj site w/ an alcohol swab, administer the inj by inserting the needle at a 90° angle into the gluteal area, anterior thigh, or deltoid; inj sites should be alternated. If a blood vessel is accidentally penetrated, aspirated blood will be visible just below the luer lock and can be seen through the transparent LuproLoc safety device. If blood is present, remove the needle immediately and do not inject the medication.
7. Inject the entire contents of the syringe.
8. Withdraw the needle; once the syringe has been withdrawn, immediately activate the LuproLoc safety device by pushing the arrow on the lock upward towards the needle tip w/ the thumb or finger until the needle cover of the safety device over the needle is fully extended and a click is heard or felt.

STORAGE

25°C (77°F); excursions permitted to 15-30°C (59-86°F). **Reconstituted Sus:** Discard if not used w/in 2 hrs.

HOW SUPPLIED

Inj: (1-Month) 7.5mg, (3-Month) 22.5mg, (4-Month) 30mg, (6-Month) 45mg

CONTRAINDICATIONS

Known hypersensitivity to GnRH agonists or any of the excipients in leuprolide acetate inj. Women who are or may become pregnant.

WARNINGS/PRECAUTIONS

May increase serum levels of testosterone during 1st weeks of treatment; transient worsening of symptoms may develop. Isolated cases of ureteral obstruction and spinal cord compression have been observed, which may contribute to paralysis

w/ or w/o fatal complications. May experience temporary increase in bone pain; manage symptomatically. Closely observe patients w/ metastatic vertebral lesions and/or urinary tract obstruction during the 1st few weeks of therapy. Hyperglycemia, increased risk of developing diabetes, MI, sudden cardiac death, and stroke reported. May prolong the QT/QTc interval; consider whether the benefits outweigh potential risks in patients w/ congenital long QT syndrome, CHF, or frequent electrolyte abnormalities, and in patients taking drugs known to prolong the QT interval. Convulsions reported in patients w/ and w/o a history of seizures, epilepsy, cerebrovascular disorders, or CNS anomalies or tumors, and in patients on concomitant medications that have been associated w/ convulsions (eg, bupropion, SSRIs). Suppresses pituitary-gonadal system; may affect diagnostic tests of pituitary gonadotropic and gonadal functions conducted during treatment and up to 3 months after discontinuation.

ADVERSE REACTIONS

Lupron Depot 7.5mg: General pain, hot flashes/sweats, GI disorders, edema, respiratory disorder, urinary disorder.
Lupron Depot 22.5mg: General pain, inj-site reaction, hot flashes/sweats, GI disorders, joint disorders, testicular atrophy, urinary disorders.
Lupron Depot 30mg: Asthenia, flu syndrome, general pain, headache, inj-site reaction, hot flashes/sweats, GI disorders, edema, skin reaction, urinary disorders.
Lupron Depot 45mg: Hot flush, inj-site pain, URI, fatigue.

PREGNANCY AND LACTATION

Pregnancy: Category X.
Lactation: Not for use in nursing.
Male Reproductive Potential: May reduce fertility based on animal studies and mechanism of action of drug.

MECHANISM OF ACTION

Synthetic GnRH; inhibitor of gonadotropin secretion. Following an initial stimulation, continuous administration results in suppression of ovarian and testicular steroidogenesis.

PHARMACOKINETICS

Absorption: Administration of various doses resulted in different parameters.
Distribution: Plasma protein binding (43-49%); V_d=27L (IV). **Elimination:** (3.75mg) Urine (<5% as parent and M-I metabolite); $T_{1/2}$=3 hrs (IV).

PATIENT CONSIDERATIONS

Assessment: Assess for hypersensitivity to the drug, metastatic vertebral lesions, urinary tract obstruction, diabetes mellitus, congenital long QT syndrome, electrolyte abnormalities, CHF, history of seizures, epilepsy, cerebrovascular disorders, CNS anomalies or tumors, and for the use of concomitant medications that have been associated w/ convulsions. Obtain baseline serum testosterone levels and prostate specific antigen (PSA) levels. Obtain baseline blood glucose and/or HbA1c levels. Correct electrolyte abnormalities.

Monitoring: Monitor response to drug and for signs/symptoms of worsening prostate cancer, ureteral obstruction, spinal cord compression, MI, stroke, QT interval prolongation, convulsions, and other adverse reactions. Monitor serum testosterone levels and PSA levels. Monitor blood glucose and/or HbA1c levels periodically. Consider periodic monitoring of ECGs and electrolytes.

Counseling: Inform of risks/benefits of therapy. Advise not to use if patient has experienced an allergic reaction to other similar drugs. Advise that therapy is usually continued, often w/ additional medication, after the development of metastatic castration-resistant prostate cancer. Inform of most common side effects associated w/ therapy. Advise that drug may cause impotence. Inform that the increase in testosterone occurring during 1st weeks of therapy may cause an increase in urinary symptoms or pain. Counsel that close medical attention during the 1st weeks of therapy is needed if metastatic cancer to the spine or urinary tract exists. Advise to notify physician if new or worsening of symptoms or adverse events occur.

LUPRON DEPOT-PED — leuprolide acetate   Rx

Class: Synthetic gonadotropin-releasing hormone (GnRH) analogue

PEDIATRIC DOSAGE
Central Precocious Puberty

≥2 Years:
Confirm clinical diagnosis prior to initiation of therapy

1-Month Administration:
Administer as a single IM inj once a month
≤25kg: 7.5mg
<25-≤37.5kg: 11.25mg
<37.5kg: 15mg

Titrate: Increase to the next available higher dose (eg, 11.25mg or 15mg at the next monthly inj) if adequate suppression is not achieved w/ the starting dose. Similarly, the dose may be adjusted w/ changes in body weight

Maint: Once a dose that results in adequate hormonal suppression is found, it can often be maintained for the duration of therapy in most children

3-Month Administration:
11.25mg or 30mg, as a single IM inj once every 3 months (12 weeks)

DOSING CONSIDERATIONS
Discontinuation
D/C at the appropriate age of onset of puberty

ADMINISTRATION
IM route

Rotate inj site periodically

Do not use partial syringes or a combination of syringes to achieve a particular dose

Reconstitution and Administration Instructions
1. Do not use the syringe if clumping or caking is evident; a thin layer of powder on the wall of the syringe is considered normal prior to mixing w/ the diluent
2. To prepare for inj, screw the white plunger into the end stopper until the stopper begins to turn
3. Hold the syringe upright and release the diluent by slowly pushing (6-8 sec) the plunger until the 1st stopper is at the blue line in the middle of the barrel
4. Keeping the syringe upright, mix the microspheres (powder) thoroughly by gently shaking the syringe until the powder forms a uniform sus; the sus will appear milky
5. If the powder adheres to the stopper or caking/clumping is present, tap the syringe w/ your finger to disperse; do not use if any of the powder has not gone into sus
6. Hold the syringe upright and pull the needle cap upward w/o twisting using the opposite hand
7. Keep the syringe upright and advance the plunger to expel the air from the syringe; now the syringe is ready for inj
8. Insert the needle at a 90° angle into the gluteal area, anterior thigh, or shoulder; alternate inj sites
NOTE: If a blood vessel is accidentally penetrated, aspirated blood would be visible just below the luer lock connection and can be seen through the transparent LuproLoc safety device; if blood is present, remove the needle immediately and do not inject the medication
9. Inject the entire contents of the syringe IM at the time of reconstitution. The sus settles very quickly following reconstitution; therefore, it should be mixed and used immediately
10. Once the syringe has been withdrawn, activate immediately the LuproLoc safety device by pushing the arrow on the lock upward towards the needle tip w/ the thumb or finger until the needle cover of the safety device is fully extended over the needle and a click is heard or felt

STORAGE
25°C (77°F); excursions permitted to 15-30°C (59-86°F). Reconstituted Sus: Discard if not used within 2 hrs.

HOW SUPPLIED
Inj: (1-Month) 7.5mg, 11.25mg, 15mg; (3-Month) 11.25mg, 30mg

CONTRAINDICATIONS
Women who are or may become pregnant. Known hypersensitivity to GnRH, GnRH agonist analogues, or any of the excipients in leuprolide acetate inj.

WARNINGS/PRECAUTIONS
Increase in clinical signs and symptoms of puberty may occur during the early phase of therapy due to initial rise in gonadotropins and sex steroids. Convulsions reported in patients with and without a history of seizures, epilepsy, cerebrovascular disorders, CNS anomalies or tumors, and in patients on concomitant medications that have been associated with convulsions (eg, bupropion, SSRIs). If noncompliant with drug regimen or dose is inadequate, gonadotropins and/or sex steroids may increase or rise above prepubertal levels. Suppresses pituitary-gonadal system; may affect diagnostic tests of pituitary gonadotropic and gonadal functions conducted during treatment and up to 6 months after discontinuation. Do not use partial syringes or combination of syringes to achieve a particular dose; each formulation and strength have different release characteristics.

ADVERSE REACTIONS
Inj-site reactions/pain, general pain, headache, acne/seborrhea, rash including erythema multiforme, emotional lability, vaginal bleeding/discharge/vaginitis, weight increase, mood altered.

PREGNANCY AND LACTATION
Category X, not for use in nursing.

MECHANISM OF ACTION
Synthetic gonadotropin-releasing hormone (GnRH) analog; potent inhibitor of gonadotropin secretion. Following an initial stimulation of gonadotropins, chronic stimulation results in suppression or "downregulation" of these hormones and consequent suppression of ovarian and testicular steroidogenesis.

PHARMACOKINETICS
Absorption: (7.5mg in adults) C_{max}=20ng/mL, T_{max}=4 hrs; (11.25mg) C_{max}=19.1ng/mL; (30mg) C_{max}=52.5ng/mL; (11.5mg and 30mg) T_{max}=1 hr. **Distribution:** Plasma protein binding (43-49%), V_d=27L (IV). **Metabolism:** M-I (major metabolite). **Elimination:** (3.75mg) Urine (<5% as parent and M-1 metabolite); $T_{1/2}$=3 hrs (1mg IV).

PATIENT CONSIDERATIONS
Assessment: Assess for history of seizures, cerebrovascular disorders, CNS anomalies or tumors. Assess for drug hypersensitivity and pregnancy status. Confirm clinical diagnosis of CPP by measuring blood concentrations of luteinizing hormone (LH) (basal or stimulated with a GnRH analog), sex steroids, and assessment of bone age versus chronological age. Obtain baseline evaluations of height and weight measurements, diagnostic imaging of the brain, pelvic/testicular/adrenal ultrasound, human chorionic gonadotropin levels, and adrenal steroid measurements to exclude congenital adrenal hyperplasia.

Monitoring: Monitor for convulsions and other adverse reactions. Monitor response with a GnRH stimulation test, basal LH or serum concentration of sex steroid levels; (1-Month) beginning 1-2 months following initiation of therapy, with changing doses, or potentially during therapy in order to confirm maintenance of efficacy or (3-Month) at months 2-3, month 6 and further as judged clinically appropriate, to ensure adequate suppression. (1-Month) Measure bone age for advancement every 6-12 months. (3-Month) Monitor height and bone age every 6-12 months.

Counseling: Counsel about the potential risk to the fetus if inadvertently used during pregnancy, or if patient becomes pregnant while taking the drug. Counsel about the importance of continuous therapy and adherence to drug administration schedule. Inform that signs of puberty (eg, vaginal bleeding) may occur during 1st few weeks of therapy; instruct to notify physician if symptoms continue beyond 2nd month. Inform about the most common side effects related to treatment. Advise that some pain and irritation is expected after inj; instruct to report if more severe or any unusual signs or symptoms occur. Advise parents/caregivers to notify physician if new or worsened symptoms develop after beginning treatment.

LUVERIS — lutropin alfa   Rx
Class: Recombinant human luteinizing hormone (LH)

ADULT DOSAGE	PEDIATRIC DOSAGE
Follicle Stimulation	Pediatric use may not have been
In Infertile Hypogonadotropic Hypogonadal Women w/ Profound Luteinizing Hormone Deficiency (<1.2 IU/L):	established
Usual: 75 IU w/ 75-150 IU of Gonal-f, given as 2 separate inj in the initial treatment cycle	
Treatment Duration: Should not exceed 14 days unless signs of imminent follicular development are present	
Administer human chorionic gonadotropin (hCG) 1 day after the last dose of lutropin alfa and Gonal-f; withhold hCG if the ovaries are abnormally enlarged or if excessive estradiol production occurs	
Max: 225 IU/day	

ADMINISTRATION
SQ route

Dissolve contents of 1 vial in 1mL sterile water for inj

Mix gently; do not shake

Administer entire contents of each vial SQ as separate inj

Use immediately after reconstitution; discard any unused reconstituted material

STORAGE
2-25°C (36-77°F). Protect from light. Use immediately after reconstitution.

HOW SUPPLIED
Inj: 75 IU

CONTRAINDICATIONS
Prior hypersensitivity to human LH preparations or one of their excipients, primary ovarian failure, uncontrolled thyroid or adrenal dysfunction, uncontrolled organic intracranial lesion (eg, pituitary tumor), abnormal uterine bleeding of undetermined origin, ovarian cyst/enlargement of undetermined origin, sex hormone dependent tumors of the reproductive tract and accessory organs, pregnancy.

WARNINGS/PRECAUTIONS
Should only be prescribed by physicians who are thoroughly familiar with infertility problems and management. Regularly monitor ovarian response with serum estradiol and ovary ultrasound. Mild to moderate uncomplicated ovarian enlargement that may be accompanied by abdominal distention and/or abdominal pain may occur; withhold hCG if ovaries are abnormally enlarged on the last day of therapy. May contribute to the development of ovarian hyperstimulation syndrome (OHSS); consider risk of treatment in women with risk factors of thromboembolic events, such as prior medical or family history, and monitor all patients for at least 2 weeks after hCG administration. Withhold hCG if there is evidence that OHSS may be developing, and d/c therapy and hospitalize patient if severe OHSS occurs. Multiple births and arterial thromboembolism may occur. Encourage couple to have intercourse daily, beginning on the day prior to hCG administration until ovulation becomes apparent.

ADVERSE REACTIONS
Headache, nausea, ovarian hyperstimulation, breast pain, abdominal pain, ovarian cyst, flatulence, inj-site reaction, pain, fatigue.

PREGNANCY AND LACTATION
Category X, caution in nursing.

MECHANISM OF ACTION
Recombinant human LH; comparable to human pituitary LH; supports follicle-stimulating hormone (FSH) induced follicular development.

PHARMACOKINETICS
Absorption: Absolute bioavailability (56%); T_{max}=4-16 hrs, C_{max}=1.1 IU/L, AUC=44hr·IU/L. **Distribution:** V_d=10L (IV). **Elimination:** Urine (<5%, unchanged); $T_{1/2}$=18 hrs.

PATIENT CONSIDERATIONS

Assessment: Assess for primary ovarian failure, uncontrolled thyroid/adrenal dysfunction or organic intracranial lesion, abnormal uterine bleeding or ovarian cyst/enlargement of undetermined origin, sex hormone dependent tumors of the reproductive tract and accessory organs, risk factors for thromboembolic events, hypersensitivity to drug, and pregnancy/nursing status.

Monitoring: Monitor for signs and symptoms of uncomplicated ovarian enlargement, OHSS, and other adverse reactions. Regularly monitor ovarian response with serum estradiol and ovary ultrasound.

Counseling: Inform of the duration of treatment and monitoring of condition that will be required. Advise of the risks of OHSS and multiple births, and other possible adverse reactions.

LYNPARZA — olaparib

Rx

Class: PARP inhibitor

ADULT DOSAGE

Advanced Ovarian Cancer

Monotherapy in Patients w/ Deleterious/Suspected Deleterious Germline BRCA Mutation Who Have Been Treated w/ ≥3 Prior Lines of Chemotherapy:

Usual: 400mg bid; continue until disease progression or unacceptable toxicity

Missed Dose

If patient misses a dose, instruct to take next dose at its scheduled time

PEDIATRIC DOSAGE

Pediatric use may not have been established

DOSING CONSIDERATIONS
Concomitant Medications
CYP3A Inhibitors:
Avoid concomitant use of strong/moderate inhibitors and consider alternatives w/ less CYP3A inhibition.
If Inhibitor Cannot Be Avoided:
Strong CYP3A Inhibitor: Reduce dose to 150mg bid
Moderate CYP3A Inhibitor: Reduce dose to 200mg bid

Adverse Reactions
To manage adverse reactions, consider dose interruption of treatment or dose reduction
Usual: 200mg bid; may reduce to 100mg bid if further dose reduction is required

ADMINISTRATION
Oral route

Swallow whole; do not chew, dissolve, or open.
Do not take if cap appears deformed or shows evidence of leakage.

STORAGE
25°C (77°F); excursions permitted to 15-30°C (59-86°F). Do not expose to >40°C (104°F); do not take the drug if it is suspected of having been exposed to >40°C (104°F).

HOW SUPPLIED
Cap: 50mg

WARNINGS/PRECAUTIONS
Myelodysplastic syndrome/acute myeloid leukemia (MDS/AML) reported. Do not start therapy until patients have recovered from hematological toxicity caused by previous chemotherapy (≤CTCAE Grade 1). For prolonged hematological toxicities, interrupt therapy and monitor blood counts weekly until recovery; if the levels have not recovered to ≤CTCAE Grade 1 after 4 weeks, refer to a hematologist for further investigations. D/C if MDS/AML is confirmed. Pneumonitis (including fatal cases) reported; interrupt treatment and initiate prompt investigation if new or worsening respiratory symptoms (eg, dyspnea, fever, cough, wheezing, radiological abnormality) occur. D/C if pneumonitis is confirmed. May cause fetal harm; avoid pregnancy while taking therapy. If contraceptive methods are being considered, use highly effective contraception during treatment and for at least 1 month following the last dose of therapy.

ADVERSE REACTIONS
Anemia, N/V, dyspepsia, abdominal pain/discomfort, decreased appetite, diarrhea, fatigue/asthenia, nasopharyngitis/URI, arthralgia/musculoskeletal pain, myalgia, lab abnormalities.

DRUG INTERACTIONS
Potentiation and prolongation of myelosuppressive toxicity w/ other myelosuppressive anticancer agents, including DNA damaging agents. Avoid w/ strong CYP3A inhibitors (eg, itraconazole, telithromycin, clarithromycin) and moderate CYP3A inhibitors (eg, amprenavir, ciprofloxacin, imatinib); if strong or moderate CYP3A inhibitors must be coadministered, reduce dose of olaparib. Avoid grapefruit and Seville oranges. Avoid w/ strong CYP3A inducers (eg, phenytoin, carbamazepine, St. John's wort) and moderate CYP3A4 inducers (eg, bosentan, efavirenz, modafinil); if a moderate CYP3A inducer cannot be avoided, be aware of a potential for decreased efficacy of olaparib.

PREGNANCY AND LACTATION
Category D, not for use in nursing.

MECHANISM OF ACTION
Poly (ADP-ribose) polymerase (PARP) inhibitor; inhibits PARP enzymes, including PARP1, PARP2, and PARP3, which are involved in normal cellular homeostasis (eg, DNA transcription, cell cycle regulation, DNA repair).

PHARMACOKINETICS
Absorption: Rapid. T_{max}=1-3 hrs. **Distribution:** V_d=167L; plasma protein binding (82%). **Metabolism:** Extensive; CYP3A4 (primary); oxidation (major) and glucuronide or sulfate conjugation. **Elimination:** Urine (44%, 15% unchanged), feces (42%, 6% unchanged); $T_{1/2}$=11.9 hrs.

PATIENT CONSIDERATIONS

Assessment: Assess pregnancy/nursing status, and for possible drug interactions. Assess for presence of deleterious or suspected deleterious germline BRCA-mutations. Obtain baseline CBC.

Monitoring: Monitor for MDS/AML, pneumonitis, and for other adverse reactions. For prolonged hematological toxicities, monitor blood counts weekly until recovery. Monitor CBC monthly.

Counseling: Instruct to take ud and to not take w/ grapefruit or Seville oranges. Advise to contact physician if experiencing any new or worsening respiratory symptoms, or signs of hematological toxicity or MDS/AML. Instruct to inform physician if patient is pregnant or becomes pregnant. Inform female patients of the risk to a fetus and potential loss of pregnancy. Advise females of reproductive potential to use effective contraception during therapy and for at least 1 month after receiving the last dose. Advise not to breastfeed while on therapy. Counsel that mild or moderate N/V is very common in patients receiving olaparib and that patients should contact their physician who will advise on available antiemetic treatment options.

MACUGEN — pegaptanib sodium

Rx

Class: Vascular endothelial growth factor (VEGF) inhibitor

ADULT DOSAGE
Neovascular (Wet) Age-Related Macular Degeneration
0.3mg once every 6 weeks into the eye to be treated

PEDIATRIC DOSAGE
Pediatric use may not have been established

ADMINISTRATION
Intravitreal route

Administer adequate anesthesia and a broad-spectrum microbicide prior to inj

STORAGE
2-8°C (36-46°F). Do not freeze or shake vigorously.

HOW SUPPLIED
Inj: 0.3mg/90µL

CONTRAINDICATIONS
Ocular or periocular infections, known hypersensitivity to pegaptanib sodium or any other excipient in this product.

WARNINGS/PRECAUTIONS
Endophthalmitis may occur; always use proper aseptic inj technique. Increases in intraocular pressure (IOP) seen within 30 min of inj; IOP and perfusion of the optic nerve head should be monitored and managed appropriately. Rare cases of anaphylaxis/anaphylactoid reactions, including angioedema, reported. For ophthalmic intravitreal inj only.

ADVERSE REACTIONS
Anterior chamber inflammation, blurred vision, cataract, conjunctival hemorrhage, corneal edema, eye discharge, eye irritation, eye pain, HTN, increased IOP, ocular discomfort, punctate keratitis, reduced visual acuity, visual disturbance, vitreous floaters.

PREGNANCY AND LACTATION
Category B, caution in nursing.

MECHANISM OF ACTION
Selective vascular endothelial growth factor (VEGF) antagonist; a pegylated modified oligonucleotide that adopts a three-dimensional conformation that enables it to bind to extracellular VEGF and thereby inhibit binding to VEGF receptors, which consequently suppresses pathological neovascularization.

PHARMACOKINETICS
Absorption: Slowly into circulation from the eye. C_{max}=80ng/mL, T_{max}=1-4 days, AUC=25mcg•hr/mL. **Metabolism:** Via endo- and exonucleases. **Elimination:** $T_{1/2}$=10 days.

PATIENT CONSIDERATIONS

Assessment: Assess for ocular or periocular infections, hypersensitivity to drug, and pregnancy/nursing status.

Monitoring: Monitor IOP and for perfusion of the optic nerve head. Monitor for signs/symptoms of endophthalmitis, anaphylaxis/anaphylactoid reactions, and other adverse events.

Counseling: Advise about risk of developing endophthalmitis following administration. Instruct to seek immediate care with ophthalmologist if eye becomes red, sensitive to light, painful, or if change in vision develops.

MAKENA — hydroxyprogesterone caproate   Rx

Class: Progestogen

ADULT DOSAGE
Preterm Birth

To reduce the risk of preterm birth in women w/ a singleton pregnancy who have a history of singleton spontaneous preterm birth

≥16 Years:
250mg (1mL) IM once weekly (every 7 days); inject slowly (over ≥1 min)

Begin treatment between 16 weeks, 0 days and 20 weeks, 6 days of gestation; continue administration once weekly until Week 37 (through 36 weeks, 6 days) of gestation or delivery, whichever occurs 1st

PEDIATRIC DOSAGE

Pediatric use may not have been established

ADMINISTRATION

IM route

Must be administered by a healthcare provider.

Instructions for Administration
1. Draw up 1mL of drug into a 3mL syringe w/ an 18-gauge needle.
2. Change the needle to a 21-gauge 1 1/2-inch needle.
3. Inject slowly (over ≥1 min) in the upper outer quadrant of the gluteus maximus; sol is viscous and oily.
4. Applying pressure to the inj site may minimize bruising and swelling.

If the 5mL multidose vial is used, discard any unused product 5 weeks after 1st use.

STORAGE

15-30°C (59-86°F). Protect from light. Store upright. **Multidose Vial:** Use w/in 5 weeks after 1st use.

HOW SUPPLIED

Inj: 250mg/mL [1mL, 5mL]

CONTRAINDICATIONS

Current/history of thrombosis or thromboembolic disorders, known/suspected/history of breast cancer or other hormone-sensitive cancer, undiagnosed abnormal vaginal bleeding unrelated to pregnancy, cholestatic jaundice of pregnancy, liver tumors (benign or malignant), active liver disease, uncontrolled HTN.

WARNINGS/PRECAUTIONS

Not intended for use in women w/ multiple gestations or other risk factors for preterm birth. D/C if an arterial/deep venous thrombotic or thromboembolic event occurs. Allergic reactions reported; consider discontinuation if such reactions occur. Decreased glucose tolerance observed; carefully monitor prediabetic/diabetic women. May cause fluid retention; carefully monitor women w/ conditions that might be influenced by this effect (eg, preeclampsia, epilepsy, migraine, asthma, cardiac/renal dysfunction). Monitor women who have a history of clinical depression; d/c if clinical depression recurs. Carefully monitor women who develop jaundice or HTN during treatment; consider whether the benefit of use warrants continuation. Not intended for use to stop active preterm labor.

ADVERSE REACTIONS

Inj-site pain/swelling/pruritus/nodule, urticaria, pruritus, nausea, diarrhea.

PREGNANCY AND LACTATION

Pregnancy: Category B.
Lactation: D/C at 37 weeks of gestation or upon delivery. Detectable amounts of progestins have been identified in the milk of mothers receiving progestin treatment.

MECHANISM OF ACTION

Synthetic progestin; has not been established.

PHARMACOKINETICS

Absorption: (Single 1000mg in non-pregnant females) C_{max}=27.8ng/mL; T_{max}=4.6 days. **Distribution:** Found in breast milk; extensive plasma protein binding. **Metabolism:** Extensive reduction, hydroxylation and conjugation via CYP3A4 and CYP3A5. **Elimination:** Feces (50%), urine (30%); (single 1000mg in non-pregnant females) $T_{1/2}$=7.8 days.

PATIENT CONSIDERATIONS

Assessment: Assess for multiple gestations or other risk factors for preterm birth, prediabetes/diabetes, conditions that might be influenced by fluid retention, history of clinical depression, and for other conditions where treatment is contraindicated or cautioned. Assess nursing status.

Monitoring: Monitor for arterial/deep venous thrombotic or thromboembolic events, allergic reactions, fluid retention, clinical depression, jaundice, HTN, and other adverse reactions. Monitor glucose levels in prediabetic and diabetic women.

Counseling: Explain that inj may cause pain, soreness, swelling, itching, or bruising. Instruct to contact physician if patient notices increased discomfort over time, oozing of blood or fluid, or if inflammatory reactions at the inj site occur.

MARQIBO — vincristine sulfate liposome   Rx

Class: Vinca alkaloid

> For IV use only; fatal if given by other routes. Death has occurred with intrathecal administration. Has different dosage recommendations than vincristine sulfate injection; verify drug name and dose prior to preparation and administration to avoid overdosage.

ADULT DOSAGE
Acute Lymphoblastic Leukemia

Philadelphia Chromosome-Negative:
In ≥2nd relapse or if disease has progressed following ≥2 antileukemia therapies

2.25mg/m² over 1 hr once every 7 days

PEDIATRIC DOSAGE

Pediatric use may not have been established

DOSING CONSIDERATIONS
Adverse Reactions
Peripheral Neuropathy:

Grade 3 or Persistent Grade 2:
Interrupt therapy
D/C therapy if peripheral neuropathy remains at Grade 3 or 4
Reduce dose to 2mg/m² if peripheral neuropathy recovers to Grade 1 or 2

Persistent Grade 2 After 1st Dose Reduction to 2mg/m²:
Interrupt therapy for up to 7 days
D/C therapy if peripheral neuropathy increases to Grade 3 or 4
Reduce dose to 1.825mg/m² if peripheral neuropathy recovers to Grade 1

Persistent Grade 2 After 2nd Dose Reduction to 1.825mg/m²:
Interrupt therapy for up to 7 days
D/C therapy if peripheral neuropathy increases to Grade 3 or 4
Reduce dose to 1.5mg/m² if peripheral neuropathy recovers to Grade 1

ADMINISTRATION

IV route

Do not use w/ in-line filters
Do not mix w/ other drugs

Preparation Instructions
1. Fill a water bath w/ water to a level of at least 8cm (3.2 inches) measured from the bottom and maintain this minimum water level throughout the procedure; water bath must remain outside of the sterile area
2. Place a calibrated thermometer in the water bath to monitor water temperature and leave it in the water bath until the procedure has been completed
3. Preheat water bath to 63-67°C; maintain this temperature until completion of the procedure using the calibrated thermometer
4. Vent the sodium phosphate inj vial w/ a sterile venting needle equipped w/ a sterile 0.2 micron filter or other suitable venting device in the biological safety cabinet; always position venting needle point well above liquid level before adding sphingomyelin/cholesterol liposome inj and vincristine sulfate inj
5. Withdraw 1mL of sphingomyelin/cholesterol liposome inj
6. Inject 1mL of sphingomyelin/cholesterol liposome inj into the sodium phosphate inj vial
7. Withdraw 5mL of vincristine sulfate inj
8. Inject 5mL of vincristine sulfate inj into the sodium phosphate inj vial
9. Remove the venting needle and gently invert the sodium phosphate inj vial 5 times to mix; do not shake
10. Fit flotation ring around the neck of the sodium phosphate inj vial
11. Confirm that the water bath temperature is at 63-67°C using the calibrated thermometer
12. Remove the sodium phosphate inj vial containing vincristine sulfate inj, sphingomyelin/cholesterol liposome inj, and sodium phosphate inj from the biological safety cabinet and place into the water bath for 10 min using the calibrated electronic timer. Monitor the temperature to ensure it is maintained at 63-67°C
13. Immediately after placing the sodium phosphate inj vial into the water bath, record the constitution start time and water temperature on the overlabel
14. At the end of the 10 min, confirm that the water temperature is 63-67°C using the calibrated thermometer and remove the vial from the water bath (use tongs to prevent burns) and remove the flotation ring
15. Record the final constitution time and the water temperature on the overlabel
16. Dry the exterior of the sodium phosphate inj vial w/ a clean paper towel, affix overlabel, and gently invert 5 times to mix; do not shake
17. Permit the constituted vial contents to equilibrate for at least 30 min to controlled room temperature
18. Vial now contains 5mg/31mL (0.16mg/mL) vincristine sulfate; return the vial back into the biological safety cabinet
19. Calculate the patient's dose based on the patient's actual BSA and remove the volume corresponding to the patient's dose from an infusion bag containing 100mL of D5 inj or 0.9% NaCl inj
20. Inject the dose into the infusion bag to result in a final volume of 100mL
21. Complete the information required on the infusion bag label and apply to the infusion bag
22. Finish administration of the diluted product w/in 12 hrs of the initiation of preparation
23. Empty, clean, and dry the water bath after each use
24. Deviations in temperature, time, and preparation procedures may fail to ensure proper encapsulation of vincristine sulfate into the liposomes. In the event that the preparation deviates from the instructions in the above steps, the components of the kit should be discarded and a new kit should be used to prepare the dose

STORAGE
2-8°C (36-46°F). Do not freeze.

HOW SUPPLIED
Inj: 5mg/31mL

CONTRAINDICATIONS
Demyelinating conditions including Charcot-Marie-Tooth syndrome, hypersensitivity to vincristine sulfate or any of the other components of this product, intrathecal administration.

WARNINGS/PRECAUTIONS
For IV use only. Administer through a secure and free-flowing venous access line only. May cause extravasation tissue injury; d/c immediately and consider local treatment measures. Sensory/motor neuropathies and orthostatic hypotension may occur; delay dose, reduce or d/c if worsening neuropathy occurs. Risk of neurologic toxicity is greater with preexisting neuromuscular disorders or when other drugs with risk of neurologic toxicity are given. Dose delay, reduction, or d/c may be necessary when severe fatigue develops. May cause myelosuppression; consider dose modification/reduction and supportive care measures if Grade 3 or 4 neutropenia, thrombocytopenia, or anemia develops. Tumor lysis syndrome reported; anticipate, monitor, and manage. Ileus, bowel obstruction, and colonic pseudo-obstruction reported; institute prophylactic bowel regimen and consider additional treatments. Fatal liver toxicity and elevated AST reported; reduce/interrupt therapy if toxicity occurs. Avoid use in pregnancy; may cause fetal harm. Caution with elderly.

ADVERSE REACTIONS
Constipation, nausea, pyrexia, fatigue, peripheral neuropathy, febrile neutropenia, diarrhea, anemia, decreased appetite, insomnia.

DRUG INTERACTIONS
Simultaneous administration of PO or IV phenytoin and antineoplastic chemotherapy combinations that include non-liposomal vincristine sulfate may reduce levels of phenytoin and increase seizure activity. Vincristine sulfate is a CYP3A and P-glycoprotein (P-gp) substrate. Avoid concomitant use with strong CYP3A inhibitors/inducers and potent P-gp inhibitors/inducers. Effect of concomitant use with potent P-gp inhibitors/inducers has not been investigated; it is likely that pharmacokinetics or pharmacodynamics will be altered.

PREGNANCY AND LACTATION
Category D, not for use in nursing.

MECHANISM OF ACTION
Vinca alkaloid; non-liposomal vincristine sulfate binds to tubulin, altering the tubulin polymerization equilibrium, resulting in altered microtubule structure and function; stabilizes spindle apparatus, preventing chromosome segregation, triggering metaphase arrest and inhibition of mitosis.

PHARMACOKINETICS
Absorption: C_{max}=1220ng/mL; AUC=14,566h•ng/mL. Elimination: Feces (69%, non-liposomal vincristine sulfate), urine (<8%).

PATIENT CONSIDERATIONS
Assessment: Assess for drug hypersensitivity, demyelinating conditions including Charcot-Marie-Tooth syndrome, preexisting neuromuscular disorders, hepatic dysfunction, pregnancy/nursing status, and possible drug interactions.

Monitoring: Monitor for symptoms of neuropathy (eg, hypoesthesia, hyperesthesia, paresthesia, hyporeflexia, areflexia, neuralgia, jaw pain, decreased vibratory sense), tumor lysis syndrome, CBC prior to each dose, LFTs, and other adverse reactions.

Counseling: Inform of the risks and benefits of therapy. Advise to report immediately any burning or local irritation during/after infusion. Instruct not to drive or operate machinery if fatigue and peripheral neuropathy are experienced. May cause constipation; advise to take with diet high in bulk fiber, fruits and vegetables, and adequate fluid intake as well as stool softener use (eg, docusate). Notify physician if constipation symptoms, fever, productive cough, decreased appetite, new or worsening symptoms of peripheral neuropathy are experienced. Advise women of childbearing potential to use effective contraceptive measures to prevent pregnancy; report immediately to physician if pregnant. Inform not to receive treatment while pregnant or breastfeeding; if wishes to restart breastfeeding after treatment, instruct to discuss appropriate timing with physician. Counsel to inform any current medications.

MATULANE — procarbazine hydrochloride   Rx

Class: Hydrazine derivative

> Administer only by or under the supervision of a physician experienced in the use of potent antineoplastic drugs. Adequate clinical and laboratory facilities should be available for proper monitoring of treatment.

ADULT DOSAGE	**PEDIATRIC DOSAGE**
Hodgkin Lymphoma	**Hodgkin Lymphoma**
Stage III/IV Hodgkin's Disease in Combination w/ other Anticancer Drugs:	**Stage III/IV Hodgkin's Disease in Combination with Other Anticancer Drugs:**
Initial: 2-4mg/kg/day as single or divided doses for 1st week (to minimize N/V), then 4-6mg/kg/day until max response is achieved or until WBC falls <4000/cmm or platelets fall <100,000/cmm	**Initial:** 50mg/m²/day for the 1st week, then 100mg/m²/day until max response is achieved or until leukopenia or thrombocytopenia occurs
Maint: 1-2mg/kg/day when max response is achieved; d/c upon	**Maint:** 50mg/m²/day when max response is achieved; d/c upon evidence of hematologic or other toxicity

evidence of hematologic or other toxicity
May resume at 1-2mg/kg/day after toxic side effects subside based on clinical evaluation and appropriate laboratory studies

MOPP (Nitrogen Mustard, Vincristine, Procarbazine, Prednisone) Regimen: 100mg/m² daily for 14 days

May resume therapy after toxic side effects have subsided

ADMINISTRATION
Oral route

STORAGE
15-30°C (59-86°F).

HOW SUPPLIED
Cap: 50mg

CONTRAINDICATIONS
Known hypersensitivity to procarbazine, inadequate marrow reserve as demonstrated by bone marrow aspiration.

WARNINGS/PRECAUTIONS
Hemolysis and appearance of Heinz-Ehrlich inclusion bodies in erythrocytes may occur. May cause fetal harm. Risks of secondary lung cancer may be multiplied by tobacco use. Allow an interval of ≥1 month without radiation/chemotherapeutic agent known to have marrow-depressant activity (determined by evidence of bone marrow recovery based on successive bone marrow studies) to elapse before initiating therapy. Undue toxicity may occur in patients with renal and/or hepatic impairment; consider hospitalization for the initial course of therapy when appropriate. Few cases of undue toxicity (eg, tremors, coma, convulsions) reported in pediatric patients. D/C promptly if CNS signs/symptoms (eg, paresthesias, neuropathies, confusion), leukopenia (WBC <4000/cmm), thrombocytopenia (platelets <100,000/cmm), hypersensitivity reaction, stomatitis, diarrhea, hemorrhage or bleeding tendencies occur. Bone marrow depression often occurs 2-8 weeks after start of therapy. If leukopenia occurs, hospitalization may be needed to prevent systemic infection.

ADVERSE REACTIONS
Leukopenia, anemia, thrombopenia, N/V.

DRUG INTERACTIONS
Avoid sympathomimetics, TCAs (eg, amitriptyline, imipramine), and other high tyramine-containing drugs/foods (eg, wine, yogurt, ripe cheese and bananas). Avoid with ethyl alcohol; Antabuse (disulfiram)-like reaction may occur. Caution with barbiturates, antihistamines, narcotics, hypotensive agents or phenothiazines to minimize CNS depression and possible potentiation. Second nonlymphoid malignancies reported with other chemotherapy and/or radiation. Azoospermia and antifertility effects reported with other chemotherapeutic agents for treating Hodgkin's disease.

PREGNANCY AND LACTATION
Category D, not for use in nursing.

MECHANISM OF ACTION
Hydrazine derivative; not established. May act by inhibition of protein, RNA, and DNA synthesis. May inhibit transmethylation of methyl groups of methionine into t-RNA. May also directly damage DNA.

PHARMACOKINETICS
Absorption: Rapid and complete; (30mg) T_{max}=60 min. Metabolism: Liver and kidney; oxidation, isomerization, hydrolysis; N-isopropylterephthalamic acid (metabolite). Elimination: (PO/IV) Urine (70% metabolite). $T_{1/2}$=10 min (IV).

PATIENT CONSIDERATIONS
Assessment: Assess for hypersensitivity to drug, leukopenia, thrombocytopenia, anemia, history of radiation or use of chemotherapeutic agent known to have marrow-depressant activity (<1 month prior to treatment initiation), pregnancy/nursing status, and possible drug interactions. Evaluate hepatic/renal function and perform bone marrow aspiration before initiating therapy.

Monitoring: Monitor for CNS signs/symptoms, leukopenia, thrombocytopenia, anemia, hypersensitivity reaction, stomatitis, diarrhea, hemorrhage or bleeding tendencies, toxicity, and other adverse reactions. Closely monitor pediatric patients for tremors, coma or convulsions. Closely monitor hematologic status (eg, Hgb, Hct, WBC, differential, reticulocytes and platelets) at least every 3 or 4 days. Repeat urinalysis, transaminase, alkaline phosphatase, and BUN tests at least weekly.

Counseling: Instruct to avoid alcoholic beverages while on therapy; inform that Antabuse (disulfiram)-like reaction may occur. Advise to avoid foods with known high tyramine content (eg, wine, yogurt, ripe cheese and bananas). Instruct to avoid OTC drugs containing antihistamines or sympathomimetics. Warn against use of prescription drugs without the knowledge and consent of physician. Advise to d/c tobacco use.

MEKINIST — trametinib   Rx

Class: Kinase inhibitor

ADULT DOSAGE	**PEDIATRIC DOSAGE**
Unresectable or Metastatic Melanoma with BRAF V600E or V600K Mutations	Pediatric use may not have been established
2mg qd, at the same time each day, as a single agent or in combination	

w/ dabrafenib until disease progression or unacceptable toxicity occurs

Missed Dose

Do not take a missed dose w/in 12 hrs of the next dose

DOSING CONSIDERATIONS

Adverse Reactions

Dose Reductions for Trametinib:

First Dose Reduction: 1.5mg qd

Second Dose Reduction: 1mg qd

Subsequent Modification: Permanently d/c if unable to tolerate 1mg qd

Febrile Drug Reaction:

Fever >104°F or Fever Complicated by Rigors, Hypotension, Dehydration, or Renal Failure: Withhold until fever resolves, then resume at same or lower dose level

Cutaneous:

Grade 3 or 4 Skin Toxicity or Intolerable Grade 2 Skin Toxicity: Withhold for up to 3 weeks; resume at a lower dose level if improved or permanently d/c if not improved

Cardiac:

Asymptomatic, Absolute Decrease in Left Ventricular Ejection Fraction (LVEF) of 10% or Greater from Baseline and Below Lower Limits of Normal (LLN) from Pretreatment Value: Withhold for up to 4 weeks. If improved to normal LVEF value, resume at a lower dose level. If not improved to normal LVEF value, permanently d/c

Symptomatic CHF/Absolute Decrease in LVEF >20% from Baseline that is Below LLN: Permanently d/c

Venous Thromboembolism (VTE):

Uncomplicated Deep Vein Thrombosis (DVT) or Pulmonary Embolism (PE): Withhold for up to 3 weeks; resume at a lower dose level if improved to Grade 0-1 or permanently d/c if not improved

Life-Threatening PE: Permanently d/c

Ocular Toxicities:

Retinal Pigment Epithelial Detachments: Withhold for up to 3 weeks. If improved, resume at same or lower dose level. If not improved, d/c or resume at a lower dose

Retinal Vein Occlusion (RVO): Permanently d/c

Pulmonary:

Interstitial Lung Disease (ILD)/Pneumonitis: Permanently d/c

Other:

Any Grade 3 Adverse Reactions or Intolerable Grade 2 Adverse Reactions: Withhold; resume at a lower dose level if improved to Grade 0-1 or permanently d/c if not improved

First Occurrence of Any Grade 4 Adverse Reaction: Withhold until adverse reaction improves to Grade 0-1, then resume at a lower dose level; or permanently d/c

Recurrent Grade 4 Adverse Reaction: Permanently d/c

Refer to dabrafenib PI for recommended dose modifications

ADMINISTRATION

Oral route

Take at least 1 hr ac or 2 hrs pc.

STORAGE

2-8°C (36-46°F). Do not freeze. Protect from moisture and light. Do not place in pill boxes.

HOW SUPPLIED

Tab: 0.5mg, 2mg

WARNINGS/PRECAUTIONS

See Dosing Considerations. Not indicated for treatment of patients who have received prior BRAF-inhibitor therapy. New primary malignancies, cutaneous and noncutaneous, may occur when therapy is administered w/ dabrafenib. Perform dermatologic evaluations prior to initiation of therapy when used w/ dabrafenib, every 2 months while on therapy, and for up to 6 months following discontinuation of the combination. Hemorrhages (eg, major hemorrhages defined as symptomatic bleeding in a critical area or organ) and VTE may occur. Cardiomyopathy, including cardiac failure, may occur; assess LVEF by echocardiogram or multigated acquisition (MUGA) scan before initiation of therapy as a single agent or w/ dabrafenib, 1 month after initiation, and then at 2- to 3-month intervals while on treatment. RVO reported and may lead to macular edema, decreased visual function, neovascularization, and glaucoma; urgently (w/in 24 hrs), perform ophthalmological evaluation for patient-reported loss of vision or other visual disturbances. Retinal pigment epithelial detachments may occur; retinal detachments may be bilateral and multifocal, occurring in the central macular region of the retina or elsewhere in the retina. Perform ophthalmological evaluation periodically and at any time a patient reports visual disturbances. ILD or pneumonitis reported; withhold therapy in patients presenting w/ new/progressive pulmonary symptoms and findings (eg, cough, dyspnea, hypoxia, pleural effusion, infiltrates) pending clinical investigations. Serious febrile reactions and fever of any severity accompanied by hypotension, rigors or chills, dehydration, or renal failure may occur when therapy is administered w/ dabrafenib. Monitor SrCr and other evidence of renal function during and following severe pyrexia. Administer antipyretics as secondary prophylaxis when resuming therapy if patient had a prior episode of severe febrile reaction or fever associated w/ complications. Administer corticosteroids (eg, prednisone 10mg daily)

for at least 5 days for second or subsequent pyrexia if temperature does not return to baseline w/in 3 days of onset of pyrexia, or for pyrexia associated w/ complications (eg, dehydration, hypotension, renal failure, severe chills/rigors), and there is no evidence of active infection. Serious skin toxicity may occur. Hyperglycemia may occur when therapy is administered w/ dabrafenib; monitor serum glucose levels upon initiation and as clinically appropriate in patients w/ preexisting diabetes or hyperglycemia. May cause fetal harm.

ADVERSE REACTIONS

Single Agent Trametinib: Rash, diarrhea, lymphedema, acneiform dermatitis, dry skin, pruritus, paronychia, stomatitis, abdominal pain, HTN, hemorrhage.

W/ Dabrafenib: Pyrexia, N/V, rash, chills, diarrhea, HTN, and peripheral edema.

PREGNANCY AND LACTATION

Pregnancy: May cause fetal harm.

Lactation: Advise women not to breastfeed during treatment and for 4 months following the last dose.

Reproductive Potential: Females of reproductive potential should use effective contraception during treatment and for 4 months after the last dose. May impair fertility in females of reproductive potential.

MECHANISM OF ACTION

Kinase inhibitor; reversible inhibitor of mitogen-activated extracellular signal regulated kinase 1 (MEK1) and MEK2 activation and of MEK1 and MEK2 kinase activity, which promote cellular proliferation. BRAF V600E mutations result in constitutive activation of the BRAF pathway, which includes MEK1 and MEK2. Inhibits BRAF V600 mutation-positive melanoma cell growth in vitro and in vivo. Use of trametinib and dabrafenib in combination resulted in greater growth inhibition of BRAF V600 mutation-positive melanoma cell lines in vitro and prolonged inhibition of tumor growth in BRAF V600 mutation positive melanoma xenografts compared w/ either drug alone.

PHARMACOKINETICS

Absorption: Absolute bioavailability (72%) (single 2mg dose); T_{max}=1.5 hrs (median). **Distribution:** Plasma protein binding (97.4%); V_d=214L. **Metabolism:** Predominantly via deacetylation alone or w/ mono-oxygenation or in combination w/ glucuronidation biotransformation pathways. Deacetylation is mediated by carboxylesterases and may also be mediated by other hydrolytic enzymes. **Elimination:** Feces (>80%), urine (<20%, <0.1% parent drug); $T_{1/2}$=3.9-4.8 days.

PATIENT CONSIDERATIONS

Assessment: Assess for diabetes, hyperglycemia, and pregnancy/nursing status. Confirm the presence of BRAF V600E or V600K mutation in tumor specimens. Assess if patient has received prior BRAF-inhibitor therapy. Perform dermatologic evaluations prior to initiation of therapy when used w/ dabrafenib. Assess LVEF by echocardiogram or MUGA scan before initiation of therapy as a single agent or w/ dabrafenib.

Monitoring: Monitor for new primary malignancies, hemorrhagic events, VTE, cardiomyopathy, retinal pigment epithelial detachment, RVO, ILD, pneumonitis, febrile reactions, skin toxicity, and other adverse reactions. When used w/ dabrafenib, perform dermatologic evaluations every 2 months while on therapy, and for up to 6 months following discontinuation of the combination. When therapy is given as a single agent or w/ dabrafenib, assess LVEF by echocardiogram or MUGA scan 1 month after initiation, and then at 2- to 3-month intervals while on treatment. Perform ophthalmological evaluation periodically and at any time a patient reports visual disturbances. Monitor serum glucose levels when therapy is used in combination w/ dabrafenib upon initiation and as clinically appropriate in patients w/ preexisting diabetes or hyperglycemia.

Counseling: Inform that evidence of BRAF V600E or V600K mutation w/in the tumor specimen is necessary to identify patients for whom treatment is indicated. Inform that combined use w/ dabrafenib may result in development of new primary cutaneous and noncutaneous malignancies, increase risk of intracranial and GI hemorrhage, increase risk of PE/DVT, and cause serious febrile reactions; advise to contact physician for signs/symptoms of malignancies, unusual bleeding/hemorrhage, venous thrombosis, or if fever develops. Advise to immediately report any signs/symptoms of heart failure, visual changes, cough or dyspnea, progressive or intolerable rash, and severe diarrhea. Advise of the need to undergo BP monitoring and to notify physician if symptoms of HTN develop. Inform of the risk of fetal harm if taken during pregnancy; instruct females of reproductive potential to use highly effective contraception during treatment and for 4 months after the last dose. Advise to contact physician if patient becomes pregnant, or if pregnancy is suspected. Instruct not to breastfeed during treatment and for 4 months after the last dose. Inform of the potential risk for impaired fertility. Instruct to take ud.

MENOPUR — menotropins Rx

Class: Follicle-stimulating hormone (FSH)/luteinizing hormone (LH)

ADULT DOSAGE	PEDIATRIC DOSAGE
Assisted Reproductive Technology	Pediatric use may not have been established
For development of multiple follicles and pregnancy in ovulatory women as part of an assisted reproductive technology cycle	
Initial: 225 IU/day starting on cycle day 2 or 3	
May be administered together w/ urofollitropin for inj; total initial dose of combined therapy should not exceed 225 IU (150 IU of menotropins	

and 75 IU of urofollitropin or 75 IU of menotropins and 150 IU of urofollitropin)
Titrate: Adjust the dose after 5 days, based on ovarian response
Do not make additional dose adjustments more frequently than every 2 days or by more than 150 IU/adjustment
Max: 450 IU (w/ or w/o urofollitropin)
Max Duration: 20 days

Continue treatment until adequate follicular development is evident, and then administer human chorionic gonadotropin (hCG)

Withhold hCG in cases where the ovarian monitoring suggests an increased risk of ovarian hyperstimulation syndrome (OHSS)

ADMINISTRATION
SQ route

Inject into the lower abdomen.

STORAGE
3-25°C (37-77°F) until dispensed. Protect from light.

HOW SUPPLIED
Inj: (Follicle stimulating hormone [FSH]/Luteinizing hormone [LH]) 75 IU/75 IU

CONTRAINDICATIONS
Prior hypersensitivity to this product or other menotropins products or one of the excipients. High levels of FSH indicating primary ovarian failure, presence of uncontrolled non-gonadal endocrinopathies (eg, thyroid, adrenal, or pituitary disorders), sex hormone dependent tumors of the reproductive tract and accessory organs, tumors of pituitary gland or hypothalamus, abnormal uterine bleeding of undetermined origin, ovarian cyst or enlargement not due to polycystic ovary syndrome, pregnancy.

WARNINGS/PRECAUTIONS
Prior to initiation of treatment, perform a complete gynecologic and endocrinologic evaluation, diagnose the cause of infertility, exclude the possibility of pregnancy or diagnosis of primary ovarian failure, and evaluate the fertility status of the male partner. Should only be used by physicians who are experienced in infertility treatment. May cause OHSS w/ or w/o pulmonary or vascular complications and multiple births. Abnormal ovarian enlargement may occur; use lowest effective dose. Prohibit intercourse in women w/ significant ovarian enlargement; hemoperitoneum resulting from rupture of ovarian cysts may occur. Hepatic dysfunction reported in association w/ OHSS. Withhold hCG if evidence of OHSS develops prior to hCG; monitor patients for at least 2 weeks after hCG administration. D/C therapy and hospitalize patient if serious OHSS occurs. Serious pulmonary conditions (eg, atelectasis, acute respiratory distress syndrome, exacerbation of asthma), thromboembolic events, ovarian torsion, and multi-fetal gestation/births reported. Risk of congenital malformations or ectopic pregnancy may be increased in women undergoing assisted reproductive technology. May increase risk of spontaneous abortions and ovarian neoplasms.

ADVERSE REACTIONS
Abdominal cramps/fullness/pain, headache, inj-site reaction/pain, nausea, OHSS.

PREGNANCY AND LACTATION
Pregnancy: Category X.
Lactation: Not for use in nursing.

MECHANISM OF ACTION
FSH/LH; produces ovarian follicular growth and maturation in women who do not have primary ovarian failure.

PHARMACOKINETICS
Absorption: (Single dose) C_{max}=8.5 mIU/mL, T_{max}=17.9 hrs, AUC=726.2 hr•mIU/mL. (Multiple dose) C_{max}=15 mIU/mL, T_{max}=8 hrs, AUC=622.7 hr•mIU/mL. **Elimination:** $T_{1/2}$=11-13 hrs (multiple dose).

PATIENT CONSIDERATIONS
Assessment: Assess for previous hypersensitivity to the drug, primary ovarian failure, uncontrolled non-gonadal endocrinopathies, tumors of pituitary gland or hypothalamus, pregnancy/nursing status, and any other conditions where treatment is contraindicated or cautioned. Perform a thorough gynecologic/endocrinologic evaluation, and diagnose the cause of infertility.

Monitoring: Monitor for OHSS, ovarian enlargement, ovarian torsion, pulmonary conditions, thromboembolic events, ectopic pregnancy, and other adverse reactions. Monitor for signs of ovulation and ovarian response. Monitor serum estradiol levels and perform vaginal ultrasound before dose adjustments.

Counseling: Instruct on the correct usage and dosing of therapy; caution not to change dosage or the schedule of administration unless instructed by the physician. Prior to therapy, inform about the time commitment and monitoring procedures necessary for treatment. Inform regarding the risks of OHSS, OHSS-associated symptoms (eg, lung, blood vessel problems), ovarian torsion, and multi-fetal gestation/birth w/ the use of the drug.

MITOMYCIN — mitomycin   Rx
Class: DNA synthesis inhibitor

> Administer under the supervision of a physician experienced in the use of cancer chemotherapeutic agents. Adequate diagnostic and treatment facilities should be readily available. Bone marrow suppression (eg, thrombocytopenia, leukopenia) is the most common and severe of the toxic effects. Hemolytic uremic syndrome (HUS) reported and may occur at any time during systemic therapy with mitomycin as a single agent or in combination with other cytotoxic drugs, mostly at doses ≥60mg of mitomycin. Blood product transfusion may exacerbate associated symptoms.

ADULT DOSAGE
Stomach/Pancreas Disseminated Adenocarcinoma

Combination w/ other approved chemotherapeutic agents and as palliative treatment when other modalities have failed

After Full Hematological Recovery from Any Previous Chemotherapy:
20mg/m² IV as a single dose via a functioning IV catheter at 6- to 8-week intervals
Max: 20mg/m²

Dose Adjustment Based on Nadir After Prior Dose:
Leukocytes 2000-2999/mm³ and Platelets 25,000-74,999/mm³: Administer 70% of prior dose
Leukocytes <2000/mm³ and Platelets <25,000/mm³: Administer 50% of prior dose

Do not repeat dose until leukocyte count has returned to 4000/mm³ and platelet count to 100,000/mm³

D/C therapy if disease continues to progress after 2 courses

PEDIATRIC DOSAGE
Pediatric use may not have been established

ADMINISTRATION
IV route

Preparation
1. Each vial contains either mitomycin 5mg and mannitol 10mg, mitomycin 20mg and mannitol 40mg, or mitomycin 40mg and mannitol 80mg; to administer, add sterile water for inj, 10mL, 40mL or 80mL respectively
2. Shake to dissolve; if product does not dissolve immediately, allow to stand at room temperature until sol is obtained

STORAGE
Dry Powder: 25°C (77°F); excursion permitted between 15-30°C (59-86°F). Protect from light. Avoid excessive heat >40°C (104°F). Reconstituted Sol: 2-8°C (36-46°F); discard after 14 days if refrigerated or after 7 days if unrefrigerated. Protect from light.

HOW SUPPLIED
Inj: 5mg, 20mg, 40mg

CONTRAINDICATIONS
Prior hypersensitivity or idiosyncratic reaction to this medication, thrombocytopenia, coagulation disorder, or an increase in bleeding tendency due to other causes.

WARNINGS/PRECAUTIONS
Not recommended as single-agent, primary therapy, or to replace appropriate surgery and/or radiotherapy. Avoid extravasation; cellulitis, ulceration, slough, and necrosis may result. Observe patient carefully and frequently during and after therapy. Monitor platelet count, WBC, differential count, and Hgb during therapy and for at least 8 weeks following therapy; if platelet count <100,000/mm³, WBC <4000/mm³, or progressive decline is seen in either, withhold further therapy until blood counts have recovered above these levels. Deaths due to septicemia as a result of leukopenia reported. Observe for evidence of renal toxicity; do not give with SrCr >1.7mg percent. Adult respiratory distress syndrome reported when given in combination with other chemotherapy and maintained at FIO_2 concentrations >50% perioperatively; exercise caution, using only enough oxygen to provide adequate arterial saturation. Monitor fluid balance; avoid overhydration. Bladder fibrosis/contraction reported with intravesical administration. Caution in elderly.

ADVERSE REACTIONS
Bone marrow suppression, HUS, inj site cellulitis, stomatitis, alopecia, fever, anorexia, N/V.

DRUG INTERACTIONS
See Boxed Warning. Acute SOB and severe bronchospasm reported following administration of vinca alkaloids in patients who had previously or simultaneously received mitomycin.

PREGNANCY AND LACTATION
Safety not known in pregnancy, not for use in nursing.

MECHANISM OF ACTION
DNA synthesis inhibitor; selectively inhibits DNA synthesis. At high concentrations, cellular RNA and protein synthesis are also suppressed.

PHARMACOKINETICS
Absorption: C_{max}=2.4mcg/mL (30mg), 1.7mcg/mL (20mg), 0.52mcg/mL (10mg).
Metabolism: Liver. **Elimination:** Urine (10% unchanged); $T_{1/2}$=17 min (30mg).

PATIENT CONSIDERATIONS

Assessment: Assess for previous hypersensitivity/idiosyncratic reaction to the drug, thrombocytopenia, coagulation disorder, increase in bleeding tendency due to other causes, renal impairment, pregnancy/nursing status, and possible drug interactions. Obtain baseline platelet count, WBC count, differential, and Hgb.

Monitoring: Monitor for bone marrow suppression, HUS, renal toxicity, adult respiratory distress syndrome, and other adverse reactions. Monitor platelet count, WBC count, differential count and Hgb during therapy and for 8 weeks following therapy. Monitor fluid balance and hydration status.

Counseling: Inform about the risks and benefits of therapy. Advise of the potential toxicities of the drug, particularly bone marrow suppression. Instruct to notify physician if pregnant/nursing. Advise to contact physician if any adverse reactions develop while on therapy.

MITOSOL — mitomycin   Rx

Class: DNA synthesis inhibitor

ADULT DOSAGE
Ocular Surgery

Adjunct to Ab Externo Glaucoma Surgery:
Usual: Apply fully saturated sponges equally to treatment area (approx 10mm x 6mm +/- 2mm), in a single layer (w/ use of surgical forceps), for 2 min

PEDIATRIC DOSAGE
Pediatric use may not have been established

ADMINISTRATION
Topical application to surgical site of glaucoma filtration surgery

Reconstitution
- Add 1mL of sterile water for inj, then shake to dissolve; if product does not dissolve immediately, allow to stand at room temperature until product dissolves into sol.
- Stable for 1 hr at room temperature.

STORAGE
20-25°C (68-77°F). Avoid excessive heat. Protect from light.

HOW SUPPLIED
Sol: 0.2mg/mL

CONTRAINDICATIONS
Pregnancy, history of hypersensitivity to mitomycin.

WARNINGS/PRECAUTIONS
Not for intraocular administration. Use in concentrations >0.2mg/mL or use for >2 min may lead to unintended corneal and/or scleral damage. Direct contact with the corneal endothelium will result in cell death. Increased risk of post-operative hypotony. May have higher risk of lenticular change and cataract formation if used in phakic patients.

ADVERSE REACTIONS
Bleb ulceration, encapsulated/cystic bleb, bleb-related infection, corneal endothelial damage, epithelial defect, cataract development, retinal pigment epithelial tear, wound dehiscence, hyphema, retinal hemorrhage, macular edema, sclera thinning/ulceration.

PREGNANCY AND LACTATION
Pregnancy: Category X.
Lactation: Not for use in nursing.

MECHANISM OF ACTION
DNA synthesis inhibitor; cellular RNA and protein synthesis may also be suppressed.

PHARMACOKINETICS
Metabolism: (Systemic) Liver. **Elimination:** (Inj) Urine (10% unchanged).

PATIENT CONSIDERATIONS

Assessment: Assess for previous hypersensitivity to the drug and pregnancy/nursing status.

Monitoring: Monitor for corneal and/or scleral damage if used in concentrations >0.2mg/mL or >2 min. Monitor for post-operative hypotony, lenticular change, cataract formation, and other adverse reactions.

Counseling: Inform of benefits and risks of therapy. Instruct to notify physician if pregnant, planning to become pregnant, or if nursing.

MITOXANTRONE — mitoxantrone   Rx

Class: Topoisomerase II inhibitor

Administer under the supervision of a physician experienced in the use of cytotoxic chemotherapy agents. Should be given slowly into a freely flowing IV infusion; never give SQ, IM, or intra-arterially. Severe local tissue damage may occur if there is extravasation. Not for intrathecal use; severe injury with permanent sequelae may occur. Except for acute nonlymphocytic leukemia (ANLL) treatment, do not give to patients with baseline neutrophil counts of <1500 cells/mm³. Perform frequent peripheral blood cell counts. Potentially fatal congestive heart failure (CHF) may occur either during therapy or months to yrs after termination of therapy. Cardiotoxicity risk increases with cumulative dose, presence or history of cardiovascular disease (CVD), radiotherapy to mediastinal/pericardial area, previous therapy with other anthracyclines or anthracenediones, or use of other cardiotoxic drugs; may occur whether or not cardiac risk factors are present. Assess for cardiac signs/symptoms by history, physical examination, and ECG prior to start of therapy. Obtain baseline quantitative evaluation of left ventricular ejection fraction (LVEF). Increases the risk of developing secondary acute myeloid leukemia. Multiple Sclerosis (MS) Patients: Assess for cardiac signs/symptoms by history, physical examination, and ECG, and perform quantitative reevaluation of LVEF prior to each dose. Avoid with a baseline LVEF below the lower limit of normal, and in patients who have experienced either a drop in LVEF to below the lower limit of normal or a clinically significant reduction in LVEF during therapy. MS patients should not receive a cumulative dose >140mg/m² and should undergo yearly quantitative LVEF evaluation after stopping therapy to monitor for late-occurring cardiotoxicity.

OTHER BRAND NAMES
Novantrone (Discontinued)

ADULT DOSAGE
Multiple Sclerosis

For reducing neurologic disability and/or frequency of clinical relapses in patients w/ secondary (chronic) progressive, progressive relapsing, or worsening relapsing-remitting multiple sclerosis

Usual: 12mg/m² as a short (approx 5-15 min) IV infusion every 3 months

Hormone-Refractory Prostate Cancer

Combination w/ corticosteroids is indicated as initial chemotherapy for the treatment of patients w/ pain related to advanced hormone-refractory prostate cancer

Usual: 12-14mg/m² as a short IV infusion every 21 days

Acute Non-Lymphocytic Leukemia

Combination w/ other approved drug(s) for initial therapy of acute nonlymphocytic leukemia; this category includes myelogenous, promyelocytic, monocytic, and erythroid acute leukemias

Induction:
Usual: 12mg/m²/day IV infusion on Days 1-3 and 100mg/m² of cytarabine as a continuous 24-hr infusion on Days 1-7

2nd induction course may be given in the event of an incomplete antileukemic response; administer for 2 days and cytarabine for 5 days using the same daily dosage levels

If severe/life-threatening nonhematologic toxicity is observed during the 1st induction course, withhold 2nd induction course until toxicity resolves

Consolidation Therapy:
12mg/m²/day IV infusion on Days 1 and 2 and cytarabine 100mg/m2 as a continuous 24-hr infusion on Days 1-5

Administer 1st course approx 6 weeks after final induction course, and the 2nd course 4 weeks after the 1st course

PEDIATRIC DOSAGE
Pediatric use may not have been established

DOSING CONSIDERATIONS
Hepatic Impairment
Multiple Sclerosis Patients:
Abnormal LFTs: Not recommended for use

ADMINISTRATION
IV route

Do not mix in the same infusion w/ other drugs
Discard unused infusion sol immediately

Dilution and Administered Instructions
1. Dilute to at least 50mL w/ either 0.9% NaCl inj or 5% dextrose inj
2. Mitoxantrone inj (concentrate) may be further diluted into D5W, normal saline, or D5 w/ normal saline and used immediately
3. Introduce the diluted sol slowly into the tubing as a freely running IV infusion of 0.9% NaCl inj or D5 inj over a period of not less than 3 min
4. Tubing should be attached to a butterfly needle or other suitable device and inserted preferably into a large vein; avoid veins over joints or in extremities w/ compromised venous or lymphatic drainage if possible

Extravasation
If any signs or symptoms of extravasation have occurred, immediately terminate the inj or infusion and restarted in another vein
Extravasation may occur w/ or w/o an accompanying stinging or burning sensation even if blood returns well on aspiration of the infusion needle; if it is known or suspected that extravasation has occurred, it is recommended that intermittent ice packs be placed over the area of extravasation and that the affected extremity be elevated

Handling Precautions
Skin accidentally exposed to mitoxantrone should be rinsed copiously w/ warm water and if the eyes are involved, standard irrigation techniques should be used immediately

STORAGE
20-25°C (68-77°F) in upright position. Do not freeze. Multidose Use: Remaining undiluted portion should be stored no longer than 7 days between 15-25°C (59-77°F) or 14 days under refrigeration. Do not freeze. Discard unused infusion sol immediately.

HOW SUPPLIED
Inj: 2mg/mL [10mL, 12.5mL, 15mL]

CONTRAINDICATIONS
Prior hypersensitivity to mitoxantrone.

WARNINGS/PRECAUTIONS
Not indicated in patients with primary progressive MS. Myelosuppression may occur at any dose. Severe myelosuppression will occur when used in high doses (>14mg/m^2/day x 3 days). Lab and supportive services must be available for hematologic and chemistry monitoring and adjunctive therapies, including antibiotics. Blood and blood products must be available to support patients during the expected period of medullary hypoplasia and severe myelosuppression. Assure full hematologic recovery before undertaking consolidation therapy and monitor patients closely during this phase. Avoid with preexisting myelosuppression resulting from prior drug therapy unless benefit warrants the risk of further medullary suppression. Local/regional neuropathy, some irreversible, following intra-arterial inj reported. Avoid in MS patients with hepatic impairment; use caution in other patients with hepatic impairment. Functional cardiac changes (eg, decreased LVEF) reported. May cause fetal harm; confirm negative pregnancy status in women with MS prior to each administration. Systemic infections should be treated concomitantly with or just prior to therapy. Hyperuricemia may occur in leukemia treatment; monitor serum uric acid levels and institute hypouricemic therapy prior to initiation of therapy. Caution in elderly.

ADVERSE REACTIONS
CHF, cardiotoxicity, nausea, alopecia, menstrual disorder, upper respiratory infection, urinary tract infection, stomatitis, arrhythmia, diarrhea, constipation, back pain, abnormal ECG, headache, sinusitis.

DRUG INTERACTIONS
See Boxed Warning. Occurrence of secondary myeloid leukemia may be more common when given in combination with deoxyribonucleic acid (DNA)-damaging antineoplastic agents. Risk of developing treatment-related acute myeloid leukemia with other cytotoxic agents and radiotherapy.

PREGNANCY AND LACTATION
Category D, not for use in nursing.

MECHANISM OF ACTION
Topoisomerase II inhibitor; intercalates into DNA through hydrogen bonding, causing crosslinks and strand breaks. Also interferes with RNA and is a potent inhibitor of topoisomerase II, an enzyme responsible for uncoiling and repairing damaged DNA.

PHARMACOKINETICS
Distribution: V$_d$>1000L/m^2; plasma protein binding (78%); found in breast milk.
Elimination: Urine (11%, 65% unchanged, 35% monocarboxylic and dicarboxylic acid derivatives and their glucuronide conjugates), feces (25%, unchanged or inactive metabolites); T$_{1/2}$=23-215 hrs.

PATIENT CONSIDERATIONS
Assessment: Assess for hypersensitivity to drug, history of CVD, mediastinal/pericardial radiotherapy, previous therapy with other anthracyclines or anthracenediones, hepatic impairment, preexisting myelosuppression, infections, pregnancy/nursing status, and possible drug interactions. Assess for cardiac signs/symptoms by history, physical examination, and ECG. Obtain baseline quantitative evaluation of LVEF, LFTs, and CBC with platelets. In leukemia patients, obtain baseline serum uric acid level.

Monitoring: Monitor for signs/symptoms of cardiotoxicity, bone marrow suppression, secondary leukemias, and other adverse reactions. Monitor for cardiac signs/symptoms by history, physical examination, ECG, quantitative evaluation of LVEF, LFTs, and CBC with platelets prior to each dose. Monitor patients closely during consolidation therapy. In patients with leukemia, monitor uric acid levels. MS patients should undergo yearly quantitative LVEF evaluation after stopping therapy to monitor for late-occurring cardiotoxicity.

Counseling: Instruct to read medication guide prior to initiating treatment and prior to each infusion. Instruct to take only ud. Advise that therapy may cause myelosuppression; inform of the signs/symptoms of myelosuppression. Advise that therapy may cause CHF that may lead to death even in people who have never had heart problems, and inform of the signs/symptoms of CHF. Advise MS patients that they should receive cardiac monitoring prior to each dose and yearly after stopping therapy. Inform that drug may impart blue-green color to urine for 24 hrs after administration and that patient should expect this during therapy. Explain that bluish discoloration of the sclera may also occur. Inform of the signs/symptoms of myelosuppression and CHF. Advise women with MS who are capable of becoming pregnant to have a pregnancy test prior to each dose, and the results known before receiving each dose.

MODERIBA — ribavirin
Class: Nucleoside analogue

Rx

Not for monotherapy treatment of chronic hepatitis C (CHC) virus infection. Primary toxicity is hemolytic anemia. Anemia associated w/ therapy may result in worsening of cardiac disease and lead to fatal and nonfatal MIs. Avoid w/ history of significant/unstable cardiac disease. Contraindicated in women who are pregnant and in male partners of pregnant women. Extreme care must be taken to avoid pregnancy during therapy and for 6 months after completion of therapy in both female patients and in female partners of male patients who are taking therapy. Use at least 2 reliable forms of effective contraception during treatment and for 6 months after discontinuation.

ADULT DOSAGE
Chronic Hepatitis C with Compensated Liver Disease
Combination w/ Peginterferon Alfa-2a:
Not Previously Treated w/ Interferon Alpha:
Monoinfection:
Genotypes 1, 4:
<75kg: 1000mg/day in 2 divided doses
≥75kg: 1200mg/day in 2 divided doses
Treatment Duration: 48 weeks
Genotypes 2, 3:
800mg/day in 2 divided doses
Treatment Duration: 24 weeks
HIV Coinfection:
800mg/day
Treatment Duration: 48 weeks
(regardless of genotype)

PEDIATRIC DOSAGE
Chronic Hepatitis C with Compensated Liver Disease
Combination w/ Peginterferon Alfa-2a:
Not Previously Treated w/ Interferon Alpha:
Monoinfection:
5-17 Years:
23-33kg: 200mg qam and 200mg qpm
34-46kg: 200mg qam and 400mg qpm
47-59kg: 400mg qam and 400mg qpm
60-74kg: 400mg qam and 600mg qpm
≥75kg: 600mg qam and 600 mg qpm
Patients who reach their 18th birthday while receiving combination therapy should remain on the pediatric dosing regimen through the completion of therapy

Treatment Duration:
Genotypes 2, 3: 24 weeks
Other Genotypes: 48 weeks

DOSING CONSIDERATIONS
Renal Impairment
Adults:
CrCl 30-50mL/min: Alternating doses, 200mg and 400mg qod
CrCl<30mL/min or Hemodialysis: 200mg/day

Adverse Reactions
W/O Cardiac Disease:
Hgb <10g/dL:
Adults: 200mg qam and 400mg qpm
Pediatrics:
23-33kg: 200mg qam
34-46kg: 200mg qam and 200mg qpm
47-59kg: 200mg qam and 200mg qpm
60-74kg: 200mg qam and 400mg qpm
≥75kg: 200mg qam and 400mg qpm

Hgb <8.5g/dL:
Adults and Pediatrics: D/C ribavirin

W/ History of Stable Cardiac Disease:
Hgb Decrease of ≥2g/dL During any 4-Week Treatment Period:
Adults: 200mg qam and 400mg qpm
Pediatrics:
23-33kg: 200mg qam
34-46kg: 200mg qam and 200mg qpm
47-59kg: 200mg qam and 200mg qpm
60-74kg: 200mg qam and 400mg qpm
≥75kg: 200mg qam and 400mg qpm

Hgb <12g/dL After 4 Weeks at Reduced Dose:
Adults and Pediatrics: D/C ribavirin

Adults:
If ribavirin has been withheld due to either a lab abnormality or clinical adverse reaction, may attempt to restart at 600mg/day and further increase to 800mg/day; not recommended to increase to the original assigned dose (1000-1200mg)
Pediatrics:
Upon resolution of a lab abnormality or clinical adverse reaction, may attempt to increase ribavirin dose to the original dose. If ribavirin has been withheld due to a lab abnormality or clinical adverse reaction, may make attempt to restart ribavirin at 1/2 the full dose

Discontinuation
Consider if at least a 2 log$_{10}$ HCV RNA reduction from baseline by Week 12 is not achieved
Consider if HCV RNA levels remain detectable after treatment Week 24
D/C if hepatic decompensation develops during treatment

ADMINISTRATION
Oral route

Take w/ food
Refer to peginterferon alfa-2a labeling for dosage and administration instructions

STORAGE
25°C (77°F); excursions permitted between 15-30°C (59-86°F).

HOW SUPPLIED
Tab: 200mg, 400mg, 600mg

CONTRAINDICATIONS
Women who are or may become pregnant, men whose female partners are pregnant, hemoglobinopathies (eg, thalassemia major, sickle cell anemia), and in combination w/ didanosine. When used w/ peginterferon alfa-2a, refer to the individual monograph.

WARNINGS/PRECAUTIONS
Combination therapy is associated w/ significant adverse reactions (eg, severe depression and suicidal ideation, hemolytic anemia, suppression of bone marrow

function, autoimmune/infectious/ophthalmologic/cerebrovascular disorders, pulmonary dysfunction, colitis, pancreatitis, diabetes). Do not start therapy unless a negative pregnancy test has been obtained immediately prior to therapy. Caution w/ baseline risk of severe anemia (eg, spherocytosis, history of GI bleeding). Caution w/ preexisting cardiac disease; suspend or d/c therapy if cardiovascular status deteriorates. Risk of hepatic decompensation and death in CHC patients w/ cirrhosis. Severe acute hypersensitivity reactions and serious skin reactions reported. D/C w/ hepatic decompensation, confirmed pancreatitis, severe hypersensitivity, or if signs/symptoms of severe skin reactions develop. Pulmonary disorders (eg, dyspnea, pulmonary infiltrates, pneumonitis, pulmonary HTN, pneumonia) reported. Closely monitor if pulmonary infiltrates/function impairment develop and d/c if appropriate. Decreases in height and weight reported in pediatric patients.

ADVERSE REACTIONS
Hemolytic anemia, fatigue/asthenia, neutropenia, headache, pyrexia, myalgia, irritability/anxiety/nervousness, insomnia, alopecia, rigors, N/V, anorexia.

DRUG INTERACTIONS
See Contraindications. Closely monitor for treatment associated toxicities (eg, hepatic decompensation) w/ nucleoside reverse transcriptase inhibitors; consider dose reduction or discontinuation of peginterferon alfa-2a and/or ribavirin. Severe neutropenia and severe anemia reported w/ zidovudine; consider discontinuation of zidovudine if appropriate. Severe pancytopenia and bone marrow suppression reported w/ azathioprine; monitor CBC, including platelet counts, weekly for the 1st month, twice monthly for the 2nd and 3rd months of treatment, then monthly or more frequently if dosage or other therapy changes are necessary; d/c peginterferon alfa-2a, ribavirin, and azathioprine if pancytopenia develops.

PREGNANCY AND LACTATION
Category X, not for use in nursing.

MECHANISM OF ACTION
Nucleoside analogue; not established. Has direct antiviral activity in tissue culture against many RNA viruses; increases mutation frequency in the genomes of several RNA viruses and ribavirin triphosphate inhibits HCV polymerase in a biochemical reaction.

PHARMACOKINETICS
Absorption: C_{max}=2748ng/mL; T_{max}=2 hrs; AUC=25,361ng•hr/mL. **Elimination:** $T_{1/2}$=120-170 hrs.

PATIENT CONSIDERATIONS
Assessment: Assess for hemoglobinopathies, autoimmune hepatitis, hepatic decompensation, baseline risk of severe anemia, history of or preexisting cardiac disease, nursing status, and possible drug interactions. Conduct pregnancy test (including in female partners of male patients), standard hematological and biochemical lab tests, ECG in patients w/ preexisting cardiac abnormalities, renal/thyroid function test, and CD4 count in HIV patients. Assess baseline height and weight in pediatric patients.

Monitoring: Monitor for hemolytic anemia, hepatic decompensation, pancreatitis, hypersensitivity/skin reactions, pulmonary infiltrates/function impairment, and other adverse reactions. Monitor cardiac status, TSH, and HCV RNA. Perform hematological tests at Weeks 2 and 4 and biochemical tests at Week 4; perform additional testing periodically. Perform pregnancy testing monthly and for 6 months after discontinuation (including female partners of male patients). Monitor height and weight in pediatric patients. In patients on concomitant therapy w/ azathioprine, monitor CBC, including platelet counts, weekly for the 1st month, twice monthly for the 2nd and 3rd months of treatment, then monthly or more frequently if dosage or other therapy changes are necessary.

Counseling: Counsel on risks/benefits associated w/ treatment. Inform of pregnancy risks; instruct to use at least 2 forms of effective contraception during therapy and for 6 months after discontinuation of therapy (including female partners of male patients). Advise to notify physician immediately in the event of pregnancy. Advise that lab evaluations are required prior to starting therapy and periodically thereafter. Advise to be well-hydrated, especially during the initial stages of treatment. Caution to avoid driving/operating machinery if dizziness, confusion, somnolence, or fatigue develops. Instruct not to drink alcohol; inform that alcohol may exacerbate CHC infection. Inform to take appropriate precautions to prevent HCV transmission.

MONOCLATE-P — antihemophilic factor (human)   Rx

Class: Antihemophilic agent

ADULT DOSAGE
Hemophilia A

Number of Antihemophilic Factor (AHF) IU Required = Weight (kg) x Desired Factor VIII (FVIII) Increase (% Normal) x 0.5

Mild Hemorrhages: Single infusion if a level of ≥30% is attained

Moderate Hemorrhage/Minor Surgery: Raise FVIII levels to 30-50% of normal
Initial: 15-25 IU/kg
Maint: 10-15 IU/kg q8-12h

Severe Hemorrhage (Near Vital Organs): Raise FVIII levels to 80-100% of normal

PEDIATRIC DOSAGE
Hemophilia A

Number of Antihemophilic Factor (AHF) IU Required = Weight (kg) x Desired Factor VIII (FVIII) Increase (% Normal) x 0.5

Mild Hemorrhages: Single infusion if a level of ≥30% is attained

Moderate Hemorrhage/Minor Surgery: Raise FVIII levels to 30-50% of normal
Initial: 15-25 IU/kg
Maint: 10-15 IU/kg q8-12h

Severe Hemorrhage (Near Vital Organs): Raise FVIII levels to 80-100% of normal

---

Initial: 40-50 IU/kg
Maint: 20-25 IU/kg q8-12h

Major Surgery:
Priming Dose: Raise FVIII levels to 80-100% of normal given 1 hr prior to surgery
Second Dose: 1/2 of priming dose 5 hrs after 1st dose
Maint: Daily minimum FVIII levels of at least 30% for 10-14 days post-op

Initial: 40-50 IU/kg
Maint: 20-25 IU/kg q8-12h

Major Surgery:
Priming Dose: Raise FVIII levels to 80-100% of normal given 1 hr prior to surgery
Second Dose: 1/2 of priming dose 5 hrs after 1st dose
Maint: Daily minimum FVIII levels of at least 30% for 10-14 days post-op

---

ADMINISTRATION
IV route
Administer sol intravenously at a rate of approximately 2 mL/minute

Reconstitution
1. Warm both the diluent and drug in unopened vials to room temperature (not above 37°C [98°F])
2. Gently swirl after combining w/ diluent
3. Administered w/in 3 hrs after reconstitution

STORAGE
2-8°C (36-46°F); may store at room temperature ≤25°C (77°F), for ≤6 months. Do not freeze.

HOW SUPPLIED
Inj: 250 IU, 500 IU, 1000 IU, 1500 IU

CONTRAINDICATIONS
Known hypersensitivity to mouse protein.

WARNINGS/PRECAUTIONS
Not effective in controlling the bleeding of patients with von Willebrand's disease. May carry risk of transmitting infectious agents (eg, viruses, Creutzfeldt-Jakob disease [CJD]). Contains trace amounts of mouse proteins; may develop possibility of hypersensitivity to mouse proteins. Monitor Hct and direct Coombs test for signs of progressive anemia with large or frequently repeated doses. Caution in elderly.

ADVERSE REACTIONS
Allergic reactions, mild chills, nausea, stinging at infusion site.

PREGNANCY AND LACTATION
Category C, safety not known in nursing.

MECHANISM OF ACTION
Antihemophilic agent; acts as a cofactor for factor IX to activate factor X in the intrinsic pathway of blood coagulation.

PHARMACOKINETICS
Elimination: $T_{1/2}$=17.5 hrs.

PATIENT CONSIDERATIONS
Assessment: Assess for hypersensitivity to mouse protein and pregnancy/nursing status.

Monitoring: Monitor Hct and direct Coombs tests for signs of progressive anemia. Monitor for hypersensitivity and transmission of infectious agents (eg, viruses).

Counseling: Inform of early signs of hypersensitivity reactions; advise to d/c and contact physician if these symptoms occur. Advise to report symptoms of hepatitis A and parvovirus B19, which most seriously affects pregnant women or the immunocompromised.

MONONINE — coagulation factor IX (human)   Rx

Class: Antihemophilic agent

ADULT DOSAGE
Hemophilia B

Prevention/Control of Bleeding:
Minor Spontaneous Hemorrhage, Prophylaxis:
Desired Factor IX (FIX) Levels for Hemostasis 15-25% or IU/dL:
Initial: Up to 20-30 IU/kg once or may repeat in 24 hrs if necessary

Major Trauma/Surgery:
Desired FIX Levels for Hemostasis 25-50% or IU/dL:
Initial: Up to 75 IU/kg q18-30h depending on $T_{1/2}$ and FIX levels for up to 10 days, depending on nature of insult

Dose Calculation:
Number of FIX IU Required = Weight (kg) x Desired FIX Increase (% or IU/dL Normal) x 1.0 IU/kg (per IU/dL)

PEDIATRIC DOSAGE
Hemophilia B

Prevention/Control of Bleeding:
Minor Spontaneous Hemorrhage, Prophylaxis:
Desired Factor IX (FIX) Levels for Hemostasis 15-25% or IU/dL:
Initial: Up to 20-30 IU/kg once or may repeat in 24 hrs if necessary

Major Trauma/Surgery:
Desired FIX Levels for Hemostasis 25-50% or IU/dL:
Initial: Up to 75 IU/kg q18-30h depending on $T_{1/2}$ and FIX levels for up to 10 days, depending on nature of insult

Dose Calculation:
Number of FIX IU Required = Weight (kg) x Desired FIX Increase (% or IU/dL Normal) x 1.0 IU/kg (per IU/dL)

DOSING CONSIDERATIONS
Concomitant Medications:
In the presence of a FIX inhibitor, higher doses may be necessary

ADMINISTRATION
IV route
Administer w/in 3 hrs of reconstitution

Reconstitution
1. Warm sol and diluent in unopened vials to room temperature (not above 37°C [98°F])
2. After combining sol and diluent, gently swirl the vial until the powder is dissolved and the sol is ready for administration

STORAGE
2-8°C (36-46°F), stable up to expiration date. May be stored at room temperature not to exceed 25°C (77°F), for up to 1 month. Do not freeze. Do not refrigerate after reconstitution.

HOW SUPPLIED
Inj: 500 IU, 1000 IU

CONTRAINDICATIONS
Known hypersensitivity to mouse protein.

WARNINGS/PRECAUTIONS
Not indicated in the treatment or prophylaxis of Hemophilia A patients with inhibitors to factor VIII. Not indicated for replacement therapy of factor II, VII, and X. Not indicated for the treatment or reversal of coumarin-induced anticoagulation or in a hemorrhagic state caused by hepatitis-induced lack of production of liver-dependent coagulation factors. May carry risk of transmitting infectious agents (eg, viruses, Creutzfeldt-Jakob disease). Associated with development of thromboembolic complications; caution in patients with liver disease, postoperative patients, neonates, patients at risk of thromboembolic phenomena or disseminated intravascular coagulation (DIC), or in patients with signs of fibrinolysis. Hypersensitivity reactions, including anaphylaxis, reported. Increased risk of inhibitor formation and acute hypersensitivity reactions in patients with major deletion mutations of the FIX gene; observe closely for signs/symptoms of acute hypersensitivity reactions, particularly during the early phases of initial exposure to product. Nephrotic syndrome reported following attempted immune tolerance induction with FIX products in Hemophilia B patients with FIX inhibitors and a history of severe allergic reactions to FIX. Administer at a rate that will permit observation of patient for any immediate reaction; d/c promptly and administer appropriate countermeasures and supportive therapy should evidence of an acute hypersensitivity reaction be observed. High doses reported to be associated with myocardial infarction, DIC, venous thrombosis, and pulmonary embolism; attempting to maintain FIX levels of >75-100% [IU/dL] during treatment is not routinely recommended or required.

ADVERSE REACTIONS
Headache, fever, chills, flushing, N/V, tingling, lethargy, hives, infusion-site stinging/burning, allergic reactions.

PREGNANCY AND LACTATION
Category C, safety not known in nursing.

MECHANISM OF ACTION
Antihemophilic agent; activated by factor XIa; in combination with factor VIII:C, activates factor X to Xa, resulting in the conversion of prothrombin to thrombin and the formation of a fibrin clot.

PHARMACOKINETICS
Elimination: $T_{1/2}$=22.6 hrs.

PATIENT CONSIDERATIONS
Assessment: Assess for known hypersensitivity to mouse protein, severity of bleeding, FIX inhibitors, liver disease, postoperative state, risk for thromboembolic phenomenon or DIC, known FIX gene deletion mutations, signs of fibrinolysis, pregnancy/nursing status, and possible drug interactions. Assess FIX level.

Monitoring: Monitor for hypersensitivity reactions, DIC, thromboembolic complications, infections, and other adverse reactions. Monitor closely during infusion. Monitor FIX levels.

Counseling: Inform of the benefits and risks of therapy. Inform of the early signs/symptoms of hypersensitivity reactions (eg, hives, generalized urticaria, chest tightness, dyspnea, wheezing, faintness, hypotension, anaphylaxis); instruct to d/c and immediately contact physician if these occur. Advise to report symptoms of hepatitis A infections (eg, poor appetite, tiredness, low-grade fever, N/V, pain in the belly, dark urine, yellowed complexion) promptly to physician.

MOZOBIL — plerixafor
Rx

Class: Hematopoietic stem cell mobilizer

ADULT DOSAGE
Hematopoietic Stem Cell Mobilization

Used in combination w/ granulocyte colony-stimulating factor (G-CSF) to mobilize hematopoietic stem cells (HSCs) to the peripheral blood for collection and subsequent autologous transplantation in patients w/ non-Hodgkin's lymphoma and multiple myeloma

Begin treatment after patient has received G-CSF qd for 4 days

≤83kg: 20mg fixed dose or 0.24mg/kg qd
>83kg: 0.24mg/kg qd
Max: 40mg/day

PEDIATRIC DOSAGE
Pediatric use may not have been established

Administer approx 11 hrs prior to initiation of each apheresis for up to 4 consecutive days

Calculation of Volume to be Administered:
Volume to be Administered (mL) = 0.012 x Actual Body Weight (kg)

DOSING CONSIDERATIONS
Concomitant Medications
Administer daily am doses of G-CSF 10mcg/kg for 4 days prior to 1st pm dose of plerixafor and on each day prior to apheresis

Renal Impairment
Moderate and Severe (CrCl ≤50mL/min):
≤83kg: 13mg or 0.16mg/kg qd
>83kg: 0.16mg/kg qd
Max: 27mg/day

ADMINISTRATION
SQ route

STORAGE
25°C (77°F); excursions permitted to 15-30°C (59-86°F).

HOW SUPPLIED
Inj: 20mg/mL [1.2mL]

CONTRAINDICATIONS
History of hypersensitivity to plerixafor.

WARNINGS/PRECAUTIONS
Serious hypersensitivity reactions, including anaphylactic-type reactions, some of which have been life-threatening w/ clinically significant hypotension and shock, reported; observe for signs and symptoms during and after administration for at least 30 min and until clinically stable following completion of each administration. May cause mobilization of tumor cells, including leukemic cells, and subsequent contamination of the apheresis product; not intended for HSC mobilization and harvest in patients w/ leukemia. Leukocytosis and thrombocytopenia reported. Evaluate patients who report left upper abdominal pain and/or scapular or shoulder pain for splenic integrity. May cause fetal harm. Caution in elderly.

ADVERSE REACTIONS
Diarrhea, N/V, inj-site reactions, fatigue, headache, arthralgia, dizziness, flatulence, insomnia.

PREGNANCY AND LACTATION
Pregnancy: Category D.
Lactation: Not for use in nursing.

MECHANISM OF ACTION
HSC mobilizer; inhibits CXCR4 chemokine receptor and blocks binding of its cognate ligand, stromal cell-derived factor-1α.

PHARMACOKINETICS
Absorption: T_{max}=30-60 min. **Distribution:** Plasma protein binding (up to 58%); V_d=0.3L/kg. **Elimination:** Urine (approx 70%, unchanged); $T_{1/2}$=3-5 hrs.

PATIENT CONSIDERATIONS
Assessment: Assess for leukemia, renal impairment, history of hypersensitivity to drug, and pregnancy/nursing status.

Monitoring: Monitor for signs/symptoms of hypersensitivity, splenic enlargement, and other adverse reactions. Monitor WBCs and platelet counts.

Counseling: Advise of the potential for anaphylactic reactions, including signs and symptoms during and following inj, and to report these symptoms immediately to physician. Instruct to inform physician immediately if symptoms of vasovagal reactions occur during or shortly after inj, or if patient experiences itching, rash, or inj-site reaction. Inform that drug may cause GI disorders; instruct on how to manage specific GI disorders and to inform physician if severe events occur following inj. Advise female patients w/ reproductive potential to use effective contraceptive methods during therapy.

MUSTARGEN — mechlorethamine hydrochloride
Rx

Class: Nitrogen mustard alkylating agent

> Administer only under the supervision of a physician experienced in the use of cancer chemotherapeutic agents. Highly toxic; handle and administer with care. Avoid inhalation of dust or vapors and contact with skin or mucous membranes (especially those of the eyes). Avoid exposure during pregnancy. Review special handling procedures prior to handling and follow diligently. Extravasation into SQ tissues results in a painful inflammation; if leakage is obvious, prompt infiltration of the area with sterile isotonic sodium thiosulfate (1/6 M) and application of an ice compress for 6-12 hrs may minimize the local reaction.

ADULT DOSAGE
Palliative Cancer Treatment

IV:
Hodgkin's disease (Stages III and IV), lymphosarcoma, chronic myelocytic or chronic lymphocytic leukemia, polycythemia vera, mycosis fungoides, and bronchogenic carcinoma

Usual: 0.4mg/kg/course given either as a single dose or in divided doses of 0.1-0.2mg/kg/day

PEDIATRIC DOSAGE
Pediatric use may not have been established

Base dose on ideal dry body weight; consider presence of edema or ascites

Do not administer subsequent courses until patient has recovered hematologically from previous course

Intracavitary:
Metastatic carcinoma resulting in effusion

Usual: 0.4mg/kg, though 0.2mg/kg (or 10-20mg) has been used by the intrapericardial route

DOSING CONSIDERATIONS
Elderly
Start at lower end of dosing range

ADMINISTRATION
IV/Intrapleural/Intraperitoneal/Intrapericardial route

Avoid use by intracavitary route when other agents that may suppress bone marrow function are being used systemically

IV Administration
Preparation of Sol:
1. Inject 10mL of sterile water for inj (SWFI) or 10mL of 0.9% NaCl inj into a vial of mechlorethamine HCl
2. W/ the needle (syringe attached) still in the rubber stopper, shake the vial several times to dissolve the drug completely
3. The resultant sol contains 1mg/mL

Technique:
1. Withdraw into the syringe the calculated volume of sol required for a single inj
2. Dispose of any remaining sol after neutralization; refer to PI for neutralization of equipment and unused sol
3. Although the drug may be injected directly into any suitable vein, it is injected preferably into the rubber or plastic tubing of a flowing IV infusion set
4. Rate of inj apparently is not critical provided it is completed w/in a few min

Intracavitary Administration
1. Add 10mL of SWFI or 10mL of 0.9% NaCl inj to the vial containing 10mg of mechlorethamine HCl; amounts of diluent of 50-100mL of normal saline have also been used
2. Change the position of the patient every 5-10 min for an hr after inj
3. Remaining fluid may be removed from the pleural or peritoneal cavity by paracentesis 24-36 hrs later
4. Follow the patient carefully by clinical and x-ray examination to detect reaccumulation of fluid

Handling Precautions
If accidental eye contact occurs, copious irrigation for at least 15 min w/ water, normal saline, or a balanced salt ophthalmic irrigating sol should be instituted immediately, followed by prompt ophthalmologic consultation
If accidental skin contact occurs, the affected part must be irrigated immediately w/ copious amounts of water, for at least 15 min while removing contaminated clothing and shoes, followed by 2% sodium thiosulfate sol; medical attention should be sought immediately and contaminated clothing should be destroyed

STORAGE
15-30°C (59-86°F). Protect from light and humidity. Prepare solutions of the drug immediately before use.

HOW SUPPLIED
Inj: 10mg

CONTRAINDICATIONS
Presence of known infectious diseases.

WARNINGS/PRECAUTIONS
Intracavitary inj is not recommended when the accumulated fluid is chylous in nature. May contribute to extensive and rapid development of amyloidosis; use only if foci of acute and chronic suppurative inflammation are absent. May cause fetal harm. Powerful vesicant; intended primarily for IV use. Caution in patients with inoperable neoplasms or in the terminal stage of the disease. Routine use in all cases of widely disseminated neoplasms is not recommended. Use in patients with leukopenia, thrombocytopenia, and anemia, due to invasion of the bone marrow by tumor carries a greater risk. Has immunosuppressive activity; may predispose patient to bacterial, viral, or fungal infection. Hyperuricemia may develop; institute adequate methods for control of hyperuricemia and ensure adequate fluid intake before treatment. Caution with chronic lymphatic leukemia; increased incidence of drug toxicity. Renal, hepatic, and bone marrow function abnormalities reported; monitor frequently. May be associated with an increased incidence of a second malignant tumor, especially when such therapy is combined with other antineoplastic agents or radiation therapy. Probable carcinogen. Caution in elderly.

ADVERSE REACTIONS
Thrombosis, thrombophlebitis, hypersensitivity reactions, N/V, anorexia, weakness, lymphocytopenia, granulocytopenia, thrombocytopenia, erythema multiforme, herpes zoster infection, oligomenorrhea, amenorrhea, impaired spermatogenesis, azoospermia.

DRUG INTERACTIONS
Caution when used in alternating courses with x-ray therapy or other chemotherapy due to potential hematologic complications; neither mechlorethamine following x-ray therapy nor x-ray therapy subsequent to the drug should be given until bone marrow function has recovered. Avoid use by the intracavitary route when other agents which may suppress bone marrow function are being used systemically.

PREGNANCY AND LACTATION
Category D, not for use in nursing.

MECHANISM OF ACTION
Nitrogen mustard alkylating agent; has a cytotoxic action which inhibits rapidly proliferating cells.

PATIENT CONSIDERATIONS
Assessment: Assess for infectious diseases, previous anaphylactic reactions to the drug, edema, ascites, foci of acute and chronic suppurative inflammation, hematologic status, pregnancy/nursing status, and possible drug interactions. Assess use in patients with inoperable neoplasms or in the terminal stage of the disease. Obtain accurate histologic diagnosis of the disease and adequate clinical history.

Monitoring: Monitor for infections, hyperuricemia, second malignant tumor, and other adverse reactions. Monitor renal, hepatic, and bone marrow functions frequently. Perform repeated blood examinations to guide subsequent therapy.

Counseling: Instruct to inform physician if pregnant, planning to become pregnant, or breastfeeding. Advise women of childbearing potential to avoid becoming pregnant. Warn of the potential risk to reproductive capacity.

MYALEPT — metreleptin

Class: Leptin analogue

Rx

> Anti-metreleptin antibodies w/ neutralizing activity have been identified; consequences may include inhibition of endogenous leptin action and/or loss of drug efficacy. Severe infection and/or worsening metabolic control reported; test for anti-metreleptin antibodies w/ neutralizing activity if severe infections or signs suspicious for loss of drug efficacy during treatment develop. T-cell lymphoma reported in patients w/ acquired generalized lipodystrophy; carefully consider the benefits and risks of treatment in patients w/ significant hematologic abnormalities and/or acquired generalized lipodystrophy. Available only through a restricted program under a Risk Evaluation and Mitigation Strategy (REMS) called the Myalept REMS Program.

ADULT DOSAGE
Leptin Deficiency

Adjunct to diet as replacement therapy to treat the complications of leptin deficiency in patients w/ congenital or acquired generalized lipodystrophy

≤40kg:
Initial:
Males and Females: 0.06mg/kg (0.012mL/kg)
Dose Adjustment: 0.02mg/kg (0.004mL/kg)
Max Daily Dose: 0.13mg/kg (0.026mL/kg)

<40kg:
Initial:
Male: 2.5mg (0.5mL)
Female: 5mg (1mL)
Dose Adjustment: 1.25-2.5mg (0.25-0.5mL)
Max Daily Dose: 10mg (2mL)

PEDIATRIC DOSAGE
Leptin Deficiency

Adjunct to diet as replacement therapy to treat the complications of leptin deficiency in patients w/ congenital or acquired generalized lipodystrophy

≤40kg:
Initial:
Males and Females: 0.06mg/kg (0.012mL/kg)
Dose Adjustment: 0.02mg/kg (0.004mL/kg)
Max Daily Dose: 0.13mg/kg (0.026mL/kg)

<40kg:
Initial:
Male: 2.5mg (0.5mL)
Female: 5mg (1mL)
Dose Adjustment: 1.25-2.5mg (0.25-0.5mL)
Max Daily Dose: 10mg (2mL)

DOSING CONSIDERATIONS
Elderly
Start at lower end of dosing range

Discontinuation
Patients at Risk for Pancreatitis:
Taper dose over a 1-week period. During tapering, monitor TG levels and consider initiating or adjusting dose of lipid-lowering medications prn

Other Important Considerations
Dose adjustments, including possible large reductions, of insulin or insulin secretagogue (eg, sulfonylurea) may be necessary; monitor blood glucose in patients on concomitant insulin therapy, especially those on high doses, or insulin secretagogue

ADMINISTRATION
SQ route
Should be administered at the same time every day.
May administer at any time of the day, w/o regard to the timing of meals.
Administer into the SQ tissue of the abdomen, thigh or upper arm; use different inj site each day when injecting in the same region.
After choosing an inj site, pinch the skin and at a 45° angle, inject the sol.
Avoid IM inj, especially in patients w/ minimal SQ adipose tissue.
Doses exceeding 1mL can be administered as 2 inj (the total daily dose divided equally) to minimize potential inj-site discomfort due to volume; when dividing doses due to volume, doses can be administered one after the other.

Reconstitution
Reconstitute w/ 2.2mL of sterile bacteriostatic water for inj (0.9% benzyl alcohol), or w/ 2.2mL of sterile water for inj.
Use w/in 3 days when stored refrigerated between 2-8°C (36-46°F) and protected from light.
For neonates and infants, reconstitute w/ preservative-free sterile water for inj and administer immediately.

Compatibility

Do not mix w/, or transfer into, the contents of another vial of metreleptin.
Do not add other medications, including insulin; use a separate syringe for insulin inj.

STORAGE

2-8°C (36-46°F). Do not freeze. Protect from light. Do not shake or vigorously agitate reconstituted vial. Refer to PI for further storage and handling instructions.

HOW SUPPLIED

Inj: 5mg/mL [11.3mg]

CONTRAINDICATIONS

General obesity not associated w/ congenital leptin deficiency, prior severe hypersensitivity reactions to metreleptin or to any of the product components.

WARNINGS/PRECAUTIONS

Not indicated for use w/ HIV-related lipodystrophy, or in patients w/ metabolic disease, including diabetes mellitus and hypertriglyceridemia, w/o concurrent evidence of congenital or acquired generalized lipodystrophy. Case of anaplastic large cell lymphoma reported. Cases of progression of autoimmune hepatitis and membranoproliferative glomerulonephritis (associated w/ massive proteinuria and renal failure) reported in patients w/ acquired generalized lipodystrophy; carefully consider the potential benefits and risks of treatment in patients w/ autoimmune disease. Generalized hypersensitivity reported; consider discontinuing if a hypersensitivity reaction occurs. Contains benzyl alcohol when reconstituted w/ Bacteriostatic Water for Inj; preservative-free Water for Inj is recommended for use in neonates and infants. Caution in elderly.

ADVERSE REACTIONS

Headache, hypoglycemia, decreased weight, abdominal pain, arthralgia, dizziness, ear infection, fatigue, nausea, ovarian cyst, URTI, anemia, back pain, diarrhea, paresthesia.

DRUG INTERACTIONS

See Dosing Considerations. Caution w/ drugs metabolized by CYP450 (eg, oral contraceptives, drugs w/ a narrow therapeutic index); effect of metreleptin on CYP450 enzymes may be clinically relevant for CYP450 substrates w/ a narrow therapeutic index, where dose is individually adjusted. Upon initiation or discontinuation of metreleptin, in patients being treated w/ CYP450 substrates w/ a narrow therapeutic index, perform therapeutic monitoring of effect (eg, warfarin) or drug concentration (eg, cyclosporine, theophylline) and adjust the individual dose of the agent PRN.

PREGNANCY AND LACTATION

Pregnancy: Category C.
Lactation: Not for use in nursing.

MECHANISM OF ACTION

Recombinant Human Leptin Analog; binds to and activates human leptin receptor, which belongs to the Class I cytokine family of receptors that signals through the JAK/STAT transduction pathway.

PHARMACOKINETICS

Absorption: (Single dose, 0.1-0.3mg/kg SQ) T_{max}=4-4.3 hrs. **Distribution:** (IV) V_d=370mL/kg (0.3mg/kg/day), 398mL/kg (1mg/kg/day), 463mL/kg (3mg/kg/day). **Elimination:** Renal (major route); (single dose, 0.01-0.3mg/mL SQ) $T_{1/2}$=3.8-4.7 hrs.

PATIENT CONSIDERATIONS

Assessment: Assess for hypersensitivity to the drug, general obesity not associated w/ congenital leptin deficiency, risk factors of pancreatitis, hematologic abnormalities, pregnancy/nursing status, and possible drug interactions.

Monitoring: Monitor for severe infections, worsening metabolic control, T-cell lymphoma in patients w/ acquired generalized lipodystrophy, hypersensitivity reactions, and other adverse events. Test for anti-metreleptin antibodies w/ neutralizing activity in patients who develop severe infections or show signs suspicious for loss of metreleptin efficacy during treatment. When discontinuing therapy in patients w/ risk factors for pancreatitis, monitor TG levels. Closely monitor blood glucose levels in patients on concomitant insulin or insulin secretagogue therapy.

Counseling: Inform about the risks/benefits of therapy. Instruct that if a dose is missed, administer dose as soon as noticed, and resume the normal dosing schedule the next day. Inform on the signs/symptoms that would warrant antibody testing. Inform on the signs/symptoms that indicate changes in hematologic status and the importance of routine lab assessment and physician monitoring. Advise that the risk of hypoglycemia is increased w/ insulin or an insulin secretagogue; instruct to closely monitor blood glucose levels. Advise patients w/ history of autoimmune disease on signs/symptoms that indicate exacerbation of underlying autoimmune disease and the importance of routine lab assessments and physician monitoring. Instruct to seek medical advice if symptoms of hypersensitivity occur. Advise nursing mothers that breastfeeding is not recommended. Inform patients/caregivers about proper preparation and administration of drug; advise that 1st dose should be administered under the supervision of a qualified healthcare professional. Instruct patients w/ a history of pancreatitis and/or severe hypertriglyceridemia to taper dose over a 1-week period when discontinuing therapy; advise that additional monitoring of TG levels and possible initiation or dose adjustment of lipid-lowering medications may be considered.

MYFORTIC — mycophenolic acid   Rx
Class: Inosine monophosphate dehydrogenase (IMPDH) inhibitor

Use during pregnancy is associated w/ increased risks of pregnancy loss and congenital malformations; counsel females of reproductive potential regarding pregnancy prevention and planning. Immunosuppression may lead to increased risk of development of lymphoma and other malignancies, particularly of the skin. Increased susceptibility to infections (bacterial, viral, fungal, protozoal, opportunistic). Only physicians experienced in immunosuppressive therapy and management of organ transplant patients should prescribe mycophenolic acid (MPA). Manage patients in facilities equipped and staffed w/ adequate lab and supportive medical resources. Physician responsible for maintenance therapy should have complete information requisite for patient follow-up.

ADULT DOSAGE

Organ Rejection Prophylaxis

Kidney Transplant:
720mg bid (1440mg/day)

Use in combination w/ cyclosporine and corticosteroids

PEDIATRIC DOSAGE

Organ Rejection Prophylaxis

≥5 Years:
At Least 6 Months Post Kidney Transplant:
400mg/m² bid
Max: 720mg bid

BSA 1.19-1.58m²: Dose either w/ three 180mg tabs, or one 180mg tab plus one 360mg tab bid (1080mg/day)
BSA >1.58m²: Dose either w/ four 180mg tabs, or two 360mg tabs bid (1440mg/day)

Use in combination w/ cyclosporine and corticosteroids

ADMINISTRATION

Oral route

Take on an empty stomach, 1 hr before or 2 hrs after food intake.
Swallow whole; do not crush, chew, or cut tabs.

STORAGE

25°C (77°F); excursions permitted to 15-30°C (59-86°F). Protect from moisture.

HOW SUPPLIED

Tab, Delayed-Release: 180mg, 360mg

CONTRAINDICATIONS

Hypersensitivity to mycophenolate sodium, mycophenolic acid, mycophenolate mofetil, or to any of its excipients.

WARNINGS/PRECAUTIONS

Should not be used interchangeably w/ mycophenolate mofetil (MMF) tabs and caps w/o medical supervision. Limit exposure to sunlight and UV light in patients at increased risk for skin cancer. Polyomavirus-associated nephropathy (PVAN), JC virus associated progressive multifocal leukoencephalopathy (PML), cytomegalovirus (CMV) infections, reactivation of hepatitis B (HBV) or hepatitis C (HCV) reported; consider reduction in immunosuppression for patients who develop evidence of new or reactivated viral infections. PVAN, especially due to BK virus infection, is associated w/ serious outcomes, including deteriorating renal function and renal graft loss. Consider PML in differential diagnosis in patients reporting neurological symptoms and consider consultation w/ a neurologist as clinically indicated. Cases of pure red cell aplasia (PRCA) reported when used w/ other immunosuppressive agents; monitor CBC weekly during the 1st month, twice monthly for the 2nd and 3rd month of therapy, and then monthly through 1st yr. Interrupt dosing or reduce dose, perform appropriate tests, and manage accordingly, if blood dyscrasias occur (neutropenia [ANC <1.3 x 10³/µL] or anemia). GI bleeding (requiring hospitalization), intestinal perforations, gastric ulcers, and duodenal ulcers reported; caution w/ active serious digestive system disease. Avoid w/ rare hereditary deficiency of hypoxanthine-guanine phosphoribosyl-transferase (HGPRT) (eg, Lesch-Nyhan and Kelley-Seegmiller syndromes). Caution in elderly.

ADVERSE REACTIONS

Anemia, leukopenia, constipation, N/V, diarrhea, dyspepsia, UTI, CMV infection, insomnia, postoperative pain.

DRUG INTERACTIONS

Caution w/ combination immunosuppressant therapy. Avoid live attenuated vaccines. Mg²⁺- and aluminum-containing antacids may decrease levels; do not administer simultaneously. Azathioprine and MMF inhibit purine metabolism; avoid concomitant use w/ azathioprine or MMF. Cholestyramine or other agents that may interfere w/ enterohepatic recirculation or drugs that may bind bile acids (eg, bile acid sequestrates or oral activated charcoal) may reduce efficacy; avoid concomitant use. Sevelamer may decrease levels; do not administer simultaneously w/ sevelamer and other Ca²⁺-free phosphate binders. Cyclosporine may decrease levels; there is a potential change of MPA levels after switching from cyclosporine to other immunosuppressive drugs or from other immunosuppressive drugs to cyclosporine. Concomitant norfloxacin and metronidazole may decrease levels; avoid w/ the combination of norfloxacin and metronidazole. Rifampin may decrease levels; avoid concomitant use unless the benefit outweighs the risk. May decrease levels and effects of hormonal contraceptives; coadminister w/ caution, and additional barrier contraceptive methods must be used. Drugs that undergo renal tubular secretion (eg, acyclovir/valacyclovir, ganciclovir/valganciclovir) may increase levels of both drugs; monitor blood cell counts. Drugs that alter the GI flora (eg, ciprofloxacin or amoxicillin plus clavulanic acid) may interact w/ MMF by disrupting enterohepatic recirculation.

PREGNANCY AND LACTATION

Pregnancy: Category D. For females using MPA during pregnancy and those becoming pregnant w/in 6 weeks of discontinuing therapy, report pregnancy to the Mycophenolate Pregnancy Registry. Strongly encourage patient to enroll in the registry. Associated w/ increased risk of 1st trimester pregnancy loss and an increased risk of congenital malformations. When appropriate, consider alternative immunosuppressants w/ less potential for embryofetal toxicity. In certain situations, the patient and her healthcare practitioner may decide that the maternal benefits outweigh the risks to the fetus.

Lactation: Not for use in nursing.

Reproductive Potential: Females of reproductive potential should have a serum or urine pregnancy test (sensitivity of at least 25 mIU/mL) immediately before starting therapy; repeat test after 8-10 days and during routine follow-up visits. In the event of a positive pregnancy test, counsel w/ regards to whether the maternal benefits may outweigh the risks to the fetus in certain situations. Females of reproductive potential should use acceptable contraception during therapy and for 6 weeks after discontinuation, unless patient chooses abstinence. Consider alternative immunosuppressants w/ less potential for embryofetal toxicity in patients considering pregnancy.

MECHANISM OF ACTION

IMPDH inhibitor; inhibits the de novo pathway of guanosine nucleotide synthesis w/o incorporation to DNA.

PHARMACOKINETICS

Absorption: Absolute bioavailability (72%); T_{max}=1.5-2.75 hrs (median).
Distribution: V_d=54L; plasma protein binding (>98% bound to albumin), (82% mycophenolic acid glucuronide [MPAG]). **Metabolism:** Glucuronyl transferase; MPAG (major metabolite). **Elimination:** Urine (>60% MPAG, 3% unchanged), bile; $T_{1/2}$=8-16 hrs, 13-17 hrs (MPAG).

PATIENT CONSIDERATIONS

Assessment: Assess for hypersensitivity to the drug, HBV or HCV infected patients, hereditary deficiency of HGPRT (eg, Lesch-Nyhan and Kelley-Seegmiller syndromes), active digestive disease, pregnancy/nursing status, and for possible drug interactions. Females of reproductive potential should have a serum or urine pregnancy test (sensitivity of at least 25 mIU/mL) immediately before starting therapy.

Monitoring: Monitor for signs/symptoms of lymphomas and other malignancies (eg, skin cancer), infections including reactivation of HBV or HCV, blood dyscrasias (eg, PRCA), GI complications, and other adverse reactions. Monitor CBC weekly during the 1st month, twice monthly for the 2nd and 3rd month of therapy, and then monthly through 1st yr. Monitor pregnancy status by doing a pregnancy test (sensitivity of at least 25 mIU/mL) 8-10 days after initiation of therapy and repeatedly during follow-up visits.

Counseling: Inform that use in pregnancy is associated w/ an increased risk of 1st trimester pregnancy loss and congenital malformation; discuss pregnancy testing, prevention (including acceptable contraception methods), and planning. Discuss appropriate alternative immunosuppressants w/ less potential for embryofetal toxicity in patients who are considering pregnancy. Advise not to breastfeed during therapy. Inform about increased risk of developing lymphomas and other malignancies; advise to limit exposure to sunlight and UV light by wearing protective clothing and using sunscreen w/ high protection factor. Inform about increased risk of developing a variety of infections, including opportunistic infections, due to immunosuppression. Inform about risk for developing blood dyscrasias. Instruct to report if experiencing any symptoms of infection, unexpected bruising, bleeding, or any other manifestation of bone marrow suppression. Inform that therapy may cause GI tract complications, including bleeding, intestinal perforations, and gastric or duodenal ulcers; advise to contact healthcare provider if symptoms of GI bleeding or sudden onset or persistent abdominal pain occurs. Inform that therapy may interfere w/ the usual response to immunizations and to avoid live vaccines. Advise to report to physician the use of any other medications while on therapy. Encourage to enroll in the pregnancy registry if patient becomes pregnant while on therapy.

MYOBLOC — rimabotulinumtoxinB   Rx

Class: Acetylcholine release inhibitor

> Distant spread of toxin effects reported hrs to weeks after inj (eg, asthenia, generalized muscle weakness, diplopia, blurred vision, ptosis, dysphagia, dysphonia, dysarthria, urinary incontinence, breathing difficulties). Swallowing and breathing difficulties can be life-threatening and there have been reports of death. Risk of symptoms is greatest in children treated for spasticity but can also occur in adults. In unapproved uses and approved indications, cases of spread of effect have been reported at doses comparable to those used to treat cervical dystonia and at lower doses.

ADULT DOSAGE

Cervical Dystonia

To reduce severity of abnormal head position and neck pain associated w/ cervical dystonia

Prior History of Tolerating Botulinum Toxin Inj:

Initial: 2500-5000 U, divided among affected muscles

Patients w/o a prior history of tolerating botulinum toxin inj should receive a lower initial dose

PEDIATRIC DOSAGE

Pediatric use may not have been established

ADMINISTRATION

IM route

STORAGE

2-8°C (36-46°F). Do not freeze or shake. Protect from light. Diluted Sol: Use within 4 hrs.

HOW SUPPLIED

Inj: 5000 U/mL [0.5mL, 1mL, 2mL]

CONTRAINDICATIONS

Infection at the proposed inj site(s), known hypersensitivity to any botulinum toxin preparation or to any of the components in the formulation.

WARNINGS/PRECAUTIONS

Not interchangeable with other botulinum toxin products; cannot be compared or converted into U of any other botulinum toxin products. Aspiration and death due to severe dysphagia reported. Serious breathing difficulties, including respiratory failure, reported. Closely monitor patients with peripheral motor neuropathic diseases, amyotrophic lateral sclerosis, or neuromuscular junctional disorders (eg, myasthenia gravis or Lambert-Eaton syndrome); patients with neuromuscular disorders may be at increased risk of severe dysphagia and respiratory compromise. Contains albumin; carries an extremely remote risk for transmission of viral diseases and Creutzfeldt-Jakob disease.

ADVERSE REACTIONS

Distant spread of toxin effects, dry mouth, dysphagia, dyspepsia, inj-site pain.

DRUG INTERACTIONS

Potentiation of toxin effect may occur with aminoglycosides or other agents interfering with neuromuscular transmission (eg, curare-like compounds); use with caution. Coadministration or overlapping administration of different botulinum toxin serotypes may potentiate neuromuscular paralysis.

PREGNANCY AND LACTATION

Category C, caution in nursing.

MECHANISM OF ACTION

Purified neurotoxin complex; inhibits acetylcholine release at the neuromuscular junction via heavy chain-mediated neurospecific binding of the toxin, internalization of the toxin by receptor-mediated endocytosis, and ATP and pH-dependent translocation of the light chain to the neuronal cytosol where it acts as a zinc-dependent endoprotease, cleaving polypeptides essential for neurotransmitter release.

PATIENT CONSIDERATIONS

Assessment: Assess for infection at the proposed inj site(s), neuromuscular disorders, preexisting swallowing or breathing difficulties, hypersensitivity to drug, pregnancy/nursing status, and possible drug interactions.

Monitoring: Monitor for spread of toxin effects, swallowing/speech/respiratory disorders, and other adverse reactions. Monitor patients with peripheral motor neuropathic disease, amyotrophic lateral sclerosis, or neuromuscular junctional disorders.

Counseling: Advise to inform physician or pharmacist if any unusual symptoms (eg, difficulty with swallowing, speaking, or breathing) develop, or if any existing symptom worsens. Counsel to avoid driving a car or engaging in other potentially hazardous activities if loss of strength, muscle weakness, or impaired vision occurs.

MYOZYME — alglucosidase alfa   Rx

Class: Enzyme

> Life-threatening anaphylactic, severe allergic, and immune mediated reactions observed during infusions; appropriate medical support should be readily available when administered. Risk of serious acute exacerbation of cardiac or respiratory compromise due to infusion reactions in patients with compromised cardiac or respiratory function; additional monitoring required.

PEDIATRIC DOSAGE

Pompe Disease

1 Month-3.5 Years:
Acid α-Glucosidase Deficiency:
Usual: 20mg/kg every 2 weeks as a 4-hr IV infusion

Administer infusions in a step-wise manner using an infusion pump; refer to PI for recommended infusion volumes and rates at each step

Infusion Rate:
Initial: ≤1mg/kg/hr
Titrate: May increase by 2mg/kg/hr every 30 min, after tolerance is established
Max: 7mg/kg/hr

Infusion rate may be slowed and/or temporarily stopped in the event of infusion reactions

ADMINISTRATION

IV route

For single use only; discard any unused product

Preparation Instructions

1. Determine the number of vials to be reconstituted based on the patient's weight and the recommended dose of 20mg/kg; refer to PI for calculation

2. If the number of vials includes a fraction, round up to the next whole number to determine the total number of vials needed

3. Remove the required number of vials from the refrigerator and allow them to reach room temperature prior to reconstitution (approx 30 min)

4. Reconstitute each alglucosidase alfa vial by slowly injecting 10.3mL of sterile water for inj to the inside wall of each vial; each vial will yield a concentration of 5mg/mL. The total extractable dose per vial is 50mg/10mL.

5. Avoid forceful impact of the water for inj on the powder and avoid foaming; this is done by slow drop-wise addition of the water for inj down the inside of the vial and not directly onto the lyophilized cake

6. Tilt and roll each vial gently; do not invert, swirl, or shake

7. Protect the reconstituted alglucosidase alfa sol from light

8. The reconstituted sol may occasionally contain some alglucosidase alfa particles (typically <10/vial) in the form of thin white strands or translucent fibers subsequent to the initial inspection and/or following dilution for infusion. These particles have been shown to contain alglucosidase alfa and may appear after the initial reconstitution step and increase over time. Studies have shown that these particles are removed via in-line filtration w/o having a detectable effect on the purity or strength

9. Dilute alglucosidase alfa in 0.9% NaCl for inj immediately after reconstitution, to a final concentration of 0.5-4mg/mL; refer to PI for recommended total infusion volume based on patient weight

10. Slowly withdraw the reconstituted sol from each vial; avoid foaming in the syringe

11. Remove airspace from the infusion bag to minimize particle formation due to the sensitivity of alglucosidase alfa to air-liquid interfaces

12. Add the reconstituted alglucosidase alfa sol slowly and directly into the NaCl sol; do not add directly into airspace that may remain w/in the infusion bag. Avoid foaming in the infusion bag

13. Gently invert or massage the infusion bag to mix; do not shake

Administration Instructions

Administer alglucosidase alfa using an in-line low-protein-binding 0.2µm filter
Do not infuse alglucosidase alfa in the same IV line w/ other product

Stability

If immediate use is not possible, the reconstituted and diluted sol is stable for up to 24 hrs at 2-8°C (36-46°F)

STORAGE

2-8°C (36-46°F). Reconstituted/Diluted Sol: 2-8°C (36-46°F); stable for up to 24 hrs. Protect from light. Do not freeze or shake.

HOW SUPPLIED

Inj: 50mg

WARNINGS/PRECAUTIONS

Anaphylaxis and severe allergic reactions reported up to 3 hrs after infusion. Severe cutaneous and systemic immune mediated reactions have occurred up to 3 yrs after initiation of therapy. Nephrotic syndrome secondary to membranous glomerulonephritis reported in patients who had persistently positive anti-rhGAA IgG antibody titers; perform periodic urinalysis. Caution with acute underlying respiratory illness and/or sepsis. Infants with cardiac dysfunction may require prolonged observation times that should be individualized based on patient's needs. Ventricular arrhythmias and bradycardia, resulting in cardiac arrest or death, or requiring cardiac resuscitation or defibrillation reported in patients with cardiac hypertrophy during general anesthesia for central venous catheter placement; use caution when administering general anesthesia. Use extreme caution if readministering in patients who have experienced anaphylactic or severe allergic, infusion, or immune mediated reactions.

ADVERSE REACTIONS

Anaphylactic/severe allergic/infusion/immune mediated reactions, respiratory failure, pneumonia, respiratory distress, catheter-related infection, respiratory syncytial virus infection, fever, rash, cough, otitis media, upper respiratory tract infection, diarrhea, gastroenteritis, decreased oxygen saturation, vomiting.

PREGNANCY AND LACTATION

Category B, caution in nursing.

MECHANISM OF ACTION

Enzyme; provides an exogenous source of GAA. Binds to mannose-6-phosphate receptors on the cell surface, and is internalized and transported into lysosomes, where it undergoes proteolytic cleavage that results in increased enzymatic activity.

PHARMACOKINETICS

Absorption: (1-7 months of age, 20mg/kg or 40mg/kg dose) C_{max}=162mcg/mL, AUC=811mcg•hr/mL. **Elimination:** $T_{1/2}$=2.3 hrs.

PATIENT CONSIDERATIONS

Assessment: Assess for acute underlying respiratory illness, compromised cardiac or respiratory function, sepsis, previous hypersensitivity, and for any drug interactions. Obtain baseline vital signs and liver enzymes.

Monitoring: Monitor for anaphylactic/allergic/infusion/immune mediated reactions, exacerbation of cardiac/respiratory compromise, and other adverse reactions. Perform periodic urinalysis and liver enzyme evaluation. Monitor for IgG antibody formation every 3 months for 2 yrs then annually thereafter. Monitor vital signs following every infusion rate increase and following the infusion.

Counseling: Encourage patients and caregivers to participate in the Pompe Registry. Inform that anaphylactic/severe allergic/immune mediated reactions have been observed in some patients receiving therapy. Inform of the risk for acute cardiorespiratory failure, cardiac arrhythmias, and infusion reactions.

NABI-HB — hepatitis B immune globulin (human) Rx

Class: Immune globulin

ADULT DOSAGE

Postexposure Prophylaxis

Acute Exposure to Blood Containing HBsAg:
0.06mL/kg IM as soon as possible after exposure and w/in 24 hrs, if possible; give a 2nd dose 1 month after 1st dose for patients who refuse hepatitis B vaccine or are known non-responders to vaccine

Refer to PI for recommendations following percutaneous or permucosal exposure

Sexual Exposure to HBsAg-Positive Person:
0.06mL/kg IM single dose w/ hepatitis B vaccine series; give w/ in 14 days of last sexual contact or if sexual contact w/ infected person will continue

Household Exposure to Persons w/ Acute Hepatitis B Virus Infection:
Prophylaxis not indicated unless there is an identifiable blood exposure to the index patient (eg, by sharing toothbrushes/razors); treat such exposures like sexual exposures

PEDIATRIC DOSAGE

Postexposure Prophylaxis

Safety/effectiveness not established

Perinatal Exposure of Infants Born to HBsAg Positive Mothers:
0.5mL IM after physiologic stabilization of infant and preferably w/in 12 hrs of birth; initiate hepatitis B vaccine series simultaneously

Household Exposure to Persons w/ Acute Hepatitis B Virus Infection: <12 Months of Age:
0.5mL IM along w/ hepatitis B vaccine Prophylaxis of other household contacts is not indicated unless there is an identifiable blood exposure to the index patient (eg, by sharing toothbrushes/razors); treat such exposures like sexual exposures

- -

ADMINISTRATION

IM route

May be administered at the same time (but at a different site), or up to 1 month preceding hepatitis B vaccination
Preferred sites are anterolateral aspect of the upper thigh and deltoid muscle

STORAGE

2-8°C (36-46°F). Do not freeze. Use within 6 hrs once opened; do not reuse or save for future use, and partially used vials should be discarded.

HOW SUPPLIED

Inj: >312 IU [1mL]; >1560 IU [5mL]

CONTRAINDICATIONS

Anaphylactic or severe systemic reaction to human globulin or IgA-deficiency disorder.

WARNINGS/PRECAUTIONS

Caution in patients with severe thrombocytopenia or coagulation disorders that contraindicate IM administration; give only if expected benefits outweigh the potential risks. Products made from human plasma may contain infectious agents and cause disease. Must be administered IM.

ADVERSE REACTIONS

Headache, erythema, myalgia, malaise, nausea, injection-site pain, elevated alkaline phosphatase levels.

DRUG INTERACTIONS

May interfere with live virus vaccines; defer until 3 months following the last dose of vaccine.

PREGNANCY AND LACTATION

Category C, caution in nursing.

MECHANISM OF ACTION

Vaccine; passive immunization from HBV exposure resulting in reduction of HBV infection rate.

PHARMACOKINETICS

Absorption: T_{max}=6.5 days. **Distribution:** V_d=11.2L. **Excretion:** $T_{1/2}$=23.1 days.

PATIENT CONSIDERATIONS

Assessment: Assess HBsAg/HBeAg, thrombocytopenia, coagulation disorder, IgA-deficiency, previous history of severe anaphylactic or systemic reaction to human globulin, live virus vaccination, and pregnancy/nursing status. Assess for acute exposure to blood of HBsAg-positive mothers, sexual contact with HBsAg-positive persons, and household persons with acute HBV infection.

Monitoring: Monitor for erythema, headache, myalgia, malaise, nausea, and elevated alkaline phosphatase levels.

Counseling: Advise to avoid live virus vaccination for 3 months after hepatitis B immune globulin administration; revaccinate persons immediately after live virus administration.

NAGLAZYME — galsulfase   Rx

Class: Enzyme

ADULT DOSAGE

Mucopolysaccharidosis VI (Maroteaux-Lamy Syndrome)

Usual: 1mg/kg administered once weekly as an IV infusion over ≥4 hrs

Infusion Rate:
Initial: 6mL/hr for the 1st hr
Titrate: If well tolerated, rate may be increased to 80mL/hr for the remaining 3 hrs

Premedication

Antihistamines (w/ or w/o antipyretics) are recommended 30-60 min prior to the start of infusion

PEDIATRIC DOSAGE

Mucopolysaccharidosis VI (Maroteaux-Lamy Syndrome)

Usual: 1mg/kg administered once weekly as an IV infusion over ≥4 hrs

Infusion Rate:
Initial: 6mL/hr for the 1st hr
Titrate: If well tolerated, rate may be increased to 80mL/hr for the remaining 3 hrs

Premedication

Antihistamines (w/ or w/o antipyretics) are recommended 30-60 min prior to the start of infusion

- -

DOSING CONSIDERATIONS

Adverse Reactions

Infusion Reactions: Extend infusion time up to 20 hrs

Other Important Considerations

Patients ≤20kg or Susceptible to Fluid Volume Overload: Consider diluting Naglazyme in a volume of 100mL; decrease infusion rate so that the total infusion duration remains ≥4 hrs

ADMINISTRATION

IV route

Preparation Instructions

Prepare using low-protein-binding containers as follows:
1. Determine the number of vials to be used based on the patient's weight and the recommended dose of 1mg/ kg; refer to PI for calculation
2. Round up to the next whole vial and remove the required number of vials from the refrigerator to allow them to reach room temperature; do not allow vials to remain at room temperature >24 hrs prior to dilution. Do not heat or microwave vials
3. From a 250mL infusion bag of 0.9% NaCl inj, withdraw and discard a volume equal to the volume of galsulfase sol to be added; if using a 100mL infusion bag, this step is not necessary
4. Slowly withdraw the calculated volume of galsulfase from the appropriate number of vials using caution to avoid excessive agitation; do not use a filter needle, as this may cause agitation
5. Slowly add the galsulfase sol to the 0.9% NaCl inj, using care to avoid agitation of the sol; do not use a filter needle
6. Gently rotate the infusion bag to ensure proper distribution; do not shake the sol

Administration Instructions

Administer the diluted sol using a low-protein-binding infusion set equipped w/ a low-protein-binding 0.2μm in-line filter
Do not infuse w/ other products in the infusion tubing

Stability

If immediate use is not possible, store the diluted sol in the refrigerator at 2-8°C (36-46°F) and administer w/in 48 hrs from the time of dilution to completion of administration

STORAGE

2-8°C (36-46°F). Do not freeze or shake. Protect from light. Diluted Sol: 2-8°C (36-46°F) and administer within 48 hrs from the time of dilution to completion of administration.

HOW SUPPLIED

Inj: 1mg/mL [5mL, vial]

WARNINGS/PRECAUTIONS

Anaphylaxis and severe allergic reactions (eg, shock, respiratory distress, dyspnea, bronchospasm, laryngeal edema, hypotension) reported; d/c immediately and initiate appropriate medical treatment if such reactions occur, and exercise caution upon rechallenge. Type III immune complex-mediated reactions, including membranous glomerulonephritis, reported; consider discontinuation and initiate appropriate medical treatment if immune-mediated reactions occur. Caution in patients susceptible to fluid volume overload (eg, patients weighing ≤20kg, patients with acute underlying respiratory illness, or with compromised cardiac and/or respiratory function); congestive heart failure may result. Consider evaluation of airway patency before initiation of treatment. Consider delaying infusions in patients who present with an acute febrile or respiratory illness; acute respiratory compromise during infusion may occur. Infusion reactions reported; d/c infusion immediately and initiate appropriate treatment if severe reactions occur. Consider risks and benefits of readministration following an immune-mediated reaction or a severe infusion reaction. Onset or worsening of spinal/cervical cord compression (SCC) requiring decompression surgery reported.

ADVERSE REACTIONS

Abdominal pain, ear pain, arthralgia, pain, conjunctivitis, dyspnea, rash, chills, chest pain, pharyngitis, areflexia, corneal opacity, gastroenteritis, HTN, malaise.

PREGNANCY AND LACTATION

Category B, caution in nursing.

MECHANISM OF ACTION

Hydrolytic lysosomal glycosaminoglycan (GAG)-specific enzyme; provides an exogenous enzyme that will be taken up into lysosomes and increase the catabolism of GAG.

PHARMACOKINETICS

Absorption: C_{max}=0.8mcg/mL (Week 1), 1.5mcg/mL (Week 24); AUC_{0-t}=2.3mcg•hr/mL (Week 1), 4.3mcg•hr/mL (Week 24). **Distribution:** V_d=103mL/kg (Week 1), 69mL/kg (Week 24). **Elimination:** $T_{1/2}$=9 min (Week 1), 26 min (Week 24).

PATIENT CONSIDERATIONS

Assessment: Assess for susceptibility to fluid volume overload, airway patency, and pregnancy/nursing status.

Monitoring: Monitor for anaphylaxis, severe allergic reactions, immune-mediated reactions, infusion reactions, SCC, and other adverse effects.

Counseling: Counsel that reactions related to administration and infusion may occur during treatment. Encourage to participate in the Clinical Surveillance Program and advise that their participation is voluntary and may involve long-term follow-up.

NATPARA — parathyroid hormone   Rx

Class: Parathyroid hormone analogue

> Potential risk of osteosarcoma; use only in patients who cannot be well-controlled on Ca^{2+} and active forms of vitamin D alone and for whom the potential benefits are considered to outweigh this risk. Avoid use w/ increased baseline risk for osteosarcoma such as patients w/ Paget's disease of bone or unexplained elevations of alkaline phosphatase, pediatric and young adult patients w/ open epiphyses, patients w/ hereditary disorders predisposing to osteosarcoma, or patients w/ a prior history of external beam or implant radiation therapy involving the skeleton. Available only through a restricted program under a Risk Evaluation and Mitigation Strategy (REMS) called the Natpara REMS program.

ADULT DOSAGE

Hypocalcemia with Hypoparathyroidism

Adjunct to Ca^{2+} and Vitamin D to Control Hypocalcemia:
Before Initiating and During Therapy:
Confirm 25-hydroxyvitamin D stores are sufficient; if insufficient, replace to sufficient levels
Confirm serum Ca^{2+} is >7.5mg/dL before initiating therapy

Initiating Therapy:
1. Initiate at 50mcg SQ qd
2. In patients using active forms of vitamin D, decrease dose of active vitamin D by 50%, if serum Ca^{2+} >7.5mg/dL
3. In patients using Ca^{2+} supplements, maintain Ca^{2+} supplement dose
4. Measure serum Ca^{2+} concentration w/in 3-7 days
5. Adjust dose of active vitamin D or Ca^{2+} supplement or both based on serum Ca^{2+} value and clinical assessment; refer to PI for suggested adjustments
6. Repeat steps 4 and 5 until target serum Ca^{2+} levels are w/in the lower 1/2 of the normal range (8-9mg/dL), active vitamin D has been discontinued, and Ca^{2+} supplementation is sufficient to meet daily requirements

Titration:
Dose Increase: May increase in increments of 25mcg every 4 weeks up to a max of 100mcg/day if serum Ca^{2+} cannot be maintained >8mg/dL w/o an active form of vitamin D and/or oral Ca^{2+} supplementation
Dose Decrease: May decrease to as low as 25mcg/day if total serum Ca^{2+} is repeatedly >9mg/dL after active form of vitamin D has been discontinued and Ca^{2+} supplement has been decreased to a dose sufficient to meet daily requirements After a dose change, monitor clinical response as well as serum Ca^{2+}; adjust active vitamin D and Ca^{2+} supplements per steps 4-6 above if indicated

Maint Dose:
Use lowest dose that achieves total serum Ca^{2+} (albumin-corrected) w/ in the lower 1/2 of normal total serum Ca^{2+} range, w/o the need for active forms of vitamin D and w/ Ca^{2+} supplementation sufficient to meet daily requirements; monitor serum

PEDIATRIC DOSAGE

Pediatric use may not have been established

Ca²⁺ and 24 hr urinary calcium once maint dose is achieved

Missed Dose
Next dose should be administered as soon as reasonably feasible and additional exogenous Ca²⁺ should be taken in the event of hypocalcemia

---

DOSING CONSIDERATIONS
Elderly
Start at low end of dosing range

Dose Interruption or Discontinuation
Abrupt interruption or discontinuation can result in severe hypocalcemia; resume treatment w/, or increase the dose of, an active form of vitamin D and Ca²⁺supplements if indicated in patients interrupting or discontinuing therapy

ADMINISTRATION
SQ route

Administer in thigh; alternate thigh every day
Refer to PI for the instructions to reconstitute using the mixing device for reconstitution and to administer using the pen delivery device (Q-Cliq pen)

STORAGE
(Cartridge) Prior to Reconstitution: 2-8°C (36-46°F). After Reconstitution: Store in the Q-Cliq pen at 2-8°C (36-46°F) and may be used for up to 14 days under these conditions; discard after 14 days. Store away from heat and light. Avoid exposure to elevated temperatures. Do not freeze or shake. (Mixing Device/Empty Q-Cliq Pen) Room temperature.

HOW SUPPLIED
Inj: 25mcg/dose, 50mcg/dose, 75mcg/dose, 100mcg/dose

WARNINGS/PRECAUTIONS
Severe hypercalcemia reported; risk is highest when starting or increasing dose of parathyroid hormone but can occur at any time. Treat hypercalcemia per standard practice and consider holding and/or lowering parathyroid hormone dose if severe hypercalcemia occurs. Severe hypocalcemia reported; risk is highest when parathyroid hormone is withheld, missed, or abruptly discontinued. Resume treatment w/, or increase dose of, an active form of vitamin D or Ca²⁺ supplements or both if indicated in patients interrupting or discontinuing therapy. Caution in elderly.

ADVERSE REACTIONS
Paresthesia, hypo/hypercalcemia, headache, N/V, hypoaesthesia, diarrhea, arthralgia, hypercalciuria, pain in extremity, URTI, upper abdominal pain, sinusitis, HTN, neck pain.

DRUG INTERACTIONS
Not recommended w/ alendronate. Concomitant use w/ cardiac glycosides (eg, digoxin) may predispose patients to digitalis toxicity if hypercalcemia develops; carefully monitor serum Ca²⁺ and digoxin levels, and for signs/symptoms of digoxin toxicity. Adjustment of digoxin and/or parathyroid hormone may be needed.

PREGNANCY AND LACTATION
Pregnancy: Category C.
Lactation: Not for use in nursing.

MECHANISM OF ACTION
Parathyroid hormone; raises serum Ca²⁺ by increasing renal tubular Ca²⁺ reabsorption, increasing intestinal Ca²⁺ absorption, and by increasing bone turnover which releases Ca²⁺ into the circulation.

PHARMACOKINETICS
Absorption: Absolute bioavailability (53%); T_{max}=5-30 min (50mcg, 100mcg); 2nd small peak at 1-2 hrs. **Distribution:** V_d=5.35L. **Metabolism:** Liver, kidneys. **Elimination:** $T_{1/2}$=3.02 hrs (50mcg), 2.83 hrs (100mcg).

PATIENT CONSIDERATIONS
Assessment: Assess for increased baseline risk for osteosarcoma, pregnancy/nursing status, and for possible drug interactions. Assess serum Ca²⁺ levels, and 25-hydroxyvitamin D stores.

Monitoring: Monitor for signs and symptoms of osteosarcoma, hypo/hypercalcemia, and other adverse reactions. Monitor serum Ca²⁺ levels and 25-hydroxyvitamin D stores.

Counseling: Inform of the risks/benefits of therapy. Inform that the drug is available only through a restricted program called the Natpara REMS program. Advise of potential risk of osteosarcoma and to promptly report signs/symptoms of possible osteosarcoma (eg, persistent localized pain, occurrence of a new tissue mass that is tender to palpation). Advise that severe hypercalcemia may occur when initiating/adjusting dose and/or making changes to coadministered drugs known to raise serum Ca²⁺; instruct to report symptoms promptly, report any changes to coadministered drugs known to influence Ca²⁺ levels, and follow recommended serum Ca²⁺ monitoring. Inform that severe hypocalcemia may occur when therapy is abruptly interrupted/discontinued; instruct to report symptoms of severe hypocalcemia promptly, report interruption in dosing, follow recommended serum Ca²⁺ monitoring, and to contact physician in the event of dose interruption as doses of active vitamin D and Ca²⁺ supplementation may need adjustment. Instruct to report use of digoxin-containing medication, and follow recommended serum Ca²⁺ monitoring. Counsel patient or caregiver on the proper technique for administering SQ inj using the mixing device and the Q-Cliq pen, including the use of aseptic technique.

NAVELBINE — vinorelbine tartrate   Rx
Class: Vinca alkaloid

> Severe myelosuppression resulting in serious infection, septic shock, hospitalization, and death may occur. Decrease the dose or withhold treatment in accordance with recommended dose modifications.

ADULT DOSAGE
Non-Small Cell Lung Cancer

Combination w/ Cisplatin:
1st-line treatment of locally advanced or metastatic non-small cell lung cancer

W/ Cisplatin 100mg/m²:
25mg/m² vinorelbine IV inj or infusion over 6-10 min on Days 1, 8, 15, and 21 of a 28-day cycle w/ cisplatin 100mg/m² on Day 1 only of each 28-day cycle

W/ Cisplatin 120mg/m²:
30mg/m² vinorelbine IV inj or infusion over 6-10 min once a week w/ cisplatin 120mg/m² on Days 1 and 29, then every 6 weeks

As a Single-Agent:
Treatment of metastatic non-small cell lung cancer
30mg/m² IV over 6-10 min once a week

PEDIATRIC DOSAGE
Pediatric use may not have been established

DOSING CONSIDERATIONS
Hepatic Impairment
Serum Total Bilirubin 2.1-3mg/dL: Administer 50% of starting dose
Serum Total Bilirubin >3mg/dL: Administer 25% of starting dose

Concurrent Hematologic Toxicity: Administer the lower of the doses based on the corresponding starting dose

Adverse Reactions
Hematologic Toxicity:
Neutrophils on Day of Treatment:
1000-1499 cells/mm³: Administer 50% of starting dose
<1000 cells/mm³: Do not administer, and repeat neutrophil count in 1 week; d/c therapy if 3 consecutive weekly doses are held because neutrophil count is <1000 cells/mm³

Fever and/or Sepsis While Neutrophil Count is <1500 cells/mm³ or 2 Consecutive Weekly Doses Held:
<1500 cells/mm³: Administer 75% of subsequent dose
1000-1499 cells/mm³: Administer 37.5% of subsequent dose
<1000 cells/mm³: Do not administer, and repeat neutrophil count in 1 week

Concurrent Hepatic Impairment: Administer the lower of the doses based on the corresponding starting dose

Neurologic Toxicity:
NCI CTCAE ≥Grade 2 Peripheral/Autonomic Neuropathy Causing Constipation: D/C therapy

ADMINISTRATION
IV route

Preparation
Dilute vinorelbine in either a syringe or IV bag using 1 of the recommended sol:
Syringe:
Dilute to a concentration between 1.5 and 3mg/mL. The following sol may be used for dilution:
1. D5 inj
2. 0.9% NaCl inj
IV Bag:
Dilute to a concentration between 0.5 and 2mg/mL. The following sol may be used for dilution:
1. D5 inj
2. 0.9% NaCl inj
3. 0.45% NaCl inj
4. D5 and 0.45% NaCl inj
5. Ringer's inj
6. Lactated Ringer's inj

Administration
Administer diluted vinorelbine into the side port of a free-flowing IV line followed by flushing w/ at least 75-125mL of 1 of the sol

Management of Suspected Extravasation
If leakage into surrounding tissue occurs or is suspected, immediately stop administration and initiate appropriate management measures in accordance w/ institutional policies

Proper Handling Procedures
If the sol contacts the skin or mucosa, immediately wash the skin or mucosa thoroughly w/ soap and water
Avoid contamination of the eye; if exposure occurs, flush the eyes w/ water immediately and thoroughly

STORAGE
2-8°C (36-46°F). Protect from light. Do not freeze. Unopened vials are stable at 25°C (77°F) for up to 72 hrs. Diluted sol may be used for up to 24 hrs under

normal room light when stored in polypropylene syringes or polyvinyl chloride bags at 5-30°C (41-86°F).

HOW SUPPLIED
Inj: 10mg/mL [1mL, 5mL]

WARNINGS/PRECAUTIONS
Drug-induced liver injury may occur. Severe and fatal paralytic ileus, constipation, intestinal obstruction, necrosis, and perforation reported; institute prophylactic bowel regimen to mitigate potential constipation, bowel obstruction, and/or paralytic ileus, considering adequate dietary fiber intake, hydration, and routine use of stool softeners. Extravasation may result in severe irritation, local tissue necrosis, and/or thrombophlebitis; d/c immediately and institute recommended management procedures if signs and symptoms occur. Sensory and motor neuropathies may occur; d/c for National Cancer Institute Common Terminology Criteria for Adverse Events ≥Grade 2 neuropathy. Pulmonary toxicity (eg, severe acute bronchospasm, interstitial pneumonitis, acute respiratory distress syndrome [ARDS]) reported. Interrupt treatment in patients who develop unexplained dyspnea, or evidence of pulmonary toxicity; permanently d/c for confirmed interstitial pneumonitis or ARDS. May cause fetal harm.

ADVERSE REACTIONS
Severe myelosuppression, leukopenia, neutropenia, anemia, increased AST, N/V, asthenia, inj-site reaction, constipation, peripheral neuropathy, diarrhea, increased total bilirubin, alopecia, thrombocytopenia, phlebitis.

DRUG INTERACTIONS
Concurrent use with CYP3A inhibitors may cause an earlier onset and/or increased severity of adverse reactions; use with caution.

PREGNANCY AND LACTATION
Category D, not for use in nursing.

MECHANISM OF ACTION
Vinca alkaloid; inhibits mitosis at metaphase via interaction with tubulin.

PHARMACOKINETICS
Distribution: V_d=25.4-40.1L/kg, plasma protein binding (79.6-91.2%). **Metabolism:** CYP3A; deacetylvinorelbine (primary metabolite), vinorelbine N-oxide. **Elimination:** Urine (18%), feces (46%); $T_{1/2}$=27.7-43.6 hrs.

PATIENT CONSIDERATIONS
Assessment: Assess for pregnancy/nursing status and possible drug interactions. Obtain baseline CBC and LFTs.

Monitoring: Monitor for paralytic ileus, constipation, intestinal obstruction, necrosis, perforation, extravasation, new/worsening signs and symptoms of sensory/motor neuropathies, pulmonary toxicity, unexplained dyspnea, and other adverse reactions. Monitor CBC prior to each dose of treatment. Monitor LFTs periodically.

Counseling: Advise to follow a diet rich in fiber, drink fluids, and use stool softeners to avoid constipation. Advise to contact physician for fever, symptoms of infection, severe constipation, abdominal pain, N/V, new onset/worsening of numbness, tingling, decreased sensation, muscle weakness, SOB, cough, wheezing, or other new pulmonary symptoms. Advise females of reproductive potential to use highly effective contraception during treatment and to contact physician if they become pregnant, or if pregnancy is suspected. Advise males to use highly effective contraception during and for 3 months after therapy.

NEORAL — cyclosporine   Rx

Class: Calcineurin-inhibitor immunosuppressant

> Should only be prescribed by physicians experienced in management of systemic immunosuppressive therapy for indicated diseases. Manage patients in facilities equipped and staffed w/ adequate lab and supportive medical resources. Increased susceptibility to infection and development of neoplasia (eg, lymphoma) may result from immunosuppression. May be coadministered w/ other immunosuppressive agents in kidney, liver, and heart transplant patients. Not bioequivalent to Sandimmune and cannot be used interchangeably w/o physician supervision. Caution in switching from Sandimmune. Monitor cyclosporine blood concentrations in transplant and rheumatoid arthritis (RA) patients to avoid toxicity due to high concentrations. Dose adjustments should be made to minimize possible organ rejection due to low concentrations in transplant patients. Increased risk of developing skin malignancies in psoriasis patients previously treated w/ PUVA, methotrexate (MTX) or other immunosuppressive agents, UVB, coal tar, or radiation therapy. May cause systemic HTN and nephrotoxicity. Monitor for renal dysfunction, including structural kidney damage, during therapy.

ADULT DOSAGE
Organ Transplant
Organ Rejection Prophylaxis in Kidney, Liver, and Heart Allogeneic Transplants:
Newly Transplanted Patients:
Initial dose may be given 4-12 hrs prior to transplant or given postoperatively; dose varies depending on transplanted organ and other immunosuppressive agents included in protocol

Suggested Initial Doses:
Renal Transplant: 9mg/kg/day ± 3mg/kg/day
Liver Transplant: 8mg/kg/day ± 4mg/kg/day
Heart Transplant: 7mg/kg/day ± 3mg/kg/day

PEDIATRIC DOSAGE
Organ Rejection Prophylaxis
Transplant recipients as young as 1 year of age have received Neoral w/ no unusual adverse effects

---

Give bid

Subsequently adjust dose to achieve a predefined blood concentration

Adjunct therapy w/ adrenal corticosteroids is recommended initially

Conversion from Sandimmune:
Start w/ same daily dose as was previously used w/ Sandimmune (1:1 dose conversion); subsequently adjust dose to attain the pre-conversion blood trough concentration. After conversion, monitor blood trough concentration every 4-7 days while adjusting to trough levels until concentration attains pre-conversion value.

Transplant Patients w/ Poor Sandimmune Absorption:
Patients tend to have higher cyclosporine concentrations after conversion to therapy; caution when converting patients at doses >10mg/kg/day.
Titrate dose individually based on trough concentrations, tolerability, and clinical response and measure blood trough concentration at least 2X a week (daily if initial dose >10mg/kg/day) until stabilized w/in desired range.

Rheumatoid Arthritis
Severe, active rheumatoid arthritis where the disease has not adequately responded to methotrexate (MTX)

W/ or w/o MTX:
Initial: 2.5mg/kg/day, taken bid
Titrate: May increase by 0.5-0.75mg/kg/day after 8 weeks and again after 12 weeks
Max: 4mg/kg/day

Salicylates, NSAIDs, and oral corticosteroids may be continued

D/C if no benefit is seen by 16 weeks

Combination w/ MTX:
Most patients can be treated w/ doses of ≤3mg/kg/day when combined w/ MTX doses of up to 15mg/week

Plaque Psoriasis
In immunocompetent patients w/ severe, recalcitrant, plaque psoriasis who failed to respond to at least 1 systemic therapy (eg, PUVA, retinoids, methotrexate) or for whom other systemic therapies are contraindicated, or cannot be tolerated

Initial: 2.5mg/kg/day, taken bid, for at least 4 weeks
Titrate: If clinical improvement does not occur, increase dose at 2-week intervals by approx 0.5mg/kg/day
Max: 4mg/kg/day

D/C if satisfactory response cannot be achieved after 6 weeks at 4mg/kg/day or the patient's max tolerated dose

- -

DOSING CONSIDERATIONS
Renal Impairment
In Kidney, Liver, and Heart Transplant:
Reduce dose if indicated
In Rheumatoid Arthritis/Plaque Psoriasis:
Not recommended for use

Hepatic Impairment
Severe: Dose reduction may be necessary

Elderly
Start at lower end of dosing range

Adverse Events
Rheumatoid Arthritis/Plaque Psoriasis:
Reduce dose by 25-50% to control adverse events; d/c therapy if dose reduction is not effective or if adverse event or abnormality is severe

Other Important Considerations
Avoid consumption of grapefruit or grapefruit juice during therapy

ADMINISTRATION

Oral route

Always administer daily dose in 2 divided doses (bid); administer on a consistent schedule w/ regard to time of day and relation to meals.

Sol

1. Dilute w/ room temperature orange or apple juice to make sol more palatable; avoid switching diluents frequently or diluting w/ grapefruit juice.
2. Take the prescribed amount of sol from the container using supplied dosing syringe, after removal of protective cover, and transfer sol to a glass of orange or apple juice (do not use a plastic container).
3. Stir well and drink at once; do not allow diluted oral sol to stand before drinking.
4. Rinse the glass w/ more diluent to ensure that the total dose is consumed.
5. After use, dry the outside of dosing syringe w/ a clean towel and replace protective cover.
6. Do not rinse dosing syringe w/ water or other cleaning agents; if syringe requires cleaning, it must be completely dry before resuming use.

STORAGE

20-25°C (68-77°F). (Sol) Use w/in 2 months upon opening. Do not refrigerate. At <20°C (68°F) may form gel; light flocculation, or formation of light sediment may occur; allow to warm to 25°C (77°F) to reverse changes.

HOW SUPPLIED

Cap: 25mg, 100mg; **Sol:** 100mg/mL [50mL]

CONTRAINDICATIONS

Hypersensitivity to cyclosporine or to any of the ingredients of the formulation. **RA/Psoriasis:** Abnormal renal function, uncontrolled HTN, malignancies. **Psoriasis:** Concomitant PUVA or UVB therapy, MTX, other immunosuppressants, coal tar, or radiation therapy.

WARNINGS/PRECAUTIONS

May cause hepatotoxicity and liver injury (eg, cholestasis, jaundice, hepatitis, liver failure). Elevations of SrCr and BUN may occur and reflect a reduction in GFR; closely monitor renal function and frequent dose adjustments may be indicated. Elevations in SrCr and BUN levels do not necessarily indicate rejection; evaluate patient before initiating dose adjustment. Thrombocytopenia and microangiopathic hemolytic anemia, resulting in graft failure, significant hyperkalemia (sometimes associated w/ hyperchloremic metabolic acidosis) and hyperuricemia reported. Avoid excessive ultraviolet light exposure. Oversuppression of the immune system may result in an increased risk of infection/malignancy; caution w/ a multiple immunosuppressant regimen. Increased risk of developing bacterial, viral, fungal, protozoal, and opportunistic infections (eg, polyomavirus infections). JC virus-associated progressive multifocal leukoencephalopathy and polyomavirus-/BK virus-associated nephropathy reported; consider reduction in immunosuppression if either develops. Convulsions, encephalopathy including posterior reversible encephalopathy syndrome, and rarely, optic disc edema reported. Evaluate before and during treatment for development of malignancies. In RA patients, monitor BP on at least 2 occasions and obtain 2 baseline SrCr levels before treatment, then monitor BP and SrCr every 2 weeks for the first 3 months of therapy, and then monthly if the patient is stable or more frequently during dose adjustments. In psoriasis patients, assess BP on at least 2 occasions and obtain baseline SrCr, BUN, CBC, Mg^{2+}, K$^+$, uric acid, and lipids before treatment, then monitor every 2 weeks for the first 3 months of therapy, and then monthly if the patient is stable or more frequently during dose adjustments. Monitor CBC and LFTs monthly w/ MTX. Monitor SrCr and BP after initiation or increases in NSAID dose for RA. Consider the alcohol content of the drug when given to patients in whom alcohol intake should be avoided or minimized (eg, pregnant or breastfeeding women, patients presenting w/ liver disease or epilepsy, alcoholic patients, or pediatric patients). HTN may occur and persist, and may require antihypertensive therapy.

ADVERSE REACTIONS

Increased susceptibility to infection, neoplasia, renal dysfunction, HTN, hirsutism/hypertrichosis, tremor, headache, gum hyperplasia, diarrhea, N/V, paresthesia, hypertriglyceridemia, hyperesthesia.

DRUG INTERACTIONS

See Boxed Warning, Dosing Considerations, and Contraindications. Avoid w/ K$^+$-sparing diuretics, aliskiren, orlistat, bosentan, or dabigatran. Vaccinations may be less effective; avoid live vaccines during therapy. Frequent gingival hyperplasia reported w/ nifedipine; avoid concomitant use w/ nifedipine in patients in whom gingival hyperplasia develops as a side effect of cyclosporine. Caution w/ rifabutin, nephrotoxic drugs, HIV protease inhibitors (eg, indinavir, nelfinavir, ritonavir, saquinavir), K$^+$-sparing drugs (eg, ACE inhibitors, ARBs), K$^+$-containing drugs, and K$^+$-rich diet. Ciprofloxacin, gentamicin, tobramycin, vancomycin, trimethoprim w/ sulfamethoxazole, melphalan, amphotericin B, ketoconazole, azapropazon, colchicine, diclofenac, naproxen, sulindac, cimetidine, ranitidine, tacrolimus, fibric acid derivatives (eg, bezafibrate, fenofibrate), MTX, and NSAIDs may potentiate renal dysfunction; closely monitor renal function and reduce dose of coadministered drug or consider alternative treatment if significant renal impairment occurs. Diltiazem, nicardipine, verapamil, fluconazole, itraconazole, ketoconazole, voriconazole, azithromycin, clarithromycin, erythromycin, quinupristin/dalfopristin, methylprednisolone, allopurinol, amiodarone, bromocriptine, colchicine, danazol, imatinib, metoclopramide, nefazodone, oral contraceptives, grapefruit, grapefruit juice, HIV protease inhibitors, boceprevir, and telaprevir may increase levels. Nafcillin, rifampin, carbamazepine, oxcarbazepine, phenobarbital, phenytoin, bosentan, octreotide, orlistat, sulfinpyrazone, terbinafine, ticlopidine, and St. John's wort may decrease levels. May increase levels of bosentan, dabigatran, and CYP3A4, P-gp, or organic anion transporter protein substrates. May increase levels of ambrisentan; do not titrate ambrisentan dose to the recommended max daily dose. CYP3A4 and/or P-gp inducers and inhibitors may alter levels; may require dose adjustments of cyclosporine if cyclosporine concentrations are significantly altered. May reduce

clearance of digoxin, colchicine, prednisolone, HMG-CoA reductase inhibitors (statins), aliskiren, bosentan, dabigatran, repaglinide, NSAIDs, sirolimus, and etoposide. Digitalis toxicity reported when used w/ digoxin; monitor digoxin levels. May increase levels and enhance toxic effects (eg, myopathy, neuropathy) of colchicine; may reduce colchicine dose. Myotoxicity cases seen w/ lovastatin, simvastatin, atorvastatin, pravastatin, and, rarely fluvastatin; temporarily withhold or d/c statin therapy if signs of myopathy develop or w/ risk factors predisposing to severe renal injury, including renal failure, secondary to rhabdomyolysis. May increase levels of repaglinide, thereby increasing the risk of hypoglycemia; closely monitor blood glucose levels. High doses of cyclosporine may increase the exposure to anthracycline antibiotics (eg, doxorubicin, mitoxantrone, daunorubicin) in cancer patients. May double diclofenac blood levels; dose of diclofenac should be in the lower end of the therapeutic range. May increase MTX levels and decrease levels of active metabolite of MTX. May elevate SrCr and increase levels of sirolimus; give 4 hrs after cyclosporine administration. Convulsions reported w/ high-dose methylprednisolone. Calcium antagonists may interfere w/ cyclosporine metabolism. Avoid in psoriasis patients receiving other immunosuppressive agents or radiation therapy (including PUVA and UVB).

PREGNANCY AND LACTATION

Category C, not for use in nursing.

MECHANISM OF ACTION

Cyclic polypeptide immunosuppressant; results from specific and reversible inhibition of immunocompetent lymphocytes in the G$_0$- and G$_1$-phase of the cell cycle. T-lymphocytes are preferentially inhibited w/ T-helper cell as main target while also possibly suppressing T-suppressor cells. Also inhibits lymphokine production and release (eg, interleukin-2).

PHARMACOKINETICS

Absorption: Incomplete; T$_{max}$=1.5-2 hrs. Pharmacokinetic parameters varied w/ different indications (renal transplant, liver transplant, RA, and/or psoriasis). **Distribution:** V$_d$=3-5L/kg (IV); plasma protein binding (90%); found in breast milk. **Metabolism:** (Extensive) Liver via CYP3A, to a lesser extent GI tract and kidneys. M1, M9, and M4N (major metabolites); oxidation and demethylation pathways. **Elimination:** Bile (primary), urine (6%, 0.1% unchanged); T$_{1/2}$=8.4 hrs.

PATIENT CONSIDERATIONS

Assessment: Assess for hypersensitivity to the drug, renal dysfunction, uncontrolled HTN, presence of malignancies, pregnancy/nursing status, and possible drug interactions. RA: Before initiating treatment, assess BP (on at least 2 occasions) and obtain 2 SrCr levels. Psoriasis: Prior to treatment, perform a dermatological and physical examination, including measuring BP. Assess for presence of occult infections and for the presence of tumors. Assess for atypical skin lesions and biopsy them. Obtain baseline SrCr (at least twice), BUN, LFTs, bilirubin, CBC, Mg^{2+}, K$^+$, uric acid, and lipid levels.

Monitoring: Monitor for signs/symptoms of hepatotoxicity, liver injury, nephrotoxicity, thrombocytopenia, microangiopathic hemolytic anemia, HTN, hyperkalemia, lymphomas and other malignancies, serious/polyoma virus infections, convulsions and other neurotoxicities, and other adverse reactions. Monitor cyclosporine blood concentrations routinely in transplant patients and periodically in RA patients. RA: Monitor BP and SrCr every 2 weeks during the initial 3 months of treatment, then monthly if patient is stable. Monitor SrCr and BP after an increase of the dose of NSAIDs and after initiation of new NSAID therapy. If coadministered w/ MTX, monitor CBC and LFTs monthly. Psoriasis: Monitor for occult infections and tumors. Monitor SrCr, BUN, BP, CBC, uric acid, K$^+$, lipids, and Mg^{2+} levels every 2 weeks during first 3 months of treatment, then monthly if stable.

Counseling: Instruct to contact physician before changing formulations of cyclosporine, which may require dose changes. Inform that repeated lab tests are required while on therapy. Advise of the potential risks if used during pregnancy and inform of the increased risk of neoplasia, HTN, and renal dysfunction. Inform that vaccinations may be less effective and to avoid live vaccines during therapy. Advise to take the medication on a consistent schedule w/ regard to time and meals, and to avoid grapefruit and grapefruit juice. Inform to avoid excessive sun exposure.

NEULASTA — pegfilgrastim   Rx

Class: Granulocyte colony-stimulating factor (G-CSF)

ADULT DOSAGE	PEDIATRIC DOSAGE
Chemotherapy-Associated Neutropenia	**Chemotherapy-Associated Neutropenia**
To decrease the incidence of infection in patients w/ nonmyeloid malignancies receiving myelosuppressive anticancer drugs associated w/ febrile neutropenia	To decrease the incidence of infection in patients w/ nonmyeloid malignancies receiving myelosuppressive anticancer drugs associated w/ febrile neutropenia
6mg SQ once per chemotherapy cycle; do not administer between 14 days before and 24 hrs after administration of cytotoxic chemotherapy	**<10kg:** 0.1mg/kg (0.01mL/kg) **10-20kg:** 1.5mg (0.15mL) **21-30kg:** 2.5mg (0.25mL) **31-44kg:** 4mg (0.40mL) **≥45kg:** Refer to adult dosing
Hematopoietic Subsyndrome of Acute Radiation Syndrome	Administer once per chemotherapy cycle; do not administer between 14 days before and 24 hrs after administration of cytotoxic chemotherapy
To increase survival in patients acutely exposed to myelosuppressive doses of radiation	

2 doses of 6mg SQ, administered 1 week apart

Administer 1st dose as soon as possible after suspected or confirmed exposure to radiation levels >2 gray (Gy)

Obtain a baseline CBC; do not delay administration if a CBC is not readily available. Estimate a patient's absorbed radiation dose (eg, level of radiation exposure) based on information from public health authorities, biodosimetry if available, or clinical findings (eg, time to onset of vomiting, lymphocyte depletion kinetics)

Hematopoietic Subsyndrome of Acute Radiation Syndrome

To increase survival in patients acutely exposed to myelosuppressive doses of radiation

<10kg: 0.1mg/kg (0.01mL/kg)
10-20kg: 1.5mg (0.15mL)
21-30kg: 2.5mg (0.25mL)
31-44kg: 4mg (0.40mL)
≥45kg: Refer to adult dosing

Administer 1st dose as soon as possible after suspected or confirmed exposure to radiation levels >2 Gy

Administer 2nd dose 1 week after the 1st dose

Obtain a baseline CBC; do not delay administration if a CBC is not readily available. Estimate a patient's absorbed radiation dose (eg, level of radiation exposure) based on information from public health authorities, biodosimetry if available, or clinical findings (eg, time to onset of vomiting, lymphocyte depletion kinetics)

ADMINISTRATION
SQ route

Administer via a single-dose prefilled syringe for manual use or w/ the On-body Injector.
Use of the On-body Injector is not recommended for patients w/ hematopoietic subsydrome of acute radiation syndrome.
Use of On-body Injector has not been studied in pediatric patients.
Prefilled syringe is not designed to allow for direct administration of doses <0.6mL (6mg).
Prior to use, remove the carton from the refrigerator and allow the prefilled syringe to reach room temperature for a minimum of 30 min; discard any prefilled syringe left at room temperature for >48 hrs.
The needle cap on the prefilled syringes contain dry natural rubber (derived from latex); persons w/ latex allergies should not administer.

Instructions for On-body Injector
For Physicians:
- Fill the On-body Injector w/ pegfilgrastim using prefilled syringe and apply to patient's skin (abdomen or back of arm).
- Use back of the arm only if a caregiver is available to monitor the status of the On-body Injector.
- Approx 27 hrs after the application, pegfilgrastim will be delivered over approx 45 min.
- May initiate administration on the same day as the administration of cytotoxic chemotherapy, as long as On-body Injector delivers pegfilgrastim no less than 24 hrs after administration of cytotoxic chemotherapy.
- Do not use On-body Injector to deliver any other drug product except pegfilgrastim prefilled syringe co-packaged w/ On-body Injector.
- Apply to intact, non-irritated skin on the arm or abdomen.
- Missed dose may occur due to an On-body Injector failure/leakage; if a dose is missed, administer new dose by single-dose prefilled syringe for manual use, as soon as possible after detection.
- Refer to Healthcare Provider Instructions for Use for the On-body Injector for Neulasta for full administration information.

STORAGE
2-8°C (36-46°F). **Prefilled Syringe for Manual Use:** Protect from light. Do not shake. Discard syringes stored at room temperature for >48 hrs. Avoid freezing; if frozen, thaw in the refrigerator before administration. Discard syringe if frozen more than once. **Onpro Kit:** Do not hold Kit at room temperature >12 hrs prior to use; discard if stored at room temperature for >12 hrs.

HOW SUPPLIED
Inj: 6mg/0.6mL [prefilled syringe for manual use, Onpro Kit]

CONTRAINDICATIONS
History of serious allergic reactions to pegfilgrastim or filgrastim.

WARNINGS/PRECAUTIONS
Not indicated for the mobilization of peripheral blood progenitor cells for hematopoietic stem cell transplantation. Splenic rupture, including fatal cases, may occur; evaluate for an enlarged spleen or splenic rupture if left upper abdominal or shoulder pain occurs. Acute respiratory distress syndrome (ARDS) may occur; evaluate for ARDS if fever and lung infiltrates or respiratory distress develops, and d/c if ARDS develops. Serious allergic reactions (eg, anaphylaxis) may occur; permanently d/c if a serious allergic reaction occurs. Use of On-body Injector may result in a significant reaction in patients who have reactions to acrylic adhesives. Severe and sometimes fatal sickle cell crises may occur in patients w/ sickle cell disorders. Glomerulonephritis reported; evaluate for cause if glomerulonephritis is suspected and consider dose reduction or interruption of pegfilgrastim if causality is likely. WBC counts of ≥100 x 10⁹/L reported; monitor CBC during therapy. May act as a growth factor for any tumor type. Capillary leak syndrome reported; closely monitor patients who develop symptoms and administer standard symptomatic treatment, which may include a need for intensive care. Increased hematopoietic activity of the bone marrow in response to therapy may result in transiently positive bone imaging changes; consider this when interpreting bone-imaging results.

ADVERSE REACTIONS
Bone pain, pain in extremity.

PREGNANCY AND LACTATION
Pregnancy: Category C.
Lactation: It is not known whether pegfilgrastim is secreted in human milk; caution in nursing.

MECHANISM OF ACTION
Granulocyte colony-stimulating factor; acts on hematopoietic cells by binding to specific cell surface receptors, thereby stimulating proliferation, differentiation, commitment, and end cell functional activation.

PHARMACOKINETICS
Elimination: $T_{1/2}$=15-80 hrs.

PATIENT CONSIDERATIONS
Assessment: Assess for history of hypersensitivity to pegfilgrastim or filgrastim, acrylic allergy, sickle cell disorders, and pregnancy/nursing status. In patients w/ hematopoietic subsyndrome of acute radiation syndrome, obtain CBC.

Monitoring: Monitor for enlarged spleen/splenic rupture, ARDS, serious allergic reactions, sickle cell crises (in patients w/ sickle cell disorders), glomerulonephritis, capillary leak syndrome, and other adverse reactions. Monitor CBC.

Counseling: Advise on the proper administration of pegfilgrastim and how to use the On-body Injector. Advise of the risks of therapy (eg, splenic rupture, ARDS, serious allergic reactions, sickle cell crisis, glomerulonephritis, capillary leak syndrome). Advise to avoid activities (eg, traveling, driving, operating heavy machinery) during 26-29 hrs following application of On-body Injector (this includes the 45-min delivery period plus 1 hr post-delivery). Advise female patients to notify physician if pregnant or nursing.

NEUMEGA — oprelvekin   Rx
Class: Thrombopoietic agent

Allergic or hypersensitivity reactions, including anaphylaxis, reported; permanently d/c if this develops.

ADULT DOSAGE
Thrombocytopenia
Prevention of severe thrombocytopenia and reduction of the need for platelet transfusions following myelosuppressive chemotherapy in adults w/ nonmyeloid malignancies who are at high risk of severe thrombocytopenia

Usual: 50mcg/kg qd
Initiate 6-24 hrs after chemotherapy completion. Continue therapy until post-nadir platelet count is ≥50,000/μL
Max: 21 days/treatment course. D/C at least 2 days before starting the next chemotherapy cycle. May give for up to 6 cycles following chemotherapy

PEDIATRIC DOSAGE
Pediatric use may not have been established

DOSING CONSIDERATIONS
Renal Impairment
Severe (CrCl <30mL/min): 25mcg/kg

ADMINISTRATION
SQ route

Administer in either the abdomen, thigh, or hip (upper arm if not self-injecting)

Preparation
1. Reconstitute using the 1mL of sterile water for inj (w/o preservative) contained in the prefilled syringe included in the kit
2. Administer oprelvekin w/in 3 hrs following reconstitution

STORAGE
2-8°C (36-46°F). Protect powder from light. Do not freeze. Reconstituted: 2-8°C (36-46°F) or up to 25°C (77°F). Do not freeze or shake.

HOW SUPPLIED
Inj: 5mg

CONTRAINDICATIONS
History of hypersensitivity to oprelvekin or any component of the product.

WARNINGS/PRECAUTIONS
Not indicated following myeloablative chemotherapy. May cause serious fluid retention; caution in congestive heart failure (CHF) patients; patients who may be susceptible to developing CHF, patients receiving aggressive hydration, patients with history of heart failure who are well-compensated and receiving appropriate medical therapy, and patients who may develop fluid retention as a result of associated medical conditions or whose medical condition may be exacerbated by fluid retention. Monitor preexisting fluid collections; consider drainage if medically indicated. Moderate decreases in Hgb, Hct, and RBCs reported. Cardiovascular events, including arrhythmias and pulmonary edema, reported. Caution with history of atrial arrhythmias. Papilledema reported; caution in patients with preexisting papilledema, or with tumors involving the CNS. Changes in visual

acuity and/or visual field defects may occur in patients with papilledema. Obtain CBC before chemotherapy and at regular intervals during therapy. Monitor platelet counts during expected nadir time and until adequate recovery has occurred (post-nadir counts ≥50,000/µL).

ADVERSE REACTIONS

Edema, dyspnea, tachycardia, conjunctival injection, palpitations, atrial arrhythmias, pleural effusions, syncope, pneumonia, neutropenic fever, headache, N/V, mucositis, diarrhea.

DRUG INTERACTIONS

Perform close monitoring of fluid and electrolyte status in patients receiving chronic diuretic therapy.

PREGNANCY AND LACTATION

Category C, not for use in nursing.

MECHANISM OF ACTION

Thrombopoietic agent; stimulates megakaryocytopoiesis and thrombopoiesis.

PHARMACOKINETICS

Absorption: Absolute bioavailability (>80%); C_{max}=17.4ng/mL; T_{max}=3.2 hrs.
Elimination: Urine; $T_{1/2}$=6.9 hrs.

PATIENT CONSIDERATIONS

Assessment: Assess for conditions where treatment is contraindicated or cautioned, pregnancy/nursing status, and possible drug interactions. Obtain baseline CBC prior to chemotherapy.

Monitoring: Monitor for signs/symptoms of hypersensitivity reactions, papilledema, fluid retention, pleural/pericardial effusion, atrial arrhythmias, and other adverse reactions. Periodically monitor CBC (including platelet counts), fluid balance, fluid and electrolyte status (chronic diuretic therapy).

Counseling: Inform of pregnancy risks. Instruct on the proper dose, method for reconstituting and administering, and importance of proper disposal of the product when used outside of the hospital or office setting. Inform of the serious and most common adverse reactions associated with the product. Advise to immediately seek medical attention if any of the signs or symptoms of allergic or hypersensitivity reactions (edema, difficulty breathing, swallowing or talking, SOB, wheezing, chest pain, throat tightness, lightheadedness), worsening of dyspnea, or symptoms attributable to atrial arrhythmia occur.

NEUPOGEN — filgrastim   Rx

Class: Granulocyte colony-stimulating factor (G-CSF)

ADULT DOSAGE

Myelosuppressive Chemotherapy

Decrease the incidence of infection, as manifested by febrile neutropenia, in patients w/ nonmyeloid malignancies receiving myelosuppressive anti-cancer drugs associated w/ a significant incidence of severe neutropenia w/ fever

Initial: 5mcg/kg/day; administer as a single SQ inj, by short IV infusion (15-30 min), or by continuous IV infusion
Titrate: May increase in increments of 5mcg/kg for each chemotherapy cycle, according to duration and severity of ANC nadir
D/C if ANC increases beyond 10,000/mm³

Administer at least 24 hrs after cytotoxic chemotherapy; do not administer w/in the 24-hr period prior to chemotherapy

Administer daily for up to 2 weeks or until the ANC has reached 10,000/mm³ following the expected chemotherapy-induced neutrophil nadir

Induction or Consolidation Chemotherapy

To reduce the time to neutrophil recovery and the duration of fever, following induction or consolidation chemotherapy treatment of patients w/ acute myeloid leukemia (AML)

Initial: 5mcg/kg/day; administer as a single SQ inj, by short IV infusion (15-30 min), or by continuous IV infusion
Titrate: May increase in increments of 5mcg/kg for each chemotherapy cycle, according to duration and severity of ANC nadir
D/C if ANC increases beyond 10,000/mm³

Administer at least 24 hrs after cytotoxic chemotherapy; do not

PEDIATRIC DOSAGE

General Dosing

Studied in pediatric patients w/ chemotherapy-associated neutropenia and in pediatric patients w/ severe chronic neutropenia; refer to PI

---

administer w/in the 24-hr period prior to chemotherapy

Administer daily for up to 2 weeks or until the ANC has reached 10,000/mm³ following the expected chemotherapy-induced neutrophil nadir

Bone Marrow Transplantation

To reduce the duration of neutropenia and neutropenia-related clinical sequelae (eg, febrile neutropenia) in patients w/ nonmyeloid malignancies undergoing myeloablative chemotherapy followed by bone marrow transplantation

10mcg/kg/day administered as an IV infusion no longer than 24 hrs; administer the first dose at least 24 hrs after cytotoxic chemotherapy and at least 24 hrs after bone marrow infusion

Dose Adjustments During Neutrophil Recovery:
When ANC >1000/mm³ for 3 Consecutive Days: Reduce to 5mcg/kg/day*
If ANC Remains >1000/mm³ for 3 More Consecutive Days: D/C therapy
If ANC Decreases to <1000/mm³: Resume at 5mcg/kg/day

*If ANC decreases to <1000/mm³ at any time during the 5mcg/kg/day administration, increase dose to 10mcg/kg/day, and follow the above steps

Hematopoietic Progenitor Cell Mobilization

Mobilization of autologous hematopoietic progenitor cells into the peripheral blood for collection by leukapheresis

10mcg/kg/day SQ inj; administer for ≥4 days before the 1st leukapheresis procedure and continue until the last leukapheresis

Administration of therapy for 6-7 days w/ leukapheresis on Days 5, 6, and 7 was found to be safe and effective

Monitor neutrophil counts after 4 days of therapy, and d/c if WBC count rises to >100,000/mm³

Severe Chronic Neutropenia

For chronic administration to reduce the incidence and duration of sequelae of neutropenia in symptomatic patients w/ congenital neutropenia, cyclic neutropenia, or idiopathic neutropenia

Initial:
Congenital Neutropenia: 6mcg/kg SQ bid
Idiopathic/Cyclic Neutropenia: 5mcg/kg SQ qd

Individualize dose based on the patient's clinical course as well as ANC; in rare instances, patients w/ congenital neutropenia have required doses ≥100mcg/kg/day

During the initial 4 weeks of therapy and during the 2 weeks following any dosage adjustment, monitor CBCs w/ differential and platelet counts. Once a patient is clinically stable, monitor CBCs w/ differential and platelet counts monthly during the first year of treatment. Thereafter, if the patient is clinically stable, less frequent routine monitoring is recommended

Hematopoietic Syndrome of Acute Radiation Syndrome

To increase survival in patients acutely exposed to myelosuppressive doses of radiation

10mcg/kg SQ qd; administer as soon as possible after suspected/confirmed exposure to radiation doses >2 gray

Obtain a baseline CBC and then serial CBCs approx every third day until the ANC remains >1000/mm³ for 3 consecutive CBCs; do not delay administration if a CBC is not readily available

Continue administration of therapy until the ANC remains >1000/mm³ for 3 consecutive CBCs or exceeds 10,000/mm³ after a radiation-induced nadir

DOSING CONSIDERATIONS
Concomitant Medications
Cytotoxic Chemotherapy: Do not use Neupogen in the period 24 hrs before through 24 hrs after the administration of cytotoxic chemotherapy

ADMINISTRATION
SQ/IV route

- Prior to use, remove the vial or prefilled syringe from the refrigerator and allow Neupogen to reach room temperature for a minimum of 30 min and a max of 24 hrs; discard any vial or prefilled syringe left at room temperature for >24 hrs.
- Discard unused portion in vials or prefilled syringes; do not re-enter the vial or save unused drug for later administration.

SQ Inj
- Inject in the outer area of upper arms, abdomen, thighs, or upper outer areas of buttocks.

Instructions for Prefilled Syringe
- Persons w/ latex allergies should not administer the prefilled syringe, because the needle cap contains dry natural rubber (derived from latex).

Dilution Instructions (Vial Only)
- If required for IV administration, vials may be diluted in D5 inj from a concentration of 300mcg/mL to 5mcg/mL; do not dilute to a final concentration <5mcg/mL.
- Sol diluted to concentrations from 5mcg/mL to 15mcg/mL should be protected from adsorption to plastic materials by the addition of albumin (human) to a final concentration of 2mg/mL.
- When diluted in D5 inj or D5 plus albumin (human), Neupogen is compatible w/ glass bottles, polyvinylchloride and polyolefin IV bags, and polypropylene syringes.
- Do not dilute w/ saline; product may precipitate.
- Store diluted sol at room temperature for up to 24 hrs; this 24-hr time period includes the time during room temperature storage of the infusion sol and the duration of the infusion.

STORAGE
2-8°C (36-46°F). Protect from light. Avoid freezing; if frozen, thaw in the refrigerator before administration. Discard if frozen more than once. Avoid shaking.

HOW SUPPLIED
Inj: 300mcg/mL, 480mcg/1.6mL [vial]; 300mcg/0.5mL, 480mcg/0.8mL [prefilled syringe]

CONTRAINDICATIONS
History of serious allergic reactions to human granulocyte colony-stimulating factors (eg, filgrastim, pegfilgrastim).

WARNINGS/PRECAUTIONS
Splenic rupture, including fatal cases, reported. Acute respiratory distress syndrome (ARDS) reported; d/c in patients w/ ARDS. Serious allergic reactions, including anaphylaxis, reported; permanently d/c in patients w/ serious allergic reactions. Sickle cell crisis, in some cases fatal, reported in patients w/ sickle cell trait/disease. Glomerulonephritis has occurred, generally resolving after dose reduction or discontinuation. If glomerulonephritis is suspected, evaluate for cause; if causality is likely, consider dose-reduction or interruption of therapy. Not approved for peripheral blood progenitor cell mobilization in healthy donors. Capillary leak syndrome (CLS) reported. Myelodysplastic syndrome (MDS) and AML reported to occur in the natural history of congenital neutropenia w/o cytokine therapy. Cytogenetic abnormalities, transformation to MDS, and AML observed in patients treated for severe chronic neutropenia (SCN); carefully consider the risks and benefits of continuing therapy if a patient w/ SCN develops abnormal cytogenetics or myelodysplasia. Thrombocytopenia and leukocytosis reported. Cutaneous vasculitis reported. Hold therapy in patients w/ cutaneous vasculitis; treatment may be started at a reduced dose when the symptoms resolve and ANC has decreased. May act as a growth factor for any tumor type. Increased hematopoietic activity of the bone marrow in response to growth factor therapy has been associated w/ transient positive bone-imaging changes; consider this when interpreting bone-imaging results.

ADVERSE REACTIONS
W/ Nonmyeloid Malignancies Receiving Myelosuppressive Anti-Cancer Drugs: Pyrexia, pain, rash, cough, dyspnea.
W/ AML: Pain, epistaxis, rash.
W/ Nonmyeloid Malignancies Undergoing Myeloablative Chemotherapy followed by BMT: Rash.
Undergoing Peripheral Blood Progenitor Cell Mobilization and Collection: Bone pain, pyrexia, headache.
W/ Severe Chronic Neutropenia: Pain, anemia, epistaxis, diarrhea, hypoesthesia, alopecia.

DRUG INTERACTIONS
Avoid simultaneous use w/ chemotherapy and radiation therapy.

PREGNANCY AND LACTATION
Pregnancy: Category C.
Lactation: Caution in nursing.

MECHANISM OF ACTION
G-CSF; acts on hematopoietic cells by binding to specific cell surface receptors and stimulating proliferation, differentiation commitment, and some end-cell functional activation.

PHARMACOKINETICS
Absorption: (SQ) Absolute Bioavailability (60-70%); C_{max}=4ng/mL (3.45mcg/kg), 49ng/mL (11.5mcg/kg); T_{max}=2-8 hrs. **Distribution:** V_d=150mL/kg (IV); crosses placenta. **Elimination:** $T_{1/2}$=231 min (34.5mcg/kg IV), 210 min (3.45mcg/kg SQ).

PATIENT CONSIDERATIONS
Assessment: Assess for hypersensitivity to the drug, latex allergy, sickle cell disorder, pregnancy/nursing status, and possible drug interactions. Obtain baseline CBC and platelet count. Confirm diagnosis of SCN prior to therapy.

Monitoring: Monitor for splenic rupture, ARDS, serious allergic reactions, sickle cell crisis, glomerulonephritis, CLS, cutaneous vasculitis, thrombocytopenia, leukocytosis, and other adverse reactions. Monitor for cytogenetic abnormalities, transformation to MDS, and AML in patients w/ SCN. In patients receiving myelosuppressive chemotherapy or induction and/or consolidation chemotherapy for AML, monitor CBC and platelet count twice weekly. Monitor CBCs and platelet counts frequently following marrow transplantation. In patients w/ SCN, monitor CBCs w/ differential and platelet counts during the initial 4 weeks of therapy and during the 2 weeks following any dose adjustment. Once patient is clinically stable, monitor CBCs w/ differential and platelet counts monthly during the 1st yr of treatment; thereafter, if clinically stable, less frequent routine monitoring is recommended. Monitor serial CBCs approx every 3rd day until the ANC remains >1000/mm³ for 3 consecutive CBCs in patients acutely exposed to myelosuppressive doses of radiation.

Counseling: Train patients/caregivers on how to measure required dose and administer inj. Instruct to contact healthcare provider if a dose is missed. Inform that rupture or enlargement of the spleen may occur; advise to immediately report to physician if symptoms develop. Advise to seek immediate medical attention if signs/symptoms of hypersensitivity reaction occur. Advise to immediately report to physician if dyspnea develops. Discuss potential risks and benefits for patients w/ sickle cell disease prior to administration. Advise to immediately report signs/symptoms of glomerulonephritis to physician. Advise to immediately report to physician signs/symptoms of vasculitis. Advise females of reproductive potential that therapy should be used during pregnancy only if the potential benefit justifies the potential risk to the fetus. Advise patients acutely exposed to myelosuppressive doses of radiation that efficacy studies of therapy for this indication could not be conducted in humans for ethical and feasibility reasons; approval of this use was based on efficacy studies conducted in animals.

NEXAVAR — *sorafenib*   Rx
Class: Kinase inhibitor

ADULT DOSAGE	PEDIATRIC DOSAGE
Hepatocellular Carcinoma **Unresectable:** 400mg (two 200mg tabs) bid Continue until patient is no longer clinically benefiting from therapy or until unacceptable toxicity occurs	Pediatric use may not have been established
Advanced Renal Cell Carcinoma 400mg (two 200mg tabs) bid Continue until patient is no longer clinically benefiting from therapy or until unacceptable toxicity occurs	
Differentiated Thyroid Carcinoma Locally recurrent or metastatic, progressive, differentiated thyroid carcinoma that is refractory to radioactive iodine treatment 400mg (two 200mg tabs) bid Continue until patient is no longer clinically benefiting from therapy or until unacceptable toxicity occurs	

DOSING CONSIDERATIONS
Adverse Reactions
Dermatologic Toxicities:
Hepatocellular/Renal Cell Carcinoma:
Grade 1 (Numbness/Dysesthesia/Paresthesia/Tingling/Painless Swelling/Erythema/Discomfort of Hands or Feet That Does Not Disrupt Normal Activities):
Any Occurrence: Continue treatment and consider topical therapy for symptomatic relief

Grade 2 (Painful Erythema and Swelling of Hands or Feet and/or Discomfort Affecting Normal Activities):
1st Occurrence: Continue treatment and consider topical therapy for symptomatic relief

No Improvement w/in 7 Days or 2nd/3rd Occurrence: Interrupt treatment until toxicity resolves to Grade 0-1; when resuming treatment, decrease dose by 1 dose level (400mg/day or 400mg qod)

4th Occurrence: D/C treatment

Grade 3 (Moist Desquamation/Ulceration/Blistering/Severe Pain of Hands or Feet, or Severe Discomfort That Causes Inability to Work or Perform Activities of Daily Living):

1st/2nd Occurrence: Interrupt treatment until toxicity resolves to Grade 0-1; when resuming treatment, decrease dose by 1 dose level (400mg/day or 400mg qod)

3rd Occurrence: D/C treatment

Differentiated Thyroid Carcinoma:

Grade 1:

Any Occurrence: Continue treatment

Grade 2:

1st Occurrence: Decrease dose to 600mg/day

No Improvement w/in 7 Days or 2nd/3rd Occurrence: Interrupt treatment until toxicity resolves or improves to Grade 1; if treatment is resumed, decrease dose as follows:

1st Dose Reduction: 600mg/day (400mg and 200mg 12 hrs apart)

2nd Dose Reduction: 400mg/day (200mg bid)

3rd Dose Reduction: 200mg qd

4th Occurrence: D/C treatment permanently

Grade 3:

1st Occurrence: Interrupt treatment until toxicity resolves or improves to Grade 1; if treatment is resumed, decrease dose to 600mg/day (400mg and 200mg 12 hrs apart)

2nd Occurrence: Interrupt treatment until toxicity resolves or improves to Grade 1; if treatment is resumed, decrease dose to 400mg/day (200mg bid)

3rd Occurrence: D/C treatment

Discontinuation

Temporary interruption or permanent discontinuation may be required for the following:
1. Cardiac ischemia or infarction
2. Hemorrhage requiring medical intervention
3. Severe or persistent HTN despite adequate anti-hypertensive therapy
4. GI perforation
5. QTc prolongation
6. Severe drug-induced liver injury

Other Important Considerations

Patients Undergoing Major Surgical Procedures: Temporarily interrupt therapy

Dose Reductions:

Hepatocellular Carcinoma/Renal Cell Carcinoma:

When dose reduction is necessary, reduce to 400mg qd; if additional dose reduction is required, reduce to a single 400mg dose qod

Differentiated Thyroid Carcinoma:

1st Dose Reduction: 600mg/day (400mg and 200mg 12 hrs apart)

2nd Dose Reduction: 400mg/day (200mg bid)

3rd Dose Reduction: 200mg qd

ADMINISTRATION

Oral route

Take w/o food (at least 1 hr ac or 2 hrs pc)

STORAGE

25°C (77°F); excursions permitted to 15-30°C (59-86°F). Store in a dry place.

HOW SUPPLIED

Tab: 200mg

CONTRAINDICATIONS

Known severe hypersensitivity to sorafenib or any other component of this medication, concomitant use w/ carboplatin and paclitaxel in patients w/ squamous cell lung cancer.

WARNINGS/PRECAUTIONS

HTN, cardiac ischemia, and/or infarction reported; consider temporary or permanent discontinuation. Increased risk of bleeding may occur; consider permanent discontinuation if bleeding necessitates medical intervention. Hand-foot skin reaction and rash reported; may require topical treatment, temporary interruption, and/or dose modification, or permanent discontinuation in severe or persistent cases. Severe dermatologic toxicities, including Stevens-Johnson syndrome (SJS) and toxic epidermal necrolysis (TEN) reported; d/c if SJS or TEN are suspected. D/C if GI perforation occurs. Temporarily interrupt therapy when undergoing major surgical procedures. May prolong the QT/QTc interval; avoid in patients w/ congenital long QT syndrome. Monitor electrolytes and ECG in patients w/ congestive heart failure (CHF), bradyarrhythmias, and in patients taking drugs known to prolong the QT interval (eg, Class Ia and III antiarrhythmics). Correct electrolyte abnormalities (Mg^{2+}, K^+, Ca^{2+}). Interrupt treatment if QTc interval is >500 msec or for an increase from baseline ≥60 msec. Drug-induced hepatitis, and increased bilirubin and INR may occur; d/c in case of significantly increased transaminases w/o alternative explanation (eg, viral hepatitis, progressing underlying malignancy). May impair exogenous thyroid suppression; monitor TSH levels monthly and adjust thyroid replacement medication as needed in patients w/ DTC. May cause fetal harm.

ADVERSE REACTIONS

HTN, fatigue, weight loss, rash, hand-foot skin reaction, alopecia, pruritus, diarrhea, N/V, abdominal pain, anorexia, constipation, hemorrhage, infection, decreased appetite.

DRUG INTERACTIONS

See Contraindications. Avoid w/ gemcitabine/cisplatin in squamous cell lung cancer patients. Avoid w/ strong CYP3A4 inducers (eg, carbamazepine, dexamethasone, St. John's wort); strong CYP3A4 inducers may decrease systemic exposure. Infrequent bleeding or increased INR w/ warfarin; monitor for changes in PT, INR, or bleeding episodes. Decreased exposure w/ oral neomycin.

PREGNANCY AND LACTATION

Category D, not for use in nursing.

MECHANISM OF ACTION

Kinase inhibitor; inhibits multiple intracellular (c-CRAF, BRAF and mutant BRAF) and cell surface kinases (KIT, FLT-3, RET, RET/PTC, VEGFR-1, VEGFR-2, VEGFR-3, and PDGFR-β) thought to be involved in tumor cell signaling, angiogenesis, and apoptosis.

PHARMACOKINETICS

Absorption: T_{max}=3 hrs. **Distribution:** Plasma protein binding (99.5%). **Metabolism:** Liver via oxidation and glucuronidation; CYP3A4, UGT1A9; pyridine N-oxide (metabolite). **Elimination:** (100mg Sol) Feces (77%, 51% unchanged), urine (19% glucuronidated metabolites). $T_{1/2}$=25-48 hrs.

PATIENT CONSIDERATIONS

Assessment: Assess for bleeding disorders, upcoming major surgical procedures, CHF, bradyarrhythmias, electrolyte abnormalities, congenital long QT syndrome, drug hypersensitivity, pregnancy/nursing status, and possible drug interactions.

Monitoring: Monitor for cardiac ischemia/infarction, hemorrhage, HTN, dermatologic toxicities, GI perforation, QT/QTc prolongation, and other adverse reactions. Monitor BP weekly during the first 6 weeks and periodically thereafter. Monitor electrolytes (eg, Mg^{2+}, Ca^{2+}, K^+) and ECG in patients w/ CHF, bradyarrhythmias, and in patients taking drugs known to prolong the QT interval. Monitor LFTs regularly, and TSH levels monthly. Monitor patients taking concomitant warfarin for changes in PT, INR, or clinical bleeding episodes.

Counseling: Inform about risks and benefits of therapy. Instruct to report to physician any episodes of bleeding or cardiac ischemia (eg, chest pain). Inform that HTN may develop, especially during the first 6 weeks; advise that BP should be monitored regularly during therapy. Inform of possible occurrence of hand-foot skin reaction and rash during therapy and appropriate countermeasures. Advise that GI perforation and drug-induced hepatitis may occur and to report signs/symptoms of hepatitis. Inform that temporary interruption of therapy is recommended in patients undergoing major surgical procedures. Counsel patients w/ a history of prolonged QT interval that drug can worsen the condition. Inform that the drug may cause birth defects or fetal loss during pregnancy; instruct both males and females to use effective birth control during treatment and for at least 2 weeks after stopping therapy. Instruct to notify physician if patient becomes pregnant while on therapy. Advise against breastfeeding while on therapy.

NEXPLANON — etonogestrel   Rx

Class: Progestin contraceptive

ADULT DOSAGE	PEDIATRIC DOSAGE
Contraception	**Contraception**
No Preceding Hormonal Contraceptive Use in the Past Month: Insert subdermally in the upper arm between Day 1 (1st day of menstrual bleeding) and Day 5 of menstrual cycle, even if patient is still bleeding	Not indicated for use premenarche; refer to adult dosing
Following Abortion or Miscarriage: **1st Trimester:** Insert w/in 5 days following 1st trimester abortion or miscarriage **2nd Trimester:** Insert between 21-28 days following 2nd trimester abortion or miscarriage	
Postpartum: **Not Breastfeeding:** Insert between 21-28 days postpartum **Breastfeeding:** Insert after the 4th postpartum week	
Remove by the end of the 3rd year; if continued contraceptive protection is desired, may replace by a new implant at the time of removal using the same incision of the previous implant	
Conversions **Switching from Combination Hormonal Contraceptives:** Insert implant on the day after the last active tab of the previous combined oral contraceptive or on the day of the removal of the vaginal ring or transdermal patch. At the latest, insert implant on the day following the usual tab-free, ring-free, patch-free or placebo tab interval of the previous combined hormonal contraceptive	

Switching from Progestin-Only Contraceptives:
Injectable Contraceptives: Insert implant on the day the next inj is due
Minipill: Insert implant on any day of the month, w/in 24 hrs after taking the last tab
Contraceptive Implant or Intrauterine System (IUS): Insert implant on the same day as the previous contraceptive implant or IUS is removed

----

ADMINISTRATION
Subdermal route

Insert implant at the inner side of the non-dominant upper arm about 8-10 cm (3-4 inches) above the medial epicondyle of the humerus, to reduce the risk of neural or vascular injury.
If inserted as recommended, backup contraception is not necessary.
If deviating from the recommended timing of insertion, advise to use a barrier method until 7 days after insertion; if intercourse has already occurred, pregnancy should be excluded.
In postpartum/breastfeeding women, advise to use a barrier method until 7 days after insertion; if intercourse has already occurred, pregnancy should be excluded.

Insertion Procedure
1. Anesthetize the insertion area (eg, w/ anesthetic spray or by injecting 2mL of 1% lidocaine).
2. Remove the transparent protection cap by sliding it horizontally in the direction of the arrow away from the needle.
3. Do not touch the purple slider until the needle is fully inserted subdermally.
4. Puncture the skin w/ the tip of the needle slightly angled <30°.
5. Lower the applicator to a horizontal position and insert needle to its full length.
6. Unlock the purple slider by pushing it slightly down and move the slider fully back until it stops.
7. Remove the applicator.
8. Verify the presence of the implant by palpation.

Refer to PI for further administration details and for removal procedure.

STORAGE
25°C (77°F); excursions permitted to 15-30°C (59-86°F). Avoid storing at temperatures >30°C (86°F).

HOW SUPPLIED
Implant: 68mg

CONTRAINDICATIONS
Known or suspected pregnancy, current/history of thrombosis or thromboembolic disorders, benign or malignant liver tumors, active liver disease, undiagnosed abnormal genital bleeding, known/suspected/personal history of breast cancer, current/history of other progestin-sensitive cancer, or allergic reaction to any of the components.

WARNINGS/PRECAUTIONS
Confirm by palpation immediately after insertion; failure to insert implant properly may lead to an unintended pregnancy. Complications related to insertion or removal procedures (eg, pain, paresthesias, bleeding, hematoma, scarring, infection) may occur. If infection develops at the insertion site, start suitable treatment; if infection persists, remove implant. Incomplete insertions or infections may lead to expulsion. Neural or vascular injury may occur if inserted too deeply. Implant removal may be difficult/impossible if inserted incorrectly, inserted too deeply, not palpable, if it is encased in fibrous tissue, or if it has migrated. Implant migration w/in the arm from the insertion site reported; may be related to a deep insertion. Reports of implants located w/in vessels of the arm and the pulmonary artery (rare); may be related to deep insertions or intravascular insertion. If at any time the implant cannot be palpated, it should be localized and removed. Failure to remove may result in continued effects of etonogestrel. May cause changes in menstrual bleeding patterns, ectopic pregnancy, thrombotic/vascular events, ovarian cysts, breast cancer, cervical cancer or intraepithelial neoplasia, hepatic adenomas, weight gain, gallbladder disease, and fluid retention. Perform appropriate measures to rule out malignancy if undiagnosed, persistent, or recurrent abnormal vaginal bleeding occurs. Carefully monitor women w/ a family history of breast cancer and those who develop breast nodules. Do not use prior to 21 days postpartum. Evaluate for retinal vein thrombosis immediately if there is unexplained loss of vision, proptosis, diplopia, papilledema, or retinal vascular lesions. Consider removal of implant if significant depression develops or in case of long-term immobilization due to surgery or illness. Remove implant in the event of thrombosis or if jaundice develops. Women w/ a history of HTN-related diseases or renal disease should be discouraged from using hormonal contraception. Remove implant if a significant increase in BP unresponsive to antihypertensive therapy or sustained HTN occurs. May induce mild insulin resistance and small changes in glucose levels; monitor prediabetic and diabetic women. May elevate LDL levels. Restart contraception immediately after removal for continued contraceptive protection. Contact lens wearers who develop visual changes or changes in lens tolerance should be assessed by an ophthalmologist. Broken or bent implants while in the patient's arm reported; broken or bent implant may slightly increase the release rate of etonogestrel. Remove implant in its entirety when it is removed. May decrease sex hormone-binding globulin (SHBG) and thyroxine levels initially, followed by gradual recovery. May be less effective in overweight women.

ADVERSE REACTIONS
Headache, vaginitis, weight increase, acne, breast pain, abdominal pain, pharyngitis, leukorrhea, influenza-like symptoms, dizziness, dysmenorrhea, back pain, emotional lability, nausea, pain.

DRUG INTERACTIONS
Drugs or herbal products that induce enzymes, including CYP3A4 that metabolize progestins (eg, barbiturates, bosentan, carbamazepine), may decrease levels of progestins and decrease the effectiveness therapy; recommended to remove implant if on long-term treatment w/ hepatic enzyme-inducing drugs. HIV protease inhibitors or non-nucleoside reverse transcriptase inhibitors have been reported in some cases to cause significant changes (increase or decrease) in plasma levels of progestins. CYP3A4 inhibitors (eg, itraconazole, ketoconazole) may increase levels of etonogestrel. May affect metabolism of other drugs and consequently may either increase (eg, cyclosporine) or decrease (eg, lamotrigine) plasma concentrations of coadministered drugs.

PREGNANCY AND LACTATION
Pregnancy: Contraindicated in pregnancy.
Lactation: May be used during breastfeeding after the 4th postpartum week. Small amounts of etonogestrel are excreted in breast milk.

MECHANISM OF ACTION
Progestin contraceptive; suppresses ovulation, increases viscosity of cervical mucus, and alters the endometrium.

PHARMACOKINETICS
Absorption: Bioavailability (100%); C_{max}=1200pg/mL; T_{max}=w/in the first 2 weeks after insertion. **Distribution:** V_d=201L; plasma protein binding [albumin (66%), SHBG (32%)]; found in breast milk. **Metabolism:** Liver via CYP3A4. **Elimination:** Urine (primary), feces; $T_{1/2}$=25 hrs.

PATIENT CONSIDERATIONS
Assessment: Assess for current or past history of thrombosis or thromboembolic disorders, benign or malignant liver tumors, active liver disease, undiagnosed abnormal genital bleeding, known/suspected/history of breast cancer or current or past history of other progestin-sensitive cancer, history of HTN-related diseases or renal disease, history of depressed mood, diabetes, hyperlipidemia, conditions that might be aggravated by fluid retention, pregnancy status, or for any other conditions where treatment is contraindicated or cautioned. Assess nursing status and for possible drug interactions.

Monitoring: Monitor for complications of insertion/removal of implant, changes in menstrual bleeding pattern, ectopic pregnancy, thrombotic/other vascular events, ovarian cysts, breast/cervical cancer, intraepithelial neoplasia, liver dysfunction, weight gain, gallbladder disease, fluid retention, and other adverse events. Monitor for visual changes or changes in lens tolerance in patients who wear contact lens and refer to an ophthalmologist if changes occur. Monitor glucose levels in diabetic and prediabetic patients, BP w/ history of HTN, lipid levels w/ a history of hyperlipidemia. Monitor for signs of depression w/ previous history. In cases of undiagnosed, persistent, or recurrent abnormal vaginal bleeding, perform appropriate measures to rule out malignancy. Perform BP check and other indicated healthcare annually.

Counseling: Inform of the risks and benefits of therapy. Counsel about insertion and removal procedure of the implant. Provide patient w/ a copy of the Patient Labeling and ensure information is understood before insertion and removal. Inform that consent form is included in the package and advise to complete consent form. Provide patient w/ the user card after insertion in order to have a record of the location of the implant in the upper arm and when it should be removed. Inform that the implant does not protect against HIV infection (AIDS) or other STDs. Advise that use may be associated w/ changes in normal menstrual bleeding patterns.

NIMODIPINE — nimodipine   **Rx**
Class: Calcium channel blocker (CCB)

> Do not administer IV or by other parenteral routes. Deaths and serious, life-threatening adverse events have occurred when the contents of caps have been injected parenterally.

OTHER BRAND NAMES
Nimotop (Discontinued)

ADULT DOSAGE
Subarachnoid Hemorrhage

Indicated for the improvement of neurological outcome by reducing the incidence and severity of ischemic deficits in patients w/ subarachnoid hemorrhage (SAH) from ruptured intracranial berry aneurysms regardless of their post-ictus neurological condition (eg, Hunt and Hess Grades I-V)

Usual: 60mg q4h for 21 days; begin therapy w/in 96 hrs of onset of SAH

PEDIATRIC DOSAGE
Pediatric use may not have been established

DOSING CONSIDERATIONS
Hepatic Impairment
Cirrhosis: Reduce to 30mg q4h; consider discontinuation of therapy, if necessary

ADMINISTRATION
Oral route

Swallow caps whole w/ a little liquid, preferably not less than 1 hr before or 2 hrs after meals
If patient cannot swallow cap, extract contents into syringe, empty into NG tube, and wash down the tube w/ 30mL of 0.9% NaCl
Do not administer nimodipine capsules IV or by other parenteral routes

STORAGE
20-25°C (68-77°F). Protect from light and freezing.

HOW SUPPLIED
Cap: 30mg

CONTRAINDICATIONS
Concomitant use with strong CYP3A4 inhibitors such as some macrolide antibiotics (eg, clarithromycin, telithromycin), some anti-HIV protease inhibitors (eg, indinavir, ritonavir, saquinavir), some azole antimycotics (eg, ketoconazole, itraconazole, voriconazole), and some antidepressants (eg, nefazodone).

WARNINGS/PRECAUTIONS
Lowering of BP reported; carefully monitor BP. Decreased metabolism in patients with impaired hepatic function; closely monitor BP and pulse rate and give a lower dose. Rare reports of intestinal pseudo-obstruction and ileus. Caution in elderly.

ADVERSE REACTIONS
Decreased BP, diarrhea.

DRUG INTERACTIONS
See Contraindications. Strong CYP3A4 inducers (eg, rifampin, phenobarbital, phenytoin) may significantly reduce levels and efficacy; avoid concomitant use. Moderate and weak CYP3A4 inhibitors (eg, amiodarone, erythromycin, valproic acid) may increase levels; monitor BP and reduce nimodipine dose if necessary. Not recommended with grapefruit/grapefruit juice. Moderate and weak CYP3A4 inducers (eg, efavirenz, pioglitazone, prednisone) may reduce efficacy; increase in nimodipine dose may be required. May increase the BP lowering effect of antihypertensives; monitor BP and dose adjustment of the BP lowering drug(s) may be necessary.

PREGNANCY AND LACTATION
Category C, not for use in nursing.

MECHANISM OF ACTION
CCB; has not been established. Inhibits Ca^{2+} ion transfer into smooth muscle cells, thereby inhibiting contractions of vascular smooth muscle.

PHARMACOKINETICS
Absorption: Rapid; T_{max}=1 hr; bioavailability (13%). Distribution: Plasma protein binding (>95%). Metabolism: Via CYP3A4. Elimination: Urine (<1% unchanged); $T_{1/2}$=8-9 hrs.

PATIENT CONSIDERATIONS

Assessment: Assess for hepatic impairment, pregnancy/nursing status, and possible drug interactions.

Monitoring: Monitor for intestinal pseudo-obstruction, ileus and other adverse reactions. Carefully monitor BP and pulse rate.

Counseling: Inform about potential risks/benefits of therapy.

NIPENT — pentostatin　　　　Rx

Class: Adenosine deaminase (ADA) inhibitor

> Should be administered under the supervision of a physician qualified and experienced in the use of cancer chemotherapeutic agents. Higher doses than specified is not recommended; dose-limiting severe renal, liver, pulmonary, and CNS toxicities reported at higher doses (20-50mg/m² in divided doses over 5 days) than recommended. Use in combination with fludarabine phosphate is not recommended; severe or fatal pulmonary toxicity may occur.

ADULT DOSAGE	**PEDIATRIC DOSAGE**
Untreated and α-Interferon-Refractory Hairy Cell Leukemia (HCL)	Pediatric use may not have been established
Hydrate with 500-1000mL of D5W in 0.5 normal saline or equivalent before drug administration and administer additional 500mL of D5W or equivalent after the drug is given	
Usual: 4mg/m² every other week as IV bolus or infusion over 20-30 min	
Give 2 additional doses after complete response is achieved	
Assess for response in patients receiving treatment at 6 months; d/c if complete/partial response is not achieved	
If partial response is achieved, continue treatment to achieve complete response; d/c if best response at the end of 12 months is a partial response	
May need to withhold or d/c individual doses when severe adverse reactions occur	

ADMINISTRATION
IV route
Refer to PI for preparation of sol

STORAGE
2-8°C (36-46°F). Reconstituted/Further Diluted Vials: Room temperature and ambient light. Use within 8 hrs.

HOW SUPPLIED
Inj: 10mg

CONTRAINDICATIONS
Hypersensitivity to pentostatin.

WARNINGS/PRECAUTIONS
Myelosuppression may occur primarily during the 1st few courses of treatment. Worsening of infection leading to death reported; control the infection before treatment is initiated or resumed. Initial courses of treatment associated with worsening of neutropenia in patients with progressive HCL; frequently monitor CBC during this time. If severe neutropenia continues beyond initial cycles, evaluate disease status, including bone marrow examination. LFTs and SrCr elevations reported; withhold dose and determine CrCl in patients with elevated SrCr. Rashes, occasionally severe, reported and may worsen with continued treatment; withholding of treatment may be required. Withhold or d/c with evidence of nervous system toxicity. Temporarily withhold treatment if absolute neutrophil count falls to <200 cells/mm³ in a patient who had an initial neutrophil count >500 cells/mm³; may resume when the count returns to predose levels. May cause fetal harm. Treat patients with infection or renal impairment only when potential benefit of treatment justifies the potential risk.

ADVERSE REACTIONS
N/V, fever, rash, fatigue, leukopenia, pruritus, cough, myalgia, chills, headache, diarrhea, abdominal pain, anorexia, upper respiratory infection.

DRUG INTERACTIONS
See Boxed Warning. Acute pulmonary edema and hypotension, leading to death, reported when used in combination with carmustine, etoposide, and high dose cyclophosphamide as part of ablative regimen for bone marrow transplant. Hypersensitivity vasculitis that resulted in death reported with concomitant allopurinol. May enhance effects of vidarabine; combined use may increase adverse reactions associated with each drug.

PREGNANCY AND LACTATION
Category D, not for use in nursing.

MECHANISM OF ACTION
Adenosine deaminase inhibitor; has not been established. Elevates intracellular levels of dATP which can block DNA synthesis through inhibition of ribonucleotide reductase. Also, inhibits RNA synthesis and causes increased DNA damage.

PHARMACOKINETICS
Distribution: Plasma protein binding (4%). Elimination: Urine (90%); $T_{1/2}$=5.7 hrs.

PATIENT CONSIDERATIONS

Assessment: Assess for hypersensitivity to the drug, infection, pregnancy/nursing status, and possible drug interactions. Obtain CBC and SrCr before each dose and at other appropriate periods during therapy.

Monitoring: Monitor for myelosuppression, worsening of infection/neutropenia, LFTs/SrCr elevations, rashes, nervous system toxicity, and other adverse reactions. Monitor hematologic parameters and blood chemistry values. Perform periodic monitoring of the peripheral blood for hairy cells to assess response to treatment. Bone marrow aspirates and biopsies may be required at 2- to 3-month intervals to assess response to treatment.

Counseling: Inform of signs and symptoms of adverse events associated with therapy. Advise women of childbearing potential to avoid becoming pregnant during therapy.

NORDITROPIN — somatropin (rDNA origin)　　　Rx

Class: Recombinant human growth hormone (hGH)

ADULT DOSAGE	**PEDIATRIC DOSAGE**
Growth Hormone Deficiency	**Growth Hormone Deficiency**
Replacement of Endogenous Growth Hormone in Patients w/ Adult-Onset or Childhood-Onset Growth Hormone Deficiency:	**Growth Failure Due to Inadequate Secretion of Endogenous Growth Hormone:** 0.024-0.034mg/kg/day SQ 6-7X/ week
Weight-Based:	**Noonan Syndrome**
Initial: ≤0.004mg/kg/day SQ	**Short Stature Associated w/ Noonan Syndrome:** Up to 0.066mg/kg/day SQ
Titrate: May increase to ≤0.016mg/kg/day after 6 weeks according to individual requirements	**Turner Syndrome**
Non-Weight Based:	**Short Stature Associated w/ Turner Syndrome:** Up to 0.067mg/kg/day SQ
Initial: 0.2mg/day SQ (range, 0.15-0.30mg/day)	**Small for Gestational Age**
Titrate: May increase gradually every 1-2 months by increments of 0.1-0.2mg/day based on response and serum insulin-like growth factor-I concentrations	**Short Stature Born Small for Gestational Age w/ No Catch-Up Growth by Age 2-4 Years:** Up to 0.067mg/kg/day SQ

DOSING CONSIDERATIONS

Elderly
Consider lower starting dose and smaller dose increments

Other Important Considerations
Estrogen-replete women may need higher doses than men

ADMINISTRATION
SQ route

Rotate inj sites to avoid lipoatrophy

STORAGE
Unused: 2-8°C (36-46°F). Do not freeze. Avoid direct light. In-use: 2-8°C (36-46°F) and use w/in 4 weeks or store at room temperature ≤25°C (77°F) for up to 3 weeks.

HOW SUPPLIED
Inj: 5mg/1.5mL, 10mg/1.5mL, 15mg/1.5mL, 30mg/3mL

CONTRAINDICATIONS
Acute critical illness due to complications following open heart surgery, abdominal surgery, multiple accidental trauma, or w/ acute respiratory failure. Pediatric patients w/ Prader-Willi syndrome (PWS) who are severely obese, have a history of upper airway obstruction or sleep apnea, or have severe respiratory impairment. Pediatric patients who have growth failure due to genetically confirmed PWS. Active malignancy or evidence of progression or recurrence of underlying intracranial tumor. Active proliferative or severe nonproliferative diabetic retinopathy. Growth promotion in pediatric patients w/ closed epiphyses. Known hypersensitivity to somatropin or any of its excipients.

WARNINGS/PRECAUTIONS
Reevaluate adults who were treated w/ somatropin for growth hormone deficiency (GHD) in childhood and whose epiphyses are closed before continuation of somatropin therapy. Treatment for short stature should be discontinued when epiphyses are fused. Implement effective weight control in patients w/ PWS and treat respiratory infections aggressively; interrupt therapy if patient shows signs of upper airway obstruction and/or new onset sleep apnea. Increased risk of a 2nd neoplasm reported in childhood cancer survivors who were treated w/ radiation to the brain/head for 1st neoplasm and who developed subsequent GHD and were treated w/ somatropin. Increased risk of developing malignancies in children w/ certain rare genetic causes of short stature; monitor for development of neoplasms if treatment is initiated. Monitor for increased growth, or potential malignant changes, of preexisting nevi. Undiagnosed impaired glucose tolerance and overt diabetes mellitus (DM) may be unmasked and new-onset type 2 DM reported. Intracranial HTN w/ papilledema, visual changes, headache, or N/V reported; d/c if papilledema is observed. If drug-induced intracranial HTN is diagnosed, may restart therapy at a lower dose after signs/symptoms resolve. Fluid retention in adults may occur. Hypothyroidism may become evident or worsen, and undiagnosed/untreated hypothyroidism may prevent optimal response. Monitor standard hormonal replacement therapy in patients w/ hypopituitarism. Slipped capital femoral epiphysis (SCFE) and progression of scoliosis may occur in pediatric patients. Increased risk of ear/hearing disorders and cardiovascular (CV) disorders in TS patients; evaluate carefully for otitis media and other ear disorders, and monitor closely for CV disorders. Tissue atrophy may occur; rotate inj site. Allergic reactions (local or systemic) may occur. Serum levels of inorganic phosphorus, alkaline phosphatase, parathyroid hormone, and insulin-like growth factor may increase. Pancreatitis reported rarely. Caution in elderly.

ADVERSE REACTIONS
Gastroenteritis, ear infection, influenza, inj-site reaction, peripheral/leg edema, arthralgia, headache, increased sweating, myalgia, bronchitis, flu-like symptoms, HTN, paresthesia, skeletal pain, laryngitis.

DRUG INTERACTIONS
Glucocorticoid therapy may attenuate growth-promoting effects in children; carefully adjust glucocorticoid replacement dosing. May inhibit 11β-hydroxysteroid dehydrogenase type 1, resulting in reduced serum cortisol concentrations; may need glucocorticoid replacement or dose adjustments of glucocorticoid therapy. May alter clearance of compounds metabolized by CYP450 liver enzymes (eg, corticosteroids, sex steroids, anticonvulsants, cyclosporine); monitor carefully. May increase clearance of antipyrine. May require greater dose w/ oral estrogen replacement. May need to adjust dose of insulin and/or oral/injectable hypoglycemic agents, and thyroid hormone replacement therapy.

PREGNANCY AND LACTATION
Category C, caution in nursing.

MECHANISM OF ACTION
Recombinant human growth hormone (GH); binds to dimeric GH receptor in cell membrane of target cells, resulting in intracellular signal transduction.

PHARMACOKINETICS
Absorption: T_{max}=4-5 hrs; C_{max}=13.8ng/mL (4mg), 17.1ng/mL (8mg). **Elimination:** $T_{1/2}$=7-10 hrs.

PATIENT CONSIDERATIONS
Assessment: Assess for PWS, preexisting DM or impaired glucose tolerance, history of scoliosis, hypothyroidism, hypopituitarism, hypersensitivity to drug, any other conditions where treatment is contraindicated or cautioned, pregnancy/nursing status, and possible drug interactions. Perform funduscopic exam.

Monitoring: Monitor growth and for clinical response, neoplasm, increased growth or malignant changes of preexisting nevi, fluid retention, intracranial HTN, allergic reactions, pancreatitis, and SCFE and progression of scoliosis in pediatric patients (eg, onset of limp, hip or knee pain). Perform periodic thyroid function tests, funduscopic exam, and monitoring of glucose levels. In patients w/ PWS, monitor weight as well as for signs of respiratory infection, sleep apnea, and upper

---

airway obstruction. Monitor patients routinely w/ a history of GHD secondary to an intracranial neoplasm while on therapy for progression/recurrence of tumor. In patients w/ TS, monitor for ear/CV disorders.

Counseling: Inform about potential benefits and risks of therapy, proper administration, and usage/disposal. Caution against any reuse of needles. Counsel to never share pen w/ another person, even if the needle is changed.

NORTHERA — droxidopa   Rx
Class: Alpha/beta adrenergic agonist

> Monitor supine BP prior to and during treatment and more frequently when increasing doses. Elevating the head of the bed lessens the risk of supine HTN, and BP should be measured in this position. Reduce or d/c treatment if supine HTN cannot be managed by elevation of the head of the bed.

ADULT DOSAGE

Neurogenic Orthostatic Hypotension
Treatment of symptomatic neurogenic orthostatic hypotension caused by primary autonomic failure (Parkinson's disease, multiple system atrophy and pure autonomic failure), dopamine β-hydroxylase deficiency, and nondiabetic autonomic neuropathy

Initial: 100mg tid; upon arising in am, at midday, and in the late afternoon at least 3 hrs prior to hs
Titrate: Titrate to symptomatic response, in increments of 100mg tid q24-48h
Max: 600mg tid (1800mg/day)

Monitor supine BP prior to initiating and after increasing the dose

PEDIATRIC DOSAGE
Pediatric use may not have been established

ADMINISTRATION
Oral route

Administer consistently, either w/ food or w/o food
Swallow cap whole
Patients who miss a dose should take their next scheduled dose

STORAGE
20-25°C (68-77°F); excursions permitted to 15-30°C (59-86°F).

HOW SUPPLIED
Cap: 100mg, 200mg, 300mg

WARNINGS/PRECAUTIONS
May cause or exacerbate supine HTN; monitor BP, both in the supine position and in the recommended head-elevated sleeping position. May increase risk of cardiovascular events if supine HTN is not well-managed. Cases of a symptom complex resembling neuroleptic malignant syndrome (NMS) reported; caution when dosage is changed or when concomitant levodopa is reduced abruptly or discontinued, especially if taking neuroleptics. May exacerbate existing ischemic heart disease, arrhythmias, and congestive heart failure (CHF). Contains tartrazine; may cause allergic-type reactions in certain susceptible persons.

ADVERSE REACTIONS
Headache, dizziness, nausea, HTN.

DRUG INTERACTIONS
Use with other agents that increase BP (eg, norepinephrine, ephedrine, midodrine) would be expected to increase the risk for supine HTN. Dopa-decarboxylase inhibitors may require dose adjustments for droxidopa.

PREGNANCY AND LACTATION
Category C, not for use in nursing.

MECHANISM OF ACTION
Synthetic amino acid precursor of norepinephrine; has not been established. Directly metabolized to norepinephrine by dopa-decarboxylase. Believed to exert pharmacological effects through norepinephrine, and not through parent molecule or other metabolites. Norepinephrine increases BP by inducing peripheral arterial and venous vasoconstriction.

PHARMACOKINETICS
Absorption: T_{max}=1-4 hrs. **Distribution:** Plasma protein binding (75%, 100ng/mL; 26%, 10,000 ng/mL); V_d=200L. **Metabolism:** Methoxylated dihydroxyphenylserine (major metabolite) by catechol-O-methyltransferase; norepinephrine by DOPA decarboxylase, or protocatechualdehyde by DOPS aldolase. **Elimination:** Kidney; $T_{1/2}$=2.5 hrs.

PATIENT CONSIDERATIONS
Assessment: Assess for ischemic heart disease, arrhythmias, CHF, hypersensitivity to tartrazine, pregnancy/nursing status, and for possible drug interactions. Obtain baseline supine BP.

Monitoring: Monitor for a symptom complex resembling NMS; exacerbation of existing ischemic heart disease, arrhythmias, or CHF; allergic reactions; and other adverse reactions. Monitor supine BP during treatment and more frequently when increasing doses. Periodically evaluate effectiveness of therapy.

Counseling: Inform that therapy causes elevation in BP and increases the risk of supine HTN, which could lead to strokes, heart attacks, and death. Instruct to rest and sleep in an upper-body elevated position and monitor BP. Instruct on how to manage observed BP elevations. Instruct to notify physician if nursing, pregnant, or planning to become pregnant. Instruct that if a dose is missed, take the next dose at the regularly scheduled time and not to double the dose.

NORVIR — ritonavir   Rx

Class: Protease inhibitor

> Coadministration w/ several classes of drugs, including sedative hypnotics, antiarrhythmics, or ergot alkaloid preparations may result in potentially serious and/or life-threatening adverse events due to possible effects of ritonavir (RTV) on the hepatic metabolism of certain drugs. Review medications taken by patients prior to prescribing RTV or when prescribing other medications to patients already taking RTV.

ADULT DOSAGE
HIV-1 Infection

In Combination w/ Other Antiretrovirals:
600mg bid; initiate at no less than 300mg bid and increase at 2- to 3-day intervals by 100mg bid
Max: 600mg bid

PEDIATRIC DOSAGE
HIV-1 Infection

In Combination w/ Other Antiretrovirals:
<1 Month of Age:
Initial: 250mg/m² bid
Titrate: Increase at 2- to 3-day intervals by 50mg/m² bid
Maint: 350-400mg/m² bid or highest tolerated dose
Max: 600mg bid

DOSING CONSIDERATIONS
Concomitant Medications
Reduce dose when used w/ other protease inhibitors

Hepatic Impairment
Mild (Child-Pugh Class A) or Moderate (Child-Pugh Class B): No dosage adjustment necessary
Severe (Child-Pugh Class C): Not recommended for use

Elderly
Start at low end of dosing range

Other Important Considerations
Do not administer oral sol to neonates before a postmenstrual age (1st day of the mother's last menstrual period to birth plus the time elapsed after birth) of 44 weeks has been attained

ADMINISTRATION
Oral route
Take w/ meals.

Tab
Swallow tab whole; do not chew, break, or crush tab.

Oral Sol
May improve the taste by mixing w/ chocolate milk, Ensure, or Advera w/in 1 hr of dosing.

STORAGE
Cap: 2-8°C (36-46°F). May not require refrigeration if used w/in 30 days and stored below 25°C (77°F). Protect from light. Avoid exposure to excessive heat.
Oral Sol: 20-25°C (68-77°F). Do not refrigerate. Avoid exposure to excessive heat.
Tab: ≤30°C (86°F). Exposure up to 50°C (122°F) for 7 days permitted. Exposure to high humidity outside the original or USP equivalent tight container (≤60mL) for >2 weeks is not recommended.

HOW SUPPLIED
Cap: 100mg; **Oral Sol:** 80mg/mL [240mL]; **Tab:** 100mg

CONTRAINDICATIONS
Known hypersensitivity (eg, toxic epidermal necrolysis or Stevens-Johnson syndrome) to RTV or any of its components. Coadministration w/ voriconazole or St. John's wort. Coadministration of RTV w/ several classes of drugs (including sedative hypnotics, antiarrhythmics, or ergot alkaloid preparations) is contraindicated and may result in potentially serious and/or life-threatening adverse events due to possible effects of RTV on the hepatic metabolism of these drugs (eg, alfuzosin HCl, amiodarone, flecainide, propafenone, quinidine, lurasidone, pimozide, dihydroergotamine, ergotamine, methylergonovine, cisapride, lovastatin, simvastatin, sildenafil when used for treatment of pulmonary arterial HTN, triazolam, oral midazolam).

WARNINGS/PRECAUTIONS
Hepatic transaminase elevations >5X ULN, clinical hepatitis, and jaundice reported; increased risk w/ underlying hepatitis B or C. Caution w/ preexisting liver diseases, liver enzyme abnormalities, or hepatitis; consider increased AST/ALT monitoring, especially during first 3 months of therapy. Pancreatitis observed; d/c if diagnosed. Allergic reactions, anaphylaxis, Stevens-Johnson syndrome, and toxic epidermal necrolysis reported; d/c if severe reactions develop. Prolonged PR interval and 2nd- or 3rd-degree atrioventricular (AV) block may occur; caution w/ underlying structural heart disease, preexisting conduction system abnormalities, ischemic heart disease, and cardiomyopathies. May elevate TGs and total cholesterol levels. New onset or exacerbation of diabetes mellitus (DM), hyperglycemia, diabetic ketoacidosis, immune reconstitution syndrome, autoimmune disorders (eg, Graves' disease, polymyositis, Guillain-Barre syndrome) in the setting of immune reconstitution, and redistribution/accumulation of body fat reported. Increased bleeding in patients w/ hemophilia type A and B reported. Various degrees of cross-resistance observed. Lab test interactions may occur. **Oral Sol:** Contains alcohol and propylene glycol. Avoid oral sol in preterm neonates in the immediate postnatal period; preterm neonates may be at increased risk of propylene glycol-associated adverse events and other

toxicities. If benefit of treating infants immediately after birth outweighs potential risk, monitor closely for increases in serum osmolality and SrCr, and for drug-related toxicity.

ADVERSE REACTIONS
Diarrhea, N/V, abdominal pain, dizziness, dysgeusia, paresthesia, peripheral neuropathy, rash, fatigue/asthenia, arthralgia, back pain, coughing, oropharyngeal pain, pruritus, flushing.

DRUG INTERACTIONS
See Boxed Warning and Contraindications. Coadministration w/ CYP3A substrates for which elevated plasma concentrations are associated w/ serious and/or life-threatening reactions is contraindicated. May increase exposure of CYP2D6 substrates. Not recommended w/ fluticasone or other glucocorticoids that are metabolized by CYP3A, salmeterol, high doses of itraconazole or ketoconazole, and simeprevir. Avoid w/ colchicine in patients w/ renal/hepatic impairment, saquinavir/rifampin/RTV combination, avanafil, and rivaroxaban. Delavirdine may increase levels and rifampin may decrease levels. May increase levels of CYP3A substrates, atazanavir, darunavir, amprenavir, saquinavir, tipranavir, maraviroc, normeperidine, disopyramide, lidocaine, mexiletine, dasatinib, nilotinib, vincristine, vinblastine, rivaroxaban, carbamazepine, clonazepam, ethosuximide, nefazodone, SSRIs, TCAs, desipramine, trazodone, dronabinol, ketoconazole, itraconazole, colchicine, clarithromycin, bedaquiline, rifabutin and rifabutin metabolite, quinine, antipsychotics (eg, quetiapine), β-blockers, calcium channel blockers, digoxin, bosentan, simeprevir, atorvastatin, rosuvastatin, cyclosporine, tacrolimus, sirolimus, fluticasone, budesonide, salmeterol, fentanyl, avanafil, sildenafil, tadalafil, vardenafil, buspirone, clorazepate, diazepam, estazolam, flurazepam, zolpidem, parenteral midazolam, dexamethasone, prednisone, and methamphetamine. May decrease levels of raltegravir, meperidine, divalproex, lamotrigine, phenytoin, bupropion, hydroxybupropion (active metabolite of bupropion), voriconazole, atovaquone, theophylline, methadone, and ethinyl estradiol. Caution w/ other drugs that prolong the PR interval, particularly w/ those drugs metabolized by CYP3A. May alter concentrations of warfarin (monitor INR) and indinavir. May need to decrease dose of tramadol and propoxyphene. RTV formulations contain alcohol; may produce disulfiram-like reactions w/ disulfiram or metronidazole. Refer to PI for dosing modifications when used w/ certain concomitant therapies.

PREGNANCY AND LACTATION
Pregnancy: Category B. An Antiretroviral Pregnancy Registry has been established to monitor maternal-fetal outcomes of pregnant women exposed to RTV.
Lactation: Not for use in nursing. The Centers for Disease Control and Prevention recommend that HIV-infected mothers not breastfeed their infants to avoid risking postnatal transmission of HIV.

MECHANISM OF ACTION
HIV-1 protease inhibitor; renders the enzyme incapable of processing the gag-pol polyprotein precursor, which leads to production of noninfectious immature HIV-1 particles.

PHARMACOKINETICS
Absorption: (Oral Sol) T_{max}=2 hrs (fasting), 4 hrs (fed); (Cap) AUC=121.7mg•hr/mL (fed), (Sol) AUC=129mg•hr/mL (fed). **Distribution:** V_d=0.41L/kg; plasma protein binding (98-99%). **Metabolism:** CYP3A (major), CYP2D6 (oxidation); isopropylthiazole (major metabolite). **Elimination:** (Oral Sol) Urine (11.3%, 3.5% unchanged), feces (86.4%, 33.8% unchanged); $T_{1/2}$=3-5 hrs.

PATIENT CONSIDERATIONS
Assessment: Assess for previous hypersensitivity to the drug, preexisting liver diseases, hepatitis, DM, hemophilia type A or B, underlying cardiac problems, lipid disorders, pregnancy/nursing status, and possible drug interactions. Obtain baseline ECG, LFTs, creatine phosphokinase (CPK), uric acid, TGs, and cholesterol levels.

Monitoring: Monitor for signs/symptoms of anaphylaxis or allergic reactions, hepatitis, jaundice, hepatic dysfunction, new onset or exacerbation of DM, hyperglycemia, pancreatitis, AV block, cardiac conduction abnormalities, immune reconstitution syndrome, fat redistribution/accumulation, and for other adverse reactions. Monitor for increased bleeding in patients w/ hemophilia type A or B. Monitor ECG, LFTs, CPK, uric acid, TGs, and cholesterol levels. Frequently monitor INR during coadministration w/ warfarin.

Counseling: Instruct to take prescribed dose ud. Instruct to inform physician if weight changes in children occur. Inform that therapy is not a cure for HIV-1 infection and illnesses associated w/ HIV-1 infection may still be experienced. Advise to practice safe sex; to use latex or polyurethane condoms; not to share personal items (eg, toothbrush, razor blades), needles, or other inj equipment; and not to breastfeed. Advise to notify physician of any use of prescription, OTC, or herbal products, particularly St. John's wort. Advise to use additional or alternative contraceptive measures if receiving estrogen-based hormonal contraceptives. Counsel about potential adverse effects; instruct to report signs/symptoms of worsening liver disease, pancreatitis, Stevens-Johnson syndrome, PR prolongation, and DM.

NOVAREL — chorionic gonadotropin   Rx

Class: Human chorionic gonadotropin

ADULT DOSAGE
Hypogonadism

Secondary to Pituitary Deficiency:
Regimen 1:
500-1000 U 3 X/week for 3 weeks, followed by the same dose 2X/week for 3 weeks

PEDIATRIC DOSAGE
Prepubertal Cryptorchidism

Not Due to Anatomical Obstruction:
4-9 Years:
Regimen 1:
4000 U 3X/week for 3 weeks

Regimen 2:
4000 U 3X/week for 6-9 months, following a dose reduction to 2000 U 3X/week for an additional 3 months

Ovulation Induction
Secondary and not due to primary ovarian failure in women who have been appropriately pretreated w/ human menotropins

Usual: 5000-10,000 U one day following the last dose of menotropins

Regimen 2:
5000 U every 2nd day for 4 inj

Regimen 3:
15 inj of 500-1000 U over a period of 6 weeks

Regimen 4:
500 U 3X/week for 4-6 weeks; if not successful, begin another 1 month later, giving 1000 U/inj

Hypogonadism
Secondary to Pituitary Deficiency: 4-9 Years:
Regimen 1:
500-1000 U 3X/week for 3 weeks, followed by the same dose 2X/week for 3 weeks

Regimen 2:
4000 U 3X/week for 6-9 months, following a dose reduction to 2000 U 3X/week for an additional 3 months

ADMINISTRATION
IM route

Reconstitution
1mL: 10000 IU/mL; administer entire dose at once
10mL: 1000 IU/mL; multiple dose administration, refrigerate between doses

STORAGE
20-25°C (68-77°F); excursions permitted between 15-30°C (59-86°F). Reconstituted Sol: 2-8°C (36-46°F). Use within 30 days.

HOW SUPPLIED
Inj: 10,000 U

CONTRAINDICATIONS
Precocious puberty, prostatic carcinoma or other androgen-dependent neoplasm, pregnancy.

WARNINGS/PRECAUTIONS
Should be used in conjunction with human menopausal gonadotropins only by physicians experienced with infertility problems. Ovarian hyperstimulation (ovarian enlargement, ascites with/without pain, and/or pleural effusion), enlargement of preexisting ovarian cysts or rupture of ovarian cysts with resultant hemoperitoneum, multiple births, and arterial thromboembolism may occur. Bacteriostatic water for inj diluent contains benzyl alcohol, which has been associated with a fatal "gasping syndrome" in premature infants. Anaphylaxis reported. May induce precocious puberty in patients treated for cryptorchidism; d/c if signs of precocious puberty occur. May cause fluid retention; caution in patients with cardiac/renal disease, epilepsy, migraine, or asthma. May cross-react in the radioimmunoassay of gonadotropins, especially luteinizing hormone.

ADVERSE REACTIONS
Headache, irritability, restlessness, depression, fatigue, edema, gynecomastia, inj-site pain, hypersensitivity reactions.

PREGNANCY AND LACTATION
Category X, caution in nursing.

MECHANISM OF ACTION
Human chorionic gonadotropin; stimulates production of gonadal steroid hormones by stimulating interstitial cells (Leydig cells) of testis to produce androgens and the corpus luteum of the ovary to produce progesterone.

PATIENT CONSIDERATIONS

Assessment: Assess for drug hypersensitivity, precocious puberty, prostatic carcinoma, androgen-dependent neoplasms, cardiac/renal disease, epilepsy, migraine, asthma, and pregnancy/nursing status.

Monitoring: Monitor for ovarian hyperstimulation, enlargement of preexisting ovarian cysts or rupture of ovarian cysts, multiple births, arterial thromboembolism, anaphylaxis, precocious puberty, fluid retention, and other adverse reactions.

Counseling: Inform of the serious adverse reactions associated with therapy and instruct to consult physician if signs/symptoms develop. Counsel about the proper disposal of needles and syringes.

NOVOEIGHT — antihemophilic factor (recombinant)   Rx

Class: Antihemophilic factor (recombinant)

ADULT DOSAGE
Hemophilia A

Dosage (IU) = Body Weight (kg) x Desired Factor VIII (FVIII) Increase (IU/dL or % normal) x 0.5

Control and Prevention of Bleeding Episodes:

Minor Bleed: FVIII Level Required:
20-40 IU/dL; repeat q12-24h for ≥1 day until bleeding resolution is achieved

PEDIATRIC DOSAGE
Hemophilia A

Dosage (IU) = Body Weight (kg) x Desired Factor VIII (FVIII) Increase (IU/dL or % normal) x 0.5

Control and Prevention of Bleeding Episodes:

Minor Bleed: FVIII Level Required:
20-40 IU/dL; repeat q12-24h for ≥1 day until bleeding resolution is achieved

Moderate Bleed: FVIII Level Required: 30-60 IU/dL; repeat q12-24h until pain and acute disability are resolved (approx 3-4 days)
Major Bleed: FVIII Level Required: 60-100 IU/dL; repeat q8-24h until resolution of bleed (approx 7-10 days)
Perioperative Management:
Minor Surgery: FVIII Level Required: 30-60 IU/dL; repeat q24h for ≥1 day until healing is achieved
Major Surgery: FVIII Level Required: 80-100 IU/dL (pre- and post-operative); repeat q8-24h until adequate wound healing, then continue therapy for ≥7 days to maintain a FVIII activity of 30-60% (IU/dL)

Routine Prophylaxis:
FVIII Dose Required: 20-50 IU/kg IV 3X/week or 20-40 IU/kg IV qod

Moderate Bleed: FVIII Level Required: 30-60 IU/dL; repeat q12-24h until pain and acute disability are resolved (approx 3-4 days)
Major Bleed: FVIII Level Required: 60-100 IU/dL; repeat q8-24h until resolution of bleed (approx 7-10 days)
Perioperative Management:
Minor Surgery: FVIII Level Required: 30-60 IU/dL; repeat q24h for ≥1 day until healing is achieved
Major Surgery: FVIII Level Required: 80-100 IU/dL (pre- and post-operative); repeat q8-24h until adequate wound healing, then continue therapy for ≥7 days to maintain a FVIII activity of 30-60% (IU/dL)

Routine Prophylaxis:
Adolescents (≥12 Years):
FVIII Dose Required: 20-50 IU/kg IV 3X/week or 20-40 IU/kg IV qod

Children (<12 Years):
FVIII Dose Required: 25-60 IU/kg IV 3X/week or 25-50 IU/kg IV qod

ADMINISTRATION
IV route

Use w/in 4 hrs after reconstitution when stored at room temperature; store the reconstituted product in the vial.
Do not administer in the same tubing or container w/ other medicinal products. Inject slowly over 2-5 min.

Refer to PI for further details on administration, preparation, and reconstitution.

STORAGE
2-8°C (36-46°F) for ≤30 months from the date of manufacture until the expiration date. W/IN the 30-month period, may also be stored at room temperature not to exceed 30°C (86°F) for ≤12 months; do not return product to the refrigerator. Do not freeze. Protect from light.

HOW SUPPLIED
Inj: 250 IU, 500 IU, 1000 IU, 1500 IU, 2000 IU, 3000 IU

CONTRAINDICATIONS
Life-threatening hypersensitivity reactions (eg, anaphylaxis) to this product, or its components (including traces of hamster proteins).

WARNINGS/PRECAUTIONS
Not indicated for the treatment of von Willebrand disease. Hypersensitivity reactions, including anaphylaxis, are possible; d/c immediately and initiate appropriate treatment if an allergic-/anaphylactic-type reaction occurs. Formation of neutralizing antibodies (inhibitors) to FVIII can occur following administration. Monitor for the development of FVIII inhibitors by appropriate clinical observation and lab testing. If expected plasma FVIII activity levels are not attained, or if bleeding is not controlled w/ an expected dose, perform testing for FVIII inhibitors. Determine inhibitor levels in Bethesda Units.

ADVERSE REACTIONS
Injection-site reactions, increased hepatic enzymes, pyrexia.

PREGNANCY AND LACTATION
Pregnancy: There are no adequate and well-controlled studies in pregnant women to determine whether there is a drug-associated risk.
Lactation: There is no information regarding the presence of the drug in human milk, the effect on the breastfed infant, and the effects on milk production; caution in nursing.

MECHANISM OF ACTION
Antihemophilic factor (recombinant); temporarily replaces the missing clotting FVIII that is needed for effective hemostasis.

PHARMACOKINETICS
Absorption: (Adults & Adolescents) AUC=14.2 IU•hr/mL (Clotting Assay), 18.7 IU•hr/mL (Chromogenic Assay); C_{max}=1.07 IU/mL (Clotting Assay), 1.54 IU/mL (Chromogenic Assay). **Distribution:** (Adults & Adolescents) V_d=53.4mL/kg (Clotting Assay), 44.3 mL/kg (Chromogenic Assay). **Elimination:** (Adults) $T_{1/2}$=10.8 hrs (Clotting Assay), 12 hrs (Chromogenic Assay). Refer to PI for pharmacokinetic parameters for patients <12 years of age.

PATIENT CONSIDERATIONS
Assessment: Assess for life-threatening hypersensitivity reactions to hamster proteins or other components of the product, von Willebrand disease, presence of FVIII inhibitors, and pregnancy/nursing status.

Monitoring: Monitor for signs/symptoms of hypersensitivity reactions and other adverse reactions. Monitor plasma FVIII activity levels by the one-stage clotting assay or the chromogenic substrate assay to confirm that adequate FVIII levels have been achieved and maintained, when clinically indicated. Perform assay to determine if FVIII inhibitor is present if expected plasma FVIII activity levels are not attained, or if bleeding is not controlled w/ the expected dose.

Counseling: Inform of benefits and risks of treatment. Advise to report any adverse reactions to healthcare provider. Inform of the early signs of hypersensitivity reactions; instruct to d/c treatment immediately, contact physician, and go to emergency department if symptoms of a hypersensitivity reaction occur. Instruct to contact physician/treatment center for further treatment and/or assessment if there is lack of clinical response to therapy. Advise on how to store the product correctly. Instruct to consult physician prior to travel and to bring an adequate supply of therapy based on current treatment regimen while traveling.

NOVOSEVEN RT — coagulation factor VIIa (recombinant)   Rx
Class: Antihemophilic agent

> Serious arterial and venous thrombotic events reported. Monitor for signs/symptoms of activation of the coagulation system and for thrombosis.

ADULT DOSAGE
Congenital Hemophilia

Congenital Hemophilia A or B w/ Inhibitors:

Acute Bleeding Episodes:
Hemostatic: 90mcg/kg IV q2h until hemostasis is achieved, or until treatment has been judged to be inadequate; adjust dose based on severity of bleeding
Post-Hemostatic: 90mcg/kg IV q3-6h for severe bleeds until after homeostasis is achieved to maintain the hemostatic plug; monitor and minimize duration

Perioperative Management:
Minor Surgery:
Initial: 90mcg/kg IV immediately before surgery and repeat q2h for the duration of surgery
Postsurgical: 90mcg/kg IV q2h for 48 hrs, then q2-6h until healing occurs

Major Surgery:
Initial: 90mcg/kg IV immediately before surgery and repeat q2h for the duration of surgery
Postsurgical: 90mcg/kg IV q2h for 5 days, then q4h until healing occurs
Administer additional bolus doses if required

Acquired Hemophilia
Acute Bleeding Episodes:
70-90mcg/kg IV q2-3h until hemostasis is achieved

Perioperative Management:
Minor/Major Surgery: 70-90mcg/kg IV immediately before surgery and repeat q2-3h for the duration of surgery, and until hemostasis is achieved

Factor VII Deficiency
Congenital:
Acute Bleeding Episodes:
15-30mcg/kg IV q4-6h until hemostasis is achieved

Perioperative Management:
Minor/Major Surgery: 15-30mcg/kg IV immediately before surgery and repeat q4-6h for the duration of surgery and until hemostasis is achieved

Effective treatment has been achieved w/ doses as low as 10mcg/kg

Glanzmann's Thrombasthenia
Refractory to platelet transfusions, w/ or w/o antibodies to platelets

Acute Bleeding Episodes:
90mcg/kg IV q2-6h in severe bleeding episodes requiring systemic hemostatic therapy until hemostasis is achieved

Perioperative Management:
Minor/Major Surgery:
Initial: 90mcg/kg IV immediately before surgery and repeat q2h for the duration of the procedure
Postsurgical: 90mcg/kg IV q2-6h to prevent postoperative bleeding

Higher average infused doses (median dose of 100mcg/kg) were noted for surgical patients who had clinical refractoriness w/ or w/o platelet-specific antibodies compared to those w/ neither

PEDIATRIC DOSAGE
Congenital Hemophilia

Congenital Hemophilia A or B w/ Inhibitors:

Acute Bleeding Episodes:
Hemostatic: 90mcg/kg IV q2h until hemostasis is achieved, or until treatment has been judged to be inadequate; adjust dose based on severity of bleeding
Post-Hemostatic: 90mcg/kg IV q3-6h for severe bleeds until after homeostasis is achieved to maintain the hemostatic plug; monitor and minimize duration

Perioperative Management:
Minor Surgery:
Initial: 90mcg/kg IV immediately before surgery and repeat q2h for the duration of surgery
Postsurgical: 90mcg/kg IV q2h for 48 hrs, then q2-6h until healing occurs

Major Surgery:
Initial: 90mcg/kg IV immediately before surgery and repeat q2h for the duration of surgery
Postsurgical: 90mcg/kg IV q2h for 5 days, then q4h until healing occurs
Administer additional bolus doses if required

Factor VII Deficiency
Congenital:
Acute Bleeding Episodes:
15-30mcg/kg IV q4-6h until hemostasis is achieved

Perioperative Management:
Minor/Major Surgery: 15-30mcg/ kg IV immediately before surgery and repeat q4-6h for the duration of surgery and until hemostasis is achieved

Effective treatment has been achieved w/ doses as low as 10mcg/kg

Glanzmann's Thrombasthenia
Refractory to platelet transfusions, w/ or w/o antibodies to platelets

Acute Bleeding Episodes:
90mcg/kg IV q2-6h in severe bleeding episodes requiring systemic hemostatic therapy until hemostasis is achieved

Perioperative Management:
Minor/Major Surgery:
Initial: 90mcg/kg IV immediately before surgery and repeat q2h for the duration of the procedure
Postsurgical: 90mcg/kg IV q2-6h to prevent postoperative bleeding

Higher average infused doses (median dose of 100mcg/kg) were noted for surgical patients who had clinical refractoriness w/ or w/o platelet-specific antibodies compared to those w/ neither

ADMINISTRATION
IV route
For IV bolus only; administer as a slow bolus inj over 2-5 min, depending on the dose administered.
Do not mix w/ other infusion sol.
Use 0.9% NaCl inj if line needs to be flushed before/after administration.
Administer w/in 3 hrs after reconstitution and discard any unused sol.

Reconstitution
Bring the powder and diluent to room temperature but not >37°C (98.6°F).
Powder and Vial of Diluent:
Add 1.1mL, 2.1mL, 5.2mL, or 8.1mL of the histidine diluent to 1mg, 2mg, 5mg, or 8mg vial of the powder respectively.
Use syringe needles w/ 20-/26-gauge size.
Do not inject the diluent directly on the powder but aim the needle against the side so that the stream of liquid runs down the vial wall.
Gently swirl until all the material dissolves.
Powder and Prefilled Diluent Syringe:
Use the 1mL, 2mL, 5mL, or 8mL of the prefilled diluent syringe for the 1mg, 2mg, 5mg, or 8mg vial respectively.
Refer to PI for further administration instructions.

STORAGE
2-25°C (36-77°F). Do not freeze. Protect from light. **Reconstituted Sol:** Room temperature or refrigerated for up to 3 hrs. Do not freeze or store in syringes.

HOW SUPPLIED
Inj: 1mg, 2mg, 5mg, 8mg

WARNINGS/PRECAUTIONS
Coagulation parameters do not necessarily correlate w/ or predict effectiveness of therapy. Increased risk of developing thromboembolic events due to circulating tissue factor or predisposing coagulopathy in patients w/ disseminated intravascular coagulation (DIC), advanced atherosclerotic disease, crush injury, septicemia, and uncontrolled postpartum hemorrhage. Caution w/ administration to patients w/ an increased risk of thromboembolic complications (eg, history of coronary artery disease [CAD], liver disease, DIC, postoperative immobilization, elderly, neonates). Reduce dose or d/c treatment depending on patient's condition if there is lab confirmation of intravascular coagulation or presence of clinical thrombosis. Hypersensitivity reactions, including anaphylaxis, reported. Administer only if clearly needed in patients w/ known hypersensitivity to the drug or any of its components, or in patients w/ known hypersensitivity to mouse, hamster, or bovine proteins; if symptoms occur, d/c treatment, administer appropriate treatment, and weigh the benefit/risks prior to restarting treatment. Antibody formation may be suspected if FVIIa activity fails to reach expected level, PT is not corrected, or bleeding is not controlled after treatment w/ recommended doses; perform analysis for antibodies. Lab test interactions may occur.

ADVERSE REACTIONS
Arterial and venous thrombotic events, fever, pain, deep thrombophlebitis, pulmonary embolism, cerebrovascular disorder, angina pectoris, anaphylactic shock, abnormal hepatic function.

DRUG INTERACTIONS
Avoid simultaneous use w/ activated prothrombin complex concentrates or prothrombin complex concentrates. Thrombosis may occur if administered concomitantly w/ coagulation factor XIII.

PREGNANCY AND LACTATION
Pregnancy: There are no adequate and well-controlled studies in pregnant women to determine whether there is a drug-associated risk.
Lactation: There is no information regarding the presence of coagulation factor VIIa (recombinant) in human milk, the effect on the breastfed infant, and the effects on milk production.

MECHANISM OF ACTION
Antihemophilic agent: Recombinant FVIIa; when complexed w/ tissue factor, can activate coagulation factor X (FX) to FXa and coagulation factor IX (FIX) to FIXa. FXa, in complex w/ other factors, then converts prothrombin to thrombin, which leads to formation of a hemostatic plug by converting fibrinogen to fibrin and thereby inducing local hemostasis. This process may also occur on the surface of activated platelets.

PHARMACOKINETICS
Distribution: (Hemophilia A or B, Non-Bleeding State) V_d (median)=106.5mL/kg (15-63 yrs of age), 128mL/kg (30-45 yrs of age), 164mL/kg (2-12 yrs of age). (Congenital FVII Deficiency) V_d=(20-43 yrs of age) 280mL/kg (15mcg/kg dose), 290mL/kg (30mcg/kg dose). **Elimination:** (Hemophilia A or B) $T_{1/2}$=2.89 hrs (15-63 yrs of age), 3.1 hrs (30-45 yrs of age), 2.6 hrs (2-12 yrs of age). (Congenital FVII Deficiency) $T_{1/2}$=(20-43 yrs of age) 2.82 hrs (15mcg/kg dose), 3.11 hrs (30mcg/kg dose).

PATIENT CONSIDERATIONS
Assessment: Assess for risk of thromboembolic complications (eg, DIC, history of CAD, liver disease, postoperative immobilization), hypersensitivity to drug, mouse, hamster, or bovine proteins, pregnancy/nursing status, and for possible drug interactions. Obtain baseline PT and FVII coagulant activity in FVII-deficient patients.

Monitoring: Monitor for development of signs/symptoms of activation of the coagulation system or thrombosis. Monitor PT, FVII activity, and for antibody formation in FVII-deficient patients. Monitor for hypersensitivity reactions, including anaphylaxis, and other adverse reactions.

Counseling: Advise to immediately seek medical help if early signs of hypersensitivity reactions (eg, hives, urticaria, tightness of chest) and signs of thrombosis (eg, new onset swelling and pain in the limbs or abdomen, new onset chest pain, SOB) occur.

NPLATE — romiplostim   Rx

Class: Thrombopoietin receptor agonist

ADULT DOSAGE

Chronic Immune Thrombocytopenia

Use in patients who have had an insufficient response to corticosteroids, immunoglobulins, or splenectomy

Initial: 1mcg/kg based on actual body weight
Titrate: Adjust weekly dose by increments of 1mcg/kg until platelet count is ≥50 x 10^9/L
Platelet Count >200 x 10^9/L for 2 Consecutive Weeks: Reduce dose by 1mcg/kg
Platelet Count >400 x 10^9/L: Do not dose; continue assessing platelet count weekly. After platelet count falls to <200 x 10^9/L, resume therapy at a dose reduced by 1mcg/kg
Max: 10mcg/kg/week

PEDIATRIC DOSAGE

Pediatric use may not have been established

DOSING CONSIDERATIONS
Concomitant Medications
Concomitant Medical Immune Thrombocytopenia (ITP) Therapies: May reduce or d/c medical ITP therapies (eg, corticosteroids, danazol, azathioprine, IV immunoglobulin, and anti-D immunoglobulin) if platelet count is ≥50 x 10^9/L

Discontinuation
D/C if platelet count does not increase to a level sufficient to avoid clinically important bleeding after 4 weeks of therapy at the max weekly dose

ADMINISTRATION
SQ route

Administer as a weekly SQ inj.
Discard any unused portion; do not pool unused portions from vials and do not administer more than 1 dose from a single vial.

Preparation
Reconstitute 250mcg vial or 500mcg vial w/ 0.72mL or 1.2mL, respectively, of preservative-free sterile water for inj.
Gently swirl and invert vial to reconstitute; do not shake.
Use a syringe w/ 0.01mL graduations.
Withdraw appropriate volume of calculated dose from vial and administer SQ. Reconstituted sol can be kept at 25°C (77°F) or 2-8°C (36-46°F) for up to 24 hrs prior to administration; protect reconstituted product from light.

STORAGE
2-8°C (36-46°F). Do not freeze. Protect from light.

HOW SUPPLIED
Inj: 250mcg, 500mcg [single-dose vial]

WARNINGS/PRECAUTIONS
Not for the treatment of thrombocytopenia due to myelodysplastic syndrome (MDS) or any cause of thrombocytopenia other than chronic ITP; progression from MDS to acute myelogenous leukemia has been observed. Use only in patients w/ ITP whose degree of thrombocytopenia and clinical condition increases the risk for bleeding. Do not use in an attempt to normalize platelet counts. Use lowest dose to achieve and maintain a platelet count ≥50 x 10^9/L. Thrombotic/thromboembolic complications may occur. Portal vein thrombosis reported in patients w/ chronic liver disease. If hyporesponsiveness or failure to maintain a platelet response occurs, search for causative factors (eg, neutralizing antibodies). Caution in elderly.

ADVERSE REACTIONS
Headache, arthralgia, dizziness, insomnia, myalgia, pain in extremity, abdominal pain, shoulder pain, dyspepsia, paresthesia.

PREGNANCY AND LACTATION
Pregnancy: Category C. Women who become pregnant during treatment are encouraged to enroll in Amgen's Pregnancy Surveillance Program.
Lactation: Not for use in nursing.

MECHANISM OF ACTION
Thrombopoietin (TPO) receptor agonist; increases platelet production through binding and activation of the TPO receptor.

PHARMACOKINETICS
Absorption: T_{max}=14 hrs (median). **Elimination:** $T_{1/2}$=3.5 days (median).

PATIENT CONSIDERATIONS
Assessment: Assess for cause and degree of thrombocytopenia, hepatic impairment, and pregnancy/nursing status.

Monitoring: Obtain CBCs, including platelet counts, weekly during dose adjustment phase, then monthly after establishment of a stable dose, and then weekly for at least 2 weeks after discontinuation. Monitor for thrombotic/thromboembolic complications, hyporesponsiveness, and failure to maintain platelet response w/ therapy.

Counseling: Inform of risks and benefits of therapy. Advise that the risks associated w/ long-term administration are unknown. Advise to avoid situations or medications that may increase risk for bleeding. Inform pregnant women that they may enroll in the surveillance program.

NUCALA — mepolizumab   Rx

Class: Monoclonal antibody/interleukin-5 (IL-5) receptor antagonist

ADULT DOSAGE
Asthma

Add-on maint treatment of severe asthma in patients w/ an eosinophilic phenotype

100mg SQ every 4 weeks into the upper arm, thigh, or abdomen

PEDIATRIC DOSAGE
Asthma

Add-on maint treatment of severe asthma in patients w/ an eosinophilic phenotype

≥12 Years:
100mg SQ every 4 weeks into the upper arm, thigh, or abdomen

ADMINISTRATION
SQ route

Reconstitution Instructions
1. Reconstitute mepolizumab in the vial w/ 1.2mL sterile water for inj (SWFI), preferably using a 2 or 3mL syringe and a 21-gauge needle; the reconstituted sol will contain a concentration of 100mg/mL. Do not mix w/ other medications.
2. Direct the stream of SWFI vertically onto the center of the lyophilized cake. Gently swirl the vial for 10 sec w/ a circular motion at 15-sec intervals until the powder is dissolved. Do not shake the reconstituted sol.
3. If a mechanical reconstitution device (swirler) is used, swirl at 450 rpm for no longer than 10 min. Alternatively, swirling at 1000 rpm for no longer than 5 min is acceptable.
4. If the reconstituted sol is not used immediately, store at <30°C (86°F), do not freeze, and discard if not used w/in 8 hrs of reconstitution.

Administration
1. For SQ administration, preferably using a 1mL polypropylene syringe fitted w/ a disposable 21- to 27-gauge x 0.5-inch (13mm) needle.
2. Just before administration, remove 1mL of reconstituted mepolizumab. Do not shake the reconstituted sol.
3. Administer the 1mL inj (equivalent to 100mg mepolizumab) SQ into the upper arm, thigh, or abdomen.

STORAGE
<25°C (77°F). Do not freeze. Store in the original package to protect from light.

HOW SUPPLIED
Inj: 100mg

CONTRAINDICATIONS
History of hypersensitivity to mepolizumab or excipients in the formulation.

WARNINGS/PRECAUTIONS
Not indicated for treatment of other eosinophilic conditions or relief of acute bronchospasm or status asthmaticus. D/C in the event of a hypersensitivity reaction. Herpes zoster reported; consider varicella vaccination if medically appropriate prior to starting therapy. Do not d/c systemic or inhaled corticosteroids abruptly upon initiation of therapy; reductions in corticosteroid dose, if appropriate, should be gradual and performed under the direct supervision of a physician. Reduction in corticosteroid dose may be associated w/ systemic withdrawal symptoms and/or unmask conditions previously suppressed by systemic corticosteroid therapy. Treat patients w/ preexisting helminth infections before initiating therapy; if patients become infected while receiving treatment and do not respond to anti-helminth treatment, d/c mepolizumab until infection resolves.

ADVERSE REACTIONS
Headache, inj-site reactions, back pain, fatigue, influenza, UTI, upper abdominal pain, pruritus, eczema, muscle spasms.

PREGNANCY AND LACTATION
Pregnancy: There is a pregnancy exposure registry that monitors pregnancy outcomes in women exposed to mepolizumab during pregnancy. Monoclonal antibodies, such as mepolizumab, are transported across the placenta in a linear fashion as pregnancy progresses; therefore, potential effects on a fetus are likely to be greater during the 2nd and 3rd trimester of pregnancy.
Lactation: There is no information regarding the presence of mepolizumab in human milk, the effects on the breastfed infant, or the effects on milk production. However, mepolizumab is a humanized monoclonal antibody (IgG1 kappa), and IgG is present in human milk in small amounts. Caution in nursing.

MECHANISM OF ACTION
IL-5 antagonist monoclonal antibody; reduces the production and survival of eosinophils by inhibiting IL-5 signaling.

PHARMACOKINETICS
Absorption: Bioavailability (approx 80%). **Distribution:** V_d=3.6L (for a 70kg individual). **Metabolism:** Degraded by proteolytic enzymes. **Elimination:** $T_{1/2}$=16-22 days.

PATIENT CONSIDERATIONS
Assessment: Assess for other eosinophilic conditions, acute bronchospasm or status asthmaticus, preexisting helminth infections, hypersensitivity to drug or excipients in the formulation, and pregnancy/nursing status.

Monitoring: Monitor for hypersensitivity reactions, acute asthma symptoms or acute exacerbations, herpes zoster, parasitic infection, and other adverse reactions.

Counseling: Inform that hypersensitivity reactions have occurred after administration and instruct to contact physician if such reactions occur. Inform that mepolizumab does not treat acute asthma symptoms or acute exacerbations. Instruct to seek medical advice if asthma remains uncontrolled or worsens after initiation of treatment. Inform that herpes zoster infections have occurred and where medically appropriate, varicella vaccination should be considered before starting treatment. Instruct not to d/c systemic or inhaled corticosteroids except under the direct supervision of a physician. Inform women there is a pregnancy exposure registry that monitors pregnancy outcomes in women exposed to mepolizumab during pregnancy.

NULOJIX — belatacept   Rx

Class: Selective costimulation modulator

> Increased risk for developing post-transplant lymphoproliferative disorder (PTLD), predominantly involving the CNS. Risk is increased in recipients without immunity to Epstein-Barr virus (EBV); use in EBV seropositive patients only. Do not use in transplant recipients who are EBV seronegative or with unknown serostatus. Should only be prescribed by physicians experienced in immunosuppressive therapy and management of kidney transplant patients. Manage patients in facilities equipped and staffed with adequate lab and supportive medical resources. Increased susceptibility to infection and the possible development of malignancies may result from immunosuppression. Use in liver transplant patients is not recommended due to an increased risk of graft loss and death.

ADULT DOSAGE

Organ Rejection Prophylaxis

Used in combination w/ basiliximab induction, mycophenolate mofetil, and corticosteroids in patients receiving a kidney transplant

The total infusion dose should be based on the actual body weight of the patient at the time of transplantation, and should not be modified during the course of therapy, unless there is a change in body weight of >10%

The prescribed dose must be evenly divisible by 12.5mg in order for the dose to be prepared accurately using the reconstituted sol and the silicone-free disposable syringe provided; evenly divisible increments are 0, 12.5, 25, 37.5, 50, 62.5, 75, 87.5, and 100

Initial Phase:
10mg/kg on Day 1 (day of transplantation, prior to implantation), Day 5 (approx 96 hrs after Day 1 dose), and end of Week 2, 4, 8, and 12 after transplantation

Maint Phase:
5mg/kg at the end of Week 16 after transplantation and every 4 weeks (± 3 days) thereafter

PEDIATRIC DOSAGE

Pediatric use may not have been established

ADMINISTRATION

IV route

Patients do not require premedication prior to administration

Preparation for Administration

1. Calculate the number of vials required to provide the total infusion dose; each vial contains 25mg of belatacept lyophilized powder
2. Reconstitute the contents of each vial w/ 10.5mL of a suitable diluent using the silicone-free disposable syringe provided w/ each vial and an 18- to 21-gauge needle; suitable diluents include: sterile water for inj (SWFI), 0.9% NaCl (NS), or D5W
Note: If the powder is accidentally reconstituted using a different syringe than the one provided, the sol may develop a few translucent particles; discard any sol prepared using siliconized syringes
3. To reconstitute the powder, insert the syringe needle into the vial through the center of the rubber stopper and direct the stream of diluent to the glass wall of the vial
4. To minimize foam formation, rotate the vial and invert w/ gentle swirling until the contents are completely dissolved; do not shake
5. The reconstituted sol contains a belatacept concentration of 25mg/mL and should be clear to slightly opalescent and colorless to pale yellow; do not use if opaque particles, discoloration, or other foreign particles are present
6. Calculate the total volume of the reconstituted 25mg/mL sol required to provide the total infusion dose
7. Prior to IV infusion, the required volume of the reconstituted sol must be further diluted w/ a suitable infusion fluid (NS or D5W). Nulojix reconstituted w/:
SWFI: Further dilute w/ either NS or D5W
NS: Further dilute w/ NS
D5W: Further dilute w/ D5W
8. From the appropriate size infusion bag or bottle, withdraw a volume of infusion fluid that is equal to the volume of the reconstituted sol required to provide the prescribed dose
9. W/ the same silicone-free disposable syringe used for reconstitution, withdraw the required amount of belatacept sol from the vial, inject it into the infusion bag or bottle, and gently rotate the infusion bag or bottle to ensure mixing
10. The final belatacept concentration in the infusion bag or bottle should range from 2-10mg/mL. Typically, an infusion volume of 100mL will be appropriate for most patients and doses, but total infusion volumes ranging from 50-250mL may be used; any unused sol remaining in the vials must be discarded
11. Administer entire infusion over a period of 30 min w/ an infusion set and a sterile, non-pyrogenic, low-protein-binding filter (w/ a pore size of 0.2-1.2µm)
12. Transfer the reconstituted sol from the vial to the infusion bag or bottle immediately; the infusion must be completed w/in 24 hrs of reconstitution of the lyophilized powder
13. Infuse in a separate line from other concomitantly infused agents; do not infuse concomitantly in the same IV line w/ other agents

STORAGE

Vial: 2-8°C (36-46°F). Protect from light by storing in the original package until time of use. Reconstituted Sol: 2-8°C (36-46°F) for up to 24 hrs. Protect from light. Max of 4 hrs of the total 24 hrs can be at room temperature (20-25°C) [68-77°F] and room light.

HOW SUPPLIED

Inj: 250mg

CONTRAINDICATIONS

Transplant recipients who are EBV seronegative or with unknown EBV serostatus.

WARNINGS/PRECAUTIONS

Administration of higher than recommended doses of drug or concomitant immunosuppressive agents or more frequent dosing is not recommended. Cytomegalovirus (CMV) infection and T-cell-depleting therapy are other known risk factors for PTLD; use T-cell depleting therapies cautiously. Patients who are EBV seropositive and CMV seronegative may also be at increased risk for PTLD. Limit exposure to sunlight and UV light. Progressive multifocal leukoencephalopathy (PML) reported at higher cumulative doses and more frequent regimens. Consider PTLD or PML if new or worsening neurological, cognitive, or behavioral signs/symptoms develop. If PML is diagnosed, consider reduction or withdrawal of immunosuppression taking into account the risk to the allograft. May increase risk of developing bacterial (tuberculosis [TB]), viral (CMV and herpes), fungal, and protozoal infections, including opportunistic infections; prophylaxis for CMV (for at least 3 months after transplantation) and *Pneumocystis jiroveci* are recommended after transplantation. Initiate treatment of latent TB infection prior to belatacept use. Polyoma virus-associated nephropathy (PVAN) reported; consider reductions in immunosuppression if evidence of PVAN develops. Increased rate and grade of acute rejection and graft loss reported with corticosteroid minimization to 5mg/day between Day 3 and Week 6 post-transplantation; corticosteroid utilization should be consistent with the belatacept clinical trial experience.

ADVERSE REACTIONS

PTLD, malignancies, anemia, diarrhea, urinary tract infection, peripheral edema, constipation, HTN, pyrexia, graft dysfunction, cough, N/V, headache, hypokalemia, hyperkalemia.

DRUG INTERACTIONS

Avoid use of live vaccines (eg, intranasal influenza, measles, mumps, rubella, oral polio, BCG, yellow fever, varicella, TY21a typhoid). Monitor for a need to adjust concomitant MMF dosage when therapy is switched between cyclosporine and belatacept, as cyclosporine decreases mycophenolic acid (MPA) exposure while belatacept does not. A higher MMF dosage may be needed after switching from belatacept to cyclosporine, since this may result in lower MPA concentrations and increase the risk of rejection. A lower MMF dosage may be needed after switching from cyclosporine to belatacept, since this may result in higher MPA concentrations and increase the risk for adverse reactions related to MPA.

PREGNANCY AND LACTATION

Category C, not for use in nursing.

MECHANISM OF ACTION

Selective T-cell costimulation blocker; binds to CD80 and CD86 on antigen-presenting cells, thereby blocking CD28 mediated costimulation of T lymphocytes.

PHARMACOKINETICS

Absorption: C_{max}=247mcg/mL (10mg/kg), 139mcg/mL (5mg/kg); AUC=22,252mcg•hr/mL (10mg/kg), 14,090mcg•hr/mL (5mg/kg). **Distribution:** V_d=0.11L/kg (10mg/kg), 0.12L/kg (5mg/kg). **Elimination:** $T_{1/2}$=9.8 days (10mg/kg), 8.2 days (5mg/kg).

PATIENT CONSIDERATIONS

Assessment: Assess for EBV serostatus, presence of infections, pregnancy/nursing status, possible drug interactions, and any other conditions where treatment is cautioned.

Monitoring: Monitor for PTLD, PML, infections, malignancies, TB, PVAN, and other adverse reactions.

Counseling: Instruct to immediately report any neurological, cognitive, or behavioral signs/symptoms during and after therapy (eg, changes in mood or usual behavior, confusion, problems thinking, memory loss, changes in walking or talking, decreased strength or weakness on one side of the body, changes in vision). Inform about increased risk of PTLD, malignancies (eg, skin cancer), PML, and infections. Advise to adhere to antimicrobial prophylaxis regimens as prescribed and to immediately report any signs/symptoms of infection during therapy. Instruct to limit exposure to sunlight and UV light by wearing protective clothing and using sunscreen with high protection factor. Instruct to look for any signs/symptoms of skin cancer (eg, suspicious moles or lesions). Advise to avoid live vaccines. Instruct to inform physician if pregnant/planning to become pregnant, or if breastfeeding.

NUPLAZID — pimavanserin

Class: Atypical antipsychotic

Rx

> Elderly patients w/ dementia-related psychosis treated w/ antipsychotic drugs are at an increased risk of death. Not approved for the treatment of patients w/ dementia-related psychosis unrelated to the hallucinations and delusions associated w/ Parkinson's disease psychosis.

ADULT DOSAGE	PEDIATRIC DOSAGE
Parkinson's Disease Psychosis Treatment of hallucinations and delusions associated w/ Parkinson's disease psychosis 34mg qd, w/o titration	Pediatric use may not have been established

DOSING CONSIDERATIONS
Concomitant Medications
Strong CYP3A4 Inhibitors:
17mg qd

Strong CYP3A4 Inducers:
Monitor for reduced efficacy; may need to increase pimavanserin dose

Renal Impairment
Severe (CrCl <30mL/min): Not recommended

Hepatic Impairment
Not recommended

ADMINISTRATION
Oral route

May take w/ or w/o food.

STORAGE
20-25°C (68-77°F); excursions permitted to 15-30°C (59-86°F).

HOW SUPPLIED
Tab: 17mg

WARNINGS/PRECAUTIONS
May prolong the QT interval; avoid in patients w/ known QT prolongation, a history of cardiac arrhythmias, and in circumstances that may increase the risk of the occurrence of torsades de pointes and/or sudden death (eg, symptomatic bradycardia, hypokalemia, hypomagnesemia, presence of congenital prolongation of the QT interval).

ADVERSE REACTIONS
Peripheral edema, confusional state.

DRUG INTERACTIONS
See Dosing Considerations. Avoid w/ other drugs known to prolong the QT interval (eg, quinidine, amiodarone, ziprasidone, chlorpromazine, thioridazine, moxifloxacin). Strong CYP3A4 inhibitors (eg, ketoconazole, clarithromycin, indinavir) may increase exposure. Strong CYP3A4 inducers (eg, carbamazepine, phenytoin, St. John's wort) may reduce exposure and result in a potential decrease in efficacy.

PREGNANCY AND LACTATION
Pregnancy: There are no data on pimavanserin use in pregnant women that would allow assessment of the drug-associated risk of major congenital malformations or miscarriage.
Lactation: There is no information regarding the presence of pimavanserin in human milk, the effects on the breastfed infant, or the effects on milk production.

MECHANISM OF ACTION
Atypical antipsychotic; mechanism not established. Effects could be mediated through a combination of inverse agonist and antagonist activity at serotonin 5-HT_{2A} receptors and to a lesser extent at serotonin 5-HT_{2C} receptors.

PHARMACOKINETICS
Absorption: T_{max}=6 hrs (median). **Distribution:** V_d=2173L; plasma protein binding (95%). **Metabolism:** Predominantly via CYP3A4 and CYP3A5, and lesser extent via CYP2J2, CYP2D6, and various other CYP and FMO enzymes; AC-279 (major active metabolite). **Elimination:** Urine (<1% of dose of pimavanserin and its active metabolite recovered, 0.55% unchanged), feces (1.53%); $T_{1/2}$=57 hrs (pimavanserin), 200 hrs (active metabolite).

PATIENT CONSIDERATIONS
Assessment: Assess for QT prolongation, history of cardiac arrhythmias, symptomatic bradycardia, hypokalemia, hypomagnesemia, renal/hepatic impairment, pregnancy/nursing status, and possible drug interactions.
Monitoring: Monitor for QT prolongation and any other adverse reaction.
Counseling: Advise to notify physician of all prescription and nonprescription medications currently taking.

NUTROPIN AQ — somatropin (rDNA origin)

Class: Recombinant human growth hormone (hGH)

Rx

ADULT DOSAGE	PEDIATRIC DOSAGE
Growth Hormone Deficiency **Adult or Childhood-Onset Etiology:** **Weight-Based:** **Initial:** ≤0.006mg/kg qd SQ **Titrate:** May increase based on individual requirements	**Growth Hormone Deficiency** Due to an inadequate secretion of endogenous growth hormone (GH) Individualize dose **Recommended Dose:** Up to 0.3mg/kg/week

Maint: Individualize dose
Max:
≤35 Years: 0.025mg/kg qd
<35 Years: 0.0125mg/kg qd
Non-Weight-Based:
Initial: 0.2mg/day SQ (range, 0.15-0.30mg/day)
Titrate: May increase gradually every 1-2 months by increments of 0.1-0.2mg/day based on clinical response and serum insulin-like growth factor-I (IGF-I) concentrations
Maint: Individualize dose

Pubertal Patients: May use up to 0.7mg/kg/week
Divide weekly dose into daily SQ inj

Idiopathic Short Stature
Treatment of idiopathic short stature defined by height standard deviation score ≤-2.25, and associated w/ growth rates unlikely to permit attainment of adult height in the normal range, in pediatric patients whose epiphyses are not closed and for whom diagnostic evaluation excludes other causes associated w/ short stature that should be observed or treated by other means

Individualize dose
Recommended Dose: Up to 0.3mg/kg/week

Divide weekly dose into daily SQ inj

Growth Failure Secondary to Chronic Kidney Disease

Individualize dose
Recommended Dose: Up to 0.35mg/kg/week
Continue therapy up to the time of renal transplantation
Divide weekly dose into daily SQ inj

Hemodialysis: Give at hs or at least 3-4 hrs after dialysis
Chronic Cycling Peritoneal Dialysis: Give in am after completion of dialysis
Chronic Ambulatory Peritoneal Dialysis: Give in pm during overnight exchange

Turner Syndrome
Treatment of short stature associated w/ Turner syndrome (TS)

Individualize dose
Recommended Dose: Up to 0.375mg/kg/week divided into equal doses 3-7X/week SQ

DOSING CONSIDERATIONS
Concomitant Medications
Oral Estrogen: May increase the dose requirements in women

Elderly
Consider lower starting dose and smaller dose increments

ADMINISTRATION
SQ route

Rotate inj sites to avoid lipodystrophy.

Reconstitution
- The Nutropin AQ Pen 10 and 20mg cartridges are color-banded to help ensure appropriate use w/ the Nutropin AQ Pen delivery device. Each cartridge must be used w/ its corresponding color-coded Nutropin AQ Pen.
- Follow the directions provided in the Nutropin AQ Pen and Nutropin AQ NuSpin 5, 10, or 20 instructions for use.

STORAGE
2-8°C (36-46°F) for 28 days after initial use. Avoid freezing. Protect from light.

HOW SUPPLIED
Inj: 10mg/2mL, 20mg/2mL [pen cartridge], 5mg/2mL, 10mg/2mL, 20mg/2mL [NuSpin]

CONTRAINDICATIONS
Acute critical illness due to complications following open-heart surgery, abdominal surgery, multiple accidental trauma, or w/ acute respiratory failure. Pediatric patients w/ Prader-Willi syndrome (PWS) who are severely obese, have a history of upper airway obstruction or sleep apnea, or have severe respiratory impairment. Pediatric patients who have growth failure due to genetically confirmed PWS. Active malignancy, or evidence of progression or recurrence of an underlying intracranial tumor. Active proliferative or severe nonproliferative diabetic retinopathy. Growth promotion in pediatric patients w/ closed epiphysis. Known hypersensitivity to somatropin, excipients, or diluent.

WARNINGS/PRECAUTIONS
Reevaluate adults who were treated w/ somatropin for growth hormone deficiency (GHD) in childhood and whose epiphyses are closed. Treatment for short stature should be discontinued when epiphyses are fused. Implement effective weight control in patients w/ PWS and treat respiratory infections aggressively. Increased risk of developing malignancies in children w/ certain rare genetic causes of short stature; monitor for development of neoplasms if treatment is initiated. Monitor for increased growth, or potential malignant changes, of preexisting nevi. Undiagnosed impaired glucose tolerance and overt diabetes mellitus (DM) may be unmasked, and new-onset type 2 DM reported. Intracranial HTN w/ papilledema, visual changes, headache, and N/V reported; d/c therapy if papilledema occurs. Fluid retention in adults may occur. Monitor other hormonal replacement treatments in patients w/ hypopituitarism. Undiagnosed/

untreated hypothyroidism may prevent optimal response. Hypothyroidism may become evident or worsen. Slipped capital femoral epiphysis (SCFE) and progression of scoliosis may occur in pediatric patients. Increased risk of ear/hearing disorders and cardiovascular (CV) disorders in TS patients. Periodically examine children w/ growth failure secondary to chronic kidney disease (CKD) for evidence of renal osteodystrophy progression. Tissue atrophy may occur; rotate inj site. Allergic reactions may occur. Serum levels of inorganic phosphorus, alkaline phosphatase, parathyroid hormone, and IGF-I may increase. Pancreatitis reported rarely. Obese individuals are more likely to manifest adverse effects when treated w/ a weight-based regimen. Estrogen replete women may need higher doses than men. Caution in elderly.

ADVERSE REACTIONS
Arthralgia, edema, joint disorders, otitis media, ear disorders, glucose intolerance, fluid retention.

DRUG INTERACTIONS
See Dosing Considerations. May inhibit 11β-hydroxysteroid dehydrogenase type 1, resulting in reduced serum cortisol concentrations; may need glucocorticoid replacement or dose adjustments of glucocorticoid therapy. Glucocorticoid therapy may attenuate growth-promoting effects in children; carefully adjust glucocorticoid replacement therapy. May increase clearance of antipyrine. May alter clearance of compounds metabolized by CYP450 liver enzymes (eg, corticosteroids, sex steroids, anticonvulsants, cyclosporine); monitor carefully. Oral estrogens may reduce IGF-1 response to treatment. May need to adjust dose of insulin, oral/injectable hypoglycemic agents, and/or thyroid hormone replacement therapy.

PREGNANCY AND LACTATION
Pregnancy: Category C.
Lactation: Caution in nursing.

MECHANISM OF ACTION
Recombinant human GH; binds to dimeric GH receptors in cell membranes of target tissue cells, resulting in intracellular signal transduction.

PHARMACOKINETICS
Absorption: Absolute bioavailability (81%); C_{max}=71.1mcg/L; T_{max}=3.9 hrs; AUC=677mcg•hr/L. **Distribution:** V_d=50mL/kg. **Metabolism:** Liver and kidneys. **Elimination:** $T_{1/2}$=2.1 hrs.

PATIENT CONSIDERATIONS
Assessment: Assess for PWS, preexisting DM or impaired glucose tolerance, hypothyroidism, hypopituitarism, history of scoliosis, hypersensitivity, any other conditions where treatment is contraindicated or cautioned, pregnancy/nursing status, and possible drug interactions. Perform funduscopic exam. Obtain x-rays of the hip in CKD patients.

Monitoring: Monitor for neoplasm, increased growth or malignant changes of preexisting nevi, fluid retention, intracranial HTN, allergic reactions, pancreatitis, and SCFE and progression of scoliosis in pediatric patients (eg, onset of limp, hip or knee pain), and for any other adverse reaction. Perform periodic thyroid function tests, funduscopic exam, and monitoring of glucose levels. In patients w/ PWS, monitor weight as well as for signs of respiratory infection, sleep apnea, and upper airway obstruction. Monitor patients w/ a history of GHD secondary to an intracranial neoplasm routinely for progression/recurrence of the tumor. In patients w/ TS, monitor for ear/CV disorders. In patients w/ CKD, periodically examine for evidence of progression of renal osteodystrophy. Monitor clinical response.

Counseling: Inform about potential benefits and risks of therapy, proper administration, and usage and disposal. Caution against any reuse of needles and syringes.

Nuwiq — antihemophilic factor (recombinant)   Rx

Class: Antihemophilic factor (recombinant)

ADULT DOSAGE
Hemophilia A
Dosing Equations:
Required (IU) = Body Weight (kg) x Desired Factor VIII (FVIII) Rise (IU/dL or % of Normal) x 0.5 (IU/kg per IU/dL)

Expected FVIII Rise (% of Normal) = 2X Administered IU / Body Weight (kg)

Dose and duration of therapy depend on the severity of the FVIII deficiency, the location and extent of the bleeding, and clinical condition

Treatment/Control of Bleeding Episodes:

Minor Bleed:
20-40 (% of Normal or IU/dL)
Required FVIII Activity: Give q12-24h for at least 1 day, until bleeding episode is resolved

Moderate to Major Bleed:
30-60 (% of Normal or IU/dL)
Required FVIII Activity: Give q12-24h for 3-4 days or more, until bleeding episode is resolved

PEDIATRIC DOSAGE
Hemophilia A
Dosing Equations:
Required (IU) = Body Weight (kg) x Desired FVIII Rise (IU/dL or % of Normal) x 0.5 (IU/kg per IU/dL)

Expected FVIII Rise (% of Normal) = 2X Administered IU / Body Weight (kg)

Dose and duration of therapy depend on the severity of the FVIII deficiency, the location and extent of the bleeding, and clinical condition

Treatment/Control of Bleeding Episodes:

Minor Bleed:
20-40 (% of Normal or IU/dL)
Required FVIII Activity: Give q12-24h for at least 1 day, until bleeding episode is resolved

Moderate to Major Bleed:
30-60 (% of Normal or IU/dL)
Required FVIII Activity: Give q12-24h for 3-4 days or more, until bleeding episode is resolved

Life-Threatening Bleed:
60-100 (% of Normal or IU/dL)
Required FVIII Activity: Give q8-24h until bleeding risk is resolved

Perioperative Management:

Minor Surgery:
30-60 (% of Normal or IU/dL)
Required FVIII Activity (Pre-/Post-Operative): Give q24 hrs for at least 1 day, until healing is achieved

Major Surgery:
80-100 (% of Normal or IU/dL)
Required FVIII Activity (Pre-/Post-Operative): Give q8-24 hrs until adequate wound healing, then continue therapy for at least another 7 days to maintain a FVIII activity of 30-60 IU/dL

Routine Prophylaxis:
30-40 IU/kg IV qod

Life-Threatening Bleed:
60-100 (% of Normal or IU/dL)
Required FVIII Activity: Give q8-24h until bleeding risk is resolved

Perioperative Management:

Minor Surgery:
30-60 (% of Normal or IU/dL)
Required FVIII Activity (Pre-/Post-Operative): Give q24h for at least 1 day, until healing is achieved

Major Surgery:
80-100 (% of Normal or IU/dL)
Required FVIII Activity (Pre-/Post-Operative): Give q8-24h until adequate wound healing, then continue therapy for at least another 7 days to maintain a FVIII activity of 30-60 IU/dL

Routine Prophylaxis:
2-11 Years: 30-50 IU/kg qod or 3X/week
12-17 Years: 30-40 IU/kg IV qod

ADMINISTRATION
IV route

Do not administer in same tubing or container as other medications.
Perform IV bolus infusion; rate of administration should be determined by comfort level, at a max rate of 4mL/min.

Reconstitution
1. Allow vial and pre-filled syringe to come to room temperature.
2. Using supplied adapter and syringe, slowly inject all liquid from syringe into the concentrate vial.
3. Without removing syringe, dissolve concentrate powder in vial by gently moving or swirling; do not shake.
4. Turn the vial and syringe upside down (still attached).
5. Slowly withdraw sol into syringe. Make sure that all liquid is transferred to the syringe.
6. Detach syringe by turning counterclockwise.
7. Do not refrigerate reconstitution; use w/in 3 hrs after reconstitution. If not used w/in this time period, discard.

STORAGE
2-8°C (35-46°F) for up to 24 months. Do not freeze. Store in the original package to protect vials from light. During shelf life, may be kept at ≤25°C (77°F) for a single period ≤3 months. After storage at room temperature, do not return the product to the refrigerator. **Reconstituted Sol:** Keep at room temperature. Do not refrigerate. Use reconstituted sol immediately or w/in 3 hrs after reconstitution; discard any remaining sol.

HOW SUPPLIED
Inj: 250 IU, 500 IU, 1000 IU, 2000 IU

CONTRAINDICATIONS
Life-threatening hypersensitivity reactions to antihemophilic factor (recombinant) or its components.

WARNINGS/PRECAUTIONS
Not indicated for the treatment of von Willebrand disease. Hypersensitivity reactions, including anaphylaxis, may occur; d/c immediately and initiate appropriate treatment. Monitor plasma FVIII activity levels by the one-stage clotting assay to confirm that adequate FVIII levels have been achieved and maintained. Formation of neutralizing antibodies may occur; monitor for development of FVIII inhibitors. If plasma FVIII level fails to increase as expected, or if bleeding is not controlled, suspect presence of an inhibitor; perform a Bethesda inhibitor assay.

ADVERSE REACTIONS
Paresthesia, headache, inj-site inflammation, inj-site pain, non-neutralizing anti-FVIII antibody formation, back pain, vertigo, dry mouth.

PREGNANCY AND LACTATION
Pregnancy: There are no data for use in pregnant women to inform of drug-associated risks; should be given to a pregnant woman only if clearly needed.
Lactation: There is no information regarding the presence in human milk, the effect on the breastfed infant, or the effects on milk production; caution in nursing.

MECHANISM OF ACTION
Antihemophilic factor (recombinant); temporarily replaces the missing clotting FVIII that is needed for effective hemostasis.

PHARMACOKINETICS
Absorption: (50 IU/kg) AUC=18h•IU/mL. **Distribution:** (50 IU/kg) V_d=59.8mL/kg. **Elimination:** (50 IU/kg) $T_{1/2}$=17.1 hrs. Refer to PI for pediatric parameters.

PATIENT CONSIDERATIONS
Assessment: Assess for life-threatening hypersensitivity reactions (including anaphylaxis), location and extent of bleeding, patient's clinical condition, and pregnancy/nursing status. Assess FVIII activity levels.

Monitoring: Monitor for signs/symptoms of hypersensitivity reactions and other adverse reactions. Monitor plasma FVIII activity levels, clinical response, and development of FVIII inhibitors.

Counseling: Inform of the early signs of hypersensitivity reactions (eg, hives, generalized urticaria, tightness of the chest); advise to stop inj, contact physician, and seek prompt emergency treatment if any of these symptoms arise. Advise to contact physician or treatment center for further treatment and/or assessment if experiencing a lack of clinical response. Advise to consult w/ healthcare provider prior to traveling; while traveling, advise to bring an adequate supply.

OBIZUR — antihemophilic factor (recombinant), porcine sequence   Rx

Class: Antihemophilic factor (recombinant)

ADULT DOSAGE
Acquired Hemophilia A

Minor and Moderate Bleeding:
Factor VII Level Required: 50-100 U/dL
Initial: 200 U/kg
Subsequent Dose: Titrate subsequent doses to maintain recommended factor VIII trough levels and individual clinical response. Dose every 4 to 12 hours; adjust frequency based on clinical response and measured factor VIII levels

Major Bleeding:
Factor VII Level Required: 100-200 U/dL (acute bleed), 50-100 U/dL (after acute bleed is controlled, if required)
Initial: 200 U/kg
Subsequent Dose: Titrate subsequent doses to maintain recommended factor VIII trough levels and individual clinical response. Dose every 4 to 12 hours, adjust frequency based on clinical response and measured factor VIII levels

PEDIATRIC DOSAGE
Pediatric use may not have been established

ADMINISTRATION
IV route

Administer reconstituted sol at 1-2mL/min
Refer to PI for reconstitution and administration instructions

STORAGE
2-8°C (36-46°F). Do not freeze. Protect from light. Use within 3 hrs after reconstitution; discard any unused reconstituted product if not used within 3 hrs after reconstitution.

HOW SUPPLIED
Inj: 500 U

CONTRAINDICATIONS
History of life-threatening hypersensitivity reactions to this product or its components (including traces of hamster proteins).

WARNINGS/PRECAUTIONS
Not indicated for the treatment of congenital hemophilia A or von Willebrand disease. Hypersensitivity reactions may occur; immediately d/c and initiate appropriate treatment if allergic or anaphylactic-type reactions occur. Inhibitory antibodies to therapy have occurred; monitor for the development of antibodies to therapy by appropriate assays. Consider other therapeutic options if such inhibitory antibodies to anti-porcine factor VIII are suspected and there is a lack of clinical response.

ADVERSE REACTIONS
Development of inhibitors to porcine factor VIII.

PREGNANCY AND LACTATION
Category C, caution in nursing.

MECHANISM OF ACTION
Antihemophilic factor (recombinant); temporarily replaces the inhibited endogenous factor VIII that is needed for effective hemostasis.

PATIENT CONSIDERATIONS
Assessment: Assess for hypersensitivity to the drug or traces of hamster proteins, severity of bleeding, and pregnancy/nursing status.

Monitoring: Monitor for hypersensitivity reactions and other adverse reactions. Monitor replacement therapy in cases of major surgery or life-threatening bleeding episodes. Perform 1-stage clotting assay to confirm that adequate factor VIII levels have been achieved and maintained. Monitor factor VIII activity 30 min and 3 hrs after initial dose and monitor factor VIII activity 30 min after subsequent doses. Monitor for the development of inhibitory antibodies to therapy; perform a Nijmegen Bethesda inhibitor assay if expected plasma factor VIII activity levels are not attained, or if bleeding is not controlled with the expected dose.

Counseling: Advise to report to physician any adverse reactions or problems following administration.

OCALIVA — obeticholic acid   Rx

Class: Farnesoid X receptor (FXR) agonist

ADULT DOSAGE
Primary Biliary Cholangitis
In combination w/ ursodeoxycholic acid (UDCA) in patients who have not achieved an adequate response to appropriate dosage of UDCA for at least 1 yr, or as monotherapy in patients who are intolerant to UDCA
Initial: 5mg qd
Titrate: Increase dose to 10mg qd if adequate reduction in alkaline phosphatase and/or total bilirubin has not been achieved after 3 months of 5mg qd dosing, and the patient is tolerating therapy.
Max: 10mg qd

PEDIATRIC DOSAGE
Pediatric use may not have been established

DOSING CONSIDERATIONS
Concomitant Medications
W/ Bile Acid Binding Resin: Take at least 4 hrs before or 4 hrs after taking bile acid binding resin, or at as great an interval as possible

Hepatic Impairment
Mild (Child-Pugh Class A): No dosage adjustment needed

Moderate (Child-Pugh Class B)/Severe (Child-Pugh Class C):
Initial: 5mg once weekly.
Titrate: Increase dose to 5mg twice weekly (at least 3 days apart) and subsequently to 10mg twice weekly (at least 3 days apart) depending on response and tolerability, if adequate reduction in alkaline phosphatase and/or total bilirubin has not been achieved after 3 months of 5mg once weekly dosing

Adverse Reactions
Intolerable Pruritus:
Consider one of the following options:
- Add an antihistamine or bile acid binding resin
- Reduce the dosage to 5mg qod for patients intolerant to 5mg once daily or to 5mg qd for patients intolerant to 10mg qd
- Temporarily interrupt therapy for up to 2 weeks followed by restarting at a reduced dosage

Increase the dosage to 10mg qd, as tolerated, to achieve optimal response

Consider discontinuing therapy in patients who continue to experience persistent, intolerable pruritus

ADMINISTRATION
Oral route

Take w/ or w/o food.

STORAGE
20-25°C (68-77°F); excursions permitted to 15-30°C (59-86°F)

HOW SUPPLIED
Tab: 5mg, 10mg

CONTRAINDICATIONS
In patients w/ complete biliary obstruction.

WARNINGS/PRECAUTIONS
Liver-related adverse reactions (eg, jaundice, worsening ascites, primary biliary cholangitis flares) observed; monitor for elevations in liver biochemical tests and liver-related adverse reactions. D/C therapy if complete biliary obstruction develops. Severe pruritus reported; management strategies include the addition of bile acid binding resins or antihistamines, dose reduction, and/or temporary interruption. Reduction in HDL-C reported; monitor for changes in serum lipid levels during treatment. Weigh potential risks against benefits of continuing treatment for patients who experience a reduction in HDL-C and do not respond to therapy after 1 yr at the highest recommended dosage that can be tolerated.

ADVERSE REACTIONS
Pruritus, fatigue, abdominal pain/discomfort, rash, arthralgia, oropharyngeal pain, dizziness, constipation, thyroid function abnormality, eczema.

DRUG INTERACTIONS
See Dosing Considerations. Bile acid binding resins (eg, cholestyramine, colestipol, colesevelam) adsorb and reduce bile acid absorption and may reduce the absorption, systemic exposure, and efficacy of Ocaliva. Potential for decreased INR; monitor INR and adjust warfarin dose, as needed. May increase the exposure to concomitant CYP1A2 substrates; monitor concentrations of CYP1A2 substrates w/ narrow therapeutic index (e.g. theophylline, tizanidine).

PREGNANCY AND LACTATION
Pregnancy: The limited available human data on the use of obeticholic acid during pregnancy are not sufficient to inform a drug-associated risk.
Lactation: There is no information on the presence of obeticholic acid in human milk, the effects on the breast-fed infant, or the effects on milk production; caution in nursing.

MECHANISM OF ACTION
FXR agonist; FXR activation decreases the intracellular hepatocyte concentrations of bile acids by suppressing *de novo* synthesis from cholesterol as well as by increased transport of bile acids out of the hepatocytes. These mechanisms limit the overall size of the circulating bile acid pool while promoting choleresis, thus reducing hepatic exposure to bile acids.

PHARMACOKINETICS

Absorption: T_{max}=1.5 hrs (obeticholic acid), 10 hrs (glyco- and tauro-obeticholic acid). **Distribution:** Plasma protein binding (>99%). V_d= 618L. **Metabolism:** Conjugated to active metabolites (glyco- and tauro-obeticholic acid [liver]), leading to enterohepatic recirculation and conversion by intestinal microbiota to obeticholic acid that can be reabsorbed or excreted. **Elimination:** Feces (-87%), urine (<3%).

PATIENT CONSIDERATIONS

Assessment: Assess for biliary obstruction, hepatic impairment, possible drug interactions, and pregnancy/nursing status. Assess baseline HDL-C.

Monitoring: Monitor for liver-related adverse reactions, elevations in liver biochemical tests, biliary obstruction, pruritus, changes in serum lipids, and other adverse reactions.

Counseling: Advise patients to report to their healthcare provider immediately if any symptoms of worsening of liver disease or complete biliary obstruction develop, or if they experience pruritus or an increase in its severity. Advise patients that they may need to undergo laboratory testing to check for changes in lipid levels while on therapy. Instruct to take at least 4 hrs before or 4 hrs after taking a bile acid binding resin, or at as great an interval as possible.

OCTAGAM 10% — immune globulin intravenous (human)   Rx

Class: Immune globulin

> Thrombosis may occur, w/ or w/o known risk factors (eg, advanced age, prolonged immobilization, hypercoagulable conditions, history of venous/arterial thrombosis, estrogen use, indwelling central vascular catheters, hyperviscosity, cardiovascular risk factors). Renal dysfunction, acute renal failure, osmotic nephrosis, and death may occur in predisposed patients (eg, those w/ a degree of preexisting renal insufficiency, diabetes mellitus, >65 years of age, volume depletion, sepsis, paraproteinemia, patients receiving nephrotoxic drugs). Administer therapy at minimum dose and infusion rate practicable for patients at risk of thrombosis, renal dysfunction, or acute renal failure. Ensure adequate hydration in patients before administration. Monitor for signs and symptoms of thrombosis and assess blood viscosity in patients at risk for hyperviscosity.

ADULT DOSAGE	PEDIATRIC DOSAGE
Chronic Immune Thrombocytopenic Purpura	Pediatric use may not have been established
To Rapidly Raise Platelet Counts to Control or Prevent Bleeding: Administer total dose of 2g/kg, divided into 2 doses of 1g/kg (10mL/kg) given on 2 consecutive days	
Rate of Administration: **First 30 min:** 1mg/kg/min (0.01mL/kg/min) **Next 30 min, if Above is Tolerated:** 2mg/kg/min (0.02mL/kg/min) **Next 30 min, if Above is Tolerated:** 4mg/kg/min (0.04mL/kg/min) **Next 30 min, if Above is Tolerated:** 8mg/kg/min (0.08mL/kg/min) **Max:** ≤12mg/kg/min (≤0.12mL/kg/min)	

ADMINISTRATION

IV route

Preparation and Handling

Do not mix w/ other medicinal products or administer simultaneously w/ other IV preparation in the same infusion set.
Do not mix w/ immune globulin IV (IGIV) products from other manufacturers.
Do not freeze; do not use sol that have been frozen.
Contains no preservative; for single use only.
Bottles may be pooled under aseptic conditions into sterile infusion bags and infused w/in 8 hrs after pooling.
Do not dilute.
Infusion line may be flushed before and after administration w/ either normal saline or D5W.

Administration

Administer therapy, which is to be at room temperature.
If an in-line filter is used, pore size should be 0.2-200 microns.
Do not use a needle of larger than 16 gauge to prevent possibility of coring. Insert needle only once, w/in the stopper area; penetrate the stopper perpendicular to its plane and w/in the ring.

STORAGE

2-8°C (36-46°F) for 24 months; w/in the first 12 months of this shelf-life, may store at ≤25°C (77°F) up to 9 months. Use or discard after storage at ≤25°C (77°F).

HOW SUPPLIED

Inj: 10% [2g, 5g, 10g, 20g]

CONTRAINDICATIONS

History of severe systemic hypersensitivity reactions (eg, anaphylaxis) to human immunoglobulin, immunoglobulin A (IgA)-deficient w/ antibodies against IgA and history of hypersensitivity.

WARNINGS/PRECAUTIONS

Infusion reactions may occur; slowing or stopping infusion usually allows symptoms to disappear promptly. May resume infusion at a lower rate once symptoms subside. Severe hypersensitivity reactions may occur; d/c infusion immediately and institute appropriate treatment if these occur. May cause hypersensitivity reactions in patients w/ corn allergy; contains maltose. For patients at risk of renal dysfunction because of preexisting renal insufficiency or predisposition to acute renal failure, administer at the minimum infusion rate practicable, not to exceed 3.3mg/kg/min (0.03mL/kg/min). D/C if renal function deteriorates. Contains maltose that may be falsely interpreted as glucose by some blood glucose monitoring systems and may result in falsely elevated glucose readings; monitor glucose levels in diabetic patients w/ a glucose-specific method only. Hyperproteinemia, increased serum viscosity and hyponatremia may occur. May contain blood group antibodies that may cause positive direct antiglobulin test (Coombs' test) result and hemolysis; consider appropriate lab testing in higher risk patients (eg, high doses [eg, ≥2g/kg] given either as a single administration or divided over several days, non-O blood group, underlying inflammatory state), including measurement of Hgb or Hct prior to infusion and w/in approx 36-96 hrs post infusion. If clinical signs/symptoms of hemolysis or a significant drop in Hgb or Hct is observed, perform confirmatory lab testing. If transfusion is indicated for patients who develop hemolysis w/ clinically compromising anemia after administration, perform adequate cross-matching to avoid exacerbating on-going hemolysis. Aseptic meningitis syndrome (AMS) may occur, more frequently following high doses (≥2g/kg) and/or rapid infusion; patients w/ a history of migraine may be more susceptible. Conduct a thorough neurological examination in patients exhibiting symptoms/signs to rule out other causes of meningitis. Noncardiogenic pulmonary edema/transfusion-related acute lung injury (TRALI) may occur; if TRALI is suspected, perform appropriate tests for the presence of anti-HLA and anti-neutrophil antibodies in the product. Made from human blood; may carry a risk of transmitting infectious agents (eg, viruses, Creutzfeldt-Jakob disease agent). The transitory rise of the various passively transferred antibodies in patient's blood may yield positive serological testing results, w/ potential for misleading interpretation. Caution in elderly.

ADVERSE REACTIONS

Headache, pyrexia, increased/decreased heart rate, HTN.

DRUG INTERACTIONS

May interfere w/ response to live viral vaccines (eg, measles, mumps, rubella); delay live viral vaccine administration ≥3 months from the time of administration.

PREGNANCY AND LACTATION

Pregnancy: Category C.
Lactation: Not known if excreted in human milk; caution in nursing.

MECHANISM OF ACTION

Immune globulin; has not been established.

PATIENT CONSIDERATIONS

Assessment: Assess for hypersensitivity reactions to human immune globulin, corn allergy, IgA-deficiency w/ antibodies against IgA, risk factors for renal dysfunction and risk of thromboembolic events, volume depletion, history of migraine, pregnancy/nursing status, and possible drug interactions. Consider baseline assessment of blood viscosity in patients at risk for hyperviscosity, including those w/ polycythemia, cryoglobulins, fasting chylomicronemia/markedly high TGs, or monoclonal gammopathies. Obtain baseline Hgb or Hct. Assess renal function, including BUN/SrCr measurement.

Monitoring: Monitor for hypersensitivity reactions, infection, thrombosis, renal dysfunction, AMS, hemolysis, pulmonary adverse reactions, hyperproteinemia, increased serum viscosity, hyponatremia, and other adverse reactions. Monitor carefully throughout the infusion. Monitor renal function and urine output periodically. Perform neurological exam including CSF studies if signs and symptoms of AMS develop. Perform tests for presence of anti-neutrophil antibodies in both product and patient serum if TRALI is suspected.

Counseling: Inform about the risks and benefits of therapy. Inform of the signs/symptoms of hypersensitivity reactions; advise to contact physician immediately if allergic symptoms occur. Instruct to immediately report to physician if signs/symptoms of renal failure, AMS, hemolysis, TRALI, or thrombosis develop. Inform that product is made from human plasma and may contain infectious agents such that can cause disease. Advise that drug may interfere w/ the response to live viral vaccines; instruct to notify immunizing physician of therapy w/ IGIV (human).

OCTAGAM 5% — immune globulin intravenous (human)   Rx

Class: Immune globulin

> Thrombosis may occur, w/ or w/o known risk factors (eg, advanced age, prolonged immobilization, hypercoagulable conditions, history of venous/arterial thrombosis, estrogen use, indwelling central vascular catheters, hyperviscosity, cardiovascular risk factors). Renal dysfunction, acute renal failure, osmotic nephrosis, and death may occur in predisposed patients (eg, those w/ a degree of preexisting renal insufficiency, diabetes mellitus, >65 years of age, volume depletion, sepsis, paraproteinemia, patients receiving nephrotoxic drugs). Administer therapy at minimum dose and infusion rate practicable for patients at risk of thrombosis, renal dysfunction, or acute renal failure. Ensure adequate hydration in patients before administration. Monitor for signs and symptoms of thrombosis and assess blood viscosity in patients at risk for hyperviscosity.

ADULT DOSAGE	PEDIATRIC DOSAGE
Primary Humoral Immunodeficiency	**Primary Humoral Immunodeficiency**
Usual: 300-600mg/kg (6-12mL/kg) every 3-4 weeks **Titrate:** May adjust over time to achieve desired trough levels and clinical responses	**6-16 Years:** **Usual:** 300-600mg/kg (6-12mL/kg) every 3-4 weeks **Titrate:** May adjust over time to achieve desired trough levels and clinical responses

Risk of Measles Exposure and Receiving Dose <400mg/kg Every 3-4 Weeks:
Increase dose to at least 400mg/kg; if exposed to measles, give dose as soon as possible after exposure

Infusion Rate:
Initial (First 30 Min): 0.5mg/kg/min (0.01mL/kg/min) for the first 30 min
Next 30 Min: If tolerated, advance to 1mg/kg/min (0.02mL/kg/min) for the second 30 min
Next 30 Min: If further tolerated, advance to 2mg/kg/min (0.04mL/min) for the third 30 min
Maint: Thereafter, may maintain at a rate up to 3.33mg/kg/min (0.07mL/kg/min)
Max: 3.33mg/kg/min (0.07mL/kg/min)

Risk of Measles Exposure and Receiving Dose <400mg/kg Every 3-4 Weeks:
Increase dose to at least 400mg/kg; if exposed to measles, give dose as soon as possible after exposure

Infusion Rate:
Initial (First 30 Min): 0.5mg/kg/min (0.01mL/kg/min) for the first 30 min
Next 30 Min: If tolerated, advance to 1mg/kg/min (0.02mL/kg/min) for the second 30 min
Next 30 Min: If further tolerated, advance to 2mg/kg/min (0.04mL/kg/min) for the third 30 min
Maint: Thereafter, may maintain at a rate up to 3.33mg/kg/min (0.07mL/kg/min)
Max: 3.33mg/kg/min (0.07mL/kg/min)

DOSING CONSIDERATIONS
Adverse Reactions
Slow or stop infusion if adverse reactions occur

Other Important Considerations
Patients at Risk for Developing Renal Dysfunction:
Administer at the minimum infusion rate practicable, not to exceed 0.07mL/kg (3.3mg/kg)/min (200mg/kg/hr)

ADMINISTRATION
IV route

Do not mix w/ other medicinal products or administer simultaneously w/ other IV preparation in the same infusion set.
Do not mix w/ immune globulin IV products from other manufacturers.
Do not freeze; do not use if frozen.
Content may be pooled under aseptic conditions into sterile infusion bags and infused w/in 8 hrs after pooling.
Do not dilute.
Product should be at room temperature during administration.
Not supplied w/ an infusion set; if an in-line filter is used, pore size should be 0.2-200 microns.
Do not use needle larger than 16 gauge; insert needle only once, w/in stopper area delineated.

STORAGE
2-25°C (36-77°F) up to 24 months from the date of manufacture. Do not freeze; do not use if frozen.

HOW SUPPLIED
Inj: 5% [1g, 2.5g, 5g, 10g, 25g]

CONTRAINDICATIONS
History of acute, severe hypersensitivity reactions to human immunoglobulin; immunoglobulin A (IgA)-deficient w/ antibodies against IgA and a history of hypersensitivity; acute hypersensitivity reaction to corn.

WARNINGS/PRECAUTIONS
Severe hypersensitivity reactions may occur; d/c infusion immediately and institute appropriate treatment. Patient should not be volume-depleted prior to initiation. Consider discontinuing therapy if renal function deteriorates. For patients judged to be at risk for developing renal dysfunction and/or at risk of developing thrombotic events, it may be prudent to reduce the amount of product infused per unit time by infusing at a max rate <0.07mL/kg (3.3mg/kg)/min (200mg/kg/hr). Contains maltose that may be falsely interpreted as glucose by some types of blood glucose monitoring systems and may result in falsely elevated glucose readings and inappropriate administration of insulin resulting in life-threatening hypoglycemia; measurement of blood glucose must be done w/ a glucose-specific method. Hyperproteinemia, increased serum viscosity, and hyponatremia may occur; distinguish true hyponatremia from pseudohyponatremia. Aseptic meningitis syndrome (AMS) reported; patients w/ a history of migraine may be more susceptible. Conduct a thorough neurological examination, including CSF studies, in patients exhibiting symptoms/signs to rule out other causes of meningitis. May contain blood group antibodies that may cause a positive direct antiglobulin reaction and hemolysis; perform appropriate confirmatory laboratory testing if signs and/or symptoms of hemolysis are present after administering the infusion. Noncardiogenic pulmonary edema/transfusion-related acute lung injury (TRALI) may occur; if TRALI is suspected, perform appropriate tests for the presence of anti-neutrophil antibodies in both the product and patient serum. Made from human blood; may carry a risk of transmitting infectious agents (eg, viruses, Creutzfeldt-Jakob disease). Various passively transferred antibodies in immunoglobulin preparations may confound the results of serological testing.

ADVERSE REACTIONS
Headache, nausea.

DRUG INTERACTIONS
See Boxed Warning. May interfere w/ response to live viral vaccines (eg, measles, mumps, rubella); delay live viral vaccine administration ≥3 months from the time of administration.

PREGNANCY AND LACTATION
Pregnancy: Category C.
Lactation: Safety not known in nursing.

MECHANISM OF ACTION
Immune globulin; not established. Supplies a broad spectrum of opsonic and neutralizing immune globulin G antibodies against bacteria or their toxins.

PHARMACOKINETICS
Absorption: C_{max}=16.7mg/mL, AUC=7022mg•h/mL. **Elimination:** $T_{1/2}$=40.7 days.

PATIENT CONSIDERATIONS
Assessment: Assess for hypersensitivity reactions to human immune globulin/corn, IgA-deficiency w/ antibodies against IgA, volume depletion, risk factors for renal dysfunction/impairment, risk of thrombotic events, history of migraine, pregnancy/nursing status, and possible drug interactions. Consider baseline assessment of blood viscosity in patients at risk for hyperviscosity, including those w/ cryoglobulins, fasting chylomicronemia/markedly high TGs, or monoclonal gammopathies. Obtain baseline BUN and SrCr levels.

Monitoring: Monitor for hypersensitivity reactions, infection, thrombotic events, renal dysfunction, AMS, hemolysis, TRALI, hyperproteinemia, increased serum viscosity, hyponatremia, and other adverse reactions. Monitor renal function and urine output periodically. Perform neurological exam including CSF studies if signs and symptoms of AMS develop. Perform tests for presence of anti-neutrophil antibodies in both the product and patient serum if TRALI is suspected.

Counseling: Inform about the risks and benefits of therapy. Advise about the early signs of hypersensitivity reactions; advise to contact physician immediately if allergic symptoms occur. Instruct to immediately report to physician if signs/symptoms of renal failure, AMS, hemolysis, TRALI, or thrombosis develop. Inform that product is made from human plasma and may contain infectious agents that can cause disease. Counsel that drug may interfere w/ the response to live viral vaccines; instruct to notify immunizing physician of therapy w/ IGIV (human).

ODEFSEY — emtricitabine/rilpivirine/tenofovir alafenamide   Rx

Class: Non-nucleoside reverse transcriptase inhibitor (NNRTI)/nucleoside reverse transcriptase inhibitor (NRTI) combination

> Lactic acidosis and severe hepatomegaly w/ steatosis, including fatal cases, reported w/ the use of nucleoside analogues in combination w/ other antiretrovirals. Not approved for the treatment of chronic hepatitis B virus (HBV) infection, and safety and efficacy has not been established in patients coinfected w/ HIV-1 and HBV. Severe acute exacerbations of hepatitis B reported in patients coinfected w/ HIV-1 and HBV and have discontinued products containing emtricitabine and/or tenofovir disoproxil fumarate, and may occur w/ discontinuation of Odefsey; closely monitor hepatic function w/ both clinical and laboratory follow-up for at least several months in patients who are coinfected w/ HIV-1 and HBV and d/c therapy. If appropriate, initiation of anti-hepatitis B therapy may be warranted.

ADULT DOSAGE	PEDIATRIC DOSAGE
HIV-1 Infection	**HIV-1 Infection**
As a complete regimen for the treatment of HIV-1 infection as initial therapy in antiretroviral-naive patients w/ HIV-1 RNA ≤100,000 copies/mL; or to replace a stable antiretroviral regimen in those who are virologically suppressed (HIV-1 RNA <50 copies/mL) for at least 6 months w/ no history of treatment failure and no known substitutions associated w/ resistance to the individual drug components	As a complete regimen for the treatment of HIV-1 infection as initial therapy in antiretroviral-naive patients w/ HIV-1 RNA ≤100,000 copies/mL; or to replace a stable antiretroviral regimen in those who are virologically suppressed (HIV-1 RNA <50 copies/mL) for at least 6 months w/ no history of treatment failure and no known substitutions associated w/ resistance to the individual drug components
Recommended Dose: 1 tab qd	**≥12 Years:**
In virologically suppressed patients, additional monitoring of HIV-1 RNA and regimen tolerability is recommended after replacing therapy to assess for potential virologic failure or rebound	**≥35kg:**
	Recommended Dose: 1 tab qd
	In virologically suppressed patients, additional monitoring of HIV-1 RNA and regimen tolerability is recommended after replacing therapy to assess for potential virologic failure or rebound

---

DOSING CONSIDERATIONS
Renal Impairment
Severe (CrCl <30mL/min): Not recommended

ADMINISTRATION
Oral route

Take w/ a meal.

STORAGE
<30°C (86°F).

HOW SUPPLIED
Tab: (Emtricitabine [FTC]/Rilpivirine [RPV]/Tenofovir Alafenamide [TAF]) 200mg/25mg/25mg

CONTRAINDICATIONS
Coadministration w/ carbamazepine, oxcarbazepine, phenobarbital, phenytoin, rifampin, rifapentine, proton pump inhibitors (eg, dexlansoprazole, esomeprazole, lansoprazole, omeprazole, pantoprazole, rabeprazole), systemic dexamethasone (more than a single dose), St. John's wort.

WARNINGS/PRECAUTIONS
Test for HBV before initiating therapy. Redistribution/accumulation of body fat reported. **FTC and TAF:** Lactic acidosis and severe hepatomegaly w/ steatosis

reported; obesity and prolonged nucleoside exposure may be risk factors. Caution w/ known risk factors for liver disease. D/C if lactic acidosis or pronounced hepatotoxicity occur. **RPV:** Severe skin and hypersensitivity reactions including cases of drug reaction w/ eosinophilia and systemic symptoms reported; d/c immediately and initiate appropriate therapy if signs/symptoms develop. Higher than recommended doses of RPV reported to prolong the QTc interval; consider therapy alternatives when administered to patients at higher risk of torsades de pointes. Depressive disorders reported; promptly evaluate if severe depressive symptoms occur. Hepatic adverse events reported; patients w/ underlying hepatitis B or C, or marked liver-associated test elevations prior to treatment, may be at increased risk for worsening/development of liver-associated test elevations. **TAF:** Renal impairment (eg, acute renal failure, Fanconi syndrome) reported; d/c in patients who develop clinically significant decreases in renal function or evidence of Fanconi syndrome. Decreased bone mineral density (BMD), increased biochemical markers of bone metabolism, and osteomalacia reported. Consider assessment of BMD in patients w/ history of pathologic bone fracture or other risk factors for osteoporosis or bone loss. **FTC and RPV:** Immune reconstitution syndrome and autoimmune disorders (eg, Graves' disease, polymyositis, Guillain-Barre syndrome) in the setting of immune reconstitution reported.

ADVERSE REACTIONS
RPV: Depressive disorders, insomnia, headache.
FTC and TAF: Nausea.

DRUG INTERACTIONS
See Contraindications. May decrease ketoconazole levels. May decrease methadone levels; monitor levels. Methadone maint therapy may need to be adjusted. **RPV:** Coadministration w/ CYP3A inducers or drugs that increase gastric pH (eg, antacids, H$_2$-receptor antagonists [H$_2$-RAs]) may result in decreased levels, loss of virologic response, and possible resistance to rilpivirine or to the class of non-nucleoside reverse transcriptase inhibitors (NNRTIs). Administer antacids at least 2 hrs before or at least 4 hrs after dosing, and H$_2$-RAs at least 12 hrs before or at least 4 hrs after dosing. CYP3A inhibitors may increase levels. Consider alternative medications in patients taking a drug w/ a known risk of torsade de pointes. Clarithromycin, erythromycin, or telithromycin may increase levels; consider alternatives (eg, azithromycin) where possible. **TAF:** P-gp inducers may decrease levels. P-gp inhibitors may increase levels. **FTC and TAF:** Drugs that reduce renal function or compete for active tubular secretion (eg, acyclovir, aminoglycosides [eg, gentamicin], high-dose or multiple NSAIDs) may increase levels of FTC, TAF, and other renally eliminated drugs. Patients taking nephrotoxic agents (eg, NSAIDs) are at increased risk of developing renal-related adverse reactions. **RPV and TAF:** Rifabutin may decrease levels; coadministration is not recommended. Azole antifungal agents may increase levels; clinically monitor for breakthrough fungal infections when azole antifungals are coadministered.

PREGNANCY AND LACTATION
Pregnancy: There are insufficient human data on the use of Odefsey during pregnancy to inform a drug-associated risk of birth defects and miscarriage. Healthcare providers are encouraged to register patients who are exposed to Odefsey during pregnancy in the Antiretroviral Pregnancy Registry. **Lactation:** FTC has been shown to be present in human breast milk; it is unknown if RPV and TAF are present in human breast milk; not for use in nursing.

MECHANISM OF ACTION
FTC: Nucleoside analogue of cytidine; inhibits activity of HIV-1 reverse transcriptase (RT) by competing w/ natural substrate deoxycytidine 5'-triphosphate and by being incorporated into nascent viral DNA, resulting in chain termination. **RPV:** NNRTI; inhibits HIV-1 replication by noncompetitive inhibition of HIV-1 RT. **TAF:** Acyclic nucleoside phosphonate analogue of adenosine 5'-monophosphate; inhibits HIV-1 replication through incorporation into viral DNA by the HIV RT, which results in DNA chain termination.

PHARMACOKINETICS
Absorption: FTC: C_{max}=2.1μg/mL, AUC=11.7μg•hr/mL, T_{max}=3 hrs. RPV: AUC=2.2μg•hr/mL, T_{max}=4 hrs. TAF: C_{max}=0.16μg/mL, AUC=0.21μg•hr/mL, T_{max}=1 hr. **Distribution:** RPV: Plasma protein binding (approx 99%). FTC: Plasma protein binding (<4%); found in breast milk. TAF: Plasma protein binding (approx 80%). **Metabolism:** RPV: CYP3A. TAF: Via cathepsin A in peripheral blood mononuclear cells and macrophages and by carboxylesterase 1 in hepatocytes, CYP3A. **Excretion:** RPV: Feces (85%), urine (6%); $T_{1/2}$=50 hrs (median). FTC: Urine (70%), feces (13.7%); $T_{1/2}$=10 hrs (median). TAF: Feces (31.7%), urine (<1%); $T_{1/2}$=0.51 hrs (median).

PATIENT CONSIDERATIONS
Assessment: Assess for obesity, prolonged nucleoside exposure, HBV infection, risk of torsades de pointes, liver dysfunction or risk factors for liver disease, renal impairment, pregnancy/nursing status, and possible drug interactions. Assess BMD in patients w/ a history of pathological bone fracture or w/ other risk factors for osteoporosis/bone loss. Assess estimated CrCl, urine glucose, and urine protein.

Monitoring: Monitor for signs/symptoms of lactic acidosis, severe hepatomegaly w/ steatosis, severe skin and hypersensitivity reactions, depressive symptoms, hepatotoxicity, fat redistribution/accumulation, immune reconstitution syndrome, autoimmune disorders, renal impairment, decreased BMD, increased biochemical markers for bone metabolism, osteomalacia, and other adverse reactions. Monitor hepatic function closely in patients coinfected w/ HBV and HIV-1 w/ clinical and lab follow-up for at least several months upon discontinuation of therapy. Monitor estimated CrCl, urine glucose, and urine protein. Monitor serum phosphorus levels in patients w/ chronic kidney disease.

Counseling: Instruct to contact physician if symptoms of lactic acidosis or pronounced hepatotoxicity, depression, or infection occurs. Inform that hepatotoxicity has been reported during treatment. Inform that severe acute exacerbations of hepatitis B may occur in patients who are coinfected w/ HBV

and HIV-1 and have discontinued therapy; advise not to d/c therapy w/o first informing physician. Instruct to immediately stop taking therapy and seek medical attention if patient develops a rash associated w/ any of the following symptoms: fever; blisters; mucosal involvement; eye inflammation (conjunctivitis); severe allergic reaction causing swelling of the face, eyes, lips, mouth, tongue, or throat; and any signs/symptoms of liver problems. Inform that laboratory tests will be performed and appropriate therapy will be initiated if severe rash occurs. Inform that fat redistribution/accumulation, renal impairment, and decreases in BMD may occur. Advise to inform physician if taking any other prescription/nonprescription medications or herbal products (eg, St. John's wort). Instruct to notify physician if pregnant or nursing.

ODOMZO — sonidegib   Rx
Class: Hedgehog pathway inhibitor

> May cause embryo-fetal death or severe birth defects when administered to a pregnant woman. Verify the pregnancy status of females of reproductive potential prior to initiating therapy. Advise females of reproductive potential to use effective contraception during treatment and for at least 20 months after the last dose. Advise males of the potential risk of exposure through semen and to use condoms w/ a pregnant partner or a female partner of reproductive potential during treatment and for at least 8 months after the last dose.

ADULT DOSAGE	PEDIATRIC DOSAGE
Basal Cell Carcinoma	Pediatric use may not have been established
Locally advanced basal cell carcinoma that has recurred following surgery or radiation therapy, or for those who are not candidates for surgery or radiation therapy	
200mg qd until disease progression or unacceptable toxicity	

DOSING CONSIDERATIONS
Adverse Reactions
Interrupt Therapy For:
- Severe or intolerable musculoskeletal adverse reactions
- First occurrence of serum creatine kinase (CK) elevation between 2.5 and 10X ULN
- Recurrent serum CK elevation between 2.5 and 5X ULN
Resume at 200mg/day upon resolution of clinical signs and symptoms

Permanently D/C Therapy For:
- Serum CK elevation >2.5X ULN w/ worsening renal function
- Serum CK elevation >10X ULN
- Recurrent serum CK elevation >5X ULN
- Recurrent severe or intolerable musculoskeletal adverse reactions

ADMINISTRATION
Oral route
Take on an empty stomach, at least 1 hr ac or 2 hrs pc.

STORAGE
25°C (77°F); excursions permitted to 15-30°C (59-86°F).

HOW SUPPLIED
Cap: 200mg

WARNINGS/PRECAUTIONS
Advise not to donate blood or blood products while taking sonidegib and for at least 20 months after the last dose. Musculoskeletal adverse reactions, which may be accompanied by serum CK elevations, reported; advise to report promptly any new unexplained muscle pain, tenderness, or weakness occurring during treatment or that persists after discontinuing therapy. Obtain baseline serum CK and creatinine levels prior to initiating therapy, periodically during treatment, and as clinically indicated (eg, if muscle symptoms are reported). Obtain SrCr and CK levels at least weekly in patients w/ musculoskeletal adverse reactions w/ concurrent serum CK elevation >2.5X ULN until resolution of clinical signs and symptoms.

ADVERSE REACTIONS
Muscle spasms, alopecia, dysgeusia, fatigue, abdominal pain, N/V, musculoskeletal pain, decreased weight, myalgia, diarrhea, decreased appetite, headache, pain, pruritus.

DRUG INTERACTIONS
Avoid w/ strong CYP3A inhibitors (eg, saquinavir, ketoconazole, nefazodone), and w/ moderate CYP3A inhibitors (eg, atazanavir, diltiazem, fluconazole). If a moderate CYP3A inhibitor must be used, administer the moderate CYP3A inhibitor for <14 days and monitor closely for adverse reactions, particularly musculoskeletal adverse reactions. Avoid w/ strong and moderate CYP3A inducers (eg, carbamazepine, efavirenz, modafinil).

PREGNANCY AND LACTATION
Pregnancy: May cause fetal harm.
Lactation: Not for use in nursing during treatment and for 20 months after the last dose.
Reproductive Potential: Advise females of reproductive potential to use effective contraception during treatment and for at least 20 months after the last dose. Advise males to use condoms, even after a vasectomy, during treatment and for at least 8 months after the last dose; advise not to donate semen during treatment and for at least 8 months after the last dose. May compromise female fertility.

MECHANISM OF ACTION

Hedgehog pathway inhibitor; binds to and inhibits smoothened, a transmembrane protein involved in hedgehog signal transduction.

PHARMACOKINETICS

Absorption: T_{max}=2-4 hrs (median); C_{max}=1030ng/mL; AUC=22mcg•h/mL. **Distribution:** V_d=9166L; plasma protein binding (>97%). **Metabolism:** Liver via CYP3A. **Elimination:** Feces (70%), urine (30%); $T_{1/2}$=28 days.

PATIENT CONSIDERATIONS

Assessment: Assess for hypersensitivity to drug, pregnancy/nursing status, and for possible drug interactions. Obtain baseline CK levels and renal function tests.

Monitoring: Monitor for musculoskeletal adverse reactions (eg, rhabdomyolysis, muscle spasms, musculoskeletal pain) and for other adverse reactions. Monitor CK and SrCr levels periodically and as clinically indicated. Obtain SrCr and CK levels at least weekly in patients w/ musculoskeletal adverse reactions w/ concurrent serum CK elevations >2.5X ULN until clinical signs/symptoms are resolved.

Counseling: Advise females of reproductive potential that drug may cause fetal harm and to use effective contraception during treatment and for at least 20 months after the last dose. Advise males, even those w/ prior vasectomy, to use condoms, to avoid potential drug exposure in both pregnant partners and female partners of reproductive potential during treatment and for at least 8 months after the last dose. Instruct female patients and female partners of male patients to contact their healthcare provider if they become pregnant or suspect that they may be pregnant. Advise females who may have been exposed to sonidegib during pregnancy, either directly or through seminal fluid, to contact the Novartis Pharmaceuticals Corporation. Instruct not to donate blood or blood products while taking sonidegib and for 20 months after stopping treatment. Advise to contact healthcare provider immediately if new or worsening signs/symptoms of muscle toxicity, dark urine, decreased urine output, or the inability to urinate develops. Instruct to take on an empty stomach, at least 1 hr ac or 2 hrs pc. Advise women not to breastfeed during treatment and for up to 20 months after the last dose.

O FEV — nintedanib   Rx

Class: Kinase inhibitor

ADULT DOSAGE

Idiopathic Pulmonary Fibrosis

Recommended: 150mg bid approx 12 hrs apart
Max: 300mg/day

Missed Dose

If a dose is missed, the next dose should be taken at the next scheduled time; do not make up for a missed dose

PEDIATRIC DOSAGE

Pediatric use may not have been established

DOSING CONSIDERATIONS

Renal Impairment
Mild to Moderate: Adjustment of starting dose is not required
Severe (CrCl<30mL/min) and ESRD: Not studied

Hepatic Impairment
Mild (Child Pugh A):
100mg bid approx 12 hrs apart

Moderate (Child Pugh B) or Severe (Child Pugh C):
Not recommended

Adverse Reactions
In addition to symptomatic treatment, if applicable, dose reduction or temporary interruption may be required until the specific adverse reaction resolves to levels that allow continuation of therapy

Treatment may be resumed at the full dosage (150mg bid), or at the reduced dosage (100mg bid), which subsequently may be increased to the full dosage. If 100mg bid is not tolerated, d/c treatment

Liver Enzyme Elevations:
AST/ALT >3X to <5X ULN w/o Signs of Severe Liver Damage:
Interrupt treatment or reduce dose to 100mg bid; once LFTs return to baseline, may reintroduce at a reduced dosage (100mg bid), which subsequently may be increased to the full dosage (150mg bid)

AST/ALT Elevations >5X ULN or >3X ULN w/ Signs/Symptoms of Severe Liver Damage:
D/C treatment

Mild Hepatic Impairment (Child Pugh A):
Consider treatment interruption/discontinuation for management of adverse reactions

ADMINISTRATION
Oral route
Take w/ food.
Swallow whole w/ liquid; do not chew or crush caps.

STORAGE
25°C (77°F); excursions permitted to 15-30°C (59-86°F). Protect from exposure to high humidity and avoid excessive heat. If repackaged, use tight container.

HOW SUPPLIED
Cap: 100mg, 150mg

WARNINGS/PRECAUTIONS

See Dosing Considerations. Associated w/ elevations of liver enzymes and bilirubin; conduct LFTs prior to treatment, monthly for 3 months, and every 3 months thereafter, and as clinically indicated. Diarrhea reported; treat at 1st signs w/ adequate hydration and antidiarrheal medication (eg, loperamide) and consider treatment interruption if diarrhea continues. D/C treatment if severe diarrhea persists despite symptomatic treatment. N/V reported; may require dose reduction or treatment interruption if N/V persists despite appropriate supportive care including antiemetic therapy. D/C treatment if severe N/V does not resolve. Can cause fetal harm. Arterial thromboembolic events (eg, MI) reported; caution when treating patients at higher cardiovascular (CV) risk including known coronary artery disease. Consider treatment interruption in patients who develop signs or symptoms of acute myocardial ischemia. May increase the risk of bleeding and GI perforation. Caution in patients who have had recent abdominal surgery, and d/c therapy in patients who develop GI perforation.

ADVERSE REACTIONS

Diarrhea, N/V, abdominal pain, liver enzyme elevation, decreased appetite, weight decreased, headache, HTN.

DRUG INTERACTIONS

P-gp and CYP3A4 inhibitors (eg, erythromycin, ketoconazole) may increase exposure; monitor closely for tolerability. P-gp and CYP3A4 inducers (eg, carbamazepine, phenytoin, St. John's wort, rifampicin) may decrease exposure; avoid coadministration. Monitor closely for bleeding if on full anticoagulation therapy and adjust anticoagulation treatment as necessary. Smoking was associated w/ decreased exposure, which may alter the efficacy profile of nintedanib.

PREGNANCY AND LACTATION

Pregnancy: Can cause fetal harm based on findings from animal studies and mechanism of action.
Lactation: Not for use in nursing.
Reproductive Potential: May reduce fertility in females of reproductive potential based on animal data. Females of reproductive potential should use effective contraception during treatment and for at least 3 months after the last dose.

MECHANISM OF ACTION

Tyrosine kinase inhibitor; inhibits receptor tyrosine kinases implicated in IPF pathogenesis (eg, vascular endothelial growth factor receptor, fibroblast growth factor receptor, platelet-derived growth factor receptor). Binds competitively to the adenosine triphosphate binding pocket of these receptors and blocks the intracellular signaling that is crucial for the proliferation, migration, and transformation of fibroblasts representing essential mechanisms of the IPF pathology.

PHARMACOKINETICS

Absorption: Absolute bioavailability (4.7%); T_{max}=2-4 hrs (fed). **Distribution:** V_d=1050L (IV); plasma protein binding (97.8%). **Metabolism:** Hydrolytic cleavage by esterases resulting in the free acid moiety BIBF 1202 is the prevalent metabolic pathway. BIBF 1202 is subsequently glucuronidated by UGT enzymes, namely UGT1A1, UGT1A7, UGT1A8, and UGT1A10 to BIBF 1202 glucuronide. **Elimination:** Urine (0.05%, unchanged [oral]), (1.4%, unchanged [IV]); feces/biliary (93.4%); $T_{1/2}$=9.5 hrs.

PATIENT CONSIDERATIONS

Assessment: Assess for CV risk, hepatic impairment, risk of bleeding/GI perforation, recent abdominal surgery, nursing status, possible drug interactions, and if smoking. Conduct LFTs and a pregnancy test prior to treatment.

Monitoring: Monitor for GI disorders, arterial thromboembolic events, bleeding events, GI perforation, and other adverse reactions. Monitor for liver enzyme elevations; conduct LFTs (ALT, AST, bilirubin) monthly for 3 months, and every 3 months thereafter, and as clinically indicated.

Counseling: Advise that liver function testing will be needed periodically. Advise to immediately report any symptoms of a liver problem. Inform that GI disorders such as diarrhea or N/V were the most commonly reported GI events; advise that physician may recommend hydration, antidiarrheal medications (eg, loperamide), or antiemetic medications to treat these side effects. Instruct to contact physician at the 1st signs of diarrhea or for any severe or persistent diarrhea or N/V. Counsel on pregnancy planning and prevention. Advise females of childbearing potential of the potential hazard to a fetus, to avoid becoming pregnant while receiving treatment, and to use effective contraception during treatment and for at least 3 months after taking the last dose of the drug. Advise to notify physician if pregnancy occurs during therapy. Advise that breastfeeding is not recommended. Advise about the signs and symptoms of acute myocardial ischemia and other arterial thromboembolic events and the urgency to seek immediate medical care for these conditions. Advise to report unusual bleeding or any signs and symptoms of GI perforation. Encourage to stop smoking prior to treatment and to avoid smoking during treatment. If a dose is missed, instruct to take the next dose at the next scheduled time and to not make up for a missed dose.

O LYSIO — simeprevir   Rx

Class: HCV NS3/4A protease inhibitor

ADULT DOSAGE

Chronic Hepatitis C

Genotype 1 or 4 Infection:
Recommended Dose: 150mg qd

May be taken in combination w/ sofosbuvir or in combination w/ peginterferon alfa (Peg-IFN-alfa)

PEDIATRIC DOSAGE

Pediatric use may not have been established

and ribavirin (RBV); for specific dosing recommendations for the antiviral drugs used in combination w/ simeprevir, refer to their respective prescribing information

Recommended Treatment Regimen and Duration:

In Combination w/ Sofosbuvir in Patients w/ Genotype 1 Infection:
Treatment-Naive and Treatment-Experienced w/o Cirrhosis:
12 weeks of simeprevir + sofosbuvir
Treatment-Naive and Treatment-Experienced w/ Cirrhosis:
24 weeks of simeprevir + sofosbuvir

In Combination w/ Peg-IFN-alfa and RBV in Patients w/ Genotype 1 or 4 Infection:
Treatment-Naive and Prior Relapsers (w/ or w/o Cirrhosis, Not Coinfected w/ HIV or w/o Cirrhosis, Coinfected w/ HIV):
Triple therapy (simeprevir/Peg-IFN-alfa/RBV) x 12 weeks; then dual therapy (Peg-IFN-alfa/RBV) x 12 weeks

Treatment-Naive and Prior Relapsers (w/ Compensated Cirrhosis, Coinfected w/ HIV):
Triple therapy x 12 weeks; then dual therapy x 36 weeks

Prior Non-Responders, Including Partial and Null-Responders (w/ or w/o Cirrhosis, w/ or w/o HIV Coinfection):
Triple therapy x 12 weeks; then dual therapy x 36 weeks

DOSING CONSIDERATIONS
Hepatic Impairment
Moderate or Severe (Child-Pugh Class B or C): Use not recommended

Discontinuation
Use w/ Sofosbuvir:
No treatment stopping rules apply to the combination of simeprevir w/ sofosbuvir

Use w/ Peg-IFN-Alfa and RBV:
HCV RNA ≥25 IU/mL at Week 4: D/C triple therapy
HCV RNA ≥25 IU/mL at Week 12: D/C dual therapy (treatment w/ simeprevir is complete at Week 12)
HCV RNA ≥25 IU/mL at Week 24: D/C dual therapy (treatment w/ simeprevir is complete at Week 12)

Do not reinitiate if treatment is discontinued because of adverse reactions or inadequate on-treatment virologic response.
D/C therapy if any of the antiviral drugs used in combination w/ simeprevir for the treatment of chronic hepatitis C infection are permanently discontinued for any reason.

Other Important Considerations
Avoid reducing dose or interrupting treatment, to prevent treatment failure.

ADMINISTRATION
Oral route
Take w/ food.
Swallow whole.

STORAGE
Room temperature <30°C (86°F). Protect from light.

HOW SUPPLIED
Cap: 150mg

CONTRAINDICATIONS
When used in combination w/ other antiviral drugs (including Peg-IFN-alfa and RBV), refer to the respective prescribing information.

WARNINGS/PRECAUTIONS
Efficacy in combination w/ Peg-IFN-alfa and RBV is substantially reduced in patients infected w/ HCV genotype 1a w/ an NS3 Q80K polymorphism at baseline; consider alternative therapy for these patients. Not recommended in patients who previously failed therapy w/ a treatment regimen that included simeprevir or other HCV protease inhibitors. Not recommended as monotherapy. Caution in patients of East Asian ancestry; may exhibit higher simeprevir plasma exposures. Fatal cardiac arrest reported w/ sofosbuvir-containing regimen (ledipasvir/sofosbuvir). Hepatic decompensation and hepatic failure, including fatal cases, reported, mostly in patients w/ advanced and/or decompensated cirrhosis; d/c therapy if bilirubin elevation is accompanied by liver transaminase increases or clinical signs/symptoms of hepatic decompensation. Photosensitivity reactions and rash observed; consider discontinuation of treatment if a photosensitivity reaction or severe rash occurs and monitor patients until resolved. Contains a sulfonamide moiety; insufficient data to exclude association between sulfa allergy and frequency/severity of adverse reactions. Refer to the respective prescribing information when used w/ other antiviral drugs.

ADVERSE REACTIONS
When Used w/ Sofosbuvir: Fatigue, headache, nausea.
When Used in Combination w/ Peg-IFN-Alfa and RBV: Rash (including photosensitivity), pruritus, nausea.

DRUG INTERACTIONS
Coadministration of amiodarone w/ simeprevir in combination w/ sofosbuvir may result in serious symptomatic bradycardia; coadministration is not recommended. If coadministration is required, cardiac monitoring is recommended in an in-patient setting for the first 48 hrs, after which outpatient or self-monitoring of HR should occur on a daily basis for at least the first 2 weeks of treatment. Caution is warranted and therapeutic drug monitoring of amiodarone, if available, is recommended for concomitant use of amiodarone w/ a simeprevir-containing regimen that does not contain sofosbuvir. Use w/ moderate or strong inducers or inhibitors of CYP3A may lead to significantly lower or higher exposure, respectively, which may result in reduced therapeutic effect or adverse reactions; coadministration is not recommended. Increased levels of amiodarone, digoxin, oral antiarrhythmics (eg, disopyramide, flecainide, mexiletine, propafenone), oral calcium channel blockers (eg, amlodipine, diltiazem, felodipine), oral midazolam, oral triazolam, and PDE-5 inhibitors (eg, sildenafil, tadalafil, vardenafil). Use w/ caution w/ oral midazolam or triazolam. Concomitant use w/ systemic erythromycin may increase levels of both agents; coadministration is not recommended. May increase cisapride or cyclosporine levels; coadministration is not recommended. May increase levels of darunavir, rosuvastatin, atorvastatin, simvastatin, pitavastatin, pravastatin, and lovastatin. May increase or decrease sirolimus levels. Levels may be decreased w/ anticonvulsants (eg, carbamazepine, oxcarbazepine, phenobarbital), rifampin, rifabutin, rifapentine, systemic dexamethasone, St. John's wort, or efavirenz; coadministration is not recommended. Levels may be increased w/ systemic clarithromycin or telithromycin, systemic antifungals (eg, itraconazole, ketoconazole, posaconazole), milk thistle (*Silybum marianum*), cobicistat-containing products, darunavir/ritonavir, ritonavir, or cyclosporine; coadministration is not recommended. Levels may be increased or decreased w/ delavirdine, etravirine, nevirapine, or other ritonavir-boosted or unboosted HIV protease inhibitors (eg, atazanavir, fosamprenavir, lopinavir); coadministration is not recommended. May increase levels of CYP3A4, OATP1B1/3, and P-gp substrates. Refer to PI for dosing modifications and monitoring parameters when used w/ certain concomitant therapies.

PREGNANCY AND LACTATION
Pregnancy: Embryofetal developmental toxicity (including fetal loss) observed in mice; potential risk to fetus.
Lactation: Detected in plasma of nursing pups in animal studies; consider developmental and health benefits of breastfeeding along w/ mother's clinical need for treatment.

Refer to prescribing information of the drugs used in combination w/ simeprevir for information regarding use in pregnancy/nursing.

MECHANISM OF ACTION
HCV NS3/4A protease inhibitor; direct-acting antiviral agent against HCV.

PHARMACOKINETICS
Absorption: AUC_{24}=57,469ng•hr/mL; T_{max}=4-6 hrs. (150mg single dose) Absolute bioavailability (62%). **Distribution:** Plasma protein binding (>99.9%). **Metabolism:** Liver via CYP3A; oxidation. **Elimination:** (200mg single dose) Feces (91%, 31% unchanged), urine (<1%), bile; $T_{1/2}$=41 hrs (HCV-infected).

PATIENT CONSIDERATIONS

Assessment: Assess for presence of HCV genotype 1a w/ NS3 Q80K polymorphism, hepatic impairment, sulfa allergy, pregnancy/nursing status, and possible drug interactions. Obtain baseline HCV-RNA levels and liver chemistry tests.

Monitoring: Monitor for signs/symptoms of hepatic decompensation, photosensitivity reactions, rash, and other adverse reactions. Monitor HCV RNA levels and liver chemistry tests as clinically indicated.

Counseling: Instruct to take ud. Inform that drug must be used in combination w/ other antiviral drugs, and that therapy should be discontinued if any of the other antiviral drugs used in combination are permanently discontinued. Counsel about the risk of serious symptomatic bradycardia when coadministered w/ amiodarone in combination w/ sofosbuvir; advise to seek medical evaluation immediately if signs/symptoms of bradycardia (eg, near-fainting or fainting, dizziness or lightheadedness, malaise) develop. Inform of the potential risk to fetus. Instruct to watch for early warning signs of liver inflammation (eg, fatigue, weakness, lack of appetite, N/V) as well as later signs (eg, jaundice, discolored feces) and to contact physician if such symptoms occur. Inform of the risk of photosensitivity reactions/rash and that these reactions may become severe; instruct to contact physician if a photosensitivity reaction or rash develops and not to stop treatment unless instructed by physician. Advise to use effective sun protection measures to limit exposure to natural sunlight and to avoid artificial sunlight (tanning beds or phototherapy) during treatment. Advise that reducing or interrupting treatment may increase possibility of treatment failure.

OMNITROPE — somatropin (rDNA origin)   Rx

Class: Recombinant human growth hormone (hGH)

ADULT DOSAGE	PEDIATRIC DOSAGE
Growth Hormone Deficiency	**Growth Hormone Deficiency**
Adult or Childhood-Onset Etiology: Weight-Based:	Due to an inadequate secretion of endogenous growth hormone
Initial: ≤0.04mg/kg/week given as daily SQ inj	Individualize dose based on growth response

Titrate: May increase at 4- to 8-week intervals based on individual requirements
Max: 0.08mg/kg/week
Non-Weight-Based:
Initial: 0.2mg/day (range, 0.15-0.30mg/day)
Titrate: May increase gradually every 1-2 months by increments of 0.1-0.2mg/day based on clinical response and serum insulin-like growth factor-I (IGF-I) concentrations
Maint: Individualize dose

Usual: 0.16-0.24mg/kg/week
Weekly dose should be divided over 6 or 7 days of SQ inj

Prader-Willi Syndrome
Individualize dose based on growth response
Usual: 0.24mg/kg/week
Weekly dose should be divided over 6 or 7 days of SQ inj

Small for Gestational Age
Treatment of growth failure in children born small for gestational age (SGA) who fail to manifest catch-up growth by age 2 years
Individualize dose based on growth response
Usual: Up to 0.48mg/kg/week
Weekly dose should be divided over 6 or 7 days of SQ inj

Turner Syndrome
Treatment of growth failure associated w/ Turner syndrome
Individualize dose based on growth response
Usual: 0.33mg/kg/week
Weekly dose should be divided over 6 or 7 days of SQ inj

Idiopathic Short Stature
Treatment of idiopathic short stature defined by height standard deviation score ≤-2.25, and associated w/ growth rates unlikely to permit attainment of adult height in the normal range, in pediatric patients whose epiphyses are not closed and for whom diagnostic evaluation excludes other causes associated w/ short stature that should be observed or treated by other means
Individualize dose based on growth response
Usual: Up to 0.47mg/kg/week
Weekly dose should be divided over 6 or 7 days of SQ inj

DOSING CONSIDERATIONS
Concomitant Medications
Oral Estrogen: May increase the dose requirements in women
Elderly
Consider lower starting dose and smaller dose increments

ADMINISTRATION
SQ route
Divide weekly dose over 6 or 7 days of SQ inj (preferably in pm)
May administer in the thigh, buttocks, or abdomen; always rotate inj sites
Preparation
Cartridge:
Each cartridge must be inserted into its corresponding pen delivery system
Vial:
Once diluent is added to powder, swirl gently; do not shake
Refer to instructions for use

STORAGE
2-8°C (36-46°F). Do not freeze. Light sensitive; store in the carton. (Cartridge) After 1st Use: Keep in the pen at 2-8°C (36-46°F) for a max of 28 days. (Vial) Reconstituted Sol: Use within 3 weeks. After 1st Inj: Store in the carton at 2-8°C (36-46°F).

HOW SUPPLIED
Inj: 5.8mg [vial], 5mg/1.5mL, 10mg/1.5mL [cartridge]

CONTRAINDICATIONS
Acute critical illness due to complications following open-heart surgery, abdominal surgery, multiple accidental trauma, or with acute respiratory failure. Pediatric patients with PWS who are severely obese, have a history of upper airway obstruction or sleep apnea, or have severe respiratory impairment. Active malignancy, or evidence of progression or recurrence of an underlying intracranial tumor. Active proliferative or severe nonproliferative diabetic retinopathy. Growth promotion in pediatric patients with closed epiphyses. Known hypersensitivity to somatropin or any of its excipients.

WARNINGS/PRECAUTIONS
Reevaluate adults who were treated with somatropin for GHD in childhood and whose epiphyses are closed. Treatment for short stature should be discontinued when the epiphyses are fused. Evaluate patients with PWS for signs of upper airway obstruction (eg, new/increased snoring) and sleep apnea before treatment and interrupt therapy if these signs occur. Implement effective weight control in patients with PWS and treat respiratory infections aggressively. Monitor all

patients with a history of GHD secondary to an intracranial neoplasm routinely while on therapy for progression/recurrence of the tumor. Increased risk of developing malignancies in children with certain rare genetic causes of short stature; monitor for development of neoplasms if treatment is initiated. Monitor for increased growth, or potential malignant changes, of preexisting nevi. Undiagnosed impaired glucose tolerance and overt diabetes mellitus (DM) may be unmasked, and new-onset type 2 DM reported. Intracranial HTN with papilledema, visual changes, headache, and/or N/V reported; d/c if papilledema occurs. Fluid retention in adults may occur. Monitor other hormonal replacement treatments in patients with hypopituitarism. Undiagnosed/untreated hypothyroidism may prevent optimal response to therapy. Hypothyroidism may become evident or worsen. Slipped capital femoral epiphysis and progression of scoliosis may occur. Increased risk of ear/hearing disorders and cardiovascular (CV) disorders in TS patients. Tissue atrophy may occur when administered at the same site over prolonged periods; avoid by rotating the inj site. Allergic reactions may occur. Serum levels of inorganic phosphorus, alkaline phosphatase, parathyroid hormone, and IGF-I may increase. Pancreatitis reported rarely. 5mg/1.5mL cartridge and diluent for 5.8mg/vial contains benzyl alcohol, which has been associated with serious adverse events and death, particularly in pediatric patients. Obese individuals are more likely to manifest adverse effects when treated w/ a weight based regimen. Estrogen replete women may need higher doses than men. Caution in elderly.

ADVERSE REACTIONS
Elevated HbA1c, eosinophilia, hematoma, hypothyroidism, headache, hypertriglyceridemia, leg pain.

DRUG INTERACTIONS
May inhibit 11β-hydroxysteroid dehydrogenase type 1, resulting in reduced serum cortisol concentrations; may need glucocorticoid replacement or dose adjustments of glucocorticoid therapy. Glucocorticoid therapy may attenuate growth-promoting effects in children; carefully adjust glucocorticoid replacement dosing. May increase clearance of antipyrine. May alter clearance of compounds metabolized by CYP450 liver enzymes (eg, corticosteroids, sex steroids, anticonvulsants, cyclosporine); monitor carefully. Oral estrogen replacement may increase somatropin dose requirements. May need to adjust dose of insulin and/or oral hypoglycemic agents, or adjust thyroid hormone replacement therapy.

PREGNANCY AND LACTATION
Category B, caution in nursing.

MECHANISM OF ACTION
Recombinant human GH; binds to a dimeric GH receptor in the cell membrane of target cells resulting in intracellular signal transduction and a host of pharmacodynamic effects.

PHARMACOKINETICS
Absorption: C_{max}=72-74mcg/L; T_{max}=4 hrs. **Metabolism:** Liver and kidneys by proteolytic degradation. **Elimination:** $T_{1/2}$=2.5-2.8 hrs.

PATIENT CONSIDERATIONS
Assessment: Assess for preexisting DM or impaired glucose tolerance, hypothyroidism, hypopituitarism, history of scoliosis, hypersensitivity to drug, any other conditions where treatment is contraindicated or cautioned, pregnancy/nursing status, and possible drug interactions. Perform funduscopic exam. In patients with TS, assess thyroid function.

Monitoring: Monitor growth and for clinical response; compliance; respiratory infection (patients with PWS); neoplasm; increased growth or malignant changes of preexisting nevi; intracranial HTN; fluid retention; allergic reactions; pancreatitis; slipped capital femoral epiphysis (eg, onset of limp, hip or knee pain) and progression of scoliosis in pediatric patients; and other adverse reactions. Perform periodic thyroid function tests, funduscopic exam, and monitoring of glucose levels. In patients with TS, monitor for ear/CV disorders. In patients with PWS, monitor weight and for signs of respiratory infection, sleep apnea, and upper airway obstruction. Monitor patients with a history of GHD secondary to an intracranial neoplasm routinely for progression/recurrence of the tumor.

Counseling: Inform about potential benefits and risks of therapy, proper administration, and usage and disposal. Caution against any reuse of needles and syringes.

ONCASPAR — pegaspargase   Rx
Class: Enzyme

ADULT DOSAGE	**PEDIATRIC DOSAGE**
Acute Lymphoblastic Leukemia	**Acute Lymphoblastic Leukemia**
As a component of a multi-agent chemotherapeutic regimen for the first-line treatment or for use in patients w/ hypersensitivity to native forms of L-asparaginase	As a component of a multi-agent chemotherapeutic regimen for the first-line treatment or for use in patients w/ hypersensitivity to native forms of L-asparaginase
2500 IU/m² IM or IV; administer no more frequently than every 14 days	2500 IU/m² IM or IV; administer no more frequently than every 14 days

ADMINISTRATION
IM/IV route
Use only 1 dose per vial; discard unused product.
IM Administration
Limit the volume at a single inj site to 2mL; if >2mL is to be administered, use multiple inj sites.

IV Administration
Administer over 1-2 hrs in 100mL of NaCl or D5 inj, through an infusion that is already running.
Use sol immediately after dilution.

Preparation and Handling
Do not administer if drug has been:
1. Frozen.
2. Stored at room temperature for >48 hrs.
3. Shaken or vigorously agitated.

STORAGE
Unopened Vial: 2-8°C (36-46°F). Do not shake or freeze. Protect from light. **Diluted Sol:** Use immediately or if not possible, store at 2-8°C (36-46°F); do not exceed 48 hrs from time of preparation to completion of administration. Protect infusion bags from direct sunlight.

HOW SUPPLIED
Inj: 3750 IU/5mL

CONTRAINDICATIONS
History of serious allergic reactions to pegaspargase; history of serious thrombosis, history of pancreatitis, or history of serious hemorrhagic events w/ prior L-asparaginase therapy.

WARNINGS/PRECAUTIONS
Anaphylaxis and serious allergic reactions, serious thrombotic events (including sagittal sinus thrombosis), pancreatitis, and glucose intolerance may occur; d/c w/ serious allergic reactions, serious thrombotic events, or pancreatitis. Observe patients for 1 hr after administration in a setting w/ resuscitation equipment and other agents necessary to treat anaphylaxis. Evaluate patients w/ abdominal pain for evidence of pancreatitis. Increased PT/PTT and hypofibrinogenemia may occur; monitor coagulation parameters at baseline and periodically during and after treatment. Initiate treatment w/ fresh frozen plasma to replace coagulation factors in patients w/ severe or symptomatic coagulopathy. Hepatotoxicity and abnormal liver function, and depression of serum albumin, and plasma fibrinogen may occur; perform appropriate monitoring.

ADVERSE REACTIONS
Allergic reactions, hyperglycemia, pancreatitis, CNS thrombosis, coagulopathy, hyperbilirubinemia, elevated transaminases.

PREGNANCY AND LACTATION
Pregnancy: Category C.
Lactation: Not for use in nursing.

MECHANISM OF ACTION
Enzyme; selectively kills leukemic cells by depleting asparagine.

PHARMACOKINETICS
Absorption: (IM) AUC=9.5 IU/mL/day (hypersensitive patients), 9.8 IU/mL/day (non-hypersensitive patients). **Elimination:** (IM) $T_{1/2}$=5.8 days (pediatric patients), 3.2 days (hypersensitive patients), 5.7 days (non-hypersensitive patients).

PATIENT CONSIDERATIONS
Assessment: Assess for history of serious allergic reactions to pegaspargase; history of serious thrombosis, history of pancreatitis, or history of serious hemorrhagic events w/ prior L-asparaginase therapy; coagulopathy; and pregnancy/nursing status. Obtain baseline coagulation parameters.

Monitoring: Monitor for anaphylaxis and serious allergic reactions, thrombotic events, pancreatitis, glucose intolerance, hepatotoxicity, and other adverse reactions. Monitor coagulation parameters periodically during and after treatment. Monitor LFTs.

Counseling: Inform of the possibility of serious allergic reactions, including anaphylaxis; instruct to seek immediate medical care for any swelling or difficulty breathing. Advise to seek immediate medical attention for severe headache, arm or leg swelling, acute SOB, chest pain, or severe abdominal pain. Instruct to immediately report excessive thirst or any increase in the volume or frequency of urination.

ONIVYDE — irinotecan liposome   Rx

Class: Topoisomerase I inhibitor

> Fatal neutropenic sepsis reported. Severe or life-threatening neutropenic fever or sepsis and severe or life-threatening neutropenia reported in patients receiving irinotecan liposome in combination w/ fluorouracil (5-FU) and leucovorin (LV). Withhold therapy for ANC <1500/mm³ or neutropenic fever. Monitor blood cell counts periodically during treatment. Severe diarrhea reported in patients receiving irinotecan liposome in combination w/ 5-FU and LV; do not administer to patients w/ bowel obstruction. Withhold therapy for diarrhea of Grade 2-4 severity. Administer loperamide for late diarrhea of any severity and administer atropine, if not contraindicated, for early diarrhea of any severity.

ADULT DOSAGE
Metastatic Pancreatic Adenocarcinoma

Treatment of metastatic adenocarcinoma of the pancreas, in combination w/ 5-FU and LV, after disease progression following gemcitabine-based therapy

Recommended Dose: 70mg/m² IV over 90 min every 2 weeks Administer prior to LV and 5-FU

PEDIATRIC DOSAGE
Pediatric use may not have been established

Homozygous for the UGT1A1*28 Allele:
Initial: 50mg/m² IV over 90 min
Titrate: Increase to 70mg/m² as tolerated in subsequent cycles

Premedication
Administer a corticosteroid and an antiemetic 30 min prior to infusion

---

DOSING CONSIDERATIONS
Adverse Reactions
NCI CTCAE Grade 3 or 4 Adverse Reactions:
Withhold drug. Initiate loperamide for late onset diarrhea of any severity. Administer IV or SQ atropine 0.25-1mg (unless contraindicated) for early onset diarrhea of any severity. Upon recovery to ≤Grade 1, resume therapy at:
1st Occurrence:
Patients Receiving 70mg/m²: 50mg/m²
Patients Homozygous for UGT1A1*28 w/o Previous Increase to 70mg/m²: 43mg/m²
2nd Occurrence:
Patients Receiving 70mg/m²: 43mg/m²
Patients Homozygous for UGT1A1*28 w/o Previous Increase to 70mg/m²: 35mg/m²
3rd Occurrence: D/C therapy
Interstitial Lung Disease (ILD): D/C therapy
Anaphylactic Reaction: D/C therapy

Refer to the full prescribing information, for recommended dose modifications for 5-FU or LV.

ADMINISTRATION
IV route
Do not substitute irinotecan liposome for other drugs containing irinotecan HCl. Do not use in-line filters.

Preparation
1. Withdraw the calculated volume from vial.
2. Dilute in 500mL D5 or 0.9% NaCl inj and mix diluted sol by gentle inversion. Protect diluted sol from light.
3. Administer diluted sol w/in 4 hrs of preparation when stored at room temperature or w/in 24 hrs of preparation when stored under refrigerated conditions (2-8°C [36-46°F]). Do not freeze.
4. Allow diluted sol to come to room temperature prior to administration.

STORAGE
2-8°C (36-46°F). Do not freeze. Protect from light.

HOW SUPPLIED
Inj: (free base) 4.3mg/mL [10mL]

CONTRAINDICATIONS
Severe hypersensitivity reaction to this medication or irinotecan HCl.

WARNINGS/PRECAUTIONS
Not indicated as a single agent for the treatment of patients w/ metastatic adenocarcinoma of the pancreas. Monitor CBC on Days 1 and 8 of every cycle and more frequently if clinically indicated. Withhold therapy for ANC <1500/mm³ or if neutropenic fever occurs; resume when the ANC is ≥1500/mm³. Reduce dose for Grade 3-4 neutropenia or neutropenic fever following recovery in subsequent cycles. May cause severe and fatal ILD; withhold in patients w/ new or progressive dyspnea, cough, and fever, pending diagnostic evaluation. D/C therapy in patients w/ confirmed diagnosis of ILD. Severe hypersensitivity reactions, including anaphylactic reactions, may occur; permanently d/c in patients who experience a severe hypersensitivity reaction. May cause fetal harm when administered to a pregnant woman.

ADVERSE REACTIONS
Diarrhea, fatigue/asthenia, N/V, decreased appetite, stomatitis, pyrexia.

DRUG INTERACTIONS
Strong CYP3A4 inducers (eg, rifampin, St. John's wort, phenytoin) reported to reduce exposure of non-liposomal irinotecan or its active metabolite, SN-38; avoid concomitant use if possible. Substitute non-enzyme inducing therapies at least 2 weeks prior to initiation of irinotecan liposome therapy. CYP3A4 inhibitors (eg, clarithromycin, indinavir, itraconazole) or UGT1A1 inhibitors (eg, atazanavir, gemfibrozil, indinavir) may increase exposure to irinotecan liposome or SN-38; avoid the use of strong CYP3A4 or UGT1A1 inhibitors if possible. D/C strong CYP3A4 inhibitors at least 1 week prior to starting irinotecan liposome therapy.

PREGNANCY AND LACTATION
Pregnancy: May cause fetal harm. Embryotoxicity and teratogenicity were observed in animals following treatment w/ irinotecan HCl, at doses resulting in irinotecan exposures lower than those achieved w/ irinotecan liposome 70mg/m² in humans. **Lactation:** There is no information regarding the presence of irinotecan liposome, irinotecan, or SN-38 in human milk, or the effects on the breastfed infant or on milk production. Not for use in nursing; nursing women should not breastfeed during treatment and for 1 month after the final dose. **Reproductive Potential:** Females of reproductive potential should use effective contraception during treatment and for 1 month after the final dose. Males w/ female partners of reproductive potential should use condoms during treatment and for 4 months after the final dose.

MECHANISM OF ACTION
Topoisomerase I inhibitor; bind reversibly to the topoisomerase I-DNA complex and prevents re-ligation of single strand DNA breaks, leading to exposure time-dependent double-strand DNA damage and cell death.

PHARMACOKINETICS

Absorption: Irinotecan: C_{max}=37.2mcg/mL; AUC=1364mcg•hr/mL. SN-38: C_{max}=5.4ng/mL; AUC=620ng•hr/mL. **Distribution:** Irinotecan: Plasma protein binding (<0.44%); V_d=4.1L **Metabolism:** Irinotecan: Liver (extensive) via esterases to SN-38 (active metabolite), and by CYP3A4 mediated oxidation. SN-38: UGT1A1 mediating glucuronidation to SN-38G. **Excretion:** Irinotecan HCl: Urine (11-20%); $T_{1/2}$=25.8 hrs. SN-38: Urine (<1%); $T_{1/2}$=67.8 hrs. SN-38G: Urine (3%).

PATIENT CONSIDERATIONS

Assessment: Assess for hypersensitivity to drug, bowel obstruction, pregnancy/nursing status, and for possible drug interactions. Assess for UGT1A1*28 allele status. Obtain baseline CBC.

Monitoring: Monitor for signs/symptoms of neutropenic sepsis, diarrhea, ILD (eg, new or progressive dyspnea, cough, fever), hypersensitivity reactions, and for any other adverse reactions. Monitor CBC on Days 1 and 8 of every cycle and more frequently if clinically indicated.

Counseling: Advise of the risk of neutropenia leading to severe and life-threatening infections and of the need for monitoring of blood counts. Instruct to contact physician if experiencing signs of infection. Inform of the risk of severe diarrhea; advise to contact physician if experiencing persistent vomiting or diarrhea, black or bloody stools, or symptoms of dehydration (eg, lightheadedness, dizziness, faintness). Inform of the risk of ILD; advise to contact physician as soon as possible for new onset cough or dyspnea. Instruct to seek immediate medical attention for signs of severe hypersensitivity reaction (eg, chest tightness; SOB; wheezing; dizziness or faintness; or swelling of the face, eyelids, or lips). Advise pregnant women of the potential risk to a fetus. Advise females of reproductive potential to use effective contraception during and for 1 month following the final dose of treatment and to inform physician of a known/suspected pregnancy. Advise males w/ female partners of reproductive potential to use condoms during and for 4 months after the final dose of treatment. Advise women not to breastfeed during treatment and for 1 month after the final dose.

OPDIVO — nivolumab   Rx

Class: Monoclonal antibody/programmed death receptor-1 (PD-1) blocker

ADULT DOSAGE

Unresectable or Metastatic Melanoma

As a Single Agent for the Treatment of BRAF V600 Wild-Type Unresectable/Metastatic Melanoma or BRAF V600 Mutation-Positive Unresectable/Metastatic Melanoma:
3mg/kg IV every 2 weeks until disease progression or unacceptable toxicity

Unresectable/Metastatic Melanoma, in Combination w/ Ipilimumab:
1mg/kg IV, followed by ipilimumab on the same day, every 3 weeks for 4 doses; the subsequent dose of nivolumab is 3mg/kg IV every 2 weeks until disease progression or unacceptable toxicity, as a single agent

Metastatic Non-Small Cell Lung Cancer

W/ Progression On or After Platinum-Based Chemotherapy:
Patients w/ epidermal growth factor receptor or anaplastic lymphoma kinase genomic tumor aberrations should have disease progression on FDA-approved therapy for these aberrations prior to receiving nivolumab

3mg/kg IV every 2 weeks until disease progression or unacceptable toxicity

Advanced Renal Cell Carcinoma

In Patients Who Have Received Prior Anti-Angiogenic Therapy:
3mg/kg IV every 2 weeks until disease progression or unacceptable toxicity

Hodgkin Lymphoma

Treatment of patients w/ classical Hodgkin lymphoma that has relapsed or progressed after autologous hematopoietic stem cell transplantation (HSCT) and post-transplantation brentuximab vedotin

3mg/kg IV every 2 weeks until disease progression or unacceptable toxicity

PEDIATRIC DOSAGE

Pediatric use may not have been established

DOSING CONSIDERATIONS

Adverse Reactions

Infusion Reactions:
Mild or Moderate: Interrupt or slow infusion rate
Severe or Life-Threatening: D/C

Colitis:
Grade 2 Diarrhea or Colitis: Withhold dose*
Grade 3 Diarrhea or Colitis: Withhold dose* (when administered as a single-agent) or permanently d/c (when administered w/ ipilimumab)
Grade 4 Diarrhea or Colitis: Permanently d/c

Pneumonitis:
Grade 2: Withhold dose*
Grade 3 or 4: Permanently d/c

Hepatitis:
AST or ALT >3 and up to 5X ULN or Total Bilirubin >1.5 and up to 3X ULN: Withhold dose*
AST or ALT >5X ULN or Total Bilirubin >3X ULN: Permanently d/c

Hypophysitis:
Grade 2 or 3: Withhold dose*
Grade 4: Permanently d/c

Adrenal Insufficiency:
Grade 2: Withhold dose*
Grade 3 or 4: Permanently d/c

Type 1 Diabetes Mellitus (DM):
Grade 3 Hyperglycemia: Withhold dose*
Grade 4 Hyperglycemia: Permanently d/c

Nephritis and Renal Dysfunction:
SrCr >1.5 and up to 6X ULN: Withhold dose*
SrCr >6X ULN: Permanently d/c

Rash:
Grade 3: Withhold dose*
Grade 4: Permanently d/c

Encephalitis:
New Onset Moderate or Severe Neurologic Signs or Symptoms: Withhold dose*
Immune-Mediated Encephalitis: Permanently d/c

Other:
Other Grade 3 Adverse Reaction:
1st Occurrence: Withhold dose*
Recurrence of Same Grade 3 Adverse Reactions: Permanently d/c
Life-Threatening or Grade 4 Adverse Reactions: Permanently d/c
Requirement for ≥10mg/day Prednisone or Equivalent for >12 Weeks: Permanently d/c
Persistent Grade 2 or 3 Adverse Reactions Lasting ≥12 Weeks: Permanently d/c

When administered w/ ipilimumab, if nivolumab is withheld, ipilimumab should also be withheld

*Resume treatment when adverse reaction returns to Grade 0 or 1

ADMINISTRATION

IV route

Preparation

1. Withdraw required volume of product and transfer into an IV container.
2. Dilute w/ either 0.9% NaCl inj or D5 inj to prepare an infusion w/ a final concentration ranging from 1-10mg/mL.
3. Mix diluted sol by gentle inversion; do not shake.
4. Discard partially used or empty vials.
5. After preparation, store infusion either at room temperature for ≤4 hrs from time of preparation (including room temperature storage of infusion in IV container and time for infusion administration) or at 2-8°C (36-46°F) for ≤24 hrs from time of infusion preparation; do not freeze.

Administration

Administer over 60 min through IV line containing a sterile, non-pyrogenic, low protein binding in-line filter (pore size 0.2-1.2μm).
Do not coadminister other drugs through the same IV line.
Flush IV line at end of infusion.
When administered w/ ipilimumab, infuse nivolumab 1st followed by ipilimumab on the same day. Use separate infusion bags and filters for each infusion.

STORAGE

2-8°C (36-46°F). Protect from light. Do not freeze or shake.

HOW SUPPLIED

Inj: 10mg/mL [4mL, 10mL]

WARNINGS/PRECAUTIONS

Refer to Dosing Considerations for recommendations to withhold or d/c therapy for the following adverse reactions. Refer to PI for corticosteroid dose in the management of the following adverse reactions. Immune-mediated pneumonitis, including fatal cases, reported; administer corticosteroids for ≥Grade 2 pneumonitis, followed by corticosteroid taper. Immune-mediated colitis may occur. Administer corticosteroids followed by corticosteroid taper for Grade 3 or 4 colitis. Administer corticosteroids followed by corticosteroid taper for Grade 2 colitis lasting >5 days; if worsening or no improvement occurs, increase corticosteroid dose. Permanently d/c therapy for recurrent colitis upon restarting therapy. Immune-mediated hepatitis may occur; administer corticosteroids for ≥Grade 2 transaminase elevations, w/ or w/o concomitant elevation in total bilirubin. Hypophysitis may occur; administer corticosteroids for ≥Grade 2 hypophysitis. Adrenal insufficiency may occur; administer corticosteroids for Grade 3 or 4 adrenal insufficiency. Thyroid disorders may occur; administer hormone replacement therapy for hypothyroidism and initiate medical management for control of hyperthyroidism. Type 1 DM may occur; administer insulin for type 1 diabetes. Immune-mediated nephritis and renal dysfunction may occur. For Grade 2 or 3 SrCr elevation, withhold therapy and administer corticosteroids followed by corticosteroid taper; if worsening or no improvement occurs, increase corticosteroid dose and permanently d/c therapy. Permanently d/c therapy and administer corticosteroids followed by corticosteroid taper for Grade 4 SrCr elevation. Immune-mediated rash may occur; administer corticosteroids for Grade 3 or 4 rash. Severe rash, including rare cases of fatal toxic epidermal necrolysis, reported. Immune-mediated encephalitis may occur; if other etiologies are ruled out, administer corticosteroids followed by corticosteroid taper. Other clinically significant immune-mediated adverse reactions (eg, uveitis, iritis, pancreatitis, facial and abducens nerve paresis, demyelination, polymyalgia rheumatica, autoimmune neuropathy) may occur during therapy and after discontinuation of therapy; exclude other causes. Based on severity of the adverse reaction, permanently d/c or withhold therapy, administer high-dose corticosteroids, and if appropriate, initiate hormone replacement therapy. Upon improvement to ≤Grade 1, initiate corticosteroid taper and continue to taper over at least 1 month. Consider restarting therapy after completion of corticosteroid taper based on the severity of the event. Severe infusion reactions reported. Complications, including fatal events, reported in patients who received allogeneic HSCT after nivolumab; follow patients closely for early evidence of transplant-related complications, such as hyperacute graft-versus-host-disease (GVHD), severe (Grade 3 to 4) acute GVHD, steroid-requiring febrile syndrome, hepatic veno-occlusive disease, and other immune-mediated adverse reactions, and intervene promptly. May cause fetal harm.

ADVERSE REACTIONS
Melanoma: (Single Agent) Fatigue, rash, musculoskeletal pain, pruritus, diarrhea, nausea. (W/ Ipilimumab) Fatigue, rash, diarrhea, N/V, pyrexia, dyspnea.
Metastatic Non-Small Cell Lung Cancer: Fatigue, musculoskeletal pain, cough, decreased appetite, constipation.
Advanced Renal Cell Carcinoma: Asthenic conditions, cough, nausea, rash, dyspnea, diarrhea, constipation, decreased appetite, back pain, arthralgia.
Classical Hodgkin Lymphoma: Fatigue, URTI, pyrexia, diarrhea, cough.

PREGNANCY AND LACTATION
Pregnancy: May cause fetal harm based on its mechanism of action and data from animal studies. Human IgG4 is known to cross the placenta and nivolumab is an IgG4; therefore, nivolumab has the potential to be transmitted from the mother to the developing fetus. Effects are likely to be greater during the 2nd and 3rd trimesters. Advise pregnant women of potential risk to fetus.
Lactation: Not for use in nursing.
Reproductive Potential: Females of reproductive potential should use effective contraception during treatment and for at least 5 months following the last dose.

MECHANISM OF ACTION
Human PD-1 blocking antibody; binds to PD-1 receptor and blocks its interaction w/ the PD-1 ligands, PD-L1 and PD-L2, releasing PD-1 pathway-mediated inhibition of the immune response, including the anti-tumor immune response. Combined nivolumab and ipilimumab (anti-CTLA-4) mediated inhibition results in enhanced T-cell function that is greater than the effects of either antibody alone, and results in improved anti-tumor responses in metastatic melanoma.

PHARMACOKINETICS
Distribution: V_d=8L, 7.92L (w/ ipilimumab); may cross placenta. **Elimination:** $T_{1/2}$=26.7 days, 24.8 days (w/ ipilimumab).

PATIENT CONSIDERATIONS
Assessment: Assess pregnancy/nursing status. Obtain baseline liver/renal (eg, SrCr)/thyroid function.
Monitoring: Monitor for signs w/ radiographic imaging and symptoms of pneumonitis. Monitor for signs/symptoms of immune-mediated colitis, hypophysitis, adrenal insufficiency, rash, encephalitis, hyperglycemia, transplant-related complications, and other adverse reactions. Monitor for abnormal liver tests, elevated SrCr, and thyroid function periodically.
Counseling: Inform of the risk of immune-mediated adverse reactions that may require corticosteroid treatment and withholding or discontinuation of therapy (eg, pneumonitis, colitis, hepatitis, endocrinopathies, nephritis and renal dysfunction, rash, encephalitis); instruct to immediately contact healthcare provider if signs/symptoms of an immune-mediated adverse reaction occur. Advise of the potential risk of infusion reaction. Advise of potential risk of posttransplant complications. Advise females of reproductive potential of the potential risk to a fetus and instruct to inform their healthcare provider of known/suspected pregnancy and to use effective contraception during treatment and for at least 5 months following the last dose of therapy. Advise women not to breastfeed while on therapy.

OPSUMIT — macitentan

Rx

Class: Endothelin receptor antagonist

> Do not administer to a pregnant female; may cause fetal harm. Exclude pregnancy before the start of treatment, monthly during treatment, and 1 month after stopping treatment. Prevent pregnancy during and for 1 month after stopping treatment; use acceptable methods of contraception. For all female patients, available only through a restricted program called the Opsumit Risk Evaluation and Mitigation Strategy (REMS).

ADULT DOSAGE
Pulmonary Arterial Hypertension

Treatment of pulmonary arterial HTN (WHO Group I) to delay disease progression

Recommended: 10mg qd
Max: 10mg qd

PEDIATRIC DOSAGE
Pediatric use may not have been established

ADMINISTRATION
Oral route
Take w/ or w/o food.
Do not split, crush, or chew tabs.

STORAGE
20-25°C (68-77°F); excursions permitted between 15-30°C (59-86°F).

HOW SUPPLIED
Tab: 10mg

CONTRAINDICATIONS
Pregnancy.

WARNINGS/PRECAUTIONS
May cause elevations of aminotransferases, hepatotoxicity, and liver failure; obtain liver enzyme tests prior to initiation of treatment and repeat during treatment as clinically indicated. D/C therapy if clinically relevant aminotransferase elevations occur, or if elevations are accompanied by an increase in bilirubin >2X ULN, or by clinical symptoms of hepatotoxicity. Consider reinitiation when hepatic enzyme levels normalize in patients who have not experienced clinical symptoms of hepatotoxicity. Decreases in Hgb concentration and Hct reported; measure Hgb prior to initiation of treatment and repeat during treatment as clinically indicated. Initiation of therapy is not recommended in patients w/ severe anemia. If signs of pulmonary edema occur, consider the possibility of associated pulmonary veno-occlusive disease (PVOD); d/c if confirmed. May decrease sperm count.

ADVERSE REACTIONS
Anemia, nasopharyngitis/pharyngitis, bronchitis, headache, influenza, UTI.

DRUG INTERACTIONS
Strong CYP3A4 inducers (eg, rifampin) may significantly reduce exposure; avoid concomitant use. Strong CYP3A4 inhibitors (eg, ketoconazole, ritonavir) may approximately double exposure; avoid concomitant use. Use other pulmonary arterial HTN treatment options when strong CYP3A4 inhibitors are needed as part of HIV treatment.

PREGNANCY AND LACTATION
Pregnancy: Category X.
Lactation: Not for use in nursing.
Reproductive Potential: Female patients must have a negative pregnancy test prior to starting treatment, and monthly pregnancy tests during treatment. Female patients must use acceptable methods of contraception during treatment and for 1 month after treatment. Patients may choose 1 highly effective form of contraception or a combination of methods; if a partner's vasectomy is the chosen method of contraception, a hormone or barrier method must be used along w/ this method. May have an adverse effect on spermatogenesis in males.

MECHANISM OF ACTION
Endothelin (ET) receptor antagonist; prevents the binding of ET-1 to both ET_A and ET_B receptors. Displays high affinity and sustained occupancy of the ET receptors in human pulmonary arterial smooth muscle cells.

PHARMACOKINETICS
Absorption: T_{max}=8 hrs. **Distribution:** V_d=50L, 40L (active metabolite); plasma protein binding (>99%). **Metabolism:** CYP3A4, CYP2C19 (minor); oxidative depropylation of the sulfamide (primary). **Elimination:** Urine (50%), feces (24%); $T_{1/2}$=16 hrs, 48 hrs (active metabolite).

PATIENT CONSIDERATIONS
Assessment: Assess pregnancy/nursing status, and for possible drug interactions. Obtain baseline liver enzyme tests and Hgb levels.
Monitoring: Monitor for signs/symptoms of pulmonary edema, PVOD, hepatic impairment, and other adverse reactions. Obtain pregnancy tests monthly during treatment and 1 month after discontinuation of treatment. Monitor liver enzyme tests and Hgb levels as clinically indicated.
Counseling: Inform of the risk of fetal harm when used during pregnancy; instruct females of reproductive potential to use effective contraception and to contact physician immediately if pregnancy is suspected. Inform female patients that they must enroll in the Opsumit REMS Program. Educate on the use of emergency contraception in the event of unprotected sex or contraceptive failure. Advise prepubertal females to immediately report to physician any reproductive status changes. Advise of the importance of Hgb testing. Educate patients on signs of hepatotoxicity.

ORALAIR — sweet vernal/orchard/perennial rye/timothy/kentucky bluegrass mixed pollens allergen extract

Rx

Class: Allergen extract

> May cause life-threatening allergic reactions (eg, anaphylaxis, severe laryngopharyngeal restriction). Do not administer to patients with severe, unstable or uncontrolled asthma. Observe patients in the office for at least 30 min following the initial dose. Prescribe auto-injectable epinephrine, instruct and train patients on its appropriate use, and instruct to seek immediate medical care upon its use. May not be suitable for patients with certain underlying medical conditions that may reduce their ability to survive a serious allergic reaction, or for patients who may be unresponsive to epinephrine or inhaled bronchodilators (eg, those taking β-blockers).

ADULT DOSAGE
Allergic Rhinitis

Immunotherapy for the treatment of grass pollen-induced allergic rhinitis w/ or w/o conjunctivitis confirmed by positive skin test or in vitro testing for

PEDIATRIC DOSAGE
Allergic Rhinitis

Immunotherapy for the treatment of grass pollen-induced allergic rhinitis w/ or w/o conjunctivitis confirmed by positive skin test or in vitro testing for

- pollen-specific IgE antibodies for any of the 5 grass species contained in this product
- Initiate treatment 4 months before the expected onset of each grass pollen season and maintain it throughout the season

≥18-≤65 Years: 300 index of reactivity daily

- pollen-specific IgE antibodies for any of the 5 grass species contained in this product
- Initiate treatment 4 months before the expected onset of each grass pollen season and maintain it throughout the season

10-17 Years:
Day 1: 100 index of reactivity (IR)
Day 2: 2X 100 IR
Day 3 and Following: 300 IR

ADMINISTRATION
SL route

Administer 1st dose in healthcare setting under supervision of physician; observe for at least 30 min and if patient tolerates the 1st dose, may take subsequent doses at home
Remove tab from blister just prior to dosing
Place tab immediately under tongue until complete dissolution for at least 1 min before swallowing
Wash hands after handling tab
Do not take tab w/ food or beverage; avoid food or beverages for 5 min following dissolution of tab

STORAGE
20-25°C (68-77°F); excursions permitted to 15-30°C (59-86°F). Protect from moisture.

HOW SUPPLIED
Tab, SL: 100 IR, 300 IR

CONTRAINDICATIONS
Severe, unstable or uncontrolled asthma; history of any severe systemic allergic reaction or local reaction to sublingual allergen immunotherapy; history of eosinophilic esophagitis; hypersensitivity to any inactive ingredients contained in the product (eg, mannitol).

WARNINGS/PRECAUTIONS
Not indicated for immediate relief of allergy symptoms. D/C if a systemic allergic reaction occurs. Reevaluate and consider discontinuation if escalating or persistent local reactions occur. May not be suitable for patients with certain medical conditions that may reduce the ability to survive a serious allergic reaction or increase the risk of adverse reaction after epinephrine (eg, markedly compromised lung function, unstable angina, uncontrolled HTN). May not be suitable for patients taking medications that can potentiate or inhibit effect of epinephrine (eg, α-adrenergic blockers, TCAs, cardiac glycosides). Eosinophilic esophagitis reported; d/c and consider a diagnosis of eosinophilic esophagitis if severe or persistent gastroesophageal symptoms (eg, dysphagia, chest pain) develop. Withhold therapy if patient is experiencing an acute asthma exacerbation; reevaluate patients who have recurrent asthma exacerbations and consider discontinuation of therapy. D/C treatment to allow complete healing of the oral cavity in patients with oral inflammation or oral wounds. Risk of therapy may be increased when treatment is initiated during the grass pollen season.

ADVERSE REACTIONS
Oral/ear/tongue pruritus, throat irritation, mouth/lip edema, cough, oropharyngeal pain, oral paraesthesia, abdominal pain, dyspepsia, pharyngeal edema.

DRUG INTERACTIONS
Concomitant dosing with other allergen immunotherapy may increase likelihood of local or systemic adverse reactions to either SQ or SL allergen immunotherapy.

PREGNANCY AND LACTATION
Category B, caution in nursing.

MECHANISM OF ACTION
Allergen extract; not established.

PATIENT CONSIDERATIONS
Assessment: Assess for hypersensitivity to drug or to any of its inactive ingredients, asthma, conditions that may reduce ability to survive a serious allergic reaction, responsiveness to epinephrine/inhaled bronchodilators, oral inflammation/wounds, any other condition where treatment is contraindicated or cautioned, pregnancy/nursing status, and for possible drug interactions.

Monitoring: Monitor for signs/symptoms of severe systemic/local allergic reactions, eosinophilic esophagitis, asthma exacerbation, and other adverse reactions.

Counseling: Educate about the signs/symptoms of a severe systemic/local allergic reaction; instruct to seek immediate medical care, d/c use, and resume treatment only at the instruction of a physician if a severe allergic reaction occurs. Inform patients that the 1st dose is administered in a healthcare setting under the supervision of a physician and that they will be monitored for at least 30 min to watch for signs/symptoms of a severe systemic/local allergic reaction. Instruct to d/c therapy and to contact physician if severe or persistent symptoms of esophagitis develop. Instruct asthma patients to d/c use and contact physician immediately if difficulty in breathing occurs or if asthma becomes difficult to control.

ORENCIA — abatacept
Class: Selective costimulation modulator   **Rx**

ADULT DOSAGE
Rheumatoid Arthritis
To reduce signs and symptoms, induce major clinical response, inhibit progression of structural damage, and improve physical function in adults w/ moderate to severe active rheumatoid arthritis; may be used as monotherapy or concomitantly w/ disease-modifying antirheumatic drugs other than TNF antagonists

IV Regimen:
Initial:
<60kg: 500mg
60-100kg: 750mg
<100kg: 1000mg
Maint: Give succeeding infusions at 2 and 4 weeks after the 1st infusion and every 4 weeks thereafter

SQ Regimen:
125mg SQ inj once weekly w/ or w/o an IV LD
If initiating w/ an IV LD, initiate w/ a single IV infusion (as per body weight categories listed in the IV regimen), followed by the first 125mg SQ inj w/in a day of the IV infusion

Switching from IV to SQ Regimen:
Give the 1st SQ dose instead of the next scheduled IV dose

PEDIATRIC DOSAGE
Juvenile Idiopathic Arthritis
To reduce signs and symptoms of moderately to severely active polyarticular juvenile idiopathic arthritis; may be used as monotherapy or concomitantly w/ methotrexate

6-17 Years:
IV Regimen:
Initial:
<75kg: 10mg/kg
≥75kg: Follow adult IV dosing regimen; not to exceed 1000mg
Maint: Give succeeding infusions at 2 and 4 weeks after the 1st infusion and every 4 weeks thereafter

---

ADMINISTRATION
IV/SQ route

IV
Give as an IV infusion over 30 min.
Do not infuse in the same IV line w/ other agents.

IV Infusion Preparation
Reconstitute w/ 10mL of sterile water for inj; only use silicone-free disposable syringe provided w/ each vial and an 18- to 21-gauge needle.
Rotate vial w/ gentle swirling until contents are completely dissolved; do not shake, and avoid prolonged/vigorous agitation.
Vent vial w/ needle to dissipate any foam after complete dissolution of powder.
Further dilute reconstituted sol w/ 0.9% NaCl inj using the same silicone-free disposable syringe to a total volume of 100mL.
Final concentration of abatacept in the bag or bottle will depend upon the amount of drug added, but will be ≤10mg/mL.
Do not shake bag or bottle.
May store fully diluted sol at room temperature or at 2-8°C (36-46°F) before use.
Infusion of fully diluted sol must be completed w/in 24 hrs of reconstitution; discard if not administered w/in 24 hrs.

SQ
Administer inj to front thigh or abdomen (except for the 2-inch area around navel) for self-inj; or outer area of the upper arm if a caregiver is administering dose.
Rotate inj site (at least 1 inch away from last inj site).
Do not inject into areas where the skin is tender, bruised, red, or hard.

STORAGE
2-8°C (36-46°F). Protect from light; store in original package until time of use. Do not allow prefilled syringe to freeze. Fully Diluted Sol: May store at room temperature or at 2-8°C (36-46°F); discard if not administered w/in 24 hrs.

HOW SUPPLIED
Inj: 125mg/mL [prefilled syringe], 250mg [vial]

WARNINGS/PRECAUTIONS
Anaphylaxis or anaphylactoid reactions reported w/ IV use; permanently d/c and institute appropriate therapy if an anaphylactic or other serious allergic reaction occurs. Serious infections, including sepsis and pneumonia, reported; caution in patients w/ history of recurrent infections, underlying conditions that may predispose to infections, or chronic, latent, or localized infections. D/C if a serious infection develops. Screen for latent tuberculosis (TB) infection and viral hepatitis prior to initiation of therapy; treat patients testing (+) for TB prior to therapy. Hepatitis B reactivation may occur. JIA patients should be brought up-to-date w/ all immunizations prior to initiation of therapy. Caution in patients w/ COPD; monitor for worsening of respiratory status. May affect host defenses against infections and malignancies. Caution in elderly. (IV) Contains maltose that may react w/ glucose dehydrogenase pyrroloquinoline quinone-based glucose monitoring and may result in falsely elevated blood glucose readings on the day of infusion; consider methods that do not react w/ maltose in patients requiring blood glucose monitoring.

ADVERSE REACTIONS
Headache, URTI, nasopharyngitis, nausea, sinusitis, UTI, influenza, bronchitis, dizziness, cough, back pain, HTN, dyspepsia, rash, pain in extremities.

DRUG INTERACTIONS
May experience more infections and serious infections w/ TNF antagonists; concurrent use is not recommended. Monitor for signs of infection while

transitioning from TNF antagonist to abatacept. Concomitant use w/ other biologic RA therapy (eg, anakinra) is not recommended. Do not give live vaccines concurrently w/ therapy or w/in 3 months of its discontinuation.

PREGNANCY AND LACTATION
Pregnancy: Category C.
Lactation: Not for use in nursing.

MECHANISM OF ACTION
Selective costimulation modulator; inhibits T-cell activation by binding to CD80 and CD86, thereby blocking interaction w/ CD28.

PHARMACOKINETICS
Absorption: (SQ) Bioavailability (78.6%). C_{max}=295mcg/mL (RA patients, IV), 48.1mcg/mL (RA patients, SQ), 217mcg/mL (JIA patients). **Distribution:** V_d=0.07L/kg (RA patients, IV), 0.11L/kg (RA patients, SQ). **Elimination:** $T_{1/2}$=13.1 days (RA patients, IV), 14.3 days (RA patients, SQ).

PATIENT CONSIDERATIONS
Assessment: Assess for previous hypersensitivity to drug, history of recurrent infections, chronic/latent/localized infections, underlying conditions that may predispose to infection, COPD, pregnancy/nursing status, and possible drug interactions. Assess immunization history in pediatric patients. Screen for latent TB infection w/ a tuberculin skin test and for viral hepatitis.

Monitoring: Monitor for signs/symptoms of hypersensitivity, infection, hepatitis B reactivation, worsening of respiratory status in COPD patients, immunosuppression, malignancies, and other adverse reactions.

Counseling: Instruct to immediately contact physician if an allergic reaction or infection occurs. Inform that may be tested for TB prior to therapy. Counsel not to receive live vaccines during therapy or w/in 3 months of its discontinuation. Inform caregivers that patients w/ JIA should be brought up-to-date w/ all immunizations prior to therapy and discuss how to best handle future immunizations once therapy has been initiated. Instruct to inform physician if pregnant/nursing or planning to become pregnant. Inform that the formulation for IV administration contains maltose, which can give falsely elevated blood glucose readings on the day of administration w/ certain blood glucose monitors; advise to discuss methods that do not react w/ maltose.

ORENITRAM — treprostinil   Rx

Class: Prostacyclin analogue

ADULT DOSAGE	PEDIATRIC DOSAGE
Pulmonary Arterial Hypertension	Pediatric use may not have been established
Treatment of pulmonary arterial HTN (PAH) (WHO Group 1) to improve exercise capacity	
Initial: 0.25mg bid (approx 12 hrs apart) or 0.125mg tid (approx 8 hrs apart)	
Titrate: Increase dose to the highest tolerated dose in increments of 0.25mg or 0.5mg bid or 0.125mg tid every 3-4 days; consider titrating slower if dose increments are not tolerated	
The appropriate maint dose is determined by tolerability. If intolerable effects occur, decrease dose in increments of 0.25mg; avoid abrupt discontinuation.	
Conversions	
Transitioning from SQ or IV Routes of Administration of Treprostinil: Decrease Remodulin dose while simultaneously increasing Orenitram dose; may reduce Remodulin dose up to 30ng/kg/min per day and increase Orenitram dose simultaneously up to 6mg/day (2mg tid) if tolerated	
Refer to PI for an equation to use to estimate a comparable total daily dose of Orenitram using a patient's dose of IV/SQ treprostinil	
Missed Dose	
If a dose is missed, take the missed dose as soon as possible, w/ food. If ≥2 doses are missed, restart at a lower dose and re-titrate.	

- -

DOSING CONSIDERATIONS
Hepatic Impairment
Mild (Child-Pugh Class A): Start at 0.125mg bid w/ 0.125mg bid dose increments every 3-4 days

Moderate (Child Pugh Class B): Avoid use
Concomitant Medications
Strong CYP2C8 Inhibitors (eg, Gemfibrozil):
Initial: 0.125mg bid w/ 0.125mg bid dose increments every 3-4 days

Discontinuation
In the event of a planned short-term treatment interruption for patients unable to take oral medications, consider a temporary infusion of SQ or IV treprostinil; refer to PI for the equation to use to calculate the total daily dose (mg) of treprostinil for the parenteral route
When discontinuing Orenitram, reduce dose in steps of 0.5-1mg/day

ADMINISTRATION
Oral route
Take w/ food.
Swallow tabs whole; do not crush, split, or chew.
STORAGE
25°C (77°F); excursions 15-30°C (59-86°F).
HOW SUPPLIED
Tab, Extended-Release: 0.125mg, 0.25mg, 1mg, 2.5mg
CONTRAINDICATIONS
Severe hepatic impairment (Child-Pugh Class C).
WARNINGS/PRECAUTIONS
Abrupt discontinuation or sudden large reductions in dosage may result in worsening of PAH symptoms. Inhibits platelet aggregation and increases the risk of bleeding. Tab shell does not dissolve; in patients w/ diverticulosis, tabs can lodge in a diverticulum. Caution in elderly.
ADVERSE REACTIONS
Headache, diarrhea, nausea, flushing, pain in jaw, pain in extremity, hypokalemia, abdominal discomfort.
DRUG INTERACTIONS
See Dosing Considerations. Coadministration w/ diuretics, antihypertensive agents, or other vasodilators increases the risk of symptomatic hypotension. Increased risk of bleeding w/ anticoagulants. Gemfibrozil (CYP2C8 inhibitor) increases exposure.
PREGNANCY AND LACTATION
Pregnancy: Category C.
Lactation: Not for use in nursing.
MECHANISM OF ACTION
Prostacyclin analogue; causes direct vasodilation of pulmonary and systemic arterial vascular beds, inhibition of platelet aggregation, and inhibition of smooth muscle cell proliferation.
PHARMACOKINETICS
Absorption: Absolute bioavailability (17%); T_{max}=4-6 hrs. **Distribution:** Plasma protein binding (96%). **Metabolism:** Extensive, via oxidation, oxidative cleavage, dehydration, and glucuronic acid conjugation; CYP2C8 (primary) and CYP2C9 (lesser extent). **Elimination:** Feces (1.13% unchanged), urine (0.19% unchanged).

PATIENT CONSIDERATIONS
Assessment: Assess for hepatic impairment, diverticulosis, pregnancy/nursing status, and possible drug interactions.
Monitoring: Monitor for bleeding and other adverse reactions.
Counseling: Instruct to avoid abrupt discontinuation and advise to take drug ud. Inform that the biologically inert components of the tab remain intact during GI transit and are eliminated in the feces as an insoluble shell.

ORFADIN — nitisinone   Rx

Class: 4-hydroxyphenylpyruvate dioxygenase (HPPD) inhibitor

ADULT DOSAGE	PEDIATRIC DOSAGE
Hereditary Tyrosinemia Type 1	**Hereditary Tyrosinemia Type 1**
In combination w/ dietary restriction of tyrosine and phenylalanine	In combination w/ dietary restriction of tyrosine and phenylalanine
Initial: 0.5mg/kg bid	**Initial:** 0.5mg/kg bid
Titrate: Titrate based on biochemical and/or clinical response; increase to 0.75mg/kg bid if succinylacetone is still detectable 1 month after the start of treatment. If the biochemical response is satisfactory, adjust dose only according to body weight gain	**Titrate:** Titrate based on biochemical and/or clinical response; increase to 0.75mg/kg bid if succinylacetone is still detectable 1 month after the start of treatment. If the biochemical response is satisfactory, adjust dose only according to body weight gain
Max: 1mg/kg bid	**Max:** 1mg/kg bid

- -

ADMINISTRATION
Oral route
Maintain dietary restriction of tyrosine and phenylalanine.
Take caps at least 1 hr ac, or 2 hrs pc; may open caps and suspend caps in a small amount of water, formula, or applesauce immediately before use for patients who have difficulty swallowing the caps and who are intolerant to the sus.
Take sus w/o regard to meals.

Preparing a Bottle w/o the Adapter Already Inserted
- Remove the bottle from the refrigerator and calculate 60 days from when the bottle is removed from the refrigerator. Write this date as the "Discard after" date on the bottle label.
- Allow the bottle to warm to room temperature (30 to 60 min).
- Shake the bottle vigorously for at least 20 sec until the solid cake at the bottom of the bottle is completely dispersed. Foam will form in the bottle.
- Insert bottle adapter.

Preparing a Bottle w/ the Adapter Inserted
- Shake bottle vigorously for at least 5 sec and check that there are no particles left at the bottom of the bottle. Foam will form in the bottle.

Measuring and Administering the Dose
- Keep bottle upright and insert the oral syringe into the adapter.
- Carefully turn bottle upside down w/ the oral syringe in place and wait for the foam to rise to the top of the bottle.
- Pull back on the syringe plunger to withdraw the dose.
- Leave the syringe in the adapter and turn the bottle upright.
- Remove the syringe from the adapter by gently twisting it out of the bottle and dispense dose.
- Do not remove the bottle adapter.
- Store bottle at room temperature (not above 25°C [77°F]).

STORAGE
Cap: 2-8°C (36-46°F). **Sus: Prior to First Use:** 2-8°C (36-46°F). Do not freeze. Store upright. **After First Opening:** Room temperature, up to 25°C (77°F) for up to 60 days. Discard unused portion if not used w/in 60 days.

HOW SUPPLIED
Cap: 2mg, 5mg, 10mg, 20mg; **Oral Sus:** 4mg/mL

WARNINGS/PRECAUTIONS
May cause an increase in plasma tyrosine levels in patients w/ hereditary tyrosinemia type 1 (HT-1); maintain concomitant reduction in dietary tyrosine and phenylalanine while on treatment. Do not adjust nitisinone dosage in order to lower the plasma tyrosine concentration. Maintain tyrosine levels <500µmol/L. Inadequate restriction of tyrosine and phenylalanine intake may increase blood tyrosine levels (>500µmol/L) and lead to ocular signs/symptoms, variable degrees of intellectual disability and developmental delay, and painful hyperkeratotic plaques on the soles and palms. If patient develops photophobia, eye pain, or signs of inflammation, perform slit-lamp reexamination and immediate measurement of plasma tyrosine concentration. Perform a clinical laboratory assessment, including plasma tyrosine levels in patients who exhibit abrupt change in neurological status. Assess dietary tyrosine and phenylalanine intake in patients w/ HT-1 treated w/ dietary restrictions and nitisinone who develop elevated plasma tyrosine levels. Transient leukopenia and thrombocytopenia reported. Sus contains 500mg/mL of glycerol; oral doses of glycerol of ≥10g have been reported to cause headache, upset stomach, and diarrhea. Consider switching patients who are unable to tolerate the oral sus to caps.

ADVERSE REACTIONS
Elevated tyrosine levels, thrombocytopenia, leukopenia, conjunctivitis, corneal opacity, keratitis, photophobia, eye pain, blepharitis, cataracts, granulocytopenia, epistaxis, pruritus, exfoliative dermatitis, dry skin.

DRUG INTERACTIONS
May increase systemic exposure of CYP2C9 substrates; additional monitoring may be warranted.

PREGNANCY AND LACTATION
Pregnancy: Limited data on nitisinone use in pregnant women are not sufficient to inform any drug-associated risk.
Lactation: There are no data on the presence of nitisinone in human milk, the effects on the breastfed infant, or the effects on milk production; caution in nursing.

MECHANISM OF ACTION
4-hydroxyphenyl-pyruvate dioxygenase inhibitor; inhibits an enzyme upstream of fumarylacetoacetate hydrolase in the tyrosine catabolic pathways, thereby preventing accumulation of the catabolic intermediates maleylacetoacetate and fumarylacetoacetate, which are converted to the toxic metabolites succinylacetone and succinylacetoacetate.

PHARMACOKINETICS
Absorption: C_{max}=10.2µmol/L (cap), 9.74µmol/L (sus); AUC=403µmol•hr/L (cap), 346µmol•hr/L (sus); T_{max}=3.5 hrs (median) (cap), 0.38 hrs (median) (sus).
Distribution: Plasma protein binding (>95%). **Metabolism:** CYP3A4 (minor).
Elimination: $T_{1/2}$=54 hrs.

PATIENT CONSIDERATIONS
Assessment: Assess for HT-1, pregnancy/nursing status, and for possible drug interactions. Perform baseline ophthalmologic examination including slit-lamp exam.

Monitoring: Monitor for ocular signs/symptoms, developmental delay, intellectual disability, painful hyperkeratotic plaques on soles and palms, transient leukopenia, thrombocytopenia, and other adverse reactions. Monitor platelet and WBC counts. Perform slit-lamp reexamination and immediate measurement of the plasma tyrosine concentration if eye pain, photophobia, or signs of inflammation occur. Monitor plasma tyrosine levels, plasma and/or urine succinylacetone concentrations, liver function parameters, and alpha-fetoprotein levels. Assess dietary tyrosine and phenylalanine intake in patients who develop elevated plasma tyrosine levels.

Counseling: Advise how to take therapy. Instruct to maintain dietary restriction of tyrosine and phenylalanine while on therapy. Inform that inadequate restriction may be associated w/ ocular signs and symptoms, intellectual disability and developmental delay, and painful hyperkeratotic plaques on the soles and palms. Advise to report any unexplained ocular, neurologic, or other symptoms promptly to physician. Advise patients receiving doses >20mL of sus that they may experience headache, upset stomach, and diarrhea and to report these symptoms to their healthcare provider.

ORKAMBI — ivacaftor/lumacaftor   Rx
Class: CFTR potentiator

ADULT DOSAGE
Cystic Fibrosis

Treatment of cystic fibrosis in patients who are homozygous for the *F508del* mutation in the *CFTR* gene

2 tabs q12h w/ fat-containing food

Missed Dose

Take missed dose w/in 6 hrs, w/ fat-containing food. If >6 hrs have passed, skip missed dose and resume at normal schedule

PEDIATRIC DOSAGE
Cystic Fibrosis

Treatment of cystic fibrosis in patients who are homozygous for the *F508del* mutation in the *CFTR* gene

≥12 Years:
2 tabs q12h w/ fat-containing food

Missed Dose

Take missed dose w/in 6 hrs, w/ fat-containing food. If >6 hrs have passed, skip missed dose and resume at normal schedule

---

DOSING CONSIDERATIONS
Concomitant Medications
Initiating a CYP3A Inhibitor in Patients Already Taking Orkambi: No dose adjustment is necessary.
Initiating Orkambi in Patients Currently Taking Strong CYP3A Inhibitors: Reduce Orkambi dose to 1 tab daily for the 1st week of treatment; following this period, continue w/ the recommended daily dose

If Orkambi is interrupted for more than 1 week and then reinitiated while taking strong CYP3A inhibitors, reduce Orkambi dose to 1 tab daily for the 1st week of treatment reinitiation; following this period, continue w/ the recommended dose

Renal Impairment
Severe (CrCl ≤30mL/min) or ESRD: Use w/ caution

Hepatic Impairment
Moderate (Child-Pugh Class B): 2 tabs in the am and 1 tab in the pm
Severe (Child-Pugh Class C): Max dose of 1 tab in the am and 1 tab in the pm, or less

ADMINISTRATION
Oral route

Appropriate fat-containing foods include eggs, avocados, nuts, butter, peanut butter, cheese pizza, and whole-milk dairy products.

STORAGE
20-25°C (68-77°F); excursions permitted to 15-30°C (59-86°F).

HOW SUPPLIED
Tab: (Lumacaftor/Ivacaftor) 200mg/125mg

WARNINGS/PRECAUTIONS
Worsening of liver function (eg, hepatic encephalopathy) in patients w/ advanced liver disease reported; use w/ caution, and monitor closely. Elevated transaminases/serum bilirubin levels reported. Monitor closely if increased transaminases/bilirubin levels develop, until abnormalities resolve, and interrupt dosing w/ ALT or AST >5X ULN or w/ ALT or AST >3X ULN and bilirubin >2X ULN; consider benefits and risks of resuming dosing. Respiratory events observed more commonly during initiation of therapy; perform additional monitoring during initiation of therapy in patients w/ percent predicted FEV₁ (ppFEV₁) <40. Increased BP reported; monitor BP periodically in all patients. Non-congenital lens opacities reported in pediatric patients; baseline and follow-up ophthalmological exams are recommended in pediatric patients. Use FDA-cleared cystic fibrosis mutation test to detect the presence of *F508del* mutation on both alleles of the *CFTR* gene if patient's genotype is unknown. Use in transplanted patients is not recommended due to potential drug-drug interactions.

ADVERSE REACTIONS
Dyspnea, nasopharyngitis, nausea, diarrhea, URTI, fatigue, abnormal respiration, blood creatine phosphokinase increased, rash, flatulence, rhinorrhea, influenza.

DRUG INTERACTIONS
See Dosing Considerations. Increased ivacaftor exposure w/ concomitant itraconazole, a strong CYP3A inhibitor. May decrease systemic exposure of CYP3A substrates, which may decrease the therapeutic effect; co-administration is not recommended w/ sensitive CYP3A substrates or CYP3A substrates w/ a narrow therapeutic index. Consider an alternative to using midazolam or triazolam. Avoid use if taking cyclosporine, everolimus, sirolimus, or tacrolimus. May alter exposure of CYP2B6, CYP2C8, CYP2C9, CYP2C19, and P-gp substrates. Strong CYP3A inducers (eg, rifampin, St. John's wort) may significantly reduce ivacaftor exposure, which may reduce therapeutic effectiveness; co-administration w/ strong CYP3A inducers is not recommended. Monitor serum concentration of digoxin and titrate digoxin dose as needed. May decrease the exposure of montelukast. May reduce the exposure/effectiveness of prednisone, methylprednisolone, ibuprofen, citalopram, escitalopram, and sertraline; may require higher doses. May decrease the exposure of clarithromycin, erythromycin, and telithromycin, which may reduce the effectiveness of these antibiotics; consider an alternative to these antibiotics (eg, ciprofloxacin, azithromycin, levofloxacin). May reduce exposure/effectiveness of itraconazole, ketoconazole, posaconazole, and voriconazole; concomitant use not recommended. Monitor patients closely for breakthrough fungal infections if use is necessary; consider an alternative (eg, fluconazole). May decrease hormonal contraceptive exposure/effectiveness and increase menstrual abnormality events; avoid concomitant use. Hormonal contraceptives should not be relied upon as an effective method of contraception when co-administered. May reduce exposure/effectiveness of repaglinide and alter the exposure of a sulfonylurea; a dose adjustment may be required. May reduce exposure/effectiveness of proton pump inhibitors (eg, omeprazole, esomeprazole, lansoprazole), and may alter the exposure of

ranitidine; a dose adjustment may be required. May alter the exposure of warfarin; monitor INR.

PREGNANCY AND LACTATION
Pregnancy: There are limited and incomplete human data from clinical trials and postmarketing reports on use of Orkambi or its individual components, lumacaftor or ivacaftor, in pregnant women to inform a drug-associated risk.
Lactation: There is no information regarding the presence of lumacaftor or ivacaftor in human milk, the effects on the breastfed infant, or the effects on milk production; caution in nursing.

MECHANISM OF ACTION
Lumacaftor: Improves conformational stability of F508del-CFTR; increases processing/trafficking of mature protein to the cell surface.
Ivacaftor: CFTR potentiator; facilitates increased Cl⁻ transport by potentiating the channel-open probability (or gating) of the CFTR protein at the cell surface.

PHARMACOKINETICS
Absorption: Lumacaftor: C_{max}=25mcg/mL, AUC=198mcg•hr/mL, T_{max}=approx 4 hrs (median). Ivacaftor: C_{max}=0.602mcg/mL, AUC=3.66mcg•hr/mL, T_{max}=approx 4 hrs (median). **Distribution:** Lumacaftor: V_d=86L; plasma protein binding (approx 99%). Ivacaftor: plasma protein binding (approx 99%). **Metabolism:** Lumacaftor: via oxidation and glucuronidation. Ivacaftor: Extensive via CYP3A; M1 and M6 (major metabolites). **Elimination:** Lumacaftor: Feces (51%, unchanged), urine (8.6%, 0.18% as unchanged); $T_{1/2}$=25.2 hrs. Ivacaftor: Feces (87.8%), urine (6.6%); $T_{1/2}$=9.34 hrs.

PATIENT CONSIDERATIONS

Assessment: Assess for history of transaminase elevations, renal/hepatic impairment, pregnancy/nursing status, and possible drug interactions. Assess baseline ALT, AST, bilirubin, and BP levels. Obtain baseline ophthalmological examinations in pediatric patients. Use an FDA-cleared CF mutation test to detect the presence of *F508del* mutation on both alleles of the *CFTR* gene if patient's genotype is unknown.

Monitoring: Monitor for respiratory events, cataracts in pediatric patients, and other adverse reactions. Monitor ALT/AST/bilirubin levels every 3 months during the 1st yr of therapy and annually thereafter. Perform follow-up ophthalmological examinations in pediatric patients. Monitor patients w/ ppFEV₁ <40 during treatment initiation. Periodically monitor BP.

Counseling: Inform that treatment may worsen liver function in patients w/ advanced liver disease. Advise that abnormalities in liver function have occurred and that blood tests will be performed prior to initiating therapy, every 3 months during the 1st yr, and annually thereafter. Explain that chest discomfort, dyspnea, and abnormal respiration may occur. Instruct to notify physician of all medications currently being taking, including herbal supplements or vitamins; instruct how to properly take concomitant drugs. Instruct patients on alternative methods of birth control. Inform that drug is best absorbed by the body when taken w/ fat-containing food. Inform about missed dosing instructions. Advise that abnormality of the eye lens has been noted in some children and adolescents receiving therapy and that baseline and follow-up ophthalmological exam and follow-up exams are recommended in pediatric patients initiating therapy.

OTEZLA — apremilast   Rx
Class: Phosphodiesterase-4 (PDE-4) inhibitor

ADULT DOSAGE
Psoriatic Arthritis

Initial Dosage Titration:
Day 1: 10mg (am)
Day 2: 10mg bid (am and pm)
Day 3: 10mg (am) and 20mg (pm)
Day 4: 20mg bid (am and pm)
Day 5: 20mg (am) and 30mg (pm)

Maint:
Day 6 and Thereafter: 30mg bid (am and pm)

Plaque Psoriasis

Patients w/ Moderate to Severe Plaque Psoriasis Who Are Candidates for Phototherapy or Systemic Therapy:

Initial Dosage Titration:
Day 1: 10mg (am)
Day 2: 10mg bid (am and pm)
Day 3: 10mg (am) and 20mg (pm)
Day 4: 20mg bid (am and pm)
Day 5: 20mg (am) and 30mg (pm)

Maint:
Day 6 and Thereafter: 30mg bid (am and pm)

PEDIATRIC DOSAGE
Pediatric use may not have been established

DOSING CONSIDERATIONS
Renal Impairment
Severe (CrCl <30mL/min):
Initial Dosage Titration:
Days 1-3: 10mg qam
Days 4 and 5: 20mg qam

Maint:
Day 6 and Thereafter: 30mg qam

ADMINISTRATION
Oral route

May be administered w/o regard to meals.
Do not crush, split, or chew.
STORAGE
<30°C (86°F).
HOW SUPPLIED
Tab: 10mg, 20mg, 30mg
CONTRAINDICATIONS
Known hypersensitivity to apremilast or to any excipients in the formulation.
WARNINGS/PRECAUTIONS
Depression or depressed mood, and suicidal ideation and behavior reported; carefully evaluate the risks and benefits of continuing treatment if such events occur. Weight decrease reported; consider discontinuation if unexplained or clinically significant weight loss occurs.
ADVERSE REACTIONS
Diarrhea, headache/tension headache, N/V, URTI.
DRUG INTERACTIONS
Decreased exposure w/ strong CYP450 inducers (eg, rifampin), which may result in loss of efficacy; not recommended w/ CYP450 inducers (eg, rifampin, phenobarbital, carbamazepine).
PREGNANCY AND LACTATION
Pregnancy: Category C.
Nursing: Caution in nursing.
MECHANISM OF ACTION
PDE-4 inhibitor; not established. PDE-4 inhibition results in increased intracellular cAMP levels.
PHARMACOKINETICS
Absorption: Absolute bioavailability (73%); T_{max}=2.5 hrs (median). **Distribution:** V_d=87L; plasma protein binding (68%). **Metabolism:** Extensive. CYP oxidative metabolism (CYP3A4 [primary], CYP1A2, and CYP2A6 [minor]) w/ subsequent glucuronidation and non-CYP mediated hydrolysis. **Elimination:** Urine (58%, 3% unchanged), feces (39%, 7% unchanged); $T_{1/2}$=6-9 hrs.

PATIENT CONSIDERATIONS

Assessment: Assess for history of depression and/or suicidal thoughts or behavior, drug hypersensitivity, renal impairment, pregnancy/nursing status, and possible drug interactions.

Monitoring: Monitor for emergence or worsening of depression, suicidal thoughts, or other mood changes, and for other adverse reactions. Monitor weight regularly and monitor renal function.

Counseling: Inform of the risks and benefits of therapy. Advise patients, their caregivers, and families to be alert for emergence or worsening of depression, suicidal thoughts, or other mood changes, and to contact physician if such changes occur. Counsel to monitor weight regularly and to notify physician if unexplained or clinically significant weight loss occurs. Instruct to take only as prescribed.

OTREXUP — methotrexate   Rx
Class: Dihydrofolic acid reductase inhibitor

Should be used only by physicians w/ knowledge and experience in the use of antimetabolite therapy. Use only in patients w/ psoriasis or rheumatoid arthritis (RA) w/ severe, recalcitrant, disabling disease not adequately responsive to other forms of therapy. Deaths reported in the treatment of malignancy, psoriasis, and RA. Closely monitor for bone marrow, liver, lung, skin, and kidney toxicities. Patients should be informed of the risks involved and be under physician's care throughout therapy. Fetal death and/or congenital anomalies reported; not recommended for females of childbearing potential unless benefits outweigh risks. Contraindicated in pregnant women. Reduced elimination w/ impaired renal function, ascites, or pleural effusions; monitor for toxicity and reduce dose or d/c in some cases. Unexpectedly severe (sometimes fatal) bone marrow suppression, aplastic anemia, and GI toxicity reported w/ coadministration of therapy (usually high dosage) w/ some NSAIDs. Causes hepatotoxicity, fibrosis, and cirrhosis (generally only after prolonged use); perform periodic liver biopsies in psoriatic patients on long-term therapy. Acutely, liver enzyme elevations frequently seen. Drug-induced lung disease may occur acutely at any time during therapy and reported at low doses. May need to interrupt therapy and carefully investigate if pulmonary symptoms (especially a dry, nonproductive cough) develop. Diarrhea and ulcerative stomatitis requires discontinuation of therapy. Malignant lymphomas, which may regress following withdrawal of treatment, may occur w/ low-dose therapy and, thus, may not require cytotoxic treatment; d/c therapy 1st and, if lymphoma does not regress, institute appropriate treatment. May induce tumor lysis syndrome in patients w/ rapidly growing tumors. Severe, occasionally fatal, skin reactions reported. Potentially fatal opportunistic infections, especially *Pneumocystis jiroveci* pneumonia, may occur. Concomitant use w/ radiotherapy may increase risk of soft tissue necrosis and osteonecrosis.

ADULT DOSAGE
Rheumatoid Arthritis

Severe, active RA (American College of Rheumatology criteria) in patients who have had an insufficient therapeutic response to, or are intolerant of, an adequate trial of 1st-line therapy including full-dose NSAIDs

Initial: 7.5mg once weekly

PEDIATRIC DOSAGE
Juvenile Idiopathic Arthritis

Active polyarticular juvenile idiopathic arthritis in patients who have had an insufficient therapeutic response to, or are intolerant of, an adequate trial of 1st-line therapy including full-dose NSAIDs

2-16 Years:
Initial: 10mg/m² once weekly

Titrate: Adjust dose gradually to achieve optimal response; significant increase in incidence and severity of serious toxic reactions, especially bone marrow suppression, reported at doses >20mg/week

Psoriasis

For symptomatic control of severe, recalcitrant, disabling psoriasis that is not adequately responsive to other forms of therapy, but only when the diagnosis has been established, as by biopsy and/or after dermatologic consultation

Initial: 10-25mg as a single weekly dose
Titrate: Adjust dose gradually to achieve optimal response; 30mg/week should not ordinarily be exceeded

Once optimal response is achieved, reduce dose to the lowest possible amount of drug and to the longest possible rest period

Titrate: Adjust dose gradually to achieve optimal response; there is experience w/ doses up to 30mg/m²/week, however there are too few published data to assess how doses >20mg/m²/week might affect the risk of serious toxicity

DOSING CONSIDERATIONS
Elderly
Consider relatively low doses and closely monitor for early signs of toxicity
ADMINISTRATION
SQ route

Patients may self-inject if determined that it is appropriate, if they have received proper training in how to prepare and administer the correct dose, and if they receive medical follow-up, as necessary; a trainer device is available for training purposes.

STORAGE
25°C (77°F); excursions permitted to 15-30°C (59-86°F). Protect from light.

HOW SUPPLIED
Inj: 7.5mg, 10mg, 12.5mg, 15mg, 17.5mg, 20mg, 22.5mg, 25mg [0.4mL]

CONTRAINDICATIONS
Pregnancy, nursing mothers, alcoholism, alcoholic liver disease, chronic liver disease, immunodeficiency syndromes, preexisting blood dyscrasias (eg, bone marrow hypoplasia, leukopenia, thrombocytopenia, significant anemia), known hypersensitivity to methotrexate (MTX).

WARNINGS/PRECAUTIONS
Use another formulation for alternative dosing in patients who require oral, IM, IV, intra-arterial, or intrathecal dosing, doses <7.5mg/week, doses >25mg/week, high-dose regimens, or dose adjustments between the available doses. Toxic effects may be related to dose/frequency of administration; if toxicity occurs, reduce dose or d/c therapy and take appropriate corrective measures, which may include use of leucovorin calcium and/or acute, intermittent hemodialysis w/ a high-flux dialyzer, if necessary. If therapy is reinstituted, carry it out w/ caution, w/ adequate consideration of further need for the drug and increased alertness as to possible recurrence of toxicity. Can suppress hematopoiesis and cause anemia, aplastic anemia, pancytopenia, leukopenia, neutropenia, and/or thrombocytopenia. Immediately d/c if there is a significant drop in blood counts; patients w/ profound granulocytopenia and fever should be evaluated immediately and usually require parenteral broad-spectrum antibiotic therapy. Neurologic toxicities may occur. May cause renal damage that may lead to acute renal failure; close attention to renal function including adequate hydration, urine alkalinization, and measurement of serum MTX and creatinine levels are essential for safe administration. Administered weekly; mistaken daily use has led to fatal toxicity. Caution in elderly/debilitated, patients w/ preexisting hematopoietic impairment, in the presence of preexisting liver damage or impaired hepatic function, and in the presence of active infection. May impair mental/physical abilities.

ADVERSE REACTIONS
Ulcerative stomatitis, leukopenia, nausea, abdominal distress, malaise, undue fatigue, chills, fever, dizziness, decreased resistance to infection.

DRUG INTERACTIONS
See Boxed Warning. NSAIDs may elevate and prolong levels; do not administer NSAIDs prior to or concomitantly w/ high doses of MTX, and use caution when NSAIDs and salicylates are administered concomitantly w/ lower doses of MTX. Proton pump inhibitors (PPIs) (eg, omeprazole, esomeprazole, pantoprazole) may elevate and prolong levels, possibly leading to toxicities; use caution if administering high-dose MTX w/ PPIs. Oral antibiotics (eg, tetracycline, chloramphenicol, nonabsorbable broad spectrum antibiotics) may decrease intestinal absorption or interfere w/ enterohepatic circulation. Penicillins may reduce renal clearance; increased serum concentrations of MTX w/ concomitant use w/ penicillins; carefully monitor. Trimethoprim/sulfamethoxazole reported rarely to increase bone marrow suppression. Closely monitor for increased risk of hepatotoxicity w/ hepatotoxins (eg, azathioprine, retinoids, sulfasalazine). May decrease theophylline clearance; monitor theophylline levels. Vitamin preparations containing folic acid or its derivatives may decrease response to systemically administered MTX; high doses of leucovorin may reduce efficacy of intrathecally administered MTX. Increases levels of mercaptopurine; may require dose adjustment. Toxicity may be increased due to displacement by salicylates, phenylbutazone, phenytoin, and sulfonamides. Renal tubular transport diminished by probenecid; carefully monitor w/ concomitant use. Combined use w/ gold, penicillamine, hydroxychloroquine, sulfasalazine, or cytotoxic agents may

increase incidence of adverse effects. Immunization may be ineffective when given during therapy; immunization w/ live virus vaccines is generally not recommended. Disseminated vaccinia infections after smallpox immunizations reported. Lesions of psoriasis may be aggravated by concomitant exposure to UV radiation.

PREGNANCY AND LACTATION
Pregnancy: Category X.
Lactation: MTX has been detected in human breast milk; not for use in nursing.
Reproductive Potential: Avoid pregnancy if either partner is receiving MTX; during and for a minimum of three months after therapy for male patients, and during and for at least one ovulatory cycle after therapy for female patients. MTX has been reported to cause impairment of fertility, oligospermia, and menstrual dysfunction during and for a short period after cessation of therapy.

MECHANISM OF ACTION
Dihydrofolic acid reductase inhibitor; interferes w/ DNA synthesis, repair, and cellular replication. Mechanism in RA not established; may affect immune function.

PHARMACOKINETICS
Absorption: (PO) Well-absorbed. Bioavailability (60%) (adults). Administration of various doses and in different disease states resulted in different parameters. **Distribution:** Plasma protein binding (50%); found in breast milk. (IV) V_d=0.18L/kg (initial), 0.4-0.8L/kg (steady-state). **Metabolism:** Hepatic and intracellular to polyglutamated forms (active); 7-hydroxymethotrexate (metabolite). (PO) Partially metabolized by intestinal flora. **Elimination:** $T_{1/2}$=3-10 hrs (psoriasis/RA/low-dose antineoplastic therapy), 8-15 hrs (high doses). (IV) Urine (80-90%, unchanged), bile (≤10%). Refer to PI for additional pharmacokinetic information.

PATIENT CONSIDERATIONS
Assessment: Assess for alcoholism, alcoholic/chronic liver disease, immunodeficiency, blood dyscrasias, ascites, pleural effusions, tumors, hypersensitivity to drug, pregnancy/nursing status, any other condition where treatment is cautioned or contraindicated, and possible drug interactions. Obtain baseline CBC w/ differential and platelet counts, hepatic enzymes, renal function tests, liver biopsy, and chest x-ray. Obtain baseline liver biopsy in psoriatic patients.
Monitoring: Monitor for toxicities of bone marrow, liver, lung, kidney, and GI tract, diarrhea, ulcerative stomatitis, malignant lymphomas, tumor lysis syndrome, skin reactions, opportunistic infections, and other adverse reactions. Monitor hematology at least monthly and renal/hepatic function every 1-2 months during therapy and more frequently during initial/changing doses, or during periods of increased risk of elevated drug levels (eg, dehydration). If drug-induced lung disease is suspected, perform pulmonary function tests. Perform periodic liver biopsies in psoriatic patients who are under long-term treatment.
Counseling: Inform of the risks of organ toxicity, the possible signs/symptoms for which the physician should be contacted, and the need for close follow-up, including periodic lab tests to monitor toxicity. Emphasize that the recommended dose is taken weekly, and that mistaken daily use of recommended dose has led to fatal toxicity. Instruct not to self-administer until trained by physician. Advise that therapy can cause fetal harm; advise that pregnancy should be avoided if either partner is receiving MTX; during and for a minimum of 3 months after therapy for male patients, and during and for at least 1 ovulatory cycle after therapy for female patients. Instruct to contact physician if pregnancy is suspected. Inform that therapy is contraindicated in nursing mothers. Discuss the risk of effects on reproduction. Inform that adverse reactions such as dizziness and fatigue may affect ability to drive or operate machinery. Inform of the need for proper disposal after use, including the use of a sharps disposal container.

OVIDREL — choriogonadotropin alfa   Rx
Class: Recombinant human chorionic gonadotropin (hCG)

ADULT DOSAGE	PEDIATRIC DOSAGE
Assisted Reproductive Technology	Pediatric use may not have been established
For induction of final follicular maturation and early luteinization in infertile women who have undergone pituitary desensitization and have been pretreated w/ follicle stimulating hormones as part of an assisted reproductive technology program	
Usual: 250mcg administered 1 day following the last dose of the follicle stimulating agent Do not administer until there is adequate follicular development Withhold in cases of excessive ovarian response	
Ovulation Induction	
In anovulatory infertile women in whom the cause of infertility is functional and not due to primary ovarian failure	
Usual: 250mcg administered 1 day following the last dose of the follicle stimulating agent Do not administer until there is adequate follicular development Withhold in cases of excessive ovarian response	

ADMINISTRATION
SQ route

STORAGE
Before Dispensing: 2-8°C (36-46°F). Following Dispensing: Refrigerate until expiry date or for no more than 30 days at room temperature up to 25°C (77°F) but must use within 30 days. Protect from light. Discard unused material.

HOW SUPPLIED
Inj: 250mcg/0.5mL

CONTRAINDICATIONS
Prior hypersensitivity to hCG preparations or one of their excipients, primary ovarian failure, uncontrolled thyroid or adrenal dysfunction, uncontrolled organic intracranial lesion (eg, pituitary tumor), abnormal uterine bleeding of undetermined origin, ovarian cyst or enlargement of undetermined origin, sex hormone dependent tumors of reproductive tract and accessory organs, pregnancy.

WARNINGS/PRECAUTIONS
Should only be used by physicians thoroughly familiar with infertility problems and their management. May cause ovarian hyperstimulation syndrome (OHSS) in women with or without pulmonary or vascular complications; risk of treatment should be considered for women with risk factors of thromboembolic events (eg, prior medical or family history). Withhold therapy if evidence of developing OHSS prior to administration. If severe OHSS occurs, d/c therapy and the patient should be hospitalized. Mild to moderate uncomplicated ovarian enlargement which may be accompanied by abdominal distention and/or abdominal pain may occur; withhold treatment if ovaries are abnormally enlarged on the last day of FSH therapy. May cause arterial thromboembolism. Multiple births and elevated ALT levels reported. Monitor ovarian response with serum estradiol and transvaginal ultrasound on a regular basis.

ADVERSE REACTIONS
Inj-site reactions (eg, pain, bruising), ovarian cyst, abdominal pain, nausea, OHSS.

PREGNANCY AND LACTATION
Category X, caution in nursing.

MECHANISM OF ACTION
Recombinant human chorionic gonadotropin; stimulates late follicular maturation and resumption of oocyte meiosis, and initiates rupture of preovulatory ovarian follicle.

PHARMACOKINETICS
Absorption: Absolute bioavailability (40%); C_{max}=121 IU/L, T_{max}=24 hrs, AUC=7701 h·IU/L. **Distribution:** (IV)V_d=5.9L. **Elimination:** Urine; $T_{1/2}$=29 hrs.

PATIENT CONSIDERATIONS
Assessment: Assess for primary ovarian failure, uncontrolled thyroid or adrenal dysfunction, uncontrolled organic intracranial lesion (eg, pituitary tumor), abnormal uterine bleeding of undetermined origin, ovarian cyst or enlargement of undetermined origin, sex hormone dependent tumors of reproductive tract and accessory organs, thromboembolic events risk factors, and pregnancy/nursing status.

Monitoring: Monitor for ovarian enlargement, OHSS, arterial thromboembolism, signs of multiple births, and other adverse reactions. Monitor ovarian response with serum estradiol and transvaginal ultrasound regularly.

Counseling: Inform about duration of therapy and the required monitoring procedures prior to therapy. Inform of the risks of OHSS, multiple pregnancies, and other possible adverse reactions.

OXSORALEN-ULTRA — methoxsalen   **Rx**

Class: Psoralen

> Should be used only by physicians who have special competence in the diagnosis/treatment of psoriasis and who have special training and experience in photochemotherapy. The use of methoxsalen and UV radiation therapy should be under constant supervision of such a physician. Photochemotherapy should be restricted to patients w/ severe, recalcitrant, disabling psoriasis that is not adequately responsive to other forms of therapy, and only when the diagnosis is certain. Because of the risks of ocular damage, aging of the skin, and skin cancer (eg, melanoma), inform patients about the risks inherent in this therapy. Do not use interchangeably w/ regular Oxsoralen or 8-MOP. Treat patients in accordance w/ the recommended dosimetry. Determine minimum phototoxic dose (MPD) and phototoxic peak time after drug administration prior to onset of photochemotherapy.

ADULT DOSAGE
Psoriasis
Symptomatic control of severe, recalcitrant, disabling psoriasis not adequately responsive to other forms of therapy and when the diagnosis has been supported by biopsy in conjunction w/ a schedule of controlled doses of long wave UV radiation

Take 1.5-2 hrs before UVA exposure

Initial:
<30kg: 10mg
30-50kg: 20mg
51-65kg: 30mg
66-80kg: 40mg
81-90kg: 50mg
91-115kg: 60mg
<115kg: 70mg

PEDIATRIC DOSAGE
Pediatric use may not have been established

Titrate: May increase by 10mg after 15 treatments if no response or only minimal response obtained

Max: Do not treat more often than once qod; number of doses/week determined by the patient's schedule of UVA exposures

Refer to PI for UVA exposure information

DOSING CONSIDERATIONS
Elderly
Start at lower end of dosing range according to body weight

ADMINISTRATION
Oral route

Take w/ low fat food or milk

STORAGE
25°C (77°F); excursions permitted to 15-30°C (59-86°F).

HOW SUPPLIED
Cap: 10mg

CONTRAINDICATIONS
Idiosyncratic reactions to psoralen compounds, history of light sensitive diseases (eg, lupus erythematosus, porphyria cutanea tarda, erythropoietic protoporphyria, variegate porphyria, xeroderma pigmentosum, albinism), invasive squamous cell carcinomas, aphakia, history/active melanoma.

WARNINGS/PRECAUTIONS
May cause serious skin burns from either UVA or sunlight if exceeded recommended dosage and/or exposure schedules. Patients should wear UVA-absorbing, wrap-around sunglasses for 24 hrs following methoxsalen ingestion. Sunlight/UV radiation exposure may cause premature skin aging. Observe and treat patients exhibiting multiple basal cell carcinomas or w/ history of basal cell carcinomas. Observe for signs of carcinoma in patients w/ history of previous x-ray, grenz ray, or arsenic therapy. Caution w/ hepatic insufficiency. Avoid vertical UVA chamber w/ cardiac diseases or if unable to tolerate prolonged standing or exposure to heat stress. Caution w/ elderly, especially w/ preexisting history of cataracts, cardiovascular conditions, kidney and/or liver dysfunction, or skin cancer. Avoid sunbathing 24 hrs before or 48 hrs post treatment. Avoid sun exposure at least 8 hrs after methoxsalen ingestion; if cannot be avoided, patient must wear protective devices (eg, hat and gloves) and/or apply sunscreens that contain ingredients that filter out UVA radiation. Sunscreens should not be applied to areas affected by psoriasis until after treatment in the UVA chamber. Total UVA-absorbing/blocking goggles must be worn during therapy; failure to do so may increase the risk of cataract formation. Protect abdominal skin, breasts, genitalia, and other sensitive areas for approx 1/3 of the initial exposure time until tanning occurs; unless affected by disease, shield male genitalia.

ADVERSE REACTIONS
Nausea, nervousness, insomnia, depression, pruritus, erythema.

DRUG INTERACTIONS
Caution w/ photosensitizers (eg, anthralin, coal tar and its derivatives, griseofulvin, phenothiazines, fluoroquinolones).

PREGNANCY AND LACTATION
Category C, not for use in nursing.

MECHANISM OF ACTION
Psoralen; not established. Upon photoactivation, conjugates and forms covalent bonds w/ DNA, which leads to the formation of both monofunctional and bifunctional adducts. May also react w/ proteins. Acts as photosensitizer; assumed to be DNA photodamage and resulting decrease in cell proliferation but other vascular, leukocyte, or cell regulatory mechanisms may also play some role.

PHARMACOKINETICS
Absorption: T_{max}=1.8 hrs. **Elimination:** Urine (approx 95%); $T_{1/2}$=approx 2 hrs.

PATIENT CONSIDERATIONS
Assessment: Assess for drug hypersensitivity, history of previous x-ray, grenz ray or arsenic therapy, any conditions where treatment is contraindicated or cautioned, pregnancy/nursing status, and possible drug interactions. Perform an ophthalmological exam and obtain routine lab tests prior to therapy.

Monitoring: Monitor for signs/symptoms of skin burning, cataract, aging of the skin, squamous cell carcinoma, basal cell carcinoma, melanoma, and other adverse reactions. Perform annual ophthalmologic exam. Regularly monitor routine lab test if on extended therapy. Determine the MPD and phototoxic peak time after administration.

Counseling: Inform of potential risks/benefits of therapy. Instruct to wear special wrap-around sunglasses that totally block or absorb UV light; instruct to put them on immediately after taking medication and to continue wearing them for 24 hrs if any light is present. Advise to not allow exposure of skin and lips to sunlight for 8 hrs after treatment. Instruct to not expose skin to either sunlight or sun lamps w/in 24 hrs of a scheduled treatment. Instruct to wear protective clothing (hat, gloves) to cover as much of body as possible after treatment as well as use a sunscreen product having a protection factor of at least 15. Notify physician if pregnant/nursing or planning to become pregnant.

Ozurdex — dexamethasone

Rx

Class: Corticosteroid

ADULT DOSAGE

Macular Edema

Following Branch Retinal Vein Occlusion or Central Retinal Vein Occlusion:

Usual: 0.7mg (1 implant) in the affected eye by intravitreal inj via Novadur drug delivery system

Diabetic Macular Edema

Usual: 0.7mg (1 implant) in the affected eye by intravitreal inj via Novadur drug delivery system

Posterior Segment Uveitis

Noninfectious Uveitis Affecting Posterior Segment of the Eye:

Usual: 0.7mg (1 implant) in the affected eye by intravitreal inj via Novadur drug delivery system

PEDIATRIC DOSAGE

Pediatric use may not have been established

ADMINISTRATION

Intravitreal route

Adequate anesthesia and a broad-spectrum microbicide applied to periocular skin, eyelid, and ocular surface are recommended prior to inj

Use each applicator only for treatment of a single eye; if contralateral eye requires treatment, use a new applicator, and change sterile field, syringe, gloves, drapes, and eyelid speculum before dexamethasone is administered to other eye

Instructions

1. Open foil pouch over a sterile field and gently drop the applicator on a sterile tray
2. Carefully remove cap from applicator; hold in 1 hand and pull safety tab straight off the applicator w/o twisting or flexing the tab
3. Hold the long axis of the applicator parallel to the limbus; the sclera should be engaged at an oblique angle w/ bevel of the needle up (away from sclera) to create a shelved scleral path
4. Advance the tip of needle w/in sclera for about 1mm (parallel to limbus), then re-direct toward center of eye and advance until penetration of the sclera is complete and vitreous cavity is entered; needle should not be advanced past point where sleeve touches conjunctiva
5. Slowly depress actuator button until an audible click is noted; remove needle in same direction as used to enter the vitreous

STORAGE

15-30°C (59-86°F).

HOW SUPPLIED

Implant: 0.7mg

CONTRAINDICATIONS

Glaucoma with cup to disc ratios of >0.8, torn or ruptured posterior lens capsule, active/suspected ocular or periocular infections including most viral diseases of the cornea and conjunctiva, including active epithelial herpes simplex keratitis (dendritic keratitis), vaccinia, varicella, mycobacterial infections, and fungal diseases. Known hypersensitivity to any components of this product.

WARNINGS/PRECAUTIONS

Intravitreal inj has been associated with endophthalmitis, eye inflammation, increased intraocular pressure (IOP), and retinal detachments; regularly monitor patients following inj. May produce posterior subcapsular cataracts, increased IOP, glaucoma, and may enhance the establishment of secondary ocular infections due to bacteria, fungi, or viruses. Not recommended in patients with history of ocular herpes simplex; potential for reactivation of the viral infection.

ADVERSE REACTIONS

IOP elevation, conjunctival hemorrhage/edema/hyperemia, eye pain, ocular HTN, cataract, headache, visual acuity reduced, conjunctivitis, dry eye, vitreous detachment/opacities/floaters, retinal aneurysm.

PREGNANCY AND LACTATION

Category C, caution in nursing.

MECHANISM OF ACTION

Corticosteroid; suppresses inflammation by inhibiting multiple inflammatory cytokines resulting in decreased edema, fibrin deposition, capillary leakage, and migration of inflammatory cells.

PHARMACOKINETICS

Distribution: Found in breast milk (systemically administered).

PATIENT CONSIDERATIONS

Assessment: Assess for hypersensitivity to product components, glaucoma, torn or ruptured posterior lens capsule, active/suspected ocular or periocular infections, history of ocular herpes simplex, and pregnancy/nursing status.

Monitoring: Monitor for eye inflammation, retinal detachments, posterior subcapsular cataracts, glaucoma, secondary ocular infections, and other adverse reactions. Monitor for elevation of IOP and for endophthalmitis by checking for perfusion of the optic nerve head immediately after inj, tonometry within 30 min following inj, and biomicroscopy between 2-7 days after inj.

Counseling: Advise that a cataract may occur after repeated treatment; if this occurs, inform that vision will decrease and that an operation to remove the cataract and restore vision will be needed. Advise that increased IOP may develop. Inform that in the days following intravitreal inj, patients are at risk for potential complications including development of endophthalmitis or elevated IOP; instruct to report any symptoms suggestive of endophthalmitis without delay. Advise to seek immediate care from an ophthalmologist if the eye becomes red, sensitive to light, painful, or if changes in vision develop. Inform that temporary visual blurring after receiving an intravitreal inj may be experienced; instruct to avoid driving/using machines until this has resolved.

Paclitaxel — paclitaxel

Rx

Class: Antimicrotubule agent

> Should be administered under supervision of a physician experienced in the use of cancer chemotherapeutic agents. Anaphylaxis and severe hypersensitivity reactions characterized by dyspnea and hypotension requiring treatment, angioedema, and generalized urticaria reported; pretreat w/ corticosteroids, diphenhydramine, and H_2 antagonists. Fatal reactions have occurred despite premedication. Do not rechallenge if severe hypersensitivity reaction occurs. Avoid in patients w/ solid tumors who have baseline neutrophil counts of <1500 cells/mm^3 and in patients w/ AIDS-related Kaposi's sarcoma if the baseline neutrophil count is <1000 cells/mm^3. Perform peripheral blood cell counts frequently to monitor occurrence of bone marrow suppression, primarily neutropenia.

ADULT DOSAGE

Ovarian Carcinoma

1st-line (in combination w/ cisplatin) and subsequent therapy for advanced carcinoma of the ovary

Previously Untreated Patients:
175mg/m^2 IV over 3 hrs, followed by cisplatin 75mg/m^2
or
135mg/m^2 IV over 24 hrs, followed by cisplatin 75mg/m^2

Administer one of the recommended regimens every 3 weeks

Previously Treated Patients:
135mg/m^2 or 175mg/m^2 IV over 3 hrs every 3 weeks

Breast Cancer

Adjuvant Treatment of Node-Positive Breast Cancer:

175mg/m^2 IV over 3 hrs every 3 weeks for 4 courses, administered sequentially to standard doxorubicin-containing combination chemotherapy

Treatment After Failure of Combination Chemotherapy for Metastatic Disease or Relapse w/in 6 Months of Adjuvant Chemotherapy:

Prior therapy should have included an anthracycline unless clinically contraindicated

175mg/m^2 IV over 3 hrs every 3 weeks

Non-Small Cell Lung Cancer

Combination w/ cisplatin for 1st-line treatment in patients who are not candidates for potentially curative surgery and/or radiation therapy

135mg/m^2 IV over 24 hrs, followed by cisplatin 75mg/m^2

Administer regimen every 3 weeks

AIDS-Related Kaposi's Sarcoma

2nd-Line Treatment:

135mg/m^2 IV over 3 hrs every 3 weeks or 100mg/m^2 IV over 3 hrs every 2 weeks

Premedication

All patients should be premedicated prior to paclitaxel inj administration in order to prevent severe hypersensitivity reactions. Such premedication may consist of dexamethasone 20mg PO approx 12 and 6 hrs before inj, diphenhydramine (or its equivalent) 50mg IV 30-60 min prior to inj, and cimetidine (300mg) or ranitidine (50mg) IV 30-60 min before inj

PEDIATRIC DOSAGE

Pediatric use may not have been established

DOSING CONSIDERATIONS

Hepatic Impairment

24-Hr Infusion:
AST/ALT 2 to <10X ULN and Bilirubin ≤1.5mg/dL: 100mg/m²
AST/ALT <10X ULN and Bilirubin 1.6-7.5mg/dL: 50mg/m²
AST/ALT ≥10X ULN and Bilirubin >7.5mg/dL: Not recommended

3-Hr Infusion:
AST/ALT <10X ULN and Bilirubin 1.26-2X ULN: 135mg/m²
AST/ALT <10X ULN and Bilirubin 2.01-5X ULN: 90mg/m²
AST/ALT ≥10X ULN and Bilirubin >5X ULN: Not recommended

Dose recommendations are for the 1st course of therapy; further dose reduction in subsequent courses should be based on individual tolerance

These recommendations are based on dosages of 135mg/m² over 24 hrs or 175mg/m² over 3 hrs; data are not available to make adjustment recommendations for other regimens (eg, AIDS-related Kaposi's sarcoma)

Adverse Reactions

Severe Neutropenia (Neutrophils <500 cells/mm³ for ≥1 Week) or Severe Peripheral Neuropathy: Reduce dose of subsequent courses by 20%

Other Important Considerations

Patients w/ Advanced HIV Disease:
1. Reduce dexamethasone dose as 1 of the 3 premedication drugs to 10mg PO (instead of 20mg PO)
2. Initiate or repeat treatment w/ paclitaxel inj only if the neutrophil count is ≥1000 cells/mm³
3. Reduce the dose of subsequent courses of paclitaxel inj by 20% for patients who experience severe neutropenia (neutrophil <500 cells/mm³ for ≥1 week)
4. Initiate concomitant hematopoietic growth factor as clinically indicated

ADMINISTRATION

IV route

Administration Precautions

The use of plasticized PVC containers and administration sets is not recommended; store diluted paclitaxel inj sol in bottles (glass, polypropylene) or plastic bags (polypropylene, polyolefin) and administer through polyethylene-lined administration sets.
Administer paclitaxel inj through an in-line filter w/ a microporous membrane not >0.22 microns; use of filter devices such as IVEX-2 filters, which incorporate short inlet and outlet PVC-coated tubing, has not resulted in significant leaching of di-(2-ethylhexyl)phthalate.

Preparation

1. Paclitaxel inj must be diluted prior to infusion. Dilute in 0.9% NaCl inj; D5 inj; D5 and 0.9% NaCl inj; or D5 in Ringer's inj to a final concentration of 0.3-1.2mg/mL.
2. Prepared sol for infusion are stable at ambient temperature (approx 25°C [77°F]) and lighting conditions for up to 27 hrs.
3. Upon preparation, sol may show haziness, which is attributed to the formulation vehicle.
4. Do not use the Chemo Dispensing Pin device or similar devices w/ spikes w/ vials of paclitaxel inj since they can cause the stopper to collapse, resulting in loss of sterile integrity of the paclitaxel inj sol.

Handling Precautions

If paclitaxel inj sol contacts the skin, wash the skin immediately and thoroughly w/ soap and water. Following topical exposure, events have included tingling, burning, and redness.
If paclitaxel inj contacts mucous membranes, the membranes should be flushed thoroughly w/ water.
Upon inhalation, dyspnea, chest pain, burning eyes, sore throat, and nausea have been reported.

STORAGE

20-25°C (68-77°F). Retain in original package to protect from light.

HOW SUPPLIED

Inj: 30mg/5mL, 100mg/16.7mL, 150mg/25mL, 300mg/50mL

CONTRAINDICATIONS

History of hypersensitivity reactions to paclitaxel or other drugs formulated in polyoxyl 35 castor oil. Patients w/ solid tumors who have baseline neutrophil counts of <1500 cells/mm³, or AIDS-related Kaposi's sarcoma patients w/ baseline neutrophil counts of <1000 cells/mm³.

WARNINGS/PRECAUTIONS

Bone marrow suppression (primarily neutropenia) is dose-dependent and is the dose-limiting toxicity. Do not retreat w/ subsequent cycles until neutrophils recover to >1500 cells/mm³ (>1000 cells/mm³ w/ Kaposi's sarcoma) and platelets recover to >100,000 cells/mm³. Severe conduction abnormalities reported (some requiring pacemaker placement); administer appropriate therapy and perform continuous cardiac monitoring during subsequent therapy. May cause fetal harm. Severe hypersensitivity reactions require immediate discontinuation of therapy and aggressive symptomatic treatment. Hypotension, bradycardia, and HTN reported; frequently monitor vital signs, particularly during 1st hour of infusion. Occasionally, infusion must be interrupted or discontinued because of initial or recurrent HTN. Contains dehydrated alcohol; consider possible CNS and other alcohol effects. Extreme caution in patients w/ bilirubin >2X ULN and in elderly. Inj-site reactions (including reactions secondary to extravasation) and peripheral neuropathy reported. Due to the possibility of extravasation, closely monitor infusion site for possible infiltration during drug administration.

ADVERSE REACTIONS

Bone marrow suppression, hypersensitivity reactions, infections, bleeding, abnormal ECG, bradycardia, hypotension, peripheral neuropathy, myalgia/arthralgia, N/V, diarrhea, alopecia, inj-site reactions, mucositis.

DRUG INTERACTIONS

Myelosuppression more profound when paclitaxel was given after cisplatin than w/ the alternate sequence. Caution w/ CYP3A4 substrates (eg, midazolam, buspirone, felodipine), inducers (eg, rifampin, carbamazepine), and inhibitors (eg, atazanavir, clarithromycin, ketoconazole). Caution w/ CYP2C8 substrates (eg, repaglinide, rosiglitazone), inhibitors (eg, gemfibrozil), and inducers (eg, rifampin). May increase levels of doxorubicin (and its active metabolite doxorubicinol).

PREGNANCY AND LACTATION

Pregnancy: Category D.
Lactation: Not for use in nursing.

MECHANISM OF ACTION

Antimicrotubule agent; promotes assembly of microtubules from tubulin dimers and stabilizes microtubules by preventing depolymerization and induces abnormal arrays or bundles of microtubules throughout the cell cycle and multiple asters of microtubules during mitosis.

PHARMACOKINETICS

Absorption: Administration of multiple doses resulted in different parameters. **Distribution:** V_d=227-688L/m²; plasma protein binding (89-98%). **Metabolism:** Liver via CYP2C8 (major), CYP3A4 (minor). 6α-hydroxypaclitaxel (major metabolite). **Elimination:** 225 or 250 mg/m² over 3 hrs: Urine (14%), feces (71%, 5% unchanged).

PATIENT CONSIDERATIONS

Assessment: Assess for hypersensitivity to drug or other drugs w/ polyoxyl 35 castor oil, hepatic impairment, bilirubin levels, pregnancy/nursing status, and possible drug interactions. Obtain baseline neutrophil counts.

Monitoring: Monitor for signs/symptoms of anaphylaxis/hypersensitivity reactions, inj-site reactions, myelosuppression, and other adverse reactions. Monitor peripheral blood cell counts frequently. Monitor vital signs frequently, particularly during 1st hr of infusion. Closely monitor infusion site for possible infiltration during administration. Monitor cardiac function in patients w/ serious conduction abnormalities and when used in combination w/ doxorubicin for the treatment of metastatic breast cancer.

Counseling: Inform about risks and benefits of therapy. Inform that drug may cause fetal harm; advise women of childbearing potential to avoid becoming pregnant. Advise to report to physician if signs of an allergic reaction or infection develop. Advise to inform physician if breastfeeding or planning to breastfeed.

PAMIDRONATE — pamidronate disodium Rx

Class: Bisphosphonate

OTHER BRAND NAMES

Aredia (Discontinued)

ADULT DOSAGE	PEDIATRIC DOSAGE
Hypercalcemia of Malignancy	Pediatric use may not have been established
In conjunction w/ adequate hydration for moderate or severe hypercalcemia associated w/ malignancy, w/ or w/o bone metastases	
Moderate Hypercalcemia (Corrected Serum Ca²⁺ 12-13.5mg/dL): **Usual:** 60-90mg single dose IV infusion over 2-24 hrs **Max:** 90mg/single dose	
Severe Hypercalcemia (Corrected Serum Ca²⁺ >13.5mg/dL): **Usual:** 90mg single dose IV infusion over 2-24 hrs **Max:** 90mg/single dose	
Longer infusions (eg, >2 hours) may reduce the risk for renal toxicity, particularly in patients w/ preexisting renal insufficiency	
Retreatment: May be carried out in patients who show complete or partial response initially, if serum Ca²⁺ does not return to normal or remain normal after initial treatment; a minimum of 7 days should elapse before retreatment, to allow for full response to initial dose. The dose and manner of retreatment is identical to that of the initial therapy	
Paget's Disease	
Moderate to Severe: **Usual:** 30mg/day as a 4-hr infusion on 3 consecutive days for a total dose of 90mg **Max:** 90mg/single dose	
Retreatment: When indicated, retreat at the dose of initial therapy	

Osteolytic Bone Metastases of Breast Cancer

In Conjunction w/ Standard Antineoplastic Therapy:
Usual: 90mg over a 2-hr infusion every 3-4 weeks
Max: 90mg/single dose

Pamidronate disodium has been frequently used w/ doxorubicin, fluorouracil, cyclophosphamide, methotrexate, mitoxantrone, vinblastine, dexamethasone, prednisone, melphalan, vincristine, megestrol, and tamoxifen

Osteolytic Bone Lesions of Multiple Myeloma

In Conjunction w/ Standard Antineoplastic Therapy:
Usual: 90mg as a 4-hr infusion given on a monthly basis
Max: 90mg/single dose

Patients with marked Bence-Jones proteinuria and dehydration should receive adequate hydration prior to pamidronate disodium infusion

---

DOSING CONSIDERATIONS

Renal Impairment
Osteolytic Bone Lesions of Multiple Myeloma/Osteolytic Bone Metastases of Breast Cancer:
Withhold treatment for renal deterioration and resume only when the creatinine returns to w/in 10% of baseline value

Renal deterioration is defined as follows:
For Patients w/ Normal Baseline Creatinine: Increase of 0.5mg/dL
For Patients w/ Abnormal Baseline Creatinine: Increase of 1mg/dL

Elderly
Start at lower end of dosing range

ADMINISTRATION
IV route

Do not mix w/ Ca^{2+}-containing infusion sol (eg, Ringer's sol)
Administer in a single IV sol and line separate from all other drugs

Hypercalcemia of Malignancy
Avoid overhydration in patients w/ potential for cardiac failure
Administer daily dose as an IV infusion over at least 2-24 hrs for 60mg and 90mg doses
Dilute recommended dose in 1000mL of sterile 0.45% or 0.9% NaCl or D5 inj
Infusion sol is stable for up to 24 hrs at room temperature

Paget's Disease
Dilute recommended daily dose of 30mg in 500mL of sterile 0.45% or 0.9% NaCl or D5 inj

Osteolytic Bone Metastases of Breast Cancer
Dilute recommended dose of 90mg in 250mL of sterile 0.45% or 0.9% NaCl or D5 inj

Osteolytic Bone Lesions of Multiple Myeloma
Dilute recommended dose of 90mg in 500mL of sterile 0.45% or 0.9% NaCl or D5 inj

STORAGE
20-25°C (68-77°F).

HOW SUPPLIED
Inj: 3mg/mL, 6mg/mL, 9mg/mL [10mL]

CONTRAINDICATIONS
Clinically significant hypersensitivity to pamidronate disodium or other bisphosphonates.

WARNINGS/PRECAUTIONS
Patients with marked Bence-Jones proteinuria and dehydration should receive adequate hydration prior to infusion. Avoid overhydration in patients with hypercalcemia of malignancy who have potential for cardiac failure. Renal deterioration, progression to renal failure, and dialysis reported in patients after the initial or a single dose administration. Focal segmental glomerulosclerosis (including the collapsing variant) with or without nephrotic syndrome, which may lead to renal failure, has been reported, particularly in the setting of multiple myeloma and breast cancer. Avoid use during pregnancy; may cause fetal harm. Cases of asymptomatic hypophosphatemia, hypokalemia, hypomagnesemia, and hypocalcemia reported; rare cases of symptomatic hypocalcemia (including tetany) reported. Short-term Ca^{2+} therapy may be necessary if hypocalcemia occurs. Patients with a history of thyroid surgery may have relative hypoparathyroidism that may predispose to hypocalcemia. Not recommended in patients with bone metastases with severe renal impairment. Osteonecrosis of the jaw (ONJ) reported, predominantly in cancer patients; maintain good oral hygiene and perform dental exam with preventive dentistry prior to treatment and if possible, avoid invasive dental procedures while on treatment. Severe and occasionally incapacitating bone, joint, and/or muscle pain reported. Atypical subtrochanteric and diaphyseal femoral fractures reported; examine contralateral femur in patients who have sustained femoral shaft fracture. Any patient with a history of bisphosphonate exposure who presents with thigh/groin pain in the absence of trauma should be suspected of having an atypical fracture and should be evaluated; consider discontinuation in patients suspected to have an atypical femur fracture. Carefully monitor patients with preexisting anemia, leukopenia, or thrombocytopenia in the first 2 weeks post-treatment. Caution in elderly.

ADVERSE REACTIONS
Infusion-site reaction (eg, redness, swelling, induration, pain on palpation), fever, N/V, anorexia, constipation, dizziness, headache, paresthesia, increased sweating, somnolence, anemia.

DRUG INTERACTIONS
Caution when used with other potentially nephrotoxic drugs. Concomitant use with thalidomide may increase the risk of renal dysfunction in multiple myeloma.

PREGNANCY AND LACTATION
Category D, caution in nursing.

MECHANISM OF ACTION
Bisphosphonate; has not been established. Adsorbs to calcium phosphate crystals in bone and may directly block dissolution of this mineral component of bone. Inhibits osteoclast activity that contributes to inhibition of bone resorption.

PHARMACOKINETICS
Elimination: Urine (46%, unchanged); $T_{1/2}$=28 hrs.

PATIENT CONSIDERATIONS

Assessment: Assess for dehydration, hypersensitivity to the drug or other bisphosphonates, cardiac failure, renal impairment, history of thyroid surgery, anemia, leukopenia, thrombocytopenia, pregnancy/nursing status, and for possible drug interactions. Assess SrCr prior to each treatment. Obtain dental exam with preventive dentistry prior to treatment in cancer patients.

Monitoring: Monitor for renal toxicity, ONJ, musculoskeletal pain, atypical femur fracture, and other adverse reactions. Monitor standard hypercalcemia-related metabolic parameters (eg, serum Ca^{2+}, phosphate, Mg^{2+}, K^+), electrolyte levels, CBC, differential, and Hct/Hgb. Monitor patients with preexisting anemia, leukopenia, or thrombocytopenia in the first 2 weeks post-treatment.

Counseling: Inform of the risks/benefits of therapy.

PANRETIN — alitretinoin   Rx

Class: Retinoid

ADULT DOSAGE	PEDIATRIC DOSAGE
AIDS-Related Kaposi's Sarcoma	Pediatric use may not have been established
Cutaneous Lesions:	
Initial: Apply bid to lesions	
Titrate: Gradually increase to tid-qid, as tolerated	
Continue as long as the patient is deriving benefit	

DOSING CONSIDERATIONS
Application-Site Toxicity:
Reduce frequency if toxicity occurs
D/C temporarily if severe irritation occurs

ADMINISTRATION
Topical route

Cover the lesion w/ a generous coating
Allow to dry for 3-5 min before covering w/ clothing
Avoid application to normal skin surrounding lesions
Avoid application on or near mucosal surfaces of the body
Do not use w/ occlusive dressings

STORAGE
25°C (77°F); excursions permitted to 15-30°C (59-86°F).

HOW SUPPLIED
Gel: 0.1% [60g]

WARNINGS/PRECAUTIONS
Avoid mucous membranes, normal skin. Not for use when systemic anti-KS therapy is required. Possible photosensitizing effects, minimize exposure of treated areas to sunlight and sunlamps. Treatment-limiting toxicities. Avoid in pregnancy.

ADVERSE REACTIONS
Rash, pain, pruritus, erythema, exfoliative dermatitis, skin disorder, paresthesia, edema.

DRUG INTERACTIONS
Avoid DEET-containing products (eg, insect repellents).

PREGNANCY AND LACTATION
Category D, not for use in nursing.

MECHANISM OF ACTION
Binds to and activates intracellular retinoid receptor subtypes that regulate the expression of genes and control the process of cellular differentiation and proliferation in both normal and neoplastic cells.

PHARMACOKINETICS
Metabolism: Liver via CYP2C9, 3A4, 1A1, and 1A2; 4-oxo-9-*cis*-retinoic acid (major metabolite).

PATIENT CONSIDERATIONS

Assessment: Assess for known hypersensitivity and pregnancy/nursing status.

Monitoring: Monitor for skin photosensitivity and signs of dermal toxicity (eg, erythema, edema).

Counseling: Advise to avoid prolonged exposure of treated areas to sunlight and sunlamps. Notify if pregnant/nursing or planning to become pregnant.

PEGASYS — peginterferon alfa-2a   Rx

Class: Biological response modifier

> May cause or aggravate fatal or life-threatening neuropsychiatric, autoimmune, ischemic, and infectious disorders. Monitor closely w/ periodic clinical and lab evaluations. D/C w/ persistently severe or worsening signs/symptoms of these conditions.

ADULT DOSAGE

Chronic Hepatitis C with Compensated Liver Disease

W/O HIV Coinfection:
Monotherapy:
180mcg once weekly for 48 weeks

Combination Treatment:
Genotypes 1, 4:
180mcg once weekly for 48 weeks (if used w/ ribavirin only)

Genotypes 2, 3:
180mcg once weekly for 24 weeks (if used w/ ribavirin only)

W/ HIV Coinfection:
180mcg once weekly for 48 weeks (if used w/ ribavirin only)

Chronic Hepatitis B with Compensated Liver Disease

HBeAg-Positive and HBeAg-Negative:
180mcg once weekly for 48 weeks

PEDIATRIC DOSAGE

Chronic Hepatitis C with Compensated Liver Disease

≥5 Years:
Combination w/ Ribavirin:
$180mcg/1.73m^2$ x BSA once weekly
Max Dose: 180mcg

Treatment Duration:
Genotypes 2, 3: 24 weeks
Other Genotypes: 48 weeks

Treatment Initiation Prior to 18 Years:
Maintain pediatric dosing through the completion of therapy

DOSING CONSIDERATIONS

Renal Impairment
Adults:
CrCl <30mL/min and/or Hemodialysis: 135mcg once weekly
If severe adverse reactions or lab abnormalities develop, dose can be reduced to 90mcg once weekly until reactions abate; d/c if intolerance persists after dosage adjustment

Hepatic Impairment
Child Pugh-Score >6 (Class B and C): D/C Pegasys

Adverse Reactions
Neutropenia:
Adults:
ANC <750 cells/mm³: Reduce dose to 135mcg once weekly
ANC <500 cells/mm³: D/C until ANC values return to >1000 cells/mm³; restart at 90mcg once weekly

Pediatrics:
ANC 750-999 cells/mm³:
Weeks 1-2: Reduce dose to $135mcg/1.73m^2$ x BSA
Weeks 3-48: No dose modification

ANC 500-749 cells/mm³:
Weeks 1-2: Hold dose until >750 cells/mm³ then resume at $135mcg/1.73m^2$ x BSA
Weeks 3-48: Reduce dose to $135mcg/1.73m^2$ x BSA

ANC 250-499 cells/mm³:
Weeks 1-2: Hold dose until >750 cells/mm³ then resume at $90mcg/1.73m^2$ x BSA
Weeks 3-48: Hold dose until >750 cells/mm³ then resume at $135mcg/1.73m^2$ x BSA

ANC <250 cells/mm³ (or Febrile Neutropenia): D/C treatment

Thrombocytopenia:
Adults:
Platelets <50,000 cells/mm³: Reduce dose to 90mcg once weekly
Platelets <25,000 cells/mm³: D/C treatment

Pediatrics:
Platelets <50,000 cells/mm³: $90mcg/1.73m^2$ x BSA

Transaminase Elevations:
Adults:
Progressive ALT Increases After Dose Reduction: D/C therapy
ALT Increases w/ Increased Bilirubin/Evidence of Hepatic Decompensation: D/C therapy

Chronic Hepatitis C Patients:
Progressive ALT Increases Above Baseline: Reduce dose to 135mcg; resume therapy after flares subside

Chronic Hepatitis B Patients:
ALT Elevations >5X ULN: Reduce dose to 135mcg or temporarily d/c; resume therapy after flares subside
Persistent, Severe Flares (ALT >10X Above ULN): Consider discontinuation

Pediatrics:
Persistent/Increasing ALT Elevations ≥5 but <10X ULN: Modify dose to $135mcg/1.73m^2$ x BSA; reduce dose further if necessary
Persistent ALT Elevations ≥10X ULN: D/C treatment

Depression:
Initial Management (4-8 Weeks):
Adults:
Moderate: Decrease dose to 135mcg or 90mcg once weekly
Severe: Permanently d/c treatment
Pediatrics:
Moderate: Decrease dose to $135mcg/1.73m^2$ x BSA or $90mcg/1.73m^2$ x BSA once weekly
Severe: Permanently d/c treatment

Worsening of Depression Severity After 8 Weeks:
Adults:
Mild: Decrease dose to 135mcg or 90mcg once weekly or d/c
Moderate: Permanently d/c treatment
Pediatrics:
Mild: Decrease dose to $135mcg/1.73m^2$ x BSA or $90mcg/1.73m^2$ x BSA once weekly
Moderate: Permanently d/c treatment
Refer to PI for psychiatric visit schedule

Discontinuation
Chronic Hepatic C Genotype 1 in Combination w/ Ribavirin or Alone:
D/C if at least a 2 log_{10} HCV RNA reduction from baseline is not achieved by Week 12
D/C if undetectable HCV RNA is not achieved after 24 weeks

ADMINISTRATION
SQ route

Administer in abdomen or thigh.
Discard unused portion in single-use vials or prefilled syringes in excess of the labeled volume.

Recommended Volume to be Administered for Different Dosages
180mcg/mL in a Vial:
90mcg Dose: Use 0.5mL
135mcg Dose: Use 0.75mL
180mcg Dose: Use entire 1mL

180mcg/0.5mL in a Prefilled Syringe:
90mcg: Use 0.25mL
135mcg: Use 0.375mL
180mcg: Use entire 0.5mL

180mcg/0.5mL in an Autoinjector:
90mcg: Do not use
135mcg: Do not use
180mcg: May use

135mcg/0.5mL in an Autoinjector:
90mcg: Do not use
135mcg: May use
180mcg: Do not use

STORAGE
2-8°C (36-46°F). Do not leave out of the refrigerator for >24 hrs. Do not freeze or shake. Protect from light.

HOW SUPPLIED
Inj: 180mcg/0.5mL [prefilled syringe]; 180mcg/0.5mL, 135mcg/0.5mL [ProClick autoinjector]; 180mcg/mL [vial]

CONTRAINDICATIONS
Known hypersensitivity reactions (eg, urticaria, angioedema, bronchoconstriction, anaphylaxis, Stevens-Johnson syndrome) to alpha interferons or any component of this medication. autoimmune hepatitis, hepatic decompensation (Child-Pugh score >6 [Class B and C]) in cirrhotic patients before treatment, hepatic decompensation w/ Child-Pugh score ≥6 in cirrhotic CHC patients coinfected w/ HIV before treatment, neonates and infants (contains benzyl alcohol). When used with other HCV antiviral drugs, including ribavirin, refer to the individual monograph(s).

WARNINGS/PRECAUTIONS
Not recommended, alone or in combination w/ ribavirin w/o additional HCV antiviral drugs, in CHC patients who previously failed therapy w/ an interferon-alfa, and in CHC patients who have had a solid organ transplantation. Avoid in combination w/ ribavirin in pregnant women or men whose female partners are pregnant. Extreme caution w/ history of depression; d/c immediately in severe cases and institute psychiatric intervention. HTN, supraventricular arrhythmias, chest pain, and MI reported; caution w/ preexisting cardiac disease. May cause bone marrow suppression and severe cytopenias; d/c, at least temporarily, if severe decrease in neutrophil or platelet count develops. May cause or aggravate hypo/hyperthyroidism, ophthalmologic disorders, and pulmonary disorders. Hypo/hyperglycemia, diabetes mellitus, and ischemic and hemorrhagic cerebrovascular events reported. CHC patients w/ cirrhosis may be at risk for hepatic decompensation and death; d/c immediately w/ hepatic decompensation. Exacerbation of hepatitis B reported; d/c immediately if hepatic decompensation, progressive ALT increases, or increased bilirubin occurs. Ulcerative or hemorrhagic/ischemic colitis, pancreatitis, and severe acute hypersensitivity reactions reported; d/c if any of these develop. Consider discontinuation of treatment and immediately start appropriate anti-infective therapy if serious and severe infections occur. D/C w/ new or worsening ophthalmologic disorders, pulmonary infiltrates or pulmonary function impairment. Peripheral neuropathy reported in combination w/ telbivudine. May inhibit growth in pediatric patients. May impair fertility in women. Caution in renal impairment and in the elderly.

ADVERSE REACTIONS
Neuropsychiatric/autoimmune/ischemic/infectious disorders, inj-site reactions, fatigue/asthenia, diarrhea, pyrexia, rigors, N/V, anorexia, myalgia, headache, irritability/anxiety/nervousness.

DRUG INTERACTIONS

May inhibit CYP1A2 and increase exposure of theophylline; monitor theophylline serum levels and consider dose adjustments. May increase levels of methadone; monitor for toxicity. Hepatic decompensation can occur w/ peginterferon alfa-2a/ribavirin in combination w/ other HCV antiviral drugs and nucleoside reverse transcriptase inhibitors (NRTIs); refer to PI for other HCV antiviral drugs and the respective NRTIs for guidance regarding toxicity management. Concomitant use of peginterferon alfa-2a/ribavirin w/ zidovudine may cause severe neutropenia and severe anemia; consider discontinuation of zidovudine as medically appropriate and also consider dose reduction or discontinuation of peginterferon alfa-2a, ribavirin or both if worsening clinical toxicities are observed, including hepatic decompensation (eg, Child-Pugh >6). Pancytopenia and bone marrow suppression reported to occur w/in 3-7 weeks after the concomitant administration of pegylated interferon/ribavirin and azathioprine; d/c peginterferon alfa-2a, ribavirin, and azathioprine for pancytopenia, and do not re-introduce pegylated interferon/ribavirin w/ concomitant azathioprine.

PREGNANCY AND LACTATION

Pregnancy: Category C, Category X (w/ ribavirin).
Lactation: Not for use in nursing.

MECHANISM OF ACTION

Pegylated virus proliferation inhibitor; binds to human type 1 interferon receptor leading to receptor dimerization, which activates multiple intracellular signal transduction pathways initially mediated by the JAK/STAT pathway. Expected to have pleiotropic biological effects in the body.

PHARMACOKINETICS

Absorption: T_{max}=72-96 hrs. **Elimination:** $T_{1/2}$=160 hrs (CHC).

PATIENT CONSIDERATIONS

Assessment: Assess for neuropsychiatric, autoimmune, ischemic or infectious disorders, hepatic/renal impairment, known hypersensitivity reactions, history of treatment failure w/ interferon alfa in CHC patients, history of solid organ transplantation in CHC patients, nursing status, possible drug interactions, or any other conditions where treatment is contraindicated or cautioned. Obtain baseline CBC, TSH, CD4+ (HIV), and eye exam. Perform ECG for preexisting cardiac diseases. Obtain pregnancy test in women of childbearing potential.

Monitoring: Monitor for signs/symptoms of neuropsychiatric, autoimmune, ischemic, infectious, cardiovascular, cerebrovascular, endocrine, and pulmonary disorders; bone marrow toxicities; colitis; pancreatitis; delayed growth in pediatric patients; and other adverse reactions. Monitor hematological (Weeks 2, 4, and periodically thereafter) and biochemical tests (Week 4 and periodically thereafter), and TSH (every 12 weeks). Perform periodic eye exams in patients w/ preexisting ophthalmologic disorders. Perform monthly pregnancy tests if on combination therapy w/ ribavirin and for 6 months after discontinuation. Monitor clinical status and hepatic/renal function.

Counseling: Counsel on benefits and risks of therapy. Advise not to use drug in combination w/ ribavirin for pregnant women or men whose female partners are pregnant. Inform of the teratogenic/embryocidal risks w/ ribavirin; instruct to use 2 forms of effective contraception during ribavirin therapy and for 6 months post-therapy. Inform that drug is not known if drug will prevent transmission of HCV/HBV infection to others. Advise that it is not known if therapy will prevent cirrhosis, liver failure or liver cancer in HBV patients. Advise that laboratory evaluations are required prior to therapy, and periodically thereafter. Counsel to avoid alcohol, and avoid driving or operating machinery if dizziness, confusion, somnolence, or fatigue occurs. Instruct to remain well hydrated, and not to switch to another brand of interferon w/o consulting physician. Instruct on the proper preparation and administration, and disposal techniques for therapy.

PEGINTRON — peginterferon alfa-2b   Rx

Class: Biological response modifier

> May cause or aggravate fatal or life-threatening neuropsychiatric, autoimmune, ischemic, and infectious disorders. Closely monitor patients w/ periodic clinical and lab evaluations. D/C w/ persistently severe or worsening signs/symptoms of these conditions. When used w/ Rebetol, refer to the individual monograph.

ADULT DOSAGE

Chronic Hepatitis C with Compensated Liver Disease

Combination Therapy w/ Rebetol w/ or w/o Hepatitis C Virus (HCV) NS3/4A Protease Inhibitor:
Use w/ HCV NS3/4A protease inhibitor w/ HCV genotype 1 infection. Use w/o HCV NS3/4A protease inhibitor in genotypes other than 1, or w/ genotype 1 infection where use of an HCV NS3/4A protease inhibitor is not warranted based on tolerability, contraindications, or other clinical factors

1.5mcg/kg/week + 800-1400mg Rebetol (based on body weight)

Refer to the PI of the specific HCV NS3/4A protease inhibitor for dosing information

PEDIATRIC DOSAGE

Chronic Hepatitis C with Compensated Liver Disease

3-17 Years:

Combination Therapy w/ Rebetol:
60mcg/m²/week + 15mg/kg/day Rebetol in 2 divided doses

Remain on pediatric dosing regimen if 18th birthday was reached during therapy

Treatment Duration:
Genotype 1: 48 weeks
Genotype 2 and 3: 24 weeks

Treatment Duration:

Interferon-Alfa-Naive Patients:
Genotype 1: 48 weeks
Genotypes 2 and 3: 24 weeks
Retreatment of Prior Treatment Failure:
48 weeks (regardless of genotype)

Monotherapy:
Monotherapy should be used only if there are contraindications to or significant intolerance of Rebetol in previously untreated patients

1mcg/kg/week (same day of the week) for 1 yr

DOSING CONSIDERATIONS

Renal Impairment
Moderate (CrCl 30-50mL/min): Reduce dose by 25%
Severe (CrCl 10-29mL/min), Including Hemodialysis: Reduce dose by 50%
Decline in Renal Function During Treatment: D/C therapy

Adverse Reactions
Dose Reduction:
Adults:
Combination Therapy w/ Rebetol: Reduce to 1mcg/kg/week, then to 0.5mcg/kg/week, if needed
Monotherapy: Reduce to 0.5mcg/kg/week
Pediatrics:
Reduce to 40mcg/m²/week, then to 20mcg/m²/week, if needed

Depression:
Initial Management (4-8 Weeks):
Moderate: Reduce dose; see dose reduction above
Severe: Permanently d/c PegIntron/Rebetol

Refer to PI for psychiatric visit schedule and for recommendations based on depression status after initial management

Lab Parameters:
Reduce PegIntron Dose If (See Dose Reduction Above):
WBCs 1 to <1.5 x 10⁹/L, neutrophils 0.5 to <0.75 x 10⁹/L, platelets 25 to <50 x 10⁹/L (adults) or 50 to <70 x 10⁹/L (pediatrics)

Reduce PegIntron Dose by Half If:
≥2g/dL decrease in Hgb during any 4-week period during treatment in patients w/ history of stable cardiac disease; pediatric patients should have weekly evaluations and hematology testing

D/C Therapy If:
WBCs <1 x 10⁹/L, neutrophils <0.5 x 10⁹/L, platelets <25 x 10⁹/L (adults) or <50 x 10⁹/L (pediatrics), creatinine >2mg/dL (pediatrics), Hgb in patients w/o history of cardiac disease <8.5g/dL, Hgb in patients w/ history of stable cardiac disease <8.5g/dL or <12g/dL after 4 weeks of dose reduction

Refer to PI for Rebetol dose reductions

Discontinuation
Adults:
Genotype 1:
Interferon-Alfa-Naive Receiving PegIntron, Alone or in Combination w/ Rebetol:
D/C if there is not at least a 2 log₁₀ drop or loss of HCV-RNA at 12 weeks of therapy.
D/C if HCV-RNA levels remain detectable after 24 weeks of therapy.

All Genotypes:
Previously Treated Patients:
D/C if HCV-RNA levels remain detectable at Week 12 or 24

Pediatrics
3-17 Years and Excluding Genotype 2 and 3:
D/C therapy at 12 weeks if treatment Week 12 HCV-RNA drops <2 log₁₀ compared to pretreatment.
D/C therapy at 24 weeks if HCV-RNA is detectable at treatment Week 24.

ADMINISTRATION
SQ route

Do not reuse the vial/prefilled pen; discard unused portion.
Refer to Rebetol and specific HCV NS3/4A protease inhibitor labeling for dosing and administration.

STORAGE
Redipen: 2-8°C (36-46°F). **Vial:** 25°C (77°F); excursions permitted to 15-30°C (59-86°F). **Redipen/Vial:** (Reconstituted Sol) Should be used immediately, but may store for up to 24 hrs at 2-8°C (36-46°F). Do not freeze. Keep away from heat.

HOW SUPPLIED
Inj: 50mcg/0.5mL, 80mcg/0.5mL, 120mcg/0.5mL, 150mcg/0.5mL [vial, Redipen]

CONTRAINDICATIONS
Known hypersensitivity reactions (eg, urticaria, angioedema, bronchoconstriction, anaphylaxis, Stevens-Johnson syndrome, toxic epidermal necrolysis) to interferon alpha or any other component of the product. Autoimmune hepatitis, hepatic decompensation (Child-Pugh score >6 [Class B and C]) in cirrhotic chronic hepatitis C (CHC) patients before or during treatment. When used w/ Rebetol, refer to the individual monograph.

WARNINGS/PRECAUTIONS
Caution w/ history of psychiatric disorders. Monitor during treatment and in the 6-month follow-up period if psychiatric problems develop; d/c if symptoms

persist or worsen, or if suicidal or homicidal ideation or aggressive behavior towards others is identified. Cases of encephalopathy reported in some w/ higher doses. Cardiovascular (CV) events reported; caution w/ CV disease (CVD) (eg, MI, arrhythmia). Hyperglycemia, diabetes mellitus, and new/worsening hypo/hyperthyroidism reported; do not begin/continue therapy in patients w/ these conditions who cannot be controlled w/ medication. Ophthalmologic disorders may be induced or aggravated; d/c if new or worsening ophthalmologic disorders develop. Ischemic and hemorrhagic cerebrovascular events reported. Suppresses bone marrow function; d/c if severe decreases in neutrophil or platelet counts develop. May rarely be associated w/ aplastic anemia. New/worsening of autoimmune disorders reported. Pancreatitis reported; suspend therapy w/ signs and symptoms suggestive of pancreatitis and d/c if diagnosed w/ pancreatitis. Ulcerative or hemorrhagic/ischemic colitis reported; d/c if signs/symptoms develop. Pulmonary disorders may be induced or aggravated; suspend combination treatment if pulmonary infiltrates or pulmonary function impairment develops. Caution w/ debilitating medical conditions (eg, history of pulmonary disease). CHC patients w/ cirrhosis may be at risk for hepatic decompensation and death. Cirrhotic CHC patients coinfected w/ HIV receiving highly active antiretroviral therapy (HAART) and alpha interferons w/ or w/o ribavirin may be at increased risk for hepatic decompensation compared to patients not receiving HAART. Increases SrCr levels in patients w/ renal insufficiency; monitor closely for signs and symptoms of interferon toxicity and adjust dose or d/c therapy. Use monotherapy w/ caution w/ CrCl <50mL/min. Serious, acute hypersensitivity reactions and cutaneous eruptions rarely reported; d/c treatment if such a reaction develops. Transient ALT increases and elevated TG levels reported; consider discontinuation in patients w/ persistently elevated TG levels (eg, TG >1000mg/dL). Dental/periodontal disorders reported w/ combination therapy w/ Rebetol. Weight loss and growth inhibition (including long-term growth inhibition) reported in pediatric patients during combination therapy w/ Rebetol.

ADVERSE REACTIONS
Adults: (Monotherapy or Combination Therapy w/ Rebetol) Inj-site inflammation/reaction, fatigue/asthenia, headache, rigors, fevers, N/V, myalgia, emotional lability/irritability. **Pediatric Patients:** Pyrexia, headache, vomiting, neutropenia, fatigue, anorexia, inj-site erythema, abdominal pain.

DRUG INTERACTIONS
Use caution when drugs w/ a narrow therapeutic range metabolized by CYP1A2 (eg, caffeine) or CYP2D6 (eg, thioridazine) are coadministered. Monitor blood cell count and suppressive effect on bone marrow function w/ zidovudine. Therapeutic monitoring of concomitant immunosuppressive agents recommended. May increase methadone, thioridazine, and theophylline levels; may need to reduce methadone dose, and monitor for thioridazine and theophylline adverse events. Closely monitor for toxicities, especially hepatic decompensation and anemia, when patient is receiving interferon w/ Rebetol and nucleoside reverse transcriptase inhibitors (NRTIs); consider dose reduction or discontinuation of interferon, Rebetol, or both if worsening clinical toxicities occur, or discontinuation of NRTI if medically appropriate. Concomitant use of peginterferon alpha and Rebetol w/ zidovudine may cause severe neutropenia and severe anemia. Peripheral neuropathy reported when used in combination w/ telbivudine.

PREGNANCY AND LACTATION
Pregnancy: Category C; recommended for use in fertile women only when they are using effective contraception. Category X (w/ Rebetol).
Lactation: Not for use in nursing.

MECHANISM OF ACTION
Pegylated virus proliferation inhibitor; binds to and activates the human type 1 interferon receptor. Upon binding, the receptor subunits dimerize and activate multiple intracellular signal transduction pathways.

PHARMACOKINETICS
Absorption: T_{max}=15-44 hrs. **Elimination:** $T_{1/2}$=40 hrs.

PATIENT CONSIDERATIONS
Assessment: Assess for history of MI, arrhythmia, and psychiatric disorders; presence of CVD, endocrine, autoimmune, and ophthalmologic disorders; debilitating medical conditions; hepatic/renal impairment; drug hypersensitivity; any other conditions where treatment is contraindicated or cautioned; pregnancy/nursing status; and possible drug interactions. Obtain baseline CBC, blood chemistry, and eye exam. Perform ECG in patients w/ preexisting cardiac abnormalities.
Monitoring: Monitor CBC, blood chemistry, TG levels, and HCV-RNA periodically. Monitor hepatic/renal function. Perform periodic ophthalmologic exams w/ preexisting ophthalmologic disorders. Patients should have regular dental exams. Monitor growth in pediatric patients. Monitor for signs/symptoms of autoimmune, cerebrovascular, infectious, endocrine, and pulmonary disorders; CV and neuropsychiatric events; bone marrow toxicity; hepatic decompensation; colitis; pancreatitis; hypersensitivity reactions; and other adverse reactions.
Counseling: Inform of benefits/risks of therapy and about proper instructions for use. Advise to report immediately to physician any symptoms of depression or suicidal ideation. Instruct females and female partners of male patients to avoid pregnancy during combination treatment w/ Rebetol and for 6 months post-therapy; instruct to use at least 2 forms of effective contraception and to have monthly pregnancy tests during and for 6 months post-therapy. Instruct to brush teeth thoroughly bid and to have regular dental examinations when used in combination w/ Rebetol; if vomiting occurs, advise to rinse out mouth afterwards. Inform that there are no data regarding whether therapy will prevent HCV infection transmission to others. Advise that lab evaluations are required prior to starting therapy and periodically thereafter. Advise to remain well hydrated. Counsel that flu-like symptoms associated w/ treatment may be minimized by hs administration of the drug or by using antipyretics. Inform that chest x-ray

or other tests may be needed if fever, cough, SOB, or other symptoms of a lung problem develop. Instruct self-administering patients on the importance of site selection, rotating inj sites, and proper disposal of needles, syringes, and Redipen.

PERJETA — pertuzumab   Rx
Class: Monoclonal antibody/HER2 blocker

> May result in subclinical and clinical cardiac failure manifesting as decreased left ventricular ejection fraction (LVEF) and CHF; evaluate cardiac function prior to and during treatment. D/C treatment for a confirmed clinically significant decrease in left ventricular function. Exposure during pregnancy may result in embryo-fetal death and birth defects; advise patients of these risks and the need for effective contraception.

ADULT DOSAGE
Breast Cancer
Metastatic:
Combination w/ trastuzumab and docetaxel for HER2-positive metastatic breast cancer in patients who have not received prior anti-HER2 therapy or chemotherapy for metastatic disease

Initial: 840mg IV infusion over 60 min, followed every 3 weeks by 420mg IV infusion over 30-60 min

Trastuzumab:
Initial: 8mg/kg IV infusion over 90 min, followed every 3 weeks by a dose of 6mg/kg IV infusion over 30-90 min

Docetaxel:
Initial: 75mg/m² IV infusion
Titrate: May increase to 100mg/m² administered every 3 weeks if initial dose is well tolerated

Neoadjuvant Treatment:
Combination w/ trastuzumab and docetaxel for the neoadjuvant treatment of patients w/ HER2-positive, locally advanced, inflammatory, or early stage breast cancer (either >2cm in diameter or node positive) as part of a complete treatment regimen for early breast cancer

Initial: 840mg IV infusion over 60 min, followed every 3 weeks by a dose of 420mg IV infusion over 30-60 min

Trastuzumab:
Initial: 8mg/kg IV infusion over 90 min, followed every 3 weeks by a dose of 6mg/kg IV infusion over 30-90 min

Administer every 3 weeks for 3-6 cycles as part of 1 of the following treatment regimens for early breast cancer:
4 preoperative cycles of pertuzumab in combination w/ trastuzumab and docetaxel, followed by 3 postoperative cycles of fluorouracil, epirubicin, and cyclophosphamide (FEC)
OR
3 preoperative cycles of FEC alone, followed by 3 preoperative cycles of pertuzumab in combination w/ docetaxel and trastuzumab
OR
6 preoperative cycles of pertuzumab in combination w/ docetaxel, carboplatin, and trastuzumab (escalation of docetaxel >75mg/m² is not recommended)

Following surgery, patients should continue to receive trastuzumab to complete 1 yr of treatment

Missed Dose
Time Between 2 Sequential Infusions is <6 Weeks:
Administer the 420mg pertuzumab dose; do not wait until the next planned dose

Time Between 2 Sequential Infusions is ≥6 Weeks:
Readminister initial dose of 840mg pertuzumab as a 60-min IV infusion, followed every 3 weeks thereafter by a dose of 420mg administered as an IV infusion over 30-60 min

PEDIATRIC DOSAGE
Pediatric use may not have been established

DOSING CONSIDERATIONS

Concomitant Medications
D/C pertuzumab if trastuzumab treatment is discontinued

Adverse Reactions
LVEF:
<45% or 45-49% w/ a ≥10% Absolute Decrease Below Pretreatment Value:
Withhold pertuzumab and trastuzumab dosing for ≥3 weeks. May resume if LVEF recovers to >49% or to 45-49% associated w/ <10% absolute decrease below pretreatment values. If after a repeat assessment w/in approx 3 weeks, LVEF has not improved or has declined further, d/c pertuzumab and trastuzumab, unless the benefits outweigh the risks
Infusion-Related Reactions:
May slow or interrupt the infusion
Hypersensitivity Reactions/Anaphylaxis:
D/C infusion immediately if serious hypersensitivity reaction occurs

ADMINISTRATION
IV route

Do not administer as IV push or bolus.
Do not mix w/ other drugs.
Administer pertuzumab, trastuzumab, and docetaxel sequentially.
Pertuzumab and trastuzumab can be given in any order; administer docetaxel after pertuzumab and trastuzumab.

Preparation
1. Withdraw the appropriate volume of pertuzumab sol from the vial(s).
2. Dilute into a 250mL 0.9% NaCl polyvinyl chloride (PVC) or non-PVC polyolefin infusion bag.
3. Mix diluted sol by gentle inversion; do not shake.
4. Administer immediately once prepared; if not used immediately, store at 2-8°C for up to 24 hrs.
5. Dilute w/ 0.9% NaCl inj only; do not use D5 sol.

STORAGE
2-8°C (36-46°F) until time of use. Protect from light. Do not freeze or shake.

HOW SUPPLIED
Inj: 30mg/mL [14mL]

CONTRAINDICATIONS
Known hypersensitivity to pertuzumab or to any of its excipients.

WARNINGS/PRECAUTIONS
Patients who have received prior anthracyclines or prior radiotherapy to the chest area may be at higher risk of decreased LVEF. Can cause fetal harm. Infusion-related reactions reported; observe closely for 60 min after the 1st infusion and for 30 min after subsequent infusions. Consider permanent discontinuation in patients w/ severe infusion reactions. Hypersensitivity/anaphylaxis reactions reported; medications/emergency equipment should be available for immediate use. Detection of HER2 protein overexpression is necessary for appropriate patient selection.

ADVERSE REACTIONS
Metastatic Breast Cancer in Combination w/ Trastuzumab and Docetaxel:
Diarrhea, alopecia, neutropenia, nausea, fatigue, rash, peripheral neuropathy.
Neoadjuvant Treatment in Combination w/ Trastuzumab and Docetaxel:
Alopecia, neutropenia, diarrhea, nausea.

PREGNANCY AND LACTATION
Pregnancy: Based on its mechanism of action and findings in animal studies, pertuzumab can cause fetal harm when administered to a pregnant woman. Monitor women who received pertuzumab in combination w/ trastuzumab during pregnancy or w/in 7 months prior to conception for oligohydramnios; if oligohydramnios occurs, perform fetal testing that is appropriate for gestational age and consistent w/ community standards of care. There is a pregnancy exposure registry that monitors pregnancy outcomes in women exposed to the drug during pregnancy. In addition, there is a pregnancy pharmacovigilance program.
Lactation: There is no information regarding the presence of pertuzumab in human milk, the effects on the breastfed infant, or the effects on milk production. Caution in nursing.
Reproductive Potential: Females of reproductive potential should use effective contraception during treatment and for 7 months following the last dose of pertuzumab in combination w/ trastuzumab. Verify the pregnancy status of females of reproductive potential prior to the initiation of therapy.

MECHANISM OF ACTION
Monoclonal antibody/HER2 blocker; inhibits ligand-initiated intracellular signaling pathways, which can result in cell growth arrest and apoptosis. Also mediates antibody-dependent cell-mediated cytotoxicity.

PHARMACOKINETICS
Elimination: $T_{1/2}$=18 days (median).

PATIENT CONSIDERATIONS
Assessment: Assess for hypersensitivity to drug and pregnancy/nursing status. Assess LVEF prior to initiation of therapy. Assess HER2 status; should be performed by laboratories w/ demonstrated proficiency in the specific technology being utilized.
Monitoring: Monitor for infusion-related reactions, hypersensitivity/anaphylaxis reactions, and other adverse reactions. Monitor LVEF at regular intervals (eg, every 3 months in the metastatic setting and every 6 weeks in the neoadjuvant setting).
Counseling: Advise to contact a healthcare professional immediately for new onset or worsening SOB, cough, swelling of the ankles/legs/face, palpitations,

weight gain of >5 lbs in 24 hrs, dizziness, or loss of consciousness. Advise pregnant women and females of reproductive potential that exposure to pertuzumab in combination w/ trastuzumab during pregnancy or w/in 7 months prior to conception can result in fetal harm; advise to contact healthcare provider w/ a known or suspected pregnancy. Advise women who are exposed to pertuzumab in combination w/ trastuzumab during pregnancy or w/in 7 months prior to conception that there is a pregnancy exposure registry and a pregnancy pharmacovigilance program that monitors pregnancy outcomes. Advise females of reproductive potential to use effective contraception during treatment and for 7 months following the last dose of pertuzumab in combination w/ trastuzumab.

PLEGRIDY — peginterferon beta-1a   Rx
Class: Biological response modifier

ADULT DOSAGE	PEDIATRIC DOSAGE
Multiple Sclerosis	Pediatric use may not have been established
Treatment of Relapsing Forms:	
Day 1: 63mcg SQ	
Day 15: 94mcg SQ	
On Day 29 and Thereafter: 125mcg SQ every 14 days	
Premedication	
Prophylactic and concurrent use of analgesics and/or antipyretics may prevent or ameliorate flu-like symptoms sometimes experienced during treatment	

ADMINISTRATION
SQ route

Rotate inj sites; usual sites are abdomen, back of the upper arm, and thigh. Prefilled pens and syringes are for a single dose only; discard after use.

STORAGE
2-8°C (36-46°F). Protect from light. Do not freeze; discard if frozen. Once removed from the refrigerator, allow to warm to room temperature (about 30 min) prior to inj; do not use external heat sources (eg, hot water) to warm the product. If refrigeration is unavailable, may store at 2-25°C (36-77°F) for up to 30 days; protect from light. May be removed from, and returned to, a refrigerator if necessary. The total combined time out of refrigeration, w/in a temperature range of 2-25°C (36-77°F), should not exceed 30 days.

HOW SUPPLIED
Inj: 125mcg/0.5mL [prefilled pen, prefilled syringe]; (Starter Pack) 63mcg/0.5mL, 94mcg/0.5mL [prefilled pen, prefilled syringe]

CONTRAINDICATIONS
History of hypersensitivity to natural or recombinant interferon beta or peginterferon, or any other component of the formulation.

WARNINGS/PRECAUTIONS
Elevations in hepatic enzymes and hepatic injury reported. Depression and suicidal ideation reported; consider discontinuation if depression or other severe psychiatric symptoms develop. Seizures reported. Anaphylaxis and other serious allergic reactions (eg, angioedema, urticaria) reported; d/c if a serious allergic reaction occurs. Inj-site reactions reported; decision to d/c therapy following necrosis at a single inj site should be based on the extent of the necrosis. If therapy is continued after inj-site necrosis has occurred, avoid administration near the affected area until it is fully healed; if multiple lesions occur, d/c until healing occurs. Cardiovascular (CV) events reported; monitor patients w/ significant cardiac disease for worsening of their cardiac condition during initiation and continuation of treatment. Decreased peripheral blood counts reported; monitor for infections, bleeding, and symptoms of anemia. Cases of thrombotic microangiopathy (TMA) (eg, thrombotic thrombocytopenia purpura, hemolytic uremic syndrome), some fatal, reported w/ interferon β products; d/c and manage if TMA occurs. Autoimmune disorders reported; consider discontinuation if a new autoimmune disorder develops. Monitor for adverse reactions due to increased drug exposure in patients w/ severe renal impairment.

ADVERSE REACTIONS
Inj-site erythema, influenza-like illness, pyrexia, headache, myalgia, chills, inj-site pain, asthenia, inj-site pruritus, arthralgia.

PREGNANCY AND LACTATION
Pregnancy: Category C. There is a pregnancy exposure registry that monitors fetal outcomes in women exposed to therapy during pregnancy.
Lactation: Caution in nursing.

MECHANISM OF ACTION
Biological response modifier; has not been established.

PHARMACOKINETICS
Absorption: T_{max}=1-1.5 days; C_{max}=280pg/mL; AUC=34.8ng•hr/mL. **Distribution:** V_d=481L. **Elimination:** Renal; $T_{1/2}$=78 hrs.

PATIENT CONSIDERATIONS
Assessment: Assess for seizure disorder, cardiac disease, myelosuppression, renal/hepatic impairment, history of hypersensitivity to drug, and pregnancy/nursing status.
Monitoring: Monitor for signs/symptoms of hepatic injury; depression, suicidal ideation, or other severe psychiatric symptoms; seizures; serious allergic reactions; inj-site reactions/necrosis; CV events or worsening of cardiac condition; TMA,

autoimmune disorders; and other adverse reactions. Monitor for infections, bleeding, and symptoms of anemia. Monitor CBCs, differential WBC count, and platelet counts; patients w/ myelosuppression may require more intensive monitoring. Monitor for adverse reactions due to increased drug exposure in patients w/ severe renal impairment.

Counseling: Advise not to change the dose or schedule of administration w/o medical consultation. Instruct on how to self-inject therapy and inform of the proper procedures to follow. Advise to rotate areas of inj w/ each dose, and not to inject into an area of the body where the skin is irritated, reddened, bruised, infected, or scarred in any way. Instruct to check the inj site after 2 hrs for redness, swelling, and tenderness, and to contact physician if a skin reaction occurs and does not clear up in a few days. Advise to inform physician if pregnant/breastfeeding. Encourage patients to enroll in the pregnancy registry if they become pregnant while taking therapy. Inform of the symptoms of hepatic dysfunction, depression, suicidal ideation, seizures, and worsening cardiac condition, and instruct to immediately report any of these symptoms to physician. Instruct to seek immediate medical attention if symptoms of allergic reactions and anaphylaxis occur. Advise that inj-site reactions may occur and to promptly report any signs of necrosis at inj site. Inform that flu-like symptoms are common following initiation of therapy.

POMALYST — pomalidomide
Rx

Class: Thalidomide analogue

> Contraindicated in pregnancy; may cause severe birth defects or embryo-fetal death. Females of reproductive potential should have 2 negative pregnancy tests before starting treatment and must use 2 forms of contraception or continuously abstain from heterosexual sex during and for 4 weeks after stopping treatment. Available only through a restricted distribution program called Pomalyst Risk Evaluation and Mitigation Strategy. Deep vein thrombosis, pulmonary embolism, MI, and stroke reported; thromboprophylaxis is recommended, and the choice of regimen should be based on assessment of the patient's underlying risk factors.

ADULT DOSAGE
Multiple Myeloma

In combination w/ dexamethasone, for patients who have received ≥2 prior therapies including lenalidomide and a proteasome inhibitor and have demonstrated disease progression on or w/in 60 days of completion of the last therapy

Initial: 4mg qd on Days 1-21 of repeated 28-day cycles until disease progression

PEDIATRIC DOSAGE
Pediatric use may not have been established

DOSING CONSIDERATIONS
Concomitant Medications
Strong CYP1A2 Inhibitors: Avoid concomitant use; consider alternative treatments. If a strong CYP1A2 inhibitor must be used, reduce pomalidomide dose by 50%

Renal Impairment
Severe Renal Impairment Requiring Dialysis:
Initial: 3mg qd (25% dose reduction); take pomalidomide after completion of dialysis procedure on hemodialysis days

Hepatic Impairment
Mild or Moderate (Child-Pugh Classes A or B):
Initial: 3mg qd (25% dose reduction)

Severe (Child-Pugh Class C):
Initial: 2mg qd (50% dose reduction)

Adverse Reactions
Neutropenia:
ANC <500/μL or Febrile Neutropenia (Fever ≥38.5°C and ANC <1000/μL): Interrupt treatment; follow CBC weekly
ANC Return to ≥500/μL: Resume treatment at 3mg/day
For Each Subsequent Drop <500/μL: Interrupt treatment
Return to ≥500/μL: Resume treatment at 1mg less than previous dose

Thrombocytopenia:
Platelets <25,000/μL: Interrupt treatment; follow CBC weekly
Platelets Return to >50,000/μL: Resume treatment at 3mg daily
For Each Subsequent Drop <25,000/μL: Interrupt treatment
Return to ≥50,000/μL: Resume treatment at 1mg less than previous dose

To initiate a new cycle, neutrophil count must be at least 500/μL and platelet count must be at least 50,000/μL; if toxicities occur after dose reductions to 1mg, then d/c treatment

Angioedema, Skin Exfoliation, Bullae, or Any Other Severe Dermatologic Reaction: Permanently d/c

Other Grade 3 or 4 Toxicities: Hold treatment and restart at 1mg less than previous dose when toxicity has resolved to ≤Grade 2

ADMINISTRATION
Oral route

May take w/ water.
May be taken w/ or w/o food.
Do not break, chew, or open caps.

STORAGE
20-25°C (68-77°F); excursions permitted to 15-30°C (59-86°F).

HOW SUPPLIED
Cap: 1mg, 2mg, 3mg, 4mg

CONTRAINDICATIONS
Pregnancy.

WARNINGS/PRECAUTIONS
See Dosing Considerations. Avoid blood donation during treatment and for 1 month following discontinuation. Greater risk of arterial thromboembolism and venous thromboembolism (VTE) may exist in patients w/ known risk factors (eg, prior thrombosis); try to minimize all modifiable factors (eg, hyperlipidemia, HTN, smoking). Neutropenia, anemia, and thrombocytopenia reported; may require dose interruption and/or modification. Monitor CBC weekly for the first 8 weeks of therapy and monthly thereafter. Hepatic failure, including fatal cases, and elevated levels of ALT and bilirubin reported; monitor LFTs monthly. D/C therapy upon elevation of liver enzymes and evaluate; after return to baseline values, consider treatment at a lower dose. Angioedema and severe dermatologic reactions reported. Dizziness, confusional state, and neuropathy reported. Cases of acute myelogenous leukemia reported in patients receiving pomalidomide as an investigational therapy outside of multiple myeloma. Tumor lysis syndrome (TLS) may occur; caution in patients w/ high tumor burden prior to treatment.

ADVERSE REACTIONS
Fatigue/asthenia, neutropenia, anemia, constipation, diarrhea, nausea, URTI, back pain, dyspnea, pyrexia.

DRUG INTERACTIONS
See Dosing Considerations. Coadministration of fluvoxamine, a strong CYP1A2 inhibitor, increased levels, which increases the risk of exposure-related toxicities. Cigarette smoking may reduce exposure due to CYP1A2 induction and may reduce efficacy.

PREGNANCY AND LACTATION
Pregnancy: Based on the mechanism of action and findings from animal studies, Pomalyst can cause embryo-fetal harm when administered to a pregnant female and is contraindicated during pregnancy. There is a pregnancy exposure registry that monitors pregnancy outcomes in females exposed to Pomalyst during pregnancy as well as female partners of male patients who are exposed to Pomalyst.

Lactation: Not for use in nursing.

Reproductive Potential:
Pregnancy Testing: Verify the pregnancy status of females of reproductive potential prior to initiating therapy and for at least 4 weeks after completing therapy; avoid pregnancy while on therapy. Females of reproductive potential must have 2 negative pregnancy tests before initiating therapy; the 1st test should be performed w/in 10-14 days, and the 2nd test w/in 24 hrs prior to prescribing Pomalyst. Once treatment has started and during dose interruptions, pregnancy testing for females of reproductive potential should occur weekly during the first 4 weeks of use, then be repeated every 4 weeks (females w/ regular menstrual cycles), or every 2 weeks (irregular menstrual cycles).
Contraception: (Females) Females of reproductive potential must commit either to abstain continuously from heterosexual sexual intercourse or to use 2 methods of reliable birth control simultaneously (1 highly effective form of contraception and 1 additional effective contraceptive method). Contraception must begin 4 weeks prior to initiating treatment and must continue during therapy, during dose interruptions, and for 4 weeks following discontinuation of therapy. (Males) Pomalidomide is present in the semen of males; must always use a latex or synthetic condom during any sexual contact w/ females of reproductive potential while on therapy and for up to 4 weeks after discontinuing therapy, even if they have undergone a successful vasectomy. Must not donate sperm.
Infertility: Based on findings in animals, female fertility may be compromised by treatment.

Refer to PI for further details on pregnancy testing/contraception.

MECHANISM OF ACTION
Thalidomide analogue; immunomodulatory agent w/ antineoplastic activity. Enhances T cell- and natural killer cell-mediated immunity and inhibits production of pro-inflammatory cytokines (eg, TNF-α and IL-6) by monocytes.

PHARMACOKINETICS
Absorption: T_{max}=2-3 hrs; AUC=860ng•hr/mL; C_{max}=75ng/mL. **Distribution:** V_d=62-138L; plasma protein binding (12-44%). **Metabolism:** Liver via CYP1A2 and CYP3A4 (major), CYP2C19 and CYP2D6 (minor). **Elimination:** Urine (73%, 2% unchanged), feces (15%, 8% unchanged); $T_{1/2}$=approx 7.5 hrs (median).

PATIENT CONSIDERATIONS
Assessment: Assess nursing status, renal/hepatic function, and for risk factors for arterial thromboembolism or VTE, high tumor burden, and possible drug interactions. Obtain pregnancy test 10-14 days before and 24 hrs prior to therapy.

Monitoring: Perform pregnancy test weekly during 1st month, then monthly thereafter (regular menstrual cycle) or every 2 weeks (irregular menstrual cycle). Monitor CBC weekly for the first 8 weeks of therapy and monthly thereafter. Monitor LFTs monthly. Monitor for signs/symptoms of arterial thromboembolism, VTE, hematologic toxicities (especially neutropenia), hypersensitivity reactions, dizziness, confusional state, neuropathy, second primary malignancies, TLS, and for other adverse reactions.

Counseling: Instruct females of reproductive potential to avoid pregnancy while on therapy and for at least 4 weeks after completing therapy, to have monthly pregnancy tests, and to use 2 different forms of contraception, including at least 1 highly effective form simultaneously during therapy, during dose interruption, and for 4 weeks after completing therapy. Instruct to immediately d/c and contact physician if patient becomes pregnant, misses her menstrual period, experiences unusual menstrual bleeding, or she stops taking birth control. Instruct males (including those w/ vasectomy) to always use latex/synthetic condoms during any sexual contact w/ females of reproductive potential during therapy and for up to 4 weeks after discontinuation. Advise males not to donate sperm. Instruct all patients not to donate blood during therapy and for 1 month following discontinuation. Inform females that there is a pregnancy exposure registry that monitors pregnancy outcomes in females exposed to pomalidomide during pregnancy. Inform of the other risks associated w/ therapy. Instruct to avoid situations where dizziness or confusional state may be a problem and not to take other medications that may cause dizziness or confusional state w/o adequate medical advice. Instruct to take ud. Advise patients that smoking tobacco may reduce the efficacy of the drug.

PORTRAZZA — necitumumab   Rx

Class: Monoclonal antibody/EGFR blocker

Cardiopulmonary arrest and/or sudden death reported. Closely monitor serum electrolytes, including serum Mg+, K+, and Ca+ w/ aggressive replacement when warranted during and after administration. Hypomagnesemia reported; monitor patients for hypomagnesemia, hypocalcemia, and hypokalemia prior to each dose during treatment and for at least 8 weeks following completion. Withhold for Grade 3 or 4 electrolyte abnormalities. Replete electrolytes as medically appropriate.

ADULT DOSAGE

Metastatic Squamous Non-Small Cell Lung Cancer

1st-Line Treatment in Combination w/ Gemcitabine and Cisplatin:
800mg IV over 60 min on Days 1 and 8 of each 3-week cycle prior to gemcitabine and cisplatin infusion

Continue until disease progression or unacceptable toxicity

Premedication

Previous Grade 1 or 2 Infusion-Related Reaction (IRR):
Premedicate w/ diphenhydramine hydrochloride (or equivalent) prior to all subsequent infusions

2nd Grade 1 or 2 Occurrence of IRR:
Premedicate for all subsequent infusions, w/ diphenhydramine hydrochloride (or equivalent), acetaminophen (or equivalent), and dexamethasone (or equivalent) prior to each infusion

PEDIATRIC DOSAGE
Pediatric use may not have been established

DOSING CONSIDERATIONS
Adverse Reactions
IRR:
Grade 1: Reduce the infusion rate by 50%
Grade 2: Stop the infusion until signs and symptoms have resolved to Grade 0 or 1; resume at 50% reduced rate for all subsequent infusions
Grade 3 or 4: Permanently d/c

Dermatologic Toxicity:
Grade 3 Rash or Acneiform Rash: Withhold until symptoms resolve to Grade ≤2, then resume at reduced dose of 400mg for at least 1 treatment cycle. If symptoms do not worsen, may increase dose to 600mg and 800mg in subsequent cycles

Permanently D/C If:
- Grade 3 rash or acneiform rash does not resolve to Grade ≤2 w/in 6 weeks
- Reactions worsen or become intolerable at a dose of 400mg
- Patient experiences Grade 3 skin induration/fibrosis
- Patient experiences Grade 4 dermatologic toxicity

ADMINISTRATION
IV route

Administer via infusion pump over 60 min through a separate infusion line; flush the line w/ 0.9% NaCl inj at the end of infusion.

Preparation for Administration
1. Dilute the required volume of necitumumab w/ 0.9% NaCl inj, in an IV infusion container to a final volume of 250mL; do not use sol containing dextrose.
2. Gently invert the container to ensure adequate mixing.
3. Do not freeze or shake the infusion sol. Do not dilute w/ other sol or co-infuse w/ other electrolytes or medication.
4. Store diluted infusion sol for no >24 hrs at 2-8°C (36-46°F), or no >4 hrs at room temperature (up to 25°C [77°F]).
5. Discard vial w/ any unused portion.

STORAGE
2-8°C (36-46°F). Protect from light. Do not freeze or shake the vial.

HOW SUPPLIED
Inj: 800mg/50mL

WARNINGS/PRECAUTIONS
See Dosing Considerations. Once electrolyte abnormalities and hypomagnesemia improve to Grade ≤2, subsequent cycles may be administered. Venous thromboembolic events (VTEs) and arterial thromboembolic events (ATEs) reported w/ combination treatment; d/c in patients w/ serious/life-threatening VTE or ATE. The most common ATEs were cerebral stroke, ischemia, and MI. Dermatologic toxicities, including rash, dermatitis acneiform, acne, dry skin,

pruritus, generalized rash, skin fissures, maculopapular rash, and erythema reported; limit sun exposure. IRR reported; d/c for serious or life-threatening IRR. Not indicated for the treatment of patients w/ non-squamous non-small cell lung cancer. May cause fetal harm.

ADVERSE REACTIONS
Rash, vomiting, diarrhea, dermatitis acneiform.

PREGNANCY AND LACTATION
Pregnancy: Can cause fetal harm.
Lactation: Do not breastfeed during treatment and for 3 months following the final dose.
Reproductive Potential: Females of reproductive potential should use effective contraception during treatment and for 3 months following the final dose.

MECHANISM OF ACTION
Recombinant human IgG1 monoclonal antibody; binds to EGFR and blocks the binding of EGFR to its ligands. Binding of necitumumab induces EGFR internalization and degradation in vitro. In vitro, binding of necitumumab also led to antibody-dependent cellular cytotoxicity in EGFR-expressing cells.

PHARMACOKINETICS
Distribution: V_d=7.0L. **Elimination:** $T_{1/2}$=14 days.

PATIENT CONSIDERATIONS
Assessment: Assess for presence or history of cardiopulmonary and dermatologic disease, pregnancy/nursing status, and for possible drug interactions. Obtain serum electrolyte levels (Mg^{2+}, K^+, Ca^{2+}).
Monitoring: Monitor for signs/symptoms of cardiopulmonary arrest, dermatologic toxicities, IRR, VTEs/ATEs, and other adverse reactions. Monitor electrolytes (eg, hypomagnesemia, hypokalemia, hypocalcemia) periodically during and for up to 8 weeks after completion of therapy.
Counseling: Advise patients of risk of decreased blood levels of Mg^{2+}, K^+, and Ca^{2+} and instruct to take medicines to replace the electrolytes exactly as advised. Inform of the increased risk of VTEs/ATEs. Instruct to minimize sun exposure w/ protective clothing and use of sunscreen. Advise to report if signs/symptoms of an infusion reaction develop. Instruct to notify physician if pregnant or nursing; inform of the potential risk to a fetus and instruct to not breastfeed during treatment and for 3 months following final dose. Advise of the need for adequate contraception in females during therapy and for 3 months after the last dose.

PRALUENT — alirocumab   Rx

Class: Proprotein Convertase Subtilisin Kexin Type 9 (PCSK9) Inhibitor

ADULT DOSAGE
Primary Hyperlipidemia
Adjunct to diet and maximally tolerated statin therapy for the treatment of patients w/ heterozygous familial hypercholesterolemia or clinical atherosclerotic cardiovascular disease, who require additional lowering of LDL-C

Initial: 75mg SQ once every 2 weeks
Titrate: May increase to max dose if LDL-C response is inadequate
Max: 150mg every 2 weeks

Missed Dose
If a dose is missed, administer the inj w/in 7 days from the missed dose and then resume the original schedule. If the missed dose is not administered w/in 7 days, wait until the next dose on the original schedule

PEDIATRIC DOSAGE
Pediatric use may not have been established

ADMINISTRATION
SQ route

Allow alirocumab to warm to room temperature for 30-40 min prior to use; use as soon as possible after it has warmed up. Do not use if it has been at room temperature for ≥24 hrs.
Administer in the thigh, abdomen, or upper arm; rotate inj site w/ each inj.
Do not inject into areas of active skin disease or injury (eg, sunburns, skin rashes, inflammation, skin infections).
Do not coadminister w/ other injectable drugs at the same inj site.

STORAGE
2-8°C (36-46°F). Store in the outer carton in order to protect from light. Do not freeze. Do not expose to extreme heat. Do not shake.

HOW SUPPLIED
Inj: 75mg/mL, 150mg/mL [prefilled pen, prefilled syringe]

CONTRAINDICATIONS
History of a serious hypersensitivity reaction to alirocumab.

WARNINGS/PRECAUTIONS
Hypersensitivity reactions, including some serious events (eg, hypersensitivity vasculitis and hypersensitivity reactions requiring hospitalization), reported; if signs/symptoms of serious allergic reactions occur, d/c treatment, treat according to the standard of care, and monitor until signs/symptoms resolve.

ADVERSE REACTIONS

Nasopharyngitis, inj-site reactions, influenza, UTI, diarrhea, bronchitis, myalgia, muscle spasms, sinusitis.

PREGNANCY AND LACTATION

Pregnancy: FDA's experience w/ monoclonal antibodies in humans indicates that they are unlikely to cross the placenta in the 1st trimester; however, they are likely to cross the placenta in increasing amounts in the 2nd and 3rd trimester. Consider the benefits and risks of alirocumab and possible risks to the fetus before prescribing to pregnant women.

Lactation: There is no information regarding the presence of alirocumab in human milk, the effects on the breastfed infant, or the effects on milk production; caution in nursing.

MECHANISM OF ACTION

Human monoclonal antibody (IgG1 isotype) that targets PCSK9; PCSK9 binds to the low-density lipoprotein receptors (LDLRs) on the surface of hepatocytes to promote LDLR degradation w/in the liver. By inhibiting the binding of PCSK9 to LDLR, alirocumab increases the number of LDLRs available to clear LDL, thereby lowering LDL-C levels.

PHARMACOKINETICS

Absorption: Absolute bioavailability (85%); T_{max}=3-7 days (median). **Distribution:** (IV) V_d=0.04-0.05L/kg. **Metabolism:** Expected to degrade to small peptides and individual amino acids. Does not affect CYP450 enzymes, P-gp, and OATP. **Elimination:** $T_{1/2}$=17-20 days (median).

PATIENT CONSIDERATIONS

Assessment: Assess for drug hypersensitivity and pregnancy/nursing status. Obtain baseline lipid levels.

Monitoring: Monitor for hypersensitivity reactions. Measure LDL-C levels w/in 4-8 weeks of initiating or titrating therapy.

Counseling: Instruct on proper inj technique, including aseptic technique, and how to use the prefilled pen/syringe correctly; inform that it may take up to 20 sec to inject alirocumab. Caution that the prefilled pen/syringe must not be reused and inform about the proper technique of disposal in a puncture-resistant container. Advise to d/c therapy and seek prompt medical attention if any signs/symptoms of serious allergic reactions occur.

PREGNYL — chorionic gonadotropin   **Rx**

Class: Human chorionic gonadotropin

ADULT DOSAGE	**PEDIATRIC DOSAGE**
Hypogonadism	**Prepubertal Cryptorchidism**
Hypogonadotropic Hypogonadism in Males:	**Not Due to Anatomical Obstruction:**
Regimen 1:	**4-9 Years:**
500-1000 U 3X/week for 3 weeks, followed by the same dose twice a week for 3 weeks	**Regimen 1:** 4000 U 3X/week for 3 weeks
Regimen 2:	**Regimen 2:** 5000 U every 2nd day for 4 inj
4000 U 3X/week for 6-9 months, followed by a reduced dose of 2000 U 3X/week for an additional 3 months	**Regimen 3:** 15 inj for 500-1000 U over a period of 6 weeks
Ovulation Induction	**Regimen 4:**
Induction of ovulation and pregnancy in anovulatory, infertile women in whom anovulation is secondary and not due to primary ovarian failure, and who have been appropriately pretreated w/ human menotropins	500 U 3X/week for 4-6 weeks; if this course is not successful, begin another series 1 month later w/ 1000 U/inj
Usual: 5000-10,000 U 1 day following the last dose of menotropins	

ADMINISTRATION

IM route

Reconstitution

Withdraw sterile air from lyophilized vial and inject into diluent vial
Remove 1-10mL from diluent and add to lyophilized vial; agitate gently until powder is completely dissolved in sol
Use completely after reconstitution

STORAGE

15-30°C (59-89°F). Reconstituted solution is stable for 60 days when refrigerated.

HOW SUPPLIED

Inj: 10,000 U [10mL]

CONTRAINDICATIONS

Precocious puberty, prostatic carcinoma, or other androgen-dependent neoplasm.

WARNINGS/PRECAUTIONS

Not effective as adjunctive therapy in the treatment of obesity. Should be used in conjunction with human menopausal gonadotropins only by experienced physicians. Anaphylaxis, ovarian hyperstimulation (ovarian enlargement, ascites with/without pain, and/or pleural effusion), rupture of ovarian cysts with resultant hemoperitoneum, multiple births, and arterial thromboembolism reported. May cause fluid retention; caution with cardiac or renal disease, epilepsy, migraine, or asthma. May induce precocious puberty in pediatrics treated for cryptorchidism; d/c if signs of precocious puberty occurs. Should only be used by physicians experienced with infertility problems.

ADVERSE REACTIONS

Headache, irritability, restlessness, depression, fatigue, edema, precocious puberty, gynecomastia, injection-site pain, hypersensitivity reactions.

PREGNANCY AND LACTATION

Safety in pregnancy and nursing not known.

MECHANISM OF ACTION

Human chorionic gonadotropin; stimulates production of gonadal steroid hormones by stimulating interstitial cells (Leydig cells) of testis to produce androgens and the ovary's corpus luteum to produce progesterone.

PATIENT CONSIDERATIONS

Assessment: Assess for drug hypersensitivity, precocious puberty, prostatic carcinoma, androgen-dependent neoplasms, cardiac/renal disease, epilepsy, migraine, asthma, pregnancy status.

Monitoring: Monitor for ovarian hyperstimulation/enlargement, ascites, pleural effusion, rupture of preexisting ovarian cysts, multiple births, arterial thromboembolism, fluid retention, precocious puberty in pediatrics, and hypersensitivity reactions.

Counseling: Counsel about potential side effects. Inform that drug is not effective as adjunct in the treatment of obesity.

PREZCOBIX — cobicistat/darunavir   **Rx**

Class: CYP3A inhibitor/protease inhibitor

ADULT DOSAGE	**PEDIATRIC DOSAGE**
HIV-1 Infection	Pediatric use may not have been established
In treatment-naive and treatment-experienced patients w/ no darunavir resistance-associated substitutions	
1 tab qd; administer in conjunction w/ other antiretroviral agents	
HIV Genotypic Testing Prior to Initiation of Therapy:	
Recommended for antiretroviral treatment-experienced patients; when genotypic testing is not feasible, therapy may be used in protease inhibitor-naive patients, but is not recommended in protease inhibitor-experienced patients	

DOSING CONSIDERATIONS

Renal Impairment

CrCl <70mL/min: Do not coadminister w/ tenofovir disoproxil fumarate (TDF)

Hepatic Impairment

Severe: Not recommended

ADMINISTRATION

Oral route

Take w/ food.

STORAGE

20-25°C (68-77°F); excursions permitted to 15-30°C (59-86°F).

HOW SUPPLIED

Tab: (Darunavir/Cobicistat) 800mg/150mg

CONTRAINDICATIONS

Concomitant use w/ alfuzosin, ranolazine, dronedarone, colchicine (in patients w/ renal and/or hepatic impairment), rifampin, lurasidone, pimozide, dihydroergotamine, ergotamine, methylergonovine, cisapride, St. John's wort, lovastatin, simvastatin, sildenafil (when used to treat pulmonary arterial HTN), oral midazolam, or triazolam due to the potential for serious and/or life-threatening events or loss of therapeutic effect.

WARNINGS/PRECAUTIONS

Redistribution/accumulation of body fat, immune reconstitution syndrome, and autoimmune disorders (eg, Graves' disease, polymyositis, Guillain-Barre syndrome) in the setting of immune reconstitution reported. Caution in elderly. **Darunavir:** Drug-induced hepatitis and liver injury, including some fatalities, reported. Consider performing increased AST/ALT monitoring in patients w/ underlying chronic hepatitis, cirrhosis, or those w/ pretreatment transaminase elevations, especially during the 1st several months of treatment. Consider interruption or discontinuation of therapy if evidence of new/worsening liver dysfunction occurs. Severe skin reactions (eg, Stevens-Johnson syndrome, toxic epidermal necrolysis, drug rash w/ eosinophilia and systemic symptoms), accompanied by fever and/or transaminase elevations in some cases, reported; d/c immediately if signs/symptoms of severe skin reactions develop. Contains a sulfonamide moiety; monitor patients w/ a known sulfonamide allergy. May develop new onset diabetes mellitus (DM), exacerbation of preexisting DM, hyperglycemia, and diabetic ketoacidosis; may require either initiation or dose adjustments of insulin or oral hypoglycemic agents. Increased bleeding including spontaneous skin hematomas and hemarthrosis reported in patients w/ hemophilia type A and B. **Cobicistat:** Decreases estimated CrCl; consider effect when interpreting changes in CrCl in patients initiating therapy particularly in patients w/ medical conditions or receiving drugs needing monitoring w/ estimated CrCl. Closely monitor patients w/ confirmed increase in SrCr >0.4mg/dL from baseline for renal safety.

ADVERSE REACTIONS
Darunavir: Diarrhea, N/V, rash, headache, abdominal pain.
Cobicistat: Refer to cobicistat PI for adverse reactions reported w/ cobicistat.

DRUG INTERACTIONS
See Dosing Considerations and Contraindications. Coadministration w/ TDF in combination w/ concomitant or recent use of a nephrotoxic agent is not recommended. Coadministration w/ drugs that are primarily metabolized by CYP3A and/or CYP2D6 or are substrates of P-gp, BCRP, OATP1B1, or OATP1B3 may increase plasma concentrations of such drugs, which could increase or prolong their therapeutic effect and can be associated w/ adverse events. CYP3A inducers may decrease levels, which may lead to loss of therapeutic effect and development of resistance. CYP3A inhibitors may increase levels. Give didanosine 1 hr before or 2 hrs after administration w/ therapy. Not recommended w/ products containing the individual components of Prezcobix, ritonavir (RTV), other antiretroviral drugs that require pharmacokinetic boosting (eg, another protease inhibitor, elvitegravir), efavirenz, etravirine, nevirapine, apixaban, dabigatran etexilate (in specific renal impairment groups), rivaroxaban, rifapentine, boceprevir, simeprevir, telaprevir, everolimus, avanafil, salmeterol, or voriconazole. Caution w/ SSRIs and w/ narcotics used for treatment of opioid dependence (buprenorphine, buprenorphine/naloxone, methadone). May increase levels of maraviroc, antiarrhythmics, digoxin, dasatinib, nilotinib, vinblastine, vincristine, anticonvulsants metabolized by CYP3A (eg, carbamazepine, clonazepam), TCAs, itraconazole, ketoconazole, trazodone, colchicine, rifabutin, antipsychotics (eg, perphenazine, risperidone, thioridazine), quetiapine, β-blockers, calcium channel blockers, corticosteroids, bosentan, atorvastatin, fluvastatin, pravastatin, rosuvastatin, immunosuppressants (cyclosporine, sirolimus, tacrolimus), narcotic analgesics metabolized by CYP3A (eg, fentanyl, oxycodone), tramadol, PDE-5 inhibitors, sedatives/hypnotics metabolized by CYP3A (eg, buspirone, diazepam, estazolam), clarithromycin, erythromycin, and telithromycin. Itraconazole, ketoconazole, posaconazole, clarithromycin, erythromycin, and telithromycin may increase levels. Monitor INR w/ warfarin. Monitor phenobarbital or phenytoin levels. Monitor for a potential decrease of antimalarial efficacy or potential QT prolongation if coadministered w/ artemether/lumefantrine. Coadministration w/ inhaled/nasal fluticasone or other corticosteroids that are metabolized by CYP3A may result in reduced serum cortisol concentrations. Coadministration w/ corticosteroids that are metabolized by CYP3A, particularly long-term use, may increase the risk of development of systemic corticosteroid effects. Coadministration w/ dexamethasone or other corticosteroids that induce CYP3A may result in loss therapeutic effect and development of resistance to darunavir. Consider additional or alternative (nonhormonal) forms of contraception if taking hormonal contraceptives. Coadministration w/ parenteral midazolam should be done in a setting that ensures close clinical monitoring and appropriate medical management in case of respiratory depression and/or prolonged sedation. Bosentan may decrease levels. **Cobicistat:** Renal impairment, including cases of acute renal failure and Fanconi syndrome, reported when used in an antiretroviral regimen w/ TDF. Anticonvulsants that induce CYP3A (eg, carbamazepine, oxcarbazepine, phenobarbital) may decrease levels; consider alternative anticonvulsant or antiretroviral therapy, and if coadministration is necessary, monitor for lack or loss of virologic response. Refer to PI for further detailed information on drug interactions, including dosing modifications required when used w/ certain concomitant therapies.

PREGNANCY AND LACTATION
Pregnancy: Category C. Physicians are encouraged to register patients in the Antiretroviral Pregnancy Registry.
Lactation: Not for use in nursing.

MECHANISM OF ACTION
Darunavir: Protease inhibitor; selectively inhibits the cleavage of HIV-1 encoded Gag-Pol polyproteins in infected cells, thereby preventing the formation of mature virus particles. **Cobicistat:** CYP3A inhibitor; inhibits CYP3A-mediated metabolism by cobicistat that enhances the systemic exposure of CYP3A substrates.

PHARMACOKINETICS
Absorption: (Fed) Darunavir: T_{max}=4-4.5 hrs. (Fed) Cobicistat: T_{max}=4-5 hrs.
Distribution: Darunavir: Plasma protein binding (95%). Cobicistat: Plasma protein binding (97-98%). **Metabolism:** Darunavir: Liver (extensive); oxidation via CYP3A. Cobicistat: CYP3A, CYP2D6 (minor). **Elimination:** Darunavir/RTV: Feces (79.5%, 41.2% unchanged), urine (13.9%, 7.7% unchanged); Darunavir: $T_{1/2}$=7 hrs (fed state). Cobicistat: Feces (86.2%), urine (8.2%); $T_{1/2}$=4 hrs (fed state).

PATIENT CONSIDERATIONS
Assessment: Assess for hypersensitivity to drug, sulfonamide allergy, liver dysfunction, autoimmune disorders, hemophilia, preexisting DM, pregnancy/nursing status, and possible drug interactions. Assess estimated CrCl. When coadministering w/ TDF, assess estimated CrCl, urine glucose, and urine protein at baseline. If feasible, perform HIV genotypic testing in antiretroviral treatment-experienced patients.

Monitoring: Monitor for signs/symptoms of hepatotoxicity, severe skin reactions, new onset/worsening renal impairment when coadministered w/ TDF, new onset/exacerbation of DM, hyperglycemia, diabetic ketoacidosis, fat redistribution/accumulation, immune reconstitution syndrome, autoimmune disorders, and other adverse reactions. In patients w/ hemophilia, monitor for bleeding events. Consider performing increased AST/ALT monitoring in patients w/ underlying chronic hepatitis, cirrhosis, or those w/ pretreatment transaminase elevations, especially during the 1st several months of treatment. Monitor INR during coadministration w/ warfarin. Perform routine monitoring of estimated CrCl, urine glucose, and urine protein when used w/ TDF. Measure serum phosphorus in patients w/ or at risk for renal impairment when used w/ TDF.

Counseling: Inform that therapy is not a cure for HIV and that patient may continue to experience illnesses associated w/ HIV-1 infection. Advise to avoid doing things that can spread HIV infection to others. Instruct to take w/ food qd as prescribed. Instruct not to alter dose or d/c w/o consulting physician. Counsel to take drug immediately for missed dose <12 hrs and to take the next dose at regular scheduled time. Instruct that if a dose is missed by >12 hrs, to take the next dose as scheduled; instruct not to double the dose. Advise about the signs/symptoms of liver problems. Inform that mild to severe skin reactions may develop; advise to immediately contact physician if signs/symptoms of severe skin reactions develop. Inform that renal impairment, including cases of acute renal failure and Fanconi syndrome, has been reported when used in combination w/ TDF-containing regimen. Instruct to notify physician of the use of any other prescription, OTC, or herbal medication. Instruct patients receiving hormonal contraceptives to use additional or alternative contraceptive (non-hormonal) measures during therapy. Inform that redistribution and accumulation of body fat may occur.

PREZISTA — darunavir   Rx
Class: Protease inhibitor

ADULT DOSAGE	PEDIATRIC DOSAGE
HIV-1 Infection	**HIV-1 Infection**
Coadministered w/ Ritonavir (RTV) and in Combination w/ Other Antiretrovirals:	**Coadministered w/ RTV and in Combination w/ Other Antiretrovirals:**
Treatment-Naive: 800mg (8mL) + RTV 100mg (1.25mL) qd	**3 to <18 Years: Treatment-Naive Patients or Treatment-Experienced Patients w/ No Darunavir Resistance Associated Substitutions:**
Treatment-Experienced: No Darunavir Resistance Associated Substitutions: 800mg (8mL) + RTV 100mg (1.25mL) qd	**Weight-Based Dose:** 35mg/kg + RTV 7mg/kg qd using the following recommendations
≥1 Darunavir Resistance Associated Substitutions or w/ No Baseline Resistance Information: 600mg (6mL) + RTV 100mg (1.25mL) bid	**≥10 to <11kg:** 350mg (3.6mL) + RTV 64mg (0.8mL) qd
	≥11 to <12kg: 385mg (4mL) + RTV 64mg (0.8mL) qd
	≥12 to <13kg: 420mg (4.2mL) + RTV 80mg (1mL) qd
	≥13 to <14kg: 455mg (4.6mL) + RTV 80mg (1mL) qd
	≥14 to <15kg: 490mg (5mL) + RTV 96mg (1.2mL) qd
	≥15 to <30kg: 600mg (6mL) + RTV 100mg (1.25mL) qd
	≥30 to <40kg: 675mg (6.8mL) + RTV 100mg (1.25mL) qd
	≥40kg: 800mg (8mL) + RTV 100mg (1.25mL) qd
	Treatment-Experienced Patients w/ ≥1 Darunavir Resistance Associated Substitution:
	Weight-Based Dose: 20mg/kg + RTV 3mg/kg bid using the following recommendations
	≥10 to <11kg: 200mg (2mL) + RTV 32mg (0.4mL) bid
	≥11 to <12kg: 220mg (2.2mL) + RTV 32mg (0.4mL) bid
	≥12 to <13kg: 240mg (2.4mL) + RTV 40mg (0.5mL) bid
	≥13 to <14kg: 260mg (2.6mL) + RTV 40mg (0.5mL) bid
	≥14 to <15kg: 280mg (2.8mL) + RTV 48mg (0.6mL) bid
	≥15 to <30kg: 375mg (3.8mL) + RTV 48mg (0.6mL) bid
	≥30 to <40kg: 450mg (4.6mL) + RTV 60mg (0.75mL) bid
	≥40kg: 600mg (6mL) + RTV 100mg (1.25mL) bid
	Dose should not exceed the recommended dose for adults

DOSING CONSIDERATIONS
Hepatic Impairment
Mild-Moderate: No dose adjustment required
Severe: Not recommended

Pregnancy
Recommended Dose: 600mg + RTV 100mg bid
Only consider 800mg + RTV 100mg qd in certain pregnant patients who are already on a stable 800mg + RTV 100mg qd regimen prior to pregnancy, are virologically suppressed (HIV-1 RNA <50 copies/mL), and in whom a change to 600mg + RTV 100mg bid may compromise tolerability or compliance

ADMINISTRATION
Oral route
Take w/ food.

Oral Sus
- Shake well before each use.
- An 8mL darunavir dose should be taken as two 4mL administrations w/ the included oral dosing syringe.
- Patients who have difficulty swallowing tabs can use the oral sus.
- Before prescribing therapy, assess children weighing ≥15kg for the ability to swallow tabs; if a child is unable to reliably swallow tab, consider the use of oral sus.
- Use oral sus for pediatric patients weighing ≤10kg.

STORAGE
25°C (77°F); excursions permitted to 15-30°C (59-86°F). **Oral Sus:** Do not refrigerate or freeze. Avoid exposure to excessive heat. Store in the original container.

HOW SUPPLIED
Oral Sus: 100mg/mL [200mL]; **Tab:** 75mg, 150mg, 600mg, 800mg

CONTRAINDICATIONS
Coadministration w/ drugs that are highly dependent on CYP3A for clearance and for which elevated plasma concentrations are associated w/ serious and/or life-threatening events (narrow therapeutic index), and w/ certain other drugs that may lead to reduced efficacy of darunavir (eg, alfuzosin, dronedarone, colchicine [in patients w/ renal and/or hepatic impairment], ranolazine, pimozide, dihydroergotamine, ergotamine, methylergonovine, cisapride, oral midazolam, triazolam, St. John's wort, lovastatin, simvastatin, rifampin, sildenafil [when used to treat pulmonary arterial HTN]). Refer to RTV PI for a description of RTV contraindications.

WARNINGS/PRECAUTIONS
Must be coadministered w/ RTV and food to achieve desired antiviral effect; refer to RTV PI for additional information on precautionary measures. Drug-induced hepatitis reported; increased risk for liver function abnormalities, including severe hepatic adverse events, in patients w/ preexisting liver dysfunction, including chronic active hepatitis B or C. Cases of liver injury reported; consider performing increased AST/ALT monitoring in patients w/ underlying chronic hepatitis, cirrhosis, or those w/ pretreatment transaminase elevations, especially during the first several months of treatment. Consider interruption or discontinuation of therapy if evidence of new/worsening liver dysfunction occurs. Severe skin reactions sometimes accompanied by fever and/or transaminase elevations, Stevens-Johnson syndrome (rare), toxic epidermal necrolysis, drug rash w/ eosinophilia and systemic symptoms, and acute generalized exanthematous pustulosis reported; d/c immediately if severe skin reactions develop. Caution in patients w/ a known sulfonamide allergy. New onset diabetes mellitus (DM), exacerbation of preexisting DM, hyperglycemia, and diabetic ketoacidosis reported. Immune reconstitution syndrome, autoimmune disorders (eg, Graves' disease, polymyositis, Guillain-Barre syndrome) in the setting of immune reconstitution, redistribution/accumulation of body fat, and increased bleeding in hemophilia type A and B reported. Caution in elderly.

ADVERSE REACTIONS
Diarrhea, N/V, headache, abdominal pain, rash.

DRUG INTERACTIONS
See Contraindications. Not recommended w/ lopinavir/RTV, saquinavir, other HIV protease inhibitors (except atazanavir), apixaban, dabigatran etexilate (in specific renal impairment groups), rivaroxaban, rifapentine, boceprevir, simeprevir, everolimus, salmeterol, and avanafil. Avoid use of tadalafil during initiation therapy; d/c tadalafil at least 24 hrs prior to starting darunavir/RTV. Not recommended w/ voriconazole unless an assessment comparing predicted benefit to risk ratio justifies use of voriconazole. May increase levels of indinavir, maraviroc, antiarrhythmics, digoxin, clarithromycin, anticoagulant, carbamazepine, amitriptyline, desipramine, imipramine, nortriptyline, trazodone, itraconazole, ketoconazole, colchicine, rifabutin, antineoplastics, quetiapine, antipsychotics, β-blockers, calcium channel blockers, systemic corticosteroids (metabolized by CYP3A), inhaled/nasal corticosteroid, bosentan, simeprevir, HMG-CoA reductase inhibitors, immunosuppressants, salmeterol, norbuprenorphine, PDE-5 inhibitors (eg, avanafil, sildenafil, vardenafil, tadalafil), sedatives/hypnotics (metabolized by CYP3A), and CYP3A, CYP2D6, and P-gp substrates. May decrease levels of warfarin, phenytoin, phenobarbital, paroxetine, sertraline, voriconazole, boceprevir, methadone, ethinyl estradiol, norethindrone, and omeprazole. CYP3A inhibitors, P-gp inhibitors, indinavir, itraconazole, ketoconazole, posaconazole, rifabutin, and simeprevir may increase levels. CYP3A inducers, lopinavir/RTV, saquinavir, rifapentine, systemic dexamethasone, and boceprevir may decrease levels. Give didanosine 1 hr before or 2 hrs after administration. Increased lumefantrine exposure may increase the risk of QT prolongation; caution w/ artemether/lumefantrine. May increase risk for development of systemic corticosteroid effects including Cushing's syndrome and adrenal suppression w/ corticosteroids metabolized by CYP3A. May require initiation or dose adjustments of insulin or oral hypoglycemics for treatment of DM. Refer to PI for dosing modifications when used w/ certain concomitant therapies.

PREGNANCY AND LACTATION
Pregnancy: There is a pregnancy exposure registry that monitors pregnancy outcomes in women exposed to Prezista during pregnancy. **Lactation:** Not for use in nursing. **Reproductive Potential:** May reduce efficacy of combined hormonal contraceptives and the progestin only pill; use an effective alternative contraceptive method or add a barrier method of contraception.

MECHANISM OF ACTION
Protease inhibitor; selectively inhibits the cleavage of HIV-1 encoded Gag-Pol polyproteins in infected cells, thereby preventing the formation of mature virus particles.

PHARMACOKINETICS
Absorption: Absolute oral bioavailability (37% darunavir), (82% darunavir/RTV); T_{max}=approx 2.5-4 hrs. **Distribution:** Plasma protein binding (approx 95%). **Metabolism:** Hepatic (extensive); oxidation via CYP3A. **Elimination:** Darunavir/RTV: Feces (approx 79.5%, approx 41.2% unchanged darunavir), urine (approx 13.9%, approx 7.7% unchanged darunavir); $T_{1/2}$=approx 15 hrs.

PATIENT CONSIDERATIONS
Assessment: Assess for sulfonamide allergy, liver dysfunction, hemophilia, preexisting DM, pregnancy/nursing status, and possible drug interactions. Assess ability to swallow tab in children ≥15kg. In treatment-experienced patients, assess treatment history and perform genotypic and/or phenotypic testing. Conduct appropriate lab testing such as serum liver biochemistries.

Monitoring: Monitor for signs/symptoms of hepatotoxicity, severe skin reactions, new onset/exacerbation of DM, diabetic ketoacidosis, fat redistribution/accumulation, immune reconstitution syndrome, autoimmune disorders, and other adverse reactions. In patients w/ hemophilia, monitor for bleeding events. Consider performing increased AST/ALT monitoring in patients w/ underlying chronic hepatitis, cirrhosis, or those w/ pretreatment transaminase elevations, especially during the first several months of treatment. Monitor INR during coadministration w/ warfarin.

Counseling: Advise to take darunavir and RTV w/ food every day on a regular dosing schedule and instruct not to alter dose, d/c RTV, or d/c therapy w/ darunavir w/o consulting physician. Advise about the signs and symptoms of liver problems. Instruct to d/c immediately if signs or symptoms of severe skin reactions develop. Advise to report to physician the use of any other prescription or nonprescription medication or herbal products, including St. John's wort. Instruct patients receiving combined hormonal contraception or the progestin only pill to use an effective alternative contraceptive method or add a barrier method during therapy because hormonal levels may decrease. Inform that redistribution/accumulation of body fat may occur. Advise to inform physician immediately of any symptoms of infection. Inform that there is an antiretroviral pregnancy registry to monitor fetal outcomes of pregnant women exposed to therapy. Instruct women w/ HIV-1 infection not to breastfeed because HIV-1 can be passed to the baby in breast milk.

PRIALT — ziconotide   Rx
Class: N-type calcium channel blocker (CCB)

> Contraindicated in patients with preexisting history of psychosis. Severe psychiatric symptoms and neurological impairment may occur during treatment. Monitor frequently for evidence of cognitive impairment, hallucinations, or changes in mood or consciousness. D/C in the event of serious neurological or psychiatric signs/symptoms.

ADULT DOSAGE	PEDIATRIC DOSAGE
Chronic Pain Severe chronic pain in patients for whom intrathecal therapy is warranted, and who are intolerant of or refractory to other treatment (eg, systemic analgesics, adjunctive therapies, or intrathecal morphine) **Initial:** Initiate dosing via intrathecal device at ≤2.4mcg/day (0.1mcg/hr) **Titrate:** Up to 2.4mcg/day at intervals of ≤2-3X/week based on analgesic response and adverse events Assess dosing requirements and adjust the pump infusion flow rate as required to achieve new dosing for each dose titration **Max:** 19.2mcg/day (0.8mcg/hr)	Pediatric use may not have been established

DOSING CONSIDERATIONS
Elderly
Use caution; start at lower end of dosing range

ADMINISTRATION
Intrathecal route

For Use w/ Medtronic SynchroMed II Infusion System:
Refer to manufacturer's manuals for specific instructions and precautions
Naive Pump Priming:
Use only the undiluted 25mcg/mL formulation for naive pump priming
Rinse internal surfaces of the pump w/ 2mL at 25mcg/mL; repeat twice for a total of 3 rinses
Initial Pump Fill:
Use only undiluted 25mcg/mL formulation for the initial pump fill
Fill the naive pump after priming w/ the appropriate volume of 25mcg/mL
Begin dosing at delivery rate of ≤2.4mcg/day
Refill pump reservoir w/in 14 days of the initial fill to ensure appropriate dose administration
Subsequent Pump Refills:
Use Medtronic refill kit to ensure aseptic transfer and empty pump contents prior to refill
Diluted: Fill pump at least every 40 days
Undiluted: Fill pump at least every 84 days

Refer to PI if the internal infusion system must be surgically replaced while person is receiving therapy

For Use in the CADD-Micro Ambulatory Infusion Pump:
Refer to manufacturer's manuals for specific instructions and precautions
Prepare sol by diluting w/ 0.9% NaCl (preservative free)
Fill pump for the 1st time w/ sol at a concentration of 5mcg/mL
Initial flow rate for external microinfusion is 0.02mL/hr to deliver initial dose rate of 2.4mcg/day

STORAGE
2-8°C (36-46°F). Refrigerate during transit. Do not freeze. Protect from light.
Diluted Sol: 2-8°C (36-46°F) for 24 hrs. Discard any solution with observed particulate matter or discoloration and any unused portion.

HOW SUPPLIED
Inj: 25mcg/mL [20mL], 100mcg/mL [1mL, 5mL]

CONTRAINDICATIONS
Any other concomitant treatment or medical condition that would render intrathecal administration hazardous, including the presence of infection at the microinfusion inj site, uncontrolled bleeding diathesis, and spinal canal obstruction that impairs circulation of CSF; preexisting history of psychosis.

WARNINGS/PRECAUTIONS
Should be administered by or under the direction of an experienced physician. Not for IV administration. May cause/worsen depression with the risk of suicide in susceptible patients. May impair mental/physical abilities. Reduce dose or d/c use if signs/symptoms of cognitive impairment develop. Risk of meningitis due to inadvertent contamination of the microinfusion device and other means (eg, CSF seeding); monitor for signs/symptoms of meningitis. Unresponsiveness or stupor may occur; if reduced levels of consciousness occur, d/c therapy until event resolves, and consider other etiologies (eg, meningitis). Elevations in serum creatine kinase (CK) levels, symptomatic myopathy, and acute renal failure associated with rhabdomyolysis and extreme CK elevations reported; monitor serum CK levels periodically. Evaluate patients clinically and obtain CK measurements in the setting of new neuromuscular symptoms or reduced physical activity; reduce dose or d/c therapy if symptoms continue and increased CK levels persist. Not an opiate and cannot prevent or relieve the symptoms associated with opiate withdrawal. Caution in elderly.

ADVERSE REACTIONS
Neuropsychiatric adverse reactions, dizziness, N/V, confusion, nystagmus, diarrhea, headache, somnolence, asthenia, vertigo, ataxia, abnormal gait, memory impairment, blurred vision, pruritus.

DRUG INTERACTIONS
Not recommended with intrathecal opiates. Coadministration with CNS depressants may increase risk of CNS adverse reactions; dosage adjustments or discontinuation of other CNS depressant drugs may be necessary as clinically appropriate, if altered consciousness occurs. Concomitant antiepileptics, neuroleptics, sedatives, or diuretics may increase risk of depressed levels of consciousness.

PREGNANCY AND LACTATION
Category C, not for use in nursing.

MECHANISM OF ACTION
N-type calcium channel blocker; has not been established. Binds/blocks N-type calcium channels, which leads to a blockade of excitatory neurotransmitter release from the primary afferent nerve terminals and antinociception.

PHARMACOKINETICS
Absorption: (1-10mcg) AUC=83.6-608ng•hr/mL, C_{max}=16.4-132ng/mL; T_{max}=1 hr.
Distribution: V_d=155mL; plasma protein binding (50%). **Metabolism:** Kidneys, liver, lungs, muscle via endopeptidases, exopeptidases, and proteases. **Elimination:** Urine (<1%) (IV), $T_{1/2}$=4.6 hrs.

PATIENT CONSIDERATIONS

Assessment: Assess for preexisting history of psychosis, presence of infection at microinfusion inj site, uncontrolled bleeding diathesis, spinal canal obstruction, drug hypersensitivity, pregnancy/nursing status, and possible drug interactions.

Monitoring: Monitor for cognitive impairment, hallucinations, or changes in mood or consciousness, serious infection or meningitis, psychiatric symptoms, decreased alertness/unresponsiveness, elevated CK, myopathy, rhabdomyolysis, neuromuscular symptoms, acute renal failure, and other adverse reactions. Monitor serum CK periodically (every other week for 1st month and monthly thereafter).

Counseling: Advise that psychiatric and cognitive symptoms may occur. Caution against engaging in hazardous activity requiring complete mental alertness or motor coordination (eg, operating machinery/driving) during treatment. Caution about possible combined effects with other CNS depressants. Instruct to contact physician immediately if patient experiences new or worsening muscle pain, soreness, weakness with or without darkened urine; change in mental status or mood; symptoms of depression or suicidal ideation; signs/symptoms of meningitis; decreased level of consciousness; unresponsiveness or stupor; withdrawal symptoms as a result of abrupt discontinuation of opioid therapy; and serious skin reactions.

PRIVIGEN — immune globulin intravenous (human)   Rx
Class: Immune globulin

> Thrombosis may occur. Renal dysfunction, acute renal failure, osmotic nephrosis, and death may occur w/ immune globulin intravenous (IGIV) products in predisposed patients. Renal dysfunction and acute renal failure occur more commonly w/ IGIV products containing sucrose; this product does not contain sucrose. For patients at risk of thrombosis (eg, using estrogens), renal dysfunction (eg, receiving known nephrotoxic drugs), or renal failure, administer at the minimum dose and infusion rate practicable. Ensure adequate hydration before administration. Monitor for signs/symptoms of thrombosis and assess blood viscosity if at risk for hyperviscosity.

ADULT DOSAGE
Primary Humoral Immunodeficiency

Replacement Therapy:
Usual: 200-800mg/kg (2-8mL/kg) every 3-4 weeks
Titrate: Adjust to achieve desired serum trough levels and clinical response
Initial Infusion Rate:
0.5mg/kg/min (0.005mL/kg/min)
Maint Infusion Rate:
Increase to 8mg/kg/min (0.08mL/kg/min) as tolerated
If a dose is missed, administer the missed dose as soon as possible, and then resume scheduled treatments every 3 or 4 weeks, as applicable

Chronic Immune Thrombocytopenic Purpura
Usual: 1g/kg (10mL/kg) daily for 2 consecutive days (total dosage of 2g/kg)
Initial Infusion Rate:
0.5mg/kg/min (0.005mL/kg/min)
Maint Infusion Rate:
Increase to 4mg/kg/min (0.04mL/kg/min) as tolerated

PEDIATRIC DOSAGE
Primary Humoral Immunodeficiency

Replacement Therapy:
≥3 Years:
Usual: 200-800mg/kg (2-8mL/kg) every 3-4 weeks
Titrate: Adjust to achieve desired serum trough levels and clinical response
Initial Infusion Rate:
0.5mg/kg/min (0.005mL/kg/min)
Maint Infusion Rate:
Increase to 8mg/kg/min (0.08mL/kg/min) as tolerated
If a dose is missed, administer the missed dose as soon as possible, and then resume scheduled treatments every 3 or 4 weeks, as applicable

Chronic Immune Thrombocytopenic Purpura
≥15 Years:
Usual: 1g/kg (10mL/kg) daily for 2 consecutive days (total dosage of 2g/kg)
Initial Infusion Rate:
0.5mg/kg/min (0.005mL/kg/min)
Maint Infusion Rate:
Increase to 4mg/kg/min (0.04mL/kg/min) as tolerated

DOSING CONSIDERATIONS
Elderly
Do not exceed recommended doses, and administer at the minimum dose and infusion rate practicable

Adverse Reactions
Slow or stop infusion if adverse reactions occur; may resume at a lower rate if symptoms subside promptly

ADMINISTRATION
IV route

Preparation and Administration
Do not shake.
Do not freeze; do not use if product has been frozen.
Should be at room temperature at the time of administration.
Infuse using a separate infusion line; prior to use, infusion line may be flushed w/ D5W or 0.9% NaCl for inj.
Do not mix w/ other IGIV products or other IV medications; may be diluted w/ D5W.
May use an infusion pump to control rate of administration.
If large doses are to be administered, several vials may be pooled using aseptic technique; begin infusion w/in 8 hrs of pooling.

STORAGE
Room temperature up to 25°C (77°F) for up to 36 months. Do not freeze; do not use if it has been frozen. Protect from light.

HOW SUPPLIED
Inj: 10% [50mL, 100mL, 200mL, 400mL]

CONTRAINDICATIONS
History of anaphylactic or severe systemic reaction to human immune globulin, hyperprolinemia, IgA-deficient patients w/ antibodies to IgA, and a history of hypersensitivity.

WARNINGS/PRECAUTIONS
Contains trace amounts of IgA; severe hypersensitivity reactions may occur. D/C infusion immediately and institute appropriate treatment if hypersensitivity develops. Ensure that patients w/ preexisting renal insufficiency are not volume depleted; consider discontinuation if renal function deteriorates. Hyperproteinemia, increased serum viscosity, and hyponatremia may occur. Distinguish true hyponatremia from pseudohyponatremia (as demonstrated by a decreased calculated serum osmolality or elevated osmolar gap); treatment aimed at decreasing serum free water in patients w/ pseudohyponatremia may lead to volume depletion, a further increase in serum viscosity, and a possible predisposition to thromboembolic events. Aseptic meningitis syndrome (AMS) reported and may occur more frequently w/ high doses (2g/kg) and/or rapid infusion; rule out other causes of meningitis. Delayed hemolytic anemia may develop; acute hemolysis reported. Severe hemolysis-related renal dysfunction/failure or disseminated intravascular coagulation reported. Noncardiogenic

pulmonary edema may occur; if transfusion-related acute lung injury (TRALI) is suspected, perform tests for presence of antineutrophil antibodies and anti-human leukocyte antigen (HLA) antibodies in both the product and patient's serum. Caution w/ high-dose regimen (for chronic ITP) in patients at increased risk of thrombosis, hemolysis, acute kidney injury, or volume overload. May carry a risk of transmitting infectious agents (eg, viruses, and, theoretically, the Creutzfeldt-Jakob disease agent). May interfere w/ some serological tests. Caution in elderly.

ADVERSE REACTIONS
Thrombosis, renal dysfunction, acute renal failure, osmotic nephrosis, headache, fatigue, N/V, chills, back pain, pain, elevated body temperature, anemia, epistaxis, blood bilirubin increased, Hct decreased.

DRUG INTERACTIONS
See Boxed Warning. May interfere w/ the response to live virus vaccines (eg, measles, mumps, rubella, varicella).

PREGNANCY AND LACTATION
Category C, safety not known in nursing.

MECHANISM OF ACTION
Immune globulin; not established. Replacement therapy for PI; supplies a broad spectrum of opsonic and neutralizing IgG antibodies against bacterial, viral, parasitic, and mycoplasma agents and their toxins.

PHARMACOKINETICS
Absorption: (3-Week Dosing Interval) C_{max}=2550mg/dL; $AUC_{0-t,0-inf}$=32,820 day•mg/dL, 79,315 day•mg/dL. (4-Week Dosing Interval) C_{max}=2260mg/dL; $AUC_{0-t,0-inf}$=36,390 day•mg/dL, 104,627 day•mg/dL. **Distribution:** Crosses placenta. (3-Week Dosing Interval) V_d=50mL/kg. (4-Week Dosing Interval) V_d=84mL/kg. **Elimination:** (3-Week Dosing Interval) $T_{1/2}$=27.6 days. (4-Week Dosing Interval) $T_{1/2}$=45.4 days.

PATIENT CONSIDERATIONS
Assessment: Assess for history of anaphylactic or severe systemic reactions to human immune globulin, hyperprolinemia, IgA deficiency, risk of thrombosis/renal dysfunction/renal failure/hemolysis/volume overload, pregnancy/nursing status, and possible drug interactions. Assess renal function. Consider baseline assessment of blood viscosity in patients at risk for hyperviscosity, including those w/ cryoglobulins, fasting chylomicronemia/markedly high TGs, or monoclonal gammopathies. Consider appropriate lab testing in patients at higher risk for hemolysis, including measurement of Hgb/Hct prior to infusion.

Monitoring: Monitor for thrombosis, hypersensitivity reactions, hyperproteinemia, hyperviscosity, hyponatremia, hemolytic anemia, pulmonary adverse reactions, infection, and other adverse reactions. Monitor renal function and urine output periodically. Perform neurological exam, including CSF studies, if AMS is suspected. Consider testing in patients at higher risk for hemolysis, including measurement of Hgb/Hct w/in 36-96 hrs post infusion. Perform confirmatory lab testing if signs/symptoms of hemolysis or a significant drop in Hgb/Hct have been observed. Perform tests for presence of antineutrophil antibodies and anti-HLA antibodies in both the product and patient's serum if TRALI is suspected. Monitor vital signs throughout the infusion.

Counseling: Instruct to immediately report to physician any signs/symptoms of hypersensitivity reactions, kidney problems, thrombosis, AMS, hemolysis, TRALI, and infection. Inform that drug is made from human blood and may contain infectious agents that can cause disease. Inform that product may interfere w/ the response to live virus vaccines; instruct to notify immunizing physician of recent therapy w/ this product.

PROCRIT — epoetin alfa   Rx

Class: Erythropoiesis-stimulating agent (ESA)

> Increased risk of death, MI, stroke, venous thromboembolism (VTE), thrombosis of vascular access, and tumor progression or recurrence. Use the lowest dose sufficient to reduce/avoid the need for RBC transfusions. Chronic Kidney Disease (CKD): Greater risks for death, serious adverse cardiovascular (CV) reactions, and stroke when administered to target Hgb level >11g/dL. Cancer: Shortened overall survival and/or increased risk of tumor progression or recurrence in patients w/ breast, non-small cell lung, head and neck, lymphoid, and cervical cancers. Must enroll in and comply w/ the ESA APPRISE Oncology Program to prescribe and/or dispense drug to patients. Use only for anemia from myelosuppressive chemotherapy. Not indicated for patients receiving myelosuppressive chemotherapy when anticipated outcome is cure. D/C following completion of chemotherapy course. Perisurgery: Due to increased risk of deep venous thrombosis (DVT), DVT prophylaxis is recommended.

ADULT DOSAGE
Anemia

Chronic Kidney Disease Associated Anemia:
Patients on Dialysis:
Initiate treatment when Hgb is <10g/dL
If Hgb approaches/exceeds 11g/dL, reduce or interrupt dose
Initial: 50-100 U/kg IV/SQ 3X weekly; IV recommended for hemodialysis patients
Patients Not on Dialysis:
Consider initiating treatment when Hgb is <10g/dL AND the following considerations apply:
1. Rate of Hgb decline indicates likelihood of requiring a RBC transfusion AND,
2. Reducing the risk of

PEDIATRIC DOSAGE
Anemia

Chronic Kidney Disease Associated Anemia:
1 Month-16 Years on Dialysis:
Initiate treatment when Hgb is <10g/dL
If Hgb approaches/exceeds 11g/dL, reduce or interrupt dose
Initial: 50 U/kg IV/SQ 3X weekly; IV recommended for hemodialysis patients
Do not increase dose more frequently than once every 4 weeks; decreases in dose may occur more frequently
If Hgb Rises Rapidly (eg, >1g/dL in any 2-Week Period): Reduce dose by ≥25% prn to reduce rapid responses

alloimmunization and/or other RBC transfusion-related risks is a goal
If Hgb exceeds 10g/dL, reduce or interrupt dose and use lowest dose sufficient to reduce the need for RBC transfusion
Initial: 50-100 U/kg IV/SQ 3X weekly
All Patients:
Do not increase dose more frequently than once every 4 weeks; decreases in dose may occur more frequently
If Hgb Rises Rapidly (eg, >1g/dL in any 2-Week Period): Reduce dose by ≥25% prn to reduce rapid responses
If Hgb Has Not Increased by >1g/dL After 4 Weeks: Increase dose by 25% If adequate response is not achieved over a 12-week escalation period, use lowest dose that will maintain a Hgb level sufficient to reduce need for RBC transfusions and evaluate other causes of anemia; d/c if responsiveness does not improve

Zidovudine Associated Anemia in HIV-Infected Patients:
Initial: 100 U/kg IV/SQ 3X weekly
Titrate:
No Hgb Increase After 8 Weeks: Increase dose by approx 50-100 U/kg at 4- to 8-week intervals until Hgb reaches level needed to avoid RBC transfusions or 300 U/kg
Hgb >12g/dL: Withhold therapy until Hgb <11g/dL; then resume at a dose 25% below previous dose
D/C therapy if an increase in Hgb is not achieved at 300 U/kg for 8 weeks

Chemotherapy Associated Anemia:
Initiate if Hgb <10g/dL and if there is a minimum of 2 additional months of planned chemotherapy
Initial: 150 U/kg SQ 3X weekly or 40,000 U SQ weekly until completion of a chemotherapy course
Dose Reduction: Reduce by 25% if:
1. Hgb increases >1g/dL in any 2-week period
2. Hgb reaches a level needed to avoid a RBC transfusion
Withhold dose if Hgb exceeds level needed to avoid RBC transfusion; reinitiate at a dose 25% below previous dose when Hgb approaches a level where RBC transfusions may be required
Dose Increase: After initial 4 weeks of therapy, if Hgb increases by <1g/dL and remains below 10g/dL increase dose to 300 U/kg 3X weekly or 60,000 U weekly
D/C therapy if there is no response in Hgb levels or if RBC transfusions are still required after 8 weeks

Surgery Patients:
300 U/kg/day SQ for 10 days before, on the day of, and for 4 days after surgery; or 600 U/kg SQ in 4 doses administered 21, 14, and 7 days before surgery and on the day of surgery
DVT prophylaxis is recommended

If Hgb Has Not Increased by >1g/dL After 4 Weeks: Increase dose by 25% If adequate response is not achieved over a 12-week escalation period, use lowest dose that will maintain a Hgb level sufficient to reduce need for RBC transfusions and evaluate other causes of anemia; d/c if responsiveness does not improve

Chemotherapy Associated Anemia: 5-18 Years:
Initiate if Hgb <10g/dL and if there is a minimum of 2 additional months of planned chemotherapy
Initial: 600 U/kg IV weekly until completion of a chemotherapy course
Dose Reduction: Reduce by 25% if
1. Hgb increases >1g/dL in any 2-week period
2. Hgb reaches a level needed to avoid a RBC transfusion
Withhold dose if Hgb exceeds level needed to avoid RBC transfusion; reinitiate at a dose 25% below previous dose when Hgb approaches a level where RBC transfusions may be required
Dose Increase: After initial 4 weeks of therapy, if Hgb increases by <1g/dL and remains below 10g/dL increase dose to 900 U/kg (max 60,000 U) weekly
D/C therapy if there is no response in Hgb levels or if RBC transfusions are still required after 8 weeks

---

ADMINISTRATION
IV/SQ route
Do not shake; do not use if shaken or frozen.
Discard unused portions in preservative-free vials; do not re-enter preservative-free vials.
Do not dilute.
Preservative-free vials may be admixed in a syringe w/ bacteriostatic 0.9% NaCl inj, w/ benzyl alcohol 0.9% in a 1:1 ratio.

STORAGE
2-8°C (36-46°F). Do not freeze; do not use if it has been frozen. Protect from light. Discard unused portions of multidose vials 21 days after initial entry.

HOW SUPPLIED
Inj: 2000 U/mL, 3000 U/mL, 4000 U/mL, 10,000 U/mL, 40,000 U/mL [single-dose vial]; 10,000 U/mL [2mL], 20,000 U/mL [1mL] [multidose vial]

CONTRAINDICATIONS
Uncontrolled HTN, pure red cell aplasia (PRCA) that begins after treatment w/ epoetin alfa or other erythropoietin protein drugs, serious allergic reactions to

epoetin alfa. (Multidose Vials) Neonates, infants, pregnant women, and nursing mothers.

WARNINGS/PRECAUTIONS

Not indicated for use in patients w/ cancer receiving hormonal agents, biologic products, or radiotherapy, unless also receiving concomitant myelosuppressive chemotherapy; in patients scheduled for surgery who are willing to donate autologous blood; in patients undergoing cardiac/vascular surgery, or as a substitute for RBC transfusions in patients requiring immediate correction of anemia. Evaluate transferrin saturation and serum ferritin prior to and during treatment; administer supplemental iron when serum ferritin is <100mcg/L or serum transferrin saturation is <20%. Correct/exclude other causes of anemia (eg, vitamin deficiency, metabolic/chronic inflammatory conditions, bleeding) before initiating therapy. Hypertensive encephalopathy and seizures reported in patients w/ CKD. Appropriately control HTN prior to initiation of and during treatment; reduce/withhold therapy if BP becomes difficult to control. PRCA and severe anemia, w/ or w/o other cytopenias that arise following development of neutralizing antibodies to erythropoietin reported. Withhold and evaluate for neutralizing antibodies to erythropoietin if severe anemia and low reticulocyte count develop; d/c permanently if PRCA develops, and do not switch to other erythropoiesis-stimulating agents. Serious allergic reactions may occur; immediately and permanently d/c therapy. Contains albumin; may carry an extremely remote risk for transmission of viral diseases or Creutzfeldt-Jakob disease. Patients may require adjustments in their dialysis prescriptions after initiation of therapy, or require increased anticoagulation w/ heparin to prevent clotting of extracorporeal circuit during hemodialysis. Multidose vial contains benzyl alcohol; benzyl alcohol is associated w/ serious adverse events and death, particularly in pediatric patients.

ADVERSE REACTIONS

MI, stroke, VTE, thrombosis of vascular access, tumor progression/recurrence, pyrexia, N/V, HTN, cough, arthralgia, pruritus, rash, headache, dizziness.

PREGNANCY AND LACTATION

Pregnancy: Category C (single-dose vials only).
Lactation: Caution in nursing (single-dose vials only).

MECHANISM OF ACTION

Erythropoiesis-stimulating glycoprotein; stimulates erythropoiesis by the same mechanism as endogenous erythropoietin.

PHARMACOKINETICS

Absorption: Adults and Pediatrics w/ CKD: (SQ) T_{max}=5-24 hrs. Anemic Cancer Patients: (SQ) T_{max}=13.3 hrs (150 U/kg), 38 hrs (40,000 U). **Elimination:** Adults and Pediatrics w/ CKD: (IV) $T_{1/2}$=4-13 hrs. Anemic Cancer Patients: (SQ) $T_{1/2}$=16-67 hrs.

PATIENT CONSIDERATIONS

Assessment: Assess for uncontrolled HTN, previous hypersensitivity to the drug, causes of anemia, pregnancy/nursing status, and other conditions where treatment is contraindicated or cautioned. Obtain baseline Hgb levels, transferrin saturation, and serum ferritin.

Monitoring: Monitor for signs/symptoms of an allergic reaction, CV/thromboembolic events, stroke, premonitory neurologic symptoms, PRCA, severe anemia, progression/recurrence of tumor, and other adverse reactions. Monitor BP, transferrin saturation, and serum ferritin. Following initiation of therapy and after each dose adjustment, monitor Hgb weekly until Hgb is stable and sufficient to minimize need for RBC transfusion.

Counseling: Inform of the risks/benefits of therapy and of the increased risks of mortality, serious CV reactions, thromboembolic reactions, stroke, and tumor progression. Advise of the need to have regular lab tests for Hgb. Inform cancer patients that they must sign the patient-physician acknowledgment form prior to therapy. Instruct to undergo regular BP monitoring, adhere to prescribed antihypertensive regimen, and follow recommended dietary restrictions. Advise to contact physician for new-onset neurologic symptoms or change in seizure frequency. Instruct regarding proper disposal of used syringes and caution against the reuse of needles, syringes, or unused portions of single-dose vials.

PROCYSBI — cysteamine bitartrate   Rx

Class: Cystine-depleting agent

ADULT DOSAGE
Nephropathic Cystinosis

Cysteamine-Naive Patients:
Start treatment immediately after diagnosis
Initial: 0.2-0.3g/m²/day (1/6 to 1/4 of the maint dose) divided q12h
Titrate: Increase gradually over 4-6 weeks until maint dose is achieved
Maint: 1.3g/m²/day divided q12h
Max: 1.95g/m²/day

Refer to PI for weight-based starting and maint doses

Switching from Immediate-Release (IR) Cysteamine Bitartrate Caps:
Initial: Total daily dose should be equal to previous total daily dose of IR cysteamine bitartrate
Max: 1.95g/m²/day

PEDIATRIC DOSAGE
Nephropathic Cystinosis

≥2 Years:
Cysteamine-Naive Patients:
Start treatment immediately after diagnosis
Initial: 0.2-0.3g/m²/day (1/6 to 1/4 of the maint dose) divided q12h
Titrate: Increase gradually over 4-6 weeks until maint dose is achieved
Maint: 1.3g/m²/day divided q12h
Max: 1.95g/m²/day

Refer to PI for weight-based starting and maint doses

Switching from IR Cysteamine Bitartrate Caps:
Initial: Total daily dose should be equal to previous total daily dose of IR cysteamine bitartrate

Dose Titration:
Target WBC cystine concentration is <1nmol 1/2 cystine/mg protein; adjust dose as needed to achieve target WBC cystine concentration. If a dose adjustment is required, increase by 10%. If adverse reactions occur, decrease dose; for patients who have initial intolerance, temporarily d/c therapy and then restart at a lower dose and gradually increase to the target dose

Lab Monitoring:
Cysteamine-Naive Patients: Measure WBC cystine concentration after reaching maint dose, then monthly for 3 months, quarterly for 1 yr, and then twice yearly, at a minimum
Patients Switching from IR Cysteamine: Measure WBC cystine concentration after 2 weeks of treatment while titrating the dose, then quarterly for 6 months, then twice yearly, at a minimum

Obtain blood samples for WBC cystine concentration measurement 12 hrs after dosing; accurately record time of the last dose, actual dose, and time the blood sample was taken

Missed Dose
If a dose is missed, take as soon as possible up to 8 hrs after the scheduled time. However, if a dose is missed and the next scheduled dose is due in <4 hrs, do not take missed dose and take the next dose at the usual scheduled time. Do not take 2 doses at one time to make up for a missed dose

Max: 1.95g/m²/day

Dose Titration:
Target WBC cystine concentration is <1nmol 1/2 cystine/mg protein; adjust dose as needed to achieve target WBC cystine concentration. If a dose adjustment is required, increase by 10%. If adverse reactions occur, decrease dose; for patients who have initial intolerance, temporarily d/c therapy and then re-start at a lower dose and gradually increase to the target dose

Laboratory Monitoring:
Cysteamine-Naive Patients: Measure WBC cystine concentration after reaching maint dose, then monthly for 3 months, quarterly for 1 yr, and then twice yearly, at a minimum
Patients Switching from IR Cysteamine: Measure WBC cystine concentration after 2 weeks of treatment while titrating the dose, then quarterly for 6 months, then twice yearly, at a minimum

Obtain blood samples for WBC cystine concentration measurement 12 hrs after dosing; accurately record time of the last dose, actual dose, and time the blood sample was taken

Missed Dose
If a dose is missed, take as soon as possible up to 8 hrs after the scheduled time. However, if a dose is missed and the next scheduled dose is due in <4 hrs, do not take missed dose and take the next dose at the usual scheduled time. Do not take 2 doses at one time to make up for a missed dose

---

DOSING CONSIDERATIONS
Concomitant Medications
Medications Containing Bicarbonate or Carbonate: Administer Procysbi at least 1 hr before or 1 hr after these agents
Alcohol: Avoid alcohol while on therapy

ADMINISTRATION
Oral route

Swallow whole; do not crush/chew caps or cap contents.
Take w/ fruit juice (except grapefruit juice).
Do not eat for at least 2 hrs before and for at least 30 min after. If unable to take w/o eating, take w/ food and limit amount of food to approx 4 oz (1/2 cup) w/in 1 hr before dose through 1 hr after.
Take in a consistent manner in regard to food; avoid high-fat food close to dosing.

Difficulty Swallowing Caps
Administration w/ Applesauce or Berry Jelly:
1. Open caps and sprinkle intact granules on 4 oz applesauce or berry jelly; mix granules.
2. Consume entire contents w/in 30 min of mixing; do not chew granules. Do not save applesauce or berry jelly and granules for later use.

Administration w/ Fruit Juice (Except Grapefruit Juice):
1. Open caps and sprinkle intact granules into 4 oz of juice; gently stir until mixed.
2. Drink entire contents w/in 30 min of mixing; do not chew granules. Do not save fruit juice and granules for later use.

Administration w/ Applesauce via a Gastrostomy Tube (14 French or larger)
A bolus (straight) feeding tube is recommended.
1. Flush the gastrostomy tube button 1st w/ 5mL of water to clear the button.
2. Open cap and empty granules into a clean container w/ approx 4 oz of applesauce (use only strained applesauce w/ no chunks). A minimum of 1 oz (1/8 cup) of applesauce may be used for children ≤25kg starting at a dose of 1 or 2 caps. Mix intact granules into applesauce.
3. Draw up the mixture into a syringe. Keep the feeding tube horizontal during administration and apply rapid and steady pressure (10mL/10 sec) to dispense the syringe contents into the tube w/in 30 min of preparation.
4. Do not save applesauce and granule mixture for later use.
5. Draw up a minimum of 10mL of fruit juice into another syringe, swirl gently, and flush the tube.

STORAGE
20-25°C (68-77°F). Prior to dispensing, store at 2-8°C (36-46°F). Protect from light and moisture.

HOW SUPPLIED
Cap, Delayed-Release: 25mg, 75mg

CONTRAINDICATIONS
Serious hypersensitivity reaction, including anaphylaxis, to penicillamine or cysteamine bitartrate.

WARNINGS/PRECAUTIONS

Skin and bone lesions that resemble Ehlers-Danlos-like syndrome may occur. Monitor for development of skin or bone lesions and interrupt dosing if these lesions develop; may restart at a lower dose under close supervision, then slowly increase to the appropriate therapeutic dose. Severe skin rashes (eg, erythema multiforme bullosa, toxic epidermal necrolysis) may occur; permanently d/c use if severe skin rashes develop. GI ulceration/bleeding and GI tract symptoms (eg, N/V, anorexia, abdominal pain) may occur; consider decreasing the dose if severe GI tract symptoms develop. CNS symptoms may occur; carefully evaluate/monitor patients who develop CNS symptoms and interrupt or adjust dose as necessary for patients w/ severe symptoms or w/ symptoms that persist or progress. May impair mental/physical abilities. Associated w/ reversible leukopenia and elevated alkaline phosphatase levels; monitor WBC counts and alkaline phosphatase levels and consider decreasing dose or discontinuing drug if tests values remain elevated, until values revert to normal. Benign intracranial HTN (pseudotumor cerebri) and/or papilledema may occur. Monitor for signs/symptoms of pseudotumor cerebri; interrupt or decrease dose and refer patient to an ophthalmologist if signs/symptoms persist and permanently d/c use if diagnosis is confirmed.

ADVERSE REACTIONS

N/V, abdominal pain/discomfort, headache, diarrhea, anorexia/decreased appetite, breath odor, fatigue, dizziness, skin odor, rash.

DRUG INTERACTIONS

See Dosing Considerations. Drugs that increase gastric pH (eg, proton pump inhibitors, medications containing bicarbonate or carbonate) may alter the pharmacokinetics of cysteamine and increase WBC cystine concentration; monitor WBC cystine concentration w/ concomitant use. Alcohol may increase the rate of cysteamine release and/or adversely alter the pharmacokinetic properties, as well as the effectiveness/safety of therapy; do not consume alcoholic beverages during treatment.

PREGNANCY AND LACTATION

Pregnancy: No available data on use in pregnant women to inform any drug-associated risks for birth defects or miscarriage. **Lactation:** Not for use in nursing.

MECHANISM OF ACTION

Cystine-depleting agent; participates w/in lysosomes in a thiol-disulfide interchange reaction converting cystine into cysteine and cysteine-cysteamine mixed disulfide, both of which can exit the lysosome in patients w/ cystinosis.

PHARMACOKINETICS

Absorption: C_{max}=3.6mg/L; T_{max}=188 min; AUC=785mg•min/L. **Distribution:** V_d=382L. Plasma protein binding (52%, predominantly to albumin). **Elimination:** $T_{1/2}$=253 min.

PATIENT CONSIDERATIONS

Assessment: Assess for hypersensitivity to the drug or to penicillamine, pregnancy/nursing status, and possible drug interactions.

Monitoring: Monitor for skin/bone lesions, severe skin rashes, GI ulceration/bleeding, GI tract symptoms, CNS symptoms, pseudotumor cerebri, and other adverse reactions. Monitor WBC counts and alkaline phosphatase levels. For cysteamine-naive patients, measure WBC cystine levels after reaching maint dose, then monthly for 3 months, quarterly for 1 yr, and then twice yearly, at a minimum. For patients switching from IR cysteamine, measure WBC cystine levels after 2 weeks of treatment while titrating dose, then quarterly for 6 months, then twice yearly, at a minimum.

Counseling: Advise that drug may cause abnormalities of the skin, bones, and joints; instruct to report any skin changes or problems w/ bones/joints to physician. Instruct to contact physician immediately if a skin rash is experienced. Inform that drug may cause ulcers/bleeding; advise to contact physician immediately if stomach pain, N/V, loss of appetite, or vomiting blood occurs. Inform that ability to perform tasks (eg, driving/operating machinery) may be impaired; instruct to contact physician immediately if seizures, lethargy, somnolence, depression, and encephalopathy are experienced. Advise that drug may cause benign intracranial HTN; advise to contact physician immediately if headache, tinnitus, dizziness, nausea, double vision, blurry vision, loss of vision, or eye pain occurs. Instruct to contact physician immediately if pregnancy is suspected. Discuss the risks/benefits of continuing therapy during pregnancy. Advise that breastfeeding is not recommended during therapy. Inform to take ud and discuss the importance of required lab testing.

PROFILNINE — factor IX complex   Rx

Class: Antihemophilic agent

ADULT DOSAGE
Hemophilia B

Prevention/Control of Bleeding:
Minor Hemorrhages:
20-30% of normal (20-30 IU of factor IX/kg) q16-24 hrs for 1-2 days; continue until hemorrhage stops and healing has been achieved

Moderate Hemorrhages:
20-30% of normal (20-30 IU of factor IX/kg) q16-24 hrs for 2-7 days; continue until hemorrhage stops and healing has been achieved

PEDIATRIC DOSAGE
Pediatric use may not have been established

Major Hemorrhages:
30-50% of normal (30-50 IU factor IX/kg) q16-24 hrs for 3-10 days Maintain factor IX levels at 20% (20 IU Factor IX/kg)

Surgery:
Prior to Surgery: 30-50% of normal (30-50 IU factor IX/kg) q16-24 hrs for 7-10 days
Dental Extractions: Raise factor IX level to 50% immediately prior to procedure

Maintain factor IX levels at 30-50% (30-50 IU factor IX/kg) until healing is achieved

Dose Calculation:
Calculation of Number of Factor IX Units Required = Wt (kg) x Desired Increase in Plasma Factor IX (%) x 1 U/kg

ADMINISTRATION
IV route

Do not administer at a rate >10mL/min
May be administered by inj (plastic disposable syringe only) or infusion Administer (at room temperature) w/in 3 hrs of reconstitution

STORAGE
≤25°C (77°F); stable for 3 yrs, up to expiration date. Do not freeze. Do not refrigerate after reconstitution.

HOW SUPPLIED
Inj: 500 IU, 1000 IU, 1500 IU

WARNINGS/PRECAUTIONS
May carry risk of transmitting infectious agents (eg, viruses, Creutzfeldt-Jakob disease). Neutralizing antibodies (inhibitors) may develop; monitor for inhibitors and quantify using Bethesda Units using appropriate lab testing. Associated w/ development of thromboembolic complications; patients undergoing surgery, post surgery, w/ known liver disease, w/ signs of fibrinolysis, thrombosis, or disseminated intravascular coagulation (DIC) are at increased risk. Monitor for early signs of consumptive coagulopathy w/ appropriate lab testing. Administer only when benefits outweigh the serious risks. Hypersensitivity, including anaphylaxis, reported. Rapid administration may result in vasomotor reactions. Packaging may contain natural rubber latex; use w/ caution in patients w/ sensitivity.

ADVERSE REACTIONS
Fever, chills, N/V, headache, lethargy, flushing, urticaria, tingling, allergic reactions.

PREGNANCY AND LACTATION
Category C, safety not known in nursing.

MECHANISM OF ACTION
Antihemophilic agent; temporarily increases plasma levels of factor IX, thus enabling a temporary correction of the factor deficiency.

PHARMACOKINETICS
Elimination: $T_{1/2}$=24.68 hrs.

PATIENT CONSIDERATIONS
Assessment: Assess for hypersensitivity to the drug, liver disease, signs of fibrinolysis, thrombosis, DIC, vaccination history for hepatitis A and B, and pregnancy/nursing status. Assess if patient has undergone any recent surgeries. Obtain baseline factor IX level.

Monitoring: Monitor for early signs of consumptive coagulopathy, thromboembolic complications, infections, hypersensitivity/allergic/vasomotor reactions, and other adverse reactions. Monitor factor IX levels frequently during replacement therapy. Monitor for development of neutralizing antibodies (inhibitors) using appropriate biological testing after repeated treatment.

Counseling: Inform of the early signs/symptoms of hypersensitivity reaction; advise to d/c use and notify physician and/or seek immediate emergency care if these symptoms occur. Advise to report any decrease in effectiveness during therapy.

PROGRAF — tacrolimus   Rx

Class: Calcineurin-inhibitor immunosuppressant

> Immunosuppression may lead to increased risk of lymphoma and other malignancies, particularly of the skin. Increased susceptibility to infections (bacterial, viral, fungal, protozoal, opportunistic). Should only be prescribed by physicians experienced in immunosuppressive therapy and management of organ transplant patients. Manage patients in facilities equipped and staffed w/ adequate lab and supportive medical resources. Physician responsible for maintenance therapy should have complete information requisite for patient follow-up.

ADULT DOSAGE
Hepatic Transplant

Prophylaxis of organ rejection in patients receiving allogeneic liver transplant; recommended to be used concomitantly w/ adrenal corticosteroids early post-transplant

PEDIATRIC DOSAGE
Hepatic Transplant

Prophylaxis of organ rejection in patients receiving allogeneic liver transplant; recommended to be used concomitantly w/ adrenal corticosteroids early post-transplant

Cap:
Initial: 0.1-0.15mg/kg/day as 2 divided doses, q12h; administer no sooner than 6 hrs after liver transplant
Titrate: Based on clinical assessments of rejection and tolerability
Maint: Lower dosages than the initial dosage may be sufficient
Observed Tacrolimus Whole Blood Trough Concentrations w/ Liver Transplant:
Months 1-12: 5-20ng/mL
IV:
Initial: 0.03-0.05mg/kg/day
If receiving tacrolimus IV infusion, give 1st oral dose 8-12 hrs after discontinuing the IV infusion

Renal Transplant
Prophylaxis of organ rejection in patients receiving allogeneic kidney transplant; recommended to be used concomitantly w/ azathioprine or mycophenolate mofetil (MMF) and adrenal corticosteroids (early post-transplant)

Cap:
Initial: 0.2mg/kg/day in combination w/ azathioprine or 0.1mg/kg/day in combination w/ MMF/Interleukin (IL)-2 receptor antagonist; give as 2 divided doses, q12h. May administer w/in 24 hrs of kidney transplant, but should be delayed until renal function has recovered
Titrate: Based on clinical assessments of rejection and tolerability
Maint: Lower dosages than the initial dosage may be sufficient
Observed Tacrolimus Whole Blood Trough Concentrations w/ Kidney Transplant:
W/ Azathioprine:
Months 1-3: 7-20ng/mL
Months 4-12: 5-15ng/mL
W/ MMF/IL-2 Receptor Antagonist:
Months 1-12: 4-11ng/mL
IV:
Initial: 0.03-0.05mg/kg/day
If receiving tacrolimus IV infusion, give 1st oral dose 8-12 hrs after discontinuing the IV infusion

Cardiac Transplant
Prophylaxis of organ rejection in patients receiving allogeneic heart transplant; recommended to be used concomitantly w/ azathioprine or mycophenolate mofetil (MMF) and adrenal corticosteroids (early post-transplant)

Cap:
Initial: 0.075mg/kg/day as 2 divided doses, q12h; administer no sooner than 6 hrs after heart transplant
Titrate: Based on clinical assessments of rejection and tolerability
Maint: Lower dosages than the initial dosage may be sufficient
Observed Tacrolimus Whole Blood Trough Concentrations w/ Heart Transplant:
Months 1-3: 10-20ng/mL
Months ≥4: 5-15ng/mL
IV:
Initial: 0.01mg/kg/day
If receiving tacrolimus IV infusion, give 1st oral dose 8-12 hrs after discontinuing the IV infusion

DOSING CONSIDERATIONS
Concomitant Medications
Cyclosporine: Do not use simultaneously; d/c tacrolimus or cyclosporine at least 24 hrs before initiating the other
Renal Impairment
Liver/Heart Transplant:
Preexisting Renal Impairment: Start at lower end of dosing range

Cap:
Initial: 0.15-0.2mg/kg/day as 2 divided doses, q12h; administer no sooner than 6 hrs after liver transplant
Observed Tacrolimus Whole Blood Trough Concentrations w/ Liver Transplant:
Months 1-12: 5-20ng/mL
IV:
Initial: 0.03-0.05mg/kg/day

Kidney Transplant:
Postoperative Oliguria: Initial dose should be administered no sooner than 6 hrs and w/in 24 hrs of transplantation, but may be delayed until renal function shows evidence of recovery
Hepatic Impairment
Severe (Child-Pugh ≥10): May require lower doses
Elderly
Start at lower end of dosing range
Other Important Considerations
Black patients may require higher doses
Do not eat grapefruit or drink grapefruit juice

ADMINISTRATION
Oral/IV route
Inj should be used only as a continuous IV infusion and when the patient cannot tolerate oral administration of cap.
Cap
Take consistently, either w/ or w/o food.
IV
Dilute product w/ 0.9% NaCl inj or D5 inj to concentration between 0.004mg/mL and 0.02mg/mL prior to use.
Diluted infusion sol should be stored in glass or polyethylene containers and should be discarded after 24 hrs; do not store in PVC container due to decreased stability and potential for extraction of phthalates; in situations where more dilute sol are utilized (eg, pediatric dosing), PVC-free tubing should likewise be used to minimize the potential for significant drug adsorption onto tubing.
Should not be mixed or co-infused w/ sol of pH ≥9 (eg, ganciclovir, acyclovir).

STORAGE
(Cap) 25°C (77°F); excursions permitted to 15-30°C (59-86°F). (Inj) 5-25°C (41-77°F).

HOW SUPPLIED
Cap: 0.5mg, 1mg, 5mg; **Inj:** 5mg/mL [1mL]

CONTRAINDICATIONS
Hypersensitivity to tacrolimus. **Inj:** Hypersensitivity to polyoxyl 60 hydrogenated castor oil (HCO-60).

WARNINGS/PRECAUTIONS
Limit exposure to sunlight and UV light in patients at increased risk for skin cancer. Increased risk for polyoma virus infections, CMV viremia, and CMV disease. Polyoma virus-associated nephropathy (PVAN) reported; may lead to renal function deterioration and kidney graft loss. Progressive multifocal leukoencephalopathy (PML) reported; consider PML in differential diagnosis in patients reporting neurological symptoms and consider consultation w/ a neurologist. Consider reductions in immunosuppression if CMV viremia, CMV disease, or if evidence of PVAN or PML develops. May cause new onset diabetes mellitus; closely monitor blood glucose concentrations. May cause acute/chronic nephrotoxicity; closely monitor patients w/ renal dysfunction. Consider changing to another immunosuppressive therapy in patients w/ persistent SrCr elevations unresponsive to dose adjustments. May cause neurotoxicity (eg, posterior reversible encephalopathy syndrome [PRES], delirium, coma); if PRES is suspected or diagnosed, maintain BP control and immediately reduce immunosuppression. Hyperkalemia and HTN reported. May prolong the QT/QTc interval and may cause torsades de pointes; avoid in patients w/ congenital long QT syndrome and consider obtaining ECGs and monitoring electrolytes (Mg^{2+}, K^+, Ca^{2+}) periodically in patients w/ CHF, bradyarrhythmias, those taking certain antiarrhythmic medications or other medicinal products that lead to QT prolongation, and those w/ electrolyte disturbances. Myocardial hypertrophy reported; consider dose reduction or discontinuation if diagnosed and consider echocardiographic evaluation in patients who develop renal failure or clinical manifestations of ventricular dysfunction. Pure red cell aplasia (PRCA) reported; consider discontinuation if diagnosed. GI perforation reported; institute appropriate medical/surgical management promptly. (Inj) Anaphylactic reactions may occur; should be reserved for patients unable to take cap orally. Patients should be under continuous observation for at least the first 30 min following the start of infusion and at frequent intervals thereafter; d/c infusion if signs/symptoms of anaphylaxis occur.

ADVERSE REACTIONS
Lymphoma, malignancies, infections, tremor, HTN, abnormal renal function, headache, insomnia, hyperglycemia, hyperkalemia, hypomagnesemia, diarrhea, N/V, paresthesia.

DRUG INTERACTIONS
See Dosing Considerations. Not recommended w/ sirolimus in liver or heart transplants; safety and efficacy not established in kidney transplant. Due to potential for additive/synergistic renal impairment, caution w/ drugs that may be associated w/ renal dysfunction (eg, aminoglycosides, ganciclovir, amphotericin B). Increased whole blood concentrations w/ CYP3A inhibitors (eg, antifungals, calcium channel blockers [CCBs], macrolide antibiotics), and magnesium and aluminum hydroxide antacids. Decreased whole blood concentrations w/ CYP3A inducers. May increase mycophenolic acid (MPA) exposure after crossover from cyclosporine to tacrolimus in patients concomitantly receiving MPA-containing products. Avoid w/ nelfinavir unless the benefits outweigh the risks. Monitor whole blood concentrations and adjust tacrolimus dose if used concomitantly w/ protease inhibitors (eg, ritonavir, telaprevir, boceprevir), CCBs (eg, verapamil, diltiazem, nifedipine), erythromycin, clarithromycin, troleandomycin, chloramphenicol, rifampin, rifabutin, phenytoin, carbamazepine, phenobarbital, St. John's wort, magnesium and aluminum hydroxide antacids, bromocriptine, nefazodone, metoclopramide, danazol, ethinyl estradiol, amiodarone, methylprednisolone, herbal products containing *Schisandra sphenanthera*

extracts, or CYP3A inhibitors/inducers. Monitor whole blood concentrations and adjust tacrolimus dose when concomitant use of antifungal drugs (eg, azoles, caspofungin) w/ tacrolimus is initiated or discontinued; initially reduce tacrolimus dose to 1/3 of the original dose when initiating therapy w/ voriconazole or posaconazole. May increase levels of phenytoin; monitor phenytoin levels and adjust phenytoin dose as needed. Caution w/ antihypertensive agents (eg, K+-sparing diuretics, ACE inhibitors, ARBs) or other agents associated w/ hyperkalemia. Reduce tacrolimus dose, closely monitor tacrolimus whole blood concentrations, and monitor for QT prolongation when coadministered w/ CYP3A4 substrates and/or inhibitors that also have the potential to prolong the QT interval. Amiodarone may increase whole blood concentrations w/ or w/o concurrent QT prolongation. Avoid live vaccines during therapy. Caution w/ concomitant immunosuppressants.

PREGNANCY AND LACTATION
Pregnancy: Category C.
Lactation: Not for use in nursing.

MECHANISM OF ACTION
Macrolide immunosuppressant; not established. Inhibits T-lymphocyte activation. Binds to an intracellular protein, FKBP-12, forming a complex of tacrolimus-FKBP-12, Ca^{2+}, calmodulin, and calcineurin, and inhibiting phosphatase activity of calcineurin. This effect may prevent dephosphorylation and translocation of nuclear factor of activated T-cells, a nuclear component thought to initiate gene transcription for the formation of lymphokines.

PHARMACOKINETICS
Absorption: (Oral) Incomplete and variable. Administration of variable doses in different populations resulted in different pharmacokinetic parameters.
Distribution: Plasma protein binding (approx 99%); crosses placenta; found in breast milk. **Metabolism:** Liver, via CYP3A (demethylation and hydroxylation); 13-demethyl tacrolimus (major metabolite); 31-demethyl (active metabolite). **Elimination:** (Oral) Feces (92.6%), urine (2.3%). (IV) Feces (92.4%); urine (<1% unchanged). Refer to PI for $T_{1/2}$ values in different populations.

PATIENT CONSIDERATIONS
Assessment: Assess for drug hypersensitivity, congenital long QT syndrome, CHF, bradyarrhythmias, electrolyte disturbances, renal/hepatic impairment, pregnancy/nursing status, and possible drug interactions. (Inj) Assess for hypersensitivity to HCO-60.

Monitoring: Monitor tacrolimus blood concentrations in conjunction w/ other laboratory and clinical parameters. Monitor for lymphomas and other malignancies, infections, neurotoxicity, HTN, QT prolongation, PRCA, GI perforation, and other adverse reactions. Monitor serum K+ and glucose concentrations. (Inj) Monitor for anaphylactic reactions.

Counseling: Inform of the risks and benefits of therapy. Advise to take medicine at the same 12-hr interval every day and not to eat grapefruit or drink grapefruit juice in combination w/ the drug. Advise to limit exposure to sunlight and UV light by wearing protective clothing and to use a sunscreen w/ a high protection factor. Instruct to contact physician if frequent urination, increased thirst or hunger, vision changes, deliriums, tremors, or any symptoms of infection develop. Advise to attend all visits and complete all blood tests ordered by medical team. Inform that therapy may cause high BP, which may require treatment w/ antihypertensive therapy. Instruct to inform physician if planning to become pregnant or breastfeed or when starting or stopping any medication (prescription and nonprescription medicines, natural/herbal remedies, nutritional supplements, vitamins). Inform that therapy may interfere w/ the usual response to immunizations and that live vaccines should be avoided.

PROLASTIN-C — alpha1-proteinase inhibitor (human)   Rx

Class: Alpha₁-proteinase inhibitor (A₁PI)

ADULT DOSAGE	**PEDIATRIC DOSAGE**
Alpha₁-Antitrypsin Deficiency	Pediatric use may not have been established
Chronic Augmentation and Maint Therapy in Patients w/ Clinically Evident Emphysema Due to Severe Deficiency of Alpha₁-Proteinase Inhibitor:	
60mg/kg IV once weekly. Infuse at 0.08mL/kg/min as determined by patient response and comfort	

ADMINISTRATION
IV route

Reconstitution
1. Allow unopened vials and diluent vials to warm to room temperature before reconstitution
2. Remove plastic cover from short end of the transfer needle, insert exposed end of the needle through the center of the stopper in the diluent vial, and then remove the cover at the other end of the transfer needle by carefully twisting
3. Invert diluent vial and insert the attached needle into drug vial at a 45° angle
4. Immediately after adding the diluent, swirl vigorously for 10-15 sec to thoroughly break up cake, then swirl continuously until the powder is completely dissolved
5. If particles are visible after reconstitution, remove by passage through a sterile filter (eg, 15 micron filter used for administering blood products)
6. Pool reconstituted product from several vials into an empty, sterile IV sol container using aseptic technique using the sterile filter needle provided

Administration
1. Administer w/in 3 hrs of reconstitution
2. Infuse separately, w/o mixing w/ other agents or diluting sol

STORAGE
≤25°C (77°F). Avoid freezing; breakage of diluent bottle might occur. After Reconstitution: Keep at room temperature for administration within 3 hrs.

HOW SUPPLIED
Inj: 1000mg

CONTRAINDICATIONS
IgA deficient patients with antibodies against IgA.

WARNINGS/PRECAUTIONS
If evidence of an acute hypersensitivity reaction is observed, promptly stop the infusion and begin appropriate therapy. May contain trace amounts of IgA. May carry a risk of transmitting infectious agents (eg, viruses, Creutzfeldt-Jakob disease agent).

ADVERSE REACTIONS
Upper respiratory tract infection, headache, pruritus, urticaria, nausea, peripheral edema, pyrexia, urinary tract infection, chest/back pain, chills, cough, dizziness, dyspnea, hot flush.

PREGNANCY AND LACTATION
Category C, caution in nursing.

MECHANISM OF ACTION
α₁-PI (α1-antitrypsin); inhibits neutrophil elastase and acts to increase and maintain serum and lung epithelial lining fluid levels of α₁-PI.

PHARMACOKINETICS
Absorption: AUC=155.9mg•hr/mL; C_{max}=1.797mg/mL. **Elimination:** $T_{1/2}$=146.3 hrs.

PATIENT CONSIDERATIONS
Assessment: Assess for IgA deficiency and pregnancy/nursing status.

Monitoring: Monitor for signs/symptoms of hypersensitivity reactions, infections, and other adverse reactions.

Counseling: Inform of the risks and benefits of therapy. Inform of the signs of hypersensitivity reactions; advise to d/c and seek immediate emergency care, depending on the severity of reaction, if symptoms occur. Inform that the product is made from human plasma and may carry risk of transmitting infectious agents.

PROLEUKIN — aldesleukin   Rx

Class: Biological response modifier

> Restrict to patients with normal cardiac and pulmonary function as defined by thallium stress testing and formal pulmonary function testing. Extreme caution with history of cardiac or pulmonary disease. Administer in a hospital setting under the supervision of a qualified physician experienced in the use of anticancer agents; intensive care facility and specialists skilled in cardiopulmonary or intensive care medicine must be available. Associated with capillary leak syndrome (CLS), impaired neutrophil function (reduced chemotaxis), and increased risk of disseminated infection (eg, sepsis, bacterial endocarditis); adequately treat pre-existing bacterial infections prior to initiation of therapy. Withhold treatment if moderate to severe lethargy or somnolence develops; continued administration may result in coma.

ADULT DOSAGE	**PEDIATRIC DOSAGE**
Metastatic Renal Cell Carcinoma	Pediatric use may not have been established
600,000 IU/kg (0.037mg/kg) q8h by a 15-min IV infusion for a max of 14 doses	
Following 9 days of rest, repeat for another 14 doses, for a max of 28 doses per course, as tolerated	
Retreatment:	
Evaluate for response approx 4 weeks after course completion and again immediately prior to start of next course; give additional courses only if there is some tumor shrinkage following last course and retreatment is not contraindicated	
Separate each treatment course by a rest period of at least 7 weeks from date of hospital discharge	
Metastatic Melanoma	
600,000 IU/kg (0.037mg/kg) q8h by a 15-min IV infusion for a max of 14 doses	
Following 9 days of rest, repeat for another 14 doses, for a max of 28 doses per course, as tolerated	
Retreatment:	
Evaluate for response approx 4 weeks after course completion and again immediately prior to start of next course; give additional courses only if there is some tumor shrinkage following last course and retreatment is not contraindicated	
Separate each treatment course by a rest period of at least 7 weeks from date of hospital discharge	

DOSING CONSIDERATIONS

Adverse Reactions

Retreatment is contraindicated in patients who have experienced the following toxicities:

1. Sustained ventricular tachycardia (≥5 beats)
2. Cardiac rhythm disturbances not controlled or unresponsive to management
3. Chest pain w/ ECG changes, consistent w/ angina or MI
4. Cardiac tamponade
5. Intubation for >72 hrs
6. Renal failure requiring dialysis >72 hrs
7. Coma or toxic psychosis lasting >48 hrs
8. Repetitive or difficult to control seizure
9. Bowel ischemia/perforation
10. GI bleeding requiring surgery

Hold Doses and Restart According to the Following:

Cardiovascular System:
Hold Dose for: A-Fb, supraventricular tachycardia, or bradycardia that requires treatment or is recurrent or persistent
May Give Subsequent Dose if: Patient is asymptomatic w/ full recovery to normal sinus rhythm

Hold Dose for: Systolic BP <90mmHg w/ increasing requirements for pressors
May Give Subsequent Dose if: Systolic BP ≥90mmHg and stable or improving requirements for pressors

Hold Dose for: Any ECG change consistent w/ MI, ischemia, or myocarditis w/ or w/o chest pain; suspicion of cardiac ischemia
May Give Subsequent Dose if: Patient is asymptomatic, MI and myocarditis have been ruled out, clinical suspicion of angina is low, there is no evidence of ventricular hypokinesia

Respiratory System:
Hold Dose for: O$_2$ saturation <90%
May Give Subsequent Dose if: O$_2$ saturation >90%

Nervous System:
Hold Dose for: Mental status changes, including moderate confusion or agitation
May Give Subsequent Dose if: Mental status changes completely resolved

Body as a Whole:
Hold Dose for: Sepsis syndrome, patient is clinically unstable
May Give Subsequent Dose if: Sepsis syndrome has resolved, patient is clinically stable, infection is under treatment

Urogenital System:
Hold Dose for: SrCr >4.5mg/dL or a SrCr ≥4mg/dL in the presence of severe volume overload, acidosis, or hyperkalemia
May Give Subsequent Dose if: SrCr <4mg/dL and fluid and electrolyte status is stable

Hold Dose for: Persistent oliguria, urine output of <10mL/hr for 16-24 hrs w/ rising SrCr
May Give Subsequent Dose if: Urine output >10mL/hr w/ a decrease of SrCr >1.5mg/dL or normalization of SrCr

Digestive System:
Hold Dose for: Signs of hepatic failure including encephalopathy, increasing ascites, liver pain, hypoglycemia
May Give Subsequent Dose if: All signs of hepatic failure have resolved; d/c all further treatment for that course. A new course of treatment, if warranted, should be initiated no sooner than 7 weeks after cessation of adverse event and hospital discharge

Hold Dose for: Stool guaiac repeatedly >3-4+
May Give Subsequent Dose if: Stool guaiac negative

Skin:
Hold Dose for: Bullous dermatitis or marked worsening of preexisting skin condition; avoid topical steroid therapy
May Give Subsequent Dose if: Resolution of all signs of bullous dermatitis

ADMINISTRATION

IV route

Vial is for single-use only; discard any unused portion

Reconstitution and Dilution Instructions

1. Reconstitute each vial w/ 1.2mL of SWFI; when reconstituted as directed, each mL contains 18 million IU (1.1mg)
2. During reconstitution, direct the SWFI at the side of the vial and gently swirl the contents to avoid excess foaming; do not shake
3. Dilute the reconstituted sol in 50mL of D5W. In cases where the total dose is ≤1.5mg (eg, a patient w/ a body weight of <40kg), the dose should be diluted in a smaller volume of D5W
4. Concentrations <0.03mg/mL and >0.07mg/mL have shown increased variability in drug delivery; avoid dilution and delivery outside of this concentration range
5. Use plastic bags as the dilution container; do not use in-line filters for administration
6. Administer w/in 48 hrs of reconstitution; bring the sol to room temperature prior to infusion

Avoid reconstitution or dilution w/ Bacteriostatic Water for inj or 0.9% NaCl inj
Do not coadminister w/ other drugs in the same container

STORAGE

2-8°C (36-46°F). Do not freeze. Protect from light. Reconstituted/Diluted: 2-25°C (36-77°F) for up to 48 hrs.

HOW SUPPLIED

Inj: 22 million IU

CONTRAINDICATIONS

Known history of hypersensitivity to interleukin-2 or any component of this medication, abnormal thallium stress test, abnormal pulmonary function tests, organ allografts. (Retreatment) Sustained ventricular tachycardia (≥5 beats), cardiac arrhythmias uncontrolled or unresponsive to management, chest pain w/ ECG changes consistent w/ angina or myocardial infarction, cardiac tamponade, intubation for >72 hrs, renal failure requiring dialysis >72 hrs, coma or toxic psychosis lasting >48 hrs, repetitive or difficult to control seizures, bowel ischemia/perforation, or GI bleeding requiring surgery.

WARNINGS/PRECAUTIONS

Exacerbation of pre-existing or initial presentation of autoimmune disease and inflammatory disorders (eg, Crohn's disease, scleroderma, thyroiditis, inflammatory arthritis, diabetes mellitus [DM], oculo-bulbar myasthenia gravis, crescentic IgA glomerulonephritis, cholecystitis, cerebral vasculitis, Stevens-Johnson syndrome, and bullous pemphigoid) reported. Confirm negative CNS metastases before treatment. New neurologic signs/symptoms and anatomic lesions reported. May cause seizures; extreme caution with known seizure disorders. Medical management of CLS begins with careful monitoring of the fluid and organ perfusion status; extreme caution with fixed requirements for large volumes of fluid (eg, hypercalcemia). Carefully balance effects of fluid shifts in the management of hypovolemia or extravascular fluid accumulation so that none of the consequences of hypovolemia (eg, impaired organ perfusion) or fluid accumulation (eg, pulmonary edema) exceed patient's tolerance. Withhold treatment for failure to maintain organ perfusion. May impair kidney/liver function. Mental status changes (eg, irritability, confusion, depression) may be indicators of bacteremia or early bacterial sepsis, hypoperfusion, occult CNS malignancy, or direct drug-induced CNS toxicity. Hypothyroidism, sometimes preceded by hyperthyroidism, reported; some may require thyroid replacement therapy. Thyroid function changes may be a manifestation of autoimmunity. Onset of symptomatic hyperglycemia and/or DM reported. May increase risk of allograft rejection in transplant patients. Serious manifestations of eosinophilia involving eosinophilic infiltration of cardiac and pulmonary tissues may occur. Refer to PI for recommended cardiac and pulmonary functions tests and laboratory tests.

ADVERSE REACTIONS

Chills, creatinine increase, bilirubinemia, hypotension, confusion, tachycardia, dyspnea, oliguria, diarrhea, N/V, anemia, rash, thrombocytopenia, immunogenicity.

DRUG INTERACTIONS

May affect CNS function, and therefore may interact with psychotropic drugs (eg, narcotics, analgesics, antiemetics, sedatives, tranquilizers). Nephrotoxic (eg, aminoglycosides, indomethacin), myelotoxic (eg, cytotoxic chemotherapy), cardiotoxic (eg, doxorubicin), or hepatotoxic (eg, methotrexate, asparaginase) drugs may increase toxicity in these organ systems. Reduced kidney/liver function secondary to treatment may delay elimination of concomitant drugs and increase risk of adverse events from those drugs. Hypersensitivity reactions reported with high-dose antineoplastic agents (dacarbazine, cis-platinum, tamoxifen, interferon-alfa). Increased myocardial injury and exacerbation or initial presentation of a number of autoimmune and inflammatory disorders may occur with interferon-alfa. Avoid preparations containing a steroid (eg, hydrocortisone). Glucocorticoids may reduce antitumor effectiveness; avoid concomitant use. β-blockers and other antihypertensives may potentiate hypotension. Acute, atypical adverse reactions reported with radiographic iodinated contrast media.

PREGNANCY AND LACTATION

Category C, not for use in nursing.

MECHANISM OF ACTION

Biological response modifier; not established. Suspected to enhance lymphocyte mitogenesis and stimulate long-term growth of human interleukin-2-dependent cell lines, enhance lymphocyte cytotoxicity, induce killer cell activity, and induce interferon-gamma production.

PHARMACOKINETICS

Metabolism: Kidneys. **Elimination:** Kidneys; T$_{1/2}$=85 min.

PATIENT CONSIDERATIONS

Assessment: Assess for pre-existing bacterial infections, autoimmune disease, or inflammatory disorders, CNS metastases, other conditions where treatment is contraindicated or cautioned, cardiac/pulmonary/renal/hepatic/CNS function, pregnancy/nursing status, and possible drug interactions. Evaluate standard hematologic tests, blood chemistries, and chest x-rays.

Monitoring: Monitor for CLS, impaired neutrophil function, disseminated infection, lethargy, somnolence, other drug toxicities, exacerbation of pre-existing conditions, and other adverse reactions. Monitor daily standard hematologic tests, blood chemistries (eg, electrolytes, renal/hepatic function), chest x-rays, vital signs, weight, fluid intake/output, and cardiac function.

Counseling: Inform about benefits/risks of therapy. Instruct to inform physician if pregnant or breastfeeding.

PROLIA — denosumab   Rx

Class: IgG$_2$ monoclonal antibody

ADULT DOSAGE

Osteoporosis

Postmenopausal Osteoporosis:
Postmenopausal women at high risk for fracture, or patients who have failed or are intolerant to other available osteoporosis therapy

PEDIATRIC DOSAGE

Pediatric use may not have been established

60mg as a single SQ inj once every 6 months

To Increase Bone Mass in Men w/ Osteoporosis:
Men at high risk for fracture, or patients who have failed or are intolerant to other available osteoporosis therapy

60mg as a single SQ inj once every 6 months

Calcium and Vitamin D Supplementation:
All patients should receive Ca^{2+} 1000mg/day and ≥400 IU vitamin D daily

Bone Loss

In Men Receiving Androgen Deprivation Therapy for Nonmetastatic Prostate Cancer:
60mg as a single SQ inj once every 6 months

In Women Receiving Adjuvant Aromatase Inhibitor Therapy for Breast Cancer:
60mg as a single SQ inj once every 6 months

Calcium and Vitamin D Supplementation:
All patients should receive Ca^{2+} 1000mg/day and ≥400 IU vitamin D daily

Missed Dose
If a dose is missed, administer as soon as patient is available, then schedule inj every 6 months from date of last inj

ADMINISTRATION
SQ route
Administer in the upper arm/thigh or abdomen.
People sensitive to latex should not handle the grey needle cap on the single-use prefilled syringe, which contains dry natural rubber (a derivative of latex).
Prior to administration, remove from the refrigerator and bring to room temperature up to 25°C (77°F), by standing in the original container for 15-30 min.
Instructions for Prefilled Syringe w/ Needle Safety Guard:
Do not slide the green safety guard forward over the needle before administering the inj; it will lock in place and prevent inj.
Insert needle and inject all the liquid SQ.
Instructions for Single-Use Vial:
Use a 27-gauge needle to withdraw and inject the 1mL dose.
Do not re-enter the vial; discard vial and any liquid remaining in the vial.
STORAGE
2-8°C (36-46°F). Do not freeze. Use w/in 14 days once removed from the refrigerator and do not expose to temperatures >25°C (77°F). Protect from direct light and heat. Avoid vigorous shaking.
HOW SUPPLIED
Inj: 60mg/mL [prefilled syringe, vial]
CONTRAINDICATIONS
Hypocalcemia, pregnancy, history of systemic hypersensitivity to any component of the product.
WARNINGS/PRECAUTIONS
Should be administered by a healthcare professional. Do not give w/ other drugs that contain the same active ingredient (eg, Xgeva). Hypersensitivity, including anaphylaxis, reported; d/c further use and initiate appropriate therapy if an anaphylactic or other clinically significant allergic reaction occurs. Hypocalcemia may be exacerbated; correct preexisting hypocalcemia prior to initiating therapy. Monitor Ca^{2+} and mineral levels (phosphorus [P] and Mg^{2+}) w/in 14 days of inj in patients predisposed to hypocalcemia and disturbances of mineral metabolism (eg, history of hypoparathyroidism, malabsorption syndromes, excision of the small intestine). Significant risk of hypocalcemia following administration w/ severe renal impairment (CrCl <30mL/min) or receiving dialysis; marked elevations of serum parathyroid hormone (PTH) may develop. Osteonecrosis of the jaw (ONJ) may occur; increased risk w/ duration of exposure to therapy. A dental examination is recommended w/ appropriate preventive dentistry prior to treatment in patients w/ risk factors for ONJ (eg, invasive dental procedures, diagnosis of cancer, concomitant therapies [eg, chemotherapy, corticosteroids, angiogenesis inhibitors]). Atypical low-energy or low-trauma fractures of the femoral shaft reported; evaluate patients w/ thigh/groin pain to rule out an incomplete femur fracture and consider interruption of therapy. Endocarditis and serious skin, abdomen, urinary tract, and ear infections leading to hospitalization reported; assess need for continued therapy if serious infections develop. Increased risk for serious infections in patients w/ an impaired immune system. Epidermal and dermal adverse events may occur; consider discontinuing therapy if severe symptoms develop. Severe and occasionally incapacitating bone, joint, and/or muscle pain reported; consider discontinuing use if severe symptoms develop. Significant suppression of bone remodeling as evidenced by markers of bone turnover and bone histomorphometry reported.

ADVERSE REACTIONS
Postmenopausal Osteoporosis: Back pain, pain in extremity, musculoskeletal pain, hypercholesterolemia, cystitis.
Men w/ Osteoporosis: Back pain, arthralgia, nasopharyngitis.
Patients Receiving Androgen Deprivation Therapy/Adjuvant Aromatase Inhibitor: Arthralgia, back pain.
DRUG INTERACTIONS
Immunosuppressant agents may increase the risk of serious infections. Concomitant administration of drugs associated w/ ONJ may increase risk of developing ONJ.
PREGNANCY AND LACTATION
Pregnancy: Category X. May cause fetal harm. Physicians are advised to recommend that pregnant patients enroll in Amgen's Pregnancy Surveillance Program.
Lactation: Not for use in nursing.
MECHANISM OF ACTION
IgG_2 monoclonal antibody; binds to receptor activator of nuclear factor kappa-B ligand (RANKL) and prevents RANKL from activating its receptor, RANK, on the surface of osteoclasts and their precursors, thereby decreasing bone resorption and increasing bone mass and strength in both cortical and trabecular bone.
PHARMACOKINETICS
Absorption: Fasting: C_{max}=6.75mcg/mL, T_{max}=10 days (median), $AUC_{0-16 weeks}$=316mcg•day/mL. **Distribution:** Crosses placenta. **Elimination:** $T_{1/2}$=25.4 days.

PATIENT CONSIDERATIONS
Assessment: Assess for drug hypersensitivity, preexisting hypocalcemia, history of hypoparathyroidism, thyroid/parathyroid surgery, malabsorption syndromes, excision of the small intestine, renal impairment, impairment of the immune system, risk factors for ONJ, pregnancy/nursing status, and possible drug interactions. Perform routine oral exam, and dental examination w/ appropriate preventive dentistry in patients w/ risk factors for ONJ.

Monitoring: Monitor for signs/symptoms of hypocalcemia, infections, hypersensitivity, dermatological reactions, serum PTH elevation, ONJ, atypical femoral fractures, delayed fracture healing, musculoskeletal pain, and other adverse reactions. Monitor Ca^{2+} and mineral levels (P and Mg^{2+}) w/in 14 days of inj in patients predisposed to hypocalcemia and disturbances of mineral metabolism.

Counseling: Advise not to take w/ other drugs w/ the same active ingredient. Inform about the importance of maintaining Ca^{2+} levels w/ adequate Ca^{2+} and vitamin D supplementation. Advise to seek prompt medical attention if signs/symptoms of hypocalcemia, infections, dermatological reactions, or hypersensitivity reactions develop. Advise to maintain good oral hygiene during treatment and to inform dentist prior to dental procedures of current treatment. Instruct to inform physician or dentist if patient experiences persistent pain and/or slow healing of the mouth or jaw after dental surgery. Advise to report new or unusual thigh, hip, or groin pain. Inform that severe bone, joint, and/or muscle pain reported during therapy; instruct to report development of severe symptoms. Inform that therapy should not be used if pregnant or nursing. Advise to adhere to proper schedule of administration.

PROMACTA — eltrombopag   Rx
Class: Thrombopoietin receptor agonist

> May increase risk of hepatic decompensation in patients w/ chronic hepatitis C when given in combination w/ interferon and ribavirin.

ADULT DOSAGE	**PEDIATRIC DOSAGE**
Chronic Immune Thrombocytopenia	**Chronic Immune Thrombocytopenia**
W/ Insufficient Response to Corticosteroids, Immunoglobulins, or Splenectomy:	**W/ Insufficient Response to Corticosteroids, Immunoglobulins, or Splenectomy:**
Initial: 50mg qd	**Initial:**
Titrate: Adjust the dose to achieve and maintain a platelet count ≥50 x 10^9/L	**1-5 Years:** 25mg qd
Max: 75mg/day	**≥6 Years:** 50mg qd
Dose Adjustment Based on Platelet Counts:	**Titrate:** Adjust the dose to achieve and maintain a platelet count ≥50 x 10^9/L
<50 x 10^9/L Following at Least 2 Weeks of Therapy:	**Max:** 75mg/day
Increase daily dose by 25mg to a max of 75mg/day; patients taking 12.5mg qd, increase to 25mg qd before increasing dose amount by 25mg	**Dose Adjustment Based on Platelet Counts:**
≥200 to ≤400 x 10^9/L at Any Time:	**<50 x 10^9/L Following at Least 2 Weeks of Therapy:**
Decrease daily dose by 25mg; wait 2 weeks to assess the effects and any subsequent dose adjustments Patients taking 25mg qd, decrease to 12.5mg qd	Increase daily dose by 25mg to a max of 75mg/day; patients taking 12.5mg qd, increase to 25mg qd before increasing dose amount by 25mg
<400 x 10^9/L:	**≥200 to <400 x 10^9/L at Any Time:**
Stop therapy and increase frequency of platelet monitoring to twice weekly; once platelet count is <150 x 10^9/L, reinitiate at a daily dose reduced by 25mg or reinitiate at a daily dose of 12.5mg for patients taking 25mg qd	Decrease daily dose by 25mg; wait 2 weeks to assess the effects and any subsequent dose adjustments Patients taking 25mg qd, decrease to 12.5mg qd
	<400 x 10^9/L:
	Stop therapy and increase frequency of platelet monitoring to twice weekly; once platelet count is <150 x 10^9/L, reinitiate at a daily dose reduced by

<400 x 10⁹/L After 2 Weeks of Therapy at Lowest Dose:
D/C therapy

Chronic Hepatitis C-Associated Thrombocytopenia

To allow the initiation and maint of interferon-based therapy

Initial: 25mg qd
Titrate: Adjust dose in 25mg increments every 2 weeks as necessary to achieve target platelet count required to initiate antiviral therapy. During antiviral therapy, adjust dose to avoid dose reductions of peginterferon
Max: 100mg/day

Dose Adjustment Based on Platelet Counts:
<50 x 10⁹/L Following at Least 2 Weeks of Therapy:
Increase daily dose by 25mg to a max of 100mg/day
≥200 to ≤400 x 10⁹/L at Any Time:
Decrease daily dose by 25mg; wait 2 weeks to assess the effects and any subsequent dose adjustments
<400 x 10⁹/L:
Stop therapy and increase frequency of platelet monitoring to twice weekly; once platelet count is <150 x 10⁹/L, reinitiate at a daily dose reduced by 25mg or reinitiate at a daily dose of 12.5mg for patients taking 25mg qd
<400 x 10⁹/L After 2 Weeks of Therapy at Lowest Dose:
D/C therapy

Severe Aplastic Anemia

W/ Insufficient Response to Immunosuppressive Therapy:
Initial: 50mg qd
Titrate: Adjust dose in 50mg increments every 2 weeks as necessary to achieve the target platelet count ≥50 x 10⁹/L
Max: 150mg/day

Dose Adjustment Based on Platelet Counts:
<50 x 10⁹/L Following at Least 2 Weeks of Therapy:
Increase daily dose by 50mg to a max of 150mg/day; patients taking 25mg qd, increase to 50mg qd before increasing dose amount by 50mg
≥200 to ≤400 x 10⁹/L at Any Time:
Decrease daily dose by 50mg; wait 2 weeks to assess the effects and any subsequent dose adjustments
<400 x 10⁹/L:
Stop therapy for 1 week; once platelet count is <150 x 10⁹/L, reinitiate therapy at a dose reduced by 50mg
<400 x 10⁹/L After 2 Weeks of Therapy at Lowest Dose:
D/C therapy

25mg or reinitiate at a daily dose of 12.5mg for patients taking 25mg qd
<400 x 10⁹/L After 2 Weeks of Therapy at Lowest Dose:
D/C therapy

Assess platelet counts weekly for 2 weeks, and then monitor monthly when switching between oral sus and tab

---

DOSING CONSIDERATIONS
Concomitant Medications
Chronic Immune Thrombocytopenia:
Modify dosage regimen of concomitant medications for therapy to avoid excessive increases in platelet counts; do not administer >1 dose of eltrombopag w/in any 24-hr period

Hepatic Impairment
≥6 Years:
Mild to Severe (Child-Pugh Class A, B, C):
Chronic Immune Thrombocytopenia:
Initial: 25mg qd; after initiating therapy or after any subsequent dosing increase, wait 3 weeks before increasing the dose
Severe Aplastic Anemia:
Initial: 25mg qd

East Asian Ancestry w/ Hepatic Impairment (Child-Pugh Class A, B, C):
Chronic Immune Thrombocytopenia:
Initial: 12.5mg qd

Discontinuation
Chronic Immune Thrombocytopenia: D/C if platelet count does not increase to a sufficient level after 4 weeks of therapy at max daily dose of 75mg
Chronic Hepatitis C-Associated Thrombocytopenia: D/C therapy when antiviral

therapy is discontinued; important liver test abnormalities may necessitate discontinuation
Severe Aplastic Anemia: D/C therapy if no hematologic response occurs after 16 weeks of therapy. Consider discontinuation if new cytogenetic abnormalities or important liver test abnormalities are observed

Other Important Considerations
≥6 Years:
Chronic Immune Thrombocytopenia/Severe Aplastic Anemia:
East Asian Ancestry:
Initial: 25mg qd

ADMINISTRATION
Oral route

- Take on empty stomach (1 hr ac or 2 hrs pc).
- Take sus/tab at least 2 hrs before or 4 hrs after other medications (eg, antacids), Ca²⁺-rich foods (eg, dairy products, Ca²⁺-fortified juices), or supplements containing polyvalent cations (eg, iron, Ca²⁺, aluminum, Mg²⁺, selenium, zinc).
- Do not crush tabs and mix w/ food or liquids.

Sus
- Administer immediately after preparation.
- Discard any sus not administered w/in 30 min after preparation.
- Prepare w/ water only; do not use hot water.
- For details on preparation and administration of sus, see Instructions for Use.

STORAGE
20-25°C (68-77°F); excursions permitted to 15-30°C (59-86°F). **Reconstituted Sus:** 20-25°C (68-77°F) for 30 min; discard if not used w/in 30 min.

HOW SUPPLIED
Sus: 25mg/pkt; **Tab:** 12.5mg, 25mg, 50mg, 75mg, 100mg

WARNINGS/PRECAUTIONS
Should not be used to normalize platelet counts. Should only be used in patients w/ immune thrombocytopenia whose degree of thrombocytopenia and clinical condition increase the risk for bleeding. Liver enzyme elevations and indirect hyperbilirubinemia may occur; if bilirubin is elevated, perform fractionation. D/C if ALT levels increase to ≥3X ULN in patients w/ normal liver function or ≥3X baseline in patients w/ pretreatment elevations in transaminases, and are progressively increasing or persistent for ≥4 weeks, or are accompanied by increased direct bilirubin or by clinical symptoms of liver injury or evidence for hepatic decompensation. Hepatotoxicity may reoccur w/ reinitiation; caution w/ reintroduction of therapy and measure LFTs weekly during the dose adjustment phase. If liver test abnormalities persist, worsen, or reoccur, then permanently d/c therapy. Thrombotic/thromboembolic complications may result from increases in platelet counts; caution in patients w/ known risk factors for thromboembolism (eg, factor V Leiden, antithrombin III deficiency, antiphospholipid syndrome, chronic liver disease). Development or worsening of cataracts reported.

ADVERSE REACTIONS
Chronic Immune Thrombocytopenia:
Adults: N/V, diarrhea, URTI, increased ALT, myalgia, UTI.
Peds >1 Year: URTI, nasopharyngitis.

Chronic Hepatitis C-Associated Thrombocytopenia: Anemia, pyrexia, fatigue, headache, nausea, diarrhea, decreased appetite, influenza-like illness, asthenia, insomnia, cough, pruritus, chills, myalgia, alopecia, peripheral edema.

Severe Aplastic Anemia: Nausea, fatigue, cough, diarrhea, headache.

DRUG INTERACTIONS
See Boxed Warning. Take at least 2 hrs before or 4 hrs after any medications or products containing polyvalent cations (eg, antacids, dairy products, mineral supplements). Increases rosuvastatin levels; recommended to reduce rosuvastatin by 50%. Caution w/ substrates of organic anion transporting polypeptide 1B1 (eg, atorvastatin, bosentan, glyburide) or breast cancer resistance protein (eg, imatinib, irinotecan, methotrexate); monitor for signs/symptoms of excessive exposure and consider dose reduction of these drugs. Lopinavir/ritonavir may decrease plasma exposure.

PREGNANCY AND LACTATION
Pregnancy: Category C.
Lactation: Not for use in nursing.

MECHANISM OF ACTION
Thrombopoietin (TPO)-receptor agonist; interacts w/ the transmembrane domain of the human TPO receptor and initiates signaling cascades that induce proliferation and differentiation from bone marrow progenitor cells.

PHARMACOKINETICS
Absorption: T_{max}=2-6 hrs; (50mg dose qd) C_{max}=7.03mcg/mL (adults), 6.8mcg/mL (12-17 yrs of age), 10.3mcg/mL (6-11 yrs of age), 11.6mcg/mL (1-5 yrs of age); AUC=101mcg•hr/mL (adults), 103mcg•hr/mL (12-17 yrs of age), 153mcg•hr/mL (6-11 yrs of age), 162mcg•hr/mL (1-5 yrs of age). **Distribution:** Plasma protein binding (>99%). **Metabolism:** Extensive; cleavage, oxidation (via CYP1A2, CYP2C8), and conjugation w/ glucuronic acid (via UGT1A1, UGT1A3), glutathione, or cysteine. **Elimination:** Urine (31%), feces (59%, 20% unchanged); $T_{1/2}$=26-35 hrs (immune thrombocytopenia), 21-32 hrs (healthy subjects).

PATIENT CONSIDERATIONS
Assessment: Assess for degree of thrombocytopenia, risk factors for thromboembolism, renal/hepatic impairment, pregnancy/nursing status, and for possible drug interactions. Obtain baseline CBCs w/ differential, including platelet count, and LFTs. Perform a baseline ocular exam.

Monitoring: Monitor for thrombotic/thromboembolic complications, hepatotoxicity, hepatic decompensation in patients w/ chronic hepatitis C, cataracts, and other adverse reactions. Closely monitor patients w/ renal impairment. Monitor LFTs every 2 weeks during dose adjustment phase, then monthly following establishment of a stable dose. If abnormal LFT levels are detected, repeat tests w/in 3-5 days. If the abnormalities are confirmed, monitor serum LFT tests weekly until resolved or stabilized. Perform a regular ocular exam. Monitor platelet counts every week prior to starting antiviral therapy in patients w/ chronic hepatitis C. Monitor CBCs w/ differentials, including platelets counts, weekly during therapy until a stable platelet count is achieved. Obtain CBCs w/ differentials, including platelet counts, monthly thereafter and then weekly for at least 4 weeks after discontinuation.

Counseling: Ensure patients or caregivers receive training on proper dosing, preparation, and administration of sus. Inform about the risks and benefits of therapy. Inform that therapy may be associated w/ hepatobiliary lab abnormalities. Advise patients w/ chronic hepatitis C and cirrhosis that hepatic decompensation may occur when receiving alfa interferon therapy. Advise to avoid situations or medications that may increase risk for bleeding and to report to physician any signs/symptoms of liver problems immediately. Inform that thrombocytopenia and risk of bleeding may reoccur upon discontinuation, particularly if therapy is discontinued while on anticoagulants/antiplatelet agents. Inform that excessive dose may result in excessive platelet counts and risk for thrombotic/thromboembolic complications. Advise to have a baseline ocular exam prior to administration of therapy and be monitored for signs/symptoms of cataracts during therapy. Advise to take sus/tab at least 2 hrs before or 4 hrs after foods, mineral supplements, and antacids which contain polyvalent cations.

PROVENGE — sipuleucel-T   Rx

Class: Immunomodulatory agent

ADULT DOSAGE	PEDIATRIC DOSAGE
Metastatic Castration-Resistant Prostate Cancer	Pediatric use may not have been established
Asymptomatic or Minimally Symptomatic, Hormone Refractory Prostate Cancer: 3 complete doses (250mL each) given at approx 2-week intervals via IV infusion over 60 min	
If unable to give scheduled infusion, additional leukapheresis is needed	
Premedication	
Oral acetaminophen and antihistamine (eg, diphenhydramine) 30 min prior to administration	

ADMINISTRATION
IV route
Begin infusion prior to expiration date and time; do not infuse expired product

Administration Instructions
1. Gently mix and resuspend contents of infusion bag; do not administer if clumps remain in the bag
2. Do not use a cell filter during infusion
3. Observe patient for at least 30 min after each infusion
4. Keep infusion bag at room temperature if infusion is interrupted
5. If infusion bag has been at room temperature >3 hrs, do not resume infusion

STORAGE
Infusion bag must remain w/in the insulated polyurethane container inside the outer cardboard shipping box until the time of administration; stable for ≤3 hrs at room temperature once removed. Do not remove from the outer cardboard shipping box. Refer to PI for complete handling instructions.

HOW SUPPLIED
Sus: 250mL

WARNINGS/PRECAUTIONS
For autologous use only. Acute infusion reactions may occur; if reactions occur, decrease the rate or stop the infusion depending on severity of reaction and administer appropriate medical therapy prn. Closely monitor patients w/ cardiac or pulmonary conditions. Thromboembolic events (eg, deep vein thrombosis [DVT], pulmonary embolism) may occur. Vascular disorders (eg, cerebrovascular disease, cardiovascular disorders) reported. Not tested for transmissible infectious diseases and may carry the risk of transmitting infectious diseases to healthcare professionals handling the product; employ universal precautions. Do not use until confirmation of product release is received.

ADVERSE REACTIONS
Chills, fatigue, fever, back pain, N/V, joint ache, headache, citrate toxicity, paresthesia, anemia, constipation, pain, dizziness, muscle ache, asthenia.

DRUG INTERACTIONS
Immunosuppressive agents may alter efficacy and/or safety; evaluate whether it is appropriate to reduce or d/c immunosuppressive agents prior to treatment.

PREGNANCY AND LACTATION
Safety in pregnancy and nursing not known.

MECHANISM OF ACTION
Immunomodulatory agent (autologous cellular immunotherapy); not established. Induces an immune response targeted against prostatic acid phosphatase, an antigen expressed in most prostate cancer.

PATIENT CONSIDERATIONS
Assessment: Assess for history of cardiac or pulmonary conditions, risk factors for thromboembolic events, and possible drug interactions.

Monitoring: Monitor for signs and symptoms of infusion reactions, especially w/ cardiac or pulmonary conditions, thromboembolic events, vascular disorders, and other adverse reactions. Monitor for infectious sequelae in patients w/ central venous catheters.

Counseling: Counsel on the importance of adhering to preparation instructions for leukapheresis procedure, possible side effects, and postprocedure care. Advise to report signs and symptoms of acute infusion reactions and symptoms suggestive of cardiac arrhythmia, cerebral ischemia, DVT, and pulmonary embolism. Instruct to notify physician if taking immunosuppressive agents. Inform of the need for a central venous catheter placement if peripheral venous access is not adequate, and counsel on the importance of catheter care; advise to inform physician if fever or any swelling or redness around the catheter site occurs. Inform of the need to undergo an additional leukapheresis if a scheduled dose is missed.

PULMOZYME — dornase alfa   Rx

Class: Enzyme

ADULT DOSAGE	PEDIATRIC DOSAGE
Cystic Fibrosis	**Cystic Fibrosis**
Improves pulmonary function in conjunction with standard therapies	Improves pulmonary function in conjunction with standard therapies
2.5mg qd via nebulizer/compressor system (may benefit with bid dosing)	**≥5 Years:** 2.5mg qd via nebulizer/compressor system (may benefit with bid dosing)

ADMINISTRATION
Inhalation route
Should not be diluted or mixed with other drugs in the nebulizer.
Squeeze each ampule prior to use to check for leaks.
Once opened, entire contents of the ampule must be used or discarded.
Refer to PI for the recommended nebulizer/compressor systems.

STORAGE
Store in the protective foil pouch at 2-8°C (36-46°F). Protect from light. Refrigerate during transport and do not expose to room temperatures for a total time of 24 hrs.

HOW SUPPLIED
Sol: 2.5mg/2.5mL

CONTRAINDICATIONS
Known hypersensitivity to dornase alfa, Chinese Hamster ovary cell products, or any component of the product.

WARNINGS/PRECAUTIONS
May consider use for pediatric patients younger than 5 years of age who may experience potential benefit in pulmonary function or who may be at risk of RTI.

ADVERSE REACTIONS
Voice alteration, pharyngitis, rash, laryngitis, chest pain, conjunctivitis, rhinitis, fever, dyspnea, dyspepsia, antibodies development.

PREGNANCY AND LACTATION
Safety not known in pregnancy/nursing.

MECHANISM OF ACTION
Enzyme; hydrolyzes the deoxyribonucleic acid in sputum of CF patients and reduces sputum viscoelasticity.

PATIENT CONSIDERATIONS
Assessment: Assess for hypersensitivity to the drug, Chinese hamster ovary cell products, or any component of the drug, and nursing status.

Monitoring: Monitor for worsening of the condition and other adverse reactions.

Counseling: Instruct on the proper techniques to store and handle therapy. Advise to squeeze each ampule prior to use in order to check for leaks. Instruct to discard sol if cloudy or discolored. Inform that entire contents of ampule must be used or discarded once opened. Instruct on the proper use and maintenance of the nebulizer and compressor system. Instruct to not dilute or mix with other drugs in the nebulizer.

PURIXAN — mercaptopurine   Rx

Class: Purine analogue

ADULT DOSAGE	PEDIATRIC DOSAGE
Acute Lymphoblastic Leukemia	**Acute Lymphoblastic Leukemia**
Component of a Multi-agent Combination Chemotherapy Maint Regimen:	**Component of a Multi-agent Combination Chemotherapy Maint Regimen:**
Initial: 1.5-2.5mg/kg (50-75mg/m²) as a single daily dose	**Initial:** 1.5-2.5mg/kg (50-75mg/m²) as a single daily dose
Continuation of appropriate dosing requires periodic monitoring of absolute neutrophil count and platelet count to assure sufficient drug exposure and to adjust for excessive hematological toxicity	Continuation of appropriate dosing requires periodic monitoring of absolute neutrophil count and platelet count to assure sufficient drug exposure and to adjust for excessive hematological toxicity

DOSING CONSIDERATIONS

Renal Impairment
Consider starting at lower end of dosing range or increasing the dosing interval to 36-48 hrs

Hepatic Impairment
Consider starting at lower end of dosing range

Elderly
Consider starting at lower end of dosing range

Other Important Considerations
Thiopurine S-Methyltransferase (TPMT) Deficiency:
Homozygous TPMT Deficiency: May require up to a 90% dosage reduction
Heterozygous TPMT Deficiency: May require dose reduction based on toxicities

ADMINISTRATION
Oral route

Shake vigorously for at least 30 sec.
Once opened, use within 6 weeks.

STORAGE
15-25°C (59-77°F) in a dry place. Do not store >25°C.

HOW SUPPLIED
Sus: 20mg/mL [100mL]

WARNINGS/PRECAUTIONS
Increased risk for severe mercaptopurine toxicity in patients with inherited little or no TPMT activity; evaluate TPMT status in patients with evidence of severe bone marrow toxicity or with repeated episodes of myelosuppression. Dose-related bone marrow suppression may occur; adjust dose for severe neutropenia and thrombocytopenia. Hepatotoxicity reported; interrupt therapy in patients with evidence of hepatotoxicity. Monitor LFTs more frequently in patients who are receiving mercaptopurine with other hepatotoxic drugs or with known pre-existing liver disease. Therapy is immunosuppressive and may impair the immune response to infectious agents. May cause fetal harm. May increase risk of secondary malignancies. Caution with renal/hepatic impairment and in elderly.

ADVERSE REACTIONS
Myelosuppression, anorexia, N/V, diarrhea, malaise, rash.

DRUG INTERACTIONS
Allopurinol inhibits 1st-pass oxidative metabolism, leading to mercaptopurine toxicity (bone marrow suppression, N/V); avoid concomitant use. May decrease anticoagulant effectiveness of warfarin; monitor PT/INR and adjust warfarin dose if necessary. Drugs that inhibit TPMT (eg, aminosalicylate derivatives [eg, olsalazine, mesalamine, sulfasalazine]), drugs whose primary or secondary toxicity is myelosuppression, and trimethoprim-sulfamethoxazole may exacerbate myelosuppression; if coadministration with aminosalicylate derivatives is necessary, use the lowest possible doses of each drug and closely monitor for bone marrow suppression. May impair the immune response to vaccines; response to all vaccines may be diminished and there is a risk of infection with live virus vaccines.

PREGNANCY AND LACTATION
Pregnancy: Category D.
Lactation: Not for use in nursing.

MECHANISM OF ACTION
Purine analogue; activation occurs via hypoxanthine-guanine phosphoribosyl transferase and several enzymes to form 6-thioguanine nucleotides (6-TGNs). Incorporation of 6-TGN into nucleic acids (instead of purine bases) results in cell-cycle arrest and cell death.

PHARMACOKINETICS
Absorption: Incomplete and variable. (Single 50mg dose, fasting conditions) AUC=136ng•hr/mL (median); C_{max}=95ng/mL (median). **Metabolism:** Thiol methylation via TPMT and oxidation via xanthine oxidase. **Elimination:** Urine; $T_{1/2}$=2 hrs.

PATIENT CONSIDERATIONS
Assessment: Assess for TPMT deficiency, renal/hepatic impairment, pregnancy/nursing status, and possible drug interactions.

Monitoring: Monitor for myelosuppression, hepatotoxicity, immunosuppression, secondary malignancies, and other adverse reactions. Monitor serum transaminase levels, alkaline phosphatase, and bilirubin levels at weekly intervals when first beginning therapy and at monthly intervals thereafter. Monitor CBC. Evaluate bone marrow in patients with prolonged or repeated marrow suppression to assess leukemia status and marrow cellularity. Evaluate TPMT status in patients with clinical or lab evidence of severe bone marrow toxicity, or with repeated episodes of myelosuppression.

Counseling: Instruct on proper handling, storage, administration, disposal and clean-up of accidental spillage of the medication; counsel regarding which syringe to use and how to administer a specified dose. Inform that the major toxicities of therapy are related to myelosuppression, hepatotoxicity, and GI toxicity; instruct to contact physician if patient experiences fever, sore throat, jaundice, N/V, signs of local infection, bleeding from any site, or symptoms suggestive of anemia. Advise women of childbearing potential to avoid becoming pregnant. Inform that the oral dispensing syringe is intended for multiple use; instruct on how to clean the syringe.

RAPAMUNE — sirolimus   Rx
Class: Immunosuppressant

> Increased susceptibility to infection and the possible development of lymphoma and other malignancies may result from immunosuppression. Only physicians experienced in immunosuppressive therapy and management of renal transplant patients should use sirolimus for prophylaxis of organ rejection in patients receiving renal transplants. Use not recommended in liver or lung transplant patients. Use in combination w/ tacrolimus was associated w/ excess mortality and graft loss in de novo liver transplant patients. Use in combination w/ cyclosporine or tacrolimus was associated w/ increased hepatic artery thrombosis in de novo liver transplant patients. Cases of bronchial anastomotic dehiscence, most fatal, reported in de novo lung transplant patients when sirolimus was used as part of an immunosuppressive regimen.

ADULT DOSAGE
Renal Transplant
Prophylaxis of Organ Rejection in Renal Transplantation:
General:
Give initial dose as soon as possible after transplantation, and 4 hrs after cyclosporine (MODIFIED)

Once maint dose is adjusted, continue on the new maint dose for ≥7-14 days before further dose adjustment

Dosage adjustment may be based on simple proportion:
New Rapamune Dose = Current Dose x (Target Concentration/Current Concentration)

LD should be considered in addition to new maint dose when it is necessary to increase sirolimus trough concentrations:
Rapamune LD = 3 x (New Maint Dose - Current Maint Dose)

Max: 40mg/day
If estimated dose is >40mg/day due to addition of LD, administer LD over 2 days; monitor trough concentrations at least 3-4 days after LD(s)

2mg of sol are clinically equivalent to 2mg tab and are interchangeable on a mg-to-mg basis; unknown if higher doses of sol are clinically equivalent to higher doses of tabs on a mg-to-mg basis

Low- to Moderate-Immunologic Risk:
LD: Give LD equivalent to 3X the maint dose
Give w/ cyclosporine and corticosteroids in de novo renal transplant patients; progressively d/c cyclosporine over 4-8 weeks at 2-4 months following transplantation
Adjust dose to maintain blood trough concentration w/in target-range

Target Sirolimus Whole Blood Trough Concentrations Following Cyclosporine Withdrawal:
1st Year: 16-24ng/mL
Thereafter: 12-20ng/mL

High-Immunologic Risk:
Give w/ cyclosporine and corticosteroids for the first 12 months following transplantation. Safety and efficacy of this combination not studied beyond first 12 months; after 12 months, consider adjustments to immunosuppressive regimen based on patient's clinical status
LD: Up to 15mg on Day 1 post-transplantation
Maint: 5mg/day beginning on Day 2; obtain trough level between Days 5 and 7 and adjust daily dose thereafter

Cyclosporine Dosing:
Initial: Up to 7mg/kg/day in divided doses; subsequently adjust to achieve target whole blood trough concentrations

Prednisone Dosing:
Minimum of 5mg/day

Antibody induction therapy may be used

Lymphangioleiomyomatosis
Initial: 2mg/day

PEDIATRIC DOSAGE
Renal Transplant
Prophylaxis of Organ Rejection in Renal Transplantation:
≥13 Years:
General:
Give initial dose as soon as possible after transplantation, and 4 hrs after cyclosporine (MODIFIED)

Once maint dose is adjusted, continue on the new maint dose for ≥7-14 days before further dose adjustment

Dosage adjustment can be based on simple proportion:
New Rapamune Dose = Current Dose x (Target Concentration/Current Concentration)

LD should be considered in addition to new maint dose when it is necessary to increase sirolimus trough concentrations:
Rapamune LD = 3 x (New Maint Dose - Current Maint Dose)

Max: 40mg/day
If estimated dose is >40mg/day due to addition of LD, administer LD over 2 days; monitor trough concentrations at least 3-4 days after LD(s)

2mg of sol are clinically equivalent to 2mg tab and are interchangeable on a mg-to-mg basis; unknown if higher doses of sol are clinically equivalent to higher doses of tabs on a mg-to-mg basis

Low- to Moderate-Immunologic Risk:
LD: Give LD equivalent to 3X the maint dose
Give w/ cyclosporine and corticosteroids in de novo renal transplant patients; progressively d/c cyclosporine over 4-8 weeks at 2-4 months following transplantation
Adjust dose to maintain blood trough concentration w/in target range

Target Sirolimus Whole Blood Trough Concentrations Following Cyclosporine Withdrawal:
1st Year: 16-24ng/mL
Thereafter: 12-20ng/mL

Measure sirolimus whole blood trough concentrations in 10-20 days, w/ a dosage adjustment to maintain concentrations between 5-15ng/mL.

Dosage adjustment may be based on simple proportion:
New Rapamune Dose = Current Dose x (Target Concentration/Current Concentration)

Once maint dose is adjusted, continue on the new maint dose for at least 7-14 days before further dose adjustment

Once a stable dose is achieved, perform therapeutic drug monitoring at least every 3 months

DOSING CONSIDERATIONS
Hepatic Impairment
Mild or Moderate: Reduce maint dose by approx 1/3
Severe: Reduce maint dose by approx 1/2

Elderly
Start at lower end of dosing range

Other Important Considerations
Low Body Weight (<40kg): Adjust initial dose based on BSA to 1mg/m²/day w/ a LD of 3mg/m²

ADMINISTRATION
Oral route

Administer qd.
Give consistently w/ or w/o food.

Tab
Do not crush, chew, or split.

Sol
Once the bottle is opened, use w/in 1 month.
Contains polysorbate 80, which is known to increase the rate of di-(2-ethylhexyl) phthalate extraction from polyvinyl chloride.
Instructions for Dilution:
1. Use amber oral dose syringe to withdraw the prescribed amount of sol from bottle.
2. Empty the correct amount of sirolimus from syringe into only a glass or plastic container holding at least 2 oz (1/4 cup, 60mL) of water or orange juice; no other liquids, including grapefruit juice, should be used for dilution.
3. Stir vigorously and drink at once.
4. Refill the container w/ an additional volume (minimum of 4 oz [1/2 cup, 120mL]) of water or orange juice, stir vigorously, and drink at once.

STORAGE
Sol: (Bottle) 2-8°C (36-46°F). Protect from light. May store at room temperatures up to 25°C (77°F) for a short period (eg, not >15 days). (Syringe) May be kept in syringe for max of 24 hrs at room temperatures up to 25°C (77°F) or at 2-8°C (36-46°F). **Tab:** 20-25°C (68-77°F). Protect from light.

HOW SUPPLIED
Sol: 1mg/mL [60mL]; **Tab:** 0.5mg, 1mg, 2mg

CONTRAINDICATIONS
Hypersensitivity to sirolimus.

WARNINGS/PRECAUTIONS
Hypersensitivity reactions reported. Associated w/ the development of angioedema. Impaired/delayed wound healing, including lymphocele and wound dehiscence, and fluid accumulation (eg, peripheral edema, lymphedema, pleural effusion, ascites, pericardial effusions) reported. May increase serum cholesterol and TGs. Long-term administration w/ cyclosporine associated w/ renal function deterioration; consider appropriate adjustment of immunosuppressive regimen w/ elevated or increasing SrCr levels. May delay recovery of renal function in patients w/ delayed graft function. Proteinuria observed in maint renal transplant patients when converting from calcineurin inhibitors (CNIs) to sirolimus; safety and efficacy of conversion in maint renal transplant patients not established. Increased risk for opportunistic infections, including activation of latent viral infections. BK virus-associated nephropathy reported. Progressive multifocal leukoencephalopathy (PML) reported. Consider reduction in immunosuppression if BK virus-associated nephropathy is suspected or if PML develops. Interstitial lung disease (ILD) (eg, pneumonitis, bronchiolitis obliterans organizing pneumonia, pulmonary fibrosis) reported. In some cases, ILD was associated w/ pulmonary HTN. Safety and efficacy of de novo use w/o cyclosporine is not established in renal transplant patients. Provide 1 yr prophylaxis for *Pneumocystis carinii* pneumonia and 3 months for CMV after transplant. Patient sample concentration values from different assays may not be interchangeable. Increased risk of skin cancer; limit exposure to sunlight and UV light.

ADVERSE REACTIONS
Peripheral edema, hypertriglyceridemia, HTN, constipation, hypercholesterolemia, increased creatinine, abdominal pain, nausea, diarrhea, headache, fever, acne, chest pain, stomatitis, nasopharyngitis.

DRUG INTERACTIONS
See Boxed Warning and Dosage. CYP3A4 and P-gp inducers may decrease concentrations. CYP3A4 and P-gp inhibitors may increase concentrations. Avoid w/ strong inhibitors (eg, ketoconazole, erythromycin, clarithromycin) and strong inducers (eg, rifampin, rifabutin) of CYP3A4 and P-gp. Cyclosporine, bromocriptine, cimetidine, cisapride, clotrimazole, danazol, diltiazem, fluconazole, protease inhibitors, metoclopramide, nicardipine, troleandomycin, and verapamil may increase levels. Carbamazepine, phenobarbital, phenytoin, rifapentine, and St. John's wort may decrease levels. May increase verapamil concentration. Vaccines may be less effective; avoid live vaccines. May increase risk of angioedema w/ drugs known to cause angioedema (eg, ACE inhibitors). Increased risk of CNIs-induced hemolytic uremic syndrome/thrombotic thrombocytopenic purpura/thrombotic microangiography w/ concomitant CNIs. Do not administer w/ grapefruit juice or use grapefruit juice for dilution. Caution w/ other nephrotoxic drugs (eg, aminoglycosides, amphotericin B). Monitor for possible development of rhabdomyolysis and other adverse effects w/ HMG-CoA inhibitors and/or fibrates.

PREGNANCY AND LACTATION
Pregnancy: Category C; effective contraception must be initiated before, during, and for 12 weeks after therapy.
Lactation: Not for use in nursing.

MECHANISM OF ACTION
Immunosuppressive agent; inhibits T-lymphocyte activation and proliferation that occurs in response to antigenic and cytokine (interleukin [IL]-2, IL-4, and IL-15) stimulation by a mechanism distinct from that of other immunosuppressants. Also inhibits antibody production. Inhibits activated mTOR pathway and proliferation of lymphangioleiomyomatosis cells.

PHARMACOKINETICS
Absorption: (Sol) Bioavailability (14%); AUC=194ng•hr/mL, C_{max}=14.4ng/mL, T_{max}=2.1 hrs. (Tab) AUC=230ng•hr/mL, C_{max}=15ng/mL, T_{max}=3.5 hrs. Different pharmacokinetic data resulted from concentration-controlled trials of pediatric renal transplants. **Distribution:** V_d=12L/kg; plasma protein binding (approx 92%). **Metabolism:** CYP3A4, P-gp; extensively in intestinal wall and liver via O-demethylation and/or hydroxylation; 7 major metabolites including hydroxy, demethyl, and hydroxydemethyl. **Elimination:** Feces (91%), urine (2.2%); $T_{1/2}$=62 hrs.

PATIENT CONSIDERATIONS
Assessment: Assess for drug hypersensitivity, immunologic risk, hepatic impairment, body weight/BMI, hyperlipidemia, infections, pregnancy/nursing status, and possible drug interactions.

Monitoring: Monitor for infections including opportunistic infections and activation of latent infections, development of PML, lymphoma, other malignancies (particularly of the skin), hypersensitivity reactions, ILD, hyperlipidemia, and other adverse reactions. Monitor trough concentrations, especially in patients w/ altered drug metabolism, in patients who weigh <40kg, in patients w/ hepatic impairment, when a change is made to sirolimus dosage form, and during concurrent administration of strong CYP3A4 inducers or inhibitors. Monitor urinary protein excretion, renal function w/ concomitant cyclosporine, hepatic function, cholesterol, TGs, and BP.

Counseling: Instruct to limit sunlight and UV light exposure by wearing protective clothing and using a sunscreen w/ a high protection. Inform about the potential risks during pregnancy and instruct to use effective contraception prior to, during, and 12 weeks after therapy has been stopped.

RASUVO — methotrexate   Rx
Class: Dihydrofolic acid reductase inhibitor

> Should be used only by physicians w/ knowledge and experience in the use of antimetabolite therapy. Use only in patients w/ psoriasis or rheumatoid arthritis (RA) w/ severe, recalcitrant, disabling disease not adequately responsive to other forms of therapy. Deaths reported in the treatment of malignancy, psoriasis, and RA. Closely monitor for bone marrow, liver, lung, skin, and kidney toxicities. Patients should be informed of the risks involved and be under physician's care throughout therapy. Fetal death and/or congenital anomalies reported; not recommended for females of childbearing potential unless benefits outweigh risks. Contraindicated in pregnant women. Reduced elimination w/ impaired renal function, ascites, or pleural effusions; monitor for toxicity and reduce dose or d/c in some cases. Unexpectedly severe (sometimes fatal) bone marrow suppression, aplastic anemia, and GI toxicity reported w/ coadministration of therapy (usually high dosage) w/ some NSAIDs. Causes hepatotoxicity, fibrosis, and cirrhosis (generally only after prolonged use); perform periodic liver biopsies in psoriatic patients on long-term therapy. Acutely, liver enzyme elevations frequently seen. Drug-induced lung disease may occur acutely at any time during therapy and reported at low doses. Pulmonary symptoms (especially a dry, nonproductive cough) may require an interruption of therapy. Diarrhea and ulcerative stomatitis require interruption of therapy. Malignant lymphomas, which may regress following withdrawal of treatment, may occur w/ low-dose therapy and, thus, may not require cytotoxic treatment; d/c therapy 1st and, if lymphoma does not regress, institute appropriate treatment. May induce tumor lysis syndrome in patients w/ rapidly growing tumors. Severe, occasionally fatal, skin reactions reported. Potentially fatal opportunistic infections, especially *Pneumocystis jiroveci* pneumonia, may occur. Concomitant use w/ radiotherapy may increase risk of soft tissue necrosis and osteonecrosis.

ADULT DOSAGE	PEDIATRIC DOSAGE
Rheumatoid Arthritis	**Juvenile Idiopathic Arthritis**
Management of selected adults w/ severe, active RA (American College of Rheumatology criteria) who have had insufficient therapeutic response to, or are intolerant of, an adequate trial of 1st-line therapy including full-dose NSAIDs	Management of children w/ active polyarticular juvenile idiopathic arthritis, who have had insufficient therapeutic response to, or are intolerant of, an adequate trial of 1st-line therapy including full-dose NSAIDs
Initial: 7.5mg as single dose once weekly	**2-16 Years:**
Titrate: May adjust gradually to achieve optimal response	**Initial:** 10mg/m² once weekly
Significant increase in incidence and	**Titrate:** May adjust gradually to achieve optimal response
	Limited data to assess how doses

severity of serious toxic reactions, especially bone marrow suppression, reported at doses >20mg/week

Psoriasis

Symptomatic control of severe, recalcitrant, disabling psoriasis not adequately responsive to other forms of therapy, but only when the diagnosis has been established, as by a biopsy and/or after dermatologic consultation

Initial: 10-25mg as single dose once weekly
Titrate: May adjust gradually to achieve optimal response
Max: 30mg/week
Maint: Once optimal response is achieved, reduce dosage to lowest possible amount of drug and to longest possible rest period

Conversions

Switching from Oral to SQ Therapy: Consider any differences in bioavailability between oral and SQ therapy

>20mg/m^2/week might affect the risk of serious toxicity; refer to PI for further information

Conversions

Switching from Oral to SQ Therapy: Consider any differences in bioavailability between oral and SQ therapy

---

DOSING CONSIDERATIONS
Renal Impairment
Reduce dose and monitor carefully for toxicity

Elderly
Consider relatively low doses and closely monitor for early signs of toxicity

Other Important Considerations
Ascites or Pleural Effusions: Reduce dose and monitor carefully for toxicity

ADMINISTRATION
SQ route
Administer in the abdomen or the thigh

Administration and Handling
Patients may self-inject if physician determines that it is appropriate, if they received proper training in how to prepare and administer the correct dose, and if they receive medical follow-up, as necessary
The patient must be explicitly informed about the once weekly dosing schedule
It is advisable to determine an appropriate fixed day of the week for the inj
Visually inspect for particulate matter and discoloration prior to administration
Do not use if the seal is broken
Handle and dispose inj consistent w/ recommendations for handling and disposal of cytotoxic drugs

Important Dosing Information
Only available in doses between 7.5-30mg in 2.5mg increments
Use another formulation of methotrexate for alternative dosing in patients who require oral, IM, IV, intra-arterial, or intrathecal dosing, doses <7.5mg/week, doses >30mg/week, high-dose regimens, or dose adjustments in increments <2.5mg

STORAGE
25°C (77°F); excursions permitted to 15-30°C (59-86°F). Protect from light.

HOW SUPPLIED
Inj: 7.5mg/0.15mL, 10mg/0.20mL, 12.5mg/0.25mL, 15mg/0.30mL, 17.5mg/0.35mL, 20mg/0.40mL, 22.5mg/0.45mL, 25mg/0.50mL, 27.5mg/0.55mL, 30mg/0.60mL

CONTRAINDICATIONS
Pregnancy, nursing mothers, alcoholism, alcoholic liver disease, chronic liver disease, immunodeficiency syndromes, preexisting blood dyscrasias (eg, bone marrow hypoplasia, leukopenia, thrombocytopenia, significant anemia), known hypersensitivity to methotrexate.

WARNINGS/PRECAUTIONS
Not indicated for the treatment of neoplastic diseases. Toxic effects may be related to dose/frequency of administration; if toxicity occurs, reduce dose or d/c therapy and take appropriate corrective measures, which may include use of leucovorin calcium and/or acute, intermittent hemodialysis w/ high-flux dialyzer, if necessary. If therapy is reinstituted, carry it out w/ caution, w/ adequate consideration of further need for the drug and increased alertness as to possible recurrence of toxicity. May cause multiple organ system toxicities (eg, GI, hematologic). Caution in debilitated patients. Avoid pregnancy if either partner is receiving therapy (during and for a minimum of 3 months after therapy for male patients, and during and for at least 1 ovulatory cycle after therapy for female patients). May cause impairment of fertility, oligospermia, and menstrual dysfunction, during and for a short period after cessation of therapy. May impair mental/physical abilities.

ADVERSE REACTIONS
Bone marrow/liver/lung/skin/kidney toxicities, diarrhea, ulcerative stomatitis, hemorrhagic enteritis, opportunistic infections, malignant lymphomas, tumor lysis syndrome, N/V, abdominal distress, malaise, undue fatigue, chills, fever, dizziness.

DRUG INTERACTIONS
See Boxed Warning. Elevated and prolonged levels w/ NSAIDs; do not administer NSAIDs prior to or concomitantly w/ high doses of therapy, and use caution when NSAIDs and salicylates are administered concomitantly w/ lower doses of therapy. Proton pump inhibitors (PPIs) (eg, omeprazole, esomeprazole, pantoprazole) may elevate and prolong levels, possibly leading to toxicities; use caution if administering high-dose therapy w/ PPIs. Oral antibiotics (eg, tetracycline, chloramphenicol, nonabsorbable broad-spectrum antibiotics) may decrease intestinal absorption or interfere w/ enterohepatic circulation. Penicillins may reduce renal clearance; hematologic and GI toxicity observed. Trimethoprim/sulfamethoxazole may increase bone marrow suppression by decreasing tubular secretion and/or an additive antifolate effect. Closely monitor for increased risk of hepatotoxicity w/ potential hepatotoxins (eg, azathioprine, retinoids, sulfasalazine). May decrease theophylline clearance; monitor theophylline levels. Vitamin preparations containing folic acid or its derivatives may decrease responses to methotrexate; high doses of leucovorin may reduce efficacy of intrathecally administered drug. Increases levels of mercaptopurine; may require dose adjustment. Toxicity may be increased due to displacement by certain drugs (eg, salicylates, phenylbutazone, phenytoin, sulfonamides). Renal tubular transport diminished by probenecid. Combined use w/ gold, penicillamine, hydroxychloroquine, sulfasalazine, or cytotoxic agents may increase incidence of adverse effects. Immunization may be ineffective when given during therapy; immunization w/ live virus vaccines is generally not recommended. Disseminated vaccinia infections after smallpox immunizations reported.

PREGNANCY AND LACTATION
Category X, not for use in nursing.

MECHANISM OF ACTION
Dihydrofolic acid reductase inhibitor; interferes w/ DNA synthesis, repair, and cellular replication. Mechanism in RA not established; may affect immune function.

PHARMACOKINETICS
Absorption: (Oral) Well-absorbed. Bioavailability (60%) (adults). Administration of various doses and in different disease states resulted in different parameters. **Distribution:** Plasma protein binding (50%); found in breast milk. (IV) V_d=0.18L/kg (initial), 0.4-0.8L/kg (steady-state). **Metabolism:** Hepatic and intracellular to polyglutamated forms (active); 7-hydroxymethotrexate (metabolite). (Oral) Partially metabolized by intestinal flora. **Elimination:** $T_{1/2}$=3-10 hrs (psoriasis/RA/low-dose antineoplastic therapy), 8-15 hrs (high doses). (IV) Urine (80-90%, unchanged), bile (≤10%). Refer to PI for additional pharmacokinetic information.

PATIENT CONSIDERATIONS

Assessment: Assess for alcoholism, alcoholic/chronic liver disease, immunodeficiency syndromes, blood dyscrasias, ascites, pleural effusions, tumors, hypersensitivity to drug, pregnancy/nursing status, any other conditions where treatment is cautioned or contraindicated, and possible drug interactions. Obtain baseline CBC w/ differential and platelet counts, hepatic enzymes, renal function tests, liver biopsy, and chest x-ray.

Monitoring: Monitor for toxicities of bone marrow, liver, lung, kidney, and GI tract; diarrhea; ulcerative stomatitis; malignant lymphoma; tumor lysis syndrome; skin reactions; opportunistic infections; and other adverse reactions. Monitor hematology at least monthly and renal/hepatic function every 1-2 months during therapy and more frequently during initial/changing doses, or during periods of increased risk of elevated drug levels (eg, dehydration). If drug-induced lung disease is suspected, perform pulmonary function tests.

Counseling: Inform of the risks of organ toxicity, the possible signs/symptoms for which physician should be contacted, and the need for close follow-up, including periodic lab tests to monitor toxicity. Emphasize that the recommended dose is taken once weekly, and that mistaken daily use of recommended dose has led to fatal toxicity. Instruct not to self-administer until trained by physician. Advise women of childbearing potential that drug should not be started until pregnancy is excluded; counsel on the serious risk to the fetus should pregnancy occur while undergoing treatment. Instruct to contact physician if pregnancy is suspected. Advise to avoid pregnancy if either partner is receiving therapy (during and for a minimum of 3 months after therapy for male patients, and during and for at least 1 ovulatory cycle after therapy for female patients). Discuss the risk of effects on reproduction. Inform that adverse reactions such as dizziness and fatigue may affect ability to drive or operate machinery. Inform of the need for proper disposal after use, including the use of a sharps disposal container.

RAVICTI — glycerol phenylbutyrate   **Rx**

Class: Urea cycle disorder agent

ADULT DOSAGE	PEDIATRIC DOSAGE
Urea Cycle Disorders	**Urea Cycle Disorders**
In patients who cannot be managed by dietary protein restriction and/or amino acid supplementation alone	In patients who cannot be managed by dietary protein restriction and/or amino acid supplementation alone
Switching from Sodium Phenylbutyrate: Should receive the dose of glycerol phenylbutyrate that contains the same amount of phenylbutyric acid; refer to PI for conversion	**≥2 Years: Switching from Sodium Phenylbutyrate:** Should receive the dose of glycerol phenylbutyrate that contains the same amount of phenylbutyric acid; refer to PI for conversion
Phenylbutyrate-Naive Patients: Initial: 4.5-11.2mL/m^2/day (5-12.4g/m^2/day); 4.5mL/m^2/day for patients w/ some residual enzyme activity who are not adequately controlled w/ protein restrictions	**Phenylbutyrate-Naive Patients: Initial:** 4.5-11.2mL/m^2/day (5-12.4g/m^2/day); 4.5mL/m^2/day for patients w/ some residual enzyme activity who are not adequately controlled w/ protein restrictions
Consider patient's residual urea synthetic capacity, dietary protein requirements, and diet adherence in determining the initial dose in treatment-naive patients	Consider patient's residual urea synthetic capacity, dietary protein requirements, and diet adherence in determining the initial dose in treatment-naive patients

For Both Subpopulations:
Administer in 3 equally divided doses, each rounded up to the nearest 0.5mL
Max: 17.5mL/day (19g/day)

For Both Subpopulations:
Administer in 3 equally divided doses, each rounded up to the nearest 0.5mL
Max: 17.5mL/day (19g/day)

DOSING CONSIDERATIONS
Hepatic Impairment
Moderate to Severe: Recommended starting dosage is at the lower end of the range

Elderly
Start at lower end of dosing range

Other Important Considerations
Adjustment Based on Plasma Ammonia: Adjust dose to produce a fasting plasma ammonia level that is <1/2 the ULN according to age

Adjustment Based on Urinary Phenylacetylglutamine (U-PAGN): Adjust dose upward if U-PAGN excretion is insufficient to cover daily dietary protein intake and the fasting ammonia is >1/2 the ULN; the amount of dose adjustment should factor in the amount of dietary protein that has not been covered, as indicated by the 24-hr U-PAGN level and the estimated Ravicti dose needed per gram of dietary protein ingested and the max total daily dose

Consider use of concomitant medications (eg, probenecid) when making dosage adjustment decisions based on U-PAGN; probenecid may result in a decrease of the U-PAGN excretion

Refer to PI for adjustment based on plasma phenylacetate

ADMINISTRATION
Oral route, NG or gastrostomy tube

Take w/ food.
Administer directly into the mouth via oral syringe or dosing cup.
Use w/ dietary protein restriction and, in some cases, dietary supplements (eg, essential amino acids, arginine, citrulline, protein-free calorie supplements).

Preparation for NG or Gastrostomy Tube Administration
1. Utilize an oral syringe to withdraw the prescribed dosage of Ravicti from the bottle.
2. Place the tip of the syringe into to the tip of the gastrostomy/NG tube.
3. Utilizing the plunger of the syringe, administer Ravicti into the tube.
4. Flush once w/ 30mL of water and allow the flush to drain.
5. Flush a 2nd time w/ an additional 30mL of water to clear the tube.

STORAGE
20-25°C (68-77°F); excursions permitted to 15-30°C (59-86°F).

HOW SUPPLIED
Liquid: 1.1g/mL [25mL]

CONTRAINDICATIONS
Pediatric patients <2 months of age.

WARNINGS/PRECAUTIONS
Not indicated for the treatment of acute hyperammonemia in patients w/ UCDs. Should be prescribed by a physician experienced in the management of UCDs. The major metabolite, phenylacetate (PAA), is associated w/ neurotoxicity; reduce dose if symptoms of N/V, headache, somnolence, confusion, or sleepiness are present in the absence of high ammonia or other intercurrent illnesses. Low or absent pancreatic enzymes or intestinal disease resulting in fat malabsorption may result in reduced or absent digestion of glycerol phenylbutyrate and/or absorption of phenylbutyrate and reduced control of plasma ammonia; monitor ammonia levels closely in patients w/ pancreatic insufficiency or intestinal malabsorption and when starting therapy in patients w/ renal impairment.

ADVERSE REACTIONS
Diarrhea, flatulence, headache.

DRUG INTERACTIONS
Use of corticosteroids may cause breakdown of body protein and increase plasma ammonia levels; monitor ammonia levels closely. Hyperammonemia may be induced by haloperidol and by valproic acid; monitor ammonia levels closely when concurrent use is necessary. Probenecid may inhibit the renal excretion of metabolites.

PREGNANCY AND LACTATION
Pregnancy: Category C. A voluntary patient registry will include evaluation of pregnancy outcomes in patients w/ UCDs.
Lactation: It is not known whether glycerol phenylbutyrate or its metabolites are present in breast milk; not for use in nursing.

MECHANISM OF ACTION
Prodrug of PBA; provides an alternate vehicle for waste nitrogen excretion.

PHARMACOKINETICS
Absorption: T_{max}=8 hrs (PBA), 12 hrs (PAA), 10 hrs (PAGN). Refer to PI for parameters in different populations. **Distribution:** Plasma protein binding (80.6-98% PBA, 37.1-65.6% PAA, 7-12% PAGN). **Metabolism:** Hydrolysis via pancreatic lipases; PBA via β-oxidation to PAA; conjugation (hepatic) and via L-glutamine-N-acetyltransferase (renal) to PAGN. **Elimination:** Urine=68.9% (PAGN [adults]); 66.4% (PAGN [pediatric patients]); <1% (PAA); <1% (PBA).

PATIENT CONSIDERATIONS
Assessment: Assess for drug hypersensitivity, acute hyperammonemia, N-acetylglutamate synthase deficiency, pancreatic insufficiency, intestinal malabsorption, renal/hepatic impairment, pregnancy/nursing status, and possible drug interactions.
Monitoring: Monitor for neurotoxicity, symptoms of N/V, headache, somnolence, confusion, or sleepiness in the absence of high ammonia or other intercurrent illnesses, and other adverse reactions. Monitor ammonia levels.

Counseling: Inform of the possible benefits/risks of therapy. Advise of the common/possible adverse reactions and instruct to call the doctor immediately if symptoms are experienced or if neurological toxicity (eg, somnolence, fatigue, lightheadedness, headache, dysgeusia, hypoacusis, disorientation, impaired memory) occurs. Encourage patients and caregivers to participate in the registry for UCD patients and advise that their participation is voluntary. Instruct to take drug exactly as prescribed and inform that treatment must be used w/ dietary protein restriction, and in some cases, dietary supplements (eg, essential amino acids, arginine, citrulline, protein-free calorie supplements).

REBETOL — ribavirin   Rx
Class: Nucleoside analogue

> Not for monotherapy treatment of chronic hepatitis C virus infection. Primary toxicity is hemolytic anemia. Anemia associated w/ therapy may result in worsening of cardiac disease and lead to fatal and nonfatal MIs. Avoid w/ history of significant/unstable cardiac disease. Contraindicated in women who are pregnant and in male partners of pregnant women. Extreme care must be taken to avoid pregnancy during therapy and for 6 months after completion of therapy in both female patients and in female partners of male patients who are taking therapy. Use at least 2 reliable forms of effective contraception during treatment and for 6 months after discontinuation.

ADULT DOSAGE
Chronic Hepatitis C with Compensated Liver Disease
Combination Therapy w/ PegIntron:
Treat w/ PegIntron 1.5mcg/kg/week SQ

<66kg: 400mg qam and 400mg qpm
66-80kg: 400mg qam and 600mg qpm
81-105kg: 600mg qam and 600mg qpm
<105kg: 600mg qam and 800mg qpm

Interferon Alfa-Naive:
Genotype 1: Treat for 48 weeks
Genotype 2 and 3: Treat for 24 weeks

Retreatment:
Treat for 48 weeks, regardless of hepatitis C virus genotype

Combination Therapy w/ Intron A:
Treat w/ Intron A 3 million IU 3X weekly SQ

≤75kg: 400mg qam and 600mg qpm
<75kg: 600mg qam and 600mg qpm

Interferon Alfa-Naive:
Treat for 24-48 weeks

Retreatment:
Treat for 24 weeks

PEDIATRIC DOSAGE
Chronic Hepatitis C with Compensated Liver Disease
Combination Therapy w/ PegIntron/Intron A:
≥3 Years:
Sol:
<47kg: 15mg/kg/day divided into two doses; may use sol regardless of body weight

Cap:
47-59kg: 400mg qam and 400mg qpm
60-73kg: 400mg qam and 600mg qpm
<73kg: 600mg qam and 600mg qpm

Treat w/ Intron A 3 million IU/m² 3X weekly SQ for 25-61kg (refer to adult dosing for >61kg) or PegIntron 60mcg/m²/week SQ

Genotype 1: Treat for 48 weeks
Genotype 2 or 3: Treat for 24 weeks

Remain on pediatric dosing while receiving therapy in combination w/ PegIntron when 18th birthday is reached

---

DOSING CONSIDERATIONS
Renal Impairment
CrCl <50mL/min: Not recommended

Elderly
Start at lower end of dosing range

Adverse Reactions
Refer to PI for dose modification/discontinuation based on lab parameters in adults and pediatric patients

Discontinuation
Adults:
Genotype 1:
Interferon-Alfa Naive:
D/C therapy if at least a 2 log$_{10}$ drop or loss of hepatitis C virus (HCV)-RNA at 12 weeks of therapy is not achieved
D/C therapy if HCV-RNA levels remain detectable after 24 weeks of therapy

All Genotypes:
Previously Treated Patients:
Consider discontinuation if fail to achieve undetectable HCV-RNA at Week 12 of therapy, or if HCV-RNA remains detectable after 24 weeks of therapy

Pediatric Patients (3-17 Years):
All Genotypes (Excluding Genotype 2 and 3):
D/C therapy at 12 weeks if treatment Week 12 HCV-RNA drops <2 log$_{10}$ compared to pretreatment
D/C therapy at 24 weeks if HCV-RNA is detectable at treatment Week 24

ADMINISTRATION
Oral route

Take w/ food.
Refer to PegIntron or Intron A PIs for further information on dosing, dosing modifications, and administration for these drugs.

Cap
Do not open, crush, or break.

STORAGE
(Cap) 25°C (77°F); excursions permitted to 15-30°C (59-86°F). (Sol) 2-8°C (36-46°F) or at 25°C (77°F); excursions permitted to 15-30°C (59-86°F).

HOW SUPPLIED
Cap: 200mg; **Sol:** 40mg/mL [100mL]

CONTRAINDICATIONS
Women who are or may become pregnant, men whose female partners are pregnant, autoimmune hepatitis, hemoglobinopathies (eg, thalassemia major, sickle cell anemia), CrCl <50mL/min, coadministration w/ didanosine. Known hypersensitivity reactions (eg, Stevens-Johnson syndrome, toxic, epidermal necrolysis, erythema multiforme) to ribavirin or any component of the product.

WARNINGS/PRECAUTIONS
Do not start therapy unless a negative pregnancy test has been obtained immediately prior to therapy. Suspend therapy in patients w/ signs and symptoms of pancreatitis; d/c therapy w/ confirmed pancreatitis. Pulmonary symptoms (eg, dyspnea, pulmonary infiltrates, pneumonitis) reported; closely monitor if pulmonary infiltrates or pulmonary function impairment develops and if appropriate, d/c therapy. Alfa interferons may induce or aggravate ophthalmologic disorders (eg, decrease or loss of vision, retinopathy); perform eye exam in all patients prior to therapy, periodically w/ preexisting ophthalmologic disorders (eg, diabetic or hypertensive retinopathy), and if ocular symptoms develop during therapy. D/C if new or worsening ophthalmologic disorders develop. Severe decreases in neutrophil and platelet counts, and hematologic, endocrine (eg, TSH), and hepatic abnormalities may occur in combination w/ PegIntron; perform hematology and blood chemistry testing prior to therapy and periodically thereafter. Dental/periodontal disorders reported in patients receiving ribavirin and interferon or peginterferon combination therapy. Weight changes and growth inhibition (including long-term growth inhibition) reported in pediatric patients during combination therapy w/ PegIntron or Intron A. Use w/ PegIntron or Intron A is associated w/ significant adverse reactions (eg, severe depression and suicidal or homicidal ideation, suppression of bone marrow function, autoimmune and infectious disorders). Caution w/ preexisting cardiac disease; d/c if cardiovascular (CV) status deteriorates.

ADVERSE REACTIONS
Hemolytic anemia, inj-site reactions, headache, fatigue, rigors, fever, N/V, anorexia, myalgia, arthralgia, insomnia, irritability, depression, neutropenia, alopecia.

DRUG INTERACTIONS
See Contraindications. Closely monitor for toxicities, especially hepatic decompensation and anemia when receiving interferon w/ribavirin and nucleoside reverse transcriptase inhibitors (NRTIs); consider dose reduction or discontinuation of interferon, ribavirin, or both, or discontinuation of NRTI if medically appropriate. May antagonize the cell culture antiviral activity of stavudine and zidovudine against HIV; caution w/ concomitant use of ribavirin with either of these drugs. Severe pancytopenia and bone marrow suppression reported w/ concomitant administration of pegylated interferon/ribavirin and azathioprine; d/c pegylated interferon/ribavirin and azathioprine if pancytopenia develops and do not reintroduce pegylated interferon/ribavirin w/ concomitant azathioprine.

PREGNANCY AND LACTATION
Category X, not for use in nursing.

MECHANISM OF ACTION
Nucleoside analogue; has not been established. Has direct antiviral activity in tissue culture against many RNA viruses; increases mutation frequency in the genomes of several viruses and ribavirin triphosphate inhibits HCV polymerase in a biochemical reaction.

PHARMACOKINETICS
Absorption: Rapid and extensive. Absolute bioavailability (64%). Multiple Dose: (Cap) (Adults) C_{max}=3680ng/mL, T_{max}=3 hrs, AUC=228,000ng•hr/mL. (Pediatrics) C_{max}=3275ng/mL, T_{max}=1.9 hrs, AUC=29,774ng•hr/mL. **Distribution:** (Adults) (Cap) Single Dose: V_d=2825L. **Metabolism:** Nucleated cells (phosphorylation); deribosylation and amide hydrolysis. **Elimination:** Urine (61%), feces (12%). (Adults) (Cap) Multiple Dose: $T_{1/2}$=298 hrs.

PATIENT CONSIDERATIONS
Assessment: Assess for autoimmune hepatitis, hemoglobinopathies, depression, preexisting ophthalmologic disorders, history of or preexisting cardiac disease, hypersensitivity, and possible drug interactions. Assess nursing status and hepatic/renal/pulmonary function. Conduct pregnancy test (including female partners of male patients), standard hematologic tests, blood chemistries, ECG in patients w/ preexisting cardiac disease, and eye examination.

Monitoring: Monitor for anemia, worsening of cardiac disease, pancreatitis, renal/hepatic dysfunction, CV deterioration, pulmonary function impairment, new/worsening ophthalmologic disorders, and other adverse reactions. Monitor height and weight in pediatric patients. Perform standard hematologic tests, blood chemistries (eg, TSH), ECG, and HCV-RNA periodically. Obtain Hct and Hgb (Week 2 and 4 of therapy, and as clinically appropriate). Perform pregnancy test monthly during therapy and for 6 months after discontinuation of therapy (including female partners of male patients). Schedule regular dental exams.

Counseling: Counsel on risk/benefits associated w/ treatment. Inform that anemia may develop. Advise that lab evaluations are required prior to starting therapy and periodically thereafter. Advise to be well-hydrated, especially during the initial stages of treatment. Inform of pregnancy risks. Instruct to use at least 2 forms of contraception and perform a monthly pregnancy test during therapy and for 6 months post-therapy (including female partners of male patients); advise to notify physician in the event of a pregnancy. Inform that appropriate precautions to prevent HCV transmission should be taken. Instruct to brush teeth bid and have regular dental exams; if vomiting occurs, advise to rinse out mouth afterwards.

REBIF — interferon beta-1a　　　Rx
Class: Biological response modifier

ADULT DOSAGE
Multiple Sclerosis
Treatment of Relapsing Forms:
22mcg or 44mcg 3X/week

Titration Schedule for 22mcg Prescribed Dose:
Week 1: 4.4mcg (half of 8.8mcg syringe)
Week 2: 4.4mcg (half of 8.8mcg syringe)
Week 3: 11mcg (half of 22mcg syringe)
Week 4: 11mcg (half of 22mcg syringe)
Week 5 and After: 22mcg
Use only prefilled syringes to titrate to the 22mcg prescribed dose

Titration Schedule for 44mcg Prescribed Dose:
Week 1: 8.8mcg
Week 2: 8.8mcg
Week 3: 22mcg
Week 4: 22mcg
Week 5 and After: 44mcg
Prefilled syringes or autoinjectors can be used to titrate to the 44mcg prescribed dose

Premedication
Concurrent use of analgesics and/or antipyretics may help ameliorate flu-like symptoms on treatment days

PEDIATRIC DOSAGE
Pediatric use may not have been established

DOSING CONSIDERATIONS
Elderly
Start at lower end of dosing range

Adverse Reactions
Decreased Peripheral Blood Counts: May necessitate dose reduction or discontinuation until toxicity is resolved
Elevated LFTs: May necessitate dose reduction or discontinuation until toxicity is resolved

ADMINISTRATION
SQ route
Administer at the same time (preferably late afternoon or pm) on the same 3 days at least 48 hrs apart each week.
Rotate site of inj w/ each dose.
Refer to PI for additional instructions.

STORAGE
2-8°C (36-46°F). Do not freeze. If needed, may store at 2-25°C (36-77°F) for up to 30 days and away from heat and light, but refrigeration is preferred.

HOW SUPPLIED
Inj: 22mcg/0.5mL, 44mcg/0.5mL [prefilled syringe, Rebidose autoinjector]; (Titration Pack) 8.8mcg/0.2mL, 22mcg/0.5mL [prefilled syringe, Rebidose autoinjector]

CONTRAINDICATIONS
History of hypersensitivity to natural or recombinant interferon beta, human albumin, or any other component of the formulation.

WARNINGS/PRECAUTIONS
Depression, suicidal ideation, and suicide attempts reported; consider cessation of treatment if depression develops. Severe liver injury reported rarely; d/c immediately if jaundice or other symptoms of liver dysfunction appear. Asymptomatic elevation of hepatic transaminases (particularly ALT) may occur; caution w/ active liver disease, alcohol abuse, increased serum ALT (>2.5X ULN), or history of significant liver disease. Consider dose reduction if ALT rises >5X ULN; may gradually re-escalate dose when enzyme levels have normalized. Anaphylaxis (rare) and other allergic reactions (eg, skin rash, urticaria) reported; d/c if anaphylaxis occurs. Inj-site reactions (eg, necrosis), decreased peripheral blood counts in all cell lines (including pancytopenia), thrombotic microangiopathy (including thrombotic thrombocytopenic purpura and hemolytic uremic syndrome), seizures, and new or worsening thyroid abnormalities reported. D/C if clinical symptoms and lab findings consistent w/ thrombotic microangiopathy occur. Caution in patients w/ preexisting seizure disorders.

ADVERSE REACTIONS
Inj-site disorders, headache, fatigue, fever, rigors, chest pain, back pain, myalgia, abdominal pain, depression, elevation of liver enzymes, hematologic abnormalities.

DRUG INTERACTIONS
Consider the potential for hepatic injury when used in combination w/ known hepatotoxic products, or when new agents are added to the regimen.

PREGNANCY AND LACTATION
Pregnancy: Category C.
Lactation: Caution in nursing.

MECHANISM OF ACTION
Biological response modifier; mechanism not established.

PHARMACOKINETICS
Absorption: (Single 60mcg SQ inj) C_{max}=5.1 IU/mL, T_{max}=16 hrs (median), AUC_{0-96h}=294 IU•hr/mL. **Elimination:** $T_{1/2}$=69 hrs.

PATIENT CONSIDERATIONS
Assessment: Assess for depression, history of or active liver disease, alcohol abuse, preexisting seizure disorder, thyroid dysfunction, myelosuppression, history of hypersensitivity to drug or to human albumin, pregnancy/nursing status, and possible drug interactions.

Monitoring: Monitor for depression, suicidal ideation, jaundice, anaphylaxis, allergic reactions, inj-site reactions, seizures, thrombotic microangiopathy, and other adverse reactions. Perform CBC and LFTs at regular intervals (1, 3, and 6 months) following initiation of therapy and then periodically thereafter in the absence of clinical symptoms; patients w/ myelosuppression may require more intensive monitoring of CBC, w/ differential and platelet counts. Perform thyroid function tests every 6 months in patients w/ a history of thyroid dysfunction, or as clinically indicated.

Counseling: Inform of the symptoms of depression, suicidal ideation, hepatic injury, decreased peripheral blood counts, and seizures, and instruct to immediately report any of these symptoms to physician. Instruct to seek immediate medical attention if symptoms of allergic reactions and anaphylaxis occur. Advise patients that inj-site reactions may occur and to promptly report any signs of necrosis at inj site. Inform that flu-like symptoms are common following initiation of therapy; advise on concurrent use of analgesics and/or antipyretics to help reduce flu-like symptoms on treatment days. Instruct on the use of aseptic technique when self-administering the drug and on the importance of rotating inj sites. Explain the importance of proper disposal of prefilled syringes and autoinjectors, and caution against reuse of these items. Inform about the risks/benefits of treatment during pregnancy.

Reclast — zoledronic acid   **Rx**

Class: Bisphosphonate

ADULT DOSAGE
Osteoporosis

Treatment in Men and Postmenopausal Women:
5mg IV once a yr

Prevention in Postmenopausal Women:
5mg IV once every 2 yrs

Glucocorticoid-Induced Osteoporosis:
In men and women who are either initiating or continuing systemic glucocorticoids in a daily dosage ≥7.5mg of prednisone and who are expected to remain on glucocorticoids for ≥12 months
Treatment/Prevention:
5mg IV once a yr

Paget's Disease

5mg IV

May consider retreatment in patients who have relapsed (based on increases in serum alkaline phosphatase), failed to achieve normalization of serum alkaline phosphatase, or those w/ symptoms

PEDIATRIC DOSAGE
Pediatric use may not have been established

DOSING CONSIDERATIONS
Other Important Considerations
Recommended Intake of Ca^{2+} and Vitamin D:
In Osteoporosis: At least 1200mg of Ca^{2+} daily and 800-1000 IU of vitamin D daily
In Paget's Disease of Bone: 1500mg of Ca^{2+} daily in divided doses (750mg bid or 500mg tid) and 800 IU of vitamin D daily, particularly in the 2 weeks following administration

ADMINISTRATION
IV route

Infuse IV over ≥15 min at a constant rate.
Hydrate patients appropriately prior to administration.
IV infusion should be followed by a 10mL normal saline flush of the IV line.
Do not allow sol to come in contact w/ any Ca^{2+} or other divalent cation-containing sol.
Administer as a single IV sol through a separate vented infusion line.
May give acetaminophen following administration to reduce incidence of acute-phase reaction symptoms.
If refrigerated, allow refrigerated sol to reach room temperature before administration.
After opening, sol is stable for 24 hrs at 2-8°C (36-46°F).

STORAGE
25°C (77°F); excursions permitted to 15-30°C (59-86°F).

HOW SUPPLIED
Inj: 5mg/100mL

CONTRAINDICATIONS
Hypocalcemia, CrCl <35mL/min, acute renal impairment, known hypersensitivity to zoledronic acid or any components of this medication.

WARNINGS/PRECAUTIONS
Consider discontinuation after 3-5 yrs of use in patients at low-risk for fracture; periodically reevaluate risk for fracture in patients who d/c therapy. Contains same active ingredient as Zometa; do not treat w/ Reclast if on concomitant therapy w/ Zometa. Treat preexisting hypocalcemia and disturbances of mineral metabolism prior to treatment. Risk of hypocalcemia in Paget's disease. Withhold therapy until normovolemic status has been achieved if history or physical signs suggest dehydration. Caution w/ chronic renal impairment. Acute renal impairment, including renal failure, reported, especially in patients w/ preexisting renal compromise, advanced age, concomitant nephrotoxic medications or diuretic therapy, or severe dehydration. Transient increase in SrCr may be greater w/ impaired renal function; interim monitoring of CrCl should be performed in at-risk patients. Assess fluid status in patients at increased risk of acute renal failure (ARF) (eg, elderly, concomitant diuretic therapy). Osteonecrosis of the jaw (ONJ) reported; risk may increase w/ duration of exposure to drug or w/ concomitant administration of drugs associated w/ ONJ. Consider a dental examination w/ appropriate preventive dentistry prior to treatment in patients w/ a history of concomitant risk factors (eg, cancer, chemotherapy, angiogenesis inhibitors, radiotherapy, corticosteroids, poor oral hygiene, preexisting dental disease or infection, anemia, coagulopathy) and if possible, avoid invasive dental procedures while on treatment. Atypical, low-energy, or low-trauma fractures of the femoral shaft reported; evaluate any patient w/ a history of bisphosphonate exposure who presents w/ thigh/groin pain to rule out an incomplete femur fracture, and consider interruption of therapy. Avoid use in pregnancy; may cause fetal harm. Severe and occasionally incapacitating bone, joint, and/or muscle pain reported; consider withholding future treatment if severe symptoms develop. Caution w/ aspirin (ASA) sensitivity; bronchoconstriction reported.

ADVERSE REACTIONS
Treatment of Osteoporosis in Postmenopausal Women: Arthralgia, pyrexia, HTN, headache, myalgia, pain in extremity, osteoarthritis, influenza-like illness, dizziness, shoulder pain, diarrhea, bone pain, fatigue, chills, asthenia.
Prevention of Osteoporosis in Postmenopausal Women: Arthralgia, pain, pyrexia, myalgia, back pain, chills, N/V, headache, fatigue, pain in extremity, abdominal pain, diarrhea, musculoskeletal pain, dizziness, dyspepsia.
Osteoporosis in Men: Myalgia, fatigue, headache, musculoskeletal pain/stiffness, pain, chills, influenza-like illness, abdominal pain, malaise, dyspnea, increased C-reactive protein, acute phase reaction, lethargy, A-fib.
Glucocorticoid-Induced Osteoporosis: Abdominal pain, musculoskeletal pain, nausea, dyspepsia.
Paget's Disease of Bone: Influenza-like illness, pyrexia, bone pain, dizziness, nausea, fatigue, rigors, myalgia, influenza, constipation, lethargy, dyspnea, dyspepsia, pain, hypocalcemia.

DRUG INTERACTIONS
Caution w/ aminoglycosides; may have an additive effect to lower serum Ca^{2+} levels for prolonged periods. Caution w/ loop diuretics; may increase risk of hypocalcemia. Caution w/ other potentially nephrotoxic drugs (eg, NSAIDs). In patients w/ renal impairment, exposure to concomitant medications that are primarily renally excreted (eg, digoxin) may increase.

PREGNANCY AND LACTATION
Pregnancy: Category D.
Lactation: Not for use in nursing.

MECHANISM OF ACTION
Bisphosphonate; acts primarily on bone. Inhibits osteoclast-mediated bone resorption.

PHARMACOKINETICS
Distribution: Plasma protein binding (28% at 200ng/mL, 53% at 50ng/mL).
Elimination: Urine (39%), feces (<3%); $T_{1/2}$=146 hrs.

PATIENT CONSIDERATIONS
Assessment: Assess for hypocalcemia, disturbances of mineral metabolism, risk factors for developing renal impairment and ONJ, ASA sensitivity, previous hypersensitivity to the drug, pregnancy/nursing status, and possible drug interactions. Obtain SrCr and calculate CrCl based on actual body weight before each dose. Assess fluid status in patients at increased risk of ARF. Perform routine oral exam, and consider appropriate preventive dentistry in patients w/ a history of risk factors for ONJ.

Monitoring: Monitor for ONJ, atypical femur fracture, musculoskeletal pain, bronchoconstriction, and other adverse events. Monitor renal function and serum Ca^{2+}/mineral levels. Reevaluate the need for continued therapy on a periodic basis.

Counseling: Inform about benefits/risks of therapy, the symptoms of hypocalcemia, and the importance of Ca^{2+} and vitamin D supplementation. Instruct to notify physician if patient had surgery to remove some or all of parathyroid glands, had sections of intestine removed, takes any other medications, or is unable to take Ca^{2+} supplements. Advise to avoid becoming pregnant during treatment. Advise to eat and drink normally (at least 2 glasses of fluid, such as water, w/in a few hrs prior to infusion) on the day of treatment, w/ in a few hrs prior to infusion. Inform of the most commonly associated side effects of therapy and instruct to consult physician if these symptoms persist. Instruct to maintain good oral hygiene and to undergo routine dental check-ups. Advise to report physician or dentist if experiencing persistent pain and/or nonhealing sore of the mouth or jaw.

RECOMBINATE — antihemophilic factor (recombinant)   Rx

Class: Antihemophilic factor (recombinant)

ADULT DOSAGE

Hemophilia A

Prevention/Control of Hemorrhagic Episodes:

Early Hemarthrosis/Muscle Bleed/Oral Bleed:

Required Factor VIII (FVIII) Level 20-40 IU/dL: Begin infusion q12-24h for 1-3 days until bleeding is resolved or healing is achieved

More Extensive Hemarthrosis/Muscle Bleed/Hematoma:

Required FVIII Level 30-60 IU/dL: Repeat infusion q12-24h for (usually) 3 days or more until pain and disability are resolved

Life-Threatening Bleeds:

Required FVIII Level 60-100 IU/dL: Repeat infusion q8-24h until threat is resolved

Perioperative Management:

Minor Surgery:

Required FVIII Level 60-80 IU/dL: Single infusion plus oral antifibrinolytic therapy w/in 1 hr

Major Surgery:

Required FVIII Level 80-100 IU/dL (Pre- and Post-Operative): Repeat infusion q8-24h depending on state of healing

Uncontrolled Bleeding Despite Recommended Dose:

Determine the plasma FVIII level and administer a sufficient dose until a satisfactory clinical response is achieved

Dose Calculation:

Expected Peak Increase of FVIII (IU/dL) = Dose (IU/kg) x 2

PEDIATRIC DOSAGE

Hemophilia A

Prevention/Control of Hemorrhagic Episodes:

Early Hemarthrosis/Muscle Bleed/Oral Bleed:

Required Factor VIII (FVIII) Level 20-40 IU/dL: Begin infusion q12-24h for 1-3 days until bleeding is resolved or healing is achieved

More Extensive Hemarthrosis/Muscle Bleed/Hematoma:

Required FVIII Level 30-60 IU/dL: Repeat infusion q12-24h for (usually) 3 days or more until pain and disability are resolved

Life-Threatening Bleeds:

Required FVIII Level 60-100 IU/dL: Repeat infusion q8-24h until threat is resolved

Perioperative Management:

Minor Surgery:

Required FVIII Level 60-80 IU/dL: Single infusion plus oral antifibrinolytic therapy w/in 1 hr

Major Surgery:

Required FVIII Level 80-100 IU/dL (Pre- and Post-Operative): Repeat infusion q8-24h depending on state of healing

Uncontrolled Bleeding Despite Recommended Dose:

Determine the plasma FVIII level and administer a sufficient dose until a satisfactory clinical response is achieved

Dose Calculation:

Expected Peak Increase of FVIII (IU/dL) = Dose (IU/kg) x 2

ADMINISTRATION

IV route

May administer at a rate up to 10mL/min when reconstituted w/ 10mL sterile water for inj or up to 5mL/min when reconstituted w/ 5mL sterile water for inj
Administer not more than 3 hrs after reconstitution
Do not refrigerate after reconstitution; administer at room temperature
Determine pulse rate before and during administration; if a significant increase in pulse rate occurs, reducing the rate of administration/temporarily halting inj usually allows the symptoms to disappear promptly
If >1 vial is to be administered, contents of multiple vials may be drawn into the same syringe; the Baxject II device is intended for single use only

STORAGE

2-8°C (36-46°F), or room temperature ≤30°C (86°F). Avoid freezing.
Reconstituted Sol: Do not refrigerate.

HOW SUPPLIED

Inj: 220-400 IU, 401-800 IU, 801-1240 IU [5mL, 10mL]; 1241-1800 IU, 1801-2400 IU [5mL]

CONTRAINDICATIONS

Life-threatening immediate hypersensitivity reactions, including anaphylaxis, to the product or its components, including bovine, mouse, or hamster proteins.

WARNINGS/PRECAUTIONS

Not indicated in von Willebrand's disease. Clinical response may vary; if bleeding is not controlled with recommended dose, determine factor VIII (FVIII) level and administer sufficient dose to achieve a satisfactory clinical response. Allergic-type hypersensitivity reactions, including anaphylaxis, reported; d/c if symptoms occur and institute immediate emergency treatment. Contains trace amounts of bovine proteins, mouse immunoglobulin G, and hamster proteins; treatment may cause development of hypersensitivity to these non-human mammalian proteins. Inhibitors (neutralizing antibodies) reported, predominantly in previously untreated and minimally treated patients. If expected plasma FVIII activity levels are not attained, or if bleeding is not controlled with an expected dose; use Bethesda Units (BU) to titer inhibitors. If inhibitor titer is <10 BU/mL, additional dose may neutralize the inhibitor and may permit an appropriate hemostatic response; if inhibitor titer is >10 BU/mL, use alternative therapeutic approaches and agents. Monitor plasma FVIII activity levels by the one-stage clotting assay to confirm the adequate FVIII levels have been achieved and maintained, when clinically indicated. Certain components used in the packaging of product contain natural rubber latex. Identification of clotting defect as a FVIII deficiency is essential before administration is initiated.

ADVERSE REACTIONS

Chills, flushing, rash, epistaxis.

PREGNANCY AND LACTATION

Category C, caution in nursing.

MECHANISM OF ACTION

Antihemophilic agent; provides an increase in plasma levels of FVIII and can temporarily correct the coagulation defect in patients with hemophilia A.

PHARMACOKINETICS

Elimination: $T_{1/2}$=14.6 hrs.

PATIENT CONSIDERATIONS

Assessment: Assess for FVIII deficiency, pregnancy/nursing status, and hypersensitivity to drug, bovine/mouse/hamster proteins, or latex. Assess FVIII activity levels and pulse rate.

Monitoring: Monitor for signs/symptoms of hypersensitivity reactions and other adverse reactions. Monitor plasma FVIII activity levels, clinical response, development of FVIII inhibitors, and pulse rate.

Counseling: Inform about the risks and benefits of therapy. Counsel about the early signs of hypersensitivity reactions; instruct to d/c therapy and contact physician if symptoms develop. Advise that local tissue irritation may occur when reconstituted with 5mL sterile water for inj. Inform that inhibitor formation may occur; advise to contact physician right away if there is lack of clinical response.

REMICADE — infliximab   Rx

Class: Monoclonal antibody/TNF blocker

Increased risk for developing serious infections (eg, active tuberculosis [TB], latent TB reactivation, invasive fungal infections, bacterial/viral infections, opportunistic infections) leading to hospitalization or death, mostly w/ concomitant use w/ immunosuppressants (eg, methotrexate [MTX], corticosteroids). D/C if serious infection or sepsis develops. Active/latent reactivation TB may present w/ disseminated or extrapulmonary disease; test for latent TB before and during therapy and initiate treatment for latent TB prior to infliximab use. Invasive fungal infections reported; consider empiric antifungal therapy in patients at risk who develop severe systemic illness. Consider risks and benefits prior to therapy in patients w/ chronic or recurrent infection. Monitor patients for development of infection during and after treatment, including development of TB in patients who tested (-) for latent TB infection prior to therapy. Lymphoma and other malignancies, some fatal, reported in children and adolescents. Postmarketing cases of aggressive and fatal hepatosplenic T-cell lymphoma (HSTCL) reported, and the majority of cases were in patients w/ Crohn's disease (CD) or ulcerative colitis (UC) and mostly in adolescent and young adult males; almost all of these patients were treated concomitantly w/ azathioprine or 6-mercaptopurine.

ADULT DOSAGE

Rheumatoid Arthritis

Moderately to Severely Active:

For reducing signs/symptoms, inhibiting progression of structural damage, and improving physical function

In Combination w/ MTX:

Induction: 3mg/kg at 0, 2, and 6 weeks

Maint: 3mg/kg every 8 weeks

Incomplete Response: May give up to 10mg/kg or treat every 4 weeks

Ankylosing Spondylitis

Active:

Induction: 5mg/kg at 0, 2, and 6 weeks

Maint: 5mg/kg every 6 weeks

Psoriatic Arthritis

For reducing signs/symptoms of active arthritis, inhibiting progression of structural damage, and improving physical function

W/ or w/o MTX:

Induction: 5mg/kg at 0, 2, and 6 weeks

Maint: 5mg/kg every 8 weeks

Plaque Psoriasis

Chronic Severe (eg, Extensive and/or Disabling):

Induction: 5mg/kg at 0, 2, and 6 weeks

Maint: 5mg/kg every 8 weeks

Crohn's Disease

Moderately to Severely Active w/ Inadequate Response to Conventional Therapy:

For reducing signs/symptoms and inducing/maintaining clinical remission

Induction: 5mg/kg at 0, 2, and 6 weeks

Maint: 5mg/kg every 8 weeks

May give 10mg/kg to patients who respond and then lose their response
Consider discontinuation if no response by Week 14

PEDIATRIC DOSAGE

Crohn's Disease

Moderately to Severely Active w/ Inadequate Response to Conventional Therapy:

For reducing signs/symptoms and inducing/maintaining clinical remission

≥6 Years:

Induction: 5mg/kg at 0, 2, and 6 weeks

Maint: 5mg/kg every 8 weeks

Ulcerative Colitis

Moderately to Severely Active w/ Inadequate Response to Conventional Therapy:

For reducing signs/symptoms and inducing/maintaining clinical remission

≥6 Years:

Induction: 5mg/kg at 0, 2, and 6 weeks

Maint: 5mg/kg every 8 weeks

Also indicated for reducing number of draining enterocutaneous and rectovaginal fistulas and maintaining fistula closure in patients w/ fistulizing Crohn's disease

Ulcerative Colitis

Moderately to Severely Active w/ Inadequate Response to Conventional Therapy:
For reducing signs/symptoms, inducing/maintaining clinical remission and mucosal healing, and eliminating corticosteroid use
Induction: 5mg/kg at 0, 2, and 6 weeks
Maint: 5mg/kg every 8 weeks

ADMINISTRATION
IV route

Do not dilute reconstituted sol w/ any other diluent.
Begin infusion w/in 3 hrs of reconstitution and dilution.
Administer infusion over a period of not less than 2 hrs.
Do not infuse concomitantly in the same IV line w/ other agents.
Refer to PI for further instructions.

STORAGE
2-8°C (36-46°F). May also be stored up to 30°C (86°F) for a single period of up to 6 months, but not exceeding the original expiration date. Do not return to refrigerated storage after removing from refrigerated storage.

HOW SUPPLIED
Inj: 100mg

CONTRAINDICATIONS
Moderate to severe heart failure (HF) (NYHA Class III/IV) w/ doses >5mg/kg, re-administration to patients who have experienced a severe hypersensitivity reaction to infliximab, known hypersensitivity to inactive components of the product or to any murine proteins.

WARNINGS/PRECAUTIONS
Do not initiate w/ an active infection. Increased risk of infection in patients >65 yrs of age and in patients w/ comorbid conditions; consider risks and benefits prior to therapy for those who have resided or traveled in areas of endemic TB or mycoses, and w/ any underlying conditions predisposing to infection. Cases of acute/chronic leukemia, melanoma, and Merkel cell carcinoma reported. Caution in patients w/ moderate to severe COPD, history of malignancy, or in continuing treatment in patients who develop malignancy during therapy. Hepatitis B virus (HBV) reactivation reported; if reactivation occurs, d/c and initiate antiviral therapy w/ appropriate supportive treatment. Severe hepatic reactions (eg, acute liver failure, jaundice, hepatitis, cholestasis) reported; d/c if jaundice or marked elevations of liver enzymes (eg, ≥5X ULN) develop. New onset (rare) HF and worsening of HF reported; d/c if new or worsening symptoms of HF occur. Leukopenia, neutropenia, thrombocytopenia, and pancytopenia reported; consider discontinuation of therapy if significant hematologic abnormalities occur. Caution in patients who have ongoing or history of significant hematologic abnormalities. Hypersensitivity reactions reported; d/c for severe hypersensitivity reactions. CNS manifestation of systemic vasculitis, seizures, and new onset/exacerbation of CNS demyelinating disorders reported (rare); caution in patients w/ these neurologic disorders and consider discontinuation if these disorders develop. Caution when switching from one biologic disease-modifying antirheumatic drug to another; overlapping biological activity may further increase risk of infection. May cause autoantibody formation and, rarely, may develop lupus-like syndrome; d/c if lupus-like syndrome develops. Live vaccines may lead to clinical infections; concurrent administration is not recommended. All pediatric patients should be up to date w/ all vaccinations prior to therapy. Fatal outcome due to disseminated BCG infection reported in infants who received BCG vaccine after in utero exposure to infliximab; wait at least 6 months following birth before administering any live vaccine to infants exposed in utero. Caution in elderly.

ADVERSE REACTIONS
Infusion reactions, nausea, abdominal pain, diarrhea, dyspepsia, URTI, sinusitis, pharyngitis, coughing, bronchitis, rash, headache.

DRUG INTERACTIONS
See Boxed Warning. Avoid w/ live vaccines or therapeutic infectious agents. Avoid use w/ tocilizumab; possible increased immunosuppression and increased risk of infection. Not recommended w/ anakinra or abatacept; may increase risk of serious infections. Not recommended w/ other biological therapeutics used to treat the same conditions. MTX may decrease the incidence of anti-infliximab antibody production and increase infliximab concentrations. Upon initiation or discontinuation of infliximab in patients being treated w/ CYP450 substrates w/ a narrow therapeutic index, monitor therapeutic effect (eg, warfarin) or drug concentration (eg, cyclosporine, theophylline) and adjust individual dose of the drug product as needed.

PREGNANCY AND LACTATION
Pregnancy: Category B.
Lactation: Not for use in nursing.

MECHANISM OF ACTION
Monoclonal antibody/TNF-α receptor blocker; neutralizes biological activity of TNF-α by binding w/ high affinity to the soluble and transmembrane forms of TNF-α and inhibits binding of TNF-α w/ its receptors.

PHARMACOKINETICS
Distribution: Crosses placenta. **Elimination:** $T_{1/2}$=7.7-9.5 days (median).

PATIENT CONSIDERATIONS
Assessment: Assess for active/chronic/recurrent infection (eg, TB, HBV), history of an opportunistic infection, recent travel to areas of endemic TB or endemic mycoses, underlying conditions that may predispose to infection, HF, history of malignancy, moderate to severe COPD, presence or history of significant hematologic abnormalities, neurologic disorders, previous hypersensitivity to drug or to murine proteins, risk factors for skin cancer, pregnancy/nursing status, and for possible drug interactions. Assess vaccination history in pediatric patients. Perform test for latent TB infection.

Monitoring: Monitor for sepsis, TB (active, reactivation, or latent), invasive fungal infections, or bacterial, viral, and other infections caused by opportunistic pathogens during and after therapy. Monitor for development of lymphoma, HSTCL, or other malignancies. Monitor for nonmelanoma skin cancers in psoriasis patients, melanoma and Merkel cell carcinoma, new or worsening symptoms of HF, HBV infection reactivation, hepatotoxicity, hematological events, hypersensitivity reactions, CNS demyelinating disorders, lupus-like syndrome, and other adverse reactions. Monitor LFTs. Perform periodic skin examination, particularly in patients w/ risk factors for skin cancer.

Counseling: Advise of potential risks and benefits of therapy. Inform that therapy may lower the ability of immune system to fight infections; instruct to immediately contact physician if any signs/symptoms of an infection develop, including TB and HBV reactivation. Inform about the risks of lymphoma and other malignancies while on therapy. Advise to report to physician signs of new or worsening medical conditions (eg, heart disease, neurological disease, autoimmune disorders) and symptoms of cytopenia.

REMODULIN — treprostinil

Rx

Class: Prostacyclin analogue

ADULT DOSAGE	PEDIATRIC DOSAGE
Pulmonary Arterial Hypertension	Pediatric use may not have been established
<16 Years:	
World Health Organization Group 1: To Diminish Symptoms Associated with Exercise: New to Prostacyclin Infusion Therapy:	
Initial: 1.25ng/kg/min; reduce rate to 0.625ng/kg/min if not tolerated	
Titrate: May increase in increments of 1.25ng/kg/min per week for the first 4 weeks, then 2.5ng/kg/min per week for the remaining duration of infusion, depending on clinical response; dosage adjustments may be undertaken more often if tolerated Restarting infusion within a few hours after an interruption may be done using the same dose rate; longer periods of interruptions may require retitration	
To Diminish the Rate of Clinical Deterioration Requiring Transition from Epoprostenol Sodium:	
Initial: 10% of current epoprostenol sodium dose	
Titrate: Individualize dose; escalate treprostinil dose as epoprostenol sodium dose is decreased Increase in PAH symptoms should be first treated with increases in treprostinil Side effects associated with prostacyclin or its analogues are to be first treated by decreasing epoprostenol sodium Refer to PI for recommended transition dose changes	

DOSING CONSIDERATIONS
Hepatic Impairment
Mild/Moderate:
Initial: 0.625ng/kg/min ideal body weight
Titrate: Increase slowly

ADMINISTRATION
SQ/IV Route

Administer SQ or IV only as a continuous infusion
Continuous SQ infusion (undiluted) is preferred mode of administration; use IV infusion (dilution required) if SQ infusion is not tolerated
Transition from epoprostenol sodium should take place in a hospital with constant observation of response (eg, walk distance, signs/symptoms of disease progression)
Refer to PI for further administration instructions

STORAGE

Unopened Vials: 25°C (77°F); excursions permitted to 15-30°C (59-86°F). Should be used for no >30 days after initial introduction into vial. Diluted with Remodulin Diluent/High-pH Glycine Diluent: 14 days at room temperature. Diluted with Sterile Water for Injection/0.9% NaCl for Injection: 4 hrs at room temperature or 24 hrs refrigerated. Refer to PI for further storage and administration time limits for the different diluents.

HOW SUPPLIED

Inj: 1mg/mL, 2.5mg/mL, 5mg/mL, 10mg/mL [20mL]

WARNINGS/PRECAUTIONS

Chronic IV infusions are delivered using an indwelling central venous catheter, which is associated with the risk of bloodstream infections (BSIs) and sepsis; continuous SQ infusion (undiluted) is preferred. Avoid abrupt withdrawal or sudden large dose reductions as these may result in a worsening of PAH symptoms. Caution with hepatic/renal insufficiency and in elderly.

ADVERSE REACTIONS

Infusion-site pain/reactions, headache, diarrhea, N/V, rash, jaw pain, vasodilation, edema, hypotension, anorexia, infusion-site infection, asthenia, abdominal pain.

DRUG INTERACTIONS

Coadministration with diuretics, antihypertensives, or other vasodilators may increase the risk of symptomatic hypotension. May increase risk of bleeding with anticoagulants. CYP2C8 inhibitors (eg, gemfibrozil) increase exposure. CYP2C8 inducers (eg, rifampin) decrease exposure.

PREGNANCY AND LACTATION

Category B, safety not known in nursing.

MECHANISM OF ACTION

Prostacyclin analogue; causes direct vasodilation of pulmonary and systemic arterial vascular beds, and inhibition of platelet aggregation.

PHARMACOKINETICS

Absorption: (SQ) Rapid, complete. Absolute bioavailability (100%). Distribution: V_d=14L/70kg ideal body weight, plasma protein binding (91%). Metabolism: Liver via CYP2C8; oxidation and glucuroconjugation. Elimination: (SQ) Urine (78.6%, 4% unchanged), feces (13.4%); $T_{1/2}$=4 hrs.

PATIENT CONSIDERATIONS

Assessment: Assess for hepatic/renal impairment, pregnancy/nursing status, and possible drug interactions.

Monitoring: Monitor for worsening of symptoms or lack of improvement, excessive pharmacologic effects, BSI, sepsis, infusion-site reactions, abrupt withdrawal symptoms, and other adverse reactions.

Counseling: Inform that drug is infused continuously through a SQ or surgically placed indwelling central venous catheter via an infusion pump. Inform patients receiving IV infusion to use an infusion set with an in-line filter. Advise that therapy may be needed for prolonged periods and the ability to accept and care for a catheter and to use an infusion pump should be considered. Inform that subsequent disease management may require the initiation of an alternative IV prostacyclin therapy, epoprostenol sodium.

REPATHA — evolocumab   Rx

Class: Proprotein Convertase Subtilisin Kexin Type 9 (PCSK9) Inhibitor

ADULT DOSAGE

Primary Hyperlipidemia

Adjunct to diet and maximally tolerated statin therapy for the treatment of adults w/ heterozygous familial hypercholesterolemia or clinical atherosclerotic cardiovascular disease, who require additional lowering of LDL-C

140mg SQ every 2 weeks or 420mg SQ once monthly

Homozygous Familial Hypercholesterolemia

Adjunct to diet and other LDL-lowering therapies (eg, statins, ezetimibe, LDL apheresis) for the treatment of patients w/ homozygous familial hypercholesterolemia who require additional lowering of LDL-C

420mg SQ once monthly

Missed Dose

If a dose is missed, administer as soon as possible if there are >7 days until the next scheduled dose. If there are <7 days until the next scheduled dose, omit the missed dose and administer the next dose according to the original schedule

PEDIATRIC DOSAGE

Homozygous Familial Hypercholesterolemia

Adjunct to diet and other LDL-lowering therapies (eg, statins, ezetimibe, LDL apheresis) for the treatment of patients w/ homozygous familial hypercholesterolemia who require additional lowering of LDL-C

13-17 Years:
420mg SQ once monthly

Missed Dose

If a dose is missed, administer as soon as possible if there are >7 days until the next scheduled dose. If there are <7 days until the next scheduled dose, omit the missed dose and administer the next dose according to the original schedule

ADMINISTRATION

SQ route

The 420mg dose can be administered over 9 min by using the single-use on-body infusor w/ prefilled cartridge, or by giving 3 inj consecutively w/in 30 min using the single-use prefilled autoinjector or single-use prefilled syringe.

Prior to use, allow to warm to room temperature for ≥30 min for the prefilled autoinjector or syringe, and for ≥45 min for the on-body infusor w/ prefilled cartridge; do not warm in any other way.

Administer into areas of the abdomen, thigh, or upper arm that are not tender, bruised, red, or indurated; rotate inj site w/ each inj.

Do not coadminister w/ other injectable drugs at the same inj site.

STORAGE

Pharmacy: 2-8°C (36-46°F) in the original carton to protect from light. Do not freeze. Do not shake. Patients/Caregivers: 2-8°C (36-46°F) in the original carton. Alternatively, can be kept at room temperature (20-25°C [68-77°F]) in the original carton; under these conditions, discard if not used w/in 30 days. Protect from direct light and do not expose to temperatures >25°C (77°F).

HOW SUPPLIED

Inj: 140mg/mL [prefilled syringe, prefilled autoinjector], 420mg/3.5mL [on-body infusor w/ prefilled cartridge]

CONTRAINDICATIONS

History of a serious hypersensitivity reaction to evolocumab.

WARNINGS/PRECAUTIONS

Hypersensitivity reactions (eg, rash, urticaria) reported; if signs/symptoms of serious allergic reactions occur, d/c treatment, treat accordingly, and monitor until signs/symptoms resolve.

ADVERSE REACTIONS

Nasopharyngitis, URTI, influenza, back pain, inj-site reactions, cough, UTI, sinusitis, headache, myalgia, dizziness, musculoskeletal pain, HTN, diarrhea, gastroenteritis.

PREGNANCY AND LACTATION

Pregnancy: There are no data available on use in pregnant women to inform a drug-associated risk.
Lactation: There is no information regarding the presence of evolocumab in human milk, the effects on the breastfed infant, or the effects on milk production; caution in nursing.

MECHANISM OF ACTION

Human monoclonal IgG2 directed against PCSK9; inhibits circulating PCSK9 from binding to the LDL receptor (LDLR), preventing PCSK9-mediated LDLR degradation and permitting LDLR to recycle back to the liver cell surface. LDL-C levels are thereby lowered by increasing the number of LDLRs available to clear LDL from the blood.

PHARMACOKINETICS

Absorption: Absolute bioavailability (72%); T_{max}=3-4 days (median). Administration of variable doses resulted in different pharmacokinetic parameters. Distribution: Crosses placenta. (IV) V_d=3.3L. Elimination: $T_{1/2}$=11-17 days.

PATIENT CONSIDERATIONS

Assessment: Assess for drug hypersensitivity and pregnancy/nursing status. Assess baseline LDL-C levels.

Monitoring: Monitor for hypersensitivity reactions and for other adverse reactions. Monitor LDL-C levels; measure LDL-C levels w/in 4-8 weeks of initiating therapy in patients w/ homozygous familial hypercholesterolemia.

Counseling: Instruct on proper administration technique; inform that it may take up to 15 sec to administer evolocumab using the single-use prefilled autoinjector or syringe, and about 9 min to administer evolocumab using the single-use on-body infusor w/ prefilled cartridge. Advise that needle cover of the prefilled autoinjector and syringe contain dry natural rubber (a derivative of latex) and may cause allergic reactions in individuals sensitive to latex.

REPRONEX — menotropins   Rx

Class: Follicle-stimulating hormone (FSH)/luteinizing hormone (LH)

ADULT DOSAGE

Ovulation Induction

To stimulate development of ovarian follicles in infertile women w/ oligo-anovulation

Initial: 150 IU/day for the first 5 days of treatment
Titrate: Adjust subsequent dosing based on response; do not adjust more frequently than every 2 days and do not exceed >75-150 IU/adjustment
Max: 450 IU/day
Max Duration: 12 days

Administer 5000-10000 U human chorionic gonadotropin (hCG) 1 day following the last dose of menotropins; withhold hCG if serum estradiol is >2000pg/mL, ovaries are abnormally enlarged, or if abdominal pain occurs

PEDIATRIC DOSAGE

Pediatric use may not have been established

Assisted Reproductive Technology

In women who have previously received pituitary suppression

Initial: 225 IU

Titrate: Adjust subsequent dosing based on response; do not adjust more frequently than every 2 days and do not exceed >75-150 IU/adjustment

Max: 450 IU/day

Max Duration: 12 days

Administer 5000-10000 U human chorionic gonadotropin (hCG) 1 day following the last dose of menotropins; withhold hCG if serum estradiol is >2000pg/mL, ovaries are abnormally enlarged, or if abdominal pain occurs

ADMINISTRATION

SQ/IM route

Dissolve contents of 1-6 vials in 1-2mL of sterile saline and administer SQ or IM immediately
Use lower abdomen (alternating sides) for SQ administration
Discard unused reconstituted material

STORAGE

3-25°C (37-77°F). Protect from light. Use immediately after reconstitution.

HOW SUPPLIED

Inj: (Follicle stimulating hormone [FSH]/Luteinizing hormone [LH]) 75 IU/75 IU

CONTRAINDICATIONS

High FSH levels indicating primary ovarian failure, uncontrolled thyroid or adrenal dysfunction, organic intracranial lesions (eg, pituitary tumor), any cause of infertility other than anovulation (unless candidate for in vitro fertilization), abnormal bleeding of undetermined origin, ovarian cysts or enlargement not due to polycystic ovary syndrome, prior hypersensitivity to menotropins, pregnancy.

WARNINGS/PRECAUTIONS

Should only be used only by physicians thoroughly familiar with infertility problems. Uncomplicated ovarian enlargement with abdominal distention and/or abdominal pain may occur; use lowest effective dose. May cause ovarian hyperstimulation syndrome (OHSS). Hepatic dysfunction reported in association with OHSS. Monitor patients for at least 2 weeks after hCG administration; d/c treatment and hospitalize patient if OHSS occurs. Withhold hCG if evidence of OHSS develops prior to hCG administration. OHSS may increase the risk of ovarian injury; avoid pelvic exam. Avoid intercourse in patients with significant ovarian enlargement; hemoperitoneum resulting from ruptured ovarian cyst may occur. Serious pulmonary conditions (eg, atelectasis, acute respiratory distress syndrome), thromboembolic events, and multiple births reported. Hypersensitivity/anaphylactic reactions reported.

ADVERSE REACTIONS

Inj-site reactions, vaginal hemorrhage, ovarian disease, pelvic pain, N/V, abdominal pain, enlarged abdomen, headache.

PREGNANCY AND LACTATION

Category X, caution in nursing.

MECHANISM OF ACTION

FSH/LH; produces ovarian follicular growth in women who do not have primary ovarian failure.

PHARMACOKINETICS

Absorption: FSH: (SQ) C_{max}=5.62 mIU/mL, T_{max}=12 hrs, AUC=385.2 mIU•h/mL. (IM) C_{max}=4.15 mIU/mL, T_{max}=18 hrs, AUC=320.1 mIU•h/mL. **Elimination:** FSH: $T_{1/2}$=53.7 hrs (SQ), 59.2 hrs (IM).

PATIENT CONSIDERATIONS

Assessment: Assess for previous hypersensitivity to the drug, primary ovarian failure, abnormal bleeding, endometrial abnormalities, thyroid/adrenal disorders, pregnancy/nursing status, partner's fertility potential, and any other conditions where treatment is contraindicated or cautioned. Perform thorough gynecologic/endocrinologic evaluation. Obtain baseline FSH and gonadotropin levels. Refer to PI for patient selection process.

Monitoring: Monitor for OHSS, pulmonary/vascular complications, ovarian enlargement, abdominal pain, and other adverse reactions. Monitor serum estradiol levels and perform vaginal ultrasound before dose adjustments. Confirm ovulation by indices of progesterone production and sonographic visualization of the ovaries.

Counseling: Inform about duration of treatment and required monitoring. Inform about risk of OHSS, other adverse reactions, and the possibility of multiple births. Encourage infertile patients with oligo-anovulation to have intercourse daily, beginning on the day prior to administration of hCG, until ovulation becomes apparent from the indices employed for determination of progestational activity.

RESCRIPTOR — delavirdine mesylate Rx

Class: Non-nucleoside reverse transcriptase inhibitor (NNRTI)

ADULT DOSAGE

HIV-1 Infection

Combination w/ at Least 2 Other Antiretrovirals:
400mg (four 100mg or two 200mg tabs) tid

PEDIATRIC DOSAGE

HIV-1 Infection

Combination with at Least 2 Other Antiretrovirals:
≥16 Years:
400mg (four 100mg or two 200mg tabs) tid

DOSING CONSIDERATIONS

Concomitant Medications

Antacids: Take at least 1 hr apart

ADMINISTRATION

Oral route

Take w/ or w/o food
Take w/ acidic beverage if achlorhydric
Take 200mg tabs intact; not dispersible in water

Dispersion of 100mg Tab

1. Add four 100mg tabs to at least 3 oz of water
2. Allow to stand for a few minutes
3. Stir until a uniform dispersion occurs
4. Consume dispersion promptly
5. Rinse glass with water and swallow the rinse

STORAGE

20-25°C (68-77°F). Protect from high humidity.

HOW SUPPLIED

Tab: 100mg, 200mg

CONTRAINDICATIONS

Known hypersensitivity to delavirdine mesylate or any components of the medication. Coadministration w/ CYP3A substrates that are associated w/ serious and/or life-threatening events at elevated plasma concentrations (eg, astemizole, terfenadine, dihydroergotamine, ergonovine, ergotamine, methylergonovine, cisapride, pimozide, alprazolam, midazolam, triazolam).

WARNINGS/PRECAUTIONS

Immune reconstitution syndrome reported. Autoimmune disorders (eg, Graves' disease, polymyositis, Guillain-Barre syndrome) have been reported to occur in the setting of immune reconstitution. Redistribution/accumulation of body fat reported. May confer cross-resistance to the other non-nucleoside reverse transcriptase inhibitors (NNRTIs). Severe rash (eg, erythema multiforme, Stevens-Johnson syndrome) reported; d/c use if this occurs. Caution with hepatic impairment and in elderly.

ADVERSE REACTIONS

Headache, fatigue, N/V, diarrhea, increased ALT/AST, rash, maculopapular rash, pruritus, erythema, insomnia, upper respiratory infection, depressive symptoms, generalized abdominal pain.

DRUG INTERACTIONS

See Contraindications. Avoid with another NNRTI. Not recommended with lovastatin, simvastatin, St. John's wort, phenytoin, phenobarbital, carbamazepine, rifabutin, rifampin, or chronic use of H_2-receptor antagonists or PPIs. Increased risk of myopathy with HMG-CoA reductase inhibitors metabolized by CYP3A4 (eg, atorvastatin, cerivastatin). May increase levels of nelfinavir, lopinavir, ritonavir, amphetamines, trazodone, antiarrhythmics, warfarin (monitor INR), calcium channel blockers, atorvastatin, cerivastatin, fluvastatin, immunosuppressants, CYP3A substrates, fluticasone, methadone, and ethinyl estradiol. May increase levels of maraviroc; maraviroc dose should be reduced. May increase levels of indinavir; consider dose reduction of indinavir. May increase levels of saquinavir; consider dose reduction of saquinavir (soft gelatin cap). May decrease levels of didanosine. Ketoconazole, fluoxetine, and CYP3A inhibitors may increase levels. Nelfinavir, didanosine, antacids, CYP3A inducers, H_2-receptor antagonists, PPIs, and dexamethasone may decrease levels. May increase levels of clarithromycin; adjust clarithromycin dose in patients with impaired renal function. May increase levels of sildenafil; do not exceed a max single sildenafil dose of 25mg in a 48-hr period. Doses of an antacid and didanosine (buffered tabs) should be separated by at least 1 hr.

PREGNANCY AND LACTATION

Category C, not for use in nursing.

MECHANISM OF ACTION

NNRTI; binds directly to reverse transcriptase and blocks RNA-dependent and DNA-dependent DNA polymerase activities.

PHARMACOKINETICS

Absorption: Rapid. (400mg tid) C_{max}=35µM, AUC=180µM•hr; T_{max}=1 hr. **Distribution:** Plasma protein binding (98%). **Metabolism:** Hepatic (N-desalkylation, pyridine hydroxylation) via CYP3A (major), 2D6. **Elimination:** (300mg tid multiple dose) Urine (51%, <5% unchanged), feces (44%); (400mg tid) $T_{1/2}$=5.8 hrs.

PATIENT CONSIDERATIONS

Assessment: Assess for hypersensitivity, achlorhydria, hepatic impairment, pregnancy/nursing status, and possible drug interactions.

Monitoring: Monitor for severe rash or rash accompanied by symptoms (eg, fever, blistering, oral lesions, conjunctivitis, swelling, muscle joint aches), immune reconstitution syndrome, cross-resistance to other NNRTIs, fat redistribution, and other adverse reactions.

Counseling: Inform patient that drug is not a cure for HIV-1 infection and that they may continue to experience illnesses associated with HIV-1 infection. Advise to avoid doing things that can spread HIV-1 infection to others. Inform to take as prescribed and to not alter the dose without consulting the physician. Advise patients with achlorhydria to take with acidic beverage (eg, orange or cranberry juice). Inform to take at least 1 hr apart if taking antacids. Advise to d/c and seek medical attention if severe rash or rash with symptoms such as fever, blistering, oral lesions, conjunctivitis, swelling, muscle or joint aches occur. Counsel that fat redistribution may occur. Advise to report use of any prescription or nonprescription medication or herbal products, particularly St. John's wort. Inform patients receiving sildenafil about increased risk of sildenafil-associated adverse events (eg, hypotension, visual changes, prolonged penile erection), and instruct to promptly report any symptoms to the physician. Counsel to notify physician if pregnant or breastfeeding.

RETISERT — fluocinolone acetonide   Rx

Class: Corticosteroid

ADULT DOSAGE	PEDIATRIC DOSAGE
Posterior Segment Uveitis	**Posterior Segment Uveitis**
Chronic Noninfectious Uveitis Affecting Posterior Segment of Eye:	**Chronic Noninfectious Uveitis Affecting Posterior Segment of Eye:**
Usual: 0.59mg surgically implanted into the posterior segment of the affected eye through a pars plana incision; may be replaced if uveitis recurs	**≥12 Years:** **Usual:** 0.59mg surgically implanted into the posterior segment of the affected eye through a pars plana incision; may be replaced if uveitis recurs

ADMINISTRATION
Intravitreal route
Handle only by the suture tab

STORAGE
15-25°C (59-77°F). Protect from freezing.

HOW SUPPLIED
Implant (Tab): 0.59mg

CONTRAINDICATIONS
Active viral diseases of the cornea and conjunctiva including epithelial herpes simplex keratitis (dendritic keratitis), vaccinia, and varicella; and also in active bacterial, mycobacterial, or fungal infections of the eyes.

WARNINGS/PRECAUTIONS
May cause complications such as cataract formation, choroidal detachment, hypotony, increased intraocular pressure (IOP), exacerbation of intraocular inflammation, retinal detachment, vitreous hemorrhage, vitreous loss, and wound dehiscence. Immediate and temporary decrease in visual acuity may occur postoperatively which last for 1-4 weeks. Late onset endophthalmitis observed; assure tight closure of scleral wound and integrity of overlying conjunctiva at the wound site. Caution in patients with a history of viral, bacterial, mycobacterial, or fungal infection of the cornea and conjunctiva (eg, epithelial herpes simplex keratitis, vaccinia, varicella). May delay healing, cause perforation of the globe where there is sclera thinning, and increase incidence of bleb formation postoperatively. May result in elevated IOP and/or glaucoma with optic nerve damage, visual acuity and fields of vision defects, and increase the hazard of secondary ocular infections (bacterial, fungal, and viral) with prolonged use. Caution with glaucoma; monitor for elevated IOP. May mask infection or enhance existing infection with acute purulent conditions of the eye. Avoid simultaneous bilateral implantation. Caution in handling to avoid damage to the implant; use aseptic technique. Should not be resterilized by any method.

ADVERSE REACTIONS
Elevated IOP, glaucoma, abnormal sensation in the eye, cataract, vitreous floaters, headache, macular edema, visual disturbance, conjunctival hemorrhage/hyperemia, eye irritation, hypotony, pruritus, maculopathy, ptosis.

PREGNANCY AND LACTATION
Category C, caution in nursing.

MECHANISM OF ACTION
Corticosteroid; has not been established. Suspected to act by induction of phospholipase A_2 inhibitory proteins, collectively called lipocortins. Inhibits the inflammatory response to a variety of inciting agents and probably delays or slows healing. Inhibits the edema, fibrin deposition, capillary dilation, leukocyte migration, capillary and fibroblast proliferation, deposition of collagen, and scar formation associated with inflammation.

PATIENT CONSIDERATIONS
Assessment: Assess for active/history of viral diseases of the cornea and conjunctiva (eg, epithelial herpes simplex keratitis, vaccinia, varicella), bacterial, mycobacterial, or fungal infections of the eye, glaucoma and pregnancy/nursing status.
Monitoring: Monitor for cataract formation, endophthalmitis, choroidal/retinal detachment, hypotony, increased IOP, exacerbation of intraocular inflammation, glaucoma, vitreous hemorrhage/loss, wound dehiscence, and other adverse reactions. Periodically monitor the integrity of the implant by visual inspection. Monitor for infection with prolonged use.
Counseling: Advise to have ophthalmologic follow-up examinations of both eyes at appropriate intervals after implantation. Counsel about possible eye complications such as cataract formation, choroidal detachment, endophthalmitis, hypotony, increased IOP, exacerbation of intraocular inflammation, retinal detachment, vitreous hemorrhage and loss, and wound dehiscence. Inform that patients will experience an immediate and temporary decrease in visual acuity in the implanted eye for 1-4 weeks post operatively. Advise that cataracts may develop.

REVATIO — sildenafil   Rx

Class: Phosphodiesterase-5 (PDE-5) inhibitor

ADULT DOSAGE	PEDIATRIC DOSAGE
Pulmonary Arterial Hypertension	Pediatric use may not have been established
Treatment of pulmonary arterial HTN (WHO Group I) to improve exercise ability and delay clinical worsening	
PO: 5mg or 20mg tid, 4-6 hrs apart **Max:** 20mg tid	
IV: For continued treatment in patients currently taking tabs/sus and who are temporarily unable to take oral medications 2.5mg or 10mg IV bolus tid	

ADMINISTRATION
Oral/IV route
Refer to PI for reconstitution of the powder for oral sus.

Incompatibilities
Do not mix w/ any other medication or additional flavoring agent.

STORAGE
(Tab/Inj) 20-25°C (68-77°F); excursions permitted to 15-30°C (59-86°F). (Sus) <30°C (86°F). Protect from moisture. Constituted: <30°C (86°F) or 2-8°C (36-46°F). Do not freeze. Shelf-life: 60 days.

HOW SUPPLIED
Inj: 10mg [12.5mL]; Sus: 10mg/mL [112mL]; Tab: 20mg

CONTRAINDICATIONS
Concomitant use of organic nitrates in any form, either regularly/intermittently, or riociguat, a guanylate cyclase stimulator. Known hypersensitivity to sildenafil or any component of the tablet, injection, or oral suspension.

WARNINGS/PRECAUTIONS
Adding sildenafil to bosentan therapy does not result in any beneficial effect on exercise capacity. Not recommended in children. Vasodilatory effects may adversely affect patients w/ resting hypotension (BP <90/50), fluid depletion, severe left ventricular outflow obstruction, or autonomic dysfunction. Not recommended w/ pulmonary veno-occlusive disease (PVOD); consider possibility of associated PVOD if signs of pulmonary edema occur. Epistaxis reported in patients w/ pulmonary HTN secondary to connective tissue disorder. When used to treat erectile dysfunction, non-arteritic anterior ischemic optic neuropathy (NAION) was reported. Caution w/ previous NAION in 1 eye and w/ retinitis pigmentosa. Cases of sudden decrease or loss of hearing, possibly accompanied by tinnitus and dizziness, reported. Caution in patients w/ anatomical penile deformation (eg, angulation, cavernosal fibrosis, Peyronie's disease) or w/ predisposition to priapism (eg, sickle-cell anemia, multiple myeloma, leukemia). Penile tissue damage and permanent loss of potency may result if priapism is not immediately treated. Vaso-occlusive crises requiring hospitalization reported in patients w/ pulmonary HTN secondary to sickle-cell disease. Caution in elderly.

ADVERSE REACTIONS
Headache, dyspepsia, gastritis, epistaxis, paresthesia, flushing, diarrhea, insomnia, dyspnea exacerbation, myalgia, nausea, sinusitis, erythema, pyrexia, rhinitis.

DRUG INTERACTIONS
See Contraindications. Vasodilatory effects may adversely affect patients on antihypertensive therapy; monitor BP when given w/ antihypertensives. Reports of epistaxis w/ oral vitamin K antagonists. Avoid w/ other PDE-5 inhibitors. Not recommended w/ ritonavir and other potent CYP3A inhibitors. Symptomatic postural hypotension w/ doxazosin reported. Additional reduction of supine BP w/ oral amlodipine reported.

PREGNANCY AND LACTATION
Pregnancy: Category B.
Lactation: Caution in nursing.

MECHANISM OF ACTION
PDE-5 inhibitor; increases cGMP w/in pulmonary vascular smooth muscle cells, resulting in relaxation and vasodilation of pulmonary vascular bed and (to a lesser degree) systemic circulation.

PHARMACOKINETICS
Absorption: (Oral)Rapid; absolute bioavailability (41%); T_{max}=60 min (median) (fasted). **Distribution:** V_d=105L; plasma protein binding (96%). **Metabolism:** CYP3A (major route) and CYP2C9 (minor route); N-desmethyl metabolite (active metabolite). **Elimination:** Feces (80% metabolites), urine (13% metabolites); $T_{1/2}$=4 hrs.

PATIENT CONSIDERATIONS
Assessment: Assess for hypotension, fluid depletion, left ventricular outflow obstruction, autonomic dysfunction, PVOD, risk factors for developing NAION,

previous NAION in 1 eye, retinitis pigmentosa, anatomical deformities of the penis, conditions predisposing to priapism, pulmonary HTN secondary to sickle-cell disease, hypersensitivity to drug, pregnancy/nursing status, and possible drug interactions. Obtain baseline BP.

Monitoring: Monitor for signs of pulmonary edema, decreased/sudden loss of vision or hearing, tinnitus, dizziness, epistaxis, priapism, vaso-occlusive crises, hypersensitivity reactions, and other adverse reactions. Monitor BP.

Counseling: Counsel about risks and benefits of the drug. Inform that drug is also marketed as Viagra for male erectile dysfunction. Advise not to take Viagra or other PDE-5 inhibitors and organic nitrates during therapy. Advise to notify physician if sudden decrease/loss of vision or hearing occurs. Instruct to seek immediate medical attention if an erection persists >4 hrs.

REVLIMID — lenalidomide

Rx

Class: Thalidomide analogue

> Do not use during pregnancy; may cause birth defects or embryo-fetal death. Females of reproductive potential should have 2 negative pregnancy tests prior to treatment and must use 2 forms of contraception or continuously abstain from heterosexual sex during and for 4 weeks after treatment. Available only through a restricted distribution program, the Revlimid REMS program. May cause significant neutropenia and thrombocytopenia. Patients on therapy for del 5q myelodysplastic syndrome (MDS) should have their CBC monitored weekly for the first 8 weeks of therapy and at least monthly thereafter; may require dose interruption and/or reduction and use of blood product support and/or growth factors. Increased risk of deep vein thrombosis (DVT) and pulmonary embolism (PE), as well as risk of MI and stroke, reported in patients w/ multiple myeloma (MM) treated w/ lenalidomide and dexamethasone; monitor for and advise patients about signs/symptoms of thromboembolism. Advise patients to seek immediate medical care if symptoms such as SOB, chest pain, or arm or leg swelling develop. Thromboprophylaxis is recommended and the choice of regimen should be based on assessment of individual's underlying risks.

ADULT DOSAGE

Multiple Myeloma

Initial: 25mg qd on Days 1-21 of repeated 28-day cycles in combination w/ dexamethasone; may reduce initial dose of dexamethasone for patients >75 yrs

Continue until disease progression or unacceptable toxicity

In Patients who are not eligible for autologous stem cell transplantation (ASCT), continue treatment until disease progression or unacceptable toxicity. For patients who are ASCT-eligible, hematopoietic stem cell mobilization should occur w/in 4 cycles of a lenalidomide-containing therapy

Myelodysplastic Syndromes

Patients w/ transfusion-dependent anemia due to low- or intermediate-1-risk myelodysplastic syndromes associated w/ a deletion 5q cytogenetic abnormality w/ or w/o additional cytogenetic abnormalities

Initial: 10mg/day

Continue or modify treatment based upon clinical and lab findings

Mantle Cell Lymphoma

Patients whose disease has relapsed or progressed after 2 prior therapies, 1 of which included bortezomib

Initial: 25mg/day on Days 1-21 of repeated 28-day cycles for relapsed or refractory disease

Continue until disease progression or unacceptable toxicity

PEDIATRIC DOSAGE

Pediatric use may not have been established

DOSING CONSIDERATIONS

Renal Impairment

Multiple Myeloma (MM):
Moderate (CrCl 30-50mL/min): Initial: 10mg q24h
Severe (CrCl <30mL/min Not Requiring Dialysis): Initial: 15mg q48h
ESRD (CrCl <30mL/min Requiring Dialysis): Initial: 5mg qd. On dialysis days, administer dose following dialysis

Myelodysplastic Syndromes (MDS):
Moderate (CrCl 30-60mL/min): Initial: 5mg q24h
Severe (CrCl <30mL/min Not Requiring Dialysis): Initial: 2.5mg q24h
ESRD (CrCl <30mL/min Requiring Dialysis): Initial: 2.5mg qd. On dialysis days, administer dose following dialysis

Mantle Cell Lymphoma (MCL):
Moderate (CrCl 30-60mL/min): Initial: 10mg q24h
Severe (CrCl <30mL/min Not Requiring Dialysis): Initial: 15mg q48h
ESRD (CrCl <30mL/min Requiring Dialysis): Initial: 5mg qd. On dialysis days, administer dose following dialysis

Adverse Reactions

MM:
Thrombocytopenia:
Platelets:
Fall to <30,000/μL: Interrupt treatment and follow CBC weekly
Return to >30,000/μL: Resume at next lower dose. Do not dose <2.5mg/day
For Each Subsequent Drop <30,000/μL: Interrupt treatment
Return to >30,000/μL: Resume at next lower dose; do not dose <2.5mg/day
Neutropenia:
Neutrophils:
Fall to <1000/μL: Interrupt treatment, follow CBC weekly
Return to >1000/μL and Neutropenia is Only Toxicity: Resume at 25mg/day or initial starting dose
Return to >1000/μL and if Other Toxicity: Resume at next lower dose. Do not dose <2.5mg/day
For Each Subsequent Drop <1000/μL: Interrupt treatment
Return to >1000/μL: Resume at next lower dose. Do not dose <2.5mg/day
Other Toxicities in MM:
For other Grade 3/4 toxicities judged to be related to treatment, hold treatment and restart at physician's discretion at next lower dose level when toxicity has resolved to <Grade 2

MDS:
Thrombocytopenia w/in 4 Weeks at Starting Dose 10mg/day (Baseline >100,000/μL):
Platelets:
Fall to <50,000/μL: Interrupt treatment
Return to >50,000/μL: Resume at 5mg/day
Thrombocytopenia w/in 4 Weeks at Starting Dose 10mg/day (Baseline <100,000/μL):
Platelets:
Falls to 50% of Baseline: Interrupt treatment
If Baseline >60,000/μL and Return to >50,000/μL: Resume at 5mg/day
If Baseline <60,000/μL and Return to >30,000/μL: Resume at 5mg/day
Thrombocytopenia after 4 Weeks at Starting Dose 10mg/day:
Platelets:
<30,000/μL or <50,000/μL w/ Platelet Transfusions: Interrupt treatment
Return to >30,000/μL (w/o Hemostatic Failure): Resume at 5mg/day
Thrombocytopenia During Treatment at 5mg/day:
Platelets:
<30,000/μL or <50,000/μL w/ Platelet Transfusions: Interrupt treatment
Return to >30,000/μL (w/o Hemostatic Failure): Resume at 2.5mg/day
Neutropenia w/in 4 Weeks of Starting Treatment at 10mg/day (Baseline ANC >1000/μL):
Neutrophils:
Fall to <750/μL: Interrupt treatment
Return to >1000/μL: Resume at 5mg/day
Neutropenia w/in 4 Weeks of Starting Treatment at 10mg/day (Baseline ANC <1000/μL):
Neutrophils:
Fall to <500/μL: Interrupt treatment
Return to >500/μL: Resume at 5mg/day
Neutropenia After 4 Weeks of Starting Treatment at 10mg/day:
Neutrophils:
<500/μL for >7 days or <500/μL Associated w/ Fever (>38.5°C): Interrupt treatment
Return to >500/μL: Resume at 5mg/day
Neutropenia During Treatment at 5mg/day:
Neutrophils:
<500/μL for >7 Days or <500/μL Associated w/ Fever (>38.5°C): Interrupt treatment
Return to >500/μL: Resume at 2.5mg/day
Other Toxicities in MDS:
For other Grade 3/4 toxicities judged to be related to treatment, hold treatment and restart at the physician's discretion at next lower dose level when toxicity has resolved to <Grade 2

MCL:
Thrombocytopenia During Treatment:
Platelets:
Fall to <50,000/μL: Interrupt treatment and follow CBC weekly
Return to >50,000/μL: Resume at 5mg less than the previous dose. Do not dose <5mg daily
Neutropenia During Treatment:
Neutrophils:
Fall to <1000/μL for at Least 7 Days or Falls to <1000/μL w/ an Associated Temperature >38.5°C or Fall to <500/μL:
Interrupt treatment and follow CBC weekly
Return to >1000/μL: Resume at 5mg less than previous dose. Do not dose <5mg/day
Other Toxicities in MCL:
For other Grade 3/4 toxicities judged to be related to treatment, hold treatment and restart at next lower dose level when toxicity has resolved to <Grade 2

ADMINISTRATION

Oral route

Take at about the same time each day, w/ or w/o food.
Swallow cap whole w/ water; do not open, crush, break, or chew.

Handling Precautions
Wash skin immediately and thoroughly w/ soap and water if powder from cap contacts the skin. If drug contacts the mucous membranes, flush thoroughly w/ water.

STORAGE
20-25°C (68-77°F); excursions permitted to 15-30°C (59-86°F).

HOW SUPPLIED
Cap: 2.5mg, 5mg, 10mg, 15mg, 20mg, 25mg

CONTRAINDICATIONS
Pregnancy, hypersensitivity (eg, angioedema, Stevens-Johnson syndrome, toxic epidermal necrolysis) to lenalidomide.

WARNINGS/PRECAUTIONS
Not indicated and not recommended for the treatment of patients w/ chronic lymphocytic leukemia outside of controlled clinical trials; increased risk of death and serious adverse cardiovascular (CV) reactions reported. Avoid pregnancy for at least 4 weeks before beginning therapy, during therapy, during dose interruptions, and for at least 4 weeks after completing therapy. Male patients (including those who had a vasectomy) must always use a latex/synthetic condom during any sexual contact w/ females of reproductive potential during therapy and for up to 28 days after discontinuing therapy. Avoid sperm donation during therapy. Avoid blood donation during treatment and for 1 month following discontinuation. Greater risk of MI or stroke in patients w/ known risk factors, including prior thrombosis; minimize all modifiable factors (eg, hyperlipidemia, HTN, smoking). Increase of invasive 2nd primary malignancies notably acute myelogenous leukemia and MDS reported in patients w/ MM, predominantly in those receiving therapy in combination w/ oral melphalan and ASCT. Hepatic failure, including fatal cases, reported in combination w/ dexamethasone. D/C treatment upon elevation of liver enzymes and consider treatment at a lower dose after values return to baseline. Angioedema and serious dermatologic reactions reported; d/c if angioedema, Stevens-Johnson syndrome (SJS), toxic epidermal necrolysis (TEN), Grade 4 rash, or exfoliative or bullous rash is suspected and do not resume following discontinuation for these reactions. Consider treatment interruption or discontinuation for Grade 2-3 skin rash. Avoid w/ a prior history of Grade 4 rash associated w/ thalidomide treatment. Contains lactose. Fatal instances of tumor lysis syndrome reported; caution in patients w/ high tumor burden prior to treatment. Tumor flare reaction (TFR) reported in patients w/ MCL; withhold treatment in patients w/ Grade 3 or 4 TFR until TFR resolves to ≤Grade 1. A decrease in the number of CD34+ cells collected after treatment (>4 cycles) reported; in patients who are ASCT candidates, referral to a transplant center should occur early in treatment to optimize the timing of the stem cell collection. Consider granulocyte-colony stimulating factor (G-CSF) w/ cyclophosphamide or the combination of G-CSF w/ a CXCR4 inhibitor in patients who received >4 cycles of a lenalidomide-containing treatment or for whom inadequate numbers of CD34+ cells have been collected w/ G-CSF alone.

ADVERSE REACTIONS
Thrombocytopenia, neutropenia, PE, pruritus, rash, diarrhea, constipation, nausea, anemia, fatigue, cough, back pain, pyrexia, muscle cramp, asthenia.

DRUG INTERACTIONS
May increase levels of digoxin; monitor digoxin levels periodically. Closely monitor PT and INR w/ warfarin in MM patients. Caution w/ erythropoietic agents or other agents that may increase the risk of thrombosis (eg, estrogen-containing therapies).

PREGNANCY AND LACTATION
Pregnancy: Category X.
Lactation: Not for use in nursing.

MECHANISM OF ACTION
Thalidomide analogue; w/ immunomodulatory, antiangiogenic, and antineoplastic properties. Inhibits proliferation and induces apoptosis of certain hematopoietic tumor cells. Immunomodulatory properties include activation of T cells and natural killer T (NKT) cells, increased numbers of NKT cells, and inhibition of proinflammatory cytokines (eg, TNF-α and IL-6) by monocytes.

PHARMACOKINETICS
Absorption: Rapid. (Single/Multiple Doses) T_{max}=0.5-6 hrs. **Distribution:** Plasma protein binding (approx 30%). **Metabolism:** 5-hydroxy-lenalidomide and N-acetyl-lenalidomide (metabolites). **Elimination:** Urine (approx 90%, approx 82% unchanged), feces (approx 4%); $T_{1/2}$=3-5 hrs.

PATIENT CONSIDERATIONS
Assessment: Assess for renal/hepatic impairment, history of Grade 4 rash, risk factors for MI and stroke, prior thrombosis, high tumor burden, lactose intolerance, hypersensitivity to the drug, pregnancy/nursing status, and possible drug interactions. Perform pregnancy test 10-14 days before and 24 hrs prior to therapy. Obtain baseline CBC.

Monitoring: Monitor for signs/symptoms of thromboembolism, neutropenia, thrombocytopenia, angioedema, SJS, TEN, tumor lysis syndrome, TFR, 2nd primary malignancies, serious adverse CV reactions, and other adverse reactions. Perform pregnancy test weekly during 1st month, then repeat monthly (regular menstrual cycle) or every 2 weeks (irregular menstrual cycle) and perform pregnancy test if period is missed or if there is any abnormal menstrual bleeding. Monitor CBC periodically; every 7 days (weekly) for the first 2 cycles, on Days 1 and 15 of cycle 3, and every 28 days (4 weeks) thereafter (MM patients taking concomitant dexamethasone); weekly for the first 8 weeks of therapy and at least monthly thereafter (MDS); and weekly for the 1st cycle (28 days), every 2 weeks during cycles 2-4, and monthly thereafter (MCL). Monitor patients w/ neutropenia for signs of infection. Monitor renal/hepatic function. Closely monitor patients w/ high tumor burden. Closely monitor PT and INR w/ warfarin in MM patients.

Counseling: Instruct females of reproductive potential to avoid pregnancy, have monthly pregnancy tests, and to use 2 different forms of contraception, including at least 1 highly effective form, simultaneously during therapy, during dose interruption, and for 4 weeks after completing therapy. Instruct to immediately d/c and contact physician if patient becomes pregnant, misses her menstrual period, experiences unusual menstrual bleeding, stops taking birth control, or believes for any reason that she is pregnant. Instruct males (including those who had a vasectomy) to always use a latex/synthetic condom during any sexual contact w/ females of reproductive potential during therapy and for up to 28 days after discontinuing therapy. Advise males not to donate sperm. Instruct not to donate blood during therapy, during dose interruptions, and for 1 month following discontinuation. Inform of the other risks associated w/ therapy. Instruct that if a dose is missed, may still take dose up to 12 hrs after the time dose is normally taken. Advise that if >12 hrs have elapsed, the dose for that day should be skipped, and the dose for the next day should be taken at the usual time. Advise to observe for bleeding/bruising, especially w/ use of concomitant medication that may increase risk of bleeding.

REYATAZ — atazanavir   Rx

Class: Protease inhibitor

ADULT DOSAGE
HIV-1 Infection
Treatment-Naive Patients:
300mg + Ritonavir (RTV) 100mg qd, or
400mg qd (w/o RTV) if intolerant to RTV

In Combination w/ Efavirenz for Treatment-Naive Patients:
400mg + RTV 100mg qd

Treatment-Experienced Patients:
300mg + RTV 100mg qd

In Combination w/ H₂-Receptor Antagonist and Tenofovir for Treatment-Experienced Patients:
400mg + RTV 100mg qd

PEDIATRIC DOSAGE
HIV-1 Infection
Powder:
≥3 Months of Age:
Treatment-Naive/Treatment-Experienced Patients:
5 to <15kg: 200mg + RTV 80mg qd
15 to <25kg: 250mg + RTV 80mg qd
≥25kg: 300mg + RTV 100mg qd
Treatment-Naive and Intolerant to 200mg Atazanavir Powder:
5 to <10kg: 150mg + RTV 80mg qd
w/ close HIV viral load monitoring

Caps:
6 to <18 Years:
Treatment-Naive/Treatment-Experienced Patients:
15 to <20kg: 150mg + RTV 100mg qd
20 to <40kg: 200mg + RTV 100mg qd
≥40kg: 300mg + RTV 100mg qd
≥13 Years:
Treatment-Naive and Intolerant to RTV:
≥40kg: 400mg qd (w/o RTV)

- -

DOSING CONSIDERATIONS
Concomitant Medications
H₂-Receptor Antagonists/Proton-Pump Inhibitors:
Dose separation may be required

Renal Impairment
ESRD w/ Hemodialysis:
Treatment-Naive: 300mg + RTV 100mg qd
Treatment-Experienced: Not recommended for use

Hepatic Impairment
Coadministration w/RTV is not recommended w/ any degree of hepatic impairment

Treatment-Naive:
Mild (Child-Pugh Class A): 400mg qd (w/o RTV)
Moderate (Child-Pugh Class B): 300mg qd (w/o RTV)
Severe (Child-Pugh Class C): Not recommended for use

Pregnancy
Treatment-Naive and Treatment-Experienced:
300mg + RTV 100mg qd
Treatment-Experienced During 2nd/3rd Trimester w/ Either H₂-Receptor Antagonist or Tenofovir:
400mg + RTV 100mg qd

ADMINISTRATION
Oral route
Take w/ food.

Cap
Do not open.
Use w/o RTV is not recommended for treatment-experienced adults/pediatric patients w/ prior virologic failure.

Powder
Must be taken w/ RTV.

Instructions for Mixing Oral Powder
Preferred Method:
1. Mix the recommended number of pkts w/ a minimum of 1 tbsp of food (eg, applesauce or yogurt).
2. Feed the mixture to the infant or young child.
3. Add an additional 1 tbsp of food to the container, mix, and feed the child the residual mixture.

For Infants Who Can Drink from a Cup:
1. Mix the recommended number of pkts w/ a minimum of 30mL of a beverage (eg, milk or water).
2. Have the child drink the mixture.
3. Add an additional 15mL of beverage to the cup, mix, and have the child drink the residual mixture. If water is used, food should also be taken at the same time.

For Infants <6 Months Who Cannot Eat Solid Food or Drink from a Cup:
1. Mix the recommended number of pkts w/ 10mL of prepared liquid infant formula.
2. Draw up the full amount of the mixture into an oral syringe and administer into either right or left inner cheek of infant.
3. Pour another 10mL of formula into the medicine cup to rinse off remaining oral powder in cup.
4. Draw up residual mixture into the syringe and administer into either inner cheek again.

Administer RTV immediately after powder administration.

Administer the entire dose of oral powder (mixed in the food or beverage) w/in 1 hr (may leave the mixture at room temperature during this 1-hr period). Ensure that the patient eats or drinks all the food or beverage that contains the powder.
Additional food may be given after consumption of the entire mixture.

STORAGE
Cap: 25°C (77°F); excursions permitted to 15-30°C (59-86°F). **Powder:** <30°C (86°F); may be kept at room temperature 20-30°C (68-86°F) for up to 1 hr prior to administration once powder is mixed w/ food/beverages. Store in original pkt and do not open until ready to use.

HOW SUPPLIED
Cap: 150mg, 200mg, 300mg; **Powder:** 50mg/pkt [30^s]

CONTRAINDICATIONS
Coadministration w/ drugs that are highly dependent on CYP3A or UGT1A1 for clearance, and for which elevated plasma concentrations are associated w/ serious and/or life-threatening events, and w/ strong CYP3A inducers (eg, alfuzosin, rifampin, irinotecan, triazolam, oral midazolam, dihydroergotamine, ergotamine, ergonovine, methylergonovine, cisapride, St. John's wort, lovastatin, simvastatin, pimozide, sildenafil when used for pulmonary arterial HTN, indinavir, nevirapine). Previously demonstrated clinically significant hypersensitivity (eg, Stevens-Johnson syndrome, erythema multiforme, or toxic skin eruptions) to any of the components of this medication.

WARNINGS/PRECAUTIONS
May prolong PR interval; consider ECG monitoring w/ preexisting conduction system disease. Rash and cases of Stevens-Johnson syndrome, erythema multiforme, and toxic skin eruptions, including drug rash w/ eosinophilia and systemic symptoms (DRESS) syndrome, reported; d/c if severe rash develops. May cause hyperbilirubinemia; dose reduction is not recommended. Powder contains phenylalanine; caution w/ phenylketonuria. Increased risk for further transaminase elevations or hepatic decompensation in patients w/ underlying hepatitis B or C infections or marked transaminase elevations before treatment; obtain LFTs prior to and during treatment. Nephrolithiasis and/or cholelithiasis reported; consider temporary interruption or discontinuation of therapy if signs/symptoms occur. New onset or exacerbation of diabetes mellitus (DM), hyperglycemia, diabetic ketoacidosis, immune reconstitution syndrome, autoimmune disorders (eg, Graves' disease, polymyositis, Guillain-Barre syndrome) in the setting of immune reconstitution, redistribution/accumulation of body fat, and increased bleeding in patients w/ hemophilia A and B reported. Various degrees of cross-resistance observed. Caution in elderly.

ADVERSE REACTIONS
N/V, jaundice/scleral icterus, rash, myalgia, headache, abdominal pain, insomnia, peripheral neurologic symptoms, diarrhea, cough, fever, AST/ALT elevations, neutropenia, hypoglycemia, extremity pain.

DRUG INTERACTIONS
See Contraindications and Dosing Considerations. Not recommended w/ salmeterol. Use w/o RTV not recommended w/ drugs highly dependent on CYP2C8 w/ narrow therapeutic indices (eg, paclitaxel, repaglinide), carbamazepine, phenytoin, phenobarbital, bosentan, and buprenorphine. ATV/RTV is not recommended w/ other protease inhibitors, voriconazole, fluticasone propionate, and boceprevir. Not recommended w/ efavirenz or proton pump inhibitors (PPIs) in treatment-experienced patients. Avoid w/ colchicine in patients w/ renal/hepatic impairment. Caution w/ oral contraceptives. CYP3A4 inducers, tenofovir, carbamazepine, boceprevir, phenytoin, phenobarbital, bosentan, efavirenz, PPIs, antacids, buffered medications, and H$_2$-receptor antagonists may decrease levels. RTV and clarithromycin may increase levels. Administer 2 hrs before or 1 hr after buffered formulations (eg, didanosine buffered or enteric-coated formulations)/antacids, ≥10 hrs after H$_2$-receptor antagonists, and 12 hrs after PPIs. May increase levels of CYP3A or UGT1A1 substrates, tenofovir, saquinavir, amiodarone, bepridil, lidocaine (systemic), quinidine, TCAs, trazodone, itraconazole, ketoconazole, colchicine, rifabutin, quetiapine, parenteral midazolam, warfarin (monitor INR), diltiazem and other calcium channel blockers, bosentan, atorvastatin, rosuvastatin, norgestimate, norethindrone, fluticasone propionate, clarithromycin, buprenorphine, norbuprenorphine, immunosuppressants, and PDE-5 inhibitors. ATV/RTV may increase levels of carbamazepine. Rosuvastatin dose should not exceed 10mg/day. May decrease levels of didanosine, and 14-OH clarithromycin (clarithromycin active metabolite). ATV/RTV may decrease levels of phenytoin, phenobarbital, and lamotrigine. Voriconazole may alter levels. May alter levels of ethinyl estradiol. Initiation of medications that inhibit or induce CYP3A may increase or decrease concentrations of ATV/RTV, respectively. Refer to PI for dosing modifications when used w/ certain concomitant therapies.

PREGNANCY AND LACTATION
Pregnancy: Physicians are encouraged to register patients in the Antiretroviral Pregnancy Registry. Lactic acidosis syndrome, symptomatic hyperlactatemia, and hyperbilirubinemia reported in pregnant women.
Lactation: Mothers should be instructed not to breastfeed due to potential for HIV-1 transmission and the potential for serious adverse reactions in breastfed infants.

MECHANISM OF ACTION
HIV-1 protease inhibitor; selectively inhibits virus-specific processing of viral Gag and Gag-Pol polyproteins in HIV-1 infected cells, preventing formation of mature virions.

PHARMACOKINETICS
Absorption: Rapid, C_{max}=3152ng/mL, T_{max}=approx 2.5 hrs, AUC=22262ng•hr/mL. **Distribution:** Plasma protein binding (86%). **Metabolism:** Liver (extensive); mono- and dioxygenation via CYP3A. **Elimination:** Urine (13%, approx 7% unchanged), feces (79%, approx 20% unchanged); $T_{1/2}$=approx 7 hrs.

PATIENT CONSIDERATIONS
Assessment: Assess for treatment history, known hypersensitivity, DM, hemophilia, conduction system disease, phenylketonuria, renal/hepatic impairment, pregnancy/nursing status, and possible drug interactions. Obtain baseline LFTs in patients w/ underlying hepatitis B or C infections or marked transaminase elevations.

Monitoring: Monitor for cardiac conduction abnormalities, PR interval prolongation, rash, DRESS, hyperbilirubinemia, nephrolithiasis, cholelithiasis, new onset or exacerbation of DM, hyperglycemia, diabetic ketoacidosis, autoimmune disorders, immune reconstitution syndrome, fat redistribution/accumulation, cross-resistance among protease inhibitors, and other adverse reactions. Monitor LFTs in patients w/ underlying hepatitis B or C infections or marked transaminase elevations. Monitor for bleeding in patients w/ hemophilia. Closely monitor for adverse events during the first 2 months postpartum.

Counseling: Inform that therapy is not a cure for HIV infection, and patients may continue to experience illnesses associated w/ HIV infections. Advise to avoid doing things that can spread HIV infection to others. Advise to take ud and to take w/ food. Instruct not to alter the dose or d/c therapy w/o consulting physician. Advise caregiver on how to mix oral powder w/ a food or beverage, and to carefully follow the instructions for use and storage of powder formulation. Inform caregivers of patients w/ phenylketonuria that oral powder contains phenylalanine, and advise to call healthcare providers if they have any questions. Instruct to report use of any other medications or herbal products. Advise to consult physician if dizziness or lightheadedness occurs. Inform that mild rashes w/o other symptoms, redistribution or accumulation of body fat, or yellowing of the skin or whites of the eyes may occur. Inform that kidney stones and/or gallstones have been reported. Advise to d/c and seek medical evaluation immediately if signs or symptoms of severe skin reactions or hypersensitivity reactions develop.

RHoGAM — rho(D) immune globulin (human)   Rx

Class: Immune globulin

OTHER BRAND NAMES
MICRhoGAM

ADULT DOSAGE
Pregnancy and Other Obstetrical Conditions

For Rh-negative women not previously sensitized to the Rh$_o$(D) factor, unless the father or baby are conclusively Rh-negative

Postpartum (In Rh-Positive Newborn):
RhoGAM: 300mcg (1500 IU) w/in 72 hrs of delivery

Antepartum Prophylaxis:
RhoGAM: 300mcg (1500 IU) at 26-28 weeks gestation; administer w/in 72 hrs of suspected/proven exposure to Rh-positive RBCs resulting from:
1. Amniocentesis, chorionic villus sampling (CVS), and percutaneous umbilical blood sampling (PUBS)
2. Abdominal trauma or obstetrical manipulation
3. Ectopic pregnancy
4. Threatened pregnancy loss after 12 weeks gestation w/ continuation of pregnancy
5. Pregnancy termination (spontaneous or induced) beyond 12 weeks gestation

If antepartum prophylaxis is indicated, it is essential that the mother receive a postpartum dose if the infant is Rh-positive

PEDIATRIC DOSAGE
Pediatric use may not have been established

Actual/Threatened Termination of Pregnancy (Up to and Including 12 Weeks Gestation):
MICRhoGAM: 50mcg (250 IU) w/ in 72 hrs; may use RhoGAM if MICRhoGAM not available

Transfusion of Rh-Incompatible Blood or Blood Products
Prevention of Rh immunization in any Rh-negative person after incompatible transfusion of Rh-positive blood or blood products

<2.5mL Rh-Positive RBCs:
MICRhoGAM: 50mcg (250 IU) w/ in 72 hrs of suspected or proven exposure to Rh-positive RBCs; may use RhoGAM if MICRhoGAM not available

2.5-15.0mL Rh-Positive RBCs:
RhoGAM: 300mcg (1500 IU) w/ in 72 hrs of suspected or proven exposure to Rh-positive RBCs

<15.0mL Rh-Positive RBCs:
RhoGAM: 300mcg (1500 IU) w/ in 72 hrs of suspected or proven exposure to Rh-positive RBCs

---

ADMINISTRATION
IM route

For single use only

RhoGAM
Each single dose prefilled syringe contains 300mcg (1500 IU) of Rh_o(D) immune globulin (human). This is the dose for the indications associated w/ pregnancy at or beyond 13 weeks unless there is clinical or laboratory evidence of a fetal-maternal hemorrhage (FMH) >15mL of Rh-positive RBCs

MICRhoGAM
Each single dose prefilled syringe of MICRhoGAM contains 50mcg (250 IU) of Rh_o(D) immune globulin (human). This dose will suppress the immune response to up to 2.5mL of Rh-positive RBCs
MICRhoGAM is indicated w/in 72 hrs after termination of pregnancy up to and including 12 weeks gestation; at or beyond 13 weeks gestation, RhoGAM should be administered

Multiple Dosage
Multiple doses of RhoGAM are required if a FMH >15mL
Administration of >20mcg of RhoGAM per mL of Rh-positive RBCs should be considered whenever a large FMH or RBC exposure is suspected/documented; multiple doses may be administered at the same time or at spaced intervals, as long as the total dose is administered w/in 3 days of exposure

Dose Frequency
Administer RhoGAM every 12 weeks to maintain an adequate level of anti-D; the exact timing for the inj is based on 12-week intervals starting from the administration of the 1st inj
If delivery of the baby does not occur 12 weeks after the administration of the standard antepartum dose (at 26-28 weeks), a 2nd dose is recommended to maximize protection antepartum
If delivery occurs w/in 3 weeks after the last antepartum dose, the postpartum dose may be withheld, but a test for FMH should be performed to determine if exposure to >15mL of RBCs has occurred

STORAGE
2-8°C. Do not freeze.

HOW SUPPLIED
Inj: (MICRhoGAM) 50mcg (250 IU); (RhoGAM) 300mcg (1500 IU) [prefilled syringe]

CONTRAINDICATIONS
Rh-positive individuals.

WARNINGS/PRECAUTIONS
For IM use only; do not inject IV. For maternal administration in postpartum use; do not inject in newborn infant. Observe patient for at least 20 min after administration. Caution in patient with prior severe systemic allergic reactions to human immune globulin. Contain a small quantity of immunoglobulin A (IgA); potential risk of hypersensitivity in IgA deficient individuals. Monitor for signs and symptoms of hemolytic reaction when used for Rh-incompatible transfusion. May carry a risk of transmitting infectious agents (eg, viruses and Creutzfeldt-Jakob disease [CJD] agent). May cause a positive antibody screening test; does not preclude further antepartum or postpartum prophylaxis. Some babies born to women given Rh_o(D) immune globulin (human) antepartum have weakly positive direct antiglobulin (Coombs') tests at birth. Fetal-maternal hemorrhage may cause false blood-typing results in the mother; use Rh_o(D) immune globulin (human) if any doubt to the patient's Rh type. Do not delay postpartum vaccination of rubella-susceptible women with rubella or MMR vaccine during the last trimester of pregnancy or at delivery.

ADVERSE REACTIONS
Injection-site reactions (eg, swelling, induration, redness, mild pain, warmth), skin rash, body aches, slight temperature elevation.

DRUG INTERACTIONS
May impair the efficacy of live vaccines (eg, measles, mumps, varicella); may inhibit immune response to live vaccines if administered within 14 days after vaccination. Delay immunization until 12 weeks after the final dose.

PREGNANCY AND LACTATION
Category C, safety not known in nursing.

MECHANISM OF ACTION
Immune globulin; has not been established. Suspected to act by suppressing immune response of Rh-negative individuals to Rh-positive RBCs.

PHARMACOKINETICS
Absorption: C_{max}=54ng/mL; T_{max}=4 days. **Distribution:** V_d=7.3L. **Elimination:** $T_{1/2}$=30.9 days.

PATIENT CONSIDERATIONS
Assessment: Assess for Rh status, IgA deficiency, prior hypersensitivity reactions to human immune globulin, pregnancy/nursing status, and possible drug interactions.

Monitoring: Monitor for signs/symptoms of hemolytic reactions, hypersensitivity reactions, viral infections, injection-site reactions, other adverse reactions, and lab test interactions.

Counseling: Discuss the risks and benefits of therapy. Inform that local reactions are common and that systemic reactions are extremely rare but allergic reactions may occur. Inform patients about the early signs of hypersensitivity reactions (eg, hives, generalized urticaria, chest tightness, wheezing, hypotension, and anaphylaxis). Inform that physician will provide a RhoGAM Patient Identification Card; advise to retain the card and present it to other healthcare providers when appropriate.

RHOPHYLAC — rho(D) immune globulin intravenous (human)   Rx

Class: Immune globulin

> Intravascular hemolysis (IVH) leading to death reported in patients treated for immune thrombocytopenic purpura (ITP). IVH can lead to anemia and multi-system organ failure (eg, acute respiratory distress syndrome, acute renal insufficiency, renal failure, disseminated intravascular coagulation [DIC]). Monitor for signs/symptoms (eg, back pain, shaking chills, fever, discolored urine, hematuria) of hemolysis in a healthcare setting for ≥8 hrs after administration; absence of these signs/symptoms w/in 8 hrs does not indicate IVH cannot occur subsequently. Perform dipstick urinalysis at baseline, 2 hrs and 4 hrs after administration, and prior to the end of the monitoring period. Perform post-treatment laboratory tests (eg, plasma Hgb, haptoglobin, lactate dehydrogenase, direct/indirect bilirubin) if IVH is present or suspected.

ADULT DOSAGE
Suppression of Rh Isoimmunization

Pregnancy and Obstetric Conditions:
Suppression of Rh isoimmunization in non-sensitized, Rh_o(D)-negative women w/ Rh-incompatible pregnancy

IV/IM:
Antepartum Prophylaxis:
1500 IU (300mcg) at 28-30 weeks of gestation

Postpartum Prophylaxis (Only if Newborn is Rh_o(D)-Positive):
1500 IU (300mcg) w/in 72 hrs of birth

Dose must be increased if exposed to >15mL of Rh_o(D)-positive RBCs; follow dosing for excessive fetomaternal hemorrhage

Obstetric Complications/Invasive Procedures During Pregnancy/Obstetric Manipulative Procedures:
1500 IU (300mcg) w/in 72 hrs of complication/procedure

Dose must be increased if exposed to >15mL of Rh_o(D)-positive RBCs; follow dosing for excessive fetomaternal hemorrhage

Excessive Fetomaternal Hemorrhage (>15mL):
1500 IU (300mcg) + 100 IU (20mcg)/mL fetal RBCs in excess of 15mL if excess transplacental bleeding is quantified or 1500 IU (300mcg) if excess transplacental bleeding cannot be quantified; administer w/in 72 hrs of complication

Incompatible Transfusions:
Suppression of Rh isoimmunization in Rh_o(D)-negative individuals transfused w/ Rh_o(D)-positive RBCs or blood components containing Rh_o(D)-positive RBCs

PEDIATRIC DOSAGE
Pediatric use may not have been established

100 IU (20mcg) per 2mL
transfused blood or per 1mL
erythrocyte concentrate w/in 72 hrs
of exposure

Chronic Immune Thrombocytopenic Purpura

To Raise Platelet Counts in $Rh_0(D)$-Positive, Non-Splenectomized Patients:
Usual: 250 IU (50mcg)/kg IV

ADMINISTRATION
IV/IM route
- Observe patients for at least 20 min following administration.
- Prior to IV use, ensure that needle-free IV administration system is compatible w/ tip of glass syringe.
- Bring to room temperature before use.
- Do not freeze.

Suppression of Rh Isoimmunization
- Do not administer SQ into fatty tissue.
- Consider IV if reaching the muscle is of concern.

ITP
- IV route only; do not give IM.

IM
- Administer in divided doses at different sites if large doses (>5mL) are required and IM inj is chosen.

IV
- Administer at a rate of 2mL/15-60 sec.

STORAGE
2-8°C (36-46°F); do not freeze. Protect from light.

HOW SUPPLIED
Inj: 1500 IU (300mcg)/2mL [prefilled syringe]

CONTRAINDICATIONS
History of anaphylactic or severe systemic reaction to human immune globulin. IgA deficiency w/ antibodies to IgA and a history of hypersensitivity to the product or any of its components. Do not administer to the newborn infant of a mother who received Rhophylac postpartum.

WARNINGS/PRECAUTIONS
Severe hypersensitivity reactions may occur; d/c immediately and institute appropriate treatment. May affect results of blood typing, antibody screening, and direct antiglobulin (Coombs') tests; antepartum administration to mother can also affect these tests in the newborn. May contain antibodies to other Rh antigens. May carry a risk of transmitting infectious agents (eg, viruses, Creutzfeldt-Jakob disease agent). **ITP:** Safety unknown in patients w/ preexisting anemia; may increase severity of anemia. If transfusions are required due to hemolysis and anemia following administration, use $Rh_0(D)$-negative packed RBCs.

ADVERSE REACTIONS
Suppression of Rh Isoimmunization: Nausea, dizziness, headache, injection-site pain, malaise.
ITP: Chills, pyrexia/increased body temperature, headache, hemolysis, increased bilirubin, decreased hemoglobin, decreased haptoglobin.

DRUG INTERACTIONS
May impair immune response to live, attenuated virus vaccines (eg, measles, mumps, rubella, varicella). Do not immunize w/ live vaccines w/in 3 months after final dose.

PREGNANCY AND LACTATION
Pregnancy: Category C.
Lactation:
Suppression of Rh Isoimmunization: Safe in nursing.
ITP: Safety not known in nursing.

MECHANISM OF ACTION
Immune globulin; not established. **ITP:** Thought to involve formation of $Rh_0(D)$ immune globulin RBC complexes removed by reticuloendothelial system (particularly spleen), resulting in Fc receptor blockade, thus sparing antibody-coated platelets.

PHARMACOKINETICS
(Suppression of Rh Isoimmunization) **Absorption:** (IV) C_{max}=62-84ng/mL. (IM) C_{max}=7-46ng/mL, T_{max}=2-7 days, absolute bioavailability (69%), **Elimination:** $T_{1/2}$=16 days (IV), 18 days (IM).

PATIENT CONSIDERATIONS
Assessment: Assess for IgA deficiency w/ antibodies to IgA and history of hypersensitivity, anaphylactic/severe systemic reactions to human immune globulin, preexisting anemia, and possible drug interactions. Perform baseline dipstick urinalysis.
Monitoring: Monitor for signs/symptoms of IVH, hypersensitivity reactions, anemia, acute renal insufficiency, renal failure, DIC, and transmission of infectious agents. Monitor patients treated for ITP for ≥8 hrs after administration. Perform a dipstick urinalysis 2 hrs and 4 hrs after administration, and prior to the end of the monitoring period.
Counseling: Instruct to immediately report symptoms of IVH, hives, chest tightness, wheezing, hypotension, anaphylaxis, and symptoms related to viral

infection. Advise to inform other healthcare providers of interference w/ response to live virus vaccines. Inform that product may contain disease-causing infectious agents.

RIASTAP — fibrinogen concentrate (human)   **Rx**
Class: Plasma glycoprotein

ADULT DOSAGE	PEDIATRIC DOSAGE
Congenital Fibrinogen Deficiency	**Congenital Fibrinogen Deficiency**
Acute bleeding episodes in patients w/ congenital fibrinogen deficiency, including afibrinogenemia and hypofibrinogenemia	Studies have included patients <16 years; the number of patients <16 years of age in this study limits statistical interpretation
Known Baseline Fibrinogen Level: Dose=[target level (mg/dL)-measured level (mg/dL)]/1.7 (mg/dL per mg/kg body weight)	
Unknown Baseline Fibrinogen Level: 70mg/kg IV	
Monitor fibrinogen level during treatment; maintain a target fibrinogen level of 100mg/dL until hemostasis is obtained	

ADMINISTRATION
IV route

Preparation
Reconstitute at room temperature. Use appropriate transfer device or syringe to transfer 50mL of sterile water for inj into vial. Gently swirl vial to ensure product is fully dissolved; do not shake vial.
Stable for 8 hours after reconstitution when stored at 20-25°C; administer w/in this time period.

Administration
Do not mix w/ other medications or IV sol; administer through separate inj site. Administer at room temperature by slow IV inj at a rate of ≤5mL/min.

STORAGE
2-25°C (36-77°F) up to 60 months. Protect from light. Do not freeze.

HOW SUPPLIED
Inj: 900mg-1300mg

CONTRAINDICATIONS
Known anaphylactic or severe systemic reactions to human plasma-derived products.

WARNINGS/PRECAUTIONS
Allergic reactions may occur; immediately d/c if signs/symptoms of anaphylaxis or hypersensitivity reactions occur. Thromboembolic events reported. Made from human plasma; may contain infectious agents (eg, viruses and, theoretically, the Creutzfeldt-Jakob disease agent) that can cause disease. All infections thought to have been transmitted by product should be reported to manufacturer.

ADVERSE REACTIONS
Fever, headache.

PREGNANCY AND LACTATION
Pregnancy: There are no studies of use in pregnant women; it is not known whether drug can cause fetal harm when administered to a pregnant woman or can affect reproduction capacity.
Lactation: There is no information regarding the presence of the drug in human milk, its effects on the breastfed infant, or its effects on milk production. Caution in nursing.

MECHANISM OF ACTION
Plasma glycoprotein; physiological substrate of thrombin, factor XIIIa, and plasmin. Replaces the missing or low coagulation factor.

PHARMACOKINETICS
Absorption: C_{max}=140mg/dL, AUC=124.3mg•hr/mL (70mg/kg dose). **Distribution:** V_d=52.7mL/kg. **Elimination:** $T_{1/2}$=78.7 hrs.

PATIENT CONSIDERATIONS
Assessment: Assess for drug hypersensitivity. Assess pregnancy/nursing status and fibrinogen levels.
Monitoring: Monitor for signs/symptoms of allergic/hypersensitivity reactions, thrombosis, and infection (eg, viruses). Monitor fibrinogen levels.
Counseling: Inform of the signs of allergic/hypersensitivity reactions (eg, hives, chest tightness, wheezing, hypotension, anaphylaxis) and thrombotic events (eg, unexplained pleuritic, chest and/or leg pain or edema, hemoptysis, dyspnea, tachypnea, neurologic symptoms) and advise to report to physician if any of these occur. Inform that therapy is made from human plasma and may contain infectious agents that can cause disease.

RIBASPHERE CAPSULES – ribavirin   Rx

Class: Nucleoside analogue

Not for monotherapy treatment of chronic hepatitis C (CHC) virus infection. Primary toxicity is hemolytic anemia. Anemia associated w/ therapy may result in worsening of cardiac disease and lead to fatal and nonfatal MIs. Avoid w/ history of significant/unstable cardiac disease. Contraindicated in women who are pregnant and male partners of pregnant women. Extreme care must be taken to avoid pregnancy during therapy and for 6 months after completion of therapy. Use at least 2 reliable forms of effective contraception during treatment and for 6 months after discontinuation.

ADULT DOSAGE

Chronic Hepatitis C with Compensated Liver Disease

Combination w/ Peginterferon Alfa-2b:
<66kg: 400mg qam and 400mg qpm
66-80kg: 400mg qam and 600mg qpm
81-105kg: 600mg qam and 600mg qpm
<105kg: 600mg qam and 800mg qpm

Treatment Duration:
Interferon Alfa-Naive Patients:
Genotype 1: 48 weeks
Genotypes 2 and 3: 24 weeks
Retreatment of Prior Treatment Failures:
48 weeks (regardless of hepatitis c virus genotype)

Combination w/ Interferon Alfa-2b:
≤75kg: 400mg qam and 600mg qpm
<75kg: 600mg qam and 600mg qpm

Treatment Duration:
Interferon Alfa-Naive Patients:
24-48 weeks
Retreatment in Relapse Patients:
24 weeks

PEDIATRIC DOSAGE

Chronic Hepatitis C with Compensated Liver Disease

Combination w/ Peginterferon Alfa-2b/Interferon Alfa-2b:
3-17 Years:
47-59kg: 400mg qam and 400mg qpm
60-73kg: 400mg qam and 600mg qpm
<73kg: 600mg qam and 600mg qpm

Recommended: 15mg/kg/day
Patients who reach their 18th birthday while receiving combination therapy should remain on the pediatric dosing regimen

Treatment Duration:
Genotype 1: 48 weeks
Genotypes 2 and 3: 24 weeks

DOSING CONSIDERATIONS

Renal Impairment
CrCl <50mL/min: Not recommended for use

Elderly
Start at lower end of dosing range

Adverse Reactions
Development of Severe Adverse Reactions/Lab Abnormalities:
Modify or d/c dose until adverse reaction abates or decreases in severity; d/c therapy if intolerance persists after dose adjustment

W/O Cardiac Disease:
Hgb 8.5-<10g/dL:
Adults: 1st dose reduction is by 200mg/day (except in patients receiving 1400mg; dose reduction should be by 400mg/day); if needed, 2nd dose reduction is by an additional 200mg/day
Patients whose dose is reduced to 600mg/day receive one 200mg cap in the am and two 200mg caps in the pm
Pediatrics: 1st dose reduction is to 12mg/kg/day, 2nd dose reduction is to 8mg/kg/day

Hgb <8.5g/dL:
D/C therapy

History of Stable Cardiac Disease:
Hgb ≥2g/dL Decrease During Any 4-Week Treatment Period: Reduce dose by 200mg/day
Hgb Remains <8.5g/dL or <12g/dL After 4 Weeks at Reduced Dose: D/C therapy
Refer to labeling for interferon alfa-2b or peginterferon alfa-2b for dose reduction information

Discontinuation
Adults:
Combination w/ Peginterferon Alfa-2b:
Interferon Alfa-Naive Patients:
Genotype 1: Consider in patients who do not achieve at least a 2log₁₀ drop or loss of HCV-RNA at 12 weeks, or if HCV-RNA remains detectable after 24 weeks of therapy
Retreatment of Prior Treatment Failures:
Consider in patients who fail to achieve undetectable HCV-RNA at week 12 of therapy, or whose HCV-RNA remains detectable after 24 weeks of therapy
Combination w/ Interferon Alfa-2b:
Interferon Alfa-Naive Patients:
Consider in any patient who has not achieved an HCV-RNA below the limit of detection of the assay by 24 weeks

Pediatrics 3-17 Years:
Combination w/ Peginterferon Alfa-2b:
Excluding Genotypes 2 and 3: D/C therapy at 12 weeks if treatment Week 12 HCV-RNA dropped less than 2log₁₀ compared to a pretreatment, or at 24 weeks if HCV-RNA is detectable at treatment Week 24

Combination w/ Interferon Alfa-2b:
Genotype 1: Consider in any patient who has not achieved an HCV-RNA below the limit of detection of the assay by 24 weeks

ADMINISTRATION
Oral route

Take w/ food.
Do not open, crush, or break caps.
Refer to labeling for interferon alfa-2b or peginterferon alfa-2b for dosage/administration information.

STORAGE
25°C (77°F); excursions permitted to 15-30°C (59-86°F).

HOW SUPPLIED
Cap: 200mg

CONTRAINDICATIONS
Women who are or may become pregnant, men whose female partners are pregnant, known hypersensitivity reactions (eg, Stevens-Johnson syndrome, toxic, epidermal necrolysis, and erythema multiforme) to ribavirin or any component of the product, autoimmune hepatitis, hemoglobinopathies (eg, thalassemia major, sickle cell anemia), CrCl <50mL/min. Coadministration w/ didanosine.

WARNINGS/PRECAUTIONS
May cause birth defects and death of unborn child; do not start therapy until a negative pregnancy test has been obtained immediately prior to initiation of therapy. Suspend therapy w/ signs and symptoms of pancreatitis; d/c therapy w/ confirmed pancreatitis. Pulmonary symptoms (eg, dyspnea, pulmonary infiltrates, pneumonitis, pulmonary HTN, pneumonia, sarcoidosis, or exacerbation of sarcoidosis) reported; closely monitor and d/c therapy if pulmonary infiltrates/impairment develops. Alfa interferons may induce or aggravate ophthalmologic disorders (eg, decrease or loss of vision, retinopathy). Perform eye exam in all patients prior to therapy, periodically w/ preexisting ophthalmologic disorders (eg, diabetic or hypertensive retinopathy), and if symptoms develop during therapy. D/C if new or worsening ophthalmologic disorders develop. Severe decreases in neutrophil and platelet counts, and hematologic, endocrine (eg, TSH), and hepatic abnormalities may occur w/ peginterferon alfa-2b; perform hematology and blood chemistry testing prior to therapy and periodically thereafter. Dental/periodontal disorders reported. Rebound growth and weight gain reported in pediatric patients following treatment. May induce a growth inhibition that results in reduced adult height in pediatric patients. Associated w/ significant adverse reactions (eg, severe depression and suicidal ideation, suppression of bone marrow function, autoimmune and infectious disorders, diabetes). Caution w/ preexisting cardiac disease; d/c if cardiovascular (CV) status deteriorates. Not for treatment of HIV infection, adenovirus, respiratory syncytial virus, parainfluenza, or influenza infections.

ADVERSE REACTIONS
Adults: hemolytic anemia, inj-site inflammation/reaction, fatigue/asthenia, headache, rigors, fevers, nausea, myalgia, anxiety, emotional lability, irritability.
Pediatrics: hemolytic anemia, pyrexia, headache, neutropenia, fatigue, anorexia, inj-site erythema, vomiting.

DRUG INTERACTIONS
See Contraindications. Closely monitor for toxicities, especially hepatic decompensation and anemia, w/ nucleoside reverse transcriptase inhibitors (NRTIs); consider dose reduction/discontinuation of therapy or discontinuation of NRTI. May inhibit phosphorylation of lamivudine, stavudine, and zidovudine. Severe pancytopenia, bone marrow suppression, and myelotoxicity reported w/ azathioprine; d/c for pancytopenia and do not reintroduce w/ concomitant azathioprine.

PREGNANCY AND LACTATION
Pregnancy: Category X. A Ribavirin Pregnancy Registry has been established to monitor maternal-fetal outcomes of pregnancies in female patients and female partners of male patients exposed to ribavirin.
Lactation: Not for use in nursing.

MECHANISM OF ACTION
Nucleoside analogue; mechanism not established. Has direct antiviral activity in tissue culture against many RNA viruses; increases mutation frequency in the genomes of several viruses and ribavirin triphosphate inhibits HCV polymerase in a biochemical reaction.

PHARMACOKINETICS
Absorption: Rapid and extensive. (Single 600mg dose) Absolute bioavailability (64%); C_{max}=782ng/mL; T_{max}=1.7 hrs; AUC=13,400ng•hr/mL. **Distribution:** V_d=2825L. **Metabolism:** Nucleated cells (phosphorylation); deribosylation and amide hydrolysis. **Elimination:** Urine (61%), feces (12%); $T_{1/2}$=43.6 hrs.

PATIENT CONSIDERATIONS
Assessment: Assess for autoimmune hepatitis, hemoglobinopathies, nursing status, hepatic/renal/pulmonary function, depression, preexisting ophthalmologic disorders, history of or preexisting cardiac disease, drug hypersensitivity, and possible drug interactions. Conduct pregnancy test (including partners of male patients), hematologic tests, TSH determination, ECG in patients w/ preexisting cardiac disease, and eye exam.

Monitoring: Monitor for anemia, worsening of cardiac disease, pancreatitis, CV deterioration, pulmonary function impairment, new/worsening ophthalmologic disorders, and other adverse reactions. Monitor CBC, LFTs, TSH, ECG, and HCV RNA periodically. Monitor growth in pediatric patients. Obtain Hct and Hgb (Week 2 and 4, more if needed). Perform pregnancy test monthly during therapy and for 6 months after discontinuation of therapy (including partners of male patients). Schedule regular dental exams.

Counseling: Inform that anemia may develop. Advise that lab evaluations are required prior to starting therapy and periodically thereafter. Advise to be well hydrated, especially during the initial stages of treatment. Inform of pregnancy risks; instruct to use at least 2 forms of contraception and perform monthly pregnancy test during therapy and for 6 months post therapy (including partners of male patients). Advise to notify physician in the event of pregnancy. Counsel on risks/benefits associated w/ treatment. Inform that appropriate precautions to prevent HCV transmission should be taken. Advise to brush teeth thoroughly twice daily and to have regular dental exams. Advise that if vomiting occurs, rinse mouth thoroughly afterwards.

RIBASPHERE TABLETS — ribavirin   Rx

Class: Nucleoside analogue

> Not for monotherapy treatment of chronic hepatitis C (CHC) virus infection. Primary toxicity is hemolytic anemia. Anemia associated w/ therapy may result in worsening of cardiac disease and lead to fatal and nonfatal MI. Avoid w/ history of significant/unstable cardiac disease. Contraindicated in women who are pregnant and male partners of pregnant women. Extreme care must be taken to avoid pregnancy during therapy and for 6 months after completion of therapy in both female patients and in female partners of male patients who are taking therapy. Use at least 2 reliable forms of effective contraception during treatment and for 6 months after discontinuation.

ADULT DOSAGE

Chronic Hepatitis C with Compensated Liver Disease

Combination w/ Peginterferon Alfa-2a:
Not Previously Treated w/ Interferon Alfa:
Monoinfection:
Genotypes 1, 4:
<75kg: 1000mg/day in 2 divided doses
≥75kg: 1200mg/day in 2 divided doses
Duration: 48 weeks

Genotypes 2, 3:
Usual: 800mg/day in 2 divided doses
Duration: 24 weeks

HIV Coinfection:
Usual: 800mg/day in 2 divided doses
Duration: 48 weeks (regardless of genotype)

PEDIATRIC DOSAGE

Chronic Hepatitis C with Compensated Liver Disease

Combination w/ Peginterferon Alfa-2a:
Not Previously Treated w/ Interferon Alfa:
Monoinfection:
≥5 Years:
23kg-33kg: 200mg qam and 200mg qpm
34kg-46kg: 200mg qam and 400mg qpm
47kg-59kg: 400mg qam and 400mg qpm
60kg-74kg: 400mg qam and 600mg qpm
≥75 kg: 600mg qam and 600mg qpm
Duration:
Genotypes 2, 3: 24 weeks
Other Genotypes: 48 weeks

Treatment Initiation Prior to 18 Years:
Maintain pediatric dosing through the completion of therapy

DOSING CONSIDERATIONS
Renal Impairment
CrCl 30-50mL/min: Alternating 200mg and 400mg qod
CrCl <30mL/min and/or Hemodialysis: 200mg/day

Adverse Reactions
Adults: May restart at 600mg/day and further increase to 800mg/day once therapy has been withheld due to a lab abnormality or clinical adverse reaction. Increasing to original dose (1000-1200mg/day) is not recommended

Pediatrics: May attempt to increase to original dose once lab abnormality or clinical adverse reaction resolve. May restart at 1/2 the full dose if therapy has been withheld due to a lab abnormality or clinical adverse reaction

W/O Cardiac Disease:
Hgb <10g/dL:
≥5 Years:
23kg-33kg: Decrease dose to 200mg qam
34kg-59kg: Decrease dose to 200mg qam and 200mg qpm
≥60kg: Decrease dose to 200mg qam and 400mg qpm
Adults:
Decrease dose to 200mg qam and 400mg qpm

Hgb <8.5g/dL:
Adults and Pediatrics ≥5 Years:
D/C Ribasphere

W/ History of Stable Cardiac Disease:
Hgb Decrease of ≥2g/dL During Any 4-Week Treatment Period:
≥5 Years:
23kg-33kg: Decrease dose to 200mg qam
34kg-59kg: Decrease dose to 200mg qam and 200mg qpm
≥60kg: Decrease dose to 200mg qam and 400mg qpm
Adults:
Decrease dose to 200mg qam and 400mg qpm

Hgb <12g/dL After 4 Weeks at Reduced Dose:
Adults and Pediatrics ≥ 5 Years:
D/C Ribasphere

Discontinuation
Consider if at least a 2 $\log_{10}$ HCV RNA reduction from baseline by Week 12 is not achieved
Consider if HCV RNA levels remain detectable after treatment Week 24
D/C if hepatic decompensation develops during treatment

ADMINISTRATION
Oral route
Take w/ food
Never administer as monotherapy
Refer to peginterferon alfa-2a labeling for dosage and administration instructions

STORAGE
25°C (77°F); excursions permitted between 15-30°C (59-86°F).

HOW SUPPLIED
Tab: 200mg, 400mg, 600mg; RibaPak [600mg/day, 800mg/day, 1000mg/day, 1200mg/day]

CONTRAINDICATIONS
Women who are or may become pregnant and men whose female partners are pregnant, hemoglobinopathies (eg, thalassemia major, sickle cell anemia), combination w/ didanosine. When used with peginterferon alfa-2a, refer to the individual monograph.

WARNINGS/PRECAUTIONS
Combination therapy is associated w/ significant adverse reactions (eg, severe depression and suicidal ideation; hemolytic anemia; suppression of bone marrow function; autoimmune, infectious, ophthalmologic, and cerebrovascular disorders; pulmonary dysfunction; colitis; pancreatitis; diabetes). Caution w/ baseline risk of severe anemia (eg, spherocytosis, history of GI bleeding). Risk of hepatic decompensation and death in CHC patients w/ cirrhosis. Severe acute hypersensitivity reactions (eg, angioedema, bronchoconstriction, anaphylaxis) and serious skin reactions reported. D/C w/ hepatic decompensation, confirmed pancreatitis, severe hypersensitivity, or if signs/symptoms of severe skin reactions develop. Pulmonary disorders (eg, dyspnea, pulmonary infiltrates, pneumonitis, pulmonary HTN, pneumonia, sarcoidosis/exacerbation of sarcoidosis) reported; closely monitor if there is evidence of pulmonary infiltrates or pulmonary function impairment, and, if appropriate, d/c therapy. Caution w/ preexisting cardiac disease; d/c if cardiovascular status deteriorates. Delay in weight and height increases in pediatric patients reported.

ADVERSE REACTIONS
Hemolytic anemia, fatigue, asthenia, neutropenia, headache, pyrexia, myalgia, irritability, anxiety, nervousness, insomnia, alopecia, rigors, N/V, influenza-like illness.

DRUG INTERACTIONS
See Contraindications. Closely monitor for toxicities (eg, hepatic decompensation) w/ nucleoside reverse transcriptase inhibitors; consider dose reduction or discontinuation of peginterferon alfa-2a, ribavirin, both. Severe pancytopenia and bone marrow suppression reported w/ azathioprine; d/c peginterferon alfa-2a, ribavirin, and azathioprine if pancytopenia develops.

PREGNANCY AND LACTATION
Category X, not for use in nursing.

MECHANISM OF ACTION
Nucleoside analogue; not established. Has direct antiviral activity in tissue culture against many RNA viruses; increases mutation frequency in the genomes of several RNA viruses and ribavirin triphosphate inhibits HCV polymerase in a biochemical reaction.

PHARMACOKINETICS
Absorption: C_{max}=2748ng/mL; T_{max}=2 hrs; AUC_{0-12h}=25,361ng•hr/mL. **Elimination:** $T_{1/2}$=120-170 hrs.

PATIENT CONSIDERATIONS

Assessment: Assess for hemoglobinopathies, autoimmune hepatitis, nursing status, hepatic/renal/pulmonary function, baseline risk of severe anemia, history of or preexisting cardiac disease, hypersensitivity, and possible drug interactions. Conduct pregnancy test (including in female partners of male patients), standard hematological and biochemical lab tests, ECG in patients w/ preexisting cardiac abnormalities, thyroid function tests, and CD4 count in HIV/AIDS patients.

Monitoring: Monitor for anemia, worsening of cardiac disease, pancreatitis, renal/hepatic dysfunction, pulmonary disorders, lab abnormalities, hypersensitivity reactions, and other adverse reactions. Perform hematological tests at Weeks 2 and 4 and biochemical tests at Week 4; perform additional testing periodically. Monitor TSH, and HCV RNA levels. Perform pregnancy test monthly during therapy and for 6 months after discontinuation (including female partners of male patients). Monitor growth in pediatric patients. In patients receiving concomitant therapy w/ azathioprine, monitor CBC, including platelet counts weekly for the first month, twice monthly for the second and third months of treatment, then monthly or more frequently if dosage or other therapy changes are necessary.

Counseling: Counsel on risks/benefits associated w/ treatment. Inform of pregnancy risks; instruct to use 2 reliable methods of birth control during therapy and for 6 months post therapy (including female partners of male patients). Advise to notify physician in the event of pregnancy. Instruct not to drink alcohol; inform that alcohol may exacerbate CHC infection. Inform to take appropriate precautions to prevent HCV transmission during treatment or in the event of treatment failure. Caution to avoid driving/operating machinery if symptoms of dizziness, confusion, somnolence, or fatigue occur. Counsel to take w/ food and keep well-hydrated. Advise that lab evaluations are required prior to starting therapy and periodically thereafter.

RILUTEK — riluzole   Rx

Class: Benzothiazole

ADULT DOSAGE	PEDIATRIC DOSAGE
Amyotrophic Lateral Sclerosis	Pediatric use may not have been established
50mg bid	

ADMINISTRATION
Oral route
Take at least 1 hr ac or 2 hrs pc.

STORAGE
20-25°C (68-77°F); protect from bright light.

HOW SUPPLIED
Tab: 50mg

CONTRAINDICATIONS
History of severe hypersensitivity reactions to riluzole or to any of its components.

WARNINGS/PRECAUTIONS
Cases of drug-induced liver injury, some fatal, and asymptomatic elevations of hepatic transaminases reported; monitor for hepatic injury every month for the first 3 months of therapy, and periodically thereafter. Not recommended in patients who develop hepatic transaminase levels >5X ULN. D/C if there is evidence of liver dysfunction. Severe neutropenia (ANC <500/mm^3) w/in the first 2 months of therapy reported. Interstitial lung disease, including hypersensitivity pneumonitis, reported; d/c if this develops. Caution in elderly. Japanese patients are more likely to have higher drug levels; risk of adverse reactions may be greater.

ADVERSE REACTIONS
Asthenia, nausea, dizziness, decreased lung function, abdominal pain.

DRUG INTERACTIONS
CYP1A2 inhibitors (eg, ciprofloxacin, enoxacin, fluvoxamine) may increase levels and the risk of riluzole-associated adverse reactions. CYP1A2 inducers may decrease levels and efficacy. Concomitant use w/ other potentially hepatotoxic drugs (eg, allopurinol, methyldopa, sulfasalazine) may increase the risk for hepatotoxicity.

PREGNANCY AND LACTATION
Pregnancy: There are no studies in pregnant women, and case reports have been inadequate to inform the drug-associated risk.
Lactation: Caution in nursing.

MECHANISM OF ACTION
Benzothiazole; mechanism not established.

PHARMACOKINETICS
Absorption: Oral bioavailability (approx 60%). **Distribution:** Plasma protein binding (96%). **Metabolism:** Oxidation via CYP1A2; direct and sequential glucuronidation via UGT-HP4. **Elimination:** Urine (90%, 2% unchanged), feces (5%); T$_{1/2}$=12 hrs.

PATIENT CONSIDERATIONS

Assessment: Assess for history of severe hypersensitivity reactions to riluzole or to any of its components, pregnancy/nursing status, and possible drug interactions. Obtain baseline LFTs.

Monitoring: Monitor for hepatic injury every month during first 3 months, then periodically thereafter. Monitor for signs/symptoms of febrile illness, neutropenia, interstitial lung disease, and for other adverse reactions.

Counseling: Instruct to notify healthcare provider if patient experiences yellowing of the whites of the eyes, fever, or respiratory symptoms (eg, dry cough, difficult or labored breathing). Advise to notify healthcare provider if pregnant, nursing, or if taking any concomitant medications.

RITUXAN — rituximab   Rx

Class: Monoclonal antibody/CD20 blocker

> Serious infusion reactions and severe mucocutaneous reactions, some fatal (death has occurred within 24 hrs of infusion), may occur. Monitor patients closely. D/C infusion for severe reaction and treat for Grade 3/4 infusion reactions. Hepatitis B virus (HBV) reactivation can occur, in some cases resulting in fulminant hepatitis, hepatic failure, and death. Screen all patients for HBV infection before treatment initiation; monitor patients during and after treatment. D/C therapy and concomitant medications in the event of HBV reactivation. Fatal progressive multifocal leukoencephalopathy (PML) may occur.

ADULT DOSAGE	PEDIATRIC DOSAGE
Non-Hodgkin's Lymphoma	Pediatric use may not have been established
375mg/m^2 as an IV infusion	

Relapsed/Refractory, Low-Grade/ Follicular, CD20-Positive, B-Cell Non-Hodgkin's Lymphoma (NHL) as a Single Agent:
Administer once weekly for 4 or 8 doses

Retreatment: Administer once weekly for 4 doses

Previously Untreated Follicular, CD20-Positive, B-Cell NHL: In Combination w/ Chemotherapy:
Administer on Day 1 of each chemotherapy cycle for up to 8 doses

Maint in Complete/Partial Responders: Administer as a single agent every 8 weeks for 12 doses; initiate 8 weeks following completion of combination treatment w/ chemotherapy

Non-Progressing, Low-Grade, CD20-Positive, B-Cell NHL as a Single Agent After 1st Line Cyclophosphamide, Vincristine, and Prednisone (CVP) Chemotherapy:
Administer once weekly for 4 doses at 6-month intervals following completion of 6-8 CVP chemotherapy cycles
Max: 16 doses

Previously Untreated Diffuse Large B-Cell, CD20-Positive NHL in Combination w/ Cyclophosphamide, Doxorubicin, Vincristine, and Prednisone (CHOP) or Other Anthracycline-Based Chemotherapy:
Administer on Day 1 of each chemotherapy cycle for up to 8 infusions

As a Component of Zevalin:
Infuse 250mg/m^2 w/in 4 hrs prior to the administration of Indium-111 (In-111) Zevalin and w/in 4 hrs prior to the administration of Yttrium-90 (Y-90) Zevalin; administer rituximab and In-111 Zevalin 7-9 days prior to rituximab and Y-90 Zevalin

Refer to the Zevalin PI for additional information

Chronic Lymphocytic Leukemia

In combination w/ fludarabine and cyclophosphamide, for previously untreated and previously treated CD20-positive chronic lymphocytic leukemia

375mg/m^2 the day prior to initiation of fludarabine and cyclophosphamide chemotherapy, then 500mg/m^2 on Day 1 of cycles 2-6 (every 28 days)

Pneumocystis jiroveci pneumonia and anti-herpetic viral prophylaxis is recommended during treatment and for up to 12 months following treatment as appropriate

Rheumatoid Arthritis

In combination w/ methotrexate for moderately to severely active rheumatoid arthritis in patients who have had an inadequate response to ≥1 TNF antagonist therapy

Two 1000mg IV infusions separated by 2 weeks

Administer subsequent courses every 24 weeks or based on evaluation, but not sooner than every 16 weeks

Granulomatosis with Polyangiitis and Microscopic Polyangiitis

In Combination w/ Glucocorticoids:
375mg/m^2 IV infusion once weekly for 4 weeks

Glucocorticoid Administration:
Methylprednisolone 1000mg/day IV for 1-3 days, followed by oral prednisone 1mg/kg/day (not to exceed 80mg/day and tapered per clinical need); begin regimen w/

in 14 days prior to or w/ initiation of rituximab and continue during and after the 4-week course of treatment

Pneumocystis jiroveci pneumonia prophylaxis is recommended during treatment and for at least 6 months following the last infusion

Premedication

Premedicate before each infusion w/ acetaminophen and an antihistamine

For patients administered rituximab according to the 90-min infusion rate, the glucocorticoid component of their chemotherapy regimen should be administered prior to infusion

Rheumatoid Arthritis Patients:

Methylprednisolone 100mg IV (or its equivalent) 30 min prior to each infusion

---

DOSING CONSIDERATIONS
Adverse Reactions
Infusion Reactions: Interrupt or slow the infusion; continue at 1/2 the previous rate upon improvement of symptoms

ADMINISTRATION
IV route

For IV infusion only; do not administer as IV push or bolus.
Do not mix or dilute w/ other drugs.
Single-use vial; discard any unused portion left in vial.

1st Infusion
Initiate at a rate of 50mg/hr; in the absence of infusion toxicity, increase rate by 50mg/hr increments every 30 min, to a max of 400mg/hr

Subsequent Infusions
Standard Infusion: Initiate at a rate of 100mg/hr; in the absence of infusion toxicity, increase by 100mg/hr increments every 30 min, to a max of 400mg/hr

Previously Untreated Follicular and Diffuse Large B-Cell Non-Hodgkin's Lymphoma Patients:
Grade 3 or 4 Infusion-Related Adverse Event Not Experienced During Cycle 1:
Administer a 90-min infusion in Cycle 2 w/ a glucocorticoid-containing chemotherapy regimen; initiate at a rate of 20% of the total dose given in the first 30 min and the remaining 80% of the total dose given over the next 60 min. If 90-min infusion is tolerated in cycle 2, use the same rate when administering the remainder of the treatment regimen (through Cycle 6 or 8)
Clinically Significant Cardiovascular Disease/Circulating Lymphocyte Count ≥5000/mm³ Before Cycle 2:
Do not administer the 90-min infusion

Preparation
1. Withdraw the necessary amount of rituximab and dilute to a final concentration of 1-4mg/mL in an infusion bag containing either 0.9% normal saline or D5W.
2. Gently invert bag to mix the sol.

STORAGE
2-8°C (36-46°F). Protect from direct sunlight. Do not freeze or shake. **Sol for Infusion:** 2-8°C (36-46°F) for 24 hrs. Stable for additional 24 hrs at room temperature; however, store diluted solutions at 2-8°C (36-46°F).

HOW SUPPLIED
Inj: 100mg/10mL, 500mg/50mL

WARNINGS/PRECAUTIONS
Should only be administered by a healthcare professional with appropriate medical support to manage severe infusion reactions that can be fatal if they occur. Not recommended for use with severe, active infections. *Pneumocystis jiroveci* pneumonia (PCP) and antiherpetic viral prophylaxis is recommended for patients with CLL during treatment and for up to 12 months following treatment as appropriate. PCP prophylaxis is recommended for patients with GPA and MPA during treatment and for at least 6 months following last infusion. Potential for immunogenicity. Acute renal failure, hyperkalemia, hypocalcemia, hyperuricemia, and/or hyperphosphatemia from tumor lysis may occur within 12-24 hrs after the 1st infusion. A high number of circulating malignant cells (≥25,000/mm³) or high tumor burden confers greater risk of tumor lysis syndrome (TLS); administer aggressive IV hydration and antihyperuricemic therapy in patients at high risk of TLS. Correct electrolyte abnormalities, monitor renal function and fluid balance, and administer supportive care, including dialysis as indicated. Serious, including fatal, bacterial, fungal, and new/reactivated viral infections may occur during and following the completion of therapy; d/c for serious infections and institute anti-infective therapy. Infections reported in some patients with prolonged hypogammaglobulinemia (>11 months after rituximab exposure). D/C if severe mucocutaneous reactions, PML, or serious/life-threatening cardiac arrhythmias occur. Perform cardiac monitoring during and after all infusions if arrhythmias develop or with history of arrhythmia/angina. Severe renal toxicity

may occur in NHL patients; d/c if SrCr rises or oliguria occurs. Abdominal pain, bowel obstruction, and perforation may occur in combination with chemotherapy. Follow current immunization guidelines and administer non-live vaccines at least 4 weeks prior to therapy for RA patients. Obtain CBC and platelet count prior to each course in lymphoid malignancy patients, at weekly to monthly intervals (more frequently if cytopenia develops) during treatment with rituximab and chemotherapy, and at 2- to 4-month intervals during therapy in RA, GPA, or MPA patients. Not recommended in patients with RA who have not had prior inadequate response to one or more TNF antagonists.

ADVERSE REACTIONS
Infusion reactions, mucocutaneous reactions, hepatitis B reactivation, PML, infections, fever, lymphopenia, chills, asthenia, neutropenia, headache, leukopenia, diarrhea, muscle spasms.

DRUG INTERACTIONS
Renal toxicity reported with cisplatin. Vaccination with live viral vaccines not recommended. Observe closely for signs of infection if biologic agents and/or disease-modifying antirheumatic drugs are used concomitantly.

PREGNANCY AND LACTATION
Pregnancy: Category C.
Lactation: Caution in nursing.

MECHANISM OF ACTION
Chimeric murine/human monoclonal IgG_1 kappa antibody/CD20 antigen blocker; binds to CD20 antigen expressed on the surface of pre-B and mature B-lymphocytes, mediates B-cell lysis, possibly by complement-dependent cytotoxicity and antibody-dependent cell-mediated cytotoxicity.

PHARMACOKINETICS
Absorption: RA: C_{max}=157mcg/mL (1st infusion), 183mcg/mL (2nd infusion), 318mcg/mL (2 x 500mg dose), 381mcg/mL (2 x 1000mg dose). **Distribution:** RA: V_d=3.1L. GPA/MPA: V_d=4.5L. **Elimination:** NHL: $T_{1/2}$=22 days, RA: $T_{1/2}$=18 days, CLL: $T_{1/2}$=32 days. GPA/MPA: $T_{1/2}$=23 days.

PATIENT CONSIDERATIONS

Assessment: Assess for severe active infections, preexisting cardiac/pulmonary conditions, prior experience of cardiopulmonary adverse reactions, high number of circulating malignant cells (≥25,000/mm³), high tumor burden, electrolyte abnormalities, risk/preexisting HBV infection, hypogammaglobulinemia, any other conditions where treatment is cautioned, pregnancy/nursing status, and possible drug interactions. Perform HBsAg and anti-HBc measurement before initiating treatment. Obtain CBC and platelet count.

Monitoring: Monitor fluid and electrolyte balance, cardiac/renal function, CBC, and platelet counts periodically. Monitor for signs/symptoms of infusion reactions, mucocutaneous reactions, hepatitis B reactivation, PML, new-onset neurologic manifestations, TLS, infections, arrhythmias, bowel obstruction/perforation, cytopenias, and other adverse reactions. Closely monitor for infusion reactions in patients with preexisting cardiac/pulmonary conditions, those who experienced prior cardiopulmonary adverse reactions, and those with high numbers of circulating malignant cells. Monitor patients with evidence of current or prior HBV infection for clinical and lab signs of hepatitis or HBV reactivation during and for several months following therapy.

Counseling: Inform of risks of therapy and importance of assessing overall health status at each visit. Inform that drug is detectable in serum for up to 6 months following completion of therapy. Advise to use effective contraception during and for 12 months after therapy.

RIXUBIS — coagulation factor IX (recombinant)   **Rx**
Class: Antihemophilic factor (recombinant)

ADULT DOSAGE	PEDIATRIC DOSAGE
Hemophilia B	Pediatric use may not have been established
Control/Prevention of Bleeding Episodes:	
Minor Bleeding:	
Required Factor IX (FIX) Level 20-30 IU/dL: q12-24h for at least 1 day, until healing is achieved	
Moderate Bleeding:	
Required FIX Level 25-50 IU/dL: q12-24h for 2-7 days, until bleeding stops and healing is achieved	
Major Bleeding:	
Required FIX Level 50-100 IU/dL: q12-24h for 7-10 days, until bleeding stops and healing is achieved	
Perioperative Management:	
Minor Surgery:	
Required FIX Level 30-60 IU/dL: q24h for at least 1 day, until healing is achieved	
Major Surgery:	
Required FIX Level 80-100 IU/dL: q8-24h for 7-10 days, until bleeding stops and healing is achieved	

Routine Prophylaxis:
40-60 IU/kg IV twice weekly; adjust dose based on response

Dosing Equation:
Initial Dose = Body Weight (kg) x Desired FIX Increase (% of normal or IU/dL) x Reciprocal of Observed Recovery (IU/kg per IU/dL)

ADMINISTRATION
IV bolus infusion route
Use a plastic syringe
Use w/in 3 hrs of reconstitution

STORAGE
2-8°C (36-46°F) for up to 24 months; do not freeze. May store at room temperature ≤30°C (86°F) for up to 12 months within the 24-month period; do not return to refrigerator after storage at room temperature.

HOW SUPPLIED
Inj: 250 IU, 500 IU, 1000 IU, 2000 IU, 3000 IU

CONTRAINDICATIONS
Known hypersensitivity to this product or its excipients, including hamster protein; disseminated intravascular coagulation (DIC); signs of fibrinolysis.

WARNINGS/PRECAUTIONS
Not indicated for induction of immune tolerance in patients with hemophilia B. Initiate therapy under the supervision of a physician experienced in the treatment of hemophilia. Hypersensitivity reactions reported; immediately d/c and initiate appropriate treatment if an allergic/anaphylactic-type reaction occurs. Contains trace amounts of Chinese hamster ovary proteins; may develop hypersensitivity to these proteins. May develop FIX inhibitors; perform an assay that measures FIX inhibitor concentration if expected FIX activity plasma levels are not attained, or if bleeding is not controlled with expected dose. Association between occurrence of FIX inhibitor and allergic reactions reported; increased risk of severe hypersensitivity reactions or anaphylaxis if these patients are re-exposed to therapy. Nephrotic syndrome reported following attempted immune tolerance induction in hemophilia B patients with FIX inhibitors. Associated with the development of thromboembolic complications; monitor for early signs of thromboembolic and consumptive coagulopathy in patients with liver disease, with signs of fibrinolysis, peri/postoperatively, or at risk for thromboembolic events or DIC.

ADVERSE REACTIONS
Dysgeusia, pain in extremity, (+) furin antibody test, FIX/furin antibodies.

PREGNANCY AND LACTATION
Category C, caution in nursing.

MECHANISM OF ACTION
Recombinant antihemophilic factor; temporarily replaces the missing coagulation FIX that is required for effective hemostasis.

PHARMACOKINETICS
Absorption: (Non-bleeding subjects) (Dose range: 71.3-79.4 IU/kg) AUC_{0-inf}=1207 IU•hrs/dL (single dose), 1305 IU•hrs/dL (repeated dose); C_{max}=66.2 IU/dL (single dose), 72.7 IU/dL (repeated dose). **Distribution:** V_d=201.9mL/kg (single dose), 178.6mL/kg (repeated dose). **Elimination:** $T_{1/2}$=26.7 hrs (single dose), 25.4 hrs (repeated dose).

PATIENT CONSIDERATIONS
Assessment: Assess for known hypersensitivity to drug or to its excipients, including hamster protein; severity of bleeding; DIC or risk for DIC; liver disease; signs of fibrinolysis; risk for thromboembolic events; presence of FIX inhibitors; and pregnancy/nursing status.

Monitoring: Monitor for hypersensitivity reactions, DIC, thromboembolic complications, nephrotic syndrome, and other adverse reactions. Monitor FIX activity plasma levels. Monitor for the development of FIX inhibitors if expected FIX activity plasma levels are not attained or if bleeding is not controlled with an expected dose.

Counseling: Advise to report to physician any adverse reactions or problems following administration. Inform of the early signs of hypersensitivity reactions and anaphylaxis; instruct to d/c and contact physician if these symptoms occur. Advise to contact physician or treatment facility for further treatment and/or assessment if experiencing a lack of clinical response to FIX replacement therapy. Instruct to follow the specific preparation and administration procedures provided by physician.

RUCONEST — C1 esterase inhibitor (recombinant)   Rx

Class: C1 esterase inhibitor

ADULT DOSAGE	PEDIATRIC DOSAGE
Hereditary Angioedema	**Hereditary Angioedema**
Treatment of Acute Attacks:	**Treatment of Acute Attacks:**
<84kg: 50 IU/kg IV over approximately 5 min	Adolescents:
>84kg: 4200 IU IV over approximately 5 min	**<84kg:** 50 IU/kg IV over approximately 5 min
Max: 4200 IU/dose	**>84kg:** 4200 IU IV over approximately 5 min

If attack symptoms persist, an additional (2nd) dose can be administered at the recommended dose level
No more than 2 doses should be administered w/in a 24-hr period

Max: 4200 IU/dose
If attack symptoms persist, an additional (2nd) dose can be administered at the recommended dose level
No more than 2 doses should be administered w/in a 24-hr period

ADMINISTRATION
IV route
Ensure that C1 esterase inhibitor vial and diluent vial are at room temperature
Using the syringe/needle or syringe/vial adapter, withdraw 14mL of sterile water for inj from the diluent vial
Remove the syringe and transfer the diluent to the C1 esterase inhibitor vial. Add the diluent slowly to avoid forceful impact on the powder Swirl the vial slowly to mix and avoid foaming
Repeat this procedure using another 14mL of diluent and a second vial of C1 esterase inhibitor
If same patient is to receive >1 vial, contents of multiple vials may be pooled into a single administration device (eg, syringe)
Do not mix w/ other medicinal products. Administer by a separate infusion line
Refer to PI for further administration, reconstitution, and preparation instructions

STORAGE
2-25°C (36-77°F), 48 months shelf life. Do not freeze. Protect from light. Reconstituted Sol: Use immediately, or w/in 8 hrs at 2-8°C (36-46°F). Do not freeze reconstituted sol.

HOW SUPPLIED
Inj: 2100 IU

CONTRAINDICATIONS
History of allergy to rabbits or rabbit-derived products, history of life-threatening immediate hypersensitivity reactions to C1 esterase inhibitor preparations, including anaphylaxis.

WARNINGS/PRECAUTIONS
Initiate treatment under the supervision of a qualified healthcare professional experienced in the treatment of HAE. Appropriately trained patients may self-administer upon recognition of an HAE attack. Severe hypersensitivity reactions may occur; d/c and institute appropriate treatment. Serious arterial and venous thromboembolic events (TE) reported in patients w/ risk factors (eg, presence of an indwelling venous catheter/access device, prior history of thrombosis, underlying atherosclerosis, use of oral contraceptives or certain androgens, morbid obesity, immobility).

ADVERSE REACTIONS
Headache, nausea, diarrhea, angioedema, back pain, vertigo.

PREGNANCY AND LACTATION
Category B, caution in nursing.

MECHANISM OF ACTION
C1 esterase inhibitor (C1INH); regulates the activation of the complement and contact system pathways by formation of complexes between the protease and the inhibitor, resulting in inactivation of both and consumption of C1INH. Exerts its inhibitory effect by irreversibly binding several proteases (target proteases) of the contact and complement systems. Suppression of contact system activation by C1INH through the inactivation of plasma kallikrein and factor XIIa is thought to modulate vascular permeability by preventing the generation of bradykinin.

PHARMACOKINETICS
Absorption: C_{max}=1.2 IU/mL (50 IU/kg), 2.3 IU/mL (100 IU/kg); T_{max}=0.31 hrs (50 IU/kg, 100 IU/kg); AUC=3.3 IU•hr/mL (50 IU/kg), 10.6 IU•hr/mL (100 IU/kg). **Distribution:** V_d=3L (50 IU/kg), 2.4L (100 IU/kg). **Elimination:** $T_{1/2}$=2.4 hrs (50 IU/kg), 2.7 hrs (100 IU/kg).

PATIENT CONSIDERATIONS
Assessment: Assess for history of allergy to rabbits or rabbit-derived products, previous hypersensitivity reactions to drug, risk factors for TE, and pregnancy/nursing status.

Monitoring: Monitor for hypersensitivity reactions, TE, and other adverse reactions. Monitor patients w/ known risk factors for TE during and after administration.

Counseling: Counsel about risks and benefits of therapy. Instruct to immediately report signs/symptoms of allergic hypersensitivity reactions, (eg, hives, urticaria, tightness of the chest, wheezing, hypotension, anaphylaxis) during or after inj. Advise to notify physician if pregnant/intending to become pregnant during treatment with C1INH. Advise to notify physician if breastfeeding/planning to breastfeed.

SABRIL — vigabatrin　　Rx

Class: GABA analogue

> Can cause permanent bilateral concentric visual field constriction including tunnel vision that can result in disability; in some cases, treatment may also damage the central retina and may decrease visual acuity. Onset of vision loss is unpredictable. Risk of vision loss increases w/ increasing dose and cumulative exposure, but there is no dose or exposure known to be free of risk of vision loss. Vision loss may not be recognized until it is severe. Vision should be assessed at baseline (no later than 4 weeks after starting therapy), at least every 3 months during therapy, and about 3-6 months after therapy is discontinued. Once detected, vision loss due to treatment is not reversible. Consider discontinuation, balancing benefit and risk, if visual loss is documented. Risk of new or worsening vision loss continues as long as therapy is used. Vision loss may worsen despite discontinuation of therapy. D/C in patients who fail to show clinical benefit w/in 2-4 weeks (infantile spasms) or 3 months (refractory complex partial seizures) of initiation, or sooner if treatment failure is obvious. Unless benefit clearly outweighs the risk, avoid use w/ other drugs associated w/ serious adverse ophthalmic effects (eg, retinopathy, glaucoma) and in patients w/, or at high risk of, other types of irreversible vision loss. Use lowest dose and shortest exposure to treatment. Available only through a restricted program under a Risk Evaluation and Mitigation Strategy (REMS) called the Sabril REMS Program.

ADULT DOSAGE

Refractory Complex Partial Seizures

Adjunctive Therapy:
≥17 Years:
Initial: 1000mg/day (500mg bid)
Titrate: May increase total daily dose in 500mg increments at weekly intervals to a recommended dose of 3000mg/day (1500mg bid)

Use lowest dose and shortest exposure to treatment

PEDIATRIC DOSAGE

Refractory Complex Partial Seizures

Adjunctive Therapy:
10-16 Years:
25-60kg:
Initial: 500mg/day (250mg bid)
Titrate: May increase weekly in 500mg/day increments to a total maint dose of 2000mg/day (1000mg bid)

<60kg: Dose according to adult recommendations

Use lowest dose and shortest exposure to treatment

Infantile Spasms

Monotherapy:
1 Month-2 Years:
Initial: 50mg/kg/day in 2 divided doses (25mg/kg bid)
Titrate: Subsequent dosing can be titrated by 25-50mg/kg/day increments every 3 days
Max: 150mg/kg/day in 2 divided doses (75mg/kg bid)

Use lowest dose and shortest exposure to treatment

DOSING CONSIDERATIONS

Renal Impairment

Infants:
Information about how to adjust the dose is unavailable

Adults and Pediatric Patients ≥10 Years:
Mild (CrCl >50-80mL/min): Decrease dose by 25%
Moderate (CrCl >30-50mL/min): Decrease dose by 50%
Severe (CrCl >10-30mL/min): Decrease dose by 75%

Discontinuation
Reduce dose gradually to d/c

ADMINISTRATION
Oral route

Take w/ or w/o food.
Either tab or powder for oral sol can be used for complex partial seizures.
Use powder for oral sol for infantile spasms; do not use tabs.

Preparation/Administration of Oral Sol
Mix powder for oral sol w/ water prior to administration.
Empty entire contents of each pkt into a clean cup, and dissolve in 10mL of cold or room temperature water per pkt.
Administer the resulting sol using the 10mL oral syringe supplied w/ medication.
The concentration of the final sol is 50mg/mL.
Each individual dose should be prepared and used immediately; discard any unused portion of sol.

STORAGE
20-25°C (68-77°F).

HOW SUPPLIED
Sol: 500mg/pkt [50⁵]; **Tab:** 500mg* *scored

WARNINGS/PRECAUTIONS
Not indicated as a 1st line agent for complex partial seizures. Abnormal MRI signal changes involving the thalamus, basal ganglia, brain stem, and cerebellum observed in some infants. May increase risk of suicidal thoughts/behavior. Withdraw therapy gradually; rapid discontinuation can be considered if withdrawal is needed because of a serious adverse event. May cause anemia, somnolence, fatigue, peripheral neuropathy, weight gain, and edema. May impair physical/mental abilities. May decrease ALT and AST plasma activity and may preclude the use of these markers, especially ALT, to detect early hepatic injury. May increase amount of amino acids in the urine, possibly leading to false (+) test for certain rare genetic metabolic diseases (eg, alpha aminoadipic aciduria). Caution in elderly.

ADVERSE REACTIONS
Refractory Complex Partial Seizures:
Adults: Fatigue, somnolence, nystagmus, tremor, blurred vision, memory impairment, weight gain, arthralgia, abnormal coordination, confusional state.
Pediatrics (10-16 Years): Weight gain, URTI, tremor, fatigue, aggression, diplopia.
Infantile Spasms:
Somnolence, bronchitis, ear infection, acute otitis media.

DRUG INTERACTIONS
See Boxed Warning. May decrease phenytoin plasma levels; consider dose adjustment of phenytoin if clinically indicated. May increase C_{max} of clonazepam resulting in an increase of clonazepam-associated adverse reactions.

PREGNANCY AND LACTATION
Pregnancy: Category C. Physicians are advised to recommend that pregnant patients taking Sabril enroll in the North American Antiepileptic Drug (NAAED) Pregnancy Registry.
Lactation: Not for use in nursing.

MECHANISM OF ACTION
GABA analogue; has not been established. Believed to be the result of its action as an irreversible inhibitor of GABA transaminase, which results in increased levels of GABA in the CNS.

PHARMACOKINETICS
Absorption: Complete. T_{max}=1 hr (adults/children), 2.5 hrs (infants). **Distribution:** V_d=1.1L/kg; found in breast milk. **Elimination:** Urine (95%, 80% parent drug); $T_{1/2}$=10.5 hrs (adults), 9.5 hrs (children), 5.7 hrs (infants).

PATIENT CONSIDERATIONS
Assessment: Assess for renal impairment, underlying suicidal behavior/ideation, pregnancy/nursing status, and possible drug interactions. Perform baseline vision assessment (no later than 4 weeks after starting therapy).

Monitoring: Monitor for abnormal MRI signal changes, suicidal thoughts/behavior, emergence/worsening of depression, unusual changes in thoughts or behavior, anemia, somnolence, fatigue, peripheral neuropathy, weight gain, edema, and other adverse reactions. Perform vision assessment at least every 3 months during therapy and about 3-6 months after discontinuation of therapy. Periodically reassess response to and continued need for treatment.

Counseling: Inform of the risk of permanent vision loss, particularly loss of peripheral vision, and the need for vision monitoring. Instruct to notify physician if changes in vision are suspected. Inform caregiver(s) of the possibility that infants may develop an abnormal MRI signal of unknown clinical significance. Counsel that therapy may increase risk of suicidal thoughts and behavior; advise of the need to be alert for the emergence or worsening of symptoms of depression, any unusual changes in mood or behavior, or the emergence of suicidal thoughts, behavior, or thoughts of self-harm. Instruct to report immediately to physician behaviors of concern. Instruct to notify physician if pregnant, intending to become pregnant during therapy, or if breastfeeding or intending to breastfeed during therapy; encourage to enroll in the NAAED Pregnancy Registry if pregnant. Advise not to drive a car or operate other complex machinery until familiar w/ the effects of therapy on ability to perform such activities. Instruct not to abruptly d/c therapy.

SAIZEN — somatropin (rDNA origin)　　Rx

Class: Recombinant human growth hormone (hGH)

ADULT DOSAGE

Growth Hormone Deficiency

Adult or Childhood Onset Etiology:
Weight-Based:
Initial: ≤0.005mg/kg qd SQ
Titrate: May increase to ≤0.01mg/kg/day after 4 weeks based on individual requirements

Non-Weight-Based:
Initial: 0.2mg/day SQ (range, 0.15-0.30mg/day)
Titrate: May increase gradually every 1-2 months by increments of 0.1-0.2mg/day based on clinical response and serum insulin-like growth factor-I (IGF-I) concentrations
Maint: Individualize dose

PEDIATRIC DOSAGE

Growth Hormone Deficiency

Due to Inadequate Secretion of Endogenous Growth Hormone:
Usual: 0.18mg/kg/week SQ divided into equal doses given either on 3 alternate days, 6X/week or daily

DOSING CONSIDERATIONS

Concomitant Medications
Oral Estrogen: Adult women may require a larger dose of somatropin

Elderly
Consider lower starting dose and smaller dose increments

ADMINISTRATION
SQ route

Reconstitution
1. Determine the appropriate patient dose 1st and then each vial should be reconstituted as follows: 5mg vial w/ 1-3mL of bacteriostatic water for inj (benzyl alcohol preserved); 8.8mg vial w/ 2-3mL of bacteriostatic water for inj (benzyl alcohol preserved)
2. If sensitivity to the diluent occurs, may reconstitute w/ sterile water for inj, the reconstituted sol should be used immediately and any unused sol should be discarded

3. Following reconstitution, swirl the vial w/ a gentle rotary motion until contents are completely dissolved; do not shake and use it only if it is clear and colorless

STORAGE
15-30°C (59-86°F). Reconstituted Sol: 2-8°C (36-46°F) for up to 14 days for vials and for up to 21 days for click.easy. Avoid freezing.

HOW SUPPLIED
Inj: 5mg [vial], 8.8mg [vial, click.easy]

CONTRAINDICATIONS
Acute critical illness due to complications following open heart surgery, abdominal surgery, multiple accidental trauma, or with acute respiratory failure. Pediatric patients with Prader-Willi syndrome (PWS) who are severely obese or have severe respiratory impairment. Long-term treatment of pediatric patients who have growth failure due to genetically confirmed PWS. Active malignancy, or evidence of progression or recurrence of an underlying intracranial tumor. Active proliferative or severe nonproliferative diabetic retinopathy. Growth promotion in pediatric patients with closed epiphysis. Known sensitivity to benzyl alcohol (bacteriostatic water for inj diluent), somatropin, or any components of the medication.

WARNINGS/PRECAUTIONS
Reevaluate adults who were treated with somatropin for GHD in childhood and whose epiphyses are closed. D/C when epiphyses are fused. Implement effective weight control in patients with PWS and treat respiratory infections aggressively. Increased risk of developing malignancies in children with certain rare genetic causes of short stature; monitor for development of neoplasms if treatment is initiated. Monitor for increased growth, or potential malignant changes of preexisting nevi. Undiagnosed impaired glucose tolerance and overt diabetes mellitus (DM) may be unmasked, and new-onset type 2 DM reported. Intracranial HTN with papilledema, visual changes, headache, N/V reported; d/c therapy if papilledema occurs. Fluid retention in adults may occur. Undiagnosed/untreated hypothyroidism may prevent optimal response. Hypothyroidism may become evident or worsen. Slipped capital femoral epiphysis (SCFE) and progression of scoliosis may occur in pediatric patients. Tissue atrophy may occur; rotate inj site. Allergic reactions may occur. Monitor other hormonal replacement treatments in patients with hypopituitarism. Serum levels of inorganic phosphorus, alkaline phosphatase, parathyroid hormone, and IGF-I may increase. Pancreatitis reported rarely. Bacteriostatic water for inj diluent contains benzyl alcohol, which has been associated with serious adverse events and death, particularly in pediatric patients. Caution in elderly.

ADVERSE REACTIONS
Arthralgia, headache, peripheral edema, myalgia, paresthesia, hypoaesthesia, skeletal pain, insomnia, carpal tunnel syndrome, generalized edema, depression, chest pain, hypothyroidism, dependent edema.

DRUG INTERACTIONS
May inhibit 11β-hydroxysteroid dehydrogenase type 1, resulting in reduced serum cortisol concentrations; may need glucocorticoid replacement or dose adjustments of glucocorticoid therapy. Glucocorticoid therapy may attenuate growth-promoting effects in children; carefully adjust glucocorticoid replacement dosing. May increase clearance of antipyrine. May alter clearance of compounds metabolized by CYP450 liver enzymes (eg, corticosteroids, sex steroids, anticonvulsants, cyclosporine); monitor carefully. Oral estrogen replacement may increase dose requirements. May need to adjust dose of insulin and/or oral/injectable hypoglycemic agents, and thyroid hormone replacement therapy.

PREGNANCY AND LACTATION
Category B, caution in nursing.

MECHANISM OF ACTION
Recombinant human GH; binds to dimeric GH receptors in cell membranes of target tissue cells resulting in intracellular signal transduction.

PHARMACOKINETICS
Absorption: Absolute bioavailability (70-90%). **Distribution:** V_d=12L (IV). **Metabolism:** Liver and kidneys. **Elimination:** $T_{1/2}$=2 hrs.

PATIENT CONSIDERATIONS
Assessment: Assess for PWS, preexisting DM or impaired glucose tolerance, hypothyroidism, hypopituitarism, history of scoliosis, hypersensitivity to drug or to benzyl alcohol, any other conditions where treatment is contraindicated or cautioned, pregnancy/nursing status, and possible drug interactions. Perform funduscopic exam.

Monitoring: Monitor growth, for clinical response, compliance, neoplasm, increased growth or malignant changes of preexisting nevi, intracranial HTN, fluid retention, allergic reactions, pancreatitis, and SCFE and progression of scoliosis in pediatric patients. Perform periodic thyroid function tests, funduscopic exam, and monitor glucose levels. In patients with PWS, monitor weight as well as for signs of respiratory infection, sleep apnea, and upper airway obstruction. Monitor patients with a history of GHD secondary to an intracranial neoplasm routinely for progression/recurrence of the tumor.

Counseling: Inform about potential benefits and risks of therapy, proper administration, usage and disposal, and caution against any reuse of needles and syringes.

SAMSCA — tolvaptan   Rx
Class: Arginine vasopressin antagonist

> Initiate and reinitiate therapy in patients only in a hospital where serum Na⁺ can be monitored closely. Osmotic demyelination resulting in dysarthria, mutism, dysphagia, lethargy, affective changes, spastic quadriparesis, seizures, coma, and death may occur due to rapid correction of hyponatremia (eg, >12mEq/L/24 hrs). Slower rates of correction may be advisable in susceptible patients (eg, with severe malnutrition, alcoholism, advanced liver disease).

ADULT DOSAGE
Hyponatremia
Hypervolemic and Euvolemic Hyponatremia:
Including Patients w/ HF and SIADH:
Initial: 15mg qd
Titrate: Increase to 30mg qd, after at least 24 hrs
Max Dose: 60mg qd
Max Duration: 30 days

Patients should be in a hospital for initiation and reinitiation of therapy

Avoid fluid restriction during the first 24 hrs of therapy; patients can continue ingestion of fluid in response to thirst. Following discontinuation, patients should be advised to resume fluid restriction

- -

DOSING CONSIDERATIONS
Concomitant Medications
Moderate CYP3A Inhibitors: Avoid coadministration
Potent CYP3A Inducers: Monitor response and adjust dose accordingly
P-gp Inhibitors: Coadministration may necessitate a decrease in tolvaptan dose

Renal Impairment
CrCl <10mL/min: Not recommended for use

Hepatic Impairment
Underlying Liver Disease: Avoid use

ADMINISTRATION
Oral route

Take w/o regard to meals

STORAGE
25°C (77°F); excursions permitted between 15-30°C (59-86°F).

HOW SUPPLIED
Tab: 15mg, 30mg

CONTRAINDICATIONS
Urgent need to raise serum Na⁺ acutely, inability to autoregulate fluid balance, hypovolemic hyponatremia, anuria, and concomitant use of strong CYP3A inhibitors (eg, clarithromycin, ketoconazole, itraconazole, ritonavir, indinavir, nelfinavir, saquinavir, nefazodone, telithromycin). Hypersensitivity (eg, anaphylactic shock, rash generalized) to tolvaptan or any component of the product.

WARNINGS/PRECAUTIONS
Frequently monitor for changes in serum electrolytes and volume during initiation and titration. Allow to continue fluid ingestion in response to thirst. Resume fluid restriction and monitor for serum Na⁺ and volume status changes following discontinuation of therapy. D/C or interrupt therapy if patient develops elevation in serum Na⁺ too rapidly; consider hypotonic fluid administration. Serious and potentially fatal liver injury may occur; avoid use in patients with underlying liver disease, including cirrhosis, and d/c therapy in patients with symptoms that may indicate liver injury. May induce copious aquaresis. Dehydration and hypovolemia may occur, especially in potentially volume-depleted patients receiving diuretics or those who are fluid restricted; interrupt or d/c therapy and provide supportive care with careful management of vital signs, fluid balance, and electrolytes if signs/symptoms of hypovolemia develop. Concomitant use with hypertonic saline is not recommended. Increased serum K⁺ levels may occur; monitor serum K⁺ levels after initiation of therapy in patients with serum K⁺ >5mEq/L and those receiving drugs known to increase serum K⁺ levels. Not recommended for patients with CrCl <10mL/min.

ADVERSE REACTIONS
Osmotic demyelination, thirst, dry mouth, pollakiuria/polyuria, nausea, asthenia, constipation, hyperglycemia, pyrexia, anorexia.

DRUG INTERACTIONS
See Contraindications. Avoid with moderate CYP3A inhibitors (eg, erythromycin, fluconazole, aprepitant, diltiazem, verapamil). Avoid with CYP3A inducers (eg, rifampin, rifabutin, rifapentin, barbiturates, phenytoin, carbamazepine, St. John's wort); if coadministered, the dose of tolvaptan may need to be increased. Dose reduction of tolvaptan may be required when coadministered with P-gp inhibitors (eg, cyclosporine). Grapefruit juice may increase exposure. Increases exposure of digoxin. Higher incidence of hyperkalemia with ARBs, ACE inhibitors, and K⁺-sparing diuretics; monitor serum K⁺ levels. Not recommended with vasopressin V_2 agonist (eg, desmopressin).

PREGNANCY AND LACTATION
Category C, not for use in nursing.

MECHANISM OF ACTION
Arginine vasopressin antagonist; antagonizes the effect of vasopressin and causes an increase in urine water excretion, resulting in an increase in free water clearance (aquaresis), a decrease in urine osmolality, and an increase in serum Na⁺ concentrations.

PHARMACOKINETICS
Absorption: T_{max}=2-4 hrs. **Distribution:** V_d=3L/kg; plasma protein binding (99%). **Metabolism:** Via CYP3A. **Elimination:** $T_{1/2}$=12 hrs.

PATIENT CONSIDERATIONS
Assessment: Assess serum Na⁺ levels, neurologic status, ability to respond to thirst, renal/hepatic function, for hypersensitivity to drug, any other conditions

PEDIATRIC DOSAGE
Pediatric use may not have been established

where treatment is cautioned or contraindicated, pregnancy/nursing status, and possible drug interactions.

Monitoring: Monitor for osmotic demyelination, changes in serum Na$^+$/electrolytes/volume, neurologic status, signs/symptoms of hypovolemia, liver injury, hypersensitivity reactions, and other adverse reactions. Monitor serum K$^+$ levels in patients with serum K$^+$ >5mEq/L and those receiving drugs known to increase serum K$^+$ levels.

Counseling: Advise to continue ingestion of fluid in response to thirst. Advise to resume fluid restriction following discontinuation of therapy. Instruct to inform physician if taking or planning to take any prescription or OTC drugs. Advise not to breastfeed during therapy.

SANDIMMUNE — cyclosporine   Rx

Class: Calcineurin-inhibitor immunosuppressant

> Should only be prescribed by physicians experienced in immunosuppressive therapy and management of organ transplant patients. Manage patients in facilities equipped and staffed w/ adequate laboratory and supportive medical resources. Give w/ adrenal corticosteroids but not w/ other immunosuppressive agents. Increased susceptibility to infection and development of lymphoma may result from immunosuppression. Not bioequivalent to Neoral; not interchangeable w/o physician supervision. Monitor cyclosporine blood concentrations at repeated intervals during chronic administration of sol/cap; adjust subsequent dose to avoid toxicity due to high levels and possible organ rejection due to low absorption.

ADULT DOSAGE

Organ Rejection Prophylaxis

Kidney, Liver, and Heart Allogeneic Transplants:

Oral:

Initial: 15mg/kg single dose given 4-12 hrs prior to transplant

Continue postoperatively for 1-2 weeks, then taper by 5%/week to a maintenance dose of 5-10mg/kg/day

IV:

For patients unable to take caps or oral sol pre- or postoperatively

Administer at 1/3 the oral dose

Initial: 5-6mg/kg/day single dose given 4-12 hrs prior to transplant

Continue postoperatively until the patient can tolerate caps or oral sol; patients should be switched to caps or oral sol as soon as possible after surgery

Adjunct therapy w/ adrenal corticosteroids is recommended

Other Indications

Treatment of chronic rejection in patients previously treated w/ other immunosuppressive agents

PEDIATRIC DOSAGE

Organ Rejection Prophylaxis

Kidney, Liver, and Heart Allogeneic Transplants:

≥6 Months of Age:

Oral:

Initial: 15mg/kg single dose given 4-12 hrs prior to transplant

Continue postoperatively for 1-2 weeks, then taper by 5%/week to a maintenance dose of 5-10mg/kg/day

Higher doses may be required in pediatric patients

IV:

For patients unable to take caps or oral sol pre- or postoperatively

Administer at 1/3 the oral dose

Initial: 5-6mg/kg/day single dose given 4-12 hrs prior to transplant

Continue postoperatively until the patient can tolerate caps or oral sol; patients should be switched to caps or oral sol as soon as possible after surgery

Higher doses may be required in pediatric patients

Adjunct therapy w/ adrenal corticosteroids is recommended

Other Indications

Treatment of chronic rejection in patients previously treated w/ other immunosuppressive agents

DOSING CONSIDERATIONS

Renal Impairment
Reduce dose if indicated

Hepatic Impairment
Severe: Dose reduction may be necessary

Elderly
Start at lower end of dosing range

ADMINISTRATION
Oral/IV route

Cap/Sol
Administer on a consistent schedule w/ regard to time of day and relation to meals

Sol
May dilute w/ milk, chocolate milk, or orange juice preferably at room temperature; avoid switching diluents frequently
Once opened, use contents w/in 2 months

Instructions:
1. Take the prescribed amount of cyclosporine from the container using the dosage syringe supplied, and transfer the sol to a glass of milk, chocolate milk, or orange juice
2. Stir well and drink at once; do not allow to stand before drinking
3. It is best to use a glass container and rinse it w/ more diluent to ensure that the total dose is taken
4. After use, replace dosage syringe in the protective cover
5. Do not rinse the dosage syringe w/ water or other cleaning agents either before or after use; if the dosage syringe requires cleaning, it must be completely dry before resuming use
6. Introduction of water into the product by any means will cause variation in dose

Inj
Immediately before use, dilute 1mL cyclosporine inj in 20-100mL 0.9% NaCl inj or D5 inj
Administer in a slow IV infusion over approx 2-6 hrs
Discard diluted infusion sol after 24 hrs
The polyoxyethylated castor oil contained in the concentrate for IV infusion can cause phthalate stripping from PVC

STORAGE
Cap: 25°C (77°F); excursions permitted to 15-30°C (59-86°F). Sol: <30°C (86°F). Do not refrigerate. Protect from freezing. Inj: <30°C (86°F). Protect from light.

HOW SUPPLIED
Cap: 25mg, 100mg; **Inj:** 50mg/mL [5mL]; **Sol:** 100mg/mL [50mL]

CONTRAINDICATIONS
(Inj) Hypersensitivity to cyclosporine and/or polyoxyethylated castor oil.

WARNINGS/PRECAUTIONS
Due to risk of anaphylaxis, only use inj if unable to take cap/sol. May cause nephrotoxicity, hepatotoxicity, and liver injury (eg, cholestasis, jaundice, hepatitis, liver failure). Elevations in SrCr and BUN levels do not necessarily indicate rejection in renal transplant patients; evaluate patient before initiating dose adjustment. Impaired renal function at any time requires close monitoring, and frequent dose adjustment may be indicated. Consider switching to other immunosuppressive therapy w/ persistent high elevations of BUN/SrCr unresponsive to dosage adjustments. Convulsions, encephalopathy (including posterior reversible encephalopathy syndrome), and rarely, optic disc edema reported. Thrombocytopenia and microangiopathic hemolytic anemia, resulting in graft failure, hyperuricemia, and hyperkalemia (sometimes associated w/ hyperchloremic metabolic acidosis) may develop. Increased risk for development of lymphomas and other malignancies. Consider the alcohol content of the drug when given to patients in whom alcohol intake should be avoided or minimized (eg, pregnant or breastfeeding women, patients presenting w/ liver disease or epilepsy, alcoholic patients, or pediatric patients). Caution w/ malabsorption. HTN may occur requiring antihypertensive therapy. Increased risk of developing bacterial, viral, fungal, protozoal, and opportunistic infections (eg, polyoma virus infections). JC virus-associated progressive multifocal leukoencephalopathy (PML) and polyoma virus-associated nephropathy (PVAN) reported; consider reduction in immunosuppression if evidence of PML or PVAN develops. (Inj) Contains polyoxyethylated castor oil. Anaphylactic reactions reported rarely w/ IV administration; observe for 30 min after start of infusion and frequently thereafter. D/C infusion if anaphylaxis occurs.

ADVERSE REACTIONS
Increased susceptibility to infection, lymphoma, renal dysfunction, tremor, hirsutism, HTN, gum hyperplasia, headache, diarrhea, hepatotoxicity, convulsions, abdominal discomfort, flushing, N/V, sinusitis.

DRUG INTERACTIONS
See Boxed Warning. Avoid w/ K$^+$-sparing diuretics, compounds that decrease drug absorption (eg, orlistat), aliskiren, grapefruit, grapefruit juice, bosentan, or dabigatran. Avoid in psoriasis patients receiving other immunosuppressive agents or radiation therapy (including PUVA and UVB). Vaccination may be less effective; avoid live vaccines during therapy. Caution w/ rifabutin, nephrotoxic drugs, HIV protease inhibitors (eg, indinavir, nelfinavir, ritonavir, saquinavir), K$^+$-sparing drugs (eg, ACE inhibitors, ARBs), K$^+$-containing drugs, and K$^+$-rich diet. Ciprofloxacin, gentamicin, tobramycin, vancomycin, trimethoprim w/ sulfamethoxazole, amphotericin B, ketoconazole, melphalan, diclofenac, azapropazon, sulindac, naproxen, colchicine, cimetidine, ranitidine, tacrolimus, fibric acid derivatives (eg, bezafibrate, fenofibrate), methotrexate (MTX), and NSAIDs may potentiate renal dysfunction; closely monitor renal function and reduce dose of cyclosporine and/or coadministered drug or consider alternative treatment. CYP3A4 or P-gp inhibitors/inducers may alter levels; adjust cyclosporine dose appropriately. Diltiazem, nicardipine, verapamil, fluconazole, itraconazole, ketoconazole, voriconazole, azithromycin, clarithromycin, erythromycin, quinupristin/dalfopristin, allopurinol, amiodarone, bromocriptine, colchicine, danazol, imatinib, nefazodone, metoclopramide, oral contraceptives, methylprednisolone, grapefruit, grapefruit juice, HIV protease inhibitors, boceprevir, and telaprevir may increase levels. St. John's wort, carbamazepine, oxcarbazepine, phenobarbital, phenytoin, bosentan, sulfinpyrazone, octreotide, orlistat, terbinafine, ticlopidine, rifampin, and nafcillin may decrease levels. May increase plasma concentration of CYP3A4, P-gp, or organic anion transporter protein substrates. May reduce clearance of digoxin, colchicine, prednisolone, HMG-CoA reductase inhibitors (statins), aliskiren, bosentan, dabigatran, repaglinide, NSAIDs, sirolimus, and etoposide. Digitalis toxicity reported when used w/ digoxin; monitor digoxin levels. May increase levels and enhance toxic effects (eg, myopathy, neuropathy) of colchicine; reduce colchicine dose. Myotoxicity cases seen lovastatin, simvastatin, atorvastatin, pravastatin, and rarely fluvastatin; temporarily withhold or d/c statin if signs of myopathy develop or w/ risk factors predisposing to severe renal injury. May increase levels of repaglinide and thereby, increasing the risk of hypoglycemia; closely monitor blood glucose levels. May increase levels of ambrisentan; do not titrate ambrisentan dose to the recommended max daily dose. May increase levels of bosentan or dabigatran. High doses of cyclosporine may increase the exposure to anthracycline antibiotics (eg, doxorubicin, mitoxantrone, daunorubicin) in cancer patients. Frequent gingival hyperplasia w/ nifedipine; avoid concomitant use w/ nifedipine in patients in whom gingival hyperplasia develops as a side effect of cyclosporine. Convulsions reported w/ high-dose methylprednisolone. Concomitant use of high-dose corticosteroids may predispose to developing encephalopathy. Increases levels of sirolimus w/ elevations of SrCr; give 4 hrs after cyclosporine. May double diclofenac blood levels. May increase levels of MTX and decrease levels of MTX metabolite. Dose adjustment may be required w/ calcium antagonists; use w/ caution.

PREGNANCY AND LACTATION
Category C, not for use in nursing.

MECHANISM OF ACTION
Cyclic polypeptide immunosuppressant; has not been established. Effectiveness due to specific and reversible inhibition of immunocompetent lymphocytes in the G_0- or G_1-phase of the cell cycle. T lymphocytes are preferentially inhibited w/ T-helper cell as main target while also possibly suppressing T-suppressor cells. Also inhibits lymphokine production and release (eg, interleukin-2, T-cell growth factor).

PHARMACOKINETICS
Absorption: Incomplete and variable. (Sol) Absolute bioavailability (approx 30%); C_{max}=approx 1ng/mL/mg; T_{max}=3.5 hrs. **Distribution:** Plasma protein binding (approx 90%); found in breast milk. **Metabolism:** Liver (Extensive). CYP3A4, hydroxylation, cyclic ether formation, and N-demethylation pathways. **Elimination:** Bile (primary), urine (6%, 0.1% unchanged); $T_{1/2}$=approx 19 hrs.

PATIENT CONSIDERATIONS
Assessment: Prior to IV administration, assess ability to take oral formulations. Assess for hypersensitivity to the drug or to polyoxyethylated castor oil, malabsorption, pregnancy/nursing status, and possible drug interactions. Obtain baseline SrCr, BUN, LFTs, and serum bilirubin.

Monitoring: Continuously monitor patients receiving IV formulation for anaphylactic reactions for at least the first 30 min following start of infusion and at frequent intervals thereafter. Monitor for signs/symptoms of hepatotoxicity, nephrotoxicity, thrombocytopenia, microangiopathic hemolytic anemia, HTN, hyperkalemia, hyperuricemia, lymphomas and other malignancies, serious/opportunistic/polyoma virus infections, convulsions and other neurotoxicities, and other adverse reactions. Frequently monitor cyclosporine blood levels, especially when converting from Neoral to Sandimmune. Monitor renal/hepatic function (eg, BUN, SrCr, serum bilirubin, LFTs).

Counseling: Instruct to contact physician before changing formulations of cyclosporine. Inform that repeated laboratory tests are required while on therapy. Advise of the potential risks if used during pregnancy and inform of the increased risk of neoplasia. Instruct patients using the oral syringe not to rinse before or after use as the introduction of water will cause variation in dosage.

SANDOSTATIN — octreotide acetate Rx

Class: Somatostatin analogue

ADULT DOSAGE

Acromegaly

To reduce blood levels of growth hormone and insulin-like growth factor-1 (IGF-I) (somatomedin C) in acromegaly patients who have had inadequate response to or cannot be treated w/ surgical resection, pituitary irradiation, and bromocriptine mesylate at maximally tolerated doses

Initial: 50mcg tid

Usual: 100mcg tid; some patients require up to 500mcg tid

If an increase in dose fails to provide additional benefit, the dose should be reduced

Withdraw yearly for approx 4 weeks from patients who have received irradiation to assess disease activity; if growth hormone or IGF-I (somatomedin C) levels increase and signs and symptoms recur, therapy may be resumed

Carcinoid Tumors

Symptomatic treatment of patients w/ metastatic carcinoid tumors where it suppresses or inhibits the severe diarrhea and flushing episodes associated w/ the disease

Usual: 100-600mcg/day in 2-4 divided doses (mean dose is 300mcg/day) for the first 2 weeks of therapy

In clinical studies, the median maint dose was approx 450mcg/day, but benefits were obtained in some patients w/ as little as 50mcg, while others required up to 1500mcg/day; experience w/ doses >750mcg/day is limited

Vasoactive Intestinal Peptide-Secreting Tumors

Treatment of the profuse watery diarrhea associated w/ vasoactive intestinal peptide-secreting tumors

PEDIATRIC DOSAGE

Pediatric use may not have been established

Usual: 200-300mcg/day in 2-4 divided doses during the initial 2 weeks of therapy (range 150-750mcg)

Titrate: Adjust dose to achieve a therapeutic response; usually doses >450mcg/day are not required

---

DOSING CONSIDERATIONS
Elderly
Start at lower end of dosing range

ADMINISTRATION
IV/SQ routes
Avoid multiple SQ inj at the same site w/in short periods of time; rotate sites in a systematic manner.
Not compatible in TPN sol.
Stable in sterile isotonic saline sol or sterile sol of D5W for 24 hrs.

Preparation and Administration
Octreotide may be diluted in volumes of 50-200mL and infused IV over 15-30 min or administered by IV push over 3 min; in emergency situations (eg, carcinoid crisis) it may be given by rapid bolus.

STORAGE
2-8°C (36-46°F) for prolonged storage. Protect from light. Stable for 14 days at 20-30°C (70-86°F) if protected from light. Do not warm artificially; sol can be allowed to come to room temperature prior administration. After initial use, multidose vials should be discarded within 14 days. Open ampuls prior to administration and discard unused portion.

HOW SUPPLIED
Inj: 50mcg/mL, 100mcg/mL, 200mcg/mL, 500mcg/mL, 1000mcg/mL

CONTRAINDICATIONS
Sensitivity to this drug or any of its components.

WARNINGS/PRECAUTIONS
May inhibit gallbladder contractility and decrease bile secretion; increased risk of gallbladder abnormalities. May alter balance between the counter-regulatory hormones, insulin, glucagon, and GH and lead to hypo- or hyperglycemia; monitor glucose tolerance periodically. May cause hypothyroidism; monitor thyroid levels periodically. Cardiac conduction and other cardiovascular abnormalities (eg, bradycardia, arrhythmias) may occur; caution in patients at risk. Risk of pregnancy with normalization of IGF-1 and GH in acromegalic women. Pancreatitis, depressed vitamin B12 levels, alteration in fat absorption, and abnormal Schilling's test reported. Caution in elderly.

ADVERSE REACTIONS
Gallbladder abnormalities, cardiac abnormalities, abdominal discomfort, diarrhea, loose stool, N/V, abdominal distention, flatulence, constipation, headache, dizziness, hypoglycemia, hyperglycemia, hypothyroidism.

DRUG INTERACTIONS
May alter absorption of orally administered drugs. May decrease blood levels of cyclosporine and may result in transplant rejection. May require dose adjustments of insulin, oral hypoglycemics, β-blockers, calcium channel blockers, or agents that control fluid and electrolyte balance. Increased availability of bromocriptine. May decrease the metabolic clearance of compounds known to be metabolized by CYP450; caution with other drugs mainly metabolized by CYP3A4 and which have a low therapeutic index (eg, quinidine, terfenadine).

PREGNANCY AND LACTATION
Pregnancy: Category B.
Lactation: Caution in nursing.

MECHANISM OF ACTION
Somatostatin analog; exerts similar pharmacologic actions to natural hormone somatostatin, but is more potent in inhibiting GH, glucagon, and insulin. Like somatostatin, it also suppresses luteinizing hormone response to gonadotropin-releasing hormone, decreases splanchnic blood flow, and inhibits release of serotonin, gastrin, vasoactive intestinal peptide (VIP), secretin, motilin, and pancreatic polypeptide.

PHARMACOKINETICS
Absorption: (SQ) Rapid and complete; (100mcg) C_{max}=5.2ng/mL, T_{max}=0.4 hrs; (Acromegaly, 100mcg SQ) C_{max}=2.8ng/mL, T_{max}=0.7 hr. **Distribution:** V_d=13.6L, plasma protein binding (65%); (Acromegaly) V_d=21.6L, plasma protein binding (41.2%). **Elimination:** Urine (32% unchanged); $T_{1/2}$=1.7-1.9 hrs. $T_{1/2}$ varies based on the severity of renal and liver disease; refer to PI for further details.

PATIENT CONSIDERATIONS
Assessment: Assess for drug hypersensitivity, renal impairment, diabetes mellitus, cardiac dysfunction, pregnancy/nursing status, and possible drug interactions. Obtain baseline thyroid function tests (TSH, total and/or free T4).

Monitoring: Monitor for biliary tract abnormalities, hypo- and hyperglycemia, hypothyroidism, cardiac conduction abnormalities, and pancreatitis. Monitor GH levels at 1-4 hr intervals for 8-12 hrs post-dose or IGF-1 levels at 2 weeks after drug initiation or dose change with acromegaly. Monitor urinary 5-hydroxyindole acetic acid, plasma serotonin, and plasma Substance P levels with carcinoid tumors. Monitor VIP levels in patients with VIPomas. Monitor thyroid function (periodically) and vitamin B12 levels with chronic therapy.

Counseling: Advise of risks and benefits of treatment. Instruct patients and other persons who may administer the medication about sterile SQ inj technique. Advise female patients of childbearing potential to use contraception during therapy.

SANDOSTATIN LAR — octreotide acetate

Rx

Class: Somatostatin analogue

ADULT DOSAGE

Acromegaly

Long-Term Maint Therapy in Patients Who Have Had an Inadequate Response to Surgery and/or Radiotherapy, or if Surgery and/or Radiotherapy is Not an Option:

Not Currently Receiving Octreotide:
Begin therapy w/ Sandostatin SQ (initial dose of 50mcg tid; most patients require doses of 100-200mcg tid but some patients require up to 500mcg tid) and maintain for at least 2 weeks to determine tolerance

Patients considered to be responders to the drug and who tolerate it may be switched to Sandostatin LAR

Currently Receiving Sandostatin Inj:
Initial: 20mg at 4-week intervals for 3 months

Titrate:
After 3 Months:
Growth Hormone (GH) ≤2.5ng/mL, Normal Insulin-Like Growth Factor-1 (IGF-1), and Controlled Clinical Symptoms: Maintain at 20mg every 4 weeks
GH >2.5ng/mL, Elevated IGF-1, and/or Uncontrolled Clinical Symptoms: Increase to 30mg every 4 weeks
GH ≤1ng/mL, Normal IGF-1, and Controlled Clinical Symptoms: Reduce to 10mg every 4 weeks
GH, IGF-1, or Symptoms Are Not Adequately Controlled at 30mg: May increase to 40mg every 4 weeks

Max: 40mg every 4 weeks

In patients who have received pituitary irradiation, withdraw therapy yearly for 8 weeks to assess disease activity; may resume therapy if GH or IGF-1 levels increase and signs/symptoms recur

Carcinoid Tumors

Long-Term Treatment of Severe Diarrhea and Flushing Episodes Associated w/ Metastatic Carcinoid Tumors:

Not Currently Receiving Octreotide:
Begin therapy w/ Sandostatin SQ (100-600mcg/day in 2-4 divided doses; some patients may require doses up to 1500mcg/day) and maintain for at least 2 weeks to determine tolerance

Patients considered to be responders to the drug and who tolerate it may be switched to Sandostatin LAR

Currently Receiving Sandostatin Inj:
Initial: 20mg at 4-week intervals for 2 months; patients should continue to receive Sandostatin SQ for at least 2 weeks in the same dosage taken before the switch

Titrate:
If Symptoms Are Adequately Controlled After 2 Months:
Consider reducing to 10mg for a trial period; if symptoms recur, then increase to 20mg every 4 weeks
If Symptoms Are Not Adequately Controlled After 2 Months:
Increase to 30mg every 4 weeks; lower to 10mg for a trial period if good control is achieved on 20mg dose and if symptoms recur, increase to 20mg every 4 weeks

Max: 30mg every 4 weeks

For exacerbation of symptoms, may give Sandostatin SQ for a few days at the dosage received prior to switching to Sandostatin LAR; d/c when symptoms are again controlled

PEDIATRIC DOSAGE

Pediatric use may not have been established

Vasoactive Intestinal Peptide-Secreting Tumors

Long-Term Treatment of Profuse Watery Diarrhea Associated w/ Vasoactive Intestinal Peptide-Secreting Tumors (VIPomas):

Not Currently Receiving Octreotide:
Begin therapy w/ Sandostatin SQ (200-300mcg in 2-4 divided doses [range 150-750mcg]; doses >450mcg/day are usually not required) and maintain for at least 2 weeks to determine tolerance

Patients considered to be responders to the drug and who tolerate it may be switched to Sandostatin LAR

Currently Receiving Sandostatin Inj:
Initial: 20mg at 4-week intervals for 2 months; patients should continue to receive Sandostatin SQ for at least 2 weeks in the same dosage taken before the switch

Titrate:
If Symptoms Are Adequately Controlled After 2 Months:
Consider reducing to 10mg for a trial period; if symptoms recur, then increase to 20mg every 4 weeks
If Symptoms Are Not Adequately Controlled After 2 Months:
Increase to 30mg every 4 weeks; lower to 10mg for a trial period if good control is achieved on 20mg dose and if symptoms recur, increase to 20mg every 4 weeks

Max: 30mg every 4 weeks

For exacerbation of symptoms, may give Sandostatin SQ for a few days at the dosage received prior to switching to Sandostatin LAR; d/c when symptoms are again controlled

---

DOSING CONSIDERATIONS

Renal Impairment
Renal Failure Requiring Dialysis:
Initial: 10mg every 4 weeks

Hepatic Impairment
Cirrhotic Patients:
Initial: 10mg every 4 weeks

Elderly
Start at lower end of dosing range

ADMINISTRATION
IM route

Administer in the gluteal region; avoid deltoid inj.
Rotate inj sites to avoid irritation.
Administer immediately after reconstitution; do not directly inject diluent w/o preparing sus.
Refer to PI for further administration instructions.

STORAGE
2-8°C (36-46°F). Protect from light until time of use. Drug product kit should remain at room temperature for 30-60 min prior to preparation of drug sus.

HOW SUPPLIED
Inj, Depot: 10mg, 20mg, 30mg

WARNINGS/PRECAUTIONS
Should be administered by a trained healthcare provider. Rotate inj sites in a systematic manner to avoid irritation. May inhibit gallbladder contractility and decrease bile secretion, which may lead to gallbladder abnormalities or sludge. Alters balance between the counter-regulatory hormones, insulin, glucagon, and GH, which may result in hypo/hyperglycemia. Hypothyroidism may occur. Bradycardia, arrhythmias, and cardiac conduction abnormalities reported. May alter dietary fat absorption. Depressed vitamin B12 levels and abnormal Schilling test reported. Serum zinc may rise excessively when fluid loss is reversed in patients on TPN. Caution in elderly.

ADVERSE REACTIONS
Acromegaly: Diarrhea, cholelithiasis, abdominal pain, flatulence.
Carcinoid Tumors and VIPomas: Back pain, fatigue, headache, abdominal pain, nausea, dizziness.

DRUG INTERACTIONS
Associated w/ nutrient absorption alterations; may alter absorption of orally administered drugs. May decrease cyclosporine levels and result in transplant rejection. May need dose adjustments of insulin, oral hypoglycemics, and drugs w/ bradycardic effects (eg, β-blockers). Increases availability of bromocriptine. May decrease metabolic clearance of drugs metabolized by CYP450; caution w/ other drugs mainly metabolized by CYP3A4 and which have a low therapeutic index (eg, quinidine, terfenadine).

PREGNANCY AND LACTATION
Pregnancy: Category B.
Lactation: Caution in nursing.

MECHANISM OF ACTION
Somatostatin analogue; long acting. Exerts similar actions to natural hormone somatostatin, but is more potent in inhibiting GH, glucagon, and insulin. Like somatostatin, it also suppresses luteinizing hormone response to gonadotropin-releasing hormone, decreases splanchnic blood flow, and inhibits release of serotonin, gastrin, vasoactive intestinal peptide, secretin, motilin, and pancreatic polypeptide.

PHARMACOKINETICS
Absorption: (Acromegaly; Day 1) C_{max}=0.3ng/mL (10mg), 0.8ng/mL (20mg), 1.3ng/mL (30mg).

PATIENT CONSIDERATIONS
Assessment: Assess for renal/hepatic impairment, cardiac dysfunction, pregnancy/nursing status, and possible drug interactions. Obtain baseline thyroid function tests (TSH, total and/or free T4) and glucose levels. Obtain baseline plasma vasoactive intestinal peptide levels in patients w/ VIPoma.

Monitoring: Monitor for signs/symptoms of gallbladder abnormalities or sludge, hypo/hyperglycemia, hypothyroidism, bradycardia, arrhythmia, cardiac conduction abnormalities, and other adverse reactions. Monitor zinc levels if receiving TPN. Monitor vitamin B12 levels. Monitor thyroid function periodically during chronic therapy. Monitor GH and IGF-1 levels in patients w/ acromegaly. Monitor urinary 5-hydroxyindole acetic acid, plasma serotonin, and plasma substance P levels in patients w/ carcinoids. Monitor glucose levels when the dose is altered.

Counseling: Inform of the risks and benefits of treatment. Advise patients w/ carcinoid tumors and VIPomas to adhere closely to scheduled return visits for reinjection to minimize exacerbation of symptoms. Instruct patients w/ acromegaly to adhere to return visit schedule to help assure steady control of GH and IGF-1 levels.

SENSIPAR — cinacalcet   Rx

Class: Calcimimetic agent

ADULT DOSAGE	**PEDIATRIC DOSAGE**
Secondary Hyperparathyroidism	Pediatric use may not have been established
In Patients w/ Chronic Kidney Disease on Dialysis:	

Initial: 30mg qd
Titrate: Increase no more frequently than every 2-4 weeks through sequential doses of 30mg, 60mg, 90mg, 120mg, and 180mg qd to target intact parathyroid (iPTH) hormone of 150-300pg/mL

Measure serum Ca^{2+} and phosphorus w/in 1 week and measure iPTH hormone 1-4 weeks after initiation/dose adjustment; serum iPTH levels should be assessed no earlier than 12 hrs after dosing

Once maint dose is established, measure serum Ca^{2+} monthly

May be used alone or in combination w/ vitamin D sterols and/or phosphate binders

Hypercalcemia

In Patients w/ Primary Hyperparathyroidism who are Unable to Undergo Parathyroidectomy and Patients w/ Parathyroid Carcinoma:
Initial: 30mg bid
Titrate: Increase every 2-4 weeks through sequential doses of 30mg bid, 60mg bid, 90mg bid, and 90mg tid-qid as necessary to normalize serum Ca^{2+} levels

Measure serum Ca^{2+} w/in 1 week after initiation/dose adjustment; once maint dose is established, measure serum Ca^{2+} every 2 months

- -

DOSING CONSIDERATIONS
Adverse Reactions
Secondary Hyperparathyroidism in Patients w/ Chronic Kidney Disease on Dialysis:
If serum Ca^{2+} falls <7.5mg/dL, or if hypocalcemia symptoms persist and vitamin D dose cannot be increased, withhold administration until Ca^{2+} levels reach 8.0mg/dL and/or symptoms of hypocalcemia resolve. Treatment should be reinitiated using next lowest dose of cinacalcet

ADMINISTRATION
Oral route

Take whole; do not divide.
Take w/ food or shortly after a meal.

STORAGE
25°C (77°F); excursions permitted to 15-30°C (59-86°F).

HOW SUPPLIED
Tab: 30mg, 60mg, 90mg

CONTRAINDICATIONS
Hypocalcemia.

WARNINGS/PRECAUTIONS
Avoid use in patients with CKD not on dialysis. Lowers serum Ca^{2+}; monitor for occurrence of hypocalcemia during treatment. Life-threatening events and fatal outcomes associated with hypocalcemia reported in patients treated with the drug, including pediatric patients. QT prolongation and ventricular arrhythmia secondary to hypocalcemia reported. Seizures reported; monitor serum Ca^{2+}, particularly in patients with history of seizure disorder. Hypotension, worsening HF, and/or arrhythmia reported in patients with impaired cardiac function. Adynamic bone disease may develop with iPTH levels <100pg/mL; reduce dose or d/c therapy if iPTH levels <150pg/mL. Monitor patients with moderate and severe hepatic impairment throughout treatment.

ADVERSE REACTIONS
N/V, diarrhea, myalgia, dizziness, HTN, asthenia, anorexia, paresthesia, fatigue, fracture, hypercalcemia, dehydration, anemia, arthralgia, depression.

DRUG INTERACTIONS
May require dose adjustment with CYP2D6 substrates (eg, desipramine, metoprolol, carvedilol) and particularly those with narrow therapeutic index (eg, flecainide, most TCAs). May require dose adjustment if a patient initiates or discontinues therapy with strong CYP3A4 inhibitors (eg, ketoconazole, itraconazole); closely monitor iPTH and serum Ca^{2+} levels.

PREGNANCY AND LACTATION
Pregnancy: Category C.
Lactation: Not for use in nursing.

MECHANISM OF ACTION
Calcimimetic agent; lowers PTH levels by increasing the sensitivity of the Ca^{2+}-sensing receptor to extracellular Ca^{2+}.

PHARMACOKINETICS
Absorption: T_{max}=2-6 hrs. **Distribution:** V_d=1000L; plasma protein binding (93-97%). **Metabolism:** Via CYP3A4, 2D6, and 1A2; hydrocinnamic acid and glucuronidated dihydrodiols (major metabolites). **Elimination:** Urine (80%), feces (15%); $T_{1/2}$=30-40 hrs.

PATIENT CONSIDERATIONS
Assessment: Assess for hypocalcemia, history of seizure disorder, hepatic impairment, cardiac function, pregnancy/nursing status, and possible drug interactions. Assess serum Ca^{2+} levels prior to administration.

Monitoring: Monitor for signs/symptoms of hypocalcemia, adynamic bone disease, and other adverse reactions. In patients with impaired cardiac function, monitor for hypotension, worsening HF, and/or arrhythmias. Monitor iPTH/Ca^{2+}/phosphorus levels with moderate and severe hepatic impairment. Monitor serum Ca^{2+} carefully for the occurrence of hypocalcemia during treatment.

Counseling: Inform of the importance of regular blood tests. Advise to report to physician if N/V and potential symptoms of hypocalcemia occur. Advise to report to their physician if taking medication to prevent seizures, have had seizures in the past, and experience any seizure episodes while on therapy. Encourage patients who are nursing during treatment to enroll in Amgen's Lactation Surveillance Program.

SEROSTIM — somatropin (rDNA origin)   Rx

Class: Recombinant human growth hormone (hGH)

ADULT DOSAGE	**PEDIATRIC DOSAGE**
HIV-associated Wasting or Cachexia	Pediatric use may not have been established

To increase lean body mass and weight, and improve physical endurance. Concomitant antiretroviral therapy is necessary

Initial: 0.1mg/kg (up to a total dose of 6mg) SQ qhs; consider 0.1mg/kg qod in patients at increased risk for adverse effects related to therapy (eg, glucose intolerance)

Weight-Based Recommendations (SQ QD):
<35kg: 0.1mg/kg
35-45kg: 4mg
45-55kg: 5mg
<55kg: 6mg

Most of the effect was apparent after 12 weeks of treatment and maintained during an additional 12 weeks of therapy; no safety or efficacy data available from controlled studies for treatment >48 weeks

- -

DOSING CONSIDERATIONS
Elderly
Consider a lower starting dose and smaller dose increments

Adverse Reactions

Consider dose reductions (eg, reducing total daily dose or number of doses/week) for side effects potentially related to therapy

ADMINISTRATION

SQ route

Therapy should be carried out under the regular guidance of a physician who is experienced in HIV infection diagnosis and management.
Rotate inj sites (thigh, upper arm, abdomen, buttock).

Reconstitution

Each vial of Serostim 5mg or 6mg is reconstituted w/ 0.5-1mL sterile water for inj (SWFI).
Each vial of Serostim 4mg is reconstituted in 0.5-1mL of bacteriostatic water for inj (0.9% benzyl alcohol preserved); for patients sensitive to benzyl alcohol, may reconstitute w/ SWFI.
When reconstituted w/ SWFI, the reconstituted sol should be used immediately and any unused portion should be discarded.
When reconstituted w/ bacteriostatic water for inj, the reconstituted sol may be refrigerated (2-8°C/36-46°F) for up to 14 days.
Approx 10% mechanical loss can be associated w/ reconstitution and administration from multidose vials.
Inject the diluent into the vial aiming the liquid against the glass vial wall. Swirl the vial w/ a gentle rotary motion until contents are dissolved completely.
Do not shake and use it only if it is clear and colorless.
Serostim can be administered using (1) a standard sterile, disposable syringe and needle, (2) a compatible Serostim needle-free inj device, or (3) a compatible Serostim needle inj device.
For proper use, refer to the instructions for use provided w/ the administration device.

STORAGE

Before Reconstitution: 15-30°C (59-86°F). **After Reconstitution w/ SWFI (Single-Use Vials):** Use immediately and discard any unused portion. **After Reconstitution w/ Bacteriostatic Water for Injection (Multi-Use Vials):** 2-8°C (36-46°F) for up to 14 days. **Reconstituted Sol:** Avoid freezing.

HOW SUPPLIED

Inj: 4mg [multi-use vial]; 5mg, 6mg [single-use vial]

CONTRAINDICATIONS

Active malignancy, active proliferative or severe nonproliferative diabetic retinopathy, and acute critical illness due to complications following open heart or abdominal surgery, multiple accidental trauma, or acute respiratory failure.

WARNINGS/PRECAUTIONS

Somatropin has been shown to potentiate HIV replication; maintain on antiretroviral therapy for the duration of treatment. New onset impaired glucose tolerance, new onset type 2 diabetes mellitus (DM), exacerbation of preexisting DM, diabetic ketoacidosis, and diabetic coma reported. Intracranial HTN w/ papilledema, visual changes, headache, and N/V reported; perform funduscopic exam before and during therapy. D/C if papilledema is observed by funduscopy; if somatropin-induced intracranial HTN is diagnosed, may restart at a lower dose after signs/symptoms have resolved. Increased tissue turgor and musculoskeletal discomfort may occur; may resolve spontaneously, w/ analgesic therapy, or after reducing frequency of dosing. Carpal tunnel syndrome may occur; d/c if symptoms do not resolve after decreasing the weekly number of doses. Tissue atrophy may result if administered SQ at the same site over a long period; rotate inj site. Local/systemic allergic reactions may occur. Monitor for the development of neoplasms in all patients and routinely monitor for progression or recurrence of a tumor in patients w/ a history of any neoplasm. Pancreatitis reported rarely. Caution in the elderly.

ADVERSE REACTIONS

Tissue turgor (swelling, particularly of hands or feet), musculoskeletal discomfort.

DRUG INTERACTIONS

Inhibits 11β-hydroxysteroid dehydrogenase type 1; patients treated w/ glucocorticoid replacement (eg, cortisone acetate, prednisone) for previously diagnosed hypoadrenalism may require an increase in maintenance or stress doses following initiation of somatropin therapy. May alter clearance of compounds metabolized by CYP450 liver enzymes (eg, corticosteroids, sex steroids, anticonvulsants, cyclosporine); careful monitoring is advised w/ concomitant use. Oral estrogens may reduce serum insulin-like growth factor-1 (IGF-1) response to somatropin; may require greater somatropin doses if taking oral estrogen replacement concomitantly. May require adjustment of doses of insulin or other hypoglycemic agents.

PREGNANCY AND LACTATION

Pregnancy: Category B.
Lactation: Caution in nursing.

MECHANISM OF ACTION

Recombinant hGH; anabolic and anticatabolic agent. Interacts w/ specific receptors on a variety of cell types, including myocytes, hepatocytes, adipocytes, lymphocytes, and hematopoietic cells. Some effects are mediated by IGF-1.

PHARMACOKINETICS

Absorption: Absolute bioavailability (70-90%). **Distribution:** (IV) V_d=12L. **Metabolism:** Liver, kidneys. **Elimination:** Urine; $T_{1/2}$=4.28 hrs (6mg SQ).

PATIENT CONSIDERATIONS

Assessment: Assess for hypersensitivity to drug or diluent; acute critical illness due to complications following open heart/abdominal surgery, multiple accidental trauma, or acute respiratory failure; active malignancy; active proliferative or severe nonproliferative diabetic retinopathy; risk factors for glucose intolerance; DM; history of any neoplasm; preexisting nevi; pregnancy/nursing status; and possible drug interactions. Obtain baseline glucose levels and perform funduscopic exam.

Monitoring: Monitor for signs/symptoms of intracranial HTN, increased tissue turgor, musculoskeletal discomfort, carpal tunnel syndrome, local/systemic reactions, glucose intolerance, pancreatitis, and other adverse reactions. Monitor glucose levels, and perform funduscopic exam periodically. Carefully monitor for development of neoplasms, progression/recurrence of tumor in patients w/ history of any neoplasm, and for increased growth, or potential malignant changes of preexisting nevi.

Counseling: Inform about benefits and risks of therapy. Instruct to contact physician if side effects or discomfort occurs. Inform about management of common side effects relating to tissue turgor, glucose intolerance, and musculoskeletal discomfort. Instruct to use sterile, disposable syringes/needles and caution against reuse; inform of the importance of proper disposal. Instruct to rotate inj sites to avoid localized tissue atrophy. Counsel to never share drug or inj devices w/ another person, even if needle/nozzle is changed; inform that sharing inj devices may pose a risk of transmission of infection. Inform that allergic reactions are possible and that prompt medical attention should be sought if these occur.

SIGNIFOR — pasireotide   Rx

Class: Somatostatin analogue

ADULT DOSAGE	PEDIATRIC DOSAGE
Cushing's Disease	Pediatric use may not have been established
In Patients for Whom Pituitary Surgery is Not an Option/Has Not Been Curative:	
Initial: 0.6mg or 0.9mg SQ bid	
Titrate: Adjust dose based on response and tolerability; if started on 0.6mg bid, may consider increasing to 0.9mg bid	
Usual Range: 0.3-0.9mg bid	

DOSING CONSIDERATIONS

Hepatic Impairment
Moderate (Child-Pugh B):
Initial: 0.3mg bid
Max: 0.6mg bid
Severe (Child-Pugh C): Avoid use

Elderly
Start at lower end of dosing range

Adverse Reactions

May require temporary dose reduction by 0.3mg decrements/inj

ADMINISTRATION

SQ route

Prior to inj, gently pinch the skin at the inj site and hold the needle/syringe at an angle of approx 45 degrees
Administer by self-inj into the top of the thigh or the abdomen; do not inject in sites showing inflammation or irritation
Do not inject multiple times at the same site w/in short periods of time, or use the same inj site for 2 consecutive inj

STORAGE

25°C (77°F); excursions permitted to 15-30°C (59-86°F). Protect from light.

HOW SUPPLIED

Inj: 0.3mg/mL, 0.6mg/mL, 0.9mg/mL [1mL]

WARNINGS/PRECAUTIONS

Hypocortisolism may occur; consider temporary dose reduction or interruption, as well as temporary exogenous glucocorticoid replacement therapy. Elevations in blood glucose levels reported; optimize intensive antidiabetic therapy prior to treatment in patients w/ uncontrolled diabetes mellitus (DM). Self-monitoring of blood glucose and/or FPG assessments should be done every week for the first 2-3 months and periodically thereafter, as well as over the first 2-4 weeks after any dose increase. Initiate or adjust antidiabetic treatment per standard of care if hyperglycemia develops. If uncontrolled hyperglycemia persists, reduce dose or d/c therapy. Bradycardia reported; carefully monitor patients w/ cardiac disease and/or risk factors for bradycardia, and correct electrolyte disturbances as necessary. Associated w/ QT prolongation; caution in patients who are at significant risk of developing QTc prolongation. Correct hypokalemia and hypomagnesemia prior to administration. ALT/AST and bilirubin elevations reported; monitor LFTs after 1-2 weeks on treatment, then monthly for 3 months, and every 6 months thereafter. Serial measures of ALT, AST, alkaline phosphatase, and total bilirubin should be done weekly, or more frequently, if any value exceeds 5X the baseline value in case of abnormal baselines or 5X the ULN in case of normal baselines. If the values are confirmed or rising, interrupt treatment and investigate for probable cause of the findings. If resolution of abnormalities to normal or near normal occurs, cautiously resume treatment w/ close observation, and only if some other likely cause has been found. Cholelithiasis reported frequently; perform ultrasonic examination of the gallbladder before, and at 6- to 12-month intervals during therapy. Inhibition of pituitary hormones, other than ACTH, may occur; monitor pituitary function (eg, TSH/free T4, growth hormone/insulin-like growth factor 1) prior to initiation of therapy and periodically during treatment. Patients who have undergone transsphenoidal surgery and pituitary irradiation are particularly at increased risk for deficiency of pituitary hormones.

ADVERSE REACTIONS

Diarrhea, nausea, hyperglycemia, cholelithiasis, headache, abdominal pain, fatigue, DM, inj-site reactions, nasopharyngitis, alopecia, asthenia, peripheral edema, decreased appetite, hypercholesterolemia.

DRUG INTERACTIONS

Carefully monitor patients w/ risk factors for bradycardia (eg, concomitant use of drugs associated w/ bradycardia); dose adjustments of β-blockers or calcium channel blockers may be necessary. Coadministration w/ drugs that prolong the QT interval may have additive effects on QT-interval prolongation; caution w/ drugs that may prolong the QT interval. May decrease relative bioavailability of cyclosporine; dose adjustment of cyclosporine may be necessary. May increase levels of bromocriptine; dose reduction of bromocriptine may be necessary.

PREGNANCY AND LACTATION

Category C, not for use in nursing.

MECHANISM OF ACTION

Somatostatin analogue; binds and activates the human somatostatin receptors resulting in inhibition of ACTH secretion, which leads to decreased cortisol secretion.

PHARMACOKINETICS

Absorption: T_{max}=0.25-0.5 hr. **Distribution:** V_d=>100L; plasma protein binding (88%). **Elimination:** Feces (48.3%), urine (7.63%); (multiple doses) $T_{1/2}$=12 hrs.

PATIENT CONSIDERATIONS

Assessment: Assess for cardiac disease, risk factors for bradycardia or QT prolongation, pituitary function, DM, pregnancy/nursing status, and possible drug interactions. Obtain baseline FPG, HbA1c, LFTs, serum K^+ and Mg^{2+} levels, ECG, and gallbladder ultrasound.

Monitoring: Monitor for hypocortisolism, bradycardia, QT prolongation, and other adverse reactions. Monitor periodically for electrolyte disturbances (eg, hypokalemia, hypomagnesemia). Monitor blood glucose and/or FPG every week for the first 2-3 months and periodically thereafter, as well as over the first 2-4 weeks after any dose increase; LFTs after 1-2 weeks on treatment, then monthly for 3 months, and every 6 months thereafter; and pituitary function periodically. Perform ultrasonic examination of the gallbladder every 6-12 months. Monitor treatment response.

Counseling: Counsel patients on possible significant adverse reactions (eg, hypocortisolism, hyperglycemia, DM, bradycardia, QT prolongation, LFT elevations, cholelithiasis, pituitary hormone deficiency). Instruct on the proper use of the drug. Instruct not to reuse unused portions of ampules and to properly dispose of ampules after use. Advise to avoid multiple inj at or near the same site w/in a short timespan.

SIGNIFOR LAR — pasireotide   Rx

Class: Somatostatin analogue

ADULT DOSAGE

Acromegaly

In Patients Who Have Had an Inadequate Response to Surgery and/or for Whom Surgery is Not an Option:

Initial: 40mg IM once every 4 weeks (28 days)

Titrate: May increase to 60mg for patients who have not normalized growth hormone and/or age and sex adjusted insulin-like growth factor-1 levels after 3 months of treatment at 40mg and who tolerate this dose. May decrease by 20mg decrements (temporarily or permanently) if adverse reactions or over-response to treatment occurs

Max: 60mg

Missed Dose

If a dose is missed and the patient returns prior to the next scheduled dose, a dose may be given up to but no later than 14 days prior to the next dose

PEDIATRIC DOSAGE

Pediatric use may not have been established

DOSING CONSIDERATIONS

Hepatic Impairment

Moderate (Child-Pugh B):

Initial: 20mg every 4 weeks

Max: 40mg every 4 weeks

Severe (Child-Pugh C): Avoid use

Elderly

Start at lower end of dosing range

ADMINISTRATION

IM route

Administer only by IM inj into the right or left gluteus immediately after reconstitution

Insert needle fully at a 90° angle to the skin; slowly pull pack plunger to check that no blood vessels have been penetrated (reposition if a blood vessel has been penetrated) and slowly depress plunger until syringe is empty. Withdraw the needle from the inj site and activate the safety guard

Reconstitution

1. Remove kit from refrigerated storage and allow to stand at room temperature for at least 30 min (but not more than 24 hrs) before starting reconstitution; kit may be re-refrigerated if needed

2. Remove plastic cap from vial and clean the rubber stopper, then remove the lid film of the vial adapter packaging, but do not remove the vial adapter from its packaging

3. Hold vial adapter packaging and position vial adapter on top of vial, then push it fully down so that it snaps in place; then lift the packaging off the vial adapter w/ a vertical movement

4. Remove cap from the prefilled diluent syringe and screw the syringe onto the vial adapter; slowly push the plunger fully to transfer diluent sol into vial

5. Keep plunger pressed and shake vial moderately in a horizontal direction for a minimum of 30 sec until powder is completely suspended; repeat moderate shaking for another 30 sec if the powder is not completely suspended

6. Turn syringe and vial upside down and slowly draw entire contents from vial into syringe; unscrew syringe from vial adapter

7. Screw safety inj needle onto syringe and pull the protective cover straight off the needle; may gently shake syringe to avoid sedimentation and maintain uniform sus, then gently tap syringe to remove any visible bubbles and expel them from the syringe

8. Reconstituted sol is now ready for immediate administration

STORAGE

2-8°C (36-46°F). Do not freeze. The product kit should remain at room temperature for a minimum of 30 min before reconstitution, but should not exceed 24 hrs at room temperature.

HOW SUPPLIED

Inj: 20mg, 40mg, 60mg

WARNINGS/PRECAUTIONS

Should only be administered by a trained healthcare professional. May cause diabetes, pre-diabetes, or increases in blood glucose levels; optimize antidiabetic treatment before initiation in patients w/ poorly controlled diabetes mellitus (DM). May require initiation or adjustment in dose or type of antidiabetic therapy(ies) per standard of care if significant hyperglycemia develops; reduce dose or d/c if hyperglycemia cannot be controlled despite medical management. After treatment discontinuation, FPG and HbA1c should be assessed if indicated; patients on antidiabetic therapy discontinuing treatment may require more frequent blood glucose monitoring and antidiabetic therapy dose adjustment to mitigate the risk of hypoglycemia. Bradycardia reported; monitor patients w/ cardiac disease and/or risk factors for bradycardia (eg, history of clinically significant bradycardia, high-grade heart block); correction of electrolyte disturbances may be necessary when initiating or during the course of treatment. QT interval prolongation reported w/ SQ administration; caution in patients who are at significant risk of developing QT interval prolongation (eg, congenital long QT prolongation, uncontrolled or significant cardiac disease [eg, recent MI, CHF, unstable angina, or clinically significant bradycardia], hypokalemia and/or hypomagnesemia). Increases in liver enzymes reported; monitor liver function until values return to pretreatment levels in patients who develop increased transaminase levels. D/C if signs/symptoms suggestive of clinically significant liver impairment develop and monitor until resolution; do not restart treatment if liver function abnormalities are suspected to be treatment-related. Cholelithiasis reported. Suppression of pituitary hormones other than growth hormoe (GH) or insulin-like growth factor-1 (IGF-1) may occur; if adrenal insufficiency is suspected, confirm and treat per standard of care w/ exogenous glucocorticoids at replacement doses. Caution w/ moderate hepatic impairment (Child-Pugh B) and in elderly.

ADVERSE REACTIONS

Hyperglycemia, DM, diarrhea, abdominal pain, N/V, abdominal distension, cholelithiasis, sinus bradycardia, arthralgia, headache, alopecia, nasopharyngitis, CPK increase, fatigue, dizziness.

DRUG INTERACTIONS

Monitor patients using concomitant drugs associated w/ bradycardia; dose adjustment of drugs known to slow HR (eg, β-blockers, calcium channel blockers) may be necessary when initiating or during the course of pasireotide treatment. Coadministration w/ drugs that prolong the QT interval may have additive effects on QT interval prolongation; caution w/ antiarrhythmics or other substances known to lead to QT prolongation; monitoring effects on QT interval at 21 days is recommended. May decrease relative bioavailability of cyclosporine; dose adjustment of cyclosporine may be necessary. May increase levels of bromocriptine; dose reduction of bromocriptine may be necessary.

PREGNANCY AND LACTATION

Category C, not for use in nursing.

MECHANISM OF ACTION

Somatostatin analogue; binds the human somatostatin receptors resulting in inhibition of GH secretion, which lowers GH and IGF-1 levels.

PHARMACOKINETICS

Distribution: V_d>100L; plasma protein binding (88%). **Elimination:** (SQ, single 0.6mg dose) Feces (48.3%), urine (7.63%).

PATIENT CONSIDERATIONS

Assessment: Assess for DM, cardiac disease, risk factors for bradycardia or QT prolongation, pregnancy/nursing status, and possible drug interactions. Obtain baseline FPG, HbA1c, LFTs, and ECG. Correct electrolyte disturbances (eg, hypokalemia, hypomagnesemia) before treatment. Assess pituitary function (eg, thyroid, adrenal, gonadal).

Monitoring: Monitor for electrolyte disturbances, cholelithiasis, and other adverse reactions. Monitor blood glucose weekly for the first 3 months after treatment initiation, the first 4-6 weeks after dose increases, and periodically thereafter, as clinically appropriate. Monitor for bradycardia in patients w/ cardiac disease and/or risk factors for bradycardia. Monitor for an effect on the QT interval at the time of maximum drug concentration (21 days after inj) in patients at risk. Monitor pituitary function periodically. Monitor liver function after the first 2 to 3 weeks of therapy, then monthly for 3 months, then as clinically indicated thereafter. Monitor treatment response.

Counseling: Counsel on possible significant adverse reactions (eg, hyperglycemia, diabetes, bradycardia, QT prolongation, LFT elevations, cholelithiasis, pituitary hormone deficiency [ies]). Instruct on the importance of adhering to return visit schedule. Inform that treatment should only be administered by a trained healthcare professional.

SIMPONI — golimumab   Rx

Class: Monoclonal antibody/TNF blocker

> Increased risk for developing serious infections (eg, active tuberculosis [TB], latent TB reactivation, invasive fungal infections, bacterial/viral infections, opportunistic infections) leading to hospitalization or death, mostly w/ concomitant use of immunosuppressants (eg, methotrexate [MTX] or corticosteroids). D/C if serious infection develops. Active TB/latent TB reactivation may present w/ disseminated or extrapulmonary disease; test for latent TB before and during therapy and initiate treatment for latent TB prior to therapy. Invasive fungal infections reported; consider empiric antifungal therapy in patients at risk who develop severe systemic illness. Consider risks and benefits prior to therapy in patients w/ chronic or recurrent infection. Monitor patients for development of infection during and after treatment, including development of TB in patients who tested (-) for latent TB infection prior to therapy. Lymphoma and other malignancies, some fatal, reported in children and adolescents.

ADULT DOSAGE

Ulcerative Colitis

Moderately to severely active ulcerative colitis (UC) in patients w/ an inadequate response or intolerant to prior treatment or in patients who have demonstrated corticosteroid dependence

Initial: 200mg SQ at Week 0, followed by 100mg SQ at Week 2
Maint: 100mg SQ every 4 weeks

Psoriatic Arthritis

Treatment of Active Psoriatic Arthritis w/ or w/o MTX or Other Nonbiologic Disease Modifying Antirheumatic Drugs (DMARDs):
50mg SQ once a month

May continue corticosteroids, non-biologic DMARDs, and/or NSAIDs during treatment

Rheumatoid Arthritis

Moderately to Severely Active in Combination w/ MTX:
50mg SQ once a month

May continue corticosteroids, non-biologic DMARDs, and/or NSAIDs during treatment

Ankylosing Spondylitis

Treatment of Active Ankylosing Spondylitis w/ or w/o MTX or Other Nonbiologic DMARDs:
50mg SQ once a month

May continue corticosteroids, non-biologic DMARDs, and/or NSAIDs during treatment

PEDIATRIC DOSAGE

Pediatric use may not have been established

ADMINISTRATION
SQ route

Allow the prefilled syringe or autoinjector to sit at room temperature outside the carton for 30 min prior to SQ inj. Do not warm in any other way.
If multiple inj are required, administer the inj at different sites on the body.
Rotate inj sites; avoid areas where skin is tender, bruised, red, or hard.
Refer to PI for further instructions.

STORAGE
2-8°C (36-46°F). Protect from light. Do not freeze or shake.

HOW SUPPLIED
Inj: 50mg/0.5mL, 100mg/mL [prefilled SmartJect autoinjector, prefilled syringe]

WARNINGS/PRECAUTIONS
Do not initiate in patients w/ an active infection. Increased risk of infection in patients >65 yrs of age and in patients w/ comorbid conditions; consider the risks and benefits prior to therapy in patients who have resided or traveled in areas of endemic TB or endemic mycoses, and w/ any underlying conditions predisposing to infection. D/C if an opportunistic infection or sepsis develops. Hepatitis B virus (HBV) reactivation reported in chronic carriers; closely monitor for signs of active HBV infection during and for several months after therapy. D/C if reactivation

occurs and initiate antiviral therapy. Consider risks and benefits prior to initiating therapy in patients w/ a known malignancy other than a successfully treated nonmelanoma skin cancer or when considering continuing therapy in patients who develop a malignancy. Cases of acute/chronic leukemia, melanoma, and Merkel cell carcinoma reported. Rare postmarketing cases of hepatosplenic T-cell lymphoma reported, and nearly all of the cases occurred in patients w/ Crohn's disease or UC and mostly in adolescent and young adult males; almost all of these patients were treated concomitantly w/ azathioprine or 6-mercaptopurine. All patients w/ UC who are at increased risk for dysplasia or colon carcinoma, or who had a prior history of dysplasia or colon carcinoma should be screened for dysplasia at regular intervals before therapy and throughout their disease course. Worsening and new onset congestive heart failure (CHF) reported; caution w/ CHF and d/c if new/worsening symptoms appear. Associated w/ rare cases of new onset or exacerbation of CNS demyelinating disorders (eg, multiple sclerosis) and peripheral demyelinating disorders (eg, Guillain-Barre syndrome); consider discontinuation if these disorders develop. May result in the formation of antinuclear antibodies and, rarely, in the development of a lupus-like syndrome; d/c treatment if symptoms suggestive of a lupus-like syndrome develop. Caution when switching from one biologic DMARD to another; overlapping biological activity may further increase risk of infection. Hematologic cytopenias (eg, pancytopenia, leukopenia, neutropenia, thrombocytopenia) reported; caution in patients who have or have had significant cytopenias. Serious systemic hypersensitivity reactions reported; d/c immediately and institute appropriate therapy if these reactions occur. Caution in elderly.

ADVERSE REACTIONS
URTI, viral infections, inj-site reactions, HTN, increased ALT/AST.

DRUG INTERACTIONS
See Boxed Warning. Not recommended w/ anakinra, abatacept, or biologics approved to treat rheumatoid arthritis, psoriatic arthritis, or ankylosing spondylitis; may increase risk of serious infections. Avoid w/ live vaccines and therapeutic infectious agents (eg, live attenuated bacteria [eg, Bacille Calmette-Guerin bladder instillation for the treatment of cancer]). Avoid administration of live vaccines to infants for 6 months following the mother's last golimumab inj during pregnancy. Upon initiation or discontinuation of therapy in patients being treated w/ CYP450 substrates w/ a narrow therapeutic index, monitor effect (eg, warfarin) or drug concentration (eg, cyclosporine, theophylline) and may adjust individual dose of the drug product as needed.

PREGNANCY AND LACTATION
Pregnancy: Category B. IgG antibodies cross placenta during pregnancy and have been detected in the serum of infants born to patients treated w/ these antibodies; infants born to women treated w/ Simponi during their pregnancy may be at increased risk of infection for up to 6 months. Administration of live vaccines to infants exposed to Simponi in utero is not recommended for 6 months following the mother's last infusion during pregnancy.
Lactation: Not for use in nursing.

MECHANISM OF ACTION
Monoclonal antibody/TNF-α receptor blocker; prevents the binding of TNF-α to its receptors, thereby inhibiting the biological activity of TNF-α.

PHARMACOKINETICS
Absorption: Absolute bioavailability (53%); C_{max}=3.2mcg/mL; T_{max}=2-6 days (median). **Distribution:** V_d=58-126mL/kg (IV); crosses the placenta. **Elimination:** (IV) $T_{1/2}$=2 weeks (median).

PATIENT CONSIDERATIONS
Assessment: Assess for active/chronic/recurrent infection, history of an opportunistic infection, recent travel to areas of endemic TB or endemic mycoses, underlying conditions that may predispose to infection, malignancies, dysplasia (in UC patients), CHF, demyelinating disorders, significant cytopenias, latex sensitivity, risk factors for skin cancer, pregnancy/nursing status, and possible drug interactions. Test for latent TB infection and for HBV infection.

Monitoring: Monitor for development of infection during and after treatment. Monitor for HBV reactivation, malignancies, dysplasia, new or worsening CHF, demyelinating disorders, hematological events, hypersensitivity reactions, and other adverse reactions. Periodically evaluate for active TB and test for latent TB infection. Perform periodic skin examination, particularly in patients w/ risk factors for skin cancer.

Counseling: Advise of the potential risks and benefits of therapy. Inform that therapy may lower the ability of immune system to fight infections; instruct to contact physician if any symptoms of infection develop. Counsel about the risk of lymphoma and other malignancies. Instruct patients sensitive to latex to not handle the needle cover on the prefilled syringe as well as the needle cover of the prefilled syringe w/in the autoinjector cap because it contains dry natural rubber (a derivative of latex). Advise to report any signs of new/worsening medical conditions (eg, CHF, demyelinating disorders, autoimmune diseases, liver disease, cytopenias, psoriasis). Inform about proper administration instructions.

SIMPONI ARIA — golimumab   Rx

Class: Monoclonal antibody/TNF blocker

> Increased risk for developing serious infections (eg, active tuberculosis [TB], latent TB reactivation, invasive fungal infections, bacterial/viral infections, and opportunistic infections) that may lead to hospitalization or death. Most patients who developed these infections were taking concomitant immunosuppressants (eg, methotrexate [MTX] or corticosteroids). D/C if serious infection develops. Patients w/ TB may present w/ disseminated or extrapulmonary disease; test for latent TB before and during therapy and initiate treatment for latent TB prior to therapy. Invasive fungal infections reported; consider empiric antifungal therapy in patients at risk who develop severe systemic illness. Consider risks and benefits prior to therapy in patients w/ chronic or recurrent infection. Monitor patients for development of signs/symptoms of infection during and after treatment, including development of TB in patients who tested (-) for latent TB infection prior to therapy. Lymphoma and other malignancies, some fatal, reported in children and adolescents treated w/ TNF-blockers.

ADULT DOSAGE
Rheumatoid Arthritis

Moderately to Severely Active in Combination w/ MTX:

2mg/kg IV infusion over 30 min at Weeks 0 and 4, then every 8 weeks thereafter

May continue other non-biologic disease-modifying antirheumatic drugs (DMARDs), corticosteroids, NSAIDs, and/or analgesics during treatment

PEDIATRIC DOSAGE
- Pediatric use may not have been established

ADMINISTRATION
IV route
1. Calculate the dosage and the number of vials needed based on the recommended dosage and the patient's weight.
2. Dilute the total volume of the Simponi Aria sol w/ 0.9% NaCl inj to a final volume of 100mL. For example, this can be accomplished by withdrawing a volume of the 0.9% NaCl inj from the 100mL infusion bag or bottle equal to the total volume of Simponi Aria. Slowly add the total volume of Simponi Aria sol to the 100mL infusion bag or bottle. Gently mix. Discard any unused sol remaining in the vials. Alternatively, Simponi Aria can be diluted using the same method described above w/ 0.45% NaCl inj.
3. Use only an infusion set w/ an in-line, sterile, non-pyrogenic, low protein-binding filter (pore size 0.22μM or less).
4. Do not infuse concomitantly in the same IV line w/ other agents.
5. Infuse diluted sol over 30 min.
6. Once diluted, the infusion sol may be stored for 4 hrs at room temperature.

STORAGE
2-8°C (36-46°F). Protect from light. Do not freeze or shake.

HOW SUPPLIED
Inj: 50mg/4mL

WARNINGS/PRECAUTIONS
Do not initiate in patients w/ an active infection. Increased risk of infection in patients >65 yrs of age and in patients w/ comorbid conditions; consider the risks and benefits prior to therapy in patients who have resided or traveled in areas of endemic TB or endemic mycoses, and w/ any underlying conditions predisposing to infection. D/C if an opportunistic infection or sepsis develops. Hepatitis B virus (HBV) reactivation reported in chronic carriers; closely monitor for signs of active HBV infection during and for several months after therapy. D/C if reactivation occurs and initiate antiviral therapy; caution when considering resuming TNF blockers. Consider risks and benefits prior to initiating therapy in patients w/ a known malignancy other than a successfully treated non-melanoma skin cancer or when considering continuing therapy in patients who develop a malignancy. Cases of acute/chronic leukemia, melanoma, and Merkel cell carcinoma reported. Rare postmarketing cases of hepatosplenic T-cell lymphoma reported, and nearly all of the cases occurred in patients w/ Crohn's disease or ulcerative colitis and mostly in adolescent and young adult males; almost all of these patients were treated concomitantly w/ azathioprine or 6-mercaptopurine. Worsening and new onset CHF reported; caution w/ CHF and d/c if new/worsening symptoms appear. Associated w/ rare cases of new onset or exacerbation of CNS demyelinating disorders (eg, multiple sclerosis) and peripheral demyelinating disorders (eg, Guillain-Barre syndrome); consider discontinuation if these disorders develop. May result in the formation of antinuclear antibodies and, rarely, in the development of a lupus-like syndrome; d/c treatment if symptoms suggestive of a lupus-like syndrome develop. Caution when switching from one biologic DMARD to another; overlapping biological activity may further increase risk of infection. Pancytopenia, leukopenia, neutropenia, and thrombocytopenia reported; caution in patients who have or have had significant cytopenias. Serious systemic hypersensitivity reactions may occur; d/c immediately and institute appropriate therapy if anaphylactic or other serious allergic reactions occur. Caution in elderly.

ADVERSE REACTIONS
URTI, viral infections, bronchitis, HTN, rash.

DRUG INTERACTIONS
See Boxed Warning. MTX decreases clearance. Not recommended w/ anakinra, abatacept, or biologics approved to treat rheumatoid arthritis; may increase risk of serious infections. Avoid w/ live vaccines and therapeutic infectious agents (eg, live attenuated bacteria [eg, bacille Calmette-Guerin bladder instillation for the treatment of cancer]). Avoid administration of live vaccines to infants for 6 months following the mother's last golimumab infusion during pregnancy. Upon initiation or discontinuation of therapy in patients being treated w/ CYP450 substrates w/ a narrow therapeutic index, monitor effect (eg, warfarin) or drug concentration (eg, cyclosporine, theophylline) and adjust individual dose of the drug product as needed.

PREGNANCY AND LACTATION
Pregnancy: Category B. IgG antibodies cross placenta during pregnancy and have been detected in the serum of infants born to patients treated w/ these antibodies; infants born to women treated w/ Simponi Aria during their pregnancy may be at increased risk of infection for up to 6 months. Administration of live vaccines to infants exposed to Simponi Aria in utero is not recommended for 6 months following the mother's last infusion during pregnancy.
Lactation: Not for use in nursing.

MECHANISM OF ACTION
Monoclonal antibody/TNF-α receptor blocker; binds to both soluble and transmembrane bioactive forms of human TNF-α. Prevents the binding of TNF-α to its receptors, thereby inhibiting the biological activity of TNF-α.

PHARMACOKINETICS
Absorption: C_{max}=44.4mcg/mL. **Distribution:** V_d=151mL/kg; crosses the placenta. **Elimination:** $T_{1/2}$=14 days.

PATIENT CONSIDERATIONS
Assessment: Assess for active/chronic/recurrent infection, history of an opportunistic infection, recent travel to areas of endemic TB or endemic mycoses, underlying conditions that may predispose to infection, malignancies, CHF, demyelinating disorders, significant cytopenias, risk factors for skin cancer, pregnancy/nursing status, and possible drug interactions. Test for latent TB infection and for HBV infection.

Monitoring: Monitor for development of infection during and after treatment. Monitor for HBV reactivation, malignancies, new or worsening CHF, demyelinating disorders, hematological events, hypersensitivity reactions, and other adverse reactions. Periodically evaluate for active TB and test for latent TB infection. Perform periodic skin examination, particularly in patients w/ risk factors for skin cancer.

Counseling: Advise of the potential risks and benefits of therapy. Inform that therapy may lower the ability of the immune system to fight infections; instruct to contact physician if any symptoms of infection develop. Inform of the risk of lymphoma and other malignancies. Advise to report any signs of new/worsening medical conditions (eg, CHF, demyelinating disorders, autoimmune diseases, liver disease, cytopenias, psoriasis).

SIMULECT — basiliximab   Rx
Class: Monoclonal antibody/interleukin-2R (IL-2R) alpha (CD25) blocker

> Should only be prescribed by physicians experienced in immunosuppressive therapy and management of organ transplant patients. Physician responsible for administration should have complete information requisite for patient follow-up. Manage patient in facilities equipped and staffed with adequate laboratory and supportive medical resources.

ADULT DOSAGE
Organ Rejection Prophylaxis

In patients receiving renal transplantation when used as part of an immunosuppressive regimen that includes cyclosporine (modified) and corticosteroids

Usual: 2 doses of 20mg each
1st Dose: Administer w/in 2 hrs prior to transplantation surgery
2nd Dose: Administer 4 days after transplantation

Withhold 2nd dose if complications (eg, severe hypersensitivity reactions or graft loss) occur

Only administer once it has been determined that the patient will receive the graft and concomitant immunosuppression

PEDIATRIC DOSAGE
Organ Rejection Prophylaxis

In patients receiving renal transplantation when used as part of an immunosuppressive regimen that includes cyclosporine (modified) and corticosteroids

<35kg:
Usual: 2 doses of 10mg each

≥35kg:
Usual: 2 doses of 20mg each
1st Dose: Administer w/in 2 hrs prior to transplantation surgery
2nd Dose: Administer 4 days after transplantation

Withhold 2nd dose if complications (eg, severe hypersensitivity reactions or graft loss) occur

Only administer once it has been determined that the patient will receive the graft and concomitant immunosuppression

ADMINISTRATION
IV (central or peripheral) route

Reconstitution of 10mg Vial
1. Add 2.5mL of sterile water for inj to the vial containing the basiliximab powder
2. Shake the vial gently to dissolve the powder
3. The reconstituted sol is isotonic and may be given either as a bolus inj or diluted to a volume of 25mL w/ normal saline or D5 for infusion
4. When mixing the sol, gently invert the bag in order to avoid foaming; do not shake

Reconstitution of 10mg Vial
1. Add 5mL of sterile water for inj to the vial containing the basiliximab powder
2. Shake the vial gently to dissolve the powder
3. The reconstituted sol is isotonic and may be given either as a bolus inj or diluted to a volume of 50mL w/ normal saline or D5 for infusion
4. When mixing the sol, gently invert the bag in order to avoid foaming; do not shake

STORAGE
Lyophilized: 2-8°C (36-46°F). Reconstituted: Use immediately. If not used immediately, store at 2-8°C (36-46°F) for 24 hrs or at room temperature for 4 hrs. Discard reconstituted solution if not used within 24 hrs.

HOW SUPPLIED
Inj: 10mg, 20mg

CONTRAINDICATIONS
Known hypersensitivity to basiliximab or any other component of the formulation.

WARNINGS/PRECAUTIONS
Efficacy for the prophylaxis of acute organ rejection in recipients of other solid organ allografts has not been demonstrated. Increased risk of developing lymphoproliferative disorders and opportunistic infections; monitor accordingly. Severe acute (onset within 24 hrs) hypersensitivity reactions (eg, hypotension, tachycardia, cardiac failure, bronchospasm, respiratory failure) including anaphylaxis observed. Exercise extreme caution in all patients previously given basiliximab when being administered a subsequent course. If severe

hypersensitivity reactions occur, permanently d/c therapy. Medications for treatment of severe hypersensitivity reactions should be available for immediate use. Long-term effects on the ability of the immune system to respond to antigens 1st encountered during basiliximab-induced immunosuppression is unknown. Antibodies may develop. Caution in elderly.

ADVERSE REACTIONS
GI effects, peripheral edema, fever, hyperkalemia, hypokalemia, hyperglycemia, hypercholesterolemia, hyperuricemia, dyspnea, upper respiratory infection, acne, HTN, headache, tremor, anemia.

PREGNANCY AND LACTATION
Category B, not for use in nursing.

MECHANISM OF ACTION
Monoclonal antibody/IL-2Rα (CD25) blocker; acts as an interleukin (IL)-2 receptor antagonist by binding to the IL-2 receptor complex and inhibiting IL-2 binding. Specifically targeted against IL-2Rα, which is selectively expressed on the surface of activated T-lymphocytes. Binding to IL-2Rα causes competitive inhibition of IL-2-mediated activation of lymphocytes, a critical pathway in the cellular immune response involved in allograft rejection.

PHARMACOKINETICS
Absorption: C_{max}=7.1mg/L (adults). **Distribution:** V_d=8.6L (adults); 4.8L (1-11 yrs); 7.8L (12-16 yrs). **Elimination:** $T_{1/2}$=7.2 days (adults); 9.5 days (1-11 yrs); 9.1 days (12-16 yrs).

PATIENT CONSIDERATIONS
Assessment: Assess use in patients who were on previous therapy with this drug, known hypersensitivity to the drug, pregnancy/nursing status, and possible drug interactions.

Monitoring: Monitor for signs/symptoms of lymphoproliferative disorders, opportunistic infections, hypersensitivity reactions (eg, hypotension, tachycardia, cardiac failure, dyspnea, wheezing, bronchospasm, pulmonary edema, respiratory failure, urticaria, rash, pruritus, and/or sneezing) and other adverse reactions.

Counseling: Advise of the potential benefits and risks of therapy. Inform that hypersensitivity reactions (eg, dyspnea, urticaria, rash) may occur during therapy. Instruct women of child-bearing potential to use an effective form of contraceptive before starting, during, and for 4 months following completion of therapy.

SKYLA — levonorgestrel   Rx

Class: Progestin contraceptive

ADULT DOSAGE
Contraception

Timing of Insertion:
Insert into the uterine cavity during the first 7 days of the menstrual cycle

Following 1st Trimester Abortion:
Insert immediately after a 1st trimester abortion

Following 2nd Trimester Abortion/ Postpartum: Postpone insertion a minimum of 6 weeks or until the uterus is fully involuted; if involution is delayed, wait until involution is complete before insertion

Timing of Removal:
Should not remain in the uterus after 3 yrs
If pregnancy is not desired, removal should be carried out during menstruation, provided the woman is still experiencing regular menses
If removal will occur at other times during the cycle, consider starting a new contraceptive method a week prior to removal

Continuation of Contraception after Removal:
If pregnancy is not desired and if a woman wishes to continue using Skyla, a new system can be inserted immediately after removal any time during the cycle

Conversions

Switching to a Different Birth Control Method:
Patients w/ Regular Cycles:
Time removal and initiation of new method to ensure continuous contraception. Either remove Skyla during the first 7 days of the menstrual cycle and start the new method, or start the new method at least 7 days prior to removing Skyla if removal is to occur at other times during the cycle

PEDIATRIC DOSAGE
Contraception

Not indicated for use premenarche; refer to adult dosing

Patients w/ Irregular Cycles or Amenorrhea:
Start the new method at least 7 days before removal

ADMINISTRATION
Intrauterine route

Should be inserted by a trained healthcare provider.
Backup contraception is not needed when inserted as directed.
Consider administering analgesics prior to insertion.
Remove Skyla if it is not positioned completely w/in the uterus; do not reinsert once it is removed.
Must be removed by the end of the 3rd yr.
Refer to PI for additional insertion and removal instructions.

STORAGE
25°C (77°F); excursions permitted to 15-30°C (59-86°F).

HOW SUPPLIED
Intrauterine Insert: 13.5mg

CONTRAINDICATIONS
Pregnancy or suspicion of pregnancy (cannot be used for post-coital contraception), congenital or acquired uterine anomaly (including fibroids if they distort the uterine cavity), acute or history of pelvic inflammatory disease (PID) (unless there has been a subsequent intrauterine pregnancy), postpartum endometritis or infected abortion in the past 3 months, known/suspected uterine or cervical neoplasia, known/suspected or history of breast cancer or other progestin-sensitive cancer, uterine bleeding of unknown etiology, untreated acute cervicitis or vaginitis (including bacterial vaginosis or other lower genital tract infections until infection is controlled), acute liver disease or liver tumor (benign or malignant), conditions associated w/ increased susceptibility to pelvic infections, and previously inserted IUD that has not been removed, hypersensitivity to any component of this product.

WARNINGS/PRECAUTIONS
Evaluate for ectopic pregnancy and remove device if pregnancy occurs w/ device in place. Increased risk of septic abortion, miscarriage, sepsis, premature delivery/labor, and possible congenital anomalies if pregnancy occurs and device is left in place. Severe infection or sepsis, including Group A streptococcal sepsis, may occur; use aseptic technique during insertion of device. Associated w/ increased risk of PID and actinomycosis. Remove device in cases of recurrent endometritis or PID, or if an acute pelvic infection is severe or does not respond to treatment. May alter bleeding pattern and result in spotting, irregular bleeding, heavy bleeding, oligomenorrhea, and amenorrhea; perform appropriate diagnostic measures to rule out endometrial pathology if bleeding irregularities develop during prolonged use. Consider possibility of pregnancy if menstruation does not occur w/in 6 weeks of the onset of a previous menstruation. Perforation may occur and may reduce contraceptive effectiveness; risk increased if inserted in lactating women and may be increased if inserted when the uterus is fixed retroverted or not completely involuted during the postpartum period. Partial or complete expulsion may occur; may be replaced w/in 7 days of a menstrual period after ruling out pregnancy. Ovarian cysts reported. Breast cancer reported w/ a levonorgestrel-releasing intrauterine system. Caution in patients w/ coagulopathy or receiving anticoagulants, migraine, focal migraine w/ asymmetrical visual loss or other symptoms indicating transient cerebral ischemia, exceptionally severe headache, marked increase in BP, and in patients w/ severe arterial disease. Consider removing device if uterine/cervical malignancy or jaundice arises during use. Consider possibility that device may have been displaced (eg, expelled or perforated the uterus) if the threads are not visible or are significantly shortened; exclude pregnancy and verify location of device. If device is displaced, remove it. May be safely scanned on MRI only under specific conditions. MRI quality may be compromised if area of interest is in exact same area or relatively close to position of the device.

ADVERSE REACTIONS
Increased bleeding, vulvovaginitis, abdominal/pelvic pain, acne/seborrhea, ovarian cyst, headache, dysmenorrhea, breast pain/discomfort, nausea.

DRUG INTERACTIONS
Drugs or herbal products that induce enzymes, including CYP3A4 that metabolize progestins (eg, barbiturates, bosentan, carbamazepine), may decrease levels. HIV protease inhibitors or non-nucleoside reverse transcriptase inhibitors may significantly increase or decrease plasma levels. CYP3A4 inhibitors (eg, itraconazole, ketoconazole) may increase plasma hormone levels.

PREGNANCY AND LACTATION
Pregnancy: Contraindicated in pregnancy.
Lactation: Small amounts of progestins reported to pass into the breast milk, resulting in detectable steroid levels in infant serum; caution in nursing.

MECHANISM OF ACTION
Progestin contraceptive; local mechanism by which continuously released levonorgestrel enhances contraceptive effectiveness has not been conclusively demonstrated. Thickens cervical mucus (preventing passage of sperm into uterus), inhibits sperm capacitation or survival, and alters endometrium.

PHARMACOKINETICS
Absorption: C_{max}=192pg/mL, T_{max}=2 days (median). **Distribution:** Plasma protein binding (bound non-specifically to serum albumin and specifically to sex hormone binding globulin); V_d=1.8L/kg; found in breast milk. **Metabolism:** Conjugation; sulfate and glucuronide (lesser extent) conjugates (metabolites). **Elimination:** Urine (45%), feces (32%, glucuronide conjugates); $T_{1/2}$=20 hrs (parenteral).

PATIENT CONSIDERATIONS

Assessment: Assess for congenital or acquired uterine anomaly, acute or history of PID, known/suspected or history of breast cancer or other progestin-sensitive cancer, acute liver disease or liver tumor, pregnancy/nursing status, any other conditions where treatment is contraindicated or cautioned, and for possible drug interactions. Perform a complete medical and social history and if indicated, a physical examination, and appropriate tests for any forms of genital or other sexually transmitted infections (STIs).

Monitoring: Monitor for intrauterine/ectopic pregnancy, sepsis, PID, actinomycosis, bleeding pattern alterations, perforation, migraine/exceptionally severe headache, jaundice, marked BP increase, and other adverse reactions. Reexamine and evaluate 4-6 weeks after insertion and once a yr thereafter, or more frequently if clinically indicated. Monitor if thread is still visible and length of thread.

Counseling: Inform that product does not protect against HIV infection (AIDS) and other STDs. Inform of the risks/benefits/side effects of the device. Inform of the risk of ectopic pregnancy, including loss of fertility; instruct to promptly report symptoms of ectopic pregnancy to physician. Inform of the possibility of PID and of the symptoms of PID; instruct to promptly notify physician if any symptoms of PID develop. Inform that irregular/prolonged bleeding and spotting, and/or cramps may occur during the 1st few weeks after insertion; instruct to report to physician if symptoms continue or are severe. Instruct on how to check if the device's threads still protrude from the cervix and caution not to pull on the threads and displace device. Inform that no contraceptive protection exists if device is displaced or expelled. Instruct to contact physician if any adverse reactions develop, if pregnancy is suspected or occurs, if HIV positive seroconversion occurs in the patient or her partner, or if possible exposure to STIs occurs. Inform that device may be safely scanned w/ MRI only under specific conditions; instruct patients who will have an MRI to notify their physician that they have an IUD.

SOLIRIS — eculizumab   Rx
Class: Monoclonal antibody/protein C5 blocker

> Life-threatening and fatal meningococcal infections reported; may become rapidly life-threatening or fatal if not recognized and treated early. Comply with the most current Advisory Committee on Immunization Practices (ACIP) recommendations for meningococcal vaccination. Immunize patients with meningococcal vaccine at least 2 weeks prior to administering the 1st dose, unless risks of delaying therapy outweigh risk of meningococcal infection development. Monitor for early signs of meningococcal infections and evaluate immediately if infection suspected. Available only through a restricted program under a Risk Evaluation and Mitigation Strategy.

ADULT DOSAGE
Paroxysmal Nocturnal Hemoglobinuria

Reduction of Hemolysis:
Initial: 600mg weekly for the first 4 weeks
Maint: 900mg for the 5th dose 1 week later, then 900mg every 2 weeks thereafter

Atypical Hemolytic Uremic Syndrome

Inhibition of Complement-Mediated Thrombotic Microangiopathy:
Initial: 900mg weekly for the first 4 weeks
Maint: 1200mg for the 5th dose 1 week later, then 1200mg every 2 weeks thereafter

Supplemental Dose After Plasmapheresis/Plasma Exchange:
If Most Recent Dose is 300mg:
300mg w/in 60 min after each plasmapheresis/plasma exchange
If Most Recent Dose is ≥600mg:
600mg w/in 60 min after each plasmapheresis/plasma exchange

Supplemental Dose After Fresh Frozen Plasma Infusion:
If Most Recent Dose is ≥300mg:
300mg w/in 60 min prior to each infusion of fresh frozen plasma

PEDIATRIC DOSAGE
Atypical Hemolytic Uremic Syndrome

Inhibition of Complement-Mediated Thrombotic Microangiopathy:
<18 Years:
5-<10kg:
Induction: 300mg weekly x 1 dose
Maint: 300mg at week 2, then 300mg every 3 weeks
10-<20kg:
Induction: 600mg weekly x 1 dose
Maint: 300mg at week 2, then 300mg every 2 weeks
20-<30kg:
Induction: 600mg weekly x 2 doses
Maint: 600mg at week 3, then 600mg every 2 weeks
30-<40kg:
Induction: 600mg weekly x 2 doses
Maint: 900mg at week 3, then 900mg every 2 weeks
≥40kg:
Induction: 900mg weekly x 4 doses
Maint: 1200mg at week 5, then 1200mg every 2 weeks

Supplemental Dose After Plasmapheresis/Plasma Exchange:
If Most Recent Dose is 300mg:
300mg w/in 60 min after each plasmapheresis/plasma exchange
If Most Recent Dose is ≥600mg:
600mg w/in 60 min after each plasmapheresis/plasma exchange

Supplemental Dose After Fresh Frozen Plasma Infusion:
If Most Recent Dose is ≥300mg:
300mg w/in 60 min prior to each infusion of fresh frozen plasma

ADMINISTRATION
IV route
Administer by IV infusion over 35 min in adults and 1-4 hrs in pediatric patients; do not administer as an IV push or bolus inj
May slow or stop infusion if an adverse reaction occurs during administration; if infusion is slowed, total infusion time should not exceed 2 hrs in adults

Monitor for at least 1 hr following completion of infusion for signs/symptoms of infusion reaction

Preparation
Withdraw required amount from vial into sterile syringe and transfer recommended dose to an infusion bag
Dilute to a final concentration of 5mg/mL by adding the appropriate amount (equal volume of diluent to drug volume) of 0.9% NaCl inj, 0.45% NaCl inj, D5W, or Ringer's inj to the infusion bag
Final admixed infusion volume is 60mL (300mg), 120mL (600mg), 180mL (900mg), or 240mL (1200mg)
Gently invert infusion bag to ensure thorough mixing of product and diluent
Discard unused portion left in vial
Prior to administration, allow admixture to adjust to room temperature; do not heat in microwave or w/ any heat source other than ambient air temperatures

STORAGE
2-8°C (36-46°F). Protect from light. Do not freeze or shake. Admixed Sol: Stable for 24 hrs at 2-8°C (36-46°F) and at room temperature.

HOW SUPPLIED
Inj: 10mg/mL [30mL]

CONTRAINDICATIONS
Patients with unresolved serious *Neisseria meningitidis* infection and patients not currently vaccinated against it.

WARNINGS/PRECAUTIONS
Not indicated for treatment of Shiga toxin *Escherichia coli*-related hemolytic uremic syndrome. May increase susceptibility to infections, especially with encapsulated bacteria. Aspergillus infections reported in immunocompromised and neutropenic patients. Administer vaccinations for the prevention of *Streptococcus pneumoniae* and *Haemophilus influenza* type b (Hib) infections according to ACIP guidelines, and use caution with any systemic infection. Monitor PNH patients for at least 8 weeks after discontinuing therapy to detect hemolysis. Monitor aHUS patients for signs/symptoms of TMA complications for at least 12 weeks after discontinuing therapy; consider reinstitution of therapy, plasma therapy, or appropriate organ-specific supportive measures if TMA complications occur after discontinuing therapy. May result in infusion reactions, including anaphylaxis or other hypersensitivity reactions; interrupt infusion and institute appropriate supportive measures if signs of cardiovascular instability or respiratory compromise occur.

ADVERSE REACTIONS
Meningococcal infections, headache, nasopharyngitis, N/V, urinary tract infection, HTN, upper respiratory tract infection, diarrhea, anemia, pyrexia, renal impairment, nasal congestion, tachycardia, abdominal pain, peripheral edema.

PREGNANCY AND LACTATION
Category C, caution in nursing.

MECHANISM OF ACTION
Monoclonal antibody/complement protein C5 blocker; specifically binds to complement protein C5 with high affinity, thereby inhibiting its cleavage to C5a and C5b and preventing the generation of the terminal complement complex C5b-9. Inhibits terminal complement-mediated intravascular hemolysis in PNH patients and complement-mediated TMA in patients with aHUS.

PHARMACOKINETICS
Absorption: C_{max}=194mcg/mL (PNH). **Distribution:** V_d=7.7L (PNH), 6.14L (aHUS); crosses the placenta; found in breast milk. **Elimination:** $T_{1/2}$=272 hrs (PNH), 291 hrs (aHUS).

PATIENT CONSIDERATIONS
Assessment: Assess for unresolved serious *N. meningitidis* infection, meningococcal vaccination status, presence of a systemic infection, and pregnancy/nursing status.

Monitoring: Monitor for signs/symptoms of meningococcal infections, other infections, infusion/hypersensitivity reactions, and other adverse reactions. Monitor PNH patients after discontinuing therapy for at least 8 weeks to detect hemolysis. Monitor aHUS patients for signs/symptoms of TMA complications for at least 12 weeks after discontinuing therapy.

Counseling: Counsel about risks/benefits of therapy, in particular, the risk of meningococcal infection, and the need to be monitored by a physician after discontinuing therapy. Inform that patients are required to receive meningococcal vaccination at least 2 weeks prior to receiving the 1st dose of treatment, if not previously vaccinated, and that they are required to be revaccinated while on therapy. Inform about the signs/symptoms of a meningococcal infection, and advise to seek immediate medical attention if these signs/symptoms occur. Instruct patients to carry the Soliris Patient Safety Information Card with them at all times, until 3 months after the last dose. Inform parents/caregivers that their child being treated for aHUS should be vaccinated against *S. pneumoniae* and Hib.

SOMATULINE DEPOT — lanreotide   Rx
Class: Somatostatin analogue

ADULT DOSAGE
Acromegaly

Inadequate Response to Surgery and/or Radiotherapy or if Surgery and/or Radiotherapy is Not an Option:
Initial: 90mg deep SQ at 4-week intervals for 3 months

PEDIATRIC DOSAGE
Pediatric use may not have been established

Titrate: After 3 months, adjust dose as follows:

If Growth Hormone (GH) >1 to ≤2.5ng/mL, Insulin-Like Growth Factor-1 (IGF-1) Normal and Clinical Symptoms Controlled:
Maintain 90mg every 4 weeks

If GH >2.5ng/mL, IGF-1 Elevated and/or Clinical Symptoms Uncontrolled:
Increase to 120mg every 4 weeks

If GH <1ng/mL, IGF-1 Normal and Clinical Symptoms Controlled:
Reduce to 60mg every 4 weeks.

Adjust dose thereafter based on response. If controlled on 60mg or 90mg dose, may be considered for an extended dosing interval of 120mg every 6 or 8 weeks

Gastroenteropancreatic Neuroendocrine Tumors
Unresectable, Well- or Moderately-Differentiated, Locally Advanced or Metastatic:
Usual: 120mg deep SQ every 4 weeks

DOSING CONSIDERATIONS
Renal Impairment
Acromegaly:
Moderate to Severe:
Initial: 60mg deep SQ at 4-week intervals for 3 months; then titrate as above

Hepatic Impairment
Acromegaly:
Moderate to Severe:
Initial: 60mg deep SQ at 4-week intervals for 3 months; then titrate as above

ADMINISTRATION
SQ route
Inject via deep SQ in the superior external quadrant of the buttock. Alternate inj site between right and left sides from 1 inj to the next.

STORAGE
2-8°C (36-46°F). Protect from light. Remove sealed pouch from refrigerator 30 min prior to inj. Keep pouch sealed until inj.

HOW SUPPLIED
Inj: 60mg/0.2mL, 90mg/0.3mL, 120mg/0.5mL

CONTRAINDICATIONS
History of hypersensitivity to lanreotide.

WARNINGS/PRECAUTIONS
Allergic reactions (eg, angioedema and anaphylaxis) reported following administration. May reduce gallbladder motility and lead to gallstone formation; may need to monitor periodically. Hypo- or hyperglycemia may occur. Slight decreases in thyroid function reported in acromegalic patients. Sinus bradycardia, bradycardia, and HTN reported in patients with acromegaly; caution in patients with bradycardia. Initiate appropriate medical management in patients who develop symptomatic bradycardia. Caution when considering acromegalic patients with moderate or severe renal/hepatic impairment for an extended dosing interval of 120mg every 6 or 8 weeks.

ADVERSE REACTIONS
Diarrhea, N/V, constipation, flatulence, abdominal pain, inj-site reactions, bradycardia, cholelithiasis, arthralgia, loose stools, headache, weight decrease, HTN, anemia, dysglycemia.

DRUG INTERACTIONS
May require dose adjustment of antidiabetic treatment. May decrease relative bioavailability of cyclosporine; may need to adjust cyclosporine dose. May reduce intestinal absorption of concomitant drugs. May increase availability of bromocriptine. Additive effect on the reduction of HR with drugs that induce bradycardia (eg, β-blockers); dose adjustment of concomitant medication may be necessary. Caution with drugs metabolized by CYP3A4 and have a low therapeutic index (eg, quinidine, terfenadine); drugs metabolized by the liver may be metabolized more slowly during lanreotide treatment and dose reductions of the concomitantly administered medications should be considered.

PREGNANCY AND LACTATION
Category C, not for use in nursing.

MECHANISM OF ACTION
Somatostatin analogue; acts mainly at the human somatostatin receptors 2 and 5 to inhibit GH. Like somatostatin, lanreotide is an inhibitor of various endocrine, neuroendocrine, exocrine, and paracrine functions.

PHARMACOKINETICS
Absorption: Administration of variable doses resulted in different parameters.
Elimination: Urine (<5%), feces (<0.5% unchanged). $T_{1/2}$=23-30 days.

PATIENT CONSIDERATIONS
Assessment: Assess for history of hypersensitivity to drug, cardiac disease, diabetes mellitus, hepatic/renal impairment, pregnancy/nursing status, and possible drug interactions. Obtain baseline blood glucose levels, and thyroid function.

Monitoring: Monitor for allergic reactions, cholelithiasis, gallbladder sludge, cardiovascular abnormalities, and other adverse reactions. Monitor blood glucose levels when treatment is initiated or dosages are adjusted, and monitor thyroid function. Monitor serum GH and IGF-1 levels 6 weeks after a dosing change, in order to evaluate persistence of patient response. Continue to monitor acromegalic patient's response with dose adjustment for biochemical and clinical symptom control, as necessary.

Counseling: Instruct to report development of any unusual symptoms, or if any known symptom persists or worsens. Advise patients with acromegaly that response to drug should be monitored by periodic measurements of GH and IGF-1 levels, with a goal of decreasing levels to normal range. Inform patients experiencing dizziness not to drive vehicles or operate machinery.

SOMAVERT — pegvisomant   Rx
Class: Growth hormone (GH) receptor antagonist

ADULT DOSAGE	PEDIATRIC DOSAGE
Acromegaly	Pediatric use may not have been established
In patients who have had an inadequate response to surgery or radiation therapy, or for whom these therapies are not appropriate	
LD: 40mg SQ	
Maint: On the next day following the LD, begin daily SQ inj of 10mg	
Titrate:	
Elevated Insulin-Like Growth Factor-I (IGF-I): Increase dose by 5mg increments every 4-6 weeks	
IGF-I Below Normal Range: Decrease dose by 5mg decrements every 4-6 weeks	
Range: 10-30mg SQ qd	
Max: 30mg SQ qd	

DOSING CONSIDERATIONS
Hepatic Impairment
Treatment Initiation Based on Baseline LFTs:
Normal: Initiate treatment; monitor LFTs at monthly intervals during the first 6 months of treatment, quarterly for the next 6 months, and then biannually for the next year.
≤3X ULN: Initiate treatment; monitor LFTs monthly for at least one year after initiation of therapy and then biannually for the next year.
<3X ULN: Do not initiate treatment until a comprehensive workup establishes the cause of liver dysfunction. If decision is made to treat, monitor LFTs and clinical symptoms very closely.
Recommendations Based on LFTs During Treatment:
≥3X but <5X ULN (w/o Signs/Symptoms of Hepatitis/Other Liver Injury/Increase in Serum Total Bilirubin):
Continue therapy; monitor LFTs weekly and perform a comprehensive hepatic workup to discern if an alternative cause of liver dysfunction is present.
≥5X ULN/Transaminase Elevations ≥3X ULN Associated w/ Any Increase in Serum Total Bilirubin (w/ or w/o Signs/Symptoms of Hepatitis/Other Liver Injury):
D/C therapy immediately; perform a comprehensive workup to determine if and when serum levels return to normal. If LFTs normalize, consider cautious reinitiation of therapy, w/ frequent LFT monitoring.
Signs/Symptoms Suggestive of Hepatitis/Other Liver Injury:
Immediately perform comprehensive hepatic workup; d/c if liver injury is confirmed.
Elderly
Start at lower end of dosing range.

ADMINISTRATION
SQ route

LD Inj Procedure
1. Before administering the LD, remove the 1st package (1 vial of lyophilized powder containing 20mg of pegvisomant and 1 vial containing the diluent) from the refrigerator about 10 min prior to planned inj time.
2. Withdraw 1mL of the supplied diluent (sterile water for inj) and inject slowly onto the sides of the vial containing lyophilized powder; do not inject the diluent directly on the powder.
3. Slowly swirl the sol to ensure that all of the lyophilized powder has gone into sol; do not invert the vial or shake the sol as this may cause denaturation of the pegvisomant protein. If foaming of the reconstituted sol is seen, the sol is likely damaged and therefore inappropriate to inject.
4. Once reconstituted, the sol will contain 20mg of pegvisomant in 1mL of sol.
5. Withdraw the 1mL reconstituted sol; administer the sol w/in 6 hrs of reconstitution.
6. Inject the 1st reconstituted sol (20mg/mL) SQ into the upper arm, upper thigh, abdomen, or buttocks using a 90° angle.
7. Repeat steps 1 to 5 to reconstitute the 2nd dose of 20mg.
8. Finally, inject the 2nd reconstituted sol (20mg/mL) SQ into the upper arm, upper thigh, abdomen, or buttocks using a 90° angle (different area than the 1st inj).

Maint Dose Inj Procedure
1. Before administering the dose, remove 1 package (1 vial of lyophilized powder containing 10, 15, 20, 25, or 30mg of pegvisomant and 1 vial containing the diluent) from the refrigerator about 10 min prior to the planned inj time.
2. Withdraw 1mL of the supplied 5mL diluent (sterile water for inj) and inject slowly onto the sides of the vial containing lyophilized powder; do not inject the diluent directly on the powder.

3. Slowly swirl the sol to ensure that all of the lyophilized powder has gone into sol; do not invert the vial or shake the sol as this may cause denaturation of the pegvisomant protein. If foaming of the reconstituted sol is seen, the sol is likely damaged and therefore inappropriate to inject.
4. Once reconstituted, the sol will contain 10, 15, 20, 25, or 30mg of pegvisomant in 1mL of sol.
5. Withdraw the 1mL reconstituted sol; administer the sol w/in 6 hrs of reconstitution.
6. Inject the reconstituted sol SQ into the upper arm, upper thigh, abdomen, or buttocks using a 90° angle.

STORAGE
2-8°C (36-46°F). Do not freeze.

HOW SUPPLIED
Inj: 10mg, 15mg, 20mg, 25mg, 30mg

WARNINGS/PRECAUTIONS
See Dosing Considerations. May improve glucose tolerance; carefully monitor patients w/ diabetes mellitus (DM). Transaminase elevations reported; obtain baseline LFTs, and monitor for development of LFT elevations or any other signs/symptoms of liver dysfunction during therapy. Cross-reactivity w/ growth hormone (GH) assays reported. Lipohypertrophy reported; rotate inj sites daily. Exercise caution and close monitoring when reinitiating therapy in patients w/ systemic hypersensitivity reactions. Administer LD under physician supervision.

ADVERSE REACTIONS
Infection, abnormal LFTs, pain, inj-site reaction, dizziness, chest/back pain, sinusitis, peripheral edema, diarrhea, flu syndrome, nausea, paresthesia, HTN.

DRUG INTERACTIONS
May need to reduce dose of insulin and/or oral hypoglycemics in DM patients. Higher doses may be needed to normalize IGF-I concentrations in patients taking opioids.

PREGNANCY AND LACTATION
Pregnancy: Category C.
Lactation: Caution in nursing.

MECHANISM OF ACTION
GH receptor antagonist; selectively binds to GH receptors on cell surfaces, where it blocks binding of endogenous GH, and thus interferes w/ GH signal transduction. Inhibition of GH action results in decreased serum IGF-I concentrations, as well as other GH-responsive serum proteins.

PHARMACOKINETICS
Absorption: Bioavailability (57%); T_{max}=33-77 hrs. Distribution: V_d=7L.
Elimination: Urine (<1%); $T_{1/2}$=60-138 hrs.

PATIENT CONSIDERATIONS
Assessment: Assess for DM, history of drug hypersensitivity, pregnancy/nursing status, and possible drug interactions. Obtain baseline LFTs.

Monitoring: Monitor for hypoglycemia (in patients w/ DM), signs/symptoms of liver dysfunction, hypersensitivity reactions, and other adverse reactions. Measure serum IGF-I concentrations every 4-6 weeks, and when a dose given in multiple inj is converted to a single daily inj. Periodically monitor LFTs.

Counseling: Inform that blood testing will be needed to check IGF-I levels and LFTs before/during treatment and that the dose may be changed based on the results of these tests. Instruct to notify physician if pregnant/breastfeeding. Advise of the most commonly reported adverse reactions (inj-site reaction, LFT elevations, pain, nausea, diarrhea). Instruct to immediately d/c therapy and contact physician if jaundice develops. Inform that GH-secreting tumors may enlarge in people w/ acromegaly and that these tumors need to be watched carefully and monitored by magnetic resonance imaging. Counsel that thickening under the skin may occur at the inj site that could lead to lumps and that switching sites may prevent or lessen this. Instruct on how to properly reconstitute and administer the drug.

SOVALDI — sofosbuvir   Rx

Class: HCV nucleotide analogue NS5B polymerase inhibitor

ADULT DOSAGE	PEDIATRIC DOSAGE
Chronic Hepatitis C	Pediatric use may not have been established
HCV Mono-Infected and HCV/HIV-1 Coinfected:	
Genotype 1 or 4: 400mg qd in combination w/ peginterferon alfa and ribavirin for 12 weeks	
Genotype 1 Ineligible for Interferon-Based Regimen: 400mg qd in combination w/ ribavirin for 24 weeks	
Genotype 2: 400mg qd in combination w/ ribavirin for 12 weeks	
Genotype 3: 400mg qd in combination w/ ribavirin for 24 weeks	
Hepatocellular Carcinoma Awaiting Liver Transplantation: 400mg qd in combination w/ ribavirin for up to 48 weeks or until time of transplant, whichever occurs 1st	

DOSING CONSIDERATIONS
Adverse Reactions
Serious Reaction Potentially Related to Peginterferon Alfa and/or Ribavirin: Reduce dose of or d/c peginterferon alfa and/or ribavirin; refer to each respective PI for instructions

ADMINISTRATION
Oral route
Take w/ or w/o food.
D/C sofosbuvir if concomitant agents are permanently discontinued.

STORAGE
Room temperature <30°C (86°F).

HOW SUPPLIED
Tab: 400mg

CONTRAINDICATIONS
Refer to the individual PIs for peginterferon alfa and ribavirin.

WARNINGS/PRECAUTIONS
Fatal cardiac arrest reported w/ sofosbuvir-containing regimen (ledipasvir/sofosbuvir).

ADVERSE REACTIONS
Fatigue, headache, nausea, insomnia, anemia, pruritus, asthenia, rash, decreased appetite, influenza-like illness, pyrexia, diarrhea, myalgia, irritability.

DRUG INTERACTIONS
Coadministration of amiodarone w/ sofosbuvir in combination w/ another direct-acting antiviral (DAA) may result in serious symptomatic bradycardia; coadministration is not recommended. If coadministration is required, cardiac monitoring is recommended in an inpatient setting for the first 48 hrs, after which outpatient or self-monitoring of HR should occur on a daily basis for at least the first 2 weeks. Intestine P-gp inducers (eg, rifampin, St. John's wort) may significantly decrease concentration and may lead to a reduced therapeutic effect; do not use w/ rifampin and St. John's wort. Carbamazepine, phenytoin, phenobarbital, oxcarbazepine, rifabutin, rifapentine, and tipranavir/ritonavir may decrease concentration, leading to reduced therapeutic effects; coadministration is not recommended. Not recommended w/ other products containing sofosbuvir.

PREGNANCY AND LACTATION
Pregnancy: Category B. If administered w/ ribavirin or peginterferon and ribavirin, combination regimen is contraindicated in pregnant women and in men whose female partners are pregnant.
Lactation: The developmental and health benefits of breastfeeding should be considered along with the mother's clinical need and any potential adverse effects on the breastfed child from the drug or from the underlying maternal condition. If sofosbuvir is administered in a regimen containing ribavirin, refer to the ribavirin PI for more information.

MECHANISM OF ACTION
HCV nucleotide analogue NS5B polymerase inhibitor; direct-acting antiviral agent against HCV.

PHARMACOKINETICS
Absorption: T_{max}=0.5-2 hrs, 2-4 hrs (GS-331007); (w/ ribavirin) AUC_{0-24}=969ng•hr/mL, 6790ng•hr/mL (GS-331007). Distribution: Plasma protein binding (approx 61-65%). Metabolism: Liver (extensive) to GS-461203 (active); dephosphorylation to GS-331007 (major). Elimination: Urine (80%; 78% GS-331007, 3.5% unchanged), feces (14%); $T_{1/2}$ (median)=0.4 hr, 27 hrs (GS-331007).

PATIENT CONSIDERATIONS
Assessment: Assess for pregnancy/nursing status and possible drug interactions.

Monitoring: Monitor for adverse reactions.

Counseling: Advise to seek medical evaluation immediately for symptoms of bradycardia. Advise patients to avoid pregnancy during combination treatment w/ sofosbuvir and ribavirin or sofosbuvir and peginterferon and ribavirin; instruct to notify physician immediately in the event of a pregnancy. Inform that the effect of treatment of hepatitis C on transmission is unknown and that appropriate precautions should be taken to prevent HCV transmission during treatment or in the event of treatment failure. Advise to take ud.

SPRYCEL — dasatinib   Rx

Class: Kinase inhibitor

ADULT DOSAGE	PEDIATRIC DOSAGE
Ph+ Chronic Phase CML	Pediatric use may not have been established
Newly Diagnosed Ph+ CML in Chronic Phase: Initial: 100mg qd Titrate: If no hematologic or cytogenetic response, increase to 140mg qd	
Chronic Phase Ph+ CML w/ Resistance or Intolerance to Prior Therapy (Including Imatinib): Initial: 100mg qd Titrate: If no hematologic or cytogenetic response, increase to 140mg qd	

Accelerated Phase CML/Myeloid or Lymphoid Blast Phase CML/Ph+ ALL

Accelerated or myeloid/lymphoid blast phase Ph+ CML w/ resistance or intolerance to prior therapy (including imatinib) and Ph+ ALL w/ resistance or intolerance to prior therapy

Initial: 140mg qd
Titrate: If no hematologic or cytogenetic response, increase to 180mg qd

---

DOSING CONSIDERATIONS
Concomitant Medications
Strong CYP3A4 Inducers:
Avoid use; if necessary, consider dose increase of dasatinib w/ careful monitoring for toxicity
Strong CYP3A4 Inhibitors:
Avoid use; if necessary, consider dose decrease of dasatinib to 20mg if taking 100mg qd, and to 40mg if taking 140mg qd
If therapy is not tolerated after dose reduction, either d/c concomitant inhibitor and allow a washout period of approx 1 week before increasing dasatinib dose, or d/c dasatinib until end of treatment w/ inhibitor
Grapefruit Juice:
Avoid grapefruit juice
Adverse Reactions
Neutropenia and Thrombocytopenia:
Chronic Phase CML:
ANC <0.5 x 10^9/L or Platelets <50 x 10^9/L:
1. Stop therapy until ANC ≥1.0 x 10^9/L and platelets ≥50 x 10^9/L
2. Resume therapy at the original starting dose if recovery occurs in ≤7 days
3. If platelets <25 x 10^9/L or recurrence of ANC <0.5 x 10^9/L for >7 days, repeat Step 1 and resume at a reduced dose of 80mg qd for 2nd episode. For 3rd episode, further reduce dose to 50mg qd (for newly diagnosed patients) or d/c (for patients resistant or intolerant to prior therapy, including imatinib)
Accelerated Phase CML, Blast Phase CML, and Ph+ ALL (Starting Dose 140mg QD):
ANC <0.5 x 10^9/L or Platelets <10 x 10^9/L:
1. If cytopenia is unrelated to leukemia, stop until ANC ≥1.0 x 10^9/L and platelets ≥20 x 10^9/L and resume at the original starting dose
2. If recurrence of cytopenia, repeat Step 1 and resume at a reduced dose of 100mg qd (2nd episode) or 80mg qd (3rd episode)
3. If cytopenia is related to leukemia, consider dose escalation to 180mg qd
Nonhematological Adverse Reactions:
If a severe nonhematological adverse reaction develops, withhold until the event has resolved or improved
May resume at a reduced dose depending on the severity and recurrence of the event

ADMINISTRATION
Oral route

Take w/ or w/o meal, either in am or pm.
Swallow whole; do not crush or cut.

STORAGE
20-25°C (68-77°F); excursions permitted between 15-30°C (59-86°F).

HOW SUPPLIED
Tab: 20mg, 50mg, 70mg, 80mg, 100mg, 140mg

WARNINGS/PRECAUTIONS
Severe thrombocytopenia, neutropenia, and anemia reported earlier and more frequently in patients w/ advanced phase CML or Ph+ ALL than in patients w/ chronic phase CML. In patients w/ chronic phase CML, perform CBCs every 2 weeks for 12 weeks, then every 3 months thereafter, or as clinically indicated. In patients w/ advanced phase CML or Ph+ ALL, perform CBCs weekly for the first 2 months and then monthly thereafter, or as clinically indicated. ≥Grade 3 CNS and GI hemorrhages, including fatalities and other cases of ≥Grade 3 hemorrhage, reported. Fluid retention may occur; perform chest x-ray if symptoms suggestive of pleural effusion or other fluid retention develop (eg, dyspnea, pleuritic chest pain, dry cough). Cardiac adverse reactions reported; monitor for signs/symptoms consistent w/ cardiac dysfunction and treat appropriately. May increase risk of developing pulmonary arterial HTN (PAH); d/c permanently if PAH is confirmed. QT prolongation reported; correct hypokalemia or hypomagnesemia prior to and during dasatinib administration. Cases of severe mucocutaneous dermatologic reactions (eg, Stevens-Johnson syndrome) reported; d/c permanently in patients who experience a severe mucocutaneous reaction during treatment if no other etiology can be identified. Tumor lysis syndrome reported; maintain adequate hydration and correct uric acid levels prior to initiating therapy w/ dasatinib, and monitor electrolyte levels. Caution w/ hepatic impairment.

ADVERSE REACTIONS
Fluid retention, diarrhea, N/V, headache, musculoskeletal pain, abdominal pain, hemorrhage, pneumonia, pyrexia, dyspnea, rash, fatigue, arthralgia, infection, muscle spasms.

DRUG INTERACTIONS
See Dosing Considerations. CYP3A4 inhibitors (eg, ketoconazole, clarithromycin, ritonavir) and grapefruit juice may increase levels. CYP3A4 inducers (eg, dexamethasone, phenytoin, carbamazepine) and St. John's wort may decrease levels. Avoid w/ antacids (eg, aluminum hydroxide/magnesium hydroxide); if use

is necessary, administer antacid dose at least 2 hrs prior to or 2 hrs after dasatinib dose. H_2 antagonists (eg, famotidine) or proton pump inhibitors (eg, omeprazole) may reduce exposure; concomitant use is not recommended. May increase levels of simvastatin (a CYP3A4 substrate); caution w/ CYP3A4 substrates w/ narrow therapeutic index (eg, alfentanil, astemizole, ergotamine). Medications that inhibit platelet function or anticoagulants may increase the risk of hemorrhage. Antiarrhythmics or other QT-prolonging agents and cumulative high-dose anthracycline therapy may increase risk of QT prolongation.

PREGNANCY AND LACTATION
Pregnancy: Can cause fetal harm; adverse pharmacologic effects (eg, hydrops fetalis, fetal leukopenia, fetal thrombocytopenia) reported w/ maternal exposure to dasatinib.
Lactation: No data are available regarding the presence of dasatinib in human milk, the effects of the drug on the breastfed infant or the effects of the drug on milk production; breastfeeding is not recommended during treatment w/ dasatinib and for 2 weeks after the final dose.
Females and Males Reproductive Potential: Females of reproductive potential should avoid pregnancy, which may include the use of effective contraceptive methods during treatment and for 30 days after the final dose. Dasatinib may result in damage to female and male reproductive tissues.

MECHANISM OF ACTION
Kinase inhibitor; inhibits BCR-ABL, SRC family, c-KIT, EPHA2, and PDGFRβ kinases.

PHARMACOKINETICS
Absorption: T_{max}=0.5-6 hrs. **Distribution:** V_d=2505L; plasma protein binding (96% [parent], 93% [active metabolite]); crosses placenta. **Metabolism:** Extensive, primarily via CYP3A4. **Elimination:** Feces (85%, 19% unchanged), urine (4%, 0.1% unchanged); $T_{1/2}$=3-5 hrs.

PATIENT CONSIDERATIONS

Assessment: Assess for signs/symptoms of underlying cardiopulmonary disease, hepatic impairment, presence or risk of QT prolongation, hypokalemia, hypomagnesemia, pregnancy/nursing status, and possible drug interactions.

Monitoring: Monitor for bleeding events, fluid retention, cardiac dysfunction, myelosuppression, QT prolongation, PAH, tumor lysis syndrome, severe mucocutaneous dermatologic reactions, and other adverse reactions. Perform chest x-ray if symptoms of pleural effusion develop. In patients w/ chronic phase CML, perform CBCs every 2 weeks for 12 weeks, then every 3 months thereafter, or as clinically indicated. In patients w/ advanced phase CML or Ph+ ALL, perform CBCs weekly for the first 2 months and then monthly thereafter, or as clinically indicated.

Counseling: Inform of pregnancy risks; instruct females of reproductive potential to avoid becoming pregnant during therapy and for 30 days after the final dose of therapy. Advise females of reproductive potential to contact physician if patient becomes pregnant, or if pregnancy is suspected, while on therapy. Instruct to seek medical attention if symptoms of hemorrhage, myelosuppression, fluid retention, significant N/V, diarrhea, headache, musculoskeletal pain, fatigue, or rash develop. Inform that product contains lactose.

STELARA — ustekinumab   Rx

Class: Monoclonal antibody/interleukin-12 (IL-12) and IL-23 antagonist

ADULT DOSAGE	PEDIATRIC DOSAGE
Psoriasis	Pediatric use may not have been established
Patients w/ Moderate to Severe Plaque Psoriasis who are Candidates for Phototherapy or Systemic Therapy:	
≤100kg (≤220 lbs): 45mg initially and 4 weeks later, followed by 45mg every 12 weeks	
<100kg (>220 lbs): 90mg initially and 4 weeks later, followed by 90mg every 12 weeks	
Psoriatic Arthritis	
Active:	
45mg initially and 4 weeks later, followed by 45mg every 12 weeks	
Coexistent Moderate to Severe Plaque Psoriasis:	
<100kg (>220 lbs): 90mg initially and 4 weeks later, followed by 90mg every 12 weeks	
Can be used alone or in combination w/ methotrexate	

ADMINISTRATION
SQ route

Administer each inj at a different anatomic location (eg, upper arms, gluteal regions, thighs, any quadrant of abdomen) than the previous inj; do not administer into areas where the skin is tender, bruised, erythematous, or indurated.
When using the single-use vial, a 27-gauge, 1/2-inch needle is recommended.

Administration Instructions
1. To prevent premature activation of the needle safety guard, do not touch the needle guard activation clips at any time during use.

2. Hold body and remove needle cover; do not hold plunger or plunger head while removing needle cover and do not use prefilled syringe if it is dropped w/o needle cover in place.

3. Inject SQ as recommended; inject all of the medication by pushing in plunger until plunger head is completely between needle guard wings; inj of entire prefilled syringe contents is necessary to activate needle guard.

4. After injection, maintain pressure on plunger head and remove needle from skin.

5. Slowly take your thumb off plunger head to allow empty syringe to move up until entire needle is covered by needle guard; discard used syringes in puncture-resistant container.

STORAGE
2-8°C (36-46°F). Store vials upright. Protect from light. Do not freeze or shake.

HOW SUPPLIED
Inj: 45mg/0.5mL, 90mg/mL [prefilled syringe, vial]

CONTRAINDICATIONS
Clinically significant hypersensitivity to ustekinumab or to any of the excipients.

WARNINGS/PRECAUTIONS
Serious bacterial, fungal, and viral infections, and infections requiring hospitalization reported. Do not give to patients with any clinically important active infection or until infection resolves or is adequately treated. Caution with chronic infection or a history of recurrent infection. Individuals genetically deficient in interleukin (IL)-12/IL-23 are particularly vulnerable to disseminated infections from mycobacteria (eg, nontuberculous, environmental mycobacteria), salmonella (eg, nontyphi strains), and Bacillus Calmette-Guerin (BCG) vaccinations; consider appropriate diagnostic testing. Evaluate for tuberculosis (TB) infection prior to, during, and after treatment; do not administer to patients with active TB. Consider anti-TB therapy prior to initiation in patients with history of latent or active TB when an adequate course of treatment cannot be confirmed. Rapid appearance of multiple cutaneous squamous cell carcinomas reported in patients who had preexisting risk factors for developing non-melanoma skin cancer; closely monitor patients with history of prolonged immunosuppressant therapy, history of PUVA treatment, and patients >60 yrs of age. Hypersensitivity reactions (eg, anaphylaxis, angioedema) reported; institute appropriate therapy and d/c. Reversible posterior leukoencephalopathy syndrome (RPLS) reported; administer appropriate treatment and d/c if suspected. Prior to initiating therapy, patients should receive all immunizations appropriate for age as recommended by current immunization guidelines. Needle cover on prefilled syringe contains dry natural rubber and should not be handled by latex-sensitive individuals. Should only be given to patients who will be closely monitored and have regular follow-up visits with a physician.

ADVERSE REACTIONS
Infection, nasopharyngitis, upper respiratory tract infection, headache, fatigue, arthralgia, nausea.

DRUG INTERACTIONS
Do not give with live vaccines; caution when administering live vaccines to household contacts of patients receiving ustekinumab. BCG vaccines should not be given during, for 1 yr prior to initiating, or 1 yr following discontinuation of treatment. Non-live vaccinations received during course of therapy may not elicit an immune response sufficient to prevent disease. Consider monitoring for therapeutic effect (eg, for warfarin) or drug concentration (eg, for cyclosporine) with concomitant CYP450 substrates, particularly those with a narrow therapeutic index; adjust individual dose prn. May decrease protective effect of allergen immunotherapy (decrease tolerance), which may increase the risk of an allergic reaction to a dose of allergen immunotherapy; caution in patients receiving or who have received allergen immunotherapy.

PREGNANCY AND LACTATION
Pregnancy: Category B.
Lactation: Caution in nursing.

MECHANISM OF ACTION
Monoclonal antibody; binds with specificity to the shared p40 protein subunit used by both the IL-12 and IL-23 cytokines.

PHARMACOKINETICS
Absorption: (Psoriasis) T_{max}=13.5 days (median, 45mg), 7 days (median, 90mg).
Distribution: (Psoriasis) V_d=161mL/kg (45mg), 179mL/kg (90mg); found in breast milk. Elimination: (Psoriasis) $T_{1/2}$=14.9-45.6 days.

PATIENT CONSIDERATIONS
Assessment: Assess for drug hypersensitivity, active/chronic/serious infections, history of recurrent infection, IL-12/IL-23 genetic deficiency, TB, immunization history, pregnancy/nursing status, and possible drug interactions.

Monitoring: Monitor for signs/symptoms of infection, appearance of non-melanoma skin cancer, TB during and after treatment, malignancies, hypersensitivity reactions, RPLS, and other adverse reactions.

Counseling: Advise that therapy may lower the ability of the immune system to fight infections. Inform of the importance of communicating any history of infections to physician and instruct to contact physician if any signs/symptoms of infection develop. Counsel about the risk of malignancies while on therapy. Advise to seek immediate medical attention if experiencing any symptoms of a serious allergic reaction. Inform of inj techniques and procedures. Advise not to reuse needles/syringes and instruct on proper disposal procedures.

STIMATE — desmopressin acetate   Rx
Class: Synthetic vasopressin analogue

ADULT DOSAGE
Hemophilia A

Use in patients w/ hemophilia A w/ factor VIII coagulant activity levels >5%

Usual: 1 spray/nostril (300mcg total dose)
<50kg: 150mcg administered as a single spray

Preoperative Use:
Administer 2 hrs prior to scheduled procedure. Repeat administration or use of any blood products for hemostasis should be determined by laboratory response and patient's clinical condition

von Willebrand's Disease

Use in patients w/ mild to moderate classic von Willebrand's disease (Type 1) w/ factor VIII levels >5%

Usual: 1 spray/nostril (300mcg total dose)
<50kg: 150mcg administered as a single spray

Preoperative Use:
Administer 2 hrs prior to scheduled procedure. Repeat administration or use of any blood products for hemostasis should be determined by laboratory response and patient's clinical condition

PEDIATRIC DOSAGE
Hemophilia A

Use in patients w/ hemophilia A w/ factor VIII coagulant activity levels >5%

≥11 Months of Age:
Usual: 1 spray/nostril (300mcg total dose)
<50kg: 150mcg administered as a single spray

Preoperative Use:
Administer 2 hrs prior to scheduled procedure. Repeat administration or use of any blood products for hemostasis should be determined by laboratory response and patient's clinical condition

von Willebrand's Disease

Use in patients w/ mild to moderate classic von Willebrand's disease (Type 1) w/ factor VIII levels >5%

≥11 Months of Age:
Usual: 1 spray/nostril (300mcg total dose)
<50kg: 150mcg administered as a single spray

Preoperative Use:
Administer 2 hrs prior to scheduled procedure. Repeat administration or use of any blood products for hemostasis should be determined by laboratory response and patient's clinical condition

---

ADMINISTRATION
Intranasal route

Prime spray pump prior to 1st use by pressing down 4X

STORAGE
≤25°C (77°F) in upright position. Discard after 25 sprays or 6 months after opening, whichever comes 1st.

HOW SUPPLIED
Spray: 1.5mg/mL [2.5mL]

WARNINGS/PRECAUTIONS
For intranasal use only. Not indicated for treatment of patients with FVIII antibodies and with evidence of an abnormal molecular form of FVIII antigen. Use DDAVP inj when intranasal route may be compromised (eg, nasal congestion/blockage/discharge, nasal mucosa atrophy, severe atrophic rhinitis) or with impaired level of consciousness. Administer a test dose to establish an appropriate change in coagulation profile prior to initiation of therapy. May cause water intoxication and/or hyponatremia; fluid restriction is recommended 1 hr prior to administration until at least 24 hrs after administration. Extreme decrease in plasma osmolality, resulting in seizures or coma, may occur. Adjust fluid intake downward particularly in pediatric patients and in elderly; caution patients not in need of antidiuretic hormone for its antidiuretic effect to ingest only enough fluid to satisfy thirst. Caution in patients with habitual or psychogenic polydipsia, conditions associated with fluid/electrolyte imbalance (eg, cystic fibrosis, heart failure, renal disorders), and in patients predisposed to thrombus formation. May produce changes in BP; caution in patients with coronary artery insufficiency and/or hypertensive cardiovascular disease (CVD). Severe allergic reactions reported rarely. Changes in nasal mucosa (eg, scarring, edema) may cause erratic, unreliable absorption; d/c until nasal problems resolve and consider DDAVP inj. Nasal spray pump can only deliver doses of 0.1mL (150mcg) or multiples of 0.1mL; may use DDAVP inj if doses other than these are required. Caution in elderly.

ADVERSE REACTIONS
Somnolence, dizziness, itchy or light-sensitive eyes, insomnia, chills, warm feeling, pain, chest pain, palpitations, tachycardia, dyspepsia, edema, vomiting, agitation, balanitis.

DRUG INTERACTIONS
Carefully monitor if used with other pressor agents. Caution with drugs that may increase the risk of water intoxication with hyponatremia (eg, TCAs, SSRIs, chlorpromazine, opiate analgesics, NSAIDs, lamotrigine, carbamazepine). Convulsions from hyponatremia (rare) reported with concomitant oxybutynin and imipramine.

PREGNANCY AND LACTATION
Category B, caution in nursing.

MECHANISM OF ACTION
Synthetic vasopressin analog; shown to be more potent than arginine vasopressin in increasing plasma levels of FVIII activity in patients with hemophilia and VWD type I.

PHARMACOKINETICS
Absorption: Bioavailability (3.3-4.1%); T_{max}=40-45 min. Elimination: $T_{1/2}$=3.3-3.5 hrs.

PATIENT CONSIDERATIONS

Assessment: Assess for hypersensitivity to drug, compromised intranasal route, impaired level of consciousness, habitual or psychogenic polydipsia, coronary artery insufficiency, hypertensive CVD, fluid/electrolyte imbalance conditions, predisposition to thrombus formation, pregnancy/nursing status, and possible drug interactions. (Hemophilia A) Assess patient status (eg, FVIII coagulant activity levels if used for hemostasis, FVIII antigen and FVIII ristocetin cofactor [von Willebrand factor (VWF)], activated PTT). (VWD) Assess patient status (eg, FVIII coagulant activity levels, VWF ristocetin cofactor and VWF antigen).

Monitoring: Monitor for signs/symptoms of hyponatremia, water intoxication, allergic reactions, and other adverse reactions. Monitor bleeding time and FVIII coagulant activity, ristocetin cofactor activity, and VWF antigen after initial administration. Monitor BP, fluid intake, and electrolyte levels.

Counseling: Inform that bottle accurately delivers 25 sprays of 150mcg each; instruct to discard any remaining solution after 25 sprays and not attempt to transfer remaining solution to another bottle. Advise to contact physician if bleeding is not controlled. Inform that water intoxication and/or hyponatremia may occur; advise that fluid restriction is recommended.

STIVARGA — regorafenib

Rx

Class: Kinase inhibitor

> Severe and sometimes fatal hepatotoxicity reported. Monitor hepatic function prior to and during treatment. Interrupt and then reduce or d/c treatment for hepatotoxicity as manifested by elevated LFTs or hepatocellular necrosis, depending upon severity and persistence.

ADULT DOSAGE

Metastatic Colorectal Cancer

Previously treated w/ fluoropyrimidine-, oxaliplatin-, and irinotecan-based chemotherapy, an antivascular endothelial growth factor therapy, and, if RAS wild-type, an anti-epidermal growth factor receptor therapy

160mg qd for the first 21 days of each 28-day cycle until disease progression or unacceptable toxicity

Locally Advanced, Unresectable or Metastatic Gastrointestinal Stromal Tumor

Previously treated w/ imatinib mesylate and sunitinib malate

160mg qd for the first 21 days of each 28-day cycle until disease progression or unacceptable toxicity

PEDIATRIC DOSAGE

Pediatric use may not have been established

DOSING CONSIDERATIONS

Renal Impairment

ESRD: Has not been studied

Hepatic Impairment

Severe (Child-Pugh Class C): Not recommended

Adverse Reactions

Interrupt For:

- Grade 2 hand-foot skin reaction (HFSR) that is recurrent or does not improve w/ in 7 days despite dose reduction; interrupt therapy for a minimum of 7 days for Grade 3 HFSR
- Symptomatic Grade 2 HTN
- Any Grade 3 or 4 adverse reaction

Reduce to 120mg:

- For the 1st occurrence of Grade 2 HFSR of any duration
- After recovery of any Grade 3 or 4 adverse reaction
- For Grade 3 AST/ALT elevation; only resume if the potential benefit outweighs the risk of hepatotoxicity

Reduce to 80mg:

- For reoccurrence of Grade 2 HFSR at the 120mg dose
- After recovery of any Grade 3 or 4 adverse reaction at the 120mg dose (except hepatotoxicity)

Discontinue For:

- Failure to tolerate 80mg dose
- Any occurrence of AST or ALT >20X ULN
- Any occurrence of AST or ALT >3X ULN w/ concurrent bilirubin >2X ULN
- Reoccurrence of AST or ALT >5X ULN despite dose reduction to 120mg
- For any Grade 4 adverse reaction; only resume if the potential benefit outweighs the risks

Other Important Considerations

A higher incidence of HFSR and LFT abnormalities occurred in Asian patients as compared w/ White patients

ADMINISTRATION

Oral route

Take at the same time each day.

Swallow tab whole w/ water after a low-fat meal that contains <600 calories and <30% fat.

Do not take 2 doses of therapy on the same day to make up for a missed dose from the previous day.

STORAGE

25°C (77°F); excursions permitted to 15-30°C (59-86°F). Store tabs in original bottle and do not remove the desiccant. Keep the bottle tightly closed after 1st opening. Discard any unused tabs 7 weeks after opening the bottle.

HOW SUPPLIED

Tab: 40mg

WARNINGS/PRECAUTIONS

See Dosing Considerations. Increased incidence of hemorrhage reported. Increased incidence of adverse reactions involving the skin and SQ tissues (eg, HFSR, toxic epidermal necrolysis, severe rash). Increased incidence of HTN reported. Avoid initiation unless BP is adequately controlled. Increased incidence of myocardial ischemia and infarction; withhold if new or acute onset cardiac ischemia or infarction develops. Resume treatment only after resolution of acute cardiac ischemic events, if benefits outweigh risks of further cardiac ischemia. Reversible posterior leukoencephalopathy syndrome (RPLS) reported; perform evaluation for RPLS in any patient presenting w/ seizures, severe headache, visual disturbances, confusion, or altered mental function. D/C if RPLS develops. GI perforation or fistula reported; permanently d/c if GI perforation or fistula develops. May impair wound healing; d/c at least 2 weeks prior to scheduled surgery. D/C in patients w/ wound dehiscence. May cause fetal harm.

ADVERSE REACTIONS

Asthenia/fatigue, HFSR, diarrhea, decreased appetite/food intake, HTN, mucositis, dysphonia, infection, pain, decreased weight, GI and abdominal pain, rash, fever, nausea.

DRUG INTERACTIONS

Strong CYP3A4 inducers may decrease plasma concentrations of regorafenib, increase plasma concentrations of the active metabolite M-5, and may lead to decreased efficacy; avoid w/ strong CYP3A4 inducers (eg, rifampin, phenytoin, carbamazepine). Strong CYP3A4 inhibitors may increase the plasma concentrations of regorafenib and decrease the plasma concentrations of the active metabolites M-2 and M-5, and may lead to increased toxicity; avoid w/ strong CYP3A4 inhibitors (eg, clarithromycin, grapefruit juice, itraconazole). Monitor INR levels more frequently in patients receiving warfarin. Coadministration w/ a BCRP substrate may increase the plasma concentrations of the BCRP substrate; monitor closely for signs/symptoms of exposure related toxicity to the BCRP substrate (eg, methotrexate, fluvastatin, atorvastatin); consult the concomitant BCRP substrate product information when considering coadministration of such products together w/ regorafenib.

PREGNANCY AND LACTATION

Pregnancy: Based on animal studies and mechanism of action, can cause fetal harm.

Lactation: Do not breastfeed during treatment and for 2 weeks after the final dose.

Reproductive Potential: Females and male patients w/ female partners of reproductive potential should use effective contraception during treatment and for 2 months after the final dose.

MECHANISM OF ACTION

Multikinase inhibitor; inhibits multiple membrane-bound and intracellular kinases involved in normal cellular functions and in pathologic processes, such as oncogenesis, tumor angiogenesis, and maintenance of the tumor microenvironment.

PHARMACOKINETICS

Absorption: (Single 160mg dose) C_{max}=2.5mcg/mL, T_{max}=4 hrs (median), AUC=70.4mcg•hr/mL. (Steady state) C_{max}=3.9mcg/mL, AUC=58.3mcg•hr/mL. **Distribution:** Plasma protein binding (99.5%). **Metabolism:** CYP3A4, UGT1A9; M-2 (N-oxide) and M-5 (N-oxide and N-desmethyl) (active metabolites). **Elimination:** Urine (19%; 17% glucuronides), feces (approx 71%; 47% parent compound, 24% metabolites); $T_{1/2}$=28 hrs (regorafenib), 25 hrs (M-2), 51 hrs (M-5).

PATIENT CONSIDERATIONS

Assessment: Assess for scheduled/recent surgical procedures, hepatic impairment, HTN, pregnancy/nursing status, and possible drug interactions. Obtain baseline LFTs (ALT, AST, and bilirubin).

Monitoring: Monitor for hepatotoxicity, hemorrhage, dermatologic toxicity, HTN, myocardial ischemia or infarction, RPLS, wound dehiscence, GI perforation or fistula, and other adverse reactions. Monitor BP weekly for the first 6 weeks of treatment and then every cycle, or more frequently, as clinically indicated. Monitor LFTs at least every 2 weeks during the first 2 months of treatment, then monthly or more frequently as clinically indicated; monitor weekly in patients experiencing elevated LFTs until improvement to <3X ULN or baseline. Monitor INR levels more frequently in patients receiving warfarin.

Counseling: Instruct to take ud. Advise of the need to undergo monitoring for liver damage and to report immediately any signs/symptoms of severe liver damage. Advise to contact physician for unusual bleeding, bruising, or symptoms of bleeding (such as lightheadedness). Advise to contact physician if patient experiences skin changes associated w/ redness, pain, blisters, bleeding, swelling, or signs/symptoms of RPLS. Advise of the need to undergo BP monitoring and to contact physician if BP is elevated or if symptoms from HTN occur (including severe headache, lightheadedness, or neurologic symptoms). Advise to seek immediate emergency help if patient experiences chest pain, SOB, feeling dizzy, or feel like passing out. Advise to contact physician immediately if patient experiences severe pain in the abdomen, persistent swelling of the abdomen, high fever, chills, N/V, or dehydration. Instruct to contact physician if patient is planning to undergo a surgical procedure or had recent surgery. Advise that drug can cause fetal harm. Instruct women and men of reproductive potential to use effective contraception during treatment and for 2 months after completion of treatment. Instruct women of reproductive potential to immediately contact physician if pregnancy is suspected or confirmed during or w/in 2 months of completing treatment. Advise nursing mothers that it is not known whether drug is present in breast milk.

STRENSIQ — asfotase alfa
Rx

Class: Enzyme

ADULT DOSAGE
Hypophosphatasia

Perinatal/Infantile-Onset Hypophosphatasia (HPP):
2mg/kg 3X/week, or 1mg/kg 6X/week (6mg/kg/week)
Titrate: May increase up to 3mg/kg 3X/week (9mg/kg/week) for lack of efficacy

Juvenile-Onset HPP:
2mg/kg 3X/week, or 1mg/kg 6X/week (6mg/kg/week)

PEDIATRIC DOSAGE
Hypophosphatasia

Perinatal/Infantile-Onset HPP:
2mg/kg 3X/week, or 1mg/kg 6X/week (6mg/kg/week)
Titrate: May increase up to 3mg/kg 3X/week (9mg/kg/week) for lack of efficacy

Juvenile-Onset HPP:
2mg/kg 3X/week, or 1mg/kg 6X/week (6mg/kg/week)

Do not use the 80mg/0.8mL vial in pediatric patients <40kg

- -

ADMINISTRATION
SQ route

Administer w/in 1 hr upon removal from refrigeration.
Rotate among the following inj sites: abdominal area, thigh, or deltoid.
Do not administer in reddened, inflamed, or swollen areas.

Preparation
1. Determine the volume needed for the dose. Follow these steps to determine the dose:
Total dose (mg)=patient's weight (kg) x dose (mg/kg)
Total inj volume (mL)=total dose (mg)/concentration (40mg/mL or 80mg/0.8mL)
*Round total inj volume to the nearest hundredth of a mL
Total number of vials=total inj volume/vial volume (mL)
2. Determine frequency of weekly inj.
3. Determine dose. Round patient weights to the nearest kg. Refer to PI for guidance on weight-based dosing.
4. When preparing an inj volume >1mL, split the volume equally between 2 syringes, and administer 2 inj at 2 separate inj sites.
5. Administer using 1mL syringes and 1/2 inch inj needles, between 25-29 gauge. For doses >1mL, split the inj volume equally between two 1mL syringes.

STORAGE
2-8°C (36-46°F). Protect from light. Do not freeze or shake.

HOW SUPPLIED
Inj: 18mg/0.45mL, 28mg/0.7mL, 40mg/mL, 80mg/0.8mL

WARNINGS/PRECAUTIONS
Hypersensitivity reactions reported; d/c and initiate appropriate medical treatment if a severe reaction occurs. Localized lipodystrophy, including lipoatrophy and lipohypertrophy, reported at inj sites after several months. Patients w/ HPP are at increased risk for developing ectopic calcifications; ectopic calcification of the eye and kidneys reported, but there is insufficient information to determine whether or not these were consistent w/ the disease or due to therapy. Monitor using ophthalmology exams and renal ultrasounds at baseline and periodically during treatment.

ADVERSE REACTIONS
Inj-site reactions, lipodystrophy, ectopic calcifications, hypersensitivity reactions.

PREGNANCY AND LACTATION
Pregnancy: There are no available human data to inform a drug associated risk. In animal studies, fetal harm was not seen.
Lactation: There are no data on the presence of asfotase alfa in human milk, the effects on the breastfed infant, or the effects on milk production; caution in nursing.

MECHANISM OF ACTION
Tissue nonspecific alkaline phosphatase (TNSALP); replaces the TNSALP enzyme and reduces the TNSALP enzyme substrate levels. HPP is caused by a deficiency in TNSALP enzyme activity, which leads to elevations in several TNSALP substrates, including inorganic pyrophosphate.

PHARMACOKINETICS
Absorption: AUC=66,042 hr•ng/mL (≤5 years of age), 89,877 hr•ng/mL (>5-12 years of age); C_{max}=1,794ng/mL (≤5 years of age), 2,108ng/mL (>5-12 years of age); T_{max}=14.9 hrs (≤5 years of age), 20.8 hrs (>5-12 years of age). **Elimination:** $T_{1/2}$=approx 5 days.

PATIENT CONSIDERATIONS
Assessment: Assess for hypersensitivity to the drug, pregnancy/nursing status, and possible drug interactions. Perform ophthalmology exams and renal ultrasounds.
Monitoring: Monitor for hypersensitivity reactions, lipodystrophy, signs and symptoms of ophthalmic and renal ectopic calcifications, and changes in vision or renal function. Obtain ophthalmology exams and renal ultrasounds periodically.
Counseling: Advise patients or caregivers on the preparation and administration of therapy. Inform that hypersensitivity reactions may occur during and after treatment; advise to seek immediate medical care if signs and symptoms occur.

Inform that lipohypertrophy and localized atrophy have been reported at inj sites after several months; advise to follow proper inj technique and to rotate inj sites. Encourage to participate in the HPP registry, which has been established to better understand HPP and to monitor and evaluate long-term treatment effects.

STRIBILD — cobicistat/elvitegravir/emtricitabine/tenofovir disoproxil fumarate
Rx

Class: CYP3A inhibitor/HIV integrase strand transfer inhibitor/nucleoside reverse transcriptase inhibitor (NRTI) combination

> Lactic acidosis and severe hepatomegaly w/ steatosis, including fatal cases, reported w/ the use of nucleoside analogues in combination w/ other antiretrovirals. Not approved for the treatment of chronic hepatitis B virus (HBV) infection. Severe acute exacerbations of hepatitis B reported in patients coinfected w/ HBV and HIV-1 upon discontinuation of therapy; closely monitor hepatic function w/ both clinical and lab follow-up for at least several months. If appropriate, initiation of anti-hepatitis B therapy may be warranted.

ADULT DOSAGE
HIV-1 Infection

For use as a complete regimen for the treatment of HIV-1 infection in adults who have no antiretroviral treatment history or to replace the current antiretroviral regimen in those who are virologically-suppressed (HIV-1 RNA <50 copies/mL) on a stable antiretroviral regimen for at least 6 months w/ no history of treatment failure and no known substitutions associated w/ resistance to the individual components of the drug

1 tab qd

PEDIATRIC DOSAGE
Pediatric use may not have been established

- -

DOSING CONSIDERATIONS
Renal Impairment
CrCl <70mL/min: Initiation of treatment not recommended
CrCl Declines <50mL/min During Treatment: D/C therapy

Hepatic Impairment
Severe (Child-Pugh Class C): Not recommended

ADMINISTRATION
Oral route

Take w/ food.

STORAGE
25°C (77°F); excursions permitted to 15-30°C (59-86°F).

HOW SUPPLIED
Tab: (Cobicistat/Elvitegravir/Emtricitabine/Tenofovir Disoproxil Fumarate [TDF]) 150mg/150mg/200mg/300mg

CONTRAINDICATIONS
Concomitant use w/ drugs that are highly dependent on CYP3A for clearance and for which elevated plasma concentrations are associated w/ serious and/or life-threatening events and w/ other drugs that may lead to reduced efficacy, and possible resistance (eg, alfuzosin, carbamazepine, phenobarbital, phenytoin, rifampin, dihydroergotamine, ergotamine, methylergonovine, cisapride, St. John's wort, lovastatin, simvastatin, pimozide, sildenafil [when dosed as Revatio for the treatment of pulmonary arterial HTN], triazolam, oral midazolam).

WARNINGS/PRECAUTIONS
Test for HBV infection and document estimated CrCl, urine glucose, and urine protein prior to initiation of therapy. Not recommended for use in patients w/ severe hepatic impairment. Renal impairment, including cases of acute renal failure and Fanconi syndrome, reported; d/c if estimated CrCl <50mL/min. Do not initiate therapy in patients w/ estimated CrCl <70mL/min. Immune reconstitution syndrome, autoimmune disorders (eg, Graves' disease, polymyositis, Guillain-Barre syndrome) in the setting of immune reconstitution, and redistribution/accumulation of body fat reported. Caution in elderly. **Cobicistat:** May cause modest increases in SrCr and modest declines in estimated CrCl w/o affecting renal glomerular function; closely monitor patients w/ confirmed increase in SrCr >0.4mg/dL from baseline for renal safety. **TDF:** Obesity and prolonged nucleoside exposure may be risk factors for lactic acidosis and severe hepatomegaly. Caution w/ known risk factors for liver disease. D/C if lactic acidosis or pronounced hepatotoxicity occurs. Decreased bone mineral density (BMD), increased biochemical markers of bone metabolism, and osteomalacia reported. Consider hypophosphatemia and osteomalacia secondary to proximal renal tubulopathy in patients at risk of renal dysfunction who present w/ persistent/worsening bone or muscle symptoms.

ADVERSE REACTIONS
Diarrhea, nausea, fatigue, headache, dizziness, insomnia, abnormal dreams, rash, creatine kinase/amylase elevation, hematuria, AST elevation.

DRUG INTERACTIONS
See Contraindications. Avoid w/ cobicistat, elvitegravir, adefovir dipivoxil, rifabutin, rifapentine, salmeterol, ledipasvir/sofosbuvir, nephrotoxic agents (eg, high-dose or multiple NSAIDs), other antiretrovirals, or w/ products containing emtricitabine, TDF, lamivudine, or ritonavir. Avoid w/ colchicine in patients w/ renal or hepatic impairment. Antacids (eg, aluminum and magnesium hydroxide) may decrease elvitegravir levels; separate administration by at least 2 hrs. May increase levels of

antiarrhythmics (eg, digoxin), clonazepam, ethosuximide, ketoconazole, itraconazole, voriconazole, colchicine, β-blockers, calcium channel blockers, inhaled or nasal fluticasone, bosentan, atorvastatin, immunosuppressants, salmeterol, neuroleptics, PDE-5 inhibitors, and sedative/hypnotics (eg, benzodiazepines). May increase levels of quetiapine; consider alternative antiretroviral therapy. Concomitant use w/ inhaled or nasal fluticasone may reduce serum cortisol concentrations. May increase norgestimate and decrease ethinyl estradiol levels; caution w/ contraceptives containing norgestimate/ethinyl estradiol. Consider alternative (nonhormonal) methods of contraception. May increase levels of buprenorphine and norbuprenorphine and may decrease levels of naloxone; monitor for sedation and cognitive effects upon coadministration w/ buprenorphine/naloxone. Monitor INR upon coadministration w/ warfarin. May increase levels of antidepressants (eg, SSRIs, TCAs, trazodone); carefully titrate antidepressant dose and monitor response. May increase levels of clarithromycin; reduce clarithromycin dose by 50% in patients w/ CrCl 50-60mL/min. Anticonvulsants (eg, oxcarbazepine, clonazepam, ethosuximide) may decrease elvitegravir and cobicistat levels; consider alternative anticonvulsants. Rifabutin, rifapentine, and dexamethasone may decrease elvitegravir and cobicistat levels. Ketoconazole, itraconazole, or voriconazole may increase levels of elvitegravir and cobicistat. May increase levels of drugs that are primarily metabolized by CYP3A/2D6, or are substrates of P-gp, breast cancer resistance protein, or organic anion transporting polypeptides 1B1/1B3. Elvitegravir may decrease levels of CYP2C9 substrates. CYP3A inducers may decrease elvitegravir and cobicistat levels and may result in loss of therapeutic effect and development of resistance. Drugs that reduce renal function or compete for active tubular secretion (eg, acyclovir, cidofovir, gentamicin) may increase levels of emtricitabine, TDF, and other renally eliminated drugs and may increase risk of adverse reactions. CYP3A inhibitors and clarithromycin may increase plasma levels of cobicistat. Cases of acute renal failure after initiation of high-dose or multiple NSAIDs reported in patients w/ risk factors for renal dysfunction who appeared stable on TDF; consider alternatives to NSAIDs, if needed, in patients at risk for renal dysfunction. Ledipasvir/sofosbuvir may increase tenofovir levels. Refer to PI for dosing modifications when used w/ certain concomitant therapies.

PREGNANCY AND LACTATION
Pregnancy: Category B. An antiretroviral pregnancy registry has been established to monitor fetal outcomes of pregnant women.
Lactation: Not for use in nursing.

MECHANISM OF ACTION
Elvitegravir: HIV-1 integrase strand inhibitor; inhibits the strand transfer activity of HIV-1 integrase, preventing the integration of HIV-1 DNA into host genomic DNA, blocking the formation of HIV-1 provirus and propagation of the viral infection. **Cobicistat:** CYP3A inhibitor; enhances the systemic exposure of CYP3A substrates (eg, elvitegravir). **Emtricitabine:** Nucleoside analogue of cytidine; inhibits the activity of HIV-1 reverse transcriptase (RT) by competing w/ the natural substrate deoxycytidine 5'-triphosphate and being incorporated into nascent viral DNA, resulting in chain termination. **TDF:** Acyclic nucleoside phosphonate diester analogue of adenosine monophosphate; inhibits the activity of HIV-1 RT by competing w/ the natural substrate deoxyadenosine 5'-triphosphate and, after incorporation into DNA, by DNA chain termination.

PHARMACOKINETICS
Absorption: Elvitegravir: C_{max}=1.7 ± 0.4mcg/mL, AUC=23 ± 7.5mcg•hr/mL, T_{max}=4 hrs. Cobicistat: C_{max}=1.1 ± 0.4mcg/mL, AUC=8.3 ± 3.8mcg•hr/mL, T_{max}=3 hrs. Emtricitabine: C_{max}=1.9 ± 0.5mcg/mL, AUC=12.7 ± 4.5mcg•hr/mL, T_{max}=3 hrs. TDF: C_{max}=0.45 ± 0.2mcg/mL, AUC=4.4 ± 2.2mcg•hr/mL, T_{max}=2 hrs.
Distribution: Elvitegravir: Plasma protein binding (approx 99%). Cobicistat: Plasma protein binding (approx 98%). Emtricitabine: Plasma protein binding (<4%); found in breast milk. TDF: Plasma protein binding (<0.7%); found in breast milk. **Metabolism:** Elvitegravir: CYP3A (major), UGT1A1/3 (minor). Cobicistat: CYP3A (major), CYP2D6 (minor). **Elimination:** Elvitegravir: Feces (94.8%), urine (6.7%); $T_{1/2}$=12.9 hrs (median). Cobicistat: Feces (86.2%), urine (8.2%); $T_{1/2}$=3.5 hrs (median). Emtricitabine: Feces (13.7%), urine (70%); $T_{1/2}$=10 hrs (median). TDF: Urine (70-80%); $T_{1/2}$=12-18 hrs (median).

PATIENT CONSIDERATIONS
Assessment: Assess for obesity, prolonged nucleoside exposure, risk factors for liver disease, renal/hepatic impairment, pregnancy/nursing status, and possible drug interactions. Assess BMD in patients who have a history of pathological bone fracture or w/ other risk factors for osteoporosis or bone loss. Obtain baseline estimated CrCl, urine glucose, and urine protein. Perform test for HBV infection prior to therapy.

Monitoring: Monitor for signs/symptoms of lactic acidosis, severe hepatomegaly w/ steatosis, new onset/worsening renal impairment, immune reconstitution syndrome, autoimmune disorders, fat redistribution/accumulation, increased biochemical markers for bone metabolism, osteomalacia, and other adverse reactions. Monitor for exacerbations of hepatitis B in patients w/ coinfection for at least several months upon discontinuation of therapy. Monitor BMD, estimated CrCl, urine glucose, and urine protein. Monitor serum phosphorus levels in patients at risk for renal impairment. Monitor INR upon coadministration w/ warfarin.

Counseling: Advise to remain under care of a physician during therapy. Inform that therapy does not cure HIV-1 infection and continuous therapy is necessary to control HIV-1 infection and decrease HIV-related illnesses. Advise to practice safe sex, to use latex or polyurethane condoms, not to share personal items (eg, toothbrush, razor blades), needles, or other inj equipment, and not to breastfeed. Instruct to take on a regular dosing schedule w/ food and to avoid missing doses. Instruct to contact physician if symptoms of lactic acidosis/pronounced hepatotoxicity, or any symptoms of infection occur. Advise that fat redistribution/accumulation, renal impairment, and decreases in BMD may occur. Inform that hepatitis B testing is recommended prior to initiating therapy. Advise to report use of any prescription or nonprescription medication or herbal products, including St. John's wort.

SUCRAID — sacrosidase   Rx
Class: Enzyme

ADULT DOSAGE
Congenital Sucrase-Isomaltase Deficiency

Replacement therapy of the genetically determined sucrase deficiency, which is part of congenital sucrase-isomaltase deficiency

2mL (17,000 IU) (2 full measuring scoops or 56 drops) per meal or snack

PEDIATRIC DOSAGE
Congenital Sucrase-Isomaltase Deficiency

Replacement therapy of the genetically determined sucrase deficiency, which is part of congenital sucrase-isomaltase deficiency

≥5 Months of Age:
≤15kg: 1mL (8500 IU) (1 full measuring scoop or 28 drops) per meal or snack
<15kg: 2mL (17,000 IU) (2 full measuring scoops or 56 drops) per meal or snack

DOSING CONSIDERATIONS
Other Important Considerations
Do not reconstitute or consume w/ fruit juice

ADMINISTRATION
Oral route

Take orally w/ each meal or snack diluted w/ 2-4 oz (60-120mL) of water, milk, or infant formula; approx 1/2 of the dosage should be taken at the beginning of meal or snack and the remainder during the meal or snack
The beverage or infant formula should be served cold or at room temperature; do not warm or heat beverage or infant formula before or after addition of drug
Dose may be measured w/ the 1mL measuring scoop (provided) or by drop count method (1mL=28 drops from the container tip)

STORAGE
2-8°C (36-46°F). Protect from heat and light. Discard four weeks after first opening due to potential for bacterial growth.

HOW SUPPLIED
Sol: 8500 IU/mL [118mL]

CONTRAINDICATIONS
Known hypersensitivity to yeast, yeast products, glycerin (glycerol), or papain.

WARNINGS/PRECAUTIONS
Severe wheezing reported. Administer initial doses near a facility where acute hypersensitivity reactions may be adequately treated. May be tested for hypersensitivity through skin abrasion testing; d/c therapy and initiate symptomatic and supportive therapy if symptoms of hypersensitivity occur. Evaluate the need for dietary starch restriction. If diagnosis is in doubt, may be warranted to conduct a short therapeutic trial (eg, 1 week) w/ sacrosidase to assess response in a patient suspected of sucrase deficiency. Caution w/ diabetes mellitus (DM). Effects not evaluated in secondary (acquired) disaccharidase deficiencies.

ADVERSE REACTIONS
Abdominal pain, N/V, diarrhea, constipation, insomnia, headache, nervousness, dehydration.

DRUG INTERACTIONS
See Dosing Considerations. Fruit juice may reduce enzyme activity.

PREGNANCY AND LACTATION
Category C, caution in nursing.

MECHANISM OF ACTION
Enzyme; provides replacement therapy for sucrase deficiency.

PATIENT CONSIDERATIONS
Assessment: Assess for hypersensitivity to yeast/yeast products/glycerin/papain, asthma, DM, and pregnancy/nursing status.

Monitoring: Monitor for severe wheezing, hypersensitivity reactions, and other adverse reactions.

Counseling: Instruct to take 1/2 of the dosage at the beginning of the meal or snack and the remainder during the meal or snack. Inform that the product is sensitive to heat; instruct not to warm or heat the beverage or infant formula. Advise to rinse measuring scoop w/ water after each use. Instruct to not reconstitute or consume w/ fruit juice. Instruct to immediately get emergency help if difficulty breathing, wheezing, or swelling of the face occurs.

SUPPRELIN LA — histrelin acetate   Rx
Class: Synthetic gonadotropin-releasing hormone (GnRH) analogue

PEDIATRIC DOSAGE
Central Precocious Puberty

≥2 Years:
Usual: 1 implant (50mg histrelin acetate) SQ in the inner aspect of upper arm every 12 months

Remove after 12 months of therapy; at the time of removal, another implant may be inserted to continue therapy

ADMINISTRATION
SQ route
Refer to PI for recommended procedure for implant insertion and removal

STORAGE
Implant in Sealed Vial, Pouch, and Carton: 2-8°C (36-46°F); excursions permitted to 25°C (77°F) for 7 days. Do not freeze. Protect from light. Implantation Kit: Room temperature. Do not refrigerate.

HOW SUPPLIED
Implant: 50mg

CONTRAINDICATIONS
Hypersensitivity to GnRH or GnRH agonist analogs, females who are or may become pregnant.

WARNINGS/PRECAUTIONS
May cause transient increase in serum concentrations of estradiol in females and testosterone in both sexes during 1st week of treatment; may experience worsening of symptoms or onset of new symptoms. Proper surgical technique is critical during implant insertion and removal; imaging techniques (eg, ultrasound, CT, magnetic resonance imaging) were used when difficult to localize and/or remove implants. Rare events of spontaneous extrusion of implant reported; evaluate for evidence of clinical and biochemical suppression of CPP manifestations. Results of diagnostic tests of pituitary gonadotropic and gonadal functions conducted during and after therapy may be affected.

ADVERSE REACTIONS
Implant-site reaction, keloid scar, scar, suture related complication, application-site pain, post-procedural pain.

PREGNANCY AND LACTATION
Category X, safety not known in nursing.

MECHANISM OF ACTION
Synthetic gonadotropin-releasing hormone (GnRH) analog; reversible down-regulation of GnRH receptors in the pituitary gland and desensitization of pituitary gonadotropes, resulting in decreased levels of luteinizing hormone (LH) and follicle-stimulating hormone (FSH).

PHARMACOKINETICS
Absorption: C_{max}=0.43ng/mL.

PATIENT CONSIDERATIONS
Assessment: Assess for hypersensitivity to the drug and pregnancy status. Confirm clinical diagnosis of CPP by measuring blood concentrations of total sex steroids, LH, and FSH following stimulation with a GnRH analog, and assessment of bone age versus chronological age. Perform baseline evaluations of height and weight measurements, diagnostic imaging of the brain (to rule out intracranial tumor), pelvic/testicular/adrenal ultrasound (to rule out steroid-secreting tumors), human chorionic gonadotropin levels (to rule out a chorionic gonadotropin-secreting tumor), and adrenal steroids to exclude congenital adrenal hyperplasia.
Monitoring: Monitor for worsening/onset of new symptoms of puberty, extrusion of implant, suppression of CPP manifestations, implant breakage, and other adverse reactions. Monitor LH, FSH, and estradiol or testosterone at 1 month post-implantation, then every 6 months thereafter. Monitor height (height velocity) and bone age every 6-12 months.
Counseling: Advise that a transient worsening of symptoms of puberty or onset of new symptoms may occur initially; however, within 4 weeks of therapy, complete suppression of gonadal steroids occurs and manifestations of puberty decrease. Instruct to refrain from getting the inserted arm wet for 24 hrs and to avoid strenuous exertion of the inserted arm for 7 days after implant insertion. Instruct to remove adhesive elastic bandage at 7 days, but not surgical strips; inform that surgical strips should be allowed to fall off on their own after several days. Advise to contact physician if any severe pain, redness, or swelling in and around implant site occurs. Instruct to monitor the incision site until it is healed. Advise patients to return for routine checks of their condition and to ensure that implant is present and functioning.

SUSTIVA — efavirenz   Rx
Class: Non-nucleoside reverse transcriptase inhibitor (NNRTI)

ADULT DOSAGE
HIV-1 Infection
Combination w/ Protease Inhibitor and/or Nucleoside Analogue Reverse Transcriptase Inhibitors:
600mg qd

PEDIATRIC DOSAGE
HIV-1 Infection
Combination w/ Other Antiretrovirals:
≥3 Months of Age:
3.5 to <5kg: 100mg qd
5 to <7.5kg: 150mg qd
7.5 to <15kg: 200mg qd
15 to <20kg: 250mg qd
20 to <25kg: 300mg qd
25 to <32.5kg: 350mg qd
32.5 to <40kg: 400mg qd
≥40kg: 600mg qd

DOSING CONSIDERATIONS
Concomitant Medications
Voriconazole: Increase voriconazole maintenance dose to 400mg q12h and decrease efavirenz dose to 300mg qd (use one 200mg and two 50mg caps or six 50mg caps)

Rifampin:
≥50kg: Increase efavirenz dose to 800mg qd

Hepatic Impairment
Moderate to Severe (Child-Pugh Class B or C): Not recommended for use

ADMINISTRATION
Oral route
Take on empty stomach, preferably hs.
Swallow caps and tabs whole w/ liquid.
Tabs must not be broken.

Cap Sprinkle Method
Use if unable to swallow caps/tabs whole:
1. Gently mix entire cap contents w/ 1-2 tsp of an age-appropriate soft food (eg, applesauce, grape jelly, yogurt) and administer.
2. Add an additional small amount (approx 2 tsp) of food to the empty mixing container, stir, and administer.
3. Administer entire mixture w/in 30 min of mixing; do not consume additional food for 2 hrs after administration.

Young Infants Receiving Cap Sprinkle-Infant Formula Mixture:
1. Gently mix entire cap contents into 2 tsp of reconstituted room temperature infant formula in a small container by carefully stirring w/ a small spoon.
2. Draw up the mixture into a 10mL oral dosing syringe for administration and administer.
3. Add an additional small amount (approx 2 tsp) of formula to the empty mixing container, stir, draw up in oral syringe, and administer.
4. Administer entire mixture w/in 30 min of mixing; do not consume additional formula for 2 hrs after administration.

STORAGE
25°C (77°F); excursions permitted to 15-30°C (59-86°F).

HOW SUPPLIED
Cap: 50mg, 200mg; Tab: 600mg

CONTRAINDICATIONS
Previously demonstrated clinically significant hypersensitivity (eg, Stevens-Johnson syndrome, erythema multiforme, or toxic skin eruptions) to any of the components of this medication.

WARNINGS/PRECAUTIONS
Do not use as monotherapy or add on as a sole agent to a failing regimen. Not recommended w/ other efavirenz-containing products, unless needed for dose adjustment. Serious psychiatric events reported; immediate medical evaluation is recommended if symptoms occur. CNS symptoms reported; dosing at hs may improve tolerability. May impair mental/physical abilities. May cause fetal harm if administered during 1st trimester of pregnancy; avoid pregnancy during use. Skin rash reported; d/c and administer appropriate treatment if severe rash associated w/ blistering, desquamation, mucosal involvement, or fever develops. Consider alternative therapy in patients who have had a life-threatening cutaneous reaction (eg, Stevens-Johnson syndrome). Consider prophylaxis w/ appropriate antihistamines before initiating therapy in pediatric patients. Caution w/ mild hepatic impairment and in elderly. Hepatotoxicity reported; monitor liver enzymes before and during treatment in patients w/ underlying hepatic disease, marked transaminase elevations, and in patients taking other medications associated w/ liver toxicity; consider monitoring in patients w/o preexisting hepatic dysfunction/risk factors. Convulsions reported; caution w/ history of seizures. Lipid elevations, immune reconstitution syndrome, fat redistribution/accumulation, and autoimmune disorders (eg, Graves' disease, polymyositis, Guillain-Barre syndrome) in the setting of immune reconstitution reported. False-(+) urine cannabinoid test results reported; confirm positive results by a more specific method.

ADVERSE REACTIONS
Impaired concentration, abnormal dreams, rash, dizziness, N/V, headache, fatigue, insomnia.

DRUG INTERACTIONS
See Dosing Considerations. Avoid w/ other non-nucleoside reverse transcriptase inhibitors (NNRTIs); may alter the levels of efavirenz and/or the other NNRTI. Avoid w/ boceprevir. Not recommended w/ atovaquone/proguanil; may increase atovaquone levels and decrease proguanil levels. Potential additive CNS effects w/ alcohol or psychoactive drugs. CYP3A substrates, inhibitors, or inducers may alter levels. May alter levels of warfarin and drugs metabolized by CYP3A or CYP2B6. Concomitant use w/ fosamprenavir may decrease amprenavir levels. Ritonavir (RTV) and voriconazole may increase levels. CYP3A inducers (eg, phenobarbital, rifampin, rifabutin), carbamazepine, and anticonvulsants may decrease levels. May increase levels of RTV and 14-OH clarithromycin (active metabolite of clarithromycin). May decrease levels of atazanavir (avoid combination in treatment-experienced patients), indinavir, lopinavir, saquinavir, maraviroc, boceprevir, simeprevir, carbamazepine, anticonvulsants (monitor levels), bupropion, sertraline, voriconazole, itraconazole, hydroxyitraconazole (active metabolite of itraconazole), ketoconazole, clarithromycin, rifabutin, artemether, dihydroartemisinin (active metabolite of artemether), lumefantrine, atorvastatin, pravastatin, simvastatin, norgestimate, norelgestromin, levonorgestrel, etonogestrel, immunosuppressants, and methadone. May decrease levels of diltiazem, desacetyl diltiazem (metabolite of diltiazem), N-monodesmethyl diltiazem (metabolite of diltiazem), or other calcium channel blockers. Not recommended w/ simeprevir. May decrease posaconazole levels; avoid concomitant use unless benefit outweighs risks. Refer to PI for further dosing modifications when used w/ certain concomitant therapies.

PREGNANCY AND LACTATION
Pregnancy: Physicians are encouraged to register patients in the Antiretroviral Pregnancy Registry. There are retrospective case reports of neural tube defects in infants whose mothers were exposed to efavirenz-containing regimens in the 1st trimester of pregnancy; avoid use of efavirenz in the 1st trimester of pregnancy. No difference seen in the risk of overall major birth defects compared to the background rate for major birth defects.

Lactation: Mothers should be advised not to breastfeed due to potential for HIV transmission.

Reproductive Potential: Females of reproductive potential should undergo pregnancy testing before initiation of therapy and should use effective contraception during treatment and for 12 weeks after discontinuing therapy. Barrier contraception should always be used in combination w/ other methods of contraception. Hormonal methods that contain progesterone may have decreased effectiveness.

MECHANISM OF ACTION
NNRTI; mediated predominantly by noncompetitive inhibition of HIV-1 reverse transcriptase.

PHARMACOKINETICS
Absorption: T_{max}=3-5 hrs; (600mg qd) C_{max}=12.9μM, AUC=184μM•hr. **Distribution:** Plasma protein binding (99.5-99.75%). **Metabolism:** Via CYP3A and 2B6 (major) to hydroxylated metabolites w/ subsequent glucuronidation. **Elimination:** Urine (14-34%, <1% unchanged), feces (16-61%); $T_{1/2}$=40-55 hrs (multiple doses), 52-76 hrs (single dose).

PATIENT CONSIDERATIONS

Assessment: Assess for underlying hepatic disease, history of inj drug use/seizures/cutaneous reaction, psychiatric history, hypersensitivity to the drug, pregnancy/nursing status, and possible drug interactions. Assess baseline LFTs and lipid profile (eg, cholesterol, TGs).

Monitoring: Monitor for psychiatric events, CNS symptoms, skin rash, convulsions, immune reconstitution syndrome (eg, opportunistic infections), fat redistribution/accumulation, and other adverse reactions. Monitor LFTs and lipid profile.

Counseling: Inform that therapy is not a cure for HIV-1 infection and illnesses associated w/ HIV-1 infection may still be experienced. Advise to practice safer sex by using latex or polyurethane condoms, not to share or reuse needles or other inj equipment or personal items (eg, toothbrush, razor blades), and not to breastfeed. Advise to take medication ud and provide appropriate instructions for missed doses. Inform that CNS symptoms may occur during 1st weeks of therapy. Counsel that rash, psychiatric symptoms, and redistribution/accumulation of body fat may occur. Advise to avoid potentially hazardous tasks if experiencing CNS symptoms. Inform of the potential additive effects of the drug when used concomitantly w/ alcohol or psychoactive drugs. Instruct to seek medical attention if symptoms of rash and/or a serious psychiatric event occur. Advise to inform physician of any history of mental illness or substance abuse. Advise females of reproductive potential to use effective contraception as well as a barrier method during treatment and for 12 weeks after discontinuing therapy; instruct to contact physician if planning to become pregnant or if pregnancy occurs or is suspected during treatment. Advise that there is a pregnancy exposure registry that monitors pregnancy outcomes in women exposed to therapy during pregnancy. Advise to report use of any prescription or OTC medication.

SUTENT — sunitinib malate   Rx

Class: Kinase inhibitor

Hepatotoxicity has been observed; may be severe, and deaths have been reported.

ADULT DOSAGE

Gastrointestinal Stromal Tumor

After Disease Progression or Intolerance to Imatinib Mesylate:
50mg qd, on a schedule of 4 weeks on, followed by 2 weeks off

Advanced Renal Cell Carcinoma
50mg qd, on a schedule of 4 weeks on, followed by 2 weeks off

Advanced Pancreatic Neuroendocrine Tumors

Progressive, Well-Differentiated Tumors w/ Unresectable Locally Advanced or Metastatic Disease:
37.5mg qd continuously w/o a scheduled off-treatment period

PEDIATRIC DOSAGE
Pediatric use may not have been established

DOSING CONSIDERATIONS
Concomitant Medications
Selection of an alternate concomitant medication w/ no or minimal enzyme inhibition/induction potential is recommended
Strong CYP3A4 Inhibitors:
GI Stromal Tumors/Advanced Renal Cell Carcinoma: Consider dose reduction to a minimum of 37.5mg qd
Advanced Pancreatic Neuroendocrine Tumors: Consider dose reduction to a minimum of 25mg qd

CYP3A4 Inducers:
GI Stromal Tumors/Advanced Renal Cell Carcinoma: Consider dose increase to a max of 87.5mg qd
Advanced Pancreatic Neuroendocrine Tumors: Consider dose increase to a max of 62.5mg qd

Renal Impairment
ESRD on Hemodialysis: May increase gradually up to 2-fold based on safety and tolerability for subsequent doses

Other Important Considerations
Interruption and/or modification in 12.5mg increments or decrements is recommended based on individual safety and tolerability

ADMINISTRATION
Oral route
Take w/ or w/o food.

STORAGE
25°C (77°F); excursions permitted to 15-30°C (59-86°F).

HOW SUPPLIED
Cap: 12.5mg, 25mg, 37.5mg, 50mg

WARNINGS/PRECAUTIONS
Interrupt therapy for Grade 3 or 4 hepatic adverse events; d/c if no resolution. Do not restart treatment if subsequent severe changes in LFTs or other signs/symptoms of liver failure occur. May cause fetal harm; avoid pregnancy. D/C in the presence of clinical manifestations of CHF, and interrupt and/or reduce dose in patients w/o clinical evidence of CHF but w/ ejection fraction <50% and >20% below baseline. Cardiovascular (CV) events, including heart failure, cardiomyopathy, myocardial ischemia, and MI reported; use w/ caution in patients who are at risk for, or have a history of, these events. Decline in left ventricular ejection fraction (LVEF) reported. Dose-dependent QT interval prolongation and torsades de pointes reported; caution w/ history of QT interval prolongation or preexisting cardiac disease, bradycardia, or electrolyte disturbances. Monitor for HTN and treat prn; temporarily suspend in cases of severe HTN until controlled. Hemorrhagic events, including tumor-related hemorrhage and pulmonary hemorrhage, reported. Serious, sometimes fatal GI complications (eg, GI perforation) reported w/ intra-abdominal malignancies. Tumor lysis syndrome (TLS) reported; closely monitor patients presenting w/ a high tumor burden prior to treatment and treat as clinically indicated. Thrombotic microangiopathy (TMA), including thrombotic thrombocytopenic purpura and hemolytic syndrome, reported; d/c if TMA develops. Proteinuria and nephrotic syndrome reported; interrupt and reduce dose for 24-hr urine protein ≥3g. D/C therapy for patients w/ nephrotic syndrome or repeat episodes of urine protein ≥3g despite dose reductions. Severe cutaneous reactions (eg, erythema multiforme, Stevens Johnson syndrome [SJS], toxic epidermal necrolysis [TEN]) reported; d/c therapy if signs/symptoms are present and do not restart treatment if a diagnosis of SJS or TEN is suspected. Necrotizing fasciitis reported; d/c therapy in patients who develop necrotizing fasciitis. Hyperthyroidism, some followed by hypothyroidism, reported; observe closely for signs/symptoms of thyroid dysfunction (eg, hypo/hyperthyroidism, thyroiditis). Associated w/ symptomatic hypoglycemia, resulting in loss of consciousness, or requiring hospitalization; reductions in blood glucose may be worse in diabetic patients. Osteonecrosis of the jaw (ONJ) reported; exposure to risk factors (eg, dental disease) may increase the risk of ONJ. Impaired wound healing reported; interrupt temporarily in patients undergoing major surgical procedures. Monitor for adrenal insufficiency in patients w/ stress, trauma, or severe infection.

ADVERSE REACTIONS
Fatigue, asthenia, fever, diarrhea, N/V, mucositis/stomatitis, dyspepsia, abdominal pain, constipation, HTN, peripheral edema, rash, hand-foot syndrome, skin discoloration.

DRUG INTERACTIONS
See Dosing Considerations. Caution w/ antiarrhythmics for QT interval prolongation/torsades de pointes. Strong CYP3A4 inhibitors (eg, ketoconazole, nefazodone, ritonavir) and grapefruit may increase levels. CYP3A4 inducers (eg, dexamethasone, phenytoin, rifampin) may decrease levels. Avoid w/ St. John's wort. TMA reported w/ bevacizumab. Concomitant use w/ bisphosphonates may increase the risk of ONJ.

PREGNANCY AND LACTATION
Pregnancy: Category D. May cause fetal harm; avoid pregnancy.
Lactation: Not for use in nursing.

MECHANISM OF ACTION
Multikinase inhibitor; inhibits multiple receptor tyrosine kinases, some of which are implicated in tumor growth, pathologic angiogenesis, and metastatic cancer progression.

PHARMACOKINETICS
Absorption: T_{max}=6-12 hrs. **Distribution:** V_d=2230L; plasma protein binding (95%, 90%[primary active metabolite]). **Metabolism:** Liver via CYP3A4. **Elimination:** Feces (61%), urine (16%); $T_{1/2}$=40-60 hrs, 80-110 hrs (primary active metabolite).

PATIENT CONSIDERATIONS

Assessment: Assess for risk/history of cardiac events, cardiac disease, bradycardia, electrolyte disturbances, dental disease, high tumor burden, diabetes, pregnancy/nursing status, and possible drug interactions. Obtain baseline LFTs, LVEF, thyroid function, CBC w/ platelet count, serum chemistries (eg, phosphate), and urinalysis.

Monitoring: Monitor for signs/symptoms of CV events, HTN, hemorrhagic events, ONJ, TLS, TMA, adrenal insufficiency, hepatotoxicity, nephrotic syndrome, severe cutaneous reactions, necrotizing fasciitis, and other adverse reactions. Monitor LFTs, LVEF (in patients w/ cardiac risk factors), ECG, electrolytes (Mg^{2+}, K^+), thyroid function, CBC w/ platelet count, and serum chemistries (eg, phosphate). Monitor blood glucose levels regularly during and after discontinuation of treatment. Perform periodic urinalysis w/ follow-up measurement of 24-hr urine protein as clinically indicated.

Counseling: Inform about the most commonly reported GI disorders and other adverse reactions that may occur. Advise that depigmentation of the hair or skin and other possible dermatologic effects may occur during treatment. Inform that severe dermatologic toxicities (eg, SJS, TEN) have been reported; advise to immediately inform physician if severe dermatologic reactions occur. Advise to consider a dental examination and appropriate preventive dentistry prior to treatment. Instruct to avoid invasive dental procedures if previously or concomitantly taking bisphosphonates. Advise of the signs, symptoms, and risks associated w/ hypoglycemia that may occur while on therapy; instruct to immediately inform physician if severe signs/symptoms of hypoglycemia occur. Inform of the signs/symptoms of TMA; instruct to inform physician if TMA occurs. Advise that urinalysis will be performed prior to and during treatment. Advise to inform physician of all concomitant medications, including OTC medications and dietary supplements. Inform of pregnancy risks; advise women of childbearing potential to avoid becoming pregnant.

SYLATRON — peginterferon alfa-2b   Rx

Class: Biological response modifier

> Increased risk of serious depression, w/ suicidal ideation and completed suicides, and other serious neuropsychiatric disorders. Permanently d/c in patients w/ persistently severe or worsening signs or symptoms of depression, psychosis, or encephalopathy; may not resolve after stopping therapy.

ADULT DOSAGE

Melanoma
Adjuvant treatment of melanoma w/ microscopic or gross nodal involvement w/in 84 days of definitive surgical resection including complete lymphadenectomy

Initial: 6mcg/kg/week SQ for 8 doses
Follow-Up: 3mcg/kg/week SQ for up to 5 yrs

Premedication
Acetaminophen 500-1000mg PO 30 min prior to 1st dose and prn for subsequent doses

PEDIATRIC DOSAGE
Pediatric use may not have been established

DOSING CONSIDERATIONS
Renal Impairment
Moderate (CrCl 30-50mL/min/1.73m²):
Initial: 4.5mcg/kg/week for 8 weeks
Follow-Up: 2.25mcg/kg/week for 5 yrs
Severe (CrCl <30mL/min/1.73m²)/ESRD on Dialysis:
Initial: 3mcg/kg/week for 8 weeks
Follow-Up: 1.5mcg/kg/week for 5 yrs

Adverse Reactions
Permanently D/C Therapy for:
- Persistent or worsening severe neuropsychiatric disorders
- Grade 4 non-hematologic toxicity
- Inability to tolerate a dose of 1mcg/kg/week
- New or worsening retinopathy

Withhold Dose for Any of the Following:
- ANC <0.5 x 10⁹/L
- Platelet count (PLT) <50 x 10⁹/L
- ECOG PS ≥2
- Non-hematologic toxicity ≥Grade 3

Resume Dosing at Reduced Dose When All of the Following Are Present:
- ANC ≥0.5 x 10⁹/L
- PLT ≥50 x 10⁹/L
- ECOG PS 0-1
- Non-hematologic toxicity has completely resolved or improved to Grade 1

Sylatron Dose Modifications:
Patients Using 6mcg/kg/week for Doses 1-8:
1st Dose Modification: 3mcg/kg/week
2nd Dose Modification: 2mcg/kg/week
3rd Dose Modification: 1mcg/kg/week
Permanently d/c if unable to tolerate 1mcg/kg/week

Patients Using 3mcg/kg/week for Doses 9-260:
1st Dose Modification: 2mcg/kg/week
2nd Dose Modification: 1mcg/kg/week
Permanently d/c if unable to tolerate 1mcg/kg/week

ADMINISTRATION
SQ route

Rotate inj sites.
If reconstituted sol is not used immediately, store at 2-8°C (36-46°F) for no more than 24 hrs; discard after 24 hrs. Do not freeze.

Preparation and Administration
1. Reconstitute w/ 0.7mL of sterile water for inj.
2. Swirl gently to dissolve the lyophilized powder; do not shake.
3. Do not withdraw >0.5mL of reconstituted sol from each vial.

STORAGE
25°C (77°F); excursions permitted to 15-30°C (59-86°F). Do not freeze.

HOW SUPPLIED
Inj: 200mcg, 300mcg, 600mcg

CONTRAINDICATIONS
History of anaphylaxis to peginterferon alfa-2b or interferon alfa-2b, autoimmune hepatitis, hepatic decompensation (Child-Pugh score >6 [class B and C]).

WARNINGS/PRECAUTIONS
Monitor and evaluate for depression and other psychiatric symptoms every 3 weeks during the first 8 weeks of therapy, every 6 months thereafter, and for at least 6 months after the last dose. Cardiac adverse reactions reported; permanently d/c for new onset of ventricular arrhythmia or cardiovascular decompensation. May cause decrease in visual acuity or blindness due to retinopathy; retinal and ocular changes may be induced or aggravated by treatment. Perform an eye exam at baseline in patients w/ preexisting retinopathy and during therapy if visual changes occur; permanently d/c if new/worsening retinopathy develops. Increases risk of hepatic decompensation and death in patients w/ cirrhosis; permanently d/c for evidence of severe (Grade 3) hepatic injury/decompensation (Child-Pugh score >6 [class B and C]). Monitor hepatic function w/ serum bilirubin, ALT, AST, alkaline phosphatase, and LDH at 2 and 8 weeks, and 2 and 3 months following initiation, then every 6 months thereafter. May cause new, onset/worsening of hypo/hyperthyroidism, and diabetes mellitus (DM); permanently d/c if any of these conditions and cannot be effectively managed. Obtain TSH levels w/in 4 weeks prior to initiation of therapy, at 3 and 6 months following initiation, then every 6 months thereafter while on therapy.

ADVERSE REACTIONS
Fatigue, increased AST/ALT, pyrexia, headache, anorexia, myalgia, nausea, chills, inj-site reaction.

DRUG INTERACTIONS
Increased exposure to caffeine (CYP1A2 substrate) or desipramine (CYP2D6 substrate) during coadministration; monitor for potential toxicities of drugs w/ a narrow therapeutic range metabolized by CYP1A2 or CYP2D6.

PREGNANCY AND LACTATION
Pregnancy: Category C.
Lactation: It is not known whether the components of Sylatron are excreted in human milk; not for use in nursing.

MECHANISM OF ACTION
Pleiotropic cytokine; mechanism not established.

PHARMACOKINETICS
Absorption: (6mcg/kg/week) C_{max}=4.4ng/mL, AUC=430ng•hr/mL; (3mcg/kg/week) C_{max}=2.5ng/mL, AUC=228ng•hr/mL. **Elimination:** $T_{1/2}$=(6mcg/kg/week) 51 hrs; (3mcg/kg/week) 43 hrs.

PATIENT CONSIDERATIONS
Assessment: Assess for history of autoimmune hepatitis, hepatic decompensation, cirrhosis, neuropsychiatric disorders, history of anaphylaxis to peginterferon alfa-2b or interferon alfa-2b, hypo/hyperthyroidism, DM, renal impairment, pregnancy/nursing status, and possible drug interactions. Perform baseline eye exam in patients w/ preexisting retinopathy. Obtain TSH levels w/in 4 weeks prior to therapy.

Monitoring: Monitor for cardiac adverse events, new/worsening retinopathy, and other adverse reactions. Obtain TSH levels at 3 and 6 months following initiation, then every 6 months thereafter while on therapy. Monitor and evaluate for depression and other psychiatric symptoms every 3 weeks during the first 8 weeks of therapy, every 6 months thereafter, and for at least 6 months after the last dose. Monitor CBC and platelet counts periodically. Monitor hepatic function w/ serum bilirubin, ALT, AST, alkaline phosphatase, and LDH at 2 and 8 weeks, and 2 and 3 months following initiation, then every 6 months thereafter. Perform eye exam if visual changes develop.

Counseling: Advise that drug may be administered w/ antipyretics at hs to minimize common flu-like symptoms, and advise to maintain hydration if symptoms occur. Instruct to report immediately any symptoms of depression or suicidal ideation to physician during treatment and up to 6 months after the last dose. Advise to notify physician in the event of pregnancy. Instruct not to reuse or share syringes and needles. Instruct on proper disposal of vials, syringes, and needles.

SYLVANT — siltuximab   Rx

Class: Monoclonal antibody/interleukin-6 (IL-6) receptor antagonist

ADULT DOSAGE
Multicentric Castleman's Disease
Treatment of patients who are HIV negative and human herpesvirus-8 negative

11mg/kg given over 1 hr as an IV infusion administered every 3 weeks until treatment failure

Perform hematology lab tests prior to each dose for the first 12 months and every 3 dosing cycles thereafter. If treatment criteria outlined below are not met, consider delaying treatment; do not reduce dose

Treatment Criteria
Requirements Prior to 1st Dose:
ANC: ≥1.0 x 10⁹/L
Platelet Count: ≥75 x 10⁹/L
Hgb: <17 g/dL

Retreatment Criteria:
ANC: ≥1.0 x 10⁹/L
Platelet Count: ≥50 x 10⁹/L
Hgb: <17 g/dL

PEDIATRIC DOSAGE
Pediatric use may not have been established

DOSING CONSIDERATIONS

Adverse Reactions
D/C in patients w/ severe infusion related reactions, anaphylaxis, severe allergic reactions, or cytokine release syndromes; do not reinstitute treatment

Other Important Considerations
Do not administer to patients w/ severe infections until the infection resolves

ADMINISTRATION
IV route

Preparation
1. Calculate the dose (mg), total volume (mL) of reconstituted sol required, and the number of vials needed. A 21-gauge 1-1/2 inch needle is recommended for preparation. Infusion bags (250mL) must contain D5W and must be made of polyvinyl chloride, polyolefin, polypropylene, or polyethylene. Alternatively, polyethylene bottles may be used.
2. Allow the vial(s) to come to room temperature over approx 30 min. Sylvant should remain at room temperature for the duration of the preparation.
3. Reconstitute each vial as follows:
100mg Vial: Reconstitute w/ 5.2mL of sterile water for inj (SWFI)
400mg Vial: Reconstitute w/ 20mL of SWFI
4. Gently swirl reconstituted vials; do not shake or swirl vigorously. The lyophilized powder should dissolve in <60 min. Reconstituted product should be kept for no more than 2 hrs prior to addition into the infusion bag.
5. Dilute the reconstituted sol dose to 250mL w/ sterile D5W by withdrawing a volume equal to the total calculated volume of reconstituted sol from the D5W, 250 mL bag.
6. Slowly add the total calculated volume (mL) of reconstituted sol to the D5W infusion bag. Gently invert the bag to mix the sol.

Administration
Administer the diluted sol by IV infusion over a period of 1 hr using administration sets lined w/ polyvinyl chloride, polyurethane, or polyethylene, containing a 0.2μm inline polyethersulfone filter. The infusion should be completed w/in 4 hrs of the dilution of the reconstituted sol to the infusion bag.
Do not infuse concomitantly in the same IV line w/ other agents.
Do not store any unused portion of the reconstituted product or of the infusion sol.

STORAGE
2-8°C (36-46°F). Protect from light.

HOW SUPPLIED
Inj: 100mg, 400mg

CONTRAINDICATIONS
Severe hypersensitivity reaction to siltuximab or any of the excipients in the product.

WARNINGS/PRECAUTIONS
May increase Hgb levels. Do not administer to patients w/ severe infections until the infection resolves. May mask signs and symptoms of acute inflammation including suppression of fever and of acute phase reactants (eg, C-reactive protein). D/C if signs of anaphylaxis or mild to moderate infusion reaction develops. If the infusion reaction resolves, may restart infusion at a lower infusion rate and consider medication w/ antihistamines, acetaminophen, and corticosteroids; d/c if the patient does not tolerate the infusion following these interventions. Administer in a setting that provides resuscitation equipment, medication, and personnel trained to provide resuscitation. GI perforation reported. Women of childbearing potential should use contraception during and for 3 months after treatment.

ADVERSE REACTIONS
Pruritus, increased weight, rash, hyperuricemia, URTI.

DRUG INTERACTIONS
Do not administer live vaccines. May increase metabolism of CYP450 substrates; upon initiation or discontinuation of siltuximab, in patients being treated w/ CYP450 substrates w/ a narrow therapeutic index, perform therapeutic monitoring of effect (eg, warfarin) or drug concentration (eg, cyclosporine, theophylline) prn and adjust dose. Caution w/ CYP3A4 substrates where a decrease in effectiveness would be undesirable (eg, oral contraceptives, lovastatin, atorvastatin).

PREGNANCY AND LACTATION
Pregnancy: Category C. Infants born to pregnant women treated w/ siltuximab may be at increased risk of infection. Women of childbearing potential should use contraception during and for 3 months after treatment.
Lactation: Not for use in nursing.

MECHANISM OF ACTION
Monoclonal antibody/IL-6 receptor antagonist; binds human IL-6 and prevents the binding of IL-6 to both soluble and membrane-bound IL-6 receptors.

PHARMACOKINETICS
Absorption: C_{max}=332mcg/mL. **Distribution:** V_d=4.5L (70kg male). **Elimination:** $T_{1/2}$=20.6 days.

PATIENT CONSIDERATIONS

Assessment: Assess for infection, risk for GI perforation, drug hypersensitivity, pregnancy/nursing status, and possible drug interactions. Perform hematology lab tests prior to each dose of therapy for the first 12 months and every 3 dosing cycles thereafter.

Monitoring: Monitor for signs/symptoms of infection, infusion-related reactions, hypersensitivity, GI perforation, and other adverse reactions.

Counseling: Inform of benefits and risks of treatment. Instruct to immediately contact physician when symptoms suggesting infection or any signs of new/worsening medical conditions appear. Advise to seek immediate medical

attention if any symptoms of a serious allergic reaction occur during the infusion. Advise patients of childbearing potential to avoid pregnancy; instruct to use contraception during and for 3 months after treatment.

SYNAGIS — palivizumab   Rx
Class: Monoclonal antibody/RSV F-protein blocker

PEDIATRIC DOSAGE
Respiratory Syncytial Virus
Prevention of serious lower respiratory tract disease in children at high risk of RSV disease

≤24 Months of Age:
15mg/kg monthly throughout RSV season; administer first dose prior to start of RSV season

Undergoing Cardiopulmonary Bypass:
Administer an additional dose as soon as possible after the procedure (even if <1 month from previous dose) then monthly thereafter, as scheduled

ADMINISTRATION
IM route
If RSV infection develops, continue monthly doses throughout RSV season.
Give inj volumes >1mL as a divided dose.
Do not dilute, shake, or vigorously agitate vial.
Administer immediately after withdrawal from vial.
Administer preferably into the anterolateral aspect of the thigh.
Refer to PI for further instructions.

STORAGE
2-8°C (36-46°F). Do not freeze.

HOW SUPPLIED
Inj: 50mg/0.5mL, 100mg/mL

CONTRAINDICATIONS
Previous significant hypersensitivity reaction to palivizumab.

WARNINGS/PRECAUTIONS
Anaphylaxis, anaphylactic shock, and other acute hypersensitivity reactions reported; permanently d/c if a significant hypersensitivity reaction occurs, and use caution during readministration if a mild hypersensitivity reaction occurs. Caution with thrombocytopenia or any coagulation disorder. May interfere with immunological-based RSV diagnostic tests and viral culture assays; diagnostic test results should be used in conjunction with clinical findings.

ADVERSE REACTIONS
Fever, rash, anaphylaxis.

PREGNANCY AND LACTATION
Pregnancy: Category C.
Lactation: Safety not known in nursing.

MECHANISM OF ACTION
Monoclonal antibody/RSV F-protein blocker; provides passive immunity against RSV. Acts by binding the RSV envelope fusion protein on the surface of the virus and blocking a critical step in the membrane fusion process. Also prevents cell-to-cell fusion of RSV-infected cells.

PHARMACOKINETICS
Absorption: Bioavailability (70%). **Elimination:** $T_{1/2}$=20 days.

PATIENT CONSIDERATIONS

Assessment: Assess for previous hypersensitivity to the drug, thrombocytopenia, and coagulation disorders. Assess if patient is undergoing cardiopulmonary bypass.

Monitoring: Monitor for anaphylaxis, hypersensitivity reactions, and other adverse reactions.

Counseling: Counsel parents/guardians about the potential risks and benefits of therapy. Inform parents/guardians of the possible side effects and of the signs/symptoms of potential allergic reactions; advise of the appropriate actions. Advise parents/guardians of the dosing schedule and the importance of compliance with the full course of therapy.

SYNAREL — nafarelin acetate   Rx
Class: Gonadotropin-releasing hormone (GnRH) analogue

PEDIATRIC DOSAGE
Central Precocious Puberty

Gonadotropin-Dependent Precocious Puberty in Children of Both Sexes:
2 sprays (400mcg)/nostril qam and qpm
Total Daily Dose: 1600mcg

Titrate:
If inadequate suppression, may increase to 1800mcg/day as 3 sprays

(600mcg) into alternating nostrils tid, for a total of 9 sprays/day

Should continue until resumption of puberty is desired if therapy has been well tolerated

May increase dose to 800mcg/day (1 spray in each nostril bid [am and pm]) if patient experiences persistent regular menstruation after 2 months of treatment

Treat for 6 months; retreatment is not recommended

DOSING CONSIDERATIONS
Concomitant Medications
Do not use a nasal decongestant for rhinitis until ≥2 hrs following dosing

ADMINISTRATION
Intranasal route

Tilt head back slightly; 30 sec should elapse between sprays. Avoid sneezing during or immediately after dosing.

STORAGE
Store upright at 25°C (77°F); excursions permitted to 15-30°C (59-86°F). Protect from light.

HOW SUPPLIED
Spray: 200mcg/spray [60 sprays]

CONTRAINDICATIONS
Hypersensitivity to GnRH, GnRH agonist analogs or any of the excipients in this medication; undiagnosed abnormal vaginal bleeding; women who are or may become pregnant, and breastfeeding.

WARNINGS/PRECAUTIONS
Establish diagnosis of central precocious puberty before initiating therapy. Monitor regularly to assess response and compliance. Begin assessment of growth velocity and bone age velocity w/in 3-6 months of treatment initiation. Some may not show suppression of the pituitary-gonadal axis due to lack of compliance w/ the recommended regimen. Reconsider possibility of gonadotropin-independent sexual precocity and conduct appropriate exams if compliance problems are excluded. In adult women w/ endometriosis, ovarian cysts reported to occur in the first 2 months of therapy w/ nafarelin.

ADVERSE REACTIONS
Acne, transient breast enlargement, vaginal bleeding, emotional lability, transient increase in pubic hair, rhinitis, body odor, seborrhea, white/brownish vaginal discharge.

PREGNANCY AND LACTATION
Pregnancy: Category X.
Lactation: Not for use in nursing.

MECHANISM OF ACTION
GnRH analogue; initially, stimulates the release of the pituitary gonadotropins, luteinizing hormone (LH) and follicle-stimulating hormone, resulting in a temporary increase in gonadal steroidogenesis. Repeated dosing abolishes the stimulatory effects on the pituitary gland. Decreased secretions of gonadal steroids cause gonadal steroid-dependent tissues and functions to become quiescent.

PHARMACOKINETICS
Absorption: Rapid; C_{max}=2.2ng/mL (400mcg single dose), 6.6ng/mL (600mcg single dose); T_{max}=10-45 min. **Distribution:** Plasma protein binding (80% at 4°C). **Metabolism:** Tyr-D(2)-Nal-Leu-Arg-Pro-Gly-NH₂(5-10) (major metabolite). **Elimination:** $T_{1/2}$=approx 2.5 hrs; (SQ, Men) Urine (44-55%), feces (18.5-44.2%).

PATIENT CONSIDERATIONS
Assessment: Assess for drug hypersensitivity, undiagnosed vaginal bleeding, pregnancy/nursing status, and for possible drug interactions. Obtain diagnosis of CPP prior to treatment. Evaluate MRI or CT scan of the brain to detect hypothalamic or pituitary tumors, or anatomical changes associated w/ increased intracranial pressure. Assess for other causes of sexual precocity (eg, congenital adrenal hyperplasia, testotoxicosis, testicular tumors, other autonomous feminizing or masculinizing disorders) prior to treatment.

Monitoring: Monitor for possible adverse reactions. Perform regular monitoring of LH response to GnRH stimulation and circulating gonadal sex steroid levels. Monitor during first 6-8 weeks for rapid suppression of pituitary gonadal function. Monitor growth velocity and bone age velocity w/in 3-6 months of initiating treatment.

Counseling: Advise about full compliance of therapy; inform that irregular or incomplete daily doses may result in stimulation of the pituitary-gonadal axis. Counsel that during the 1st month of treatment, signs of puberty (eg, vaginal bleeding or breast enlargement) may occur; instruct to notify physician if symptoms do not resolve w/in first 2 months of treatment. Instruct to consult a physician about use of a topical decongestant for intercurrent rhinitis. If topical nasal decongestant is required, do not use decongestant until ≥2 hrs following therapy. Instruct to avoid sneezing during or immediately after dosing.

SYNAREL (GYN) — nafarelin acetate   Rx
Class: Gonadotropin-releasing hormone (GnRH) analogue

ADULT DOSAGE	PEDIATRIC DOSAGE
Endometriosis	Pediatric use may not have been established
For Pain Relief and Reduction of Endometriotic Lesions:	
Initiate therapy between Days 2 and 4 of the menstrual cycle	
1 spray (200mcg) in 1 nostril qam and 1 spray into the other nostril qpm	

DOSING CONSIDERATIONS
Concomitant Medications
Do not use a nasal decongestant for rhinitis until ≥2 hrs following dosing

ADMINISTRATION
Intranasal route

Avoid sneezing during or immediately after dosing.

STORAGE
Store upright at 25°C (77°F); excursions permitted to 15-30°C (59-86°F). Protect from light.

HOW SUPPLIED
Spray: 200mcg/spray [60 sprays]

CONTRAINDICATIONS
Hypersensitivity to GnRH, GnRH agonist analogs or any of the excipients in this medication; undiagnosed abnormal vaginal bleeding; women who are or may become pregnant, and breastfeeding.

WARNINGS/PRECAUTIONS
Pregnancy must be excluded before starting treatment; d/c therapy if patient becomes pregnant during treatment. Use nonhormonal methods of contraception during therapy. Ovarian cysts reported during first 2 months of treatment. Cystic enlargements may resolve by about 4-6 weeks of therapy, but in some cases may require discontinuation of drug and/or surgical intervention. Suppression of the pituitary-gonadal system reported; diagnostic tests of pituitary gonadotropic and gonadal functions conducted during treatment and up to 4 to 8 weeks after discontinuation of therapy may be misleading.

ADVERSE REACTIONS
Hot flashes, decreased libido, vaginal dryness, headache, emotional lability, acne, myalgia, nasal irritation, reduced breast size, insomnia, edema, seborrhea, weight gain, depression, hirsutism.

PREGNANCY AND LACTATION
Pregnancy: Category X.
Lactation: Not for use in nursing.

MECHANISM OF ACTION
GnRH analogue; initially, stimulates release of the pituitary gonadotropins, luteinizing hormone and follicle-stimulating hormone, resulting in a temporary increase of ovarian steroidogenesis. Repeated dosing abolishes the stimulatory effects on the pituitary gland. Decreased secretions of gonadal steroids cause gonadal steroid-dependent tissues and functions to become quiescent.

PHARMACOKINETICS
Absorption: Rapid; C_{max}=0.6ng/mL (200mcg single dose), 1.8ng/mL (400mcg single dose); T_{max}=10-40 min. **Distribution:** Plasma protein binding (80% at 4°C). **Metabolism:** Tyr-D(2)-Nal-Leu-Arg-Pro-Gly-NH₂(5-10) (major metabolite). **Elimination:** $T_{1/2}$=approx 3 hrs; (SQ, Men) Urine (44-55%), feces (18.5-44.2%).

PATIENT CONSIDERATIONS
Assessment: Assess for drug hypersensitivity, polycystic ovary disease, undiagnosed vaginal bleeding, pregnancy/nursing status, and possible drug interactions. Assess use in patients who have major risk factors for decreased bone density.

Monitoring: Monitor for the occurrence of ovarian cysts during the first 2 months of therapy and other adverse reactions.

Counseling: Instruct to notify physician if regular menstruation persists. Counsel to avoid use if pregnant, breastfeeding, have undiagnosed abnormal vaginal bleeding, or allergic to any of the ingredients. Advise to use nonhormonal method of contraception and that breakthrough bleeding or ovulation may occur if successive doses are missed. Instruct to d/c and consult physician if patient becomes pregnant. Instruct to consult a physician about use of a topical decongestant for intercurrent rhinitis. If a topical decongestant is required, do not use the decongestant until ≥2 hrs following administration. Instruct to avoid sneezing during or immediately after dosing.

SYNRIBO — omacetaxine mepesuccinate   Rx
Class: Protein synthesis inhibitor

ADULT DOSAGE	PEDIATRIC DOSAGE
Chronic Myeloid Leukemia	Pediatric use may not have been established
Chronic or accelerated phase w/ resistance and/or intolerance to ≥2 tyrosine kinase inhibitors	
Induction: 1.25mg/m² bid (approx 12-hr intervals) for 14 consecutive days every 28 days, over a 28-day cycle; repeat cycle every 28 days until hematologic response is achieved	
Maint: 1.25mg/m² bid (approx 12-hr intervals) for 7 consecutive days every 28 days, over a 28-day cycle	

DOSING CONSIDERATIONS

Adverse Reactions

Hematologic Toxicity:

Grade 4 Neutropenia (ANC <0.5 x 10⁹/L) or Grade 3 Thrombocytopenia (Platelet Counts <50 x 10⁹/L) During a Cycle:
Delay starting next cycle until ANC ≥1.0 x 10⁹/L and platelet count ≥50 x 10⁹/L; reduce number of dosing days by 2 days for next cycle

Non-Hematologic Toxicity:
Manage symptomatically; interrupt and/or delay therapy until toxicity is resolved

ADMINISTRATION
SQ route

Reconstitution Instructions
1. Reconstitute w/ 1mL of 0.9% NaCl inj prior to SQ inj.
2. After addition of diluent, gently swirl until a clear sol is obtained; lyophilized powder should be completely dissolved in <1 min.
3. The resulting sol contains 3.5mg/mL.

Handling Precautions
If contact w/ skin occurs, immediately and thoroughly wash affected area w/ soap and water.
If contact w/ the eyes occurs, thoroughly flush the eyes w/ water.

STORAGE
20-25°C (68-77°F); excursions permitted from 15-30°C (59-86°F). Protect from light. **Reconstituted Sol:** Use w/in 12 hrs if stored at 20-25°C (68-77°F) or use w/in 6 days if stored at 2-8°C (36-46°F).

HOW SUPPLIED
Inj: 3.5mg

WARNINGS/PRECAUTIONS
Severe and fatal myelosuppression (eg, thrombocytopenia, neutropenia, anemia) reported; delay next cycle and/or reduce the number of days of treatment. Increased risk of infection in neutropenic patients; monitor frequently. Monitor CBC weekly during induction and initial maintenance cycles, and every 2 weeks during later maintenance cycles, as clinically indicated. Cerebral hemorrhage and severe, nonfatal GI hemorrhages observed; monitor platelet counts. Glucose intolerance and hyperglycemia, including hyperosmolar non-ketotic hyperglycemia reported; monitor blood glucose levels frequently, especially in patients w/ diabetes mellitus (DM) or risk factors for DM. Avoid w/ poorly controlled DM until glycemic control is established. May cause fetal harm if administered during pregnancy.

ADVERSE REACTIONS
Thrombocytopenia, anemia, neutropenia, lymphopenia, bone marrow failure, infections/infestations, diarrhea, N/V, inj-site related reactions, fatigue, pyrexia, asthenia, arthralgia.

DRUG INTERACTIONS
Increased risk of bleeding w/ anticoagulants, aspirin, and NSAIDs; avoid when platelet count is <50,000/μL.

PREGNANCY AND LACTATION
Pregnancy: Category D.
Lactation: Not for use in nursing.

MECHANISM OF ACTION
Protein synthesis inhibitor; not fully elucidated. Binds to the A-site cleft in the peptidyl-transferase center of the large ribosomal subunit from a strain of archaeabacteria. In vitro, reduces protein levels of the Bcr-Abl oncoprotein and Mcl-1, an antiapoptotic Bcl-2 family member.

PHARMACOKINETICS
Absorption: T_{max}=30 min. **Distribution:** V_d=141L; plasma protein binding (≤50%). **Metabolism:** Hydrolyzed via plasma esterases; 4'-DMHHT (metabolite). **Elimination:** Urine (<15%, unchanged); $T_{1/2}$=6 hrs.

PATIENT CONSIDERATIONS
Assessment: Assess for thrombocytopenia, neutropenia, anemia, hemorrhage, DM, risk factors for DM, pregnancy/nursing status, and possible drug interactions.

Monitoring: Monitor for signs and symptoms of myelosuppression, hemorrhage, infection, and other adverse reactions. Monitor CBC and blood glucose levels.

Counseling: Advise patient to read medication guide and provide instructions for appropriate use. Advise of the possibility of serious bleeding due to low platelet counts; instruct to report immediately any signs/symptoms suggestive of hemorrhage. Instruct to report in advance if patients plan to have any dental or surgical procedures. Inform that hematological parameters (eg, WBCs, platelets, RBCs) will need to be monitored. Instruct to report if fever or any signs/symptoms of infection (eg, SOB, significant fatigue, bleeding) develop. Advise diabetic patients of the possibility of hyperglycemia and the need to monitor blood glucose levels carefully. Advise females of reproductive potential to avoid pregnancy/nursing while on treatment. Inform that N/V, diarrhea, abdominal pain, and constipation may develop; instruct to seek medical attention if symptoms persist. Instruct to avoid driving/operating any dangerous tools or machinery if tiredness is experienced. Inform that skin rash may occur and to immediately report severe/worsening rash or itching. Inform that hair loss may be experienced.

SYPRINE — trientine hydrochloride

Class: Chelating agent

Rx

ADULT DOSAGE	PEDIATRIC DOSAGE
Wilson's Disease	**Wilson's Disease**
Intolerant of Penicillamine:	**Intolerant of Penicillamine:**
Initial: 750-1250mg/day in divided doses bid, tid, or qid	**6-12 Years:**
Titrate: May be increased to a max of 2000mg/day; increase only when clinical response is not adequate or if concentration of free serum copper is persistently >20mcg/dL	**Initial:** 500-750mg/day in divided doses bid, tid, or qid
	Titrate: May be increased to a max of 1500mg/day; increase only when clinical response is not adequate or if concentration of free serum copper is persistently >20mcg/dL
Determine optimal long-term maint dose at 6- to 12-month intervals	Determine optimal long-term maint dose at 6- to 12-month intervals

DOSING CONSIDERATIONS
Elderly
Start at lower end of dosing range

ADMINISTRATION
Oral route

Take on an empty stomach
Swallow caps whole w/ water; do not open or chew
Take 1 hr ac or 2 hrs pc and at least 1 hr apart from any other drug, food, or milk

STORAGE
2-8°C (36-46°F). Keep container tightly closed.

HOW SUPPLIED
Cap: 250mg

CONTRAINDICATIONS
Hypersensitivity to this product.

WARNINGS/PRECAUTIONS
Regular medical supervision recommended throughout therapy. Closely monitor patients, especially women, for iron deficiency anemia. Asthma, bronchitis, and dermatitis reported after prolonged environmental exposure in workers who use trientine hydrochloride as a hardener of epoxy resins; observe for possible hypersensitivity. Caution in elderly.

ADVERSE REACTIONS
Iron deficiency, systemic lupus erythematosus, dystonia, muscular spasm, myasthenia gravis.

DRUG INTERACTIONS
Avoid mineral supplements. Two hrs should elapse between coadministration with iron. Take 1 hr apart from any other drugs.

PREGNANCY AND LACTATION
Category C, caution in nursing.

MECHANISM OF ACTION
Chelating agent; binds to and facilitates removal of excess copper from the body.

PATIENT CONSIDERATIONS
Assessment: Assess for drug hypersensitivity, cystinuria, rheumatoid arthritis, serum copper levels, pregnancy/nursing status, and possible drug interactions.

Monitoring: Monitor for hypersensitivity reactions, iron deficiency anemia, serum free copper and temperature nightly for first month. Monitor with a 24-hr urinary copper analysis periodically (every 6-12 months).

Counseling: Advise to take on an empty stomach, at least 1 hr ac or 2 hrs pc, and at least 1 hr apart from any other drug, food, or milk. Instruct to swallow caps whole with water; do not open or chew. Advise to wash any site exposed to capsule contents promptly. Advise to take temperature nightly for the first month of treatment and to report any symptoms such as fever or skin eruption.

TAFINLAR — dabrafenib

Class: Kinase inhibitor

Rx

ADULT DOSAGE	PEDIATRIC DOSAGE
Unresectable or Metastatic Melanoma with BRAF V600E Mutation	Pediatric use may not have been established
150mg bid, approx 12 hrs apart, as a single agent until disease progression or unacceptable toxicity occurs	
Unresectable or Metastatic Melanoma with BRAF V600E or V600K Mutations	
150mg bid, approx 12 hrs apart, in combination w/ trametinib until disease progression or unacceptable toxicity occurs	
Missed Dose	
Do not take a missed dose w/in 6 hrs of the next dose	

DOSING CONSIDERATIONS

Adverse Reactions
Dose Reductions for Dabrafenib:
First Dose Reduction: 100mg bid
Second Dose Reduction: 75mg bid
Third Dose Reduction: 50mg bid
Subsequent Modification: Permanently d/c if unable to tolerate 50mg bid

New Primary Noncutaneous Malignancies:
Permanently d/c if RAS mutation-positive noncutaneous malignancies develop

Febrile Drug Reaction:
Fever of 101.3-104°F: Withhold until fever resolves, then resume at same or lower dose level

Fever >104°F or Fever Complicated by Rigors, Hypotension, Dehydration, or Renal Failure: Withhold until fever resolves, then resume at a lower dose level or permanently d/c

Cutaneous:
Grade 3 or 4 Skin Toxicity or Intolerable Grade 2 Skin Toxicity: Withhold for up to 3 weeks; resume at a lower dose level if improved or permanently d/c if not improved

Cardiac:
Symptomatic CHF: Withhold; if improved, then resume at the same dose
Absolute Decrease in Left Ventricular Ejection Fraction (LVEF) >20% from Baseline That is Below Lower Limit of Normal: Withhold; if improved, then resume at the same dose

Uveitis Including Iritis and Iridocyclitis:
If mild or moderate uveitis does not respond to ocular therapy, or for severe uveitis, withhold for up to 6 weeks; resume at the same or at a lower dose level if improved to Grade 0-1, or permanently d/c if not improved

Other:
Any Grade 3 Adverse Reaction or Intolerable Grade 2 Adverse Reactions: Withhold; resume at a lower dose level if improved to Grade 0-1, or permanently d/c if not improved
First Occurrence of Any Grade 4 Adverse Reaction: Withhold until adverse reaction improves to Grade 0-1, then resume at a lower dose level; or permanently d/c
Recurrent Grade 4 Adverse Reaction: Permanently d/c
Refer to trametinib PI for trametinib modifications

ADMINISTRATION
Oral route
Take at least 1 hr ac or 2 hrs pc.
Do not open, crush, or break caps.

STORAGE
25°C (77°F); excursions permitted to 15-30°C (59-86°F).

HOW SUPPLIED
Cap: 50mg, 75mg

WARNINGS/PRECAUTIONS
See Dosing Considerations. Not indicated for treatment of patients w/ wild-type BRAF melanoma. New primary cutaneous and noncutaneous malignancies may occur when dabrafenib is administered alone or in combination w/ trametinib; perform dermatologic evaluations prior to initiation, every 2 months while on therapy, and for up to 6 months following discontinuation. Increased cell proliferation may occur in BRAF wild-type cells exposed to BRAF inhibitors; confirm evidence of BRAF V600E or V600K mutation status prior to treatment initiation. Hemorrhages (eg, major hemorrhages) may occur when administered w/ trametinib; permanently d/c for all Grade 4 hemorrhagic events and for any persistent Grade 3 hemorrhagic events. Cardiomyopathy may occur; assess LVEF by echocardiogram or multigated acquisition (MUGA) scan before initiation of dabrafenib w/ trametinib, 1 month after initiation, and then at 2- to 3-month intervals while on treatment. Uveitis may occur; monitor for visual signs/symptoms (eg, change in vision, photophobia, eye pain). Permanently d/c for persistent Grade 2 or greater uveitis of >6 weeks duration. Serious febrile reactions and fever of any severity complicated by hypotension, rigors/chills, dehydration, or renal failure may occur; incidence and severity of pyrexia are increased w/ trametinib. Monitor SrCr and other evidence of renal function during and following severe pyrexia. Serious skin toxicity may occur. Hyperglycemia may occur; monitor serum glucose levels upon initiation and as clinically appropriate in patients w/ preexisting diabetes or hyperglycemia. Potential risk of hemolytic anemia in patients w/ G6PD deficiency; closely monitor such patients for signs of hemolytic anemia. May cause fetal harm.

ADVERSE REACTIONS
Single Agent Dabrafenib: Hyperkeratosis, headache, pyrexia, arthralgia, papilloma, alopecia, palmar-plantar erythrodysesthesia syndrome.
W/ Trametinib: Pyrexia, rash, chills, headache, arthralgia, cough.

DRUG INTERACTIONS
Strong inhibitors of CYP3A4 or CYP2C8 may increase concentrations and strong inducers of CYP3A4 or CYP2C8 may decrease concentrations; substitution of these medications is recommended during treatment. If concomitant use of strong inhibitors (eg, ketoconazole, nefazodone, clarithromycin, gemfibrozil) or strong inducers (eg, rifampin, phenytoin, carbamazepine, phenobarbital, St. John's wort) of CYP3A4 or CYP2C8 is unavoidable, monitor closely for adverse reactions when taking strong inhibitors or loss of efficacy when taking strong inducers. May decrease systemic exposures of midazolam (CYP3A4 substrate), S-warfarin (CYP2C9 substrate), and R-warfarin (CYP3A4/CYP1A2 substrate). Monitor INR levels more frequently in patients receiving warfarin during initiation or discontinuation of dabrafenib. Coadministration w/ CYP3A4 and CYP2C9 substrates (eg, dexamethasone, hormonal contraceptives) may result in decreased concentrations and loss of efficacy; substitute for these medications or monitor for loss of efficacy if use of these medications is unavoidable.

PREGNANCY AND LACTATION
Pregnancy: May cause fetal harm.
Lactation: Advise women not to breastfeed during treatment and for 2 weeks following the last dose.
Reproductive Potential: Females of reproductive potential should use effective nonhormonal contraception during treatment and for 2 weeks after the last dose. May impair fertility in females of reproductive potential. Potential risk for impaired spermatogenesis that may be irreversible in males.

MECHANISM OF ACTION
Kinase inhibitor; inhibits BRAF V600 mutation-positive melanoma cell growth. Use of dabrafenib and trametinib in combination resulted in greater growth inhibition of BRAF V600 mutation-positive melanoma cell lines in vitro and prolonged inhibition of tumor growth in BRAF V600 mutation-positive melanoma xenografts compared w/ either drug alone.

PHARMACOKINETICS
Absorption: Absolute bioavailability (95%); T_{max}=2 hrs (median). **Distribution:** Plasma protein binding (99.7%); V_d=70.3L. **Metabolism:** Via CYP2C8 and CYP3A4 to hydroxy-dabrafenib (active), hydroxy-dabrafenib is oxidized via CYP3A4 to carboxy-dabrafenib, carboxy-dabrafenib is decarboxylated to desmethyl-dabrafenib (active), desmethyl-dabrafenib via CYP3A4 to oxidative metabolites. **Elimination:** Feces (71%), urine (23%, metabolites); $T_{1/2}$=8 hrs, 10 hrs (hydroxy-dabrafenib), 21-22 hrs (carboxy- and desmethyl-dabrafenib).

PATIENT CONSIDERATIONS
Assessment: Assess for diabetes, hyperglycemia, G6PD deficiency, pregnancy/nursing status, and possible drug interactions. Assess for presence of BRAF V600E or V600K mutation in tumor specimens. Perform dermatologic evaluations. Assess LVEF by echocardiogram or MUGA scan before initiation of dabrafenib w/ trametinib.

Monitoring: Monitor for new primary malignancies, hemorrhagic events, cardiomyopathy, uveitis, febrile reactions, fever, skin toxicity, hyperglycemia, and other adverse reactions. Perform dermatologic evaluations every 2 months during therapy and for up to 6 months following discontinuation. Monitor LVEF by echocardiogram and MUGA scan 1 month after initiation and then at 2- to 3-month intervals during therapy. Monitor SrCr and other evidence of renal function during and following severe pyrexia. Monitor serum glucose levels upon initiation and as clinically appropriate in patients w/ preexisting diabetes or hyperglycemia. Closely monitor patients w/ G6PD deficiency for signs of hemolytic anemia. Monitor INR levels more frequently in patients receiving warfarin during initiation or discontinuation.

Counseling: Inform that evidence of BRAF V600E or V600K mutation in the tumor specimen is necessary to identify patients for whom treatment is indicated. Inform of increased risk of developing new primary cutaneous and noncutaneous malignancies; instruct to contact healthcare provider immediately for any new lesions, changes to existing lesions on the skin, or signs/symptoms of other malignancies. Inform that combined use w/ trametinib may increase risk of intracranial and GI hemorrhage; advise to contact healthcare provider or seek immediate medical attention for unusual bleeding or hemorrhage. Advise that therapy may cause cardiomyopathy and to report signs/symptoms of heart failure. Advise that therapy may cause uveitis and to contact healthcare provider if changes in vision occur. Inform that therapy may cause pyrexia, including serious febrile reactions, and that incidence and severity are increased w/ trametinib; advise to contact healthcare provider if fever develops. Advise of risk of serious skin reactions and to contact healthcare provider for progressive or intolerable rash. Advise diabetic patients that therapy may impair glucose control and to report severe hyperglycemia symptoms to healthcare provider. Advise patients w/ known G6PD deficiency to contact healthcare provider to report signs/symptoms of anemia or hemolysis. Instruct female patients to use effective nonhormonal contraception during treatment and for 2 weeks after discontinuation of dabrafenib; advise to contact healthcare provider if pregnancy occurs, or is suspected, while on therapy. Advise breastfeeding mothers to d/c nursing while on therapy and for 2 weeks after the last dose. Inform males and females of reproductive potential that treatment may impair fertility.

TAGRISSO — osimertinib   Rx

Class: Kinase inhibitor

ADULT DOSAGE	PEDIATRIC DOSAGE
Metastatic Non-Small Cell Lung Cancer	Pediatric use may not have been established
Treatment of patients w/ metastatic epidermal growth factor receptor (EGFR) T790M mutation-positive non-small cell lung cancer (NSCLC), as detected by an FDA-approved test, who have progressed on or after EGFR tyrosine kinase inhibitor therapy	
80mg qd until disease progression or unacceptable toxicity	
Missed Dose	
If a dose is missed, do not make up the missed dose and take the next dose as scheduled	

DOSING CONSIDERATIONS
Concomitant Medications
Strong CYP3A4 Inducers: If concurrent use is unavoidable, increase osimertinib dose to 160mg qd when coadministering w/ a strong CYP3A inducer; resume at 80mg 3 weeks after discontinuation of the strong CYP3A4 inducer

Adverse Reactions
Pulmonary:
Interstitial Lung Disease (ILD)/Pneumonitis: Permanently d/c
Cardiac:
QTc Interval >500 msec on at Least 2 Separate ECGs: Withhold until QTc interval is <481 msec or recovery to baseline if baseline QTc is ≥481 msec, then resume at 40mg dose
QTc Interval Prolongation w/ Signs/Symptoms of Life-Threatening Arrhythmia: Permanently d/c
Asymptomatic, Absolute Decrease in Left Ventricular Ejection Fraction (LVEF) of 10% from Baseline and <50%: Withhold for up to 4 weeks. Resume if LVEF improves to baseline, or permanently d/c if LVEF does not improve to baseline
Symptomatic CHF: Permanently d/c
Other:
Grade ≥3 Adverse Reaction: Withhold for up to 3 weeks
If Improvement to Grade 0-2 w/in 3 Weeks: Resume at 80mg or 40mg qd
If No Improvement w/in 3 Weeks: Permanently d/c

ADMINISTRATION
Oral route

Take w/ or w/o food.

Administration to Patients Who Have Difficulty Swallowing Solids
1. Disperse tab in 60mL (2 oz) of non-carbonated water only; stir until tab is dispersed into small pieces.
2. Swallow immediately.
3. Do not crush, heat, or ultrasonicate during preparation.
4. Rinse container w/ 120-240mL (4-8 oz) of water and immediately drink.

If administering via NG tube, disperse the tab as above in 15mL of non-carbonated water, and then use an additional 15mL of water to transfer any residues to the syringe; the resulting 30mL liquid should be administered as per NG tube instructions w/ appropriate water flushes (approx 30mL).

STORAGE
25°C (77°F); excursions permitted to 15-30°C (59-86°F).

HOW SUPPLIED
Tab: 40mg, 80mg

WARNINGS/PRECAUTIONS
See Dosing Considerations. ILD/pneumonitis reported; withhold therapy and promptly investigate for ILD in any patient who presents w/ worsening of respiratory symptoms. QTc interval prolongation reported; periodically monitor ECGs and electrolytes in patients w/ congenital long QTc syndrome, CHF, or electrolyte abnormalities. Cardiomyopathy reported; assess LVEF before initiation and then at 3-month intervals while on treatment. May cause fetal harm.

ADVERSE REACTIONS
Diarrhea, rash, dry skin, nail toxicity.

DRUG INTERACTIONS
Coadministration w/ a strong CYP3A4 inducer decreased exposure; may lead to reduced efficacy. Avoid coadministration w/ strong CYP3A inducers (eg, phenytoin, rifampin, carbamazepine, St. John's wort); increase osimertinib dose if concurrent use is unavoidable. Coadministration w/ a breast cancer resistance protein (BCRP) substrate increased exposure of the BCRP substrate; may increase risk of exposure-related toxicity. Monitor for adverse reactions of the BCRP substrate (eg, rosuvastatin, sulfasalazine, topotecan). Periodically monitor ECGs and electrolytes in patients taking medications known to prolong the QTc interval.

PREGNANCY AND LACTATION
Pregnancy: Based on data from animal studies and its mechanism of action, can cause fetal harm.
Lactation: Lactating women should not breastfeed during treatment and for 2 weeks after final dose.
Reproductive Potential: Females of reproductive potential should use effective contraception during treatment and for 6 weeks after the final dose. Male patients w/ female partners of reproductive potential should use effective contraception during treatment and for 4 months following the final dose. May impair fertility in females and males of reproductive potential.

MECHANISM OF ACTION
Kinase inhibitor; binds irreversibly to certain mutant forms of EGFR. Exhibits anti-tumor activity against NSCLC lines harboring EGFR-mutations (T790M/L858R, L858R, T790M/exon 19 deletion, and exon 19 deletion) and, to a lesser extent, wild-type EGFR amplifications.

PHARMACOKINETICS
Absorption: T_{max}=6 hrs (median). **Distribution:** V_d=986L. Plasma protein binding is likely high. **Metabolism:** Oxidation (predominantly CYP3A) and dealkylation. AZ7550 and AZ5104 (active metabolites). **Elimination:** Feces (68%), urine (14%), unchanged (2%). $T_{1/2}$=48 hrs.

PATIENT CONSIDERATIONS
Assessment: Assess for congenital long QTc syndrome, CHF, and electrolyte abnormalities. Assess LVEF, pregnancy/nursing status, and for possible drug interactions.

Monitoring: Monitor for ILD, pneumonitis, QTc interval prolongation, and cardiomyopathy. Periodically monitor ECGs and electrolytes in patients w/ congenital long QTc syndrome, CHF, electrolyte abnormalities, or who are taking medications known to prolong the QTc interval. Assess LVEF at 3-month intervals.

Counseling: Inform of the risks of severe or fatal ILD, including pneumonitis; advise to contact physician immediately to report new or worsening respiratory symptoms. Inform patients of symptoms that may be indicative of significant QTc prolongation (eg, dizziness, lightheadedness, syncope) and advise to report these symptoms. Advise to inform physician about the use of any heart or BP medications. Advise to immediately report any signs or symptoms of heart failure. Inform that drug can cause fetal harm if taken during pregnancy. Advise pregnant women of the potential risk to a fetus. Advise females to inform physician if they become pregnant or if pregnancy is suspected while on therapy. Instruct females of reproductive potential to use effective contraception during treatment and for 6 weeks after the final dose. Instruct males w/ female partners of reproductive potential to use effective contraception during treatment and for 4 months after the final dose. Advise women not to breastfeed during treatment and for 2 weeks after the final dose.

TALTZ — ixekizumab   Rx
Class: Monoclonal antibody/IL-17A antagonist

ADULT DOSAGE	PEDIATRIC DOSAGE
Plaque Psoriasis	Pediatric use may not have been established
In Patients Who Are Candidates for Systemic/Phototherapy:	
Moderate to Severe:	
160mg (two 80mg inj) at Week 0, followed by 80mg at Weeks 2, 4, 6, 8, 10, and 12, then 80mg every 4 weeks	

ADMINISTRATION
SQ route

Administer each inj at a different anatomic location (eg, upper arms, thighs, any quadrant of abdomen) than previous inj.
Do not inject into areas where the skin is tender, bruised, erythematous, indurated, or affected by psoriasis.
Before inj, remove from refrigerator and allow to reach room temperature (30 min) w/o removing needle cap.
Product does not contain preservatives; discard any unused product remaining in the autoinjector or prefilled syringe.
Refer to prescribing information for further instructions for administration.

STORAGE
2-8°C (36-46°F). Protect from light. Do not freeze; do not use if product has been frozen. Do not shake.

HOW SUPPLIED
Inj: 80mg/mL [autoinjector, prefilled syringe]

CONTRAINDICATIONS
Previous serious hypersensitivity reaction to ixekizumab or to any of the excipients in the product.

WARNINGS/PRECAUTIONS
Intended for use under the guidance and supervision of a physician. May increase risk of infection. If a serious infection develops or if not responding to standard therapy, monitor the patient closely and d/c therapy until the infection resolves. Evaluate for tuberculosis (TB) infection prior to initiating treatment; do not administer to patients w/ active TB infection. Initiate treatment of latent TB prior to administering therapy; consider anti-TB therapy prior to initiation in patients w/ a past history of latent or active TB in whom an adequate course of treatment cannot be confirmed. Serious hypersensitivity reactions (eg, angioedema, urticaria) reported; d/c immediately and initiate appropriate therapy if a serious hypersensitivity reaction occurs. Crohn's disease and ulcerative colitis, including exacerbations, reported. Prior to initiating therapy, consider completion of all age-appropriate immunizations according to current immunization guidelines.

ADVERSE REACTIONS
Inj-site reactions, URTIs, nausea, tinea infections.

DRUG INTERACTIONS
Avoid w/ live vaccines. May normalize formation of CYP450 enzymes; upon initiation or discontinuation of therapy in patients who are receiving concomitant CYP450 substrates, particularly those w/ a narrow therapeutic index, consider monitoring for therapeutic effect (eg, warfarin) or drug concentration (eg, cyclosporine) and consider dosage modification of the CYP450 substrate.

PREGNANCY AND LACTATION
Pregnancy: There are no available data on ixekizumab use in pregnant women to inform any drug-associated risks. Human IgG is known to cross the placental barrier; therefore, ixekizumab may be transmitted from the mother to the developing fetus.
Lactation: There are no data on the presence of ixekizumab in human milk, the effects on the breastfed infant, or the effects on milk production; caution in nursing.

MECHANISM OF ACTION
Monoclonal antibody/interleukin-17A (IL-17A) antagonist; selectively binds to the IL-17A cytokine and inhibits its interaction w/ the IL-17 receptor. Inhibits the release of proinflammatory cytokines and chemokines.

PHARMACOKINETICS
Absorption: Bioavailability (60-81%); C_{max}=16.2mcg/mL (160mg); T_{max}=4 days.
Distribution: V_d=7.11L. **Elimination:** $T_{1/2}$=13 days.

PATIENT CONSIDERATIONS
Assessment: Assess for previous hypersensitivity to the drug or to any of the excipients of the product, infection including TB infection, inflammatory bowel

disease, immunization status, pregnancy/nursing status, and possible drug interactions.

Monitoring: Monitor for signs/symptoms of infection, inflammatory bowel disease, hypersensitivity reactions, and other adverse reactions. Monitor for signs/symptoms of active TB during and after treatment.

Counseling: Advise of the potential benefits and risks of therapy. Instruct on proper SQ inj technique, including aseptic technique, and how to use the autoinjector or prefilled syringe correctly. Inform that drug may lower the ability of immune system to fight infections; instruct to contact physician if any symptoms of infection develop. Advise to seek immediate medical attention if any symptoms of a serious hypersensitivity reaction occur.

TARCEVA — erlotinib　　　　　　　　　　Rx

Class: Kinase inhibitor

ADULT DOSAGE
Non-Small Cell Lung Cancer

1st-line treatment of patients w/ metastatic non-small cell lung cancer (NSCLC) whose tumors have epidermal growth factor receptor (EGFR) exon 19 deletions or exon 21 (L858R) substitution mutations; treatment of locally advanced or metastatic NSCLC after failure of at least 1 prior chemotherapy regimen; maint treatment of locally advanced or metastatic NSCLC that has not progressed after 4 cycles of platinum-based 1st-line chemotherapy

Recommended Dose: 150mg qd; continue until disease progression or unacceptable toxicity occurs

Pancreatic Cancer

1st-line treatment of locally advanced, unresectable, or metastatic pancreatic cancer

Recommended Dose: 100mg qd in combination w/ gemcitabine; continue until disease progression or unacceptable toxicity occurs

PEDIATRIC DOSAGE
Pediatric use may not have been established

DOSING CONSIDERATIONS
Concomitant Medications
Reduce by 50mg Decrements If:
If severe reactions occur w/ concomitant use of strong CYP3A4 inhibitors or when using concomitantly w/ an inhibitor of both a CYP3A4 and CYP1A2 (eg, ciprofloxacin); avoid concomitant use if possible

Increase by 50mg Increments As Tolerated For:
- Concomitant use w/ CYP3A4 inducers; increase by 50mg increments at 2-week intervals to a max of 450mg; avoid concomitant use if possible
- Concurrent cigarette smoking; increase by 50mg increments at 2-week intervals to a max of 300mg; immediately reduce the dose to the recommended dose (150mg or 100mg qd) upon cessation of smoking

Drugs Affecting Gastric pH:
- Avoid concomitant use w/ proton pump inhibitors if possible
- If treatment w/ an H$_2$-receptor antagonist is required, dose must be taken 10 hrs after the H$_2$-receptor antagonist dosing and at least 2 hrs before the next dose of the H$_2$-receptor antagonist
- If an antacid is necessary, antacid dose and erlotinib dose should be separated by several hrs

Renal Impairment
No clinical studies have been conducted in patients w/ compromised renal function

Hepatic Impairment
Total Bilirubin >ULN or Child-Pugh A, B, and C: Closely monitor; use w/ extra caution in patients w/ total bilirubin >3X ULN

Adverse Reactions:
D/C For:
- Interstitial Lung Disease (ILD)
- Severe hepatic toxicity that does not improve significantly or resolve w/in 3 weeks
- GI perforation
- Severe bullous, blistering, or exfoliating skin conditions
- Corneal perforation or severe ulceration
Withhold For:
- During diagnostic evaluation for possible ILD
- For severe (CTCAE Grade 3-4) renal toxicity, and consider discontinuation
- In patients w/o preexisting hepatic impairment for total bilirubin levels >3X ULN or transaminases >5X ULN, and consider discontinuation
- In patients w/ preexisting hepatic impairment or biliary obstruction for doubling of bilirubin or tripling of transaminases values over baseline and consider discontinuation
- For persistent severe diarrhea not responsive to medical management (eg, loperamide)

- For severe rash not responsive to medical management
- For keratitis of (NCI-CTC version 4.0) Grade 3-4 or for Grade 2 lasting more than 2 weeks
- For acute/worsening ocular disorders such as eye pain, and consider discontinuation
Reduce by 50mg Decrements:
When restarting therapy following withholding treatment for a dose-limiting toxicity that has resolved to baseline or Grade ≤1

ADMINISTRATION
Oral route

Take on an empty stomach (at least 1 hr ac or 2 hrs pc).

STORAGE
25°C (77°F); excursions permitted to 15-30°C (59-86°F).

HOW SUPPLIED
Tab: 25mg, 100mg, 150mg

WARNINGS/PRECAUTIONS
See Dosing Considerations. Not recommended for use in combination w/ platinum-based chemotherapy. Cases of serious ILD may occur; withhold for acute onset of new/progressive unexplained pulmonary symptoms and permanently d/c therapy if ILD is confirmed. Hepatorenal syndrome; severe acute renal failure; renal insufficiency; hepatotoxicity w/ or w/o hepatic impairment; bullous, blistering, and exfoliative skin conditions (eg, Stevens-Johnson syndrome/toxic epidermal necrolysis); MI/ischemia; cerebrovascular accidents (CVAs); microangiopathic hemolytic anemia w/ thrombocytopenia; and fetal harm may occur. Decreased tear production, abnormal eyelash growth, keratoconjunctivitis sicca, or keratitis may occur and can lead to corneal perforation/ulceration. GI perforation may occur; increased risk in patients w/ prior history of peptic ulceration or diverticular disease.

ADVERSE REACTIONS
Rash, diarrhea, anorexia, asthenia, dyspnea, cough, N/V.

DRUG INTERACTIONS
See Dosing Considerations. Concomitant use w/ antiangiogenic agents, corticosteroids, NSAIDs, and/or taxane-based chemotherapy may increase risk of GI perforation. Increased levels w/ potent CYP3A4 inhibitors (eg, ketoconazole), and w/ inhibitors of both CYP3A4 and CYP1A2 (eg, ciprofloxacin). Decreased levels w/ CYP3A4 inducers (eg, rifampicin). Cigarette smoking and drugs affecting gastric pH (eg, omeprazole, ranitidine) may decrease levels. INR elevations and bleeding events reported w/ coumarin-derived anticoagulants (eg, warfarin); monitor PT/INR regularly.

PREGNANCY AND LACTATION
Pregnancy: Category D; based on its mechanism of action, erlotinib can cause fetal harm when administered to a pregnant woman.
Lactation: Not for use in nursing.
Reproductive Potential: Females of reproductive potential should use effective contraception during treatment and for at least 2 weeks after the last dose.

MECHANISM OF ACTION
EGFR tyrosine kinase inhibitor; reversibly inhibits the kinase activity of EGFR, preventing autophosphorylation of tyrosine residues associated w/ the receptor and thereby inhibiting further downstream signaling.

PHARMACOKINETICS
Absorption: Bioavailability (60% w/o food, 100% w/ food); T$_{max}$=4 hrs.
Distribution: V$_d$=232L; plasma protein binding (93%). **Metabolism:** CYP3A4 (major); 1A2, 1A1 (minor). **Elimination:** Feces (83%; 1% parent drug), urine (8%; 0.3% parent drug); T$_{1/2}$=36.2 hrs (median).

PATIENT CONSIDERATIONS
Assessment: Assess for hepatic/renal impairment, dehydration, history of peptic ulceration or diverticular disease, pregnancy/nursing status, and possible drug interactions.
Monitoring: Monitor for signs and symptoms of ILD, hepatotoxicity, GI perforation, MI/ischemia, renal failure/insufficiency, CVAs, microangiopathic hemolytic anemia w/ thrombocytopenia, ocular disorders, bullous and exfoliative skin disorders, and other adverse reactions. Monitor LFTs, renal function, and serum electrolytes periodically.
Counseling: Inform of risks/benefits of therapy. Instruct to notify physician if onset or worsening of skin rash or development of bullous lesions or desquamation; severe/persistent diarrhea, N/V, or anorexia; unexplained SOB or cough; or eye irritation occurs. Instruct to stop smoking and advise to contact physician for any changes in smoking status. Advise on the presentation of skin, hair, and nail disorders. Instruct on initial management of rash or diarrhea. Counsel on pregnancy planning and prevention; advise females of reproductive potential to use highly effective contraception during treatment and for at least 2 weeks after the last dose. Advise to contact physician if pregnant or if pregnancy is suspected and to d/c nursing during treatment.

TARGRETIN CAPSULES — bexarotene　　　　Rx

Class: Retinoid

> Associated w/ birth defects. Do not administer to a pregnant woman.

ADULT DOSAGE
Cutaneous T-Cell Lymphoma

Treatment of cutaneous manifestations of cutaneous T-cell lymphoma in patients who are refractory to at least 1 prior systemic therapy

PEDIATRIC DOSAGE
Pediatric use may not have been established

Initial: 300mg/m²/day
Titrate: If no tumor response after 8 weeks of treatment and if initial dose of 300mg/m²/day is well-tolerated, may increase to 400mg/m²/day w/ careful monitoring

Continue as long as the patient is deriving benefit (administered for up to 97 weeks in clinical trials)

DOSING CONSIDERATIONS

Adverse Reactions
May adjust the 300mg/m²/day dose level to 200mg/m²/day then to 100mg/m²/day, or temporarily suspend, if necessitated by toxicity. When toxicity is controlled, may carefully readjust upward

ADMINISTRATION
Oral route

Take as a single daily dose.
Take w/ a meal.

STORAGE
2-25°C (36-77°F). Avoid exposing to high temperatures and humidity after bottle is opened. Protect from light.

HOW SUPPLIED
Cap: 75mg

CONTRAINDICATIONS
Females who are pregnant, known serious hypersensitivity to bexarotene or other components of the product.

WARNINGS/PRECAUTIONS
May induce substantial elevations in lipids; if fasting TGs are elevated or become elevated during treatment, institute antilipemic therapy, and if necessary, reduce or interrupt dose of bexarotene. Fasting TGs should be normal or normalized w/ appropriate intervention prior to initiating therapy; maintain TG levels <400mg/dL to reduce risk of clinical sequelae. Acute pancreatitis (including a fatal case) reported; interrupt therapy and evaluate if pancreatitis is suspected. May be at greater risk for pancreatitis if risk factors exist (eg, prior pancreatitis, uncontrolled hyperlipidemia, excessive alcohol consumption, uncontrolled diabetes mellitus, biliary tract disease, medications known to increase TG levels or to be associated w/ pancreatic toxicity). Elevations in LFTs, cholestasis, and liver failure reported; obtain baseline LFTs and monitor LFTs after 1, 2 and 4 weeks of treatment initiation, and if stable, at least every 8 weeks thereafter during treatment. Interrupt or d/c therapy if test results exceed >3X ULN values for AST, ALT, or bilirubin. Hypothyroidism reported; consider treatment w/ thyroid hormone supplementation. Leukopenia and neutropenia reported. New cataracts or worsening of previous cataracts reported; perform ophthalmologic evaluation if visual difficulties occur. May cause photosensitivity; minimize exposure to sunlight and artificial UV light. Lab test interactions may occur.

ADVERSE REACTIONS
Hyperlipemia, hypercholesterolemia, headache, hypothyroidism, asthenia, leukopenia, rash, diarrhea, anemia, N/V, peripheral edema, infection, abdominal pain, exfoliative dermatitis, dry skin.

DRUG INTERACTIONS
Limit vitamin A supplements to avoid potential additive toxic effects. May enhance action of insulin, agents enhancing insulin secretion (eg, sulfonylureas), or insulin-sensitizers (eg, thiazolidinedione class), resulting in hypoglycemia. Gemfibrozil increased bexarotene concentrations; coadministration is not recommended. May reduce concentrations of CYP3A4 substrates (eg, oral/systemic hormonal contraceptives); strongly consider using a non-hormonal contraception if treatment w/ bexarotene is intended for a female w/ reproductive potential.

PREGNANCY AND LACTATION
Pregnancy: May cause fetal harm. Must not be given to a pregnant female or a female who intends to become pregnant. If pregnancy does occur during treatment, immediately d/c the drug and advise the pregnant female of the potential risk to a fetus.
Lactation: There is no information regarding the presence of bexarotene in human milk, the effects on the breast fed infant, or the effects on milk production; not for use in nursing.
Reproductive Potential: Obtain a negative pregnancy test w/ a sensitivity of at least 50 mIU/L w/in 1 week prior to therapy; obtain another pregnancy test at monthly intervals while the patient remains on therapy. Females must use effective contraception for 1 month prior to the initiation of therapy, during therapy, and for ≥1 month following discontinuation of therapy; use 2 reliable forms of contraception simultaneously (1 of which should be nonhormonal) unless abstinence is the chosen method. Initiate therapy on the 2nd or 3rd day of a normal menstrual period. No more than a 1 month supply of therapy should be given to female patients to allow assessment of pregnancy test and reinforcement of counseling regarding avoidance of pregnancy and birth defects. Male patients w/ sexual partners who are pregnant, possibly pregnant, or who could become pregnant must use condoms during sexual intercourse while on therapy and for ≥1 month after the last dose.

MECHANISM OF ACTION
Retinoid; has not been established. Selectively binds and activates retinoid X receptor subtypes. Once activated, these receptors function as transcription factors that regulate the expression of genes that control cellular differentiation and proliferation. Inhibits the growth in vitro of some tumor cell lines of hematopoietic and squamous cell origin.

PHARMACOKINETICS
Absorption: T_{max}=2 hrs. **Distribution:** Plasma protein binding (>99%). **Metabolism:** Oxidation by CYP3A4; 6- and 7-hydroxy-bexarotene and 6- and 7-oxo-bexarotene (metabolites). **Elimination:** Urine (<1% unchanged); $T_{1/2}$=7 hrs.

PATIENT CONSIDERATIONS
Assessment: Assess for risk factors for pancreatitis, hepatic insufficiency, hypersensitivity to bexarotene or other components of the product, nursing status, and possible drug interactions. Obtain a negative pregnancy test w/ a sensitivity of at least 50 mIU/L w/in 1 week prior to therapy. Perform fasting blood lipid determinations before therapy. Obtain baseline LFTs, thyroid function tests, and CBC (including WBC count w/ differential).

Monitoring: Monitor for pancreatitis, visual difficulties, photosensitivity, and other adverse reactions. Perform pregnancy test at monthly intervals. Perform fasting blood lipid determinations weekly until lipid response is established (usually occurs w/in the initial 2-4 weeks), and monitor at 8-week intervals thereafter. Monitor LFTs after 1, 2, and 4 weeks of treatment initiation, and if stable, at least every 8 weeks thereafter during treatment. Monitor thyroid function tests as indicated, and CBC (including WBC count w/ differential) periodically during treatment.

Counseling: Inform of the risks/benefits of therapy. Inform that drug may cause fetal harm; instruct to d/c use immediately and notify physician if pregnancy occurs. Instruct females of reproductive potential on the importance of monthly pregnancy testing while taking therapy. Instruct females of reproductive potential to use effective contraception for 1 month prior to initiation of therapy, during therapy, and for at least 1 month following discontinuation of therapy; advise to use 2 reliable forms of contraception simultaneously, one of which should be non-hormonal. Instruct male patients w/ sexual partners who are pregnant, possibly pregnant, or who could become pregnant to use condoms during sexual intercourse while on therapy and for at least 1 month after the last dose. Instruct to notify physician if signs/symptoms of pancreatitis, hepatotoxicity, or neutropenia develop. Instruct to inform physician about any changes in vision during treatment. Advise patients to limit vitamin A intake to ≤15,000 IU/day to avoid potential additive toxic effects. Advise to minimize exposure to sunlight and artificial UV light. Inform of the possibility of developing hypoglycemia when using insulin, agents enhancing insulin secretion, or insulin-sensitizers while on therapy; instruct patients on these medications to check their blood sugar frequently and to notify physician of any changes in blood sugar level. Instruct to take w/ a meal. Advise patients of laboratory testing that will occur during therapy.

TARGRETIN GEL — bexarotene   Rx

Class: Retinoid

ADULT DOSAGE	PEDIATRIC DOSAGE
Cutaneous T-Cell Lymphoma	Pediatric use may not have been established
In patients who have stage IA and IB lymphoma, who have refractory or persistent disease after other therapies or who have not tolerated other therapies	
Initial: Apply once qod for the 1st week	
Titrate: Increase application frequency at weekly intervals to qd, then bid, then tid, and finally qid according to lesion tolerance; continue treatment as long as patient is deriving benefit	

DOSING CONSIDERATIONS

Adverse Reactions
May reduce frequency if application-site toxicity occurs, and may temporarily d/c for a few days until symptoms subside if severe irritation occurs

ADMINISTRATION
Topical route

Apply sufficient gel to cover lesion with a generous coating
Allow gel to dry before covering with clothing
Do not use occlusive dressings with gel

STORAGE
25°C (77°F); excursions permitted to 15-30°C (59-86°F). Avoid exposing to high temperatures and humidity after the tube is opened. Protect from light.

HOW SUPPLIED
Gel: 1% [60g]

CONTRAINDICATIONS
Pregnant woman or a woman who intends to become pregnant, known hypersensitivity to bexarotene or other components of the product.

WARNINGS/PRECAUTIONS
Obtain negative pregnancy test with a sensitivity of at least 50 mIU/L within 1 week prior to therapy; repeat pregnancy test monthly during therapy. Effective contraception must be used for 1 month prior to initiation of and during therapy, and for at least 1 month following discontinuation of therapy; use 2 reliable forms of contraception simultaneously unless abstinence is the chosen method. Male patients with sexual partners who are pregnant, possibly pregnant, or who could become pregnant must use condoms during sexual intercourse while on therapy and for at least 1 month after last dose. Initiate therapy on the 2nd or 3rd

day of normal menstrual period. No more than a 1 month supply of drug should be given to allow assessment of pregnancy test results and reinforcement of counseling regarding avoidance of pregnancy and birth defects. Caution with hypersensitivity to other retinoids. Associated with photosensitivity; minimize exposure to sunlight and artificial UV light. Pharmacokinetics may be altered in patients with renal/hepatic insufficiency. May irritate unaffected skin; avoid application to normal skin and near mucosal surfaces. Do not use occlusive dressings.

ADVERSE REACTIONS
Rash, pruritus, pain, skin disorder, infection, contact dermatitis, headache, edema, hyperlipemia, asthenia, cough increased, sweating, leukopenia, lymphadenopathy, paresthesia.

DRUG INTERACTIONS
Avoid with products containing N,N-diethyl-m-toluamide (DEET), a common component of insect repellent products. Drugs that affect levels or activity of CYP3A4 may potentially affect disposition; ketoconazole, itraconazole, erythromycin, gemfibrozil, and grapefruit juice may increase levels. However, increases are unlikely to result in adverse effects due to low systemic exposure after low to moderately intense gel regimens. Limit vitamin A intake to ≤15,000 IU/day to avoid potential additive toxic effects.

PREGNANCY AND LACTATION
Category X, not for use in nursing.

MECHANISM OF ACTION
Retinoid; has not been established. Selectively binds and activates retinoid X receptor subtypes. Once activated, these receptors function as transcription factors that regulate the expression of genes that control cellular differentiation and proliferation.

PHARMACOKINETICS
Distribution: Plasma protein binding (>99%). **Metabolism:** Oxidation via CYP3A4; 6- and 7-hydroxy-bexarotene, 6- and 7-oxo-bexarotene (metabolites). **Elimination:** (PO) Urine (<1%).

PATIENT CONSIDERATIONS
Assessment: Assess for retinoid hypersensitivity, renal/hepatic insufficiency, pregnancy/nursing status, and possible drug interactions. Obtain negative pregnancy test with a sensitivity of at least 50 mIU/L within 1 week prior to therapy.

Monitoring: Monitor for application-site toxicity, irritation, photosensitivity, and other adverse reactions. Perform monthly pregnancy test.

Counseling: Advise to avoid pregnancy during therapy. Instruct to notify physician if pregnant/nursing or planning to become pregnant. Advise to continuously use effective contraception starting 1 month prior to until at least 1 month after therapy; instruct to use 2 reliable forms of contraception simultaneously. Instruct male patients with sexual partners who are pregnant or capable of becoming pregnant to use condoms during sexual intercourse while on therapy and for at least 1 month after last dose. Inform of the need for monthly pregnancy tests. Advise to minimize exposure to sunlight and artificial UV light, not to exceed recommended daily dietary allowance of vitamin A, and not to use insect repellents containing DEET. Instruct to use exactly ud, not to use occlusive dressings, and to avoid scratching treated areas. Advise to avoid bathing or swimming until at least 3 hrs after any application, and to wait 20 min before application if applying after a shower or bath. Instruct not to apply on or near mucosal surfaces of body. Inform that drug takes time to work; counsel not to stop at 1st sign of improvement.

TASIGNA — nilotinib   Rx
Class: Kinase inhibitor

> Prolongs QT interval. Monitor for hypokalemia or hypomagnesemia and correct deficiencies prior to administration and periodically. Obtain ECGs to monitor QTc at baseline, 7 days after initiation, and periodically thereafter, and following any dose adjustments. Sudden deaths reported. Do not administer to patients w/ hypokalemia, hypomagnesemia, or long QT syndrome. Avoid w/ drugs known to prolong the QT interval and strong CYP3A4 inhibitors. Avoid food 2 hrs before and 1 hr after taking the dose.

ADULT DOSAGE
Ph+ Chronic Myeloid Leukemia

Newly Diagnosed Philadelphia Chromosome-Positive Chronic Myeloid Leukemia (Ph+ CML)-Chronic Phase (CP):
300mg bid

Resistant or Intolerant Ph+ CML-CP and CML-Accelerated Phase (AP):
In patients resistant/intolerant to prior therapy that included imatinib
400mg bid

May be given in combination w/ hematopoietic growth factors (eg, erythropoietin, granulocyte colony-stimulating factor), hydroxyurea, or anagrelide if clinically indicated

PEDIATRIC DOSAGE
Pediatric use may not have been established

DOSING CONSIDERATIONS
Concomitant Medications
Strong CYP3A4 Inhibitors (eg, Ketoconazole, Clarithromycin, Atazanavir):
- Avoid concomitant use
- If treatment w/ any of these agents is required, interrupt nilotinib treatment
- If coadministration is a must, consider dose reduction to 300mg qd w/ resistant or intolerant Ph+ CML or to 200mg qd w/ newly diagnosed Ph+ CML; closely monitor for QT interval prolongation in patients who cannot avoid use of strong inhibitor
- If the strong inhibitor is discontinued, allow a washout period before nilotinib dose is adjusted upward to the indicated dose
- Avoid grapefruit products

Strong CYP3A4 Inducers (eg, Dexamethasone, Phenytoin, Carbamazepine):
- Avoid concomitant use
- Avoid St. John's wort

Hepatic Impairment
Newly Diagnosed Ph+ CML:
Mild, Moderate, or Severe (Child-Pugh Class A, B, or C): 200mg bid initially, followed by dose escalation to 300mg bid based on tolerability

Resistant or Intolerant Ph+ CML:
Mild or Moderate (Child-Pugh Score A or B): 300mg bid initially, followed by dose escalation to 400mg bid based on tolerability
Severe (Child-Pugh Score C): 200mg bid initially, followed by sequential dose escalation to 300mg bid and then to 400mg bid based on tolerability

Adverse Reactions
ECGs w/ a QTc >480 msec:
1. Withhold nilotinib, and perform an analysis of serum K^+ and Mg^{2+}, and if below lower limit of normal, correct w/ supplements to w/in normal limits. Concomitant medication usage must be reviewed
2. Resume w/in 2 weeks at prior dose if QTcF returns to <450 msec and to w/in 20 msec of baseline
3. If QTcF is between 450 msec and 480 msec after 2 weeks, reduce dose to 400mg qd
4. If, following dose reduction to 400mg qd, QTcF returns to >480 msec, d/c therapy
5. An ECG should be repeated approx 7 days after any dose adjustment

Neutropenia and Thrombocytopenia (Not Related to Underlying Leukemia):
ANC <1.0 x 10⁹/L and/or Platelet Counts <50 x 10⁹/L:
1. Stop nilotinib, and monitor blood counts
2. Resume w/in 2 weeks at prior dose if ANC >1.0 x 10⁹/L and platelets >50 x 10⁹/L
3. If blood counts remain low for >2 weeks, reduce dose to 400mg qd

Selected Nonhematologic Lab Abnormalities:
Elevated Serum Lipase or Amylase ≥Grade 3:
1. Withhold nilotinib, and monitor serum lipase or amylase
2. Resume at 400mg qd if serum lipase or amylase returns to ≤Grade 1

Elevated Bilirubin ≥Grade 3:
1. Withhold nilotinib, and monitor bilirubin
2. Resume at 400mg qd if bilirubin returns to ≤Grade 1

Elevated Hepatic Transaminases ≥Grade 3:
1. Withhold nilotinib, and monitor hepatic transaminases
2. Resume at 400mg qd if hepatic transaminases returns to ≤Grade 1

Other Nonhematologic Toxicities:
Grade 3 to 4 Lipase Elevations, Grade 3 to 4 Bilirubin, or Hepatic Transaminase Elevations:
Withhold dose and may resume at 400mg qd

Other Significant Moderate or Severe Toxicities:
Withhold dose and resume at 400mg qd when the toxicity has resolved. If clinically appropriate, consider escalating dose back to 300mg bid (newly diagnosed Ph+ CML) or 400mg bid (resistant or intolerant Ph+ CML).

ADMINISTRATION
Oral route
Take on an empty stomach.
Avoid food for at least 2 hrs before and 1 hr after taking the dose.
Take at approx 12-hr intervals.
Swallow whole w/ water.
May disperse contents of each cap in 1 tsp of applesauce if unable to swallow; take immediately (w/in 15 min) and do not store for future use.

STORAGE
25°C (77°F); excursions permitted between 15-30°C (59-86°F).

HOW SUPPLIED
Cap: 150mg, 200mg

CONTRAINDICATIONS
Hypokalemia, hypomagnesemia, long QT syndrome.

WARNINGS/PRECAUTIONS
May cause myelosuppression (eg, Grade 3/4 thrombocytopenia, neutropenia, and anemia); perform CBCs every 2 weeks for the first 2 months, then monthly thereafter, or as clinically indicated. Cardiovascular (CV) events, including arterial vascular occlusive events, reported; evaluate CV status and monitor and actively manage CV risk factors during therapy. May increase serum lipase; increased risk in patients w/ history of pancreatitis. Interrupt dosing and consider appropriate diagnostics to exclude pancreatitis if lipase elevations are accompanied by abdominal symptoms. May result in hepatotoxicity as measured by elevations in bilirubin, AST/ALT, and alkaline phosphatase. May cause hypophosphatemia, hypo/hyperkalemia, hypocalcemia, and hyponatremia; correct electrolyte abnormalities prior to initiation and during therapy. Exposure is increased in patients w/ impaired hepatic function; monitor QT interval frequently. Tumor

lysis syndrome cases reported in patients w/ resistant or intolerant CML; maintain adequate hydration and correct uric acid levels prior to initiation. Hemorrhage reported in patients w/ newly diagnosed Ph+ CML. Reduced exposure in patients w/ total gastrectomy; perform more frequent monitoring and consider dose increase or alternative therapy. Contains lactose; not recommended for patients w/ rare hereditary problems of galactose intolerance, severe lactase deficiency w/ a severe degree of intolerance to lactose-containing products, or of glucose-galactose malabsorption. May cause fetal harm. Severe (Grade 3 or 4) fluid retention, effusions (eg, pleural effusion, pericardial effusion, ascites) or pulmonary edema reported w/ newly diagnosed Ph+ CML-CP. Monitor patients for signs of severe fluid retention and for symptoms of respiratory/cardiac compromise during treatment; evaluate etiology and treat patients accordingly. Caution w/ relevant cardiac disorders.

ADVERSE REACTIONS
Non-Hematologic: Rash, pruritus, headache, N/V, fatigue, alopecia, myalgia, upper abdominal pain, constipation, diarrhea.
Hematologic: Myelosuppression (thrombocytopenia, neutropenia, anemia).

DRUG INTERACTIONS
See Boxed Warning and Dosing Considerations. May increase concentrations of drugs eliminated by CYP3A4 (eg, midazolam, certain HMG-CoA reductase inhibitors), CYP2C8, CYP2C9, CYP2D6, and UGT1A1 enzymes; dose adjustment may be necessary for CYP3A4 substrates, especially those that have narrow therapeutic indices (eg, alfentanil, cyclosporine, dihydroergotamine). May decrease concentrations of drugs eliminated by CYP2B6, CYP2C8, and CYP2C9 enzymes; monitor patients closely when nilotinib is coadministered w/ drugs that have a narrow therapeutic index and are substrates for these enzymes. May increase concentrations of P-gp substrates; use w/ caution. Concomitant administration of strong CYP3A4 inhibitors or inducers may increase or decrease nilotinib concentrations significantly. Decreased solubility and reduced bioavailability w/ drugs that inhibit gastric acid secretion to elevate the gastric pH; concomitant use w/ proton pump inhibitors is not recommended. When the concurrent use of a H$_2$ blocker is necessary, administer approx 10 hrs before and 2 hrs after the dose of nilotinib. If antacid administration is necessary, administer approx 2 hrs before or 2 hrs after the dose of nilotinib. P-gp inhibitors may increase concentrations; use w/ caution. Avoid w/ drugs that may prolong the QT interval (eg, antiarrhythmic drugs), and grapefruit products and other foods that inhibit CYP3A4.

PREGNANCY AND LACTATION
Pregnancy: Category D. May cause fetal harm when administered to a pregnant woman. Women of childbearing potential should avoid becoming pregnant while on therapy.
Lactation: Not for use in nursing.

MECHANISM OF ACTION
Kinase inhibitor; inhibits BCR-ABL kinase. Binds to and stabilizes the inactive conformation of the kinase domain of ABL protein.

PHARMACOKINETICS
Absorption: T_{max}=3 hrs. **Distribution:** Plasma protein binding (98%). **Metabolism:** Via oxidation and hydroxylation. **Elimination:** Feces (93%, 69% unchanged); $T_{1/2}$=17 hrs.

PATIENT CONSIDERATIONS
Assessment: Assess for electrolyte abnormalities, history of pancreatitis, long QT syndrome, cardiac disorders, total gastrectomy, hepatic impairment, galactose intolerance, lactase deficiency, glucose-galactose malabsorption, pregnancy/nursing status, and possible drug interactions. Obtain baseline ECG, uric acid levels, and chemistry panels, including lipid profile and glucose.

Monitoring: Monitor for myelosuppression; perform CBCs every 2 weeks for the first 2 months of therapy, then monthly thereafter or as clinically indicated. Perform chemistry panels, including electrolytes and liver enzymes periodically. Monitor lipid profiles and glucose periodically during 1st yr of therapy and at least yearly during chronic therapy. Monitor for signs/symptoms of QT prolongation; obtain ECG 7 days after initiation, periodically thereafter, and after any dose adjustments. Maintain adequate hydration, evaluate CV status, and monitor CV risk factors. Monitor serum lipase levels and LFTs monthly or as clinically indicated. Monitor for signs of severe fluid retention, symptoms of respiratory/cardiac compromise, tumor lysis syndrome, hemorrhage, and other adverse reactions.

Counseling: Instruct to take ud. Advise to seek immediate medical attention w/ any symptoms suggestive of a CV event. Instruct not to consume grapefruit products at any time during treatment. Instruct to inform physician of other medicines being taken, including OTC drugs or herbal supplements (eg, St. John's wort). Advise that use of drug during pregnancy may cause harm to the fetus and that nilotinib should not be taken during pregnancy unless necessary. Instruct women of childbearing potential to use highly effective contraceptives while on therapy. Instruct not to d/c or change dose w/o consulting physician.

TECENTRIQ — atezolizumab   Rx
Class: Monoclonal antibody/programmed death ligand-1 (PD-L1) blocker

ADULT DOSAGE
Locally Advanced or Metastatic Urothelial Carcinoma

Use in patients w/ disease progression during or following platinum-containing chemotherapy or disease progression w/in 12 months of

PEDIATRIC DOSAGE
Pediatric use may not have been established

neoadjuvant or adjuvant treatment w/ platinum-containing chemotherapy

1200mg q3wks until disease progression or unacceptable toxicity

---

DOSING CONSIDERATIONS
Adverse Reactions
Withhold for Any of the Following:
- Grade 2 pneumonitis
- AST or ALT >3-5X ULN or total bilirubin >1.5-3X ULN
- Grade 2 or 3 diarrhea or colitis
- Symptomatic hypophysitis, adrenal insufficiency, hypothyroidism, hyperthyroidism, or Grade 3 or 4 hyperglycemia
- Grade 2 ocular inflammatory toxicity
- Grade 2 or 3 pancreatitis, or Grade 3 or 4 increases in amylase or lipase levels (>2X ULN)
- Grade 3 or 4 infection
- Grade 2 infusion-related reactions
- Grade 3 rash

Permanently D/C for Any of the Following:
- Grade 3 or 4 pneumonitis
- AST or ALT >5X ULN or total bilirubin >3X ULN
- Grade 4 diarrhea or colitis
- Grade 4 hypophysitis
- Myasthenic syndrome/myasthenia gravis, Guillain-Barre syndrome, or meningoencephalitis (all grades)
- Grade 3 or 4 ocular inflammatory toxicity
- Grade 4 or any grade of recurrent pancreatitis
- Grade 3 or 4 infusion-related reactions
- Grade 4 rash

ADMINISTRATION
IV route
- Administer initial infusion over 60 min through an IV line w/ or w/o a sterile, non-pyrogenic, low-protein binding in-line filter (pore size of 0.2-0.22 micron).
- If first infusion is tolerated, all subsequent infusions may be delivered over 30 min.
- Do not coadminister other drugs through the same IV line.
- Do not administer as an IV push or bolus.

Preparation
1. Withdraw 20mL from vial.
2. Dilute into a 250 mL polyvinyl chloride, polyethylene, or polyolefin infusion bag containing 0.9% NaCl inj.
3. Dilute w/ 0.9% NaCl inj only.
4. Mix diluted sol by gentle inversion; do not shake.
5. Discard partially used or empty vials.
6. Administer immediately once prepared.

If diluted infusion sol is not used immediately, it can be stored either:
- At room temperature for ≤6 hrs from the time of preparation (including time for administration).
- Under refrigeration at 2-8°C (36-46°F) for ≤24 hrs.
Do not shake or freeze.

STORAGE
2-8°C (36-46°F) in original carton to protect from light. Do not freeze. Do not shake.

HOW SUPPLIED
Inj: 1200mg/20mL

WARNINGS/PRECAUTIONS
See Dosing Considerations. Refer to PI for corticosteroid dose in the management of the following adverse reactions. Immune-mediated pneumonitis or interstitial lung disease reported; monitor for signs w/ radiographic imaging and symptoms of pneumonitis. Immune-mediated hepatitis reported; monitor AST, ALT, and bilirubin prior to and periodically during treatment. Withhold for Grade 2 and permanently d/c for Grade 3 or 4 immune-mediated hepatitis. Immune-mediated colitis or diarrhea reported. Immune-related thyroid disorders, adrenal insufficiency, hypophysitis, and type 1 diabetes mellitus (DM), including diabetic ketoacidosis, reported. Initiate treatment w/ insulin for type 1 DM. Other immune-related adverse reactions (eg, meningoencephalitis, myasthenic syndrome/myasthenia gravis, Guillain-Barre, ocular inflammatory toxicity, pancreatitis) reported. Monitor for clinical signs/symptoms of meningitis or encephalitis, symptoms of motor and sensory neuropathy, hepatitis, diarrhea or colitis, endocrinopathies, and acute pancreatitis. Severe infections, (eg, sepsis, herpes encephalitis, mycobacterial infection leading to retroperitoneal hemorrhage) reported; monitor for signs/symptoms of infection and treat w/ antibiotics for suspected or confirmed bacterial infections. Severe infusion reactions reported; interrupt or slow rate of infusion w/ mild or moderate infusion reactions. May cause fetal harm.

ADVERSE REACTIONS
Fatigue, decreased appetite, nausea, UTI, pyrexia, constipation.

PREGNANCY AND LACTATION
Pregnancy: May cause fetal harm.
Lactation: Not for use in nursing and for at least 5 months after last dose.
Reproductive Potential: Females of reproductive potential should use effective contraception during treatment and for at least 5 months following the last dose. May impair fertility in females while receiving treatment.

MECHANISM OF ACTION

Monoclonal antibody/programmed death ligand-1 (PD-L1) blocker; binds to PD-L1 and blocks its interactions w/ both PD-1 and B7.1 receptors, releasing the PD-L1/PD-1 mediated inhibition of the immune response, including activation of the anti-tumor immune response w/o inducing antibody-dependent cellular cytotoxicity.

PHARMACOKINETICS

Distribution: V_d=6.9L. **Elimination:** $T_{1/2}$=27 days.

PATIENT CONSIDERATIONS

Assessment: Assess pregnancy/nursing status. Obtain baseline thyroid function and AST, ALT, and bilirubin levels.

Monitoring: Monitor for signs of immune-mediated pneumonitis w/ radiographic imaging and monitor for symptoms of pneumonitis. Monitor for signs/symptoms of immune-mediated hepatitis, diarrhea/colitis, hypophysitis, thyroid disorders, adrenal insufficiency, meningitis/encephalitis, hyperglycemia, motor and sensory neuropathy, pancreatitis, severe infections, infusion-related reactions, and other adverse reactions. Periodically monitor thyroid function and AST, ALT, and bilirubin levels.

Counseling: Inform of the risk of immune-related adverse reactions that may require corticosteroid treatment and interruption or discontinuation of atezolizumab. Advise to contact healthcare provider immediately for any new or worsening cough, chest pain, SOB, jaundice, severe N/V, pain on the right side of abdomen, lethargy, easy bruising or bleeding, diarrhea, severe abdominal pain, and signs/symptoms of hypophysitis, hyperthyroidism, hypothyroidism, adrenal insufficiency, type 1 DM, meningitis, myasthenic syndrome/myasthenia gravis, Guillain-Barre syndrome, ocular inflammatory toxicity, pancreatitis, infection, infusion-related reactions, and rash. Advise that treatment may cause fetal harm. Instruct females of reproductive potential to use effective contraception during treatment and for at least 5 months after the last dose. Advise not to breastfeed while on therapy and for at least 5 months after the last dose.

TECFIDERA — dimethyl fumarate   Rx

Class: Immunomodulatory agent

ADULT DOSAGE	PEDIATRIC DOSAGE
Multiple Sclerosis	Pediatric use may not have been established
Relapsing Forms:	
Initial: 120mg bid	
Titrate: Increase to 240mg bid after 7 days	
Maint: 240mg bid. Consider temporary dose reductions to 120mg bid for individuals who do not tolerate the maint dose; resume the recommended dose of 240mg bid w/in 4 weeks. Consider discontinuation for patients unable to tolerate return to maint dose	

ADMINISTRATION

Oral route

Take w/ or w/o food.
Swallow whole and intact; do not crush or chew.
Do not sprinkle cap contents on food.
To reduce flushing, take w/ food or take up to 325mg of non-enteric coated aspirin 30 min prior to therapy.

STORAGE

15-30°C (59-86°F). Protect from light.

HOW SUPPLIED

Cap, Delayed-Release: 120mg, 240mg

CONTRAINDICATIONS

Known hypersensitivity to dimethyl fumarate (DMF) or to any of the excipients of this medication.

WARNINGS/PRECAUTIONS

May cause anaphylaxis and angioedema; d/c if signs/symptoms occur. Progressive multifocal leukoencephalopathy (PML) reported; withhold treatment and perform appropriate diagnostic evaluation at the 1st sign/symptom suggestive of PML. May decrease lymphocyte counts; obtain CBC, including lymphocyte count, before initiating treatment, after 6 months of starting treatment, and then every 6-12 months thereafter, and as clinically indicated. Consider interruption of therapy w/ lymphocyte counts <0.5 x 10⁹/L persisting for >6 months; continue to obtain lymphocyte counts until their recovery if therapy is discontinued or interrupted due to lymphopenia. Consider withholding treatment in patients w/ serious infections until resolution; decisions about whether or not to restart therapy should be individualized based on clinical circumstances. May cause flushing; administration w/ food may reduce the incidence of flushing. Alternatively, administration of non-enteric coated aspirin (up to a dose of 325mg) 30 min prior to dosing may reduce the incidence or severity of flushing.

ADVERSE REACTIONS

Flushing, abdominal pain, diarrhea, nausea.

PREGNANCY AND LACTATION

Pregnancy: Category C. Encourage pregnant patients to enroll in the Tecfidera Pregnancy Registry.
Lactation: Caution in nursing.

MECHANISM OF ACTION

Immunomodulatory agent; not established. DMF and the metabolite (monomethyl fumarate [MMF]) have been shown to activate the nuclear factor (erythroid-derived 2)-like 2 (Nrf2) pathway. Nrf2 pathway is involved in the cellular response to oxidative stress.

PHARMACOKINETICS

Absorption: MMF: C_{max}=1.87mg/L (w/ food), AUC=8.21mg•hr/L (w/ food), T_{max}=2-2.5 hrs (median). **Distribution:** MMF: V_d=53-73L; plasma protein binding (27-45%). **Metabolism:** Extensive via rapid presystemic hydrolysis by esterases to MMF (active metabolite). **Elimination:** Primary Route: Exhalation of CO_2 (60%). Minor Route: Urine (16%), feces (1%); $T_{1/2}$=1 hr (MMF).

PATIENT CONSIDERATIONS

Assessment: Assess for known hypersensitivity to drug or any of the excipients, and pregnancy/nursing status. Obtain baseline CBC including lymphocyte count.

Monitoring: Monitor for anaphylaxis, angioedema, PML, lymphopenia, flushing, and other adverse reactions. Monitor CBC including lymphocyte count after 6 months of treatment, every 6-12 months thereafter, and as clinically indicated.

Counseling: Instruct to take ud. Advise to d/c therapy and seek medical care if signs/symptoms of anaphylaxis or angioedema develop. Inform that PML has occurred in patients who received therapy and is characterized by progression of deficits and usually leads to death or severe disability; instruct to contact physician if any symptoms suggestive of PML develop. Inform that therapy may decrease lymphocyte counts. Advise to contact physician if patient experiences persistent and/or severe flushing or GI reactions. Inform patients experiencing flushing that taking w/ food or taking a non-enteric coated aspirin prior to taking therapy may help. Instruct to inform physician if patient is pregnant or plans to become pregnant while on therapy; encourage enrollment in the Tecfidera pregnancy registry if patient becomes pregnant while on therapy.

TECHNIVIE — ombitasvir/paritaprevir/ritonavir   Rx

Class: CYP3A inhibitor/HCV NS5A inhibitor/HCV NS3/4A protease inhibitor

ADULT DOSAGE	PEDIATRIC DOSAGE
Chronic Hepatitis C (Genotype 4)	Pediatric use may not have been established
Combination w/ Ribavirin (RBV) in Patients w/o Cirrhosis:	
2 tabs qd (am) w/ RBV at 1000mg/day (<75kg) and 1200mg/day (≥75kg) in 2 divided doses for 12 weeks	
May be given w/o RBV for 12 weeks for treatment-naive patients who cannot take or tolerate RBV	

DOSING CONSIDERATIONS

Hepatic Impairment
Moderate to Severe (Child-Pugh B and C): Contraindicated

ADMINISTRATION

Oral route

Take in the am w/ a meal w/o regard to fat or calorie content.

STORAGE

≤30°C (86°F).

HOW SUPPLIED

Tab: (Ombitasvir/Paritaprevir/Ritonavir [RTV]) 12.5mg/75mg/50mg

CONTRAINDICATIONS

Moderate to severe hepatic impairment (Child-Pugh Class B and C). Drugs that are highly dependent on CYP3A for clearance and for which elevated plasma concentrations are associated w/ serious and/or life-threatening events, and drugs that are moderate or strong inducers of CYP3A and may lead to reduced efficacy (alfuzosin HCl, colchicine, ranolazine, dronedarone, carbamazepine, phenytoin, phenobarbital, rifampin, lurasidone, pimozide, ergotamine, dihydroergotamine, methylergonovine, ethinyl estradiol-containing medications such as combined oral contraceptives, cisapride, St. John's wort, lovastatin, simvastatin, efavirenz, sildenafil [when dosed as Revatio for the treatment of pulmonary arterial hypertension], triazolam, oral midazolam). Known hypersensitivity to RTV (eg, toxic epidermal necrolysis, Stevens-Johnson syndrome). Refer to the RBV prescribing information for a list of contraindications for RBV.

WARNINGS/PRECAUTIONS

Hepatic decompensation and hepatic failure, including liver transplantation or fatal outcomes, reported; d/c treatment in patients who develop evidence of hepatic decompensation. ALT elevations to >5X ULN reported; occurred during first 4 weeks of treatment and declined w/in 2-8 weeks w/ continued dosing. Perform hepatic lab testing during first 4 weeks of treatment and as clinically indicated thereafter. Monitor closely if ALT is elevated above baseline. Consider discontinuing if ALT levels remain persistently >10X ULN. D/C if ALT elevation is accompanied by signs/symptoms of liver inflammation or increasing direct bilirubin, alkaline phosphatase, or INR. Any hepatitis C virus (HCV)/HIV-1 coinfected patients should also be on a suppressive antiretroviral drug regimen to reduce the risk of HIV-1 protease inhibitor drug resistance. Refer to the RBV prescribing information for a full list of the warnings and precautions for RBV.

ADVERSE REACTIONS

Asthenia, fatigue, nausea, insomnia, pruritus, skin reactions, serum bilirubin elevations.

DRUG INTERACTIONS

See Contraindications. ALT elevation reported more frequently w/ ethinyl estradiol-containing medications (eg, combined oral contraceptives, contraceptive patches, contraceptive vaginal rings); d/c ethinyl estradiol-containing medications prior to starting therapy. Alternative methods of contraception (eg, progestin only contraception, nonhormonal methods) are recommended during therapy; ethinyl estradiol-containing medications can be restarted approx 2 weeks following completion of treatment. Caution w/ estrogens other than ethinyl estradiol (eg, estradiol and conjugated estrogens) used in hormone replacement therapy. Coadministration w/ drugs that are substrates of CYP3A, P-gp, BCRP, OATP1B1, or OATP1B3 may result in increased plasma concentrations of such drugs. Coadministration w/ strong inhibitors of CYP3A may increase paritaprevir and RTV concentrations. Inhibition of P-gp, BCRP, OATP1B1, or OATP1B3 may increase the plasma concentrations of the various components of Technivie. May increase levels of angiotensin receptor blockers, digoxin, antiarrhythmics, ketoconazole, quetiapine, calcium channel blockers, inhaled/nasal fluticasone, furosemide (C_{max}), rilpivirine, pravastatin, cyclosporine, tacrolimus, salmeterol, buprenorphine, norbuprenorphine, hydrocodone, or alprazolam. Concomitant use w/ inhaled or nasal fluticasone may reduce serum cortisol concentrations. May decrease levels of carisoprodol, cyclobenzaprine, norcyclobenzaprine, diazepam, nordiazepam, omeprazole, darunavir (C_{trough}), or voriconazole. Atazanavir, atazanavir/RTV, or lopinavir/RTV may increase paritaprevir levels. Not recommended w/ voriconazole, atazanavir, atazanavir/RTV, lopinavir/RTV, rilpivirine once daily, or salmeterol. Refer to PI for further information on drug interactions, including dosing modifications when used w/ certain concomitant therapies.

PREGNANCY AND LACTATION

Pregnancy: Category B. When therapy is administered w/ RBV, the combination regimen is contraindicated in pregnant women and in men whose female partners are pregnant.

Lactation: It is not known whether any of the components of the drug or their metabolites are present in human milk. Caution in nursing.

MECHANISM OF ACTION

Ombitasvir: Inhibitor of HCV NS5A, which is essential for viral RNA replication and virion assembly. **Paritaprevir:** Inhibitor of HCV NS3/4A protease which is necessary for the proteolytic cleavage of the HCV encoded polyprotein (into mature forms of the NS3, NS4A, NS4B, NS5A, and NS5B proteins) and is essential for viral replication. **RTV:** Not active against HCV but it is a potent CYP3A inhibitor that increases peak and trough plasma drug concentrations of paritaprevir and overall drug exposure.

PHARMACOKINETICS

Absorption: Absolute bioavailability (48% [ombitasvir], 53% [paritaprevir]). AUC_{0-24}=1239 (ombitasvir), 2276 (paritaprevir), 6072 (RTV) ng•hr/mL (median); C_{max}=82 (ombitasvir), 194 (paritaprevir), 543 (RTV) ng/mL (median); T_{max}=4-5 hrs. **Distribution:** Plasma protein binding (99.9%, ombitasvir), (97-98.6%, paritaprevir), (>99%, RTV); V_d=173L (ombitasvir), 103L (paritaprevir). **Metabolism:** Ombitasvir: Amide hydrolysis followed by oxidative metabolism. Paritaprevir: Via CYP3A4 (major), CYP3A5. RTV: Via CYP3A (major), CYP2D6. **Elimination:** Ombitasvir: Feces (90.2%, 87.8% unchanged), Urine (1.91%, 0.03% unchanged); $T_{1/2}$=21-25 hrs. Paritaprevir: Feces (88%, 1.1% unchanged), Urine (8.8%, 0.05% unchanged); $T_{1/2}$=5.5 hrs. RTV: Feces (86.4%, 33.8% unchanged), Urine (11.3%, 3.5% unchanged); $T_{1/2}$=4 hrs.

PATIENT CONSIDERATIONS

Assessment: Assess for cirrhosis, hepatic impairment, pregnancy/nursing status, hypersensitivity to any component in drug, and possible drug interactions. Assess baseline hepatic laboratory and clinical parameters. Assess HCV genotype.

Monitoring: Monitor for signs/symptoms of hepatic decompensation, hepatic failure, liver inflammation, ALT elevations, and other adverse reactions. Perform hepatic lab testing during first 4 weeks of treatment and as clinically indicated thereafter.

Counseling: Advise to take ud. Inform patients to watch for signs of liver inflammation or failure (eg, fatigue, weakness, lack of appetite); instruct to notify physician w/o delay if such symptoms develop. Advise to avoid pregnancy during treatment and w/in 6 months of stopping treatment w/ Technivie w/ RBV; instruct to notify physician immediately in the event of a pregnancy. Inform of drug interactions that may occur; instruct to report to physician use of any prescription, nonprescription medication, or herbal products. Inform that contraceptives containing ethinyl estradiol should not be used.

TEMODAR — temozolomide

Rx

Class: Alkylating agent

ADULT DOSAGE

Newly Diagnosed High Grade Glioblastoma Multiforme

Concomitant Phase:
75mg/m² /day for 42 days concomitant w/ focal radiotherapy

Dose should be continued throughout the 42-day concomitant period up to 49 days if all of the following conditions are met:
- ANC ≥1.5 x 10⁹/L
- Platelet count ≥100 x 10⁹/L
- Common toxicity criteria (CTC) nonhematological toxicity ≤Grade 1 (except for alopecia, N/V)

PEDIATRIC DOSAGE

Pediatric use may not have been established

Maint Phase:
Four weeks after completing the concomitant phase, temozolomide is administered for an additional 6 cycles of maint treatment

Cycle 1: 150mg/m² qd for 5 days followed by 23 days w/o treatment
Cycles 2-6: May increase to 200mg/m² at start of Cycle 2 if nonhematologic toxicity for Cycle 1 is ≤Grade 2 (except alopecia, N/V), ANC ≥1.5 x 10⁹/L, and platelet count ≥100 x 10⁹/L. The dose remains at 200mg/m²/day for the first 5 days of each subsequent cycle unless toxicity occurs; if the dose was not escalated at Cycle 2, do not escalate in subsequent cycles.

Refractory Anaplastic Astrocytoma

Patients Who Have Experienced Disease Progression on a Drug Regimen Containing Nitrosourea and Procarbazine:
Initial: 150mg/m² qd for 5 consecutive days per 28-day cycle
Titrate: May increase to 200mg/m²/day for 5 consecutive days per 28-day treatment cycle if both the nadir and day of dosing (Day 29, Day 1 of next cycle) ANC are ≥1.5 x 10⁹/L (1500/μL) and both the nadir and Day 29, Day 1 of next cycle platelet counts are ≥100 x 10⁹/L (100,000/μL)

Therapy may be continued until disease progression

DOSING CONSIDERATIONS

Adverse Reactions

Glioblastoma Multiforme (GBM) During Concomitant Radiotherapy:
Interrupt Dose If:
1. ANC ≥0.5 and <1.5 x 10⁹/L
2. Platelet count ≥10 and <100 x 10⁹/L
3. Nonhematologic toxicity (except alopecia, N/V) CTC Grade 2

D/C Therapy If:
1. ANC <0.5 x 10⁹/L
2. Platelet count <10 x 10⁹/L
3. Nonhematologic toxicity (except alopecia, N/V) CTC Grade 3 or 4

GBM During Maint Treatment:
Dose Levels for Maint Treatment:
Dose Level -1 (Reduction for Prior Toxicity): 100mg/m²/day
Dose Level 0 (Dose During Cycle 1): 150mg/m²/day
Dose Level 1 (Dose During Cycles 2-6 in Absence of Toxicity): 200mg/m²/day

Reduce by 1 Dose Level If:
1. ANC <1.0 x 10⁹/L
2. Platelet count <50 x 10⁹/L
3. Nonhematologic toxicity (except alopecia, N/V) CTC Grade 3

D/C Therapy If:
1. Dose reduction to <100mg/m² is required
2. The same Grade 3 nonhematological toxicity (except for alopecia, N/V) recurs after dose reduction
3. Nonhematologic toxicity (except alopecia, N/V) CTC Grade 4

Refractory Anaplastic Astrocytoma:
Refer to PI for dose modification

Other Important Considerations

Dose must be adjusted according to nadir neutrophil and platelet counts in the previous cycle and the neutrophil and platelet counts at the time of initiating the next cycle

ADMINISTRATION

Oral/IV route

Cap

Take on an empty stomach; bedtime administration may be advised.
Swallow whole w/ a glass of water; do not open or chew.
Antiemetic therapy may be administered prior to and/or following administration.

Inj

Infuse IV over 90 min.

When reconstituted w/ 41mL sterile water for inj, the resulting sol will contain 2.5mg/mL temozolomide.
Bring vial to room temperature prior to reconstitution.
Gently swirl the vials; do not shake.
Do not further dilute the reconstituted sol.
After reconstitution, store at room temperature (25°C [77°F]) and use w/in 14 hrs, including infusion time.

Withdraw up to 40mL from each vial to make up the total dose and transfer into an empty 250mL infusion bag.
Infuse IV using a pump over 90 min; flush the lines before and after each infusion.

May be administered in the same IV line w/ 0.9% NaCl inj only.
Do not infuse other medications simultaneously through the same IV line.

STORAGE
Cap: 25°C (77°F); excursions permitted to 15-30°C (59-86°F). **Inj:** 2-8°C (36-46°F). After reconstitution, store reconstituted product at 25°C (77°F); must be used w/ in 14 hrs, including infusion time.

HOW SUPPLIED
Cap: 5mg, 20mg, 100mg, 140mg, 180mg, 250mg; **Inj:** 100mg

CONTRAINDICATIONS
History of hypersensitivity reaction (eg, urticaria, allergic reaction including anaphylaxis, toxic epidermal necrolysis, and Stevens-Johnson syndrome) to any components of the product. History of hypersensitivity to dacarbazine (DTIC).

WARNINGS/PRECAUTIONS
See Dosing Considerations. Myelosuppression, including prolonged pancytopenia, which may result in aplastic anemia, may occur. Prior to dosing, patients must have an ANC≥1.5 x 10^9/L and a platelet count ≥100 x 10^9/L. For the concomitant treatment phase w/ radiotherapy, obtain a CBC prior to initiation of treatment and weekly during treatment. For the 28-day treatment cycles, obtain a CBC prior to treatment on Day 1 and on Day 22 (21 days after the first dose) of each cycle or w/in 48 hrs of that day, and weekly until the ANC is >1.5 x 10^9/L and platelet count exceeds 100 x 10^9/L. Greater risk of myelosuppression in women and elderly patients. Cases of myelodysplastic syndrome and secondary malignancies, including myeloid leukemia, observed. *Pneumocystis carinii* pneumonia (PCP) prophylaxis is required in all patients w/ newly diagnosed GBM who are receiving concomitant radiotherapy for 42-day regimen, and should be continued in patients who develop lymphocytopenia until recovery from lymphocytopenia (CTC ≤Grade 1); higher occurrence of PCP when temozolomide is administered during a longer dosing regimen. Fatal and severe hepatotoxicity reported; perform LFTs at baseline, midway through 1st cycle, prior to each subsequent cycle, and approx 2-4 weeks after last dose. May cause fetal harm. Caution w/ severe renal/hepatic impairment and in elderly. **Inj:** Bioequivalence established only when inj is given over 90 min; infusion over a shorter or longer period may result in suboptimal dosing and may increase possibility of infusion related adverse reactions.

ADVERSE REACTIONS
Alopecia, N/V, anorexia, headache, constipation, fatigue, convulsions, thrombocytopenia.

DRUG INTERACTIONS
Valproic acid may decrease oral clearance.

PREGNANCY AND LACTATION
Pregnancy: Category D. May cause fetal harm.
Lactation: Not for use in nursing.

MECHANISM OF ACTION
Alkylating agent (imidazotetrazine derivative); not directly active but undergoes rapid nonenzymatic conversion at physiologic pH to the reactive compound 5-(3-methyltriazen-1-yl)-imidazole-4-carboxamide (MTIC). Cytotoxicity of MTIC is thought to be primarily due to alkylation of DNA. Alkylation (methylation) occurs mainly at the O^6 and N^7 positions of guanine.

PHARMACOKINETICS
Absorption: (PO) Rapid and complete, T_{max}=1 hr (median); C_{max}=7.5mcg/mL, 282ng/mL; AUC=23.4mcg•hr/mL, 864ng•hr/mL (MTIC). (IV) C_{max}=7.3mcg/mL, 276ng/mL (MTIC); AUC=24.6mcg•hr/mL, 891ng•hr/mL (MTIC). **Distribution:** V_d=0.4L/kg; plasma protein binding (15%). **Metabolism:** Spontaneous hydrolysis to the active species, MTIC, and to temozolomide acid metabolite. MTIC is further hydrolyzed to 5-amino-imidazole-4-carboxamide and methylhydrazine. **Elimination:** Urine (37.7%, 5.6% unchanged), feces (0.8%); $T_{1/2}$=1.8 hrs.

PATIENT CONSIDERATIONS
Assessment: Assess for previous hypersensitivity to drug or DTIC, myelosuppression, hepatic/renal impairment, pregnancy/nursing status, and possible drug interactions. Obtain baseline LFTs, CBC, and ANC.

Monitoring: Monitor for myelosuppression, PCP, myelodysplastic syndrome, secondary malignancies, and other adverse reactions. For the concomitant treatment phase w/ radiotherapy, obtain a CBC weekly during treatment. For the 28-day treatment cycles, obtain a CBC on Day 22 (21 days after the first dose) of each cycle or w/in 48 hrs of that day. If ANC falls <1.5 x 10^9/L and the platelet count falls <100 x 10^9/L, obtain blood counts weekly until recovery. Perform LFTs midway through the 1st cycle, prior to each subsequent cycle, and approx 2-4 weeks after the last dose. **Inj:** Monitor for infusion-related reactions.

Counseling: Instruct to take exactly as prescribed. Instruct to take rigorous precautions to avoid inhalation or contact w/ skin or mucous membranes if caps or vials are accidentally opened or damaged. Inform about the most frequently occurring adverse effects (eg, N/V).

THALOMID — thalidomide   Rx
Class: Immunomodulatory agent

> **Severe birth defects or embryo-fetal death may occur if taken during pregnancy. Should never be used by pregnant women or females who could become pregnant. Approved for marketing only through a special restricted distribution program called the "THALOMID REMS program." May increase risk of venous thromboembolism in patients w/ multiple myeloma (MM), especially w/ standard chemotherapeutic agents including dexamethasone; observe for signs/symptoms of thromboembolism. Instruct patients to seek medical care if symptoms such as SOB, chest pain, or arm or leg swelling develop. Consider thromboprophylaxis based on assessment of individual's underlying risk factors.**

ADULT DOSAGE
Multiple Myeloma

Newly Diagnosed:
200mg qd; administer in combination w/ dexamethasone 40mg PO on Days 1-4, 9-12, and 17-20, every 28 days

Erythema Nodosum Leprosum

Acute Treatment of Cutaneous Manifestations:
Initial: 100-300mg qd

Patients <50kg:
Start at low end of dosing range

Patients w/ Severe Cutaneous Reaction or Who Previously Required Higher Doses to Control Reaction:
May initiate at higher doses up to 400mg/day qhs or in divided doses w/ water, at least 1 hr after meals

Moderate-Severe Neuritis Associated w/ Severe Cutaneous Reaction:
May initiate corticosteroids concomitantly w/ thalidomide; taper steroid usage and d/c when neuritis has ameliorated

Continue dosing w/ thalidomide until signs and symptoms of active reaction have subsided, usually at least 2 weeks; patients may then be tapered off medication in 50mg decrements every 2-4 weeks

Maint Therapy for Prevention/ Suppression of Recurrence:
Use the minimum dose necessary to control reaction; attempt tapering off medication every 3-6 months, in decrements of 50mg every 2-4 weeks

PEDIATRIC DOSAGE
Multiple Myeloma

≥12 Years:
Newly Diagnosed:
200mg qd; administer in combination w/ dexamethasone 40mg PO on Days 1-4, 9-12, and 17-20, every 28 days

Erythema Nodosum Leprosum

≥12 Years:
Acute Treatment of Cutaneous Manifestations:
Initial: 100-300mg qd

Patients <50kg:
Start at low end of dosing range

Patients w/ Severe Cutaneous Reaction or Who Previously Required Higher Doses to Control Reaction:
May initiate at higher doses up to 400mg/day qhs or in divided doses w/ water, at least 1 hr after meals

Moderate-Severe Neuritis Associated w/ Severe Cutaneous Reaction:
May initiate corticosteroids concomitantly w/ thalidomide; taper steroid usage and d/c when neuritis has ameliorated

Continue dosing w/ thalidomide until signs and symptoms of active reaction have subsided, usually at least 2 weeks; patients may then be tapered off medication in 50mg decrements every 2-4 weeks

Maint Therapy for Prevention/ Suppression of Recurrence:
Use the minimum dose necessary to control reaction; attempt tapering off medication every 3-6 months, in decrements of 50mg every 2-4 weeks

DOSING CONSIDERATIONS
Adverse Reactions
Consider dose reduction, delay, or discontinuation in patients who develop NCI CTC Grade 3 or 4 adverse reactions and/or based on clinical judgment

MM: Patients who develop reactions (eg, constipation, somnolence, peripheral neuropathy) may benefit by either temporarily discontinuing the drug or continuing at a lower dose; drug may be started at a lower dose or at the previous dose w/ the abatement of these adverse reactions

ADMINISTRATION
Oral route

Take w/ water, preferably hs and at least 1 hr after evening meal.
Do not open/crush caps.

Handling Precautions
If powder contacts the skin, wash immediately and thoroughly w/ soap and water. If powder contacts mucous membranes, flush thoroughly w/ water.

STORAGE
20-25°C (68-77°F); excursions permitted to 15-30°C (59-86°F). Store in blister packs until ingestion. Protect from light.

HOW SUPPLIED
Cap: 50mg, 100mg, 150mg, 200mg

CONTRAINDICATIONS
Pregnancy, hypersensitivity to thalidomide or its components.

WARNINGS/PRECAUTIONS
Females of reproductive potential should avoid contact w/ caps. Healthcare providers or other caregivers should utilize appropriate precautions to prevent potential cutaneous exposure. Females of reproductive potential must avoid pregnancy and must commit either to completely abstain from heterosexual intercourse or to use 2 methods of reliable birth control (at least 1 highly effective method required even w/ history of infertility, unless due to hysterectomy) for at least 4 weeks before beginning therapy, during therapy, during dose interruptions, and for at least 4 weeks after completing therapy. Perform appropriate pregnancy tests prior to and during therapy. Male patients (including those w/ vasectomy) w/ female partners of reproductive potential must always use a latex/synthetic condom during any sexual contact during therapy and for up to 28 days after discontinuation of therapy. Male patients must not donate sperm. Patients must not donate blood during treatment and for 1 month following discontinuation. Ischemic heart disease, including MI, and stroke reported in patients w/ previously untreated MM. May impair physical/mental ability; dose reductions may be required. May cause irreversible peripheral neuropathy; d/c therapy if drug-induced neuropathy develops. May cause dizziness and orthostatic hypotension. Decreased WBC counts, including neutropenia, reported. Do not initiate if ANC is <750/mm³; reevaluate therapy and consider withholding thalidomide. Thrombocytopenia, including Grade 3 or 4 occurrences reported; dose reduction, delay, or discontinuation may be required. May increase plasma HIV RNA levels in HIV-seropositive patients. Bradycardia reported; dose reduction or discontinuation may be required. May cause serious dermatologic reactions

(eg, Stevens-Johnson syndrome [SJS], toxic epidermal necrolysis [TEN]); d/c if skin rash occurs and do not resume therapy if the rash is exfoliative, purpuric, or bullous or if SJS or TEN is suspected. Seizures, including grand mal convulsions, reported. Caution in patients at risk of tumor lysis syndrome. Consider risks of adverse effects in choosing contraceptive methods. Hypersensitivity reported; may necessitate interruption of therapy if a severe hypersensitivity reaction occurs. D/C if the reaction recurs when dosing is resumed. Not indicated as monotherapy for cutaneous manifestations of moderate/severe erythema nodosum leprosum (ENL) in the presence of moderate/severe neuritis.

ADVERSE REACTIONS
MM: Fatigue, hypocalcemia, edema, constipation, sensory neuropathy, dyspnea, muscle weakness, leukopenia, neutropenia, rash/desquamation, confusion, anorexia, nausea, anxiety.
ENL: Somnolence, rash, headache.

DRUG INTERACTIONS
See Boxed Warning. Avoid w/ medications that may cause drowsiness (eg, opioids, antihistamines, antipsychotics, antianxiety agents, CNS depressants). Caution w/ drugs that may cause additive bradycardic effect (eg, calcium channel blockers, β-blockers, digoxin, lithium). Caution w/ drugs associated w/ peripheral neuropathy (eg, amiodarone, docetaxel, vincristine). Concomitant use of HIV-protease inhibitors, griseofulvin, modafinil, penicillins, rifampin, rifabutin, phenytoin, carbamazepine, or certain herbal supplements (eg, St. John's wort) w/ hormonal contraceptive agents may reduce effectiveness of the contraception up to 1 month after discontinuation of these concomitant therapies; females requiring treatment w/ 1 or more of these drugs must use two other effective or highly effective methods of contraception while taking thalidomide. Caution w/ erythropoietic agents or other agents that may increase the risk of thromboembolism (eg, estrogen-containing therapies) in patients w/ MM.

PREGNANCY AND LACTATION
Pregnancy: Category X.
Lactation: Not for use in nursing.

MECHANISM OF ACTION
Immunomodulatory agent; not established. Possesses immunomodulatory, anti-inflammatory, and antiangiogenic properties. Immunologic effects may be caused by suppression of excessive TNF-α production and down-modulation of selected cell surface adhesion molecules involved in leukocyte migration. May suppress macrophage involvement in prostaglandin synthesis and modulation of interleukin-10 and -12 production by peripheral blood mononuclear cells. In MM, increased numbers of circulating natural killer cells and plasma levels of interleukin-2 and interferon-gamma are also seen. Angiogenesis inhibition may include the proliferation of endothelial cells.

PHARMACOKINETICS
Absorption: Slow. Administration of variable doses resulted in different parameters. **Distribution:** Plasma protein binding (55%, [+]-[R]-thalidomide and 66%, [-]-[S]-thalidomide). **Metabolism:** Hydrolysis. **Elimination:** Feces (<2%); urine (91.9%, <3.5% unchanged); $T_{1/2}$=5.5-7.3 hrs.

PATIENT CONSIDERATIONS
Assessment: Assess use in those capable of reproduction. Assess that patients are committed to either abstaining from heterosexual contact or willing to use a latex/synthetic condom for males or 2 forms of reliable contraception, including 1 highly effective method and 1 additional effective method for females, and beginning 4 weeks prior to treatment for females. Assess pregnancy status w/ in 10-14 days and w/in 24 hrs prior to therapy. Assess for moderate to severe neuritis, history/risk factors for seizures, hypersensitivity to drug, nursing status, and possible drug interactions. Consider electrophysiological testing. Obtain baseline neutrophil counts.

Monitoring: Monitor for venous thromboembolism, ischemic heart disease, MI, stroke, drowsiness, somnolence, peripheral neuropathy, dizziness, orthostatic hypotension, neutropenia, hypersensitivity reactions, bradycardia, syncope, seizures, serious dermatological reactions, missed periods or abnormal menstrual bleeding, and other adverse reactions. Monitor for signs/symptoms of bleeding, especially if on concomitant medication that may increase the risk of bleeding. Perform pregnancy test weekly during 1st month, then repeat monthly (regular menstrual cycle) or every 2 weeks (irregular menstrual cycle). Monitor for use of reliable methods of birth control (2 methods for females) during therapy, during dose interruptions, and continuing for 4 weeks after completing therapy. Perform electrophysiologic testing every 6 months, and WBC w/ differential count periodically. In HIV patients, monitor viral load after 1st and 3rd months of therapy and every 3 months thereafter. Monitor patients at risk of tumor lysis syndrome. Examine for early signs of neuropathy at monthly intervals for the first 3 months of therapy.

Counseling: Inform that drug is only available through a restricted distribution program and only from certified pharmacies; patients must sign a patient-prescriber agreement form and comply w/ the requirements. Inform that drug is contraindicated in pregnancy and can cause serious birth defects or embryo-fetal death; advise females of reproductive potential to avoid pregnancy during and for at least 4 weeks after therapy. Advise of the importance of monthly pregnancy tests and to use 2 different forms of contraception, including at least 1 highly effective form, simultaneously during therapy, during dose interruptions, and for 4 weeks after completing therapy. Instruct patients to immediately d/c and contact physician if they become pregnant, miss their menstrual period, experience unusual menstrual bleeding, or if they stop birth control. Advise males (including those w/ vasectomy) to use latex/synthetic condoms during any sexual contact during and up to 28 days after discontinuation of therapy; advise also not to donate sperm during therapy. Instruct not to donate blood during therapy and for 1 month following discontinuation. Inform of the potential risk of venous thromboembolism (eg, deep vein thrombosis, pulmonary embolism), ischemic

heart disease (eg, MI), and stroke, and of need for prophylactic treatment. Inform of the risk of dizziness and orthostatic hypotension w/ therapy; advise to sit upright for a few minutes prior to standing up from a recumbent position. Inform of other risks associated w/ therapy.

THERACYS — BCG live

Class: Attenuated live BCG culture

Rx

> **Contains live, attenuated mycobacteria. Potential risk for transmission; prepare, handle, and dispose as a biohazard material. Bacillus Calmette-Guerin (BCG) dissemination may occur when administered by the intravesical route. Serious infections, including fatal infections reported. BCG may persist in the urinary tract for several months after BCG instillations and delayed manifestations of disseminated BCG may develop months or years after BCG therapy.**

ADULT DOSAGE
Bladder Cancer

Treatment and prophylaxis of carcinoma in situ of the urinary bladder and for the prophylaxis of primary or recurrent stage Ta and/or T1 papillary tumors following transurethral resection (TUR)

Induction: 1 dose (81mg) each week intravesically for 6 consecutive weeks
Maint: 1 dose at 3, 6, 12, 18, and 24 months following the initial dose

Begin a minimum of 14 days after biopsy or TUR

PEDIATRIC DOSAGE
Pediatric use may not have been established

ADMINISTRATION
Intravesical route

Wear gloves and eye protection and take precautions to avoid contact of BCG w/ broken skin.
If the preparation cannot be performed in a biocontainment hood, wear a mask and gown.
Do not expose reconstituted product to sunlight, direct or indirect; keep exposure to artificial light to a minimum.

Preparation
1. Mix freeze-dried material w/ 3mL of sterile, preservative-free saline sol.
2. Shake the vial gently until a fine, even sus results; avoid foaming.
3. Withdraw entire contents (approx 3mL) of the reconstituted material into the syringe.
4. Further dilute the reconstituted material from the vial (1 dose) in sterile, preservative-free saline to a final volume of 50mL.
5. Use immediately after reconstitution; any delay between reconstitution and administration must not exceed 2 hrs at a temperature 2-25°C (35-77°F).

Administration
1. Insert a urethral catheter into bladder, drain bladder, instill 50mL of the drug slowly by gravity, and then withdraw catheter.
2. Have patient retain the sus for as long as possible for up to 2 hrs.
3. During the first 15 min following instillation, the patient should lie prone; thereafter, allow the patient to be in an upright position.
4. At the end of 2 hrs, have the patient void in a seated position for safety reasons.
5. Instruct patient to increase fluid intake in order to flush the bladder in the hours following treatment.

STORAGE
2-8°C (35-46°F).

HOW SUPPLIED
Inj: 81mg

CONTRAINDICATIONS
Known systemic hypersensitivity reaction to any component of this product or after a previous administration of this product or a medicinal product containing the same substances. Immunosuppressed persons w/ congenital/acquired immune deficiencies, whether due to concurrent disease (eg, AIDS, leukemia, lymphoma), cancer therapy (eg, cytotoxic drugs, radiation), or immunosuppressive therapy (eg, corticosteroids). Current symptoms or a previous history of systemic BCG reaction. A minimum of 14 days must elapse before therapy is administered following biopsy, TUR, or traumatic catheterization. Concurrent febrile illness, UTI, macroscopic hematuria, or active tuberculosis (TB).

WARNINGS/PRECAUTIONS
Not recommended for Stage Ta low-grade papillary tumors, unless at high risk of recurrence. Caution w/ preexisting arterial aneurysms or prosthetic devices (eg, arterial grafts, cardiac devices, artificial joints); ectopic BCG infection may occur. Systemic BCG reaction may occur. Avoid trauma and/or introduction of contaminants to the urinary tract. Monitor for signs/symptoms of toxicity after each intravesical treatment. Permanently d/c therapy, evaluate and treat immediately for BCG infection, and seek an infectious diseases consultation if persistent fever or an acute febrile illness consistent w/ BCG infection develops. If a bacterial UTI occurs during treatment, withhold instillation until complete resolution of the bacterial UTI. Stopper of vial contains natural rubber latex that may cause allergic reactions. Increased risk of bladder contracture in patients w/ small bladder capacity. Carefully consider treatment decisions in patients w/ a condition that may require future mandatory immunosuppression (eg, awaiting an organ transplant, myasthenia gravis). May induce a positive response to a tuberculin skin test (tuberculin purified protein derivative [PPD]); conduct

tuberculin skin test before administration if a patient's reactivity to PPD needs to be determined.

ADVERSE REACTIONS
Transient dysuria, urinary frequency/urgency, malaise, hematuria, fever, chills, cystitis, mild nausea.

DRUG INTERACTIONS
See Contraindications. Not sensitive to pyrazinamide. Immunosuppressants, myelosuppressants, or radiation interfere w/ the development of immune response to therapy and increase the risk of disseminated BCG infection. Antimicrobial drugs, including antimycobacterial agents (eg, isoniazid), may interfere w/ the effectiveness; do not use antimycobacterial agents prophylactically to prevent local, irritative side effects of therapy.

PREGNANCY AND LACTATION
Pregnancy: Category C. Do not become pregnant while on therapy.
Lactation: Not for use in nursing.

MECHANISM OF ACTION
Attenuated, live BCG culture; has not been established. Antitumor effect appears to be T-lymphocyte dependent. Promotes a local acute inflammatory and subacute granulomatous reaction w/ macrophage and lymphocyte infiltration in the urothelium and lamina propria of the urinary bladder.

PATIENT CONSIDERATIONS

Assessment: Assess for drug or latex hypersensitivity, immunosuppression, symptoms/history of systemic BCG reaction, febrile illness, UTI, macroscopic hematuria, active TB, any other conditions where treatment is contraindicated or cautioned, pregnancy/nursing status, and possible drug interactions.

Monitoring: Monitor for signs/symptoms of infections, systemic BCG reaction, and other adverse reactions. Monitor for signs/symptoms of toxicity after each intravesical treatment.

Counseling: Instruct to notify physician if patient has any symptoms (eg, fever, chills, malaise) that last >48 hrs or increase in severity, or if an increased urinary urgency or frequency of urination, blood in urine, joint pain, eye pain/irritation/redness, cough, skin rash, jaundice, or vomiting occurs. Advise that for 6 hrs after treatment, to void while seated to minimize splashing of urine, and to disinfect voided urine by adding an approximately equal volume of household bleach (5% hypochlorite sol) into the toilet bowl and allowing the bleach and urine to stand for 15 min prior to flushing. Inform that family and close contacts should avoid contact w/ voided urine. Instruct to increase fluid intake to flush the bladder for several hrs after treatment, unless medically contraindicated. Advise women not to become pregnant while on therapy.

THYMOGLOBULIN — anti-thymocyte globulin (rabbit)   Rx

Class: Immune globulin

> Should only be used by physicians experienced in immunosuppressive therapy for management of renal transplant.

ADULT DOSAGE
Renal Transplant Acute Rejection

In Conjunction w/ Concomitant Immunosuppression:
Recommended: 1.5mg/kg/day for 7-14 days via IV infusion using a high-flow vein over a minimum of 6 hrs for 1st infusion, and over at least 4 hrs on subsequent days of therapy

Administration of antiviral prophylactic therapy is recommended

Premedication

Corticosteroids, acetaminophen, and/or an antihistamine administration is recommended 1 hr prior to the infusion

PEDIATRIC DOSAGE
Pediatric use may not have been established

DOSING CONSIDERATIONS
Adverse Reactions
WBC Count 2000-3000 cells/mm³ or Platelet Count 50,000-75,000 cells/mm³: Reduce dose by 50%
WBC Count <2000 cells/mm³ or Platelet Count <50,000 cells/mm³: Consider discontinuing therapy

ADMINISTRATION
IV route

Reconstitution
Reconstituted Thymoglobulin is physically and chemically stable for up to 24 hrs at room temperature; however, room temperature storage is not recommended. As Thymoglobulin contains no preservatives, reconstituted product should be used immediately.
1. Allow vials to reach room temperature before reconstituting the lyophilized product.
2. Aseptically reconstitute each vial w/ 5mL of sterile water for inj.
3. Rotate vial gently until powder is completely dissolved; each reconstituted vial contains 25mg or 5mg/mL of Thymoglobulin.

Dilution
1. Transfer the contents of the calculated number of Thymoglobulin vials into the bag of infusion sol (saline or dextrose); use 50mL of infusion sol per 1 vial of Thymoglobulin (total volume usually between 50-500mL).
2. Mix the sol by inverting the bag gently only once or twice.

Infusion
1. Infuse through an in-line 0.22µm filter.
2. Set the flow rate to deliver the dose over a minimum of 6 hrs for the 1st dose, and over at least 4 hrs for subsequent doses.

STORAGE
2-8°C (36-46°F). Protect from light. Do not freeze.

HOW SUPPLIED
Inj: 25mg

CONTRAINDICATIONS
Active acute/chronic infections.

WARNINGS/PRECAUTIONS
Medical surveillance required during infusion. Serious immune-mediated reactions (eg, anaphylaxis, severe cytokine release syndrome [CRS]) reported. D/C infusion immediately if anaphylactic reaction occurs. Medical personnel, emergency treatment (eg, epinephrine 1:1000 dilution) and other resuscitative measures should be available. Infections (eg, bacterial, fungal, viral, protozoal), reactivation of infection (particularly CMV), and sepsis reported in combination w/ multiple immunosuppressive agents; careful patient monitoring and appropriate anti-infective prophylaxis are recommended. CRS reported w/ rapid infusion rates. Thrombocytopenia and/or leukopenia (including lymphopenia, neutropenia) have been identified and are reversible after dose adjustment. May increase incidence of malignancies (eg, lymphoma, lymphoproliferative disorders [which may be virally mediated]). Infusion-site reactions (eg, pain, swelling, erythema) may occur. May interfere w/ rabbit antibody-based immunoassays and w/ cross-match or panel-reactive antibody cytotoxicity assays.

ADVERSE REACTIONS
Chills, leukopenia, headache, abdominal pain, HTN, nausea, dyspnea, hyperkalemia, myalgia, insomnia, hypotension, rash, sweating, malaise, acne.

DRUG INTERACTIONS
Immunization w/ attenuated live vaccines is not recommended for patients who have recently received therapy. May predispose patients to over-immunosuppression w/ standard immunosuppressive regimen; may decrease maintenance immunosuppression therapy during period of antibody therapy. May stimulate antibody production, which cross-reacts w/ rabbit immune globulins.

PREGNANCY AND LACTATION
Pregnancy: Category C.
Lactation: Not for use in nursing.

MECHANISM OF ACTION
Gamma immune globulin; not established. Possibly induces immunosuppression in vivo via T-cell clearance from the circulation and modulation of T-cell activation, homing, and cytotoxic activities.

PHARMACOKINETICS
Elimination: $T_{1/2}$=2-3 days.

PATIENT CONSIDERATIONS

Assessment: Assess for history of allergy or anaphylaxis to rabbit proteins, active acute/chronic infections, pregnancy/nursing status, and possible drug interactions. Obtain baseline lymphocyte, and WBC and platelet counts.

Monitoring: Monitor for signs/symptoms of infusion reactions, severe infections, malignancies, CRS, anaphylactic reactions, and other adverse reactions. Monitor lymphocyte (total lymphocytes and/or T-cell subset), WBC and platelet counts.

Counseling: Inform of the potential benefits/risks of treatment.

TIKOSYN — dofetilide   Rx

Class: Class III antiarrhythmic

> To minimize risk of induced arrhythmia, for a minimum of 3 days, place patients initiated or reinitiated on therapy in a facility that can provide calculations of CrCl, continuous ECG monitoring, and cardiac resuscitation.

ADULT DOSAGE
Atrial Fibrillation

Conversion of A-Fib/A-Flutter to Normal Sinus Rhythm and Maint of Normal Sinus Rhythm in Patients w/ Highly Symptomatic A-Fib/A-Flutter of >1 Week Duration Who Were Converted to Normal Sinus Rhythm:

Reserve for patients in whom A-fib/A-flutter is highly symptomatic. Hypokalemia should be corrected before initiation; maintain serum K⁺ levels >3.6-4.0mEq/L.

Initial:
Individualize dose based on CrCl and QTc (use QT interval if HR <60bpm); QTc must be ≤440 msec to proceed
CrCl >60mL/min: 500mcg bid
CrCl 40-60mL/min: 250mcg bid

PEDIATRIC DOSAGE
Pediatric use may not have been established

CrCl 20 to <40mL/min: 125mcg bid
CrCl <20mL/min: Contraindicated
Post Dose Adjustment:
After 2-3 hrs if the QTc has increased ≤15%, continue current dose; if QTc has increased >15% compared to the baseline or if the QTc is >500 msec (550 msec w/ ventricular conduction abnormalities), adjust subsequent doses as such:
Initial Dose of 500mcg bid: Reduce dose to 250mcg bid
Initial Dose of 250mcg bid: Reduce dose to 125mcg bid
Initial Dose of 125mcg bid: Reduce dose to 125mcg qd
Maint:
If at any time after the 2nd dose the QTc increases >500 msec (550 msec in patients w/ ventricular conduction abnormalities), d/c dofetilide
If renal function deteriorates, adjust dose based on CrCl as seen above
Max:
CrCl >60mL/min: 500mcg bid
Cardioversion:
If patients do not convert to normal sinus rhythm w/in 24 hrs of initiation, electrical conversion should be considered. Patients continuing on dofetilide after successful electrical cardioversion should continue to be monitored by ECG for 12 hrs post cardioversion, or a minimum of 3 days after initiation of dofetilide therapy, whichever is greater

Conversions
Switching from Class I or Other Class III Antiarrhythmics:
Withdraw previous antiarrhythmic therapy under careful monitoring for a minimum of 3 plasma half-lives before initiating therapy; do not initiate dofetilide following amiodarone therapy until amiodarone plasma levels are <0.3mcg/mL or until withdrawn for at least 3 months

----

DOSING CONSIDERATIONS
Discontinuation
If dofetilide needs to be discontinued to allow dosing of other potentially interacting drugs, a washout period of ≥2 days should be followed before starting the other drug

ADMINISTRATION
Oral route
Take PO w/ or w/o food.
Initiate/titrate in presence of continuous ECG monitoring and personnel trained in management of serious ventricular arrhythmias.

STORAGE
15-30°C (59-86°F). Protect from humidity and moisture.

HOW SUPPLIED
Cap: 125mcg, 250mcg, 500mcg

CONTRAINDICATIONS
Congenital or acquired long QT syndromes, baseline QT interval or QTc >440 msec (500 msec w/ ventricular conduction abnormalities), severe renal impairment (CrCl <20mL/min), known hypersensitivity to the drug. Concomitant verapamil, HCTZ (alone/in combinations [eg, triamterene]), and inhibitors of renal cation transport system (eg, cimetidine, trimethoprim [alone/combination w/ sulfamethoxazole], ketoconazole, prochlorperazine, dolutegravir, megestrol).

WARNINGS/PRECAUTIONS
May cause serious ventricular arrhythmias, primarily torsades de pointes (TdP); risk of TdP can be reduced by controlling the plasma concentration through adjustment of the initial dofetilide dose according to CrCl and by monitoring the ECG. Calculate CrCl before 1st dose. Caution in patients w/ severe hepatic impairment. Do not discharge patients w/in 12 hrs of conversion to normal sinus rhythm. Maintain normal K⁺ levels prior to and during administration. Patients w/ A-fib should be anticoagulated prior to cardioversion and may continue to use after cardioversion. Rehospitalize patient for 3 days anytime dose is increased. Consider electrical cardioversion if patient does not convert to normal sinus rhythm w/in 24 hrs of initiation of therapy. If dofetilide needs to be discontinued to allow dosing of other potentially interacting drug(s), a washout period of at least 2 days should be followed before starting the other drug(s). Caution in elderly.

ADVERSE REACTIONS
Headache, chest pain, dizziness, ventricular arrhythmia, ventricular tachycardia, TdP, respiratory tract infection, dyspnea, nausea, flu syndrome, insomnia, back pain, diarrhea, rash, abdominal pain.

DRUG INTERACTIONS
See Contraindications. Hypokalemia or hypomagnesemia may occur w/ K⁺-depleting diuretics, increasing the potential for TdP. CYP3A4 inhibitors (eg, macrolides, protease inhibitors, serotonin reuptake inhibitors) and drugs actively secreted by cationic secretion (eg, triamterene, metformin, amiloride) may increase levels; caution when coadministered. Not recommended w/ drugs that prolong the QT interval (eg, phenothiazines, TCAs, certain oral macrolides). Withhold Class I and III antiarrhythmics for at least 3 half-lives prior to dosing w/ dofetilide. Do not initiate therapy until amiodarone levels are <0.3mcg/mL or until amiodarone has been withdrawn for at least 3 months. Higher occurrence of TdP w/ digoxin.

PREGNANCY AND LACTATION
Pregnancy: Category C.
Lactation: Not for use in nursing.

MECHANISM OF ACTION
Class III antiarrhythmic; blocks cardiac ion channel carrying rapid component of delayed rectifier K⁺ current, I_{Kr}.

PHARMACOKINETICS
Absorption: T_{max}=2-3 hrs (fasted). **Distribution:** V_d=3L/kg; plasma protein binding (60-70%). **Metabolism:** Liver via CYP3A4 through N-dealkylation and N-oxidation pathways. **Elimination:** Urine (80% unchanged, 20% metabolites); $T_{1/2}$=10 hrs.

PATIENT CONSIDERATIONS
Assessment: Assess for previous hypersensitivity to drug, congenital or acquired long QT syndrome, renal/hepatic impairment, pregnancy/nursing status, and possible drug interactions. Correct K⁺ levels prior to therapy. Obtain baseline ECG and CrCl prior to therapy.

Monitoring: Monitor serum K⁺ levels and for development of ventricular arrhythmias (eg, TdP). After initiation or cardioversion, continuously monitor by ECG for a minimum of 3 days, or for a minimum of 12 hrs after electrical/pharmacological conversion to normal sinus rhythm, whichever is greater. Reevaluate renal function and QTc every 3 months, as medically warranted.

Counseling: Inform about risks/benefits, need for compliance w/ prescribed dosing, potential drug interactions, and the need for periodic monitoring of QTc and renal function. Instruct to notify physician of any changes in medications and supplements or if hospitalized or prescribed a new medication for any condition. Counsel to report immediately any symptoms associated w/ electrolyte imbalance (eg, excessive/prolonged diarrhea, sweating, vomiting, loss of appetite, thirst). Instruct not to double the next dose if a dose is missed and to take the next dose at the usual time.

TIVICAY — dolutegravir   Rx

Class: HIV-integrase strand transfer inhibitor

ADULT DOSAGE	PEDIATRIC DOSAGE
HIV-1 Infection	**HIV-1 Infection**
Used in combination w/ other antiretrovirals	Used in combination w/ other antiretrovirals
Treatment-Naive/Treatment-Experienced Integrase Strand Transfer Inhibitor (INSTI)-Naive: 50mg qd	**Treatment-Naive/Treatment-Experienced Integrase Strand Transfer Inhibitor (INSTI)-Naive:** 30 to <40kg: 35mg qd ≥40kg: 50mg qd
INSTI-Experienced w/ Certain INSTI-Associated Resistance Substitutions or Clinically Suspected INSTI Resistance: 50mg bid	

DOSING CONSIDERATIONS
Concomitant Medications
Treatment-Naive/Treatment-Experienced INSTI-Naive in Combination w/ Certain UGT1A/CYP3A Inducers (eg, Efavirenz, Fosamprenavir/Ritonavir [RTV], Tipranavir/RTV, Carbamazepine, Rifampin):
Adults:
50mg bid
Pediatric Patients:
30 to <40kg:
35mg bid
≥40kg:
50mg bid

Hepatic Impairment
Severe (Child-Pugh Score C): Not recommended
Mild to Moderate (Child-Pugh Score A or B): No dose adjustment needed

ADMINISTRATION
Oral route
Take w/ or w/o food.

STORAGE
25°C (77°F); excursions permitted to 15-30°C (59-86°F).

HOW SUPPLIED
Tab: 10mg, 25mg, 50mg

CONTRAINDICATIONS
Previous hypersensitivity reaction to dolutegravir, coadministration w/ dofetilide.

WARNINGS/PRECAUTIONS

Hypersensitivity reactions reported; d/c therapy and other suspect agents immediately if signs/symptoms develop, monitor clinical status (eg, liver aminotransferases), and initiate appropriate therapy. Patients w/ underlying hepatitis B or C may be at increased risk for worsening or development of transaminase elevations. Redistribution/accumulation of body fat observed. Immune reconstitution syndrome reported. Autoimmune disorders (eg, Graves' disease, polymyositis, Guillain-Barre syndrome) reported in the setting of immune reconstitution and can occur many months after initiation of treatment. Caution in elderly. Caution in INSTI-experienced patients (w/ certain INSTI-associated resistance substitutions or clinically suspected INSTI resistance) w/ severe renal impairment.

ADVERSE REACTIONS

Insomnia, fatigue, headache.

DRUG INTERACTIONS

See Dosing Considerations and Contraindications. Drugs that induce/inhibit UGT1A1, CYP3A, UGT1A3, UGT1A9, breast cancer resistance protein, and P-gp may decrease/increase levels, respectively. Decreased levels w/ etravirine; etravirine use w/o coadministration of atazanavir/RTV, darunavir/RTV, or lopinavir/RTV is not recommended. Decreased levels w/ carbamazepine, efavirenz, fosamprenavir/RTV, and tipranavir/RTV; use alternative combinations that do not include metabolic inducers where possible for INSTI-experienced patients w/ certain INSTI-associated resistance substitutions or clinically suspected INSTI resistance. Decreased levels w/ nevirapine, oxcarbazepine, phenytoin, phenobarbital, and St. John's wort; avoid coadministration. Administer 2 hrs before or 6 hrs after taking medications containing polyvalent cations (eg, cation-containing antacids/laxatives, sucralfate, buffered medications) and oral Ca^{2+} or iron supplements (eg, multivitamins); alternatively, dolutegravir and supplements containing Ca^{2+} or iron can be taken together w/ food. May increase levels of drugs eliminated via renal organic cation transporters, OCT2, or multidrug and toxin extrusion transporter 1 (eg, metformin); limit the total daily dose of metformin to 1000mg when starting metformin or dolutegravir. When stopping dolutegravir, the metformin dose may require an adjustment; monitor blood glucose when initiating concomitant use and after withdrawal of dolutegravir. Decreased levels w/ rifampin; use alternatives to rifampin where possible for INSTI-experienced patients w/ certain INSTI-associated resistance substitutions or clinically suspected INSTI resistance.

PREGNANCY AND LACTATION

Pregnancy: There are insufficient human data on the use of dolutegravir during pregnancy. Physicians are encouraged to register patients in the Antiretroviral Pregnancy Registry.
Lactation: Not for use in nursing.

MECHANISM OF ACTION

HIV-1 INSTI; inhibits HIV integrase by binding to integrase active site and blocking the strand transfer step of retroviral DNA integration, which is essential for the HIV replication cycle.

PHARMACOKINETICS

Absorption: Adults: AUC_{0-24}=53.6mcg•hr/mL (50mg qd), 75.1mcg•hr/mL (50mg bid); C_{max}=3.67mcg/mL (50mg qd), 4.15mcg/mL (50mg bid); T_{max}=2-3 hrs. Pediatrics: 30 to <40kg (35mg qd): C_{max}=4.4mcg/mL, AUC_{0-24}=64.6mcg•hr/mL. ≥40kg (50mg qd): C_{max}=3.89mcg/mL, AUC_{0-24}=50.1mcg•hr/mL. **Metabolism:** Via UGT1A1, CYP3A. **Elimination:** Urine (31%, <1% unchanged), feces (53% unchanged); $T_{1/2}$=approx 14 hrs.

PATIENT CONSIDERATIONS

Assessment: Assess for previous hypersensitivity to the drug, hepatitis B or C infection, renal/hepatic impairment, pregnancy/nursing status, and possible drug interactions.

Monitoring: Monitor for signs/symptoms of hypersensitivity reactions, redistribution/accumulation of body fat, immune reconstitution syndrome, autoimmune disorders, and other adverse reactions. If a hypersensitivity reaction develops, monitor clinical status, including liver aminotransferases. In patients w/ underlying hepatic disease, monitor for hepatotoxicity.

Counseling: Instruct to d/c immediately and seek medical attention if rash develops and is associated w/ other symptoms of hypersensitivity. Advise patients w/ underlying hepatitis B or C to have lab testing before and during therapy. Inform that fat redistribution/accumulation may occur. Advise to inform physician immediately of any symptoms of infection. Advise that therapy is not a cure for HIV-1 infection and that patients may continue to experience illnesses associated w/ HIV-1 infection, including opportunistic infections. Advise to take all HIV medications exactly as prescribed. Advise to avoid doing things that can spread HIV to others. Instruct to inform physician if any unusual symptom develops, or if any known symptom persists or worsens. Counsel patients on missed dose instructions. Advise not to breastfeed.

TOBI — tobramycin

Rx

Class: Aminoglycoside

OTHER BRAND NAMES

TOBI Podhaler

ADULT DOSAGE

Cystic Fibrosis

Management of Cystic Fibrosis w/ *Pseudomonas aeruginosa*:

Sol:
300mg bid (as close to 12 hrs apart as possible; not <6 hrs apart) for 28 days by inh over approx 15 min, using a nebulizer

Cap:
Inh of four 28mg caps bid (as close to 12 hrs apart as possible; not <6 hrs apart) for 28 days using the Podhaler device

After 28 days of therapy, stop for the next 28 days, then resume for the next 28 day on and 28 day off cycle

PEDIATRIC DOSAGE

Cystic Fibrosis

Management of Cystic Fibrosis w/ *Pseudomonas aeruginosa*:
≥6 Years:

Sol:
300mg bid (as close to 12 hrs apart as possible; not <6 hrs apart) for 28 days by inh over approx 15 min, using a nebulizer

Cap:
Inh of four 28mg caps bid (as close to 12 hrs apart as possible; not <6 hrs apart) for 28 days using the Podhaler device

After 28 days of therapy, stop for the next 28 days, then resume for the next 28 day on and 28 day off cycle

---

ADMINISTRATION

Oral inh route

Sol

Do not dilute or mix w/ dornase alfa or other medications in the nebulizer
Use w/ handheld PARI LC PLUS reusable nebulizer w/ a DeVilbiss Pulmo-Aide compressor

Cap

Do not swallow cap
Use w/ Podhaler device only; always use the new Podhaler device provided w/ each weekly pack
Only remove cap from blister immediately before use
Refer to PI for preparation and administration instructions

STORAGE

(Sol) 2-8°C (36-46°F). Upon removal from the refrigerator, or if refrigeration is unavailable, may be stored at room temperature (up to 25°C [77°F]) for up to 28 days. Do not expose to intense light. (Cap) 25°C (77°F); excursions permitted to 15-30°C (59-86°F). Protect from moisture.

HOW SUPPLIED

Sol, Inhalation: 300mg/5mL; **Cap, Inhalation (Podhaler):** 28mg [8, 56, 224 caps]

CONTRAINDICATIONS

Known hypersensitivity to any aminoglycoside.

WARNINGS/PRECAUTIONS

Ototoxicity (eg, tinnitus), nephrotoxicity, or bronchospasm may occur. May aggravate muscle weakness. If ototoxicity or nephrotoxicity occurs, d/c therapy until serum concentrations fall <2mcg/mL. May cause fetal harm.

ADVERSE REACTIONS

Cough, lung disorder, dyspnea, hemoptysis, N/V, pulmonary function test decreased, headache, fever, chest pain, diarrhea, dysgeusia, dysphonia.

DRUG INTERACTIONS

Avoid concurrent and/or sequential use w/ other drugs w/ neurotoxic, nephrotoxic, or ototoxic potential. Some diuretics may enhance toxicity by altering concentrations in serum and tissue; do not administer w/ ethacrynic acid, furosemide, urea, or IV mannitol.

PREGNANCY AND LACTATION

Category D, not for use in nursing.

MECHANISM OF ACTION

Aminoglycoside; acts primarily by disrupting protein synthesis, leading to altered cell membrane permeability, progressive disruption of the cell envelope, and eventual cell death.

PHARMACOKINETICS

Absorption: (Sol) C_{max}=1.04mcg/mL; T_{max}=1 hr (median); AUC=4.8mcg•hr/mL. (Cap) C_{max}=1.02mcg/mL (single dose), 1.48-1.99mcg/mL (multiple dose); T_{max}=1 hr (median); AUC=4.6mcg•hr/mL. **Distribution:** Crosses placenta. (Cap) V_d=85.1L. **Elimination:** Urine (unchanged). (Sol) Expectorated sputum (unabsorbed). (Cap) $T_{1/2}$=3 hrs.

PATIENT CONSIDERATIONS

Assessment: Assess for auditory, vestibular, renal, or neuromuscular dysfunction, drug hypersensitivity, pregnancy/nursing status, and possible drug interactions. Consider an audiogram at baseline, particularly for patients at increased risk of auditory dysfunction.

Monitoring: Monitor for ototoxicity, nephrotoxicity, neuromuscular effects, bronchospasm, and other adverse reactions. Consider an audiogram for patients who show any evidence of auditory dysfunction.

Counseling: Instruct to take drug ud, and to complete a full 28-day course of therapy even if feeling better. Inform of adverse reactions associated w/ therapy, such as ototoxicity, bronchospasm, nephrotoxicity, and neuromuscular disorders; instruct to inform physician if new or worsening symptoms develop, or if ringing in the ears, dizziness, or any changes in hearing occur. Inform of the need to monitor hearing, serum concentrations, or renal function during treatment. Advise to inform physician if patient has any history of kidney problems, is pregnant/nursing, or plans to become pregnant. (Cap) Advise that tobramycin inhalation sol or alternative therapeutic options may be considered if coughing that may be experienced w/ therapy becomes bothersome or cannot be tolerated. Advise to count each day of use towards the 28 day on-treatment part of the cycle if prescribed a 1-day or 7-day pack either immediately before or during a 28-day treatment w/ therapy; instruct to take only a total of 28 consecutive days of treatment during a cycle.

TORISEL — temsirolimus

Class: Kinase inhibitor

Rx

ADULT DOSAGE

Advanced Renal Cell Carcinoma

25mg infused over a 30- to 60-min period once a week until disease progression or unacceptable toxicity occurs

Premedication

Give prophylactic IV diphenhydramine 25-50mg (or similar antihistamine) approx 30 min before the start of each dose

PEDIATRIC DOSAGE

Pediatric use may not have been established

DOSING CONSIDERATIONS

Concomitant Medications

Strong CYP3A4 Inhibitors: Avoid use; if necessary, consider dose reduction to 12.5mg/week. If strong inhibitor is discontinued, allow a washout period of approx 1 week before dose is adjusted back to the dose used prior to initiation of the inhibitor. Avoid grapefruit juice.

Strong CYP3A4 Inducers: Avoid use; if necessary, consider dose increase from 25mg/week up to 50mg/week. If strong inducer is discontinued, return to dose used prior to initiation of the inducer.

Hepatic Impairment

Mild (Bilirubin >1-1.5X ULN or AST >ULN but Bilirubin ≤ULN): Reduce to 15mg/week

Other Important Considerations

Interruption/Adjustment:

ANC <1000/mm³, Platelet Count <75,000/mm³, or NCI CTCAE ≥Grade 3 Adverse Reactions: Hold therapy

Toxicities Resolve to ≤Grade 2: May restart therapy w/ the dose reduced by 5mg/week to a dose no lower than 15mg/week

ADMINISTRATION

IV route

- Complete administration of the final diluted sol w/in 6 hrs from the time that drug is first added to 0.9% NaCl inj.
- Infusion pump is the preferred method of administration.
- Appropriate administration materials should be composed of glass, polyolefin, or polyethylene, and consist of non-diethylhexylphthalate (DEHP), non-polyvinylchloride (PVC) tubing w/ appropriate filter (pore size ≤5 microns).
- If PVC administration set must be used, it should not contain DEHP.
- If administration set does not have an in-line filter, add a polyethersulfone end-filter (pore size 0.2-5 microns).
- Diluted inj contains polysorbate 80, which is known to increase rate of DEHP extraction from PVC.
- Avoid addition of other drugs/nutritional agents to admixture and avoid combination w/ agents capable of modifying sol pH.
- Protect from excessive room light/sunlight.
- Store in bottles (glass, polypropylene) or plastic bags (polypropylene, polyolefin) and administer through polyethylene-lined administration sets.
- Concentrate-diluent mixture is stable <25°C for up to 24 hrs.

Dilution Process

1. Mix each vial w/ 1.8mL of enclosed diluent for a resultant sol containing 30mg/3mL; mix well by inversion and allow sufficient time for air bubbles to subside.
2. Withdraw required amount of concentrate-diluent mixture and further dilute into an infusion bag containing 250mL of 0.9% NaCl inj; stability in other infusion sol has not been evaluated. Mix by inversion of bag/bottle and avoid excessive shaking.

STORAGE

2-8°C (36-46°F). Protect from light.

HOW SUPPLIED

Inj: 25mg/mL

CONTRAINDICATIONS

Bilirubin >1.5X ULN.

WARNINGS/PRECAUTIONS

Hypersensitivity/infusion reactions may occur. D/C infusion and observe for at least 30-60 min if hypersensitivity reaction develops; treatment may be resumed w/ the administration of an H₁ receptor antagonist, if not previously administered, and/or an H₂ receptor antagonist approx 30 min before restarting infusion. Assess benefit-risk prior to the continuation of therapy w/ severe or life-threatening reactions. Caution w/ mild hepatic impairment, known hypersensitivity to polysorbate 80 or an antihistamine, or patients who cannot receive an antihistamine for other medical reasons. Hyperglycemia reported; may need an increase in the dose of, or initiation of, insulin and/or oral hypoglycemic agents. May cause immunosuppression; observe for infections. *Pneumocystis jiroveci* pneumonia (PJP) reported; consider prophylaxis of PJP when concomitant use of corticosteroids or other immunosuppressive agents is required. Interstitial lung disease (ILD) reported; withhold therapy and consider empiric treatment w/ corticosteroids and/or antibiotics if clinically significant respiratory symptoms develop. Increases in serum TGs and cholesterol reported; may require initiation, or increase in the dose, of lipid-lowering agents. Fatal bowel perforation reported. Rapidly progressive and sometimes fatal acute renal failure not clearly related to disease progression reported. Associated w/ abnormal wound healing; caution during perioperative period. Increased risk of intracerebral bleeding in patients w/ CNS tumors. Avoid close contact w/ those who have received live vaccines. May cause fetal harm. Elderly may be more likely to experience certain adverse reactions (eg, diarrhea, edema, pneumonia).

ADVERSE REACTIONS

Rash, asthenia, mucositis, nausea, edema, anorexia, lab abnormalities (anemia, hyperglycemia, hyperlipemia, hypertriglyceridemia, lymphopenia, elevated alkaline phosphatase, elevated SrCr, hypophosphatemia, thrombocytopenia, elevated AST, leukopenia).

DRUG INTERACTIONS

See Dosing Considerations. Avoid w/ St. John's wort, grapefruit juice, or live vaccines. Strong inducers of CYP3A4/5 (eg, dexamethasone, phenytoin, rifampin) may decrease exposure of sirolimus. Strong CYP3A4 inhibitors (eg, atazanavir, clarithromycin, itraconazole) may increase levels of sirolimus. Dose-limiting toxicity reported w/ sunitinib. Increased risk of intracerebral bleeding w/ anticoagulants.

PREGNANCY AND LACTATION

Pregnancy: Category D. Avoid becoming pregnant throughout treatment and for 3 months after therapy has stopped. Men w/ partners of childbearing potential should use reliable contraception throughout treatment and for 3 months after the last dose. **Lactation:** Not for use in nursing.

MECHANISM OF ACTION

Mammalian target of rapamycin (mTOR) inhibitor; binds to an intracellular protein (FKBP-12) and the protein-drug complex inhibits the activity of mTOR that controls cell division, resulting in a G1 growth arrest in treated tumor cells, inability to phosphorylate p70S6k and S6 ribosomal protein, and reduced levels of hypoxia-inducible factors HIF-1 and HIF-2α and the vascular endothelial growth factor.

PHARMACOKINETICS

Absorption: C_{max}=585ng/mL, AUC=1627ng•h/mL. **Distribution:** V_d=172L. **Metabolism:** Liver via CYP3A4; sirolimus (active major metabolite). **Elimination:** Urine (4.6%), feces (78%); $T_{1/2}$=17.3 hrs, 54.6 hrs (sirolimus).

PATIENT CONSIDERATIONS

Assessment: Assess for CNS tumors, drug hypersensitivity, pregnancy/nursing status, and possible drug interactions. Obtain baseline hepatic function (eg, AST, bilirubin levels), lung radiograph, and serum glucose, cholesterol, and TG levels.

Monitoring: Monitor for hypersensitivity/infusion reactions, infections, ILD, clinical respiratory symptoms, bowel perforation, renal failure, wound healing complications, intracerebral bleeding, and other adverse reactions. Monitor hepatic function, CBCs, chemistry panels, and serum glucose, cholesterol, and TG levels.

Counseling: Counsel about the risks and benefits of therapy. Inform of possible serious allergic reactions despite premedication w/ antihistamines. Instruct to report to physician if any facial swelling, difficulty of breathing, excessive thirst or frequency of urination, new/worsening respiratory symptoms or abdominal pain, or blood in stools occurs. Advise to inform physician of all medications currently being taken. Advise that vaccinations may be less effective while on therapy; instruct to avoid use of live vaccines and close contact w/ people who have received live vaccines. Instruct women of childbearing potential and men w/ partners of childbearing potential to use reliable contraception throughout treatment and for 3 months after the last dose. Advise elderly patients that they may be more likely to experience certain adverse reactions.

TRACLEER — bosentan

Class: Endothelin receptor antagonist

Rx

Available only through a restricted program called the Tracleer REMS Program, a component of the Tracleer Risk Evaluation and Mitigation Strategy (REMS); prescribers, patients, and pharmacies must enroll in the program. Elevation of liver aminotransferases (ALT and AST) and bilirubin reported; measure serum aminotransferase levels prior to initiation of treatment and then monthly. Hepatic cirrhosis (after prolonged therapy in patients w/ multiple comorbidities and drug therapies) and liver failure reported. Avoid w/ elevated aminotransferases (>3X ULN) at baseline; d/c if liver aminotransferase elevations are accompanied by clinical symptoms of hepatotoxicity (eg, N/V, fever, jaundice) or increases in bilirubin ≥2X ULN. Likely to cause major birth defects if used during pregnancy; exclude pregnancy before start of treatment. Throughout treatment, and for 1 month after discontinuing, females of reproductive potential must use 2 reliable methods of contraception unless the patient has an IUD or tubal sterilization, in which case, no other contraception is needed. Hormonal contraceptives, including oral, injectable, transdermal, and implantable contraceptives, may not be effective in patients receiving bosentan; do not use as the sole means of contraception. Obtain monthly pregnancy tests.

ADULT DOSAGE

Pulmonary Arterial Hypertension

Treatment of pulmonary arterial HTN (WHO Group 1) to improve exercise ability and to decrease clinical worsening

Initial: 62.5mg bid (in am and pm) for 4 weeks
Maint/Max: 125mg bid

Low Body Weight:
<40kg and >12 Years:
Initial/Maint: 62.5mg bid
There is limited information about the safety and efficacy of therapy in children between 12-18 yrs of age

PEDIATRIC DOSAGE

Pediatric use may not have been established

DOSING CONSIDERATIONS
Concomitant Medications
Patients on Ritonavir for at Least 10 Days:
Initial: 62.5mg qd or qod based on individual tolerability

Adding Ritonavir:
D/C bosentan at least 36 hrs prior to initiation of ritonavir.
After at least 10 days following initiation of ritonavir, resume therapy at 62.5mg qd or qod based on individual tolerability.

Hepatic Impairment
Preexisting Impairment:
Moderate/Severe: Not recommended
Aminotransferases >3X ULN: Not recommended

Development of Aminotransferase Elevations:
D/C treatment if aminotransferase elevations are accompanied by clinical symptoms of hepatotoxicity (eg, N/V, abdominal pain, jaundice) or increases in bilirubin ≥2X ULN

ALT/AST >3 and ≤5X ULN:
Confirm by another aminotransferase test; if confirmed, reduce daily dose to 62.5mg bid or interrupt treatment. Monitor aminotransferase levels at least every 2 weeks thereafter.
If the aminotransferase levels return to pretreatment values, continue/reintroduce the treatment as appropriate. Reintroduce at the starting dose and check aminotransferase levels w/in 3 days and every 2 weeks thereafter.

ALT/AST >5 and ≤8X ULN:
Confirm by another aminotransferase test; if confirmed, stop treatment and monitor aminotransferase levels at least every 2 weeks thereafter.
Once aminotransferase levels return to pretreatment values, consider reintroduction of treatment. Reintroduce at the starting dose and check aminotransferase levels w/in 3 days and every 2 weeks thereafter.

ALT/AST >8X ULN:
D/C treatment; reintroduction of treatment should not be considered

Discontinuation
Consider gradual dose reduction (62.5mg bid for 3-7 days)

ADMINISTRATION
Oral route
Take w/ or w/o food

STORAGE
20-25°C (68-77°F); excursions permitted to 15-30°C (59-86°F).

HOW SUPPLIED
Tab: 62.5mg, 125mg

CONTRAINDICATIONS
Females who are or may become pregnant. Coadministration w/ cyclosporine A or w/ glyburide. Hypersensitivity to bosentan or any component of product.

WARNINGS/PRECAUTIONS
Not recommended w/ moderate or severe liver impairment. Fluid retention and peripheral edema reported. If clinically significant fluid retention develops, evaluate further to determine cause and possible need for treatment or discontinuation of therapy. If signs of pulmonary edema occur, consider possibility of associated pulmonary veno-occlusive disease (PVOD) and consider discontinuing therapy. Decreased sperm counts reported. May cause a dose-related decrease in Hgb and Hct; check Hgb concentrations after 1 and 3 months, and every 3 months thereafter.

ADVERSE REACTIONS
Respiratory tract infection, headache, edema, chest pain, syncope, flushing, hypotension, sinusitis, arthralgia, abnormal serum aminotransferases, palpitations, anemia.

DRUG INTERACTIONS
See Boxed Warning, Contraindications, and Dosing Considerations. Coadministration w/ both a CYP2C9 inhibitor (eg, fluconazole, amiodarone) and a strong CYP3A inhibitor (eg, ketoconazole, itraconazole) or a moderate CYP3A inhibitor (eg, amprenavir, erythromycin, fluconazole) may largely increase levels; coadministration of such combinations is not recommended. Increased levels w/ ketoconazole; increased effects of bosentan should be considered. May decrease levels of CYP3A/CYP2C9 substrates; estrogens and progestins in hormonal contraceptives; oral hypoglycemic agents predominantly metabolized by CYP2C9/CYP3A; simvastatin and other statins significantly metabolized by CYP3A (eg, lovastatin, atorvastatin); S-warfarin (a CYP2C9 substrate) and R-warfarin (a CYP3A substrate); and sildenafil. Monitor cholesterol levels after bosentan is initiated in patients using CYP3A-metabolized statins to see whether the statin dose needs adjustment. Increased trough levels w/ lopinavir/ritonavir; adjust dose of bosentan when initiating lopinavir/ritonavir. Rifampin may increase trough levels after 1st concomitant dose, but decrease levels at steady-state; measure serum aminotransferases weekly for first 4 weeks before reverting to normal monitoring. Caution w/ tacrolimus. Increased levels w/ sildenafil.

PREGNANCY AND LACTATION
Pregnancy: Category X. Females of reproductive potential should have a negative pregnancy test before treatment initiation; a urine or serum pregnancy test should be performed during the first 5 days of a normal menstrual period and at least 11 days after the last unprotected act of sexual intercourse. Obtain follow-up urine or serum pregnancy tests monthly in females of reproductive potential. Females of reproductive potential must use acceptable methods of contraception during treatment and for 1 month after treatment; patient must choose 1 highly effective form of contraception (IUD or tubal sterilization) or a combination of methods (hormone method w/ a barrier method or 2 barrier methods). If partner's vasectomy is chosen, a hormone or barrier method must be used along w/ this method.
Lactation: Not for use in nursing.

MECHANISM OF ACTION
Endothelin receptor antagonist; specific and competitive antagonist at endothelin receptor types ET_A and ET_B w/ slightly higher affinity for ET_A receptors than ET_B receptors.

PHARMACOKINETICS
Absorption: Absolute bioavailability (50%); T_{max}=3-5 hrs. **Distribution:** V_d=18L; plasma protein binding (>98%). **Metabolism:** Liver via CYP2C9 and CYP3A. **Elimination:** Biliary, urine (<3%); $T_{1/2}$=5 hrs.

PATIENT CONSIDERATIONS
Assessment: Assess for liver impairment, hypersensitivity, pregnancy/nursing status, and possible drug interactions. Obtain baseline serum aminotransferase levels.

Monitoring: Monitor for clinical symptoms of hepatotoxicity, increases in bilirubin ≥2X ULN, fluid retention, signs of pulmonary edema, PVOD, and other adverse reactions. Monitor serum aminotransferase levels monthly. Obtain monthly pregnancy tests. Check Hgb concentrations after 1 and 3 months of therapy and then every 3 months thereafter.

Counseling: Advise that drug is only available through a restricted access program called the Tracleer REMS Program and from specialty pharmacies enrolled in the Tracleer REMS Program. Inform of hepatotoxicity risk; discuss the requirement for monthly monitoring of serum aminotransferases. Inform that drug may cause serious birth defects if used by pregnant women. Inform females of reproductive potential to have monthly pregnancy tests and to use 2 reliable methods of contraception during and for 1 month after treatment discontinuation. Inform females who have an IUD or tubal sterilization that they can use these forms of contraception alone. Instruct to immediately contact physician if pregnancy is suspected. Educate regarding use of emergency contraception in the event of unprotected sex or contraceptive failure. Advise prepubertal females to report changes in reproductive status to prescriber. Inform that patient must sign the Tracleer Patient Enrollment and Consent Form to confirm the patient's understanding of the risks. Inform of other risks associated w/ therapy (eg, decreases in Hgb, Hct, and sperm count; fluid retention). Advise of the importance of Hgb testing.

TREANDA — bendamustine hydrochloride   Rx

Class: Alkylating agent

ADULT DOSAGE	PEDIATRIC DOSAGE
Chronic Lymphocytic Leukemia	Pediatric use may not have been established
100mg/m² IV over 30 min on Days 1 and 2 of a 28-day cycle, up to 6 cycles	
B-Cell Non-Hodgkin Lymphoma	
Indolent B-Cell Non-Hodgkin Lymphoma That Has Progressed During or w/in 6 Months of Treatment w/ Rituximab or a Rituximab-Containing Regimen:	
120mg/m² IV over 60 min on Days 1 and 2 of a 21-day cycle, up to 8 cycles	

DOSING CONSIDERATIONS
Renal Impairment
CrCl <40mL/min: Not recommended for use

Hepatic Impairment
Moderate (AST or ALT 2.5-10X ULN and Total Bilirubin 1.5-3X ULN): Not recommended for use
Severe (Total Bilirubin >3X ULN): Not recommended for use

Adverse Reactions
Chronic Lymphocytic Leukemia:
Grade 4 Hematologic Toxicity: Delay
Clinically Significant ≥Grade 2 Nonhematologic Toxicity: Delay
Nonhematologic Toxicity Has Recovered to ≤Grade 1 and/or the Blood Counts Have Improved (ANC ≥1 x 10⁹/L, Platelets ≥75 x 10⁹/L): Reinitiate; dose reduction may be warranted
≥Grade 3 Hematologic Toxicity: Reduce to 50mg/m² on Days 1 and 2 of each cycle
≥Grade 3 Hematologic Toxicity Recurs: Reduce to 25mg/m² on Days 1 and 2 of each cycle
≥Grade 3 Nonhematologic Toxicity: Reduce to 50mg/m² on Days 1 and 2 of each cycle

May consider dose re-escalation in subsequent cycles

B-Cell Non-Hodgkin Lymphoma:
Grade 4 Hematologic Toxicity: Delay
Clinically Significant ≥Grade 2 Nonhematologic Toxicity: Delay
Nonhematologic Toxicity Has Recovered to ≤Grade 1 and/or the Blood Counts Have Improved (ANC ≥1 x 10⁹/L, Platelets ≥75 x 10⁹/L): Reinitiate; dose reduction may be warranted
Grade 4 Hematologic Toxicity: Reduce to 90mg/m² on Days 1 and 2 of each cycle
Grade 4 Hematologic Toxicity Recurs: Reduce to 60mg/m² on Days 1 and 2 of each cycle
≥Grade 3 Nonhematologic Toxicity: Reduce to 90mg/m² on Days 1 and 2 of each cycle
≥Grade 3 Nonhematologic Toxicity Recurs: Reduce to 60mg/m² on Days 1 and 2 of each cycle

ADMINISTRATION
IV route

Selection/Preparation
Do not mix or combine the 2 formulations.
Admixture should be prepared as close as possible to the time of patient administration.

Sol:
Withdraw and transfer for dilution in a biosafety cabinet or containment isolator using only a polypropylene syringe w/ a metal needle and a polypropylene hub. Do not use w/ devices containing polycarbonate or acrylonitrile-butadiene-styrene (ABS) (eg, closed system transfer devices [CSTDs], adapters, syringes) prior to dilution in the infusion bag.
After dilution of into the infusion bag, devices that contain polycarbonate or ABS, including infusion sets, may be used.

1. Withdraw the volume needed for the required dose (from the 90mg/mL sol).
2. Immediately transfer to a 500mL infusion bag of 0.9% NaCl. As an alternative, a 500mL infusion bag of 2.5% dextrose/0.45% NaCl may be considered. The resulting final concentration should be w/in 0.2-0.7mg/mL.
3. Administer diluted sol w/in 24 hrs when stored at 2-8°C (36-46°F) or w/in 2 hrs when stored at 15-30°C (59-86°F).

Powder:
Only use powder for inj if a CSTD or adapter that contains polycarbonate or ABS is used as supplemental protection during preparation.

1. Reconstitute 25mg vial w/ 5mL of sterile water for inj (SWFI) and 100mg vial w/ 20mL of SWFI.
2. Shake well to yield a clear, colorless to a pale yellow sol w/ a concentration of 5mg/mL; should completely dissolve in 5 min and transfer reconstituted sol to infusion bag w/in 30 min of reconstitution.
3. Withdraw the volume needed for the required dose and immediately transfer to 500mL infusion bag of 0.9% NaCl; as an alternative, a 500mL infusion bag of 2.5% dextrose/0.45% NaCl may be considered.
4. The resulting final concentration should be w/in 0.2-0.6mg/mL; thoroughly mix the contents of the infusion bag after transferring.
5. Administer w/in 24 hrs when stored at 2-8°C (36-46°F) or w/in 3 hrs when stored at 15-30°C (59-86°F).

STORAGE
Sol: 2-8°C (36-47°F). Protect from light. **Powder:** Up to 25°C (77°F); excursions permitted up to 30°C (86°F). Protect from light.

HOW SUPPLIED
Inj: (Powder) 25mg, 100mg; (Sol) 45mg/0.5mL, 180mg/2mL

CONTRAINDICATIONS
Known hypersensitivity to bendamustine.

WARNINGS/PRECAUTIONS
Severe myelosuppression reported; may require dose delays and/or subsequent dose reductions if recovery to the recommended values has not occurred by the 1st day of the next scheduled cycle. Monitor leukocytes, platelets, Hgb, and neutrophils frequently if treatment-related myelosuppression occurs. Infection (eg, pneumonia, sepsis, hepatitis) and death reported. Increased risk for reactivation of infections (eg, hepatitis B, cytomegalovirus, herpes zoster); patients should undergo appropriate measures for infection and infection reactivation prior to administration. Infusion reactions and severe anaphylactic/anaphylactoid reactions reported; monitor clinically and d/c for severe reactions. Consider measures to prevent severe reactions (eg, antihistamines, antipyretics, corticosteroids) in subsequent cycles in patients who have experienced Grade 1 or 2 infusion reactions. Consider discontinuation for Grade 3 infusion reactions as clinically appropriate; d/c for Grade 4 infusion reactions. Do not rechallenge in patients who experience ≥Grade 3 allergic-type reactions. Tumor lysis syndrome reported; preventive measures include vigorous hydration and close monitoring of blood chemistry, particularly K+ and uric acid levels. Skin reactions (eg, rash, toxic skin reactions, bullous exanthema) reported; monitor closely and withhold or d/c if skin reactions are severe or progressive. Premalignant and malignant diseases (eg, myelodysplastic syndrome, myeloproliferative disorders, acute myeloid leukemia, bronchial carcinoma) reported. Extravasations reported; assure good venous access prior to starting infusion and monitor for infusion-site redness, swelling, pain, infection, and necrosis during and after administration. May cause fetal harm. Caution w/ mild/moderate renal impairment and w/ mild hepatic impairment.

ADVERSE REACTIONS
Chronic Lymphocytic Leukemia: Pyrexia, N/V.
Non-Hodgkin Lymphoma: N/V, fatigue, diarrhea, pyrexia.

DRUG INTERACTIONS
CYP1A2 inhibitors (eg, fluvoxamine, ciprofloxacin) may increase plasma concentrations of bendamustine and may decrease plasma concentrations of active metabolites. CYP1A2 inducers (eg, omeprazole, smoking) may decrease plasma concentrations of bendamustine and may increase plasma concentrations of active metabolites. Use caution or consider alternative treatments if treatment w/ CYP1A2 inhibitors/inducers is needed. May increase risk of severe skin toxicity w/ allopurinol.

PREGNANCY AND LACTATION
Pregnancy: Category D.
Lactation: Not for use in nursing.

MECHANISM OF ACTION
Alkylating agent; has not been established. Bifunctional mechlorethamine derivative containing a purine-like benzimidazole ring; forms electrophilic alkyl groups that form covalent bonds w/ electron-rich nucleophilic moieties, resulting in interstrand DNA crosslinks. Bifunctional covalent linkage can lead to cell death via several pathways. Active against both quiescent and dividing cells.

PHARMACOKINETICS
Distribution: Plasma protein binding (94-96%); V_d=20-25L. **Metabolism:** Extensive via hydrolytic (primary), oxidative, and conjugative pathways; gamma-hydroxy-bendamustine (M3), N-desmethyl-bendamustine (M4) (active minor metabolites) via CYP1A2. **Elimination:** Urine (50%, 3.3% unchanged, <1% as M3 and M4), feces (25%); $T_{1/2}$=40 min, 3 hrs (M3), 30 min (M4).

PATIENT CONSIDERATIONS
Assessment: Assess for renal/hepatic impairment, hypersensitivity to drug, pregnancy/nursing status, and possible drug interactions.

Monitoring: Monitor for signs/symptoms of myelosuppression, infections, anaphylaxis/infusion reactions, tumor lysis syndrome, skin reactions, premalignant/malignant diseases, extravasation, lab abnormalities, and other adverse reactions. Monitor CBCs and blood chemistry, particularly K+ and uric acid levels.

Counseling: Inform of the possibility of mild/serious allergic reactions and instruct to immediately report rash, facial swelling, or difficulty breathing during or soon after infusion. Inform that therapy may cause a decrease in WBC counts, platelets, and RBC counts, and of the need for frequent monitoring of blood counts; instruct to report SOB, significant fatigue, bleeding, fever, or other signs of infection. Advise that therapy may cause tiredness; instruct to avoid driving or operating dangerous tools or machinery if tiredness occurs. Inform that therapy may cause N/V, diarrhea, and mild rash or itching; instruct to report any adverse reactions immediately to physician. Advise women to avoid becoming pregnant and men to use reliable contraception throughout treatment and for 3 months after discontinuation of therapy; instruct to immediately report pregnancy and to avoid nursing while on therapy.

TRELSTAR — triptorelin pamoate   **Rx**
Class: Synthetic gonadotropin-releasing hormone (GnRH) analogue

ADULT DOSAGE	PEDIATRIC DOSAGE
Advanced Prostate Cancer	Pediatric use may not have been established
Palliative Treatment:	
3.75mg: 1 inj every 4 weeks	
11.25mg: 1 inj every 12 weeks	
22.5mg: 1 inj every 24 weeks	

ADMINISTRATION
IM route

Administer by a single inj in either buttock

Alternate inj site periodically

Reconstitution Instructions
1. Using a syringe fitted w/ a sterile 21-gauge needle, withdraw 2mL sterile water for inj, and inject into the vial
2. Shake well to thoroughly disperse particles to obtain a uniform sus; the sus will appear milky
3. Slowly withdraw the entire contents of the reconstituted sus into the syringe
4. Administer the sus immediately after reconstitution
5. Inject in either buttock w/ the contents of the syringe

Refer to PI for reconstitution instructions w/ MIXJECT system

STORAGE
20-25°C (68-77°F). Do not freeze with Mixject.

HOW SUPPLIED
Inj: 3.75mg, 11.25mg, 22.5mg [vial, Mixject delivery system]

CONTRAINDICATIONS
Known hypersensitivity to triptorelin pamoate, any other components of the product, or other gonadotropin-releasing hormone (GnRH) agonists or GnRH. Women who are or may become pregnant.

WARNINGS/PRECAUTIONS
Administer under the supervision of a physician. Dosage strengths are not additive; select strength based on desired dosing schedule. Anaphylactic shock, hypersensitivity, and angioedema reported; d/c immediately and administer appropriate supportive and symptomatic care if these occur. May cause transient increase in serum testosterone levels; worsening or onset of new symptoms (eg, bone pain, neuropathy, hematuria, urethral/bladder outlet obstruction) may occur during the 1st few weeks of treatment. Spinal cord compression reported; institute standard treatment or consider immediate orchiectomy in extreme cases if spinal cord compression or renal impairment develops. Closely monitor patients with metastatic vertebral lesions and/or with upper or lower urinary tract obstruction during 1st few weeks of therapy. Androgen deprivation therapy may prolong QT/QTc interval; consider whether benefits outweigh potential risks in patients with congenital long QT syndrome, congestive heart failure (CHF), frequent electrolyte abnormalities, and in patients taking drugs known to prolong QT interval. Correct electrolyte abnormalities and consider periodic monitoring of electrocardiograms and electrolytes. Hyperglycemia and an increased risk of developing diabetes reported; monitor blood glucose and/or HbA1c periodically. Sudden cardiac death, stroke, and an increased risk of developing myocardial infarction (MI) reported; monitor for signs/symptoms of cardiovascular disease (CVD). Monitor response by measuring serum testosterone levels periodically or as indicated. Chronic or continuous administration in therapeutic doses may suppress pituitary-gonadal

axis; diagnostic tests of pituitary-gonadal function conducted during treatment and after cessation of therapy may be misleading.

ADVERSE REACTIONS

Hot flush, HTN, headache, skeletal pain, dysuria, leg edema, erectile dysfunction, testicular atrophy, inj-site pain, leg pain, pain.

DRUG INTERACTIONS

Avoid with hyperprolactinemic drugs.

PREGNANCY AND LACTATION

Category X, not for use in nursing.

MECHANISM OF ACTION

Synthetic GnRH agonist analogue; initially increases circulating levels of luteinizing hormone (LH), follicle-stimulating hormone (FSH), testosterone, and estradiol. Chronic and continuous administration causes a sustained decrease in LH and FSH secretion and marked reduction of testicular steroidogenesis.

PHARMACOKINETICS

Absorption: (IM) C_{max}=28.4ng/mL (3.75mg), 38.5ng/mL (11.25mg), 44.1ng/mL (22.5mg); T_{max}=1-3 hrs. **Distribution:** (0.5mg IV) V_d=30-33L. **Elimination:** (IV) Urine (41.7%, unchanged), $T_{1/2}$=3 hrs.

PATIENT CONSIDERATIONS

Assessment: Assess for hypersensitivity to drug/other GnRH agonists/GnRH, metastatic vertebral lesions, urinary tract obstruction, diabetes, congenital long QT syndrome, electrolyte abnormalities, CHF, and possible drug interactions. Obtain baseline serum testosterone levels.

Monitoring: Monitor response to drug and for signs/symptoms of worsening prostate cancer, spinal cord compression, renal impairment, anaphylactic shock, hypersensitivity, angioedema, CVD, and other adverse reactions. Periodically monitor serum testosterone, blood glucose and/or HbA1c, electrocardiograms, and electrolytes.

Counseling: Inform that patients may experience worsening of symptoms of prostate cancer during the 1st weeks of treatment and that these symptoms should decline 3-4 weeks following administration of therapy. Inform of the increased risk of developing diabetes, MI, sudden cardiac death, and stroke. Advise that allergic reactions could occur and that serious reactions require immediate treatment. Instruct to report any previous hypersensitivity to drug, other GnRH agonists, or GnRH.

TRETTEN — coagulation factor XIII A-subunit (recombinant)   Rx

Class: Factor XIII subunits

ADULT DOSAGE
Factor XIII Deficiency

Routine prophylaxis for bleeding in patients w/ congenital factor XIII A-subunit deficiency

35 IU/kg IV once monthly to achieve a target trough level of FXIII activity ≥10% using a validated assay; consider dose adjustment if adequate coverage is not achieved with the recommended dose

PEDIATRIC DOSAGE
Factor XIII Deficiency

Routine prophylaxis for bleeding in patients w/ congenital factor XIII A-subunit deficiency

35 IU/kg IV once monthly to achieve a target trough level of FXIII activity ≥10% using a validated assay; consider dose adjustment if adequate coverage is not achieved with the recommended dose

---

ADMINISTRATION
IV route

Reconstitution
Draw back the plunger of the sterile syringe and admit a volume of 3.2mL air into the syringe
Screw the syringe onto the vial adapter on the diluent vial
Inject the air from the syringe into the diluent vial until resistance is felt. Then hold the syringe with the diluent vial upside down and withdraw 3.2mL water into the syringe
Attach the syringe w/ the vial adapter to the powder vial. Hold the syringe slightly tilted with vial facing downwards. Push the plunger slowly to inject all water (3.2mL) into the powder vial. Do not inject the diluent directly on the powder to avoid foaming
Gently swirl the vial until all material is dissolved. Do not shake the vial
For larger dose that requires multiple vials, reconstitute each additional vial using the same procedure with a separate syringe
For smaller dose that requires less than the full volume in the vial, reconstituted sol may be diluted with 0.9% NS to facilitate measurement of small volumes

Administration
Administer at a rate not exceeding 1-2mL/min
Use the reconstituted sol immediately
Do not administer with other infusion sol
Do not administer as drip

STORAGE
2-8°C (36-46°F). Do not freeze. Protect from light. Reconstituted Sol: If not used immediately, store refrigerated or at room temperature not to exceed 25°C (77°F) for up to 3 hrs.

HOW SUPPLIED
Inj: 2000-3125 IU

CONTRAINDICATIONS
Known hypersensitivity to the active substance or to any of the excipients.

WARNINGS/PRECAUTIONS

May cause allergic reactions; d/c immediately and institute appropriate treatment if signs/symptoms of anaphylaxis or hypersensitivity reactions occur. Thromboembolic complications may occur; monitor patients with conditions that predispose to thrombosis for signs/symptoms of thrombosis after administration. Inhibitory antibodies may occur; patients with inhibitory antibodies may manifest as an inadequate response to treatment. If expected plasma FXIII activity levels are not attained, or if breakthrough bleeding occurs while receiving prophylaxis, perform an assay that measures FXIII inhibitory antibody concentrations.

ADVERSE REACTIONS

Headache, pain in the extremities, inj-site pain, increase in fibrin D dimer levels.

DRUG INTERACTIONS

Thrombosis may occur if administered concomitantly with factor VIIa.

PREGNANCY AND LACTATION

Category C, caution in nursing.

MECHANISM OF ACTION

Protransglutaminase (recombinant FXIII [rFXIII]-A_2 homodimer); binds to free human FXIII B-subunit, resulting in a heterotetramer [rA_2B_2] with a similar $T_{1/2}$ to [A_2B_2]. rFXIII has been shown to be activated by thrombin in the presence of Ca^{2+}. Activated rFXIII has been shown in dose-dependent manner to increase mechanical strength of fibrin clots, retard fibrinolysis, and rFXIII has been shown to enhance platelet adhesion to the site of injury.

PHARMACOKINETICS

Absorption: C_{max}=0.71 IU/mL; AUC=128.3 IU•hr/mL. 1-<6 Yrs: C_{max}=0.48 IU/mL; AUC=107.8 IU•hr/mL. **Distribution:** V_d=65.9mL/kg. 1-<6 Yrs: V_d=61.2mL/kg. **Elimination:** $T_{1/2}$=5.1 days. 1-<6 Yrs: $T_{1/2}$=7.1 days.

PATIENT CONSIDERATIONS

Assessment: Assess for hypersensitivity to drug, conditions that predispose to thrombosis, pregnancy/nursing status, and possible drug interactions.

Monitoring: Monitor for signs/symptoms of hypersensitivity reactions, thromboembolic complications, development of inhibitory antibodies, and other adverse reactions. Monitor trough FXIII activity level.

Counseling: Inform of the signs/symptoms of allergic hypersensitivity reactions (eg, urticaria, rash, chest tightness) and thrombosis (eg, limb or abdomen swelling and/or pain, chest pain, SOB). Inform that breakthrough bleeding may be the sign and symptom of inhibitor formation.

TRISENOX — arsenic trioxide   Rx

Class: DNA fragmentation agent

> Patients treated for acute promyelocytic leukemia (APL) have experienced symptoms similar to retinoic-acid-APL or APL differentiation syndrome, which can be fatal; immediately initiate high-dose steroids (dexamethasone 10mg IV bid) at 1st signs of syndrome, and continue for ≥3 days until signs/symptoms have abated. Before initiating therapy, perform a 12-lead ECG, assess SrCr and electrolytes, correct preexisting electrolyte abnormalities, and consider discontinuing drugs known to prolong QT interval. May cause QT interval prolongation and complete atrioventricular (AV) block; QT prolongation can lead to a torsades de pointes-type ventricular arrhythmia. Risk of torsades de pointes is related to extent of QT prolongation, use of concomitant QT prolonging drugs, history of torsades de pointes, preexisting QT interval prolongation, CHF, use of K⁺-wasting diuretics, or other conditions that result in hypokalemia or hypomagnesemia. Torsades de pointes reported in a patient also receiving amphotericin B during induction of therapy for relapsed APL.

ADULT DOSAGE
Refractory or Relapsed Acute Promyelocytic Leukemia (APL)

Induction of remission and consolidation in patients w/ APL who are refractory to, or have relapsed from, retinoid and anthracycline chemotherapy, and whose APL is characterized by presence of the t(15;17) translocation or PML/RAR-alpha gene expression

Induction: 0.15mg/kg IV qd until bone marrow remission
Max: 60 doses
Consolidation: 0.15mg/kg IV qd for 25 doses over period up to 5 weeks
Begin consolidation treatment 3-6 weeks after completion of induction therapy

PEDIATRIC DOSAGE
Refractory or Relapsed Acute Promyelocytic Leukemia (APL)

Induction of remission and consolidation in patients w/ APL who are refractory to, or have relapsed from, retinoid and anthracycline chemotherapy, and whose APL is characterized by presence of the t(15;17) translocation or PML/RAR-alpha gene expression

≥4 Years:
Induction: 0.15mg/kg IV qd until bone marrow remission
Max: 60 doses
Consolidation: 0.15mg/kg IV qd for 25 doses over period up to 5 weeks
Begin consolidation treatment 3-6 weeks after completion of induction therapy

---

DOSING CONSIDERATIONS
Renal Impairment
Severe (CrCl <30mL/min): Dose reduction may be warranted

Adverse Reactions
Severe Nonhematologic Adverse Reactions (eg, Neurologic/Dermatologic Toxicity): Consider delaying infusion until the event has resolved (≤Grade 1)

ADMINISTRATION
IV route
Infuse over 1-2 hrs (up to 4 hrs if acute vasomotor reactions occur)
Discard unused portions of each ampule
Do not mix w/ other medications

Reconstitution
Dilute w/ 100-250mL D5 Inj or 0.9% NaCl inj immediately after withdrawal from the ampule

STORAGE
25°C (77°F); excursions permitted to 15-30°C (59-86°F). Do not freeze. After Dilution: Chemically and physically stable when stored for 24 hrs at room temperature and 48 hrs when refrigerated.

HOW SUPPLIED
Inj: 1mg/mL [10mL]

CONTRAINDICATIONS
Hypersensitivity to arsenic.

WARNINGS/PRECAUTIONS
Monitor ECG weekly; monitor more frequently if clinically unstable. If QTc >500 msec, complete corrective measures and reassess QTc w/ serial ECGs prior to initiating therapy. Maintain K^+ concentrations >4mEq/L and Mg^{2+} concentrations >1.8mg/dL during therapy. Reassess if absolute QT interval value >500 msec and immediately correct concomitant risk factors, if any, while the risk/benefit of continuing versus suspending should be considered. Potentially carcinogenic; monitor for the development of 2nd primary malignancies. Monitor electrolyte, glucose levels, hepatic, renal, hematologic, and coagulation profiles at least 2X weekly; monitor more frequently if clinically unstable during induction and at least weekly during consolidation. Caution w/ hepatic impairment. Monitor for toxicity w/ severe hepatic (Child-Pugh Class C)/renal impairment (CrCl<30mL/min).

ADVERSE REACTIONS
APL differentiation syndrome, QT interval prolongation, complete AV block, torsades de pointes, leukocytosis, N/V, diarrhea, abdominal pain, fatigue, edema, hyperglycemia, hypokalemia, cough, headache, dizziness.

DRUG INTERACTIONS
See Boxed Warning. Monitor ECGs more frequently when it is not feasible to avoid concomitant use w/ drugs that prolong the QT/QTc interval. Avoid w/ drugs that can lead to electrolyte abnormalities (eg, amphotericin B, diuretics); monitor electrolytes more frequently if concomitant use must occur.

PREGNANCY AND LACTATION
Pregnancy: May cause fetal harm.
Lactation: Excreted in human milk; not for use in nursing.
Reproductive Potential: Females and males w/ female partners of reproductive potential should use effective contraception during and after treatment.

MECHANISM OF ACTION
DNA fragmentation agent; not established. Causes morphological changes and DNA fragmentation, characteristic of apoptosis in NB4 human promyelocytic leukemia cells in vitro. Also causes damage or degradation of fusion protein PML/RAR-α.

PHARMACOKINETICS
Absorption: Arsenious Acid (As^{III}): T_{max}=2 hrs; AUC=194ng•hr/mL (Day 1 of Cycle 1), 332ng•hr/mL (Day 25 of Cycle 1). **Distribution:** V_d=562L (As^{III}); found in breast milk. **Metabolism:** Converted to As^{III} (active) upon dilution; then via methylation into monomethylarsonic acid (MMA^V) and dimethylarsinic acid (DMA^V) (main metabolites) in the liver; or via oxidation into arsenic acid (metabolite). **Elimination:** Urine (approx 15%, unchanged As^{III}); $T_{1/2}$=10-14 hrs (As^{III}), 32 hrs (MMA^V), 72 hrs (DMA^V).

PATIENT CONSIDERATIONS
Assessment: Assess for previous hypersensitivity to the drug, history of torsades de pointes, preexisting QT interval prolongation, and CHF. Assess WBC count, renal and hepatic function, ECG, electrolytes (K^+, Ca^{2+}, and Mg^{2+}), pregnancy/nursing status, and possible drug interactions.

Monitoring: Monitor for hypersensitivity reactions, APL differentiation syndrome (eg, unexplained fever, dyspnea, weight gain, abnormal chest auscultatory findings or radiographic abnormalities), torsades de pointes, QT interval prolongation, AV block, secondary primary malignancies, toxicity in severe hepatic/renal impairment, and other adverse reactions. Monitor electrolyte levels, glucose levels, hepatic/renal function, hematologic and coagulation profile at least twice weekly, and more frequently for clinically unstable patients during the induction phase and at least weekly during the consolidation phase. Monitor ECG weekly, and more frequently for clinically unstable patients.

Counseling: Inform about benefits/risks of therapy. Counsel about symptoms of APL differentiation syndrome and instruct to immediately notify physician if any symptoms of APL differentiation develop. Inform that drug may cause ECG abnormalities, including QT prolongation; instruct to immediately notify physician if any symptoms of QT prolongation develop (eg, fainting, irregular heart beat). Instruct to immediately call physician if any treatment-related adverse reactions occur. Inform females of reproductive potential of the risk to a fetus and instruct to inform their physician if they are or may be pregnant. Advise females and males of reproductive potential to use effective contraception during and after treatment. Counsel females to d/c breastfeeding during treatment.

TRIUMEQ — abacavir/dolutegravir/lamivudine   Rx
Class: Integrase strand transfer inhibitor/nucleoside reverse transcriptase inhibitor (NRTI) combination

> Lactic acidosis and severe hepatomegaly w/ steatosis, including fatal cases, reported w/ nucleoside analogues; d/c if clinical or lab findings suggestive of lactic acidosis or pronounced hepatotoxicity occur. **Abacavir:** Serious and sometimes fatal hypersensitivity reactions, w/ multiple organ involvement, reported; d/c immediately if a hypersensitivity reaction is suspected and never restart therapy or any other abacavir-containing product. Patients who carry the HLA-B*5701 allele are at a higher risk of a hypersensitivity reaction; screen all patients for HLA-B*5701 allele prior to initiating or reinitiating therapy, unless patient has a previously documented HLA-B*5701 allele assessment. **Lamivudine:** Severe acute exacerbations of hepatitis B reported in patients coinfected w/ hepatitis B virus (HBV) and HIV-1 and have discontinued therapy; closely monitor hepatic function for at least several months. If appropriate, initiation of antihepatitis B therapy may be warranted.

ADULT DOSAGE	PEDIATRIC DOSAGE
HIV-1 Infection	Pediatric use may not have been
1 tab qd	established

DOSING CONSIDERATIONS
Concomitant Medications
Efavirenz, Fosamprenavir/Ritonavir (RTV), Tipranavir/RTV, Carbamazepine, or Rifampin: Take an additional dolutegravir 50mg tab, separated by 12 hrs from therapy

Renal Impairment
CrCl <50mL/min: Not recommended

Hepatic Impairment
Mild (Child-Pugh Score A): Not recommended
Moderate (Child-Pugh Class B) or Severe (Child-Pugh Class C): Contraindicated

ADMINISTRATION
Oral route
Take w/ or w/o food.
Screen for the HLA-B*5701 allele prior to initiating therapy.

STORAGE
25°C (77°F); excursions permitted to 15-30°C (59-86°F). Protect from moisture.

HOW SUPPLIED
Tab: (Abacavir/Dolutegravir/Lamivudine) 600mg/50mg/300mg

CONTRAINDICATIONS
Patients w/ HLA-B*5701 allele; prior hypersensitivity reaction to abacavir, dolutegravir, or lamivudine; coadministration w/ dofetilide; moderate or severe hepatic impairment.

WARNINGS/PRECAUTIONS
Not recommended for use w/ current or past history of resistance to any components of therapy. Therapy alone is not recommended w/ resistance-associated integrase substitutions or clinically suspected integrase strand transfer inhibitor resistance. Immune reconstitution syndrome reported. Autoimmune disorders (eg, Graves' disease, polymyositis, Guillain-Barre syndrome) reported to occur in the setting of immune reconstitution and may occur many months after initiation of treatment. Redistribution/accumulation of body fat may occur. Caution in elderly. **Abacavir:** May increase risk of MI. Consider underlying risk of coronary heart disease (CHD) when prescribing therapy; minimize all modifiable risk factors. **Dolutegravir:** Hypersensitivity reactions reported; d/c therapy and other suspect agents immediately if signs/symptoms develop. May be at increased risk for worsening or development of transaminase elevations in patients w/ underlying hepatitis B or C. **Lamivudine:** Emergence of lamivudine-resistant HBV reported.

ADVERSE REACTIONS
Insomnia, headache, fatigue.

DRUG INTERACTIONS
See Dosing Considerations and Contraindications. Closely monitor for treatment-associated toxicities, especially hepatic decompensation in patients receiving interferon alfa w/ or w/o ribavirin; consider dose reduction or discontinuation of interferon alfa, ribavirin, or both if worsening clinical toxicities are observed, including hepatic decompensation (eg, Child-Pugh >6); consider discontinuation of Triumeq as medically appropriate. Not recommended w/ other abacavir- or lamivudine-containing products. **Abacavir:** May increase oral methadone clearance; an increased methadone dose may be required in a small number of patients. **Dolutegravir:** Drugs that induce/inhibit UGT1A1, CYP3A, UGT1A3, UGT1A9, breast cancer resistance protein, and P-gp may decrease/increase levels, respectively. Decreased levels w/ etravirine; use of Triumeq w/ etravirine w/o coadministration of atazanavir/RTV, darunavir/RTV, or lopinavir/RTV is not recommended. Decreased levels w/ efavirenz, fosamprenavir/RTV, tipranavir/RTV, rifampin, and carbamazepine. Decreased levels w/ nevirapine, oxcarbazepine, phenytoin, phenobarbital, and St. John's wort; avoid coadministration w/ Triumeq. Administer 2 hrs before or 6 hrs after taking medications containing polyvalent cations (eg, cation-containing antacids/laxatives, sucralfate, buffered medications) or taking oral Ca^{2+} or iron supplements (eg, multivitamins); alternatively, therapy and supplements containing Ca^{2+} or iron can be taken together w/ food. May increase levels of drugs eliminated via organic cation transporter 2 or multidrug and toxin extrusion transporter 1 (eg, metformin); limit the total daily dose of metformin to 1000mg when starting either metformin or Triumeq; monitoring of blood glucose when initiating concomitant use and after withdrawal of Triumeq is recommended. When stopping Triumeq, metformin dose may require adjustment.

PREGNANCY AND LACTATION
Pregnancy: Category C.
Lactation: Not for use in nursing.

MECHANISM OF ACTION
Abacavir: Carbocyclic synthetic nucleoside analogue; inhibits HIV-1 reverse transcriptase (RT) activity by competing w/ natural substrate deoxyguanosine-5'-triphosphate and by incorporating into viral DNA. **Dolutegravir:** HIV-1 integrase strand transfer inhibitor; inhibits HIV integrase by binding to integrase active site and blocking the strand transfer step of retroviral DNA integration, which is essential for the HIV replication cycle. **Lamivudine:** Synthetic nucleoside analogue; inhibits RT via DNA chain termination after incorporation of the nucleotide analogue.

PHARMACOKINETICS
Absorption: Abacavir: Rapid. C_{max}=4.26mcg/mL; AUC=11.95mcg•hr/mL. Dolutegravir: AUC_{0-24}=53.6mcg•hr/mL; C_{max}=3.67mcg/mL; T_{max}=2-3 hrs. Lamivudine: Rapid. C_{max}=2.04mcg/mL; AUC=8.87mcg•hr/mL.

Distribution: Abacavir: Plasma protein binding (50%). Dolutegravir: V_d=17.4L; plasma protein binding (≥98.9%). Lamivudine: Found in breast milk. **Metabolism:** Abacavir: Via alcohol dehydrogenase and glucuronyl transferase; 5'-carboxylic acid, 5'-glucuronide (metabolites). Dolutegravir: Via UGT1A1, CYP3A. Lamivudine: Trans-sulfoxide (metabolite). **Elimination:** Abacavir: $T_{1/2}$=1.54 hrs. Dolutegravir: Urine (31%, <1% unchanged), feces (53% unchanged); $T_{1/2}$=14 hrs. Lamivudine: Urine (70%, unchanged) (IV); $T_{1/2}$=5-7 hrs.

PATIENT CONSIDERATIONS

Assessment: Assess for previous hypersensitivity to the drug, hepatic/renal impairment, hepatitis B or C infection, risk factors for CHD, pregnancy/nursing status, and possible drug interactions. Screen for HLA-B*5701 allele prior to initiation/reinitiation of therapy. Assess medical history for prior exposure to any abacavir-containing product.

Monitoring: Monitor for signs/symptoms of hypersensitivity reactions, lactic acidosis, hepatomegaly w/ steatosis, immune reconstitution syndrome, autoimmune disorders, fat redistribution/accumulation, MI, and other adverse reactions. Monitor hepatic function. Monitor for exacerbations of hepatitis B in patients who are coinfected w/ HBV; closely monitor hepatic function for at least several months after stopping therapy in patients coinfected w/ HBV.

Counseling: Inform about the risks and benefits of therapy. Advise to report the use of any prescription or nonprescription medication or herbal products. Advise about hypersensitivity reactions; instruct to contact physician immediately if symptoms develop and not to restart or replace w/ any drug containing abacavir w/o medical consultation. Inform that the drug may cause lactic acidosis and severe hepatomegaly w/steatosis. Inform patients w/ underlying hepatitis B or C that they may be at increased risk of worsening or development of transaminase elevations. Inform that hepatic decompensation has occurred in HIV-1/HCV-coinfected patients receiving combination antiretroviral therapy and interferon alfa w/ or w/o ribavirin. Inform that fat redistribution/accumulation may occur. Advise that drug is not a cure for HIV-1 infection and that illness associated w/ HIV-1 infection may continue, including opportunistic infections. Instruct to take all HIV medications exactly as prescribed. Advise to avoid doing things that can spread HIV-1 infection to others. Advise to inform physician immediately of any symptoms of infection or if any unusual symptom develops, or if any known symptom persists or worsens. Explain missed dose instructions.

TRIZIVIR = abacavir/lamivudine/zidovudine   Rx

Class: Nucleoside reverse transcriptase inhibitor (NRTI) combination

> Lactic acidosis and severe hepatomegaly w/ steatosis, including fatal cases, reported w/ nucleoside analogues and other antiretrovirals. D/C if clinical or lab findings suggestive of lactic acidosis or pronounced hepatotoxicity occur. **Abacavir:** Serious and sometimes fatal hypersensitivity reactions w/ multiple organ involvement reported; d/c immediately if a hypersensitivity reaction is suspected and never restart therapy or any other abacavir-containing product. Patients who carry the HLA-B*5701 allele are at a higher risk of a hypersensitivity reaction; screen all patients for HLA-B*5701 allele prior to initiating or reinitiating therapy, unless patient has a previously documented HLA-B*5701 allele assessment. **Zidovudine:** Associated w/ hematologic toxicity (eg, neutropenia, severe anemia), particularly w/ advanced HIV-1 disease. Symptomatic myopathy associated w/ prolonged use. **Lamivudine:** Severe acute exacerbations of hepatitis B reported in patients coinfected w/ hepatitis B virus (HBV) and HIV-1 and have discontinued therapy; closely monitor hepatic function w/ both clinical and lab follow-up for at least several months. If appropriate, initiation of antihepatitis B therapy may be warranted.

ADULT DOSAGE	PEDIATRIC DOSAGE
HIV-1 Infection	**HIV-1 Infection**
1 tab bid	**<40kg:**
	1 tab bid

DOSING CONSIDERATIONS

Renal Impairment
CrCl <50mL/min: Not recommended for use

Hepatic Impairment
Mild: Not recommended for use
Moderate/Severe: Contraindicated

ADMINISTRATION

Oral route

Take w/ or w/o food.
Screen for the HLA-B*5701 allele prior to initiating therapy.

STORAGE

25°C (77°F); excursions permitted to 15-30°C (59-86°F).

HOW SUPPLIED

Tab: (Abacavir Sulfate/Lamivudine/Zidovudine) 300mg/150mg/300mg

CONTRAINDICATIONS

Prior hypersensitivity reaction to Trizivir, moderate or severe hepatic impairment, patients w/ HLA-B*5701 allele.

WARNINGS/PRECAUTIONS

Obesity and prolonged nucleoside exposure may be risk factors for lactic acidosis and severe hepatomegaly w/ steatosis; suspend therapy if clinical or lab findings suggestive of lactic acidosis or pronounced hepatotoxicity develop. Immune reconstitution syndrome reported. Autoimmune disorders (eg, Graves' disease, polymyositis, Guillain-Barre syndrome) reported to occur in the

setting of immune reconstitution and can occur many months after initiation of treatment. Redistribution/accumulation of body fat may occur. Cross-resistance potential w/ nucleoside reverse transcriptase inhibitors reported. Caution w/ any known risk factors for liver disease and in elderly. Avoid use in adolescents weighing <40kg and in patients requiring dose adjustments (eg, renal impairment [CrCl <50mL/min]). **Abacavir:** Consider underlying risk of coronary heart disease (CHD) when prescribing therapy. **Lamivudine:** Emergence of lamivudine-resistant HBV reported. **Zidovudine:** Caution w/ compromised bone marrow evidenced by granulocyte count <1000 cells/mm³ or Hgb <9.5g/dL; monitor blood counts frequently w/ advanced HIV-1 disease and periodically in other HIV-1 infected patients. Interrupt therapy if anemia or neutropenia develops.

ADVERSE REACTIONS

N/V, headache, malaise, fatigue, hypersensitivity reaction, diarrhea, fever, chills, depressive disorders, musculoskeletal pain, skin rashes, anxiety, ear/nose/throat infections.

DRUG INTERACTIONS

Avoid w/ other abacavir-, lamivudine-, zidovudine-, and/or emtricitabine-containing products. Closely monitor for treatment associated toxicities, especially hepatic decompensation, neutropenia, and anemia, in patients receiving interferon alfa w/ or w/o ribavirin and Trizivir; consider discontinuation of Trizivir as medically appropriate and consider dose reduction or discontinuation of interferon alfa, ribavirin, or both if worsening clinical toxicities are observed. **Abacavir:** Ethanol may decrease elimination, causing an increase in overall exposure. May increase oral methadone clearance; an increased methadone dose may be required in a small number of patients. **Zidovudine:** Avoid w/ stavudine, doxorubicin, and nucleoside analogues (eg, ribavirin). May increase hematologic toxicity w/ ganciclovir, interferon alfa, ribavirin, and other bone marrow suppressive or cytotoxic agents.

PREGNANCY AND LACTATION

Pregnancy: Category C.
Lactation: Not for use in nursing.

MECHANISM OF ACTION

Abacavir: Carbocyclic synthetic nucleoside analogue; inhibits HIV-1 reverse transcriptase (RT) by competing w/ natural substrate deoxyguanosine-5'-triphosphate and by incorporating into viral DNA. **Lamivudine/Zidovudine:** Synthetic nucleoside analogue; inhibits RT via DNA chain termination after incorporation of the nucleotide analogue.

PHARMACOKINETICS

Absorption: Rapid. Abacavir: Oral Bioavailability: (86%); C_{max}=3 mcg/mL; AUC=6.02mcg•hr/mL. Lamivudine: Oral Bioavailability: (86%). Zidovudine: Oral Bioavailability: (64%). **Distribution:** Abacavir: V_d=0.86L/kg; plasma protein binding (50%). Lamivudine: V_d=1.3L/kg; plasma protein binding (low). Zidovudine: V_d=1.6L/kg; plasma protein binding (low); crosses the placenta. **Metabolism:** Abacavir: Via alcohol dehydrogenase and glucuronyl transferase; 5'-carboxylic acid, 5'-glucuronide (metabolites). Lamivudine: Trans-sulfoxide (metabolite). Zidovudine: Hepatic via glucuronyl transferase; 3'-azido-3'-deoxy-5'-O-β-D-glucopyranuronosylthymidine (GZDV) (major metabolite). **Elimination:** Abacavir: $T_{1/2}$=1.45 hrs. Lamivudine: (IV) Urine (70%, unchanged); $T_{1/2}$=5-7 hrs. Zidovudine: Urine (14% unchanged, 74% GZDV); $T_{1/2}$=0.5-3 hrs.

PATIENT CONSIDERATIONS

Assessment: Assess for history of hypersensitivity reactions, advanced HIV disease, hepatic/renal impairment, risk factors for lactic acidosis, risk factors for CHD, bone marrow compromise, HBV infection, pregnancy/nursing status, and possible drug interactions. Screen for HLA-B*5701 allele prior to initiation of therapy. Assess medical history for prior exposure to any abacavir-containing product.

Monitoring: Monitor for signs/symptoms of hypersensitivity reactions, hematologic toxicity, lactic acidosis, hepatomegaly w/ steatosis, myopathy, immune reconstitution syndrome, autoimmune disorders, fat redistribution/accumulation, MI, and other adverse reactions. Monitor hepatic/renal function. Monitor hepatic function closely for at least several months in patients who d/c therapy and are coinfected w/ HIV-1 and HBV. Perform frequent blood counts in patients w/ advanced HIV-1 disease and perform periodic blood counts for other HIV-1-infected patients.

Counseling: Inform about hypersensitivity reactions; instruct to contact physician immediately if symptoms develop and not to restart or replace w/ any drug containing abacavir w/o medical consultation. Inform about risk for hematologic toxicities and advise on importance of close blood count monitoring while on therapy. Counsel about the possible occurrence of myopathy and myositis w/ pathological changes during prolonged use and that therapy may cause a rare but serious condition called lactic acidosis w/ hepatomegaly. Inform patients coinfected w/ HBV that deterioration of liver disease has occurred in some cases when treatment was discontinued; instruct to discuss any changes in regimen w/ physician. Inform that hepatic decompensation has occurred in HIV-1/hepatitis C virus coinfected patients receiving combination antiretroviral therapy and interferon alfa w/ or w/o ribavirin. Inform that redistribution/accumulation of body fat may occur. Advise that drug is not a cure for HIV-1 infection and that illness associated w/ HIV-1 may still be experienced. Advise to avoid doing things that can spread HIV-1 infection to others. Inform patients to take all HIV medications exactly as prescribed.

TRUVADA — emtricitabine/tenofovir disoproxil fumarate   Rx

Class: Nucleoside reverse transcriptase inhibitor (NRTI) combination

> Lactic acidosis and severe hepatomegaly w/ steatosis, including fatal cases, reported w/ the use of nucleoside analogues in combination w/ other antiretrovirals. Not approved for treatment of chronic hepatitis B virus (HBV) infection. Severe acute exacerbations of hepatitis B reported in patients coinfected w/ HBV and HIV-1 and who have discontinued therapy; closely monitor hepatic function w/ both clinical and lab follow-up for at least several months. If appropriate, initiation of anti-hepatitis B therapy may be warranted. Drug-resistant HIV-1 variants have been identified w/ use for preexposure prophylaxis (PrEP) indication following undetected acute HIV-1 infection. PrEP use must only be prescribed to individuals confirmed to be HIV-negative immediately prior to initiating and periodically (at least every 3 months) during use; do not initiate if signs/symptoms of acute HIV-1 infection are present unless negative infection status is confirmed.

ADULT DOSAGE

HIV-1 Infection

Combination w/ Other Antiretrovirals:
1 tab (200mg/300mg) qd

HIV-1 Pre-Exposure Prophylaxis

Combination w/ Safer Sex Practices for High-Risk Patients:
1 tab (200mg/300mg) qd

PEDIATRIC DOSAGE

HIV-1 Infection

Combination w/ Other Antiretrovirals:
17 to <22kg: 1 tab (100mg/150mg) qd
22 to <28kg: 1 tab (133mg/200mg) qd
28 to <35kg: 1 tab (167mg/250mg) qd
≥35kg: 1 tab (200mg/300mg) qd

Monitor weight periodically and adjust dose accordingly

DOSING CONSIDERATIONS

Renal Impairment
HIV-1 Infection:
CrCl 30-49mL/min: 1 tab q48h
CrCl <30mL/min (Including Hemodialysis): Not recommended for use

HIV-1 PrEP:
CrCl <60mL/min: Not recommended for use

ADMINISTRATION

Oral route

Take w/ or w/o food.
Swallow tab whole.

STORAGE

25°C (77°F); excursions permitted to 15-30°C (59-86°F).

HOW SUPPLIED

Tab: (Emtricitabine/Tenofovir Disoproxil Fumarate [TDF]) 100mg/150mg, 133mg/200mg, 167mg/250mg, 200mg/300mg

CONTRAINDICATIONS

Individuals w/ unknown or positive HIV-1 status when used for PrEP. Use in HIV-infected patients w/o other concomitant antiretroviral agents.

WARNINGS/PRECAUTIONS

Obesity and prolonged nucleoside exposure may be risk factors for lactic acidosis and severe hepatomegaly w/ steatosis. Caution w/ known risk factors for liver disease. D/C if findings suggestive of lactic acidosis or pronounced hepatotoxicity develop. Test for the presence of chronic HBV before initiating therapy; offer vaccination to HBV-uninfected individuals. Redistribution/accumulation of body fat and immune reconstitution syndrome reported. Autoimmune disorders (eg, Graves' disease, polymyositis, Guillain-Barre syndrome) reported in the setting of immune reconstitution and can occur many months after initiation of treatment. Early virological failure and high rates of resistance substitutions reported w/ certain regimens that only contain 3 nucleoside reverse transcriptase inhibitors; consider treatment modification in these patients. Use for PrEP only as part of a comprehensive prevention strategy that includes other prevention measures (eg, safer sex practices). Delay starting PrEP therapy for at least 1 month and reconfirm HIV-1 status or use an FDA-approved test to diagnose acute or primary HIV-1 infection if symptoms of acute viral infection are present and recent (<1 month) exposures are suspected. D/C PrEP therapy if symptoms of acute HIV-1 infection develop following potential exposure event until negative status is confirmed using an FDA-approved test. Caution in elderly. **TDF:** Renal impairment (eg, acute renal failure, Fanconi syndrome) reported; caution in patients at risk of renal dysfunction, including patients who have previously experienced renal events while receiving adefovir dipivoxil. Promptly evaluate renal function in at-risk patients w/ persistent/worsening bone pain, pain in extremities, fractures, and/or muscular pain/weakness. Decreased bone mineral density (BMD) and increased biochemical markers of bone metabolism reported. Osteomalacia associated w/ proximal renal tubulopathy reported; consider hypophosphatemia and osteomalacia secondary to proximal renal tubulopathy in patients at risk of renal dysfunction who present w/ persistent or worsening bone/muscle symptoms.

ADVERSE REACTIONS

HIV-1 Infected Patients: Diarrhea, nausea, fatigue, headache, dizziness, depression, insomnia, abnormal dreams, rash.
HIV-1 Uninfected Patients: Headache, abdominal pain, decreased weight.

DRUG INTERACTIONS

Avoid w/ concurrent or recent use of nephrotoxic agents (eg, high-dose or multiple NSAIDs). Do not coadminister w/ emtricitabine-, TDF-, or tenofovir alafenamide-containing products, drugs containing lamivudine, or w/ adefovir dipivoxil. Coadministration w/ drugs eliminated by active tubular secretion (eg, acyclovir, cidofovir, ganciclovir, valacyclovir, aminoglycosides [eg, gentamicin], high-dose or multiple NSAIDs) may increase levels of emtricitabine, TDF, and/or the coadministered drug. Drugs that decrease renal function may increase levels of emtricitabine and/or TDF. Refer to PI for dosing modifications when used w/ concomitant therapies. **TDF:** May increase levels of didanosine; d/c

didanosine if didanosine-associated adverse effects develop. Decreases atazanavir levels; do not coadminister w/ atazanavir w/o ritonavir (RTV). Lopinavir/ RTV, atazanavir w/ RTV, and darunavir w/ RTV may increase TDF levels; d/c treatment if TDF-associated adverse reactions develop. P-gp and breast cancer resistance protein transporter inhibitors may increase absorption. Ledipasvir/ sofosbuvir may increase exposure; monitor for adverse reactions in patients receiving concomitant therapy w/ ledipasvir/sofosbuvir w/o an HIV-1 protease inhibitor/RTV or an HIV-1 protease inhibitor/cobicistat combination. Consider an alternative hepatitis C virus or antiretroviral therapy in patients receiving concomitant therapy w/ ledipasvir/sofosbuvir and an HIV-1 protease inhibitor/ RTV or an HIV-1 protease inhibitor/cobicistat combination. If coadministration is necessary, monitor for adverse reactions associated w/ TDF. Refer to PI for dosing modifications when used w/ concomitant therapies.

PREGNANCY AND LACTATION

Pregnancy: Category B. Physicians are encouraged to register pregnant patients in the Antiretroviral Pregnancy Registry.
Lactation: Excreted in human milk; not for use in nursing.

MECHANISM OF ACTION

Emtricitabine: Nucleoside analogue of cytidine; inhibits activity of HIV-1 reverse transcriptase (RT) by competing w/ natural substrate deoxycytidine 5'-triphosphate and by being incorporated into nascent viral DNA, which results in chain termination. **TDF:** Acyclic nucleoside phosphonate diester analogue of adenosine monophosphate; inhibits activity of HIV-1 RT by competing w/ the natural substrate deoxyadenosine 5'-triphosphate and, after incorporation into DNA, by DNA chain termination.

PHARMACOKINETICS

Absorption: Emtricitabine: Rapid. (Fasted) Bioavailability (92%) (median); C_{max}=1.8mcg/mL; T_{max}=1-2 hrs; AUC=10mcg•hr/mL. TDF: (Fasted) Bioavailability (25%) (median); C_{max}=0.3mcg/mL; T_{max}=1 hr; AUC=2.29mcg•hr/mL. **Distribution:** Found in breast milk. Emtricitabine: Plasma protein binding (<4%). TDF: Plasma protein binding (<0.7%). **Metabolism:** Emtricitabine: 3'-sulfoxide diastereomers and their glucuronic acid conjugate (metabolites). **Elimination:** Emtricitabine: Urine (86%; 13% metabolites); $T_{1/2}$=10 hrs (median). TDF: Urine (70-80%, unchanged) (IV); $T_{1/2}$=17 hrs (median).

PATIENT CONSIDERATIONS

Assessment: Assess for risk factors for lactic acidosis or liver disease, renal dysfunction, HBV infection, pregnancy/nursing status, and possible drug interactions. Confirm a negative HIV-1 test immediately prior to initiating PrEP therapy. In patients at risk of renal dysfunction, assess CrCl, serum phosphorus (P), urine glucose, and urine protein. Assess BMD in patients w/ history of pathologic bone fracture or other risk factors for osteoporosis or bone loss.

Monitoring: Monitor for signs/symptoms of lactic acidosis, hepatomegaly w/ steatosis, hepatotoxicity, new onset or worsening renal impairment, bone effects, redistribution/accumulation of body fat, immune reconstitution syndrome, autoimmune disorders, and other adverse reactions. Closely monitor hepatic function w/ both clinical and laboratory follow-up for at least several months in patients coinfected w/ HBV and HIV-1 and who have discontinued therapy. Screen for HIV-1 infection at least once every 3 months when using for PrEP. In patients at risk of renal dysfunction or w/ mild renal impairment, monitor CrCl, serum P, urine glucose, and urine protein periodically.

Counseling: Inform about the risks/benefits of therapy. Inform that medication is not a cure for HIV-1 and patients may continue to experience illness associated w/ HIV-1 infection (eg, opportunistic infections). Advise about the importance of adhering to recommended dosing schedule. Inform about safe sex practices. Instruct not to breastfeed, share needles or personal items that can have blood or body fluids on them, or d/c w/o informing physician. For PrEP, inform patients/ partners about the importance of knowing their HIV-1 status, obtaining HIV-1 test at least every 3 months, getting tested for other sexually transmitted infections, and immediate reporting to physician if any symptoms of acute HIV-1 infection develop. Monitor weight periodically in pediatric patients.

TYBOST — cobicistat   Rx

Class: CYP3A inhibitor

ADULT DOSAGE

HIV-1 Infection

To increase systemic exposure of atazanavir or darunavir (once daily dosing regimen) in combination w/ other antiretroviral agents

Treatment-Naive/Experienced:
150mg qd + atazanavir 300mg qd

Treatment-Naive; Treatment-Experienced w/ No Darunavir Resistance-Associated Substitutions:
150mg qd + darunavir 800mg qd

PEDIATRIC DOSAGE

Pediatric use may not have been established

DOSING CONSIDERATIONS

Renal Impairment
CrCl <70mL/min: Do not coadminister w/ tenofovir disoproxil fumarate (TDF)

ADMINISTRATION

Oral route

Take w/ food.
Must be coadministered at the same time as atazanavir or darunavir.

STORAGE
25°C (77°F); excursions permitted to 15-30°C (59-86°F). Keep tightly closed.

HOW SUPPLIED
Tab: 150mg

CONTRAINDICATIONS
Concomitant use w/ alfuzosin, ranolazine, dronedarone, carbamazepine, phenobarbital, phenytoin, colchicine (in patients w/ renal and/or hepatic impairment), rifampin, irinotecan (when coadministered w/ atazanavir only), lurasidone, pimozide, dihydroergotamine, ergotamine, methylergonovine, cisapride, St. John's wort, lovastatin, simvastatin, nevirapine (when coadministered w/ atazanavir only), sildenafil (when used to treat pulmonary arterial HTN), indinavir (when coadministered w/ atazanavir only), triazolam, and oral midazolam.

WARNINGS/PRECAUTIONS
Not interchangeable w/ ritonavir to increase systemic exposure of darunavir 600mg bid, fosamprenavir, saquinavir, or tipranavir. Decreases estimated CrCl due to inhibition of tubular secretion of creatinine w/o affecting actual renal glomerular function; consider this effect when interpreting changes in estimated CrCl in patients initiating therapy, particularly in patients w/ medical conditions or receiving drugs needing monitoring w/ estimated CrCl. Consider alternative medications that do not require dosage adjustments in patients w/ renal impairment. Closely monitor patients who experience a confirmed increase in SrCr of >0.4mg/dL from baseline for renal safety.

ADVERSE REACTIONS
Jaundice, rash.

DRUG INTERACTIONS
See Contraindications. Renal impairment, including cases of acute renal failure and Fanconi syndrome, reported w/ TDF; coadministration is not recommended in patients w/ estimated CrCl <70mL/min. Coadministration w/ TDF in combination w/ concomitant or recent use of a nephrotoxic agent is not recommended. Not recommended w/ >1 antiretroviral that requires pharmacokinetic enhancement (eg, 2 protease inhibitors or a protease inhibitor in combination w/ elvitegravir); darunavir in combination w/ efavirenz, nevirapine, or etravirine; atazanavir in combination w/ etravirine; atazanavir in combination w/ efavirenz in treatment-experienced patients; darunavir 600mg bid; other HIV-1 protease inhibitors (eg, fosamprenavir, saquinavir, tipranavir); fixed-dose combination tablets that contain cobicistat; and lopinavir/ritonavir or regimens containing ritonavir. Not recommended w/ boceprevir, simeprevir, salmeterol, avanafil, or voriconazole. May increase concentration of drugs that are primarily metabolized by CYP3A (eg, maraviroc, clonazepam, corticosteroids [eg, dexamethasone, inhaled/nasal fluticasone or budesonide], cyclosporine, everolimus, sirolimus, tacrolimus) or CYP2D6, or are substrates of P-gp, BCRP, OATP1B1, or OATP1B3. Coadministration w/ inhaled or nasal fluticasone or other corticosteroids that are metabolized by CYP3A may result in reduced serum cortisol concentrations. Coadministration w/ dexamethasone or other corticosteroids that induce CYP3A may result in decreased concentrations of cobicistat, atazanavir, and darunavir, which may lead to loss of therapeutic effect and possible development of resistance. CYP3A inhibitors may increase concentrations, which may lead to clinically significant adverse reactions. Coadministration w/ atazanavir in combination w/ antacids (eg, aluminum and magnesium hydroxide) may decrease atazanavir levels; administer a minimum of 2 hrs apart. May increase levels of antiarrhythmics (eg, amiodarone, quinidine, digoxin), dasatinib, nilotinib, vinblastine, vincristine, itraconazole, ketoconazole, colchicine, rifabutin, β-blockers, calcium channel blockers, bosentan, HMG-CoA reductase inhibitors (eg, atorvastatin, rosuvastatin), fentanyl, tramadol, antipsychotic (eg, perphenazine, risperidone, thioridazine, quetiapine), PDE-5 inhibitors (eg, sildenafil, tadalafil), and sedatives/hypnotics (eg, buspirone, diazepam, parenteral midazolam). When coadministering w/ digoxin, titrate digoxin dose and monitor digoxin concentrations. Coadministration w/ macrolide/ketolide antibiotics (clarithromycin, erythromycin, telithromycin) may increase levels of the antibiotic and of cobicistat, atazanavir, and darunavir; consider alternative antibiotics. Monitor for hematologic or GI side effects w/ vincristine and vinblastine. Monitor INR w/ warfarin. Avoid w/ rivaroxaban. Clinical monitoring of anticonvulsants that are metabolized by CYP3A (eg, clonazepam) is recommended. Coadministration w/ anticonvulsants w/ CYP3A induction effects that are not contraindicated (eg, eslicarbazepine, oxcarbazepine) may decrease cobicistat and atazanavir level; consider alternative anticonvulsant or antiretroviral therapy to avoid potential changes in exposures and monitor for lack or loss of virologic response if coadministration is necessary. Caution w/ SSRIs (eg, paroxetine), TCAs (eg, amitriptyline, desipramine), and trazodone; may increase levels of TCAs and trazodone. Bosentan may decrease levels. Coadministration w/ atazanavir in combination w/ H₂-receptor antagonists (eg, famotidine) may decrease atazanavir levels; administer atazanavir/cobicistat coadministration at either the same time or a minimum of 10 hrs after administering H₂-receptor antagonists. Consider additional or alternative (nonhormonal) forms of contraception if to be used w/ hormonal contraceptives. Caution w/ buprenorphine, buprenorphine/naloxone, and methadone. Coadministration w/ atazanavir in combination w/ proton pump inhibitors (eg, omeprazole), may decrease atazanavir levels; administer cobicistat w/ atazanavir a minimum of 12 hrs after administering proton pump inhibitors (PPIs) in treatment-naive patients; coadministration w/ PPIs, w/ or w/o tenofovir, is not recommended in treatment-experienced patients. Refer to PI for further information including dosing modifications when used w/ certain concomitant therapies.

PREGNANCY AND LACTATION
Pregnancy: There are no data w/ cobicistat in pregnant women to inform a drug-associated risk. There is a pregnancy exposure registry that monitors fetal outcomes in women exposed to therapy during pregnancy.
Lactation: Not for use in nursing.

MECHANISM OF ACTION
CYP3A inhibitor; increases the systemic exposure of CYP3A substrates atazanavir and darunavir.

PHARMACOKINETICS
Absorption: (W/ Darunavir) T_{max}=3.5 hrs (median); C_{max}=0.99mcg/mL; AUC=7.6mcg•hr/mL. **Distribution:** Plasma protein binding (97-98%). **Metabolism:** CYP3A, CYP2D6 (minor). **Elimination:** Feces (86.2%), urine (8.2%); $T_{1/2}$=3-4 hrs.

PATIENT CONSIDERATIONS
Assessment: Assess pregnancy/nursing status and for possible drug interactions. Assess estimated CrCl. When used w/ TDF, assess estimated CrCl, urine glucose, and urine protein.

Monitoring: Monitor for adverse reactions. Monitor CrCl. When used w/ TDF, perform routine monitoring of estimated CrCl, urine glucose, and urine protein and measure serum phosphorus in patients w/ or at risk for renal impairment.

Counseling: Inform of the risks and benefits of therapy. Inform patients that they should remain under the care of a physician when using therapy. Counsel about the risks of developing resistance to HIV-1 medications. Instruct that if a dose of the drug and atazanavir or darunavir is missed by <12 hrs, to take the missed dose of the drug w/ atazanavir or darunavir together right away, and the next dose together as usual; if a dose of the drug w/ atazanavir or darunavir is missed by >12 hrs, instruct to wait and take the next dose at the usual time. If a dose of the drug w/ atazanavir or darunavir is skipped, instruct not to double the next dose. Inform that therapy may interact w/ many drugs w/ potential serious implications and that some drugs should not be taken w/ therapy; advise to report to physician the use of any other prescription or nonprescription medication or herbal products, including St. John's wort. Inform patients that there is a pregnancy exposure registry that monitors pregnancy outcomes in women exposed to cobicistat during pregnancy. Instruct mothers not to breastfeed while on therapy.

TYKERB — lapatinib Rx
Class: Kinase inhibitor

Hepatotoxicity observed; may be severe and deaths have been reported.

ADULT DOSAGE	PEDIATRIC DOSAGE
HER2-Positive Metastatic Breast Cancer In combination w/ capecitabine in patients who have received prior therapy, including an anthracycline, a taxane, and trastuzumab 1250mg qd on Days 1-21 continuously w/ capecitabine 2000mg/m²/day (administered PO in 2 doses approx 12 hrs apart) on Days 1-14 in a repeating 21-day cycle; take capecitabine w/ food or w/in 30 min after food Continue until disease progression or unacceptable toxicity occurs **Hormone Receptor-Positive, HER2-Positive Metastatic Breast Cancer** In combination w/ letrozole for the treatment of postmenopausal women for whom hormonal therapy is indicated 1500mg qd continuously w/ letrozole 2.5mg qd	Pediatric use may not have been established

DOSING CONSIDERATIONS
Concomitant Medications
Strong CYP3A4 Inhibitors:
Avoid use; if coadministration is required, reduce lapatinib dose to 500mg/day
If strong inhibitor is discontinued, a washout period of approx 1 week should be allowed before the lapatinib dose is adjusted upward to the indicated dose
Avoid w/ grapefruit

Strong CYP3A4 Inducers:
Avoid use; if coadministration is required, titrate dose gradually as follows:
HER2-Positive Metastatic Breast Cancer: Titrate up to 4500mg/day
Hormone Receptor-Positive, HER2-Positive Metastatic Breast Cancer: Titrate up to 5500mg/day
If strong inducer is discontinued, reduce lapatinib dose to the indicated dose

Hepatic Impairment
Severe (Child-Pugh Class C):
HER2-Positive Metastatic Breast Cancer: Reduce dose to 750mg/day
Hormone Receptor-Positive, HER2-Positive Metastatic Breast Cancer: Reduce dose to 1000mg/day

Adverse Reactions
Cardiac Events:
D/C Therapy in Patients w/:
1. Decreased left ventricular ejection fraction (LVEF) ≥Grade 2 by National Cancer Institute Common Terminology Criteria for Adverse Events (NCI CTCAE v3)
2. LVEF that drops below the lower limit of normal

If LVEF Recovers to Normal and Patient is Asymptomatic for ≥2 Weeks:
In Combination w/ Capecitabine: Restart dose at 1000mg/day
In Combination w/ Letrozole: Restart dose at 1250mg/day
Diarrhea:
NCI CTCAE Grade 3 or Grade 1 or 2 w/ Complicating Features: Interrupt therapy
When Diarrhea Resolves to ≤Grade 1:
HER2-Positive Metastatic Breast Cancer: Reduce dose to 1000mg/day
Hormone Receptor-Positive, HER2-Positive Metastatic Breast Cancer: Reduce dose to 1250mg/day
NCI CTCAE Grade 4: Permanently d/c therapy
Other Toxicities:
≥Grade 2 NCI CTCAE Toxicity: Consider discontinuation/dose interruption
When Toxicity Improves to ≤Grade 1: Restart at standard dose
If Toxicity Recurs:
In Combination w/ Capecitabine: Restart at 1000mg/day
In Combination w/ Letrozole: Restart at 1250mg/day

ADMINISTRATION
Oral route

Take at least 1 hr ac or 1 hr pc
Do not divide the daily dose

STORAGE
25°C (77°F); excursions permitted to 15-30°C (59-86°F).

HOW SUPPLIED
Tab: 250mg

CONTRAINDICATIONS
Known severe hypersensitivity (eg, anaphylaxis) to lapatinib or any components of the medication.

WARNINGS/PRECAUTIONS
Patients should have disease progression on trastuzumab prior to initiation of treatment w/ lapatinib in combination w/ capecitabine. Decreased LVEF reported; confirm normal LVEF prior to therapy. D/C if severe liver function changes occur, and do not retreat. Diarrhea, including severe cases and deaths, reported; early identification and intervention is critical. Prompt treatment of diarrhea w/ antidiarrheals (eg, loperamide) after the 1st unformed stool is recommended. Severe diarrhea may require administration of oral or IV electrolytes/fluids, use of antibiotics such as fluoroquinolones (especially if diarrhea persists >24 hrs, there is fever, or Grade 3 or 4 neutropenia), and interruption or discontinuation of therapy. Associated w/ interstitial lung disease and pneumonitis; d/c if pulmonary symptoms indicative of interstitial lung disease/pneumonitis (≥Grade 3) occur. QT prolongation observed; caution in patients who have or may develop prolongation of QTc (eg, taking antiarrhythmics or other drugs that prolong the QT interval, cumulative high-dose anthracycline therapy). Correct hypokalemia and hypomagnesemia before administration. Severe cutaneous reactions reported; d/c treatment if life-threatening reactions (eg, erythema multiforme, Stevens-Johnson syndrome, toxic epidermal necrolysis) are suspected. May cause fetal harm.

ADVERSE REACTIONS
Hepatotoxicity, diarrhea, N/V, stomatitis, dyspepsia, palmar-plantar erythrodysesthesia, rash, dry skin, mucosal inflammation, pain in extremity, back pain, dyspnea, fatigue, headache, alopecia.

DRUG INTERACTIONS
See Dosing Considerations. Caution w/ substrates of CYP3A4, CYP2C8, and P-gp; consider dose reduction of the concomitant substrate drug when dosing lapatinib concurrently w/ concomitant substrate drugs w/ narrow therapeutic windows. Increased levels w/ P-gp inhibitors; use w/ caution. Increased levels w/ grapefruit. May increase exposure of paclitaxel and midazolam. May increase exposure of digoxin; monitor serum digoxin concentrations prior to initiation of lapatinib and throughout coadministration. If digoxin level is >1.2ng/mL, reduce digoxin dose by 1/2.

PREGNANCY AND LACTATION
Category D, not for use in nursing.

MECHANISM OF ACTION
Kinase inhibitor; inhibits both epidermal growth factor receptor (ErbB1) and HER2 (ErbB2), resulting in tumor cell growth inhibition.

PHARMACOKINETICS
Absorption: Incomplete and variable. C_{max}=2.43mcg/mL (1250mg daily); T_{max}=approx 4 hrs; AUC=36.2mcg•hr/mL (1250mg daily). **Distribution:** Plasma protein binding (>99%). **Metabolism:** Liver (extensive); (major) CYP3A4, CYP3A5; (minor) CYP2C19, CYP2C8. **Elimination:** Feces (27% [median] parent), urine (<2%); $T_{1/2}$=14.2 hrs (single dose).

PATIENT CONSIDERATIONS

Assessment: Assess for severe hepatic impairment, decreased LVEF or conditions that may impair left ventricular function, QT prolongation, hypokalemia, hypomagnesemia, pregnancy/nursing status, drug hypersensitivity, and possible drug interactions. Obtain baseline ECG, LFTs, serum K+, and Mg2+ levels.

Monitoring: Monitor for hepatotoxicity, diarrhea, bowel changes, pulmonary symptoms indicative of interstitial lung disease or pneumonitis, decreased LVEF, QT prolongation, severe cutaneous reactions, and other adverse reactions. Consider ECG and electrolyte monitoring. Monitor LFTs every 4-6 weeks during therapy and as clinically indicated.

Counseling: Instruct to notify physician if SOB, palpitations, or fatigue occurs. Advise that diarrhea is a common side effect and instruct on how it should be managed/prevented; instruct to contact physician immediately if any change in bowel patterns or severe diarrhea occurs. Counsel to report use of any prescription/nonprescription drugs or herbal products. Instruct not to take w/ grapefruit products. Advise women not to become pregnant while on therapy.

TYSABRI — natalizumab   Rx
Class: Monoclonal antibody/integrin receptor antagonist

> Increases risk of progressive multifocal leukoencephalopathy (PML). Risk factors for development of PML include duration of therapy, prior use of immunosuppressants, and presence of anti-JC virus (JCV) antibodies. Monitor for any new signs/symptoms of PML; withhold dosing immediately at the 1st sign/symptom suggestive of PML. For diagnosis, an evaluation that includes a gadolinium-enhanced MRI scan of the brain and, when indicated, CSF analysis for JC viral DNA are recommended. Due to the risk of PML, available only through a restricted program under a Risk Evaluation and Mitigation Strategy (REMS) called the TOUCH Prescribing Program.

ADULT DOSAGE
Multiple Sclerosis

Monotherapy for the Treatment of Relapsing Forms of Multiple Sclerosis (MS):
300mg IV infusion over 1 hr every 4 weeks

Crohn's Disease

To induce and maintain clinical response and remission in patients w/ moderately to severely active Crohn's disease (CD) w/ evidence of inflammation who have had an inadequate response to, or are unable to tolerate, conventional CD therapies and TNF-α inhibitors

300mg IV infusion over 1 hr every 4 weeks

- Aminosalicylates may be continued during treatment
- D/C therapy if therapeutic benefit is not experienced by 12 weeks of induction therapy
- For patients starting therapy while on chronic oral corticosteroids, commence steroid tapering as soon as a therapeutic benefit has occurred; if patient cannot be tapered off of oral corticosteroids w/in 6 months of starting therapy, d/c natalizumab
- Consider discontinuation for patients who require additional steroid use that exceeds 3 months in a calendar year to control their CD

PEDIATRIC DOSAGE
Pediatric use may not have been established

ADMINISTRATION
IV route

Dilution
1. To prepare sol, withdraw 15mL from the vial and inject the concentrate into 100mL of 0.9% NaCl inj; no other IV diluents may be used to prepare the sol.
2. Gently invert sol to mix completely; do not shake.
3. The final dosage sol has a concentration of 2.6mg/mL.
4. Following dilution, infuse sol immediately, or refrigerate at 2-8°C (36-46°F), and use w/in 8 hrs; if refrigerated, allow sol to warm to room temperature prior to infusion. Do not freeze.

Administration
1. Infuse 300mg in 100mL 0.9% NaCl inj, over approx 1 hr (infusion rate approx 5mg/min).
2. Do not administer as an IV push or bolus inj.
3. Observe patients during infusion and for 1 hr after completion of infusion.
4. After the infusion is complete, flush w/ 0.9% NaCl inj.
5. Do not inject other medications into infusion set side ports or mix w/ therapy. Use of filtration devices during administration has not been evaluated.

STORAGE
2-8°C (36-46°F). Do not shake or freeze. Protect from light.

HOW SUPPLIED
Inj: 300mg/15mL

CONTRAINDICATIONS
PML or history of PML. Hypersensitivity reaction to natalizumab.

WARNINGS/PRECAUTIONS
Anti-JCV antibody testing should not be used to diagnose PML. Avoid anti-JCV antibody testing during and for at least 2 weeks following plasma exchange due to the removal of antibodies from the serum. Retest patients w/ negative anti-JCV antibody test result periodically. PML reported following discontinuation in patients who did not have findings suggestive of PML at the time of discontinuation; monitor for any new signs or symptoms that may be suggestive of PML for at least 6 months following discontinuation. Immune reconstitution inflammatory syndrome (IRIS) reported in patients who developed PML and subsequently discontinued therapy; monitor for development of IRIS and treat appropriately. Increases the risk of developing encephalitis and meningitis caused by herpes simplex and varicella zoster viruses; d/c and treat appropriately if herpes encephalitis or meningitis occurs. Liver injury, including acute liver failure requiring transplant, reported; d/c in patients w/ jaundice or other evidence of significant liver injury (eg, lab

evidence). Hypersensitivity reactions, including serious systemic reactions (eg, anaphylaxis) reported; d/c administration, initiate appropriate therapy, and do not retreat. Patients who receive natalizumab for a short exposure (1 to 2 infusions) followed by an extended period w/o treatment are at higher risk of developing anti-natalizumab antibodies and/or hypersensitivity reactions on re-exposure; consider testing for the presence of antibodies in patients who wish to recommence therapy following a dose interruption. May increase risk for infections. Avoid in patients w/ systemic medical conditions resulting in significantly compromised immune system function. Induces increases in circulating lymphocytes, monocytes, eosinophils, basophils, and nucleated RBCs or transient decreases in Hgb levels.

ADVERSE REACTIONS
MS: Headache, fatigue, arthralgia, UTI, lower respiratory tract infection, gastroenteritis, vaginitis, depression, pain in extremity, abdominal discomfort, diarrhea, rash.
CD: Headache, fatigue, URTI, nausea.

DRUG INTERACTIONS
Avoid w/ immunomodulatory therapy, immunosuppressants (eg, 6-mercaptopurine, azathioprine, cyclosporine, methotrexate) or TNF-α inhibitors. Concurrent use of antineoplastic, immunosuppressant, or immunomodulating agents may further increase risk of infections, including PML and other opportunistic infections.

PREGNANCY AND LACTATION
Pregnancy: Category C.
Lactation: Detected in human milk. The effects of this exposure on infants are unknown.

MECHANISM OF ACTION
Monoclonal antibody/integrin receptor antagonist; specific mechanisms by which natalizumab exerts its effects in MS and CD have not been fully defined. Binds to the α4-subunit of α4β1 and α4β7 integrins expressed on the surface of all leukocytes except neutrophils, and inhibits the α4-mediated adhesion of leukocytes to their counter-receptor(s).

PHARMACOKINETICS
Absorption: (MS) C_{max}=110mcg/mL; (CD) C_{max}=101mcg/mL. **Distribution:** Found in breast milk; (MS) V_d=5.7L; (CD) V_d=5.2L. **Elimination:** (MS) $T_{1/2}$=11 days; (CD) $T_{1/2}$=10 days.

PATIENT CONSIDERATIONS
Assessment: Assess for risk of PML, immunosuppression, drug hypersensitivity, pregnancy/nursing status, and possible drug interactions. Obtain MRI prior to initiating therapy. Test for anti-JCV antibody status; retest periodically in patients w/ negative result.

Monitoring: Monitor for PML, IRIS, encephalitis, meningitis, hepatotoxicity, hypersensitivity/antibody formation, infections, and other adverse reactions. Evaluate patients 3 and 6 months after the 1st infusion, every 6 months thereafter, and for at least 6 months after discontinuing treatment. Consider periodic monitoring for radiographic signs consistent w/ PML to allow for an early diagnosis of PML.

Counseling: Educate on risks/benefits of therapy. Instruct to promptly report any new or continuously worsening symptoms that persist over several days to physician. Advise patients to inform all of their physicians that they are receiving natalizumab. Counsel about the follow-up schedule (3 and 6 months after 1st infusion, every 6 months thereafter, and for at least 6 months after discontinuation). Instruct to seek medical attention if symptoms suggestive of PML develop, including progressive weakness on one side of the body or clumsiness of the limbs, disturbance of vision, and changes in thinking, memory, and orientation leading to confusion and personality changes. Instruct patients to continue to look for new signs and symptoms suggestive of PML for approx 6 months following treatment discontinuation. Advise that therapy is only available through a restricted program called the TOUCH Prescribing Program and inform about requirements. Instruct to report symptoms of infections, hypersensitivity reactions, hepatotoxicity, and herpes encephalitis/meningitis.

TYVASO — treprostinil   Rx
Class: Prostacyclin analogue

ADULT DOSAGE
Pulmonary Arterial Hypertension
Treatment of pulmonary arterial HTN (WHO Group 1) to improve exercise ability

Dose in 4 separate, equally spaced treatment sessions (approx 4 hrs apart) per day, during waking hrs

Initial: 3 breaths (18mcg) per treatment session, qid.
If 3 breaths are not tolerated, reduce to 1 or 2 breaths and subsequently increase to 3 breaths, as tolerated.

Maint: Increase dose by an additional 3 breaths at approx 1- to 2-week intervals, if tolerated, until the target dose of 9 breaths (54mcg) is reached per treatment session, qid.

PEDIATRIC DOSAGE
Pediatric use may not have been established

If adverse effects preclude titration to target dose, continue at the highest tolerated dose.
Max: 9 breaths per treatment session, qid

Missed Dose
If scheduled treatment session is missed/interrupted, resume therapy as soon as possible at usual dose

---

DOSING CONSIDERATIONS
Renal Impairment
Titrate slowly
Hepatic Impairment
Titrate slowly

ADMINISTRATION
Oral inh route
Use only w/ the Tyvaso Inhalation System.
Do not mix w/ other medications in the inh system.
Avoid skin or eye contact w/ sol. Do not orally ingest Tyvaso sol.

The inh system should be prepared for use each day according to the instructions for use.
One ampule of Tyvaso contains a sufficient volume of medication for all 4 treatment sessions in a single day.
Prior to the 1st treatment session, the patient should twist the top off a single ampule and squeeze the entire contents into the medicine cup.
Between each of the 4 daily treatment sessions, the device should be capped and stored upright w/ the remaining medication inside.
Discard medicine cup and any remaining medicine at the end of each day.
Refer to PI for further administration instructions.

STORAGE
25°C (77°F); excursions permitted to 15-30°C (59-86°F). Use w/in 7 days once the foil pack is opened; store unopened ampules in the foil pouch. After an ampule is opened and transferred to the medicine cup, the sol should remain in the device for no more than 1 day (24 hrs).

HOW SUPPLIED
Sol, Inhalation: 0.6mg/mL [2.9mL]

WARNINGS/PRECAUTIONS
Effects diminish over the minimum recommended dosing interval of 4 hrs; treatment timing can be adjusted for planned activities. Efficacy not established w/ significant underlying lung disease; carefully monitor patients w/ acute pulmonary infections to detect any worsening of lung disease and loss of drug effect. May produce symptomatic hypotension in patients w/ low systemic arterial pressure. Titrate slowly in patients w/ hepatic or renal insufficiency. Inhibits platelet aggregation and increases risk of bleeding. Caution in elderly.

ADVERSE REACTIONS
Cough, throat irritation, headache, GI effects, muscle/jaw/bone pain, flushing, syncope.

DRUG INTERACTIONS
Coadministration w/ diuretics, antihypertensive agents, or other vasodilators may increase risk of symptomatic hypotension. May increase risk of bleeding w/ anticoagulants. CYP2C8 inhibitors (eg, gemfibrozil) may increase exposure. CYP2C8 inducers (eg, rifampin) may decrease exposure.

PREGNANCY AND LACTATION
Pregnancy: Category B.
Lactation: It is not known whether treprostinil is excreted in human milk.

MECHANISM OF ACTION
Prostacyclin analogue; causes direct vasodilation of pulmonary and systemic arterial vascular beds and inhibition of platelet aggregation.

PHARMACOKINETICS
Absorption: Absolute bioavailability (64%) (18mcg), (72%) (36mcg), (54mcg) C_{max}=0.91 or 1.32ng/mL, T_{max}=0.25 or 0.12 hr, AUC=0.81 or 0.97ng·hr/mL. **Distribution:** (IV) V_d=14L/70kg ideal body weight; plasma protein binding (91%). **Metabolism:** Liver via CYP2C8; oxidation and glucuroconjugation. **Elimination:** (SQ) Urine (79% metabolites, 4% unchanged), feces (13% metabolites); $T_{1/2}$=4 hrs.

PATIENT CONSIDERATIONS
Assessment: Assess for pulmonary disease/infections, low systemic arterial pressure, hepatic/renal insufficiency, pregnancy/nursing status, and possible drug interactions.

Monitoring: Monitor for worsening of lung disease, loss of drug effect, symptomatic hypotension, bleeding, and other adverse reactions.

Counseling: Counsel on proper administration process, including dosing, set up, operation, cleaning, and maintenance. Advise to have access to a backup Tyvaso Inhalation System device to avoid potential interruptions in drug delivery because of equipment malfunction. Inform to resume therapy as soon as possible if a scheduled treatment session is missed or interrupted. Instruct to avoid skin or eye contact w/ the sol and to rinse immediately w/ water if sol comes in contact w/ the skin or eyes.

TYZEKA — telbivudine   Rx

Class: Nucleoside reverse transcriptase inhibitor (NRTI)

> Lactic acidosis and severe hepatomegaly with steatosis, including fatal cases, reported with nucleoside analogues alone or in combination with other antiretrovirals. Severe acute exacerbations of hepatitis B reported in patients who discontinued therapy; monitor hepatic function closely for at least several months. If appropriate, resumption of anti-hepatitis B therapy may be warranted.

ADULT DOSAGE	PEDIATRIC DOSAGE
Chronic Hepatitis B	**Chronic Hepatitis B**
Tab:	**≥16 Years:**
600mg qd	**Tab:**
Sol:	600mg qd
30mL qd	**Sol:**
	30mL qd

DOSING CONSIDERATIONS
Renal Impairment
CrCl 30-49mL/min:
Tab: 600mg q48h
Sol: 20mL qd
CrCl <30mL/min (Not Requiring Dialysis):
Tab: 600mg q72h
Sol: 10mL qd
ESRD:
Tab: 600mg q96h; administer after hemodialysis, when administered on hemodialysis days
Sol: 6mL qd; administer after hemodialysis, when administered on hemodialysis days
Other Important Considerations
HBV DNA ≥300 copies/mL After 24 Weeks of Treatment:
Institute alternate therapy

ADMINISTRATION
Oral route
Take with or without food

STORAGE
25°C (77°F); excursions permitted to 15-30°C (59-86°F). (Sol) Use within 2 months after opening. Do not freeze.

HOW SUPPLIED
Sol: 100mg/5mL [300mL]; **Tab:** 600mg

CONTRAINDICATIONS
Combination with pegylated interferon alfa-2a.

WARNINGS/PRECAUTIONS
Initiate only if pretreatment HBV DNA and ALT levels are known. HBV DNA should be <9 log_{10} copies/mL and ALT should be ≥2X ULN in HBeAg-positive patients prior to therapy. HBV DNA should be <7 log_{10} copies/mL in HBeAg-negative patients prior to therapy. Institute alternate therapy in patients with incomplete viral suppression (HBV DNA ≥300 copies/mL) after 24 weeks of treatment or if patients test positive for HBV DNA at any time after initial response. Female gender, obesity, and prolonged nucleoside exposure may be risk factors for developing lactic acidosis and hepatomegaly with steatosis; d/c therapy if lactic acidosis or hepatotoxicity develops. Caution with known risk factors for liver disease. Myopathy/myositis and peripheral neuropathy reported; interrupt therapy if suspected and d/c if confirmed. Rhabdomyolysis and uncomplicated myalgia reported. Caution in elderly.

ADVERSE REACTIONS
Fatigue, creatinine kinase increase, headache, cough, diarrhea, abdominal pain, nausea, pharyngolaryngeal pain, arthralgia, pyrexia, rash, lactic acidosis, severe hepatomegaly with steatosis, back pain, dizziness.

DRUG INTERACTIONS
See Contraindications. Drugs that alter renal function may alter plasma concentrations. Combination with interferons may be associated with risk of peripheral neuropathy.

PREGNANCY AND LACTATION
Category B, not for use in nursing.

MECHANISM OF ACTION
Thymidine nucleoside analogue; inhibits HBV DNA polymerase (reverse transcriptase) by competing with the natural substrate thymidine 5'-triphosphate and causing DNA chain termination after incorporation into viral DNA.

PHARMACOKINETICS
Absorption: (600mg qd) C_{max}=3.69mcg/mL, T_{max}=2 hrs, AUC=26.1mcg•h/mL. Administration with varying degrees of renal function resulted in different pharmacokinetic parameters. **Distribution:** Plasma protein binding (3.3%). **Elimination:** (600mg single dose) Urine (42%), $T_{1/2}$=40-49 hrs.

PATIENT CONSIDERATIONS
Assessment: Assess for renal/hepatic impairment, use in women, obesity, nucleoside exposure duration, risk factors for liver disease, pregnancy/nursing status, and possible drug interactions. Obtain HBV DNA and ALT levels prior to therapy.

Monitoring: Monitor hepatic function periodically and for several months after discontinuation. Monitor for exacerbation of HBV after discontinuation, lactic acidosis, hepatomegaly, hepatotoxicity, myopathy, and peripheral neuropathy. Monitor HBV DNA levels at 24 weeks of therapy and every 6 months thereafter.

Monitor renal function in elderly patients. Closely monitor for any signs/symptoms of unexplained muscle pain, tenderness, or weakness when initiating with any drug associated with myopathy.

Counseling: Advise patients to remain under care of a physician during therapy and to discuss any new symptoms or concurrent medications. Advise to report promptly unexplained muscle weakness, tenderness or pain, numbness, tingling, and/or burning sensations in the arms and/or legs with or without difficulty walking. Inform that medication is not a cure for hepatitis B and long-term treatment benefits are unknown. Inform that deterioration of liver disease may occur in some cases if treatment is discontinued; advise to discuss any changes in regimen with physician. Inform that therapy has not shown to reduce risk of transmission of HBV to others through sexual contact or blood contamination and counsel on HBV prevention strategies. Advise patients on low-sodium diet that sol contains 47mg sodium/600mg. Advise to dispose of unused/expired drug properly, and to remove all identifying information from the original container prior to disposal.

UNITUXIN — dinutuximab   Rx

Class: GD2-binding monoclonal antibody

> Serious and potentially life-threatening infusion reactions reported; administer required prehydration and premedication including antihistamines prior to each infusion. Monitor closely for signs/symptoms of an infusion reaction during and for at least 4 hrs following completion of each infusion. Immediately interrupt therapy for severe infusion reactions and permanently d/c for anaphylaxis. May cause severe neuropathic pain; administer IV opioid prior to, during, and for 2 hrs following completion of infusion. Grade 3 peripheral sensory neuropathy reported. Severe motor neuropathy reported in adults. D/C therapy for severe unresponsive pain, severe sensory neuropathy, or moderate to severe peripheral motor neuropathy.

PEDIATRIC DOSAGE
Neuroblastoma
In combination w/ granulocyte-macrophage colony-stimulating factor, interleukin-2 and 13-cis-retinoic acid, for the treatment of patients w/ high-risk neuroblastoma who achieve at least a partial response to prior 1st-line multiagent, multimodality therapy

Usual: 17.5mg/m²/day as IV infusion over 10-20 hrs for 4 consecutive days for a max of 5 cycles
Initiate at an infusion rate of 0.875mg/ m²/hr for 30 min; may gradually increase as tolerated to a max rate of 1.75mg/m²/hr

Schedule of Administration:
Cycles 1, 3, and 5:
Take on Days 4, 5, 6, and 7
Cycles 1, 3, and 5 are 24 days in duration

Cycles 2 and 4:
Take on Days 8, 9, 10, and 11
Cycles 2 and 4 are 32 days in duration

Required Pretreatment and Guidelines for Pain Management:
IV Hydration: Administer 10mL/kg IV infusion of 0.9% NaCl inj over 1 hr just prior to initiating each dinutuximab infusion

Analgesics: Administer 50mcg/kg morphine sulfate IV immediately prior to initiation of dinutuximab, then continue as a morphine sulfate drip at an infusion rate of 20-50mcg/ kg/hr during and for 2 hrs following completion of dinutuximab. Administer additional 25-50mcg/ kg IV doses of morphine sulfate prn for pain for up to once q2h followed by an increase in morphine sulfate infusion rate in clinically stable patients.
Consider using fentanyl or hydromorphone if morphine sulfate is not tolerated.
If pain is inadequately managed w/ opioids, consider use of gabapentin or lidocaine in conjunction w/ IV morphine.

Antihistamines/Antipyretics:
Administer 0.5-1mg/kg (max dose of 50mg) of antihistamine (eg, diphenhydramine) IV over 10-15 min starting 20 min prior to initiation of dinutuximab and as tolerated q4-6h during dinutuximab infusion.

Administer 10-15mg/kg (max dose of 650mg) of acetaminophen 20 min prior to each dinutuximab infusion and q4-6h prn for fever or pain. Administer 5-10mg/kg of ibuprofen q6h prn for control of persistent fever or pain.

DOSING CONSIDERATIONS
Adverse Reactions
Infusion-Related Reactions:
Mild to moderate adverse reactions (eg, transient rash, fever, rigors, localized urticaria) that respond promptly to symptomatic treatment
Onset of Reaction: Reduce infusion rate to 50% of the previous rate and monitor closely
After Resolution: Gradually increase infusion rate up to a max rate of 1.75mg/m²/hr

Prolonged or Severe Adverse Reactions (eg, Mild Bronchospasm w/o Other Symptoms, Angioedema That Does Not Affect the Airway):
Onset of Reaction: Interrupt immediately
After Resolution: Resume at 50% of the previous rate and observe closely, if signs and symptoms resolve rapidly
1st Recurrence: D/C until the following day. If symptoms resolve and continued treatment is warranted, premedicate w/ 1mg/kg (max dose of 50mg) hydrocortisone IV and administer dinutuximab at a rate of 0.875mg/m²/hr in an intensive care unit
2nd Recurrence: D/C permanently

Capillary Leak Syndrome:
Moderate to Severe but Not Life-Threatening:
Onset of Reaction: Interrupt immediately
After Resolution: Resume at 50% of the previous rate

Life-Threatening:
Onset of Reaction: D/C for the current cycle
After Resolution: Administer at 50% of the previous rate in subsequent cycles
1st Recurrence: D/C permanently

Hypotension Requiring Medical Intervention:
Symptomatic Hypotension, Systolic BP (SBP) < Lower Limit of Normal for Age, or SBP Decreased by >15% Compared to Baseline:
Onset of Reaction: Interrupt infusion
After Resolution: Resume infusion at 50% of the previous rate. Increase infusion rate as tolerated up to a max rate of 1.75mg/m²/hr if BP remains stable for at least 2 hrs

Severe Systemic Infection or Sepsis:
Onset of Reaction: D/C until resolution of infection, and then proceed w/ subsequent cycles of therapy

Neurological Disorders of the Eye:
Onset of Reaction: D/C infusion until resolution
After Resolution: Reduce dose by 50%
1st Recurrence or if Accompanied by Visual Impairment: D/C permanently

Permanently Discontinue w/ the Following:
- Grade 3 or 4 anaphylaxis
- Grade 3 or 4 serum sickness
- Grade 3 pain unresponsive to max supportive measures
- Grade 4 sensory neuropathy or Grade 3 sensory neuropathy that interferes w/ daily activities for >2 weeks
- Grade 2 peripheral motor neuropathy
- Subtotal or total vision loss
- Grade 4 hyponatremia despite appropriate fluid management

ADMINISTRATION
IV route

Administer as a diluted IV infusion only; do not administer as an IV push or bolus. Verify that patients have adequate hematologic, respiratory, hepatic, and renal function prior to initiating each course of therapy.

Preparation
Aseptically withdraw the required volume from the single-use vial and inject into a 100mL bag of 0.9% NaCl inj.
Mix by gentle inversion; do not shake.
Initiate infusion w/in 4 hrs of preparation.
Discard diluted sol 24 hrs after preparation.

STORAGE
2-8°C (36-46°F). Do not freeze or shake the vial. Protect from light.

HOW SUPPLIED
Inj: 3.5mg/mL [5mL]

CONTRAINDICATIONS
History of anaphylaxis to dinutuximab.

WARNINGS/PRECAUTIONS
Pain reported; decrease infusion rate to 0.875mg/m²/hr for severe pain. Capillary leak syndrome reported; immediately interrupt or d/c therapy and institute supportive management in patients w/ symptomatic or severe capillary leak syndrome. Hypotension, infection, neurological disorders of the eye, bone marrow suppression, and electrolyte abnormalities reported. Atypical hemolytic uremic syndrome reported; permanently d/c therapy and institute supportive management for signs of hemolytic uremic syndrome. May cause fetal harm.

ADVERSE REACTIONS
Infusion reactions, neuropathy, pain, pyrexia, thrombocytopenia, lymphopenia, hypotension, hyponatremia, anemia, vomiting, diarrhea, hypokalemia, neutropenia, urticaria, hypoalbuminemia.

PREGNANCY AND LACTATION
Pregnancy: May cause fetal harm. Monoclonal antibodies are transported across the placenta as pregnancy progresses, w/ the largest amount transferred during the 3rd trimester.
Lactation: It is not known if dinutuximab is present in human milk; not for use in nursing.
Reproductive Potential: Females of reproductive potential should use effective contraception during treatment and for 2 months after the last dose of dinutuximab.

MECHANISM OF ACTION
Glycolipid disialoganglioside (GD2)-binding monoclonal antibody; binds to cell surface of GD2 and induces cell lysis of GD2-expressing cells through antibody-dependent cell-mediated cytotoxicity and complement-dependent cytotoxicity.

PHARMACOKINETICS
Absorption: C_{max}=11.5mcg/mL. **Distribution:** V_d=5.4L. **Elimination:** $T_{1/2}$=10 days.

PATIENT CONSIDERATIONS
Assessment: Assess for hematologic/respiratory/hepatic/renal dysfunction, history of anaphylaxis to drug, and pregnancy/nursing status.

Monitoring: Monitor for neuropathy, pain, capillary leak syndrome, hypotension, infection, neurological disorders of the eye, atypical hemolytic uremic syndrome, and other adverse reactions. Monitor closely for signs/symptoms of an infusion reaction during and for at least 4 hrs following completion of each infusion. Monitor serum electrolytes (daily) and peripheral blood counts.

Counseling: Inform of the risk of serious infusion reactions and anaphylaxis; severe pain and peripheral sensory and motor neuropathy; capillary leak syndrome; hypotension; infection; neurological disorders of the eye; bone marrow suppression; electrolyte abnormalities; and hemolytic uremic syndrome. Instruct to promptly report to physician if any signs/symptoms of any of these conditions develop. Advise women of reproductive potential of the potential risk to the fetus if administered during pregnancy and the need for use of effective contraception during and for at least 2 months after completing therapy.

UPTRAVI — selexipag   Rx
Class: Prostacyclin receptor agonist

ADULT DOSAGE	PEDIATRIC DOSAGE
Pulmonary Arterial Hypertension Treatment of pulmonary arterial HTN (WHO Group I) to delay disease progression and reduce risk of hospitalization **Initial:** 200mcg bid **Titrate:** Increase in increments of 200mcg bid, usually at weekly intervals **Max:** 1600mcg bid If a patient reaches a dose that cannot be tolerated, the dose should be reduced to previously tolerated dose **Missed Dose** If a dose is missed, take as soon as possible unless next dose is w/in the next 6 hrs If treatment is missed for ≥3 days, restart at a lower dose and then retitrate	Pediatric use may not have been established

---

DOSING CONSIDERATIONS
Hepatic Impairment
Moderate (Child-Pugh Class B):
Initial: 200mcg qd
Titrate: Increase in increments of 200mcg qd at weekly intervals, as tolerated
Severe (Child-Pugh Class C): Avoid use

ADMINISTRATION
Oral route

Tolerability may be improved when taken w/ food.
Do not split, crush, or chew tabs.

STORAGE
20-25°C (68-77°F); excursions permitted between 15-30°C (59-86°F).

HOW SUPPLIED
Tab: 200mcg, 400mcg, 600mcg, 800mcg, 1000mcg, 1200mcg, 1400mcg, 1600mcg

WARNINGS/PRECAUTIONS
Consider the possibility of associated pulmonary veno-occlusive disease if signs of pulmonary edema occur; d/c therapy if confirmed.

ADVERSE REACTIONS
Headache, diarrhea, jaw pain, N/V, myalgia, pain in extremity, flushing, arthralgia, anemia, decreased appetite, rash.

DRUG INTERACTIONS
Strong CYP2C8 inhibitors (eg, gemfibrozil) may significantly increase exposure to selexipag and its active metabolite; avoid concomitant administration.

PREGNANCY AND LACTATION

Pregnancy: There are no adequate and well-controlled studies in pregnant women.

Lactation: It is not known if selexipag is present in human milk; not for use in nursing.

MECHANISM OF ACTION

Prostacyclin receptor (IP receptor) agonist; selective for the IP receptor versus other prostanoid receptors.

PHARMACOKINETICS

Absorption: T_{max}=1-3 hrs; 3-4 hrs (active metabolite). **Distribution:** Plasma protein binding (approx 99%). **Metabolism:** Enzymatic hydrolysis of the acylsulfonamide by hepatic carboxylesterase 1, to yield the active metabolite. Oxidative metabolism via CYP3A4 and CYP2C8 leads to the formation of hydroxylated and dealkylated products. UGT1A3 and UGT2B7 are involved in the glucuronidation of the active metabolite. **Elimination:** Feces (93%); urine (12%); $T_{1/2}$=0.8-2.5 hrs; 6.2-13.5 hrs (active metabolite).

PATIENT CONSIDERATIONS

Assessment: Assess pregnancy/nursing status, and for possible drug interactions.

Monitoring: Monitor for signs of pulmonary edema and other adverse events.

Counseling: Inform not to split, crush, or chew tablets. Advise patients what to do in case of a missed dose.

UVADEX — methoxsalen   Rx

Class: Psoralen

> Should be used only by physicians who have special competence in the diagnosis/treatment of cutaneous T-cell lymphoma and who have special training and experience in the UVAR XTS or THERAKOS CELLEX Photopheresis System.

ADULT DOSAGE

Cutaneous T-Cell Lymphoma

Palliative Treatment of Skin Manifestations of Cutaneous T-Cell Lymphoma Unresponsive to Other Forms of Treatment:

Dosage Per Treatment Calculated According to Treatment Volume:
Treatment volume x 0.017 = mL of methoxsalen for each treatment
Inject prescribed amount into recirculation bag prior to photoactivation phase

Normal Treatment Schedule:
Give on 2 consecutive days every 4 weeks for a minimum of 7 treatment cycles (6 months)

Accelerated Treatment Schedule:
May increase frequency of treatment to 2 consecutive treatments every 2 weeks if the assessment during the 4th treatment cycle (approx 3 months) reveals an increased skin score from the baseline score

If 25% improvement in the skin score is attained after 4 consecutive weeks, may resume the regular treatment schedule

Patients maintained in the accelerated treatment schedule may receive a max of 20 cycles

PEDIATRIC DOSAGE
Pediatric use may not have been established

ADMINISTRATION
Extracorporeal route

Do not dilute
Contents of vial should be injected into THERAKOS UVAR XTS or THERAKOS CELLEX photopheresis system immediately after being drawn up into syringe; do not inject directly into patients
Once drawn into plastic syringe, immediately inject into photoactivation bag; discard methoxsalen exposed to plastic syringe for >1 hr
Vials are single use only; discard any unused portion
Can adsorb onto PVC and plastics; only THERAKOS UVAR XTS or THERAKOS CELLEX photopheresis procedural kits supplied for use w/ the instrument should be used to administer this product

STORAGE
15-30°C (59-86°F).

HOW SUPPLIED
Inj: 20mcg/mL [10mL]

CONTRAINDICATIONS
Idiosyncratic or hypersensitivity reactions to methoxsalen, other psoralen compounds or any of the excipients; patients w/ aphakia; contraindications to the photopheresis procedure; or history of light sensitive disease (eg, lupus erythematosus, porphyria cutanea tarda, erythropoietic protoporphyria, variegate porphyria, xeroderma pigmentosum, albinism).

WARNINGS/PRECAUTIONS

Cutaneous squamous cell cancers reported with oral methoxsalen administration. May cause fetal harm. Sunlight/UV radiation exposure after administration may cause premature skin aging. May increase risk of skin cancers; closely monitor patients who exhibit multiple basal cell carcinomas or who have a history of basal cell carcinoma. Serious burns from either UVA/sunlight (even through window glass) can result if recommended dose is exceeded or precautions are not followed. Avoid all exposure to sunlight during the 24 hrs after treatment. Patients should wear UVA-absorbing, wrap-around sunglasses for 24 hrs after treatment to avoid cataractogenicity.

ADVERSE REACTIONS

Hypotension, cardiovascular effects, infections.

DRUG INTERACTIONS

Increased risk for photosensitivity reactions with known photosensitizing agents (eg, anthralin, coal tar and its derivatives, griseofulvin, phenothiazines, nalidixic acid, halogenated salicylanilides [bacteriostatic soaps], sulfonamides, tetracyclines, thiazides, and certain organic staining dyes [eg, methylene blue, toluidine blue, rose bengal, methyl orange]).

PREGNANCY AND LACTATION

Category D, caution in nursing.

MECHANISM OF ACTION

Psoralen; has not been established. Upon photoactivation, conjugates and forms covalent bonds with DNA, which leads to the formation of both monofunctional and bifunctional adducts. May also react with proteins. The formation of photoadducts results in inhibition of DNA synthesis, cell division, and epidermal turnover.

PHARMACOKINETICS

Metabolism: Rapid. **Elimination:** Urine (95% metabolites).

PATIENT CONSIDERATIONS

Assessment: Assess for idiosyncratic/hypersensitivity reaction, any conditions where treatment is contraindicated or cautioned, pregnancy/nursing status, and possible drug interactions.

Monitoring: Monitor for signs/symptoms of skin burning, skin cancer (eg, cutaneous squamous cell cancers), cataracts, and premature aging of skin. Monitor closely those patients who exhibit multiple basal cell carcinomas or who have a history of basal cell carcinomas.

Counseling: Instruct emphatically to wear UVA-absorbing, wrap-around sunglasses, and cover exposed skin or use a sunblock (SP 15 or higher) for the 24-hr period following treatment, whether exposed to direct or indirect sunlight in the open or through a window glass. Advise women of childbearing potential to avoid becoming pregnant during therapy.

VALCHLOR — mechlorethamine   Rx

Class: Nitrogen mustard alkylating agent

ADULT DOSAGE

Cutaneous T-Cell Lymphoma

Stage IA and IB Mycosis Fungoides-Type Cutaneous T-Cell Lymphoma in Patients Who Have Received Prior Skin-Directed Therapy:
Apply a thin film qd to affected areas of the skin

PEDIATRIC DOSAGE
Pediatric use may not have been established

DOSING CONSIDERATIONS

Adverse Reactions

Skin Ulceration, Blistering, or Moderately-Severe or Severe Dermatitis (Marked Skin Redness with Edema):
D/C for any grade; upon improvement, restart at a reduced frequency of once every 3 days.
If reintroduction is tolerated for at least 1 week, increase frequency of application to qod for at least 1 week and then to qd application if tolerated.

ADMINISTRATION
Topical route

Caregivers must wear disposable nitrile gloves when applying gel to patients and wash hands thoroughly with soap and water after removal of gloves.
If there is accidental skin exposure to gel, caregivers must immediately wash exposed areas thoroughly with soap and water for at least 15 minutes and remove contaminated clothing.
Do not use occlusive dressings on areas of the skin where product was applied.

STORAGE
Prior to Dispensing: -25 to -15°C (-13-5°F). **Once Dispensed:** 2-8°C (36-46°F). Keep in its original box and avoid contact with food when storing in refrigerator. Discard unused product after 60 days.

HOW SUPPLIED
Gel: 0.016% [60g]

CONTRAINDICATIONS
Known severe hypersensitivity to mechlorethamine.

WARNINGS/PRECAUTIONS
Exposure to eyes causes pain, burns, inflammation, photophobia, and blurred vision; blindness and severe irreversible anterior eye injury may occur. If eye exposure occurs, immediately irrigate for at least 15 min with copious amounts of water, normal saline, or a balanced salt ophthalmic irrigating solution and obtain immediate

medical (eg, ophthalmologic) consultation. Exposure of mucous membranes (eg, oral mucosa, nasal mucosa) causes pain, redness, and ulceration, which may be severe; should mucosal contact occur, immediately irrigate for at least 15 min with copious amounts of water, followed by immediate medical consultation. Avoid direct skin contact with product in individuals other than the patient; risks of secondary exposure include dermatitis, mucosal injury, and secondary cancers. Dermatitis reported; monitor for redness, swelling, inflammation, itchiness, blisters, ulceration, and secondary skin infections. Non-melanoma skin cancer reported; monitor for non-melanoma skin cancers during and after treatment. May cause fetal harm. Flammable; avoid fire, flame, and smoking until medication has dried.

ADVERSE REACTIONS
Dermatitis, pruritus, bacterial skin infection, skin ulceration/blistering, skin hyperpigmentation.

PREGNANCY AND LACTATION
Pregnancy: Category D.
Lactation: Not for use in nursing.

MECHANISM OF ACTION
Nitrogen mustard alkylating agent; inhibits rapidly proliferating cells.

PATIENT CONSIDERATIONS
Assessment: Assess for drug hypersensitivity, and pregnancy/nursing status.

Monitoring: Monitor for dermatitis (redness, swelling, inflammation, itchiness, blisters, ulceration, secondary skin infections), non-melanoma skin cancers (during and after treatment), and other adverse reactions. Monitor if eye exposure or mucosal contact occurs.

Counseling: Instruct to wash hands thoroughly with soap and water after handling or applying the product. Instruct caregivers to wear disposable nitrile gloves when applying the product to patients and to wash hands thoroughly with soap and water after removal of gloves; advise that if there is accidental skin exposure to the product, to immediately wash exposed areas thoroughly with soap and water for at least 15 min and remove contaminated clothing. Instruct not to use occlusive (air or water-tight) dressings on areas of the skin where product was applied. Advise to discard unused product, empty tubes, and used application gloves in household trash in a manner that prevents accidental application or ingestion by others, including children and pets. Advise that adherence to the recommended storage condition will ensure the product will work as expected; instruct to consult a pharmacist prior to using product that has been left at room temperature for >1 hr/day. Counsel on what to do in case of eye exposure or mucosal contact. Instruct to consult with physician if skin irritation occurs after applying the product. Instruct to notify physician of any new skin lesions and to undergo periodic assessment for signs and symptoms of skin cancer. Advise of the potential hazard to a fetus and to avoid pregnancy while using the product. Advise women to d/c nursing due to the potential for topical or systemic exposure to product. Instruct to avoid fire, flame, and smoking until medication has dried.

VALCYTE — valganciclovir hydrochloride   Rx

Class: Synthetic guanine derivative nucleoside analogue

> Severe leukopenia, neutropenia, anemia, thrombocytopenia, pancytopenia, bone marrow aplasia, and aplastic anemia reported. Based on animal data, temporary or permanent inhibition of spermatogenesis may occur and there is a potential for birth defects and cancers in humans.

ADULT DOSAGE
Cytomegalovirus Retinitis
Treatment in Patients w/ AIDS:
Tab:
Induction: 900mg (two 450mg tabs) bid for 21 days
Maint: 900mg qd following induction treatment, or in patients w/ inactive CMV retinitis

Cytomegalovirus Disease
Tab:
Prevention in Heart or Kidney-Pancreas Transplant:
Usual: 900mg (two 450mg tabs) qd starting w/in 10 days of transplant until 100 days post-transplant
Prevention in Kidney Transplant:
Usual: 900mg qd starting w/in 10 days of transplant until 200 days post-transplant

PEDIATRIC DOSAGE
Cytomegalovirus Disease
Tab/Sol:
Once daily dosage is based on BSA and CrCl derived from a modified Schwartz formula; refer to PI
Prevention in Kidney Transplant:
4 Months-16 Years:
Start qd dose (7 x BSA x CrCl) w/in 10 days of transplant until 200 days post-transplant
Prevention in Heart Transplant:
1 Month-16 Years:
Start qd dose (7 x BSA x CrCl) w/in 10 days of transplant until 100 days post-transplant

---

DOSING CONSIDERATIONS
Renal Impairment
Dosing for Adult Patients:
CrCl 40-59mL/min:
Induction: 450mg bid
Maint/Prevention: 450mg qd

CrCl 25-39mL/min:
Induction: 450mg qd
Maint/Prevention: 450mg every 2 days

CrCl 10-24mL/min:
Induction: 450mg every 2 days
Maint/Prevention: 450mg 2X/week

CrCl <10mL/min (on Hemodialysis):
Induction: Not recommended for use
Maint/Prevention: Not recommended for use
Elderly
Start at lower end of dosing range

ADMINISTRATION
Oral route
Take w/ food
Tab
Do not break or crush

Handling
Avoid direct skin or mucous membrane contact w/ broken or crushed tabs, the powder for oral sol, or the constituted oral sol; if contact occurs, wash thoroughly w/ soap and water, and rinse eyes thoroughly w/ plain water

STORAGE
Tab/Dry Powder: 25°C (77°F); excursions permitted to 15-30°C (59-86°F). Constituted Sol: 2-8°C (36-46°F) for no longer than 49 days. Do not freeze.

HOW SUPPLIED
Sol: 50mg/mL [88mL deliverable volume]; **Tab:** 450mg

CONTRAINDICATIONS
Clinically significant hypersensitivity reaction (eg, anaphylaxis) to valganciclovir, ganciclovir, or any component of the formulation.

WARNINGS/PRECAUTIONS
Avoid if ANC <500 cells/μL, platelet count <25,000/μL, or Hgb <8g/dL. Cytopenia may occur and may worsen w/ continued dosing; caution w/ preexisting cytopenias. May cause suppression of fertility in females. Avoid pregnancy in female patients and in females w/ male partners taking the drug. Acute renal failure may occur in elderly and patients w/o adequate hydration; maintain adequate hydration in all patients.

ADVERSE REACTIONS
Hematologic toxicity, diarrhea, N/V, pyrexia, tremor, HTN, URTI, UTI, graft rejection, headache.

DRUG INTERACTIONS
May increase levels of mycophenolate mofetil metabolites (w/ renal impairment), zidovudine, and didanosine (monitor for toxicity). Probenecid (monitor for toxicity) and mycophenolate mofetil (w/ renal impairment) may increase levels. Zidovudine and didanosine may decrease levels. Caution w/ nephrotoxic drugs, myelosuppressive drugs, or irradiation.

PREGNANCY AND LACTATION
Pregnancy: Ganciclovir caused maternal and fetal toxicity and embryo-fetal mortality in pregnant mice and rabbits as well as teratogenicity in rabbits at exposures greater than human exposure. Advise pregnant woman of the potential risk to the fetus.
Lactation: Breastfeeding is not recommended during treatment because of the potential for serious adverse events in nursing infants and because of the potential for transmission of HIV.
Reproductive Potential: Females of reproductive potential should use effective contraception during treatment and for at least 30 days following treatment. Males should be advised to practice barrier contraception during and for at least 90 days following treatment. Temporary or permanent female and male infertility may occur.

MECHANISM OF ACTION
Synthetic guanine derivative nucleoside analogue; inhibits viral DNA polymerase synthesis, resulting in inhibition of human CMV replication.

PHARMACOKINETICS
Absorption: (Tab) Ganciclovir: Absolute bioavailability (59.4%); C_{max}=5.61mcg/mL; T_{max}=1-3 hrs; AUC=29.1mcg•h/mL. **Distribution:** Ganciclovir: V_d=0.703L/kg (IV); plasma protein binding (1-2%). **Metabolism:** Intestinal wall, liver; valganciclovir (prodrug) hydrolyzed to ganciclovir. **Elimination:** Ganciclovir: Renal; $T_{1/2}$=4.08 hrs (Tab). Refer to PI for different parameters.

PATIENT CONSIDERATIONS
Assessment: Assess for renal impairment, preexisting cytopenia, prior/current irradiation, hydration status, pregnancy/nursing status, and possible drug interactions. Obtain baseline ANC, platelet count, and Hgb.

Monitoring: Monitor for signs/symptoms of hematologic toxicity, infertility, renal dysfunction, and other adverse reactions. Monitor CBC w/ differential and platelet counts frequently. Monitor SrCr or CrCl regularly. Perform ophthalmologic exams at a minimum of every 4-6 weeks during therapy.

Counseling: Inform that drug may cause granulocytopenia (neutropenia), anemia, thrombocytopenia, and elevated creatinine levels; dose modification or discontinuation of dosing may be required. Advise that CBC, platelet counts, and creatinine levels should be performed frequently during therapy. Advise females of reproductive potential to use effective contraception during and for at least 30 days following treatment, and advise males to practice barrier contraception during and for at least 90 days following treatment. Advise that drug is considered a potential carcinogen. Inform patients that tasks requiring alertness may be affected, including the ability to drive and operate machinery; convulsions, sedation, dizziness, ataxia, and/or confusion have been reported w/ the use of the drug. Inform that the drug is not a cure for CMV retinitis and patients may continue to experience progression of retinitis during or following treatment. Advise to have ophthalmologic follow-up exams at a minimum of every 4-6 weeks while being treated. Inform adult patients that they should use tabs, not oral sol.

VALSTAR — valrubicin　　　Rx

Class: Anthracycline

ADULT DOSAGE	PEDIATRIC DOSAGE
BCG-Refractory Bladder Carcinoma in Situ	Pediatric use may not have been established
In patients for whom immediate cystectomy would be associated w/ unacceptable morbidity/mortality	
800mg once a week for 6 weeks	
Delay administration at least 2 weeks after transurethral resection and/or fulguration	

ADMINISTRATION

Intravesical route

- Do not mix w/ other drugs.
- Prepare and store in glass, polypropylene, or polyolefin containers and tubing; use non-di(2-ethylhexyl) phthalate containing administration sets (eg, those that are polyethylene-lined).

Instillation Instructions
1. Allow four 5mL vials to warm slowly to room temperature; do not heat.
2. Withdraw 20mL from the 4 vials and dilute w/ 55mL of 0.9% NaCl inj, providing 75mL of a diluted sol; stable for 12 hrs at ≤25°C (77°F).
3. Insert a urethral catheter into the patient's bladder, drain the bladder, and slowly instill the diluted 75mL sol via gravity flow over several min.
4. Withdraw the catheter; the patient should retain the drug for 2 hrs before voiding.
5. At the end of 2 hrs, patient should void (some patients will be unable to retain the drug for the full 2 hrs).
6. Patients should maintain adequate hydration following treatment.

STORAGE
Unopened Vials: 2-8°C (36-46°F). Do not heat or freeze.

HOW SUPPLIED
Sol: 40mg/mL [5mL]

CONTRAINDICATIONS
Perforated bladder, known hypersensitivity to anthracyclines or polyoxyl castor oil, active UTI, small bladder capacity and unable to tolerate a 75mL instillation.

WARNINGS/PRECAUTIONS
Risk of metastatic bladder cancer w/ delayed cystectomy; reconsider cystectomy if there is not a complete response of carcinoma in situ (CIS) to treatment after 3 months or if CIS recurs. Avoid in patients w/ a perforated bladder or in whom the integrity of the bladder mucosa has been compromised; delay administration until bladder integrity has been restored. Evaluate the status of the bladder before instillation in patients undergoing transurethral resection of the bladder (TURB); delay administration at least two weeks after transurethral resection and/ or fulguration. Caution w/ severe irritable bladder symptoms. Bladder spasm and spontaneous discharge of the intravesical instillate may occur; clamping of urinary catheter is not advised. May cause fetal harm.

ADVERSE REACTIONS
Urinary frequency, dysuria, urinary urgency, bladder spasm, hematuria, bladder pain, urinary incontinence, cystitis, UTI, nocturia, local burning symptoms, abdominal pain, nausea.

PREGNANCY AND LACTATION
Pregnancy: May cause fetal harm.
Lactation: Lactating women should not breastfeed during treatment and for 2 weeks after the final dose.
Reproduction Potential: Females of reproductive potential should use effective contraception during treatment and for 6 months after the final dose. Men w/ female partners of reproductive potential should use effective contraception during treatment and for 3 months following the final dose. May impair fertility in males of reproductive potential.

MECHANISM OF ACTION
Anthracycline; inhibits the incorporation of nucleosides into nucleic acids, causing extensive chromosomal damage, and arrests the cell cycle in G_2. Interferes w/ the normal DNA breaking-sealing action of DNA topoisomerase II.

PHARMACOKINETICS
Absorption: $AUC_{0-6\ hrs}$=78nmol/L•hr (900mg). **Metabolism:** N-trifluoroacetyladriamycin and N-trifluoroacetyladriamycinol (major metabolites). **Elimination:** Urine (98.6%, 0.4% metabolites).

PATIENT CONSIDERATIONS
Assessment: Assess for hypersensitivity to anthracyclines or polyoxyl castor oil, UTI, small bladder capacity and unable to tolerate a 75mL instillation, integrity of the bladder, perforated bladder, severe irritable bladder symptoms, and pregnancy/nursing status.

Monitoring: Monitor for bladder spasm, spontaneous discharge of the intravesical instillate, disease recurrence or progression, and other adverse reactions.

Counseling: Counsel about risks and benefits of therapy. Advise that delaying cystectomy could lead to development of metastatic bladder cancer. Inform that red-tinged urine is typical for the first 24 hrs following administration; advise to report prolonged irritable bladder symptoms or prolonged passage of red-colored urine to physician immediately. Instruct to maintain adequate hydration following treatment. Advise females of reproductive potential of the potential risk to a

---

fetus and to use effective contraception during treatment and for 6 months after the last dose. Instruct females to inform their physician of a known or suspected pregnancy. Advise male patients w/ female partners of reproductive potential to use effective contraception during treatment and for 3 months after the last dose. Counsel females not to breastfeed during treatment and for 2 weeks after the last dose.

VANTAS — histrelin acetate　　　Rx

Class: Synthetic gonadotropin-releasing hormone (GnRH) analogue

ADULT DOSAGE	PEDIATRIC DOSAGE
Advanced Prostate Cancer	Pediatric use may not have been established
Palliative Treatment:	
1 implant for 12 months; implant is inserted SQ in the inner aspect of the upper arm	
Remove after 12 months of therapy; at the time an implant is removed, another implant may be inserted to continue therapy	

ADMINISTRATION
SQ route
Refer to PI for recommended procedure for implant insertion and removal.

STORAGE
Implant: 2-8°C (36-46°F); excursions permitted to 25°C (77°F) for 7 days. Refrigerate until the day of insertion. Do not open vial until just before the time of insertion. Protect from light. Do not freeze. Implantation Kit: 20-25°C (68-77°F).

HOW SUPPLIED
Implant: 50mg

CONTRAINDICATIONS
Hypersensitivity to GnRH, GnRH agonist analogs, or any of the components in this product; women who are or may become pregnant.

WARNINGS/PRECAUTIONS
Causes a transient increase in serum concentrations of testosterone during the 1st week of treatment; may experience worsening of symptoms or onset of new symptoms (eg, bone pain, neuropathy, hematuria, ureteral or bladder outlet obstruction). Spinal cord compression, which may result in paralysis, and ureteral obstruction, which may cause renal impairment, reported; closely observe patients w/ metastatic vertebral lesions and/or w/ urinary tract obstruction during the 1st few weeks of therapy. Difficulty in locating or removing implant reported; carefully adhere to recommended procedure of implant insertion/ removal to minimize the potential for complications and for implant expulsion. Hyperglycemia and an increased risk of developing diabetes reported; monitor blood glucose and/or HbA1c periodically. Increased risk of developing MI, sudden cardiac death, and stroke reported; monitor for signs/symptoms of cardiovascular disease (CVD). Results of diagnostic tests of pituitary gonadotropic and gonadal functions conducted during and after therapy may be affected. May prolong QT/ QTc interval; caution w/ congenital long QT syndrome, CHF, frequent electrolyte abnormalities, and in patients taking drugs known to prolong the QT interval. Correct electrolyte abnormalities.

ADVERSE REACTIONS
Hot flashes, fatigue, implant-site reaction (bruising/pain/soreness/tenderness), testicular atrophy, renal impairment, gynecomastia, constipation, erectile dysfunction.

PREGNANCY AND LACTATION
Category X, not for use in nursing.

MECHANISM OF ACTION
Synthetic gonadotropin-releasing hormone analog; acts as a potent inhibitor of gonadotropin secretion when given continuously in therapeutic doses. Desensitizes responsiveness of pituitary gonadotropin, causing a reduction in testicular steroidogenesis.

PHARMACOKINETICS
Absorption: C_{max}=1.1ng/mL; T_{max}=12 hrs (median). **Distribution:** V_d=58.4L (500mcg SQ bolus). **Metabolism:** C-terminal dealkylation and hydrolysis. **Elimination:** $T_{1/2}$=3.92 hrs (SQ bolus).

PATIENT CONSIDERATIONS
Assessment: Assess for hypersensitivity to drug, metastatic vertebral lesions, urinary tract obstruction, and risk for diabetes and CVD.

Monitoring: Monitor for worsening or onset of new symptoms, signs/symptoms of spinal cord compression, ureteral obstruction, CVD, and other adverse reactions. Monitor response by measuring serum concentrations of testosterone and prostate-specific antigen periodically, especially if the anticipated clinical or biochemical response to treatment has not been achieved. Monitor blood glucose and/or HbA1c periodically. Consider periodic monitoring of ECG and electrolytes.

Counseling: Inform of risks and benefits of therapy. Instruct to refrain from wetting the inserted arm for 24 hrs and from heavy lifting or strenuous exertion of the arm for 7 days after implant insertion. Instruct to contact physician if implant was expelled from the body or if any adverse reactions develop.

VARITHENA — polidocanol   Rx

Class: Sclerosing agent

ADULT DOSAGE
Varicose Veins

Incompetent Great Saphenous Veins, Accessory Saphenous Veins, and Visible Varicosities of the Great Saphenous Vein System Above and Below the Knee:
Up to 5mL/inj
Max: 15mL/session

May repeat treatment if the size and extent of the veins to be treated require >15mL; separate treatment sessions by ≥5 days

PEDIATRIC DOSAGE
Pediatric use may not have been established

ADMINISTRATION
IV route; administer via a single cannula into the lumen of the target incompetent trunk veins or by direct inj into varicosities.

Activate using the oxygen canister and polidocanol canister. Once a transfer unit is in place, foam can be generated and transferred to a syringe. Discard syringe contents if there are any visible bubbles. Administer injectable foam w/in 75 sec of extraction from the canister. Use a new syringe after each inj, and use a new transfer unit for each treatment session.

Local anesthetic may be administered prior to cannula insertion.

Cannulate the vein using ultrasound guidance to confirm venous access.

Inject slowly (1mL/sec in the great saphenous vein [GSV] and 0.5mL/sec in accessory veins or varicosities) while monitoring using ultrasound. Confirm venospasm of treated vein using ultrasound.

When treating proximal GSV, stop inj when polidocanol is 3-5cm distal to the saphenofemoral junction.

Apply compression bandaging and stockings and have patient walk for ≥10 min, while being monitored. Maintain compression for 2 weeks after treatment.

STORAGE
20-25°C (68-77°F); excursions permitted between 15-30°C (59-86°F). Do not shake canisters and do not refrigerate or freeze. Store in a well-ventilated place and away from sources of heat, including strong light conditions. **Pressurized Oxygen:** Store away from combustible materials. **Activated Canister:** Use w/in 7 days. Store upright, w/ the Transfer Unit attached, under the same temperature conditions as the convenience box.

HOW SUPPLIED
Inj: 180mg/18mL

CONTRAINDICATIONS
Known allergy to polidocanol, acute thromboembolic disease.

WARNINGS/PRECAUTIONS
Physicians administering the drug must be experienced w/ venous procedures and be trained in the administration of the drug. Retained coagulum may be removed by aspiration (microthrombectomy) to improve comfort and reduce skin staining. Severe allergic reactions, including anaphylactic reactions, reported; monitor for at least 10 min following inj and be prepared to treat anaphylaxis appropriately. Intra-arterial inj or extravasation of drug may cause severe necrosis, ischemia, or gangrene; increased risk for tissue ischemia in patients w/ underlying arterial disease (eg, marked peripheral arteriosclerosis or thromboangiitis obliterans [Buerger's disease]). Consult a vascular surgeon immediately if intra-arterial inj occurs. May cause venous thrombosis; increased risk in patients w/ reduced mobility, history of deep vein thrombosis (DVT) or pulmonary embolism, recent (w/in 3 months) major surgery, or prolonged hospitalization, or who are pregnant. Follow administration instructions closely and monitor for signs of venous thrombosis after treatment. Avoid contact w/ eyes.

ADVERSE REACTIONS
Pain/discomfort in extremity, infusion-site thrombosis (retained coagulum), inj-site hematoma/pain, thrombophlebitis superficial, extravasation.

PREGNANCY AND LACTATION
Pregnancy: Category C. Do not use during pregnancy.
Lactation: Not for use in nursing.

MECHANISM OF ACTION
Sclerosing agent; foam displaces blood from the vein to be treated, then polidocanol scleroses the endothelium. The hydrophobic pole of the polidocanol molecule attaches to the lipid cell membrane of the venous endothelium, resulting in disruption of the osmotic barrier, destruction of the venous endothelium, and vasospasm. Following exposure to polidocanol, the interior surface of the vein becomes thrombogenic, which leads to thrombus formation and venous occlusion.

PHARMACOKINETICS
Absorption: T_{max}=15 min (1st inj), 5 min (2nd inj). **Distribution:** V_d=35-82L.
Elimination: $T_{1/2}$=102-153 min.

PATIENT CONSIDERATIONS
Assessment: Assess for known allergy to polidocanol, acute thromboembolic disease, arterial disease, risk for venous thrombosis, and pregnancy/nursing status.
Monitoring: Monitor for anaphylactic/allergic reactions, tissue ischemia/necrosis, venous thrombosis, and other adverse reactions.

Counseling: Advise to keep post-treatment bandages dry and in place for 48 hrs and to wear thigh- or knee-high compression stockings on the treated legs continuously for 2 weeks. Advise to walk for at least 10 min immediately after the procedure and daily for the next month. Advise to avoid heavy exercise for 1 week and extended periods of inactivity for 1 month, following treatment.

VARIZIG — varicella zoster immune globulin (human)   Rx

Class: Immune globulin

ADULT DOSAGE
Postexposure Prophylaxis of Varicella

Reduces the severity of varicella in high-risk individuals

≥40.1kg: 625 IU or 6mL
Max: (>40kg) 625 IU

Refer to pediatric dosing section for patients weighing ≤40kg
Consider a 2nd full dose of treatment for high-risk patients who have additional exposures to varicella >3 weeks after initial administration

PEDIATRIC DOSAGE
Postexposure Prophylaxis of Varicella

Reduces the severity of varicella in high-risk individuals

≤2kg: 62.5 IU or 0.6mL
2.1-10kg: 125 IU or 1.2mL
10.1-20kg: 250 IU or 2.4mL
20.1-30kg: 375 IU or 3.6mL
30.1-40kg: 500 IU or 4.8mL
≥40.1kg: 625 IU or 6mL

Minimum: (<2kg) 62.5 IU
Max: (>40kg) 625 IU

Consider a 2nd full dose of treatment for high-risk patients who have additional exposures to varicella >3 weeks after initial administration

ADMINISTRATION
IM route

Administer as soon as possible following varicella zoster virus exposure, ideally w/in 96 hrs
Divide the IM dose and administer in ≥2 inj sites, depending on patient size
Do not exceed 3mL/inj site
Inject into the deltoid muscle or the anterolateral aspects of the upper thigh
Due to the risk of sciatic nerve injury, do not use the gluteal region as a routine inj site
If the gluteal region is used, only use the upper, outer quadrant

STORAGE
2-8°C (36-46°F). Do not freeze.

HOW SUPPLIED
Inj: ≥125 IU/1.2mL

CONTRAINDICATIONS
Anaphylactic or severe systemic (hypersensitivity) reactions to human immune globulin preparations, IgA-deficient patients w/ antibodies against IgA and a history of hypersensitivity.

WARNINGS/PRECAUTIONS
Thrombotic events may occur during or following treatment; caution w/ a history of atherosclerosis, multiple cardiovascular (CV) risk factors, advanced age, impaired cardiac output, coagulation disorders, prolonged periods of immobilization, and/or known/suspected hyperviscosity. Consider baseline assessment of blood viscosity in patients at risk for hyperviscosity including those w/ cryoglobulins, fasting chylomicronemia/markedly high triacylglycerols (TGs), or monoclonal gammopathies. In patients who have severe thrombocytopenia or any coagulation disorder that would contraindicate IM inj, only administer if expected benefits outweigh potential risks. Severe hypersensitivity reactions may occur; d/c immediately and provide appropriate treatment if hypersensitivity occurs. Administer in a setting w/ appropriate equipment, medication, and personnel trained in the management of hypersensitivity, anaphylaxis, and shock. Made from human plasma; may carry a risk of transmitting infectious agents (eg, viruses, variant Creutzfeldt-Jakob disease agent and Creutzfeldt-Jakob disease agent). Caution in elderly who are judged to be at increased risk of thrombotic events.

ADVERSE REACTIONS
Pyrexia, N/V, inj-site pain, headache, rash.

DRUG INTERACTIONS
Passive transfer of antibodies may impair the efficacy of live attenuated virus vaccines (eg, measles, rubella, mumps, and varicella). Defer vaccination w/ live virus vaccines until approx 3 months after administration.

PREGNANCY AND LACTATION
Category C, caution in nursing.

MECHANISM OF ACTION
Immune globulin; provides passive immunization for non-immune individuals exposed to varicella zoster virus, reducing the severity of varicella infections.

PHARMACOKINETICS
Absorption: AUC_{0-28}=2472 mIU•day/mL; AUC_{0-84}=4087 mIU•day/mL; C_{max}=136 mIU/mL; T_{max}=4.5 days. **Elimination:** $T_{1/2}$=26.2 days.

PATIENT CONSIDERATIONS
Assessment: Assess for IgA-deficient patients w/ antibodies against IgA, hypersensitivity to human immune globulin preparations, severe thrombocytopenia or any coagulation disorder, risk factors for thrombotic events (eg, history of atherosclerosis, multiple CV risk factors, advanced age, impaired cardiac output, prolonged periods of immobilization, known/suspected hyperviscosity), any other conditions where treatment is contraindicated or

cautioned, pregnancy/nursing status, and possible drug interactions. Consider baseline assessment of blood viscosity in patients at risk for hyperviscosity.

Monitoring: Monitor for thrombotic events, severe hypersensitivity reactions, infection, and other adverse reactions.

Counseling: Inform about the risks and benefits of treatment. Advise that treatment is intended to reduce the severity of chickenpox infections and to consult physician if signs and symptoms of varicella develop. Inform that drug may contain infectious agents such as viruses that may cause disease. Inform that persons known to have severe, potentially life-threatening reactions to human immune globulin products should not receive the drug. Instruct to notify physician immediately if any signs or symptoms of an allergic reaction develop. Inform that drug can interfere w/ immune response to live virus vaccines (eg, measles, mumps, rubella, and varicella); instruct patients to notify their immunizing physician of recent therapy.

VECTIBIX — panitumumab   Rx

Class: Monoclonal antibody/EGFR blocker

> Dermatologic toxicities reported and were severe (NCI-CTC ≥Grade 3) in patients receiving drug monotherapy.

ADULT DOSAGE	**PEDIATRIC DOSAGE**
Metastatic Colorectal Cancer	Pediatric use may not have been established
Wild-Type *KRAS* (Exon 2 in Codons 12 or 13):	
As 1st line therapy in combination w/ FOLFOX, and as monotherapy following disease progression after prior treatment w/ fluoropyrimidine-, oxaliplatin-, and irinotecan-containing chemotherapy	
Usual: 6mg/kg IV infusion over 60 min, every 14 days	
If the 1st infusion is tolerated, administer subsequent infusions over 30-60 min	
Administer doses >1000mg over 90 min	

DOSING CONSIDERATIONS

Adverse Reactions

Infusion Reactions:

Mild or Moderate (Grade 1 or 2): Reduce infusion rate by 50% for the duration of that infusion

Severe: Terminate infusion; permanently d/c therapy depending on severity and/or persistence of the reaction

Dermatologic Toxicity:

Grade 3 (NCI-CTC/CTCAE) Reaction:

1st Occurrence: Withhold 1-2 doses; if reaction improves to <Grade 3, reinitiate at the original dose

2nd Occurrence: Withhold 1-2 doses; if reaction improves to <Grade 3, reinitiate at 80% of the original dose

3rd Occurrence: Withhold 1-2 doses; if reaction improves to <Grade 3, reinitiate at 60% of the original dose

4th Occurrence: Permanently d/c therapy

Grade 3 (NCI-CTC/CTCAE) Reaction Not Recovering After Withholding 1 or 2 Doses/Grade 4 Reaction: Permanently d/c therapy

ADMINISTRATION

IV infusion

Do not administer as IV push or bolus

Do not mix w/, or administer as an infusion w/, other medicinal products

Do not add other medications to sol containing panitumumab

Preparation

1. Withdraw the necessary amount of panitumumab for a dose of 6mg/kg
2. Dilute to a total volume of 100mL w/ 0.9% NaCl inj; doses >1000mg should be diluted to 150mL w/ 0.9% NaCl inj
3. Do not exceed a final concentration of 10mg/mL
4. Mix diluted sol by gentle inversion; do not shake

Administration

1. Administer using a low-protein-binding 0.2μm or 0.22μm in-line filter
2. Administer via infusion pump; flush line before and after administration w/ 0.9% NaCl inj
3. Infuse doses ≤1000mg over 60 min through a peripheral IV line or indwelling IV catheter; if 1st infusion is tolerated, administer subsequent infusions over 30-60 min
4. Administer doses >1000mg over 90 min
5. Discard any unused portion remaining in the vial

Use diluted sol w/in 6 hrs of preparation if stored at room temperature, or w/in 24 hrs of dilution if stored at 2-8°C (36-46°F)

STORAGE

2-8°C (36-46°F). Protect from direct sunlight. Do not freeze.

HOW SUPPLIED

Inj: 20mg/mL [5mL, 10mL, 20mL]

WARNINGS/PRECAUTIONS

Not indicated for treatment of patients w/ *RAS*-mutant mCRC or for whom *RAS* mutation status is unknown. Monitor for the development of inflammatory or infectious sequelae in patients who develop dermatologic or soft tissue toxicities. Life-threatening and fatal infectious complications (eg, necrotizing fasciitis, abscesses, sepsis) and bullous mucocutaneous disease w/ blisters, erosions, and skin sloughing observed. Withhold or d/c therapy for dermatologic or soft tissue toxicity associated w/ severe or life-threatening inflammatory or infectious complications. Increased tumor progression/mortality, or lack of benefit reported in patients w/ *RAS*-mutant mCRC. Hypomagnesemia and other electrolyte disturbances reported (eg, hypokalemia); replete Mg^{2+} and other electrolytes as appropriate. Severe diarrhea and dehydration, leading to acute renal failure and other complications observed in combination w/ chemotherapy. Fatal and nonfatal pulmonary fibrosis and interstitial lung disease (ILD) reported; interrupt therapy for acute onset or worsening of pulmonary symptoms, and d/c if ILD is confirmed. Exposure to sunlight may exacerbate dermatologic toxicity; limit sun exposure during therapy. Keratitis and ulcerative keratitis reported; interrupt or d/c therapy for acute or worsening keratitis.

ADVERSE REACTIONS

Skin disorders (eg, erythema, acneiform dermatitis, pruritus, exfoliation, rash), anorexia, hypomagnesemia, paronychia, fatigue, stomatitis, N/V, diarrhea, dyspnea, cough.

DRUG INTERACTIONS

Increased mortality and toxicity in combination w/ bevacizumab and chemotherapy.

PREGNANCY AND LACTATION

Category C, not for use in nursing.

MECHANISM OF ACTION

IgG2 kappa monoclonal antibody/EGFR blocker; binds specifically to EGFR on both normal and tumor cells, and competitively inhibits binding of ligands for EGFR.

PHARMACOKINETICS

Absorption: C_{max}=213mcg/mL, AUC_{0-tau}=1306mcg•day/mL. **Elimination:** $T_{1/2}$=7.5 days.

PATIENT CONSIDERATIONS

Assessment: Assess for presence or history of interstitial pneumonitis or pulmonary fibrosis, pregnancy/nursing status, and for possible drug interactions. Obtain serum electrolyte levels (Mg^{2+}, K^+, Ca^{2+}). Assess *RAS*-mutational status in colorectal tumors and confirm the absence of a *RAS* mutation.

Monitoring: Monitor for signs/symptoms of dermatologic and soft tissue toxicities, infusion reactions, ILD, pulmonary fibrosis, keratitis/ulcerative keratitis, and other adverse reactions. Monitor electrolytes (eg, hypomagnesemia, hypocalcemia) periodically during and for up to 8 weeks after completion of therapy.

Counseling: Advise to contact physician if signs/symptoms of an infusion reaction, persistent/recurrent coughing, wheezing, dyspnea, new onset facial swelling, diarrhea, dehydration, or skin/ocular changes develop. Instruct to notify physician if pregnant or nursing. Advise of the need for adequate contraception in both males and females during and for 6 months after the last dose of therapy. Instruct to limit sun exposure (eg, use sunscreen, wear hats) during and for 2 months after the last dose of therapy.

VELCADE — bortezomib   Rx

Class: Proteasome inhibitor

ADULT DOSAGE	**PEDIATRIC DOSAGE**
Multiple Myeloma	Pediatric use may not have been established
Initial: 1.3mg/m² IV bolus (3-5 sec) at a concentration of 1mg/mL, or SQ at a concentration of 2.5mg/mL	
Previously Untreated Multiple Myeloma:	
Administer in combination w/ oral melphalan and oral prednisone for nine 6-week cycles	
Cycles 1-4: Administer twice weekly (Days 1, 4, 8, 11, 22, 25, 29, and 32)	
Cycles 5-9: Administer once weekly (Days 1, 8, 22, and 29)	
Relapsed Multiple Myeloma:	
Administer twice weekly for 2 weeks (Days 1, 4, 8, and 11), followed by 10-day rest period (Days 12-21)	
For extended therapy of >8 cycles, may administer on standard schedule or on a maint schedule of once weekly for 4 weeks (Days 1, 8, 15, and 22), followed by 13-day rest period (Days 23-35)	
Retreatment of Relapsed Multiple Myeloma:	
May start at the last tolerated dose. Administer twice weekly (Days 1, 4, 8, and 11) every 3 weeks	
Max: 8 cycles	

May administer either as a single agent or in combination w/ dexamethasone

At least 72 hrs should elapse between consecutive doses

Mantle Cell Lymphoma

Initial: 1.3mg/m^2 IV bolus (3-5 sec) at a concentration of 1mg/mL, or SQ at a concentration of 2.5mg/mL

Previously Untreated Mantle Cell Lymphoma:
Administer in combination w/ IV rituximab, cyclophosphamide, doxorubicin, and oral prednisone (VcR-CAP) for six 3-week cycles
Administer bortezomib 1st followed by rituximab
Administer twice weekly for 2 weeks (Days 1, 4, 8, and 11), followed by a 10-day rest period on Days 12-21
For patients w/ a response 1st documented at Cycle 6, two additional VcR-CAP cycles are recommended

Relapsed Mantle Cell Lymphoma:
Administer twice weekly for 2 weeks (Days 1, 4, 8, and 11), followed by 10-day rest period (Days 12-21)
For extended therapy of >8 cycles, may administer on standard schedule

At least 72 hrs should elapse between consecutive doses

DOSING CONSIDERATIONS

Hepatic Impairment
Moderate (Bilirubin >1.5-3X ULN)-Severe (Bilirubin >3X ULN): Reduce to 0.7mg/m^2 in the 1st cycle
Consider escalation to 1.0mg/m^2 or further reduction to 0.5mg/m^2 in subsequent cycles based on tolerability

Adverse Reactions
Combination Bortezomib, Melphalan, and Prednisone:
Prolonged Grade 4 Neutropenia or Thrombocytopenia/Thrombocytopenia w/ Bleeding Observed in Previous Cycle: Consider reduction of melphalan dose by 25% in next cycle
Platelets <30 x 10^9/L or ANC <0.75 x 10^9/L on a Bortezomib Dosing Day (Other Than Day 1): Withhold bortezomib dose
Several Bortezomib Doses in Consecutive Cycles Withheld Due to Toxicity:
Reduce dose by 1 dose level (from 1.3mg/m^2 to 1mg/m^2, or from 1mg/m^2 to 0.7mg/m^2)
≥Grade 3 Nonhematological Toxicities:
Withhold therapy until symptoms resolve to Grade 1 or baseline; may be reinitiated w/ 1 dose level reduction (from 1.3mg/m^2 to 1mg/m^2, or from 1mg/m^2 to 0.7mg/m^2)

Days 4, 8, and 11 During Cycles of Combination Bortezomib, Rituximab, Cyclophosphamide, Doxorubicin, and Prednisone Therapy:
≥Grade 3 Neutropenia, or Platelet <25 x 10^9/L:
Withhold therapy for up to 2 weeks until the patient has an ANC ≥0.75 x 10^9/L and platelets ≥25 x 10^9/L
If, after bortezomib has been withheld, the toxicity does not resolve, d/c
If toxicity resolves such that the patient has an ANC ≥0.75 x 10^9/L and platelets ≥25 x 10^9/L, dose should be reduced by 1 dose level (from 1.3mg/m^2 to 1mg/m^2, or from 1mg/m^2 to 0.7mg/m^2)
≥Grade 3 Nonhematological Toxicities:
Withhold therapy until symptoms of the toxicity have resolved to Grade 2 or better; may reinitiate w/ 1 dose level reduction (from 1.3mg/m^2 to 1mg/m^2, or from 1mg/m^2 to 0.7mg/m^2)
Neuropathic Pain and/or Peripheral or Motor Neuropathy:
Grade 1 (Asymptomatic; Loss of Deep Tendon Reflexes or Paresthesia) w/o Pain or Loss of Function: No action
Grade 1 w/ Pain or Grade 2 (Moderate Symptoms; Limiting Instrumental Activities of Daily Living [ADL]): Reduce to 1mg/m^2
Grade 2 w/ Pain or Grade 3 (Severe Symptoms; Limiting Self Care ADL):
Withhold therapy until toxicity resolves, then reinitiate w/ a reduced dose at 0.7mg/m^2 once per week
Grade 4 (Life-Threatening Consequences; Urgent Intervention Indicated): D/C therapy

Refer to PI for further dosing guidelines

ADMINISTRATION
IV/SQ route

Reconstitution
Reconstitute only w/ 0.9% NaCl; should be administered w/in 8 hrs of preparation.
Different volumes of 0.9% NaCl are used to reconstitute the product for the different routes of administration.
Because each route of administration has a different reconstituted concentration, caution should be used when calculating the volume to be administered.
The reconstituted concentration for SQ administration is 2.5mg/mL when diluted w/ 1.4mL 0.9% NaCl.

The reconstituted concentration for IV administration is 1mg/mL when diluted w/ 3.5mL 0.9% NaCl.
Refer to PI for further reconstitution/preparation instructions.

STORAGE
25°C (77°F); excursions permitted to 15-30°C (59-86°F). Protect from light.
Reconstituted Sol: 25°C (77°F). May be stored in the original vial and/or the syringe prior to administration. May be stored for up to 8 hrs in a syringe; total storage time must not exceed 8 hrs when exposed to normal indoor lighting.

HOW SUPPLIED
Inj: 3.5mg

CONTRAINDICATIONS
Intrathecal administration, hypersensitivity (not including local reactions) to bortezomib, boron, or mannitol.

WARNINGS/PRECAUTIONS
Severe sensory and motor peripheral neuropathy reported; consider starting SQ therapy for patients w/ preexisting or at high risk of peripheral neuropathy. Hypotension reported. Acute development or exacerbation of CHF and new onset of decreased left ventricular ejection fraction (LVEF) reported. Isolated cases of QT interval prolongation reported. Acute respiratory distress syndrome (ARDS), acute diffuse infiltrative pulmonary disease of unknown etiology (eg, pneumonitis, interstitial pneumonia, lung infiltration), and pulmonary HTN reported; consider interrupting therapy until a prompt and comprehensive diagnostic evaluation is conducted if new or worsening cardiopulmonary symptoms develop. Posterior reversible encephalopathy syndrome (PRES) reported; d/c if PRES develops. May cause N/V, diarrhea, constipation, and ileus; antiemetic and antidiarrheal medications may be necessary. Administer fluid/electrolyte replacement therapy to prevent dehydration; interrupt for severe symptoms. Thrombocytopenia and neutropenia reported. GI and intracerebral hemorrhage occurred during thrombocytopenia; support w/ transfusions and supportive care. Tumor lysis syndrome reported. Acute liver failure reported in patients receiving multiple concomitant medications and w/ serious underlying medical conditions. Hepatic reactions, including hepatitis, increases in liver enzymes, and hyperbilirubinemia, reported; interrupt therapy to assess reversibility. Women of reproductive potential should avoid becoming pregnant while on therapy. Administer therapy after dialysis procedure. Consider retreatment in patients w/ multiple myeloma who had previously responded to treatment and have relapsed at least 6 months after completing prior therapy. Caution in elderly.

ADVERSE REACTIONS
Thrombocytopenia, neutropenia, N/V, peripheral neuropathy, diarrhea, anemia, constipation, pyrexia, anorexia, paresthesia, headache, dyspnea, leukopenia, fatigue.

DRUG INTERACTIONS
Avoid w/ St. John's wort. Efficacy may be reduced w/ strong CYP3A4 inducers (eg, rifampin); concomitant use is not recommended. Oral antidiabetic agents may require dosage adjustment. Ketoconazole may increase exposure; monitor for signs of bortezomib toxicity and consider bortezomib dose reduction when given w/ strong CYP3A4 inhibitors (eg, ketoconazole, ritonavir). May increase exposure to drugs that are CYP2C19 substrates.

PREGNANCY AND LACTATION
Pregnancy: Category D.
Lactation: Not for use in nursing.

MECHANISM OF ACTION
Proteasome inhibitor; reversibly inhibits chymotrypsin-like activity of the 26S proteasome in cells.

PHARMACOKINETICS
Absorption: Administration via different routes resulted in different pharmacokinetic parameters. **Distribution:** V_d=498-1884L/m^2; plasma protein binding (83%). **Metabolism:** Oxidation via CYP3A4, 2C19, 1A2; 2D6, 2C9 (minor); deboronation (major pathway). **Elimination:** (IV) $T_{1/2}$ =40-193 hrs (1mg/m^2), 76-108 hrs (1.3mg/m^2).

PATIENT CONSIDERATIONS

Assessment: Assess for peripheral neuropathy, history of syncope, dehydration, risk factors for or existing heart disease, diabetes mellitus, hepatic/renal impairment, any conditions where treatment is contraindicated or cautioned, pregnancy/nursing status, and possible drug interactions. Obtain baseline BP, CBCs, and then platelet count prior to each dose.

Monitoring: Monitor for signs/symptoms of new/worsening peripheral neuropathy, hypotension, CHF, decreased LVEF, new or worsening cardiopulmonary symptoms, PRES, N/V, diarrhea, constipation, ileus, tumor lysis syndrome, hepatic toxicity, and other adverse reactions. Closely monitor patients w/ risk factors for or existing heart disease. Monitor LFTs. Monitor CBCs and blood glucose levels (in diabetics) frequently.

Counseling: Inform that therapy may cause fatigue, dizziness, syncope, orthostatic/postural hypotension; advise not to drive or operate heavy machinery if any of these symptoms develop. Advise how to avoid dehydration. Instruct to seek medical advice if symptoms of dizziness, lightheadedness, fainting spells, or muscle cramps are experienced. Advise to use effective contraceptive measures to prevent pregnancy and instruct to inform physician immediately if patient becomes pregnant. Advise that treatment should not be received while pregnant/breastfeeding. Advise to check blood sugar frequently if taking oral antidiabetic medications and instruct to notify physician if any changes in blood sugar levels occur. Instruct to contact physician if symptoms of new/worsening peripheral neuropathy, PRES or progressive multifocal leukoencephalopathy, cardiac/respiratory/hepatic toxicity, dermal reactions, an increase in BP, bleeding, fever, constipation, or decreased appetite develops.

VELETRI — epoprostenol

Rx

Class: Prostacyclin analogue

ADULT DOSAGE	PEDIATRIC DOSAGE
Pulmonary Arterial Hypertension	Pediatric use may not have been established
Improvement of Exercise Capacity (WHO Group I):	
Initial: 2ng/kg/min IV chronic infusion	
Titrate: Increase in increments of 2ng/kg/min every 15 min or longer until a tolerance limit to the drug is established or further increases in the infusion rate are not clinically warranted. Use a lower dose if initial infusion rate is not tolerated	
If symptoms of PAH persist or recur, adjust the infusion by 1-2ng/kg/min increments at intervals of at least 15 min	

DOSING CONSIDERATIONS
Elderly
Start at lower end of dosing range

Adverse Reactions
Dose-Limiting Pharmacological Effects:
Decrease gradually in 2ng/kg/min decrements every 15 min or longer until effects resolve

Other Important Considerations
Taper doses after initiation of cardiopulmonary bypass in patients receiving lung transplants

ADMINISTRATION
IV route

Administer by continuous IV infusion via a central venous catheter using an ambulatory infusion pump; may administer peripherally during initiation of treatment
Reconstitute only ud using sterile water for inj or NaCl 0.9% inj
Do not dilute reconstituted sol or administer w/ other parenteral sol or medications; consider a multi-lumen catheter if other IV therapies are routinely administered
Refer to PI for further reconstitution, administration, and infusion rate instructions

STORAGE
20-25°C (68-77°F). Do not expose to direct sunlight. Refer to PI for storage of reconstituted sol.

HOW SUPPLIED
Inj: 0.5mg, 1.5mg

CONTRAINDICATIONS
Chronic use in patients w/ CHF due to severe left ventricular systolic dysfunction, chronic use in patients who develop pulmonary edema during dose initiation, known hypersensitivity to the drug or to structurally related compounds.

WARNINGS/PRECAUTIONS
Should be used only by clinicians experienced in the diagnosis and treatment of pulmonary HTN. Initiate therapy in a setting w/ adequate personnel and equipment for physiologic monitoring and emergency care. During dose initiation, asymptomatic increases in pulmonary artery pressure coincident w/ increases in cardiac output occurred rarely; consider dose reduction in such cases. Deliver continuously on an ambulatory basis through a permanent indwelling central venous catheter during chronic use. Unless contraindicated, administer anticoagulant therapy to reduce risk of pulmonary thromboembolism or systemic embolism through a patent foramen ovale. Abrupt withdrawal (including interruptions in drug delivery) or sudden large reductions in dosage may result in symptoms associated w/ rebound pulmonary HTN (eg, dyspnea, dizziness, asthenia); avoid abrupt withdrawal or sudden large reductions in infusion rates.

ADVERSE REACTIONS
Flushing, headache, N/V, hypotension, anxiety, nervousness, agitation, chest pain, abdominal pain, dizziness, bradycardia, anorexia, musculoskeletal pain, chills/fever/sepsis/flu-like symptoms, diarrhea.

DRUG INTERACTIONS
Additional BP reductions may occur w/ diuretics, antihypertensive agents, or other vasodilators. May increase risk of bleeding w/ other antiplatelet agents or anticoagulants. May elevate levels of digoxin.

PREGNANCY AND LACTATION
Category B, caution in nursing.

MECHANISM OF ACTION
Prostacyclin analogue; causes direct vasodilation of pulmonary and systemic arterial vascular beds and inhibition of platelet aggregation.

PHARMACOKINETICS
Metabolism: Hydrolysis, enzymatic degradation; 6-keto-PGF$_1$α and 6,15-diketo-13,14-dihydro-PGF$_1$α (primary metabolites). **Elimination:** Urine (82%), feces (4%); $T_{1/2}$≤6 min.

PATIENT CONSIDERATIONS
Assessment: Assess for hypersensitivity to drug, CHF due to severe left ventricular systolic dysfunction, pregnancy/nursing status, and possible drug interactions. Assess patient's capacity to accept and care for permanent IV catheter and infusion pump.

Monitoring: Monitor for signs of recurrence or worsening of pulmonary HTN, pulmonary edema, and other adverse reactions. Monitor standing and supine BP and HR closely for several hrs following dose adjustments.

Counseling: Counsel about proper reconstitution and administration of the drug; advise to adhere to sterile technique in preparing the drug and in the care of the catheter. Inform that therapy will likely be needed for prolonged periods, possibly yrs.

VELTASSA — patiromer

Rx

Class: Potassium binder

> Patiromer binds to many orally administered medications, which could decrease their absorption and reduce their effectiveness. Administer other oral medications at least 6 hrs before or 6 hrs after patiromer. If adequate dosing separation is not possible, choose patiromer or the other oral medication.

ADULT DOSAGE	PEDIATRIC DOSAGE
Hyperkalemia	Pediatric use may not have been established
Initial: 8.4g qd	
Titrate: May increase or decrease to reach desired serum K$^+$ concentration; may increase in increments of 8.4g based on serum K$^+$ levels at 1-week or longer intervals	
Max: 25.2g qd	

ADMINISTRATION
Oral route

Administer at least 6 hrs before or 6 hrs after other oral medications.
Take w/ food.
Do not heat (eg, microwave) or add to heated foods or liquids.
Do not take medication in its dry form.
Prepare each dose immediately prior to administration.

Preparation
1. Measure 1/3 cup of water. Pour half of the water into a glass, then add patiromer and stir.
2. Add the remaining half of the water and stir thoroughly; the powder will not dissolve and the mixture will look cloudy.
3. Add more water to the mixture as needed for desired consistency.
4. Drink mixture immediately; if powder remains after drinking, add more water, stir, and drink immediately. Repeat prn to ensure the entire dose is administered.

STORAGE
2-8°C (36-46°F). If stored at room temperature 25°C (77°F), use w/in 3 months of being taken out of the refrigerator. Avoid exposure to excessive heat >40°C (104°F).

HOW SUPPLIED
Powder: 8.4g, 16.8g, 25.2g

CONTRAINDICATIONS
History of a hypersensitivity reaction to patiromer or any components of the medication.

WARNINGS/PRECAUTIONS
Not for use as an emergency treatment for life-threatening hyperkalemia. Avoid use in patients w/ severe constipation, bowel obstruction or impaction, including abnormal postoperative bowel motility disorders; may be ineffective and worsen GI conditions. May lead to hypomagnesemia; monitor serum Mg^{2+} and consider Mg^{2+} supplementation w/ low serum Mg^{2+} levels.

ADVERSE REACTIONS
Constipation, hypomagnesemia, diarrhea, nausea, abdominal discomfort, flatulence.

DRUG INTERACTIONS
See Boxed Warning.

PREGNANCY AND LACTATION
Pregnancy: Not absorbed systemically and maternal use is not expected to result in fetal risk.
Lactation: Not absorbed systemically by the mother; breastfeeding is not expected to result in risk to infant.

MECHANISM OF ACTION
Cation-exchange polymer; increases fecal K$^+$ excretion through binding of K$^+$ in the lumen of the GI tract, which reduces the concentration of free K$^+$ in the GI lumen, resulting in a reduction of serum K$^+$ levels.

PATIENT CONSIDERATIONS
Assessment: Assess for severe constipation, bowel obstruction/impaction, pregnancy/nursing status, and possible drug interactions.

Monitoring: Monitor for hypersensitivity reactions, worsening of GI motility, serum Mg^{2+} and K$^+$ levels, and other adverse reactions.

Counseling: Advise to separate dosing of other oral medications by at least 6 hrs before or after administration of therapy. Instruct to take ud w/ food and to adhere to prescribed diets. Instruct not to heat, add to heated foods or liquids, or take in its dry form.

VENCLEXTA — venetoclax   Rx

Class: BCL-2 inhibitor

ADULT DOSAGE

Chronic Lymphocytic Leukemia

Treatment of patients w/ chronic lymphocytic leukemia (CLL) w/ 17p deletion, as detected by an FDA-approved test, who have received at least 1 prior therapy

Administer according to a weekly ramp-up schedule

Week 1: 20mg qd
Week 2: 50mg qd
Week 3: 100mg qd
Week 4: 200mg qd
Week 5 and Beyond: 400mg qd

Continue until disease progression or unacceptable toxicity is observed

Missed Dose

If a dose is missed w/in 8 hrs of the time it is usually taken, take the missed dose as soon as possible and resume the normal daily dosing schedule

If a dose is missed by >8 hrs, do not take the missed dose; resume the usual dosing schedule the next day

If vomiting occurs following dosing, no additional dose should be taken; take next dose at the usual time

PEDIATRIC DOSAGE

Pediatric use may not have been established

DOSING CONSIDERATIONS

Concomitant Medications

Strong CYP3A Inhibitors:
Initiation and Ramp-Up Phase: Contraindicated
Steady Daily Dose (After Ramp-Up Phase): Avoid inhibitor use or reduce venetoclax dose by at least 75%

Moderate CYP3A Inhibitors/P-gp Inhibitors: Avoid inhibitor use or reduce venetoclax dose by at least 50%

Resume dose that was used prior to initiating CYP3A/P-gp inhibitor 2-3 days after discontinuation of the inhibitor

Renal Impairment

CrCl <80mL/min: Increased risk of tumor lysis syndrome (TLS); may require more intensive prophylaxis and monitoring to reduce the risk of TLS when initiating therapy
Severe (CrCl <30mL/min) or on Dialysis: Recommended dose has not been determined

Hepatic Impairment

Mild or Moderate: Monitor more closely for signs of toxicity during the initiation and dose ramp-up phase
Severe: Recommended dose has not been determined

Adverse Reactions

Dose Modification for Toxicity During Treatment:

Interruption at 400mg: Restart at 300mg
Interruption at 300mg: Restart at 200mg
Interruption at 200mg: Restart at 100mg
Interruption at 100mg: Restart at 50mg
Interruption at 50mg: Restart at 20mg
Interruption at 20mg: Restart at 10mg

Continue the reduced dose for 1 week before increasing the dose during the ramp-up phase

TLS:
- Withhold the next day's dose if blood chemistry changes or symptoms suggestive of TLS develop
- Resume at the same dose if resolved w/in 24-48 hrs of the last dose
- Resume at a reduced dose if blood chemistry changes require >48 hrs to resolve
- Resume at a reduced dose following resolution for any events of clinical TLS
- Consider discontinuing venetoclax for patients who require dose reductions to <100mg for more than 2 weeks

Non-Hematologic Toxicities (Grade 3 or 4):
First Occurrence: Interrupt venetoclax; once the toxicity has resolved to Grade 1 or baseline level, may resume at the same dose; no dose modification is required
Second and Subsequent Occurrences: Interrupt venetoclax; follow "dose modification for toxicity" instructions listed above when resuming treatment w/ venetoclax after resolution; a larger dose reduction may occur at the discretion of the physician

Consider discontinuing venetoclax for patients who require dose reductions to <100mg for more than 2 weeks

Hematologic Toxicities:
Grade 3 or 4 Neutropenia w/ Infection or Fever; or Grade 4 Hematologic Toxicities (Except Lymphopenia):
First Occurrence: Interrupt venetoclax. If clinically indicated, may administer granulocyte-colony stimulating factor (G-CSF) w/ venetoclax to reduce infection

risk associated w/ neutropenia. May resume at the same dose once toxicity is resolved to Grade 1 or baseline
Second and Subsequent Occurrences: Interrupt venetoclax. Consider using G-CSF as clinically indicated. Follow "dose modification for toxicity" instructions listed above when resuming treatment w/ venetoclax after resolution; a larger dose reduction may occur at the discretion of the physician

Consider discontinuing venetoclax for patients who require dose reductions to <100mg for more than 2 weeks

ADMINISTRATION

Oral route

- Take w/ a meal and water at approx the same time each day.
- Swallow tab whole; do not chew, crush, or break prior to swallowing.
- Refer to prescribing information for TLS prophylaxis recommendations.

STORAGE

≤30°C (86°F).

HOW SUPPLIED

Tab: 10mg, 50mg, 100mg

CONTRAINDICATIONS

Concomitant use w/ strong CYP3A inhibitors at initiation and during ramp-up phase.

WARNINGS/PRECAUTIONS

See Dosing Considerations. Patients w/o 17p deletion at diagnosis should be retested at relapse; acquisition of 17p deletion may occur. TLS, including fatal events and renal failure requiring dialysis, reported in previously treated CLL patients w/ high tumor burden. Assess TLS risk and administer appropriate prophylaxis for TLS. Monitor blood chemistries and manage abnormalities promptly; interrupt dosing if needed. Employ more intensive measures (IV hydration, frequent monitoring, hospitalization) as overall risk increases. Grade 3 or 4 neutropenia reported; interrupt dosing or reduce dose for severe neutropenia. Consider supportive measures including antimicrobials for signs of infection and use of growth factors (eg, G-CSF). May cause embryo-fetal harm.

ADVERSE REACTIONS

Neutropenia, diarrhea, nausea, anemia, URTI, thrombocytopenia, fatigue.

DRUG INTERACTIONS

See Dosing Considerations and Contraindications. Concomitant use w/ strong (eg, ketoconazole, conivaptan, indinavir) or moderate CYP3A inhibitors (eg, erythromycin, ciprofloxacin, diltiazem) and P-gp inhibitors (eg, amiodarone, captopril, felodipine) increases exposure and may increase the risk of TLS at initiation and during ramp-up phase. Resume the venetoclax dose that was used prior to initiating the CYP3A inhibitor or P-gp inhibitor 2-3 days after discontinuing the inhibitor. Vaccinations may be less effective; do not administer live attenuated vaccines prior to, during, or after treatment until B-cell recovery occurs. Avoid grapefruit products, Seville oranges, and starfruit during treatment. Coadministration w/ multiple doses of rifampin, a strong CYP3A inducer, decreased levels; avoid w/ strong CYP3A inducers (eg, carbamazepine, phenytoin, St. John's wort) or moderate CYP3A inducers (eg, bosentan, efavirenz, modafinil) and consider alternative treatments w/ less CYP3A induction. May increase warfarin levels; closely monitor INR. Avoid P-gp substrates w/ a narrow therapeutic index (eg, digoxin, everolimus, sirolimus); take at least 6 hrs before venetoclax if coadministration must occur.

PREGNANCY AND LACTATION

Pregnancy: May cause fetal harm.
Lactation: There are no data on the presence of venetoclax in human milk, the effects on the breastfed child, or the effects on milk production; not for use in nursing.
Reproductive Potential: Females of reproductive potential should undergo pregnancy testing before initiation of therapy and use effective contraception during treatment and for at least 30 days after the last dose. Male fertility may be compromised by treatment.

MECHANISM OF ACTION

BCL-2 inhibitor; helps restore the process of apoptosis by binding directly to the BCL-2 protein, displacing pro-apoptotic proteins like BIM, triggering mitochondrial outer membrane permeabilization and the activation of caspases.

PHARMACOKINETICS

Absorption: T_{max}=5-8 hrs (fed); C_{max}=2.1µg/mL (low-fat meal), AUC=32.8µg•hr/mL (low-fat meal). **Distribution:** Highly bound to human plasma protein; V_d=256-321L. **Metabolism:** Predominantly via CYP3A4/5; M27 (major active metabolite). **Elimination:** Feces (>99.9%, 20.8% unchanged), urine (<0.1%); $T_{1/2}$=26 hrs.

PATIENT CONSIDERATIONS

Assessment: Assess for risk of TLS, renal/hepatic impairment, pregnancy/nursing status, and for possible drug interactions. Assess for the presence of 17p deletions in blood specimens.

Monitoring: Monitor for TLS, neutropenia, and any other adverse reaction. Monitor blood chemistries and CBC.

Counseling: Advise of the risk of TLS; instruct to immediately report to physician any signs/symptoms of TLS (eg, fever, chills, N/V, confusion, shortness of breath, seizure). Advise to adequately hydrate every day (approx 6-8 glasses or 56 oz of water per day) when taking therapy; instruct to drink water starting 2 days before and on the day of the first dose, and every time the dose is increased. Inform of the importance of keeping scheduled appointments for blood work or other lab tests. Inform that it may be necessary to take in the presence of a doctor to allow monitoring for TLS. Advise to contact physician immediately if a fever or any signs of infection develop. Instruct to avoid consuming grapefruit products, Seville oranges, or starfruit during treatment. Instruct to inform physician of the use of any prescription medication, OTC drugs, vitamins, and herbal products. Advise to avoid vaccination w/ live vaccines. Inform women of the potential risk to the fetus and to avoid pregnancy during treatment; instruct to contact physician if the patient becomes pregnant, or if pregnancy is suspected, during treatment. Instruct female patients of reproductive potential to use effective contraception during therapy and for at least 30 days after completing therapy. Advise not to breastfeed while taking therapy. Inform males of reproductive potential of the possibility of infertility and the possible use of sperm banking. Instruct to take ud. Advise to keep tabs in the original packaging during the first 4 weeks of treatment, and not to transfer the tabs to a different container.

VENTAVIS — iloprost   Rx

Class: Prostacyclin analogue

ADULT DOSAGE
Pulmonary Arterial Hypertension

Treatment of pulmonary arterial HTN (WHO Group 1) to improve exercise tolerance, symptoms (NYHA Class), and lack of deterioration

Intended to be inhaled using the I-neb AAD System
Initial: 2.5mcg
Titrate: If 2.5mcg is well tolerated, increase to 5mcg and maintain at that dose; otherwise maintain at 2.5mcg
Give 6-9X/day (no more than once q2h) during waking hrs, according to individual need and tolerability
Max: 45mcg/day (5mcg 9X/day)

PEDIATRIC DOSAGE
Pediatric use may not have been established

DOSING CONSIDERATIONS
Hepatic Impairment
Child-Pugh Class B or C: Consider increasing dosing interval (eg, 3-4 hrs between doses depending on response at the end of the dose interval)

Elderly
Start at lower end of dosing range

ADMINISTRATION
Oral inh route

Use w/ I-neb AAD system only
Do not mix w/ other medications in the delivery system
For each inh session, the entire contents of each opened ampule should be transferred into the I-neb AAD system medication chamber immediately before use
Discard any sol remaining in the medication chamber after each inh session
Refer to PI for detailed instructions

STORAGE
20-25°C (68-77°F); excursions permitted to 15-30°C (59-86°F).

HOW SUPPLIED
Sol, Inhalation: 10mcg/mL, 20mcg/mL [1mL]

WARNINGS/PRECAUTIONS
Do not allow solution to come into contact with the skin or eyes; avoid oral ingestion. Do not initiate in patients with systolic BP (SBP) <85mmHg. Occurrence of exertional syncope may reflect a therapeutic gap or insufficient efficacy; consider the need to adjust dose or change therapy. D/C immediately if signs of pulmonary edema occur; this may be a sign of pulmonary venous HTN. May induce bronchospasm, which may be more severe or frequent in patients with a history of hyperreactive airways. Caution in elderly.

ADVERSE REACTIONS
Increased cough, headache, vasodilation/flushing, flu syndrome, N/V, trismus, hypotension, syncope, insomnia, palpitations, back pain, alkaline phosphatase/gamma-glutamyl transpeptidase increased, muscle cramps.

DRUG INTERACTIONS
May increase hypotensive effect of vasodilators and antihypertensive agents. Increased risk of bleeding with anticoagulants or platelet inhibitors.

PREGNANCY AND LACTATION
Category C, not for use in nursing.

MECHANISM OF ACTION
Prostacyclin PGI_2 analogue; dilates systemic and pulmonary arterial vascular beds.

PHARMACOKINETICS
Absorption: C_{max}=150pg/mL. **Distribution:** (IV) V_d=0.7-0.8L/kg (healthy); plasma protein binding (60%). **Metabolism:** β-oxidation of the carboxyl side chain; tetranor-iloprost (main metabolite). **Elimination:** (IV/PO, Healthy) Urine (68%), feces (12%); (IV) $T_{1/2}$=20-30 min.

PATIENT CONSIDERATIONS
Assessment: Assess for SBP <85mmHg, history of hyperreactive airways, hepatic impairment, pregnancy/nursing status, and possible drug interactions.

Monitoring: Monitor for exertional syncope, pulmonary edema, bronchospasm, and other adverse reactions. Monitor vital signs while initiating treatment.

Counseling: Advise to use only as prescribed; instruct on proper preparation and administration techniques. Inform that a fall in BP may occur and may cause dizziness or fainting; advise to stand up slowly when getting out of a chair or bed, and to consult physician about dose adjustment if fainting worsens. Advise that

---

medication should be inhaled at intervals of not less than 2 hrs and that the acute benefits of therapy may not last 2 hrs; inform that times of administration may be adjusted to cover planned activities. Instruct to have easy access to a back-up I-neb Adaptive Aerosol Delivery (AAD) System to avoid potential interruptions in drug delivery. Instruct not to allow solution to come into contact with the skin or eyes, and to avoid oral ingestion.

VIDAZA — azacitidine   Rx

Class: Pyrimidine nucleoside analogue

ADULT DOSAGE
Myelodysplastic Syndromes

Treatment of the following French-American-British (FAB) myelodysplastic syndrome subtypes: refractory anemia or refractory anemia w/ ringed sideroblasts (if accompanied by neutropenia or thrombocytopenia or requiring transfusions), refractory anemia w/ excess blasts, refractory anemia w/ excess blasts in transformation, and chronic myelomonocytic leukemia

1st Treatment Cycle:
Initial: 75mg/m²/day SQ or IV for 7 days

Subsequent Treatment Cycles:
Repeat cycle every 4 weeks
Dose may be increased to 100mg/m² if no beneficial effect is seen after 2 cycles and if no toxicity other than N/V has occurred

Treat for a minimum of 4-6 cycles; complete or partial response may require additional cycles

Treatment may be continued as long as the patient continues to benefit

Premedication
Premedicate for N/V

PEDIATRIC DOSAGE
Pediatric use may not have been established

DOSING CONSIDERATIONS
Adverse Reactions
Hematology Lab Values:
For patients w/ baseline WBC ≥3.0 x 10⁹/L, ANC ≥1.5 x 10⁹/L, and platelets ≥75.0 x 10⁹/L, adjust the dose as follows, based on nadir counts for any given cycle:
ANC <0.5 x 10⁹/L or Platelets <25 x 10⁹/L: Administer 50% of dose in next course
ANC <0.5-1.5 x 10⁹/L or Platelets 25-50 x 10⁹/L: Administer 67% of dose in next course

For patients whose baseline counts are WBC <3.0 x 10⁹/L, ANC<1.5 x 10⁹/L, or platelets <75.0 x 10⁹/L, dose adjustments should be based on nadir counts and bone marrow biopsy cellularity at the time of the nadir as noted below, unless there is clear improvement in differentiation at the time of the next cycle, in which case the dose of the current treatment should be continued
WBC or Platelet 50-75% Decrease in Counts from Baseline:
Bone Marrow Biopsy Cellularity 15-30%: Administer 50% of dose in next course
Bone Marrow Biopsy Cellularity <15%: Administer 33% of dose in next course
WBC or Platelet >75% Decrease in Counts from Baseline:
Bone Marrow Biopsy Cellularity 30-60%: Administer 75% of dose in next course
Bone Marrow Biopsy Cellularity 15-30%: Administer 50% of dose in next course
Bone Marrow Biopsy Cellularity <15%: Administer 33% of dose in next course
If a nadir as defined above has occurred, the next course of treatment should be given 28 days after the start of the preceding course, provided that both the WBC and the platelet counts are >25% above the nadir and rising
If a >25% Increase is Not Seen by Day 28: Reassess counts every 7 days
If a 25% Increase is Not Seen by Day 42: Treated w/ 50% of the scheduled dose

Serum Electrolytes and Renal Toxicity:
Unexplained Reductions in Serum Bicarbonate Levels to <20mEq/L: Reduce dose by 50% on next course
Unexplained Elevations of BUN/SrCr: Delay next cycle until values return to normal or baseline, and reduce dose by 50% on next course

ADMINISTRATION
IV/SQ route

The vial is single-use and does not contain any preservatives; discard unused portions of each vial properly.

Instructions for SQ Administration
1. Reconstitute w/ 4mL of sterile water for inj (SWFI).
2. Inject the diluents slowly into the vial.
3. Vigorously shake or roll the vial until a uniform sus is achieved; the sus will be cloudy.
4. The resulting sus will contain azacitidine 25mg/mL.
5. Do not filter the sus after reconstitution; doing so could remove the active substance.
6. To provide a homogeneous sus, the contents of the dosing syringe must be re-suspended immediately prior to administration; to re-suspend, vigorously roll the syringe between the palms until a uniform, cloudy suspension is achieved.

7. Doses >4mL should be divided equally into 2 syringes and injected into 2 separate sites; rotate sites for each inj (thigh, abdomen, or upper arm). New inj should be given ≥1 inch from an old site and never into areas where the site is tender, bruised, red, or hard.

Immediate SQ Administration:
Administer w/in 1 hr after reconstitution.

Delayed SQ Administration:
Reconstituted product may be kept in the vial or drawn into a syringe. The product must be refrigerated immediately; after removal from refrigerated conditions, the sus may be allowed to equilibrate to room temperature for up to 30 min prior to administration.

Instructions for IV Administration
1. Reconstitute the appropriate number of vials to achieve the desired dose; reconstitute each vial w/ 10mL SWFI.
2. Vigorously shake or roll the vial until all solids are dissolved.
3. The resulting sol will contain azacitidine 10mg/mL.
4. Withdraw the required amount of azacitidine sol to deliver the desired dose and inject into a 50-100mL infusion bag of either 0.9% NaCl inj or lactated Ringer's inj.
5. Administer the total dose over a period of 10-40 min; administration must be completed w/in 1 hr of reconstitution of the azacitidine vial.

IV Sol Incompatibility:
Azacitidine is incompatible w/:
1. D5 sol
2. Hespan
3. Sol containing bicarbonate

Handling Precautions
If reconstituted azacitidine comes into contact w/ the skin, immediately and thoroughly wash w/ soap and water; if it comes into contact w/ mucous membranes, flush thoroughly w/ water.

STORAGE
25°C (77°F); excursions permitted to 15-30°C (59-86°F). Reconstituted Sus: Using Non-refrigerated Water for Inj: 25°C (77°F) for up to 1 hr or 2-8°C (36-46°F) for up to 8 hrs. Using Refrigerated (2-8°C [36-46°F]) Water for Inj: 2-8°C (36-46°F) for up to 22 hrs. Reconstituted Sol: 25°C (77°F) for up to 1 hr.

HOW SUPPLIED
Inj: 100mg

CONTRAINDICATIONS
Advanced malignant hepatic tumors, hypersensitivity to azacitidine or mannitol.

WARNINGS/PRECAUTIONS
Obtain CBC, liver chemistries, and SrCr prior to 1st dose. Anemia, neutropenia, and thrombocytopenia may occur; monitor CBC frequently for response and/or toxicity (at a minimum, before each cycle). Potentially hepatotoxic in patients w/ severe preexisting hepatic impairment; caution w/ liver disease. Monitor patients w/ renal impairment for toxicity. May cause fetal harm; women of childbearing potential should avoid pregnancy, while men should not father a child during treatment. Caution in elderly.

ADVERSE REACTIONS
N/V, anemia, thrombocytopenia, pyrexia, leukopenia, diarrhea, inj-site erythema, constipation, neutropenia, ecchymosis, petechiae, rigors, weakness, hypokalemia.

DRUG INTERACTIONS
Renal toxicity reported w/ IV azacitidine in combination w/ other chemotherapeutic agents (eg, etoposide).

PREGNANCY AND LACTATION
Pregnancy: Category D.
Lactation: Not for use in nursing.

MECHANISM OF ACTION
Pyrimidine nucleoside analog; believed to cause hypomethylation of DNA and direct cytotoxicity on abnormal hematopoietic cells in the bone marrow.

PHARMACOKINETICS
Absorption: (SQ) Rapid. Absolute bioavailability (89%); C_{max}=750ng/mL; T_{max}=0.5 hr.
Distribution: (IV) V_d=76L. **Elimination:** (IV) Urine (85%), feces (<1%). (SQ) Urine (50%); $T_{1/2}$=41 min.

PATIENT CONSIDERATIONS
Assessment: Assess for advanced malignant hepatic tumors, hypersensitivity to drug or to mannitol, renal/hepatic impairment, pregnancy/nursing status, and possible drug interactions. Obtain baseline CBC, LFTs, and SrCr.

Monitoring: Monitor CBC frequently for response and/or toxicity (at a minimum, before each cycle). Monitor LFTs, renal function, and serum electrolytes.

Counseling: Instruct to inform physician of any underlying liver or renal disease, or if pregnant/breastfeeding. Advise women of childbearing potential to avoid becoming pregnant, and men not to father a child while on therapy.

VIDEX EC — didanosine   Rx

Class: Nucleoside reverse transcriptase inhibitor (NRTI)

> **Fatal and nonfatal pancreatitis reported when used alone or in combination regimens. Suspend therapy in patients with suspected pancreatitis and d/c with confirmed pancreatitis. Lactic acidosis and severe hepatomegaly with steatosis, including fatal cases, reported with the use of nucleoside analogues alone or in combination. Fatal lactic acidosis reported in pregnant women who received the combination of didanosine and stavudine with other antiretroviral agents; use with caution.**

OTHER BRAND NAMES
Videx

ADULT DOSAGE
HIV-1 Infection

Combination with Other Antiretrovirals:
Cap:
20-<25kg: 200mg qd
25-<60kg: 250mg qd
≥60kg: 400mg qd
Sol:
<60kg:
Preferred Dosing: 125mg bid
Once-Daily Dosing Requirement: 250mg qd
≥60kg:
Preferred Dosing: 200mg bid
Once-Daily Dosing Requirement: 400mg qd

PEDIATRIC DOSAGE
HIV-1 Infection

Combination with Other Antiretrovirals:
Cap:
≥2 Weeks of Age:
20-<25kg: 200mg qd
25-<60kg: 250mg qd
≥60kg: 400mg qd
Sol:
2 Weeks-8 Months of Age:
100mg/m^2 bid
<8 Months of Age:
120mg/m^2 bid
Not to exceed adult dosing recommendation

DOSING CONSIDERATIONS
Renal Impairment
Cap:
CrCl 30-59mL/min:
<60kg: 125mg qd
≥60kg: 200mg qd
CrCl 10-29mL/min:
<60kg: 125mg qd
≥60kg: 125mg qd
CrCl <10mL/min or Continuous Ambulatory Peritoneal Dialysis/Hemodialysis:
≥60kg: 125mg qd
Sol:
CrCl 30-59mL/min:
<60kg: 150mg qd or 75mg bid
≥60kg: 200mg qd or 100mg bid
CrCl 10-29mL/min:
<60kg: 100mg qd
≥60kg: 150mg qd
CrCl <10mL/min or Continuous Ambulatory Peritoneal Dialysis/Hemodialysis:
<60kg: 75mg qd
≥60kg: 100mg qd

Concomitant Medications
Tenofovir Disoproxil Fumarate:
CrCl ≥60mL/min:
<60kg: Reduce dose to 200mg qd
≥60kg: Reduce dose to 250mg qd

ADMINISTRATION
Oral route

Take on an empty stomach
Swallow caps whole

Sol
Administer at least 30 min ac or 2 hrs pc

Reconstitution Instructions:
20mg/mL Initial Sol:
Add 100mL or 200mL of purified water to the 2g or 4g bottle of powder, respectively

10mg per mL Final Admixture:
1. Immediately mix one part of the 20mg/mL initial sol with one part of an antacid containing aluminum hydroxide (400mg /5mL), magnesium hydroxide (400mg /5mL), and simethicone (40mg/ 5mL) for a final concentration of 10mg/mL
2. Shake thoroughly prior to use

STORAGE
(Cap) 25°C (77°F); excursions permitted between 15-30°C (59-86°F). Store in tightly closed containers. (Sol) 15-30°C (59-86°F). Admixture: 2-8°C (36-46°F) for up to 30 days.

HOW SUPPLIED
Cap, Delayed-Release (EC): 125mg, 200mg, 250mg, 400mg; **(Videx) Sol:** 2g, 4g

CONTRAINDICATIONS
Coadministration with allopurinol or ribavirin.

WARNINGS/PRECAUTIONS
Increased risk of pancreatitis in patients with advanced HIV-1 infection, especially elderly. Obesity and prolonged nucleoside exposure may be risk factors for lactic acidosis and severe hepatomegaly with steatosis. Caution in patients with known risk factors for liver disease. Suspend treatment in any patient who develops clinical signs/symptoms with/without lab findings consistent with symptomatic hyperlactatemia, lactic acidosis, or pronounced hepatotoxicity. Increased frequency of liver function abnormalities in patients with preexisting liver dysfunction; consider interruption or discontinuation of therapy with evidence of worsening liver disease. Noncirrhotic portal HTN reported, including cases leading to liver transplantation or death; d/c with evidence of noncirrhotic portal HTN. Peripheral neuropathy reported and occurred more frequently in patients with advanced HIV disease or history of neuropathy; consider discontinuation if peripheral neuropathy develops. Retinal changes and optic neuritis reported. Immune reconstitution syndrome reported. Autoimmune disorders (eg, Graves' disease, polymyositis, Guillain-Barre syndrome) reported in the setting of immune reconstitution and can occur many months after initiation of treatment. Body fat redistribution/accumulation reported. Caution in elderly.

ADVERSE REACTIONS
Pancreatitis, lactic acidosis, severe hepatomegaly with steatosis, diarrhea, peripheral neurologic symptoms/neuropathy, headache, N/V, rash, abdominal pain, serum AST/ALT/alkaline phosphatase/amylase/lipase/bilirubin elevation.

DRUG INTERACTIONS
See Boxed Warning and Contraindications. Avoid with hydroxyurea with or without stavudine; may increase risk for pancreatitis, hepatotoxicity, and peripheral neuropathy. Caution with drugs that may cause pancreatic toxicity or neurotoxicity (eg, stavudine). Administer nelfinavir 1 hr after didanosine. Ganciclovir and tenofovir may increase levels. Methadone may decrease levels. (Sol) Avoid with methadone. Caution with aluminum- or Mg^{2+}-containing antacids. May decrease levels of delavirdine, indinavir, azole antifungals, and quinolone and tetracycline antibiotics.

PREGNANCY AND LACTATION
Category B, not for use in nursing.

MECHANISM OF ACTION
Synthetic purine nucleoside analogue; inhibits the activity of HIV-1 reverse transcriptase both by competing with the natural substrate, deoxyadenosine 5'-triphosphate, and by its incorporation into viral DNA causing termination of viral DNA chain elongation.

PHARMACOKINETICS
Absorption: Rapid. Oral bioavailability (42%, adults; 25%, pediatric patients 8 months-19 yrs of age [sol]); T_{max}=0.25-1.5 hrs. **Distribution:** Plasma protein binding (<5%). Refer to PI for other parameters in adult and pediatric patients. **Metabolism:** Cellular enzymes to dideoxyadenosine 5'-triphosphate (active metabolite). **Elimination:** Urine (18%). Refer to PI for $T_{1/2}$.

PATIENT CONSIDERATIONS
Assessment: Assess for risk factors for pancreatitis, lactic acidosis, or liver disease, renal/hepatic impairment, history of peripheral neuropathy, pregnancy/nursing status, and possible drug interactions.

Monitoring: Monitor for signs/symptoms of pancreatitis, lactic acidosis, hepatotoxicity, worsening of liver disease, noncirrhotic portal HTN, peripheral neuropathy, immune reconstitution syndrome, autoimmune disorders, fat redistribution/accumulation, and other adverse reactions. Monitor renal function. Consider appropriate lab testing, including liver enzymes, serum bilirubin, albumin, CBC, INR, and ultrasonography, if noncirrhotic portal HTN is suspected. Consider periodic retinal examinations.

Counseling: Inform of risks and benefits of therapy. Caution about the use of medications or other substances, including alcohol, which may exacerbate drug toxicities. Inform that treatment is not a cure for HIV and patients may continue to experience illnesses associated with HIV. Advise to avoid doing things that can spread HIV to others.

VIEKIRA PAK — dasabuvir; ombitasvir/paritaprevir/ritonavir   Rx

Class: CYP3A inhibitor/HCV NS5A inhibitor/HCV non-nucleoside NS5B palm polymerase inhibitor/
HCV NS3/4A protease inhibitor

ADULT DOSAGE
Chronic Hepatitis C (Genotype 1)

2 tabs (ombitasvir, paritaprevir, ritonavir [RTV]) qd (am) and 1 dasabuvir tab bid (am and pm)

Coadministration w/ Ribavirin (RBV):
<75kg: 1000mg/day RBV divided and administered bid w/ food
≥75kg: 1200mg/day RBV divided and administered bid w/ food

Genotype 1a, w/o Cirrhosis:
2 tabs (ombitasvir, paritaprevir, RTV) qd (am) + 1 dasabuvir tab bid (am and pm) + RBV for 12 weeks

Genotype 1a, w/ Compensated Cirrhosis (Child-Pugh A):
2 tabs (ombitasvir, paritaprevir, RTV) qd (am) + 1 dasabuvir tab bid (am and pm) + RBV for 24 weeks. 12-week treatment duration may be considered for some patients based on prior treatment history

Genotype 1b, w/ or w/o Compensated Cirrhosis (Child-Pugh A):
2 tabs (ombitasvir, paritaprevir, RTV) qd (am) + 1 dasabuvir tab bid (am and pm) for 12 weeks

Follow the genotype 1a dosing recommendations in patients w/ an unknown genotype 1 subtype or w/ mixed genotype 1 infection

Liver Transplant Recipients w/ Normal Hepatic Function and Mild Fibrosis (Metavir Fibrosis Score ≤2):
2 tabs (ombitasvir, paritaprevir, RTV) qd (am) + 1 dasabuvir tab bid (am and pm) + RBV for 24 weeks, irrespective of hepatitis C virus genotype 1 subtype. If calcineurin inhibitor used concomitantly, calcineurin inhibitor dosage adjustment is needed

PEDIATRIC DOSAGE
Pediatric use may not have been established

DOSING CONSIDERATIONS
Hepatic Impairment
Mild (Child-Pugh A): No dose adjustment needed
Moderate to Severe (Child-Pugh B and C): Contraindicated

ADMINISTRATION
Oral route
Take w/ a meal w/o regard to fat or calorie content.

STORAGE
≤30°C (86°F).

HOW SUPPLIED
Tab: (Ombitasvir/Paritaprevir/RTV) 12.5mg/75mg/50mg, (Dasabuvir) 250mg

CONTRAINDICATIONS
Moderate to severe hepatic impairment (Child-Pugh B and C). Coadministration w/ drugs that are highly dependent on CYP3A for clearance and for which elevated plasma concentrations are associated w/ serious and/or life-threatening events; coadministration w/ moderate or strong inducers of CYP3A and strong inducers of CYP2C8 that may lead to reduced efficacy of therapy; and coadministration w/ strong inhibitors of CYP2C8 that may increase dasabuvir plasma concentrations and the risk of QT prolongation. Coadministration w/ alfuzosin, ranolazine, dronedarone, carbamazepine, phenytoin, phenobarbital, colchicine, gemfibrozil, rifampin, lurasidone, ergotamine, dihydroergotamine, methylergonovine, ethinyl estradiol-containing medications (eg, combined oral contraceptives), cisapride, St. John's wort, lovastatin, simvastatin, pimozide, efavirenz, sildenafil (when used to treat pulmonary arterial HTN), triazolam, or oral midazolam. Known hypersensitivity (eg, toxic epidermal necrolysis, Stevens-Johnson syndrome) to RTV. When used w/ RBV, refer to the individual PI.

WARNINGS/PRECAUTIONS
Hepatic decompensation and hepatic failure including liver transplantation or fatal outcomes reported; monitor for signs and symptoms of hepatic decompensation and d/c if evidence of hepatic decompensation develops. Elevations of ALT to >5X ULN reported. Perform hepatic lab testing during the first 4 weeks of starting treatment and as clinically indicated thereafter. If ALT is found to be elevated above baseline levels, repeat and monitor closely. Consider discontinuing if ALT levels remain persistently >10X ULN. D/C if ALT elevation is accompanied by signs or symptoms of liver inflammation or increasing direct bilirubin, alkaline phosphatase, or INR. If coadministered w/ RBV, the warnings and precautions for RBV, in particular the pregnancy avoidance warning, apply to this combination regimen; refer to RBV PI for a full list of warnings/precautions for RBV. Any HCV/HIV-1 coinfected patients being treated should also be on a suppressive antiretroviral drug regimen to reduce the risk of HIV-1 protease inhibitor drug resistance.

ADVERSE REACTIONS
W/ RBV: Fatigue, nausea, pruritus, skin reactions, insomnia, asthenia. **W/O RBV:** Nausea, pruritus, insomnia, asthenia.

DRUG INTERACTIONS
See Contraindications. Not recommended w/ darunavir/RTV, lopinavir/RTV, rilpivirine (qd dosing), and salmeterol. Not recommended w/ voriconazole unless an assessment of the benefit-to-risk ratio justifies the use of voriconazole. Not recommended w/ metformin in patients w/ renal insufficiency or hepatic impairment. Monitor for signs of lactic acidosis (eg, respiratory distress, somnolence, non-specific abdominal distress, worsening renal function) w/ metformin. If taking quetiapine, consider alternative anti-HCV therapy. Therapeutic monitoring is recommended w/ antiarrhythmics. May increase levels of drugs that are substrates of CYP3A, UGT1A1, breast cancer resistance protein (BCRP), OATP1B1, or OATP1B3. May increase levels of ARBs, quetiapine, antiarrhythmics, calcium channel blockers (eg, amlodipine), ketoconazole, inhaled/nasal fluticasone, furosemide (C_{max}), rilpivirine, rosuvastatin, pravastatin, cyclosporine, tacrolimus, salmeterol, buprenorphine, norbuprenorphine, hydrocodone, and alprazolam. Concomitant use w/ inhaled/nasal fluticasone may reduce serum cortisol concentrations; consider alternative corticosteroids. May decrease levels of voriconazole, darunavir (C_{trough}), carisoprodol, cyclobenzaprine, norcyclobenzaprine, omeprazole, diazepam, and nordiazepam. Inhibition of P-gp, BCRP, OATP1B1, or OATP1B3 may increase levels of the various components of Viekira Pak. ALT elevation reported more frequently w/ ethinyl estradiol-containing medications (eg, combined oral contraceptives, contraceptive patches, contraceptive vaginal rings); alternative methods of contraception (eg, progestin-only contraception, nonhormonal methods) are recommended during therapy. Ethinyl estradiol-containing medications can be restarted approx 2 weeks following completion of treatment. **Paritaprevir:** Atazanavir/RTV (qd dosing), and lopinavir/RTV may increase levels. **Paritaprevir/RTV:** Strong CYP3A inhibitors may increase levels. **Dasabuvir:** CYP2C8 inhibitors may increase levels. Refer to PI for further information on drug interactions, including dosing modifications when used w/ certain concomitant therapies.

PREGNANCY AND LACTATION
Pregnancy: No adequate human data are available to establish whether or not Viekira Pak poses a risk to pregnancy outcomes.
Lactation: It is not known whether Viekira Pak and its metabolites are present in human breast milk, affect human milk production, or have effects on the breastfed infant; caution in nursing.

If administered w/ ribavirin, refer to the prescribing information of ribavirin for additional information.

MECHANISM OF ACTION

Ombitasvir: Inhibitor of HCV NS5A, which is essential for viral RNA replication and virion assembly. **Paritaprevir:** Inhibitor of HCV NS3/4A protease, which is necessary for the proteolytic cleavage of the HCV encoded polyprotein (into mature forms of the NS3, NS4A, NS4B, NS5A, and NS5B proteins) and is essential for viral replication. **Dasabuvir:** Non-nucleoside inhibitor of the HCV RNA-dependent RNA polymerase encoded by the NS5B gene, which is essential for replication of the viral genome. **RTV:** Potent CYP3A inhibitor; increases peak and trough plasma drug concentrations of paritaprevir and overall drug exposure.

PHARMACOKINETICS

Absorption: T_{max}=4-5 hrs. Dasabuvir: Absolute bioavailability (70%). C_{max}=667ng/mL (median); AUC_{0-12}=3240ng•hr/mL (median). Ombitasvir: Absolute bioavailability (48%). C_{max}=68ng/mL (median); AUC_{0-24}=1000ng•hr/mL (median). Paritaprevir: Absolute bioavailability (53%). C_{max}=262ng/mL (median); AUC_{0-24}=2220ng•hr/mL (median). RTV: C_{max}=682ng/mL (median); AUC_{0-24}=6180ng•hr/mL (median). **Distribution:** Dasabuvir: Plasma protein binding (>99.5%); V_d=149L. Ombitasvir: Plasma protein binding (99.9%); V_d=173L. Paritaprevir: Plasma protein binding (97-98.6%); V_d=103L. RTV: Plasma protein binding (>99%); V_d=21.5L (apparent). **Metabolism:** Ombitasvir: Via amide hydrolysis followed by oxidative metabolism. Paritaprevir: Via CYP3A4 (major), CYP3A5. RTV: Via CYP3A (major), CYP2D6. Dasabuvir: Via CYP2C8 (major), CYP3A. **Elimination:** Dasabuvir: Feces (94.4%, 26% unchanged), urine (<2%, 0.03% unchanged); $T_{1/2}$=5.5-6 hrs. Ombitasvir: Feces (90.2%, 87.8% unchanged), urine (1.91%, 0.03% unchanged); $T_{1/2}$=21-25 hrs. Paritaprevir: Feces (88%, 1.1% unchanged), urine (8.8%, 0.05% unchanged); $T_{1/2}$=5.5 hrs. RTV: Feces (86.4%, 33.8 unchanged), urine (11.3%, 3.5 unchanged); $T_{1/2}$=4 hrs.

PATIENT CONSIDERATIONS

Assessment: Assess for drug hypersensitivity, hepatic decompensation, hepatic impairment, pregnancy/nursing status, and possible drug interactions. Assess LFTs.

Monitoring: Monitor for hepatic decompensation, ALT elevation, and other adverse reactions. Perform hepatic lab testing (eg, direct bilirubin levels) during the first 4 weeks of starting treatment and as clinically indicated thereafter. If ALT is found to be elevated above baseline levels, repeat and monitor closely.

Counseling: Inform to watch for early warning signs of liver inflammation or failure (eg, fatigue, lack of appetite, N/V); instruct to contact physician w/o delay if such symptoms occur. Advise to avoid pregnancy during treatment w/ RBV and w/in 6 months of stopping RBV; instruct to notify physician immediately in the event of a pregnancy. Inform that therapy may interact w/ some drugs; advise to report to physician the use of any prescription, nonprescription medication, or herbal products. Inform that contraceptives containing ethinyl estradiol are contraindicated w/ therapy. Advise patients to take therapy every day at the regularly scheduled time w/ a meal w/o regard to fat or calorie content. Inform patients that it is important not to miss or skip doses and to take therapy for the duration that is recommended by physician.

VIEKIRA XR — dasabuvir/ombitasvir/paritaprevir/ritonavir   Rx

Class: CYP3A inhibitor/HCV NS5A inhibitor/HCV non-nucleoside NS5B palm polymerase inhibitor/ HCV NS3/4A protease inhibitor

ADULT DOSAGE

Chronic Hepatitis C (Genotype 1)

3 tabs qd

Coadministration w/ Ribavirin (RBV):
<75kg: 1000mg/day RBV divided and administered bid w/ food
≥75kg: 1200mg/day RBV divided and administered bid w/ food

Genotype 1a, w/o Cirrhosis:
Viekira XR (3 tabs) qd + RBV bid for 12 weeks

Genotype 1a, w/ Compensated Cirrhosis (Child-Pugh A):
Viekira XR (3 tabs) qd + RBV bid for 24 weeks. 12-week treatment duration may be considered for some patients based on prior treatment history

Genotype 1b, w/ or w/o Compensated Cirrhosis (Child-Pugh A):
Viekira XR (3 tabs) qd for 12 weeks

Follow the genotype 1a dosing recommendations in patients w/ an unknown genotype 1 subtype or w/ mixed genotype 1 infection

Liver Transplant Recipients w/ Normal Hepatic Function and Mild Fibrosis (Metavir Fibrosis Score ≤2):
Viekira XR (3 tabs) qd + RBV bid for 24 weeks, irrespective of hepatitis C virus genotype 1 subtype. If calcineurin inhibitor used concomitantly, calcineurin inhibitor dosage adjustment is needed

PEDIATRIC DOSAGE

Pediatric use may not have been established

DOSING CONSIDERATIONS

Hepatic Impairment
Mild (Child-Pugh A): No dose adjustment needed
Moderate to Severe (Child-Pugh B and C): Contraindicated

ADMINISTRATION

Oral route

Take w/ a meal.
Swallow tab whole.
Do not consume alcohol w/in 4 hrs of taking Viekira XR.

STORAGE

≤30°C (86°F).

HOW SUPPLIED

Tab, Extended-Release: (Dasabuvir/Ombitasvir/Paritaprevir/Ritonavir [RTV]) 200mg/8.33mg/50mg/33.33mg

CONTRAINDICATIONS

Moderate to severe hepatic impairment (Child-Pugh B and C). Coadministration w/ drugs that are highly dependent on CYP3A for clearance and for which elevated plasma concentrations are associated w/ serious and/or life-threatening events; coadministration w/ moderate or strong inducers of CYP3A and strong inducers of CYP2C8 that may lead to reduced efficacy of therapy; and coadministration w/ strong inhibitors of CYP2C8 that may increase dasabuvir plasma concentrations and the risk of QT prolongation. Coadministration w/ alfuzosin, ranolazine, dronedarone, carbamazepine, phenytoin, phenobarbital, colchicine, gemfibrozil, rifampin, lurasidone, pimozide, ergotamine, dihydroergotamine, methylergonovine, ethinyl estradiol-containing medications (eg, combined oral contraceptives), cisapride, St. John's wort, lovastatin, simvastatin, efavirenz, sildenafil (when used to treat pulmonary arterial HTN), triazolam, or oral midazolam. Known hypersensitivity (eg, toxic epidermal necrolysis, Stevens-Johnson syndrome) to RTV. When used w/ RBV, refer to the individual PI.

WARNINGS/PRECAUTIONS

Hepatic decompensation and hepatic failure including liver transplantation or fatal outcomes reported; monitor for signs and symptoms of hepatic decompensation and d/c if evidence of hepatic decompensation develops. Elevations of ALT to >5X ULN reported. Perform hepatic lab testing during the first 4 weeks of starting treatment and as clinically indicated thereafter. If ALT is found to be elevated above baseline levels, repeat and monitor closely. Consider discontinuing if ALT levels remain persistently >10X ULN. D/C if ALT elevation is accompanied by signs or symptoms of liver inflammation or increasing direct bilirubin, alkaline phosphatase, or INR. If coadministered w/ RBV, the warnings and precautions for RBV, in particular the pregnancy avoidance warning, apply to this combination regimen; refer to RBV PI for a full list of warnings/precautions for RBV. Any HCV/HIV-1 coinfected patients being treated should also be on a suppressive antiretroviral drug regimen to reduce the risk of HIV-1 protease inhibitor drug resistance.

ADVERSE REACTIONS

W/ RBV: Fatigue, nausea, pruritus, skin reactions, insomnia, asthenia. **W/O RBV:** Nausea, pruritus, insomnia, asthenia.

DRUG INTERACTIONS

See Contraindications. Not recommended w/ darunavir/RTV, lopinavir/RTV, rilpivirine (qd dosing), and salmeterol. Not recommended w/ voriconazole unless an assessment of the benefit-to-risk ratio justifies the use of voriconazole. Not recommended w/ metformin in patients w/ renal insufficiency or hepatic impairment. Monitor for signs of lactic acidosis (eg, respiratory distress, somnolence, non-specific abdominal distress, worsening renal function) w/ metformin. If taking quetiapine, consider alternative anti-HCV therapy. Therapeutic monitoring is recommended w/ antiarrhythmics. May increase levels of drugs that are substrates of CYP3A, UGT1A1, breast cancer resistance protein (BCRP), OATP1B1, or OATP1B3. May increase levels of ARBs, quetiapine, antiarrhythmics, calcium channel blockers (eg, amlodipine), ketoconazole, inhaled/nasal fluticasone, furosemide (C_{max}), rilpivirine, rosuvastatin, pravastatin, cyclosporine, tacrolimus, salmeterol, buprenorphine, norbuprenorphine, hydrocodone, and alprazolam. Concomitant use w/ inhaled/nasal fluticasone may reduce serum cortisol concentrations; consider alternative corticosteroids, particularly for long-term use. May decrease levels of voriconazole, darunavir (C_{trough}), carisoprodol, cyclobenzaprine, norcyclobenzaprine, omeprazole, diazepam, and nordiazepam. Inhibitors of P-gp, BCRP, OATP1B1, or OATP1B3 may increase levels of the various components of Viekira XR. ALT elevation reported more frequently w/ ethinyl estradiol-containing medications (eg, combined oral contraceptives, contraceptive patches, contraceptive vaginal rings); these agents must be discontinued prior to starting therapy and alternative methods of contraception (eg, progestin-only contraception, nonhormonal methods) are recommended during therapy. Ethinyl estradiol-containing medications can be restarted approx 2 weeks following completion of treatment. **Paritaprevir:** Atazanavir/RTV (qd dosing), and lopinavir/RTV may increase levels. **Paritaprevir/RTV:** Strong CYP3A inhibitors may increase levels. **Dasabuvir:** CYP2C8 inhibitors may increase levels. Refer to PI for further information on drug interactions, including dosing modifications when used w/ certain concomitant therapies.

PREGNANCY AND LACTATION

Pregnancy: No adequate human data are available to establish whether or not Viekira XR poses a risk to pregnancy outcomes. If Viekira XR is administered w/ RBV, the combination regimen is contraindicated in pregnant women and in men whose female partners are pregnant if administered w/ RBV.
Lactation: It is not known whether Viekira XR and its metabolites are present in human breast milk, affect human milk production, or have effects on the breastfed infant; caution in nursing.

Refer to the prescribing information of RBV for additional information.

MECHANISM OF ACTION

Ombitasvir: Inhibitor of HCV NS5A, which is essential for viral RNA replication and virion assembly. **Paritaprevir:** Inhibitor of HCV NS3/4A protease, which is necessary for the proteolytic cleavage of the HCV encoded polyprotein (into mature forms of the NS3, NS4A, NS4B, NS5A, and NS5B proteins) and is essential for viral replication. **Dasabuvir:** Non-nucleoside inhibitor of the HCV RNA-dependent RNA polymerase encoded by the NS5B gene, which is essential for replication of the viral genome. **RTV:** Potent CYP3A inhibitor; increases peak and trough plasma drug concentrations of paritaprevir and overall drug exposure.

PHARMACOKINETICS

Absorption: Dasabuvir: Absolute bioavailability (70%); T_{max}=8 hrs (median). Ombitasvir: Absolute bioavailability (48%); T_{max}=5 hrs (median). Paritaprevir: Absolute bioavailability (53%); T_{max}=5 hrs (median). RTV: T_{max}=4 hrs (median). **Distribution:** Dasabuvir: Plasma protein binding (>99.5%); V_d=149L. Ombitasvir: Plasma protein binding (99.9%); V_d=173L. Paritaprevir: Plasma protein binding (97-98.6%); V_d=103L. RTV: Plasma protein binding (>99%); V_d=21.5L (apparent). **Metabolism:** Ombitasvir: Via amide hydrolysis followed by oxidative metabolism. Paritaprevir: Via CYP3A4 (major), CYP3A5. RTV: Via CYP3A (major), CYP2D6. Dasabuvir: Via CYP2C8 (major), CYP3A. **Elimination:** Dasabuvir: Feces (94.4%, 26.2% unchanged), urine (~2%, 0.03% unchanged); $T_{1/2}$=5.5-6 hrs. Ombitasvir: Feces (90.2%, 87.8% unchanged), urine (1.91%, 0.03% unchanged); $T_{1/2}$=21-25 hrs. Paritaprevir: Feces (88%, 1.1% unchanged), urine (8.8%, 0.05% unchanged); $T_{1/2}$=5.5 hrs. RTV: Feces (86.4%, 33.8% unchanged), urine (11.3%, 3.5% unchanged); $T_{1/2}$=4 hrs.

PATIENT CONSIDERATIONS

Assessment: Assess for drug hypersensitivity, hepatic decompensation/impairment, pregnancy/nursing status, and possible drug interactions. Assess LFTs.

Monitoring: Monitor for hepatic decompensation, ALT elevation, and other adverse reactions. Perform hepatic lab testing (eg; direct bilirubin levels) during the first 4 weeks of starting treatment and as clinically indicated thereafter. If ALT is found to be elevated above baseline levels, repeat and monitor closely.

Counseling: Inform to watch for early warning signs of liver inflammation or failure (eg, fatigue, lack of appetite, N/V); instruct to contact physician w/o delay if such symptoms occur. Advise to avoid pregnancy during treatment w/ RBV and w/in 6 months of stopping RBV; instruct to notify physician immediately in the event of a pregnancy. Inform that therapy may interact w/ some drugs; advise to report to physician the use of any prescription, nonprescription medication, or herbal products. Inform that contraceptives containing ethinyl estradiol are contraindicated w/ therapy. Advise patients to take therapy every day at the regularly scheduled time w/ a meal and not to consume alcohol w/in 4 hrs of their dose. Inform that it is important not to miss or skip doses and to take therapy for the duration that is recommended by physician.

VIMIZIM — elosulfase alfa   Rx

Class: Enzyme

Life-threatening anaphylactic reactions observed during infusion. Anaphylaxis (eg, cough, erythema, throat tightness, urticaria, flushing, cyanosis, hypotension, rash, dyspnea, chest discomfort, GI symptoms) in conjunction with urticaria reported during infusions, regardless of duration of treatment; closely observe patients during and after administration. Inform patients of the signs/symptoms of anaphylaxis and instruct to seek immediate medical care should symptoms occur. Patients with acute respiratory illness may be at risk of serious acute exacerbation of their respiratory compromise due to hypersensitivity reactions; additional monitoring required.

ADULT DOSAGE

Mucopolysaccharidosis IVA (Morquio A Syndrome)

Usual: 2mg/kg IV over a minimum range of 3.5-4.5 hrs, based on infusion volume, once every week

Premedication

Pretreat w/ antihistamines (w/ or w/o antipyretics) 30-60 min prior to start of infusion

PEDIATRIC DOSAGE

Mucopolysaccharidosis IVA (Morquio A Syndrome)

≥5 Years:

Usual: 2mg/kg IV over a minimum range of 3.5-4.5 hrs, based on infusion volume, once every week

Premedication

Pretreat w/ antihistamines (w/ or w/o antipyretics) 30-60 min prior to start of infusion

DOSING CONSIDERATIONS

Adverse Reactions

Hypersensitivity Reactions: Slow, temporarily stop, or d/c infusion rate for that visit

ADMINISTRATION

IV route

Preparation Instructions

1. Determine the number of vials to be diluted based on the patient's weight and the recommended dose.
2. Dilute the calculated dose to a final volume of 100mL or 250mL using 0.9% NaCl inj; the final volume is based on the patient's weight as follows:
Patients <25kg: Final volume should be 100mL
Patients ≥25kg: Final volume should be 250mL
3. The sol should be clear to slightly opalescent and colorless to pale yellow when diluted; a sol w/ slight flocculation (eg, thin translucent fibers) is acceptable for administration.
4. Gently rotate the bag to ensure proper distribution; avoid agitation during preparation and do not shake the sol.
5. Administration should be completed w/in 48 hrs from the time of dilution.

Administration Instructions

Administer the diluted sol using a low-protein binding infusion set equipped w/ a low-protein binding 0.2μm in-line filter.

Patients <25kg:

Initial Infusion Rate: 3mL/hr for the first 15 min

Titrate: If tolerated, increase to 6mL/hr for the next 15 min; if this rate is tolerated, then the rate may be increased every 15 min in 6mL/hr increments

Max Infusion Rate: 36mL/hr

Total volume of the infusion should be delivered over a minimum of 3.5 hrs.

Patients ≥25kg:

Initial Infusion Rate: 6mL/hr for the first 15 min

Titrate: If tolerated, increase to 12mL/hr for the next 15 min; if this rate is tolerated, then the rate may be increased every 15 min in 12mL/hr increments

Max Infusion Rate: 72mL/hr

Total volume of the infusion should be delivered over a minimum of 4.5 hrs.

Do not infuse w/ other products in the infusion tubing.

Stability Information

If immediate use is not possible, store the diluted product for up to 24 hrs at 2-8°C (36-46°F), followed by up to 24 hrs at 23-27°C (73-81°F).

STORAGE

2-8°C (36-46°F). Do not freeze or shake. Protect from light. Diluted Sol: Store for up to 24 hrs at 2-8°C (36-46°F) followed by up to 24 hrs at 23-27°C (73-81°F). Complete administration within 48 hrs from the time of dilution.

HOW SUPPLIED

Inj: 1mg/mL [5mL]

WARNINGS/PRECAUTIONS

Spinal/cervical cord compression (SCC) reported. Anaphylaxis and hypersensitivity reactions reported; d/c infusion immediately and initiate appropriate treatment if severe allergic reactions occur. Caution with readministration in patients who have severe allergic reactions. Increased risk of life-threatening complications from hypersensitivity reactions in patients with acute febrile or respiratory illness at the time of infusion; consider patient's clinical status prior to administration and consider delaying the infusion. Sleep apnea is common in MPS IVA patients; evaluate airway patency prior to initiation of treatment.

ADVERSE REACTIONS

Pyrexia, N/V, headache, abdominal pain, chills, fatigue.

PREGNANCY AND LACTATION

Pregnancy: Category C.

Lactation: Caution in nursing.

MECHANISM OF ACTION

Hydrolytic lysosomal glycosaminoglycan (GAG)-specific enzyme; provides exogenous N-acetylgalactosamine-6-sulfatase that is taken up into lysosomes and increases the catabolism of GAGs KS and C6S.

PHARMACOKINETICS

Absorption: C_{max}=1.49mcg/mL (Week 0), 4.04mcg/mL (Week 22); AUC_{0-t}=238mcg•min/mL (Week 0), 577mcg•min/mL (Week 22). **Distribution:** V_d=396mL/kg (Week 0), 650mL/kg (Week 22). **Elimination:** $T_{1/2}$=7.52 min (Week 0), 35.9 min (Week 22).

PATIENT CONSIDERATIONS

Assessment: Assess for respiratory illness, clinical status, airway patency, and pregnancy/nursing status.

Monitoring: Monitor for anaphylaxis/severe allergic reactions, SCC, and other adverse reactions.

Counseling: Counsel that reactions (eg, life-threatening anaphylaxis) related to administration and infusion may occur during treatment. Inform patients of the signs and symptoms of anaphylaxis and to seek immediate medical care should symptoms occur. Inform patients and pregnant/nursing women of the Morquio A Registry and advise that their participation is voluntary and may involve long-term follow-up.

VINBLASTINE — vinblastine sulfate   Rx

Class: Vinca alkaloid

Should be administered by individuals experienced in the administration of therapy. Extremely important to properly position IV needle or catheter before inj; may cause considerable irritation if leakage into surrounding tissue occurs. D/C immediately if extravasation occurs and introduce any remaining portion of the dose into another vein. Local hyaluronidase inj and moderate heat application to the area of leakage help disperse the drug and minimize discomfort and possibility of cellulitis. For IV use only; fatal if given by other routes. Intrathecal administration usually results in death; after inadvertent intrathecal administration, immediate neurosurgical intervention is required to prevent ascending paralysis leading to death.

OTHER BRAND NAMES

Velban (Discontinued)

ADULT DOSAGE

Palliative Cancer Treatment

Frequently Responsive Malignancies:
Generalized Hodgkin's disease (Stages III and IV, Ann Arbor modification of Rye staging system)
Lymphocytic lymphoma (nodular and diffuse, poorly and well differentiated)
Histiocytic lymphoma
Mycosis fungoides (advanced stages)

PEDIATRIC DOSAGE

Letterer-Siwe disease

Initial: 6.5mg/m² BSA

Hodgkin Lymphoma

Combination Therapy:
Initial: 6mg/m² BSA

Germ Cell Testicular Cancer

Combination Therapy:
Initial: 3mg/m² BSA

Advanced carcinoma of the testis
Kaposi's sarcoma
Letterer-Siwe disease (histiocytosis X)

Less Frequently Responsive Malignancies:
Choriocarcinoma resistant to other chemotherapeutic agents
Carcinoma of the breast, unresponsive to appropriate endocrine surgery and hormonal therapy

Dose at weekly intervals; give no more frequently than once every 7 days
Do not increase dose after that dose which reduces WBC count to approx 3000 cells/mm³
When the dose of vinblastine that will produce the above degree of leukopenia has been established, a dose of 1 increment smaller than that dose should be administered at weekly intervals for maintenance
Do not give next dose until WBC count has returned to at least 4000 cells/mm³

1st Dose: 3.7mg/m² BSA; check WBC count to determine sensitivity to therapy
2nd Dose: 5.5mg/m² BSA
3rd Dose: 7.4mg/m² BSA
4th Dose: 9.25mg/m² BSA
5th Dose: 11.1mg/m² BSA
Max: 18.5mg/m² BSA
Usual Weekly Dose: 5.5-7.4mg/m² BSA

- -

DOSING CONSIDERATIONS
Hepatic Impairment
Direct Serum Bilirubin >3mg/100mL: Reduce by 50%

Other Important Considerations
Pediatric Patients: Dose modifications should be guided by hematologic tolerance

ADMINISTRATION
IV route

Inject either into the tubing of a running IV infusion or directly into a vein; inj may be completed in about 1 min
Rinse syringe and needle w/ venous blood before withdrawal of the needle in order to minimize possibility of extravasation
Dose should not be diluted in large volumes of diluent (eg, 100-250mL) or given IV for prolonged periods (30 to ≥60 min)
Enhanced possibility of thrombosis; avoid injecting into an extremity in which the circulation is impaired or potentially impaired by such conditions as compressing/invading neoplasm, phlebitis, or varicosity

STORAGE
2-8°C (36-46°F). Protect from light.

HOW SUPPLIED
Inj: 1mg/mL [10mL]

CONTRAINDICATIONS
Significant granulocytopenia (unless result of disease being treated), bacterial infections.

WARNINGS/PRECAUTIONS
Avoid pregnancy; may cause fetal harm. Aspermia reported in males. Leukopenia (granulocytopenia) may reach dangerously low levels following administration of the higher recommended doses. Stomatitis and neurologic toxicity, although not common or permanent, can be disabling. Toxicity may be enhanced in the presence of hepatic insufficiency. Monitor for evidence of infection until WBC count has returned to a safe level if leukopenia w/ WBC count <2000 cells/mm³ occurs. Avoid w/ malignant-cell infiltration of bone marrow, or in older persons w/ cachexia or ulcerated areas of the skin surface. Acute SOB and severe bronchospasm reported. Progressive dyspnea requiring chronic therapy may occur; do not readminister the drug. Caution w/ ischemic cardiac disease or hepatic dysfunction. Administering small daily amounts for long periods is not advised; strict adherence to the recommended dosage schedule is very important. Avoid eye contamination.

ADVERSE REACTIONS
Leukopenia (granulocytopenia), constipation, HTN, malaise, bone pain, pain in tumor-containing tissue, jaw pain.

DRUG INTERACTIONS
Simultaneous oral or IV phenytoin and antineoplastic chemotherapy combinations that include vinblastine may reduce levels of phenytoin and increase seizure activity; dosage adjustment should be based on serial blood level monitoring. Caution w/ drugs known to inhibit drug metabolism by the CYP3A subfamily; may cause earlier onset and/or an increased severity of side effects. Enhanced toxicity reported w/ erythromycin. Acute SOB and severe bronchospasm reported most frequently w/ mitomycin-C; do not readminister vinblastine.

PREGNANCY AND LACTATION
Category D, not for use in nursing.

MECHANISM OF ACTION
Vinca alkaloid; inhibits microtubule formation in mitotic spindle, resulting in an arrest of dividing cells at the metaphase stage.

PHARMACOKINETICS
Metabolism: Liver via CYP3A. **Elimination:** Biliary (major), feces (10%), urine (14%); $T_{1/2}$=24.8 hrs.

PATIENT CONSIDERATIONS
Assessment: Assess for significant granulocytopenia (unless result of disease being treated), bacterial infections, cachexia or ulcerated areas of the skin surface (in older persons), malignant-cell infiltration of bone marrow, ischemic cardiac disease, pulmonary/hepatic dysfunction, pregnancy/nursing status, and possible drug interactions. Obtain WBC count prior to planned dose.

Monitoring: Monitor for signs/symptoms of extravasation, leukopenia, infection, acute SOB, severe bronchospasm, and other adverse reactions. Monitor WBC counts to determine sensitivity to drug.

Counseling: Instruct to avoid pregnancy during therapy. Instruct to report immediately the appearance of sore throat, fever, chills, sore mouth, or any other serious medical event. Counsel on how to avoid constipation while on therapy. Inform that alopecia may occur and that scalp hair will regrow to its pretreatment extent even w/ continued treatment. Inform that jaw pain, in organs containing tumor tissue, and N/V may occur. Caution to avoid eye contamination; if accidental contamination occurs, instruct to wash w/ water immediately and thoroughly.

VINCRISTINE — vincristine sulfate
Class: Vinca alkaloid

Rx

> Should be administered by individuals experienced in the administration of therapy. It is extremely important to properly position IV needle or catheter before inj; may cause considerable irritation if leakage occurs into surrounding tissue. D/C immediately if extravasation occurs; introduce any remaining portion of the dose into another vein. Local hyaluronidase inj and moderate heat application to the area of leakage may help disperse the drug and minimize discomfort and possibility of cellulitis. For IV use only; fatal if given by other routes. Should be diluted in a flexible plastic container and prominently labeled as indicated for IV use only to reduce the potential for fatal medication errors due to incorrect route of administration.

ADULT DOSAGE
Acute Leukemia
Usual: 1.4mg/m² at weekly intervals

Other Indications
Combination w/ other oncolytic agents in Hodgkin's disease, non-Hodgkin's malignant lymphomas, rhabdomyosarcoma, neuroblastoma, and Wilms' tumor

PEDIATRIC DOSAGE
Acute Leukemia
Usual: 1.5-2mg/m² at weekly intervals
≤10kg:
Initial: 0.05mg/kg once weekly

Other Indications
Combination w/ other oncolytic agents in Hodgkin's disease, non-Hodgkin's malignant lymphomas, rhabdomyosarcoma, neuroblastoma, and Wilms' tumor

- -

DOSING CONSIDERATIONS
Concomitant Medications
Combination w/ L-Asparaginase: Administer vincristine 12-24 hrs before administration of the enzyme in order to minimize toxicity

Hepatic Impairment
Direct Serum Bilirubin >3mg/100mL: Reduce dose by 50%

ADMINISTRATION
IV route

Do not add extra fluid to the vial prior to removal of the dose
Withdraw the sol into an accurate dry syringe, measuring the dose carefully
Do not add extra fluid to the vial in an attempt to empty it completely
Administer via an intact, free-flowing IV needle or catheter
Sol may be injected either directly into a vein or into the tubing of a running IV infusion; inj should be accomplished w/in 1 min
Do not dilute in sol that raise or lower the pH outside the range of 3.5 to 5.5
Do not mix w/ anything other than normal saline or glucose in water

Preparation for Flexible Plastic Container
When diluted w/ 0.9% NaCl inj in concentrations from 0.0015-0.08mg/mL, vincristine is stable for up to 24 hrs when protected from light or 8 hours under normal light at 25°C

Management of Extravasation
1. Immediately d/c the inj and introduce any remaining portion of the dose into another vein
2. Local inj of hyaluronidase and application of moderate heat to the area of leakage will help disperse the drug and may minimize discomfort and the possibility of cellulitis

STORAGE
2-8°C (36-46°F); store upright. Protect from light.

HOW SUPPLIED
Inj: 1mg/mL [1mL, 2mL]

CONTRAINDICATIONS
Demyelinating form of Charcot-Marie-Tooth syndrome.

WARNINGS/PRECAUTIONS
Avoid use during pregnancy; may cause fetal harm. Acute uric acid nephropathy reported; determine serum uric acid levels frequently during first 3-4 weeks of therapy or take appropriate preventative measures. Carefully consider administration of next dose in the presence of leukopenia or complicating

infection. May require additional agents if CNS leukemia is diagnosed. Monitor dosage and neurologic side effects if given in patients with preexisting neuromuscular disease. Acute SOB and severe bronchospasm reported; may require aggressive treatment, particularly with preexisting pulmonary dysfunction. Progressive dyspnea requiring chronic therapy may occur; do not readminister therapy. Avoid eye contact. Caution with hepatic dysfunction. Neurotoxicity appears to be dose related; caution when calculating and administering the dose.

ADVERSE REACTIONS
Hair loss, leukopenia, neuritic pain, constipation, sensory loss, paresthesia, difficulty walking, slapping gait, loss of deep-tendon reflexes, muscle wasting, generalized sensorimotor dysfunction.

DRUG INTERACTIONS
See Dosage. Simultaneous administration of oral or IV phenytoin and antineoplastic chemotherapy combinations including vincristine may reduce levels of phenytoin and increase seizure activity. Caution with drugs known to inhibit drug metabolism by the CYP3A subfamily. Concurrent administration with itraconazole may cause earlier onset and/or increased severity of neuromuscular side effects. Acute SOB and severe bronchospasm reported, most frequently with concomitant mitomycin-C. Caution with drugs with neurotoxic potential or agents known to be ototoxic (eg, platinum-containing oncolytics). D/C drugs known to cause urinary retention for the 1st few days following administration of therapy. Coronary artery disease and myocardial infarction reported with previous treatment of mediastinal radiation and chemotherapy combinations that include vincristine. Do not administer while receiving radiation therapy through ports that include the liver. Administration of L-asparaginase before therapy may reduce hepatic clearance.

PREGNANCY AND LACTATION
Category D, not for use in nursing.

MECHANISM OF ACTION
Vinca alkaloid; has not been established. Related to the inhibition of microtubule formation in mitotic spindle, resulting in an arrest of dividing cells at metaphase stage.

PHARMACOKINETICS
Metabolism: Via CYP3A subfamily. **Elimination:** Feces (80%), urine (10-20%); $T_{1/2}$=85 hrs.

PATIENT CONSIDERATIONS
Assessment: Assess for demyelinating form of Charcot-Marie-Tooth syndrome, CNS leukemia, hepatic dysfunction, preexisting neuromuscular disease/pulmonary dysfunction, pregnancy/nursing status, and possible drug interactions. Perform CBC before each dose administration.

Monitoring: Monitor for acute SOB, severe bronchospasm, progressive dyspnea, neurotoxicity, and other adverse reactions. Monitor serum uric acid levels frequently during first 3-4 weeks of treatment.

Counseling: Inform of the risks and benefits of therapy. Advise women of childbearing potential to avoid becoming pregnant while on therapy. Instruct to avoid eye contact with drug; severe irritation may occur. Instruct to wash eye immediately and thoroughly if accidental contamination occurs.

VIRACEPT — nelfinavir mesylate   Rx

Class: Protease inhibitor

ADULT DOSAGE
HIV-1 Infection

Combination w/ Other Antiretrovirals:
Tab:
1250mg (five 250mg or two 625mg tabs) bid or 750mg (three 250mg tabs) tid
Max: 2500mg/day

PEDIATRIC DOSAGE
HIV-1 Infection

Combination w/ Other Antiretrovirals:
2-<13 Years:
Oral Powder:
9-<16kg: 45-55mg/kg bid or 25-35mg/kg tid
16->23kg: 25-35mg/kg tid
Max: 2500mg/day
250mg Tab:
10->21kg: 45-55mg/kg bid or 25-35mg/kg tid
Max: 2500mg/day
>13 Years:
Tab:
1250mg (five 250mg or two 625mg tabs) bid or 750mg (three 250mg tabs) tid
Max: 2500mg/day

DOSING CONSIDERATIONS
Hepatic Impairment
Moderate or Severe (Child-Pugh B or C, Score ≥7): Not recommended for use

ADMINISTRATION
Oral route
Take all doses w/ meals

Patients Unable to Swallow Tabs
1. Place tab(s) in a small amount of water
2. Once dissolved, mix the liquid well and consume immediately
3. Rinse the glass w/ water and swallow the rinse to ensure entire dose is consumed

Oral Powder
1. Mix oral powder w/ a small amount of water, milk, formula, soy formula, soy milk, or dietary supplements; do not reconstitute w/ water in original container or mix w/ acidic food or juice (eg, orange juice, apple juice, apple sauce)

---

2. Once mixed, consume entire contents in order to obtain the full dose; if mixture is not consumed immediately, store under refrigeration for up to 6 hrs

STORAGE
15-30°C (59-86°F). (Powder) If mixture is not consumed immediately, store under refrigeration, but must not exceed 6 hrs.

HOW SUPPLIED
Powder: 50mg/g [144g]; **Tab:** 250mg, 625mg

CONTRAINDICATIONS
Concomitant use w/ drugs that are highly dependent on CYP3A for clearance and for which elevated concentrations are associated w/ serious and/or life-threatening events (eg, alfuzosin, amiodarone, quinidine, dihydroergotamine, ergotamine, methylergonovine, cisapride, lovastatin, simvastatin, pimozide, sildenafil [for treatment of pulmonary arterial HTN], triazolam, oral midazolam), and drugs that may lead to reduced efficacy of nelfinavir (eg, St. John's wort, rifampin).

WARNINGS/PRECAUTIONS
Powder contains phenylalanine; caution w/ phenylketonuria. New onset or exacerbation of diabetes mellitus (DM), hyperglycemia, and diabetic ketoacidosis reported. Increased bleeding, including spontaneous skin hematomas and hemarthrosis, in patients w/ hemophilia type A and B reported. Redistribution/ accumulation of body fat reported. Immune reconstitution syndrome reported. Autoimmune disorders (eg, Graves' disease, polymyositis, and Guillain-Barre syndrome) reported in the setting of immune reconstitution and can occur many months after initiation of treatment.

ADVERSE REACTIONS
Diarrhea, nausea, flatulence, rash, abdominal pain, anorexia, leukopenia, neutropenia.

DRUG INTERACTIONS
See Contraindications. Avoid w/ colchicine in patients w/ renal/hepatic impairment. Not recommended w/ salmeterol. May increase levels of dihydropyridine calcium channel blockers, indinavir, saquinavir, trazodone, rifabutin, bosentan, colchicine, HMG-CoA reductase inhibitors (eg, atorvastatin, rosuvastatin), immunosuppressants, fluticasone, azithromycin, PDE-5 inhibitors, quetiapine, and CYP3A substrates. May decrease levels of delavirdine, phenytoin, methadone, ethinyl estradiol, and norethindrone. CYP3A or CYP2C19 inhibitors, delavirdine, indinavir, ritonavir, saquinavir, cyclosporine, tacrolimus, and sirolimus may increase levels. CYP3A or CYP2C19 inducers (eg, rifampin), omeprazole, nevirapine, carbamazepine, phenobarbital, phenytoin, and rifabutin may decrease levels. May affect warfarin concentrations; monitor INR. Give didanosine 1 hr before or 2 hrs after administration. Coadministration w/ proton pump inhibitors may lead to a loss of virologic response and development of resistance. May require initiation or dose adjustments of insulin or oral hypoglycemics for treatment of DM. Refer to PI for dosing modifications when used w/ certain concomitant therapies.

PREGNANCY AND LACTATION
Category B, not for use in nursing.

MECHANISM OF ACTION
HIV-1 protease inhibitor; prevents cleavage of gag and gag-pol polyprotein, resulting in production of immature, noninfectious virus.

PHARMACOKINETICS
Absorption: 28 days: (1250mg bid) C_{max}=4mg/L; AUC=52.8mg•hr/L. (750mg tid) C_{max}=3mg/L; AUC=43.6mg•hr/L. 14 days: (1250mg bid) C_{max}=4.7mg/L; AUC=35.3mg•hr/L. **Distribution:** V_d=2-7L/kg; plasma protein binding (>98%). **Metabolism:** Liver via CYP3A, 2C19 (oxidation). **Elimination:** Feces (78% metabolites, 22% unchanged), urine (1-2%); $T_{1/2}$=3.5-5 hrs.

PATIENT CONSIDERATIONS
Assessment: Assess for previous hypersensitivity to the drug, hepatic impairment, DM, hemophilia, pregnancy/nursing status, and possible drug interactions. Assess for phenylketonuria if planning to use the powder formulation.

Monitoring: Monitor for new onset or exacerbation of DM, hyperglycemia, diabetic ketoacidosis, immune reconstitution syndrome, autoimmune disorders, fat redistribution/accumulation, and other adverse reactions. In patients w/ hemophilia, monitor for bleeding events.

Counseling: Instruct to take ud. Inform that therapy is not a cure for HIV and that illnesses associated w/ HIV may continue. Advise to avoid doing things that can spread HIV to others. Instruct not to alter the dose or d/c therapy w/o consulting physician. Instruct to notify physician if using any other prescription/nonprescription medication, or herbal products, particularly St. John's wort. Advise to use alternative or additional contraceptive measures if taking oral contraceptives. Inform that most frequent adverse event is diarrhea, which can usually be controlled w/ nonprescription drugs (eg, loperamide). Inform that fat redistribution/accumulation may occur. Alert patients w/ phenylketonuria that powder formulation contains phenylalanine.

VIRAMUNE XR — nevirapine   Rx

Class: Non-nucleoside reverse transcriptase inhibitor (NNRTI)

Severe, life-threatening, and in some cases fatal, hepatotoxicity (particularly in the first 18 weeks) and skin reactions (eg, Stevens-Johnson syndrome, toxic epidermal necrolysis, hypersensitivity reactions) reported. Increased risk of hepatotoxicity reported in women and patients with higher CD4+ cell counts, including pregnant women. Hepatic failure reported in patients without HIV taking nevirapine for postexposure prophylaxis (PEP). Use for occupational and non-occupational PEP is contraindicated. D/C therapy and seek medical evaluation immediately if hepatitis, transaminase elevations combined with rash or other systemic symptoms, severe skin rash, or hypersensitivity reactions develop; do not restart therapy. The 14-day lead-in period with 200mg daily dosing must be followed; may decrease the incidence of rash. Monitor intensively during the first 18 weeks of therapy, especially the first 6 weeks.

OTHER BRAND NAMES
Viramune

ADULT DOSAGE
HIV-1 Infection

Combination w/ Other Antiretrovirals:
Tab (Immediate-Release [IR]):
Initial: 200mg qd for the first 14 days
Maint: 200mg bid

Tab, Extended-Release (ER):
Not Currently Taking IR Nevirapine:
Initial: One 200mg IR tab qd for first 14 days
Maint: One 400mg ER tab qd

Switching from IR Tab to ER Tab:
Switch to 400mg ER tab qd w/o 14-day lead-in period

PEDIATRIC DOSAGE
HIV-1 Infection

Combination w/ Other Antiretrovirals:
Tab/Oral Sus:
≥15 Days of Age:
Initial: 150mg/m² qd for the first 14 days
Maint: 150mg/m² bid
Max: 400mg/day

Tab, Extended-Release (ER):
6-<18 Years:
Initial:
150mg/m² IR tab/oral sus qd for first 14 days
Max: 200mg/day
Maint:
BSA 0.58-0.83m²: Two 100mg ER tabs qd
BSA 0.84-1.16m²: Three 100mg ER tabs qd
BSA ≥1.17m²: One 400mg ER tab qd
Max: 400mg/day

DOSING CONSIDERATIONS
Renal Impairment
Requiring Dialysis: Administer additional 200mg IR dose after each dialysis treatment
Hepatic Impairment
Moderate or Severe (Child-Pugh Class B or C): Not recommended for use
Symptomatic Hepatic Event Occurrence: Permanently d/c; do not restart after recovery

Adverse Reactions
Severe Rash/Rash Accompanied by Constitutional Findings: D/C
Mild to Mod Rash w/o Constitutional Symptoms During Lead-In Period: Do not initiate XR therapy until rash has resolved; duration of lead-in period should not exceed 28 days, at which point an alternative regimen should be sought

Other Important Considerations
Dose Interruption for >7 Days: Restart using lead-in dosing

ADMINISTRATION
Oral route

Take w/ or w/o food

Tab, ER
Swallow whole; do not chew, crush, or divide

Oral Sus
Shake gently prior to administration
Administer the entire measured dose by using an oral dosing syringe or dosing cup

STORAGE
25°C (77°F); excursions permitted to 15-30°C (59-86°F).

HOW SUPPLIED
[IR] Sus: 50mg/5mL [240mL]. **Tab:** 200mg*; **Tab, ER:** 100mg, 400mg *scored

CONTRAINDICATIONS
Moderate or severe (Child-Pugh Class B or C) hepatic impairment. Use as part of occupational and non-occupational PEP regimens.

WARNINGS/PRECAUTIONS
Not recommended for adult females with CD4⁺ cell counts >250 cells/mm³ or in adult males with CD4⁺ cell counts >400 cells/mm³. Coinfection with hepatitis B or C and/or increased transaminase elevations at the start of therapy may increase risk of later symptomatic events (≥6 weeks after starting therapy) and asymptomatic increases in AST/ALT. Caution with hepatic fibrosis/cirrhosis; monitor for drug-induced toxicity. Rhabdomyolysis reported in some patients with skin and/or liver reactions. Monitor closely if isolated rash of any severity occurs; delay in stopping treatment after the onset of rash may result in a more serious reaction. Do not use as single agent to treat HIV-1 or add on as a sole agent to a failing regimen; resistant virus emerges rapidly when administered as monotherapy. Consider potential for cross-resistance in the choice of new antiretroviral agents to be used in combination with therapy. Take into account the half-lives of the combination antiretroviral drugs when discontinuing the regimen; nevirapine has a long half-life and resistance may develop if antiretrovirals with shorter half-lives are stopped concurrently. Immune reconstitution syndrome, autoimmune disorders (eg, Graves' disease, polymyositis, Guillain-Barre syndrome) in the setting of immune reconstitution, and redistribution/accumulation of body fat reported. Caution in elderly.

ADVERSE REACTIONS
Hepatotoxicity, skin reactions, diarrhea, nausea, headache, fatigue, abdominal pain.

DRUG INTERACTIONS
Avoid with atazanavir, boceprevir, telaprevir, ketoconazole, itraconazole, and rifampin. Not recommended with fosamprenavir (without ritonavir), efavirenz, and St. John's wort or St. John's wort-containing products; avoid coadministration. Increased incidence and severity of rash with prednisone during the first 6 weeks of therapy; not recommended to prevent nevirapine-associated rash. May increase levels of 14-OH clarithromycin and rifabutin. May increase levels of antithrombotics (eg, warfarin); monitor anticoagulation levels. May decrease levels of CYP3A/2B6 substrates, clarithromycin, ethinyl estradiol, norethindrone, efavirenz, atazanavir, amprenavir, indinavir, lopinavir, methadone, nelfinavir, boceprevir, telaprevir, antiarrhythmics, anticonvulsants, ketoconazole, itraconazole, calcium channel blockers, cancer chemotherapy, ergot alkaloids, immunosuppressants, motility agents, and opiate agonists. Fluconazole may increase levels and rifampin may decrease levels. Refer to PI for further information when used with certain concomitant therapies.

PREGNANCY AND LACTATION
Category B, not for use in nursing.

MECHANISM OF ACTION
NNRTI; binds directly to reverse transcriptase and blocks RNA-dependent and DNA-dependent DNA polymerase activities by causing a disruption of the enzyme's catalytic site.

PHARMACOKINETICS
Absorption: Readily absorbed. IR: Absolute bioavailability (93%, tab), (91%, sus); C_{max}=2mcg/mL; T_{max}=4 hrs. ER (single dose): AUC=161,000ng•hr/mL; C_{max}=2060ng/mL; T_{max}=24 hrs (median). **Distribution:** V_d=1.21L/kg (IV, healthy); plasma protein binding (60%). Crosses placenta; found in breast milk. **Metabolism:** Liver (extensive); glucuronide conjugation, oxidative metabolism via CYP3A and CYP2B6. **Elimination:** $T_{1/2}$=45 hrs (single dose), 25-30 hrs (multiple dosing). IR: Urine (81.3%; <3%, parent drug), feces (10.1%).

PATIENT CONSIDERATIONS

Assessment: Assess for hepatic fibrosis/cirrhosis, hepatitis B or C coinfection, pregnancy/nursing status, and possible drug interactions. Obtain baseline LFTs. (ER) Assess the ability to swallow tabs in pediatric patients.

Monitoring: Monitor for hepatotoxicity, skin or hypersensitivity reactions, immune reconstitution syndrome, autoimmune disorders, fat redistribution/accumulation, rhabdomyolysis, and other adverse reactions. Perform intensive clinical and lab monitoring, including LFTs, during the first 18 weeks of therapy and frequently throughout treatment. Measure serum transaminases immediately if signs/symptoms of hepatitis, hypersensitivity reactions, and rash develop. Monitor anticoagulation levels with antithrombotics (eg, warfarin).

Counseling: Inform about the risks and benefits of therapy. Inform that severe liver disease/skin reactions may occur. Counsel about signs/symptoms of hepatotoxicity, skin reactions, and other adverse reactions, and advise to d/c and seek medical evaluation immediately if any occur. Inform to take drug as prescribed. Instruct not to alter the dose without consulting physician. Inform that therapy is not a cure for HIV-1 infection and that illnesses associated with HIV-1 infection, including opportunistic infections, may still occur. Advise to avoid doing things that can spread HIV-1 infection to others (eg, sharing needles or other inj equipment, sharing personal items that can have blood or body fluids on them [toothbrush, razor blades], breastfeeding). Instruct not to have any kind of sex without protection; inform to always practice safe sex by using a latex or polyurethane condom to lower the chance of sexual contact with semen, vaginal secretions, or blood. Advise to notify physician of the use of any other prescription/OTC medication, or herbal products, particularly St. John's wort. Inform women taking therapy that hormonal methods of birth control should not be used as the sole method of contraception. Inform that fat redistribution may occur. Instruct not to take IR tabs/sus and ER tabs at the same time. (ER) Advise that soft remnants of the drug may be seen in stool.

VIREAD — tenofovir disoproxil fumarate   Rx
Class: Nucleoside reverse transcriptase inhibitor (NRTI)

> Lactic acidosis and severe hepatomegaly w/ steatosis, including fatal cases, reported w/ the use of nucleoside analogues in combination w/ other antiretrovirals. Severe acute exacerbations of hepatitis reported in hepatitis B virus (HBV)-infected patients who have discontinued therapy; closely monitor hepatic function w/ both clinical and lab follow-up for at least several months. If appropriate, resumption of antihepatitis B therapy may be warranted.

ADULT DOSAGE
HIV-1 Infection

In Combination w/ Other Antiretroviral Agents:
300mg tab qd; may use oral powder (7.5 scoops) if unable to swallow tabs

Chronic Hepatitis B
300mg tab qd; may use oral powder (7.5 scoops) if unable to swallow tabs

PEDIATRIC DOSAGE
HIV-1 Infection

In Combination w/ Other Antiretroviral Agents:
2 to <12 Years:
8mg/kg qd as tabs or oral powder
Max: 300mg qd

≥12 Years (≥35kg):
300mg tab qd; may use oral powder (7.5 scoops) if unable to swallow tabs

Dosing Recommendations for Pediatric Patients ≥2 Years Using Oral Powder:
10 to <12kg: 2 scoops qd
12 to <14kg: 2.5 scoops qd
14 to <17kg: 3 scoops qd
17 to <19kg: 3.5 scoops qd
19 to <22kg: 4 scoops qd
22 to <24kg: 4.5 scoops qd
24 to <27kg: 5 scoops qd
27 to <29kg: 5.5 scoops qd
29 to <32kg: 6 scoops qd
32 to <34kg: 6.5 scoops qd
34 to <35kg: 7 scoops qd
≥35kg: 7.5 scoops qd

Dosing Recommendations for Pediatric Patients ≥2 Years and Weighing ≥17kg Using Tabs:
17 to <22kg: 150mg qd
22 to <28kg: 200mg qd
28 to <35kg: 250mg qd
≥35kg: 300mg qd

Chronic Hepatitis B

≥12 Years (≥35kg):
300mg tab qd; may use oral powder (7.5 scoops) if unable to swallow tabs

DOSING CONSIDERATIONS
Renal Impairment
Adults:
CrCl ≥50mL/min: 300mg tab q24h
CrCl 30-49mL/min: 300mg tab q48h
CrCl 10-29mL/min: 300mg tab q72-96h
Hemodialysis: 300mg tab every 7 days or after a total of approx 12 hrs of dialysis; administer following completion of dialysis

ADMINISTRATION
Oral route

Take tabs w/o regard to food.

Oral Powder
Measure only w/ the supplied dosing scoop.
One level scoop contains 40mg of tenofovir disoproxil fumarate.
Mix w/ 2-4 oz of soft food not requiring chewing (eg, applesauce, baby food, yogurt) and administer entire mixture immediately.
Do not administer in a liquid.

STORAGE
25°C (77°F); excursions permitted to 15-30°C (59-86°F).

HOW SUPPLIED
Oral Powder: 40mg/g [60g]; **Tab:** 150mg, 200mg, 250mg, 300mg

WARNINGS/PRECAUTIONS
Obesity and prolonged nucleoside exposure may be risk factors for lactic acidosis and severe hepatomegaly w/ steatosis. Caution w/ known risk factors for liver disease. D/C if findings suggestive of lactic acidosis or pronounced hepatotoxicity develop. Renal impairment (eg, acute renal failure, Fanconi syndrome) reported; assess CrCl prior to initiating and as clinically appropriate during therapy. In patients at risk of renal dysfunction, including patients who have previously experienced renal events while receiving adefovir dipivoxil, assess CrCl, serum phosphorus (P), urine glucose, and urine protein prior to initiation and periodically during therapy. Promptly evaluate renal function in at-risk patients w/ persistent/worsening bone pain, pain in extremities, fractures, and/or muscular pain/weakness. Use only in HIV-1 and HBV coinfected patients as part of an appropriate antiretroviral combination regimen. Before initiating therapy, offer HIV-1 antibody testing to all HBV-infected patients and test all patients w/ HIV-1 for presence of chronic hepatitis B. Decreased bone mineral density (BMD) and increased biochemical markers of bone metabolism reported; consider assessment of BMD for patients w/ history of pathologic bone fracture or other risk factors for osteoporosis or bone loss. Osteomalacia associated w/ proximal renal tubulopathy reported; consider hypophosphatemia and osteomalacia secondary to proximal renal tubulopathy in patients at risk of renal dysfunction who present w/ persistent or worsening bone or muscle symptoms. Redistribution/accumulation of body fat and immune reconstitution syndrome reported. Autoimmune disorders (eg, Graves' disease, polymyositis, Guillain-Barre syndrome) reported in the setting of immune reconstitution and can occur many months after initiation of treatment. Early virological failure and high rates of resistance substitutions reported w/ certain regimens that only contain 3 nucleoside reverse transcriptase inhibitors; use triple nucleoside regimens w/ caution. Caution in elderly.

ADVERSE REACTIONS
HIV-1 Infection: Rash, diarrhea, headache, pain, depression, asthenia, nausea.
Chronic Hepatitis B and Compensated Liver Disease: Nausea.
Chronic Hepatitis B and Decompensated Liver Disease: Abdominal pain, N/V, insomnia, pruritus, dizziness, pyrexia.

DRUG INTERACTIONS
Avoid w/ concurrent or recent use of nephrotoxic agents (eg, high-dose or multiple NSAIDs). Do not coadminister w/ tenofovir disoproxil fumarate (TDF)-containing products or w/ adefovir dipivoxil. May increase levels of didanosine; d/c didanosine if didanosine-associated adverse reactions develop. Decreases levels of atazanavir; do not coadminister w/ atazanavir w/o ritonavir. Lopinavir/ritonavir, atazanavir w/ ritonavir, and darunavir w/ ritonavir may increase levels; d/c treatment if TDF-associated adverse reactions develop. P-gp and breast cancer resistance protein transporter inhibitors may increase absorption. Coadministration w/ Harvoni may increase tenofovir exposure; monitor for TDF-associated adverse reactions w/ concomitant Harvoni w/o HIV-1 protease inhibitor/ritonavir or an HIV-1 protease inhibitor/cobicistat combination. Consider alternative hepatitis C virus or antiretroviral therapy in patients receiving concomitant Harvoni and an HIV-1 protease inhibitor/ritonavir or an HIV-1 protease inhibitor/cobicistat combination); if coadministration is necessary, monitor for TDF-associated adverse reactions. Coadministration w/ drugs that reduce renal function or compete for active tubular secretion (eg, cidofovir, acyclovir, aminoglycosides [eg, gentamicin], high-dose or multiple NSAIDs) may increase levels of tenofovir and/or the levels of other renally eliminated drugs. Refer to PI for dosing modifications when used w/ certain concomitant therapies.

PREGNANCY AND LACTATION
Pregnancy: Category B. Physicians are encouraged to register patients in the Antiretroviral Pregnancy Registry.
Lactation: Mothers should be instructed not to breastfeed due to potential for HIV-1 transmission.

MECHANISM OF ACTION
Nucleotide analogue reverse transcriptase inhibitor; inhibits activity of HIV-1 reverse transcriptase and HBV reverse transcriptase by competing w/ natural substrate deoxyadenosine 5'-triphosphate and, after incorporation into DNA, by DNA chain termination.

PHARMACOKINETICS
Absorption: Adults: (Fasted) Bioavailability (25%); (Fasted, 300mg single dose) C_{max}=0.30mcg/mL, T_{max}=1 hr, AUC=2.29mcg•hr/mL. Pediatric Patients: (12 to <18 yrs of age, 300mg tab) C_{max}=0.38mcg/mL, AUC=3.39mcg•hr/mL; (2 to <12 yrs of age, 8mg/kg oral powder) C_{max}=0.24mcg/mL, AUC=2.59mcg•hr/mL.
Distribution: Plasma or serum protein binding (less than 0.7 and 7.2%, respectively); V_d=1.3L/kg (1mg/kg IV dose), 1.2L/kg (3mg/kg IV dose); found in breast milk.
Elimination: (Fed, 300mg qd multiple doses) Urine (32%); (Single dose) $T_{1/2}$=17 hrs.

PATIENT CONSIDERATIONS
Assessment: Assess for risk factors for lactic acidosis or liver disease, renal dysfunction, pregnancy/nursing status, and possible drug interactions. In patients at risk of renal dysfunction, assess CrCl, serum P, urine glucose, and urine protein. Test for HIV-1 antibody (in HBV-infected patients) and presence of chronic hepatitis B (in patients w/ HIV-1). Assess BMD in patients w/ history of pathologic bone fracture or other risk factors for osteoporosis or bone loss.
Monitoring: Monitor for signs/symptoms of lactic acidosis, hepatomegaly w/ steatosis, hepatotoxicity, renal impairment, bone effects, redistribution/accumulation of body fat, immune reconstitution syndrome (eg, opportunistic infections), autoimmune disorders, and other adverse reactions. Closely monitor hepatic function w/ both clinical and lab follow-up for at least several months in HBV-infected patients who have discontinued therapy. In patients at risk of renal dysfunction, monitor CrCl, serum P, urine glucose, and urine protein periodically. Periodically monitor weight in pediatric patients to guide dose adjustment.
Counseling: Inform about risks and benefits of therapy. Inform that therapy is not a cure for HIV-1 and patients may continue to experience illness associated w/ HIV-1 infection (eg, opportunistic infections). Instruct to avoid doing things that can spread HIV or HBV to others (eg, sharing of needles/inj equipment or personal items that can have blood/body fluids on them). Advise to always practice safer sex by using latex or polyurethane condoms. Instruct not to breastfeed. Instruct not to d/c w/o 1st informing physician. Counsel about the importance of adhering to regular dosing schedule and to avoid missing doses.

VISTIDE — cidofovir

Rx

Class: Viral DNA synthesis inhibitor

Renal impairment is the major toxicity. Cases of acute renal failure resulting in dialysis and/or contributing to death reported with as few as 1 or 2 doses; prehydrate with IV normal saline (NS) and administer probenecid with each dose. Monitor renal function (SrCr and urine protein) within 48 hrs prior to each dose. Modify dose with renal function changes. Contraindicated with nephrotoxic agents. Neutropenia reported; monitor neutrophil counts. Carcinogenic, teratogenic, and hypospermatic in animal studies.

ADULT DOSAGE
Cytomegalovirus Retinitis

Treatment in Patients w/ AIDS:
Initial: 5mg/kg once weekly for 2 consecutive weeks
Maint: 5mg/kg once every 2 weeks

Probenecid must be administered PO w/ each dose of cidofovir; administer 2g 3 hrs prior to cidofovir dose, and 1g at 2 hrs and again at 8 hrs after completion of the 1-hr infusion (for a total of 4g)

PEDIATRIC DOSAGE
Pediatric use may not have been established

DOSING CONSIDERATIONS
Renal Impairment
SrCr 0.3-0.4mg/dL Above Baseline: Reduce maint dose to 3mg/kg
SrCr ≥0.5mg/dL Above Baseline or Development of ≥3+ Proteinuria: D/C therapy

ADMINISTRATION
IV route

Preparation and Administration
1. Extract the appropriate volume of cidofovir from the vial and transfer the dose to an infusion bag containing 100mL 0.9% NS sol.
2. Infuse the entire volume into the patient at a constant rate over a 1-hr period; use of a standard infusion pump for administration is recommended.

Hydration
Administer at least 1L of 0.9% NS sol IV w/ each infusion of cidofovir. Infuse NS over a 1- to 2-hr period immediately before cidofovir infusion. Patients who can tolerate additional fluid load should receive a 2nd liter; if administered, the 2nd liter should be initiated either at the start of the cidofovir infusion or immediately afterwards, and infused over a 1- to 3-hr period.

STORAGE
Vial: 20-25°C (68-77°F). **Admixture:** Under refrigeration, 2-8°C (36-46°F), for no more than 24 hrs. If refrigerated, allow admixture to equilibrate to room temperature prior to use.

HOW SUPPLIED
Inj: 75mg/mL

CONTRAINDICATIONS
Initiation of therapy in patients w/ SrCr >1.5mg/dL, CrCl ≤55mL/min, or urine protein ≥100mg/dL (≥2+ proteinuria). Nephrotoxic agents (d/c at least 7 days before therapy). Direct intraocular use. Hypersensitivity to cidofovir. History of clinically severe hypersensitivity to probenecid or other sulfa-containing medications.

WARNINGS/PRECAUTIONS
Decreased intraocular pressure (IOP) and visual acuity reported; monitor IOP. Decreased serum bicarbonate associated with proximal tubule injury and renal wasting syndrome (including Fanconi's syndrome) reported. Cases of metabolic acidosis in association with liver dysfunction and pancreatitis resulting in death reported. Do not administer doses greater than recommended or exceed frequency or rate of administration. Uveitis or iritis reported; consider treatment with topical corticosteroids with or without topical cycloplegic agents. Monitor for signs and symptoms of uveitis/iritis.

ADVERSE REACTIONS
Renal toxicity, N/V, neutropenia, proteinuria, decreased IOP, uveitis/iritis, pneumonia, dyspnea, infection, fever, creatinine elevation ≥2mg/dL, decreased serum bicarbonate.

DRUG INTERACTIONS
See Contraindications.

PREGNANCY AND LACTATION
Category C, not for use in nursing.

MECHANISM OF ACTION
Viral DNA synthesis inhibitor; suppresses CMV replication by selective inhibition of viral DNA synthesis.

PHARMACOKINETICS
Absorption: Administration of variable doses (with or without probenecid) resulted in different parameters. **Distribution:** V_d=537mL/kg (without probenecid), 410mL/kg (with probenecid); plasma protein binding (<6%). **Elimination:** Urine (80-100% unchanged).

PATIENT CONSIDERATIONS
Assessment: Assess renal function (SrCr and urine protein) within 48 hrs prior to each dose, history of clinically severe hypersensitivity to probenecid or other sulfa-containing agents, pregnancy/nursing status, and possible drug interactions.

Monitoring: Monitor renal function and adjust dose as required. Give IV hydration to patients with proteinuria and repeat test as necessary. Monitor WBC counts with differential (prior to each dose), and neutrophil count. IOP, visual acuity, and ocular symptoms should be monitored periodically.

Counseling: Inform that drug does not cure CMV retinitis and that patient may continue to experience progression of retinitis during and following treatment. Advise to have regular follow-up ophthalmologic examinations. Advise to temporarily d/c zidovudine administration, or decrease zidovudine dose by 1/2, on days of cidofovir administration only. Inform of the major toxicity of the drug. Counsel on importance of completing a full course of probenecid with each cidofovir dose. Warn of potential adverse events caused by probenecid. Inform that drug may cause tumors in humans. Advise men that testes weight reduction and hypospermia may occur and may cause infertility. Inform of embryotoxicity in animal studies; advise women of childbearing potential to use effective contraception during and for 1 month following therapy and for men to practice barrier contraceptive methods during and for 3 months after therapy.

VISUDYNE — verteporfin   Rx

Class: Photosensitizing agent

ADULT DOSAGE	PEDIATRIC DOSAGE

ADULT DOSAGE

Subfoveal Choroidal Neovascularization

Treatment of patients w/ predominantly classic subfoveal choroidal neovascularization due to age-related macular degeneration, pathologic myopia, or presumed ocular histoplasmosis

6mg/m² IV, diluted in D5 for inj (30mL total volume), over 10 min at 3mL/min.
Initiate 689nm wavelength laser light therapy w/ nonthermal diode laser 15 min after start of 10-min IV infusion; in choroidal neovascularization, recommended light dose is 50J/cm² of neovascular lesion at an intensity of 600mW/cm² over 83 sec

Reevaluate after 3 months and repeat if choroidal neovascular leakage is detected on fluorescein angiography

PEDIATRIC DOSAGE
Pediatric use may not have been established

Concurrent Bilateral Treatment: Patients w/ Previous Verteporfin Therapy in 1 Eye w/ Acceptable Safety Profile:
Both eyes can be treated concurrently after a single administration of verteporfin.
More aggressive lesion should be treated 1st at 15 min after start of infusion; immediately at end of light application to 1st eye, adjust laser settings to introduce treatment parameters for 2nd eye, w/ same light dose and intensity as for 1st eye, starting no later than 20 min from start of infusion.

Patients w/o Prior Verteporfin Therapy:
Treat only 1 eye (most aggressive lesion) at 1st course; 1 week after the 1st course, if no significant safety issues are identified, treat the 2nd eye using the same treatment regimen after a 2nd verteporfin infusion. Evaluate after 3 months and start concurrent therapy following a new infusion if both lesions still show evidence of leakage.

Refer to PI for more information

ADMINISTRATION
IV route
- Reconstitute each vial w/ 7mL of sterile water for inj to provide 7.5mL containing 2mg/mL.
- Dilute reconstituted sol in D5 for inj (30mL total volume).
- Inject via syringe pump and in-line filter over 10 min at 3mL/min.
- Do not use NS or other parenteral sol, except D5 for inj, for dilution.
- Do not mix w/ other drugs in the same sol.
- Protect from light and use w/in 4 hrs of reconstitution.
- Only use compatible lasers.

STORAGE
20-25°C (68-77°F).

HOW SUPPLIED
Inj: 15mg

CONTRAINDICATIONS
Porphyria, known hypersensitivity to any component of this preparation.

WARNINGS/PRECAUTIONS
Avoid extravasation; if extravasation occurs, d/c infusion immediately; protect area from direct light until swelling and discoloration fade. Avoid exposure of skin or eyes to direct sunlight or bright indoor light for 5 days following inj. Protect from intense light if surgery w/in 48 hrs after therapy is necessary. Do not retreat if severe vision decrease of ≥4 lines w/in 1 week after therapy occurs; consider retreatment after vision completely recovers to pretreatment levels and benefits outweigh risks. Reduced effects w/ increasing age.

ADVERSE REACTIONS
Inj-site reactions (including pain, edema, inflammation), visual disturbances (including blurred vision, flashes of light, decreased visual acuity).

DRUG INTERACTIONS
Calcium channel blockers, polymyxin B, and radiation therapy may enhance rate of uptake by vascular endothelium. Other photosensitizing agents (eg, tetracyclines, sulfonamides, phenothiazines) may increase the potential for skin photosensitivity reactions. Compounds that quench active oxygen species or scavenge radicals (eg, dimethyl sulfoxide, β-carotene, ethanol, formate, mannitol) may decrease activity. Drugs that decrease clotting, vasoconstriction, or platelet aggregation (eg, thromboxane A_2 inhibitors) may decrease efficacy.

PREGNANCY AND LACTATION
Pregnancy: Should be used during pregnancy only if potential benefit justifies potential risk to fetus.
Lactation: Verteporfin and its diacid metabolite have been found in human breast milk; not for use in nursing.

MECHANISM OF ACTION
Photosensitizing agent; activated by light in presence of oxygen; light activation causes local damage to neovascular endothelium, subsequently leading to vessel occlusion. Damaged endothelium releases procoagulant and vasoactive factors through lipo-oxygenase and cyclo-oxygenase pathways, resulting in platelet aggregation, fibrin clot formation, and vasoconstriction.

PHARMACOKINETICS
Distribution: Found in breast milk. **Metabolism:** Liver and plasma esterases; diacid metabolite. **Elimination:** Feces (major), urine (<0.01%); $T_{1/2}$=5-6 hrs.

PATIENT CONSIDERATIONS
Assessment: Assess for drug hypersensitivity, porphyria, pregnancy/nursing status, and possible drug interactions.

Monitoring: Monitor for signs/symptoms of extravasation or inj-site reactions, severe decreases in vision, and hypersensitivity reactions. Monitor that IV line is free flowing.

Counseling: Advise that temporary photosensitivity will occur after infusion. Advise to wear wrist band reminder to avoid direct sunlight for 5 days; advise to avoid exposure of unprotected skin, eyes, or other body organs to direct sunlight or bright indoor light. Advise that prolonged exposure to light from light-emitting medical devices (eg, pulse oximeters) should also be avoided for 5 days. Advise to protect all parts of skin and eyes by wearing protective clothing and dark sunglasses. Advise to not stay in the dark and encourage to expose skin to ambient indoor light. Advise that visual disturbances may develop that may interfere w/ ability to drive or use machines; advise not to drive or use machines as long as symptoms persist.

VITEKTA — elvitegravir   Rx

Class: HIV-integrase strand transfer inhibitor

ADULT DOSAGE

HIV-1 Infection

In combination w/ an HIV protease inhibitor coadministered w/ ritonavir (RTV) and other antiretroviral drug(s) in treatment-experienced patients

85mg Dose:
85mg qd + atazanavir 300mg qd + RTV 100mg qd
or
85mg qd + lopinavir 400mg bid + RTV 100mg bid

150mg Dose:
150mg qd + darunavir 600mg bid + RTV 100mg bid
or
150mg qd + fosamprenavir 700mg bid + RTV 100mg bid
or
150mg qd + tipranavir 500mg bid + RTV 200mg bid

PEDIATRIC DOSAGE
Pediatric use may not have been established

DOSING CONSIDERATIONS
Hepatic Impairment
Severe: Not recommended for use

ADMINISTRATION
Oral route
Take w/ food.

STORAGE
Room temperature <30°C (86°F).

HOW SUPPLIED
Tab: 85mg, 150mg

CONTRAINDICATIONS
Refer to the individual PIs for coadministered protease inhibitor and RTV.

WARNINGS/PRECAUTIONS
Immune reconstitution syndrome reported. Autoimmune disorders (eg, Graves' disease, polymyositis, Guillain-Barre syndrome) reported in the setting of immune reconstitution and can occur many months after initiation of treatment. Caution in elderly.

ADVERSE REACTIONS
Diarrhea, nausea, headache, hyperbilirubinemia, hematuria, increased serum amylase/creatine kinase/GGT, hypercholesterolemia, hypertriglyceridemia, hyperglycemia, glucosuria, neutropenia.

DRUG INTERACTIONS
Coadministration w/ HIV-1 protease inhibitors other than RTV, atazanavir, lopinavir, darunavir, fosamprenavir, or tipranavir is not recommended. Use w/ elvitegravir-containing drugs (eg, Stribild) is not recommended. Use in combination w/ a protease inhibitor and cobicistat is not recommended; may result in suboptimal levels of elvitegravir and/or the protease inhibitor, leading to loss of therapeutic effect and development of resistance. Coadministration w/ efavirenz, nevirapine, St. John's wort, rifampin, rifapentine, phenobarbital, phenytoin, carbamazepine, or oxcarbazepine is not recommended; may decrease elvitegravir levels. Coadministration w/ boceprevir is not recommended; may reduce levels of boceprevir and may alter levels of HIV protease inhibitors. CYP3A inducers may increase the clearance of elvitegravir, as well as RTV; may result in decreased plasma levels of elvitegravir and/or a concomitantly administered protease inhibitor and lead to loss of therapeutic effect and to possible resistance. Atazanavir/RTV, lopinavir/RTV, and ketoconazole may increase elvitegravir levels. Administer didanosine at least 1 hr before or 2 hrs after elvitegravir. Antacids may decrease levels; separate elvitegravir and antacid administration by at least 2 hrs. Coadministration w/ systemic dexamethasone may decrease levels; consider alternative corticosteroids. Rifabutin or bosentan may decrease levels. May increase levels of ketoconazole, bosentan, rifabutin, or 25-O-desacetylrifabutin. May increase norgestimate and decrease ethinyl estradiol levels; alternative methods of nonhormonal contraception are recommended. May increase levels of buprenorphine and norbuprenorphine and may decrease levels of naloxone and methadone. Closely monitor for sedation and cognitive effects when coadministered w/ buprenorphine/naloxone. Refer to PI for further information on drug interactions, including dose modifications required when used w/ certain concomitant therapies.

PREGNANCY AND LACTATION
Pregnancy: Category B. Physicians are encouraged to register patients in the Antiretroviral Pregnancy Registry.
Lactation: Not for use in nursing.

MECHANISM OF ACTION
HIV-1 integrase strand transfer inhibitor; prevents the integration of HIV-1 DNA into host genomic DNA, blocking the formation of the HIV-1 provirus and propagation of the viral infection.

PHARMACOKINETICS
Absorption: T_{max}=4 hrs; C_{max}=1.2mcg/mL (85mg), 1.5mcg/mL (150mg); AUC_{tau}=18mcg•hr/mL. **Distribution:** Plasma protein binding (98-99%). **Metabolism:** Oxidation via CYP3A; glucuronidation via UGT1A1/3. **Elimination:** Feces (94.8%), urine (6.7% as metabolites); $T_{1/2}$=8.7 hrs (median).

PATIENT CONSIDERATIONS
Assessment: Assess for severe hepatic impairment, pregnancy/nursing status, and for possible drug interactions.
Monitoring: Monitor for signs/symptoms of immune reconstitution syndrome, autoimmune disorders, and for other adverse reactions.
Counseling: Advise patients to remain under the care of a healthcare provider during therapy. Inform that drug is not a cure for HIV-1 infection and continuous therapy is necessary to control HIV-1 infection and decrease HIV-related illnesses. Advise to continue to practice safer sex, to use latex or polyurethane condoms, and to not reuse/share needles. Instruct to take ud, on a regular dosing schedule w/ food, and to avoid missing doses. Inform that therapy may interact w/ many drugs; advise to notify physician if using any other prescription or nonprescription medication or herbal product (eg, St. John's wort). Advise to inform physician immediately if any symptoms of infection develop.

VIVITROL — naltrexone   Rx

Class: Opioid antagonist

ADULT DOSAGE

Alcohol Dependence

Treatment of Alcohol Dependence in Patients Who are Able to Abstain from Alcohol in an Outpatient Setting Prior to Initiation of Therapy:
380mg IM every 4 weeks or once a month

Prior to initiating therapy, an opioid-free duration of a minimum of 7-10 days is recommended

Opioid Dependence

Prevention of Relapse to Opioid Dependence, Following Opioid Detoxification:
380mg IM every 4 weeks or once a month

Prior to initiating therapy, an opioid-free duration of a minimum of 7-10 days is recommended

Conversions

Switching from Buprenorphine, Buprenorphine/Naloxone, or Methadone:
Be prepared to manage withdrawal symptomatically w/ nonopioid medications

PEDIATRIC DOSAGE
Pediatric use may not have been established

ADMINISTRATION
IM route

Administer as IM gluteal inj, alternating buttocks for each subsequent inj. Must be suspended only in the diluent supplied in the carton and must be administered only w/ 1 of the administration needles supplied in the carton; do not substitute any other components for the components of the carton.
For patients w/ a larger amount of subcutaneous tissue overlying the gluteal muscle, may utilize the supplied 2-inch needle to help ensure that the injectate reaches the IM mass.
For very lean patients, the 1.5-inch needle may be appropriate to prevent the needle contacting the periosteum.
Either needle may be used for patients w/ average body habitus.
Prior to preparation, allow drug to reach room temperature (approx 45 min).
Refer to PI for further preparation and administration instructions.

STORAGE
2-8°C (36-46°F). Do not freeze. Can be stored at ≤25°C (77°F) for no more than 7 days prior administration.

HOW SUPPLIED
Inj, Extended-Release: 380mg

CONTRAINDICATIONS
Concomitant opioid analgesics; current physiologic opioid dependence; acute opioid withdrawal; failure of naloxone challenge test or positive urine screen for opioids; previous hypersensitivity to naltrexone, polylactide-co-glycolide, carboxymethylcellulose, or any other components of the diluent.

WARNINGS/PRECAUTIONS
Patients may have reduced tolerance to opioids after opioid detoxification; may result in potentially life-threatening opioid intoxication with use of previously tolerated opioid doses. Potential risk to patients attempting to overcome the antagonism by

taking opioids; may lead to life-threatening opioid intoxication or fatal overdose. Inj-site reactions reported; inadvertent SQ inj may increase likelihood of severe inj-site reactions. Withdrawal syndrome, severe enough to require hospitalization, may occur when withdrawal is precipitated abruptly by the administration of an opioid antagonist to an opioid-dependent patient. Opioid-dependent patients, including those being treated for alcohol dependence, should be opioid-free before starting treatment to reduce risk of either precipitated withdrawal in patients dependent on opioids or exacerbation of a preexisting subclinical withdrawal syndrome; an opioid-free interval of a minimum of 7-10 days is recommended for patients previously dependent on short-acting opioids. May experience severe manifestations of precipitated withdrawal when being switched from opioid agonist to opioid antagonist therapy; patients transitioning from buprenorphine or methadone may be vulnerable to precipitation of withdrawal symptoms for as long as 2 weeks. A naloxone challenge test may be helpful to determine if patient is opioid-free; however, precipitated withdrawal may occur despite having negative urine toxicology screen or tolerating a naloxone challenge test. Cases of hepatitis, clinically significant liver dysfunction, and transient, asymptomatic hepatic transaminase elevations reported; d/c in the event of symptoms and/or signs of acute hepatitis. Depression and suicidality reported. In emergency situations, suggested plan for pain management is regional analgesia or use of nonopioid analgesics. If opioid therapy is required, monitor continuously in an anesthesia care setting. Cases of eosinophilic pneumonia and hypersensitivity reactions, including anaphylaxis, reported. As with any IM inj, caution with thrombocytopenia or any coagulation disorder (eg, hemophilia, severe hepatic failure). Does not eliminate or diminish alcohol withdrawal symptoms. May cross-react with certain immunoassay methods for the detection of drugs of abuse in urine. Caution with moderate to severe renal impairment.

ADVERSE REACTIONS
N/V, diarrhea, insomnia, depression, inj-site reactions, somnolence, anorexia, muscle cramps, dizziness, syncope, appetite disorder, hepatic enzyme abnormalities, nasopharyngitis, toothache, headache.

DRUG INTERACTIONS
See Contraindications. Antagonizes effects of opioid-containing medicines (eg, cough and cold remedies, antidiarrheals, opioid analgesics).

PREGNANCY AND LACTATION
Pregnancy: Category C.
Lactation: Not for use in nursing.

MECHANISM OF ACTION
Opioid antagonist; blocks the effects of opioids by competitive binding at opioid receptors, with the highest affinity for the mu opioid receptor.

PHARMACOKINETICS
Absorption: T_{max}=2 hrs (1st peak), 2-3 days (2nd peak). Distribution: Plasma protein binding (21%); (PO) found in breast milk. Metabolism: Extensive, via dihydrodiol dehydrogenase; 6β-naltrexol (primary metabolite). Elimination: Urine; $T_{1/2}$=5-10 days.

PATIENT CONSIDERATIONS
Assessment: Assess for opioid use, acute opioid withdrawal, thrombocytopenia, coagulation disorders, renal impairment, any other conditions where treatment is contraindicated or cautioned, pregnancy/nursing status, and possible drug interactions. Assess patients, including patients treated for alcohol dependence, for underlying opioid dependence, and for any recent use of opioids. Assess body habitus to assure that needle length is adequate.

Monitoring: Monitor for opioid intoxication/overdose, severe inj-site reactions, precipitation of opioid withdrawal, signs/symptoms of acute hepatitis, depression, suicidality, hypersensitivity reactions, and other adverse reactions.

Counseling: Advise that if they previously used opioids, they may be more sensitive to lower doses of opioids and at risk of accidental overdose if they use opioids when their next dose is due, if they miss a dose, or after treatment is discontinued. Advise that patients will not perceive any effect if they attempt to self-administer heroin or any other opioid drug in small doses while on therapy. Inform that administration of large doses of heroin or any other opioid to try to bypass the blockade may lead to serious injury, coma, or death. Inform that patient may not experience the expected effects from opioid-containing analgesic, antidiarrheal, or antitussive medications. Advise that inj-site reactions may occur and instruct to seek medical attention for worsening skin reactions. Instruct to be off all opioids for a minimum of 7-10 days before starting therapy in order to avoid precipitation of opioid withdrawal. Advise not to take therapy if they have any symptoms of opioid withdrawal. Advise all patients, including those with alcohol dependence, to notify physician of any recent use of opioids or any history of opioid dependence before starting therapy. Inform that drug may cause liver injury; instruct to immediately notify physician if symptoms and/or signs of liver disease develop. Inform the patient, family members, and caregivers that the patient may experience depression while taking therapy and to contact physician if the patient becomes depressed or symptoms of depression are experienced. Instruct to carry documentation to alert medical personnel to therapy. Advise that drug may cause an allergic pneumonia; instruct to immediately notify physician if signs and symptoms of pneumonia develop. Inform that drug may cause nausea, which tends to subside within a few days post-inj. Advise that they may also experience tiredness, headache, vomiting, decreased appetite, painful joints, and muscle cramps. Advise that therapy has been shown to treat alcohol and opioid dependence only when used as part of a treatment program that includes counseling and support. Advise that dizziness may occur; instruct to avoid driving or operating heavy machinery. Advise to notify physician if pregnant or intending to become pregnant during treatment, breastfeeding, or experiencing unusual or significant side effects while on therapy.

VORAXAZE — glucarpidase   Rx
Class: Enzyme

ADULT DOSAGE	PEDIATRIC DOSAGE
Methotrexate Toxicity	**Methotrexate Toxicity**
Methotrexate (MTX) concentrations (>1µmol/L) in patients w/ delayed MTX clearance due to impaired renal function	Methotrexate (MTX) concentrations (>1µmol/L) in patients w/ delayed MTX clearance due to impaired renal function
Usual: 50 U/kg as a single IV bolus inj over 5 min	**Usual:** 50 U/kg as a single IV bolus inj over 5 min

ADMINISTRATION
IV route

Administer IV as a bolus inj over 5 min
Flush IV line before and after administration

Preparation
Reconstitute contents of vial w/ 1mL of sterile saline for inj
Roll and tilt vial gently to mix; do not shake
Discard any unused product

STORAGE
2-8°C (36-46°F). Do not freeze. Reconstituted Sol: Use immediately or store at 2-8°C (36-46°F) for up to 4 hrs.

HOW SUPPLIED
Inj: 1000 U [vial]

WARNINGS/PRECAUTIONS
Not for use in patients who exhibit expected clearance of MTX or those with normal or mildly impaired renal function because of the potential risk of subtherapeutic exposure to MTX. Serious allergic reactions reported. MTX concentrations within 48 hrs following glucarpidase administration can only be reliably measured by a chromatographic method; measurement of MTX using immunoassays is unreliable for samples collected within 48 hrs following glucarpidase administration. Continue to administer leucovorin after glucarpidase; do not administer leucovorin within 2 hrs before or after a dose of glucarpidase. For the first 48 hrs after glucarpidase, administer the same leucovorin dose as given prior to glucarpidase; beyond 48 hrs after glucarpidase, administer leucovorin based on the measured MTX concentration. Do not d/c therapy with leucovorin based on the determination of a single MTX concentration below the leucovorin treatment threshold. Continue leucovorin until MTX concentration has been maintained below the leucovorin treatment threshold for a minimum of 3 days. Continue hydration and alkalinization of the urine as indicated.

ADVERSE REACTIONS
Paresthesia, flushing, N/V, hypotension, headache.

DRUG INTERACTIONS
May interact with potential exogenous glucarpidase substrates such as reduced folates and folate antimetabolites.

PREGNANCY AND LACTATION
Category C, caution in nursing.

MECHANISM OF ACTION
Carboxypeptidase enzyme; hydrolyzes the carboxyl-terminal glutamate residue from folic acid and classical antifolates such as MTX, and converts MTX to its inactive metabolites. Provides an alternative nonrenal pathway for MTX elimination in patients with renal dysfunction during high-dose MTX treatment.

PHARMACOKINETICS
Absorption: C_{max}=3.3mcg/mL, AUC=23.3mcg•hr/mL. Distribution: V_d=3.6L. Elimination: $T_{1/2}$=5.6 hrs.

PATIENT CONSIDERATIONS
Assessment: Assess for renal impairment, pregnancy/nursing status, and for possible drug interactions. Assess MTX concentrations.

Monitoring: Monitor for serious allergic reactions and other adverse reactions. Monitor MTX concentrations (using a chromatographic method when measuring within 48 hrs following administration) and renal function.

Counseling: Inform that allergic reactions, including potentially serious reactions, may occur during treatment. Advise to immediately report to physician any signs/symptoms of an infusion reaction (eg, fever, chills, flushing, feeling hot, rash, hives, itching, throat tightness/breathing problems, tingling, numbness, headache). Inform of the importance of continued monitoring of MTX blood concentrations and renal status at the appropriate times after discharge from the hospital.

VOTRIENT — pazopanib   Rx
Class: Kinase inhibitor

> Severe and fatal hepatotoxicity reported; monitor hepatic function and interrupt, reduce, or d/c dosing as recommended.

ADULT DOSAGE	PEDIATRIC DOSAGE
Advanced Renal Cell Carcinoma	Pediatric use may not have been established
Initial: 800mg qd w/o food (≥1 hr ac or 2 hrs pc)	
Max: 800mg	
Initial Dose Reduction: 400mg	
Additional Dose Decrease/Increase: Should be in 200mg steps	

Advanced Soft Tissue Sarcoma
Patients Who Have Received Prior Chemotherapy:
Initial: 800mg qd w/o food (≥1 hr ac or 2 hrs pc)
Max: 800mg

Dose Decrease/Increase: Should be in 200mg steps

Missed Dose
If a dose is missed, it should not be taken if it is <12 hrs until the next dose

---

DOSING CONSIDERATIONS
Concomitant Medications
Strong CYP3A4 Inhibitors: Avoid concomitant use; consider an alternate concomitant medication w/ no or minimal potential to inhibit CYP3A4. If coadministration is warranted, reduce pazopanib dose to 400mg; further dose reductions may be needed if adverse effects occur during therapy.
Strong CYP3A4 Inducers: Avoid concomitant use; consider an alternate concomitant medication w/ no or minimal enzyme induction potential. Do not use pazopanib if chronic use of strong CYP3A4 inducers cannot be avoided.

Hepatic Impairment
Mild: No dose adjustment is required.
Moderate: Consider alternative therapy or reduce dose to 200mg/day
Severe: Not recommended for use

ADMINISTRATION
Oral route

Do not crush tabs.
Take w/o food (≥1 hr ac or 2 hrs pc).

STORAGE
20-25°C (68-77°F); excursions permitted to 15-30°C (59-86°F).

HOW SUPPLIED
Tab: 200mg

WARNINGS/PRECAUTIONS
Patients >65 yrs of age are at greater risk for hepatotoxicity. QT prolongation and torsades de pointes reported. Cardiac dysfunction (eg, decreased left ventricular ejection fraction [LVEF], CHF) reported. Hemorrhagic events reported; avoid w/ history of hemoptysis, cerebral hemorrhage, or clinically significant GI hemorrhage in the past 6 months. Arterial thromboembolic events (ATEs) reported; caution in patients at increased risk for these events or who have had a history of these events and avoid use if an ATE has occurred w/in the past 6 months. Venous thromboembolic events (VTEs) (eg, pulmonary embolism [PE]) and GI perforation/fistula reported. Thrombotic microangiopathy (TMA), including thrombotic thrombocytopenic purpura (TTP) and hemolytic uremic syndrome (HUS), reported; permanently d/c in patients developing TMA. Interstitial lung disease (ILD)/pneumonitis reported and can be fatal; d/c therapy if ILD or pneumonitis occurs. Reversible posterior leukoencephalopathy syndrome (RPLS) reported; permanently d/c in patients developing RPLS. HTN and hypertensive crisis reported; d/c if evidence of hypertensive crisis or if HTN is severe and persistent despite antihypertensive therapy and dose reduction. May impair wound healing; d/c therapy w/ wound dehiscence and ≥7 days prior to scheduled surgery. Hypothyroidism reported. Proteinuria reported; interrupt therapy and reduce dose for 24-hr urine protein ≥3g; d/c for repeat episodes despite dose reductions. Serious infections reported; institute appropriate anti-infective therapy promptly and consider interruption or discontinuation if serious infections develop. May cause serious adverse effects on organ development in pediatric patients; not for use in pediatric patients. May cause fetal harm if used during pregnancy.

ADVERSE REACTIONS
Renal Cell Carcinoma: Diarrhea, HTN, hair color changes (depigmentation), N/V, anorexia, fatigue.
Soft Tissue Sarcoma: Fatigue, diarrhea, N/V, decreased weight/appetite, HTN, hair color changes, tumor pain, dysgeusia, headache, musculoskeletal pain, myalgia, GI pain, dyspnea, skin hypopigmentation.

DRUG INTERACTIONS
See Dosing Considerations. Concomitant use w/ proton pump inhibitors (PPIs) (eg, esomeprazole) decreased exposure; avoid concomitant use w/ drugs that raise gastric pH. If such drugs are needed, consider short-acting antacids in place of PPIs and H_2-receptor antagonists; separate antacid and pazopanib dosing by several hrs. Do not use in combination w/ other cancer therapy; increased toxicity and mortality reported w/ pemetrexed and lapatinib. Strong CYP3A4 inhibitors (eg, ketoconazole, ritonavir, clarithromycin) may increase concentrations. Avoid grapefruit or grapefruit juice. CYP3A4 inducers (eg, rifampin) may decrease plasma concentrations; consider an alternate concomitant medication w/ no or minimal enzyme induction potential. Avoid use w/ strong inhibitors of P-gp or breast cancer resistance protein (BCRP), and consider alternative concomitant medicinal products w/ no or minimal potential to inhibit P-gp or BCRP. Not recommended w/ agents w/ narrow therapeutic windows that are metabolized by CYP3A4, CYP2D6, or CYP2C8. Simvastatin may increase incidence of ALT elevations; follow pazopanib dosing guidelines or consider alternatives to pazopanib or consider discontinuing simvastatin. Caution in patients taking antiarrhythmics or other medications that may prolong the QT interval.

PREGNANCY AND LACTATION
Pregnancy: Category D.
Lactation: Not for use in nursing.
Reproductive Potential: Use effective contraception during treatment and for at least 2 weeks after last dose.

MECHANISM OF ACTION
Tyrosine kinase inhibitor; inhibits vascular endothelial growth factor receptor (VEGFR)-1, VEGFR-2, VEGFR-3, platelet-derived growth factor receptor-α and -β, fibroblast growth factor receptor-1 and -3, cytokine receptor, interleukin-2 receptor inducible T-cell kinase, leukocyte-specific protein tyrosine kinase, and transmembrane glycoprotein receptor tyrosine kinase.

PHARMACOKINETICS
Absorption: T_{max}=2-4 hrs (median); (800mg dose) AUC=1037mcg•hr/mL, C_{max}=58.1mcg/mL. **Distribution:** Plasma protein binding (>99%). **Metabolism:** CYP3A4 (major), CYP1A2/CYP2C8 (minor). **Elimination:** Feces (primary), urine (<4% administered dose); (800mg dose) $T_{1/2}$=30.9 hrs.

PATIENT CONSIDERATIONS
Assessment: Assess for history of QT interval prolongation, cardiac disease, hepatic impairment, pregnancy/nursing status, and for possible drug interactions. Assess for history of hemoptysis/cerebral hemorrhage, clinically significant GI hemorrhage, or an ATE in the past 6 months. Assess if patient is planning to undergo any surgical procedure. Assess thyroid function. Obtain baseline BP, LFTs, ECG, electrolytes, and urinalysis. Obtain baseline LVEF in patients at risk of cardiac dysfunction.

Monitoring: Monitor for signs/symptoms of hepatotoxicity, QT prolongation, torsades de pointes, cardiac dysfunction, hemorrhagic events, ATEs, VTEs, TMA, TTP, HUS, PE, RPLS, GI perforation or fistula, ILD/pneumonitis, HTN/hypertensive crisis, impaired wound healing, proteinuria, infections, and other adverse reactions. Monitor BP early after starting treatment and then frequently to ensure BP control. Perform periodic urinalysis w/ follow-up measurement of 24-hr urine protein as clinically indicated. Monitor ECG, thyroid function tests, and serum electrolytes. Monitor LFTs at Weeks 3, 5, 7, and 9, at Months 3 and 4, as clinically indicated, and periodically after Month 4. Periodically monitor LVEF in patients at risk of cardiac dysfunction.

Counseling: Advise the patient to read the FDA-approved patient labeling (Medication Guide). Advise that lab monitoring will be required prior to and while on therapy. Instruct to report any signs/symptoms of liver dysfunction, HTN, CHF, unusual bleeding, arterial thrombosis, new onset of dyspnea, chest pain, localized limb edema, GI perforation/fistula, infection, worsening of neurologic function consistent w/ RPLS, and pulmonary signs/symptoms indicative of ILD or pneumonitis. Advise to d/c treatment ≥7 days prior to a scheduled surgery. Inform that thyroid function testing and urinalysis will be performed during treatment. Advise on how to manage diarrhea and to notify healthcare provider if moderate to severe diarrhea occurs. Advise women of childbearing potential to avoid becoming pregnant during therapy. Advise to inform healthcare provider of all concomitant medications, vitamins, or dietary and herbal supplements. Advise that depigmentation of the hair or skin may occur during treatment. Advise females of childbearing potential to use effective contraception during treatment and for at least 2 weeks after last dose.

VPRIV — velaglucerase alfa   **Rx**
Class: Enzyme

ADULT DOSAGE	PEDIATRIC DOSAGE
Type 1 Gaucher Disease	**Type 1 Gaucher Disease**
Naive to Enzyme Replacement Therapy:	**≥4 Years:**
Initial: 60 U/kg administered every other week as a 60-min IV infusion	**Naive to Enzyme Replacement Therapy:**
Titrate: Adjust dose based on achievement and maint of therapeutic goals	**Initial:** 60 U/kg administered every other week as a 60-min IV infusion
	Titrate: Adjust dose based on achievement and maint of therapeutic goals
Switching from Imiglucerase: Initiate treatment at the previous imiglucerase dose 2 weeks after the last imiglucerase dose	**Switching from Imiglucerase:** Initiate treatment at the previous imiglucerase dose 2 weeks after the last imiglucerase dose
Premedication	**Premedication**
Consider pretreatment w/ antihistamines and/or corticosteroids in patients who exhibited symptoms of hypersensitivity associated w/ prior Vpriv infusions	Consider pretreatment w/ antihistamines and/or corticosteroids in patients who exhibited symptoms of hypersensitivity associated w/ prior Vpriv infusions

---

ADMINISTRATION
IV route

Reconstitution of Lyophilized Powder
1. Determine the number of vials to be reconstituted based on the individual patient's weight and the prescribed dose
2. Inject 4.3mL of sterile water for inj into a vial containing lyophilized powder
3. Mix gently; do not shake. The reconstituted sol will have a 100 U/mL concentration
4. If additional vials are needed, repeat steps 2 and 3

5. W/ a single syringe, withdraw the calculated dose of drug from the appropriate number of vials

6. Using a separate syringe, withdraw air from a bag of 100mL of 0.9% NaCl sol suitable for IV administration, then dilute the calculated dose of Vpriv directly into the NaCl sol

7. Mix gently; do not shake. Slight flocculation (white irregular shaped particles) may occasionally occur; diluted sol w/ slight flocculation is acceptable for administration

8. Use reconstituted sol and diluted sol immediately. If immediate use is not possible, the reconstituted sol or diluted sol may be stored for up to 24 hrs at 2-8°C (36-46°F). Do not freeze and protect from light. Complete the infusion w/in 24 hrs of reconstitution of vials

9. Vials are for single use only. Discard any unused sol

Administration Instructions

Administer the diluted sol through an in-line low protein-binding 0.2μm filter over 60 min

Do not infuse w/ other products in the same infusion tubing

STORAGE

2-8°C (36-46°F). Do not freeze. Protect from light.

HOW SUPPLIED

Inj: 400 U

WARNINGS/PRECAUTIONS

Hypersensitivity reactions, including anaphylaxis, reported; have appropriate medical support readily available. If anaphylactic or other acute reactions occur, d/c infusion immediately and initiate appropriate medical treatment. Manage based on the severity of the reaction (eg, slowing infusion rate; treatment w/ antihistamines, antipyretics, and/or corticosteroids; stopping and resuming treatment w/ increased infusion time). Caution in elderly.

ADVERSE REACTIONS

Hypersensitivity reaction, headache, dizziness, abdominal pain, nausea, back pain, joint pain (knee), prolonged activated PTT, pyrexia, asthenia/fatigue.

PREGNANCY AND LACTATION

Category B, caution in nursing.

MECHANISM OF ACTION

Hydrolytic lysosomal glucocerebroside-specific enzyme; catalyzes the hydrolysis of glucocerebroside, reducing the amount of accumulated glucocerebroside.

PHARMACOKINETICS

Distribution: V_d=82-108mL/kg. **Elimination:** $T_{1/2}$=11-12 min.

PATIENT CONSIDERATIONS

Assessment: Assess for previous hypersensitivity to the drug/other ERT and for pregnancy/nursing status.

Monitoring: Monitor for symptoms of hypersensitivity reactions and other adverse reactions.

Counseling: Advise that treatment is given IV every other week. Advise that treatment may cause hypersensitivity reactions.

VUMON — teniposide   Rx

Class: Podophyllotoxin derivative

> Cytotoxic; administer only under the supervision of a qualified physician experienced in the use of cancer chemotherapeutic agents. Severe myelosuppression with resulting infection or bleeding may occur. Hypersensitivity reactions (eg, anaphylaxis-like symptoms) may occur with initial dosing or at repeated exposure to the drug. Epinephrine, with or without corticosteroids, and antihistamines may be used to alleviate hypersensitivity reaction symptoms.

PEDIATRIC DOSAGE
Refractory Childhood Acute Lymphoblastic Leukemia

Induction Therapy:
165mg/m² w/ cytarabine 300mg/m² twice weekly for 8-9 doses; or 250mg/m² with vincristine 1.5mg/m² IV weekly for 4-8 weeks and prednisone 40mg/m² PO for 28 days

---

DOSING CONSIDERATIONS
Renal Impairment
Dose adjustments may be necessary

Hepatic Impairment
Dose adjustments may be necessary

ADMINISTRATION
IV route

Administer with non-di(2-ethylhexyl) phthalate containing IV administration sets

Refer to PI for preparation for IV administration and administration precautions

STORAGE
2-8°C. Protect from light. Solutions prepared in 0.9% NaCl and D5W 5% at concentrations of 0.1mg/mL, 0.2mg/mL, or 0.4mg/mL are stable at room temperature for up to 24 hrs.

HOW SUPPLIED
Inj: 10mg/mL [5mL]

CONTRAINDICATIONS

Previous hypersensitivity to teniposide and/or Cremophor EL (polyoxyethylated castor oil).

WARNINGS/PRECAUTIONS

If retreating patient with earlier hypersensitivity reaction, pretreat with corticosteroid and antihistamine. Continuously observe for at least the first 60 min after starting infusion and frequently thereafter. D/C immediately if signs or symptoms of anaphylaxis occurs. Give only by slow IV infusion (lasting at least 30-60 min); hypotension reported with rapid IV inj. D/C infusion if significant hypotension develops and administer fluids or other supportive therapy as appropriate. If infusion is restarted, use slower administration rate and monitor patient carefully. Reduce dose or d/c if severe reactions occur; caution with reinstitution of therapy and consider further need for the drug and alertness to possible recurrence of toxicity. Improper administration may result in extravasation causing local tissue necrosis and/or thrombophlebitis. May cause fetal harm when administered during pregnancy. May compromise male patients' ability to father a child or cause birth defects if they do so. Caution with hepatic dysfunction.

ADVERSE REACTIONS

Myelosuppression, hypersensitivity reactions, leukopenia, neutropenia, thrombocytopenia, anemia, mucositis, diarrhea, N/V, infection, alopecia, bleeding, rash, fever.

DRUG INTERACTIONS

Acute CNS depression, hypotension, and metabolic acidosis reported in patients receiving high-dose teniposide who were pretreated with antiemetic drugs. Caution with tolbutamide, sodium salicylate, and sulfamethizole; may potentiate toxicity. May increase plasma clearance of methotrexate. May result in severe myelosuppression with other chemotherapeutic agents. Neurotoxicity including severe neuropathy, reported with vincristine sulfate.

PREGNANCY AND LACTATION

Category D, not for use in nursing.

MECHANISM OF ACTION

Podophyllotoxin derivative; acts in the late S or early G_2 phase of the cell cycle, thus preventing cells from entering mitosis. Inhibits topoisomerase II, causing dose-dependent single- and double-stranded breaks in DNA and DNA-protein cross-links.

PHARMACOKINETICS

Absorption: C_{max}=>40mcg/mL, T_{max}=1-2 hrs. **Distribution:** V_d=3.1L/m²; plasma protein binding (>99%). **Elimination:** Urine, feces; $T_{1/2}$=5 hrs.

PATIENT CONSIDERATIONS

Assessment: Assess for hypersensitivity to the drug and/or polyoxyethylated castor oil, Down syndrome, hypoalbuminemia, renal/hepatic dysfunction, pregnancy/nursing status, and for possible drug interactions. Obtain baseline CBC, Hgb, WBC with differential, platelet count, renal function, and LFTs.

Monitoring: Monitor for myelosuppression, hypersensitivity reactions, extravasation, and CNS depression. Monitor CBC, Hgb, WBC with differential, platelet count, BP, and renal/hepatic function. Perform repeat bone marrow examination prior to continuation of therapy in severe myelosuppression setting. Carefully monitor patients with hypoalbuminemia.

Counseling: Inform of risks/benefits of therapy. Advise women of childbearing potential to avoid becoming pregnant during therapy. Advise men of reproductive age that the drug may compromise their ability to father a child and that there is some possibility for birth defects if they do; counsel on the possibility of storing sperm for future artificial insemination.

WILATE — coagulation factor VIII complex (human)/von Willebrand factor (human)   Rx

Class: von Willebrand factor (vWF)/coagulation factor VIII

ADULT DOSAGE
von Willebrand's Disease

For on-demand treatment and control of bleeding episodes and for perioperative management of bleeding

Dosing for Hemorrhages:
Minor Hemorrhage:
von Willebrand Factor: Ristocetin Cofactor Assay (VWF:RCo) and Factor VIII (FVIII) Activity Trough Levels: >30%
LD: 20-40 IU/kg IV
Maint: 20-30 IU/kg IV q12-24h prn for up to 3 days

Major Hemorrhage:
VWF:RCo and FVIII Activity Trough Levels: >50%
LD: 40-60 IU/kg IV
Maint: 20-40 IU/kg IV q12-24h prn for up to 5-7 days

Repeat doses as needed

Dosing for Surgeries:
Minor (eg, Tooth Extraction):
LD: 30-60 IU/kg w/in 3 hours before surgery
VWF:RCo Peak Levels: 50%

PEDIATRIC DOSAGE
von Willebrand's Disease

For on-demand treatment and control of bleeding episodes and for perioperative management of bleeding

Dosing for Hemorrhages:
VWF:RCo and FVIII Activity Trough Levels: >30%
Minor Hemorrhage:
LD: 20-40 IU/kg IV
Maint: 20-30 IU/kg IV q12-24h prn for up to 3 days

Major Hemorrhage:
VWF:RCo and FVIII Activity Trough Levels: >50%
LD: 40-60 IU/kg IV
Maint: 20-40 IU/kg IV q12-24h prn for up to 5-7 days

Repeat doses as needed

Dosing for Surgeries:
Minor (eg, Tooth Extraction):
LD: 30-60 IU/kg w/in 3 hours before surgery
VWF:RCo Peak Levels: 50%
Maint: 15-30 IU/kg or half the LD q12-24h until wound healing is achieved, up to 3 days

Maint: 15-30 IU/kg or half the LD q12-24h until wound healing is achieved, up to 3 days
VWF:RCo Trough Levels: >30%

Major:
LD: 40-60 IU/kg w/in 3 hours before surgery
VWF:RCo Peak Levels: 100%
Maint: 20-40 IU/kg or half the LD q12-24h (at least 2 doses w/in the first 24 hours after the start of surgery) until wound healing is achieved, up to 6 days or more
VWF:RCo Trough Levels: >50%

Do not exceed FVIII activity levels of 250%

Refer to PI for LD calculations based on patient's individual (in vivo recovery) IVR which is to be determined pre-surgery

Measure pulse rate before/during inj; if a marked increase in pulse rate occurs, reduce inj speed or interrupt admin

VWF:RCo Trough Levels: >30%
Major:
LD: 40-60 IU/kg w/in 3 hours before surgery
VWF:RCo Peak Levels: 100%
Maint: 20-40 IU/kg or half the LD q12-24h (at least 2 doses w/in the first 24 hours after the start of surgery) until wound healing is achieved, up to 6 days or more
VWF:RCo Trough Levels: >50%

Do not exceed FVIII activity levels of 250%

Refer to PI for LD calculations based on patient's individual IVR which is to be determined pre-surgery

Measure pulse rate before/during inj; if a marked increase in pulse rate occurs, reduce inj speed or interrupt admin

ADMINISTRATION
IV route

Do not mix w/ other medicinal products or administer simultaneously w/ other IV preparations in the same infusion set.
Only reconstitute powder directly before inj; use immediately after reconstitution.
Inject IV at a slow speed of 2-4mL/min.

Reconstitution/Administration:
1. Warm the concentrate and diluent vials to room temperature.
2. Peel away lid of outer package of Mix2Vial transfer set; leave device in clear outer packaging to maintain sterility.
3. Place diluent vial on level surface and hold firmly; invert Mix2Vial over diluent vial and push the blue plastic cannula firmly through the rubber stopper of the diluent vial.
4. Remove outer package from Mix2Vial, quickly invert over product vial and push transparent plastic cannula end of the Mix2Vial firmly through the product vial stopper.
5. W/ both sides still attached, gently swirl concentrate vial to ensure complete dissolution; do not shake the vial in order to avoid foaming.
6. Once contents are fully dissolved, unscrew the Mix2Vial into 2 separate pieces; discard empty diluent vial and blue Mix2Vial piece.
7. Attach plastic disposable syringe to Mix2Vial w/ vial upright, invert system and draw reconstituted sol into syringe.
8. Firmly hold barrel of syringe (keeping syringe plunger facing down) and detach Mix2Vial from syringe and discard empty product vial.
9. Attach suitable infusion needle to syringe and inject into intended inj site.

STORAGE
2-8°C (36-46°F) for up to 36 months. W/IN this period, may store for up to 6 months at ≤25°C (77°F). Once stored at room temperature, do not return to the refrigerator. Do not freeze. Store in the original container to protect from light.

HOW SUPPLIED
Inj: [VWF:RCo/FVIII] 500 IU/500 IU [5mL], 1000 IU/1000 IU [10mL]

CONTRAINDICATIONS
Known hypersensitivity reactions (eg, anaphylactic or severe systemic reactions) to human plasma-derived products, any ingredient of the formulation, or components of the container.

WARNINGS/PRECAUTIONS
Not indicated for treatment of hemophilia A. Initiate under the supervision of a physician experienced in treatment of coagulation disorders. Hypersensitivity reactions may occur; monitor closely and observe for any symptoms throughout infusion period. Inhibitor antibodies may occur w/ anaphylactic reactions; evaluate for presence of inhibitors in patients experiencing anaphylactic reactions. Avoid sustained excessive VWF and FVIII activity levels; may increase risk of thrombotic events. Patients w/ von Willebrand disease, especially type 3, may develop neutralizing antibodies (inhibitors) to VWF and FVIII. If expected VWF activity plasma levels are not attained, or if bleeding is not controlled w/ adequate dosing or repeated dosing, determine if VWF inhibitor is present. May carry risk of transmitting infectious agents (eg, viruses, Creutzfeldt-Jakob disease).

ADVERSE REACTIONS
Urticaria, dizziness, hypersensitivity reactions.

PREGNANCY AND LACTATION
Pregnancy: There is no data w/ use in pregnant women to inform a drug-associated risk.
Lactation: There is no information regarding the presence in human milk, the effect on the breastfed infant, and the effects on milk production. Caution in nursing.

MECHANISM OF ACTION
VWF and FVIII; constituents of normal plasma. VWF promotes platelet aggregation and platelet adhesion on damaged vascular endothelium; also serves as a stabilizing carrier protein for the procoagulant protein FVIII, an essential cofactor in activation of factor X leading to formation of thrombin and fibrin. Temporarily replaces missing VWF and FVIII that are needed for effective hemostasis.

PHARMACOKINETICS
Absorption: VWF:RCo: $AUC_{(0-inf)}$=1235 IU•hr/dL, C_{max}=76 IU/dL; FVIII: $AUC_{(0-inf)}$=2290 IU•hr/dL, C_{max}=112 IU/dL. **Distribution:** VWF:RCo: V_d=69.7mL/kg; FVIII: V_d=72.4mL/kg. **Elimination:** VWF:RCo: $T_{1/2}$=15.8 hrs. FVIII: $T_{1/2}$=19.6 hrs.

PATIENT CONSIDERATIONS
Assessment: Assess for known hypersensitivity, especially to plasma-derived products or components of the container, and pregnancy/nursing status.
Monitoring: Monitor for hypersensitivity reactions, thromboembolic events, VWF:RCo and FVIII activity levels, development of VWF and FVIII inhibitors, and infection.
Counseling: Inform of early signs of hypersensitivity reactions (eg, hives, wheezing, hypotension); advise to d/c immediately if allergic and to contact physician if allergic symptoms occur. Inform that undergoing multiple treatments may increase risk of thrombotic events thereby requiring frequent monitoring of plasma VWF:RCo and FVIII. Inform that there is a potential of developing inhibitors to VWF, leading to an inadequate clinical response. Contact physician if expected VWF activity plasma levels are not attained or if bleeding is not controlled w/ an adequate dose or repeated dosing. Inform that despite procedures for screening donors and plasma as well as those for inactivation or removal of infectious agents, the possibility of transmitting infective agents w/ plasma-derived products cannot be totally excluded.

WinRho SDF — rho(D) immune globulin intravenous (human) Rx
Class: Immune globulin

> Intravascular hemolysis (IVH) leading to death reported in patients treated for immune thrombocytopenic purpura (ITP). IVH can lead to anemia and multisystem organ failure including acute respiratory distress syndrome (ARDS). Serious complications including severe anemia, acute renal insufficiency, renal failure, and disseminated intravascular coagulation (DIC) reported. Closely monitor patients treated for ITP for ≥8 hrs after administration for signs/symptoms of IVH (eg, back pain, shaking chills, fever, discolored urine, hemoglobinuria, or hematuria); absence of these signs/symptoms within 8 hrs does not indicate IVH cannot occur subsequently. Perform a dipstick urinalysis at baseline, 2 hrs, 4 hrs after administration, and prior to the end of the monitoring period. Perform post-treatment laboratory tests (eg, plasma Hgb, haptoglobin, LDH, direct and indirect bilirubin) if IVH is present or suspected.

ADULT DOSAGE
Immune Thrombocytopenic Purpura

To Increase Platelet Count to Prevent Excessive Hemorrhage in Non-Splenectomized, Rh₀(D)-Positive Patients w/ Chronic Immune Thrombocytopenic Purpura (ITP) or w/ ITP Secondary to HIV Infection:
IV:
Initial: 250 IU/kg (50mcg/kg) as single dose or in 2 divided doses on separate days
Hgb <10g/dL: 125-200 IU/kg (25-40mcg/kg)

Subsequent Dosing:
Maint: 125-300 IU/kg (25-60mcg/kg)

If Patient Does Not Respond to Initial Dose, Administer Subsequent Dose Based on Hgb:
<8g/dL: Use alternative treatments
8-10g/dL: 125-200 IU/kg (25-40mcg/kg)
<10g/dL: 250-300 IU/kg (50-60mcg/kg)

Administer over 3-5 min

Suppression of Rh Isoimmunization
Pregnancy and Other Obstetric Conditions:
Suppression of Rh isoimmunization in non-sensitized, Rh₀(D)-negative women w/ Rh-incompatible pregnancy
IV/IM:
Antepartum Prophylaxis:
1500 IU (300mcg) at 28 weeks gestation; if administered early in pregnancy, give at 12-week intervals
Postpartum (if Newborn is Rh₀(D)-Positive):
600 IU (120mcg) w/in 72 hrs of birth

If Rh status of baby is unknown at 72 hrs, administer to mother at 72 hrs after delivery; if >72 hrs have elapsed, do not withhold, but administer as soon as possible up to 28 days after delivery

Abortion/Amniocentesis/Other Manipulation After 34 Weeks Gestation:
600 IU (120mcg) w/in 72 hrs

Amniocentesis/Chorionic Villus Sampling Before 34 Weeks

PEDIATRIC DOSAGE
Immune Thrombocytopenic Purpura

To Increase Platelet Count to Prevent Excessive Hemorrhage in Non-Splenectomized, Rh₀(D)-Positive Patients w/ Chronic/Acute Immune Thrombocytopenic Purpura (ITP) or w/ ITP Secondary to HIV Infection:
IV:
Initial: 250 IU/kg (50mcg/kg) as single dose or in 2 divided doses on separate days
Hgb <10g/dL: 125-200 IU/kg (25-40mcg/kg)

Subsequent Dosing:
Maint: 125-300 IU/kg (25-60mcg/kg)

If Patient Does Not Respond to Initial Dose, Administer Subsequent Dose Based on Hgb:
<8g/dL: Use alternative treatments
8-10g/dL: 125-200 IU/kg (25-40mcg/kg)
<10g/dL: 250-300 IU/kg (50-60mcg/kg)

Administer over 3-5 min

Gestation:
1500 IU (300mcg) immediately after procedure; repeat every 12 weeks during pregnancy

Threatened Abortion:
1500 IU (300mcg) immediately

Incompatible Transfusions:
Suppression of Rh isoimmunization in $Rh_0(D)$-negative individuals transfused w/ $Rh_0(D)$-positive RBCs or blood components containing $Rh_0(D)$-positive RBCs

Usual: 3000 IU (600mcg) IV q8h or 6000 IU (1200mcg) IM q12h; administer w/in 72 hours after exposure

If Exposed to $Rh_0(D)$-Positive Whole Blood:
45 IU (9mcg)/mL blood IV or 60 IU (12mcg)/mL blood IM

If Exposed to $Rh_0(D)$-Positive RBCs:
90 IU (18mcg)/mL cells IV or 120 IU (24mcg)/mL cells IM

DOSING CONSIDERATIONS
Elderly
Start at lower end of dosing range

ADMINISTRATION
IV/IM route

Bring to room temperature prior to use
Reconstitution not required; sol is ready to use
Remove entire contents of vial to obtain dosage; if partial vials are required for dosage calculation, withdraw entire contents of vial to ensure accurate calculation of dose requirement

IM
Administer into deltoid muscle of upper arm or anterolateral aspect of upper thigh; avoid gluteal region

IV
Administer separately from other drugs
Administer at a rate of 2mL/5-15 sec

Immune Thrombocytopenic Purpura
Administer entire dose IV over 3-5 min
Use normal saline as diluent, if dilution is preferred prior to IV administration; do not use D5W

STORAGE
2-8°C (36-46°F). Do not freeze.

HOW SUPPLIED
Inj: 600 IU (120mcg), 1500 IU (300mcg), 2500 IU (500mcg), 5000 IU (1000mcg), 15000 IU (3000mcg).

CONTRAINDICATIONS
Known anaphylactic or severe systemic reaction to human immune globulin products, autoimmune hemolytic anemia w/ pre-existing hemolysis/high risk for hemolysis, IgA deficiency w/ antibodies against IgA and a history of hypersensitivity, and suppression of isoimmunization in infants.

WARNINGS/PRECAUTIONS
Allergic or hypersensitivity reactions may occur; d/c immediately and institute appropriate treatment. Not for use as immunoglobulin replacement therapy for immune globulin deficiency syndromes. May carry a risk of transmitting infectious agents (eg, viruses, Creutzfeldt-Jakob disease agent). Liquid formulation contains maltose; may falsely elevate blood glucose levels. Thromboembolic events, acute renal dysfunction/failure, osmotic nephropathy, and death reported. Caution with pre-existing renal insufficiency, diabetes mellitus, advanced age, volume depletion, sepsis, paraproteinemia, or patients at risk of developing thromboembolic events (eg, history of atherosclerosis, cardiovascular risk factors, impaired cardiac output, advanced age, coagulation disorders, prolonged immobilization, and hyperviscosity); administer drug at minimum infusion rate practicable. Assess renal function (eg, BUN, SrCr) prior to therapy; assess renal function periodically in patients at risk for renal failure. Consider baseline assessment of blood viscosity in patients at risk for hyperviscosity. May lead to positive serological testing results (eg, positive direct/indirect Coombs' test); potential for misleading interpretation. Administer to mother if uncertain about father's Rh group or immune status. May cause transfusion-related acute lung injury (TRALI) and noncardiogenic pulmonary edema; monitor for pulmonary adverse reactions. If TRALI is suspected, perform appropriate tests for presence of anti-neutrophil and anti-HLA antibodies in both product and patient's serum. Caution in elderly. (Suppression of Rh Isoimmunization) Avoid use in $Rh_0(D)$ negative patients who are Rh immunized, evidenced by indirect anti-globulin (Coombs') test with presence of anti-$Rh_0(D)$ (anti-D) antibody. For postpartum use following an Rh-incompatible pregnancy, administer to mother only. (ITP) May decrease Hgb levels (extravascular hemolysis); do not administer if Hgb is <8g/dL. If transfusions are required, use $Rh_0(D)$-negative RBCs.

ADVERSE REACTIONS
IVH, anemia, multisystem organ failure, ARDS, acute renal insufficiency, renal failure, DIC, headache, chills, fever, asthenia, dizziness.

DRUG INTERACTIONS
May impair response to live, attenuated virus vaccines (eg, measles, mumps, rubella, and varicella); immunization with live vaccines should not be given for 3 months following administration. Administer at the minimum infusion rate practicable in patients at risk of renal dysfunction/failure including those receiving known nephrotoxic drugs.

PREGNANCY AND LACTATION
Category C. (Suppression of Rh Isoimmunization) Caution in nursing. (ITP) Safety not known in nursing.

MECHANISM OF ACTION
Immune globulin; not established. (ITP) Thought to involve formation of anti-$Rh_0(D)$-coated RBC complexes that are removed by reticuloendothelial system (spleen), resulting in Fc receptor blockade, sparing antibody coated platelets.

PHARMACOKINETICS
Absorption: (600 IU, IV) C_{max}=36-48ng/mL, T_{max}=2 hrs; (600 IU, IM) C_{max}=18-19ng/mL, T_{max}=5-10 days. **Elimination:** (IV) $T_{1/2}$= 24 days, (IM) $T_{1/2}$= 30 days.

PATIENT CONSIDERATIONS
Assessment: Assess for autoimmune hemolytic anemia, pre-existing hemolysis/high risk of hemolysis, IgA deficiency with antibodies to IgA and history of hypersensitivity, anaphylactic/severe systemic reactions to human immune globulin, history of atherosclerosis, multiple CV risk factors, advanced age, impaired cardiac output, coagulation disorders, prolonged immobilization, hyperviscosity, risk factors for thromboembolic events, pregnancy/nursing status, and possible drug interactions. Assess renal function (eg, BUN and creatinine) and for risk factors for renal dysfunction/failure. Perform blood type, blood count, reticulocyte count, and dipstick urinalysis in ITP patients. Obtain baseline assessment of blood viscosity in patients at risk for hyperviscosity. Assess for the presence of anti $Rh_0(D)$ (anti-D) antibodies via an indirect antiglobulin (Coombs') test.

Monitoring: Monitor for hypersensitivity reactions, transmission of infectious agents, IVH, renal dysfunction, thromboembolic events, pulmonary adverse reactions, and other adverse events. Monitor patients treated for ITP for ≥8 hrs after administration; perform dipstick urinalysis 2 hrs and 4 hrs after administration, and prior to the end of monitoring period. Monitor for clinical response in patients treated for ITP (eg, platelet counts, RBCs, Hgb, reticulocyte levels). If IVH is suspected, perform CBC (eg, Hgb, platelet counts), haptoglobin, urine dipstick, renal function tests, LFTs, and DIC specific tests. If TRALI is suspected, perform tests for presence of anti-neutrophil antibodies and anti-HLA antibodies.

Counseling: Inform about benefits and risks of therapy. Inform to immediately report symptoms of IVH, anemia, hypersensitivity reactions, hives, generalized urticaria, chest tightness, wheezing, hypotension, anaphylaxis, and symptoms related to viral infection. Instruct to self monitor for signs/symptoms of IVH for 72 hrs, especially for discoloration of urine. Advise to use only glucose specific tests to monitor blood glucose levels since interference due to maltose could result in falsely elevated glucose readings. Inform that product may contain disease causing infectious agents. Advise to inform other physicians of interference with response to live virus vaccines.

XALKORI — crizotinib   Rx
Class: Kinase inhibitor

ADULT DOSAGE	PEDIATRIC DOSAGE
Metastatic Non-Small Cell Lung Cancer	Pediatric use may not have been established

ADULT DOSAGE

Metastatic Non-Small Cell Lung Cancer

Metastatic non-small cell lung cancer (NSCLC) w/ anaplastic lymphoma kinase (ALK)-positive tumors as detected by an FDA-approved test

Also indicated for metastatic NSCLC w/ ROS1-positive tumors

250mg bid until disease progression or no longer tolerated

Missed Dose

If a dose is missed, make up that dose unless the next dose is due w/in 6 hrs

PEDIATRIC DOSAGE
Pediatric use may not have been established

DOSING CONSIDERATIONS
Renal Impairment
Severe (CrCl <30mL/min) Not Requiring Dialysis: 250mg qd

Hepatic Impairment
Has not been studied; use w/ caution

Adverse Reactions
Reduce dose as below, if ≥1 dose reduction is necessary due to Grade 3 or 4 adverse reactions:
1st Dose Reduction: 200mg bid
2nd Dose Reduction: 250mg qd
Permanently D/C: If unable to tolerate 250mg qd

Hematologic Toxicities*:
CTCAE Grade 3: Withhold therapy until recovery to ≤Grade 2, then resume at the same dose schedule
CTCAE Grade 4: Withhold therapy until recovery to ≤Grade 2, then resume at next lower dose
*Except lymphopenia (unless associated w/ clinical events such as opportunistic infections)

Nonhematologic Toxicities:
ALT or AST Elevation:
<5X ULN w/ Total Bilirubin ≤1.5X ULN: Withhold therapy until recovery to baseline or ≤3X ULN, then resume at reduced dose

<3X ULN w/ Total Bilirubin >1.5X ULN (In the Absence of Cholestasis or Hemolysis): Permanently d/c therapy

Drug-Related Interstitial Lung Disease (ILD)/Pneumonitis:
Any Grade: Permanently d/c therapy

QTc Interval:
>500 msec on at Least 2 Separate ECGs: Withhold therapy until recovery to baseline or to a QTc <481 msec, then resume at reduced dose
<500 msec or ≥60 msec Change from Baseline w/ Torsades de Pointes or Polymorphic Ventricular Tachycardia or Signs/Symptoms of Serious Arrhythmia: Permanently d/c therapy

Bradycardia:
Symptomatic, May Be Severe and Medically Significant, Medical Intervention Indicated:
1. Withhold therapy until recovery to asymptomatic bradycardia or to a HR of ≥60bpm
2. Evaluate concomitant medications known to cause bradycardia, as well as anti-hypertensive medications
3. If contributing concomitant medication is identified and discontinued, or its dose is adjusted, resume at previous dose upon recovery to asymptomatic bradycardia or to a HR of ≥60bpm
4. If no contributing concomitant medication is identified, or if contributing concomitant medications are not discontinued or dose modified, resume at reduced dose upon recovery to asymptomatic bradycardia or to a HR of ≥60bpm
Life-Threatening Consequences, Urgent Intervention Indicated:
1. Permanently d/c if no contributing concomitant medication is identified
2. If contributing concomitant medication is identified and discontinued, or its dose is adjusted, resume at 250mg qd upon recovery to asymptomatic bradycardia or to a HR of ≥60bpm, w/ frequent monitoring

Visual Loss:
Grade 4 Ocular Disorder: D/C during evaluation of severe vision loss

ADMINISTRATION
Oral route

Take w/ or w/o food.
Swallow caps whole.
If vomiting occurs after taking a dose, take the next dose at the regular time.

STORAGE
20-25°C (68-77°F); excursions permitted between 15-30°C (59-86°F).

HOW SUPPLIED
Cap: 200mg, 250mg

WARNINGS/PRECAUTIONS
See Dosing Considerations. Hepatotoxicity w/ fatal outcome reported. Concurrent elevations in ALT or AST ≥3X ULN and total bilirubin ≥2X ULN, w/ normal alkaline phosphatase, reported. Elevations in ALT or AST >5X ULN reported. Severe, life-threatening, or fatal ILD/pneumonitis may occur. QTc prolongation may occur; avoid use w/ congenital long QT syndrome. Monitor ECGs and electrolytes in patients w/ CHF, bradyarrhythmias, electrolyte abnormalities, or who are taking medications known to prolong the QT interval. Symptomatic bradycardia may occur. Visual field defect w/ vision loss reported. D/C in patients w/ new onset of severe visual loss (best corrected vision <20/200 in one or both eyes); perform an ophthalmological evaluation consisting of best corrected visual acuity, retinal photographs, visual fields, optical coherence tomography (OCT) and other evaluations as appropriate for new onset of severe visual loss. Can cause fetal harm if used during pregnancy.

ADVERSE REACTIONS
Vision disorders, N/V, diarrhea, edema, constipation, elevated transaminases, fatigue, decreased appetite, URI, dizziness, neuropathy.

DRUG INTERACTIONS
Increased plasma concentrations w/ strong CYP3A inhibitors (eg, clarithromycin, ketoconazole, ritonavir) and grapefruit/grapefruit juice; avoid use. Caution w/ moderate CYP3A inhibitors. Decreased plasma concentrations w/ strong CYP3A inducers (eg, carbamazepine, phenytoin, rifampin); avoid use. Avoid w/ CYP3A substrates w/ narrow therapeutic range (eg, cyclosporine, fentanyl, tacrolimus); may require dose reductions of the CYP3A substrates if concomitant use is required. Avoid w/ other agents known to cause bradycardia (eg, β-blockers, nondihydropyridine calcium channel blockers, clonidine, digoxin) to the extent possible.

PREGNANCY AND LACTATION
Pregnancy: Can cause fetal harm.
Lactation: Do not breastfeed during therapy and for 45 days after the final dose.
Reproductive Potential: Females of reproductive potential should use effective contraception during therapy and for at least 45 days after the final dose. Males w/ female partners of reproductive potential should use condoms during therapy and for at least 90 days after the final dose. May cause reduced fertility in females and males of reproductive potential.

MECHANISM OF ACTION
Tyrosine kinase inhibitor; inhibits receptor tyrosine kinases, including ALK, hepatocyte growth factor receptor, ROS1, and recepteur d'origine nantais.

PHARMACOKINETICS
Absorption: Absolute bioavailability (43%); T_{max}=4-6 hrs (median). **Distribution:** V_d=1772L (IV); plasma protein binding (91%). **Metabolism:** Liver (extensive) via CYP3A4/5; oxidation and O-dealkylation (primary), and conjugation. **Elimination:** Feces (63%, 53% unchanged), urine (22%, 2.3% unchanged); $T_{1/2}$=42 hrs.

PATIENT CONSIDERATIONS
Assessment: Assess for congenital long QT syndrome, CHF, bradyarrhythmias, electrolyte abnormalities, hepatic/renal impairment, pregnancy/nursing status, and possible drug interactions. Assess for presence of ALK or ROS1 positivity in tumor specimens.

Monitoring: Monitor for signs/symptoms of ILD, pneumonitis, QTc prolongation, bradycardia, visual loss, and other adverse reactions. Monitor LFTs including ALT and total bilirubin every 2 weeks during the first 2 months, then once a month and as clinically indicated, w/ more frequent repeat testing if transaminase elevations develop. Monitor ECGs and electrolytes in patients w/ CHF, bradyarrhythmias, electrolyte abnormalities, or who are taking medications known to prolong the QT interval. Monitor HR and BP regularly. Monitor CBCs including differential WBC counts monthly and as clinically indicated, w/ more frequent repeat testing if Grade 3 or 4 abnormalities are observed, or if fever or infection occurs. Perform an ophthalmological evaluation consisting of best corrected visual acuity, retinal photographs, visual fields, OCT, and other evaluations as appropriate for new onset of severe visual loss.

Counseling: Instruct to immediately report symptoms of hepatotoxicity or any new or worsening pulmonary symptoms. Advise to report symptoms of bradycardia and to inform physician about the use of any heart or BP medications. Inform of potential risk of severe visual loss and to immediately contact physician if severe visual loss develops. Inform that visual changes (eg, perceived flashes of light, blurry vision, light sensitivity, floaters) are commonly reported adverse events and may occur while driving or operating machinery. Instruct to avoid grapefruit or grapefruit juice while on therapy; advise to inform physician of all concomitant medications, including prescription medicines, OTC drugs, vitamins, and herbal products. Advise on what to do if a dose is missed or if vomiting occurs after taking a dose. Inform of potential risk to a fetus. Advise to inform physician of known/suspected pregnancy, and not to breastfeed during therapy and for 45 days after the final dose. Advise females of reproductive potential and males w/ female partners of reproductive potential on effective contraception use. Advise females and males of reproductive potential of potential for reduced fertility.

XELJANZ — tofacitinib   Rx

Class: Kinase inhibitor

> Increased risk for developing serious infections (eg, active tuberculosis [TB], invasive fungal infections, bacterial/viral infections due to opportunistic pathogens) that may lead to hospitalization or death. Most patients who developed these infections were taking concomitant immunosuppressants (eg, methotrexate [MTX], corticosteroids). If a serious infection develops, interrupt treatment until infection is controlled. Test for latent TB prior to and during therapy; initiate latent TB treatment prior to therapy. Consider risks and benefits prior to initiating therapy in patients w/ chronic or recurrent infection. Monitor for development of signs and symptoms of infection during and after treatment. Lymphoma and other malignancies reported. Increased rate of Epstein-Barr virus-associated post-transplant lymphoproliferative disorder observed in renal transplant patients w/ concomitant immunosuppressive medications.

OTHER BRAND NAMES
Xeljanz XR

ADULT DOSAGE
Rheumatoid Arthritis

As monotherapy or in combination w/ methotrexate (MTX) or other nonbiologic disease-modifying antirheumatic drugs (DMARDs) for moderately to severely active rheumatoid arthritis in patients who have had an inadequate response or intolerance to MTX

Tab:
5mg bid
Tab, Extended-Release (ER):
11mg qd

Conversions

Switching From Tab to Tab, ER:
Patients treated w/ Xeljanz 5mg bid may be switched to Xeljanz XR 11mg qd following the last dose of Xeljanz 5mg

PEDIATRIC DOSAGE
Pediatric use may not have been established

DOSING CONSIDERATIONS
Concomitant Medications
Potent CYP3A4 Inhibitors:
Tab: Reduce dose to 5mg qd
≥1 Concomitant Medication Resulting in Both Moderate CYP3A4 Inhibition and Potent CYP2C19 Inhibition:
Tab: Reduce dose to 5mg qd
Potent CYP3A4 Inducers:
Tab/Tab, ER: Not recommended for use
Renal Impairment
Moderate or Severe:
Tab: Reduce dose to 5mg qd
Hepatic Impairment
Moderate:
Tab: Reduce dose to 5mg qd
Severe:
Tab/Tab, ER: Not recommended for use
Adverse Reactions
Lymphopenia:
Absolute Lymphocyte Count <500 cells/mm³: Do not initiate treatment
Absolute Lymphocyte Count ≥500 cells/mm³: Maintain dose

Absolute Lymphocyte Count <500 cells/mm³ (Confirmed by Repeat Testing):
D/C treatment

Neutropenia:
ANC <1000 cells/mm³: Do not initiate treatment
ANC >1000 cells/mm³: Maintain dose
ANC 500-1000 cells/mm³: For persistent decreases in this range, interrupt dosing until ANC is >1000; when ANC is >1000, resume at Xeljanz 5mg bid/Xeljanz XR 11mg qd
ANC <500 cells/mm³ (Confirmed by Repeat Testing): D/C treatment

Anemia:
Hgb <9g/dL: Do not initiate treatment
Hgb ≤2g/dL Decrease and ≥9g/dL: Maintain dose
Hgb >2g/dL Decrease or <8g/dL (Confirmed by Repeat Testing): Interrupt administration until Hgb values have normalized

ADMINISTRATION
Oral route

Take w/ or w/o food.
Swallow ER tabs whole and intact; do not crush, split, or chew.

STORAGE
20-25°C (68-77°F).

HOW SUPPLIED
Tab: (Xeljanz) 5mg; **Tab, ER:** (Xeljanz XR) 11mg

WARNINGS/PRECAUTIONS
See Dosing Considerations. Avoid w/ active, serious infection, including localized infections. Caution in patients w/ chronic/recurrent infections, who have been exposed to TB, w/ a history of a serious/opportunistic infection, who have resided in/traveled to areas of endemic TB/mycoses, or w/ predisposing factors to infection. Interrupt treatment if an opportunistic infection or sepsis occurs. Viral reactivation, including herpes virus reactivation (eg, herpes zoster), reported; screen for viral hepatitis before starting therapy. Increased risk of herpes zoster; risk appears to be higher in patients treated in Japan. Consider risks and benefits of treatment in patients w/ a known malignancy other than a successfully treated non-melanoma skin cancer or when considering continuing treatment in patients who develop a malignancy. Non-melanoma skin cancers reported; periodic skin examination is recommended for patients at increased risk for skin cancer. GI perforation reported; caution in patients w/ increased risk for GI perforation (eg, history of diverticulitis). Promptly evaluate for early identification of GI perforation in patients presenting w/ new onset of abdominal symptoms. Associated w/ initial lymphocytosis, neutropenia, increases in lipid parameters, and liver enzyme elevations. Interrupt treatment if drug-induced liver injury is suspected until this diagnosis has been excluded. Caution in elderly and diabetes patients. **Tab, ER:** Caution w/ preexisting severe GI narrowing (pathologic or iatrogenic).

ADVERSE REACTIONS
Infections (eg, URTIs, nasopharyngitis), diarrhea, headache.

DRUG INTERACTIONS
See Boxed Warning and Dosing Considerations. Avoid w/ live vaccines. Increased immunosuppression w/ potent immunosuppressive drugs (eg, azathioprine, tacrolimus, cyclosporine); concurrent use w/ potent immunosuppressants (eg, azathioprine, cyclosporine) or biologic DMARDs is not recommended. Increased exposure w/ potent CYP3A4 inhibitors (eg, ketoconazole), and drugs that are both moderate CYP3A4 inhibitors and potent CYP2C19 inhibitors (eg, fluconazole). Decreased exposure resulting in loss of or reduced clinical response to treatment w/ potent CYP3A4 inducers (eg, rifampin).

PREGNANCY AND LACTATION
Pregnancy: Category C. Physicians are encouraged to register pregnant patients in the pregnancy registry.
Lactation: Not for use in nursing.

MECHANISM OF ACTION
Kinase inhibitor; inhibits Janus kinase, which transmits signals arising from cytokine or growth factor-receptor interactions on the cellular membrane to influence cellular processes of hematopoiesis and immune cell function.

PHARMACOKINETICS
Absorption: (Tab) Absolute bioavailability (74%); T_{max}=0.5-1 hr. (Tab, ER) T_{max}=4 hrs. **Distribution:** (IV) V_d=87 L; plasma protein binding (40%). **Metabolism:** Liver via CYP3A4 (primary) and CYP2C19 (minor). **Elimination:** Urine (30% unchanged); $T_{1/2}$=3 hrs (Tab), 6 hrs (Tab, ER).

PATIENT CONSIDERATIONS
Assessment: Assess for infections (eg, bacteria, fungi, viruses), including latent or active TB, predisposing factors to infection, active hepatic disease or impairment, known malignancy, risk of GI perforation, diabetes, preexisting GI narrowing, pregnancy/nursing status, and possible drug interactions. Obtain baseline absolute lymphocyte count, ANC, and lipid and Hgb levels.

Monitoring: Monitor for TB (active, reactivation, or latent), invasive fungal infections, or bacterial, viral, and other opportunistic infections during and after therapy. Monitor for viral reactivation, lymphoma, malignancy, lymphoproliferative disorders, GI perforations, and other adverse reactions. Monitor absolute lymphocyte counts every 3 months. Monitor neutrophil counts and Hgb after 4-8 weeks of treatment and every 3 months thereafter. Routinely monitor LFTs. Monitor lipid parameters approx 4-8 weeks following initiation. Perform periodic skin examination in patients at increased risk of skin cancer.

Counseling: Advise about potential risks/benefits of therapy. Inform that therapy may lower resistance to infection; advise patients not to start taking medication if they have an active infection. Instruct to contact physician immediately if symptoms suggesting an infection appear during treatment to ensure rapid evaluation and appropriate treatment. Advise that the risk of herpes zoster is increased in patients treated w/ therapy. Inform that medication may increase risk of lymphoma and other cancers; instruct to inform physician of any type of cancer that they have ever had. Inform that certain lab tests may be affected and that blood tests are required before and during treatment. Inform that medication should not be used during pregnancy unless clearly necessary; advise to inform physician right away if pregnant. Advise to enroll in the pregnancy registry for pregnant women who have taken medication during pregnancy. **Tab, ER:** Inform that an inert tablet shell may pass in the stool or via colostomy and that the active medication has already been absorbed by the time the inert tablet shell is seen.

XELODA — capecitabine   Rx
Class: Fluoropyrimidine carbamate

> Altered coagulation parameters and/or bleeding, including death, reported w/ concomitant coumarin-derivative anticoagulants (eg, warfarin, phenprocoumon). Monitor PT and INR frequently in order to adjust anticoagulant dose accordingly. Postmarketing reports showed clinically significant increases in PT and INR in patients who were stabilized on anticoagulants at start of therapy. Age >60 yrs and a diagnosis of cancer independently predispose to an increased risk of coagulopathy.

ADULT DOSAGE
Metastatic Colorectal Cancer
1st-line treatment of metastatic colorectal carcinoma and as a single agent for adjuvant treatment in patients w/ Dukes' C colon cancer who have undergone complete resection of the primary tumor when treatment w/ fluoropyrimidine therapy alone is preferred

Monotherapy:
Usual: 1250mg/m² bid for 2 weeks followed by a 1-week rest period, given as 3-week cycles

Adjuvant to Dukes' C Colon Cancer: 1250mg/m² bid for 2 weeks followed by 1-week rest period, given as 3-week cycles for total of 8 cycles (24 weeks)
Refer to PI for dose calculations based on BSA

Metastatic Breast Cancer
Treatment of metastatic breast cancer in combination w/ docetaxel after failure of prior anthracycline-containing chemotherapy. Monotherapy treatment of metastatic breast cancer in patients resistant to both paclitaxel and anthracycline-containing chemotherapy regimen or resistant to paclitaxel and for whom further anthracycline therapy is not indicated

Monotherapy:
1250mg/m² bid for 2 weeks followed by a 1-week rest period, given as 3-week cycles

Combination w/ Docetaxel:
Usual: 1250mg/m² bid for 2 weeks followed by 1-week rest period, combined w/ docetaxel at 75mg/m² as a 1-hr IV infusion every 3 weeks
Premedication:
Start prior to docetaxel administration
Refer to PI for dose calculations based on BSA

PEDIATRIC DOSAGE
Pediatric use may not have been established

DOSING CONSIDERATIONS
Concomitant Medications
Phenytoin and Coumarin-Derivative Anticoagulants: May need to reduce dose of phenytoin and coumarin-derivative anticoagulants

Renal Impairment
Moderate (CrCl 30-50mL/min): Reduce to 75% of starting dose when used as monotherapy or in combination w/ docetaxel (from 1250mg/m² to 950mg/m² bid)

Adverse Reactions
Toxicity NCIC Grade 2:
1st Appearance: Interrupt until resolved to Grade 0-1, then give 100% of dose
2nd Appearance: Interrupt until resolved to Grade 0-1, then give 75% of dose
3rd Appearance: Interrupt until resolved to Grade 0-1, then give 50% of dose
4th Appearance: D/C treatment permanently

Toxicity NCIC Grade 3:
1st Appearance: Interrupt until resolved to Grade 0-1, then give 75% of dose
2nd Appearance: Interrupt until resolved to Grade 0-1, then give 50% of dose
3rd Appearance: D/C treatment permanently

Toxicity NCIC Grade 4:
1st Appearance: D/C permanently or if physician deems it to be in the best interest to continue, interrupt until resolved to Grade 0-1, then give 50% of dose

Refer to PI for docetaxel dose reductions when used in combination w/ capecitabine

ADMINISTRATION
Oral route
Swallow tabs whole w/ water w/in 30 min pc; do not cut or crush.

STORAGE
25°C (77°F); excursions permitted to 15-30°C (59-86°F). Keep tightly closed.

HOW SUPPLIED
Tab: 150mg, 500mg

CONTRAINDICATIONS
Severe renal impairment (CrCl <30mL/min); known hypersensitivity to capecitabine, any components of the medication, or 5-fluorouracil (5-FU).

WARNINGS/PRECAUTIONS
May induce diarrhea; give fluid and electrolyte replacement w/ severe diarrhea. Cardiotoxicity (eg, MI/ischemia, angina) observed; may be more common in patients w/ a prior history of coronary artery disease (CAD). Increased risk for acute early-onset of toxicity and severe, life-threatening, or fatal adverse reactions (eg, mucositis, diarrhea, neutropenia, neurotoxicity) in patients w/ certain homozygous or certain compound heterozygous mutations in the dihydropyrimidine dehydrogenase (DPD) gene that results in complete or near complete absence of DPD activity; withhold or permanently d/c therapy based on clinical assessment of the onset, duration, and severity of the observed toxicities. Patients w/ partial DPD activity may also have increased risk of severe, life-threatening, or fatal adverse reactions. Dehydration reported and may cause acute renal failure; patients w/ preexisting compromised renal function are at higher risk. Patients w/ anorexia, asthenia, N/V, or diarrhea may rapidly become dehydrated; monitor during administration and do not restart treatment until patient is rehydrated and any precipitating causes have been corrected or controlled. Caution w/ mild and moderate renal impairment. Severe mucocutaneous reactions (eg, Stevens-Johnson syndrome, toxic epidermal necrolysis) may occur; permanently d/c in patients who experience a severe mucocutaneous reaction possibly attributable to treatment. Hand-and-foot syndrome may occur. Hyperbilirubinemia reported; interrupt therapy if drug-related Grade 3 or 4 elevations in bilirubin occur until the hyperbilirubinemia decreases to ≤3X ULN. Necrotizing enterocolitis, neutropenia, thrombocytopenia, anemia, and decreases in Hgb reported. Avoid w/ baseline neutrophil counts of <1.5 x 10⁹/L and/or thrombocyte counts of <100 x 10⁹/L. Caution in elderly; patients ≥80 yrs of age may experience greater incidence of Grade 3 or 4 adverse events. Caution w/ mild to moderate hepatic dysfunction due to liver metastases. May cause fetal harm.

ADVERSE REACTIONS
Diarrhea, hand-and-foot syndrome, asthenia, pyrexia, anemia, N/V, fatigue, dermatitis, thrombocytopenia, constipation, taste disturbance, stomatitis, alopecia, abdominal pain, decreased appetite.

DRUG INTERACTIONS
See Boxed Warning and Dosing Considerations. Higher risk of dehydration w/ known nephrotoxic agents. May increase the mean AUC of S-warfarin. May increase phenytoin levels. Leucovorin may increase levels and toxicity of 5-FU. Caution w/ CYP2C9 substrates.

PREGNANCY AND LACTATION
Pregnancy: Category D.
Lactation: Not for use in nursing.

MECHANISM OF ACTION
Fluoropyrimidine carbamate; binds to thymidylate synthase to form a covalently bound ternary complex that inhibits the formation of thymidylate from 2'-deoxyuridylate, which inhibits DNA synthesis/cell division, and interferes w/ RNA processing and protein synthesis.

PHARMACOKINETICS
Absorption: T_{max}=1.5 hrs. **Distribution:** Plasma protein binding (<60%); primarily bound to human albumin (approx 35%). **Metabolism:** Extensive enzymatic conversion to 5-FU; hydrogenated to the much less toxic 5-fluoro-5, 6-dihydro-fluorouracil by DPD; cleavage of the pyrimidine ring to 5-fluoro-ureido-propionic acid; cleavage to α-fluoro-β-alanine. **Elimination:** Urine (95.5%, 3% unchanged), feces (2.6%); $T_{1/2}$=0.75 hr.

PATIENT CONSIDERATIONS

Assessment: Assess for hypersensitivity to drug or to 5-FU, complete or near complete absence of DPD activity, partial DPD activity, renal/hepatic dysfunction, history of CAD, pregnancy/nursing status, and possible drug interactions. Obtain baseline neutrophil/thrombocyte counts.

Monitoring: Monitor for severe diarrhea, necrotizing enterocolitis, cardiotoxicity, acute early-onset of toxicity, severe/life-threatening/fatal adverse reactions, hand-and-foot syndrome, hyperbilirubinemia, neutropenia, thrombocytopenia, anemia, decreases in Hgb, severe toxicity, dehydration, acute renal failure, severe mucocutaneous reactions, and other adverse reactions. Monitor PT and INR frequently w/ concomitant oral coumarin-derivative anticoagulant therapy.

Counseling: Instruct to d/c therapy and contact physician immediately if moderate/severe toxicity, Grade ≥2 diarrhea/stomatitis, or severe bloody diarrhea w/ severe abdominal pain and fever is experienced. Advise to notify physician if patient has known DPD deficiency; inform that patient is at an increased risk of acute early-onset of toxicity and severe, life-threatening, or fatal adverse reactions if patient has complete or near complete absence of DPD activity. Instruct to d/c therapy immediately in patients experiencing Grade ≥2 dehydration/nausea/vomiting/hand-and-foot syndrome. Instruct to contact physician immediately if fever or infection occurs. Counsel about pregnancy risks; instruct to avoid pregnancy during therapy.

XENAZINE — tetrabenazine   Rx
Class: Monoamine depletor

> Increased risk of depression and suicidal thoughts and behavior (suicidality) in patients w/ Huntington's disease. Balance the risks of depression and suicidality w/ the clinical need for control of chorea. Closely observe for emergence or worsening of depression, suicidality, or unusual changes in behavior. Particular caution in patients w/ history of depression, suicide attempts, or ideation. Contraindicated in actively suicidal patients and in those w/ untreated or inadequately treated depression.

ADULT DOSAGE
Huntington's Disease

Treatment of Chorea Associated w/ Huntington's Disease:

Dosing Recommendations Up to 50mg/day:
Initial: 12.5mg qam
Titrate: Increase to 12.5mg bid (25mg/day) after 1 week; slowly titrate up at weekly intervals by 12.5mg/day. If 37.5-50mg/day is needed, give in a tid regimen
Max Single Dose: 25mg

Dosing Recommendations >50mg/day:
Patient should be 1st tested and genotyped to determine if they are poor or extensive metabolizers by their ability to express CYP2D6

Extensive/Intermediate CYP2D6 Metabolizers:
Titrate: Increase slowly at weekly intervals by 12.5mg/day. Doses >50mg/day should be given in a tid regimen
Max Single Dose: 37.5mg
Max Daily Dose: 100mg

Poor CYP2D6 Metabolizers:
Titrate: Increase slowly at weekly intervals by 12.5mg/day
Max Single Dose: 25mg
Max Daily Dose: 50mg

Resumption of Treatment:
Following treatment interruption of >5 days, re-titrate therapy when resumed
For short-term treatment interruption of <5 days, resume therapy at previous maint dose w/o titration

PEDIATRIC DOSAGE
Pediatric use may not have been established

DOSING CONSIDERATIONS
Concomitant Medications
Concomitant Strong CYP2D6 Inhibitor:
Max Single Dose: 25mg
Max Daily Dose: 50mg

Adverse Reactions
If adverse reactions occur, stop titration and reduce dose; if unresolved, consider discontinuing therapy

Discontinuation
May d/c treatment w/o tapering

ADMINISTRATION
Oral route
Take w/o regard to food

STORAGE
25°C (77°F); excursions permitted to 15-30°C (59-86°F).

HOW SUPPLIED
Tab: 12.5mg, 25mg* *scored

CONTRAINDICATIONS
Patients who are actively suicidal; w/ untreated or inadequately treated depression; w/ hepatic impairment; taking MAOIs (should not be used w/ or w/in a minimum of 14 days of discontinuing an MAOI) and reserpine (wait ≥20 days after stopping reserpine before starting therapy).

WARNINGS/PRECAUTIONS
May worsen mood, cognition, rigidity, and functional capacity. Neuroleptic malignant syndrome (NMS) reported; d/c immediately and institute proper treatment if NMS occurs. Monitor for signs/symptoms of akathisia, restlessness, agitation, and parkinsonism; reduce dose or may need to d/c therapy. Dysphagia may occur; may be associated w/ aspiration pneumonia. May impair mental/physical activities. May cause QT prolongation; avoid w/ congenital long QT syndrome and history of cardiac arrhythmias. Postural dizziness reported; monitor vital signs on standing if vulnerable to hypotension. May elevate serum prolactin levels; perform lab tests and consider discontinuation. May cause extrapyramidal symptoms and tardive dyskinesia (TD); consider discontinuation if signs/symptoms of TD occur. May cause toxicity in melanin-containing tissues w/ extended use and there may be the possibility of long-term ophthalmologic effects.

ADVERSE REACTIONS

Depression, suicidality, sedation/somnolence, fatigue, insomnia, anxiety/anxiety aggravated, irritability, akathisia, parkinsonism/bradykinesia, falls, URTI, N/V, balance difficulty, laceration, ecchymosis.

DRUG INTERACTIONS

See Dosing Considerations and Contraindications. Dose reduction may be necessary when adding a strong CYP2D6 inhibitor (eg, quinidine, fluoxetine, paroxetine) in patients maintained on a stable dose. Concomitant use w/ alcohol or other sedating drugs may have additive effects and worsen sedation and somnolence. Avoid other drugs known to cause QTc prolongation, including antipsychotics (eg, chlorpromazine, haloperidol, thioridazine, ziprasidone), antibiotics (eg, moxifloxacin), Class 1A (eg, quinidine, procainamide) and Class III (eg, amiodarone, sotalol) antiarrhythmic agents. Concomitant use w/ dopamine antagonists or antipsychotics may increase risk for parkinsonism, NMS, and akathisia.

PREGNANCY AND LACTATION

Category C, not for use in nursing.

MECHANISM OF ACTION

Monoamine depletor; not established. Suspected to reversibly inhibit the human vesicle monoamine transporter type-2, resulting in decreased uptake of monoamines into synaptic vesicles and depletion of monoamine stores.

PHARMACOKINETICS

Absorption: T_{max}=1-1.5 hrs (α and β-HTBZ), 2 hrs (9-desmethyl-β-DHTBZ). **Distribution:** Plasma protein binding (82-85%, tetrabenazine) (60-68%, α-HTBZ) (59-63%, β-HTBZ). **Metabolism:** Rapid, extensive; liver via carbonyl reductase to α-HBTZ and β-HBTZ (major metabolites), O-dealkylation of α-HBTZ and β-HBTZ via CYP2D6 (primary) to 9-desmethyl-α-DHTBZ (minor metabolite) and 9-desmethyl-β-DHTBZ (major metabolite). **Elimination:** Urine (75%; metabolites), feces (7-16%); $T_{1/2}$=7 hrs (α-HTBZ), 5 hrs (β-HTBZ), 12 hrs (9-desmethyl-β-DHTBZ).

PATIENT CONSIDERATIONS

Assessment: Assess for history of depression/suicidality, active suicidality, untreated or inadequately treated depression, alcohol intake, hepatic impairment, congenital long QT syndrome, history of cardiac arrhythmias, risk of aspiration pneumonia, pregnancy/nursing status, and possible drug interactions. Obtain CYP2D6 genotype if dose >50mg/day is required, baseline vital signs, and serum prolactin levels.

Monitoring: Monitor for emergence or worsening of depression, suicidality, unusual changes in behavior, NMS, akathisia, restlessness, agitation, parkinsonism, dysphagia, sedation/somnolence, hyperprolactinemia, TD, dizziness, QT prolongation, and other adverse effects. Periodically reevaluate the need for therapy by assessing effectiveness and adverse effects.

Counseling: Advise patient, patient's families, and caregivers to be alert for the risk of suicidal ideation, depression or worsening of depression, withdrawal, insomnia, irritability, aggressiveness, akathisia (psychomotor restlessness), anxiety, agitation, panic attacks, sedation, parkinsonism, difficulty swallowing; instruct to inform physician immediately if any adverse reactions occur. Advise that therapy may impair the ability to perform tasks that require complex motor and mental skills and to caution when performing activities requiring mental alertness until effect of drug is known. Advise that alcohol may potentiate sedation. Instruct to notify physician if pregnant, intending to become pregnant, or if breastfeeding or intending to breastfeed.

Xeomin — incobotulinumtoxinA   Rx

Class: Acetylcholine release inhibitor

> Distant spread of toxin effects (eg, asthenia, generalized muscle weakness, diplopia, blurred vision, ptosis, dysphagia, dysphonia, dysarthria, urinary incontinence, breathing difficulties) reported hrs to weeks after inj. Swallowing and breathing difficulties can be life threatening and there have been reports of death. Risk of symptoms is greatest in children treated for spasticity but can also occur in adults treated for spasticity and other conditions, particularly in patients who have underlying conditions that would predispose them to these symptoms. In unapproved uses and approved indications, cases of spread of effect have been reported at doses comparable to those used to treat cervical dystonia and at lower doses.

ADULT DOSAGE

Upper Limb Spasticity

Dosage, frequency, and number of inj sites should be tailored to the individual patient based on the size, number, and location of muscles to be treated, severity of spasticity, presence of local muscle weakness, patient's response to previous treatment, and adverse event history w/ incobotulinumtoxinA

Frequency of treatments should be no sooner than every 12 weeks

If not previously treated w/ botulinum toxins, initial dosing should begin at the low end of the recommended dosing range and titrated as clinically necessary

Recommended Dose per Muscle:

Clenched Fist

Flexor Digitorum Superficialis/Flexor Digitorum Profundus: 25-100 U divided in 2 sites

PEDIATRIC DOSAGE

Pediatric use may not have been established

Flexed Wrist

Flexor Carpi Radialis: 25-100 U divided in 1-2 sites
Flexor Carpi Ulnaris: 20-100 U divided in 1-2 sites

Flexed Elbow

Brachioradialis: 25-100 U divided in 1-3 sites
Biceps: 50-200 U divided in 1-4 sites
Brachialis: 25-100 U divided in 1-2 sites

Pronated Forearm

Pronator Quadratus: 10-50 U in 1 site
Pronator Teres: 25-75 U divided in 1-2 sites

Thumb in Palm

Flexor Pollicis Longus: 10-50 U in 1 site
Adductor Pollicis: 5-30 U in 1 site
Flexor Pollicis Brevis/Opponens Pollicis: 5-30 U in 1 site

Cervical Dystonia

Initial: 120 U; usually injected into the sternocleidomastoid, levator scapulae, splenius capitis, scalenus, and/or the trapezius muscle(s)

Frequency of repeat treatments should be determined by clinical response, but should generally be no more frequent than every 12 weeks

Blepharospasm

In patients previously treated w/ onabotulinumtoxinA

Initial: Same dose as previous onabotulinumtoxinA treatment; if the previous onabotulinumtoxinA dose is unknown, administer 1.25-2.5 U/inj site
Total Initial: 70 U (35 U/eye)

Frequency of repeat treatments should be determined by clinical response, but should generally be no more frequent than every 12 weeks

Glabellar Lines

Temporary improvement in the appearance of moderate to severe glabellar lines associated w/ corrugator and/or procerus muscle activity

20 U per treatment session, divided into 5 equal IM inj of 4 U each

The 5 inj sites are: 2 inj in each corrugator muscle and 1 inj in the procerus muscle

Retreatment should be administered no more frequently than every 3 months

---

ADMINISTRATION

IM route

Max cumulative dose for any indication should not exceed 400 U in a treatment session.

After reconstitution, use for only 1 inj session and for only 1 patient.

Reconstituted sol should be administered w/in 24 hours after dilution; during this time period, should be stored at 2-8°C (36-46°F).

If proposed inj sites are marked w/ a pen, product must not be injected through the pen marks; otherwise, a permanent tattooing effect may occur.

Number of inj sites is dependent upon size of muscle to be treated and volume of reconstituted sol injected.

Inject carefully when injected at sites close to sensitive structures (eg, carotid artery, lung apices, esophagus).

Preparation and Reconstitution

1. Prior to inj, reconstitute each vial w/ sterile, preservative-free 0.9% NaCl inj.
2. Use a 20- to 27-gauge short bevel needle and draw up an appropriate amount of preservative-free 0.9% NaCl inj into a syringe; refer to PI for diluent volumes for reconstitution.
3. Gently inject saline sol into vial.
4. If vacuum does not pull the solvent into the vial, then incobotulinumtoxinA must be discarded.
5. Mix w/ the saline by carefully swirling and inverting/flipping the vial; do not shake vigorously.

Upper Limb Spasticity and Cervical Dystonia

A suitable sterile needle (eg, 26-gauge [0.45mm diameter], 37mm length for superficial muscles; or 22-gauge [0.70mm diameter], 75mm length for inj into deeper muscles) should be used.

Localization of involved muscles w/ electromyographic guidance or nerve stimulation techniques may be useful.

Blepharospasm

A suitable sterile needle (eg, 30-gauge [0.40mm diameter], 12.5mm length should be used.

Glabellar Lines
A suitable sterile needle 30- to 33-gauge (0.3-0.2mm diameter), 13mm length should be used.

STORAGE
Unopened Vial: 20-25°C (68-77°F), 2-8°C (36-46°F), or -20 to -10°C (-4 to 14°F).

HOW SUPPLIED
Inj: 50 U, 100 U, 200 U

CONTRAINDICATIONS
Known hypersensitivity to any botulinum toxin preparation or to any of the components in the formulation. Infection at the proposed inj site(s).

WARNINGS/PRECAUTIONS
Not interchangeable w/ other botulinum toxin products; cannot be compared to or converted into U of any other botulinum toxin products. Hypersensitivity reactions reported; d/c and immediately institute appropriate medical therapy if serious and/or immediate hypersensitivity reactions occur. Increased risk of dysphagia in patients w/ smaller neck muscle mass and patients who require bilateral inj into the sternocleidomastoid muscles; limiting the dose injected into the sternocleidomastoid muscle may decrease the occurrence of dysphagia. Patients w/ neuromuscular disorders w/ peripheral motor neuropathic diseases, amyotrophic lateral sclerosis, or neuromuscular junctional disorders (eg, myasthenia gravis or Lambert-Eaton syndrome) may be at increased risk for severe dysphagia and respiratory compromise. Reduced blinking from inj in the orbicularis muscle can lead to corneal exposure, persistent epithelial defect, and corneal ulceration, especially in patients w/ VII nerve disorders; carefully test corneal sensation in eyes previously operated upon, avoid inj into the medial lower lid area to avoid ectropion, and vigorously treat any epithelial defect. Caution in patients at risk of developing narrow-angle glaucoma. Ecchymosis easily occurs in the soft tissues of the eyelid; immediate gentle pressure at the inj site can limit that risk. Risk of ptosis in patients treated for glabellar lines; avoid inj near the levator palpebrae superioris, particularly in patients w/ larger brow depressor complexes, and place corrugator inj at least 1cm above bony supraorbital ridge. Contains albumin; carries an extremely remote risk for transmission of viral diseases and Creutzfeldt-Jakob disease.

ADVERSE REACTIONS
Upper Limb Spasticity: Seizure, nasopharyngitis, dry mouth, URTI.
Cervical Dystonia: Dysphagia, neck pain, muscle weakness, inj-site pain, musculoskeletal pain.
Blepharospasm: Eyelid ptosis, dry eye, dry mouth, diarrhea, headache, visual impairment, dyspnea, nasopharyngitis, respiratory tract infection.
Glabellar Lines: Headache, facial paresis, inj-site hematoma, eyelid edema.

DRUG INTERACTIONS
Potentiation of toxin effect may occur w/ aminoglycosides or other agents interfering w/ neuromuscular transmission (eg, tubocurarine-type muscle relaxants); use w/ caution. Use of anticholinergic drugs after administration may potentiate systemic anticholinergic effects. Excessive neuromuscular weakness may be exacerbated by administration of another botulinum toxin prior to the resolution of the effects of a previously administered botulinum toxin. Use of a muscle relaxant before or after administration may exaggerate excessive weakness.

PREGNANCY AND LACTATION
Pregnancy: Category C.
Lactation: Caution in nursing.

MECHANISM OF ACTION
Acetylcholine release inhibitor; blocks cholinergic transmission at the neuromuscular junction by inhibiting the release of acetylcholine from peripheral cholinergic nerve endings.

PATIENT CONSIDERATIONS
Assessment: Assess for hypersensitivity to any botulinum toxin preparation or to any of the components in the formulation, infection at the proposed inj site(s), compromised swallowing or respiratory function, neuromuscular disorders w/ peripheral motor neuropathic diseases, amyotrophic lateral sclerosis, risk of developing narrow-angle glaucoma, pregnancy/nursing status, and possible drug interactions.

Monitoring: Monitor for spread of toxin effects, hypersensitivity reactions, swallowing/speech/respiratory disorders, and other adverse reactions.

Counseling: Advise to seek immediate medical care if swallowing, speech, or respiratory disorders arise. Remind previously immobile or sedentary patients to gradually resume activities following the inj of the drug. Inform that the drug may cause dyspnea, or mild to severe dysphagia, w/ risk of aspiration. Instruct to avoid driving or engaging in other potentially hazardous activities if loss of strength, muscle weakness, blurred vision, or drooping eyelids occur. Inform that the drug may cause reduced blinking or effectiveness of blinking; instruct to seek immediate medical attention if eye pain or irritation occurs following treatment.

Xgeva — denosumab   Rx
Class: IgG$_2$ monoclonal antibody

ADULT DOSAGE
Bone Metastasis from Solid Tumors
Prevention of Skeletal-Related Events:
120mg SQ every 4 weeks

Giant Cell Tumor of Bone
Treatment of tumor that is unresectable or where surgical resection is likely to result in severe morbidity

PEDIATRIC DOSAGE
Giant Cell Tumor of Bone
Treatment of tumor that is unresectable or where surgical resection is likely to result in severe morbidity

Adolescents (Skeletally Mature):
120mg SQ every 4 weeks w/ additional 120mg doses on Days 8 and 15 of the 1st month of therapy

120mg SQ every 4 weeks w/ additional 120mg doses on Days 8 and 15 of the 1st month of therapy

Hypercalcemia of Malignancy
Refractory to Bisphosphonate Therapy:
120mg SQ every 4 weeks w/ additional 120mg doses on Days 8 and 15 of the 1st month of therapy

----

ADMINISTRATION
SQ route
Administer in the upper arm, upper thigh, or abdomen.
Remove from refrigerator and bring to room temperature (up to 25°C [77°F]) prior to administration; do not warm any other way.
Avoid vigorous shaking.
Use 27-gauge needle to withdraw and inject entire vial contents.
Do not re-enter vial; discard vial after single-use or entry.

STORAGE
2-8°C (36-46°F). Do not freeze. Once removed from the refrigerator, do not expose to >25°C (77°F) or direct light; use w/in 14 days. Protect from direct light and heat.

HOW SUPPLIED
Inj: 120mg/1.7mL

CONTRAINDICATIONS
Hypocalcemia, known clinically significant hypersensitivity to denosumab.

WARNINGS/PRECAUTIONS
Do not give w/ other drugs that contain the same active ingredient (eg, Prolia). Hypersensitivity, including anaphylaxis, reported; initiate appropriate treatment and d/c therapy permanently if an anaphylactic or other clinically significant allergic reaction occurs. May cause severe symptomatic hypocalcemia, and fatal cases reported; increased risk in patients w/ increasing renal dysfunction, and w/ inadequate/no Ca^{2+} supplementation. Correct preexisting hypocalcemia prior to treatment, monitor Ca^{2+} levels throughout therapy especially in 1st weeks of initiation, and administer Ca^{2+}, Mg^{2+}, and vitamin D as necessary. Osteonecrosis of the jaw (ONJ) may occur; perform an oral exam and appropriate preventive dentistry prior to initiation of therapy and periodically during therapy. Avoid invasive dental procedures during therapy; consider temporary discontinuation of therapy if an invasive dental procedure must be performed. Atypical femoral fractures reported; evaluate patients w/ thigh/groin pain to rule out an incomplete femur fracture and consider interruption of therapy. Clinically significant hypercalcemia reported in patients w/ growing skeletons weeks to months following treatment discontinuation. May cause fetal harm.

ADVERSE REACTIONS
Fatigue/asthenia, hypophosphatemia, nausea.

DRUG INTERACTIONS
Monitor Ca^{2+} levels more frequently w/ other drugs that can lower Ca^{2+} levels.

PREGNANCY AND LACTATION
Pregnancy: Category D. Effects are likely to be greater during the 2nd and 3rd trimesters of pregnancy. Report pregnancies to Amgen.
Lactation: Not for use in nursing.
Reproductive Potential: Females of reproductive potential should use highly effective contraception during therapy, and for at least 5 months after the last dose of therapy. There is potential for fetal exposure when a male treated w/ therapy has unprotected sexual intercourse w/ a pregnant partner.

MECHANISM OF ACTION
IgG$_2$ monoclonal antibody; binds to RANK ligand (RANKL), a transmembrane or soluble protein essential for the formation, function, and survival of osteoclasts (cells responsible for bone resorption), thereby modulating Ca^{2+} release from bone. It prevents RANKL from activating its receptor, RANK, on the surface of osteoclasts, their precursors, and osteoclast-like giant cells.

PHARMACOKINETICS
Absorption: Bioavailability (62%). **Distribution:** Crosses placenta. **Elimination:** T$_{1/2}$=28 days.

PATIENT CONSIDERATIONS
Assessment: Assess for preexisting or risk of hypocalcemia, drug hypersensitivity, pregnancy/nursing status, and possible drug interactions. Perform an oral exam and appropriate preventive dentistry.

Monitoring: Monitor for anaphylactic/hypersensitivity reaction, ONJ, atypical femoral fracture, and other adverse reactions. Monitor Ca^{2+} levels. Perform an oral exam and appropriate preventive dentistry periodically.

Counseling: Advise to contact physician if experiencing symptoms of hypersensitivity reaction, hypocalcemia, ONJ, or atypical femoral fracture; persistent pain or slow healing of the mouth or jaw after dental surgery; or if pregnant/nursing. Advise to contact physician if symptoms of hypercalcemia following treatment discontinuation in patients w/ growing skeletons occur. Advise of the need for proper oral hygiene and routine dental care, to inform dentist that patient is receiving the drug, and to avoid invasive dental procedures during treatment. Advise females of reproductive potential to use highly effective contraception during and for at least 5 months after treatment. Advise that denosumab is also marketed as Prolia; instruct to inform physician if taking Prolia.

XIAFLEX — collagenase clostridium histolyticum   Rx

Class: Collagenase

> Corporal rupture (penile fracture), penile ecchymoses or hematoma, sudden penile detumescence, and/ or a penile "popping" sound or sensation reported. Promptly evaluate signs/symptoms to assess for corporal rupture or severe penile hematoma that may require surgical intervention. Available for the treatment of Peyronie's disease only through a restricted program under a Risk Evaluation and Mitigation Strategy (REMS) called the Xiaflex REMS Program.

ADULT DOSAGE

Dupuytren's Contracture

W/ a Palpable Cord:

0.58mg per inj administered into a palpable cord w/ a contracture of a metacarpophalangeal (MP) or a proximal interphalangeal (PIP) joint

Approx 24-72 hrs after inj, perform a finger extension procedure if a contracture persists to facilitate cord disruption; refer to PI for instructions

4 weeks after inj and finger extension procedure, if a MP or PIP contracture remains, the cord may be re-injected w/ a single dose of 0.58mg and the finger extension procedure may be repeated (approx 24-72 hrs after inj); inj and finger extension procedures may be administered up to 3X per cord at approx 4-week intervals

Perform up to 2 inj in the same hand according to the inj procedure during a treatment visit; 2 palpable cords affecting 2 joints may be injected or 1 palpable cord affecting 2 joints in the same finger may be injected at 2 locations during a treatment visit

If patient has other palpable cords w/ contractures of MP or PIP joints, these cords may be injected at other treatment visits approx 4 weeks apart

Peyronie's Disease

Treatment of adult men w/ a palpable plaque and curvature deformity of at least 30° at the start of therapy

0.58mg per inj administered into a Peyronie's plaque; if >1 plaque is present, inject into the plaque causing the curvature deformity

A treatment course consists of a max of 4 treatment cycles; each treatment cycle consists of 2 inj procedures. The 2nd inj procedure is performed 1-3 days after the 1st

The penile modeling procedure is performed 1-3 days after the 2nd inj of the treatment cycle; refer to PI for instructions

The interval between treatment cycles is approx 6 weeks. The treatment course, therefore, consists of a max of 8 inj procedures and 4 modeling procedures

If the curvature deformity is <15° after the 1st, 2nd, or 3rd treatment cycle, or if further treatment is not clinically indicated, then the subsequent treatment cycles should not be administered

PEDIATRIC DOSAGE

Pediatric use may not have been established

ADMINISTRATION

Intralesional route

Dupuytren's Contracture

Each vial and sterile diluent should only be used for a single inj; if 2 joints on the same hand are to be treated during a treatment visit, separate vials and syringes should be used for each reconstitution and inj.

Reconstitution of Lyophilized Powder:

1. Before use, allow the vial containing the lyophilized powder and the vial containing the diluent for reconstitution to stand at room temperature for at least 15 min and no longer than 60 min.
2. Use only the supplied diluent for reconstitution; the diluent contains Ca^{2+}, which is required for the activity of Xiaflex.
3. Using a 1mL syringe w/ 0.01mL graduations and a 27-gauge 1/2-inch needle (not supplied), withdraw a volume of the diluent supplied, as follows:

For Cords Affecting a MP Joint: 0.39mL
For Cords Affecting a PIP Joint: 0.31mL

4. Inject the diluent slowly into the sides of the vial containing the lyophilized powder.
5. Slowly swirl the sol to ensure that all of the lyophilized powder has gone into sol; do not invert the vial or shake the sol.
6. The reconstituted sol can be kept at room temperature for up to 1 hr or refrigerated for up to 4 hrs prior to administration; if the sol is refrigerated, allow it to return to room temperature for approx 15 min before use.
7. Discard the syringe and needle used for reconstitution and the diluent vial.

Preparation Prior to Inj:

1. Administration of a local anesthetic agent prior to inj is not recommended, as it may interfere w/ proper placement of the Xiaflex inj.
2. If injecting into a cord affecting the PIP joint of the 5th finger, care should be taken to inject as close to the palmar digital crease as possible (as far proximal to the digital PIP joint crease), and the needle insertion should not be >2-3mm in depth. Tendon ruptures occurred after inj near the digital PIP joint crease.
3. Reconfirm the cord(s) to be injected; the site chosen for each inj should be the area where the contracting cord is maximally separated from the underlying flexor tendons and where the skin is not intimately adhered to the cord.
4. Apply an antiseptic at the inj site and allow the skin to dry.

Inj Procedure:

1. Using a new 1mL hubless syringe that contains 0.01mL graduations w/ a permanently fixed, 27-gauge 1/2-inch needle (not supplied), withdraw a volume of reconstituted sol (containing 0.58mg of Xiaflex) as follows:

For Cords Affecting a MP Joint: 0.25 mL
For Cords Affecting a PIP Joint: 0.20mL

2. W/ your non-dominant hand, secure the patient's hand to be treated while simultaneously applying tension to the cord, and w/ your dominant hand, place the needle into the cord, using caution to keep the needle w/in the cord.
3. Avoid having the needle tip pass completely through the cord to help minimize the potential for inj into tissues other than the cord.
4. After needle placement, if there is any concern that the needle is in the flexor tendon, apply a small amount of passive motion at the distal interphalangeal joint.
5. If insertion of the needle into a tendon is suspected or paresthesia is noted by the patient, withdraw the needle and reposition it into the cord; if the needle is in the proper location, there will be some resistance noted during the inj procedure.
6. After confirming that the needle is correctly placed in the cord, inject approx 1/3 of the dose.
7. Withdraw the needle tip from the cord and reposition it in a slightly more distal location (approx 2-3mm) to the initial inj in the cord and inject another 1/3 of the dose.
8. Again withdraw the needle tip from the cord and reposition it a 3rd time proximal to the initial inj (approx 2-3mm) and inject the final portion of the dose into the cord.
9. When administering 2 inj in the same hand during a treatment visit, use a new syringe and separate vial of reconstituted sol for each inj. Repeat steps 1-9.
10. When administering 2 inj in the same hand during a treatment visit, begin w/ the affected finger in the most lateral aspect of the hand and continue toward the medial aspect (eg, 5th finger to index finger).
11. When administering 2 inj in a cord affecting 2 joints in the same finger, begin w/ the affected joint in the most proximal aspect of the finger and continue toward the distal aspect (eg, MP to PIP).
12. Wrap the patient's treated hand w/ a soft, bulky, gauze dressing.
13. Instruct the patient to limit motion of the treated finger(s) and to keep the injected hand elevated until hs.
14. Instruct the patient not to attempt to disrupt the injected cord(s) by self-manipulation and to return to the healthcare provider's office the next day for follow-up and a finger extension procedure(s), if needed.
15. Discard the unused portion of the reconstituted sol and diluent after inj; do not store, pool, or use any vials containing unused reconstituted sol or diluent.

Peyronie's Disease

Reconstitution of Lyophilized Powder:

1. Before use, allow the vial containing the lyophilized powder and the vial containing the diluent for reconstitution to stand at room temperature for at least 15 min and no longer than 60 min.
2. Use only the supplied diluent for reconstitution; the diluent contains Ca^{2+}, which is required for the activity of Xiaflex.
3. Using a 1mL syringe w/ 0.01mL graduations and a 27-gauge 1/2-inch needle (not supplied), withdraw a volume of 0.39mL of the diluent supplied.
4. Inject the diluent slowly into the sides of the vial containing the lyophilized powder.
5. Slowly swirl the sol to ensure that all of the lyophilized powder has gone into sol; do not invert the vial or shake the sol.
6. The reconstituted sol can be kept at room temperature for up to 1 hr or refrigerated for up to 4 hrs prior to administration; if the sol is refrigerated, allow it to return to room temperature for approx 15 min before use.
7. Discard the syringe and needle used for reconstitution and the diluent vial.

Identification of Treatment Area:

Prior to each treatment cycle, identify the treatment area as follows:
1. Induce a penile erection; a single intracavernosal inj of 10 or 20mcg of alprostadil may be used for this purpose. Apply antiseptic at inj site and allow the skin to dry prior to intracavernosal inj.
2. Locate the plaque at the point of max concavity (or focal point) in bend of the penis.
3. Mark the point w/ a surgical marker; this indicates target area in the plaque for Xiaflex deposition.

Inj Procedure:

1. Apply antiseptic at the inj site and allow the skin to dry.
2. Administer suitable local anesthetic, if desired.

3. Using a new hubless syringe containing 0.01mL graduations w/ a permanently fixed 27-gauge 1/2-inch needle (not supplied), withdraw a volume of 0.25mL of reconstituted sol (containing 0.58mg of Xiaflex).
4. The penis should be in a flaccid state before inj.
5. Place the needle tip on the side of the target plaque in alignment w/ the point of maximal concavity.
6. Orient the needle so that it enters the edge of the plaque and advance the needle into the plaque itself from the side; do not advance the needle beneath the plaque nor perpendicularly towards the corpora cavernosum.
7. Insert and advance the needle transversely through the width of the plaque, towards the opposite side of the plaque w/o passing completely through it.
8. Proper needle position is tested and confirmed by carefully noting resistance to minimal depression of the syringe plunger.
9. W/ the tip of the needle placed w/in the plaque, initiate inj, maintaining steady pressure to slowly inject Xiaflex into the plaque.
10. Withdraw the needle slowly so as to deposit the full dose along the needle track w/in the plaque; for plaques that are only a few mm in width, the distance of withdrawal of the syringe may be very minimal.
11. Upon complete withdrawal of the needle, apply gentle pressure at the inj site.
12. Apply a dressing as necessary.
13. Discard the unused portion of the reconstituted sol and diluent after each inj; do not store, pool, or use any vials containing unused reconstituted sol or diluent.
14. The 2nd inj of each treatment cycle should be made approx 2-3mm apart from the 1st inj.

STORAGE
2-8°C (36-46°F). Do not freeze. **Reconstituted Sol:** May keep at room temperature of 20-25°C (68-77°F) for up to 1 hr or refrigerate at 2-8°C (36-46°F) for up to 4 hrs.

HOW SUPPLIED
Inj: 0.9mg

CONTRAINDICATIONS
Treatment of Peyronie's plaques that involve the penile urethra, history of hypersensitivity to the medication or to collagenase used in any other therapeutic application or application method.

WARNINGS/PRECAUTIONS
Should be administered by a healthcare provider experienced in inj procedures of the hand and treatment of Dupuytren's contracture, or experienced in treatment of male urological diseases who has completed required training for use of collagenase clostridium histolyticum in the treatment of Peyronie's disease. Inj into collagen-containing structures (eg, tendons/ligaments of the hand, corpora cavernosa of the penis) may result in damage to those structures and possible permanent injury (eg, tendon rupture, ligament damage). Avoid injecting into the urethra, corpora cavernosa, tendons, nerves, blood vessels, or other collagen-containing structures. Other serious local reactions (eg, pulley rupture, ligament injury, complex regional pain syndrome, sensory abnormality of the hand) reported. Severe allergic reactions (eg, anaphylaxis) may occur. Avoid in patients w/ coagulation disorders.

ADVERSE REACTIONS
Dupuytren's Contracture: Peripheral edema, contusion, injection-site hemorrhage, injection-site reaction, pain in the injected extremity.
Peyronie's Disease: Penile hematoma, penile swelling, penile pain.

DRUG INTERACTIONS
Avoid in patients receiving concomitant anticoagulants, except low-dose aspirin (eg, ≤150mg/day).

PREGNANCY AND LACTATION
Pregnancy: Category B.
Lactation: Caution in nursing.

MECHANISM OF ACTION
Collagenase; hydrolyzes collagen, resulting in lysis of collagen deposits.

PHARMACOKINETICS
Absorption: (Peyronie's Disease) C_{max}= <29ng/mL (collagenase AUX-I), <71ng/mL (collagenase AUX-II); T_{max}=10 min.

PATIENT CONSIDERATIONS
Assessment: Assess for history of hypersensitivity to drug or to collagenase in other therapeutic applications, Peyronie's plaque involving the penile urethra, coagulation disorders, pregnancy/nursing status, and possible drug interactions.
Monitoring: Monitor for signs/symptoms of hypersensitivity reactions, tendon rupture, ligament damage, corporal rupture, penile ecchymoses/hematoma, sudden penile detumescence, penile "popping" sound or sensation, and other adverse reactions.
Counseling: Dupuytren's Contracture: Advise of serious complications that may result in inability to fully bend finger and may require surgery. Inform that inj is likely to result in swelling, bruising, bleeding, and/or pain of injected site and surrounding tissue. After inj, instruct not to flex/extend the fingers of injected hand, not to disrupt injected cord(s) by self-manipulation, to elevate injected hand until hs, and to promptly contact physician if there is evidence of infection, sensory changes in treated finger(s), trouble bending finger(s) after the swelling goes down, or skin laceration. Instruct to return for follow up 1-3 days after the inj visit. Instruct not to perform strenuous activity w/ injected hand until advised to do so, to wear splint at hs for up to 4 months, and to perform a series of finger flexion and extension exercises each day. **Peyronie's Disease:** Advise of serious complications that may require surgery to correct. Inform that penis may appear bruised and/or swollen, and that they may have mild to moderate penile pain that can be relieved by taking OTC medications. Instruct to promptly contact physician if they have severe pain, swelling, purple bruising/swelling of the penis, difficulty urinating or blood in the urine, or sudden loss of ability to maintain an erection; inform that these may be accompanied by a popping or cracking sound from the penis. Instruct to return to physician's office when directed for further inj(s) and/or penile modeling procedure(s), and to wait 2 weeks after 2nd inj of a treatment

cycle before resuming sexual activity, provided pain and swelling have subsided. Advise not to have sex between the 1st and 2nd inj of a treatment cycle.

XOLAIR — omalizumab   Rx
Class: Monoclonal antibody/IgE blocker

> Anaphylaxis, presenting as bronchospasm, hypotension, syncope, urticaria, and/or angioedema of throat or tongue, reported as early as after the 1st dose and beyond 1 yr of therapy; closely observe patients. Inform of the signs/symptoms of anaphylaxis and instruct to seek immediate medical care should symptoms occur.

ADULT DOSAGE
Asthma
Moderate to Severe Persistent Asthma w/ a (+) Skin Test or In Vitro Reactivity to a Perennial Aeroallergen and Inadequately Controlled w/ Inhaled Corticosteroids:
75-375mg SQ every 2 or 4 weeks, based on body weight (kg) and pretreatment serum total IgE level (IU/mL)

Periodically reassess the need for continued therapy based upon the patient's disease severity and level of asthma control

Refer to PI for dose determination charts and further information

Chronic Idiopathic Urticaria
Symptomatic Despite H1 Antihistamine Treatment:
150mg or 300mg SQ every 4 weeks

Periodically reassess the need for continued therapy

PEDIATRIC DOSAGE
Asthma
Moderate to Severe Persistent Asthma w/ a (+) Skin Test or In Vitro Reactivity to a Perennial Aeroallergen and Inadequately Controlled w/ Inhaled Corticosteroids:
≥6 Years:
75-375mg SQ every 2 or 4 weeks, based on body weight (kg) and pretreatment serum total IgE level (IU/mL)

Periodically reassess the need for continued therapy based upon the patient's disease severity and level of asthma control

Refer to PI for dose determination charts and further information

Chronic Idiopathic Urticaria
Symptomatic Despite H1 Antihistamine Treatment:
≥12 Years:
150mg or 300mg SQ every 4 weeks

Periodically reassess the need for continued therapy.

ADMINISTRATION
SQ route
The inj may take 5-10 sec to administer.
Do not administer more than 150mg (contents of one vial) per inj site.

Number of Inj and Total Inj Volume
75mg inj involves 1 inj (0.6mL total volume inj).
150mg inj involves 1 inj (1.2mL total volume inj).
225mg inj involves 2 inj (1.8mL total volume inj).
300mg inj involves 2 inj (2.4mL total volume inj).
375mg inj involves 3 inj (3.0mL total volume inj).

Reconstitution for Single Vial
Before reconstitution, determine the number of vials that will need to be reconstituted.
1. Reconstitute w/ sterile water for inj (SWFI).
2. Draw 1.4mL of SWFI into a 3mL syringe equipped w/ a 1-inch, 18-gauge needle.
3. Insert the needle and inject the SWFI directly onto the product.
4. Gently swirl the upright vial for approx 1 min; do not shake.
5. Gently swirl the vial for 5-10 sec approx every 5 min in order to dissolve any remaining solids. The lyophilized product takes 15-20 min to dissolve.
6. If it takes longer than 20 min to dissolve completely, gently swirl the vial for 5-10 sec approx every 5 min until there are no visible gel-like particles in the sol. Do not use if the contents of the vial do not dissolve completely by 40 min.
7. Invert the vial for 15 sec in order to allow the sol to drain toward the stopper.
8. Using a new 3mL syringe equipped w/ a 1-inch, 18-gauge needle, draw the sol into the syringe.
9. Replace the 18-gauge needle w/ a 25-gauge needle for SQ inj.

STORAGE
2-8°C (36-46°F). **Reconstituted:** 2-8°C (36-46°F) for up to 8 hrs, or 4 hrs at room temperature. Protect from direct sunlight.

HOW SUPPLIED
Inj: 150mg

CONTRAINDICATIONS
Severe hypersensitivity reaction to omalizumab or any ingredient of this medication.

WARNINGS/PRECAUTIONS
Not indicated for treatment of other forms of urticaria, relief of acute bronchospasm or status asthmaticus, or other allergic conditions. Administer only in a healthcare setting prepared to manage anaphylaxis and observe patients for an appropriate period after administration. D/C if a severe hypersensitivity reaction occurs. Malignant neoplasms reported. Do not abruptly d/c systemic or inhaled corticosteroids when initiating therapy. Eosinophilic conditions reported; be alert to eosinophilia, vasculitic rash, worsening pulmonary symptoms, cardiac complications, and/or neuropathy, especially upon reduction of oral corticosteroids. Monitor patients at high risk for geohelminth infections (eg, roundworm, hookworm). Signs/symptoms similar to those seen in patients w/ serum sickness, including arthritis/arthralgia, rash, fever, and lymphadenopathy, reported; d/c if these symptoms develop. Serum total IgE levels increase due to formation of Xolair:IgE complexes and may persist for up to 1 yr following discontinuation of therapy; do not use serum total

IgE levels obtained <1 yr following discontinuation to reassess dosing regimen for asthma patients.

ADVERSE REACTIONS
Asthma: ≥12 Years: Arthralgia, pain (general), leg pain, fatigue, dizziness, fracture, arm pain, pruritus, dermatitis, earache.
Asthma: 6 to <12 Years: Nasopharyngitis, headache, pyrexia, upper abdominal pain, pharyngitis streptococcal, otitis media, viral gastroenteritis, arthropod bites, epistaxis.
Chronic Idiopathic Urticaria (CIU): Nausea, nasopharyngitis, sinusitis, URTI, viral URTI, arthralgia, headache, cough.

PREGNANCY AND LACTATION
Pregnancy: The data w/ Xolair use in pregnant women are insufficient to inform on drug-associated risk. Monoclonal antibodies (eg, omalizumab) are transported across the placenta in a linear fashion as pregnancy progresses; potential effects on a fetus are likely to be greater during the 2nd and 3rd trimesters of pregnancy.
Lactation: Caution in nursing.

MECHANISM OF ACTION
Monoclonal antibody/IgE blocker; (asthma) inhibits binding of IgE to the high-affinity IgE receptor on the surface of mast cells and basophils, limiting the degree of release of mediators of allergic response. **CIU:** Has not been established; binds to IgE and lowers free IgE levels; IgE receptors on cells down-regulate.

PHARMACOKINETICS
Absorption: Slow. Absolute bioavailability (62%); T_{max}=7-8 days. **Distribution:** V_d=78mL/kg. **Elimination:** $T_{1/2}$=26 days (asthma), 24 days (CIU).

PATIENT CONSIDERATIONS
Assessment: Assess for acute bronchospasm or status asthmaticus, malignancies, hypersensitivity reaction to drug or any of its ingredients, risk of geohelminth infections, and pregnancy/nursing status. Obtain baseline body weight and serum IgE levels.

Monitoring: Monitor for anaphylaxis, hypersensitivity reactions, inj-site reactions, malignancies, viral/geohelminth infections, URTIs, eosinophilia, vasculitic rash, worsening pulmonary symptoms, cardiac complications, neuropathy, arthritis/arthralgia, rash, fever, lymphadenopathy, and other adverse reactions. Periodically reassess need for continued therapy. Monitor body weight, CBC, and IgE levels prn.

Counseling: Instruct to read the medication guide before treatment. Inform of the risk of life-threatening anaphylaxis; instruct to seek immediate medical care if symptoms of anaphylaxis occur. Instruct not to decrease dose of or stop taking any other asthma or CIU medications unless otherwise instructed. Inform that immediate improvement of asthma or CIU symptoms may not be seen after beginning therapy. Instruct to notify physician if pregnant or breastfeeding.

Xtandi — enzalutamide   Rx

Class: Antiandrogen

ADULT DOSAGE	PEDIATRIC DOSAGE
Metastatic Castration-Resistant Prostate Cancer	Pediatric use may not have been established
160mg (four 40mg caps) qd	

DOSING CONSIDERATIONS
Concomitant Medications
Strong CYP2C8 Inhibitors: Avoid concomitant use; if coadministration is necessary, reduce enzalutamide dose to 80mg qd. If coadministration of the strong inhibitor is discontinued, return to enzalutamide dose used prior to initiation of the strong CYP2C8 inhibitor

Strong CYP3A4 Inducers: Avoid concomitant use; if coadministration is necessary, increase enzalutamide dose from 160mg to 240mg qd. If coadministration of the strong inducer is discontinued, return to enzalutamide dose used prior to initiation of the strong CYP3A4 inducer

Adverse Reactions
≥Grade 3 Toxicity/Intolerable Side Effect: Withhold dosing for 1 week or until symptoms improve to ≤Grade 2, then resume at the same or a reduced dose (120mg or 80mg), if warranted

ADMINISTRATION
Oral route

Take w/ or w/o food.
Swallow caps whole; do not chew, dissolve, or open.

STORAGE
20-25°C (68-77°F); excursions permitted from 15-30°C (59-86°F). Store in a dry place; keep container tightly closed.

HOW SUPPLIED
Cap: 40mg

CONTRAINDICATIONS
Women who are or may become pregnant.

WARNINGS/PRECAUTIONS
Seizures reported; caution in engaging in any activity where sudden loss of consciousness could cause serious harm to patient or to others. D/C permanently if seizures develop during treatment. Posterior reversible encephalopathy syndrome (PRES) reported; d/c if PRES develops. Caution in elderly.

ADVERSE REACTIONS
Asthenia/fatigue, back pain, decreased appetite, constipation, arthralgia, diarrhea, hot flush, URTI, peripheral edema, dyspnea, musculoskeletal pain, decreased weight, headache, HTN, dizziness/vertigo.

DRUG INTERACTIONS
See Dosing Considerations. Coadministration of a strong CYP2C8 inhibitor (gemfibrozil) increased exposure of enzalutamide. Coadministration of rifampin (strong CYP3A4 inducer and moderate CYP2C8 inducer) decreased exposure. St John's wort may decrease exposure and should be avoided. May reduce plasma exposure of midazolam (CYP3A4 substrate), warfarin (CYP2C9 substrate), and omeprazole (CYP2C19 substrate). Avoid concomitant use w/ narrow therapeutic index drugs that are metabolized by CYP3A4 (eg, alfentanil, cyclosporine, dihydroergotamine, sirolimus), CYP2C9 (eg, phenytoin, warfarin), and CYP2C19 (eg, S-mephenytoin); enzalutamide may decrease their exposure. If coadministration w/ warfarin cannot be avoided, conduct additional INR monitoring.

PREGNANCY AND LACTATION
Pregnancy: Category X.
Lactation: Not for use in nursing.

MECHANISM OF ACTION
Nonsteroidal antiandrogen; acts on different steps in the androgen receptor signaling pathway. Competitively inhibits androgen binding to androgen receptors and inhibits androgen receptor nuclear translocation and interaction w/ DNA.

PHARMACOKINETICS
Absorption: C_{max}=16.6mcg/mL, 12.7mcg/mL (major active metabolite); T_{max}=1 hr (median). **Distribution:** V_d=110L; plasma protein binding (97-98%, 95% active metabolite). **Metabolism:** Hepatic via CYP2C8 and CYP3A4; N-desmethyl enzalutamide (major active metabolite). **Elimination:** Urine (71%), feces (14%, 0.4% unchanged, 1% active metabolite); $T_{1/2}$=5.8 days, 7.8-8.6 days (major active metabolite).

PATIENT CONSIDERATIONS
Assessment: Assess pregnancy/nursing status and for possible drug interactions.

Monitoring: Monitor for seizures, PRES, and other adverse reactions. Conduct additional INR monitoring if coadministration w/ warfarin cannot be avoided.

Counseling: Instruct to take dose at the same time each day. Inform those receiving a gonadotropin-releasing hormone analogue to maintain such treatment during the course of therapy. Inform that therapy has been associated w/ increased risk of seizures; discuss conditions that may predispose to seizures and medications that may lower seizure threshold. Advise of risk of engaging in any activity where sudden loss of consciousness could cause serious harm to self or others. Inform patients to contact physician right away if they have loss of consciousness or seizures. Inform to contact physician right away if rapidly worsening symptoms possibly indicative of PRES are experienced. Instruct not to interrupt, modify dose, or d/c therapy w/o 1st consulting physician. Instruct not to take more than the prescribed dose per day. Apprise of the common side effects associated w/ therapy. Inform that drug may cause infections, falls and fall-related injuries, and HTN. Instruct to use a condom if having intercourse w/ a pregnant woman, and to use a condom and another effective birth control method if having intercourse w/ a woman of childbearing potential; advise that these measures are required during and for 3 months after treatment.

Xyntha — antihemophilic factor (recombinant)   Rx

Class: Antihemophilic factor (recombinant)

OTHER BRAND NAMES
Xyntha Solofuse

ADULT DOSAGE	PEDIATRIC DOSAGE
Congenital Hemophilia A	**Congenital Hemophilia A**
Dosage (IU) = Body weight (kg) x desired factor VIII (FVIII) rise (IU/dL or % of normal) x 0.5 (IU/kg per IU/dL)	Dosage (IU) = Body weight (kg) x desired factor VIII (FVIII) rise (IU/dL or % of normal) x 0.5 (IU/kg per IU/dL)
Control and Prevention of Bleeding Episodes:	**Control and Prevention of Bleeding Episodes:**
Minor Bleed: Dose to maintain plasma FVIII activity at 20-40 IU/dL, given q12-24h for at least 1 day, depending upon the severity of the bleeding episode	**Minor Bleed:** Dose to maintain plasma FVIII activity at 20-40 IU/dL, given q12-24h for at least 1 day, depending upon the severity of the bleeding episode
Moderate Bleed: Dose to maintain plasma FVIII activity at 30-60 IU/dL, given q12-24h for 3-4 days or until adequate local hemostasis is achieved	**Moderate Bleed:** Dose to maintain plasma FVIII activity at 30-60 IU/dL, given q12-24h for 3-4 days or until adequate local hemostasis is achieved
Major Bleed: Dose to maintain plasma FVIII activity at 60-100 IU/dL; given q8-24h until bleeding is resolved	**Major Bleed:** Dose to maintain plasma FVIII activity at 60-100 IU/dL, given q8-24h until bleeding is resolved
Perioperative Management:	**Perioperative Management:**
Minor Operations: Dose to maintain plasma FVIII activity at 30-60 IU/dL, given q12-24h for 3-4 days or until adequate local hemostasis is achieved; a single infusion + oral antifibrinolytic therapy w/in 1 hr may be sufficient for a tooth extraction	**Minor Operations:** Dose to maintain plasma FVIII activity at 30-60 IU/dL, given q12-24h for 3-4 days or until adequate local hemostasis is achieved; a single infusion + oral antifibrinolytic therapy w/in 1 hr may be sufficient for a tooth extraction
Major Operations: Dose to maintain plasma FVIII activity at 60-100 IU/dL, given q8-24h until threat is resolved, or in the case of surgery, until adequate local hemostasis and wound healing are achieved	**Major Operations:** Dose to maintain plasma FVIII activity at 60-100 IU/dL, given q8-24h until threat is resolved, or in the case of surgery, until adequate local hemostasis and wound healing are achieved

ADMINISTRATION
IV route

Do not administer in the same tubing or container as other medications

If using 1 vial of Xyntha w/ 1 Xyntha Solofuse, use a separate ≥10mL luer lock syringe to draw back the reconstituted contents of the vial and the syringe

If using multiple syringes/vials of the medication, reconstitute each syringe/vial according to the instructions using a separate ≥10mL luer lock syringe to draw back the reconstituted contents of each syringe/vial

Administer w/in 3 hrs after reconstitution or after removal of grey rubber tip cap from Solofuse

Refer to PI for further details on administration, preparation, and reconstitution

STORAGE
2-8°C (36-46°F) for up to 36 months from the date of manufacture until the expiration date. May also store at room temperature not to exceed 25°C (77°F) for up to 3 months. Avoid freezing. Avoid prolonged exposure to light. (Solofuse) At the end of 3-month period, immediately use or discard the product. Do not put back into the refrigerator. (Xyntha) At the end of 3-month period, immediately use, discard, or return product to refrigerated storage. May return to the refrigerator until the expiration date after room temperature storage. Do not store at room temperature and return it to the refrigerator more than once. Diluent Syringe: 2-25°C (36-77°F).

HOW SUPPLIED
Inj: 250 IU, 500 IU, 1000 IU, 2000 IU; (Solofuse) 250 IU, 500 IU, 1000 IU, 2000 IU, 3000 IU

CONTRAINDICATIONS
Life-threatening immediate hypersensitivity reactions, including anaphylaxis, to the product or its components, including hamster proteins.

WARNINGS/PRECAUTIONS
Not indicated in patients w/ von Willebrand's disease. Initiate therapy under the supervision of a physician experienced in the treatment of hemophilia A. Allergic-type hypersensitivity reactions, including anaphylaxis, reported; d/c if symptoms occur and administer emergency treatment. FVIII inhibitors reported; perform an assay that measures FVIII inhibitor concentration if expected FVIII activity levels are not attained or if bleeding is not controlled w/ an appropriate dose.

ADVERSE REACTIONS
Headache, arthralgia, N/V, diarrhea, asthenia, pyrexia, cough.

PREGNANCY AND LACTATION
Category C, caution in nursing.

MECHANISM OF ACTION
Antihemophilic factor (recombinant); temporarily replaces the missing clotting FVIII that is needed for effective hemostasis.

PHARMACOKINETICS
Absorption: (Initial visit) C_{max}=1.08 IU/mL; AUC=13.5 IU•hr/mL. (Month 6) C_{max}=1.24 IU/mL; AUC=15 IU•hr/mL. (Pre-surgery) C_{max}=1.08 IU/mL; AUC= 16 IU•hr/mL. (Adolescents) C_{max}=0.97 IU/mL; AUC=8.5 IU•hr/mL. (Young Children) C_{max}=0.78 IU/mL; AUC=12.2 IU•hr/mL. **Distribution:** V_d= 66.1mL/kg (initial visit), 67.4mL/kg (month 6), 69mL/kg (pre-surgery), 67.1mL/kg (adolescents), 66.9mL/kg (young children). **Elimination:** $T_{1/2}$=11.2 hrs (initial visit), 11.8 hrs (month 6), 16.7 hrs (pre-surgery), 6.9 hrs (adolescents), 8.3 hrs (young children).

PATIENT CONSIDERATIONS
Assessment: Assess for hypersensitivity to drug or hamster proteins or other constituents of the product, location and extent of bleeding, patient's clinical condition, and pregnancy/nursing status. Assess plasma FVIII activity levels.

Monitoring: Monitor for development of FVIII inhibitors, plasma FVIII activity levels, clinical response, signs/symptoms of hypersensitivity reactions, and other adverse reactions.

Counseling: Advise to report physician if any adverse reactions develop, if pregnant or intending to become pregnant, or if breastfeeding. Inform about early signs/symptoms of hypersensitivity reactions (eg, hives, generalized urticaria, chest tightness) and anaphylaxis; instruct to d/c use and contact physician if symptoms occur. Advise to contact physician if lack of clinical response to FVIII replacement therapy is experienced. Advise to consult physician prior to travel and to bring adequate supply based on patient's current regimen of treatment when traveling. (Solofuse) Inform that local irritation may occur.

XYREM — sodium oxybate
CIII

Class: CNS depressant

> Obtundation and clinically significant respiratory depression occurred at recommended doses; almost all patients in trials were receiving CNS stimulants. Sodium oxybate is the Na⁺ salt of gamma hydroxybutyrate (GHB); abuse of GHB, alone or in combination w/ other CNS depressants, is associated w/ CNS adverse reactions, including seizure, respiratory depression, decreased level of consciousness, coma, and death. Available only through a restricted distribution program (Xyrem REMS Program).

ADULT DOSAGE
Narcolepsy

Treatment of Cataplexy and Excessive Daytime Sleepiness:
Initial: 4.5g/night administered in 2 equally divided doses (2.25g qhs and 2.25g taken 2.5-4 hrs later)
Titrate: Increase by 1.5g/night at weekly intervals (additional 0.75g qhs and 0.75g taken 2.5-4 hrs later)
Effective Dose Range: 6-9g/night
Max: 9g/night

PEDIATRIC DOSAGE
Pediatric use may not have been established

DOSING CONSIDERATIONS
Concomitant Medications
Divalproex Sodium:
Patients Already Stabilized on Xyrem: Addition of divalproex sodium should be accompanied by an initial reduction in the nightly dose of Xyrem by at least 20%
Patients Already Taking Divalproex Sodium: Use lower starting dose of Xyrem; monitor patient response and adjust dose accordingly

Hepatic Impairment
Initial: 2.25g/night administered in 2 equally divided doses (approx 1.13g qhs and approx 1.13g taken 2.5-4 hrs later)

Elderly
Start at lower end of dosing range

ADMINISTRATION
Oral route

Take 1st dose at least 2 hrs after eating
Prepare both doses prior to bedtime
Prior to ingestion, dilute each dose w/ approx 1/4 cup (approx 60mL) of water in the empty pharmacy vials provided
Take both doses while in bed and lie down immediately after dosing
Remain in bed following ingestion of the 1st and 2nd doses; an alarm may need to be set to awaken for 2nd dose

STORAGE
25°C (77°F); excursions permitted to 15-30°C (59-86°F).

HOW SUPPLIED
Oral Sol: 0.5g/mL [180mL]

CONTRAINDICATIONS
Concomitant use w/ sedative hypnotic agents and alcohol. Succinic semialdehyde dehydrogenase deficiency.

WARNINGS/PRECAUTIONS
May impair physical/mental abilities. Evaluate for history of drug abuse and monitor closely for signs of misuse/abuse. May impair respiratory drive, especially in patients w/ compromised respiratory function. Increased central apneas, oxygen desaturation events, and sleep-related breathing disorders may occur. Sleep-related breathing disorders tend to be more prevalent in obese patients, postmenopausal women not on hormone replacement therapy, and narcolepsy patients. Caution w/ history of depressive illness and/or suicide attempt; monitor for emergence of depressive symptoms. Confusion, anxiety, and other neuropsychiatric reactions (eg, hallucinations, paranoia) reported; carefully evaluate emergence of confusion, thought disorders, and/or behavior abnormalities. Parasomnias reported; fully evaluate episodes of sleepwalking. Contains high salt content; consider amount of daily Na⁺ intake in each dose in patients sensitive to salt intake.

ADVERSE REACTIONS
N/V, dizziness, diarrhea, somnolence, enuresis, tremor, attention disturbance, pain, sleep paralysis, paresthesia, disorientation, irritability, hyperhidrosis.

DRUG INTERACTIONS
See Dosing Considerations and Contraindications. Concurrent use w/ other CNS depressants (eg, opioid analgesics, sedating antidepressants/antipsychotics/antiepileptic drugs, muscle relaxants) may increase risk of respiratory depression, hypotension, profound sedation, syncope, and death; consider dose reduction or discontinuation of ≥1 CNS depressants (including sodium oxybate) if combination therapy is required. Consider interruption of treatment w/ sodium oxybate if short-term use of an opioid (eg, post- or perioperative) is required. Concomitant use w/ divalproex sodium resulted in a 25% mean increase in systemic exposure to sodium oxybate; monitor response closely and adjust dose accordingly if concomitant use is warranted.

PREGNANCY AND LACTATION
Category C, caution in nursing.

MECHANISM OF ACTION
CNS depressant; has not been established. Hypothesized that the therapeutic effects are mediated through $GABA_B$ actions at noradrenergic, dopaminergic, and thalamocortical neurons.

PHARMACOKINETICS
Absorption: Rapid; absolute bioavailability (88%); T_{max}=0.5-1.25 hr.
Distribution: V_d=190-384mL/kg; plasma protein binding (<1%). **Metabolism:** GHB dehydrogenase catalyzes the conversion of sodium oxybate to succinic semialdehyde, which is biotransformed to succinic acid by succinic semialdehyde dehydrogenase. Succinic acid enters the Krebs cycle. β-oxidation (secondary). **Elimination:** Lungs, urine (<5% unchanged); $T_{1/2}$=0.5-1 hr.

PATIENT CONSIDERATIONS
Assessment: Assess for succinic semialdehyde dehydrogenase deficiency, alcohol intake, history of drug abuse, compromised respiratory function, history of depressive illness and/or suicide attempt, hepatic impairment, sensitivity to salt intake, pregnancy/nursing status, and possible drug interactions.

Monitoring: Monitor for obtundation, respiratory depression, CNS depression, signs of abuse/misuse, sleep-disordered breathing, depression and suicidality, confusion, anxiety, other neuropsychiatric reactions, parasomnias, and other possible adverse reactions.

Counseling: Inform about the Xyrem REMS Program. Instruct to see prescriber frequently (every 3 months) to review therapy. Instruct to store drug in a secure place, out of reach of children/pets. Inform that patients are likely to fall asleep quickly (w/in 5-15 min) after taking the drug; instruct to remain in bed after taking 1st and 2nd doses. Advise not to drink alcohol or take other sedative hypnotics while on therapy. Inform that therapy can be associated w/ respiratory depression. Instruct to avoid operating hazardous machinery until patients are reasonably certain that therapy does not affect them adversely and for at least 6 hrs after the 2nd nightly dose. Advise to contact physician if depressed mood, markedly diminished interest or pleasure in usual activities, significant change in weight and/or appetite, psychomotor agitation or retardation, increased fatigue, feelings of guilt or worthlessness, slowed thinking or impaired concentration, or suicidal ideation develops. Inform that sleepwalking may occur; instruct to notify physician if this occurs. Inform patients who are sensitive to salt intake that the drug contains a significant amount of Na⁺ and they should limit their Na⁺ intake.

YERVOY — ipilimumab   Rx
Class: Monoclonal antibody/CTLA-4 blocker

> Can result in severe and fatal immune-mediated adverse reactions, and may involve any organ system; the most common reactions are enterocolitis, hepatitis, dermatitis (eg, toxic epidermal necrolysis [TEN]), neuropathy, and endocrinopathy. The majority of these reactions initially manifested during treatment; however, a minority occurred weeks to months after discontinuation of therapy. Permanently d/c therapy and initiate systemic high-dose corticosteroid therapy for severe immune-mediated reactions. Assess for signs/symptoms of enterocolitis, dermatitis, neuropathy, and endocrinopathy, and evaluate clinical chemistries (eg, LFTs, ACTH level, thyroid function tests) at baseline and before each dose.

ADULT DOSAGE

Unresectable or Metastatic Melanoma
3mg/kg IV over 90 min every 3 weeks for a max of 4 doses

In the event of toxicity, doses may be delayed, but all treatment must be administered w/in 16 weeks of the first dose

Cutaneous Melanoma
Adjuvant treatment of patients w/ pathologic involvement of regional lymph nodes of >1mm who have undergone complete resection, including total lymphadenectomy

10mg/kg IV over 90 min every 3 weeks for 4 doses followed by 10mg/kg every 12 weeks for up to 3 years

In the event of toxicity, doses are omitted, not delayed

PEDIATRIC DOSAGE
Pediatric use may not have been established

DOSING CONSIDERATIONS
Hepatic Impairment
Mild (Total Bilirubin >1-1.5X ULN or AST >ULN): No dose adjustment needed
Moderate (Total Bilirubin >1.5-3X ULN and Any AST) or Severe (Total Bilirubin >3X ULN and Any AST): Not studied

Adverse Reactions
Endocrine:
Symptomatic Endocrinopathy: Withhold therapy; resume in patients w/ complete or partial resolution of adverse reactions (Grade 0 to 1) and who are receiving <7.5mg prednisone or equivalent per day.
Symptomatic Reactions Lasting ≥6 Weeks: Permanently d/c.
Inability to Reduce Corticosteroid Dose to 7.5mg Prednisone or Equivalent per Day: Permanently d/c.
Ophthalmologic:
Grade 2 through 4 Reactions Not Improving to Grade 1 w/in 2 Weeks While Receiving Topical Therapy: Permanently d/c.
Grade 2 through 4 Reactions Requiring Systemic Treatment: Permanently d/c.
All Other:
Grade 2: Withhold therapy; resume in patients w/ complete or partial resolution of adverse reactions (Grade 0 to 1) and who are receiving <7.5mg prednisone or equivalent per day.
Grade 2 Reactions Lasting ≥6 Weeks: Permanently d/c.
Inability to Reduce Corticosteroid Dose to 7.5mg Prednisone or Equivalent per Day: Permanently d/c.
Grade 3 or 4: Permanently d/c.

ADMINISTRATION
IV route
Administer diluted sol over 90 min through an IV line containing a sterile, non-pyrogenic, low-protein-binding in-line filter.
Flush the IV line w/ 0.9% NaCl inj or D5 inj after each dose.
Do not mix w/, or administer as an infusion w/, other medicinal products.

Preparation of Sol
1. Allow the vials to stand at room temperature for approx 5 min prior to preparation of infusion.
2. Withdraw the required volume of ipilimumab and transfer into an IV bag.
3. Dilute w/ 0.9% NaCl inj or D5 inj to prepare a diluted sol, w/ a final concentration ranging from 1-2mg/mL.
4. Mix diluted sol by gentle inversion; do not shake.
5. Store diluted sol for no more than 24 hrs at 2-8°C (36-46°F) or at 20-25°C (68-77°F).
6. Discard partially used vials or empty vials.

STORAGE
2-8°C (36-46°F). Do not freeze. Protect from light.

HOW SUPPLIED
Inj: 5mg/mL [10mL, 40mL]

WARNINGS/PRECAUTIONS
Refer to Dosing Considerations for recommendations to withhold or d/c therapy for the following adverse reactions. Refer to PI for corticosteroid dose in the management of the following adverse reactions. Immune-mediated enterocolitis, including fatal cases, can occur. Permanently d/c in patients w/ severe enterocolitis and initiate corticosteroids; initiate corticosteroid taper upon improvement to ≤Grade 1. Withhold therapy for moderate enterocolitis; administer antidiarrheal treatment and, if persistent for >1 week, initiate corticosteroids. Immune-mediated hepatitis, including fatal cases, can occur. Permanently d/c in patients w/ Grade 3 or 4 hepatotoxicity and administer corticosteroids; when LFTs show sustained improvement or return to baseline, initiate corticosteroid taper. Withhold therapy in patients w/ Grade 2 hepatotoxicity. Immune-mediated dermatitis, including fatal cases, can occur. Permanently d/c in patients w/ Stevens-Johnson syndrome, TEN, or rash complicated by full thickness dermal ulceration, or necrotic, bullous, or hemorrhagic manifestations. Administer corticosteroids; when dermatitis is controlled, initiate corticosteroid taper. Withhold in patients w/ moderate to severe signs/symptoms. Immune-mediated neuropathies, including fatal cases, can occur. Permanently d/c in patients w/ severe neuropathy (eg, Guillain-Barre-like syndromes). Consider initiation of corticosteroids. Withhold in patients w/ moderate neuropathy (not interfering w/ daily activities). Immune-mediated endocrinopathies, including life-threatening cases, can occur. Withhold in symptomatic patients; initiate corticosteroids and appropriate hormone replacement therapy. Permanently d/c for clinically significant or severe immune-mediated adverse reactions; initiate corticosteroids for severe immune-mediated adverse reactions. Administer corticosteroid eye drops to patients who develop uveitis, iritis, or episcleritis; permanently d/c for immune-mediated ocular disease that is unresponsive to local immunosuppressive therapy. Can cause fetal harm.

ADVERSE REACTIONS
Unresectable/Metastatic Melanoma: Diarrhea, colitis, pruritus, rash, fatigue.
Adjuvant Treatment of Melanoma: Rash, pruritus, diarrhea, N/V, colitis, weight decreased, fatigue, pyrexia, headache, decreased appetite, insomnia.

DRUG INTERACTIONS
Increased transaminases w/ or w/o concomitant increases in total bilirubin reported in patients who received concurrent vemurafenib (960mg bid or 720mg bid).

PREGNANCY AND LACTATION
Pregnancy: Ipilimumab can cause fetal harm based on its mechanism of action and data from animal studies. Human IgG1 is known to cross the placental barrier; therefore, ipilimumab has the potential to be transmitted from the mother to the developing fetus. Effects are likely to be greater during the 2nd and 3rd trimesters. Advise pregnant women of potential risk to fetus. A Pregnancy Safety Surveillance Study has been established to collect information about pregnancies in women who have received ipilimumab; advise pregnant women to enroll.
Lactation: D/C nursing during treatment and for 3 months following the final dose.
Reproductive Potential: Females of reproductive potential should use effective contraception during treatment and for 3 months following the last dose.

MECHANISM OF ACTION
Human monoclonal antibody/CTLA-4 blocker; binds to CTLA-4 and blocks its interaction w/ its ligands, CD80/CD86. Blockade of CTLA-4 has been shown to augment T-cell activation and proliferation, including the activation and proliferation of tumor infiltrating T-effector cells and reduction of T-regulatory cell function, which may contribute to a general increase in T-cell responsiveness, including the antitumor immune response.

PHARMACOKINETICS
Distribution: Crosses placenta. **Elimination:** $T_{1/2}$=15.4 days.

PATIENT CONSIDERATIONS
Assessment: Assess pregnancy/nursing status. Evaluate clinical chemistries, including LFTs, ACTH level, and thyroid function tests, at baseline.
Monitoring: Monitor for signs/symptoms of immune-mediated enterocolitis, hepatitis, dermatitis, motor or sensory neuropathy, hypophysitis, adrenal insufficiency, hypo/hyperthyroidism, and other adverse reactions. Monitor clinical chemistries, including LFTs, ACTH level, and thyroid function tests before each dose, and as clinically indicated based on symptoms.
Counseling: Inform of the potential risk of immune-mediated adverse reactions. Advise female patients that therapy can cause fetal harm. Instruct females of reproductive potential to use effective contraception during treatment and for 3 months after the last dose. Advise to contact physician if pregnant or if pregnancy is suspected. Advise females who may have been exposed to drug during pregnancy to contact Bristol-Myers Squibb; advise pregnant women to enroll in the Pregnancy Safety Surveillance Study. Advise women not to breastfeed during treatment and for 3 months after the last dose.

YONDELIS — trabectedin   Rx
Class: Alkylating agent

ADULT DOSAGE

Unresectable or Metastatic Liposarcoma or Leiomyosarcoma
In patients who received a prior anthracycline-containing regimen

Recommended: 1.5mg/m² as an IV infusion every 21 days, until disease progression or unacceptable toxicity, in patients w/ normal bilirubin and AST or ALT ≤2.5X ULN

PEDIATRIC DOSAGE
Pediatric use may not have been established

Premedication
Administer dexamethasone 20mg IV 30 min prior to each dose

DOSING CONSIDERATIONS
Renal Impairment
Mild (CrCl 60-89mL/min) or Moderate (CrCl 30-59mL/min): No dose adjustment recommended
Severe (CrCl <30mL/min) or ESRD: Has not been evaluated

Hepatic Impairment
Moderate (Bilirubin Levels 1.5X to 3X ULN, and AST and ALT <8X ULN):
Recommended Dose: $0.9mg/m^2$
Severe (Bilirubin Levels >3X to 10X ULN, and Any AST and ALT): Do not administer

Adverse Reactions
Permanently D/C For:
- Persistent adverse reactions requiring a delay in dosing of >3 weeks
- Adverse reactions requiring dose reduction following trabectedin administered at $1mg/m^2$ for patients w/ normal hepatic function or at $0.3mg/m^2$ for patients w/ preexisting moderate hepatic impairment
- Severe liver dysfunction (all of the following: bilirubin 2X ULN and AST/ALT 3X ULN w/ alkaline phosphatase <2X ULN) in the prior treatment cycle for patients w/ normal liver function at baseline
- Exacerbation of liver dysfunction in patients w/ preexisting moderate hepatic impairment

Delay Next Dose for Up to 3 Weeks:
- Platelets <100,000 platelets/μL
- ANC <1500 neutrophils/μL
- Total bilirubin >ULN
- AST/ALT >2.5X ULN
- Alkaline phosphatase >2.5X ULN
- Creatine phosphokinase >2.5X ULN
- Decreased left ventricular ejection fraction (LVEF): less than lower limit of normal or clinical evidence of cardiomyopathy
- Other nonhematologic Grade 3 or 4 adverse reactions

Reduce Next Dose by One Dose Level for Adverse Reaction(s) During Prior Cycle:
- Platelets <25,000 platelets/μL
- ANC <1000 neutrophils/μL w/ fever/infection or <500 neutrophils/μL lasting >5 days
- Total bilirubin >ULN
- AST/ALT >5X ULN
- Alkaline phosphatase >2.5X ULN
- Creatine phosphokinase >5X ULN
- Decreased LVEF: absolute decrease of ≥10% from baseline and less than lower limit of normal or clinical evidence of cardiomyopathy
- Other nonhematologic Grade 3 or 4 adverse reactions

Dose Reductions for Patients w/ Normal Hepatic Function or Mild Hepatic Impairment (Including Patients w/ Bilirubin 1 to 1.5X ULN, and Any AST or ALT) Prior to Initiation of Treatment:
1st Dose Reduction: $1.2mg/m^2$ every 3 weeks
2nd Dose Reduction: $1mg/m^2$ every 3 weeks

Dose Reductions for Patients w/ Moderate Hepatic Function Prior to Initiation of Treatment:
1st Dose Reduction: $0.6mg/m^2$ every 3 weeks
2nd Dose Reduction: $0.3mg/m^2$ every 3 weeks

The dose should not be increased in subsequent treatment cycles once the dose is reduced for adverse reactions.

ADMINISTRATION
IV route
Infuse reconstituted, diluted sol over 24 hrs through a central venous line using an infusion set w/ a 0.2 micron polyethersulfone in-line filter.
Complete infusion w/in 30 hrs of initial reconstitution; discard any unused portion of the product or of the infusion sol.
Do not mix w/ other drugs.
Discard any remaining sol w/in 30 hrs of reconstituting the lyophilized powder.

Preparation:
1. Inject 20mL of sterile water for inj into the vial; shake the vial until complete dissolution.
2. Immediately following reconstitution, withdraw the calculated volume of drug and further dilute in 500mL of 0.9% NaCl and D5 inj.

Compatibility:
Type 1 colorless glass vials
PVC and polyethylene bags and tubing
Polyethylene and polypropylene mixture bags
Polyethersulfone in-line filters
Titanium, platinum, or plastic ports
Silicone and polyurethane catheters
Pumps having contact surfaces made of PVC, polyethylene, or polyethylene/polypropylene

STORAGE
2-8°C (36-46°F).

HOW SUPPLIED
Inj: (Powder) 1mg

CONTRAINDICATIONS
Severe hypersensitivity (eg, anaphylaxis) to trabectedin.

WARNINGS/PRECAUTIONS
See Dosing Considerations. Neutropenic sepsis, rhabdomyolysis, musculoskeletal toxicity, hepatotoxicity, and cardiomyopathy can occur. Extravasation, resulting in tissue necrosis requiring debridement, can occur. Can cause fetal harm.

ADVERSE REACTIONS
N/V, fatigue, constipation, decreased appetite, diarrhea, peripheral edema, dyspnea, headache.

DRUG INTERACTIONS
Ketoconazole may increase systemic exposure; avoid use of strong CYP3A inhibitors (eg, oral ketoconazole, itraconazole, clarithromycin). Avoid grapefruit or grapefruit juice. If a strong CYP3A inhibitor for short-term use (eg, <14 days) must be used, administer the strong CYP3A inhibitor 1 week after infusion, and d/c the day prior to the next infusion. Rifampin may decrease systemic exposure; avoid strong CYP3A inducers (eg, rifampin, phenobarbital, St. John's wort).

PREGNANCY AND LACTATION
Pregnancy: Can cause fetal harm based on mechanism of action.
Lactation: There are no data on the presence of trabectedin in human milk, the effects on the breastfed infant, or the effects on milk production; not for use during nursing.
Reproductive Potential: Female patients of reproductive potential should use effective contraception during and for 2 months after the last dose of therapy. Males w/ a female sexual partner of reproductive potential should use effective contraception during and for 5 months after the last dose of therapy. May result in decreased fertility in males and females.

MECHANISM OF ACTION
Alkylating agent; binds guanine residues in the minor groove of DNA, forming adducts and resulting in a bending of the DNA helix towards the major groove. Adduct formation triggers a cascade of events that can affect the subsequent activity of DNA binding proteins, including some transcription factors, and DNA repair pathways, resulting in perturbation of the cell cycle and eventual cell death.

PHARMACOKINETICS
Distribution: V_d>5000L; plasma protein binding (approx 97%). **Metabolism:** Hepatic metabolism via CYP3A (extensive). **Elimination:** Urine (6%), feces (58%). $T_{1/2}$=approx 175 hrs.

PATIENT CONSIDERATIONS
Assessment: Assess for drug hypersensitivity, LVEF, pregnancy/nursing status, and for possible drug interactions. Assess neutrophil count, creatine phosphokinase levels, and LFTs prior to each dose.

Monitoring: Monitor for rhabdomyolysis, hepatotoxicity, extravasation, and for other adverse reactions. Monitor neutrophil count periodically, and LVEF at 2- to 3-month intervals.

Counseling: Inform of the risks of myelosuppression; instruct to contact physician immediately for fever or unusual bruising, bleeding, tiredness, or paleness. Advise to contact physician immediately if experiencing symptoms of rhabdomyolysis, hepatotoxicity, cardiomyopathy, hypersensitivity, or extravasation. Inform pregnant women of the potential risk to fetus and advise to contact physician if pregnant or suspected to be pregnant during treatment. Advise females of reproductive potential to use effective contraception during treatment and for at least 2 months after last dose. Advise males w/ female partners of reproductive potential to use effective contraception during treatment and for at least 5 months after last dose. Advise females not to breastfeed during treatment.

ZALTRAP — ziv-aflibercept   Rx
Class: Vascular endothelial growth factor (VEGF) inhibitor

> Severe and sometimes fatal hemorrhage, including GI hemorrhage, reported in combination w/ 5-fluorouracil, leucovorin, and irinotecan (FOLFIRI). Monitor for signs and symptoms of GI bleeding and other severe bleeding. Do not administer in patients w/ severe hemorrhage. Nonfatal/fatal GI perforation may occur; d/c therapy in patients who experience GI perforation. Severe compromised wound healing may occur in combination w/ FOLFIRI; d/c in patients w/ compromised wound healing. Suspend for at least 4 weeks prior to elective surgery; do not resume for at least 4 weeks following major surgery and until the surgical wound is fully healed.

ADULT DOSAGE
Metastatic Colorectal Cancer
In combination w/ FOLFIRI for patients w/ cancer that is resistant to or has progressed following an oxaliplatin-containing regimen

4mg/kg IV infusion over 1 hr every 2 weeks until disease progression or unacceptable toxicity

Administer prior to any component of the FOLFIRI regimen on day of treatment

PEDIATRIC DOSAGE
Pediatric use may not have been established

DOSING CONSIDERATIONS
Discontinuation
D/C Therapy For:
- Severe hemorrhage
- GI perforation
- Compromised wound healing
- Fistula formation
- Hypertensive crisis or hypertensive encephalopathy
- Arterial thromboembolic events

- Nephrotic syndrome or thrombotic microangiopathy
- Reversible posterior leukoencephalopathy syndrome (RPLS)

Temporarily Suspend Therapy:
- At least 4 weeks prior to elective surgery
- For recurrent or severe hypertension, until controlled; upon resumption, permanently reduce dose to 2mg/kg
- For proteinuria of 2g/24 hrs; resume when proteinuria is <2g/24 hrs. For recurrent proteinuria, suspend therapy until proteinuria is <2g/24 hrs and then permanently reduce dose to 2mg/kg

ADMINISTRATION
IV route

Preparation
- Do not re-enter the vial after the initial puncture; discard any unused portion left in the vial.
- Withdraw the prescribed dose and dilute in 0.9% NaCl sol or 5% dextrose sol for inj; final concentration is 0.6-8mg/mL.
- Use polyvinyl chloride (PVC) infusion bags containing bis (2-ethylhexyl) phthalate (DEHP) or polyolefin infusion bags.

Administration
- Administer through a 0.2μm polyethersulfone filter.
- Do not use filters made of polyvinylidene fluoride or nylon.
- Do not administer as an IV push or bolus.
- Do not combine w/ other drugs in the same infusion bag or IV line.
- Store diluted sol at 2-8°C (36-46°F) for up to 24 hrs, or at 20-25°C (68-77°F) for up to 8 hrs.

Administer using an infusion set made of 1 of the following materials:
- PVC containing DEHP
- DEHP-free PVC containing trioctyl-trimellitate
- Polypropylene
- Polyethylene-lined PVC
- Polyurethane

STORAGE
2-8°C (36-46°F). Keep vials in original carton to protect from light.

HOW SUPPLIED
Inj: 25mg/mL [4mL, 8mL]

WARNINGS/PRECAUTIONS
For minor surgery (eg, central venous access port placement, biopsy, tooth extraction), may initiate/resume therapy once surgical wound is fully healed. Fistula formation, involving GI and non-GI sites, reported; d/c in patients who develop fistula. Increased risk of Grade 3-4 HTN; treat w/ appropriate antihypertensives and continue monitoring BP regularly. Arterial thromboembolic events (ATEs) (eg, transient ischemic attack, cerebrovascular accident, angina pectoris); severe proteinuria; nephrotic syndrome; and thrombotic microangiopathy (TMA) reported. Higher incidence of neutropenic complications (eg, febrile neutropenia, neutropenic infection) reported; delay therapy until neutrophil count is ≥1.5 x 10⁹/L. Diarrhea and dehydration reported; closely monitor elderly for diarrhea and dehydration. RPLS reported; confirm diagnosis of RPLS w/ MRI and d/c if RPLS develops.

ADVERSE REACTIONS
Leukopenia, diarrhea, neutropenia, proteinuria, increased AST, stomatitis, fatigue, thrombocytopenia, increased ALT, hypertension, decreased weight, decreased appetite, epistaxis, abdominal pain, dysphonia, increased SrCr, headache.

PREGNANCY AND LACTATION
Pregnancy: Category C.
Lactation: Not for use in nursing.
Reproduction Potential: Male and female reproductive function and fertility may be compromised during treatment; females and males of reproductive potential should use highly effective contraception during and up to a minimum of 3 months after the last dose.

MECHANISM OF ACTION
VEGF inhibitor; binds to human VEGF-A, to human VEGF-B, and to human PlGF, and thereby inhibits the binding and activation of their cognate receptors. This inhibition can result in decreased neovascularization and decreased vascular permeability.

PHARMACOKINETICS
Elimination: $T_{1/2}$=6 days.

PATIENT CONSIDERATIONS
Assessment: Assess for recent surgery, severe hemorrhage, compromised wound healing, HTN, proteinuria, history of ATEs, neutropenia, and pregnancy/nursing status. Obtain baseline CBC w/ differential count.

Monitoring: Monitor for signs/symptoms of bleeding, GI perforation, fistula formation, compromised wound healing, hypertensive crisis/encephalopathy, ATEs, nephrotic syndrome, TMA, diarrhea, dehydration, RPLS, and other adverse reactions. Monitor BP every 2 weeks or more frequently as indicated. Monitor proteinuria by urine dipstick analysis and/or urinary protein creatinine ratio (UPCR) for the development or worsening of proteinuria; obtain a 24-hr urine collection in patients w/ a dipstick of ≥2+ for protein or UPCR >1. Monitor CBC w/ differential count prior to initiation of each cycle.

Counseling: Advise to contact physician if bleeding/symptoms of bleeding, elevated BP/symptoms from HTN, severe diarrhea, vomiting, severe abdominal pain, or fever or other signs of infection occur. Inform of the increased risk of compromised wound healing and instruct not to undergo surgery or procedures, including tooth extractions, w/o discussing 1st w/ the physician. Inform of an increased risk of ATEs. Inform of the potential risks to the fetus or neonate during pregnancy or nursing; instruct to use highly effective contraception in both males and females during and for at least 3 months following last dose of therapy; advise to immediately contact physician if patient or their partner becomes pregnant during treatment.

ZANOSAR — streptozocin   Rx

Class: DNA synthesis inhibitor

> Administer only under the supervision of a physician experienced in use of cancer chemotherapeutic agents. A patient should have access to a facility with laboratory and supportive resources sufficient to monitor drug tolerance, and to protect and maintain a patient compromised by drug toxicity. Renal toxicity is dose-related, cumulative, and may be severe or fatal. Other toxicities reported include N/V, liver dysfunction, diarrhea, and hematological changes. Streptozocin is mutagenic. The physician must judge the possible benefit against the known toxic effects of the drug in considering the advisability of therapy.

ADULT DOSAGE
Metastatic Islet Cell Carcinoma
Daily Schedule:
500mg/m² for 5 consecutive days every 6 weeks until max benefit or treatment-limiting toxicity occurs
Dose escalation not recommended

Weekly Schedule:
Initial: 1000mg/m² at weekly intervals for first 2 courses
Titrate: May increase dose in subsequent courses if therapeutic response is not achieved and if significant toxicity w/ the previous course of treatment is not experienced
Max: 1500mg/m²/dose

PEDIATRIC DOSAGE
Pediatric use may not have been established

ADMINISTRATION
IV route
Administer by rapid inj or short/prolonged infusion

Preparation
1. Reconstitute w/ 9.5mL of dextrose inj or 0.9% NaCl inj
2. Resulting pale-gold sol will contain 100mg of streptozocin and 22mg of citric acid per mL
3. Where more dilute infusion sol are desirable, further dilution in dextrose inj or 0.9% NaCl inj is recommended

Handling Precautions
If the sterile powder or a sol prepared from streptozocin contacts the skin or mucosae, immediately wash the affected area w/ soap and water

STORAGE
2-8°C. Protect from light. May store reconstituted sol for ≤12 hrs.

HOW SUPPLIED
Inj: 1g

WARNINGS/PRECAUTIONS
Limit use to patients with symptomatic or progressive metastatic disease. Monitor renal function before and after each course of therapy. Obtain serial urinalysis, BUN, plasma creatinine, serum electrolytes, and CrCl prior to, at least weekly during, and for 4 weeks after administration. Reduce dose or d/c therapy if significant renal toxicity is present. Risk of serious renal damage with preexisting renal disease. Irritating to tissue; extravasation may cause severe tissue lesions and necrosis. Monitor CBCs and LFTs at least weekly. Caution in elderly.

ADVERSE REACTIONS
Renal toxicity, N/V, diarrhea, liver dysfunction, hematological changes, glucose tolerance abnormalities, nephrogenic diabetes insipidus, local inflammation.

DRUG INTERACTIONS
May demonstrate additive toxicity with other cytotoxic drugs. Avoid with other potential nephrotoxins. May prolong doxorubicin half-life leading to severe bone marrow suppression; consider reducing doxorubicin dose. Coadministration with phenytoin may reduce streptozocin cytotoxicity.

PREGNANCY AND LACTATION
Category D, not for use in nursing.

MECHANISM OF ACTION
DNA synthesis inhibitor; inhibits cell proliferation and progression of cells into mitosis.

PATIENT CONSIDERATIONS
Assessment: Assess for symptomatic or progressive metastatic disease, preexisting renal disease, pregnancy/nursing status, and possible drug interactions. Obtain serial urinalysis, BUN, plasma creatinine, serum electrolytes, and CrCl prior to therapy.

Monitoring: Monitor for adverse events such as renal toxicity (eg, azotemia, anuria, hypophosphatemia, glycosuria, and renal tubular acidosis), hematopoietic toxicity, severe N/V, hepatotoxicity, and injection-site reactions. Monitor CBC and LFTs at least weekly. Obtain serial urinalysis, BUN, plasma creatinine, serum electrolytes, and CrCl prior to, at least weekly during, and for 4 weeks after administration.

Counseling: Inform that confusion, lethargy, and depression have been reported in limited number of patients receiving continuous IV infusion for 5 days. Use caution while operating machinery/driving.

ZARXIO — filgrastim-sndz   Rx

Class: Granulocyte colony-stimulating factor (G-CSF)

ADULT DOSAGE

Chemotherapy-Associated Neutropenia

Decreases incidence of infection, as manifested by febrile neutropenia, in patients w/ nonmyeloid malignancies receiving myelosuppressive anticancer drugs associated w/ a significant incidence of severe neutropenia w/ fever. Also reduces the time to neutrophil recovery and duration of fever, following induction or consolidation chemotherapy treatment of patients w/ acute myeloid leukemia (AML)

Receiving Myelosuppressive Chemotherapy or Induction and/or Consolidation Chemotherapy for AML:
Initial: 5mcg/kg/day qd
Titrate: May increase in increments of 5mcg/kg for each chemotherapy cycle, according to duration and severity of ANC nadir
D/C if ANC increases beyond 10,000/mm^3

To reduce the duration of neutropenia and neutropenia-related clinical sequelae in patients w/ nonmyeloid malignancies undergoing myeloablative chemotherapy followed by marrow transplantation

Receiving Bone Marrow Transplant:
10mcg/kg/day by IV infusion no longer than 24 hrs
Titrate:
When ANC >1000/mm^3 for 3 Consecutive Days: Reduce to 5mcg/kg/day, then
If ANC Remains >1000/mm^3 for 3 More Consecutive Days: D/C therapy, then
If ANC Decreases to <1000/mm^3: Resume at 5mcg/kg/day
If ANC decreases to <1000/mm^3 at any time during the 5mcg/kg/day administration, increase to 10mcg/kg/day, and retitrate following the above steps

Hematopoietic Progenitor Cell Mobilization

Mobilizes autologous hematopoietic progenitor cells into the peripheral blood for collection by leukapheresis

10mcg/kg/day SQ for ≥4 days before the 1st leukapheresis procedure and continued until the last leukapheresis

Monitor neutrophil counts after 4 days of therapy, and d/c if WBC count rises to >100,000/mm^3

Administration of therapy for 6-7 days w/ leukapheresis on Days 5, 6, and 7 was found to be safe and effective

Severe Chronic Neutropenia

Reduces incidence and duration of sequelae

Initial:
Congenital: 6mcg/kg SQ bid
Idiopathic/Cyclic: 5mcg/kg SQ qd
Titrate: Adjust dose based on clinical course and ANC

PEDIATRIC DOSAGE
General Dosing
Refer to prescribing information for information on pediatric dosing

ADMINISTRATION
SQ/IV route

- Direct administration to patients requiring doses <0.3mL (180mcg) is not recommended due to potential for dosing errors.
- Avoid administration of prefilled syringe in persons w/ latex allergies; needle cap contains natural rubber latex.
- Prior to use, remove prefilled syringe from the refrigerator and allow therapy to reach room temperature for a minimum of 30 min and a max of 24 hrs.
- Discard any prefilled syringe left at room temperature for >24 hrs.

SQ Administration
- Inject in the outer area of upper arms, abdomen, thighs, or upper outer areas of buttocks.

Chemotherapy-Associated Neutropenia
Cancer Patients Receiving Myelosuppressive Chemotherapy or Induction and/or Consolidation Chemotherapy for Acute Myeloid Leukemia:
- May administer by SQ inj, by short IV infusion (15-30 min), or by continuous IV infusion.
- Administer at least 24 hrs after cytotoxic chemotherapy.
- Do not administer w/in the 24-hr period prior to chemotherapy.
- Administer daily for up to 2 weeks or until ANC has reached 10,000/mm^3 following the expected chemotherapy-induced neutrophil nadir.
Cancer Patients Receiving Bone Marrow Transplant:
- Administer 1st dose at least 24 hrs after cytotoxic chemotherapy and at least 24 hrs after bone marrow infusion.

Dilution
- May dilute in D5 to concentrations between 5-15mcg/mL.
- Protect diluted concentrations between 5-15mcg/mL from adsorption to plastic materials by the addition of albumin (human) to a final concentration of 2mg/mL.
- When diluted in D5 or D5 plus albumin (human), compatible w/ glass bottles, polyvinylchloride, polyolefin, and polypropylene.
- Do not dilute w/ saline; product may precipitate.
- May store at room temperature for up to 24 hrs; the 24-hr time period includes the time during room temperature storage of the infusion sol and the duration of the infusion.

STORAGE
2-8°C (36-46°F). Protect from light. Do not shake. Avoid freezing; if frozen, thaw in the refrigerator before administration. Discard if frozen more than once.

HOW SUPPLIED
Inj: 300mcg/0.5mL, 480mcg/0.8mL

CONTRAINDICATIONS
History of serious allergic reactions to human granulocyte colony-stimulating factors such as filgrastim or pegfilgrastim products.

WARNINGS/PRECAUTIONS
Splenic rupture, including fatal cases, reported. Acute respiratory distress syndrome (ARDS) reported; d/c in patients w/ ARDS. Serious allergic-type reactions, including anaphylaxis, reported; permanently d/c in patients w/ serious allergic reactions. Sickle cell crisis, in some cases fatal, reported in patients w/ sickle cell trait/disease. Glomerulonephritis reported; evaluate for cause if glomerulonephritis is suspected, and consider dose reduction or interruption of therapy if causality is likely. Not approved for peripheral blood progenitor cell collection mobilization in healthy donors; alveolar hemorrhage manifesting as pulmonary infiltrates and hemoptysis reported. Capillary leak syndrome (CLS) reported. Myelodysplastic syndrome (MDS) and AML reported to occur in the natural history of congenital neutropenia w/o cytokine therapy. Cytogenetic abnormalities, transformation to MDS, and AML observed in patients treated for severe chronic neutropenia (SCN); carefully consider the risks and benefits of continuing therapy if a patient w/ SCN develops abnormal cytogenetics or myelodysplasia. Thrombocytopenia and leukocytosis reported. Cutaneous vasculitis reported; hold therapy w/ cutaneous vasculitis and may start therapy at a reduced dose when the symptoms resolve and the ANC has decreased. May act as a growth factor for any tumor type. Consider transient positive bone-imaging changes when interpreting bone-imaging results.

ADVERSE REACTIONS
Nonmyeloid Malignancies Receiving Myelosuppressive Anti-Cancer Drugs: Pyrexia, pain, rash, cough, dyspnea.
AML: Pain, epistaxis, rash.
Nonmyeloid Malignancies Undergoing Myeloablative Chemotherapy Followed by Bone Marrow Transplantation: Rash.
Undergoing Peripheral Blood Progenitor Cell Mobilization and Collection: Bone pain, pyrexia, headache.
Severe Chronic Neutropenia: Pain, anemia, epistaxis, diarrhea, hypoesthesia, alopecia.

DRUG INTERACTIONS
Do not use in the period 24 hrs before through 24 hours after the administration of cytotoxic chemotherapy. Avoid simultaneous use w/ chemotherapy and radiation therapy.

PREGNANCY AND LACTATION
Pregnancy: Category C.
Lactation: Caution in nursing.

MECHANISM OF ACTION
Granulocyte colony-stimulating factor; acts on hematopoietic cells by binding to specific cell surface receptors and stimulating proliferation, differentiation commitment, and some end-cell functional activation.

PHARMACOKINETICS
Absorption: (SQ) Absolute Bioavailability (60-70%); C_{max}=4ng/mL (3.45mcg/kg), 49ng/mL (11.5mcg/kg); T_{max}=2-8 hrs. **Distribution:** (IV) V_d=150mL/kg; crosses placenta. **Elimination:** $T_{1/2}$=3.5 hrs (IV), 231 min (34.5mcg/kg IV), 210 min (3.45mcg/kg SQ).

PATIENT CONSIDERATIONS

Assessment: Assess for hypersensitivity to the drug, latex allergy, sickle cell disorder, pregnancy/nursing status, and possible drug interactions. Confirm diagnosis of SCN prior to therapy. Obtain baseline CBC and platelet count in patients receiving myelosuppressive chemotherapy/induction, and/or consolidation chemotherapy for AML.

Monitoring: Monitor for serious allergic-type reactions, splenic rupture, ARDS, sickle cell crisis, glomerulonephritis, CLS, cutaneous vasculitis, thrombocytopenia, leukocytosis, and other adverse reactions. Monitor for cytogenetic abnormalities, transformation to MDS, and AML in patients w/ SCN. In patients receiving myelosuppressive chemotherapy/induction, and/or consolidation chemotherapy for AML, monitor CBC and platelet count twice weekly. In patients w/ SCN, monitor CBC w/ differential and platelet counts during the initial 4 weeks of therapy and during the 2 weeks following any dose adjustment, and, once patient is clinically stable, monthly during the 1st yr of treatment; thereafter, if clinically stable, less frequent routine monitoring is recommended. Frequently monitor CBCs and platelet counts following marrow transplantation.

Counseling: Instruct patient and caregiver on direct patient administration, including how to measure the required dose, particularly if on a dose other than the entire syringe. Inform that rupture or enlargement of the spleen may occur; advise to immediately report to physician if symptoms develop. Advise to seek immediate medical attention if signs/symptoms of a hypersensitivity reaction occur. Advise to immediately report to physician if dyspnea or signs/symptoms of vasculitis develop. Discuss potential risks and benefits for patients w/ sickle cell disease prior to administration. Advise female of reproductive potential that therapy should be used during pregnancy only if the potential benefit justifies the potential risk to the fetus.

ZAVESCA — miglustat　　　Rx

Class: Glucosylceramide synthase inhibitor

ADULT DOSAGE	PEDIATRIC DOSAGE
Type 1 Gaucher Disease	Pediatric use may not have been established
As monotherapy for mild to moderate type 1 Gaucher disease when enzyme replacement therapy is not a therapeutic option	
Recommended Dose: 100mg tid at regular intervals	

DOSING CONSIDERATIONS
Renal Impairment
Mild (CrCl 50-70mL/min):
Initial: 100mg bid
Moderate (CrCl 30-50mL/min):
Initial: 100mg qd
Severe (CrCl <30mL/min):
Not recommended for use
Elderly
Start at lower end of dosing range
Adverse Reactions
Tremor, Diarrhea, Other: May be necessary reduce dose to one 100mg cap qd or bid in some patients
ADMINISTRATION
Oral route
Therapy should be directed by physicians who are knowledgeable in the management of Gaucher disease.
STORAGE
20-25°C (68-77°F); brief exposure to 15-30°C (59-86°F) permitted.
HOW SUPPLIED
Cap: 100mg
WARNINGS/PRECAUTIONS
Peripheral neuropathy reported; perform baseline and repeat neurological evaluations at 6-month intervals. Reassess risks/benefits of therapy if symptoms of peripheral neuropathy develop; may consider cessation of treatment. Tremor or exacerbation of existing tremor reported; reduce dose to ameliorate tremor or d/c if tremor does not resolve w/in days of dose reduction. Diarrhea and weight loss commonly reported; avoid high carbohydrate content foods if diarrhea occurs. Evaluate for significant underlying GI disease in patients w/ persistent GI events that continue during treatment, and in those who do not respond to usual interventions. Caution w/ significant GI disease (eg, inflammatory bowel disease), and in elderly. Mild reductions in platelet counts may occur.
ADVERSE REACTIONS
Diarrhea, weight decrease, abdominal pain/distention, flatulence, N/V, tremor, dizziness, headache, leg cramps, unsteady gait, back pain, generalized weakness, constipation, dry mouth.
DRUG INTERACTIONS
May increase clearance of imiglucerase.
PREGNANCY AND LACTATION
Pregnancy: Category C.
Lactation: Not for use in nursing.
MECHANISM OF ACTION
Glucosylceramide synthase inhibitor; helps reduce the rate of glycosphingolipid biosynthesis so that the amount of glycosphingolipid substrate is reduced to a level which allows the residual activity of the deficient glucocerebrosidase enzyme to be more effective (substrate reduction therapy). Can reduce the synthesis of glucosylceramide-based glycosphingolipids.
PHARMACOKINETICS
Absorption: T_{max}=2-2.5 hrs. **Distribution:** V_d=83-105L. **Elimination:** Urine (83%, 67% unchanged), feces (12%); $T_{1/2}$=6-7 hrs.

PATIENT CONSIDERATIONS
Assessment: Assess for renal impairment, existing tremor, GI disease, pregnancy/ nursing status, and possible drug interactions. Obtain baseline neurological evaluation.

Monitoring: Monitor for signs/symptoms of peripheral neuropathy, tremor/ exacerbation of tremor, diarrhea, weight loss, and other adverse reactions. Perform neurological evaluations at 6-month intervals. Monitor platelet counts.
Counseling: Instruct to promptly report any signs/symptoms of peripheral neuropathy (eg, numbness, tingling, pain, burning in hands/feet), and the development of tremor or worsening in an existing tremor. Advise that diarrhea and weight loss may occur; instruct to adhere to dietary instructions, and to avoid high carbohydrate content foods during treatment if diarrhea occurs. Inform of the potential risks and benefits of therapy and of alternative modes of therapy.

ZECUITY — sumatriptan　　　Rx

Class: 5-HT$_{1B/1D}$ agonist (triptans)

ADULT DOSAGE	PEDIATRIC DOSAGE
Migraine	Pediatric use may not have been established
Acute Treatment w/ or w/o Aura: Apply 1 patch for 4 hrs or until red light emitting diode light goes off. If headache relief is incomplete, a 2nd patch may be applied ≥2 hrs after activation of the 1st patch to a different site	
Max: 1 patch/dose or 2 patches/24 hrs	
The safety of using >4 patches in 1 month has not been established	

DOSING CONSIDERATIONS
Elderly
Start at lower end of dosing range
ADMINISTRATION
Transdermal route
Apply to dry intact, non-irritated skin on upper arm or thigh on a site that is relatively hair free and w/o scars, tattoos, abrasions, or other skin conditions; may secure the system w/ medical tape if needed.
Do not apply to a previous application site until the site remains erythema free for at least 3 days.
Once applied, push the activation button to turn on the red light emitting diode (LED) w/in 15 min.
When the LED light turns off, dosing is complete and the system can be removed. After use, fold the system so the adhesive side sticks to itself and safely discard away from children and pets.
STORAGE
20-25°C (68-77°F); excursions permitted to 15-30°C (59-86°F). Do not refrigerate or freeze. Contains lithium-manganese dioxide batteries; dispose in accordance with state and local regulations.
HOW SUPPLIED
Iontophoretic Transdermal System: 6.5mg/4 hrs
CONTRAINDICATIONS
Ischemic coronary artery disease (CAD) (eg, angina pectoris, history of MI, documented silent ischemia), coronary artery vasospasm (eg, Prinzmetal's angina), Wolff-Parkinson-White syndrome or arrhythmias associated with other cardiac accessory conduction pathway disorders, history of stroke, transient ischemic attack, history of hemiplegic or basilar migraine, peripheral vascular disease, ischemic bowel disease, uncontrolled HTN, severe hepatic impairment, or allergic contact dermatitis to sumatriptan. Recent (within 24 hrs) use of ergotamine-containing medication, ergot-type medication (eg, dihydroergotamine, methysergide) or another 5-hydroxytryptamine$_1$ agonist. Concurrent administration of an MAO-A inhibitor or recent (within 2 weeks) use of an MAO-A inhibitor. Known hypersensitivity to sumatriptan or components of this medication.
WARNINGS/PRECAUTIONS
For transdermal use only. Use only if a clear diagnosis of migraine has been established. Reconsider the diagnosis of migraine before giving a 2nd dose if patient does not respond to the 1st dose of therapy. No evidence of benefit for the use of a 2nd transdermal system (TDS) to treat headache recurrence or incomplete headache relief during a migraine attack. Contains metal parts; remove before an MRI procedure. Do not apply in areas near or over electrically-active implantable or body-worn medical devices (eg, implantable cardiac pacemaker, body-worn insulin pump, implantable deep brain stimulator). May lead to allergic contact dermatitis; d/c if suspected. Systemic sensitization or other systemic reactions may develop if other sumatriptan-containing products are taken via other routes (eg, PO, SQ); administer 1st subsequent dose under close medical supervision. May cause coronary artery vasospasm (Prinzmetal's angina) and sensations of tightness, pain, pressure, and heaviness in the chest, throat, neck, and jaw, usually of noncardiac origin. Perform cardiovascular (CV) evaluation in triptan-naive patients who have multiple CV risk factors before treatment; if negative, consider 1st administration in a medically supervised setting and perform an ECG upon activation of TDS. Consider periodic CV evaluation in intermittent long-term users. Life-threatening cardiac rhythm disturbances reported; d/c if these occur. Cerebral hemorrhage, subarachnoid hemorrhage, and stroke may occur; exclude other potentially serious neurological conditions prior to therapy in patients not previously diagnosed as migraineurs, and in migraineurs who present with atypical symptoms. May cause noncoronary vasospastic reactions (eg, peripheral vascular ischemia, GI vascular ischemia/infarction, splenic infarction, Raynaud's syndrome). Transient/permanent blindness and significant partial vision

loss reported. Overuse may lead to exacerbation of headache; detoxification including drug withdrawal, and treatment of withdrawal symptoms may be necessary. Serotonin syndrome may occur; d/c if suspected. Significant elevation in BP, including hypertensive crisis with acute impairment of organ systems, reported. Anaphylactic/anaphylactoid reactions may occur. Seizures reported; caution in patients with a history of epilepsy or conditions associated with a lowered seizure threshold.

ADVERSE REACTIONS
Application-site reactions (pain, paresthesia, pruritus, warmth, discomfort, irritation, discoloration, vesicles).

DRUG INTERACTIONS
See Contraindications. Serotonin syndrome reported with SSRIs, SNRIs, TCAs, or MAOIs.

PREGNANCY AND LACTATION
Category C, not for use in nursing.

MECHANISM OF ACTION
Selective 5-HT$_{1B/1D}$ agonist; thought to be due to the agonist effects at the 5HT$_{1B/1D}$ receptors on intracranial blood vessels (including arteriovenous anastomoses) and sensory nerves of the trigeminal system, which result in cranial vessel constriction and inhibition of proinflammatory neuropeptide release.

PHARMACOKINETICS
Absorption: C_{max}=22ng/mL, AUC_{0-inf}=110 hr•ng/mL, T_{max} =1.1 hrs (median). **Distribution:** (Healthy) V_d=2.4L/kg; plasma protein binding (14-21%). **Metabolism:** via MAO-A; indole acetic acid (IAA) (major metabolite). **Elimination:** Urine (11%, unchanged, 69% IAA), $T_{1/2}$=3.1 hrs.

PATIENT CONSIDERATIONS

Assessment: Assess for cardiovascular disease, HTN, hemiplegic/basilar migraine, ECG changes, and any other conditions where treatment is cautioned or contraindicated, hepatic function, pregnancy/nursing status, and for possible drug interactions. Confirm diagnosis of migraine and exclude other potentially serious neurologic conditions prior to therapy. Perform CV evaluation in patients who have CV risk factors.

Monitoring: Monitor for signs/symptoms of cardiac events, cerebrovascular events, peripheral vascular ischemia, GI vascular ischemia/infarction, serotonin syndrome, allergic contact dermatitis, anaphylactic/anaphylactoid reactions, visual disturbances, HTN, and other adverse reactions. Perform ECG immediately after administration of therapy and monitor CV function in intermittent long-term users. Monitor for medication overuse; exacerbation of headache may occur.

Counseling: Instruct to use TDS ud; instruct not to bathe, shower, or swim while wearing TDS. Inform that most patients experience some skin redness under the TDS upon removal, which usually disappears within 24 hrs. Inform patients that the TDS contains metal parts and must be removed before an MRI procedure. Inform that treatment may cause serious CV adverse reactions (eg, MI or stroke) that may result in hospitalization and even death. Instruct patients to be alert for signs/symptoms of chest pain, SOB, weakness, and slurring of speech; instruct to notify physician if these symptoms and other symptoms of vasospastic reactions occur. Inform patients of the signs and symptoms of allergic contact dermatitis, and instruct to seek medical advice if skin lesions suggestive of allergic contact dermatitis develop. Counsel about the possible drug interactions and the risk of anaphylactic/anaphylactoid reactions. Inform patients that the use of therapy ≥10 days per month may lead to exacerbation of headache; encourage to record headache frequency and drug use. Advise to notify physician if pregnant/nursing or planning to become pregnant. Instruct patients to evaluate their ability to perform complex tasks during migraine attacks and after using therapy.

ZELBORAF — vemurafenib   Rx

Class: Kinase inhibitor

ADULT DOSAGE

Unresectable or Metastatic Melanoma with BRAF V600E Mutation

960mg q12h until disease progression or unacceptable toxicity occurs

Missed Dose

Missed dose can be taken up to 4 hrs prior to next dose

PEDIATRIC DOSAGE
Pediatric use may not have been established

- -

DOSING CONSIDERATIONS
Adverse Reactions
Permanently D/C If:
Grade 4 adverse reaction, 1st appearance (if clinically appropriate) or 2nd appearance
QTc prolongation >500 msec and increased by >60 msec from pretreatment values

Withhold for:
NCI CTCAE Grade 2 or greater adverse reactions

Upon Recovery to Grade 0-1, Restart at a Reduced Dose as Follows:
720mg bid for 1st appearance of intolerable Grade 2 or Grade 3 adverse reactions
480mg bid for 2nd appearance of Grade 2 (if intolerable) or Grade 3 adverse reactions or for 1st appearance of Grade 4 adverse reaction (if clinically appropriate)

Do not reduce dose to below 480mg bid

ADMINISTRATION
Oral route
Take w/ or w/o meal.
Do not crush or chew.
Do not take an additional dose if vomiting occurs after therapy; continue w/ the next scheduled dose.

STORAGE
20-25°C (68-77°F); excursions permitted between 15-30°C (59-86°F).

HOW SUPPLIED
Tab: 240mg

WARNINGS/PRECAUTIONS
See Dosing Considerations. Not indicated for wild-type BRAF melanoma. Cutaneous malignancies (eg, cutaneous squamous cell carcinoma [SCC], keratoacanthoma, melanoma) reported and non-cutaneous SCC of the head and neck may occur; monitor closely for signs or symptoms of new non-cutaneous SCC or other malignancies. Potential risk factors associated w/ cutaneous SCC include ≥65 yrs of age, prior skin cancer, and chronic sun exposure. May promote malignancies associated w/ activation of renin-angiotensin system through mutation or other mechanisms. Increased cell proliferation in BRAF wild-type cells can occur w/ BRAF inhibitors; confirm evidence of BRAF V600E mutation in tumor specimens prior to initiating therapy. Anaphylaxis and other serious hypersensitivity/dermatological reactions may occur; d/c permanently if severe hypersensitivity/dermatological reactions occur. QT prolongation leading to an increased risk of ventricular arrhythmias (eg, torsades de pointes) may occur. Do not initiate therapy in patients w/ uncorrectable electrolyte abnormalities, QTc >500 msec, long QT syndrome, or who are taking medicines known to prolong the QT interval. Liver injury leading to functional hepatic impairment (eg, coagulopathy or other organ dysfunction) may occur. Uveitis, blurred vision, photophobia, and mild to severe photosensitivity may occur. May cause fetal harm. Radiation sensitization and recall reported in patients treated w/ radiation prior to, during, or subsequent to therapy; fatal cases have been reported in patients w/ visceral organ involvement. Renal failure (eg, acute interstitial nephritis, acute tubular necrosis) may occur.

ADVERSE REACTIONS
Arthralgia, rash, alopecia, fatigue, photosensitivity reaction, nausea, pruritus, skin papilloma.

DRUG INTERACTIONS
Strong CYP3A4 inhibitors (eg, ketoconazole, nefazodone, clarithromycin) and inducers (eg, phenytoin, carbamazepine, rifampin) may alter vemurafenib concentrations; avoid concomitant use and replace these drugs w/ alternative drugs when possible. Administration w/ tizanidine (a sensitive CYP1A2 substrate) increased tizanidine systemic exposure; avoid w/ drugs w/ a narrow therapeutic window that are predominantly metabolized by CYP1A2. If coadministration cannot be avoided, closely monitor and consider dose reduction of concomitant CYP1A2 substrates. Increases in transaminases and bilirubin occurred w/ concurrent ipilimumab. Administration w/ digoxin (a sensitive P-gp substrate) increased digoxin systemic exposure; avoid concurrent use of P-gp substrates known to have narrow therapeutic indices. If use is unavoidable, consider dose reduction of P-gp substrates w/ narrow therapeutic indices.

PREGNANCY AND LACTATION
Pregnancy: Category D. Women of childbearing age and men should use contraception during and for at least 2 months after discontinuation of therapy. **Lactation:** Not for use in nursing.

MECHANISM OF ACTION
Kinase inhibitor; inhibits some mutated forms of BRAF serine-threonine kinase (eg, BRAF V600E). BRAF V600E can cause cell proliferation in the absence of growth factors that would normally be required for proliferation.

PHARMACOKINETICS
Absorption: T_{max}=3 hrs (median); C_{max}=62mcg/mL; AUC_{0-12}=601mcg•hr/mL. **Distribution:** Plasma protein binding (>99%); V_d=106L. **Elimination:** Feces (approx 94%), urine (approx 1%); $T_{1/2}$=57 hrs (median).

PATIENT CONSIDERATIONS

Assessment: Assess for BRAF V600E mutation, prior skin cancer, chronic sun exposure, electrolyte abnormality, long QT syndrome, prior treatment w/ radiation, pregnancy/nursing status, and possible drug interactions. Perform dermatologic evaluation and obtain baseline ECG, electrolyte levels, LFTs, and SrCr.

Monitoring: Monitor for development of new primary malignancies, new non-cutaneous SCC, other malignancies, severe dermatologic and hypersensitivity reactions, photosensitivity, uveitis, renal failure, and other adverse reactions. Perform dermatologic evaluation every 2 months during treatment and consider for 6 months after discontinuation. Monitor for QTc prolongation during treatment and after dose modification of therapy; evaluate ECG and electrolytes after 15 days, monthly during the first 3 months, then every 3 months thereafter, or as clinically indicated. Monitor LFTs monthly or as clinically needed. Monitor closely when administered concomitantly or sequentially w/ radiation treatment. Periodically monitor SrCr levels.

Counseling: Inform about the potential benefits and risks of treatment. Inform that BRAF V600E mutation assessment is required for patient selection. Inform about the increased risk of developing new primary cutaneous malignancies and advise on the importance of immediately reporting any skin changes. Inform about the risk of QT prolongation, which may result in ventricular arrhythmias; advise on the importance of monitoring ECG and electrolytes during treatment. Inform about the risk of photosensitivity and advise to avoid sun exposure and to wear protective clothing, sunscreen, and lip balm w/ SPF ≥30 when outdoors. Inform that anaphylaxis, other serious hypersensitivity reactions, and severe dermatologic reactions can occur. Advise to stop taking therapy and to seek immediate medical attention/contact healthcare provider if these occur. Inform that liver injury can occur, and advise of the importance of laboratory monitoring of their liver during treatment. Advise to contact healthcare provider immediately for ophthalmologic symptoms. Advise of risk of fetal harm;

instruct women of childbearing age and men to use contraception during and for at least 2 months after ending therapy. Advise patients to inform healthcare provider if they have had or are planning to receive radiation therapy. Inform that renal failure may occur; inform about the importance of monitoring SrCr prior to and during treatment.

ZEMAIRA — alpha1-proteinase inhibitor (human)   Rx

Class: Alpha₁-proteinase inhibitor (A₁PI)

ADULT DOSAGE

__Alpha₁-Antitrypsin Deficiency__

__Chronic Augmentation and Maint Therapy in Patients w/ Alpha₁-Proteinase Inhibitor (A₁-PI) Deficiency and Clinical Evidence of Emphysema:__
60mg/kg IV once weekly. Administer at a rate of approx 0.08mL/kg/min as determined by response and comfort of patient

PEDIATRIC DOSAGE
Pediatric use may not have been established

DOSING CONSIDERATIONS
__Adverse Reactions__
Slow or stop infusion if adverse reactions occur; if symptoms subside promptly, may resume infusion at a lower rate that is comfortable for the patient

ADMINISTRATION
IV route
__Preparation and Reconstitution__
1. Ensure that drug and diluent vials are at room temperature.
2. Remove protective cover from the white (diluent) end of the transfer device; insert the white end of the transfer device into the center of the stopper of the upright diluent vial.
3. Remove protective cover from the green (drug) end of the transfer device. Invert diluent vial w/ attached transfer device and, using minimum force, insert green end of transfer device into the center of the rubber stopper of the upright drug vial (green top). The flange of the transfer device should rest on the surface of the stopper so that the diluent flows into drug vial.
4. Allow the vacuum in the drug vial to pull diluent into vial.
5. During diluent transfer, wet the lyophilized cake completely by gently tilting the vial. Do not allow the air inlet filter to face downward; use caution not to lose the vacuum.
6. After diluent transfer is complete, the transfer device will allow filtered air into vial through the air filter; additional venting is not required. Withdraw the transfer device from the diluent vial and discard the diluent vial and transfer device.
7. Gently swirl vial until powder is completely dissolved; do not shake.
8. If >1 drug vial is needed to achieve required dose, use aseptic technique to transfer reconstituted sol from vials into the administration container (eg, empty IV bag or glass bottle).

__Administration__
Do not mix w/ other medicinal products; administer through a separate dedicated infusion line.
Administer at room temperature w/in 3 hrs after reconstitution.
Filter reconstituted sol during administration; use IV administration set w/ a suitable 5 micron infusion filter to ensure proper filtration.

STORAGE
≤25°C (77°F). Avoid freezing.

HOW SUPPLIED
__Inj:__ 1000mg

CONTRAINDICATIONS
History of anaphylaxis/severe systemic reactions to Zemaira or A₁-PI protein, IgA-deficient patients w/ antibodies against IgA.

WARNINGS/PRECAUTIONS
Not indicated as therapy for lung disease patients in whom severe A₁-PI deficiency has not been established. May contain trace amounts of IgA. D/C infusion immediately if an anaphylactic or severe anaphylactoid reaction occurs. May carry a risk of transmitting infectious agents (eg, viruses, Creutzfeldt-Jakob disease).

ADVERSE REACTIONS
Headache, sinusitis, URI, bronchitis, asthenia, increased cough, fever, inj-site hemorrhage, rhinitis, sore throat, vasodilation.

PREGNANCY AND LACTATION
__Pregnancy:__ Category C.
__Lactation:__ Caution in nursing.

MECHANISM OF ACTION
A₁-PI; acts to increase and maintain serum levels and lung epithelial lining fluid levels of A₁-PI. A₁-PI is the primary antiprotease in the lower respiratory tract, where it inhibits neutrophil elastase.

PHARMACOKINETICS
__Absorption:__ AUC=144μM x day; C_{max}=44.1μM. __Distribution:__ V_d=3.8L. __Elimination:__ $T_{1/2}$=5.1 days.

PATIENT CONSIDERATIONS
__Assessment:__ Assess for drug/A₁-PI protein hypersensitivity, IgA deficiency, and pregnancy/nursing status.
__Monitoring:__ Monitor for anaphylactic/anaphylactoid reactions, infection, and other adverse reactions. Monitor closely the infusion rate and clinical state, including vital signs, during the infusion.

__Counseling:__ Inform of the early signs of a hypersensitivity reaction; advise to d/c and contact physician and/or seek immediate emergency care if these symptoms occur. Inform that the product is made from human blood and may carry a risk of transmitting infectious agents. Inform that dizziness may occur following administration and advise to exercise caution immediately following an infusion.

ZEPATIER — elbasvir/grazoprevir   Rx

Class: HCV NS5A inhibitor/HCV NS3/4A protease inhibitor

ADULT DOSAGE

__Chronic Hepatitis C__

__Treatment of Chronic Hepatitis C Virus (HCV) Genotypes 1 or 4 Infection w/ or w/o Ribavirin (RBV):__
1 tab qd

__Treatment Regimen and Duration of Therapy in Patients w/ or w/o Cirrhosis:__
Test patients w/ HCV genotype 1a infection for presence of virus w/ NS5A resistance-associated polymorphisms prior to initiation of treatment to determine dosage regimen and duration

__Genotype 1a: Treatment-Naive or Peginterferon Alfa (PegIFN)/RBV-Experienced w/o Baseline NS5A Polymorphisms:__
Zepatier for 12 weeks

__Genotype 1a: Treatment-Naive or PegIFN/RBV-Experienced w/ Baseline NS5A Polymorphisms:__
Zepatier + RBV for 16 weeks

__Genotype 1b: Treatment-Naive or PegIFN/RBV-Experienced:__
Zepatier for 12 weeks

__Genotype 1a or 1b: PegIFN/RBV/ Protease Inhibitor-Experienced:__
Zepatier + RBV for 12 weeks

__Genotype 4: Treatment-Naive:__
Zepatier for 12 weeks

__Genotype 4: PegIFN/RBV-Experienced:__
Zepatier + RBV for 16 weeks

PEDIATRIC DOSAGE
Pediatric use may not have been established

ADMINISTRATION
Oral route
Take w/ or w/o food.
Refer to RBV labeling for dosing and administration instructions.

STORAGE
20-25°C (68-77°F); excursions permitted between 15-30°C (59-86°F). Protect from moisture.

HOW SUPPLIED
__Tab:__ (Elbasvir/Grazoprevir) 50mg/100mg

CONTRAINDICATIONS
Moderate or severe hepatic impairment (Child-Pugh B or C). Coadministration w/ OATP1B1/3 inhibitors or w/ strong CYP3A inducers. Coadministration w/ phenytoin, carbamazepine, rifampin, St. John's wort, efavirenz, atazanavir, darunavir, lopinavir, saquinavir, tipranavir, or cyclosporine. If administered w/ RBV, refer to the RBV prescribing information for a list of contraindications for RBV.

WARNINGS/PRECAUTIONS
ALT elevations reported; perform hepatic laboratory testing prior to therapy, at treatment week 8, and as clinically indicated. Additional hepatic laboratory testing should be performed at treatment week 12 in patients receiving 16 weeks of therapy. Consider discontinuing therapy if ALT levels remain persistently >10X ULN. D/C if ALT elevation is accompanied by signs/symptoms of liver inflammation or increasing conjugated bilirubin, alkaline phosphatase, or INR. Refer to the RBV prescribing information for a full list of warnings and precautions for RBV.

ADVERSE REACTIONS
__Zepatier for 12 Weeks:__ Fatigue, headache, nausea.
__Zepatier + Ribavirin for 16 Weeks:__ Anemia, headache.

DRUG INTERACTIONS
See Contraindications. Moderate or strong CYP3A inducers may decrease levels and therapeutic effect; not recommended w/ moderate CYP3A inducers. Strong CYP3A inhibitors may increase levels. Not recommended w/ nafcillin, ketoconazole, bosentan, etravirine, modafinil, or elvitegravir/cobicistat/emtricitabine/tenofovir (disoproxil fumarate or alafenamide). Nafcillin, bosentan, etravirine, and modafinil may decrease levels. Systemic ketoconazole may increase levels and may increase the overall risk of hepatotoxicity. Coadministration w/ systemic tacrolimus may increase tacrolimus levels; upon initiation of coadministration w/ Zepatier, frequently monitor tacrolimus whole blood concentrations, changes in renal function, and for tacrolimus-associated adverse events. Elvitegravir/cobicistat/ emtricitabine/tenofovir disoproxil (fumarate or alafenamide) may increase levels. May increase atorvastatin levels; atorvastatin dose should not exceed 20mg/day. May increase rosuvastatin

levels; rosuvastatin dose should not exceed 10mg/day. May increase fluvastatin, lovastatin, and simvastatin levels; monitor for statin-associated adverse events and use lowest necessary dose. **Grazoprevir:** OATP1B1/3 inhibitors may increase levels.

PREGNANCY AND LACTATION

Pregnancy: No adequate human data are available to establish whether or not Zepatier poses a risk to pregnancy outcomes. If Zepatier is administered w/ RBV, the combination regimen is contraindicated in pregnant women and in men whose female partners are pregnant; refer to the RBV prescribing information for more information on use in pregnancy.

Lactation: It is not known whether Zepatier is present in human breast milk, affects human milk production, or has effects on the breastfed infant; caution in nursing. If Zepatier is administered w/ RBV, the information for RBV w/ regard to nursing mothers also applies to this combination regimen; refer to the RBV prescribing information for information on use during lactation.

Females and Males of Reproductive Potential: If Zepatier is administered w/ RBV, the information for RBV w/ regard to pregnancy testing, contraception, and infertility also applies to this combination regimen; refer to RBV prescribing information for additional information.

MECHANISM OF ACTION

Elbasvir: Inhibitor of HCV NS5A, which is essential for viral RNA replication and virion assembly. **Grazoprevir:** An inhibitor of the HCV NS3/4A protease which is necessary for the proteolytic cleavage of the HCV encoded polyprotein (into mature forms of the NS3, NS4A, NS4B, NS5A, and NS5B proteins) and is essential for viral replication.

PHARMACOKINETICS

Absorption: Elbasvir: T_{max}=3 hrs (median); AUC_{0-24}=1920ng•hr/mL; C_{max}=121ng/mL. Grazoprevir: T_{max}=2 hrs (median); AUC_{0-24}=1420ng•hr/mL; C_{max}=165ng/mL. **Distribution:** Elbasvir: Plasma protein binding (>99.9%); V_d=680L. Grazoprevir: Plasma protein binding (>98.8%); V_d=1250L. **Metabolism:** Oxidative metabolism via CYP3A (partial). **Excretion:** Feces (>90%), urine (<1%). Elbasvir: $T_{1/2}$=24 hrs. Grazoprevir: $T_{1/2}$=31 hrs.

PATIENT CONSIDERATIONS

Assessment: Assess for hypersensitivity to drug, pregnancy/nursing status, and for possible drug interactions. Test patients w/ HCV genotype 1a infection for the presence of virus w/ NS5A resistance-associated polymorphisms. Perform baseline hepatic laboratory testing.

Monitoring: Monitor for ALT elevations and for any other adverse reaction. Perform hepatic laboratory testing at treatment week 8, and as clinically indicated; perform additional hepatic laboratory testing at treatment week 12 for patients receiving 16 weeks of therapy.

Counseling: Instruct to observe for warning signs of liver inflammation (eg, fatigue, weakness, lack of appetite, N/V, jaundice, discolored feces) and to contact physician w/o delay if such symptoms occur. Advise to notify physician if pregnant or nursing. Advise to report the use of any prescription, non-prescription medication, or herbal products to physician. Inform that therapy should be taken every day at the regularly scheduled time w/ or w/o food.

ZERIT — stavudine   Rx

Class: Nucleoside reverse transcriptase inhibitor (NRTI)

> Lactic acidosis and severe hepatomegaly with steatosis, including fatal cases, reported with nucleoside analogues. Fatal lactic acidosis reported in pregnant women who received the combination of stavudine and didanosine with other antiretroviral agents; use with caution. Fatal and nonfatal pancreatitis reported when used as part of a combination regimen that included didanosine.

ADULT DOSAGE
HIV-1 Infection

Combination with Other Antiretrovirals:
<60kg: 30mg q12h
≥60kg: 40mg q12h

PEDIATRIC DOSAGE
HIV-1 Infection

Combination with Other Antiretrovirals:
Birth-13 Days of Age:
0.5mg/kg q12h

≥14 Days of Age:
<30kg: 1mg/kg q12h
≥30kg: Use adult dose

DOSING CONSIDERATIONS
Renal Impairment
CrCl 26-50mL/min:
<60kg: 15mg q12h
≥60kg: 20mg q12h

CrCl 10-25mL/min or on Hemodialysis:
<60kg: 15mg q24h
≥60kg: 20mg q24h

Administer after completion of hemodialysis on dialysis days and at the same time of day on non-dialysis days

ADMINISTRATION
Oral route

Take with or without food
Shake oral sol vigorously prior to measuring each dose

STORAGE
25°C (77°F); excursions permitted between 15-30°C (59-86°F). (Sol) Protect from excessive moisture. After Constitution: 2-8°C (36-46°F). Discard any unused portion after 30 days.

HOW SUPPLIED
Cap: 15mg, 20mg, 30mg, 40mg; **Sol:** 1mg/mL [200mL]

CONTRAINDICATIONS
Clinically significant hypersensitivity to stavudine or to any components contained in the formulation.

WARNINGS/PRECAUTIONS
Female gender, obesity, and prolonged nucleoside exposure may be risk factors for lactic acidosis and severe hepatomegaly with steatosis. Caution in patients with known risk factors for liver disease. Suspend treatment if findings suggestive of symptomatic hyperlactatemia, lactic acidosis, or pronounced hepatotoxicity develop; consider permanent discontinuation with confirmed lactic acidosis. Increased frequency of liver function abnormalities, including severe and potentially fatal hepatic adverse events in patients with preexisting liver dysfunction; monitor accordingly and consider interruption or discontinuation if worsening of liver disease is evident. Motor weakness reported rarely; d/c if this develops. Dose-related peripheral sensory neuropathy reported; occurs more frequently in patients with advanced HIV-1 disease, history of peripheral neuropathy, or receiving other drugs associated with neuropathy (eg, didanosine). Consider permanent discontinuation if peripheral neuropathy develops. Redistribution/accumulation of body fat reported; monitor for signs/symptoms of lipoatrophy or lipodystrophy. Immune reconstitution syndrome reported. Autoimmune disorders (eg, Graves' disease, polymyositis, Guillain-Barre syndrome) reported in the setting of immune reconstitution and can occur many months after initiation of treatment. Caution with renal impairment and in elderly.

ADVERSE REACTIONS
Lactic acidosis, severe hepatomegaly with steatosis, peripheral neurologic symptoms/neuropathy, headache, diarrhea, rash, N/V, increased AST/ALT/amylase.

DRUG INTERACTIONS
See Boxed Warning. Suspend combination of stavudine and didanosine and any other agents that are toxic to the pancreas in patients with suspected pancreatitis; caution with reinstitution of stavudine and avoid use in combination with didanosine if pancreatitis is confirmed. Avoid with zidovudine or hydroxyurea with or without didanosine. Hepatic decompensation may occur in combination with interferon and ribavirin in HIV-1/HCV coinfected patients; monitor for clinical toxicities and consider discontinuation if this occurs. Caution with doxorubicin or ribavirin.

PREGNANCY AND LACTATION
Category C, not for use in nursing.

MECHANISM OF ACTION
Synthetic thymidine nucleoside analogue; inhibits activity of HIV-1 reverse transcriptase by competing with natural substrate thymidine triphosphate and by causing DNA chain termination following its incorporation into viral DNA. Inhibits cellular DNA polymerases β and gamma and markedly reduces synthesis of mitochondrial DNA.

PHARMACOKINETICS
Absorption: Rapid. Oral bioavailability (86.4%) (adults), (76.9%) (pediatrics); C_{max}=536ng/mL (adults); T_{max}=1 hr; AUC_{0-24}=2568ng•hr/mL. **Distribution:** (IV) V_d=46L (adults), 0.73L/kg (pediatrics). **Metabolism:** Oxidized stavudine, glucuronide conjugates, and N-acetylcysteine conjugate (minor metabolites). **Elimination:** Urine (42%) (IV, adults), (34%) (pediatrics); $T_{1/2}$=1.6 hrs (adults), 0.96 hr (pediatrics).

PATIENT CONSIDERATIONS

Assessment: Assess for drug hypersensitivity, risk factors for lactic acidosis or liver disease, renal/hepatic impairment, history of peripheral neuropathy, pregnancy/nursing status, and possible drug interactions.

Monitoring: Monitor for signs/symptoms of lactic acidosis, hepatotoxicity, worsening of liver disease, motor weakness, peripheral neuropathy, pancreatitis, fat redistribution/accumulation, lipoatrophy/lipodystrophy, immune reconstitution syndrome (eg, opportunistic infections), and autoimmune disorders.

Counseling: Inform that therapy is not a cure for HIV and patients may continue to experience illnesses associated with HIV. Advise to avoid doing things that can spread HIV to others (eg, sharing needles, other inj equipment, or personal items that can have blood or body fluids on them; sex without protection; breastfeeding). Advise diabetic patients that oral sol contains 50mg of sucrose/mL. Advise to seek medical attention immediately if symptoms of hyperlactatemia or lactic acidosis syndrome (eg, unexplained weight loss, abdominal discomfort, N/V, fatigue, dyspnea, motor weakness) develop. Instruct to report symptoms of peripheral neuropathy to physician. Advise to avoid alcohol while on therapy. Inform that fat redistribution/accumulation may occur.

ZIAGEN — abacavir   Rx

Class: Nucleoside reverse transcriptase inhibitor (NRTI)

> Serious and sometimes fatal hypersensitivity reactions w/ multiple organ involvement reported; d/c immediately if a hypersensitivity reaction is suspected and never restart therapy or any other abacavir-containing product. Patients who carry the HLA-B*5701 allele are at a higher risk of a hypersensitivity reaction; screen all patients for HLA-B*5701 allele prior to initiating or reinitiating therapy, unless patient has a previously documented HLA-B*5701 allele assessment. Lactic acidosis and severe hepatomegaly w/ steatosis, including fatal cases, reported w/ the use of nucleoside analogues and other antiretrovirals. D/C if clinical or lab findings suggestive of lactic acidosis or pronounced hepatotoxicity occur.

ADULT DOSAGE

HIV-1 Infection

Combination w/ Other Antiretrovirals:
300mg bid or 600mg qd

PEDIATRIC DOSAGE

HIV-1 Infection

Combination w/ Other Antiretrovirals:
≥3 Months of Age:
Sol:
8mg/kg bid or 16 mg/kg qd
Max: 600mg/day

Tab:
14 to <20kg:
QD Dosing:
300mg (1 tab)
BID Dosing:
AM Dose: 150mg (1/2 tab)
PM Dose: 150mg (1/2 tab)

≥20 to <25kg:
QD Dosing:
450mg (1 1/2 tabs)
BID Dosing:
AM Dose: 150mg (1/2 tab)
PM Dose: 300mg (1 tab)

≥25kg:
QD Dosing:
600mg (2 tabs)
BID Dosing:
AM Dose: 300mg (1 tab)
PM Dose: 300mg (1 tab)

DOSING CONSIDERATIONS

Hepatic Impairment
Mild (Child-Pugh Class A): 200mg (10mL) bid

ADMINISTRATION
Oral route

Take w/ or w/o food.
Screen for the HLA-B*5701 allele prior to initiating therapy.

STORAGE
20-25°C (68-77°F). **Sol:** Do not freeze. May be refrigerated.

HOW SUPPLIED
Sol: (Abacavir Sulfate) 20mg/mL [240mL]; **Tab:** (Abacavir Sulfate) 300mg* *scored

CONTRAINDICATIONS
Prior hypersensitivity reaction to abacavir, moderate or severe hepatic impairment, patients w/ HLA-B*5701 allele.

WARNINGS/PRECAUTIONS
Obesity and prolonged nucleoside exposure may be risk factors for lactic acidosis and severe hepatomegaly w/ steatosis; caution w/ known risk factors for liver disease. Suspend therapy if clinical or lab findings suggestive of lactic acidosis or pronounced hepatotoxicity develop. Immune reconstitution syndrome reported. Autoimmune disorders (eg, Graves' disease, polymyositis, Guillain-Barre syndrome) reported to occur in the setting of immune reconstitution and can occur many months after initiation of treatment. Redistribution/accumulation of body fat reported. Consider the underlying risk of coronary heart disease when prescribing therapy. Caution in elderly.

ADVERSE REACTIONS
Dreams/sleep disorders, drug hypersensitivity, N/V, headache/migraine, malaise, fatigue, diarrhea, rashes, abdominal pain, gastritis, depressive disorders, dizziness, fever.

DRUG INTERACTIONS
Not recommended w/ other products containing abacavir. Ethanol decreases elimination, causing an increase in overall exposure. May increase oral methadone clearance; an increased methadone dose may be required in a small number of patients.

PREGNANCY AND LACTATION
Pregnancy: Physicians are encouraged to register patients in the Antiretroviral Pregnancy Registry. Fetal harm has been seen in animal studies; relevance to human pregnancy registry data is unknown.
Lactation: Mothers should be instructed not to breastfeed due to potential for HIV-1 transmission.

MECHANISM OF ACTION
Carbocyclic nucleoside analogue; inhibits HIV-1 reverse transcriptase activity by competing w/ the natural substrate deoxyguanosine-5'-triphosphate and by its incorporation into viral DNA.

PHARMACOKINETICS
Absorption: Rapid and extensive. Absolute bioavailability (83%) (tab). (300mg bid) C_{max}=3mcg/mL; AUC_{0-12h}=6.02mcg•hr/mL. (600mg qd) C_{max}=4.26mcg/mL; AUC=11.95mcg•hr/mL. **Distribution:** (IV) V_d=0.86L/kg; plasma protein binding (50%). **Metabolism:** Via alcohol dehydrogenase and glucuronyl transferase; carbovir triphosphate (active metabolite). **Elimination:** Urine (1.2% unchanged, 81% metabolites), feces (16%); $T_{1/2}$=1.54 hrs.

PATIENT CONSIDERATIONS
Assessment: Assess for previous hypersensitivity to the drug, hepatic impairment, risk factors for lactic acidosis or liver disease, risk of coronary heart disease, pregnancy/nursing status, and possible drug interactions. Screen for HLA-B*5701 allele prior to initiation of therapy. Assess medical history for prior exposure to any abacavir-containing product.

Monitoring: Monitor for hypersensitivity reactions, lactic acidosis, hepatotoxicity, immune reconstitution syndrome, autoimmune disorders, fat redistribution/accumulation, MI, and other adverse reactions.

Counseling: Inform about the risk of hypersensitivity reactions; instruct to contact physician immediately if symptoms develop, and not to restart therapy or any other abacavir-containing product w/o medical consultation. Inform that lactic acidosis (w/ liver enlargement) and fat redistribution/accumulation may occur. Inform that drug is not a cure for HIV-1 infection and that illnesses associated w/ HIV-1 may still be experienced. Advise to avoid doing things that can spread HIV-1 to others (eg, sharing needles, other inj equipment, or personal items that can have blood or body fluids on them; having sex w/o protection; breastfeeding). Instruct to take all HIV medications exactly as prescribed.

ZIDOVUDINE — zidovudine   Rx
Class: Nucleoside reverse transcriptase inhibitor (NRTI)

> Associated w/ hematologic toxicity (eg, neutropenia, severe anemia), particularly w/ advanced HIV-1 disease. Symptomatic myopathy associated w/ prolonged use. Lactic acidosis and severe hepatomegaly w/ steatosis, including fatal cases, reported w/ nucleoside analogues; suspend treatment if lactic acidosis or pronounced hepatotoxicity occurs.

OTHER BRAND NAMES
Retrovir

ADULT DOSAGE

Prevention of Maternal-Fetal HIV Transmission

<14 Weeks of Pregnancy:
PO:
100mg 5X/day until start of labor
During Labor and Delivery:
IV:
2mg/kg over 1 hr followed by continuous infusion of 1mg/kg/hr until clamping of umbilical cord

HIV-1 Infection

Combination w/ Other Antiretrovirals:
PO:
300mg bid
IV:
1mg/kg at a constant rate over 1 hr q4h

PEDIATRIC DOSAGE

HIV-1 Infection

Combination w/ Other Antiretrovirals:
4 Weeks-<18 Years:
Weight Based:
4-<9kg: 12mg/kg bid or 8mg/kg tid (24mg/kg/day)
≥9-<30kg: 9mg/kg bid or 6mg/kg tid (18mg/kg/day)
≥30kg: 300mg bid or 200mg tid (600mg/day)

BSA Based:
240mg/m² bid or 160mg/m² tid (480mg/m²/day)

Prevention of Maternal-Fetal HIV Transmission

Neonates:
Start w/in 12 hrs after birth and continue through 6 weeks of age
PO: 2mg/kg q6h (8mg/kg/day)
IV: 1.5mg/kg over 30 min q6h (6mg/kg/day)

DOSING CONSIDERATIONS

Renal Impairment
Hemodialysis/Peritoneal Dialysis/CrCl <15mL/min:
PO: 100mg q6-8h
IV: 1mg/kg q6-8h

Adverse Reactions
Significant Anemia (Hgb <7.5g/dL or Reduction >25% of Baseline)/Neutropenia (Granulocyte Count <750 cells/mm³ or Reduction >50% from Baseline):
May require dose interruption until evidence of marrow recovery occurs; if marrow recovery occurs following dose interruption, may resume dose using adjunctive measures (eg, epoetin alfa), depending on hematologic indices and patient tolerance

ADMINISTRATION
Oral/IV route

Administer IV infusion only until oral therapy can be administered

PO
Take w/ or w/o food

IV
Avoid rapid infusion and bolus inj
Infusion must be diluted prior to administration

Dilution Instructions
1. Remove calculated dose from the 20mL vial and add to D5 inj sol to a concentration ≤4mg/mL
2. Administer diluted sol w/in 8 hrs if stored at 25°C (77°F) or 24 hrs if stored at 2-8°C (36-46°F), to minimize contamination

STORAGE
(Tab) 20-25°C (68-77°F). (Retrovir) 15-25°C (59-77°F). (Cap) Protect from moisture. (Inj) Protect from light. Diluted Sol: Stable for 24 hrs at room temperature and for 48 hrs if refrigerated at 2-8°C (36-46°F).

HOW SUPPLIED
Tab: 300mg; **(Retrovir) Cap:** 100mg; **Inj:** 10mg/mL [20mL]; **Syrup:** 10mg/mL [240mL]

CONTRAINDICATIONS
Life-threatening hypersensitivity reaction (eg, anaphylaxis, Stevens-Johnson syndrome) to any of the components of the formulation.

WARNINGS/PRECAUTIONS

Caution w/ granulocyte count <1000 cells/mm³ or Hgb <9.5g/dL; monitor blood counts frequently in patients w/ poor bone marrow reserve, particularly w/ advanced HIV-1 disease and periodically w/ other HIV-infected patients and w/ asymptomatic/ early HIV-1 disease. Vial stoppers for inj contain natural rubber latex which may cause allergic reactions in latex-sensitive individuals. Obesity and prolonged nucleoside exposure may be risk factors for lactic acidosis and severe hepatomegaly w/ steatosis. Caution w/ any known risk factors for liver disease and in elderly. Pancytopenia and immune reconstitution syndrome reported. Autoimmune disorders (eg, Graves' disease, polymyositis, Guillain-Barre syndrome) reported to occur in the setting of immune reconstitution and can occur many months after initiation of treatment. May cause redistribution/accumulation of body fat.

ADVERSE REACTIONS

Hematologic toxicity, myopathy, lactic acidosis, severe hepatomegaly w/ steatosis, headache, N/V, malaise, anorexia, asthenia, constipation, abdominal pain/cramps, arthralgia, chills.

DRUG INTERACTIONS

Avoid w/ stavudine, nucleoside analogues affecting DNA replication (eg, ribavirin), doxorubicin, and other combination products containing zidovudine. Hepatic decompensation may occur in HIV/hepatitis C virus (HCV) coinfected patients receiving interferon alfa w/ or w/o ribavirin; closely monitor for treatment-associated toxicities. May increase risk of hematologic toxicities w/ ganciclovir, interferon alfa, ribavirin, and other bone marrow suppressive or cytotoxic agents.

PREGNANCY AND LACTATION

Category C, not for use in nursing.

MECHANISM OF ACTION

Synthetic nucleoside analogue; inhibits reverse transcriptase via DNA chain termination after incorporation of the nucleotide analogue.

PHARMACOKINETICS

Absorption: (Oral) Rapid. Bioavailability (64%); T_{max}=0.5-1.5 hrs. (IV) C_{max}=1.1mcg/mL. **Distribution:** V_d=1.6L/kg; plasma protein binding (<38%); crosses the placenta; found in breast milk. **Metabolism:** Hepatic. 3'-azido-3'-deoxy-5'-O-β-D-glucopyranuronosylthymidine (major metabolite). **Elimination:** Urine (14% unchanged, 74% metabolite [oral]; 18% unchanged, 60% metabolite [IV]); $T_{1/2}$=0.5-3 hrs. Refer to PI for pediatric patients and patients w/ renal impairment pharmacokinetic parameters.

PATIENT CONSIDERATIONS

Assessment: Assess for previous hypersensitivity reaction to the drug, advanced HIV disease, latex sensitivity, risk factors for lactic acidosis/liver disease, bone marrow compromise, renal/hepatic impairment, pregnancy/nursing status, and possible drug interactions. (Oral) Assess ability to swallow cap/tab in children.

Monitoring: Monitor for signs/symptoms of hematologic toxicity, lactic acidosis, hepatomegaly w/ steatosis, myopathy, immune reconstitution syndrome, autoimmune disorders, fat redistribution/accumulation, and other adverse reactions. Monitor blood counts/hematologic indices periodically and the need for dosage adjustment.

Counseling: Inform that potentially life-threatening hypersensitivity reactions can occur; instruct to immediately contact physician if rash develops. Inform about risk for hematologic toxicities and advise on importance of close blood count monitoring while on therapy. Counsel about the possible occurrence of myopathy and myositis w/ pathological changes during prolonged use and that therapy may cause a rare but serious condition called lactic acidosis w/ liver enlargement (hepatomegaly). Inform that hepatic decompensation has occurred in HIV-1/HCV coinfected patients receiving combination antiretroviral therapy and interferon alfa w/ or w/o ribavirin. Inform that immune reconstitution syndrome may occur; advise to inform physician immediately of any symptoms of infection. Inform that redistribution/accumulation of body fat may occur. Instruct to report any other adverse events that occur. Instruct not to breastfeed to prevent postnatal transmission. Inform that drug is not a cure for HIV-1 infection and that illness associated w/ HIV-1 may still be experienced. Inform to take all HIV medications exactly as prescribed. Advise to avoid doing things that can spread HIV-1 infection to others; instruct to continue to practice safe sex.

ZINBRYTA — daclizumab Rx

Class: Monoclonal antibody/interleukin-2R (IL-2R) alpha (CD25) blocker

> May cause severe liver injury including life-threatening events, liver failure, and autoimmune hepatitis; can occur at any time during treatment and seen up to 4 months after last dose. Contraindicated in patients w/ preexisting hepatic disease or hepatic impairment. Obtain ALT, AST, and bilirubin levels prior to initiation of therapy. Test transaminase levels and total bilirubin monthly and assess before the next dose. Follow transaminase levels and total bilirubin monthly for 6 months after the last dose. In case of elevation in transaminases or total bilirubin, treatment interruption or discontinuation may be required. Immune-mediated disorders (eg, skin reactions, lymphadenopathy, noninfectious colitis) reported. Reported that some patients required systemic corticosteroids or other immunosuppressant treatment for autoimmune hepatitis/immune-mediated disorders and continued this treatment after the last dose of therapy. Only available through a restricted program under a Risk Evaluation and Mitigation Strategy (REMS) called the Zinbryta REMS Program.

ADULT DOSAGE
Multiple Sclerosis
Relapsing forms of multiple sclerosis (MS) in patients who have had an inadequate response to ≥2 drugs indicated for the treatment of MS

150mg once monthly

PEDIATRIC DOSAGE
Pediatric use may not have been established

DOSING CONSIDERATIONS

Hepatic Impairment

ALT or AST >5X ULN or Total Bilirubin >2X ULN or ALT or AST ≥3 but <5X ULN and Total Bilirubin >1.5 but <2X ULN:
- Interrupt therapy and investigate for other etiologies of abnormal lab values
- If no other etiologies are identified, then d/c
- If other etiologies are identified, reassess overall risk-benefit profile of treatment and consider whether to resume daclizumab when both AST or ALT are <2X ULN and total bilirubin is ≤ULN

Other Dosing Considerations
- Evaluate patients at high risk for tuberculosis (TB) infection prior to initiating treatment
- If positive for TB, treat tuberculosis by standard medical practice prior to therapy
- Avoid initiating in patients w/ TB or other severe active infection
- Prior to initiation, screen for hepatitis B and C
- Consider any necessary immunization w/ live vaccines prior to treatment; live vaccines are not recommended during treatment and up to 4 months after discontinuation of treatment

ADMINISTRATION

SQ route

- Remove from the refrigerator 30 min before administration, to allow drug to warm to room temperature. Do not use external heat sources. Do not place back into refrigerator after allowing it to warm to room temperature.
- Inject into thigh, abdomen, or back of the upper arm.
- Use each prefilled syringe one time and then discard appropriately.

STORAGE

2-8°C (36-46°F). Store in the original carton to protect from light. Do not freeze or expose to temperatures >30°C (86°F). Discard if frozen. If refrigeration is unavailable, may store protected from light up to 30°C (86°F) for a period up to 30 days. Discard after 30 days w/o refrigeration.

HOW SUPPLIED

Inj: 150mg/mL

CONTRAINDICATIONS

Preexisting hepatic disease or hepatic impairment, including ALT or AST at least 2X ULN; history of autoimmune hepatitis or other autoimmune condition involving the liver; history of hypersensitivity to daclizumab or any other components of the formulation.

WARNINGS/PRECAUTIONS

See Dosing Considerations. If clinical signs or symptoms suggestive of hepatic dysfunction develop (eg, unexplained N/V, abdominal pain, fatigue, anorexia, jaundice, dark urine), promptly measure serum transaminases and total bilirubin and interrupt or d/c treatment. D/C if autoimmune hepatitis is suspected. Ensure adequate evaluation to confirm etiology or to exclude other causes if immune-mediated disorders are suspected; consider discontinuing treatment and refer to an appropriate specialist for further evaluation and treatment if a serious immune-mediated disorder develops. May cause anaphylaxis, angioedema, and urticaria after the first dose or at any time during treatment; d/c and do not restart treatment if anaphylaxis or other allergic reactions occur. Increases the risk for infections. Avoid initiating in patients w/ severe active infection until the infection is fully controlled. If serious infection develops, consider withholding treatment until the infection resolves. Depression-related events (eg, suicidal ideation, suicide attempt) reported; caution w/ previous or current depressive disorders. Consider discontinuing therapy if severe depression and/or suicidal ideation develops.

ADVERSE REACTIONS

Nasopharyngitis, URTI, rash, influenza, dermatitis, oropharyngeal pain, bronchitis, eczema, lymphadenopathy, depression, pharyngitis, increased ALT.

DRUG INTERACTIONS

See Dosing Considerations. Caution w/ hepatotoxic drugs; carefully consider need for herbal products or dietary supplements that can cause hepatotoxicity.

PREGNANCY AND LACTATION

Pregnancy: Administration to monkeys during gestation resulted in embryofetal death and reduced fetal growth at maternal exposures >30X than expected clinically. In monkeys administered 50mg/kg weekly from gestation day 50 to birth, there were no effects on pre- or postnatal development for up to 6 months after birth. **Lactation:** There are no data on the presence of daclizumab in human milk, the effects on the breastfed child, or the effects of the drug on milk production; caution in nursing.

MECHANISM OF ACTION

Monoclonal antibody; precise mechanism unknown but presumed to involve modulation of IL-2 mediated activation of lymphocytes through binding to CD25, a subunit of the high-affinity IL-2 receptor.

PHARMACOKINETICS

Absorption: Absolute bioavailability (approx 90%); T_{max}=5-7 days; C_{max}=30μg/mL; AUC=640μg-days/mL. **Distribution:** V_d=6.34L. **Metabolism:** Undergoes catabolism to peptides and amino acids w/o renal elimination. **Elimination:** $T_{1/2}$=21 days.

PATIENT CONSIDERATIONS

Assessment: Assess for history of hypersensitivity to daclizumab or any other components of the formulation, hepatitis B and C, preexisting hepatic disease or hepatic impairment, history of autoimmune hepatitis or other autoimmune condition involving the liver, TB or other severe active infection, previous or current depressive disorders, pregnancy/nursing status, and for possible drug interactions. Obtain baseline ALT, AST, and bilirubin levels.

Monitoring: Monitor for hepatic injury, immune-mediated disorders, anaphylaxis, angioedema, urticaria, infections, new or worsening depression, suicidal ideation, and other adverse reactions. Monitor transaminase levels and total bilirubin monthly and assess before the next dose. Monitor transaminase levels and total bilirubin monthly for 6 months after the last dose.

Counseling: Advise of symptoms of allergic reactions/anaphylaxis, hepatic dysfunction, lymphadenopathy, GI reactions (eg, colitis), and dermatologic reactions; instruct to report such symptoms to healthcare provider immediately. Discuss the importance of monitoring hepatic lab values monthly and for up to 6 months after the last dose of therapy. Inform patients that they will be given a Zinbryta Patient Wallet Card that they should carry w/ them at all times; advise to show card to other treating healthcare providers. Advise that therapy can cause the immune system to attack healthy cells in the body and this can affect any organ system. Inform that treatment is only available through a REMS program and that the patient must enroll in the program and comply w/ ongoing monitoring requirements. Inform that there is an increased risk of developing infections during treatment; instruct to contact healthcare provider if symptoms of infection develop. Advise of the symptoms of depression and suicidal ideation and instruct to report symptoms of depression or thoughts of suicide to healthcare provider immediately. Provide appropriate instruction for methods of self-inj.

ZINECARD — dexrazoxane   Rx
Class: EDTA derivative

ADULT DOSAGE	PEDIATRIC DOSAGE
Doxorubicin-Induced Cardiomyopathy	Pediatric use may not have been established
For reducing the incidence and severity of cardiomyopathy associated w/ doxorubicin administration in women w/ metastatic breast cancer who have received a cumulative doxorubicin dose of 300 mg/m² and who will continue to receive doxorubicin therapy to maintain tumor control. Do not use w/ the initiation of doxorubicin therapy	
Usual: 10:1 ratio of dexrazoxane:doxorubicin (eg, 500mg/m²:50mg/m²)	

DOSING CONSIDERATIONS
Renal Impairment
Moderate to Severe (CrCl <40mL/min): Reduce dexrazoxane dose by 50% (5:1 ratio of dexrazoxane:doxorubicin)

Hepatic Impairment
Reduce dose proportionately (maintaining the 10:1 ratio)

Elderly
Start at lower end of dosing range

ADMINISTRATION
IV route

Do not administer via IV push
Do not mix w/ other drugs
Administer via IV infusion over 15 min
Give doxorubicin w/in 30 min after completion of dexrazoxane infusion

Preparation and Handling of Infusion Sol
Reconstitute w/ 25mL of sterile water for inj for a 250mg vial and 50mL for a 500mg vial
Dilute the reconstituted sol further w/ lactated Ringer's inj to a concentration of 1.3 to 3.0 mg/mL in IV infusion bags for IV infusion

STORAGE
25°C (77°F); excursions permitted to 15-30°C (59-86°F). Reconstituted Sol: Stable for 30 min at room temperature or 2-8°C (36-46°F) for up to 3 hrs. Diluted Infusion Sol: Stable for 1 hr at room temperature or 2-8°C (36-46°F) for up to 4 hrs.

HOW SUPPLIED
Inj: 250mg, 500mg

CONTRAINDICATIONS
Concomitant use with non-anthracycline chemotherapy regimens.

WARNINGS/PRECAUTIONS
Do not use with the initiation of doxorubicin therapy. Treatment does not completely eliminate the risk of anthracycline-induced cardiac toxicity. Monitor cardiac function before and periodically during therapy to assess left ventricular ejection fraction (LVEF); if results indicate deterioration in cardiac function associated with doxorubicin, carefully evaluate the benefit of continued therapy against the risk of irreversible cardiac damage. Secondary malignancies (eg, acute myeloid leukemia, myelodysplastic syndrome) reported in combination with chemotherapy. May cause fetal harm. Caution in elderly.

ADVERSE REACTIONS
Alopecia, N/V, fatigue, anorexia, stomatitis, fever, infection, diarrhea, pain on inj, sepsis, neurotoxicity, streaking/erythema, phlebitis, esophagitis, dysphagia.

DRUG INTERACTIONS
See Contraindications. Avoid during initiation of fluorouracil, doxorubicin, and cyclophosphamide therapy; may interfere with the antitumor efficacy of the regimen. May add to myelosuppression caused by chemotherapeutic agents; obtain CBC prior to and during each course of therapy, and administer dexrazoxane and chemotherapy only when adequate hematologic parameters are met.

PREGNANCY AND LACTATION
Category D, not for use in nursing.

MECHANISM OF ACTION
EDTA derivative; not established. Suspected to interfere with iron-mediated free radical generation thought to be responsible, in part, for anthracycline-induced cardiomyopathy.

PHARMACOKINETICS
Absorption: (500mg/m²) C_{max}=36.5mcg/mL, T_{max}=15 min. **Distribution:** (500mg/m²) V_d=22.4L/m²; (600mg/m²) V_d=22L/m². **Elimination:** (500mg/m²) Urine (42%); $T_{1/2}$=2.5 hrs. (600mg/m²) $T_{1/2}$=2.1 hrs.

PATIENT CONSIDERATIONS
Assessment: Assess for renal/hepatic impairment, pregnancy/nursing status, and possible drug interactions. Monitor cardiac function to assess LVEF. Obtain baseline CBC.

Monitoring: Monitor for secondary malignancies and other adverse reactions. Obtain CBC during each course of chemotherapy. Monitor cardiac function periodically during therapy to assess LVEF.

Counseling: Inform about the risks/benefits of therapy. Advise women of reproductive potential that drug may cause fetal harm; instruct to use highly effective contraception during treatment.

ZOLADEX 10.8MG — goserelin acetate   Rx
Class: Synthetic gonadotropin-releasing hormone (GnRH) analogue

ADULT DOSAGE	PEDIATRIC DOSAGE
Prostate Carcinoma	Pediatric use may not have been established
Combination w/ Flutamide for Locally Confined Stage T2b-T4 Prostate Carcinoma (Stage B2-C): One 3.6mg implant SQ, followed in 28 days by one 10.8mg implant SQ	
Start treatment 8 weeks prior to initiating radiotherapy and continue during radiation therapy	
Palliative Treatment for Advanced Prostate Carcinoma: One 10.8mg implant SQ every 12 weeks; intended for long-term administration unless clinically inappropriate	

DOSING CONSIDERATIONS
Other Important Considerations
Zoladex 10.8mg implant is not indicated in women; for female patients requiring treatment w/ goserelin, refer to prescribing information for Zoladex 3.6mg implant

ADMINISTRATION
SQ route

Administer every 12 weeks into the anterior abdominal wall below the navel line under the supervision of a physician; while a delay of a few days is permissible, every effort should be made to adhere to the 12-week schedule.

Administration Instructions
1. Put patient in comfortable position w/ upper part of body slightly raised; prepare an area of the anterior abdominal wall below navel line w/ alcohol swab. Caution while injecting into the anterior abdominal wall due to the proximity of underlying inferior epigastric artery and its branches.
2. Remove syringe from foil pouch and hold it at a slight angle to the light to check that at least part of implant is visible.
3. Remove the plastic safety tab and needle cover. Unlike liquid inj, do not attempt to remove air bubbles; attempts to do so may displace the implant.
4. Holding syringe around protective sleeve, pinch skin of anterior abdominal wall below navel line, and insert needle, bevel side up, at a 30-45° angle into skin in 1 continuous, deliberate motion until protective sleeve touches the patient's skin.
5. Depress plunger until it cannot be depressed any further. If plunger is not depressed fully, protective sleeve will not activate. When protective sleeve "clicks," it will automatically begin to slide to cover the needle.
6. Withdraw needle and allow protective sleeve to slide and cover needle.
7. Do not use syringe for aspiration. If the hypodermic needle penetrates a large vessel, blood will be seen instantly in syringe chamber; withdraw needle and inject w/ a new syringe elsewhere.
8. Do not penetrate into muscle or peritoneum.

STORAGE
Room temperature; do not exceed 25°C (77°F).

HOW SUPPLIED
Implant: 10.8mg

CONTRAINDICATIONS
Known hypersensitivity to GnRH, GnRH agonist analogues, or any components in the medication; pregnancy.

WARNINGS/PRECAUTIONS
Initially, may cause transient increases in serum testosterone levels; worsening or onset of new symptoms of prostate cancer may occur during the 1st few weeks of treatment. May experience temporary increase in bone pain; manage symptomatically. Ureteral obstruction and spinal cord compression reported; institute standard treatment if spinal cord compression or renal impairment secondary to ureteral obstruction develops, and in extreme cases, consider an immediate

orchiectomy. Hypersensitivity, antibody formation, and acute anaphylactic reactions reported. Hyperglycemia and increased risk of developing diabetes reported. Increased risk of developing MI, sudden cardiac death, and stroke reported. Androgen deprivation therapy may prolong QT/QTc interval; consider whether benefits outweigh potential risks in patients w/ congenital long QT syndrome, CHF, or frequent electrolyte abnormalities, and in patients taking drugs known to prolong the QT interval. Correct electrolyte abnormalities. Inj-site injury and vascular injury including pain, hematoma, hemorrhage, and hemorrhagic shock, requiring blood transfusions and surgical intervention, reported; caution w/ low BMI and/or in patients receiving full anticoagulation. Closely monitor testosterone levels in obese patients who have not responded clinically. Lab test interactions may occur.

ADVERSE REACTIONS
Hot flashes, sexual dysfunction, decreased erections.

PREGNANCY AND LACTATION
Pregnancy: Category X.
Lactation: Not for use in nursing.

MECHANISM OF ACTION
Synthetic GnRH analogue; inhibits pituitary gonadotropin secretion. Initially increases serum luteinizing hormone and follicle-stimulating hormone levels w/ subsequent increases in serum levels of testosterone. Chronic administration leads to suppression of pituitary gonadotropins, and a fall in testosterone levels.

PHARMACOKINETICS
Absorption: Rapid. C_{max}=8.85ng/mL; T_{max}=1.8 hrs. **Distribution:** (250mcg aqueous sol SQ) V_d=44.1L. Plasma protein binding (27%). **Metabolism:** Hydrolysis of C-terminal amino acids. **Elimination:** Urine (>90%, 20% unchanged).

PATIENT CONSIDERATIONS
Assessment: Assess for hypersensitivity to the drug, diabetes, cardiovascular (CV) risk factors, congenital long QT syndrome, CHF, electrolyte abnormalities, and low BMI. Obtain baseline serum testosterone, blood glucose and/or HbA1c levels. Assess if patient is receiving full anticoagulation.

Monitoring: Monitor for worsening or occurrence of signs/symptoms of prostate cancer, bone pain, ureteral obstruction, spinal cord compression, renal impairment, hypersensitivity/acute anaphylactic reactions, antibody formation, CV disease, inj-site injury, and other adverse reactions. Periodically monitor serum testosterone, blood glucose, and/or HbA1c levels. Consider periodic monitoring of ECGs and electrolytes.

Counseling: Inform of risks and benefits of therapy. Inform of the risk of developing ureteral obstruction, spinal cord compression, reduction in bone mineral density, diabetes, loss of glycemic control in patients w/ preexisting diabetes, MI, sudden cardiac death, and stroke. Advise to contact physician immediately if experiencing any symptoms of inj-site injury or if any other adverse events (eg, abdominal pain/distension, dyspnea, dizziness, hypotension, any altered levels of consciousness) develop.

ZOLINZA — vorinostat   Rx
Class: Histone deacetylase (HDAC) inhibitor

ADULT DOSAGE	PEDIATRIC DOSAGE
Cutaneous T-Cell Lymphoma	Pediatric use may not have been established
Cutaneous Manifestations in Progressive, Persistent or Recurrent Disease on or Following 2 Systemic Therapies: 400mg qd	
Intolerant to Therapy: May reduce to 300mg qd; may further reduce to 300mg qd for 5 consecutive days each week, as necessary	
Treatment may be continued as long as there is no evidence of progressive disease or unacceptable toxicity	

DOSING CONSIDERATIONS
Hepatic Impairment
Mild to Moderate (Bilirubin 1-3X ULN/AST>ULN): Reduce starting dose to 300mg qd
Severe (Bilirubin>3X ULN): There is insufficient evidence to recommend a starting dose for patients w/ severe hepatic impairment; patients w/ severe hepatic impairment have not been treated at doses >200mg/day

ADMINISTRATION
Oral route
Take w/ food.
Do not open or crush cap.
Avoid direct contact of powder w/ skin or mucous membranes; wash thoroughly if such contact occurs.
Avoid exposure to crushed and/or broken cap.

STORAGE
20-25°C (68-77°F); excursions permitted between 15-30°C (59-86°F).

HOW SUPPLIED
Cap: 100mg

WARNINGS/PRECAUTIONS
Pulmonary embolism (PE) and deep vein thrombosis (DVT) reported; monitor for signs and symptoms of these events, particularly w/ prior history of thromboembolic events. Dose-related thrombocytopenia and anemia may occur;

---

adjust dosage or d/c treatment as clinically appropriate. GI disturbances (eg, N/V, diarrhea) reported. Adequately control preexisting N/V and diarrhea before beginning therapy. Hyperglycemia observed. Monitor blood cell counts and chemistry tests, including serum electrolytes, Mg^{2+}, Ca^{2+}, glucose, and SrCr every 2 weeks during the first 2 months of therapy and monthly thereafter. Correct hypokalemia and hypomagnesemia prior to therapy. Monitor K^+ and Mg^{2+} more frequently in symptomatic patients (eg, patients w/ N/V, diarrhea, fluid imbalance, cardiac symptoms). May cause fetal harm. Caution w/ renal/hepatic impairment and in elderly.

ADVERSE REACTIONS
Diarrhea, fatigue, N/V, thrombocytopenia, anemia, anorexia, dysgeusia, decreased weight, dry mouth, increased blood creatinine, chills, constipation, dizziness.

DRUG INTERACTIONS
Prolongation of PT and INR observed w/ coumarin-derivative anticoagulants; monitor PT and INR more frequently. Severe thrombocytopenia and GI bleeding reported w/ concomitant use w/ other histone deacetylase inhibitors (eg, valproic acid); monitor platelet counts every 2 weeks for the first 2 months.

PREGNANCY AND LACTATION
Pregnancy: Category D.
Lactation: Not for use in nursing.

MECHANISM OF ACTION
Histone deacetylase (HDAC) inhibitor; inhibits HDAC enzymes, HDAC1, HDAC2, HDAC3, and HDAC6, which catalyze the removal of acetyl groups from the lysine residues of proteins, including histones and transcription factors. HDAC inhibition results in accumulation of acetyl groups on the histone lysine residues resulting in an open chromatin structure and transcriptional activation; cell growth is terminated and apoptosis occurs.

PHARMACOKINETICS
Absorption: (Fasted, single 400mg dose) C_{max}=1.2μM, T_{max}=1.5 hrs (median), AUC=4.2μM•hr; (High-fat meal, single 400mg dose) C_{max}=1.2μM, T_{max}=4 hrs (median), AUC=5.5μM•hr. (Fed, multiple 400mg doses) C_{max}=1.2μM, T_{max}=4 hrs (median), AUC=6.0μM•hr. **Distribution:** Plasma protein binding (71%). **Metabolism:** Liver via glucuronidation, hydrolysis, and β-oxidation. **Elimination:** Urine (<1% unchanged); $T_{1/2}$=2 hrs.

PATIENT CONSIDERATIONS
Assessment: Assess for renal/hepatic impairment, history of thromboembolic events, GI disturbances, fluid imbalance, cardiac symptoms, diabetes, hypokalemia, hypomagnesemia, pregnancy/nursing status, and possible drug interactions.

Monitoring: Monitor for signs/symptoms of PE and DVT, thrombocytopenia, anemia, GI disturbances, dehydration, hyperglycemia, and other adverse reactions. Monitor blood cell counts, chemistry tests, electrolytes, serum glucose, and SrCr every 2 weeks for the first 2 months and monthly thereafter. Monitor K^+ and Mg^{2+} more frequently in symptomatic patients.

Counseling: Inform about risks and benefits of therapy. Instruct to drink at least 2L/day of fluids to prevent dehydration. Advise to promptly report to physician if excessive vomiting or diarrhea, unusual bleeding, signs of DVT, or any other adverse events develop.

ZOMACTON — somatropin (rDNA origin)   Rx
Class: Recombinant human growth hormone (hGH)

	PEDIATRIC DOSAGE
	Growth Hormone Deficiency
	Due to Inadequate Secretion of Endogenous Growth Hormone: Up to 0.1mg/kg SQ 3X/week (up to 0.3mg/kg/week)

ADMINISTRATION
SQ route

Reconstitution
- Reconstitute 5mg vial w/ 1-5mL of bacteriostatic 0.9% NaCl for inj (benzyl alcohol preserved); reconstitute w/ sterile normal saline for inj and use only one dose per vial when administering to newborns.
- Reconstitute 10mg vial w/ 1mL syringe of bacteriostatic water for inj containing 0.33% metacresol.
- Swirl vial w/ a gentle rotary motion until contents are completely dissolved and the sol is clear.
- Do not shake; shaking or vigorous mixing will cause sol to be cloudy.
- Some cloudiness may occur after refrigeration; allow product to warm to room temperature and do not use if cloudiness persists or particulate matter is noted.
- May be administered using a standard sterile disposable syringe or a Zoma-Jet Needle-Free inj device.
- For proper use, refer to user's manual provided w/ administration device.

STORAGE
2-8°C (36-46°F). Avoid freezing the accompanying diluent. **Reconstituted Sol:** 2-8°C (36-46°F) for up to 14 days when reconstituted w/ bacteriostatic 0.9% NaCl and for up to 28 days when reconstituted w/ bacteriostatic water for inj. Do not freeze.

HOW SUPPLIED
Inj: 5mg, 10mg

CONTRAINDICATIONS
Hypersensitivity to somatropin or to any of the excipients, closed epiphyses, active proliferative or severe nonproliferative diabetic retinopathy, active

malignancy or evidence of progression or recurrence of an underlying intracranial tumor. Acute critical illness due to complications following open heart surgery, abdominal surgery or multiple accidental trauma, or w/ acute respiratory failure. Prader-Willi syndrome (PWS) w/ severe obesity or w/ severe respiratory impairment. Growth failure due to genetically confirmed PWS. Known sensitivity to benzyl alcohol (found in bacteriostatic 0.9% NaCl diluent) or allergy to metacresol (found in bacteriostatic water for inj diluent).

WARNINGS/PRECAUTIONS
Evaluate patients w/ PWS for signs of upper airway obstruction (eg, new/increased snoring) and sleep apnea before treatment and interrupt therapy if these signs occur. Implement effective weight control in patients w/ PWS and treat respiratory infections aggressively. Pancreatitis reported rarely. Bacteriostatic 0.9% NaCl diluent contains benzyl alcohol, which has been associated w/ serious adverse events and death, particularly in pediatric patients; reconstitute w/ sterile normal saline for inj when administering the 5mg inj to newborns. Carry out therapy under the guidance of a physician experienced in the diagnosis and management of pediatric patients w/ growth hormone deficiency (GHD). Monitor all patients w/ a history of GHD secondary to an intracranial neoplasm routinely while on therapy for progression/recurrence of the tumor. Increased risk of developing malignancies in children w/ certain rare genetic causes of short stature; monitor for development of neoplasms. Monitor for increased growth or potential malignant changes of preexisting nevi. May decrease insulin sensitivity and unmask undiagnosed impaired glucose tolerance and overt diabetes mellitus (DM). New onset type 2 DM reported. Monitor standard hormonal replacement therapy in patients w/ hypopituitarism. Undiagnosed/untreated hypothyroidism may prevent optimal response. Central (secondary) hypothyroidism may become evident or worsen during treatment; may need to initiate thyroid hormone replacement therapy. Increased incidence of slipped capital femoral epiphysis and progression of scoliosis may occur. Intracranial HTN w/ papilledema, visual changes, headache, and/or N/V reported; d/c therapy if papilledema is observed by funduscopy. Monitor bone age, especially in patients who are pubertal and/or receiving thyroid hormone replacement therapy. Tissue atrophy may occur when administered at the same site over a long period; rotate inj site. Local/systemic allergic reactions may occur. Serum levels of inorganic phosphorus, alkaline phosphatase, and insulin-like growth factor-1 (IGF-1) may increase after therapy.

ADVERSE REACTIONS
Headache, gynecomastia, inj-site reactions (eg, pain, bruise), pancreatitis.

DRUG INTERACTIONS
May need to adjust dose of antihyperglycemic agents (eg, insulin, oral agents), and thyroid hormone replacement therapy. May inhibit 11β-hydroxysteroid dehydrogenase type 1, resulting in reduced serum cortisol concentrations; may need glucocorticoid replacement or dose adjustments of glucocorticoid therapy. Glucocorticoid therapy may attenuate growth-promoting effects in children; carefully adjust glucocorticoid replacement dosing. May increase clearance of antipyrine. May alter clearance of compounds metabolized by CYP450 liver enzymes (eg, corticosteroids, sex steroids, anticonvulsants, cyclosporine); monitor carefully.

PREGNANCY AND LACTATION
Pregnancy: Category C.
Lactation: Caution in nursing.

MECHANISM OF ACTION
Recombinant human growth hormone; stimulates linear growth in children who lack adequate levels of endogenous growth hormone. Produces increased growth rates and IGF-1 concentrations that are similar to those seen after therapy w/ human growth hormone of pituitary origin.

PHARMACOKINETICS
Absorption: Absolute bioavailability (approx 70%); C_{max}=80ng/mL; T_{max}=approx 7 hrs. **Elimination:** $T_{1/2}$=approx 2.7 hrs.

PATIENT CONSIDERATIONS
Assessment: Assess for PWS, preexisting DM or impaired glucose tolerance, hypothyroidism, hypopituitarism, history of scoliosis, hypersensitivity to drug/benzyl alcohol/metacresol, any other conditions where treatment is contraindicated or cautioned, pregnancy/nursing status, and possible drug interactions. Perform funduscopic exam.

Monitoring: Monitor for neoplasms, respiratory infection (patients w/ PWS), increased growth or malignant changes of preexisting nevi, slipped capital femoral epiphysis, progression of scoliosis, intracranial HTN, allergic reactions, pancreatitis, and other adverse reactions. Routinely monitor all patients w/ a history of GHD secondary to an intracranial neoplasm for progression or recurrence of the tumor. Perform periodic thyroid function tests, funduscopic exam, and monitoring of glucose levels and bone age. Monitor growth of patient.

Counseling: Inform about potential benefits and risks of therapy. Instruct on proper administration and disposal of therapy.

ZOMETA — zoledronic acid   Rx
Class: Bisphosphonate

ADULT DOSAGE
Hypercalcemia of Malignancy
Albumin-Corrected Serum Ca^{2+} ≥12mg/dL (3.0mmol/L):
Max: 4mg as a single-dose; infuse IV over no less than 15 min
May consider retreatment if serum Ca^{2+} does not return to normal or remain normal after initial treatment; wait for a minimum of 7 days before retreatment

PEDIATRIC DOSAGE
Pediatric use may not have been established

Vigorous saline hydration should be initiated promptly and an attempt should be made to restore the urine output to about 2L/day throughout treatment; adequately hydrate patients throughout treatment, but avoid overhydration, especially in patients w/ cardiac failure

Multiple Myeloma and Metastatic Bone Lesions of Solid Tumors

In Conjunction w/ Standard Antineoplastic Therapy:
4mg IV infusion over no less than 15 min every 3-4 weeks

Prostate cancer should have progressed after treatment w/ at least 1 hormonal therapy

---

DOSING CONSIDERATIONS
Renal Impairment
Multiple Myeloma and Metastatic Bone Lesions of Solid Tumors:
CrCl >60mL/min: 4mg
CrCl 50-60mL/min: 3.5mg
CrCl 40-49mL/min: 3.3mg
CrCl 30-39mL/min: 3mg
Withhold treatment for renal deterioration

Other Important Considerations
Multiple Myeloma and Metastatic Bone Lesions of Solid Tumors:
Administer oral Ca^{2+} supplement of 500mg and a multiple vitamin containing 400 IU of vitamin D daily

ADMINISTRATION
IV route
Infuse IV over no less than 15 min.
Do not mix w/ Ca^{2+} or other divalent cation-containing infusion sol (eg, lactated Ringer's sol), and administer as a single IV sol in a line separate from all other drugs.

4mg/100mL Single-Use Ready-to-Use Bottle
This sol is ready-to-use and may be administered directly to the patient w/o further preparation.

Preparation of Reduced Doses from Ready-to-Use Bottle (4mg/100mL):
- Remove 12mL, 18mL, or 25mL from bottle and replace w/ an equal volume of sterile 0.9% NaCl or D5 inj for a dose of 3.5mg, 3.3mg, or 3mg, respectively.
- If not used immediately after dilution, refrigerate sol at 2-8°C (36-46°F).
- Equilibrate refrigerated sol to room temperature prior to administration; total time between dilution, storage in refrigerator, and end of administration must not exceed 24 hrs.

4mg/5mL Single-Use Vial
This concentrate should immediately be diluted in 100mL of sterile 0.9% NaCl or D5 inj. Do not store undiluted concentrate in a syringe, to avoid inadvertent inj.

Preparation of Reduced Doses from Single-Use Vial (4mg/5mL):
- Remove 4.4mL (3.5mg), 4.1mL (3.3mg), or 3.8mL (3mg) from vial and immediately dilute in 100mL of sterile 0.9% NaCl or D5 inj.
- If not used immediately after dilution, refrigerate sol at 2-8°C (36-46°F).
- Equilibrate refrigerated sol to room temperature prior to administration; total time between dilution, storage in refrigerator, and end of administration must not exceed 24 hrs.

STORAGE
25°C (77°F); excursions permitted to 15-30°C (59-86°F).

HOW SUPPLIED
Inj: 4mg/5mL, 4mg/100mL

CONTRAINDICATIONS
Hypersensitivity to zoledronic acid or any components of Zometa.

WARNINGS/PRECAUTIONS
Contains same active ingredient as Reclast; do not treat concomitantly w/ Reclast or other bisphosphonates. Adequately rehydrate patients w/ hypercalcemia of malignancy prior to administration and throughout treatment. Carefully monitor standard hypercalcemia-related metabolic parameters (eg, serum levels of Ca^{2+}, phosphate, and Mg^{2+}) as well as SrCr, following initiation of therapy; if hypocalcemia, hypophosphatemia, or hypomagnesemia occur, short-term supplemental therapy may be necessary. Caution in patients w/ hypercalcemia of malignancy w/ severe renal impairment. Not recommended in patients w/ bone metastases w/ severe renal impairment. Osteonecrosis of the jaw (ONJ) reported; risk may increase w/ duration of exposure to drug. Perform dental examination w/ preventive dentistry prior to treatment and if possible, avoid invasive dental procedures while on treatment. Severe and occasionally incapacitating bone, joint, and/or muscle pain reported; d/c if severe symptoms develop. Atypical subtrochanteric and diaphyseal femoral fractures reported; examine contralateral femur in patients who have sustained femoral shaft fracture. Any patient w/ a history of bisphosphonate exposure who presents w/ thigh/groin pain in the absence of trauma should be suspected of having an atypical fracture and should be evaluated; consider discontinuation in patients suspected to have an atypical femur fracture. Bronchoconstriction may occur in aspirin-sensitive patients. May cause fetal harm. Hypocalcemia and cardiac arrhythmias/neurologic adverse events secondary to cases of severe hypocalcemia reported; correct hypocalcemia before initiating treatment and adequately supplement w/ Ca^{2+} and vitamin D. Caution in elderly.

ADVERSE REACTIONS
Bone pain, N/V, insomnia, fatigue, pyrexia, anemia, constipation, dyspnea, diarrhea, weakness, myalgia, cough, arthralgia, edema (lower limb).

DRUG INTERACTIONS
Caution w/ aminoglycosides or calcitonin; may have an additive effect to lower serum Ca^{2+} level for prolonged periods. Caution w/ drugs known to cause hypocalcemia; severe hypocalcemia may develop. Caution w/ loop diuretics due to an increased risk of hypocalcemia; do not use in patients w/ hypercalcemia of malignancy until patient is adequately rehydrated. Caution w/ other potentially nephrotoxic drugs.

PREGNANCY AND LACTATION
Pregnancy: Category D. May cause fetal harm when administered to a pregnant woman.
Lactation: Not for use in nursing.

MECHANISM OF ACTION
Bisphosphonate; not established. Inhibits bone resorption by inhibiting osteoclastic activity and inducing osteoclast apoptosis. Also blocks osteoclastic resorption of mineralized bone and cartilage through its binding to bone.

PHARMACOKINETICS
Elimination: Urine (39%); $T_{1/2}$=146 hrs.

PATIENT CONSIDERATIONS
Assessment: Assess for hypocalcemia, risk factors for ONJ, hypersensitivity to drug, aspirin sensitivity, renal impairment, pregnancy/nursing status, and possible drug interactions. Assess hydration status and SrCr prior to each treatment. Perform dental exam w/ preventive dentistry. Measure serum Ca^{2+}.

Monitoring: Monitor renal function, standard hypercalcemia-related metabolic parameters (eg, serum Ca^{2+}, phosphate, Mg^{2+}), and hydration status. Monitor for ONJ, musculoskeletal pain, atypical femur fracture, bronchoconstriction, hypocalcemia, and other adverse reactions.

Counseling: Instruct to notify physician of kidney problems, if pregnant/planning to become pregnant, if breastfeeding, or if aspirin-sensitive. Inform of the importance of getting blood tests during the course of therapy. Advise to have dental exam prior to treatment and avoid invasive dental procedures during treatment. Inform of the importance of good dental hygiene, routine dental care, and regular dental check-ups. Advise to immediately notify physician about any oral symptoms (eg, loosening of a tooth, pain, swelling, or non-healing of sores or discharge) during treatment. Advise patients w/ multiple myeloma or bone metastasis of solid tumors to take an oral Ca^{2+} supplement of 500mg and a multiple vitamin containing 400 IU of vitamin D daily. Instruct to report any thigh, hip, or groin pain. Inform of the most common side effects that may develop.

ZORBTIVE — somatropin (rDNA origin)   Rx

Class: Human growth hormone (hGH)

ADULT DOSAGE	PEDIATRIC DOSAGE
Short Bowel Syndrome	Pediatric use may not have been established
In Patients Receiving Specialized Nutritional Support: 0.1mg/kg qd SQ for 4 weeks **Max:** 8mg/day	

DOSING CONSIDERATIONS
Concomitant Medications
Changes to concomitant medications should be avoided

Elderly
Start at a lower dose

Adverse Reactions
Treat moderate fluid retention and arthralgias symptomatically or reduce dose by 50%
D/C for up to 5 days for severe toxicities; upon resolution of symptoms, resume at 50% of original dose
Permanently d/c if severe toxicity recurs or does not disappear w/in 5 days

ADMINISTRATION
SQ route

Rotate inj site

Reconstitution
Each vial of 8.8mg is reconstituted in 1-2mL of bacteriostatic water for inj (0.9% benzyl alcohol)
Approx 10% mechanical loss can be associated w/ reconstitution and administration from multidose vials
Inject the diluent into the vial aiming the liquid against the glass vial wall to reconstitute
Swirl the vial w/ a gentle rotary motion until contents are dissolved completely
The sol should be clear immediately after reconstitution. Do not inject if the reconstituted product is cloudy immediately after reconstitution or after refrigeration
The reconstituted sol can be refrigerated for up to 14 days. Allow refrigerated sol to come to room temperature prior to administration
A standard insulin-type SQ syringe is recommended for administration

STORAGE
Before Reconstitution: 15-30°C (59-86°F). After Reconstitution with Bacteriostatic Water for Inj: 2-8°C (36-46°F) for up to 14 days. Avoid freezing.

HOW SUPPLIED
Inj: 8.8mg

CONTRAINDICATIONS
Acute critical illness due to complications following open heart or abdominal surgery, multiple accidental trauma, or acute respiratory failure; active neoplasia (either newly diagnosed or recurrent); benzyl alcohol sensitivity; known hypersensitivity to growth hormone.

WARNINGS/PRECAUTIONS
Benzyl alcohol associated with toxicity in newborns. If sensitivity occurs, may reconstitute with sterile water for inj; use immediately and discard any unused portion. Allergic reactions may occur. Associated with acute pancreatitis. Cases of new-onset impaired glucose intolerance, new-onset type 2 diabetes mellitus (DM), exacerbation of preexisting DM, diabetic ketoacidosis, and diabetic coma reported. Syndrome of intracranial HTN with papilledema, visual changes, headache, and N/V reported in small number of children with growth failure treated with growth hormone products; perform funduscopic evaluation at the initiation and periodically during therapy. Increased tissue turgor and musculoskeletal discomfort may occur during therapy but may resolve spontaneously with analgesic therapy, or after reducing the frequency of dosing. Carpal tunnel syndrome may occur; d/c if symptoms do not resolve after reducing the dose or frequency. Caution in elderly.

ADVERSE REACTIONS
Edema, melena, rectal hemorrhage, arthritis, fungal infection, inflammation at the inj site, paresthesia, phantom pain, bronchospasm, dyspnea, purpura, skin disorder, insomnia, hypomagnesemia, dysuria.

DRUG INTERACTIONS
May impact cortisol and cortisone metabolism. May unmask previously undiagnosed primary (and secondary) hypoadrenalism requiring glucocorticoid therapy. Use of glucocorticoid replacement therapy for previously diagnosed hypoadrenalism, especially cortisone acetate or prednisone, may require an increase in maint or stress doses. Dose adjustment of antidiabetics may be required.

PREGNANCY AND LACTATION
Category B, caution in nursing.

MECHANISM OF ACTION
Human growth hormone; anabolic and anticatabolic agent that exerts influence by interacting with specific receptors on a variety of cell types. On gut, actions may be direct or mediated via local or systemic production of insulin-like growth factor-1; also enhances transmucosal transport of water, electrolytes, and nutrients.

PHARMACOKINETICS
Absorption: Absolute bioavailability (70-90%). **Distribution:** (IV) V_d=12L. **Metabolism:** Liver, kidneys. **Elimination:** $T_{1/2}$=3.94 hrs (SQ), 0.58 hrs (IV).

PATIENT CONSIDERATIONS
Assessment: Assess for acute critical illness, active neoplasia, hypersensitivity to benzyl alcohol, pregnancy/nursing status, and possible drug interactions. Perform baseline funduscopic examination.

Monitoring: Monitor for hypersensitivity/allergic reactions, acute pancreatitis, impaired glucose intolerance, new-onset type 2 DM, exacerbation of preexisting DM, diabetic ketoacidosis, diabetic coma, carpal tunnel syndrome, increased tissue turgor, musculoskeletal discomfort, and other adverse reactions. Perform funduscopic examination periodically.

Counseling: Inform about the risks and benefits associated with the treatment. Instruct to notify physician if they experience any side effects or discomfort during treatment. Advise to properly dispose the needles and syringes using an appropriate container; advise not to reuse the needles and syringes. Instruct to rotate inj sites to avoid localized tissue atrophy.

ZORTRESS — everolimus   Rx

Class: Immunosuppressant

> Should only be prescribed by physicians experienced in immunosuppressive therapy and management of organ transplant patients. Immunosuppression may lead to increased susceptibility to infection and possible development of malignancies (eg, lymphoma, skin cancer). Increased risk of kidney arterial and venous thrombosis leading to graft loss was reported, mostly w/in the first 30 days post-transplantation. Increased nephrotoxicity may occur in combination w/ standard doses of cyclosporine; reduce dose of cyclosporine to reduce renal dysfunction, and monitor cyclosporine and everolimus whole blood trough concentrations. Increased mortality w/in the first 3 months post-transplantation in heart transplant patients on immunosuppressive regimens w/ or w/o induction therapy; not recommended in heart transplantation.

ADULT DOSAGE	PEDIATRIC DOSAGE
Renal Transplant	Pediatric use may not have been established
Prophylaxis of Organ Rejection in Kidney Transplant: **Initial:** 0.75mg bid, in combination w/ basiliximab induction and concurrently w/ reduced dose of cyclosporine; give as soon as possible after transplantation. Initiate oral prednisone once oral medication is tolerated. **Titrate:** May require dose adjustment based on blood concentrations achieved, tolerability, individual response, change in concomitant medications, and clinical situation; optimal dose adjustments should be based on trough levels obtained 4 or 5 days after a previous dosing change	

Recommended Therapeutic Range:
3-8ng/mL (based on LC/MS/MS assay method); if trough level is <3ng/mL, double total daily dose, or if trough level is >8ng/mL on 2 consecutive measures, decrease by 0.25mg bid

Refer to PI for further drug monitoring instructions and for cyclosporine therapeutic drug monitoring parameters

Hepatic Transplant
Prophylaxis of Allograft Rejection w/ a Liver Transplant:
Initial: 1mg bid, in combination w/ reduced dose of tacrolimus; start at least 30 days post-transplant
Titrate: May require dose adjustment based on blood concentrations achieved, tolerability, individual response, change in concomitant medications, and clinical situation; optimal dose adjustments should be based on trough levels obtained 4 or 5 days after a previous dosing change

Recommended Therapeutic Range: 3-8ng/mL (based on LC/MS/MS assay method); if trough level is <3ng/mL, double total daily dose, or if trough level is >8ng/mL on 2 consecutive measures, decrease by 0.25mg bid

Refer to PI for further drug monitoring instructions and for tacrolimus therapeutic drug monitoring parameters

----

DOSING CONSIDERATIONS
Hepatic Impairment
Mild (Child-Pugh Class A): Reduce initial daily dose by 1/3 of normal daily dose
Moderate or Severe (Child-Pugh Class B or C): Reduce initial daily dose to 1/2 of the normal daily dose

ADMINISTRATION
Oral route

Do not crush; swallow whole w/ water.
Administer consistently approx 12 hrs apart w/ or w/o food and at the same time as cyclosporine or tacrolimus.

STORAGE
25°C (77°F); excursions permitted to 15-30°C (59-86°F). Protect from light and moisture.

HOW SUPPLIED
Tab: 0.25mg, 0.5mg, 0.75mg

CONTRAINDICATIONS
Known hypersensitivity to everolimus, sirolimus, or to components of the drug product.

WARNINGS/PRECAUTIONS
Limit exposure to sunlight and UV light. Prophylaxis for *Pneumocystis jiroveci (carinii)* pneumonia and CMV recommended. Increased risk of hepatic artery thrombosis (HAT), which may lead to graft loss or death; do not give earlier than 30 days after liver transplant. Consider switching to other immunosuppressive therapies if renal function does not improve after dose adjustments or if dysfunction is thought to be drug related. Angioedema, increased risk of delayed wound healing, increased occurrence of wound-related complications, and generalized fluid accumulation reported. Interstitial lung disease (ILD), implying lung intraparenchymal inflammation (pneumonitis) and/or fibrosis of noninfectious etiology, some w/ pulmonary HTN as a secondary event reported; resolution may occur upon drug interruption w/ or w/o glucocorticoid therapy. Consider diagnosis of ILD for symptoms of infectious pneumonia that do not respond to antibiotic therapy and in whom non-drug causes have been ruled out. Increased risk of hyperlipidemia and proteinuria w/ higher whole blood trough concentrations; use of anti-lipid therapy may not normalize lipid levels. Reevaluate the risk/benefit of continuing therapy in patients w/ severe refractory hyperlipidemia. Increased risk of polyoma virus infections, including polyoma virus-associated nephropathy (PVAN) and progressive multiple leukoencephalopathy (PML), may occur; consider reductions in immunosuppression if evidence of PVAN or PML develops. Concomitant use w/ cyclosporine may increase risk of thrombotic microangiopathy/TTP/hemolytic uremic syndrome. May increase risk of new-onset diabetes mellitus (DM) after transplant. Azoospermia or oligospermia may be observed. Avoid w/ rare hereditary problems of galactose intolerance (Lapp lactase deficiency, glucose-galactose malabsorption); diarrhea and malabsorption may occur.

ADVERSE REACTIONS
Kidney Transplantation: Peripheral edema, constipation, HTN, nausea, anemia, urinary tract infection, hyperlipidemia.
Liver Transplantation: Diarrhea, headache, peripheral edema, HTN, nausea, pyrexia, abdominal pain, leukopenia.

DRUG INTERACTIONS
See Boxed Warning. Caution w/ drugs known to impair renal function. May increase risk of angioedema w/ drugs known to cause angioedema (eg, ACE inhibitors). Monitor for development of rhabdomyolysis w/ HMG-CoA reductase inhibitors and/or fibrates; use of simvastatin and lovastatin are strongly discouraged in patients receiving everolimus w/ cyclosporine. Coadministration w/ strong CYP3A4 inhibitors (eg, ketoconazole, clarithromycin, ritonavir) and strong CYP3A4 inducers (eg, rifampin, rifabutin) is not recommended w/o close monitoring of everolimus whole blood trough concentrations. Avoid w/ live vaccines, grapefruit, and grapefruit juice. Inhibitors of P-gp (eg, digoxin, cyclosporine), moderate inhibitors of CYP3A4 and P-gp (eg, fluconazole, macrolide antibiotics, nicardipine), and verapamil may increase levels. If coadministered w/ erythromycin or verapamil, monitor everolimus blood concentrations and if necessary, make a dose adjustment. Caution w/ CYP3A4 and CYP2D6 substrates w/ a narrow therapeutic index. Increased levels w/ cyclosporine; dose adjustment may be needed if cyclosporine dose is altered. CYP3A4 inducers (eg, St. John's wort, carbamazepine, phenobarbital) may decrease levels. Combination immunosuppressant therapy should be used w/ caution. May increase octreotide C_{min} levels.

PREGNANCY AND LACTATION
Pregnancy: Category C.
Lactation: Not for use in nursing.

MECHANISM OF ACTION
Macrolide immunosuppressant; inhibits antigenic and interleukin (IL-2 and IL-15) stimulated activation and proliferation of T and B lymphocytes. Binds to a cytoplasmic protein, the FK506 binding protein-12 (FKBP-12), to form an immunosuppressive complex (everolimus: FKBP-12) that binds to and inhibits the mammalian target of rapamycin, a key regulatory kinase in cells.

PHARMACOKINETICS
Absorption: (0.75mg bid) AUC=75ng•hr/mL, C_{max}=11.1ng/mL, T_{max}=1-2 hrs.
Distribution: Plasma protein binding (74%); (0.75mg bid) V_d=110L. **Metabolism:** Via CYP3A4 and P-gp. **Elimination:** Feces (80%), urine (5%). (0.75mg bid) $T_{1/2}$=30 hrs.

PATIENT CONSIDERATIONS
Assessment: Assess for hereditary problems of galactose intolerance, hepatic impairment, hypersensitivity to the drug or to sirolimus, pregnancy/nursing status, and possible drug interactions. Obtain baseline lipid and glucose levels.

Monitoring: Monitor for infections, angioedema, thrombosis, wound-related complications, fluid accumulation, lymphomas and other malignancies, hyperlipidemia, hepatic impairment, proteinuria, PVAN, HAT, ILD, pneumonitis, and other adverse reactions. Monitor everolimus and cyclosporine or tacrolimus whole blood trough concentrations, lipid profile, blood glucose concentrations, renal function, and hematologic parameters.

Counseling: Counsel to avoid grapefruit and grapefruit juice. Inform of the risk of developing lymphomas and other malignancies, particularly of the skin; instruct to limit exposure to sunlight and UV light. Advise that therapy has been associated w/ an increased risk of kidney arterial and venous thrombosis, resulting in graft loss, usually occurring w/in the first 30 days post-transplantation. Inform of the risks of impaired kidney function w/ concomitant cyclosporine as well as the need for routine blood concentration monitoring for both drugs; advise of the importance of SrCr monitoring. Inform of risk of hyperlipidemia and the importance of lipid profile monitoring. Advise women to avoid pregnancy throughout treatment and for 8 weeks after discontinuation. Instruct to notify physician of all medications and herbal/dietary supplements being taken. Inform that therapy has been associated w/ impaired or delayed wound healing, and fluid accumulation. Inform of increased risk of proteinuria, DM, infections, noninfectious pneumonitis, and angioedema; advise to contact physician if symptoms develop. Instruct to avoid receiving live vaccines.

ZYDELIG — idelalisib   Rx

Class: Kinase inhibitor

> **Fatal and/or serious hepatotoxicity reported; monitor hepatic function prior to and during treatment; interrupt and then reduce or d/c as recommended. Fatal and/or serious and severe diarrhea or colitis reported; monitor for the development of severe diarrhea or colitis; interrupt and then reduce or d/c as recommended. Fatal and serious pneumonitis may occur; monitor for pulmonary symptoms and bilateral interstitial infiltrates; interrupt or d/c as recommended. Fatal and serious intestinal perforation may occur; d/c therapy for intestinal perforation.**

ADULT DOSAGE
Relapsed Small Lymphocytic Lymphoma

In Patients Who Have Received at Least 2 Prior Systemic Therapies:
Max Initial: 150mg bid

Relapsed Chronic Lymphocytic Leukemia

Combination w/ Rituximab:
Max Initial: 150mg bid

Relapsed Follicular B-cell non-Hodgkin Lymphoma

In Patients Who Have Received at Least 2 Prior Systemic Therapies:
Max Initial: 150mg bid

PEDIATRIC DOSAGE
Pediatric use may not have been established

DOSING CONSIDERATIONS
Adverse Reactions
Pneumonitis:
D/C in patients w/ any severity of symptomatic pneumonitis
ALT/AST:
<3-5X ULN: Maintain dose; monitor at least weekly until ≤1X ULN

<5-20X ULN: Withhold treatment; monitor at least weekly until ≤1X ULN, then resume at 100mg bid
<20X ULN: D/C permanently
Bilirubin:
<1.5-3X ULN: Maintain dose; monitor at least weekly until ≤1X ULN
<3-10X ULN: Withhold treatment; monitor at least weekly until ≤1X ULN, then resume at 100mg bid
<10X ULN: D/C permanently
Diarrhea:
Moderate (Increase of 4-6 stools/day): Maintain dose; monitor at least weekly until resolved
Severe (Increase of ≥7 stools/day)/Hospitalization: Withhold treatment; monitor at least weekly until resolved, then resume at 100mg bid
Life-Threatening: D/C permanently

Neutropenia:
ANC 1-<1.5 Gi/L: Maintain dose
ANC 0.5-<1 Gi/L: Maintain dose; monitor at least weekly
ANC <0.5 Gi/L: Interrupt treatment; monitor at least weekly until ANC >0.5 Gi/L, then resume at 100mg bid
Thrombocytopenia:
Platelets 50-<75 Gi/L: Maintain dose
Platelets 25-<50 Gi/L: Maintain dose; monitor at least weekly
Platelets >25 Gi/L: Interrupt treatment; monitor at least weekly, then resume at 100mg bid when platelets ≥25 Gi/L

ADMINISTRATION
Oral route
Swallow tab whole.
Take w/ or w/o food.

STORAGE
20-30°C (68-86°F); excursions permitted to 15-30°C (59-86°F).

HOW SUPPLIED
Tab: 100mg, 150mg

CONTRAINDICATIONS
History of serious allergic reactions, including anaphylaxis and toxic epidermal necrolysis (TEN).

WARNINGS/PRECAUTIONS
TEN reported with rituximab and bendamustine; other severe or life-threatening (Grade ≥3) cutaneous reactions (eg, exfoliative dermatitis, erythematous rash, maculopapular rash, skin disorder) reported in idelalisib-treated patients; monitor for development of severe cutaneous reactions and d/c therapy. Serious allergic reactions (eg, anaphylaxis) reported; d/c permanently and institute appropriate therapy if serious allergic reactions develop. Treatment-emergent Grade 3 or 4 neutropenia reported; monitor blood counts at least every 2 weeks for the first 3 months, and at least weekly while neutrophil counts are <1 Gi/L. May cause fetal harm. If contraceptive methods are being considered, females of reproductive potential should use effective contraception during treatment, and for at least 1 month after the last dose. Monitor for signs of idelalisib toxicity in patients with baseline hepatic impairment.

ADVERSE REACTIONS
Hepatotoxicity, colitis, diarrhea, pneumonitis, intestinal perforation, pyrexia, sepsis, febrile neutropenia, N/V, GERD, stomatitis, headache, chills, pain, rash.

DRUG INTERACTIONS
Avoid with drugs that may cause liver toxicity and drugs that cause diarrhea. Decreased exposure with strong CYP3A inducers (eg, rifampin, phenytoin, St. John's wort, carbamazepine); avoid coadministration. May increase exposure of a sensitive CYP3A substrate; avoid with CYP3A substrates. Increased exposure with strong CYP3A inhibitors; monitor for signs of idelalisib toxicity.

PREGNANCY AND LACTATION
Pregnancy: Category D.
Lactation: Not for use in nursing.

MECHANISM OF ACTION
Phosphatidylinositol 3-kinase inhibitor; induces apoptosis and inhibits proliferation in cell lines derived from malignant B-cells and in primary tumor cells. Inhibits several cell signaling pathways, including B-cell receptor signaling and the CXCR4 and CXCR5 signaling, which are involved in trafficking and homing of B-cells to the lymph nodes and bone marrow. Treatment of lymphoma cells resulted in inhibition of chemotaxis and adhesion, and reduced cell viability.

PHARMACOKINETICS
Absorption: T_{max}=1.5 hrs (fasted, median). **Distribution:** V_d=23L; plasma protein binding (>84%). **Metabolism:** Via aldehyde oxidase and CYP3A, GS-563117 (major metabolite); UGT1A4 (minor metabolism). **Elimination:** (150mg single dose) Urine (14%, 49% [GS-563117]), feces (78%, 44% [GS-563117]); $T_{1/2}$=8.2 hrs.

PATIENT CONSIDERATIONS
Assessment: Assess for history of serious allergic reactions, pregnancy/nursing status, and possible drug interactions. Assess hepatic function.
Monitoring: Monitor for diarrhea, colitis, pulmonary symptoms and bilateral interstitial infiltrates, intestinal perforation, neutropenia, thrombocytopenia, new/worsening abdominal pain, chills, fever, N/V, severe cutaneous reactions, serious allergic reactions, and other adverse reactions. Monitor ALT and AST every 2 weeks for the first 3 months of treatment, every 4 weeks for the next 3 months, then every 1-3 months thereafter. Monitor weekly for liver toxicity if the ALT or AST rises above 3X ULN until resolved. Monitor blood counts at least every 2 weeks for the first 3 months of therapy, and at least weekly in patients while neutrophil counts are <1.0 Gi/L. Monitor for signs of idelalisib toxicity in patients with baseline hepatic impairment.
Counseling: Advise that significant elevations in liver enzymes may occur, and that serial testing of serum liver tests (ALT, AST, bilirubin) are recommended while taking the drug. Instruct to report liver dysfunction symptoms to physician. Advise that severe diarrhea or colitis may occur and to notify physician immediately if bowel movements increase by ≥6/day. Advise of the possibility of pneumonitis, intestinal perforation, severe cutaneous reactions, and anaphylaxis; instruct to contact physician if any signs/symptoms of these conditions develop. Advise of the need for periodic monitoring of blood counts; instruct to notify physician if fever or any signs of infection develop. Advise women of the potential hazard to fetus and to avoid pregnancy during therapy; instruct to use adequate contraception during therapy and for at least 1 month after completing therapy. Advise not to breastfeed during treatment. Instruct to take exactly as prescribed and not to change dose or stop therapy unless told to do so by physician. Advise that if a dose is missed by <6 hrs, to take missed dose right away and take next dose as usual. If a dose is missed by >6 hrs, advise to wait and take next dose at the usual time.

ZYKADIA — ceritinib   Rx

Class: Kinase inhibitor

ADULT DOSAGE	**PEDIATRIC DOSAGE**
Metastatic Non-Small Cell Lung Cancer	Pediatric use may not have been established
Treatment of patients w/ anaplastic lymphoma kinase-positive metastatic non-small cell lung cancer who have progressed on or are intolerant to crizotinib	
750mg qd until disease progression or unacceptable toxicity	
Missed Dose	
If a dose is missed, make up that dose unless the next dose is due w/in 12 hrs	

DOSING CONSIDERATIONS
Concomitant Medications
Strong CYP3A Inhibitors:
Avoid concurrent use; if unavoidable, reduce ceritinib dose by approx 1/3, rounded to the nearest 150mg dose strength.
After discontinuation of a strong CYP3A inhibitor, resume ceritinib dose that was taken prior to initiating the strong CYP3A4 inhibitor.

Adverse Reactions
Unable to Tolerate 300mg/day: D/C therapy

ALT or AST Elevation:
<5X ULN w/ Total Bilirubin ≤2X ULN: Withhold therapy until recovery to baseline or ≤3X ULN, then resume w/ a 150mg dose reduction
<3X ULN w/ Total Bilirubin >2X ULN (in the Absence of Cholestasis or Hemolysis): Permanently d/c therapy

Treatment-Related Interstitial Lung Disease (ILD)/Pneumonitis:
Any Grade: Permanently d/c therapy

QTc Interval:
>500 msec on ≥2 Separate ECGs: Withhold therapy until QTc interval is <481 msec or recovery to baseline if baseline QTc is ≥481 msec, then resume w/ a 150mg dose reduction
Prolongation w/ Torsades de Pointes or Polymorphic Ventricular Tachycardia or Signs/Symptoms of Serious Arrhythmia: Permanently d/c therapy

Severe or Intolerable N/V or Diarrhea (Despite Optimal Antiemetic/ Antidiarrheal Therapy):
Withhold therapy until improved, then resume w/ a 150mg dose reduction

Persistent Hyperglycemia >250mg/dL (Despite Optimal Antihyperglycemic Therapy):
1. Withhold therapy until hyperglycemia is adequately controlled, then resume w/ a 150mg dose reduction
2. D/C therapy if adequate hyperglycemic control cannot be achieved w/ optimal medical management

Bradycardia:
Symptomatic, Not Life Threatening:
1. Withhold therapy until recovery to asymptomatic bradycardia or to a HR of ≥60 bpm
2. Evaluate concomitant medications known to cause bradycardia and adjust ceritinib dose
Clinically Significant, Requiring Intervention or Life Threatening in Patients Taking a Concomitant Medication Also Known to Cause Bradycardia or Hypotension:
1. Withhold therapy until recovery to asymptomatic bradycardia or to a HR of ≥60 bpm
2. If concomitant medication can be adjusted or discontinued, resume ceritinib w/ a 150mg dose reduction, w/ frequent monitoring
Life Threatening in Patients Not Taking a Concomitant Medication Also Known to Cause Bradycardia or Hypotension:
Permanently d/c therapy

Lipase/Amylase Elevation:
<2X ULN: Withhold and monitor serum lipase and amylase; resume w/ a 150mg dose reduction after recovery to <1.5X ULN

ADMINISTRATION
Oral route
Take on an empty stomach (do not administer w/in 2 hrs of a meal).
If vomiting occurs during treatment, do not administer an additional dose and continue w/ the next scheduled dose.

STORAGE
25°C (77°F); excursions permitted between 15-30°C (59-86°F).

HOW SUPPLIED
Cap: 150mg

WARNINGS/PRECAUTIONS
See Dosing Considerations. Diarrhea, N/V, and abdominal pain reported; monitor and manage appropriately. Drug-induced hepatotoxicity reported; monitor LFTs including ALT, AST, and total bilirubin once a month and as clinically indicated, w/ more frequent testing if transaminase elevations occur. Severe, life-threatening, or fatal ILD/pneumonitis may occur; monitor for pulmonary symptoms and exclude other potential causes. QTc interval prolongation may occur; avoid use w/ congenital long QT syndrome. Conduct periodic monitoring w/ ECGs and electrolytes in patients w/ CHF, bradyarrhythmias, and electrolyte abnormalities. Hyperglycemia may occur; initiate or optimize anti-hyperglycemic medications as indicated. Bradycardia may occur. Pancreatitis reported. May cause fetal harm.

ADVERSE REACTIONS
Increased ALT/AST, N/V, diarrhea, abdominal pain, constipation, fatigue, decreased appetite.

DRUG INTERACTIONS
See Dosing Considerations. Caution w/ medications known to prolong QTc interval. Avoid w/ other agents known to cause bradycardia (eg, β-blockers, non-dihydropyridine calcium channel blockers, clonidine). Increased systemic exposure w/ ketoconazole. Avoid w/ strong CYP3A inhibitors. Decreased systemic exposure w/ rifampin. Avoid w/ strong CYP3A inducers (eg, carbamazepine, phenytoin, rifampin). Avoid w/ grapefruit and grapefruit juice. Avoid concurrent use of CYP3A substrates (eg, alfentanil, cyclosporine, tacrolimus) and CYP2C9 substrates (eg, phenytoin, warfarin) w/ narrow therapeutic indices; consider dose reduction of substrates if concomitant use is unavoidable.

PREGNANCY AND LACTATION
Pregnancy: Category D.
Lactation: Not for use in nursing.
Reproductive Potential: Females of reproductive potential should use effective contraception during treatment and for at least 2 weeks following completion of therapy.

MECHANISM OF ACTION
Tyrosine kinase inhibitor; inhibits anaplastic lymphoma kinase, insulin-like growth factor 1 receptor, insulin receptor, and ROS1.

PHARMACOKINETICS
Absorption: T_{max}=4-6 hrs. **Distribution:** V_d=4230L (single 750mg dose); plasma protein binding (97%). **Metabolism:** Liver via CYP3A. **Elimination:** (single 750mg dose) Feces (92.3%, 68% unchanged), urine (1.3%); $T_{1/2}$=41 hrs.

PATIENT CONSIDERATIONS
Assessment: Assess for congenital long QT syndrome, CHF, bradyarrhythmias, electrolyte abnormalities, pregnancy/nursing status, and possible drug interactions. Obtain baseline LFTs, fasting serum glucose, ECG, and lipase and amylase levels.

Monitoring: Monitor for signs/symptoms of GI toxicity, ILD, pneumonitis, QTc interval prolongation, and other adverse reactions. Monitor LFTs once a month and as clinically indicated. Conduct periodic monitoring of ECGs and electrolytes in patients w/ CHF, bradyarrhythmias, or electrolyte abnormalities, or who are taking medications known to prolong the QTc interval. Monitor lipase, amylase, and glucose levels, HR, and BP regularly.

Counseling: Advise to take ud. Inform that diarrhea, N/V, and abdominal pain are the most commonly reported adverse reactions; advise to contact physician for severe or persistent GI symptoms and inform of supportive care options (eg, antiemetics, antidiarrheal medications). Instruct to contact physician immediately for signs/symptoms of hepatotoxicity and hyperglycemia. Inform of the risks of severe or fatal ILD/pneumonitis; advise to immediately report new or worsening respiratory symptoms. Inform of the risks of QTc interval prolongation and bradycardia; advise to contact physician immediately to report new signs/symptoms or changes in/new use of heart/BP medications. Inform of the signs/symptoms of pancreatitis. Advise to inform physician if pregnant. Inform females of reproductive potential of the risk to fetus; advise to use effective contraception during treatment and for at least 2 weeks following completion of therapy. Advise not to breastfeed and not to consume grapefruit and grapefruit juice during treatment.

ZYTIGA — abiraterone acetate   Rx
Class: Antiandrogen

ADULT DOSAGE	PEDIATRIC DOSAGE
Metastatic Castration-Resistant Prostate Cancer 1000mg qd w/ prednisone 5mg PO bid	Pediatric use may not have been established

DOSING CONSIDERATIONS
Concomitant Medications
Strong CYP3A4 Inducers (eg, Phenytoin, Carbamazepine, Rifampin):
Avoid concomitant strong CYP3A4 inducers during treatment
If a strong CYP3A4 inducer must be coadministered, increase the abiraterone dosing frequency to bid only during the coadministration period (eg, from 1000mg qd to 1000mg bid); reduce dose back to the previous dose/frequency if inducer is discontinued

Hepatic Impairment
Moderate (Child-Pugh Class B): Reduce dose to 250mg qd
Severe (Child-Pugh Class C): Not recommended

Adverse Reactions
Elevations in ALT and/or AST >5X ULN or Total Bilirubin >3X ULN w/ Baseline Moderate Hepatic Impairment:
D/C use and do not retreat

Development of Hepatotoxicity During Treatment (ALT and/or AST >5X ULN or Total Bilirubin >3X ULN):
Interrupt treatment; may restart at a reduced dose of 750mg qd following return of LFTs to baseline or to AST and ALT ≤2.5X ULN and total bilirubin ≤1.5X ULN
If hepatotoxicity recurs at 750mg qd, may restart retreatment at 500mg qd, following return of LFTs to baseline or to AST and ALT ≤2.5X ULN and total bilirubin ≤1.5X ULN
If hepatotoxicity recurs at 500mg qd, d/c treatment
Permanently d/c for patients who develop a concurrent elevation of ALT >3X ULN and total bilirubin >2X ULN in the absence of biliary obstruction or other causes responsible for the concurrent elevation

ADMINISTRATION
Oral route

Swallow tab whole w/ water; do not crush or chew.
Take on an empty stomach; no food should be consumed for at least 2 hrs before and 1 hr after the dose is taken.
Women who are pregnant or may be pregnant should not handle drug w/o protection (eg, gloves).

STORAGE
20-25°C (68-77°F); excursions permitted from 15-30°C (59-86°F).

HOW SUPPLIED
Tab: 250mg

CONTRAINDICATIONS
Women who are or may become pregnant.

WARNINGS/PRECAUTIONS
See Dosing Considerations. May cause HTN, hypokalemia, and fluid retention; caution w/ history of cardiovascular disease (CVD) or w/ underlying medical conditions that might be compromised by increases in BP, hypokalemia, or fluid retention. Adrenocortical insufficiency reported in patients receiving abiraterone in combination w/ prednisone, following interruption of daily steroids and/or w/ concurrent infection or stress; use caution and monitor for signs/symptoms, particularly if patients are withdrawn from prednisone, have prednisone dose reductions, or experience unusual stress. Signs/symptoms of adrenocortical insufficiency may be masked by adverse reactions associated w/ mineralocorticoid excess. Increased dosage of corticosteroids may be indicated before, during, and after stressful situations. ALT/AST increases, severe hepatic toxicity, including fulminant hepatitis, acute liver failure and deaths reported; promptly measure serum total bilirubin, AST, and ALT if signs/symptoms suggestive of hepatotoxicity develop. Safety of retreatment of patients who develop AST or ALT ≥20X ULN and/or bilirubin ≥10X ULN is unknown.

ADVERSE REACTIONS
Fatigue, joint swelling/discomfort, edema, hot flush, diarrhea, vomiting, cough, HTN, dyspnea, UTI, contusion, hypertriglyceridemia, elevated AST/ALT.

DRUG INTERACTIONS
See Dosing Considerations. Rifampin (strong CYP3A4 inducer) reported to decrease exposure. Increased levels of dextromethorphan (CYP2D6 substrate) reported. Avoid coadministration w/ CYP2D6 substrates w/ narrow therapeutic index (eg, thioridazine); if alternative treatments cannot be used, exercise caution and consider dose reduction of the concomitant CYP2D6 substrate. Increased exposure of pioglitazone (CYP2C8 substrate) reported; monitor closely for signs of toxicity related to a CYP2C8 substrate w/ narrow therapeutic index if used concomitantly.

PREGNANCY AND LACTATION
Pregnancy: Category X, may cause fetal harm.
Lactation: Not for use in nursing.

MECHANISM OF ACTION
Androgen biosynthesis inhibitor; inhibits 17 α-hydroxylase/C17,20-lyase (CYP17), an enzyme expressed in testicular, adrenal, and prostatic tumor tissues and required for androgen biosynthesis.

PHARMACOKINETICS
Absorption: T_{max}=2 hrs (median); C_{max}=226ng/mL; AUC=993ng•hr/mL. **Distribution:** V_d=19,669L; plasma protein binding (>99%). **Metabolism:** Hydrolysis via esterase to abiraterone (active metabolite). **Elimination:** Feces (approx 88%, approx 55% unchanged), urine (approx 5%); $T_{1/2}$=12 hrs.

PATIENT CONSIDERATIONS
Assessment: Assess for hepatic impairment, history of CVD and underlying medical conditions that might be compromised by increases in BP, hypokalemia, or fluid retention, and for possible drug interactions. Obtain baseline AST, ALT, and bilirubin levels. Control HTN and correct hypokalemia before treatment.

Monitoring: Monitor for HTN, hypokalemia, and fluid retention at least monthly, signs/symptoms of adrenocortical insufficiency, and other adverse reactions. Monitor ALT, AST, and bilirubin levels every 2 weeks for the first 3 months (or weekly for the 1st month, then every 2 weeks for the following 2 months in patients w/ baseline moderate hepatic impairment), and monthly thereafter. For patients who resume treatment after development of hepatotoxicity, monitor serum transaminases and bilirubin at a minimum of every 2 weeks for 3 months, and monthly thereafter.

Counseling: Inform that drug is used together w/ prednisone and instruct to take ud and not to interrupt or stop either of these medications w/o consulting a physician. Inform those receiving gonadotropin-releasing hormone agonists to maintain such treatment during therapy. Instruct that if a daily dose is missed, to take the normal dose the following day, but if >1 daily dose is skipped, advise to inform physician. Counsel about the common side effects (eg, peripheral edema, hypokalemia, HTN, elevated LFTs, UTI). Inform that liver function will be monitored using blood tests. Advise that drug may harm a developing fetus and that women who are pregnant or may be pregnant should not handle the drug w/o protection (eg, gloves). Instruct to use a condom if having sex w/ a pregnant woman, and to use a condom and another effective method of birth control if having sex w/ a woman of childbearing potential; advise that these measures are required during and for 1 week after treatment.

DRUGS THAT SHOULD NOT BE CRUSHED

Listed below are various slow-release as well as enteric-coated products that should not be crushed or chewed. Slow-release (sr) represents products that are controlled-release, extended-release, long-acting, or timed-release. Enteric-coated (ec) represents products that are delayed-release.

In general, capsules containing slow-release or enteric-coated particles may be opened and their contents administered on a spoonful of soft food. Instruct patients not to chew particles, though. (Patients should, in fact, be discouraged from chewing any medication unless it is specifically formulated for that purpose.)

This list should not be considered all-inclusive. Generic and alternate brands of some products may exist. Tablets intended for sublingual or buccal administration (not included in this list) should be administered only as intended, in an intact form.

DRUG	MANUFACTURER	FORM	DRUG	MANUFACTURER	FORM
Aciphex	Eisai	ec	Cardizem LA	Valeant	sr
Actoplus Met XR	Takeda	sr	Cardura XL	Roerig	sr
Adalat CC	Bayer Healthcare	sr	Cartia XT	Actavis	sr
Adderall XR	Shire U.S.	sr	Cipro XR	Bayer Healthcare	sr
Adenovirus Type 4 and Type 7 Vaccine	Teva Women's Health, Inc.	ec	Clarinex-D 12 Hour	Merck Sharp & Dohme	sr
			Clarinex-D 24 Hour	Merck Sharp & Dohme	sr
Advicor	AbbVie Inc.	sr	Claritin-D 12 Hour	MSD Consumer Care	sr
Afeditab CR	Actavis Pharma	sr	Claritin-D 24 Hour	MSD Consumer Care	sr
Aggrenox	Boehringer Ingelheim	sr	Cometriq	Exelixis, Inc.	sr
Aleve-D Cold & Sinus	Bayer Healthcare	sr	Concerta	Ortho-McNeil-Janssen	sr
Aleve-D Sinus & Headache	Bayer Healthcare	sr	Coreg CR	GlaxoSmithKline	sr
			Covera-HS	Pfizer	sr
Allegra-D 12 Hour	sanofi-aventis	sr	Creon	AbbVie Inc.	ec
Allegra-D 24 Hour	sanofi-aventis	sr	Cymbalta	Eli Lilly	ec
Alophen	Numark	ec	Dairycare	Plainview	ec
Altoprev	Shionogi Inc.	sr	Delzicol	Warner Chilcott	ec
Ambien CR	sanofi-aventis	sr	Depakote	AbbVie Inc.	ec
Ampyra ER	Acorda Therapeutics	sr	Depakote ER	AbbVie Inc.	sr
Amrix	Cephalon	sr	Depakote Sprinkles	AbbVie Inc.	ec
Aplenzin	Valeant	sr	Detrol LA	Pharmacia and Upjohn	sr
Apriso	Salix	sr	Dexedrine Spansules	Amedra	sr
Arthrotec	Pfizer	ec	Dexilant	Takeda	ec
Asacol	Warner Chilcott	ec	Diamox Sequels	Teva Women's Health	sr
Asacol HD	Warner Chilcott	ec	Diclegis	Duchesnay USA	ec
Astagraf XL	Astellas	sr	Dilacor XR	Watson	sr
Augmentin XR	Dr. Reddy's	sr	Dilantin	Pfizer	sr
Avinza	Pfizer	sr	Dilatrate-SR	Actient	sr
Azulfidine EN-tabs	Pfizer	ec	Diltia XT	Watson	sr
Bayer Aspirin Regimen	Bayer Healthcare	ec	Ditropan XL	Ortho-McNeil Janssen	sr
Biaxin XL	AbbVie Inc.	sr	Donnatal Extentabs	PBM	sr
Budeprion SR	Teva	sr	Doryx	Warner Chilcott	ec
Cabometyx	Exelixis, Inc.	sr	Duavee	Wyeth	ec
Calan SR	Pfizer	sr	Dulcolax	Boehringer Ingelheim	ec
Campral	Forest	ec	EC Naprosyn	Genentech	ec
Carbatrol	Shire U.S.	sr	Ecotrin 81 mg	GlaxoSmithKline	ec
Cardene SR	EKR Therapeutics	sr	Ecotrin 325 mg	GlaxoSmithKline	ec
Cardizem CD	Valeant	sr	Effexor-XR	Wyeth	sr

(Continued)

DRUG	MANUFACTURER	FORM	DRUG	MANUFACTURER	FORM
Elepsia XR	Sun Pharma	sr	Lialda	Shire	ec
Embeda	Pfizer	sr	Liptruzet	Merck	ec
Enablex	Warner Chilcott	sr	Lithobid	Ani	sr
Entocort EC	AstraZeneca	ec	Luvox CR	Jazz Pharmaceuticals	sr
Envarsus XR	Veloxis	sr	Mag64	Rising	ec
Equetro	Validus	sr	MagDelay	Major	ec
ERYC	Warner Chilcott	ec	Mag-Tab SR	Niche	sr
Ery-Tab	Arbor	ec	Maxifed	MCR American	sr
Exalgo	Mallinckrodt	sr	Maxifed DM	MCR American	sr
Ferro-Sequels	Inverness Medical	sr	Maxifed DMX	MCR American	sr
Fetzima	Forest	sr	Maxifed-G	MCR American	sr
Flagyl ER	Pfizer	sr	Menopause Relief Trio	Mason Vitamins	sr
Fleet Bisacodyl	Fleet, C.B.	ec	Mestinon Timespan	Valeant	sr
Focalin XR	Novartis	sr	Metadate CD	Unither	sr
Folitab 500	Rising	sr	Metadate ER	Upstate Pharma	sr
Forfivo XL	Edgemont	sr	Methylin	Shionogi	sr
Fortamet	Shionogi Pharma	sr	Micro-K	Ther-Rx	sr
Fulyzaq	Salix	ec	Micro-K 10	Ther-Rx	sr
Fumatinic	Laser	sr	Mild-C	Carlson, J.R.	sr
Galzin	Teva	ec	Mirapex ER	Boehringer Ingelheim	sr
Gilphex TR	Gil	sr	Moxatag	Pragma	sr
Glucophage XR	Bristol-Myers-Squibb	sr	MS Contin	Purdue	sr
Glucotrol XL	Roerig	sr	Mucinex	Reckitt Benckiser	sr
Glumetza	Santarus	sr	Mucinex D	Reckitt Benckiser	sr
Hemax	Pronova	sr	Mucinex DM	Reckitt Benckiser	sr
Horizant	XenoPort	sr	Myfortic	Novartis	ec
Imbruvica	Pharmacyclics	ec	Myrbetriq	Astellas	sr
Inderal LA	Akrimax	sr	Namenda XR	Forest	sr
Innopran XL	Akrimax	sr	Namzaric	Forest	sr
Intuniv	Shire	sr	Naprelan	Almatica	sr
Invega	Ortho-McNeil-Janssen	sr	Nexium	AstraZeneca	ec
Janumet XR	Merck Sharp & Dohme	sr	Nexium 24H	Pfizer Consumer	ec
Jentadueto XR	Boehringer Ingelheim	sr	Niaspan	AbbVie Inc.	sr
Kadian	Actavis	sr	Nifediac CC	Teva	sr
Kapvay ER	Concordia	sr	Nifedical XL	Teva	sr
Keppra XR	UCB	sr	Nitro-Time	Time-Cap	sr
Khedezla ER	Pernix Therapeutics	sr	Norel AD	U.S. Pharmaceutical	sr
Klor-Con 8	Upsher-Smith	sr	Norpace CR	Pfizer	sr
Klor-Con 10	Upsher-Smith	sr	Nucynta ER	Janssen	sr
Klor-Con M10*	Upsher-Smith	sr	Oleptro	Angelini Pharma	sr
Klor-Con M15*	Upsher-Smith	sr	Olysio	Janssen	ec
Klor-Con M20*	Upsher-Smith	sr	Opana ER	Endo	sr
Kombiglyze XR	BMS/AstraZeneca	sr	Opsumit	Actelion	ec
K-Tab	AbbVie Inc.	sr	Oracea	Galderma	ec
Lamictal XR	GlaxoSmithKline	sr	Orenitram	United Therapeutics Corp.	sr
Lescol XL	Novartis	sr	Oxtellar XR	Supernus	sr
Levbid	Alaven	sr	Oxycontin	Purdue	sr

DRUG	MANUFACTURER	FORM	DRUG	MANUFACTURER	FORM
Pancreaze	Ortho-McNeil-Janssen	ec	Tarka	AbbVie Inc.	sr
Paser	Jacobus	ec	Taztia XT	Watson	sr
Paxil CR	Apotex	sr	Tecfidera	biogen	ec
PCE	Arbor	ec	Tegretol-XR	Novartis	sr
Pentasa	Shire U.S.	sr	Theo-24	Actient	sr
Pentoxil	Upsher-Smith	sr	Tiazac	Valeant	sr
Phenytek	Mylan	sr	Toprol XL†	AstraZeneca	sr
Poly Hist Forte	Poly	sr	Toviaz	Pfizer	sr
Poly-Vent DM	Poly	sr	Treximet	Pernix Therapeutics	ec
Prevacid	Takeda	ec	Trilipix	AbbVie Inc.	ec
Prilosec	AstraZeneca	ec	Trokendi XR	Supernus	sr
Prilosec OTC	Procter & Gamble	sr	Tussicaps	Valeant	sr
Pristiq	Wyeth	sr	Tuzistra XR	Vernalis Therapeutics	sr
Procardia XL	Pfizer	sr	Tylenol Arthritis	McNeil Consumer	sr
Protonix	Wyeth	ec	Uceris	Santarus, Inc.	sr
Prozac Weekly	Eli Lilly	ec	Ultram ER	Janssen	sr
Qsymia	Vivus	sr	Uptravi	Actelion	ec
Ranexa	Gilead	sr	Urocit-K	Mission	sr
Rayaldee	Opko	sr	Uroxatral	Concordia	sr
Rayos	Horizon	ec	Verelan	Kremers Urban	ec
Razadyne ER	Ortho-McNeil-Janssen	sr	Verelan PM	Kremers Urban	sr
Requip XL	GlaxoSmithKline	sr	Videx EC	Bristol-Myers-Squibb	ec
Rescon	Capellon	sr	Vimovo	Horizon	ec
Ritalin LA	Novartis	sr	Voltaren-XR	Novartis	sr
Ritalin-SR	Novartis	sr	Vospire ER	Dava	sr
Rodex Forte	Legere	sr	Votrient	GlaxoSmithKline	ec
Rytary	Impax	sr	Wellbutrin SR	GlaxoSmithKline	sr
Rythmol SR	GlaxoSmithKline	sr	Wellbutrin XL	Valeant	sr
SAM-e	Pharmavite	ec	Wobenzym N	Marlyn	ec
Sanctura XR	Allergan	sr	Xanax XR	Pharmacia and Upjohn	sr
Seroquel XR	AstraZeneca	sr	Xtampza ER	Patheon Inc.	sr
Simcor	AbbVie Inc.	sr	Zenpep	Aptalis Pharma	ec
Sinemet CR	Merck Sharp & Dohme	sr	Zohydro ER	Pernix Therapeutics	sr
Sitavig	Cipher	ec	Zyban	GlaxoSmithKline	sr
Slo-Niacin	Upsher-Smith	sr	Zyflo CR	Chiesi	sr
Slow Fe	Novartis Consumer	sr	Zyrtec-D	McNeil Consumer	sr
Slow-Mag	Purdue	ec	*May split in half or dissolve in water.		
Solodyn	Medicis	sr	†May divide tablet.		
St. Joseph Pain Reliever	McNeil Consumer	ec			
Stavzor	Noven	ec			
Sudafed 12 hour	McNeil Consumer	sr			
Sudafed 24 hour	McNeil Consumer	sr			
Sular	Shionogi Pharma	sr			
Sulfasalazine DR	Qualitest	ec			
Symax Duotab	Capellon	sr			
Symax-SR	Capellon	sr			
Tafinlar	GlaxoSmithKline	ec			

ABBREVIATIONS, ACRONYMS, AND SYMBOLS

ABBREVIATIONS	DESCRIPTIONS
- (eg, 6-8)	to (eg, 6 to 8)
/	per
<	less than
>	greater than
≤	less than or equal to
≥	greater than or equal to
α	alpha
β	beta
μL	microliter
μm	micrometer
μM	micromolar
μmol	micromole
5-FU	5-fluorouracil
5-HT	5-hydroxytryptamine (serotonin)
aa	of each
ABECB	acute bacterial exacerbation of chronic bronchitis
ac	before meals
ACE inhibitor	angiotensin converting enzyme inhibitor
ACTH	adrenocorticotropic hormone
ad	right ear
ADHD	attention-deficit hyperactivity disorder
A-fib	atrial fibrillation
A-flutter	atrial flutter
AIDS	acquired immunodeficiency syndrome
ALK	anaplastic lymphoma kinase
ALT	alanine transaminase (SGPT)
am or AM	morning
AMI	acute myocardial infarction
ANA	antinuclear antibody
ANC	absolute neutrophil count
APAP	acetaminophen
Apo B	apolipoprotein B
ARB	angiotensin II receptor blocker
as	left ear
ASA	aspirin

(Continued)

ABBREVIATIONS	DESCRIPTIONS
AST	aspartate transaminase (SGOT)
au	each ear
AUC	area under the curve
AV	atrioventricular
BCG	bacillus Calmette-Guerin
BCRP	breast cancer resistance protein
bid	twice daily
BMI	body mass index
BP	blood pressure
BPH	benign prostatic hypertrophy
bpm	beats per minute
BSA	body surface area
BUN	blood urea nitrogen
Ca^{2+}	calcium
CABG	coronary artery bypass graft
CAD	coronary artery disease
cAMP	cyclic-3',5'-adenosine monophosphate
cap	capsule or gelcap
CAP	community-acquired pneumonia
CBC	complete blood count
CCB	calcium channel blocker
CF	cystic fibrosis
cGMP	cyclic guanosine monophosphate
CHF	congestive heart failure
CK	creatine kinase
Cl^-	chloride
cm	centimeter
C_{max}	peak plasma concentration
CMV	cytomegalovirus
CNS	central nervous system
COMT inhibitor	catechol-O-methyl transferase inhibitor
COPD	chronic obstructive pulmonary disease
COX-2 inhibitor	cyclooxygenase-2 inhibitor
CPK	creatine phosphokinase
CR	controlled-release
CrCl	creatinine clearance
cre	cream
CRF	chronic renal failure
CSF	cerebrospinal fluid

ABBREVIATIONS	DESCRIPTIONS
cSSSI	complicated skin and skin structure infection
CTC	common toxicity criteria
CV	cardiovascular
CVA	cerebrovascular accident
CVD	cardiovascular disease
CYP450	cytochrome P450
D5	dextrose 5%
D5W	dextrose 5% in water
d/c or D/C	discontinue
DHEA	dehydroepiandrosterone
DM	diabetes mellitus
DMARD	disease modifying antirheumatic drug
DNA	deoxyribonucleic acid
DR	delayed-release
DVT	deep vein thrombosis
ECG	electrocardiogram
EDTA	edetate disodium
EEG	electroencephalogram
eg	for example
EGFR	epidermal growth factor receptor
EPS	extrapyramidal symptom
ER	extended-release
ESRD	end-stage renal disease
fl oz	fluid ounce
FPG	fasting plasma glucose
FSH	follicle-stimulating hormone
g	gram
G6PD	glucose-6-phosphate dehydrogenase
GABA	gamma-aminobutyric acid
GAD	general anxiety disorder
GERD	gastroesophageal reflux disease
GFR	glomerular filtration rate
GGT	gamma-glutamyl transpeptidase
GI	gastrointestinal
GnRH	gonadotropin-releasing hormone
GVHD	graft-versus-host disease
HbA1c	hemoglobin A1c
hCG	human chorionic gonadotropin

(Continued)

ABBREVIATIONS	DESCRIPTIONS
Hct	hematocrit
HCTZ	hydrochlorothiazide
HDL	high-density lipoprotein
HER2	human epidermal growth factor receptor 2
HF	heart failure
Hgb	hemoglobin
HIV	human immunodeficiency virus
HMG-CoA	3-hydroxy-3-methylglutaryl-coenzyme A
HR	heart rate
hr, hrs	hour, hours
hs	bedtime
HSV	herpes simplex virus
HTN	hypertension
IBD	inflammatory bowel disease
IBS	irritable bowel syndrome
ICH	intracranial hemorrhage
ICP	intracranial pressure
IgG	immunoglobulin G
IM	intramuscular/intramuscularly
INH	isoniazid
inh	inhalation
inj	injection
INR	international normalized ratio
IOP	intraocular pressure
IR	immediate-release
IU*	international unit
IUD	intrauterine device
IV	intravenous/intravenously
K+	potassium
kg	kilogram
KIU	kallikrein inhibitor unit
L	liter
lb, lbs	pound, pounds
LD	loading dose
LDL	low-density lipoprotein
LFT	liver function test
LH	luteinizing hormone
LHRH	luteinizing-hormone releasing hormone
lot	lotion

ABBREVIATIONS	DESCRIPTIONS
loz	lozenge
LVEF	left ventricular ejection fraction
LVH	left ventricular hypertrophy
M	molar
MAC	*Mycobacterium avium* complex
maint	maintenance
MAOI	monoamine oxidase inhibitor
max	maximum
mcg	microgram
mEq	milliequivalent
mg	milligram
Mg^{2+}	magnesium
MI	myocardial infarction
min	minute (usually as mL/min)
mL	milliliter
mm	millimeter
mM	millimolar
MRI	magnetic resonance imaging
MS*	multiple sclerosis
msec	millisecond
MTX	methotrexate
N/A	not applicable or not available
Na^+	sodium
NaCl	sodium chloride
NG	nasogastric
NKA	no known allergies
NMS	neuroleptic malignant syndrome
NPO	nothing by mouth
NSAID	nonsteroidal anti-inflammatory drug
NV or N/V	nausea and vomiting
NYHA Class	New York Heart Association Class
OA	osteoarthritis
OCD	obsessive-compulsive disorder
od	right eye
oint	ointment
os	left eye
OTC	over-the-counter
ou	each eye

(Continued)

ABBREVIATIONS	DESCRIPTIONS
oz	ounce
P	phosphorus
PAT	paroxysmal atrial tachycardia
pc	after meals
PCN	penicillin
PCP	*Pneumocystis carinii* pneumonia
PD	Parkinson's disease
PDE-5 inhibitor	phosphodiesterase-5 inhibitor
PE	pulmonary embolism
P-gp	P-glycoprotein
PID	pelvic inflammatory disease
pkt, pkts	packet, packets
pm or PM	evening
po or PO	orally
PONV	postoperative nausea and vomiting
postop	postoperative/postoperatively
PPI	proton pump inhibitor
pr	rectally
preop	preoperative/preoperatively
prn or PRN	as needed
PSA	prostate-specific antigen
PSVT	paroxysmal supraventricular tachycardia
PT	prothrombin time
PTSD	post-traumatic stress disorder
PTT	partial thromboplastin time
PTU	propylthiouracil
PUD	peptic ulcer disease
PVD	peripheral vascular disease
q4h, q6h, q8h, etc.	every four hours, every six hours, every eight hours, etc.
qam	once every morning
qd*	once daily
qh	every hour
qhs	every night at bedtime/before retiring
qid	four times daily
qod*	every other day
qpm	once every evening
qs	a sufficient quantity
qs ad	a sufficient quantity to make

ABBREVIATIONS	DESCRIPTIONS
RA	rheumatoid arthritis
RAAS	renin-angiotensin-aldosterone system
RAS	renin-angiotensin system
RBC	red blood cell
RDS	respiratory distress syndrome
REM	rapid eye movement
RNA	ribonucleic acid
Rx	prescription
SA	sinoatrial
SAH	subarachnoid hemorrhage
SBP	systolic blood pressure
sec	second
SGOT	serum glutamic-oxaloacetic transaminase (AST)
SGPT	serum glutamic-pyruvic transaminase (ALT)
SIADH	syndrome of inappropriate antidiuretic hormone secretion
SJS	Stevens-Johnson syndrome
SL	sublingual/sublingually
SLE	systemic lupus erythematosus
SNRI	serotonin and norepinephrine reuptake inhibitor
SOB	shortness of breath
sol	solution
SQ, SC	subcutaneous/subcutaneously
SR	sustained-release
SrCr	serum creatinine
SSRI	selective serotonin reuptake inhibitor
SSSI	skin and skin structure infection
STD	sexually transmitted disease
sup or supp	suppository
sus	suspension
SVT	supraventricular tachycardia
SWFI	sterile water for injection
$T_{1/2}$	half-life
T3	triiodothyronine
T4	thyroxine
tab	tablet or caplet
tab, SL	sublingual tablet

(Continued)

ABBREVIATIONS	DESCRIPTIONS
TB	tuberculosis
TBG	thyroxine-binding globulin
tbl or tbsp	tablespoonful
TCA	tricyclic antidepressant
TD	tardive dyskinesia
TEN	toxic epidermal necrolysis
TFT	thyroid function test
TG	triglyceride
tid	three times daily
T_{max}	time to maximum concentration
TNF	tumor necrosis factor
total-C	total cholesterol
TPN	total parenteral nutrition
TSH	thyroid-stimulating hormone
tsp	teaspoonful
TTP	thrombotic thrombocytopenic purpura
U*	unit
UC	ulcerative colitis
ud	as directed
ULN	upper limit of normal
URTI/URI	upper respiratory tract infection
UTI	urinary tract infection
UV	ultraviolet
V_d	volume of distribution
VEGF	vascular endothelial growth factor
VLDL	very low density lipoprotein
VTE	venous thromboembolism
w/ or W/	with
w/in or W/IN	within
w/o or W/O	without
WBC	white blood cell
WHO	World Health Organization
X	times (eg, >2X ULN)
yr, yrs	year, years

*The Joint Commission cautions use of these abbreviations on orders and medication-related documentation that is handwritten (including free-text computer entry) or on pre-printed forms. Visit www.jointcommission.org for more information.